SABISTON TEXTBOOK *of* SURGERY

The BIOLOGICAL BASIS of MODERN SURGICAL PRACTICE

SABISTON TEXTBOOK *of* SURGERY

The BIOLOGICAL BASIS of MODERN SURGICAL PRACTICE

20TH EDITION

COURTNEY M. TOWNSEND, JR., MD
Professor
Robertson-Poth Distinguished Chair in General Surgery
Department of Surgery
University of Texas Medical Branch
Galveston, Texas

R. DANIEL BEAUCHAMP, MD
J.C. Foshee Distinguished Professor and Chairman, Section of Surgical Sciences
Professor of Surgery and Cell and Developmental Biology and Cancer Biology
Vanderbilt University School of Medicine
Surgeon-in-Chief, Vanderbilt University Hospital
Nashville, Tennessee

B. MARK EVERS, MD
Professor and Vice-Chair for Research, Department of Surgery
Director, Lucille P. Markey Cancer Center
Markey Cancer Foundation Endowed Chair
Physician-in-Chief, Oncology Service Line UK Healthcare
University of Kentucky
Lexington, Kentucky

KENNETH L. MATTOX, MD
Professor and Vice Chairman
Michael E. DeBakey Department of Surgery
Baylor College of Medicine
Chief of Staff and Chief of Surgery
Ben Taub General Hospital
Houston, Texas

ELSEVIER

ELSEVIER

1600 John F. Kennedy Blvd.
Ste 1800
Philadelphia, PA 19103-2899

ISBN: 978-0-323-29987-9
International Edition ISBN: 978-0-323-40162-3

Notices

Knowledge and best practice in this field are constantly changing. As new research and experience broaden our understanding, changes in research methods, professional practices, or medical treatment may become necessary.

Practitioners and researchers must always rely on their own experience and knowledge in evaluating and using any information, methods, compounds, or experiments described herein. In using such information or methods they should be mindful of their own safety and the safety of others, including parties for whom they have a professional responsibility.

With respect to any drug or pharmaceutical products identified, readers are advised to check the most current information provided (i) on procedures featured or (ii) by the manufacturer of each product to be administered, to verify the recommended dose or formula, the method and duration of administration, and contraindications. It is the responsibility of practitioners, relying on their own experience and knowledge of their patients, to make diagnoses, to determine dosages and the best treatment for each individual patient, and to take all appropriate safety precautions.

To the fullest extent of the law, neither the Publisher nor the authors, contributors, or editors, assume any liability for any injury and/or damage to persons or property as a matter of products liability, negligence or otherwise, or from any use or operation of any methods, products, instructions, or ideas contained in the material herein.

Please change to the following:

Library of Congress Cataloging-in-Publication Data

Sabiston textbook of surgery : the biological basis of modern surgical practic / [edited by] Courtney M. Townsend, Jr, R. Daniel Beauchamp, B. Mark Evers, Kenneth L. Mattox.—20th edition.
p. ; cm.
Textbook of surgery
Preceded by Sabiston textbook of surgery / [edited by] Courtney M. Townsend Jr. … [et al.]. 19th ed. 2012.
Includes bibliographical references and index.
ISBN 978-0-323-29987-9 (hardcover : alk. paper)—ISBN 978-0-323-40162-3 (international edition : alk. paper)
I. Townsend, Courtney M., Jr., editor. II. Beauchamp, R. Daniel, editor. III. Evers, B. Mark, 1957-, editor. IV. Mattox, Kenneth L., 1938-, editor. V. Title: Textbook of surgery.
[DNLM: 1. Surgical Procedures, Operative. 2. General Surgery. 3. Perioperative Care. WO 500]
RD31
617—dc23

2015035365

Executive Content Strategist: Michael Houston
Content Development Specialist: Joanie Milnes
Publishing Services Manager: Patricia Tannian
Senior Project Manager: Cindy Thoms
Book Designer: Renee Duenow

Printed in Canada

Last digit is the print number: 9 8 7 6 5 4 3 2 1

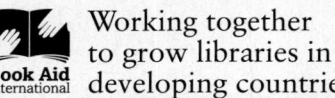

To our patients, who grant us the privilege of practicing our craft;
to our students, residents, and colleagues, from whom we learn;
and to our wives—Mary, Shannon, Karen, and June—without
whose support this would not have been possible.

CONTRIBUTORS

Cary B. Aarons, MD
Assistant Professor of Clinical Surgery
University of Pennsylvania
Philadelphia, Pennsylvania

Andrew B. Adams, MD, PhD
Assistant Professor
Emory Transplant Center
Department of Surgery
Emory University School of Medicine
Atlanta, Georgia

Charles A. Adams, Jr., MD
Chief
Division of Trauma and Surgical Critical Care
Rhode Island Hospital
Associate Professor of Surgery
Alpert Medical School of Brown University
Providence, Rhode Island

Ahmed Al-Mousawi, MD
Shriners Hospitals for Children
Department of Surgery
University of Texas Medical Branch
Galveston, Texas

Jatin Anand, MD
Resident in Cardiothoracic Surgery
Division of Cardiovascular and Thoracic Surgery
Department of Surgery
Duke University Medical Center
Durham, North Carolina

Nancy Ascher, MD, PhD
Professor and Chair
Department of Surgery
University of California at San Francisco
San Francisco, California

Stanley W. Ashley, MD
Chief Medical Officer and Senior Vice President for Medical Affairs
Brigham and Women's Hospital
Frank Sawyer Professor of Surgery
Harvard Medical School
Boston, Massachusetts

Paul S. Auerbach, MD
Professor of Emergency Medicine
Redlich Family Professor
Stanford University
Stanford, California

Brian Badgwell, MD
Associate Professor of Surgery
MD Anderson Cancer Center
Houston, Texas

Faisal G. Bakaeen, MD, FACS
Staff Surgeon
Department of Thoracic and
Cardiovascular Surgery
Heart and Vascular Institute
Cleveland, Ohio
Adjunct Professor
The Michael E. DeBakey Department of Surgery
Baylor College of Medicine
Houston, Texas

Philip S. Barie, MD, MBA, FIDSA, FACS, FCCM
Professor of Surgery and Public Health
Weill Cornell Medical College
New York, New York

B. Timothy Baxter, MD
Vice-Chairman, Department of Surgery
Professor, Vascular Surgery
Department of Surgery
University of Nebraska Medical Center
Omaha, Nebraska

R. Daniel Beauchamp, MD
J.C. Foshee Distinguished Professor and Chairman
Section of Surgical Sciences
Professor of Surgery and Cell and Developmental Biology and Cancer Biology
Vanderbilt University School of Medicine
Surgeon-in-Chief
Vanderbilt University Hospital
Nashville, Tennessee

Yolanda Becker, MD, FACS
Professor and Director of Kidney and Pancreas Transplant
Division of Transplantation
Department of Surgery
University of Chicago
Pritzker School of Medicine
Chicago, Illinois

Joshua I.S. Bleier, MD
Program Director
Division of Colon and Rectal Surgery
University of Pennsylvania Health System
Associate Professor of Clinical Surgery
University of Pennsylvania
Philadelphia, Pennsylvania

Howard Brody, MD, PhD
Former Director
Institute for the Medical Humanities
University of Texas Medical Branch
Galveston, Texas

Carlos V.R. Brown, MD, FACS
Associate Professor and Vice Chairman of Surgery
University of Texas Southwestern—Austin
Trauma Medical Director
University Medical Center Brackenridge
Austin, Texas

Bruce D. Browner, MD, MS
Gray-Gossling Chair
Professor and Chairman Emeritus
Department of Orthopaedic Surgery
University of Connecticut
Farmington, Connecticut
Director
Department of Orthopaedics
Hartford Hospital
Hartford, Connecticut

Brian B. Burkey, MD
Vice-Chairman
Head and Neck Institute
Cleveland Clinic
Cleveland, Ohio

Joshua Carson, MD
Shriners Hospitals for Children
Department of Surgery
University of Texas Medical Branch
Galveston, Texas

Steven N. Carter, MD
Clinical Assistant Professor of Surgery
Department of Surgery
University of Oklahoma Health Sciences Center
Oklahoma City, Oklahoma

Howard C. Champion, MD
Professor of Surgery
Uniformed Service University of the Health Sciences
Bethesda, Maryland

Faisal Cheema, MD, FACS
Assistant Professor
Division of Vascular Surgery and Endovascular Therapy
Department of Surgery
University of Texas Medical Branch
Galveston, Texas

Charlie C. Cheng, MD, FACS
Assistant Professor
Division of Vascular Surgery and Endovascular Therapy
Department of Surgery
University of Texas Medical Branch
Galveston, Texas

Kenneth J. Cherry, MD
Edwin P. Lehman Professor of Surgery
Division of Vascular and Endovascular Surgery
University of Virginia Medical Center
Charlottesville, Virginia

John D. Christein, MD
Associate Professor
Department of Surgery
University of Alabama School of Medicine
Birmingham, Alabama

Dai H. Chung, MD
Professor and Chairman
Janie Robinson and John Moore Lee Chair
Department of Pediatric Surgery
Vanderbilt University Medical Center
Nashville, Tennessee

William G. Cioffi, MD
Chief
Department of Surgery
Rhode Island Hospital
Professor and Chairman of Surgery
Alpert Medical School of Brown University
Providence, Rhode Island

Michael Coburn, MD
Professor and Chairman
Scott Department of Urology
Baylor College of Medicine
Houston, Texas

Carlo M. Contreras, MD
Assistant Professor of Surgery
University of Alabama at Birmingham
Birmingham, Alabama

Lorraine D. Cornwell, MD
Assistant Professor
Cardiothoracic Surgery
Baylor College of Medicine
Michael E. DeBakey VA Medical Center
Houston, Texas

Marion E. Couch, MD, PhD, MBA, FACS
Richard T. Miyamoto Professor and Chair of Head and Neck Surgery
Physician Executive
Surgical Services for IU Health Physicians
Indiana University School of Medicine
Indianapolis, Indiana

Merril T. Dayton, MD
Salt Lake City, Utah

Bradley M. Dennis, MD
Assistant Professor of Surgery
Division of Trauma and Surgical Critical Care
Department of Surgery
Vanderbilt University Medical Center
Nashville, Tennessee

Sohum K. Desai, MD
Resident
Division of Neurosurgery
Department of Surgery
University of Texas Medical Branch
Galveston, Texas

Rajeev Dhupar, MD, MBA
Assistant Professor
Department of Cardiothoracic Surgery
Division of Thoracic and Foregut Surgery
University of Pittsburgh Medical Center
Pittsburgh, Pennsylvania

Jose J. Diaz, MD, CNS, FACS, FCCM
Professor of Surgery
Chief Acute Care Surgery
R. Adams Cowley Shock Trauma Center
University of Maryland Medical Center
Baltimore, Maryland

Zachary C. Dietch, MD
Department of Surgery
The University of Virginia Health System
Charlottesville, Virginia

Roger Dmochowski, MD, MMHC, FACS
Professor of Urology
Director, Pelvic Medicine and Reconstruction Fellowship
Department of Urology
Professor of Obstetrics and Gynecology
Vice Chair, Section of Surgical Sciences
Vanderbilt University Medical Center
Associate Director of Quality and Safety
Executive Director of Risk Prevention
Vanderbilt Health System
Executive Medical Director for Patient Safety and Quality (Surgery)
Associate Chief of Staff
Medical Director of Risk Management
Vanderbilt University Hospital
Nashville, Tennessee

Vikas Dudeja, MD
Assistant Professor
Division of Surgical Oncology
Department of Surgery
University of Miami
Miller School of Medicine
Miami, Florida

Quan-Yang Duh, MD
Professor of Surgery
University of California—San Francisco
Surgical Service
San Francisco VA Medical Center
San Francisco, California

Timothy J. Eberlein, MD
Bixby Professor and Chairman
Department of Surgery
Spencer T. and Ann W. Olin Distinguished Professor
Director, Alvin J. Siteman Cancer Center
Washington University School of Medicine
St. Louis, Missouri

James S. Economou, MD, PhD
Beaumont Professor of Surgery
Professor of Microbiology, Immunology, and Molecular Genetics
Professor of Medical and Molecular Pharmacology
University of California—Los Angeles
Los Angeles, California

E. Christopher Ellison, MD
Professor
Department of Surgery
Ohio State University
Columbus, Ohio

Stephen R.T. Evans, MD
Professor of Surgery
Georgetown University Medical Center
Executive Vice President and Chief Medical Officer
MedStar Health
Washington, DC

B. Mark Evers, MD
Professor and Vice-Chair for Research
Department of Surgery
Director
Lucille P. Markey Cancer Center
Markey Cancer Foundation Endowed Chair
Physician-in-Chief
Oncology Service Line UK Healthcare
University of Kentucky
Lexington, Kentucky

Grant Fankhauser, MD
Assistant Professor
Division of Vascular Surgery and Endovascular Therapy
Department of Surgery
University of Texas Medical Branch
Galveston, Texas

Farhood Farjah, MD, MPH
Division of Cardiothoracic Surgery
Surgical Outcomes Research Center
University of Washington
Seattle, Washington

Celeste C. Finnerty, PhD
Shriners Hospitals for Children
Department of Surgery
Sealy Center for Molecular Medicine
Institute for Translational Sciences
University of Texas Medical Branch
Galveston, Texas

Nicholas A. Fiore II, MD
Private Practice
Houston, Texas

David R. Flum, MD, MPH
Professor and Association Chair for Research Surgery
Director, Surgical Outcomes Research Center
University of Washington
Seattle, Washington

Yuman Fong, MD
Chairman
Department of Surgery
City of Hope Medical Center
Duarte, California

Mandy Ford, PhD
Associate Professor
Emory Transplant Surgery
Department of Surgery
Emory University School of Medicine
Atlanta, Georgia

Charles D. Fraser, Jr., MD
Chief and The Donovan Chair in Congenital Heart Surgery
Surgeon-in-Chief, Texas Children's Hospital
Professor of Surgery and Pediatrics
Susan V. Clayton Chair in Surgery
Baylor College of Medicine
Houston, Texas

Julie A. Freischlag, MD
Professor of Surgery
Vice Chancellor
Human Health Services
Dean, School of Medicine
University of California—Davis
Sacramento, California

Gerald M. Fried, MD, CM, FRCSC, FACS
Edward W. Archibald Professor and Chairman of Surgery
McGill University
Montreal, Quebec, Canada

Robert D. Fry, MD
Emilie and Roland DeHellebranth Professor of Surgery Emeritus
University of Pennsylvania
Philadelphia, Pennsylvania

Nasrin Ghalyaie, MD
Assistant Professor of Surgery
Department of Surgery
University of Arizona College of Medicine
Tucson, Arizona

S. Peter Goedegebuure, PhD
Research Associate Professor
Department of Surgery
Washington University School of Medicine
St. Louis, Missouri

Oliver L. Gunter, MD, MPH
Associate Professor of Surgery
Division of Trauma and Surgical Critical Care
Vanderbilt University School of Medicine
Nashville, Tennessee

Jennifer L. Halpern, MD
Assistant Professor
Department of Orthopaedic Surgery
Vanderbilt Orthopaedic Institute
Nashville, Tennessee

John B. Hanks, MD
C. Bruce Morton Professor and Chief
Division of General Surgery
Department of Surgery
University of Virginia
Charlottesville, Virginia

Laura R. Hanks, MD
Resident in Obstetrics and Gynecology
Department of Obstetrics and Gynecology
University of Rochester
School of Medicine and Dentistry
Rochester, New York

Jennifer W. Harris, MD
General Surgery Resident
Post-Doctoral Research Fellow
Markey Cancer Center
Lexington, Kentucky

Jennifer A. Heller, MD
Assistant Professor of Surgery
Director
Johns Hopkins Vein Center
Department of Surgery
Johns Hopkins Medical Institutions
Baltimore, Maryland

Jon C. Henry, MD
Fellow
Vascular Surgery
University of Pittsburgh Medical Center
Pittsburgh, Pennsylvania

Antonio Hernandez, MD
Associate Professor
Department of Anesthesiology
Vanderbilt University Medical Center
Nashville, Tennessee

David N. Herndon, MD, FACS
Chief of Staff
Shriners Hospitals for Children
Department of Surgery
University of Texas Medical Branch
Galveston, Texas

Martin J. Heslin, MD, MSHA
Professor and Director
Division of Surgical Oncology
Department of Surgery
University of Alabama at Birmingham
Birmingham, Alabama

Asher Hirshberg, MD
Director of Emergency Vascular Surgery
Kings County Hospital Center
Brooklyn, New York

Wayne Hofstetter, MD
Professor of Surgery
Deputy Chair
Department of Thoracic and Cardiovascular Surgery
University of Texas
MD Anderson Cancer Center
Houston, Texas

Ginger E. Holt, MD
Associate Professor
Department of Orthopaedic Surgery
Vanderbilt Orthopaedic Institute
Nashville, Tennessee

Michael D. Holzman, MD, MPH
Professor of Surgery
Department of Surgery
Vanderbilt University Medical Center
Nashville, Tennessee

Michael S. Hu, MD, MPH, MS
Post-Doctoral Fellow
Division of Plastic and Reconstructive Surgery
Department of Surgery
Stanford University School of Medicine
Stanford, California
General Surgery Resident
Department of Surgery
John A. Burns School of Medicine
University of Hawaii
Honolulu, Hawaii

Eric S. Hungness, MD, FACS
Associate Professor of Surgery and Medical Education
S. David Stulberg Research Professor
Northwestern University
Feinberg School of Medicine
Chicago, Illinois

Kelly K. Hunt, MD
Professor
Department of Breast Surgical Oncology
University of Texas
MD Anderson Cancer Center
Houston, Texas

Jeffrey Indes, MD, FACS
Assistant Professor of Surgery and Radiology
Associate Program Director, Vascular Surgery
Yale University School of Medicine
New Haven, Connecticut

Patrick G. Jackson, MD, FACS
Assistant Professor of Surgery
Chief, Division of General Surgery
MedStar Georgetown University Hospital
Washington, DC

Eric H. Jensen, MD
Assistant Professor of Surgery
University of Minnesota
Minneapolis, Minnesota

Marc G. Jeschke, MD, PhD, FACS, FCCM, FRCS(c)
Director, Ross Tilley Burn Centre
Department of Surgery
Division of Plastic Surgery
University of Toronto
Sunnybrook Health Sciences Centre
Toronto, Ontario, Canada

Howard W. Jones III, MD
Professor and Chairman
Department of Obstetrics and Gynecology
Vanderbilt University School of Medicine
Nashville, Tennessee

Bellal Joseph, MD
Associate Professor of Surgery
University of Arizona
Tucson, Arizona

Lauren C. Kane, MD
Associate Surgeon
Texas Children's Hospital
Assistant Professor of Surgery and Pediatrics
Baylor College of Medicine
Houston, Texas

Jae Y. Kim, MD
Assistant Professor
Division of Thoracic Surgery
City of Hope Cancer Center
Duarte, California

Charles W. Kimbrough, MD
The Hiram C. Polk, Jr., MD Department of Surgery
University of Louisville School of Medicine
Louisville, Kentucky

Mahmoud N. Kulaylat, MD
Associate Professor
Department of Surgery
Jacobs School of Medicine and Biomedical Sciences
University of New York—Buffalo
Buffalo, New York

Terry C. Lairmore, MD
Professor of Surgery
Director, Division of Surgical Oncology
Baylor Scott and White Healthcare
Texas A&M University System Health Science Center
College of Medicine
Temple, Texas

Christian P. Larsen, MD, DPhil
Dean and Vice President for Health Affairs
Mason Professor of Transplantation Surgery
Emory Transplant Center
Department of Surgery
Emory University School of Medicine
Atlanta, Georgia

David W. Larson, MD, MBA
Chair, Colon and Rectal Surgery
Professor of Surgery
Mayo Clinic
Rochester, Minnesota

Mimi Leong, MD, MS
Staff Physician, Section of Plastic Surgery
Operative Care Line
Michael E. DeBakey Department of Surgery
Veterans Affairs Medical Center
Clinical Assistant Professor
Division of Plastic Surgery
Michael E. DeBakey Department of Surgery
Baylor College of Medicine
Houston, Texas

Lillian F. Liao, MD, MPH
Assistant Professor of Surgery
Pediatric Trauma Medical Director
University of Texas Health Science Center—San Antonio
San Antonio, Texas

Masha J. Livhits, MD
Clinical Instructor
Section of Endocrine Surgery
University of California—Los Angeles
David Geffen School of Medicine
Los Angeles, California

Michael T. Longaker, MD, MBA, FACS
Deane P. and Louise Mitchell Professor and Vice-Chair in Department of Surgery
Co-Director of Stanford Institute for Stem Cell Biology and Regenerative Medicine
Director of Program in Regenerative Medicine
Stanford University School of Medicine
Stanford, California

H. Peter Lorenz, MD
Professor of Surgery (Plastic and Reconstructive)
Stanford University School of Medicine
Fellowship Director, Craniofacial Surgery
Service Chief, Plastic Surgery
Lucile Packard Children's Hospital at Stanford
Stanford, California

Robert R. Lorenz, MD, MBA
Medical Director Payment Reform, Risk and Contracting
Head and Neck Surgery
Laryngotracheal Reconstruction and Oncology
Head and Neck Institute
Cleveland Clinic
Cleveland, Ohio

Najjia N. Mahmoud, MD
Chief, Division of Colon and Rectal Surgery
University of Pennsylvania Health System
Associate Professor of Surgery
University of Pennsylvania
Philadelphia, Pennsylvania

David M. Mahvi, MD
James R. Hines Professor of Surgery
Chief, GI and Oncologic Surgery
Department of Surgery
Northwestern University
Feinberg School of Medicine
Chicago, Illinois

Mark A. Malangoni, MD, FACS
Associate Executive Director
American Board of Surgery
Adjunct Professor of Surgery
University of Pennsylvania
Perelman School of Medicine
Philadelphia, Pennsylvania

Silas T. Marshall, MD
Orthopaedic Traumatology and Fracture Care
Proliance Orthopaedics and Sports Medicine
University of Connecticut
Farmington, Connecticut

R. Shayn Martin, MD, FACS
Assistant Professor of Surgery
Department of Surgery
Wake Forest School of Medicine
Executive Director, Critical Care Services
Wake Forest Baptist Health
Winston-Salem, North Carolina

Kenneth L. Mattox, MD
Professor and Vice Chairman
Michael E. DeBakey Department of Surgery
Baylor College of Medicine
Chief of Staff and Chief of Surgery
Ben Taub General Hospital
Houston, Texas

Addison K. May, MD
Professor of Surgery and Anesthesiology
Division of Trauma and Surgical Critical Care
Department of Surgery
Vanderbilt University Medical Center
Nashville, Tennessee

Mary H. McGrath, MD, MPH, FACS
Professor of Surgery
Division of Plastic Surgery, Department of Surgery
University of California—San Francisco
San Francisco, California

Kelly M. McMasters, MD, PhD
Ben A. Reid, Sr., MD Professor and Chair
The Hiram C. Polk, Jr., MD Department of Surgery
University of Louisville
Louisville, Kentucky

Amit Merchea, MD
Assistant Professor of Surgery
Colon and Rectal Surgery
Mayo Clinic
Jacksonville, Florida

J. Wayne Meredith, MD, FACS
Richard T. Meyers Professor and Chair
Department of Surgery
Wake Forest School of Medicine
Chief of Clinical Chairs
Chief of Surgery
Wake Forest Baptist Health
Winston-Salem, North Carolina

Dean J. Mikami, MD
Associate Professor
General Surgery
The Ohio State University
Wexner Medical Center
Columbus, Ohio

Richard Miller, MD, FACS
Professor of Surgery
Chief, Division of Trauma and Surgical Critical Care
Department of Surgery
Section of Surgical Sciences
Vanderbilt University Medical Center
Nashville, Tennessee

Elizabeth A. Mittendorf, MD, PhD
Associate Professor
Department of Breast Surgical Oncology
University of Texas
MD Anderson Cancer Center
Houston, Texas

Jason Mizell, MD
Professor of Surgery
Division of Colon and Rectal Surgery
University of Arkansas for Medical Sciences
Little Rock, Arkansas

Aaron Mohanty, MD
Associate Professor
Division of Neurosurgery
Department of Surgery
University of Texas Medical Branch
Galveston, Texas

Jeffrey F. Moley, MD
Professor of Surgery
Chief, Section of Endocrine and Oncologic Surgery
Washington University School of Medicine
Associate Chief
Surgical Services
St. Louis VA Medical Center
St. Louis, Missouri

Carmen L. Mueller, BSc(H), MD, FRCSC, Med
Assistant Professor of Surgery
General Surgery
McGill University
Montreal, Quebec, Canada

Kevin D. Murphy, MD, MCH, FRCS(PLAST.)
Assistant Professor
Division of Plastic Surgery
Department of Surgery
University of Texas Medical Branch
Galveston, Texas

Elaine E. Nelson, MD
Medical Director of the Emergency Department
Regional Medical Center of San Jose
San Jose, California

David Netscher, MD
Clinical Professor
Division of Plastic Surgery
Department of Orthopedic Surgery
Baylor College of Medicine
Adjunct Professor of Clinical Surgery
Weill Medical College
Cornell University
Houston, Texas

Leigh Neumayer, MD, MS
Professor and Chair of Surgery
Department of Surgery
University of Arizona College of Medicine
Tucson, Arizona

Robert L. Norris, MD
Professor of Emergency Medicine
Stanford University Medical Center
Stanford, California

Brant K. Oelschlager, MD
Professor of Surgery
Byers Endowed Professor in Esophageal Research
Department of Surgery
University of Washington
Seattle, Washington

Shuab Omer, MD
Assistant Professor
Department of Cardiothoracic Surgery
Michael E. DeBakey VAMC
Baylor College of Medicine
Houston, Texas

Juan Ortega-Barnett, MD, FAANS
Assistant Professor
Department of Surgery
Division of Neurosurgery
University of Texas Medical Branch
Galveston, Texas

Joel T. Patterson, MD, FAANS, FACS
Associate Professor and Chief
Division of Neurosurgery
Department of Surgery
University of Texas Medical Branch
Galveston, Texas

E. Carter Paulson, MD, MSCE
Assistant Professor of Clinical Surgery
University of Pennsylvania
Philadelphia, Pennsylvania

Carlos A. Pellegrini, MD
Chief Medical Officer
UW Medicine Vice President for Medical Affairs
University of Washington
Seattle, Washington

Linda G. Phillips, MD
Truman G. Blocker Distinguished Professor and Chief
Division of Plastic Surgery
Department of Surgery
University of Texas Medical Branch
Galveston, Texas

Iraklis I. Pipinos, MD
Professor, Vascular Surgery
Department of Surgery
University of Nebraska Medical Center
Omaha, Nebraska

Jason H. Pomerantz, MD
Associate Professor of Surgery
Division of Plastic Surgery
Department of Surgery
University of California—San Francisco
San Francisco, California

Russell G. Postier, MD
John A. Schilling Professor and Chairman
Department of Surgery
University of Oklahoma Health Sciences Center
Oklahoma City, Oklahoma

Benjamin K. Poulose, MD, MPH
Associate Professor of Surgery
Department of Surgery
Vanderbilt University Medical Center
Nashville, Tennessee

Karen L. Powers, MD
Stonegate Plastic Surgery
Lakeland Regional Medical Center
St. Joseph, Michigan

Joe B. Putnam, Jr., MD
Medical Director
Baptist MD Anderson Cancer Center
Jacksonville, Florida

Courtney E. Quinn, MD, MS
Assistant Professor
Department of Surgery
Section of Endocrine Surgery
Yale-New Haven Hospital
Yale University School of Medicine
New Haven, Connecticut

Aparna Rege, MD
Clinical Associate
Surgery
Duke University Medical Center
Durham, North Carolina

Peter Rhee, MD, MPH
Professor of Surgery and Molecular Cellular Biology
University of Arizona
Tucson, Arizona

Taylor S. Riall, MD, PhD
Professor
Chief
Division of General Surgery and Surgical Oncology
University of Arizona
Tucson, Arizona

William O. Richards, MD
Professor and Chair
Department of Surgery
University of South Alabama College of Medicine
Mobile, Alabama

Bryan Richmond, MD, MBA, FACS
Professor of Surgery
Section Chief, General Surgery
West Virginia University, Charleston Division
Charleston, West Virginia

Noe A. Rodriguez, MD
Shriners Hospitals for Children
Department of Surgery
University of Texas Medical Branch
Galveston, Texas

Michael J. Rosen, MD
Professor of Surgery
Lerner College of Medicine
Cleveland Clinic Foundation
Cleveland, Ohio

Todd K. Rosengart, MD, FACS
Professor and Chairman
DeBakey Bard Chair of Surgery
Michael E. DeBakey Department of Surgery
Baylor College of Medicine
Houston, Texas

Ronnie A. Rosenthal, MS, MD
Professor of Surgery
Yale University School of Medicine
New Haven, Connecticut
Chief, Surgical Service
VA Connecticut Health Care System
West Haven, Connecticut

Ira Rutkow, MD, DrPH
Independent Scholar
New York, New York

Leslie J. Salomone, MD
Clinical Practitioner
Endocrinology and Metabolism
Baptist Health System
Jacksonville, Florida

Warren S. Sandberg, MD, PhD
Professor and Chair
Department of Anesthesiology
Professor of Anesthesiology, Surgery, and Biomedical Informatics
Vanderbilt University School of Medicine
Nashville, Tennessee

Dominic E. Sanford, MD, MPHS
Resident in General Surgery
Department of Surgery
Washington University School of Medicine
St. Louis, Missouri

Robert G. Sawyer, MD, FACS
Department of Surgery
Division of Patient Outcomes
Policy and Population Research
Department of Public Health Sciences
The University of Virginia Health System
Charlottesville, Virginia

Herbert S. Schwartz, MD
Professor and Chairman
Department of Orthopaedic Surgery
Vanderbilt Orthopaedic Institute
Nashville, Tennessee

Boris Sepesi, MD, FACS
Assistant Professor
Department of Thoracic and Cardiovascular Surgery
University of Texas
MD Anderson Cancer Center
Houston, Texas

Puja M. Shah, MD
Department of Surgery
The University of Virginia Health System
Charlottesville, Virginia

Skandan Shanmugan, MD
Assistant Professor of Clinical Surgery
University of Pennsylvania
Philadelphia, Pennsylvania

Edward R. Sherwood, MD, PhD
Professor
Department of Anesthesiology
Vanderbilt University Medical Center
Nashville, Tennessee

Michael B. Silva, Jr., MD, FACS
The Fred J. and Dorothy E. Wolma Professor in Vascular Surgery
Professor in Radiology
Chief, Division of Vascular Surgery and Endovascular Therapy
Director, Texas Vascular Center
University of Texas Medical Branch
Galveston, Texas

Vlad V. Simianu, MD, MPH
Resident, Surgery
Research Fellow
Surgical Outcomes Research Center
University of Washington
Seattle, Washington

Michael J. Sise, MD
Clinical Professor
Department of Surgery
University of California—San Diego Medical Center
Medical Director, Division of Trauma
Scripps Mercy Hospital
San Diego, California

Philip W. Smith, MD
Assistant Professor of Surgery
Department of Surgery
University of Virginia
Charlottesville, Virginia

Thomas Gillispie Smith III, MD
Assistant Professor
Scott Department of Urology
Baylor College of Medicine
Houston, Texas

Jonathan D. Spicer, MD, PhD, FRCS
Assistant Professor
Division of Thoracic Surgery
Dr. Ray Chiu Distinguished Scientist in Surgical Research
McGill University
Montreal, Quebec, Canada

Ronald Squires, MD
Professor
Department of Surgery
University of Oklahoma Health Sciences Center
Oklahoma City, Oklahoma

Michael Stein, MD, FACS
Director of Trauma
Department of General Surgery
Rabin Medical Center—Beilinson Hospital
Petach-Tikva, Israel

Andrew H. Stephen, MD
Division of Trauma and Surgical Critical Care
Rhode Island Hospital
Assistant Professor of Surgery
Alpert Medical School of Brown University
Providence, Rhode Island

Ronald M. Stewart, MD
Professor and Chair of Surgery
Dr. Witten B. Russ Endowed Chair in Surgery
Department of Surgery
University of Texas Health Science Center San Antonio
San Antonio, Texas

Debra L. Sudan, MD
Professor of Surgery
Department of Surgery
Duke University Medical Center
Durham, North Carolina

Ali Tavakkoli, MD, FACS, FRCS
Associate Professor of Surgery
Minimally Invasive and GI Surgery
Brigham and Women's Hospital
Harvard Medical School
Boston, Massachusetts

Ezra N. Teitelbaum, MD
Chief Resident
Department of Surgery
Northwestern University
Feinberg School of Medicine
Chicago, Illinois

James S. Tomlinson, MD, PhD
Associate Professor of Surgery
Executive Associate Dean for Clinical Affairs
Division of Surgical Oncology
University of California—Los Angeles
Los Angeles, California

Courtney M. Townsend, Jr., MD
Professor
Robertson-Poth Distinguished Chair in General Surgery
Department of Surgery
University of Texas Medical Branch
Galveston, Texas

Margaret C. Tracci, MD, JD
Associate Professor of Surgery
Division of Vascular and Endovascular Surgery
University of Virginia Medical Center
Charlottesville, Virginia

Richard H. Turnage, MD
Professor of Surgery
University of Arkansas for Medical Sciences
Little Rock, Arkansas

Robert Udelsman, MD, MBA
William H. Carmalt Professor of Surgery and Oncology
Chairman of Surgery
Department of Surgery
Yale University School of Medicine
New Haven, Connecticut

Marshall M. Urist, MD
Professor of Surgery
Department of Surgery
Division of Surgical Oncology
University of Alabama at Birmingham
Birmingham, Alabama

Cheryl E. Vaiani, PhD
Clinical Ethics Consultant, Ethics Service
Institute for the Medical Humanities
University of Texas Medical Branch
Galveston, Texas

Selwyn M. Vickers, MD, FACS
Senior Vice President and Dean
School of Medicine
University of Alabama at Birmingham
Birmingham, Alabama

Graham G. Walmsley, BA
Medical Scientist Training Program Student
Stanford University School of Medicine
Stanford, California

Rebekah White, MD
Associate Professor
Department of Surgery
Duke University School of Medicine
Durham, North Carolina

Piotr Witkowski, MD
Associate Professor and Director of Islet Transplant
Department of Surgery
Division of Transplantation
University of Chicago
Pritzker School of Medicine
Chicago, Illinois

Daniel K. Witmer, MD
Resident
Department of Orthopaedic Surgery
University of Connecticut
Farmington, Connecticut

James C. Yang, MD
Senior Investigator, Surgery Branch
Center for Cancer Research
National Cancer Institute
Bethesda, Maryland

Robert B. Yates, MD
Clinical Assistant Professor
Department of Surgery
University of Washington
Seattle, Washington

Michael W. Yeh, MD
Associate Professor of Surgery and Medicine (Endocrinology)
Chief
Section of Endocrine Surgery
University of California—Los Angeles
David Geffen School of Medicine
Los Angeles, California

Heather Yeo, MD, MHS
Assistant Professor of Surgery
Assistant Professor of Healthcare Policy and Research
Department of Surgery
NYP-Weill Cornell Medical Center
New York, New York

A SCORE OF SCORES

This 20th or "Score" edition of *Sabiston's Textbook of Surgery* represents both a culmination and the continuation of the record of the 19 preceding editions, each of which scored their goal of serving as surgery's English language evidence-based reference work. The tradition of providing expansive update information, including detailed exposition of surgical pathophysiology to assist the surgeon in his/her adaptation of generic data for an innovative solution of an atypical clinical problem, has been maintained in this edition. The first two sections of this edition characterize, in detail, the systemic and organ specific responses to injury, describe perioperative management (including anesthesia), and cover the diagnosis and treatment of surgical infections and other surgical complications. The third section is devoted to trauma and critical care in recognition of the fact that surgical intervention is in itself a controlled form of trauma and that critical care expertise is essential to optimize surgical outcomes. Those initial three sections also contain chapters on ethics and professionalism, critical analysis of outcomes, patient safety issues, surgical aspects of mass casualty incidents, and a preview of the potential benefits of emerging technologies such as informatics, electronics, and robotics. Collectively the information in those sections prepares the reader to evaluate and use the current best-evidence-based recommendations for the management of surgical disease of organ systems and tissues as presented in the subsequent nine sections. The last section consists of seven chapters in which essential subspecialty-specific principles are enunciated and related to general surgery practice to complete the picture of surgery as a medical discipline.

This new edition, which is designed to meet the information format preferences of medical students, residents, fellows, and practicing surgeons of all ages, is available in both print and electronic format including that for e-readers such as Kindle. Additionally, this edition has a website called Expert Consult (www.expertconsult.com), which enables the reader to obtain enhanced content such as interactive images that can be used to generate slideshow presentations and annotated test-yourself material, and, with variable magnification, optimize visualization of specific image details.

Dr. Townsend, the editorial descendant of Christopher, Davis, and Sabiston, and his associate editors have generated an effective mix of authoritative senior authors, with voices heard in previous editions and thoroughly updated in this volume, and carefully chosen rising stars to promote clinically useful understanding of the principles guiding surgical intervention. In the aggregate this textbook promotes the concept of "precision surgery," which has developed during the eight decades since 1936 when Frederick Christopher published the first edition of his *Textbook of Surgery* from which this volume has descended. As such, this new edition will enhance the reader's ability to optimize the diagnosis of surgical disease and the treatment of surgical patients. In short, this new "Score" edition has scored again by extending the reign of *Sabiston's Textbook of Surgery* as the "...definitive treatise on surgical practice" as cited by a perceptive reviewer of the 18th edition in 2008.

Basil A. Pruitt, Jr., MD, FACS, FCCM, MCCM
Clinical Professor of Surgery
Betty and Bob Kelso Distinguished Chair in Burn and Trauma Surgery
Dr. Ferdinand P. Herff Chair in Surgery
University of Texas Health Science Center at San Antonio

Dries DJ. Book review. *Sabiston's Textbook of Surgery: The biological basis of modern surgical practice,* 18th edition. Shock 2008; 29: 650.

PREFACE

Surgery continues to evolve as new technology, techniques, and knowledge are incorporated into the care of surgical patients. The 20th edition of *Sabiston Textbook of Surgery* reflects these exciting changes and new knowledge. We have incorporated more than 50 new authors to ensure that the most current information is presented. This new edition has revised and enhanced the current chapters to reflect these changes.

The primary goal of this new edition is to remain the most thorough, useful, readable, and understandable textbook presenting the principles and techniques of surgery. It is designed to be equally useful to students, trainees, and experts in the field. We are committed to maintaining this tradition of excellence begun in 1936. Surgery, after all, remains a discipline in which the knowledge and skill of a surgeon combine for the welfare of our patients.

Courtney M. Townsend, Jr., MD

ACKNOWLEDGMENTS

We would like to recognize the invaluable contributions of Karen Martin, Steve Schuenke, and Eileen Figueroa, and administrator Barbara Petit. Their dedicated professionalism, tenacious efforts, and cheerful cooperation are without parallel. They accomplished whatever was necessary, often on short or instantaneous deadlines, and were vital for the successful completion of the endeavor.

Our authors, respected authorities in their fields and busy physicians and surgeons, all did an outstanding job in sharing their wealth of knowledge.

We would also like to acknowledge the professionalism of our colleagues at Elsevier: Michael Houston, Executive Content Strategist; Joanie Milnes, Content Development Specialist; Patricia Tannian, Publication Services Manager; and Cindy Thoms, Senior Project Manager.

CONTENTS

VIDEO CONTENTS

SECTION I

Surgical Basic Principles

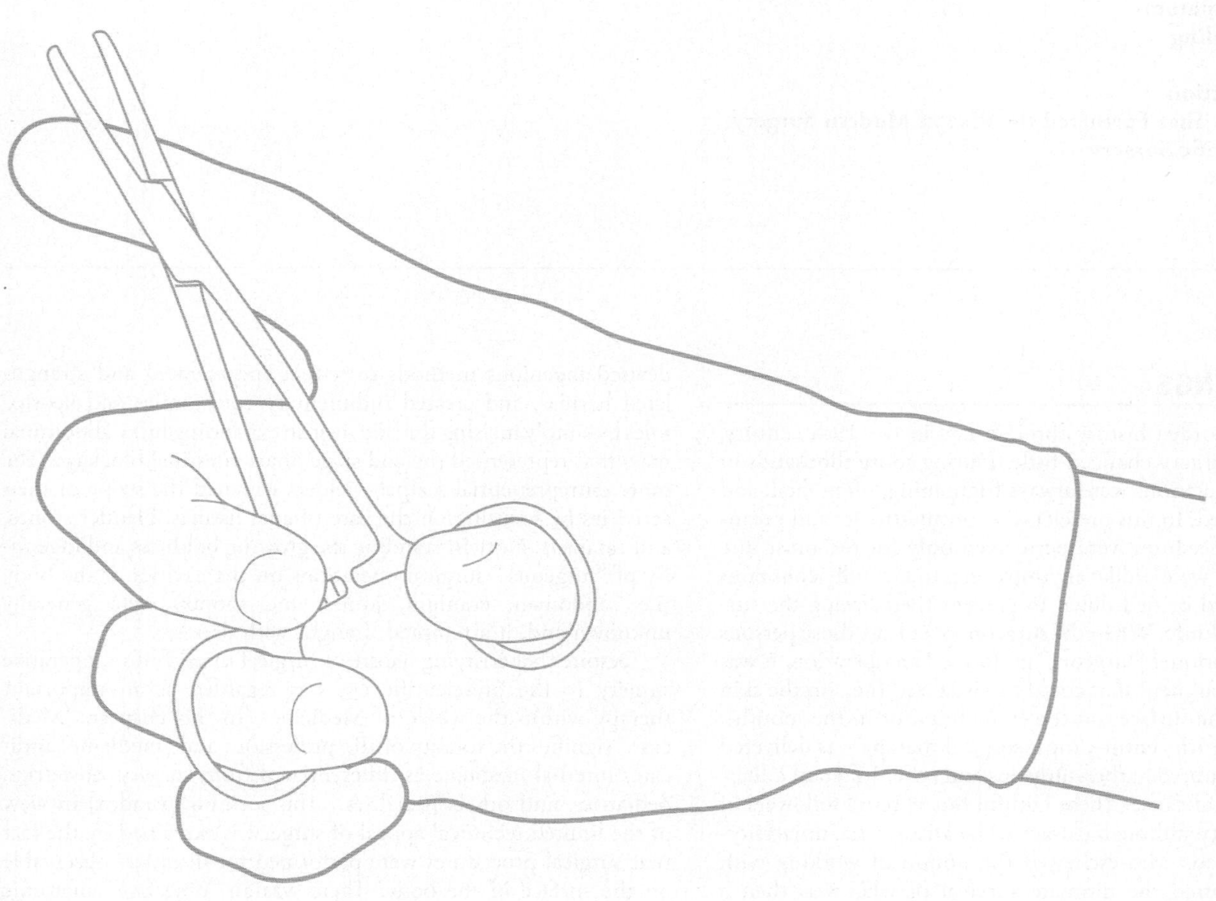

1 CHAPTER

The Rise of Modern Surgery: An Overview

Ira Rutkow

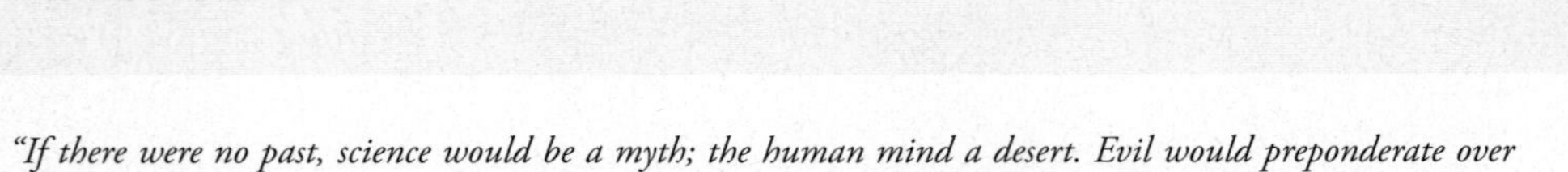

"If there were no past, science would be a myth; the human mind a desert. Evil would preponderate over good, and darkness would overspread the face of the moral and scientific world."

Samuel D. Gross (Louisville Review 1:26–27, 1856)

CHAPTER OUTLINE

THE BEGINNINGS

From earliest recorded history through late in the 19th century, the manner of surgery changed little. During those thousands of years, surgical operations were always frightening, often fatal, and frequently infected. In this prescientific, preanesthetic, and preantiseptic time, procedures were performed only for the most dire of necessities and were unlike anything seen today; fully conscious patients were held or tied down to prevent their fleeing the surgeon's unsparing knife. When the surgeon, or at least those persons who used the sobriquet "surgeon," performed an operation, it was inevitably for an ailment that could be visualized (i.e., on the skin and just below the surface, on the extremities, or in the mouth).

Through the 14th century, most surgical therapy was delivered by minimally educated barber-surgeons and other itinerant adherents of the surgical cause. These faithful but obscure followers of the craft of surgery, although ostracized by aristocratic, university-educated physicians who eschewed the notion of working with one's hands, ensured the ultimate survival of what was then a vocation passed on from father to son. The roving "surgeons" mainly lanced abscesses; fixed simple fractures; dressed wounds; extracted teeth; and, on rare occasions, amputated a digit, limb, or breast. Around the 15th century, the highborn physicians began to show an interest in the art of surgery. As surgical techniques evolved, knife bearers, whether privileged physicians or wandering vagabonds, ligated arteries for readily accessible aneurysms, excised large visible tumors, performed trephinations, devised ingenious methods to reduce incarcerated and strangulated hernias, and created rudimentary colostomies and ileostomies by simply incising the skin over an expanding intra-abdominal mass that represented the end stage of an intestinal blockage. The more entrepreneurial scalpel wielders widened the scope of their activities by focusing on the care of anal fistulas, bladder stones, and cataracts. Notwithstanding the growing boldness and ingenuity of "surgeons," surgical operations on the cavities of the body (i.e., abdomen, cranium, joints, and thorax) were generally unknown and, if attempted, fraught with danger.

Despite the terrifying nature of surgical intervention, operative surgery in the prescientific era was regarded as an important therapy within the whole of Medicine. (In this chapter, "Medicine" signifies the totality of the profession, and "medicine" indicates internal medicine as differentiated from surgery, obstetrics, pediatrics, and other specialties.) This seeming paradox, in view of the limited technical appeal of surgery, is explained by the fact that surgical procedures were performed for disorders observable on the surface of the body: There was an "objective" anatomic diagnosis. The men who performed surgical operations saw what needed to be fixed (e.g., inflamed boils, broken bones, bulging tumors, grievous wounds, necrotic digits and limbs, rotten teeth) and treated the problem in as rational a manner as the times permitted.

For individuals who practiced medicine, care was rendered in a more "subjective" manner involving diseases whose etiologies were neither seen nor understood. It is difficult to treat the symptoms of illnesses such as arthritis, asthma, diabetes, and heart failure when there is no scientific understanding as to what constitutes their pathologic and physiologic underpinnings. It was not until the 19th century and advances in pathologic anatomy and experimental physiology that practitioners of medicine were able to embrace a therapeutic viewpoint more closely approximating that of surgeons. There was no longer a question of treating signs and symptoms in a blind manner. Similar to surgeons who operated on maladies that could be physically described, physicians now cared for patients using clinical details based on "objective" pathophysiologic findings.

Surgeons never needed a diagnostic and pathologic/physiologic revolution in the style of the physician. Despite the imperfection of their knowledge, prescientific surgeons with their unwavering amputation/extirpation approach to treatment sometimes did cure with technical confidence. Notwithstanding their dexterity, it required the spread of the revolution in Medicine during the 1880s and 1890s and the implementation of aseptic techniques along with other soon-to-come discoveries, including the x-ray, blood transfusion, and frozen section, to allow surgeons to emerge as specialists. It would take several more decades, well into the 20th century, for administrative and organizational events to occur before surgery could be considered a bona fide profession.

The explanation for the slow rise of surgery was the protracted elaboration of four key elements (knowledge of anatomy, control of bleeding, control of pain, and control of infection) that were more critical than technical skills when it came to the performance of a surgical procedure. These prerequisites had to be understood and accepted before a surgical operation could be considered a viable therapeutic option. The first two elements started to be addressed in the 16th century, and although surgery greatly benefited from the breakthroughs, its reach was not extended beyond the exterior of the body, and pain and infection continued to be issues for the patient and the surgical operation. Over the ensuing 300 years, there was little further improvement until the discovery of anesthesia in the 1840s and recognition of surgical antisepsis during the 1870s and 1880s. The subsequent blossoming of scientific surgery brought about managerial and socioeconomic initiatives (standardized postgraduate surgical education and training programs; experimental surgical research laboratories; specialty journals, textbooks, monographs, and treatises; and professional societies and licensing organizations) that fostered the concept of professionalism. By the 1950s, the result was a unified profession that was practical and scholarly in nature. Some of the details of the rise of modern surgery follow—specifically how the four key elements that allowed a surgical operation to be viewed as a practical therapeutic choice came to be acknowledged.

KNOWLEDGE OF ANATOMY

Although knowledge of anatomy is the primary requirement of surgery, it was not until the mid-1500s and the height of the European Renaissance that the first great contribution to an understanding of the structure of the human body occurred. This came about when Popes Sixtus IV (1414-1484) and Clement VII (1478-1534) reversed the church's long-standing ban of human dissection and sanctioned the study of anatomy from the cadaver. Andreas Vesalius (1514-1564) (Fig. 1-1) stepped to the forefront of anatomic studies along with his celebrated treatise, *De Humani Corporis Fabrica Libri Septem* (1543). The *Fabrica* broke with the past and provided more detailed descriptions of the human body

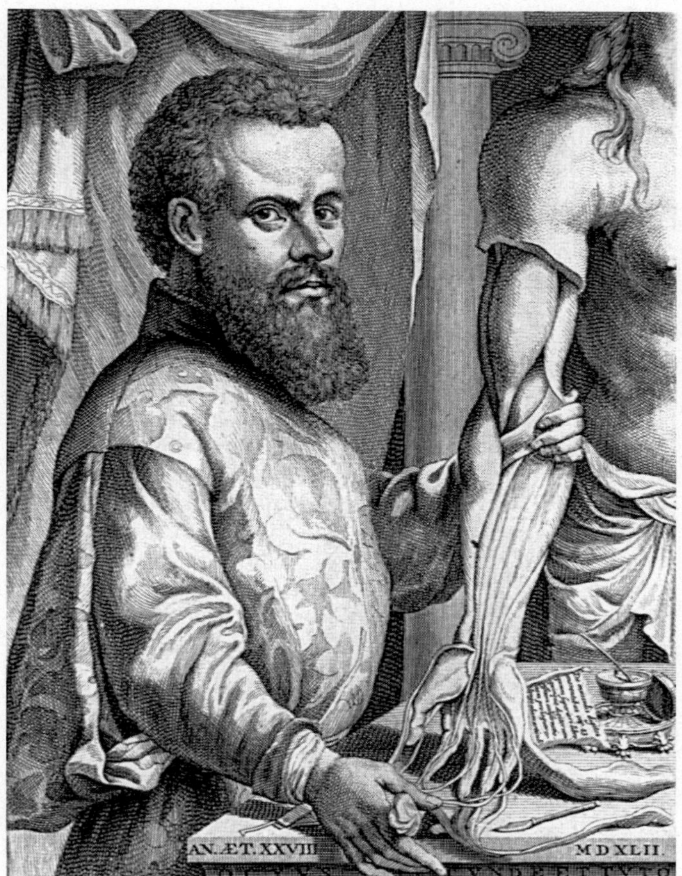

FIGURE 1-1 Andreas Vesalius (1514-1564).

than any of its predecessors. It corrected errors in anatomy that were propagated thousands of years earlier by Greek and Roman authorities, especially Claudius Galen (129-199 AD), whose misleading and later church-supported views were based on animal rather than human dissection. Just as groundbreaking as his anatomic observations was Vesalius' blunt assertion that dissection had to be completed hands-on by physicians themselves. This was a direct repudiation of the long-standing tradition that dissection was a loathsome task to be performed only by individuals in the lower class while the patrician physician sat on high reading out loud from a centuries-old anatomic text.

Vesalius was born in Brussels to a family with extensive ties to the court of the Holy Roman Emperors. He received his medical education in France at universities in Montpellier and Paris and for a short time taught anatomy near his home in Louvain. Following several months' service as a surgeon in the army of Charles V (1500-1558), the 23-year-old Vesalius accepted an appointment as professor of anatomy at the University of Padua in Italy. He remained there until 1544, when he resigned his post to become court physician to Charles V and later to Charles' son, Philip II (1527-1598). Vesalius was eventually transferred to Madrid, but for various reasons, including supposed trouble with authorities of the Spanish Inquisition, he planned a return to his academic pursuits. However, first, in 1563, Vesalius set sail for a year-long pilgrimage to the Holy Land. On his return voyage, Vesalius' ship was wrecked, and he and others were stranded on the small Peloponnesian island of Zakynthos. Vesalius died there as a result of exposure, starvation, and the effects of a severe illness, probably typhoid.

The 7 years that Vesalius spent in Padua left an indelible mark on the evolution of Medicine and especially surgery. His well-publicized human dissections drew large crowds, and Vesalius was in constant demand to provide anatomic demonstrations in other Italian cities, all of which culminated in the publication of the *Fabrica*. Similar to most revolutionary works, the book attracted critics and sympathizers, and the youthful Vesalius was subjected to vitriolic attacks by some of the most renowned anatomists of that era. To his many detractors, the impassioned Vesalius often responded with intemperate counterattacks that did little to further his cause. In one fit of anger, Vesalius burned a trove of his own manuscripts and drawings.

The popularity of Vesalius' *Fabrica* rested on its outstanding illustrations. For the first time, detailed drawings of the human body were closely integrated with an accurate written text. Artists, believed to be from the school of Titian (1477-1576) in Venice, produced pictures that were scientifically accurate and creatively beautiful. The woodcuts, with their majestic skeletons and flayed muscled men set against backgrounds of rural and urban landscapes, became the standard for anatomic texts for several centuries.

The work of Vesalius paved the way for wide-ranging research into human anatomy, highlighted by a fuller understanding of the circulation of blood. In 1628, William Harvey (1578-1657) showed that the heart acts as a pump and forces blood along the arteries and back via veins, forming a closed loop. Although not a surgeon, Harvey's research had enormous implications for the evolution of surgery, particularly its relationship with anatomy and the conduct of surgical operations. As a result, in the 17th century, links between anatomy and surgery intensified as skilled surgeon-anatomists arose.

During the 18th century and first half of the 19th century, surgeon-anatomists made some of their most remarkable observations. Each country had its renowned individuals: In The Netherlands were Govard Bidloo (1649-1713), Bernhard Siegfried Albinus (1697-1770), and Pieter Camper (1722-1789); Albrecht von Haller (1708-1777), August Richter (1742-1812), and Johann Friedrich Meckel (1781-1833) worked in Germany; Antonio Scarpa (1752-1832) worked in Italy; and in France, Pierre-Joseph Desault (1744-1795), Jules Cloquet (1790-1883), and Alfred Armand Louis Marie Velpeau (1795-1867) were the most well known. Above all, however, were the efforts of numerous British surgeon-anatomists who established a well-deserved tradition of excellence in research and teaching.

William Cowper (1666-1709) was one of the earliest and best known of the English surgeon-anatomists, and his student, William Cheselden (1688-1752), established the first formal course of instruction in surgical anatomy in London in 1711. In 1713, *Anatomy of the Human Body* by Cheselden was published and became so popular that it went through at least 13 editions. Alexander Monro *(primus)* (1697-1767) was Cheselden's mentee and later established a center of surgical-anatomic teaching in Edinburgh, which was eventually led by his son Alexander (*secundus*) (1737-1817) and grandson Alexander *(tertius)* (1773-1859). In London, John Hunter (1728-1793) (Fig. 1-2), who is considered among the greatest surgeons of all time, gained fame as a comparative anatomist-surgeon, while his brother, William Hunter (1718-1783), was a successful obstetrician who authored the acclaimed atlas, *Anatomy of the Human Gravid Uterus* (1774). Another brother duo, John Bell (1763-1820) and Charles Bell (1774-1842), worked in Edinburgh and London, where their exquisite anatomic engravings exerted a lasting influence. By the middle of the 19th century, surgical anatomy as a scientific discipline was well established. However, as surgery evolved into a more demanding profession, the anatomic atlases and illustrated surgical textbooks were less likely to be written by the surgeon-anatomist and instead were written by the full-time anatomist.

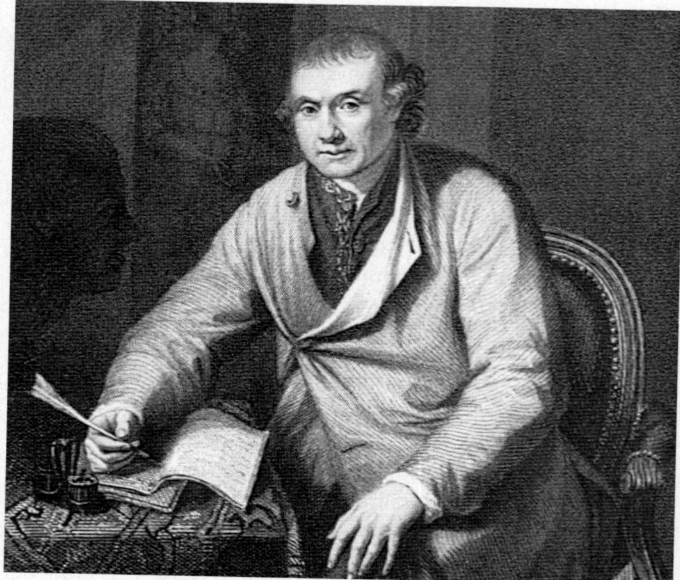

FIGURE 1-2 John Hunter (1728-1793).

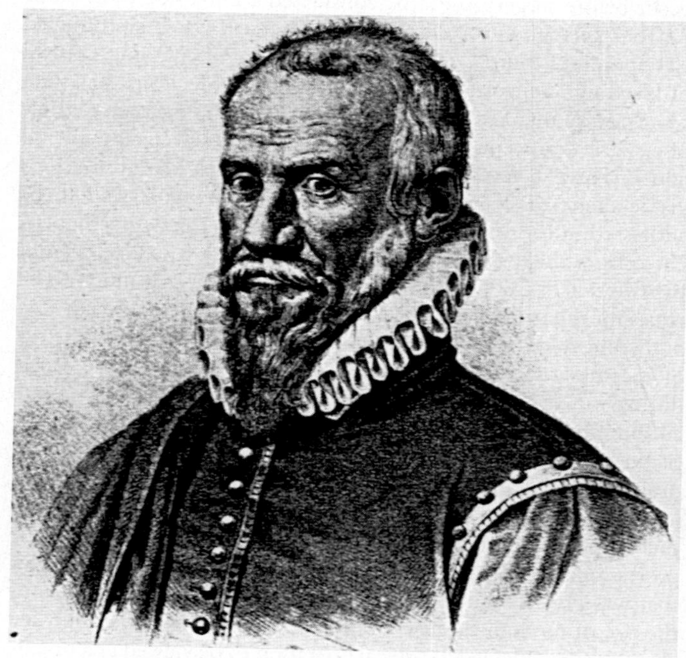

FIGURE 1-3 Ambroise Paré (1510-1590).

CONTROL OF BLEEDING

Although Vesalius brought about a greater understanding of human anatomy, one of his contemporaries, Ambroise Paré (1510-1590) (Fig. 1-3), proposed a method to control hemorrhage during a surgical operation. Similar to Vesalius, Paré is important to the history of surgery because he also represents a severing of the final link between the surgical thoughts and techniques of the ancients and the push toward a more modern era. The two men were acquaintances, both having been summoned to treat Henry II (1519-1559), who sustained what proved to be a fatal lance blow to his head during a jousting match.

Paré was born in France and, at an early age, apprenticed to a series of itinerant barber-surgeons. He completed his indentured education in Paris, where he served as a surgeon's assistant/wound dresser in the famed Hôtel Dieu. From 1536 until just before his death, Paré worked as an army surgeon (he accompanied French armies on their military expeditions), while also maintaining a civilian practice in Paris. Paré's reputation was so great that four French kings, Henry II, Francis II (1544-1560), Charles IX (1550-1574), and Henry III (1551-1589) selected him as their surgeon-in-chief. Despite being a barber-surgeon, Paré was eventually made a member of the Paris-based College of St. Côme, a self-important fraternity of university-educated physician/surgeons. On the strength of Paré's personality and enormity of his clinical triumphs, a rapprochement between the two groups ensued, which set a course for the rise of surgery in France.

In Paré's time, applications of a cautery or boiling oil or both were the most commonly employed methods to treat a wound and control hemorrhage. Their use reflected belief in a medical adage dating back to the age of Hippocrates: Those diseases that medicines do not cure, iron cures; those that iron cannot cure, fire cures; and those that fire cannot cure are considered incurable. Paré changed such thinking when, on a battlefield near Turin, his supply of boiling oil ran out. Not knowing what to do, Paré blended a concoction of egg yolk, rose oil (a combination of ground-up rose petals and olive oil), and turpentine and treated the remaining injured. Over the next several days, he observed that the wounds of the soldiers dressed with the new mixture were neither as inflamed nor as tender as the wounds treated with hot oil. Paré abandoned the use of boiling oil not long afterward.

Paré sought other approaches to treat wounds and staunch hemorrhage. His decisive answer was the ligature, and its introduction proved a turning point in the evolution of surgery. The early history of ligation of blood vessels is shrouded in uncertainty, and whether it was the Chinese and Egyptians or the Greeks and Romans who first suggested the practice is a matter of historical conjecture. One thing is certain: The technique was long forgotten, and Paré considered his method of ligation during an amputation to be original and nothing short of divine inspiration. He even designed a predecessor to the modern hemostat, a pinching instrument called the bec de corbin, or "crow's beak," to control bleeding while the vessel was handled.

As with many ground-breaking ideas, Paré's suggestions regarding ligatures were not readily accepted. The reasons given for the slow embrace range from a lack of skilled assistants to help expose blood vessels to the large number of instruments needed to achieve hemostasis—in preindustrial times, surgical tools were handmade and expensive to produce. The result was that ligatures were not commonly used to control bleeding, especially during an amputation, until other devices were available to provide temporary hemostasis. This did not occur until the early 18th century when Jean-Louis Petit (1674-1750) invented the screw compressor tourniquet. Petit's device placed direct pressure over the main artery of the extremity to be amputated and provided the short-term control of bleeding necessary to allow the accurate placement of ligatures. Throughout the remainder of the 18th and 19th centuries, the use of new types of sutures and tourniquets increased in tandem as surgeons attempted to ligate practically every blood vessel in the body. Nonetheless, despite the abundance of elegant instruments and novel suture materials (ranging from buckskin to horsehair), the satisfactory control of bleeding, especially in delicate surgical operations, remained problematic.

Starting in the 1880s, surgeons began to experiment with electrified devices that could cauterize. These first-generation electrocauteries were ungainly machines, but they did quicken the conduct of a surgical operation. In 1926, Harvey Cushing (1869-1939), professor of surgery at Harvard, experimented with a less cumbersome surgical device that contained two separate electric circuits, one to incise tissue without bleeding and the other simply to coagulate. The apparatus was designed by a physicist, William Bovie (1881-1958), and the two men collaborated to develop interchangeable metal tips, steel points, and wire loops that could be attached to a sterilizable pistol-like grip used to direct the electric current. As the electrical and engineering snags were sorted out, the Bovie electroscalpel became an instrument of trailblazing promise; almost a century later, it remains a fundamental tool in the surgeon's armamentarium.

CONTROL OF PAIN

In the prescientific era, the inability of surgeons to perform pain-free operations was among the most terrifying dilemmas of Medicine. To avoid the horror of the surgeon's merciless knife, patients often refused to undergo a needed surgical operation or repeatedly delayed the event. That is why a scalpel wielder was more concerned about the speed with which he could complete a procedure than the effectiveness of the dissection. Narcotic and soporific agents, such as hashish, mandrake, and opium, had been used for thousands of years, but all were for naught. Nothing provided any semblance of freedom from the misery of a surgical operation. This was among the reasons why the systematic surgical exploration of the abdomen, cranium, joints, and thorax had to wait.

As anatomic knowledge and surgical techniques improved, the search for safe methods to render a patient insensitive to pain became more pressing. By the mid-1830s, nitrous oxide had been discovered, and so-called laughing gas frolics were coming into vogue as young people amused themselves with the pleasant side effects of this compound. After several sniffs, individuals lost their sense of equilibrium, carried on without inhibition, and felt little discomfort as they clumsily knocked into nearby objects. Some physicians and dentists realized that the pain-relieving qualities of nitrous oxide might be applicable to surgical operations and tooth extractions.

A decade later, Horace Wells (1815-1848), a dentist from Connecticut, had fully grasped the concept of using nitrous oxide for inhalational anesthesia. In early 1845, he traveled to Boston to share his findings with a dental colleague, William T.G. Morton (1819-1868), in the hopes that Morton's familiarity with the city's medical elite would lead to a public demonstration of painless tooth-pulling. Morton introduced Wells to John Collins Warren (1778-1856), professor of surgery at Harvard, who invited the latter to show his discovery before a class of medical students, one of whom volunteered to have his tooth extracted. Wells administered the gas and grasped the tooth. Suddenly, the supposedly anesthetized student screamed in pain. An uproar ensued as catcalls and laughter broke out. A disgraced Wells fled the room followed by several bystanders who hollered at him that the entire spectacle was a "humbug affair." For Wells, it was too much to bear. He returned to Hartford and sold his house and dental practice.

However, Morton understood the practical potential of Wells' idea and took up the cause of pain-free surgery. Uncertain about the reliability of nitrous oxide, Morton began to test a compound that one of his medical colleagues, Charles T. Jackson (1805-1880), suggested would work better as an inhalational anesthetic—sulfuric ether. Armed with this advice, Morton studied the properties of the substance while perfecting his inhalational techniques. In fall 1846, Morton was ready to demonstrate the results of his experiments to the world and implored Warren to provide him a public venue. On October 16, with the seats of the operating amphitheater of Massachusetts General Hospital filled to capacity, a tense Morton, having anesthetized a 20-year-old man, turned to Warren and told him that all was ready. The crowd was silent and set their gaze on the surgeon's every move. Warren grabbed a scalpel, made a 3-inch incision, and excised a small vascular tumor on the patient's neck. For 25 minutes, the spectators watched in stunned disbelief as the surgeon performed a painless surgical operation.

Whether the men in the room realized that they had just witnessed one of the most important events in Medical history is unknown. An impressed Warren, however, slowly uttered the five most famous words in American surgery: "Gentlemen, this is no humbug." No one knew what to do or say. Warren turned to his patient and repeatedly asked him whether he felt anything. The answer was a definitive no—no pain, no discomfort, nothing at all. Few medical discoveries have been so readily accepted as inhalational anesthesia. News of the momentous event spread swiftly as a new era in the history of surgery began. Within months, sulfuric ether and another inhalational agent, chloroform, were used in hospitals worldwide.

The acceptance of inhalational anesthesia fostered research on other techniques to achieve pain-free surgery. In 1885, William Halsted (1852-1922) (Fig. 1-4), professor of surgery at the Johns

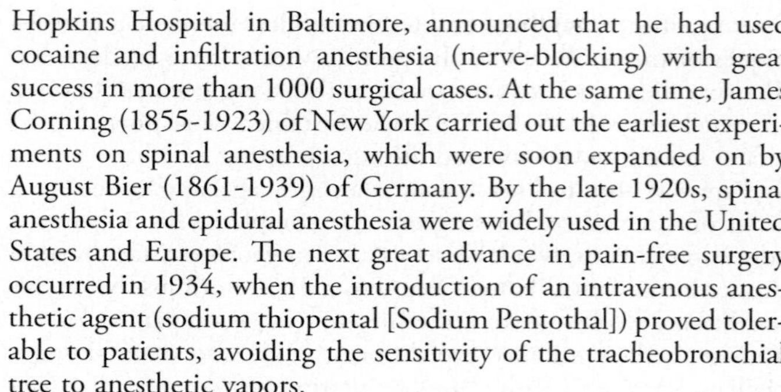

Hopkins Hospital in Baltimore, announced that he had used cocaine and infiltration anesthesia (nerve-blocking) with great success in more than 1000 surgical cases. At the same time, James Corning (1855-1923) of New York carried out the earliest experiments on spinal anesthesia, which were soon expanded on by August Bier (1861-1939) of Germany. By the late 1920s, spinal anesthesia and epidural anesthesia were widely used in the United States and Europe. The next great advance in pain-free surgery occurred in 1934, when the introduction of an intravenous anesthetic agent (sodium thiopental [Sodium Pentothal]) proved tolerable to patients, avoiding the sensitivity of the tracheobronchial tree to anesthetic vapors.

CONTROL OF INFECTION

Anesthesia helped make the potential for surgical cures more seductive. Haste was no longer of prime concern. However, no matter how much the discovery of anesthesia contributed to the relief of pain during surgical operations, the evolution of surgery could not proceed until the problem of postoperative infection was resolved. If ways to deaden pain had never been conceived, a surgical procedure could still be performed, although with much difficulty. Such was not the case with infection. Absent antisepsis and asepsis, surgical procedures were more likely to end in death rather than just pain.

In the rise of modern surgery, several individuals and their contributions stand out as paramount. Joseph Lister (1827-1912) (Fig. 1-5), an English surgeon, belongs on this select list for his efforts to control surgical infection through antisepsis. Lister's research was based on the findings of the French chemist Louis Pasteur (1822-1895), who studied the process of fermentation and showed that it was caused by the growth of living microorganisms. In the mid-1860s, Lister hypothesized that these invisible

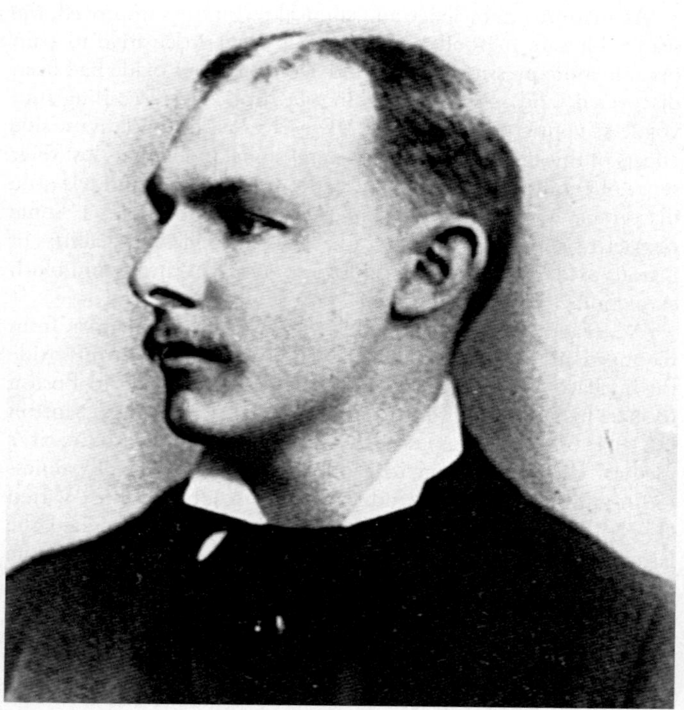

FIGURE 1-4 William Halsted (1852-1922).

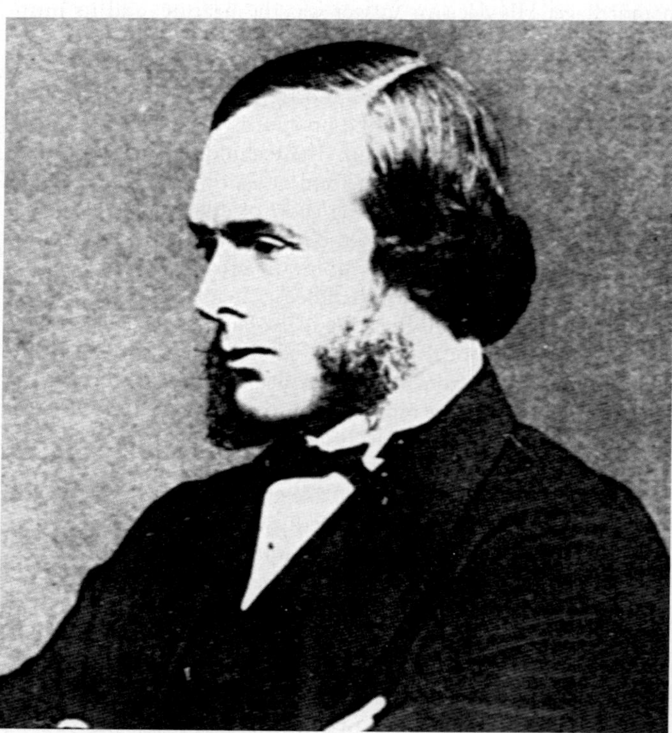

FIGURE 1-5 Joseph Lister (1827-1912).

"germs," or, as they became known, bacteria, were the cause of wound healing difficulties in surgical patients. He proposed that it was feasible to prevent suppuration by applying an antibacterial solution to a wound and covering the site in a dressing saturated with the same germicidal liquid.

Lister was born into a well-to-do Quaker family from London. In 1848, he received his medical degree from University College. Lister was appointed a fellow of the Royal College of Surgeons 4 years later. He shortly moved to Edinburgh, where he became an assistant to James Syme (1799-1870). Their mentor/mentee relationship was strengthened when Lister married Syme's daughter Agnes (1835-1896). At the urging of his father-in-law, Lister applied for the position of professor of surgery in Glasgow. The 9 years that he spent there were the most important period in Lister's career as a surgeon-scientist.

In spring 1865, a colleague told Lister about Pasteur's research on fermentation and putrefaction. Lister was one of the few surgeons of his day who, because of his familiarity with the microscope (his father designed the achromatic lens and was one of the founders of modern microscopy), had the ability to understand Pasteur's findings about microorganisms on a first-hand basis. Armed with this knowledge, Lister showed that an injury was already full of bacteria by the time the patient arrived at the hospital.

Lister recognized that the elimination of bacteria by excessive heat could not be applied to a patient. Instead, he turned to chemical antisepsis and, after experimenting with zinc chloride and sulfites, settled on carbolic acid (phenol). By 1866, Lister was instilling pure carbolic acid into wounds and onto dressings and spraying it into the atmosphere around the operative field and table. The following year, he authored a series of papers on his experience in which he explained that pus in a wound (these were the days of "laudable pus," when it was mistakenly believed the more suppuration the better) was not a normal part of the healing process. Lister went on to make numerous modifications in his technique of dressings, manner of applying them, and choice of antiseptic solutions—carbolic acid was eventually abandoned in favor of other germicidal substances. He did not emphasize hand scrubbing but merely dipped his fingers into a solution of phenol and corrosive sublimate. Lister was incorrectly convinced that scrubbing created crevices in the palms of the hands where bacteria would proliferate.

A second major advance by Lister was the development of sterile absorbable sutures. Lister believed that much of the suppuration found in wounds was created by contaminated ligatures. To prevent the problem, Lister devised an absorbable suture impregnated with phenol. Because it was not a permanent ligature, he was able to cut it short, closing the wound tightly and eliminating the necessity of bringing the ends of the suture out through the incision, a surgical practice that had persisted since the days of Paré.

For many reasons, the acceptance of Lister's ideas about infection and antisepsis was an uneven and slow process. First, the various procedural changes that Lister made during the evolution of his method created confusion. Second, listerism, as a technical exercise, was complicated and time-consuming. Third, early attempts by other surgeons to use antisepsis were abject failures. Finally, and most importantly, acceptance of listerism depended on an understanding of the germ theory, a hypothesis that many practical-minded scalpel wielders were loath to recognize.

As a professional group, German-speaking surgeons were the earliest to grasp the importance of bacteriology and Lister's ideas. In 1875, Richard von Volkmann (1830-1889) and Johann Nussbaum (1829-1890) commented favorably on their treatment of compound fractures with antiseptic methods. In France, Just Lucas-Championière (1843-1913) was not far behind. The following year, Lister traveled to the United States, where he spoke at the International Medical Congress held in Philadelphia and gave additional lectures in Boston and New York. Lister's presentations were memorable, sometimes lasting more than 3 hours, but American surgeons remained unconvinced about his message. American surgeons did not begin to embrace the principles of antisepsis until the mid-1880s. The same was also true in Lister's home country, where he initially encountered strong opposition led by the renowned gynecologist Lawson Tait (1845-1899).

Over the years, Lister's principles of antisepsis gave way to principles of asepsis, or the complete elimination of bacteria. The concept of asepsis was forcefully advanced by Ernst von Bergmann (1836-1907), professor of surgery in Berlin, who recommended steam sterilization (1886) as the ideal method to eradicate germs. By the mid-1890s, less clumsy antiseptic and aseptic techniques had found their way into most American and European surgical amphitheaters. Any lingering doubts about the validity of Lister's concepts of wound infection were eliminated on the battlefields of World War I. Aseptic technique was virtually impossible to attain on the battlefield, but the invaluable principle of wound treatment by means of surgical débridement and mechanical irrigation with an antiseptic solution was developed by Alexis Carrel (1873-1944) (Fig. 1-6), the Nobel prize-winning French-American surgeon, and Henry Dakin (1880-1952), an English chemist.

Once antiseptic and aseptic techniques had been accepted as routine elements of surgical practice, it was inevitable that other antibacterial rituals would take hold, in particular, the use of caps, hats, masks, drapes, gowns, and rubber gloves. Until the 1870s, surgeons did not use gloves because the concept of bacteria on the hands was not recognized. In addition, no truly functional glove had ever been designed. This situation changed in 1878, when an employee of the India-Rubber Works in Surrey, England, received British and U.S. patents for the manufacture of a surgical glove

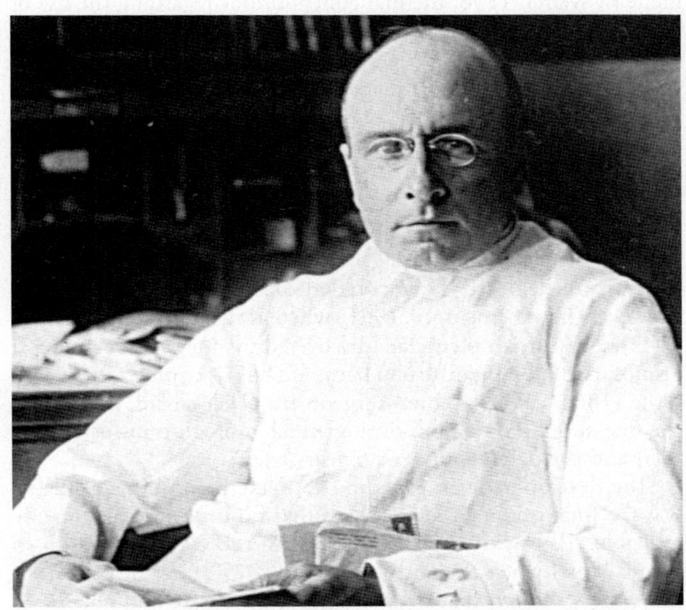

FIGURE 1-6 Alexis Carrel (1873-1944).

that had a "delicacy of touch." The identity of the first surgeon who required that flexible rubber gloves be consistently worn for every surgical operation is uncertain. Halsted is regarded as the individual who popularized their use, although the idea of rubber gloves was not fully accepted until the 1920s.

In 1897, Jan Mikulicz-Radecki (1850-1905), a Polish-Austrian surgeon, devised a single-layer gauze mask to be worn during a surgical operation. An assistant modified the mask by placing two layers of cotton-muslin onto a large wire frame to keep the gauze away from the surgeon's lips and nose. This modification was crucial because a German microbiologist showed that bacteria-laden droplets from the mouth and nose enhanced the likelihood of wound infection. Silence in the operating room became a cardinal feature of surgery in the early 20th century. At approximately the same time, when it was also determined that masks provided less protection if an individual was bearded, the days of surgeons sporting bushy beards and droopy mustaches went by the wayside.

OTHER ADVANCES THAT FURTHERED THE RISE OF MODERN SURGERY

X-Rays

Most prominent among other advances that furthered the rise of modern surgery was the discovery by Wilhelm Roentgen (1845-1923) of x-rays. He was professor of physics at Würzburg University in Germany, and in late December 1895, he presented to that city's medical society a paper on electromagnetic radiation. Roentgen was investigating the photoluminescence from metallic salts that had been exposed to light when he noticed a greenish glow coming from a screen painted with a phosphorescent substance located on a shelf over nine feet away. He came to realize there were invisible rays (he termed them *x-rays*) capable of passing through objects made of wood, metal, and other materials. Significantly, these rays also penetrated the soft tissues of the body in such a way that more dense bones were revealed on a specially treated photographic plate. Similar to the discovery of inhalational anesthesia, the importance of x-rays was realized immediately. By March 1896, the first contributions regarding the use of roentgenography in the practice of Medicine in the United States were reported. In short order, numerous applications were developed as surgeons rapidly applied the new finding to the diagnosis and location of dislocations and fractures, the removal of foreign bodies, and the treatment of malignant tumors.

Blood Transfusion

Throughout the late 19th century, there were scattered reports of blood transfusions, including one by Halsted on his sister for postpartum hemorrhage with blood drawn from his own veins. However, it was not until 1901, when Karl Landsteiner (1868-1943), an Austrian physician, discovered the major human blood groups, that blood transfusion became a less risky practice. George Crile (1864-1943), a noted surgeon from Cleveland, performed the first surgical operation during which a blood transfusion was used and the patient survived 5 years later.

The development of a method to make blood noncoagulable was the final step needed to ensure that transfusions were readily available. This method was developed in the years leading up to World War I when Richard Lewisohn (1875-1962) of New York and others showed that by adding sodium citrate and glucose as an anticoagulant and refrigerating the blood, it could be stored for several days. Once this was known, blood banking became feasible as demonstrated by Geoffrey Keynes (1887-1982), a noted British surgeon (and younger brother of the famed economist John Maynard Keynes), who built a portable cold-storage unit that enabled transfusions to be carried out on the battlefield. In 1937, Bernard Fantus (1874-1940), director of the pharmacology and therapeutics department at Cook County Hospital in Chicago, took the concept of storing blood one step further when he established the first hospital-based "blood bank" in the United States.

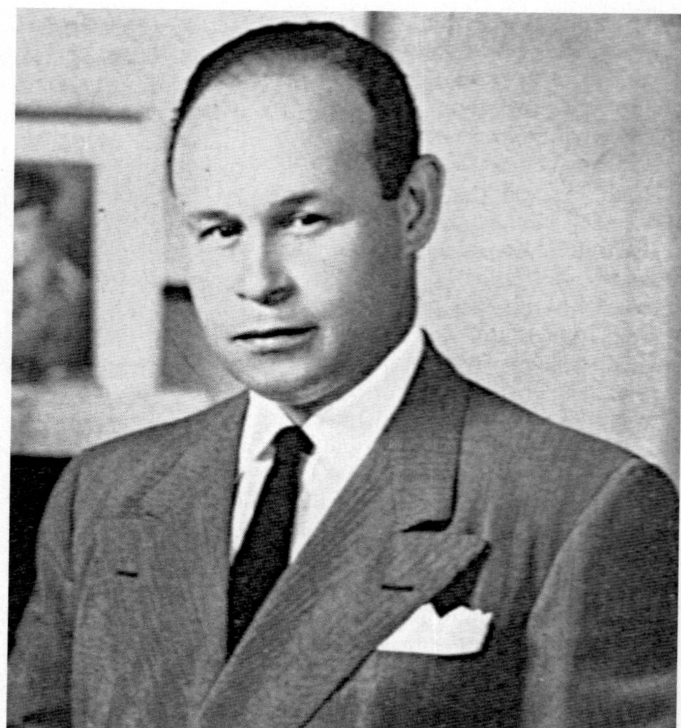

FIGURE 1-7 Charles Drew (1904-1950).

Despite the success in storing and crossmatching blood, immune-related reactions persisted. In this regard, another important breakthrough came in 1939, when Landsteiner identified the Rh factor (so named because of its presence in the rhesus monkey). At the same time, Charles Drew (1904-1950) (Fig. 1-7), a surgeon working at Columbia University, showed how blood could be separated into two main components, red blood cells and plasma, and that the plasma could be frozen for long-term storage. His discovery led to the creation of large-scale blood banking, especially for use by the military during World War II. The storing of blood underwent further refinement in the early 1950s when breakable glass bottles were replaced with durable plastic bags.

Frozen Section

The introduction of anesthesia and asepsis allowed surgeons to perform more technically demanding surgical operations. It also meant that surgeons had to refine their diagnostic capabilities. Among the key additions to their problem-solving skills was the technique of frozen section, an innovation that came to be regarded as one of the benchmarks of scientific surgery. In the late 19th century and early years of the 20th century, "surgical pathology" consisted of little more than a surgeon's knowledge of gross pathology and his ability to recognize lesions on the surface of the

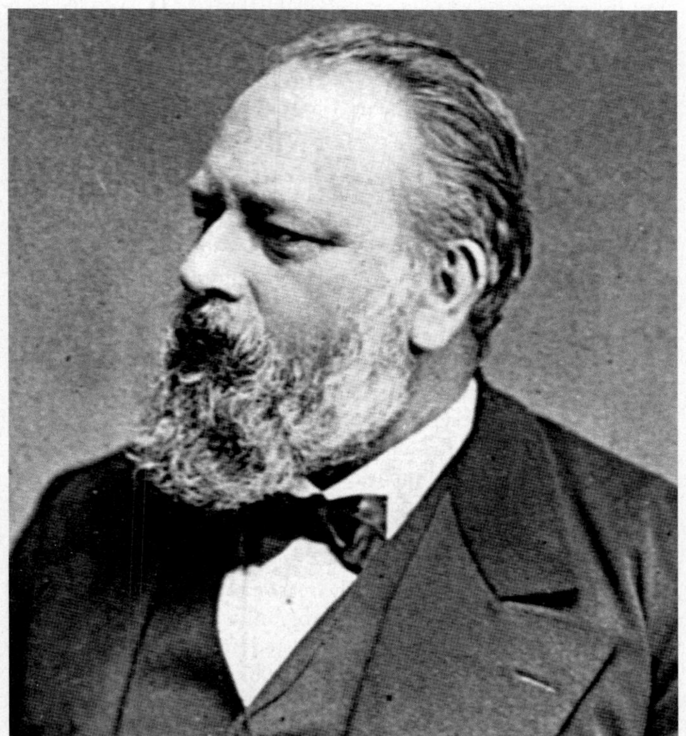

FIGURE 1-8 Theodor Billroth (1829-1894).

body. Similar to the notion of the surgeon-anatomist, the surgeon-pathologist, exemplified by James Paget (1814-1899) of London and the renowned Theodor Billroth (1829-1894) (Fig. 1-8) of Vienna, authored the major textbooks and guided the field.

In 1895, Nicholas Senn (1844-1908), professor of pathology and surgery at Rush Medical College in Chicago, recommended that a "freezing microtome" be used as an aid in diagnosis during a surgical operation. However, the early microtomes were crude devices, and freezing led to unacceptable distortions in cellular morphology. This situation was remedied as more sophisticated methods for hardening tissue evolved, particularly systems devised by Thomas Cullen (1868-1953), a gynecologist at the Johns Hopkins Hospital, and Leonard Wilson (1866-1943), chief of pathology at the Mayo Clinic. During the late 1920s and early 1930s, a time when pathology was receiving recognition as a specialty within Medicine and the influence of the surgeon-pathologist was on the decline, the backing by Joseph Bloodgood (1867-1935), a distinguished surgeon from Baltimore and one of Halsted's earliest trainees, led to the routine use of frozen section during a surgical operation.

ASCENT OF SCIENTIFIC SURGERY

By the first decades of the 20th century, the interactions of politics, science, socioeconomics, and technical advances set the stage for what would become a spectacular showcasing of the progress of surgery. Surgeons wore antiseptic-appearing white caps, gowns, and masks. Patients donned white robes, operating tables were draped in white cloth, and instruments were bathed in white metal basins that contained new and improved antiseptic solutions. All was clean and tidy, with the conduct of the surgical operation no longer a haphazard affair. So great were the innovations that the foundation of basic surgical procedures, including procedures involving the abdomen, cranium, joints, and thorax, was completed by the end of World War I (1918). This transformation was successful not only because surgeons had fundamentally changed but also because Medicine and its relationship to science had been irrevocably altered. Sectarianism and quackery, the consequences of earlier medical dogmatism, were no longer tenable within the confines of scientific inquiry.

Nonetheless, surgeons retained a lingering sense of professional and social discomfort and continued to be pejoratively described by some physicians as nonthinkers who worked in an inferior manual craft. The result was that scalpel bearers had no choice but to allay the fear and misunderstanding of the surgical unknown of their colleagues and the public by promoting surgical procedures as an acceptable part of the new armamentarium of Medicine. This was not an easy task, particularly because the negative consequences of surgical operations, such as discomfort and complications, were often of more concern to patients than the positive knowledge that devastating disease processes could be thwarted.

It was evident that theoretical concepts, research models, and clinical applications were necessary to demonstrate the scientific basis of surgery. The effort to devise new surgical operations came to rely on experimental surgery and the establishment of surgical research laboratories. In addition, an unimpeachable scientific basis for surgical recommendations, consisting of empirical data collected and analyzed according to nationally and internationally accepted standards and set apart from individual assumptions, had to be developed. Surgeons also needed to demonstrate managerial and organizational unity, while conforming to contemporary cultural and professional norms.

These many challenges involved new administrative initiatives, including the establishment of self-regulatory and licensing bodies. Surgeons showed the seriousness of their intent to be viewed as specialists within the mainstream of Medicine by establishing standardized postgraduate surgical education and training programs and professional societies. In addition, a new type of dedicated surgical literature appeared: specialty journals to disseminate news of surgical research and technical innovations promptly. The result of these measures was that the most consequential achievement of surgeons during the mid-20th century was ensuring the social acceptability of surgery as a legitimate scientific endeavor and the surgical operation as a bona fide therapeutic necessity.

The history of the socioeconomic transformation and professionalization of modern surgery varied from country to country. In Germany, the process of economic and political unification under Prussian dominance presented new and unlimited opportunities for physicians and surgeons, particularly when government officials decreed that more than a simple medical degree was necessary for the right to practice. A remarkable scholastic achievement occurred in the form of the richly endowed state-sponsored university where celebrated professors of surgery administered an impressive array of surgical training programs (other medical disciplines enjoyed the same opportunities). The national achievements of German-speaking surgeons soon became international, and from the 1870s through World War I, German universities were the center of world-recognized surgical excellence.

The demise of the status of Austria-Hungary and Germany as the global leader in surgery occurred with the end of the World War I. The conflict destroyed much of Europe—if not its physical features, then a large measure of its passion for intellectual and scientific pursuits. The result was that a vacuum existed internationally in surgical education, research, and therapeutics. It was only natural that surgeons from the United States, the industrialized nation least affected psychologically and physically by the outcome of the war, would fill this void. So began the ascent of American surgery to its current position of worldwide leadership. Some details about the transformation and professionalization of modern American surgery follow.

Standardized Postgraduate Surgical Education and Training Programs

For the American surgeon of the late 19th century, any attempt at formal learning was a matter of personal will with limited practical opportunities. There were a few so-called teaching hospitals but no full-time academic surgeons. To study surgery in these institutions consisted of assisting surgeons in their daily rounds and observing the performance of surgical operations; there was minimal hands-on operative experience. Little, if any, integration of the basic sciences with surgical diagnosis and treatment took place. In the end, most American surgeons were self-taught and, consequently, not eager to hand down hard-earned and valuable skills to younger men who were certain to become competitors.

Conversely, the German system of surgical education and training brought the basic sciences together with practical clinical teaching coordinated by full-time academicians. There was a competitiveness among the young surgeons-in-training that began in medical school with only the smartest and strongest willed being rewarded. At the completion of an internship, which usually included a stint in a basic science laboratory, the young physician would, if fortunate, be asked to become an assistant to a professor of surgery. At this point, the surgeon-to-be was thrust into the thick of an intense contest to become the first assistant (called the chief resident today). There was no regular advancement from the bottom to the top of the staff, and only a small number ever became the first assistant. The first assistant would hold his position until called to a university's chair of surgery or until he tired of waiting and went into practice. From this labyrinth of education and training programs, great surgeons produced more great surgeons, and these men and their schools of surgery offered Halsted the inspiration and philosophies he needed to establish an American system of education and training in surgery.

Halsted was born into a well-to-do New York family and received the finest educational opportunities possible. He had private elementary school tutors, attended boarding school at Phillips Andover Academy, and graduated from Yale in 1874. Halsted received his medical degree 3 years later from the College of Physicians and Surgeons in New York (now Columbia University) and went on to serve an 18-month internship at Bellevue Hospital. With the accomplishments of the German-speaking medical world attracting tens of thousands of American physicians to study abroad, Halsted joined the pilgrimage and spent 1878 through 1880 at universities in Berlin, Hamburg, Kiel, Leipzig, Vienna, and Würzburg. He could not help but notice the stark difference between the German and American manner of surgical education and training.

The surgical residency system that Halsted implemented at the Johns Hopkins Hospital in 1889 was a consolidation of the German approach. In his program, the first of its kind in the United States, Halsted insisted on a more clearly defined pattern of organization and division of duties. The residents had a larger volume of operative material at their disposal, a more intimate contact with practical clinical problems, and a graduated concentration of clinical authority and responsibility in themselves rather than the professor. Halsted's aim was to train outstanding surgical teachers, not merely competent operating surgeons. He showed his residents that research based on anatomic, pathologic, and physiologic principles, along with animal experimentation, made it possible to develop sophisticated operative procedures.

Halsted proved, to an often leery profession and public, that an unambiguous sequence of discovery to implementation could be observed between the experimental research laboratory and the clinical operating room. In so doing, he developed a system of surgery so characteristic that it was termed a "school of surgery." More to the point, Halsted's principles of surgery became a widely acknowledged and accepted scientific imprimatur. More than any other surgeon, it was the aloof and taciturn Halsted, who moved surgery from the melodramatics and grime of the 19th century surgical theater to the silence and cleanliness of the 20th century operating room.

Halsted is regarded as "Adam" in American surgery, but he trained only 17 chief residents. The reason for this was that among the defining features of Halsted's program was an indefinite time of tenure for his first assistant. Halsted insisted that just one individual should survive the steep slope of the residency pyramid and only every few years. Of these men, several became professors of surgery at other institutions where they began residency programs of their own, including Harvey Cushing at Harvard, Stephen Watts (1877-1953) at Virginia, George Heuer (1882-1950) and Mont Reid (1889-1943) at Cincinnati, and Roy McClure (1882-1951) at Henry Ford Hospital in Detroit. By the 1920s, there were a dozen or so Halsted-style surgical residencies in the United States. However, the strict pyramidal aspect of the Halsted plan was so self-limiting (i.e., one first assistant/chief resident with an indefinite length of appointment) that in an era when thousands of physicians clamored to be recognized as specialists in surgery, his restrictive style of surgical residency was not widely embraced. For that reason, his day-to-day impact on the number of trained surgeons was less significant than might be thought.

There is no denying that Halsted's triad of educational principles—knowledge of the basic sciences, experimental research, and graduated patient responsibility—became a preeminent and permanent feature of surgical training programs in the United States. However, by the end of World War II, most surgical residencies were organized around the less severe rectangular structure of advancement employed by Edward Churchill (1895-1972) at the Massachusetts General Hospital beginning in the 1930s. This style of surgical education and training was a response to newly established national standards set forth by the American Medical Association (AMA) and the American Board of Surgery.

In 1920, for the first time, the AMA Council on Medical Education published a list of 469 general hospitals with 3000 "approved" internships. The annual updating of this directory became one of the most important and well-publicized activities of the AMA and provided health care planners with their earliest detailed national database. The AMA expanded its involvement in postgraduate education and training 7 years later when it issued a registry of 1700 approved residencies in various medical and surgical specialties, including anesthesia, dermatology, gynecology and obstetrics, medicine, neuropsychiatry, ophthalmology, orthopedics, otolaryngology, pathology, pediatrics, radiology, surgery, tuberculosis, and urology. By this last action, the AMA publicly declared support for the concept of specialization, a key policy decision that profoundly affected the professional future of physicians in the United States and the delivery of health care.

Experimental Surgical Research Laboratories

Halsted believed that experimental research provided residents with opportunities to evaluate surgical problems in an analytic fashion, an educational goal that could not be achieved solely by treating patients. In 1895, he organized an operative course on animals to teach medical students how to handle surgical wounds and use antiseptic and aseptic techniques. The classes were popular, and, several years later, Halsted asked Cushing, who had recently completed his residency at Hopkins and then spent time in Europe sharpening his experimental research skills with the future Nobel laureates Theodor Kocher (1841-1917) (Fig. 1-9) and Charles Sherrington (1857-1952), to assume responsibility for managing the operative surgery course as well as his experimental laboratory.

Cushing, the most renowned of Halsted's assistants, was a graduate of Yale College and Harvard Medical School. He would go on to become professor of surgery at Harvard and first surgeon-in-chief of the newly built Peter Bent Brigham Hospital. Cushing's clinical accomplishments are legendary and include describing basophil adenomas of the pituitary gland, discovering the rise in systemic blood pressure that resulted from an increase in intracranial pressure, and devising ether charts for the surgical operating room. Just as impressive are Cushing's many achievements outside the world of medical science, the foremost being a Pulitzer Prize in Biography or Autobiography in 1926 for his two-volume work *Life of Sir William Osler*.

Cushing found the operative surgery classroom space to be limited, and he persuaded university trustees to authorize funds to construct the first animal laboratory for surgical research in the United States, the Hunterian Laboratory of Experimental Medicine, named after the famed Hunter. Halsted demanded the same excellence of performance in his laboratory as in the hospital's operating room, and Cushing assured his mentor that this request would be respected. Similar to Halsted, Cushing was an exacting and demanding taskmaster, and he made certain that the Hunterian, which included indoor and outdoor cages for animals, cordoned-off areas for research projects, and a large central room with multiple operating tables, maintained a rigorous scholarly environment where students learned to think like surgical investigators while acquiring the basics of surgical technique. As for the residents in Halsted's program, time in the Hunterian became an integral part of their surgical education and training.

Other American surgeons at the turn of the century demonstrated an interest in experimental surgical research (Senn's book, *Experimental Surgery*, the first American book on the subject, was published in 1889, and Crile's renowned treatise, *An Experimental Research into Surgical Shock*, was published in 1899), but their scientific investigations were not conducted in as formal a setting as the Hunterian. Cushing went on to use the Hunterian for his own neurosurgical research and later took the concept of a surgical research laboratory to Boston where, several surgical generations later, Joseph Murray (1919-2012), working alongside the Brigham's Moseley Professor of Surgery, Francis D. Moore (1913-2001) (Fig. 1-10), won the 1990 Nobel Prize in Physiology or Medicine for his work on organ and cell transplantation in the treatment of human disease, specifically kidney transplant.

One other American surgeon has been named a Nobel laureate. Charles Huggins (1901-1997) (Fig. 1-11) was born in Canada but graduated from Harvard Medical School and received his surgical training at the University of Michigan. While working at the surgical research laboratory of the University of Chicago, Huggins found that antiandrogenic treatment, consisting of orchiectomy or the administration of estrogens, could produce long-term regression in patients with advanced prostatic cancer.

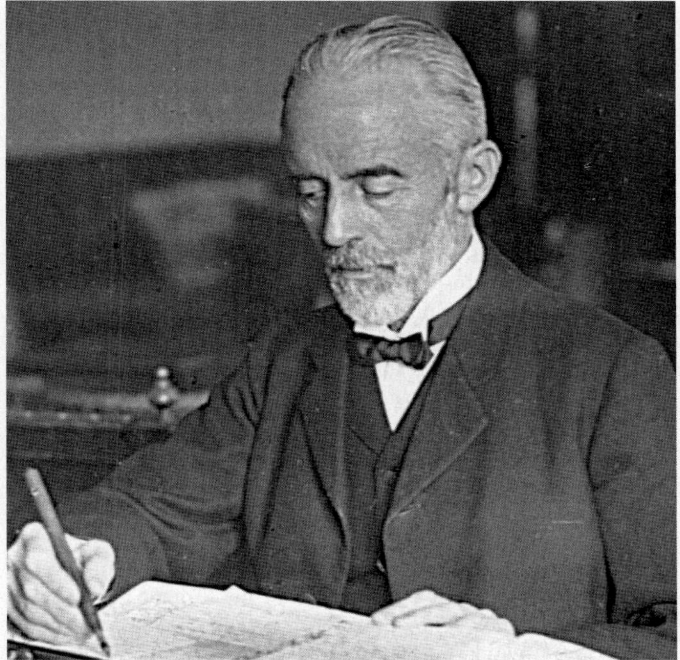

FIGURE 1-9 Theodor Kocher (1841-1917).

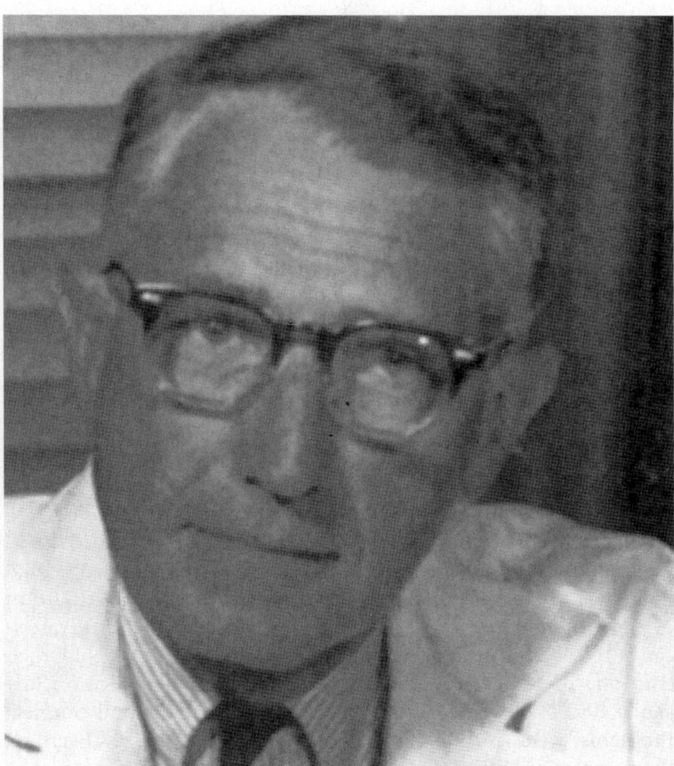

FIGURE 1-10 Francis D. Moore (1913-2001).

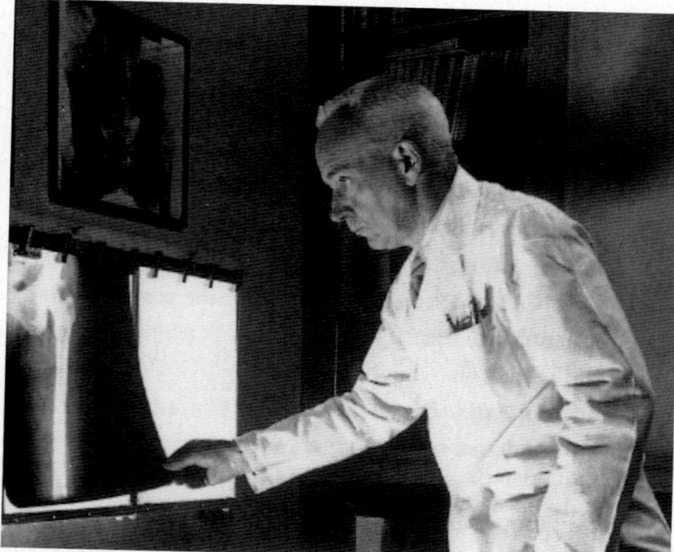

FIGURE 1-11 Charles Huggins (1901-1997).

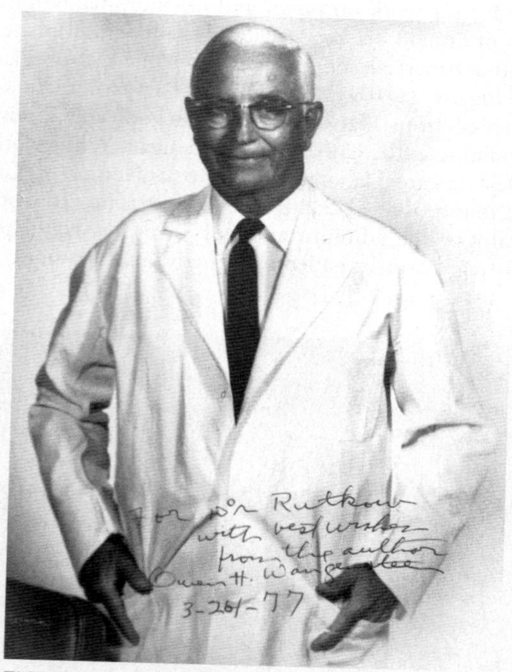
For Dr Rutkow
with best wishes
from the author
Owen H. Wangensteen
3-26-77

FIGURE 1-12 Owen H. Wangensteen (1898-1981).

These observations formed the basis for the treatment of malignant tumors by hormonal manipulation and led to his receiving the Nobel Prize in Physiology or Medicine in 1966.

Regarding the long-term influence of the Hunterian, it served as a model that was widely embraced by many university hospital officials and surgical residency directors. Thus began a tradition of experimental research that remains a feature of modern American surgical education and training programs, the results of which continue to be seen and heard at the American College of Surgeons Owen H. Wangensteen Forum on Fundamental Surgical Problems, held during the annual Clinical Congress. Owen H. Wangensteen (1898-1981) (Fig. 1-12) was the long-time professor of surgery at the University of Minnesota where he brought his department to prominence as a center for innovative experimental and clinical surgical research.

Specialty Journals, Textbooks, Monographs, and Treatises

Progress in science brought about an authoritative and rapidly growing body of medical and surgical knowledge. The timely dissemination of this information into the clinical practice of surgery became dependent on weekly and monthly medical journals. Physicians in the United States proved adept at promoting this new style of journalism, and by the late 1870s, more health-related periodicals were published in the United States than almost all of Europe. However, most medical magazines were doomed to early failure because of limited budgets and a small number of readers. Despite incorporating the words "Surgery," "Surgical," or "Surgical Sciences" in their masthead, none of these journals treated surgery as a specialty. There were simply not enough physicians who wanted to or could afford to practice surgery around the clock. Physicians were unable to operate with any reasonable anticipation of success until the mid-to-late 1880s and the acceptance of the germ theory and Lister's concepts of antisepsis. Once this occurred, the push toward specialization gathered speed, as numbers of surgical operations increased along with a cadre of full-time surgeons.

For surgeons in the United States, the publication of the *Annals of Surgery* in 1885 marked the beginning of a new era, one guided in many ways by the content of the specialty journal. The *Annals* became intimately involved with the advancement of the surgical sciences, and its pages record the story of surgery in the United States more accurately than any other written source. The magazine remains the oldest continuously published periodical in English devoted exclusively to surgery. Other surgical specialty journals soon appeared, and they, along with the published proceedings and transactions of emerging surgical specialty societies, proved crucial in establishing scientific and ethical guidelines for the profession.

As important as periodicals were to the spread of surgical knowledge, American surgeons also communicated their know-how in textbooks, monographs, and treatises. Similar to the rise of the specialty journal, these massive, occasionally multivolume works first appeared in the 1880s. When David Hayes Agnew (1818-1892), professor of surgery at the University of Pennsylvania, wrote his three-volume, 3000-page *Principles and Practice of Surgery*, he was telling the international surgical world that American surgeons had something to say and were willing to stand behind their words. At almost the same time, John Ashhurst (1839-1900), soon-to-be successor to Agnew at the University of Pennsylvania, was organizing his six-volume *International Encyclopedia of Surgery* (1881-1886), which introduced the concept of a multiauthored surgical textbook. The *Encyclopedia* was an instant publishing success and marked the first time that American and European surgeons worked together as contributors to a surgical text. Ashhurst's effort was shortly joined by Keen's *An American Text-Book of Surgery* (1892), which was the first surgical treatise written by various authorities all of whom were American.

These tomes are the forebears of the present book. In 1936, Frederick Christopher (1889-1967), an associate professor of surgery at Northwestern University and chief surgeon to the Evanston Hospital in Evanston, Illinois, organized a *Textbook of Surgery*. The *Textbook*, which Christopher described as a "cross-sectional presentation of the best in American surgery," quickly became one

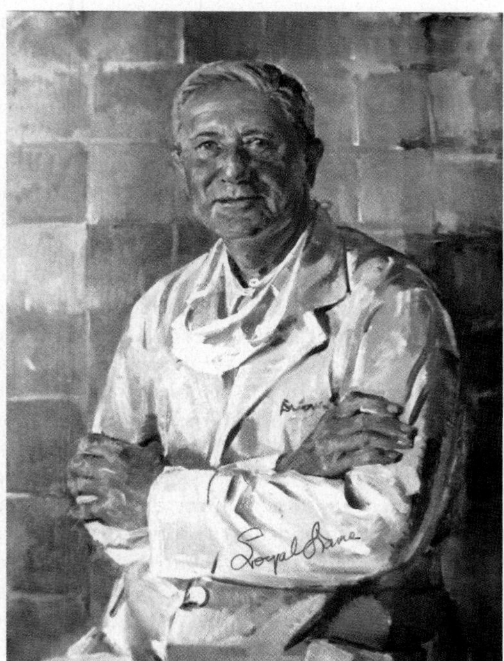

FIGURE 1-13 Loyal Davis (1896-1982).

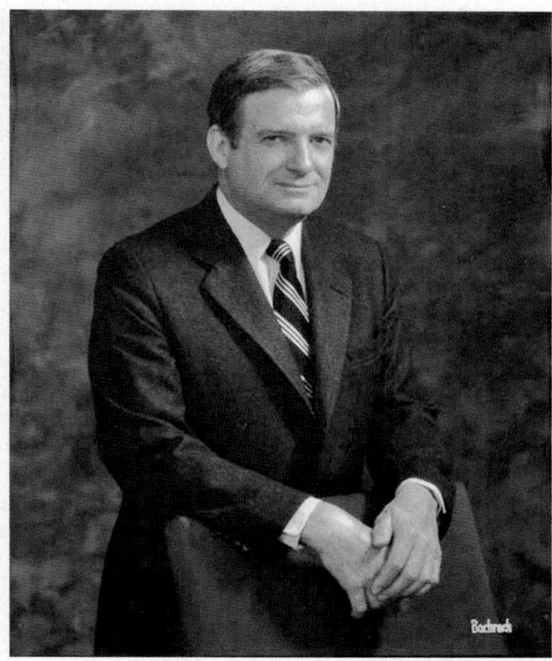

FIGURE 1-14 David Sabiston (1924-2009).

of the most popular of the surgical primers in the United States. He remained in charge for four more editions and, in 1956, was succeeded by Loyal Davis (1896-1982) (Fig. 1-13), professor of surgery at Northwestern University. Davis, who also held a Ph.D. in the neurologic sciences and had studied with Cushing in Boston, was an indefatigable surgical researcher and prolific author. Not only did he edit the sixth, seventh, eighth, and ninth editions of what became known as *Christopher's Textbook of Surgery*, but from 1938 to 1981, Davis also was editor-in-chief of the renowned journal, *Surgery, Gynecology and Obstetrics*. (In the last years of his life, Davis gained further recognition as the father-in-law of President Ronald Reagan.) In 1972, David Sabiston (1924-2009) (Fig. 1-14), professor of surgery at Duke, assumed editorial control of the renamed *Davis-Christopher Textbook of Surgery*. Sabiston was an innovative vascular and cardiac surgeon who held numerous leadership roles throughout his career, including President of the American College of Surgeons, the American Surgical Association, the Southern Surgical Association, and the American Association for Thoracic Surgery. Not only did Sabiston guide editions 10 through 15 of the *Davis-Christopher Textbook*, but he also served as editor-in-chief of the *Annals of Surgery* for 25 years. Starting in 2000 with the 16th edition, Courtney M. Townsend, Jr. (1943-), professor of surgery at the University of Texas Medical Branch in Galveston, took over editorial responsibility for the retitled *Sabiston Textbook of Surgery: The Biological Basis of Modern Surgical Practice*. He has remained in charge through the current 20th edition, and the now legendary work, which Christopher first organized more than 8 decades ago, holds the record for having been updated more times and being the longest lived of any American surgical textbook.

Professional Societies and Licensing Organizations

By the 1920s, surgery was at a point in American society where it was becoming "professionalized." The ascent of scientific surgery had led to technical expertise that gave rise to specialization. However, competence in the surgical operating room alone was not sufficient to distinguish surgery as a profession. Any discipline that looks to be regarded as a profession must assert exclusive control over the expertise of its members and convince the public that these skills are unique and dependable (i.e., act as a monopoly). For the community at large, the notion of trustworthiness is regarded as a fundamental criterion of professional status. To gain and maintain that trust, the professional group has to have complete jurisdiction over its admission policies and be able to discipline and force the resignation of any associate who does not meet rules of acceptable behavior. In their quest for professionalization and specialization, American surgeons created self-regulating professional societies and licensing organizations during the first half of the 20th century.

Around 1910, conflicts between general practitioners and specialists in surgery reached a fever pitch. As surgical operations became more technically sophisticated, inadequately trained or incompetent physicians-cum-surgeons were viewed as endangering patients' lives as well as the reputation of surgery as a whole. That year, Abraham Flexner (1866-1959) issued his now famous report that reformed medical education in the United States. Much as Flexner's manifesto left an indelible mark on more progressive and trustworthy medical schooling, the establishment of the American College of Surgeons 3 years later was meant to impress on general practitioners the limits of their surgical abilities and to show the public that a well-organized group of specialist surgeons could provide dependable and safe operations.

The founding of the American College of Surgeons fundamentally altered the course of surgery in the United States. Patterned after the Royal Colleges of Surgeons of England, Ireland, and Scotland, the American College of Surgeons established professional, ethical, and moral guidelines for every physician who practiced surgery and conferred the designation Fellow of the American College of Surgeons (FACS) on its members. For the first time, there was a national organization that united surgeons by exclusive membership in common educational, socioeconomic, and political causes. Although the American Surgical Association had been founded more than 3 decades earlier, it was composed of a small group of elite senior surgeons and was not meant to serve as a national lobbying front. There were also regional surgical societies, including the Southern Surgical Association (1887) and the Western Surgical Association (1891), but they had less restrictive membership guidelines than the American College of Surgeons, and their geographic differences never brought about national unity.

Because the integrity of the medical profession is largely assured by the control it exercises over the competency of its members, the question of physician licensing and limits of specialization, whether mandated by the government or by voluntary self-regulation, became one of crucial importance. State governments had begun to establish stricter licensing standards, but their statutes did not adequately delineate generalist from specialist. This lack of rules and regulations for specialty practice was a serious concern. Leaders in Medicine realized that if the discipline did not move to regulate specialists, either federal or state agencies would be forced to fill this role, a situation that few physicians wanted. There was also lay pressure. Patients, increasingly dependent on physicians for scientific-based medical and surgical care, could not determine who was qualified to do what—state licensure only established a minimum standard, and membership in loosely managed professional societies revealed little about competency.

By the end of World War I, most surgical (and medical) specialties had established nationally recognized fraternal organizations, such as the American College of Surgeons. In the case of the American College of Surgeons, although its founders hoped to distinguish full-time surgeons from general practitioners, the organization initially set membership guidelines low in its haste to expand enrollment—10 years after its creation, there were more than 7000 Fellows. The American College of Surgeons emphasized an applicant's ability to perform a surgical operation and was less concerned about the depth of overall medical knowledge that sustained an individual's surgical judgment. Furthermore, membership did not depend on examinations or personal interviews. Despite these flaws, the American College of Surgeons did begin to clarify the concept of a surgical specialist to the public. The sheer presence of the American College of Surgeons implied that full-time surgeons outperformed general practitioners and their part-time approach to surgery, while reinforcing the professional authority and clinical expertise of the surgical specialist.

Even with the presence of organizations such as the American College of Surgeons, without a powerful centralized body to coordinate activities, attempts to regulate the push toward specialization in Medicine progressed in a confused and desultory manner. In response to this haphazard approach as well as mounting external pressures and internal power struggles, specialties began to form their own organizations to determine who was a bona fide specialist. These self-governed and self-regulated groups became known as "boards," and they went about evaluating candidates with written and oral examinations as well as face-to-face interviews.

The first board was created in 1917 for ophthalmology and was followed by boards for otolaryngology (1924), obstetrics and gynecology (1930), pediatrics (1933), psychiatry and neurology (1934), radiology (1934), and pathology (1936). Certification by a board indicated a practitioner's level of expertise; thus the limits of specialization set by the board delineated the clinical boundaries of the specialty. For example, in 1936, practitioners of medicine organized a board to cover the whole of internal medicine. In doing so, the specialty exerted firm control over its budding subspecialties, including cardiology, endocrinology, gastroenterology, hematology, and infectious disease. Surgery took a more difficult and divisive path. Before surgeons were able to establish a board for the overall practice of surgery, surgical subspecialists had organized separate boards in otolaryngology, colon and rectal (1935), ophthalmology, orthopedics (1935), and urology (1935). The presence of these surgical subspecialty boards left an open and troubling question: What was to become of the general surgeon?

In the mid-1930s, a faction of younger general surgeons, led by Evarts Graham (1883-1957), decided to set themselves apart from what they considered the less than exacting admission standards of the American College of Surgeons. Graham was professor of surgery at Washington University in St. Louis and the famed discoverer of cholecystography. He demonstrated the link between cigarettes and cancer and performed the first successful one-stage pneumonectomy (as fate would have it, the chain-smoking Graham died of lung cancer). Graham would go on to dominate the politics of American surgery from the 1930s through the 1950s. For now, Graham and his supporters told the leaders of the American College of Surgeons about their plans to organize a certifying board for general surgeons. Representatives of the American College of Surgeons reluctantly agreed to cooperate, and the American Board of Surgery was organized in 1937.

Despite optimism that the American Board of Surgery could formulate a certification procedure for the whole of surgery, its actual effect was limited. Graham attempted to restrain the surgical subspecialties by brokering a relationship between the American Board of Surgery and the subspecialty boards. It was a futile effort. The surgical subspecialty boards pointed to the educational and financial rewards that their own certification represented as reason enough to remain apart from general surgeons. The American Board of Surgery never gained control of the surgical subspecialties and was unable to establish a governing position within the whole of surgery. To this day, little economic or political commonality exists between general surgery and the various subspecialties. The consequence is a surgical lobby that functions in a divided and inefficient manner.

Although the beginning of board certification was a muddled and contentious process, the establishment of the various boards did bring about important organizational changes to Medicine in the United States. The professional status and clinical authority that board certification afforded helped distinguish branches and sub-branches of Medicine and facilitated the rapid growth of specialization. By 1950, almost 40% of physicians in the United States identified themselves as full-time specialists, and of this group, greater than 50% were board certified. It was not long before hospitals began to require board certification as a qualification for staff membership and admitting privileges.

THE MODERN ERA

The 3 decades of economic expansion after World War II had a dramatic impact on the scale of surgery, particularly in the United States. Seemingly overnight, Medicine became big business with health care rapidly transformed into society's largest growth industry. Spacious hospital complexes were built that epitomized not only the scientific advancement of the healing arts but also demonstrated the strength of America's postwar boom. Society gave surgical science unprecedented recognition as a prized national asset, noted by the vast expansion of the profession and the extensive distribution of surgeons throughout the United States. Large

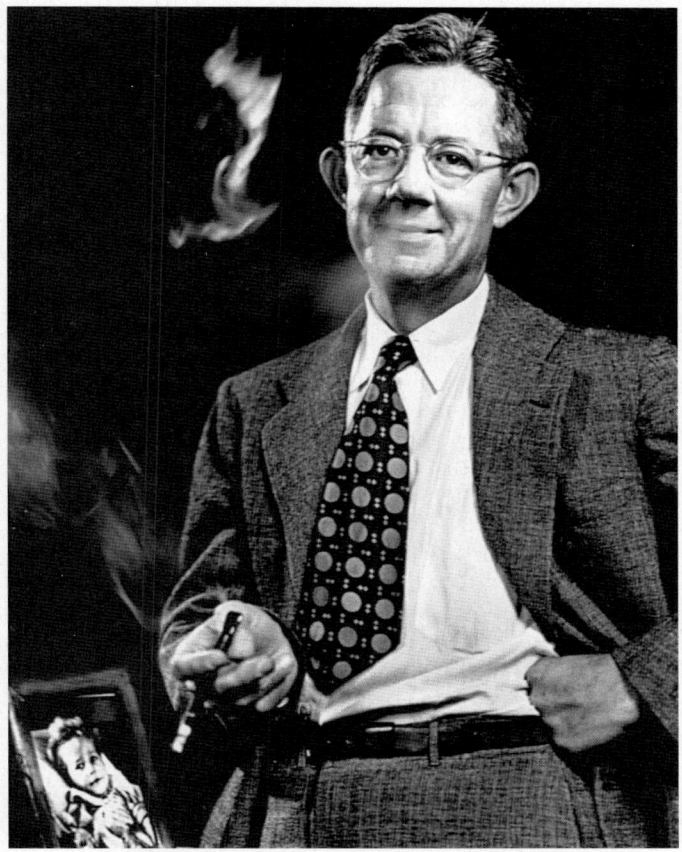

FIGURE 1-15 Alfred Blalock (1899-1964).

urban and community hospitals established surgical education and training programs and found it relatively easy to attract residents. Not only would surgeons command the highest salaries, but also Americans were enamored with the drama of the operating room. Television series, movies, novels, and the more than occasional live performance of a heart operation on television beckoned the lay individual.

It was an exciting time for American surgeons, with important advances made in the operating room and the basic science laboratory. This progress followed several celebrated general surgical firsts from the 1930s and 1940s, including work on surgical shock by Alfred Blalock (1899-1964) (Fig. 1-15), the introduction of pancreaticoduodenectomy for cancer of the pancreas by Allen Oldfather Whipple (1881-1963), and decompression of mechanical bowel obstruction by a suction apparatus by Owen Wangensteen. Among the difficulties in identifying the contributions to surgery after World War II is a surfeit of famous names—so much so that it becomes a difficult and invidious task to attempt any rational selection of representative personalities along with their significant writings. This dilemma was remedied in the early 1970s, when the American College of Surgeons and the American Surgical Association jointly sponsored SOSSUS (Study on Surgical Services for the United States). It was a unique and vast undertaking by the surgical profession to examine itself and its role in the future of health care in the United States. Within the study's three-volume report (1975) is an account from the surgical research subcommittee that named the most important surgical advances in the 1945-1970 era.

In this effort, a group of American surgeons, from all specialties and academic and private practice, attempted to appraise the relative importance of advances in their area of expertise. General surgeons considered kidney transplantation, the replacement of arteries by grafts, intravenous hyperalimentation, hemodialysis, vagotomy and antrectomy for peptic ulcer disease, closed chest resuscitation for cardiac arrest, the effect of hormones on cancer, and topical chemotherapy of burns to be of first-order importance. Of second-order importance were chemotherapy for cancer, identification and treatment of Zollinger-Ellison syndrome, the technique of portacaval shunt, research into the metabolic response to trauma, and endocrine surgery. Colectomy for ulcerative colitis, endarterectomy, the Fogarty balloon catheter, continuous suction drainage of wounds, and development of indwelling intravenous catheters were of third-order importance.

Among the other surgical specialties, research contributions deemed of first-order importance were as follows: Pediatric surgeons chose combined therapy for Wilms tumor; neurosurgeons chose shunts for hydrocephalus, stereotactic surgery and microneurosurgery, and the use of corticosteroids and osmotic diuretics for cerebral edema; orthopedists chose total hip replacement; urologists chose ileal conduits and the use of hormones to treat prostate cancer; otorhinolaryngologists selected surgery for conductive deafness; ophthalmologists selected photocoagulation and retinal surgery; and anesthesiologists selected the development of nonflammable anesthetics, skeletal muscle relaxants, and the use of arterial blood gas and pH measurements.

Additional innovations of second-order and third-order value consisted of the following: Pediatric surgeons chose understanding the pathogenesis and treatment of Hirschsprung's disease, the development of abdominal wall prostheses for omphalocele and gastroschisis, and surgery for imperforate anus; plastic surgeons chose silicone and Silastic implants, surgery of cleft lip and palate, and surgery of craniofacial anomalies; neurosurgeons chose percutaneous cordotomy and dorsal column stimulation for treatment of chronic pain and surgery for aneurysms of the brain; orthopedic surgeons chose Harrington rod instrumentation, compression plating, pelvic osteotomy for congenital dislocation of the hip, and synovectomy for rheumatoid arthritis; urologists selected the treatment of vesicoureteral reflux, diagnosis and treatment of renovascular hypertension, and surgery for urinary incontinence; otorhinolaryngologists selected translabyrinthine removal of acoustic neuroma, conservation surgery for laryngeal cancer, nasal septoplasty, and myringotomy and ventilation tube for serous otitis media; ophthalmologists selected fluorescein fundus angiography, intraocular microsurgery, binocular indirect ophthalmoscopy, cryoextraction of lens, corneal transplantation, and the development of contact lenses; and anesthesiologists chose progress in obstetric anesthesia and an understanding of the metabolism of volatile anesthetics.

All these advances were important to the rise of surgery, but the clinical developments that most captivated the public imagination and showcased the brilliance of post–World War II surgery were the growth of cardiac surgery and organ transplantation. Together, these two fields stand as signposts along the new surgical highway. Fascination with the heart goes far beyond that of clinical medicine. From the historical perspective of art, customs, literature, philosophy, religion, and science, the heart has represented the seat of the soul and the wellspring of life itself. Such reverence also meant that this noble organ was long considered a surgical untouchable.

Although suturing of a stab wound to the pericardium in 1893 by Daniel Hale Williams (1856-1931) and successful treatment of an injury that penetrated a cardiac chamber in 1902 by Luther

Hill (1862-1946) were significant triumphs, the development of safe cardiothoracic surgery that could be counted on as something other than an occasional event did not occur until the 1940s. During World War II, Dwight Harken (1910-1993) gained extensive battlefield experience in removing bullets and shrapnel in or near the heart and great vessels. Building on his wartime experience, Harken and other pioneering surgeons, including Charles Bailey (1910-1993), expanded intracardiac surgery by developing operations for the relief of mitral valve stenosis. In 1951, Charles Hufnagel (1916-1989), working at Georgetown University Medical Center, designed and inserted the first workable prosthetic heart valve in a man. The following year, Donald Murray (1894-1976) completed the first successful aortic valve homograft.

At approximately the same time, Alfred Blalock, professor of surgery at Johns Hopkins, working with Helen Taussig (1898-1986), a pediatrician, and Vivien Thomas (1910-1985), director of the hospital's surgical research laboratories, developed an operation for the relief of congenital defects of the pulmonary artery. The Blalock-Taussig-Thomas subclavian artery–pulmonary artery shunt for increasing blood flow to the lungs of a "blue baby" proved to be an important event in the rise of modern surgery. Not only was it a pioneering technical accomplishment, but it also managed to give many very ill children a relatively normal existence. The salutary effect of such a surgical feat, particularly its public relations value, on the growth of American surgery cannot be overstated.

Despite mounting successes, surgeons who operated on the heart had to contend not only with the quagmire of blood flowing through the area of dissection but also with the unrelenting to-and-fro motion of a beating heart. Technically complex cardiac repair procedures could not be developed further until these problems were solved. John H. Gibbon, Jr. (1903-1973) (Fig. 1-16), addressed this problem by devising a machine that would take on the work of the heart and lungs while the patient was under anesthesia, in essence pumping oxygen-rich blood through the circulatory system while bypassing the heart so that the organ could be more easily operated on. The first successful open heart operation in 1953, conducted with the use of a heart-lung machine, was a momentous surgical contribution.

The surgical treatment of coronary artery disease gained momentum during the 1960s, and by 1980, more cardiac operations were completed annually for coronary artery insufficiency than for all other types of cardiac disease. Although the performance of a coronary artery bypass procedure at the Cleveland Clinic in 1967 by René Favaloro (1923-2000) is commonly regarded as the first successful surgical approach to coronary artery disease, Michael DeBakey (1908-2008) (Fig. 1-17) had completed a similar procedure 3 years earlier but did not report the case until 1973. DeBakey is probably the best-known American surgeon of the modern era. He was a renowned cardiac and vascular surgeon, clinical researcher, medical educator, and international medical statesman as well as the long-time Chancellor of Baylor College of Medicine. He pioneered the use of Dacron grafts to replace or repair blood vessels, invented the roller pump, developed ventricular assist devices, and created an early version of what became the Mobile Army Surgical Hospital (MASH) unit. DeBakey was an influential advisor to the federal government about health care policy and served as chairman of the President's Commission on Heart Disease, Cancer, and Stroke during the Lyndon Johnson administration.

As reported in SOSSUS, when cardiothoracic surgeons were queried about first-order advances in their specialty for the 1945-1970 time period, they selected cardiopulmonary bypass, open and closed correction of congenital cardiovascular disease, the development of prosthetic heart valves, and the use of cardiac pacemakers. Of second-order significance was coronary bypass for coronary artery disease.

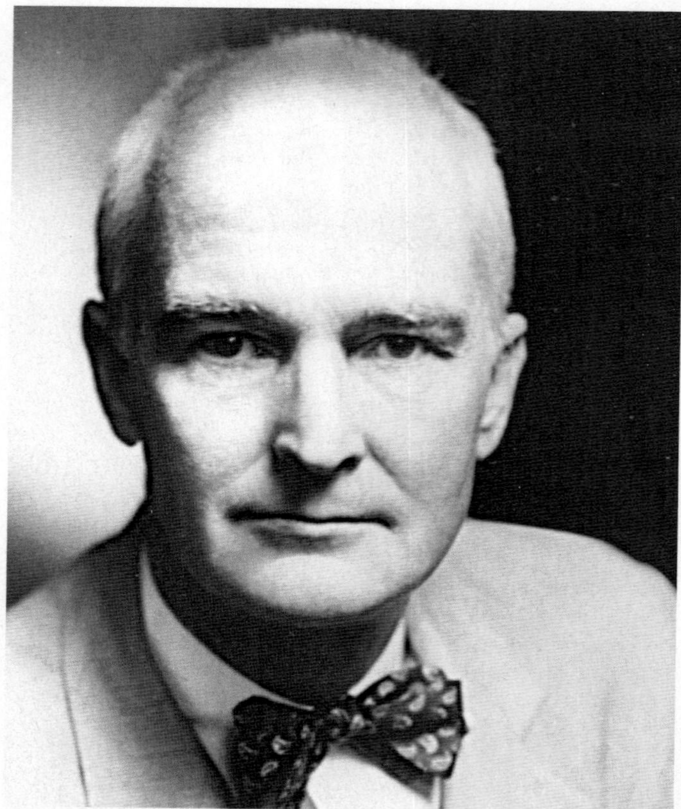

FIGURE 1-16 John H. Gibbon, Jr. (1903-1973).

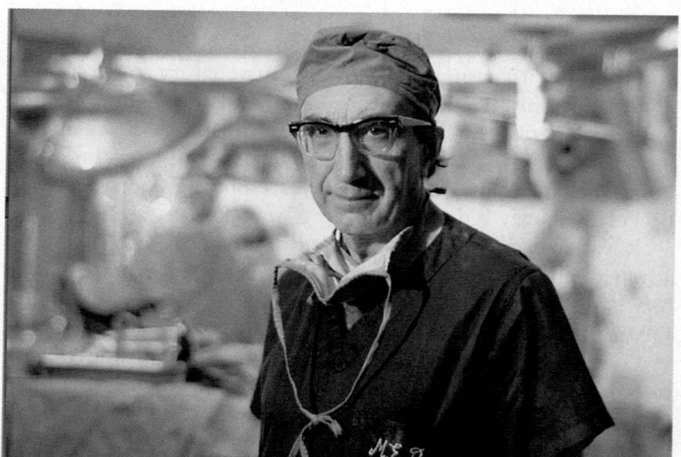

FIGURE 1-17 Michael DeBakey (1908-2008).

What about the replacement of damaged or diseased organs? Even in the mid-20th century, the thought of successfully transplanting worn-out or unhealthy body parts verged on scientific fantasy. At the beginning of the 20th century, Alexis Carrel had developed revolutionary new suturing techniques to anastomose the smallest blood vessels. Using his surgical élan on experimental animals, Carrel began to transplant kidneys, hearts, and spleens.

His research was a technical success, but some unknown biologic process always led to rejection of the transplanted organ and death of the animal. By the middle of the 20th century, medical researchers began to clarify the presence of underlying defensive immune reactions and the necessity of creating immunosuppression as a method to allow the host to accept the foreign transplant. In the 1950s, using high-powered immunosuppressant drugs and other modern modalities, David Hume (1917-1973), John Merrill (1917-1986), Francis Moore, and Joseph Murray blazed the way with kidney transplants. In 1963, the first human liver transplant occurred; 4 years later, Christiaan Barnard (1922-2001) successfully completed a human heart transplant.

DIVERSITY

The evolution of surgery has been influenced by ethnic, gender, racial, and religious bias. Every segment of society is affected by such discrimination, particularly African Americans, women, and certain immigrant groups, who were victims of injustices that forced them into struggles to attain competency in surgery. In the 1930s, Arthur Dean Bevan (1861-1943), professor of surgery at Rush Medical College and an important voice in American surgery, urged that restrictive measures be taken against individuals with Jewish-sounding surnames to decrease their presence in Medicine. It would be historically wrong to deny the long-whispered belief held by the Jewish medical community that anti-Semitism was particularly rife in general surgery before the 1950s compared with the other surgical specialties.

In 1868, a department of surgery was established at Howard University. However, the first three chairmen all were white Anglo-Saxon Protestants. Not until 1928, when Austin Curtis (1868-1939) was appointed professor of surgery, did the department have its first African American head. Similar to all black physicians of his era, Curtis was forced to train at a so-called Negro hospital, Provident Hospital in Chicago, where he came under the tutelage of Daniel Hale Williams, the most influential and highly regarded of that era's African American surgeons.

With little likelihood of obtaining membership in the AMA or its related societies, African American physicians joined together in 1895 to form the National Medical Association. Black surgeons identified an even more specific need when the Surgical Section of the National Medical Association was created in 1906. From its start, the Surgical Section held "hands-on" surgical clinics, which represented the earliest example of organized, so-called "show me" surgical education in the United States. When Williams was named a Fellow of the American College of Surgeons in 1913, the news spread rapidly throughout the African American surgical community. Still, applications of African American surgeons for the American College of Surgeons were often acted on slowly, which suggests that denials based on race were clandestinely conducted throughout much of the United States.

In the mid-1940s, Charles Drew, chairman of the Department of Surgery at Howard University School of Medicine, acknowledged that he refused to accept membership in the American College of Surgeons because this supposedly representative surgical society had, in his opinion, not yet begun to accept routinely capable and well-qualified African American surgeons. Strides toward more racial equality within the profession have been taken since that time, as noted in the career of Claude H. Organ, Jr. (1926-2005) (Fig. 1-18), a distinguished editor, educator, and historian. Among his books, the two-volume *A Century of Black Surgeons: The U.S.A. Experience* and the authoritative *Noteworthy Publications by African-American Surgeons* underscored the numerous contributions made by African American surgeons to the U.S. health care system. In addition, as the long-standing editor-in-chief of the *Archives of Surgery* as well as serving as president of the American College of Surgeons and chairman of the American Board of Surgery, Organ wielded enormous influence over the direction of American surgery.

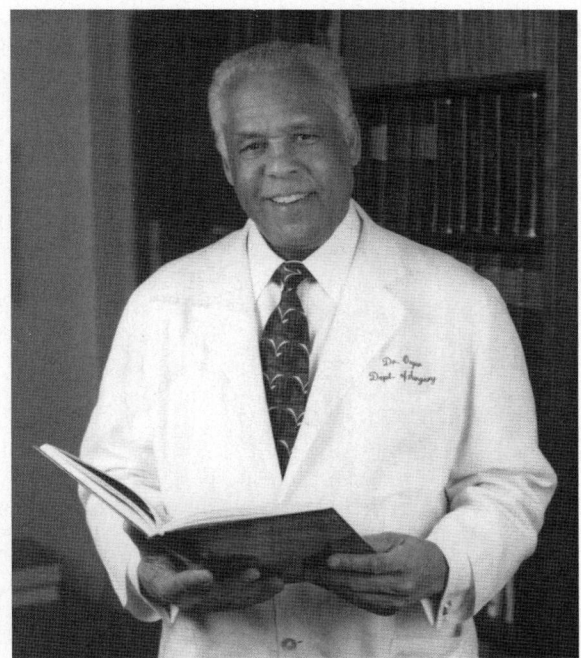

FIGURE 1-18 Claude H. Organ, Jr. (1926-2005).

One of the many overlooked areas of surgical history concerns the involvement of women. Until more recent times, options for women to obtain advanced surgical training were severely restricted. The major reason was that through the mid-20th century, only a handful of women had performed enough operative surgery to become skilled mentors. Without role models and with limited access to hospital positions, the ability of the few practicing female physicians to specialize in surgery seemed an impossibility. Consequently, women surgeons were forced to use different career strategies than men and to have more divergent goals of personal success to achieve professional satisfaction.

Through it all and with the aid of several enlightened male surgeons, most notably William Williams Keen of Philadelphia and William Byford (1817-1890) of Chicago, a small cadre of female surgeons did exist in turn-of-the-century America, including Mary Dixon Jones (1828-1908), Emmeline Horton Cleveland (1829-1878), Mary Harris Thompson (1829-1895), Anna Elizabeth Broomall (1847-1931), and Marie Mergler (1851-1901). The move toward full gender equality is seen in the role that Olga Jonasson (1934-2006) (Fig. 1-19), a pioneer in clinical transplantation, played in encouraging women to enter the modern, male-dominated world of surgery. In 1987, when she was named chair of the Department of Surgery at Ohio State University College of Medicine, Jonasson became the first woman in the United States to head an academic surgery department at a coeducational medical school.

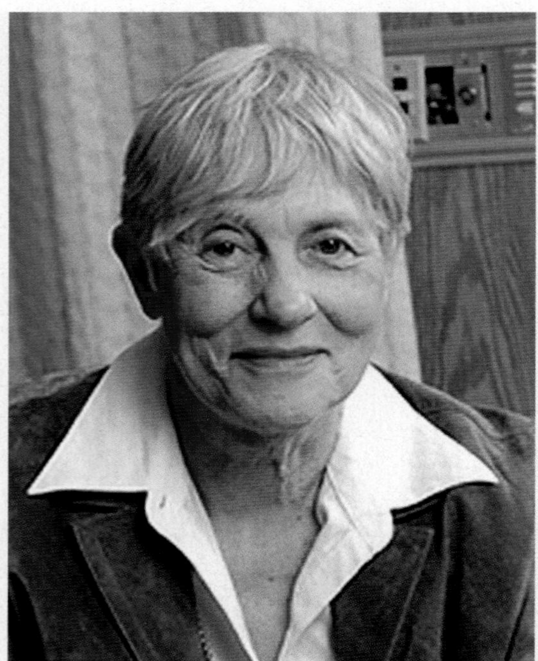

FIGURE 1-19 Olga Jonasson (1934-2006).

THE FUTURE

History is easiest to write and understand when the principal story has already finished. However, surgery continues to evolve. As a result, drawing neat and tidy conclusions about the future of the profession is a difficult task fraught with ill-conceived conclusions and incomplete answers. Nonetheless, several millennia of history provide plentiful insights on where surgery has been and where it might be going.

Throughout its rise, the practice of surgery has been largely defined by its tools and the manual aspects of the craft. The last decades of the 20th century and beginning years of the 21st century saw unprecedented progress in the development of new instrumentation and imaging techniques. Advancement will assuredly continue; if the study of surgical history offers any lesson, it is that progress can always be expected, at least relative to technology. There will be more sophisticated surgical operations with better results. Automation will robotize the surgeon's hand for certain procedures. Still, the surgical sciences will always retain their historical roots as fundamentally a manually based art and craft.

Despite the many advances, these refinements have not come without noticeable social, economic, and political costs. These dilemmas frequently overshadow clinical triumphs, and this suggests that going forward, the most difficult challenges of surgeons may not be in the clinical realm but, instead, in better understanding the sociologic forces that affect the practice of surgery. The most recent years can be seen as the beginnings of a schizophrenic existence for surgeons in that newly devised complex and lifesaving operations are met with innumerable accolades, whereas criticism of the economics of surgery portrays the surgeon as a financially driven selfish individual.

Although they are philosophically inconsistent, the very dramatic and theatrical features of surgery, which make surgeons heroes from one perspective and symbols of mendacity and greed from the opposite point of view, are the very reasons why society demands so much of surgeons. There is the precise and definitive nature of surgical intervention, the expectation of success that surrounds every operation, the short time frame in which outcomes are realized, the high income levels of most surgeons, and the insatiable inquisitiveness of lay individuals about every aspect of consensually cutting into another human's flesh. These phenomena, ever more sensitized in this age of mass media and instantaneous communication, make surgeons seem more accountable than their medical colleagues and, simultaneously, symbolic of the best and worst in Medicine. In ways that were previously unimaginable, this vast economic, political, and social transformation of surgery controls the fate of the individual surgeon to a much greater extent than surgeons as a collective force can manage through their own profession.

National political aims have become overwhelming factors in securing and shepherding the future growth of surgery. Modern surgery is an arena of tradeoffs, a balance between costs, organization, technical advances, and expectations. Patients will be forced to confront the reality that no matter how advanced surgery becomes, it cannot solve all the health-related problems in life. Society will need to come to terms with where the ethical lines should be drawn on everything from face transplants to robotized surgery to gene therapy for surgical diseases. The ultimate question remains: How can the advance of science, technology, and ethics be brought together in the gray area between private and public good?

Studying the fascinating history of our profession, with its many magnificent personalities and outstanding scientific achievements, may not help us predict the future of surgery. Recall Theodor Billroth's remark at the end of the 19th century, "A surgeon who tries to suture a heart wound deserves to lose the esteem of his colleagues." The surgical crystal ball is a cloudy one at best. However, to understand our past does shed some light on current and future clinical practices. Still, if history teaches us anything, it is that surgery will advance and grow inexorably. If surgeons in the future wish to be regarded as more than mere technicians, members of the profession need to appreciate the value of its past glories better. Study our history. Understand our past. Do not allow the rich heritage of surgery to be forgotten.

SELECTED REFERENCES

Earle AS: *Surgery in America: from the colonial era to the twentieth century*, New York, 1983, Praeger.

This is a fascinating compilation of journal articles by well-known surgeons that traces the development of the art and science of surgery in the United States.

Hurwitz A, Degenshein GA: *Milestones in modern surgery*, New York, 1958, Hoeber-Harper.

The numerous chapters contain biographical information and a reprinted or translated excerpt of each surgeon's most important surgical contribution.

Leonardo RA: *History of surgery*, New York, 1943, Froben.

Leonardo RA: *Lives of master surgeons*, New York, 1948, Froben.

Leonardo RA: *Lives of master surgeons, supplement 1*, New York, 1949, Froben.

These three texts together provide an in-depth description of the whole of surgery, from ancient times to the mid-20th century. Especially valuable are the countless biographies of famous and near-famous surgeons.

Meade RH: *A history of thoracic surgery*, Springfield, Ill, 1961, Charles C Thomas.
Meade RH: *An introduction to the history of general surgery*, Philadelphia, 1968, Saunders.

With extensive bibliographies, these two books are among the most ambitious of such systematic works.

Porter R: *The greatest benefit to mankind, a medical history of humanity*, New York, 1997, WW Norton.

Although more a history of the whole of medicine than of surgery, this text became an instantaneous classic and should be required reading for all physicians and surgeons.

Rutkow I: *The history of surgery in the United States, 1775–1900*, vol 1, San Francisco, 1988, Norman Publishing.
Rutkow I: *The history of surgery in the United States, 1775–1900*, vol 2, San Francisco, 1992, Norman Publishing.
Rutkow I: *Surgery, an illustrated history*, St. Louis, 1993, Mosby-Year Book.
Rutkow I: *American surgery, an illustrated history*, Philadelphia, 1998, Lippincott-Raven.
Rutkow I: *Seeking the cure: a history of medicine in America*, New York, 2010, Scribner.

Using biographical compilations, colored illustrations, and detailed narratives, these five books explore the evolution of surgery.

Thorwald J: *The century of the surgeon*, New York, 1956, Pantheon.
Thorwald J: *The triumph of surgery*, New York, 1960, Pantheon.

In dramatic fashion, in these two books, the author uses a fictional eyewitness narrator to create continuity in the story of surgery during its most important decades of growth, the late 19th and early 20th centuries.

Wangensteen OH, Wangensteen SD: *The rise of surgery, from empiric craft to scientific discipline*, Minneapolis, 1978, University of Minnesota Press.

This is not a systematic history but an assessment of various operative techniques and technical innovations that contributed to or slowed the evolution of surgery.

Zimmerman LM, Veith I: *Great ideas in the history of surgery*, Baltimore, 1961, Williams & Wilkins.

Well-written biographical narratives accompany numerous readings and translations from the works of almost 50 renowned surgeons of varying eras.

2 CHAPTER

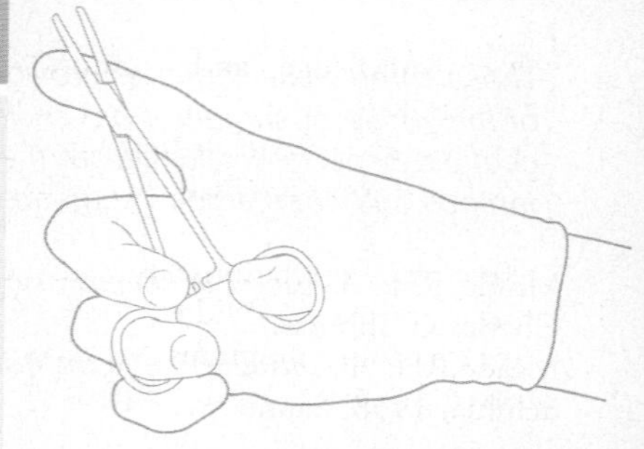

Ethics and Professionalism in Surgery

Cheryl E. Vaiani, Howard Brody

OUTLINE

THE IMPORTANCE OF ETHICS IN SURGERY

Although the ethical precepts of respect for persons, beneficence, nonmaleficence, and justice have been fundamental to the practice of medicine since ancient times, ethics has assumed an increasingly visible and codified position in health care over the past 50 years. The Joint Commission, the courts, presidential commissions, medical school and residency curriculum planners, professional organizations, the media, and the public all have grappled with determining the right course of action in health care matters. The explosion of medical technology and knowledge, changes in the organizational arrangement and financing of the health care system, and challenges to traditional precepts posed by the corporatization of medicine all have created new ethical questions.

The practice of medicine or surgery is, at its center, a moral enterprise. Although clinical proficiency and surgical skill are crucial, so are the moral dimensions of a surgeon's practice. According to Bosk,[1] a sociologist, the surgeon's actions and patient outcome are more closely linked in surgery than in medicine, and that linkage dramatically changes the relationship between the surgeon and the patient. Little,[2] a surgeon and humanist, suggested that there is a distinct moral domain within the surgeon-patient relationship. According to Little, "testing and negotiating the reality of the category of rescue, negotiating the inherent proximity of the relationship, revealing the nature of the ordeal, offering and providing support through its course, and being there for the other in the aftermath of the surgical encounter, are ideals on which to build a distinctively surgical ethics."[2] Because surgery is an extreme experience for the patient, surgeons have a unique opportunity to understand their patients' stories and provide support for them. The virtue and duty of engaged presence as described by Little extends beyond a warm, friendly personality and can be taught by precept and example. Although Little does not specifically identify trust as a component of presence, it seems inherent to the moral depth of the surgeon-patient relationship. During surgery, the patient is in a totally vulnerable position, and a high level of trust is demanded for the patient to place his or her life directly in the surgeon's hands. Such trust requires that the surgeon strive to act always in a trustworthy manner.

From the Hippocratic Oath to the 1847 American Medical Association statement of medical principles through the present, the traditional ethical precepts of the medical profession have included the primacy of patient welfare. The American College of Surgeons was founded in 1913 on the principles of high-quality care for the surgical patient and the ethical and competent practice of surgery. The preamble to its Statement on Principles states the following[3]:

> The American College of Surgeons has had a deep and effective concern for the improvement of patient care and for the ethical practice of medicine. The ethical practice of medicine establishes and ensures an environment in which all individuals are treated with respect and tolerance; discrimination or harassment on the basis of age, sexual preference, gender, race, disease, disability, or religion, are proscribed as being inconsistent with the ideals and principles of the American College of Surgeons.

The Code of Professional Conduct continues[4]:

> As Fellows of the American College of Surgeons, we treasure the trust that our patients have placed in us, because trust is integral to the practice of surgery. During the continuum of pre-, intra-, and postoperative care, we accept responsibilities to:
>
> - Serve as effective advocates of our patients' needs.
> - Disclose therapeutic options, including their risks and benefits.
> - Disclose and resolve any conflict of interest that might influence decisions regarding care.
> - Be sensitive and respectful of patients, understanding their vulnerability during the perioperative period.
> - Fully disclose adverse events and medical errors.
> - Acknowledge patients' psychological, social, cultural, and spiritual needs.
> - Encompass within our surgical care the special needs of terminally ill patients.

- Acknowledge and support the needs of patients' families.
- Respect the knowledge, dignity, and perspective of other health care professionals.

The same expectations are echoed in the Accreditation Council for Graduate Medical Education core competencies that medical-surgical training programs are expected to achieve: compassion, integrity, respect, and responsiveness that supersedes self-interest, accountability, and responsiveness to a diverse patient population.[5]

Historically, the surgeon's decisions were often unilateral ones. Surgeons made decisions about medical benefit with little, if any, acknowledgment that patient benefit might be a different matter. Current surgical practice recognizes the patient's increasing involvement in health care decision making and grants that the right to choose is shared between the surgeon and patient. A focus on informed consent, confidentiality, and advance directives acknowledges this changed relationship of the surgeon and patient. However, the moral dimensions of a surgeon's practice extend beyond those issues to ask how the conscientious, competent, ethical surgeon should reveal damaging mistakes to a family when they have occurred, balance the role of patient advocate with that of being a gatekeeper, handle a colleague who is too old or too impaired to operate safely, or think about surgical innovation. Jones and colleagues,[6] in a helpful casebook of surgical ethics, have noted that even a matter as mundane as the order of patients in a surgical schedule may conceal important ethical decisions.

END-OF-LIFE CARE

Care of patients at the end of life has garnered increasing attention in recent years.[7] In the first of a series of articles concerning palliative care by the surgeon in the *Journal of the American College of Surgeons,* Dunn and Milch[8] explained that palliative care provides the surgeon with a "new opportunity to rebalance decisiveness with introspection, detachment with empathy." They also suggested that although surgeons might appreciate cognitively the need for palliative care, it also presents surgeons with difficult emotional challenges and ambiguities. In recognition of his leadership in the areas of hospice and palliative care, Robert A. Milch received the inaugural Hastings Center Cunniff-Dixon Physician Award in 2010 for leadership in care near the end of life. In accepting the award, Dr. Milch stated, "to the extent that we are able to play a part in that wonder, helping to heal even when we cannot cure, tending the wounds of body and spirit, we are ourselves elevated and transformed."[9] Gawande[10] noted that physicians too often suffer the emotional reaction of failure when dying patients seek quality rather than quantity of life and often make decisions that worsen the problem by failing to ask patients their basic wishes. In one controlled study of patients with advanced lung cancer, patients randomly assigned to receive a palliative care intervention had better quality of life and lived an additional 2 months on average.[11]

Resuscitation in the Operating Room

One of the most difficult issues in end-of-life care for the surgical patient concerns resuscitation. Informed decisions about cardiopulmonary resuscitation (CPR) require that patients have an accurate understanding of their diagnosis, prognosis, likelihood of success of CPR in their situation, and the risks involved. Surgeons sometimes are reluctant to honor a patient's request not to be resuscitated when the patient is considering an operative procedure. Patients with terminal illness may desire surgery for palliation, pain relief, or vascular access yet not desire resuscitation if they experience cardiac arrest. The American College of Surgeons and the American Society of Anesthesiologists have rejected the unilateral suspension of orders not to resuscitate in surgery without a discussion with the patient, but some physicians believe that patients cannot have surgery without being resuscitated and view a do not resuscitate (DNR) order as "as an unreasonable demand to lower the standard of care."[12] Providers may worry that an order to forgo CPR may be extended inappropriately to withholding other critical interventions, such as measures required to control bleeding and maintain blood pressure. They also may fear being prevented from resuscitating patients for whom the cardiac arrest is the result of a medical error.

Discussions with the patient or surrogate about his or her goal for care and desires in various scenarios can help guide decision making. Such conversations allow a mutual decision that respects the patient's autonomy and the physician's professional obligations. On one hand, a patient who refuses resuscitation because the current health status is burdensome can clearly be harmed by intervening to resuscitate while in the operating room. On the other hand, a patient who refuses because of the (presumed) low likelihood of success may change this decision once he or she understands the more favorable outcomes of intraoperative resuscitation.[13] A physician can choose to transfer the care of the patient to another physician if he or she is uncomfortable with the patient's decision about interventions but should not impose this decision on the patient. CPR is not appropriate for every patient who has a cardiac or pulmonary arrest, even if the patient is in the operating room. Physicians need to develop skills in communicating accurate information about the risks and benefits of resuscitation with patients and families in light of the patient's condition and prognosis, make this discussion a routine part of the plan of care, and develop an appropriate team relationship between the surgeon and anesthesiologist to implement the decision.

CULTURAL SENSITIVITY

Much has been said about the culture of surgery and the personality type of surgeons. The slogan "when in doubt, cut it out" is representative of the surgeon's imperative to act. Harsh generalizations of surgeons as egotistical, having a "God complex," and acting as "playground bullies" are frequent. As an often-stereotyped specialty, surgeons should have an astute appreciation for the impact of culture in the clinical encounter. The interaction between the surgeon who recommends operative treatment and the patient who believes that the pain is from a spiritual source and cannot be treated by surgery is unlikely to go well unless the surgeon has the tools to understand and respect the patient's cultural beliefs, values, and ways of doing things.

Training for cultural competence in health care is an essential clinical skill in the increasingly diverse U.S. population and has been recognized and integrated into the current education of medical professionals. Strong evidence of racial and ethnic disparities in health care supports the critical need for such training. Patient-centered care must recognize culture as a major force in shaping an individual's expectations of a physician, perceptions of good and bad health, understanding of the cause of a disease, methods of preventive care, interpretation of symptoms, and recognition of appropriate treatment. Being a culturally competent surgeon is more than having knowledge about specific cultures; cultural knowledge must be carefully handled to avoid stereotyping or oversimplification. Instead, cultural competence involves the "exploration, empathy, and responsiveness to patients' needs, values, and preferences."[14] Self-assessment is often the first step to developing the attitude and skill of cultural competence. Honest and insightful inquiry into one's own feelings, beliefs, and values, including assumptions, biases, and stereotypes, is essential to awareness of the impact of culture on care.

The Association of American Medical Colleges' statement on education for cultural competence lists the following clinical skills as essential for medical students to acquire[15]:

1. Knowledge, respect, and validation of differing values, cultures, and beliefs, including sexual orientation, gender, age, race, ethnicity, and class
2. Dealing with hostility and discomfort as a result of cultural discord
3. Eliciting a culturally valid social and medical history
4. Communication, interaction, and interviewing skills
5. Understanding language barriers and working with interpreters
6. Negotiating and problem-solving skills
7. Diagnosis, management, and patient-adherent skills leading to patient compliance

Various models for effective cross-cultural communication and negotiation exist[16-20] to assist the physician in discovering and understanding the patient's cultural frame of reference. The BELIEF instrument by Dobbie and colleagues[21] is one such model:

Beliefs about health: What caused your illness/problem?
Explanation: Why did it happen at this time?
Learn: Help me to understand your belief/opinion.
Impact: How is this illness/problem impacting your life?
Empathy: This must be very difficult for you.
Feelings: How are you feeling about it?

These models demand the skills of good listening, astute observation, and skillful communication used within the framework of respect and flexibility on the part of the physician. Bridging the cultural divide uses the same skills and traits that engender patient trust and satisfaction and improve quality of care. As Kleinman and associates[17] explained in a classic article, BELIEF types of questions are excellent to ask during every patient encounter, not only those with patients from markedly different cultures. These questions stress the usefulness of regarding every patient interaction as a type of cross-cultural experience.

SHARED DECISION MAKING

Ethically and legally, informed consent is at the heart of the relationship between the surgeon and the patient. The term *informed consent* originated in the legal sphere and still conveys a sense of legalism and bureaucracy to many physicians. The term *shared decision making* has become more popular in more recent times. It is, for all purposes, essentially synonymous with the idea of informed consent, but it suggests a clinical and educational context that most physicians find more congenial.

Shared decision making is the process of educating the patient and assessing that he or she has understood and given permission for diagnostic or therapeutic interventions. The underlying ethical principle is respect for persons, or autonomy. Informed consent reflects the legal and ethical rights people have to make choices about what happens to their body in accordance with their values and goals and the ethical duty of the physician to enhance the patient's well-being.

There is no absolute formula for obtaining informed consent for a procedure, treatment plan, or therapy. A common error is to confuse the signing of a consent form with the process of informed consent. At best, the form is documentation that the process of shared decision making has occurred; it is not a substitute for that process. The process should include explanations from the physician in language the patient can understand and provide the opportunity for the patient to ask questions and consult with others, if necessary. Clarification of the patient's understanding is an important part of the decision making process. Asking patients to explain in their own words what they expect to happen and possible outcomes gives a much better indication of their understanding than having them merely repeat what the physician has stated ("What do you understand about the surgery that has been recommended to you?"). Ideally, the process allows the physician and patient to work together to choose a course of treatment using the physician's expertise and the patient's values and goals.

Determining a patient's capacity to participate in decision making is an important role of the physician and inherent in the process of informed consent. Although capacity is generally assumed in adult patients, there are numerous occasions when the capacity for decision making is questionable or absent. Illness, medication, and altered mental status may result in an inability to participate independently in medical decision making. Capacity for decision making occurs along a continuum, and the more serious the consequences of the decision, the higher the level of capacity that it is prudent to require. Decision making capacity also may change; an individual may be capable of medical decisions one day and not another day or even at a particular time of day but not at another time. Probably the most common reason for questioning a patient's capacity is patient refusal of a treatment, procedure, or plan that the physician thinks is indicated. A patient's refusal raises a red flag and may be an appropriate indicator for an evaluation of capacity, but it should not be the only one. Determination of capacity should be an essential part of the informed consent process for any decision.

How does a physician best evaluate a patient's capacity? There is no one definitive assessment tool for capacity. Although there are many guides and standards for evaluating capacity, it is most generally a common sense judgment that arises from a clinician's interaction with the patient. Mental status tests that assess orientation to person, place, and time are less useful than direct assessment of a patient's ability to make a particular medical decision. Simple questions such as the following assess the evaluation of capacity in the clinical setting more directly[22,23]:

- What do you understand about what is going on with your health right now?
- What treatment (or diagnostic test or procedure) has been proposed to you?
- What are the benefits and risks?
- Why have you decided …?

PROFESSIONALISM

Within medical ethics, the topic of professionalism has received increasing attention more recently. Although the more usual approaches to ethics focus on what decisions one ought to make in a particular situation, professionalism instead addresses questions of enduring moral character—what sort of physician one is, rather than only what one does or does not do.

A common way to address professionalism is to list a series of desirable character traits.[24] However, almost all discussions of professionalism ultimately rely heavily on two simple points.[25] First, physicians are presumed, by virtue of entering into practice, to have made a moral commitment to place the interests of their patients above their own self-interests, at least to a considerable degree. Second, approaching medicine as a profession is commonly contrasted with viewing medical practice as merely a business.

Common challenges to surgeons' professionalism arise during interactions with the pharmaceutical and medical device industries, in which one may earn a substantial monetary reward for activities that promote the marketing interests of companies, even if those activities fail to promote better health for patients. If care is to remain affordable for most patients, the need to control U.S. health care costs represents another major challenge to professionalism. Will physicians and their professional societies act like special interest lobbies, mainly interested in maintaining generous reimbursements for their favored procedures, regardless of evidence about the efficacy of procedures? Or will physicians rise to the challenge of supporting evidence-based medicine and take leadership in identifying low-efficacy procedures the restricted use of which could conserve scarce health care resources?[26]

CONCLUSION

The challenges of contemporary surgical practice not only necessitate attention to the lessons of the past but also contemplation of the future. Traditional codes and oaths provide guidance, but reflection, self-assessment, and deliberation about what it means to be a good surgeon are essential. Educational efforts must inculcate the professional attitudes, values, and behaviors that recognize and support a culture of integrity and ethical accountability.

A good deal of the discussion in this chapter might be summarized in the following sentence: "Have a searching conversation with the patient and discover what he or she really wants." Surgical practice today is marked by more busyness, as bureaucratic tasks such as electronic medical records constantly distract physicians from meaningful contact with their patients. Some people have even proposed "slow medicine" as a necessary corrective.[27] Ethics and professionalism in surgery will require a firm commitment and a willingness to make sacrifices and not merely the desire to fit in with everyday practice.

SELECTED REFERENCES

Brody H: *Hooked: ethics, the medical profession, and the pharmaceutical industry*, Lanham, Md, 2007, Rowman & Littlefield.

This book examines the relationships between physicians and the pharmaceutical industry and how the integrity of the profession of medicine is threatened by those relationships.

Cassell EJ: *The nature of healing: the modern practice of medicine*, New York, 2013, Oxford University Press.

An experienced internist reflects on the relationship between patient and physician.

Chen PW: *Final exam: a surgeon's reflections on mortality*, New York, 2007, Alfred A. Knopf.

A transplant surgeon writes about her own fears and doubts about confronting death and how she helps her patients face the same issues.

Gawande A: *Being mortal: medicine and what matters in the end*, Toronto, 2014, Doubleday Canada.

A surgeon offers his thoughts on end-of-life care.

Jones JW, McCullough LB, Richman BW: *The ethics of surgical practice: cases, dilemmas, and resolutions*, New York, 2008, Oxford University Press.

Case studies of surgical ethics are presented, varying from principles and practice through research and innovation to finances and institutional relationships.

Jonsen AR, Siegler M, Winslade WJ: *Clinical ethics: a practical approach to ethical decisions in clinical medicine*, ed 7, New York, 2010, McGraw-Hill.

This is the standard physician's pocket guide to clinical and ethical decision making.

May WF: *The physician's covenant: images of the healer in medical ethics*, Philadelphia, 1983, Westminster John Knox Press.

This book offers reflections on the physician as parent, fighter, technician, and teacher.

Nuland SB: *How we die: reflections on life's final chapter*, New York, 1994, Vintage Books.

This national bestseller is by a senior surgeon, writer, and historian of medicine.

Selzer R: *Letters to a young doctor*, New York, 1982, Simon & Schuster.

A seasoned surgeon-writer offers sage advice for young surgeons.

REFERENCES

1. Bosk CL: *Forgive and remember: managing medical failure*, ed 2, Chicago, 2003, University of Chicago Press.
2. Little M: Invited commentary: Is there a distinctively surgical ethics? *Surgery* 129:668–671, 2001.
3. American College of Surgeons: Statements on principles, 2008 <http://www.facs.org/fellows_info/statements/stonprin.html>.
4. American College of Surgeons: Code of professional conduct, 2003 <http://www.facs.org/memberservices/codeofconduct.html>.

5. Accreditation Council for Graduate Medical Education (ACGME): Common program requirements: General competencies, 2007 <http://www.acgme.org/outcome/comp/GeneralCompetenciesStandards21307.pdf>.
6. Jones JW, McCullough LB, Richman BW: *The ethics of surgical practice: cases, dilemmas, and resolutions*, New York, 2008, Oxford University Press.
7. American College of Surgeons' Committee on Ethics: Statement on principles guiding care at the end of life. *Bull Am Coll Surg* 83:46, 1998.
8. Dunn GP, Milch RA: Introduction and historical background of palliative care: Where does the surgeon fit in? *J Am Coll Surg* 193:325–328, 2001.
9. Hastings Center: Surgeon and hospice founder accepts Hastings Center Cunniff-Dixon Physician Award, 2011 <http://www.thehastingscenter.org/News/Detail.aspx?id=4422>.
10. Gawande A: *Being mortal: medicine and what matters in the end*, Toronto, 2014, Doubleday Canada.
11. Temel JS, Greer JA, Muzikansky A, et al: Early palliative care for patients with metastatic non-small-cell lung cancer. *N Engl J Med* 363:733–742, 2010.
12. Youngner SJ, Cascorbi HF, Shuck JM: DNR in the operating room. Not really a paradox. *JAMA* 266:2433–2434, 1991.
13. Girardi LN, Barie PS: Improved survival after intraoperative cardiac arrest in noncardiac surgical patients. *Arch Surg* 130: 15–18, 1995.
14. Betancourt JR: Cultural competence—marginal or mainstream movement? *N Engl J Med* 351:953–955, 2004.
15. Association of American Medical Colleges: Cultural competence education, 2005 <https://www.aamc.org/download/54338/data/culturalcomped.pdf>.
16. Levin SJ, Like RC, Gottlieb JE: ETHNIC: A framework for culturally competent ethical practice. *Patient Care* 34:188–189, 2000.
17. Kleinman A, Eisenberg L, Good B: Culture, illness, and care: Clinical lessons from anthropologic and cross-cultural research. *Ann Intern Med* 88:251–258, 1978.
18. Green AR, Betancourt JR, Carrillo JE: Integrating social factors into cross-cultural medical education. *Acad Med* 77:193–197, 2002.
19. Flores G: Culture and the patient-physician relationship: Achieving cultural competency in health care. *J Pediatr* 136:14–23, 2000.
20. Expert Panel on Cultural Competence Education for Students in Medicine and Public Health: *Cultural competence education for students in medicine and public health: report of an expert panel*, Washington, D.C., 2012, Association of American Medical Colleges and Association of Schools of Public Health. <https://members.aamc.org/eweb/upload/Cultural%20Competence%20Education_revisedl.pdf>.
21. Dobbie AE, Medrano M, Tysinger J, et al: The BELIEF Instrument: A preclinical teaching tool to elicit patients' health beliefs. *Fam Med* 35:316–319, 2003.
22. Boyle RJ, et al: The process of informed consent. In Fletcher JC, Lombardo PA, Marshall MF, editors: *Introduction to clinical ethics*, ed 2, Hagerstown, Md, 1997, University Publishing Group, pp 89–105.
23. Lo B: *Resolving ethical dilemmas: a guide for clinicians*, ed 3, New York, 2005, Lippincott Williams & Wilkins.
24. Medical Professionalism Project: Medical professionalism in the new millennium: A physician's charter. *Lancet* 359:520–522, 2002.
25. Brody H, Doukas D: Professionalism: A framework to guide medical education. *Med Educ* 48:980–987, 2014.
26. Brody H: Medicine's ethical responsibility for health care reform—the Top Five list. *N Engl J Med* 362:283–285, 2010.
27. Bauer JL: Slow medicine. *J Altern Complement Med* 14: 891–892, 2008.

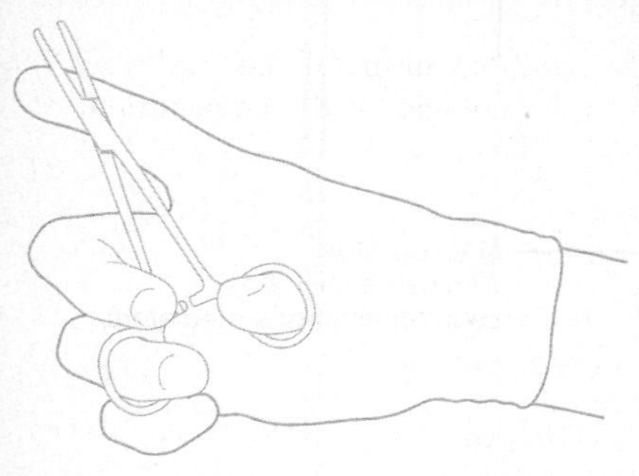

CHAPTER 3

The Inflammatory Response

Puja M. Shah, Zachary C. Dietch, Robert G. Sawyer

OUTLINE

Components of the Immune System
Acute Inflammation
Chronic Inflammation

Inflammation represents the body's response to injury or an invasion by foreign microbes. The body's responses are protective mechanisms that serve to initiate repair of injured tissue and rid the body of invading microbes and are essential for survival. At the same time, unchecked or dysregulated inflammation may cause severe morbidity and potentially fatal complications. Numerous autoimmune conditions, including many seen in surgical patients, represent disorders of the inflammatory system. A comprehensive review of the immune system is beyond the scope of this chapter; rather, the purpose of this chapter is to provide a concise and clinically relevant overview for surgeons.

The inflammatory process can be broadly distinguished by acute and chronic responses, which are each characterized by their own unique environmental milieu. Clinically, surgeons encounter many conditions that are characterized by the coexistence of acute and chronic inflammatory responses. A distinction between acute and chronic inflammation implies that a clear division exists between the cellular components and mediators of inflammation involved in each phase. However, the mechanisms regulating the initiation, maintenance, and characteristics of the inflammatory response are exceedingly complex and interrelated, and many details remain incompletely understood.

COMPONENTS OF THE IMMUNE SYSTEM

The immune response is mediated by innate and adaptive immune mechanisms. Innate immunity is an evolutionarily primitive system, the elements of which dominate the early response to foreign pathogenic invaders and tissue injury in a nonspecific manner. The adaptive immune system, which was a later evolutionary development, responds more slowly but adds a specialized response to immunologic insults through differentiation of lymphocytes. Adaptive immunity consists of two responses: humoral immunity and cell-mediated immunity. Together, these systems characterize the various clinical manifestations of acute and chronic inflammatory responses. A review of key cellular and molecular elements of the immune system is presented in Figure 3-1.

ACUTE INFLAMMATION

The acute inflammatory process can be triggered rapidly after injury or invasion by foreign microbes and is characterized by vascular permeability, edema, and a cellular response dominated by neutrophils. Insults that may trigger the acute inflammatory response include infections (bacterial, viral, fungal, parasitic), trauma, tissue necrosis and ischemia, foreign bodies, and hypersensitivity reactions.

Recognition of Stimuli and Activation of the Acute Inflammatory Response

Classic teaching in immunology postulated that the immune system was activated by recognition of foreign stimuli, such as invading microbes. However, this model failed to explain many observed phenomena in which the body failed to mount a vigorous response to clear nonself stimuli such as mammalian fetuses or tumors with mutated proteins.

The self-nonself theory has since been discarded in favor of Matzinger's danger hypothesis, which proposed that the immune system is activated by various recognizable danger signals, broadly *termed danger (or damage)-associated molecular patterns* (DAMPs) (Fig. 3-2). Matzinger's hypothesis provided a plausible explanation for how the immune system can be activated by foreign microbes such as viruses and bacteria as well as other nonforeign stimuli such as tissue necrosis secondary to trauma. Nonhost invaders such as bacterial pathogens contain unique biochemical properties recognized by the immune system, termed *pathogen-associated molecular patterns* (PAMPs). These PAMPs represent a subset of DAMPs.

Trauma, which causes tissue destruction and the release of endogenous intracellular proteins, triggers a receptor-mediated immune response. The host proteins that trigger this response are a subset of DAMPs and are termed *alarmins*. Alarmins can be released during nonprogrammed cell death—but not during apoptosis—and by cells of the immune system as a mechanism to recruit other cells of the innate immune system.

PAMPs and alarmins can be recognized by Toll-like receptors (TLRs), which are microbial sensors located in the plasma membrane and endosomes of various cells, including phagocytes and

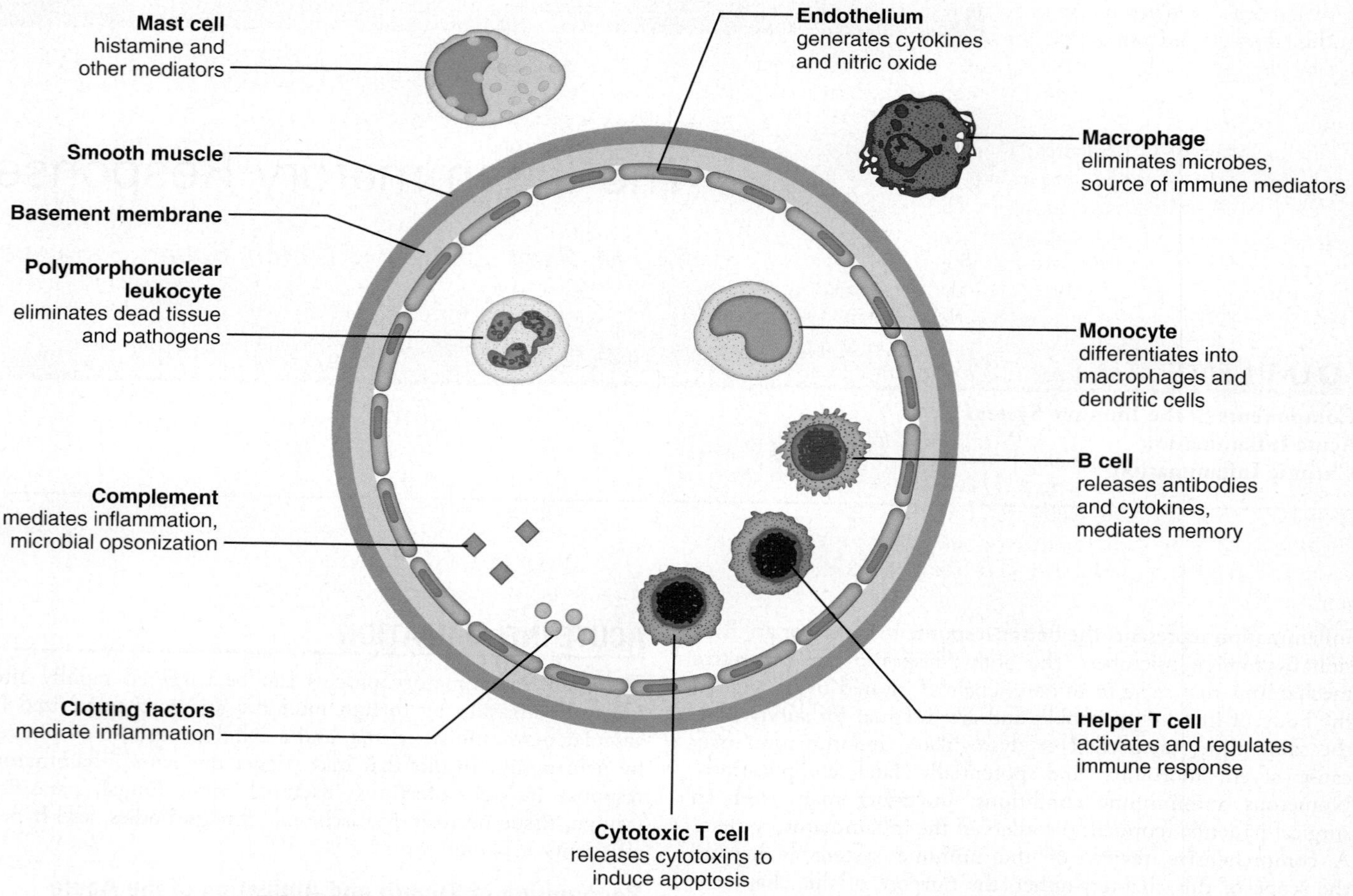

Mast cell
histamine and other mediators
Smooth muscle
Basement membrane
Polymorphonuclear leukocyte
eliminates dead tissue and pathogens
Complement
mediates inflammation, microbial opsonization
Clotting factors
mediate inflammation
Endothelium
generates cytokines and nitric oxide
Macrophage
eliminates microbes, source of immune mediators
Monocyte
differentiates into macrophages and dendritic cells
B cell
releases antibodies and cytokines, mediates memory
Helper T cell
activates and regulates immune response
Cytotoxic T cell
releases cytotoxins to induce apoptosis

FIGURE 3-1 Basic components of the immune system and their respective functions.

Pathogens
PAMPS
NLR agonists and inflammasome activators
TLR
DAMPS
Endogenous TLR agonists
NLR
TLR
TLR
Injury and tissue damage
Alarmins (IL-1α, etc)
Inflammatory response

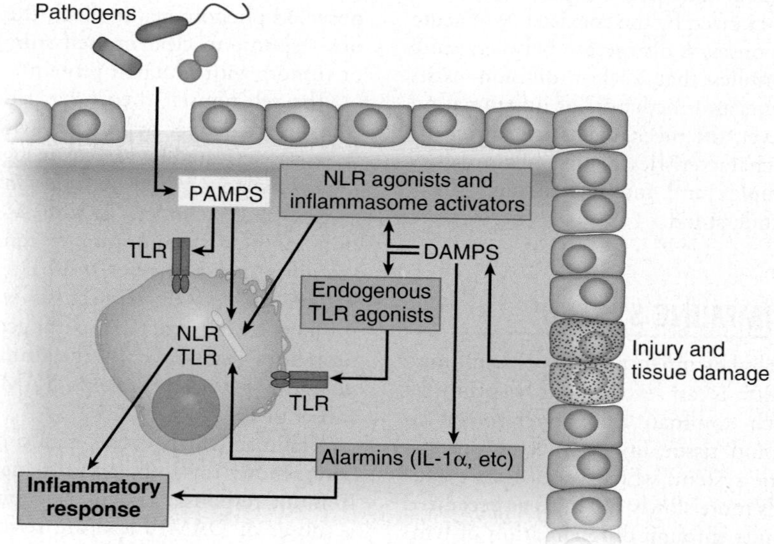

FIGURE 3-2 Recognition of pathogen-associated molecular patterns (PAMPs), which include ligands to Toll-like receptors (TLR) and NOD-like receptors (NLR) ligands, results in production of proinflammatory cytokines. This response to infection initiates inflammation and further release of damage-associated molecular patterns (DAMPs), resulting in synergistic activation of innate immune cells and inflammatory cascades. Injury and tissue damage cause release of DAMPs or alarmins, including TLR agonists and inflammasome activators that generate production of proinflammatory cytokine mediators.

epithelial cells, involved in the immune response. TLRs include a binding domain and a signaling domain, and recognition of extracellular danger signals from microbes or dead tissue triggers the production of numerous proteins that further stimulate the immune response.

The discovery of TLRs, named after the initial protein Toll that was identified in *Drosophila melanogaster,* marked a major leap in the understanding of innate immunity. The search for TLRs began with the identification of interleukin-1 receptor (IL-1R), a receptor for the proinflammatory cytokine interleukin-1 (IL-1) known to cause fever, T cell activation, and the acute-phase response. However, the signaling pathway for interleukin-1 receptor antagonist (IL-1Ra) was a mystery because the function of the receptor's cytosolic domain was unknown. A key development was the discovery that this motif was homologous to that of the *D. melanogaster* protein Toll. At the time, Toll was known to have nuclear factor-κB (NF-κB)–dependent roles in a *Drosophila* development pathway promoting dorsoventral polarity, whereas an NF-κB-dependent pathway in B cells was known to be activated in response to lipopolysaccharide (LPS), a component in the gram-negative bacterial cell wall. IL-1 also had been demonstrated to activate NF-κB signaling.[1]

This evidence suggested that IL-1R and mammalian inflammatory pathways shared NF-κB-dependent pathways similar to that of Toll in *D. melanogaster*. Later discoveries revealed that activation of the Toll^{10b} receptor induced antimicrobial peptide production through an NF-κB-dependent pathway.[1] The first mammalian TLR, hToll, later renamed TLR4, was identified in 1997 and found to induce CD80, which provides costimulation for T cell–mediated immune responses via CD28.

This discovery provided some of the first evidence of a link between the innate and adaptive immune systems; however, the function of TLRs in mammals remained unclear.[1] The role of TLRs in mammalian immunity finally became evident through study of LPS, the component of endotoxin found in gram-negative bacteria that causes severe sepsis. At the time, mice with knockout for *Lps^d* were known to be resistant to the effects of LPS, suggesting that expression of the knockout gene was necessary to generate an immune response to LPS. In 1998, Beutler cloned *Lps^d* and definitively identified it as TLR4. Subsequent work showed that TLR4, in concert with a coreceptor MD2, functioned as an LPS receptor.[1] In addition to LPS, TLR4 recognizes other endogenous alarmins, including heat shock protein 70, high mobility group box 1 protein (HMGB1), saturated fatty acids, and fibronectin type III extra domain A. In addition, TLR4 been implicated as a mediator of sterile inflammation in animal models of hemorrhagic shock, ischemia reperfusion injury, and wound repair. For example, hemorrhage-induced lung injury in mice has been shown to be dependent on the activation of TLR4.

TLRs activate antipathogen cascades in response to extracellular DAMPs, whereas another complex referred to as the inflammasome responds to intracellular danger signals. Inflammasomes are large cytoplasmic complexes that contain NOD-like receptors (NLRs). NLRs are cytoplasmic leucine rich repeat–containing proteins that serve as the scaffolding and sensing elements of the inflammasome. Similar to TLRs, some NLRs respond to foreign microbes as well as endogenous signals. Recognition of an intracellular danger signal by the inflammasome activates caspases, intracellular proteases produced as inactive zymogens, which trigger inflammatory cascades expressing IL-1β and IL-18.

Cell disruption occurring as a result of trauma causes release of intracellular contents, such as adenosine triphosphate and uric acid, which are known to activate inflammasomes. For example, uric acid, which forms monosodium urate crystals in the joint disease gout, activates the NALP3 inflammasome, resulting in IL-1 production and acute inflammation. The discovery of mutations in IL-1-regulating genes in two early-onset autoinflammatory syndromes, cryopyrin-associated periodic syndrome and deficiency of IL-1Ra, led to the successful use of drugs targeting IL-1 in both syndromes and later in four randomized controlled trials evaluating IL-1 antagonism in gout. Research showing that inflammasome pathways are activated by cholesterol crystals and free fatty acids has generated interest in IL-1 antagonist therapy for diabetes and atherosclerosis; however, the data are less clear.

Early Manifestations of Acute Inflammation

For the purpose of this discussion, the pathophysiology of sepsis is examined to illustrate the acute inflammatory response. The innate immune system initiates the inflammatory response by detecting invading foreign microbes via pattern recognition receptors (PRRs), which are germline-encoded receptors expressed by epithelial cells and cells of the innate immune system, including dendritic cells and macrophages. PRRs differ from receptors of the adaptive immune system in that they recognize specific PAMPs that are essential to the survival of the foreign microbe and that cannot be easily modified to avoid detection. A classic, well-described PAMP is LPS, the main virulence factor of gram-negative bacteria. Others include peptidoglycan, lipoteichoic acid, flagellin, and bacterial DNA.[2]

Activation of PRRs, which include TLRs or NLRs, by PAMPs results in transcription of NF-κB-dependent pathways leading to the production of various inflammatory mediators. Important cytokines, including cellular origins and biologic effects, are listed in Tables 3-1 and 3-2. Historically, the early immune response to a pathogen was thought to involve the production of proinflammatory cytokines, such as IL-1, tumor necrosis factor-α (TNF-α), IL-6, IL-12, interferon-γ (IFN-γ), and macrophage migration inhibitory factor (MIF). Early deaths from sepsis were hypothesized to result from an overwhelming proinflammatory response, not the infection itself.[3] Late deaths in infected patients were attributed to a compensatory anti-inflammatory response in which patients died of overwhelming infection because of downregulation of the immune response.[3] These events were thought to be separate, distinct phases of the immune response, and the evidence to support these theories arose from several sources. Patients with meningococcal septicemia were shown to have high circulating levels of TNF-α; high levels of TNF-α were found after injecting endotoxin in animals and humans, and studies in animal models showed that blocking TNF activity improved survival in endotoxin infection.[3]

More recent research challenged these theories by demonstrating that the early cytokine milieu in acute inflammation involves a complex balance between proinflammatory and an array of anti-inflammatory mediators and that these counteracting processes are not distinct.[2] These anti-inflammatory mediators serve to check uncontrolled inflammation and the tissue damage that would result and include soluble TNF receptors (TNFRs), IL-1Ra, IL-1 receptor type II (IL-1R2), inactivators of the complement cascade, IL-10, transforming growth factor-β (TGF-β), and IL-4.[2,4]

Tumor Necrosis Factor-α and Interleukin-1

The actions of TNF-α and IL-1 have been described extensively in infectious and noninfectious inflammatory disorders. Although

TABLE 3-1 Cellular Sources and Important Biologic Effects of Selected Cytokines

CYTOKINE	ABBREVIATION	MAIN SOURCES	IMPORTANT BIOLOGIC EFFECTS
Tumor necrosis factor	TNF	Mφ, others	See Table 3-2
Lymphotoxin-α	LT-α	Th1, NK	Same as TNF
Interferon-α	IFN-α	Leukocytes	Increases expression of cell surface class I MHC molecules; inhibits viral replication
Interferon-β	IFN-β	Fibroblasts	Same as IFN-α
Interferon-γ	IFN-γ	Th1	Activates Mφ; promotes differentiation of CD4⁺ T cells into Th1 cells; inhibits differentiation of CD4⁺ T cells into Th2 cells
Interleukin-1α	IL-1α	Keratinocytes, others	See Table 3-2
Interleukin-1β	IL-1β	Mφ, NK, DC	See Table 3-2
Interleukin-2	IL-2	Th1	In combination with other stimuli, promotes proliferation of T cells; promotes proliferation of activated B cells; stimulates secretion of cytokines by T cells; increases cytotoxicity of NK cells
Interleukin-3	IL-3	T cells, NK	Stimulates pluripotent bone marrow stem cells to increase production of leukocytes, erythrocytes, and platelets
Interleukin-4	IL-4	Th2	Promotes growth and differentiation of B cells; promotes differentiation of CD4⁺ T cells into Th2 cells; inhibits secretion of proinflammatory cytokines by Mφ
Interleukin-5	IL-5	T cells, mast cells, Mφ	Induces production of eosinophils from myeloid precursor cells
Interleukin-6	IL-6	Mφ, Th2, EC, enterocytes	Induces fever; promotes B cell maturation and differentiation; stimulates hypothalamic-pituitary-adrenal axis; induces hepatic synthesis of acute-phase proteins
Interleukin-8	IL-8	Mφ, EC, enterocytes	Stimulates chemotaxis by PMNs; stimulates oxidative burst by PMNs
Interleukin-9	IL-9	Th2	Promotes proliferation of activated T cells; promotes immunoglobulin secretion by B cells
Interleukin-10	IL-10	Th2, Mφ	Inhibits secretion of proinflammatory cytokines by Mφ
Interleukin-11	IL-11	DC, bone marrow	Increases production of platelets; inhibits proliferation of fibroblasts
Interleukin-12	IL-12	Mφ, DC	Promotes differentiation of CD4⁺ T cells into Th1 cells; enhances IFN-γ secretion by Th1 cells
Interleukin-13	IL-13	Th2, others	Inhibits secretion of proinflammatory cytokines by Mφ
Interleukin-17A	IL-17A	Th17	Stimulates production of proinflammatory cytokines by Mφ and many other cell types
Interleukin-18	IL-18	Mφ, others	Costimulation with IL-12 of IFN-γ secretion by Th1 cells and NK cells
Interleukin-21	IL-21	Th2, Th17	Modulation of B cell survival; inhibition of IgE synthesis; inhibition of proinflammatory cytokine production by Mφ
Interleukin-23	IL-23	Mφ, DC	In conjunction with TGF-β, promotes differentiation of naïve T cells into Th17 cells
Interleukin-27	IL-27	Mφ, DC	Suppresses effector functions of lymphocytes and Mφ
Monocyte chemotactic protein-1	MCP-1	EC, others	Stimulates chemotaxis by monocytes; stimulates oxidative burst by Mφ
Granulocyte-macrophage colony-stimulating factor	GM-CSF	T cells, Mφ, EC, others	Enhances production of granulocytes and monocytes by bone marrow; primes Mφ to produce proinflammatory mediators after activation by another stimulus
Granulocyte colony-stimulating factor	G-CSF	Mφ, fibroblasts	Enhances production of granulocytes by bone marrow
Erythropoietin	EPO	Kidney cells	Enhances production of erythrocytes by bone marrow
Transforming growth factor-β	TGF-β	T cells, Mφ, platelets, others	Stimulates chemotaxis by monocytes and induces synthesis of extracellular proteins by fibroblasts; promotes differentiation of naïve T cells into Treg cells; with IL-6 or IL-23, promotes differentiation of naïve T cells into Th17 cells; inhibits immunoglobulin secretion by B cells; downregulates activation of NK cells

DC, Dendritic cells; *EC,* endothelial cells; *Mφ,* cells of the monocyte-macrophage lineage; *MHC,* major histocompatibility complex; *NK,* natural killer cells; *PMNs,* polymorphonuclear neutrophils; *Th1, Th2, Th17,* subsets of differentiated CD4⁺ helper T cells; *Treg,* T-regulatory.

these cytokines are structurally distinct, their biologic functions in the inflammatory response overlap considerably. In animal and human models, IL-1 and TNF-α have been shown to act synergistically to mediate the early inflammatory response and induce a shocklike state characterized by vascular permeability, loss of vascular tone, pulmonary edema, and hemorrhage. In addition, both cytokines are pyrogenic.

TNF-α is produced by a wide variety of cells, most notably monocytes and macrophages, and mediates a broad array of downstream inflammatory processes. It is initially synthesized as a membrane-bound 26-kDa molecule that is subsequently cleaved by a TNF converting enzyme to form a soluble 17-kDa protein. TNF-α binds to two distinct receptors, TNFR1 and TNFR2, which initiate a broad cascade of proinflammatory events leading

TABLE 3-2 Partial List of Physiologic Effects Induced by Infusing Interleukin-1 or Tumor Necrosis Factor into Human Subjects

EFFECT	IL-1	TNF
Fever	+	+
Headache	+	+
Anorexia	+	+
Increased plasma adrenocorticotropic hormone level	+	+
Hypercortisolemia	+	+
Increased plasma nitrite-nitrate levels	+	+
Systemic arterial hypotension	+	+
Neutrophilia	+	+
Transient neutropenia	+	+
Increased plasma acute-phase protein levels	+	+
Hypoferremia	+	+
Hypozincemia	−	+
Increased plasma level of IL-1Ra	+	+
Increased plasma level of TNF-R1 and TNF-R2	+	+
Increased plasma level of IL-6	+	+
Increased plasma level of IL-8	+	+
Activation of coagulation cascades	−	+
Increased platelet count	+	−
Pulmonary edema	−	+
Hepatocellular injury	−	+

IL-1, Interleukin-1; *IL-1Ra,* interleukin-1 receptor antagonist; *IL-6,* interleukin-6; *IL-8,* interleukin-8; *TNF,* tumor necrosis factor; *TNF-R1,* tumor necrosis factor type 1 receptor; *TNF-R2,* tumor necrosis factor type 1 receptor.

to the production and release of downstream inflammatory mediators. TNF-α is rapidly transcribed and translated and released within 30 minutes of an inciting event. In studies using injections of TNF-α, animal and human subjects manifest a clinical response resembling systemic inflammatory response syndrome or septic shock. TNF-α has been dubbed the "master regulator" of inflammatory cytokine production because of its early and broad role in mediating downstream cytokine production. Bacterial endotoxin is a powerful stimulus for TNF-α release, along with the IL-1 family of cytokines, and has been extensively studied in animal and human models of sepsis. Similar to IL-1, TNF-α acts on macrophages, neutrophils, and endothelial cells. TNF-α causes increased production of macrophages, stimulates macrophage activity, and prolongs macrophage survival.[2] In endothelial cells, TNF-α increases the expression of adhesion molecules, including intercellular adhesion molecule-1, vascular cell adhesion molecule-1, and chemokines.[2] TNF-α also promotes extravasation of neutrophils into tissue by increasing adhesion via integrins.[2] Along with IL-1, TNF-α is a main mediator of a hypercoagulable state in sepsis, in part by upregulating endothelial expression of procoagulant.[2] Together with IL-1, TNF-α activates macrophages to secrete additional inflammatory cytokines such as IL-6 and IL-8 and other mediators such as nitric oxide, which contributes to vascular instability and may depress myocardial function in sepsis.[4]

The clinical significance of TNF-α in sepsis may depend in part on the concentration of its receptors, soluble TNFRs. Soluble TNFRs have been found to be elevated in healthy volunteers given endotoxin and in septic patients, in whom soluble TNFR levels correlated with mortality. It has been proposed that the ratio between TNF-α and soluble TNFRs may have more prognostic value in patients than concentrations of either protein alone.[2]

IL-1 was the first interleukin identified and includes a family of 11 ligands—seven agonists (IL-1α, IL-1β, IL-18, IL-33, IL-36α, IL-36β, and IL-36γ), three receptor antagonists (IL-1Rα, IL-36Ra, and IL-38), and the anti-inflammatory cytokine IL-37.[5] These ligands bind to a family of 11 receptors, the IL-1R family. IL-1 affects virtually all cells in the mammalian body and has important roles in mediating many inflammatory processes, including infectious, autoimmune, autoinflammatory, and degenerative conditions.[5] Its effects on the immune system are indirect—for example, by inducing gene expression of proinflammatory mediators and expression of adhesion molecules on mesenchymal and endothelial cells to promote migration of immune effector cells into tissue.

IL-1 mediates a broad response in the acute inflammatory process and activates functions of the adaptive immune system. The IL-1 family of proteins is synthesized by many different immune and nonimmune cell types, including macrophages, monocytes, neutrophils, B and T lymphocytes, natural killer (NK) cells, dendritic cells, keratinocytes, fibroblasts, endothelial cells, and enterocytes.

IL-1 is a pyrogen that mediates fever in the central nervous system, increasing leukocyte recruitment, adhesion, and migration to facilitate resistance to infection. IL-1 also activates the hypothalamic-pituitary-adrenal axis, which results in increased cortisol production, an important feature of the innate immune system in acute inflammation.[5] In addition, IL-1 increases the life span of the primary effector cells of innate immunity—neutrophils and macrophages—and it facilitates the differentiation of the innate and adaptive responses.[5]

The functions of IL-1α and IL-1β are essentially identical, despite notable structural differences. Cells typically produce either IL-1α or IL-1β but not both. The precursor to IL-1α can be found in epithelial layers throughout the body, including the gastrointestinal tract, kidneys, lungs, and endothelial cells, and it mediates a rapid inflammatory response when released under certain conditions. Its release is regulated; cellular necrosis (e.g., as a result of ischemia) stimulates IL-1α to move from the nucleus to the cellular cytoplasm and remain unbound, until it is released during cell disintegration. The extracellular IL-1α precursor binds to IL-1R on adjacent cells or to resident tissue macrophages, triggering the production of IL-1β, which mediates much of the subsequent inflammatory response. In this sense, IL-1α functions as an alarmin and is responsible for early inflammation after cellular necrosis. In contrast, apoptosis causes IL-1α to bind chromatin in the cytoplasm. As the apoptotic cell shrinks during programmed cell death, macrophages take up the cell in endocytic vesicles, where IL-1α remains unavailable to initiate inflammation.[5]

In contrast to IL-1α and its precursor, pro-IL-1α, the precursor to IL-1β, pro-IL-1β, is not biologically active and requires cleavage by the intracellular protease IL-1β converting enzyme, or caspase-1, of which the precursor, procaspase-1, is first activated with cleavage by the inflammasome before IL-1β is released to the extracellular environment.[5] IL-1β can be found in tissue macrophages, monocytes, skin dendritic cells, and brain microglia in response to TLR activation, activated complement, other cytokines, and IL-1.[5]

The importance of IL-1β to host defense against foreign microbial invaders and its role in conditions characterized by dysregulated inflammation are illustrated by studies in caspase-1-deficient mice. These mice demonstrate susceptibility to bacterial infections with *Escherichia coli, Shigella flexneri, Salmonella typhimurium, Francisella tularensis, Listeria monocytogenes,* and *Candida albicans.* In an experimental model of sepsis using knockout mice, a threefold to fourfold decrease in the median lethal dose of *E. coli* was observed when caspase-1-deficient mice were injected with bacteria.[6] In addition, caspase-1-deficient mice fail to mount a severe inflammatory response in multiple inflammatory models, including endotoxemia, peritonitis, pancreatitis, and colitis. Caspase-1 also has been implicated in many inflammatory diseases, including acute renal failure, metastatic melanoma, cutaneous T cell lymphoma, multiple sclerosis, arthritis, and asthma. These observations demonstrate that IL-1β has a crucial role in host defense against bacterial pathogens, but that it also mediates pathologic inflammation in numerous commonly observed conditions.

High-Mobility Group Box 1

HMGB1 is a potent mediator of LPS-induced lethality that was first identified in 1973 as a DNA-binding protein that facilitates gene expression and DNA replication.[7] Its role as a cytokine-like mediator was not recognized until 1999, when Tracey and colleagues identified HMGB1 as a late mediator of lethal endotoxemia in mice.

Normally a nuclear DNA protein, HMGB1 may be released to the extracellular space by immune cells in response to infection or after cellular injury to stimulate the immune responses.[7] HMGB1 is commonly released after immune cell activation but requires post-translational modification before translocation from the nucleus to cytoplasmic lysosomes. Extracellular secretion occurs when HMGB1-containing lysosomes fuse with plasma membranes, stimulating subsequent inflammatory responses mediated by specific receptors, including TLR2, TLR4, TLR7, TLR9, and receptor for advanced glycoprotein end-products (RAGE), among others.[7]

HMGB1 also may augment the actions of other antigens and inflammatory cytokines, such as IL-1β and LPS, by forming complexes with these mediators.[7] In addition, HMGB1 may be secreted passively during cellular necrosis with rapid breakdown of cellular barriers to the extracellular environment. However, secretion of HMGB1 is not seen in cells undergoing apoptosis, an evolutionarily adaptive mechanism to prevent immunologic activation during programmed cell death.

In sepsis, peak levels of HMGB1 are observed well after peak concentrations of other predominant mediators such as TNF-α, IL-6, and IFN-γ. In mice, peak levels are observed 16 to 32 hours after the onset of endotoxemia and correlate with the timing of death.[7] Administration of purified recombinant HMGB1 to mice is lethal, whereas administration of neutralizing anti-HMGB1 antibodies to septic mice confers protection against death.[7] In humans with sepsis, higher HMGB1 concentrations are typically observed among nonsurvivors over survivors. Production of autoantibodies to HMGB1 also has been associated with survival in patients with septic shock.

Interleukin-18

IL-18 was first described as a factor produced by macrophages in response to stimulation with LPS and subsequently was dubbed "IFN-γ-inducing factor" because of its influence on IFN-γ production. Later renamed IL-18, this cytokine is produced by a wide variety of hematopoietic and nonhematopoietic cells, including osteoblasts, keratinocytes, intestinal epithelial cells, microglia, and synovial fibroblasts.[8] Similar to IL-1β, IL-18 is produced as an inactive precursor and requires activation by caspase-1 before secretion into the extracellular space.[8] IL-18 is known to upregulate the helper T cell subclass Th1–mediated cellular immune response to bacterial infection in conjunction with IL-12 by activating NK cells, natural killer T (NKT) cells, and CD4 T cells to produce IFN-γ, a powerful proinflammatory cytokine. For example, mice injected with exogenous IL-18 before injection with *E. coli* demonstrate enhanced IFN-γ production.[8] IFN-γ then acts on macrophages to phagocytose foreign bacteria. In addition, IL-18 may upregulate the Th2 response to bacterial infection by stimulating Th2 cytokine and antibody production and by activating neutrophils.[8]

Interleukin-6

IL-6 is a 21-kDa glycoprotein that is found in high concentrations after tissue injury, such as burns and major surgery, and in sepsis and septic shock. Similar to IL-1 and TNF, IL-6 is produced by a wide variety of cellular lineages, including monocytes, macrophages, dendritic cells, lymphocytes, endothelial cells, fibroblasts, and smooth muscle cells. Similarly, IL-6 production is activated in response to an array of stimuli, such as LPS, IL-1, TNF-α, platelet-activating factor, and reactive oxygen metabolites. Concentrations of IL-6 peak after TNF-α and IL-1 concentrations and have been shown to correlate with Acute Physiology and Chronic Health Evaluation (APACHE) scores, injury severity, surgical stress, septic shock, and mortality. The biologic effects of IL-6 include stimulation of B cell and T cell production, maturation, and differentiation; activation of coagulation; and stimulation of hematopoiesis. In addition, IL-6 contributes to host defense by activating the production of the acute-phase response by inducing fever; leukocytosis; and the production of hepatic acute-phase proteins, such as C-reactive protein, complement, fibrinogen, and ferritin. The net effect of IL-6 appears to be predominantly proinflammatory, although it also exerts anti-inflammatory influence. For example, the deletion of the gene for IL-6 in mice was shown to protect against acute lung injury after injection of carrageenan into the pleural space, and absence of the IL-6 gene was shown to protect against the development of peritonitis and mortality after peritoneal injection of zymosan. IL-6 also has been identified as a negative inotropic factor in a model of meningococcal sepsis using rat myocytes. Cardiac depression, which is frequently seen in sepsis, exacerbates tissue and organ malperfusion. Conversely, IL-6 has been shown to mediate anti-inflammatory effects in other studies by inhibiting TNF and IL-1 production and by enhancing production of other anti-inflammatory cytokines, such as IL-1Ra, TNFRs, IL-10, TGF-β, and cortisol.[2] For example, in a murine model of acute pancreatitis, deficiency of the IL-6 gene in knockout mice enhanced the inflammatory response compared with wild-type mice.[9] Although the precise balance of these counterregulatory processes has not been fully elucidated, the cumulative impact of IL-6 appears to be proinflammatory.

Interleukin-8

IL-8 is a cytokine with potent chemoattractant properties, making it one member of a small superfamily of approximately 40 cytokines also known as chemokines. IL-8 is a powerful attractant and stimulator of neutrophils, a hallmark feature of the body's inflammatory response. In addition to attracting neutrophils, IL-8 stimulates neutrophil degranulation, upregulates expression of adhesion molecules, and increases production of reactive oxygen species (ROS). IL-8 is produced by various cells, notably monocytes, macrophages, and endothelial cells. Similarly, IL-8 production is upregulated by numerous stimuli, including other cytokines such as TNF, PAMPs such as bacterial and viral products, and cellular stress. Levels of IL-8 increase rapidly following an appropriate stimulus and have been demonstrated to correlate with important clinical parameters in patients with sepsis. In particular, IL-8 is thought to play a key role in the epithelial and physiologic dysfunction observed in acute lung injury and acute respiratory distress syndrome.

Interleukin-12

The most significant role of IL-12 in the inflammatory process is as a bridge between the innate and adaptive immune responses to pathogens. IL-12 is produced by monocytes and macrophages, neutrophils, and dendritic cells and binds to receptors expressed by T cells and NK cells. Binding of IL-12 stimulates IFN-γ production and release, which upregulates bactericidal activity of macrophages and further enhances production of Th1 cytokines. In addition, IL-12 promotes differentiation of naïve T cells into Th1 cells, which augments resistance to antigen-induced apoptosis and expands the pool of IFN-γ-producing cells. The role of IL-12 in upregulating the cellular immune response is essential for defense against intracellular pathogens. Mice deficient in IL-12 demonstrate greater susceptibility to infection by intracellular pathogens, such as avian *Mycoplasma* species.

However, the role of IL-12 in sepsis is uncertain despite much research. Early murine models using cecal ligation and puncture (CLP) suggested that immunoneutralization or deletion of the IL-12 gene resulted in increased mortality, indicating that IL-12 exerts a protective effect in sepsis through its induction of IFN-γ and stimulation of phagocytic and microbicidal activities. However, a separate murine model evaluating endotoxemia reported improved survival with neutralization of IL-12 and increased mortality in mice with overexpression of IL-12.[10] In humans, one study of patients with postoperative sepsis reported that IL-12 was significantly reduced in sepsis versus controls, and cytokine levels were not significantly associated with outcome.[11] In another prospective study of patients undergoing major visceral surgery, the authors reported that a selective preoperative defect in monocyte IL-12 production causing impaired monocyte function was predictive for a lethal outcome in postoperative sepsis.[12] Likewise, studies of peripheral blood mononuclear cells correlated LPS-stimulated IL-12 production with survival in patients with sepsis.

Interleukin-17

IL-17 is produced by a subset of Th cells, Th17 cells, which were first identified approximately 1 decade ago. An important function of Th17 cells is the clearance of pathogens not adequately handled by Th1 or Th2 cells.[13] In addition to IL-17, Th17 cells produce various other cytokines that act in concert to induce a potent inflammatory response observed in autoimmune and inflammatory conditions. IL-17 also is produced by other cells of the innate and adaptive immune systems, including NKT cells, neutrophils, eosinophils, and others.[13] IL-17 and related cytokines act broadly to induce the expression of various cytokines (TNF, IL-1β, IL-6), chemokines, and metalloproteinases and serve as key cytokines in the recruitment and activation of neutrophils.[13] IL-17 appears to be a critical mediator in the defense of certain pathogens. In knockout mice lacking the IL-17 receptor, host defense against *Klebsiella* and *Candida* is greatly compromised largely as a result of impaired neutrophil trafficking to the site of inflammation. In contrast, infection with *Pseudomonas aeruginosa* or *Aspergillus fumigatus* does not appear to depend on the production of IL-17, despite increased production. IL-17 may be responsible for pathologic inflammation in this scenario and risk of autoimmunity.[13]

Interferon-γ

The interferon family of cytokines is a powerful mediator of the innate response to invading pathogens. Type I interferons, which include IFN-α subtypes, IFN-β, IFN-ω, and IFN-τ, are primarily involved in innate response to viral pathogens. IFN-γ, which has a prominent role in responding to bacterial invaders, is the lone type II interferon. It is structurally distinct from type I interferons, binds to a separate receptor, and is encoded separately from other interferon types.[14] IFN-γ is mainly produced by CD4 Th1 cells, CD8 cytotoxic cells, and NK cells but is also produced to a lesser degree by B cells, NKT cells, and antigen-presenting cells. Its production is stimulated by macrophage-derived cytokines, including TNF-α, IL-12, and IL-18.[2]

IFN-γ is a powerful proinflammatory mediator and can participate in a positive proinflammatory feedback loop while downregulating anti-inflammatory mediators. IFN-γ orchestrates many early responses of the immune system by directing specific immune cells to the site of inflammation—through upregulation of adhesion molecules, promotion of blood stasis, expression of cytokines, and promotion of extravasation—and coordinates a transition between innate and adaptive immune functions.

In conjunction with IL-12, IFN-γ plays a crucial role in promoting differentiation of naïve CD4 cells to the Th1 phenotype. Recognition of PAMPs and alarmins by macrophages, dendritic cells, and neutrophils triggers production of IL-12, which stimulates naïve CD4 T cells and NK cells to produce IFN-γ. This pathway establishes a positive feedback loop whereby IL-12-stimulated IFN-γ acts on monocytes and macrophages to upregulate IL-12 production.[14] Further augmenting its proinflammatory effects are the actions of IFN-γ to downregulate anti-inflammatory mediators by inhibiting the differentiation of lymphocytes into Th2 cells. Th2 cells produce anti-inflammatory mediators—notably, IL-4 and IL-10—and suppression of these cytokines contributes to the proinflammatory effects of IFN-γ activity.

One of the most important functions of IFN-γ is to enhance the microbicidal activity of macrophages. Two important microbicidal effector functions on macrophages include the reduced nicotinamide adenine dinucleotide phosphate (NADPH)–dependent phagocyte oxidase system and inducible nitrogen oxide synthase (iNOS), which produce ROS and reactive nitrogen intermediates, respectively.[14] ROS and reactive nitrogen intermediates are small molecules that attack microbial invaders by penetrating the cell wall/coat. Mice lacking NADPH oxidase and iNOS have been shown to be highly susceptible to foreign pathogens, illustrating the importance of these systems to host defense. IFN-γ is approved for use in patients with chronic granulomatous disease, a life-threatening disease caused by an inherited defect in NADPH oxidase, and has been shown to reduce the incidence of infections significantly in these patients.

Macrophage Migration Inhibitory Factor

MIF was the first cytokine discovered approximately 50 years ago in studies of delayed-type hypersensitivity reactions. Its name was derived after the unidentified factor was noted to inhibit the migration of peritoneal exudate cells.[15] It was subsequently observed to mediate a variety of cellular responses during inflammation.

MIF protein and messenger RNA are constitutively expressed by many tissues and cells, including monocytes, macrophages, dendritic cells, T and B lymphocytes, eosinophils, mast cells, basophils, and neutrophils. The cytokine is stored as preformed pools within cells, enabling rapid release after exposure to a proinflammatory stimulus. Stores of MIF are quickly replenished through MIF gene transcription and RNA translation. Macrophage MIF is released after exposure to various bacterial stimuli, including bacterial endotoxin, exotoxins, gram-negative and gram-positive bacteria, cytokines such as TNF-α and interferon-γ, and other stimuli.[15] Release of the proinflammatory MIF also is stimulated in the presence of low concentrations of anti-inflammatory glucocorticoid hormones, in contrast to the inhibitory effects of steroid hormones on most other cytokines.

Among its effects, MIF upregulates antimicrobial activity by prolonging macrophage survival, increasing TLR4 expression on macrophages, and promoting macrophage recruitment.[2] Consequently, MIF release causes secretion of TNF-α, IFN-γ, IL-1, and other downstream cytokines. MIF-deficient mice have been shown to have a broad reduction in the production of inflammatory mediators, illustrating that MIF has an upstream regulatory influence in the inflammatory cascade.

The role of MIF in sepsis has been studied extensively. Early studies suggested that MIF contributed to the pathologic manifestations of the early immune response in sepsis, whereas more recent research suggests that high MIF concentrations are protective. In an early study of the role of MIF in sepsis, coinjections of MIF and LPS in mice significantly enhanced lethality over LPS injection alone, whereas other studies reported that neutralization of MIF reduced cytokine production and organ damage and increased survival in murine models of sepsis.[2]

MIF was suggested as an early predictor of mortality in sepsis after studies in humans with severe sepsis or septic shock demonstrated an association between MIF concentration and mortality. In a large cohort study investigating the association of MIF alleles with disease progression among patients with community-acquired pneumonia and control subjects, overexpression of MIF as a result of a specific polymorphism was associated with a 50% survival benefit.[16] In humans, a second, MIF-like ligand, *D*-dopachrome tautomerase, has been identified and shown to activate the same extracellular signal-regulated kinase 1,2 mitogen-activated protein kinase and downstream inflammatory pathways as MIF. *D*-dopachrome tautomerase concentrations have been shown to correlate with disease severity in sepsis, and immunoneutralization in mice protects mice from mortality resulting from endotoxemia.[17]

Interleukin-4

The exact role of IL-4 in the immune response to inflammation is unclear. IL-4 is a 15- to 20-kDa glycoprotein and is produced by Th2 cells, mast cells, basophils, and eosinophils. IL-4 opposes proinflammatory cytokines by downregulating the release of proinflammatory mediators, such as TNF, IL-1, IL-8, and PGE2, from monocytes and macrophages and downregulates endothelial activity regulated by TNF. IL-4 also promotes differentiation of naïve CD4 T cells into Th2 cells, which produce additional IL-4 and other anti-inflammatory cytokines, and limits differentiation of CD4 T cells into Th1 cells, which limits synthesis and release of proinflammatory cytokines.

By promoting Th2 differentiation and inhibiting Th1 differentiation, IL-4 upregulates the humoral immune response mediated by B cells and downregulates cell-mediated immune responses. In humans, one study reported that IL-4 expression correlated with survival in patients with severe sepsis, although IL-4 concentrations on admission did not differ significantly among survivors and nonsurvivors.[18] A more recent study suggested that a polymorphism in the promoter region for IL-4 may affect the balance between Th1 and Th2 differentiation and the risk for sepsis in severely injured trauma patients.[19]

Interleukin-10

IL-10 is another anti-inflammatory pleiotropic cytokine that inhibits the inflammatory immune response through various mechanisms. IL-10 is a 35-kDa homodimeric cytokine produced primarily by Th2 cells but also by many other immune cell types, including monocytes, macrophages, B lymphocytes, and NK cells.[2] IL-10 has been demonstrated to inhibit the expression of TNF-α, IL-1, IL-6, IL-8, and IL-12 by monocytes and macrophages, while increasing the expression of IL-1Ra and TNFRs to neutralize the proinflammatory actions of IL-1 and TNF. IL-10 also inhibits IL-12 production, which reduces expression of IFN-γ and IL-2 by downregulating the activity of Th1 cells. These findings were supported in murine models of sepsis in which injections of recombinant IL-10 conferred protection from lethal endotoxemia, whereas injections of anti-IL-10 neutralizing antibodies reduced the protective effect of IL-10.

However, in other murine models of polymicrobial sepsis using CLP, the same protective effect of IL-10 was not as evident. These models suggested that the timing of IL-10 activity may mediate important transitions in the early and late immune responses to sepsis. For example, an early murine model of sepsis using CLP demonstrated that pretreatment with anti-IL-10 antibodies resulted in enhanced lethality after CLP versus controls.[20] Similarly, another study observed a nonsignificant increase in mortality among mice administered neutralizing IL-10 antibodies early after CLP and, more importantly, that late administration of IL-10 improved survival in septic mice. Another study supported these earlier findings, showing again that IL-10 deficiency provokes more rapid lethality after CLP, whereas administration of recombinant IL-10 delayed the transition to irreversible septic shock.[21] IL-10 may regulate a transition from early reversible sepsis to irreversible septic shock.

Transforming Growth Factor-β

TGF-β is a pleiotropic cytokine that was classically recognized to have anti-inflammatory effects on the immune response, although more recent research revealed that the cytokine has a proinflammatory role during the acute-phase response. TGF-β is produced as a 100-kDa dimeric precursor protein that undergoes intracellular cleavage to generate a complex consisting of an active form of TGF-β and a precursor protein, latency-associated protein (LAP). In a manner unique to cytokines, this complex is secreted to the extracellular environment, where it remains until activation by various stimuli. TGF-β can be activated through proteolysis or conformational changes that liberate it from LAP. This may occur when LAP binds to vascular endothelium or to integrins on epithelial cells and dendritic cells, or secondary to activity of free radicals, or in the presence of low pH.[13]

The predominant influence of TGF-β is on T lymphocytes. Activated TGF-β binds to cell-surface receptors and initiates signal transduction pathways regulating leukocyte proliferation, differentiation, and survival and influences inflammatory responses by regulating chemotaxis; activation; and survival of lymphocytes, NK cells, dendritic cells, macrophages, and other immune cells.

TGF-β has been shown to have important roles in wound healing and tissue repair, inflammation, and carcinogenesis. Much early work in vitro demonstrated the anti-inflammatory role of TGF-β, which was shown to suppress the release of proinflammatory mediators such as IL-1, TNF-α, and HMGB1 and to upregulate anti-inflammatory mediators such as soluble TNFRs and IL-1Ra.[2] Similarly, TGF-β was shown to downregulate IL-2 production and T cell differentiation, while promoting differentiation of immunosuppressive T-regulatory cells.

In multiple murine models of sepsis, administration of TGF-β prevented endotoxin-induced hypotension and reduced mortality. In patients, lower levels of TGF-β after major trauma are associated with renal and hepatic insufficiency, and higher levels correlate with an increased risk of sepsis. TGF-β also has been shown to block depression of cardiac myocytes by proinflammatory cytokines produced during sepsis and in serum from patients with sepsis.

More recently, the discovery of Th17 cells marked a major advance in the understanding of T cell differentiation. TGF-β was shown to promote Th17 cell differentiation, which results in the expression of proinflammatory cytokines, including IL-17A and IL-17F, and promotion of B cell class switching to IgG antibody production. Although controversy remains about the importance of TGF-β in promoting Th17 differentiation, the preponderance of evidence suggests that TGF-β is activated by IL-6 production in the early immune response to promote proinflammatory Th17 differentiation while downregulating T-regulatory cell differentiation.

Complement

The complement system has been classically described as an important component of the innate immune system, but it has been recognized more recently to support adaptive immunity. Appropriate activation of the complement cascade results in opsonization of pathogens that are subsequently cleared by phagocytes.[22] However, inappropriate activation and complement deficiencies may result in inflammatory disease and dysregulated inflammation. Complement was first recognized in the late 1800s as a component that aided in the humoral killing of bacteria by heat-stable antibodies in serum.[22] More than 30 proteins are known to be involved in the complement system and are found as soluble serum proteins or as membrane-associated proteins.[22] Activation of the complement system occurs through three distinct pathways that each converge to a common pathway resulting in the activation of C3a and C5a and the C5b-C9 membrane attack complex (MAC), which mediate an array of physiologic responses (Fig. 3-3).[22]

The anaphylotoxins C3a and C5a exert numerous effects in inflammatory responses by binding to their respective receptors, C3aR, C5aR, and C5a receptor-like 2 receptor. They serve as chemoattractants for phagocytes, cause degranulation of histamine from mast cells, induce oxidative bursts from neutrophils, stimulate smooth muscle cell contraction, and mediate vasodilation.[22]

The classical pathway is activated by immune complexes after IgG or IgM antibodies bind to antigens. The C1 complex, which consists of C1q, C1r, and C1s molecules, cleaves C4 and C2 to form the classical pathway C3 convertase, C4bC2a. From this point, the pathway converges at C3 and results in the activation of C3a and C5a. The alternative pathway is activated by recognition of certain bacterial surface markers, such as carbohydrates, lipids, and proteins, and generates C3a and C5a. The lectin-binding pathway is activated when mannose-binding lectin or ficolin bind to pathogen surfaces, triggering C4a and C5a before joining the common pathway to produce the MAC. The MAC, or terminal complement complex, forms a pore in target cells, resulting in cell lysis.

In addition to the classically described role of complement in innate immunity, the complement system has been recognized more recently to influence adaptive immunity, including B cell and T cell biology. B cells, follicular dendritic cells, and a subset of T cells express the complement receptors, CR1 and CR2, which mediate complement-associated B cell functions and regulate the amplitude of B cell responses.[22] Similarly, complement affects T cell responses, including activation, proliferation, differentiation, and induction of regulatory T cells.[22]

Complement mutations and deficiencies are responsible for many serious and debilitating diseases and pathologic conditions. Hemolytic uremic syndrome, characterized by hemolytic anemia, thrombocytopenia, and acute renal failure, results from mutant complement factors that cause intravascular fibrin deposition.[22] Deficiency or mutation of C1 inhibitor causes dysregulated bradykinin production, leading to profound increases in vascular permeability that characterize hereditary angioedema. Paroxysmal nocturnal hemoglobinuria, characterized by hemolytic anemia and thrombosis, occurs when a mutation in the gene *PIG-A* impairs complement inhibition, leading to intense complement-mediated lysis of red and white blood cells. Other diseases, including systemic lupus erythematosus, also involve defects in complement function.

Just as complement mutations and deficiencies can cause serious disease, excessive complement activation and dysregulated activity also are observed in certain diseases, including multiple sclerosis, Alzheimer disease, asthma, chronic obstructive pulmonary disease (COPD), sepsis, and hyperacute organ rejection.[22] In sepsis, excessive C5a has been implicated as a particularly harmful mediator, contributing to immunoparalysis, multiorgan failure, thymocyte and adrenal medullary cell apoptosis, consumptive coagulopathy, and septic cardiomyopathy.

Pathogens have evolved various mechanisms to avoid detection and attack by the complement system. The bacterium *Staphylococcus aureus* is one example of a pathogen with sophisticated adaptations to elude the complement system. For example, *S. aureus* expresses two proteins, staphylococcal protein A and staphylococcal immunoglobulin-binding protein A that bind to the Fc portion of IgG and prevent complement activation and phagocytosis.[22] *S. aureus* also produces a staphylokinase that cleaves plasminogen to plasmin and degrades IgG and the opsonin C3b, allowing the bacteria to evade the complement system.[22] Additionally, *S. aureus* secretes complement inhibitors that bind to C3 convertases and block complement activation. Pathogens, including viruses, have evolved mechanisms to thwart every stage of the complement system, including activation, opsonization, chemotaxis, and phagocytosis.[22]

Immunotherapy for Sepsis

Despite decades of research and numerous clinical trials, the promise of immunomodulatory therapy in sepsis has largely remained unrealized. This section provides a brief, albeit incomplete, overview of notable attempted therapeutic interventions for sepsis and several promising areas of investigation.

Sepsis has classically been described in two stages—a predominant, proinflammatory stage characterized by cytokine production to mobilize the host immune response to combat infection

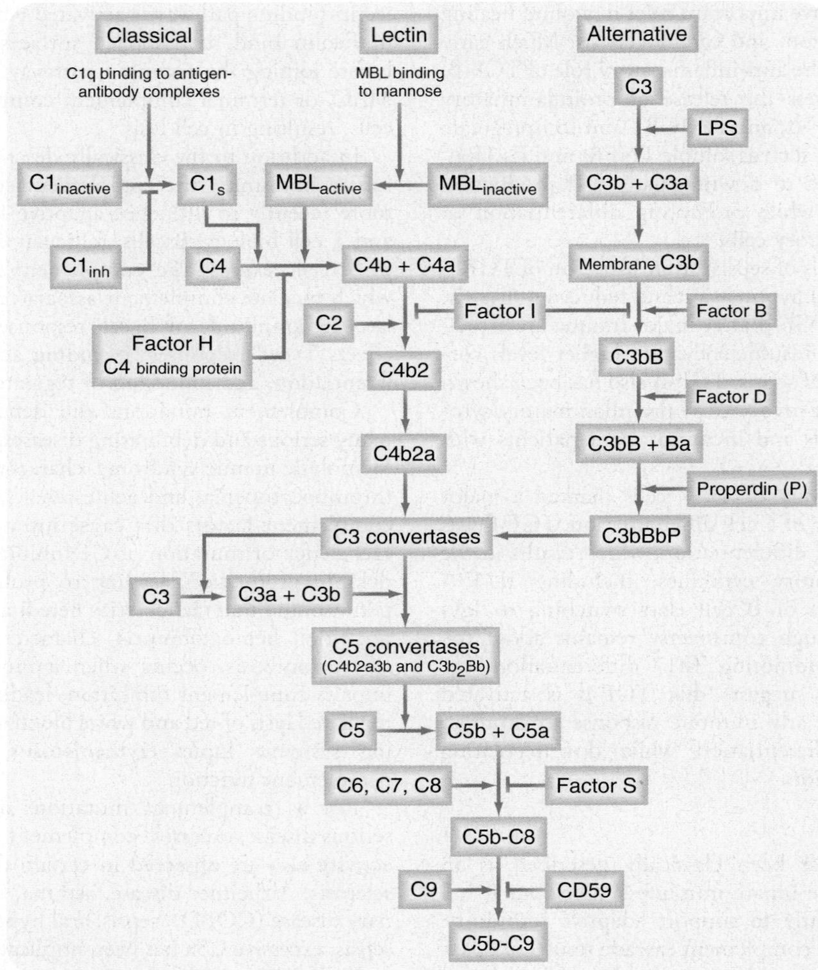

FIGURE 3-3 Activation of the complement cascade via the classical, lectin, or alternative pathways leads to formation of the membrane attack complex (C5b through C9). Various complement inhibitors antagonize several steps in the cascade: C1 inhibitor (C1inh), factor I, factor H, C4-binding protein, factor S, and CD59, among others not shown here. *MBL,* Mannose-binding lectin.

followed by an anti-inflammatory response marked by the body's inability to respond to an infectious challenge. Most experimental therapies have targeted the first stage of immune response because proinflammatory cytokines have been thought to be largely responsible for most septic morbidity. However, following the failures of targeted therapies to proinflammatory mediators, interest has shifted to targeted immunomodulating therapies for the anti-inflammatory stage of sepsis.

Because of their importance as mediators in sepsis, IL-1 and TNF-α were logical targets for early investigation and clinical trials. Various targeting strategies have included monoclonal antibodies to TNF-α, soluble TNFRs, IL-1Ra, and soluble IL-1 receptors. Although results of experimental models were promising, these therapies unexpectedly failed to improve mortality among septic patients in clinical trials.[2] Similar therapies have proven successful in other inflammatory conditions, such as Crohn's disease, rheumatoid arthritis, and psoriatic arthritis, where anti-IL-1 and anti-TNF-α pharmaceuticals have been approved for use. For example, infliximab is a monoclonal anti-TNF antibody used to induce long-term remission in patients with Crohn's disease. Other agents, including adalimumab (monoclonal anti-TNF antibody) and anakinra (recombinant human IL-1Ra) have been approved for use in rheumatoid arthritis, and etanercept (TNFR2 fusion protein), originally intended for use in sepsis, is approved for use in psoriatic arthritis. One potential explanation offered for the failure of anti-IL-1 and anti-TNF-α therapies in sepsis is that high concentrations of these cytokines are observed only in the early hours of sepsis, potentially representing a very narrow window for intervention.[2]

Interest in the use of glucocorticoid therapy in sepsis has varied considerably in recent decades. Glucocorticoids are thought to reduce harmful proinflammatory cytokine production and counteract harmful vasodilation by increasing vascular responsiveness to catecholamines.[23] Most studies have failed to demonstrate a benefit in mortality; however, evidence suggests that hydrocortisone therapy reduces time to reversal of shock.[23] The Surviving Sepsis Campaign recommends hydrocortisone therapy for patients with septic shock unresponsive to fluid resuscitation and vasopressor therapy.

Perhaps the most disappointing failure in immunomodulating therapy for sepsis was the experience with recombinant human activated protein C (rhAPC). Protein C is a thrombolytic protein that inactivates coagulation factors Va and VIIIa, resulting in decreased thrombin production and inhibition of thrombin-induced platelet activation. In addition, activated protein C was demonstrated to possess other anti-inflammatory properties beyond the scope of this discussion. On the strength of results from the PROWESS trial[24] showing reduced mortality among septic patients, rhAPC was approved for use in humans despite increased risks of bleeding. Subgroup analysis demonstrated that the mortality benefits were limited to patients with severe disease, and guidelines recommended that the use of rhAPC be limited to patients with high risk of death. However, the subsequent PROWESS-SHOCK trial[25] failed to demonstrate a difference in mortality versus placebo among patients with septic shock, and rhAPC was ultimately withdrawn from the market.

Other cytokines with later roles in sepsis, such as MIF and HMGB1, have gained interest as alternative therapeutic targets as well as specific chemical antagonists against the proinflammatory mediator platelet-activating factor. Platelet-activating factor receptor antagonist therapy was studied in septic patients, and post-hoc subgroup analysis suggested a mortality benefit in patients with gram-negative sepsis. However, a subsequent randomized trial showed no difference in mortality and, notably, no differences in circulating concentrations of TNF-α, TNFR, and IL-6 among treatment groups.[23] MIF has been investigated as a therapeutic target in sepsis because of its broad, complex role in sepsis. Small molecules such as ISO-1 have been found to interact with MIF and inhibit its proinflammatory downstream effects. Administration of ISO-1 has improved mortality in murine models of sepsis using a CLP method, and interest exists in evaluating human anti-MIF agents for use in sepsis. Similarly, antagonism of HMGB1 has proven effective in reducing mortality in murine models of sepsis and remains an active area of interest for potential human applications.[7]

More recently, interest in immunomodulatory therapy for sepsis has shifted to strategies to alter the immunosuppressive state, which is now recognized to account for more septic morbidity than the proinflammatory phase. Two immunostimulative therapies that have been studied in humans are IFN-γ and granulocyte-macrophage colony-stimulating factor (GM-CSF). In small clinical trials, these immune stimulants showed promising results in reversing immunoparalysis, and larger clinical trials are currently underway to explore these potential therapeutic options further. Another immunostimulative candidate of interest is IL-7, a potent antiapoptotic cytokine that enhances lymphocyte development and survival and effector cell function. IL-7 has been shown to enhance survival in murine models of sepsis and to restore immune function in patients ex vivo.[26]

CHRONIC INFLAMMATION

Inflammation is the body's protective response to immune reactions, acute injury, or infection and seeks to reach a homeostatic equilibrium.[27] Occasionally, the inflammatory response continues longer than weeks to months. It occurs as a persistent, abnormal response to normal stimuli leading to chronic activation of the immune system and a prolonged inflammatory state.[27,28] It can occur de novo or as a continuation of the acute inflammatory response. Chronic inflammatory states are a varying combination of inflammation, tissue repair, and injury occurring simultaneously.[28] Chronic immune activation can lead to various physiologic changes, alter metabolic requirements of individual cells, and predispose to chronic comorbidities.[27] Chronic immune cell activity may alter the transcriptomics, metabolomics, and microbiota of the body.[27,29,30]

A relatively new and large entity, the "omics" comprise genomics, transcriptomics, proteomics, metabolomics, lipidomics, and interactomics, all of which seek to identify individual elements and pathways in cellular processes.[30] Understanding these components may allow for targeted alterations at the cellular level to improve disease states. A key focus in inflammatory states is on the metabolome, which analyzes the altered levels of low-molecular-weight compounds that are produced as a result of the changes occurring in DNA and RNA transcription from chronic immune activation. Metabolomics profiling involves nuclear magnetic resonance or mass spectrometry analysis of blood, urine, serum, stool, or other tissue samples with a resultant metabolomics profile containing peaks. Peaks correspond to the amount of the particular metabolite present in the sample. Similarly, the microbiome encompasses the bacterial organisms living within the human body contributing to diverse biologic processes. The microbiome, similar to the metabolomics profile, changes in response to inflammation and activation of the immune response.[27] "Genetic dysbiosis" refers to the hypothesis that aberrancies in host recognition of microbial flora lead to altered recognition of these organisms ultimately causing various inflammatory disease states.[29] The remainder of this section explains the various chronic inflammatory states by organ system and the modulators involved in these processes.

Chronic Inflammation by Organ System

Pulmonary

COPD is an increasingly common respiratory diagnosis with a multifactorial cause. COPD decreases the amount of airflow to and from the pulmonary alveoli. More than 5% of the population is affected, and this number is likely to increase in ensuing years, killing approximately 120,000 individuals each year. COPD is defined as a "common preventable and treatable disease, characterized by airflow limitation that is usually progressive and associated with an enhanced chronic inflammatory response in the airways and the lung to noxious particles or gases," by the Global Initiative for Chronic Obstructive Lung Disease.[31]

Pathophysiologic changes and immune reactions. The pathophysiologic basis for COPD consists of chronic inflammation causing increased number of mucous glands, goblet cells, and degradation of the alveolar cell wall with loss of pulmonary recoil.[31] Additionally, the parenchyma of the lung is destroyed along with chronic inflammation of large and small airways.

Macrophages, neutrophils, T lymphocytes (primarily $CD8^+$), dendritic cells, and B lymphocytes are increased in COPD, with macrophages playing a vital role in the chronic inflammatory response. Macrophages, activated by cigarette smoke and other pollutants, secrete various mediators such as TNF-α, IL-6, IL-8, monocyte chemotactic peptide, and leukotriene B_4. Additionally, proteolytic enzymes are secreted by ROS, which participate in the alveolar wall and pulmonary parenchyma destruction. IL-8 and leukotriene B_4 cause the migration of neutrophils to the respiratory tract, which subsequently cause a surge in mucous glands and goblet cells.[31,32]

Biopsy specimens of bronchial specimens from patients with COPD also have demonstrated $CD4^+$ and $CD8^+$ T lymphocytes, suggesting that these cells play a role in the chronic inflammation. The number of T lymphocytes correlates positively with the extent of and rate of alveolar and airway destruction. $CD8^+$ T lymphocytes may cause lysis of alveolar epithelial cells through perforin, granzyme B, and TNF-α secretion, although this mechanism is not clearly understood.

The epithelial cells of airways play a large role in the inflammatory response because they store a large variety of inflammatory mediators. When toxins such as smoke stimulate these cells, factors such as TNF-α, TGF-β, IL-1β, IL-8, and GM-CSF are secreted. These factors go on to cause small airway fibrosis through fibroblast activation.[31]

Additionally, TNF-α upregulates monocyte chemotactic protein, a potent stimulator of monocytes, eosinophils, basophils, and T lymphocytes. TNF-α also induces airway remodeling through activation of epithelial cells, smooth muscle cells, and other inflammatory cells. Monocytes, macrophages, and fibroblasts produce IL-1, which is important for mounting a response to bacterial infection, along with tissue destruction leading to inflammation. IL-6 is a key cytokine causing increasing severity in COPD progression. Additionally, IL-6 stimulates C-reactive protein production by the liver (an acute-phase reactant) and may be important in pulmonary autoimmune disease.[32]

Diagnosis of chronic obstructive pulmonary disease. Traditionally, diagnosis of airway inflammation was made with techniques such as bronchoalveolar lavage or transbronchial/intrabronchial biopsy. These techniques are invasive and not clinically feasible to establish a diagnosis. Induced sputum is a newer technique in which nebulized isotonic or hypertonic saline is administered. Expectorated secretions are then analyzed for diagnosis.

Exhaled fraction of nitrous oxide is another biomarker study that can be used in diagnosis. Nitrous oxide is produced in respiratory epithelium; however, one limitation with this method is that smoking reduces the concentration of exhaled nitrous oxide present.[31]

Therapeutic approaches to chronic obstructive pulmonary disease. Bronchodilators, steroids, and anticholinergics are the hallmark of traditional COPD management. A newer treatment strategy involves roflumilast, a phosphodiesterase 4 inhibitor, which may be helpful in reducing severe airflow obstruction. Aside from this, there have been few trials with medications that may block cytokines in the inflammatory response for COPD. There have been trials of anti-TNF-α, but the results have not been promising. Ongoing studies are aimed at specific cytokines through monoclonal antibody administration; however, these are still in trial phases.[32]

Pancreas

The pancreas is unique in that it has endocrine and exocrine functions involved in glycemic regulation and nutrient digestion, respectively. Acute and chronic pancreatitis are similar symptomatically but occur over varying durations. The distinguishing features of acute and chronic pancreatitis are in histologic diagnosis. Acute pancreatitis is characterized by acinar degranulation and fat necrosis, whereas chronic pancreatitis is defined by acinar loss, fibrotic changes, and invasion with immune cells. This chronic inflammation occurs with uncontrolled acinar cell activation causing pancreatic autodigestion. Acute pancreatitis typically leads to chronic pancreatitis, which is a progressive and fibrotic disease. Chronic inflammatory changes lead to parenchymal destruction and ultimately loss of endocrine and exocrine functions resulting in diabetes and nutrient malabsorption. Chronic pancreatitis is a predisposing condition for pancreatic ductal adenocarcinoma, which can occur 10 to 20 years after initial diagnosis of chronic pancreatitis diagnosis. Acute pancreatitis typically is associated with elevations of lipase and amylase as a result of pancreatic cell damage. In chronic pancreatitis, these enzymes are normal or only mildly elevated.[33,34]

The etiology of chronic pancreatitis is not fully understood but is thought to be a combination of genetic, environmental, and metabolic abnormalities. The pancreas contains pancreatic stellate cells (PSCs), which are normally dormant. PSCs are stellate cells that surround the pancreatic ducts, vasculature, and acini. When PSCs are exposed to toxins such as alcohol or inflammatory cytokines, these cells transform into myofibroblast-like cells. Activated macrophages at the site of pancreatic injury induce collagen and fibronectin synthesis by PSCs. Cell-mediated immunity plays a role in chronic pancreatitis. A preponderance of $CD4^+$ T cells, $CD8^+$ T cells, and B lymphocytes has been demonstrated in murine models.[33,34] Although acute and chronic pancreatitis demonstrate differences, it is believed that acute pancreatitis leads to eventual development of chronic pancreatitis as a two-step process known as the "sentinel acute pancreatitis event hypothesis" as described by Whitcomb. The process begins with a "sentinel event" initiating an immune response. The second step is prolonged inflammation causing pancreatic destruction over time.[35]

The first phase begins when toxins or insults activate macrophages and secrete TNF-α, which causes conversion of PSCs to myofibroblast-like cells. In the second phase, TGF-β replaces TNF-α, which has anti-inflammatory properties. The stellate cells produce matrix proteins as part of the healing phase, and when the matrix proteins are chronically activated, fibrosis and scarring result. The toxic insult additionally activates NF-κB, a transcription factor important in cell signaling. It translocates to the nucleus where proinflammatory cytokines are transcribed. NF-κB causes upregulation of IL-10, which causes inflammatory changes in chronic pancreatitis. Ultimately, patients with chronic pancreatitis present with pain, have recurrent hospital admissions, and are at increased risk for pancreatic cancer over time. Treatment is aimed at alleviating pain, replacing loss of exocrine and endocrine function through exogenous digestive enzymes, and providing hypoglycemic medications. Therapy aimed at immune regulation is under investigation at the present time. Surgical management of chronic pancreatitis is limited to a selected patients and is not the mainstay of therapy.[34,35]

Inflammatory Bowel Disease

Inflammatory bowel disease (IBD) is an autoimmune condition encompassing ulcerative colitis and Crohn's disease. The exact etiology is not well understood. IBD is thought to be multifactorial including a combination of genetic, environmental, and intestinal causes, which prompt a prolonged immune response. In particular, the immune system attacks bacteria that normally live in a symbiotic relationship with the host lumen. Secretion of proinflammatory mediators occurs indefinitely and alters the microbiota perturbing gastrointestinal homeostasis.[36,37]

Pathophysiologic Changes

The bowel wall consists of four layers—mucosa, submucosa, muscularis propria, and adventitia. The mucosal layer creates a barrier between gastrointestinal contents and the abdominal organs. This layer is composed of epithelial cells and mucus-secreting goblet cells, along with endocrine glands secreting various digestive hormones. A breakdown of this layer along with disruption of mucous secretion is the general feature of IBD. Crohn's disease occurs anywhere along the gastrointestinal tract; "from mouth to anus" is a common adage used to describe Crohn's disease. Ulcerative colitis is chronic inflammation generally confined to the large bowel with some "backwash ileitis." Crohn's disease generally occurs as a transmural process, affecting all layers of the bowel wall. Crohn's disease also manifests with granulomas more often than ulcerative colitis. Ulcerative colitis occurs as a more superficial process, affecting the epithelial layer primarily. Hemorrhagic changes and disordered crypt architecture are hallmark features.[37]

Clinical Presentation and Diagnosis

Symptomatically, ulcerative colitis and Crohn's disease have similar clinical presentations with some distinct differences. All patients experience abdominal pain and weight loss; patients with ulcerative colitis tend to have bloody diarrhea and left lower quadrant pain, whereas patients with Crohn's disease experience obstruction more often with right lower quadrant pain.[37]

IBD can be diagnosed in several ways including colonoscopy with mucosal biopsy or capsule endoscopy to evaluate the health of the mucosa. Biopsies can be helpful in discerning Crohn's disease from ulcerative colitis based on the depth of inflammation and the presence of granulomas. Computed tomography and magnetic resonance imaging are useful in evaluation for other intra-abdominal manifestations of IBD.

Immune Activation in Inflammatory Bowel Disease

The translocation of gut bacteria and chemicals across the mucosal layer initiates a proinflammatory cascade. The cycle begins with differentiation and proliferation of T lymphocytes into Th cells. Th cells can be of either the Th1 subclass, which generally secretes proinflammatory cytokines, or the Th2 subclass, which secretes anti-inflammatory cytokines. Th1 cells are part of the cell-mediated immunity pathway, whereas Th2 cells constitute part of humoral immunity. Th1 and Th2 also negatively regulate each other; Th1 cytokines inhibit the Th2 pathway and vice versa. IBD is driven primarily by a Th1 immune response.

TNF-α is arguably the most important cytokine involved in the IBD pathway. Mononuclear cells produce TNF-α, IL-6, IL-12, and IL-23 after activation of TLRs (such as occurs when gram-negative bacteria bind to these receptors). TNF-α secretion then upregulates mitogen-activated protein kinase and NF-κB, which participate in a positive feedback pathway wherein TNF-α production is increased further.[37] This TNF-α pathway also upregulates caspase 8 production, an important mediator of intestinal cell apoptosis; this suggests that although disruption of mucosal integrity causes an inflammatory response, the response itself causes further interruption of the protective barrier.[36]

The Janus kinase (JAK)/signal transducer and activator of transcription (STAT) pathway is another important cascade in the production of IBD. Four members of the JAK pathway—JAK1, JAK2, JAK3, and tyrosine kinase 2—use STAT transcription factors (STAT1, STAT2, STAT3, STAT4, STAT5A, STAT5B, STAT6) to regulate cytokine responses. JAKs phosphorylate STATs, which upregulate certain genes involved in the inflammatory response. The JAK/STAT pathway regulates IL-6, IL-12, and IL-23, which are highly involved in IBD. IL-12 causes differentiation of T cells into Th1 cells and triggers TNF-α production by NK cells. IL-23 induces propagation of a subset of Th cells known as Th17 cells, which yield TNF-α and IL-6. Studies suggest that IL-6 is important in the chronic inflammatory response, particularly in autoimmune diseases. IL-12 and IL-23 are important for systemic immune activation and intestinal inflammation, respectively.[36,37]

Immune Therapy for Inflammatory Bowel Disease

Current treatments available for IBD are aimed at modulating the chronic immune response. Anti-TNF-α antibodies, such as infliximab, adalimumab, and certolizumab, have been shown to decrease the inflammatory response associated with IBD. Tofacitinib is a JAK inhibitor, and although it is approved only for treating rheumatoid arthritis at the present time, several ongoing trials are evaluating its efficacy for IBD. Ustekinumab binds to IL-12 and IL-23 effectively blocking their activity and is similarly undergoing clinical trials to determine its usefulness in IBD.[36]

Chronic Gastritis

The most common cause of chronic gastritis worldwide is infection with *Helicobacter pylori,* a microbial pathogen that infects approximately 50% of the world. *H. pylori* is a gram-negative spirochete that lives within gastric crypts. It secretes urease, causing conversion of urea to ammonia, neutralizing hydrochloric acid in the stomach. G cells in the gastric antrum produce gastrin, which is inhibited by the normally acidic environment of the stomach. The loss of a low pH diminishes the negative feedback mechanism, and gastrin levels remain elevated. Various inflammatory cells and cytokines are recruited, leading to chronic gastritis. The resultant chronic inflammation perpetuates acid suppression through cellular atrophy. A small percentage of patients (<15%)—patients with chronic inflammation in the gastric antrum—have decreased somatostatin production. Somatostatin is responsible for inhibiting gastrin production. When this feedback is removed, gastrin levels increase.[38-40]

Histologic Changes

The Correa pathway describes the distinct steps in the changes occurring from normal tissue to gastric cancer.[40] Initially, an individual has normal gastric mucosa, which develops into superficial gastritis, perhaps under the influence of *H. pylori* or salt. Next, chronic inflammation gradually occurs and recruits various immune cells. The chronic inflammation is termed *atrophic gastritis* after certain histologic changes occur. Bacterial overgrowth occurs during this phase because of the achlorhydria and hypergastrinemia. The development of atrophic gastritis is the critical step in developing cancer. The mucosal cells then undergo metaplastic followed by dysplastic changes. Carcinoma ultimately develops as a result of these alterations.[40]

Mucosal cells that undergo changes to atrophic cells lose their oxyntic glands. Oxyntic glands contain parietal cells, which are responsible for the secretion of hydrochloric acid and intrinsic factor. The changes occurring in atrophy are termed *pseudopyloric metaplasia* or *spasmolytic polypeptide expressing metaplasia*. The loss of parietal cells is thought to alter gastric cell growth and differentiation. This loss of regulation causes cells to undergo further intestinal metaplasia. The gastric glands are replaced by straight tubular crypts, which contain goblet and absorptive cells. The lamina propria demonstrates a histologic infiltration of inflammatory cells in gastric metaplasia.

Clinical Manifestations

Individuals who acquire *H. pylori* tend to acquire the bacterium early in life, and it then persists. Most individuals who are infected remain asymptomatic throughout their lifetime. Patients may seek treatment if the infection causes symptoms. There is generally a long phase of chronic gastritis with minimal symptoms. If ulcer disease occurs, prevalence historically peaks in the third or fourth decade of life. Approximately 10% develop ulcer disease (duodenal or gastric). Of these, 1% to 3% go on to develop gastric carcinoma several decades later by the previously described pathway. Patients who develop duodenal ulcers appear to be protected from gastric cancer from higher acid levels. *H. pylori* infection alone is insufficient to cause gastric cancer. Of gastric and duodenal ulcers, 85% are due to infection with *H. pylori*. These patients also are 3.5 times more likely to develop peptic ulcer disease. The infection ultimately causes an intense inflammatory response with an inability to resolve the infection.[40,41] *H. pylori* also is thought to be the cause of mucosa-associated lymphoid tissue (MALT).[42]

Immunologic Changes

Th1 cells are significantly increased during infection with *H. pylori*, which causes epithelial cell death through various mechanisms. The resultant cytokines and proinflammatory molecules enhance apoptosis induced by *H. pylori* bacteria.

TNF-α-related apoptosis-inducing ligand (TRAIL) is a T cell ligand that normally causes cell death in transformed cell lines but not in normal primary cells. When gastric cells are exposed to *H. pylori*, TRAIL-mediated apoptosis occurs, suggesting that infiltrating T cells play a role in immune-mediated gastric cell death during infection with *H. pylori*. This pathway upregulated caspase 8, which sends death signals to mitochondria.

The chronic gastric mucosal inflammation that occurs in *H. pylori* infection is due largely to T lymphocyte activation and infiltration. Gastric epithelial cell interaction with the bacteria recruits neutrophils and lymphocytes; this causes release of IL-1, IL-6, IL-8, IL-12, TNF-α, and IFN-γ. The TNF-α and IL-1 that are released induce upregulation of CCL20 in gastric epithelial cells. CCL20 interacts with its ligand, CCR6, present on dendritic cells and some memory T cells. This interaction recruits CD45 memory T cells to the inflammatory sites; this implies that the infiltrating T cells are activated CD4 cells, which cause chronic gastritis secondary to *H. pylori* infection.

Two genetic loci in *H. pylori* are associated with chronic inflammation and progression to cancer—CagA and VacA. CagA is a gene product from CagA-positive *H. pylori* bacteria. The CagA product is internalized in epithelial cells by a translocation system. Tyrosine is phosphorylated by Src kinases. The phosphorylated CagA induces epithelial cell changes. Infections with these particular strains are associated with gastric neoplasms and MALT lymphomas. MALT lymphomas require *H. pylori* infection for development—the bacterial colonization recruits lymphocytes as previously mentioned. Eradication of *H. pylori* bacteria causes remission of MALT lymphomas. The lymphomas are of a B cell lineage through CD40 and CD40L interaction, although the exact mechanism of this interaction is unknown.[40,41] Similarly, VacA is a protein that causes vacuolization in certain cell lines including gastric cells. It blocks multiplication of T cells by stopping the cell cycle in the G_1/S interphase.[40]

Treatment

Treatment strategies for *H. pylori*–induced gastritis are aimed at eradicating the organism. Some studies demonstrate reversal of atrophic gastric and restoration of the normal glandular architecture with infection resolution.[40]

Chronic Vascular Inflammation

Myocardial infarction, the leading cause of morbidity and mortality in the Western world, occurs as a result of atherosclerosis, hypertension, diabetes mellitus, or dysfunctional lipid metabolism leading to coronary artery vasoconstriction. Innate immunity contributes to the initiation and progression of atherosclerosis.[43]

Atherosclerosis is a chronic inflammatory condition of large and medium-sized arteries. There are two mechanisms by which chronic vascular inflammation causes atherosclerosis. The first, known as the direct mechanism, occurs when lipoproteins become trapped in the subendothelial space of the arterial wall and undergo various changes. This mechanism instigates an inflammatory response, which recruits macrophages and T cells. Macrophages scavenge these molecules and form intracellular lipid-filled vacuoles (foam cells). These foam cells form atherosclerotic plaques. As time progresses, the foam cells die, leaving behind plaques with acellular, necrotic centers. A fibrous cap covers the necrotic center, and when this capsule ruptures, a thrombus develops as a result of debris interaction with the coagulation system. The indirect mechanism occurs when the vasculature is exposed to microorganisms or pollution. In both of these mechanisms, thrombi develop, which cause myriad complications including stroke and myocardial infarction.[44,45]

Cellular Differentiation Involved in Chronic Vascular Inflammation

Lipid molecules, either oxidized or free cholesterol molecules, appear to initiate endothelial and adhesion molecule activation triggering the inflammatory cascade.[45] After initiation of the inflammatory response in vessels (usually by infection or injury), polymorphonuclear neutrophils, mainly neutrophils, infiltrate the affected area, followed by monocytes. CD14 and CD16 monocytes are the key leukocytes involved in this reaction. These two cell types secrete varying levels of TNF-α and IL-10. The monocytes then differentiate into macrophages after migrating to the site of inflammation. The M1 macrophages produce IL-1β and TNF-α and participate in a Th1 response. The M2 macrophages produce IL-10 and IL-12 and contribute to a Th2 reaction.[43]

IL-12 secreted by monocytes and macrophages stimulates NK cells. NK cells also are activated by direct cell-to-cell contact between monocytes or macrophages and NK receptors. NK cells go on to produce IFN-γ, which creates a positive feedback loop by causing further differentiation of monocytes into macrophages. Similarly, IFN-γ produces oxidative stress in the vessel wall, further inflammatory cell recruitment, and angiotensin II vascular dysfunction.[43]

The monocytes, differentiated macrophages, and NK cells all contribute to plaque formation. These plaques are known to contain TLR2 and TLR4. Absence or diminished number of TLR2 and TLR4 decreases the growth of atherosclerotic lesions. Furthermore, these lesions can regress by de-recruitment of monocytes and macrophages—these cells present antigens from the plaque to native T and B cells in the spleen. The antigens form oxidation-specific epitopes, which become a target for macrophages, antibodies, and innate plasma proteins.[46] The innate immune system causes plaque regression.[45]

Indirect Mechanism of Activation

Patients with autoimmune disease, smokers, and individuals exposed to high levels of pollution are at higher risk for death from myocardial infarction. All these states lead to increased levels of inflammatory cytokines. These cytokines are believed to be perpetuated in the systemic circulation, taken up by vessel walls causing plaque formation initiation. Smoking and pollution also may contribute to oxidization of lipid particles, initiating the indirect mechanism of vascular inflammation.

The next mechanism of indirect activation is related to dysfunctional high-density lipoprotein (HDL) particles. HDL historically has been thought of cardioprotective by transporting plaque cholesterol to the liver, where it is converted to bile and subsequently excreted. HDL also carries the enzyme paraoxonase, which is an anti-inflammatory and antioxidant and may prevent atherosclerosis. Patients with autoimmune diseases have dysfunction of this enzyme, along with dysfunctional expression of adhesion molecules. These patients are thought to oxidize low-density lipoprotein particles at a higher rate. Patients with cardiovascular disease also have dysfunctional HDL, although the mechanism of this is unclear.

The last known mechanism of indirect activation of atherosclerotic plaques is dependent on humoral immunity. Patients with atherosclerosis generate autoantibodies against oxidized phospholipids within atherosclerotic plaques. These antibodies appear to be generated from interaction with bacterial cell wall (PAMPs) or apoptotic (DAMPs) cells. Just as air pollution increases cytokines, some authors believe this exposure contributes to production of the autoantibodies.[45]

Therapeutic Options

Oxidization of LDL is the primary inciting mechanism for the chronic vascular inflammatory cascade. Several other important mediators include oxidation-specific epitopes, TNF-α, and $CD4^+$ T cells and B cells. Many of the therapeutic options available at the present time are still under investigation.

Antibodies to oxidation-specific epitopes are being used to explore reduction in atherogenesis in murine models. TNF-α antibodies are similarly applied to evaluate improvement in cardiovascular disease in trials. A clinical trial involving canakinumab is ongoing at the present time.[46] This monoclonal antibody deactivates IL-1β, which reduces cardiovascular disease in patients with existing disease. The trial has demonstrated reduced C-reactive protein levels but has yet to show decreased levels of lipoprotein. Oxidation of lipids is the main mechanism of activation, and reducing lipoprotein levels from the outset is the most effective prevention method. Further investigation is needed to determine optimal therapy when chronic vascular inflammation has already been established.[46]

Chronic Hepatic Inflammation and Cirrhosis

Overview of Cirrhosis and Hepatic Immune Cell Organization

The liver exerts many important functions on systemic immune homeostasis. A key function includes immune surveillance and production of molecules that participate in an immune response. Chronic inflammation of the liver results in cirrhosis and develops as a result of immune-mediated inflammation. Furthermore, cirrhosis impairs hepatic participation in immune surveillance leading to decreased immune activation. Immunodeficiency and chronic systemic inflammation subsequently develop.

The liver is uniquely organized in a manner whereby immune cells are arranged to monitor for systemic and intestinal pathogens. Primary hepatic immune cells include Kupffer cells (similar to macrophages), sinusoidal endothelial cells, and dendritic cells. Kupffer cells and sinusoidal endothelial cells comprise the hepatic reticuloendothelial system. Kupffer cells reside within vascular spaces on the intraluminal side and engulf pathogens as they pass by. Kupffer cells also bind to complement component 3b. Kupffer cells and sinusoidal endothelial cells are antigen-presenting cells and contain MHC class I and II receptors. Hepatic dendritic cells drive activation of T cells, some of which may reside in the liver. The liver is crucial to the development of the systemic immune system (innate and adaptive) through production of complement proteins, pattern recognition receptors, acute-phase proteins, and proinflammatory cytokines.[47]

Hepatic fibrosis occurs as a result of chronic hepatic injury by mechanisms such as excess alcohol intake or lipid accumulation. In particular, hepatic fibrosis results from altered wound healing strategies as a method to reduce cellular damage. Extracellular matrix proteins accrue from increased production and deposition, which causes scar formation. When this accrual of extracellular matrix proteins occurs over prolonged duration, fibrotic septa develop around hepatic nodules and altered vasculature. Hepatocytes degenerate, and Kupffer cells are lost. In the initial phases of cirrhosis, there is not a significant increase in morbidity. However, as cirrhosis progresses, liver failure and portal hypertension may develop. Hepatic encephalopathy, varices, hepatorenal syndrome, and hepatocellular carcinoma all can occur as consequences of hepatic cirrhosis.[48]

Immune-Mediated Hepatic Degradation

Autophagy is an important component of normal hepatic homeostatic mechanisms. Autophagy is the degradation of cellular components via uptake through a vacuole, fusion with a lysosome, and digestion of contents. This process allows removal of degenerating mitochondria and regulation of metabolic processes. Alterations of this pathway lead to alcoholic cirrhosis, nonalcoholic fatty liver disease, and fibrosis.

When the liver undergoes damage from any cause, myofibroblasts migrate and accumulate at the site of injury. Some myofibroblasts also develop from hepatic stellate cells. They begin secreting extracellular matrix proteins such as fibrillar collagen and enzymes such as metalloproteinase. Additionally, cytokines involved in liver regeneration and angiogenesis are secreted (Fig. 3-4).

As mentioned earlier, injury activates Kupffer cells, which aid in initiation of the fibrotic process. Kupffer cells contribute to activation of hepatic stellate cells. $CD4^+$ T lymphocytes (Th2) secrete IL-13 and IL-17, both of which promote fibrosis. Th1 lymphocytes secrete IFN-γ, which reduce liver fibrosis.[48]

Systemic Immune System Effects of Cirrhosis

The liver is intimately associated with the systemic immune system because it produces many proteins and inflammatory molecules involved in immune activation. Cirrhosis has damaging effects on systemic inflammation. Neutrophils have decreased phagocytic activity against opsonized pathogens along with impaired chemotaxis to injured sites. Function, number, and differentiation of monocytes are altered in cirrhotic states. B lymphocyte number decreases significantly, and IgG production is inhibited. T lymphocytes do not proliferate as rapidly, and NK cells are defective in cirrhosis. In addition, certain proinflammatory systemic cytokines such as TNF-α and IL-6 are upregulated.[47]

Clinical Manifestations of Cirrhosis

Gut-associated lymphoid tissue is the first defense layer against enteric pathogens. Gastric mucosa–associated lymphoid tissue undergoes damage in cirrhosis as a result of increased intestinal permeability. The constant bacterial load continuously activates monocytes, dendritic cells, and T lymphocytes, which secrete cytokines; this causes systemic inflammation as a result of the activated immune cells and cytokine production. Cirrhosis-induced inflammation and systemic inflammation are the primary

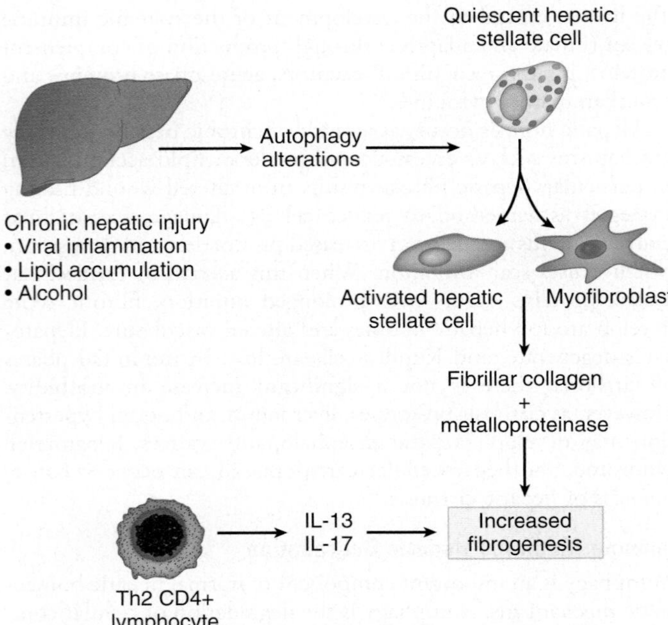

FIGURE 3-4 Hepatic fibrosis is driven by autophagy and cellular alterations. Autophagy, a generally well-regulated process, undergoes alterations when hepatic cell injury occurs through alcohol, viral inflammation, or accumulation of lipids that cause oxidative stress. Quiescent hepatic stellate cells acquire myofibroblast properties or become "activated stellate cells" under these conditions. Fibrogenesis occurs as a result of fibrillar collagen and metalloproteinase deposition from these two cell types. Interleukin-13 (IL-13) and interleukin-17 (IL-17), secreted from helper T cells (Th2), contribute to fibrogenesis.

factors causing the clinical manifestations. Chronic hepatic inflammation causes a paucity of an immune response to bacterial pathogens, leading to higher bacterial susceptibility; this may lead to multiorgan dysfunction and increased mortality.

Patients also may experience alteration of vascular tone because of higher levels of proinflammatory cytokines and higher nitric oxide levels. Splanchnic and peripheral vascular tone is diminished in cirrhotic patients.

Encephalopathy is caused by two mechanisms. It is caused directly by inflammatory cytokines stimulating various receptors. Activated immune cells such as macrophages also are recruited to the brain. These two in concert increase levels of TNF-α in the brain causing fatigue and encephalopathy.

Renal function is decreased by decreased glomerular filtration rate (GFR). GFR is decreased through damaged microvasculature as a result of elevated levels of circulating cytokines.[47]

Advanced cirrhosis typically is treated with a liver transplant, pending a patient's eligibility. Treatments for alleviating chronic hepatic dysfunction burden are aimed at the specific underlying causes of cirrhosis.

Chronic Renal Inflammation

The kidneys have several important roles in homeostasis, including acid-base balance, controlling blood pressure through salt and water balance, calcium regulation, and production of red blood cells. Renal disease is increasing in the United States and causes dysfunction in the aforementioned processes. Renal disease is the eighth leading cause of death in the United States. It causes significant morbidity within the population, and understanding the pathophysiology can help with prevention. Renal disease typically is categorized as acute or chronic. Acute kidney injury may progress to chronic kidney disease (CKD). CKD also is caused by complications of diabetes, obesity, and autoimmune conditions. Underlying both of these mechanisms are the chronic inflammatory states that lead to persistent renal alterations.[49]

Role of Innate Immunity in the Development of Chronic Renal Disease

Complement proteins appear to be involved in development of and protection against renal disease. Murine models have demonstrated a protective effect of C3 and C5 on glomerular damage and reduction in albuminuria. Conversely, mice deficient in C1q or C4 have a risk of developing lupus nephritis, a form of chronic autoimmune renal inflammation.

Dendritic cells that reside within the kidney present antigens to T cells, which lead to glomerular inflammation. T cells and complement complexes activate macrophages as a secondary inflammatory mediator; this suggests that macrophages are not a primary mediator of inflammation in the renal system. The macrophages that are involved in chronic renal inflammation are activated by IFN-γ or TNF-α. The macrophages then release other inflammatory cytokines, such as IL-1, IL-6, and IL-23, leading to renal fibrosis.[49]

Adaptive Immunity in Renal Inflammation

Cell-mediated mechanisms direct the adaptive immune system through T lymphocytes, whereas antibody-mediated immunity is directed by B lymphocytes. B lymphocytes contribute to renal disease when autoantibodies are formed causing systemic lupus erythematosus, Goodpasture syndrome, and IgA nephropathy. The key contributors to cell-mediated immunity in renal disease are $CD8^+$ cytotoxic T cells and $CD4^+$ Th cells. Cytotoxic T cells are activated by autoantigens, which not only cause inflammation but also release further renal-specific autoantigens, perpetuating the inflammatory cycle. $CD4^+$ Th cells are activated by cytokines and APCs, stimulating Th differentiation into Th1, Th2, or Th17 cells.

Th1 cells produce IFN-γ, IL-2, TNF-α, and lymphotoxin-α. These substrates activate macrophages and $CD8^+$ cells and cause tissue injury. Th2 cells produce IL-4, IL-5, and IL-10, which are generally considered anti-inflammatory cytokines. In renal disease, these cytokines can induce B cell maturation and production of renal-directed autoantibodies. Th17 cells produce IL-17, IL-21, and IL-22, all of which lead to TNF-α production. TNF-α is an important inflammatory molecule leading to autoimmune-mediated nephritis.[49]

Pathophysiologic Changes Caused by Chronic Renal Inflammation

Chronic renal inflammation reduces renal blood flow and ultimately causes hypertensive states. The decreased renal blood flow causes a reduction in GFR, eventually producing end-stage renal disease. The cytokines TNF-α, TGF-β, and interleukins also act to change sodium regulation. TNF-α generally decreases renal blood flow and GFR and subsequently increases natriuresis. TGF-β inhibits renal vasculature autoregulatory systems. IL-1 directly influences renal epithelial cells to cause sodium excretion.[49]

Fibrosis, sclerosis, and tubulointerstitial alterations are the hallmark changes in CKD. Glomerular injury is caused by vascular endothelial growth factor directed at podocytes, leading to sclerosis and fibrosis along with hypertrophy and hyperfiltration. Mesangial cells become activated during the inflammatory response forming a fibroblast phenotype. These fibroblast-like cells secrete extracellular matrix proteins contributing to fibrosis. Adhesion molecules are upregulated by endothelial cell activation; this allows macrophages to infiltrate the glomerulus, resulting in thrombi, hyaline deposition, and basement membrane destruction.

Tubulointerstitial damage occurs as a result of glomerular hypertrophy and deregulation of blood flow. The altered tubular cells convert to a fibroblast-like state. They secrete collagen and participate in fibrosis formation. These fibroblasts eventually undergo regulated cell death, leaving behind an acellular renal scar.[49]

Immune Therapy for Chronic Renal Disease

Treatment for CKD is aimed at controlling diabetes, hypertension, and hypercholesterolemia. Novel approaches for treatment are aimed at the immune pathways involved in formation of CKD. The renin-angiotensin-aldosterone system is commonly targeted through angiotensin-converting enzyme inhibitors and angiotensin receptor blockers for management of hypertension. There is newer evidence that angiotensin-converting enzyme inhibitors and angiotensin receptor blockers decrease urinary protein excretion, circulating T cells, cytokine production, and ultimately renal inflammation. Corticosteroids are used as a mainstay treatment for systemic lupus erythematosus and other chronic autoimmune renal diseases. They protect against glomerular injury, complement activation, and proteinuria.

Immune-mediated therapies include cyclosporine and mycophenolate mofetil. They target purine synthesis, which inhibits T cell and B cell growth and proliferation. Adalimumab, infliximab, and etanercept are antibodies directed against TNF-α that decrease renal inflammation in models and are currently in experimental phases for use in humans.[49]

Sterile Inflammation

Examples of Sterile Inflammation

There are instances in which inflammation is not triggered by a microbial pathogen, but rather through the body's innate mechanisms. Ischemic reperfusion injury, trauma, crystal-induced inflammation, and toxins all can cause a sterile immune response. Cellular necrosis is unplanned cell death, from either acute or chronic inflammation, which releases factors and reinforces an inflammatory cascade. Triggers of sterile inflammation are typically classified as intracellular or extracellular. Examples of intracellular activators include heat shock proteins, mitochondrial DNA, and other cellular chaperones. Extracellular matrix pieces, such as hyaluronan, are thought to be activators of sterile inflammation. All cells produce uric acid as a result of purine metabolism. When a cell undergoes necrosis, it releases uric acid, which combines with sodium to produce monosodium urate crystals. These crystals trigger release of proinflammatory cytokines such as IL-1β and TNF-α.

Pathways Involved in Sterile Inflammation

TLRs are thought to be a primary mediator of sterile inflammation. TLR2 and TLR4 have been shown in murine models to be involved in the response to ischemia reperfusion injury through the MyD88 adapter.

The inflammasome is a multiprotein complex residing within cells. Patients with acute myocardial infarction with associated ischemia reperfusion injury have activation of the inflammasome receptors. These receptors cause recruitment of apoptosis-associated specklike caspase, which triggers caspase-1 and IL-1β production.

The aforementioned receptors can be activated in either sterile or nonsterile inflammation; however, there are receptors specific to sterile inflammation. RAGE is one such receptor. RAGE is a transmembrane receptor expressed in endothelial cells, myocardium, and various immune cells. This receptor responds to a plethora of ligands causing release of inflammatory cytokines.

Natural Progression of Sterile Inflammation

Neutrophils are the first cells to respond in the sterile inflammatory pathway and create clusters. Necrotic cells release mediators, such as annexin A1, which prevent further recruitment of neutrophils. Neutrophils cause uptake of necrotic debris by macrophages in a process known as efferocytosis. Macrophages secrete vascular endothelial growth factor, which helps with resolution of tissue hypoxia and activates angiogenesis. Lastly, macrophages secrete mediators such as lipoxin, which is known to participate in sterile inflammation resolution.[50]

SELECTED REFERENCES

Bernard GR, Vincent JL, Laterre PF, et al: Efficacy and safety of recombinant human activated protein C for severe sepsis. *N Engl J Med* 344:699–709, 2001.

The landmark PROWESS trial offered convincing evidence that the antithrombotic, anti-inflammatory, and profibrinolytic properties of rhAPC reduced mortality in severe sepsis, despite increased risks of bleeding. Based on this evidence, rhAPC became the first treatment for severe sepsis approved by the U.S. Food and Drug Administration.

Matzinger P: The danger model: a renewed sense of self. *Science* 296:301–305, 2002.

Matzinger challenged the conventional belief that the immune system distinguished between self and nonself and postulated that the immune system is more concerned with danger signals, which may originate from foreign pathogens or from dead or dying cells.

Ranieri VM, Thompson BT, Barie PS, et al: Drotrecogin alfa (activated) in adults with septic shock. *N Engl J Med* 366:2055–2064, 2012.

The PROWESS-SHOCK trial addressed controversy about the efficacy of rhAPC by randomly assigning patients with septic shock and high risk of death to rhAPC versus placebo. At 28 and 90 days, rhAPC failed to demonstrate a mortality benefit, and it was subsequently withdrawn from the market.

Shen H, Kreisel D, Goldstein DR: Processes of sterile inflammation. *J Immunol* 191:2857–2863, 2013.

Sterile inflammation occurs in the absence of microorganisms but causes significant morbidity each year. Ischemia, hypotension, reperfusion injury, and chronic diseases all trigger sterile inflammation. The inflammatory pathways involved in infections are well known. Although these pathways contribute to sterile inflammation, less is known about the distinct pathways that cause sterile inflammation. Unique treatment strategies, separate from strategies required in systemic inflammatory response syndrome or sepsis, are required. Understanding these pathways helps guide clinical decision making in patients with this condition.

Wang D, Bodovitz S: Single cell analysis: the new frontier in "omics". *Trends Biotechnol* 28:281–290, 2010.

Single-cell analysis of the interactions between genes, proteins, and metabolites historically has been unavailable because of a lack of technology. With the advent of transcriptomics, genomics, proteomics, and metabolomics, single-cell examination has become a new trend. Mass spectrometry and advanced automated DNA sequencers have the potential to identify individual cell alterations occurring in disease states. This advancement has the ability to transform treatment strategies and allows the creation of tailored treatment plans to individual patients based on cellular changes.

Zheng L, Xue J, Jaffee EM, et al: Role of immune cells and immune-based therapies in pancreatitis and pancreatic ductal adenocarcinoma. *Gastroenterology* 144:1230–1240, 2013.

Many patients with chronic pancreatitis previously experienced bouts of acute pancreatitis, and recurrent acute pancreatitis is generally the inciting factor for chronic pancreatitis. A small percentage of patients with chronic pancreatitis progress to pancreatic ductal carcinoma. The inflammatory reaction in these patients is almost identical to the reaction seen in patients with chronic pancreatitis. It is not well understood why some patients progress, whereas most patients do not. Although the distinction is unclear, much can be learned about the inflammatory pathways that are activated in chronic pancreatitis by examining histologic changes during acute and chronic pancreatitis.

REFERENCES

1. O'Neill LA, Golenbock D, Bowie AG: The history of Toll-like receptors—redefining innate immunity. *Nat Rev Immunol* 13:453–460, 2013.
2. Schulte W, Bernhagen J, Bucala R: Cytokines in sepsis: Potent immunoregulators and potential therapeutic targets—an updated view. *Mediators Inflamm* 2013:165974, 2013.
3. King EG, Bauza GJ, Mella JR, et al: Pathophysiologic mechanisms in septic shock. *Lab Invest* 94:4–12, 2014.
4. Cohen J: The immunopathogenesis of sepsis. *Nature* 420:885–891, 2002.
5. Garlanda C, Dinarello CA, Mantovani A: The interleukin-1 family: Back to the future. *Immunity* 39:1003–1018, 2013.
6. Joshi VD, Kalvakolanu DV, Hebel JR, et al: Role of caspase 1 in murine antibacterial host defenses and lethal endotoxemia. *Infect Immun* 70:6896–6903, 2002.
7. Diener KR, Al-Dasooqi N, Lousberg EL, et al: The multifunctional alarmin HMGB1 with roles in the pathophysiology of sepsis and cancer. *Immunol Cell Biol* 91:443–450, 2013.
8. Kinoshita M, Miyazaki H, Ono S, et al: Immunoenhancing therapy with interleukin-18 against bacterial infection in immunocompromised hosts after severe surgical stress. *J Leukoc Biol* 93:689–698, 2013.
9. Cuzzocrea S, Mazzon E, Dugo L, et al: Absence of endogenous interleukin-6 enhances the inflammatory response during acute pancreatitis induced by cerulein in mice. *Cytokine* 18:274–285, 2002.
10. Zisman DA, Kunkel SL, Strieter RM, et al: Anti-interleukin-12 therapy protects mice in lethal endotoxemia but impairs bacterial clearance in murine *Escherichia coli* peritoneal sepsis. *Shock* 8:349–356, 1997.
11. Emmanuilidis K, Weighardt H, Matevossian E, et al: Differential regulation of systemic IL-18 and IL-12 release during postoperative sepsis: High serum IL-18 as an early predictive indicator of lethal outcome. *Shock* 18:301–305, 2002.
12. Weighardt H, Heidecke CD, Westerholt A, et al: Impaired monocyte IL-12 production before surgery as a predictive factor for the lethal outcome of postoperative sepsis. *Ann Surg* 235:560–567, 2002.
13. Korn T, Bettelli E, Oukka M, et al: IL-17 and Th17 cells. *Annu Rev Immunol* 27:485–517, 2009.
14. Schroder K, Hertzog PJ, Ravasi T, et al: Interferon-gamma: An overview of signals, mechanisms and functions. *J Leukoc Biol* 75:163–189, 2004.
15. Calandra T, Froidevaux C, Martin C, et al: Macrophage migration inhibitory factor and host innate immune defenses against bacterial sepsis. *J Infect Dis* 187(Suppl 2):S385–S390, 2003.
16. Yende S, Angus DC, Kong L, et al: The influence of macrophage migration inhibitory factor gene polymorphisms on outcome from community-acquired pneumonia. *FASEB J* 23:2403–2411, 2009.
17. Merk M, Zierow S, Leng L, et al: The D-dopachrome tautomerase (DDT) gene product is a cytokine and functional homolog of macrophage migration inhibitory factor (MIF). *Proc Natl Acad Sci U S A* 108:E577–E585, 2011.
18. Wu HP, Wu CL, Chen CK, et al: The interleukin-4 expression in patients with severe sepsis. *J Crit Care* 23:519–524, 2008.
19. Gu W, Zeng L, Zhang LY, et al: Association of interleukin 4-589T/C polymorphism with T(H)1 and T(H)2 bias and sepsis in Chinese major trauma patients. *J Trauma* 71:1583–1587, 2011.
20. van der Poll T, Marchant A, Buurman WA, et al: Endogenous IL-10 protects mice from death during septic peritonitis. *J Immunol* 155:5397–5401, 1995.
21. Latifi SQ, O'Riordan MA, Levine AD: Interleukin-10 controls the onset of irreversible septic shock. *Infect Immun* 70:4441–4446, 2002.
22. Sarma JV, Ward PA: The complement system. *Cell Tissue Res* 343:227–235, 2011.
23. Webster NR, Galley HF: Immunomodulation in the critically ill. *Br J Anaesth* 103:70–81, 2009.
24. Bernard GR, Vincent JL, Laterre PF, et al: Efficacy and safety of recombinant human activated protein C for severe sepsis. *N Engl J Med* 344:699–709, 2001.
25. Ranieri VM, Thompson BT, Barie PS, et al: Drotrecogin alfa (activated) in adults with septic shock. *N Engl J Med* 366: 2055–2064, 2012.

26. Boomer JS, Green JM, Hotchkiss RS: The changing immune system in sepsis: Is individualized immuno-modulatory therapy the answer? *Virulence* 5:45–56, 2014.
27. Fitzpatrick M, Young SP: Metabolomics—a novel window into inflammatory disease. *Swiss Med Wkly* 143:w13743, 2013.
28. Kumar V, Abbas AK, Aster JC: Inflammation and Repair. In *Robbins and cotran pathologic basis of disease*, ed 9, Philadelphia, 2015, Saunders, pp 69–111. <https://www-clinicalkey-com.proxy.its.virginia.edu/#!/ContentPlayerCtrl/doPlayContent/3-s2.0-B9781455726134000037/>. Accessed September 20, 2014.
29. Nibali L, Henderson B, Sadiq ST, et al: Genetic dysbiosis: The role of microbial insults in chronic inflammatory diseases. *J Oral Microbiol* 6, 2014.
30. Wang D, Bodovitz S: Single cell analysis: The new frontier in "omics". *Trends Biotechnol* 28:281–290, 2010.
31. Angelis N, Porpodis K, Zarogoulidis P, et al: Airway inflammation in chronic obstructive pulmonary disease. *J Thorac Dis* 6(Suppl 1):S167–S172, 2014.
32. Caramori G, Adcock IM, Di Stefano A, et al: Cytokine inhibition in the treatment of COPD. *Int J Chron Obstruct Pulmon Dis* 9:397–412, 2014.
33. Zheng L, Xue J, Jaffee EM, et al: Role of immune cells and immune-based therapies in pancreatitis and pancreatic ductal adenocarcinoma. *Gastroenterology* 144:1230–1240, 2013.
34. Inman KS, Francis AA, Murray NR: Complex role for the immune system in initiation and progression of pancreatic cancer. *World J Gastroenterol* 20:11160–11181, 2014.
35. Whitcomb DC: Risk, Etiology, and Pathology of Chronic Pancreatitis. In Forsmark CE, editor: *Pancreatitis and its complications*, Totowa, NJ, 2005, Humana Press, pp 149–171. <http://download.springer.com/static/pdf/970/chp%3A10.1385%2F1-59259-815-3%3A149.pdf!auth66=1411730022_20972324c3a9f590b04994f79a820a8f&ext=.pdf>. Accessed September 24, 2014.
36. Pedersen J, Coskun M, Soendergaard C, et al: Inflammatory pathways of importance for management of inflammatory bowel disease. *World J Gastroenterol* 20:64–77, 2014.
37. Fakhoury M, Negrulj R, Mooranian A, et al: Inflammatory bowel disease: Clinical aspects and treatments. *J Inflamm Res* 7:113–120, 2014.
38. Chao C, Hellmich MR: Gastrin, inflammation, and carcinogenesis. *Curr Opin Endocrinol Diabetes Obes* 17:33–39, 2010.
39. De Preter V, Verbeke K: Metabolomics as a diagnostic tool in gastroenterology. *World J Gastrointest Pharmacol Ther* 4: 97–107, 2013.
40. Fox JG, Wang TC: Inflammation, atrophy, and gastric cancer. *J Clin Invest* 117:60–69, 2007.
41. Tsai HF, Hsu PN: Interplay between *Helicobacter pylori* and immune cells in immune pathogenesis of gastric inflammation and mucosal pathology. *Cell Mol Immunol* 7:255–259, 2010.
42. Beswick EJ, Suarez G, Reyes VE: *H pylori* and host interactions that influence pathogenesis. *World J Gastroenterol* 12:5599–5605, 2006.
43. Knorr M, Munzel T, Wenzel P: Interplay of NK cells and monocytes in vascular inflammation and myocardial infarction. *Front Physiol* 5:295, 2014.
44. Tsiantoulas D, Diehl CJ, Witztum JL, et al: B cells and humoral immunity in atherosclerosis. *Circ Res* 114:1743–1756, 2014.
45. Rosenfeld ME: Inflammation and atherosclerosis: Direct versus indirect mechanisms. *Curr Opin Pharmacol* 13:154–160, 2013.
46. Lichtman AH, Binder CJ, Tsimikas S, et al: Adaptive immunity in atherogenesis: New insights and therapeutic approaches. *J Clin Invest* 123:27–36, 2013.
47. Albillos A, Lario M, Alvarez-Mon M: Cirrhosis-associated immune dysfunction: Distinctive features and clinical relevance. *J Hepatol* 61:1385–1396, 2014.
48. Mallat A, Lodder J, Teixeira-Clerc F, et al: Autophagy: A multifaceted partner in liver fibrosis. *Biomed Res Int* 2014: 869390, 2014.
49. Imig JD, Ryan MJ: Immune and inflammatory role in renal disease. *Compr Physiol* 3:957–976, 2013.
50. Shen H, Kreisel D, Goldstein DR: Processes of sterile inflammation. *J Immunol* 191:2857–2863, 2013.

4 CHAPTER

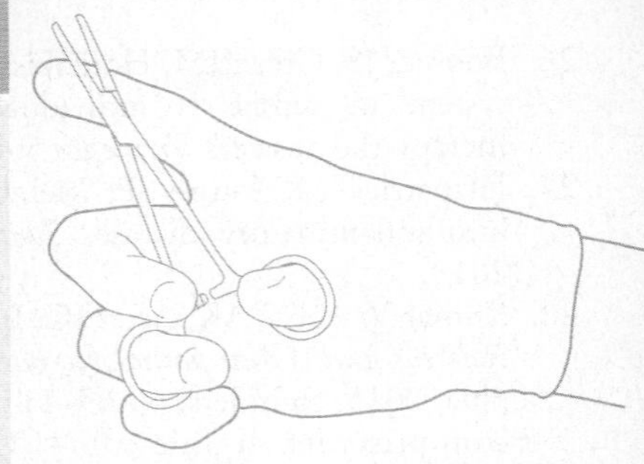

Shock, Electrolytes, and Fluid

Peter Rhee, Bellal Joseph

OUTLINE

Surgeons are the masters of fluids because they need to be. They care for patients who cannot eat or drink for various reasons; for example, they have hemorrhaged, undergone surgery, or lost fluids from tubes, drains, or wounds. Surgeons are obligated to know how to care for these patients, who put their lives in their hands. This topic might appear simple only for those who do not understand the complexities of the human body and its ability to regulate and compensate fluids. In reality, the task of managing patients' blood volume is one of the most challenging burdens surgeons face, often requiring complete control of the intake and output of fluids and electrolytes, often in the presence of blood loss. Surgeons do not yet completely understand the physiology of shock and resuscitation, and their knowledge is superficial. Given the nature of the profession, they have studied those topics and dealt with patients who bleed and exsanguinate. Historically, wartime experience has always helped them move ahead in their knowledge of the management of fluids and how to better resuscitate. The recent wars in Iraq and Afghanistan are no exception as we have learned much from these wars.

Constant attention to and titration of fluid loss therapy is required because the human body is dynamic. The key to treatment is to realize what an individual patient's initial condition is and to understand that the fluid status is constantly changing. Bleeding, sepsis, neuroendocrine disturbances, and dysfunctional regulatory systems can all affect patients who are undergoing the dynamic changes of illness and healing. The correct management of blood volume is highly time dependent. If it is managed well, surgeons are afforded the chance to manage other aspects of surgery, such as nutrition, administration of antibiotics, drainage of abscesses, relief of obstruction and of incarceration, treatment of ischemia, and resection of tumors. Knowing the difference between dehydration, anemia, hemorrhage, and over-resuscitation is vital.

The human body is predominantly water, which resides in the intravascular, intracellular, and interstitial (or third) space. The water moves between these spaces and depends on many variables. Because surgeons can only directly control the intravascular space, this chapter concentrates on the correct management of the intravascular space as this is the only means to control the other two fluid compartments.

This chapter also examines historical aspects of shock, fluids, and electrolytes—not just to note interesting facts or to pay tribute to deserving physicians but also to try to understand how our knowledge was gained. Doing so is vital to understand past changes in management as well as to accept future changes. We are often awed at the discoveries made yet also astounded by how wrong we often were and why. Certainly, in turn, future surgeons will look back at our current body of knowledge and be amazed at how little we knew. A consequence of not studying the past will mean that we may repeat the errors of the past.

After the historical highlights, this chapter discusses various fluids that are now used along with potential fluids under development. Finally, caring for perioperative patients is explored from a daily needs perspective.

HISTORY

History is disliked by those who are in a hurry to just learn the bottom line. Learning from the past, however, is essential to know which treatments have worked and which have not. Dogma must always be challenged and questioned. Were the current treatments based on science? Studying the history of shock is important for at least three reasons. First, physicians and physiologists have been fascinated with blood loss out of necessity. Second, we need to assess what experiments have or have not been done. Third, we need to know more, because our current understanding of shock is elementary.

Resuscitation

One of the earliest authenticated resuscitations in the medical literature is the "miraculous deliverance of Anne Green," who was

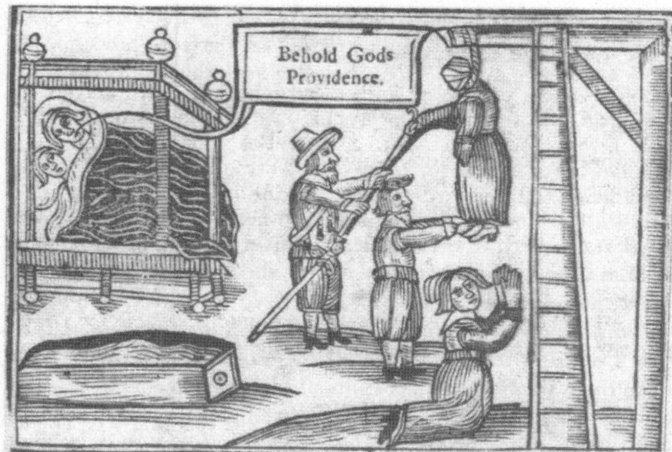

FIGURE 4-1 Miraculous deliverance of Anne Green, who was executed in 1650. (From Hughes JT: Miraculous deliverance of Anne Green: An Oxford case of resuscitation in the seventeenth century. *Br Med J [Clin Res Ed]* 285:1792–1793, 1982; by kind permission of the Bodleian Library, Oxford.)

executed by hanging on December 14, 1650.[1] Green was executed in the customary way by "being turned off a ladder to hang by the neck." She hanged for half an hour, during which time some of her friends pulled "with all their weight upon her legs, sometimes lifting her up, and then pulling her down again with a sudden jerk, thereby the sooner to dispatch her out of her pain" (Fig. 4-1). When everyone thought she was dead, the body was taken down, put in a coffin, and taken to the private house of Dr. William Petty, who, by the King's orders, was allowed to perform autopsies on the bodies of all persons who had been executed.

When the coffin was opened, Green was observed to take a breath, and a rattle was heard in her throat. Petty and his colleague, Thomas Willis, abandoned all thoughts of dissection and proceeded to revive their patient. They held her up in the coffin and then, by wrenching her teeth apart, poured hot cordial into her mouth, which caused her to cough. They rubbed and chafed her fingers, hands, arms, and feet; after a quarter of an hour of such effort, they put more cordial into her mouth. Then, after tickling her throat with a feather, she opened her eyes momentarily.

At that stage, they opened a vein and bled her of 5 ounces of blood. They continued administering the cordial and rubbing her arms and legs. Next, they applied compressing bandages to her arms and legs. Heating plasters were put to her chest, and another plaster was inserted as an enema "to give heat and warmth to her bowels." They then placed Green in a warm bed, with another woman to lie with her to keep her warm. After 12 hours, Green began to speak; 24 hours after her revival, she was answering questions freely. At 2 days, her memory was normal, apart from her recollection of her execution and the resuscitation.

Shock

Hemorrhagic shock has been extensively studied and written about for many years. Injuries, whether intentional or not, have occurred so frequently that much of the understanding of shock has been learned by surgeons taking care of the injured.

What is shock? The current widely accepted definition is inadequate perfusion of tissue. However, many subtleties lie behind this statement. Nutrients for cells are required, but which nutrients are not well defined at this point. Undoubtedly the most critical nutrient is oxygen, but concentrating on just oxygenation alone probably represents very elemental thinking. Blood is highly complex and carries countless nutrients, buffers, cells, antibodies, hormones, chemicals, electrolytes, and antitoxins. Even if we think in an elemental fashion and try to optimize the perfusion of tissue, the delivery side of the equation is affected by blood volume, anemia, and cardiac output. Moreover, the use of nutrients is affected by infection and drugs. The vascular tone plays a role as well; for example, in neurogenic shock, the sympathetic tone is lost, and in sepsis, systemic vascular resistance decreases because of a broken homeostatic process or possibly because of evolutionary factors.

Many advances in medicine have been achieved by battlefield observations. Unfortunately, in both military and civilian trauma, hemorrhagic shock is the leading cause of preventable death. Repeatedly, wounded patients have survived their initial injuries, with adequate control of the hemorrhage, only to undergo malaise and deterioration, resulting in death. Such cases led to many explanations; most observers theorized a circulating toxic agent, thought to be secondary to the initial insult. The first record available that shows an understanding of the need for fluid in injured patients was apparently from Ambroise Paré (1510-1590), who urged the use of clysters (enemas to administer fluid into the rectum) to prevent "noxious vapors from mounting to the brain." Yet he also wrote that phlebotomy is "required in great wounds when there is fear of deflexion, pain, delirium, raving, and unquietness"; he and others practiced bloodletting during that era because shock accompanying injury was thought to be from "toxins."

The term *shock* appears to have been first employed in 1743 in a translation of the French treatise of Henri Francois Le Dran regarding battlefield wounds. He used the term to designate the act of impact or collision, rather than the resulting functional and physiologic damage. However, the term can be found in the book *Gunshot Wounds of the Extremities*, published in 1815 by Guthrie, who used it to describe the physiologic instability.

Humoral theories persisted until the late 19th century, but in 1830, Herman provided one of the first clear descriptions of intravenous (IV) fluid therapy. In response to a cholera epidemic, he attempted to rehydrate patients by injecting 6 ounces of water into the vein. In 1831, O'Shaughnessy also treated cholera patients by administering large volumes of salt solutions intravenously and published his results in *Lancet*.[2] Those were the first documented attempts to replace and to maintain the extracellular internal environment or the intravascular volume. Note, however, that the treatment of cholera and dehydration is not the ideal treatment of hemorrhagic shock.

In 1872, Gross defined shock as "a manifestation of the rude unhinging of the machinery of life." His definition, given its accuracy and descriptiveness, has been repeatedly quoted in the literature. Theories on the cause of shock persisted through the late 19th century; although it was unexplainable, it was often observed. George Washington Crile investigated it and concluded, at the beginning of his career, that the lowering of the central venous pressure in the shock state in animal experiments was due to a failure of the autonomic nervous system.[3] Surgeons witnessed a marked change in ideas about shock between 1888 and 1918. In the late 1880s, there were no all-encompassing theories, but most surgeons accepted the generalization that shock resulted from a malfunctioning of some part of the nervous system. Such a malfunctioning has now been shown to *not* be the main reason—but surgeons are still perplexed by the mechanisms of hemorrhagic shock, especially regarding the complete breakdown of the circulatory system that occurs in the later stages of shock.

In 1899, using contemporary advances with sphygmomanometers, Crile proposed that a profound decline in blood pressure (BP) could account for all symptoms of shock. He also helped alter the way physicians diagnosed shock and followed its course. Before Crile, most surgeons relied on respiration, pulse, or a declining mental status when evaluating the condition of patients. After Crile's first books were published, many surgeons began measuring BP. In addition to changing how surgeons thought about shock, Crile was a part of the therapeutic revolution. His theories remained generally accepted for nearly 2 decades, predominantly in surgical circles. Crile's work persuaded Harvey Cushing to measure BP in all operations, which in part led to the general acceptance of BP measurement in clinical medicine. Crile also concluded that shock was not a process of dying but rather a marshaling of the body's defenses in patients struggling to live. He later deduced that the reduced volume of circulating blood, rather than the diminished BP, was the most critical factor in shock.

Crile was instrumental in forming numerous theories of shock but was also known for the "anoci-association" theory of shock, which accounted for pain and its physiologic response during surgery. He realized that the constant administration of nitrous oxide during operations was required and that doing so necessitated an additional professional person at the operating table—the skilled nurse anesthetist. In 1908, he trained Agatha Hodgins, one of his nurses at Western Reserve, who later founded the American Association of Nurse Anesthetists.

Crile's theories evolved as he continued his experimentations; in 1913, he proposed the kinetic system theory. He was interested in thyroid hormone and its response to wounds but realized that epinephrine was a key component of the response to shock. He relied on experiments by Walter B. Cannon, who found that epinephrine was released in response to pain or emotion, shifting blood from the intestines to the brain and extremities. Epinephrine release also stimulated the liver to convert glycogen to sugar for release into the circulation. Cannon argued that all the actions of epinephrine aided the animal in its effort to defend itself.[4]

Crile incorporated Cannon's study into his theory. He proposed that impulses from the brain after injury stimulated glands to secrete their hormones, which in turn effected sweeping changes throughout the body. Crile's kinetic system included a complex interrelationship among the brain, heart, lungs, blood vessels, muscles, thyroid gland, and liver. He also noted that if the body received too much stress, the adrenal glands would run out of epinephrine, the liver of glycogen, the thyroid of its hormone, and the brain itself of energy, accounting for autonomic changes. Once the kinetic system ran out of energy, BP would fall, and the animal would go into shock.

At the end of the 19th century, surgeons for the most part employed a wide variety of tonics, stimulants, and drugs. Through careful testing, Crile demonstrated that most of those agents were ineffective, stressing that only saline solutions, epinephrine, blood transfusions, and safer forms of anesthesia were beneficial in shock. In addition, he vigorously campaigned against the customary approach of polypharmacy, instead promoting only drugs of proven value. He stated that stimulants, long a mainstay of treatment in shock, did not raise BP and should be discarded: "A surgeon should not stimulate an exhausted vasomotor center with strychnine. That would be as futile as flogging a dead horse."

Henderson recognized the importance of decreased venous return and its effect on cardiac output and arterial pressure. His work was aided by advances in techniques that allowed careful recording of the volume curves of the ventricles. Fat embolism also led to a shocklike state, but its possible contribution was questioned because study results were difficult to reproduce. The vasomotor center and its contributions in shock were heavily studied in the early 1900s. In 1914, Mann noted that unilaterally innervated vessels of the tongues of dogs, ears of rabbits, and paws of kittens appeared constricted during shock compared with contralaterally denervated vessels.

Battlefield experiences continued to intensify research on shock. During the World War I era, Cannon used clinical data from the war as well as data from animal experiments to examine the shock state carefully. He theorized that toxins and acidosis contributed to the previously described lowering of vascular tone. He and others then focused on acidosis and the role of alkali in preventing and prolonging shock. The adrenal gland and the effect of cortical extracts on adrenalectomized animals were of fascination during this period.

Then, in the 1930s, a unique set of experiments by Blalock[5] determined that almost all acute injuries are associated with changes in fluid and electrolyte metabolism. Such changes were primarily the result of reductions in the effective circulating blood volume. Blalock showed that those reductions after injury could be the result of several mechanisms (Box 4-1). He clearly showed that fluid loss in injured tissues was loss of extracellular fluid (ECF) that was unavailable to the intravascular space for maintaining circulation. The original concept of a "third space," in which fluid is sequestered and therefore unavailable to the intravascular space, evolved from Blalock's studies.

Carl John Wiggers first described the concept of "irreversible shock."[6] His 1950 textbook, *Physiology of Shock,* represented the attitudes toward shock at that time. In an exceptionally brilliant summation, Wiggers assembled the various signs and symptoms of shock from various authors in that textbook (Fig. 4-2), along with his own findings.

His experiments used what is now known as the Wiggers prep. In his most common experiments, he used previously splenectomized dogs and cannulated the arterial system. He took advantage of an evolving technology that allowed him to measure the pressure within the arterial system, and he studied the effects of lowering BP through blood withdrawal. After removing the dogs' blood to an arbitrary set point (typically, 40 mm Hg), he noted that their BP soon spontaneously rose as fluid was spontaneously recruited into the intravascular space.

BOX 4-1 Causes of Shock According to Blalock in 1930

- Hematogenic (oligemia)
- Neurogenic (caused primarily by nervous influences)
- Vasogenic (initially decreased vascular resistance and increased vascular capacity as in sepsis)
- Cardiogenic (failure of the heart as a pump as in cardiac tamponade or myocardial infarction)
- Large volume loss (extracellular fluid, as occurs in patients with diarrhea, vomiting, and fistula drainage)

Data from Blalock A: Principles of surgical care: Shock and other problems, St. Louis, 1940, CV Mosby.

SYMPTOM COMPLEX OF SHOCK

General appearance and reactions

Mental state
Apathy
Delayed responses
Depressed cerebration
Weak voice
Listless or restlessness

Countenance
Drawn–anxious
Lusterless eyes
Sunken eyeballs
Ptosis of upper lids (slight)
Upward rotation of eyeballs (slight)

Neuromuscular state
Hypotonia
Muscular weakness
Tremors and twitchings
Involuntary muscular movements
Difficulty in swallowing

Neuromuscular tests
Depressed tendon reflexes
Depressed sensibilities
Depressed visual and auditory reflexes

General but variable symptoms
Thirst
Vomiting
Diarrhea
Oliguria
Visible or occult blood in vomitus, and stools

Skin and mucous membranes

Skin
Pale, livid, ashen gray
Slightly cyanotic
Moist, clammy
Mottling of dependent parts
Loose, dry, inelastic, cold

Mucous membranes
Pale, livid, slightly cyanotic

Conjunctiva
Glazed, lusterless

Tongue
Dry, pale, parched, shriveled

Respiration and metabolism

Respiration
Variable but not dyspneic
Usually increased rate
Variable depth
Occasional deep sighs
Sometimes irregular or phasic

Temperature
Subnormal, normal, supernormal

Basal metabolic rate
reduced (?)

Circulation and blood

Superficial veins
Collapsed and invisible
Failure to fill on compression or massage
Inconspicuous jugular pulsations

Heart
Apex sounds feeble
Rate, usually rapid

Radial pulse
Usually rapid
Small volume
"feeble,"
"thready"

Brachial blood pressures
Lowered
Pulse pressure small

Retinal vessels
Narrowed

Blood volume
Reduced

Blood chemistry
Hemoconcentration or hemodilution
Venous O_2 decreased
A-V O_2 difference increased
Arterial CO_2 reduced
Alkali reserve reduced

FIGURE 4-2 Wiggers' description of symptom complex of shock. (From Wiggers CJ: Present status of shock problem. *Physiol Rev* 22:74, 1942.)

To keep the dogs' BP at 40 mm Hg, Wiggers had to continually withdraw additional blood during this "compensated" stage of shock. During compensated shock, the dogs could use their reserves to survive. Water was recruited from the intracellular compartment as well as from the extracellular space. The body tried to maintain the vascular flow necessary to survive. However, after a certain period, he found that to keep the dogs' BP at the arbitrary set point of 40 mm Hg, he had to reinfuse shed blood; he termed this phase uncompensated or irreversible shock. Eventually, after a period of irreversible shock, the dogs died.

If the dogs had not yet gone into the uncompensated phase, any type of fluid used for resuscitation would have made survival likely. In fact, most dogs at that stage, even without resuscitation, would self-resuscitate by going to a water source. Once they entered the uncompensated phase of shock, however, their reserves were exhausted; even if blood was given back, the survival rates were better if additional fluid of some sort was administered. Uncompensated shock is surely what Gross meant by "unhinging of the machinery of life." Currently, hemorrhagic shock models are classified as involving either controlled or uncontrolled hemorrhage. The Wiggers prep is controlled hemorrhage and is referred to as pressure-controlled hemorrhage.

Another animal model that uses controlled hemorrhage is the volume-controlled model. Arguments against this model include the inconsistency of the blood volume from one animal to another and the variability in response. Calculation of blood volume is usually based on a percentage of body weight (typically, 7% of body weight), but such percentages are not exact and result in variability from one animal to another. However, proponents of the volume model and critics of the pressure model argue that a certain pressure during hypotension elicits a different response from one animal to another. Even in the pressure-controlled hemorrhage model, animals vary highly in regard to when they go from compensated shock to uncompensated shock. The pressure typically used in the pressure-controlled model is 40 mm Hg; the volume used in the volume-controlled model is 40%. The variance in the volume-controlled model can be minimized by specifying a narrow weight range for the animals (e.g., rats within 10 g, large animals within 5 pounds). It is also important to have the same experimenters doing the exact same procedure at the same time of the day in animals that were prepared and hydrated the exact same way.

The ideal model is uncontrolled hemorrhage, but its main problem is that the volume of hemorrhage is uncontrolled by the nature of the experiment. Variability is the highest in this model even though it is the most realistic. Computer-assisted pressure models can be used that mimic the pressures during uncontrolled shock to reduce the artificiality of the pressure-controlled model.

Fluids

How did the commonly used IV fluids, such as normal saline, enter medical practice? It is often taken for granted, given the vast body of knowledge in medicine, that they were adopted through a rigorous scientific process, but that was not necessarily the case.

Normal saline has a long track record and is extremely useful, but we now know that it also can be harmful. Hartog Jakob Hamburger, in his in vitro studies of red cell lysis in 1882, incorrectly suggested that 0.9% saline was the concentration of salt in human blood. This fluid is often referred to as physiologic or normal saline, but it is neither physiologic nor normal. Supposedly, 0.9% normal saline originated during the cholera pandemic that afflicted Europe in 1831, but an examination of the composition of the fluids used by physicians of that era found no resemblance to normal saline. The origin of the concept of normal saline remains unclear.[7]

In 1831, O'Shaughnessy described his experience in the treatment of cholera:

> Universal stagnation of the venous system, and rapid cessation of the arterialization of the blood, are the earliest, as well as the most characteristic effects. Hence the skin becomes blue—hence animal heat is no longer generated—hence the secretions are suspended; the arteries contain black blood, no carbonic acid is evolved from the lungs, and the returned air of expiration is cold as when it enters these organs.[8]

O'Shaughnessy wrote those words at the age of 22, having just graduated from Edinburgh Medical School. He tested his new method of infusing IV fluids on a dog and observed no ill effects. Eventually, he reported that the aim of his method was to restore blood to its natural specific gravity and to restore its deficient saline matters. His experience with human cholera patients taught him that the practice of bloodletting, then highly common, was good for "diminishing the venous congestion" and that nitrous oxide (laughing gas) was not useful for oxygenation.

In 1832, Robert Lewins reported that he witnessed Thomas Latta injecting extraordinary quantities of saline into veins, with the immediate effects of "restoring the natural current in the veins and arteries, of improving the color of the blood, and [of] recovering the functions of the lungs." Lewins described Latta's saline solution as consisting of "two drachms of muriate, and two scruples of carbonate, of soda, to sixty ounces of water." Later, however, Latta's solution was found to equate to having 134 mmol/liter of Na^+, 118 mmol/liter of Cl^-, and 16 mmol/liter of HCO_3^-.

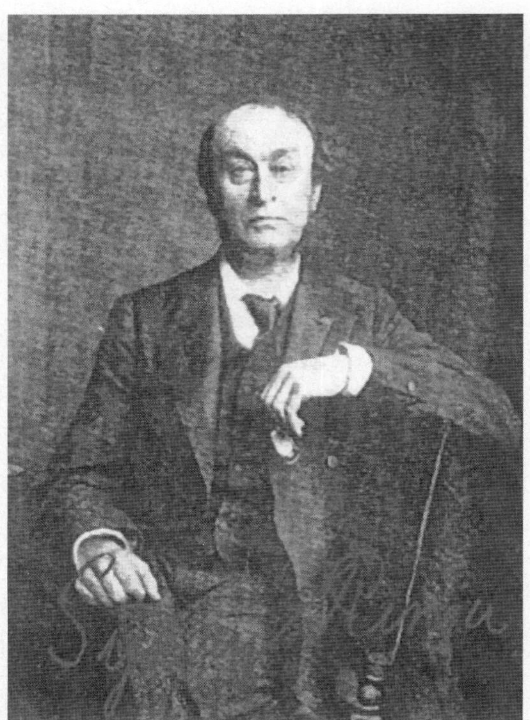

FIGURE 4-3 Sydney Ringer, credited for the development of lactated Ringer's solution. (From Baskett TF: Sydney Ringer and lactated Ringer's solution. *Resuscitation* 58:5–7, 2003.)

During the next 50 years, many reports cited various recipes used to treat cholera, but none resembled 0.9% saline. In 1883, Sydney Ringer reported on the influence exerted by the constituents of the blood on the contractions of the ventricle (Fig. 4-3). Studying hearts cut out of frogs, he used 0.75% saline and a blood mixture made from dried bullocks' blood.[9] In his attempts to identify which aspect of blood caused better results, he found that a "small quantity of white of egg completely obviates the changes occurring with saline solution." He concluded that the benefit of "white of egg" was because of the albumin or the potassium chloride. To show what worked and what did not, he described endless experiments with alterations of multiple variables.

However, Ringer later published another article stating that his previously reported findings could not be repeated; through careful study, he realized that the water used in his first article was actually not distilled water, as reported, but rather tap water from the New River Water Company. It turned out that his laboratory technician, who was paid to distill the water, took shortcuts and used tap water instead. Ringer analyzed the water and found that it contained many trace minerals (Fig. 4-4). Through careful and diligent experimentation, he found that calcium bicarbonate or calcium chloride—in doses even smaller than in blood—restored good contractions of the frog ventricles. The third component that he found essential to good contractions was sodium bicarbonate. He knew the importance of the trace elements. He also stated that fish could live for weeks unfed in tap water but would die in distilled water in a few hours, minnows, for instance, died in an average of 4.5 hours. Thus, the three ingredients that he found essential were potassium, calcium, and bicarbonate. Ringer's solution soon became ubiquitous in physiologic laboratory experiments.

In the early 20th century, fluid therapy by injection under the skin (hypodermoclysis) and infusion into the rectum

They consist of:		
Calcium	38.3	per million.
Magnesium	4.5	"
Sodium	23.3	"
Potassium	7.1	"
Combined carbonic acid	78.2	"
Sulfuric acid	55.8	"
Chlorine	15	"
Silicates	7.1	"
Free carbonic acid	54.2	"

FIGURE 4-4 Sidney Ringer's report of contents in water from the New River Water Company. (From Baskett TF: Sydney Ringer and lactated Ringer's solution. *Resuscitation* 58:5–7, 2003.)

(proctoclysis) became routine. Hartwell and Hoguet reported its use in intestinal obstruction in dogs, laying the foundation for saline therapy in human patients with intestinal obstruction.

As IV crystalloid solutions were developed, Ringer's solution was modified, most notably by pediatrician Alexis Hartmann. In 1932, wanting to develop an alkalinizing solution to administer to his acidotic patients, Hartmann modified Ringer's solution by adding sodium lactate. The result was lactated Ringer's (LR) or Hartmann's solution. He used sodium lactate (instead of sodium bicarbonate); the conversion of lactate into sodium bicarbonate was sufficiently slow to lessen the danger posed by sodium bicarbonate, which could rapidly shift patients from compensated acidosis to uncompensated alkalosis.

In 1924, Rudolph Matas, regarded as the originator of modern fluid treatment, introduced the concept of the continued IV drip but also warned of potential dangers of saline infusions. He stated, "Normal saline has continued to gain popularity but the problems with metabolic derangements have been repeatedly shown but seem to have fallen on deaf ears." In healthy volunteers, modern-day experiments have shown that normal saline can cause abdominal discomfort and pain, nausea, drowsiness, and decreased mental capacity to perform complex tasks.

The point is that normal saline and LR solutions have been formulated for conditions other than the replacement of blood, and the reasons for the formulation are archaic. Such solutions have been useful for dehydration; when they are used in relatively small volumes (1 to 3 liters per day), they are well tolerated and relatively harmless; they provide water, and the human body can tolerate the amounts of electrolytes they contain. Over the years, LR has attained widespread use for treatment of hemorrhagic shock. However, normal saline and LR are mostly permeable through the vascular membrane, but they are poorly retained in the vascular space. After a few hours, only about 175 to 200 mL of a 1-liter infusion remains in the intravascular space. In countries other than the United States, LR is often referred to as Hartmann's solution, and normal saline is referred to as physiologic (sometimes even spelled *fisiologic*) solution. With the advances in science in the last 50 years, it is difficult to understand why advances in resuscitation fluids have not been made.

Blood Transfusions

Concerned about the blood that injured patients lost, Crile began to experiment with blood transfusions. As he stated, "After many accidents, profuse hemorrhage often led to shock before the patient reached the hospital. Saline solutions, adrenalin, and precise surgical technique could substitute only up to a point for the lost blood." At the turn of the 19th century, transfusions were seldom used. Their use waxed and waned in popularity because of transfusion reactions and difficulties in preventing clotting in donated blood. Through his experiments in dogs, Crile showed that blood was interchangeable: he transfused blood without blood group matching. Alexis Carrel was able to sew blood vessels together with his triangulation technique, using it to connect blood vessels from one person to another for the purpose of transfusions. However, Crile found Carrel's technique too slow and cumbersome in humans, so he developed a short cannula to facilitate transfusions.

By the time World War II occurred, shock was recognized as the single most common cause of treatable morbidity and mortality. At the time of the Japanese attack on Pearl Harbor on December 7, 1941, no blood banks or effectual blood transfusion facilities were available. Most military locations had no stocks of dried pooled plasma. Although the wounded of that era were evacuated quickly to a hospital, the mortality rate was still high. IV fluids of any kind were essentially unavailable, except for a few liters of saline manufactured by means of a still in the operating room. IV fluid was usually administered by an old Salvesen flask and reused rubber tube. Often, a severe febrile reaction resulted from the use of that tubing.

The first written documentation of resuscitation in World War II patients was 1 year after Pearl Harbor, in December 1942, in notes from the 77th Evacuation Hospital in North Africa. E. D. Churchill stated, "The wounded in action had for the most part either succumbed or recovered from any existing shock before we saw them. However, later cases came to us in shock, and some of the early cases were found to be in need of whole blood transfusion. There was plenty of reconstituted blood plasma available. However, some cases were in dire need of whole blood. We had no transfusion sets, although such are available in the United States: no sodium citrate; no sterile distilled water; and no blood donors."

The initial decision to rely on plasma rather than on blood appears to have been based in part on the view held in the Office of the Surgeon General of the Army and in part on the opinion of the civilian investigators of the National Research Council. Those civilian investigators thought that in shock, the blood was thick and the hematocrit level high. On April 8, 1943, the Surgeon General stated that no blood would be sent to the combat zone. Seven months later, he again refused to send blood overseas because of the following: (1) his observation of overseas theaters had convinced him that plasma was adequate for resuscitation of wounded men; (2) from a logistics standpoint, it was impractical to make locally collected blood available farther forward than general hospitals in the combat zone; and (3) shipping space was too sparse. Vasoconstricting drugs such as epinephrine were condemned because they were thought to decrease blood flow and tissue perfusion as they dammed the blood in the arterial portion of the circulatory system.

During World War II, out of necessity, efforts to make blood transfusions available heightened and led to the institution of blood banking for transfusions. Better understanding of hypovolemia and inadequate circulation led to the use of plasma as a favored resuscitative solution, in addition to whole blood replacement. Thus, the treatment of traumatic shock greatly improved. The administration of whole blood was thought to be extremely effective, so it was widely used. Mixed with sodium citrate in a 6:1 ratio to bind the calcium in the blood, which prevented clotting, worked well.

However, no matter what solution was used—blood, colloids, or crystalloids—the blood volume seemed to increase by only a fraction of what was lost. In the Korean War era, it was recognized that more blood had to be infused for the blood volume lost to be adequately regained. The reason for the need for more blood was unclear, but it was thought to be due to hemolysis, pooling of blood in certain capillary beds, and loss of fluid into tissues. Considerable attention was given to elevating the feet of patients in shock.

PHYSIOLOGY OF SHOCK

Bleeding

Research and experience have both taught us much about the physiologic responses to bleeding. The Advanced Trauma Life Support (ATLS) course defines four classes of shock (Table 4-1). In general, that categorization has helped point out the physiologic responses to hemorrhagic shock, emphasizing the identification of blood loss and guiding treatment. Shock can be thought of anatomically at three levels (Fig. 4-5). It can be cardiogenic with extrinsic abnormalities (such as tension pneumothorax, hemothorax, or tamponade) or intrinsic abnormalities (such as pump failure due to infarct, cardiac failure, contusion, cardiac laceration). Injury to large vessels can cause shock if they are bleeding. At the level of the small vessels, shock is due to neurogenic dysfunction or sepsis.

The four classes of shock as taught in the ATLS course are problematic as they were not rigorously tested and proven. Those who generated the ATLS table admit that the classes were fairly arbitrary and were not necessarily based on rigorous scientific

TABLE 4-1 ATLS Classes of Hemorrhagic Shock

	CLASS I	CLASS II	CLASS III	CLASS IV
Blood loss (%)	0-15	15-30	30-40	>40
Central nervous system	Slightly anxious	Mildly anxious	Anxious or confused	Confused or lethargic
Pulse (beats/min)	<100	>100	>120	>140
Blood pressure	Normal	Normal	Decreased	Decreased
Pulse pressure	Normal	Decreased	Decreased	Decreased
Respiratory rate	14-20/min	20-30/min	30-40/min	>35/min
Urine (mL/hr)	>30	20-30	5-15	Negligible
Fluid	Crystalloid	Crystalloid	Crystalloid + blood	Crystalloid + blood

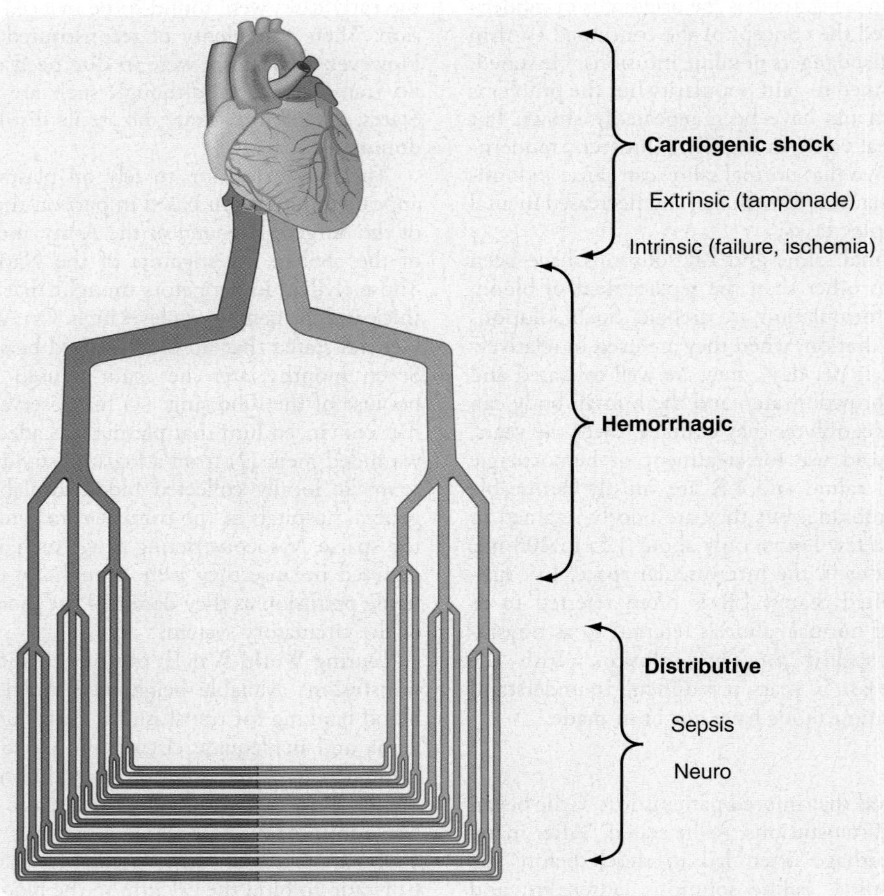

FIGURE 4-5 Types of shock.

data. Patients in shock do not always have the physiologic changes as taught in the ATLS course, and a high degree of variance exists among patients, particularly in children and older patients. Children, in general, seem to be able to compensate, even after large volumes of blood loss, because of the higher water composition of their bodies. However, when they decompensate, it can be rapid. Progression into hemorrhagic shock can be a large step off the cliff rather than a gradual decent. Older patients do not compensate well; when they start to collapse physiologically, the process can be devastating because their ability to recruit fluid is not as good and their cardiac reserves are less.

The problem with the signs and symptoms classically shown in the ATLS classes is that in reality, the manifestations of shock can be confusing and difficult to assess. For example, is an individual patient's change in mental status caused by blood loss, traumatic brain injury (TBI), pain, or illicit drugs? The same dilemma applies for respiratory rate and skin changes. Are alterations in a patient's respiratory rate or skin caused by pneumothorax, rib fractures, or inhalation injury?

To date, despite the many potential methods of monitoring shock, none has been found as clinically useful as BP. As clinicians, we all know that there is a wide range of normal BPs. The question often is this: What is the baseline BP of the patient being treated? When a seemingly normal BP is found, is that hypotension or hypertension compared with the patient's normal BP? How do we know how much blood has been lost? Even if blood volume is measured directly (relatively faster bedside methods are now available using tagged red cells), what was the patient's baseline blood volume? To what blood volume should the patient be resuscitated? The end point of resuscitation has been elusive. The variance in all of the variables makes assessment and treatment a challenge.

One important factor to recognize is that clinical symptoms are relatively few in patients who are in class I shock. The only change in class I shock is anxiety according to the ATLS course. Is the anxiety after injury from blood loss, pain, trauma, or drugs? A heart rate higher than 100 beats/min has been used as a physical sign of bleeding, but evidence of its significance is minimal. Brasel and collegues[10] have shown that heart rate was neither sensitive nor specific in determining the need for emergent intervention, the need for packed red blood cell (PRBC) transfusions in the first 2 hours after an injury, or the severity of the injury. Heart rate was not altered by the presence of hypotension (systolic BP < 90 mm Hg).

In patients who are in class II shock, we are taught that their heart rate is increased, but again, this is a highly unreliable marker; pain and mere nervousness can also increase heart rate. The change in pulse pressure—the difference between systolic and diastolic pressure—is also difficult to identify because the baseline BP of patients is not always known. The change in pulse pressure is thought to be caused by an epinephrine response constricting vessels, resulting in higher diastolic pressures. It is important to recognize that the body compensates well.

Not until patients are in class III shock does BP supposedly decrease. At this stage, patients have lost 30% to 40% of their blood volume; for an average man weighing 75 kg (168 pounds), this equates to 2 liters of blood loss (Fig. 4-6). It is helpful to remember that a can of soda or beer is 355 mL; a six-pack is 2130 mL. Theoretically, if a patient is hypotensive from blood loss, we are looking for a six-pack of blood. Small amounts of blood loss should not result in hypotension. Whereas intracranial bleeding can cause hypotension in the last stages of herniation, it is almost impossible that it is the result of a large volume of blood loss intracranially as there is not enough space there. It is critical to recognize uncontrolled bleeding and even more critical to stop bleeding before patients go into class III shock. It is more important to recognize blood loss than it is to replace blood loss. A common mistake is to think that trauma patients are often hypotensive; the reality is that hypotension is rare in trauma patients (occurring less than 6% of the time).

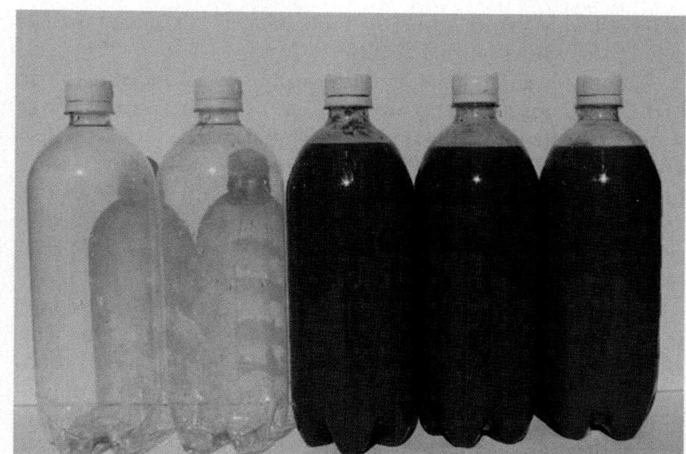

FIGURE 4-6 Liters of blood lost for class III shock, or 40% of 5 liters, according to the ATLS.

In addition, the ATLS course, which is designed for physicians who are not surgeons, does not recognize many subtle but important aspects of bleeding. The concepts of the course are relatively basic. However, surgeons know that there are some nuances of the varied responses to injuries in both animals and humans. In the case of arterial hemorrhage, for example, we know that animals do not necessarily manifest tachycardia as their first response when bleeding but actually become bradycardic. It is speculated that this is a teleologically developed mechanism because bradycardic response reduces cardiac output and minimizes free uncontrolled exsanguination. A bradycardic response to bleeding is not consistently shown in all animals, including humans. Some evidence shows that this response, termed relative bradycardia, does often occur in humans. Relative bradycardia is defined as a heart rate below 100 beats/min when the systolic BP is below 90 mm Hg. When bleeding patients have relative bradycardia, their mortality rate is lower. Up to 44% of hypotensive patients who are not bleeding have relative bradycardia. However, patients with a heart rate below 60 beats/min are usually moribund. Bleeding patients with a heart rate of 60 to 90 beats/min have the highest survival rate compared with patients who are tachycardic (a heart rate of more than 90 beats/min).[11]

The physiologic response to bleeding also subtly differs according to whether the source of bleeding is arterial or venous. Arterial bleeding is obviously a problem, but it often stops temporarily on its own; the human body has evolved to trap the blood loss in adventitial tissues, and the transected artery will spasm and thrombose. A lacerated artery can actually bleed more than a transected artery as the spasm of the lacerated artery can enlarge the hole in the vessel. Thrombosis of the artery sometimes does *not* occur in transected or lacerated vessels. Arterial bleeding, when constantly monitored, can result in rapid hypotension as there is a leak in the arterial system. Because the arterial system does not have valves, the recorded BP can drop early even before large-volume loss has occurred. In these patients with arterial bleeding, hypotension may occur soon, but because ischemia has not yet had a chance to occur, measurements of lactate or base deficit often yield normal results.

Venous bleeding, however, is typically slower, and the human body can compensate. It provides the time for recruitment of water from the intracellular and interstitial spaces. Large volumes of blood can be lost before hypotension ensues. Because venous or capillary bed bleeding is slower and the body has a chance to compensate, there is more time for ischemia, and thus there is time for lactate and base deficit results to be abnormal. Venous blood loss can be massive before hypotension occurs.

It is generally taught that the hematocrit or hemoglobin level is not reliable in predicting blood loss. That is true for patients with a high hematocrit or hemoglobin level, but in patients resuscitated with fluids, a rapid drop in the hematocrit and hemoglobin levels can occur immediately. Bruns and associates[12] have shown that the hemoglobin level can be low within the first 30 minutes after patients arrive at trauma centers. Therefore, although patients with a high or normal hemoglobin level may have significant bleeding, a low hemoglobin level, because it occurs rapidly, can reflect the true extent of blood loss. Infusion of acellular fluids often will dilute the blood and decrease the hemoglobin levels even further.

The lack of good indicators to distinguish which patients are bleeding has led many investigators to examine heart rate variability or complexity as a potential new vital sign. Many clinical studies have shown that heart rate variability or complexity is associated with poor outcome, but this has yet to catch on, perhaps because of the difficulty of calculating it. Heart rate variability or complexity would have to be calculated using software, with a resulting index on which clinicians would have to rely. This information would not be available by merely examining patients. Another issue with heart rate variability or complexity is that the exact physiologic mechanism for its association with poor outcome has yet to be elucidated.[13] This new vital sign may be programmable into currently used monitors, but its usefulness has yet to be confirmed.

Hypotension has been traditionally set, arbitrarily, at 90 mm Hg and below. Eastridge and coworkers[14] have suggested that hypotension be redefined as below 110 mm Hg. In 2008, Bruns and colleagues[15] confirmed the concept, showing that a prehospital BP below 110 mm Hg was associated with a sharp increase in mortality and that 15% of patients with BP below 110 mm Hg would eventually die in the hospital. As a result, they recommended redefining prehospital triage criteria. In older patients, normal vital signs may miss occult hypoperfusion as these patients often have increased lactate and base deficit levels.

Shock Index

Because heart rate and systolic BP independently are not accurate at identifying hemorrhagic shock and because the increase in heart rate does not always accompany a decrease in systolic BP, the shock index (SI), which uses these two variables together, has been studied to determine if it would be of use. SI is defined as heart rate divided by systolic BP. It has been shown to be a better marker for assessing severity of shock than heart rate and BP alone. It has utility not only in trauma patients but also in sepsis, obstetrics, myocardial infarction, stroke, and other acute critical illnesses. In the trauma population, it has been shown to be more useful than heart rate and BP alone, and it has also been shown to be of benefit specifically in the pediatric and geriatric populations. It has been correlated with need for interventions such as blood transfusion and invasive procedures including operations. SI is known as a hemodynamic stability indicator. However, SI does not take into account the diastolic BP, and thus a modified SI (MSI) was created. MSI is defined as heart rate divided by mean arterial pressure. High MSI indicates a value of stroke volume and low systemic vascular resistance, a sign of hypodynamic circulation. In contrast, low MSI indicates a hyperdynamic state. MSI has been considered a better marker than SI for mortality rate prediction. Although SI or MSI is better than heart rate and systolic BP alone, the combination of these variables will undoubtedly be more useful. There are additional studies showing that more complex calculations with more variables are more useful than simpler ones. For example, taking into account the age, mechanism of injury, Glasgow Coma Scale (GCS) score, lactate levels, hemoglobin levels, and other physiologic parameters will result in statistically better prediction than with one individual vital sign. It is intuitive that the addition of variables would be more predictive of outcome. That is why the presence of an experienced surgeon is critical; in a few seconds, the astute clinician will quickly take into account multiple variables, including gender, age, GCS score, mechanism of injury, and other parameters. Whereas SI and MSI are statistically more accurate than one individual parameter, there is no substitute for the experienced clinician at the bedside. This may be the reason that these parameters, such as SI and MSI, have not been widely adopted.

Lactate and Base Deficit

Lactate has been an associated marker of injury, and possibly ischemia, and has stood the test of time.[16] However, new data question the cause and role of lactate. The emerging information is confusing; it suggests that we may not understand lactate for what it truly implies. Lactate has long been thought to be a byproduct of anaerobic metabolism and is routinely perceived to be an end waste product that is completely unfavorable. Physiologists are now questioning this paradigm and have found that lactate behaves more advantageously than not. An analogy would be that firefighters are associated with fires, but that does not mean that firefighters are bad, nor does it mean that they caused the fires.

Research has shown that lactate increases in muscle and blood during exercise. It is at its highest level at or just after exhaustion. Accordingly, it was assumed that lactate was a waste product. We also know that lactic acid appears in response to muscle contraction and continues in the absence of oxygen. In addition, accumulated lactate disappears when an adequate supply of oxygen is present in tissues.

Recent evidence indicates that lactate is an active metabolite, capable of moving between cells, tissues, and organs, where it may be oxidized as fuel or reconverted to form pyruvate or glucose. It now appears that increased lactate production and concentration, as a result of anoxia or dysoxia, are often the exception rather than the rule. Lactate seems to be a shuttle for energy; the lactate shuttle is now the subject of much debate. The end product of glycolysis is pyruvic acid. Lack of oxygen is thought to convert pyruvate into lactate. However, lactate formation may allow carbohydrate metabolism to continue through glycolysis. It is postulated that lactate is transferred from its site of production in the cytosol to neighboring cells and to a variety of organs (e.g., heart, liver, and kidney), where its oxidation and continued metabolism can occur.

Lactate is also being studied as a pseudohormone as it seems to regulate the cellular redox state, through exchange and conversion into pyruvate and through its effects on the ratio of nicotinamide adenine dinucleotide to nicotinamide adenine dinucleotide (reduced)—the NAD^+/NADH ratio. It is released into the systemic circulation and taken up by distal tissues and organs, where it also affects the redox state in those cells. Further evidence has shown that it affects wound regeneration, with promotion of increased collagen deposition and neovascularization. Lactate may also induce vasodilation and catecholamine release and stimulate fat and carbohydrate oxidation.

Lactate levels in blood are highly dependent on the equilibrium between production and elimination from the bloodstream. The liver is predominantly responsible for clearing lactate, and acute or chronic liver disease affects lactate levels. Lactate was always thought to be produced from anaerobic tissues, but it now seems that a variety of tissue beds that are not undergoing anaerobic metabolism produce lactate when they are signaled of distress.

In canine muscle, lactate is produced by moderate-intensity exercise when the oxygen supply is ample. A high adrenergic stimulus also causes a rise in lactate as the body prepares for or responds to stress. A study of climbers of Mount Everest showed that the resting PO_2 on the summit was about 28 mm Hg and decreased even more during exercise. The blood lactate level in those climbers was essentially the same as at sea level even though they were in a state of hypoxia.[17] Such facts have allowed us to question lactate and its true role.

In humans, lactate may be the preferred fuel in the brain and heart; in these tissues, infused lactate is used before glucose at rest and during exercise. Because it is glucose sparing, lactate allows glucose and glycogen levels to be maintained. In addition to lactate's being preferred in the brain, evidence seems to indicate that lactate also has a role as being protective to brain tissues in TBI.[18] Lactate fuels the human brain during exercise. The level of lactate, whether it is a waste product or a source of energy, seems to signify tissue distress from anaerobic conditions or other factors.[19] During times of stress, there is a release of epinephrine and other catecholamines, which also causes a release of lactate.

Base deficit, a measure of the number of millimoles of base required to correct the pH of a liter of whole blood to 7.4, seems to correlate well with lactate level, at least in the first 24 hours after an injury. Rutherford, in 1992, showed that a base deficit of 8 was associated with a 25% mortality rate in patients older than 55 years without a head injury or in patients younger than 55 years with a head injury. When base deficit remains elevated, most clinicians believe that it is an indication of ongoing shock.

One of the problems with base deficit is that it is commonly influenced by the chloride from various resuscitation fluids, resulting in a hyperchloremic nongap acidosis. In patients with renal failure, base deficit can also be a poor predictor of outcome; in the acute stage of renal failure, a base deficit of less than 6 mmol/liter is associated with poor outcome.[20] With the use of hypertonic saline (HTS), which has three to eight times the sodium chloride concentration as normal saline, depending on the concentration used, in trauma patients, the hyperchloremic acidosis has been shown to be relatively harmless. However, when HTS is used, base deficit should be interpreted with caution.

Compensatory Mechanisms

When needed, blood flow to less critical tissues is diverted to more critical tissues. The earliest compensatory mechanism in response to a decrease in intravascular volume is an increase in sympathetic activity. Such an increase is mediated by pressure receptors or baroreceptors in the aortic arch, atria, and carotid bodies. A decrease in pressure inhibits parasympathetic discharge while norepinephrine and epinephrine are liberated and causes adrenergic receptors in the myocardium and vascular smooth muscle to be activated. Heart rate and contractility are increased; peripheral vascular resistance is also increased, resulting in increased BP. However, the various tissue beds are not affected equally; blood is shunted from less critical organs (e.g., skin, skeletal muscle, and splanchnic circulation) to more critical organs (e.g., brain, liver, and kidneys).

Then, the juxtaglomerular apparatus in the kidney—in response to the vasoconstriction and decrease in blood flow—produces the enzyme renin, which generates angiotensin I. The angiotensin-converting enzyme located on the endothelial cells of the pulmonary arteries converts angiotensin I to angiotensin II. In turn, angiotensin II stimulates an increased sympathetic drive, at the level of the nerve terminal, by releasing hormones from the adrenal medulla. In response, the adrenal medulla affects intravascular volume during shock by secreting catechol hormones—epinephrine, norepinephrine, and dopamine—which are all produced from phenylalanine and tyrosine. They are called *catecholamines* because they contain a catechol group derived from the amino acid tyrosine. The release of catecholamines is thought to be responsible for the elevated glucose level in hemorrhagic shock. Although the role of glucose elevation in hemorrhagic shock is not fully understood, it does not seem to affect outcome.[21]

Cortisol, also released from the adrenal cortex, plays a major role in that it controls fluid equilibrium. In the adrenal cortex, the zona glomerulosa produces aldosterone in response to stimulation by angiotensin II. Aldosterone is a mineralocorticoid that modulates renal function by increasing recovery of sodium and excretion of potassium. Angiotensin II also has a direct action on the renal tubules: reabsorbing sodium. The control of sodium is a primary way that the human body controls water absorption or secretion in the kidneys. One of the problems in shock is that the release of hormones is not infinite; the supply can be exhausted.

This regulation of intravascular fluid status is further affected by the carotid baroreceptors and the atrial natriuretic peptides. Signals are sent to the supraoptic and paraventricular nuclei in the brain. Antidiuretic hormone (ADH) is released from the pituitary, causing retention of free water at the level of the kidney. Simultaneously, volume is recruited from the extravascular and cellular spaces. A shift of water occurs as hydrostatic pressures fall in the intravascular compartment. At the capillary level, hydrostatic pressures are also reduced because the precapillary sphincters are vasoconstricted more than the postcapillary sphincters.

Lethal Triad

The triad of acidosis, hypothermia, and coagulopathy is common in resuscitated patients who are bleeding or in shock from various factors. Our basic understanding is that inadequate tissue perfusion results in acidosis caused by lactate production. In the shock state, the delivery of nutrients to the cells is thought to be inadequate, so adenosine triphosphate (ATP) production decreases. The human body relies on ATP production to maintain homeostatic temperatures. ATP is the source of heat in all homeothermic (warm-blooded) animals. Thus, if ATP production is inadequate to maintain body temperature, the body will trend toward the ambient temperature. For most human patients, this is 22° C (72° F), the temperature inside typical hospitals. The resulting hypothermia then affects the efficiency of enzymes, which work best at 37° C. For surgeons, the critical problem with hypothermia is that the coagulation cascade depends on enzymes that are affected by hypothermia. If enzymes are not functioning optimally because of hypothermia, coagulopathy worsens, which, in surgical patients, can contribute to uncontrolled bleeding from injuries or the surgery itself. Further bleeding continues to fuel the triad. The optimal method to break the "vicious circle of death" is to stop the bleeding and the causes of hypothermia. In most typical scenarios, hypothermia is not spontaneous from ischemia but is induced because of use of room temperature fluid or cold blood products.

Acidosis

Bleeding causes a host of responses. During the resuscitative phase, the lethal triad (acidosis, hypothermia, and coagulopathy) is frequent in severely bleeding patients, most likely because of two major factors. First is the decreased perfusion causing lactic acidosis, and consumptive coagulopathy. The second is the resuscitation injury from the amount and type of fluid infused contributing to hypothermia if the fluid is not warmed and dilutional coagulopathy. Some believe that the acidotic state is not necessarily undesirable because the body tolerates acidosis better than alkalosis. Oxygen is more easily offloaded from the hemoglobin molecules in the acidotic environment. Basic scientists who try to preserve tissue ex vivo find that cells live longer in an acidotic environment. Correcting acidosis with sodium bicarbonate has classically been avoided as it is treating a number or symptom when the cause needs to be addressed. Treating the pH alone has shown no benefit, but it can lead to complacency. The patients may appear to be better resuscitated, but the underlying cause of the acidosis has not been adequately addressed. It is also argued that rapidly injecting sodium bicarbonate can worsen intracellular acidosis because of the diffusion of the converted CO_2 into the cells.

The best fundamental approach to metabolic acidosis from shock is to treat the underlying cause of shock. In the surgeon's case, it is blood loss or ischemic tissue. However, some clinicians believe that treating the pH has advantages because the enzymes necessary for the coagulation cascade work better at an optimal temperature and optimal pH. Coagulopathy can contribute to uncontrolled bleeding, so some have recommended treating acidosis with bicarbonate infusion for patients in dire scenarios. Treating acidosis with sodium bicarbonate may have a benefit in an unintended and unrecognized way. Rapid infusion of bicarbonate is usually accompanied by a rise in BP in hypotensive patients. This rise is usually attributed to correcting the pH; however, sodium bicarbonate in most urgent scenarios is given in ampules. The 50-mL ampule of sodium bicarbonate has 1 mEq/mL—in essence, similar to giving a hypertonic concentration of sodium, which quickly draws fluid into the vascular space. Given its high sodium concentration, a 50-mL bolus of sodium bicarbonate has physiologic results similar to 325 mL of normal saline or 385 mL of LR. Essentially, it is like giving small doses of HTS. Sodium bicarbonate quickly increases CO_2 levels by its conversion in the liver, so if the minute ventilation is not increased, respiratory acidosis can result.

THAM (tromethamine; tris[hydroxymethyl] aminomethane) is a biologically inert amino alcohol of low toxicity that buffers CO_2 and acids. It is sodium free and limits the generation of CO_2 in the process of buffering. At 37° C, the pK_a of THAM is 7.8, making it a more effective buffer than sodium bicarbonate in the physiologic range of blood pH. In vivo, THAM supplements the buffering capacity of the blood bicarbonate system by generating sodium bicarbonate and decreasing the partial pressure of CO_2. It rapidly distributes to the extracellular space and slowly penetrates the intracellular space, except in the case of erythrocytes and hepatocytes, and it is excreted by the kidney. Unlike sodium bicarbonate, which requires an open system to eliminate CO_2 to exert its buffering effect, THAM is effective in a closed or semiclosed system, and it maintains its buffering ability during hypothermia. THAM acetate (0.3 M, pH 8.6) is well tolerated, does not cause tissue or venous irritation, and is the only formulation available in the United States. THAM may induce respiratory depression and hypoglycemia, which may require ventilatory assistance and the administration of glucose.

The initial loading dose of THAM acetate (0.3 M) for the treatment of acidemia may be estimated as follows:

$$\text{THAM (in mL of 0.3 M solution)} = \text{lean body weight (in kilograms)} \times \text{the base deficit (in mmol/liter)}$$

The maximal daily dose is 15 mmol per kilogram per day for an adult (3.5 liters of a 0.3 M solution in a patient weighing 70 kg). It is indicated in the treatment of respiratory failure (acute respiratory distress syndrome [ARDS] and infant respiratory distress syndrome) and has been associated with the use of hypothermia and permissive hypercapnia (controlled hypoventilation). Other indications are diabetic and renal acidosis, salicylate and barbiturate intoxication, and increased intracranial pressure (ICP) associated with brain trauma. It is used in cardioplegic solutions and during liver transplantation. Despite these attributes, THAM has not been documented clinically to be more efficacious than sodium bicarbonate.

Hypothermia

Hypothermia can be both beneficial and detrimental. A fundamental knowledge of hypothermia is of vital importance in the care of surgical patients. The beneficial aspects of hypothermia are mainly a result of decreased metabolism. Injury sites are often iced, creating vasoconstriction and decreasing inflammation through decreased metabolism. This concept of cooling to slow metabolism is also the rationale behind using hypothermia to decrease ischemia during cardiac, transplant, pediatric, and neurologic surgery. Also, amputated extremities are iced before reimplantation. Cold water near-drowning victims have higher survival rates, thanks to preservation of the brain and other vital organs. The Advanced Life Support Task Force of the International Liaison Committee of Resuscitation now recommends cooling (to 32° C to 34° C for 12 to 24 hours) of unconscious adults who have spontaneous circulation after out-of-hospital cardiac arrest caused by ventricular fibrillation. Induced hypothermia is vastly different from spontaneous hypothermia, which is typically from shock, inadequate tissue perfusion, or cold fluid infusion.

Medical or accidental hypothermia is vastly different from trauma-associated hypothermia (Table 4-2). The survival rates after accidental hypothermia range from about 12% to 39%. The average temperature drop is to about 30° C (range, 13.7° C to 35.0° C). That lowest recorded temperature in a survivor of accidental hypothermia (13.7° C, or 56.7° F) was in an extreme skier in Norway; she was trapped under the ice and eventually fully recovered neurologically.

TABLE 4-2 Classification of Hypothermia

	TRAUMA	ACCIDENTAL
Mild	36°-34° C	35°-32° C
Moderate	34°-32° C	32°-28° C
Severe	<32° C (<90° F)	<28° C (<82° F)

The data in patients with trauma-associated hypothermia differ. Their survival rate falls dramatically with their core temperature, reaching 100% mortality when it reaches 32° C at any point—whether it is in the emergency department, operating room, or intensive care unit (ICU). In trauma patients, hypothermia is due to shock and is thought to perpetuate uncontrolled bleeding because of the associated coagulopathy. Trauma patients with a postoperative core temperature below 35° C have a fourfold increase in death; below 33° C, a sevenfold increase in death. Hypothermic trauma patients tend to be more severely injured and older, with bleeding as indicated by blood loss and transfusions.[22]

Surprisingly, in a study using the National Trauma Data Base, Shafi and colleagues showed that hypothermia and its associated poor outcome were not related to the state of shock. It was previously thought that a core temperature below 32° C was uniformly fatal in trauma patients who have the additional insult of tissue injury and bleeding. However, a small number of trauma patients have now survived, despite a recorded core temperature below 32° C. Beilman and coworkers demonstrated that hypothermia was associated with more severe injuries, bleeding, and a higher rate of multiple-organ dysfunction in the ICU,[23] but not with death.

To understand hypothermia, we have to remember that humans are homeothermic (warm-blooded) animals, in contrast to poikilothermic (cold-blooded) animals such as snakes and fish. To maintain a body temperature of 37° C, our hypothalamus uses a variety of mechanisms to tightly control core body temperature. We use oxygen as the key ingredient or fuel to generate heat in the mitochondria in the form of ATP. When ATP production is below its lowest threshold, one of the side effects is the lowering of body temperature to the ambient temperature, which typically is less than core body temperature. In contrast, during exercise, we use more oxygen, as more ATP is required and we produce excess heat. In an attempt to modulate core temperature, we start perspiring to use the cooling properties of evaporation.

Hypothermia, although potentially beneficial, is detrimental in trauma patients mainly because it causes coagulopathy. Cold affects coagulopathy by decreasing enzyme activity, enhancing fibrinolytic activity, and causing platelet dysfunction. Platelets are affected by the inhibition of thromboxane B_2 production, resulting in decreased aggregation. A heparin-like substance is released, causing diffuse intravascular coagulation–like syndrome. Hageman factor and thromboplastin are some of the enzymes most affected. Even a drop in core temperature of just a few degrees results in 40% inefficiency in some of the enzymes.

Heat affects the coagulation cascade so much that when blood is drawn in cold patients and sent to the laboratory, the sample is heated to 37° C, because even 1° or 2° of cold delays clotting and renders test results inaccurate. Thus, in a cold and coagulopathic patient, if the coagulation profile obtained from the laboratory shows an abnormality, the result represents the level of coagulopathy if the patient (and not just the sample) had been warmed to 37° C. Therefore, a cold patient is always even more coagulopathic than indicated by the coagulation profile. A normal coagulation profile does not necessarily represent what is going on in the body.

Heat is measured in calories. One calorie is the amount of energy required to raise the temperature of 1 mL of water (which has, by definition, a specific heat of 1.0). It takes 1 kcal to raise the temperature of 1 liter of water by 1° C. If an average man (weight, 75 kg) consisted of pure water, it would take 75 kcal to raise his temperature by 1° C. However, we are not made of pure water, and blood has a specific heat coefficient of 0.87. Thus, the human body as a whole has a specific heat coefficient of 0.83. Therefore, it actually takes 62.25 kcal (75 kg × 0.83) to raise body temperature by 1° C. If a patient were to lose 62.25 kcal, body temperature would drop by 1° C. This basic science is important in choosing methods to retain heat or to treat hypothermia or hyperthermia. It allows one to compare the efficacy of one method with another.

The normal basal metabolic heat generation is about 70 kcal/hr. Shivering can increase this to 250 kcal/hr. Heat is transferred to and from the body by contact or conduction (as in a frying pan and Jacuzzi), air or convection (as in an oven and sauna), radiation, and evaporation. Convection is an extremely inefficient way to transfer heat as the air molecules are so far apart compared with liquids and solids. Conduction and radiation are the most efficient ways to transfer heat. However, heating the patient with radiation is fraught with inconsistencies and technical challenges, and thus it is difficult to apply clinically, so we are left with conduction to transfer energy efficiently.

Warming or cooling through manipulation of the temperature of IV fluids is useful as it uses conduction to transfer heat. Although IV fluids can be warmed, the U.S. Food and Drug Administration (FDA) allows fluid warmers to be set at a maximum of 40° C. Therefore, the differential between a cold trauma patient (34° C) and warmed fluid is only 6°. Thus, 1 liter of warmed fluids can transfer only 6 kcal to the patient. As previously calculated, one needs about 62 kcal to raise the core temperature by 1°. Therefore, we need 10.4 liters of warmed fluids to raise the core temperature by 1° to 35° C. Once that has been achieved, the differential is now only 5° between the patient and the warmed fluid, so it actually takes 12.5 liters of warmed fluids to raise the patient from 35° C to 36° C. A cold patient at 32° C needs to be given 311 kcal (75 kg × 0.83) to be warmed to 37° C. Note that a liter of fluid must be given at the highest rate possible because if the infusion rate is slow, it cools to room temperature as the IV line is exposed to ambient room temperature. To avoid IV line cooling, devices that warm fluids up to the point of insertion into the body should be used.

Warming of patients by infusion of warmed fluids is difficult, but fluid warmers are still critically important; the main reason to warm fluids is so that patients are not cooled. Cold fluids can cool patients quickly. The fluids that are typically infused are either at room temperature (22° C) or 4° C if the fluids were refrigerated. The internal temperature of a refrigerator is 4° C, and this is where PRBCs are stored. Therefore, it takes 5 liters of 22° C fluid or 2 liters of cold blood products to cool a patient by 1°. Again, the main reason for using fluid warmers is not necessarily to warm patients but to prevent cooling them during resuscitation.

Rewarming techniques are classified as passive or active. Active warming is further classified as external or internal (Table 4-3). Passive warming involves *preventing* heat loss. An example of passive warming is drying the patient to minimize evaporative cooling, giving warm fluids to prevent cooling, or covering the patient so that the ambient air temperature immediately around the patient can be higher than the room temperature. Covering the patient's head helps reduce a tremendous amount of heat loss. Aluminum-lined head covers are preferred; they reflect back the infrared radiation that is normally lost through the scalp. Warming of the room technically helps reduce the heat loss gradient, but the surgical staff is usually unable to work in a humidified room of 37° C. Passive warming also includes closing an open body

TABLE 4-3 Classification of Warming Techniques

PASSIVE	ACTIVE EXTERNAL	ACTIVE INTERNAL
Dry the patient	Bair Hugger	Warmed fluids
Warm fluids	Heated warmers	Heat ventilator
Warm blankets and sheets	Lamps	Cavity lavage, chest tube, abdomen, bladder
Head covers	Radiant warmers	Continuous arterial or venous rewarming
Warm the room	Clinitron bed	Full or partial bypass

TABLE 4-4 Calories Delivered by Active Warming

METHOD	KCAL/HR
Airway from vent	9
Overhead radiant warmers	17
Heating blankets	20
Convective warmers	15-26
Body cavity lavages	35
Continuous arteriovenous rewarming	92-140
Cardiopulmonary bypass	710

cavity, such as the chest or abdomen, to prevent evaporative heat loss. The most important way to prevent heat loss is to treat hemorrhagic shock by controlling bleeding. Once shock has been treated, metabolism will heat the patient from his or her core. This point cannot be overemphasized.

Active warming actively transfers calories to the patient, either externally through the skin or internally. Skin and fat are designed to be highly efficient in preventing heat transfer. Whereas the fat is insulating against loss of heat, it is also the reason that transfer of heat past the skin is difficult. Active external warming is thus inefficient because of our built-in insulation compared with internal warming. External active warming with forced-air heating, such as with Bair Hugger temperature management therapy (Arizant Healthcare Inc., Eden Prairie, Minn), is technically classified as active warming, but air is a terribly inefficient medium, so not many calories are provided to patients. Forced-air heating increases only the patient's ambient temperature, but it can actually cool the patient initially because it increases evaporative heat loss if the patient is wet from blood, fluids, clothes, or sweat. Warming the skin may feel good to the patient and the surgeon, but it actually decreases shivering (a highly efficient method of internal warming that tricks the thermoregulatory nerve input on the skin). Because forced-air heating uses convection, the actual amount of active warming is estimated to be only 10 kcal/hr.

Active external warming is better performed by placing patients on heating pads, which use conduction to transfer heat. Beds are available that can warm patients faster, such as the Clinitron bed (Hill-Rom, Batesville, Ind), which uses heated air-fluidized beads. Such beds are not practical in the operating room but are applicable in the ICU. Removal of wet sheets and wet clothes remains an essential aspect of rewarming. Heating pads that use heated water use countercurrent heat exchange; placed under the patient during surgery, they can be effective in minimizing mild hypothermia. The amount of kilocalories per hour depends on the extent of dilation or vasoconstriction of the blood vessels in the skin. This countercurrent heat exchange system can also be used to cool the patient if so desired.

The best method to warm patients is to deliver the calories internally (Table 4-4). Heating the air used for ventilators is technically internal active warming, but it is inefficient because, again, the heat transfer method is convection. The surface area of the lungs is massive, but the energy is mainly transferred through humidified water droplets, mostly by convection and not conduction. The amount of heat transferred through warmed humidified air is also minimal by comparison to methods that use conduction. Body cavities can be lavaged by infusing warmed fluids through chest tubes or by merely irrigating the abdominal cavity with hot fluids. Other means written about but rarely used in practice include gastric lavage and esophageal lavage with special tubes. If gastric lavage is desired, one method is continuous lavage by infusion of warmed fluids through the sump port while the fluid is sucked out of the main tube. Bladder irrigation with an irrigation Foley catheter is also useful. Instruments to warm the hand through conduction show much promise but are not yet readily available.

The best means to deliver heat is through a countercurrent exchange system, using conduction to transfer calories. Again, heating the IV fluids and then infusing the warmed fluids is technically active internal warming, but again, because of the limitations of how hot we can heat the fluids, it is relatively inefficient. Heating fluids before infusion is to minimize cooling rather than to actively warm. Full cardiopulmonary bypass is unmatched; it delivers more than 5 liters/min of heated blood to every place in the body where there are capillaries. If full cardiopulmonary bypass is not available or not desired, alternatives include continuous venous or arterial rewarming. Venous-venous rewarming is most easily accomplished using the roller pump of a dialysis machine (which is often more available to the average surgeon). A prospective study showed arterial-venous rewarming to be highly effective. It can warm patients to 37° C in about 39 minutes, compared with an average warming time of 3.2 hours with standard techniques. Special Gentilello arterial warming catheters are inserted into the femoral artery, and a second line is inserted into the opposite femoral vein. The pressure from the artery produces flow, which is then directed to a fluid warmer and back into the vein. This method depends highly on the patient's BP because flow is directly related to BP. There are also commercially available central line catheters that directly heat the blood; a countercurrent exchange system heats the tip of the catheter with warmed fluids, and as blood passes over this warmed catheter, it can directly transfer kilocalories.

During the last decades, with the changes in resuscitation methods, the incidence of hypothermia has decreased, and it is now less of a problem. Dilutional coagulopathy also occurs less frequently as the volume of crystalloids has been minimized, and particular attention has been paid to ensure that all resuscitation fluids and blood are warmed before infusion.

Coagulopathy

Coagulopathy in surgical patients is multifactorial. In addition to acidosis and hypothermia, the other main usual cause of coagulopathy is decreased clotting factors. This decrease is caused by consumption (from the innate attempt to stop bleeding), dilution (from infused fluids devoid of clotting factors), and genetic (hemophilia) factors.

Coagulopathy often needs to be corrected. The most commonly used tests for coagulopathy are prothrombin time, partial thromboplastin time, and international normalized ratio. However, these tests have been shown to be inaccurate in detecting coagulopathy in surgical patients. One of the major reasons is that coagulopathy is a dynamic state that evolves through different stages of hypocoagulability, hypercoagulability, and fibrinolysis. The traditional tests of blood clotting lack the ability to detect the evolution of coagulopathy through these stages. Moreover, the traditional tests are performed at normal pH and temperature, so they cannot take into account the effects of hypothermia and acidosis on coagulation. The traditional tests of coagulation are performed on serum and not on whole blood, so they are unable to measure the interaction of coagulation factors with platelets.

More recently, thromboelastography and rotational thromboelastometry have emerged as dynamic measures of coagulation that provide a more sensitive and accurate measure of the coagulation changes seen in trauma patients. Thromboelastography and rotational thromboelastometry are based on similar principles of detecting clot strength, which is the final product of the coagulation cascade. They are also performed on whole blood, so they take into account the functional interaction of coagulation factors and platelets.

Thromboelastography parameters include R, reaction time; α, alpha angle; and MA, maximum amplitude. The R time reflects the latent time until fibrin formation begins. An increase in this time may result from factor deficiency or decreased factor activity, whereas a decrease in R time reflects a hypercoagulable state. The steepness of the α angle reflects the rate of fibrin formation. The measure of clot strength is MA, which reflects clot elasticity. The value of MA is a measure of the strength of interaction between the coagulation factors and platelets. Qualitative or quantitative defects in either of these would result in decreased MA. Thromboelastography provides the additional ability to measure the fibrinolytic arm of the coagulation cascade. LY30 and LY60 indices provide a measure of the fibrinolysis rate by calculating the decrease in clot strength at 30 and 60 minutes, respectively. A large lysis index reflects rapid fibrinolysis and may help guide the use of antifibrinolytic therapy in these patients, which has been shown to reduce mortality if it is used within 3 hours of injury. These tests are routinely used in cardiac surgery and are becoming more popular in trauma in the form of point-of-care testing, but they are not widely available in most hospitals (Fig. 4-7).

The methods to define and to treat coagulopathy are still varied. Hypothermia has a vital role in coagulopathy as the coagulation cascade is dependent on enzymatic activities. Thus, coagulopathy is associated with shock and increased mortality. Bleeding from coagulopathy or any other reason perpetuates hemorrhagic shock, which induces more acidosis, more hypothermia, and more consumption and use of fluids. The only way to break this vicious circle is to stop the bleeding.

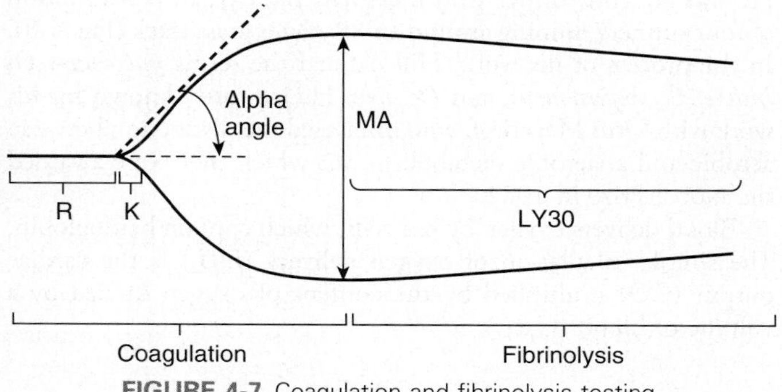

FIGURE 4-7 Coagulation and fibrinolysis testing.

In recent years, interest in using drugs to stop bleeding and to correct coagulopathy has increased. Recombinant factor VIIa (rFVIIa) was developed for use in hemophiliacs. It works with tissue factor and activated platelets. Tissue factor is ubiquitous, but with tissue injury, it is released at high levels at the site of injury, as are activated platelets. Theoretically, because rFVIIa targets the site of tissue injury, it is ideal in surgery. For example, if a patient had blunt injuries to the spleen and a femur fracture and was infused rFVIIa, the drug would work predominantly at the site of injury but would not create a systemic state of thrombotic or embolic problems. It was used off-label in patients with massive bleeding with coagulopathy, so case reports started to emerge in the literature. Case series then appeared, and eventually reports with recommendations of how and when to use it were published.

Boffard and colleagues[24] then showed, in a randomized, double-blinded, placebo-controlled trial, that blunt trauma patients who received rFVIIa had a significantly lower blood transfusion requirement and a lower incidence of massive transfusion. The trial also showed similar trends in penetrating trauma patients as well as improved early outcome in both blunt and penetrating trauma patients. However, the difference was not statistically significant. In addition, the trial showed a trend toward a lower incidence of multiple-organ failure and ARDS. In a post hoc analysis, Rizoli and associates examined the efficacy of rFVIIa in coagulopathic patients, stating that it significantly reduced the need for blood transfusions and the incidence of multiple-organ failure and ARDS. Enthusiasm for its use has waned, however, because the cost of the drug is high and prospective trials did not show a statistical survival advantage. The average cost for the drug is \$1/μg/kg; for a 75-kg person, that equates to \$7500 per dose.

The military began using rFVIIa during the war in Iraq and reported a decreased 30-day mortality rate without an increased risk of severe thrombotic events. Caution started to emerge as thromboembolic events were being reported. It seems that injured vessels were at risk for thrombosis. The ideal dose of the drug is still unclear, as is the optimal timing of administration.

Selecting the correct population of patients for rFVIIa is also a major factor. Some reports did not show significant survival benefit, but this could be a result of the drug's being used only in moribund patients, for whom no medical therapy would have improved outcome. The reason for not using it early or in nonmoribund patients was the high cost of the drug. A large multicenter prospective trial of rFVIIa was initiated, but it was difficult to implement, and eventually the study was terminated early as enrollment was difficult and the study was determined to be futile. Early analysis of the study showed that the overall mortality in both the control group and the group that received the drug was lower than predicted. Thus, the chance of showing statistical difference in 30-day mortality was low because the study was underpowered. Although rFVIIa probably does decrease the need for blood transfusions, it may or may not save lives. Mortality is often affected by much more than blood transfusions.

Although rFVIIa is not yet shown to be beneficial in traumatic shock, it may be particularly useful in patients with TBI.[25] It may not be the ultimate solution to coagulopathy, but rFVIIa has certainly garnered interest in use of drugs to combat coagulopathy after trauma. Other drugs have recently been identified to possibly have a role in the treatment of coagulopathy after trauma. Factor IX or prothrombin complex concentrate (PCC) has become popular for the treatment of surgical coagulopathy. For patients taking warfarin, PCC is the recommended treatment of choice. This is of particular benefit in elderly patients with TBI, in whom treatment with fresh-frozen plasma (FFP) can potentially be a problem if the patient has comorbid cardiac disease and could induce cardiac heart failure from volume overload. Additional benefit of using PCC is that the time to reversal of coagulopathy is shorter than when FFP is used.[26] PCC actually has many factors (factors II, VII, IX, X) in it, including variable amounts of factor VIIa, depending on the brand of PCC used. It also has the advantage of costing only one-tenth the cost of rFVIIa. The use of blood-based component therapy is paramount in treating coagulopathy (see later, "Evolution of Modern Resuscitation"). However, the concept of treating traumatic bleeding with a drug needs to be thoroughly tested and developed. If there were a drug that, when administered, would stop or reduce bleeding, treat coagulopathy at a low cost, and not cause serious complications, it would be a real contribution to medicine. Again, the problem is that current modes are expensive, and the adverse events from administering such a drug are still not fully elucidated.

Tranexamic acid (TXA) is a synthetic analogue of the amino acid lysine. It is an antifibrinolytic that competitively inhibits the activation of plasminogen to plasmin. Thus, it prevents degradation of fibrin, which is a protein that forms the framework of blood clots. TXA has about eight times the antifibrinolytic activity of an older analogue, ε-aminocaproic acid. It is used to treat or to prevent excessive blood loss during surgical procedures, such as on the heart, liver, and vascular system, and in large orthopedic procedures. It seems that topical TXA is effective and safe after total knee and hip replacement surgery, reducing bleeding and the need for blood transfusions. Studies have shown similar results in children undergoing craniofacial surgery, spinal surgery, and others. It is even used for heavy menstrual bleeding in oral tablet form and in dentistry as a 5% mouthwash. Recently, it is advocated for use in trauma. It seems to be effective in reducing rebleeding in spontaneous intracranial bleeding. A small double-blinded, placebo-controlled, randomized study of 238 patients resulted in reducing progressive intracranial bleeding after trauma, but because of the small sample size, it was not statistically significant. TXA is used to treat primary fibrinolysis, which is integral in the pathogenesis of the acute coagulopathy of trauma.

The CRASH-2 (Clinical Randomization of an Antifibrinolytic in Significant Hemorrhage) trial, a multicenter randomized controlled civilian trial of 20,211 patients, showed that TXA reduced all-cause mortality versus placebo (14.5% versus 16.0%).[27] The risk of death caused by bleeding was also reduced (4.9% versus 5.7%). CRASH-2 also suggested that TXA was less effective and could even be harmful if treatment was delayed more than 3 hours after admission. This was confirmed in the retrospective MATTERs (Military Application of Tranexamic Acid in Trauma Emergency Resuscitation) study and rapidly incorporated into military practice guidelines and subsequently for civilians worldwide.[28] The PED-TRAX study demonstrated that in children treated at a military hospital in Afghanistan, TXA administration to 66 of the 766 children was independently associated with decreased mortality and improved neurologic and pulmonary outcomes. TXA has had other retrospective studies showing worse outcome. Although the CRASH-2 trial was a randomized study with placebo, the critics of the study point out that the study was in 270 hospitals

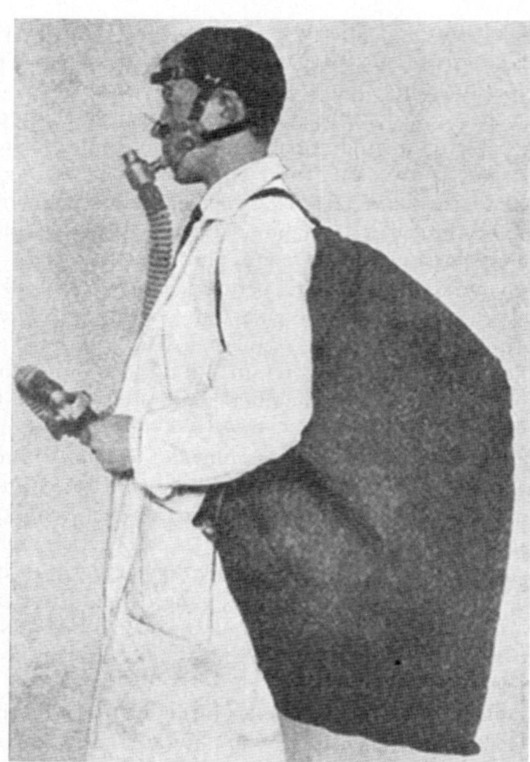

FIGURE 4-8 Bag with side tube, low on the left-hand side, for use while running. The tap is carried in the left hand. (From Hill AV, Lupton H: Muscular exercise, lactic acid, and the supply and utilization of oxygen. *Q J Med* 16:135–171, 1923.)

in 40 countries, and the large sample size may result in a beta 1 error, meaning that the study was statistically significant because of the large number of patients in the study, but the small differences in outcome may not necessarily be clinically significant. The absolute risk reduction was approximately 1.5% with an estimated number needed to treat of 68. The CRASH-3 trial is currently being conducted to assess the effect of TXA on risk of death or disability in patients with TBI. The key will be dosing, timing, and patient selection. The drug is attractive because it is inexpensive ($5.70 per dose) and easy to use with seemingly minimal side effects.

Oxygen Delivery

The definition of shock is inadequate tissue perfusion, but many clinicians have incorrectly simplified it to inadequate tissue oxygenation. Much of what we know about oxygen delivery and consumption started with a physiologist named Archibald V. Hill. He was an avid runner who measured the oxygen consumption of four runners running around an 88-meter grass track (Fig. 4-8). In the process of his work, Hill defined the terms *maximum* O_2 *intake*, O_2 *requirement*, and O_2 *debt*. He is mostly known for his work with Otto Meyerhof, who unraveled the distinction between aerobic and anaerobic metabolism, for which they were awarded the Nobel Prize in 1922.

Blood delivers oxygen by red cells, which contain hemoglobin. The simple calculation of oxygen delivery (DO_2) is the cardiac output (CO) multiplied by the content of oxygen carried by a volume of blood (CaO_2):

$$DO_2 = CO \times CaO_2$$

The average hemoglobin carries 1.34 mL of oxygen per gram, depending on the arterial hemoglobin (Hgb) oxygen saturation (SaO_2) of the red cell. In addition, a minor amount of oxygen is dissolved in plasma. This amount is calculated by multiplying the solubility constant 0.003 times the partial pressure of oxygen in the arterial blood (PaO_2). The CaO_2 of arterial blood is calculated as follows:

$$CaO_2 = (1.34 \times Hgb \times SaO_2) + (0.003 \times PaO_2)$$

where hemoglobin is in grams per deciliter. Cardiac output is heart rate multiplied by the stroke volume. In a normal state, the stroke volume can be increased by shunting blood from one tissue bed to the central vasculature, but most of the change in cardiac output is due to increased heart rate. In states of hemorrhage and resuscitation, the stroke volume is affected by infusion of fluids. As blood volume is decreased, it will ultimately affect stroke volume and is compensated by an increase in heart rate.

Oxygen consumption (VO_2) by cells is calculated by subtracting the content of oxygen in the venous system (CvO_2) from delivered oxygen content in the arterial blood (CaO_2):

$$VO_2 = CO \times (CaO_2 - CvO_2)$$

After simplifying the terms and converting the units, the result is as follows:

$$VO_2 = CO \times 1.34 \times Hgb \times (SaO_2 - SvO_2)$$

The most conventional method of sampling the venous oxygen content is by drawing blood from the most distal port of a pulmonary artery catheter. The sample is taken from the pulmonary artery because venous blood is mixed there from all parts of the body. Oxygen content in the inferior vena cava is typically higher than in the superior vena cava, which is higher than in the coronary sinus. The average mixed venous sample is 75% saturated, so the oxygen consumption is thought to be on average 25% of the oxygen delivered (Fig. 4-9). Thus, teleologically, there is ample reserve of oxygen delivered.

With advancements in technology, catheters are now available that can continuously measure the venous saturation in the pulmonary artery. These use technology similar to the pulse oximeter built into the tip of a pulmonary artery catheter, which uses near-infrared light waves to measure the oxygen saturation state of hemoglobin. These advanced catheters can also provide cardiac output continuously. In the past, cardiac output was inferred by measuring the rate of change in temperature in the heart, at the distal aspect of a pulmonary artery catheter, by infusing a standard volume of iced or room temperature water into the proximal port and measuring the change in temperature.

Cardiac output and oxygen delivery are also affected by the end-diastolic volume of the left ventricle. As described by Starling in 1915, cardiac output increases when the ventricular fibers increase in length. There is a maximum filling point, then cardiac output no longer increases (Fig. 4-10). Left ventricular end-diastolic (LVED) volume can be inferred by using a pulmonary artery catheter and measuring the wedge pressure. This reflects the pressure in the left ventricle because the vessels from the pulmonary artery to the left ventricle have no valves. Alternative approaches can help optimize the filling volume in the left ventricle. Pulmonary artery catheters for calculating the right ventricular end-diastolic volume are now available. Echocardiography using transthoracic or esophageal probes can directly estimate the filling volumes in the heart. However, variations in volume and heart size can distort results. Heart size is also affected by medical conditions that can stress and dilate the heart. The interpretation of heart size and adequate resuscitation data is thus subjective.

Optimization (Supernormalization)

During the late 1980s, surgical critical care evolved into a specialty, focusing heavily on ventilator support and optimizing oxygen delivery to tissues. One of the pioneers of modern surgical critical care, William Shoemaker, theorized that during shock, because of a lack of oxygen delivery, there was anaerobic metabolism and an oxygen debt that needed to be repaid. He showed that after volume loading, if oxygen delivery increased, consumption would also increase—until a certain point, when an additional increase in oxygen delivery did not result in increased consumption. This increased oxygen consumption was thought to be the process of paying back the oxygen debt that occurred during ischemia throughout the body. Patients in shock were found to have a hyperdynamic stage, in which increased oxygen delivery resulted in increased consumption. The assumption was

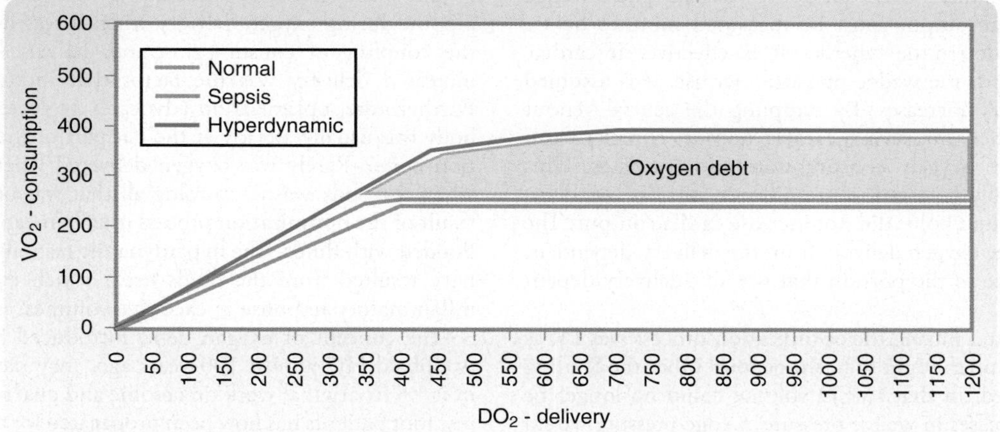

FIGURE 4-9 Oxygen Delivery and Consumption. During normal states, oxygen delivery is approximately 1000 mL/min of O_2. The oxygen consumption in a normal state is 25% of delivery and is approximately 250 mL/min. At very low oxygen delivery, it is believed that consumption is delivery dependent and occurs in shock. There is oxygen debt during shock and during recovery, and there is a hyperdynamic stage during which the circulatory system is paying back its oxygen debt.

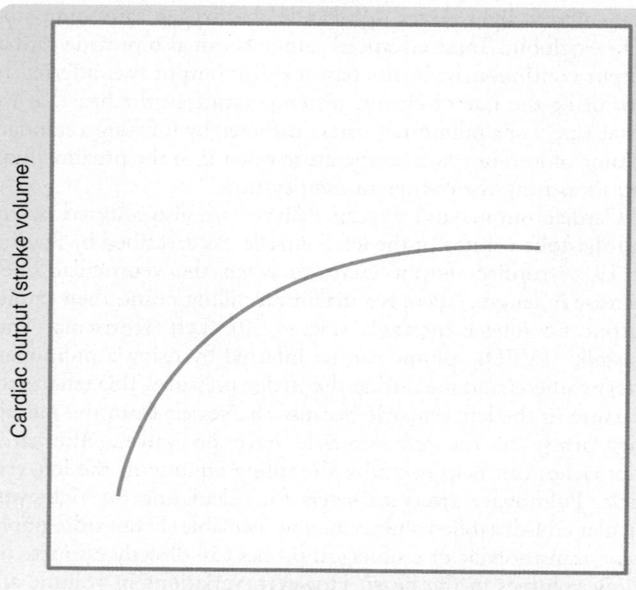

FIGURE 4-10 Starling Curve. As LVED pressure is increased, the fibers of the heart muscle are lengthened, resulting in increased contraction and increased cardiac output. This occurs to a certain point, at which increases in volume and length do not result in increases in cardiac output.

that increased consumption was replenishing the oxygen debt that the body had incurred.

Shoemaker popularized the concept of optimization or supernormalization of oxygen delivery, which means that oxygen delivery is maximized or increased until its consumption no longer increases but instead levels off. The optimization process involved administering a rapid bolus of fluid and confirming that it raised wedge pressure. Because the response to fluid infusion was dynamic, the infusion process had to occur during a short period, such as 20 minutes. If it took longer, changes in the vascular space and specifically the heart may be due to other variables in addition to the fluids used. Also, if the response was not measured immediately after infusion, the effect of the infusion was known to degrade quickly as fluids moved out of the vascular space. Wedge pressure and cardiac output must be measured minutes before fluid infusion to determine whether it is effective. If cardiac output increases with the wedge pressure increase, it is assumed that oxygen delivery increases. By sampling the central venous oxygen content when measuring cardiac output, clinicians can determine whether oxygen consumption also increases. This process was originally repeated, over and over, until it was demonstrated that the fluid bolus did not increase cardiac output. The goal was to optimize oxygen delivery from the delivery-dependent portion of the curve to the portion that was not delivery dependent (see Fig. 4-9).

The preferred fluid during the optimization process was LR as it was inexpensive and thought to be innocuous. Once the Starling curve was optimized, in that LVED volume could no longer be increased with increases in wedge pressure, wedge pressure would be kept at that maximal level. Further increases in wedge pressure, without increasing LVED volume, meant that patients might suffer from unnecessary pulmonary edema.

Once fluid infusion maximized cardiac output and oxygen delivery, an inotropic agent would be added to further push cardiac output to a higher level. The agent recommended at that time was dobutamine. The dose was increased, and its effect on cardiac output was documented. With each maneuver, oxygen consumption was measured and cardiac output "optimized" to meet the consumption demands. This optimizing process maximized oxygen delivery to ensure that all tissue beds were being fed adequately. Shoemaker's earlier clinical trials had shown that patients resuscitated in this manner had a lower incidence of multiple organ dysfunction syndrome (MODS) and death. During this optimizing era, ARDS and MODS were the leading causes of late death in trauma patients.

However, subsequent clinical studies failed to repeat Shoemaker's success. Randomized prospective trials showed that the optimization of oxygen delivery and consumption did not improve outcome.[29] In general, patients who responded to the optimization process did well, but those who could not have their oxygen delivery augmented to a higher level did poorly. Thus, although response to optimization was prognostic of outcome, the process itself did not seem to change outcome. One of the reasons that the earlier studies succeeded may have been because the control patients were not adequately resuscitated. With the later trials, when patients were adequately resuscitated, the optimization process did not improve outcome. In fact, the aggressive use of fluids to achieve supranormal oxygen delivery could cause abdominal compartment syndrome from excessive crystalloid infusions.[30] Over time, the widely used pulmonary artery catheter fell out of favor. Studies have shown that the discontinued use of the pulmonary artery catheter has not adversely affected outcome. Because of the invasive nature of the pulmonary artery and concern that the data derived from the catheter were often misinterpreted, its use has virtually disappeared from the modern-day surgical ICU.

Moreover, oxygen delivery in hyperdynamic patients could not be driven to a point at which consumption seemed to level off. One theory was that as the heart was being pushed with the supernormalization process, the heart's metabolism increased such that it was the major organ seemingly consuming all of the excess oxygen being delivered. The harder the heart worked to deliver the oxygen, the more it had to use. Normal cardiac output for an average man is about 5 liters/min, yet patients were often driven to a cardiac output of 15 liters/min or more for days at a time.

The critics of the optimization process asserted that there was a point during oxygen delivery when it was flow dependent, but the coupling of consumption and delivery made it seem like increased delivery was the factor that increased consumption. Furthermore, optimization advocates neglected the fact that the body was usually already at the flat part of the oxygen consumption curve. Rarely was oxygen delivered when it was critical or when the body was consuming all that was being delivered. The result of the optimization process usually meant that patients were flooded with fluids. The hyperdynamic response and MODS may have resulted from the fluids used, which may have caused an inflammatory response at excessive volumes.

The concept of oxygen debt, introduced by the physiologist Archibald Hill almost 100 years ago, may have some vital flaws in it.[31] His original work on aerobic and anaerobic metabolism in just four patients has now been propagated for a century. However, modern exercise physiology studies have shown that oxygen debt is repaid during a short period; it does not take days. In contrast, the optimization process showed oxygen debt for long periods.

During massive hemorrhage, some ischemia to some tissues is theoretically possible. However, in acute hemorrhage, when the

BP falls to 40 mm Hg, cardiac output and thus oxygen delivery are typically reduced by only 50%. Before resuscitation with acellular fluids, the hemoglobin level does not fall significantly. In this state, oxygen delivery is cut by only half, and the body is designed to have plenty of reserves (cells consume only 25% of the delivered oxygen in the normal state). Whether any ongoing anaerobic metabolism is actually occurring is questionable as the oxygen delivery has to fall to 25% of baseline to theoretically be anaerobic. When resuscitation takes place without blood to restore the vascular volume to the original volume, the hemoglobin level theoretically may fall by 50%, but cardiac output is usually restored to the original state. Again, oxygen delivery is only halved, with plenty of oxygen still being delivered to avoid ongoing anaerobic metabolism. It is difficult to reduce cardiac output and hemoglobin level to a level at which oxygen delivery is reduced by 75%, that is, to below the anaerobic threshold.

In hypovolemic shock states, it was thought that even though global oxygen delivery may be adequate, regional hypoxia is ongoing. Different organs and tissue beds are not similar in their oxygen needs or consumption. Hypoxic insult may be experienced by the critical organs, whose flow is usually preserved, whereas nonessential organs are sacrificed in terms of oxygen delivery. Yet such patients are not actively moving and their oxygen demand is minimal. Thus, the theory of oxygen debt is in question. In exercise states, even if there is oxygen debt, it is paid back quickly and does not take days.

To optimize oxygen delivery, one of the most efficient ways, according to past calculations, was to add hemoglobin. If the hemoglobin level increased from 8.0 to 10 g/dL, by transfusing 2 units of blood, oxygen delivery would increase by 25%. Blood transfusions were part of the optimization process because they also increased wedge pressure and LVED volume and thus cardiac output, but it was rarely noted that transfusions placed patients on the flat part of the consumption curve.

Decades ago, it was also thought that an increased hematocrit level would reduce flow in the capillaries, so clinicians had reservations about transfusing too much blood. Studies in the 1950s demonstrated better flow at the capillary level with diluted blood. However, the small amount of decreased flow with the higher viscosity was in the range of a few percentage points and did not compare to the 25% increase in oxygen delivery with a transfusion of a couple of units of PRBCs. Blood transfusions by calculations would be the most efficient way of increasing oxygen delivery, if that were the goal.

Current exercise physiology studies have shown that professional athletes perform better when their hemoglobin levels are above normal. The athletes who blood dope, by undergoing autologous blood transfusions or by taking red cell production enhancers such as erythropoietin or testosterone, are now banned for illegal performance enhancement. Such athletes have cardiac outputs of more than 20 to 50 liters/min. They do not seem to have any problems with blood sludging from the higher flow and more viscous blood than normal. The argument against this analogy of athletes and their capability to deliver oxygen despite a high hematocrit level is that injured patients have capillaries that are not vasodilated and are often plugged with white and red cells.

Global Perfusion versus Regional Perfusion

Gaining the ability to measure BP was revolutionary. However, because the main functions of the vascular system are to deliver needed nutrients and to carry out excreted substances from the cells, clinicians constantly ask whether BP or flow is more important. During sepsis, systemic vascular resistance is low. A malfunction somewhere in the autoregulatory system is assumed.

A teleologic explanation is also possible. Lower systemic vascular resistance could be a way our body evolved so that cardiac output can be easily increased as afterload is reduced. Some shunting is believed to occur at the capillary level; however, should BP be augmented with exogenous administration of pressor agents, normalizing BP at the expense of capillary flow? High doses of pressor agents most likely worsen flow because lactate levels rise if the pressor dose is too high. That rise in lactate levels could be caused by a stress response as catecholamines are known to increase lactate levels, or it could also be caused by decreased flow at the capillary bed.

Purists would prefer to have lower pressure, as long as flow is adequate, but some organs are somewhat sensitive to pressure. For example, the brain and kidneys are traditionally thought to be pressure dependent; however, when early experiments were done, it was difficult to isolate flow from pressure because those two values are interrelated. With the concept that flow might be more important than just pressure, technology developed to focus on measuring flow of nutrients rather than pressure.

During hemorrhage or hypovolemia, blood is redirected to organs such as the brain, liver, and kidneys—at the expense of tissue beds such as the skin, muscle, and gut. Thus, the search ensued to find the consequences of this shunting process. The gastrointestinal (GI) tract became the focus of much of this research. Two main methods were developed, gastric tonometry and near-infrared (NIR) technology.

Gastric tonometry measures the adequacy of blood flow in the GI tract through placement of a CO_2-permeable balloon, filled with saline, in the stomach of a patient after gastric acid suppression. The balloon is left in contact with the mucosa of the stomach for 30 minutes, allowing the CO_2 of the gastric mucosa to pass into the balloon and equilibrate. The saline and gas are then withdrawn from the balloon, and the partial pressure of the CO_2 is measured. That value, in conjunction with the arterial bicarbonate (HCO_3^-), is used in the Henderson-Hasselbalch equation to calculate the pH of the gastric mucosa and, by inference, to determine the adequacy of blood flow to the splanchnic circulation.

The logistic difficulties of gastric tonometry are concerning. Data on its use have suggested that even though it can help predict survival, resuscitating patients to an improved value had no survival benefit. Most clinicians have now abandoned gastric tonometry. A multicenter trial showed that in patients with septic shock, gastric tonometry was predictive of outcome, but implementing this technology was no better than using the cardiac index as a resuscitation goal.[32] Regional variables of organ dysfunction are thought to be better monitoring variables than global pressure-related hemodynamic variables. However, the data seem to indicate consistently that initial resuscitation of critically ill patients with shock does not require monitoring of regional variables. After stabilization, regional variables are, at best, merely predictors of outcome.

The optimal device for monitoring the adequacy of resuscitation should be noninvasive, simple, cheap, and portable. NIR spectroscopy uses the NIR region of the electromagnetic spectrum from about 800 nm to 2500 nm. Typical applications are wide ranging: physics, astronomy, chemistry, pharmaceuticals, medical diagnostics, and food and agrochemical quality control. The main attraction of NIR is that light, at those wavelengths, can penetrate skin and bone. This is why your hand looks red when it is placed over a flashlight; the other visible light waves are absorbed or reflected, but red light and infrared light pass through skin and bone readily.

A common device using NIR technology that has now become standard in the medical industry is the pulse oximeter. Using slightly different light waves, it yielded correlations with such variables as the cytochrome aa_3 status by adding a third light wave in the 800-nm region. When the oxygen supply is less than adequate, the rate of electron transport is reduced, and oxidative phosphorylation decreases, leading ultimately to anaerobic metabolism. Optical devices that use NIR wavelengths can determine the redox potential of copper atoms on cytochrome aa_3 and have been used to study intracellular oxidative processes noninvasively. Thus, with NIR technology, the metabolic rate of tissue can be directly determined to assess whether it is being adequately perfused. Animal models of hemorrhagic shock have validated the potential use of NIR technology in that they showed changes in regional tissue beds (Fig. 4-11). The superiority of NIR results over conventional measurements of shock has been shown in animal and human studies.

To test the utility of this potentially ideal monitoring device, a multicenter prospective study was conducted to determine whether NIR technology could detect patients at risk of hemorrhagic shock and its sequelae. Performed in seven level I trauma centers, the study enrolled 383 patients who were in severe traumatic shock with hypotension and who required blood transfusions. A probe similar to a pulse oximeter was placed on the thenar muscle of patients' hands, continuously gathering NIR values. The NIR probe was found to be as sensitive as base deficit in predicting death and MODS in hypotensive trauma patients.[33] The receiver operating characteristic curves show that it also may be somewhat better than BP in predicting outcome. More important, the negative predictive value was 90% (Fig. 4-12). The noninvasive and continuous NIR probe was able to demonstrate perfusion status. Note, however, that MODS developed in only 50 patients in that study. This was probably because the method of resuscitating trauma patients changed during this period, and this reduced MODS and death rates. The changes that took place are discussed later in this chapter but, in brief, were due to damage control resuscitation.

NIR technology may be able to show when a patient is in shock or even when a patient is doing well. Occult hypoperfusion can be detected or even ruled out reliably with NIR. In the trauma setting, a noninvasive method that can continuously detect trends in parameters such as regional oxygenation status, base deficit, or BP will surely find a role. Will this technology change how patients are treated? The debate now centers on this issue and raises some questions. Once a patient's hypoperfusion status has been determined, whether by BP, NIR technology, or some other device, what should we do with that information? Is it necessary to increase oxygen delivery to regional tissue beds that are inadequately oxygenated? Previous studies have shown that optimizing global oxygen delivery is not useful and that regional tissue monitoring with gastric tonometry has also failed to show benefit, so will NIR technology be helpful or harmful? An example of harm is over-resuscitating a patient to fix an abnormal value that may or may not mean much clinically. The end point of resuscitation is constantly being debated. Because NIR results correlate well with base deficit, we may one day use NIR technology to infer the base deficit value indirectly.

NIR technology has other promising uses in surgery, such as direct monitoring of flow and tissue oxygenation in high-risk patients (e.g., in those undergoing organ transplantation; for free

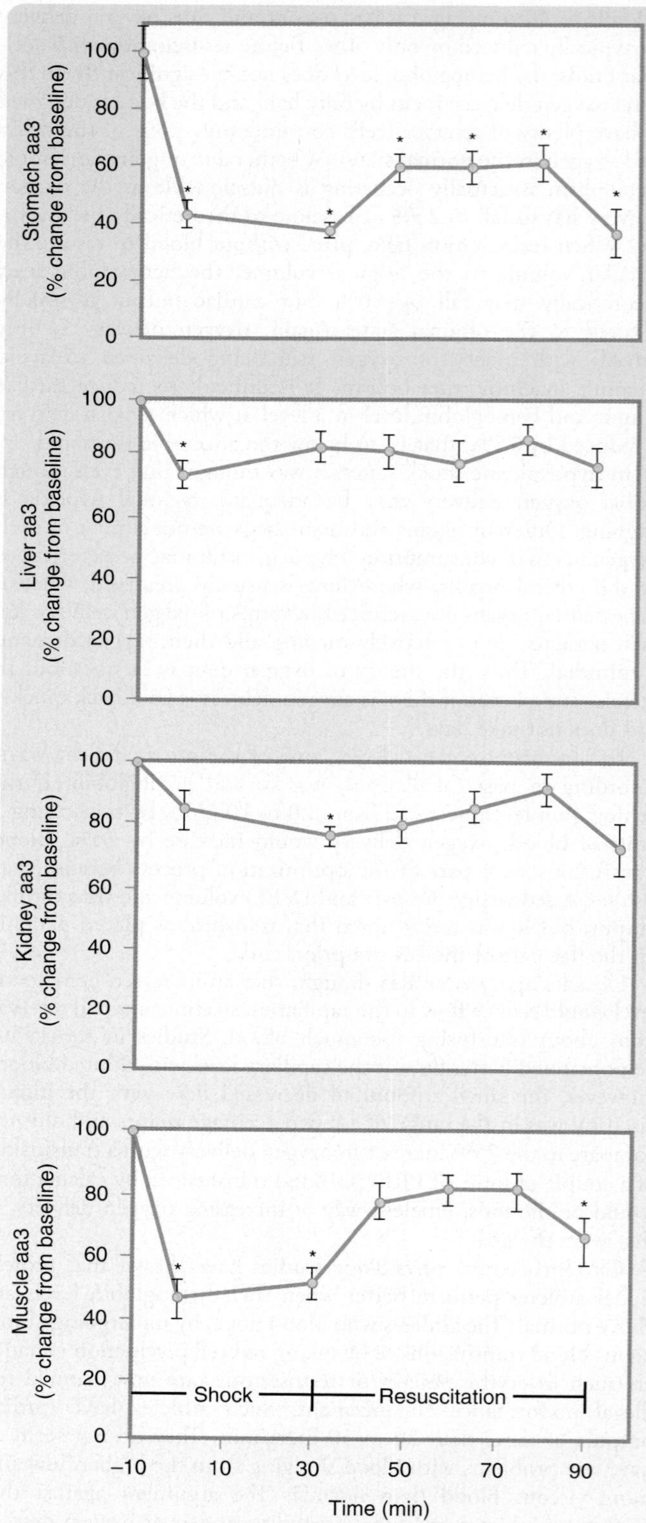

FIGURE 4-11 Cytochrome *aa*3 measurements in rabbits during hemorrhagic shock. Shown are regional tissue beds and implied tissue oxygenation. Oxygenation at the mitochondrial level is preserved in kidney and liver compared with muscle and stomach. (From Rhee P, Langdale L, Mock C, et al: Near-infrared spectroscopy: Continuous measurement of cytochrome oxidation during hemorrhagic shock. *Crit Care Med* 25:166–170, 1997.)

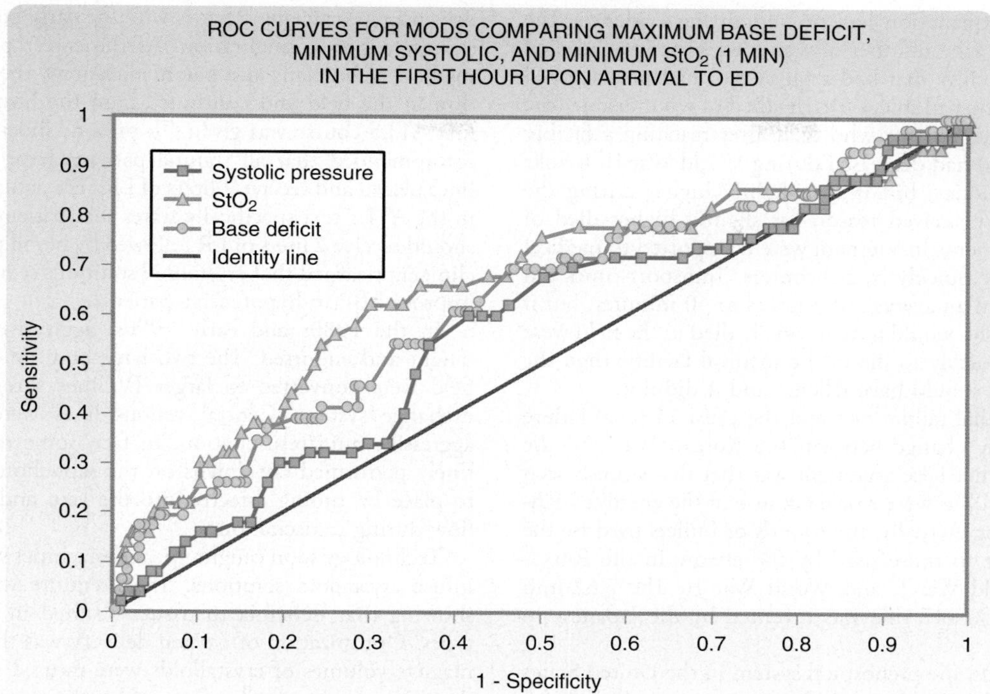

FIGURE 4-12 NIR spectroscopy in 383 patients with traumatic hemorrhagic shock with hypotension who required blood transfusion. NIR measured tissue oxygenation levels in the thenar muscle noninvasively and was found to correlate well with arterial base deficit. (From Cohn SM, Nathens AB, Moore FA, et al: Tissue oxygen saturation predicts the development of organ dysfunction during traumatic shock resuscitation. *J Trauma* 62:44–55, 2007.)

flap perfusion; for classification of burn injuries; in intraoperative assessment of bowel ischemia; with compartment syndrome or even subdural and epidural hematomas). Perhaps the most useful application will be in the ICU in septic shock patients at risk for multiple-organ failure.

Septic Shock

In 2001, Rivers and colleagues reported that among patients with severe sepsis or septic shock in a single urban emergency department, mortality was significantly lower among those who were treated according to a 6-hour protocol of early goal-directed therapy than among those who were given standard therapy (30.5% versus 46.5%). The premise was that usual care was not aggressive or timely. Early goal-directed therapy addressed this as it called for central venous catheterization to monitor central venous pressure and central venous oxygen saturation, which were used to guide the use of IV fluids, vasopressors, PRBC transfusions, and dobutamine to achieve prespecified physiologic targets. Based on this type of research, the Surviving Sepsis Campaign clinical guidelines were published in 2004 and updated in 2008 and 2014.[34] The various methods of therapy were graded by a panel of international experts.[35] A randomized prospective study has now shown that protocol-based care for early septic shock does not seem to improve outcome.[36] The newer study was not identical to the original Rivers study as the survival rates were much higher, but this study may just show that the usual therapy may have already adopted many of the principles of early goal-directed therapy, and thus the difference is negligible. This study also found no significant benefit of the mandated use of central venous catheterization and central hemodynamic monitoring in all patients.

PROBLEMS WITH RESUSCITATION

Lessons learned from the Korean War showed that resuscitation with blood and blood products was useful. Throughout that war, the concept prevailed that a limited amount of salt and water should be given to patients after injuries. By the time of the Vietnam War, volume resuscitation in excess of replacement of shed blood became an acceptable practice. That practice may have been influenced by studies of hemorrhagic shock performed by Tom Shires. In his classic study, Shires used the Wiggers model and bled 30 dogs to a mean BP of 50 mm Hg for 90 minutes. He then infused LR (5% of body weight) followed by blood in 10 dogs, plasma (10 mL/kg) followed by blood in another 10 dogs, and shed blood alone in the remaining 10 dogs. The dogs that received LR had the best survival rate. Shires concluded that although the replacement of lost blood with whole blood remains the primary treatment of shock, adjunctive replacement of the coexisting functional volume deficit with a balanced salt solution appears to be of value.

Soon the surgical community went from being judicious with crystalloid solutions to being aggressive. Surgeons returning from the Vietnam War advocated the use of crystalloids, a seemingly cheap and easy method of resuscitating patients. They touted that lives were saved. However, what evolved from this method of resuscitation was the so-called Da Nang lung, eventually known as ARDS. (The U.S. Navy had its field hospital in Da Nang, Vietnam.) The explanation for the evolution of the new condition was that battlefield patients were now living long enough to develop ARDS because their lives were saved with aggressive resuscitation and better critical care, including a greater capability to treat renal failure.

However, that explanation had no supporting evidence. The killed in action rate (the number of wounded patients who died before reaching a facility that had a physician) had not changed for more than a century (Table 4-5). The died of wounds rate (the number of wounded patients who died after reaching a facility that had a physician) had decreased during World War II, thanks to the use of antibiotics, but it was slightly higher during the Vietnam War. The perceived reason for slightly higher died of wounds was that patients in Vietnam were transported to medical facilities much more quickly by helicopters. Transport times did indeed decrease from an average of 4 hours to 40 minutes, but if the sicker patients who would have normally died in the field were transported more quickly to die in the medical facility, then the killed in action rate should have fallen—and it did not.

Moreover, the renal failure rate and the cause of renal failure did not significantly change between the Korean War and the Vietnam War. Another false argument was that the wounds seen during the Vietnam War were worse because of the enemy's high-velocity AK-47 rifles. Actually, the rounds or bullets used by the AK-47 were similar to those used by the enemy in the Russo-Japanese War, World War I, and World War II. The 7.62-mm round used in the AK-47 rifle was invented by the Japanese in the 1890s.

In the early 1970s, the prehospital system in the United States started to evolve. Previously, ambulances were usually hearses driven by morticians. That is why the early ambulances were the station wagon configuration. As the career paths of emergency medical technicians and paramedics grew, they started resuscitation in the field and continued it to the hospital. In 1978, the first ATLS course was given. To prevent shock, the ATLS course recommended that all trauma patients have two large-bore IV lines placed and receive 2 liters of LR. The actual recommendation in the ATLS text specifically states that patients in class III shock should receive 2 liters of LR followed by blood products. However, clinicians learned that crystalloid solutions seemed innocuous and improved BP in hypotensive patients.

In the 1980s and early 1990s, aggressive resuscitation was taught and endorsed. The two large-bore IV lines started in the field were converted to larger IV lines through a wire-guided exchange system. Central venous lines were placed early for aggressive fluid resuscitation. In fact, some trauma centers routinely performed cut-downs on the saphenous vein at the ankle to place IV tubing directly into the vein and thereby maximize flow during resuscitation.

Technology soon caught up, and machines were built to rapidly infuse crystalloid solutions. The literature was filled with data showing that ischemia to tissues resulted in disturbances of all types. Optimization of oxygen delivery was the goal. As a result, massive volumes of crystalloids were infused into patients. Residents were encouraged to "pound" patients with fluids. If trauma patients did not develop ARDS, it was taught that the patients were not adequately resuscitated, but many clinical trials eventually showed that prehospital fluids did not improve outcome (Table 4-6).

TABLE 4-5 Mortality Rates

	KILLED IN ACTION (%)	DIED OF WOUNDS (%)
Civil War	16.0	13.0
Russo-Japanese War	20.0	9.0
World War I	19.6	8.1
World War II	19.8	3.0
Korean War	19.5	2.4
Vietnam War	20.2	3.5

Bleeding

One of the most influential studies on hemorrhagic shock was performed by Ken Mattox, and in 1994, the results were reported by Bickell and coworkers.[37] The aim of Mattox's study, a prospective clinical trial, was to determine whether withholding of prehospital fluids affected outcome in hypotensive patients after a penetrating torso injury. IV lines were started in patients with penetrating torso trauma with BP lower than 90 mm Hg. On

TABLE 4-6 Prehospital Fluid Studies in Trauma Patients

ARTICLE	SUMMARY OF FINDINGS
Aprahamian C, Thompson BM, Towne JB, et al: The effect of a paramedic system on mortality of major open intra-abdominal vascular trauma. *J Trauma* 23:687–690, 1983.	Paramedic system Open intra-abdominal vascular trauma
Kaweski SM, Sise MJ, Virgilio RW: The effect of prehospital fluids on survival in trauma patients. *J Trauma* 30:1215–1218, 1990.	Prehospital fluids Trauma patients
Bickell WH, Wall MJ Jr, Pepe PE, et al: Immediate versus delayed fluid resuscitation for hypotensive patients with penetrating torso injuries. *N Engl J Med* 331:1105–1109, 1994.	Presurgery fluids Hypotensive penetrating torso injuries
Turner J, Nicholl J, Webber L, et al: A randomised controlled trial of prehospital intravenous fluid replacement therapy in serious trauma. *Health Technol Assess* 4:1–57, 2000.	Prehospital 1309 serious trauma patients
Kwan I, Bunn F, Roberts I: Timing and volume of fluid administration for patients with bleeding following trauma. *Cochrane Database Syst Rev* 1:CD002245, 2001.	Prehospital Bleeding trauma patients
Dula DJ, Wood GC, Rejmer AR, et al: Use of prehospital fluids in hypotensive blunt trauma patients. *Prehosp Emerg Care* 6:417–420, 2002.	Prehospital Hypotensive blunt trauma patients
Greaves I, Porter KM, Revell MP: Fluid resuscitation in pre-hospital trauma care: a consensus view. *J R Coll Surg Edinb* 47:451–457, 2002.	Prehospital A consensus view
Dutton RP, Mackenzie CF, Scalea TM: Hypotensive resuscitation during active hemorrhage: impact on in-hospital mortality. *J Trauma* 52:1141–1146, 2002.	Presurgery fluids Hypotensive active hemorrhage
Dula DJ, Wood GC, Rejmer AR, et al: Use of prehospital fluids in hypotensive blunt trauma patients. *Prehosp Emerg Care* 6:417–420, 2002.	Prehospital fluids Hypotensive patients

alternating days, patients received standard fluid therapy in the field or had fluids withheld until they reached the hospital. Withholding of prehospital fluids conferred a statistically significant survival advantage—a revolutionary, counterintuitive finding that shocked surgeons. To reiterate, if no fluids were given in the prehospital setting to hypotensive patients, they would survive more often than if they were given fluids in the field.

One criticism of this study was that patients who were already dead in the field when paramedics arrived were excluded from analysis. It made sense that fluids would not help those who had already died in the field and thus they should not be counted, yet purists asserted that those patients should have been included in the final analysis. Critics of Mattox's study claimed that reanalysis of the data using the methodology of intention to treat made the statistical significance no longer valid as the *P* value for survival was higher than .05. Even if that assertion were accounted for, Mattox's study would still show that patients who did not receive fluids had a survival advantage, albeit the difference would no longer be statistically significant. Everything that surgeons had been taught before 1994 stressed that not treating hypotensive patients with fluids would certainly and surely lead to death, yet Mattox's study showed the opposite.

That 1994 article popularized the concept of permissive hypotension, that is, allowing hypotension during uncontrolled hemorrhage. The fundamental rationale for permissive hypotension was that restoration of BP with fluids would increase bleeding from uncontrolled sources. In fact, Cannon in 1918 had stated that "inaccessible or uncontrolled sources of blood loss should not be treated with IV fluids until the time of surgical control."

Animal studies have validated the idea of permissive hypotension. Burris and colleagues have shown that moderate resuscitation results in best outcome compared with no resuscitation or aggressive resuscitation. In a swine model of uncontrolled hemorrhage, Sondeen showed that raising BP with either fluids or pressors could lead to increased bleeding. The idea was that increasing BP would dislodge the clot that had formed. The study also found that the pressure that would cause rebleeding was a mean arterial pressure of 64 ± 2 mm Hg, with a systolic pressure of 94 ± 3 mm Hg and diastolic pressure of 45 ± 2 mm Hg. Other animal studies have confirmed these concepts.

The next question was whether the continued strategy of permissive hypotension in the operating room would result in improved survival. Dutton and associates randomized one group of patients to a target systolic BP of higher than 100 mm Hg and another group to a target systolic BP of 70 mm Hg. Fluid therapy was titrated until definitive hemorrhage control was achieved. However, despite attempts to maintain BP at 70 mm Hg, the average BP was 100 mm Hg in the low-pressure group and 114 mm Hg in the high-pressure group. Patients' BP rose spontaneously. Titrating patients' BP to the low target was difficult, even with less use of fluids. The survival rate did not differ between the two groups.

The idea of permissive hypotension was slow to catch on. The argument against allowing anything besides aggressive resuscitation was dismissed. Critics continued to emphasize that the Mattox trial focused only on penetrating injuries and should not be extrapolated to blunt trauma. Clinicians feared that patients with traumatic blunt head injuries would be harmed without a normalized BP. However, Shafi and Gentilello examined the National Trauma Data Bank and found that hypotension was an independent risk factor for death, but it did not increase the mortality rate in patients with TBIs any more than in patients without TBIs. The risk of death quadrupled in patients with hypotension, in both the TBI group (odds ratio, 4.1; 95% confidence interval, 3.5 to 4.9) and the non-TBI group (odds ratio, 4.6; 95% confidence interval, 3.4 to 6.0). Furthermore, in 2006, Plurad and coworkers showed that emergency department hypotension was not an independent risk factor for acute renal dysfunction or failure.

Trauma Immunology and Inflammation

The 1990s witnessed an explosion of information regarding alterations of homeostasis and cellular physiochemistry during shock. The scientific investigations of Shires, Carrico, Baue, and countless others shed light on the basic mechanisms underlying resuscitation of patients in shock. The pathophysiologic process has been identified as having an aberrant inflammatory status, resulting in the body's immune system damaging the endothelial tissues and ultimately the end organ. This inflammatory state leads to a spectrum of conditions, including fluid sequestration, which leads to edema and progresses to acute lung injury, systemic inflammatory response syndrome, ARDS, and MODS.[38] Such conditions were in every surgical ICU. Attention focused on biochemical perturbations and altered mediators as sites for possible interventions. The fundamental cause was thought to be that ischemia and reperfusion as shown in animal models would create a state of damage to the capillary endothelium and subsequent changes to the end organ. It was generally accepted that the reason for the reperfusion injury was mediated by activated neutrophils that emitted deleterious cytokines and released free oxygen radicals. The animal models used to study these concepts were actually ischemia-reperfusion models in which the superior mesenteric artery that supplied blood to the intestines was clamped for a prolonged time before the clamp was removed. Later it was thought that this was not an appropriate model to study hemorrhagic shock. It was found that there was a difference in pathophysiologic mechanisms between ischemia-reperfusion injury and resuscitation injury.

Death after traumatic injury was described as trimodal. Some patients died within a short time after injury, some died in the hospital within a few hours, and many died late in the hospital course. However, a study in trauma patients has shown that deaths occur in a logarithmic decay fashion and follow the rule of biology; no grouping of deaths can be seen, unless the data are represented or lumped together as immediate, early, or late. The only reason for the initial trimodal distribution was that patients who died after 24 hours were labeled under late deaths.[39]

According to the traditional (although now discredited) trimodal pattern, the patients who typically died first could be aided by a better prehospital system and, more important, by injury prevention. For the second group of patients, better resuscitation was thought to be a potentially lifesaving intervention. For the third group (the late deaths), immunomodulation was considered to be key. The cause was thought to be the inflammatory adaptive aberrancy after successful resuscitation. When there is prolonged end-arteriole cessation of flow producing tissue ischemia for a time, followed by reperfusion, it is termed reperfusion injury. For example, with an injury to the femoral artery that requires 4 to 6 hours for circulation to be restored, muscle cells undergo ischemia and reperfusion, and the cells will start to swell, which can result in compartment syndrome in the lower leg. This ischemia and reperfusion was thought to occur after a period of hypotension. However, it is now known that the pathophysiologic change is due to resuscitation injury rather than to reperfusion injury.

With improved technology, the immunologic response after trauma was heavily researched. In the past, we were limited to studying physiology. A theory started to evolve that shock caused an aberrant inflammatory response, which then needed to be modulated and suppressed. Many studies during this era showed that the inflammatory system was upregulated or activated after shock. The white cells in the blood became activated. Neutrophils were identified as the key mediators in the acute phase of shock, whereas lymphocytes are typically key players in chronic diseases (e.g., cancer and viral infections). Shock, caused by various mechanisms, was thought to induce ischemia to tissues and, after reperfusion, to set off an inflammatory response, which primarily affected the microcirculation and caused leaks (Fig. 4-13).

Typically, neutrophils are rapidly transported through capillaries. However, when they are signaled by chemokines, neutrophils will start to roll, firmly adhere to the endothelium, and migrate out of the capillaries to find the body's foes and initiate healing. Early researchers thought that neutrophils would battle invaders (e.g., bacteria) through phagocytic activity and the release of oxygen free radicals; this was thought to be the reason for the leak in the capillary system (Fig. 4-14). Because neutrophils can be primed to have an enhanced response, a massive search took place to identify causes of neutrophil priming and downregulation. The many cytokines targeted included interleukin types 1 through 18, tumor necrosis factor (TNF), and adhesion molecules, such as intercellular adhesion molecules, vascular cell adhesion molecules, E-selectin, L-selectin, P-selectin, and platelet-activating factor.

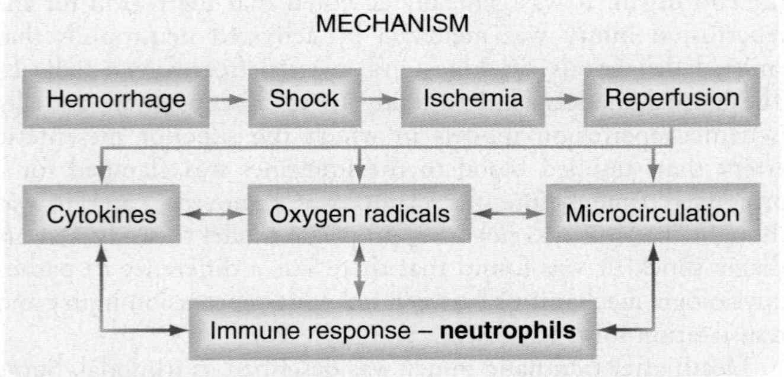

FIGURE 4-13 Hemorrhage causing neutrophil activation.

That research had much overlap with the research being performed in the arenas of reimplantation, vascular ischemia, and reperfusion. Clinically, it was already known that the implantation of severed extremities would have pathophysiologic results similar to those from ischemia, reperfusion, and swelling caused by leaky capillaries. The immune response was described as bimodal. The first response was the priming by trauma or shock, followed by an exaggerated response when hit with a second insult (e.g., infection).

In the late 1990s, other researchers focused on the role of the alimentary tract. They knew that the splanchnic circulation was shunted of blood by vasoconstriction during hemorrhagic shock, so the gut suffers the most ischemia during shock and is the most susceptible to reperfusion injury. The animal model most often used to study the gut's role in inflammation was a rat model of superior mesenteric artery occlusion and reperfusion. Because systemic inflammatory response syndrome is a sterile phenomenon, the gut was implicated as a potential player in the development of MODS. Animals were shown to have a translocation of bacteria into the portal system, and this initiation of the inflammatory cascade was investigated as the source of MODS. Investigators also knew that the release of *Escherichia coli* bacteria in the blood released endotoxins that further initiated release of cytokines (e.g., TNF, cachectin). However, studies in humans failed to demonstrate translocation of bacteria in intraoperative samples of portal vein during resuscitation. The problem was that although complete occlusion of the superior mesenteric artery for hours followed by reperfusion does result in swollen, necrotic, injured bowel, these findings were extrapolated to humans undergoing hemorrhagic shock. Again, during hemorrhagic shock, the superior mesenteric artery is not occluded, and even at severe states, there is trickle flow of blood to the splanchnic organs.

Because patients in shock bleed and receive blood transfusions, transfusion of PRBCs was also implicated as the cause of MODS. Patients who required massive amounts of PRBCs were most

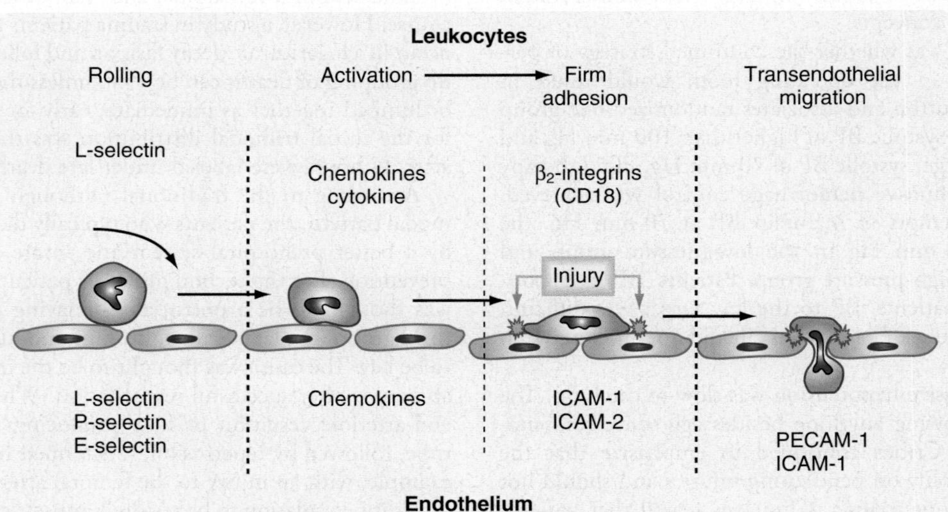

FIGURE 4-14 Intravascular neutrophils that are activated will adhere and roll until another set of mechanisms causes firm adherence, and transendothelial migration out of the vascular system occurs. It is believed that this transmigration process injures the endothelium, with the release of an oxygen free radical. This could result in fluid leaks out of the vascular system. *ICAM,* Intercellular adhesion molecules; *PECAM,* platelet–endothelial cell adhesion molecule.

likely to develop MODS. Researchers in this elucidating area found that the use of older PRBCs was an independent risk factor for the development of MODS. PRBCs have a shelf life of 42 days in the refrigerated state. As blood ages, changes occur in the fluid that have been shown to affect the immune response negatively. However, clinical trials in cardiac patients have failed to find the age of the blood as a significant problem.

In the past, when technology was limited, PRBCs were mainly tested for the red cells' capability to carry oxygen and their viability under the microscope and in the body. Most major trauma centers now have learned to use leukoreduced PRBCs, that is, the small number of white cells that can release oxygen free radicals and cytokines are now routinely filtered, before the PRBCs are stored. Leukoreduction removes 99.9% of donor white cells and, in one large Canadian study, reduced the mortality rate from 7.03% to 6.19%. Other trauma studies have shown no reduction in the mortality rate but still showed a decrease in rates of infection, infectious complications, and late ARDS. To date, the largest study of leukoreduction in trauma patients has not shown any reduction in the rates of infection, organ failure, or mortality.[40]

Numerous trials have examined the blockage of cytokines to treat septic patients. Two prospective, randomized, multicenter, double-blinded trials, the North American Sepsis Trial (NORASEPT) and the International Sepsis Trial (INTERSEPT), studied the 28-day mortality rate of critically ill patients who received anti-TNF antibody. Neither trial showed any benefit. Other trials testing other potential cytokines were disappointing as well. The cytokines tested included CD11/CD18,[41] anti–interleukin 1 receptor, antiendotoxin antibodies, bradykinin antagonists, and platelet-activating factor receptor antagonists. The search continues for one key mediator that could be manipulated to solve the "toxemia" of shock.[42] However, such attempts to simplify the events and to find one solution may be the main problem because there is no simple answer and no simple solution. The answer may lie in cocktails of substances. The humoral and endocrine systems, which are always mediated by blood, are exceedingly complex. Shock has many causes and mechanisms. Understanding this is crucial as we look for solutions.

EVOLUTION OF MODERN RESUSCITATION

Detrimental Impact of Fluids

As early as 1996, the U.S. Navy used a swine model to study the effects of fluids on neutrophil activation after hemorrhagic shock and resuscitation. It was shown that neutrophils are activated after a 40% blood volume hemorrhage when followed by resuscitation with LR. That finding was not surprising. What was enlightening was that the level of neutrophil activation was similar in control animals that did not undergo hemorrhagic shock but merely received LR (Fig. 4-15). In other control animals that did not receive LR but instead were resuscitated with shed blood or HTS after hemorrhagic shock, the neutrophils were not activated. The implication was that the inflammatory process was not caused by shock and resuscitation but by LR itself.

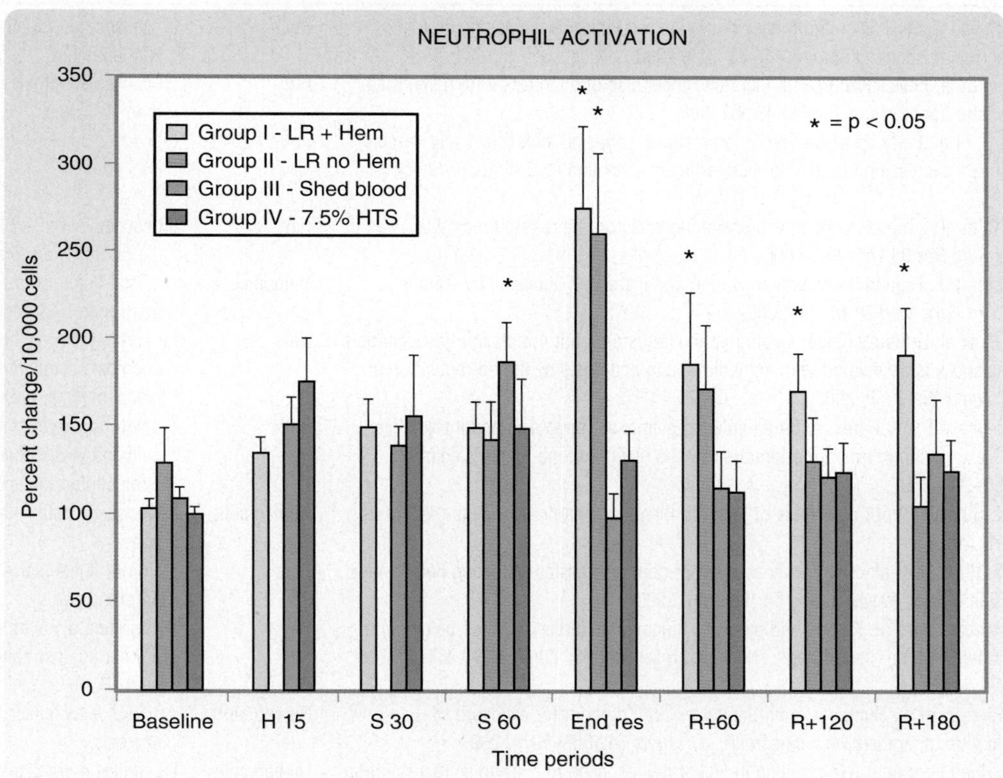

FIGURE 4-15 Neutrophil activation in whole blood of swine measured by flow cytometry. The highest neutrophil activation followed hemorrhagic shock and resuscitation using LR. Similar neutrophil activation occurred when the animal was not resuscitated but was infused with LR. No activation occurred when shocked animals were resuscitated with whole blood or 7.5% HTS. (From Rhee P, Burris D, Kaufmann C, et al: Lactated Ringer's resuscitation causes neutrophil activation after hemorrhagic shock. *J Trauma* 44:313–319, 1998.)

Those findings were repeated over several years in a series of experiments using human blood as well as in experiments in small and large animal models of hemorrhagic shock. When the blood was diluted with various resuscitation fluids, the inflammatory changes depended on the fluid used; despite similar physiologic results in vivo, the immunologic results were different (Fig. 4-16). The response was ubiquitous throughout the entire inflammatory response system, including at the levels of DNA and RNA expression.

Ultimately, it was recognized that the inflammatory response was due to the various resuscitation fluids. The type and amount of fluids directly caused inflammation. All the artificial fluids used to raise BP could cause the inflammatory sequelae of shock. The type of fluids and the amount were responsible for the inflammatory response (Table 4-7). What might be obvious today was not obvious then and was unrecognized for decades. It was not recognized that blood is extremely complex and replacement or resuscitation with simple fluids other than blood had consequences. Blood does more than raise BP and carry red cells. In the past, we studied the complexity of the body's immune response but failed to realize that fluids such as LR and normal saline that

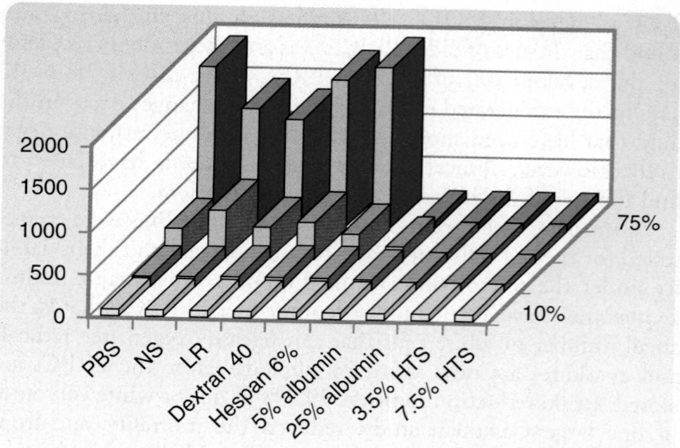

FIGURE 4-16 Human neutrophil activation using whole blood diluted with various resuscitation fluids, as measured by flow cytometry. Phosphate-buffered saline (PBS) was used because it has a pH of 7.4. (From Rhee P, Wang D, Ruff P, et al: Human neutrophil activation and increased adhesion by various resuscitation fluids. *Crit Care Med* 28:74–78, 2000.)

TABLE 4-7 Summary of Studies by U.S. Navy Demonstrating Fluids Causing Inflammation After Resuscitation

ARTICLE	MODEL	SUMMARY OF FINDINGS
Rhee P, Burris D, Kaufmann C, et al: Lactated Ringer's solution resuscitation causes neutrophil activation after hemorrhagic shock. *J Trauma* 44:313–319, 1998.	Swine	LR causes neutrophil activation; blood HTS does not.
Deb S, Martin B, Sun L, et al: Resuscitation with lactated Ringer's solution in rats with hemorrhagic shock induces immediate apoptosis. *J Trauma* 46:582–588, 1999.	Rat	LR causes apoptosis in liver and gut more than HTS does.
Sun LL, Ruff P, Austin B, et al: Early up-regulation of intercellular adhesion molecule-1 and vascular cell adhesion molecule-1 expression in rats with hemorrhagic shock and resuscitation. *Shock* 11:416–422, 1999.	Rat	LR causes cytokine release more than HTS does.
Alam HB, Sun L, Ruff P, et al: E- and P-selectin expression depends on the resuscitation fluid used in hemorrhaged rats. *J Surg Res* 94:145–152, 2000.	Rat	LR causes increased E- and P-selectin expression more than HTS does.
Rhee P, Wang D, Ruff P, et al: Human neutrophil activation and increased adhesion by various resuscitation fluids. *Crit Care Med* 28:74–78, 2000.	Human cells	Artificial fluids cause neutrophil activation more than HTS and albumin do.
Deb S, Sun L, Martin B, et al: Lactated Ringer's solution and hetastarch but not plasma resuscitation after rat hemorrhagic shock is associated with immediate lung apoptosis by the up-regulation of the Bax protein. *J Trauma* 49:47–53, 2000.	Rats	LR and hetastarch increase lung apoptosis compared with plasma whole blood, plasma, and albumin.
Alam HB, Austin B, Koustova E, et al: Resuscitation-induced pulmonary apoptosis and intracellular adhesion molecule-1 expression in rats are attenuated by the use of ketone Ringer's solution. *J Am Coll Surg* 193:255–263, 2001.	Rats	Substituting ketones for lactate reduces pulmonary apoptosis and release of intercellular adhesion molecules.
Koustova E, Stanton K, Gushchin V, et al: Effects of lactated Ringer's solutions on human leukocytes. *J Trauma* 52:872–878, 2002.	Human cells	D-LR causes inflammation more than L-LR does.
Alam HB, Stegalkina S, Rhee P, et al: cDNA array analysis of gene expression following hemorrhagic shock and resuscitation in rats. *Resuscitation* 54:195–206, 2002.	Rats	Different fluids cause gene expression at different levels.
Koustova E, Rhee P, Hancock T, et al: Ketone and pyruvate Ringer's solutions decrease pulmonary apoptosis in a rat model of severe hemorrhagic shock and resuscitation. *Surgery* 134:267–274, 2003.	Rats	Ketone and pyruvate Ringer's solutions protect against apoptosis compared with LR.
Stanton K, Alam HB, Rhee P, et al: Human polymorphonuclear cell death after exposure to resuscitation fluids in vitro: apoptosis versus necrosis. *J Trauma* 54:1065–1074, 2003.	Human cells	Artificial fluids cause apoptosis and necrosis.
Gushchin V, Alam HB, Rhee P, et al: cDNA profiling in leukocytes exposed to hypertonic resuscitation fluids. *J Am Coll Surg* 197:426–432, 2003.	Human cells	LR causes more cytokine release by gene expression than HTS does.
Alam HB, Stanton K, Koustova E, et al: Effect of different resuscitation strategies on neutrophil activation in a swine model of hemorrhagic shock. *Resuscitation* 60:91–99, 2004.	Swine	Artificial fluids cause neutrophil activation despite resuscitation rates.
Jaskille A, Alam HB, Rhee P, et al: D-Lactate increases pulmonary apoptosis by restricting phosphorylation of bad and eNOS in a rat model of hemorrhagic shock. *J Trauma* 57:262–269, 2004.	Rats	D-Lactate in fluids causes more apoptosis than L-lactate does.

TABLE 4-8 Components of Ketone Ringer's Solution

COMPONENT	NORMAL SALINE (mEq/L)	D-LR (mEq/L)	L-LR (mEq/L)	KETONE RINGER'S (mEq/L)
D-Lactate	–	14	–	–
L-Lactate	–	14	28	–
3-D-β-Hydroxybutyrate	–	–	–	28
Sodium	154	130	130	130
Potassium	–	4	4	4
Calcium	–	3	3	3
Chloride	154	109	109	109

Replacing lactate with an alternative fuel source such as ketone affected the immunologic response after resuscitation.

were developed more than 100 years ago are not an ideal substitute for blood when used in massive quantities.

Further investigations showed that when the lactate in LR was replaced with other sources of energy that could be better used by the mitochondria, the inflammatory aspects were attenuated. One such novel fluid was ketone Ringer's solution (Table 4-8). Lactic acid occurs in two stereoisomeric forms as well as in a true racemic mixture of the isomers. In biologic systems, the true racemic mixture or equal molarity of the isomers rarely occurs. Usually, one or the other isomer predominates. The stereoisomers are named L(+) and D(−) lactic acid. L(+)-Lactate is a normal intermediary of mammalian metabolism. The isomer D(−)-lactate is produced when tissue glyoxalase converts methylglyoxal into a lactic acid of the D form, such as in lactose-fermenting bacteria. L(+)-Lactate has low toxicity as a consequence of the rapid metabolism. D(−)-Lactate, however, has higher toxic potential. Psychoneurotic disturbances have been described with pure D(−)-lactate. Increasing evidence has indicated a connection between high plasma concentration of racemic lactate and anxiety and panic disorders. Racemic dialysis fluids have reportedly been associated with clinical cases of D-lactate toxicity. Experiments with the isomers have shown that D(−)-lactate causes significant inflammatory changes in rats and swine as well as activation of human neutrophils.

In 1999, with the new information implicating LR as the cause of ARDS and MODS, the U.S. Navy contracted with the Institute of Medicine to review the topic of the optimal resuscitation fluid.[43] The report made many recommendations; key recommendations were that LR be manufactured with only the L(+) isomer of lactate and that researchers continue to search for alternative resuscitation fluids that do not contain lactate but rather other nutrients, such as ketones. It stated that the optimal resuscitation fluid is 7.5% HTS because of the decreased inflammation associated with it as well as its logistic advantage in terms of weight and size. Although the Institute of Medicine had been asked to make recommendations for the military, the report's authors thought that the evidence was applicable to civilian injuries as well. The U.S. military also requested Baxter, among others manufacturers of LR, to eliminate D(−)-lactate in LR, which it has done. The LR from Baxter currently contains only the L(+)-lactate isomer.

HTS has a long record of research and development. It has been used in humans for decades and has been consistently shown to be less inflammatory than LR. This showed from an immunologic point of view that HTS is better than LR and that LR is worse than HTS. Although this is stating the same thing, it is a paradigm shift in recognizing that LR and normal saline may be detrimental. Again, blood is complex, and the fluids used in the past were a poor replacement.

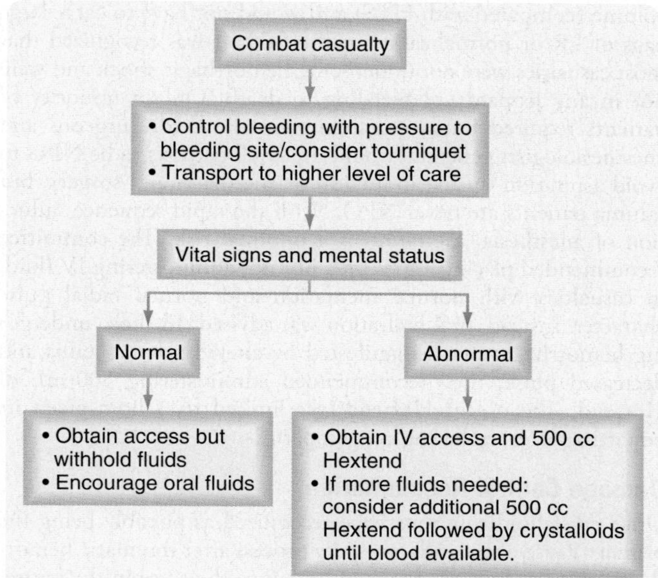

FIGURE 4-17 New recommendation for fluid resuscitation from the U.S. military by the Committee on Tactical Combat Casualty Care. (From Rhee P, Koustova E, Alam H: Searching for the optimal resuscitation method: Recommendations for the initial fluid resuscitation in combat casualties. *J Trauma* 54:S52-S62, 2003.)

It was also being recognized that PRBCs are different from whole blood and a poor replacement of whole blood lost during hemorrhage. PRBCs are separated by centrifuge, washed, and then filtered. Much of the plasma and its content are decanted out. Clotting factors, glucose, hormones, and cytokines crucial for signaling are not in PRBCs or in most of the fluids formerly used for resuscitation. Evidence that the fluid type affects the inflammatory response is now growing and has been confirmed in a number of studies.[44]

The Committee on Tactical Combat Casualty Care was formed in 2000 by the U.S. Navy and now sets policy on the prehospital management of combat casualties. Their recommendations and algorithm for resuscitation were revolutionary compared with the civilian recommendations (Fig. 4-17). The algorithm was formed with the following points in mind:

1. Most combat casualties do not require fluid resuscitation.
2. Oral hydration is an underused option as most combat casualties require resuscitation.
3. Aggressive resuscitation has not been shown to be beneficial in civilian victims of penetrating trauma.

4. Moderate resuscitation in animal models of uncontrolled hemorrhage offers the best outcome.
5. Large volumes of LR are not safe.
6. Colloid or HTS offers a significant advantage in terms of less weight and cube for the military medic or corpsman.

As crystalloids were being recognized as potentially harmful to bleeding patients, a consensus panel of military experts recommended that a plasma volume expander, 6% hetastarch, should be the fluid of choice for the military.[45] The rationale was that even though the Institute of Medicine recommended 7.5% HTS, it was not commercially available and it was not approved by the FDA for use in bleeding patients. The panel believed that a colloid offered the benefit of less weight and cube, meaning that the average medic could resuscitate patients with one third of the volume (compared with HTS) and would not have to carry large bags of LR or normal saline in the field. It was recognized that most casualties were not undergoing hemorrhagic shock and were not in any jeopardy of bleeding to death. Only a minority of patients required fluid resuscitation in the field. Surgeons and anesthesiologists generally would prefer all patients to be NPO to avoid aspiration during induction of anesthesia and surgery, but trauma patients are never NPO. With the rapid sequence induction of anesthesia, aspiration is a minimal risk. The committee recommended placing an IV line, but not administering IV fluid, in casualties with normal mentation and normal radial pulse character. Instead, oral hydration was advised. In those undergoing hemorrhagic shock manifested by altered mental status and decreased pulse, they recommended administering 500 mL of Hextend. The use of Hextend was limited to 1 liter, given its potential for exacerbating coagulopathy.

Damage Control Resuscitation

Once crystalloid solutions were recognized as possibly being the primary cause of the inflammatory process after traumatic hemorrhagic shock, efforts were made to reduce their use in the battlefield. Abdominal compartment syndrome (Fig. 4-18), which had been described after aggressive resuscitation, was also found to be directly associated with the volume of crystalloid infused. Thus, the concept of damage control resuscitation or hemostatic resuscitation was developed.[46] It involved concentrating on rapid control of bleeding as the highest priority; using permissive hypotension, because this would minimize the use of acellular fluids as well as potential disruption of natural clot formation; minimizing the use of crystalloid solutions; using HTS to reduce the total volume of crystalloid necessary; using blood products early; and considering the use of drugs, such as rFVIIa or factor IX, to stop bleeding and to reduce coagulopathy (Box 4-2). The rationale for the early use of blood products was that large volumes of crystalloids were detrimental; because fresh whole blood was not available, component therapy with PRBCs, thawed plasma, and platelets would approximate whole blood and minimize the use of acellular fluids. Component therapy was not ideal compared with fresh whole blood. However, because of logistic problems, it was not readily available, and component therapy was to be used empirically for massively bleeding patients with ongoing uncontrolled hemorrhage. Mental status was thought to be a useful guide to determine who needed care; the use of the radial pulse was preferred to BP cuffs, which are not practical when personnel are under fire in the combat setting.

With the promotion of damage control resuscitation, clinical studies indicated that aggressive early use of blood products, such as PRBCs and FFP, actually reduced the total volume of PRBCs used by 25%.[47] These studies also used permissive hypotension and focused on surgical control of hemorrhage rather than on resuscitation before surgical control of hemorrhage. Other studies have shown that with damage control resuscitation, the incidence of ARDS decreases, from 25% of ICU admissions to 9%.[48] ARDS now occurs in patients with pulmonary contusion, pneumonia, or sepsis, but it is no longer a routine complication in trauma patients who undergo damage control resuscitation.

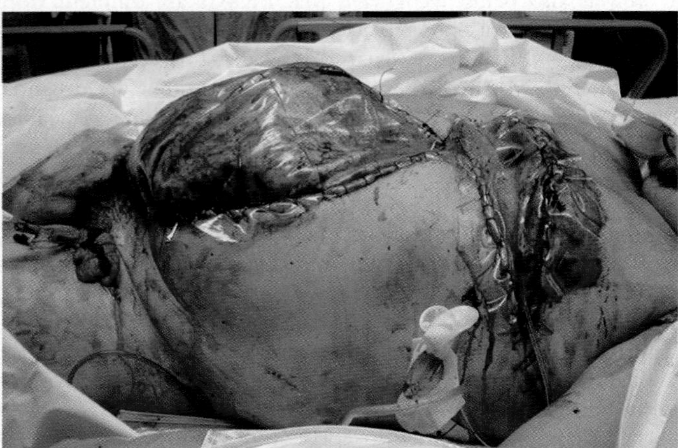

FIGURE 4-18 Patient after damage control surgery with abdominal and thoracic compartment syndrome caused by massive fluid resuscitation. (Courtesy Dr. Demetri Demetriades, Trauma Recovery Surgical Critical Care Program, USC University Hospital, Los Angeles.)

Whole Blood Resuscitation

Damage control resuscitation was developed because surgeons in the recent war in Iraq came back and stated that fresh whole blood was useful for massively bleeding soldiers. Although the surgeons early in this war were hesitant and reluctant to try the walking blood bank (see later) that was used to obtain fresh whole blood from noncombat soldiers, eventually it was tried and found to be highly successful and easy. Returning military surgeons repeatedly noted that patients resuscitated with whole blood did not seem to have the coagulation or pulmonary problems seen previously. After operative procedures, even patients who underwent several blood volume replacement procedures were warm, not acidotic, and not coagulopathic. Trauma surgeons were starting to recognize that crystalloid resuscitation should and could be avoided by using damage control resuscitation. Because they had only recently started to recognize that currently used fluids had an impact on outcome, they had not yet had a chance to develop the optimal resuscitation fluid to replace blood. As a result, military surgeons

BOX 4-2 Components of Damage Control or Hemostatic Resuscitation

- Permissive hypotension until definitive surgical control
- Minimize crystalloid use
- Initial use of 5% hypertonic saline
- Early use of blood products (PRBCs, FFP, platelets, cryoprecipitates)
- Consider drugs to treat coagulopathy (rFVIIa, prothrombin concentrate, TXA)

From Dellinger RP, Levy MM, Carlet JM, et al: Surviving Sepsis Campaign: International guidelines for management of severe sepsis and septic shock: 2008. *Crit Care Med* 36:296–327, 2008.

advocated the aggressive use of FFP, not because it was ideal but because it was probably better than crystalloid or colloidal solutions.

The military has a logistic advantage that the civilian sector does not yet have. When casualties arrive, military surgeons activate the walking blood bank, resulting in hundreds of noncombatant soldiers on the base coming to the medical facility to donate their blood. Given the relative safety of these donors from an infectious aspect as they were all prescreened and they had been previously blood typed as denoted on their dog tags, fresh whole blood was readily available. In the military, when surgical units are available, it is usually at a base where many do not go out on patrol and can donate blood. Obviously, those in combat roles are not eligible to donate because they would no longer be fit to be combatants. Bleeding patients were transfused with PRBCs and given HTS and crystalloid solution until fresh whole blood was available, usually within about 30 minutes after activation of the walking blood bank.

When military surgeons receive a warning about incoming casualties, they can activate the walking blood bank ahead of their arrival even sooner. The blood is withdrawn and mixed with 50 to 100 mL of citrate-phosphate-dextrose, which binds calcium and prevents clotting in the bag. The bag of fresh whole blood is then transfused within minutes after donation. Hypocalcemia can occur from citrate-phosphate-dextrose, and it is recommended that ionized calcium levels be monitored and 10 mL of 10% calcium chloride be administered if needed as hypocalcemia can contribute to coagulopathy.

When the military started its practice of using whole blood, no data supported it. Reports eventually emerged showing its safety and efficacy, even when PRBCs were readily available,[49] and now coalition forces have also started the practice of whole blood transfusions. The controversy about the use of fresh whole blood will continue because randomized prospective studies are not logistically feasible in the war zone. It is important to note that fresh whole blood is different from banked refrigerated whole blood.

Resuscitation With 1:1:1

As news of these successful battlefield practices spread, the civilian literature started to echo the benefits of surgical hemorrhage control before resuscitation and the aggressive use of PRBCs and FFP, summarized in Table 4-9. Because whole blood was not available in the civilian sector, efforts focused on trying to re-create whole blood by transfusing components of blood together. It had been thought that component therapy needed to be directed by laboratory results. Surgeons could transfuse only patients with documented coagulopathy and could transfuse only the necessary components. Empirical use was discouraged.

Whole blood is separated into its various components by centrifugation. The plasma is drawn off and separated into fibrinogen and platelets. PRBCs, with a hematocrit level of 60% to 70%, are washed, anticoagulants and preservatives are added, and then they are stored. Component separation has made the best use of whole blood, reducing waste. However, component therapy is analogous to eating coffee beans, sugar, cream, and hot water separately to make coffee internally.

The U.S. Army reported its success with the aggressive use of FFP, largely because of the efforts of Colonel Holcomb, who had access to the Military Trauma Registry. Registry data have consistently confirmed the benefits of transfusing blood components in a ratio of 1 unit of PRBCs to 1 unit of FFP to 1 unit of platelets, a ratio now termed 1 : 1 : 1. In a civilian setting, Maegele and colleagues have reported that the aggressive use of FFP also resulted in improved outcome. Duchesne and associates wondered whether they might have been wrong for 60 years by not being aggressive with FFP and showed in another study that it reduced mortality and coagulopathy.

Tiexaira and coworkers have shown that although it is better to be aggressive, the ratio of 1 unit of PRBCs to 2 units of FFP may be equivalent. The previous studies had a tendency to place patients with a 1 : 2 ratio into the aggressive group and could not clearly distinguish among 1 : 1 versus 1 : 2 versus 1 : 3. Other studies also failed to find a survival benefit with FFP but showed that it reduces coagulopathy. Aggressive use of platelets[50] and fibrinogen[51] has also been shown to improve outcome. In a six-center retrospective study, Zink and associates[52] have shown that the early administration of a high ratio of FFP and platelets improves survival and decreases overall need for PRBCs in massively transfused patients. The largest difference in mortality occurred during the first 6 hours after admission, suggesting that the early administration of FFP and platelets is critical. Most hospitals use apheresis platelets, which are pooled platelets; 1 unit is equivalent to what was previously called a six-pack of platelets.

There have been multiple studies using large databases and prospective studies trying to determine if aggressive use of FFP and platelets can lead to improved outcome. It was argued that the studies showing an advantage were flawed in that they suffered from selection bias, whereby early survivors lived long enough to be given blood products. The PROMMTT study demonstrated that clinicians were transfusing patients with a blood product ratio of 1 : 1 : 1 or 1 : 1 : 2 and that early transfusion of plasma was associated with improved 6-hour survival.[53]

The most recent addition to this debate is the PROPPR trial. This study was a prospective randomized multicenter clinical trial. It was an effectiveness and safety study in severe bleeding trauma patients using plasma, platelets, and red blood cells in a 1 : 1 : 1 ratio to 1 : 1 : 2 ratio.[54] The primary outcomes were 24-hour and 30-day all-cause mortality. It showed that there was no significant difference in mortality at 24 hours ($P = .12$) or at 30 days ($P = .26$). However, more patients in the 1 : 1 : 1 group achieved hemostasis and fewer experienced death as a result of exsanguination by 24 hours. There were no safety differences between the two groups. The 1 : 1 : 1 group received more blood product but did not experience high rates of ARDS or MODS, infection, venous thromboembolism, or sepsis. Holcomb and colleagues suggested that clinicians should consider using a 1 : 1 : 1 transfusion protocol, starting with the initial units transfused while patients are actively bleeding and then transitioning to laboratory-guided treatment once hemorrhage control is achieved. The authors also noted that the 1 : 1 : 2 group approached a cumulative ratio of 1 : 1 : 1 after the initial ratio-driven protocol ended as they used laboratory-guided treatment, which caused them to catch up to the 1 : 1 : 1 group.

Massive Transfusion Protocol

Studies have led to the development of the massive transfusion protocol (MTP), which calls for the aggressive use of component therapy. The protocol was designed to enable a hospital's blood bank to improve logistic systems for the empirical use of blood components. A number of studies have shown that implementing an MTP improves survival in trauma patients.[55] To qualify as a trauma center, the American College of Surgeons Verification

TABLE 4-9 Summaries of Recent Retrospective Studies on the Use of Fresh-Frozen Plasma

ARTICLE	SUMMARY OF FINDINGS
Borgman MA, Spinella PC, Perkins JG, et al: The ratio of blood products transfused affects mortality in patients receiving massive transfusions at a combat support hospital. *J Trauma* 63:805–813, 2007.	Retrospective study of 246 patients; PRBC : FFP ratio group of 1 : 1.4 had better survival rates.
Gonzalez EA, Moore FA, Holcomb JB, et al: Fresh frozen plasma should be given earlier to patients requiring massive transfusion. *J Trauma* 62:112–119, 2007.	Retrospective study of 97 patients; they recommended early use of FFP before ICU admission.
Kashuk JL, Moore EE, Johnson JL, et al: Postinjury life threatening coagulopathy: Is 1:1 fresh frozen plasma:packed red blood cells the answer? *J Trauma* 65:261–270, 2008.	Retrospective study of 133 patients; logistic regression showed improved coagulopathy but no improvement in survival.
Gunter OL, Jr, Au BK, Isbell JM, et al: Optimizing outcomes in damage control resuscitation: Identifying blood product ratios associated with improved survival. *J Trauma* 65:527–534, 2008.	Retrospective study of 259 patients; increased use of FFP and platelets improved survival after major trauma.
Holcomb JB, Wade CE, Michalek JE, et al: Increased plasma and platelet to red blood cell ratios improves outcome in 466 massively transfused civilian trauma patients. *Ann Surg* 248:447–458, 2008.	Retrospective study of 467 patients undergoing transfusion of 10 units of PRBCs or more; survival was better with increased use of FFP and platelets.
Spinella PC, Perkins JG, Grathwohl KW, et al: Effect of plasma and red blood cell transfusions on survival in patients with combat related traumatic injuries. *J Trauma* 64:S69–S77, 2008.	708 patients undergoing transfusion showed that FFP use was associated with improved survival.
Maegele M, Lefering R, Paffrath T, et al: Red-blood-cell to plasma ratios transfused during massive transfusion are associated with mortality in severe multiple injury: A retrospective analysis from the Trauma Registry of the Deutsche Gesellschaft für Unfallchirurgie. *Vox Sang* 95:112–119, 2008.	Retrospective study of 713 patients showed improved survival with increased aggressive use of FFP in patients undergoing massive transfusion.
Duchesne JC, Hunt JP, Wahl G, et al: Review of current blood transfusions strategies in a mature level I trauma center: Were we wrong for the last 60 years? *J Trauma* 65:272–276, 2008.	Retrospective study of 135 patients with massive transfusions who had better outcome with 1 : 1.
Sperry JL, Ochoa JB, Gunn SR, et al: An FFP : PRBC transfusion ratio ≥1 : 1.5 is associated with a lower risk of mortality after massive transfusion. *J Trauma* 65:986–993, 2008.	Multicenter prospective cohort study with 415 patients showed that higher FFP use was associated with less mortality.
Moore FA, Nelson T, McKinley BA, et al: Is there a role for aggressive use of fresh frozen plasma in massive transfusion of civilian trauma patients? *Am J Surg* 196:948–958, 2008.	Retrospective study of 93 patients; concluded that damage control resuscitation with FFP may have a role in civilian trauma.
Teixeira PG, Inaba K, Shulman I, et al: Impact of plasma transfusion in massively transfused trauma patients. *J Trauma* 66:693–697, 2009.	Retrospective study of 383 patients showing that high FFP use was associated with better survival.
Duchesne JC, Islam TM, Stuke L, et al: Hemostatic resuscitation during surgery improves survival in patients with traumatic-induced coagulopathy. *J Trauma* 67:33–37, 2009.	Seven-year retrospective study with 435 patients showed survival advantage in patients receiving FFP : RBC ratio of 1 : 1 compared with 1 : 4.
Snyder CW, Weinberg JA, McGwin G Jr, et al: The relationship of blood product ratio to mortality: Survival benefit or survival bias? *J Trauma* 66:358–362, 2009.	Retrospective study of 134 patients showed improved survival with higher use of FFP, but the advantage was not persistent when adjusted for survival bias.
Watson GA, Sperry JL, Rosengart MR, et al: Fresh frozen plasma is independently associated with a higher risk of multiple organ failure and acute respiratory distress syndrome. *J Trauma* 67:221–227, 2009.	Prospective multicenter cohort study of blunt trauma patients showed that FFP was associated with increased risk of multiple-organ failure and ARDS.
Zink KA, Sambasivan CN, Holcomb JB, et al: A high ratio of plasma and platelets to packed red blood cells in the first 6 hours of massive transfusion improves outcomes in a large multicenter study. *Am J Surg* 197:565–570, 2009.	Retrospective multicenter (16) study with 466 patients who had lower mortality if FFP and platelets were used early and as 1 : 1.
Riskin DJ, Tsai TC, Riskin L, et al: Massive transfusion protocols: The role of aggressive resuscitation versus product ratio in mortality reduction. *J Am Coll Surg* 209:198–205, 2009.	Retrospective study of 77 patients; concluded that massive transfusion protocol was associated with improved survival.

Review Committee recommends that all trauma centers have their own MTP in place.

An example of an MTP directive is that for severely injured patients, the blood bank should bring a cooler with 2 units of unmatched O-negative blood that can be immediately used for resuscitation (Table 4-10). Most patients do not require massive transfusion, usually defined as a transfusion of more than 10 units of PRBCs in 24 hours. If possible, a patient's blood sample should be drawn before the uncrossmatched blood is transfused; even 1 unit of PRBCs can sometimes interfere with crossmatching. If a patient requires more PRBCs before crossmatched blood is available, an additional 4 units of O-negative blood should be made available. If crossmatched blood is available, the next 4 units transfused should be crossmatched blood.

Because most patients do not require more than 6 units of PRBCs, most do not receive FFP. For patients who require more PRBCs, 7 to 12 units of PRBCs should be delivered along with 6 units of FFP and 1 unit of apheresis platelets. Preferably, the FFP and platelets should be transfused first, before the next 6 units of PRBCs are transfused. Thus, for a severely injured patient who will require massive transfusion, the ratio now starts to approach the preferred 1 : 1 : 1 ratio. The "trick" that has gained popularity is to attach a large visible label on the back of all the blood products and to number them sequentially; thus, the

TABLE 4-10 Massive Transfusion Protocol at the University of Arizona

	COOLER 1	COOLER 2	COOLER 3	COOLER 4	COOLER 5	COOLER 6
Units of PRBCs	2	4	6	6	6	6
Units of FFP			6	6	6	6
Units of platelets			1	1		1
Units of cryoprecipitate				20		10

Platelets are pooled and are equivalent to a six-pack of platelets. The sample is immediately sent for type and cross and coagulation profile. Coolers 3 and higher have crossmatched PRBCs. Coolers 7, 9, 11, 13, and 15 have the same contents as cooler 5. Coolers 8, 10, 12, and 14 have the same contents as cooler 6. Each unit has a large label with the number on it.

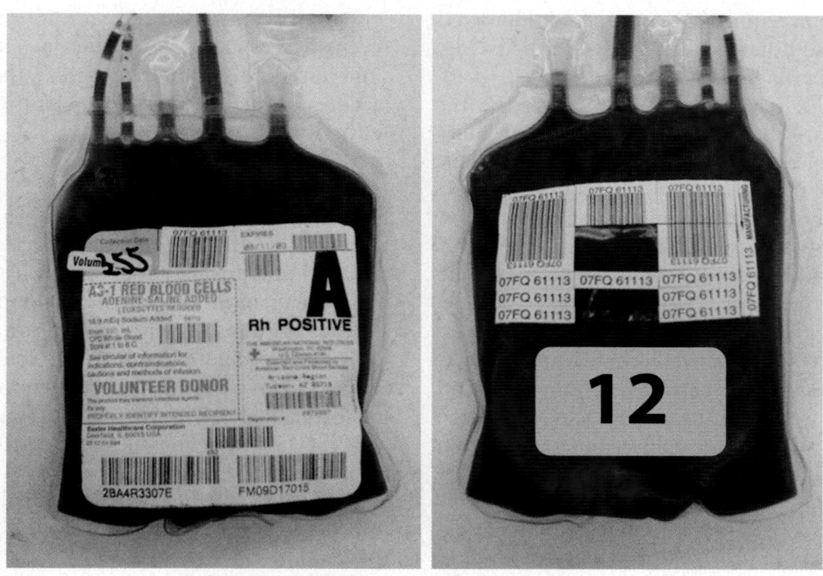

FIGURE 4-19 Label on back of transfused unit.

emergency department, operating room, or ICU personnel can always quickly determine which unit of PRBCs, FFP, or platelets is being transfused (Fig. 4-19). The use of uncrossmatched blood is a predictor of the need for the MPT, but it has also been associated with complications such as ARDS and sepsis.[56]

Our current approach—namely, allowing permissive hypotension, minimizing crystalloid resuscitation, using HTS, and aggressively using blood and blood products—may seem obvious now, but it is different from the approach used 15 years ago. It is now becoming recognized that whole blood is highly complex and that crystalloids do not resemble blood in any way. Crystalloids are acceptable when they are used for rehydrating patients, for providing daily water needs, and for delivering electrolytes into the veins, but they can be harmful when they are used to replace liters of lost blood in the massive quantities formerly used. Not that long ago, more than 30 liters of fluid might have been administered within a few hours after a trauma patient arrived at the trauma center.

CURRENT STATUS OF FLUID TYPES

Crystalloids

The mechanism responsible for acidosis, after large volumes of normal saline are infused, is the dilution of serum bicarbonate (HCO_3^-) through the replacement of lost plasma with fluids that do not contain bicarbonate. Normally, chloride and bicarbonate ions are reciprocated up or down with each other. Often, the result of massive normal saline infusion is a hyperchloremic anion gap metabolic acidosis. At extreme levels, acidosis can impair cardiac performance and decrease responsiveness to cardiac inotropic drugs. Many would argue that for cellular protection, the human body offloads oxygen more easily from hemoglobin in the acidotic state and that acidosis, at least to a degree, is actually better for a patient than alkalosis.

Regardless of the theoretical advantages and disadvantages of induced metabolic acidosis, no clinical evidence exists that it makes a difference. Surgeons with experience using HTS sometimes encounter induced metabolic acidosis but have found it to be of minimal clinical consequence. Induced metabolic hyperchloremic acidosis is different from spontaneous metabolic acidosis and from hypovolemic lactic acidosis. No evidence exists that hyperchloremic acidosis does anything more than confuse the interpretation of the metabolic state. Given the lack of any significant proven benefit of one crystalloid over another, many trauma systems use normal saline in the prehospital setting. This is because stocking just one form of fluid is convenient. Another reason is that when transfusion is required, the LR has to be switched to normal saline as LR contains calcium and is contraindicated. This is a regulatory policy even though studies have shown that the use of LR as a carrier in the same IV line as blood has no relevant side effects.

Plasma-Lyte (Baxter, Deerfield, Ill), a balanced crystalloid solution, was developed more than 20 years ago and contains additional electrolytes, such as acetate and gluconate. The overall chloride level is also lower. Plasma-Lyte also contains magnesium, so care should be taken in patients with renal failure. It may also affect peripheral vascular resistance and heart rate, and it may worsen organ ischemia. It is similar to other crystalloids in that it can cause lung edema and increase ICP and generalized edema. The numerous reports of its use have addressed its safety during the priming of extracorporeal circulation pumps and its use in cold ischemia, circulatory arrest, organ transplantation, and organ preservation.

In a study examining the use of HTS with dextran (HTSD), patients were randomized to receive 7.5% HTSD or Plasma-Lyte A. The 2-hour sodium, bicarbonate, CO_2, and pH values were comparable. The HTSD group required less crystalloid. However, the volumes infused were also different. In a study by McFarlane, 30 patients undergoing hepatobiliary or pancreatic surgery were randomized to 0.9% normal saline or Plasma-Lyte 148 at 15 mL/kg/hr. During surgery, Plasma-Lyte was found to be more efficacious. It was balanced, with less hyperchloremia and base deficit. However, no significant difference in sodium, potassium, or blood lactate level was found in either group. In a kidney transplantation study, Plasma-Lyte A did not increase lactate levels (like LR) and did not cause acidosis (like normal saline); the best metabolic profile was maintained in patients receiving Plasma-Lyte A. Plasma-Lyte is also favored in various cell preparations and as a storage medium for platelets. Compared with LR and normal saline, Plasma-Lyte may be a better balanced solution, but no studies exist that show it is safe or more efficacious in large volumes. It may be an ideal solution for daily maintenance fluid, but it does not offer a significant benefit for resuscitation more than other crystalloids. A randomized trial by Young and colleagues showed that compared with normal saline, patients resuscitated with Plasma-Lyte A had improved acid-base status and less hyperchloremia at 24 hours after injury.[57] The components of the various crystalloids are shown in Table 4-11. In summary, there are advantages and disadvantages for various crystalloids. Plasma-Lyte has the advantage in that it has magnesium, and studies have shown that this reduces the need for magnesium replacement, although there are concerns of infusing large volumes of Plasma-Lyte as it can infuse too much magnesium. From the chloride point of view, LR may be better than Plasma-Lyte, which may be better than normal saline. In a large volume, there may be advantages of resuscitating with LR as it has the least amount of chloride. There seems to be no studies showing survival advantage with any crystalloids. In short-term hemorrhagic shock studies in swine using large volumes of crystalloids, LR was shown to be better than normal saline and Plasma-Lyte. In most institutions, the costs of LR, normal saline, and Plasma-Lyte are similar, which is about $3.00. If LR is to be used, it should be the LR manufactured by Baxter, which currently makes LR with only the L(+)-lactate isomer, and it does not contain the D(−)-lactate isomer. Human studies from Asia are reporting better outcome with LR with L(+)-lactate isomer. D(−)-Lacate but not L(+)-lactate was significantly associated with increased mortality. Mechanical ventilation, irrespective of whether it was started within or beyond 48 hours of admission, explained most of the variation in morality. L(+)-Lactate decreased and D(−)-lactate increased the use of mechanical ventilation starting later than 48 hours after admission. Physicians should recognize the harmful effects of D(−)-lactate and the beneficial effects of L(+)-lactate in real-life clinical settings.[58]

Hypertonic Saline

HTS has been extensively studied. In summary, the studies have shown that sodium is the main electrolyte that controls intravascular volume. Investigators who have worked with HTS in bleeding animals have learned that to obtain a physiologic response, the same response as with an infusion of large volumes of crystalloids can be achieved with a much smaller volume as long as the sodium load is the same. For example, in an animal model of hemorrhagic shock, if 1 liter of normal saline is required to achieve a BP of 120 mm Hg, the same result can be obtained with an infusion of 120 mL of 7.5% normal saline. For 5% HTS, only 182 mL would be needed. In animal studies, HTS draws water into the intravascular space from the intracellular and interstitial spaces.

HTS has consistently been shown to reduce the inflammatory response and is thus considered to be immunomodulatory (Fig. 4-20). Immunosuppression from HTS may thus be beneficial and detrimental, depending on when and how it is used. In randomized prospective studies with HTS alone or with a colloid such as hetastarch or dextran, results show that HTS is equivalent to crystalloid solutions in terms of mortality. The concentration that has been studied the most is 7.5% HTS. From 1995 to 2005, when inflammation was being extensively studied, the theoretical advantages of HTS were a decrease in the inflammatory response and potentially a reduction in ARDS and MODS. Thus, it was

TABLE 4-11 Commercially Available Crystalloids and Their Composition

	NORMAL SALINE	LACTATED RINGER'S	PLASMA-LYTE A	NORMOSOL	PLASMA
Positive Ions					
Sodium	154	130	140	140	134-145
Potassium		4	5	5	3.4-5
Calcium		3			2.25-2.65
Magnesium			3	3	0.7-1.1
Negative Ions					
Chloride	154	109	98	98	98-108
Lactate		28	27	27	
Bicarbonate					22-32
Gluconate			23	23	
pH	5.4-7.0	6.5	7.4	7.4	7.4
Osmolarity	308	273	294	295	280-295

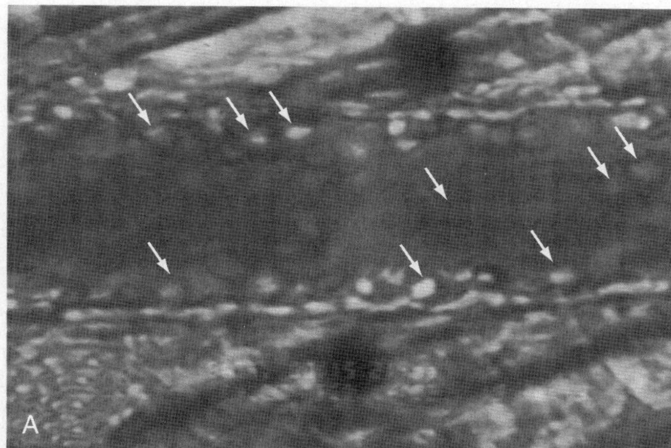

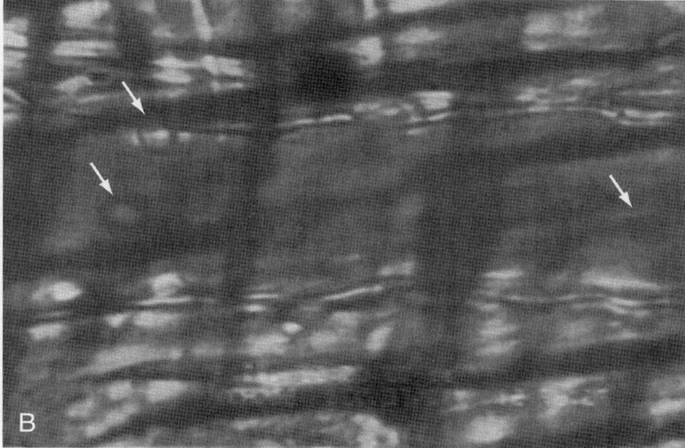

FIGURE 4-20 Immunologic response from hypertonic resuscitation is less than that after LR has been given. (From Pascual JL, Khwaja KA, Ferri LE, et al: Hypertonic saline resuscitation attenuates neutrophil lung sequestration and transmigration by diminishing leukocyte-endothelial interactions in a two-hit model of hemorrhagic shock and infection. *J Trauma* 54:121–132, 2003.)

thought to be potentially the ideal fluid of choice in hemorrhagic shock resuscitation. One of the main problems with 7.5% HTS is that there is no manufacturer that makes and sells it. This is because it is extremely difficult and expensive to obtain FDA approval, and there is probably no profit in selling salt water. In Europe, 7.5% HTS with dextran is available.

The Resuscitation Outcomes Consortium (ROC), which is composed of 10 trauma centers in the United States and Canada, has been funded to participate in trauma and emergency medicine trials. ROC is a federally funded organization to examine potential prehospital interventions.

The first trauma trial by ROC examined HTS. This prospective randomized trial enrolled hypotensive patients (systolic BP <70 mm Hg) with blunt or penetrating trauma, with and without traumatic head injury. Patients were randomized into one of three arms by dose and fluid: (1) 250-mL bolus of normal saline; (2) 250-mL bolus of 7.5% HTS; and (3) 250-mL of 7.5% HTS with 6% dextran 70. The HTS trial enrolled 2221 patients using a community consent process. There were two studies in this trial. One enrolled 894 patients into the hemorrhagic shock study and 1327 patients into the TBI study. The TBI trial enrolled patients with or without hypotension; the main enrollment criterion was a GCS score of 8 or less.

The HTS shock trial showed that patients receiving HTS had only a mild elevation in their sodium level (147 mEq/liter versus 140 mEq/liter in the normal saline group) as the infusion volume was small and only in the prehospital setting. The admission hemoglobin level was also significantly different. The patients who received HTS with or without dextran had a hemoglobin level of 10.2 g/dL compared with 11.1 g/dL in the normal saline group. This may reflect the amount of intravascular resuscitation from HTS versus normal saline. The overall 28-day survival rates were almost identical: HTS patients, 73%; HTS with dextran patients, 74.5%; and normal saline patients, 74.4% ($P = .91$).

However, the HTS trial was stopped before the end of its planned enrollment by the Drug Safety and Monitoring Board for two main reasons. First, interim analysis showed futility because the outcomes were so similar. Second, a detailed subgroup analysis found a potential for harm in a subgroup of patients who did not receive PRBC transfusion in the first 24 hours. For unexplained reasons, their mortality rate was significantly higher if they received HTS or HTS with dextran. HTS and HTS with dextran patients who received more than 10 units of PRBCs within the first 24 hours had a lower mortality rate, although the difference was not statistically significant.

The main criticism of this study was that it allowed only a small dose in the prehospital phase, and HTS infusion did not continue at the hospital. Also, the sodium level was raised to only 147 mEq/liter, signifying that not enough HTS was used to affect the immunomodulatory capability of HTS as some feel that the sodium level needs to be much higher to achieve that affect. In hypotensive patients, 250 mL of normal saline is clinically irrelevant, but because 250 mL of HTS with dextran D or HTS is approximately equivalent to 2 liters of normal saline, the group of patients who received HTS were being resuscitated more, whereas the normal saline group was not. Thus, the trial seemed to compare 250 mL of normal saline to the equivalent of 2 liters of normal saline. Support for this theory is that the hemoglobin level was lower in the group of patients who received HTS. The trial of HTS in patients with TBI was also halted; the interim analysis also showed futility, meaning that the primary outcome was almost identical between the normal saline and HTS groups. Such an outcome can also be interpreted as showing that HTS is safe, but technically the trial was not powered to show noninferiority.

HTS was studied in TBI because preliminary studies had shown promise. HTS infusion is highly effective in decreasing ICP and can do this while increasing blood volume, BP, and blood flow to the brain. Compared with mannitol, which is customarily used for lowering ICP, HTS might do this without dehydrating patients or putting them at further risk for secondary brain injury caused by hypotension or renal failure from mannitol. Patients receiving high-dose mannitol drips are also susceptible to pulmonary insufficiency, causing longer ICU stays. Infusion of mannitol requires high daily volumes. Mannitol is safe if it is used carefully in patients with isolated TBIs, but in hypotensive multitrauma patients, it can be detrimental and might cause hypotension.

Commercially, HTS comes in 23%, 5%, and 3% concentrations in the United States. Curiously, all the human studies used 7.5% HTS, which is not commercially available. This could be the main strategic mistake of the HTS studies. Most animal and human studies have used 7.5% HTS, an arbitrary concentration as 10% HTS was found to be highly irritating to peripheral veins. HTS injected rapidly into human volunteers causes pain at the infusion site. Thus, the preferred route is through the central vein.

In animal studies, if 7.5% HTS is given through the interosseous route, osteomyonecrosis and compartment syndrome can ensue. Some nontrauma studies have used 3% and 23% concentrations, but minimal clinical experience has been reported with 5%. There are two studies reporting their experience using 5% HTS in trauma patients, with or without TBI, and it has been found to be safe.[59] This finding is logical because the 7.5% HTS studies have shown it to be safe. Using 5% HTS may be the best strategy to recruit intravascular volume compared with crystalloid resuscitation. The method used in trauma patients is to give 5% HTS in 250-mL infusions and, if more than 500 mL is needed, to check sodium levels. The sodium content of 250 mL of 5% HTS is equivalent to 1645 mL of LR. Thus, a bolus can be given quickly, without having to use hypotonic solutions such as LR. If 500 mL of 5% HTS is used in acute trauma patients, some believe that can resuscitate patients without having to give 3 liters of a crystalloid solution. That belief complies with the concept of damage control resuscitation, in which one of the goals is to minimize crystalloid use.

Colloids

Human albumin (4% to 5%) in saline is considered to be the reference colloidal solution. It is fractionated from blood and heat treated to prevent transmission of viruses. It has many theoretical advantages, especially in animal studies, but clinical studies have not been able to show outcome differences. Its main theoretical advantage is that compared with crystalloids, it is less inflammatory. This may be because it is a natural molecule, not artificial. Other than its dilutional effect, albumin is associated with minimal coagulopathy. No clinical evidence has shown that albumin is better than other colloids, but the SAFE study in Australia has shown 4% albumin to be safe, compared with normal saline, in ICU patients.[60] The SAFE study, whose main intent was to show equivalency, found no difference in the primary outcome (28-day mortality rate) or in any secondary outcome. The Committee on Tactical Combat Casualty Care has recommended a low-volume resuscitation fluid using 500 mL of Hextend, for tactical reasons. The reason for that choice was that 7.5% HTS is not commercially available. The adoption of damage control or hemostatic resuscitation has been thought to result in improved outcome, decreased blood use, and decreased incidence of ARDS.[61] ARDS and MODS still occur, but at a much lower rate than previously seen. They seem to occur only in trauma patients with a pulmonary contusion or an infectious process, whereas ARDS and MODS were rampant in trauma patients.

There are still other advantages of 25% albumin over artificial colloids. It has a proven immunologic anti-inflammatory effect and five times less volume than current artificial colloids. Unlike artificial colloids, it does not potentially lead to coagulopathic side effects. It has been proven safe from infectious and clinical standpoints. The volume of fluid that has to be carried is obviously much less (Fig. 4-21). Albumin costs approximately 30 times more than crystalloids and three times more than dextran or Hextend, but those comparisons were made against 5% human albumin. The cost of 100 mL of 25% albumin, compared with 500 mL of Hextend on a physiologic basis, is only approximately three times as much. During the Vietnam War, 25% albumin was first made available, and it seemed to have worked well. It was packaged in a green can that could be transported without damage, had a long shelf life, and was easy to use.

The commonly used synthetic colloids are plasma, albumin, dextran, gelatin, and starch-based colloids. Hetastarch solutions are produced from amylopectin obtained from sorghum, maize, or potatoes. Extensive randomized controlled trials have examined the safety and efficacy of 5% albumin, 6% hetastarch, and 6% dextran. However, no evidence has shown that one colloid is superior to another or that colloids are better or worse than crystalloids.[62] Colloids such as hetastarch can have proinflammatory effects similar to those of crystalloids. In some cases, colloids will do more harm in large volumes than crystalloids, but not all colloids should be considered the same. It is well known that artificial colloids can perpetuate coagulopathy; dextran is used specifically to help prevent clotting after vascular surgery. The inflammatory system is tightly interwoven with the coagulation process. Hetastarch, particularly the high-molecular-weight preparations, is associated with alterations in coagulation, specifically resulting in changes in the viscoelastic measurements and fibrinolysis. Studies have questioned the safety of concentrated (10%) hetastarch solutions with a molecular weight of more than 200 and a molar substitution ratio of more than 0.5 in patients with severe sepsis, citing increased rates of death, acute kidney injury, and use of renal replacement therapy. To prolong intravascular expansion, a high degree of substitution on glucose molecules protects against hydrolysis by nonspecific amylases in the blood. However, this results in accumulation in reticuloendothelial tissues such as skin, liver, and kidneys. Because of the potential for accumulation in tissues, the recommended maximal daily dose of hetastarch is 33 to 55 mL/kg/day. Thus, it would be prudent to limit the use of Hextend to 1 liter in trauma patients, who are often harmed if they have coagulopathy from increased bleeding. Studies in trauma patients have shown an association between acute kidney injury and death after blunt trauma. Patients with severe sepsis

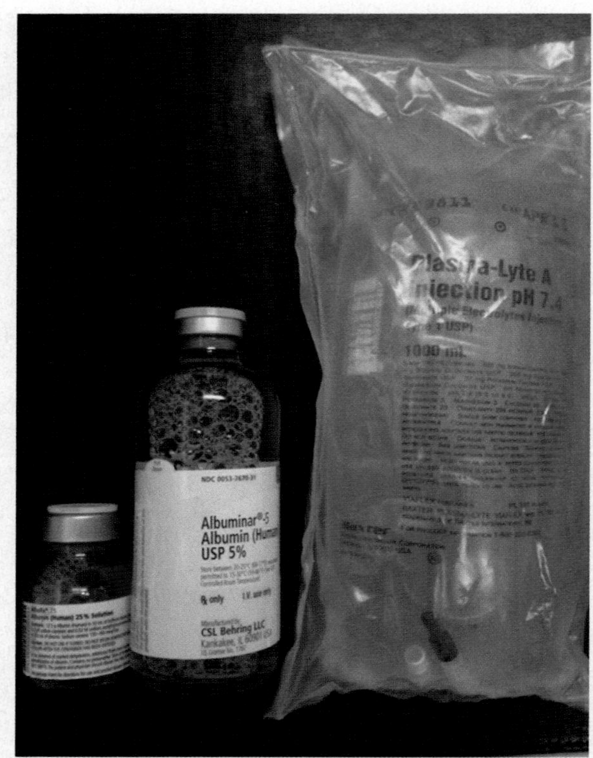

FIGURE 4-21 Comparison of container sizes: 50 mL of 25% albumin, 500 mL of 5% albumin, and 1 liter of LR. The 50 mL of 25% albumin is physiologically equivalent to approximately 2000 to 2500 mL of crystalloids.

assigned to fluid resuscitation with hydroxyethyl starch 130/0.4 had an increased risk of death at day 90 and were more likely to require renal replacement therapy compared with those receiving Ringer's acetate. In animal models, albumin seems to be better for preventing inflammation, whereas hetastarch and dextran, in high doses, appear to cause inflammation and coagulopathy.

FUTURE RESUSCITATION RESEARCH

Blood Substitutes

In contrast to volume expanders, blood substitutes refer to fluids that can carry oxygen. Each year in the United States, 15 million units of PRBCs are transfused. Methods to decrease the need for blood transfusions include preoperative autologous donation, intraoperative blood retrieval and reinfusion, and isovolemic hemodilutions. Such methods allow withdrawing of a patient's blood at the start of surgery, replacing it with volume expanders, and then, at the end of surgery, retransfusing the patient with his or her donated blood. Because of blood supply limitations, infectious and transfusion complications, and storage limitations, the need for blood substitutes remains. The ideal blood substitute would do the following:

- Deliver oxygen
- Require no compatibility testing
- Have few side effects
- Have prolonged storage capabilities
- Persist in the circulation
- Be cost-effective

Currently, blood substitutes are either hemoglobin based or nonhemoglobin based. Research on hemoglobin-based fluids dates back to the 1920s when the stroma of the cells was lysed to obtain hemoglobin. Purification and sterilization were hurdles that took decades to overcome, but it was soon realized that free hemoglobin had toxic effects (because of the breakdown products). Problems with free hemoglobin include osmotic diuretic effects, renal toxicity, coagulation abnormalities, short half-life, and vasoactive effect (which is known to be caused by hemoglobin solutions scavenging nitric oxide).

During the next 3 decades (the 1930s, 1940s, and 1950s), efforts concentrated on stabilizing the hemoglobin molecule to increase its persistence in the circulation and to prevent toxic effects. Such strategies included cross-linking the molecule between the tetramer subunits, polymerizing it, encapsulating it in an artificial red cell or in liposomes, and using microsphere technology to form a million stable micromolecules. Development of some hemoglobin substitutes advanced to clinical trials.

Blood substitutes are referred to as hemoglobin oxygen carriers (HBOCs). Current second-generation HBOCs are pasteurized and thus free of communicable pathogens; they also have no ABO/Rh or other blood antigens. They are universally compatible and require no blood banking. They can be easily administered without special training or expertise. The problems of a short half-life and renal toxicity have now been overcome, but some troublesome side effects remain: free radical generation and exacerbation of reperfusion injury, methemoglobin production, and immunologic effects (including immunosuppression and potentiation of endotoxin-related pathogenicity).

The hemoglobin for blood substitutes comes from a variety of sources, such as outdated donated human blood, bovine or swine blood, and transgenic *E. coli*. Each source has its benefits (availability, cost) as well as its side effects (infections, other complications). Human hemoglobin has the advantage of being a naturally occurring product that has been extensively studied. Its obvious disadvantage is lack of availability. About 2 units of discarded blood are required to make 1 unit of the HBOC. Even if we were to capture all of the discarded human blood, the numbers of units made would only be half of what was discarded.

The potential advantages of animals as a source of hemoglobin are tremendous; they are a relatively cheap source, and their supply is ample. Yet despite efforts at controlling a herd, problems such as bovine spongiform encephalitis will inevitably surface. Recombinant hemoglobin has problems as well. Volumes of bacterial culture and the stringent processing methods are costly. It is estimated that only 0.1 g of hemoglobin can be generated from 1 liter of *E. coli* culture. This equates to 750 liters to make 1 unit. Production of 3 million units would require more than 1.125 billion liters of culture.

One of the first HBOC products tested was manufactured by Baxter in 1999. Diaspirin cross-linked hemoglobin (DCLHb), known as HemAssist, was tested. This chemically modified human hemoglobin solution was used in a highly publicized trial in patients with traumatic hemorrhagic shock, one of the first trials to use community consent (instead of individual patient consent). Baxter terminated the trial early because the patients who received the test product had a higher 28-day mortality rate (47%) than those who received normal saline (25%) ($P < .015$). The trial brought disappointment to investigators anticipating the success of the first red cell substitute.

A recent analysis compared data from the Baxter trial with the 17 U.S. emergency departments and the parallel 27 European Union prehospital systems now using DCLHb. This analysis did not show any difference in outcome. The authors reported that neither mean BP readings nor elevated BP readings correlated with DCLHb treatment of traumatic hemorrhagic shock patients. As such, no clinically demonstrable DCLHb pressor effect could be directly related to the adverse mortality outcome observed in the Baxter trial.

Two other products currently have potential for clinical use. Both are polymerized rather than tetramerized. Polymerization is thought to be better because the molecular masses are higher (130 kDa) than with tetramerization (65 kDa), resulting in longer intravascular presence. Some investigators have proposed that polymerization avoids contact with nitric oxide, attenuating the vasoconstriction seen with previous products.

One of those products is HBOC-201 (Hemopure; Biopure Corporation), made from bovine blood. It is universally compatible and is stable at room temperature for up to 3 years. Animal studies showed great promise. Human trials involving orthopedic patients also showed promise, but safety issues were a concern; patients who received Hemopure had an increased number of serious adverse events. The vasoconstrictive properties of Hemopure may have caused myocardial infarction in susceptible patients. Biopure Corporation went bankrupt and was taken over by OPK Biotech, which has a product called Oxyglobin (HBOC-301) for veterinary use. FDA approval for Hemopure is still pending. OPK Biotech has continued to develop Hemopure for human use; the U.S. Navy is supporting research for potential use in the military setting. Studies have been proposed to coinfuse a nitric oxide donor such as nitroglycerin in a fixed ratio, in a single-bag compound or as separate infusions. However, there is little likelihood that surgeons will accept a product to treat shock that requires coinfusion of a vasodilator.

The more promising hemoglobin-based product is PolyHeme. The way it is produced removes nearly all of the cross-linked tetrameric hemoglobin (<1%). PolyHeme is made from outdated human donated blood and has a shelf life of about a year at room temperature. Of several human trials, the most recent was a multicenter study in trauma patients with the need for informed consent waived.[63] Patients were randomized to receive PolyHeme or to receive crystalloids and PRBCs. A total of 29 trauma centers enrolled 714 patients. They reported that patients can be resuscitated with PolyHeme, without using stored blood, for up to 6 units in 12 hours after injury; outcomes between the two groups were comparable (30-day mortality rate: 13.4%, PolyHeme group; 9.6%, control group). However, the PolyHeme group had more serious adverse events, specifically, an increased number of myocardial infarctions. Nonetheless, the benefit-risk ratio of PolyHeme is favorable when blood is needed but not available.

A meta-analysis of 16 HBOC trials, including 4 trauma trials involving HemAssist or PolyHeme, showed that HBOC patients had a significantly increased risk of myocardial infarctions and death compared with controls. The problem of vasoconstriction will have to be further worked out. Vasodilators can be added to mitigate vasoconstriction, but whether enthusiasm for HBOCs persists remains to be seen. Without doubt, however, they have a real potential benefit for patients who do not have access to PRBCs, such as in rural areas or the military.

Third-generation hemoglobin substitutes have begun to address the deficiencies of earlier formulations. The encapsulation of hemoglobin in liposomes is an innovation, but efforts to make it ideal continue. The mixing of phospholipids and cholesterol in the presence of free hemoglobin forms a sphere with hemoglobin in the center. These liposomes have oxygen dissociation curves similar to red cells, and administration can transiently achieve high circulating levels of hemoglobin and oxygen-carrying capacity. Research is still in the preclinical testing stage; progress in prolonging the half-life and elucidating the effects on the immune system, particularly reticuloendothelial sequestration, is crucial before clinical testing can begin.

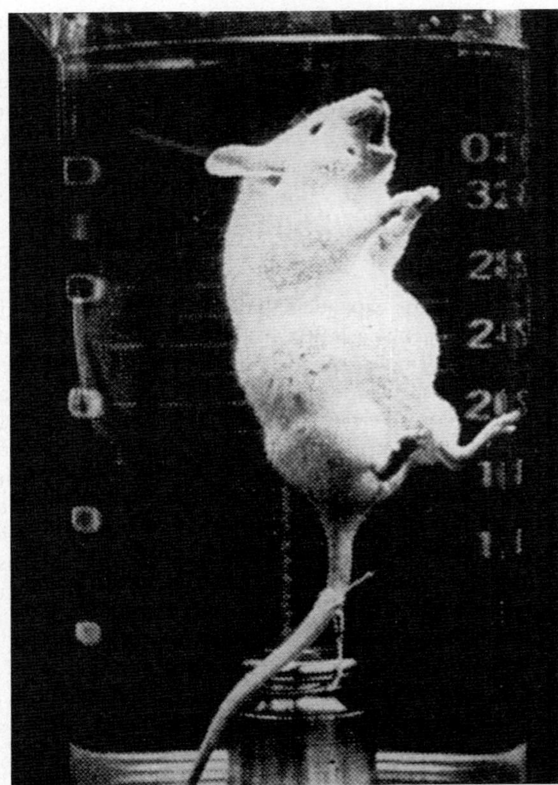

FIGURE 4-22 Mouse surviving while submerged in perfluorocarbons. (From Shaffer TH, Wolfson MR: Liquid ventilation. In Polin RA, Fox WW, Abman SH, editors: *Fetal and neonatal physiology*, ed 3, WB Saunders, 2003, Philadelphia.)

Perfluorocarbons

Perfluorocarbons (PFCs) are completely inert biologically and similar to Teflon or Gore-Tex. Altering the molecule (by fluoridating the ring structure) lowers the melting point and thus makes it a liquid at room temperature. PFCs captured the imagination of many in 1966 when photographs were introduced of a mouse completely submerged in the liquid form but breathing and surviving in it (Fig. 4-22). PFCs dissolve larger quantities of oxygen and CO_2 than plasma. They have yet to find a purpose in liquid form, but enthusiasm has increased for their use in partial liquid ventilation. Trials in adults with ARDS have shown no benefit, but trials are still ongoing in children with hyaline membrane disease.

PFCs have two challenges to overcome for use as blood substitutes. The first is that the liquid form is immiscible in water; thus, PFCs must be suspended as microdroplets with the use of emulsifying agents. The second is that unlike hemoglobin, the oxygen that is dissolved in PFCs has a linear relationship to the partial pressure of oxygen, whereas hemoglobin has a sigmoidal disassociation curve favoring full loading at normal atmospheric oxygen levels. Thus, the FIO_2 that has to be applied is too high.

Second-generation PFCs have been formulated to allow more oxygen-carrying capacities, with alterations in the emulsion properties. Such new compounds can also be stored at 4°C, whereas previous solutions had to be frozen. Oxygent (Alliance Pharmaceutical Corp./Baxter Healthcare Corp.) is a 60% perflubron emulsion with a median particle diameter of less than 0.2 µm. The use of lecithin as an emulsifier eliminated the adverse effects of complement activation observed in earlier studies of PFCs. Possible current scenarios for its use include cardiopulmonary bypass with normovolemic hemodilution and balloon angioplasty (to provide oxygenated blood past the catheter while it is inflated). In a phase 3 study, Oxygent was shown to reduce the need for red blood cell transfusion in patients undergoing noncardiac surgery (16%, Oxygent group; 26%, control group; $P < .05$). Oxygent patients, however, had more serious adverse events (32% in the Oxygent group versus 21% in the control group; $P < .05$). In another phase 3 study, in patients undergoing cardiac bypass, Oxygent possibly increased the incidence of strokes. All further studies were halted.

Two other PFC products have been introduced. In early-phase clinical trials, OxyFluor (HemaGen) produced mild thrombocytopenia and influenza-like symptoms in healthy volunteers. Baxter International has withdrawn support for further development. Phase 2 trials of Oxycyte (Synthetic Blood International) have been suspended; it has been taken over by Oxygen Biotherapeutics, Inc., and is being sold over the counter as a cosmetic product known as Dermacyte, an oxygen concentrate gel for wound healing. Dermacyte is also being investigated for the treatment of cancer during chemotherapy or radiation therapy because oxygen free radicals are thought to kill cancer cells. PFCs are not free of side effects and are not efficacious for oxygen delivery and use.

Novel Fluids

The recognition that currently available fluids are not a replacement for blood and that they in fact can be harmful if used in large amounts to expand blood volume has initiated exciting research for better fluids. Blood is so highly complex that the ultimate goal is to develop artificial whole blood, but doing so will take much time. The ideal method would be to manufacture whole blood with a bioreactor using stem cells, but this development would take decades.

The permutations of future fluid development are endless. Novel crystalloids are being tested, as are hypertonic solutions with and without oxygen carriers, hypertonic colloids, freeze-dried plasma (FDP), and drug therapy.

The Institute of Medicine in 1999 recommended research to eliminate lactate in LR and to investigate the use of alternative energy substrates in resuscitation fluids. It recognized that although reperfusion injury can occur in shock resuscitation, a separate entity called resuscitation injury is a result of the method of resuscitation and the fluids used.

Two substances have since been identified that may alter the inflammatory response after resuscitation. In small and large animal models, studies found that simply replacing the lactate in LR with either ketones or pyruvate reduced the inflammatory response after hemorrhagic shock resuscitation. Other investigators have concentrated on various forms of pyruvate to minimize resuscitation injury; ethyl pyruvate seems promising.[64] Studies in animals show that pyruvate Ringer's solution corrects lactic acidosis and prolongs survival during hemorrhagic shock in rats. From a cellular level, a combination of anti-inflammatory constituents in fluids seems more efficacious. Since the introduction of the idea that there is a difference between fluids containing the isomers D-lactate and L-lactate, studies have demonstrated that there is outcome difference in terms of survival and mechanical ventilation. L-Lactate is superior to D-lactate.

Studies of the mechanisms behind such improved results found that monocarboxylate-supplemented resuscitation provides energy substrates, with minimal alteration in the conventionally used fluids such as LR. Replacing the lactate in LR with either pyruvate or ketones protected the brain and other tissues after shock.[65] That finding led to research on the reasons for this protective effect and on the potential of using drugs alone to treat hemorrhagic shock.

Dried Plasma

Clinical data showing better outcomes with the combination of minimizing crystalloids and aggressively using blood products led to the development of dried plasma. This approach was used in World War II and the Korean War but became less popular over time (Fig. 4-23). Part of the reason was probably research showing that crystalloids and colloids did not make a difference as well as concern about possible transmission of infection. However, the capability of removing potential infectious agents along with the improved technology for manufacturing of dried plasma resurrected research in this field. Dried plasma is prepared in one of two ways. It can be freeze dried (FDP) or lyophilized with a combination of low temperature and low pressure and low-moisture circulating air. It can also be spray dried in a high-temperature chamber, where it is aerosolized. The product can be stored in either of these forms with minimal protein degradation until it is reconstituted, pH adjusted, and then administered. The advantages of dried plasma are the long shelf life and that it does not need refrigeration and tight temperature control. It avoids the difficult logistics of keeping fresh-frozen products and the preparation time of thawing FFP. Modern-day dried plasma has been treated so that the historical concerns of transmitting viruses are minimized.

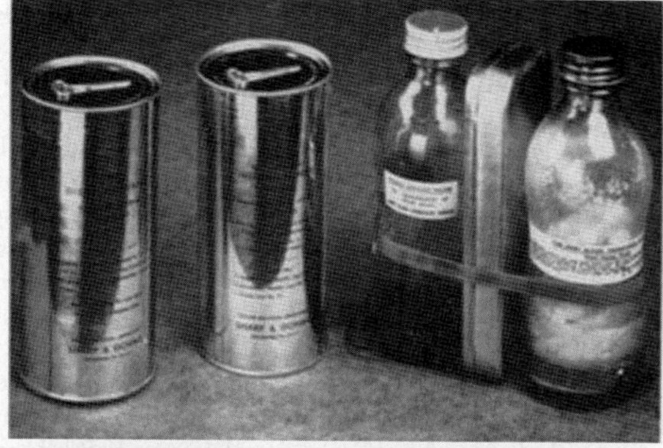

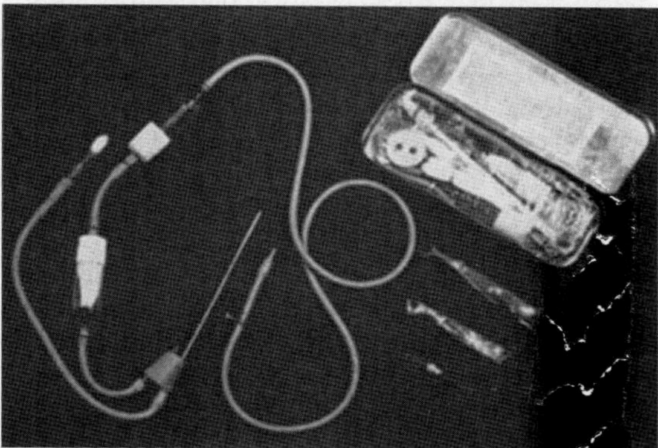

FIGURE 4-23 Freeze-dried plasma used during World War II. (Courtesy Office of Medical History, U.S. Army Medical Department, Center of History and Heritage, Washington, DC.)

Through funding by the U.S. Navy, plasma separated from fresh porcine blood was lyophilized to produce FDP and then compared with FFP. After a 60% blood volume hemorrhage, pigs were resuscitated with reconstituted FDP, which was just as efficacious as thawed plasma and had an identical coagulation profile. A multi-institutional polytrauma animal trial found that FDP was better than Hextend (which led to anemia and coagulopathy).[66] Currently, this area of research and development is exciting and promising. FDP is currently available in Europe but not in the United States.

The French Army has been using freeze-dried and secured plasma (FDSP) since 1994. It is made from fresh deleukocyted blood of up to 10 volunteers. Blood type selection allows the dilution and neutralization of natural anti-A and anti-B hemagglutinins. This FDSP is thus compatible with any blood type. It is also shelf stable in ambient temperatures for 2 years and is easily rehydrated with 200 mL of water for use in less than 3 minutes. FDSP contains all clotting factors and proteins. The fibrinogen and clotting factor levels of FDSP are equivalent to FFP. Early reports of using FDP in 87 battlefield casualties show that it is effective for preventing or treating coagulopathy in a French ICU in Afghanistan. Germany also has FDP (LyoPlas N-w), which comes from a single donor screened for blood-borne pathogens. Unlike FFP, LyoPlas N-w undergoes filtration to further remove cellular remnants to reduce the risk of infection or transfusion immune reactions. It remains efficient for 12 months when it is maintained at a temperature range of 4° C to 25° C. Germany has fielded more than 500,000 units of LyoPlas N-w without unusual or significant adverse effects compared with FFP. In addition to the ability to prevent or to treat coagulopathy, it is an excellent way to restore volume as it is a colloid. The Israel Defense Forces Medical Corps policy is that plasma is the fluid of choice for selected, severely wounded patients, and thus it included FDP as part of its armamentarium for use at the point of injury by advanced lifesavers across the entire military. The U.S. special forces are attempting to secure FDP for their use. Because the thawing of FFP takes a long time and with up to a third of the thawed FFP having fractured bags, the idea of dried plasma is logical, especially to the military.

From the military perspective, a method of developing artificial whole blood was needed that was practical and not harmful. Again, fresh whole blood is so complex that simple fluids are not a replacement. The reality of artificial whole blood is many years away, but FDP is just around the corner in terms of being able to treat hemorrhagic shock without causing as much harm as currently available colloids and crystalloids do. FDP can also undo physiologic derangements by restoring intravascular volume and treating coagulopathy. The logistic advantages of a product that can be easily reconstituted would be a tremendous advance. Much research is looking at oxygen carriers and small-volume resuscitation, so the concept that FDP can be reconstituted with less water—and initial resuscitation performed with a hypertonic, hyperoncotic resuscitation fluid—is exciting.

There has been research to develop freeze-dried red blood cells, but the challenge has been to overcome the freezing, drying, and rehydration process without stressful injury to the red blood cells. Although freeze-dried red blood cells have been shown to have acceptable viscoelastic deformability properties, with storage times to about 1 week by adding trehalose, a sugar molecule, this product is still in very early stages of development. Freeze-dried platelets and platelet-derived particles are also being developed. Frozen platelets are cryopreserved in 6% dimethyl sulfoxide and can be stored for up to 10 years at −80° C. Freeze-died platelets have been in development for more than 50 years, but preserving functionality has been a challenge. Modern preparations, which are treated with 1.8% paraformaldehyde, frozen in 5% albumin, and then lyophilized, have been more encouraging. Once rehydrated, they seem structurally intact, contain most of the glycoproteins, and are capable of supporting thrombin generation and fibrin deposition. However, in vivo testing shows that the duration of hemostatic activity is brief, approximately 4 to 6 hours, and sometimes limited to 15 minutes. Recent studies of human freeze-dried platelets in a swine liver injury model have demonstrated improved survival and reduced blood loss, but 13% of the surviving animals were found to have thrombotic complications. The idea of freeze-dried plasma, red blood cells, and platelets would mean reconstitutable whole blood.

Pharmacologic Agents

Resuscitation fluids simply replace the lost intravascular volume but have no inherent prosurvival properties. Therefore, a body of work is investigating whether it would be logical to design therapies promoting a prosurvival phenotype. Among patients resuscitated from hemorrhagic shock, a wide spectrum of responses is observed. Although some patients recover without any complications, others develop multiple organ failure. This unpredictable response is not caused by a widespread variation in the human genome. Since the decoding of the human genome, it has become apparent that only 20,000 to 35,000 protein-coding genes are responsible for millions of different phenotypes. The rapidly expanding field of epigenetics focuses on mechanisms and phenomena that affect the phenotype of a cell or an organism without affecting the genotype. Over the years, many pharmacologic agents have been tested as possible adjuncts (or substitutes) to conventional fluid resuscitation. These drugs cover a wide spectrum, including neuroendocrine agents, calcium channel blockers, ATP pathway modifiers, prostaglandins, sex steroids, antioxidants, anti-inflammatory agents, and immune modulators. Although there is strong laboratory evidence of their beneficial effects on tissue perfusion, myocardial contractility, reticuloendothelial function, cell survival, oxidative injury, and immune activation, most of these agents are not yet in clinical use as resuscitative agents.

This area of work is an example of translational research that is novel and could be revolutionary. DNA transcription is regulated, in part, by acetylation of nuclear histones that are controlled by two groups of enzymes: histone deacetylases (HDACs) and histone acetyltransferases (HATs). Animal experiments showed that hemorrhagic shock and resuscitation were associated with HDAC/HAT activity misbalance and that the acetylation status of cardiac histones is influenced by the choice of resuscitation strategy. Shock-induced changes can be reversed through the infusion of a pharmacologic HDAC inhibitor, even when it is administered for only a limited period after the insult. Animal experiments have shown tremendous promise in elucidating mechanisms behind the success of using an HDAC inhibitor to prolong life after shock.[65]

Alam and colleagues have been investigating the role of HDAC inhibitors, such as valproic acid (VPA, an anticonvulsant) and suberoylanilide hydroxamic acid. They hypothesized that they may be useful in the treatment of shock through restoration of normal cellular acetylation. In their experiments, large swine subjected to trauma (femur and liver injury) and to severe hemorrhage (60% blood loss) were randomized into one of three groups: no treatment (control group), treatment with fresh whole blood, or treatment with VPA (400 mg/kg) without resuscitation. The early survival rate was 100% in the fresh whole blood group, 86% in the VPA group, and 25% in the control group.[67] Impressively, this survival improvement was achieved without conventional fluid resuscitation or blood transfusion, which makes this approach appealing for the logistically constrained prehospital and battlefield environments. It appears that HDAC inhibitors rapidly activate nuclear histones as well as numerous cellular proteins to create a prosurvival phenotype in hemorrhagic and septic shock. This group has also reported that VPA is neuroprotective and is promising for the treatment of TBI. It has also been shown to be beneficial in sepsis. A number of these HDAC inhibitors are being tested in phase 1 and 2 clinical trials (nontraumatic situations).

Given concerns that inflammation after trauma might be a pathologic event, another unique approach is to use estrogen and progesterone to treat patients after traumatic hemorrhagic shock. A number of independent laboratory studies have pointed to the use of estrogen and progesterone as a promising method to reduce secondary injury in hemorrhagic shock and other similar processes. Those studies have shown that the early administration of estrogen (a strong antioxidant, anti-inflammatory, and mitochondrial stabilizer as well as an antiapoptotic agent) significantly decreased the severity of injury caused by early, devastating cell death. The use of estrogen has now been tested in 60 clinical trials, mostly in the fields of prostate cancer, uremic bleeding, liver transplantation, spine surgery, cardiology, cardiac surgery, and

TBI. Its safety record is good. However, human trials in TBI have failed to show any efficacy.

Suspended Animation

The military has supported research to develop a technique to prevent patients from dying of exsanguination. Repairable torso hemorrhage is still a major cause of potentially preventable death in the battlefield, so research is being conducted to identify a method of preserving a patient's life long enough to later repair the sources of hemorrhage. This concept is termed suspended animation. Rather than resuscitation, the goal is to stop cellular death, either with induced hypothermia or by chemical means.

Initially, animal studies focused on identifying hibernation inducers that chemically signal cells to decrease metabolism. Serum from hibernating squirrels can be injected into nonhibernating squirrels and induce hibernation. Metabolism slows, heart rate decreases, and life seems to be suspended. Many mammals are highly tolerant of ischemia, such as diving seals, which can remain underwater for 45 minutes at a time. Bears hibernate in the cold, and turtles can bury themselves in mud without dying. The search continues for the answer to this question: How can human life persist without oxygenation at the rate we are accustomed to? This fascinating area of research should help us understand the meaning of life at the cellular level, but the clinical use of hibernating inducers is many years away.

Hypothermia or cooling reduces the metabolic needs of cells. Thus, induced hypothermia has been studied to determine whether it can put life on hold. Once metabolic demands are decreased, life can be slowed or "suspended." This metabolic suspension can be effectively achieved with hypothermia as well as with various chemical infusions. Interestingly, life or metabolism does not seem to end with the cessation of perfusion; rather, it actually ends during reperfusion, when irreversible cellular damage is done. Reperfusion of cells that have exhausted their supply of nutrients can damage cells and thus end life. The mechanisms are complex, but calcium exchange may be a key component.

Because exsanguination is a major cause of death both in the battlefield and in civilian trauma, the suspension of life with hypothermia or chemical cellular arrest could buy time to transport patients to a hospital where their vascular injuries can be repaired and their life restored. Animal work has been performed to perfect a method of inducing suspended animation and then successfully restoring life without neurologic injury. Clinically, induced hypothermic arrest is actually already being used in cardiothoracic surgery and neurosurgery, but the current length of time that flow to the brain can be halted is only about 45 minutes. In cardiac surgery, the heart is arrested and cooled while the rest of the body is perfused with a pump. The idea is to take the methods that are used to preserve the heart and apply them to the whole body, including the brain. However, such methods are complex and require extensive preparation and immense teamwork; whether they can be simplified for emergencies, such as unexpected exsanguination, is unknown.

Animal work on this topic has been performed for 60 years. The late Peter Safar, the father of modern-day cardiopulmonary resuscitation, studied induced profound hypothermic arrest in dogs and rats under controlled conditions. Research funded by the U.S. Navy involved a series of experiments showing that profound hypothermia to 10° C can be induced by infusing cold fluids containing massive doses of potassium. Essentially, the process is similar to achieving cardioplegia except that a solution is infused to arrest not only the heart but the entire body. The solution used to induce such massive hypothermic and chemical arrest is an organ preservation fluid (HypoThermosol) that contains 70 mEq/liter of potassium.

Patients who have in effect died of exsanguinating traumatic hemorrhage typically undergo a resuscitative thoracotomy in the emergency department to stop their bleeding and to attempt to resuscitate them. However, this is a desperate maneuver with dismal results; only 7.4% of such patients survive. The U.S. Navy developed a new method; once the chest is opened, instead of trying to resuscitate patients, they are infused with cold HypoThermosol.

Large animal (swine) models have been used to develop the techniques that induce suspended animation in the emergent setting; studies have repeatedly shown that swine could be put into whole body arrest and then rapidly (within 20 to 30 minutes) made hypothermic to 10° C. During this process, all the blood is removed from the swine; they are left in that state for about 1 to 3 hours. This, by clinical definition, "kills" the swine; no metabolism occurs during that state, no brain or heart activity can be detected, and no blood is in the body. These animal studies have shown feasibility of this approach in a clinically realistic model with a variety of injuries including hemorrhagic shock with soft tissue injuries, vascular injuries below the diaphragm, and solid organ injuries. The survival is better than 75% long term, and the animals recover neurologically intact with normal cognitive function.

Theoretically, this is the period during which human patients could be taken to the operating room for vascular repairs; such patients almost always have suffered major vascular injury causing exsanguination. Because the vascular repairs would be done in an asanguineous state, no blood loss during the repairs would occur. Such repairs have been accomplished with portable pumps that are smaller than a can of soda.[67] This is also the period during which human patients could be put on a standard bypass machine by a second team of surgeons; that machine would be used to revive patients by flushing out the potassium and warming them while blood is infused. In the swine model, this entire process has been shown to be feasible, even after extended periods of shock and even with associated vascular, solid organ, and hollow visceral injuries.

Research on this concept by the military has advanced to a point at which a multicenter clinical trial is now planned. The mechanisms and methods to suspend life and then to restart it have clearly been identified. The traditional teaching has been that hypothermia during trauma care is bad, but the difference between spontaneous hypothermia and induced hypothermia is huge. Spontaneous hypothermia indicates hemorrhagic shock and is often associated with massive resuscitation with cold or room temperature fluids. Such severely injured patients will do poorly, given their blood loss and the dilutional coagulopathy (which is obviously detrimental when patients have uncontrolled bleeding). Appropriately induced hypothermia, however, can be beneficial.

PERIOPERATIVE FLUID MANAGEMENT

Body Water

Humans are made predominantly of water (50% to 70% of body weight). The precise percentage is affected by gender, body fat, and age. The human body can do without many things for long periods, but water is essential. In the body, water resides in three compartments or spaces: (1) intracellular, (2) intravascular, and (3) interstitial. The intracellular compartment has the largest volume of water, constituting about 30% to 40% of body weight (two thirds of the body's total water). The intravascular volume is usually calculated as 5% to 7% of body weight. Water shifts rapidly between the three compartments. Large resources of water can be pulled from the intracellular compartment into the intravascular compartment; large volumes of water can be stored in the interstitial compartment. Water in the interstitial compartment is recirculated by the lymphatics and eventually returns into the intravascular compartment.

A fixed amount of water is in bones and dense connective tissue, but this water is relatively stable and not considered to be in circulation. Water is secreted by various cells in the skin, cerebrospinal fluid, and intraocular, synovial, renal, and GI systems; this water is also not considered to be in circulation.

Clinical tools are available to accurately measure the volume of water in the body. One method is bioimpedance spectroscopy, which measures electrical current impedance that is imperceptible to the person to estimate total body water. The method is best used to calculate body fat.

Methods to measure intravascular volume are also commercially available. They usually involve injecting a known concentration of tagged molecules (such as potassium-40 or albumin) that remain intravascular for a known period. Potassium is predominantly an intracellular solute, and albumin is predominantly extracellular. Sampling the blood and calculating the volume based on the decreased concentration of the injected tracer is fairly accurate. This method has not caught on for clinical use because the baseline volume is not known; even if it were known, the intravascular volume is contractible and expandable, so the desired intravascular target volume is not yet known. During injuries and illnesses, when homeostasis has not been maintained, normal values may not be applicable or desirable during resuscitation. The practicality of measuring these spaces has not been identified, yet research has shown that a person's extracellular volume can be expanded even if he or she is dehydrated intracellularly.

The main intracellular electrolytes are potassium and magnesium. Intracellularly, they are the principal cations; phosphates and proteins are the principal anions. Extracellularly, in contrast, sodium is the predominant cation; chloride and bicarbonate are the predominant anions. In plasma (given its higher protein content, which is due to organic anions), the total concentrations of cations are higher and the concentrations of inorganic anions are lower than in the interstitial fluids. The Gibbs-Donnan equilibrium equation states that the product of the concentrations of any pair of diffusible cations and anions on one side of a semipermeable membrane will equal the product of the same pair of ions on the other side. Cell walls are semipermeable membranes; the flow of water is determined by the osmotically active particles (about 290 to 310 mOsm). The effective osmotic pressure depends on those substances that fail to pass through the pores of the semipermeable membrane.

The unit of milliequivalents (mEq) per liter refers to the number of electrical charges; milliosmoles (mOsm) per liter, to the number of osmotically active particles or ions. A milliequivalent in a solution must be precisely balanced by the same number of milliequivalents of a cation and anion. The balance affects the direction of water as it equilibrates. The osmotic pressure of a solution refers to the actual number of osmotically active particles present in the solution, but it does not depend on the chemical-combining capacities of the substances. For example, sodium chloride dissociates to 2 mOsm, whereas sodium sulfate (Na_2SO_4) dissociates into three particles: 2 mOsm of sodium and 1 mOsm of sulfate. However, 1 mOsm of an un-ionized substance such as glucose is equal to 1 mOsm of the substance.

The dissolved proteins in the plasma are responsible for the effective osmotic pressure between the plasma and the interstitial fluid, frequently referred to as the colloid osmotic pressure. Sodium is pumped outside the cell and potassium inside the cell. Thus, sodium is the major electrolyte responsible for the osmotic pressure, but glucose and urea (which do not easily penetrate the cell membrane) also increase the effective osmotic pressure. Water passes across the cell membrane freely, so sodium has a highly important impact on the movement of water. However, the concentration of sodium is not necessarily related to the volume status of ECF. A severe extracellular volume deficit can occur with a low or high sodium concentration over time.

The osmotic gradient is also important in controlling water. The number of osmotic particles is the key. The size of the osmotic particle does not matter. For example, transfusion of PRBCs will actually cause water to pass from the intravascular space to the interstitial space. Immediately after transfusion of PRBCs, hydrostatic pressure increases inside the vascular space, and water is pushed out. Although the hematocrit level of PRBCs is 60% to 70%, the red cells act as one osmotic particle. Because the size difference between red cells and proteins in the blood is so significant, fewer osmotic particles are in a given volume of blood compared with normal whole blood. Therefore, the osmotic pressure intravascularly is actually reduced after transfusion of PRBCs. PRBCs are prepared by centrifuging the red cells and removing the plasma. Thus, the number of osmotic particles in PRBCs is markedly reduced.

The size difference between a red cell and albumin is huge (like a soccer ball versus a grain of sand), but each will act as one osmotic particle. The number of soccer balls that can fit into a stadium is limited, but the number of grains of sand that can fit is many orders of magnitude higher. Similarly, with a transfusion of PRBCs, water is pushed out of the intravascular space into either the interstitial or intercellular space because of the decrease in the number of osmotic particles per volume.

Maintenance Fluids

In surgical patients, assessing the intravascular status is a pivotal task but one of the most difficult. Surgical patients have blood loss from trauma, operations, and diseases. In addition, volume deficits occur from losses of GI fluids because of vomiting, diarrhea, nasogastric suctioning, fistulas, and drains. Fluid also shifts out of the intravascular space because of burns, inflammation (as in pancreatitis), intestinal obstruction, infection, and sepsis.

Nonetheless, the main daily task of perioperative patient care is assessing the intravascular status. Is it where it needs to be? It is safer for surgeons to assume that a patient is hypovolemic or hypervolemic than normal; the normovolemic band is very small. Normovolemia occurs only as patients pass from hypervolemia to hypovolemia. The maintenance fluid should constantly be adjusted, depending on the individual patient's current status. Surgeons must pay attention to each patient's fluid status and body needs rather than infuse maintenance fluid at the same rate.

For the routine preoperative care of patients about to undergo elective surgery, the customary approach is to start a maintenance drip of crystalloids. Note, however, that patients who undergo same-day surgery have little need for preoperative fluids. All preoperative patients are asked to not take in any fluids by mouth starting the night before surgery, a directive that typically does not result in any problems. Remember that all of us (whether or

BOX 4-3 Maintenance Fluid Calculation

Maintenance IV Fluid Calculation
- 4 mL/kg/hr for first 10 kg
- 2 mL/kg/hr for next 10 kg
- 1 mL/kg/hr for every kg over 20 kg

Sample Calculation for 45-kg Patient
10 kg × 4 mL/kg/hr = 40 mL/hr
10 kg × 2 mL/kg/hr = 20 mL/hr
25 kg × 1 mL/kg/hr = 25 mL/hr
Maintenance rate = 85 mL/hr

Sample Calculation for 73-kg Patient
- 10 kg × 4 mL/kg/hr = 40 mL/hr
- 10 kg × 2 mL/kg/hr = 20 mL/hr
- 53 kg × 1 mL/kg/hr = 53 mL/hr

Maintenance rate = 113 mL/hr

not we are surgical patients) are NPO (Latin for *nil per os* or nothing by mouth) when we go to sleep; we do not normally wake up hypotensive or in renal failure. Thus, for patients about to undergo major surgery requiring inpatient hospitalization after surgery, IV fluids the night before are not necessary; they typically will receive plenty of fluids from the anesthesiologist during the operation.

In patients who underwent a colectomy, a small prospective randomized study showed that minimizing crystalloids during surgery led to a better outcome; such patients had less nausea and vomiting, decreased hospital length of stay, and faster return of GI function. However, starting such patients on a maintenance fluid is safe, mainly to provide water (Box 4-3). In adult patients weighing more than 40 kg, the simple rule for calculating the fluid rate is 40 plus the weight in kilograms; that is, a 73-kg patient's maintenance rate would be 113 kg/hr (73 + 40).

Maintenance fluids have not been rigorously tested, so the ideal fluid is unknown. The current standard is to use 5% dextrose in half-normal saline with 40 mEq/liter of potassium. The source of the standard's formulation remains unclear. For a 70-kg NPO man, it would provide sodium and potassium, yet it is not what the average person requires (Table 4-12). The average 70-kg man's requirements are listed in Table 4-13.

The average salt intake per day in American men has been difficult to assess; the median is an estimated 7.8 to 11.8 g/day. Because that range does not include salt added at the table, it is probably an underestimate. The U.S. Department of Agriculture recommends a salt intake of less than 2.3 g/day. Normal saline contains 9 g of sodium chloride in 1 liter of water. The amount of fluids and electrolytes infused into patients with the standard formulation is highly inaccurate. The decision to give 5% dextrose in maintenance fluid is thought to derive from fasting studies of Harvard medical students in the 1920s. Those studies found that providing about 100 g of glucose decreased protein spillage in the urine. The rationale for the use of half-normal saline and 20 mEq/liter of potassium is unknown. A survey of critical care intensivists showed that most did not know the daily recommended intake of sodium or potassium.

Surgeons fear that an insufficient volume of fluid will lead to renal failure. Oliguria in a 70-kg man is defined by less than 400 mL of urine produced and excreted in a 24-hour period. That is the minimum volume required to maintain normal serum blood urea nitrogen and creatinine levels so that the kidney is able to maximally function. That volume equates to 0.24 mL/kg/hr. Historically, surgical residents were mandated to give patients enough IV maintenance fluid to produce 0.5 mL/kg/hr, probably to build in a safety margin to ensure enough volume. Today, it is not uncommon to see residents give patients a liter fluid bolus of crystalloids for urine output of less than 50 mL/kg/hr, a practice that will usually lead to overhydration. The kidneys are marvelous at protecting the body from physicians who have not studied physiology. In general, overhydration has not been typically seen as a problem, and anasarca has been seen as harmless; however, that view is accurate only for patients who are not on a ventilator. Studies suggest that excess fluids may delay the return of bowel function.

TABLE 4-12 Contents of Maintenance Solution*

	TOTAL IN 24 HOURS
Water	2760 mL
Dextrose	132 g
Sodium	11.8 g (203 mEq)
Potassium	1.9 g (53 mEq)

*With 5% dextrose in half-normal saline with 40 mEq/liter of potassium in a 70-kg patient during 24 hours.

TABLE 4-13 Normal Needs for 70-kg Man per Day

	TOTAL IN 24 HOURS
Water	2000 mL
Urine	1500 mL
Sodium	2-4 g
Potassium	100 mEq

Postoperatively, in general, patients are more often hypervolemic initially. Because of the bleeding from surgery and the need for IV infusion, anesthesiologists often give patients too much blood and fluid during surgery. Giving a few liters of blood and fluid is probably inconsequential. For patients who have lost liters of blood, however, accurate measurement is impossible; inferences have to be made as to what the volume status is. Patients who have lost a minimal amount of blood during elective surgery, who have received liters of crystalloids, and who have adequate urine output do not necessarily need IV maintenance fluids. For typical patients on the surgical ward, normal functioning kidneys will generally make up for any errors in the amount of blood and fluid given. However, for ICU patients on a ventilator who have severe traumatic injuries, sepsis, or blood loss, there is less room for error.

For ICU patients, in general, too much intravascular volume is better than too little. Too much volume equates to increased time on the ventilator, according to practicing intensivists; too little equates to renal insufficiency or renal failure. Pulmonary failure has an associated mortality rate of 20% to 25%, whereas renal failure has an associated mortality rate of 48%. Managing volume correctly would equate to a perfect number of days on the ventilator and to no days on dialysis.

Immediately after surgery, volume requirements are vastly different than during the next day. Again, for ICU patients, it is generally better to err on the conservative side with increased IV volume postoperatively for a predetermined period. Most surgeons do not have an issue with giving several 1-liter boluses of fluids but are terribly afraid of having an IV rate of 500 mL for 4 hours even though the total volume of fluid may be the same. When fluids are given as a bolus, the body has a tendency to be confused; hormone releases will wildly fluctuate as it tries to compensate for such wide swings in pressure and volume in the vascular system.

Surgical patients are often hypovolemic intravascularly, despite being overhydrated during the operation. The body can be dramatically overloaded by many liters (at least per calculations of how much fluid has been infused) yet still be hypovolemic intravascularly. The total daily water input in such patients may be up, but determining the current intravascular volume is vital to try to predict volume status over time as the water shifts from the interstitial space to the intravascular space.

Especially for ICU patients, the same maintenance rate over days can be a problem. Again, determining their fluid status is difficult. Surgeons need to gather as much information as possible to guess what the IV maintenance rate should be. Knowing the blood urea nitrogen to creatinine ratio is helpful. A ratio higher than 20 is generally thought to be on the dry side; a ratio lower than 10, on the wet side. Such generalizations are true only for patients with normal renal function. Urine output is an excellent way to determine what the kidneys' opinion is. High output generally will mean that the body is trying to rid itself of water; surgeons should assist it by decreasing the maintenance fluid rate. Anasarca is a helpful clue, as are the customary vital signs.

In older patients with heart failure or sepsis who are intravascularly hypovolemic, anasarca can be profound. Many such patients will need more IV fluids despite having anasarca. To help estimate vascular volume, central venous pressure and data from pulmonary artery catheters (if available) are useful. However, caution should be taken in interpreting heart rate. Central venous pressure, wedge pressure from pulmonary artery catheter, stroke volume, cardiac output, and volume status all roughly correlate, but heart rate and intravascular volume are difficult to correlate. Heart rate is affected by many known and unknown variables, including pain, anxiety, hormone levels, and temperature.

For patients with arterial blood gases, the PaO_2 to FIO_2 (P/F) ratio is extremely helpful. The P/F ratio is the arterial oxygen concentration divided by the inspired percentage of oxygen. In a healthy young patient without heart disease, the arterial oxygen content is about 100; because room air is 0.21% oxygen, the P/F ratio is about 500 (100/0.21). If that same patient is placed on 100% oxygen, arterial oxygen content would be 500 with a P/F ratio of 500. In a healthy patient who does not have pneumonia, sepsis, or pulmonary contusion, the P/F ratio can reflect interstitial or lung water status; it will help direct what the maintenance rate should be.

If patients have a calculated maintenance IV rate, the surgeon evidently thinks that the intravascular volume rate is ideal and that the water shifts that occur all the time are not expected to be an issue (because the total water content is deemed ideal).

In surgical patients with low urine output, the most common error is to provide furosemide as an IV bolus. In most if not all such patients, low urine output postoperatively means that they have deceased renal blood flow from insufficient intravascular volume. When blood flow to the kidneys is decreased, the kidneys sense inadequate intravascular volume; therefore, the renin-angiotensin system, ADH, atrial natriuretic peptide, carotid baroreceptors, and other mechanisms will be put into play in an effort to preserve water. If furosemide as a bolus is injected, it poisons the distal Henle loop, rendering it unable to hold in water and thus increasing urine output. Increased urine output in patients with an intravascular volume deficit worsens the deficit. An entire set of compensatory mechanisms will kick in again in an effort to preserve more water.

Low urine output is a signal that the maintenance rate should be higher; high urine output is usually a signal that the maintenance rate should be lower. If surgeons are forced to pull water out of a patient's body because of life-threatening hypoxia, diuretics such as dopamine or furosemide can be used in a drip form, which does not result in the toxic side effects seen with a bolus of furosemide. Still, decreasing intravascular volume status will have multiple effects on many organs.

For resuscitation of patients, our knowledge of biochemistry and physiology might suggest that one particular fluid would make much more sense than another. For example, fluids such as Plasma-Lyte and Normosol-R resemble the contents of the electrolytes in blood more than solutions such as LR or normal saline. Solutions resembling serum may be optimal in that they lessen the chance of hyperchloremic acidosis caused by the higher concentrations of chloride in normal saline. In the body, chloride and bicarbonate seem to be in equilibrium; in the presence of high levels of chloride, a non–anion gap acidosis will result. However, advocates of normal saline argue that even though acidosis due to anaerobic metabolism is not generally desired, hyperchloremic acidosis is not necessarily harmful. It may help offload oxygen at the tissue level from the hemoglobin molecule.

Despite all those arguments, no evidence shows any clinical benefit of one crystalloid solution over another. The cheapest and most readily available fluid may make the most sense. The hospital costs of most all crystalloids are relatively the same. Because the difference in cost is so small, the cost-saving argument is probably invalid.

Fluids devoid of some elements that require later replacement, for example, of potassium, raise a more pertinent issue. They may not be cost-effective in the long run, even if they are initially cheaper. The costs of monitoring and replacing electrolytes can add up to significant amounts. Normal saline has issues with the chloride load, and the balanced fluids like Plasma-Lyte reduce the need for frequent replacement of electrolytes such as calcium, potassium, and magnesium. None of the crystalloids are truly balanced, and they all have some advantages and disadvantages. These solutions can also be problematic when the patient is in renal failure. High doses of magnesium are also a potential issue in certain circumstances. Because surgical patients often require blood transfusions, purists will urge the use of crystalloids as carriers without calcium because there is fear that calcium will cause blood to clot in the IV lines. LR contains 3 mEq/liter of calcium, which will exceed the chelating capability of the citrate in the blood bag. Whole blood or PRBCs mixed with an equal volume of LR have not increased clot formation in vitro compared with saline reconstitution. These are tools in the armamentarium, and there are times for all of them. For daily maintenance needs of a few liters a day in a patient without renal failure, Plasma-Lyte or Normosol may be better than LR or saline.

Adrenal Gland

The adrenal medulla affects intravascular volume during shock by secreting catechol hormones. They are called catecholamines because they contain a catechol group derived from the amino acid tyrosine. The most abundant catecholamines are epinephrine, norepinephrine, and dopamine, all of which are produced from phenylalanine and tyrosine. Cortisol is also released from the adrenal cortex and plays a major role in that it controls fluid equilibrium. From the adrenal cortex and the zona glomerulosa, aldosterone is produced in response to stimulation by angiotensin II. Aldosterone is a mineralocorticoid that modulates renal function by increasing recovery of sodium and excretion of potassium. One of the problems in shock is that the release of all of these hormones is not infinite; they can be exhausted.

Many other organs are involved in the control of hormones, including the hypothalamic-pituitary interface, which leads to the release of adrenocorticotropic hormone (ACTH) from the anterior pituitary gland. This system is affected by a variety of circumstances, including intravascular pressure, intravascular volume, and electrolytes such as sodium. The juxtaglomerular apparatus of the kidney produces the enzyme renin, which generates angiotensin I. Then, angiotensin I is converted to angiotensin II by the angiotensin-converting enzyme located on the endothelial cells of the pulmonary arteries. This regulation of intravascular fluid status is further affected by the carotid baroreceptors and the atrial natriuretic peptides. To infuse any of these hormones or to block them leads to compensatory mechanisms and perturbations within this complicated system.

The system is also affected by many other factors that we have recently found—and will be affected by others that we have yet to discover. For example, TBI has shown us that the hypothalamic-pituitary interface can be directly affected by mechanical trauma or by ICP. For such patients, treatment becomes difficult to control as they go through a wide range of physiologic responses. Patients undergoing brain herniation will go from a bradycardic hypertensive state to a profoundly tachycardic and hypotensive state. During that roller coaster ride, urine output is also affected, and diabetes insipidus (DI) can occur. Most likely, the human body has teleologically evolved to try to reduce brain edema at all costs; high-volume urine output often results, requiring vasopressin infusions. Patients whose regulating system is malfunctioning or whose adrenal glands have been exhausted also have a need for high-dose pressors. However, studies have shown that the infusion of cortisol and thyroid hormone in drip form can decrease such instability and minimize the need for fluid infusion and pressors. Patients undergoing brain herniation illustrate how complex the regulatory system is; surgeons must be cognizant of the minute-to-minute changes that can occur.

Adrenal glucocorticoid insufficiency, but not complete failure, occurs in patients with impaired function of the hypothalamic-pituitary-adrenal axis. Such patients produce limited amounts of corticosteroids. Clinical problems develop when patients are stressed by hypovolemia from hemorrhage, onset of an infection, fear, or hypothermia. In evaluating patients during a surgical emergency, chronic adrenal insufficiency may be initially diagnosed after intractable hypotension is found. Pathologic causes of chronic adrenal insufficiency include autoimmune destruction of the adrenal gland and adrenalitis, in which cytotoxic lymphocytes gradually destroy cortisol-synthesizing cells in the adrenal cortex. Patients with adrenalitis gradually develop symptoms of fatigue, inanition, weight loss, and postural dizziness. Their chief complaint may be vague cramping abdominal pain, nausea, and a change in bowel habits. Laboratory findings suggesting adrenal insufficiency are hyperkalemia, acidemia, hyponatremia, and elevated serum creatinine levels. The diagnosis of adrenal insufficiency secondary to end-organ failure is established by disproportionately elevated ACTH levels (compared with cortisol levels).

Clinical findings in patients with sudden acute adrenal insufficiency can be nonspecific. If plasma cortisol levels precipitously decline to nil, patients will have abdominal pain syndrome, vomiting, and a tender abdomen and then will progress to prostration, coma, and hypotension unresponsive to catecholamine infusion. Signs and symptoms of a gradual reduction in cortisol function include malaise, fatigue, and hyponatremia with hyperkalemia. Patients with a complete loss of circulating glucocorticoids can die within hours after irreversible hypotension.

In critically ill patients, quickly establishing the diagnosis of adrenal insufficiency is difficult. Laboratory tests can confirm that plasma levels of the hormones are depressed, but test results take hours to obtain. Pending the laboratory test results, surgeons treat such patients with hormone replacement therapy. Treatment of glucocorticoid deficiency in adults consists of an IV infusion of 100 mg of hydrocortisone, which has an onset of action within 1 to 2 hours and a duration of action of 8 hours. Thus, the commonly recommended replacement dose in an adult is 100 mg of IV hydrocortisone, infused every 8 hours and then rapidly tapered during the subsequent days as the patient's condition stabilizes and the laboratory test results become available.

Other glucocorticoids used for IV replacement therapy include methylprednisolone and dexamethasone. Methylprednisolone has an anti-inflammatory milligram-per-milligram potency of 5; dexamethasone, of 25 (relative to 1.0 for hydrocortisone). Patients whose adrenal glands are destroyed may also require replacement of mineralocorticoids. Patients with primary adrenal failure should be treated with 50 to 200 μg/day of fludrocortisone.

Antidiuretic Hormone and Water

ADH causes water to be reabsorbed and thus reduces urine output. The pituitary releases ADH or arginine vasopressin (AVP). Synthesized in the hypothalamic region, ADH is stored in the pituitary. Excess production or release of ADH causes overhydration; water is retained and thus sodium levels are lowered. Because serum osmolality is predominantly related to sodium, it will be lower than normal (285 mmol/kg) with excess ADH.

One example of overhydration is a syndrome called SIADH (syndrome of inappropriate ADH). Despite being overhydrated because of too much ADH production, the kidneys are signaled to hold onto water. Therefore, urine osmolality will be high (>300 mmol/kg) even though serum osmolality is low.

Yet if ADH is not synthesized or released, such as in patients with TBI, the kidneys will start to put out high volumes of water; urine osmolality will be as low as 100 mmol/kg. The resulting dehydration will lead to elevated serum sodium levels. In patients with TBI, the development of DI is associated with significant brain injury and poor prognosis. In patients with DI or SIADH, the body's thermostat or regulator is dysfunctional; close attention needs to be paid to maintain volume control. Treatment of patients with DI should include desmopressin (1-desamino-8-D-AVP or DDAVP); of patients with SIADH, water restriction.

ELECTROLYTES

Sodium

Sodium is vital for homeostasis and the action potential in the body. It is the predominant molecule that controls water movement in and out of the vascular system. The normal range of serum sodium concentration is 135 to 145 mEq/liter. Hyponatremia and hypernatremia, heavily controlled by ADH, are common problems in surgical patients. In general, mild forms of hyponatremia and hypernatremia are not a problem, but hyponatremia is more concerning than hypernatremia. Of the many signs and symptoms associated with each, none of them is specific; none of the signs or symptoms alone would lead a clinician to diagnose a sodium abnormality. A blood test is always required.

Hyponatremia

Hyponatremia can be mild (130 to 138 mEq/liter), moderate (120 to 130 mEq/liter), or severe (<120 mEq/liter). Both mild hyponatremia and moderate hyponatremia are common but only rarely symptomatic. Severe hyponatremia, however, can cause headaches and lethargy; patients can become comatose or have seizures, although chronic severe hyponatremia can often be asymptomatic. Hyponatremia is a problem when cells swell as a result of the body's decreased ability to maintain homeostatic osmolality outside the cells. Typically, hyponatremia is caused by pathologic processes in the brain or lungs.

Assessing the cause of hyponatremia is important as patients are usually classified on the basis of their volume status. Patients with hyponatremia are usually hypotonic; on occasion, they may be hypertonic, with high serum glucose or mannitol levels. In severe hyperglycemia, osmolality of the ECF rises and exceeds that of the intracellular fluid. The reason is that glucose penetrates cell membranes slowly when insulin is absent, so hyperglycemia pulls water out of the cells into the ECF. Serum sodium concentrations fall in proportion to the dilution caused by the hyperglycemia. The measured sodium level is lowered by 1.6 mEq/liter for every 100 mg/dL of glucose above 100. That phenomenon is referred to as transitional hyponatremia because no net change in body water occurs. No specific therapy is required; artificially lowered sodium concentrations will return to normal once the plasma glucose level is normalized. The most common formulas for sodium are shown in Box 4-4.

The patient's fluid volume status is critical in assessing hyponatremia. In general, hyponatremia is thought of as either renal or extrarenal. Excretion of sodium by the kidneys is due to renal failure or to problems with ADH or diuretics. Extrarenal causes include sodium loss due to wounds, burns, sweating, congestive heart failure, cirrhosis, hypothyroidism, GI losses, and cerebral salt-wasting syndrome. Acute hyponatremia can also occur if dehydrated patients are infused with fluids free of sodium. In patients who have bled or who are intravascularly depleted of water (e.g., because of vomiting, diarrhea, pancreatitis, or burns), IV infusion of 5% dextrose in water can rapidly cause hyponatremia. As the normal response to hyponatremia is the suppression of ADH to secrete water to increase the sodium concentration in the serum, the problem is exacerbated in hypovolemic patients because the hypothalamus is secreting ADH in an effort to preserve water. Thus, hyponatremic patients should have undetectable levels of ADH. However, ADH release can be stimulated both by elevated ECF osmolality and by reduced ECF volume. ADH secretion commonly occurs transiently after trauma or burns and even in the early postoperative period, causing euvolemic hyponatremia. In hypovolemic patients, baroreceptors also stimulate the hypothalamus to retain water through ADH release.

Diuresis with furosemide or mannitol, in addition to causing intravascular fluid loss, can cause hyponatremia. It also increases sodium loss by the kidneys and increases ADH release as the body tries to counteract the rapid fluid loss by preserving water. Hyperglycemia, if it is high enough for glucose to be spilled in the urine, will also induce an osmotic diuresis that depletes extracellular water and also leads to hyponatremia. Along with diuresis, hyperglycemia can lead to a variety of electrolyte imbalances (many regulatory mechanisms are involved) and can cause wild hormonal swings and imbalances.

Renal loss of sodium can lead to hyponatremia and to excessive release of natriuretic peptides related to brain injury or disease. One particularly difficult condition to treat is cerebral salt-wasting syndrome. Even when such patients are treated with salt, the regulatory mechanisms cause high urine output (up to 4 to 6 liters per day) with consequent urine sodium losses. Those losses correlate with elevated brain natriuretic peptide levels in plasma. The lost sodium must be replaced either through an IV line or by enteral intake.

In patients with a brain injury, hyponatremia that is normally well tolerated may be devastating; it is thought to cause cerebral intracellular swelling as osmolality is reduced. In such patients, infusion of HTS may be required. HTS is available commercially (in 3%, 5%, or 23% concentrations). A pharmacist can also make HTS at any desired concentration without much difficulty. Depending on the electrolyte imbalances, salt infusions can take a variety of forms; sodium can be provided as sodium chloride, sodium acetate, or sodium bicarbonate or in combinations.

If HTS is to be infused at concentrations higher than 5%, the preferred route is through central IV catheters; higher concentrations can be caustic to peripheral veins and can also cause pain. In general, no more than 10 mEq/day of sodium should be provided. The volume of fluids needed should be taken into consideration when the concentration is chosen. If a patient requires a large volume of fluids in a 4-hour period, 0.9% normal saline will elevate the sodium level. In hypervolemic patients, the goal is to minimize the volume infused, so a higher concentration, such as 5%, can be used. The reason for elevating sodium levels slowly is to avoid central pontine myelinolysis, which can occur 1 to 6 days later; it is manifested as pseudobulbar palsy, quadriparesis, seizures, movement disorders, and decreased level of consciousness.

If urologic or gynecologic surgery is performed with hypo-osmotic irrigation, acute hyponatremia can occur. During endometrial resection as well as in transurethral resection of the prostate, acute water intoxication has been reported as a complication.

BOX 4-4 Sodium Equations for Clinical Use

Sodium Deficit

Sodium deficit (mEq) = ([Na] goal − [Na] plasma) × TBW

TBW = (weight × 60%)

Free Water Deficit

Free water deficit = (([Na]/140) − 1) × TBW

Corrected Sodium

Corrected sodium = [Na] + 0.016 × (glucose − 100)

Serum Osmolality (Calculated)

2 × [Na] + BUN/2.8 + glucose/18

Fractional Excretion of Sodium

FeNa = [Na] urine + creatinine plasma /[Na] plasma + creatinine urine

<1% = prerenal (hypovolemia)

>2% = intrinsic renal disorder

BUN, Blood urea nitrogen; *TBW,* total body water.

In surgical ICU patients, a frequent cause of hyponatremia is SIADH. This syndrome can be acute or chronic. In hypovolemic patients, the body's natural response is to release ADH; however, if the body is euvolemic and yet releases ADH inappropriately, the diagnosis of SIADH can be made. Therefore, the diagnosis of SIADH should be made only in euvolemic patients. In addition, the urine osmolarity is usually above 150 mmol/kg and the urine sodium above 20 mmol/liter. Given the aberrant release of ADH, the serum osmolality is often less than 270 mmol, and yet the kidneys still excrete concentrated urine. It is usually managed with fluid restrictions. Furthermore, it is important to differentiate SIADH from adrenal insufficiency, in which hypokalemia also does occur.

A hyponatremic patient with a urine osmolality of 350 mmol is producing ADH, and the kidneys are concentrating it as they should; the source of hyponatremia is usually extrarenal. ADH-secreting tumors (such as carcinoid tumors or small cell carcinomas of the lung) can cause chronic SIADH. These lung tumors usually cause euvolemic hyponatremia. Up to 35% of patients with active acquired immunodeficiency syndrome (AIDS) who are admitted for hospitalization have SIADH. Hyponatremia can also be caused by renal dysfunction in patients with conditions that impair the capability to retain sodium, such as medullary cystic disease, polycystic kidney disease, analgesic nephropathy, chronic pyelonephritis, and obstructive uropathy after decompression syndrome.

Hypernatremia

Hypernatremia is usually defined as serum sodium concentration above 145 mEq/liter. Moderate hypernatremia (146 to 159 mEq/liter) is fairly well tolerated, whereas severe hypernatremia (>160 mEq/liter) can be detrimental. Hypernatremia is associated with muscle weakness, restlessness, lethargy, insomnia, and, in severe cases, central pontine myelinolysis or coma. The common causes of hypernatremia include endocrine syndromes (in which ADH synthesis or release fails), failure of renal tubular cells to respond to ADH, increased salt intake or infusion, and loss of water. Hypernatremia can be a problem in that it pulls water out of the cells; the primary concern is that it is thought to contract the cerebral cells. However, recent experience with HTS has shown that acutely elevated sodium levels are relatively safe. HTS is used to contract cerebral intracellular volume in patients with TBI to reduce the total brain volume when intracranial swelling or mass effect is a factor. The normal response to hypernatremia is for the kidneys to generate hyperosmolar urine and to retain water. Renal correction of hypernatremia depends on the patient's having access to water.

Hypernatremia is associated with hypertonicity and should be classified in the context of hypovolemia, euvolemia, or hypervolemia. Hypovolemic hypernatremia commonly occurs in dehydrated patients with low water intake, high fluid losses such as vomiting, nasogastric tube loss, vomiting, or diarrhea. Euvolemic hypernatremia is seen in patients with DI (nephrogenic or neurogenic) because of excess loss of urinary free water. Hypervolemic hypernatremia is usually iatrogenic caused by resuscitation with hypertonic solutions or a result of excess mineralocorticoid in Conn or Cushing syndrome.

Hypernatremia (like hyponatremia) is thought of as either renal or extrarenal. Renal fluid losses are due to diuretics, the polyuric phase of acute tubular necrosis, or postobstructive diuresis of the kidney. After decompression of a chronically obstructed ureter, renal tubular cells seem to respond less to ADH. Nephrogenic DI is defined as an impaired capacity of the renal tubules to respond to ADH and to concentrate urine. Moderate hypernatremia develops in patients with nephrogenic DI when they lose water in dilute urine, despite elevated plasma levels of ADH. If an infusion of ADH does not increase urine osmolality, DI is the likely diagnosis. Drugs such as lithium, glyburide, demeclocycline, and amphotericin B can induce DI. The treatment of patients with lithium-induced nephrogenic DI is amiloride (5 to 10 mg daily).

Hypercalcemia or severe hypokalemia also impairs the capacity of renal tubular cells to absorb sodium. Patients with end-stage renal dysfunction and low glomerular filtration rates may produce a fixed volume of 2 to 4 liters/day of iso-osmotic urine. In hot and arid environments, such patients are particularly susceptible to dehydration and hypernatremia.

The extrarenal causes of hypernatremia include loss of water from vomiting, diarrhea, nasogastric tube suctioning, burns, sweating, fever, or problems with insufficient ADH levels. Infusion of sodium (like HTS) can also cause hypernatremia; the duration depends on the amount of crystalloids infused for resuscitation during 24 hours. A study on the use of 5% HTS in trauma patients showed that sodium levels rose above 150 mEq/liter and stayed elevated for days. In contrast, previous studies on the use of 7.5% HTS infusions found that the hypernatremia was brief. The transient hypernatremia was probably caused by aggressive use of other crystalloids for resuscitation after the HTS infusion, which quickly diluted the hypernatremia.

In dealing with hypernatremia, it is again important to first assess volume status. Correcting the hypernatremia depends on volume status. In hypovolemic patients, offsetting the volume deficit with isotonic fluids is sufficient. However, nonhypovolemic patients need free water replacement with hypotonic solutions. In hypervolemic patients, diuretics may be used—carefully. In general, in asymptomatic patients, sodium levels should not be corrected too rapidly; doing so could cause cerebral edema. In patients with acute hypernatremia, the rate is usually no more than 1 to 2 mEq/hr; with chronic hyponatremia, no more than 0.5 mEq/hr. Sodium levels should not be corrected at a rate of more than 8 mEq/day. Careful and frequent sodium monitoring is often required.

Patients with DI are producing dilute urine at hundreds of milliliters per hour. They should be treated with DDAVP, a synthetic analogue of ADH that has a half-life of several hours. DDAVP increases water movement out of the collecting duct, but it does not have the vasoconstrictive properties of ADH. Patients with mild DI can be treated with intranasal DDAVP and water intake. DDAVP can be administered orally, intranasally, subcutaneously, or intravenously. The intranasal dose is 10 μg once or twice daily. In ICU patients, IV administration is preferred for control and accuracy.

Potassium

Potassium is the main intracellular ion; sodium, the main extracellular ion. The normal potassium concentration in serum is 4.5 mmol/liter. Small changes in serum reflect large intracellular changes that may cause significant morbidity and mortality. The daily average intake of potassium is 50 to 100 mmol/day. The kidneys control the daily excretion, which ranges widely from 20 to 400 mmol. The renin-angiotensin-aldosterone hormone axis is the key regulator of potassium clearance. As aldosterone increases in plasma, so does potassium excretion.

Hypokalemia

Patients with hypokalemia have a [K^+] lower than 3.5 mmol/liter. Hypokalemia is commonly a result of hyperpolarization of the resting potential of the cell. Hyperpolarization interferes with neuromuscular function. Hypokalemia is associated with generalized fatigue and weakness, ileus, atrial arrhythmia, and acute renal insufficiency. On occasion, rhabdomyolysis occurs in patients whose [K^+] drops below 2.5 mmol/liter. Flaccid paralysis with respiratory compromise can occur as [K^+] decreases to less than 2 mmol/liter.

Hypokalemia is caused by renal losses, extrarenal losses, or intracellular shifts from medications or hyperthyroidism. Extrarenal losses can be caused by persistent vomiting, gastric tubes, diarrhea, alkalosis, catecholamine secretion, insulin administration, or high-output enteric or pancreatic fistulas. Hypokalemia is a common problem in patients with congestive heart failure who are receiving multiple drugs. It can also develop in patients treated with diuretics that force renal function to excrete urine with an elevated potassium concentration. Long-term diuretic therapy can produce a sustained negative potassium balance. Patients with a chronic potassium deficiency can develop a cardiac rhythm disturbance. The electrocardiogram of patients with hypokalemia will show depressed T waves and U waves. Hypokalemia leads to cardiac arrhythmia, particularly atrial tachycardia with or without block, atrioventricular dissociation, ventricular tachycardia, and ventricular fibrillation. The risk for hypokalemia-associated arrhythmia is higher in patients treated with digoxin, even when potassium concentrations are in the low-normal range. Hypokalemia not caused by diuretics may be due to a rare endocrine disorder, including primary hyperaldosteronism and renin-secreting tumors. Hypokalemia is also frequently associated with hypomagnesemia and acidemia.

Treatment of acute hypokalemia. Hypokalemic patients require potassium replacement, which can be achieved by oral or IV routes. Oral supplementation is generally 40 to 100 mEq/day, in two to four doses. The IV rate is 10 to 20 mEq/hr; if potassium is infused at rates of more than 10 mEq/hr, cardiac monitoring is required. In emergency situations, the rate can be as high as 40 mEq/hr, but then a central vein should be used; high concentrations of potassium in IV fluids can be irritating to peripheral veins. In patients with renal dysfunction, whose potassium excretion is reduced, both the IV rate of potassium replacement and the total dose should be lower.

After treatment, frequent monitoring of potassium levels is necessary. Because hypokalemia represents large intracellular deficits, replenishing total body levels may take days. Potassium therapy is given as the chloride salt because hypokalemia is commonly associated with a contraction in the extracellular water, in which chloride is the predominant anion. Potassium in foods is linked to phosphate. Potassium phosphate salts may need to be given by the IV route, particularly when expansion of intracellular water is anticipated. To reduce the risk of serious cardiac arrhythmia with cardiac disease or after cardiac surgery in patients who have a serum value below 3.5 mmol/liter, serum [K^+] should be promptly corrected to a level higher than 4.0 mmol/liter. Patients with substantial and continuing GI loss of potassium require extraordinary potassium replacement to achieve correction of hypokalemia.

Magnesium levels should be concomitantly monitored; hypomagnesemia can produce refractory hypokalemia. Magnesium is an important cofactor for potassium uptake and for maintenance of intracellular potassium levels. In addition, supplemental magnesium reduces the risk of arrhythmia.

Hypokalemic patients with concurrent acidemia are treated with potassium replacement, before their pH is corrected by bicarbonate administration. Diabetic patients with ketoacidosis may initially have normal [K^+], but hypokalemia rapidly develops as insulin is administered and as glucose shifts into cells; for such patients, potassium supplements should be added to the resuscitation fluid, once the physician is confident that renal function is adequate. If hypokalemia develops while patients are undergoing diuretic therapy, additional drugs can reduce the renal loss of potassium. For example, triamterene or spironolactone blocks the effect of aldosterone and reduces potassium loss in urine.

Hyperkalemia

Hyperkalemia is defined as [K^+] of more than 5.0 mmol/liter. If levels exceed 6 mmol/liter, perturbations in the resting cell membrane potential occur, and normal depolarization and repolarization are impaired. The most common cause of hyperkalemia is renal failure in hospitalized patients. The transport of potassium is passive, but the transport of sodium requires energy. This difference across the cell is maintained by Na^+,K^+-adenosinetriphosphatase (ATPase) activity, which requires energy. The energy is in the form of cellular ATP. Its levels are highly variable in different stages of shock when nutrients are not available (whether carbohydrates or oxygen). When cellular ATP levels fall, the sodium pump is impaired. If either sodium or potassium levels are severely high or low, the membrane potential will be affected. Eventually, without energy, cell death occurs, and the sodium-potassium gradient cannot be maintained; the sodium gradient is needed to maintain the membrane potential. Pseudohyperkalemia also may occur when red blood cells lyse in tubes. In such cases, determination of the potassium level may be repeated.

The primary clinical problem is cardiac arrhythmia, which can be lethal. Hyperkalemia is associated with peaked T waves; dangerous hyperkalemia (6 to 7 mmol/liter) is indicated by T waves higher than R waves (Fig. 4-24).

The most common cause of hyperkalemia is acute onset of renal dysfunction or failure. Cellular injury (such as sepsis or ischemia-reperfusion) can also release potassium from its intracellular source, which can overwhelm the kidneys' ability to clear potassium. At least 20% of normal renal function is required to respond to ADH and to maintain normal potassium levels. The reperfusion of ischemic tissues resulting in rhabdomyolysis causes

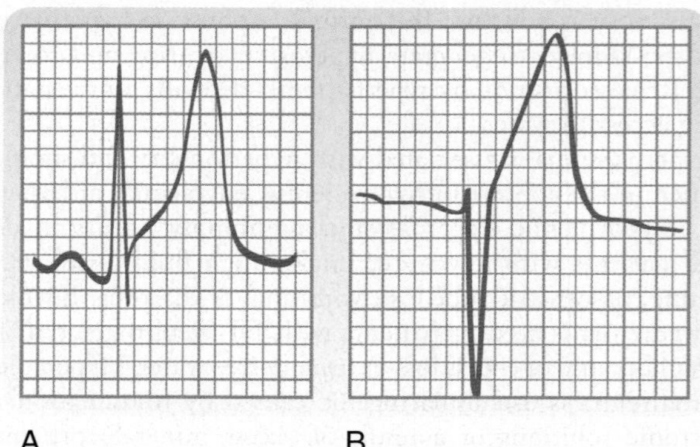

FIGURE 4-24 **Electrocardiographic Changes.** **A,** Indicating hyperkalemia. The T wave is tall, narrow, and symmetrical. **B,** Indicating acute myocardial infarction. The T wave is tall but broad based and asymmetrical. (From Somers MP, Brady WJ, Perron AD, et al: The prominent T wave: Electrocardiographic differential diagnosis. *Am J Emerg Med* 20:243–251, 2002.)

high potassium levels; to prevent cardiac arrest, a bolus of IV sodium bicarbonate may be of some benefit. The bicarbonate shifts potassium intracellularly. Note that impaired aldosterone levels (as with infarction of bilateral adrenal glands) can activate other renal mechanisms and stimulate potassium excretion, resulting in moderate levels of hyperkalemia.

Drugs can have a direct effect on the renal tubules and on potassium excretion; examples include triamterene, spironolactone, beta blockers, cyclosporine, and tacrolimus. They are usually a contributing factor but not a primary cause. Succinylcholine, a depolarizing paralytic agent, is used in patients with muscle atrophy from disuse, prolonged bed rest, neurologic denervation syndromes, severe burns, direct muscle trauma, or rhabdomyolysis; it can cause severe hyperkalemia, resulting in cardiac arrest. When drawing blood samples from patients, clinicians must recognize that sample hemolysis can release potassium, so laboratory test results could be spurious. If the sample or test results are suspect, another sample should be taken before drastic efforts are made to treat hyperkalemia.

In addition, ischemia-reperfusion injury is associated with hyperkalemia. Revascularization after an ischemic injury may cause severe hyperkalemia based on duration of the ischemic episode, ranging from 4 to 6 hours. As a result, it is usually recommended to administer bicarbonate before reperfusion.

Treatment of hyperkalemia. In patients at risk for development of cardiac arrhythmia from hyperkalemia, several interventions are useful. IV calcium can immediately reduce the risk of arrhythmia; it antagonizes the depolarization effect of elevated [K^+]. Sodium bicarbonate infusion buffers extracellular protons and allows net transfer of cytosolic protons across the cell membrane through carbonic acid. The shift of protons out of the cell is associated with a shift of potassium into the cells. Bicarbonate therapy is most effective in hyperkalemic patients with metabolic acidemia. Insulin and glucose infusions prompt an increase in Na^+,K^+-ATPase activity and a decline in extracellular water potassium concentration as the extracellular water potassium is pumped into the cell.

In patients with both aldosterone deficiency and hyperkalemia, a mineralocorticoid drug such as 9α-fludrocortisone will increase renal excretion of potassium. In patients with acute renal failure, hemodialysis is the most reliable method to control hyperkalemia. Continuous filtration methods clear potassium at a slower rate than hemodialysis does. Chronic hyperkalemia associated with renal dysfunction can be managed by oral or rectal administration of sodium polystyrene sulfonate, a cation exchange resin that binds potassium in the gut lumen. Rectally administered binding resins are particularly effective because the colonic mucosa can excrete mucus with large amounts of potassium. Surgeons should clearly establish a process for managing hyperkalemia because rapidly escalating potassium levels pose an immediate threat and require rapidly delivered effective therapy (Box 4-5). Dysfunctional renal handling of potassium from mineralocorticoid deficiency or resistance leads to hyperkalemia. Renal failure is commonly associated with tubular defects and potassium management problems along with hyperaldosteronism. However, in patients with normal renal function, assessing levels of aldosterone, renin, and cortisol can help differentiate between mineralocorticoid deficiency and resistance. In patients with aldosterone deficiency, fludrocortisone is useful.

BOX 4-5 Guidelines for Treatment of Adult Patients With Hyperkalemia

First: Stop all infusion of potassium.

Electrocardiographic Evidence of Pending Arrest

Loss of P wave and broad slurring of QRS; immediate effective therapy indicated

1. IV infusion of calcium salts
   10 mL of 10% calcium chloride during a 10-minute period
   or
   10 mL of 10% calcium gluconate during a 3- to 5-minute period
2. IV infusion of sodium bicarbonate
   50-100 mEq during a 10- to 20-minute period; benefit proportional to extent of pretherapy acidemia

Electrocardiographic Evidence of Potassium Effect

Peaked T waves; prompt therapy needed

1. Glucose and insulin infusion
   IV infusion of 50 mL of $D_{50}W$ and 10 units of regular insulin; monitor glucose
2. Immediate hemodialysis

Biochemical Evidence of Hyperkalemia and No Electrocardiographic Changes

Effective therapy needed within hours

1. Potassium-binding resins into the GI tract, with 20% sorbitol
2. Promotion of renal kaliuresis by loop diuretic

$D_{50}W$, 50% dextrose in water.

Calcium

Calcium, a divalent cation, is a critical component of many extracellular and intracellular reactions. It is the most abundant electrolyte in the body overall. About 99% of it is found in the bones; the remaining 1% circulates in the blood. For surgeons, it is of particular interest; it is an essential cofactor in the coagulation cascade, and intracellular ionized calcium (iCa^{2+}) participates in the regulation of neuronal, hormonal, muscular, and renal cellular function. Total serum calcium concentration (normally, 8.5 to 10.5 mg/dL) is present in three molecular forms: protein-bound calcium, diffusible calcium bound to anions (bicarbonate, phosphate, and acetate), and freely diffusible calcium as iCa^{2+}.

The biochemically active species is iCa^{2+}, which constitutes about 45% of total serum calcium. More than 80% of protein-bound calcium is attached to albumin, so the total calcium concentration in serum will decrease in patients with hypoalbuminemia. Physiologically, the total plasma calcium level must be corrected relative to the albumin level. Normal calcium levels may range from 8.5 to 10.5 mg/day, assuming an albumin level of 4.5 g/dL. The calcium concentration [Ca] usually changes by 0.8 mg/dL for every change of 1.0 g/dL in plasma albumin concentration. This formula estimates the actual total plasma calcium level:

$$\text{Corrected } [iCa^{2+}] = \text{Total } [Ca] + (0.8 \times [4.5 - \text{albumin level}])$$

Acidosis decreases the amount of calcium bound to albumin, whereas alkalosis increases the bound fraction of calcium. A small amount of calcium (about 6%) is bound to anions such as citrate and sulfate. The remainder is [iCa^{2+}] that is biologically active.

The increase in [iCa^{2+}] is controlled by cell membrane enzymes that transport calcium out of the cell. In muscle cells, [iCa^{2+}] is stored in the sarcoplasmic reticulum. It can be quickly released into intracellular fluid, in which it has a key role in the molecular events that cause muscle contraction. Tight control of [iCa^{2+}] in ECF is essential. The serum calcium concentration is controlled by the interaction of parathyroid hormone (PTH), calcitonin, and vitamin D. PTH and calcitonin are hormones subject to regulatory release by endocrine cells, whereas vitamin D is either consumed in the diet or formed in the skin as cholecalciferol in response to ultraviolet irradiation. Bone contains an enormous reservoir of calcium in the form of a matrix of calcium and other molecules. Turnover of calcium salts in bone is constant and integral to maintaining a stable [iCa^{2+}] in ECF. Receptors in the membranes of parathyroid cells release PTH when [iCa^{2+}] in ECF declines. PTH activates osteoclasts in bones, which release calcium from the structural matrix of bone. PTH stimulates tubule cells in the proximal nephron both to absorb calcium from the filtrate and to excrete phosphates. PTH with vitamin D enhances calcium absorption from the lumen of the gut.

Calcitonin has the opposite effects on calcium metabolism (compared with PTH). As calcitonin levels in ECF increase because of its excretion from type C cells of the thyroid, [iCa^{2+}] declines as more calcium is bound to bone matrix. Vitamin D circulating in blood is converted in the liver to 25-hydroxycholecalciferol. Then, 25-hydroxycholecalciferol circulating in blood encounters kidney cells that further hydroxylate the sterol to 1,25-dihydroxycholecalciferol, which is the most potent calcium-modulating hormone. Next, 1,25-dihydroxycholecalciferol increases the transport of calcium and phosphate from the lumen of the bowel into the ECF of the intestine. Furthermore, in conjunction with PTH, 1,25-dihydroxycholecalciferol increases bone resorption, increasing the calcium concentration in ECF. In summary, multiple hormonal mechanisms produce a balance of influences on the concentration of calcium in ECF.

Hypocalcemia

Hypocalcemia is defined as total serum concentration below 8.4 mg/dL or ionized calcium concentration below 4.5 mg/dL. It varies from an asymptomatic biochemical abnormality to a life-threatening disorder, depending on its duration, severity, and rapidity of development. It is caused by loss of calcium from the circulation or by insufficient entry of calcium into the circulation.

Acute hypocalcemia can be life-threatening. It impairs transmembrane depolarization; [iCa^{2+}] below 0.8 mEq/liter can lead to central nervous system dysfunction. Hypocalcemic patients can have paresthesias, muscle spasms (including tetany), and seizures. As [iCa^{2+}] declines, patients can notice numbness, paresthesias of the distal extremities, and painful muscle spasms. If patients hyperventilate, a respiratory alkalosis may exacerbate their condition and further reduce [iCa^{2+}]. Cardiac dysfunction is also common. Patients with low [iCa^{2+}] may require IV infusion of calcium to restore cardiac function. Hypocalcemic patients have a prolonged QT interval on electrocardiograms that may progress to complete heart block or ventricular fibrillation.

Hypoparathyroidism, the most common cause of hypocalcemia, often develops because of surgery in the central neck, such as radical resection of head and neck cancers. It develops in 1% to 2% of patients after a total thyroidectomy. The hypocalcemia may be transient, permanent, or intermittent, as with vitamin D deficiency during the winter. Autoimmune hypoparathyroidism can be an isolated defect or part of polyglandular autoimmune syndrome type I in association with adrenal insufficiency and mucocutaneous candidiasis; most of these patients have autoantibodies directed against the calcium-sensing receptor. Congenital causes of hypocalcemia include activation of mutations of the calcium-sensing receptor, which resets the calcium-PTH relation to a lower serum calcium level. Mutations affecting intracellular processing of the pre-pro-PTH molecule can lead to hypoparathyroidism, hypocalcemia, or both. Finally, some cases of hypoparathyroidism are associated with hypoplasia or aplasia of the parathyroid glands; the best known is DiGeorge syndrome.

Pseudohypoparathyroidism is a group of disorders characterized by postreceptor resistance to PTH. One classic variant is Albright hereditary osteodystrophy, associated with low stature, round facies, short digits, and mental retardation. Hypomagnesemia induces PTH resistance and also affects PTH production. Severe hypermagnesemia (>6 mg/dL) can lead to hypocalcemia by inhibiting PTH secretion. When it is associated with decreased dietary calcium intake, vitamin D deficiency leads to hypocalcemia. The low calcium level stimulates PTH secretion (secondary hyperparathyroidism), leading to hypophosphatemia.

Rhabdomyolysis and tumor lysis syndrome cause loss of calcium from the circulation when large amounts of intracellular phosphate are released, thereby increasing calcium levels in bone and extraskeletal tissues. A similar mechanism causes hypocalcemia with phosphate administration.

Acute pancreatitis results in calcium sequestration in the abdomen, causing hypocalcemia. After surgery for hyperparathyroidism, patients with severe prolonged disease (such as those with secondary or tertiary hyperparathyroidism who are in renal failure) can develop a form of hypocalcemia known as hungry bone syndrome, in which serum calcium is rapidly deposited into the bone. The syndrome is rarely seen after correction of long-standing metabolic acidosis or after thyroidectomy for hyperthyroidism.

Several medications (such as ethylenediaminetetraacetic acid [EDTA], citrate present in transfused blood, lactate, and foscarnet) chelate calcium in the circulation, sometimes producing hypocalcemia in which the iCa^{2+} level is decreased even though the total calcium level may be normal. Acute hypocalcemia in the postoperative period can occur in response to rapid blood transfusions. In the past, stored blood contained a higher concentration of citrate, which binds to and chelates serum calcium. Now that citrate has been eliminated from blood-banking techniques, this is rarely seen. Extensive osteoblastic skeletal metastases (such as from prostate and breast cancers) may also cause hypocalcemia. Chemotherapy, including cisplatin, 5-fluorouracil, and leucovorin, causes hypocalcemia mediated through hypomagnesemia. In patients with sepsis, hypocalcemia is usually associated with hypoalbuminemia.

Tumor lysis syndrome is a constellation of electrolyte abnormalities that include hypocalcemia, hyperphosphatemia, hyperuricemia, and hyperkalemia. Such abnormalities occur when antineoplastic therapy causes a sudden surge in tumor cell death and a release of cytosolic contents. Solid tumors and lymphomas have been implicated. Acute renal failure occurs in patients with tumor lysis syndrome and prevents spontaneous correction of the electrolyte abnormalities; emergency dialysis may be the only way to comprehensively correct the abnormalities.

Acute hypocalcemia is frequent after resuscitation from shock. In a study of patients in burn shock, Wray and associates hypothesized that a major factor contributing to the development of hypocalcemia was depressed levels of 1,25-dihydroxycholecalciferol, perhaps caused by a sudden lack of vitamin D in the diet. In patients with severe pancreatitis, the fall in calcium is speculated to be the consequence of ionized extracellular calcium becoming linked to fats in the peripancreatic inflammatory phlegmon. Rapid infusion of a citrate load during the transfusion of blood products (particularly platelet concentrates and FFP) may also lead to acute severe hypocalcemia ([iCa^{2+}] < 0.62 mmol/liter) and to hypotension. Rapid increases in serum phosphate can occur after improper administration or excessive dosing of phosphate-containing cathartics; as the phosphate concentration increases, severe hypocalcemia ensues.

Treatment of hypocalcemia. Patients with acute symptomatic hypocalcemia (calcium level < 7.0 mg/dL, iCa^{2+} level < 0.8 mmol/liter) should be treated promptly with IV calcium. Calcium may be given orally or intravenously in the form of calcium gluconate or calcium chloride. Calcium gluconate, preferred to calcium chloride, causes less tissue necrosis if it is extravasated, so it should be given through the central vein route. The first 100 to 200 mg of elemental calcium (1 to 2 g calcium gluconate) should be given during 10 to 20 minutes. Faster administration may result in cardiac dysfunction and even arrest. Those first 100 to 200 mg should then be followed by a slow calcium infusion at 0.5 to 1.5 mg/kg/hr. Calcium infusion should continue until the patient is receiving effective doses of oral calcium and vitamin D. Calcium for infusion should be diluted in saline or dextrose solution to avoid vein irritation. The infusion should not contain bicarbonate or phosphate, either of which can form an insoluble calcium salt. If bicarbonate or phosphate administration is necessary, a separate IV line should be used.

Coexisting hypomagnesemia should be corrected in every patient. Care should be taken in patients with renal insufficiency because they cannot excrete excess magnesium. Magnesium is given by infusion, initiated with 2 g of magnesium sulfate during 10 to 15 minutes, followed by 1 g/hr. In patients with severe hyperphosphatemia (such as those with tumor lysis syndrome, rhabdomyolysis, or chronic renal failure), treatment is focused on correcting the hyperphosphatemia.

Acute hyperphosphatemia usually resolves in patients with intact renal function. Phosphate excretion may be aided by saline infusion (caution: this can lead to worsening of hypocalcemia); in addition, acetazolamide, a carbonic anhydrase inhibitor, can be given at 10 to 15 mg/kg every 3 to 4 hours. Hemodialysis may be necessary for patients with symptomatic hypocalcemia and hyperphosphatemia, especially if renal function is impaired. Chronic hyperphosphatemia is managed by a low-phosphate diet and by use of phosphate binders with meals.

Chronic hypocalcemia (hypoparathyroidism) is treated by oral calcium administration and, if that is insufficient, vitamin D supplementation. The serum calcium level should be targeted to about 8.0 mg/dL. Most patients will be entirely asymptomatic at that level. Further elevation will lead to hypercalciuria because of the lack of PTH effect on the renal tubules. Chronic hypercalciuria carries the risks of nephrocalcinosis, nephrolithiasis, and renal impairment.

Several oral calcium preparations are available. Calcium carbonate is the cheapest form, but it may be poorly absorbed, especially in older patients and those with achlorhydria. Similarly, various forms of vitamin D are available. If oral calcium preparations cannot achieve adequate calcium repletion, vitamin D should be added. The usual initial daily dose is 50,000 IU of 25-hydroxyvitamin D (or 0.25 to 0.5 mg of 1,25-hydroxyvitamin D). Calcium and vitamin D doses are established by gradual titration. When adequate calcemia is achieved, urinary calcium excretion is measured. If hypercalciuria is detected, a thiazide diuretic may be added to diminish calciuria and to further increase the serum calcium level. The serum calcium level should be monitored. If the phosphorus level is higher than 6.0 mg/dL when the calcium level is satisfactory, an unabsorbable phosphate binder should be added. Once calcium and phosphorus levels are controlled, the patient should be monitored every 3 to 6 months for both levels and for urinary calcium excretion.

Special consideration is necessary for the treatment of women with hypoparathyroidism who are pregnant or nursing. During pregnancy, vitamin D requirements gradually increase, up to three times as high as the prepregnancy requirements. Supplementary doses of vitamin D should be titrated, using frequent serum calcium level measurements. After delivery, if the baby is to be bottle fed, the dose should be decreased to the prepregnancy dose. If the baby is to be nursed, the dose of calcitriol should be decreased to 50% of the prepregnancy dose[4] because endogenous calcitriol production is stimulated by prolactin and by increased production of PTH-related peptide (PTHrP), which is also stimulated by prolactin.

Several reports have described successful control of hypocalcemia with synthetic PTH (1,34-PTH, teriparatide) by twice-daily subcutaneous administration, with a lower risk of hypercalciuria.

Hypercalcemia

Mild hypercalcemia is suspected when total serum calcium levels are in the range of 10.5 to 12 mg/dL. Patients with a serum calcium concentration of 12 to 14.5 mg/dL have moderate hypercalcemia. Patients with transient hypercalcemia are generally asymptomatic. Those with sustained elevations in renal calcium excretion are susceptible to the development of renal lithiasis. Patients have severe hypercalcemia when serum calcium levels exceed 15 mg/dL; such patients have symptoms of weakness, stupor, and central nervous system dysfunction. In hypercalcemic patients, a renal concentrating defect also occurs, leading to polyuria and to loss of sodium and water. Indeed, many hypercalcemic patients are dehydrated. Hypercalcemic crisis is a syndrome in which total serum calcium levels exceed 17 mg/dL; such patients are subject to life-threatening cardiac tachyarrhythmia, coma, acute renal failure, and ileus with abdominal distention.

The most common cause of hypercalcemia (in fact, in 90% of all patients) is primary hyperparathyroidism; other causes include unregulated PTH secretion and malignant disease. It occurs most commonly with malignant diseases in hospitalized patients and with hyperparathyroidism in the general population. Breast cancer is the most common malignant cause. Other rare causes include thyrotoxicosis, vitamin A and D overdose, granulomatous diseases, and commonly used drugs like thiazide diuretics and lithium. Another rare cause of hypercalcemia is familial hypocalciuric hypercalcemia, which is due to an autosomal dominant mutation in the calcium-sensing receptor causing increased calcium and magnesium retention by the kidneys. Signs and symptoms of hypercalcemia are nonspecific and include nausea, vomiting, altered mental status, constipation, depression, lethargy, myalgias, arthralgias, polyuria, headache, abdominal and flank pain (renal stones), and coma. They are sometimes described as abdominal groans, psychic moans, and renal stones. However, most of these symptoms are manifested after chronic hypercalcemia and not after acute hypercalcemia. Usually, a patient's clinical presentation is recognized as related to hypercalcemia only after it has been diagnosed by blood test results. It is extremely difficult to diagnose hypercalcemia by a patient's history alone.

Bone demineralization is found in patients with severe and prolonged hyperparathyroidism. The majority (85%) of such patients have a solitary hyperfunctioning adenoma in one parathyroid gland; the remaining 15% have excessive PTH release as a result of hyperplasia of all four glands. PTH induces phosphaturia and depresses serum phosphate concentrations; such a laboratory finding corroborates the diagnosis of primary hyperparathyroidism. Secondary hyperparathyroidism, an endocrine disease characterized by hyperplasia of the parathyroid glands, develops in patients with chronic renal failure. Decreased renal function results in impaired synthesis of 1,25-dihydroxycholecalciferol. Although patients have low serum calcium levels, their osteomalacia indicates excessive PTH secretion. To control elevated PTH levels in patients with secondary hyperparathyroidism, surgical removal of most of the parathyroid tissue may be required.

Humoral hypercalcemia of malignancy (HHM) is a clinical syndrome in which elevated calcium levels are caused by synthesis of the humoral factor by the tumoral process. Usually, HHM is applied to patients with excessive tumoral production of PTHrP. However, rare cases characterized by excessive production of PTH and calcitriol have also been described. Patients with HHM constitute about 80% of all patients with hypercalcemia associated with malignant disease. PTHrP and PTH share the same receptor, but the clinical presentation differs. HHM patients have a markedly larger degree of renal calcium excretion; PTH potently stimulates tubular calcium resorption, and hypercalciuria is less pronounced. HHM is usually associated with low serum calcitriol levels; PTH stimulates calcitriol production, and its level is usually elevated. PTHrP stimulates only bone resorption, with very low osteoblastic activity and therefore usually normal alkaline phosphatase levels; PTH stimulates bone resorption and formation.

HHM patients usually have a clinically obvious malignant disease and a poor prognosis. The only exceptions to this rule are patients with small, well-differentiated endocrine tumors (such as pheochromocytomas or islet cell tumors). However, such tumors constitute a minority of cases. HHM is most commonly seen with squamous cell carcinomas (e.g., of the lung, esophagus, cervix, or head and neck) and with renal, bladder, and ovarian cancers. Treatment of HHM patients is aimed at reducing the tumor burden, reducing osteoclastic resorption of the bone, and increasing calcium excretion through the urine.

Most cases of hypercalcemia are associated with Hodgkin disease. The other third of cases are associated with non-Hodgkin lymphoma and are caused by increased production of calcitriol by the malignant cells. Hypercalcemia usually responds well to treatment with corticosteroids. Multiple myeloma, lymphoma, and solid tumors metastatic to bone (particularly breast, lung, and prostate cancer) cause hypercalcemia by excessive osteoclastic activity. Drugs can also cause hypercalcemia, including theophylline, lithium, thiazide diuretics, and extraordinarily high doses of vitamin A and D. In addition, hypercalcemia can develop in young, normally active patients with high bone turnover rates who are suddenly forced into immobility, such as during forced bed rest after injury or major illness. This hypercalcemia of immobilization resolves with return to normal activity.

Another cause of hypercalcemia is milk-alkali syndrome, a rare condition caused by ingestion of large amounts of calcium together with sodium bicarbonate. It is currently associated with ingestion of calcium carbonate in over-the-counter antacid preparations and in drugs used to prevent and to treat osteoporosis. Features of the syndrome include hypercalcemia, renal failure, and metabolic alkalosis. The exact pathophysiologic mechanism is unknown. In rare cases, the amount of calcium ingested may be as low as 2000 to 3000 mg/day, but in most patients, the amount is between 6000 and 15,000 mg/day. Treatment consists of rehydration, diuresis, and cessation of calcium and antacid ingestion. If diuresis is impossible because of renal failure, dialysis using a dialysate with a low calcium concentration is effective. Renal failure usually resolves in patients with short-term hypercalcemia but may persist in those with chronic hypercalcemia.

Treatment of hypercalcemia. Definitive management of hypercalcemia depends on correction of the primary problem. Thus, patients with hyperparathyroidism secondary to a parathyroid adenoma or hyperplasia are cured of hypercalcemia by excision of the diseased parathyroid tissue. Hypercalcemic patients taking thiazide drugs should be converted to alternative therapies. Patients with a malignant neoplasm and hypercalcemia may respond to surgical excision, radiation therapy, or chemotherapy. Symptomatic patients with severe hypercalcemia related to malignant disease can be quickly and effectively treated by saline infusion to expand intravascular volume, followed by the administration of a loop diuretic (i.e., furosemide) to induce saline diuresis with associated urinary calcium clearance. Patients with severe hypercalcemia frequently have a contracted extracellular volume, so isotonic saline infusion is essential. Hypercalcemic patients in renal failure who cannot benefit from drug-induced diuresis can be treated by hemodialysis.

Severe hypercalcemia referred to as hypercalcemic crisis occurs with serum calcium concentration above 14 mg/dL and is related to release of calcium from bone by tumor; it can be managed by administration of bisphosphonates. Such drugs have a potent capacity to reduce osteoclast-mediated release of calcium from bone. Several formulations of bisphosphonates are available (in order of preference, zoledronic acid, pamidronate disodium, and etidronate disodium), all of which produce a slow decline in $[iCa^{2+}]$ during several days. In patients with metastatic breast cancer, bisphosphonates given as long-term prophylactic agents at a regular dosage have been shown to effectively prevent hypercalcemia.

Administration of exogenous calcitonin is often initially effective in patients with hypercalcemia. Calcitonin (4 U/kg subcutaneously every 12 hours) inhibits bone resorption and decreases renal tubular resorption of calcium, with a shorter onset of action than bisphosphonates; therefore, it is the better choice for short-term control of calcium. However, long-term treatment frequently leads to tachyphylaxis, possibly related to the development of antibodies to the exogenous calcitonin. Chelating agents (EDTA or phosphate salts) that bind and neutralize $[iCa^{2+}]$ are rarely indicated. Such agents are associated with the complications of metastatic calcification and acute renal failure and with the risk of depressing $[iCa^{2+}]$ to hypocalcemic levels.

Magnesium

Magnesium, an essential cation in the cell, is the second most prevalent cation. It is a critical cofactor in any reaction powered by ATP, so deficiencies can affect metabolism. It also acts as a calcium channel antagonist and plays a key role in the modulation of any activity involving calcium, such as muscle contraction and insulin release. The normal concentration of magnesium $[Mg^{2+}]$ in plasma ranges between 1.5 and 2.0 mEq/liter. Like calcium, it exists in three states: protein bound (30%, bound mostly to albumin), bound to anions (10%), and ionized (60%).

Magnesium is primarily intracellular, with less than 1% of body stores in the ECF. Measured plasma magnesium levels often do not reflect total body magnesium content. Clinical sequelae of altered magnesium content depend more on tissue magnesium levels than on the blood magnesium concentration. Consequently, it is often difficult to consistently correlate symptoms to specific plasma magnesium levels. One method to infer the tissue magnesium level is a physiologic test that measures the renal response to a magnesium load. Patients who retain more than 30% of an 800-mg load of IV magnesium are thought to be magnesium depleted, whereas those who retain less than 20% are said to be magnesium replete.

The kidneys are responsible for maintaining magnesium balance by excreting the absorbed magnesium. The ionized and bound forms of magnesium are freely filtered at the glomerulus. The distal tubule resorbs 10% of the filtered magnesium and plays an important role in calcium-independent magnesium homeostasis. The hormonal regulation of magnesium homeostasis has not been completely determined. PTH, glucagon, and ADH increase the resorption of magnesium in the Henle loop. In the distal convoluted tubule, aldosterone, ADH, and glucagon are thought to increase magnesium resorption. To maintain magnesium homeostasis, renal resorption of magnesium varies widely. Fractional resorption of filtered magnesium can decline to nearly zero in the presence of hypermagnesemia or reduced glomerular filtration rate. In contrast, in response to magnesium depletion or decreased intake, the fractional resorption of magnesium can rise to 99.5% to minimize urinary losses.

Hypomagnesemia

In ICU patients, the prevalence of hypomagnesemia ranges from 11% to 65%, but it is usually asymptomatic. Some studies have shown little significance to hypomagnesemia; other studies have shown an association with mortality. Any association with mortality is not necessarily causal, of course, and may merely reflect the patient's state of health. Symptoms of hypomagnesemia have been reported at modest degrees of depletion, but in general, symptoms become more common as the serum magnesium level falls below 1.2 mg/dL. Associating specific symptoms with hypomagnesemia is difficult. However, severe hypomagnesemia in postsurgical patients can lead to life-threatening ventricular arrhythmias such as torsades de pointes.

Hypokalemia is commonly associated with hypomagnesemia and reportedly occurs in 40% of patients with hypomagnesemia. The converse is also true; 60% of patients with hypokalemia are hypomagnesemic. The causes of hypomagnesemia are multiple, including renal, GI, and skin losses as well as hungry bone syndrome. Skin losses can be due to burns or toxic epidermal necrolysis. Renal losses can be due to a long list of drugs, but the most common are diuretics.

Hypomagnesemia also causes a specific disorder of renal potassium wasting that is refractory to potassium supplementation until magnesium is adequately replete. Recently, the mechanism whereby magnesium depletion results in renal potassium loss has been elucidated. Decreased intracellular magnesium slows ATP production. Throughout the body, such slowed ATP production has a negative effect on Na^+,K^+-ATPase activity. The result is loss of intracellular potassium, which flows downs its concentration gradient into the tubule and is lost in the urine.

Hypocalcemia, hyponatremia, and hypophosphatemia are also common in patients with hypomagnesemia. Intracellular hypomagnesemia can develop in patients with chronic diarrhea syndrome or in those who undergo prolonged aggressive diuretic therapy. Magnesium deficiency is also common in patients with heavy ethanol intake. Diabetic patients with persistent osmotic diuresis from glycosuria commonly have hypomagnesemia.

Treatment of hypomagnesemia. Patients with mild hypomagnesemia can be treated with oral replacement; symptomatic hypomagnesemia should be treated with IV magnesium. The most common formulation is magnesium sulfate; 1 g of magnesium sulfate contains 0.1 g of elemental magnesium. No trials have been done to determine the optimal regimen for magnesium replacement, but consensus statements suggest 8 to 12 g of magnesium sulfate in the first 24 hours followed by 4 to 6 g/day for 3 or 4 days to replete body stores. IV magnesium therapy is advocated in some acutely ill patients without documented magnesium depletion. The American College of Cardiology and the American Heart Association recommend 1 to 2 g of magnesium sulfate as an IV bolus during 5 minutes for torsades de pointes therapy. Emerging data have suggested that magnesium may also play a role in reducing reperfusion injury and decreasing infarct size in patients with acute myocardial infarction. Currently, the American Heart Association recommends 2 g of magnesium sulfate during 15 minutes, followed by 18 g during 24 hours in patients with suspected myocardial infarction who have hypomagnesemia.

Magnesium replacement should be done cautiously in patients with renal insufficiency, and recommendations call for dose reductions of 50% to 75% of baseline. During infusions, patients should be monitored closely for decreased deep tendon reflexes. Magnesium levels should be checked at regular intervals. Oral supplementation has been shown to successfully correct increased magnesium retention. Potassium-sparing diuretics may be helpful in patients with chronic renal magnesium wasting. Diuretics that block the sodium channel in the distal convoluted tubule, such as amiloride and triamterene, reduce magnesium wasting in some patients. Severe hypomagnesemia (<1.0 mEq/liter) requires sustained therapy because of the slow equilibration of extracellular magnesium with intracellular stores. Correction of hypomagnesemia can also reduce the risk of cardiac arrhythmia. The magnitude of magnesium deficiency frequently parallels the magnitude of hypocalcemia. Hypocalcemia in patients with magnesium deficiency is resistant to calcium replacement alone, so such patients should receive magnesium concurrently.

Hypermagnesemia

Hypermagnesemia is a common abnormality in patients with renal failure but is otherwise uncommon among other patients. Theophylline toxicity, now rare, was associated with hypermagnesemia in the past. Hypermagnesemia can be exacerbated by the ingestion of magnesium-containing drugs, particularly antacids; Epsom salts also contain magnesium, as does magnesium citrate, which is often used in surgical care. High levels of magnesium seem to be tolerated well and, in general, without sequelae. In one report, a patient in diabetic ketoacidosis with hypomagnesemia received 50 g of magnesium sulfate during 6 hours, rather than the intended 2 g. Despite a documented magnesium level of 24 mg/dL and significant short-term morbidity, the patient completely recovered.

IV magnesium overdoses may be better tolerated than oral overdoses. Hypermagnesemia due to oral ingestion of magnesium is unusual in the absence of renal insufficiency. A fatal case of hypermagnesemia was documented in a developmentally disabled child who was given magnesium to relieve constipation. Despite calcium infusions and dialysis, the child died. The chronic ingestion of magnesium likely made the child's condition refractory to treatment, perhaps because of greater total body magnesium burden from chronic overload. Hypermagnesemia has also been repeatedly reported after the use of magnesium-containing enemas. In postsurgical patients who are oliguric, hypermagnesemia may occur because of magnesium retention, particularly if the patient is acidotic.

Magnesium can block synaptic transmission of nerve impulses. It also causes the initial loss of deep tendon reflexes and may lead to flaccid paralysis and apnea. Neuromuscular toxicity also affects smooth muscle, resulting in ileus and urinary retention. In cases of oral intoxication, the development of ileus can slow intestinal transit times, further increasing absorption of magnesium. Hypermagnesemia has also been reported to cause a parasympathetic blockade resulting in fixed and dilated pupils, mimicking brainstem herniation. Other neurologic signs include lethargy, confusion, and coma.

Magnesium blocks the shift of calcium into myocardial cells and can act as a calcium channel blocker. In cardiac tissue, it also blocks potassium channels needed for repolarization. Patients with severe hypermagnesemia can show evidence of heart failure. Other cardiac manifestations of hypermagnesemia, at least initially, include bradycardia and hypotension. Higher magnesium levels cause a prolonged PR interval, increased QRS duration, and prolonged QT interval. Extreme cases can result in complete heart block or cardiac arrest.

Metabolic disturbances due to hypermagnesemia have been less recognized than those due to hypomagnesemia. Hypocalcemia can occur, although it is typically mild and asymptomatic. Symptomatic hypermagnesemia (despite normal renal function) has been reported with magnesium infusions, typically during treatment of patients who are in preterm labor or who have preeclampsia or eclampsia. Routine magnesium measurements are often not performed, although the infusion protocols (a load of 4 to 6 g, followed by 1 to 2 g/hr) result in serum magnesium levels of 4 to 8 mg/dL. Obstetric patients who experience accidental overdoses of magnesium usually have good outcomes, despite magnesium levels as high as 19 mg/dL.

Treatment of hypermagnesemia. The principles for treatment of hypermagnesemia are similar to those for treatment of hypercalcemia. Calcium is given to stabilize the heart, normal saline is given for fluid expansion, and diuretics are given to hasten renal excretion. In patients with hypermagnesemia and intact renal function, stopping the infusion or supply of magnesium will allow them to recover. Severe hypermagnesemia is treated with IV calcium gluconate 10% (10 to 20 mL during 10 minutes). Patients are typically given 100 to 200 mg of IV elemental calcium during 5 to 10 minutes. To speed the renal clearance of magnesium, loop diuretics and saline diuresis are intuitive options, but no literature explicitly supports this use.

In critically ill patients, disorders of magnesium homeostasis can have dramatic effects. Yet such disorders often go unrecognized. In ICU patients, hypomagnesemia is common and associated with poor outcomes, so measurement of serum magnesium should be routine. Unlike magnesium depletion, hypermagnesemia is a rare but frequently iatrogenic and fatal problem.

In patients with renal insufficiency, dialysis rapidly corrects hypermagnesemia and is the only way to acutely lower magnesium levels. Aggressive use of dialysis may improve survival. In patients with severe renal dysfunction, dialysis offers a way to rapidly clear magnesium. Both peritoneal dialysis and hemodialysis are effective at lowering magnesium levels. Intermittent hemodialysis corrects hypermagnesemia more rapidly than peritoneal dialysis or continuous renal replacement therapy.

SELECTED REFERENCES

Awad S, Allison SP, Lobo DN: The history of 0.9% saline. *Clin Nutr* 27:179–188, 2008.

Summary of how saline was developed, noting that the science behind its development is lacking.

Bickell WH, Wall MJ, Jr, Pepe PE, et al: Immediate versus delayed fluid resuscitation for hypotensive patients with penetrating torso injuries. *N Engl J Med* 331:1105–1109, 1994.

Classic study, probably the most referenced paper in trauma, showing that despite their being hypotensive in the field after penetrating torso injury, treating these patients with crystalloid solutions resulted in worse outcome and not infusing fluids improved outcome.

Cohn SM, Nathens AB, Moore FA, et al: Tissue oxygen saturation predicts the development of organ dysfunction during traumatic shock resuscitation. *J Trauma* 62:44–54, 2007.

Multicenter prospective study using seven busy level I trauma centers to determine usefulness of measuring tissue oxygenation. It showed that this noninvasive tool, which attaches to the thenar muscle, correlates well with base excess and can predict poor outcome. However, the study selected out the most severely injured patients with bleeding requiring transfusions, and the ability to predict that these patients will do poorly was obvious. It also showed that the number of patients who developed multiple organ failure was small.

Committee on Fluid Resuscitation for Combat Casualties: *Fluid resuscitation: State of the science for treating combat casualties and civilian injuries.* Report of the Institute of Medicine, Washington, DC, 1999, National Academy Press.

Considered a white paper by the Institute of Medicine, it was considered radical in that it did not recommend lactated Ringer's as the fluid of choice for civilians and the military. It recommended hypertonic saline and additional research to eliminate d-isomer lactate from lactated Ringer's and to investigate other metabolites, such as ketones, as an alternative.

Finfer S, Bellomo R, Boyce N, et al: A comparison of albumin and saline for fluid resuscitation in the intensive care unit. *N Engl J Med* 350:2247–2256, 2004.

Prospective multicenter study designed to show that albumin is safe in the intensive care unit. However, it used 4% albumin and showed that the outcome was no different.

Fluid resuscitation of combat casualties: Conference proceedings. June 2001 and October 2001. *J Trauma* 54(Suppl):S1–S234, 2003.

This entire supplement summarizes the rationale for the changes recommended for the treatment of combat casualties.

Holcomb JB, Jenkins D, Rhee P, et al: Damage control resuscitation: Directly addressing the early coagulopathy of trauma. *J Trauma* 62:307–310, 2007.

This paper describes the evolution of damage control resuscitation and rationale behind the recommendation of permissive hypotension, reduction of crystalloid use, use of hypertonic saline, and aggressive use of blood products early and often for best results.

Moore EE, Moore FA, Fabian TC, et al: PolyHeme Study Group: Human polymerized hemoglobin for the treatment of hemorrhagic shock when blood is unavailable: The USA multicenter trial. *J Am Coll Surg* 208:1–13, 2009.

Study showing that artificial hemoglobin made from expired human blood could be used safely and as a replacement of blood in the field and in the hospital.

Plurad D, Martin M, Green D, et al: The decreasing incidence of late post-traumatic acute respiratory distress syndrome: The potential role of lung protective ventilation and conservative transfusion practice. *J Trauma* 63:1–7, 2007.

This paper shows the decreasing incidence of ARDS in trauma and its association with decreased crystalloid use.

Spinella PC, Perkins JG, Grathwohl KW, et al: Warm fresh whole blood is independently associated with improved survival for patients with combat-related traumatic injuries. *J Trauma* 66:S69–S76, 2009.

Describes the usefulness of whole blood transfusion practice found by the military.

Velmahos GC, Demetriades D, Shoemaker WC, et al: End points of resuscitation of critically injured patients: Normal or supranormal? A prospective randomized trial. *Ann Surg* 232:409–418, 2000.

Excellent study showing in a prospective manner that increasing oxygen delivery through increasing content and cardiac output did not improve survival in trauma patients in the intensive care unit.

REFERENCES

1. Hughes JT: Miraculous deliverance of Anne Green: an Oxford case of resuscitation in the seventeenth century. *Br Med J (Clin Res Ed)* 285:1792–1793, 1982.
2. O'Shaughnassy WB: Experiments on the blood in cholera. *Lancet* 32:490, 1831.
3. Crile GW: *An experimental research into surgical shock*, Philadelphia, 1899, JB Lippincott.
4. Cannon WB: The emergency function of the adrenal medulla in pain and the major emotions. *Am J Physiol* 33:356–372, 1914.
5. Blalock A: Experimental shock: The cause of low blood pressure caused by muscle injury. *Arch Surg* 20:959–996, 1930.
6. Wiggers CJ: The present status of shock problem. *Physiol Rev* 22:74–123, 1942.
7. Awad S, Allison SP, Lobo DN: The history of 0.9% saline. *Clin Nutr* 27:179–188, 2008.
8. O'Shaughnessy WB: Proposal of a new method of treating the blue epidemic cholera by the injection of highly-oxygenated salts into the venous system. *Lancet* 17:366–371, 1831.
9. Ringer S: Concerning the influence exerted by each of the constituents of the blood on the contraction of the ventricle. *J Physiol* 3:380–393, 1882.
10. Brasel KJ, Guse C, Gentilello LM, et al: Heart rate: Is it truly a vital sign? *J Trauma* 62:812–817, 2007.
11. Ley EJ, Salim A, Kohanzadeh S, et al: Relative bradycardia in hypotensive trauma patients: a reappraisal. *J Trauma* 67:1051–1054, 2009.
12. Bruns B, Lindsey M, Rowe K, et al: Hemoglobin drops within minutes of injuries and predicts need for an intervention to stop hemorrhage. *J Trauma* 63:312–315, 2007.
13. Riordan WP, Jr, Norris PR, Jenkins JM, et al: Early loss of heart rate complexity predicts mortality regardless of mechanism, anatomic location, or severity of injury in 2178 trauma patients. *J Surg Res* 156:283–289, 2009.
14. Eastridge BJ, Salinas J, McManus JG, et al: Hypotension begins at 110 mm Hg: Redefining "hypotension" with data. *J Trauma* 63:291–297, 2007.
15. Bruns B, Gentillelo L, Elliot A, et al: Prehospital hypotension redefined. *J Trauma* 65:1217–1221, 2008.
16. Krishna U, Joshi SP: Modh M: An evaluation of serial blood lactate measurement as an early predictor of shock and its outcome in patients of trauma or sepsis. *Indian J Crit Care Med* 13:66–73, 2009.
17. Grocott MP, Martin DS, Levett DZ, et al: Arterial blood gases and oxygen content in climbers on Mount Everest. *N Engl J Med* 360:140–149, 2009.
18. Cureton EL, Kwan RO, Dozier KC, et al: A different view of lactate in trauma patients: protecting the injured brain. *J Surg Res* 159:468–473, 2010.
19. Reynolds PS, Barbee RW, Ward KR: Lactate profiles as a resuscitation assessment tool in a rat model of battlefield hemorrhage resuscitation. *Shock* 30:48–54, 2008.
20. Bilello JF, Davis JW, Lemaster D, et al: Prehospital hypotension in blunt trauma: Identifying the "crump factor.". *J Trauma* 70:1038–1042, 2011.
21. Sperry JL, Frankel HL, Nathens AB, et al: Characterization of persistent hyperglycemia: What does it mean postinjury? *J Trauma* 66:1076–1082, 2009.
22. Inaba K, Teixeira PG, Rhee P, et al: Mortality impact of hypothermia after cavitary explorations in trauma. *World J Surg* 33:864–869, 2009.
23. Beilman GJ, Blondet JJ, Nelson TR, et al: Early hypothermia in severely injured trauma patients is a significant risk factor for multiple organ dysfunction syndrome but not mortality. *Ann Surg* 249:845–850, 2009.
24. Boffard KD, Riou B, Warren B, et al: Recombinant factor VIIa as adjunctive therapy for bleeding control in severely injured trauma patients: Two parallel randomized, placebo-controlled, double-blind clinical trials. *J Trauma* 59:8–15, 2005.
25. Mayer SA, Brun NC, Begtrup K, et al: Recombinant activated factor VII for acute intracerebral hemorrhage. *N Engl J Med* 352:777–785, 2005.
26. Joseph B, Aziz H, Pandit V, et al: Prothrombin complex concentrate versus fresh-frozen plasma for reversal of

coagulopathy of trauma: Is there a difference? *World J Surg* 38:1875–1881, 2014.

27. CRASH-2 trial collaborators, Shakur H, Roberts I, et al: Effects of tranexamic acid on death, vascular occlusive events, and blood transfusion in trauma patients with significant haemorrhage (CRASH-2): A randomised, placebo-controlled trial. *Lancet* 376:23–32, 2010.
28. Morrison JJ, Dubose JJ, Rasmussen TE, et al: Military Application of Tranexamic Acid in Trauma Emergency Resuscitation (MATTERs) Study. *Arch Surg* 147:113–119, 2012.
29. Velmahos GC, Demetriades D, Shoemaker WC, et al: Endpoints of resuscitation of critically injured patients: Normal or supranormal? A prospective randomized trial. *Ann Surg* 232:409–418, 2000.
30. Madigan MC, Kemp CD, Johnson JC, et al: Secondary abdominal compartment syndrome after severe extremity injury: are early, aggressive fluid resuscitation strategies to blame? *J Trauma* 64:280–285, 2008.
31. Noakes TD: How did AV Hill understand the VO_{2max} and the "plateau phenomenon"? Still no clarity? *Br J Sports Med* 42:574–580, 2008.
32. Palizas F, Dubin A, Regueira T, et al: Gastric tonometry versus cardiac index as resuscitation goals in septic shock: A multicenter, randomized, controlled trial. *Crit Care* 13:R44, 2009.
33. Cohn SM, Nathens AB, Moore FA, et al: Tissue oxygen saturation predicts the development of organ dysfunction during traumatic shock resuscitation. *J Trauma* 62:44–54, 2007.
34. Dellinger RP, Levy MM, Rhodes A, et al: Surviving Sepsis Campaign: International guidelines for management of severe sepsis and septic shock: 2012. *Crit Care Med* 41:580–637, 2013.
35. Dellinger RP, Levy MM, Carlet JM, et al: Surviving Sepsis Campaign: International guidelines for management of severe sepsis and septic shock: 2008. *Crit Care Med* 36:296–327, 2008.
36. Yealy DM, Kellum JA, Huang DT, et al: A randomized trial of protocol-based care for early septic shock. *N Engl J Med* 370:1683–1693, 2014.
37. Bickell WH, Wall MJ, Jr, Pepe PE, et al: Immediate versus delayed fluid resuscitation for hypotensive patients with penetrating torso injuries. *N Engl J Med* 331:1105–1109, 1994.
38. Eiseman B, Beart R, Norton L: Multiple organ failure. *Surg Gynecol Obstet* 144:323–326, 1977.
39. Demetriades D, Kimbrell B, Salim A, et al: Trauma deaths in a mature urban trauma system: Is "trimodal" distribution a valid concept? *J Am Coll Surg* 201:343–348, 2005.
40. Englehart MS, Cho SD, Morris MS, et al: Use of leukoreduced blood does not reduce infection, organ failure, or mortality following trauma. *World J Surg* 33:1626–1632, 2009.
41. Rhee P, Morris J, Durham R, et al: Recombinant humanized monoclonal antibody against CD18 (rhuMAb CD18) in traumatic hemorrhagic shock: results of a phase II clinical trial. Traumatic Shock Group. *J Trauma* 49:611–619, 2000.
42. Todd SR, Kao LS, Catania A, et al: Alpha-melanocyte stimulating hormone in critically injured trauma patients. *J Trauma* 66:465–469, 2009.
43. Committee on Fluid Resuscitation for Combat Casualties: *Fluid Resuscitation: State of the Science for Treating Combat Casualties and Civilian Injuries*. Report of the Institute of Medicine, Washington, DC, 1999, National Academy Press.
44. Gao J, Zhao WX, Xue FS, et al: Effects of different resuscitation fluids on acute lung injury in a rat model of uncontrolled hemorrhagic shock and infection. *J Trauma* 67:1213–1219, 2009.
45. Fluid resuscitation of combat casualties. Conference proceedings. June 2001 and October 2001. *J Trauma* 54:S1–S234, 2003.
46. Holcomb JB, Jenkins D, Rhee P, et al: Damage control resuscitation: directly addressing the early coagulopathy of trauma. *J Trauma* 62:307–310, 2007.
47. Teixeira PG, Oncel D, Demetriades D, et al: Blood transfusions in trauma: six-year analysis of the transfusion practices at a Level I trauma center. *Am Surg* 74:953–957, 2008.
48. Plurad D, Martin M, Green D, et al: The decreasing incidence of late posttraumatic acute respiratory distress syndrome: the potential role of lung protective ventilation and conservative transfusion practice. *J Trauma* 63:1–7, 2007.
49. Spinella PC, Perkins JG, Grathwohl KW, et al: Warm fresh whole blood is independently associated with improved survival for patients with combat-related traumatic injuries. *J Trauma* 66:S69–S76, 2009.
50. Perkins JG, Cap AP, Spinella PC, et al: An evaluation of the impact of apheresis platelets used in the setting of massively transfused trauma patients. *J Trauma* 66:S77–S84, 2009.
51. Stinger HK, Spinella PC, Perkins JG, et al: The ratio of fibrinogen to red cells transfused affects survival in casualties receiving massive transfusions at an army combat support hospital. *J Trauma* 64:S79–S85, 2008.
52. Zink KA, Sambasivan CN, Holcomb JB, et al: A high ratio of plasma and platelets to packed red blood cells in the first 6 hours of massive transfusion improves outcomes in a large multicenter study. *Am J Surg* 197:565–570, 2009.
53. Holcomb JB, del Junco DJ, Fox EE, et al: The prospective, observational, multicenter, major trauma transfusion (PROMMTT) study: comparative effectiveness of a time-varying treatment with competing risks. *JAMA Surg* 148:127–136, 2013.
54. Holcomb JB, Tilley BC, Baraniuk S, et al: Transfusion of plasma, platelets, and red blood cells in a 1 : 1 : 1 vs a 1 : 1 : 2 ratio and mortality in patients with severe trauma: the PROPPR randomized clinical trial. *JAMA* 313:471–482, 2015.
55. Dente CJ, Shaz BH, Nicholas JM, et al: Improvements in early mortality and coagulopathy are sustained better in patients with blunt trauma after institution of a massive transfusion protocol in a civilian level I trauma center. *J Trauma* 66:1616–1624, 2009.
56. Inaba K, Branco BC, Rhee P, et al: Impact of ABO-identical vs ABO-compatible nonidentical plasma transfusion in trauma patients. *Arch Surg* 145:899–906, 2010.
57. Young JB, Utter GH, Schermer CR, et al: Saline versus Plasma-Lyte A in initial resuscitation of trauma patients. A randomized trial. *Ann Surg* 259:255–262, 2014.
58. Kuwabara K, Hagiwara A, Matsuda S, et al: A community-based comparison of trauma patient outcomes between D- and L-lactate fluids. *Am J Emerg Med* 31:206–214, 2013.
59. Joseph B, Aziz H, Snell M, et al: The physiological effects of hyperosmolar resuscitation: 5% vs 3% hypertonic saline. *Am J Surg* 208:697–702, 2014.
60. Finfer S, Bellomo R, Boyce N, et al: A comparison of albumin and saline for fluid resuscitation in the intensive care unit. *N Engl J Med* 350:2247–2256, 2004.

61. Martin M, Salim A, Murray J, et al: The decreasing incidence and mortality of acute respiratory distress syndrome after injury: a 5-year observational study. *J Trauma* 59:1107–1113, 2005.
62. Annane D, Siami S, Jaber S, et al: Effects of fluid resuscitation with colloids vs crystalloids on mortality in critically ill patients presenting with hypovolemic shock: the CRISTAL randomized trial. *JAMA* 310:1809–1817, 2013.
63. Moore EE, Moore FA, Fabian TC, et al: Human polymerized hemoglobin for the treatment of hemorrhagic shock when blood is unavailable: The USA multicenter trial. *J Am Coll Surg* 208:1–13, 2009.
64. Cruz RJ, Jr, Harada T, Sasatomi E, et al: Effects of ethyl pyruvate and other α-keto carboxylic acid derivatives in a rat model of multivisceral ischemia and reperfusion. *J Surg Res* 165:151–157, 2011.
65. Lin T, Chen H, Koustova E, et al: Histone deacetylase as therapeutic target in a rodent model of hemorrhagic shock: Effect of different resuscitation strategies on lung and liver. *Surgery* 141:784–794, 2007.
66. Alam HB, Bice LM, Butt MU, et al: Testing of blood products in a polytrauma model: Results of a multi-institutional randomized preclinical trial. *J Trauma* 67:856–864, 2009.
67. Alam HB, Casas F, Chen Z, et al: Development and testing of portable pump for the induction of profound hypothermia in a swine model of lethal vascular injuries. *J Trauma* 61:1321–1329, 2006.

5 CHAPTER

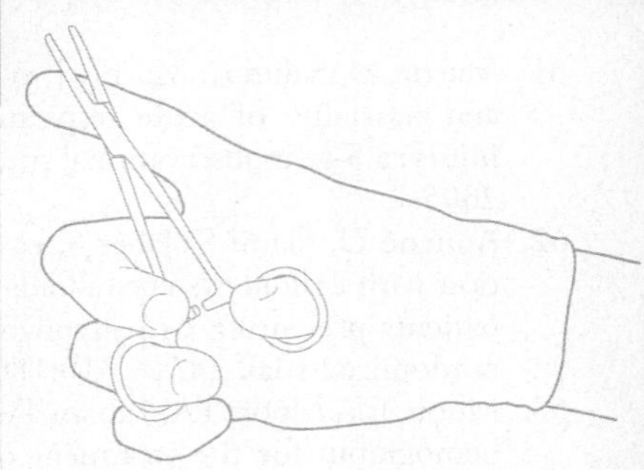

Metabolism in Surgical Patients

Joshua Carson, Ahmed Al-Mousawi, Noe A. Rodriguez, Celeste C. Finnerty, David N. Herndon

OUTLINE

 **Please access ExpertConsult.com to view the corresponding videos for this chapter.**

Metabolism, the process by which the body assimilates and modifies substrate to yield the energy and materials required to sustain human structure and function, engages a plethora of chemical processes to sustain life and enable growth, healing, development, reproduction, homeostasis, and adaptation and response to the environment. Through these metabolic pathways, nutrients are absorbed, transformed, and broken down to release energy. The nutritional status of an individual depends on an adequate diet, function of the alimentary tract, and physiologic condition. In surgical patients and critically ill patients, energy requirements, alimentation, and metabolic processes may be altered as a consequence of environmental, pathologic, or traumatic factors. Development and implementation of nutritional support represents one of the main advances of the last century that has led to improved patient care and surgical outcomes. This chapter addresses the basic physiology of human metabolism and nutrition in health and healing, the pathophysiology of malnutrition, the metabolic response to injury, and the basic principles of nutritional therapy for surgical patients.

SUBSTRATE METABOLISM

The primary goal of nutritional support is to provide an adequate energy supply and all the nutrients necessary to support life and function. Nutrients obtained from the diet are ingested, digested, and absorbed before the released substrates can be stored or expended for energy. The major components of the diet are carbohydrates, lipids, and proteins (Fig. 5-1). As a source of calories, 1 g of carbohydrate yields 3.4 kcal (16 kJ) of protein, and 4 kcal (17 kJ) yields 9 kcal (37 kJ) of fat. Cells and tissues use different fuel sources preferentially. Erythrocytes and neurons use glucose, muscle and cardiac myocytes can also use fat, and enterocytes and lymphocytes can metabolize the amino acid glutamine. Adaptation to different fuels can occur under circumstances of starvation.

At the cellular level, adenosine triphosphate (ATP) is the main source of energy that drives reactions and metabolic processes. Hydrolysis of the two high-energy anhydride phosphate bonds within the molecule releases energy that fuels cellular work. A continuous supply of ATP is synthesized by reactions that use glucose, amino acids, and fatty acids to phosphorylate and recycle ATP from adenosine diphosphate (ADP) and adenosine monophosphate.

The glycolytic pathway converts the six-carbon molecule glucose into two three-carbon molecules of pyruvate, with net production of ATP and reduced nicotinamide adenine dinucleotide (NADH). In cells with mitochondria and sufficient oxygen supply, pyruvate is metabolized to carbon dioxide through aerobic metabolism. If there is a lack of mitochondria or oxygen, glycolysis occurs anaerobically, producing lactate. Anaerobic metabolism occurs in cells during states of hypoperfusion, in muscle cells during bursts of increased activity, and in cells without mitochondria such as red blood cells, in which anaerobic glycolysis is the only energy-producing pathway.

Phosphorylation of ADP to form ATP occurs in the cytoplasm during glycolysis (anaerobic, substrate-level phosphorylation) and in mitochondria in the tricarboxylic acid (aerobic, TCA) cycle. Oxidative phosphorylation of NADH and succinate, products of the TCA cycle, generates further ATP within mitochondria through aerobic respiration, a more efficient pathway than anaerobic glycolysis. Two molecules of pyruvate are produced from each molecule of glucose that enters glycolysis, yielding two ATP molecules. In comparison, a single molecule of glucose yields approximately 32 molecules of ATP through glycolysis, subsequent oxidation of pyruvate to acetyl coenzyme A (acetyl-CoA), and progression into the TCA cycle with oxidative phosphorylation of the products.

Lipolysis involves hydrolysis of triacylglycerol (TAG) stored in adipose tissue to release fatty acids and glycerol. Although glycerol

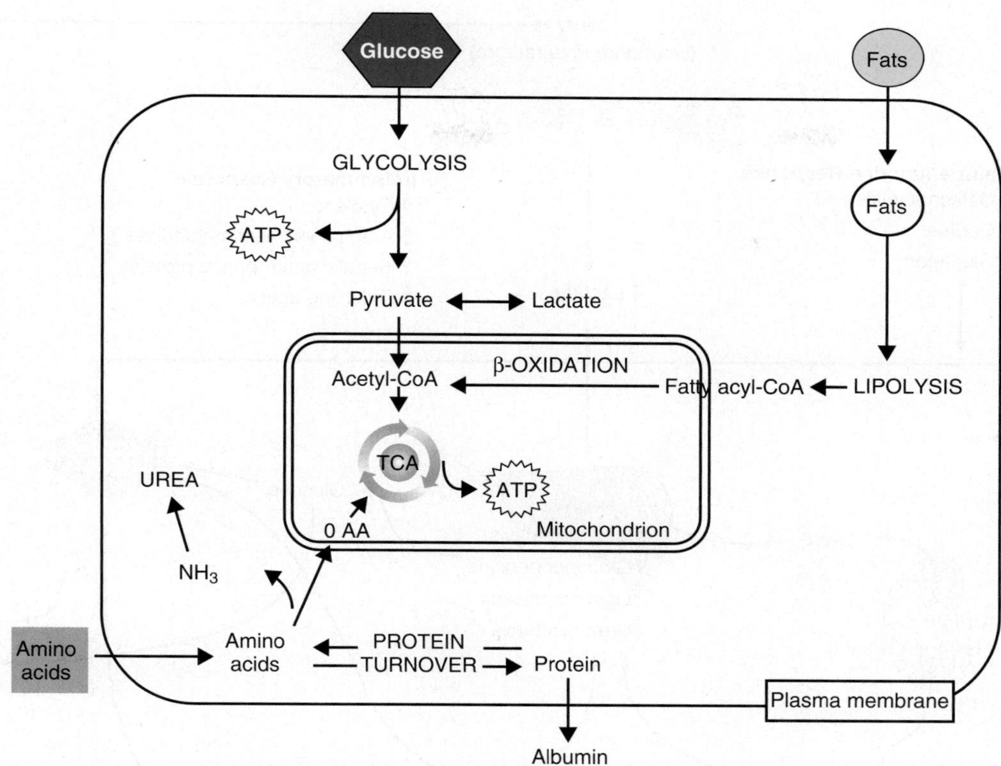

FIGURE 5-1 Metabolic response to injury and trauma.

can be used by the liver to synthesize glucose, fatty acids cannot be used to synthesize glucose in humans. As a result, during periods of stress or prolonged starvation, proteolysis occurs to maintain glucose homeostasis after depletion of glycogen stores. Proteolysis occurs primarily through degradation of muscle protein or solid organs.

β-Oxidation is the oxidative degradation of saturated fatty acids, whereby two carbon units are sequentially removed to form acetyl-CoA and electron donor molecules (NADH and reduced flavin adenine dinucleotide) used to generate ATP by oxidative phosphorylation. Fats represent a dense source of calories because this process has an extremely high energy yield, with 129 molecules of ATP being formed from 1 molecule of the fatty acid palmitate.

Carbohydrate Metabolism

Carbohydrates are a primary source of calories and are divided into simple carbohydrates and complex carbohydrates. Simple carbohydrates include monosaccharides (1 sugar unit) and disaccharides (2 sugar units), and complex carbohydrates include oligosaccharides (3 to 10 sugar units) and polysaccharides (>10 sugar units).

Carbohydrate digestion begins in the mouth with the action of salivary amylase, which hydrolyzes polysaccharide bonds in the amylose and amylopectin molecules that constitute starch. Breakdown continues in the gut through the action of pancreatic amylase and the enzymes sucrase, lactase, maltase, and isomaltase from intestinal epithelial cells to yield monosaccharides. Bacteria in normal gut flora enable the breakdown of certain polysaccharides and starches, which humans lack the enzymes to digest, and help prevent the invasion of pathogenic strains in the intestine.

The products of intestinal digestion yield the monosaccharides glucose, fructose, and galactose. These sugars are rapidly absorbed and transported to the liver. Approximately 90% of portal venous glucose is removed from the blood by hepatocytes through carrier-facilitated diffusion. Carrier molecules on the sinusoidal domain of hepatocytes are capable of binding and transferring the sugars into the cytoplasm.

Glycogen is the stored form of carbohydrate in the liver and skeletal muscle. The liver plays a key role in processes that synthesize and degrade glycogen (glycogenesis and glycogenolysis) as well as in the endogenous synthesis of glucose (gluconeogenesis). Glycogen can be stored in the liver, at concentrations of up to 65 g/kg of tissue, and is stored in muscle for its exclusive use. Hepatic synthesis of glycogen begins with a core composed of a high-density protein (glycogenin) and the action of a rate-determining enzyme, glycogen synthase. This enzyme is activated by insulin and glucose, both of which are elevated in the postprandial state, leading to elongation of the glycogen chain by the addition of glucose units. Conversely, glycogen synthase is inhibited by glucagon and epinephrine. During fasting, glycogenolysis leads to the release of glucose, with the rate-limiting enzyme glycogen phosphorylase being activated by glucagon and epinephrine and being inhibited by insulin. Glycogen stores are exhausted within 48 hours of fasting, and body protein stores must be mobilized to maintain an adequate glucose supply to the brain.

Glucose levels are maintained not only through glycogenolysis, but also through the conversion of noncarbohydrate substrates by gluconeogenesis, which occurs primarily in the liver and, to a lesser extent, in the renal cortex. Substrates for this pathway include all amino acids derived from the proteolysis of skeletal muscle (except lysine and leucine), glycerol derived from the degradation of triglycerides (TGs) in adipose tissue, and lactate produced from anaerobic glycolysis (Fig. 5-2). The enzyme-catalyzed reactions of the gluconeogenic pathway include the reversal of several steps of glycolysis and four irreversible reactions.

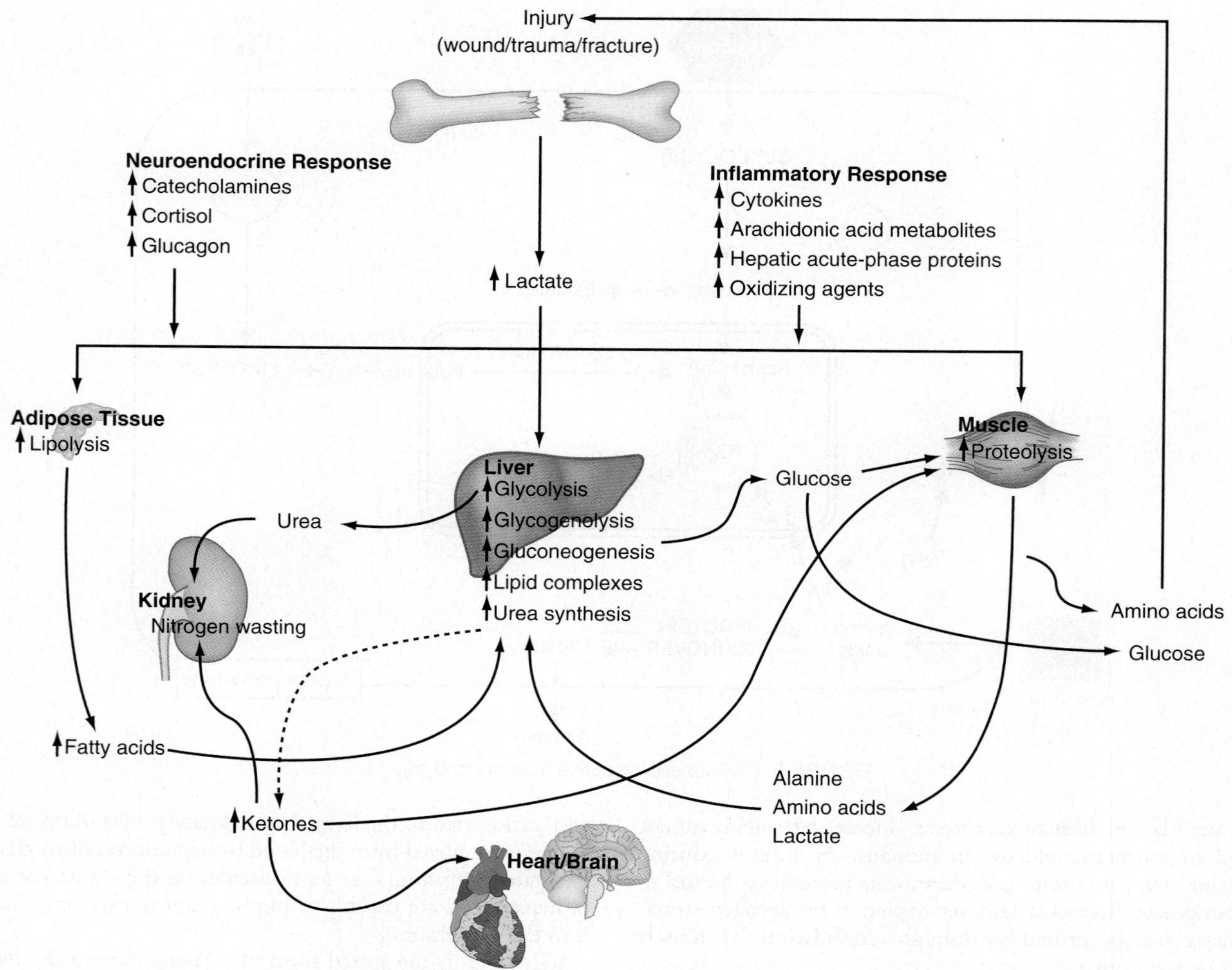

FIGURE 5-2 Simplified overview of metabolic pathways.

Lipid Metabolism

Lipids are hydrophobic molecules that include fatty acids, phospholipids, glycerolipids, sphingolipids, eicosanoids, and vitamins. Lipids play key roles in cell structure and function, including energy storage and expenditure, formation of biologic membranes, and cell signaling. If lipids are not immediately used by cells, they can be stored in the form of TGs. TGs are the most potent caloric stores in the body—1 g of fat delivers 9 kcal (37.7 kJ).

Dietary TGs are unable to pass through intestinal epithelial cells and must first be emulsified and hydrolyzed to monoacylglycerols (MAGs) or free fatty acids. This process is mediated by a mixture of lipases found primarily in biliary, pancreatic, and intestinal secretions from glands positioned along the gastrointestinal (GI) tract (tongue, stomach, pancreas, glycocalyx of intestinal wall). The stomach plays two important roles: (1) secretion of gastric lipase, responsible for the digestion and absorption of up to 20% of total TGs, and (2) initiation of emulsification. Fat then enters the upper duodenum, 80% in the form of TGs and the rest in the form of partially hydrolyzed compounds. Emulsified TGs stimulate the contraction of the gallbladder and the release of bile and pancreatic fluid containing lipase, colipase, phospholipase A_2, and cholesteryl esterase. Bile acids and colipase enable pancreatic lipase to act on TGs to produce diacylglycerols (DAGs), MAGs, and free fatty acids.

Lipolysis occurs within the cytosolic lipid droplets of adipocytes, where a series of lipases initiate the breakdown of TAG into free fatty acids and glycerol. Until more recently, hormone-sensitive lipase (HSL) was thought to be the only enzyme that hydrolyzed TGs in adipose tissue. A second enzyme, adipose triglyceride lipase (ATGL), is now believed to catalyze the first step in the hydrolysis of TGs (Fig. 5-3).

In the postabsorptive state, adipose tissue releases free fatty acids and glycerol to the circulation for use as energy. Hepatic β-oxidation of fatty acids produces ketone bodies, acetoacetate, and 3-hydroxybutyrate, which can be used directly as fuel sources by cardiac muscle, skeletal muscle, and renal cortex as well as cerebral tissue after 1 week of fasting. This switch of the central nervous system during starvation away from the primary use of carbohydrates to the use of ketone bodies as a fuel represents a critical adaptive step that has a secondary sparing effect on body protein.

Desnutrin-ATGL initiates lipolysis by hydrolyzing TAG to DAG. HSL hydrolyzes DAG to MAG, which is subsequently hydrolyzed by MAG lipase to generate glycerol and three fatty acids. Fatty acids generated during lipolysis can be released into the circulation for use by other organs or oxidized within

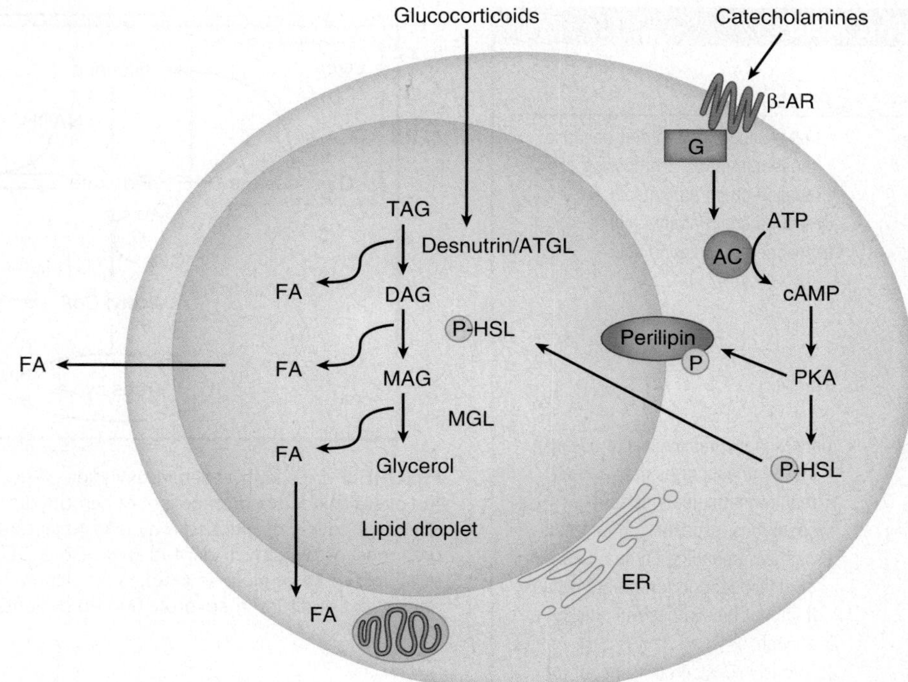

FIGURE 5-3 Regulation of lipolysis within adipocytes. (Adapted from Ahmadian M, Wang Y, Sul HS: Lipolysis in adipocytes. *Int J Biochem Cell Biol* 42:555–559, 2010.)

adipocytes. During fasting, glucocorticoids increase the expression of desnutrin-ATGL. Furthermore, fasting induces binding of catecholamines to Gαs-coupled β-adrenergic receptors (β-ARs), allowing them to activate adenylate cyclase to increase cyclic adenosine monophosphate and activate protein kinase A (PKA). PKA phosphorylates the lipid droplet–associated protein perilipin and HSL, resulting in the translocation of HSL from the cytosol to the lipid droplet to induce hydrolysis of the lipid droplet.

Protein Metabolism

Proteins are essential to the structure and function of every cell and participate in cell adhesion, signaling, and immunogenicity. The digestion of protein into peptides begins in the stomach through acid denaturation and the enzymatic action of pepsin. Digestion of peptides into tripeptides, dipeptides, and amino acids takes place at the level of the duodenum through proteases secreted from the pancreas and peptidases associated with the glycocalyx of the intestinal wall. Dipeptides, oligopeptides, and single amino acids are absorbed in the small intestine.

Human protein synthesis requires 20 amino acids; 8 are termed *essential amino acids* because they cannot be synthesized de novo from other amino acids (there are 10 essential amino acids if arginine and histidine are included as essential in infants) and must be obtained in the diet. Six amino acids are termed *conditionally essential amino acids* because they may not be synthesized at rates that meet requirements during childhood, illness, and other conditions and may need to be supplemented. The remaining six amino acids are termed *nonessential amino acids* because they can be synthesized internally (Table 5-1).

Various tissues, including liver, muscle, kidney, lung, and adipose, share regulatory roles in amino acid metabolism, although the catabolism of most essential amino acids occurs in the liver. The three branched-chain amino acids (BCAAs)—leucine, isoleucine, and valine—are an exception because these are poorly metabolized during first-pass metabolism in the liver and are degraded by skeletal muscle. The breakdown of BCAAs in muscle generates alanine and glutamine.

Alanine is released from skeletal muscle, in addition to lactate, during the anaerobic glycolysis of glucose, which generates ATP. In the Cori cycle, the liver converts lactate produced by muscle back to glucose for muscle fuel in an ATP-dependent manner. Similarly, alanine can be used by the liver and is a preferred precursor for hepatic gluconeogenesis as part of the glucose-alanine cycle (see Fig. 5-2). Alanine is provided by either muscle during protein turnover or amino acids in the diet.

Metabolism of nitrogen-containing compounds in the body, including amino acids, produces ammonia, which is converted to urea, a less toxic substance, by a series of reactions that comprise the urea cycle. The urea cycle generates urea from ammonia produced from amino acid oxidation, with certain amino acids, including arginine, entering the urea cycle directly as intermediates. Increased catabolism of protein and the release of amino acids for gluconeogenesis lead to excess nitrogen production, negative nitrogen balance, and increased excretion of urea by the kidneys (see Fig. 5-2). Liver failure can lead to hepatic encephalopathy as a result of buildup of nitrogenous compounds, including ammonia. Inborn errors of metabolism also give rise to disorders from dysfunction of the urea cycle.

Regulation of the Amino Acid Pool

Anabolic or catabolic hormonal signaling, various pathophysiologic mechanisms, type and availability of nutrients, and routes of their administration all are factors that regulate the pool of free amino acids. During enteral nutrition (EN), the portal venous system delivers ingested amino acids to the liver; 25% of these reach the general circulation to supply the plasma pool of amino

TABLE 5-1 Amino Acids

AMINO ACID GROUP (ABBREVIATION)	FEATURES
Essential Amino Acids	Must be contained in diet because these cannot be synthesized
Valine (Val)	Branched-chain amino acid
Leucine (Leu)	Branched-chain amino acid
Isoleucine (Ile)	Branched-chain amino acid
Lysine (Lys)	
Methionine (Met)	
Threonine (Thr)	
Phenylalanine (Phe)	
Tryptophan (Trp)	
Conditionally Essential	Conditionally indispensable because low synthesis rates may exceed requirements under certain conditions, especially in infants
Arginine (Arg)	Essential depending on health status of individual and for infants because it cannot be synthesized quickly enough
Histidine (His)	Previously considered essential for infants; now also considered essential for adults
Tyrosine (Tyr)	Can be synthesized from phenylalanine
Cysteine (Cys)	Can be synthesized from methionine
Glutamine (Gln)	Major energy source for intestinal mucosa
Proline (Pro)	
Nonessential Amino Acids	Needs can be fully met by synthesis
Alanine (Ala)	
Asparagine (Asn)	
Aspartate (Asp)	
Glutamate (Glu)	
Glycine (Gly)	
Serine (Ser)	

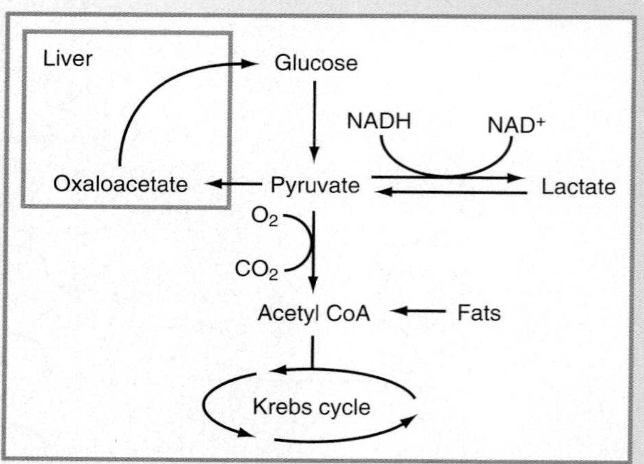

FIGURE 5-4 Oxidative decarboxylation of pyruvate is a pivotal step in the overall oxidative metabolism of carbohydrates and fats. Overwhelmingly high levels of glucose may lead to lactate production, even in the presence of oxygen. (Adapted from Gore DC, Ferrando A, Barnett J, et al: Influence of glucose kinetics on plasma lactate concentration and energy expenditure in severely burned patients. *J Trauma* 49:673–677, 2000.)

acids, 55% are converted to urea, 6% are used for the synthesis of constitutive plasma proteins (e.g., albumin, prealbumin), and 14% become liver protein. In a severe hypermetabolic response to surgery or trauma, there is a significant increase in demand for amino acids and proteins. Similarly, increase in demand is noted during growth, physical activity, pregnancy, and lactation.

Glucose-Alanine and Glucose-Lactate Amino Acid Cycles

After severe injury or major surgery, the rates of glucose uptake, glycolysis, and oxidation of BCAAs in muscle are increased. Stimulated by glucagon, the liver transfers the amino group from alanine via the urea cycle to produce pyruvate.

Pyruvate enters the gluconeogenesis pathway via the mitochondrial enzyme pyruvate carboxylase. Glucose is then synthesized and released back to the circulation. Of the 20 amino acids, 18 are gluconeogenic, with alanine being the most frequent source incorporated via the glucose-alanine cycle.

Lactate is a byproduct of anaerobic metabolism of glucose. In physiologic states, it is produced by red blood cells (anaerobic cells) and skeletal muscle and taken up by the liver, where it is initially converted to pyruvate and subsequently to glucose via the gluconeogenic pathway. This is commonly known as the glucose-lactate, or Cori, cycle. The reactions that convert lactate back to glucose require a great deal of energy, which is supplied through lipolysis and β-oxidation of fat (see Fig. 5-2).

In critically ill patients, lactate serves as a global marker of tissue hypoperfusion and insufficient oxygen delivery. However, there are additional mechanisms to explain lactate accumulation in these patients; elevations in plasma lactate levels in severely injured patients may be partly related to increases in glucose flux and may not totally reflect a deficit in oxygen availability (Fig. 5-4).

Protein Turnover

Protein turnover is continuously altered by dietary intake, protein synthesis, and protein breakdown. Amino acids are removed from the free pool of amino acids during protein synthesis and conversion to urea in a dynamic balance termed *protein turnover*. Net synthesis of protein is indicative of an anabolic state, whereas degradation of protein is indicative of a catabolic state. During critical illness, sepsis, trauma, or severe burn injury, there are increased rates of synthesis and breakdown of muscle protein, although the magnitude of the latter is more significant and leads to a catabolic state. Increased proteolysis initiates an imbalance in the supply and demand of free amino acids; if protein breakdown persists, net protein catabolism leads to significant muscle wasting.

Proteolysis

The triggers and cellular signaling pathways that induce proteolysis and muscle catabolism are incompletely understood and are areas of intense research interest, along with therapeutic targets and therapies to prevent muscle wasting. Proteolysis may be induced to varying degrees by a range of conditions including fasting, cancer, neurologic genetic disorders, diabetes, sepsis, AIDS, burns, trauma, hyperthyroidism, and excess glucocorticoids. The terminal biochemical process involves conjugation of ubiquitin to the amino group of lysine residues in proteins

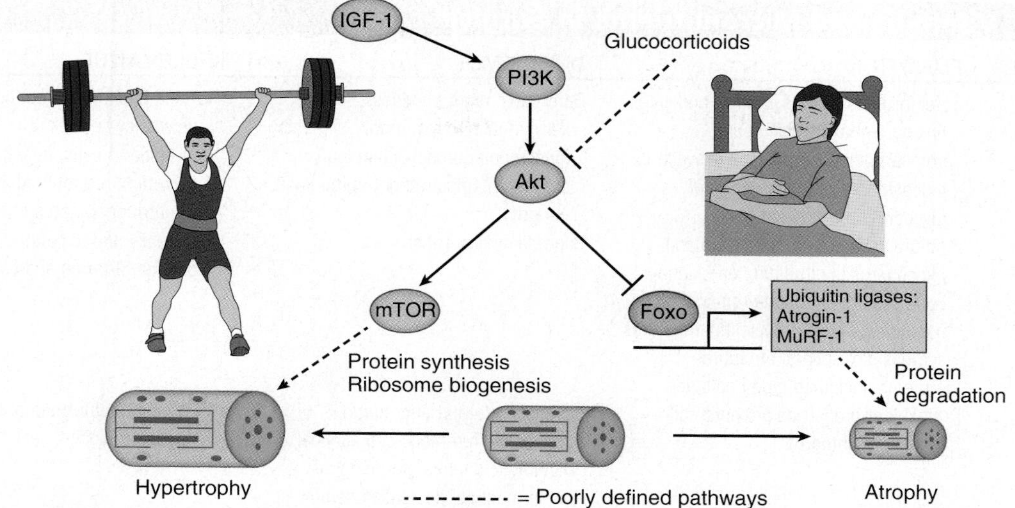

FIGURE 5-5 The proteins Akt1 and Foxo at the decision point of atrophy versus hypertrophy. (Redrawn from Hoffman EP, Nader GA: Balancing muscle hypertrophy and atrophy. *Nat Med* 10:584–585, 2004.)

through a series of enzymes: (1) E1 ubiquitin–activating enzyme, (2) E2 ubiquitin–conjugating enzyme, and (3) E3 ubiquitin ligases. The key enzymes in this process are the E3 ligases. Three E3 ubiquitin ligases are expressed in muscle: atrogin-1 (also known as MAFbx), muscle RING finger protein 1 (MuRF1), and E3α-I. Approximately 85 specialized proteases that act on ubiquitin are encoded in human genes. Nuclear factor κB is a major transcription factor that triggers muscle protein degradation via ubiquitination.

Studies suggest that Akt1 is the balancing force between muscle atrophy and hypertrophy. Insulin-like growth factor 1 (IGF-1) and other anabolic stimuli activate the PI3K-Akt1 pathway, leading to the activation of downstream targets (mammalian target of rapamycin [mTOR] and S6K1) that stimulate muscle protein synthesis and hypertrophy (Fig. 5-5). Conversely, Akt1 is responsible for the phosphorylation status of the Foxo family of transcription factors. If Foxo is phosphorylated by Akt1, it leaves the nucleus and becomes inactive, preventing the induction of atrophy. However, if Akt1 activity is suppressed, Foxo becomes dephosphorylated and transcriptionally active, allowing it to bind directly to the key atrogin-1 ubiquitination gene, among others, and increase protein degradation and muscle atrophy.

Vitamins and Micronutrients

In addition to requiring macronutrients, proteins, carbohydrates, and fats, numerous cellular processes and enzymes require small quantities of vitamins, minerals, and trace elements (Table 5-2). Decreased levels of vitamins and trace elements have been implicated in impaired wound healing, depressed immune dysfunction, and an increased systemic inflammatory response to illness.[1] Micronutrient and vitamin deficiencies are uncommon in otherwise healthy subjects; however, studies of critically ill patients have noted significant incidences of various vitamin and micronutrient deficiencies in intensive care unit (ICU) settings, although more recent studies suggest that such deficiencies vary significantly by geographic region.[1-3]

Although deficiencies are avoidable with adequate supplementation, some vitamins and micronutrients require portal passage for conversion or activation, a step that is potentially bypassed with parenteral infusion and may be disabled by various disease processes. In patients with short bowel syndrome or extensive ileal resection, vitamins and micronutrients that normally require enterohepatic circulation are not adequately absorbed or activated. Patients with adult-onset pernicious anemia or atrophic gastritis with hypochlorhydria can have vitamin B_{12} deficiency. Fat malabsorption induced by pancreatic insufficiency can lead to inadequate uptake of fat-soluble micronutrients. Severe or protracted inflammatory bowel disease can result in iron and vitamin deficiencies. Plasma levels of trace elements also are significantly decreased for prolonged periods after injury because of increased urinary excretion and significant cutaneous losses.

MALNUTRITION AND STARVATION

Of patients admitted to the hospital, 50% may be malnourished, and an additional 25% to 30% become malnourished during their hospital stay. Malnutrition can occur as a result of the following, either in singly or in combination: protein deficits, calorie deficits, excessive calorie consumption, or inefficient calorie consumption. *Malnutrition can be understood as a pathophysiologic dysfunction resulting from a failure to consume or to metabolize sufficient nutrients to support the body's structural and functional integrity.*

From a pathophysiology standpoint, malnutrition is driven by two processes, either alone or in combination: (1) starvation (a state in which nutrient intake does not meet the body's metabolic demands) and (2) metabolic dysfunction (a state in which the body fails to metabolize available nutrients effectively in a manner that effectively meets its immediate needs). Clinically, malnutrition may be due to an underlying illness, inadequate intake, or both. These two aspects of malnutrition (starvation and metabolic dysregulation) frequently reinforce one another. For example, a patient who is acutely injured may fail to maintain adequate nutritional intake secondary to the traumatic injuries (e.g., pain or lethargy can inhibit self-feeding, GI dysfunction from abdominal injury can limit enteral intake of nutrition). Likewise, starvation can often exacerbate disease states, worsening metabolic dysfunction. Treatment of underlying disease processes is as

TABLE 5-2 **Vitamins and Micronutrients in Surgical Care**

MICRONUTRIENT	FUNCTION	DEFICIENCY	RELEVANCE
Vitamin A	Cofactor in collagen synthesis and cross linking; antioxidant; immune stimulation; macrophage extravasation; mucosal integrity; regulation of glycoprotein synthesis	Dermatitis, night blindness, xerophthalmia, respiratory ailments (pneumonia, bronchopulmonary dysplasia), impaired gut epithelial integrity	Wound healing and epithelial regeneration; deficiency can result in diminished activity of helper T cells, impaired mucous secretion; retinol-binding protein sensitive to nutritional status of individuals
Vitamin D	Promotes absorption of calcium and phosphorus (by intestine and kidney), bone growth, and bone remodeling (by osteoblasts and osteoclasts); regulates synthesis of several structural proteins, including type I collagen	Bone demineralization	Deficiency and impairment, causing bone demineralization and osteopenia
Vitamin E	Antioxidant properties promote cell membrane integrity	Increased platelet aggregation, decreased red blood cell survival, hemolytic anemia, neurologic abnormalities, decreased serum creatinine level, excessive creatinuria	Prolonged steatorrhea and neuronal degeneration
Vitamin K	Essential for coagulation; prerequisite for wound healing	Bruising, hemorrhage	Deficiency reported in long-term antibiotic therapy, TPN lacking fat emulsions, malabsorption
Vitamin B_1 (thiamine)	Cofactor in collagen cross linking; facilitates entry of glucose into TCA cycle	Beriberi, lactic acidosis, anorexia, fatigue, peripheral neuropathy, Wernicke-Korsakoff syndrome, cardiomegaly	Deficiency reported in depleted patients who receive sudden load of carbohydrates; wound healing; treated with 25-100 mg thiamine/day
Vitamin B_5 (pantothenic acid)	Component of coenzymes involved in energy release from macronutrients and synthesis of heme and fat	Fatigue, sleep disturbances, nausea, abdominal cramps, vomiting, diarrhea, muscle cramps, mental depression, hypoglycemia	Deficiency leading to poor wound healing and skin graft take
Biotin	Coenzyme in carboxylation reactions (gluconeogenesis, fatty acid, propionate synthesis)	Glossitis, dermatitis, pallor, hair loss	Long-term TPN, alcoholism, postgastrectomy
Vitamin C	Antioxidant, protects against free radical damage; collagen cross linking and hydroxylation of lysine and proline during collagen formation; immune-mediated and antibacterial functions of white blood cells; DNA and RNA replication; lymphocyte function	Fatigue, anorexia, muscular pain, scurvy (anemia, hemorrhagic disorders, defective collagen in bone, cartilage, teeth, connective tissues, muscle degeneration, gingivitis, capillary weakness, impaired wound healing)	Crucial in wound healing; facilitates tissue regeneration and collagen formation in bone, teeth, connective tissue
Calcium	Remodeling and degradation of collagen rely on calcium-dependent collagenases	Osteoporosis	Important in reducing osteopenia and function of collagenases; deficiency leading to hypotension, cardiovascular collapse, unresponsiveness to fluids and pressors, PTH end-organ resistance, arrhythmias
Copper	Promotes cross linking of collagen and elastin synthesis; scavenges free radicals	Skeletal demineralization, impaired glucose tolerance, anemia, neutropenia, leukopenia, changes in skin and hair pigmentation; linked to fatal arrhythmias and poorer outcomes	Significant wound exudate; losses of copper and zinc known to occur in pediatric burn patients[51]
Iron	Essential in heme-containing molecules for oxygen transport (hemoglobin) and storage (myoglobin), electron transport, and redox reactions (cytochromes)	Anemia, cheilosis, glossitis, hair loss, brittle fingernails, koilonychias, pallor, tissue hypoxia, exertional dyspnea, heart enlargement	Deficiency may occur because of anemia and blood loss; inadequacy leading to reduced resistance to infection and cold intolerance
Magnesium	Cofactor in protein and collagen synthesis	Nausea, muscle weakness, irritability, mental derangement	Deficiency can lead to cardiac arrhythmia, increased nervous system irritability, tetany
Selenium	Reduces intracellular hydroperoxides; protects membrane lipids from oxidative damage; may reduce mortality in critically ill patients	Growth retardation, muscle pain and weakness, myopathy, cardiomyopathy	Important in cell-mediated immune function; deficiency can lead to altered thyroid hormone metabolism, increased plasma glutathione levels

TABLE 5-2 Vitamins and Micronutrients in Surgical Care—cont'd

MICRONUTRIENT	FUNCTION	DEFICIENCY	RELEVANCE
Zinc	Essential cofactor in wide range of enzyme systems involved in protein synthesis, metalloenzymes, DNA replication, immune function, collagen formation, cross linking	Hair loss, dermatitis, growth retardation, delayed sexual maturation, testicular atrophy, decreased appetite, depressed smell and taste acuity, depression, diarrhea	Deficiency can cause impaired wound healing; may affect bone formation; wound exudate losses

Adapted from Norbury WB, Situ E, Herndon DN: Nutritional support in the critically ill. In Cameron JL, editor: *Current surgical therapy*, ed 9, Philadelphia, 2007, Mosby, pp 1234–1245.
PTH, Parathyroid hormone.

critical to nutritional therapy as nutritional therapy is to the treatment of the underlying disease.

Functionally, malnutrition results in impairment of multiple organ systems. Severe malnutrition and prolonged starvation eventually lead to reduced GI barrier function, respiratory insufficiency, skeletal muscle wasting, decreased myocardial mass, renal atrophy, diastolic cardiac dysfunction, and decreased sensitivity to inotropic agents. In a surgical patient, malnutrition manifests most prominently as immunosuppression (an attendant infection) and delayed wound healing. The time course of these complications depends on the specific deficiency, and their severity is typically the cumulative product of the degree and duration of deficiency. The ubiquity of malnutrition (in individual subtypes and combinations thereof) in the ICU is perhaps most clearly manifest in the epidemic of lean muscle wasting seen in critically ill and injured patients.[4]

Malnutrition Subtypes

Although malnutrition traditionally was considered a single disease process, evolving insights into diverse pathophysiologic processes that can be seen in various settings have led to a more nuanced understanding of malnutrition as something more similar to a set of interrelated syndromes than a monolithic process.[5] In 2010, the International Guideline Committee formed under the auspices of the American Society for Parenteral and Enteral Nutrition and the European Society for Clinical Nutrition and Metabolism proposed dividing the diagnosis of "malnutrition" into three distinct syndromes:

1. Starvation-associated malnutrition: Malnutrition resulting purely from prolonged starvation.
2. Chronic disease–associated malnutrition: Malnutrition that develops when a patient is exposed to prolonged nutrient deficit attributable to metabolic derangements caused by a sustained disease process.
3. Acute disease–associated or injury-associated malnutrition: Malnutrition manifesting acutely as an effective nutrient deficit that results from an overwhelming metabolic derangement.

Starvation

Starvation represents a mismatch between nutritional supply and demand, driven by limited nutritional intake. Specifically, starvation can result from a relative deficiency of total energy supplied, select nutrients, or a combination of these. (This deficit is defined in relation to real-time nutritional requirement needs of the individual patient—not to any fixed quantity.) Starvation-associated malnutrition is frequently encountered in surgical patients whose primary illness interferes with their ability to maintain nutrient intake. Common examples include oral intolerance as a result of nausea or postprandial pain, dysphagia in esophageal obstruction, or decreased feeding in a bed-bound patient with pain or altered mental status. Even in the absence of these limitations, surgical patients are frequently subjected to iatrogenic starvation malnutrition. Patients repeatedly placed on NPO restrictions in anticipation of or preparation for invasive tests and procedures can rapidly accumulate a profound nutritional deficit. Every effort should be made to coordinate care in a fashion that minimizes such starvation.

In the metabolic response to starvation-associated malnutrition, endogenous material is converted to available nutritional substrate. Glycogen serves as the primary body fuel for the first 12 to 24 hours. When glycogen stores are depleted, gluconeogenesis increases, and amino acids are degraded as fuel. Over time, ketone bodies from fat can serve as the primary oxidative fuel source. Malnutrition caused by starvation responds to restoration of nutrition.

Kwashiorkor and Marasmus

Kwashiorkor is a chronic condition that develops after long-term protein-energy malnutrition. In developing countries, kwashiorkor is more commonly caused by famine or an insufficient food supply. In the developed world, most cases are an indication of severe neglect or abuse. Less commonly, protein-energy malnutrition can be secondary to gastric surgery, anorexia nervosa, or diseases involving significant loss of ingested nutrients (e.g., pancreatic insufficiency, celiac disease, ulcerative colitis, cystic fibrosis, renal failure, malignancies). Features of kwashiorkor include pedal edema, apathy, hepatic enlargement, skin atrophy and depigmentation, and decreased muscle mass. The World Health Organization devised a three-phase management approach. In phase 1, the patient is resuscitated and stabilized; in phase 2, the patient undergoes nutritional rehabilitation; and phase 3 involves final follow-up evaluation and recurrence prevention.

Marasmus is another chronic condition caused by a sustained deficiency in dietary calories. It is a serious worldwide problem, particularly affecting children in developing countries. In surgical patients, marasmus is commonly associated with infections and GI tract disturbances. The changes in metabolism seen during marasmus are similar to changes in starvation discussed earlier. Marasmus can result from decreased energy intake, increased loss of ingested calories (diarrhea, emesis), or increased energy expenditure. The response to energy deficiency is a decrease in basal energy metabolism, slowing of growth, and loss of muscle mass and subcutaneous fat deposits. Management of marasmus involves cautious nutritional rehabilitation; correction of electrolyte imbalance; and aggressive treatment of complications such as infections, dehydration, anemia, and heart failure. During treatment, these

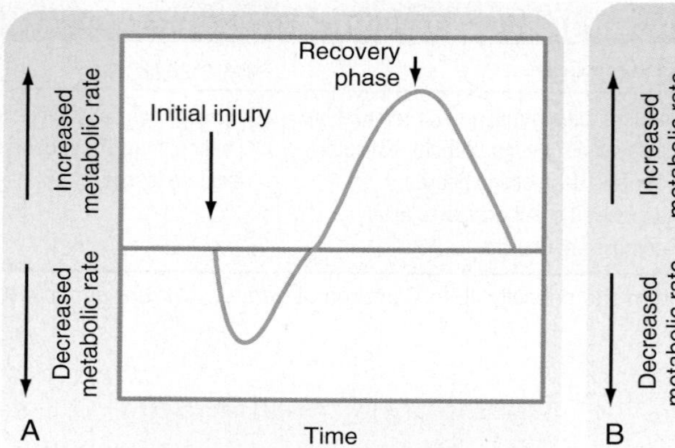

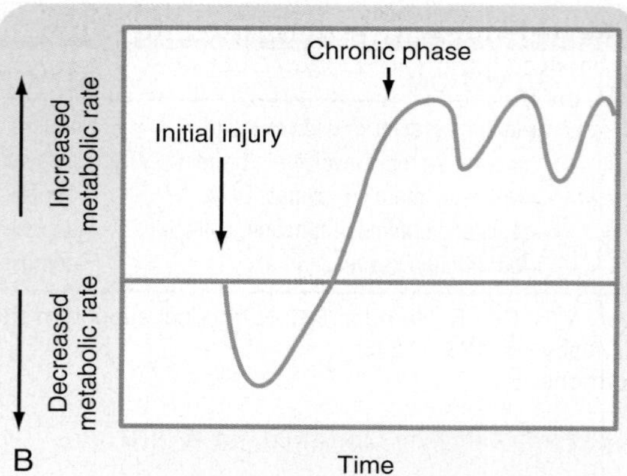

FIGURE 5-6 **A,** Classic ebb and flow phases of the acute stress response. The metabolic rate initially falls below normal and then increases to supranormal levels before returning to normal. **B,** Ebb and flow revisited. In chronically ill patients in critical care, the classic ebb and flow pattern is altered. Recurrent bouts of sepsis and other proinflammatory stimuli result in a fluctuating metabolic demand, which remains chronically elevated. (Adapted from Ball S, Baudouin SV: Endocrine disorders in the critically ill: The endocrine response to critical illness. In Hall GM, Hunter JM, Cooper MS, editors: *Core topics in endocrinology in anaesthesia and critical care,* Cambridge, England, 2010, Cambridge University Press, pp 126–131.)

patients are at significant risk of developing potentially fatal refeeding syndrome, particularly if weight loss of more than 10% has recently occurred.

Stress-Induced Changes in Substrate Metabolism

The inflammatory response to trauma and injury profoundly alters patterns of substrate metabolism. These changes reflect an evolved, adaptive response to trauma in which the entire metabolic profile of the organism is modulated to facilitate immediate response to the acute injury or threat. In the immediate response to trauma, catecholamines surge, glucose stores are released to the bloodstream, fatty acids are mobilized through lipolysis, and resource-intensive maintenance processes such as digestion and protein synthesis are suppressed—all facilitating a complete mobilization of resources to support the fight-or-flight response. The phenomenon of the prolonged systemic inflammatory response to trauma seen in patients who are supported through major injury by modern critical care is not an evolved response but represents a novel byproduct of modern medicine. In this setting, the initially adaptive acute stress response, sustained over days, becomes a pathologic process (Fig. 5-6).

The stress response is characterized by a rapid mobilization of fat stores through catecholamine activation of triglyceride lipase. The acute stress response also is accompanied by insulin resistance, with peripheral glucose intolerance and hepatic gluconeogenesis. Meanwhile, in contrast to starvation, inflammatory states appear to suppress ketogenesis with a direct correlation being seen between the severity of injury and the degree of ketogenesis inhibition. Particularly problematic in the surgical patient, the prolonged injury response induces a state of pronounced, refractory protein catabolism. This catabolic state drives a significant decline in lean body mass, the clinical hallmark of stress-associated malnutrition.

The most remarkable aspect of malnutrition associated with the metabolic response to trauma or inflammation is that in contrast to starvation, the catabolic state and other metabolic derangements associated with acute injury or inflammation cannot be entirely corrected or reversed simply by feeding adequate calories. Starvation-associated changes in metabolism represent a temporary adaptation to a lack of nutrition, whereas the catabolic response to acute injury occurs independently of feeding status.

Nonetheless, the consequences of this catabolism are exacerbated by calorie deprivation—starving a patient in the midst of a trauma-associated "metabolic storm" can result in precipitous loss of lean body mass. Multiple studies of acutely ill and injured patients treated with aggressive nutritional therapy to match estimated energy expenditure have demonstrated that these increased calories translate into increased adipogenesis rather than a reversal of lean body mass wasting.[6,7]

The metabolic response to systemic infection yields changes similar to the changes seen in the trauma response. Following the onset of sepsis, proinflammatory cytokines stimulate the secretion of cortisol, glucagon, and catecholamines. These hormones promote glycogenolysis and gluconeogenesis. When glycogen stores are exhausted, lipid and protein become the major sources of energy. Infection causes modifications in the production and uptake of glucose, resulting in hyperglycemia. As sepsis progresses, visceral blood flow is reduced and leads to the development of hypoglycemia. Sepsis can be associated with an increase in metabolic rate of 50% above basal energy expenditure.

Protein metabolism also is deranged during sepsis. There is increased synthesis of certain proteins that is associated with a reprioritization of hepatic protein synthesis and an increase in the synthesis of acute-phase proteins such as C-reactive protein. In contrast, synthesis of constitutive proteins such as albumin and prealbumin is decreased. Increased synthesis of glutamine occurs during sepsis. Glutamine serves as a primary fuel for the immune system and gut epithelium, maintaining the protective barrier function of the gut mucosa and increasing blood flow to the intestine. The excretion of muscle breakdown products such as urea, creatinine, uric acid, and ammonia is increased. The net protein loss in severe sepsis can exceed 2 g/kg/day. Even when given aggressive nutritional support, septic patients can lose more than 10% of total body protein in 3 weeks.[8] If the catabolic state is not modified, tissue repair and immune response are impaired, with severe loss of skeletal and visceral proteins also occurring.

The catabolic hormones induce lipolysis of TAG stores in adipose tissue to generate glycerol and free fatty acids. In severe sepsis, hyperlipidemia and hyperlactemia are present, with a discrepancy occurring between lactate production and lactate uptake. This response results in increased plasma lactate concentrations that are associated with severe sepsis.

NUTRITIONAL ASSESSMENT AND MONITORING

Goal-directed nutritional support is essential for improving outcomes after trauma and surgery and should be based on repeated assessment of response to feeding. Underfeeding in the setting of a stress-induced catabolic surge can result in a precipitous decline in nutritional status. Overfeeding is detrimental, leading to hypercapnia and metabolic acidosis, hyperglycemia, hypertriglyceridemia, hepatic dysfunction, and azotemia. An ongoing nutritional assessment is the starting point for any nutritional therapy.

Global Assessment and Nutritional Risk Screening

Nutritional assessment of surgical patients includes evaluation of preexisting malnutrition, medical conditions and metabolic disorders, malabsorption, dental disease, drug dependency, and alcoholism. In addition to requiring a comprehensive medical history and physical examination, nutritional assessment may include relevant laboratory tests, anthropometric measurements, and other assessments of body composition and energy expenditure, combined with the serial evaluation of results and response to therapy (Box 5-1). In surgical patients, wounds can serve as a unique indicator of functional nutritional status. In the absence of wound-specific confounders (e.g., wound infection, arterial insufficiency), the ability of a patient's wound to heal in a timely fashion is convincing evidence of adequate nutrition. Although this measure is extremely useful to an experienced physician, it is difficult to apply in research or on a systems-wide basis because the "normal" timeline for healing is a subjective estimate based on the examining physician applying his or her experience with similar wounds in healthy patients.

Multiple formal clinical survey tools have been created to assess nutritional status and screen for malnutrition. Nutritional risk screening incorporates patient and disease factors to determine nutritional risk. It is the only widely used nutritional screening tool based on grade I clinical evidence and the only tool shown to predict morbidity and mortality reliably in acute care and GI surgery patients.[9-11]

Anthropometry

Anthropometric measurements comprise a range of physical body measurements that are compared with standard values or used to evaluate individual changes in nutritional status over time. These measurements are frequently incorporated into mathematical models designed to predict nutritional status, energy needs, or both.

Body Weight

Body weight reflects fluid balance and nutritional status. Day-to-day changes typically reflect acute fluid balance. In the setting of acute illness or injury, massive fluid retention and shifts tend to mask weight loss from skeletal muscle. However, sustained weight gain or weight loss generally indicates a nutrition or malnutrition phenomenon. Significant weight loss over a broader period of time (weeks to months) is a powerful predictor of mortality, particularly if the loss is rapid or unplanned. In the absence of pathologic fluid retention, sustained weight gain is a classic hallmark of a return to anabolism. Overprovision of calories and protein does not avert persistence of muscle protein breakdown, and weight gains may be caused by increases in body fat, particularly in obese patients. Overweight and obese patients may be unable to use fat stores after injury and may not be as well nourished as is often assumed, with low muscle mass in relation to their weight.

Ideal Body Weight

A practical anthropometric approach is the calculation of ideal body weight (IBW), particularly when the usual body weight or weight of the patient before the onset of illness is unknown. Values for IBW can be found in standardized tables that relate height to expected weight, or IBW can be estimated by the following equations:

- Men: 48 kg for the first 152 cm and 2.7 kg for each additional 2.54 cm
- Women: 45 kg for the first 152 cm and 2.3 kg for each additional 2.54 cm

Although sometimes useful as a reference point, the concept of "ideal body weight" is outdated, and it is probably better understood as an approximation of lean body mass.

Lean Body Mass

"Lean body mass" refers to nonadipose tissue mass, exclusive of any added mass from acute shifts in water content. The term *ideal* is not appropriate because there is not a specific limit to how much lean body mass a patient can healthfully maintain. Malnutrition (ongoing or recent) can be identified by either a low lean body mass or a persistent decline in lean body mass. Malnourished obese patients provide a telling example of the importance of lean body mass. Multiple studies have identified critical malnutrition in obese patients who, despite generous fat stores, show markedly low lean body mass on sophisticated measurements. In patients with this type of obesity, termed *sarcopenic obesity,* surgical morbidity and mortality rates correlate far more closely with lean body mass than with gross mass or any calculated "ideal" weight.[5,12]

Body Mass Index

Body mass index (BMI) is a statistical index that uses height and weight to provide an estimate of body fat in males and females of all ages. However, individual variation can occur, and BMI should not be used as the sole means of classifying a person as obese or malnourished. The U.S. National Health and Nutrition Examination Survey of 2007 indicated that 63% of Americans are overweight, with 26% in the obese category (BMI $\geq$30 kg/m^2). In children, BMI percentile allows for comparison of children with

BOX 5-1 Methods of Nutritional Assessment

- Clinical history
- Body weight
- Anthropometric measurements: IBW, BMI, skinfold thickness
- Indirect calorimetry
- Oxygen consumption, determination of respiratory quotient
- Body composition analysis: Dual-energy x-ray absorptiometry
- Biochemical measurements: Albumin, transferrin, prealbumin
- Measurement of nitrogen balance
- Measurements of immunologic function

BOX 5-2 Interpretation of Body Mass Index

- Severely underweight: <16.5 kg/m^2
- Underweight: 16.5-18.4 kg/m^2
- Normal weight: 18.5-24.9 kg/m^2
- Overweight: 25-29.9 kg/m^2
- Obesity grade I: 30-34.9 kg/m^2
- Obesity grade II: 35-39.9 kg/m^2
- Obesity grade III: ≥40 kg/m^2

the same sex and age. A BMI that is less than the 5th percentile is considered underweight, and a BMI above the 95th percentile is considered obese. In adults, BMI is interpreted based on consensus-based cutoff levels (Box 5-2).[13]

$$\text{BMI} = \text{weight (in kg)}/\text{height}^2 \text{ (in m}^2\text{)}$$

Clinical Imaging

Dual-Energy X-Ray Absorptiometry

Dual-energy x-ray absorptiometry (DEXA) is a useful technique for monitoring long-term nutritional progress by measuring changes in body tissue composition, including lean body mass, fat mass, and bone density. Tissue density values are derived from quantitative measures of the attenuation of two x-ray beams. These measurements are compared with standard models used for bone and soft tissue, and they are used to calculate lean body mass, fat mass, and bone mineral content. Maintaining and enhancing skeletal muscle as lean body mass is a principal objective of nutritional support, so these measurements are useful in nutritional assessment.

Computed Tomography and Ultrasound

Although DEXA is well established as an accurate and precise tool for assessing body composition, availability issues limit its application. High-resolution CT scanners have been shown to predict DEXA assessments reliably; however, significant cost, radiation exposure, and need for patient transport are barriers to widespread clinical use. More recently, multiple groups have shown that measurements from a limited bedside ultrasound examination predict total body composition with excellent intraoperator and interoperator reliability.[14,15] Given its ubiquitous availability, low cost, ease of use, and minimally invasive nature, bedside ultrasound has significant potential for widespread clinical application in nutritional assessment and monitoring.

Serum Albumin Level

Albumin accounts for more than 50% of the total protein in serum and is the major contributor to colloid osmotic pressure (Table 5-3). Albumin requires significant energy stores for synthesis, is inhibited by inflammation, and has a long half-life of approximately 20 days. For these reasons, serum albumin levels are useful in detecting and quantifying malnutrition. In patients undergoing elective surgery, preoperative albumin levels have been found to be a better prognostic indicator of morbidity and mortality than anthropometric measurements.[16] Preoperative albumin levels less than 3 g/dL are independently associated with an increased risk of developing serious complications within 30 days of surgery, including sepsis, acute renal failure, coma, failure to wean from ventilation, cardiac arrest, pneumonia, and wound infection.

TABLE 5-3 Surgical Risk by Serum Albumin Level*

SERUM ALBUMIN (g/dL)	30-DAY MORTALITY RATE (%)	30-DAY MORBIDITY RATE (%)
>4.5	≤1	≤10
3.5	5	25
3.0	9	35
2.5	15	45
<2.1	≈30	65

Adapted from Gibbs J, Cull W, Henderson W, et al: Preoperative serum albumin level as a predictor of operative mortality and morbidity: Results from the National VA Surgical Risk Study. *Arch Surg* 134:36–42, 1999.

*Perioperative levels of serum albumin have been shown to be powerful predictors of morbidity and mortality.

Albumin levels also are useful in detecting protein-energy malnutrition, which is frequently difficult to recognize in patients not presenting with low body weight and results from increased demands associated with the stress of illness, injury, or infection. If these requirements are not met from dietary sources, body protein stores are depleted, leading to complications (e.g., malabsorption, impaired immunologic response, and reduced production of other constitutive proteins).

The value of serum protein level as an indicator of nutritional status is limited in the acute phase following injury, inflammation, infection, and surgical stress. Fluid shifts and increased capillary permeability lead to protein leakage from the intravascular compartment, which results in hemodilution and false hypoproteinemia. In critical and acute care settings, short-term changes in albumin levels should not be interpreted as being indicative of nutritional progress.

Pediatric Assessment

In children, nutritional assessment includes a clinical history, physical examination, and analysis of biochemical markers as well as plotting growth on percentile charts. The U.S. Centers for Disease Control and Prevention has published revised, standard, gender-specific percentile charts for growth, including stature and weight for age and BMI. These charts are demographically representative of the U.S. population from age 2 to 20 years, with charts available for younger children as well (Fig. 5-7). These charts are used to monitor a patient's long-term nutritional progress. A patient's position on the growth chart is the best simple tool to evaluate overall nutritional status in the acute setting. A value below the fifth percentile or a trend line crossing two major percentile lines indicates a serious failure to thrive.

EVALUATING METABOLISM AND ENERGY REQUIREMENTS

Determining nutritional requirements of critically ill patients is essential because the provision of inadequate or excess calories can adversely affect outcome. Estimates of caloric requirements can be made using several different equations, calculated using blood gas measurements with the Fick equation. In surgical patients, direct measurement of resting energy expenditure (REE) or basal metabolic rate (BMR) can have distinct benefits over empirical estimates

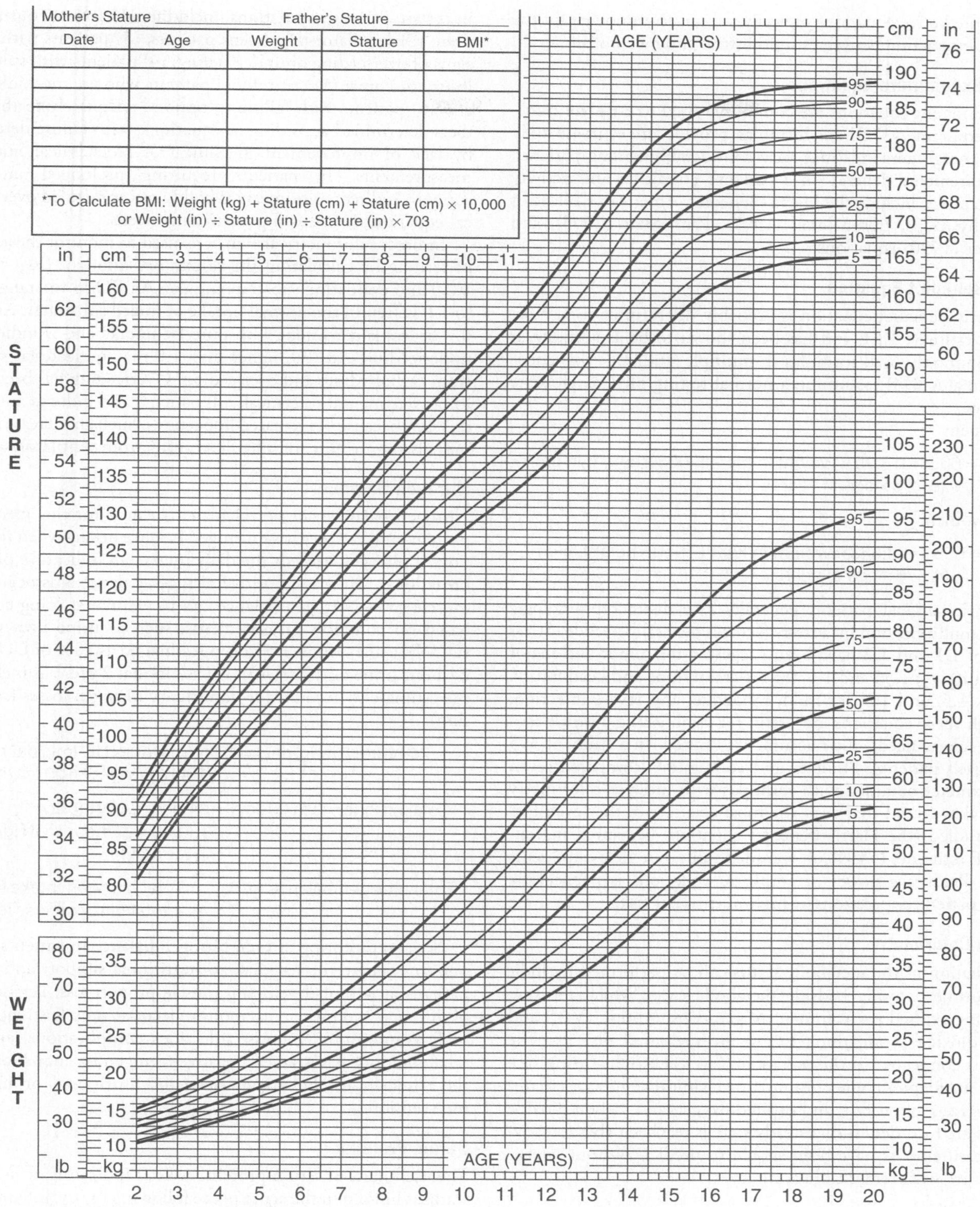

Published May 30.2000 (modified 11/21/00).
SOURCE: Developed by the National Center for Health Statistics in collaboration with the National Center for Chronic Disease Prevention and Health Promotion (2000).
http://www.edc.gov/growthcharts

FIGURE 5-7 Stature-for-age and weight-for-age percentile charts for boys 2 to 20 years. (From Centers for Disease Control and Prevention: Growth charts, 2000, http://www.cdc.gov/growthcharts.)

because predictive equations typically fail to accommodate for the complex interaction between surgical stress and metabolism.

Energy Expenditure Equations

Several different equations are commonly used to estimate nutritional requirements. These formulas provide an estimate only because energy demands may vary considerably among patients, and requirements depend on a patient's condition and activity level. Examples include the Harris-Benedict, American College of Chest Physicians, Ireton-Jones (1997), Penn State (2003), and Swinamer (1990) equations.

Harris-Benedict Equation

The Harris-Benedict equation is probably the formula used most often to estimate REE and has been shown to be as accurate as other commonly used formulas in multiple studies.[17] This equation estimates BMR assuming a normal resting physiologic state as follows.

For men:

$$\text{BMR} = 66.5 + (13.75 \times \text{weight in kg}) + (5.003 \times \text{height in cm}) - (6.775 \times \text{age in years})$$

For women:

$$\text{BMR} = 655.1 + (9.563 \times \text{weight in kg}) + (1.850 \times \text{height in cm}) - (4.676 \times \text{age in years})$$

Because surgical patients generally face distinct physiologic stresses, multiplication by a stress factor is generally needed. Stress factors of 1.1 and 1.2 have been suggested for minor and major elective surgery; 1.35 and 1.6, for skeletal trauma and head injury; and 1.1, 1.5, and 1.8, for mild, moderate, and severe infection. Although these equations are useful for establishing a quick estimate of caloric needs, their accuracy is limited. In a study of 395 hospitalized patients, Boullata and colleagues[17] compared seven REE estimates obtained with formulas with indirect calorimetry results. They found that even the most accurate of the seven formulas studied (the Harris-Benedict equation) generated inaccurate REE estimates (>10% off recorded values) in 40% of patients studied. Predictive power of empirical equations is particularly poor in patient populations at high nutritional risk.

Indirect Calorimetry

An evaluation of the metabolic status can be performed by indirect calorimetry using bedside metabolic carts, which measure REE using expired gas volumes; oxygen consumption ($\dot{V}O_2$) and carbon dioxide production ($\dot{V}CO_2$) are measured directly. The patient is connected to the metabolic cart via a tight-fitting face mask or an adapter connection to a mechanical ventilator circuit. The patient is left at rest, and expired oxygen and carbon dioxide volumes are recorded until a steady state is reached. These steady-state measurements have been shown to predict 24-hour energy expenditure with remarkable accuracy.

$$\text{REE (in kcal/day)} = 1.44\,(3.9\,\dot{V}O_2\ [\text{in mL/min}] + 1.1\,\dot{V}CO_2\ [\text{in mL/min}])$$

Measurements obtained are generally reliable and reproducible over a wide range of catabolic conditions, metabolic rates, and values of FIO_2. Poor agreement between measured and predicted REEs has been reported in certain circumstances, with average differences between measured and predicted REE being as high as 635 ± 526 kcal/day in severely burned children. Bedside carts are recommended to calculate optimal nutritional requirements in certain patient populations, including (1) severely burned children; (2) ventilator-dependent patients; (3) patients with clinical signs of overfeeding or underfeeding; (4) patients with spinal cord injury or coma; (5) critically ill patients who are morbidly obese; and (6) patients with failure to respond adequately to the use of diets determined according to equations, with failure determined by lack of improvement in clinical or biochemical nutritional measurements. In patients requiring prolonged nutritional support, indirect calorimetry is highly recommended over empirical equations for assessing nutritional needs.

Indirect calorimetry also may be used to monitor the adequacy of feeding by calculating the respiratory quotient ($RQ = \dot{V}CO_2/\dot{V}O_2$) and evaluating substrate uptake. An RQ in the range of 0.7 to 1.0 is seen in the normal uptake of mixed substrates. An RQ of 0.7 or less is consistent with pure fat uptake and is indicative of underfeeding. An RQ higher than 1.0 may indicate fat synthesis from carbohydrate and overfeeding. Overfeeding has been shown to be detrimental to critically ill patients and induces an increase in $\dot{V}CO_2$ because of increased lipogenesis. Such an increase in $\dot{V}CO_2$ may also contribute to difficult weaning from ventilatory support.

Nitrogen Balance

Nitrogen balance can be calculated to monitor the adequacy of protein intake. A negative nitrogen balance occurs when the excretion of nitrogen exceeds the daily intake, an indication of muscle breakdown, whereas a positive nitrogen balance is associated with muscle gain. Nitrogen balance can be estimated using equations based on common measurements, such as urine urea nitrogen (UUN), urine nonurea nitrogen (estimated as 20% of UUN), and 24-hour urine output (UO). An additional 2 g/day is included in the estimate to account for nonurinary nitrogen losses (stool and skin).

$$\text{24-hour UUN (g/day)} = \text{UUN (mg/dL)} \times \text{UO (mL/day)} \times 1/1000\ (\text{g/mg}) \times 1/100\ (\text{dL/mL})$$

$$\text{Total nitrogen loss (g/day)} = \text{24-hour UUN (g/day)} + (0.20 \times \text{24-hour UUN [g/day]}) + 2\ (\text{g/day})$$

$$\text{Total nitrogen balance (g/day)} = \text{Total nitrogen intake (g/day)} - \text{total nitrogen loss (g/day)}$$

Serial monitoring of total nitrogen balance in patients permits one to evaluate the response to nutritional support and identify patients at risk of developing muscle protein loss. Persistent loss of nitrogen and protein catabolism decrease muscle strength, alter body composition, increase infectious complications, and delay rehabilitation. A sustained negative nitrogen balance should alert the clinician to the urgent need for nutritional or metabolic intervention.

Serum Proteins

The usefulness of serum protein levels as indicators of nutritional status is limited in the acute phase following injury, inflammation, infection, and surgical stress. Fluid shifts and increased capillary permeability lead to protein leakage from the intravascular compartment, which results in hemodilution and false hypoproteinemia.

NUTRITIONAL SUPPORT

Surgical patients with suboptimal nutritional support have impaired wound healing, altered immune responses, accelerated

BOX 5-3 Criteria to Initiate Perioperative Nutritional Support[54-56]

Severe nutritional risk expected with at least one of the following:

- Past medical history: Severe undernutrition, chronic disease
- Involuntary loss >10%-15% of usual body weight within 6 mo or >5% within 1 mo
- Expected blood loss >500 mL during surgery
- Weight 20% less than IBW or BMI <18.5 kg/m^2
- Failure to thrive on pediatric growth and development curves (<5th percentile or a trend line crossing two major percentile lines)
- Serum albumin <3.0 g/dL or transferrin <200 mg/dL in the absence of an inflammatory state, hepatic dysfunction, or renal dysfunction
- Anticipate that patient will be unable to meet caloric requirements within 7-10 days perioperatively
- Catabolic disease (e.g., significant burns or trauma, sepsis, and pancreatitis)

catabolism, increased organ dysfunction, delayed recovery, and increased morbidity and mortality. Patients who are inadequately fed after surgery become critically undernourished within 10 days and have a markedly increased risk of death. The ultimate goal of perioperative nutritional management is to meet caloric and nutrient-specific requirements safely to promote wound healing, diminish risk of infection, and prevent loss of muscle protein.

Nutritional support should be considered for all patients according to clinical assessments and guidelines over the perioperative period (Box 5-3). If a surgical intervention can be delayed, 10 to 14 days of preoperative nutritional support for patients with severe nutritional risk has been shown to be beneficial before surgery.[9]

Preoperative Nutrition

Nonmalnourished Patients

In elective operations, the metabolic insult begins well before the incision, when the patient is asked to adhere to "NPO past midnight" in anticipation of elective surgery. Even in non-GI surgeries, postoperative nausea can last for hours, leading to a cumulative starvation period greater than 24 hours. This period can significantly tax the starvation response of the healthiest patients. The duration of starvation can be curtailed by minimizing the "NPO" window. Clear liquid intake can safely be allowed 2 hours before surgery and can significantly dampen the metabolic insult of surgery.[18]

Augmenting glycogen stores through carbohydrate supplementation in the immediate preoperative period can mitigate the physiologic impact of starvation. Multiple studies have shown that oral ingestion of adequate volumes of carbohydrate-rich solution in the 24-hour preoperative period leads to decreased muscle wasting, insulin resistance, and tissue glycolyzation postoperatively.[11,19-21]

Patients undergoing elective surgery also have been shown to benefit from preoperative initiation of immunonutrition. Responses have been found to be optimal when therapy is initiated 5 to 7 days preoperatively. This likely corresponds to the time required to increase effective tissue concentrations of the micronutrients used. The foundations and applications of immunonutrition are discussed in depth further on.

Malnourished Patients

It has long been established that preoperative malnutrition is associated with poor surgical outcomes.[11,22] Nutritional status should be assessed in all patients considered for elective surgery (see "Global Assessment and Nutritional Risk Screening"). Although full correction of malnutrition in a patient before surgery may not be feasible, preoperative intervention can mitigate its impact in select cases. As with any therapy, the efficacy of preoperative nutritional therapy relies on patient selection (see Box 5-3). In a large multicenter trial, Jie and colleagues[9] analyzed outcomes in patients undergoing abdominal surgery with or without preoperative nutritional therapy, which was defined as at least 7 days of goal-directed EN or parenteral nutrition (PN). They reported that in patients with a nutritional risk screening malnutrition score of 5 or higher, preoperative nutritional intervention halved the complications rate; in patients with a score of 4 or lower, preoperative therapy was not associated with any significant difference in complication rates.[9] Whether the benefit of preoperative nutritional therapy outweighs the risks of delaying surgery is a highly complex patient-specific decision and is determined through the surgeon's assessment of various factors, including (1) the patient's level of malnutrition, (2) the nutritional options available to the patient preoperatively (e.g., enteric feeds at goal, limited enteric feeds, total parenteral nutrition [TPN]), (3) the likelihood of the malnutrition responding to preoperative nutrition, and (4) the relative risk of delaying the particular surgery considered.

Principles Guiding Routes of Nutrition: Enteral, Parenteral, or Both

For decades, surgical and critical care literature documented significant morbidity and mortality risks associated with the use of PN. This emphasis on the risks of PN led to the widespread dogma that the beneficial impact of PN can outweigh its risks only when applied to patients who are otherwise facing prolonged total starvation. However, more recent reassessments of PN in the setting of contemporary critical care practices suggest that the risk profile of PN has declined significantly over the past 20 years.

Although PN undoubtedly involves significant risks and morbidity, it is believed that more recent advances in critical care (e.g., improved glycemic control practices, increased evidence on infection control techniques) have significantly mitigated these risks. Perhaps most convincingly, Harvey and colleagues[23] randomly assigned 2400 patients in the ICU to receive either EN or PN and found no indication of increased 30-day morbidity or mortality in the PN group.

There has been a trend in the surgical and critical care literature to broaden the indications for TPN. Challenging the consensus recommendation that initiation of PN in patients intolerant of EN be delayed until the patient has demonstrated persistent intolerance over several days, Doig and associates[24] demonstrated that early initiation of PN improved outcomes in patients with contraindications to enteral feeding (Box 5-4). Going one step further, multiple large trials evaluated the use of PN as a supplement to, rather than replacement for, EN, with variable results.[25-27] As opposed to conventional TPN, supplemental PN is used to augment nutrition in patients who are able to tolerate significant amounts of EN, but not in quantities sufficient to meet their calculated protein-caloric requirements. In these patients, the dose of supplemental PN is calculated to equal the difference between projected protein-caloric requirements and protein-caloric value of the EN tolerated.

The utility of supplemental PN (applied liberally) is a matter of considerable debate. We believe that supplemental nutrition

BOX 5-4 Contraindications to Enteral Nutrition

Intractable vomiting, diarrhea refractory to medical management
Paralytic ileus
High-output intestinal fistulas (too distal to bypass with feeding tube)
GI obstruction, ischemia
Diffuse peritonitis
Severe shock or hemodynamic instability
Severe GI hemorrhage
Severe short bowel syndrome (<100 cm of small bowel remaining)
Severe GI malabsorption (e.g., EN failed, as evidenced by progressive deterioration in nutritional status)
Inability to gain access to GI tract
Need for EN is expected for <7 days

Adapted from Villet S, Chiolero RL, Bollmann MD, et al: Negative impact of hypocaloric feeding and energy balance on clinical outcome in ICU patients. *Clin Nutr* 24:502–509, 2005.

can be quite helpful when applied selectively, based on the clinician's assessment of the metabolic needs and nutritional status of the individual patient. As our previous discussion indicates (see "Malnutrition and Starvation" and "Nutritional Assessment and Monitoring"), patients' ability to tolerate undernourishment differs markedly, depending on their current metabolic profile and their nutritional status before injury. For example, it is our practice to use supplemental PN in the acute phase of burn injury response in patients unable to tolerate enteral feeds at quantities sufficient to meet (or at least approach) protein-caloric requirements. Alternatively, among patients who manifest enteral feeding intolerance in the subacute phase of their burn injury response, we typically prescribe supplemental PN only to patients with evidence of preexisting malnutrition at the time of burn. Considerations for selecting the optimal route of nutrition are listed in Box 5-5.

Enteral Nutrition

Benefits of Enteral Nutrition (Trophic Feeding)

In addition to serving as a means for systemic delivery of nutrients, EN performs a critical function in supporting the alimentary tract itself. Mucosal exposure to feeds provides direct high-concentration nutrients (e.g., glutamine, alanine), stimulates enteric blood flow, maintains barrier function by preserving tight-junction integrity, and induces production and release of mucosal immunoglobulin and critical endogenous growth factors. These functions are not replaced with PN.[28] After dietary ingestion, polysaccharides such as fiber and starch undergo bacterial fermentation in the colonic lumen. Bacterial fermentation is essential for two major reasons: (1) support of the normal flora of the gut lumen, which prevents colonization and subsequent infection (e.g., *Clostridium difficile*), and (2) production of acetoacetate, propionate, and butyrate (a short-chain fatty acid). Butyrate appears to be the preferred fuel of colonic mucosa cells and is essential for mucosal integrity.

Animal and human studies show that the presence of enteral feeds (in addition to or in place of PN) is associated with increased mucosal mass, mucosal oxygenation, brush-border enzyme synthesis, and villus height compared with PN alone.[28,29] Significant evidence suggests that, in certain clinical settings, early intestinal feeding minimizes ileus by facilitating gut motility.[30]

BOX 5-5 Considerations for Selecting Routes

1. Use the oral route if the GI tract is fully functional and there are no other contraindications to oral feeding.
2. In patients who do not have any absolute contraindication to EN and who are expected to be unable to take adequate nutrition orally within 24-48 hours, initiate or attempt direct EN as soon as possible.[57] This includes patients who are physically capable of PO nutrition but fail to take in food orally because of appetite suppression or behavioral challenges.
3. If the enteral route is contraindicated or not tolerated,
   a. Initiate TPN within 24-48 hours in all critically ill or injured patients who are not expected to be able to tolerate significant EN within 48-72 hours.
   b. Initiate TPN within 24-48 hours in all patients (regardless of injury or illness severity) who are not expected to be able to tolerate significant EN within 3-4 days.
   c. Consider initiating supplemental PN in any critically ill or injured patient who can tolerate only limited enteral feeding and who is not expected to tolerate sufficient enteral feeds to meet 60%-80% of projected protein-caloric needs within 48-72 hours.
4. Administer at least 20% of the caloric and protein requirements enterally while reaching the required goal with additional PN.
5. Maintain PN until the patient is able to tolerate 75% of calories through the enteral route, and maintain EN until the patient is able to tolerate 75% of calories via the oral route.

Early Initiation of Enteral Nutrition

Copious data support the safety and benefit of initiating EN early in the postoperative period, including in the setting of GI surgeries.[31,32] EN is frequently delayed unnecessarily because of concerns of exacerbating postoperative ileus or damaging fresh GI anastomosis, although repeated studies and expert panels have concluded that such practices are misguided.[11] Full feeds should not be delivered in the setting of marked hemodynamic instability or high-dose vasopressor requirements because of risk of inducing or exacerbating nonobstructive mesenteric ischemia. However, complete EN can be delivered safely to patients on low-to-moderate doses of vasopressors with stable or decreasing vasopressor requirements.[11,33]

Delivering Enteral Nutrition

Oral Feeding

For a conscious patient with an intact appetite and swallowing function, direct oral intake is the preferred feeding modality (Fig. 5-8). Swallowing function must be sufficient to avoid food aspiration and the attendant risks of pneumonitis and pneumonia. Indicators of compromised swallow function include neurologic impairment (cognitive or oral-motor), coughing or choking with feeds, or symptoms indicating a possible aspiration-associated pathology (e.g., chronic cough, recurrent pneumonia). Assessment of swallow function can range from bedside observation to formal speech pathology consultation and imaging-based swallow studies.

When prescribing an oral diet, the physician must continuously monitor for adequate intake. In the acute surgical setting, patients may fail to take in adequate calories because of decreased appetite, depressed mental status, pain, or any other practical obstacle to eating. Should a patient consistently fail to meet estimated caloric needs with an oral diet, supplemental feeds via nasoenteric tube should be considered.

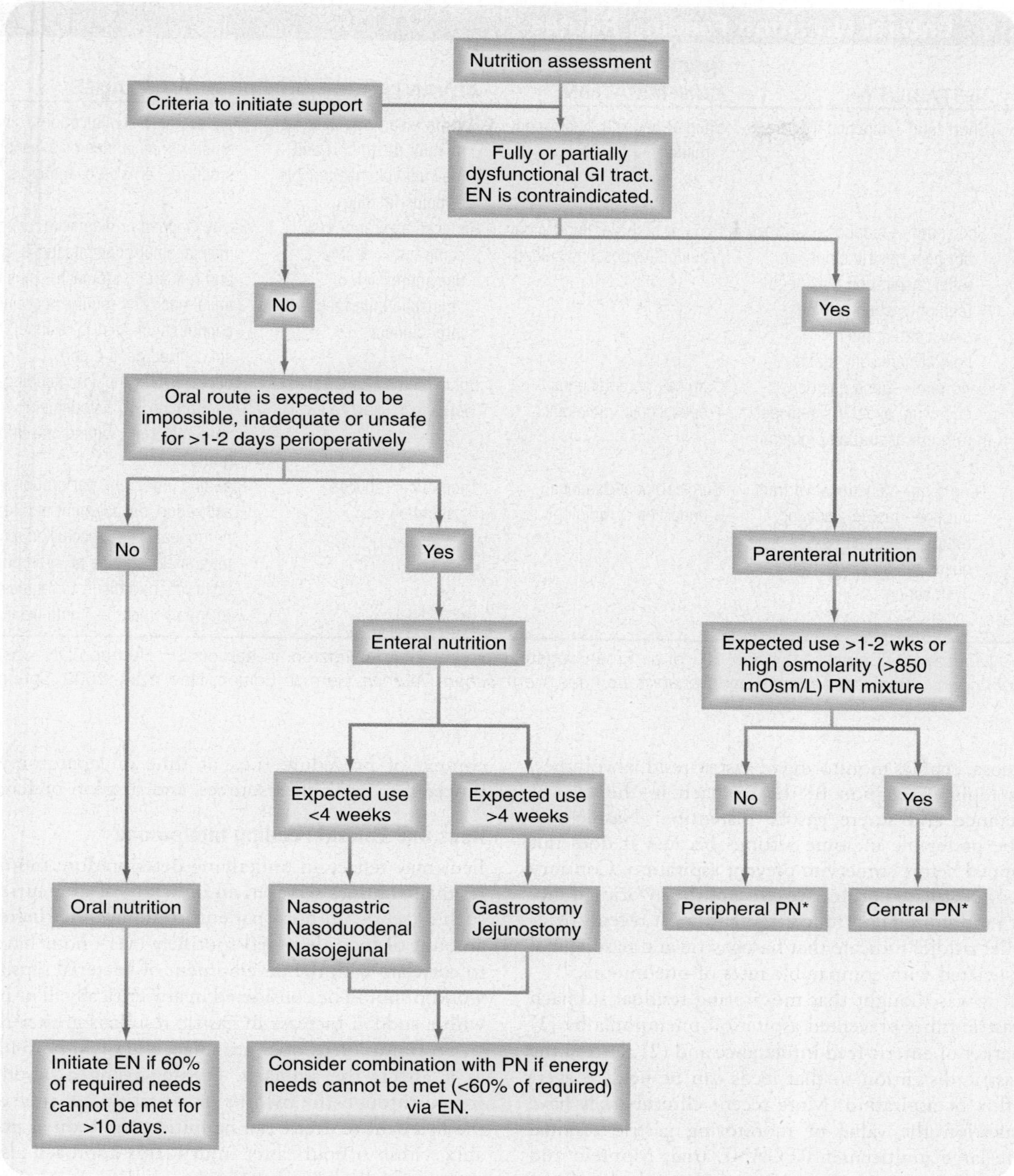

FIGURE 5-8 Algorithm for route of nutritional support in surgical patients.

Enteral Access for Feeding

In patients incapable of oral feeding, administration of EN can be accomplished via various routes (Table 5-4). Nasogastric, nasoduodenal, and nasojejunal tubes (Fig. 5-9) are used in patients who are expected to require support for a short time (<4 weeks). Other surgical options include open or percutaneous gastrostomy and jejunostomy, usually for patients who are expected to require long-term EN (>4 weeks).

The practice of checking the positioning of tubes by x-ray before their use is a time-consuming process that has been motivated partly by the unintended placement of small-diameter tubes into lower airways. However, nasogastric tubes may be placed with confidence by auscultation over the stomach while quickly delivering 50 mL of air with an irrigation syringe. Nasojejunal and duodenal tubes may be too small for this procedure. With nasoenteric feeding beyond the stomach, the tube should be advanced through the duodenum. Although drainage nasogastric tubes are used to prevent aspiration and vomiting in patients with obstruction, any nasoenteric tube in which suction is left off or obstructive loses protective properties and increases the aspiration risk by stenting open the lower esophageal sphincter. For this reason, it is recommended that the head of the bed be raised to 35 degrees whenever nasoenteric tubes are in place and that the functioning of nasogastric tubes is checked regularly.

Either gastric or small bowel tubes can be used for delivering EN. Gastric feeding access allows for direct (trophic) feeding of

TABLE 5-4 **Enteral Nutrition Feeding Routes**

ROUTE	SUITABILITY	INSERTION METHOD, CONFIRMATION	ADVANTAGES	DISADVANTAGES
Nasogastric	Short term—functional GI tract	Blind at bedside; fluoroscopy guided	Easy to insert, replace; can monitor gastric pH and residual volume; capable of bolus feeding	Misplacement complications, sinusitis, epistaxis, nasal necrosis, esophageal strictures, erosive esophagitis
Nasoduodenal, nasojejunal	Short term—functional GI tract but poor gastric emptying, reflux, aspiration risk; begin feed only when volume resuscitated and hemodynamically stable	Blind at bedside; fluoroscopy guided, endoscopy guided	Reduced aspiration risk; some tubes enable decompression of stomach while feeding into jejunum	Easily clogged or displaced, aspiration risk, misplacement complications, displacement and reflux into stomach, sinusitis, epistaxis, nasal necrosis; requires continuous infusion; cannot check gastric residuals except with specialized gastric port
Gastrostomy	Long term—good gastric emptying; avoid if significant reflux or aspiration problem	Surgical, percutaneous, endoscopic, radiologic	Bolus feeding; large-bore tube less likely to block	Procedure risks include bleeding, perforation, aspiration risk, dislodgment with peritoneal contamination, wound site infection, granulation
Jejunostomy	Long term—functional GI tract but poor gastric emptying, reflux, aspiration risk, gastroparesis or gastric dysfunction	Surgical, percutaneous, endoscopic, radiologic	Theoretical reduced aspiration risk	Bleeding, infection, perforation, migration, aspiration, dislodgment and leakage into peritoneal cavity, occlusion, pneumatosis, intestinal ischemia or infarction, bowel obstruction; difficult to replace; cannot check residuals; requires continuous infusion

Adapted from Al-Mousawi A, Branski LK, Andel HL, et al: Ernährungstherapie bei Brandverletzten. In Kamolz LP, Herndon DN, Jeschke MG, editors: *Verbrennungen: Diagnose, Therapie und Rehabilitation des thermischen Traumas*, German Edition, New York, 2009, Springer-Verlag, pp 183–194.

the gastric mucosa, enables monitoring of gastric residual volumes, and facilitates rapid evacuation of the stomach in the case of feeding intolerance and severe gastric distention. Nasojejunal feeding may be preferable in some settings because it does not need to be stopped before surgery to prevent aspiration. Contrary to the previously postulated protective effect of the pyloric sphincter, the largest randomized controlled trial and most recent meta-analysis of earlier studies indicate that nasogastric and nasojejunal feeding are associated with comparable rates of pneumonia.[34]

In the past, it was thought that monitoring residual stomach volumes via gastric tubes prevented aspiration pneumonia by (1) serving as a marker of enteric feed intolerance and (2) alerting the clinician to gastric distention so that feeds can be held to avert impending reflux or aspiration. More recent clinical trials have called into question the value of monitoring gastric residual volume. In the large multicenter REGANE trial, Montejo and coworkers[35] found that increasing the gastric residual volume threshold for holding tube feeds from 200 mL to 500 mL had no effect on the rate of pneumonia, time on ventilator, or length of ICU stay. In a randomized clinical trial involving 449 patients in multiple French ICUs, Reignier and colleagues[36] found that patients managed without any monitoring of gastric residual volume showed no increase in pneumonia rates or length of mechanical ventilation compared with patients managed with strict gastric residual volume limits. In both studies, increasing or eliminating gastric residual volume threshold led to significantly improved nutritional intakes.

Surgical feeding access options should be considered if a patient requires nasal tube feeding for a prolonged period beyond 2 or 3 weeks. Procedural approaches include percutaneous endoscopic gastrostomy, fluoroscopic-guided gastrostomy or jejunostomy, or surgical (open or laparoscopic) enteral access. Procedure selection depends on multiple factors, including patient anatomy, context of procedure (i.e., at time of laparotomy for separate procedure), available resources, and surgeon preference.

Ileus and Enteral Feeding Intolerance

Ileus may reflect an underlying deterioration; monitoring gastric residual volumes serves as an indicator of intercurrent conditions such as sepsis. In burn patients, residuals that increase above the amount of food delivered routinely every hour have been shown to correlate with the development of bacterial sepsis. A full sepsis workup should be considered in any critically ill or injured patient with a sudden increase in gastric residuals greater than 200 mL.

Postinjury ileus does not affect the small bowel as profoundly as it affects the stomach. Feeding using a nasoduodenal tube passed through the pylorus or a nasojejunal tube advanced past the ligament of Treitz can be initiated as soon as possible, preferably within 6 hours after injury. This approach also allows continuous feeding during surgeries and physical therapy sessions. Some authorities recommend attempting gastric feeds before resorting to postpyloric feeding, reasoning that gastric feeds may minimize the risk of gastric ileus.

Early Initiation of Enteral Feeding

Early (24 to 48 hours) institution of EN after major surgery minimizes the risk of undernutrition and can abate the hypermetabolic response seen after surgery. In a critically ill patient, EN should be initiated within 48 hours of injury or admission; average daily intake delivered within the first week should be at least 60% to 70% of the total estimated energy requirements, as determined by the assessment. Provision of EN in this time frame and at this level may be associated with decreased length of hospital stay, days on mechanical ventilation, and infectious complications.

Ileus associated with severe injury is not as common as previously thought. Ileus derived from mesenteric hypoperfusion

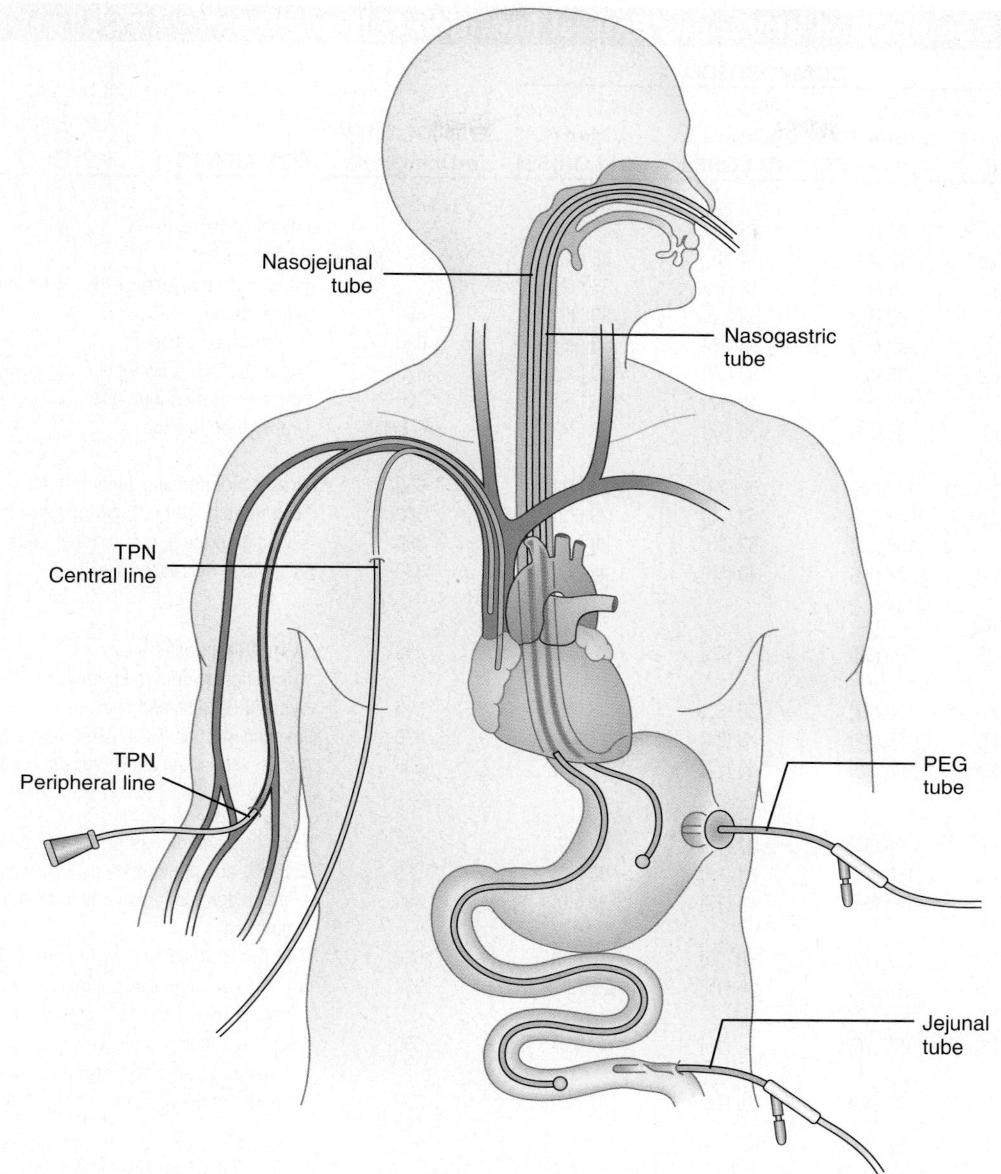

FIGURE 5-9 Nasogastric and nasojejunal tube positions. *PEG,* percutaneous endoscopic gastrostomy. (From Norbury WB, Herndon DN: Modulation of the hypermetabolic response after burn injury. In Herndon DN, editor: *Total burn care,* ed 3, Edinburgh, 2007, Saunders, p 423.)

before adequate resuscitation is reversed once the patient has been resuscitated. Conversely, over-resuscitation leads to GI edema and should be avoided. The initiation of immediate enteral feeding allows the delivery of full calculated caloric requirements by the third day after injury. Reduction of hypermetabolism by initiating enteral feeding soon after injury is possible, with this reduction in metabolic rate being associated with less intense elevations in glucagon, cortisol, and catecholamine levels.

Formulations

Numerous enteral formulations are available and can be classified according to their composition. Standard formulas are sterile, nutritionally complete, and intended for patients with a normal GI tract who cannot ingest adequate nutrients and calories by regular oral diets. Specialty formulations may be more efficiently absorbed in patients with short gut syndrome, severe trauma, burn injury, and chronic malabsorptive diarrhea. Whole-protein formulations are appropriate for most patients. Peptide-based or free amino acid formulations may be considered for patients with a severely compromised GI tract or severe protein-fat malabsorption. Modular formulas consist of a singular macronutrient as a source of calories (e.g., fiber, protein) and are generally used by mixing with standard or specialty formulas. Immune-enhancing formulas consist of nutritional components enriched with arginine, glutamine, nucleotides, and omega-3 fatty acids. Although most formulations are hyperosmolar at full strength, dilution by 25% to 50% to make isotonic and hypotonic formulas is initially preferred to minimize the possibility of diarrhea from excess osmotic load and to facilitate absorption (Table 5-5).

Continuous enteral feeding with milk or a soy-based milk substitute can maintain total body weight throughout the hospital course but may be unable to maintain lean body mass. In patients

TABLE 5-5 Composition of Various Enteral Nutrition Formulations*

FORMULA	COMPOSITION kcal/mL	CHO, g/liter (% CALORIES)	PRO, g/liter (% CALORIES)	FAT, g/liter (% CALORIES)	OSMOLALITY (mOsm/liter)	COMMENTS
Standard						
Similac	0.67	72 (43)	15 (8)	36 (49)		Infant nutrition
Enfamil	0.67	73 (44)	14 (8)	35 (48)		Infant nutrition
Isomil	0.67	68 (41)	18 (10)	37 (49)		Infant nutrition, lactose-free, used in cow protein allergy
Isosource HN	1.2	160 (53)	53 (18)	39 (29)	490	High nitrogen
Ensure Plus	1.5	208 (57)	54 (15)	46 (28)	680	Concentrated calories
Pediasure Enteral	1.0	133 (53)	30 (12)	40 (35)	335	For ages 1-13 yr, with fiber, not easily digestible
Jevity 1 Cal	1.06	155 (54)	44 (17)	35 (29)	300	Isotonic nutrition with fiber
Boost Kid Essential	1.0	135 (54)	30 (12)	38 (34)	550-600	Oral or tube feeding
Boost HP	1.0	137 (55)	62 (24)	25 (21)	650	Oral or tube feeding, high protein
Promote	1.0	130 (52)	62 (25)	26 (23)	340	High protein, oral or tube feeding
Promote w/Fiber	1.0	138 (50)	62 (25)	28 (25)	380	Very high protein, oral or tube feeding
Nutren 1.0	1.0	127 (51)	40 (16)	38 (33)	370	With fiber, decreases diarrhea
Immune-Enhancing						
Crucial	1.5	89 (36)	63 (25)	45 (39)	490	With ARG, critical illness, major surgery, transitional feedings, hydrolyzed protein
Impact	1.0	130 (53)	56 (22)	28 (25)	375	With ARG, GLN, and fiber
Impact GLN	1.3	150 (46)	78 (24)	43 (30)	630	Immunonutrition, GLN, ARG, omega-3 PUFA, nucleic acids
Oxepa	1.5	105 (28)	63 (17)	94 (55)	535	ARDS, acute lung injury, sepsis; concentrated
Specialty						
Glucerna	1.0	96 (34)	42 (17)	54 (49)	355	For glucose-intolerant or diabetic patients, low CHO
Nepro	1.8	167 (34)	81 (18)	96 (48)	585	For CKD and patients on dialysis; concentrated
Osmolite 1 Cal	1.06	144 (54)	44 (17)	35 (29)	300	Isotonic, for use in patients intolerant to hyperosmolar nutrition
Vivonex RTF	1.0	175 (70)	50 (20)	12 (10)	630	Transitional feeding, low fat, easily digestible
Vivonex TEN	1.0	210 (82)	38 (15)	2.8 (3)	630	100% free amino acids, very low fat, used for severe trauma (e.g., burns) or surgery, transitional feeding
Vivonex Plus	1.0	190 (76)	45 (18)	6.7 (6)	650	100% free amino acids, very low fat, used for severe trauma (e.g., burns) or surgery, transitional feeding
Elecare	0.67	72 (43)	20 (15)	32 (42)	350	Prepared at 9.4 g/60 mL; amino acid–based nutrition
Modular						
Resource Benefiber	0.27	66 (100)	0	0	—	Prepared at 4 g/60 mL; tasteless, odorless, soluble fiber, used for constipation
Resource Beneprotein	0.83	0	200 (100)	0	—	Prepared at 7 g/30 mL; whey protein, mixed in foods, protein-calorie malnutrition

Adapted from Al-Mousawi A, Branski LK, Andel HL, et al: Ernährungstherapie bei Brandverletzten. In Kamolz LP, Herndon DN, Jeschke MG, editors: *Verbrennungen: Diagnose, Therapie und Rehabilitation des thermischen Traumas*, German edition, New York, 2009, Springer-Verlag, pp 183–194.

ARDS, acute respiratory distress syndrome; *ARG,* arginine; *CHO,* carbohydrate; *CKD,* chronic kidney disease; *GLN,* glutamine; *PRO,* protein; *PUFA,* polyunsaturated fatty acid.

*Data extrapolated from Nestle Clinical Nutrition: Enteral product reference guide, Nestle, 2010, Minneapolis; and Abbott Laboratories: Abbott nutrition pocket guide, Abbott Park, Ill, 2009, Abbott Laboratories.

with a severe hypermetabolic response, peripheral breakdown of fat is increased. Fatty acids are delivered to the liver and undergo re-esterification; their accumulation leads to fatty liver changes. The use of high-fat diets such as milk, which consists of 44% fat, 42% carbohydrate, and 14% protein, needs to be carefully considered because additional fat may lead to increased fat in the liver. In a subset of distinctly hypermetabolic patients, the use of high-sugar, high-protein diets consisting of 3% fat, 82% carbohydrate, and 15% protein stimulates protein synthesis, increases endogenous insulin production, and improves lean body mass accretion.[37]

Muscle protein degradation is markedly decreased with the administration of a high-carbohydrate diet compared with fat-containing diets. Endogenous insulin concentration is increased, improving the net balance of skeletal muscle protein by decreasing protein breakdown.

Immunonutrition

Major injury, whether traumatic or induced by surgery, results in significant suppression of immune function, which may influence a patient's recovery. Specific nutrients, including arginine, omega-3 polyunsaturated fatty acids, glutamine, and nucleotides, have been shown to modulate the host response in animal and clinical experiments, with potential improvements in immune function. Clinically, arginine supplementation is intended to support T lymphocytes and provides a substrate for the generation of nitric oxide. The administration of omega-3 fatty acids promotes the synthesis of more favorable prostaglandins, and inclusion of nucleotides nonspecifically enhances immune competence. Long-chain omega-3 fatty acids decrease the production of inflammatory eicosanoids, cytokines, and adhesion molecules; this occurs directly by replacing arachidonic acid as an eicosanoid substrate, inhibiting arachidonic acid metabolism, and giving rise to anti-inflammatory resolvins. The indirect effect occurs through the modulation of transcription factors that regulate the expression of inflammatory genes. Omega-3 polyunsaturated fatty acids are potentially useful anti-inflammatory agents and may be beneficial for patients at risk of acute and chronic inflammatory conditions (Table 5-6).

Numerous clinical trials have evaluated the efficacy of immune-enhancing enteral formulas and have shown superior outcomes compared with standard formulations in certain patient populations. Their use has been recommended from 7 days before to 7 days after surgery in the following patients:

- Patients undergoing major neck surgery for cancer (e.g., laryngectomy, pharyngectomy)
- Severely malnourished patients (serum albumin level <2.8 g/dL) or patients undergoing major oncologic GI surgery (e.g., esophagus, stomach, pancreas, duodenum, hepatobiliary tree)
- Patients with severe trauma to two or more body systems (e.g., abdomen, chest, head, spinal cord, extremities) and an injury severity score of 18 or greater or an abdominal trauma index of 20 or greater, which generally includes grade 3 pancreatoduodenal, grade 4 colonic, and grade 4 hepatic or gastric injuries
- Patients with mild sepsis (Acute Physiology and Chronic Health Evaluation II score <15; possibly harmful and not recommended for patients with severe sepsis)
- Patients with acute respiratory distress syndrome

Potential benefits of nutritional supplementation with fish oil–derived omega-3 fatty acids compared with the more common omega-6 fatty acids from plant sources include improved immune responses and outcomes. These benefits may derive from a reduced incidence of hyperglycemia and decreased production of proinflammatory cytokines such as prostaglandin E_2 and leukotrienes. These are derived from metabolism of arachidonic acid, which is metabolized via the same pathways as omega-6 fatty acids.[38]

TABLE 5-6 Effect of Omega-3 Polyunsaturated Fatty Acids on Eicosanoid Synthesis*

METABOLITE	PHYSIOLOGIC ACTION	OMEGA-3 EFFECT
AA Eicosanoid		
PGE_2	Proinflammatory, vasodilator†	↓
TXA_2	Potent platelet aggregation and vasoconstrictor	↓
LTB_4	Proinflammatory, neutrophil chemotaxis	↓
EPA Eicosanoid		
TXA_3	Mild platelet aggregation	↑
PGI_3	Mild platelet disaggregation	↑
RvE1	Potent anti-inflammatory	↑
DHA Docosanoid		
RvD1	Potent anti-inflammatory	↑
NPD1	Potent anti-inflammatory, neuroprotective bioactivity	↑

AA, arachidonic acid; *DHA,* docosahexaenoic acid; *EPA,* eicosapentaenoic acid; *LT,* leukotriene; *NP,* neuroprotectin; *PG,* prostaglandin; *PGI,* prostacyclin; *Rv,* resolvin; *TX,* thromboxane.
*Biochemical basis of a less inflammatory phenotype.
†Prostaglandin E_2 has been reported to have dual proinflammatory and anti-inflammatory activity. The latter, although weak, has been reported to be the effect of the induced production of lipoxins.

Complications

Complications of nasogastric and enteric feeding include nausea and vomiting, epistaxis, sinusitis, nasal necrosis, aspiration leading to pneumonia, tube malpositioning, dislodgment, and feeding-associated diarrhea (Table 5-7). Fine-bore tubes are more comfortable but can become blocked easily. Auscultation examination of gastric fluid aspirate and pH testing can be used to confirm tube position, particularly for large-bore nasal tubes, although many units prefer radiologic confirmation. Tubes also can be inserted under endoscopic or fluoroscopic guidance. Monitoring guidelines for EN are given in Table 5-8.

Refeeding syndrome can be precipitated by prolonged fasting and IV fluid administration in chronically malnourished patients. Clinically, refeeding syndrome is heralded by the development of refractory hypokalemia, hypomagnesemia, and hypophosphatemia. The transition from metabolizing body fat to carbohydrate in the feed can cause an abrupt increase in insulin and disturbances of intracellular electrolytes. Electrolyte abnormalities can result in cardiac failure and dysrhythmias, respiratory failure, neurologic disturbances, and renal and hepatic dysfunction. With all nutritional support, the rate of feeding should begin slowly to prevent abrupt metabolic changes.

Aside from mechanical issues related to the feeding tube, the most common complications of enteral feedings result from solute overload. Inappropriately rapid administration of hyperosmolar solutions may result in diarrhea; dehydration; electrolyte imbalance; hyperglycemia; and loss of potassium, magnesium, and other ions through diarrhea. If aggressive administration of hyperosmolar solute continues, pneumatosis intestinalis with bowel necrosis and perforation can result. Hyperosmolar nonketotic coma also can occur with enteral feedings, as with PN.

Parenteral Nutrition

The development of PN in the 1960s represented a major advance in surgical care, allowing for nutrition in and survival of patients with a nonfunctioning GI tract. PN involves IV infusion of nutrients in an elemental form, bypassing the usual processes of digestion. When long-term delivery of hyperosmolar regimens is required, TPN is facilitated through a dedicated central line (see Fig. 5-9). A peripheral line can be used to provide lower osmolar solutions during shorter periods of time. To promote gut integrity

TABLE 5-7 Complications of Enteral Feeding

PROBLEM	COMMON CAUSES	MANAGEMENT
Diarrhea	Medications (e.g., antibiotics, H_2 blockers, laxatives, hyperosmotic, hypertonic solutions), feeding intolerance (osmolarity, fat), acquired lactase deficiency	Measure stool output. Rule out infection (bacterial, viral, parasitic). Supply fiber. Change medication or formula. Check osmolarity and infusion rate. Replace lost fluids as needed. Administer antimotility medications (e.g., loperamide, codeine). Note: Do not administer antimotility medications until *Clostridium difficile* colitis has been ruled out.
Nausea and vomiting	Delayed stomach emptying, constipation, medications, odor and appearance of formulations	Administer feedings at room temperature. Use isotonic formulations. Use closed system when possible. Reduce doses of narcotics. Use gastroprokinetic agents (metoclopramide, erythromycin). Monitor gastric residuals and stool output.
Constipation, fecal impaction	Dehydration, lack or excess of fiber	Monitor fluid balance daily. Rectal disimpaction. Consider use of cathartics, stool softeners, laxatives, or enemas.
Aspiration pneumonitis	Long-term supine position, delayed stomach emptying, altered mental status, malpositioned feeding tube, vomiting, nonfunctional nasogastric drainage tube	Place head of bed at 45 degrees during feedings. Stop EN if gastric residual volume is >200 mL. Use of nasoduodenal or nasojejunal tubes has not been shown to decrease aspiration risk (compared with gastric feeding).
Hypervolemic hyponatremia (overhydration)	Excess fluid intake, refeeding syndrome, organ failure (e.g., liver, heart, kidney)	Monitor fluid balance and body weight daily. Consider fluid restriction. Change formula (avoid low-sodium intake). Initiate diuretic therapy.
Hypernatremia	Dehydration, inadequate fluid intake	Increase free water.
Dehydration	Diarrhea, inadequate fluid intake	Determine cause. Increase fluid intake.
Hyperglycemia	High content of carbohydrate in feedings, insulin resistance	Evaluate and adjust feeding formula. Consider insulin regimen. Check for dextrose-based carriers in IV medications.
Hypokalemia, hypomagnesemia, hypophosphatemia	Diarrhea, refeeding syndrome	Correct electrolyte abnormalities. Determine cause. Reduce rate if refeeding syndrome is present and monitor patient.
Hyperkalemia	Excess potassium intake, renal impairment	Change feeding formula. Reduce potassium intake. Consider insulin regimen.

and motility in patients receiving PN alone, one should use small volumes of EN, when possible.

The use of PN is vital for patients with partial or complete GI dysfunction and who are unable to digest and absorb sufficient nutrients, including patients with bowel obstruction, enteritis, fistulas, or short bowel syndrome and patients with chemotherapy toxicity. Based on extensive literature documenting negligible or negative impact on outcomes, the use of PN has been contraindicated in any patient able to tolerate significant amounts of EN. However, in the time leading up to the publication of this chapter, several large multi-institutional clinical trials have suggested that more recent advances in critical care have significantly increased the safety of PN, forcing a reconsideration of indications (see "Principles Guiding Routes of Nutrition: Enteral, Parenteral, or Both").

Before receiving PN, patients should be hemodynamically stable and able to tolerate the fluid volume and nutrient content of parenteral formulations; PN should be used with caution in patients with congestive heart failure, pulmonary disease, diabetes mellitus, and other metabolic disorders because the significant amounts of fluid and sugar may be difficult for patients to tolerate (Table 5-9). Although there has been some debate regarding the optimal timing for initiating TPN in patients unable to tolerate adequate EN, results of more recent large randomized controlled trials suggest that early initiation of TPN is an appropriate general strategy in such patients.[6,39,40]

Formulations

PN includes all IV formulations, emulsions, or admixtures of nutrients that are administered in an elemental form. In the United States, PN formulations are traditionally composed of 60% to 70% dextrose and 10% to 20% amino acids, administered daily, and combined as two-in-one solutions. Formulations also may include 10% to 30% lipid emulsion, which may be combined into a single

TABLE 5-8 Suggested Monitoring Schedule for Enteral Feeding

PARAMETER	ACUTE PATIENT	STABLE PATIENT
Electrolytes	Daily	1-2×/wk
Complete blood count	Daily	1-2×/wk
Glucose level	3×/day; more often if poor control	3×/day; less often if good control
Creatinine and urea levels	Daily	Weekly or twice weekly
Nitrogen balance	As needed for concern of underfeeding or protein malnutrition	As needed for concern of underfeeding or protein malnutrition
Input and output	Daily	Daily
Body weight	Daily	2-3×/wk
Urine output	Hourly	Every 4 hr

TABLE 5-9 Clinical Conditions Requiring Cautious Use of Parenteral Nutrition

CONDITION	SUGGESTED CRITERIA
Hyperglycemia	Glucose >300 mg/dL
Azotemia	BUN >100 mg/dL
Hyperosmolality	Serum osmolality >350 mOsm/kg
Hypernatremia	Sodium >150 mEq/L
Hypokalemia	Potassium <3 mEq/L
Hyperchloremic metabolic acidosis	Chloride >115 mEq/L
Hypophosphatemia	Phosphorus <2 mg/dL
Hypochloremic metabolic alkalosis	Chloride <85 mEq/L

From Mirtallo JM, In Gottschlich MM, DeLegge MH, Guenter P, editors: *The A.S.P.E.N. nutrition support core curriculum*, Silver Spring, Md, 2012, American Society for Parenteral and Enteral Nutrition, p 268.
BUN, Blood urea nitrogen.

TABLE 5-10 Composition of Parenteral Nutrition Formulations

SAMPLE NUTRITION*	CALORIC CONTENT g/dL	kcal/g	kcal/mL	mOsm/liter
2-in-1 Solutions				
Dextrose				
DW 10%	10	3.4 (CHO)	0.34	505
DW 30%	30	3.4 (CHO)	1.02	1510
DW 70%	70	3.4 (CHO)	2.38	3530
Amino acids				
Aminosyn RF 5.2%	5.2	4 (PRO)	0.2	427
Travasol 10%	10	4 (PRO)	0.4	998
Prosol 20%	20	4 (PRO)	0.8	1835
Lipid emulsion				
Intralipid 10%	10	11 (fat)†	1.1	300
Intralipid 20%	20	10 (fat)†	2	350
Intralipid 30%	30	10 (fat)†	3	310

CHO, carbohydrate; *PRO*, protein.
*3-in-1 solutions: Total nutrient admixture.
†Estimated at 9 kcal/g for fat plus additional calories from glycerol.

formulation (three-in-one solution) or supplemented separately, usually less often (once or twice weekly). Parenteral formulations can be ordered in solutions in a wide range of concentrations, including 10% to 70% dextrose, 5.2% to 20% amino acids, and 10% to 30% lipid emulsions (Table 5-10).

In addition to sterile water, electrolytes, vitamins, and minerals, PN formulations can include medications such as insulin and histamine$_2$ (H_2) blockers. Various combinations of these components are incorporated into the regimen for IV administration based on the patient's individual requirements.

Ordering Parenteral Nutrition

In general, minimal fluid requirements in the absence of GI or other losses are 25 to 35 mL/kg/day. Feeding volume is built up slowly over a few days. Using the example of a 70-kg person, one first calculates the overall caloric goal and the proportion contributed by protein, usually as follows:

$$\text{Total kilocalories (25 to 35 kcal/kg/day)} = 30\ \text{kcal/kg/day} \times 70\ \text{kg} = 2100\ \text{kcal}$$

$$\text{Protein (1.5 g/kg/day)} = 1.5\ \text{kcal/kg/day} \times 70\ \text{kg} = 105\ \text{g protein}$$

1. For TPN formulated without lipid (two-in-one solution; in our practice, we recommend lipid infusion at least every 1 to 2 weeks for most patients to prevent essential fatty acid deficiency):

$$\text{Total kilocalories} = 2100\ \text{kcal}$$

$$\text{Calories from amino acids} = 105\ \text{g} \times 4\ \text{kcal/g} = 420\ \text{kcal}$$

$$\text{Remaining calories} = 2100 - 420 = 1680\ \text{kcal}$$

Then make up the difference with dextrose:

$$1680\ \text{kcal}/(3.4\ \text{kcal/g}) = 494\ \text{g dextrose}$$

2. For TPN formulated with lipid (three-in-one solution):

$$\text{Total kilocalories} = 2100\ \text{kcal}$$

Provide 20% of the total calories as lipid:

$$\text{Lipid} = 2100\ \text{kcal} \times 0.2 = 420\ \text{kcal}$$

$$420\ \text{kcal}/(9\ \text{kcal/g}) = 47\ \text{g lipid}$$

Calories from amino acids:

$$105\ \text{g} \times 4\ \text{kcal/g} = 420\ \text{kcal}$$

Remaining calories:

$$2100 - 420 - 420 = 1260\ \text{kcal}$$

Then make up the difference with dextrose:

$$1260\ \text{kcal}/(3.4\ \text{kcal/g}) = 370\ \text{g dextrose}$$

Final volume (for three-in-one, maximally concentrated):

$$\text{Amino acids (10\% stock solution)} = 105\ \text{g} = 1050\ \text{mL}$$

$$\text{Dextrose (70\% stock solution)} = 370\ \text{g} = 528\ \text{mL}$$

$$\text{Lipids (20\% stock solution)} = 47\ \text{g} = 235\ \text{mL}$$

$$\text{Total volume} = 1813\ \text{mL/day}$$

The final concentrations (wt/vol) are 5.8% amino acids, 20.4% dextrose, and 2.6% lipid.

An example of an adult PN order form is provided in Figure 5-10.

Physician Orders
PARENTERAL NUTRITION (PN) - ADULT

Primary Diagnosis: ______________________ **Ht:** ________ cm **Dosing Wt:** ________ kg

PN Indication: ______________________ **Allergies:** ______________________

Instructions: This form must be completed for a new order or continuation of PN and faxed to the Pharmacy by **[Insert Time]** to receive same day preparation. PN administration begins at **[Insert Time]**. Contact the Nutrition Support Service at: (XXX)-XXX-XXXX for additional information.

Administration Route: ☐ CVC or PICC *Note: Proper tip placement of the CVC or PICC must be confirmed prior to PN infusion*

☐ Peripheral IV (PIV) *(Final PN Osmolarity ≤________ mOsm/L)*

Monitoring: Daily weights, strict input & output, bedside glucose monitoring every ______ hours

☐ Na, K, Cl, CO_2, glucose, BUN, Scr, Mg, PO_4, every ________________

☐ T. Bili, Alk Phos, AST, ALT, Albumin, Triglycerides, Calcium every ________________

Base Solution: *Select one* — *Parenteral nutrition **MUST** be administered through a dedicated infusion port and filtered with a 1.2-micron in-line filter at all times. Discard any unused volume after 24 hours.*

☐ **PERIPHERAL 2-in-1**	☐ **CENTRAL 2-in-1**	☐ **CENTRAL 3-in-1**
Dextrose ______ g	Dextrose ______ g	Dextrose ______ g
Amino Acids (*Brand* __________) ______ g	Amino Acids (*Brand* __________) ______ g	Amino Acids (*Brand* __________) ______ g
For patients with PIV and established glucose tolerance: Provides _____ *kcal; Maximum Rate not to exceed* ______ *mL/hour*	*For patients with CVC or PICC and established glucose tolerance: Provides* _____ *kcal; Maximum Rate not to exceed* ______ *mL/hour*	Fat Emulsion (*Brand* __________) ______ g
		For patients with CVC or PICC and established glucose/fat emulsion tolerance: Provides _____ *kcal; Maximum Rate not to exceed* ______ *mL/hour*
		Use of additional fat emulsion not required with 3-in-1 base solution

RATE & VOLUME: ______ mL/hour for ______ hours = ______ mL/day
Must specify

or **CYCLIC INFUSION:** ______ mL/hour for ______ hours, then ______ mL/hour for ______ hours = ______ mL/day

Fat Emulsion (*Brand* __________) ***- via PIV or CVC with 2-in-1 base solutions*** *(Select caloric density & volume)*

☐ 10% ☐ 250 mL Infuse at ______ mL/hour over ______ hours Frequency __________

☐ 20% ☐ 500 mL *(Note: Infusions <4 or >12 hours not recommended)* *Discard any unused volume after 12 hours.*

Additives: (per day)			***Normal Dosages***
Sodium Chloride	______	mEq	*1–2 mEq Sodium/kg/day*
as Acetate	______	mEq	*pH or CO_2 dependent*
as Phosphate	______	mmol of PO_4	*Consider if hyperkalemic*
Potassium Chloride	______	mEq	*1–2 mEq Potassium/kg/day*
as Acetate	______	mEq	*pH or CO_2 dependent*
as Phosphate	______	mmol of PO_4	*20–40 mmol/day (1 mmol Phos = 1.5 mEq K)*
Calcium **Gluconate**	______	mEq	*5–15 mEq/day*
Magnesium **Sulfate**	______	mEq	*8–24 mEq/day*
Adult **Multivitamins**	______	mL/day	*Contains Vitamin K 150 mcg*
Adult **Trace Elements**	______	mL/day	*Zn ___ mg, Cu ___ mg, Mn ___ mg, Cr ___ mcg, Se ___ mcg (with normal hepatic function)*
H_2 **Antagonist** ______	______	mg	*___ mg/day with normal renal function*
Other:			

Additives: (per day)
Regular Insulin ______ units
Recommend if hyperglycemic, start with 1 unit for every 10 g of dextrose

***Pharmacy Use Only:* Ca/PO_4 Limit checked** ___
(Note: Some brands of amino acids contain phosphate)

Physician's Signature: ______________________ **PagerNumber:** ______________ **Date/time:** __________

Orders transcribed by: ______________ **Date/time:** __________ **Orders verified by:** ______________ **Date/time:** __________

SEND COMPLETED ORDERS TO PHARMACY

FIGURE 5-10 Adult PN order form. This template can serve as a guide to meet the criteria for mandatory and strongly recommended components of a PN order form. These components are not intended to be guidelines for formulas or monitoring. The PN order form content should be adapted to meet the needs of the individual institution based on patient population, prescribing patterns, and judgment by health care professionals. See text. (Adapted from Mirtallo J, Canada T, Johnson D, et al: Safe practices for parenteral nutrition. *JPEN J Parenter Enteral Nutr* 28(Suppl):S39–S70, 2004.)

Complications

Parenteral feeding is associated with complications arising from line insertion and infection, including pneumothorax, hematoma, bacteremia, endocarditis, damage to vessels and other structures, air embolism, and thrombosis. In contrast to EN, TPN has been associated with increased rates of bacterial translocation. TPN also has been associated with increased proinflammatory cytokine levels and increased pulmonary dysfunction. The use of TPN, even as a simple supplement of maximally tolerated enteral feeding to reach nutritional requirements, has been associated with impairment of hepatic function and immune response.[41] However, much of the literature documenting this often-cited association predates the era of tight glycemic control. It remains unclear how much of the morbidity associated with TPN can be attributed to secondary hyperglycemia.

Overfeeding patients can lead to major complications. The overfeeding of carbohydrates results in elevated respiratory quotients, increased fat synthesis, and increased carbon dioxide elimination, leading to difficulty in weaning from ventilator support. Excess carbohydrate or fat also can lead to fat deposition in the liver. Excess protein replacement leads to elevations in blood urea nitrogen levels (Table 5-11).

Carbohydrate Content

Designated chemically as D-glucose, dextrose is the most commonly used carbohydrate substrate and provides 3.4 kcal/g (16 kJ). Dextrose solutions come in a wide range of concentrations and can be diluted as required to provide calories and adjust blood glucose levels. PN may contain dextrose or other carbohydrates as part of the formulation, or these may be administered separately. Concentrated hypertonic dextrose solutions of 20% to 70% are usually administered via central lines because these solutions cause irritation if administered into peripheral veins and can lead to thrombophlebitis. Contraindications to the use of concentrated dextrose solutions include alcohol withdrawal and delirium tremens in a dehydrated patient and suspected intracranial or intraspinal hemorrhage. Once metabolized, carbohydrates are ultimately oxidized to carbon dioxide and water, so caution should be used to control infusion rates to avoid hyperglycemia and hypercapnia when weaning patients from ventilator support.

In the acute setting, supplying sufficient carbohydrate reduces liver glycogen breakdown; it also may exert a protein-sparing effect by supplying an alternative fuel to amino acids. Endogenous glucose production has been shown to be significantly suppressed when glucose is infused at a rate of 1 mg/kg/min and maximally suppressed at 4 mg/kg/min, with or without exogenous insulin infusion—infusion at a faster rate does not suppress gluconeogenesis further.

Glucose infusion rates require greater monitoring and caution in pediatric patients because of the increased risk of hyperglycemia and hypoglycemia. A suggested guideline maximum concentration is 25% dextrose at an infusion rate of up to 7 mg/kg/min.

When calculating TPN requirements, one usually calculates protein requirements first and subtracts these from total calories, with remaining calorie requirements being met with carbohydrate, with or without lipids. Formulations are often concentrated because patients in a critical care setting often may be at risk of volume overload.

TABLE 5-11 Complications of Parenteral Nutrition

PROBLEM	COMMON CAUSES	MANAGEMENT
Hypoglycemia	Excess insulin administration, sudden cessation of PN infusion	Stop insulin. Start IV 10% dextrose. Give 50% dextrose ampule before resuming central line feeding.
Hyperglycemia	Excess dextrose concentration, stress-associated (e.g., sepsis), chromium deficiency	0.1-0.2 U insulin/g dextrose therapy, SQ or IV insulin sliding scale, limit dextrose content, consider discontinuing PN until improved blood glucose control.
Hypertriglyceridemia (acceptable concentrations <400 mg/dL)	Dextrose overfeeding, rapid administration of IV fat emulsion (>110 mg/kg/hr)	Infusion of IV fat emulsion should be restricted to <30% of total calories or 1 g/kg/day, given slowly over no less than 8-10 hr, if administered separately.
Essential fatty acid deficiency (e.g., dermatitis, alopecia, hepatomegaly, thrombocytopenia, anemia)	1- to 3-wk administration of PN lacking linoleic and alpha-linolenic fatty acid emulsions	2%-4% daily energy requirements should be derived from linoleic acid, 0.5% from alpha-linolenic acid[52] (500 mL of 10% IV fat emulsion over 8-10 hr, twice weekly).
Electrolyte and mineral abnormalities	Inadequate monitoring	Electrolytes should be checked daily, and PN formulas should be adjusted daily until electrolytes are stabilized.
	Inadequate supplementation in TPN formula	Parenteral iron uncommonly increases risk of anaphylactic reactions.
Azotemia	Dehydration, excess protein, inadequate carbohydrate calories	Free water, 5% dextrose via a peripheral vein.
Metabolic bone disease (osteoporosis in 41% of patients on long-term home PN)	Unclear, multifactorial (e.g., postmenopausal, long-term PN, Cushing syndrome, Crohn's disease, malabsorption, multiple myeloma, osteogenesis imperfecta, corticosteroids, heparin, immobilization)	Early screening of risk factors, DEXA, management of premorbid conditions. Special PN considerations: Supplement calcium, phosphorus, magnesium, copper. Minimize aluminum contamination, treat metabolic acidosis, avoid heparin.
Elevated liver function parameters (increased transaminase, bilirubin, alkaline phosphatase levels)	Common after initiation; usually temporary	If persistent, usually caused by amino acid load; reduce protein delivery.

DEXA, Dual-energy x-ray absorptiometry.

Lipid Content

IV fat emulsions provide a dense source of calories and are particularly useful when carbohydrate administration approaches maximal limits or blood glucose control is an issue. They are also useful in preventing essential fatty acid deficiency. However, the optimal use of lipid emulsions during parenteral feeding is controversial, especially with regard to critically ill surgical patients and patients under metabolic stress because changes in fatty acid metabolism after severe injuries may predispose these particular patients to the adverse effects of lipid infusions. Delivery of lipid emulsion has been associated with immunosuppression, modulation of the inflammatory response, and adverse clinical outcomes. In polytrauma patients, infusion of IV fat emulsion in the early postinjury period has been associated with increased length of ICU and hospital stays, prolonged mechanical ventilation, and increased susceptibility to infection compared with patients not given IV fat emulsion until after 10 days. However, it is uncertain whether these differences are attributable to withholding lipid or provision of fewer total calories.

Commercially available parenteral regimens in the United States are composed of soybean oil rich in the omega-6 fatty acid linoleic acid, a precursor of arachidonic acid used in the synthesis pathway of prostaglandins, thromboxanes, and leukotrienes. Because of this proinflammatory potential, there is a trend toward limiting omega-6 content and switching to lipids such as fish oil or to lipids rich in omega-3 fatty acids such as eicosapentaenoic acid, which competes to reduce cell membrane availability of arachidonic acid and its products. Reduced prostaglandin and leukotriene levels lead to decreased chemotaxis, cytokine production, platelet aggregation, coagulation, and smooth muscle contraction. Another potential effect of excessive long-chain omega-6 fatty acids is depletion of available antioxidants in plasma lipoproteins.

Polyunsaturated omega-3 fatty acids found in fish oil have been shown to prevent the development of inflammatory conditions by modulating the synthesis of eicosanoids and other inflammatory mechanisms. A meta-analysis examining the use of fish oil emulsions in randomized controlled trials in patients undergoing elective surgery showed a significant reduction in infectious complications and shortened hospital stay, although no mortality benefit overall was demonstrated. However, an earlier meta-analysis of the immunologic effects of lipid emulsions found no clear evidence that long-chain triglycerides detrimentally affect immune function.

Potential deficiency of essential fatty acids may occur after the first week of parenteral feeding, although patients with large adipose stores can go for much longer periods without supplementation. In our practice, we do not begin administering parenteral lipids within the first week of PN. Patients receiving prolonged PN are administered a minimum of 500 mL of lipid emulsion every 2 weeks to avoid essential fatty acid deficiency during parenteral feeding.

Protein Content

The recommended daily amount of protein intake for most healthy adults is 0.8 g/kg body weight/day (46 to 56 g/day). Muscle protein degradation following severe injury leads to loss of lean mass, which persists for months after visible wound healing, and at least approximately 20% of total energy requirements need to be in the form of protein intake to limit this loss. This is equivalent to 1.5 to 2.0 g protein/kg IBW/day in fasted surgical patients and up to 3.0 g/kg/day in severely injured patients. Most standard enteral and parenteral feeding mixtures provide this increased quantity of protein if sufficient volume of formula is delivered to meet the patient's increased caloric requirements. Traditionally, the nitrogen-to-calorie ratio for most feeding formulas prepared for surgical patients has been 1 : 150 (i.e., 1 g of nitrogen for every 150 kcal). For PN, a protein-fat-glucose caloric ratio has generally approximated 20 : 30 : 50. Patients with chronic renal failure and hepatic failure have conventionally been treated with low-protein diets.

Fluid and Electrolytes

Patients with GI disorders, particularly disorders leading to extensive bowel resection, may experience demanding water and electrolyte imbalances. These patients require extra vigilance; monitoring is critical for the prevention, early diagnosis, and treatment of these imbalances. In adult patients with PN, at least 30 to 40 mL/kg of fluid, 1 to 2 mEq/kg of sodium and potassium, 10 to 15 mEq of calcium, 8 to 20 mEq of magnesium, and 20 to 40 mmol of phosphate should be administered daily. Patients who are rapidly anabolic, including patients who were previously malnourished, may require additional potassium, magnesium, and phosphorus, whereas patients with renal impairment may require restriction.

DISEASE-SPECIFIC CONCERNS

This section considers nutritional support in relation to numerous surgical conditions and describes current metabolic and nutritional strategies.

Antioxidant Therapy

Acute injury and critical illness are often associated with depletion of endogenous antioxidants, which has been associated with worsening of clinical outcomes. Critical antioxidants shown to be situationally deficient in clinical illness include glutamine, selenium, zinc, copper, and manganese. Myriad clinical trials have assessed the effect of antioxidant micronutrient supplementation in critically ill patients, with a range of results. Antioxidant supplements have been found to mitigate systemic inflammatory responses, prevent nosocomial pneumonia, and decrease mortality in various critical care settings.[42-44] However, a large multicenter randomized controlled trial with more than 1000 patients found no effect on outcomes associated with antioxidant vitamin supplementation and (surprisingly) that increased mortality was associated with glutamine supplementation.[3] Subsequent post-hoc subgroup analysis suggested that the negative effect of glutamine supplementation is more pronounced in patients with multiorgan dysfunction syndrome, particularly patients with renal failure.[3] Considering the literature in aggregate, identifying exactly which combination of antioxidants is likely to be helpful as nutritional supplements is difficult, and it does not appear that any and all can be administered with sanguine effects. However, the benefit of perioperative antioxidant therapy in elective surgery remains well established. We recommend supplementing antioxidant trace elements in the setting of acute injury and critical illness but only in patients with identified deficiencies on screening.

Burn Injury and the Metabolic Stress Response

Following all forms of major trauma, inflammatory and hormonal responses are activated and greatly influence metabolic pathways and mechanisms. Nutrient intake, absorption, and substrate uptake are affected during the different stages of the stress response.

Elevated metabolic rate is a common feature of critical illness, arising in conditions of trauma, major surgery, severe burns, and sepsis. The stress response leads to activation of an array of physiologic processes that respond to altered metabolic requirements and attempt to restore homeostasis. Although these changes initially may be beneficial, in critical illness and sepsis, inflammation and associated changes are often exaggerated and prolonged, leading to clinical complications, delayed recovery, and increased mortality. Nutrient requirements increase and become more difficult to predict, and enteral or parenteral feeding often is necessary to meet vastly increased nutritional requirements.

Severe burns affecting approximately 30% or more of the total body surface area are associated with a major elevation in metabolic rate. The inflammatory and hormonal mechanisms underlying this response are complex but are known to include a prolonged increase in circulating catecholamine, glucocorticoid, and glucagon levels, leading to elevated rates of gluconeogenesis, glycogenolysis, and protein catabolism. Other features of metabolic dysfunction include insulin resistance and increased peripheral lipolysis.

Burns are classified according to their size, mechanism, and depth of injury. They range from superficial (first-degree) burns affecting only the epidermis to partial-thickness (second-degree) burns that involve the dermis and full-thickness (third-degree) burns extending through all layers of the skin. An estimate of the body surface burned can be obtained using the rule of nines (modified for pediatric use according to age) or a Lund-Browder chart.

Patients with severe burns need fluid resuscitation to prevent hypovolemic shock, with resuscitation being guided by the percentage of body surface area burned and body weight. Several different formulas are used to calculate requirements over the first 24 hours. Urine output remains the best indicator of volume status, with minimum target values of 0.5 mL/kg/hr in adults and 1 mL/kg/hr in children. Over-resuscitation should be avoided to prevent complications of fluid overload, including pulmonary edema and cardiac dysfunction.

Early resuscitation of severely burned patients is crucial. In circumstances in which medical care is not immediately available (e.g., in isolated locations or in mass casualty situations), this may be possible through oral rehydration and basic electrolyte replacement because most patients will initially be able to drink.

Nutritional support should be initiated as early as possible to supply vastly elevated caloric and protein demands. Patients usually have a functioning GI tract but may be incapable of sufficient oral intake to meet requirements, particularly after larger burns, and enteral feeding is the route of choice to supplement or replace oral intake. Although nutritional support aims to offset losses and maintain energy requirements, nutritional supplementation alone has not been found to be completely effective for arresting loss of muscle mass. Strategies to counteract the features of hypermetabolism and catabolism include pharmacologic, surgical, and environmental interventions.

Caloric requirements in patients with severe burns can be difficult to predict accurately because energy expenditure is drastically increased and varies with the condition of the patient, operative interventions, and septic episodes. Various formulas can be used to estimate caloric requirements in burn patients, although indirect calorimetry (if available) provides a superior estimate of energy needs and can be used to determine the respiratory quotient to detect overfeeding (Tables 5-12 and 5-13). Indirect calorimetry provides a value for REE, with this measurement typically being increased by 10% to 20% when used to guide feeding to allow for variability and activity.

TABLE 5-12 Formulas for Estimating Caloric Requirements in Adult Burn Patients

FORMULA	EQUATION	COMMENTS
Harris-Benedict[53]		
Men	BEE (kcal/day) = 66.5 + (13.75 × W) + (5.00 × H) − (6.76 × A)	Multiply BEE by stress factor of 1.2-2.0 (1.2-1.5 sufficient for most burns) to estimate caloric requirement.
Women	BEE (kcal/day) = 655 + (9.56 × W) + (1.85 × H) − (4.68 × A)	
Curreri		
Age, 16-59 yr	Calories (kcal/day) = (25 × W) + (40 × %BSAB)	Specific for burns; may significantly overestimate energy requirements; maximum 50% BSAB.
Age >60 yr	Calories (kcal/day) = (20 × W) + (65 × %BSAB)	

A, Age (yr); *BEE,* basal energy expenditure; *%BSAB,* percentage of total body surface area burned; *H,* height (cm); *W,* weight (kg).

TABLE 5-13 Formulas for Estimating Caloric Requirements in Pediatric Burn Patients

FORMULA	SEX/AGE (yr)	EQUATION (DAILY REQUIREMENT IN kcal)
WHO	Boys 0-3	(60.9 × W) − 54
	3-10	(22.7 × W) + 495
	10-18	(17.5 × W) + 651
	Girls 0-3	(61.0 × W) − 51
	3-10	(22.5 × W) + 499
	10-18	(12.2 × W) + 746
RDA	0-6 mo	108 × W
	6 mo-1 yr	98 × W
	1-3	102 × W
	4-10	90 × W
	11-14	55 × W
Curreri junior	<1	RDA + (15 × %BSAB)
	1-3	RDA + (25 × %BSAB)
	4-15	RDA + (40 × %BSAB)
Galveston infant	0-1	2100 kcal/m^2 BSA + 1000 kcal/m^2 BSAB
Galveston revised	1-11	1800 kcal/m^2 BSA + 1300 kcal/m^2 BSAB
Galveston adolescent	≥12	1500 kcal/m^2 BSA + 1500 kcal/m^2 BSAB

Adapted from Al-Mousawi A, Branski LK, Andel HL, et al: Ernährungstherapie bei Brandverletzten. In Kamolz LP, Herndon DN, Jeschke MG, editors: *Verbrennungen: Diagnose, Therapie und Rehabilitation des thermischen Traumas,* German Edition. New York, 2009, Springer-Verlag/Wien, pp 183–194.
BSA, body surface area; *RDA,* recommended dietary allowance; *W,* weight (kg); *WHO,* World Health Organization.

Severe burn injuries covering 30% or more of the total body surface area represent one of the most severe forms of trauma, and extreme and prolonged muscle wasting is seen in these patients. Negative nitrogen balance, insulin resistance, lipolysis, and protein wasting may persist for 1 year after severe injuries, leading to a significant delay in rehabilitation.

A wide range of treatment modalities can be applied to mitigate the catabolic response to major burn injury. Pharmacologic treatments have been investigated for their potential to counteract catabolic effects and attenuate the metabolic response in the acute and rehabilitation phases. These include anabolic agents such as recombinant human growth hormone (in children), oxandrolone, insulin, IGF-1, and β-AR blockers such as propranolol. Early excision of full-thickness burn wounds and application of skin grafts or substitutes is known to decrease metabolic rates to a much greater degree than delaying surgery to 1 week after injury. Keeping ambient temperatures at 33° C also reduces the metabolic rate in patients with large burns. Providing a structured exercise program in conjunction with occupational and physical therapy during rehabilitation improves passive and active range of motion, muscle strength, and lean body mass.[45] Modulation of the stress response also includes pain and anxiety control through the administration of analgesics and anxiolytics as well as psychological therapy. Surgery, pharmacology, infection control, environmental thermoregulation, nutrition, and rehabilitative physiotherapy all are used to minimize the massive catabolic response to major burn.

Propranolol is a nonselective β-AR antagonist that has been shown to reduce thermogenesis, tachycardia, and REE in burn patients. Catecholamines trigger peripheral lipolysis in injured patients; propranolol may help reduce the pro-lipolytic effect of excessive circulating catecholamines and substantially decrease fatty infiltration of the liver.

In children with severe burns, recombinant human growth hormone and oxandrolone, a synthetic testosterone analogue and anabolic agent, have shown promising results during hypermetabolic states, significantly improving growth and lean body mass. However, a European multicenter trial in adult patients found significantly greater mortality in critical care patients administered growth hormone. For this reason, it is considered for use only in children.

Organ Transplantation

In organ transplantation, consideration must be given to the assessment of the patient's nutritional status and preparation for metabolic disturbances in the postoperative period. Although organ recipients do not have a propensity to develop high metabolic rates unless secondary conditions are present (e.g., sepsis, other surgical complications), elevated REEs have been reported following surgery; REEs up to 42% above predicted values have been reported 10 days after liver transplantation. Also, REE is persistently increased up to 1 year posttransplantation. To prevent loss of weight and lean body mass in these patients, one should provide 1.3 to 1.5 times the calculated basal energy expenditure, or 30 to 35 kcal/kg. Numerous immunosuppressive medications are used to prevent and treat rejection of newly transplanted organs. The side effects of these drugs often affect nutrient intake and digestion, most commonly in the form of GI disorders (e.g., constipation, diarrhea, nausea, vomiting, dyspepsia, pancreatitis). Malnutrition is an important factor influencing outcome after organ transplantation, and optimization of overall nutritional status before and after surgery is critical for the living donor and the recipient.

Inflammatory Bowel Disease

Patients with inflammatory bowel disease often experience a range of complications during the course of their disease that impair their nutritional status, including significant weight loss caused by sitophobia (aversion to food), diarrhea, protein-wasting enteropathy, GI bleeding, development of fistulas, and abdominal pain. Acute exacerbations also may increase energy demands and worsen these complications. In patients with Crohn's disease, criteria to initiate nutritional support are similar to criteria for other patients (see earlier). When EN is indicated, formulas low in fat content have better efficacy than elemental or semielemental formulas. PN usually does not have a primary role unless EN is contraindicated. Additionally, PN may be used temporarily (<2 weeks) in combination with antibiotics with the intention of allowing the GI mucosa to heal to facilitate surgery further. In patients with Crohn's disease and severe short bowel syndrome, home PN is particularly suitable.

Short Bowel Syndrome

Short bowel syndrome results from the resection of functioning gut to a length below that necessary for adequate digestion and absorption of nutrients. In adults, resection is most commonly performed because of Crohn's disease, mesenteric thrombosis, or volvulus; in infants, necrotizing enterocolitis is the most common cause. Within 24 to 48 hours after resection, the intestinal adaptation process begins with epithelial hyperplasia in the intestinal crypts. If a patient is left with 1.5 feet of small bowel anastomosed to the left colon, hypertrophy of the remaining small bowel in most cases enables survival, while reducing the need for daily PN support to twice weekly. The goal of nutritional support in patients with short bowel syndrome is to maximize intestinal adaptation through aggressive EN, while limiting complications. EN has a potent trophic effect on the intestinal mucosa, resulting in lengthening of intestinal villi, increasing absorptive surface area, and improving digestive and absorptive function. Patients receiving home TPN commonly survive for 10 to 20 years or longer, which was impossible before the development of TPN. Some patients undergo sufficient hypertrophy of the remaining small bowel that the need for home TPN is ultimately decreased or removed. Efforts to promote more rapid hypertrophy of the small bowel by using gut-specific hormones, fiber, fuels, and isotonic solutions have been reported. More randomized prospective trials are needed to determine the efficacy of nutrient and non-nutrient stimuli in maximizing intestinal adaptation and optimizing the management of short bowel syndrome.

Hepatic Insufficiency

The liver has a remarkable ability to recover and compensate, with 80% to 90% impairment required for features of hepatic insufficiency to appear (e.g., decreased albumin, prolonged prothrombin time, mental confusion). Hepatic insufficiency results in a catabolic state similar to sepsis. Cytokines have been implicated in this catabolic state. Increases occur in levels of tumor necrosis factor, interleukin-1, and interleukin-6, which have catabolic effects on muscle, adipose tissue, and liver. Lipids and proteins replace carbohydrates as primary sources of energy, resulting in depletion of lipid and protein reserves. There is a derangement of carbohydrate, lipid, and protein metabolism. Glucose intolerance occurs, along with decreased storage of glycogen in the liver and muscle. Fatty acid levels, ketone body levels, and ketone body production are increased. Inhibition of lipoprotein lipase affects lipid storage, resulting in an imbalance between fat synthesis and catabolism. There is an increase in urine nitrogen losses with normal renal function. The increased protein catabolism does not return to normal with feeding. The net effect of these metabolic abnormalities is protein-calorie malnutrition.

A serum amino acid imbalance also is seen with increased levels of phenylalanine, tyrosine, and tryptophan (aromatic amino acids) and decreased levels of the BCAAs leucine, valine, and isoleucine. This imbalance results in abnormal amine neurotransmitter products in which norepinephrine and dopamine are replaced by compounds such as octopamine and phenylethanolamine. This imbalance is a possible basis for hepatic encephalopathy. Treatment involves monitoring protein intake. The quantity of amino acid in the diet is reduced to 20 to 40 g/day. If encephalopathy worsens or does not improve, formulations with greater concentrations of BCAAs and reduced concentrations of aromatic amino acids are administered. In general, parenteral formulations are tolerated better than enteral formulations.

Most patients with hepatic failure have increased losses of potassium, magnesium, and zinc, so close attention to fluid and electrolyte management is necessary. Significant ascites can be treated with fluid restriction.

Gastric Bypass Surgery

In a Roux-en-Y gastric bypass, the stomach volume is reduced by creating a small pouch at the top of the stomach using surgical staples or a plastic band. The stomach is connected directly to the middle portion of the small intestine (jejunum), bypassing the rest of the stomach, duodenum, and proximal portion of jejunum. GLP-1, produced by L cells in the distal intestinal tract, is a powerful incretin. Patients who have a Roux-en-Y gastric bypass have increased levels of GLP-1 with improvement in diabetes; these results are not seen after restrictive bariatric procedures. After gastric bypass and jejunointestinal bypass, a pleiotropic endocrine response may contribute to improved glycemic control, appetite reduction, and long-term changes in body weight.[46]

Intensive Insulin and Glycemic Control

In diabetic and nondiabetic surgical patients, hyperglycemia and hypoglycemia have been associated with increased morbidity and mortality. Hyperglycemia increases inflammation and has deleterious effects on the immune, respiratory, renal, and nervous systems. Hyperglycemia decreases the rate of wound healing and increases infection rates, length of hospital stay, ventilator dependence, and mortality.[47] Hypoglycemia has detrimental effects, especially in the central and autonomic nervous systems and circulatory system. Clinically, hypoglycemia is manifested by dizziness, drowsiness, fatigue, tachycardia, seizures, and coma. Control of systemic and local glucose levels is critical to local wound healing and overall outcomes.

Using intensive insulin protocols to maintain tight glycemic control has emerged as an important therapy in improving outcomes and reducing complications in critical care patients. The severe stress response to critical illness leads to insulin resistance and impaired glucose uptake, and these protocols help reduce the incidence of hyperglycemic episodes by maintaining normoglycemia. Although early enthusiasts for intensive glucose control advocated protocols to maintain blood glucose levels in ranges as narrow as 81-108 mg/dL, the NICE-SUGAR trial established that a slightly more moderate approach (i.e., maintaining blood glucose levels <180 mg/dL) yielded much of the benefits of tighter protocols, without decreased morbidity and mortality from hypoglycemia.[48]

Pancreatitis

The incidence of acute pancreatitis, currently 35 per 100,000, continues to increase worldwide and correlates with increasing alcohol consumption. Mortality reaches 40% in severe cases and up to 80% in septic patients with multiorgan failure. Severe cases of pancreatitis are associated with the development of sepsis and prolonged organ failure; however, patients have traditionally been kept NPO to minimize pancreatic stimulation and decrease subsequent pancreatic inflammation. This practice is known to lead to intestinal ischemia, bacterial translocation, and potential sepsis. A meta-analysis of 291 patients revealed that patients with acute pancreatitis who received EN had significantly reduced infectious complications, although no significant differences were observed in mortality.[49] At the present time, no evidence suggests that the addition of prokinetics is beneficial in patients with severe acute pancreatitis.

In patients with acute pancreatitis, initial volume resuscitation and pain control should be followed by early postpyloric enteral feeding starting within 24 hours of admission. This approach has been shown to reduce complications, length of stay, and mortality. Patients with mild acute pancreatitis may begin a low-fat oral diet.

The pancreas manifests signs of endocrine or exocrine insufficiency only after 90% of its cell mass has been destroyed. In patients with chronic pancreatitis, pain and continued alcoholism are mainly associated with the development of early malnutrition before organ damage reaches criteria for insufficiency. It is essential that nutritional management in these patients begin with abstinence from alcohol and relief from abdominal pain, with the addition of pancreatic enzymes as necessary, management of nutrient-specific deficiencies, and initiation of PN when indicated.

Obesity

The prevalence of obesity in the industrialized world is increasing and has resulted in a growing number of obese patients. Extensive research in humans and animals provides evidence that obesity is caused by dietary and genetic factors. Gene defects in the coding sequences for leptin and the melanocortin-4 receptor have been identified as being contributory to the occurrence of clinically severe obesity. However, these gene defects are very rare, and there are currently 600 candidate genes under investigation that are suspected to be involved in a polygenic manner in the development of obesity. Nevertheless, genetic factors are only contributory and susceptibility factors in obesity, with dietary behavior being the main factor responsible for the huge increase.

Imbalance between caloric intake and energy needs is one of the leading factors leading to weight gain. In recent decades, altered nutritional behaviors in the industrialized world, including larger portions of processed high-calorie foods, sugar-sweetened drinks, and increasingly sedentary lifestyles, have contributed significantly to the pandemic development of obesity. Even small, consistent, daily excesses in caloric intake have major long-term effects because this positive balance accumulates over time.

In addition to presenting technical challenges in anesthesia and surgical procedures, obese patients can have additional nutritional needs because of metabolic alterations, necessitating greater perioperative care. Obesity is associated with an increased incidence of preexisting comorbidities, including endocrine disorders, cardiovascular disease and risk factors, GI conditions, and immune dysfunction. Consequently, obese patients are predisposed to a higher incidence of clinical complications, morbidity, and

TABLE 5-14 Body Weight Classification*

CLASSIFICATION	BMI (kg/m^2)	WAIST CIRCUMFERENCE: MEN, ≤40 INCHES; WOMEN, ≤35 INCHES	WAIST CIRCUMFERENCE: MEN, >40 INCHES; WOMEN, >35 INCHES
Underweight	<18.5		
Normal	18.5-24.9		
Overweight	25.0-29.9	Increased	High
Obesity I	30.0-34.9	High	Very high
Obesity II	35.0-39.9	Very high	Very high
Obesity III	>39.9	Extremely high	Extremely high

Adapted from National Heart, Lung, and Blood Institute: The practical guide: Identification, evaluation, and treatment of overweight and obesity in adults, 2000 (http://www.nhlbi.nih.gov/guidelines/obesity/prctgd_c.pdf.)

*Based on BMI and relative risk of type 2 diabetes, hypertension, and cardiovascular disease compared with normal weight individuals, according to waist measurement.

mortality. For this reason, additional clinical care requirements need to be considered and addressed during the operative stay.

Assessment of the BMI was described earlier. BMI has been shown to compare relatively accurately with the percentage of total body fat and morbidity. The classification of body weight with respect to underweight, normal weight, overweight, and obesity is shown in Table 5-14. This classification is commonly applied to the whole population, although it has some limitations. There are two exceptions. Total body fat can be overestimated in trained athletes because they have a higher percentage of lean body mass, and total body fat may be underestimated in older individuals because of muscle loss. For children and adolescents, the BMI needs to be adjusted because boys and girls have different growth characteristics, with the distribution of fat, muscle mass, and bone mineral content varying with growth. The body mass indices in this population are compared against growth charts, taking into account age and gender. Body mass is expressed as a BMI for age percentile. Underweight is classified as lower than the 5th percentile; healthy weight, from the 5th to 85th percentile; overweight, from the 85th to the 95th percentile; and obese, equal to or higher than the 95th percentile. Evaluation of weight status according to a patient's BMI is important because this can provide information regarding the patient's potential comorbidities and risk for complications during hospitalization.

Although one might think obese patients are at a nutritional advantage, clinical and basic research demonstrates that these patients are often at a distinct metabolic and nutritional disadvantage compared with nonobese cohorts. Although the reasons for this disadvantage are incompletely understood, obesity is associated with distinct changes in metabolic response to trauma.[50] Furthermore, obesity should not be interpreted as a sign of robust or even adequate nutritional stores. Despite the intuitive tendency to perceive these patients as "overnourished," metabolic and anthropometric studies of obese patients have established that even with excess fat stores, these patients demonstrate a high degree of protein-malnutrition. This deceptive combination of excess body fat and lean body mass wasting has been termed *sarcopenic obesity*.[5] The best way to provide nutritional support to such patients during acute illness is a matter of active research and considerable debate. There is considerable evidence to support the strategy of "hypocaloric nutrition" in critically ill obese patients. However, the terms *hypocaloric nutrition* and *hypoalimentation* often lead to extremely problematic misinterpretation of the approach described. Contrary to the common misunderstanding, hypocaloric nutrition is not meant to imply simply providing fewer feeds than needed to meet metabolic needs. Rather, this strategy involves application of protein-rich, low-fat nutrition so that patients are provided with adequate nutrition to meet or exceed their active protein requirements, while leaving a deficit in carbohydrate-based and fat-based calories to encourage mobilization of existing fat-calorie stores.

Comorbidities and Preexisting Conditions

Patients with a BMI greater than 30 kg/m^2 are considered at especially high risk and require special consideration during their hospital stay because of preexisting comorbidities and increased incidence of clinical complications. In most cases, more than one comorbidity is present in an obese patient. The most important related factors that need to be considered in surgical patients are presented here.

Type 2 Diabetes Mellitus

Almost 80% of obese patients have type 2 diabetes mellitus. A strong causality between obesity and diabetes mellitus type 2 has been shown. Type 2 diabetes can lead to obesity, and obesity can induce diabetes. Type 2 diabetes is caused by insulin resistance in peripheral cells and a decreased production of insulin in the pancreas. Insulin resistance can lead to diminished liver function and impaired wound healing. It is molecularly linked with the inflammatory response.

Cardiovascular Disease

Obesity is associated with an increased incidence of cardiovascular disease, including coronary heart disease, cardiomyopathy, congestive heart failure, sudden death, and stroke. These factors need to be considered when planning surgical procedures requiring anesthesia and during the perioperative hospital stay.

Deep Vein Thrombosis and Embolism

Hospitalized patients are at high risk for thromboses and consequently for embolic events. Obesity independently increases the risk of these events. The major contributing factors are abdominal fat distribution, venous insufficiency, congestive heart failure, and systemic hyperlipidemia. Moreover, obesity is thought to contribute to the development of thrombotic complications by increasing prothrombotic factors. These factors need to be considered especially in immobilized patients, and patients should be closely monitored and given prophylactic treatment.

Hepatobiliary Disease

The metabolic state in obese patients has been shown to be associated with several conditions in the hepatobiliary tract. Obesity is one of the most common causes of nonalcoholic liver disease. This can range from nonsymptomatic hepatic steatosis to inflammatory steatosis, fatty infiltration, and liver cirrhosis. This liver damage results in altered metabolism and severe changes in the production of liver proteins. There is an association among the development of gallstones, cholelithiasis, and obesity. With these adverse changes in liver metabolism, it is necessary to substitute essential proteins. Moreover, the dosages of these drugs need to be adjusted because of their altered rate of metabolism.

Osteoarthritis

The incidence of osteoarthritis is increased in obesity because of functional effects on weight-bearing joints. Pain in weight-bearing joints can range from functional limitations to invalidism. These circumstances have to be considered in the differential diagnosis, especially in patients susceptible to trauma. Joint pain also needs to be considered as a differential diagnosis in patients with tumors, who are susceptible to bone metastases.

Metabolic Syndrome

Metabolic syndrome refers to a special form of obesity. Metabolic syndrome is a combination of simultaneous risk factors associated with central obesity that lead to a greatly increased risk of coronary artery disease, stroke, and type 2 diabetes. Underlying causes are similar to the causes of regular obesity, including genetic factors, physical inactivity, and age. Around 20% to 25% of the world's population is estimated to have metabolic syndrome. This high incidence also needs to be addressed in the treatment of surgical patients.

A key feature of metabolic syndrome is body fat distribution in a central (abdominal) pattern. According to the International Diabetes Federation, a waist circumference more than 40 inches for men and 35 inches for women meets the criteria for metabolic syndrome (see Table 5-14) when at least two of the following criteria are also met:

- Increased triglyceride level: ≥150 mg/dL (>1.70 mmol/liter) (or receiving specific treatment)
- Decreased high-density lipoprotein cholesterol: <40 mg/dL (<1.03 mmol/liter) for men and <50 mg/dL (<1.29 mmol/liter) for women (or receiving specific treatment)
- Systolic blood pressure ≥130 mm Hg or diastolic blood pressure ≥85 mm Hg (or hypertension previously diagnosed and treated)
- Fasting plasma glucose level ≥100 mg/dL (5.6 mmol/liter) or diagnosed type 2 diabetes mellitus

The metabolic syndrome has a high prevalence in middle-aged and older patients (30% to 40%). It is associated with increased cardiovascular morbidity and mortality, including arterial hypertonia, and in most cases is associated with subclinical organ damage, such as microalbuminuria, decreased glomerular filtration rate, left ventricular hypertrophy, diastolic dysfunction, and arterial thickening.

Obese Surgical Patients

The characteristics of obese surgical patients need to be considered at admission and during the course of the hospital stay. Secondary metabolic changes only rarely require a special enteric or parenteral treatment regimen. During catabolic phases especially, hyperinsulinemia is normalized rapidly. In general, some weight loss should be considered before the admission of obese patients. Weight reduction by 10% of the total body weight should be considered before planned elective admissions, if feasible, because it can result in significant improvements in lung function parameters and a vast normalization of metabolism. Some studies have indicated that after operative procedures and during the hospital stay, a moderate, hypocaloric, protein-rich balanced diet should be given. This diet results in the mobilization of endogenous fat depots; the high protein content helps protect lean body mass from catabolic breakdown.

Only a few studies have been conducted despite the high incidence of problems related to overweight and obesity. Current knowledge and specialized treatment regimens are limited. However, overweight and obese patients need special attention throughout their entire hospital stay.

SUMMARY

Recognition of the importance of nutritional support for optimal outcomes in surgical patients and critically ill patients has prompted research on and development of a wide variety of regimens and strategies. Surgery, trauma, and sepsis lead to the release of inflammatory mediators and systemic hormonal and metabolic adaptations from the stress response. Nutritional support is a key component of modern surgical care, and collaboration with nutrition specialists can assist in providing appropriate support while avoiding complications. When nutritional support is required and no contraindications are present, EN is the first choice for most patients, with calculations being based on individual patient requirements. Various methods are available for the delivery of nutritional support; PN should be used, when necessary, in patients with contraindications to EN. In addition to being managed by operative interventions to address underlying pathology, catabolism and hypermetabolism can be managed by prompt treatment of infection and through environmental and pharmacologic strategies to diminish these factors, with nutritional support being started as early as possible to meet increased demands.

SELECTED REFERENCES

Cuthbertson DP: Post-shock metabolic response (Arris-Gale Lecture to the Royal College of Surgeons of England). *Lancet* 239:433–437, 1942.

In this landmark article on the hypermetabolic response, Cuthbertson characterized the metabolic response of surgical and trauma patients as observed during his experiments in animal models.

Fischer JE: *Nutrition and metabolism in the surgical patient*, ed 2, Boston, 1996, Little, Brown.

This work encompasses the background biochemistry and practical knowledge of surgical nutrition and metabolism.

Gottschlich MM, DeLegge MH, Guenter P, editors: *The A.S.P.E.N. nutrition support core curriculum*, Silver Spring, Md, 2008, American Society for Parenteral and Enteral Nutrition.

This comprehensive text covers all aspects of nutritional support in depth. Numerous case studies and examples are provided.

Herndon DN: *Total burn care*, ed 3, Edinburgh, 2007, Saunders.

This book is written by surgeons, anesthesiologists, residents, nurses, and allied health professionals dedicated to the management of surgical patients with the most severe hypermetabolic and hypercatabolic condition—burn patients.

Moore FD: *Metabolic care of the surgical patient*, Philadelphia, 1959, Saunders.

This book is a classic of surgical metabolism, with great contributions to the understanding of fluids and nutrition.

Wilmore DW, Long JM, Mason AD, Jr, et al: Catecholamines: Mediator of the hypermetabolic response to thermal injury. *Ann Surg* 180:653–669, 1974.

This classic work introduced catecholamines, not thyroid hormones, as the primary mediators of the hypermetabolic response. This was among the first studies to suggest the possibility of a pharmacologic intervention.

REFERENCES

1. Forceville X, Vitoux D, Gauzit R, et al: Selenium, systemic immune response syndrome, sepsis, and outcome in critically ill patients. *Crit Care Med* 26:1536–1544, 1998.
2. Angstwurm MW, Engelmann L, Zimmermann T, et al: Selenium in Intensive Care (SIC): Results of a prospective randomized, placebo-controlled, multiple-center study in patients with severe systemic inflammatory response syndrome, sepsis, and septic shock. *Crit Care Med* 35:118–126, 2007.
3. Heyland D, Muscedere J, Wischmeyer PE, et al: A randomized trial of glutamine and antioxidants in critically ill patients. *N Engl J Med* 368:1489–1497, 2013.
4. Puthucheary ZA, Rawal J, McPhail M, et al: Acute skeletal muscle wasting in critical illness. *JAMA* 310:1591–1600, 2013.
5. Jensen GL, Mirtallo J, Compher C, et al: Adult starvation and disease-related malnutrition: A proposal for etiology-based diagnosis in the clinical practice setting from the International Consensus Guideline Committee. *JPEN J Parenter Enteral Nutr* 34:156–159, 2010.
6. Casaer MP, Langouche L, Coudyzer W, et al: Impact of early parenteral nutrition on muscle and adipose tissue compartments during critical illness. *Crit Care Med* 41:2298–2309, 2013.
7. Hart DW, Wolf SE, Herndon DN, et al: Energy expenditure and caloric balance after burn: Increased feeding leads to fat rather than lean mass accretion. *Ann Surg* 235:152–161, 2002.
8. Plank LD, Hill GL: Sequential metabolic changes following induction of systemic inflammatory response in patients with severe sepsis or major blunt trauma. *World J Surg* 24:630–638, 2000.
9. Jie B, Jiang ZM, Nolan MT, et al: Impact of preoperative nutritional support on clinical outcome in abdominal surgical patients at nutritional risk. *Nutrition* 28:1022–1027, 2012.
10. Kondrup J, Rasmussen HH, Hamberg O, et al: Nutritional risk screening (NRS 2002): A new method based on an analysis of controlled clinical trials. *Clin Nutr* 22:321–336, 2003.
11. McClave SA, Kozar R, Martindale RG, et al: Summary points and consensus recommendations from the North American Surgical Nutrition Summit. *JPEN J Parenter Enteral Nutr* 37:99S–105S, 2013.
12. Choban P, Dickerson R, Malone A, et al: A.S.P.E.N. Clinical guidelines: Nutrition support of hospitalized adult patients with obesity. *JPEN J Parenter Enteral Nutr* 37:714–744, 2013.
13. National Heart Blood, and Lung Institute in cooperation with the National Institute on Diabetes and Digestive and Kidney Diseases: Clinical Guidelines on the Identification, Evaluation, and Treatment of Overweight and Obesity in Adults: The Evidence Report. NIH Publication No. 98-4083, 1998.
14. Gruther W, Benesch T, Zorn C, et al: Muscle wasting in intensive care patients: Ultrasound observation of the M. quadriceps femoris muscle layer. *J Rehabil Med* 40:185–189, 2008.
15. Tillquist M, Kutsogiannis DJ, Wischmeyer PE, et al: Bedside ultrasound is a practical and reliable measurement tool for assessing quadriceps muscle layer thickness. *JPEN J Parenter Enteral Nutr* 38:886–890, 2014.
16. Gibbs J, Cull W, Henderson W, et al: Preoperative serum albumin level as a predictor of operative mortality and morbidity: Results from the National VA Surgical Risk Study. *Arch Surg* 134:36–42, 1999.
17. Boullata J, Williams J, Cottrell F, et al: Accurate determination of energy needs in hospitalized patients. *J Am Diet Assoc* 107:393–401, 2007.
18. Faria MS, de Aguilar-Nascimento JE, Pimenta OS, et al: Preoperative fasting of 2 hours minimizes insulin resistance and organic response to trauma after video-cholecystectomy: A randomized, controlled, clinical trial. *World J Surg* 33:1158–1164, 2009.
19. Noblett SE, Watson DS, Huong H, et al: Pre-operative oral carbohydrate loading in colorectal surgery: A randomized controlled trial. *Colorectal Dis* 8:563–569, 2006.
20. Soop M, Nygren J, Myrenfors P, et al: Preoperative oral carbohydrate treatment attenuates immediate postoperative insulin resistance. *Am J Physiol Endocrinol Metab* 280:E576–E583, 2001.
21. Yuill KA, Richardson RA, Davidson HI, et al: The administration of an oral carbohydrate-containing fluid prior to major elective upper-gastrointestinal surgery preserves skeletal muscle mass postoperatively—a randomised clinical trial. *Clin Nutr* 24:32–37, 2005.
22. McClave SA, Martindale RG, Vanek VW, et al: Guidelines for the Provision and Assessment of Nutrition Support Therapy in the Adult Critically Ill Patient: Society of Critical Care Medicine (SCCM) and American Society for Parenteral and Enteral Nutrition (A.S.P.E.N.). *JPEN J Parenter Enteral Nutr* 33:277–316, 2009.
23. Harvey SE, Parrott F, Harrison DA, et al: Trial of the route of early nutritional support in critically ill adults. *N Engl J Med* 371:1673–1684, 2014.
24. Doig GS, Simpson F, Sweetman EA, et al: Early parenteral nutrition in critically ill patients with short-term relative contraindications to early enteral nutrition: A randomized controlled trial. *JAMA* 309:2130–2138, 2013.
25. Heidegger CP, Berger MM, Graf S, et al: Optimisation of energy provision with supplemental parenteral nutrition in critically ill patients: A randomised controlled clinical trial. *Lancet* 381:385–393, 2013.
26. Kutsogiannis J, Alberda C, Gramlich L, et al: Early use of supplemental parenteral nutrition in critically ill patients: Results of an international multicenter observational study. *Crit Care Med* 39:2691–2699, 2011.
27. Singer P, Anbar R, Cohen J, et al: The tight calorie control study (TICACOS): A prospective, randomized, controlled pilot study of nutritional support in critically ill patients. *Intensive Care Med* 37:601–609, 2011.

28. Alverdy JC, Aoys E, Moss GS: Total parenteral nutrition promotes bacterial translocation from the gut. *Surgery* 104:185–190, 1988.
29. Groos S, Hunefeld G, Luciano L: Parenteral versus enteral nutrition: Morphological changes in human adult intestinal mucosa. *J Submicrosc Cytol Pathol* 28:61–74, 1996.
30. Boelens PG, Heesakkers FF, Luyer MD, et al: Reduction of postoperative ileus by early enteral nutrition in patients undergoing major rectal surgery: Prospective, randomized, controlled trial. *Ann Surg* 259:649–655, 2014.
31. Barlow R, Price P, Reid TD, et al: Prospective multicentre randomised controlled trial of early enteral nutrition for patients undergoing major upper gastrointestinal surgical resection. *Clin Nutr* 30:560–566, 2011.
32. Osland E, Yunus RM, Khan S, et al: Early versus traditional postoperative feeding in patients undergoing resectional gastrointestinal surgery: A meta-analysis. *JPEN J Parenter Enteral Nutr* 35:473–487, 2011.
33. Khalid I, Doshi P, DiGiovine B: Early enteral nutrition and outcomes of critically ill patients treated with vasopressors and mechanical ventilation. *Am J Crit Care* 19:261–268, 2010.
34. Davies AR, Morrison SS, Bailey MJ, et al: A multicenter, randomized controlled trial comparing early nasojejunal with nasogastric nutrition in critical illness. *Crit Care Med* 40:2342–2348, 2012.
35. Montejo JC, Minambres E, Bordeje L, et al: Gastric residual volume during enteral nutrition in ICU patients: The REGANE study. *Intensive Care Med* 36:1386–1393, 2010.
36. Reignier J, Mercier E, Le Gouge A, et al: Effect of not monitoring residual gastric volume on risk of ventilator-associated pneumonia in adults receiving mechanical ventilation and early enteral feeding: A randomized controlled trial. *JAMA* 309:249–256, 2013.
37. Hart DW, Wolf SE, Zhang XJ, et al: Efficacy of a high-carbohydrate diet in catabolic illness. *Crit Care Med* 29:1318–1324, 2001.
38. Pontes-Arruda A, Martins LF, de Lima SM, et al: Enteral nutrition with eicosapentaenoic acid, gamma-linolenic acid and antioxidants in the early treatment of sepsis: Results from a multicenter, prospective, randomized, double-blinded, controlled study: The INTERSEPT study. *Crit Care* 15:R144, 2011.
39. Casaer MP, Mesotten D, Hermans G, et al: Early versus late parenteral nutrition in critically ill adults. *N Engl J Med* 365:506–517, 2011.
40. Doig GS, Heighes PT, Simpson F, et al: Early enteral nutrition reduces mortality in trauma patients requiring intensive care: A meta-analysis of randomised controlled trials. *Injury* 42:50–56, 2011.
41. Herndon DN, Barrow RE, Stein M, et al: Increased mortality with intravenous supplemental feeding in severely burned patients. *J Burn Care Rehabil* 10:309–313, 1989.
42. Allingstrup MJ, Esmailzadeh N, Wilkens Knudsen A, et al: Provision of protein and energy in relation to measured requirements in intensive care patients. *Clin Nutr* 31:462–468, 2012.
43. Berger MM, Eggimann P, Heyland DK, et al: Reduction of nosocomial pneumonia after major burns by trace element supplementation: Aggregation of two randomised trials. *Crit Care* 10:R153, 2006.
44. Berger MM, Soguel L, Shenkin A, et al: Influence of early antioxidant supplements on clinical evolution and organ function in critically ill cardiac surgery, major trauma, and subarachnoid hemorrhage patients. *Crit Care* 12:R101, 2008.
45. Neugebauer CT, Serghiou M, Herndon DN, et al: Effects of a 12-week rehabilitation program with music and exercise groups on range of motion in young children with severe burns. *J Burn Care Res* 29:939–948, 2008.
46. le Roux CW, Aylwin SJ, Batterham RL, et al: Gut hormone profiles following bariatric surgery favor an anorectic state, facilitate weight loss, and improve metabolic parameters. *Ann Surg* 243:108–114, 2006.
47. van den Berghe G, Wouters P, Weekers F, et al: Intensive insulin therapy in critically ill patients. *N Engl J Med* 345:1359–1367, 2001.
48. Finfer S, Chittock DR, Su SY, et al: Intensive versus conventional glucose control in critically ill patients. *N Engl J Med* 360:1283–1297, 2009.
49. McClave SA, Chang WK, Dhaliwal R, et al: Nutrition support in acute pancreatitis: A systematic review of the literature. *JPEN J Parenter Enteral Nutr* 30:143–156, 2006.
50. Jeevanandam M, Young DH, Schiller WR: Obesity and the metabolic response to severe multiple trauma in man. *J Clin Invest* 87:262–269, 1991.
51. Vorungati VS, Klein GL, Lu HX, et al: Impaired zinc and copper status in children with burn injuries: Need to reassess nutritional requirements. *Burns* 31:711–716, 2005.
52. Mirtallo J, Canada T, Johnson D, et al: Safe practices for parenteral nutrition. *JPEN J Parenter Enteral Nutr* 28(Suppl):S39–S70, 2004.
53. Harris JA, Benedict VS: *Biometric studies of basal metabolism in man*, Washington, DC, 1919, Carnegie Institute of Washington.
54. ASPEN Board of Directors and the Clinical Guidelines Task Force: Guidelines for the use of parenteral and enteral nutrition in adult and pediatric patients. *JPEN J Parenter Enteral Nutr* 26(Suppl):1SA–138SA, 2002.
55. Gottschlich MM, DeLegge MH, Guenter P, editors: *The A.S.P.E.N. nutrition support core curriculum*, Silver Spring, Md, 2008, American Society for Parenteral and Enteral Nutrition.
56. Weimann A, Braga M, Harsanyi L, et al: EPSEN Guidelines on Enteral Nutrition: Surgery including organ transplantation. *Clin Nutr* 25:224–244, 2006.
57. Kreymann KG, Berger MM, Deutz NE, et al: EPSEN Guidelines on Enteral Nutrition: Intensive care. *Clin Nutr* 25:210–223, 2006.

6 CHAPTER

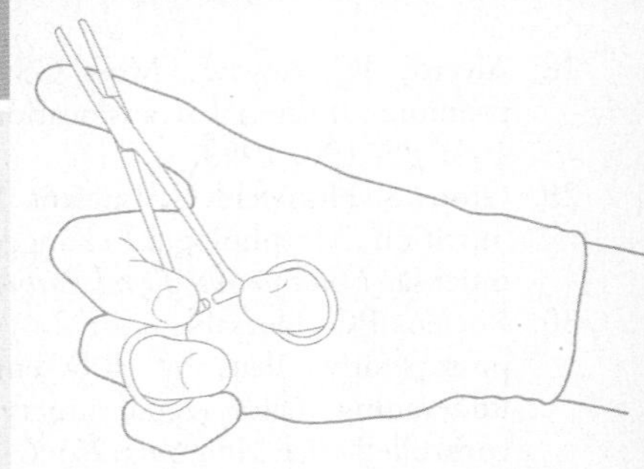

Wound Healing

Mimi Leong, Kevin D. Murphy, Linda G. Phillips

OUTLINE

Although the treatment and healing of wounds are some of the oldest subjects discussed in the medical literature, and although there have been numerous advances in understanding the steps involved in wound healing, the exact mechanisms underlying wound healing remain unclear.

TISSUE INJURY AND RESPONSE

Injured tissues attempt to restore their normal function and structural integrity after injury. Attempts to restore mechanical integrity and to restore barriers to fluid loss and infection and to reestablish normal blood and lymphatic flow patterns are termed *wound repair*. During wound repair, flawless repair is sacrificed because of the urgency to return to function. In contrast, regeneration, which is the goal of wound healing, is the perfect restoration of the preexisting tissue architecture without scar formation; regeneration is achievable only during embryonic development; in lower organisms; or in certain tissues, such as bone and liver.

All wounds undergo the same basic steps of repair. Acute wounds proceed in an orderly and timely reparative process to achieve sustained restoration of structure and function. A chronic wound stalls during a sustained inflammatory phase and fails to heal.

WOUND-HEALING PHASES

The three phases of wound healing are inflammation, proliferation, and maturation. In a large wound such as a pressure sore, the eschar or fibrinous exudate reflects the inflammatory phase, the granulation tissue is part of the proliferative phase, and the contracting or advancing edge is part of the maturational phase. All three phases may occur simultaneously, and the phases may overlap with their individual processes (Fig. 6-1).

Inflammatory Phase

During the immediate reaction of the tissue to injury, hemostasis occurs quickly and is rapidly followed by inflammation. This phase represents an attempt to limit damage by stopping bleeding; sealing the wound surface; and removing necrotic tissue, foreign debris, and bacteria. The inflammatory phase is characterized by increased vascular permeability, migration of cells into the wound by chemotaxis, secretion of cytokines and growth factors into the wound, and activation of the migrating cells.

Hemostasis and Inflammation

Blood vessel injury results in intense local arteriolar and capillary vasoconstriction followed by vasodilation and increased vascular permeability (Fig. 6-2). Erythrocytes and platelets adhere to the damaged capillary endothelium, resulting in plugging of capillaries and leading to cessation of hemorrhage. Platelet adhesion to the endothelium is primarily mediated through the interaction between high-affinity glycoprotein receptors and the integrin receptor GPIIb-IIIa ($\alpha_{IIb}\beta_3$). Platelets also express other integrin receptors that mediate direct binding to collagen ($\alpha_2\beta_1$) and laminin ($\alpha_6\beta_1$) or indirect binding to subendothelial matrix-bound fibronectin ($\alpha_5\beta_1$), vitronectin ($\alpha_v\beta_3$), and other ligands. Platelet activation occurs by binding to exposed type IV and type V collagen from the damaged endothelium, resulting in platelet aggregation. The initial contact between platelets and collagen requires von Willebrand factor VIII, a heterodimeric protein synthesized by megakaryocytes and endothelial cells.

Increased Vascular Permeability

Platelet binding results in conformational changes in platelets that trigger intracellular signal transduction pathways that lead to platelet activation and the release of biologically active proteins. Platelet alpha granules are storage organelles that contain platelet-derived growth factor (PDGF), transforming growth factor-β (TGF-β), insulin-like growth factor I (IGF-I), fibronectin, fibrinogen, thrombospondin, and von Willebrand factor. The dense

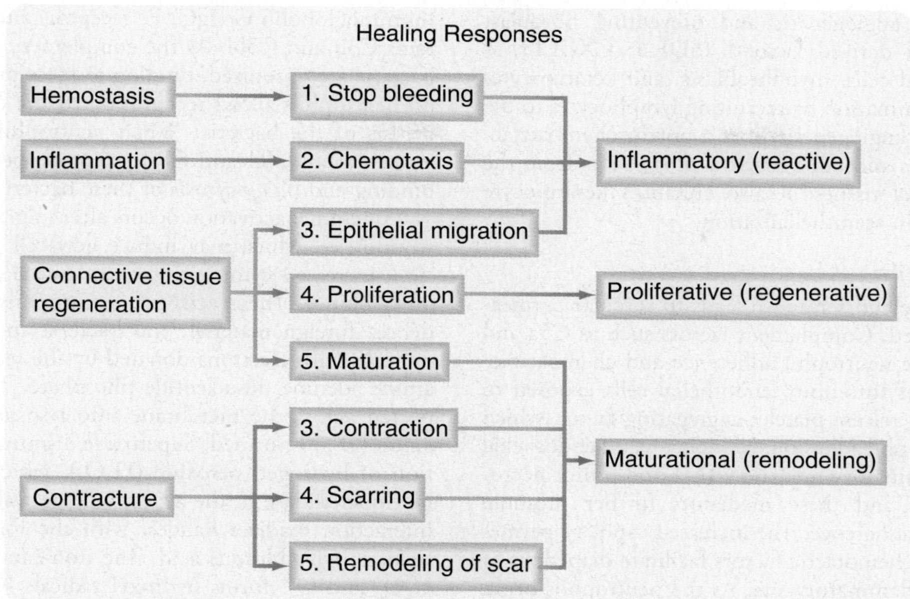

FIGURE 6-1 Schematic diagram of the wound-healing continuum.

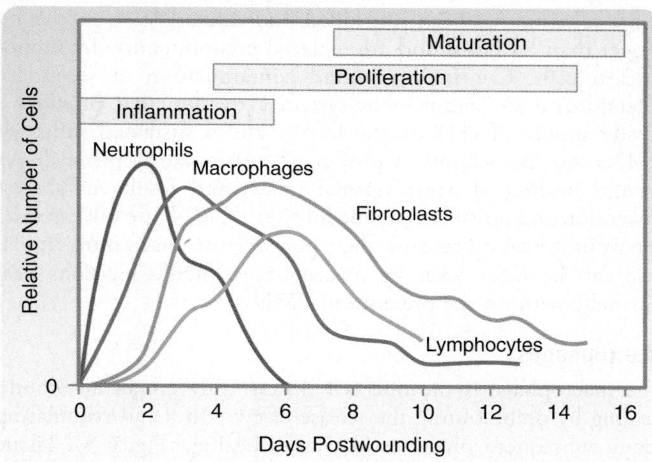

FIGURE 6-2 Time course of the appearance of different cells in the wound during healing. Macrophages and neutrophils are predominant during the inflammatory phase (peak at days 3 and 2, respectively). Lymphocytes appear later and peak at day 7. Fibroblasts are the predominant cells during the proliferative phase. (Adapted from Witte MB, Barbul A: General principles of wound healing. *Surg Clin North Am* 77:509–528, 1997.)

bodies contain vasoactive amines, such as serotonin, that cause vasodilation and increased vascular permeability. Mast cells adherent to the endothelial surface release histamine and serotonin, resulting in increased permeability of endothelial cells and causing leakage of plasma from the intravascular space to the extracellular compartment.

The clotting cascade is initiated through the intrinsic and extrinsic pathways. As the platelets become activated, the membrane phospholipids bind factor V, which allows interaction with factor X. Membrane-bound prothrombinase activity is generated and potentiates thrombin production exponentially. The thrombin itself activates platelets and catalyzes the conversion of fibrinogen to fibrin. The fibrin strands trap red blood cells to form the clot and seal the wound. The resulting lattice framework is the scaffold for endothelial cells, inflammatory cells, and fibroblasts to repair the damaged vessel.

Thromboxane A2 and prostaglandin F2α, formed from the degradation of cell membranes in the arachidonic acid cascade, also assist in platelet aggregation and vasoconstriction. Although these activities serve to limit the amount of injury, they can also cause localized ischemia, resulting in further damage to cell membranes and the release of more prostaglandin F2α and thromboxane A2.

Chemokines

Chemokines stimulate the migration of different cell types, particularly inflammatory cells, into the wound and are active participants in the regulation of the different phases of wound healing. The CXC, CC, and C ligand families bind to G protein–coupled surface receptors called CXC receptors and CC receptors.

Macrophage chemoattractant protein (MCP-1 or CCL2) is induced in keratinocytes after injury. It is a potent chemoattractant for monocytes/macrophages, T lymphocytes, and mast cells. Expression of this chemokine is sustained in chronic wounds and results in the prolonged presence of polymorphonuclear cells (PMNs) and macrophages, leading to the prolonged inflammatory response. CXCL1 (GRO-α) is a potent PMN chemotactic regulator and is increased in acute wounds. It is also involved in reepithelialization. Interleukin-8 (IL-8; CXCL8) expression is increased in acute and chronic wounds. It is involved in reepithelialization and induces the leukocyte expression of matrix metalloproteinases (MMPs), which stimulates remodeling. It is also a strong chemoattractant for PMNs and participates in inflammation. Relatively low levels of IL-8 are found in fetal wounds and may be why fetal wounds have decreased inflammation and heal without scars. Expression of the keratinocyte-produced chemokine interferon inducible protein 10 (CXCL10) is elevated in acute wounds and chronic inflammatory conditions. It impairs wound healing by increasing inflammation and recruiting lymphocytes to the wound. It also inhibits proliferation by decreasing reepithelialization and angiogenesis and preventing fibroblast migration. Stromal cell–derived factor-1 (SDF-1; CXCL12) is expressed by endothelial cells, myofibroblasts, and keratinocytes and is involved in inflammation by recruiting lymphocytes to the wound and promoting angiogenesis. It is a potent chemoattractant for endothelial cells and bone marrow progenitors from the circulation to peripheral tissues. It also enhances keratinocyte proliferation, resulting in reepithelialization.

Polymorphonuclear Cells

The release of histamine and serotonin leads to vascular permeability of the capillary bed. Complement factors such as C5a and leukotriene B4 promote neutrophil adherence and chemoattraction. In the presence of thrombin, endothelial cells exposed to leukotriene C4 and D4 release platelet-aggregating factor, which further enhances neutrophil adhesion. Monocytes and endothelial cells produce the inflammatory mediators IL-1 and tumor necrosis factor-α (TNF-α), and these mediators further promote endothelial-neutrophil adherence. The increased capillary permeability and the various chemotactic factors facilitate diapedesis of neutrophils into the inflammatory site. As the neutrophils begin their migration, they release the contents of their lysosomes and enzymes such as elastase and other proteases into the extracellular matrix (ECM), which further facilitates neutrophil migration. The combination of intense vasodilation and increased vascular permeability leads to clinical findings of inflammation, rubor (redness), tumor (swelling), calor (heat), and dolor (pain). Local tissue swelling is further promoted by the deposition of fibrin, a protein end product of coagulation, and the fibrin becomes entrapped in lymphatic vessels.

Evidence suggests that the migration of PMNs requires sequential adhesive and de-adhesive interactions between β_1 and β_2 integrins and ECM components. Integrin molecules are a family of cell surface receptors that are closely coupled with the cell's cytoskeleton. These molecules interact with components of the ECM, such as fibronectin, to provide adhesion and to transduce signal to the interior of the cell.

Integrins are crucial for cell motility and are required in inflammation and normal wound healing as well as in embryonic development and tumor metastases. After extravasation, PMNs, attracted by chemotaxins, migrate through the ECM via transient interactions between integrin receptors and their ligands. Four phases of integrin-mediated cell motility have been described: adhesion, spreading, contractility or traction, and retraction. Activation of specific integrins through ligand binding has been shown to increase cell adhesion and activate reorganization of the cell's actin cytoskeleton. Spreading is characterized by the development of lamellipodia and filopodia. Traction at the leading edge of the cell develops through binding of integrin, followed by translocation of the cell over the adherent segment of the plasma membrane. The integrin is shifted to the rear of the cell and releases its substrate, permitting cell advancement. Regulation of integrin function by adhesive substrates offers a mechanism for local control of migrant cells. Within the assembled framework of the ECM, binding sites for integrins have been identified on collagen, laminin, and fibronectin.

The chemotactic agent mediates the PMN response through signal transduction as the chemotaxin binds to receptors on the cell surface. Bacterial products such as *N*-formyl-methionyl-leucyl-phenylalanine bind to induce cyclic adenosine monophosphate, but if there is maximal receptor occupancy, superoxide is produced at peak rates. Neutrophils also possess receptors for immunoglobulin G (IgG; Fc receptor) and the complement proteins C3b and C3bi. As the complement cascade is released and bacteria are opsonized, binding of these proteins to cell receptors on neutrophils allows recognition by the neutrophils and phagocytosis of the bacteria. When neutrophils are stimulated, they express more CR1 and CR3 receptors, permitting more efficient binding and phagocytosis of these bacteria.

Functional activation occurs after migration of PMNs into the wound site, which may induce new cell surface antigen expression, increased cytotoxicity, or enhanced production and release of cytokines. These activated neutrophils scavenge for necrotic debris, foreign material, and bacteria and generate free oxygen radicals, with electrons donated by the reduced form of nicotinamide adenine dinucleotide phosphate. The electrons are transported across the membrane into lysosomes, where superoxide anion (O_2^-) is formed. Superoxide dismutase catalyzes the formation of hydrogen peroxide (H_2O_2), which is then degraded by myeloperoxidase in the azurophilic granules of neutrophils. This interaction oxidizes halides, with the formation of byproducts such as hypochlorous acid. The iron-catalyzed reaction between H_2O_2 and O_2^- forms hydroxyl radicals (OH·). This potent free radical is bactericidal as well as toxic to neutrophils and surrounding viable tissues.

Migration of PMNs stops after several days or when wound contamination has been controlled. Individual PMNs survive no longer than 24 hours and are replaced predominantly by mononuclear cells. Continuing wound contamination or secondary infection causes complement system activation that provides a steady supply of chemotactic factors and a sustained influx of PMNs into the wound. A prolonged inflammatory phase delays wound healing, destroys normal tissue, and results in abscess formation and possibly systemic infection. PMNs are not essential for wound healing because their phagocytosis and antimicrobial role can be taken over by macrophages. Sterile incisions heal normally without the presence of PMNs.

Macrophages

The macrophage is the one cell that is truly crucial to wound healing by orchestrating the release of cytokines and stimulating many subsequent processes in wound healing (Fig. 6-3). Tissue macrophages are derived from chemotaxis of migrating monocytes and appear within 24 to 48 hours of injury. When neutrophils start to disappear, macrophages appear and induce PMN apoptosis. Monocyte chemotactic factors include bacterial products, complement degradation products (C5a), thrombin, fibronectin, collagen, TGF-β, and PDGF-BB. Monocyte chemotaxis occurs as a result of the interaction of integrin receptors on the monocyte surface with ECM fibrin and fibronectin. The β integrin receptor also transduces the signal to initiate macrophage phagocytic activity. Activated integrin expression mediates monocyte transformation into wound macrophages. Transformation results in increased phagocytic activity and selective expression of cytokines and signal transduction elements by messenger RNA (mRNA), including the early growth response genes *EGR2* and *c-fos*. Macrophages have specific receptors for IgG, C3b (CR1 and CR3), and fibronectin (integrin receptors) that permit surface recognition and phagocytosis of opsonized pathogens.

Bacterial debris, such as lipopolysaccharide, activates monocytes to release free radicals and cytokines that mediate angiogenesis and fibroplasia. The presence of IL-2 increases free radical release and enhances bactericidal activity. Activity of the free radicals is potentiated by IL-2. Free radicals generate bacterial debris,

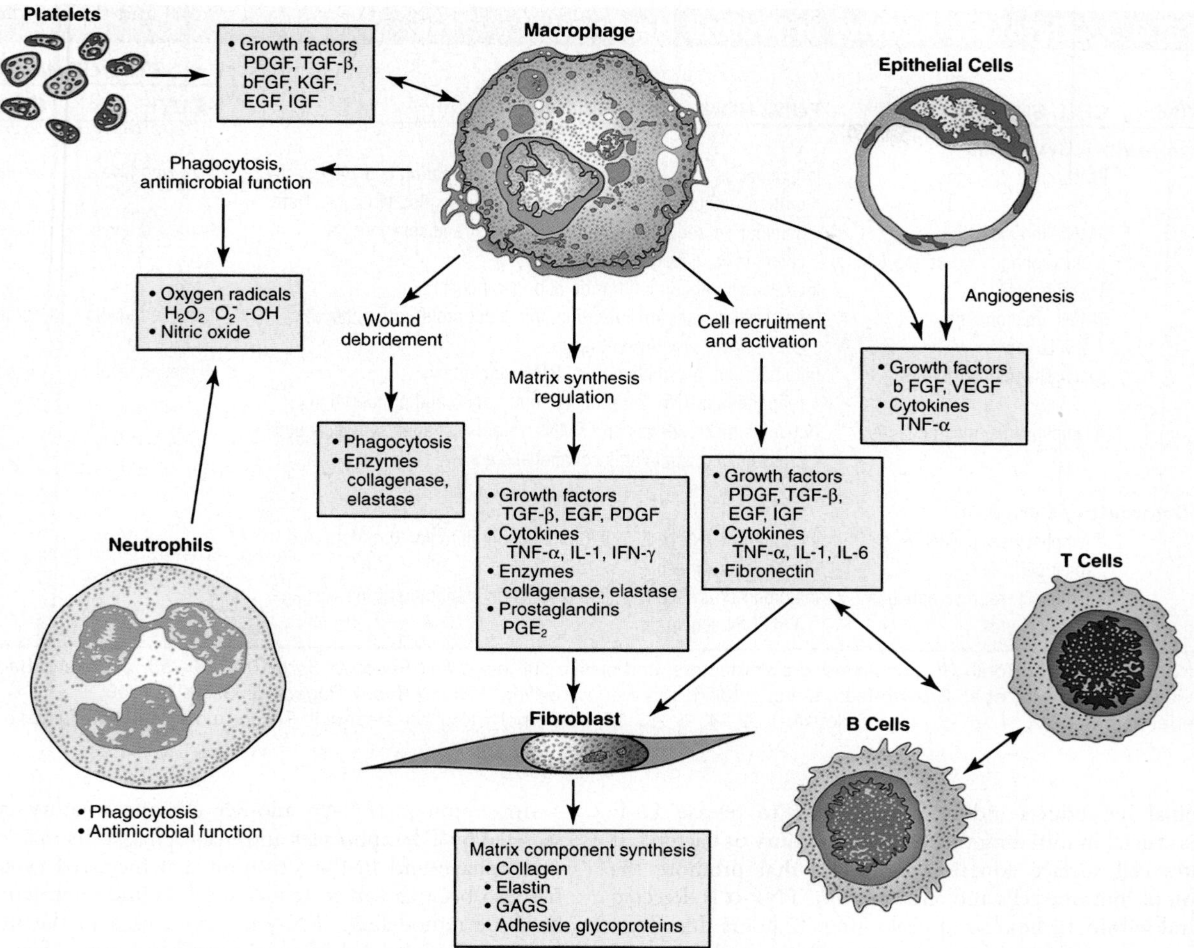

FIGURE 6-3 Interaction of cellular and humoral factors in wound healing. Note the key role of the macrophage. *bFGF,* basic fibroblast growth factor; *EGF,* epidermal growth factor; *GAGs,* glycosaminoglycans; *H_2O_2,* hydrogen peroxide; *IFN-γ,* interferon-γ; *IGF,* insulin-like growth factor; *IL-1,* interleukin-1; *IL-6,* interleukin-6; *KGF,* keratinocyte growth factor; *O_2^-,* superoxide; *–OH,* hydroxyl radical; *PDGF,* platelet-derived growth factor; *PGE_2,* prostaglandin E2; *TGF-β,* transforming growth factor-β; *TNF-α,* tumor necrosis factor-α; *VEGF,* vascular endothelial growth factor. (Adapted from Witte MB, Barbul A: General principles of wound healing. *Surg Clin North Am* 77:509–528, 1997.)

which further potentiates the activation of monocytes. Activated wound macrophages also produce nitric oxide (NO), a substance that has been demonstrated to have many functions other than antimicrobial properties.

As the monocyte or macrophage is activated, phospholipase is induced, cell membrane phospholipids are enzymatically degraded, and thromboxane A2 and prostaglandin F2α are released. The macrophage also releases leukotrienes B4 and C4 and 15-hydroxyeicosatetraenoic acid and 5-hydroxyeicosatetraenoic acid. Leukotriene B4 is a potent chemotaxin for neutrophils and increases their adherence to endothelial cells.

Wound macrophages release proteinases, including MMPs (MMP-1, MMP-2, MMP-3, and MMP-9), which degrade the ECM and are crucial for removing foreign material, promoting cell movement through tissue spaces, and regulating ECM turnover. This activity is dependent on the cyclic adenosine monophosphate pathway and can be blocked by nonsteroidal anti-inflammatory drugs or glucocorticoid drugs. Colchicine and retinoic acid appear to decrease collagenase production as well.

Macrophages secrete numerous cytokines and growth factors (Tables 6-1 and 6-2). IL-1, a proinflammatory cytokine, is an acute-phase response cytokine. This endogenous pyrogen causes lymphocyte activation and stimulation of the hypothalamus, inducing the febrile response. It also directly affects hemostasis by inducing the release of vasodilators and stimulating coagulation. Its effect is further amplified as endothelial cells produce it in the presence of TNF-α and endotoxin. IL-1 has numerous effects, such as enhancement of collagenase production, stimulation of cartilage degradation and bone reabsorption, activation of neutrophils, regulation of adhesion molecules, and promotion of chemotaxis. It stimulates other cells to secrete proinflammatory cytokines. Its effects extend into the proliferative phase, during which it increases fibroblast and keratinocyte growth and collagen synthesis. Studies have demonstrated increased levels of IL-1 in chronic nonhealing wounds, suggesting its role in the pathogenesis of poor wound healing. The early beneficial responses of IL-1 in wound healing appear to be maladaptive if elevated levels last beyond the first week after injury.

TABLE 6-1 Cytokine Activity in Wound Healing

CYTOKINE	CELL SOURCE	FUNCTION	TYPE OF WOUND: ACUTE	TYPE OF WOUND: CHRONIC
Proinflammatory Cytokines				
TNF-α	PMNs, macrophages	Inflammation, reepithelialization, PMN margination and cytotoxicity, with or without collagen synthesis; provides metabolic substrate	Increased levels	Increased levels
IL-1	PMNs, monocytes, macrophages, keratinocytes	Inflammation, reepithelialization, fibroblast and keratinocyte chemotaxis, collagen synthesis	Increased levels	Increased levels
IL-2	T lymphocytes	Increases fibroblast infiltration and metabolism		
IL-6	PMNs, macrophages, fibroblasts	Inflammation, reepithelialization, fibroblast proliferation, hepatic acute-phase protein synthesis	Increased levels	Increased levels
IL-8	Macrophages, fibroblasts	Inflammation, macrophage and PMN chemotaxis; reepithelialization, keratinocyte maturation and proliferation	Increased levels	Increased levels
IFN-γ	T lymphocytes, macrophages	Activates macrophages and PMNs, retards collagen synthesis and cross linking, stimulates collagenase activity		
Anti-inflammatory Cytokines				
IL-4	T lymphocytes, basophils, mast cells	Inhibition of TNF-α, IL-1, IL-6 production; fibroblast proliferation, collagen synthesis		
IL-10	T lymphocytes, macrophages, keratinocytes	Inhibition of TNF-α, IL-1, IL-6 production, inhibition of macrophage and PMN activation		

Adapted from Rumalla VK, Borah GL: Cytokines, growth factors, and plastic surgery. *Plast Reconstr Surg* 108:719–733, 2001; and Barrientos S, Stojadinovic O, Golinko MS, et al: Growth factors and cytokines in wound healing. *Wound Repair Regen* 16:585–601, 2008.
IFN-γ, Interferon-γ; *IL-1, -2, -4, -6, -8, -10,* interleukin-1, -2, -4, -6, -8, -10; *PMN,* polymorphonuclear cell; *TNF-α,* tumor necrosis factor-α.

Microbial byproducts induce macrophages to release TNF. TNF-α is crucial in initiating the response to injury or bacteria. It upregulates cell surface adhesion molecules that promote the interaction of immune cells and endothelium. TNF-α is detected in a wound within 12 hours and peaks after 72 hours. Its effects include hemostasis, increased vascular permeability, and enhanced endothelial proliferation. Similar to IL-1, TNF-α induces fever, increased collagenase production, reabsorption of cartilage and bone, and release of PDGF as well as the production of more IL-1. However, excessive production of TNF-α has been associated with multisystem organ failure and increased morbidity and mortality in inflammatory disease states, partly through its effects on activating macrophages and neutrophils. Studies have noted elevated levels of TNF-α in nonhealing versus healing chronic venous ulcers. As in the case of IL-1, TNF-α appears to be essential in the early inflammatory response required for wound healing, but local and systemic persistence of this cytokine may lead to impaired wound maturation.

IL-6, which is produced by monocytes and macrophages, is involved in stem cell growth, activation of B cells and T cells, and regulation of the synthesis of hepatic acute-phase proteins. Within acute wounds, IL-6 is also secreted by PMNs and fibroblasts, and increase in IL-6 parallels the increase in the PMN count locally. IL-6 is detectable within 12 hours of experimental wounding and may persist at high concentrations for longer than 1 week. It also works synergistically with IL-1, TNF-α, and endotoxins. It is a potent stimulator of fibroblast proliferation and is decreased in aging fibroblasts and fetal wounds.

IL-8 (also called CXCL8) is secreted primarily by macrophages and fibroblasts in the acute wound, with peak expression within the first 24 hours. Its major effects have already been discussed and include increased PMN and monocyte chemotaxis, PMN degranulation, and expression of endothelial cell adhesion molecules.

Interferon-γ (IFN-γ), another proinflammatory cytokine, is secreted by T lymphocytes and macrophages. Its major effects are macrophage and PMN activation and increased cytotoxicity. It has also been shown to reduce local wound contraction and aid in tissue remodeling. IFN-γ has been used in the treatment of hypertrophic and keloid scars, possibly by its effect in slowing collagen production and cross linking, whereas collagenase (MMP-1) production increases. Experimentally, it has been shown to impair reepithelialization and wound strength in a dose-dependent manner when applied locally or systemically. These findings suggest that administration of IFN-γ may improve scar hypertrophy by decreasing the strength of the wound.

Macrophages also release growth factors that stimulate fibroblast, endothelial cell, and keratinocyte proliferation and are important in the proliferative phase (see Table 6-2). Macrophage-secreted PDGF stimulates collagen and proteoglycan synthesis. PDGF exists as three isomers—PDGF-AA, PDGF-AB, and PDGF-BB. The PDGF-BB isomer is the only growth factor preparation approved by the U.S. Food and Drug Administration (FDA) and is the most widely studied clinically.

TGF-α and TGF-β are released by activated monocytes. TGF-α stimulates epidermal growth and angiogenesis. TGF-β itself stimulates monocytes to express other peptides, such as TGF-α, IL-1, and PDGF. TGF-β, which is also released by platelets and fibroblasts within wounds, exists as at least three isomers—$β_1$, $β_2$, and $β_3$—and its effects include fibroblast migration and maturation and ECM synthesis. TGF-$β_1$ has been shown to play an important role in collagen metabolism and healing of gastrointestinal injuries and anastomoses. In experimental models, TGF-$β_1$ accelerates wound healing in normal, steroid-impaired, and irradiated animals.

TGF-β is the most potent stimulant of fibroplasia, and its strong mitogenic effects have been implicated in the fibrogenesis seen in disease states such as scleroderma and interstitial

TABLE 6-2 Growth Factors That Affect Wound Healing

GROWTH FACTOR	CELL SOURCE	FUNCTION	TYPE OF WOUND: ACUTE	TYPE OF WOUND: CHRONIC
PDGF	Platelets, macrophages, endothelial cells, keratinocytes, fibroblasts	Inflammation; granulation tissue formation; reepithelialization; matrix formation and remodeling; chemotactic for PMNs, macrophages, fibroblasts, and smooth muscle cells; activates PMNs, macrophages, and fibroblasts; mitogenic for fibroblasts, endothelial cells; stimulates production of MMPs, fibronectin, and HA; stimulates angiogenesis and wound contraction	Increased levels	Decreased levels
TGF-β (including isoforms β_1, β_2, and β_3)	Platelets, T lymphocytes, macrophages, endothelial cells, keratinocytes, fibroblasts	Inflammation; granulation tissue formation; reepithelialization; matrix formation and remodeling; chemotactic for PMNs, macrophages, lymphocytes, fibroblasts; stimulates TIMP synthesis, keratinocyte migration, angiogenesis, and fibroplasia; inhibits production of MMPs and keratinocyte proliferation; induces TGF-β production	Increased levels	Decreased levels
EGF	Platelets, macrophages, fibroblasts	Mitogenic for keratinocytes and fibroblasts; stimulates keratinocyte migration	Increased levels	Decreased levels
FGF-1 and FGF-2 family	Macrophages, mast cells, T lymphocytes, endothelial cells, fibroblasts, keratinocytes, smooth muscle cells, chondrocytes	Granulation tissue formation; reepithelialization; matrix formation and remodeling; chemotactic for fibroblasts, mitogenic for fibroblasts and keratinocytes; stimulates keratinocyte migration; angiogenesis; wound contraction and matrix deposition	Increased levels	Decreased levels
KGF (also called FGF-7)	Fibroblasts, keratinocytes, smooth muscle cells, chondrocytes, endothelial cells, mast cells	Stimulate proliferation and migration of keratinocytes, increase transcription of factors involved in detoxification of ROS, potent mitogen for vascular endothelial cells; upregulates VEGF, stimulates endothelial cell production of UPA	Increased levels	Decreased levels
VEGF	Keratinocytes, platelets, PMNs, macrophages, endothelial cells, smooth muscle cells, fibroblasts	Granulation tissue formation; increases vasopermeability; mitogenic for endothelial cells	Increased levels	Decreased levels
TGF-α	Macrophages, T lymphocytes, keratinocytes, platelets, fibroblasts, lymphocytes	Reepithelialization; increase keratinocyte migration and proliferation		
IGF-I	Macrophages, fibroblasts	Stimulates elastin production and collagen synthesis, fibroblast proliferation		

Adapted from Schwartz SI (ed): *Principles of Surgery*, ed 7, New York, 1999, McGraw-Hill, p 269; and Barrientos S, Stojadinovic O, Golinko MS, et al: Growth factors and cytokines in wound healing. *Wound Repair Regen* 16:585–601, 2008.

EGF, Epidermal growth factor; *FGF-1, -2, -7,* fibroblast growth factor-1, -2, -7; *HA,* hyaluronic acid; *IGF-I,* insulin-like growth factor I; *KGF,* keratinocyte growth factor; *MMP,* matrix metalloproteinase; *PDGF,* platelet-derived growth factor; *PMN,* polymorphonuclear cell; *ROS,* reactive oxygen species; *TGF-α,-β,* transforming growth factor-α, -β; *TIMP,* tissue inhibitors of metalloproteinase; *UPA,* urokinase-type plasminogen activator; *VEGF,* vascular endothelial growth factor.

pulmonary fibrosis. Enhanced expression of TGF-β_1 mRNA is found in keloid and hypertrophic scars. In contrast, fetal wounds have been demonstrated to have a paucity of TGF-β, suggesting that the scarless repair seen in utero occurs because of low or absent amounts of TGF-β. Studies of the three isomers have suggested that although TGF-β_1 and TGF-β_2 play an important role in tissue fibrosis and postinjury scarring, TGF-β_3 may limit scarring. As the concentration of TGF-β increases in the inflammatory site, fibroblasts are directly stimulated to produce collagen and fibronectin, leading to the proliferative phase.

Wound macrophages exhibit different functional phenotypes—M1 (classically activated) and M2 (alternatively activated)—that are at the extremes of a continuum of macrophage function. Lipopolysaccharide and IFN-γ stimulate the differentiation into M1 macrophages that release TNF-α, NO, and IL-6. These mediators are responsible for host defense but at the expense of significant collateral tissue damage. M2 macrophages are activated by IL-4 and IL-13; suppress inflammatory reactions and adaptive immune responses; and play an important role in wound healing, angiogenesis, and defense against parasitic infections. However, despite their beneficial functions, M2 macrophages can also be involved in different diseases, such as allergy, asthma, and fibrosis, which is the result of a helper T cell (Th2) response, which is predominated by IL-4 or IL-10. Both phenotypes are important when correctly balanced during the different phases of wound healing. In the inflammatory phase, greater M1 macrophage activity is required for macrophage debris scavenging and invading pathogen destruction. In the proliferative phase, M2 macrophages predominate. The balance between M1 and M2 macrophages is likely disturbed during abnormal wound-healing responses.

Several studies have demonstrated the importance of macrophages in wound healing by macrophage depletion. Macrophage depletion delays wound infiltration by fibroblasts and decreased wound fibrosis. Newborn animals that lacked macrophages, mast cells, and functional neutrophils as a result of defective myelopoiesis healed without scarring at the same speed as wild-type animals if their wounds were protected by antibiotic coverage, suggesting that inflammatory cells are not essential for wound closure. However, several models of specific inducible macrophage depletion based on genetically modified mice resulted in a detrimental effect of preinjury depletion of macrophages.[1-3] Mice depleted before injury typically showed a defect in reepithelialization, granulation tissue formation, angiogenesis, wound cytokine production, and myofibroblast-associated wound contraction. Macrophage depletion 9 days after injury did not result in any morphologic or biologic differences between control and treatment mice, suggesting that macrophages may not be required at later stages of wound healing.[2]

Lymphocytes

Significant numbers of T lymphocytes appear by day 5 after injury and peak on day 7. B lymphocytes appear to be principally involved in downregulating healing as the wound closes. Lymphocytes stimulate fibroblasts with cytokines (IL-2 and fibroblast-activating factor). Lymphocytes also secrete inhibitory cytokines (TGF-β, TNF-α, and IFN-γ). Antigen-presenting macrophages present bacterial "debris" or enzymatically degraded host proteins to lymphocytes, stimulating lymphocyte proliferation and cytokine release. T cells produce IFN-γ, which stimulates the macrophage to release TNF-α and IL-1. IFN-γ decreases prostaglandin synthesis enhancing the effect of inflammatory mediators, suppressing collagen synthesis, and inhibiting macrophage exodus. IFN-γ appears to be an important mediator of chronic nonhealing wounds, and its presence suggests that T lymphocytes are primarily involved in chronic wound healing.

Drugs that suppress T-lymphocyte function and proliferation (steroids, cyclosporine, tacrolimus) result in impaired wound healing in experimental wound models, possibly through decreased NO synthesis. In vivo lymphocyte depletion suggests the existence of an incompletely characterized T cell lymphocyte population that is neither $CD4^+$ nor $CD8^+$ that seems to be responsible for the promotion of wound healing.

Proliferative Phase

As the acute responses of hemostasis and inflammation begin to resolve, the scaffolding is laid for repair of the wound through angiogenesis, fibroplasia, and epithelialization. This stage is characterized by the formation of granulation tissue, which consists of a capillary bed; fibroblasts; macrophages; and a loose arrangement of collagen, fibronectin, and hyaluronic acid. Numerous studies have used growth factors to modify granulation tissue, particularly fibroplasia. Adenoviral transfer, topical application, and subcutaneous injection of PDGF, TGF-β, keratinocyte growth factor (KGF), vascular endothelial growth factor (VEGF), and epidermal growth factor (EGF) have been tested to increase the proliferation of granulation tissue.

Angiogenesis

Angiogenesis is the process of new blood vessel formation and is necessary to support a healing wound environment. After injury, activated endothelial cells degrade the basement membrane of postcapillary venules, allowing the migration of cells through this gap. Division of these migrating endothelial cells results in tubule or lumen formation. Eventually, deposition of the basement membrane occurs and results in capillary maturation.

After injury, the endothelium is exposed to numerous soluble factors and comes in contact with adhering blood cells. These interactions result in upregulation of the expression of cell surface adhesion molecules, such as vascular cell surface adhesion molecule-1. Matrix-degrading enzymes, such as plasmin and the metalloproteinases, are released and activated and degrade the endothelial basement membrane. Fragmentation of the basement membrane allows migration of endothelial cells into the wound, promoted by fibroblast growth factor (FGF), PDGF, and TGF-β. Injured endothelial cells express adhesion molecules, such as the integrin $\alpha_v\beta_3$, which facilitates attachment to fibrin, fibronectin, and fibrinogen and facilitates endothelial cell migration along the provisional matrix scaffold. Platelet endothelial cell adhesion molecule-1 (PECAM-1), also found on endothelial cells, modulates their interaction with each other as they migrate into the wound.

Capillary tube formation is a complex process that involves cell-cell and cell-matrix interactions, modulated by adhesion molecules on endothelial cell surfaces. PECAM-1 has been observed to mediate cell-cell contact, whereas β_1 integrin receptors may aid in stabilizing these contacts and forming tight junctions between endothelial cells. Some of the new capillaries differentiate into arterioles and venules, whereas others undergo involution and apoptosis, with subsequent ingestion by macrophages. Regulation of endothelial apoptosis is not well understood.

Angiogenesis appears to be stimulated and manipulated by various cytokines predominantly produced by macrophages and platelets. As the macrophage produces TNF-α, it orchestrates angiogenesis during the inflammatory phase. Heparin, which can stimulate the migration of capillary endothelial cells, binds with high affinity to a group of angiogenic factors.

VEGF, a member of the PDGF family of growth factors, has potent angiogenic activity. It is produced in large amounts by keratinocytes, macrophages, endothelial cells, platelets, and fibroblasts during wound healing. Cell disruption and hypoxia, hallmarks of tissue injury, appear to be strong initial inducers of potent angiogenic factors at the wound site, such as VEGF and its receptor. VEGF family members include VEGF-A, VEGF-B, VEGF-C, VEGF-D, VEGF-E, and placental growth factor (PlGF). VEGF-A promotes early events in angiogenesis and subsequently is crucial to wound healing. It binds to tyrosine kinase surface receptors Flt-1 (VEGF receptor-1, or VEGFR-1) and KDR (VEGF receptor-2, or VEGFR-2). Flt-1 is required for blood vessel organization, whereas KDR is important for endothelial cell chemotaxis, proliferation, and differentiation. Animal studies have shown that VEGF-A administration restores impaired angiogenesis found in diabetic ischemic limbs; however, other studies have shown that exogenous VEGF results in vascular leakage and disorganized blood vessel formation. VEGF-C, which is also elevated during wound healing, is primarily released by macrophages and is important during the inflammatory phase of wound healing. Although it works primarily through VEGF receptor-3 (VEGFR-3), which is expressed in macrophages and lymphatic endothelium, it can also activate VEGFR-2, increasing vascular permeability. In vivo administration of VEGF-C in an animal model using an adenoviral vector to genetically diabetic mice resulted in accelerated healing. PlGF is another proangiogenic factor that is elevated after wounding. It is involved in inflammation and expressed by keratinocytes and endothelial cells. It is believed to work synergistically with VEGF, potentiating its proangiogenic function.

Both acidic and basic FGFs (FGF-1 and FGF-2) are released from disrupted parenchymal cells and are early stimulants of angiogenesis. FGF-2 provides the initial angiogenic stimulus within the first 3 days of wound repair, followed by a subsequent prolonged stimulus mediated by VEGF from days 4 through 7. There is a dose-dependent effect of VEGF and FGF-2 on angiogenesis. Both TGF-α and EGF stimulate endothelial cell proliferation. TNF-α is chemotactic for endothelial cells; it promotes formation of the capillary tube and may mediate angiogenesis through its induction of hypoxia-inducible factor 1 (HIF-1). It regulates the expression of other hypoxia-responsive genes, including inducible NO synthase and VEGF. HIF-1α mRNA is prominently present in wound inflammatory cells during the initial 24 hours, and HIF-1α protein is present in cells isolated from the wound 1 and 5 days after injury in vitro. Data also suggest that there is a positive interaction between endogenous NO and VEGF, with endogenous NO enhancing VEGF synthesis. Similarly, VEGF has been shown to promote NO synthesis in angiogenesis, suggesting that NO mediates aspects of VEGF signaling required for endothelial cell proliferation and organization.

TGF-β is a chemoattractant for fibroblasts and probably assists in angiogenesis by signaling the fibroblast to produce FGFs. Other factors that have been shown to induce angiogenesis include angiogenin, IL-8, and lactic acid. Several of the matrix materials, such as fibronectin and hyaluronic acid from the wound site, are angiogenic. Fibronectin and fibrin are produced by macrophages and damaged endothelial cells. Collagen appears to interact by causing the tubular formation of endothelial cells in vitro. Angiogenesis results from the complex interaction of ECM material and cytokines.

Fibroplasia

Fibroblasts are specialized cells that differentiate from resting mesenchymal cells in connective tissue; they do not arrive in the wound cleft by diapedesis from circulating cells. After injury, the normally quiescent and sparse fibroblasts are chemoattracted to the inflammatory site, they divide and produce the components of the ECM. After stimulation by macrophage-derived and platelet-derived cytokines and growth factors, the fibroblast, which is normally arrested in the G_0 phase, undergoes replication and proliferation. Platelet-derived TGF-β stimulates fibroblast proliferation indirectly by releasing PDGF. The fibroblast can also stimulate replication in an autocrine manner by releasing FGF-2. To continue proliferating, fibroblasts require further stimulation by factors such as EGF or IGF-I. Although fibroblasts require growth factors for proliferation, they do not need growth factors to survive. Fibroblasts can live quiescently in growth factor–free media in monolayers or three-dimensional cultures.

The primary function of fibroblasts is to synthesize collagen, which they begin to produce during the cellular phase of inflammation. The time required for undifferentiated mesenchymal cells to differentiate into highly specialized fibroblasts accounts for the delay between injury and the appearance of collagen in a healing wound. This period, generally 3 to 5 days, depending on the type of tissue injured, is termed the *lag phase* of wound healing. Fibroblasts begin to migrate in response to chemotactic substances such as growth factors (PDGF, TGF-β), C5 fragments, thrombin, TNF-α, eicosanoids, elastin fragments, leukotriene B4, and fragments of collagen and fibronectin.

The rate of collagen synthesis declines after 4 weeks and eventually balances the rate of collagen destruction by collagenase (MMP-1). At this point, the wound enters a phase of collagen maturation. The maturation phase continues for months or years. Glycoprotein and mucopolysaccharide levels decrease during the maturation phase, and new capillaries regress and disappear. These changes alter the appearance of the wound and increase its strength.

Epithelialization

The epidermis serves as a physical barrier to prevent fluid loss and bacterial invasion. Tight cell junctions within the epithelium contribute to its impermeability, and the basement membrane zone gives structural support and provides attachment between the epidermis and the dermis. The basement membrane zone consists of several layers: (1) lamina lucida (electron clear), consisting of laminin and heparan sulfate; (2) lamina densa (electron dense), containing type IV collagen; and (3) anchoring fibrils, consisting of type IV collagen, which secure the epidermodermal interface and connect the lamina densa to the dermis.

The basal layer of the epidermis attaches to the basement membrane zone by hemidesmosomes. Reepithelialization of wounds begins within hours after injury. Initially, the wound is rapidly sealed by clot formation and then by epithelial (epidermal) cell migration across the defect. Keratinocytes located at the basal layer of the residual epidermis or in the depths of epithelium-lined dermal appendages migrate to resurface the wound. Epithelialization involves a sequence of changes in wound keratinocytes—detachment, migration, proliferation, differentiation, and stratification. If the basement membrane zone is intact, epithelialization proceeds more rapidly. The cells are stimulated to migrate. Attachments to neighboring and adjoining cells and to the dermis are loosened, as demonstrated by intracellular tonofilament retraction, dissolution of intercellular desmosomes and hemidesmosomes linking the epidermis to the basement membrane, and formation of cytoplasmic actin filaments.

Epidermal cells express integrin receptors that allow them to interact with ECM proteins such as fibronectin. The migrating cells dissect the wound by separating the desiccated eschar from viable tissue. This path of dissection is determined by the integrins that the epidermal cells express on their cell membranes. Degradation of the ECM, required if epidermal cells are to migrate between the collagenous dermis and fibrin eschar, is driven by epidermal cell production of collagenase (MMP-1) and plasminogen activator, which activates collagenase and plasmin. The migrating cells are also phagocytic and remove debris in their path. Cells behind the leading edge of migrating cells begin to proliferate. The epithelial cells move in a leapfrog and tumbling fashion until the edges establish contact. If the basement membrane zone is not intact, it will be repaired first. The absence of neighboring cells at the wound margin may be a signal for the migration and proliferation of epidermal cells. Local release of EGF, TGF-α, and KGF and increased expression of their receptors may also stimulate these processes. Topical application of KGF-2 in young and aged animals accelerates reepithelialization. Basement membrane proteins, such as laminin, reappear in a highly ordered sequence from the margin of the wound inward. After the wound is completely reepithelialized, the cells become columnar and stratified again, while firmly attaching to the reestablished basement membrane and underlying dermis.

Extracellular Matrix

The ECM exists as a scaffold to stabilize the physical structure of tissues, but it also plays an active and complex role by regulating the behavior of cells that contact it. Cells within it produce the macromolecular constituents, including (1) glycosaminoglycans (GAGs), or polysaccharide chains, usually found covalently linked to protein in the form of proteoglycans, and (2) fibrous proteins such as collagen, elastin, fibronectin, and laminin.

In connective tissue, proteoglycan molecules form a gel-like ground substance. This highly hydrated gel allows the matrix to withstand compressive force while permitting rapid diffusion of nutrients, metabolites, and hormones between blood and tissue cells. Collagen fibers within the matrix serve to organize and strengthen it, whereas elastin fibers give it resilience, and matrix proteins have adhesive functions.

The wound matrix accumulates and changes in composition as healing progresses, balanced between new deposition and degradation (Fig. 6-4). The provisional matrix is a scaffold for cellular migration and is composed of fibrin, fibrinogen, fibronectin, and vitronectin. GAGs and proteoglycans are synthesized next and support further matrix deposition and remodeling. Collagens, which are the predominant scar proteins, are the end result. Attachment proteins, such as fibrin and fibronectin, provide linkage to the ECM through binding to cell surface integrin receptors.

Stimulation of fibroblasts by growth factors induces upregulated expression of integrin receptors, facilitating cell-matrix interactions. Ligand binding induces clustering of integrin into focal adhesion sites. Regulation of integrin-mediated cell signaling by the extracellular divalent cations Mg^{2+}, Mn^{2+}, and Ca^{2+} perhaps is caused by induction of conformational changes in the integrins.

A dynamic and reciprocal relationship exists between fibroblasts and the ECM. Cytokine regulation of fibroblast responses is altered by variations in the composition of the ECM. For example, expression of matrix-degrading enzymes, such as the MMPs, is upregulated after cytokine stimulation of fibroblasts. Collagenolytic MMP-1 is induced by IL-1 and downregulated by TGF-β. Activation of plasminogen to plasmin by plasminogen activator and procollagenase to collagenase by plasmin results in matrix degradation and facilitates cell migration. Modulation of these processes provides additional mechanisms whereby the cell-matrix interaction can be regulated during wound healing. Matrix modulation is also seen in tumor metastasis. Neoplastic cells lose their dependence on anchorage, mediated mainly by integrins; this is probably caused by decreased production of fibronectin and subsequent decreased adhesion and, as a result, these cells can break away from the primary tumor and metastasize.

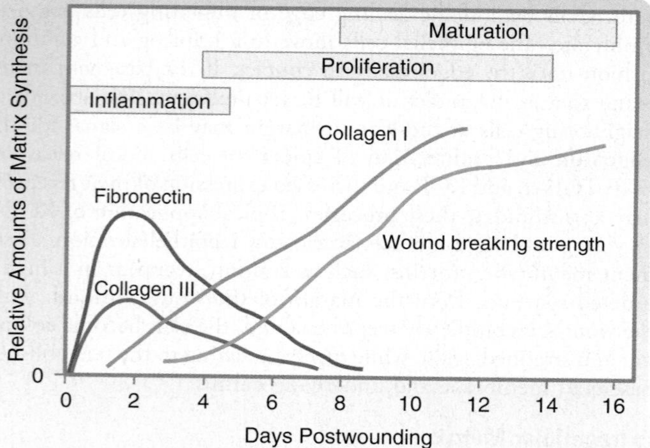

FIGURE 6-4 Wound matrix deposition over time. Fibronectin and type III collagen constitute the early matrix. Type I collagen accumulates later and corresponds to the increase in wound-breaking strength. (Adapted from Witte MB, Barbul A: General principles of wound healing. *Surg Clin North Am* 77:509–528, 1997.)

An example of the necessary dynamic interactions occurring in the provisional matrix during wound healing is the effect of TGF-β on incisional wounds sealed with fibrin sealant. Fibrin sealant is a derivative of plasma components that mimics the last step in the coagulation cascade. Commercially available fibrin sealant has an approximately 10-fold greater concentration of fibrin than plasma and consequently provides a more airtight, waterproof seal. Fibrin sealant may serve as a mechanical barrier to the early cell-mediated events occurring in wound healing. Supplementation of fibrin sealant with TGF-β has been demonstrated to reverse the inhibitory effects of fibrin sealant on wound healing and increase tensile strength compared with sutured wounds. The increased tensile strength may be a result of improved cell migration into the wound site, more rapid clearance of fibrin sealant, suppression of gelatinase (MMP-9), and enhancement of ECM synthesis in TGF-β–supplemented wounds.

Collagen structure. Collagens are found in all multicellular animals and are secreted by various cell types. They are a major component of skin and bone and constitute 25% of the total protein mass in mammals. The proline-rich and glycine-rich collagen molecule is a long, stiff, triple-stranded helical structure that consists of three collagen polypeptide α chains wound around one another in a ropelike superhelix. With its ringlike structure, proline provides stability to the helical conformation in each α chain, whereas glycine, because of its small size, allows tight packing of the three α chains to form the final superhelix. There are at least 20 types of collagen, the main constituents of connective tissue being types I, II, III, V, and XI. Type I is the principal collagen of skin and bone and is the most common. In adults, the skin is approximately 80% type I and 20% type III. In newborns, the content of type III collagen is greater than that found in adults. In early wound healing, there is also increased expression of type III collagen. Type I collagens are the fibrillar, or fibril-forming, collagens. They are secreted into the extracellular space, where they assemble into collagen fibrils (10 to 300 nm in diameter), which then aggregate into larger, cable-like bundles called collagen fibers (several micrometers in diameter).

Other types of collagens include types IX and XII (fibril-associated collagens) and types IV and VII (network-forming collagens). Types IX and XII are found on the surface of collagen fibrils and serve to link the fibrils to one another and to other components in the ECM. Type IV molecules assemble into a meshlike pattern and are a major part of the mature basal lamina. Dimers of type VII form anchoring fibrils that help attach the basal lamina to the underlying connective tissue and are especially abundant in the skin.

Type XVII and type XVIII collagens are two of a number of collagen-like proteins. Type XVII has a transmembrane domain and is found in hemidesmosomes. Type XVIII is located in the basal laminae of blood vessels. The peptide endostatin, which inhibits angiogenesis and shows promise as an anticancer drug, is formed by cleavage of the C-terminal domain of type XVIII collagen.

Collagen synthesis. Collagen polypeptide chains are synthesized on membrane-bound ribosomes and enter the endoplasmic reticulum (ER) lumen as pro–α chains (Fig. 6-5). These precursors have amino-terminal signal peptides to direct them to the ER as well as propeptides at the N-terminal and C-terminal ends. Within the lumen of the ER, some of the prolines and lysines undergo hydroxylation to form hydroxyproline and

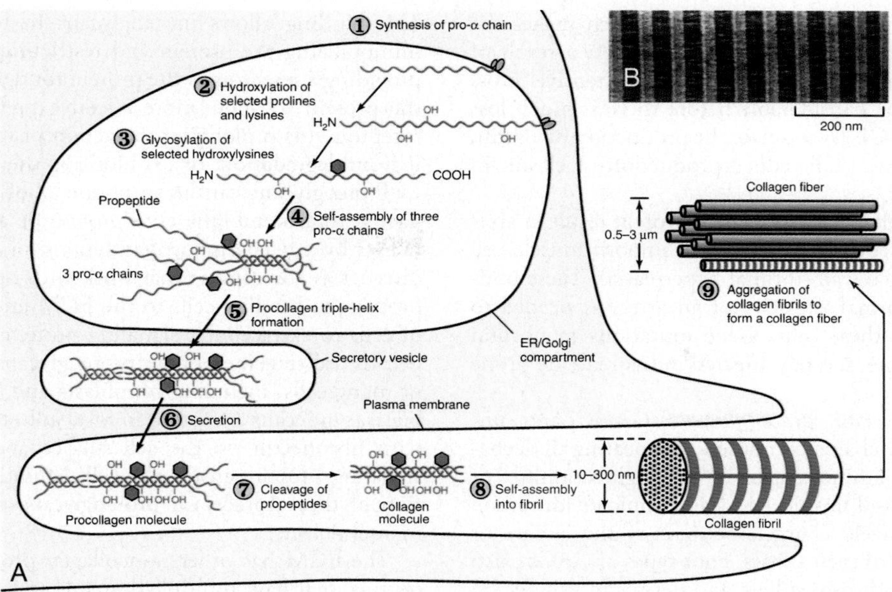

FIGURE 6-5 Intracellular and extracellular events in the formation of a collagen fibril. **A,** Collagen fibrils are shown assembling in the extracellular space contained within a large infolding in the plasma membrane. As one example of how collagen fibrils can form ordered arrays in the extracellular space, they are shown further assembling into large collagen fibers, which are visible with a light microscope. The covalent cross links that stabilize the extracellular assemblies are not shown. **B,** Electron micrograph of a negatively stained collagen fibril revealing its typical striated appearance. *ER,* Endoplasmic reticulum. (**A,** From Alberts B, Johnson A, Lewis J, et al [eds]: *Molecular biology of the cell,* ed 4, New York, 2002, Garland, p 1100; **B,** Courtesy Robert Horne.)

hydroxylysine. Hydroxylation results in the stable triple-stranded helix through the formation of interchain hydrogen bonds. The pro–α chain then combines with two others to form procollagen, a hydrogen-bonded, triple-stranded helical molecule. In conditions such as vitamin C (ascorbic acid) deficiency (scurvy), proline hydroxylation is prevented, resulting in the formation of unstable triple helices secondary to the synthesis of defective pro–α chains. Vitamin C deficiency is characterized by the gradual loss of preexisting normal collagen, which leads to fragile blood vessels and loose teeth.

After secretion into the ECM, specific proteases cleave the propeptides of the procollagen molecules to form collagen monomers. These monomers assemble to form collagen fibrils in the ECM, driven by the tendency of collagen to self-assemble. Covalent cross linking of the lysine residues provides tensile strength. The extent and type of cross linking vary from tissue to tissue. In tissues such as tendons, in which tensile strength is crucial, collagen cross linking is extremely high. In mammalian skin, the fibrils are organized in a basketweave pattern to resist multidirectional tensile stress. In tendons, fibrils are in parallel bundles aligned along the major axis of tension.

Numerous factors can affect collagen synthesis. Vitamin C (ascorbic acid), TGF-β, IGF-I, and IGF-II increase collagen synthesis. IFN-γ decreases type I procollagen mRNA synthesis, and glucocorticoids inhibit procollagen gene transcription, leading to decreased collagen synthesis.

Several genetic disorders are caused by abnormalities in collagen fibril formation. In osteogenesis imperfecta, deletion of one procollagen α_1 allele results in weak, easily fractured bones. Ehlers-Danlos syndrome is a result of mutations affecting type III collagen and is characterized by fragile skin and blood vessels and hypermobile joints.

Elastic fibers. Tissues such as skin, blood vessels, and lungs require strength and elasticity to function. Elastic fibers in the ECM of these tissues provide the resilience to allow recoil after transient stretching.

Elastic fibers are predominantly composed of elastin, a highly hydrophobic protein (≈750 amino acids long). Soluble tropoelastin is secreted into the extracellular space, where it forms lysine cross links to other tropoelastin molecules to generate a large network of elastin fibers and sheets. Elastin is composed of hydrophobic and alanine-rich and lysine-rich α-helical segments that alternate along the polypeptide chain. The hydrophobic segments are responsible for the elastic properties of the molecule. The alanine-rich and lysine-rich α-helical segments form cross links between adjacent molecules. Although the proposed conformation of elastin molecules is controversial, the predominant theory is that the elastin polypeptide chain adopts a random coil conformation that allows the network to stretch and recoil like a rubber band. Elastic fibers consist of an elastin core covered by a sheath of microfibrils, which are composed of several distinct glycoproteins such as fibrillin. Elastin-binding fibrillin is essential for integrity of the elastic fibers.

Microfibrils appear before elastin in developing tissues and seem to form a scaffold on which the secreted elastin molecules are deposited. Elastin is produced early in life, stabilizes, and does not undergo much further synthesis or degradation, with a turnover that approaches the life span. Age-related modification is a result of progressive degradation as the elastic fibers gradually become tortuous, frayed, and porous. Scanning electron microscopy shows that, in humans, the elastic meshwork grows largely undistorted during postnatal growth, during which fibers seem to enlarge in synchrony with growth of the tissue. In circumstances not involving a wound, there is little elastin degradation, probably because of the hydrophobic nature of elastin, which makes the interior of this highly folded protein inaccessible. As a result of this high degree of three-dimensionality and extensive cross linking, cleavage must be considerable before there is much loss of elasticity. IGF-I and TGF-β stimulate the production of elastin. Glucocorticoids and basic FGF reduce production of elastin in adult skin cells.

Mutations causing a deficiency of elastin protein result in arterial narrowing as a consequence of excessive smooth muscle cell proliferation in the arterial wall (intimal hyperplasia). These findings suggest that the normal elasticity of an artery is needed to prevent proliferation of these cells. Gene mutations in fibrillin result in Marfan syndrome; severely affected individuals are prone to aortic rupture.

Glycosaminoglycans and proteoglycans. GAGs are unbranched polysaccharide chains composed of repeating disaccharide units, a sulfated amino sugar (*N*-acetylglucosamine or *N*-acetylgalactosamine) and uronic acid (glucuronic or iduronic). GAGs are highly negatively charged because of the sulfate or carboxyl groups on most of their sugars. Four types of GAGs exist: (1) hyaluronan, (2) chondroitin sulfate and dermatan sulfate, (3) heparan sulfate, and (4) keratan sulfate.

GAGs in connective tissue usually constitute less than 10% of the weight of fibrous proteins. Their highly negative charge attracts osmotically active cations, such as Na^+, which causes large amounts of water to be incorporated into the matrix. This results in porous hydrated gels and is responsible for the turgor that enables the matrix to withstand compressive force.

Hyaluronan is the simplest GAG. It is composed of repeating nonsulfated disaccharide units and is found in adult tissues, but it is especially prevalent in fetal tissues. Its abundance in fetal wounds is believed to be a factor in the scarless wound healing seen in fetal tissues. In contrast to the other GAGs, hyaluronan is not covalently attached to any protein and is synthesized directly from the cell surface by an enzyme complex embedded in the plasma membrane.

Hyaluronan plays several different roles because of its large hydration shell. It is produced in large quantities during wound healing, during which it facilitates cell migration by physically expanding the ECM and allowing cells additional space for migration; it also reduces the strength of adhesion of migrating cells to matrix fibers. Hyaluronan synthesized from the basal side of epithelium creates a cell-free space for cell migration, such as during embryogenesis and formation of the heart and other organs. When cell migration is finished, the excess hyaluronan is degraded by hyaluronidase. Studies using hyaluronic acid derivative have suggested that these derivatives can accelerate wound healing in burns, surgical wounds, and chronic wounds.[4]

Proteoglycans are a diverse group of glycoproteins with functions mediated by their core proteins and GAG chains. The number and types of GAGs attached to the core protein can vary greatly, and the GAGs themselves can be modified by sulfonation. Because of their GAGs, proteoglycans provide hydrated space around and between cells. They also form gels of different pore size and charge density to regulate the movement of cells and molecules. Perlecan, a heparan sulfate proteoglycan, plays this role in the basal lamina of the kidney glomerulus. Decreased levels of perlecan are believed to play a role in diabetic albuminuria.

Proteoglycans function in chemical signaling by binding various secreted signal molecules, such as growth factors, and modulating their signaling activity. Proteoglycans also can bind other secreted proteins, such as proteases and protease inhibitors. This binding allows proteoglycans to regulate proteins by (1) immobilizing the protein and restricting its range of action, (2) providing a reservoir of the protein for delayed release, (3) altering the protein to allow more effective presentation to cell surface receptors, (4) prolonging the action of the protein by protecting it from degradation, or (5) blocking the activity of the protein.

Proteoglycans can be components of plasma membranes and have a transmembrane core protein or are attached to the lipid bilayer by a glycosylphosphatidylinositol anchor. These proteoglycans act as coreceptors that work with other cell surface receptor proteins in binding cells to the ECM and initiating the response of cells to extracellular signaling proteins. For example, the syndecans are transmembrane proteoglycans located on the surface of many cells, including fibroblasts and epithelial cells. In fibroblasts, syndecans are found in focal adhesions, where they interact with fibronectin on the cell surface and with cytoskeletal and signaling proteins inside the cell. Mutations leading to inactivation of these coreceptor proteoglycans result in severe developmental defects.

The ECM has other noncollagen proteins, such as the fibronectins, that have multiple domains and can bind to other matrix macromolecules and cell surface receptors. These interactions help organize the matrix and facilitate cell attachment. Fibronectin is important in animal embryogenesis.

Fibronectin exists as soluble and fibrillar isoforms. Soluble plasma fibronectin circulates in various body fluids and enhances blood clotting, wound healing, and phagocytosis. The highly insoluble fibrillar forms assemble on cell surfaces and are deposited in the ECM. The fibronectin fibrils that form on the surface of fibroblasts are usually coupled with neighboring intracellular actin stress fibers. The actin filaments promote assembly of the fibronectin fibril and influence fibril orientation. Integrin transmembrane adhesion proteins mediate these interactions. The contractile actin and myosin cytoskeleton pulls on the fibronectin matrix and generates tension.

Basal lamina. Basal laminae are flexible, thin (40 to 120 nm) mats of specialized ECM that separate cells and epithelia from the underlying or surrounding connective tissue. In skin, the basal lamina is tethered to the underlying connective tissue by specialized anchoring fibrils. This composite of basal lamina and collagen is the basement membrane.

The basal lamina acts in numerous ways: (1) as a molecular filter to prevent the passage of macromolecules (i.e., in the kidney glomerulus), (2) as a selective barrier to certain cells (i.e., the lamina beneath the epithelium prevents fibroblasts from contacting epithelial cells but does not stop macrophages or lymphocytes), (3) as a scaffold for regenerating cells to migrate, and (4) as an important element in tissue regeneration in locations where the basal lamina survives.

Although composition may vary from tissue to tissue, most mature basal laminae contain type IV collagen, perlecan, and the glycoproteins laminin and nidogen. Type IV collagen has a more flexible structure than the fibrillar collagens; its triple-stranded helix is interrupted, allowing multiple bends.

Laminins generally consist of three long polypeptide chains (α, β, and γ). Mice lacking the laminin γ_1 chain die during embryogenesis because they cannot make a basal lamina. The laminin in basement membranes consists of several domains that bind to perlecan, nidogen, and laminin receptor proteins found on cell surfaces. The type IV collagen and laminin networks are connected by nidogen and perlecan, which act as stabilizing bridges. Many of the cell surface receptors for type IV collagen and laminin are members of the integrin family. Another important type of laminin receptor is dystroglycan, a transmembrane protein that together with integrins may organize assembly of the basal lamina.

Degradation of the extracellular matrix. Regulated turnover of the ECM is crucial to many biologic processes. ECM degradation occurs during metastasis when neoplastic cells migrate from their site of origin to distant organs via the bloodstream or lymphatics. In injury or infection, localized degradation of the ECM occurs so that cells can migrate across the basal lamina to reach the site of injury or infection. Locally secreted cellular proteases, such as MMPs or serine proteases, degrade the ECM components. Matrix proteolysis helps the cell migrate by (1) clearing a path through the matrix; (2) exposing binding sites, promoting cell binding or migration; (3) facilitating cell detachment so that a cell can move forward; and (4) releasing signal proteins that promote cell migration.

Proteolysis is tightly regulated. Many proteases are secreted as inactive precursors that are activated when required. In addition, cell surface receptors bind these proteases to ensure that they act only on sites where they are needed. Finally, protease inhibitors, such as tissue inhibitors of metalloproteinase (TIMP), can bind these enzymes and block their activity.

Maturational Phase

Wound contraction occurs by centripetal movement of the whole thickness of the surrounding skin and reduces the amount of disorganized scar. In contrast, wound contracture is a physical constriction or limitation of function and is a result of the process of wound contraction. Contractures occur when excessive scar exceeds normal wound contraction, and it results in a functional disability. Examples of contractures are scars that traverse joints and prevent extension and scars that involve the eyelid or mouth and cause an ectropion.

Wound contraction appears to take place as a result of a complex interaction of the extracellular materials and fibroblasts that is not completely understood. Using a fibroblast-populated collagen lattice, Ehrlich demonstrated that aborted cell locomotion appears to cause bunching and contraction of the collagen fibers. In this in vitro model, trypsinized collagen is populated by fibroblasts that adhere to it in culture. If normal dermal fibroblasts are cultured, they attempt to move but are trapped by the collagen fibers. The tractional forces cause the lattice to bunch and contract.

Numerous studies have shown that fibroblasts in a contracting wound undergo change to stimulated cells, termed *myofibroblasts*. These cells have function and structure in common with fibroblasts and smooth muscle cells and express alpha smooth muscle actin in bundles termed *stress fibers*. The actin appears at day 6 after wounding, persists at high levels for 15 days, and is gone by 4 weeks, when the cell undergoes apoptosis. It appears that a stimulated fibroblast develops contractile ability related to the formation of cytoplasmic actin-myosin complexes. When this stimulated cell is placed in the fibroblast-populated collagen lattice, contraction occurs even more quickly. The tension that is exerted by the fibroblasts' attempt at contraction appears to stimulate the actin-myosin structures in their cytoplasm. If colchicine, which inhibits microtubules, or cytochalasin D, which inhibits microfilaments, is added to the tissue culture, the result is minimal contraction of the collagen gels. Fibroblasts develop a linear arrangement in the line of tension that, when removed, causes the cells to round up.

Stimulated fibroblasts, or myofibroblasts, are found to be a constant feature present in abundance in diseases involving excessive fibrosis, including hepatic cirrhosis, renal and pulmonary fibrosis, Dupuytren's contracture, and desmoplastic reactions induced by neoplasia. The actin microfilaments are arranged linearly along the long axis of the fibroblast. They are associated with dense bodies that allow attachment to the surrounding ECM. Fibronexus is the attachment entity that connects the cytoskeleton to the ECM and spans the cell membrane in doing so.

MMPs also appear to be important for wound contraction. It has been demonstrated that stromelysin-1 (MMP-3) strongly affects wound contraction. MMPs may be necessary to allow cleavage of the attachment between the fibroblast and the collagen so that the lattice can be made to contract. Different populations of fibroblasts, from different organs, respond to the contraction stimulus in a heterogeneous fashion. It is likely that the stromelysin-1, with the participation of β_1 integrins, allows modification of attachment sites between fibroblasts and the collagen fibrils. Similarly, cytokines such as TGF-β_1 affect contraction by increasing the expression of β_1 integrin.

Remodeling

The fibroblast population decreases, and the dense capillary network regresses. Wound strength increases rapidly within 1 to 6 weeks and then appears to plateau up to 1 year after the injury (see Fig. 6-5). Compared with nonwounded skin, tensile strength is only 30% in the scar. An increase in breaking strength occurs after approximately 21 days, mostly as a result of cross linking. Although collagen cross linking causes further wound contraction and an increase in strength, it also results in a scar that is more brittle and less elastic than normal skin. In contrast to normal skin, the epidermodermal interface in a healed wound is devoid of rete pegs, the undulating projections of epidermis that penetrate into the papillary dermis. Loss of this anchorage results in increased fragility and predisposes the neoepidermis to avulsion after minor trauma.

ABNORMAL WOUND HEALING

In such a complex series of interweaving events as wound healing, many factors can impede the outcome (Box 6-1). The amount of tissue lost or damaged, amount of foreign material or bacterial inoculation, and length of exposure to toxic factors can affect the time to recovery. Intrinsic factors such as age, chemotherapeutic agents, atherosclerosis, cardiac or renal failure, and location on the body all affect wound healing. Ultimately, the type of scar—whether it is adequate, inadequate, or proliferative—is dictated by the amount of collagen deposition and balanced by the amount of collagen degradation. If the balance is tipped in either direction, the result is poor.

Hypertrophic Scars and Keloids

Keloids and hypertrophic scars are proliferative scars characterized by excessive net collagen deposition (Fig. 6-6). Keloids, by definition, grow beyond the borders of the original wounds and rarely regress with time; they are more prevalent in darkly pigmented skin, developing in 15% to 20% of African Americans, Asians, and Hispanics. There is strong evidence suggesting a genetic susceptibility, including familial heritability, common occurrence in twins, and high prevalence in certain ethnic populations. Shih and Bayat[5] suggest a strong multigenetic disposition to keloid

BOX 6-1 Factors That Inhibit Wound Healing

Infection
Ischemia
- Circulation
- Respiration
- Local tension

Diabetes mellitus
Ionizing radiation
Advanced age
Malnutrition
Vitamin deficiencies
- Vitamin C
- Vitamin A

Mineral deficiencies
- Zinc
- Iron

Exogenous drugs
- Doxorubicin (Adriamycin)
- Glucocorticosteroids

formation with a varied inheritance pattern that is predominantly autosomal dominant. Proposed pathways include apoptosis, mitogen-activated protein kinase, TGF-β, IL-6, and plasminogen activator inhibitor-1.

Keloids occur above the clavicles, on the trunk, on the upper extremities, and on the face. They cannot be prevented and are frequently refractory to medical and surgical intervention. Hypertrophic scars are raised scars within the confines of the original wound and frequently regress spontaneously.

Keloids and hypertrophic scars differ histologically from normal scars. Hypertrophic scars primarily contain well-organized type III collagen, whereas keloids contain disorganized type I and type III collagen bundles.[6] Keloids and hypertrophic scars have stretched collagen bundles aligned in the same plane as the epidermis, whereas collagen bundles are randomly arrayed and relaxed in normal scars. Keloid scars have thicker, abundant collagen bundles that form acellular nodelike structures in the deep dermis with a paucity of cells centrally. Hypertrophic scars, in contrast, contain islands composed of aggregates of fibroblasts, small vessels, and collagen fibers throughout the dermis.[5]

Hypertrophic scars are often preventable. Prolonged inflammation and insufficient resurfacing, (e.g., burn wounds) promote hypertrophic scarring. Scars perpendicular to the underlying muscle fibers tend to be flatter and narrower, with less collagen formation than when they are parallel to the underlying muscle fibers. Tension appears to signal the formation of activated fibroblasts resulting in excessive collagen deposition. The position of an elective scar can be chosen to induce a narrower, less obvious healed scar. As muscle fibers contract, the wound edges become reapproximated when they are perpendicular to the underlying muscle and tend to gape if placed parallel to it, leading to greater wound tension and scar formation.

Hypertrophic scars represent a reversible hyperproliferative scar phenotype that regresses when the original stimulus (skin tension, stimulatory growth factors) are removed. Keloids appear to be genetically predisposed and switched on irreversibly by factors such as TGF-β. Expression of the isoforms TGF-β_1 and TGF-β_2 is increased in human keloid cells compared with normal human dermal fibroblasts. Hypertrophic scar fibroblasts produce more TGF-β_1. In addition, in these scars, collagen synthesis is elevated, whereas collagen degradation is low. MMPs are also affected in these scars: MMP-1 (collagenase) and MMP-9 (gelatinase, early tissue repair) are decreased, whereas MMP-2 (gelatinase, late tissue remodeling) is significantly elevated. Blocking TGF-β activity with antibodies decreases scar fibrosis. Growth factors have also been implicated in fibrosis and have been studied as targets for the blockade of fibrosis. IFN-γ, which suppresses collagen synthesis, has been tested clinically in keloid scars and has produced an average 30% reduction in scar thickness.

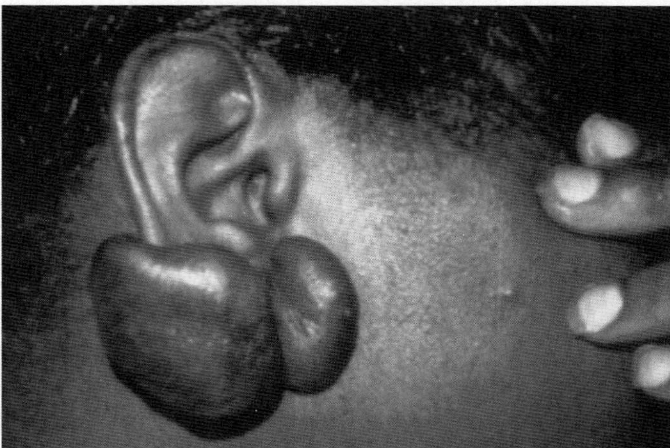

FIGURE 6-6 Keloids caused by ear piercing.

Prevention of Hypertrophic or Keloid Scars

The three strategies that reduce adverse scarring immediately after wound closure are tension relief, hydration/occlusion, and use of taping/pressure garments. Wounds with greater tension (perpendicular to Langer's lines), with excessive tension on closure, and in certain anatomic locations (deltoid and sternal) are at a higher risk of adverse scarring. Scarring can be reduced by postsurgical taping of the wound for 3 months. Moisturizing lotions and moisture-retentive dressings (silicone sheets and gels) can reduce the thickness, discomfort, and itching and improve the appearance of the scar. After wound healing, water still evaporates more rapidly through scar tissue and may take more than a year to recover to prewound levels. Silicone products may ameliorate evaporative losses and assist hydration of the stratum corneum. These strategies need to be employed soon after initial wound healing. Pressure garments should be used prophylactically in wounds that are wide (e.g., burns); these wounds may take more than 2 or 3 weeks to heal. Garments should be applied as soon as the wound is closed and the patient can tolerate the pressure.[7] Avoidance of sun exposure and use of SPF 50+ sunscreens for 1 year postoperatively reduces scar hyperpigmentation and improves clinical appearance.

Linear Hypertrophic Scars

Early linear scar hypertrophy (e.g., after trauma or surgery) at 6 weeks to 3 months should be treated with pressure therapy. After 6 months, silicone therapy should be continued for as long as necessary if there is further scar maturation. Ongoing hypertrophy may be treated with intralesional corticosteroids (triamcinolone acetonide, 10 to 40 mg/mL) injected into the papillary dermis every 2 to 4 weeks until flat.[8] This is the only invasive management option that has enough supporting evidence to be recommended in evidence-based guidelines. Approximately 50% to 100% of patients respond, and 9% to 50% experience recurrence.[8] Adverse steroid effects include skin atrophy, hypopigmentation, telangiectasias,[8] and excessive pain during injections. Injections should be limited to the scar itself to minimize adjacent fat atrophy.

Surgical scar revision may be considered for permanent linear hypertrophic scars present after 1 year.[9] Simple resection and primary closure may be combined with adjacent tissue undermining, subcutaneous sutures, adjunctive Z-plasty, and postsurgical taping and silicone therapy.

Hypertrophic scars also can be seen in conjunction with a scar contracture. Scar contractures are abnormal shortening of nonmatured scars resulting in functional impairment, particularly if the scar is across a joint. Correction of a scar contracture generally requires surgery with Z-plasty, skin graft, or flap to release tension in the scar to restore function and reduce scar hypertrophy.

Widespread Hypertrophic Scars

Severe burns, mechanical trauma, necrotizing infections, wounds requiring more than 2 to 3 weeks to heal, or wounds healed with skin grafting require early application of silicone and compression therapy.[7] This therapy should be initiated as soon as the wound is closed and the patient can tolerate the pressure.

The mechanism of action of pressure therapy is poorly understood but may involve reduction of wound oxygen tension by occlusion of small blood vessels resulting in a decrease of myofibroblast proliferation and collagen synthesis. Pressure therapy is believed to act on cellular mechanoreceptors that are involved in cellular apoptosis and linked to the ECM. The increased pressure regulates apoptosis of dermal fibroblasts and diminishes hypertrophic scarring. In addition, sensory nerve cells transduce mechanical pressure into intracellular biochemical and gene expression, synthesizing and releasing different cytokines involved in the physiopathogenesis of proliferative scarring.[10]

Pressure and silicone therapy should be continued or intensified and combined with selective localized corticosteroid injections in resistant areas. Bleomycin, 5-fluorouracil, and verapamil have been used as adjuncts to corticosteroid therapy.[11] Laser therapy, although invasive, is another potentially useful adjunct to reduce scar thickness; resurface scar texture; and treat residual redness, telangiectasias, or hyperpigmentation.

Early surgery is indicated for functional impairment. Burn scar contracture release procedures in the neck and axilla are best performed with flaps to improve functional and cosmetic outcomes further that may not be achievable with skin grafts. Widespread large hypertrophic scars may require serial excision or tissue expansion.

Keloids

First-line treatments include silicones in combination with pressure therapy and intralesional corticosteroid injections. Intralesional 5-fluorouracil, bleomycin, and verapamil should be used in accordance with established treatment protocols.[8] Refractory cases after 12 months of therapy should be considered for surgical excision in combination with adjuvant therapy. Excision alone results in a high recurrence rate of 50% to 100% and enlargement of the keloid.[8] Immediate postoperative electron beam irradiation or brachytherapy with iridium-192 reduces recurrence rates[12] but may hypothetically be associated with radiation damage to adjacent tissues or induction of malignancy. However, in an extensive review of the literature, Ogawa and colleagues[13] concluded that the risk of malignancy attributable to keloid radiation therapy is minimal. An additional promising new invasive treatment modality is internal cryotherapy, in which a metal rod is introduced into the keloid and the subsequent extreme cooling leads to tissue necrosis; one study demonstrated a 54% reduction in scar volume without recurrence. Finally, imiquimod 5%, a topical immunomodulator that stimulates interferon production to increase collagen degradation, has been shown, in combination with surgical excision, to result in low keloid recurrence rates (0 to 29%) in some studies but high recurrence rates (89%) in others.[14]

Although existing strategies for the management of hypertrophic scars and keloids are broadly similar, the histologic differences between the two scars suggest that, in the future, therapeutic approaches could be developed that are specifically tailored for these different types of scars. However, at the present time, there is no single proven best therapy for the management of these excessive healing scars, and the large number of treatment options reflects this (Table 6-3).[8]

Chronic Nonhealing Wounds

By definition, chronic wounds are wounds that have failed to proceed through an orderly and timely reparative process to produce anatomic and functional integrity over a period of 3 months. In the United States, it is estimated that 2 to 3 million patients per year are at risk of developing diabetic ulcers, 600,000 patients per year develop chronic leg ulcers secondary to venous insufficiency, and 1 to 3 million patients per year develop pressure ulcers secondary to immobility. These numbers are likely to increase as a result of an aging population and the rising incidence of risk factors for atherosclerotic disease, such as diabetes mellitus and smoking. These wounds are a significant challenge to health care professionals and an immense burden on health care systems and the economy. Patients also report reduced quality of life and social isolation.

Numerous common factors promote adverse wound healing conditions (see Fig. 6-1). Systemic factors, such as malnutrition, aging, tissue hypoxia, and diabetes, contribute significantly to the pathogenesis of chronic wounds. A combination of systemic and localized adverse wound factors collectively overwhelm the normal healing processes, resulting in a hostile wound healing environment (Fig. 6-7).[15]

Chronic wounds do not occur in animals, and understanding of chronic wounds has come from human studies limited to observation, biopsy, and wound exudate analyses. Chronic wounds have derangements in the various stages of wound healing and have unusually elevated or depressed levels of cytokines, growth factors, or proteinases. Chronic wound fluid, in contrast to acute wound fluid, has been shown to have greater levels of IL-1, IL-6, and TNF-α; levels of these proinflammatory cytokines decreased as the wound healed. An inverse relationship between TNF-α and essential growth factors, such as EGF and PDGF, has been demonstrated.

Chronic wounds typically exhibit powerful proinflammatory stimuli, including bacterial colonization, necrotic tissue, foreign bodies, and localized tissue hypoxia. Tissue edema is significant, and the distance between capillaries is increased, reducing oxygen diffusion to individual cells. Chronic wounds typically have high bacterial counts, which stimulates an inflammatory host response with PMNs expressing reactive oxygen species and proteases resulting in a highly pro-oxidant environment. Disturbed oxidant balance is the likely key factor in the amplification and persistence

TABLE 6-3 Prevention and Treatment Options for Keloids and Hypertrophic Scars

MODALITY OR TREATMENT OPTION	RESPONSE RATE (%)	RECURRENCE RATE (%)	COMMENTS	STUDY DESIGN
Prevention				
Preventive silicone sheeting (postsurgery)	0-75	25-36	Multiple preparations available; tolerated by children; expensive; avoid on open wounds; poor study design	Review of multiple case studies
Postsurgical intralesional corticosteroid injection (triamcinolone acetonide [Kenalog], 10-40 mg/mL at 6-wk intervals)	NA	0-100 (mean, 50)	Patient acceptance and safety; may cause hypopigmentation, skin atrophy, telangiectasia	Review of multiple case studies
Postsurgical topical imiquimod, 5% cream (Aldara)	NA	28	May cause hyperpigmentation, irritation	Case study
Postsurgical fluorouracil, triamcinolone acetonide, and pulsed dye lasers (best outcomes)	70 at 12 wk	NA	Effective; may cause hyperpigmentation, wound ulceration	Clinical trial
First-Line Treatment				
Cryotherapy	50-76	NA	Useful on small lesions; easy to perform; may cause hypopigmentation, pain	Review of multiple case studies
Intralesional corticosteroid injection (triamcinolone acetonide [Kenalog], 10-40 mg/mL at 6-wk intervals)	50-100	9-50	Inexpensive, requires multiple injections; may cause discomfort, skin atrophy, telangiectasia	Review of multiple case studies
Silicone elastomer sheeting	50-100	NA	Multiple preparations available; tolerated by children; expensive; poor study design	Review of multiple case studies
Pressure dressing (24-30 mm Hg) worn for 6-12 mo	90-100	NA	Inexpensive; difficult schedule; poor adherence	Review of multiple case studies
Surgical excision	NA	50-100	Z-plasty option for burns; immediate postsurgical treatment needed to prevent regrowth	Review of multiple case studies
Combined cryotherapy and intralesional corticosteroid injection	84	NA	See benefits of individual treatments; may cause hypopigmentation	Case study
Triple-keloid therapy (surgery, corticosteroids, silicone sheeting)	88 at 13 mo	12.5 at 13 mo	Tedious; time-intensive; expensive	Case study
Pulsed dye laser	NA	NA	Specialist referral needed; expensive; variable results depending on trial (controversial)	Case studies
Second-Line and Alternative Treatment				
Verapamil, 2.5 mg/mL, intralesional injection combined with perilesional excision and silicone sheeting	54 at 18 mo	NA	Repeated injections; limited experience; may cause discomfort	Clinical trial
Fluorouracil, 50 mg/mL, intralesional injection 2-3 times/wk	88	0	Effective; may cause hyperpigmentation, wound ulceration	Review of multiple case studies
Bleomycin tattooing, 1.5 IU/mL	92, 88	NA	Effective; may cause pulmonary fibrosis, cutaneous reactions	Review of case study; control trial
Postsurgical interferon-α2b, 1.5 million IU, intralesional injection bid for 4 days	30-50	8-19	Expensive; may cause pruritus, altered pigmentation, pain	Review of multiple case studies
Radiation therapy alone	56 (mean)	NA	Local growth inhibition; may cause cancer, hyperpigmentation, paresthesias	Review of multiple case studies
Postsurgical radiation therapy	76	NA	Local growth inhibition; may cause cancer	Review of multiple case studies
Onion extract topical gels (Mederma)	NA	NA	Limited effect alone, better in combination with silicone sheeting	Prospective case study

Adapted from Juckett G, Hartman-Adams H: Management of keloids and hypertrophic scars. *Am Fam Physician* 80:253–260, 2009.
NA, Not available.

of the inflammatory state in chronic wounds. In addition to direct cell membrane and ECM protein damage, PMN-derived reactive oxygen species, such as superoxide, hydroxyl radicals, and hydrogen peroxide, can selectively activate signaling pathways leading to activation of transcription factors that control expression of proinflammatory chemokines and cytokines such as IL-1, IL-6, TNF-α, and proteolytic enzymes such as MMPs and serine proteases. Bacterial components, including formyl methionyl peptides and extracellular adherence proteins, may also contribute to the upregulation of the inflammatory response.

The amount of normal wound ECM is determined by a dynamic balance among overall matrix synthesis, deposition, and

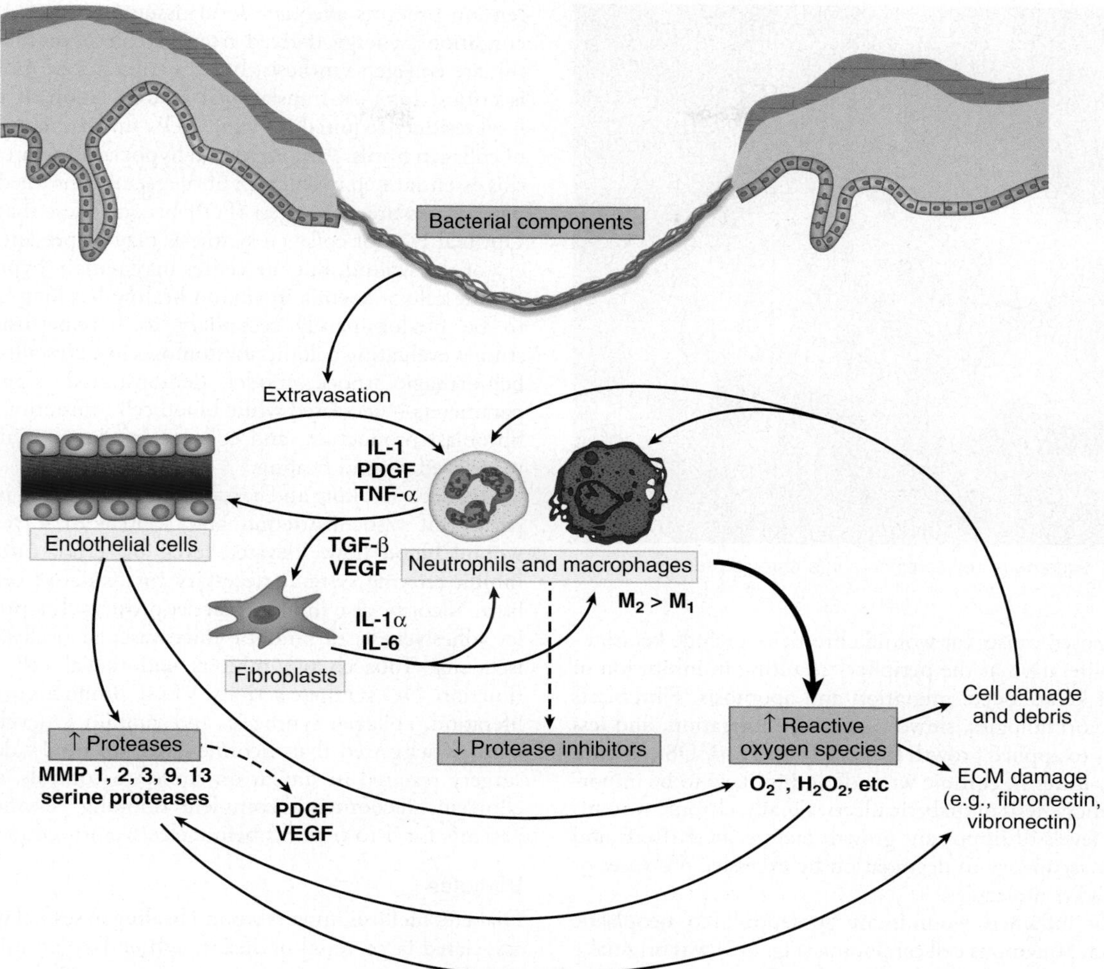

FIGURE 6-7 Mechanisms involved in the development and persistence of chronic wounds. Chronic wounds do not adequately complete the "normal" phases of wound healing. A state of chronic inflammation develops as many of the cells recruited to the wound in the proliferative phase of healing adopt a proinflammatory secretory profile. Inflammatory cells, particularly neutrophils and macrophages (M_1 phenotype > M_2 phenotype), persist in the wound, creating a highly pro-oxidant, protease-rich environment with an abundance of proinflammatory cytokines such as interleukin-1 (*IL-1*), interleukin-6 (*IL-6*), and tumor necrosis factor-α (*TNF-α*). The result is a hostile environment with downregulation of protease inhibitors and direct damage to extracellular matrix (*ECM*), cellular components, and protective growth factors such as platelet-derived growth factor (*PDGF*) and vascular endothelial growth factor (*VEGF*). Reactive oxygen species and proteases, such as matrix metalloproteinases (*MMP 1, 2, 3, 9, 13*), are the most significant deleterious influences. *Solid lines* indicate upregulation, and *dashed lines* indicate downregulation. Width of the line is proportional to the effect of the influence. *H_2O_2,* Hydrogen peroxide; *O_2^-,* superoxide; *TGF-β,* transforming growth factor-β. (From Greaves NS, Iqbal SA, Baguneid M, et al: The role of skin substitutes in the management of chronic cutaneous wounds. *Wound Repair Regen* 21:194–210, 2013.)

degradation. A defining feature of chronic wounds is unbalanced activity, which overwhelms tissue protective mechanisms. Although activated keratinocytes, fibroblasts, and endothelial cells have been shown to increase expression of proteases, incoming neutrophils and macrophages are considered to be the source of proteases, particularly cathepsin G, urokinase-type plasminogen activator, and neutrophil elastase. The expression and activity of gelatinases (MMP-2, MMP-9), collagenases (MMP-1, MMP-8), stromelysins (MMP-3, MMP-10, MMP-11), and membrane-type MMP (MT1-MMP) are upregulated in chronic venous ulcers.

Proinflammatory cytokines are potent inducers of MMP expression in chronic wounds, while also reducing TIMP expression, resulting in a relative excess of MMP activity. For example, α_1-proteinase inhibitor, α_2-macroglobulin, and components of the ECM, such as fibronectin and vibronectin, are downgraded or inactivated within chronic wounds. Growth factors, such as PDGF and VEGF, are also targeted when there is excess protease activity.

Shih and colleagues[16] demonstrated that genes such as insulin-like growth factor binding protein 2, collagen type XI alpha 1, inhibin beta A (*INHBA*), and thrombospondin 1 (*THBS1*) are dysregulated in chronic wounds. They found *INHBA* and *THBS1* upregulation to be characteristic biomarkers of senescent wounds or wounds that overexpress TGF-β. Both result in significant delays in wound healing.[16]

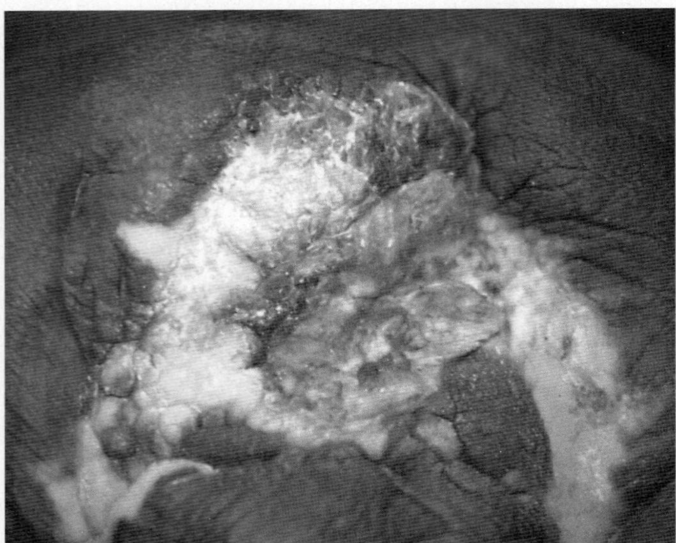

FIGURE 6-8 Squamous cell carcinoma in a chronic pressure sore.

Other proposed causes for wound chronicity include keratinocyte hyperproliferation at the periphery resulting in inhibition of fibroblast and keratinocyte migration and apoptosis. Fibroblasts have altered morphologies, slower rates of proliferation, and less responsiveness to applied growth factors. The CD4/CD8 cell ratio is significantly lower in chronic wounds and is likely to be important in the pathogenesis of diabetic ulcers. Finally, chronic wounds have reduced levels of important growth factors (FGF, EGF, and TGF-β) likely secondary to degradation by excessive proteases or trapping by ECM molecules.

Chronically inflamed wounds are susceptible to neoplastic transformation. Squamous cell carcinoma (Fig. 6-8) was originally reported in chronic burn scars by Marjolin. Chronic osteomyelitis, pressure sores, venous stasis ulcers, and hidradenitis may also develop neoplastic change. Biopsies should be performed in cases of chronic wounds that appear clinically atypical. Cutaneous wounds may first exhibit pseudoepitheliomatous hyperplasia—a premalignant condition. Such a diagnosis on biopsy should prompt additional biopsies to exclude squamous cell carcinoma, which may already be present in other areas of the wound.

Infection

Wound infection is the most common cause of healing delays. Bacterial counts exceeding 10^5 organisms per gram of tissue obtained by quantitative biopsy or the presence of virulent organisms, typically beta-hemolytic streptococci, would prevent wounds from healing by any means, including flap closure, skin graft placement, or primary suture. Bacterial infection prolongs the inflammatory phase and interferes with epithelialization, wound contraction, and collagen deposition. Bacterial endotoxins stimulate phagocytosis and release of collagenase, which degrades collagen and promotes destruction of surrounding normal tissue. Mechanical and antibiotic treatment is required to decrease the bacterial count, reduce inflammation, and allow wound closure to occur.

Other Causes of Abnormal Wound Healing

Hypoxia

Molecular oxygen is essential for collagen formation. Ischemia secondary to cardiac failure, arterial disease, or simple wound tension prevents adequate local tissue perfusion. Under hypoxic conditions, energy derived from glycolysis may be sufficient to initiate collagen synthesis, but the presence of molecular oxygen is critical for post-translational hydroxylation of the prolyl and lysyl residues required for triple-helix formation and cross linking of collagen fibrils. Although mild hypoxia stimulates angiogenesis, this essential step in collagen fibril assembly proceeds poorly when partial pressure of oxygen (PO_2) becomes less than 40 mm Hg. Optimal PO_2 for collagen synthesis may be present at the periphery of the wound, but the center may remain hypoxic.

The role of anemia in wound healing has long been attributed to be predominantly secondary to hypoperfusion. However, studies evaluating colonic anastomoses in a crystalloid-resuscitated hemorrhagic shock model demonstrated altered histologic parameters—decreased white blood cell infiltration, angiogenesis, fibroblast production, and collagen production, all contributing to delayed wound healing.

Tobacco smoking and consumption of tobacco products causes peripheral vasoconstriction and a 30% to 40% reduction in wound blood flow. Elevated levels of serum carbon monoxide inhibit enzyme systems necessary for oxidative cellular metabolism. Nicotine also inhibits platelet prostacyclin, promoting platelet adhesiveness, thrombotic microvascular occlusion, and tissue ischemia. Tobacco use inhibits endothelial cell and fibroblast function, NO synthase activity, VEGF production, fibroblast proliferation, collagen synthesis, and vitamin C levels.[17] Studies in animals suggested that nicotine cessation for 14 days before flap surgery resulted in similar outcomes to controls, although most clinicians recommend complete smoking cessation in human patients for 4 to 6 weeks before elective procedures.

Diabetes

Diabetes mellitus impairs wound healing in several ways. Diabetes-associated large vessel occlusion and end-organ microangiopathy each lead to tissue ischemia and infection. Diabetic sensory neuropathy leads to repeated trauma and unrelieved wound pressure. Tissue hypoxia can be demonstrated by reduced dorsal foot transcutaneous oxygen tension (TcO_2). The thickened capillary basement membrane decreases perfusion in the microenvironment, and elevated perivascular localization of albumin suggests increased capillary leak.

VEGF upregulation in patients with diabetes is also impaired.[18] Hypoxia is normally a potent upregulator of VEGF, but cells from patients with diabetes do not upregulate VEGF expression in response to hypoxia. Diabetic animals are unable to increase VEGF production after soft tissue ischemia[18] because of deficient transactivation by the transcription factor HIF-1α. HIF-1α mediates hypoxia-stimulated VEGF expression. With high glucose levels, decreased binding of HIF-1α to its coactivator p300 resulted in decreased HIF-1α functional activity. Covalent binding of the dicarbonyl metabolite methylglyoxal to p300 resulted in modification of p300 and was responsible for the decreased association of HIF-1α and p300. Administration of deferoxamine, an inhibitor of methylglyoxal conjugation, to diabetic mice resulted in normalization of HIF-1α–p300 interaction and transactivation of HIF-1α, with increased neovascularization and enhanced wound healing.

Sensory neuropathy in patients with diabetes predisposes them to repeated trauma. They are susceptible to infection because of an attenuated inflammatory response, impaired chemotaxis, and inefficient bacterial killing. Infection further increases local tissue metabolism, placing an additional burden on the tenuous blood supply, amplifying the risk for tissue necrosis. Lymphocyte and leukocyte function are impaired. Collagen degradation is increased, whereas collagen deposition is impaired. Collagen is brittle secondary to glycosylation in the ECM. In addition, collagen glycation diminishes focal adhesion formation between fibroblast and matrix resulting in decreased fibroblast migration.

Hyperglycemia causes increased advanced glycation end-products, which induce the production of inflammatory molecules (TNF-α, IL-1) and interfere with collagen synthesis. High glucose exposure also results in changes in cellular morphology, decreased proliferation, and abnormal differentiation of keratinocytes. Decreased chemotaxis, phagocytosis, bacterial killing, and reduced heat shock protein expression impair the early phase of wound healing in patients with diabetes. Altered leukocyte infiltration and wound fluid IL-6 characterize the late inflammatory phases of wound healing in these patients. Growth factors are abnormally expressed, degraded rapidly in wound fluids as a result of increased insulin degrading enzyme activity. Insulin degrading enzyme activity in wound fluid is positively correlated with hemoglobin A_{1c} levels. Elevated MMP and reduced TIMP levels are seen in diabetic wounds in a pattern similar to chronic wounds. Finally, there is increasing evidence that resident cells in chronic wounds undergo phenotypic changes that render them senescent and impair their capacity for proliferation and movement.

Ionizing Radiation

Ionizing radiation has its greatest effect on rapidly dividing cells in phases G_2 through M of the cell cycle. Injury to keratinocytes and fibroblasts impairs epithelialization and formation of granulation tissue during wound healing. Radiation injury in endothelial cells results in endarteritis, atrophy, fibrosis, and delayed tissue repair. Repetitive radiation injury results in repetitive inflammatory responses and ongoing cellular regeneration. Early side effects include erythema, dry desquamation, skin hyperpigmentation, and local hair loss. Late effects include skin atrophy, dryness, telangiectasia, dyschromia, dyspigmentation, fibrosis, and ulceration.[19] The inflammatory and proliferative phases may be disrupted by the early effects of radiation. Affected factors include TGF-β, VEGF, TNF-α, IFN-γ, and cytokines such as IL-1 and IL-8. These cytokines are overexpressed after the radiation injury leading to uncontrolled matrix accumulation and fibrosis. NO, which induces collagen deposition, is decreased in irradiated wounds; this may explain the impaired wound strength seen in irradiated wounds. Decreased MMP-1 may contribute to inadequate soft tissue reconstitution (Table 6-4). Keratinocytes, which are crucial for wound epithelialization, demonstrate a shift in expression from the high molecular keratins 1 and 10 to the low molecular keratins 5 and 14 after radiation injury.

In nonhealing ulcers, keratinocytes display decreased expression of TGF-α, TGF-β_1 FGF-1, FGF-2, KGF, VEGF, and hepatocyte growth factor (HFG). Expression of MMP-2, MMP-12, and MMP-13 has been shown to be elevated in irradiated human keratinocytes and fibroblasts.[20] Fibroblasts play a central role in wound healing through deposition and remodeling of collagen fibers. In irradiated tissue, fibroblasts generate disorganized collagen bundles from dysregulation of MMP and TIMP. Because TGF-β regulates MMPs and TIMP, it may be of particular relevance to radiogenic ulcers (see Table 6-4).[21]

Strategies for treating problematic radiogenic ulcers include standard wound care, negative pressure wound therapy, nutritional optimization, and optimized blood and oxygen delivery. Hyperbaric oxygen (HBO) therapy may improve tissue oxygen partial pressure in the treatment of osteoradionecrosis[22-24] via increased capillary density and more complete neovascularization. Hyperbaric treatment of cell cultures resulted in the downregulation of nine genes involved in adhesion, angiogenesis, inflammation, and oxidative stress.[25] IL-8 mRNA levels were suppressed in endothelial cells with daily HBO therapy.[25] HBO therapy is used clinically in patients with chronic diabetic ulcers and wound-healing complications after radiotherapy, and randomized clinical trials demonstrated efficacy when HBO therapy was used in conjunction with standard wound care in cases of recalcitrant, diabetic, and radiation-induced wounds.[26]

TABLE 6-4 Possible Key Wound-Healing Factors Affected by Radiotherapy With Respect to the Phases of Wound Healing

PHASE OF WOUND HEALING	FACTORS AFFECTED BY RADIATION THERAPY
Inflammation	TGF-β, VEGF, IL-1, IL-8, TNF-α, IFN-γ
Proliferation	TGF-β, VEGF, EGF, FGF, PDGF, NO
Remodeling	MMP-1, MMP-2, MMP-12, MMP-13, TIMP

From Haubner F, Ohmann E, Pohl F, et al: Wound healing after radiation therapy: Review of the literature. *Radiat Oncol* 7:162, 2012.
EGF, Epidermal growth factor; *FGF,* fibroblast growth factor; *IFN-γ,* interferon-γ; *IL-1, -8,* interleukin-1, -8; *MMP-1, -2, -12, -13,* matrix metalloproteinase-1, -2, -12, -13; *NO,* nitric oxide; *PDGF,* platelet-derived growth factor; *TGF-β,* transforming growth factor-β; *TIMP,* tissue inhibitors of metalloproteinase; *TNF-α,* tumor necrosis factor-α; *VEGF,* vascular endothelial growth factor.

Aging

Older patients are more likely to experience delayed healing and surgical wound dehiscence. The aging epidermis has fewer Langerhans cells and melanocytes and flattening of the dermal-epidermal junction. Keratinocyte proliferation is reduced, and the turnover time is increased by 50%. The dermis has fewer fibroblasts, macrophages, and mast cells; reduced vascularity; and less collagen and GAGs. There is a quantitative imbalance between collagen production and degradation and a qualitative alteration of the remaining collagen, which has fewer ropelike bundles and shows greater disorganization. Skin elasticity is decreased because of altered elastin morphology. Diminished light touch and pressure reduced nociceptive receptors and dermal atrophy increase susceptibility to injury by mechanical forces. Immunosenescence (reduced Langerhans cells and fibroblast activity) impairs wound healing and increases the likelihood of chronic wounds. Microvascular disturbances predispose to ischemic ulcers. Finally, there is reduced sebum secretion and vitamin D_3 production.[27]

MMP-2 and MMP-9 are upregulated after experimental wounding in healthy elderly subjects versus younger controls. Decreased reepithelialization, depressed collagen synthesis, impaired angiogenesis, and decreased growth factors (especially proangiogenic FGF-2 and VEGF) are seen in studies of older animals. The early inflammatory phase appears to be altered in older adults. Impaired macrophage activity (reduced phagocytosis and delayed infiltration) and impaired B lymphocyte activity also have been demonstrated in animal studies. Decreased MMP activation and decreased TGF-β_1 receptor expression in response to hypoxia were demonstrated in keratinocytes isolated from aged donors.

Malnutrition

Protein catabolism delays wound healing and promotes wound dehiscence, particularly when serum albumin levels are less than 2.0 g/dL. Protein supplements can reverse this deficiency.

Vitamin deficiencies affect wound healing primarily as a result of their effect as cofactors. Delayed healing can occur 3 months after vitamin C deprivation and can be reversed by supplements of 10 mg/day and no more than 2000 g/day. Deficiency of vitamin A impedes monocyte activation and deposition of fibronectin, affecting cellular adhesion, and impairs TGF-β receptors. Vitamin A contributes to lysosomal membrane destabilization and directly counteracts the effect of glucocorticoids. Vitamin K deficiency limits the synthesis of prothrombin and factors VII, IX, and X. Vitamin K metabolism is impeded by antibiotics; patients who have chronic or recurrent infections need to have clotting parameters checked before surgical procedures.

Zinc is a necessary cofactor for RNA polymerase and DNA polymerase. Zinc deficiency impairs early wound healing, but it is rare except with large burns, severe polytrauma, and hepatic cirrhosis. Iron deficiency anemia is a debatable cause of delayed wound healing. Although ferrous ion is a cofactor needed to convert proline to hydroxyproline, reports are conflicting regarding the effects of acute and chronic anemia on wound healing. In general, patients should have a well-rounded diet consisting of adequate protein intake and caloric value plus vitamin and mineral supplementation.

Drugs

Some exogenously administered drugs directly impair wound healing. Chemotherapeutic agents, such as doxorubicin (Adriamycin), nitrogen mustard, cyclophosphamide, methotrexate, and bis-chloroethylnitrosourea, are potent wound inhibitors in animal models and interfere with uncomplicated wound healing clinically. They reduce mesenchymal cell proliferation, platelet and inflammatory cell counts, and availability of growth factors, particularly if given preoperatively. Tamoxifen, an antiestrogen, decreases cellular proliferation, with a decrease in wound-breaking strength that is dose dependent and may be secondary to decreased TGF-β production. Glucocorticosteroids impair fibroblast proliferation and collagen synthesis, resulting in decreased granulation tissue formation. Furthermore, steroids stabilize lysosomal membranes. Administration of vitamin A can reverse this particular effect. Diminished wound-breaking strength caused by exogenous steroids is time and dose related. High doses of nonsteroidal anti-inflammatory drugs have been reported to delay healing, but doses in the therapeutic range are unlikely to have an effect.

Treatment of Chronic Wounds

The management of a chronic wound depends on its etiology. Currently available therapies are slow, labor-intensive, and expensive without any guarantee of healing if all local and systemic factors are not addressed. Wound-healing research identified key structural proteins and molecules in normal and disordered wound healing as possible targets for future interventions. This research led to the application of topical growth factors to chronic wounds, which, although initially promising, almost universally failed to produce clinically significant improvements in wound healing. The reason for the failure is presumed to be a result of degradation of the growth factors by proteases in the wound fluid. This failure highlighted the complex nature of wound healing, where simply replacing one element is not enough.

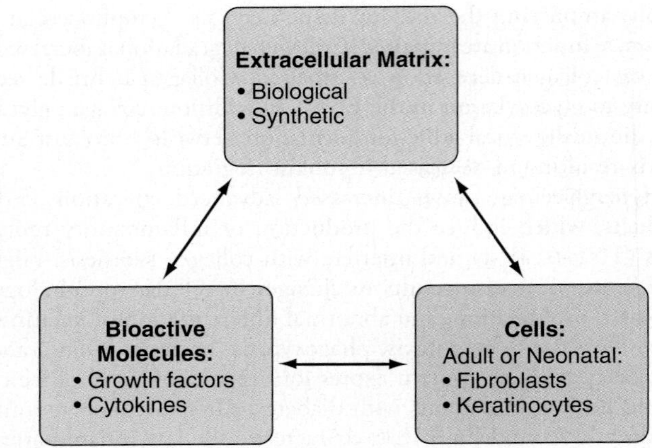

FIGURE 6-9 The "dynamic reciprocity" model of wound healing. Interactions are dynamic as they vary with time and location within the wound site. Products of any one element influence the actions of the others. Inappropriate downregulation of any one element can result in conversion from an acute to a chronic wound. (From Greaves NS, Iqbal SA, Baguneid M, et al: The role of skin substitutes in the management of chronic cutaneous wounds. *Wound Repair Regen* 21:194–210, 2013.)

Skin substitutes (discussed later) provide multiple factors that may alter the nature of the wound microenvironment in favor of and allow healing to occur. Split-thickness skin grafting is the surgical substitution of native epidermis and partial dermis to assist wound closure, and it has a strong evidence base from treatment of acute burn wounds and chronic nonhealing wounds.[28] Skin is harvested from the patient and transferred to an adequately prepared wound bed. The graft provides wound coverage by providing a favorable healing environment through exclusion of pathogenic bacteria and provision of ECM, cells (keratinocytes and fibroblasts), and bioactive molecules (cytokines, chemokines, and growth factors) that facilitate wound repair through a process of "dynamic reciprocity" (Fig. 6-9).[15] However, autologous skin grafts occasionally are limited or unavailable. Biologic skin substitutes have been used for many years and include cadaveric skin allografts and porcine and bovine xenografts.[28] These grafts are not durable because they do not integrate into the host, and they are associated with rejection and disease transfer. However, they provide adequate temporary wound cover, limiting complications until autologous grafts or other definitive management strategies are available.

WOUND DRESSINGS

Wound dressings—present since antiquity—evolved very little for many years until 1867, when Lister introduced antiseptic dressings by soaking lint and gauze in carbolic acid. Since then, numerous more sophisticated products have become available; however, certain characteristics in wound dressings should be considered in the nonsurgical treatment of a wound (Box 6-2). Wound healing is most successful in a moist, clean, and warm environment. Not all dressings can provide all of these characteristics, and not all wounds require all of them; hence, the choice of dressing should match the prevailing wound conditions.

Two concepts that are critical when selecting appropriate dressings for wounds are occlusion and absorption. Studies have demonstrated that the rate of epithelialization under a moist occlusive

BOX 6-2 Characteristics of Ideal Dressing

Creates a moist environment
Removes excess exudate
Prevents desiccation
Allows for gaseous exchange
Impermeable to microorganisms
Thermally insulating
Prevents particulate contamination
Nontoxic to beneficial host cells
Provides mechanical protection
Nontraumatic
Easy to use
Cost-effective

Adapted from Morin RJ, Tomaselli NL: Interactive dressings and topical agents. *Clin Plast Surg* 34:643–658, 2007.

dressing is twice that of a wound that is left uncovered and allowed to dry. An occlusive dressing provides a mildly acidic pH and low oxygen tension on the wound surface, which is conducive for fibroblast proliferation and formation of granulation tissue. However, wounds that produce significant amounts of exudate or have high bacterial counts require a dressing that is absorptive and prevents maceration of the surrounding skin. These dressings also need to reduce the bacterial load while absorbing the exudate produced. Placement of a pure occlusive dressing without bactericidal properties would allow bacterial overgrowth and worsen the infection.

Dressings can be categorized into four classes: (1) nonadherent fabrics; (2) absorptive dressings; (3) occlusive dressings; and (4) creams, ointments, and solutions (Table 6-5). Briefly, nonadherent fabrics are fine-mesh gauze supplemented with a substance to augment their occlusive properties or antibacterial abilities, such as Scarlet Red, a relatively nonocclusive dressing that is impregnated with *O*-tolylazo-*O*-tolylazo-β-naphthol that is used on skin graft harvest sites in burn care. Xeroform is a relatively occlusive, hydrophobic dressing containing 3% bismuth tribromophenate in a petrolatum base, which helps mask wound odors and has antimicrobial activity against *Staphylococcus aureus* and *Escherichia coli.*

Occlusive dressings provide moisture retention, mechanical protection, and a barrier to bacteria. These dressings can be divided into biologic and nonbiologic dressings. Examples of biologic dressings are allograft, xenograft, amnion, and skin substitutes. An allograft is a graft transplanted between genetically unique humans, whereas a xenograft is a graft, such as pigskin, transplanted between species. Allografts and xenografts are temporary dressings; both will be rejected if left on a wound for an extended period. Amnion is derived from human placentas and is another effective biologic wound dressing. Initially, these dressings were most often used in the treatment of burn wounds; however, they can be used as a temporary measure in other wounds.

Absorptive dressings are useful for wounds with a significant amount of exudate. Leg ulcers can produce 12 g/10 cm^2/24 hours of exudate. Examples include wide-mesh gauze, the oldest of this type of dressing, which loses its effectiveness when saturated, and newer materials, such as foam dressings, which provide the absorbent qualities for removing large quantities of exudate and have a nonadherent quality to prevent disruption of newly formed granulation tissue on removal. Examples include Lyofoam (ConvaTec, Skillman, NJ), Allevyn (Smith & Nephew, Largo, FL), and Curafoam (Kendall Company, Mansfield, MA). Wound healing beneath absorptive dressings appears to be slower than under occlusive dressings, possibly because of wicking of cytokines from the wound bed or decreased keratinocyte migration.

The final class of wound dressings consists of creams, ointments, and solutions. This is a broad category that extends from traditional materials, such as zinc oxide paste, to preparations containing growth factors. Various categories include dressings with antibacterial properties such as acetic acid, Dakin's solution, silver nitrate, mafenide (Sulfamylon), silver sulfadiazine (Silvadene), iodine-containing ointments (Iodosorb), and bacitracin. Application of these products is indicated when clinical signs of infection are present or if quantitative culture demonstrates more than 10^5 organisms per gram of tissue.

The number of available wound products is staggering. The surgeon must have information about available dressings to allow effective wound management (Box 6-3).

OTHER THERAPIES

Hyperbaric Oxygen Therapy

Wound ischemia is the most common cause of wound-healing failure. HBO therapy uses oxygen as a drug and the hyperbaric chamber as a delivery system to increase PO_2 at the target area. HBO therapy is used for myriad disease processes, including bacterial infections, decompression sickness, improvement of split-thickness skin graft take, flap survival and salvage, acute thermal burns, necrotizing fasciitis, chronic wounds, hypoxic wounds, osteoradionecrosis, and radiation injuries.[29] Ischemia or tissue hypoxia (PO_2 <30 mm Hg) significantly impairs normal metabolic activity and decreases wound healing by impairing fibroblast proliferation, collagen synthesis, and epithelialization. HBO therapy involves inhalation of 100% oxygen at 1.9 to 2.5 atm, which can increase tissue PO_2 10 times higher than usual. The higher PaO_2 is sufficient to supply the tissue with all its metabolic requirements, even in the absence of hemoglobin; this elevated level lasts for 2 to 4 hours after termination of HBO therapy and induces synthesis of endothelial cell NO synthase as well as angiogenesis. Oxygen has been reported to stimulate angiogenesis, enhance fibroblast and leukocyte function, and normalize cutaneous microvascular reflexes.[30,31]

Evaluation of the vascular supply to the target area is essential, and revascularization before HBO therapy is an essential prerequisite to HBO therapy. Patients will likely benefit from adjuvant HBO therapy if improvement in tissue oxygenation can be demonstrated in a hypoxic wound while breathing oxygen under hyperbaric conditions.[29] Transcutaneous oxygen pressure ($TcPO_2$) is used to assess wound perfusion and oxygenation. A wound $TcPO_2$ less than 35 mm Hg in room air indicates a hypoxic wound. In-chamber $TcPO_2$ of 200 mm Hg or more suggests potential benefit from HBO therapy.

HBO treatments for hypoxic wounds are usually delivered at 1.9 to 2.5 atm for sessions of 90 to 120 minutes each, with the patient breathing 100% oxygen during the treatment. Treatments are given once daily, five to six times per week and should be given as an adjunct to surgical or medical therapies. Clinical evidence of wound improvement should be noted after 15 to 20 treatments.

Complications of HBO therapy are caused by changes in atmospheric pressure and elevated PO_2. Middle ear barotrauma, ranging from tympanic membrane hyperemia to eardrum

TABLE 6-5 Types of Dressings

CATEGORY	COMPOSITION AND CHARACTERISTICS	FUNCTION	EXAMPLES	COMMENTS
Nonadherent fabrics	Fine-mesh gauze with supplement to augment occlusive and nonadherent properties, healing-facilitating capabilities, and antibacterial characteristics	Protection, moist environment	Scarlet Red, Vaseline gauze, Xeroform, Xeroflo, Mepitel, Adaptic, Telfa	Scarlet Red, Xeroform, Telfa, Vaseline gauze—hydrophobic, more occlusive; Xeroflo, Mepitel, Adaptic—less occlusive, allow drainage of fluid into overlying dressing layers
Absorptive				
Gauze	Wide mesh gauze	Removing exudates, prevents maceration	Wide-mesh gauze	Not effective when saturated; can be used for wound débridement if in contact with wound
Foams	Hydrophobic polyurethane sheets	Protection, absorption of exudate	Lyofoam, Allevyn, Curafoam, Flexzan, Vigifoam	Advantages—comfortable, can expand and conform to wound, easily removed for cleansing Disadvantages—need to be replaced as wounds heal, custom shapes are labor-intensive to make, limited protection from bacteria, cannot be used while bathing
Occlusive				
Nonbiologic		Insulation, moisture retention, protective barrier acts against bacteria		
Films	Clear polyurethane membranes with acrylic adhesive on one side	See above	Tegaderm, Mefilm, Carrafilm, Bioclusive, Transeal, Opsite	Waterproof; permeable to oxygen, carbon dioxide, and water vapor; do not interfere with patient function; allow visualization of wound; nonabsorptive, can leak; require intact skin around wound area; wound contraction may be slowed, removal may disrupt new epithelium
Hydrocolloids	Hydrocolloid matrix (gelatin, pectin, carboxymethylcellulose)	As above; absorbs water from wound exudates, swells, liquefies to form moist gel	Duoderm, NuDerm, Comfeel, Hydrocol, Cutinova, Tegasorb	Available as adhesive wafers, paste, powders; similar features as films, but bulkier; more protection, but may interfere more with function
Alginates	Cellulose-like polysaccharide fibers derived from calcium salt of alginate (seaweed)	As above; calcium alginate conversion to soluble sodium salt after contact with wound exudates results in hydrophilic gel	Algiderm, Algosteril, Kaltostat, Curasorb, Carasorb, Melgisorb, SeaSorb, Kalginate, Sorbsan	Occlusive environment; various forms—ropes, ribbons, pads
Hydrogels	Polyethylene oxide or carboxymethylcellulose polymer and water (80%)	As above; rehydrating agents for dry wounds; little water absorption (high water content)	Vigilon, Nu-gel, Tegagel, FlexiGel, Curagel, Flexderm	Available as gels, sheets, impregnated gauze; occlusive environment
Biologic		Similar to nonbiologics		
Homograft	Derived from genetically unique humans		Cadaver skin	Temporary dressing; is rejected if left on wound for extended period
Xenograft	Interspecies graft (e.g., pig)		Pigskin	Same as above
Amnion	Human placenta			Good biologic dressing
Skin substitutes	Different compositions		Integra, Alloderm, Apligraf, Biobrane, Transcyte	Integra—bilayered membrane skin substitute; AlloDerm—acellular cadaveric dermis; Apligraf—living, bilayered, biologic dressing composed of neonatal dermal fibroblasts on collagen matrix

TABLE 6-5 Types of Dressings—cont'd

CATEGORY	COMPOSITION AND CHARACTERISTICS	FUNCTION	EXAMPLES	COMMENTS
Creams, Ointments, and Solutions				
Antibacterial	Different compositions	Used to treat infected wounds	Acetic acid (gram-negative, *Pseudomonas*); Dakin's solution (broad antibacterial spectrum); iodine-containing antibacterials (Iodosorb, Iodoflex, Betadine; broad antibacterial and antifungal spectrum); silver nitrate (broad antibacterial spectrum); mafenide acetate (Sulfamylon; broad antibacterial spectrum) silver sulfadiazine (Silvadene; broad antibacterial, antifungal, and antiviral spectrum); Acticoat (broad antibacterial spectrum)	Acetic acid—impairs wound healing; Dakin's—toxic to fibroblasts; iodine-containing solutions—toxic to fibroblasts, impairs wound healing; silver nitrate—treats burns, slows epithelialization, hyponatremia, stains clothes black; mafenide acetate—penetrates eschar, painful application, inhibits reepithelialization, carbonic anhydrase inhibitor; silver sulfadiazine—transient neutropenia, accelerates epithelialization of partial-thickness burns, neovascularization, commonly used for burns; Acticoat—silver-impregnated occlusive dressing, antibacterial activity lasts 3 days
Antibacterial ointments	Different compositions	Used to treat infected wounds; soothing to apply; lubricates wound surface; occlusive; antibacterial activity lasts 12 hr	Bacitracin (gram-positive cocci and bacilli); neomycin (gram-negative) polymyxin B sulfate (gram-negative); Polysporin (polymyxin B, bacitracin); Neosporin (polymyxin B, bacitracin, neomycin); triple antibiotic ointment (polymyxin B, bacitracin, neomycin)	Neosporin—increased reepithelialization in experimental wounds by 25% compared with wounds with no dressing
Enzymatic	Different compositions; uses naturally occurring enzymes	Removal of necrotic tissue	Sutilains (derived from *Bacillus subtilis*); collagenase (Santyl; derived from *Clostridium histolyticum*); papain (derived from vegetable pepsin)	Sutilains—digests denatured collagen; collagenase—digests denatured and native collagen; papain—effective against collagen in presence of cofactor containing sulfhydryl group; addition of urea doubles enzymatic action of papain
Other	Normal saline wet to dry gauze dressing	Removal of necrotic tissue		Nondiscriminating—necrotic and newly formed granulation tissue and epithelium removed; can be painful

Adapted from Lionelli GT, Lawrence WT: Wound dressings. *Surg Clin North Am* 83:617–638, 2003.

perforation, is the most common complication. Pneumothorax (particularly tension pneumothorax) is far less common but potentially life-threatening. Other complications associated with increased PO_2 include brain oxygen toxicity, manifested by convulsions resembling grand mal seizures; oxygen lung toxicity, resulting from damage from oxygen free radicals to lung parenchyma and airways and ranging from tracheobronchitis to full-blown respiratory distress syndrome; and transient myopia. Absolute contraindications to HBO therapy are (1) uncontrolled pneumothorax, (2) current or recent treatment with bleomycin or doxorubicin (potential aggravation of cardiac and pulmonary toxicity), and (3) treatment with disulfiram (increases risk of developing oxygen toxicity).

Randomized clinical trials demonstrated that HBO is a useful adjunctive therapy for diabetic ischemic foot ulcers and reduces the rate of extremity amputation. In addition, the Cochrane Collaborative in 2004 reviewed HBO therapy for chronic wounds and concluded that HBO therapy reduces the risk of amputation for patients with diabetic foot ulcers and increases the chance of healing at 1 year. These studies are difficult to interpret because of the length of time chronic wounds take to heal and the variability among wounds that cannot be controlled. Furthermore, the Cochrane Collaborative noted that the recommendations were based on small, underpowered studies and that further randomized studies were greatly needed to clarify the benefits of this costly therapy. Despite the obvious potential scientific biases, medical insurance companies have decided to support HBO therapy as an adjunct treatment for perfused, chronic, nonhealing lower extremity wounds, provided that the limbs have already undergone revascularization.

BOX 6-3 Dressing Options for Noninfected Clean Wounds

- Incisional wound
  - Three-layer dressings
  - Ointments
  - Occlusive dressings
- Partial-thickness wounds (e.g., abrasions, donor sites)
  - No dressing (scab)
  - Impregnated gauze
  - Creams, ointments
  - Occlusive dressings
- Full-thickness wounds (e.g., pressure sores)
  - Alginates or hydrogels—rarely applicable
  - Creams, gels (e.g., Silvadene)
  - Wet to dry dressing changes
  - Vacuum-assisted closure device

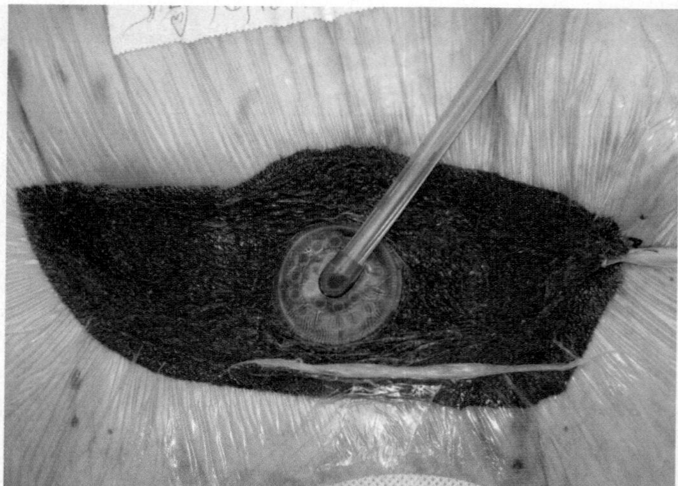

FIGURE 6-10 Negative pressure–assisted wound closure sponge in place on a patient's abdomen.

Despite evidence suggesting potential benefit of HBO therapy on healing chronic wounds, its cost is high. Patients often travel long distances for daily treatments at great cost to themselves and their families. Although reported protocols for treatment of ischemic limb ulcers vary significantly, most involve a total cost of $15,000 to $40,000. HBO therapy is not recommended as a primary treatment for patients with uncomplicated diabetic or ischemic ulcers; however, in selected more complicated cases, HBO therapy may have a role.[32]

Negative Pressure–Assisted Wound Therapy

One of the most significant discoveries in wound management in recent decades was the improvement in wounds with negative pressure–assisted wound therapy (NPWT) (Fig. 6-10). With this technology, the surgeon has options in addition to immediate closure of wounds (i.e., adjunctive therapy before or after surgery or an alternative to surgery in extremely ill patients).

Argenta and associates originally described the use of negative pressure to assist in wound closure in 1997. By applying subatmospheric pressure to wounds, they demonstrated removal of chronic edema, an increase in local blood flow, and stimulation of granulation tissue. This technique may be used on acute, subacute, and chronic wounds. Additional studies demonstrated significant improvement in wound depth in chronic wounds treated with NPWT compared with wounds treated with saline wet to moist dressings. In addition, treatment with negative pressure results in faster healing times, with fewer associated complications.

The exact mechanism of the improvement in healing with NPWT has yet to be determined. Many investigators initially believed that the reason for increased wound healing is the removal of wound exudates while keeping the wound moist. As originally hypothesized by Argenta and associates, with NPWT, there is a fivefold increase in blood flow to cutaneous tissues. Further studies showed an increase in capillary caliber and stimulated endothelial proliferation and angiogenesis. It is well known that increased bacterial loads result in slowed wound healing; however, despite increased wound healing with NPWT, it has been shown to result in increased bacterial counts. Other studies suggested that NPWT produces three-dimensional stress within the cells (microstrain) and across the whole area of the wound (macrostrain), resulting in changes such as increased cellular proliferation and higher microvessel density. Evidence also suggests that NPWT alters wound fluid composition by removing potentially deleterious proteinases and inflammatory cytokines, such as MMP-1, MMP-2, MMP-9, and TNF-α.

Although the mechanisms responsible for the improvement achieved with NPWT have yet to be clearly elucidated, this treatment represents a significant improvement in cost-effectiveness and has decreased length of stay after acute and chronic wounds. There have been reports of a 78% decrease in hospital stay and a 76% decrease in cost with NPWT. This cost decrease and effectiveness of wound treatment with NPWT have translated to home health care treatment of Medicare patients.

Clinical benefits of NPWT have been demonstrated in randomized controlled trials and include a decrease in wound volume or size, accelerated wound bed preparation, accelerated wound healing, improved rate of graft take, decreased drainage time for acute wounds, reduction of complications, enhancement of response to first-line treatment, increased patient survival, and decreased cost. Trials published more recently have further demonstrated the wound-healing efficacy of NPWT. A 16-week, 18-center, randomized clinical trial conducted by Armstrong and Lavery comprising 162 patients with diabetes with larger and more complex wounds than in previous randomized trials found that NPWT healed more wounds after partial foot amputation versus the standard of care (43 [56%] versus 33 [39%]; $P = .040$). The authors noted that NPWT produced faster wound-healing rates ($P = .005$) and faster granulation tissue formation rates versus standard of care based on the time needed to complete closure ($P = .002$). Resource utilization for patients treated with NPWT was evaluated in the same study population. Apelqvist reported that patients randomly assigned to the NPWT group required fewer surgical procedures (including débridement) than the control group (43 versus 120; $P < .001$), fewer average number of dressing changes (41 [range, 6-140] in the NPWT group versus 118.0 [range, 12-226] in the control group; $P < .0001$), and fewer outpatient treatment visits (4 [range, 0-47] in the NPWT group versus 11 [range, 0-106] in the control group; $P < .05$). A cost savings greater than $12,800 resulted compared with standard therapy. Combined with the clinical data, these analyses provide compelling evidence that appropriate use of NPWT is efficacious and cost-effective in achieving healing of properly selected wounds on an inpatient and outpatient basis.

FETAL WOUND HEALING

Fetal skin wounds heal rapidly without the scarring and inflammation characteristic of adult skin wounds. In adult cutaneous healing, dermal appendages (hair follicles, sweat and sebaceous glands) fail to regenerate. In addition, healed adult wounds have densely packed collagen bundles oriented perpendicularly to the wound surface, whereas collagen in uninjured and fetal skin retains a reticular pattern. Fetal wounds reepithelialize faster, with less neovascularization and a faster increase in strength. Fetal wounds differ in inflammatory responses, ECM components, growth factor expression, and biologic responses to growth factor expression. It was thought that fetal wound healing represented ideal tissue repair and that understanding fetal wound healing would provide surgeons the tools to regulate and control the different steps in adult wound healing.

Fetal repair depends on gestational age and wound size. The wound size threshold (diameter of excised skin at which 50% of wounds heal without scarring at a given gestational age) appears to be 6 to 10 mm for 60-day-gestation and 70-day-gestation animals and 4 to 6 mm for 80-day-gestation and 90-day-gestation animals. Larger wounds may extend the time to healing and expose wound tissue to a different ECM and growth factor profile. Larger excisional wounds may also stimulate the formation of myofibroblasts resulting in scar formation. The transition from scarless to scarring repair occurs near the end of the second trimester. Wounds heal faster in a fetus than in a neonate, and they heal more slowly in adults compared with neonates.

Skin appendages are formed when dermal fibroblasts induce the epithelium to form hair follicles or glands. Wounds created early in gestation heal without scarring and with dermal appendages, suggesting tissue regeneration versus repair. In contrast, late gestation wounds heal with scarring and without dermal appendages. The transition from scarless healing to healing without dermal appendages suggests that fetal fibroblasts lose their ability to induce the epithelium to form dermal appendages with advancing gestational age.

Intrinsic differences (oxygen tension of the human fetus) rather than extrinsic differences (amniotic fluid environment) are more likely determinants of whether wounds will heal with scars. Oxygen tension is markedly decreased in fetal sheep (mean PaO_2 = 20 mm Hg) compared with adult sheep (mean PaO_2 of 116 mm Hg); this is partially compensated by the relative affinity of fetal hemoglobin for oxygen.

The fetal environment, an extrinsic difference between fetal and adult wounds, is characterized by a hyaluronic acid–rich amniotic fluid. The increased number of hyaluronic acid receptors and increased amount of hyaluronic acid may create a permissive environment in which fibroblast movement is facilitated, resulting in the increased rate and efficiency of fetal healing.

Much of fetal wound-healing research has focused on fetal fibroblasts. Fetal fibroblasts appear to have characteristics quite different from adult fibroblasts. Proline hydroxylation is a rate-limiting step in collagen synthesis by dermal cells. Early-gestation fetal human fibroblasts have increased prolyl hydroxylase activity that gradually decreases to adult levels after 20 weeks of gestation. Collagen types I, III, V, and VI appear earlier, and the ratio of type III to type I is greater in fetal wounds, which is consistent with the higher prevalence of type III collagen in normal fetal tissue. Fetal fibroblasts in vitro have higher collagen production than their adult counterparts. This higher collagen production may be secondary to the unique regulatory mechanism for prolyl hydroxylase and may explain why there is higher fibroblast activity in fetuses younger than 20 weeks' gestation.

Collagen synthesis decreases to adult levels after 20 weeks' gestation, and collagen degradation increases with gestational age. Increased gene expression of MMP-1, MMP-3, and MMP-9 correlates with the onset of scar formation in nonwounded fetal skin. These findings suggest that late-gestation fetal rat skin undergoes an adult type of tissue remodeling after wounding that leads to the scarring seen in adult skin.

There are also differences in the components of the ECM of fetal and adult wounds. After injury, fibronectin levels are similar in adults and fetuses, but tenascin, an inhibitor of fibronectin, increases earlier and returns to normal more rapidly in the fetus. Larger amounts of fibronectin in fetal wounds stimulate immediate cell attachment, whereas the more rapid deposition of tenascin in the fetus allows cells to migrate and fully epithelialize the wound more rapidly and decrease wound-healing time.

Hyaluronic acid is persistently elevated in fetal wounds. During gestation, decreasing levels of hyaluronic acid correlate with increasing scarring potential. The unique ECM composition of fetal tissues may influence collagen fibril deposition by facilitating cell mobility and migration, leading to the loose collagen pattern seen in healed fetal wounds as opposed to the dense collagenous pattern seen in adult scars. However, few studies have examined the effect of modifying the ECM components.

In addition, the fetus exhibits a reduced inflammatory response with a lack of neutrophil infiltration and decreased infiltration of endogenous immunoglobulins. The paucity of macrophages and a difference in the temporal appearance of macrophages in fetal wounds may explain differences in growth factor profiles and the reduced inflammatory response. These studies cite a direct correlation between increased macrophage recruitment in older fetuses and the development of increased scarring.

Fetal wounds have minimal levels of TGF-β and FGF-2. TGF-β is the growth factor that has been most extensively studied in fetal wound repair. TGF-β_1 induces rapid healing and scar formation when added to adult rat wounds and induces inflammation and fibrosis when added to fetal rabbit wounds. TGF-β production may be blunted in hypoxemic conditions, leading to the theory that the decreased oxygen tension in the fetal environment inhibits TGF-β production and results in decreased scar formation. It has been suggested that differential expression of the different TGF-β isoforms, rather than the presence of TGF-β, may be important in explaining the differences in repair.

PDGF also disappears more rapidly in fetal wounds. The paucity of growth factors may be explained by decreased inflammatory cell recruitment. Normal inflammatory (adult-type) wound healing may have evolved to reduce the risk of infection at the expense of healing quality. Growth factor manipulation to make wounds more fetal-like has failed to result in completely scarless healing and has failed to regenerate dermal appendages. In addition, some inconsistencies in fetal wound healing are not clearly understood. There are differences in species with regard to scarless fetal wound healing, and not all fetal tissues are capable of scarless healing. For example, fetal lamb diaphragm and gastric wounds scar, whereas concurrent skin wounds heal without scarring.

The presence of myofibroblasts and concurrent scar formation suggests that a transition in fibroblast phenotype may contribute to scarring. Excisional wounds in 75-day-gestation fetal lambs showed an absence of scar formation and alpha smooth muscle actin expression. Alpha smooth muscle actin appears after 100 days of gestation along with scar formation.

Focus has shifted more recently to multiple pluripotent stem cells, such as epithelial stem cells (EpSCs), mesenchymal stem cells (MSCs), and "small dot" cells, and their role in fetal wound healing. The slowly proliferating EpSCs, which are interspersed throughout the basal layers, are surrounded by more quickly proliferating basal cells and their suprabasal progeny to form epidermal proliferative units. EpSCs are also found within the bulge area of hair follicles and are believed to migrate to the epidermis after injury and differentiate into dermal, vascular, and neural components.

MSCs play a role in regenerative healing, including immunomodulation, antifibrosis, antiapoptosis, and angiogenesis,[33] as well as preventing excessive inflammation. They immunoregulate through multiple independent pathways, including the induction of IL-10 secretion by macrophages.[34]

"Small dot" cells also have been identified to play a role in fetal wound healing. There is a 20-fold greater increase of these cells in fetal blood than postnatal blood. Fluorescence-labeled "small dot" cells transplanted into a postnatal murine incisional wound model migrated to the wound bed and decreased scarring.[35] Further investigations should help to elucidate the importance of these stem cell populations in fetal wound healing and in treating abnormal wound healing (Table 6-6).[36]

TABLE 6-6 Comparison of Fetal Regenerative Wound Healing Profile With Postnatal Wound Healing

	FETAL	POSTNATAL
Phenotype	Regenerative	Scar formation
Growth Factors		
bFGF	Lower	Higher
PDGF	Lower	Higher
VEGF	Higher	Lower
TGF-β		
TGF-β_1	Low levels	High levels
TGF-β_2	Low levels	High levels
TGF-β_3	High levels	Low levels
Inflammatory Response		
Inflammatory cell	Minimal	High levels leukocytes, macrophages, mast cells infiltrate
Cytokines		
Proinflammatory: IL-6, IL-8	Low levels	High levels
Anti-inflammatory: IL-10	High levels	Low levels
Extracellular Matrix		
Collagen		
Histology	Fine, reticular weave	Thick, ropelike bundles
Type III collagen	High levels	Low levels
Deposition	Immediate	Delayed
Cross linking	Low levels	High levels
TGF-β_1-stimulated deposition	Absent	Present
Hyaluronan		
Expression	High levels Persistent expression	Low levels Transient expression
Molecular weight	High	Low
HA receptors (fibroblast)	High levels	Low levels
Mechanical force		
Myofibroblast (day 14)	Absent	Present
Stem cells		
MSC	High levels	Lower levels
Dot cells	Present	Absent

From Leung A, Crombleholme TM, Keswani SG: Fetal wound healing: Implications for minimal scar formation. *Curr Opin Pediatr* 24:371–378, 2012.

bFGF, Basic fibroblast growth factor; *HA*, hyaluronan; *IL-6, -8, -10*, interleukin-6, -8, -10; *MSC*, mesenchymal stem cell; *PDGF*, platelet-derived growth factor; *TGF-β*, transforming growth factor-β; *VEGF*, vascular endothelial growth factor.

NEW HORIZONS

Tissue Engineering

In 1987, the National Science Foundation bioengineering panel defined tissue engineering as "the application of the principles and methods of engineering and the life sciences toward the development of biologic substitutes to restore, maintain, or improve function." These principles and methods have been used toward the creation of skin products made of cells, ECM components, or combinations of the two. This tissue-engineered skin has developed and progressed rapidly over the past 20 years, mainly because of the limitations associated with autografts, and may function by providing the cellular or matrix components that could be necessary for wounds to heal. These new skin substitutes more accurately mimic native tissues to promote sustained healing without rejection. The use of biologic dressings, scaffolds, stem cell therapy, and gene therapy are a few examples of tissue engineering, in which new tissues are created rather than transferred.

Bioengineered skin substitutes can potentially save millions of dollars a year for health care delivery services through reduced spending on dressings and treatment of wound-induced complications, particularly in the treatment of venous, diabetic, and pressure ulcers that form 90% of all chronic wounds. Bioengineered skin substitutes act as protective dressings, by limiting bacterial colonization and fluid loss, but they also stimulate healing (Fig. 6-11).[15] Their design is variable and dependent on the layer of skin they are designed to replace.

Bioengineered Skin Substitutes

Epidermal replacements are created by expansion of patient-derived keratinocytes in the laboratory.[37] These are fragile constructs that are attached to a carrier material to facilitate application to the wound. Dermal substitutes are based on a structural three-dimensional matrix material, which behaves similar to ECM, and may incorporate cells or bioactive molecules. Provision of these key factors to the wound bed may provide the necessary stimulus to rebalance the wound microenvironment in favor of healing. Bilayer materials represent a combination of features seen in epidermal and dermal models.

Epidermal Substitutes

The gold standard epidermal substitute is an autograft derived from split-thickness skin grafting or from cell line bioreactor expansion. Epidermal replacements are created by expansion of patient-derived cells in the laboratory until enough cell mass is generated to be transferred to the wound. Autologous

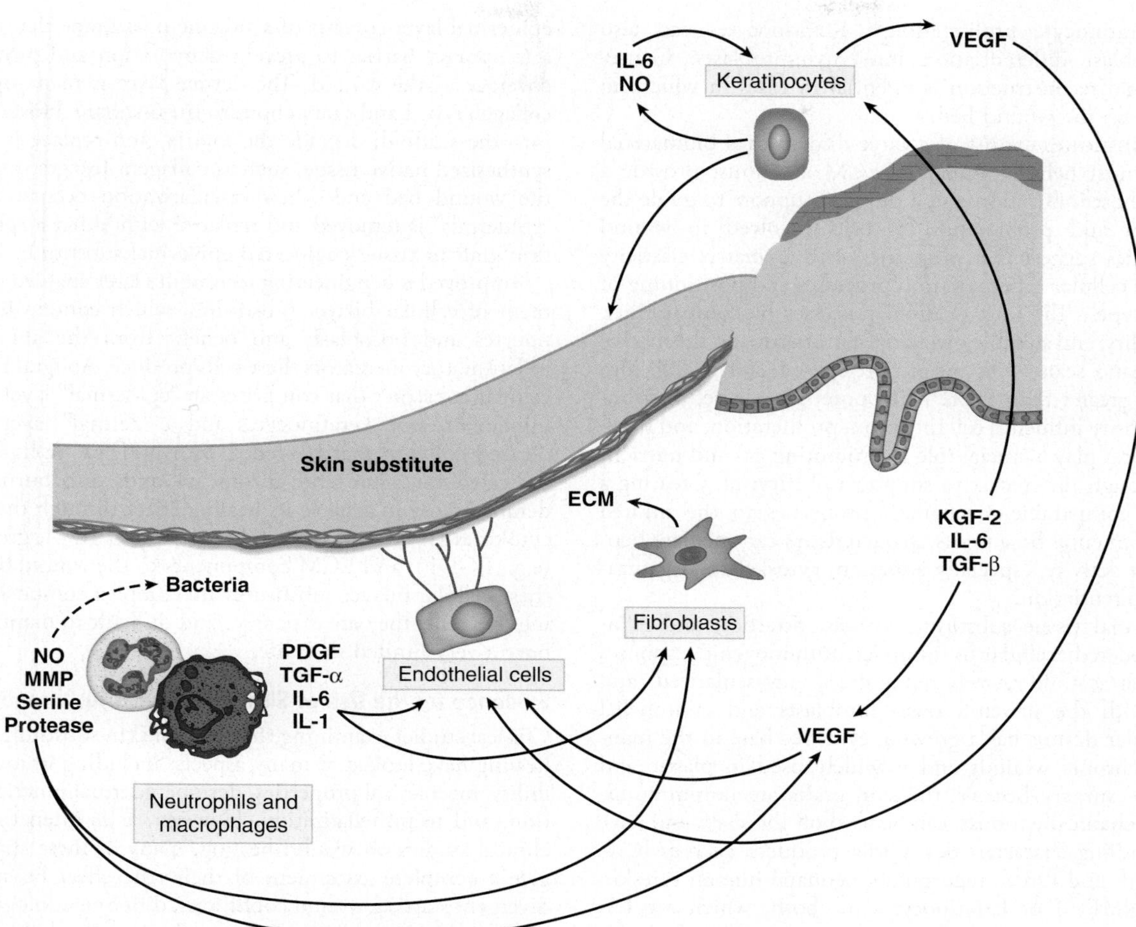

FIGURE 6-11 The effect of skin substitutes in the wound bed. Skin substitutes have variable structures and cellular content. They may be cellular or acellular, but both forms induce the influx of endogenous cells, including fibroblasts, keratinocytes, endothelial cells, macrophages, and neutrophils into the wound bed. These cells secrete various cytokines and growth factors that stimulate angiogenesis, extracellular matrix (*ECM*) deposition, and reepithelialization via the process of dynamic reciprocity. The skin substitute is replaced by native tissues eventually resulting in a healed wound. *Solid lines* indicate upregulation, and *dashed lines* indicate downregulation. *IL-1,* Interleukin-1; *IL-6,* interleukin-6; *KGF-2,* keratinocyte growth factor-2; *MMP,* matrix metalloproteinase; *NO,* nitric oxide; *PDGF,* platelet-derived growth factor; *TGF-α,* transforming growth factor-α; *TGF-β,* transforming growth factor-β; *VEGF,* vascular endothelial growth factor. (From Greaves NS, Iqbal SA, Baguneid M, et al: The role of skin substitutes in the management of chronic cutaneous wounds. *Wound Repair Regen* 21:194–210, 2013.)

keratinocytes were first cultured in the laboratory 35 years ago; this progressed into production of cultured epithelial autografts (small sheets of cells two to three layers thick) that were initially used to treat burn victims. Although these grafts are not subject to rejection, there may be a 2- to 3-week delay to generate enough tissue to cover a defect. Epicel, Epidex, Myskin, Bioseed, and Cellspray are epidermal replacements that use autologous keratinocytes.[38] Cryoskin and Celaderm contain allogeneic keratinocytes. Delivery systems include application as cultured epithelial autografts (e.g., Epicel), carrier dressings ranging from bovine collagen to a chemically defined polymer (e.g., Myskin), and conversion into a suspension that can be sprayed onto wound sites (e.g., Cellspray). Limitations of human donor-derived epidermal replacements include (1) need for a well-vascularized dermal bed, (2) low expansion capabilities, and (3) adaptation of phenotypes to in vitro conditions, limiting their ability to form new tissue.

In addition, other epidermal replacements, such as allografts, xenografts, inert membranes (e.g., silicone), and epidermal or bilayer substitutes that do not provide autologous keratinocytes, can provide only temporary wound coverage.[28] As a result, these replacements are primarily used for patients with major burns or tissue loss to limit the immediate complications of the injury until definitive coverage can be provided.

Dermal Substitutes

When the dermis is destroyed, epidermal substitutes are not enough to ensure wound healing.[37] The dermis is essential for skin elasticity and mechanical resistance and epithelial-mesenchymal communications facilitate many complex ex vivo functions of epidermal cells.[38] The absence of the dermis has been associated with increased frequency of developing fibrotic conditions.[38] Keratinocytes and fibroblasts participate in double paracrine signaling: Keratinocytes initiate growth factors in fibroblasts, which stimulate keratinocyte proliferation.[37] Keratinocytes can also control fibroblast differentiation into myofibroblasts. Consequently, dermal reconstruction is essential in cases in which no dermis is left on the wound bed.

Dermal substitutes consist of a three-dimensional biomaterial matrix that must behave similar to ECM and must provide a template for host infiltration and a physical support to guide the differentiation and proliferation of cells involved in wound healing. Studies suggest that properties such as matrix elasticity can influence cellular differentiation processes and positioning of specific cell types. The ideal scaffold possesses biocompatibility, biodegradability, and suitable mechanical properties on the macro, micro, and nano scale, with mean pore size of 100 to 200 mm and porosity greater than 90%. Micropore size, shape, distribution, and porosity influence cell intrusion, proliferation, and function. Nanopores play a crucial role in promoting gas and nutrient diffusion through the matrix to support cell survival. Creating a matrix with comparable mechanical properties to the injured tissue is fundamental because its characteristics can mediate beneficial cellular activity, especially adhesion, cytoskeletal organization, and differentiation.

Many dermal tissue substitutes (Oasis, Strattice, and Alloderm) are rendered acellular to minimize immunogenic responses and provide a scaffold that is repopulated, revascularized, and remodeled with the patient's own fibroblasts and endothelial cells.[38] Acellular dermis has a growing evidence base in the management of chronic wounds and is widely used in plastic and reconstructive surgery because the skin grafts are nonimmunogenic, are mechanically robust, can be used off the shelf, and have favorable handling characteristics. Other products, such as ICX-SKN, Apligraf, and Orcel, incorporate neonatal human foreskin fibroblasts (NHFFs) or keratinocytes, or both, which are less immunogenic than their adult counterparts, to provide substitutes containing living cells.[28,38]

There is some clinical evidence to suggest that cellular products may be superior to acellular products in terms of wound healing. The presence of live cells impregnated onto the matrix material ensures that important growth factors can be secreted in sufficient concentrations to replace the growth factors that are absent or downregulated in the wound. Compton and colleagues demonstrated that tissue-engineered dermal matrices combined with seeded cells could lead to true dermal regeneration when they observed in vivo regeneration of organized skin at 35 days using a biodegradable collagen GAG matrix seeded with a suspension of autologous keratinocytes. Yannas also found that dermal substitutes with living dermal fibroblasts resulted in better wound healing with less myofibroblastic activity. In addition, autologous cells were preferable to allogeneic ones, and fibroblasts from dermis produced better results than fibroblasts from adipose tissue. Studies with Dermagraft, which contains NHFFs, yielded good results for patients with chronic wounds of various etiologies by stimulating cellular infiltration, angiogenesis, and epithelialization. Tremblay and colleagues demonstrated that cellular dermal substitutes promoted more rapid vascularization than acellular counterparts (4 days versus 14 days) in a mouse model.

Bilayer Substitutes

Bilayer substitutes—available in cellular and acellular varieties—are the most advanced class in terms of structural mimicry of natural skin and are the most expensive available substitutes. Integra, developed in 1981, was the first acellular bilayer and has been used successfully to treat burns and chronic wounds. The epidermal layer consists of a silicone membrane that functions as a temporary barrier to prevent dehydration and provide flexible coverage of the wound. The dermal layer is made up of bovine collagen type I and shark chondroitin-6-sulfate. Host cells migrate into the scaffold, degrade the matrix, and replace it with newly synthesized native tissue, such as collagen. Integra is grafted onto the wound bed and when vascularization occurs, the silicone "epidermis" is removed and replaced with either a split-thickness skin graft or tissue-engineered epidermal substitute.

Improved bioengineering techniques later enabled the development of cellular bilayer substitutes, which contain living keratinocytes and fibroblasts and benefit from the angiogenic and inflammatory mediators these cells produce. Apligraf is a bilayered cellular construct that comprises an "epidermal" layer of neonatal human foreskin keratinocytes and a "dermal" layer of bovine-derived collagen matrix seeded with NHFFs. Apligraf, which is indicated for acute and chronic wounds and burns, has been demonstrated to achieve its healing effect through the delivery of cytokines (IFN-α, IFN-β, IL-1, IL-6, and IL-8), growth factors (e.g., PGDF), and ECM components to the wound bed. Because these cellular bilayer substitutes are complex composites containing live cells, they are expensive and difficult to manufacture and have a very limited shelf life.

Evidence for the Use of Skin Substitutes in Chronic Wounds

Clinical studies examining the effect of skin substitutes on wound healing have looked at many aspects, including immunocompatibility, mechanical properties, dermoepidermal junction regeneration, and reepithelialization. However, as is often the case with clinical studies on wound healing, many of these studies do not give a complete assessment of their true effect because of their divergent starting wound conditions, differing etiologies, and lack of controls. In many instances, qualitative morphologic examination of regenerated tissue is overlooked in favor of a quantitative assessment of wound closure, such as time to closure. Furthermore, much of the evidence is based on low-quality case series and case controls, but there have been a few significant randomized controlled trials to date that have suggested that skin substitutes are useful in accelerating wound healing in chronic wounds, such as diabetic ulcers and venous leg ulcers, and reducing the incidence of osteomyelitis and amputation.

Risks Associated With Skin Substitutes

In contrast to the use of allografts and xenografts, which can result in graft rejection and transfer of disease from graft to host, modern tissue substitutes have rare instances of rejection. The reasons why rejection is rare in these instances are as follows: (1) Cultured epidermal cells do not express major histocompatibility class II HLA-DR antigens and are not contaminated with Langerhans cells, which are the antigen-presenting cells of the skin; (2) many of these tissue substitutes are acellular, leaving only a protein scaffold[38]; and (3) substitutes that are cellular are populated with fetal cells (e.g., NHFF) that are less likely to trigger an immune response.[28]

Although there is a small risk of disease transmission to the host of bloodborne pathogens, such as HIV, syphilis, hepatitis B, and hepatitis C, all skin substitutes are rigorously tested to reduce the risk of disease transmission to the host. They all must obtain Human Tissue Act or FDA approval, or both, before clinical application.

Cellular tissue substitutes benefit from the early release of various cytokines and growth factors that accelerate wound healing. However, this beneficial effect may be offset or outweighed by a proinflammatory macrophage response to their cellular content. Two macrophage phenotypes (M1 and M2) were discussed previously.[39] The presence of intact cells within implanted scaffolds can be associated with adverse remodeling.[40] Sandor and colleagues demonstrated that the presence of cells within a scaffold was associated with increased amounts of proinflammatory cytokines, increased M1 macrophage polarization, and a poor remodeling outcome in a primate model. Similarly, Brown and colleagues[39] found that implantation of a xenogeneic ECM scaffold containing a cellular component resulted in the classic cascade of inflammatory processes with infiltration of predominantly M1 macrophages at 3 days postimplantation, with eventual scar tissue formation in a rat model. When the same scaffold materials were prepared by methods that remove the cellular component, the mononuclear cell response was marked by primarily M2 macrophages.[39] Other studies also showed that thoroughly decellularized biologic ECM scaffolds promote a host response that is polarized toward the M2 macrophage phenotype and associated with constructive tissue remodeling.[39,41]

Future of Bioengineered Skin Substitutes

At the present time, the most advanced skin substitutes cannot fully mimic the properties of normal skin and lack dermal appendages. They lack glands; pilosity; and specialized cells for the perception of cold, heat, pain, pressure, and vibration.[38] Skin pigmentation is discrepant. Future constructs should induce an environment so that wounds heal quickly without scarring or more ideally so that skin regenerates, preserving function and cosmesis. The ideal substitute would be composed of all three components involved in dynamic skin reciprocity—cells, ECM, and bioactive molecules. No FDA-approved products of this type exist at the present time, although a highly porous alginate scaffold, seeded with murine myoblasts and impregnated with FGF-2 and HGF, has demonstrated promise in promoting repopulation of native muscle cells in the wound site.

Gene and Stem Cell Therapy

Gene and stem cell therapy are emerging as promising approaches for the treatment of acute and chronic wounds. Embryonic stem cells were discovered in 1981, and it was quickly recognized that their regenerative properties could potentially be harnessed for treating chronic wounds. However, because of ethical issues, research and their use have been limited. This situation led to the investigation and subsequent discovery of self-renewing multipotent adult progenitor cells (MAPCs), which do not have the same ethical limitations.

Whole bone marrow was first investigated as a possible candidate for cellular therapy because of the ease of harvest and because it is a source of autologous MAPCs. Studies demonstrated that bone marrow can increase vascularity and accelerate closure of chronic wounds. However, because bone marrow is composed of different cell types, including MAPCs, which make up a very small portion of the bone marrow, it is unclear which cell populations are beneficial for wound healing. Isolation of MSCs, a heterogeneous group of MAPCs, from bone marrow and their use in wound-healing studies demonstrated that MSCs result in improved granulation tissue formation and neovascularization compared with whole bone marrow.

MSCs are self-renewing and can differentiate into different mesenchymal lineages, including adipocytes and chondrocytes. They have been isolated in vivo from many different tissues, including bone marrow, skeletal muscle, adipose, and blood. They have been shown to improve acute and chronic wound healing in human and animal models. Although it was thought that the mechanism of action was totally understood, studies have suggested that MSCs act through many mechanisms, including cell differentiation, growth factor and cytokine production, immune system modulation, maintenance of the ECM, and wound contraction.

Although differences in gene and cytokine expression can be observed in MSCs derived from different origins,[42] a set of core genes are preserved and expressed by all MSCs. MSCs from different tissues share properties, allowing identification of these cells as MSCs. There are no data at the present time to suggest that MSCs from one tissue origin should be used preferentially over another for wound-healing applications, although placental-derived MSCs have become a popular target for research. Bone marrow–derived MSCs and placental-derived MSCs showed minimal differences of cell phenotype, differentiation, and immunomodulative properties, and similar to other MSCs, placental-derived MSCs are immune-privileged, allowing for allogeneic use.

Multiple mechanisms are involved in MSC-mediated wound healing, including anti-inflammatory and antimicrobial, immunomodulative, and tissue reparative activities. MSCs play an important role in mediating each phase of the wound-healing process (Fig. 6-12).[43] During the inflammatory phase, MSCs coordinate the effects of inflammatory cells and inhibit the effects of inflammatory cytokines such as TNF and IFN-γ. MSCs also decrease wound infection by secreting antimicrobial factors and by stimulating immune cell phagocytosis. In addition, MSCs promote the transition from the inflammatory to the proliferative phase. In the proliferative phase, MSCs express growth factors such as VEGF, basic FGF, and KGF to promote granulation and epithelialization. Finally, MSCs regulate remodeling of the wound by promoting organized ECM deposition. The benefits of MSCs in wound healing have been demonstrated in several preclinical and clinical studies.

Methods of MSC delivery into the wound include direct injection of a single cell suspension, gel or matrix delivery systems, and synthetic bio-inspired polymers. Recruitment of endogenous MSCs is another method to deliver these cells to the wound. Clinical results using MSCs topically or systemically to enhance the healing of wounds have been promising. Badiavas demonstrated that direct topical application of bone marrow–derived cells to chronic nonhealing wounds can lead to wound closure and rebuilding of tissues. Falanga and colleagues also administered MSCs topically by developing a delivery system using fibrin glue in treating acute and chronic wounds. Bone marrow–derived MSCs, combined with a fibrin spray, were applied topically up to three times. Surgical defects created from excision of nonmelanoma skin cancers healed within 8 weeks, suggesting that MSCs contributed to accelerated resurfacing. Chronic lower-extremity wounds present for longer than 1 year significantly decreased in size or healed completely by 20 weeks. The study also found a correlation between the surface density of MSCs and the reduction in ulcer size.

Systemic administration of MSCs also was observed to promote healing in chronic wounds, particularly when there is an underlying condition such as diabetes and other systemic disorders. In a randomized controlled study of 24 patients with nonhealing ulcers of lower extremities by Dash and colleagues, the authors simultaneously administered cultured autologous bone marrow–derived MSCs intramuscularly into the affected limb and topically

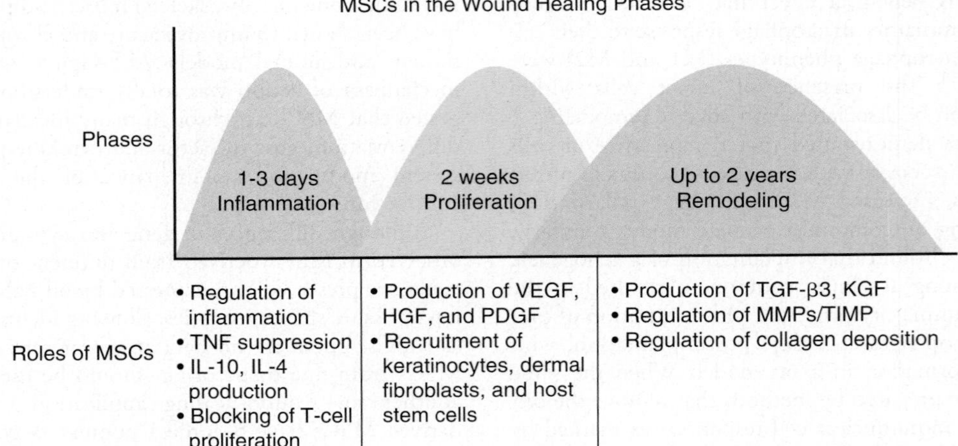

FIGURE 6-12 Mesenchymal stem cell (*MSC*) roles in each phase of the wound-healing process. *HGF,* Hepatocyte growth factor; *IL-4,* interleukin-4; *IL-10,* interleukin-10; *KGF,* keratinocyte growth factor; *MMPs,* matrix metalloproteinases; *PDGF,* platelet-derived growth factor; *TGF-β3,* transforming growth factor-β3; *TIMP,* tissue inhibitors of metalloproteinase; *TNF,* tumor necrosis factor; *VEGF,* vascular endothelial growth factor. (From Maxson S, Lopez EA, Yoo D, et al: Concise review: Role of mesenchymal stem cells in wound repair. *Stem Cells Transl Med* 1:142–149, 2012.)

directly onto the ulcer.[44] Within 12 weeks, significant improvement in pain and a greater decrease in wound size (72% versus 25%) were observed in the MSC-treated group compared with the control group. Clinical benefit of systemic administration of MSCs was also observed in a randomized controlled study conducted by Lu and colleagues.[45] Briefly, one limb of the patient was injected intramuscularly with cultured autologous bone marrow–derived MSCs or fresh nonculture bone marrow–derived mononuclear cells. The contralateral leg was injected with normal saline as a control for each patient. Compared with control groups, MSC injections and mononuclear cell injections resulted in marked improvement in pain-free walking at 24 weeks and significant increase in ulcer healing rate. Furthermore, the MSC-treated group demonstrated significantly greater increase in ulcer healing rate compared with the group injected with mononuclear cells. Although these studies have shown promising results, there are still numerous areas of future study, including the effect of the source of the MSCs, the benefits of MSCs alone or within a matrix, the timing and frequency of MSC administration, and the number of cells administered.

Although the use of placental-derived MSCs is a popular target for research at the present time, the use of placental tissue for wound treatment started more than 100 years ago. The first reported case series used amnion membrane and chorionic membrane as skin substitutes for burns and ulcers. More recently, placental tissue has been studied as an alternative source of MSCs, providing multipotent differentiation and beneficial immunosuppressive capabilities similar to MSCs derived from other tissues, such as bone marrow–derived MSCs, in terms of morphology, growth, membrane markers, and differentiation potential. MSCs from placenta presented the same morphology and growth characteristics as well as markers such as CD105, CD29, and CD44. No expression of the hematopoietic markers CD34, CD45, and HLA-DR was detected. The authors also demonstrated differentiation potential of placental MSCs into endothelial and neuronal cells. Other studies confirmed the MSC markers, such as CD44, CD73, CD90, and CD105 membrane markers, in cells derived from placental membranes. Additional studies demonstrated trilineage differentiation capabilities of placental-derived MSCs as well as their lack of immunogenicity and positive immunomodulatory effects in vitro.

Native placenta tissue cells also provide ECM and numerous growth factors important in wound healing. Analysis of cryopreserved amnion membrane growth factor and growth factor receptor content by reverse transcriptase polymerase chain reaction and enzyme-linked immunosorbent assay identified EGF, KGF, HGF, basic FGF, and the family of TGFs. All of these factors are critical in the wound-healing process.

Skin substitutes containing human MSCs have been characterized to identify critical components necessary for wound healing. A unique feature of these skin substitutes is the presence of viable cells, including MSCs, fibroblasts, and epithelial cells. Fluorescence-activated cell sorting analysis of cells within the skin substitutes reveals the expression of MSC markers, CD105 and CD166, and the absence of CD45, confirming their stem cell identity. Because $CD45^+$ cells are potentially immunogenic, the absence of this antigen indicates a lack of cell-mediated immunogenicity. The number of MSCs present within the skin substitutes is unpublished. However, the published cell concentration within placental membranes ranges from 1 to 4×10^4 cells/cm^2.[2,46] The viability of cells within the skin substitute is also confirmed, ensuring that functioning cells are delivered at the time of use. Post-thaw, the product's cell viability must be determined to be greater than 70% before it can be released for clinical use. Although the presence of viable MSCs within the skin substitute is beneficial for wound repair,[47,48] it is the combination of viable MSCs, native ECM, and growth factors within the skin substitute that is integral in promoting wound repair.

A protein profile of the skin substitute reveals the presence of growth factors needed to carry out the phases of normal healing—inflammatory, proliferative, and remodeling (Table 6-7).[43] Several anti-inflammatory and antimicrobial factors are present in the placental-derived MSC–containing skin substitute, including defensins, neutrophil gelatinase-associated lipocalin, interleukin-1

TABLE 6-7 Functional Classes of Wound-Healing Proteins in Human Mesenchymal Stem Cell–Containing Skin Substitutes

SPECIFIC PROTEINS	PRIMARY FUNCTION
MMP-1, MMP-2, MMP-3, MMP-7, MMP-8, MMP-9, MMP-10, MMP-13	Matrix and growth factor degradation, facilitate cell migration
TIMP-1 and TIMP-2	Inhibit activity of MMPs, angiogenic
Ang-2, HB-EGF, EGF, FGF-7 (also known as KGF), PIGF, PEDF, TPO, TGF-α, IGF	Stimulate growth and migration
bFGF, PDGF-AA, PDGF-AB, PDGF-BB, VEGF, VEGF-C, VEGF-D	Promote angiogenesis, also proliferative and migration stimulatory effects
TGF-β_3, HGF	Inhibit scar and contracture formation
IFN-α_2	Prevent fibrosis by decreasing TGF-β_1 and TGF-β_2
α_2-Macroglobulin	Inhibit protease activity, coordinate growth factor bioavailability
Acrp-30	Regulate growth and activity of keratinocytes
IL-1Ra	Anti-inflammatory
N-GAL	Antibacterial
LIF	Support of angiogenic growth factors
SDF-1β	Recruit cells to site of tissue damage
IGFBP-1, IGFBP-2, IGFBP-3	Regulate IGF and its proliferative effects

From Maxson S, Lopez EA, Yoo D, et al: Concise review: Role of mesenchymal stem cells in wound repair. *Stem Cells Transl Med* 1:142–149, 2012.

Acrp-30, Adiponectin; *Ang-2,* angiotensin-2; *bFGF,* basic fibroblast growth factor; *EGF,* epidermal growth factor; *FGF-7,* fibroblast growth factor-7; *HB-EGF,* heparin-bound epidermal growth factor; *HGF,* hepatocyte growth factor; *IFN-α_2,* interferon-α_2; *IGF,* insulin-like growth factor; *IGFBP-1, -2, -3,* insulin-like growth factor binding protein-1, -2, -3; *IL-1Ra,* interleukin-1 receptor antagonist; *KGF,* keratinocyte growth factor; *LIF,* leukemia inhibitory factor; *MMP-1, -2, -3, -7, -8, -9, 10, -13,* matrix metalloproteinase-1, -2, -3, -7, -8, -9, 10, -13; *N-GAL,* neutrophil gelatinase-associated lipocalin; *PDGF,* platelet-derived growth factor; *PEDF,* pigment epithelium-derived factor; *PIGF,* placenta growth factor; *SDF-1β,* stromal cell–derived factor 1β; *TGF-α,* transforming growth factor-α; *TIMP-1, -2,* tissue inhibitor of matrix metalloproteinase-1, -2; *TPO,* thrombopoietin; *VEGF,* vascular endothelial growth factor.

receptor antagonist, and several others. These factors help to transition from the inflammatory phase to the proliferative phase of wound healing and to clear infected wounds. Also present are the angiogenic proteins VEGF, basic FGF, and PDGF; the epithelial cell stimulatory proteins KGF and EGF; and the antiscarring proteins TGF-β_3, IFN-α_2, and HGF. Physiologic levels of growth factors and cytokines are critical to ensure healing of chronic wounds. The unique population of viable cells allows for the sustained release of a cocktail of growth factors, persisting at physiologic levels over extended periods and eliminating the need for frequent reapplication. Functionally, the skin substitutes have been shown to promote cell migration and wound closure in in vitro wound-healing assays.

Further investigation is also needed to elucidate the interactions between MSCs and the various immune and wound-healing cell types that are present in the wound bed because these studies would be useful to optimize the timing and dosage of MSC delivery to the wound for maximal efficacy. The use of MSCs as a therapy presents advantages over pharmaceuticals, protein/growth factors, and committed progenitor cells because MSCs are able to interact with the surrounding cell types and biochemical environment to express in a regulated manner the appropriate trophic factors for enhanced dermal wound healing. MSCs will likely emerge as an important therapy to reduce the formation of fibrotic tissue and the appearance of scars after cutaneous injury (Fig. 6-13).[49]

Bone marrow–derived or whole blood–derived endothelial progenitor cells are endothelial precursors and play a role in angiogenesis and vasculogenesis. These cells improve tissue perfusion by increasing neovascularization. Subsequently, these cells, which can secrete angiogenic factors such as VEGF, are potentially important in the treatment of numerous disease processes, including wound healing, myocardial infarction, vascular disease, and cancer.

Skin has also been shown to be a large repository of MAPCs. These MAPCs can arise from the epidermis, dermis, hair follicle bulge, dermal sheath, and dermal papillae. In particular, the hair follicle bulge area is considered an abundant, easily accessible source of actively growing MAPCs. Hair follicle MAPCs have been shown to differentiate into neurons, glial cells, keratinocytes, and smooth muscle cells. Because of their location, skin-derived MAPCs are present in the wound and are accessible for harvest.

Gene therapy, or the insertion of a gene into recipient cells, has the potential to affect wound healing by recruiting MAPCs to the wound in vivo or through ex vivo modification of MAPCs; the modified cell can then be used for cellular therapy. Gene therapy using vectors has been used experimentally to improve wound healing through overexpression of chemokine genes known to have effects on MAPC homing. Gene therapy allows for the continuous production of the desired protein into the wound by the transduced cells. Direct administration of proteins into the wound could potentially result in degradation of the proteins by wound proteases. Gene therapy–mediated overexpression of HIF-1α and SDF-1α have been used to improve wound healing in a diabetic mouse model.

Although much is still unknown about the use of gene therapy in wound healing, a great deal of research is underway. As more is learned about the molecular biology of wound healing, there will likely be greater use of gene therapy to accelerate wound healing.

The therapy of choice needs to be based on the basics of wound bed preparation and modified according to the characteristics of the wound. Despite the availability of many dressings and alternative therapies, no substantial studies have shown a difference in healing between therapies of the same category. The cost-benefit ratio of some therapeutic modalities is still unclear. A systematic approach that addresses débridement, exudate

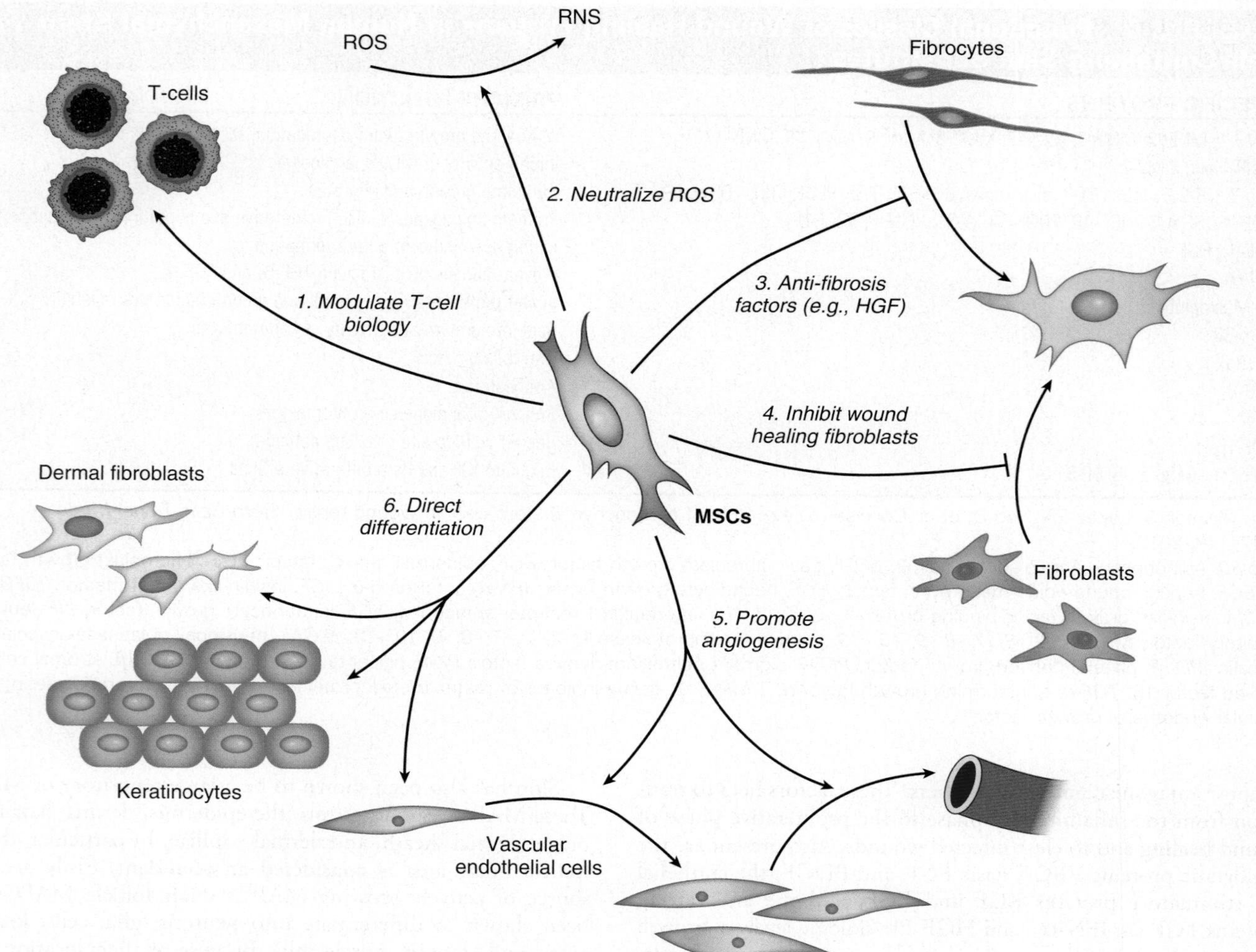

FIGURE 6-13 Mesenchymal stem cells (*MSCs*) can influence cutaneous regeneration by multiple distinct mechanisms acting on multiple cell types. *HGF,* Hepatic growth factor; *RNS,* reactive nitrogen species; *ROS,* reactive oxygen species. (From Jackson WM, Nesti LJ, Tuan RS: Mesenchymal stem cell therapy for attenuation of scar formation during wound healing. *Stem Cell Res Ther* 3:20, 2012.)

management, and bacterial burden should be the standard of clinical practice and can be accomplished even in situations with limited resources.

SELECTED REFERENCES

Alberts B, Johnson A, Lewis J, et al, editors: Cell junctions, cell adhesion, and the extracellular matrix. In *The Molecular Biology of the Cell*, ed 4, New York, 2002, Garland, pp 1091–1114.

This chapter provides a comprehensive review of matrix and integrin biology and the critical role of these in biologic processes, including tissue repair.

Barrientos S, Stojadinovic O, Golinko MS, et al: Growth factors and cytokines in wound healing. *Wound Repair Regen* 16:585–601, 2008.

This article reviews cytokines, growth factors, and chemokines in wound healing.

Bello YM, Falabella AF, Eaglstein WH: Tissue-engineered skin. Current status in wound healing. *Am J Clin Dermatol* 2:305–313, 2001.

This article discusses the various skin substitutes available and their uses in wound healing.

Dang C, Ting K, Soo C, et al: Fetal wound healing current perspectives. *Clin Plast Surg* 30:13–23, 2003.

This review article discusses the morphologic, cellular, and molecular aspects of scarless fetal wound healing.

Eming SA, Hammerschmidt M, Krieg T, et al: Interrelation of immunity and tissue repair or regeneration. *Semin Cell Dev Biol* 20:517–527, 2009.

This article reviews the complex role of the immune system in tissue repair and tissue regeneration.

Herdrich BJ, Lind RC, Liechty KW: Multipotent adult progenitor cells: Their role in wound healing and the treatment of dermal wounds. *Cytotherapy* 10:543–550, 2008.

This article provides a comprehensive review of the current state of stem cell therapy in wound healing.

Hunter JE, Teot L, Horch R, et al: Evidence-based medicine: Vacuum-assisted closure in wound care management. *Int Wound J* 4:256–269, 2007.

This article reviews negative-pressure wound closure using evidence-based medicine.

Juckett G, Hartman-Adams H: Management of keloids and hypertrophic scars. *Am Fam Physician* 80:253–260, 2009.

This article discusses current evidence-based treatment of keloids and hypertrophic scars.

Kulikovsky M, Gil T, Mettanes I, et al: Hyperbaric oxygen therapy for non-healing wounds. *Isr Med Assoc J* 11:480–485, 2009.

Negative-pressure wound closure topics and uses are reviewed.

Lionelli GT, Lawrence WT: Wound dressings. *Surg Clin North Am* 83:617–638, 2003.

This article provides a thorough discussion of classes and uses of wound dressings.

Singer AJ, Clark RAF: Cutaneous wound healing. *N Engl J Med* 341:738–746, 1999.

This article provides a comprehensive review of the cellular and molecular aspects of wound healing.

REFERENCES

1. Goren I, Allmann N, Yogev N, et al: A transgenic mouse model of inducible macrophage depletion: Effects of diphtheria toxin-driven lysozyme M-specific cell lineage ablation on wound inflammatory, angiogenic, and contractive processes. *Am J Pathol* 175:132–147, 2009.
2. Lucas T, Waisman A, Ranjan R, et al: Differential roles of macrophages in diverse phases of skin repair. *J Immunol* 184:3964–3977, 2010.
3. Mirza R, DiPietro LA, Koh TJ: Selective and specific macrophage ablation is detrimental to wound healing in mice. *Am J Pathol* 175:2454–2462, 2009.
4. Voigt J, Driver VR: Hyaluronic acid derivatives and their healing effect on burns, epithelial surgical wounds, and chronic wounds: A systematic review and meta-analysis of randomized controlled trials. *Wound Repair Regen* 20:317–331, 2012.
5. Shih B, Bayat A: Genetics of keloid scarring. *Arch Dermatol Res* 302:319–339, 2010.
6. Gauglitz GG, Korting HC, Pavicic T, et al: Hypertrophic scarring and keloids: Pathomechanisms and current and emerging treatment strategies. *Mol Med* 17:113–125, 2011.
7. Engrav LH, Heimbach DM, Rivara FP, et al: 12-Year within-wound study of the effectiveness of custom pressure garment therapy. *Burns* 36:975–983, 2010.
8. Juckett G, Hartman-Adams H: Management of keloids and hypertrophic scars. *Am Fam Physician* 80:253–260, 2009.
9. Cooper JS, Lee BT: Treatment of facial scarring: Lasers, filler, and nonoperative techniques. *Facial Plast Surg* 25:311–315, 2009.
10. Yagmur C, Akaishi S, Ogawa R, et al: Mechanical receptor-related mechanisms in scar management: A review and hypothesis. *Plast Reconstr Surg* 126:426–434, 2010.
11. Davison SP, Dayan JH, Clemens MW, et al: Efficacy of intralesional 5-fluorouracil and triamcinolone in the treatment of keloids. *Aesthet Surg J* 29:40–46, 2009.
12. Rio E, Bardet E, Peuvrel P, et al: Perioperative interstitial brachytherapy for recurrent keloid scars. *Plast Reconstr Surg* 124:180e–181e, 2009.
13. Ogawa R, Yoshitatsu S, Yoshida K, et al: Is radiation therapy for keloids acceptable? The risk of radiation-induced carcinogenesis. *Plast Reconstr Surg* 124:1196–1201, 2009.
14. Cacao FM, Tanaka V, Messina MC: Failure of imiquimod 5% cream to prevent recurrence of surgically excised trunk keloids. *Dermatol Surg* 35:629–633, 2009.
15. Greaves NS, Iqbal SA, Baguneid M, et al: The role of skin substitutes in the management of chronic cutaneous wounds. *Wound Repair Regen* 21:194–210, 2013.
16. Shih B, Sultan MJ, Chaudhry IH, et al: Identification of biomarkers in sequential biopsies of patients with chronic wounds receiving simultaneous acute wounds: A genetic, histological, and noninvasive imaging study. *Wound Repair Regen* 20:757–769, 2012.
17. Sorensen LT, Toft BG, Rygaard J, et al: Effect of smoking, smoking cessation, and nicotine patch on wound dimension, vitamin C, and systemic markers of collagen metabolism. *Surgery* 148:982–990, 2010.
18. Thangarajah H, Yao D, Chang EI, et al: The molecular basis for impaired hypoxia-induced VEGF expression in diabetic tissues. *Proc Natl Acad Sci U S A* 106:13505–13510, 2009.
19. Hom DB, Ho V, Lee CKK: Irradiated skin and its postsurgical management. In Hom DB, Hebda PA, Gosain AK, editors: *Essential Tissue Healing of the Face and the Neck*, Shelton, CT, 2009, BC Decker and People's Medical Publishing House, pp 224–238.
20. Goessler UR, Bugert P, Kassner S, et al: In vitro analysis of radiation-induced dermal wounds. *Otolaryngol Head Neck Surg* 142:845–850, 2010.
21. Haubner F, Ohmann E, Pohl F, et al: Wound healing after radiation therapy: Review of the literature. *Radiat Oncol* 7:162, 2012.
22. Delanian S, Chatel C, Porcher R, et al: Complete restoration of refractory mandibular osteoradionecrosis by prolonged treatment with a pentoxifylline-tocopherol-clodronate combination (PENTOCLO): A phase II trial. *Int J Radiat Oncol Biol Phys* 80:832–839, 2011.
23. Freiberger JJ, Yoo DS, de Lisle Dear G, et al: Multimodality surgical and hyperbaric management of mandibular osteoradionecrosis. *Int J Radiat Oncol Biol Phys* 75:717–724, 2009.
24. Jacobson AS, Buchbinder D, Hu K, et al: Paradigm shifts in the management of osteoradionecrosis of the mandible. *Oral Oncol* 46:795–801, 2010.
25. Kendall AC, Whatmore JL, Harries LW, et al: Changes in inflammatory gene expression induced by hyperbaric oxygen

treatment in human endothelial cells under chronic wound conditions. *Exp Cell Res* 318:207–216, 2012.
26. Thom SR: Hyperbaric oxygen: Its mechanisms and efficacy. *Plast Reconstr Surg* 127(Suppl 1):131S–141S, 2011.
27. Sgonc R, Gruber J: Age-related aspects of cutaneous wound healing: A mini-review. *Gerontology* 59:159–164, 2013.
28. Macri L, Clark RA: Tissue engineering for cutaneous wounds: Selecting the proper time and space for growth factors, cells and the extracellular matrix. *Skin Pharmacol Physiol* 22:83–93, 2009.
29. Kulikovsky M, Gil T, Mettanes I, et al: Hyperbaric oxygen therapy for non-healing wounds. *Isr Med Assoc J* 11:480–485, 2009.
30. Goldman RJ: Hyperbaric oxygen therapy for wound healing and limb salvage: A systematic review. *PM R* 1:471–489, 2009.
31. Kuffler DP: Hyperbaric oxygen therapy: An overview. *J Wound Care* 19:77–79, 2010.
32. Wu SC, Marston W, Armstrong DG: Wound care: The role of advanced wound healing technologies. *J Vasc Surg* 52:59S–66S, 2010.
33. Wang S, Qu X, Zhao RC: Mesenchymal stem cells hold promise for regenerative medicine. *Front Med* 5:372–378, 2011.
34. Prockop DJ, Oh JY: Mesenchymal stem/stromal cells (MSCs): Role as guardians of inflammation. *Mol Ther* 20:14–20, 2012.
35. Kong W, Li S, Lorenz HP: Germ plasm-like Dot cells maintain their wound regenerative function after in vitro expansion. *Clin Exp Pharmacol Physiol* 37:e136–e144, 2010.
36. Leung A, Crombleholme TM, Keswani SG: Fetal wound healing: Implications for minimal scar formation. *Curr Opin Pediatr* 24:371–378, 2012.
37. Lazic T, Falanga V: Bioengineered skin constructs and their use in wound healing. *Plast Reconstr Surg* 127(Suppl 1):75S–90S, 2011.
38. Auger FA, Lacroix D, Germain L: Skin substitutes and wound healing. *Skin Pharmacol Physiol* 22:94–102, 2009.
39. Brown BN, Valentin JE, Stewart-Akers AM, et al: Macrophage phenotype and remodeling outcomes in response to biologic scaffolds with and without a cellular component. *Biomaterials* 30:1482–1491, 2009.
40. Keane TJ, Londono R, Turner NJ, et al: Consequences of ineffective decellularization of biologic scaffolds on the host response. *Biomaterials* 33:1771–1781, 2012.
41. Valentin JE, Stewart-Akers AM, Gilbert TW, et al: Macrophage participation in the degradation and remodeling of extracellular matrix scaffolds. *Tissue Eng Part A* 15:1687–1694, 2009.
42. Hwang JH, Shim SS, Seok OS, et al: Comparison of cytokine expression in mesenchymal stem cells from human placenta, cord blood, and bone marrow. *J Korean Med Sci* 24:547–554, 2009.
43. Maxson S, Lopez EA, Yoo D, et al: Concise review: Role of mesenchymal stem cells in wound repair. *Stem Cells Transl Med* 1:142–149, 2012.
44. Dash NR, Dash SN, Routray P, et al: Targeting nonhealing ulcers of lower extremity in human through autologous bone marrow-derived mesenchymal stem cells. *Rejuvenation Res* 12:359–366, 2009.
45. Lu D, Chen B, Liang Z, et al: Comparison of bone marrow mesenchymal stem cells with bone marrow-derived mononuclear cells for treatment of diabetic critical limb ischemia and foot ulcer: A double-blind, randomized, controlled trial. *Diabetes Res Clin Pract* 92:26–36, 2011.
46. Bieback K, Brinkmann I: Mesenchymal stromal cells from human perinatal tissues: From biology to cell therapy. *World J Stem Cells* 2:81–92, 2010.
47. Wolbank S, Hildner F, Redl H, et al: Impact of human amniotic membrane preparation on release of angiogenic factors. *J Tissue Eng Regen Med* 3:651–654, 2009.
48. Yew TL, Hung YT, Li HY, et al: Enhancement of wound healing by human multipotent stromal cell conditioned medium: The paracrine factors and p38 MAPK activation. *Cell Transplant* 20:693–706, 2011.
49. Jackson WM, Nesti LJ, Tuan RS: Mesenchymal stem cell therapy for attenuation of scar formation during wound healing. *Stem Cell Res Ther* 3:20, 2012.

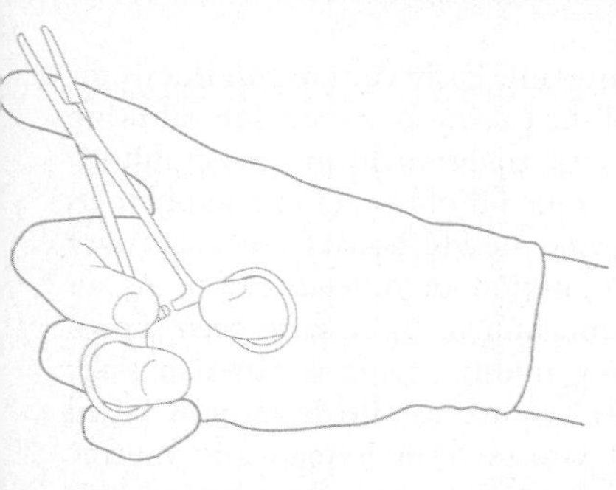

CHAPTER 7

Regenerative Medicine

Michael S. Hu, Graham G. Walmsley, H. Peter Lorenz, Michael T. Longaker

OUTLINE

Regeneration is the restoration of normal tissue and organ architecture and function after injury or disease. Although many complex organisms retain the capacity for substantial regrowth of limbs and organ repair throughout adult life, humans have sacrificed regenerative potential for speed and strength of repair. This trade-off leaves humans vulnerable to significant scarring with accompanying loss of functionality and esthetic appeal. Developing the technology to induce true tissue regeneration promises to enhance dramatically the effectiveness of normal wound healing, while simultaneously reducing the negative sequelae of scar formation.

Although surgeons have understood the dynamics of wound healing for decades, comprehensive tissue and organ regeneration remains clinically elusive. The field of regenerative medicine combines diverse disciplines ranging from cell and molecular biology to tissue engineering and biomaterial science in the continuing search for regenerative therapies. Current emphasis is largely on stem cells—undifferentiated cells that have the ability to self-renew and give rise to specialized cell types. As basic scientific research continues to elucidate mechanisms underlying stem cell biology, translational opportunities for stem cell–based therapies have become increasingly tenable. This chapter provides an overview of the current status of stem cell biology, tissue engineering, and clinical application and highlights future steps required for incorporation of regenerative medicine into clinical practice.

STEM CELL SOURCES

Stem cells are characterized by the ability to self-renew and differentiate into multiple functional cell types (Table 7-1). Traditionally, stem cells are divided into two main groups based on their differentiation potential: pluripotent and multipotent (Fig. 7-1). Pluripotent stem cells, or embryonic stem cells (ESCs), can differentiate into any cell in the body, whereas multipotent stem cells, or adult stem cells, are limited to multiple cell lineages, but not all. In addition to the traditional stem cell classification, the advent of reprogramming technology introduced a new class of stem cells termed *induced pluripotent stem cells* (iPSCs). First described in 2007 by Yamanaka and Thomson in two independent studies, human iPSCs are derived by manipulating the genetic expression of terminally differentiated multipotent stem cells to convert them into pluripotent stem cells. Together, these diverse stem cell populations hold the promise of a versatile armamentarium for researchers and clinicians to address a wide-ranging spectrum of human disease and dysfunction.

Embryonic Stem Cells

In embryologic development, two distinct lineages emerge during the transition from morula to blastocyst: trophoectoderm and inner cell mass. ESCs are derived from the inner cell mass. ESCs are characterized by the capacity for unlimited self-renewal and the ability to differentiate into any somatic cell type.[1] The former characteristic is maintained by numerous transcription factors, most prominently Oct4, Sox2, and Nanog, which act as essential gene expression regulators to preserve ESC pluripotency, while suppressing differentiation.[2] Two glycolipid antigens, SSEA3 and SSEA4, are cell surface markers used to identify and isolate human ESCs.[3]

ESC potential in regenerative medicine has been widely demonstrated.[4] For instance, when cultured under specific growth factor conditions, mouse and human ESCs have demonstrated the capacity in vitro to form a diverse array of terminally differentiated cells, including cardiomyocytes, hematopoietic progenitors, neurons, skeletal myocytes, adipocytes, osteocytes, chondrocytes, and pancreatic islet cells.[5,6] However, many limitations curtail the use of human ESCs in regenerative medicine. Although pluripotentiality and unlimited ability for self-renewal make ESCs attractive for cell replacement therapy, these traits also enable dysregulated growth, which can lead to the formation of teratomas and teratocarcinomas. Teratomas and associated tumors contain undifferentiated pluripotent stem cells and differentiated cells from all three primary germ layers. A tendency for ESCs to form tumors has been observed when human ESCs are transplanted into mice, raising the concern that human ESC–based therapy may also lead to unwanted tumor formation.[1] Until this risk can be addressed, the clinical use of ESC-derived tissue remains limited.

In addition, any cell-based therapy must be free of animal contaminants that can elicit an immune reaction or pathogens

TABLE 7-1 Definitions of Stem Cell–Related Terms

TERM	DEFINITION
Totipotent	Ability to form all cell types and lineages of organism (e.g., fertilized egg)
Pluripotent	Ability to form all lineages of the body (e.g., embryonic stem cells)
Multipotent	Ability of adult stem cells to form multiple cell types of one lineage (e.g., mesenchymal stem cells)
Unipotent	Cells form one cell type (e.g., follicular bulge skin stem cells)
Reprogramming	Dedifferentiation into an embryonic state; can be induced by nuclear transfer, genetic manipulation, viral transduction, and related methods

that transmit disease after transplant. Early culture conditions for human ESC lines were established using protocols for culturing mouse ESCs.[7] Human ESCs were traditionally grown on mitotically inactivated murine embryonic fibroblasts (also referred to as *feeder layers*). Feeder layers provide the additional factors necessary for ESC proliferation and inhibition of differentiation. As an example of animal contaminant, human ESCs have been shown to be capable of incorporating immunogenic nonhuman sialic acid from murine feeder cells.[8] Concerns also have been raised over the possible transfer of viruses from human and murine feeder layers to ESCs.[9] Many laboratories are working to solve this problem, with studies demonstrating the ability to culture human ESCs under serum-free and feeder-free conditions.[8]

Lastly, there are significant political and ethical hurdles that hinder further investigations of human ESCs. At the present time, the limited number of ESC lines available and the restrictions

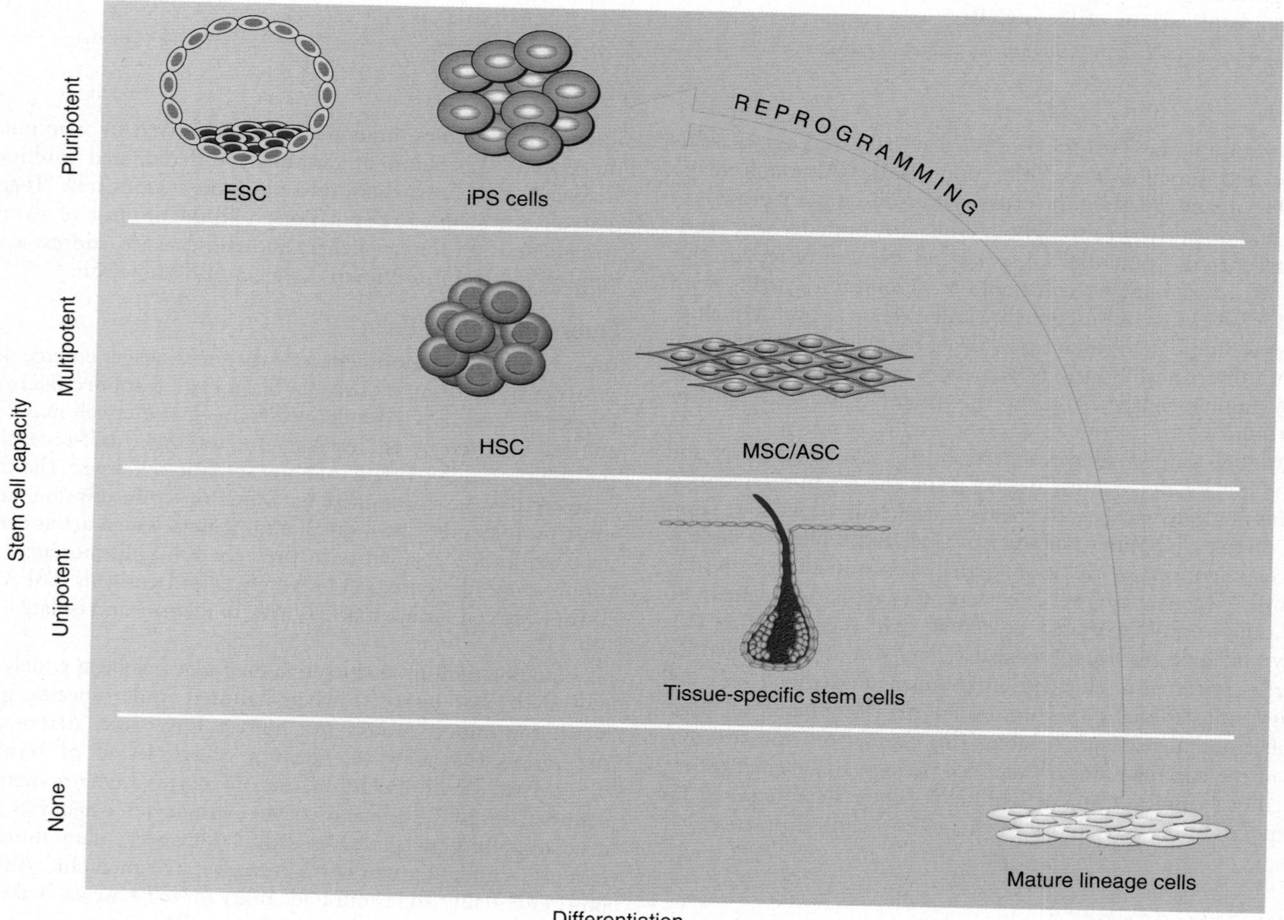

FIGURE 7-1 Schematic of stem cell organization. Embryonic stem cells (ESCs), derived from the inner cell mass of the blastocyst, have the highest stem cell capacity (pluripotent) and are the least committed to any tissue lineage. Adult stem cells such as hematopoietic stem cells (HSCs) and mesenchymal stem cells (MSCs) are multipotent and are limited to certain tissue lineages, although they remain in a relatively undifferentiated state at rest. Tissue-specific stem cells, such as skin follicular bulge cells, are limited to producing a single cell and tissue type (unipotent), although they retain considerable proliferative capacity to regenerate their specific tissue. Mature lineage cells, such as mature epithelium, do not have regenerative potential. Induced pluripotent stem (iPS) cells are mature lineage cells or adult stem cells that have been reprogrammed to a state of relative pluripotency and have much of the same regenerative potential as ESCs. *ASC,* adipose stem cell.

placed on their use have precluded major progress in ESC-based applications.

Somatic Cell Nuclear Transfer

Somatic cell nuclear transfer (SCNT), a technique for creating viable embryos, involves the transfer of a nucleus from a somatic cell containing the desired genetic profile into an enucleated ovum. Mitotic divisions of the resultant cell in culture lead to the generation of a blastocyst capable of yielding a complete organism. Major landmarks in this field include the 1997 production of a normal sheep (Dolly)—the first mammal to be cloned from a somatic cell.[10] This procedure has been reproduced in other mammals, including mice, cattle, pigs, cats, and dogs.[11]

These experimental studies suggest that a similar approach using SCNT might work in humans for therapeutic cloning, whereby human ESCs produced by this approach could be subsequently differentiated into therapeutically useful cells and transplanted back into patients with degenerative diseases. A more recent SCNT study combined the nucleus from a patient with type 1 diabetes with a donated enucleated oocyte and successfully differentiated the resultant stem cell into beta cells capable of producing insulin. This study marks an important step toward the use of SCNT in regenerative therapies.[12]

However, cells that result from SCNT are imperfect copies of the cells of the nucleus donor. The enucleated ovum contains mitochondrial DNA in the cytoplasm that is genetically distinct from the mitochondrial DNA of the nucleus donor. Research has suggested that mismatched mitochondrial DNA in these hybrid cells generates allogenicity and subjects transplanted stem cells to immune rejection.[13] In addition, the low differentiation efficiency of this procedure continues to hinder progress in the field, with several studies reporting less than 10% efficiency in the derivation of SCNT-generated ESCs.[14] Despite these hurdles, SCNT and therapeutic cloning may be a promising means to generate genetically matched stem cell lines. Long-lasting cell lines from patients can be used to screen potentially useful drugs or other treatments and may provide replacement cells for damaged organs.

Induced Pluripotent Stem Cells

In light of the impediments surrounding SCNT technology, alternatives that recapitulate the reprogramming process in vitro while avoiding the need for donated oocytes altogether are ultimately preferable. A groundbreaking study published in 2006 by Takahashi and Yamanaka[15] defined a specific set of transcription factors (Oct4, Sox2, Klf4, and cMyc) that could be manipulated to reprogram adult mouse fibroblasts back into a pluripotent state, creating ESC-like iPSCs. In 2007, Yu and colleagues[16] from Thomson's laboratory and Takahashi and coworkers[17] from Yamanaka's laboratory published articles separately demonstrating that similar transcription factors are sufficient for the pluripotent induction of human somatic cells as well. The ease and reproducibility of generating iPSCs compared with SCNT gave rise to the hope that iPSCs might fulfill much of the promise of human ESCs in regenerative medicine.

In terms of molecular and developmental features, mouse and human iPSCs closely resemble blastocyst-derived ESCs.[15,18] Similar to ESCs, iPSCs injected into immunodeficient mice can generate teratomas that contain derivatives of all three embryonic germ layers. In addition, when combined with diploid blastocysts, iPSCs generated viable high-contribution chimeras (mice that show major tissue contributions of the injected iPSCs in the host mouse). Germline contribution was confirmed by mating chimeras generated from two iPSC lines.[15,18] Lastly, studies using reverse transcriptase polymerase chain reaction (RT-PCR) assays and immunocytochemistry showed that iPSCs express key markers of ESCs.

However, more recent studies also have suggested that iPSCs are not identical to ESCs. Global gene expression analysis comparing iPSCs with ESCs using microarrays demonstrated that approximately 4% of the more than 32,000 analyzed genes had more than a fivefold difference in expression.[19] Furthermore, chimeras and progeny mice derived from iPSCs had higher than normal rates of tumor formation than those derived from ESCs, which in some cases may have been caused by reactivation of the transfected *c-Myc* oncogene.[20] These key differences need to be explored further to confirm the safety of iPSC use in regenerative medicine.

In addition, generation of iPSCs has been complicated by the use of retroviral and lentiviral vectors to activate necessary reprogramming transcription factors. Viral genome is inserted near endogenous genes, resulting in either gene activation or silencing. This insertional mutagenesis can lead to uncontrolled modification of the genome, with the potential development of cancer. Much progress has been made in generating integration-free murine iPSCs, and numerous laboratories are actively investigating alternatives to viral integration with adenoviral, plasmid-based, and recombinant protein–based strategies.[21,22] Even without viral integration, the safety of iPSCs needs to be rigorously tested because many essential reprogramming factors are proto-oncogenic, and their overexpression has been linked with tumorigenesis.[23] The characterization of iPSCs may be enhanced by high-resolution analysis of genomic integrity to identify minor deletions, inversions, or loss of individual alleles.

Derived from the patient's own cells, iPSCs hold promise to eliminate the need for immunosuppressive therapies after transplantation. Ideally, they represent the perfect therapy with which to restore lost organ function and have the potential to create a major impact on regenerative medicine. Human iPSCs can be generated from adipose-derived stem cells (ASCs) in a feeder-free environment with greater speed and higher efficiency than comparable strategies targeting adult human fibroblasts.[24] Given the ease of isolating a large quantity of ASCs from lipoaspirates, ASCs could be an ideal autologous source of cells for generating individual-specific iPSCs.

The therapeutic potential of iPSCs has been demonstrated in several preclinical models. For example, Wernig and colleagues[25] demonstrated that neurons derived from reprogrammed fibroblasts could alleviate the disease phenotype in a rat model of Parkinson disease. Using a humanized sickle cell anemia mouse model, Hanna and associates[26] showed that the genetic defect could be corrected using transplantation of hematopoietic stem cells (HSCs) derived from iPSCs (reprogrammed from fibroblasts of those mice) that had homologous recombination of an intact wild-type β-globin gene.

In 2014, the first human clinical trial using iPSCs to treat age-related macular degeneration was launched in Japan. Scientists across the globe are waiting to see if this procedure halts degeneration and what, if any, adverse effects may result. If this clinical trial is successful, it will allay some of the major safety concerns and pave the way for further iPSC-based clinical trials.

Fetal Stem Cells

Although less prominently discussed, fetal stem cells represent another potential source for regenerative cell-based therapies.

Fetal stem cells can be derived from fetal blood, liver, bone marrow, amniotic fluid, and placenta.[27,28] Fetal stem cells have similar immunophenotype as ESCs but are more restricted in the variety of mature cell types into which they can differentiate. They have been found to be capable of expanding in culture for at least 20 passages, and their capacity for adipogenic, osteogenic, and chondrogenic differentiation has been demonstrated under appropriate growth conditions.[29] In addition, transplantation into a xenogeneic sheep model established the ability of these cells to engraft and undergo site-specific tissue differentiation.

Despite these promising findings, significant debate exists over the use of fetal tissue and the attendant risks associated with intrauterine collection of fetal blood. Nonetheless, fetal stem cells may provide a novel means whereby future autogenous in utero cellular and genetic therapies can be devised.

Adult Stem Cells

When embryonic development is completed, humans and other complex organisms lose their store of pluripotent stem cells. During adult life, the regenerative capacity of tissues and organs is maintained by adult stem cells. In contrast to ESCs and iPSCs, adult stem cells are multipotent, which means that they can differentiate into some, but not all, tissue lineages and are typically confined to a certain tissue type and microenvironment, termed a *stem cell niche*.[30] Adult stem cells exist in these tissue-specific reservoirs and retain the ability to form many different cellular lineages (Fig. 7-2). Although the differentiation potential of these cells is not as complete as that of ESCs or iPSCs, their relative abundance and ease of isolation from adult patients establishes adult stem cells as a highly relevant cell type for potential clinical

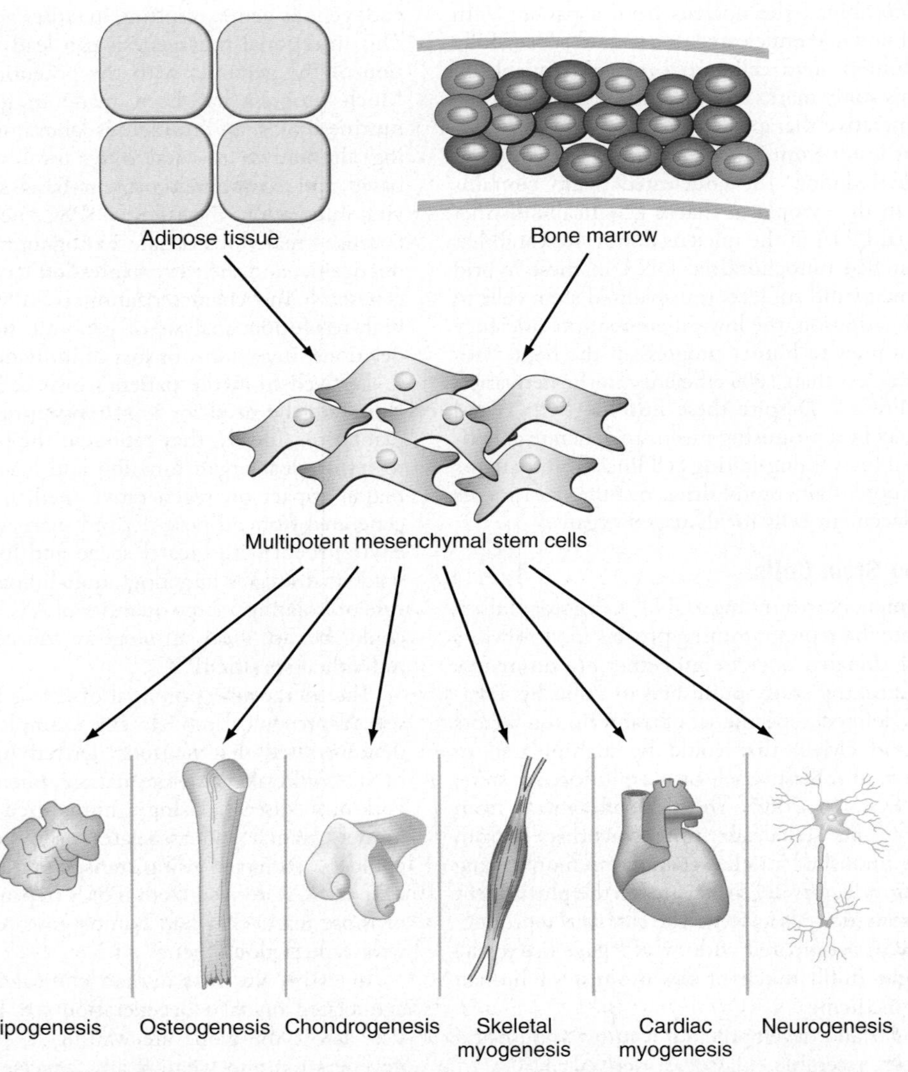

FIGURE 7-2 Adult multipotent mesenchymal stem cells can be isolated from adipose tissue (adipose stem cells) or from bone marrow (mesenchymal stem cells). These cells have been shown to differentiate into multiple tissue types in vitro, including adipose tissue (apidogenesis), bone (osteogenesis), cartilage (chondrogenesis), skeletal and cardiac muscle (skeletal and cardiac myogenesis), and nerve (neurogenesis) tissues. There has been varying success in differentiating these cells into these tissue types in vivo, which will be necessary before adult multipotent stem cells can be clinically useful for regenerative medicine applications.

applications. Adult multipotent stem cells have been a focus of intensive research efforts over the past several decades.

The most studied and best characterized type of adult stem cell is the HSC, which has served as the experimental paradigm for basic studies into the biology of adult stem cells.[31] Additional insight has been gained into the organization and function of two other categories of adult stem cells, mesenchymal stem cells (MSCs) and adipose stromal cells, which show considerable promise for use in regenerative medicine.

Hematopoietic Stem Cells

Since being definitively isolated in mice several decades ago, HSCs have been the most studied and best characterized type of adult multipotent stem cell.[32] These blood-forming cells reside in specialized niches within adult bone marrow and maintain homeostasis of all lineages of hematopoietic cells. At the present time, the most widely used stem cell therapy is bone marrow transplantation for hematologic malignancies. In this therapy, transplanted HSCs replace ablated host bone marrow and subsequently repopulate all lineages of the hematopoietic system.[31] Despite the enormous ability of HSCs to regenerate the hematopoietic system, HSCs have not been proven to be able to transdifferentiate into other tissue lineages, limiting their usefulness in cell-based therapeutic interventions outside of the hematopoietic system.[33] Additionally, HSCs are difficult to maintain in vitro, further limiting their usefulness for regenerative medicine applications. In light of these limitations, a more promising avenue involves investigating a possible role for HSCs in the induction of tolerance before organ transplantation.[34]

Skeletal Stem Cells

Since the isolation and characterization of HSCs in 1988,[32] the hematopoietic niche has undergone extensive characterization and is the best characterized stem cell niche to date. More recently, a population of postnatal skeletal stem cells in mice were prospectively isolated and mapped to their downstream progenitors of bone, cartilage, and stromal tissue.[35] Furthermore, specific combinations of niche factors were defined and used to activate skeletal stem cell programs in situ to form cartilage or bone and bone marrow stroma. This work has important implications for potential therapies across a wide range of skeletal disorders, such as osteosarcoma, fractures, and damaged cartilage.

Mesenchymal Stem Cells

The stromal fraction of adult bone marrow contains a heterogeneous population of cells that were originally described as supportive cells for hematopoietic cells and later termed MSCs. This group of multipotent cells can differentiate into mesenchymal-derived structures, such as bone, fat, cartilage, and muscle.[36] MSCs are rare in the bone marrow because they make up only approximately 1 in 10,000 bone marrow cells. They have traditionally been isolated by their ability to adhere to polystyrene tissue culture plastic. However, this isolation method produces a heterogeneous mix of cells, which has made comparison of experimental protocols and standardization of results difficult. Reports of human MSC surface antigen expression profiles vary widely; there is no consensus at the present time on the surface markers that can be used for prospective isolation protocols. A comprehensive review of the literature suggested that proposed MSC surface markers can be categorized into two groups: sole markers and stemness markers.[37,38] Sole markers may present an alternative isolation method to traditional adherence protocols and have been successfully used to purify MSC-like cells from an in vivo environment. Examples of sole markers include Stro-1 and CD271. Stemness markers identify cells with ESC-like qualities of self-renewal and potential for differentiation down multiple lineages. Examples of stemness markers include CD146 and SSEA-3. However, there are numerous limitations with the aforementioned surface markers. For example, Stro-1 is also found on enucleated erythroid cells and is not expressed by MSCs universally. Further development of a standardized isolation protocol for MSCs is an active area of ongoing research.

MSCs have been widely studied for use in the regeneration of cartilage and skeletal defects, and results from animal models of both metabolic and traumatic skeletal injuries have been encouraging.[39] MSCs play a supportive role in tissue regeneration by creating a favorable local environment through secretion of growth factors and angiogenic signals. For example, MSCs have been shown to increase wound healing in chronic wounds, although the cells do not persist in the wounds over time.[40] MSCs also have been shown to improve myocardial function after infarction in animal models,[41] although results in human trials using systemic injection of bone marrow cells after myocardial infarction have been mixed.[42,43] Also, because infarcted myocardium and other damaged tissues often present environments hostile to the engraftment and proliferation of stem cells, promoting MSC survival in these settings presents a significant hurdle to the therapeutic efficacy of MSCs.[44]

Adipose-Derived Stromal Cells

There is growing excitement in the field of regenerative medicine concerning the use of the stromal vascular fraction of subcutaneous adipose tissue, which contains a heterogeneous group of undifferentiated cells that are collectively referred to as *adipose stem cells* (ASCs). These cells also have been referred to as *processed lipoaspirate cells, adipose-derived stem cells,* and *adipose-derived mesenchymal cells.* Zuk and colleagues[45] demonstrated that these cells can be coaxed to differentiate into bone, adipose tissue, cartilage, and muscle in vitro. In addition, there have been several reports of limited differentiation of ASCs into neural tissue[46] and cardiac myocytes.[47] The major advantage of ASCs is their relative abundance and ease of isolation from subcutaneous adipose tissue through standard lipoaspirate techniques. Approximately 1 billion ASCs per liter of lipoaspirate specimen can be isolated. More studies to characterize thoroughly the heterogeneous mixture of cells that are present in adipose tissue are ongoing, but unpublished data from our group have suggested that ASCs may contain multiple subpopulations with distinct differential abilities to produce specific tissue types. By applying different growth factors, such as bone morphogenetic protein or fibroblast growth factor, ASCs can be induced to form different tissues for therapeutic use.[48] When fully characterized, appropriately selected ASCs treated with specific growth factors could have profoundly important tissue-specific applications.

Endothelial Progenitor Cells

Circulating cells that express hematopoietic and endothelial surface markers have been isolated from the peripheral blood in animals and humans. These cells are called *endothelial progenitor cells* (EPCs) because there is substantial evidence that they are recruited from the bone marrow and traffic to sites of vascular injury and ischemia to participate in vasculogenesis, the growth of new blood vessels from circulating progenitors, in response to hypoxia and tissue ischemia.[49] Similar to MSCs and ASCs, these cells appear to be mesenchymal or stromal in origin, but there is no widely agreed on profile of surface antigen expression or isolation protocol for these cells. Furthermore, it is unclear whether these cells differentiate into mature endothelial cells or merely serve as supportive perivascular cells during the process of vasculogenesis.

Miscellaneous Adult Stem Cells

Although a thorough discussion of each tissue-specific stem cell type is beyond the scope of this chapter, a limited description of a few additional cell types relevant to surgery is warranted. In the skin, stem cells reside in two general niches: (1) along the hair follicles in the bulge region deep to the sebaceous glands and (2) in the deep interfollicular epidermis.[50] The follicular bulge cells proliferate and form the hair shaft as it grows. These multipotent adult stem cells are believed to contribute to epidermal regeneration after trauma or injury. To maintain normal homeostasis of the epidermis, the deep interfollicular epidermal cells migrate upward to replenish the layers of the epidermis in a process that replaces all skin cells every 3 to 4 weeks.

In the small intestine, proliferative cells reside at the base of the crypts and send differentiating cells upward to repopulate the mature gut epithelium, with complete turnover every 4 to 5 days. Although intestine-specific stem cells exist, the lack of specific antigens for cell isolation has made precise identification of the putative intestinal stem cell elusive and the structure of the intestinal stem cell compartment controversial.[51]

Given the frequent cell turnover and significant regenerative capacity of epithelial organs such as the cornea, small intestine, and skin,[52] it is not surprising that these tissues harbor robust resident adult stem cell populations. However, adult stem cells also have been isolated from organ systems that were previously thought to have little or no regenerative capacity, including cardiac[53] and neural tissue.[54] These findings suggest that most or all mature mammalian tissues and organs have corresponding adult stem cell populations actively involved in local tissue homeostasis and organ regeneration. More experimental work is needed before these populations of tissue-specific resident stem cells can be effectively exploited for medical applications.

Stem Cells and Cancer

The tremendous self-renewal and regenerative potential of stem cells comes with a price. If the asymmetrical division and self-renewal process of stem cells become dysregulated, the risk of malignant transformation increases significantly.[55] Mutations and dysregulation of stem cell self-renewal underlie most hematopoietic malignancies and have been implicated in cancers of the breast, gastrointestinal system, central nervous system, and many other solid tumors.[56] Even microscopic disease left behind after resection of a cancerous lesion can cause recurrent disease. Thus, one of the major risks with stem cell–based therapy is that small numbers of dysregulated stem cells can, if implanted, become a clinically significant tumor. As stem cell–based therapy is adapted for clinical use, cancer biologists have made clear that controls to mitigate risk of potential stem cell dysregulation, such as verifying the genetic stability of therapeutic stem cells, must be prioritized.

BIOENGINEERING FOR REGENERATIVE MEDICINE

Research Applications

Stem cells are profoundly influenced by their surroundings, as evidenced by the importance of the niche to stem cell populations in vivo. This aspect of stem cell physiology has prompted the field of regenerative medicine to expand from pure stem cell biology to include engineering of biomaterials and mechanical systems. The goal is to provide therapeutic platforms to deliver therapeutic stem cells by creating synthetic niches in vitro (Fig. 7-3).[57] Some of the most important biomaterials are biomimetic, mimicking the normal anatomic or physiologic environment in which stem cells are found to encourage more efficient cellular engraftment and proliferation. A basic application of this principle involves designing complex culture systems to provide a more physiologic environment than standard two-dimensional rigid polystyrene plastic for studying stem cell growth in vitro. For example, by coating a culture dish with the ligand leukemia inhibitory factor bound to a thin polymer, Alberti and colleagues[58] demonstrated a significant increase in mouse ESC proliferation. Additionally, a group in Switzerland demonstrated that ASCs expanded in a three-dimensional ceramic scaffold–based perfusion culture system had improved osteogenic capabilities compared with ASCs expanded on traditional two-dimensional tissue culture dishes.[59] An offshoot of the incorporation of engineering concepts into the field of regenerative medicine has resulted in an increasing awareness of the influence of mechanical forces on stem cell behavior and the importance of understanding and controlling the mechanical environment of these cells in engineered tissue grafts developed for use in regenerative therapies.

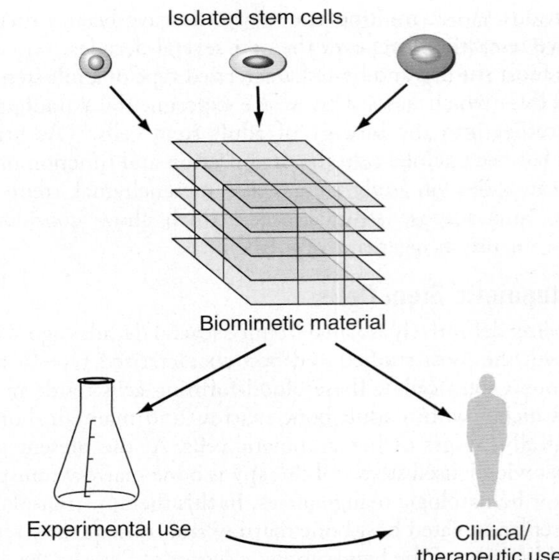

FIGURE 7-3 Biomimetic materials are engineered to create favorable stem cell niches for in vitro experimental stem cell biology studies and for clinical use in regenerative medicine applications. Because all stem cells are exquisitely sensitive to environmental cues, the bioengineering component of regenerative medicine will be crucial to modulate and control stem cell behavior to allow effective cell–based therapies to be used clinically.

Biomaterials as Constructs for Cell Delivery and Directed Differentiation

In addition to experimental tools, bioengineered materials may be particularly valuable as platforms for cell delivery in regenerative medicine applications. To date, most efforts have centered on the use of biomaterials such as collagen polymers, polyglycolic acid, polylactic glycolic acid, and polyethylene glycol hydrogels, which are porous and allow cell ingress. These polymers can be easily molded and shaped to a desired configuration. Several groups also have used modified ink jet printers to create precisely patterned scaffolds and hydrogels to devise finely tuned systems for cellular support and growth factor delivery.[60] A frequently articulated goal of these biomaterial studies is the development of synthetic systems that mimic physiologic extracellular matrix and promote directed proliferation and differentiation of stem cells in vivo after delivery. This approach would allow implantation of a relatively small number of stem cells within a bioengineered construct that would then encourage targeted stem cell expansion and differentiation to regenerate the desired tissue.[61] Although much of this research is still in the early stages of discovery and development, significant advances have moved us much closer to the day when bioengineered constructs will facilitate stem cell–based therapies for regenerative medicine applications.

Organ-Level Tissue Engineering

In addition to creating mimetic scaffolds for cell-based therapies and custom culture systems, the fields of biomaterials science and tissue engineering have expanded their focus to include organ-level engineering—that is, to construct a synthetic or partially engineered organ for transplantation into a patient with end-stage organ failure. Because of the severe limitations on donor organ availability, the prospect of engineering replacement organs from a patient's own cells is a highly appealing solution to the problem of organ scarcity. Urology has taken the lead in this field because urologic structures such as the bladder and urethra lend themselves well to organ engineering. For example, Atala[60] demonstrated the clinical feasibility of urethral and bladder grafts engineered from collagen matrices and seeded cells. Although organ engineering appears to be on the verge of clinical viability for hollow organs such as the bladder, ex vivo engineering of solid organs with complex physiology, such as the liver and kidney, represents a much more difficult challenge.

The kidney presents an enormous challenge to organ engineering because of its complex three-dimensional architecture and the diverse functional requirements of each cellular component. Nonetheless, several groups have reported limited success with a bioartificial kidney containing living tubule cells and connected through standard hemodialysis access lines.[62] Although this is a nonimplanted temporary ex vivo solution, these early studies suggest that an engineered cell-scaffold construct may be able to supplant long-term renal replacement therapy. Ongoing studies using collagen matrices and in vitro expansion of renal cells to create anatomically and physiologically appropriate glomerulotubular units have shown some promise in animal studies.[63]

The liver is also difficult to engineer because of the inherent complexity of hepatic anatomy and physiology. Isolated hepatocyte transplantation has shown some short-term effectiveness in treating Crigler-Najjar syndrome and other metabolic disorders of the liver, but whole organ replacement has not been achieved.[64] Several groups are working to seed expanded or immortalized human liver cells on biomimetic scaffolds, but these experiments are in the preliminary stages of development.[65] Although organ-level engineering has significant potential, much more work is required before this field will achieve clinical applicability.

CLINICAL APPLICATIONS OF STEM CELLS

Since the first successful isolation of human ESCs in 1998 by Thomson and colleagues,[1] stem cell–mediated therapies have transformed the field of regenerative medicine with the promise of enhanced tissue repair and tremendous potential for the treatment of degenerative diseases. Many novel cell-based treatments are under careful evaluation at the present time. The preliminary outcomes of these initial clinical experiences with stem cell therapy are summarized in Table 7-2. These studies are geared toward evaluating the safety and efficacy of stem cell–based therapies to treat many diseases. Many of the studies have attempted to expand on the success of bone marrow HSC transplantation in treating blood disorders and cancer.

Embryonic Stem Cells

Clinical studies on the use of pluripotent stem cells began in 2009, when the U.S. Food and Drug Administration approved the first clinical trial using ESCs. The study, led by the biotechnology company Geron, evaluated the use of ESCs in the treatment of complete spinal cord injury.[65,66] Although the trial was suspended in 2011 when Geron announced that the corporation would be focusing instead on cancer research, many other applications using ESCs are beginning to enter clinical trials. Regulatory approval has been obtained for the use of ESCs to treat blindness associated with retinal loss based on encouraging in vitro and in vivo preclinical studies, and β-islet cells derived from ESCs are also being tested clinically for the correction of type 1 diabetes.[66]

Induced Pluripotent Stem Cells

The first clinical study using autologous iPSCs was approved by the Japan Ministry of Health in 2013 and began recruiting patients on August 1, 2014. As part of the study, skin cells obtained from patients with age-related macular degeneration were converted into iPSCs and differentiated into retinal pigment epithelium cells. The epithelial cells were grown into thin sheets that were subsequently transplanted back into the patient, in the damaged retina. Patients will be closely monitored for potential adverse reactions and transplant sites will be closely monitored for functional integration for the next 1 to 3 years.

Multipotent Adult Stem Cells

Because of the ethical and political concerns related to the use of embryonic and fetal cells as the basis of clinical treatments, the field of regenerative medicine has begun to emphasize the potential of adult multipotent stem cells as the foundation for stem cell–based therapies. MSCs and ASCs readily differentiate into the mesenchymal lineages of bone, cartilage, fat, and muscle, which make them ideal candidates for regeneration of those tissues in adult patients. There have been several case reports of ASCs and MSCs used to repair bone defects, but no rigorous clinical trials performed to our knowledge as of this writing. Based on promising results in animal models, there has been considerable interest in the implantation of bone marrow cells in the setting of myocardial infarction and ischemic cardiomyopathy.[41] Several trials have been performed using intramyocardial or intracoronary injection of bone marrow–derived cells. These studies have generated mixed results, with modest increases in left ventricular ejection fraction but little evidence of long-term survival benefits. More studies are needed to determine the role of stem cell–based treatments in ischemic myocardial pathologies.

Overall, there is much promise for stem cell–based therapies, but this potential has been largely unrealized to date. Despite this, regenerative medicine seems poised to become clinically relevant in the near term, which likely will considerably expand the tools available to surgeons and patients.

TABLE 7-2 Reported Clinical Applications of Stem Cells

CLINICAL APPLICATION	CELL TYPE	DELIVERY METHOD
Inflammatory bowel disease (Crohn's disease)[a]	ASC	Surgical implantation into perianal fistulas
Muscular dystrophy[b]	Muscle-derived progenitors, $CD133^+$	Local injection
Ischemic cardiomyopathy (MAGNUM Trial)[c]	BM MSC	Surgically implanted three-dimensional collagen matrix
Acute myocardial infarction (BOOST Trial)[d]	Total BM	Intracoronary injection
Acute myocardial infarction (REPAIR-AMI Trial)[e]	Total BM	Intracoronary injection
Acute myocardial infarction (ASTAMI Trial)[f]	BM MNC	Intracoronary injection
Ischemic cardiomyopathy[g]	Total BM	Systemic injection
Tracheobronchomalacia[h]	BM MSC	Differentiated to chondrocytes and surgically implanted
Traumatic calvarial defect[i]	ASC	Surgical implantation in fibrin glue
Achondroplasia[j]	BM MSC	Transplantation concurrently with distraction osteogenesis

ASC, adipose stem cell; *BM,* bone marrow; *MNC,* mononuclear cell; *MSC,* mesenchymal stem cell.
[a]From Garcia-Olmo D, Herreros D, Pascual M, et al: Treatment of enterocutaneous fistula in Crohn's disease with adipose-derived stem cells: A comparison of protocols with and without cell expansion. Int J Colorectal Dis 24:27–30, 2009.
[b]From Torrente Y, Belicchi M, Marchesi C, et al: Autologous transplantation of muscle-derived $CD133^+$ stem cells in Duchenne muscle patients. Cell Transplant 16:563–577, 2007.
[c]From Chachques JC, Trainini JC, Lago N, et al: Myocardial assistance by grafting a new bioartificial upgraded myocardium (MAGNUM trial): Clinical feasibility study. Ann Thorac Surg 85:901–908, 2008.
[d]From Wollert KC, Meyer GP, Lotz J, et al: Intracoronary autologous bone-marrow cell transfer after myocardial infarction: The BOOST randomised controlled clinical trial. Lancet 364:141–148, 2004.
[e]From Schächinger V, Erbs S, Elsässer A, et al; REPAIR-AMI Investigators: Intracoronary bone marrow-derived progenitor cells in acute myocardial infarction. N Engl J Med 355:1210–1221, 2006.
[f]From Lunde K, Solheim S, Aakhus S, et al: Intracoronary injection of mononuclear bone marrow cells in acute myocardial infarction. N Engl J Med 355:1199–1209, 2006.
[g]From Meyer GP, Wollert KC, Lotz J, et al: Intracoronary bone marrow cell transfer after myocardial infarction: 5-year follow-up from the randomized-controlled BOOST trial. Eur Heart J 30:2978–2984, 2009.
[h]From Macchiarini P, Jungebluth P, Go T, et al: Clinical transplantation of a tissue-engineered airway. Lancet 372:2023–2030, 2008.
[i]From Lendeckel S, Jödicke A, Christophis P, et al: Autologous stem cells (adipose) and fibrin glue used to treat widespread traumatic calvarial defects: Case report. J Craniomaxillofac Surg 32:370–373, 2004.
[j]From Kitoh H, Kitakoji T, Tsuchiya H, et al: Transplantation of marrow-derived mesenchymal stem cells and platelet-rich plasma during distraction osteogenesis—a preliminary result of three cases. Bone 35:892–898, 2004.

SELECTED REFERENCES

Atala A: Engineering organs. *Curr Opin Biotechnol* 20:575–592, 2009.

This excellent review from a leader in the field of regenerative medicine outlines the progress made and challenges faced by tissue and organ engineering as it relates to regenerative medicine.

Beltrami AP, Barlucchi L, Torella D, et al: Adult cardiac stem cells are multipotent and support myocardial regeneration. *Cell* 114:763–776, 2003.

This article discusses the isolation of resident cardiac stem cells and their potential uses in myocardial regeneration. Resident cardiac stem cells are a prime example of the limits of tissue-specific stem cell populations for use in regenerative medicine.

Blanpain C, Horsley V, Fuchs E: Epithelial stem cells: Turning over new leaves. *Cell* 128:445–458, 2007.

This excellent review describes the current understanding of epithelial stem cells and discusses their potential applications for regenerative medicine.

Kiel MJ, He S, Ashkenazi R, et al: Haematopoietic stem cells do not asymmetrically segregate chromosomes or retain BrdU. *Nature* 449:238–242, 2007.

This important article demonstrates that asymmetrical cell division does not occur in hematopoietic stem cells. This establishes the concept that not all adult stem cells are clonal populations and that heterogeneity of transcription is likely the normal state of a stem cell population.

Lutolf MP, Gilbert PM, Blau HM: Designing materials to direct stem cell fate. *Nature* 462:433–441, 2009.

This comprehensive review describes the role of bioengineering in stem cell biology research and regenerative medicine.

Pittenger MF, Mackay AM, Beck SC, et al: Multilineage potential of adult human mesenchymal stem cells. *Science* 284:143–147, 1999.

This article provided the first description of human mesenchymal stem cells. The authors demonstrated the existence of a nonhematopoietic cell population in the bone marrow with multipotent differentiation ability.

Spangrude GJ, Heimfeld S, Weissman IL: Purification and characterization of mouse hematopoietic stem cells. *Science* 241:58–62, 1988.

This article provided the original description of hematopoietic stem cell isolation, which established the paradigm for adult stem cell research.

Takahashi K, Yamanaka S: Induction of pluripotent stem cells from mouse embryonic and adult fibroblast cultures by defined factors. *Cell* 126:663–676, 2006.

This was the original description of the creation of induced pluripotent stem cells by viral transfection with four genes. Subsequent studies generated induced pluripotent stem cells from human skin cells and adipose-derived stem cells. Because the original transfection methods involved genomic integration of viral particles, much work is ongoing to allow the safe induction of pluripotency in cells by using techniques that would allow these cells to be used clinically.

Thomson JA, Itskovitz-Eldor J, Shapiro SS, et al: Embryonic stem cell lines derived from human blastocysts. *Science* 282:1145–1147, 1998.

These authors were the first to isolate and describe human embryonic stem cells. This article created much interest in embryonic stem cells as potential sources of cell-based therapies for regenerative medicine but also raised several important ethical concerns that are the source of ongoing debate in the scientific and broader community.

Zuk PA, Zhu M, Ashjian P, et al: Human adipose tissue is a source of multipotent stem cells. *Mol Biol Cell* 13:4279–4295, 2002.

In this seminal description of adipose stromal cells, the authors demonstrated that multipotent mesenchymal stem cells could be isolated from the stromal vascular fraction of human adipose tissue. This was the first account of an adult stem cell population isolated from a tissue other than the bone marrow.

REFERENCES

1. Thomson JA, Itskovitz-Eldor J, Shapiro SS, et al: Embryonic stem cell lines derived from human blastocysts. *Science* 282:1145–1147, 1998.
2. Boyer LA, Lee TI, Cole MF, et al: Core transcriptional regulatory circuitry in human embryonic stem cells. *Cell* 122:947–956, 2005.
3. International Stem Cell Initiative, Adewumi O, Aflatoonian B, et al: Characterization of human embryonic stem cell lines by the International Stem Cell Initiative. *Nat Biotechnol* 25:803–816, 2007.
4. Martin GR: Isolation of a pluripotent cell line from early mouse embryos cultured in medium conditioned by teratocarcinoma stem cells. *Proc Natl Acad Sci U S A* 78:7634–7638, 1981.
5. Poliard A, Nifuji A, Lamblin D, et al: Controlled conversion of an immortalized mesodermal progenitor cell towards osteogenic, chondrogenic, or adipogenic pathways. *J Cell Biol* 130:1461–1472, 1995.
6. Wu DC, Boyd AS, Wood KJ: Embryonic stem cell transplantation: Potential applicability in cell replacement therapy and regenerative medicine. *Front Biosci* 12:4525–4535, 2007.
7. Villa-Diaz LG, Ross AM, Lahann J, et al: Concise review: The evolution of human pluripotent stem cell culture: From feeder cells to synthetic coatings. *Stem Cells* 31:1–7, 2013.
8. Martin MJ, Muotri A, Gage F, et al: Human embryonic stem cells express an immunogenic nonhuman sialic acid. *Nat Med* 11:228–232, 2005.
9. Stacey GN, Cobo F, Nieto A, et al: The development of "feeder" cells for the preparation of clinical grade hES cell lines: Challenges and solutions. *J Biotechnol* 125:583–588, 2006.
10. Amit M, Shariki C, Margulets V, et al: Feeder layer- and serum-free culture of human embryonic stem cells. *Biol Reprod* 70:837–845, 2004.
11. Wilmut I, Schnieke AE, McWhir J, et al: Viable offspring derived from fetal and adult mammalian cells. *Nature* 385:810–813, 1997.
12. Yamada M, Johannesson B, Sagi I, et al: Human oocytes reprogram adult somatic nuclei of a type 1 diabetic to diploid pluripotent stem cells. *Nature* 510:533–536, 2014.
13. Deuse T, Wang D, Stubbendorff M, et al: SCNT-derived ESCs with mismatched mitochondria trigger an immune response in allogeneic hosts. *Cell Stem Cell* 16:33–38, 2015.
14. Perry AC: Progress in human somatic-cell nuclear transfer. *N Engl J Med* 353:87–88, 2005.
15. Takahashi K, Yamanaka S: Induction of pluripotent stem cells from mouse embryonic and adult fibroblast cultures by defined factors. *Cell* 126:663–676, 2006.
16. Yu J, Vodyanik MA, Smuga-Otto K, et al: Induced pluripotent stem cell lines derived from human somatic cells. *Science* 318:1917–1920, 2007.
17. Takahashi K, Tanabe K, Ohnuki M, et al: Induction of pluripotent stem cells from adult human fibroblasts by defined factors. *Cell* 131:861–872, 2007.
18. Wernig M, Meissner A, Foreman R, et al: In vitro reprogramming of fibroblasts into a pluripotent ES-cell-like state. *Nature* 448:319–324, 2007.
19. Chin MH, Mason MJ, Xie W, et al: Induced pluripotent stem cells and embryonic stem cells are distinguished by gene expression signatures. *Cell Stem Cell* 5:111–123, 2009.
20. Okita K, Ichisaka T, Yamanaka S: Generation of germline-competent induced pluripotent stem cells. *Nature* 448:313–317, 2007.
21. Stadtfeld M, Nagaya M, Utikal J, et al: Induced pluripotent stem cells generated without viral integration. *Science* 322:945–949, 2008.
22. Zhou H, Wu S, Joo JY, et al: Generation of induced pluripotent stem cells using recombinant proteins. *Cell Stem Cell* 4:381–384, 2009.
23. Liu SV: iPS cells: A more critical review. *Stem Cells Dev* 17:391–397, 2008.
24. Sun N, Panetta NJ, Gupta DM, et al: Feeder-free derivation of induced pluripotent stem cells from adult human adipose stem cells. *Proc Natl Acad Sci U S A* 106:15720–15725, 2009.
25. Wernig M, Zhao JP, Pruszak J, et al: Neurons derived from reprogrammed fibroblasts functionally integrate into the fetal brain and improve symptoms of rats with Parkinson's disease. *Proc Natl Acad Sci U S A* 105:5856–5861, 2008.

26. Hanna J, Wernig M, Markoulaki S, et al: Treatment of sickle cell anemia mouse model with iPS cells generated from autologous skin. *Science* 318:1920–1923, 2007.
27. Guillot PV, O'Donoghue K, Kurata H, et al: Fetal stem cells: Betwixt and between. *Semin Reprod Med* 24:340–347, 2006.
28. De Coppi P, Bartsch G, Jr, Siddiqui MM, et al: Isolation of amniotic stem cell lines with potential for therapy. *Nat Biotechnol* 25:100–106, 2007.
29. Götherström C, Ringdén O, Tammik C, et al: Immunologic properties of human fetal mesenchymal stem cells. *Am J Obstet Gynecol* 190:239–245, 2004.
30. Moore KA, Lemischka IR: Stem cells and their niches. *Science* 311:1880–1885, 2006.
31. Orkin SH, Zon LI: Hematopoiesis: An evolving paradigm for stem cell biology. *Cell* 132:631–644, 2008.
32. Spangrude GJ, Heimfeld S, Weissman IL: Purification and characterization of mouse hematopoietic stem cells. *Science* 241:58–62, 1988.
33. Balsam LB, Wagers AJ, Christensen JL, et al: Haematopoietic stem cells adopt mature haematopoietic fates in ischaemic myocardium. *Nature* 428:668–673, 2004.
34. Weissman IL, Shizuru JA: The origins of the identification and isolation of hematopoietic stem cells, and their capability to induce donor-specific transplantation tolerance and treat autoimmune diseases. *Blood* 112:3543–3553, 2008.
35. Chan CK, Seo EY, Chen JY, et al: Identification and specification of the mouse skeletal stem cell. *Cell* 160:285–298, 2015.
36. Pittenger MF, Mackay AM, Beck SC, et al: Multilineage potential of adult human mesenchymal stem cells. *Science* 284:143–147, 1999.
37. Lv FJ, Tuan RS, Cheung KM, et al: Concise review: The surface markers and identity of human mesenchymal stem cells. *Stem Cells* 32:1408–1419, 2014.
38. Kolf CM, Cho E, Tuan RS: Mesenchymal stromal cells. Biology of adult mesenchymal stem cells: Regulation of niche, self-renewal and differentiation. *Arthritis Res Ther* 9:204, 2007.
39. El Tamer MK, Reis RL: Progenitor and stem cells for bone and cartilage regeneration. *J Tissue Eng Regen Med* 3:327–337, 2009.
40. Falanga V, Iwamoto S, Chartier M, et al: Autologous bone marrow-derived cultured mesenchymal stem cells delivered in a fibrin spray accelerate healing in murine and human cutaneous wounds. *Tissue Eng* 13:1299–1312, 2007.
41. Orlic D, Kajstura J, Chimenti S, et al: Bone marrow cells regenerate infarcted myocardium. *Nature* 410:701–705, 2001.
42. Rosenzweig A: Cardiac cell therapy—mixed results from mixed cells. *N Engl J Med* 355:1274–1277, 2006.
43. Gersh BJ, Simari RD, Behfar A, et al: Cardiac cell repair therapy: A clinical perspective. *Mayo Clin Proc* 84:876–892, 2009.
44. Hosoda T, Kajstura J, Leri A, et al: Mechanisms of myocardial regeneration. *Circ J* 74:13–17, 2010.
45. Zuk PA, Zhu M, Ashjian P, et al: Human adipose tissue is a source of multipotent stem cells. *Mol Biol Cell* 13:4279–4295, 2002.
46. Ashjian PH, Elbarbary AS, Edmonds B, et al: In vitro differentiation of human processed lipoaspirate cells into early neural progenitors. *Plast Reconstr Surg* 111:1922–1931, 2003.
47. Léobon B, Roncalli J, Joffre C, et al: Adipose-derived cardiomyogenic cells: In vitro expansion and functional improvement in a mouse model of myocardial infarction. *Cardiovasc Res* 83:757–767, 2009.
48. An C, Cheng Y, Yuan Q, et al: IGF-1 and BMP-2 induces differentiation of adipose-derived mesenchymal stem cells into chondrocyte-like cells. *Ann Biomed Eng* 38:1647–1654, 2010.
49. Asahara T, Murohara T, Sullivan A, et al: Isolation of putative progenitor endothelial cells for angiogenesis. *Science* 275:964–967, 1997.
50. Gurtner GC, Werner S, Barrandon Y, et al: Wound repair and regeneration. *Nature* 453:314–321, 2008.
51. Garrison AP, Helmrath MA, Dekaney CM: Intestinal stem cells. *J Pediatr Gastroenterol Nutr* 49:2–7, 2009.
52. Blanpain C, Horsley V, Fuchs E: Epithelial stem cells: Turning over new leaves. *Cell* 128:445–458, 2007.
53. Beltrami AP, Barlucchi L, Torella D, et al: Adult cardiac stem cells are multipotent and support myocardial regeneration. *Cell* 114:763–776, 2003.
54. Gross CG: Neurogenesis in the adult brain: Death of a dogma. *Nat Rev Neurosci* 1:67–73, 2000.
55. Morrison SJ, Kimble J: Asymmetric and symmetric stem-cell divisions in development and cancer. *Nature* 441:1068–1074, 2006.
56. Rossi DJ, Jamieson CH, Weissman IL: Stems cells and the pathways to aging and cancer. *Cell* 132:681–696, 2008.
57. Lutolf MP, Gilbert PM, Blau HM: Designing materials to direct stem-cell fate. *Nature* 462:433–441, 2009.
58. Alberti K, Davey RE, Onishi K, et al: Functional immobilization of signaling proteins enables control of stem cell fate. *Nat Methods* 5:645–650, 2008.
59. Scherberich A, Galli R, Jaquiery C, et al: Three-dimensional perfusion culture of human adipose tissue-derived endothelial and osteoblastic progenitors generates osteogenic constructs with intrinsic vascularization capacity. *Stem Cells* 25:1823–1829, 2007.
60. Atala A: Engineering organs. *Curr Opin Biotechnol* 20:575–592, 2009.
61. Xu Y, Shi Y, Ding S: A chemical approach to stem-cell biology and regenerative medicine. *Nature* 453:338–344, 2008.
62. Song JH, Humes HD: The bioartificial kidney in the treatment of acute kidney injury. *Curr Drug Targets* 10:1227–1234, 2009.
63. Humes HD, Buffington DA, MacKay SM, et al: Replacement of renal function in uremic animals with a tissue-engineered kidney. *Nat Biotechnol* 17:451–455, 1999.
64. Dalgetty DM, Medine CN, Iredale JP, et al: Progress and future challenges in stem cell-derived liver technologies. *Am J Physiol Gastrointest Liver Physiol* 297:G241–G248, 2009.
65. Kobayashi N: Life support of artificial liver: Development of a bioartificial liver to treat liver failure. *J Hepatobiliary Pancreat Surg* 16:113–117, 2009.
66. Couzin J: Biotechnology. Celebration and concern over U.S. trial of embryonic stem cells. *Science* 323:568, 2009.

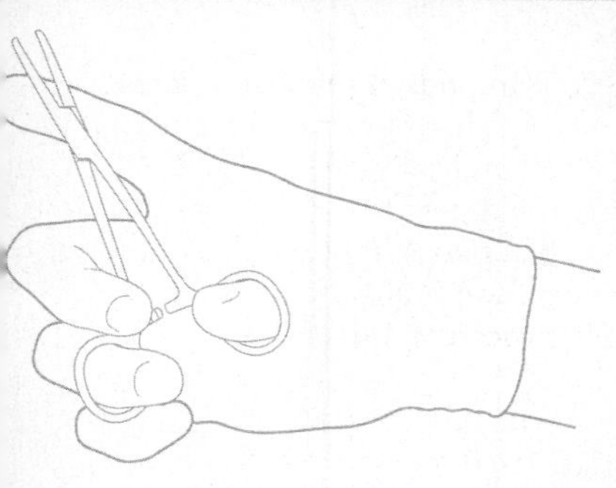

CHAPTER 8

Evidence-Based Surgery: Critically Assessing Surgical Literature

Vlad V. Simianu, Farhood Farjah, David R. Flum

OUTLINE

With the growing recognition that almost everyone requires surgery at some point in their lives, surgical disease is being increasingly considered from the perspective of populations using the research tools and vocabulary of public health. Over the last decade, surgical health services and outcomes research has emerged as an essential approach to infusing the field of surgery with a more rigorous evidence base. Current surgical investigations employ a broad range of research methods with the goal of more rapidly integrating the best available evidence into the practice of surgeons in all communities.

In an era of increasing regulatory oversight and focus on more accountable care, it is essential that surgeons understand the evidence (or lack thereof) that drives their decisions about who should have operations, the techniques used, and the outcomes expected so that they can optimize the care of their patients and lead in health policy and quality improvement activities. This chapter provides a pragmatic guide to the critical evaluation of published studies relating to surgery to advance the use of evidence in surgical practice. To that end, this chapter is structured around questions that a critical reader should ask when reading a research study and the issues that should be considered as part of that evaluation.

WHAT IS THE PURPOSE OF THE STUDY?

The purpose of a study should drive the selection of study groups, outcomes of interest, data sources, study design, and analytic plan. Lack of clarity in the study purpose or objectives can confuse subsequent interpretation of the data and lead to unsupported conclusions.

The purpose of a study falls into two general categories: hypothesis generating or hypothesis testing (Fig. 8-1). Descriptive studies should be considered hypothesis generating—identifying possible associations and serving as an impetus for future investigations. Hypothesis-testing studies must make every attempt to exclude the influence of chance and bias in evaluating a discrete hypothesis and clarify whether the hypothesis concerns superiority, inferiority, or equivalence (noninferiority). Studies that fall short in linking purpose and methodology not only are confusing but also may lead to erroneous interpretation of the findings. For example, a study was intended to describe trends in the misdiagnosis of appendicitis and use of imaging. A decrease in misdiagnosis coincident with an increase in imaging may lead to the hypothesis that imaging reduces the misdiagnosis of appendicitis. However, because the study was never intended to rule out bias (i.e., other unmeasured variables that could influence the use of imaging and the misdiagnosis of appendicitis), one must avoid the temptation to conclude that increasing imaging over time is causally related to decreasing rates of misdiagnosed appendicitis.[1]

IS THE STUDY USING THE RIGHT DATA?

Many sources of information exist to conduct clinical research. Data sources are diverse, and all have advantages and disadvantages. A balance between study purpose, resources (i.e., money), and feasibility (i.e., acceptance, ethics, and time) should drive the optimal selection of a data source. Table 8-1 provides a synopsis of the advantages, disadvantages, and examples of some commonly used data sources.

Research using administrative data, such as Medicare claims, has become particularly prevalent owing to the availability and affordability of these large data sets. However, these data are collected for billing, not research, and there are often important issues with completeness (likely to reliably include only metrics related to discretely billable aspects of care) and specification (clinical variables such as laterality of an operation or intention of a treatment). In addition, administrative data are often not

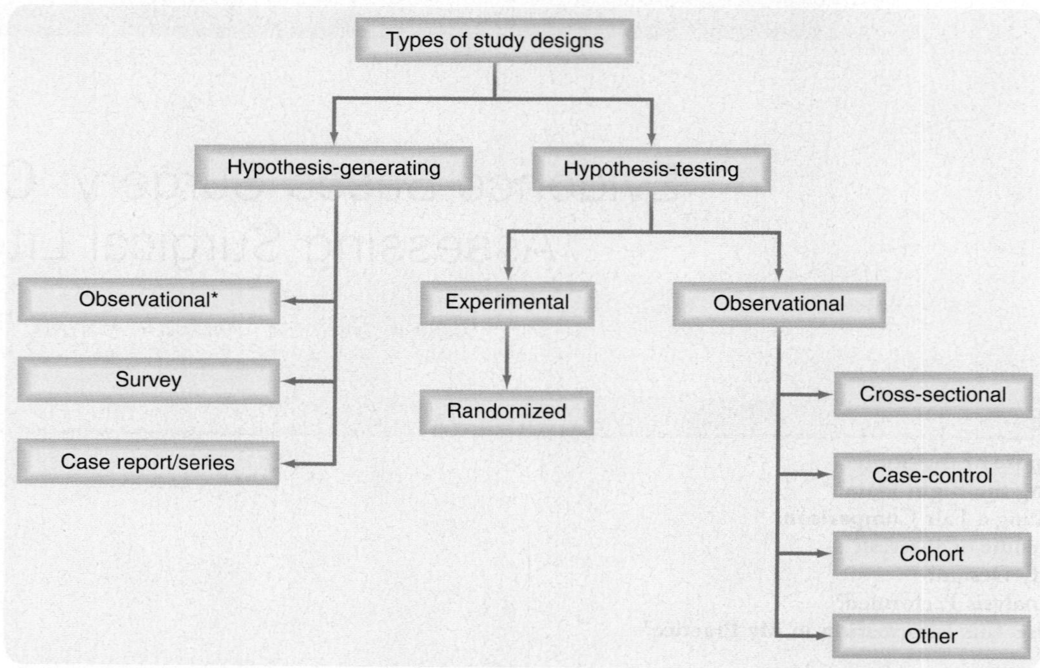

FIGURE 8-1 Hierarchy of study designs. The asterisk indicates that the same study designs found in the other branch apply.

linked longitudinally, making it difficult to measure outcomes beyond an index event. When data are linked longitudinally, they are often representative of unique populations, such as individuals insured by the same payer, within a single system of health care delivery, or uncharacteristically similar in age (e.g., Medicare) or sex (e.g., Department of Veterans Affairs).

IS THE STUDY MAKING A FAIR COMPARISON?

Many surgical studies compare outcomes or end points across groups of patients, surgeons, or hospitals. Defining comparison groups is straightforward most of the time, but sometimes it can be an elusive task. Inattention to the nuances of defining comparison groups can lead to a biased study. Several common challenges in defining comparison groups are outlined subsequently. A common problem is related to comparisons with "usual care." Usual care comprises an ill-defined group of activities that when left unspecified may or may not reflect care in a given community. There also may be circumstances where randomly assigning a patient to "usual care" poses an ethical challenge, especially if usual care includes fewer checks for safety and is widely believed to be inferior to the intervention.

Misclassification

Misclassification is the incorrect categorization of a subject into a study group and can lead to bias even when the study design and analysis are appropriate. There are two types of misclassification, nondifferential and differential. Nondifferential misclassification indicates an equal and random chance that any one subject will be misclassified (or included as part of the wrong study group). If a difference in outcome truly exists across groups, nondifferential misclassification biases the results toward the null hypothesis, a conservative bias. Differential misclassification indicates nonrandom misclassification. With differential misclassification, the bias may be conservative or anticonservative, depending on the manner in which patients were misclassified and the true relationship between group assignment and outcome. Differential misclassification is the more serious concern and may not always be predictable (discoverable).

The Will Rogers phenomenon—based on the famous quote, *"When the Okies left Oklahoma and moved to California, they raised the average intelligence level in both states"*—is better known as stage migration and is a classic example of misclassification.[2] Cancer stage predicts long-term survival. Patients may be staged by clinical examination or imaging or both, although these techniques are not as accurate as pathologic tissue examination (the gold standard). Some patients may be understaged—categorized as having early-stage disease when they have advanced/late-stage disease—and others may be overstaged. To the extent that patients are understaged and overstaged, their cancer stage is misclassified. If all patients in a study undergo suboptimal staging, misclassification occurs at random (nondifferential). A comparison of survival rates across stage would be blunted despite the fact that cancer stage is one of the strongest predictors of survival. Stage migration can also lead to nondifferential misclassification. A hypothesis-generating study compared stage-based survival across patients with lung cancer who underwent more versus less intense use of diagnostic staging modalities.[3] Patients undergoing more diagnostic procedures would be expected to have more accurate staging and less misclassification. A strong association was observed between more intense use of diagnostic staging modalities and longer stage-based survival. In this case, the nondifferential misclassification was predictable. The authors appropriately cited stage migration as a possible explanation, among others, for their findings.

Time-Varying Exposures

Time-varying (or time-dependent) exposures refer to groups whose populations vary with time. Failure to account for time-varying exposures may lead to biased results and incorrect

TABLE 8-1 Data Sources for Outcomes and Health Services Research

DATA SOURCE	ADVANTAGES	DISADVANTAGES	EXAMPLE
Medical records	Easy to obtain Useful for hypothesis generation	Missing data Time-consuming Inability to measure certain information (e.g., intent) Limited scientific value	Case reports Case series
PRO	Unique data on symptoms, function, and health status	Time-consuming: interviews or questionnaires	SF-36 Health Survey
	Global (multidimensional) or specific (unidimensional)	Unique instruments can have validity issues when population broadened Change/effect can be difficult to interpret	PROMIS
Administrative	Large numbers Real-world data Often generalizable Easy to obtain Affordable	Limited clinical variables Data collected for billing, not research	Medicare State discharge data
Registry	Often contains clinical data	Built for limited reasons, so has restricted data Often has missing data because information captured from usual care rather than research visits	SEER National Cancer Database
		Often include only cross-sectional data and need linkage to other data sources for follow-up	Device registries (TAVR)
	Population-based real-world data not restricted to tertiary or referral centers		
Linked data sets	Richer source of data than either registry or administrative alone	Missing data	SEER-Medicare
	Allows longitudinal assessment of episodes of care	Inability to capture intent of therapy	
Quality Improvement and Surveillance Project	Prospectively collected data	Overrepresentation of tertiary or referral centers	National Surgical Quality Improvement Project
	Rich in clinical, laboratory, and demographic patient data	Random sample of patients, not comprehensive	Society of Thoracic Surgeons database
National surveys	National sample Some longitudinal diagnoses and health care claims data	May overrepresent certain racial groups in survey sample	Medical expenditure panel survey

Adapted from Rosenthal R, Schafer J, Briel M, et al: How to write a surgical clinical research protocol: Literature review and practical guide. *Am J Surg* 207:299–312, 2014.
PRO, patient reported outcomes; *PROMIS*, Patient-Reported Outcomes Measurement Information System; *SEER*, Surveillance, Epidemiology and End Results; *SF-36*, 36-item short-form health survey; *TAVR*, Transcatheter Aortic Valve Replacement.

conclusions. An example of potential bias arising from time-varying covariates is an analysis of heart transplantation survival data.[4] The impact of heart transplantation on survival was assessed by comparing patients who received a transplant with patients who did not receive a transplant. Although the initial analysis revealed a survival benefit associated with transplantation, the manner in which patients were grouped (treating transplantation as a fixed variable) led to bias in favor of patients with transplants.

Transplantation wait times are often long, and many patients die while awaiting a donor organ; patients on the transplantation waitlist who died a short time after being listed did not have a chance to undergo transplantation. When the investigators retrospectively assigned patients to these two study groups (transplanted versus not transplanted), the patients who survived long enough to receive a new heart introduced selection bias in favor of transplantation because their survival times were on average longer than in the nontransplantation group. In actuality, each subject's exposure status (transplanted versus not transplanted) was time dependent. While on the waitlist and before transplantation, a subject could contribute survival time to the nontransplantation group; after transplantation, the same subject could contribute survival time to the transplantation group. Reanalysis of the data evaluating exposure status in a time-dependent fashion revealed no association between transplantation and survival.[5]

WHAT IS THE OUTCOME OF INTEREST?

Concluding that intervention A is better than intervention B must be supported by evidence of a difference in outcomes. But what does "better" mean? What if operation A is better with regard to one type of outcome but worse in terms of another? Outcomes assessment cannot determine which intervention is better for the patient, but it can inform patients and providers about differences between two or more competing diagnostic or therapeutic options. Readers judging the value of a study should determine which outcomes were assessed, from what perspective, and whether the chosen outcomes were consistent with the study's purpose. Outcomes may be objective (e.g., death) or subjective (e.g., patient satisfaction).

Patient-Reported Outcomes

Patient-reported outcomes (PROs) measure experiences or events that are best reported by the patient. Sometimes PROs are called subjective outcomes because the response cannot be verified by a provider or researcher. Examples of common PRO concepts are health-related quality of life, satisfaction with care, functional status, well-being, and health status. PROs usually consist of several more discrete concepts (or domains). For example, health-related quality of life measures domains such as physical (e.g., pain), psychological (e.g., depression), and social functioning (e.g., the ability to carry out activities of daily living). Specific examples of items contained within these domains are related to pain, sleep problems, sexual function, vitality and energy, and pain.

PRO data are collected through the use of survey instruments and may be measured repeatedly over time. These instruments are composed of individual questions, statements, or tasks evaluated by a patient. PRO instruments use a clearly defined method for administration; data are collected using a standardized format; and the scoring, analysis, and interpretation of results should have been validated in the study population. In general, researchers are advised to use existing instruments to measure PROs (rather than creating their own) because the appropriate development of an instrument requires significant time, resources, testing, and validation before application.[6] PRO instruments are categorized as general instruments (e.g., the 36-item short-form health survey) because they broadly describe physical, mental, and social health, or disease-specific instruments (e.g., the diverticulitis quality of life instrument) because they target a unique condition.

Many clinicians confuse PROs and patient-centered outcomes. A patient-centered outcome is one that is important to a patient. For example, among patients with cancer, long-term survival and recurrence are both very important to patients, but these outcomes can be observed to occur by individuals other than the patient. Survival and recurrence are patient-centered outcomes but not PROs.

Costs, Charges, and Resource Utilization

Charges are the amount of money requested for health services and supplies. By comparison, costs are the actual amount of money spent to deliver care. The perspective of the study defines which costs are necessary to ascertain and include in the analysis. For example, although a societal perspective would include the costs of care and the direct and indirect monetary costs associated with care (e.g., travel and boarding expenses, lost productivity at work, caretaker expenses), a hospital's perspective would be more selective, not considering the patient's out-of-pocket expenses but including payer reimbursement.

There are three common approaches to comparing cost outcomes. A cost-benefit analysis quantifies health benefit in terms of dollars. The great challenge with this approach is assigning a dollar value to a life or a specific health outcome. A cost-utility analysis quantifies health benefits in terms of quality-adjusted life-years (QALYs). Utilities are a measure of overall quality of life, usually scaled between 0 and 1, with 1 being perfect health, and are multiplied by survival time to determine QALYs. When this outcome metric is evaluated as a cost per QALY, it is readily comparable between interventions. An intervention with an associated cost per QALY of $50,000 or less has typically been considered cost-effective, although there is ongoing debate about the validity of this metric, and a range of costs/QALY of $20,000 to $100,000 has been proposed as more reasonable.[7] Cost-effectiveness analyses measure health benefit in terms of an outcome metric called the incremental cost-effectiveness ratio, which is the difference in costs between two competing therapeutic options divided by the difference in health outcome. If the incremental cost-effectiveness ratio comparing a new treatment with a standard treatment reveals that the new treatment is more expensive and less efficacious, it is considered to be dominated by the standard and not favored, whereas a less expensive and more efficacious new treatment dominates the standard and is favored. Circumstances in which an intervention is both more expensive and efficacious or both less expensive and efficacious represent "trade-offs" and are not as clear-cut to policymakers.

Resource utilization refers to the use of health services related to an intervention. In the context of surgical care, this includes utilization of prehospital resources—clinic visits, preoperative testing, optimization, and diagnostics—as well as hospital resources—length of stay; hospital readmission; use of outpatient, pharmacy, and durable medical equipment (e.g., wheelchairs and oxygen) services; and post–hospital care emergency department use, skilled nursing facilities, and home care. It can be challenging to determine how much resource utilization is related to the intervention or procedure under study and how much is attributable to a patient's baseline clinical conditions (e.g., chronic disease, adverse events) and nonclinical factors (e.g., patient-level social support, patient preference for in-hospital versus out-of-hospital care, insurance status precluding use of home nursing). For example, an investigator might study readmission after pancreatic resection for cancer. Although readmission events are readily identified, it may be impossible (depending on the data source) to know whether the readmission was planned (e.g., for chemotherapy administration) or unplanned (e.g., because of a complication) or appropriate (e.g., because a complication requires inpatient treatment).

Safety

Safety end points attempt to address the risks of a diagnostic procedure or intervention (e.g., bile duct injury or surgical site infection) or delivery of care (e.g., wrong-site surgery). Operative mortality and postoperative complications (morbidity) are the most commonly measured markers of safety. Safety endpoints are often used in studies because they are relatively easy to measure and require only a short follow-up period. Safety studies often need to be quite large in size because of the relative infrequency of the event. Most randomized controlled trials (RCT) and small series are not sufficient to evaluate for infrequent outcomes.

Appropriateness

With increasing health care expenditures, there has been an emerging effort to focus on the proportion of patients who do not meet the "appropriate" indications for an interventional procedure, determined by professional societies and research studies. A series of cohort studies performed in the 1990s and repeated in the 2000s searched medical records and diagnostic images for evidence of standard indications for carotid endarterectomy, coronary artery bypass grafting, and percutaneous revascularization and found that one in three did not meet standard criteria.[8,9] In response, many groups increased their production of guidelines and appropriateness criteria.[10] Compliance with established appropriate care guidelines in surgery is an increasingly reported outcome, although the impact of such guidelines in reducing rates of procedures that are truly unnecessary has been mixed.[11]

Surrogate End Points

Interest in surrogate end points has emerged because certain clinical outcomes may be difficult to assess secondary to the infrequency of a clinical event, the cost of ascertainment, or a long lag time to development. Surrogate end points are commonly used in studies of new pharmaceutical interventions when efficient data gathering about treatment effect is essential to move a product to the marketplace rapidly.[12] The true clinical benefits of an intervention may take years to recognize, and it may be desirable to identify an intermediate outcome that could serve as a surrogate for the actual clinical effect. One problem with using surrogate end points is that an intervention may influence an outcome through various, potentially unintended or unanticipated, pathways. When evaluating a study, the reader must ask not only whether the selected outcome can answer the research question but also whether that outcome is a meaningful clinical end point or simply a more easily measured surrogate. Criteria for validating a surrogate end point have been proposed—the surrogate end point should be correlated with the clinical end point of interest and fully capture the net effect of the intervention on the end point of interest. Unless a chosen surrogate outcome has been validated and vetted in other surgical studies, the results and conclusions should be interpreted with caution.

A classic example of a surrogate end point is detection of venous thromboembolism (VTE).[13] In this RCT, the authors sought to evaluate the efficacy and safety of thromboprophylaxis with dalteparin administered for 28 days after major abdominal surgery compared with 7 days of treatment. The primary efficacy end point was objectively verified VTE on venography (not necessarily symptomatic and most were not) occurring between 7 and 28 days after surgery. In the 7-day dalteparin group, 29 VTE events were identified (4 of which were symptomatic, so 25 were found only by imaging). The 28-day dalteparin group had 12 VTE events, all asymptomatic. Herein lies the major problem with this study—asymptomatic VTE, identified solely by imaging, is a surrogate end point. Although it is biologically plausible that asymptomatic VTE progresses to symptomatic VTE, the rate of this is unknown, and, more importantly, the underlying rates of *asymptomatic* VTE are unknown. The proper measure would have been efficacy at reducing symptomatic VTE. This is a rare event (4 of 178 or 2% in the 7-day group and 0 of 165 or 0% in the 28-day group), and this study is underpowered to show this difference.

Composite End Points

Sometimes there is no single optimal outcome, or, as just discussed, events are rare resulting in insufficient power to evaluate outcomes. In these situations, studies may report composite end points. For example, a composite end point for efficacy VTE measurement may include symptomatic deep vein thrombosis, symptomatic pulmonary embolism, major complications, and death from any cause during treatment. However, for composite end points to be meaningful, they should be of similar importance and frequency. Imbalance in the components does not allow reviewers to judge which individual outcome contributed most to the composite end point.

WHAT IS THE STUDY DESIGN?

Several study designs are commonly used in surgical research. Selecting the appropriate study design depends on the study purpose (hypothesis generating versus hypothesis testing as in Fig. 8-1) and the availability of resources for and feasibility of conducting the research. The informed reader should ensure that the investigators have used an acceptable study design to address the research question. A summary of the most common study designs in surgical literature is provided in Table 8-2.

TABLE 8-2 Important Considerations in Design Types

STUDY TYPE	EXPOSURE/OUTCOME RELATIONSHIP	CONSIDERATIONS	EXAMPLE
Randomized controlled trial	Randomly assigned an exposure and followed for outcome	Equipoise? Choice of control (e.g., placebo vs. standard of care) Generalizability? Blinding? Intention to treat? Superiority vs. noninferiority	Randomized trial of watchful waiting versus repair of inguinal hernia in adult men[17]
Cross-sectional	Exposure and outcome are assessed at the same point in time	Not suitable if disease has short duration or is rare	Cross-sectional study evaluating variation in receipt of VTE prophylaxis in hospitalized medical and surgical patients in 32 countries[26]
Cohort	Identified by exposure, followed for outcome (prospective or retrospective)	One exposure, multiple outcomes Confounding Inefficient for rare outcomes or outcomes that occur long after exposure	Cohort of patients who underwent endoscopic vs. open saphenous vein harvest during CABG, followed over time for rates of death and composite adverse events[27]
Case-control	Identified by outcome, assessed for exposure (prospective or retrospective)	One outcome, multiple exposures How was control group chosen? Confounding Recall bias	Study identifying risk factors (exposures) associated with retained foreign bodies after surgery (cases) vs. controls that did not have retained foreign body[28]
Case report/series		Generalizability	Case series of port-site metastasis, highlighting a rare but potentially serious risk[29]

CABG, coronary artery bypass graft; *VTE*, venous thromboembolism.

Randomized Controlled Trials

RCTs provide the highest level of evidence supporting causality. If randomization is performed properly and if the number of randomly assigned individuals is sufficiently large, confounding variables are distributed equally between groups, which is the main advantage of an RCT. That is, outcomes between two or more groups can be compared without concern for bias. However, conducting an RCT is challenging because of issues concerning equipoise, ethics, willingness to be randomly assigned, costs, and generalizability.

In an RCT, subjects are randomly assigned to an intervention group, where they receive an experimental intervention (a given trial may randomly assign subjects to one or more interventions), or to a control group, where they receive a controlled measurable alternative (placebo or a standard form of existing therapy). Subjects are followed to measure the occurrence of the outcomes of interest. Successful randomization eliminates systematic differences in potential confounding variables between the study groups. Subjects (single-blind) and in some cases the investigators (double-blind) may be blinded to which study intervention individual subjects are assigned. In open-label studies, neither subjects nor investigators are blinded. Blinding of study subjects is intended to mitigate the influence of a placebo effect, whereas blinding the investigators reduces bias from differential delivery of care and outcomes assessment between study groups. Blinding in surgery can be challenging. Sham or placebo surgery has been previously conducted[14] but requires special ethical justification.

An important analytic issue with RCTs is intent to treat (ITT). When an analysis is conducted following the ITT principle, outcome comparisons between control and treatment groups are based on the initial randomization and disregard any crossover—that is, subjects who were randomly assigned to control but received the study intervention or subjects who were assigned to an intervention but received the control. If analytic approaches other than ITT are used, an equal balance of confounders across comparison groups cannot be guaranteed, and the benefits of randomization may be lost. For example, an investigator who is an advocate of an intervention might prefer that only patients in an RCT who underwent that procedure be included in the analysis (known as a per-protocol analysis), excluding patients randomly assigned to the treatment but who crossed over to the control group or grouping the crossovers with the control group. ITT analysis is essential because it allows surgeons and patients to discuss whether choosing that intervention is best for that particular patient. When considering whether the patient should or should not undergo a procedure, neither the patient nor the surgeon knows whether the patient will be able to complete the intervention or strategy or will require a more conventional approach, perhaps because of the patient's inability to tolerate the procedure. ITT provides information about how the intervention compares at the moment the decision is being made.

The purpose of the RCT—superiority, equivalence, or noninferiority—has particular importance when interpreting its results. If two interventions are compared under a hypothesis of superiority and a statistically significant difference is not identified, the reader may be tempted to conclude that the two therapies are equivalent in terms of that outcome. However, the absence of an observable difference in outcomes is not the same as having evidence that outcomes are identical between two groups.[15] It is mathematically impossible to design a study with sufficient power to prove no difference in outcomes. Instead, investigators specify a priori the minimum difference in outcome that would be clinically important. The analysis is then designed to determine whether differences in outcomes are greater than this least important meaningful difference. Although noninferiority designs have clear value in surgical research, they are uncommon. To rule out small differences in outcomes, a very large number of patients must be enrolled to ensure sufficient statistical power.[16]

One noninferiority RCT evaluated whether watchful waiting of minimally symptomatic hernia provided equivalent pain score outcomes compared with conventional hernia repair.[17] In minimally symptomatic patients, the basis of recommending surgical hernia repair is to prevent complications related to the hernia (incarceration or strangulation or both), although these are rare events. The ITT results of the trial showed that the least important meaningful differences of 10% between pain-limiting activities and 8 points in pain score improvement over baseline at 2 years were not met. The authors concluded that delaying surgical repair until symptoms increase is equally efficacious, especially as acute hernia incarcerations were so infrequent.

Efficacy and Effectiveness

It is important to distinguish between efficacy and effectiveness. Efficacy refers to the extent to which a treatment intervention achieves its purported benefit and the durability of that result. Efficacy usually relates to outcomes in the context of controlled research studies (e.g., RCTs) and ideal patient care conditions, whereas effectiveness relates to outcomes in usual practice. Many patients encountered in usual practice would not qualify to be included in RCTs because of age, comorbid conditions, willingness to be randomly assigned, compliance, or other reasons. Effectiveness studies are conducted among larger populations inclusive of sufficient heterogeneity ideally to evaluate the way an intervention performs in the average community with average patients and clinicians. The best effectiveness studies would include all the patients in a very large population, but that is often not feasible, and so effectiveness researchers must balance concerns about generalizability of findings with the practical issues of conducting large trials. However, it is critical that effectiveness studies be conducted because real-world evaluations change our understanding of something we see in an RCT. For example, an RCT of more than 800 patients concluded that preoperative skin cleansing with chlorhexidine has superior efficacy to iodine in preventing surgical site infection.[18] These results could not be replicated in effectiveness studies, perhaps because of the differential selection of skin-cleansing agents and varied approaches to measuring infections in real practice.[19,20]

Variations on Randomized Trials

Although RCTs can offer the strongest evidence pointing toward causality, they are not ideal for all research questions. Numerous variations in the RCT design exist to allow assessment of effectiveness of an intervention across broad populations of patients and practice environments. The pragmatic RCT, in which the traditional "control" arm is replaced with "usual practice," is a contemporary methodology that capitalizes on the benefits of randomization but also accounts for variable practice environments and settings. In cluster-randomized trials, groups of subjects, rather than individuals, are randomly assigned. Cluster-randomized trials permit researchers to study interventions that cannot be directed toward selected individuals (e.g., implementing a surgical safety checklist as a hospital policy) and can control for "contamination" across individuals in the same cluster (e.g., one surgeon's use of preoperative antibiotics may influence another surgeon to do the same). In step-wedge randomized trials, the study intervention is sequentially rolled out to individuals or clusters of participants. The order in which participants receive the intervention is random, but all participants have received it by the end of the study. Step-wedge designs are used in situations in which a true RCT parallel design may be impractical for logistical or financial reasons or the intervention is thought to cause more good than harm (so withholding it in a true RCT would be unethical). In factorial RCTs, participants are assigned to a group that receives a combination of interventions (or noninterventions), allowing researchers to compare multiple effects with a smaller sample size than a traditional RCT. Finally, adaptive trials allow for key trial characteristics (e.g., treatment arms, eligibility, and sample size) to evolve in response to information accrued in the trial itself. This trial methodology (sometimes termed *personalized medicine trials*) is increasingly being applied to patient-centered outcomes research where focus on certain subpopulations may evolve with the trial.

To increase the quality and transparency of studies, online study registration with the International Standard Randomized Controlled Trial Number registry is essential. Study registration means that the research questions, study population, and analytic plan are detailed before the study begins, which prevents publication bias of reporting only positive studies. Registration also requires use of established methods and reporting standards. For example, the Consolidated Standards of Reporting Trials (CONSORT) guidelines require that details about various methodologic issues pertinent to the conduct of RCTs (e.g., randomization, blinding, ITT) be included in the final article.[21,22]

Meta-Analysis

Any one study may be underpowered to answer a given research question or reflect a particular degree of heterogeneity that might mislead the reader. Meta-analysis is a technique that pools available published data in an effort to increase the statistical power of an analysis. Meta-analysis is not applicable only to RCT data; it can also be used to pool results from observational studies. Similar to the CONSORT criteria for randomized trials, the Quality of Reporting of Meta-Analyses[23] and Meta-Analysis of Observational Studies in Epidemiology[24] guidelines have been developed to ensure the quality and validity of results obtained through meta-analysis. These guidelines should be considered when evaluating the quality of evidence provided by a pooled analysis.

For example, several randomized trials have questioned the surgical dogma of vigorous mechanical bowel preparation (MBP) before colorectal surgery. Several small RCTs suggested that MBP was associated with higher risk of anastomotic leakage and should be abandoned ($N = 47$ to 380 subjects in the published studies). More recent and larger RCTs suggested similar risk of anastomotic leakage with MBP but a higher risk of deep abdominal abscess without MBP (approximately 1350 subjects). However, no one study was powered to examine all outcomes of interest. A meta-analysis combining all the trials (4859 patients, 2452 who had MBP and 2407 who did not), showed no difference between the groups in terms of anastomotic leakage or deep abscesses and showed a significantly lower rate of all surgical site infections when MBP was omitted.[25]

Regardless of the type of pooled data, in all cases, an important consideration in appraising a meta-analysis is the homogeneity of the pooled studies. If the included studies evaluated similar end points, patient populations, and comparison groups, using similar definitions of variables and methods of outcome ascertainment, the pooled results may be informative. Significant heterogeneity indicates more variation in study outcomes than chance alone can explain, a sign that the designs or results of the included studies may not be compatible and should not be pooled. This heterogeneity is particularly a concern when observational data have been aggregated because these studies tend to have less control of variability and minimal control of confounding and bias. One approach to increasing the transparency of pooled results from observational studies is to pool the baseline characteristics of the comparison groups also.

Cross-Sectional Study

Cross-sectional studies include data collected at a single point in time. The data from cross-sectional studies are most commonly used to explore relationships between variables and disease burden or stacked over time to look at temporal trends. These studies are best used for hypothesis generation. Limitations that arise from how a population is sampled, lack of multiple time points, and detection or recall bias do not allow this type of study to make causal links. For example, the ENDORSE (Epidemiologic International Day for the Evaluation of Patients at Risk for Venous Thromboembolism in the Acute Hospital Care Setting) study assessed more than 68,000 patients from 32 countries for variation in VTE prophylaxis. The study found 35,000 patients (52%) were at risk for VTE. Of those, 59% of surgical patients and 40% of medical patients received appropriate prophylaxis.[26] The description of variation in practice motivated subsequent studies comparing different types of VTE prophylaxis and interventions to improve adherence with established guidelines.

Cohort Study

Cohort studies follow patients nonrandomly assigned to different groups to determine whether outcomes vary across groups. Data may be examined prospectively or retrospectively, but the onset of observation is with the exposure (i.e., group assignment) and extends over time to determine if a particular event occurs or not. The advantages of cohort studies are the ability to estimate the incidence (or rate) of exposures and outcomes, assess multiple outcomes simultaneously, and study rare exposures. Cohort studies are inefficient for evaluating outcomes that are rare or occur a long time after exposure.

For example, in a secondary analysis of the PREVENTION VI trial data, outcome differences between patients who underwent endoscopic versus open saphenous vein harvesting during coronary artery bypass grafting were evaluated.[27] After adjusting for potential confounding factors, the authors found that rates of death and two composite end points were more frequent in the endoscopic harvesting group. This study highlighted two advantages of the cohort design—it allowed an estimation of the rate of adverse events associated with competing interventions and the simultaneous assessment of multiple outcomes.

Case-Control Study

Case-control studies compare the frequency of exposures between patients who have and have not experienced an outcome of interest. These studies begin by enrolling subjects with and without the outcome of interest and then look back in time to search for differences in potential risk factors. Case-control designs are infrequently used in the surgical literature. One example involved an evaluation of risk factors associated with retained foreign bodies after surgery.[28] Researchers reviewed the medical records of all patients who made claims or provided incident reports to a large, statewide malpractice insurer ($n = 54$). Each case was matched to four control patients ($n = 235$) who did not make such claims. Risk factors for retained foreign bodies included emergency surgery, unplanned change in the operation, and body mass index. This study highlighted two advantages of the case-control design—the ability to evaluate risk factors for a rare outcome and to assess multiple risk factors simultaneously.

Case-control studies sometimes are confused with cohort studies, perhaps because of difficulty regarding the meaning of case and control in the research context. In health services and epidemiologic research, a case refers to a subject who has experienced an outcome of interest, whereas a control refers to a patient who has not experienced that outcome. All patients experiencing the outcome should be included in a case-control study, particularly when that outcome is rare. It is unnecessary to sample all patients without the outcome because there is no statistical benefit for including more than four controls for each case. However, sampled patients without the outcome should be representative of the overall population to which they belong. Because of the manner in which subjects are sampled in a case-control study, it is impossible to estimate the frequency of the exposure in the population at large from case-control studies. Advantages of the case-control design include efficiency in evaluating the factors associated with rare outcomes or outcomes occurring a long time after exposure and the ability to evaluate multiple exposures simultaneously. When measurement of an exposure is expensive or time-consuming (e.g., costly laboratory assays, detailed interviews), this can be a much more efficient way to use resources because those resources need to be expended only on subjects with the outcome of interest and the limited number of controls.

Case Reports and Case Series

A case report aims to highlight an unusual or unexpected procedure or event, whereas a case series demonstrates that such events can happen more than once. A benefit of these studies is that they can reveal a potentially unrecognized benefit or adverse effect of surgical therapy and may generate new hypotheses, prompting more rigorous scientific evaluation. Laparoscopic radical prostatectomy is an established approach for treating localized prostate cancer and reportedly offers oncologic benefit equivalent to open resection. However, since 1994, surgeons have reported 14 total cases of port site metastasis, highlighting a rare but potentially serious risk of a minimally invasive surgery (MIS) approach to prostatectomy.[29] These studies are distinct from cohort investigations because there is no comparison made between competing strategies or interventions.

WAS THE RIGHT ANALYSIS PERFORMED?

The statistical analysis of any study should stem from the study aims, design, and data sources. An understanding of several methodologic concepts serves as a foundation for reviewing the literature critically.

Variable Types and Descriptive Statistics

Table 8-3 provides a summary of commonly used variables and associated measures of central tendency and statistical tests. A continuous variable is one that can take on any number of values within a specified range of possibilities. Age and length of stay are examples of continuous variables. Descriptive statistics are used to describe the central tendency of continuous variables. The arithmetic mean provides a good estimate of central tendency for normally distributed (gaussian or bell-shaped) data. If the data are skewed (not normally distributed), the mean is a biased estimator of the central tendency. In these cases, the median or geometric mean provides a better estimate.

Categorical variables have discrete values. The simplest categorical variable is a binary variable that can take on only one of two values, such as sex (male, female). Ordinal variables are ordered categorical variables. Cancer stage is a classic example of an ordinal categorical variable. Nominal variables are unordered categorical variables, such as race. Categorical variables are described in terms of proportions.

Time-to-event variables consist of two variables—a continuous variable that measures the time interval from an established start point (e.g., date of diagnosis or therapy) to a failure event (e.g., death or disease recurrence) or the end of the observation period and a binary variable, which indicates whether the failure event occurred. Long-term survival is a classic example of a time-to-event variable. The Kaplan-Meier method is the most common way to provide a description of the probability of an event occurring at a certain point in time (e.g., survival at 5 years). This method takes into consideration that over time the number of patients at risk for an event decreases; as patients drop out of a study or experience the outcome event, there will be progressively fewer patients at risk for having the outcome (a patient who dies cannot die again). The Kaplan-Meier method may overestimate risk in the setting of competing risks. For example, time to re-intervention has competing risks—the disease process may evolve prompting re-intervention; over time, a contraindication to re-intervention may develop; or death may occur, in which case a patient is no longer at risk. However, methods exist for handling time-to-event variables in the setting of competing risks.[30]

TABLE 8-3 Commonly Used Parameters in Surgical Outcomes and Health Services Research

TYPE OF VARIABLE	MEASUREMENT	DESCRIPTIVE STATISTIC	MULTIVARIABLE REGRESSION MODEL
Continuous	Mean Median	Unpaired t-test Paired t-test for repeated measures ANOVA for two or more groups	Linear
Categorical	Proportion	Chi-square test Mantel-Haenszel odds	Logistic
Time-to-event	Kaplan-Meier	Log-rank test	Cox hazard

ANOVA, analysis of variance.

Hypothesis Testing

Hypothesis testing uses statistics to determine whether observed differences between two or more groups are true or are attributable to chance. Foremost, the reader should know whether the goal is to show superiority, equivalence, or noninferiority of the treatments being compared because this guides the type of hypothesis testing performed (equivalence = two-sided hypothesis; noninferiority = one-sided hypothesis). The *P* value is a statistical summary measure for hypothesis testing. A significance level of 5% ($P = .05$) is widely used to indicate a statistically significant finding, although the 5% threshold is arbitrary, and for some measures a lower (with large databases where false-positive findings are to be avoided) or higher (when a higher noise-to-signal ratio is acceptable as in safety evaluations) level may be appropriate. A *P* value is interpreted as the probability that the observed difference in outcomes between groups is the result of chance (i.e., the difference is not based on the effect of the intervention). The smaller the *P* value, the less likely the difference could represent a false-positive finding. As a general rule, the larger the difference being compared and the larger the sample size for a given comparison, the lower the *P* value and the less likely that the finding is the result of chance alone.

Two types of errors can occur with hypothesis testing. An α (or type I) error occurs when one observes a difference in outcomes when such a difference does not actually exist. If the research question and analysis have not been specified a priori or numerous statistical tests are performed on many subgroups, a type I error can occur. For example, if a threshold of 5% were considered statistically significant, 5 of 100 statistical tests could potentially demonstrate a statistically significant finding that is attributable to chance alone (a false-positive finding). If one repeats a comparative analysis in different subgroups (i.e., multiple comparisons), there are more opportunities to observe a false-positive result.[31] When multiple comparisons are necessary, corrections (e.g., Bonferroni correction) to the *P* value can be made in an attempt to safeguard against type I errors. A β (or type II) error occurs when no difference in outcomes is observed when a difference truly exists (a false-negative finding). This type of error occurs when a study has insufficient power to detect true differences in outcomes between groups. Power is directly related to sample size and the size of the observed difference.

Hypothesis testing is also possible by examining confidence interval (CI). Summary measures of the difference between groups are provided as an estimated ratio (outcomes in the study group divided by outcomes in the standard or control group) or as an absolute difference, with a 95% CI. The CI provides an estimate of the uncertainty around a given value; a wide CI indicates a lack of precision, whereas a tight (small) interval would be indicative of minimal uncertainty. When the summary measure is an odds or relative risk ratio, a CI inclusive of 1.0 indicates no statistical difference in outcomes. If the summary measure is the absolute difference or relative risk, a CI inclusive of 0 indicates no statistically significant difference.

Table 8-3 provides a summary of statistical tests that are often used for hypothesis testing by variable type. The unpaired t-test is used to compare two independent groups that have continuous outcome variables. A paired t-test is used to compare two dependent groups that have continuous outcome variables. An example of a dependent group comparison is serial blood pressure measurements on the same person. An analysis of variance is used when comparing more than two groups with a continuous outcome variable. The chi-square test is often used to compare the distributions of two or more groups with categorical outcome variables. Fisher exact test is more appropriate for such comparisons when the sample size is small. A log-rank test is used to compare two groups with time-to-event outcome variables.

Multivariable Analysis

Multivariable regression models are among the most commonly used methods to evaluate the relationship between variables and outcomes while controlling for the influence of other measured variables. Linear regression is used to evaluate the relationship between factors potentially associated with a continuous outcome variable, such as length of stay. The output of this model is a risk difference. This model assumes the outcome variable is normally distributed. In the case of most health services end points, such as length of stay, normal distribution is not the case. To deal with non-normal outcomes, a mathematical "transformation" of the data might be used to create a new variable that more closely approximates a normal distribution—for example, taking the logarithm of the length of stay.

Logistic regression is used when the outcome variable is binary (e.g., operative mortality). Probabilities and odds, although calculated differently, are both measures of risk and are usually presented in the form of a ratio (the odds or risk in the study group divided by the control group). Understanding the difference between these measures is important because the odds will overestimate the probability if the outcome occurs frequently in the population. When the outcome is rare, the odds generally provide a good approximation of the probability. It is particularly relevant when conducting multivariable analysis that a minimum number of events are included to achieve a reliable estimate. As rules of thumb, a minimum of 10 events (and equivalent number of nonevents) per variable are required for logistic regression (binary outcome),[32] and 10 to 15 observations per variable are required for linear regression (continuous outcome).[33]

Cox proportional hazard regression is used for the evaluation of time-to-event outcomes. The summary measure of risk provided by this model is also in the form of a ratio. A hazard refers to the instantaneous risk of an event at any time. The proportional hazards assumption must be valid to interpret the results of this type of regression and requires that the differences in risks of an event between groups remain constant over time.

Propensity Score Analysis

Propensity score analysis is an alternative method of risk adjustment. When two groups are being compared, logistic regression is used to calculate a subject's probability of having an exposure of interest (e.g., MIS compared with open surgery). That probability is the propensity score (propensity to undergo MIS). The outcomes of interest for patients who do and do not undergo MIS (but have a similar propensity to undergo MIS) can be compared through matching, stratified analyses, or regression (adjusting only for propensity).

Propensity score analyses are appealing because they seem intuitive; they compare outcomes across groups that have a similar probability of receiving the therapy of interest. This analysis is often described as being "similar to an RCT" in the sense that it compares outcomes between groups at equal propensity for receiving the therapy of interest. This analogy often leads people to believe that propensity score analyses provide advantages in risk adjustment over standard techniques such as regression. This belief is generally unsubstantiated because the analytic approach has no bearing on a key measurement issue—the ability to measure all confounders, known or unknown, using observational data. The informed reader should be aware of three circumstances in which the use of propensity scores may be appropriate: (1) there are many confounders relative to the number of events (i.e., <10 events per covariate) resulting in an unpowered regression analysis, (2) there is no interest in the association between the adjustment factors and outcome, and (3) the relationship between the exposure and propensity for treatment can be estimated more accurately than the relationship between the exposure and outcome.[34] For example, in a cohort study looking at mortality and readmission associated with hepatocellular cancer, patients were grouped based on treatment as undergoing resection, radiofrequency ablation, or no treatment. Because of multiple confounders, the authors used liver-associated comorbid conditions to create a propensity score for receipt of treatment. The three groups of patients were matched to determine the adjusted risk ratios for mortality and readmission based on each treatment group.[35]

Instrumental Variable Analysis

Instrumental variable analysis is another method of controlling bias. The principle underlying this type of analysis is that there are unmeasured confounders that might bias the results of a study. Selecting a variable exogenous to the study subject, one over which the study subject has no control, that is strongly associated with the exposure but not associated with the outcome (except possibly through the causal pathway involving the exposure) controls for any and all confounding factors associated with the outcome and exposure of interest.

As an example, consider distance from a cardiac specialty center as an instrumental variable. In this case, the instrumental variable is strongly associated with the exposure under study (patients who live further away are less likely to have cardiac catheterization) but not associated with the measured outcome (having a myocardial infarction). The best instruments are instruments that act as a surrogate for randomization. However, well-selected instrumental variables are hard to find in surgical research. For example, the association between treatment and outcome is confounded if causes of noncompliance with a therapy are also independent risk factors for the outcome, and bias can actually be accentuated.[36] Readers must decide whether they agree with the choice of the instrumental variable and whether they will believe the results. A publication evaluating the association between cardiac catheterization and mortality provides a good demonstration of the use of an instrumental variable compared with other common risk adjustment techniques.[37]

Missing Data

A common problem in research is missing data, especially when using observational data. If the study is small and the investigator ignores (throws out) subjects with missing data, the power of the study is compromised. More importantly, if data are missing in a systematic way (e.g., related to the exposure and outcome), excluding subjects with missing data will likely bias the analysis. Missing data can fall into one of three categories—missing completely at random (MCAR), missing at random (MAR), and missing not at random (MNAR).

Data that are MCAR are missing for random reasons unrelated to the exposure, covariate, or outcome. A good example of how MCAR may occur is when a research assistant accidentally drops a test tube of blood from a study subject. The reason for the lost data has nothing to do with the treatment that the patient received; the outcome that the patient may experience; or the patient's sex, race, or social status. When data are MAR, the data are missing conditional on some other measured value. For example, women may be less willing to give information about their weight. As such, one could predict the likelihood of missing weight data based on sex. When data are MNAR, the data are missing conditional on an unmeasured value. For example, a patient may be unwilling to offer information about his or her income, perhaps because he or she considers it to be too high or too low. In this case, the reason for missing information about income is the level of the income itself.

It is difficult to establish whether missing data are MCAR, MAR, or MNAR, and investigators must make informed assumptions. If missing data do not vary across factors associated with an outcome, and the authors are unaware of any systematic reason for missing data, it would be reasonable to assume MCAR. If missing data occur more frequently across certain groups of patients, one might assume MAR, although the possibility of MNAR cannot be excluded. If the investigator is aware of MNAR, there is no good solution for handling missing data. With MCAR and MAR, there are numerous methods for handling missing data, including the missing data indicator method (in which missing data points are coded as a separate category instead of missing) as well as various methods of imputation, or using models to estimate the value of missing data. Of these, multiple imputation appears to introduce the least bias.[38] Finally, with MCAR, one could conduct a case-complete analysis (i.e., throw out subjects with missing data), although dropping patients can reduce the study size enough to affect other analyses.

Correlated Data

Correlated data have implications for statistical inference in studies that make repeated measures of an outcome over time (longitudinal study) and studies that examine subjects that cluster within groups. In general, methods used to handle correlated data in the context of repeated outcome measures account for similarity in characteristics or outcome or both within a subject and between subjects. For example, clustering refers to the notion that patients treated by the same surgeons or at the same medical center are likely to be more similar to each other than patients treated by a different surgeon. Similarly, surgeons working at a particular type of hospital are more likely to be similar to each other than surgeons working at a different hospital. Under such circumstances, the outcomes of patients under the care of a particular surgeon and a surgeon working at a particular hospital are more likely to be similar (or correlated). Statistical methods accounting for correlated data may include hierarchical regression models, bayesian analysis, or clustering adjustment. For example, investigators examined the relationship between surgeon volume and operative mortality for several different procedures, after adjusting for patient characteristics and hospital volume.[39] Their analysis involved three levels of variables—pertaining to patients (age, sex, comorbidity), surgeons (procedural volume), and hospitals (procedural volume). For most procedures, higher surgeon volume was associated with lower adjusted operative mortality rates. The authors used statistical modeling (binary mixed effects) to account for clustering of patients within surgeons and clustering of surgeons within hospitals. Surgeons reading published studies should be aware of situations in which correlated data may exist and look for how the authors chose to handle the correlation.

HOW SHOULD I USE THIS INFORMATION IN MY PRACTICE?

To summarize the research question that the study aims to address, the reader might find it helpful to use the "PICOT framework," an acronym that stands for the study **P**opulation, independent variables (i.e., **I**ntervention/exposure, covariates), a **C**omparator group if applicable, dependent variable (i.e., **O**utcome, end point), and **T**ime frame of outcomes assessment. Thinking of research studies through a PICOT lens guides a systematic assessment of the study's quality,[40,41] and all the pertinent points needed to support the PICOT framework should be readily available to guide the reader through an appraisal of the study (Table 8-4).[17,42]

Confounding

One of the most important issues to consider in the evaluation and conduct of outcomes research using observational data is confounding. A confounder is a measured or unmeasured variable associated with the exposure of interest and associated with the outcome. This dual relationship can influence the degree and direction of, or even completely mitigate, an observed association between exposure and outcome. As an example, consider a hypothetical study aiming to determine whether there is an association between insurance status and long-term survival among patients with resected colon cancer. The results demonstrate a significantly lower survival rate among uninsured patients compared with insured patients. However, the authors did not measure and adjust for cancer stage, a well-known and strong determinant of long-term survival. Patients without insurance may present with later stage cancer because of limited access to care. Without controlling for the higher proportion of patients with higher stage cancer in the uninsured groups, the results are likely biased such that the uninsured would appear to have worse outcomes than they actually do. A comprehensive report about the direction of bias resulting from confounding is available.[43]

In RCTs, if randomization is performed properly and the number of randomly assigned individuals is large, confounders should be balanced in the different treatment arms.[44] Investigators who perform observational studies can address confounding with analytic approaches and in their discussion of the study's limitations. Multivariable regression, propensity score, and instrumental variable analysis all are analytic methods of addressing confounding using measured variables. For variables that were not measured or cannot be measured, the authors of a study should describe these variables, describe their relationship with the exposure and the outcome, and discuss the potential direction and magnitude of confounding bias.

Generalizability

Generalizability refers to the ability to take research findings and apply them to clinical practice. For example, RCTs are conducted in a highly controlled setting, with strict inclusion and exclusion criteria, staff dedicated to follow-up, and protocol adherence. Although RCTs provide the highest level of evidence about the efficacy of competing interventions, the environment in which they take place may limit the ability of other providers to reproduce the delivery of care and outcomes in a clinical (nonresearch) setting.

Issues concerning generalizability are also associated with observational studies. For example, Medicare data are limited to older or disabled patients. Practice patterns and outcomes among

TABLE 8-4 PICOT Research Question

WHAT IS THE ... ?	CONSIDER	EXAMPLE[17] AND *IMPLICATION(S)*
Patient/population	Age? Sex? Diagnosis? Inpatient/outpatient? Emergency/elective?	Men ≥18 years old, presenting with asymptomatic or minimally symptomatic inguinal hernia *Focus on minimally symptomatic patients affects the generalizability of the study and selection of the appropriate research design.*
Intervention/exposure	Surgical? Pharmaceutical? Diagnostic? Prophylactic? Management processes?	Watchful waiting *"Watchful waiting" for hernia is a description of nonsurgical care, but study needs to specify other interventions, such as diagnostic testing, follow-up that solicits symptoms, or passive follow-up that relies on patients initiating a complaint.*
Comparison	Another intervention? Standard of care? No intervention? Placebo?	Lichtenstein open tension-free repair *How does the study handle patients who crossed over between study arms?*
Outcome	Safety (e.g., surgical site infection) Effectiveness vs. efficacy (e.g., recurrence) Patient-reported outcome (e.g., pain score) Resource utilization (e.g., length of stay) Cost	Primary: pain and discomfort scores Secondary: complications, functional status, satisfaction with care *Some of these outcomes are "subjective," and it is important to know what is considered an important difference.*
Time frame for evaluation	One vs. several time points? Continuous? Does time to end point matter?	At baseline, 6 months, and annually *If the results change over time, which time point should I pay attention to?*

Adapted from Richardson WS, Wilson MC, Nishikawa J, et al: The well-built clinical question: A key to evidence-based decisions. *ACP J Club* 123:A12–13, 1995; and Rosenthal R, Schafer J, Briel M, et al: How to write a surgical clinical research protocol: Literature review and practical guide. *Am J Surg* 207:299–312, 2014.

Medicare patients may or may not be generalizable to non-Medicare patients. Critical readers should consider why care patterns and outcomes described in research studies might not be reproducible in other clinical settings and patient populations.

Determining Causality Using Observational Data

Observational data may reveal associations between exposures (i.e., competing therapies) and outcomes. Investigators often infer a causal relationship between exposures and outcomes based on such associations.[45] Several criteria have been proposed for inferring causality from observational studies; these are often termed the *Bradford Hill criteria*. One criterion for inferring causality is that the exposure must happen before the outcome. Otherwise, the exposure cannot plausibly lead to the outcome. Although an obvious criterion, it is frequently omitted. Next, the association and hypothesized causal relationship must also be biologically (clinically) plausible. Finally, the magnitude of association between the exposure and outcome must be large, and if there are varying degrees of exposure, there should also be matching varying magnitudes of association between exposure and outcome (e.g., dose-response relationship).

For example, a cohort study evaluating the relationship between preoperative hematocrit levels and adverse events found an increased risk of death and postoperative cardiac events when hematocrit levels were below normal thresholds. Although the authors appropriately acknowledge that a causal relationship could not be established from their observational study, their exposure (preoperative low hematocrit) preceded the outcome (postoperative cardiac event); there was a strong "dose-response" association between hematocrit level and adverse events and a biologically plausible mechanism of impaired cardiac physiology.[46,47]

Is There Conflict of Interest?

Surgeons and investigators commonly serve in advisory roles for pharmaceutical companies or device manufacturers. Such associations may affect a researcher's objectivity if a study hypothesis addresses the effect of that company's product, constituting a conflict of interest. These considerations loom largest over industry-sponsored trials. When reading an RCT supported by the corporation that makes a given drug or device, it is crucial to read the methods, results, and conclusions with a critical eye to ensure that any potential influence from the sponsor has not affected study validity. Furthermore, it is the responsibility of all investigators to disclose all associations fully (for themselves or their families) that could conceivably be construed as a conflict of interest. Without such disclosures, the objectivity and validity of a given study must be even more closely scrutinized. As part of the Affordable Care Act, the Physician Payments Sunshine Act requires manufacturers to disclose payments given to physicians and hospitals. This information is publically available at http://cms.gov/openpayments/.

Evolving With the Evidence

The "information overload" associated with new and evolving evidence poses a unique challenge to surgeons, who have long been considered leaders in adapting and improving their practice (e.g., weekly morbidity and mortality conferences). Numerous knowledge management strategies exist to help cope with the growing amount of data. When appropriate, surgeons can participate in multidisciplinary teams, conferences, or education focused on spreading the most important contemporary evidence. Professional societies (local, national, or international) are a good source of "best" evidence, and membership in these groups allows surgeons to access and incorporate evidence-based practice in a timely manner. For example, the American College of Surgeons publishes a highly regarded literature review called "Selected Readings in General Surgery." In addition, engagement in a growing number of free-to-use "web-portals" (e.g., General Surgery—Medscape, available at http://www.medscape.com/generalsurgery/) and medical media communication (e.g., General Surgery News, available at http://www.generalsurgerynews.com/) can highlight the newest evidence. Lastly, surgeons are increasingly becoming part of "learning health care systems," whether by practicing in integrated health care delivery systems (e.g., Kaiser, Geisinger) or through community collaboratives (e.g., Surgical Care and Outcomes Assessment Program). Such learning health care systems create surveillance of practice change and give more real-time evidence about what is most effective in health care. Through these methods, surgeons can create the "evidence-based culture" needed to achieve the best outcomes in future generations.

CONCLUSIONS

The delivery of patient care using the best available evidence is the responsibility of all surgeons. Interpreting the evidence from published reports requires an understanding of the terms and methods of clinical outcomes and health services research. The questions posed in this chapter should serve as a guide for critically examining the surgical literature. Critical readers of the surgical literature are better able to embrace the promise of evidence-based surgery.

SELECTED REFERENCES

Austin PC: An introduction to propensity score methods for reducing the effects of confounding in observational studies. *Multivariate Behav Res* 46:399–424, 2011.

The propensity score is essentially a balancing score that allows design and analysis of an observational study so that it mimics characteristics of a randomized controlled trial. This article provides a practical discussion of different propensity score–based methods of analysis and their interpretation.

Bridges JF, Onukwugha E, Mullins CD: Healthcare rationing by proxy: Cost-effectiveness analysis and the misuse of the $50,000 threshold in the US. *Pharmacoeconomics* 28:175–184, 2010.

The benchmark of $50,000 per quality-adjusted life-year is often used in cost-effectiveness assessments. This article provides an excellent review of the accuracy and appropriateness of this cost per quality-adjusted life-year metric and includes a timely discussion regarding health care cost-effectiveness research.

Brookhart MA, Rassen JA, Schneeweiss S: Instrumental variable methods in comparative safety and effectiveness research. *Pharmacoepidemiol Drug Saf* 19:537–554, 2010.

This study provides several examples including comparison and discussion of several commonly used instrumental variable methodologic techniques in health services research.

Fleming TR, Powers JH: Biomarkers and surrogate endpoints in clinical trials. *Stat Med* 31:2973–2984, 2012.

The selection of appropriate end points is perhaps the most important issue in the design of any research study, in particular, randomized controlled trials. This article provides a thorough contemporary discussion of surrogate end points and how such end points can influence study results.

Mehio-Sibai A, Feinleib M, Sibai TA, et al: A positive or a negative confounding variable? A simple teaching aid for clinicians and students. *Ann Epidemiol* 15:421–423, 2005.

Confounding can introduce conservative (inappropriately accepting the null hypothesis) or anticonservative (inappropriately rejecting the null hypothesis) bias. This simple model can help the reader think about the directionality of the confounding bias and help with interpretation of the magnitude reported effects.

Rubin DB: The design versus the analysis of observational studies for causal effects: Parallels with the design of randomized trials. *Stat Med* 26:20–36, 2007.

Although randomized controlled trials are considered the gold standard for estimating causal effects, they are often not feasible because of time, ethics, or cost. Observational studies can and should be used in appropriate situations to infer causality, and this article provides the framework for how studies can be structured to do so.

REFERENCES

1. Drake FT, Florence MG, Johnson MG, et al: Progress in the diagnosis of appendicitis: A report from Washington State's Surgical Care and Outcomes Assessment Program. *Ann Surg* 256:586–594, 2012.
2. Basu S, Alavi A: Staging with PET and the "Will Rogers" effect: Redefining prognosis and survival in patients with cancer. *Eur J Nucl Med Mol Imaging* 35:1–4, 2008.
3. Farjah F, Flum DR, Ramsey SD, et al: Multi-modality mediastinal staging for lung cancer among Medicare beneficiaries. *J Thorac Oncol* 4:355–363, 2009.
4. Clark DA, Stinson EB, Griepp RB, et al: Cardiac transplantation in man. VI. Prognosis of patients selected for cardiac transplantation. *Ann Intern Med* 75:15–21, 1971.
5. Crowley J, Hu M: Covariance analysis of heart-transplant survival data. *J Am Stat Assoc* 72:27–36, 1977.
6. Spiegel BM, Reid MW, Bolus R, et al: Development and validation of a disease-targeted quality of life instrument for chronic diverticular disease: The DV-QOL. *Qual Life Res* 24:163–179, 2015.
7. Bridges JF, Onukwugha E, Mullins CD: Healthcare rationing by proxy: Cost-effectiveness analysis and the misuse of the $50,000 threshold in the US. *Pharmacoeconomics* 28:175–184, 2010.
8. Brook RH, Park RE, Chassin MR, et al: Predicting the appropriate use of carotid endarterectomy, upper gastrointestinal endoscopy, and coronary angiography. *N Engl J Med* 323:1173–1177, 1990.
9. Kahan JP, Park RE, Leape LL, et al: Variations by specialty in physician ratings of the appropriateness and necessity of indications for procedures. *Med Care* 34:512–523, 1996.
10. Coronary Revascularization Writing Group, Patel MR, Dehmer GJ, et al: ACCF/SCAI/STS/AATS/AHA/ASNC/HFSA/SCCT 2012 appropriate use criteria for coronary revascularization focused update: A report of the American College of Cardiology Foundation Appropriate Use Criteria Task Force, Society for Cardiovascular Angiography and Interventions, Society of Thoracic Surgeons, American Association for Thoracic Surgery, American Heart Association, American Society of Nuclear Cardiology, and the Society of Cardiovascular Computed Tomography. *J Thorac Cardiovasc Surg* 143:780–803, 2012.
11. Brodie BR, Stuckey T, Downey W, et al: Outcomes and complications with off-label use of drug-eluting stents: Results from the STENT (Strategic Transcatheter Evaluation of New Therapies) group. *JACC Cardiovasc Interv* 1:405–414, 2008.
12. Fleming TR, Powers JH: Biomarkers and surrogate endpoints in clinical trials. *Stat Med* 31:2973–2984, 2012.
13. Rasmussen MS, Jorgensen LN, Wille-Jorgensen P, et al: Prolonged prophylaxis with dalteparin to prevent late thromboembolic complications in patients undergoing major abdominal surgery: A multicenter randomized open-label study. *J Thromb Haemost* 4:2384–2390, 2006.
14. Moseley JB, O'Malley K, Petersen NJ, et al: A controlled trial of arthroscopic surgery for osteoarthritis of the knee. *N Engl J Med* 347:81–88, 2002.
15. Alderson P, Roberts I: Should journals publish systematic reviews that find no evidence to guide practice? Examples from injury research. *BMJ* 320:376–377, 2000.
16. Farjah F, Flum DR: When not being superior may not be good enough. *JAMA* 298:924–925, 2007.
17. Fitzgibbons RJ, Jr, Giobbie-Hurder A, Gibbs JO, et al: Watchful waiting vs repair of inguinal hernia in minimally symptomatic men: A randomized clinical trial. *JAMA* 295:285–292, 2006.
18. Darouiche RO, Wall MJ, Jr, Itani KM, et al: Chlorhexidine-alcohol versus povidone-iodine for surgical-site antisepsis. *N Engl J Med* 362:18–26, 2010.
19. Swenson BR, Hedrick TL, Metzger R, et al: Effects of preoperative skin preparation on postoperative wound infection rates: A prospective study of 3 skin preparation protocols. *Infect Control Hosp Epidemiol* 30:964–971, 2009.
20. Hakkarainen TW, Dellinger EP, Evans HL, et al: Comparative effectiveness of skin antiseptic agents in reducing surgical site infections: A report from the Washington State Surgical Care and Outcomes Assessment Program. *J Am Coll Surg* 218:336–344, 2014.
21. Turner L, Shamseer L, Altman DG, et al: Consolidated standards of reporting trials (CONSORT) and the completeness of reporting of randomised controlled trials (RCTs) published in medical journals. *Cochrane Database Syst Rev* 11: MR000030, 2012.
22. Nagendran M, Harding D, Teo W, et al: Poor adherence of randomised trials in surgery to CONSORT guidelines for non-pharmacological treatments (NPT): A cross-sectional study. *BMJ Open* 3:e003898, 2013.
23. Moher D, Cook DJ, Eastwood S, et al: Improving the quality of reports of meta-analyses of randomised controlled trials: The QUOROM statement. Quality of Reporting of Meta-analyses. *Lancet* 354:1896–1900, 1999.

24. Stroup DF, Berlin JA, Morton SC, et al: Meta-analysis of observational studies in epidemiology: A proposal for reporting. Meta-analysis Of Observational Studies in Epidemiology (MOOSE) group. *JAMA* 283:2008–2012, 2000.
25. Slim K, Vicaut E, Launay-Savary MV, et al: Updated systematic review and meta-analysis of randomized clinical trials on the role of mechanical bowel preparation before colorectal surgery. *Ann Surg* 249:203–209, 2009.
26. Cohen AT, Tapson VF, Bergmann JF, et al: Venous thromboembolism risk and prophylaxis in the acute hospital care setting (ENDORSE study): A multinational cross-sectional study. *Lancet* 371:387–394, 2008.
27. Lopes RD, Hafley GE, Allen KB, et al: Endoscopic versus open vein-graft harvesting in coronary-artery bypass surgery. *N Engl J Med* 361:235–244, 2009.
28. Gawande AA, Studdert DM, Orav EJ, et al: Risk factors for retained instruments and sponges after surgery. *N Engl J Med* 348:229–235, 2003.
29. Savage SJ, Wingo MS, Hooper HB, et al: Pathologically confirmed port site metastasis after laparoscopic radical prostatectomy: Case report and literature review. *Urology* 70:1222.e9–1222.e11, 2007.
30. Resche-Rigon M, Azoulay E, Chevret S: Evaluating mortality in intensive care units: Contribution of competing risks analyses. *Crit Care* 10:R5, 2006.
31. Assmann SF, Pocock SJ, Enos LE, et al: Subgroup analysis and other (mis)uses of baseline data in clinical trials. *Lancet* 355:1064–1069, 2000.
32. Peduzzi P, Concato J, Kemper E, et al: A simulation study of the number of events per variable in logistic regression analysis. *J Clin Epidemiol* 49:1373–1379, 1996.
33. Babyak MA: What you see may not be what you get: A brief, nontechnical introduction to overfitting in regression-type models. *Psychosom Med* 66:411–421, 2004.
34. Austin PC: An introduction to propensity score methods for reducing the effects of confounding in observational studies. *Multivariate Behav Res* 46:399–424, 2011.
35. Massarweh NN, Park JO, Yeung RS, et al: Comparative assessment of the safety and effectiveness of radiofrequency ablation among elderly medicare beneficiaries with hepatocellular carcinoma. *Ann Surg Oncol* 19:1058–1065, 2012.
36. Brookhart MA, Rassen JA, Schneeweiss S: Instrumental variable methods in comparative safety and effectiveness research. *Pharmacoepidemiol Drug Saf* 19:537–554, 2010.
37. Stukel TA, Fisher ES, Wennberg DE, et al: Analysis of observational studies in the presence of treatment selection bias: Effects of invasive cardiac management on AMI survival using propensity score and instrumental variable methods. *JAMA* 297:278–285, 2007.
38. Donders AR, van der Heijden GJ, Stijnen T, et al: Review: A gentle introduction to imputation of missing values. *J Clin Epidemiol* 59:1087–1091, 2006.
39. Birkmeyer JD, Stukel TA, Siewers AE, et al: Surgeon volume and operative mortality in the United States. *N Engl J Med* 349:2117–2127, 2003.
40. Richardson WS, Wilson MC, Nishikawa J, et al: The well-built clinical question: A key to evidence-based decisions. *ACP J Club* 123:A12–A13, 1995.
41. Schardt C, Adams MB, Owens T, et al: Utilization of the PICO framework to improve searching PubMed for clinical questions. *BMC Med Inform Decis Mak* 7:16, 2007.
42. Rosenthal R, Schafer J, Briel M, et al: How to write a surgical clinical research protocol: Literature review and practical guide. *Am J Surg* 207:299–312, 2014.
43. Mehio-Sibai A, Feinleib M, Sibai TA, et al: A positive or a negative confounding variable? A simple teaching aid for clinicians and students. *Ann Epidemiol* 15:421–423, 2005.
44. Altman DG, Bland JM: Statistics notes. Treatment allocation in controlled trials: Why randomise? *BMJ* 318:1209, 1999.
45. Rubin DB: The design versus the analysis of observational studies for causal effects: Parallels with the design of randomized trials. *Stat Med* 26:20–36, 2007.
46. Farjah F, Flum DR: Hematocrit level and postsurgical outcome: Powers of observation. *JAMA* 297:2525–2526, 2007.
47. Wu WC, Schifftner TL, Henderson WG, et al: Preoperative hematocrit levels and postoperative outcomes in older patients undergoing noncardiac surgery. *JAMA* 297:2481–2488, 2007.

CHAPTER 9

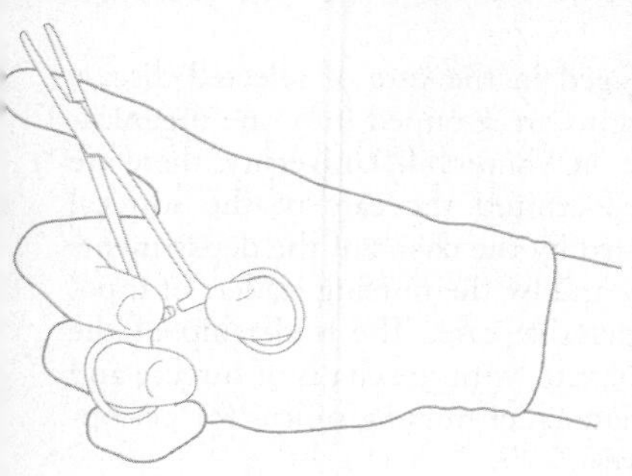

Safety in the Surgical Environment

Warren S. Sandberg, Roger Dmochowski, R. Daniel Beauchamp

OUTLINE

The intent of surgery is to improve health, so it was galvanizing when a series of eye-opening reports published in the 1990s provided clear evidence of high rates of serious adverse events that resulted in serious harm to hospitalized patients. In its landmark report "To Err is Human," published in 1999, the Institute of Medicine[1] estimated that 1 million people per year were injured and 98,000 per year died as a result of medical errors. When the focus was specifically turned to surgical patients, surgical care accounted for 48% to 66% of adverse events among nonpsychiatric hospital discharges.[2] Adverse events occurred in 3% of operative procedures and deliveries, and surgical adverse events were associated with a 5.6% mortality rate, accounting for 12.2% of hospital deaths. Furthermore, 54% of surgical adverse events were judged to be preventable.

Adverse events in surgical patients encompass adverse events common to all hospitalized patients, such as adverse drug events, falls, missed diagnoses, deep venous thrombosis, pulmonary embolism, aspiration events, respiratory failure, nosocomial pneumonia, myocardial infarction, and cardiac arrhythmias. In addition, adverse events specific to surgery include technique-related complications, wound infections, and postoperative bleeding. In 2000, the Institute of Medicine called for a national effort to reduce medical errors by 50% within 5 years; however, progress has fallen far short of that goal despite numerous private and public initiatives aimed at finding solutions.[3] Leape and colleagues[3] proposed that these efforts have fallen short because health care organizations have not undertaken the major cultural changes that are required to accomplish true and lasting improvements in performance. Leape and colleagues[3] proposed that "health care entities must become 'high reliability organizations' that hold themselves accountable to consistently offer safe, effective patient centered care." These authors put forward the following five transforming concepts for adoption by health care organizations seeking such transformative change in culture: (1) Transparency must be a practiced value in everything we do; (2) care must be delivered by multidisciplinary teams working in integrated care platforms; (3) patients must become full partners in all aspects of health care; (4) health care workers need to find joy and meaning in their work; and (5) medical education must be redesigned to prepare new physicians to function in this new environment.

Since the publication of the position paper by Leape and colleagues,[3] much has been accomplished, but there remains much to do. Mortality among patients hospitalized for surgery remains high. In an observational sampling study of 7-day mortality in Europe, there was enormous heterogeneity around a high (mean 3.6%) mortality rate, even in places such as Great Britain.[4] Most of the deaths occurred on hospital wards in patients not expected to need care in an intensive care unit (ICU). A reproducibility test of this study in the United States is in the data analysis phase. There is no reason to expect a different result. In a prospective study in a similar patient population by the same research group,[5] the mortality was much lower. Assessing the differences between these works is illustrative: In the prospective work, one of the study assessments was postoperative oxygen saturation determination. The mortality in this prospective study was much lower, only about 1%. Of that mortality, 40% was in the ICU. One speculation as to the driver of the difference is that in the prospective study, an investigator physically interacts with patients. The investigator recognizes deteriorating patients, and sends them to the ICU, where they either die or recover, having been rescued.

Another secular trend that may drive the persistently high perioperative mortality is the shift of more and more patients to ambulatory surgery, creating a population of hospitalized patients with the most severe pathophysiology and increasing morbidity and mortality. In such a situation, no improvement may be a victory.

When trying to estimate a rate for perioperative mortality, the observational study is the most trustworthy. It is more "environmentally valid," representing routine practice without unusual oversight or extra observation. The picture remains challenging, but the simple solution of "paying more attention"—through leadership commitment to improving the quality of care through education and creating robust multidisciplinary systems of care supported by technology as appropriate—can produce real surgical quality improvements across the arc of perioperative medicine.

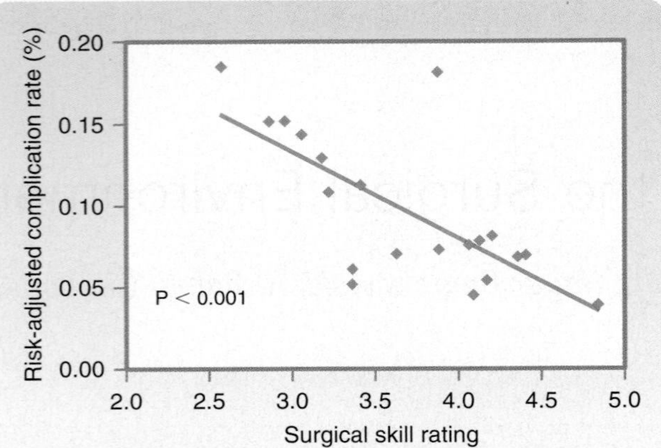

FIGURE 9-1 Relationship between summary peer rating of technical skill and risk-adjusted complication rates after laparoscopic gastric bypass. (From Birkmeyer JD, Finks JF, O'Reilly A, et al: Surgical skill and complication rates after bariatric surgery. *N Engl J Med* 369:1434–1442, 2013.)

Throughout the consideration of system-level efforts to improve safety in the surgical environment, it is important to remember that the individual surgeon's technique still influences outcomes. For example, in a study of 20 bariatric surgeons, there was a strong relationship between summary peer rating of technical skill (derived by expert review of blinded recordings of procedures) and risk-adjusted complication rates after laparoscopic gastric bypass.[6] Each diamond in Figure 9-1 represents 1 of 20 practicing bariatric surgeons. Technical skill was assigned on a 1-to-5 scale (5 being better) by blinded review performed by at least 10 other surgeons unaware of the identity of the operating surgeon. Complication rates were obtained from a prospective, externally audited clinical outcomes registry after adjustment for patient comorbidities.[6] Surgical skill was predictive of the rate of surgical complications, nonsurgical (medical) complications, reoperations, readmissions, and emergency department visits, indicating that the technical skill of the surgeon is a potential driver of many of the system-level performance domains currently receiving much attention in the area of quality improvement.

How then do we create an environment where it is acceptable to acknowledge differences in performance as the first step toward across-the-board performance improvement? Also, how do we collect and report back the data required to assess current performance and monitor progress toward the desired state?

FOSTERING A CULTURE OF SAFETY THROUGH LEADERSHIP

Creating a culture of safety in the perioperative system requires leadership investment from surgeons. In the perioperative system, just as in the operating room (OR) and procedure suite, the surgeon sets the tone, but he or she cannot achieve success alone. Creating a joint governance structure in the perioperative system wherein nursing staff, advance practice nurses, anesthesiologists, and other medical consultants are fully engaged in leadership is vital to being able to capture the engagement and expertise of these clinicians in the patient safety effort. Health systems are recognizing this fact and trying to cement the multidisciplinary approach by creating service lines wherein all the clinician and nonclinician individuals engaged in the care of selected disease categories or patient populations are grouped into one organizational structure. For example, at Vanderbilt University, there are major service lines organized around the care of the surgical patient, and these are jointly led by the chairs of the departments of surgery and anesthesiology and by the nursing leaders of inpatient, outpatient, and perioperative care. The leadership of the perioperative enterprise is tripartite, with the chairs of surgery and anesthesiology and the associate chief nursing officer for perioperative services as co-executives.

These leadership teams create transparency and fair adjudication of conflicts over scarce resources such as OR time and access to hospital beds, which builds trust and reduces conflict. The tripartite leadership executive models expected behavior by example. The leaders articulate the expectation of engagement with quality initiatives such as hand hygiene[7] by fully participating themselves and by using executive authority to encourage good performance in subordinates. They also demonstrate commitment to patient safety by investing departmental and institutional resources into the creation and operation of quality and safety organizations within their respective departments and across the service line.

At Vanderbilt University, there is a perioperative chief quality officer who works with clinical leadership, nursing, and administration within the patient care areas to identify priorities and to identify necessary resources to support quality improvement and to address safety issues promptly. The Center for Clinical Improvement in the institution provides assistance with resources to support root cause analyses of patient deaths, adverse outcomes, and near misses. Reporting of adverse outcomes and near misses is encouraged in a "blame-free" environment, both in person and via a confidential web-based reporting tool. Within the Perioperative Enterprise, there is a Surgical Site Infection Collaborative and a Perioperative Quality and Safety Committee that collaborate with one another and that receive inputs from the various surgical services, perioperative nursing services, and infection control services. Each surgical service conducts weekly to biweekly morbidity, mortality, and improvement (MMI) conferences. Cases identified in these service-level MMI conferences that exemplify "systems" concerns or issues are referred to a multidisciplinary MMI committee that selects cases for presentation at an institution-wide MMI conference that is held on a quarterly basis. System-level quality projects identified in these various venues are "worked" by quality improvement teams until the quality problems are solved, usually as evidenced by diminution or elimination of the problem for an extended period or number of cases.

LOCAL ORGANIZATIONAL STRUCTURES TO PROMOTE PERIOPERATIVE SAFETY

When considering the local working environment, procedures, and policies in any health care organization, it is important to remember that almost every step, check, and double-check in the perioperative process, no matter how apparently redundant or pointless, was almost certainly developed as a reaction to a near miss or an event involving patient harm. Nevertheless, it is important to revisit continually and optimize patient care processes in a proactive way to engineer systems deliberately to ensure patient and personnel safety.

Effective health care organizations develop and maintain a multidisciplinary ongoing patient safety program that operates in

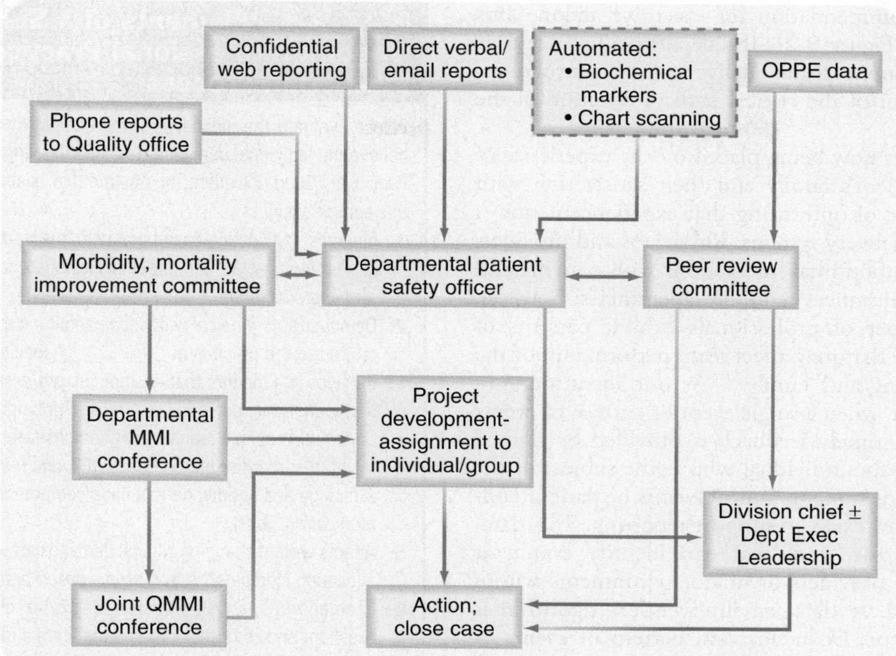

FIGURE 9-2 Patient safety officer (PSO) inputs and relationships. The *red arrows* indicate pathways by which information about patient safety events and system quality functions and opportunities for improvements are routed to the PSO. The *blue arrows* indicate communication pathways and potential issue routing between the PSO and the various quality, safety, and performance improvement functions in a procedural department. The *green arrows* indicate information flow and directives to executive and leadership functions for action items developed by the quality and safety functions. The *dashed outline box* indicates a new information input function that is being implemented as of writing. *MMI,* Morbidity, Mortality Improvement; *OPPE,* ongoing professional practice evaluation; *QMMI,* Quality, Morbidity, Mortality Improvement.

a blame-free culture where deference to expertise is one of the norms of behavior. Input to the program includes proactive scans for opportunities to improve systems but importantly features many routes for reporting nonroutine events, near misses, and critical events for analysis and system redesigns when needed. At Vanderbilt, each of the major role groups has an appointed patient safety officer (PSO), operating in concert with the perioperative Chief Quality Officer. These individuals are chosen for their discretion and effectiveness at taking in and appropriately routing information about safety problems and for their ability to shepherd such investigations and process improvements through to completion. The quality management structure created in the Department of Anesthesiology at Vanderbilt can serve as one illustration of an effective and equitable system (Fig. 9-2). The PSO can receive reports from the confidential web-based reporting system, reports from self-disclosures as part of routine medical documentation, and in-person reports. Institutional Risk Management is also included in report review so as to integrate risk mitigation with improvement activities. In a foreshadowing of future capability expectations, the Vanderbilt Anesthesia PSO also receives surveillance reports suggesting patient injury from automated scans of the electronic medical record (EMR). These searches include abnormal laboratory values such as new postoperative elevations of serum creatinine or troponin or chart entries and orders indicating unplanned escalations of care. The surgical departments have an almost identical quality and safety organizational structure. The surgical and anesthetic organizational structures are closely associated, and continuous communication links surveillance and intervention activities.

The PSO serves as the primary input point and clearing-house for safety considerations and can refer issues to a Quality, Morbidity, Mortality Improvement (QMMI) Committee to deal with system-of-care problems amenable to structural, procedural, and technical solutions or to a Peer Review Committee to deal with events related more to individual performance, knowledge, and decision making, or both. The departmental PSO collaborates with PSOs from other professional departments and from Perioperative Services, all under the umbrella of a Multidisciplinary QMMI Committee co-chaired by the surgery and anesthesiology PSOs.

Projects referred to the QMMI Committee have included refreshing protocols for cardiac implantable electronic device management and multidisciplinary development of policies and procedures for management of surgical patients receiving dual antiplatelet therapy for maintenance of drug-eluting intracoronary stents. These are public projects. Alternatively, most of the work of the Peer Review Committee is confidential, protected from discovery by legal statute. The Peer Review Committee comprises individual clinicians selected for their clinical acumen, probity, and discretion.

The departmental PSO maintains a confidential database of reports, analyses, projects, and dispositions of QMMI projects as well as Peer Review Committee referrals. Because of the sensitive nature of the work and the need to preserve a safe environment for reporting, the entire safety reporting and peer review process is firewalled from operational leadership (i.e., the people who make decisions about OR access, team assignments, salaries) unless there is a QMMI Committee recommendation or a Peer

Review Committee recommendation for executive action. This process is illustrated in Figure 9-2—the departmental executive leadership charters and supports the quality and safety structures, but they are depicted out of the critical path of function of the structures they sponsor.

Increasing emphasis is now being placed on the experience of the patient and the patient's family and their satisfaction with care, and the importance of optimizing that experience is now a priority for health care delivery systems. Physicians and providers may occasionally have suboptimal interactions with patients and families. Most of these instances represent aberrancies; however, a relatively small number of professionals exhibit patterns of behavior or performance that may affect team performance or the experience of the patient and family.[8,9] At our institution, to promote professionalism, when a single event or pattern of events is observed or reported, timely feedback is provided by trained physician messengers to the individual who is the subject of the report. To facilitate the documentation of events or patient concerns, an electronic record exists to support reporting. This database provides a surveillance tool that can identify events or patterns associated with providers or microenvironments within the institution. Using these data, an intervention algorithm is applied based on the type, frequency, and pattern of events or concerns. Using this accountability model, a nonjudgmental, nondirective conversation occurs between a "concerned professional" and a colleague regardless of hierarchy.

This system has been associated with a substantial improvement in patient satisfaction and a significant reduction in malpractice-related costs. This system has been expanded more recently to include concerns of other members of the team about providers that may have adverse consequences for health care team interactions and care outcomes. The team-based concerns have identified numerous areas for improvement in provider behaviors and have increased within-team functionality.

BOX 9-1 Elements of a Survey-Based Ongoing Professional Practice Evaluation Process

Please evaluate the individual in the context of patient care. Rate how you believe the individual demonstrates the following competencies. Choices are: Poor, Fair, Good, Excellent, or Abstain (No basis for knowledge to evaluate this competency).

1. Engages in evidence-based practice. Integrates new evidence to improve his/her own patient care practices (competency in *practice-based learning and improvement*).
2. Demonstrates *medical knowledge* about established and evolving science related to the practice of _________ (specialty).
3. Behaves in a manner that exemplifies *professionalism* (honesty and integrity, work ethic, punctuality, altruism, bringing honor to the profession).
4. Communicates in a manner that demonstrates respect toward coworkers, facilitates interdisciplinary teamwork, and results in effective information exchange and optimal patient care (competency in *interpersonal and communication skills*).
5. Adapts well to changing clinical demands affecting workload and resource allocation (competency in *systems-based practice*).
6. Is organized and well-prepared for his/her clinical assignment. Provides excellent and compassionate patient care and demonstrates excellence in clinical skills (competency in *patient care*).
7. Appropriately seeks and accepts consultation from colleagues (competencies in *practice-based learning and improvement, professionalism,* and *interpersonal and communication skills*).
8. Makes you comfortable handing over care of a patient to, accepting a hand-over of care from, or sharing responsibility for the care of a patient with him/her (*all* competencies)
9. Makes you comfortable referring a friend or loved one for clinical care by him/her (*all* competencies).

NATIONAL AND HEALTH CARE SYSTEM–LEVEL SAFETY INITIATIVES

High-performing organizations also create an efficient bureaucracy to monitor clinician quality and apply expected standards of performance fairly and consistently. Many of these structures, such as the organized medical staff, are mandated by accrediting bodies such as The Joint Commission (TJC), and they serve meaningful purposes in terms of ensuring a consistent level of quality in the medical staff. For example, the requirement for ongoing professional practice evaluation is intended to ensure that all members of the medical staff are frequently evaluated in their specialty practice by methods that are objective and applied more frequently than annually. These evaluations take many forms, ranging from document review to direct observation. Key features of a well-designed ongoing professional practice evaluation process include direct mapping to the clinician's unique medical practice, frequent review, and objective criteria for identifying clinicians whose practice falls outside of normative expectations.

Frequent peer-to-peer assessment via survey is a middle ground between the nonspecific nature of chart reviews and the substantial effort required by direct observations. Box 9-1 demonstrates the series of nine peer-to-peer questions used in the Vanderbilt University Department of Anesthesiology (but transferable to virtually any specialty) to assess specific performance elements that map to the six Accreditation Council for Graduate Medical Education general competencies. There are also summative, general questions. In the Vanderbilt Department of Anesthesiology, these questions are automatically assigned (by a program that runs within the EMR) to clinician pairs who have worked together recently. Confidential responses are collected by the same software, and the data are presented to designated individuals (the Peer Review Committee Chair in our case). The Vanderbilt system handles all of the transactions automatically and electronically, but other practices operate such systems using e-mail, for example.

Clinicians who are new members of the medical staff, clinicians who request new or expanded privileges, and clinicians identified as differing from normative expectations all are subject to a focused professional practice evaluation. TJC allows the medical staff organization substantial latitude in the construction of a focused professional practice evaluation; however, in most instances, a focused professional practice evaluation involves some form of direct proctoring in the identified area of medical practice. In addition to a robust and efficient bureaucracy focused on normative expectations of practice, high-performing organizations establish quality and safety improvement teams (see earlier) that operate autonomously but with the support of the departmental or practice hierarchies.

Major government and third-party payers are becoming increasingly interested in quality and safety in health care, and much attention at the present time focuses on high criticality environments such as perioperative and periprocedural systems. Payers now regularly collect process outcomes (e.g., timely preoperative antibiotic administration) and health outcomes (e.g., surgical site infection) and report them publically (HospitalCompare.gov). Accrediting bodies, specialty boards, and government payers all are applying pressure to clinicians to focus on quality and safety in their practices (Table 9-1).

Perioperative team building has parallels in the aviation industry in that teams intermittently come together for relatively short, defined periods of time to accomplish a complex task, requiring the specialized skills of each team member, under potentially stressful conditions in which there is inherent danger. Haynes and colleagues[10] demonstrated the impact of implementing a standardized surgical safety checklist on patient outcomes. In a study of more than 3700 surgical patients from eight major hospitals in eight cities worldwide, they found that implementing the

TABLE 9-1 Major Perioperative and Surgical Data Registries and Quality Improvement Initiatives

PROJECT NAME	ACRONYM	SPONSOR ORGANIZATIONS	MAJOR INITIATIVES	KEY RESULTS	REFERENCES
Surgical Care Improvement Project	SCIP	CMS, CDC, AHRQ, ACS, AHA, ASA, AORN, VA, IHI, TJC	(1) Reduce incidence and impact of SSIs through timely administration and discontinuation of appropriate antibiotics, appropriate glucose control in selected patient populations, hair removal by clipping, maintenance of normothermia, and appropriate removal of urinary catheters (2) Reduce incidence of perioperative major cardiac events by continuing beta blockade in patients with previous beta blockade (3) Reduce venous thromboembolism and pulmonary embolism by use of thromboprophylaxis when indicated	SCIP process measure compliance is publically reported, sorted by hospital Better compliance with timely antibiotic administration and selection of appropriate antibiotic was associated with a robust reduction in SSI rates[36] Compliance with the overall process bundle, assessed as an all-or-none score, was associated with an adjusted odds ratio for infection of 0.85 (95% confidence interval, 0.76-0.95), but none of the individual SCIP measures alone were significantly associated with reduced probability of infection[37]	Fry[38]; http://www.jointcommission.org/assets/1/6/Surgical%20Care%20Improvement%20Project.pdf
National Surgical Quality Improvement Project	VA-NSQIP, ACS-NSQIP	VA, ACS	Risk-adjusted outcomes databases comprising up to 135 clinical variables including perioperative risk factors, intraoperative and postoperative events, morbidities, and 30-day mortality, all prospectively abstracted from the medical record by dedicated nursing personnel	Sampling methodology: Hospitals abstract data and send to ACS for analysis. Data reported back to hospitals along with risk-adjusted comparison to all other hospitals. Hospitals act on data and use subsequent NSQIP performance to monitor (hoped for) performance improvements ACS NSQIP risk calculator (http://riskcalculator.facs.org/) can be used to estimate risks of complications, death, and length of stay	http://site.acsnsqip.org/ For a review of the history, function, and evidence that feedback quality and between-hospital comparisons improve hospital performance and patient outcomes, see Maggard-Gibbons[39]
Society of Thoracic Surgeons National Database	STS National Database	STS	Prospective, self-reported clinical variables reported to a national database. Three distinct areas of focus are maintained: adult cardiac surgery, general thoracic surgery, and congenital heart surgery. Performance outcomes reports fed back to participant organizations in risk-adjusted format to allow comparison with local, regional, and national norms	STS public reporting online for CABG, AVR, and AVR+CABG; first public reporting of hospital and surgeon group level performance. Reports are published online and in the consumer journal *Consumer Reports*. Current data are incomplete—not all hospitals and groups have reported data in a form suitable to be listed	http://www.sts.org/national-database

Continued

TABLE 9-1 Major Perioperative and Surgical Data Registries and Quality Improvement Initiatives—cont'd

PROJECT NAME	ACRONYM	SPONSOR ORGANIZATIONS	MAJOR INITIATIVES	KEY RESULTS	REFERENCES
Metabolic and Bariatric Surgery Accreditation and Quality Improvement Program	MBSAQIP	ACS, ASMBS	Accreditation standard setting and monitoring for bariatric surgery programs. All accredited centers report outcomes to MBASQIP database using a prospective, longitudinal data collection system based on standardized definitions and collected by trained data reviewers, analogous to NSQIP. Provides semiannual, risk-adjusted comparative performance reports to participating centers	In 2011, published comparative morbidity and effectiveness of the major gastric volume reduction procedures based on data gathered from 109 participating centers[40] Periodically publishes Resources for Optimal Care of the Bariatric Surgery Patient	https://www.facs.org/quality-programs/mbsaqip
American College of Surgeons National Trauma Databank	ACS-NTDB	ACS			
Hospital Compare		CMS	Data gathered from multiple mandatory reporting sources or gathered independently by CMS. Includes survey data about experiences as reported by recently discharged patients	Public reporting site that allows individual patients to view and compare hospital performance data within their area as well as regionally and nationally. Ostensibly, patients could use such comparisons to make decisions about where to seek elective care for specific conditions	http://www.medicare.gov/hospitalcompare

ACS, American College of Surgeons; *AHA,* American Heart Association; *AHRQ,* Agency for Healthcare Research and Quality; *AORN,* American of Perioperative Registered Nurses; *ASA,* American Society of Anesthesiologists; *ASMBS,* American Society for Metabolic and Bariatric Surgery; *AVR,* aortic valve replacement; *CABG,* coronary artery bypass grafting; *CDC,* U.S. Centers for Disease Control and Prevention; *CMS,* Centers for Medicare & Medicaid Services; *IHI,* Institute for Healthcare Improvement; *MBSAQIP,* Metabolic and Bariatric Surgery Accreditation and Quality Improvement Program; *NTDB,* National Trauma Databank; *NSQIP,* National Surgical Quality Improvement Project; *SCIP,* Surgical Care Improvement Project; *SSI,* surgical site infection; *STS,* Society of Thoracic Surgeons; *TJC,* The Joint Commission; *VA,* Department of Veterans Affairs.

checklist reduced complication rates from 11% to 7% and reduced postoperative death rate from 1.5% to 0.8%.

Shortly after the landmark study by Haynes and colleagues,[10] de Vries and coworkers[11] reported that implementation of a comprehensive, multidisciplinary surgical safety checklist that included medications, marking of the operative site, and postoperative management plans in six hospitals in the Netherlands resulted in a significant decrease in complication rates and in-hospital mortality. These results were compared with data from a control group of five hospitals. When compared with a 3-month baseline period, the rates of total complications in surgical patients were reduced from 27.3 per 100 to 16.7 per 100. The proportion of patients with one or more complications decreased from 15.4% to 10.6%, and the inpatient mortality rate decreased from 1.5% to 0.8% in the surgical population among the study group of hospitals. Control hospitals did not experience a change in these outcomes over the same time intervals.

Neily and associates[12] demonstrated that implementation of a medical team training program with intraoperative briefings and debriefings in 74 Department of Veterans Affairs hospitals resulted in 18% improvement in annual risk-adjusted surgical mortality compared with a 7% decrease in mortality among 34 facilities that had not received such training. The mortality rates did not begin to show improvement until the second quarter after such training was completed and improved more through the third quarter. Other improvements reported during structured interviews of participants in the team training included improved communication among OR staff, increased staff awareness, improved overall efficiency, and improved overall teamwork.

In contrast to the aforementioned positive observational studies, Urbach and colleagues[13] reported the results of a group of 101 surgical hospitals in Ontario, Canada, using administrative health data to compare operative mortality, rates of surgical complications, and other 30-day postdischarge outcomes before and after adoption of a surgical safety checklist. In assessment of the 3 months before and after adoption of the surgical safety checklist including more than 100,000 procedures for each time interval, they observed that adjusted risk of death within 30 days of an operation was 0.71% before implementation and 0.65% after implementation of the checklist, a non–statistically significant difference. Also, there was no significant difference in the adjusted risk of surgical complications in comparing the time periods before and after implementation. On the surface, this study did not support the efficacy of surgical safety checklists, but the study has several important limitations, including the short study intervals of only 3 months, resulting in inadequate levels of adoption of the checklists and inadequate assessment of the compliance and quality of the practice of the checklists. Also, the study included a skewed, and likely low-acuity, patient population of 60.8% ambulatory cases with 20% of all cases being eye cases and 28.7% being musculoskeletal cases. This low acuity is likely to have contributed to the low rates of complications and deaths observed in both periods in this study.

A different but important focus for checklist deployment is the prevention of rare, devastating events. Nearly half of surgical "never" events resulting in indemnity payments in the United States result from "wrong surgeries"—a concept encompassing a wrong procedure, wrong site, or surgery on the wrong person. Wrong surgery often results in patient death and is devastating to the care team. Estimates of wrong surgery incidence range from 1 : 112,994[14] to 1 : 5000[15] and may be increasing. Checklist application[10,16] has reduced the frequency of complications resulting in injury and death. TJC has made the implementation of the Universal Protocol for the prevention of wrong-site, wrong-patient, and wrong-procedure surgery, including the preprocedural time-out, an accreditation requirement.[17] The Universal Protocol includes the following elements: preprocedural verification, site marking, and final verification during the preprocedural time-out. Preprocedural verification includes verification of the appropriate history and physical examination in the medical record, the presence of a signed consent form, nursing assessment, and preanesthesia assessment (when applicable). At Vanderbilt, a nonemergency patient cannot be transported to the OR without completing these components of the preprocedural verification. This preprocedural verification continues in the OR, including verification that the necessary diagnostic laboratory, radiology, and other test results are present and properly displayed. The requirement for and presence of blood products, implants, devices, or special equipment is also confirmed in the preprocedural verification process.

The time-out that occurs immediately before initiation of the procedure provides a final verification of the correct patient, correct site, and correct procedure. The time-out is most effective when it is standardized and conducted consistently in all procedural areas of the hospital; it should be conducted immediately before starting an invasive procedure or making the incision. It is initiated by a designated member of the procedural team and involves the immediate members of the procedure team. During the time-out, other activities are suspended so that team members may focus on active confirmation of the patient, site, and procedure. Any new team members should be introduced. At a minimum, the team members must agree on the correct patient identity, correct procedural site (with the site marking verified when laterality or level is a concern), and correct procedure to be done. Finally, completion of the time-out should be documented for the patient medical record.

This description of the surgical time-out defines the minimal criteria to satisfy TJC requirements; however, if these are the only elements included in the process, the positive impact is limited. The Crew Resource Management training and discipline of the Universal Protocol enables organizations to enhance communication between health care professionals in the perioperative management teams and to incorporate process improvement measures, such as those defined by the Surgical Care Improvement Project, into the checklists. These evidence-based interventions include timely administration of perioperative antibiotics, administration of beta blockers in patients at risk of ischemic heart disease, venous thromboembolism prophylaxis, and intraoperative normothermia. The time-out checklist may also include availability and sterility of instrumentation and implantable devices. The conclusion of the optimal surgical time-out should include an open invitation for any member of the team to speak up at any time during the procedure if he or she recognizes a problem that poses risk to the patient or health care team. Box 9-2 summarizes elements of surgical safety checklists.

Checklists must be performed reliably to be effective, which requires the care team to achieve optimal performance consistently. This is a potential vulnerability. To create a technologic backstop to team performance, Vanderbilt University has used automated process monitoring and process control as well as forced function concepts to implement an electronic time-out checklist to reduce the wrong surgery rate. We created an electronic preprocedural briefing and time-out checklist mediated via the intraoperative nursing documentation module of our OR documentation system. Checklist questions are sequentially displayed to the entire care team on a large in-room monitor (Fig. 9-3) interposed as a required documentation step between the "patient-in-OR" and "incision" events. In our assessment of system effectiveness, all 118,472 main campus OR cases between July 30, 2010, and February 28, 2013, were subject to the electronic time-out procedure. Total development costs were $34,000 and used existing hardware. In a de novo installation, the additional hardware cost would have been $2500 per OR. Since the implementation of this process, there have been no wrong surgeries (0 in 118,472 cases in the formal observation period; Clopper-Pearson 95% confidence interval 0.0 to 3.11×10^{-5} wrong surgeries per case) in Vanderbilt ORs. This finding is encouraging given the expected rate of wrong surgery based on current national performance (1 wrong surgery per 23,600 cases, or 4.24×10^{-5} wrong surgeries per case). Since implementation of this electronically mediated hard-stop time-out system, no wrong surgeries have occurred either during the observation period or afterward at Vanderbilt.

Implementation of a surgical continuum of care (SCoC) model and continuum of care (CoC) for medical/surgical populations within the Geisinger Health Systems hospitals resulted in improvements in mortality rates, reduction in length of stay, and cost savings.[18] These models of care were implemented based on the hypothesis "that a surgical patient with physiological deterioration during the hospital course would have had a variable period of occult deterioration before the 'critical event' that results in activation of code team for cardiopulmonary arrest." The SCoC and CoC models involved redesign of care delivery to include hospitalist comanagement of adult surgical patients in the SCoC model and the hospital-wide adult population in the CoC model. Central elements of the redesigned models of care included multidisciplinary floor-based team building; unit cohort-based placement of patients according to degree of physiologic derangement and

BOX 9-2 Elements of the Surgical Safety Checklist

Sign In

Before induction of anesthesia, members of the team (at least the nurse and an anesthesia professional) state that the following have been done:

- The patient has verified his or her identity, surgical site and procedure, and consent.
- The surgical site is marked or site marking is not applicable.
- The pulse oximeter is on the patient and functioning.
- All members of the team are aware of whether the patient has a known allergy.
- The patient's airway and risk of aspiration have been evaluated, and appropriate equipment and assistance are available.
- If there is a risk of blood loss of at least 500 mL (or 7 mL/kg body weight in children), appropriate access and fluids are available.

Time-Out

Before skin incision, the entire team (nurses, surgeons, anesthesia professionals, and any others participating in the care of the patient) or specific members state aloud the following:

- Team confirms that all team members have been introduced by name and role.
- Team confirms the patient's identity, surgical site, and procedure.
- Team reviews the anticipated critical events.
  - Surgeon reviews critical and unexpected steps, operative duration, and anticipated blood loss.
  - Anesthesia professionals review concerns specific to patient.
  - Nurses review confirmation of sterility, equipment availability, and other concerns.
- Team confirms that prophylactic antibiotics have been administered ≤60 minutes before incision is made or that antibiotics are not indicated.
- Team confirms that all essential imaging results for correct patient are displayed in operating room.

Sign Out

Before the patient leaves the operating room, the following are done:

- Nurse reviews the following aloud with the team:
  - Name of procedure, as recorded
  - That needle, sponge, and instrument counts are complete (or not applicable)
  - That specimen (if any) is correctly labeled, including patient's name
  - Whether there are any issues with equipment that need to be addressed
- The surgeon, nurse, and anesthesia professional review aloud the key concerns for the recovery and care of the patient.

Adapted from Haynes AB, Weiser TG, Berry WR, et al: A surgical safety checklist to reduce morbidity and mortality in a global population. *N Engl J Med* 360:491–499, 2009.

anticipated risk of deterioration; the creation of a safety-net unit called the Progressive Care Unit; and intensivist/hospitalist staffing of the Progressive Care Unit. In addition, the care teams organized acuity-stratified rounding on higher risk patients at periodic intervals and implemented a real-time communication technology system. In a study of more than 100,000 admissions, the above-described interventions resulted in a decrease in the risk-adjusted mortality index from 1.16 before intervention to 0.77 by 6 months after intervention with an unchanged case mix index. The interventions also significantly decreased length of stay and resulted in cost savings in the high-risk and high-acuity populations of patients. Simpler interventions can also improve outcomes. For example, implementation of structured handoffs of care between residents led to a reduction in medical errors and preventable adverse events.[19]

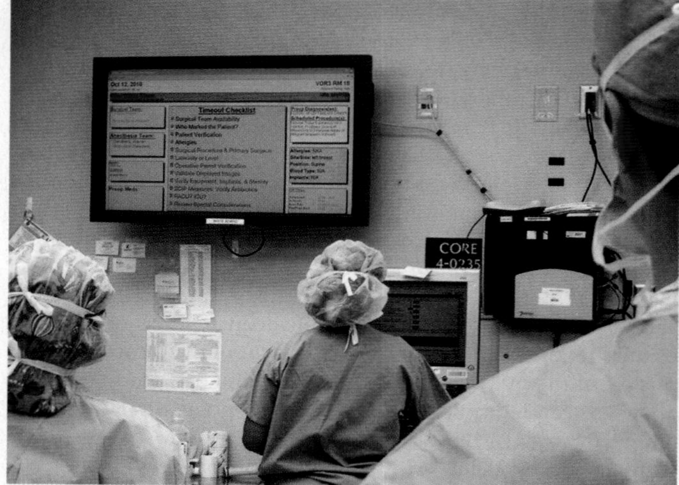

FIGURE 9-3 Electronic white-board mediated time-out. Attention of personnel is focused on the display on which the time-out questions are being sequentially addressed. The display serves as a framing system for this important safety step. The view is from the anesthesiologist's position at the head of the bed, with (from left to right) the scrub technician, the circulator nurse, and the surgeon. The circulator's computer (visible to the lower right of the large display) shows the questions on the large display and captures the responses entered by the circulator.

When evaluating the results and impact of quality improvements resulting from mandates or public reporting, it is important to consider the source of the data being reported and the incentives of all of the reporting individuals. Farmer and colleagues[20] drew attention to the precipitous decrease in rates of central line-associated bloodstream infections (CLABSIs) in the course of one quarter after the Centers for Medicare & Medicaid Services (CMS) terminated reimbursement for CLABSI treatment (Fig. 9-4).[20] These CLABSI rates were derived from a national sample of administrative data used for billing, which heretofore have been assumed to reflect the care provided accurately. However, Lee and associates,[21] using an outcomes data source (outcomes data reported by institutions to a national quality database), saw essentially no immediate change in CLABSI rates around the period when CMS stopped reimbursements (Fig. 9-4*B*).[21] Similarly, Lee and associates[21] saw no change in catheter-associated urinary tract infection or ventilator-associated pneumonia around the time of cessation of reimbursement by CMS for these complications, whereas Farmer and colleagues[20] detected a precipitous decrease in administrative coding for another surgical complication, retained foreign body, exactly concomitant with the cessation of reimbursement.

Continuous effort to improve surgical outcomes is consistent with the ethos of the surgeon and the right thing to do. However, in the current reimbursement environment, there can be perverse incentives that may limit the impact of quality improvement initiatives. For example, when conducting a complete financial margin analysis of initiatives to reduce complications, a study demonstrated that successful programs may result in a negative cash flow to a hospital unless the hospital's surgical volume is growing sufficiently to fill beds vacated by patients who avoid

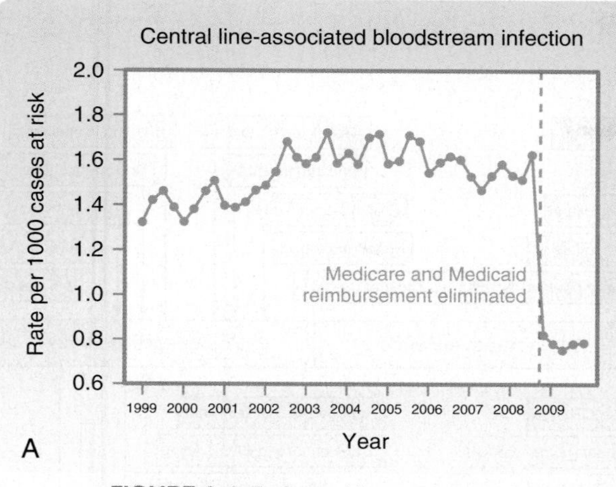

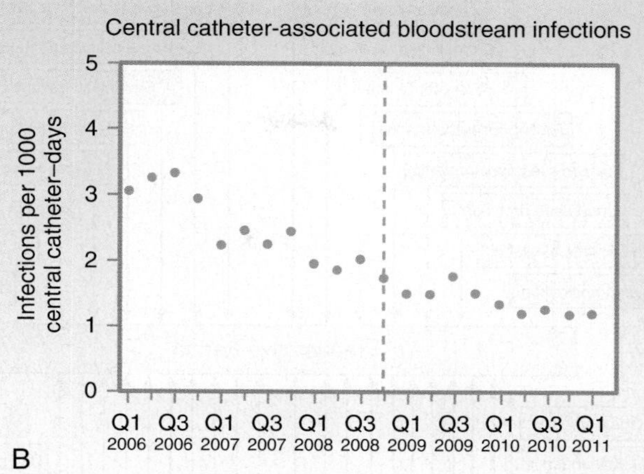

FIGURE 9-4 **A,** Central line–associated bloodstream infection. **B,** Central catheter–associated bloodstream infections. The *red dashed lines* mark the end of reimbursement for patients with central line–associated bloodstream infections. (**A,** From Farmer SA, Black B, Bonow RO: Tension between quality measurement, public quality reporting, and pay for performance. *JAMA* 309:349–350, 2013; **B,** from Lee GM, Kleinman K, Soumerai SB, et al: Effect of nonpayment for preventable infections in U.S. hospitals. *N Engl J Med* 367:1428–1437, 2012.)

complications.[22] This finding drives home the importance of sharing the financial benefits of successful quality improvement efforts between the providers and the payers.

SYSTEM-LEVEL INTERVENTIONS IMPROVE SAFETY

The goal of all efforts to improve quality and safety in the perioperative environment is to create systems of care that work efficiently; that rarely, if ever, fail; that alert clinicians of their incipient failure; and that fail into a safe mode. Clinicians working in perioperative systems to improve quality and safety must think of themselves, their plans, their actions, and their quality improvement work as part of an integrated system of care. A useful construct is the notion of perioperative systems design.

Perioperative systems design describes a rational approach to managing the convergent flow of patients having procedures from disparate physical and temporal starting points (frequently home), through the OR, and then to such a place and time (e.g., home or hospital bed) where future events pertaining to the patient have no further impact on OR operations.[23] This process for an individual patient can be envisioned as a set of interdependent activities beginning with the decision to perform an operation and ending when the patient definitively recovers from surgery. The risk of disruption is briefly illustrated in Figure 9-5,[23] which shows approximately the steps required to bring a patient through an operation and some of the common roadblocks. At each point, physical infrastructure and work processes affect patient progress, quality, safety, and system efficiency. The perioperative process is extremely vulnerable to perturbations, particularly during the critical intraoperative portion. Problems in a single patient's care, regardless of where in the care trajectory they occur, frequently propagate upstream and downstream and ripple across the OR suite or health system as well (e.g., consider the impact of overrunning the booked procedure length for the first case in a room with three cases). Although the perioperative process is commonly conceptualized as a consistent system, workflow analyses reveal that even "defined" workflows have so many exceptions as to be essentially chaotic.[24] Frequently, improvements in one aspect of a perioperative system design highlight fragilities elsewhere. For example, improving OR throughput often unmasks limits to postanesthesia care unit (PACU) capacity.[25] In practice, many steps in the perioperative process are completely dependent on the successful completion of the preceding steps. This tight linkage implies that perioperative systems must be considered globally when making changes to one facet. In particular, upstream and downstream issues must be addressed in an effective perioperative systems design. Any proposed quality, safety, or efficiency improvement effort should be evaluated in terms of its likely and potential positive and negative impacts on the overall perioperative process.

Much hope has been pinned on the propagation of EMRs into the perioperative environment. EMRs allow rapid searches for apparently rare patient safety events within single institutions[26,27] and across multiple facilities.[28] Consortia of major medical facilities (Multicenter Perioperative Outcomes Group [https://www.mpogresearch.org/]) and national professional society efforts (e.g., the Anesthesia Quality Institute of the American Society of Anesthesiologists) now focus on aggregating perioperative EMR data with the aim of estimating incidence and, more importantly, identifying controllable risk factors for poor perioperative outcomes.

The convergence of EMRs and the perioperative system holds out a more proactive possibility for creating a system that performs reliably and fails safely. Specifically, the EMR can serve as the substrate for electronic monitoring of patient progress through the therapeutic encounter and compare this progress with the desired plan. Current technology is insufficient to achieve this ideal in its totality, but there are tractable subtasks that are amenable to electronic process monitoring and process control.[29,30] For example, important perioperative documentation tasks, process steps such as timely administration of perioperative antibiotics, and improvements in intraoperative monitoring have been achieved using systems with computerized ongoing continuous monitoring of the perioperative process and automatic reminders sent directly to the bedside provider when process exceptions are detected.[31-33] At Vanderbilt University, electronic systems integrate data from multiple sources and update themselves over time to monitor the status of patients who might meet criteria for preventive interventions. For example, patients who

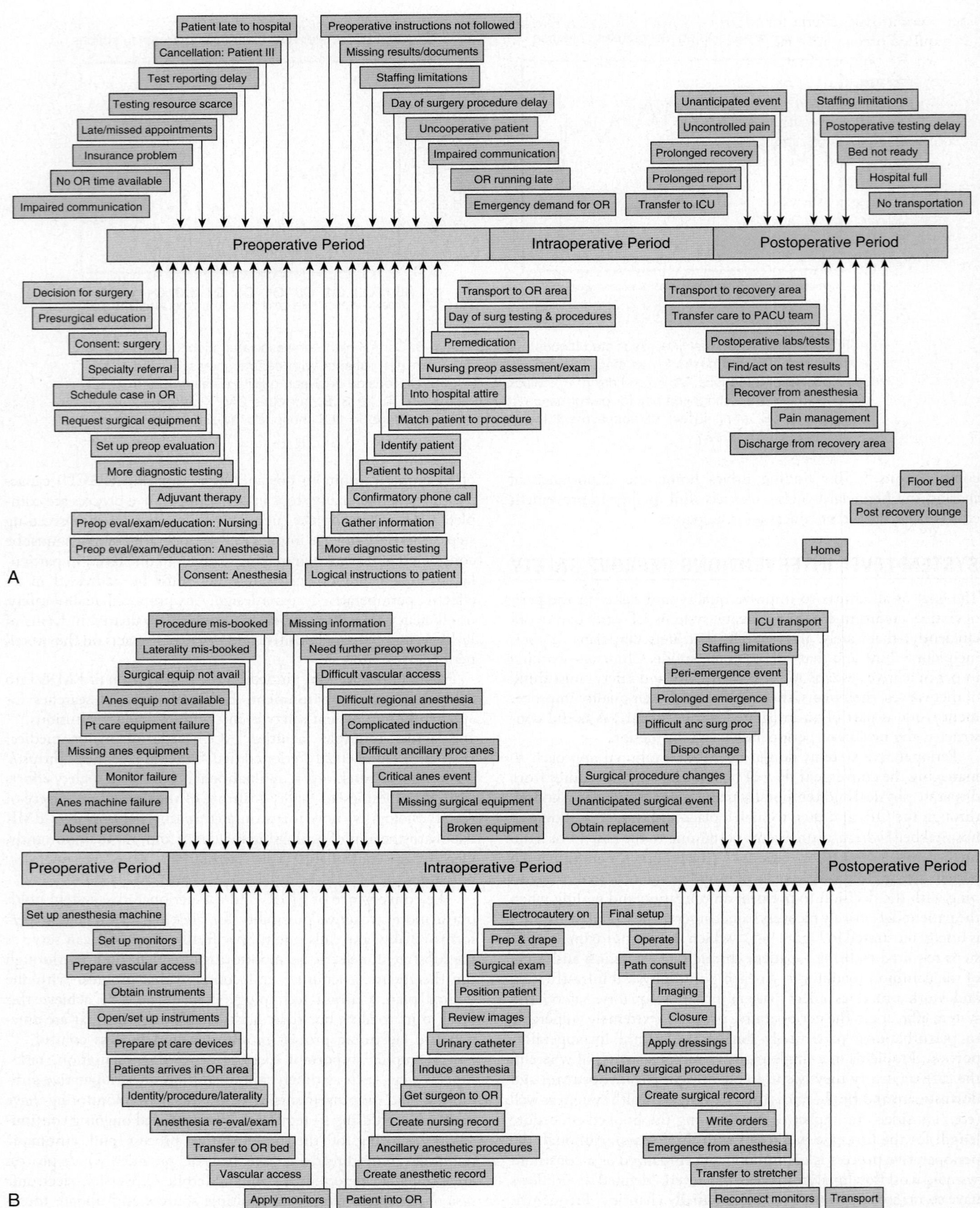

FIGURE 9-5 Timeline for intraoperative period. *ICU,* intensive care unit; *OR,* operating room; *PACU,* post-anesthesia care unit. (From Sandberg WS, Ganous TJ, Steiner C: Setting a research agenda for perioperative systems design. *Semin Laparosc Surg* 10:57–70, 2003.)

meet certain risk criteria for obstructive sleep apnea (as assessed by required preoperative electronic data collection) automatically trigger a Respiratory Therapy assessment for continuous positive airway pressure in the PACU after surgery. Similarly, electronic systems continually scan for diabetic patients (denoted by diagnosis or oral hypoglycemic agents or insulin in the electronic medication list). The hospital laboratory system is monitored for regular glucose checks for these diabetic patients during the perioperative period. If a diabetic patient is not monitored according to expectations per protocol, a reminder to monitor is sent to the bedside provider. Implementation of this system coincided with reduced 14-day readmission rates and deep wound infections for diabetic patients undergoing surgery (Sandberg W, et al: Unpublished results).

Technology can move electronic decision support even closer to the patient. For example, investigators at Dartmouth were able to reduce the rate of unplanned ICU transfers by the simple expedient of placing a pulse oximeter connected to a system that propagated SpO_2 alarms from the patient's room to the nurse on all patients in the monitored units.[34] The system was so successful that Dartmouth implemented continuous pulse oximetry for all inpatients.

Automatic process monitoring and process control using electronic records and clinical information systems hold substantial promise, but even simple tasks require careful attention to design detail. Figure 9-6 provides a simple example from a system implemented at Vanderbilt to ensure that all patients entering the recovery room have a set of postoperative orders by the time handover is complete. In the top workflow, the system is set up to notify the physician to write orders if no PACU orders are found in the computerized physician order entry (CPOE) system by the time the patient enters the PACU. Consequently, the notification, if it fires, technically gives its notification after it is needed and notifies a provider who may have moved on to another task, creating an interruption. The lower workflow in Figure 9-6 illustrates what was actually implemented at Vanderbilt. The system monitors the routine OR clinical documentation workflow and the CPOE system, awaiting the indication that a surgical procedure has moved to the "closing" phase. The system fires only if there are no PACU orders by the time "closing" is documented. An example of the system output is shown in the figure inset. In the Dartmouth oximetry example, the design team eventually implemented a system in which the SpO_2 trigger was SpO_2 less than 80% for 30 seconds to achieve an acceptably low false-positive rate.[34] Careful attention to system design was required, and the choice of limits was not intuitively obvious.

Electronic process monitoring and process control for simple tasks such as the electronic time-out described in Figure 9-3 can help to eliminate wrong surgery related to site, side, and patient identification in environments where it is deployed. Similarly, in our system, when an anesthesiologist opens an OR medical record to create a chart for a surgical operation or procedure, he or she is first greeted by a splash screen of all abnormal and critical laboratory values for that patient, descending chronologically. However, such electronic process monitoring and process control systems are rarely, if ever, part of the feature set of commercial EMRs. Rather, they are either the constructs of the quality improvement teams at the institutions that created them or customizations created for users who insisted on them.

What are some of the core feature requirements of an EMR that allow it to facilitate improved perioperative quality and safety? The benefit of a "findable," legible, comprehensive record of all the events that have happened to a patient cannot be overemphasized. Current EMRs may have room for improvement in terms of usability, but they are vastly superior to the paper records they replaced in terms of availability, legibility, and aggregating data. However, these advantages accrue only to the degree that the EMR has access to all of the information about a patient. Most hospital systems still operate their own implementations of commercial EMRs and limit data sharing to comply with patient privacy regulations. Interoperability between commercially available systems is an important goal to achieve greater sharing of currently fragmented data.

CPOE systems are another major component of EMRs. The creation of legible orders by a person with an identifiable signature and contact information is, on its face, a major safety advance, although there have been notable problematic implementations.[35] Order writing is, by its nature, a potential point of risk for patients. A misplaced decimal point is sufficient to cause harm through underdose or overdose. Drug allergies, interactions, and side effects are common. Duplicate orders and orders creating unwanted drug-drug interactions are problematic. However, because CPOE systems are typically self-contained, there is substantial opportunity to mitigate risk through robust decision support. A well-designed and implemented CPOE system should allow writing preoperative orders that can be activated when the patient reports for surgery. Specific orders for the PACU should add to the preoperative orders, but the system should readily suspend (and fence off from the main, active order set) any existing general care orders. Similarly, the PACU orders should automatically expire or "sunset" as the patient moves back to the general care population. Finally, a CPOE system should automatically check for patient-specific drug allergies and drug-drug interactions each time a new entry is made. The system must challenge the clinician to justify orders that violate allergy and drug interaction rules or standard dosing parameters.

CONCLUSIONS

Perioperative care is in the midst of a transformative renaissance. A major aspect of this change is an evolution in the culture of care. That evolutionary change is being reflected in multiple, somewhat articulated contemporaneous improvement processes being developed or used at the present time. Health care culture must be changed to focus on quality care and patient safety as a societal mandate. As noted earlier, Leape and coworkers[3] have provided the health care system with the critical elements and foundational attributes to promulgate this cultural progression.

Organizational transparency is a key aspect of the progression. Internal and external reporting structures currently exist to accomplish the aim of transparent outcomes and systems reporting (e.g., NSQIP). However, these structures will need to adjust and evolve in consonance with improvements in care and recognition of previously unappreciated or underappreciated factors that disrupt care processes or in other ways affect outcomes. Perioperative provider involvement in the maturation of these reporting structures is of utmost importance. Internal control processes such as standardized adverse event reporting and investigation, coupled to multidisciplinary venues for discussion and education (e.g., MMI meetings), and with linkage of findings to "just in time" improvement processes overseen by entities such as the Perioperative Quality Improvement committee provide real-time institutional process control and improvement.

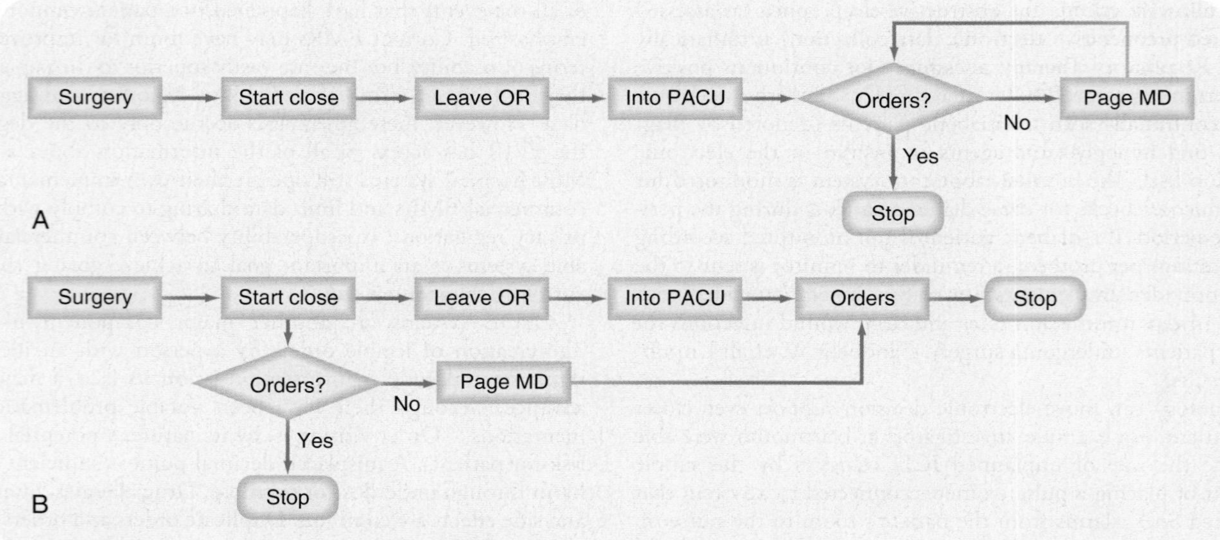

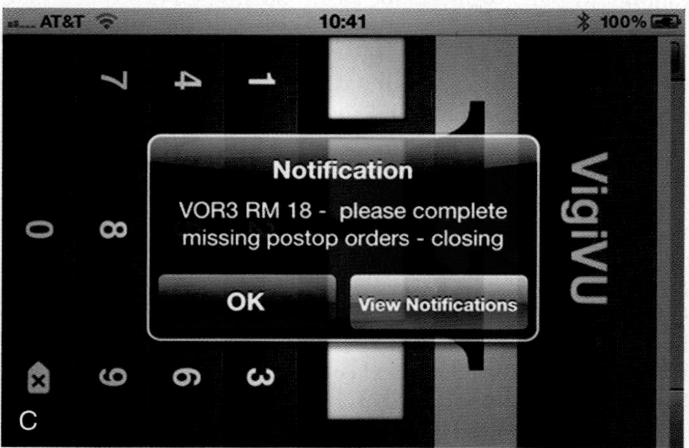
AT&T
10:41
100%
Notification
VOR3 RM 18 - please complete
missing postop orders - closing
OK
View Notifications
VigiVU
C

FIGURE 9-6 A, Flow chart of business logic designed to detect and notify a clinician when a process step (in this case, recovery room orders) has been missed. This is the logic flow frequently used in manual process checking and results in many phone calls, pages, and texts related to missing documentation, instructions, and information. It creates at least two interruptions and halts of progress: one for the person detecting the lapse and one for the recipient of the notification. Electronic medical records enable automation of the check for missing process steps, but the flow of work for the physician (MD) still creates an interruption as well as a stop in work as the postanesthesia care unit (PACU) awaits instructions. **B,** Flow chart of business logic wherein the check for complete information needed for the next step is tied to a predicate indicator, in this case, the notion that virtually every case has a detectable "beginning of the end" as the team begins to close the wound. In the specific example, it is reasonable to expect that as the team begins wound closure, most or all of the planned PACU interventions have been specified, and orders can be written by the anesthesiologist for PACU care during the end of the operation and before emergence from anesthesia begins. This avoids both interruptions associated with a traditional workflow. **C,** Output of the automated system for missed process step detection and notification developed at Vanderbilt University. Communication is via alphanumeric pages, commonly forwarded to mobile phones. *OR,* operating room.

The importance of team-based care throughout the perioperative episode is vital to integrity of process. Essential to effective team-based care is coherent communication within and among care teams. Checklists and information technology provide components and critical supplements to the process, but other elements are also vital to the care delivery process. All of these processes must be built with the patient's well-being and wishes as the central guiding elements. The process must also seek and respond to feedback from the patient and the patient's family that reflects their experience with the health care environment. Optimized patient literacy, education, and effective communication strategies can substantively improve the overall experience. The recognition that physician and surgeon behaviors can have an impact on the care process has led to the development of methods and tools to identify suboptimal occurrences and initiate specific interventions using structured algorithms. Furthermore, the use of team-based training tools incorporating universal time-out and huddles/debriefs improves caregiver job satisfaction and has been shown to have a positive impact on the culture of safety measures.

The importance of perioperative goals and efforts that harmonize with institutional goals cannot be underemphasized.

Leadership commitment to clearly enunciated goals is vital to success. Continuous education links evidence and experience to all members of the care team. Each member of the team contributes to quality care and safety, and this is incorporated into the medical and nursing curriculum.

Just as the last decade has brought tremendous change to the perioperative care arena, it is reasonable to assume that further evolution to our current systems will occur in the near future. The recent concept that any adverse event equates to a "never event" provides a sentinel philosophy for our continued efforts to ensure that perioperative care is of the highest quality and reproducibility.

SELECTED REFERENCES

Birkmeyer JD, Finks JF, O'Reilly A, et al: Surgical skill and complication rates after bariatric surgery. *N Engl J Med* 369:1434–1442, 2013.

Surgeon technique has been an infrequently assessed variable in the assessment of surgical outcomes. The authors review the observed technique during surgery of a group of bariatric surgeons with analysis of outcomes related to the procedures.

Fry DE: Surgical site infections and the Surgical Care Improvement Project (SCIP): Evolution of national quality measures. *Surg Infect (Larchmt)* 9:579–584, 2008.

This is a comprehensive review of the national Surgical Care Improvement Project effort to reduce surgical site infections. The national Surgical Infection Prevention Project was an initiative sponsored jointly by the Centers for Medicare and Medicaid Services and the U.S. Centers for Disease Control and Prevention to decrease the incidence of surgical site infections in major surgical procedures.

Ghaferi AA, Birkmeyer JD, Dimick JB: Variation in hospital mortality associated with inpatient surgery. *N Engl J Med* 361:1368–1375, 2009.

This is a landmark study of 84,730 patients who underwent inpatient general and vascular surgery from 2005 through 2007 that used data from the American College of Surgeons National Surgical Quality Improvement Program.

Haynes AB, Weiser TG, Berry WR, et al: A surgical safety checklist to reduce morbidity and mortality in a global population. *N Engl J Med* 360:491–499, 2009.

Surgery has become an integral part of global health care, with an estimated 234 million operations performed yearly. The article assesses surgical outcomes before and after safety checklist implementation.

Leape L, Berwick D, Clancy C, et al: Transforming healthcare: A safety imperative. *Qual Saf Health Care* 18:424–428, 2009.

Improvement in surgical care and outcomes will require substantial cultural transformation. The elements of the transformative principles are defined and summarized.

Maggard-Gibbons M: The use of report cards and outcome measurements to improve the safety of surgical care: The American College of Surgeons National Surgical Quality Improvement Program. *BMJ Qual Saf* 23:589–599, 2014.

The use of standardized, institution-specific and provider-specific, reporting is expanding. Many entities are calculating these reports including governmental and payer groups. Physician involvement is critical to ensure integrity, fairness, and value to these reporting systems.

REFERENCES

1. Institute of Medicine: *To err is human: building a safer healthcare system*, Washington, DC, 1999, National Academy Press.
2. Gawande AA, Thomas EJ, Zinner MJ, et al: The incidence and nature of surgical adverse events in Colorado and Utah in 1992. *Surgery* 126:66–75, 1999.
3. Leape L, Berwick D, Clancy C, et al: Transforming healthcare: A safety imperative. *Qual Saf Health Care* 18:424–428, 2009.
4. Pearse RM, Moreno RP, Bauer P, et al: Mortality after surgery in Europe: A 7 day cohort study. *Lancet* 380:1059–1065, 2012.
5. Mazo V, Sabate S, Canet J, et al: Prospective external validation of a predictive score for postoperative pulmonary complications. *Anesthesiology* 121:219–231, 2014.
6. Birkmeyer JD, Finks JF, O'Reilly A, et al: Surgical skill and complication rates after bariatric surgery. *N Engl J Med* 369:1434–1442, 2013.
7. Kenney C: *Transforming healthcare: virginia mason medical center's pursuit of the perfect patient experience*, New York, 2011, CRC Press.
8. Pichert JW, Hickson G, Moore I: Using patient complaints to promote patient safety. In Henriksen K, Battles JB, Keyes MA, et al, editors: *Advances in patient safety: new directions and alternative approaches*, (Vol 2: Culture and Redesign). Rockville, Md, 2008, Agency for Healthcare Research and Quality.
9. Sanfey H, Darosa DA, Hickson GB, et al: Pursuing professional accountability: An evidence-based approach to addressing residents with behavioral problems. *Arch Surg* 147:642–647, 2012.
10. Haynes AB, Weiser TG, Berry WR, et al: A surgical safety checklist to reduce morbidity and mortality in a global population. *N Engl J Med* 360:491–499, 2009.
11. de Vries EN, Prins HA, Crolla RM, et al: Effect of a comprehensive surgical safety system on patient outcomes. *N Engl J Med* 363:1928–1937, 2010.
12. Neily J, Mills PD, Young-Xu Y, et al: Association between implementation of a medical team training program and surgical mortality. *JAMA* 304:1693–1700, 2010.
13. Urbach DR, Govindarajan A, Saskin R, et al: Introduction of surgical safety checklists in Ontario, Canada. *N Engl J Med* 370:1029–1038, 2014.
14. Kwaan MR, Studdert DM, Zinner MJ, et al: Incidence, patterns, and prevention of wrong-site surgery. *Arch Surg* 141:353–357, discussion 357–358, 2006.
15. Rothman G: Wrong-site surgery. *Arch Surg* 141:1049–1050, author reply 1050, 2006.

16. Pronovost P, Needham D, Berenholtz S, et al: An intervention to decrease catheter-related bloodstream infections in the ICU. *N Engl J Med* 355:2725–2732, 2006.
17. The Joint Commission: 2015 National Patient Safety Goals. 2015. Available at: <http://www.jointcommission.org/standards_information/npsgs.aspx>. Accessed July 29, 2015.
18. Ravikumar TS, Sharma C, Marini C, et al: A validated value-based model to improve hospital-wide perioperative outcomes: Adaptability to combined medical/surgical inpatient cohorts. *Ann Surg* 252:486–496, discussion 496–498, 2010.
19. Starmer AJ, Spector ND, Srivastava R, et al: Changes in medical errors after implementation of a handoff program. *N Engl J Med* 371:1803–1812, 2014.
20. Farmer SA, Black B, Bonow RO: Tension between quality measurement, public quality reporting, and pay for performance. *JAMA* 309:349–350, 2013.
21. Lee GM, Kleinman K, Soumerai SB, et al: Effect of nonpayment for preventable infections in U.S. hospitals. *N Engl J Med* 367:1428–1437, 2012.
22. Krupka DC, Sandberg WS, Weeks WB: The impact on hospitals of reducing surgical complications suggests many will need shared savings programs with payers. *Health Aff (Millwood)* 31:2571–2578, 2012.
23. Sandberg WS, Ganous TJ, Steiner C: Setting a research agenda for perioperative systems design. *Semin Laparosc Surg* 10:57–70, 2003.
24. Meyer MA, Seim AR, Fairbrother P, et al: Automatic time-motion study of a multistep preoperative process. *Anesthesiology* 108:1109–1116, 2008.
25. Schoenmeyr T, Dunn PF, Gamarnik D, et al: A model for understanding the impacts of demand and capacity on waiting time to enter a congested recovery room. *Anesthesiology* 110:1293–1304, 2009.
26. Hobai IA, Gauran C, Chitilian HV, et al: The management and outcome of documented intraoperative heart rate-related electrocardiographic changes. *J Cardiothorac Vasc Anesth* 25: 791–798, 2011.
27. Ehrenfeld JM, Agarwal AK, Henneman JP, et al: Estimating the incidence of suspected epidural hematoma and the hidden imaging cost of epidural catheterization: A retrospective review of 43,200 cases. *Reg Anesth Pain Med* 38:409–414, 2013.
28. Bateman BT, Mhyre JM, Ehrenfeld J, et al: The risk and outcomes of epidural hematomas after perioperative and obstetric epidural catheterization: a report from the Multicenter Perioperative Outcomes Group Research Consortium. *Anesth Analg* 116:1380–1385, 2013.
29. Rothman B, Sandberg WS, St Jacques P: Using information technology to improve quality in the OR. *Anesthesiol Clin* 29:29–55, 2011.
30. Wanderer JP, Sandberg WS, Ehrenfeld JM: Real-time alerts and reminders using information systems. *Anesthesiol Clin* 29:389–396, 2011.
31. St Jacques P, Sanders N, Patel N, et al: Improving timely surgical antibiotic prophylaxis redosing administration using computerized record prompts. *Surg Infect (Larchmt)* 6:215–221, 2005.
32. Sandberg WS, Sandberg EH, Seim AR, et al: Real-time checking of electronic anesthesia records for documentation errors and automatically text messaging clinicians improves quality of documentation. *Anesth Analg* 106:192–201, 2008.
33. Ehrenfeld JM, Epstein RH, Bader S, et al: Automatic notifications mediated by anesthesia information management systems reduce the frequency of prolonged gaps in blood pressure documentation. *Anesth Analg* 113:356–363, 2011.
34. Taenzer AH, Pyke JB, McGrath SP, et al: Impact of pulse oximetry surveillance on rescue events and intensive care unit transfers: a before-and-after concurrence study. *Anesthesiology* 112:282–287, 2010.
35. Han YY, Carcillo JA, Venkataraman ST, et al: Unexpected increased mortality after implementation of a commercially sold computerized physician order entry system. *Pediatrics* 116:1506–1512, 2005.
36. Cataife G, Weinberg DA, Wong HH, et al: The effect of Surgical Care Improvement Project (SCIP) compliance on surgical site infections (SSI). *Med Care* 52:S66–S73, 2014.
37. Stulberg JJ, Delaney CP, Neuhauser DV, et al: Adherence to surgical care improvement project measures and the association with postoperative infections. *JAMA* 303:2479–2485, 2010.
38. Fry DE: Surgical site infections and the surgical care improvement project (SCIP): Evolution of national quality measures. *Surg Infect (Larchmt)* 9:579–584, 2008.
39. Maggard-Gibbons M: The use of report cards and outcome measurements to improve the safety of surgical care: The American College of Surgeons National Surgical Quality Improvement Program. *BMJ Qual Saf* 23:589–599, 2014.
40. Hutter MM, Schirmer BD, Jones DB, et al: First report from the American College of Surgeons Bariatric Surgery Center Network: Laparoscopic sleeve gastrectomy has morbidity and effectiveness positioned between the band and the bypass. *Ann Surg* 254:410–420, discussion 420–422, 2011.

SECTION II

Perioperative Management

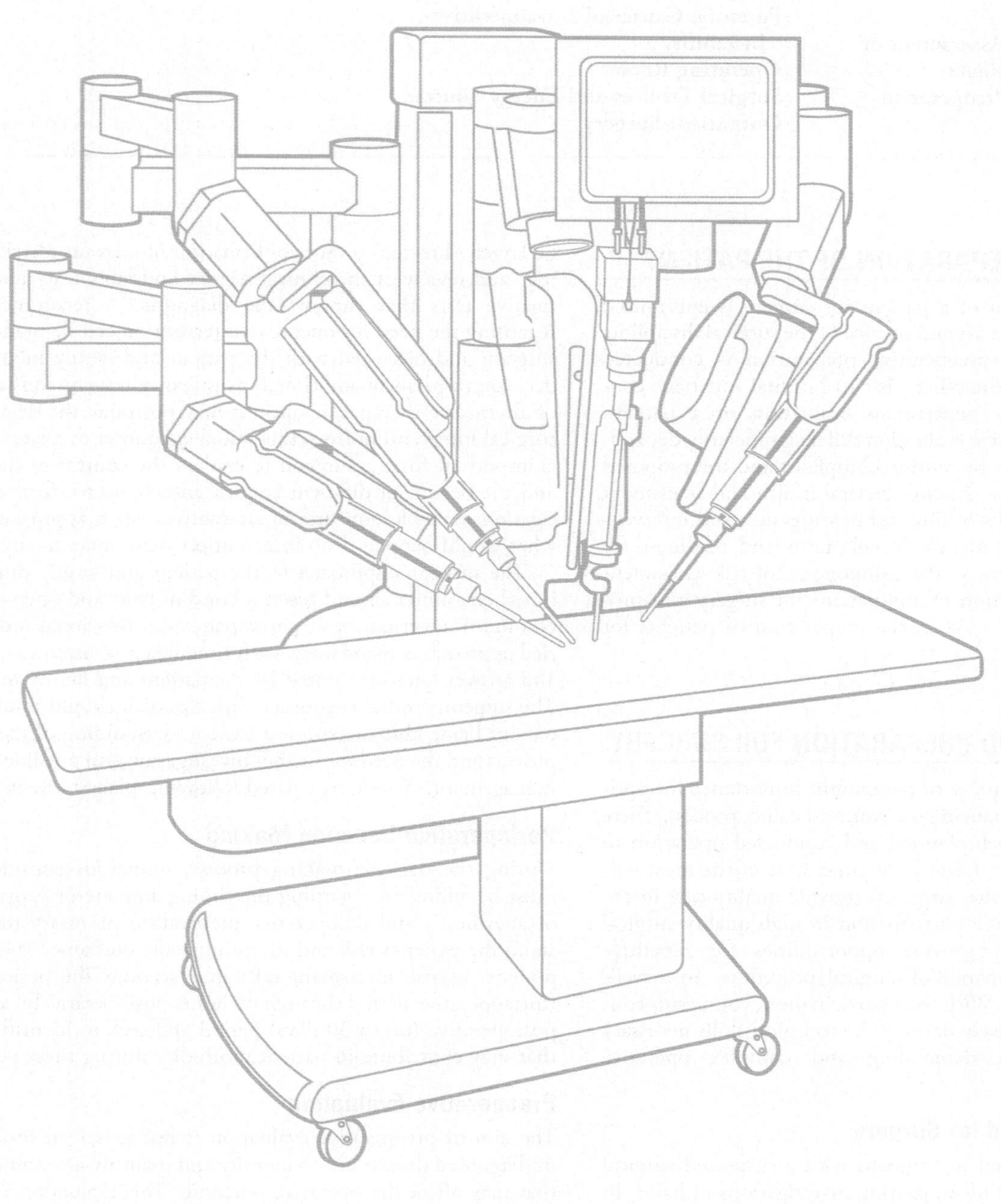

10 CHAPTER

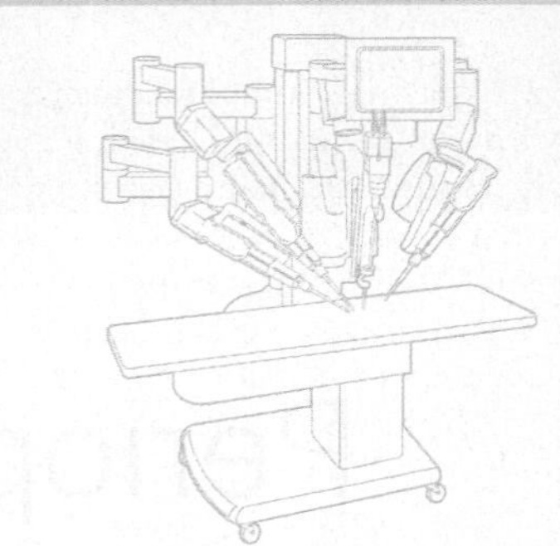

Principles of Preoperative and Operative Surgery

Leigh Neumayer, Nasrin Ghalyaie

OUTLINE

PREOPERATIVE PREPARATION OF THE PATIENT

The modern preparation of a patient for surgery is epitomized by the convergence of the art and science of the surgical discipline. The context in which preoperative preparation is conducted ranges from an outpatient office visit to hospital inpatient consultation to emergency department evaluation of a patient. Approaches to preoperative evaluation differ significantly depending on the nature of the presenting complaint and the proposed surgical intervention, the patient's general health and assessment of risk factors, and results of directed investigation and interventions to optimize the patient's overall status and readiness for surgery. This chapter reviews the components of risk assessment applicable to the evaluation of any patient for surgery and provides basic algorithms to aid in the preparation of patients for surgery.

PRINCIPLES OF AND PREPARATION FOR SURGERY

Proper operative technique is of paramount importance for optimizing outcome and enhancing the wound-healing process. There is no substitute for a well-planned and conducted operation to provide the best possible surgical outcome. One of the most reliable means of ensuring that surgeons provide quality care in the operating room is through participation in high-quality surgical training programs that provide opportunities for repetitive observation and performance of surgical procedures in a well-structured environment. With their participation, young surgeons in training can progressively develop the technical skills necessary to perform the most demanding and complex operative procedures.

Determining the Need for Surgery

Patients are often referred to surgeons with a suspected surgical diagnosis and the results of supporting investigations in hand. In this context, the surgeon's initial encounter with the patient may be largely directed toward confirmation of relevant physical findings and review of the clinical history and laboratory and investigative tests that support the diagnosis. A recommendation regarding the need for operative intervention can be made by the surgeon and discussed with the patient and family members. A decision to perform additional investigative tests or consideration of alternative therapeutic options may postpone the decision for surgical intervention from this initial encounter to a later time. It is important for the surgeon to explain the context of the illness and the benefit of different surgical interventions, further investigation, possible nonsurgical alternatives when appropriate, and what would happen if no intervention were undertaken.

The surgeon's approach to the patient and family during the initial encounter should foster a bond of trust and open a line of communication among all participants. A professional and unhurried approach is mandatory, with time taken to listen to concerns and answer questions posed by the patient and family members. The surgeon's initial encounter with a patient should result in the patient being able to express a basic understanding of the disease process and the need for further investigation and possible surgical management. A well-articulated follow-up plan is essential.

Perioperative Decision Making

During the decision-making process, numerous considerations must be addressed regarding the timing and site of surgery, type of anesthesia, and preoperative preparation necessary to understand the patient's risk and to optimize the outcome. These components of risk assessment take into account the perioperative (intraoperative period through 48 hours postoperatively) and later postoperative (up to 30 days) period and seek to identify factors that may contribute to patient morbidity during these periods.

Preoperative Evaluation

The aim of preoperative evaluation is not to screen broadly for undiagnosed disease but to identify and quantify any comorbidity that may affect the operative outcome. This evaluation is driven by findings on the history and physical examination suggestive of organ system dysfunction or by epidemiologic data suggesting the benefit of evaluation based on age, sex, or patterns of disease progression. The goal is to uncover problem areas that may require further investigation or be amenable to preoperative optimization (Table 10-1).[1] Routine preoperative testing is not cost-effective and, even in older adults, is less predictive of perioperative morbidity than the American Society of Anesthesiologists (ASA) status or American Heart Association (AHA)/American College of Cardiology (ACC) guidelines for surgical risk.

The preoperative evaluation is determined in light of the risk of the planned procedure (low, medium, or high), planned anesthetic technique, and postoperative disposition of the patient (outpatient or inpatient, ward bed, or intensive care). In addition, the preoperative evaluation is used to identify patient risk factors for postoperative morbidity and mortality. Along with being a generally accepted program for risk adjustment to monitor and improve surgical outcomes, the American College of Surgeons National Surgical Quality Improvement Program (ACS NSQIP) has been used to develop predictive models for postoperative morbidity and mortality, and several factors have consistently been found to be independent predictors of postoperative events. The ACS NSQIP has been validated as an excellent quality improvement tool by accounting for the influence of patient risk on outcomes from surgery and allowing hospitals to compare their outcomes with the outcomes of their peers. Understanding the risks of surgery is important for patients and surgeons in the shared decision-making process. Informed consent requires that patients have a thorough understanding of the potential risks of surgery. However, predicting postoperative risks and identifying patients at a higher risk of adverse events have traditionally been based on individual surgeon experience and augmented by published rates in the literature from single-institution studies or clinical trials.

The ACS NSQIP collects high-quality, standardized clinical data on preoperative risk factors and postoperative complications from more than 500 hospitals in the United States. These data are

TABLE 10-1 Suggestions for Adult Preoperative Testing

TEST	BASIC: MINOR SURGERY IN HEALTHY PATIENT (WITHIN 90 DAYS)				Additive Surgical and Medical Factors: SURGICAL PROCEDURES (WITHIN 90 DAYS)							CLINICALLY SIGNIFICANT AND CHANGING DISORDERS AND/OR MEDICATIONS (SHADED = WITHIN 90 DAYS; LIGHT = TEST FOR DISORDER PROBABLY SHOULD BE PERFORMED WITHIN 30 DAYS)																			
	Healthy Adult <45 y/o	45-54 y/o	55-69 y/o	>70 y/o	Cardiac/Thoracic	Vascular	Major Intraperitoneal/Abdominal	Anticipated >2 U EBL	Intracranial	Orthopedic Prosthesis	TURP, Hysterostomy	Hypertension	Smoking	Morbid Obesity	h/o Stroke	Cancer (?Metastatic)	Seizure Medications	Cardiovascular	Respiratory	Diabetes	Hepatic	Renal	Fluid or Electrolyte Loss	Autoimmune/Lupus	EtOH/Drug Abuse	Steroids/Cushing's Syndrome	HIV	Parathyroid	Unstable Thyroid	Anticoagulant/Bleeding	Suspected Pregnancy
ECG		M	Y	Y	Y	Y	Y	Y	Y			Y	Y	Y	Y	Y		Y	Y	Y	Y	Y	±	Y	Y	Y	Y	Y	Y		
CBC + platelets			Y	Y	Y	Y	Y	Y	Y	Y	Y			Y	Y	Y	Y	Y	Y	Y	Y	Y	Y	Y	Y	Y	Y	Y	Y	Y	
Electrolytes				Y	Y	Y	Y	Y	Y	Y	Y	Y		Y	Y	Y		Y	Y	Y	Y	Y	Y	Y	Y	Y	Y	Y	Y		
BUN/creatinine				Y	Y	Y	Y	Y	Y	Y	Y	Y			Y	Y		Y	Y	Y	Y	Y		Y	Y	Y	Y	Y	Y		
Glucose				Y	Y	Y	Y	Y	Y	Y	Y			Y	Y	Y		Y		Y	Y	Y			Y	Y	Y	Y	Y		
LFTs							±									Y	Y				Y				Y		Y				
Calcium																												Y			
PT/PTT					Y			Y	Y												Y	Y		Y	Y					Y	
U/A, culture										S																					
CXR					Y											S			Y								S				
Hormone levels																													Y		
Bleeding time									S																					±	
Pregnancy																															Y*
Drug levels									S								S								±						
Tumor markers																S															
Clot	Depends primarily on extensiveness of proposed surgery, as per Blood Bank MSBOS guidelines																														

Adapted from Halaszynski TM, Juda R, Silverman DG: Optimizing postoperative outcomes with efficient preoperative assessment and management. *Crit Care Med* 32:S76–S86, 2004.

NOTE: (1) Times and test listings are suggestions; they are not absolute and should not preclude other testing in given settings or prevent a case from proceeding if the anesthesiologist and surgeon deem it to be appropriate. (2) Testing for a given disorder depends on the severity of the disorder in the context of the planned surgery; that is, are the tests likely to generate potentially clinically significant information and provide information that would be an important component of the history and physical examination?

Shaded area indicates timing of test is not typically critical; results from 90 days (and possibly 180 days) may be acceptable. Unshaded area indicates it is typically best to obtain test within 30 days of surgery.

BUN, blood urea nitrogen; *CXR,* chest x-ray; *EBL,* estimated blood loss; *EtOH,* ethanol; *h/o,* history of; *LFTs,* liver function tests; *M,* usually indicated for male patient; *MSBOS,* maximum surgical blood order schedule; *PT/PTT,* prothrombin time/partial thromboplastin time; *S,* may be requested (and reviewed) by the surgeon as part of surgical workup; *TURP,* transurethral resection of the prostate; *U/A,* urinalysis; *Y,* usually indicated; *±,* if situation acute or severe.

*At a minimum, a urine pregnancy test should be performed on the morning of surgery in any woman of childbearing age, unless the uterus or ovaries are surgically absent.

used to provide hospitals with risk-adjusted 30-day outcomes comparisons. The intended use would be to counsel patients and facilitate decision making for elective surgery in an office-based setting or to discuss risks for more emergent or urgent surgery in the inpatient setting.

Universal Surgical Risk Calculator

The ACS NSQIP surgical risk calculator is a decision-support tool based on reliable multi-institutional clinical data, which can be used to estimate the risks of most operations.[2] The goal of the ACS NSQIP risk calculator is to provide accurate, patient-specific risk information to guide surgical decision making and informed consent. The risk calculator uses 21 patient predictors (e.g., age, ASA class, body mass index [BMI], hypertension) and the planned procedure (Current Procedural Terminology code) to predict the chance that patients will have any of nine different outcomes within 30 days after surgery (Table 10-2). The outcomes include the following:

- Death
- Any complication—superficial incisional surgical site infection (SSI), deep incisional SSI, organ space SSI, wound disruption, pneumonia, unplanned intubation, pulmonary embolism (PE), ventilator use for more than 48 hours, progressive renal insufficiency, acute renal failure, urinary tract infection, stroke, cardiac arrest, myocardial infarction (MI), proximal deep venous thrombosis (DVT), systemic sepsis
- Serious complication—death, cardiac arrest, MI, pneumonia, progressive renal insufficiency, acute renal failure, PE, DVT, return to the operating room, deep incisional SSI, organ space SSI, systemic sepsis, unplanned intubation, urinary tract infection, wound disruption
- Pneumonia
- Cardiac event (cardiac arrest or MI)
- SSI
- Urinary tract infection
- Venous thromboembolism (VTE)
- Renal failure (progressive renal insufficiency or acute renal failure)

The risk calculator was built using data collected from more than 1.4 million operations from 393 hospitals participating in the ACS NSQIP during the period 2009-2012. Entering the most complete and accurate patient information provides the most precise risk information. However, the estimates can still be calculated if some of the patient information is unknown.

If preoperative evaluation uncovers significant comorbidity or evidence of poor control of an underlying disease process, consultation with an internist or medical subspecialist may be required to facilitate the workup and direct management. In this process,

TABLE 10-2 ACS NSQIP Variables Used in the Prior Colon-Specific and the New Universal Surgical Risk Calculators

VARIABLE	CATEGORIES	COLON-SPECIFIC	UNIVERSAL
Age group, yr	<65/65-74/75-84/≥85	X	X
Sex	Male/female	X	X
Functional status	Independent/partially dependent/totally dependent	X	X
Emergency case	Yes/no	X	X
ASA class	I or II/III/IV/V	X	X
Steroid use for chronic condition	Yes/no	X	X
Ascites within 30 days preoperatively	Yes/no	X	X
Systemic sepsis within 48 hr preoperatively	None/SIRS/sepsis/septic shock	X	X
Ventilator dependent	Yes/no	X	X
Disseminated cancer	Yes/no	X	X
Diabetes	No/oral/insulin	X	X
Hypertension requiring medication	Yes/no	X	X
Previous cardiac event	Yes/no	X	X
Congestive heart failure in 30 days preoperatively	Yes/no	X	X
Dyspnea	Yes/no	X	X
Current smoker within 1 yr	Yes/no	X	X
History of COPD	Yes/no	X	X
Dialysis	Yes/no	X	X
Acute renal failure	Yes/no	X	X
BMI class	Underweight/normal/overweight/obese 1/obese 2/obese 3	X	X
Colon surgery group (colectomy)	Partial laparoscopic with anastomosis/partial laparoscopic with ostomy/partial open with anastomosis/partial open with ostomy/total laparoscopic with ostomy/total open with ostomy	X	
Indication for colon surgery	Diverticulitis/enteritis or colitis/hemorrhage/neoplasm/obstruction or perforation/vascular insufficiency/volvulus/other	X	
CPT-specific linear risk	2,805 values		X

From Bilimoria KY, Liu Y, Paruch JL, et al: Development and evaluation of the universal ACS NSQIP surgical risk calculator: A decision aid and informed consent tool for patients and surgeons. *J Am Coll Surg* 217:833–842.e1–e3, 2013.

ACS NSQIP, American College of Surgeons National Surgical Quality Improvement Program; *ASA,* American Society of Anesthesiologists; *BMI,* body mass index; *COPD,* chronic obstructive pulmonary disease; *CPT,* Current Procedural Terminology; *SIRS,* systemic inflammatory response syndrome.

communication between the surgeon and consultants is essential to define realistic goals for this optimization process and to expedite surgical management.

For all patients, their general risk should be categorized using the ASA classification, which is one of the first risk categorization systems. It has six stratifications:

I. Normal healthy patient
II. Patient with mild systemic disease
III. Patient with severe systemic disease that limits activity but is not incapacitating
IV. Patient who has incapacitating disease that is a constant threat to life
V. Moribund patient not expected to survive 24 hours with or without an operation
VI. A declared brain-dead patient whose organs are being removed for donor purposes

The letter "E" is added to any of the above-listed stratifications for an emergency operation. Although the system seems subjective, it continues to be a significant independent predictor of mortality. Although the ASA class should be determined for each patient, a more in-depth assessment of risk is indicated for procedures more involved than a skin biopsy.

Perioperative Mortality Predictor

Accurate estimation of the risk of death can help patients and physicians to make decisions and to manage expectations.[3] Various scoring systems to assess perioperative mortality have been reported in the literature, including the Physiologic and Operative Severity Score for the enumeration of Mortality and Morbidity, Surgical Risk Score, Biochemistry and Haematology Outcome Models,[4] Acute Physiology and Chronic Health Evaluation (APACHE II score does not predict multiorgan failure or mortality in postoperative surgical patients), Cleveland Clinic Foundation Colorectal Cancer Model,[5] and the French Association of Surgery colorectal scale.[6,7] However, these scores are not easily calculated at the bedside. None of these scoring systems has the ability to predict accurately death or survival solely on the basis of preoperative variables, and they do not account for variability in perioperative outcomes.

The ACS NSQIP database has been described by the Institute of Medicine as the best in the United States for measuring and for reporting surgical quality and outcomes. The ACS NSQIP assesses surgical quality at more than 500 hospitals in the United States by collecting detailed data on preoperative risk factors and postoperative morbidity and mortality. Comprehensive computerized procedures and on-site auditing ensure data integrity. The NSQIP also has a reliable postdischarge mortality predictor (PMP). The PMP is an accurate, simple, effective, and clinically meaningful tool to calculate the risk of perioperative death using only preoperative variables. Risk can be easily calculated at the bedside without any laboratory values. Use of the PMP would give physicians the ability to report the risk of death reliably for a wide range of patients undergoing common elective and emergent general surgery procedures. It would be helpful in providing accurate information about the risk of death and in obtaining informed consent. In addition to being a useful counseling tool, the PMP could provide data on the performance of surgeons and hospitals.

Inpatient status had the greatest contribution to PMP score (Tables 10-3 and 10-4). The practice of ambulatory surgery is increasing in the United States, but inpatient surgery is still required for sicker patients and for more complex operations. Inpatient status exposes patients to hospital-acquired infections,

TABLE 10-3 Characteristics Associated With 30-Day Mortality in 202,741 Patients

CHARACTERISTIC	*P*	OR	95% CI
Inpatient	<.001	4.943	3.909-6.249
Age ≥80 yr	<.001	3.884	3.490-4.322
Liver morbidity	<.001	3.181	2.792-3.626
Functional status	<.001	3.138	2.869-3.433
Disseminated cancer	<.001	3.080	2.706-3.507
Renal morbidity	<.001	2.879	2.523-3.287
Sepsis	<.001	2.824	2.584-3.086
Pulmonary morbidity	<.001	2.517	2.301-2.752
DNR	<.001	2.335	1.966-2.772
Age 70-79 yr	<.001	2.189	1.973-2.429
Steroid	<.001	1.729	1.534-1.949
Age 65-69 yr	<.001	1.649	1.446-1.880
Cardiac morbidity	<.001	1.622	1.465-1.796
Weight loss*	<.001	1.572	1.387-1.782
Bleeding disorder	<.001	1.465	1.321-1.625
Open pancreas surgery	<.001	1.396	1.206-1.617
Obese	.159	0.931	0.842-1.029

From Vaid S, Bell T, Grim R, et al: Predicting risk of death in general surgery patients on the basis of preoperative variables using American College of Surgeons National Surgical Quality Improvement Program data. *Perm J* 16:10–17, 2012.
CI, confidence interval; *DNR,* do not resuscitate; *OR,* odds ratio.
*>10% body weight in the last 6 months.

TABLE 10-4 30-Point Bedside Preoperative Mortality Predictor Scoring System

PATIENT VARIABLE	SCORE
Inpatient	6
Sepsis	4
Poor functional status*	3
Disseminated cancer	1
Age, yr	
≥80	2
70-79	1
65-69	0.5
Comorbidities	
Cardiac	5
Pulmonary	3
Renal	1
Liver	1
Steroid for chronic condition	1
Weight loss†	1
Bleeding disorder	1
DNR	1
Obesity	−1
Highest possible score	30

From Vaid S, Bell T, Grim R, et al: Predicting risk of death in general surgery patients on the basis of preoperative variables using American College of Surgeons National Surgical Quality Improvement Program data. *Perm J* 16:10–17, 2012.
DNR, do not resuscitate.
*Total assistance required for all daily activities.
†>10% body weight in last 6 months.

which contributes indirectly to mortality. Advanced age independently predicted death or survival. Poor functional status and do-not-resuscitate directives were independent predictors of mortality. Cirrhosis and renal failure were independent risk factors of death. Medical comorbidities, such as cardiac problems, pulmonary dysfunction, and bleeding disorders, also independently predicted death. Preoperative optimization of these conditions may be an avenue for risk reduction. Sepsis was an independent predictor of death. The mortality rate associated with emergency laparotomies is greater than mortality for elective operations. Steroid use in the preoperative phase was an independent predictor of death. The presence of disseminated cancer also independently predicted death. Surgical complexity was only minimally predictive and only in very complex procedures, such as pancreatectomy (see Tables 10-3 and 10-4).

OPTIMAL PREOPERATIVE ASSESSMENT OF GERIATRIC SURGICAL PATIENTS

By 2007, the percentage of persons 65 years old and older increased modestly to 13%, yet hospital use among older individuals increased drastically to 37% of hospital discharges and 43% of the days of care.[8] Older individuals have significantly higher rates per population of inpatient and outpatient surgical and nonsurgical procedures compared with other age groups. It is imperative that strategies are developed to meet these growing demands and to ensure higher quality care for geriatric surgical patients.

The ACS NSQIP/American Geriatrics Society Best Practices Guidelines focus on the optimal preoperative assessment of the geriatric surgical patient. These guidelines are a compilation of the most current and evidence-based recommendations for improving the perioperative care of this vulnerable population (Box 10-1).

BOX 10-1 Checklist for Optimal Preoperative Assessment of Geriatric Surgical Patients

In addition to conducting a complete history and physical examination of the patient, the following assessments are strongly recommended:

- ☐ Assess patient's **cognitive ability** and **capacity** to understand anticipated surgery.
- ☐ Screen patient for **depression.**
- ☐ Identify patient's risk factors for developing postoperative **delirium.**
- ☐ Screen for **alcohol** and other **substance abuse/dependence.**
- ☐ Perform a preoperative **cardiac** evaluation according to the American College of Cardiology/American Heart Association algorithm for patients undergoing noncardiac surgery.
- ☐ Identify patient's risk factors for postoperative **pulmonary** complications, and implement appropriate strategies for prevention.
- ☐ Document **functional status** and history of **falls.**
- ☐ Determine baseline **frailty** score.
- ☐ Assess patient's **nutritional status,** and consider preoperative interventions if patient is at severe nutritional risk.
- ☐ Take an accurate and detailed **medication history,** and consider appropriate perioperative adjustments. Monitor for **polypharmacy.**
- ☐ Determine patient's **treatment goals** and **expectations** in the context of possible treatment outcomes.
- ☐ Determine patient's **family** and **social support system.**
- ☐ Order appropriate preoperative **diagnostic tests** focused on elderly patients.

BOX 10-2 Cognitive Assessment With the Mini-Cog™: 3 Item Recall and Clock Draw

1. Get the patient's attention, then say:
   "I am going to say three words that I want you to remember now and later. The words are: *banana, sunrise, chair.* Please say them for me now."
   Give the patient three tries to repeat the words. If unable after three tries, go to next item.
2. Say all the following phrases in the order indicated:
   "Please draw a clock in a circle on this paper. Put all the numbers in the circle and set the hands to show 11:10 (10 past 11)."
   If subject has not finished clock drawing in 3 minutes, discontinue and ask for recall items.
3. Say: "What were the three words I asked you to remember?"

Adapted from Borson S, Scanlan J, Brush M, et al: The Mini-Cog: a cognitive "vital signs" measure for dementia screening in multi-lingual elderly. *J Geriatr Psychiatry* 15(11):1021–1027, 2000.

Cognitive Impairment and Dementia

For any patient without a known history of cognitive impairment or dementia, obtaining a detailed history and performing a cognitive assessment, such as the Mini-Cog,[9] is strongly recommended (Box 10-2 and Table 10-5). If knowledgeable informants (e.g., spouse or family members) are available, interviewing them about the evolution of any cognitive or functional decline in the patient is recommended. If the patient has experienced a decline, referral to a primary care physician, geriatrician, or mental health specialist should be considered for further evaluation. Careful documentation of the patient's preoperative cognitive status is strongly recommended because postoperative cognitive dysfunction is common but difficult to quantify without a record of the baseline cognitive status.

Assessing the patient's decision-making capacity is critical in determining his or her ability to provide informed surgical consent. The four legally relevant criteria for decision-making capacity are as follows: (1) patient can clearly indicate his or her treatment choice; (2) patient understands the relevant information communicated by the physician; (3) patient acknowledges his or her medical condition, treatment options, and the likely outcomes; and (4) patient can engage in a rational discussion about the treatment options.

Depression

Screening patients for depression is strongly recommended. The physician may use simple tools, such as the Patient Health Questionnaire-2 (Box 10-3). If the patient answers yes to either question, further evaluation by a primary care physician, geriatrician, or mental health specialist is recommended. Preoperative depression has been associated with increased mortality after coronary artery bypass grafting (CABG)[10,11] and longer postoperative length of stay after CABG and valve operations.[12] Depression also has been associated with higher pain perception and increased postoperative analgesic use.

Postoperative Delirium

Postoperative delirium is a common complication in elderly patients. In one prospective study of patients undergoing major elective and noncardiac operations, 9% of patients developed postoperative delirium.[13] In another study of patients undergoing surgery and requiring a postoperative intensive care unit (ICU)

TABLE 10-5 Interpretation of the Mini-Cog™

Scoring:

3-item recall (0-3 points):	1 point for each correct word
Clock draw (0 or 2 points):	0 points for abnormal clock
	2 points for normal clock

A Normal Clock Has All of the Following Elements:

All numbers 1-12, each only once, are present in correct order and direction (clockwise) inside the circle.

Two hands are present, one pointing to 11 and one pointing to 2, hand length is not scored.

Any Clock Missing Any of These Elements Is Scored Abnormal

Refusal to Draw a Clock Is Scored Abnormal:

Total score of 0, 1, or 2 suggests possible impairment.

Total score of 3, 4, or 5 lower likelihood of dementia.

Adapted from Borson S, Scanlan J, Brush M, et al: The Mini-Cog: a cognitive "vital signs" measure for dementia screening in multi-lingual elderly. *J Geriatr Psychiatry* 15(11):1021–1027, 2000.

BOX 10-3 Screening for Depression With Patient Health Questionnaire-2

1. In the past 12 months, have you ever had a time when you felt sad, blue, depressed, or down for most of the time for at least 2 weeks?
2. In the past 12 months, have you ever had a time, lasting at least 2 weeks, when you didn't care about things that you usually care about or when you didn't enjoy the things that you usually enjoy?

Interpretation

If the patient says *yes* to either question, further evaluation by a primary care physician, geriatrician, or mental health specialist is recommended.

NOTE: This screening test has not been validated in extremely frail elderly patients, patients with severe concurrent medical illnesses, patients experiencing medication side effects, or patients with impaired communication skills.

stay, 44% of the patients experienced postoperative delirium.[14] Risk factors for postoperative delirium are listed in Box 10-4; the strongest predisposing factor is preexisting cognitive impairment and dementia.[14]

The surgeon should identify the patient's risk factors for developing postoperative delirium (see Box 10-4). For patients at risk for postoperative delirium, administration of benzodiazepines and antihistamines (e.g., diphenhydramine [Benadryl; McNeil]) should be avoided except in certain circumstances. Postoperative delirium is associated with higher mortality and complications.

Alcohol and Substance Abuse

Preoperative alcohol abuse and dependence are associated with increased rates of postoperative mortality and complications, including pneumonia, sepsis, wound infection and disruption, and prolonged length of hospital stay.[15] Patients can be screened for alcohol and substance abuse and dependence using the modified CAGE (Cut down, Annoyed, Guilty, and Eye-opener) questionnaire. For patients who answer yes to any of these questions, perioperative prophylaxis should be considered for withdrawal syndromes. If the operation can be delayed, motivated patients can be referred to a substance abuse specialist for preoperative abstinence or medical detoxification. It is recommended that patients with alcohol use disorder receive perioperative daily multivitamins (with folic acid) and high-dose oral or parenteral thiamine (100 mg).

BOX 10-4 Risk Factors for Postoperative Delirium

Cognitive and behavioral disorders
Cognitive impairment and dementia
Untreated or inadequately controlled pain
Depression
Alcohol use
Sleep deprivation
Disease or illness related
Severe illness or comorbidities
Renal insufficiency
Anemia
Hypoxia
Metabolic
Poor nutrition
Dehydration
Electrolyte abnormalities
Functional impairments
Poor functional status
Immobilization
Hearing or vision impairment
Other
Older age (≥70 yr)
Polypharmacy and use of psychotropic medications (benzodiazepines, anticholinergics, and antihistamines)
Risk of urinary retention or constipation, presence of urinary catheter

Cardiac Evaluation

All patients should be evaluated for perioperative cardiac risk according to the ACC/AHA algorithm for noncardiac surgery (Fig. 10-1).[16] Postoperative MI is associated with hospital mortality rates of 15% to 25%; these patients also are at greater risk for cardiovascular death and nonfatal MI during the 6 months after surgery.[17]

Older patients are more vulnerable to perioperative cardiac adverse events, and it is imperative to identify elderly patients with higher risk of cardiac complications and communicate operative risk effectively. An easy and inexpensive method to determine cardiopulmonary functional status for noncardiac surgery is the patient's ability or inability to climb two flights of stairs. Two flights of stairs are needed because it demands more than 4 metabolic equivalents. In a review of all studies of stair climbing as preoperative assessment, prospective studies showed it to be a good predictor of mortality associated with thoracic surgery.[1] In major noncardiac surgery, an inability to climb two flights of stairs is an independent predictor of perioperative morbidity, but not mortality.

Pulmonary Evaluation

Postoperative pulmonary complications are common and contribute considerably to overall morbidity and mortality. The *ACS NSQIP Best Practices Guidelines: Prevention of Postoperative Pulmonary Complications* identifies perioperative risk factors for postoperative pulmonary complications and prevention strategies (Box 10-5).[18] The surgeon should consider implementing appropriate preoperative strategies to reduce risk for postoperative pulmonary

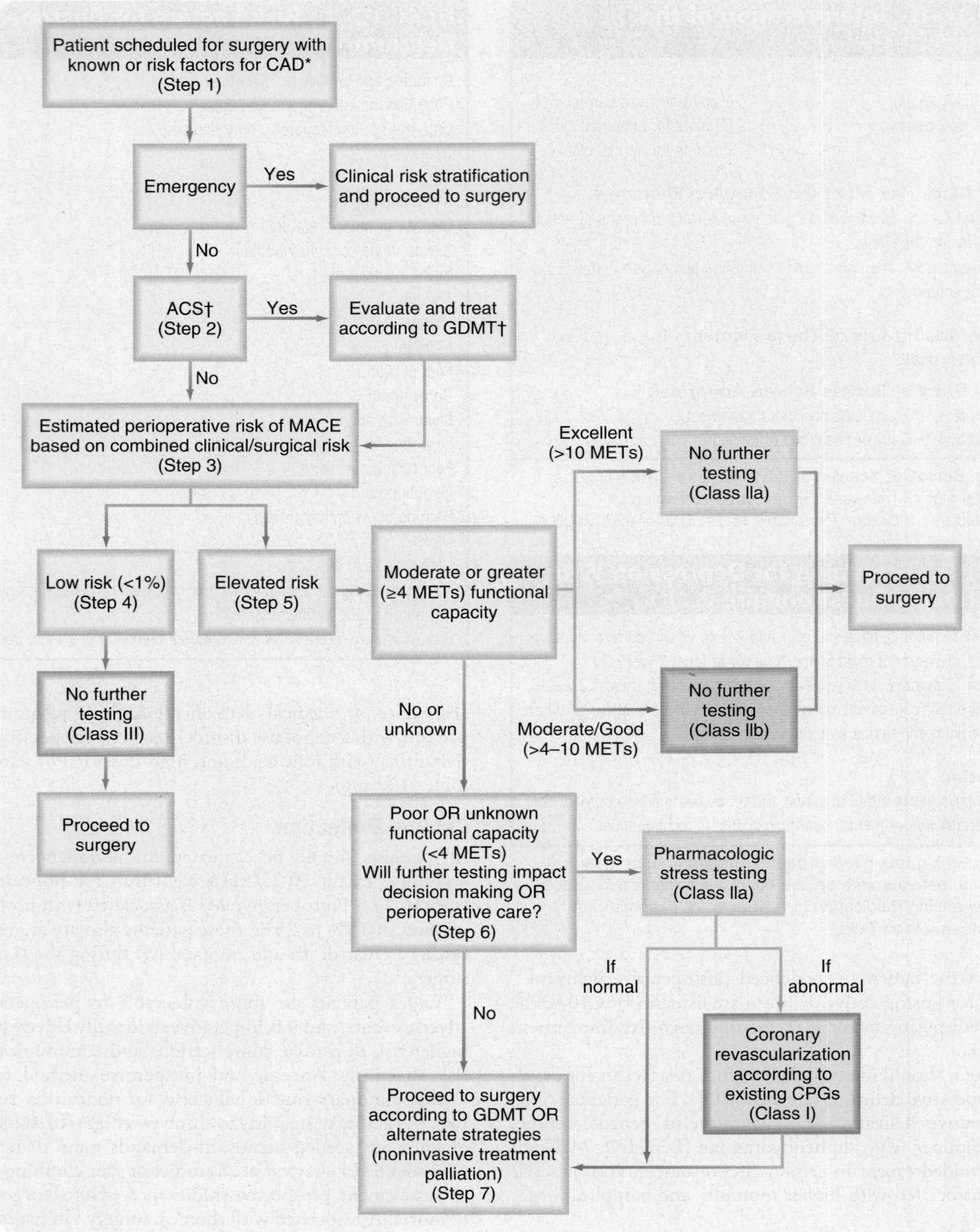
Patient scheduled for surgery with known or risk factors for CAD* (Step 1)
Emergency
Yes
Clinical risk stratification and proceed to surgery
No
ACS† (Step 2)
Yes
Evaluate and treat according to GDMT†
No
Estimated perioperative risk of MACE based on combined clinical/surgical risk (Step 3)
Low risk (<1%) (Step 4)
Elevated risk (Step 5)
Moderate or greater (≥4 METs) functional capacity
Excellent (>10 METs)
No further testing (Class IIa)
Proceed to surgery
No further testing (Class IIb)
Moderate/Good (>4–10 METs)
No or unknown
No further testing (Class III)
Proceed to surgery
Poor OR unknown functional capacity (<4 METs) Will further testing impact decision making OR perioperative care? (Step 6)
Yes
Pharmacologic stress testing (Class IIa)
If normal
If abnormal
No
Coronary revascularization according to existing CPGs (Class I)
Proceed to surgery according to GDMT OR alternate strategies (noninvasive treatment palliation) (Step 7)

complications, including preoperative optimization of pulmonary function in patients with uncontrolled chronic obstructive pulmonary disease and asthma, smoking cessation, preoperative intensive inspiratory muscle training, and selective chest radiograph and pulmonary function tests.

BOX 10-5 Risk Factors for Postoperative Pulmonary Complications

Patient-Related Factors
Age >60 yr
COPD
ASA class II or greater
Functional dependence
Congestive heart failure
Obstructive sleep apnea
Pulmonary hypertension
Current cigarette use
Impaired sensorium
Preoperative sepsis
Weight loss >10% in 6 months
Serum albumin <3.5 mg/dL
BUN ≥7.5 mmol/liter (≥21 mg/dL)
Serum creatinine >133 μmol/liter (>1.5 mg/dL)

Surgery-Related Factors
Prolonged operation >3 hr
Surgical site
Emergency operation
General anesthesia
Perioperative transfusion
Residual neuromuscular blockade after an operation

Not Risk Factors
Obesity
Well-controlled asthma
Diabetes

ASA, American Society of Anesthesiologists; *BUN,* blood urea nitrogen; *COPD,* chronic obstructive pulmonary disease.

Functional Status, Mobility, and Fall Risk

All patients should be assessed for their ability to perform daily activities (functional status). Box 10-6 presents a short, simple screening test for assessing baseline and current functional status in ambulatory patients. If the patient answers no to any of these questions, a more in-depth evaluation should be considered, including full screening of activities of daily living and instrumental activities of daily living. Any functional limitations should be documented and may prompt perioperative interventions (i.e., referral to occupational or physical therapy) and proactive discharge planning. Any reported deficits in vision, hearing, or swallowing should be documented. All patients should be asked about history of falls and be evaluated for limitations in gait and mobility using the Timed Up and Go Test (Box 10-7).

Frailty

Frailty is a syndrome of decreased physiologic reserve and resistance to stressors, which leaves patients more vulnerable to poor

BOX 10-6 Short Simple Screening Test for Functional Assessment

Ask the patient the following questions:

1. "Can you get out of bed or a chair yourself?"
2. "Can you dress and bathe yourself?"
3. "Can you make your own meals?"
4. "Can you do your own shopping?"

If *no* to any of these questions, more in-depth evaluation should be performed, including full screening of activities of daily living and instrumental activities of daily living.

Deficits should be documented and may prompt perioperative interventions (i.e., referral to occupational therapy or physical therapy) and proactive discharge planning.

From Woolger JM: Preoperative testing and medication management. *Clin Geriatr Med* 24:573–583, vii, 2008; and Lachs MS, Feinstein AR, Cooney LM Jr, et al: A simple procedure for general screening for functional disability in elderly patients. *Ann Intern Med* 112:699–706, 1990.

FIGURE 10-1 Stepwise approach to perioperative cardiac assessment for coronary artery disease (CAD). Step 1: In patients scheduled for surgery with risk factors for or known CAD, determine the urgency of surgery. If an emergency, determine the clinical risk factors that may influence perioperative management and proceed to surgery with appropriate monitoring and management strategies based on the clinical assessment. *See full publication for recommendations for patients with symptomatic HF, VHD, or arrythmias. Step 2: If surgery is urgent or elective, determine if the patient has an acute coronary syndrome (ACS). If yes, refer patient for cardiology evaluation and management according to guideline-directed medical therapy (GDMT) according to the unstable angina/non–ST segment elevation myocardial infarction (UA/NSTEMI) and ST segment elevation myocardial infarction (STEMI) clinical practice guidelines (CPGs). †See full publication for recommendations in patients with UA/NSTEMI and STEMI CPGs. Step 3: If the patient has risk factors for stable CAD, estimate the perioperative risk of a major adverse cardiac event (MACE) on the basis of the combined clinical/surgical risk. This estimate can use the American College of Surgeons National Surgical Quality Improvement Program risk calculator or incorporate the Revised Cardiac Risk Index with an estimation of surgical risk. For example, a patient undergoing very-low-risk surgery (e.g., ophthalmologic surgery), even with multiple risk factors, would have a low risk of MACE, whereas a patient undergoing major vascular surgery with few risk factors would have an elevated risk of MACE. Step 4: If the patient has a low risk of MACE (<1%), no further testing is needed, and the patient may proceed to surgery. Step 5: If the patient is at elevated risk of MACE, determine functional capacity with an objective measure or scale such as the Duke Activity Status Index. If the patient has moderate, good, or excellent functional capacity (≥4 metabolic equivalents [METs]), then proceed to surgery without further evaluation. Step 6: If the patient has poor (<4 METs) or unknown functional capacity, the clinician should consult with the patient and perioperative team to determine whether further testing would affect patient decision making (e.g., decision to perform original surgery or willingness to undergo coronary artery bypass grafting or percutaneous coronary intervention, depending on the results of the test) or perioperative care. If yes, pharmacologic stress testing is appropriate. In patients with unknown functional capacity, exercise stress testing may be reasonable to perform. If the stress test is abnormal, consider coronary angiography and revascularization depending on the extent of the abnormal test. The patient can proceed to surgery with GDMT or consider alternative strategies, such as noninvasive treatment of the indication for surgery (e.g., radiation therapy for cancer) or palliation. If the test is normal, proceed to surgery according to GDMT. Step 7: If testing would not affect decision making or care, proceed to surgery according to GDMT or consider alternative strategies, such as noninvasive treatment of the indication for surgery (e.g., radiation therapy for cancer) or palliation. *HF,* heart failure; *VHD,* valvular heart disease. (From Fleisher LA, Fleischmann KE, Auerbach AD, et al: 2014 ACC/AHA guideline on perioperative cardiovascular evaluation and management of patients undergoing noncardiac surgery: A report of the American College of Cardiology/American Heart Association Task Force on Practice Guidelines. *J Am Coll Cardiol* 64:e77–e137, 2014.)

BOX 10-7 Assessment of Gait and Mobility Limitations With the Timed Up and Go Test

Patients should sit in a standard armchair with a line 10 feet in length in front of the chair. They should use standard footwear and walking aids and should not receive any assistance.

Have the patient perform the following commands:

1. Rise from the chair (if possible, without using the armrests)
2. Walk to the line on the floor (10 feet)
3. Turn
4. Return to the chair
5. Sit down again

From Panel on Prevention of Falls in Older Persons, American Geriatrics Society and British Geriatrics Society: Summary of the Updated American Geriatrics Society/British Geriatrics Society clinical practice guideline for prevention of falls in older persons. *J Am Geriatr Soc* 59:148–157, 2011.

TABLE 10-6 Frailty Score (Operational Definition)

CRITERIA	DEFINITION
Shrinkage	Unintentional weight loss ≥10 past year
Weakness	Decreased grip strength
Exhaustion	Self-reported poor energy and endurance
Low physical activity	Low weekly energy expenditure
Slowness	Slow walking

From Bergman H, Ferrucci L, Guralnik J, et al: Frailty: An emerging research and clinical paradigm—issues and controversies. *J Gerontol A Biol Sci Med Sci* 62:731–737, 2007; and Makary MA, Segev DL, Pronovost PJ, et al: Frailty as a predictor of surgical outcomes in older patients. *J Am Coll Surg* 210:901–908, 2010.

NOTE: The patient receives 1 point for each criterion met: 0-1, not frail; 2-3, intermediate frail (prefrail); 4-5, frail.

health outcomes, including falls, worsening mobility and activities of daily living disability, hospitalizations, and death. It is a clinically distinct entity from comorbidity and disability. Frailty in elderly surgical patients has been shown to predict independently higher rates of postoperative adverse events, increased length of stay, and higher likelihood of discharge to a skilled or assisted-living facility. In addition, patients with intermediate frailty have elevated risk for postoperative complications and more than a twofold increased risk of becoming frail over 3 years compared with nonfrail patients (Table 10-6).

Nutritional Status

Poor nutritional status is associated with increased risk of postoperative adverse events, mostly infectious complications (e.g., SSIs, pneumonia, urinary tract infections) and wound complications (e.g., dehiscence and anastomotic leaks), and increased length of stay for patients undergoing elective gastrointestinal surgery. All patients should be evaluated for their nutritional status by documenting height and weight and calculating BMI, measuring baseline serum albumin and prealbumin levels, and inquiring about unintentional weight loss in the last year. Risk factors for severe nutritional risk are BMI less than 18.5 kg/m^2, serum albumin less than 3.0 g/dL (with no evidence of hepatic or renal dysfunction), and unintentional weight loss greater than 10% to 15% within 6 months. Patients at severe nutritional risk should, if feasible, undergo a full nutritional assessment by a dietitian to design a perioperative nutritional plan to address deficits and should be considered for preoperative nutritional support.[19]

Medication Management

The patient's complete medication list, including use of nonprescription agents (over-the-counter, nonsteroidal anti-inflammatory drugs [NSAIDs], vitamins, eye drops, topical agents) and herbal products, should be reviewed and documented. The patient's risk for adverse drug reactions can be minimized by identifying medications that should be discontinued before surgery or should be avoided and by reducing dosage or substituting potentially inappropriate medications. The physician should also consider which medications should be started or continued preoperatively to reduce perioperative risks of adverse events.

Beta blockers should be continued in patients undergoing a noncardiac operation who are taking the medication for angina, symptomatic arrhythmia, hypertension, or other cardiac indications. Perioperative beta blockade started within 1 day or less before noncardiac surgery prevents nonfatal MI but increases risks of stroke, death, hypotension, and bradycardia and is not recommended.[20]

Patient Counseling

It is very important that a discussion occur between the physician and the patient to determine explicitly the patient's preferences and expectations from the treatment. It is strongly recommended that the surgeon ensure that the patient has an advance directive and a designated health care proxy or surrogate decision makers. These documents should be placed in the medical chart. In the absence of documented preferences, physicians often rely on health care proxies to make end-of-life decisions for patients.

Preoperative Testing

Routine sets of preoperative *screening* tests are *not* recommended. Three exceptions are hemoglobin, renal function tests, and albumin, which are indicated for all geriatric surgical patients. Preoperative *diagnostic* tests including coagulation studies, serum electrolytes, urinalysis, chest radiograph, and electrocardiogram (ECG) should be performed selectively and limited to higher risk patients who can be identified based on history and physical examination, known comorbidities, and the type of procedure to be performed.[13]

SYSTEMS APPROACH TO PREOPERATIVE EVALUATION

Cardiovascular System

Cardiovascular disease is the leading cause of death in the industrialized world, and its contribution to perioperative mortality during noncardiac surgery is significant. Of the 27 million patients undergoing surgery in the United States every year, 8 million, or almost 30%, have significant coronary artery disease or other cardiac comorbid conditions. Perioperative cardiac complications occur in 1 million of these patients, with substantial morbidity, mortality, and cost. Consequently, much of the preoperative risk assessment and patient preparation centers on the cardiovascular system.

Assessment tools for stratification of the cardiovascular portion of anesthetic risk have been available for some time. The premiere

TABLE 10-7 Cardiac Risk Indices

CARDIAC RISK INDEX WITH VARIABLES	POINTS	COMMENTS
Goldman Cardiac Risk Index, 1977		**Cardiac Complication Rate**
1. Third heart sound or jugular venous distention	11	0-5 points = 1%
2. Recent myocardial infarction	10	6-12 points = 7%
3. Nonsinus rhythm or PAC on ECG	7	13-25 points = 14%
4. >5 premature ventricular contractions	7	>26 points = 78%
5. Age >70 yr	5	
6. Emergency operations	4	
7. Poor general medical condition	3	
8. Intrathoracic, intraperitoneal, or aortic surgery	3	
9. Important valvular aortic stenosis	3	
Detsky Modified Multifactorial Index, 1986		**Cardiac Complication Rate**
1. Class 4 angina	20	>15 = high risk
2. Suspected critical aortic stenosis	20	
3. MI within 6 mo	10	
4. Alveolar pulmonary edema within 1 wk	10	
5. Unstable angina within 3 mo	10	
6. Class 3 angina	10	
7. Emergency surgery	10	
8. MI >6 mo ago	5	
9. Alveolar pulmonary edema resolved >1 wk ago	5	
10. Rhythm other than sinus or PACs on ECG	5	
11. >5 PVCs any time before surgery	5	
12. Poor general medical status	5	
13. Age >70 yr	5	
Eagle Criteria for Cardiac Risk Assessment, 1989		
1. Age >70 yr	1	<1, no testing
2. Diabetes	1	1-2, send for noninvasive test
3. Angina	1	≥3, send for angiography
4. Q waves on ECG	1	
5. Ventricular arrhythmias	1	
Revised Cardiac Risk Index		
1. History of ischemic heart disease	1	Risk for cardiac death, nonfatal myocardial infarction, and nonfatal cardiac arrest:
2. History of congestive heart failure	1	0 predictors = 0.4%
3. History of cerebrovascular disease (stroke or transient ischemic attack)	1	1 predictor = 0.9%
4. History of diabetes requiring preoperative insulin use	1	2 predictors = 6.6%
5. Chronic kidney disease (creatinine >2 mg/dL)	1	≥3 predictors = >11%
6. Undergoing suprainguinal vascular, intraperitoneal, or intrathoracic surgery	1	

From Akhtar S, Silverman DG: Assessment and management of patients with ischemic heart disease. *Crit Care Med* 32:S126–136, 2004; and Fleisher LA, Beckman JA, Brown KA, et al: ACC/AHA 2007 Guidelines on perioperative cardiovascular evaluation and care for noncardiac surgery: Executive summary: A report of the American College of Cardiology/American Heart Association Task Force on Practice Guidelines (Writing Committee to Revise the 2002 Guidelines on Perioperative Cardiovascular Evaluation for Noncardiac Surgery) developed in collaboration with the American Society of Echocardiography, American Society of Nuclear Cardiology, Heart Rhythm Society, Society of Cardiovascular Anesthesiologists, Society for Cardiovascular Angiography and Interventions, Society for Vascular Medicine and Biology, and Society for Vascular Surgery. *J Am Coll Cardiol* 50:1707–1732, 2007.

ECG, electrocardiogram; *MI,* myocardial infarction; *PAC,* Premature atrial contraction; *PVC,* premature ventricular contraction.

example is Goldman's criteria of cardiac risk for noncardiac surgery (Table 10-7).[1] This strategy, designed decades ago by multivariate analysis, assigns points to easily reproducible characteristics. The points are added to yield a total, which has been correlated with perioperative cardiac risk. One important contribution of this work was the inclusion of functional capacity, clinical signs and symptoms, and operative risk assessment to estimate the patient's overall risk and plan preoperative interventions. This concept has been refined further in the Revised Cardiac Risk Index (RCRI), which uses six predictors of complications to estimate cardiac risk in noncardiac surgical patients and is shown in Table 10-7.[21] In addition, several other investigators have proposed cardiac risk indices; however, many were found to be expensive and time-consuming.

In an attempt to assess and optimize the cardiac status of patients undergoing noncardiac surgery, a joint committee of the

ACC and AHA developed an easily used tool (see Fig. 10-1).[16] This methodology takes into account previous coronary revascularization and evaluation and clinical risk assessment divided into major, intermediate, and minor clinical predictors. The next factor taken into account is the patient's functional capacity, which is estimated by obtaining a history of the patient's daily activities. The earlier mentioned variables and type of surgery are used to determine whether the pretest probability can be altered by noninvasive testing.

The standard exercise stress test, with or without thallium for perfusion imaging, can be limited by the functional capacity of the patient. Patients unable to exercise to an acceptable stress level may require pharmacologic stress testing with dipyridamole; thereafter, perfusion defects can be assessed via thallium or a dobutamine-induced stress, followed by functional evaluation with echocardiography. Angiography can be used to define the exact anatomic abnormalities contributing to the ischemia.

When these data have been obtained, the surgeon and consultants need to weigh the benefits of surgery against the risks and determine whether any perioperative intervention would reduce the probability of a cardiac event. The intervention usually centers on coronary revascularization via CABG or percutaneous coronary intervention (PCI). Performing PCI before noncardiac surgery should be limited to (1) patients with left main disease whose comorbidities preclude bypass surgery without undue risk and (2) patients with unstable coronary artery disease who would be appropriate candidates for emergency or urgent revascularization.[22,23]

Patients with ST segment elevation MI or non–ST segment elevation acute coronary syndrome benefit from early invasive management, in whom balloon angioplasty or bare-metal stent (BMS) implantation should be considered. Elective noncardiac surgery should be delayed 14 days after balloon angioplasty and 30 days after BMS implantation. Elective noncardiac surgery should not be performed in patients within 12 months after implantation of a drug-eluting stent (DES) because of risks of discontinuing dual antiplatelet therapy for many procedures.

Based on the 2014 ACC/AHA guidelines, timing of elective noncardiac surgery in patients with previous PCI is as follows:

- Elective noncardiac surgery should be delayed 14 days after balloon angioplasty and 30 days after BMS implantation.[22,24]
- Elective noncardiac surgery should optimally be delayed 365 days after DES implantation.[25]
- Elective noncardiac surgery after DES implantation may be considered after 180 days if the risk of further delay is greater than the expected risks of ischemia and stent thrombosis.[25,26]

Elective noncardiac surgery should not be performed within 30 days after BMS implantation or within 12 months after DES implantation in patients in whom dual antiplatelet therapy will need to be discontinued perioperatively. Elective noncardiac surgery should not be performed within 14 days of balloon angioplasty in patients in whom aspirin will need to be discontinued perioperatively.

The optimal timing of a surgical procedure after MI depends on the duration of time since the event and assessment of the patient's risk for ischemia by clinical symptoms or noninvasive study. Any patient can be evaluated as a surgical candidate after an acute MI (within 7 days of evaluation) or a recent MI (within 7 to 30 days of evaluation). The infarction event is considered a major clinical predictor in the context of ongoing risk for ischemia. General recommendations are to wait 4 to 6 weeks after MI to perform elective surgery.[1]

Perioperative Beta Blocker Therapy Recommendation

"A Systematic Review for the 2014 ACC/AHA Guideline on Perioperative Cardiovascular Evaluation and Management of Patients Undergoing Noncardiac Surgery" adds some clarity around the controversial issue of beta blocker therapy.[20] The systematic review suggests that preoperative use of beta blockers was associated with a reduction in cardiac events, but few data support the effectiveness of preoperative administration of beta blockers to reduce the risk of surgical death. There is a consistent and clear association between beta blocker administration and adverse outcomes, such as bradycardia and stroke. These findings were consistent when the DECREASE studies or POISE (Perioperative Ischemic Evaluation Study) was excluded.[27-30] Exclusion of these studies did not substantially affect estimates of the risk or benefit.

Per new recommendations, beta blockers should be continued in patients undergoing surgery who have been taking long-term beta blockers. Management of beta blockers after surgery should be guided by clinical circumstances, independent of when the agent was started. In patients with intermediate-risk or high-risk myocardial ischemia noted in preoperative risk stratification tests, it may be reasonable to begin perioperative beta blockers.[31]

In patients with three or more RCRI risk factors (e.g., diabetes mellitus, heart failure, coronary artery disease, renal insufficiency, cerebrovascular accident), it may be reasonable to begin beta blockers before surgery.[32] However, in patients with a long-term indication for beta blocker therapy but no other RCRI risk factors, the benefit of initiating beta blockers in the perioperative setting is uncertain. Beta blocker therapy should not be started on the day of surgery. In patients in whom beta blocker therapy is initiated, it may be reasonable to begin perioperative beta blockers far enough in advance to assess safety and tolerability, preferably 2 to 7 days before surgery.[29]

Clinical assessments for tolerability are a key element of perioperative strategies. The decision to begin beta blockers should be influenced by whether a patient has other relative contraindications (e.g., uncompensated heart failure) or is at risk for stroke.[33]

Pulmonary System

Preoperative evaluation of pulmonary function may be necessary for thoracic or general surgical procedures. Although extremity, neurologic, and lower abdominal surgical procedures have little effect on pulmonary function and do not routinely require pulmonary function studies, thoracic and upper abdominal procedures can decrease pulmonary function and predispose to pulmonary complications. It is prudent to consider assessment of pulmonary function for all lung resection cases, for thoracic procedures requiring single-lung ventilation, and for major abdominal and thoracic cases in patients who are older than 60 years, have significant underlying medical disease, smoke, or have overt pulmonary symptoms. Necessary tests include forced expiratory volume in 1 second (FEV_1), forced vital capacity, and diffusing capacity of carbon monoxide. Adults with an FEV_1 less than 0.8 liter/sec or 30% of predicted, have a high risk for complications and postoperative pulmonary insufficiency; nonsurgical solutions are sought. Pulmonary resections need to be planned so that the postoperative FEV_1 is higher than 0.8 liter/sec, or 30% of predicted. Such planning can be done with the aid of quantitative lung scans, which can indicate which segments of the lung are functional.

Postoperative pulmonary complications carry with them great cost—estimated to be more than $50,000—and increased short-term and long-term mortality.[1] Risk factors for the development of postoperative pulmonary complications were identified in a large population of patients from Department of Veterans Affairs centers (Tables 10-8 and 10-9) and more recently confirmed in a mixed population. Although the Department of Veterans Affairs population was fairly homogeneous, the Patient Safety in Surgery study[1] included a more diverse group. Even with the diversity, the rates of pulmonary complications were not much different, and the risk factors were very similar. Preoperative pulmonary assessment determines not only factors that confer increased risk but also potential targets to reduce the risk for pulmonary complications. General factors that increase risk for postoperative pulmonary complications include increasing age, reduced albumin level, dependent functional status, weight loss, and possibly obesity. Concurrent comorbid conditions such as impaired sensorium, previous stroke, congestive heart failure, acute renal failure, long-term steroid use, and blood transfusion are also associated with increased risk for postoperative pulmonary complications. Specific pulmonary risk factors include chronic obstructive pulmonary disease, smoking, preoperative sputum production, pneumonia, dyspnea, and obstructive sleep apnea.

Preoperative interventions that may decrease postoperative pulmonary complications include smoking cessation (within 2 months before the planned procedure), bronchodilator therapy, antibiotic therapy for preexisting infection, and pretreatment of asthmatic patients with steroids. In addition, encouraging exercise preoperatively may improve a patient's recovery postoperatively. A reasonable recommendation would be to encourage patients to walk 3 miles in less than 1 hour several times weekly. Perioperative strategies include the use of epidural anesthesia, vigorous pulmonary toilet and rehabilitation, and continued bronchodilator therapy.

Renal System

Approximately 5% of the adult population has some degree of renal dysfunction that can affect the physiology of multiple organ systems and cause additional morbidity in the perioperative period. A preoperative creatinine level of 2.0 mg/dL or greater is an independent risk factor for cardiac complications. The goal of preoperative evaluation in these patients is to identify coexisting cardiovascular, circulatory, hematologic, and metabolic derangements secondary to renal dysfunction.

A patient with known renal insufficiency undergoes a thorough history and physical examination, with particular questioning about previous MI and symptoms consistent with ischemic heart disease. The cardiovascular examination seeks to document signs of fluid overload. The patient's functional status and exercise tolerance are carefully elicited. Diagnostic testing for a patient with renal dysfunction includes an ECG, serum chemistry panel, and complete blood count (CBC). If physical examination findings are suggestive of heart failure, a chest radiograph may be helpful. Urinalysis and urinary electrolyte studies are not often helpful in the setting of established renal insufficiency, although they may be diagnostic in patients with new-onset renal dysfunction.

Laboratory abnormalities are often seen in a patient with advanced renal insufficiency. Some metabolic derangements in a patient with advanced renal failure may be mild and asymptomatic and are revealed by electrolyte or blood gas analysis. Anemia, when present in these patients, may be mild and asymptomatic or associated with fatigue, low exercise tolerance, and exertional angina. Such anemia can be treated with erythropoietin or darbepoietin preoperatively or perioperatively. Because the platelet dysfunction associated with uremia is often a qualitative one, platelet counts are usually normal. A safe course is to communicate with the anesthesiologist about the potential need for agents to be available in the operating room to assist in improving platelet function. A patient with end-stage renal disease frequently requires additional attention in the perioperative period. Pharmacologic manipulation of hyperkalemia, replacement of calcium for symptomatic hypocalcemia, and use of phosphate-binding antacids for hyperphosphatemia are often required. Sodium bicarbonate is used in the setting of metabolic acidosis not caused by hypoperfusion when serum bicarbonate levels are less than 15 mEq/liter. It can be administered in intravenous fluid as 1 to 2 ampules in 1 liter of a 5% dextrose solution. Hyponatremia is treated by volume restriction, although dialysis is commonly required during the perioperative period for control of volume and electrolyte abnormalities.

Patients with chronic end-stage renal disease undergo dialysis before surgery to optimize their volume status and control the potassium level. Intraoperative hyperkalemia can result from surgical manipulation of tissue or transfusion of blood. These patients often undergo dialysis on the day after surgery as well. In the acute setting, patients who have a stable volume status can undergo surgery without preoperative dialysis, provided that no other indication exists for emergency dialysis.[1] Prevention of secondary renal insults in the perioperative period includes the avoidance of nephrotoxic agents and maintenance of adequate intravascular volume throughout this period. In the postoperative period, the pharmacokinetics of many drugs may be unpredictable, and adjustments in dosage need to be made according to pharmacy recommendation. Narcotics used for postoperative pain control may have prolonged effects despite hepatic clearance, and nonsteroidal agents are avoided in patients with renal insufficiency.

Hepatobiliary System

Hepatic dysfunction may reflect the common pathway of numerous insults to the liver, including viral-mediated, drug-mediated, and toxin-mediated disease. A patient with liver dysfunction requires careful assessment of the degree of functional impairment as well as a coordinated effort to avoid additional insult in the perioperative period (Fig. 10-2).[1]

A history of any exposure to blood and blood products or exposure to hepatotoxic agents is obtained. Patients frequently know whether hepatitis has been diagnosed and need to be questioned about when the diagnosis was made and what activity led to the infection. Although such a history may not affect further patient evaluation, it is important to obtain in case an operative team member is injured during the planned surgical procedure. A review of systems specifically inquires about symptoms such as pruritus, fatigability, excessive bleeding, abdominal distention, and weight gain. Evidence of hepatic dysfunction may be seen on physical examination. Jaundice and scleral icterus may be evident with serum bilirubin levels greater than 3 mg/dL. Skin changes include spider angiomas, caput medusae, palmar erythema, and clubbing of the fingertips. Abdominal examination may reveal distention, evidence of fluid shift, and hepatomegaly. Encephalopathy or asterixis may be evident. Muscle wasting or cachexia can be prominent.

A patient with liver dysfunction should undergo standard liver function tests. Elevations in hepatocellular enzyme levels may suggest a diagnosis of acute or chronic hepatitis, which can be investigated by serologic testing for hepatitis A, B, and C. Alcoholic hepatitis is suggested by decreased transaminase levels and an aspartate aminotransferase-to-alanine transaminase ratio

TABLE 10-8 **Risk Factors for Development of Postoperative Pneumonia and Respiratory Failure**

RISK FACTOR	POSTOPERATIVE PNEUMONIA RISK INDEX, OR (95% CI)	POINT VALUE	RESPIRATORY FAILURE RISK INDEX, OR (95% CI)	POINT VALUE
Type of Surgery				
AAA repair	4.29 (3.34-5.50)	15	14.3 (12.0-16.9)	27
Thoracic	3.92 (3.36-4.57)	14	8.14 (7.17-9.25)	21
Upper abdominal	2.68 (2.38-3.03)	10	4.21 (3.80-4.67)	14
Neck	2.30 (1.73-3.05)	8	3.10 (2.40-4.01)	11
Neurosurgical	2.14 (1.66-2.75)	8	4.21 (3.80-4.67)	14
Vascular	1.29 (1.10-1.52)	3	4.21 (3.80-4.67)	14
Emergency surgery	1.33 (1.16-1.54)	3	3.12 (2.83-3.43)	11
General anesthesia	1.56 (1.36-1.80)	4	1.91 (1.64-2.21)	—
Age, yr				
>80	5.63 (4.62-6.84)	17	—	—
70-79	3.58 (2.97-4.33)	13	—	—
60-69	2.38 (1.98-2.87)	9	—	—
50-59	1.49 (1.23-1.81)	4	—	—
<50	1.00 (referent)	—	—	—
60-69	—	—	1.51 (1.36-1.69)	4
<60	—	—	1.00 (referent)	—
≥70	—	—	1.91 (1.71-2.13)	6
Functional Status				
Totally dependent	3.83 (2.33-3.43)	10	1.92 (1.74-2.11)	7
Partially dependent	1.83 (1.63-2.06)	6	1.92 (1.74-2.11)	7
Independent	1.00 (referent)	—	1.00 (referent)	—
Albumin Level				
<3.0 g/dL	—	—	2.53 (2.28-2.80)	9
>3.0 g/dL	—	—	1.00 (referent)	—
Weight loss >10% (within 6 mo)	1.92 (1.68-2.18)	7	1.37 (1.19-1.57)*	—
Long-term steroid use	1.33 (1.12-1.58)	3	—	—
Alcohol, >2 drinks/day (within 2 wk)	1.24 (1.08-1.42)	2	1.19 (1.07-1.33)*	—
Diabetes, treated with insulin	—	—	1.15 (1.00-1.33)*	—
History of COPD	1.72 (1.55-1.91)	5	1.81 (1.66-1.98)	6
Current Smoker				
Within 1 yr	1.28 (1.17-1.42)	3	—	—
Within 2 wk	—	—	1.24 (1.14-1.36)*	—
Preoperative pneumonia	—	—	1.70 (1.24-2.13)*	—
Dyspnea				
At rest	—	—	1.69 (1.36-2.09)*	—
With minimal exertion	—	—	1.21 (1.09-1.34)*	—
	—	—	1.00 (referent)	—
No Dyspnea				
Impaired sensorium	1.51 (1.26-1.82)	4	1.22 (1.04-1.43)*	—
History of CVA	1.47 (1.28-1.68)	4	1.20 (1.05-1.38)*	—
History of CHF	—	—	1.25 (1.07-1.47)*	—
BUN Level				
<8 mg/dL	1.47 (1.26-1.72)	4	1.00 (referent)	—
8-21 mg/dL	1.00 (referent)	—	1.00 (referent)	—
22-30 mg/dL	1.24 (1.11-1.39)	2	1.00 (referent)	—
>30 mg/dL	1.41 (1.22-1.64)	3	2.29 (2.04-2.56)	8
Preoperative renal failure	—	—	1.67 (1.23-2.27)*	—
Preoperative transfusion (>4 units)	1.35 (1.07-1.72)	3	1.56 (1.28-1.91)*	—

From Arozullah AM, Khuri SF, Henderson WG, et al: Development and validation of a multifactorial risk index for predicting postoperative pneumonia after major noncardiac surgery. *Ann Intern Med* 135:847–857, 2001; and Arozullah AM, Daley J, Henderson WG, et al: Multifactorial risk index for predicting postoperative respiratory failure in men after major noncardiac surgery. The National Veterans Administration Surgical Quality Improvement Program. *Ann Surg* 232:242–253, 2000.

AAA, Abdominal aortic aneurysm; *BUN,* blood urea nitrogen; *CHF,* congestive heart failure; *CI,* confidence interval; *COPD,* chronic obstructive pulmonary disease; *CVA,* cerebrovascular accident; *OR,* odds ratio.

*The risk factor was statistically significant in multivariable analysis but was not included in the respiratory failure risk index.

TABLE 10-9 Pulmonary Risk Class Assignment

RISK CLASS	POSTOPERATIVE PNEUMONIA RISK INDEX (POINT TOTAL)	PREDICTED PROBABILITY OF PNEUMONIA (%)	RESPIRATORY FAILURE RISK INDEX (POINT TOTAL)	PREDICTED PROBABILITY OF RESPIRATORY FAILURE (%)
1	0-15	0.2	0-10	0.5
2	16-25	1.2	11-19	2.2
3	26-40	4.0	20-27	5.0
4	41-55	9.4	28-40	11.6
5	>55	15.3	>40	30.5

From Arozullah AM, Khuri SF, Henderson WG, et al: Development and validation of a multifactorial risk index for predicting postoperative pneumonia after major noncardiac surgery. *Ann Intern Med* 135:847–857, 2001; and Arozullah AM, Daley J, Henderson WG, et al: Multifactorial risk index for predicting postoperative respiratory failure in men after major noncardiac surgery. The National Veterans Administration Surgical Quality Improvement Program. *Ann Surg* 232:242–253, 2000.

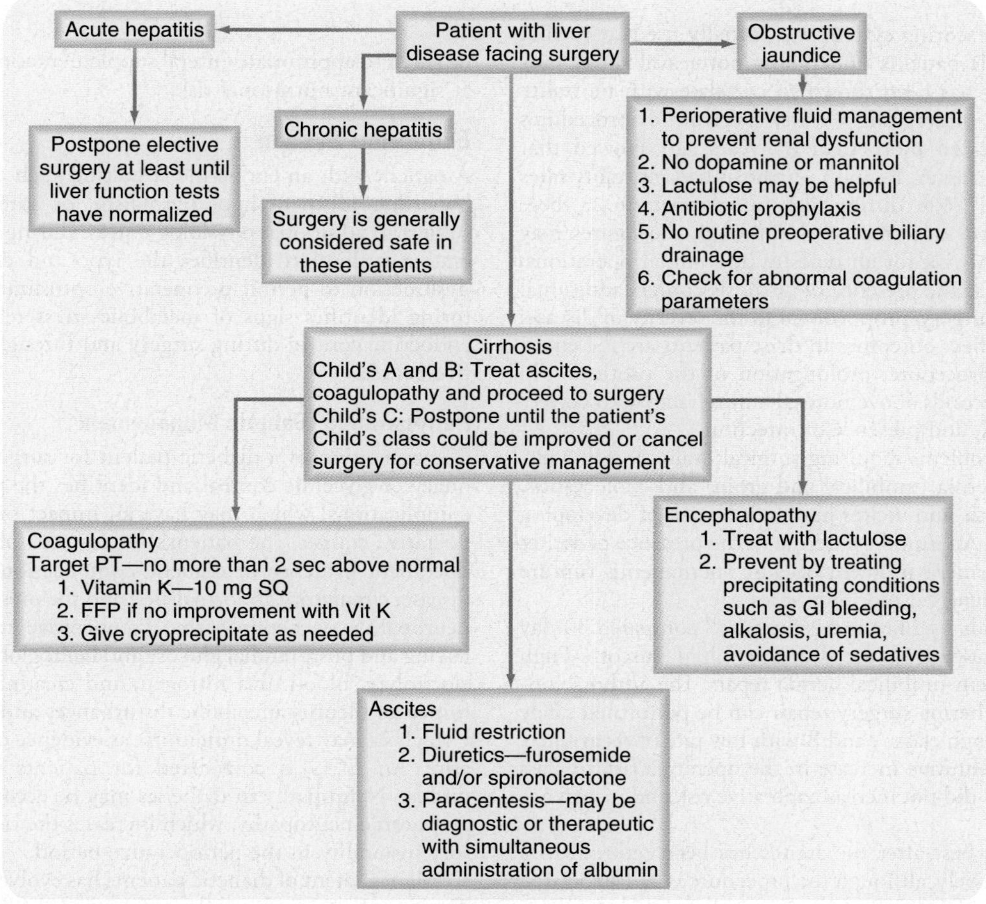

FIGURE 10-2 Approach to a patient with liver disease. *FFP,* fresh-frozen plasma; *GI,* gastrointestinal; *PT,* prothrombin time; *SQ,* subcutaneous. (From Rizvon MK, Chou CL: Surgery in the patient with liver disease. *Med Clin North Am* 87:211–227, 2003.)

greater than 2. Laboratory evidence of chronic hepatitis or clinical findings consistent with cirrhosis is investigated with tests of hepatic synthetic function, notably serum albumin, prothrombin, and fibrinogen levels. Patients with evidence of impaired hepatic synthetic function also have a CBC and serum electrolyte analysis. Type and screen are indicated for any procedure in which blood loss could be more than minimal.

In the event of an emergency situation requiring surgery, such an investigation may be impossible. A patient with acute hepatitis and elevated transaminase levels is managed nonoperatively, when feasible, until several weeks after normalization of laboratory values. Urgent or emergency procedures in these patients are associated with increased morbidity and mortality. A patient with evidence of chronic hepatitis may often safely undergo surgery. A patient with cirrhosis may be assessed with the Child-Pugh classification, which stratifies operative risk according to a score based on abnormal albumin and bilirubin levels, prolongation of the prothrombin time, and degree of ascites and encephalopathy

TABLE 10-10 Child-Pugh Scoring System

PARAMETER	POINTS 1	2	3
Encephalopathy	None	Stage I or II	Stage III or IV
Ascites	Absent	Slight (controlled with diuretics)	Moderate despite diuretic treatment
Bilirubin (mg/dL)	<2	2-3	>3
Albumin (g/liter)	>3.5	2.8-3.5	<2.8
PT (prolonged seconds)	<4	4-6	>6
INR	<1.7	1.7-2.3	>2.3

Class A, 5-6 points; class B, 7-9 points; class C, 10-15 points.
INR, international normalized ratio; *PT*, prothrombin time.

TABLE 10-11 Insulin Types

TYPE OF INSULIN	ONSET OF ACTION	PEAK EFFECT	DURATION OF ACTION
Rapid-acting (lispro, NovoLog, Apidra)	10-30 min	30-90 min	3-4 hr
Short-acting (regular, Humulin, Novolin)	30-60 min	2-5 hr	6-10 hr
Intermediate-acting (NPH, Lente)	1-4 hr	4-12 hr	12-24 hr
Long-acting (glargine [Lantus])	1-2 hr	3-20 hr	24-30 hr

From Ahmed Z, Lockhart CH, Weiner M, et al: Advances in diabetic management: Implications for anesthesia. *Anesth Analg* 100:666–669, 2005.

(Table 10-10). This scoring system was initially used to predict mortality in cirrhotic patients undergoing portacaval shunt procedures, although it has been shown to correlate with mortality in cirrhotic patients undergoing a wider spectrum of procedures as well. Data generated more than 25 years ago showed that patients with Child class A, B, and C cirrhosis had mortality rates of 10%, 31%, and 76% during abdominal operations; these figures were validated more recently.[1] Although the figures may not represent current risk for all types of abdominal operations, little doubt exists that the presence of cirrhosis confers additional risk for abdominal surgery, proportional to the severity of disease. Other factors that affect outcomes in these patients are the emergency nature of a procedure, prolongation of the prothrombin time more than 3 seconds above normal and refractory to correction with vitamin K, and presence of infection.

Two common problems requiring surgical evaluation in a cirrhotic patient are hernia (umbilical and groin) and cholecystitis. Patients with cirrhosis and ascites have a 20% risk of developing an umbilical hernia. An umbilical hernia in the presence of ascites is a difficult management problem because spontaneous rupture is associated with increased mortality rates.

A prospective study by Eker and colleagues[34] compared 30-day mortality among patients in the different Child-Turcotte-Pugh classes who underwent umbilical hernia repair. The authors concluded that elective hernia surgery repair can be performed safely in Child-Turcotte-Pugh class A and B with low rate of recurrence, and there was no definitive increase in the operative risk in class C. Refractory ascites did not increase operative risk and recurrence rate.

Elective repair is best after the ascites has been reduced to a minimum preoperatively, although the procedure is still associated with mortality rates of 14%. Repair of groin hernias in the presence of ascites is less risky in terms of recurrence and mortality. Patients with cirrhosis who have incidental gallstones on ultrasonography should not undergo cholecystectomy unless they are symptomatic. Several reports have shown decreased rates of complications with laparoscopic procedures performed in cirrhotic patients. Among the best-described procedures is laparoscopic cholecystectomy performed in patients with Child class A through C. Compared with open cholecystectomy, lower morbidity in terms of blood loss and wound infection has been observed.[1]

Malnutrition is common in cirrhotic patients and is associated with a reduction in hepatic glycogen stores and reduced hepatic protein synthesis. Patients with advanced liver disease often have a poor appetite, tense ascites, and abdominal pain. Attention must be given to appropriate enteral supplementation, as for all patients at significant nutritional risk.

Endocrine System

A patient with an endocrine condition such as diabetes mellitus, hyperthyroidism or hypothyroidism, or adrenal insufficiency is subject to additional physiologic stress during surgery. The preoperative evaluation identifies the type and degree of endocrine dysfunction to permit preoperative optimization. Careful monitoring identifies signs of metabolic stress related to inadequate endocrine control during surgery and throughout the postoperative course.

Perioperative Diabetic Management

The evaluation of a diabetic patient for surgery assesses the adequacy of glycemic control and identifies the presence of diabetic complications, which may have an impact on the patient's perioperative course. The patient's history and physical examination document evidence of diabetic complications including cardiac disease; circulatory abnormalities; and the presence of retinopathy, neuropathy, or nephropathy. Preoperative testing may include fasting and postprandial glucose and hemoglobin A_{1c} levels. Serum electrolyte, blood urea nitrogen, and creatinine levels are determined to identify metabolic disturbances and renal involvement. Urinalysis may reveal proteinuria as evidence of diabetic nephropathy. An ECG is considered for patients with long-standing disease. Neuropathy in diabetics may be accompanied by cardiac autonomic neuropathy, which increases the risk for cardiorespiratory instability in the perioperative period.

Management of diabetic patients has evolved in the last decade. The introduction of new drugs for non–insulin-dependent diabetes, in addition to new types of insulin and new insulin delivery systems for insulin-dependent diabetes, has changed how these patients are approached in the perioperative period.

Insulin is available in several types and is typically classified by its length of action (Table 10-11). Rapid-acting and short-acting insulin preparations are usually withheld when the patient stops oral intake and are used for acute management of hyperglycemia during the NPO period. Intermediate-acting and long-acting insulin preparations are administered at two thirds the normal evening dose the night before surgery and half the normal morning dose the day of surgery, with frequent bedside glucose determinations and treatment with short-acting insulin as needed. An infusion of 5% dextrose is initiated the morning of surgery.

Insulin pumps are used by some patients as their method of glucose management. These pumps use short-acting insulin (Velosulin) and have a variable delivery rate that can be programmed to simulate endogenous insulin production more closely. On the day of surgery, the patient continues with the basal insulin infusion. The pump is used to correct the glucose level as it is measured. Patients generally have a correction or sensitivity factor that decreases their glucose by 50 mg/dL. It is important to know this factor before the planned surgical procedure so that glucose can be managed in the operating room.[1]

Patients who take oral hypoglycemic agents (sulfonylureas, such as chlorpropamide and glyburide) typically withhold their normal dose the day of surgery. Patients can resume their oral agent when diet is resumed. An exception is metformin. If the patient has altered renal function, this agent needs to be discontinued until renal function normalizes or stabilizes to avoid potential lactic acidosis.[1] Coverage for hyperglycemia is with a short-acting insulin preparation based on blood glucose monitoring.

Management of Other Endocrinopathies

A patient with known or suspected thyroid disease is evaluated with a thyroid function panel; in particular, thyroid-stimulating hormone (TSH) level is measured. Evidence of hyperthyroidism (very low TSH level) is addressed preoperatively, and surgery is deferred until a euthyroid state has been achieved, when feasible. These patients need to have electrolyte levels determined and an ECG performed as part of the preoperative evaluation. In addition, if the physical examination suggests signs of airway compromise from a large goiter, further imaging may be warranted. A patient with hyperthyroidism who takes antithyroid medication such as propylthiouracil or methimazole is instructed to continue this regimen on the day of surgery. The patient's usual doses of beta blockers or digoxin are also continued. In the event of urgent surgery in a thyrotoxic patient at risk for thyroid storm, a combination of adrenergic blockers and glucocorticoids may be required; these are administered in consultation with an endocrinologist. Patients with newly diagnosed hypothyroidism generally do not require preoperative treatment, although they may be subject to increased sensitivity to medications, including anesthetic agents and narcotics. Severe hypothyroidism (high TSH level) can be associated with myocardial dysfunction, coagulation abnormality, and electrolyte imbalance, notably hypoglycemia. Severe hypothyroidism needs to be corrected before elective operations. Hypothyroidism should also be considered in a severely ill patient who is not recovering from surgery in a normal fashion.

A patient with a history of steroid use may require supplementation for a presumed abnormal adrenal response to perioperative stress (Box 10-8). Patients who have taken more than 5 mg of prednisone (or equivalent) per day for more than 3 weeks within the past year are considered at risk when undergoing major surgery. Lower doses of steroid or minor procedures are not generally associated with adrenal suppression.

The adequacy of the hypothalamic-pituitary response to adrenocorticotropic hormone can be tested in any patient who may have some degree of suppression secondary to long-term or intermittent steroid use. A low-dose (1 μg) adrenocorticotropic hormone stimulation test may demonstrate abnormal response to adrenal stimulation and suggest the need for perioperative steroid supplementation. More recent guidelines suggest titrating the dosage of glucocorticoid replacement to the degree of surgical stress (see Box 10-8). Minor operations such as hernia repair under local anesthesia may not require any additional steroid. Moderate operations such as open cholecystectomy or lower extremity revascularization require 50 mg bolus and 75 mg/day of hydrocortisone equivalent for 1 or 2 days. Major operations such as colectomy or cardiac surgery are covered with 100 mg bolus and 150 mg/day of hydrocortisone equivalent for 2 to 3 days. Inadequacy of the hypothalamic-pituitary-adrenal axis in the perioperative period can lead to unexplained hypotension.

BOX 10-8 Perioperative Supplemental Glucocorticoid Regimens

No HPAA Suppression

<5 mg of prednisone or equivalent/day for any duration

Alternate-day single morning dose of short-acting glucocorticoid of any dose or duration

Any dose of glucocorticoid for <3 wk

Treatment: Give usual daily glucocorticoid dose during perioperative period

HPAA Suppression Documented or Presumed

>20 mg of prednisone or equivalent/day for ≥3 wk

Cushingoid appearance

Biochemical adrenal insufficiency on a low-dose ACTH stimulation test

Minor procedures or local anesthesia

Treatment: Give usual glucocorticoid dose before surgery

No supplementation unless signs or symptoms of adrenal insufficiency, then 25 mg hydrocortisone IV

Moderate surgical stress

Treatment: 50 mg hydrocortisone IV before induction of anesthesia, 25 mg hydrocortisone every 8 hr thereafter for 24-48 hr, then resume usual dose

Major surgical stress

Treatment: 100 mg hydrocortisone IV before induction of anesthesia, 50 mg hydrocortisone every 8 hr thereafter for 48-72 hr, then resume usual dose

HPAA Suppression Uncertain

5-20 mg of prednisone or its equivalent for ≥3 wk

≥5 mg of prednisone or its equivalent for ≥3 wk in the year before surgery

Minor procedures or local anesthesia

Treatment: Give usual glucocorticoid dose before surgery

No supplementation

Moderate or major surgical stress

Check low-dose ACTH stimulation test to determine HPAA suppression, *or*

Give supplemental glucocorticoids as though suppressed.

Adapted from Schiff RL, Welsh GA: Perioperative evaluation and management of the patient with endocrine dysfunction. *Med Clin North Am* 87:175–192, 2003; and Kohl BA, Schwartz S: Surgery in the patient with endocrine dysfunction. *Med Clin North Am* 93:1031–1047, 2009.

ACTH, adrenocorticotropic hormone; *HPAA*, hypothalamic-pituitary-adrenal axis; *IV*, intravenously.

Patients with pheochromocytoma require preoperative pharmacologic management to prevent intraoperative hypertensive crises or hypotension leading to cardiovascular collapse. The state of catecholamine excess associated with pheochromocytoma is controlled by a combination of α-adrenergic and β-adrenergic blockade before surgery. To achieve adequate therapeutic effect by alpha blockade, 1 to 2 weeks is generally required; this can be accomplished with a nonselective agent such as phenoxybenzamine or a selective α_1-adrenergic agent such as prazosin. Alpha blockade usually uncovers a vascular volume deficit that is not apparent clinically. In addition, patients have generally been placed on a sodium-restricted diet as part of hypertension management. Liberalization of sodium in the diet may aid in replenishing plasma volume. Beta blockade is initiated several days after the α-adrenergic agent is begun and serves to inhibit the tachycardia that accompanies nonselective alpha blockade and to control arrhythmia. Patients with pheochromocytoma may undergo surgery when pharmacologic blood pressure control is achieved.

Immune System

The approach to a patient with suspected immunosuppression is the same, regardless of whether this state results from antineoplastic drugs in a cancer patient or immunosuppressive therapy in a transplant patient or is the result of advanced disease in a patient with AIDS. The goal is to optimize immunologic function before surgery and to minimize the risk for infection and wound breakdown.

Preoperative assessment includes the following: A thorough history is obtained, including the patient's underlying disease and current functional status; a history of immunosuppressive treatment, including names of medications and duration of treatment; and a history of recent changes in weight. The physical examination documents signs of organ dysfunction that may underlie progression of the disease or be related to its treatment. Laboratory assessment includes a CBC with differential and platelet count, electrolyte determination, and liver function tests; an ECG and a chest radiograph are obtained when age or physical findings suggest risk. Possible sites of infection must be investigated, including examination of any indwelling catheters, and a complete workup of any suspected infectious focus may be warranted. Additional studies of T cell, B cell, polymorphonuclear, or complement function may be helpful to delineate the degree of immune system compromise. Neutropenia, anemia, or thrombocytopenia may accompany the underlying disease process or result from treatment of the condition with immunosuppressive medication. Decisions regarding red blood cell transfusion or the use of synthetic erythropoietin or colony-stimulating factors are often based on the degree of dysfunction and other patient risk factors. Careful attention is paid to nutritional deficiency in this patient population, with supplementation indicated in the perioperative period. Appropriate antibiotic prophylaxis is critical.

Immunocompromised patients may be at risk for wound complications, especially if they are receiving exogenous steroid therapy. When taken within 3 days of surgery, steroids reduce the degree of wound inflammation, epithelialization, and collagen synthesis, which can lead to wound breakdown and infection. In addition, patients receiving sirolimus as part of their antirejection protocol can have difficulties with wound healing, so this drug should be discontinued if possible before operation.

HIV-Infected Patients and Surgery

As morbidity and mortality continue to decrease with improved medical management of HIV infection, more HIV-infected patients are requiring surgery. It is important to understand how the agents used to treat HIV affect the patient during surgery.

HIV treatment involves antiretroviral drugs from one of four classes: protease inhibitors, fusion inhibitors, nucleoside reverse transcriptase inhibitors, and non-nucleoside reverse transcriptase inhibitors. These agents are not immunosuppressive agents but work directly on the pathway of HIV cell integration and reproduction. For this reason, they do not have a significant effect on wound healing or infection rates. The patient's white blood cell count or, more specifically, the absolute neutrophil count, in addition to the direct HIV titer, is more predictive of postoperative complications. Lactic acidosis as a result of mitochondrial toxicity is one specific finding with nucleoside reverse transcriptase inhibitors.[1] This condition needs to be added to the differential diagnosis of a critically ill patient with known HIV infection who has a persistently elevated lactate concentration. Hypoperfusion is ruled out initially, but drug complication needs to be investigated. Treatment is discontinuation of the agent.

Hematologic System

Hematologic assessment may lead to the identification of disorders such as anemia, inherited or acquired coagulopathy, or a hypercoagulable state. Substantial morbidity may result from failure to identify these abnormalities preoperatively. The need for perioperative prophylaxis for VTE must be carefully reviewed in every surgical patient.

Anemia is the most common laboratory abnormality encountered in preoperative patients. It is often asymptomatic and may require further investigation to understand its cause. The history and physical examination may uncover subjective symptoms of energy loss, dyspnea, or palpitations, and pallor or cyanosis may be evident. Patients are evaluated for lymphadenopathy, hepatomegaly, or splenomegaly, and pelvic and rectal examinations are performed. A CBC; reticulocyte count; and serum iron, total iron-binding capacity, ferritin, vitamin B_{12}, and folate levels are obtained to investigate the cause of anemia. Preoperative treatment and optimization are appropriate for an anemic patient. Transfusion guidelines have been published by different societies. In general, transfusion is not indicated in a hemodynamically stable patient with hemoglobin greater than 10 g/dL and no signs of active bleeding. However, the lower threshold for transfusion varies from 6 g/dL to 8 g/dL. The AABB (formerly the American Association of Blood Banks) developed a guideline to provide clinical recommendations about hemoglobin concentration thresholds and other clinical variables that trigger red blood cell transfusions in hemodynamically stable patients.[35]

The AABB recommends adhering to a restrictive transfusion strategy. In adult and pediatric patients in the ICU, transfusion should be considered at hemoglobin concentrations of 7 g/dL or less. In postoperative surgical patients, transfusion should be considered at hemoglobin concentrations of 8 g/dL or less or for symptoms (chest pain, orthostatic hypotension, tachycardia unresponsive to fluid resuscitation, or congestive heart failure). A Cochrane systematic review and a meta-analysis of clinical trials suggested a restrictive policy of transfusion at a hemoglobin concentration of 7 to 8 g/dL in most patients.[36,37]

The use of transfusion thresholds is safe in most patient populations, and they may improve clinical outcomes, while reducing unnecessary transfusion. However, every patient should be assessed clinically. For patients in the ICU, including patients with septic shock, blood transfusion is recommended to maintain hemoglobin at greater than 7 g/dL rather than a higher threshold. An individualized approach is necessary in patients with acute coronary syndromes. In patients with symptoms or ongoing ischemia, it is recommended to maintain hemoglobin at 10 g/dL or greater.[38]

Acute Bleeding and Trauma

Acute bleeding is a challenging clinical setting for evaluating red cell transfusion thresholds. For patients with massive bleeding or hemodynamic instability, transfusion should be guided by the severity of the bleeding and the ability to control the

TABLE 10-12 Decisional Criteria for Transfusion in Acute Anemia

CLASS OF HEMORRHAGE	PERCENTAGE REDUCTION IN BLOOD VOLUME	mL*	INDICATION FOR TRANSFUSION OF RBCs	GoR
I	<15%	<750	Unnecessary, unless preexisting anemia	2C+
II	15%-30%	750-1500	Unnecessary, unless preexisting anemia or cardiopulmonary disease	2C+
III	30%-40%	1500-2000	Probably necessary	2C+
IV	>40%	>2000	Necessary	2C+

From Liumbruno G, Bennardello F, Lattanzio A, et al: Recommendations for the transfusion of red blood cells. *Blood Transfus* 7:49–64, 2009.
GoR, grade of recommendation; *RBC,* red blood cell.
*In an adult weighing 70 kg with a circulatory volume of 5000 mL.

bleeding. Use of massive transfusions in hemodynamically unstable patients cannot be guided by hemoglobin levels alone and often cannot be delayed by interval measurements of hemoglobin (Table 10-12).

All patients undergoing surgery are questioned to assess their bleeding risk. Coagulopathy may result from inherited or acquired platelet or factor disorders or may be associated with organ dysfunction or medications. The inquiry begins with direct questioning about a personal or family history of abnormal bleeding. Supporting information includes a history of easy bruising or abnormal bleeding associated with minor procedures or injury. A history of liver or kidney dysfunction or recent common bile duct obstruction needs to be elicited, and an assessment of nutritional status must be done. Medications are carefully reviewed, and the use of anticoagulants, salicylates, NSAIDs, and antiplatelet drugs is noted. Physical examination may reveal bruising, petechiae, or signs of liver dysfunction. Patients with thrombocytopenia may have qualitative or quantitative defects as a result of immune-related disease, infection, drugs, or liver or kidney dysfunction. Qualitative defects may respond to medical management of the underlying disease process, whereas quantitative defects may require platelet transfusion when counts are less than 50,000/mL in a patient at risk for bleeding. Coagulation studies are not routinely ordered, but patients with a history suggestive of coagulopathy should undergo coagulation studies before surgery. Coagulation studies are also done before the procedure if considerable bleeding is anticipated or any significant bleeding would be catastrophic. Patients with documented disorders of coagulation may require perioperative management of factor deficiencies, often in consultation with a hematologist.

Antiplatelet Management in Noncardiac Surgery Patients

The value of aspirin in preventing ischemic complications in patients without stents is unclear. Aspirin use was associated with an increased risk of major perioperative bleeding. Aspirin continuation may still be reasonable in patients with high-risk coronary artery disease or cerebrovascular disease, in which the risks of potential cardiovascular events outweigh the risks of perioperative bleeding. Antiplatelet management in patients with PCI and noncardiac surgery has always been challenging. Discontinuation of dual antiplatelet therapy in the early period after stent implantation is a strong risk factor for stent thrombosis. Should urgent or emergency noncardiac surgery be required, a decision to continue aspirin or dual antiplatelet therapy should be individualized, with the risk weighed against the benefits of continuing therapy. New practice guidelines advise that elective noncardiac surgery be delayed for at least 30 days after BMS implantation and at least 12 months after DES implantation. Independently of the time frame between DES implantation and surgery, single antiplatelet therapy (preferably with aspirin) should be continued (Fig. 10-3).[16,39]

Anticoagulation Management in Noncardiac Surgery Patients

The management of anticoagulation in patients undergoing surgical procedures is challenging because interrupting anticoagulation transiently increases the risk of a thromboembolism event. However, surgery and invasive procedures have associated bleeding risks that are increased by anticoagulants administered for prevention of thromboembolism. A balance between reducing the risk of thromboembolism and preventing excessive bleeding must be assessed clinically for the individual patient. Additionally, the specific anticoagulant used must be considered. For patients taking a vitamin K antagonist (VKA) (e.g., warfarin), it takes several days to reduce the anticoagulant effect and then to reestablish it postoperatively. The newer target-specific oral anticoagulants (e.g., direct thrombin inhibitor dabigatran and factor Xa inhibitors rivaroxaban, edoxaban, apixaban) have shorter half-lives and are easier to discontinue and resume rapidly preoperatively. However, they lack a specific antidote or reversal strategy.

The American College of Chest Physicians Evidence-Based Clinical Practice Guidelines (2012) addresses the management of patients who are receiving anticoagulant or antiplatelet therapy and require an elective surgery or procedure.[1] The Guidelines recommend stopping VKAs 5 days before elective surgery in patients requiring a VKA for various reasons. Stopping a VKA allows the international normalized ratio to fall to the range of 1.5 or less, assuming that the patient is maintained at an international normalized ratio of 2.0 to 3.0. For all patients but those undergoing procedures that carry a high risk of postoperative bleeding, warfarin can be restarted the day of or day after surgery because it takes up to five doses to become therapeutic.

Additional recommendations for specific diagnoses requiring long-term anticoagulation are based on risk-benefit analysis. Bridging anticoagulation is recommended during VKA interruption only in patients with a mechanical heart valve, atrial fibrillation, stroke or transient ischemic attack, acute arterial embolism, or VTE at high risk for thromboembolism. This bridging may be achieved by therapeutic dose low-molecular-weight heparin (LMWH) or perioperative intravenous heparinization. For patients taking LMWH, it is recommended to give the last dose 24 hours before surgery and restart approximately 48 to 72 hours postoperatively. For patients requiring systemic heparinization, it should be stopped within 6 hours of surgery and restarted within 12 to 24 hours postoperatively. For patients undergoing procedures with a high risk of postoperative bleeding or in which large surfaces have been dissected, one should consider using prophylactic-dose LMWH for the dosing regimen for several days and then switch

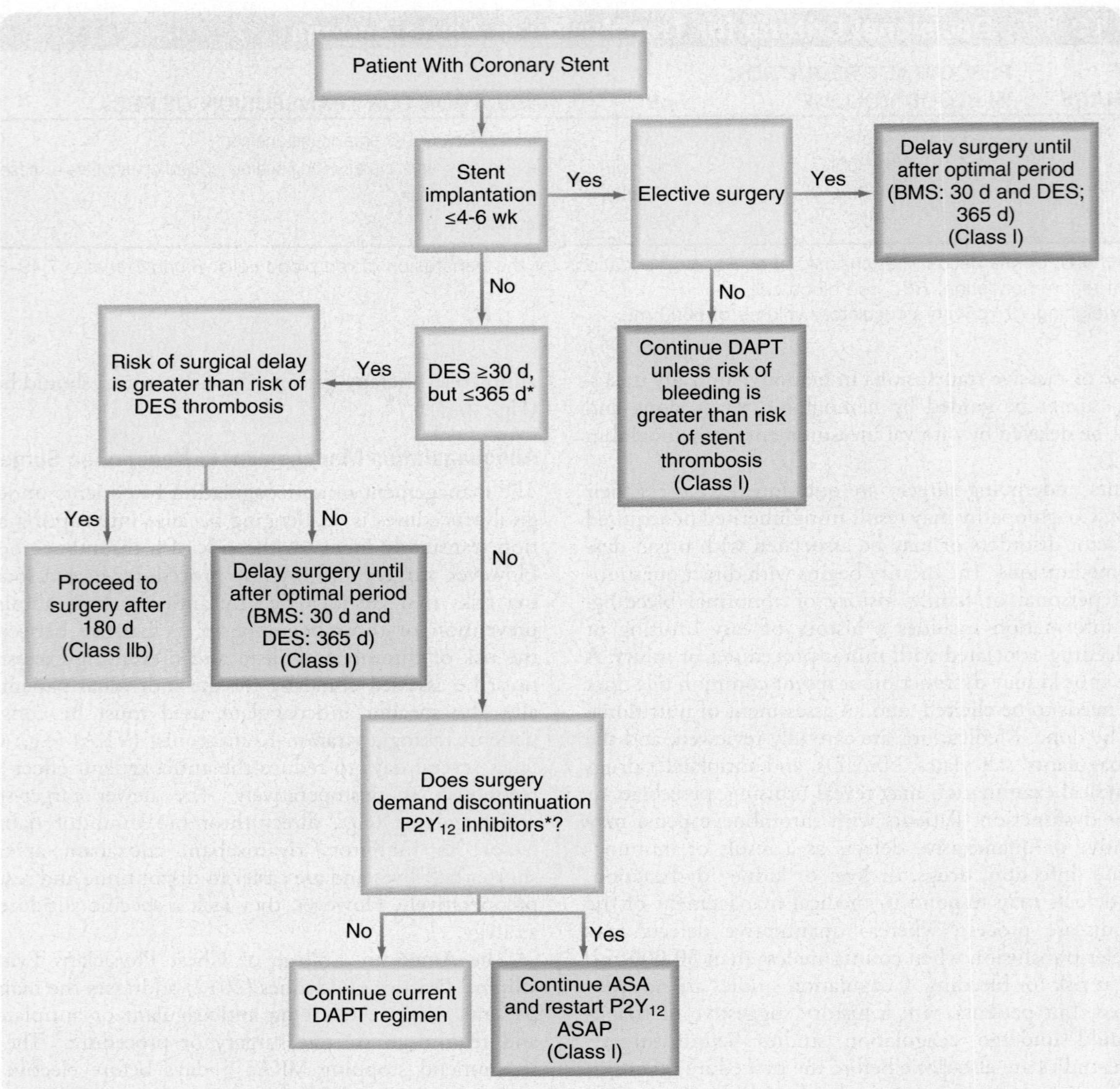

FIGURE 10-3 Algorithm for antiplatelet management in patients with percutaneous coronary intervention and noncardiac surgery. *Assuming patient is currently on dual antiplatelet therapy (DAPT). *ASA,* aspirin; *ASAP,* as soon as possible; *BMS,* bare-metal stent; *DES,* drug-eluting stent. (From Fleisher LA, Fleischmann KE, Auerbach AD, et al: 2014 ACC/AHA guideline on perioperative cardiovascular evaluation and management of patients undergoing noncardiac surgery: A report of the American College of Cardiology/American Heart Association Task Force on Practice Guidelines. *J Am Coll Cardiol* 64:e77–e137, 2014.)

back to therapeutic dosing. When possible, surgery is postponed in the first month after an episode of VTE or arterial thromboembolism. Patients taking anticoagulants for less than 2 weeks for PE or DVT or patients for whom the risk of perioperative bleeding is high should be considered for retrievable inferior vena cava filter placement before surgery (Table 10-13).

In moderate-risk to high-risk patients who are receiving acetylsalicylic acid and require noncardiac surgery, continuing acetylsalicylic acid around the time of surgery is suggested instead of stopping acetylsalicylic acid 7 to 10 days before surgery. In patients with a coronary stent who require surgery, deferring surgery for more than 6 weeks after BMS placement and for more than 6 months after DES placement is highly recommended. In patients requiring surgery within 6 weeks of BMS placement or within 6 months of DES placement, continuing antiplatelet therapy perioperatively is highly recommended.

Oral Direct Thrombin and Factor Xa Inhibitors[40]

Dabigatran

Dabigatran (Pradaxa) is a direct thrombin inhibitor. It prevents thrombus development through direct, competitive inhibition of thrombin in converting fibrinogen to fibrin (factor IIa). A dose adjustment is required in patient with renal insufficiency. If possible, dabigatran should be discontinued 1 to 2 days (creatinine clearance ≥50 mL/min) or 3 to 5 days (creatinine clearance <50 mL/min) before invasive or surgical procedures because of the increased risk of bleeding. Drug discontinuation for a longer time should be considered for patients undergoing major surgery,

TABLE 10-13 Recommendations for Perioperative Management of Patients on Long-Term Anticoagulation

INDICATION FOR LONG-TERM ANTICOAGULATION	PATIENT CHARACTERISTICS	PERIOPERATIVE MANAGEMENT
Prosthetic heart valves	High risk Recent (<6 mo) stroke or TIA Any mitral valve Caged ball or tilting disc aortic valve	Strongly recommend bridging
	Moderate risk—bileaflet aortic valve with ≥2 risk factors for stroke*	Consider bridging based on individual
	Low risk—bileaflet aortic valve with <2 risk factors for stroke*	No bridging
Chronic atrial fibrillation	High risk Recent (within 3 mo) stroke or TIA Rheumatic valvular heart disease	Strongly recommend bridging
	Moderate risk—chronic atrial fibrillation with ≥2 risk factors for stroke*	Consider bridging
	Low risk—chronic atrial fibrillation with <2 risk factors for stroke*	No bridging
VTE	High risk Recent (≤3 mo) VTE Severe thrombophilia (e.g., deficiency of protein C, protein S, or antithrombin; antiphospholipid antibody†) Major comorbid disease (cardiac or pulmonary)	Strongly recommend bridging
	Moderate risk VTE within the past 3-12 mo Recurrent VTE Nonsevere thrombophilia (e.g., heterozygous factor V Leiden or prothrombin gene mutation) Active cancer (treated within 6 mo or palliative)	Consider bridging
	Low risk—VTE >12 mo previous and no other risk factor	No bridging

From Douketis JD, Spyropoulos AC, Spencer FA, et al: Perioperative management of antithrombotic therapy: Antithrombotic Therapy and Prevention of Thrombosis, 9th ed: American College of Chest Physicians Evidence-Based Clinical Practice Guidelines. *Chest* 141:e326S–350S, 2012.
TIA, transient ischemic attack; *VTE,* venous thromboembolism.
*Risk factors for stroke include atrial fibrillation, previous stroke, TIA, or systemic embolism; age >75 yr; hypertension, diabetes mellitus, left ventricular dysfunction.
†Antiphospholipid antibodies—anticardiolipin antibody, lupus anticoagulant.

spinal puncture, or placement of a spinal or epidural catheter or port, in whom complete hemostasis may be required. Dabigatran may be restarted promptly after surgery. There is no routine coagulation test to evaluate dabigatran coagulation effect. A normal or near-normal activated partial thromboplastin time may be used in selected patients to evaluate blood clearance before surgery. Dabigatran is approved in the United States for stroke prevention in nonvalvular atrial fibrillation and is being reviewed for secondary prevention of VTE.

Rivaroxaban

Rivaroxaban (Xarelto) is a highly selective direct factor Xa inhibitor in converting prothrombin to thrombin with oral bioavailability and rapid onset of action. Given the partial renal elimination of rivaroxaban, dosing adjustments are required in renal insufficiency. It can be discontinued approximately 2 to 3 days before a procedure. There is no routine coagulation test at the present time to evaluate rivaroxaban anticoagulant effect. A normal or near-normal anti–factor Xa activity level may be used in selected patients to evaluate the drug blood clearance before surgery. Rivaroxaban is approved in the United States for VTE prevention after major orthopedic surgery and for stroke prevention in atrial fibrillation and is approved in Europe and Canada for secondary prevention of VTE.

Apixaban

Apixaban (Eliquis) is a highly selective oral direct factor Xa inhibitor in converting prothrombin to thrombin. Because apixaban is predominately eliminated by nonrenal mechanisms, dose adjustment is likely not required in moderate renal dysfunction, although use in patients with severe renal insufficiency (creatinine clearance <15 mL/min) or dialysis dependence is not recommended. There are no data available at the present time to guide the use of apixaban in elderly patients, patients with extremes of body weight, or patients with hepatic insufficiency. It can be discontinued approximately 2 to 3 days before a procedure. There is no routine coagulation test to evaluate apixaban coagulation effect. A normal or near-normal anti–factor Xa activity level may be used in selected patients to evaluate blood clearance before surgery. Apixaban is approved by the U.S. Food and Drug Administration for stroke prevention in patients with atrial fibrillation and is approved in Europe for VTE prevention after major orthopedic surgery.

Venous Thromboembolism Prophylaxis in Surgical Patients

VTE is a common cause of preventable death in hospitalized patients. All surgical patients should be assessed for VTE risk. In patients undergoing general and abdominopelvic surgery, the risk of VTE varies depending on patient-specific and

TABLE 10-14 **Caprini Risk Assessment Model for Venous Thromboembolism in General Surgical Patients**

1 POINT	2 POINTS	3 POINTS	4 POINTS
Age 41-60 yr	Age 61-74 yr	Age ≥75 yr	Stroke <1 mo
BMI >25 kg/m^2	Arthroscopic surgery	Prior episodes of VTE	Fracture of hip, pelvis, or leg
Minor surgery	Laparoscopy >45 min	Family history for VTE	Elective arthroplasty
Edema in the lower extremities	Major open surgery >45 min	Prothrombin 20210 A	Acute spinal cord injury <1 mo
Varicose veins	Cancer	Factor V Leiden	
Pregnancy or postpartum	Plaster cast	Lupus anticoagulants	
Oral contraceptive	Bed bound for >72 hr	Anticardiolipin antibodies	
Hormonal therapy	Central venous access	High homocysteine in the blood	
Unexplained or recurrent abortion		Heparin-induced thrombocytopenia	
Sepsis (<1 mo)		Other congenital or acquired thrombophilia	
Serious lung disease such as pneumonia (<1 mo)			
Abnormal pulmonary function test			
Acute myocardial infarction			
Congestive heart failure (<1 mo)			
Bed rest			
Inflammatory bowel disease			

From Caprini JA: Thrombosis risk assessment as a guide to quality patient care. *Dis Mon* 51:70–78, 2005; and Bahl V, Hu HM, Henke PK, et al: A validation study of a retrospective venous thromboembolism risk scoring method. *Ann Surg* 251:344–350, 2010.
BMI, body mass index; *VTE,* venous thromboembolism.

procedure-specific factors. Patient risk factor stratification is achieved by considering many factors such as age older than 60 years, prior VTE, anesthesia lasting 2 or more hours, and bed rest lasting 4 or more days; older age, male sex, longer length of hospital stay, and higher Charlson Comorbidity Score[41]; and sepsis, pregnancy or postpartum state, central venous access, malignancy, and inpatient hospital stay longer than 2 days. Examples of relatively low-risk procedures include laparoscopic cholecystectomy, appendectomy, transurethral prostatectomy, inguinal herniorrhaphy, and unilateral or bilateral mastectomy. Open-abdominal and open-pelvic procedures are associated with a higher risk of VTE. Patients undergoing abdominal or pelvic surgery for cancer have the highest risk of VTE.

The American College of Chest Physicians Evidence-Based Clinical Practice Guidelines (2012)[42] recommend using the Caprini Risk Assessment Model or risk assessment model from the Patient Safety in Surgery Study (Rogers score) as a guide for decision making. The Caprini score estimates VTE risk by adding points for various VTE risk factors, as shown in Table 10-14.[43,44] In the published American College of Chest Physicians guidelines, VTE risk is categorized as being very low (0 to 1 point), low (2 points), moderate (3 to 4 points), or high (≥5 points). This model is relatively easy to use and appears to discriminate reasonably well among patients at low, moderate, and high risk for VTE. The risk assessment model from the Patient Safety in Surgery Study is shown in Table 10-15.[45] This model assigned points (Rogers score) to variables that were found to be independent predictors of VTE risk, including type of operation, work relative value units, patient characteristics, and laboratory values (see Table 10-15). Using this model, the risk of symptomatic VTE varied from very low (0.1%) to low (approximately 0.5%) to moderate (approximately 1.5%) in development and validation samples.

Current guidelines related to VTE prophylaxis in adult surgical patients undergoing nonorthopedic abdominal and pelvic procedures are shown in Table 10-16. Numerous regimens may be appropriate for prophylaxis of VTE, depending on assessed risk coupled with the perceived risk of perioperative bleeding, including early ambulation, application of intermittent compression devices, and use of unfractionated heparin or LMWH. Initial prophylactic doses of heparin can be given preoperatively, within 2 hours of surgery, and with compression devices in place before induction of anesthesia.

Optimal thromboprophylaxis in nonorthopedic surgical patients considers the risks of VTE and bleeding complications as well as the values and preferences of individual patients. There are various relative contraindications for pharmacologic anticoagulation, such as presence of active hemorrhage; thrombocytopenia; hypertensive crisis; and recent intracranial, intraocular, or spinal surgery. Mechanical prophylaxis (intermittent pneumatic compression) is relatively contraindicated in the presence of leg edema more than 3+; pulmonary edema; severe peripheral vascular disease; and local condition of the leg, which may be worsened by a compression sleeve.

Neuraxial blockade (spinal or epidural anesthesia) is not a contraindication for pharmacologic thromboprophylaxis if the medication is used in an adequate time interval. However, neuraxial blockade should be avoided in patients with a clinical bleeding disorder because of the rare but serious complication of perispinal hematoma.

ADDITIONAL PREOPERATIVE CONSIDERATIONS

Nutritional Status

Evaluation of the patient's nutritional status is part of the preoperative evaluation. BMI less than 18.5 kg/m^2, serum albumin less than 3 g/dL, and unintentional weight loss greater than 10% to 15% over a 6-month period are significant findings. Assessing protein status is particularly important in surgical patients and is affected by oral intake, gastrointestinal absorption, muscle mass, duration of current illness, or infection. The degree of malnutrition is estimated on the basis of weight loss, physical findings, and plasma protein level assessment. The adequacy of a nutritional regimen can be confirmed with many serum markers. These serum components do not directly indicate nutritional status, but they

TABLE 10-15 Risk Assessment Model from the Patient Safety in Surgery Study

FACTOR	RISK SCORE POINTS
Operation type other than endocrine	
Respiratory and hernia	9
Thoracoabdominal aneurysm, embolectomy/thrombectomy, venous reconstruction, and endovascular repair	7
Aneurysm	4
Mouth, palate	4
Stomach, intestines	4
Integument	3
Hernia	2
ASA physical status classification	
III, IV, or V	2
2	1
Female sex	1
Work RVUs	
>17	3
10-17	2
2 points for each of the following conditions	2
Disseminated cancer	
Chemotherapy for malignancy within 30 days of operation	
Preoperative serum sodium >145 mmol/liter	
Transfusion >4 units packed RBCs 72 hr before operation	
Ventilator dependent	
1 point for each of the following conditions	1
Wound class (clean/contaminated)	
Preoperative hematocrit level ≤38%	
Preoperative bilirubin level >1.0 mg/dL	
Dyspnea	
Albumin level ≤3.5 mg/dL	
Emergency	
0 points for each of the following conditions	0
ASA physical status class I	
Work RVUs <10	
Male sex	

From Rogers SO, Jr, Kilaru RK, Hosokawa P, et al: Multivariable predictors of postoperative venous thromboembolic events after general and vascular surgery: Results from the patient safety in surgery study. *J Am Coll Surg* 204:1211–1221, 2007.
ASA, American Society of Anesthesiologists; *RBC*, red blood cell; *RVU*, relative value unit.

reflect the severity of illness and may be used in conjunction with other clinical findings. Albumin (longest half-life, 18 to 20 days), transferrin (intermediate half-life, 8 to 9 days), and prealbumin (transthyretin; shortest half-life, 2 to 3 days) levels can be determined on a regular basis in hospitalized patients. Low serum albumin (<2.2 g/dL) is a marker of a negative catabolic state and is a predictor of poor outcome.[46]

Serum transferrin reflects protein status and iron storage in the body. A low transferrin level should be considered an indicator of protein deficiency only in the setting of a normal serum iron study. Serum prealbumin responds quickly to the onset of malnutrition, and the level increases rapidly with adequate protein intake. However, in the setting of acute or chronic inflammation or renal or hepatic disease, prealbumin level is affected and is not helpful for assessing overall nutritional status.

These proteins are responsive to stress conditions, and their synthesis may be inhibited in the immediate perioperative period. When a patient is on a stable regimen and in the anabolic phase of recovery, these markers reflect the adequacy of nutritional efforts. The effect of perioperative nutritional support on outcomes has been studied in many trials. Patients with severe malnutrition—as defined by a combination of weight loss, visceral protein indicators, and prognostic indices—appear to benefit most from preoperative nutrition (enteral, if possible). Well-nourished patients undergoing surgery do not appear to benefit from aggressive perioperative nutritional support. Generally, nutritional support begins within 7 to 10 days after surgery in patients unable to resume their normal diet. The exception is trauma victims (including burn victims), who, because of their persistent catabolic state, benefit from much earlier initiation of nutritional support if it is anticipated that they will be unable to manage oral intake within a few days.

Nutritional Interventions

Nutritional interventions may include oral supplementation, enteral (tube) feeding, or parenteral (intravenous) feeding. For all patients, an enteral route of feeding is preferred because of safety, relative simplicity, reduced complications, lower cost, and the ability to maintain mucosal barrier function. However, in circumstances in which the patient cannot tolerate enteral feeds or they are contraindicated, the parenteral route is used.

Early postoperative enteral feeding may decrease the incidence of infectious complications and is a component of most enhanced recovery after surgery (ERAS) protocols.[47] ERAS, also known as "fast-track" programs, is the evidence-based care protocol developed by the ERAS Society. It is designed to standardize medical care to reduce health care costs and improve overall outcomes. The ERAS protocol describes the perioperative care pathway with recommendations for patient care at various steps in the perioperative process. Approximately 20 care elements have been shown to influence care time and postoperative complications.

Preoperative pathway strategies include preadmission counseling; fluid and carbohydrate loading; antibiotic prophylaxis; thromboprophylaxis; and elimination of prolonged fasting, mechanical bowel preparation, or premedication. Fasting policies are in place to reduce the risk of aspiration of gastric contents during a general anesthetic. Practice guidelines have been established by the ASA for preoperative fasting. Recommendations are 8 hours or more fasting after intake of fried or fatty foods or meat and 6 hours or more fasting after ingestion of a light meal, nonhuman milk, or infant formula. The ASA recommends fasting at least 2 hours from clear liquid intake, including medicines.[48] This approach to fasting helps to avoid symptoms of dehydration, hypoglycemia, or caffeine withdrawal. Many fast-track protocols suggest a carbohydrate-rich drink 2 hours before surgery in order to convert the patient from the "fasted" to the "fed" state causing reduction in postoperative insulin resistance. There is limited evidence to support carbohydrate-rich drinks in patients undergoing elective colon surgery.

Intraoperative strategies include maintenance of normothermia (body warmer/warm intravenous fluids) and use of short-acting anesthetic agents, midthoracic epidural anesthesia, fluid management, and minimally invasive surgical techniques. Postoperative strategies include prevention and relief of pain especially with nonopioid oral analgesia; avoidance of nasogastric tube placement, nausea and vomiting, or fluid overload; and early mobilization, urinary catheter removal, and enteral nutrition.

TABLE 10-16 Venous Thromboembolism Prophylaxis Guidelines in Adult Surgical Patients*

VTE RISK CATEGORY	LOW BLEEDING RISK	HIGH RISK FOR MAJOR BLEEDING
Very low risk (0.5%; Caprini score 0, Roger score <7)	Early ambulation	Early ambulation
Low risk (~1.5%; Caprini score 1-2, Rogers score, 7-10)	Mechanical prophylaxis (IPC)	IPC
Moderate risk (~3.0%; Caprini score 3-4, Rogers score >10)	LMWH or LDUH *or* IPC	IPC
High risk (~6.0%; Caprini score ≥5)	LMWH or LDUH *and* mechanical prophylaxis with elastic stockings *or* IPC	IPC until risk of bleeding diminishes and pharmacologic thromboprophylaxis can be initiated
High risk (~6.0%; with contraindications to LMWH/UFH)	Low-dose aspirin, fondaparinux or mechanical prophylaxis with IPC	IPC until risk of bleeding diminishes and pharmacologic thromboprophylaxis can be initiated
Cancer surgery (abdominal/pelvic cancers)	Extended-duration pharmacologic prophylaxis (4 wk) with LMWH	

From Gould MK, Garcia DA, Wren SM, et al: Prevention of VTE in nonorthopedic surgical patients: Antithrombotic Therapy and Prevention of Thrombosis, 9th ed: American College of Chest Physicians Evidence-Based Clinical Practice Guidelines. *Chest* 141:e227S–277S, 2012.
IPC, intermittent pneumatic compression; *LDUH,* low-dose unfractionated heparin; *LMWH,* low-molecular-weight heparin; *UFH,* unfractionated heparin; *VTE,* venous thromboembolism.
*Nonorthopedic general and abdominal pelvic surgery including gastrointestinal, genitourinary, bariatric, vascular, reconstructive, cardiothoracic, and gynecologic surgery hospitalized surgical patients.

Fast-track programs suggest starting a clear liquid diet within a few hours after surgery, followed by high-calorie drinks to minimize the negative protein balance postoperatively.

Obesity

The perioperative mortality rate is significantly increased in patients with clinically severe obesity (BMI >40 kg/m^2 or >35 kg/m^2 with significant comorbid conditions). The goal of preoperative evaluation of an obese patient is to identify risk factors that might modify perioperative care of the patient. Clinically severe obesity is associated with a higher frequency of essential hypertension, pulmonary hypertension, left ventricular hypertrophy, congestive heart failure, and ischemic heart disease. Obese patients are at increased risk for adverse cardiovascular events at the time of noncardiac surgery. The AHA has recommended performing at least a chest radiograph and a 12-lead ECG in all obese patients with at least one risk factor for coronary heart disease (diabetes, smoking, hypertension, or hyperlipidemia) or poor exercise tolerance. Obesity is also a risk factor for postoperative wound infection. The rate of wound infections is much lower with laparoscopic surgery in this group, which could have a bearing on selection of the operative approach. Obesity is an independent risk factor for DVT and PE, and appropriate prophylaxis is instituted in obese patients.

PREOPERATIVE CHECKLIST

The preoperative evaluation concludes with a review of all pertinent studies and information obtained from investigative tests. This review is documented in the chart, which represents an opportunity to ensure that all necessary and pertinent data have been obtained and appropriately interpreted. Informed consent after discussion with the patient and family members regarding the indication for the anticipated surgical procedure and its risks and proposed benefits is documented in the chart. The preoperative checklist also gives the surgeon an opportunity to review the need for beta blockade, DVT prophylaxis, and prophylactic antibiotics.

Preoperative orders are written and reviewed. The patient receives written instructions regarding the time of surgery and management of special perioperative issues such as fasting, bowel preparation, and medication use.

Antibiotic Prophylaxis

Appropriate antibiotic prophylaxis in surgery depends on the most likely pathogens encountered during the surgical procedure. The expected wound classification of the planned operative procedure (Table 10-17) is helpful for deciding the appropriate antibiotic spectrum and is considered before ordering or administering any preoperative medication. Prophylactic antibiotics are not generally required for clean (class I) cases except in the setting of indwelling prosthesis placement or when bone is incised. Patients who undergo class II procedures benefit from a single dose of an appropriate antibiotic administered before the skin incision. For abdominal (hepatobiliary, pancreatic, gastroduodenal) cases, cefazolin is generally used. Contaminated (class III) cases require mechanical preparation or parenteral antibiotics with aerobic and anaerobic activity. Dirty or infected cases often require the same antibiotic spectrum, which can be continued into the postoperative period in the setting of ongoing infection or delayed treatment (Table 10-18).

The appropriate antibiotic is chosen before surgery and administered within 60 minutes before surgical incision (120 minutes for vancomycin or fluoroquinolones) (Table 10-19).[49] Although single-dose prophylaxis is usually sufficient, the duration of prophylaxis for all procedures should be less than 24 hours. Repeat dosing occurs at an appropriate interval, usually 3 hours for abdominal cases or twice the half-life of the antibiotic, although the patient's renal function may alter the timing (Table 10-20). If an agent with a short half-life is used (e.g., cefazolin, cefoxitin), it should be readministered if the procedure duration exceeds the recommended redosing interval (from the time of initiation of the preoperative dose). Readministration may also be warranted if prolonged or excessive bleeding occurs or if there are other factors that may shorten the half-life of the prophylactic agent (e.g., extensive burns). Readministration may not be warranted in patients in whom the half-life of the agent may be prolonged (e.g., patients with renal insufficiency or failure). For patients with methicillin-resistant *Staphylococcus aureus* colonization, it is reasonable to add a single preoperative dose of vancomycin to the recommended agent or agents. With an infected biliary tract,

TABLE 10-17 Surgical Wound Classifications as Defined by ACS NSQIP*

Clean	Uninfected operative wounds in which no inflammation is encountered and the respiratory, alimentary, genital, and uninfected urinary tracts are not entered
Clean/contaminated	Operative wounds in which the respiratory, alimentary, genital, or urinary tract is entered under controlled conditions and without unusual contamination
Contaminated	Open, fresh, accidental wounds; operations with major breaks in sterile technique or gross spillage from the gastrointestinal tract; and incisions in which acute, nonpurulent inflammation is encountered
Dirty	Old traumatic wounds with retained devitalized tissue and wounds that involve existing clinical infection or perforated viscera.

From Eisenberg D: Surgical site infections: Time to modify the wound classification system? *J Surg Res* 175:54–55, 2012.
ACS NSQIP, American College of Surgeons National Surgical Quality Improvement Program.
*User Guide for the 2008 ACS NSQIP Participant Use Data File.

TABLE 10-18 Analysis of Postoperative Surgical Site Infections Stratified by Wound Classification (Traditional versus ACS NSQIP)

	CLEAN (%)	CLEAN/CONTAMINATED (%)	CONTAMINATED (%)	DIRTY (%)
Traditional	1-5	3-11	10-17	>27
ACS NSQIP SSI	2.58	6.67	8.61	11.80
Superficial SSI	1.76	3.94	4.75	5.16
Deep incisional SSI	0.54	0.86	1.31	2.10
Organ/space SSI	0.28	1.87	2.55	4.54

From Ortega G, Rhee DS, Papandria DJ, et al: An evaluation of Surgical Site Infection by wound classification system using the ACS-NSQIP. *J Surg Res* 174:33–38, 2012.
ACS NSQIP, American College of Surgeons National Surgical Quality Improvement Program; *SSI,* surgical site infection.

additional antimicrobial coverage should be considered. Fluoroquinolones are associated with an increased risk of tendinitis and tendon rupture in all ages. Ceftriaxone use should be limited to patients requiring antimicrobial treatment for acute cholecystitis or acute biliary tract infections and not cases with biliary colic or dyskinesia without infection.

Factors that indicate a high risk of infectious complications in laparoscopic cholecystectomy include emergency procedures, diabetes, long procedure duration, intraoperative gallbladder rupture, age older than 70 years, and conversion from laparoscopic to open cholecystectomy. It is reasonable to give a single dose of antimicrobial prophylaxis to all patients undergoing laparoscopic cholecystectomy.

Prophylaxis is not routinely indicated for brachiocephalic procedures. Although there are no data to support it, patients undergoing brachiocephalic procedures involving vascular prostheses or patch implantation (e.g., carotid endarterectomy) may benefit from prophylaxis. These guidelines reflect recommendations for perioperative antibiotic prophylaxis to prevent SSIs and do not provide recommendations for prevention of opportunistic infections in immunosuppressed transplantation patients (e.g., for antifungal or antiviral medications).

Review of Medications

Careful review of the patient's home medications is part of the preoperative evaluation before any operation; the goal is to use medications that control the patient's medical illnesses appropriately, while minimizing the risk associated with anesthetic-drug interactions or the hematologic or metabolic effects of some commonly used medications and therapies. The patient is asked to name all medications, including psychiatric drugs, hormones, and alternative or herbal medications, and to provide dosages and frequency.

In general, patients taking cardiac drugs including beta blockers and antiarrhythmics, pulmonary drugs such as inhaled or nebulized medications, anticonvulsants, antihypertensives, or psychiatric drugs are advised to take their medications with a sip of water on the morning of surgery. Parenteral forms or substitutes are available for many drugs and may be used if the patient remains NPO for any significant period postoperatively. It is important to return patients to their normal medication regimen as soon as possible. Two notable examples are the additional cardiovascular morbidity associated with the perioperative discontinuation of beta blockers and rebound hypertension with abrupt cessation of the antihypertensive clonidine. Medications such as lipid-lowering agents or vitamins can be omitted on the day of surgery.

Some drugs are associated with an increased risk for perioperative bleeding and are withheld before surgery. Drugs that affect platelet function are withheld for variable periods; clopidogrel (Plavix) is withheld for 7 to 10 days, whereas NSAIDs are withheld between 1 day (ibuprofen and indomethacin) and 3 days (naproxen and sulindac), depending on the drug's half-life. Because the use of estrogen and tamoxifen has been associated with an increased risk for thromboembolism, they probably need to be withheld for 4 weeks preoperatively.[1]

The widespread use of herbal medications has prompted review of the effects of some commonly used preparations and their potential adverse outcomes during the perioperative period. These substances may fail to be recorded in the preoperative evaluation, although important metabolic and hematologic effects can result from their regular use (Table 10-21).[1] Generally, the use of herbal medications is stopped preoperatively, but this needs to be done with caution in patients who report the use of valerian, which may be associated with a benzodiazepine-like withdrawal syndrome.

TABLE 10-19 Recommendations for Surgical Antimicrobial Prophylaxis

TYPE OF PROCEDURE	RECOMMENDED AGENTS[a,b]	ALTERNATIVE AGENTS IN PATIENTS WITH β-LACTAM ALLERGY	STRENGTH OF EVIDENCE[c]
Cardiac coronary artery bypass	Cefazolin, cefuroxime	Clindamycin,[d] vancomycin[d]	A
Cardiac device insertion procedures (e.g., pacemaker implantation)	Cefazolin, cefuroxime	Clindamycin, vancomycin	A
Ventricular assist devices	Cefazolin, cefuroxime	Clindamycin, vancomycin	C
Thoracic noncardiac procedures, including lobectomy, pneumonectomy, lung resection, and thoracotomy	Cefazolin, ampicillin-sulbactam	Clindamycin,[d] vancomycin[d]	A
Video-assisted thoracoscopic surgery	Cefazolin, ampicillin-sulbactam	Clindamycin,[d] vancomycin[d]	C
Gastroduodenal[e] procedures involving entry into lumen of gastrointestinal tract (bariatric, pancreaticoduodenectomy[f])	Cefazolin	Clindamycin or vancomycin + aminoglycoside[g] or aztreonam or fluoroquinolone[h-j]	A
Procedures without entry into gastrointestinal tract (antireflux, highly selective vagotomy) for high-risk patients	Cefazolin	Clindamycin or vancomycin + aminoglycoside[g] or aztreonam or fluoroquinolone[h-j]	A
Biliary tract open procedure	Cefazolin, cefoxitin, cefotetan, ceftriaxone,[k] ampicillin-sulbactam[h]	Clindamycin or vancomycin + aminoglycoside[g] or aztreonam or fluoroquinolone,[h-j] metronidazole + aminoglycoside[g] or fluoroquinolone[h-j]	A
Laparoscopic procedure			
Elective, low-risk[l]	None	None	A
Elective, high-risk[l]	Cefazolin, cefoxitin, cefotetan, ceftriaxone,[k] ampicillin-sulbactam[h]	Clindamycin or vancomycin + aminoglycoside[g] or aztreonam or fluoroquinolone,[h-j] metronidazole + aminoglycoside[g] or fluoroquinolone[h-j]	A
Appendectomy for uncomplicated appendicitis	Cefoxitin, cefotetan, cefazolin + metronidazole	Clindamycin + aminoglycoside[g] or aztreonam or fluoroquinolone,[h-j] metronidazole + aminoglycoside[g] or fluoroquinolone[h-j]	A
Small intestine			
Nonobstructed	Cefazolin	Clindamycin + aminoglycoside[g] or aztreonam or fluoroquinolone[h-j]	C
Obstructed	Cefazolin + metronidazole, cefoxitin, cefotetan	Metronidazole + aminoglycoside[g] or fluoroquinolone[h-j]	C
Hernia repair (hernioplasty and herniorrhaphy)	Cefazolin	Clindamycin, vancomycin	A
Colorectal[m]	Cefazolin + metronidazole, cefoxitin, cefotetan, ampicillin-sulbactam,[h] ceftriaxone + metronidazole,[n] ertapenem	Clindamycin + aminoglycoside[g] or aztreonam or fluoroquinolone,[h-j] metronidazole + aminoglycoside[g] or fluoroquinolone[h-j]	A
Head and neck clean	None	None	B
Clean with placement of prosthesis (excludes tympanostomy tubes)	Cefazolin, cefuroxime	Clindamycin[d]	C
Clean-contaminated cancer surgery	Cefazolin + metronidazole, cefuroxime + metronidazole, ampicillin-sulbactam	Clindamycin[d]	A
Other clean-contaminated procedures with the exception of tonsillectomy and functional endoscopic sinus procedures	Cefazolin + metronidazole, cefuroxime + metronidazole, ampicillin-sulbactam	Clindamycin[d]	B
Neurosurgery elective craniotomy and cerebrospinal fluid–shunting procedures	Cefazolin	Clindamycin,[d] vancomycin[d]	A
Implantation of intrathecal pumps	Cefazolin	Clindamycin,[d] vancomycin[d]	C
Cesarean delivery	Cefazolin	Clindamycin + aminoglycoside[g]	A
Hysterectomy (vaginal or abdominal)	Cefazolin, cefotetan, cefoxitin, ampicillin-sulbactam[h]	Clindamycin or vancomycin + aminoglycoside[g] or aztreonam or fluoroquinolone,[h-j] metronidazole + aminoglycoside[g] or fluoroquinolone[h-j]	A

TABLE 10-19 Recommendations for Surgical Antimicrobial Prophylaxis—cont'd

TYPE OF PROCEDURE	RECOMMENDED AGENTS[a,b]	ALTERNATIVE AGENTS IN PATIENTS WITH β-LACTAM ALLERGY	STRENGTH OF EVIDENCE[c]
Ophthalmic	Topical neomycin-polymyxin B-gramicidin or fourth-generation topical fluoroquinolones (gatifloxacin or moxifloxacin) given as 1 drop every 5-15 min for 5 doses.[o] Addition of cefazolin 100 mg by subconjunctival injection or intracameral cefazolin 1-2.5 mg or cefuroxime 1 mg at the end of procedure is optional	None	B
Orthopedic clean operations involving hand, knee, or foot and not involving implantation of foreign materials	None	None	C
Spinal procedures with and without instrumentation	Cefazolin	Clindamycin,[d] vancomycin[d]	A
Hip fracture repair	Cefazolin	Clindamycin,[d] vancomycin[d]	A
Implantation of internal fixation devices (e.g., nails, screws, plates, wires)	Cefazolin	Clindamycin,[d] vancomycin[d]	C
Total joint replacement	Cefazolin	Clindamycin,[d] vancomycin[d]	A
Urologic lower tract instrumentation with risk factors for infection (includes transrectal prostate biopsy)	Fluoroquinolone,[h-j] trimethoprim-sulfamethoxazole, cefazolin	Aminoglycoside[g] with or without clindamycin	A
Clean without entry into urinary tract	Cefazolin (addition of a single dose of an aminoglycoside may be recommended for placement of prosthetic material [e.g., penile prosthesis])	Clindamycin,[d] vancomycin[d]	A
Involving implanted prosthesis	Cefazolin ± aminoglycoside, cefazolin ± aztreonam, ampicillin-sulbactam	Clindamycin ± aminoglycoside or aztreonam, vancomycin ± aminoglycoside or aztreonam	A
Clean with entry into urinary tract	Cefazolin (addition of a single dose of an aminoglycoside may be recommended for placement of prosthetic material [e.g., penile prosthesis])	Fluoroquinolone,[h-j] aminoglycoside[g] ± clindamycin	A
Clean-contaminated	Cefazolin + metronidazole, cefoxitin	Fluoroquinolone,[h-j] aminoglycoside[g] + metronidazole or clindamycin	A
Vascular[p]	Cefazolin	Clindamycin,[d] vancomycin[d]	A
Heart, lung, heart-lung transplantation[q]; heart transplantation[r]	Cefazolin	Clindamycin,[d] vancomycin[d]	A (based on cardiac procedures)
Lung and heart-lung transplantation[r,s]	Cefazolin	Clindamycin,[d] vancomycin[d]	A (based on cardiac procedures)
Liver transplantation[q,t]	Piperacillin-tazobactam, cefotaxime + ampicillin	Clindamycin or vancomycin + aminoglycoside[g] or aztreonam or fluoroquinolone[h-j]	B
Pancreas and pancreas-kidney transplantation[r]	Cefazolin, fluconazole (for patients at high risk of fungal infection [e.g., patients with enteric drainage of the pancreas])	Clindamycin or vancomycin + aminoglycoside[g] or aztreonam or fluoroquinolone[h-j]	A
	Cefazolin	Clindamycin or vancomycin + aminoglycoside[g] or aztreonam or fluoroquinolone[h-j]	A
Plastic surgery clean with risk factors or clean-contaminated	Cefazolin, ampicillin-sulbactam	Clindamycin,[d] vancomycin[d]	C

From Bratzler DW, Dellinger EP, Olsen KM, et al: Clinical practice guidelines for antimicrobial prophylaxis in surgery. *Am J Health Syst Pharm* 70:195–283, 2013.

Continued

TABLE 10-19 Recommendations for Surgical Antimicrobial Prophylaxis—cont'd

[a]The antimicrobial agent should be started within 60 min before surgical incision (120 min for vancomycin or fluoroquinolones). Although single-dose prophylaxis is usually sufficient, the duration of prophylaxis for all procedures should be <24 hr. If an agent with a short half-life is used (e.g., cefazolin, cefoxitin), it should be readministered if the procedure duration exceeds the recommended redosing interval (from the time of initiation of the preoperative dose). Readministration may also be warranted if prolonged or excessive bleeding occurs or if there are other factors that may shorten the half-life of the prophylactic agent (e.g., extensive burns). Readministration may not be warranted in patients in whom the half-life of the agent may be prolonged (e.g., patients with renal insufficiency or renal failure).
[b]For patients known to be colonized with methicillin-resistant *Staphylococcus aureus*, it is reasonable to add a single preoperative dose of vancomycin to the recommended agents.
[c]Strength of evidence that supports the use or nonuse of prophylaxis is classified as A (levels I-III), B (levels IV-VI), or C (level VII). Level I evidence is from large, well-conducted, randomized controlled clinical trials. Level II evidence is from small, well-conducted, randomized controlled clinical trials. Level III evidence is from well-conducted cohort studies. Level IV evidence is from well-conducted case-control studies. Level V evidence is from uncontrolled studies that were not well conducted. Level VI evidence is conflicting evidence that tends to favor the recommendation. Level VII evidence is expert opinion.
[d]For procedures in which pathogens other than staphylococci and streptococci are likely, an additional agent with activity against those pathogens could be considered. For example, if there are surveillance data showing that gram-negative organisms are a cause of surgical site infections for the procedure, practitioners may consider combining clindamycin or vancomycin with another agent (cefazolin if the patient is not allergic to β-lactam antibiotics; aztreonam, gentamicin, or single-dose fluoroquinolone if the patient is allergic to β-lactam antibiotics).
[e]Prophylaxis should be considered for patients at highest risk for postoperative gastroduodenal infections, such as patients with increased gastric pH (e.g., patients receiving histamine H_2 receptor antagonists or proton pump inhibitors), gastroduodenal perforation, decreased gastric motility, gastric outlet obstruction, gastric bleeding, morbid obesity, or cancer. Antimicrobial prophylaxis may not be needed when the lumen of the intestinal tract is not entered.
[f]Consider additional antimicrobial coverage with infected biliary tract.
[g]Gentamicin or tobramycin.
[h]Because of increasing resistance of *Escherichia coli* to fluoroquinolones and ampicillin-sulbactam, local population susceptibility profiles should be reviewed before use.
[i]Ciprofloxacin or levofloxacin.
[j]Fluoroquinolones are associated with an increased risk of tendinitis and tendon rupture in patients of all ages. However, this risk would be expected to be quite small with single-dose antibiotic prophylaxis. Although the use of fluoroquinolones may be necessary for surgical antibiotic prophylaxis in some children, they are not first-choice drugs in pediatric patients because of an increased incidence of adverse events compared with control subjects in some clinical trials.
[k]Ceftriaxone use should be limited to patients requiring antimicrobial treatment for acute cholecystitis or acute biliary tract infections that may not be determined before incision; ceftriaxone should not be used in patients undergoing cholecystectomy for noninfected biliary conditions, including biliary colic or dyskinesia without infection.
[l]Factors that indicate a high risk of infectious complications in laparoscopic cholecystectomy include emergency procedures, diabetes, long procedure duration, intraoperative gallbladder rupture, age >70 years, conversion from laparoscopic to open cholecystectomy, American Society of Anesthesiologists classification of ≥3, episode of colic within 30 days before the procedure, reintervention in <1 month for noninfectious complication, acute cholecystitis, bile spillage, jaundice, pregnancy, nonfunctioning gallbladder, immunosuppression, and insertion of prosthetic device. Because many of these risk factors are impossible to determine before surgical intervention, it may be reasonable to give a single dose of antimicrobial prophylaxis to all patients undergoing laparoscopic cholecystectomy.
[m]For most patients, a mechanical bowel preparation combined with oral neomycin sulfate plus oral erythromycin base or with oral neomycin sulfate plus oral metronidazole should be given in addition to intravenous prophylaxis.
[n]In cases in which there is increasing resistance to first-generation and second-generation cephalosporins among gram-negative isolates from SSIs, a single dose of ceftriaxone plus metronidazole may be preferred over the routine use of carbapenems.
[o]The necessity of continuing topical antimicrobials postoperatively has not been established.
[p]Prophylaxis is not routinely indicated for brachiocephalic procedures. Although there are no data to support it, patients undergoing brachiocephalic procedures involving vascular prostheses or patch implantation (e.g., carotid endarterectomy) may benefit from prophylaxis.
[q]These guidelines reflect recommendations for perioperative antibiotic prophylaxis to prevent surgical site infections and do not provide recommendations for prevention of opportunistic infections in immunosuppressed transplantation patients (e.g., for antifungal or antiviral medications).
[r]Patients who have left ventricular assist devices as a bridge and who experience chronic infection might also benefit from coverage of the infecting microorganism.
[s]The prophylactic regimen may need to be modified to provide coverage against any potential pathogens, including gram-negative (e.g., *Pseudomonas aeruginosa*) or fungal organisms, isolated from the donor lung or the recipient before transplantation. Patients undergoing lung transplantation with negative cultures before transplantation should receive antimicrobial prophylaxis as appropriate for other types of cardiothoracic surgeries. Patients undergoing lung transplantation for cystic fibrosis should receive 7-14 days of treatment with antimicrobials selected according to culture before transplantation and susceptibility results. This treatment may include additional antibacterial or antifungal agents.
[t]The prophylactic regimen may need to be modified to provide coverage against any potential pathogens, including vancomycin-resistant enterococci, isolated from the recipient before transplantation.

Preoperative Fasting

The standard order of "NPO past midnight" for preoperative patients is based on the theory of reduction of volume and acidity of the stomach contents during surgery. Aspiration may occur during all types of anesthesia in nonfasted patients because of the effect of the anesthetic and sedative medications on decreasing the airway protective reflexes. Guidelines have recommended a shift to allow a period of restricted fluid intake for up to a few hours before surgery. The ASA recommends that adults stop intake of solids for at least 6 hours and clear fluids for 2

TABLE 10-20 Clinical Practice Guidelines for Antimicrobial Prophylaxis in Surgery

ANTIMICROBIAL	RECOMMENDED DOSE: ADULTS[a]	RECOMMENDED DOSE: CHILDREN[b]	HALF-LIFE IN ADULTS WITH NORMAL RENAL FUNCTION (hr)[19]	RECOMMENDED REDOSING INTERVAL (FROM INITIATION OF PREOPERATIVE DOSE) (hr)[c]
Ampicillin-sulbactam	3 g (ampicillin 2 g/ sulbactam 1 g)	50 mg/kg of ampicillin component	0.8-1.3	2
Ampicillin	2 g	50 mg/kg	1-1.9	2
Aztreonam	2 g	30 mg/kg	1.3-2.4	4
Cefazolin	2 g, 3 g for patients weighing ≥120 kg	30 mg/kg	1.2-2.2	4
Cefuroxime	1.5 g	50 mg/kg	1-2	4
Cefotaxime	1 g[d]	50 mg/kg	0.9-1.7	3
Cefoxitin	2 g	40 mg/kg	0.7-1.1	2
Cefotetan	2 g	40 mg/kg	2.8-4.6	6
Ceftriaxone	2 g[e]	50-75 mg/kg	5.4-10.9	NA
Ciprofloxacin[f]	400 mg	10 mg/kg	3-7	NA
Clindamycin	900 mg	10 mg/kg	2-4	6
Ertapenem	1 g	15 mg/kg	3-5	NA
Fluconazole	400 mg	6 mg/kg	30	NA
Gentamicin[g]	5 mg/kg based on dosing weight (single dose)	2.5 mg/kg based on dosing weight	2-3	NA
Levofloxacin[f]	500 mg	10 mg/kg	6-8	NA
Metronidazole	500 mg	15 mg/kg; neonates weighing <1200 g should receive a single 7.5-mg/kg dose	6-8	NA
Moxifloxacin[f]	400 mg	10 mg/kg	8-15	NA
Piperacillin-tazobactam	3.375 g	Infants 2-9 mo: 80 mg/kg of piperacillin component Children >9 mo and ≤40 kg: 100 mg/kg of piperacillin component	0.7-1.2	2
Vancomycin	15 mg/kg	15 mg/kg	4-8	NA
Oral Antibiotics for Colorectal Surgery Prophylaxis (Used in Conjunction With Mechanical Bowel Preparation)				
Erythromycin base	1 g	20 mg/kg	0.8-3	NA
Metronidazole	1 g	15 mg/kg	6-10	NA
Neomycin	1 g	15 mg/kg	2-3 (3% absorbed under normal gastrointestinal conditions)	NA

From Bratzler DW, Dellinger EP, Olsen KM, et al: Clinical practice guidelines for antimicrobial prophylaxis in surgery. *Am J Health Syst Pharm* 70:195–283, 2013.
NA, not applicable.
[a]Adult doses are obtained from different studies.
[b]The maximum pediatric dose should not exceed the usual adult dose.
[c]For antimicrobials with a short half-life (e.g., cefazolin, cefoxitin) used before long procedures, redosing in the operating room is recommended at an interval of approximately two times the half-life of the agent in patients with normal renal function. Recommended redosing intervals marked as NA are based on typical case length; for unusually long procedures, redosing may be needed.
[d]Although Food and Drug Administration–approved package insert labeling indicates 1 g, experts recommend 2 g for obese patients.
[e]When used as a single dose in combination with metronidazole for colorectal procedures.
[f]Although fluoroquinolones have been associated with an increased risk of tendinitis or tendon rupture in patients of all ages, use of these agents for single-dose prophylaxis is generally safe.
[g]In general, gentamicin for surgical antibiotic prophylaxis should be limited to a single dose given preoperatively. Dosing is based on the patient's actual body weight. If the patient's actual weight is more than 20% above ideal body weight (IBW), the dosing weight (DW) can be determined as follows: DW = IBW + 0.4 (actual weight − IBW).

hours. When the literature was reviewed by the Cochrane group, they found 22 trials in healthy adults that provided 38 controlled comparisons.[1] There was no evidence that the volume or pH of gastric contents differed with the length and type of fasting. Although not reported in all the trials, there appeared to be no increased risk for aspiration or regurgitation with a shortened period of fasting. Very few trials have investigated the fasting routine in patients at higher risk for regurgitation or aspiration (pregnant patients, older patients, obese patients, or patients with stomach disorders). There has also been increasing evidence that preoperative carbohydrate supplementation is safe and may improve a patient's response to perioperative stress.[1] Surgeons

TABLE 10-21 Perioperative Concerns and Recommendations for Herbal Medicines

COMMON NAME OF HERB	PERIOPERATIVE CONCERNS	RELEVANT PHARMACOLOGIC EFFECT	PREOPERATIVE RECOMMENDATIONS
Echinacea	Allergic reactions; decreased effectiveness of immunosuppressants; potential for immunosuppression with long-term use	Activation of cell-mediated immunity	No data
Ephedra	Risk for myocardial ischemia and stroke from tachycardia and hypertension; ventricular arrhythmias with halothane; long-term use depletes endogenous catecholamines and may cause intraoperative hemodynamic instability; life-threatening interaction with monoamine oxidase inhibitors	Increased heart rate and blood pressure through direct and indirect sympathomimetic effects	Discontinue at least 24 hr before surgery
Garlic	Potential to increase risk for bleeding, especially when combined with other medications that inhibit platelet aggregation	Inhibition of platelet aggregation (may be irreversible); increased fibrinolysis; equivocal hypertensive activity	Discontinue at least 7 days before surgery
Ginkgo	Potential to increase risk for bleeding, especially when combined with other medications that inhibit platelet aggregation	Inhibition of platelet-activating factor	Discontinue at least 36 hr before surgery
Ginseng	Hypoglycemia; potential to increase risk for bleeding; potential to decrease anticoagulative effect of warfarin	Lowers blood glucose; inhibition of platelet aggregation (may be irreversible); increased PT/PTT in animals	Discontinue at least 7 days before surgery
Kava	Potential to increase sedative effect of anesthetics; potential for addiction, tolerance, and withdrawal after abstinence unstudied	Sedation, anxiolysis	Discontinue at least 24 hr before surgery
St. John's wort	Induction of cytochrome P450 enzymes, with effect on cyclosporine, warfarin, steroids, and protease inhibitors and possibly benzodiazepines, calcium channel blockers, and many other drugs; decreased serum digoxin levels	Inhibition of neurotransmitter uptake; monoamine oxidase inhibition is unlikely	Discontinue at least 5 days before surgery
Valerian	Potential to increase sedative effect of anesthetics; benzodiazepine-like acute withdrawal; potential to increase anesthetic requirements with long-term use	Sedation	No data

From Ang-Lee MK, Moss J, Yuan CS: Herbal medicines and perioperative care. *JAMA* 286:208–216, 2001.
PT/PTT, prothrombin time/partial thromboplastin time.

and anesthesiologists should evaluate the evidence and consider adjusting their standard fasting policies.

POTENTIAL CAUSES OF INTRAOPERATIVE INSTABILITY

A patient who is under anesthesia can have physiologic derangements that need to be addressed. Some of these derangements can be dramatic and require immediate attention; others allow for investigation before introduction of therapy. These derangements are usually of a cardiac or pulmonary nature or are related to the administration of anesthesia.

Myocardial Infarction

It has been estimated that 1.5% of patients who undergo noncardiac surgery experience a perioperative MI.[1] Some of these events occur in the operating room. The typical presentation is of new-onset ECG changes, dysrhythmias, or hypotension. If the patient has reasonable hemodynamics and no evidence of decreased perfusion, the procedure can usually be completed. However, any evidence of instability should lead to termination of the procedure and cardiac evaluation. Temporary abdominal closure techniques can be used, if needed. Intervention decisions for MI should be made in conjunction with a cardiologist.

Pulmonary Embolism

Depending on the procedure, PE can be a significant source of intraoperative instability. It has been estimated that 2% of patients undergoing hip surgery experience a PE during the procedure. Signs of intraoperative PE include new tachycardia, evidence of right heart strain, hypotension, and complete cardiovascular collapse. The onset is sudden, and rapid diagnosis and treatments are paramount.

Transesophageal echocardiography is commonly used in the operating room. Intraoperative transesophageal echocardiography can be used to identify the PE directly or to show the physiologic effects on cardiac function and allow for an inferred diagnosis.[1] Right ventricular dysfunction, tricuspid regurgitation, and leftward bowing of the interatrial septum are the typical findings. If an embolism is suspected, management depends on the stability of the patient. If the patient is unstable, the procedure should be aborted and efforts to address the PE instituted. Such efforts include cardiovascular support, thrombolytics, and pulmonary embolectomy in severe cases.

Pneumothorax

Pneumothorax is a known complication of laparoscopy. As more procedures are approached with minimally invasive techniques, especially esophageal procedures, the risk of pneumothorax increases. The main risk of pneumothorax with laparoscopy is development of a tension pneumothorax and associated cardiovascular collapse. Clinically, ballooning of the diaphragm can be seen. Physiologic changes include deoxygenation, hypercarbia, and hypotension. ECG changes can also be noted.

Diagnosis and treatment are straightforward. If the patient is decompensating and there are decreased breath sounds in one hemithorax, abdominal insufflation should be released. Needle decompression or tube thoracostomy should be performed. Confirmation with chest radiograph is unnecessary and can delay treatment, leading to further instability. After a chest tube has been placed, pneumoperitoneum can be reintroduced, and patient physiology can be followed. If no derangements are noted, the procedure can be completed.

Anaphylaxis and Latex Allergy

Intraoperative anaphylactic reactions may occur in 1 in 4500 surgical procedures and carry a 3% to 6% risk for mortality.[1] Causative agents are most often muscle relaxants, latex, anesthetic induction agents such as etomidate and propofol, and narcotic drugs. Additional agents administered while patients are under anesthesia that may be associated with anaphylaxis include dyes (e.g., isosulfan blue dye for sentinel node procedures), colloid solutions, antibiotics, blood products, protamine, and mannitol.

The manifestations of anaphylactic reactions occurring under anesthesia may range from mild cutaneous eruptions to hypotension, cardiovascular collapse, bronchospasm, and death. When an anaphylactic reaction is suspected, use of the offending agent is discontinued, and the patient is given epinephrine, 0.3 to 0.5 mL of a 1 : 1000 solution subcutaneously. With severe anaphylaxis, epinephrine is given intravenously and repeated at 5- to 10-minute intervals as needed. Histamine 1 (H_1) blockade with diphenhydramine, 50 mg intravenously or intramuscularly, plus histamine 2 (H_2) blockade with ranitidine, 50 mg intravenously, as well as hydrocortisone, 100 to 250 mg intravenously every 6 hours, is usually required. Additional supportive measures in the setting of hemodynamic or respiratory collapse may include fluid boluses, pressors, orotracheal intubation, and nebulized β_2-adrenergic agonists or racemic epinephrine. Postoperative monitoring in the ICU is generally required for a patient who has had a severe intraoperative anaphylactic reaction.

Latex sensitivity is the second most common cause of anaphylactic reactions (after muscle relaxants) and must be screened for in the medical history. Although the incidence of such sensitivity may be less than 5% in the general population, higher risk groups, including individuals with a genetic predisposition (atopic conditions) or chronic exposure to latex and individuals with spina bifida, may have rates of 72%. Patients who give a history consistent with possible latex sensitivity undergo skin testing before anticipated operative procedures. Appropriate intraoperative measures to ensure a latex-free environment obviate most perioperative risk in a patient with latex allergy.

Malignant Hyperthermia

The incidence of malignant hyperthermia (MH) is higher in children and young adults than in adults; a rate of 1 in 15,000 has been estimated in the group at highest risk—boys younger than 15 years old.[1] MH represents an acute episode of hypermetabolism and muscle injury related to the administration of halogenated anesthetic agents or succinylcholine. Susceptibility to MH is inherited according to an autosomal dominant pattern, with apparent incomplete penetrance. The patient may fail to reveal familial knowledge of the trait, and a personal history of muscle disorder may not be evident.

An acute episode of MH may be recognized by increased sympathetic nervous system activity, muscle rigidity, and high fever. Associated derangements include hypercapnia, arrhythmia, acidosis, hypoxemia, and rhabdomyolysis. When suspected, MH is treated by discontinuing inhalational anesthetic agents and succinylcholine, completely changing the anesthesia circuit, and administering dantrolene sodium at doses of 2 to 3 mg/kg intravenously. This drug may be titrated to the abatement of symptoms. Additional supportive measures include active or passive cooling and pharmacologic treatment of arrhythmia, hyperkalemia, and acidosis.

Wrong-Site Surgery and Universal Protocol

In 2004, The Joint Commission adopted, as a national patient safety goal, the elimination of wrong-site, wrong-procedure, wrong-patient procedures.[1] A Universal Protocol was developed, and the concept of the time-out was instituted. The protocol includes preoperative marking of the surgical site; confirming the site by comparing physician notes, consent, mark, and patient identification; and ensuring that the proper implants or devices are available for the procedure. Many institutions add other pieces of information to their time-out, such as antibiotic and VTE prophylaxis. An example of such a time-out process is shown in Figure 10-4. Implementation of surgical checklists are associated with overall reduction in rates of death and complications.

OPERATING ROOM

Preparation for surgery does not end with evaluation of the patient and selection of the operative procedure. The surgeon is responsible for ensuring that everything needed for the procedure is available on the day of surgery, including special equipment required to carry out the operation and implants, blood, blood products, or special medications.

Well-trained surgeons, anesthesiologists, and operating room staff along with a space equipped with an easily maneuverable operating table, good lighting, and ample space for personnel and equipment are required to run an operating room efficiently. The room is cleaned and the table is checked for malfunction before and after each case. It is extremely costly and stressful to replace the operating table or other equipment with the patient already in the operating room. Preoperative communication among surgeons, anesthesiologists, and operating room staff is vitally important. Such communication helps save time, prevents confusion and undue frustration in the management of equipment use, accounts for patient needs and personnel requirements, and makes planned procedures progress safely and efficiently. The modern operating room for a trauma service has a temperature control panel that allows the room temperature to be modified rapidly to avoid hypothermia. Patients are positioned and secured on the table. Position-related neuromuscular or orthopedic injury can be prevented with careful positioning and padding. Barriers consisting of sterile drapes and gowns are established between the surgeon, patient, and other operating room staff. The barriers need to be impermeable to water and other body fluids. Finally, a hands-free communication system (e.g., intercom, voice-activated speaker phone) must be functioning in the room to facilitate communication among surgeons and pathologists, radiologists, blood bank, pharmacy, and the patient's family members. Most importantly, if an unexpected situation arises, help can be summoned immediately.

Maintenance of Normothermia

Hypothermia averaging only 1.5° C below normal is associated with adverse outcomes that add hospitalization costs of $2500 to $7000 for each surgical patient. Many factors increase the risk for perioperative hypothermia—extremes of age, female sex, ambient

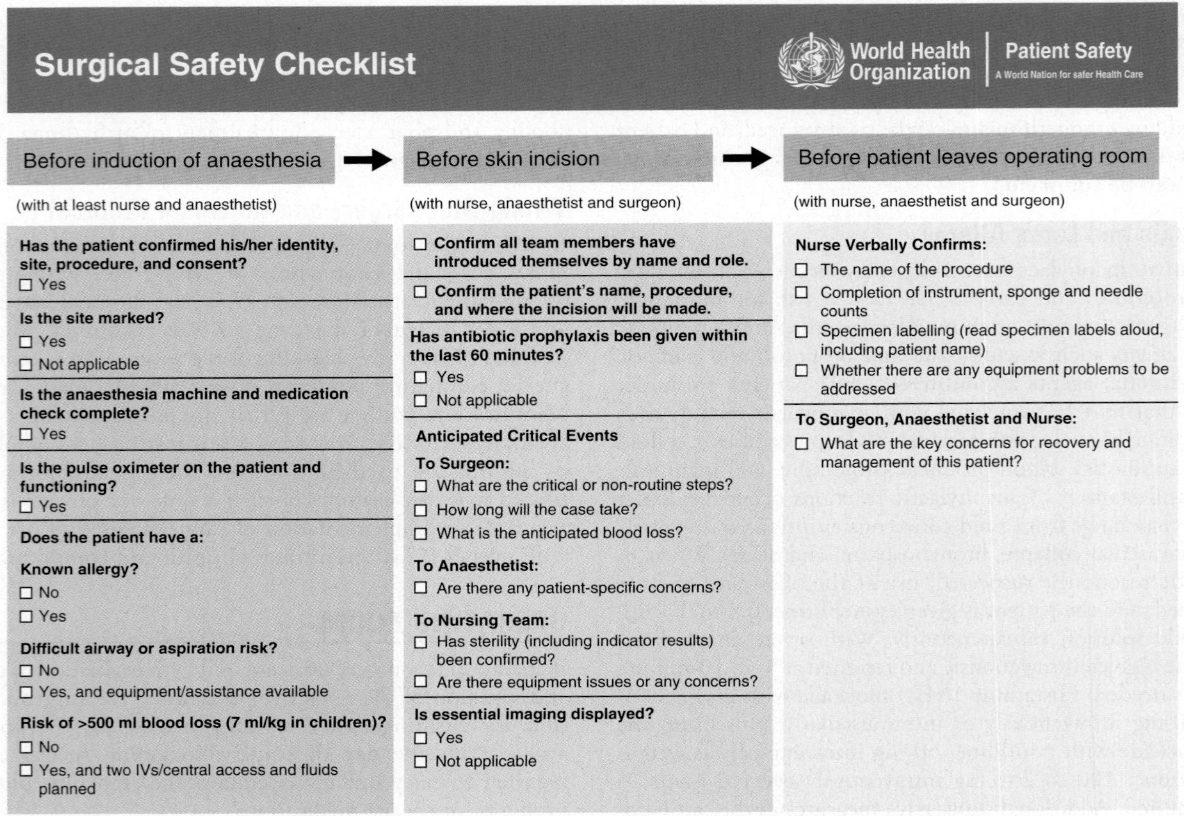

Surgical Safety Checklist

World Health Organization | Patient Safety — A World Alliance for safer Health Care

Before induction of anaesthesia → **Before skin incision** → **Before patient leaves operating room**

Before induction of anaesthesia

(with at least nurse and anaesthetist)

Has the patient confirmed his/her identity, site, procedure, and consent?
- ☐ Yes

Is the site marked?
- ☐ Yes
- ☐ Not applicable

Is the anaesthesia machine and medication check complete?
- ☐ Yes

Is the pulse oximeter on the patient and functioning?
- ☐ Yes

Does the patient have a:

Known allergy?
- ☐ No
- ☐ Yes

Difficult airway or aspiration risk?
- ☐ No
- ☐ Yes, and equipment/assistance available

Risk of >500 ml blood loss (7 ml/kg in children)?
- ☐ No
- ☐ Yes, and two IVs/central access and fluids planned

Before skin incision

(with nurse, anaesthetist and surgeon)

- ☐ **Confirm all team members have introduced themselves by name and role.**
- ☐ **Confirm the patient's name, procedure, and where the incision will be made.**

Has antibiotic prophylaxis been given within the last 60 minutes?
- ☐ Yes
- ☐ Not applicable

Anticipated Critical Events

To Surgeon:
- ☐ What are the critical or non-routine steps?
- ☐ How long will the case take?
- ☐ What is the anticipated blood loss?

To Anaesthetist:
- ☐ Are there any patient-specific concerns?

To Nursing Team:
- ☐ Has sterility (including indicator results) been confirmed?
- ☐ Are there equipment issues or any concerns?

Is essential imaging displayed?
- ☐ Yes
- ☐ Not applicable

Before patient leaves operating room

(with nurse, anaesthetist and surgeon)

Nurse Verbally Confirms:
- ☐ The name of the procedure
- ☐ Completion of instrument, sponge and needle counts
- ☐ Specimen labelling (read specimen labels aloud, including patient name)
- ☐ Whether there are any equipment problems to be addressed

To Surgeon, Anaesthetist and Nurse:
- ☐ What are the key concerns for recovery and management of this patient?

FIGURE 10-4 Surgical safety checklist published by the World Health Organization. www.who.int/patientsafety/safesurgery/checklist/en.

room temperature, length and type of surgical procedure, cachexia, preexisting conditions, significant fluid shifts, use of cold irrigants, and use of general or regional anesthesia. The term *normothermia* is defined as a core temperature between 36° C and 38° C. Preventive warming measures are used to avoid hypothermia. Passive insulation includes warmed cotton blankets, socks, head covering, limited skin exposure, circulating water mattresses, and increase in ambient room temperature (68° F to 75° F). Some patients may require active warming, which includes use of a forced air convection warming system, humidified and warmed anesthetic gases, and warmed intravenous fluids. The greatest temperature decline occurs during the first hour of surgery. Therefore, temperature monitoring is indicated even for short procedures.[1]

Preoperative Skin Preparation

Preoperative skin preparation of the patient and surgeon is important in preventing SSIs. The effectiveness of the preparation depends on the type of antiseptic used and the method of application. The U.S. Centers for Disease Control and Prevention recommends that the size of the area prepared be sufficient; the solution applied in concentric circles; the applicator discarded once the periphery has been reached; and time allowed for the solution to dry, especially when alcoholic solutions are used because they are flammable. The Association of Operating Room Nurses has added that the applicator needs to be sterile, and the solution needs to be applied with the use of friction and extend from the incision site to the periphery. A review of this subject has revealed six evaluable studies; however, all described a unique comparison and could not be combined for meta-analysis.[1] It was concluded at that time that there was insufficient evidence to recommend one skin preparation antiseptic over another. A more recent randomized, controlled study investigated chlorhexidine-alcohol versus povidone-iodine for the prevention of SSIs.[1] In this study, 849 patients were randomly assigned, and at 30 days, there were significantly fewer wound infections in the chlorhexidine-alcohol group. The results were significant for superficial and deep SSIs. There were no differences in adverse events related to the solution used. Hair removal, if needed, is accomplished by clipping with electric clippers rather than shaving with a razor.

Hemostasis

Minimizing blood loss is an important technical aspect of surgery. Increased blood loss exacerbates the stress of surgery and resuscitation; less blood loss allows the performance of a technically superior operation. In the presence of adequate hemostasis, one can conduct a more precise dissection and shorten operating and recovery times for the patient. Avoidance of blood transfusion obviates the risk for transfusion-related complications and the transmission of bloodborne diseases.[1]

Essential operative technique dictates that larger vessels (<1 mm in diameter) be tied, clipped, or sealed with monopolar or bipolar electrocautery or high-frequency ultrasonic devices. Major named vessels, in particular, are not only tied but also undergo suture ligation. Hemoclip application is acceptable, especially in an operating field with an extremely confined space or when dealing with delicate vessels, such as portal vein branches. With limited access procedures, such as those performed with minimal access techniques, clip application seems to be a better choice than knot tying. It is sometimes necessary to use hemoclips, such as when performing an oncologic procedure in which outlining of the margins provides a radiopaque marker for postoperative irradiation.

In the event of catastrophic bleeding, such as when confronted with an unexpected intraoperative major vessel injury, intraperitoneal rupture of an aortic aneurysm, or bleeding from major intra-abdominal trauma, temporary occlusion of the aorta at the esophageal hiatus with a compression device such as a sponge on a stick or vascular clamp or manual compression is considered. Such a maneuver may be lifesaving by allowing the anesthesia staff to catch up with blood loss by aggressive resuscitation. It also allows the surgeon to remove intraperitoneal blood and clots with lap sponges or suction devices until the exact bleeding site can be identified, controlled, and repaired primarily or with an interposition graft. Occasionally, a partial vascular injury may need to be extended or converted to a complete transection to allow a better repair. This approach is particularly applicable to injury of the aorta and vena cava.

Bleeding that occurs from multiple sites in a trauma patient, such as liver laceration, pelvic fracture, or both, especially in a hypothermic patient, may best be treated with packing alone or in conjunction with angiographic embolization to achieve temporary control followed by a second-look operation. This maneuver of damage control is of paramount importance. It may be the only way that a patient's life can be saved. This principle of damage control can and should be applied beyond trauma patients to all surgical patients when unexpected bleeding is encountered or a second-look laparotomy will be necessary. Other adjunctive measures that may be helpful in dealing with wide areas of surface tissue oozing include microwave coagulation, laser coagulation, and application of topical hemostatic agents (e.g., Surgicel, thrombin, Gelfoam, and fibrin glue).

Wound Closure

Wound closure can be temporary or permanent; the latter can be primary or secondary. Critical factors in making this decision are the patient's condition, clinical setting, area of the body involved, condition of the wound itself, and disease process or injury that led to surgical intervention.

Various methods can be chosen to close wounds in different parts of the body, depending on the clinical circumstance. In general, clean noncontaminated wounds with healthy local tissue conditions are best closed by primary permanent closure. In a patient with a condition requiring re-exploration or a patient with abdominal compartment syndrome, temporary closure is preferable. Heavily contaminated extremity or trunk wounds are left open with packing. Heavily contaminated abdominal wounds are best served by fascial closure alone, with the skin left open and packed. The principle of eliminating dead space to reduce the risk for seroma and hematoma formation is important, and this can be achieved internally with sutures or a suction device or externally with a compression appliance.

Permanent closure can be achieved with running or interrupted sutures. Suture can be monofilament or multifilament, braided or nonbraided, and dissolvable or nondissolvable (Tables 10-22 and 10-23). In general, when proven infection or contamination is a concern, monofilament nonbraided suture is preferred. For abdominal wall closure in a debilitated, malnourished patient with cancer, permanent closure with nondissolvable suture seems prudent. In a cirrhotic patient with established ascites or a patient with potential for the development of postoperative ascites, the abdomen is closed with running suture, and a multilayer watertight closure must be achieved.

Temporary closure of the abdominal wall may be appropriate in the setting of a multiply injured patient or a patient with intra-abdominal hypertension. This closure can be achieved with a vacuum suction device or a prosthesis bridging technique using a sterile intravenous bag or polypropylene mesh (Table 10-24). The vacuum suction technique (Vac-Pac) involves using a two-sided temporary closing material made of a Ioban over a blue towel. The Ioban faces the intestine and prevents adhesion to the blue towel. The membrane is tucked beneath the abdominal wall, with the blue towel side facing up to provide retention and prevent potential loss of domain. The central portion of the drape is fenestrated before placement. Suction catheters and gauze dressings are placed beneath a second Biodrape that covers the entire abdominal wall and seals the closure (Fig. 10-5). This technique has many advantages; it is quick and easy to use, the temporary closure can be constructed from materials that are readily available in the operating room, no suturing is required (and therefore the integrity of the abdominal fascia is maintained for later permanent closure), and the applied suction prohibits fluid from accumulating in the abdominal cavity. Disadvantages include an inability to inspect the intestine (as with an intravenous bag) at the bedside and increased complexity of fluid and electrolyte balance because of potentially large fluid losses. It has been our practice to return these patients to the operating room every 3 to 4 days for replacement of the temporary closure. If possible, interrupted permanent fascial closure sutures are placed at the superior and inferior ends

TABLE 10-22 Comparison of Absorbable Sutures

SUTURE	TYPES	RAW MATERIAL	TENSILE STRENGTH RETENTION IN VIVO	TISSUE REACTION
Surgical gut	Chromic	Collagen derived from healthy cattle and sheep	Individual patient characteristics can affect rate of tensile strength loss	Moderate reaction
Monocryl (poliglecaprone 25)	Monofilament	Copolymer of glycolide and epsilon-caprolactone	≈50%-60% (violet, 60%-70%) remains at 1 wk ≈20%-30% (violet, 30%-40%) remains at 2 wk Lost within 3 wk (violet, 4 wk)	Minimal acute inflammatory reaction
Coated Vicryl (polyglactin 910)	Braided, monofilament	Glycolide and L-lactide coated with copolymer of lactide and calcium stearate	≈75% remains at 2 wk ≈50% remains at 3 wk 25% remains at 4 wk	Minimal acute inflammatory reaction
PDS II (polydioxanone)	Monofilament	Polyester polymer	≈70% remains at 2 wk ≈50% remains at 4 wk ≈25% remains at 6 wk	Slight reaction

Adapted from Ethicon: Wound closure manual, Somerville, NJ, 2007, Ethicon.

TABLE 10-23 Comparison of Nonabsorbable Sutures

SUTURE	TYPES	RAW MATERIAL	TENSILE STRENGTH RETENTION IN VIVO	TISSUE REACTION
Perma-Hand—silk suture	Braided	Organic protein called fibroin	Progressive degradation of fiber may result in gradual loss of tensile strength over time	Acute inflammatory reaction
Ethilon—nylon suture	Monofilament	Long-chain aliphatic polymers Nylon 6 or Nylon 6,6	Progressive hydrolysis may result in gradual loss of tensile strength over time	Minimal acute inflammatory reaction
Nurolon—nylon suture	Braided	Long-chain aliphatic polymers Nylon 6 or Nylon 6,6	Progressive hydrolysis may result in gradual loss of tensile strength over time	Minimal acute inflammatory reaction
Mersilene—polyester fiber suture	Braided monofilament	Polyethylene terephthalate	No significant change known to occur in vivo	Minimal acute inflammatory reaction
Ethibond Excel—polyester fiber suture	Braided	Polyethylene terephthalate coated with polybutilate	No significant change known to occur in vivo	Minimal acute inflammatory reaction
Prolene—polypropylene suture	Monofilament	Isotactic crystalline stereoisomer of polypropylene	Not subject to degradation or weakening by action of tissue enzymes	Minimal acute inflammatory reaction
ProNova—poly (hexafluoropropylene-VDF) suture	Monofilament	Polymer blend of poly (vinylidene fluoride) and poly (vinylidene fluoride–cohexafluoropropylene)	Not subject to degradation or weakening by action of tissue enzymes	Minimal acute inflammatory reaction

Adapted from Ethicon: Wound closure manual, Somerville, NJ, 2007, Ethicon.

TABLE 10-24 Types of Synthetic Mesh and Their Uses

TYPE OF MESH	TRADE NAME	TYPE	COMMENTS
Nonabsorbable			
Polypropylene	Marlex, Prolene, Atrium	Monofilament	Highly elastic, withstands infection well; widely used for abdominal wall reconstruction, hernia repair
PTFE	Teflon	Multifilament	Nonexpanded mesh; associated with many complications; limited usefulness
Expanded PTFE	Gore-Tex	Multifilament	Greatest elongation compared with other nonabsorbable meshes; minimal tissue incorporation; multiple uses in abdominal, vascular reconstruction
Polyethylene terephthalate	Mersilene, Dacron	Multifilament	Polyester fiber mesh with broad usefulness in abdominal wall, hernia repair; less extensively used than polypropylene
Absorbable			
Polyglycolic acid	Dexon	Multifilament	Useful for temporary abdominal closure; resists infection
Polyglactin 910	Vicryl	Multifilament	Useful for temporary abdominal closure; resists infection

Adapted from Fenner DE: New surgical mesh. *Clin Obstet Gynecol* 43:650–658, 2000.
PTFE, polytetrafluoroethylene.

of the fascia to close the fascia gradually, over the course of up to four trips to the operating room.

Two more recent concepts in abdominal surgery include the use of adhesion reduction barriers and synthetic biomembranes for abdominal wall closure. Two types of adhesion reduction barriers are available, hyaluronic acid–carboxymethylcellulose and oxidized regenerated cellulose. Both of these materials are applied to the raw surface of the bowel before abdominal closure, and they turn to a gelatinous substance within 1 hour.[1] Although the use of these membranes does not obviate adhesions totally, they have been demonstrated in clinical trials to decrease their severity.[1] The second innovation involves using engineered tissue matrices for abdominal wall closure. These materials are constructed from donor integumentary tissue and processed to remove the epidermal and dermal cellular portions and the antigenic component of the allograft. The resulting product is a collagen-based matrix with its native tensile strength intact but its capacity to generate an immune response abrogated. The interstices of the allograft are colonized by cellular populations from the recipient.[1] This material promises to yield an adjunct to closure of a complex abdominal wall defect that has good strength and is more resistant to infection than the use of synthetic materials such as polypropylene mesh.

Staplers

Surgical staplers have changed the practice of surgery in a profound way, most notably within the field of minimally invasive technology. Several different devices are available for stapling, as follows:

1. Skin staplers
2. Ligating and dividing staplers
3. Gastrointestinal anastomosis (GIA) staplers
4. Thoracoabdominal staplers
5. End-to-end anastomosis staplers
6. Laparoscopic hernia mesh tackers
7. Open hernia mesh staplers
8. Endo-GIA staplers

A modification of the GIA stapler for laparoscopic use, the endo-GIA, has particularly broad usefulness. It can facilitate the ligation and transection of major vascular pedicles in laparoscopy, as in the performance of splenectomy, nephrectomy, or hepatectomy, or facilitate GIA or transection of solid organs such as the pancreas. In a video-assisted thoracoscopic surgical procedure, it can aid in wedge resection of an injured or diseased lung. The GIA (endo-GIA or standard version) stapler may aid in the transection of thick or indurated mesentery during intestinal resection in patients with inflammatory bowel disease.

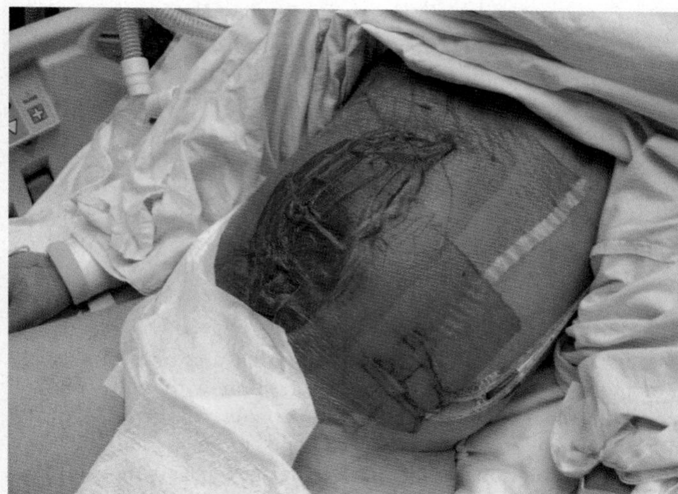

FIGURE 10-5 Vac-Pac temporary abdominal wound closure. This closure method allows easy reentry into the abdomen and does not compromise the fascia. To fashion, place a surgical towel between two medium sticky drapes, and place it in the abdomen; tuck the edges underneath the fascia with an overlap of several centimeters. Closed suction drains are placed along the edges and brought out through the skin. Another surgical towel is placed over the open portion of the wound, and a large sticky drape is used to cover the entire abdomen. The drains are immediately connected to wall suction to provide adequate compression of the dressing.

Surgical Adhesives

Surgical adhesives have been widely used in modern surgery. They can be used for a simple task such as skin closure or for more complex wound problems. Many agents are clinically available and are used for various purposes. Fibrin seal adhesive has been used to close fistulas; prevent lymphatic leakage after complete lymphadenectomy in the axilla or groin; and prevent leakage from tissue surfaces that have been newly transected, such as staple lines of the lung or pancreatic resection. It also has been adapted to seal the terminal bronchus via bronchoscopy as a noninvasive means for treating a small subset of patients with pneumothorax. Fibrin seal adhesive has become the preferred way to treat pseudoaneurysms in the groin or axilla that result from arterial puncture. Ultrasound-guided direct injection into such lesions has been reported to be successful, with low complication rates.[1] Adhesives can also be used as an adjunct to reinforce and provide a watertight seal to a delicate GIA, such as one involving the biliary tract or pancreas.

Surgical adhesives work by admixing a two-component agent derived from whole blood; each is secured in separate containers for shipping and storage. When mixed, the components form a viscous semiliquid tissue glue that can be applied onto a suture line, fistula tract or cavity, or other raw tissue surface or potential small dead space. When set, it becomes a solid adhesive biomembrane, sealant, or plug that is self-retained. Major obstacles to its widespread use are cost and the potential for complications related to disease transmission with the use of blood products.

Two other commonly used agents are 2-octyl cyanoacrylate (Dermabond) and butyl-2-cyanoacrylate (Histoacryl). Cyanoacrylate has been used for repair of organs and as an adhesive in many orthopedic procedures. Dermabond has been demonstrated to be an adequate replacement for the traditional suture closure of simple skin lacerations. Dermabond also allows the patient to resume showering within a few hours of wound closure.

SURGICAL DEVICES AND ENERGY SOURCES

Electrosurgery and Electrocautery

In 1928, Cushing first published a series of 500 neurosurgical procedures performed with an electrocautery device that was developed by Bovie. Since then, electrocautery and electrosurgery have become the most important and basic surgical tools in the operating room.

High-frequency alternating current can be delivered in unipolar or bipolar fashion. The unipolar (or monopolar) device is composed of a generator, electrode for application, and electrode for the returning current to complete the circuit. The patient's body becomes part of the circuit when the system is activated. Because the effectiveness of energy conversion into heat is inversely related to the area of contact, the application electrode is designed to be small to generate heat efficiently, and the returning electrode is designed to be large to disperse energy and prevent burn injury. The heat generated depends on three other factors in addition to the size of the contact area: (1) the power setting or frequency of the current, (2) the length of activation time, and (3) whether the waveform released from the generator is continuous or intermittent. Unipolar devices can be used to incise tissue when activated with a constant waveform and to coagulate when activated with an intermittent waveform. In the cutting mode, much heat is generated relatively quickly over the target, with minimal lateral thermal spread. As a result, the device cuts through tissue without coagulating any underlying vessels. In contrast, in the coagulation mode, electrocautery generates less heat on a slower frequency, with the potential for large lateral thermal spread. Such spread results in tissue dehydration and vessel thrombosis. A blended waveform can be chosen that is able to take advantage of the cutting and coagulation modes. A large grounding pad must be placed securely on the patient for the unipolar electrosurgical or electrocautery device to function properly and prevent thermal burn injury at the current reentry electrode site.

Bipolar electrocautery establishes a short circuit between the tips of the instrument, whether a tissue grasper or forceps, without the requirement for a grounding pad. The tissue grasped between the tips of the instrument completes the circuit. In generating heat that affects only the tissue within the short circuit, it provides precise thermal coagulation. Bipolar electrocautery is more effective than the monopolar instrument in coagulating vessels because it adds the mechanical advantage of compression of tissue between the tips of the instrument to the thermal coagulation. Bipolar electrocautery is particularly useful when conducting a procedure in which lateral thermal injury or an arcing phenomenon needs to be avoided.

Lasers

Lasers use photons to excite the chromophore molecules within target tissue and generate kinetic energy that is released as heat, which causes protein denaturation and coagulation necrosis. This effect occurs without much collateral damage to surrounding tissue. It can be applied to the surface of target tissue or interstitially with a fiberoptic probe placed under precision image guidance. The energy generated and the depth of tissue penetration can be varied with the power setting selected and the photon chosen for the particular task. The laser effect can be enhanced by photosensitizing agents. The most common lasers in use are the argon, carbon dioxide, and neodymium:yttrium-aluminum-garnet (Nd-YAG) lasers. The depth of energy penetration within the target organ is least with the argon laser, moderate with the carbon dioxide laser, and deepest with the Nd-YAG laser.

Interstitial laser photocoagulation is a more recently adopted laser treatment technology. With a precisely placed optic fiber (or fibers) inside the target tissue, laser light is delivered and absorbed by the surrounding structure and tissue. The degree of absorption within and around the target tissue depends on the wavelength of the laser chosen and specific optical properties of the tissue. The optical properties of different tumors or tissues are markedly different and depend on their tissue composition and density, degree of parenchymal fibrosis, vascularity, and presence or absence of necrosis.

Argon Beam Coagulator

The argon beam coagulator creates a monopolar electrical circuit between a hand-held probe and the target tissue by establishing a steady flow of electrons through a channel of electrically activated and ionized argon gas. This high-flow argon gas conducts electrical current to the target tissue and generates thermal coagulation of this tissue. The depth of the thermal penetration of tissue ranges from fractions of a millimeter to a maximum of 6 mm, depending on three factors:

1. Power setting
2. Distance between the probe and the target
3. Length of application

The hand-held control is usually combined with the regular Bovie, which can provide much more focused tissue coagulation for any identifiable vessels. The argon gas blows blood away from the surface of the target, so argon beam coagulation is more effective for the bleeding parenchyma of an organ. Visibility is improved by the same mechanism. It is most commonly used to treat parenchymal hemorrhage of an organ, particularly the liver, but can be used on the spleen, kidney, or any other solid organ with surface oozing.

Photodynamic Therapy

Photodynamic therapy allows destruction of cancer cells and has been expanded to the eradication of metaplastic cells. It begins with the administration of a target-specific photosensitizer that is eventually concentrated in the target tissue. The photosensitizing agent is activated with a wavelength-specific light energy source, which leads to the generation of free radicals cytotoxic to the target tissue. Photodynamic therapy has been used to treat different types of late-stage cancers, mainly in a palliative setting, but it has also been used for the treatment of some chemoresistant tumors. Applications reported in the literature include treating early radiographically detected non–small cell lung cancer, pancreatic cancer, squamous cell and basal cell carcinoma of the skin, recurrent superficial bladder cancer, chest wall involvement from breast cancer, and chest wall recurrence of breast cancer. Its usefulness has been expanded to include the treatment of noncancer conditions, such as Barrett esophagus and psoriasis.[1]

High-Frequency Sound Wave Techniques

Ultrasound has had a strong impact on the practice of modern medicine. It has different functions, depending on the frequency of ultrasound generated by the machine. At a low power level, it causes no tissue damage and is mainly used for diagnostic purposes. With a high-frequency setting, ultrasound can be used to dissect, cut, and coagulate. Several high-frequency ultrasonic devices are available for use in surgical practice.

Another beneficial manipulation of acoustic wave technology is extracorporeal shock wave lithotripsy. It has been used in treating cholelithiasis and nephrolithiasis. The patient is placed in a water bath, and a high-energy acoustic shock wave is generated by piezoelectric or electromagnetic technology and focused. The water-tissue interface allows the wave to pass through normal tissue without injuring it. The energy of the shock wave is focused on the offending stone by ultrasound and causes disruption and fragmentation of the calculus, which is subsequently passed via the ureter.

Harmonic Scalpel

The harmonic scalpel is an instrument that uses ultrasound technology to dissect tissue in bipolar fashion with only minimal collateral tissue damage. The device vibrates at a high frequency, approximately 55,000 times per second, to cut tissue. The high-frequency vibration of tissue molecules generates stress and friction in the tissue, which generates heat and denaturation of protein. Because of this unique capability to dissect tissue and coagulate small blood vessels all at once, with minimal energy transfer to surrounding tissue, the device has gained recognition among surgeons. It has been used in many different types of minimally invasive surgery, and its application has been extended to many open procedures.

Ultrasonic Cavitation Devices

The Cavitron ultrasonic surgical aspirator uses lower frequency ultrasound energy to fragment and dissect tissue of low fiber content. It is basically an ultrasound probe combined with an aspirator, so it functions as an acoustic vibrator and suction device at the same time. The Cavitron has various applications. Because the instrument fragments and aspirates tissue of low collagen and high water content, it can be effective surgically for liver and pancreatic procedures without causing damage to surrounding tissue. Compared with the dissection technique of other instruments, such as the scalpel or cautery, the advantages of using this device are less blood loss, improved visibility, and reduced collateral tissue injury. It has been used for resecting lesions in noncirrhotic liver and pancreatic tumors, especially small endocrine tumors within a soft normal pancreas, without fibrosis. It has also been used for partial nephrectomy, salvage splenectomy, head and neck procedures, and treatment of many gynecologic tumors.

Radiofrequency Ablation

Radiofrequency energy can be used for tissue ablation in curative or palliative treatment of different cancers. It is also effective for treating benign conditions such as neuralgia, bone pain, and cardiac arrhythmias (e.g., atrial fibrillation). The basic method of radiofrequency application is to place an electrode (or electrodes) into or over the target tissue to transmit a high-frequency alternating current to the tissue in the range of 350 to 500 kHz. Rapid alternating directional movement of ions results in the release of kinetic energy. It can increase the temperature of the target tissue to greater than 100° C and cause protein denaturation, desiccation, and coagulation necrosis; it has a built-in sensor for automatically terminating transmission of the current at a particular set-point to prevent overheating and unwanted collateral damage. The main use of this modality is for tumors in the liver parenchyma. Its applications have been expanded to tumors in the lung, kidney, adrenal gland, breast, thyroid, pancreas, and bone. The indications for radiofrequency ablation are continuing to grow because it is inexpensive and can be reliably used to destroy a larger tumor mass.

Cryoablation

Cryotherapy can be applied topically to treat skin conditions or tumors or interstitially for the ablation of liver lesions. It destroys cells by freezing and thawing. With liquid nitrogen or argon circulating through a probe placed over or within the target lesion, the tissue can be frozen to a temperature of −35° C or lower. Cell damage occurs as a result of disruption of subcellular structures, with ice crystal formation in the freezing phase and degradation during the thawing process. Ischemia of the tissue from focal disruption of the circulation, shifting of water and electrolyte content in situ, and protein denaturation also contribute to the tissue damage induced by cryotherapy. However, lesions that contact major vessels can be difficult to treat with this modality because of the heat sink effect introduced by circulating blood. Nonetheless, it has been reported to be effective in treating primary and secondary lesions of the liver that are unresectable. The major disadvantage of interstitial cryotherapy is its cost. Patients usually need general anesthesia for the procedure, the equipment is more expensive than a radiofrequency system, and the process itself is time-consuming. Complications such as hemorrhage from tissue fracture are a concern. Cryoablation is currently used to treat solid tumors in the lung, liver, breast, kidney, and prostate.

Microwave Ablation and Radiosurgery

Microwave coagulation is achieved by using a generator to transmit microwave energy at a frequency of 2450 MHz via a probe placed under image guidance within target organs or tissue. A rapidly alternating electrical field is created in the target tissue to induce motion of polar molecules in the tissue, such as water. Kinetic energy is dissipated as heat, which causes coagulation necrosis. It was initially used for lesions in the liver; however, its applications have been expanded to treatment of cardiac rhythm disturbances, prostatic hyperplasia, endometrial bleeding, sterilization of bony margins, and partial nephrectomy. The major limiting factor is that the area that can be ablated with the current equipment is very small, necessitating multiple insertions of the microwave probe to treat a single lesion.[37]

The premier tool in radiosurgery is the Gamma Knife; its principal area of use is in neurosurgery. This tool allows more than 200 separate sources of high-energy gamma radiation, arranged in a circular fashion, to be focused stereotactically onto a minute area in the brain. Avoiding injury to normal brain tissue requires that the head be held motionless by an external fixation device. This ability to destroy finite areas within the brain has been applied to the treatment of benign and malignant brain neoplasms, arteriovenous malformations, and epilepsy.

OUTPATIENT SURGERY

Over the past 25 years, outpatient surgery has become more commonplace. It is estimated that 75% of elective surgical procedures are now performed in an outpatient setting, which means that patients do not experience an overnight stay around the time of the procedure. Even patients who will need a postoperative inpatient stay after the procedure are usually admitted to the hospital after the surgery. Outpatient surgery can be performed in an operating room associated with a large hospital, in a freestanding outpatient surgery center, or in a physician's office. Preoperative evaluation of the patient usually takes place on an ambulatory basis, and more coordination is required by the surgeon to ensure that the evaluation is completed and acted on in a timely fashion. Patients with significant comorbid conditions are evaluated by the anesthesia staff at least 1 day before the planned procedure (Box 10-9).[1] The standards for perioperative monitoring are similar regardless of the setting and are tailored to the complexity of the procedure and comorbid conditions of the patient. In addition,

BOX 10-9 Conditions for Which Preoperative Evaluation May Be Recommended before Day of Surgery

General

Medical condition inhibiting patient's ability to engage in normal daily activity
Medical condition necessitating continual assistance or monitoring at home within past 6 mo
Admission within past 2 mo for acute condition or exacerbation of a chronic condition

Cardiocirculatory

History of angina, coronary artery disease, myocardial infarction
Symptomatic arrhythmias
Poorly controlled hypertension (diastolic >110 mm Hg, systolic >160 mm Hg)
History of congestive heart failure

Respiratory

Asthma, chronic obstructive pulmonary disease requiring long-term medication or with acute exacerbation and progression within past 6 mo
History of major airway surgery or unusual airway anatomy
Upper or lower airway tumor or obstruction
History of chronic respiratory distress requiring home ventilator assistance or monitoring

Endocrine

Insulin-dependent diabetes mellitus
Adrenal disorders
Active thyroid disease

Neuromuscular

History of seizure disorder or other significant central nervous system disease (e.g., multiple sclerosis)
History of myopathy or other muscle disorder

Hepatic

Any active hepatobiliary disease or compromise

Musculoskeletal

Kyphosis or scoliosis causing functional compromise
Temporomandibular joint disorder
Cervical or thoracic spine injury

Oncology

Patients receiving chemotherapy
Other oncology process with significant physiologic residual or compromise

Gastrointestinal

Massive obesity (<140% ideal body weight)
Hiatal hernia
Symptomatic gastroesophageal reflux

the patient's postoperative disposition takes into account the distance from the place of surgery as well as who will be available to monitor the patient.

In general, patients can be discharged home under their own recognizance after procedures performed under local anesthesia without sedation. The need for postoperative pain control with narcotic-based agents may alter the suitability of patients transporting themselves and is considered when making decisions about disposition. Any patient who receives sedation, general anesthetic, or both at a minimum needs to have a ride home. Ideally, the patient would have a responsible individual staying overnight in the same residence. The patient's ability to perform tasks at home also would be influenced by the need for narcotics as well as any restrictions or limitations dictated by the procedure. Patients unable to maintain oral intake after surgery, because of the operation itself or the need for postoperative ventilator support, or who need intravenous or other nonoral pain medication require postoperative hospitalization. The need for postoperative care has a bearing on the type of facility in which the surgeon chooses to perform the procedure.

SELECTED REFERENCES

Bilimoria KY, Liu Y, Paruch JL, et al: Development and evaluation of the universal ACS NSQIP surgical risk calculator: A decision aid and informed consent tool for patients and surgeons. *J Am Coll Surg* 217:833–842.e1–3, 2013.

The American College of Surgeons National Surgical Quality Improvement Program surgical risk calculator was developed to estimate the risks of most operations and allow clinicians and patients to make decisions using empirically derived, patient-specific postoperative risks.

Chow WB, Rosenthal RA, Merkow RP, et al: Optimal preoperative assessment of the geriatric surgical patient: A best practices guideline from the American College of Surgeons National Surgical Quality Improvement Program and the American Geriatrics Society. *J Am Coll Surg* 215:453–466, 2012.

Best practices guidelines concerning optimal perioperative care of geriatric surgical patients were developed by the American College of Surgeons National Surgical Quality Improvement Program and the American Geriatrics Society.

Douketis JD, Spyropoulos AC, Spencer FA, et al: Perioperative management of antithrombotic therapy: Antithrombotic Therapy and Prevention of Thrombosis, 9th ed: American College of Chest Physicians Evidence-Based Clinical Practice Guidelines. *Chest* 141:e326S–e350S, 2012.

Evidence-based practice guidelines are presented for management of patients on anticoagulant or antiplatelet therapy who require elective surgery.

Fleisher LA, Fleischmann KE, Auerbach AD, et al: 2014 ACC/AHA guideline on perioperative cardiovascular evaluation and management of patients undergoing noncardiac surgery: A report of the American College of Cardiology/American Heart Association Task Force on practice guidelines. *J Am Coll Cardiol* 64:e77–e137, 2014.

Evidence-based guidelines for perioperative cardiovascular evaluation of patients undergoing noncardiac surgery were updated in 2014 by the American College of Cardiology/American Heart Association Task Force on Practice Guidelines.

Vaid S, Bell T, Grim R, et al: Predicting risk of death in general surgery patients on the basis of preoperative variables using American College of Surgeons National Surgical Quality Improvement Program data. *Perm J* 16:10–17, 2012.

The preoperative mortality predictor is a quick bedside or office tool to determine the risk of perioperative death in patients undergoing common general surgical procedures using only preoperative variables.

Wijeysundera DN, Duncan D, Nkonde-Price C, et al: Perioperative beta blockade in noncardiac surgery: A systematic review for the 2014 ACC/AHA guideline on perioperative cardiovascular evaluation and management of patients undergoing noncardiac surgery: A report of the American College of Cardiology/American Heart Association Task Force on practice guidelines. *J Am Coll Cardiol* 64:2406–2425, 2014.

A systematic review and meta-analysis was performed by the American College of Cardiology and American Heart Association to establish new recommendations for perioperative beta blockade in patients undergoing noncardiac surgery.

REFERENCES

1. Neumayer L, Vargo D: Principles of preoperative and operative surgery. In Townsend CM, Beauchamp RD, Evers BM, et al, editors: *Sabiston textbook of surgery: the biological basis of modern surgical practice*, ed 19, Philadelphia, 2012, Saunders.
2. Bilimoria KY, Liu Y, Paruch JL, et al: Development and evaluation of the universal ACS NSQIP surgical risk calculator: A decision aid and informed consent tool for patients and surgeons. *J Am Coll Surg* 217:833–842, e1–e3, 2013.
3. Vaid S, Bell T, Grim R, et al: Predicting risk of death in general surgery patients on the basis of preoperative variables using American College of Surgeons National Surgical Quality Improvement Program data. *Perm J* 16:10–17, 2012.
4. Neary WD, Prytherch D, Foy C, et al: Comparison of different methods of risk stratification in urgent and emergency surgery. *Br J Surg* 94:1300–1305, 2007.
5. Fazio VW, Tekkis PP, Remzi F, et al: Assessment of operative risk in colorectal cancer surgery: The Cleveland Clinic Foundation colorectal cancer model. *Dis Colon Rectum* 47:2015–2024, 2004.
6. Duval H, Dumont F, Vibert E, et al: The Association Francaise de Chirurgie (AFC) colorectal index: A reliable preoperative prognostic index in colorectal surgery [in French]. *Ann Chir* 131:34–38, 2006.
7. Alves A, Panis Y, Mantion G, et al: The AFC score: Validation of a 4-item predicting score of postoperative mortality after colorectal resection for cancer or diverticulitis: Results of a prospective multicenter study in 1049 patients. *Ann Surg* 246:91–96, 2007.

8. Hall MJ, DeFrances CJ, Williams SN, et al: National Hospital Discharge Survey: 2007 summary. *Natl Health Stat Report* 29:1–20, 24, 2010.
9. Corrada MM, Brookmeyer R, Berlau D, et al: Prevalence of dementia after age 90: Results from the 90+ study. *Neurology* 71:337–343, 2008.
10. De Cosmo G, Congedo E, Lai C, et al: Preoperative psychologic and demographic predictors of pain perception and tramadol consumption using intravenous patient-controlled analgesia. *Clin J Pain* 24:399–405, 2008.
11. Taenzer P, Melzack R, Jeans ME: Influence of psychological factors on postoperative pain, mood and analgesic requirements. *Pain* 24:331–342, 1986.
12. Li C, Friedman B, Conwell Y, et al: Validity of the Patient Health Questionnaire 2 (PHQ-2) in identifying major depression in older people. *J Am Geriatr Soc* 55:596–602, 2007.
13. McGory ML, Kao KK, Shekelle PG, et al: Developing quality indicators for elderly surgical patients. *Ann Surg* 250:338–347, 2009.
14. Woolger JM: Preoperative testing and medication management. *Clin Geriatr Med* 24:573–583, 2008.
15. Devereaux PJ, Goldman L, Yusuf S, et al: Surveillance and prevention of major perioperative ischemic cardiac events in patients undergoing noncardiac surgery: a review. *CMAJ* 173:779–788, 2005.
16. Fleisher LA, Fleischmann KE, Auerbach AD, et al: 2014 ACC/AHA guideline on perioperative cardiovascular evaluation and management of patients undergoing noncardiac surgery: A report of the American College of Cardiology/American Heart Association Task Force on practice guidelines. *J Am Coll Cardiol* 64:e77–e137, 2014.
17. Davenport DL, Ferraris VA, Hosokawa P, et al: Multivariable predictors of postoperative cardiac adverse events after general and vascular surgery: Results from the patient safety in surgery study. *J Am Coll Cardiol* 204:1199–1210, 2007.
18. Chow WB, Rosenthal RA, Merkow RP, et al: Optimal preoperative assessment of the geriatric surgical patient: A best practices guideline from the American College of Surgeons National Surgical Quality Improvement Program and the American Geriatrics Society. *J Am Coll Surg* 215:453–466, 2012.
19. Weimann A, Braga M, Harsanyi L, et al: ESPEN guidelines on enteral nutrition: Surgery including organ transplantation. *Clin Nutr* 25:224–244, 2006.
20. Wijeysundera DN, Duncan D, Nkonde-Price C, et al: Perioperative beta blockade in noncardiac surgery: A systematic review for the 2014 ACC/AHA guideline on perioperative cardiovascular evaluation and management of patients undergoing noncardiac surgery: A report of the American College of Cardiology/American Heart Association Task Force on practice guidelines. *J Am Coll Cardiol* 64:2406–2425, 2014.
21. Fleisher LA, Beckman JA, Brown KA, et al: ACC/AHA 2007 guidelines on perioperative cardiovascular evaluation and care for noncardiac surgery: Executive summary: A report of the American College of Cardiology/American Heart Association Task Force on Practice Guidelines (Writing Committee to Revise the 2002 Guidelines on Perioperative Cardiovascular Evaluation for Noncardiac Surgery) developed in collaboration with the American Society of Echocardiography, American Society of Nuclear Cardiology, Heart Rhythm Society, Society of Cardiovascular Anesthesiologists, Society for Cardiovascular Angiography and Interventions, Society for Vascular Medicine and Biology, and Society for Vascular Surgery. *J Am Coll Cardiol* 50:1707–1732, 2007.
22. Hillis LD, Smith PK, Anderson JL, et al: 2011 ACCF/AHA guideline for coronary artery bypass graft surgery. A report of the American College of Cardiology Foundation/American Heart Association Task Force on Practice Guidelines. Developed in collaboration with the American Association for Thoracic Surgery, Society of Cardiovascular Anesthesiologists, and Society of Thoracic Surgeons. *J Am Coll Cardiol* 58:e123–e210, 2011.
23. Gersh BJ, Maron BJ, Bonow RO, et al: 2011 ACCF/AHA guideline for the diagnosis and treatment of hypertrophic cardiomyopathy: Executive summary: A report of the American College of Cardiology Foundation/American Heart Association Task Force on Practice Guidelines developed in collaboration with the American Association for Thoracic Surgery, American Society of Echocardiography, American Society of Nuclear Cardiology, Heart Failure Society of America, Heart Rhythm Society, Society for Cardiovascular Angiography and Interventions, and Society of Thoracic Surgeons. *J Am Coll Cardiol* 58:2703–2738, 2011.
24. Kaluza GL, Joseph J, Lee JR, et al: Catastrophic outcomes of noncardiac surgery soon after coronary stenting. *J Am Coll Cardiol* 35:1288–1294, 2000.
25. Nuttall GA, Brown MJ, Stombaugh JW, et al: Time and cardiac risk of surgery after bare-metal stent percutaneous coronary intervention. *Anesthesiology* 109:588–595, 2008.
26. Cruden NL, Harding SA, Flapan AD, et al: Previous coronary stent implantation and cardiac events in patients undergoing noncardiac surgery. *Circ Cardiovasc Interv* 3:236–242, 2010.
27. Grines CL, Bonow RO, Casey DE, Jr, et al: Prevention of premature discontinuation of dual antiplatelet therapy in patients with coronary artery stents: A science advisory from the American Heart Association, American College of Cardiology, Society for Cardiovascular Angiography and Interventions, American College of Surgeons, and American Dental Association, with representation from the American College of Physicians. *Circulation* 115:813–818, 2007.
28. Dunkelgrun M, Boersma E, Schouten O, et al: Bisoprolol and fluvastatin for the reduction of perioperative cardiac mortality and myocardial infarction in intermediate-risk patients undergoing noncardiovascular surgery: A randomized controlled trial (DECREASE-IV). *Ann Surg* 249:921–926, 2009.
29. Poldermans D, Schouten O, Vidakovic R, et al: A clinical randomized trial to evaluate the safety of a noninvasive approach in high-risk patients undergoing major vascular surgery: The DECREASE-V Pilot Study. *J Am Coll Cardiol* 49:1763–1769, 2007.
30. Devereaux PJ, Yang H, Guyatt GH, et al: Rationale, design, and organization of the PeriOperative ISchemic Evaluation (POISE) trial: A randomized controlled trial of metoprolol versus placebo in patients undergoing noncardiac surgery. *Am Heart J* 152:223–230, 2006.
31. Le Manach Y, Collins GS, Ibanez C, et al: Impact of perioperative bleeding on the protective effect of beta-blockers during infrarenal aortic reconstruction. *Anesthesiology* 117:1203–1211, 2012.
32. Barrett TW, Mori M, De Boer D: Association of ambulatory use of statins and beta-blockers with long-term mortality after vascular surgery. *J Hosp Med* 2:241–252, 2007.

33. Bateman BT, Schumacher HC, Wang S, et al: Perioperative acute ischemic stroke in noncardiac and nonvascular surgery: Incidence, risk factors, and outcomes. *Anesthesiology* 110:231–238, 2009.
34. Eker HH, van Ramshorst GH, de Goede B, et al: A prospective study on elective umbilical hernia repair in patients with liver cirrhosis and ascites. *Surgery* 150:542–546, 2011.
35. Carson JL, Grossman BJ, Kleinman S, et al: Red blood cell transfusion: A clinical practice guideline from the AABB. *Ann Intern Med* 157:49–58, 2012.
36. Carson JL, Carless PA, Hebert PC: Transfusion thresholds and other strategies for guiding allogeneic red blood cell transfusion. *Cochrane Database Syst Rev* 4:CD002042, 2012.
37. Carson JL, Carless PA, Hebert PC: Outcomes using lower vs higher hemoglobin thresholds for red blood cell transfusion. *JAMA* 309:83–84, 2013.
38. Carson JL, Brooks MM, Abbott JD, et al: Liberal versus restrictive transfusion thresholds for patients with symptomatic coronary artery disease. *Am Heart J* 165:964–971, e1, 2013.
39. Kristensen SD, Knuuti J, Saraste A, et al: 2014 ESC/ESA Guidelines on non-cardiac surgery: Cardiovascular assessment and management: The Joint Task Force on non-cardiac surgery: Cardiovascular assessment and management of the European Society of Cardiology (ESC) and the European Society of Anaesthesiology (ESA). *Eur Heart J* 35:2383–2431, 2014.
40. King CS, Holley AB, Moores LK: Moving toward a more ideal anticoagulant: The oral direct thrombin and factor Xa inhibitors. *Chest* 143:1106–1116, 2013.
41. Spyropoulos AC, Hussein M, Lin J, et al: Rates of venous thromboembolism occurrence in medical patients among the insured population. *Thromb Haemost* 102:951–957, 2009.
42. Gould MK, Garcia DA, Wren SM, et al: Prevention of VTE in nonorthopedic surgical patients: Antithrombotic Therapy and Prevention of Thrombosis, 9th ed: American College of Chest Physicians Evidence-Based Clinical Practice Guidelines. *Chest* 141(2 Suppl):e227S–e277S, 2012.
43. Caprini JA: Thrombosis risk assessment as a guide to quality patient care. *Dis Mon* 51:70–78, 2005.
44. Bahl V, Hu HM, Henke PK, et al: A validation study of a retrospective venous thromboembolism risk scoring method. *Ann Surg* 251:344–350, 2010.
45. Rogers SO, Jr, Kilaru RK, Hosokawa P, et al: Multivariable predictors of postoperative venous thromboembolic events after general and vascular surgery: Results from the patient safety in surgery study. *J Am Coll Surg* 204:1211–1221, 2007.
46. van Stijn MF, Korkic-Halilovic I, Bakker MS, et al: Preoperative nutrition status and postoperative outcome in elderly general surgery patients: A systematic review. *JPEN J Parenter Enteral Nutr* 37:37–43, 2013.
47. Aarts MA, Okrainec A, Glicksman A, et al: Adoption of enhanced recovery after surgery (ERAS) strategies for colorectal surgery at academic teaching hospitals and impact on total length of hospital stay. *Surg Endosc* 26:442–450, 2012.
48. American Society of Anesthesiologists Committee: Practice guidelines for preoperative fasting and the use of pharmacologic agents to reduce the risk of pulmonary aspiration: Application to healthy patients undergoing elective procedures: An updated report by the American Society of Anesthesiologists Committee on Standards and Practice Parameters. *Anesthesiology* 114:495–511, 2011.
49. Bratzler DW, Dellinger EP, Olsen KM, et al: Clinical practice guidelines for antimicrobial prophylaxis in surgery. *Am J Health Syst Pharm* 70:195–283, 2013.

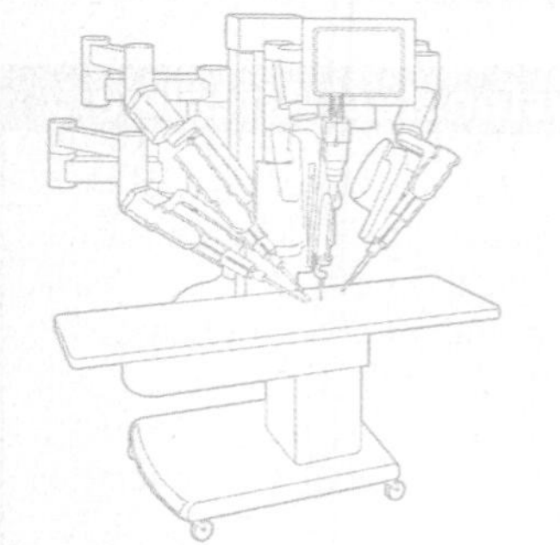

CHAPTER 11

Surgical Infections and Antibiotic Use

Philip S. Barie

OUTLINE

Traditionally, surgical infections have been considered to be those that require surgical therapy (e.g., complicated intra-abdominal infections and skin or soft tissue infections). However, surgical patients are particularly vulnerable to nosocomial infections, so a more expansive definition includes any infection that affects surgical patients. Examples of infections that may complicate perioperative care include surgical site infections (SSIs), central line–associated bloodstream infections (CLABSIs), urinary tract infections (UTIs), and hospital- or ventilator-associated pneumonia (HAP, VAP). This chapter takes the more encompassing view, recognizing that the surgical patient is at particular risk for nosocomial infections for numerous reasons.

Surgery's inherent invasiveness creates portals of entry for pathogens to invade the host through natural epithelial barriers. Surgical illness is immunosuppressive (e.g., trauma, burns, malignant tumors), as is therapeutic immunosuppression after solid organ transplantation. General anesthesia almost always means a period of endotracheal intubation and mechanical ventilation and a period of reduced consciousness during emergence that poses a risk of pulmonary aspiration of gastric contents; both increase the risk of pneumonia. Considering that the development of a postoperative infection has a negative impact on surgical outcomes, recognizing and minimizing risk and an aggressive approach to the diagnosis and treatment of these infections are crucial.

Although morbid and costly, infection is preventable to some degree, and every physician who has patient contact must do his or her utmost to prevent infection. An ensemble of prevention methods is required because no single method is universally effective. Infection control is paramount. Surgical incisions and traumatic wounds must be handled gently, inspected daily, and dressed if necessary using strict asepsis. Drains and catheters must be avoided, if possible, and removed as soon as practicable. Prophylactic and therapeutic antibiotics, whether empirical or directed against a known infection, should be used sparingly to minimize antibiotic selection pressure on the development of multidrug-resistant (MDR) pathogens. Each of these aspects is discussed in detail.

RISK FACTORS FOR INFECTION

Host Factors

The host is defined by genotype, expressed phenotypically as characteristic traits. Innate immunity provides continuous surveillance against tissue invasion by foreign antigens in the interstitial spaces just beneath epithelial barriers. Potential pathogens are ubiquitous in the environment, but although colonization of epithelia occurs even in healthy hosts, invasion generally requires a portal of entry, which for surgical patients might include injured tissue, incision, puncture site for vascular access, or indwelling catheter. Injury also stimulates a repair response (inflammation), which may cause a wide-ranging autodestructive augmentation of the inflammatory response.

The phenotypic stress response augments cardiovascular function through the autonomic nervous system, promotes glycogenolysis, catabolizes peripheral lean tissue and fat for gluconeogenesis, enhances coagulation to stanch hemorrhage, and stimulates a proinflammatory cytokine response to begin the tissue repair process (Box 11-1).[1] Innate immunity and adaptive immunity are depressed in large part by the actions of cortisol (Table 11-1 and Box 11-2).[2]

Older age (generally, age ≥65 years) is a definite risk factor for adverse outcomes from infection,[3] related to immune senescence and an increased incidence of nosocomial infection. Hyperglycemia induces immune cell dysfunction (Box 11-3) and is a recognized risk factor for infection (Box 11-4). Even transitory hyperglycemia is associated with an increased risk of SSIs[4-7] and other nosocomial infections and translates into increased mortality after trauma[8,9] and critical surgical illness[10,11] for diabetic and nondiabetic patients.

BOX 11-1 Overview of the Stress Response to Injury

Activation of the autonomic nervous system
Activation of hypophyseal-pituitary-adrenal axis
Peripheral insulin resistance
Production of proinflammatory and anti-inflammatory cytokines and lipid mediators
Production of reactive oxygen and nitrogen intermediates
Acute-phase changes of hepatic protein synthesis
Recruitment and activation of neutrophils, monocytes-macrophages, and lymphocytes
Upregulation of procoagulant activity

TABLE 11-1 Principal Hormonal Responses to Surgical Stress

ENDOCRINE GLAND	HORMONES	CHANGE IN SECRETION
Anterior pituitary	Corticotropin	Increased
	Growth hormone	Increased
	Thyrotropin	Variable
	Follicle-stimulating hormone, luteinizing hormone	Variable
Posterior pituitary	Arginine vasopressin	Increased
Adrenal cortex	Cortisol	Increased
	Aldosterone	Increased
Pancreas	Insulin	Decreased
	Glucagon	Increased
Thyroid	Thyroxine	Decreased
	Triiodothyronine	Decreased

Genetics and Genomics of Trauma and Sepsis

It is controversial as to whether gender makes a difference in outcome after infection and sepsis. Androgens are immunosuppressive in vitro and in animal studies, and male animals have higher mortality after trauma and sepsis,[12,13] but human data are conflicting. Population-based studies have cast doubt on the clinical importance of the laboratory observations of gender-based differences. Gannon and colleagues[14] have found no gender-based difference of mortality among 18,892 trauma patients; of interest, male patients were more likely to develop pneumonia, but female patients were more likely to succumb. Angus and associates[15] were unable to detect any adverse outcomes from sepsis among female patients in a nationwide U.S. population-based study.

Modern high-throughput, multiplexed assays allow the molecular characterization of pathologic conditions. Most genes have hundreds or thousands of nucleotides, but only a relatively short sequence is needed for the precise identification of each. The DNA microarray, minute quantities of vast numbers (i.e., many thousands) of short, gene-specific probe nucleotides affixed to a slide chip, can be used to identify messenger RNA that can be isolated from cells or tissues and labeled to produce complementary nucleotides (cDNA or cRNA). When incubated with the microarray, the cDNA or cRNA will bind by conventional base pairing. With a scanner and the aid of computational biomedicine, the label signal intensity (mRNA abundance) may be calculated and compared, generating an expression profile called the

BOX 11-2 Immune Dysfunction After Injury

Lymphopenia
Helper to suppressor T cell ratio <1
Downregulated
- T and B cell proliferation
- NK cell activity
- IL-2 receptor expression
- IL-4 and IL-10 production
- HLA-DR expression
- DTH skin test response

Nonspecific Immunity
Monocytosis
Upregulated
- Acute-phase proteins
- Inflammatory cytokine production
- Eicosanoid production

Downregulated
- Neutrophil function

DTH, delayed-type hypersensitivity; *HLA,* human leukocyte antigen; *IL,* interleukin; *NK,* natural killer cell.

BOX 11-3 Glucose Dyshomeostasis During Stress and Effects on Cellular Immunity

Effects of Hyperglycemia on Immune Cell Function
- Decreased respiratory burst of alveolar macrophages
- Decreased insulin-stimulated chemokinesis
- Glucose-induced protein kinase C activation
- Increased adherence
- Increased adhesion molecule generation
- Spontaneous activation of neutrophils

Effects of Stress Response on Carbohydrate Metabolism
- Enhanced peripheral glucose uptake
- Hyperlactatemia
- Increased gluconeogenesis
- Depressed glycogenolysis
- Peripheral insulin resistance

BOX 11-4 Medical Conditions Known to Increase Risk of Postoperative Infection

- Extremes of age (neonates, very old adults)
- Malnutrition
- Obesity
- Diabetes mellitus
- Prior site irradiation
- Hypothermia
- Hypoxemia
- Coexisting infection remote to surgical site
- Corticosteroid therapy
- Recent operation, especially of chest or abdomen
- Chronic inflammation
- Hypocholesterolemia

transcriptome for the cell or tissue of interest. Such techniques have furthered the understanding of host predisposition and response to sepsis[16,17]; application of related techniques of cell separation, genome-wide expression, and cell-specific pathway analyses may be useful to characterize alterations in human disease or the presence of specific microbes. However, their presence does not distinguish whether the microbe is a colonist or a pathogen.

In infection, genomic variability may correlate with disease susceptibility. Single-nucleotide polymorphisms, single point mutations in the nucleotide structures of genes related to inflammation (e.g., tumor necrosis factor-α [TNF-α], interleukin [IL]-1, IL-6, and IL-8), the anti-inflammatory response (e.g., IL-10, IL-1 receptor antagonist), the innate immune response (e.g., Toll-like receptor 4), and the coagulation system (e.g., factor V, plasminogen activator inhibitor 1), have been associated with a predisposition to sepsis.[18] However, heterogeneity in the immune response and predisposition to infection as well as the severity of infections and resultant mortality make conclusions difficult to determine, which makes it unlikely that a single single-nucleotide polymorphism will be identifiable in an individual patient to characterize risk.

Interactions Between the Host and Therapy

The risk of infection may exist as the result of injury itself, impairment of host defenses, resuscitation, or definitive care. Hypothermia may occur as the result of exposure, large-volume infusion of unwarmed fluids or blood products, or evaporative losses during intracavitary surgery, especially if the chest and abdomen are opened. Peripheral and cutaneous vasoconstriction occurs to preserve core heat, but vasoconstriction decreases microcirculatory blood flow, which may also be disrupted by hypovolemia, inflammatory response, activation of coagulation, and decreased deformability of transfused red blood cells (see later).[19] Hypothermia is immunosuppressive, affects cardiovascular performance adversely, and increases mortality after trauma and surgery.[20,21]

Tissue hypoxia after trauma may result from injury to the face, airways, lungs, or chest wall and from inability to secure the airway, massive blood loss, cardiovascular instability, disruption of the microcirculation, or acute respiratory distress syndrome (ARDS). Tissue hypoxia appears to predispose to SSI.[22] Administration of supplemental oxygen ($FIO_2 = 0.8$) reduces the risk of SSI after elective surgery (meta-analysis).[21]

The manner of resuscitation may influence outcome. Fluids are necessary to restore hemodynamics and microcirculatory perfusion, but the quantity and type of fluid that should be administered are still debated. Historically, crystalloid fluids were preferred to colloids, being less expensive and with results that were at least equivalent.[23] Although some trials, such as that of the SAFE investigators,[24] have led to a reappraisal, the question remains controversial. Delaney and coworkers[25] have conducted a meta-analysis of 17 trials (1977 subjects); eight trials were specifically of colloid versus crystalloid for resuscitation of patients with sepsis. Colloid resuscitation was associated with reduced mortality in a fixed-effects model (odds ratio [OR], 0.82; 95% confidence interval [CI], 0.67-1.0; $P = .047$) but not when a more robust random-effects model was used for the meta-analysis (OR, 0.84; 95% CI, 0.69-1.02; $P = .08$). However, six of the trials included, by a single investigator, have been called into question for scientific misconduct[26]; omission of those results from the meta-analysis still produced a significant result by fixed-effects meta-analysis (OR, 0.76; 95% CI, 0.62-0.95; $P = .015$). Functionally, resuscitation of the immune system may be the crucial determinant, as evidenced by observations that a persistent systemic inflammatory response after injury is associated with an increased risk of nosocomial infection and death.[27]

Blood Transfusion

Blood transfusion can be lifesaving after trauma or hemorrhage, but increased risk of infection is the consequence. Transfusions express immunosuppression through altered leukocyte antigen presentation and a shift to the T helper 2 phenotype.[28] Claridge and colleagues[29] have identified an exponential relationship between transfusion and infection risk among trauma patients, detectable after even 1 unit of transfusion and becoming a near certainty after more than 15 units of transfused blood (relative risk [RR], 1.084; 95% CI, 1.028-1.142). Hill and associates[30] have estimated by meta-analysis that the risk of infection related to blood transfusion is increased for trauma patients by more than fivefold (OR, 5.26; 95% CI, 5.03-5.43) and for surgical patients by more than threefold. This increased risk for infection by transfusion has also been identified for critically ill patients in general[31] and for CLABSI[32] and VAP[33] specifically. Loss of membrane high-energy phosphates associated with prolonged storage of banked blood leads to impaired erythrocyte deformability, disruption of the microcirculation, and impaired oxygen offloading.[34] Consequently, blood transfusion does not increase oxygen consumption in severe sepsis[35] and may actually increase organ dysfunction.[36] It is safe to be conservative in the administration of red blood cell concentrates to stable patients in the intensive care unit (ICU).[37]

Control of Blood Glucose Concentration

Not only does hyperglycemia impair host immune function, it also reflects the catabolism and insulin resistance associated with surgical stress. Poor perioperative glycemic control increases the risk of infection and worsens outcomes from sepsis for diabetic and nondiabetic patients. Cardiac surgery patients have a higher risk of infection of sternal incision and lower extremity donor sites. Moderate hyperglycemia (>200 mg/dL) at any time on the first postoperative day increases the risk of SSI fourfold after cardiac[6] and noncardiac surgery.[7] Insulin infusion to keep the blood glucose level below 110 mg/dL was associated with a 40% decrease in mortality among critically ill postoperative patients (≈70% of whom had undergone cardiac surgery) and also fewer nosocomial infections and less organ dysfunction.[38] However, glycemic control has become somewhat controversial because of nonconfirmation of a salutary effect in critically ill medical patients. Moreover, concern about an increased incidence of hypoglycemia (≈6%, <60 mg/dL) in patients treated with intensive insulin therapy and resultant increased mortality has led to relaxation of glycemic control targets to approximately 140 to 180 mg/dL.[39] Nonetheless, a meta-analysis of recent trials by Griesdale and associates[10] has indicated that the risk of mortality is decreased significantly for patients treated with intensive insulin therapy in dedicated surgical ICUs (RR, 0.63; 95% CI, 0.44-0.91), regardless of whether the patients had diabetes mellitus. However, countervailing opinion as to the usefulness and safety of intensive insulin therapy is prevalent.[21]

Nutritional support is crucial, considering that restoration of anabolism requires calories and nitrogen in excess of basal requirements of 25 to 30 kcal and 1 g nitrogen/kg/day. It is challenging to provide adequate calories and protein while simultaneously avoiding hyperglycemia. Parenteral nutrition may convey no advantage over not feeding the patient at all,[40] perhaps because of the inherent morbidity of central intravenous (IV) feeding (i.e., the risks of CLABSI and hyperglycemia). By contrast, early enteral feeding within the first 48 hours, perhaps immediately if the gut is functional, is clearly beneficial, with the possible exceptions of intestinal ischemia and pneumonia prevention (see later). The risk of infection was reduced by 55% (OR, 0.45; 95% CI, 0.30-0.66) in a meta-analysis of 15 randomized trials of early enteral feeding after surgery, trauma, or burns.[41]

INFECTION CONTROL

General principles of surgical care, critical care, and infection control must be adhered to at all times. Resuscitation must be rapid yet precise; overresuscitation and underresuscitation increase the risk of infection. Pathologic changes must be identified and treated as soon as possible. Central venous catheters inserted under suboptimal barrier precautions (e.g., lack of cap, mask, sterile gown, and sterile gloves for the operator and a full bed drape for the patient) must be removed and replaced, if necessary, by a new puncture at a new site as soon as the patient's condition permits. Drains should be avoided and removed as soon as possible, if required.[42] Detailed evidence-based guidelines for the general prevention of SSIs,[43] CLABSIs,[44,45] and VAP have been published.[46,47]

Infection control is an individual and collective responsibility. Hand hygiene is the most effective means to reduce the spread of infection, but compliance is a continual challenge.[48] Alcohol gel hand cleansers are effective,[49] except against the spores of *Clostridium difficile,* which requires cleansing with soap and water.[50] Universal precautions—cap, mask, gown, gloves, and protective eyewear—must be observed whenever there is a risk of splashing of body fluids.

Endogenous flora are the source of most bacterial pathogens. Skin surfaces, artificial airways, gut lumen, wounds, catheters, and inanimate surfaces (e.g., bed rails, computer terminals)[51] may become colonized. Any break in natural epithelial barriers (e.g., incisions, percutaneous catheters, airway or urinary catheters) creates a portal of entry for invasion of pathogens. The fecal-oral route is the most common manner whereby pathogens reach the portal, but health care workers facilitate the transmission of pathogens on their hands.

Contact isolation is an important part of infection control and should be used selectively to prevent the spread of pathogens such as methicillin-resistant *Staphylococcus aureus* (MRSA), vancomycin-resistant enterococci (VRE), or MDR gram-negative bacilli. However, contact isolation may decrease the amount of direct patient contact.[52] An appropriate balance must be struck because reduced nurse staffing of ICUs has been independently associated with an increased risk of a number of nosocomial infections.[53]

Catheter Care

Optimal catheter care includes avoidance when unnecessary; appropriate skin preparation and barrier protection during insertion; proper catheter selection (e.g., antimicrobial or antiseptic coated); proper dressing of indwelling catheters; and removal as soon as no longer needed, or as is practicable, but no longer than 24 hours after insertion under less than ideal circumstances (e.g., trauma bay, cardiac resuscitation).

Risks and benefits must be weighed in deciding to place any catheter, including the risk of infection. Almost all indwelling catheters carry such a risk, but nontunneled central venous catheters and pulmonary artery catheters pose the highest risk, including local site infections and CLABSIs. Other catheters that pose increased infection risk include endotracheal tubes, intercostal thoracostomy catheters (inserted as an emergency), ventriculostomy catheters for intracranial pressure monitoring, and urinary bladder catheters. Each day of endotracheal intubation and mechanical ventilation increases the risk of pneumonia by 1% to 3%[54]; it is controversial whether tracheostomy decreases that risk.[55]

Chlorhexidine gluconate, a phenolic biguanide derivative, is used in concentrations of 0.5% to 4.0% alone or in lower concentrations in combination with an alcohol as a skin antiseptic. The microbicidal action, which is bactericidal, viricidal, and fungicidal, is somewhat slow but persistent. Chlorhexidine should be used preferentially for skin preparation for vascular catheter insertion; it is superior to povidone-iodine solution[56] and is also recommended for surgical skin preparation,[57] for topical bathing of critically ill patients,[58,59] and as an antiseptic coating for indwelling central vascular catheters.[60] If povidone-iodine solution is used for surgical site preparation, it must be allowed to dry for microbicidal effect. Note that its use is discouraged unless a mucous membrane is to be prepared. Full barrier precautions are mandatory for all bedside catheterization procedures, except arterial and urinary bladder catheterization, for which sterile gloves and a sterile field suffice if they are maintained meticulously. Whenever a central venous catheter is inserted under suboptimal conditions, it must be removed—and replaced at a different site if it is still needed—as soon as permitted by the patient's hemodynamic status but no longer than 24 hours after insertion. A single dose of a first-generation cephalosporin (e.g., cefazolin) may prevent some infections after emergency tube thoracostomy or ventriculostomy, but it is not indicated for vascular or bladder catheterizations.

It is crucial to maintain dressings carefully, which can be challenging if the patient is agitated or the body surface is irregular (e.g., the neck [internal jugular vein catheterization] as opposed to the chest wall [subclavian vein catheterization]). Marking the dressing clearly with the date and time of each change is simple and effective. Dressing carts or similar equipment should not be brought from patient to patient; instead, sufficient supplies should be kept in each patient's room. The potential for transmission of pathogens on inanimate fomites (e.g., scissors) must be borne in mind. Implementation of care bundles and dedicated catheter care teams substantially reduce the risk of CLABSIs and UTIs.[61,62]

The choice of catheter may play a role in decreasing the risk of infection related to endotracheal tubes, central venous catheters, and urinary catheters. Continuous aspiration of subglottic secretions through an endotracheal tube with an extra lumen that opens to the airway just above the balloon facilitates the removal of secretions that accumulate below the vocal cords but above the endotracheal tube balloon, an area that cannot be reached by routine suctioning. The incidence of VAP is decreased by 50% by continuous aspiration of subglottic secretions.[63] Silver-impregnated endotracheal tubes are effective in reducing airway colonization[64] and may reduce the incidences of VAP and mortality.[65] Antibiotic-coated (e.g., minocycline, rifampin) or antiseptic-coated (e.g., chlorhexidine, silver sulfadiazine) central venous catheters can reduce the incidence of catheter-related bloodstream infections,[44,66] especially in high-prevalence units; minocycline- or rifampin-coated catheters may be more effective. Urinary bladder catheters coated with ionic silver reduce the incidence of catheter-related bacterial cystitis by a similar amount.[67,68]

Ventilator weaning by protocol, including daily sedation holidays and spontaneous breathing trials, allows endotracheal extubation sooner and decreases the risk of VAP (see later).[69] An even better strategy may be avoidance of endotracheal intubation entirely. Respiratory failure can sometimes be managed with noninvasive positive pressure ventilation delivered by mask (e.g., continuous positive airway pressure).[70] Improved resuscitation and noninvasive monitoring techniques have decreased the use of pulmonary artery catheters, which pose a particularly high risk of infection.[71] Most drains do not decrease the risk of infection; in fact, the risk is probably increased[72] because the catheters hold open a portal for invasion by bacteria.

SPECIFIC INFECTIONS

Surgical Site Infection

The spectrum of bacterial contamination of the surgical site is well described.[72] Clean surgical procedures affect only skin structures and other soft tissues. Clean-contaminated procedures open a hollow viscus under controlled circumstances (e.g., elective aerodigestive or genitourinary tract surgery). Contaminated procedures introduce a large inoculum of bacteria into a normally sterile body cavity, but too briefly for infection to become established during surgery (e.g., penetrating abdominal trauma, enterotomy during adhesiolysis for mechanical bowel obstruction). Dirty procedures are those performed to control established infection (e.g., colon resection for perforated diverticulitis).

The microbiology of SSI depends on the nature of the procedure, location of the incision, and whether a body cavity or hollow viscus is entered during surgery. Most SSIs are caused by skin flora inoculated into the incision during surgery; therefore, the most common SSI pathogens are all gram-positive cocci—*Staphylococcus epidermidis, S. aureus,* and *Enterococcus* spp. For infrainguinal incisions and intracavitary surgery, gram-negative bacilli such as *Escherichia coli* and *Klebsiella* spp. are potential pathogens. When surgery is performed on the pharynx, lower gastrointestinal tract, or female genital tract, anaerobic bacteria become potential SSI pathogens. Antibiotic prophylaxis should be suitably directed against likely pathogens (see later).

The incidence of SSIs has been estimated to be about 3% in the United States, although the incidence varies greatly from less than 5% for clean surgery to more than 20% for emergency colon surgery, which is often performed in a dirty field. Moreover, the overall estimate is almost certainly an underestimate, considering that SSI after ambulatory surgery, which now represents more than 70% of all operations in the United States, is seldom reported. Numerous factors determine whether a patient will develop an SSI, including those related to the patient, environment, and treatment (Box 11-5).[72] As incorporated in the National Nosocomial Infections Surveillance (NNIS) System and its successor program, the National Healthcare Safety Network (NHSN),[73-75] the most recognized factors are wound classification, American Society of Anesthesiologists class 3 or higher (class 3 is chronic active medical illness), and prolonged operative time, where time is longer than the 75th percentile for the given procedure. According to the NNIS System–NHSN, the risk of SSI increases as the number of risk factors present increases, irrespective of the type of operation.[76] Laparoscopic surgery is associated with a decreased incidence of SSI under most circumstances. There are several possible reasons that laparoscopic surgery decreases the risk of SSI, including decreased wound size, limited use of cautery in the abdominal wall, and diminished stress response to tissue injury.

BOX 11-5 Risk Factors for the Development of Surgical Site Infections

Patient Factors
Ascites (for abdominal surgery)
Chronic inflammation
Corticosteroid therapy (controversial)
Obesity
Diabetes
Extremes of age
Hypocholesterolemia
Hypoxemia
Peripheral vascular disease (for lower extremity surgery)
Postoperative anemia
Prior site irradiation
Recent operation
Remote infection
Skin or nasal carriage of staphylococci
Skin disease in the area of infection (e.g., psoriasis)
Undernutrition

Environmental Factors
Contaminated medications
Inadequate disinfection or sterilization
Inadequate skin antisepsis
Inadequate ventilation

Treatment Factors
Drains
Emergency procedure
Hypothermia
Inadequate antibiotic prophylaxis
Oxygenation (controversial)
Prolonged preoperative hospitalization
Prolonged operative time

Host-derived factors contribute importantly to the risk of SSI, including increased age,[77] obesity, malnutrition, diabetes mellitus,[7] hypocholesterolemia,[78] and several other factors not accounted for specifically by the NNIS System–NHSN (see Box 11-5). In a study of 5031 noncardiac surgical patients, the incidence of SSI was 3.2%.[79] Independent risk factors for the development of SSI included ascites, diabetes mellitus, postoperative anemia, and recent weight loss but not chronic obstructive pulmonary disease, tobacco use, or corticosteroid use. In another prospective study of 9016 patients, 12.5% of patients developed an infection of some type within 28 days after surgery.[80] Multivariable analysis revealed that decreased serum albumin concentration, increased age, tracheostomy, and amputations were associated with an early infection, whereas a dialysis shunt, vascular repair, and early infection were associated with hospital readmission. Factors associated with 28-day mortality included increased age, low serum albumin concentration, increased serum creatinine concentration, and early infection.

Hypothermia during surgery is common if patients are not warmed actively because of evaporative water loss, administration of room temperature fluids, and other factors.[81] Maintenance of normal core body temperature is unequivocally important for decreasing the incidence of SSIs. Mild intraoperative hypothermia is associated with an increased incidence of SSIs after elective colon surgery[82] and diverse operations.[83]

It is controversial whether perioperative oxygen administration is beneficial for the prevention of infection.[84] The ischemic milieu of the fresh surgical incision is vulnerable to bacterial invasion. Moreover, oxygen has been postulated to have a direct antibacterial effect.[85,86] Although clinical trials have had conflicting results,[87,88] one meta-analysis has suggested a benefit of supplemental oxygen administration specifically to reduce the incidence of SSIs,[21] but further studies may be needed before the practice becomes routine.

Skin closure of a contaminated or dirty incision is believed to increase the risk of SSIs, but few good studies exist to evaluate the multiplicity of wound closure techniques available to surgeons. Open abdomen techniques of temporary abdominal closure for management of trauma or severe peritonitis are increasingly being used. Retrospective data have indicated that antibiotics are not indicated for prophylaxis of the open abdomen,[89] although an inability to achieve primary abdominal closure is associated with several infectious complications (e.g., pneumonia, bloodstream infection, SSIs). Infectious complications, in turn, significantly increase costs from prolonged length of stay but not mortality.[90]

Drains placed in incisions probably cause more infections than they prevent. Epithelialization of the wound is prevented and the drain becomes a conduit, holding open a portal for invasion by pathogens colonizing the skin. Several studies of drains placed into clean or clean-contaminated incisions have shown that the rate of SSI is not reduced[91,92]; in fact, the rate is increased.[93-96] Considering that drains pose this risk, they should be used as little as possible and removed as soon as possible.[97] Under no circumstances should prolonged antibiotic prophylaxis be administered to cover indwelling drains (see later).

Wound irrigation is a controversial means to reduce the risk of SSIs. Routine low-pressure saline irrigation is ineffective,[98] but high-pressure (i.e., pulsed) irrigation may be beneficial.[99] Intraoperative topical antibiotics can minimize the risk of SSIs,[100-102] but the use of antiseptics rather than antibiotics might minimize the development of resistance.

SSI remains a clinical diagnosis. Presenting signs and symptoms depend on the depth of infection, typically as early as postoperative day 4 or 5, although rare necrotizing SSIs caused by *Streptococcus pyogenes* or *Clostridium perfringens* may develop within 24 hours after surgery. Clinical signs range from local induration only to the hallmarks of infection (e.g., erythema, edema, tenderness, warmth, pain-related immobility), which may be manifested before wound drainage. In cases of deep incisional SSIs, tenderness may extend beyond the margin of erythema, and crepitus, cutaneous vesicles, or bullae may be present. With ongoing infection, signs of systemic inflammatory response syndrome (SIRS; two or more of fever, leukocytosis, tachycardia, or tachypnea) herald the development of sepsis. In intracavitary (organ, space) SSIs, symptoms specific to the involved organ system will usually predominate, such as ileus, respiratory distress or failure, or altered sensorium.

Cultures are not mandatory for the management of superficial incisional SSIs, particularly if drainage and wound care alone will suffice without antibiotics and if superficial swab cultures are collected, which are susceptible to contamination by nearby skin colonists. In cases of deeper infection or hospital-acquired infection, exudates or drainage specimens should be sent for analysis from the surgically opened wound as opposed to the already opened wound, which becomes colonized.

More severe SSIs, especially the dangerous forms of necrotizing soft tissue infection (NSTI), are true emergencies that need immediate surgical attention. Even modest delays can increase mortality substantially. Freischlag and coworkers[103] have shown that mortality increases from 32% to 70% when therapy is delayed longer than 24 hours. Immediate widespread débridement is indicated for established NSTIs without waiting for identification of the causative pathogen or development of a specific symptom. Sequential surgical débridements may be needed to control the infection.

The first steps in the treatment of SSIs are to open and to examine the suspicious portion of the incision and to decide about further surgical treatment.[104] If the infection is confined to the skin and superficial underlying subcutaneous tissue, opening the incision and providing local wound care may be all the treatment that is necessary. Antibiotic therapy of superficial incisional SSIs is indicated only for erythema extending beyond the wound margin or for systemic signs of infection. Deeper SSIs may require formal surgical exploration and débridement to obtain local control of the infection. SSI must also be considered as a cause of delayed or failed wound healing and prompt the same decisions as described earlier.

Organ or space SSIs occur within a body cavity (e.g., intra-abdominal, intrapleural, intracranial) and are directly related to a surgical procedure. These deep infections may remain occult or be manifested with few symptoms, mimicking incisional SSIs and leading to inadequate initial treatment; they become apparent only when a major complication ensues. The diagnosis of organ or space SSIs usually requires some form of imaging to confirm the site and extent of infection. Adequate source control requires a drainage procedure, whether open or percutaneous.

Vacuum-assisted wound closure (VAC) was first appraised experimentally by Morykwas and colleagues[105] in a porcine model in 1997. Therapy by VAC optimizes blood flow, decreases edema, and aspirates accumulated fluid, thereby facilitating bacterial clearance. Negative pressure promotes wound contraction to cover the defect and may trigger intracellular signaling that increases cellular proliferation.[106] The clinical usefulness of VAC has been described only anecdotally, mostly for sternal infections after cardiac surgery, abdominal wall dehiscence, management of complex perineal wounds, or securing skin grafts.[107,108]

Many general and specific tactics for the prevention of SSIs have been brought together in a bundle known as the Surgical Care Improvement Project (SCIP), the effectiveness of which has been called into question.[109,110] A predecessor program, the National Surgical Infection Prevention Project, focused primarily on the quality of antibiotic prophylaxis, including choice of agent, timing of administration, and duration of prophylaxis. A national audit found that the agents being prescribed for prophylaxis were often inappropriate, the effectiveness of prophylaxis was decreased because the timing of administration was suboptimal, and only 40% of patients administered surgical antibiotic prophylaxis had the antibiotic discontinued within 24 hours, risking adverse events (e.g., superinfection, development of bacterial resistance).[111] It was advised that antibiotic administration should occur within 60 minutes before incision and that prophylaxis should continue for no longer than 24 hours.[112] Implementation demonstrated improved adherence to process measures.[113]

The National Surgical Infection Prevention Project was incorporated into the SCIP, with additional process measures added (Box 11-6), including recommendations for agents to be used for prophylaxis in specific circumstances (Table 11-2). As a U.S. federal program, the SCIP includes reporting mandates, with financial incentives for compliance that will eventually become

BOX 11-6 Surgical Care Improvement Project Performance Measures*

Antibiotic Prophylaxis

Proportion of patients who have their antibiotic dose initiated within 1 hour before surgical incision (2 hours for vancomycin or a fluoroquinolone)

Proportion of patients who receive an approved antibiotic agent for prophylaxis consistent with current recommendations (published guidelines; see Table 11-2)

Proportion of patients whose prophylactic antibiotics were discontinued within 24 hours of the surgery end time (48 hours for cardiac surgery)

Clindamycin use is preferred for patients allergic to β-lactam antibiotics.

Vancomycin is allowed for prophylaxis of cardiac, vascular, and orthopedic surgery if there is a physician-documented reason in the medical record or documented β-lactam allergy.

Glucose Control (Cardiac Surgery Patients)

Blood glucose concentration must be maintained <200 mg/dL for the first 2 days after surgery.

Blood glucose determination closest to 6 AM on postoperative days 1 and 2 (surgery end date is postoperative day 0) is monitored.

Hair Removal

No hair removal should be performed; if hair is removed, clippers or a depilatory agent should be used immediately before surgery. Razors are not to be used.

Normothermia (Colorectal Surgery Patients)

Core body temperature should be between 96.8° F and 100.4° F within the first hour after leaving the operating room.

*Relevant to prevention of surgical site infection.

penalties for noncompliance.[114] Perhaps not unexpectedly, several studies have reported that the incidence of SSIs has not decreased under the SCIP,[109,110] possibly for several reasons.[115] Baseline infection rates may have increased as a result of improved reporting, masking any decrease from process improvement. The inherent assumption that a focus on process improvement will result in an improved outcome may be flawed. Causes and prevention of SSIs are complex and multifactorial, and compartmentalization by the SCIP may be an oversimplification. Moreover, the SCIP is not a smorgasbord of tactics from which the clinician may pick and choose; prevention of SSIs requires the flawless execution of an ensemble of prevention tactics,[116] not all of which are included in the SCIP. For example, correction of patient factors is notably missing. Nonetheless, all the SCIP measures are supported by ample, good-quality evidence, and the search for processes that lead to meaningful improvements in outcome must continue.

Postoperative Pneumonia

Surgical patients are particularly susceptible to pneumonia, particularly if they require mechanical ventilation (Table 11-3). VAP, defined as pneumonia occurring 48 to 72 hours after endotracheal intubation, is the most common ICU infection among surgical and trauma patients. The incidence appears to be decreasing, but unfortunately, VAP is partially iatrogenic and sometimes associated with difficult to treat MDR pathogens. Increasingly ill patients, nonspecific diagnostic criteria, indiscriminate antibiotic use, and unclear therapeutic end points have all contributed to the increased prevalence of VAP caused by MDR pathogens. In turn, MDR pathogens increase the likelihood of inadequate initial antimicrobial therapy, which exerts further selection pressure for these pathogens and results in higher mortality.

Distinction is sometimes made between early-onset VAP (occurring <5 days after intubation) and late-onset VAP (occurring ≥5 days after intubation). Early-onset VAP, to which trauma

TABLE 11-2 Surgical Care Improvement Program: Approved Antibiotic Prophylactic Regimens for Elective Surgery

TYPE OF OPERATION	ANTIBIOTICS
Cardiac (including coronary artery bypass grafting),[a] vascular[b]	Cefazolin or cefuroxime or vancomycin[c]
Hip or knee arthroplasty[b]	Cefazolin or cefuroxime or vancomycin[c]
Colon[d,e]	Oral: Neomycin sulfate plus erythromycin base or metronidazole, administered for 18 hours before surgery Parenteral: Cefoxitin or cefotetan or ertapenem or cefazolin plus metronidazole or ampicillin-sulbactam
Hysterectomy[f]	Cefazolin or cefoxitin or cefotetan or cefuroxime or ampicillin-sulbactam

[a]Prophylaxis may be administered for up to 48 hours for cardiac surgery; for all other cases, the limit is 24 hours.

[b]For β-lactam allergy, clindamycin and vancomycin are acceptable substitutes for cardiac, vascular, and orthopedic surgery.

[c]Vancomycin is acceptable with a physician-documented justification for use in the patient's medical record.

[d]For β-lactam allergy, acceptable choices are the following: clindamycin plus gentamicin, a fluoroquinolone, or aztreonam; and metronidazole plus gentamicin or a fluoroquinolone.

[e]For colon surgery, oral or parenteral prophylaxis alone or both combined is acceptable.

[f]For β-lactam allergy, acceptable choices are the following: clindamycin plus gentamicin, a fluoroquinolone, or aztreonam; metronidazole plus gentamicin or a fluoroquinolone; and clindamycin monotherapy.

TABLE 11-3 Rates of Health Care–Associated Pneumonia Among Various ICU Types*

	TT USE		VAP RATE (MEAN/MEDIAN)	
ICU TYPE	1992-2004	2006-2008	1992-2004	2006-2008
Medical	0.46	0.48	4.9/3.7	2.4/2.2
Pediatric	0.39	0.42	2.9/2.3	1.8/0.7
Surgical	0.44	0.39	9.3/8.3	4.9/3.8
Cardiovascular	0.43	0.39	7.2/6.3	3.9/2.6
Neurosurgical	0.39	0.36	11.2/6.2	5.3/4.0
Trauma	0.56	0.57	15.2/11.4	8.1/5.2

From National Nosocomial Infections Surveillance (NNIS) System Report, data summary from January 1992 through June 2004, issued October 2004. *Am J Infect Control* 32:470–485, 2004; and Edwards JR, Peterson KD, Mu Y, et al: National Healthcare Safety Network (NHSN) report: Data summary for 2006 through 2008, issued December 2009. *Am J Infect Control* 37:783–805, 2009.

TT use is the number of days of indwelling endotracheal tube or tracheostomy per 1000 patient-days in ICU; *VAP*, ventilator-associated pneumonia.

*Infection rates are indexed per 1000 patient-days.

BOX 11-7 Risk Factors for the Development of Ventilator-Associated Pneumonia

Age ≥60 years
Acute respiratory distress syndrome
Chronic obstructive pulmonary disease or other underlying pulmonary disease
Coma or impaired consciousness
Serum albumin level <2.2 g/dL
Burns, trauma
Blood transfusion
Organ failure
Supine position
Large-volume gastric aspiration
Sinusitis
Immunosuppression
Prolonged mechanical ventilation

patients are particularly prone, is often a result of aspiration of gastric contents and is usually caused by antibiotic-sensitive bacteria such as methicillin-sensitive *S. aureus, Streptococcus pneumoniae,* and *Haemophilus influenzae.*[46,117,118] Conversely, patients with late-onset VAP are at increased risk for infection with MDR pathogens (e.g., *Pseudomonas aeruginosa, Acinetobacter* spp.).

The incidence of VAP depends on the diagnostic criteria used and therefore varies in published reports. Clinical criteria alone (e.g., those of the Centers for Disease Control and Prevention, which do not require the identification of a pathogen) underestimate the incidence of VAP compared with microbiologic or histologic data.[119,120] A systematic review of 89 studies of mechanically ventilated patients with VAP[121] has reported a pooled incidence of VAP of 22.8% (95% CI, 18.8-26.9). The risk for trauma patients, especially those with traumatic brain injury, is especially high. The incidence of VAP increases with the duration of mechanical ventilation at a rate of 3%/day during the first 5 days, 2%/day during days 5 to 10, and 1%/day after that.[54]

Risk factors for VAP are summarized in Box 11-7. Perhaps most important is airway intubation itself. The risk of HAP increases 6- to 20-fold in mechanically ventilated patients[121,122]; VAP is especially common in patients with ARDS because of prolonged mechanical ventilation and devastated local airway host defenses.[123]

Several evidence-based strategies can prevent VAP, but to be used effectively, a thorough understanding of modifiable risk factors is required (Table 11-4).[124] Prevention of VAP begins with the minimization of endotracheal intubation and duration of mechanical ventilation. Noninvasive positive pressure ventilation should be used when possible (e.g., awake patient with intact airway reflexes) because it is associated with a lower incidence of VAP.[125] When the airway must be secure, orotracheal intubation is preferred to the nasotracheal route; orotracheal intubation decreases the risk of VAP by 50%[126] by decreasing the risk of nosocomial sinusitis, a known antecedent of VAP. Evidence-based strategies to decrease the duration of mechanical ventilation include daily assessment for readiness to be extubated by interruption of sedation and spontaneous breathing trials,[127] standardized weaning protocols, and adequate ICU staffing.[128]

After intubation, most VAP preventive measures aim to decrease the risk of aspiration. Maintenance of endotracheal cuff pressure more than 20 cm H_2O, new balloon cuff materials and technology that facilitate a better seal between balloon and

TABLE 11-4 Strategies to Prevent Ventilator-Associated Pneumonia

STRATEGY	RECOMMENDED	INSUFFICIENT EVIDENCE
Universal infection control precautions	+	
Orotracheal intubation (versus nasotracheal)	+	
Maintenance of endotracheal cuff pressure >20 cm H_2O	+	
Continuous aspiration of subglottic secretions	+	
Semirecumbent positioning	+	
Modified cuff technology	+	
Sliver-impregnated endotracheal tube	+	
Postpyloric feeding		+
Postponement of enteral feeding for at least 48 hours after intubation	+	
Selective decontamination of the digestive tract		?
Topical chlorhexidine (pharynx or bathing)	+	
Transfusion restriction	+	
Antibiotic cycling		+

tracheal side wall,[129] and continuous aspiration of subglottic secretions[63] reduce the incidence of VAP significantly. Semirecumbent positioning (30 to 45 degrees, head up) is also protective compared with supine positioning, especially during enteral feeding.[130] Postpyloric feeding may decrease the risks of gastroesophageal reflux and aspiration. A meta-analysis of 11 randomized trials has reported a RR of 0.77 (95% CI, 0.60-1.00; $P = .05$) for VAP with postpyloric feeding compared with gastric feedings,[131] but promotility agents such as erythromycin facilitate safe intragastric feeding.[132] However, early enteral feedings may increase the risk of VAP. Shorr and colleagues[33] have reported that enteral nutrition begun 48 hours or less after the initiation of mechanical ventilation is independently associated with the development of VAP (OR, 2.65; 95% CI, 1.93-3.63; $P < .0001$).

Pharmacologic strategies to minimize the risk of VAP include stress ulcer prophylaxis and selective decontamination of the digestive tract (SDD) with topical or systemic antibiotics or antiseptics. Many clinical trials have examined the effect of SDD on the incidence of VAP, but the literature is limited by questionable study methodology,[133] study in ICUs in which MDR pathogens were rare, and increased number of infections caused by MDR bacteria observed in the SSD groups,[134,135] especially gram-positive cocci. For these reasons, the use of SDD remains controversial for the routine prevention of VAP. However, a meta-analysis of studies of oropharyngeal decontamination with topical chlorhexidine has provided sufficient evidence to recommend the practice,[136] especially for cardiac surgical patients.

Ample data document the relationship between blood transfusion and infection risk in surgical, trauma, and critically ill patients.[28-32] Shorr and associates[33] have found red blood cell transfusion to be an independent risk factor for VAP (OR, 1.89; 95% CI, 1.33-2.68; $P = .0004$). Earley and coworkers[137] have documented a 90% decreased incidence of VAP in a surgical ICU after implementation of an anemia management protocol that resulted in fewer blood transfusions.

The diagnosis of VAP is challenging to make accurately because noninfectious processes that produce abnormal chest radiographs and gas exchange (e.g., congestive heart failure, atelectasis, ARDS, pulmonary embolism, pulmonary hemorrhage) may coexist. Intubated sedated patients cannot mobilize respiratory secretions without assistance. Moreover, immunocompromised patients, such as solid organ transplant recipients, may have pneumonia without fever, cough, sputum production, or leukocytosis.[138] The diagnosis of VAP requires not only determination if the patient has pneumonia but also determination of the causative agent. Poor specificity (false-positive results) is a problem because it exposes patients to risk from overtreatment with antibiotics and also increases the risk of emergence of MDR bacteria.[139,140] Conversely, inadequate initial therapy is associated with increased mortality that cannot be reduced by subsequent modification of the antibiotic regimen.[141]

According to the Centers for Disease Control and Prevention criteria, the diagnosis of VAP requires one or more of the following: fever, leukocytosis or leukopenia, purulent sputum, hypoxemia, or a new or evolving chest radiograph infiltrate. No pathogen need be identified. However, noninfectious processes mimic these nonspecific signs, so clinical criteria alone are unreliable. A new chest radiograph infiltrate, along with two of the criteria mentioned, is only 69% sensitive and 75% specific for VAP compared with postmortem histology.[142] Subsequent reports have confirmed the low specificity of the clinical diagnosis of VAP[143]; microbiologic confirmation occurs in less than 50% of cases.[144] Computed tomography has only a fair correlation with the diagnosis of pneumonia in complex patients.[145]

The clinical pulmonary infection score (CPIS) incorporates clinical, radiographic, and microbiologic criteria (e.g., temperature, leukocyte count, chest radiograph infiltrates, appearance and volume of tracheal secretions, PaO_2, FIO_2, culture, and Gram stain of tracheal aspirate—0 to 2 points each) to yield a maximum score of 12 points.[146] A CPIS higher than 6 points indicates a high probability of VAP. However, the specificity of CPIS is no better than clinical acumen alone compared with lower respiratory tract cultures obtained through bronchoscopic bronchoalveolar lavage (BAL) or protected specimen brush (PSB)[147,148] and is inaccurate for use on trauma patients.[149] However, the negative predictive value of a negative Gram stain from a stable patient is almost 100%.[150]

Because of the low specificity of traditional diagnostic criteria, culture of lower respiratory tract samples is mandatory for nosocomial pneumonia before the administration of antibiotics to minimize false-negative results. The methods of specimen collection (invasive versus noninvasive) and specimen analysis (semiquantitative versus quantitative) have been debated. Noninvasive techniques include endotracheal suction aspiration, blinded plugged telescoping catheter, blinded PSB, and mini-BAL. Endotracheal aspirates are less specific because of an increased likelihood of contamination by oropharyngeal flora, reflecting colonization rather than infection, which is the crucial issue in diagnosis.

Invasive techniques (BAL or PSB) collect samples by fiberoptic bronchoscopy and allow direct inspection of the airways but are more expensive and resource-intensive. Whereas semiquantitative microbiology reports growth in ordinal categories (e.g., light, moderate, heavy), quantitative microbiology reports growth in terms of colony-forming units (CFU) per milliliter of aliquot; a threshold value is assigned to distinguish colonization from infection. Commonly used thresholds are 10^3 CFU/mL for PSB, 10^4 CFU/mL for BAL, and 10^5 CFU/mL for endotracheal suction aspiration. Any threshold should be lowered by one order of magnitude for antibiotic therapy before sample acquisition.[151]

Bronchoscopic specimen techniques are more specific than blinded techniques, and both techniques are superior to endotracheal suction aspiration, although it is unclear whether this makes a difference clinically. Shorr and colleagues[152] have performed a meta-analysis of randomized trials that compared outcomes of patients with VAP managed with invasive versus noninvasive sampling when both samples were cultured quantitatively. Although the pooled OR suggested a survival advantage to the invasive approach (OR, 0.62), the result was not significant. However, patients in the invasive group were significantly more likely to undergo changes in the antimicrobial regimen, whether narrowing of therapy or cessation.

Organisms that may be pathogens in VAP or contaminants when recovered from the airway include *P. aeruginosa,* Enterobacteriaceae, *S. pneumoniae, S. aureus,* and *H. influenzae.* Conversely, enterococci, viridans streptococci, coagulase-negative staphylococci, and *Candida* spp. are rarely if ever a cause of respiratory dysfunction.

Central Line–Associated Bloodstream Infection

Critically ill patients often require reliable large-bore central venous access (e.g., femoral, internal jugular, subclavian vein), but the catheters are prone to infection. Strict adherence to infection control, proper insertion technique, and catheter care are crucial for prevention (see earlier) because surgical and trauma patients are at high risk (Table 11-5). When catheters are placed under elective (controlled) circumstances, optimal technique includes chlorhexidine skin preparation (not povidone-iodine), maximum barrier precautions (i.e., draping the entire bed into the sterile field; donning a cap, mask, and sterile gown and gloves), and implementation of a formal catheter care protocol. If insertion

TABLE 11-5 Rates of Central Venous Catheter Use and Central Line–Associated Bloodstream Infection Among Various ICU Types*

	CVC USE		CLABSI RATE (MEAN/MEDIAN)	
ICU TYPE	1992-2004	2006-2008	1992-2004	2006-2008
Medical	0.52	0.45	5.0/3.9	1.9/1.0
Pediatric	0.46	0.48	6.6/5.2	3.0/2.5
Surgical	0.61	0.59	4.6/3.4	2.3/1.7
Cardiovascular	0.79	0.71	2.7/1.8	1.4/0.8
Neurosurgical	0.48	0.44	4.6/3.1	2.5/1.9
Trauma	0.61	0.63	7.4/5.2	3.6/3.0

From National Nosocomial Infections Surveillance (NNIS) System Report, data summary from January 1992 through June 2004, issued October 2004. *Am J Infect Control* 32:470–485, 2004; and Edwards JR, Peterson KD, Mu Y, et al: National Healthcare Safety Network (NHSN) report: Data summary for 2006 through 2008, issued December 2009. *Am J Infect Control* 37:783–805, 2009.

CVC use is the number of days of central venous catheter placement per 1000 patient-days in ICU.

*Infection rates are indexed per 1000 patient-days.

technique is breached, the risk of infection increases exponentially, and the catheter should be removed and replaced (if it is still needed) at a different site using strict asepsis and antisepsis as soon as the patient's condition permits but certainly within 24 hours. Infection risk is highest for femoral vein catheters and lowest for catheters placed through the subclavian route.[153] Peripheral vein catheters, peripherally placed central catheters, and tunneled central venous catheters (e.g., Hickman, Broviac) pose less risk of infection than percutaneous central venous catheters. Bundles and checklists are effective measures to decrease the risk of CLABSIs when they are implemented and adhered to rigorously.[154-157] Antibiotic- and antiseptic-coated catheters are controversial but may help decrease the risk of infection in units that have a high rate of infection.[44]

All intravascular devices and insertion sites must be assessed daily to determine ongoing need and whether signs of local infection are present (e.g., inflammation or purulence at the exit site or along the tunnel). Contaminated catheter hubs are common portals of entry for organisms colonizing the endoluminal surface of the catheter. Infusate (e.g., fluid, blood products, IV medications) can become contaminated and cause bacteremia or fungemia, which is likely to result in septic shock. Abrupt onset of signs and symptoms of sepsis or shock in patients with an indwelling vascular catheter should prompt suspicion of catheter infection. Positive blood cultures for staphylococci or *Candida* spp. strongly suggest infection of a vascular catheter, which should prompt removal and culture of the catheter. Studies have demonstrated the reliability of semiquantitative or quantitative catheter tip culture methods for the diagnosis of a colonized catheter.[158] The predictive value of a positive catheter culture is low when there is a low pretest probability of catheter-related line sepsis, and catheters removed from ICU patients should be cultured only if there is strong clinical suspicion of CLABSI. For patients undergoing evaluation for fever who do not have SIRS, there is usually no need to remove or to change all indwelling catheters immediately; however, this would be prudent in a patient with a prosthetic heart valve or fresh arterial graft and is strongly recommended for severe sepsis or septic shock, peripheral embolization, disseminated intravascular coagulation, or ARDS.

Suppurative phlebitis of a central vein caused by a centrally placed catheter is unusual. With suppurative phlebitis, bloodstream infection characteristically originates from a peripheral vein catheter site with an infected intravascular thrombus, producing a picture of overwhelming sepsis with high-grade bacteremia or fungemia. This syndrome is encountered most often in burn patients or other ICU patients who develop catheter-related infection that goes unrecognized, permitting microbes to proliferate. In patients with persistent *S. aureus* bacteremia or fungemia, echocardiography is appropriate to assess for endocarditis and to guide further therapy.[159]

Urinary Tract Infection

Catheter-associated bacteriuria or candiduria usually represents colonization, is rarely symptomatic, and is an unlikely cause of fever or secondary bloodstream infection,[160,161] even in immunocompromised patients,[162] unless there is urinary tract obstruction or a history of recent urologic manipulation, injury, or surgery and neutropenia.[163,164] As such, there has been relatively little emphasis until recently on the prevention of nosocomial UTIs compared with VAP or CLABSIs.[165] As effective prevention tactics, emphasis is now being placed on avoidance or brief duration of catheterization (e.g., <48 hours for elective surgery patients)[157,165] and the use of silver alloy–coated catheters[67,68] when instrumentation is required.

Traditional signs and symptoms (e.g., dysuria, urgency, pelvic or flank pain, fever or chills) that correlate with bacteriuria in noncatheterized patients are rarely reported in ICU patients with documented catheter-associated bacteriuria or candiduria (>10^5 CFU/mL).[166,167] In the ICU, most UTIs are related to urinary catheters and are caused by multiresistant, nosocomial, gram-negative bacilli other than *E. coli, Enterococcus* spp., and yeasts.[165]

When clinical evaluation suggests the urinary tract as a possible source of fever, a urine specimen should be evaluated by direct microscopy, Gram stain, and quantitative culture.[161] The specimen should be aspirated from the catheter sampling port after disinfection of the port with 70% to 90% alcohol, not collected from the drainage bag. Urine collected for culture should reach the laboratory promptly to prevent multiplication of bacteria within the receptacle, which might lead to the misdiagnosis of infection; any delay should prompt refrigeration of the specimen.

In contrast to community-acquired UTIs, in which pyuria is highly predictive of important bacteriuria, pyuria may be absent with catheter-associated UTI. Even if it is present, pyuria is not a reliable predictor of UTI in the presence of a catheter.[167] The concentration of urinary bacteria or yeast needed to cause symptomatic UTI or fever is unclear. Whereas it is clear that counts higher than 10^3 CFU/mL represent true bacteriuria or candiduria in catheterized patients,[168] no evidence has shown that higher counts are more likely to represent symptomatic infection.

Whereas it is appropriate to collect urine specimens in the investigation of fever (see later), routine monitoring or surveillance cultures of urine contribute little to patient management. Rapid dipstick tests, which detect leukocyte esterase and nitrite, are unreliable in the setting of a catheter-related UTI. The leukocyte esterase test correlates with the degree of pyuria, which may or may not be present in a catheter-related UTI. The nitrite test reflects Enterobacteriaceae, which convert nitrate to nitrite, and is therefore unreliable to screen for *Enterococcus, Candida,* and *Staphylococcus* spp.

Intra-abdominal Infection

Intra-abdominal infections (IAIs) represent a diverse group of diseases commonly encountered in surgical practice. Such infections are dichotomized traditionally and for clinical research purposes into uncomplicated (uIAI) and complicated (cIAI)[169] and, more recently, as to whether they arose in the community-associated (CA-IAI) or hospital-associated (HA-IAI) setting (e.g., associated with a colon anastomotic dehiscence) and whether they are low, moderate, or high risk for clinical failure, morbidity, or death. In uIAIs, infection is contained within a single organ, and there may be no perforation of the gastrointestinal tract. The uIAIs almost never cause serious illness and are not considered further here, although a complicating nosocomial infection could make matters worse.[170]

By contrast, cIAIs extend beyond the source organ and into the peritoneal cavity through a perforated viscus, thereby stimulating a greater SIRS response. The extent of infection depends on containment by local intraperitoneal host defenses. Contained infection results in the formation of an abscess, which is facilitated by foreign bodies to lower the inoculum size and microbial synergy, and creates a low pH environment that impairs phagocyte function and impedes permeation of immune cells and antibiotics. Uncontained spread of infection leads to diffuse peritonitis, a condition characterized by higher mortality that necessitates urgent celiotomy.[171]

Most IAIs may be controlled effectively, with low associated morbidity, through removal or repair of the infected focus, treatment with narrow-spectrum and pathogen-specific antimicrobial therapy (if indicated), and restoration of anatomy if resection is performed for definitive source control. However, in cases of high-risk or hospital-acquired cIAI, broad-spectrum empirical antimicrobial therapy is indicated because of an increased risk of causative MDR pathogens.[172,173] Inappropriate initial antimicrobial therapy of high-risk patients with cIAIs leads to increased rates of clinical failure and death,[174,175] often caused by multiorgan dysfunction syndrome. In cases of severe sepsis or septic shock secondary to IAI, termed *abdominal sepsis,* mortality is approximately 25% to 35%[176,177] but may exceed 70%.[178,179] Treatment of abdominal sepsis is predicated on adequate physical drainage or resection of the infected focus (termed *source control*), which may range from percutaneous drainage to serial laparotomies and open abdominal wound management in severe cases.[180]

Mortality is higher from HA-IAIs than from CA-IAIs.[181,182] Health care–associated nonpostoperative IAIs, which arise in patients hospitalized for reasons unrelated to abdominal disease, portend a particularly poor prognosis.[183] In these cases, diagnosis is often delayed because of a low index of suspicion, poor underlying health status, and altered sensorium. Health care–associated IAIs are significantly more likely to involve pathogens that are resistant to narrow-spectrum agents[173] and therefore are more likely to be treated inadequately compared with patients with CA-IAIs, contributing to treatment failures and a higher incidence of morbidity and mortality.[175]

ANTIBIOTIC USE

Pharmacokinetic and Pharmacodynamic Principles

Pharmacokinetics (PK) involves the principles of drug absorption, distribution, and metabolism.[184] Dose-response relationships are influenced by dose, dosing interval, and route of administration. Plasma and tissue drug concentrations are influenced by absorption, distribution, and elimination, which in turn depend on drug metabolism and excretion. Serum drug concentrations may be correlated, depending on tissue penetration, but to the extent that they are correlated, relationships between local drug concentration and effect are defined by pharmacodynamic (PD) principles (see later).

Basic concepts of PK include *bioavailability*, the percentage of drug dose that reaches the systemic circulation. Bioavailability is 100% after IV administration but is affected by absorption, intestinal transit time, and degree of hepatic metabolism after oral administration. The *half-life* ($t_{1/2}$), the time required for the serum drug concentration to be reduced by half, reflects *clearance* and *volume of distribution* (V_D)[184] and is useful to estimate for the interpretation of drug concentration data. V_D, a derived proportionality constant of no particular physiologic significance that is independent of a drug's clearance or $t_{1/2}$, is useful for estimating the plasma drug concentration achievable from a given dose. V_D varies substantially because of pathophysiologic processes; a reduced V_D causes a higher plasma drug concentration for a given dose, whereas fluid overload and hypoalbuminemia, which decrease drug binding, increase V_D, making dosing more complex.

Clearance refers to the volume of liquid from which a drug is eliminated completely per unit of time, whether by tissue distribution, metabolism, or elimination. Knowledge of drug clearance is important for determining the dose of drug necessary to maintain a steady-state concentration. Drug elimination may be by metabolism, excretion, or dialysis. Most drugs are metabolized by the liver to polar compounds for eventual renal excretion, which may occur by filtration or active or passive transport. The degree of filtration is determined by molecular size and charge and by the number of functional nephrons. In general, if 40% or more of administered drug or its active metabolites is eliminated unchanged in the urine, decreased renal function will require a dosage adjustment.

PD is unique for antibiotic therapy because drug-patient, drug-microbe, and microbe-patient interactions must be accounted for.[184] In contrast to most drug treatment, the key drug interaction is not with the host but with the microbe. Microbial physiology, inoculum size, microbial growth phase, mechanisms of resistance, microenvironment (e.g., local pH), and host response are important factors to consider. Because of microbial resistance, the mere administration of a drug may not be microbicidal if an adequate concentration is not achieved.

Antibiotic PD parameters determined by laboratory analysis include the minimal inhibitory concentration (MIC), the lowest serum drug concentration that inhibits bacterial growth (MIC_{90} refers to 90% inhibition). However, some antibiotics may suppress bacterial growth at subinhibitory concentrations *(postantibiotic effect).* Appreciable postantibiotic effect can be observed with aminoglycosides and fluoroquinolones for gram-negative bacteria and with some β-lactam drugs (notably carbapenems) against *S. aureus*. However, MIC testing may not detect resistant bacterial subpopulations within the inoculum (e.g., heteroresistance of *S. aureus*).[185] Moreover, in vitro results may be irrelevant if bacteria are inhibited only by drug concentrations that cannot be achieved clinically.

Sophisticated analytic strategies use both PK and PD, for example, by determination of the peak serum concentration to MIC ratio, duration of time (T) that plasma concentration remains above the MIC (T > MIC), and area of the plasma concentration time curve above the MIC (area under the curve). Accordingly, aminoglycosides exhibit concentration-dependent killing,[186] whereas β-lactam agents exhibit efficacy determined by time above the MIC.[187] For β-lactam antibiotics with a short $t_{1/2}$, it may be efficacious to administer them by continuous infusion.[188,189] Some agents (e.g., fluoroquinolones) exhibit both properties; bacterial killing increases as drug concentration increases up to a saturation point, after which the effect becomes concentration independent.

Antibiotic Prophylaxis

Prophylactic antibiotics are used most often to prevent infection of a surgical incision. Preoperative antibiotic prophylaxis is proved to reduce the risk of postoperative SSIs in many circumstances. However, only the incision itself is protected, and only while it is open and thus vulnerable to inoculation. If it is not administered properly, antibiotic prophylaxis is ineffective and may be harmful. Antibiotic prophylaxis of surgery does not prevent postoperative nosocomial infections, which actually occur at an increased rate after prolonged prophylaxis,[190] selecting for more resistant pathogens when infection does develop.[42]

Antibiotic prophylaxis is indicated for most clean-contaminated and contaminated (or potentially contaminated) operations. An example of a clean-contaminated operation in which antibiotic prophylaxis is usually not indicated is elective laparoscopic cholecystectomy.[191] A meta-analysis of five trials (899 patients) revealed no benefit compared with placebo for prevention of SSIs (OR, 0.68; 95% CI, 0.24-1.91), major infection, or distant infection. Antibiotic prophylaxis is indicated for high-risk biliary surgery; high risk is conferred by age older than 70 years, diabetes mellitus, or a recently instrumented biliary tract (e.g., biliary stent).

Elective colon surgery is a clean-contaminated procedure in which preparatory practices are in evolution,[192,193] although the evidence of benefit of systemic antibiotic prophylaxis is unequivocal. Antibiotic bowel preparation, standardized in the 1970s by the oral administration of nonabsorbable neomycin and erythromycin base in addition to mechanical cleansing, reduced the risk of SSIs to the present rate of approximately 15%. However, mechanical bowel preparation and preoperative oral antibiotics are omitted increasingly according to the belief that there is no additive benefit beyond parenteral antibiotic prophylaxis and that the risk of anastomotic dehiscence and *C. difficile*–associated disease (CDAD) may be increased. Current SCIP guidelines for antibiotic prophylaxis of elective colon surgery give equal weighting to oral prophylaxis alone, parenteral prophylaxis alone, or the combination (see Table 11-2), despite the fact that two meta-analyses (that asked different questions) are in conflict about the efficacy of oral prophylaxis for colorectal surgery. Song and Glenny[194] have compared oral antibiotics alone with oral or systemic antibiotic prophylaxis (five trials) and found a higher SSI rate with oral prophylaxis alone (OR, 3.34; 95% CI, 1.66-6.72). In contrast, Lewis[192] performed a meta-analysis of 13 randomized trials of systemic versus combined oral and systemic prophylaxis and showed significant benefit for the combined approach (RR, 0.51; 95% CI, 0.24-0.78).

Antibiotic prophylaxis of clean surgery is controversial. When bone is incised (e.g., craniotomy, sternotomy) or a prosthesis is inserted, antibiotic prophylaxis is generally indicated. Some controversy persists with clean surgery of soft tissues (e.g., breast, hernia). Meta-analysis of randomized controlled trials has shown some benefit of antibiotic prophylaxis of breast cancer surgery without immediate reconstruction[195,196] but no decrease of SSI rate for groin hernia surgery,[197,198] even when nonabsorbable mesh is implanted.

Arterial reconstruction with a prosthetic graft is an example of clean surgery in which the risk of infection is high, especially infra-inguinal. In a meta-analysis[199] of 23 randomized controlled trials of prophylactic systemic antibiotics for peripheral arterial reconstruction (Table 11-6), it was found that prophylactic systemic antibiotics reduced the risk of SSI by approximately 75% and of early graft infection by about 69%. There was no benefit to prophylaxis for longer than 24 hours of antibiotic bonding to the graft material itself or preoperative bathing with an antiseptic agent compared with unmedicated bathing.

Four principles guide the administration of an antimicrobial agent for prophylaxis[112]:

1. Safety
2. An appropriate narrow spectrum of coverage of relevant pathogens
3. Little or no reliance on the agent for therapy of infection (because of the possible induction of resistance with heavy use)
4. Administration within 1 hour before surgery and for a defined brief period thereafter (no longer than 24 hours, 48 hours for cardiac surgery, and ideally, a single dose)

According to these principles, quinolones or carbapenems are undesirable agents for surgical prophylaxis, although prophylaxis with ertapenem and quinolone has been endorsed by the SCIP for prophylaxis of colon surgery (the latter with metronidazole for penicillin-allergic patients; see Table 11-2).

TABLE 11-6 Meta-analysis of Measures to Prevent Infection After Arterial Reconstruction

INTERVENTION	NO. OF TRIALS	ODDS RATIO	95% CI
Systemic antibiotic prophylaxis			
Surgical site infection	10	0.25	0.17-0.38
>24 hours prophylaxis	3	1.28	0.82-1.98
Early graft infection	5	0.31	0.11-0.85
Rifampicin bonding of polyester grafts			
Graft infection (1 month)	3	0.63	0.27-1.49
Graft infection (2 years)	2	1.05	0.46-2.40
Suction wound drainage, groin			
Surgical site infection	2	0.96	0.50-1.86
Preoperative antiseptic bath			
Surgical site infection	3	0.97	0.70-1.36
In situ surgical technique			
Surgical site infection	2	0.48	0.31-0.74

From Stewart A, Eyers PS, Earnshaw JJ: Prevention of infection in arterial reconstruction. *Cochrane Database Syst Rev* 3:CD003073, 2006.

Most SSIs are caused by gram-positive cocci, so prophylaxis should be directed primarily against staphylococci for clean cases and for high-risk, clean-contaminated, elective biliary, and gastric surgery cases. A first-generation cephalosporin is preferred in almost all circumstances (Table 11-7), with clindamycin used for penicillin-allergic patients.[112] If gram-negative or anaerobic coverage is required, a second-generation cephalosporin or the combination of a first-generation agent plus metronidazole is the first-choice regimen of most experts. Vancomycin prophylaxis is generally appropriate only in institutions in which the incidence of MRSA infection is high (>20% of all SSIs caused by MRSA).

The optimal time to give parenteral antibiotic prophylaxis is within 1 hour before incision.[200] Antibiotics given sooner are ineffective, as are agents given after the incision is closed. A 2001 audit of prescribing practices in the United States indicated that only 56% of patients who received prophylactic antibiotics did so within 1 hour before the skin incision; timeliness was documented in only 76% of cases in a 2005 audit in Department of Veterans Affairs hospitals.[201] Most inappropriately timed first doses of prophylactic antibiotic occur too early; changing institutional processes to administer the drug in the operating room can improve compliance with best practices. Antibiotics with short half-lives ($t_{1/2} < 2$ hours; e.g., cefazolin or cefoxitin) should be redosed every 3 to 4 hours during surgery if the operation is prolonged or bloody.[202] Even though the SCIP specifies a 24-hour limit for prophylaxis, single-dose prophylaxis (with intraoperative redosing, if indicated) is equivalent to multiple doses for the prevention of SSI.[203] Unfortunately, excessively prolonged antibiotic prophylaxis is pervasive and potentially harmful. Prolonged prophylaxis increases the risk of nosocomial infections unrelated to the surgical site and of the emergence of MDR pathogens. Pneumonia and vascular catheter–related infections have been associated with prolonged prophylaxis,[204,205] as has the emergence of SSI caused by MRSA.[42]

TABLE 11-7 Appropriate Cephalosporin Prophylaxis for Selected Types of Surgery*

PROCEDURE	ALTERNATIVE PROPHYLAXIS IN SERIOUS PENICILLIN ALLERGY
First-Generation Cephalosporin	
Cardiovascular and Thoracic	
Median sternotomy	Clindamycin (for all cardiovascular and thoracic cases except amputation)
Pacemaker insertion	
Vascular reconstruction involving abdominal aorta, insertion of prosthesis, or groin incision (except carotid endarterectomy, which requires no prophylaxis)	
Implantable defibrillator	
Pulmonary resection	
Lower limb amputation	Gentamicin and metronidazole
General	
Cholecystectomy (high risk only)	Gentamicin
Gastrectomy (high risk only; not uncomplicated chronic duodenal ulcer)	Gentamicin and metronidazole
Hepatobiliary	Gentamicin and metronidazole
Major débridement of traumatic wound	Gentamicin
Genitourinary (ampicillin plus gentamicin is a reasonable alternative)	Ciprofloxacin
Gynecologic	
Cesarean section (stat)	Metronidazole or doxycycline, after cord clamping
Hysterectomy (cefoxitin is a reasonable alternative)	Doxycycline
Head and Neck, Oral Cavity	
Major procedures entering oral cavity or pharynx	Gentamicin and clindamycin or metronidazole
Neurosurgery	
Craniotomy	Clindamycin, vancomycin
Orthopedics	
Major joint arthroplasty	Vancomycin[†]
Open reduction of closed fracture	Vancomycin[†]
Second-Generation Cephalosporin[‡]	
Appendectomy	Metronidazole plus gentamicin
Colon surgery[§]	
Surgery for penetrating abdominal trauma	

*Should be given as a single IV dose just before the operation. Consider an additional dose if the operation is prolonged longer than 3 to 4 hours.

[†]Primary prophylaxis with vancomycin (i.e., for the non–penicillin-allergic patient) may be appropriate for cardiac valve replacement, placement of a nontissue peripheral vascular prosthesis, or total joint replacement in institutions in which a high rate of infections with MRSA or MRSE has occurred. The precise definition of high rate is debated. A single dose administered immediately before surgery is sufficient unless the procedure lasts for more than 6 hours, in which case the dose should be repeated. Prophylaxis should be discontinued after a maximum of two doses but may be continued for up to 48 hours.

[‡]An intraoperative dose should be given if cefoxitin is used and the duration of surgery exceeds 3 to 4 hours because of the short half-life of the drug. A postoperative dose is not necessary but is permissible for up to 24 hours.

[§]Benefit beyond that provided by bowel preparation with mechanical cleansing and oral neomycin and erythromycin base is debatable.

Evidence has shown that only 40% of patients who receive antibiotic prophylaxis do so for less than 24 hours.[111] As a result of ischemia caused by surgical hemostasis, antibiotic penetration into the incision immediately after surgery is questionable until neovascularization occurs (24 to 48 hours). Antibiotics should not be given to cover indwelling drains or catheters, in lavage or irrigation fluid, or as a substitute for poor surgical technique.

Principles of Antibiotic Therapy

Antimicrobial therapy is a mainstay of the treatment of infections, but widespread overuse and misuse of antibiotics have led to an alarming increase in MDR pathogens. New agents may allow shorter courses of therapy and prophylaxis, which are desirable for cost savings and control of microbial flora. Effective therapy with no toxicity requires a careful but expeditious search for the source of infection and an understanding of the principles of PK (see earlier).

Evaluation of Possible Infection

Absent a fever, any hypotension, tachycardia, tachypnea, confusion, rigors, skin lesions, respiratory manifestations, oliguria, lactic acidosis, leukocytosis, leukopenia, immature neutrophils (i.e., bands >10%), or thrombocytopenia may indicate a workup for infection and immediate empirical therapy. Although the

BOX 11-8 Miscellaneous Causes of Fever Related to Noninfectious States

Acalculous cholecystitis
Acute myocardial infarction
Acute respiratory distress syndrome (fibroproliferative phase)
Adrenal insufficiency
Cytokine release syndrome
Fat embolism
Gout
Hematoma
Heterotopic ossification
Immune reconstitution inflammatory syndrome
Infarction of any tissue
Intracranial hemorrhage (trauma or vascular cause)
Myocardial infarction
Pancreatitis
Pericarditis
Pulmonary infarction
Stroke
Thyroid storm
Transfusion of blood or blood products
Transplant rejection
Tumor lysis syndrome
Venous thromboembolic disease
Withdrawal syndromes (e.g., drug, alcohol)

initial manifestation may be the development of organ dysfunction in some cases, new temperature elevation is usually the trigger for an evaluation for the presence of infection (fever workup). However, some infected patients do not become febrile and may even be hypothermic. Hypothermic or euthermic patients may have a life-threatening infection. These include older patients, those with open abdominal wounds or with end-stage liver disease or chronic renal failure, and patients taking anti-inflammatory or antipyretic drugs. Moreover, fever, especially in the postoperative period, may have a noninfectious cause; therefore, fever does not equate with infection (Box 11-8).[206]

The definition of fever is arbitrary and depends on how and when temperature was measured. In addition to host biology, a variety of environmental forces in an ICU can alter body temperature, such as specialized mattresses, lighting, heating or air conditioning, peritoneal lavage, and renal replacement therapy.[207] Thermoregulatory mechanisms can be disrupted by drugs or by injury to the central nervous system. Thus, it is often difficult to determine whether an abnormal temperature is a reflection of a physiologic process, drug, or environmental influence. Moreover, in surgical patients, the substantial possibility (≈50%) that a fever has a noninfectious cause must be considered.[206]

Many ICUs consider any patient with a core temperature of 38.3° C or higher (≥101° F) to be febrile and to warrant evaluation for possible infection. However, a lower threshold may be decided on for immunocompromised patients. Laboratory tests or imaging studies should be performed only after a clinical assessment (history and physical examination) indicates that infection may be present. Fever is common during the initial 72 hours after surgery and is usually noninfectious in origin.[207] Muscle compression injury (direct trauma or as a result of compartment syndrome) and tetanus are two rare complications of traumatic wounds that may cause fever. Other potentially serious noninfectious causes of postoperative fever include deep venous thrombosis, tissue ischemia or necrosis, pulmonary embolism, adrenal insufficiency, drug-induced fever, anesthesia-induced malignant hyperthermia, and acute allograft rejection. However, once a patient is more than 96 hours after surgery, fever is more likely to represent infection.

Drug fever is decidedly unusual in surgical patients and must be considered a diagnosis of exclusion. Some drugs cause fever by producing local infusion site inflammation (e.g., phlebitis, sterile abscesses, soft tissue reaction), such as amphotericin B, erythromycin, and potassium chloride. Some drugs may also stimulate heat production (e.g., thyroxine), limit heat dissipation (e.g., atropine, epinephrine), or alter thermoregulation (e.g., butyrophenone tranquilizers, phenothiazines, antihistamines, antiparkinson drugs). Drug fever in surgical ICUs is most often attributed to antimicrobial agents (e.g., vancomycin, β-lactams) and anticonvulsants (especially phenytoin). Malignant hyperthermia and neuroleptic malignant syndrome deserve consideration when fever is especially high because the results can be devastating if they are left untreated.[208] Malignant hyperthermia can be delayed in onset for as long as 24 hours, especially if the patient is receiving corticosteroids. Malignant hyperthermia is a genetically determined response mediated by a dysregulation of cytoplasmic calcium flux in skeletal muscle, resulting in intense muscle contraction, fever, and increased creatine kinase concentration. It can be caused by succinylcholine and inhalational anesthetics. The neuroleptic malignant syndrome is slightly more common than malignant hyperthermia and more often identified in the ICU. It has been associated with phenothiazines, thioxanthenes, and butyrophenones. It also is manifested as muscle rigidity, fever, and increasing creatine kinase concentration. However, unlike in malignant hyperthermia, the initiator of muscle contraction is central, the syndrome is often less intense, and mortality is lower.

Drug withdrawal syndromes may be associated with fever, tachycardia, diaphoresis, and hyperreflexia, including those caused by alcohol, opioids, barbiturates, and benzodiazepines. A history of use of these drugs may not be available when the patient is admitted to the ICU. Withdrawal and related fever may therefore occur several hours or days after admission.

Fever can be related to hematoma or SSI. SSI is rare in the first few days after operation, except for group A streptococcal infections and clostridial infections that can develop within hours to 1 to 3 days after surgery. These causes should be suspected on the basis of inspection of the incision. Thus, it is mandatory to remove the surgical dressing to inspect the incision as part of any fever evaluation. However, if an incision is opened and cultured, a deep culture specimen should be collected; swabbing an open wound superficially or collecting fluid from drains (if present) for culture is unhelpful because the likelihood of colonization is high.

A chest radiograph is optional for evaluation of postoperative fever unless long-term mechanical ventilation, respiratory rate, auscultation, abnormal blood gas levels, or pulmonary secretions suggest a high yield. The clinician must be alert to the possibility that the patient could have aspirated during the perioperative period or of the uncommon event that the patient was incubating a community-acquired pneumonia before the operation caused, for example, by pneumococci or influenza A. A urinalysis or culture is not mandatory to evaluate fever during the initial 3 days postoperatively unless there is reason, by history or examination, to suspect a UTI. After trauma, UTI is common only after injury to the urinary tract.

Blood Cultures

Blood culture specimens should be obtained from patients with a new fever when clinical evaluation does not suggest strongly a noninfectious cause. The site of venipuncture should be cleaned with 2% chlorhexidine gluconate in 70% isopropyl alcohol or 1% to 2% tincture of iodine. Povidone-iodine (10%), although acceptable, is not bactericidal until dry; some false-positive blood cultures may be caused by premature specimen collection.[209] One blood culture specimen is defined as a 20- to 30-mL sample of blood drawn at a single time from a single site, regardless of how many bottles or tubes are filled for processing; the minimum inoculum for an adult blood culture should be 10 mL/bottle. The sensitivity of blood culturing for detection of true bacteremia or fungemia is related to many factors, most importantly the volume of blood drawn and obtaining the culture specimens before the initiation of anti-infective therapy.[210]

Evidence has suggested that the cumulative yield of pathogens is optimized when three blood culture specimens with adequate volume (20 to 30 mL each) are drawn.[210] Each culture specimen should ideally be drawn by separate venipuncture or through a separate intravascular device but not through multiple ports of the same intravascular catheter. There is no evidence that the yield of culture samples drawn from an artery or vein is different. Drawing of two or three blood culture samples with appropriate volume from separate sites of access at the onset of fever is the most effective way to discern whether an organism found on blood culture represents a true pathogen (multiple cultures are often positive), a contaminant (only one of multiple blood cultures is positive for an organism commonly found on skin and clinical correlation does not support infection), or a bacteremia or fungemia from an infected catheter (one culture sample from the source catheter is positive, often with a positive catheter tip, and other culture samples are not).[211]

Empirical Antibiotic Therapy

Empirical antibiotic therapy must be administered judiciously. Injudicious therapy could result in undertreatment of established infection or unnecessary therapy when the patient has only inflammation or bacterial colonization; either may be deleterious. Inappropriate treatment (e.g., delay,[212,213] therapy misdirected against usual pathogens, failure to treat MDR pathogens) leads unequivocally to increased mortality.[141,214,215]

Strategies have been promulgated to optimize antibiotic administration, including reliance on physician prescribing patterns, computerized decision support, administration by protocol, and formulary restriction programs. These are considered under the general framework of antibiotic stewardship.[216] Because of the increasing prevalence of MDR pathogens, it is crucial for initial empirical antibiotic therapy to be targeted appropriately, administered in a sufficient dosage to ensure bacterial killing, narrowed in spectrum (de-escalation)[217] as soon as possible on the basis of microbiology data and clinical response, and continued only as long as necessary.[218] Appropriate antibiotic prescribing not only optimizes patient care but supports infection control practices and preserves microbial ecology.

Choice of Antibiotic

Antibiotic choice is based on several interrelated factors (Box 11-9). Paramount is activity against identified or likely (for empirical therapy) pathogens, presuming that infecting and colonizing organisms can be distinguished, and narrow-spectrum coverage is always desired. Estimation of likely pathogens depends on the

BOX 11-9 Factors Influencing Antibiotic Choice

Activity against known or suspected pathogens
Disease believed responsible
Distinguish infection from colonization
Narrow-spectrum coverage most desirable
Antimicrobial resistance patterns
Patient-specific factors
- Severity of illness (?)
- Age (?)
- Immunosuppression
- Organ dysfunction
- Allergy

Institutional guidelines and restrictions

disease process believed responsible; whether the infection is community, health care, or hospital acquired; and whether MDR organisms are present or likely to be. Local knowledge of antimicrobial resistance patterns is essential, even at the unit-specific level. Patient-specific factors of importance include age, debility, immunosuppression, intrinsic organ function, prior allergy or other adverse reaction, and recent antibiotic therapy. Institutional factors of importance include guidelines that could specify a particular therapy, formulary availability of specific agents, outbreaks of infections caused by MDR pathogens, and antibiotic control programs.

A number of agents are available for therapy (Box 11-10).[219] Agents may be chosen on the basis of spectrum, whether broad or targeted (e.g., antipseudomonal, antianaerobic), in addition to the factors noted. If a nosocomial gram-positive pathogen is suspected (e.g., wound infection, SSI, CLABSI, HAP, VAP) or MRSA is endemic, empirical vancomycin (or linezolid) is appropriate. Some authorities recommend dual-agent therapy for serious *Pseudomonas* infections (an antipseudomonal β-lactam drug plus an aminoglycoside), but evidence of efficacy is mixed.[220-222] Combination therapy for a specific pathogen (e.g., double coverage of *Pseudomonas*) may, in fact, worsen outcomes. A meta-analysis of β-lactam monotherapy versus β-lactam–aminoglycoside combination therapy for immunocompetent patients with sepsis (64 trials, 7586 patients) found no difference in mortality (RR, 0.90; 95% CI, 0.77-1.06) or development of resistance.[221] In fact, clinical failure was more common with combination therapy, as was the incidence of acute kidney injury. However, it is important for empirical therapy of any infection that might be caused by a gram-positive or gram-negative organism (e.g., HAP, VAP, HA-IAI) to include activity against all likely pathogens.[47,223]

Duration of Therapy

The end point of antibiotic therapy is largely undefined, in part because quality data are few. If cultures are negative, empirical antibiotic therapy should usually be stopped after no more than 48 to 72 hours. Unnecessary antibiotic therapy increases the risk of MDR infection, so prolonged therapy with negative cultures is usually unjustifiable. The morbidity of antibiotic therapy also includes allergic reactions, development of nosocomial superinfections (e.g., fungal, enterococcal, and *C. difficile*–related infections), organ toxicity, reduced yield from subsequent cultures, and vitamin K deficiency with coagulopathy or accentuation of warfarin effect.

If infection is evident, treatment is continued as indicated clinically. Some infections can be treated for 5 days or less. Every

BOX 11-10 Antibacterial Agents for Empirical Use

Antipseudomonal
Piperacillin-tazobactam
Cefepime, ceftazidime
Imipenem-cilastatin, meropenem, doripenem
Ciprofloxacin, levofloxacin (depending on local susceptibility patterns)
Aminoglycosides
Polymyxins (polymyxin B, colistin [polymyxin E])

Targeted Spectrum
Gram-Positive
Glycopeptide (e.g., vancomycin, telavancin)
Lipopeptide (e.g., daptomycin; not for known or suspected pneumonia)
Oxazolidinone (e.g., linezolid)

Gram-Negative
Third-generation cephalosporin (not ceftriaxone)
Monobactam
Polymyxins (polymyxin B, colistin [polymyxin E])

Antianaerobic
Metronidazole

Broad Spectrum
Piperacillin-tazobactam
Carbapenems
Fluoroquinolones (depending on local susceptibility patterns)
Tigecycline (plus an antipseudomonal agent)

Antianaerobic
Metronidazole
Carbapenems
β-Lactam and β-lactamase combination agents
Tigecycline

Anti-MRSA
Ceftaroline
Daptomycin (not for use against pneumonia)
Minocycline (oral only)
Linezolid
Telavancin
Tigecycline (not in pregnancy or for children younger than 8 years)
Vancomycin

decision to start antibiotics must be accompanied by an a priori decision about the duration of therapy. A reason to continue therapy beyond the predetermined end point must be compelling. Bacterial killing is rapid in response to effective agents, but the host response may not subside immediately. Therefore, the clinical response of the patient should not be the sole determinant. If a patient still has SIRS at the predetermined end point, it is more useful to stop therapy and to reevaluate for persistent or new infection, MDR pathogens, and noninfectious causes of SIRS than to continue therapy uninformed.

DISEASE-, PATHOGEN-, AND ANTIBIOTIC-SPECIFIC CONSIDERATIONS

Pneumonia

After initiation of therapy for suspected VAP, lower respiratory tract cultures may reveal no growth or growth below the predetermined threshold value, substantial (above threshold) growth of a susceptible pathogen, or growth of an MDR pathogen. Under the first scenario, antimicrobial therapy may be discontinued if the patient has not deteriorated.[224] Under the second scenario, therapy is de-escalated[225] to a narrow-spectrum agent active against the pathogen. In the third scenario, the initial broad-spectrum agent active against the pathogen is continued or therapy is escalated to target the MDR pathogen.

Once pathogen-specific therapy has been initiated, its duration must be determined, with the goal of avoiding prolonged unnecessary administration. Resolution of clinical and radiographic parameters typically lags behind the eradication of infection.[47] Dennesen and colleagues[226] have noted a clinical response to therapy (e.g., normalization of temperature, white blood cell count, and arterial oxygen saturation and decreased bacterial count in sputum) within 6 days of therapy of VAP. A randomized multicenter trial of 401 patients (VAP proved by bronchoscopy and quantitative microbiology)[227] showed an 8-day course (versus 15 days) of initially appropriate antimicrobial therapy to be effective, provided the patient was stable and the pathogen was not a nonfermenting gram-negative bacillus. In select patients (i.e., those unlikely to have VAP based on a CPIS ≤ 6), a 3-day course of therapy may be sufficient.[228]

Nonresponders to therapy for VAP pose a dilemma.[47] Inadequate therapy, misdiagnosis, or a pneumonia-related complication (e.g., empyema, lung abscess) must be considered. The evaluation should be repeated, including quantitative sputum cultures using a quantitative diagnostic threshold one log lower, given recent antibiotic exposure. Broadened empirical antibiotic coverage should be reinstituted thereafter until new data become available.

Central Line–Associated Bloodstream Infection

The pathogens of CLABSI are predominantly gram-positive cocci, most commonly methicillin-resistant *Staphylococcus epidermidis* (MRSE), MRSA, and enterococci. Unfortunately, MRSE is the most common cause of catheter-related bloodstream infections and of false-positive blood cultures because of contamination during the collection process. Most authorities consider the isolation of MRSE from a single blood culture to be a contaminant and do not treat, especially if the patient has no indwelling hardware that might become infected secondarily (e.g., prosthetic joint, heart valve). Gram-negative bacillary pathogens are less common but are seldom contaminants. Fungal CLABSIs are less common in surgical patients than in medical patients but must be treated empirically in critically ill patients at risk.

Treatment is by catheter removal (for peripheral or percutaneous central venous catheters) and parenteral antibiotics, at least initially.[3,229] It is unclear whether a positive catheter culture requires therapy beyond catheter removal without local signs of infection or a true positive blood culture. Bloodstream infections caused by *S. aureus* probably require at least 2 weeks of therapy regardless of cause, although some argue for a longer course (4 to 6 weeks) because of the risk of metastatic infection (e.g., pneumonia, endocarditis). Vancomycin or linezolid may be chosen for MRSA CLABSIs (or MRSE when treatment is indicated), with daptomycin as an alternative. Therapy for enterococcal or gram-negative CLABSIs is dictated by bacterial susceptibility, with no clear consensus about the duration of therapy. Beyond removal of the catheter, treatment of fungal CLABSIs is controversial; some recommend at least 2 weeks of systemic antifungal therapy. MDR fungal pathogens are less common in surgical patients, except for solid organ transplant recipients, so initial empirical therapy with an echinocandin is often de-escalated to fluconazole after susceptibility is reported.[230]

Intra-abdominal Infection

Only approximately 15% of patients with secondary peritonitis are ill enough to require ICU care. Severe secondary peritonitis may follow penetrating intestinal injury that is not recognized or treated promptly (>12-hour delay). Other causes include dehiscence of a bowel anastomosis with leakage or development of an intra-abdominal abscess. Secondary peritonitis is polymicrobial, with anaerobic gram-negative bacilli (e.g., *Bacteroides fragilis*) predominating and *E. coli* and *Klebsiella* spp. commonly isolated from community-onset infections. Various antibiotic regimens of an appropriate spectrum may be prescribed.[223] Enterococci, *Pseudomonas*, and other bacteria may be isolated but do not require specific therapy if the patient is otherwise healthy (e.g., not immunocompromised) and responding to therapy as prescribed.

When HA-IAI is a complication of disease or therapy, the flora is more likely to reflect MDR pathogens,[173,175] and outcomes are worsened if empirical therapy is not appropriate. For example, enterococci, *Enterobacter*, and *Pseudomonas* are more prevalent, whereas *E. coli* and *Klebsiella* are less common.[231] Antibiotic therapy must be adjusted accordingly, and surgical source control must be achieved. Failure of two source control procedures with persistent intra-abdominal collections is referred to as *tertiary peritonitis*. Tertiary peritonitis is also characterized by complete failure of intra-abdominal host defenses.[232] There is debate about whether tertiary peritonitis is a true invasive infection or peritoneal colonization with incompetent local host defenses, so whether antibiotic therapy is indicated is controversial. Bacteria isolated in tertiary peritonitis are avirulent opportunists, such as MRSE, enterococci, *Pseudomonas*, and *Candida albicans*, supporting the incompetent host defense hypothesis. Some authorities recommend management with an open abdomen technique, so that peritoneal toilet can be provided manually—at the bedside in some cases—under sedation or anesthesia, until local host defenses recover. There may be no alternative to open abdomen management if the infection extends to involve the abdominal wall, and extensive débridement is required.

Clostridium difficile–Associated Disease

CDAD, or *C. difficile* infection, develops because antibiotic therapy disrupts the balance of colonic flora, allowing the overgrowth of *C. difficile*, which is present in the fecal flora of approximately 3% of normal hosts. Any antibiotic can induce this selection pressure, even when it is given appropriately as surgical prophylaxis, although clindamycin, third-generation cephalosporins, and fluoroquinolones have a predilection.[233] Paradoxically, even antibiotics used to treat CDAD (e.g., metronidazole) have been associated with CDAD. Restriction of cephalosporin and fluoroquinolone prescribing can reduce the rate of infection.[234]

CDAD is unquestionably a nosocomial infection. Spores persist on inanimate surfaces for prolonged periods and can be transmitted patient to patient by contaminated equipment (e.g., bedpans, rectal thermometers) or by health care workers as fomites. Alcohol gel hand disinfection is not active against spores of *C. difficile*, so hand washing with soap and water is necessary in caring for an infected patient or generally during outbreaks.

The clinical spectrum of CDAD is wide, ranging from asymptomatic (8% of affected patients do not have diarrhea) to life-threatening transmural pancolitis with perforation and severe sepsis or septic shock. The typical patient will have fever, abdominal distention with or without tenderness, copious diarrhea, and leukocytosis. Colon hemorrhage is rare and, if observed, should prompt consideration of an alternative diagnosis.

Treatment of mild cases consists of withdrawal of the putative offending antibiotic; oral antibiotic therapy is often prescribed but may not be necessary. More severe cases may require parenteral metronidazole or oral or enteral vancomycin (by gavage or enema, if ileus precludes oral therapy); parenteral vancomycin is ineffective. The new oral macrolide fidaxomicin is noninferior to vancomycin and may reduce the risk of relapsed disease, a major clinical problem.[235] Some patients with severe or fulminating disease may require a colectomy, usually a total abdominal colectomy.[236] The prevalence of severe disease has increased markedly with the emergence of a new strain of *C. difficile*. The new strain has undergone mutation of a gene that suppresses toxin production so that far more toxin is elaborated, resulting in clinically severe disease.[237] More of these patients will require surgery, but it remains to be determined whether or how antibiotic therapy should be modified to combat this dangerous bacterium.

Complicated Skin and Soft Tissue Infections

The complicated skin and soft tissue infections (cSSTIs) involve deeper tissues or require major surgical intervention. Infection in the presence of medical comorbidities, particularly chronic kidney disease, diabetes mellitus, or peripheral arterial disease, also defines a cSSTI. Examples include major abscesses, deep space infections, diabetic foot infections (DFIs), some postoperative SSIs (those with systemic signs of infection), infected decubitus ulcers, and NSTIs. In randomized controlled trials, comparable outcomes of antibiotic therapy for cSSTIs (except NSTIs, which are usually [≈80%] polymicrobial) are achieved by agents that treat only gram-positive cocci (e.g., vancomycin, linezolid, daptomycin, telavancin). Because of the heterogeneity of these infections, the reader is referred to comprehensive treatment guidelines for the management of cSSTI (Box 11-11).[238]

Patients with diabetes mellitus are at risk for considerable morbidity as a result of chronic foot ulceration and foot infection, including limb loss. DFIs are usually a consequence of skin ulceration from ischemia or trauma to a neuropathic foot. The compartmentalized anatomy of the foot, with its various spaces, tendon sheaths, and neurovascular bundles, allows ischemic necrosis to affect tissues within a compartment or to spread along anatomic tissue planes. Recurrent infections are common, and 10% to 30% of affected patients eventually require amputation. Diabetic patients are predisposed to foot infections not only because of the portal of entry and poor blood supply but also because of defects in humoral immunity (e.g., impaired neutrophil chemotaxis, phagocytosis, intracellular killing) and impaired monocyte-macrophage function, which correlate with the adequacy of glycemic control. Cell-mediated immunity and complement function may also be impaired.

Acute infections are usually caused by gram-positive cocci. *S. aureus* is the most important pathogen in DFIs. It is often present as a monomicrobial infection, but usually it is also an important pathogen in polymicrobial infections. Chronic wounds, recurrent infections, and infections in hospitalized patients are more likely to harbor complex flora, including aerobic and anaerobic flora. Among gram-negative bacilli, bacteria of the family Enterobacteriaceae are common, and *P. aeruginosa* may be isolated from wounds that have been treated with hydrotherapy or wet dressings. Enterococci may be recovered from patients treated

BOX 11-11 Recommendations from Guidelines for Treatment of Complicated Skin and Soft Tissue Infections

Non-Necrotizing Cellulitis

Most frequent causative agent is *Streptococcus pyogenes;* other agents include *Haemophilus influenzae* and pneumococcus.

Parenteral penicillin is treatment of choice; treatment failures may occur in severe disease.

Protein synthesis inhibitory agents alone or in combination with cell wall–active agents should be given in severe cases, but macrolide resistance is increasing.

Other regimens may include antistaphylococcal penicillins, cefazolin, ceftaroline, and ceftriaxone.

Complicated Skin and Soft Tissue Infections

Involve a broad variety of pathogens; frequently polymicrobial

S. aureus is most common isolate; community-acquired (CA) MRSA is increasingly common.

Simple abscesses may respond to incision and drainage alone.

Complex abscesses and abscesses with cellulitis require adjuvant antibiotics.

Empirical antibiotic therapy should be directed toward the most likely pathogens, including CA-MRSA in most settings.

Suspected polymicrobial infections should be managed with coverage of enteric gram-negative and anaerobic pathogens.

Necrotizing Soft Tissue Infections

Delays in diagnosis increase morbidity and mortality.

Presence of gas in soft tissue is specific for necrotizing infections but insensitive.

Computed tomography and magnetic resonance imaging improve detection of soft tissue gas, but radiographic findings of tissue fluid and edema are neither sensitive nor specific.

Clinical features suggestive of NSTIs are

- Pain disproportionate to physical examination findings
- Tense edema
- Bullae
- Skin ecchymosis, necrosis
- Cutaneous anesthesia
- Systemic toxicity
- Progression despite antibiotic therapy

Predictive laboratory values

- White blood cell count >14 × 10^9/L
- Serum sodium level <135 mmol/L
- Blood urea nitrogen level >15 mg/dL

Early antibiotic coverage of likely pathogens is indicated; this depends on the clinical setting, inciting pathophysiologic process, and previous antibiotic exposure.

Timely, wide surgical débridement of involved tissue improves outcome.

Frequent reevaluation or return to the operating room within 24 hours ensures adequacy of débridement and lack of progression.

Necrotizing infections are usually polymicrobial; they may involve anaerobic and aerobic gram-positive and gram-negative pathogens.

Possible single-agent regimens include imipenem-cilastatin, meropenem, ertapenem, piperacillin-tazobactam, ticarcillin–clavulanic acid, and tigecycline.

Diabetic Foot Infections

These may involve a wide variety of pathogens; separating colonizing bacteria from pathogens may be difficult.

Gram-positive cocci are most common, but gram-negative bacilli and anaerobes may be involved. Chronic wounds may have resistant pathogens.

Empirical therapy should take local susceptibility patterns, previous antibiotic exposure, and prior pathogens into consideration.

Adequate tissue culture specimens should be obtained.

Possible antibiotic regimens include cefazolin, ceftriaxone, cefoxitin, ceftaroline, ampicillin-sulbactam, piperacillin-tazobactam, and a carbapenem; daptomycin and linezolid can be used with the addition of gram-negative coverage.

For MRSA infections, vancomycin, telavancin, ceftaroline, daptomycin, tigecycline, and linezolid can be considered.

Adapted from May AK, Stafford RE, Bulger EM, et al: Treatment of complicated skin and soft tissue infections. *Surg Infect (Larchmt)* 10:467–499, 2009.

previously with a cephalosporin. Anaerobic bacteria seldom cause DFIs as the sole pathogen but may be isolated from deep infections or necrotic tissue. Antibiotic-resistant bacteria, especially MRSA, may be isolated from patients who have received antibiotics previously or who have been hospitalized or reside in long-term care facilities. Agents that have been shown to be effective for therapy of DFIs in clinical trials include cephalosporins, β-lactamase inhibitor combination antibiotics, fluoroquinolones, clindamycin, carbapenems, vancomycin, and linezolid. The optimal duration of therapy for DFIs has not been determined; common practice is to treat mild infections for 1 week, whereas serious infections may require up to a 2-week course of therapy. Adequate débridement, resection, or amputation can shorten the necessary duration of therapy.

Antibiotic Activity Spectra

Susceptibility testing of specific organisms is necessary for the treatment of serious infections, including all nosocomial infections. Recommendations will focus on agents useful for the treatment of nosocomial infections. Recommended agents for specific organisms are guidelines only because in vitro susceptibilities may not correlate with clinical efficacy. Exposure to certain agents has been associated with the emergence of specific MDR bacteria, which require a different empirical antibiotic choice or modification of a regimen if they are identified or suspected (Table 11-8).

Cell Wall–Active Agents

β-Lactam antibiotics. The β-lactam antibiotic group consists of penicillins, cephalosporins, monobactams, and carbapenems. Within this group, several agents have been combined with β-lactamase inhibitors to broaden the spectrum of activity. Several subgroups of antibiotics are recognized within the group, notably several generations of cephalosporins and penicillinase-resistant penicillins.

Penicillins. Penicillinase-resistant semisynthetic penicillins include methicillin, nafcillin, oxacillin, cloxacillin, and dicloxacillin. These agents are used primarily as therapy for sensitive strains of staphylococci. Hospitalized patients should not be treated empirically with these agents because of high rates of MRSA, and almost all enterococcal strains are resistant. However, if the *S. aureus* isolate is susceptible, these drugs are the treatment of choice.

With the exception of carboxy penicillins and ureidopenicillins, penicillins retain little or no activity against most gram-negative bacilli. Carboxypenicillins (ticarcillin and carbenicillin) and ureidopenicillins (azlocillin, mezlocillin, and piperacillin,

TABLE 11-8 Causes and Consequences of Bacterial Resistance as Related to Empirical Antibiotic Choices

INITIAL THERAPEUTIC AGENT	EMERGENT RESISTANT BACTERIA	TREATMENT OF RESISTANT BACTERIA
Fluoroquinolones	MRSA	Vancomycin, others (see Box 11-10)
	MDR gram-negative bacilli*	Carbapenem or polymyxin or tigecycline (not for *Pseudomonas*)
	Clostridium difficile infection	Vancomycin or metronidazole or fidaxomicin
Vancomycin	VRE	Tigecycline, linezolid, daptomycin
	VISA	Ceftaroline, tigecycline, linezolid, daptomycin
Cephalosporins	VRE	Tigecycline, linezolid, daptomycin
	MDR gram-negative bacilli	Carbapenem or polymyxin or tigecycline (not for *Pseudomonas*)
	Clostridium difficile infection	Vancomycin or metronidazole or fidaxomicin
Carbapenems	MDR gram-negative bacilli	Carbapenem or polymyxin or tigecycline (not for *Pseudomonas*)
	Stenotrophomonas maltophilia	Trimethoprim-sulfamethoxazole
	Clostridium difficile infection	Vancomycin or metronidazole or fidaxomicin

VISA, Vancomycin intermediate-resistant *Staphylococcus aureus.*
*MDR gram-negative bacilli include producers of extended-spectrum β-lactamases, metallo-β-lactamases, and carbapenemases.

sometimes referred to as acylampicillins) have some activity against gram-negative bacteria and *P. aeruginosa*. Ureidopenicillins have greater intrinsic activity against *Pseudomonas*, but none are used widely any more without a β-lactamase inhibitor in combination (BLIC). Combination with a β-lactamase inhibitor (e.g., sulbactam, tazobactam, clavulanic acid) enhances the effectiveness of the parent β-lactam agent (piperacillin > ticarcillin > ampicillin) and, to a lesser extent, the inhibitor (tazobactam > sulbactam ~ clavulanic acid). The spectrum of activity varies within the class, so the treating clinician needs to be familiar with each of the drugs. All the BLIC drugs are effective against streptococci and MRSA and highly effective against anaerobes (except for *C. difficile*). Piperacillin-tazobactam has the widest spectrum of activity against gram-negative bacteria and the most potency among β-lactam drugs against *P. aeruginosa*. Ampicillin-sulbactam is unreliable against *E. coli* and *Klebsiella* (resistance rate ≅ 50%), but it has useful activity against *Acinetobacter* spp. because of the sulbactam moiety.

Cephalosporins. More than 20 cephalosporins compose the class; the characteristics of the drugs vary widely but are similar within four broad generations. First- and second-generation agents are useful only for prophylaxis, uncomplicated infections, or de-escalation therapy when results of susceptibility testing are known. Third-generation agents have enhanced activity against gram-negative bacilli (some have specific antipseudomonal activity), but most are ineffective against gram-positive cocci and none are effective against anaerobes. Cefepime, the fourth-generation cephalosporin available in the United States, has enhanced antipseudomonal activity and has regained activity against most gram-positive cocci but not against MRSA. Ceftaroline (usual dose, 600 mg IV every 12 hours) has not been classified but has anti-MRSA activity unique among the cephalosporins while retaining modest activity comparable to that of first-generation agents against gram-negative bacilli.[239] None of the cephalosporins are active against enterococci. The heterogeneity of spectra, especially among third-generation agents, requires broad familiarity with all these drugs.

Third-generation cephalosporins. Third-generation cephalosporins include cefoperazone, cefotaxime, cefpodoxime, cefprozil, ceftazidime, ceftibuten, ceftizoxime, ceftriaxone, and locarbacef. They possess a modestly extended spectrum of activity against gram-negative bacilli but not against gram-positive bacteria (except for ceftriaxone) or anaerobic bacteria. Third-generation cephalosporins, particularly ceftazidime, have been associated with the induction of extended-spectrum β-lactamase (ESBL) production among many of the Enterobacteriaceae (see Table 11-8). Their activity is reliable only against non–ESBL-producing species of Enterobacteriaceae, including *Enterobacter, Citrobacter, Providencia,* and *Morganella,* but they are no longer reliable for empirical use as monotherapy against nonfermenting gram-negative bacilli (e.g., *Acinetobacter* spp., *P. aeruginosa, Stenotrophomonas maltophilia*).

Fourth-generation cephalosporins. The gram-negative spectrum of cefepime is broader than that of the third-generation cephalosporins (the antipseudomonal activity exceeds that of ceftazidime), whereas the anti–gram-positive activity is comparable to that of a first-generation cephalosporin. The safety profile is excellent, and the potential for induction of ESBL production is less. There is no activity against enterococci or enteric anaerobes. Similar to the carbapenems, cefepime appears to be intrinsically more resistant to hydrolysis by β-lactamases, but not enough for its activity to be reliable against ESBL-producing bacteria.

Monobactams. The single available agent of this class, aztreonam, has a spectrum of activity against gram-negative bacilli similar to that of the third-generation cephalosporins, with no activity against gram-positive organisms or anaerobes. Aztreonam is not a potent inducer of β-lactamases. Resistance to aztreonam is widespread, but the drug may be useful for directed therapy against known susceptible strains and may be used safely for penicillin-allergic patients because the incidence of cross-reactivity is low (see later).

Carbapenems. Carbapenems have a five-carbon ring attached to the β-lactam nucleus. The alkyl groups are oriented in a *trans* configuration rather than in the *cis* configuration characteristic of other β-lactam agents, making these drugs resistant to β-lactamases. Four drugs, imipenem-cilastatin, meropenem, doripenem, and ertapenem, are available in the United States. Imipenem-cilastatin, meropenem, and doripenem have the widest (and generally comparable) antibacterial spectrum of any antibiotics, with excellent activity against aerobic and anaerobic streptococci, methicillin-sensitive staphylococci, and almost all gram-negative bacilli except *Acinetobacter, Legionella, P. cepacia,* and *S. maltophilia.*[240] Activity against the Enterobacteriaceae exceeds that of all antibiotics, with the possible exceptions of piperacillin-tazobactam and cefepime, and activities of meropenem and doripenem against *P. aeruginosa* are approached only by that of amikacin. All carbapenems are superlative antianaerobic agents, so there is no reason to combine a carbapenem with metronidazole except, for example, to treat concurrent mild *C. difficile* colitis in a patient with a life-threatening infection that mandates carbapenem therapy.

Meropenem and doripenem have less potential for neurotoxicity than imipenem-cilastatin, which is contraindicated in patients with active central nervous system disease or injury (except the spinal cord), because of the rare (≈0.5%) appearance of myoclonus or generalized seizures in patients who have received high doses (with normal renal function) or inadequate dosage reductions with renal insufficiency. With all carbapenems, widespread disruption of host microbial flora may lead to superinfections (e.g., fungi, *C. difficile, Stenotrophomonas,* resistant enterococci).

Ertapenem is not useful against *Pseudomonas, Acinetobacter, Enterobacter* spp., or MRSA, but its long half-life permits once-daily dosing.[241] Ertapenem is highly active against ESBL-producing Enterobacteriaceae and also has less potential for neurotoxicity.

Lipoglycopeptides. Vancomycin, a soluble lipoglycopeptide, is bactericidal, but only on dividing organisms. Unfortunately, tissue penetration of vancomycin is universally poor, which limits its effectiveness. Both *S. aureus* and *S. epidermidis* are usually susceptible to vancomycin, although MICs for *S. aureus* are increasing, requiring higher doses for effect[242,243] and leading to rates of clinical failure that have exceeded 50% in some reports (Table 11-9).[244] *Streptococcus pyogenes,* group B streptococci, *S. pneumoniae* (including penicillin-resistant *S. pneumoniae*), and *C. difficile* are also susceptible. Most strains of *Enterococcus faecalis* are inhibited (but not killed) by attainable concentrations, but *Enterococcus faecium* is increasingly vancomycin resistant.

It is important for public health that widespread inappropriate use of vancomycin be curtailed. Actual indications include serious infections caused by MRSA or MRSE, gram-positive infections in patients with serious penicillin allergy, and oral therapy (or by enema in patients with ileus) for serious cases of *C. difficile* infection. Parenteral vancomycin (a starting dose of 15 mg/kg is now recommended for patients with normal renal function to achieve a minimum trough concentration of 15 to 20 μg/mL)[242,243] must be infused during at least 1 hour to avoid toxicity (e.g., red man syndrome). Despite concern about MRSA as a causative pathogen for SSIs, properly designed randomized trials are lacking, and routine vancomycin prophylaxis is not recommended.[245]

Telavancin, a synthetic derivative of vancomycin, has been approved for the treatment of cSSTIs.[246] The drug is active against MRSA, pneumococci including penicillin-resistant *S. pneumoniae,* and vancomycin-susceptible enterococci, with MICs generally lower than 1 μg/mL. There appears to be a dual mechanism of action, including cell membrane disruption and inhibition of cell wall synthesis. The most common side effects are taste disturbance, nausea, vomiting, and headache. There may be a small increased risk of acute kidney injury. The usual dose is 10 mg/kg, infused intravenously during 60 minutes, every 24 hours for 7 to 14 days; dosage reductions are necessary in renal insufficiency. No information is available about dosing during renal replacement therapy.

Cyclic lipopeptides. Daptomycin has potent, rapid bactericidal activity against most gram-positive organisms. The mechanism of action is by rapid membrane depolarization, potassium efflux, arrest of DNA and RNA synthesis, arrest of protein synthesis, and cell death. Daptomycin exhibits concentration-dependent killing and has a long half-life (8 hours). A dose of 4 mg/kg once daily is recommended for cSSTIs versus 6 mg/kg/day for bacteremia. Daptomycin is excreted in the urine, so the dosing interval should be increased to 48 hours when creatinine clearance is lower than 30 mL/min. No antagonistic drug interactions have been observed.

Daptomycin is active against many aerobic and anaerobic gram-positive bacteria, including MDR strains such as MRSA, MRSE, and VRE. Furthermore, daptomycin is also effective against a variety of anaerobes, including *Peptostreptococcus* spp., *C. perfringens,* and *C. difficile.* Resistance to daptomycin has been reported for MRSA and VRE.

Importantly, daptomycin must not be used for the treatment of pneumonia or as empirical therapy when pneumonia is in the differential diagnosis, even when it is caused by a susceptible organism, because daptomycin penetrates lung tissue poorly and is also inactivated by pulmonary surfactant.[247]

Polymyxins. Polymyxins are cyclic, cationic peptide antibiotics that have fatty acid residues[248]; of the five polymyxins described originally (polymyxins A to E), two (B and E) have been used clinically. Polymyxin B and polymyxin E (colistin) differ by a single amino acid. Polymyxins bind to the anionic bacterial outer membrane, leading to a deterrent effect that disrupts membrane integrity. High-affinity binding to the lipid of a moiety of lipopolysaccharide may have an endotoxin-neutralizing effect. Commercial preparations of polymyxin B are standardized, but those of colistimethate (a less toxic prodrug of colistin that is administered clinically) are not, so dosing depends on which preparation is being supplied. Most recent reports have described colistimethate use, but the drugs are therapeutically equivalent.

Dosing of polymyxin B is 1.5 to 2.5 mg/kg (15,000 to 25,000 U/kg) daily in divided doses, whereas dosing of colistimethate ranges from 2.5 to 6 mg/kg/day, also in divided doses. The diluent is voluminous, adding substantially to daily fluid intake. Data on PK are scant, but the drugs exhibit rapid concentration-dependent bacterial killing against a wide variety of gram-negative bacilli, including most isolates of *E. coli, P. aeruginosa, S. maltophilia, Klebsiella* spp., *Enterobacter* spp., and *Acinetobacter* spp. Activity has remained generally excellent despite the widespread emergence of MDR pathogens. Combinations of polymyxin B or colistimethate and rifampin exhibit synergistic activity in vitro. Uptake into tissue is poor, but intrathecal and inhalational administration has been described. Clinical response rates for respiratory tract infections appear to be lower than for other sites of infection.

TABLE 11-9 Causes of Vancomycin Failure*

PARAMETER PREDICTING FAILURE	ADJUSTED ODDS RATIO	95% CI
Infective endocarditis	4.55	2.26-9.15
Nosocomial acquisition of infection	2.19	1.21-3.97
Initial vancomycin trough concentration <15 μg/mL	2.00	1.25-3.22
Vancomycin MIC >1 μg/mL	1.52	1.09-2.49

From Kullar R, Davis SL, Levine DP, et al: Impact of vancomycin exposure on outcomes in patients with methicillin-resistant *Staphylococcus aureus* bacteremia: Support for consensus guidelines suggested targets. *Clin Infect Dis* 52:975–981, 2011.

*In a single-center cohort of 320 patients with documented MRSA bacteremia, using logistic regression analysis.

Polymyxins had fallen out of favor because of nephrotoxicity and neurotoxicity issues, but the emergence of MDR pathogens has returned them to clinical use. Up to 40% of colistimethate-treated patients (5% to 15% for polymyxin B) will have an increase of serum creatinine levels, but renal replacement therapy is seldom required. Neurotoxicity (5% to 7% for both) usually becomes manifested as muscle weakness or polyneuropathy.

Protein Synthesis Inhibitors

Several classes of antibiotics, although dissimilar structurally and having divergent spectra of activity, exert their antibacterial effects by binding to bacterial ribosomes and inhibition of protein synthesis. This classification is valuable mechanistically, linking several classes of antibiotics conceptually that have few clinically useful members.

Aminoglycosides. Once disdained for their toxicity, aminoglycosides have had a resurgence in use as resistance to newer antibiotics (especially third-generation cephalosporins and fluoroquinolones) has developed. Gentamicin, tobramycin, and amikacin are still used frequently. Aminoglycosides bind to the bacterial 30S ribosomal subunit, inhibiting protein synthesis. With the exception of gentamicin's modest activity against gram-positive cocci, the spectrum of activity for the various agents is almost identical. Prescribing decisions should be based on toxicity and local resistance patterns.

Nevertheless, the potential toxicity is real, and aminoglycosides are now seldom used as first-line therapy, except in a synergistic combination to treat a serious *Pseudomonas* infection, enterococcal endocarditis, or infection caused by an MDR gram-negative bacillus. As second-line therapy, these drugs are highly efficacious against the Enterobacteriaceae, but there is less activity against *Acinetobacter* and limited activity against *P. cepacia, Aeromonas* spp., and *S. maltophilia.*

Aminoglycosides kill bacteria most effectively with a concentration peak to MIC ratio higher than 12, so a loading dose is necessary and serum drug concentration must be monitored. Synergistic therapy with a β-lactam agent is theoretically effective because bacterial cell wall damage caused by the β-lactam drug enhances intracellular penetration of the aminoglycoside; however, evidence of improved clinical outcomes is controversial,[220-222,249] especially with conventional dosing. Conventional dosing for serious infections requires 5 mg/kg/day of gentamicin or tobramycin after a loading dose of 2 mg/kg, or 15 mg/kg/day of amikacin after a loading dose of 7.5 mg/kg. PK is variable and unpredictable in critically ill patients, and higher doses are sometimes necessary (e.g., for burn patients). High doses (e.g., gentamicin, 7 mg/kg/day; amikacin, 20 mg/kg/day) given once daily can obviate these problems in many patients. Marked dosage reductions are necessary in renal insufficiency, but the drugs are dialyzed and a maintenance dose should be given after each hemodialysis treatment.

Tetracyclines. Tetracyclines bind irreversibly to the 30S ribosomal subunit, but unlike aminoglycosides, they are bacteriostatic. Widespread resistance limits their usefulness in the hospital setting (with two exceptions, doxycycline and tigecycline). Tetracyclines are active against anaerobes; *Actinomyces* can be treated successfully. Doxycycline is active against *B. fragilis* but is seldom used for this purpose. All tetracyclines are contraindicated in pregnancy and for children younger than 8 years because of dental toxicity.

Tigecycline is a rather new glycylcycline derived from minocycline.[250] With the major exceptions of *Pseudomonas* spp. and *Proteus mirabilis,* the spectrum of activity is broad, including many MDR gram-positive and gram-negative bacteria, including MRSA, VRE, and *Acinetobacter* spp. Tigecycline overcomes typical bacterial resistance to tetracyclines because of a modification at position 9 of its core structure, which enables high-affinity binding to the 30S ribosomal unit. Tigecycline is active against aerobic and anaerobic streptococci, staphylococci, MRSA, MRSE, and enterococci including VRE. Activity against gram-negative bacilli is directed against Enterobacteriaceae, including ESBL-producing strains, *Pasteurella multocida, Aeromonas hydrophila, S. maltophilia, Enterobacter aerogenes,* and *Acinetobacter* spp. Antianaerobic activity is excellent. The drug is approved for therapy of cIAIs and cSSTIs.

Concern has been raised recently by a post hoc analysis indicating that the mortality of tigecycline-treated patients is higher in pooled phase 3 and 4 clinical trials, including unpublished registration trials.[251] The adjusted risk difference for all-cause mortality based on a random-effects model stratified by trial weight was 0.6% (95% CI, 0.1-1.2) between tigecycline and comparator agents. However, an independent meta-analysis has found no such survival disadvantage in an analysis of eight published randomized controlled trials (4651 patients).[252] Overall, no difference was identified for the pooled clinically (OR, 0.92; 95% CI, 0.76-1.12) or microbiologically (OR, 0.86; 95% CI, 0.69-1.07) evaluable populations from these trials.

Oxazolidinones. Oxazolidinones bind to the ribosomal 50S subunit, preventing complexing with the 30S subunit. Assembly of a functional initiation complex for protein synthesis is blocked, preventing translation of mRNA. This mode of action is novel compared with that of other protein synthesis inhibitors that permit mRNA translation but then inhibit peptide elongation. Prevention of the initiation of protein synthesis is inherently no more lethal than prevention of peptide elongation; therefore, linezolid is bacteriostatic against most susceptible organisms. The ribosomes of *E. coli* are as susceptible to linezolid as those of gram-positive cocci, but with minor exceptions, gram-negative bacteria are oxazolidinone resistant because oxazolidinones are excreted by efflux pumps.

Linezolid is equally active against methicillin-susceptible *S. aureus* and MRSA, vancomycin-susceptible enterococci and VRE, and susceptible and penicillin-resistant pneumococci. Most gram-negative bacteria are resistant, but *Bacteroides* spp. are susceptible. Linezolid requires no dosage reduction in renal insufficiency and exhibits excellent tissue penetration, but it is uncertain whether this provides clinical benefit in the treatment of cSSTIs, HAP, and VAP.[253] A meta-analysis has suggested that linezolid is equivalent to vancomycin for HAP and VAP,[254] but some clinicians believe that linezolid should supplant vancomycin as first-line therapy for serious infections caused by gram-positive cocci.

Macrolide-lincosamide-streptogramin family

Clindamycin. The only lincosamide in active clinical use is clindamycin, which also binds to the 50S ribosome. Clindamycin has good antianaerobic activity (although *B. fragilis* resistance is increasing) and reasonably good activity against susceptible gram-positive cocci, not MRSA or VRE. Clindamycin is used occasionally for anaerobic infections and is preferred to vancomycin for prophylaxis of clean surgical cases in penicillin-allergic patients (see Box 11-6).[112] Because clindamycin inhibits exotoxin production in vitro, it has been advocated in preference to penicillin as first-line therapy for invasive *S. pyogenes* infections. The use of clindamycin has been associated with the development of *C. difficile* infection.

Drugs That Disrupt Nucleic Acids

Fluoroquinolones. Fluoroquinolones inhibit bacterial DNA synthesis by inhibiting DNA gyrase, which folds DNA into a superhelix in preparation for replication. The fluoroquinolones exhibit a broad spectrum of activity and excellent oral absorption and bioavailability, and they are generally well tolerated (except for photosensitivity and cartilage [especially in children] and tendon damage). These are potent agents with an unfortunate propensity to develop (and to induce) resistance rapidly (see Table 11-8). Agents with parenteral and oral formulations include ciprofloxacin, levofloxacin, and moxifloxacin, which has some anti-anaerobic activity. Several others have been withdrawn from the market or have never been approved because of toxicity.

Fluoroquinolones are most active against enteric gram-negative bacteria, particularly the Enterobacteriaceae and *Haemophilus* spp. There is some activity against *P. aeruginosa, S. maltophilia,* and gram-negative cocci. Activity against gram-positive cocci is variable; it is least for ciprofloxacin and best for the so-called respiratory quinolones (e.g., moxifloxacin). Ciprofloxacin is most active against *P. aeruginosa.* However, rampant overuse of fluoroquinolones is rapidly causing resistance that might severely limit the future usefulness of these agents.[255] Fluoroquinolone use has been associated with the emergence of resistant *E. coli, Klebsiella* spp., *P. aeruginosa,* and MRSA.[256,257] Fluoroquinolones prolong the QTc interval and may precipitate the ventricular dysrhythmia torsades de pointes, so electrocardiographic measurement of the QTc interval before and during fluoroquinolone therapy is important. Also, fluoroquinolones interact with warfarin to cause a rapid marked prolongation of the international normalized ratio, so anticoagulation must be monitored closely during therapy.

Cytotoxic Antibiotics

Metronidazole. Metronidazole is active against almost all anaerobes and against many protozoa that parasitize human beings. Metronidazole has potent bactericidal activity, including activity against *B. fragilis, Prevotella* spp., *Clostridium* spp. (including *C. difficile*), and anaerobic cocci, although it is ineffective against actinomycosis. Resistance remains rare and is of negligible clinical significance.

Metronidazole causes DNA damage after intracellular reduction of the nitro group of the drug. Acting as a preferential electron acceptor, it is reduced by low redox potential electron transport proteins, decreasing the intracellular concentration of the unchanged drug and maintaining a transmembrane gradient that favors uptake of additional drug. The drug therefore penetrates well into almost all tissues, including neural tissue, making it effective for deep-seated infections and bacteria that are not multiplying rapidly. Absorption after oral or rectal administration is rapid and almost complete. The $t_{1/2}$ of metronidazole is 8 hours because of an active hydroxy metabolite. Increasingly, IV metronidazole is administered every 8 to 12 hours in recognition of the active metabolite, but once-daily dosing is possible.[258] No dosage reduction is required for renal insufficiency, but the drug is dialyzed effectively and administration should be timed to follow dialysis if twice-daily dosing is used. PK in patients with hepatic insufficiency suggests a dosage reduction of 50% with marked impairment.

Trimethoprim-sulfamethoxazole. Sulfonamides exert bacteriostatic activity by interfering with bacterial folic acid synthesis, a necessary step in DNA synthesis. Resistance is widespread, thus limiting its use. The addition of sulfamethoxazole to trimethoprim, which prevents the conversion of dihydrofolic acid to tetrahydrofolic acid by the action of dihydrofolate reductase (downstream from the action of sulfonamides), accentuates the bactericidal activity of trimethoprim.

The combination of trimethoprim-sulfamethoxazole (TMP-SMX) is active against *S. aureus, S. pyogenes, S. pneumoniae, E. coli, P. mirabilis, Salmonella* and *Shigella* spp., *Yersinia enterocolitica, S. maltophilia, Listeria monocytogenes,* and *Pneumocystis jirovecí.* Used for UTIs, acute exacerbations of chronic bronchitis, and *Pneumocystis* infections, TMP-SMX is a treatment of choice for infections caused by *S. maltophilia* and outpatient and sometimes inpatient treatment of infections caused by community-acquired MRSA.

A fixed-dose combination of TMP-SMX (1 : 5) is available for parenteral administration. The standard oral formulation is 80 mg of trimethoprim and 400 mg of sulfamethoxazole, but lesser and greater strength tablets are available. Oral absorption is rapid, and bioavailability is almost 100%. Tissue penetration is excellent. The parenteral formulation, 10 mL, contains 160 mg of trimethoprim and 800 mg of sulfamethoxazole. Full doses (150 to 300 mg of trimethoprim in three or four divided doses) may be given if creatinine clearance is higher than 30 mL/min, but the drug is not recommended when the creatinine clearance is less than 15 mL/min.

ANTIBIOTIC TOXICITIES

β-Lactam Allergy

Allergic reaction is the most common toxicity of β-lactam antibiotics. The incidence is approximately 7 to 40 per 1000 treatment courses of penicillin.[259] Parenteral therapy is more likely to provoke an allergic reaction. Most serious reactions occur in patients with no history of penicillin allergy, simply because a history of penicillin allergy is commonly sought and is reported by 5% to 20% of patients, far in excess of the true incidence. Patients with a prior reaction have a fourfold to sixfold increased risk of another reaction compared with the general population. However, this risk decreases with time, from 80% to 90% skin test reactivity at 2 months to 20% reactivity at 10 years. The risk of cross-reactivity between penicillins and carbapenems and cephalosporins is approximately 5%, being highest for first-generation cephalosporins. There is negligible cross-reactivity to monobactams.

Red Man Syndrome

Tingling and flushing of the face, neck, or thorax may occur with parenteral vancomycin therapy but is less common than fever, rigors, or local phlebitis. Although a hypersensitivity reaction, it is not an allergic phenomenon because of the clear association with too rapid infusion of the drug (<1 hour, which can also cause hypotension). The cause is believed to be histamine release induced by local hyperosmolality. A maculopapular rash caused by hypersensitivity occurs in approximately 5% of patients.

Nephrotoxicity

There is little difference among aminoglycosides in terms of nephrotoxic potential. Aminoglycosides do not provoke inflammation; thus, there are no allergic components to any manifestation of aminoglycoside toxicity. The mechanisms of clinical toxicity relate to ischemia and toxicity to the renal proximal tubular cell.[259] Ultimately, injury is manifested by necrosis of the proximal tubular cell, reduction of the glomerular filtration rate, and decreased creatinine clearance but is usually reversible, and progression to dialysis dependence is rare. Aminoglycoside nephrotoxicity is accentuated by several cofactors, including frequent dosing, older age, sodium and volume depletion, acidemia, hypokalemia, hypomagnesemia, and coexistent liver disease. The risk of injury is ameliorated by single daily dose therapy. If renal function deteriorates, it is advisable to discontinue therapy unless treatment is for a life-threatening infection.

Vancomycin nephrotoxicity is increasing because of higher dosing and concurrent administration of other nephrotoxins. Nephrotoxicity of polymyxins may be an unavoidable consequence of the need to use an agent with known nephrotoxic potential to treat serious infections cause by MDR gram-negative bacilli when there are few alternatives, if any.

Ototoxicity

Aminoglycosides cause cochlear or vestibular toxicity that is usually irreversible and may develop after the cessation of therapy.[260] Repeated exposures create cumulative risk. Most patients develop cochlear toxicity or a vestibular lesion; rarely are both organs injured. Cochlear toxicity can be subtle because few patients have baseline audiograms, and formal screening programs are seldom undertaken. Few patients complain of hearing loss, but when it is sought, the incidence of cochlear toxicity may be more than 60%. Clinical hearing loss may occur in 5% to 15% of patients.

Ototoxicity caused directly by vancomycin is accepted as fact but has been poorly documented in the literature. Hearing loss attributed to vancomycin is better described as neurotoxicity, manifested as auditory nerve damage, tinnitus, and loss of acuity for high-frequency tones. Synergistic injury is possible with coadministration of other ototoxic drugs, especially aminoglycosides and furosemide. There is no correlation between ototoxicity and nephrotoxicity for drugs that cause both (e.g., aminoglycosides, vancomycin).

Avoiding Toxicity: Adjustment of Antibiotic Dosage

Hepatic Insufficiency

The liver metabolizes and eliminates drugs that are too lipophilic for renal excretion. The cytochromes P450 (a gene superfamily consisting of >300 different enzymes) oxidize lipophilic compounds to water-soluble products. Other enzymes convert drugs or metabolites by conjugating them with sugars, amino acids, sulfate, or acetate to facilitate biliary or renal excretion, whereas enzymes such as esterases and hydrolases act by other distinct mechanisms. Oxidation, in particular, is disrupted when liver function is impaired.

Drug dosing in hepatic insufficiency is complicated by insensitivity of clinical assessments to quantify liver function and changing metabolism as the degree of impairment fluctuates (e.g., resolving cholestasis). Changes in renal function with progressive hepatic impairment add considerable complexity. Renal blood flow is decreased in cirrhosis, and glomerular filtration is decreased in cirrhosis with ascites. Adverse drug reactions are more frequent with cirrhosis than with other forms of liver disease.

The effect of liver disease on drug disposition is difficult to predict in individual patients; none of the usual tests of liver function can be used to guide dosage.[261] In general, a dosage reduction of up to 25% of the usual dose is considered if hepatic metabolism is 40% or lower and renal function is normal (Box 11-12). Greater dosage reductions (up to 50%) are advisable if the drug is administered chronically, there is a narrow therapeutic index, protein binding is significantly reduced, or the drug is excreted renally and renal function is severely impaired.

BOX 11-12 Antibiotics Requiring Dosage Reduction for Hepatic and Renal Insufficiency

Hepatic

Aztreonam
Cefoperazone
Chloramphenicol
Clindamycin
Erythromycin
Isoniazid
Linezolid
Metronidazole
Nafcillin
Quinupristin-dalfopristin
Rifampin
Tigecycline

Renal

Aminoglycosides
Aztreonam
Carbapenems
Cephalosporins (most)
Chloramphenicol
Fluoroquinolones
Macrolides (except erythromycin and fidaxomicin)
Penicillins
Polymyxins
Sulfonamides
Trimethoprim-sulfamethoxazole
Vancomycin

Renal Insufficiency

Renal drug elimination depends on glomerular filtration, tubular secretion, and reabsorption, any of which may be altered with renal dysfunction. Renal failure may affect hepatic and renal drug metabolic pathways. Drugs whose hepatic metabolism is likely to be disrupted in renal failure include aztreonam, several cephalosporins, macrolides, and carbapenems.

Accurate estimates of renal function are important in patients with mild to moderate renal dysfunction because the clearance of many drugs by dialysis actually makes management easier. Factors influencing drug clearance by hemofiltration include molecular size, aqueous solubility, plasma protein binding, equilibration kinetics between plasma and tissue, and the apparent V_D. New high-flux polysulfone dialysis membranes can clear molecules up to 5 kDa efficiently (the molecular mass of vancomycin is 1.486 kDa). The need to dose patients during or after renal replacement therapy must be borne in mind; during continuous renal replacement therapy, the estimated creatinine clearance is approximately 15 to 25 mL/min in addition to the patient's intrinsic clearance.[262] Cefaclor, cefoperazone, ceftriaxone, chloramphenicol, clindamycin, cloxacillin, dicloxacillin, doxycycline, erythromycin, linezolid, methicillin, nafcillin, oxacillin, metronidazole, rifampin, and tigecycline do not require dosage reductions in renal failure (see Box 11-12).

IMPORTANT PATHOGENS OF CRITICALLY ILL PATIENTS

Vancomycin-Resistant Enterococci

VRE are predominantly *E. faecium* and thus usually manifest high-level resistance to ampicillin as well, which limits therapeutic options. Patients at risk include those with prolonged hospitalizations, multiple ICU admissions, and multiple or prolonged courses of antibiotics, especially cephalosporins and vancomycin (see Table 11-8). Although many isolates of VRE reflect colonization rather than invasive infection, isolation of VRE from the bloodstream or purulent closed space collections in symptomatic patients merits antimicrobial treatment. At present, there are four approved agents for VRE infection—daptomycin, linezolid, quinupristin-dalfopristin, and tigecycline—although chloramphenicol also has activity. Although there are no direct comparative trials of these agents, the side effect profiles of the other three agents appear favorable compared with quinupristin-dalfopristin. Linezolid-resistant VRE strains are being reported, particularly in patients with inadequately drained or nonremovable foci of infection who receive protracted therapy.

Staphylococcus aureus

With the advent of effective infection control procedures, the incidence of MRSA infections may be decreasing.[263,264] Nonetheless, MRSA remains a formidable and dangerous pathogen. Vancomycin has been the traditional first-line therapy of choice for most serious MRSA infections; however, there is increasing awareness of its limitations.[243,265] Vancomycin achieves only slow bactericidal activity, has poor lung and central nervous system penetration, and has poor activity in prosthetic biofilms. Heteroresistance to vancomycin has been detected in high-inoculum infections, and intermediate and complete vancomycin resistance has been described recently, although it remains rare. Combination therapy with gentamicin may enhance its bactericidal activity; however, this use does not alter clinical cure rates. In vancomycin-intolerant patients or vancomycin-refractory MRSA infections (i.e., vancomycin failures),[244] linezolid and quinupristin-dalfopristin have shown modest efficacy as a salvage option.[266] Daptomycin is bactericidal rapidly against *S. aureus* (including MRSA), but whether rapid bacterial killing confers a clinical advantage for therapy of most infections is debatable. Tigecycline is active (bacteriostatic) against MRSA, which does not confer a clinical disadvantage in most therapeutic situations. Ceftaroline is the newest option for the treatment of MRSA infections.

Pseudomonas aeruginosa

P. aeruginosa is a ubiquitous, avirulent opportunist whose virulence is enhanced in critically ill patients.[267] It is the second most common isolate from ICU infections, and infections caused by *P. aeruginosa* are the leading cause of death from nosocomial infection in the ICU, with infection-associated mortality as high as 70% in patients with pneumonia or bacteremia. Therapy is complex because of intrinsic and acquired resistance to a diverse spectrum of antimicrobial agents. Resistance is mediated through chromosomal-mediated β-lactamases, aminoglycoside-modifying enzymes, and mutations of outer membrane porin channels, which impede entry of carbapenems into the periplasmic space. A prominent characteristic is a high rate (20% to 40%) of de novo resistance developing during antipseudomonal therapy, a major cause of failed therapy.[268] Meropenem and doripenem may provide slightly higher activity than imipenem-cilastatin, with a lower propensity for central nervous system toxicity.

Multidrug-Resistant Enterobacteriaceae, Including *Klebsiella* Species

Resistance to β-lactams and other antibiotics in the Enterobacteriaceae family is increasingly associated with plasmid-mediated resistance determinants that are transferred easily among species, including ESBLs and carbapenemases, specifically the CTX-M family of ESBLs, KPC family of serine carbapenemases, and VIM, IMP, and NDM-1 metallo-β-lactamases.[269-271] These enzymes are now appearing worldwide in multiple combinations of ESBLs and carbapenemases, thereby conferring resistance to almost all β-lactam antibiotics. The increasing prevalence of carbapenem-resistant gram-negative bacteria is particularly disconcerting.

Klebsiella spp. and other Enterobacteriaceae are notable for exhibiting chromosome-mediated inducible β-lactamases, which deactivate antipseudomonal penicillins (e.g., ticarcillin, piperacillin), aztreonam, and cephalosporins. Ceftazidime is a potent inducer of chromosomal β-lactamase expression and is increasingly avoided as monotherapy or combination therapy of infections caused by even susceptible organisms. Cefepime does not appear to induce this type of chromosome-mediated resistance to the same degree but itself is susceptible to the action of ESBLs. Because most ESBL-producing strains also coexpress resistance to other agents (e.g., aminoglycosides, fluoroquinolones), there are few antimicrobials available to treat infections with these organisms, and data regarding agents in development are limited to in vitro studies. Therapeutic options are limited to carbapenems (the mainstay of therapy for ESBL producers) and tigecycline.

Stenotrophomonas maltophilia

At present, there are no clinical laboratory standards for the interpretation of disk diffusion susceptibilities for *S. maltophilia*. In the absence of broth dilution testing results, the most reliable agents have been TMP-SMX alone or TMP-SMX and ticarcillin–clavulanic acid in combination. The use of other agents has been associated with high rates of clinical failure despite in vitro susceptibility.

Acinetobacter baumannii Complex

Acinetobacter baumannii is a pleomorphic, aerobic, gram-negative bacillus (referred to sometimes as a coccobacillus) that is isolated commonly from the hospital environment and hospitalized patients. *A. baumannii* colonizes aquatic environments preferentially and is not part of normal fecal flora. This organism is often cultured from hospitalized patients' respiratory secretions, wounds or surgical sites, and urine. Historically, most *Acinetobacter* isolates recovered from hospitalized patients represented colonization rather than infection, especially in the ICU setting, being particularly common with endotracheal intubation, multiple IV catheters, monitoring devices, surgical drains, urinary catheters, or prior antimicrobial therapy with agents that have little or no activity against *Acinetobacter*. Colonization of the gastrointestinal tract by *Acinetobacter* is uncommon.

Although *A. baumannii* is avirulent, it is capable of causing infection of the seriously ill host.[272,273] *Acinetobacter* infections are increasingly common; when they occur, they usually involve organ systems with a high fluid content (e.g., sputum, cerebrospinal fluid, peritoneal fluid, urine), manifesting most commonly as pneumonia, catheter-associated bacteriuria, or bloodstream infection. *Acinetobacter* pneumonias have a predilection to occur in outbreaks. Nosocomial meningitis may occur in colonized neurosurgical patients with externalized ventricular drains (i.e., ventriculostomy). *Acinetobacter* is rarely associated with meningitis, endocarditis (native and prosthetic valve infections), peritonitis, UTIs, community-acquired pneumonia, or cholangitis.

A. baumannii is inherently resistant to several antibiotics, but MDR strains have emerged that are susceptible to relatively few antibiotics. Antibiotics to which MDR *Acinetobacter* is usually susceptible include meropenem, doripenem, amikacin, tigecycline, colistin, and polymyxin B, with one of the last two agents increasingly being used. There are no clinical laboratory standards for the interpretation of disk diffusion susceptibilities for tigecycline against *A. baumannii.* Mortality and morbidity resulting from *A. baumannii* infection relate to the underlying immune status of the host rather than to the inherent virulence of the organism.

FUNGAL INFECTIONS

Fungi are ubiquitous heterotrophic eukaryotes, resilient to environmental stress and adaptable to diverse environments. The most important human pathogens are the yeasts and molds. Invasive mycoses have emerged as a major cause of morbidity and mortality in hospitalized surgical patients. The U.S. incidence of nosocomial candidemia is approximately 8 per 100,000 population, at a cost of approximately $1 billion per year. Fungemia is the fourth most common type of bloodstream infection in the United States, but many surgical patients develop invasive infections without positive blood cultures. Host or therapeutic immunosuppression, organ transplantation, implantable devices, and human immunodeficiency virus infection have all changed the landscape of fungal pathogenicity.

Risk Factors

Whereas the incidence of hospital-acquired fungal infections almost doubled in the past decade, the greatest increase occurred in critically ill surgical patients, making the surgical ICU population an extremely high risk group.[274] Several conditions (patient dependent and disease specific) are independent predictors for invasive fungal infection, including ICU length of stay, extent of medical comorbidity, host immune suppression, and number of medical devices present. Neutropenia, diabetes mellitus, new-onset renal replacement therapy, total parenteral nutrition, broad-spectrum antibiotic administration, bladder catheterization, azotemia, diarrhea, and corticosteroid therapy have also been associated with candidemia.[275,276]

Diabetes Mellitus

Diabetes mellitus is an independent predictor for mucosal candidiasis, invasive candidiasis, and aspergillosis. Diabetic ketoacidosis has a strong association with rhinocerebral *Mucor* (produced by Zygomycetes) and other atypical fungal infections, with hyperglycemia being the strongest predictor of candidemia after liver transplantation and cardiopulmonary bypass. Glycosylation of cell surface receptors facilitates fungal binding and subsequent internalization and apoptosis of targeted cells. Glycosylation of opsonins disables fungal antigen recognition. The serum of diabetic patients has diminished capacity to bind iron, therefore making it available to the pathogen. Altered Th1 (helper phenotype) lymphocyte recognition of fungal targets impairs the production of interferon-γ. *Candida* spp. overexpress a C3 receptor–like protein that facilitates adhesion to endothelium and mucosal surfaces.

Neutropenia

There is a direct correlation between the degree of neutropenia and risk of invasive fungal infection.[277] Although a meta-analysis has concluded that there is little benefit from prophylaxis in neutropenic cancer patients, empirical antifungal therapy is standard for febrile neutropenia patients after chemotherapy or bone marrow transplantation. When profound neutropenia exists, the risk for breakthrough candidemia during antifungal therapy is significantly higher.

Organ Transplantation and Immunosuppression

The two most common opportunistic fungal pathogens of transplant patients are *Candida* and *Aspergillus* spp. The risk of fungal infection decreases 6 months after transplantation, unless a rejection episode requires intensification of the immunosuppression. In the solid organ transplant recipient, the graft itself is often affected. In liver transplantation, the risk of fungemia increases with the duration of the operation and number of transfusions. Other risk factors include the type of bile duct anastomosis (Roux-en-Y), tissue ischemia, cytomegalovirus infection, and graft-versus-host disease. *Aspergillus* tracheobronchitis in lung transplant patients is most likely to occur at the bronchial anastomosis. Surveillance bronchoscopy is recommended in this setting. *Aspergillus* is also the main organism responsible for fungemia after heart transplantation and is second only to cytomegalovirus as the cause of pneumonia in the first month after surgery.

Infectious complications are the primary cause of morbidity and mortality after pancreas and kidney-pancreas transplantation. The most common pathogens are gram-positive cocci, followed by gram-negative bacilli and *Candida.* Risk factors for fungal infections in this setting include bladder rather than enteric drainage (in cases of pancreas transplantation) and the use of muromonab-CD3 for antirejection therapy. Kidney recipients have the lowest incidence of infectious complications of all solid organ transplants, but the risk is sufficiently high that all solid organ transplant recipients (kidney recipients included) receive fungal prophylaxis with fluconazole (see later).

Malignant Disease

Cancer and chemotherapy produce three types of immune dysfunction that render the patient vulnerable to opportunistic infections: neutropenia (see earlier), deficits in lymphocyte-mediated innate immunity (e.g., lymphoma and during corticosteroid treatment), and adaptive immunodeficiency (e.g., multiple myeloma, Waldenström macroglobulinemia, and after splenectomy). As many as one third of cases of febrile neutropenia after chemotherapy for malignant disease are caused by invasive fungemia (see later). The type of lymphopenia is as important as the nadir of the lymphocyte count. Whereas Th1-type responses (TNF-α, interferon-γ, and IL-12) confer protection, Th2 (IL-4 and IL-10) suppressor phenotype responses are associated with progression of disease. Corticosteroids have anti-inflammatory properties related to their inhibitory effects on the activation of various transcription factors, in particular nuclear factor κB. In murine models, steroid treatment increases the production of IL-10 and decreases the recruitment of mononuclear cells in response to a fungal challenge. However, IL-8–mediated neutrophil recruitment is unaffected.

Central Venous Catheters

Many episodes of candidemia represent a CLABSI. Isolation of *Candida parapsilosis* from blood is strongly associated with CLABSI, parenteral nutrition, and prosthetic devices. In non-neutropenic subjects, the most common portals of entry for catheter contamination and subsequent infection are the skin during catheter placement, manipulation of an indwelling catheter, and cross-infection among ICU patients attributed to health care workers. Other possible sources for primary catheter colonization include contaminated parenteral nutrition solution, multidrug administration with repetitive violation of the sterile fluid path, and presence of other medical devices. The secondary route of contamination for devices in direct contact with the bloodstream (e.g., pacemakers, cardiac valves, joint prostheses) is candidemia originating from the gastrointestinal tract. Endogenous flora are also the most common source in neutropenic and other immunosuppressed patients. Once the catheter is contaminated, a stereotypical series of events occurs. Yeast adhere to the catheter surface and develop hyphae that integrate into a biofilm that increases in size and tridimensional complexity. A biofilm is the main reservoir for candidemia secondary to contaminated medical devices because it induces stasis and sequesters the fungi from antimycotic medication and the immune response.

In general, catheter removal is indicated after the diagnosis of systemic fungal infections and fungemia. Antifungal agents are usually continued after the catheter is removed, and *Candida* endophthalmitis should be ruled out (see later).

Prediction of Invasive *Candida* Infection

Overgrowth and recovery of *Candida* spp. from multiple sites, even from asymptomatic patients, carries a high likelihood of invasive candidiasis. Risk factors for the development of *Candida* colonization include female gender, antibiotic therapy before an ICU admission, prolonged stay in the ICU, and multiple gastrointestinal operations.[278] The source of the pathogen in the surgical context is usually the gastrointestinal tract.

Because colonization with *Candida* spp. presages invasive disease, it is desirable to identify and to characterize patients further in terms of risk. Surveillance cultures may be used to screen ICU patients. Several scoring systems have been proposed to quantify the risk of invasive fungal infection (Box 11-13). Pittet and colleagues[279] have proposed the colonization index, which has been validated in surgical patients. A threshold index of 0.5 or higher has been proposed for the initiation of empirical antifungal therapy in critically ill patients (see later). The *Candida* score, developed by Leon and associates,[280] considers dynamic patient factors that are present before the fact of colonization is identified and thus may be an earlier indicator. A threshold score of 2.5 points is indicative of high risk. Comparisons between the two are few, but the *Candida* Score may perform better.[281,282] The colonization index developed[283] and modified[284] by Ostrosky-Zeichner and coworkers suggests high risk in patients who remain in the ICU for 4 days or longer, have a central venous catheter in place, or are treated with antibiotics and in the presence of two of the following: use of total parenteral nutrition, need for dialysis, recent major surgery, diagnosis of pancreatitis, and treatment with systemic corticosteroids or other immunosuppressive agents.

Shorr and colleagues[285] have described a score to predict candidemia specifically, using data present on hospital admission (not specifically for surgical patients). This simple model assesses six factors (see Box 11-13), including age, absence of fever, recent hospitalization, admission from another health care facility, and need for mechanical ventilation; it differentiates patients' risk for candidemia in a graded fashion (e.g., no risk factors, 0.4%; three risk factors, 3.2%; six risk factors, 27.3%; $P < .0001$) on presentation to the hospital.

The use of broad-spectrum antibiotics is a well-documented risk factor for fungal colonization and subsequent infection. Interrelations between bacteria and fungi in human disease are complex. Antibiotics that have some antianaerobic therapy are associated with substantial increases in colony counts of yeast flora of the

BOX 11-13 Scoring Systems for Risk Stratification for Invasive Candidiasis

Candida Colonization Index[279]

This is the number of culture sites positive for the identical yeast isolate, divided by the number of sites cultured. At least three sites should be cultured (oral mucosa, axillae, rectum, gastric contents, urine). A score ≥0.5 point is considered high risk for subsequent infection. Discrimination statistics were not reported.

***Candida* Score**[280]

Four dichotomous variables are awarded points. A summed total score ≥2.5 points is strongly predictive of invasive fungal infection (sensitivity, 81%; specificity, 74%; C statistic = 0.847).

Total parenteral nutrition: 1 point
Surgery on ICU admission: 1 point
Multifocal *Candida* species colonization: 1 point
Severe sepsis: 2 points

Ostrosky-Zeichner Score (2007)[283]

This is a prediction rule that provides a dichotomous risk assessment based on the presence of at least three risk factors: relative risk, 5; sensitivity, 0.27, specificity; 0.93, positive predictive value; 0.13, negative predictive value; 0.97, accuracy, 0.90.

Any systemic antibiotic (days 1-3 of the ICU stay) *or*
Central venous catheter (days 1-3) *and*
At least two of the following:

- Total parenteral nutrition (days 1-3)
- Any renal replacement therapy (days 1-3)
- Any major surgery (days −7 to 0)
- Pancreatitis (days −7 to 0)
- Any steroid use (days −7 to −3)

Any other immunosuppression (days −7 to 0)

Ostrosky-Zeichner Modified Score (2011)[284]

This is a prediction rule that provides a dichotomous risk assessment based on the presence of at least three risk factors: relative risk, 4; sensitivity, 0.50; specificity, 0.83; positive predictive value, 0.10; negative predictive value, 0.97; accuracy, 0.81.

Mechanical ventilation >48 hours (days 1-4) *and*
Any systemic antibiotic (days 1-3 of the ICU stay) *and*
Central venous catheter (days 1-3) *and*
At least one of the following:

- Total parenteral nutrition (days 1-3)
- Any renal replacement therapy (days 1-3)
- Any major surgery (days −7 to 0)
- Pancreatitis (days −7 to 0)
- Any steroid or other immunosuppression (days −7 to 0)

Shorr Candidemia Score[285]

A simple, equal-weight score (1 point each) differentiated reasonably well among patients admitted with a bloodstream infection, with a C statistic of 0.70.

Age <65 years
Temperature ≤98° F or severe altered mental status
Cachexia
Hospitalization within the previous 30 days
Admission from another health care facility
Need for mechanical ventilation

gut, whereas antibiotics with poor anaerobic activity are less likely to produce this effect. Sawyer and associates[286] have demonstrated that *C. albicans* induces bacterial translocation into abscesses, but the relationship is one of direct competency rather than synergy or cooperation. The precise mechanism of action for this observation is unknown but is probably related to fungi to microbe competence and growth suppression. *Candida* may enhance the pathogenicity of certain bacteria but not of others; this interaction remains to be elucidated.

Intensive Care Unit and Invasive Mechanical Ventilation

Epidemiologic observations have correlated the duration of mechanical ventilation and amount of intensive care required with the occurrence of fungal colonization and invasive infections. Other factors related to susceptibility for systemic candidiasis are total parenteral nutrition, prophylaxis of stress-related gastric mucosal hemorrhage, radiation therapy, previous bacteremia, abdominal surgery, renal replacement therapy, extremes of age, recurrent mucocutaneous candidiasis, and duration of cardiopulmonary bypass longer than 120 minutes.

Fungal Pathogens

Candida albicans

C. albicans is a common cause of human disease, which can be focal or disseminated.[287] *C. albicans* accounts for about 60% of *Candida* isolates, followed by *Candida glabrata* (15% to 25% of all *Candida* infections). The incidence of candidemia has increased during the past 30 years, representing 8% to 15% of all nosocomial bloodstream infections, with mortality rates reported in some series to be as high as 80%. *Candida* bloodstream infection carries an independent increased risk of death in adult ICU patients.[288]

A morphologic transition from yeast to hyphal forms is the most important determinant of dissemination of *C. albicans*; the mycelial phase is invasive[289] because of upregulated elaboration of proteinases. Host and pathogen play a role in this dimorphism. Phenotypic switching accompanied by changes in antigen expression, colony morphology, and tissue affinities is recognized, but the inducer mechanisms and triggering stimuli are unknown.

Multifocal candidiasis is the simultaneous isolation of *Candida* from two or more of the following normally sterile locations: respiratory, digestive, and urinary tracts; wounds; or drainage. Disseminated candidiasis requires microbiologic evidence of yeast in fluids from normally sterile sites (such as cerebrospinal, pleural, pericardial, or peritoneal fluid), histologic samples from viscera, or a diagnosis of endophthalmitis or candidemia with negative catheter tip cultures. Disseminated candidiasis and true fungemia can lead to septic shock, similar to that seen with bacterial pathogens. The dimorphic transition results in shock and end-organ failure in susceptible individuals, mechanistically independent of TNF-α.

The diagnosis of fungemia as the cause of a patient's sepsis depends on a strong clinical suspicion because fungemia and bacteremia are indistinguishable on the basis of clinical criteria.[290] Blood cultures for *Candida* are falsely negative more than 50% of the time; moreover, bacterial pathogens may interfere with the recovery of *Candida.* Biomarkers including the fungal cell wall component (1→3)-β-D-glucan,[291] anti-*Candida* immunoglobulin G antibodies,[292] and procalcitonin[293] are suggestive of but not sufficiently accurate for diagnosis. There are no reliable laboratory tests to identify the presence of *Candida* or to differentiate between *Candida* colonization and invasive candidiasis. No single site of isolation is superior to others in predicting which patients have systemic infection. Purpura fulminans and unexplained myalgias are suggestive of candidiasis in the appropriate clinical context. Three or more colonized sites or two positive blood cultures at least 24 hours apart, with one obtained after the removal of any central venous catheter, are strong indicators of fungemia.[294] Whereas asymptomatic recovery of *Candida* in urine rarely requires therapy, candiduria should be treated if it is symptomatic, after instrumentation or renal transplantation, or if the patient is neutropenic. Removal or changing of the bladder drainage catheter is required.

Fungal endophthalmitis usually is a result of hematogenous spread from systemic fungemia.[295] *Candida* spp. are the most common offenders, although *Aspergillus, Cryptococcus, Fusarium, Scedosporium,* and others are known causes of endophthalmitis. Retinal involvement has been diagnosed in 28% to 45% of all patients with known candidemia and may be the first sign of hitherto undetected fungemia. Early treatment of invasive fungal infection decreases the incidence of endophthalmitis. All patients with invasive candidiasis or fungemia must undergo a formal ophthalmologic assessment to rule out eye involvement. The observation of a classic three-dimensional, retina-based, cotton-wool vitreal inflammatory process is diagnostic of *Candida* endophthalmitis.

Treatment of endophthalmitis consists of IV antifungal therapy and may require intraocular injections of amphotericin B, caspofungin, or voriconazole. In patients in whom extension to the vitreous or pars anterior is evident, surgical débridement or vitrectomy may be required. Delay in treatment frequently leads to blindness.

Non-*albicans Candida*

The incidence of non-*Candida* fungemia and sepsis is increasing, accounting for up to 50% of non-*albicans Candida* adult ICU infections. Undoubtedly, the pressure of antifungal therapy is an explanation for the emergence of *C. glabrata* and *C. krusei* as pathogens.[296] Other species of yeast are related to specific events, such as *C. parapsilosis* in the presence of an indwelling central venous catheter. An increased incidence of *C. tropicalis* in oncology patients is secondary to the inherent invasiveness of the organism, especially through damaged gastrointestinal mucosa. Clinically, the features of these infections are indistinguishable from those of *C. albicans.*

Aspergillus

Noninvasive types of aspergillosis include allergic bronchopulmonary aspergillosis, a form of hypersensitivity reaction in asthmatics, and aspergilloma. These entities, without tissue invasion, usually do not require antifungal therapy. However, invasive aspergillosis is increasing in incidence and has become a major cause of death among patients with liquid tumors. Although invasive *Aspergillus* infections usually occur through inhalation of conidia, the fungus may also be ingested on food (e.g., pepper, regular and herbal teas, fruits, corn, rice). Spores of *Aspergillus* and other filamentous fungi are thermotolerant, are difficult to eradicate, and threaten the immunocompromised host. Conidia that are not cleared by alveolar macrophages germinate in the alveoli; hyphal forms invade the pulmonary parenchyma, with prominent vascular invasion and early dissemination.[297]

Other Emerging Fungal Pathogens

Zygomycetes *(Mucor)* are becoming increasingly important in ICU patients. The portal of entry in the immunocompromised host is usually inhalation of aerosolized thermotolerant spores, although percutaneous exposure (surgical or traumatic wounds and burns) has been reported. The source of these spores is usually decaying organic matter in soil, but they can be found in hospital food, including fruit, bread, cookies, crackers, regular and herbal tea, and pepper. The major risk factors for mucormycosis are diabetic ketoacidosis, neutropenia, iron overload, deferoxamine therapy, and protein-calorie malnutrition. Infection may cause extensive tissue necrosis; treatment includes surgical débridement, depending on the extent of the disease.

Prophylaxis

The substantial morbidity and mortality of invasive fungal infections have led to the practice of administering prophylactic antifungal agents, usually fluconazole, to critically ill patients. Early on, concern was raised that increasing the use of azole antifungals would lead to increased resistance to the agents.[298,299] A prospective, randomized, placebo-controlled trial of enteral fluconazole, 400 mg/day, was conducted among 260 critically ill surgical patients with a length of stay of 3 days or longer in a tertiary care surgical ICU.[300] After adjustment for potentially confounding effects of the Acute Physiology and Chronic Health Evaluation (APACHE) III score, days to first dose, and fungal colonization at enrollment, the risk of fungal infection was reduced by 55% in the fluconazole group, but no difference in mortality was observed. In a follow-up prospective, observational study,[301] subjects admitted for 3 days or longer to the surgical ICU underwent surveillance fungal cultures of rectal-fecal swabs, urine, and endotracheal aspirates on admission, once weekly thereafter, and on ICU discharge while fluconazole prophylaxis of high-risk surgical patients continued as usually carried out. *C. glabrata* colonization was not more common among patients in the later cohort compared with earlier (adjusted odds ratio [AOR], 0.90; 95% CI, 0.57-1.41). Patients with invasive candidiasis in the later cohort were not more likely than those in the earlier trial to have infection caused by *C. glabrata* (AOR, 1.93; 95% CI, 0.20-18.98), whereas patients with invasive candidiasis in the 2003 cohort were less likely than patients in the 1998 trial to have acquired invasive candidiasis in the ICU (AOR, 0.08; 95% CI, 0.01-0.82).

Four randomized studies comparing fluconazole to placebo for the prevention of fungal infections in the surgical ICU were subjected to meta-analysis.[302] The studies enrolled 626 patients but used differing dosing regimens of fluconazole. All trials were double-blinded and two were multicenter studies. Fluconazole prophylaxis significantly reduced the incidence of fungal infections (pooled OR, 0.44; 95% CI, 0.27-0.72; $P < .001$). However, fluconazole prophylaxis was not associated with a survival advantage (pooled OR for mortality, 0.87; 95% CI, 0.59-1.28). Fluconazole did not alter the rate of candidemia, perhaps because it developed in only 2.2% of all participants. Data were insufficient to allow comment on the impact of fluconazole prophylaxis on resource use, distribution of non-*albicans* species of *Candida,* or emergence of resistance.

Prophylactic fluconazole administration in general surgical ICU patients appears to decrease the incidence of mycotic infections but does not improve survival. The absence of a survival advantage may reflect the paucity of data in this area and the possibility that this issue requires further study. Current guidelines recommend fluconazole prophylaxis for high-risk patients (Box 11-14).[303]

Antifungal Prophylaxis of Solid Organ Transplant Recipients

Solid organ transplantation is lifesaving for end-stage organ failure, but post-transplantation invasive fungal infections remain a major cause of morbidity and mortality. To improve outcomes, various prevention strategies have been tested, including antifungal prophylaxis with systemic and topical nonabsorbable agents. Currently, data support the use of antifungal prophylaxis in liver, lung, small bowel, and pancreas transplant recipients (see Box 11-14).[303]

In a meta-analysis of randomized placebo-controlled trials with fluconazole prophylaxis, the incidence of fungal infections was significantly reduced; however, there was no survival advantage, similar to antifungal prophylaxis of critically ill general surgical patients.[304] For liver transplant patients, the number needed to treat to prevent one infection is 14, given an incidence of 10%. The meta-analysis also concluded that for lower risk recipients (i.e., renal homograft recipients), the number needed to treat increases to 28.

A systematic review and meta-analysis of antifungal prophylaxis in liver transplant recipients evaluated 10 randomized trials (1106 patients) of any prophylactic antifungal regimen versus no antifungal agent or another antifungal regimen.[305] In general, results were consistent across trials, despite clinical and methodologic heterogeneity. Antifungal prophylaxis did not reduce mortality (RR, 0.84; 95% CI, 0.54-1.30), but fluconazole prophylaxis reduced invasive fungal infections (RR, 0.28; 95% CI, 0.13-0.57). Fluconazole prophylaxis did not significantly increase colonization or infection with azole-resistant fungi, although data were limited.

Antifungal Therapy

Candidemia is defined as the following: (1) one blood culture that grows *Candida* spp. and histologically documented invasive candidiasis or an ophthalmic examination consistent with candidal endophthalmitis; (2) at least two blood cultures obtained at different times from a peripheral vein that grow the same *Candida* sp.; or (3) one blood culture obtained peripherally and one blood culture obtained through an indwelling central line, both of which grow identical *Candida* sp. Patients with one positive blood culture drawn through an IV line and a positive semiquantitative catheter tip culture are not considered infected unless they satisfy one of these criteria.

Severe non-bloodstream candidal infections are defined as *Candida* spp. isolated from a normally sterile body site and the presence of at least one of the following: fever (>38.5° C [101.3° F]) or hypothermia (<36° C [96.8° F]); unexplained prolonged hypotension (systolic blood pressure <80 mm Hg for >2 hours, unresponsive to volume challenge); and absence of response to adequate antibiotic treatment for a suspected bacterial infection. *Candida* spp. pneumonia, which some authorities believe does not exist in immunocompetent hosts, requires the recovery of more than 10^5 CFU/mL of *Candida* spp. in BAL fluid in addition to the appearance of a new infiltrate on the chest radiograph. Invasive fungal infections in non-neutropenic ICU patients are treated if histology or cytopathology shows yeast cells or pseudohyphae from a needle aspiration or biopsy specimen (excluding mucous membranes), a positive culture obtained aseptically from a normally sterile and clinically or radiologically abnormal site is consistent with infection (excluding urine, sinuses, and mucous membranes), or a positive percutaneous blood culture in patients with temporally related clinical signs and symptoms is compatible with the relevant organism. Survival is more likely from candidemia than from other forms of invasive candidiasis and is strongly influenced negatively by critical illness.[306]

BOX 11-14 Synopsis of Clinical Practice Guidelines for the Management of Candidiasis*

Antifungal Prophylaxis for Solid Organ Transplant Recipients and ICU Patients

Solid Organ Transplant Recipients

Postoperative antifungal prophylaxis for liver (A-I), pancreas (B-II), and small bowel (B-III) transplant recipients at high risk of candidiasis, daily for 7-14 days.

- Fluconazole (200-400 mg [3-6 mg/kg] daily)
- Liposomal amphotericin B (L-AmB) (1-2 mg/kg)

Patients Hospitalized in the ICU

Fluconazole (400 mg [6 mg/kg] daily) is recommended for high-risk patients in adult units that have a high incidence of invasive candidiasis (B-I).

Treatment of Identified Candidemia in Non-Neutropenic Patients

Initial Therapy for Most Adult Patients (A-I)

Fluconazole (loading dose of 800 mg [12 mg/kg], then 400 mg [6 mg/kg] daily) *or*

Echinocandin

- Caspofungin: loading dose of 70 mg, then 50 mg daily, *or*
- Micafungin: 100 mg daily, *or*
- Anidulafungin: loading dose of 200 mg, then 100 mg daily is recommended

An echinocandin is favored for patients with moderate to severe illness or for patients who have had recent azole exposure (A-III). Fluconazole is recommended for patients who are less critically ill and who have had no recent azole exposure (A-III). The same therapeutic approach is advised for children, with attention to differences in dosing.

Transition from an echinocandin to fluconazole is recommended for patients who have isolates likely to be susceptible to fluconazole (e.g., *C. albicans*) and who are clinically stable (A-II).

For infection caused by *C. glabrata,* an echinocandin is preferred (B-III). Transition to fluconazole or voriconazole therapy is not recommended without confirmation of isolate susceptibility (B-III). For patients who received fluconazole or voriconazole initially, have improved clinically, and have negative follow-up cultures, continuation of the azole to completion of therapy is reasonable (B-III).

For infection caused by *C. parapsilosis,* treatment with fluconazole is recommended (B-III). For patients who have received an echinocandin initially, have improved clinically, and have negative follow-up cultures, continuation of the echinocandin to completion of therapy is reasonable (B-III).

Amphotericin B deoxycholate (AmB-d), 0.5-1.0 mg/kg daily, or a lipid formulation of AmB (LFAmB), 3-5 mg/kg daily, is an alternative if there is intolerance to or limited availability of other antifungal agents (A-I). Transition from AmB-d or LFAmB to fluconazole is recommended if isolates are likely to be susceptible to fluconazole (e.g., *C. albicans*) and the patient is stable clinically (A-I).

Voriconazole, 400 mg (6 mg/kg) twice daily for two doses and then 200 mg (3 mg/kg) twice daily thereafter, is effective for candidemia (A-I), but there is little advantage over fluconazole, and is recommended as step-down oral therapy for selected cases of candidiasis caused by *C. krusei* or voriconazole-susceptible *C. glabrata* (B-III).

The recommended duration of therapy for candidemia without obvious metastatic complications is for 2 weeks after documented clearance of *Candida* from the bloodstream and resolution of symptoms attributable to candidemia (A-III).

IV catheter removal is strongly recommended (A-II).

Empirical Treatment for Suspected Invasive Candidiasis in Non-Neutropenic Patients

Empirical therapy for suspected candidiasis in non-neutropenic patients is similar to that for proven candidiasis (B-III):

- Fluconazole (loading dose of 800 mg [12 mg/kg], then 400 mg [6 mg/kg] daily)
- Caspofungin (loading dose of 70 mg, then 50 mg daily)
- Anidulafungin (loading dose of 200 mg, then 100 mg daily)
- Micafungin (100 mg daily)

An echinocandin is preferred for patients who have had recent azole exposure, whose illness is moderately severe or severe, or who are at high risk of infection caused by *C. glabrata* or *C. krusei* (B-III).

AmB-d (0.5-1.0 mg/kg daily) and LFAmB (3-5 mg/kg daily) are alternatives if there is intolerance to or limited availability of other antifungals (B-III).

Empirical antifungal therapy should be considered for critically ill patients with risk factors for invasive candidiasis and no other known cause of fever, based on clinical assessment of risk, serologic markers for invasive candidiasis, or culture data from nonsterile sites (B-III).

Adapted from Playford EG, Webster AC, Sorrell TC, et al: Systematic review and meta-analysis of antifungal agents for preventing fungal infections in liver transplant recipients. *Eur J Clin Microbiol Infect Dis* 25:549–561, 2006.

*Infectious Diseases Society of America, 2009; strength of evidence-based recommendations is shown in parentheses.

The repertoire of antifungal agents has expanded with the introduction of less toxic formulations of amphotericin B, improved triazoles, echinocandins, and other agents that target the fungal cell wall.[307] Table 11-10 lists available antifungal agents. Amphotericin B is a natural polyene macrolide that binds primarily to ergosterol, the principal sterol in the fungal cell membrane, leading to disruption of ion channels, production of oxygen free radicals, and apoptosis. It is active against most fungi, including in cerebrospinal fluid. Because of its high level of protein binding, tissue concentrations are not usually affected by hemodialysis. Infusion-related reactions can occur in up to 73% of patients with the first dose and often diminish during continued therapy. Amphotericin B–associated nephrotoxicity can lead to azotemia and hypokalemia, although acute potassium release with rapid infusion can occur and lead to cardiac arrest. Amphotericin B lipid formulations allow higher dose administration with lessened nephrotoxicity, but whether outcomes are enhanced is unproved. Nystatin is a polyene similar in structure to amphotericin B and is currently used topically for *C. albicans.* Flucytosine is a fluorinated pyrimidine analogue that is converted to 5-fluorouracil, which causes RNA miscoding and inhibits DNA synthesis. It is available in the United States in oral form only and has been used with amphotericin B for synergism against *Candida* spp. However, in general, there is scant evidence that dual-agent therapy for fungal infections is beneficial.[308]

The azoles inhibit the cytochrome P450–dependent enzyme 14α-reductase, altering fungal cell membranes through the accumulation of abnormal 14α-methyl sterols. Ketoconazole is available only in tablet form and is indicated for candidiasis and candiduria. Fluconazole and itraconazole are available in oral and parenteral formulations and are active against *Candida* spp., except *C. krusei,* and *Fusarium* spp. Itraconazole is active against *Aspergillus* spp. As noted, *C. glabrata* and *C. krusei* resistance has been observed with fluconazole. The tissue concentration of both

TABLE 11-10 Antifungal Agents

ANTIFUNGAL AGENT	INDICATIONS	ROUTE AND DOSAGE
Amphotericin B	*Candida albicans* (>95%), *C. glabrata* (95%), *C. parapsilosis* (>95%), *C. krusei* (>95%), *C. tropicalis* (99%), *C. guilliermondii, C. lusitaniae* Variable activity: *Aspergillus* spp., ferrous *Trichosporon beigelii, Fusarium* spp., *Blastomyces dermatitidis*	IV: 0.5-1.0 mg/kg/day during 2-4 hr Oral: 1 mL oral suspension, swish and swallow 4× daily, ×2 wk
Amphotericin B liposomal (less nephrotoxicity)	*C. albicans* (>95%), *C. glabrata* (>95%), *C. parapsilosis* (>95%), *C. krusei* (>95%), *C. tropicalis* (99%), *C. guilliermondii, C. lusitaniae* Variable activity: *Aspergillus* spp.	IV: 3-5 mg/kg/day
Amphotericin B colloidal dispersion	*C. albicans* (>95%), *C. glabrata* (>95%), *C. parapsilosis* (>95%), *C. krusei* (>95%), *C. tropicalis* (99%), *C. guilliermondii, C. lusitaniae* Variable activity: *Aspergillus* spp.	IV: 3-5 mg/kg/day
Amphotericin B lipid complex	*C. albicans* (>95%), *C. glabrata* (>95%), *C. parapsilosis* (>95%), *C. krusei* (>95%), *C. tropicalis* (99%), *C. guilliermondii, C. lusitaniae* Variable activity: *Aspergillus* spp.	IV: 5 mg/kg/day
Ketoconazole	*C. albicans*	PO: 200-400 mg/daily
Voriconazole	*Aspergillus* spp., *Fusarium* spp., *C. albicans* (99%), *C. glabrata* (99%), *C. parapsilosis* (99%), *C. tropicalis* (99%), *C. krusei* (99%), *C. guilliermondii* (>95%), *C. lusitaniae* (95%)	IV: 6 mg/kg q12h ×2, then 4 mg/kg IV every 12 hr PO: >40 kg, 200 mg every 12 hr; <40 kg, 100 mg every 12 hr
Fluconazole	*C. albicans* (97%), *C. glabrata* (85%-90% resistant, intermediate), *C. parapsilosis* (99%) *C. tropicalis* (98%), *C. krusei* (5%) Fungistatic against *Aspergillus* spp.	Candidiasis: prophylaxis (IV or oral), 100-400 mg/day; invasive, 400-800 mg/day Oropharyngeal: 200 mg day 1, then 100 daily for 2 wk
Itraconazole	Fungicidal to *Aspergillus* spp., *C. albicans* (93%), *C. glabrata* (50%), *C. parapsilosis* (45%), *C. tropicalis* (58%), *C. krusei* (69%), *C. guilliermondii, C. lusitaniae* Blastomycoses, histoplasmosis, chromomycosis	IV: Load 200 mg IV 2× daily ×4 doses, then 200 mg 4× daily maximum 14 days Oral: 200 mg daily or 2× daily Life-threatening: Load 600-800/day ×3-5/days, then 400-600 mg/day
Caspofungin	*C. albicans, C. glabrata, C. parapsilosis, C. tropicalis, C. krusei, C. guilliermondii, C. lusitaniae*	IV: 70 mg IV, then 50 mg IV every day
Micafungin	*C. albicans, C. glabrata, C. parapsilosis, C. tropicalis, C. krusei, C. guilliermondii, C. lusitaniae*	IV: 100-200 mg IV daily
Anidulafungin	*C. albicans, C. glabrata, C. parapsilosis, C. tropicalis, C. krusei, C. guilliermondii, C. lusitaniae*	Esophageal candidiasis: 100 mg IV day 1, 50 mg/day thereafter Candidemia: 200 mg IV day 1, 100 mg/day thereafter
Flucytosine	Not effective for *C. krusei* Effective for *C. albicans, C. tropicalis, C. parapsilosis, C. lusitaniae*	PO: 50-150 mg/kg/day divided qid
Nystatin	*C. albicans*	100,000 U swish and swallow qid
Clotrimazole	Thrush (usually not cultured)	Oral troches daily for 14 days

drugs is influenced by many agents, such as antacids, H_2 antagonists, isoniazid, phenytoin, and phenobarbital. Biofilms produced by *Candida* spp. are penetrated by fluconazole and most other antifungal agents.[309,310]

Second-generation antifungal triazoles include posaconazole, ravuconazole, and voriconazole. They are active against *Candida* spp., including fluconazole-resistant strains, and *Aspergillus* spp. For the latter, voriconazole is emerging as the treatment of choice.[311,312]

The echinocandins include caspofungin, micafungin, and anidulafungin, each of which is approved therapy for candidiasis and candidemia but is third-line treatment for invasive aspergillosis.[313] Because of their distinct mechanism of action, disrupting the fungal cell wall by inhibiting (1→3)-β-D-glucan synthesis, the echinocandins can theoretically be used in combination with other standard antifungal agents.[308] The echinocandins have activity against *Candida* and *Aspergillus* spp. but are not reliably active against other fungi. Echinocandin activity is excellent against most *Candida* spp. but moderate against *C. parapsilosis, C. guilliermondii,* and *C. lusitaniae.* Echinocandins exhibit no cross-resistance with azoles or polyenes.[314] Prospective randomized trials have demonstrated that micafungin is noninferior to caspofungin for therapy of invasive candidiasis[315] and as effective as liposomal amphotericin B.[316] Micafungin may be cost-effective in comparison to fluconazole therapy.

With the proliferation of non-*albicans Candida* infections caused by the widespread use of fluconazole, empirical therapy regimens recommend an echinocandin or lipid formulation of amphotericin B as the first-line agent for therapy of seriously or critically ill patients (see Box 11-14 and Table 11-10).[305,317] Once the pathogen has been identified as *Candida,* therapy may be de-escalated to fluconazole, except for *C. glabrata* and *C. krusei,* for which continuation therapy with an echinocandin may be indicated (Table 11-11).

TABLE 11-11 Usual Susceptibilities of *Candida* Species to Selected Antifungal Agents

CANDIDA SPP	FLUCONAZOLE	ITRACONAZOLE	VORICONAZOLE (NOT STANDARDIZED)	AMPHOTERICIN B	CASPOFUNGIN (NOT STANDARDIZED)
C. albicans	S	S	S	S	S
C. tropicalis	S	S	S	S	S
C. parapsilosis	S	S	S	S	S to I (?R)
C. glabrata	S-DD to R	S-DD to R	S to I	S to I	S
C. krusei	R	S-DD to R	S to I	S to I	S
C. lusitaniae	S	S	S	S to R	S

I, intermediate; *R*, resistant; *S*, susceptible; *S-DD*, susceptible dose-dependent (increased MIC may be overcome by higher dosing, such as 12 mg/kg/day fluconazole).

REFERENCES

1. Desborough JP: The stress response to trauma and surgery. *Br J Anaesth* 85:109–117, 2000.
2. Napolitano LM, Faist E, Wichmann MW, et al: Immune dysfunction in trauma. *Surg Clin North Am* 79:1385–1416, 1999.
3. Gardner EM, Murasko DM: Age-related changes in type 1 and type 2 cytokine production in humans. *Biogerontology* 3:271–290, 2002.
4. Latham R, Lancaster AD, Covington JF, et al: The association of diabetes and glucose control with surgical-site infections among cardiothoracic surgery patients. *Infect Control Hosp Epidemiol* 22:607–612, 2001.
5. Cheadle WG: Risk factors for surgical site infection. *Surg Infect (Larchmt)* 7(Suppl 1):S7–S11, 2006.
6. Zerr KJ, Furnary AP, Grunkemeier GL, et al: Glucose control lowers the risk of wound infection in diabetics after open heart operations. *Ann Thorac Surg* 63:356–361, 1997.
7. Pomposelli JJ, Baxter JK, 3rd, Babineau TJ, et al: Early postoperative glucose control predicts nosocomial infection rate in diabetic patients. *JPEN J Parenter Enteral Nutr* 22:77–81, 1998.
8. Yendamuri S, Fulda GJ, Tinkoff GH: Admission hyperglycemia as a prognostic indicator in trauma. *J Trauma* 55:33–38, 2003.
9. Bochicchio GV, Bochicchio KM, Joshi M, et al: Acute glucose elevation is highly predictive of infection and outcome in critically injured trauma patients. *Ann Surg* 252:597–602, 2010.
10. Griesdale DE, de Souza RJ, van Dam RM, et al: Intensive insulin therapy and mortality among critically ill patients: A meta-analysis including NICE-SUGAR study data. *CMAJ* 180:821–827, 2009.
11. Eachempati SR, Hydo LJ, Shou J, et al: Implementation of tight glucose control for critically ill surgical patients: A process improvement analysis. *Surg Infect (Larchmt)* 10:523–531, 2009.
12. Wichmann MW, Zellweger R, DeMaso CM, et al: Enhanced immune responses in females, as opposed to decreased responses in males following haemorrhagic shock and resuscitation. *Cytokine* 8:853–863, 1996.
13. Diodato MD, Knoferl MW, Schwacha MG, et al: Gender differences in the inflammatory response and survival following haemorrhage and subsequent sepsis. *Cytokine* 14:162–169, 2001.
14. Gannon CJ, Napolitano LM, Pasquale M, et al: A statewide population-based study of gender differences in trauma: Validation of a prior single-institution study. *J Am Coll Surg* 195:11–18, 2002.
15. Angus DC, Linde-Zwirble WT, Lidicker J, et al: Epidemiology of severe sepsis in the United States: Analysis of incidence, outcome, and associated costs of care. *Crit Care Med* 29:1303–1310, 2001.
16. Laudanski K, Miller-Graziano C, Xiao W, et al: Cell-specific expression and pathway analyses reveal alterations in trauma-related human T cell and monocyte pathways. *Proc Natl Acad Sci U S A* 103:15564–15569, 2006.
17. Arcaroli J, Fessler MB, Abraham E: Genetic polymorphisms and sepsis. *Shock* 24:300–312, 2005.
18. Gunderson KL, Steemers FJ, Lee G, et al: A genome-wide scalable SNP genotyping assay using microarray technology. *Nat Genet* 37:549–554, 2005.
19. Machiedo GW, Powell RJ, Rush BF, Jr, et al: The incidence of decreased red blood cell deformability in sepsis and the association with oxygen free radical damage and multiple-system organ failure. *Arch Surg* 124:1386–1389, 1989.
20. Danks RR: Triangle of death. How hypothermia acidosis and coagulopathy can adversely impact trauma patients. *JEMS* 27:61–66, 68–70, 2002.
21. Dickinson A, Qadan M, Polk HC, Jr: Optimizing surgical care: A contemporary assessment of temperature, oxygen, and glucose. *Am Surg* 76:571–577, 2010.
22. Ives CL, Harrison DK, Stansby GS: Tissue oxygen saturation, measured by near-infrared spectroscopy, and its relationship to surgical-site infections. *Br J Surg* 94:87–91, 2007.
23. Cochrane Injuries Group Albumin Reviewers: Human albumin administration in critically ill patients: Systematic review of randomised controlled trials. *BMJ* 317:235–240, 1998.
24. Finfer S, Bellomo R, Boyce N, et al: A comparison of albumin and saline for fluid resuscitation in the intensive care unit. *N Engl J Med* 350:2247–2256, 2004.
25. Delaney AP, Dan A, McCaffrey J, et al: The role of albumin as a resuscitation fluid for patients with sepsis: A systematic review and meta-analysis. *Crit Care Med* 39:386–391, 2011.
26. Shafer SL: Notice of retraction. *Anesth Analg* 111:1567, 2010.
27. Bochicchio GV, Napolitano LM, Joshi M, et al: Persistent systemic inflammatory response syndrome is predictive of nosocomial infection in trauma. *J Trauma* 53:245–250, 2002.
28. Nathens AB, Nester TA, Rubenfeld GD, et al: The effects of leukoreduced blood transfusion on infection risk following injury: A randomized controlled trial. *Shock* 26:342–347, 2006.

29. Claridge JA, Sawyer RG, Schulman AM, et al: Blood transfusions correlate with infections in trauma patients in a dose-dependent manner. *Am Surg* 68:566–572, 2002.
30. Hill GE, Frawley WH, Griffith KE, et al: Allogeneic blood transfusion increases the risk of postoperative bacterial infection: A meta-analysis. *J Trauma* 54:908–914, 2003.
31. Taylor RW, O'Brien J, Trottier SJ, et al: Red blood cell transfusions and nosocomial infections in critically ill patients. *Crit Care Med* 34:2302–2308, quiz 2309, 2006.
32. Shorr AF, Jackson WL, Kelly KM, et al: Transfusion practice and bloodstream infections in critically ill patients. *Chest* 127:1722–1728, 2005.
33. Shorr AF, Duh MS, Kelly KM, et al: Red blood cell transfusion and ventilator-associated pneumonia: A potential link? *Crit Care Med* 32:666–674, 2004.
34. Scharte M, Fink MP: Red blood cell physiology in critical illness. *Crit Care Med* 31:S651–S657, 2003.
35. Fernandes CJ, Jr, Akamine N, De Marco FV, et al: Red blood cell transfusion does not increase oxygen consumption in critically ill septic patients. *Crit Care* 5:362–367, 2001.
36. Moore FA, Moore EE, Sauaia A: Blood transfusion. An independent risk factor for postinjury multiple organ failure. *Arch Surg* 132:620–624, 1997.
37. Offner PJ, Moore EE, Biffl WL, et al: Increased rate of infection associated with transfusion of old blood after severe injury. *Arch Surg* 137:711–716, 2002.
38. van den Berghe G, Wouters P, Weekers F, et al: Intensive insulin therapy in the critically ill patients. *N Engl J Med* 345:1359–1367, 2001.
39. Krinsley JS: Understanding glycemic control in the critically ill: 2011 update. *Hosp Pract (Minneapolis)* 39:47–55, 2011.
40. Heyland DK, MacDonald S, Keefe L, et al: Total parenteral nutrition in the critically ill patient: A meta-analysis. *JAMA* 280:2013–2019, 1998.
41. Marik PE, Zaloga GP: Early enteral nutrition in acutely ill patients: A systematic review. *Crit Care Med* 29:2264–2270, 2001.
42. Manian FA, Meyer PL, Setzer J, et al: Surgical site infections associated with methicillin-resistant *Staphylococcus aureus:* Do postoperative factors play a role? *Clin Infect Dis* 36:863–868, 2003.
43. Mangram AJ, Horan TC, Pearson ML, et al: Guideline for prevention of surgical site infection, 1999. Hospital Infection Control Practices Advisory Committee. *Infect Control Hosp Epidemiol* 20:250–278, 1999.
44. O'Grady NP, Alexander M, Burns LA, et al: Guidelines for the prevention of intravascular catheter-related infections. *Clin Infect Dis* 52:e162–e193, 2011.
45. Mermel LA, Allon M, Bouza E, et al: Clinical practice guidelines for the diagnosis and management of intravascular catheter–related infection: 2009 update by the Infectious Diseases Society of America. *Clin Infect Dis* 49:1–45, 2009.
46. Minei JP, Nathens AB, West M, et al: Inflammation and the host response to injury, a large-scale collaborative project: Patient-oriented research core-standard operating procedures for clinical care. II. Guidelines for prevention, diagnosis and treatment of ventilator-associated pneumonia (VAP) in the trauma patient. *J Trauma* 60:1106–1113, 2006.
47. American Thoracic Society; Infectious Diseases Society of America: Guidelines for the management of adults with hospital-acquired, ventilator-associated, and healthcare-associated pneumonia. *Am J Respir Crit Care Med* 171:388–416, 2005.
48. Erasmus V, Daha TJ, Brug H, et al: Systematic review of studies on compliance with hand hygiene guidelines in hospital care. *Infect Control Hosp Epidemiol* 31:283–294, 2010.
49. Prospero E, Barbadoro P, Esposto E, et al: Extended-spectrum beta-lactamases *Klebsiella pneumoniae:* Multimodal infection control program in intensive care units. *J Prev Med Hyg* 51:110–115, 2010.
50. Oughton MT, Loo VG, Dendukuri N, et al: Hand hygiene with soap and water is superior to alcohol rub and antiseptic wipes for removal of *Clostridium difficile. Infect Control Hosp Epidemiol* 30:939–944, 2009.
51. Dancer SJ: The role of environmental cleaning in the control of hospital-acquired infection. *J Hosp Infect* 73:378–385, 2009.
52. Evans HL, Shaffer MM, Hughes MG, et al: Contact isolation in surgical patients: A barrier to care? *Surgery* 134:180–188, 2003.
53. Stone PW, Pogorzelska M, Kunches L, et al: Hospital staffing and health care–associated infections: A systematic review of the literature. *Clin Infect Dis* 47:937–944, 2008.
54. Cook DJ, Walter SD, Cook RJ, et al: Incidence of and risk factors for ventilator-associated pneumonia in critically ill patients. *Ann Intern Med* 129:433–440, 1998.
55. Harrington DT, Phillips B, Machan J, et al: Factors associated with survival following blunt chest trauma in older patients: Results from a large regional trauma cooperative. *Arch Surg* 145:432–437, 2010.
56. Milstone AM, Passaretti CL, Perl TM: Chlorhexidine: Expanding the armamentarium for infection control and prevention. *Clin Infect Dis* 46:274–281, 2008.
57. Darouiche RO, Wall MJ, Jr, Itani KM, et al: Chlorhexidine-alcohol versus povidone-iodine for surgical-site antisepsis. *N Engl J Med* 362:18–26, 2010.
58. Evans HL, Dellit TH, Chan J, et al: Effect of chlorhexidine whole-body bathing on hospital-acquired infections among trauma patients. *Arch Surg* 145:240–246, 2010.
59. Dixon JM, Carver RL: Daily chlorohexidine gluconate bathing with impregnated cloths results in statistically significant reduction in central line–associated bloodstream infections. *Am J Infect Control* 38:817–821, 2010.
60. Weber DJ, Rutala WA: Central line–associated bloodstream infections: Prevention and management. *Infect Dis Clin North Am* 25:77–102, 2011.
61. Bonello RS, Fletcher CE, Becker WK, et al: An intensive care unit quality improvement collaborative in nine Department of Veterans Affairs hospitals: Reducing ventilator-associated pneumonia and catheter-related bloodstream infection rates. *Jt Comm J Qual Patient Saf* 34:639–645, 2008.
62. Jain M, Miller L, Belt D, et al: Decline in ICU adverse events, nosocomial infections and cost through a quality improvement initiative focusing on teamwork and culture change. *Qual Saf Health Care* 15:235–239, 2006.
63. Muscedere J, Rewa O, McKechnie K, et al: Subglottic secretion drainage for the prevention of ventilator-associated pneumonia: A systematic review and meta-analysis. *Crit Care Med* 39:1985–1991, 2011.
64. Rello J, Kollef M, Diaz E, et al: Reduced burden of bacterial airway colonization with a novel silver-coated endotracheal

tube in a randomized multiple-center feasibility study. *Crit Care Med* 34:2766–2772, 2006.
65. Afessa B, Shorr AF, Anzueto AR, et al: Association between a silver-coated endotracheal tube and reduced mortality in patients with ventilator-associated pneumonia. *Chest* 137:1015–1021, 2010.
66. Hanna HA, Raad II, Hackett B, et al: Antibiotic-impregnated catheters associated with significant decrease in nosocomial and multidrug-resistant bacteremias in critically ill patients. *Chest* 124:1030–1038, 2003.
67. Beattie M, Taylor J: Silver alloy vs. uncoated urinary catheters: A systematic review of the literature. *J Clin Nurs* 20:2098–2108, 2011.
68. Johnson JR, Kuskowski MA, Wilt TJ: Systematic review: Antimicrobial urinary catheters to prevent catheter-associated urinary tract infection in hospitalized patients. *Ann Intern Med* 144:116–126, 2006.
69. Ely EW, Baker AM, Dunagan DP, et al: Effect on the duration of mechanical ventilation of identifying patients capable of breathing spontaneously. *N Engl J Med* 335:1864–1869, 1996.
70. Esteban A, Frutos-Vivar F, Ferguson ND, et al: Noninvasive positive-pressure ventilation for respiratory failure after extubation. *N Engl J Med* 350:2452–2460, 2004.
71. Shah MR, Hasselblad V, Stevenson LW, et al: Impact of the pulmonary artery catheter in critically ill patients: Meta-analysis of randomized clinical trials. *JAMA* 294:1664–1670, 2005.
72. Barie PS: Surgical site infections: Epidemiology and prevention. *Surg Infect (Larchmt)* 3(Suppl 1):S9–S21, 2002.
73. National Nosocomial Infections Surveillance (NNIS): System Report, Data Summary from January 1992–June 2001, issued August 2001. *Am J Infect Control* 29:404–421, 2001.
74. National Nosocomial Infections Surveillance (NNIS): System Report, data summary from January 1992 through June 2004, issued October 2004. *Am J Infect Control* 32:470–485, 2004.
75. Edwards JR, Peterson KD, Mu Y, et al: National Healthcare Safety Network (NHSN) report: Data summary for 2006 through 2008, issued December 2009. *Am J Infect Control* 37:783–805, 2009.
76. Garibaldi RA, Cushing D, Lerer T: Risk factors for postoperative infection. *Am J Med* 91:158S–163S, 1991.
77. Raymond DP, Pelletier SJ, Crabtree TD, et al: Surgical infection and the aging population. *Am Surg* 67:827–832, 2001.
78. Delgado-Rodriguez M, Medina-Cuadros M, Martinez-Gallego G, et al: Total cholesterol, HDL-cholesterol, and risk of nosocomial infection: A prospective study in surgical patients. *Infect Control Hosp Epidemiol* 18:9–18, 1997.
79. Malone DL, Genuit T, Tracy JK, et al: Surgical site infections: Reanalysis of risk factors. *J Surg Res* 103:89–95, 2002.
80. Scott JD, Forrest A, Feuerstein S, et al: Factors associated with postoperative infection. *Infect Control Hosp Epidemiol* 22:347–351, 2001.
81. Hedrick TL, Heckman JA, Smith RL, et al: Efficacy of protocol implementation on incidence of wound infection in colorectal operations. *J Am Coll Surg* 205:432–438, 2007.
82. Kurz A, Sessler DI, Lenhardt R: Perioperative normothermia to reduce the incidence of surgical-wound infection and shorten hospitalization. Study of Wound Infection and Temperature Group. *N Engl J Med* 334:1209–1215, 1996.
83. Flores-Maldonado A, Medina-Escobedo CE, Rios-Rodriguez HM, et al: Mild perioperative hypothermia and the risk of wound infection. *Arch Med Res* 32:227–231, 2001.
84. Brar MS, Brar SS, Dixon E: Perioperative supplemental oxygen in colorectal patients: A meta-analysis. *J Surg Res* 166:227–235, 2011.
85. Knighton DR, Halliday B, Hunt TK: Oxygen as an antibiotic. A comparison of the effects of inspired oxygen concentration and antibiotic administration on in vivo bacterial clearance. *Arch Surg* 121:191–195, 1986.
86. Gottrup F: Oxygen in wound healing and infection. *World J Surg* 28:312–315, 2004.
87. Greif R, Akca O, Horn EP, et al: Supplemental perioperative oxygen to reduce the incidence of surgical-wound infection. *N Engl J Med* 342:161–167, 2000.
88. Pryor KO, Fahey TJ, 3rd, Lien CA, et al: Surgical site infection and the routine use of perioperative hyperoxia in a general surgical population: A randomized controlled trial. *JAMA* 291:79–87, 2004.
89. Miller RS, Morris JA, Jr, Diaz JJ, Jr, et al: Complications after 344 damage-control open celiotomies. *J Trauma* 59:1365–1371, 2005.
90. Vogel TR, Diaz JJ, Miller RS, et al: The open abdomen in trauma: Do infectious complications affect primary abdominal closure? *Surg Infect (Larchmt)* 7:433–441, 2006.
91. Al-Inany H, Youssef G, Abd ElMaguid A, et al: Value of subcutaneous drainage system in obese females undergoing cesarean section using Pfannenstiel incision. *Gynecol Obstet Invest* 53:75–78, 2002.
92. Magann EF, Chauhan SP, Rodts-Palenik S, et al: Subcutaneous stitch closure versus subcutaneous drain to prevent wound disruption after cesarean delivery: A randomized clinical trial. *Am J Obstet Gynecol* 186:1119–1123, 2002.
93. Siegman-Igra Y, Rozin R, Simchen E: Determinants of wound infection in gastrointestinal operations: The Israeli study of surgical infections. *J Clin Epidemiol* 46:133–140, 1993.
94. Noyes LD, Doyle DJ, McSwain NE, Jr: Septic complications associated with the use of peritoneal drains in liver trauma. *J Trauma* 28:337–346, 1988.
95. Magee C, Rodeheaver GT, Golden GT, et al: Potentiation of wound infection by surgical drains. *Am J Surg* 131:547–549, 1976.
96. Vilar-Compte D, Mohar A, Sandoval S, et al: Surgical site infections at the National Cancer Institute in Mexico: A case-control study. *Am J Infect Control* 28:14–20, 2000.
97. Barie PS: Are we draining the life from our patients? *Surg Infect (Larchmt)* 3:159–160, 2002.
98. Platell C, Papadimitriou JM, Hall JC: The influence of lavage on peritonitis. *J Am Coll Surg* 191:672–680, 2000.
99. Cervantes-Sanchez CR, Gutierrez-Vega R, Vazquez-Carpizo JA, et al: Syringe pressure irrigation of subdermic tissue after appendectomy to decrease the incidence of postoperative wound infection. *World J Surg* 24:38–41, 2000.
100. Andersen B, Bendtsen A, Holbraad L, et al: Wound infections after appendicectomy. I. A controlled trial on the prophylactic efficacy of topical ampicillin in non-perforated appendicitis. II. A controlled trial on the prophylactic efficacy of delayed primary suture and topical ampicillin in perforated appendicitis. *Acta Chir Scand* 138:531–536, 1972.

101. Yoshii S, Hosaka S, Suzuki S, et al: Prevention of surgical site infection by antibiotic spraying in the operative field during cardiac surgery. *Jpn J Thorac Cardiovasc Surg* 49:279–281, 2001.
102. O'Connor LT, Jr, Goldstein M: Topical perioperative antibiotic prophylaxis for minor clean inguinal surgery. *J Am Coll Surg* 194:407–410, 2002.
103. Freischlag JA, Ajalat G, Busuttil RW: Treatment of necrotizing soft tissue infections. The need for a new approach. *Am J Surg* 149:751–755, 1985.
104. Turina M, Cheadle WG: Management of established surgical site infections. *Surg Infect (Larchmt)* 7:S33–S41, 2006.
105. Morykwas MJ, Argenta LC, Shelton-Brown EI, et al: Vacuum-assisted closure: A new method for wound control and treatment: Animal studies and basic foundation. *Ann Plast Surg* 38:553–562, 1997.
106. Venturi ML, Attinger CE, Mesbahi AN, et al: Mechanisms and clinical applications of the vacuum-assisted closure (VAC) device: A review. *Am J Clin Dermatol* 6:185–194, 2005.
107. Heller L, Levin SL, Butler CE: Management of abdominal wound dehiscence using vacuum-assisted closure in patients with compromised healing. *Am J Surg* 191:165–172, 2006.
108. Schaffzin DM, Douglas JM, Stahl TJ, et al: Vacuum-assisted closure of complex perineal wounds. *Dis Colon Rectum* 47:1745–1748, 2004.
109. Stulberg JJ, Delaney CP, Neuhauser DV, et al: Adherence to Surgical Care Improvement Project measures and the association with postoperative infections. *JAMA* 303:2479–2485, 2010.
110. Ingraham AM, Cohen ME, Bilimoria KY, et al: Association of Surgical Care Improvement Project infection-related process measure compliance with risk-adjusted outcomes: Implications for quality measurement. *J Am Coll Surg* 211:705–714, 2010.
111. Bratzler DW, Houck PM, Richards C, et al: Use of antimicrobial prophylaxis for major surgery: Baseline results from the National Surgical Infection Prevention Project. *Arch Surg* 140:174–182, 2005.
112. Bratzler DW, Houck PM: Antimicrobial prophylaxis for surgery: An advisory statement from the National Surgical Infection Prevention Project. *Am J Surg* 189:395–404, 2005.
113. Dellinger EP, Hausmann SM, Bratzler DW, et al: Hospitals collaborate to decrease surgical site infections. *Am J Surg* 190:9–15, 2005.
114. Barie PS: No pay for no performance. *Surg Infect (Larchmt)* 8:421–433, 2007.
115. Dellinger EP: Adherence to Surgical Care Improvement Project measures: The whole is greater than the parts. *Future Microbiol* 5:1781–1785, 2010.
116. Lee JT: Nonmagical tools. *Infect Control Hosp Epidemiol* 24:769–771, 2003.
117. Kollef MH, Shorr A, Tabak YP, et al: Epidemiology and outcomes of health-care-associated pneumonia: Results from a large US database of culture-positive pneumonia. *Chest* 128:3854–3862, 2005.
118. Rello J, Ollendorf DA, Oster G, et al: Epidemiology and outcomes of ventilator-associated pneumonia in a large U.S. database. *Chest* 122:2115–2121, 2002.
119. Fagon JY, Chastre J, Wolff M, et al: Invasive and noninvasive strategies for management of suspected ventilator-associated pneumonia. A randomized trial. *Ann Intern Med* 132:621–630, 2000.
120. Safdar N, Dezfulian C, Collard HR, et al: Clinical and economic consequences of ventilator-associated pneumonia: A systematic review. *Crit Care Med* 33:2184–2193, 2005.
121. Celis R, Torres A, Gatell JM, et al: Nosocomial pneumonia. A multivariate analysis of risk and prognosis. *Chest* 93:318–324, 1988.
122. Torres A, Aznar R, Gatell JM, et al: Incidence, risk, and prognosis factors of nosocomial pneumonia in mechanically ventilated patients. *Am Rev Respir Dis* 142:523–528, 1990.
123. Markowicz P, Wolff M, Djedaini K, et al: Multicenter prospective study of ventilator-associated pneumonia during acute respiratory distress syndrome. Incidence, prognosis, and risk factors. ARDS Study Group. *Am J Respir Crit Care Med* 161:1942–1948, 2000.
124. Pieracci FM, Barie PS: Strategies in the prevention and management of ventilator-associated pneumonia. *Am Surg* 73:419–432, 2007.
125. Antonelli M, Conti G, Rocco M, et al: A comparison of noninvasive positive-pressure ventilation and conventional mechanical ventilation in patients with acute respiratory failure. *N Engl J Med* 339:429–435, 1998.
126. Holzapfel L, Chevret S, Madinier G, et al: Influence of long-term oro- or nasotracheal intubation on nosocomial maxillary sinusitis and pneumonia: Results of a prospective, randomized, clinical trial. *Crit Care Med* 21:1132–1138, 1993.
127. Kress JP, Pohlman AS, O'Connor MF, et al: Daily interruption of sedative infusions in critically ill patients undergoing mechanical ventilation. *N Engl J Med* 342:1471–1477, 2000.
128. Marelich GP, Murin S, Battistella F, et al: Protocol weaning of mechanical ventilation in medical and surgical patients by respiratory care practitioners and nurses: Effect on weaning time and incidence of ventilator-associated pneumonia. *Chest* 118:459–467, 2000.
129. Zanella A, Scaravilli V, Isgro S, et al: Fluid leakage across tracheal tube cuff, effect of different cuff material, shape, and positive expiratory pressure: A bench-top study. *Intensive Care Med* 37:343–347, 2011.
130. Drakulovic MB, Torres A, Bauer TT, et al: Supine body position as a risk factor for nosocomial pneumonia in mechanically ventilated patients: A randomised trial. *Lancet* 354:1851–1858, 1999.
131. Heyland DK, Dhaliwal R, Drover JW, et al: Canadian clinical practice guidelines for nutrition support in mechanically ventilated, critically ill adult patients. *JPEN J Parenter Enteral Nutr* 27:355–373, 2003.
132. Berne JD, Norwood SH, McAuley CE, et al: Erythromycin reduces delayed gastric emptying in critically ill trauma patients: A randomized, controlled trial. *J Trauma* 53:422–425, 2002.
133. van Nieuwenhoven CA, Buskens E, van Tiel FH, et al: Relationship between methodological trial quality and the effects of selective digestive decontamination on pneumonia and mortality in critically ill patients. *JAMA* 286:335–340, 2001.
134. Verwaest C, Verhaegen J, Ferdinande P, et al: Randomized, controlled trial of selective digestive decontamination in 600 mechanically ventilated patients in a multidisciplinary intensive care unit. *Crit Care Med* 25:63–71, 1997.

135. Lingnau W, Berger J, Javorsky F, et al: Changing bacterial ecology during a five-year period of selective intestinal decontamination. *J Hosp Infect* 39:195–206, 1998.
136. Chlebicki MP, Safdar N: Topical chlorhexidine for prevention of ventilator-associated pneumonia: A meta-analysis. *Crit Care Med* 35:595–602, 2007.
137. Earley AS, Gracias VH, Haut E, et al: Anemia management program reduces transfusion volumes, incidence of ventilator-associated pneumonia, and cost in trauma patients. *J Trauma* 61:1–5, 2006.
138. Sawyer RG, Crabtree TD, Gleason TG, et al: Impact of solid organ transplantation and immunosuppression on fever, leukocytosis, and physiologic response during bacterial and fungal infections. *Clin Transplant* 13:260–265, 1999.
139. Neuhauser MM, Weinstein RA, Rydman R, et al: Antibiotic resistance among gram-negative bacilli in US intensive care units: Implications for fluoroquinolone use. *JAMA* 289:885–888, 2003.
140. Niederman MS: Appropriate use of antimicrobial agents: Challenges and strategies for improvement. *Crit Care Med* 31:608–616, 2003.
141. Alvarez-Lerma F: Modification of empirical antibiotic treatment in patients with pneumonia acquired in the intensive care unit. ICU-Acquired Pneumonia Study Group. *Intensive Care Med* 22:387–394, 1996.
142. Fabregas N, Ewig S, Torres A, et al: Clinical diagnosis of ventilator associated pneumonia revisited: Comparative validation using immediate post-mortem lung biopsies. *Thorax* 54:867–873, 1999.
143. Mabie M, Wunderink RG: Use and limitations of clinical and radiologic diagnosis of pneumonia. *Semin Respir Infect* 18:72–79, 2003.
144. Fagon JY, Chastre J, Domart Y, et al: Nosocomial pneumonia in patients receiving continuous mechanical ventilation. Prospective analysis of 52 episodes with use of a protected specimen brush and quantitative culture techniques. *Am Rev Respir Dis* 139:877–884, 1989.
145. Winer-Muram HT, Steiner RM, Gurney JW, et al: Ventilator-associated pneumonia in patients with adult respiratory distress syndrome: CT evaluation. *Radiology* 208:193–199, 1998.
146. Fartoukh M, Maitre B, Honore S, et al: Diagnosing pneumonia during mechanical ventilation: The clinical pulmonary infection score revisited. *Am J Respir Crit Care Med* 168:173–179, 2003.
147. Luyt CE, Chastre J, Fagon JY: Value of the clinical pulmonary infection score for the identification and management of ventilator-associated pneumonia. *Intensive Care Med* 30:844–852, 2004.
148. Veinstein A, Brun-Buisson C, Derrode N, et al: Validation of an algorithm based on direct examination of specimens in suspected ventilator-associated pneumonia. *Intensive Care Med* 32:676–683, 2006.
149. Croce MA, Swanson JM, Magnotti LJ, et al: The futility of the clinical pulmonary infection score in trauma patients. *J Trauma* 60:523–527, 2006.
150. Blot F, Raynard B, Chachaty E, et al: Value of Gram stain examination of lower respiratory tract secretions for early diagnosis of nosocomial pneumonia. *Am J Respir Crit Care Med* 162:1731–1737, 2000.
151. Torres A, El-Ebiary M: Bronchoscopic BAL in the diagnosis of ventilator-associated pneumonia. *Chest* 117:198S–202S, 2000.
152. Shorr AF, Sherner JH, Jackson WL, et al: Invasive approaches to the diagnosis of ventilator-associated pneumonia: A meta-analysis. *Crit Care Med* 33:46–53, 2005.
153. McGee DC, Gould MK: Preventing complications of central venous catheterization. *N Engl J Med* 348:1123–1133, 2003.
154. Pronovost P: Interventions to decrease catheter-related bloodstream infections in the ICU: The Keystone Intensive Care Unit Project. *Am J Infect Control* 36:S171.e1–S171.e5, 2008.
155. Pronovost PJ, Goeschel CA, Colantuoni E, et al: Sustaining reductions in catheter related bloodstream infections in Michigan intensive care units: Observational study. *BMJ* 340:c309, 2010.
156. Furuya EY, Dick A, Perencevich EN, et al: Central line bundle implementation in US intensive care units and impact on bloodstream infections. *PLoS ONE* 6:e15452, 2011.
157. Miller RS, Norris PR, Jenkins JM, et al: Systems initiatives reduce healthcare-associated infections: A study of 22,928 device days in a single trauma unit. *J Trauma* 68:23–31, 2010.
158. Clinical and Laboratory Standards Institute: Principles and procedures for blood cultures; approved guideline, 2007. <http://www.clsi.org/source/orders/free/m47-a.pdf>.
159. Mermel LA, Farr BM, Sherertz RJ, et al: Guidelines for the management of intravascular catheter-related infections. *Clin Infect Dis* 32:1249–1272, 2001.
160. Tambyah PA, Maki DG: Catheter-associated urinary tract infection is rarely symptomatic: A prospective study of 1,497 catheterized patients. *Arch Intern Med* 160:678–682, 2000.
161. Golob JF, Jr, Claridge JA, Sando MJ, et al: Fever and leukocytosis in critically ill trauma patients: It's not the urine. *Surg Infect (Larchmt)* 9:49–56, 2008.
162. Safdar N, Slattery WR, Knasinski V, et al: Predictors and outcomes of candiduria in renal transplant recipients. *Clin Infect Dis* 40:1413–1421, 2005.
163. Bryan CS, Reynolds KL: Hospital-acquired bacteremic urinary tract infection: Epidemiology and outcome. *J Urol* 132:494–498, 1984.
164. Quintiliani R, Klimek J, Cunha BA, et al: Bacteraemia after manipulation of the urinary tract. The importance of pre-existing urinary tract disease and compromised host defences. *Postgrad Med J* 54:668–671, 1978.
165. Ksycki MF, Namias N: Nosocomial urinary tract infection. *Surg Clin North Am* 89:475–481, ix–x, 2009.
166. Laupland KB, Bagshaw SM, Gregson DB, et al: Intensive care unit–acquired urinary tract infections in a regional critical care system. *Crit Care* 9:R60–R65, 2005.
167. Schwartz DS, Barone JE: Correlation of urinalysis and dipstick results with catheter-associated urinary tract infections in surgical ICU patients. *Intensive Care Med* 32:1797–1801, 2006.
168. Schiotz HA: The value of leucocyte stix results in predicting bacteriuria and urinary tract infection after gynaecological surgery. *J Obstet Gynaecol* 19:396–398, 1999.
169. Solomkin JS, Hemsell DL, Sweet R, et al: Evaluation of new anti-infective drugs for the treatment of intra-abdominal

infections. Infectious Diseases Society of America and the Food and Drug Administration. *Clin Infect Dis* 15(Suppl 1):S33–S42, 1992.

170. Merlino JI, Yowler CJ, Malangoni MA: Nosocomial infections adversely affect the outcomes of patients with serious intraabdominal infections. *Surg Infect (Larchmt)* 5:21–27, 2004.
171. Nathens AB, Rotstein OD, Marshall JC: Tertiary peritonitis: Clinical features of a complex nosocomial infection. *World J Surg* 22:158–163, 1998.
172. Pacelli F, Doglietto GB, Alfieri S, et al: Prognosis in intra-abdominal infections. Multivariate analysis on 604 patients. *Arch Surg* 131:641–645, 1996.
173. Roehrborn A, Thomas L, Potreck O, et al: The microbiology of postoperative peritonitis. *Clin Infect Dis* 33:1513–1519, 2001.
174. Sturkenboom MC, Goettsch WG, Picelli G, et al: Inappropriate initial treatment of secondary intra-abdominal infections leads to increased risk of clinical failure and costs. *Br J Clin Pharmacol* 60:438–443, 2005.
175. Montravers P, Gauzit R, Muller C, et al: Emergence of antibiotic-resistant bacteria in cases of peritonitis after intra-abdominal surgery affects the efficacy of empirical antimicrobial therapy. *Clin Infect Dis* 23:486–494, 1996.
176. Barie PS, Hydo LJ, Shou J, et al: Efficacy and safety of drotrecogin alfa (activated) for the therapy of surgical patients with severe sepsis. *Surg Infect (Larchmt)* 7(Suppl 2):S77–S80, 2006.
177. Barie PS, Vogel SB, Dellinger EP, et al: A randomized, double-blind clinical trial comparing cefepime plus metronidazole with imipenem-cilastatin in the treatment of complicated intra-abdominal infections. Cefepime Intra-abdominal Infection Study Group. *Arch Surg* 132:1294–1302, 1997.
178. Farthmann EH, Schoffel U: Principles and limitations of operative management of intraabdominal infections. *World J Surg* 14:210–217, 1990.
179. Garcia-Sabrido JL, Tallado JM, Christou NV, et al: Treatment of severe intra-abdominal sepsis and/or necrotic foci by an "open-abdomen" approach. Zipper and zipper-mesh techniques. *Arch Surg* 123:152–156, 1988.
180. Marshall JC, Maier RV, Jimenez M, et al: Source control in the management of severe sepsis and septic shock: An evidence-based review. *Crit Care Med* 32:S513–S526, 2004.
181. Wittmann DH, Aprahamian C, Bergstein JM: Etappenlavage: Advanced diffuse peritonitis managed by planned multiple laparotomies utilizing zippers, slide fastener, and Velcro analogue for temporary abdominal closure. *World J Surg* 14:218–226, 1990.
182. Ohmann C, Wittmann DH, Wacha H: Prospective evaluation of prognostic scoring systems in peritonitis. Peritonitis Study Group. *Eur J Surg* 159:267–274, 1993.
183. Gajic O, Urrutia LE, Sewani H, et al: Acute abdomen in the medical intensive care unit. *Crit Care Med* 30:1187–1190, 2002.
184. DiPiro JT, Edmiston CE, Jr, Bohnen JM: Pharmacodynamics of antimicrobial therapy in surgery. *Am J Surg* 171:615–622, 1996.
185. Anstead GM, Owens AD: Recent advances in the treatment of infections due to resistant *Staphylococcus aureus*. *Curr Opin Infect Dis* 17:549–555, 2004.
186. Kashuba AD, Bertino JS, Jr, Nafziger AN: Dosing of aminoglycosides to rapidly attain pharmacodynamic goals and hasten therapeutic response by using individualized pharmacokinetic monitoring of patients with pneumonia caused by gram-negative organisms. *Antimicrob Agents Chemother* 42:1842–1844, 1998.
187. Thomas JK, Forrest A, Bhavnani SM, et al: Pharmacodynamic evaluation of factors associated with the development of bacterial resistance in acutely ill patients during therapy. *Antimicrob Agents Chemother* 42:521–527, 1998.
188. Benko AS, Cappelletty DM, Kruse JA, et al: Continuous infusion versus intermittent administration of ceftazidime in critically ill patients with suspected gram-negative infections. *Antimicrob Agents Chemother* 40:691–695, 1996.
189. Lau WK, Mercer D, Itani KM, et al: Randomized, open-label, comparative study of piperacillin-tazobactam administered by continuous infusion versus intermittent infusion for treatment of hospitalized patients with complicated intra-abdominal infection. *Antimicrob Agents Chemother* 50:3556–3561, 2006.
190. Velmahos GC, Toutouzas KG, Sarkisyan G, et al: Severe trauma is not an excuse for prolonged antibiotic prophylaxis. *Arch Surg* 137:537–541, 2002.
191. Al-Ghnaniem R, Benjamin IS, Patel AG: Meta-analysis suggests antibiotic prophylaxis is not warranted in low-risk patients undergoing laparoscopic cholecystectomy. *Br J Surg* 90:365–366, 2003.
192. Lewis RT: Oral versus systemic antibiotic prophylaxis in elective colon surgery: A randomized study and meta-analysis send a message from the 1990s. *Can J Surg* 45:173–180, 2002.
193. Centers for Medicare & Medicaid Services: Anticipated public reporting of National Hospital Quality Measure SIP-2 (SCIP Infection 2), appropriate antibiotic selection for surgical prophylaxis, 2006. <http://www.cms.hhs.gov/HospitalQualityInits/Downloads/HospitalSDPSMemoRandum.pdf>.
194. Song F, Glenny AM: Antimicrobial prophylaxis in colorectal surgery: A systematic review of randomized controlled trials. *Br J Surg* 85:1232–1241, 1998.
195. Tejirian T, DiFronzo LA, Haigh PI: Antibiotic prophylaxis for preventing wound infection after breast surgery: A systematic review and meta-analysis. *J Am Coll Surg* 203:729–734, 2006.
196. Cunningham M, Bunn F, Handscomb K: Prophylactic antibiotics to prevent surgical site infection after breast cancer surgery. *Cochrane Database Syst Rev* (2):CD005360, 2006.
197. Aufenacker TJ, Koelemay MJ, Gouma DJ, et al: Systematic review and meta-analysis of the effectiveness of antibiotic prophylaxis in prevention of wound infection after mesh repair of abdominal wall hernia. *Br J Surg* 93:5–10, 2006.
198. Sanchez-Manuel FJ, Seco-Gil JL: Antibiotic prophylaxis for hernia repair. *Cochrane Database Syst Rev* (4):CD003769, 2004.
199. Stewart A, Eyers PS, Earnshaw JJ: Prevention of infection in arterial reconstruction. *Cochrane Database Syst Rev* (3):CD003073, 2006.
200. Classen DC, Evans RS, Pestotnik SL, et al: The timing of prophylactic administration of antibiotics and the risk of surgical-wound infection. *N Engl J Med* 326:281–286, 1992.

201. Hawn MT, Gray SH, Vick CC, et al: Timely administration of prophylactic antibiotics for major surgical procedures. *J Am Coll Surg* 203:803–811, 2006.
202. Zanetti G, Giardina R, Platt R: Intraoperative redosing of cefazolin and risk for surgical site infection in cardiac surgery. *Emerg Infect Dis* 7:828–831, 2001.
203. McDonald M, Grabsch E, Marshall C, et al: Single-versus multiple-dose antimicrobial prophylaxis for major surgery: A systematic review. *Aust N Z J Surg* 68:388–396, 1998.
204. Namias N, Harvill S, Ball S, et al: Cost and morbidity associated with antibiotic prophylaxis in the ICU. *J Am Coll Surg* 188:225–230, 1999.
205. Fukatsu K, Saito H, Matsuda T, et al: Influences of type and duration of antimicrobial prophylaxis on an outbreak of methicillin-resistant *Staphylococcus aureus* and on the incidence of wound infection. *Arch Surg* 132:1320–1325, 1997.
206. Barie PS, Hydo LJ, Eachempati SR: Causes and consequences of fever complicating critical surgical illness. *Surg Infect (Larchmt)* 5:145–159, 2004.
207. O'Grady NP, Barie PS, Bartlett JG, et al: Guidelines for evaluation of new fever in critically ill adult patients: 2008 update from the American College of Critical Care Medicine and the Infectious Diseases Society of America. *Crit Care Med* 36:1330–1349, 2008.
208. Caroff SN, Mann SC: Neuroleptic malignant syndrome and malignant hyperthermia. *Anaesth Intensive Care* 21:477–478, 1993.
209. Trautner BW, Clarridge JE, Darouiche RO: Skin antisepsis kits containing alcohol and chlorhexidine gluconate or tincture of iodine are associated with low rates of blood culture contamination. *Infect Control Hosp Epidemiol* 23:397–401, 2002.
210. Cockerill FR, 3rd, Wilson JW, Vetter EA, et al: Optimal testing parameters for blood cultures. *Clin Infect Dis* 38:1724–1730, 2004.
211. Mermel LA, Maki DG: Detection of bacteremia in adults: Consequences of culturing an inadequate volume of blood. *Ann Intern Med* 119:270–272, 1993.
212. Kumar A, Roberts D, Wood KE, et al: Duration of hypotension before initiation of effective antimicrobial therapy is the critical determinant of survival in human septic shock. *Crit Care Med* 34:1589–1596, 2006.
213. Barie PS, Hydo LJ, Shou J, et al: Influence of antibiotic therapy on mortality of critical surgical illness caused or complicated by infection. *Surg Infect (Larchmt)* 6:41–54, 2005.
214. Kollef MH, Ward S, Sherman G, et al: Inadequate treatment of nosocomial infections is associated with certain empirical antibiotic choices. *Crit Care Med* 28:3456–3464, 2000.
215. Garnacho-Montero J, Garcia-Garmendia JL, Barrero-Almodovar A, et al: Impact of adequate empirical antibiotic therapy on the outcome of patients admitted to the intensive care unit with sepsis. *Crit Care Med* 31:2742–2751, 2003.
216. Dellit TH, Owens RC, McGowan JE, Jr, et al: Infectious Diseases Society of America and the Society for Healthcare Epidemiology of America guidelines for developing an institutional program to enhance antimicrobial stewardship. *Clin Infect Dis* 44:159–177, 2007.
217. Kollef MH, Micek ST: Strategies to prevent antimicrobial resistance in the intensive care unit. *Crit Care Med* 33:1845–1853, 2005.
218. Hayashi Y, Paterson DL: Strategies for reduction in duration of antibiotic use in hospitalized patients. *Clin Infect Dis* 52:1232–1240, 2011.
219. Giamarellou H: Treatment options for multidrug-resistant bacteria. *Expert Rev Anti Infect Ther* 4:601–618, 2006.
220. Aarts MA, Hancock JN, Heyland D, et al: Empiric antibiotic therapy for suspected ventilator-associated pneumonia: A systematic review and meta-analysis of randomized trials. *Crit Care Med* 36:108–117, 2008.
221. Paul M, Benuri-Silbiger I, Soares-Weiser K, et al: Beta lactam monotherapy versus beta lactam-aminoglycoside combination therapy for sepsis in immunocompetent patients: Systematic review and meta-analysis of randomised trials. *BMJ* 328:668, 2004.
222. Kumar A, Zarychanski R, Light B, et al: Early combination antibiotic therapy yields improved survival compared with monotherapy in septic shock: A propensity-matched analysis. *Crit Care Med* 38:1773–1785, 2010.
223. Solomkin JS, Mazuski JE, Bradley JS, et al: Diagnosis and management of complicated intra-abdominal infection in adults and children: Guidelines by the Surgical Infection Society and the Infectious Diseases Society of America. *Surg Infect (Larchmt)* 11:79–109, 2010.
224. Kollef MH, Kollef KE: Antibiotic utilization and outcomes for patients with clinically suspected ventilator-associated pneumonia and negative quantitative BAL culture results. *Chest* 128:2706–2713, 2005.
225. Eachempati SR, Hydo LJ, Shou J, et al: The pathogen of ventilator-associated pneumonia does not influence the mortality rate of surgical intensive care unit patients treated with a rotational antibiotic system. *Surg Infect (Larchmt)* 11:13–20, 2010.
226. Dennesen PJ, van der Ven AJ, Kessels AG, et al: Resolution of infectious parameters after antimicrobial therapy in patients with ventilator-associated pneumonia. *Am J Respir Crit Care Med* 163:1371–1375, 2001.
227. Chastre J, Wolff M, Fagon JY, et al: Comparison of 8 vs 15 days of antibiotic therapy for ventilator-associated pneumonia in adults: A randomized trial. *JAMA* 290:2588–2598, 2003.
228. Singh N, Rogers P, Atwood CW, et al: Short-course empirical antibiotic therapy for patients with pulmonary infiltrates in the intensive care unit. A proposed solution for indiscriminate antibiotic prescription. *Am J Respir Crit Care Med* 162:505–511, 2000.
229. Pappas PG, Rex JH, Sobel JD, et al: Guidelines for treatment of candidiasis. *Clin Infect Dis* 38:161–189, 2004.
230. O'Grady NP, Chertow DS: Managing bloodstream infections in patients who have short-term central venous catheters. *Cleve Clin J Med* 78:10–17, 2011.
231. Pieracci FM, Barie PS: Intra-abdominal infections. *Curr Opin Crit Care* 13:440–449, 2007.
232. Buijk SE, Bruining HA: Future directions in the management of tertiary peritonitis. *Intensive Care Med* 28:1024–1029, 2002.
233. Pepin J, Saheb N, Coulombe MA, et al: Emergence of fluoroquinolones as the predominant risk factor for *Clostridium difficile*–associated diarrhea: A cohort study during an epidemic in Quebec. *Clin Infect Dis* 41:1254–1260, 2005.
234. Price J, Cheek E, Lippett S, et al: Impact of an intervention to control *Clostridium difficile* infection on hospital- and

community-onset disease: An interrupted time series analysis. *Clin Microbiol Infect* 16:1297–1302, 2010.
235. Louie TJ, Miller MA, Mullane KM, et al: Fidaxomicin versus vancomycin for *Clostridium difficile* infection. *N Engl J Med* 364:422–431, 2011.
236. Lamontagne F, Labbe AC, Haeck O, et al: Impact of emergency colectomy on survival of patients with fulminant *Clostridium difficile* colitis during an epidemic caused by a hypervirulent strain. *Ann Surg* 245:267–272, 2007.
237. McDonald LC, Killgore GE, Thompson A, et al: An epidemic, toxin gene-variant strain of *Clostridium difficile. N Engl J Med* 353:2433–2441, 2005.
238. May AK, Stafford RE, Bulger EM, et al: Treatment of complicated skin and soft tissue infections. *Surg Infect (Larchmt)* 10:467–499, 2009.
239. Kaushik D, Rathi S, Jain A: Ceftaroline: A comprehensive update. *Int J Antimicrob Agents* 37:389–395, 2011.
240. Rodloff AC, Goldstein EJ, Torres A: Two decades of imipenem therapy. *J Antimicrob Chemother* 58:916–929, 2006.
241. Zhanel GG, Johanson C, Embil JM, et al: Ertapenem: Review of a new carbapenem. *Expert Rev Anti Infect Ther* 3:23–39, 2005.
242. Liu C, Bayer A, Cosgrove SE, et al: Clinical practice guidelines by the Infectious Diseases Society of America for the treatment of methicillin-resistant *Staphylococcus aureus* infections in adults and children: Executive summary. *Clin Infect Dis* 52:285–292, 2011.
243. Rybak MJ, Lomaestro BM, Rotschafer JC, et al: Vancomycin therapeutic guidelines: A summary of consensus recommendations from the Infectious Diseases Society of America, the American Society of Health-System Pharmacists, and the Society of Infectious Diseases Pharmacists. *Clin Infect Dis* 49:325–327, 2009.
244. Kullar R, Davis SL, Levine DP, et al: Impact of vancomycin exposure on outcomes in patients with methicillin-resistant *Staphylococcus aureus* bacteremia: Support for consensus guidelines suggested targets. *Clin Infect Dis* 52:975–981, 2011.
245. Falagas ME, Alexiou VG, Peppas G, et al: Do changes in antimicrobial resistance necessitate reconsideration of surgical antimicrobial prophylaxis strategies? *Surg Infect (Larchmt)* 10:557–562, 2009.
246. Chang MH, Kish TD, Fung HB: Telavancin: A lipoglycopeptide antimicrobial for the treatment of complicated skin and skin structure infections caused by gram-positive bacteria in adults. *Clin Ther* 32:2160–2185, 2010.
247. Silverman JA, Mortin LI, Vanpraagh AD, et al: Inhibition of daptomycin by pulmonary surfactant: In vitro modeling and clinical impact. *J Infect Dis* 191:2149–2152, 2005.
248. Landman D, Georgescu C, Martin DA, et al: Polymyxins revisited. *Clin Microbiol Rev* 21:449–465, 2008.
249. Bailey JA, Virgo KS, DiPiro JT, et al: Aminoglycosides for intra-abdominal infection: Equal to the challenge? *Surg Infect (Larchmt)* 3:315–335, 2002.
250. Stein GE, Craig WA: Tigecycline: A critical analysis. *Clin Infect Dis* 43:518–524, 2006.
251. U.S. Food and Drug Administration: FDA drug safety communication: Increased risk of death with Tygacil (tigecycline) compared with other antibiotics used to treat similar infections, 2010. <www.fda.gov/Drugs/DrugSafety/ucm224370.htm>.
252. Cai Y, Wang R, Liang B, et al: Systematic review and meta-analysis of the effectiveness and safety of tigecycline for treatment of infectious disease. *Antimicrob Agents Chemother* 55:1162–1172, 2011.
253. Eckmann C, Dryden M: Treatment of complicated skin and soft-tissue infections caused by resistant bacteria: Value of linezolid, tigecycline, daptomycin and vancomycin. *Eur J Med Res* 15:554–563, 2010.
254. Walkey AJ, O'Donnell MR, Wiener RS: Linezolid vs glycopeptide antibiotics for the treatment of suspected methicillin-resistant *Staphylococcus aureus* nosocomial pneumonia: A meta-analysis of randomized controlled trials. *Chest* 139:1148–1155, 2011.
255. Nseir S, Di Pompeo C, Soubrier S, et al: First-generation fluoroquinolone use and subsequent emergence of multiple drug-resistant bacteria in the intensive care unit. *Crit Care Med* 33:283–289, 2005.
256. Livermore DM, Woodford N: The beta-lactamase threat in Enterobacteriaceae, *Pseudomonas* and *Acinetobacter. Trends Microbiol* 14:413–420, 2006.
257. Charbonneau P, Parienti JJ, Thibon P, et al: Fluoroquinolone use and methicillin-resistant *Staphylococcus aureus* isolation rates in hospitalized patients: A quasi experimental study. *Clin Infect Dis* 42:778–784, 2006.
258. Sprandel KA, Drusano GL, Hecht DW, et al: Population pharmacokinetic modeling and Monte Carlo simulation of varying doses of intravenous metronidazole. *Diagn Microbiol Infect Dis* 55:303–309, 2006.
259. De Broe ME, Giuliano RA, Verpooten GA: Aminoglycoside nephrotoxicity: Mechanism and prevention. *Adv Exp Med Biol* 252:233–245, 1989.
260. Bates DE: Aminoglycoside ototoxicity. *Drugs Today (Barc)* 39:277–285, 2003.
261. Roberts JA, Lipman J: Antibacterial dosing in intensive care: Pharmacokinetics, degree of disease and pharmacodynamics of sepsis. *Clin Pharmacokinet* 45:755–773, 2006.
262. Trotman RL, Williamson JC, Shoemaker DM, et al: Antibiotic dosing in critically ill adult patients receiving continuous renal replacement therapy. *Clin Infect Dis* 41:1159–1166, 2005.
263. Centers for Disease Control and Prevention (CDC): Vital signs: Central line–associated bloodstream infections—United States, 2001, 2008, and 2009. *MMWR Morb Mortal Wkly Rep* 60:243–248, 2011.
264. Burton DC, Edwards JR, Horan TC, et al: Methicillin-resistant *Staphylococcus aureus* central line–associated bloodstream infections in US intensive care units, 1997-2007. *JAMA* 301:727–736, 2009.
265. Moellering RC, Jr: Vancomycin: A 50-year reassessment. *Clin Infect Dis* 42(Suppl 1):S3–S4, 2006.
266. Tverdek FP, Crank CW, Segreti J: Antibiotic therapy of methicillin-resistant *Staphylococcus aureus* in critical care. *Crit Care Clin* 24:249–260, vii–viii, 2008.
267. Wu LR, Zaborina O, Zaborin A, et al: Surgical injury and metabolic stress enhance the virulence of the human opportunistic pathogen *Pseudomonas aeruginosa. Surg Infect (Larchmt)* 6:185–195, 2005.
268. Driscoll JA, Brody SL, Kollef MH: The epidemiology, pathogenesis and treatment of *Pseudomonas aeruginosa* infections. *Drugs* 67:351–368, 2007.
269. Tenover FC: Mechanisms of antimicrobial resistance in bacteria. *Am J Med* 119:S3–S10, 2006.

270. Bush K: Bench-to-bedside review: The role of beta-lactamases in antibiotic-resistant gram-negative infections. *Crit Care* 14:224, 2010.
271. Patel G, Bonomo RA: Status report on carbapenemases: Challenges and prospects. *Expert Rev Anti Infect Ther* 9:555–570, 2011.
272. Bonomo RA, Szabo D: Mechanisms of multidrug resistance in *Acinetobacter* species and *Pseudomonas aeruginosa*. *Clin Infect Dis* 43(Suppl 2):S49–S56, 2006.
273. Grupper M, Sprecher H, Mashiach T, et al: Attributable mortality of nosocomial *Acinetobacter* bacteremia. *Infect Control Hosp Epidemiol* 28:293–298, 2007.
274. Vincent JL, Anaissie E, Bruining H, et al: Epidemiology, diagnosis and treatment of systemic *Candida* infection in surgical patients under intensive care. *Intensive Care Med* 24:206–216, 1998.
275. Blumberg HM, Jarvis WR, Soucie JM, et al: Risk factors for candidal bloodstream infections in surgical intensive care unit patients: The NEMIS prospective multicenter study. The National Epidemiology of Mycosis Survey. *Clin Infect Dis* 33:177–186, 2001.
276. Paphitou NI, Ostrosky-Zeichner L, Rex JH: Rules for identifying patients at increased risk for candidal infections in the surgical intensive care unit: Approach to developing practical criteria for systematic use in antifungal prophylaxis trials. *Med Mycol* 43:235–243, 2005.
277. Ziakas PD, Kourbeti IS, Voulgarelis M, et al: Effectiveness of systemic antifungal prophylaxis in patients with neutropenia after chemotherapy: A meta-analysis of randomized controlled trials. *Clin Ther* 32:2316–2336, 2010.
278. Chow JK, Golan Y, Ruthazer R, et al: Risk factors for *albicans* and non-*albicans* candidemia in the intensive care unit. *Crit Care Med* 36:1993–1998, 2008.
279. Pittet D, Monod M, Suter PM, et al: *Candida* colonization and subsequent infections in critically ill surgical patients. *Ann Surg* 220:751–758, 1994.
280. Leon C, Ruiz-Santana S, Saavedra P, et al: A bedside scoring system ("Candida score") for early antifungal treatment in nonneutropenic critically ill patients with *Candida* colonization. *Crit Care Med* 34:730–737, 2006.
281. Leon C, Ruiz-Santana S, Saavedra P, et al: Usefulness of the "Candida score" for discriminating between *Candida* colonization and invasive candidiasis in non-neutropenic critically ill patients: A prospective multicenter study. *Crit Care Med* 37:1624–1633, 2009.
282. Kratzer C, Graninger W, Lassnigg A, et al: Design and use of Candida scores at the intensive care unit. *Mycoses* 54:467–474, 2011.
283. Ostrosky-Zeichner L, Sable C, Sobel J, et al: Multicenter retrospective development and validation of a clinical prediction rule for nosocomial invasive candidiasis in the intensive care setting. *Eur J Clin Microbiol Infect Dis* 26:271–276, 2007.
284. Ostrosky-Zeichner L, Pappas PG, Shoham S, et al: Improvement of a clinical prediction rule for clinical trials on prophylaxis for invasive candidiasis in the intensive care unit. *Mycoses* 54:46–51, 2011.
285. Shorr AF, Tabak YP, Johannes RS, et al: Candidemia on presentation to the hospital: Development and validation of a risk score. *Crit Care* 13:R156, 2009.
286. Sawyer RG, Adams RB, May AK, et al: Development of *Candida albicans* and *C. albicans/Escherichia coli/Bacteroides fragilis* intraperitoneal abscess models with demonstration of fungus-induced bacterial translocation. *J Med Vet Mycol* 33:49–52, 1995.
287. Eggimann P, Garbino J, Pittet D: Epidemiology of *Candida* species infections in critically ill non-immunosuppressed patients. *Lancet Infect Dis* 3:685–702, 2003.
288. Felk A, Kretschmar M, Albrecht A, et al: *Candida albicans* hyphal formation and the expression of the Efg1-regulated proteinases Sap4 to Sap6 are required for the invasion of parenchymal organs. *Infect Immun* 70:3689–3700, 2002.
289. Prowle JR, Echeverri JE, Ligabo EV, et al: Acquired bloodstream infection in the intensive care unit: Incidence and attributable mortality. *Crit Care* 15:R100, 2011.
290. Shorr AF, Lazarus DR, Sherner JH, et al: Do clinical features allow for accurate prediction of fungal pathogenesis in bloodstream infections? Potential implications of the increasing prevalence of non-*albicans* candidemia. *Crit Care Med* 35:1077–1083, 2007.
291. Mohr JF, Sims C, Paetznick V, et al: Prospective survey of (1→3)-beta-D-glucan and its relationship to invasive candidiasis in the surgical intensive care unit setting. *J Clin Microbiol* 49:58–61, 2011.
292. Pitarch A, Nombela C, Gil C: Prediction of the clinical outcome in invasive candidiasis patients based on molecular fingerprints of five anti-*Candida* antibodies in serum. *Mol Cell Proteomics* 10:2011. M110.004010.
293. Charles PE, Castro C, Ruiz-Santana S, et al: Serum procalcitonin levels in critically ill patients colonized with *Candida* spp: New clues for the early recognition of invasive candidiasis? *Intensive Care Med* 35:2146–2150, 2009.
294. Dean DA, Burchard KW: Surgical perspective on invasive *Candida* infections. *World J Surg* 22:127–134, 1998.
295. Riddell JT, Comer GM, Kauffman CA: Treatment of endogenous fungal endophthalmitis: Focus on new antifungal agents. *Clin Infect Dis* 52:648–653, 2011.
296. Meersseman W, Vandecasteele SJ, Wilmer A, et al: Invasive aspergillosis in critically ill patients without malignancy. *Am J Respir Crit Care Med* 170:621–625, 2004.
297. Eggimann P, Pittet D: Postoperative fungal infections. *Surg Infect (Larchmt)* 7(Suppl 2):S53–S56, 2006.
298. Rocco TR, Reinert SE, Simms HH: Effects of fluconazole administration in critically ill patients: Analysis of bacterial and fungal resistance. *Arch Surg* 135:160–165, 2000.
299. Gleason TG, May AK, Caparelli D, et al: Emerging evidence of selection of fluconazole-tolerant fungi in surgical intensive care units. *Arch Surg* 132:1197–1201, 1997.
300. Pelz RK, Hendrix CW, Swoboda SM, et al: Double-blind placebo-controlled trial of fluconazole to prevent candidal infections in critically ill surgical patients. *Ann Surg* 233:542–548, 2001.
301. Magill SS, Swoboda SM, Shields CE, et al: The epidemiology of *Candida* colonization and invasive candidiasis in a surgical intensive care unit where fluconazole prophylaxis is utilized: Follow-up to a randomized clinical trial. *Ann Surg* 249:657–665, 2009.
302. Shorr AF, Chung K, Jackson WL, et al: Fluconazole prophylaxis in critically ill surgical patients: A meta-analysis. *Crit Care Med* 33:1928–1935, quiz 1936, 2005.
303. Pappas PG, Kauffman CA, Andes D, et al: Clinical practice guidelines for the management of candidiasis: 2009 update by the Infectious Diseases Society of America. *Clin Infect Dis* 48:503–535, 2009.

304. Brizendine KD, Vishin S, Baddley JW: Antifungal prophylaxis in solid organ transplant recipients. *Expert Rev Anti Infect Ther* 9:571–581, 2011.
305. Playford EG, Webster AC, Sorrell TC, et al: Systematic review and meta-analysis of antifungal agents for preventing fungal infections in liver transplant recipients. *Eur J Clin Microbiol Infect Dis* 25:549–561, 2006.
306. Horn DL, Ostrosky-Zeichner L, Morris MI, et al: Factors related to survival and treatment success in invasive candidiasis or candidemia: A pooled analysis of two large, prospective, micafungin trials. *Eur J Clin Microbiol Infect Dis* 29:223–229, 2010.
307. Chen SC, Playford EG, Sorrell TC: Antifungal therapy in invasive fungal infections. *Curr Opin Pharmacol* 10:522–530, 2010.
308. Ostrosky-Zeichner L: Combination antifungal therapy: A critical review of the evidence. *Clin Microbiol Infect* 14(Suppl 4):65–70, 2008.
309. Mukherjee PK, Zhou G, Munyon R, et al: *Candida* biofilm: A well-designed protected environment. *Med Mycol* 43:191–208, 2005.
310. Al-Fattani MA, Douglas LJ: Penetration of *Candida* biofilms by antifungal agents. *Antimicrob Agents Chemother* 48:3291–3297, 2004.
311. Herbrecht R, Denning DW, Patterson TF, et al: Voriconazole versus amphotericin B for primary therapy of invasive aspergillosis. *N Engl J Med* 347:408–415, 2002.
312. Kullberg BJ, Sobel JD, Ruhnke M, et al: Voriconazole versus a regimen of amphotericin B followed by fluconazole for candidaemia in non-neutropenic patients: A randomised non-inferiority trial. *Lancet* 366:1435–1442, 2005.
313. Glöckner A: Treatment and prophylaxis of invasive candidiasis with anidulafungin, caspofungin and micafungin: Review of the literature. *Eur J Med Res* 16:167–179, 2011.
314. Anidulafungin (Eraxis) for *Candida* infections. *Med Lett Drugs Ther* 48:43–44, 2006.
315. Pappas PG, Rotstein CM, Betts RF, et al: Micafungin versus caspofungin for treatment of candidemia and other forms of invasive candidiasis. *Clin Infect Dis* 45:883–893, 2007.
316. Kuse ER, Chetchotisakd P, da Cunha CA, et al: Micafungin versus liposomal amphotericin B for candidaemia and invasive candidosis: A phase III randomised double-blind trial. *Lancet* 369:1519–1527, 2007.
317. Zilberberg MD, Kothari S, Shorr AF: Cost-effectiveness of micafungin as an alternative to fluconazole empirical treatment of suspected ICU-acquired candidemia among patients with sepsis: A model simulation. *Crit Care* 13:R94, 2009.

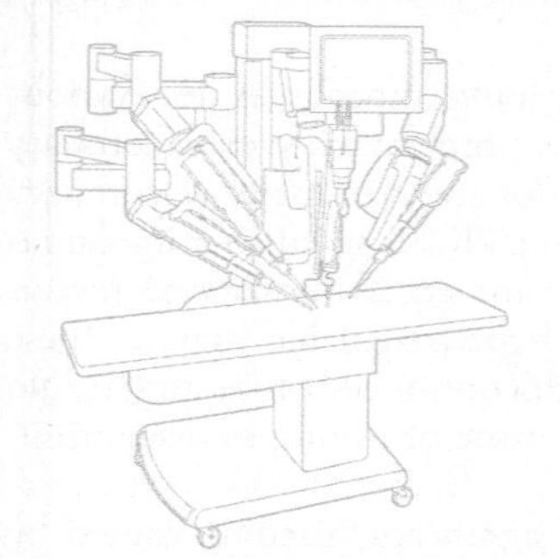

CHAPTER 12

Surgical Complications

Mahmoud N. Kulaylat, Merril T. Dayton

OUTLINE

Surgical complications constitute a frustrating and difficult aspect of the operative treatment of patients. Regardless of how technically gifted and capable surgeons are, all must deal with complications that occur after operative procedures. The cost of surgical complications in the United States is equal to millions of dollars; in addition, surgical complications are associated with lost work productivity, disruption of family life, and stress to employers and society in general. The functional results of the operation are frequently compromised by complications; in some cases, the patient never recovers to the preoperative level of function. The most significant and difficult part of complications is the suffering experienced by a patient who enters the hospital anticipating an uneventful operation but who suffers and is compromised by the complication.

Complications can occur for various reasons. A surgeon can perform a technically sound operation in a patient who is severely compromised by the disease process and have a complication. A surgeon who is sloppy or careless or hurries through an operation can make technical errors that account for the operative complications. Finally, the patient can be healthy nutritionally, have an operation performed meticulously, and yet experience a complication because of the nature of the disease. The possibility of postoperative complications remains part of every surgeon's mental preparation for a difficult operation.

Surgeons can do much to avoid complications by careful preoperative screening. When the surgeon sees the surgical candidate for the first time, numerous questions need to be addressed, such as the nutritional status of the patient and the health of the heart and lungs. The surgeon must make a decision regarding performing the appropriate operation for the known disease. Similarly, the timing of the operation is often an important issue. Some operations can be performed in a purely elective fashion, whereas others must be done in an urgent fashion. Occasionally, the surgeon requires that the patient lose weight before the operation to enhance the likelihood of a successful outcome. The surgeon may request preoperative consultation from a cardiologist or pulmonary specialist to ensure that the patient will be able to tolerate the stress of a particular procedure.

Once the operation has begun, the surgeon can do much to influence the postoperative outcome. Surgeons must handle tissues gently, dissect meticulously, and honor tissue planes. Performing the technical portions of the operation carefully lowers the risk for a significant complication. At all costs, surgeons must avoid the temptation to rush, cut corners, or accept marginal technical results. Similarly, the judicious use of antibiotics and other preoperative medications can influence the outcome. For a seriously ill patient, adequate resuscitation may be necessary before giving a general anesthetic.

Compulsive postoperative surveillance is mandatory after the operation is completed. Performing thorough and careful checks on patients on a regular basis postoperatively gives the operating surgeon an opportunity to be vigilant and seek postoperative complications at an early stage, when they can be most effectively addressed. During this process, the surgeon carefully checks all wounds, evaluates intake and output, checks temperature profiles, ascertains what the patient's activity levels have been, evaluates nutritional status, and checks pain levels. With years of experience, the clinician is able to assess these parameters and detect deviations from the normal postoperative course. Expeditious response to a complication makes the difference between a brief, inconvenient complication and a devastating, disabling one. A wise surgeon deals with complications quickly, thoroughly, and appropriately.

SURGICAL WOUND COMPLICATIONS

Seroma

Causes

A seroma is a collection of liquefied fat, serum, and lymphatic fluid under the incision. The fluid is usually clear, yellow, and viscous and is found in the subcutaneous layer of the skin. Seromas represent the most benign complication after an operative procedure and are particularly likely to occur when large skin flaps are developed in the course of the operation, as is often seen with mastectomy, axillary dissection, groin dissection, and large ventral hernias or when a prosthetic mesh (polytetrafluoroethylene) is used in the repair of a ventral hernia.

Presentation and Management

A seroma usually manifests as a localized and well-circumscribed swelling, pressure, or discomfort and occasional drainage of clear liquid from the immature surgical wound. Prevention of seroma formation may be achieved with placement of suction drains under the flaps. Premature removal of suction drains often results in large seromas that require aspiration under sterile conditions, followed by placement of a pressure dressing. A seroma that reaccumulates after at least two aspirations is evacuated by opening the incision and packing the wound with saline-moistened gauze to allow healing by secondary intention. In the presence of synthetic mesh, open drainage is best performed in the operating room, the incision is best closed to avoid exposure and infection of the mesh, and suction drains are placed. An infected seroma is also treated with open drainage. The presence of synthetic mesh in these cases prevents the wound from healing. Management of the mesh depends on the severity and extent of infection. In the absence of severe sepsis and spreading cellulitis and in the presence of localized infection, the mesh can be left in situ and removed later when the acute infectious process has resolved. Otherwise, the mesh must be removed, and the wound must be managed with open wound care.

Hematoma

Causes

A hematoma is an abnormal collection of blood, usually in the subcutaneous layer of a recent incision or in a potential space in the abdominal cavity after extirpation of an organ (e.g., splenic fossa hematoma after splenectomy or pelvic hematoma after proctectomy). Hematomas are more worrisome than seromas because of the potential for secondary infection. Hematoma formation is related to inadequate hemostasis, depletion of clotting factors, or the presence of coagulopathy. Numerous disease processes can contribute to coagulopathy, including myeloproliferative disorders, liver disease, renal failure, sepsis, clotting factor deficiencies, and medications. Medications most commonly associated with coagulopathy are antiplatelet drugs, such as acetylsalicylic acid (aspirin), clopidogrel, ticlopidine, eptifibatide, and abciximab, and anticoagulants, such as unfractionated heparin (UFH), low-molecular-weight heparin (LMWH; e.g., enoxaparin, dalteparin sodium, tinzaparin), and vitamin K antagonist (VKA; e.g., warfarin sodium).

Presentation and Management

The clinical manifestations of a hematoma may vary with its size, location, and presence of infection. A hematoma may manifest as an expanding, unsightly swelling or pain in the area of a surgical incision. In the neck, a large hematoma may cause compromise of the airway; in the retroperitoneum, it may cause a paralytic ileus, anemia, and ongoing bleeding caused by local consumptive coagulopathy; and in the extremity and abdominal cavity, it may result in compartment syndrome. On physical examination, the hematoma appears as a localized soft swelling with purplish blue discoloration of the overlying skin. The swelling varies from small to large and may be tender to palpation or associated with drainage of dark red fluid from the fresh wound.

Hematoma formation is prevented preoperatively by correcting any clotting abnormalities and discontinuing medications that alter coagulation. Antiplatelet medications and anticoagulants may be given to patients undergoing procedures for various reasons. Clopidogrel is given after implantation of a coronary stent; acetylsalicylic acid is given for the treatment of coronary artery disease (CAD) and stroke; and VKA is given after implantation of a mechanical mitral valve for atrial fibrillation, venous thromboembolism (VTE), and hypercoagulable states. These medications must be temporarily discontinued before surgery. No specific studies have addressed the issue of timing of discontinuation of such medications.

One must balance the risk of significant bleeding caused by uncorrected medication-induced coagulopathy and the risk of thromboembolic events after discontinuation of therapy. The risk of bleeding varies with the type of surgery or procedure and adequacy of hemostasis; the risk of thromboembolism depends on the indication for antithrombotic therapy and the presence of comorbid conditions.[1] In patients at high risk for thromboembolism (e.g., patients with a mechanical mitral valve or older generation aortic valve prosthesis, VTE within 3 months, severe thrombophilia, recent atrial fibrillation [within 6 months], stroke, or transient ischemic attack who are scheduled to undergo an elective major surgical procedure involving a body cavity), VKA must be discontinued 4 to 5 days before surgery to allow the international normalized ratio (INR) to be less than 1.5. In patients whose INR is still elevated (>1.5), low-dose vitamin K (1 to 2 mg) is given orally. Patients are then given bridging anticoagulation—that is, a therapeutic dose of rapidly acting anticoagulant, intravenous (IV) UFH or LMWH. Patients receiving IV UFH (half-life, 45 minutes) can have the medication discontinued 4 hours before surgery, and patients receiving therapeutic dose LMWH subcutaneously (variable half-life) can have the medication discontinued 16 to 24 hours before surgery. VKA is resumed 12 to 24 hours after surgery (it takes 2 to 3 days for anticoagulant effect to begin after start of VKA) and when there is adequate hemostasis. In patients at high risk of bleeding (major surgery or surgery with high bleeding risk) for whom postoperative therapeutic LMWH or UFH is planned, initiation of therapy is delayed for 48 to 72 hours, low-dose LMWH or UFH is administered, or the therapy is completely avoided. Patients at low risk for thromboembolism do not require heparin therapy after discontinuation of VKA. Patients receiving acetylsalicylic acid or clopidogrel must have the medication withheld 6 to 7 days before surgery; otherwise, the surgery must be delayed until the patient has completed the course of treatment. Antiplatelet therapy is resumed approximately 24 hours after surgery. In patients with a bare metal coronary stent who require surgery within 6 weeks of stent placement, acetylsalicylic acid and clopidogrel are continued in the perioperative period. In patients who are receiving VKA and require urgent surgery, immediate reversal of anticoagulant effect requires transfusion with fresh-frozen plasma or other prothrombin concentrate and low-dose IV or oral vitamin K. During surgery, adequate hemostasis must be achieved with ligature, electrocautery, fibrin glue, or topical bovine thrombin before closure. Closed suction drainage systems are placed in large potential spaces and removed postoperatively when the output is not bloody and scant.

Evaluation of a patient with a hematoma, especially one that is large and expanding, includes assessment of preexisting risk factors and coagulation parameters (e.g., prothrombin time, activated partial thromboplastin time, INR, platelet count, bleeding time) and appropriate treatment. A small hematoma does not require any intervention and eventually resorbs. Most retroperitoneal hematomas can be managed by expectant waiting after correction of associated coagulopathy (platelet transfusion if bleeding time is prolonged, desmopressin in patients who have renal failure, and fresh-frozen plasma in patients who have an increased INR). A large or expanding hematoma in the neck is managed in a similar fashion and best evacuated in the operating room urgently after securing the airway if there is any respiratory compromise. Similarly, hematomas detected soon after surgery, especially hematomas developing under skin flaps, are best evacuated in the operating room.

Acute Wound Failure (Dehiscence)

Causes

Acute wound failure (wound dehiscence or a burst abdomen) refers to postoperative separation of the abdominal musculoaponeurotic layers. Wound dehiscence is among the most dreaded complications faced by surgeons and is of great concern because of the risk of evisceration; the need for some form of intervention; and the possibility of repeat dehiscence, surgical wound infection, and incisional hernia formation.

Acute wound failure occurs in approximately 1% to 3% of patients who undergo an abdominal operation. Dehiscence most often develops 7 to 10 days postoperatively but may occur anytime after surgery (range, 1 to >20 days). Numerous factors may contribute to wound dehiscence (Box 12-1). Acute wound failure is often related to technical errors in placing sutures too close to the edge, too far apart, or under too much tension. Local wound complications such as hematoma and infection can also predispose to localized dehiscence. A deep wound infection is one of the most common causes of localized wound separation. Increased intra-abdominal pressure (IAP) is often blamed for wound disruption, and factors that adversely affect wound healing are cited as contributing to this complication. In healthy patients, the rate of wound failure is similar whether closure is accomplished with a continuous or an interrupted technique. In high-risk patients, continuous closure is worrisome because suture breakage in one place weakens the entire closure.

Presentation and Management

Acute wound failure may occur without warning; evisceration makes the diagnosis obvious. A sudden, dramatic drainage of a large volume of clear, salmon-colored fluid precedes dehiscence in 25% of patients. More often, patients report a ripping sensation. Probing the wound with a sterile, cotton-tipped applicator or gloved finger may detect a partial dehiscence.

BOX 12-1 Factors Associated With Wound Dehiscence

- Technical error in fascial closure
- Emergency surgery
- Intra-abdominal infection
- Advanced age
- Wound infection, hematoma, and seroma
- Elevated intra-abdominal pressure
- Obesity
- Long-term corticosteroid use
- Previous wound dehiscence
- Malnutrition
- Radiation therapy and chemotherapy
- Systemic disease (uremia, diabetes mellitus)

Acute wound failure is prevented by careful attention to technical detail during fascial closure, such as proper spacing of the suture, adequate depth of bite of the fascia, relaxation of the patient during closure, and achieving a tension-free closure. For very high-risk patients, interrupted closure is often the wisest choice. Alternative methods of closure must be selected when primary closure is impossible without undue tension. Although retention sutures were used extensively in the past, their use is less common today, with many surgeons opting to use a synthetic mesh or bioabsorbable tissue scaffold.

Treatment of dehiscence depends on the extent of fascial separation and the presence of evisceration or significant intra-abdominal pathology (e.g., intestinal leak, peritonitis). A small dehiscence, especially in the proximal aspect of an upper midline incision 10 to 12 days postoperatively, can be managed conservatively with saline-moistened gauze packing of the wound and use of an abdominal binder. In the event of evisceration, the eviscerated intestines must be covered with a sterile, saline-moistened towel, and preparations must be made to return to the operating room after a very short period of fluid resuscitation. Similarly, if probing of the wound reveals a large segment of the wound that is open to the omentum and intestines, or if there is peritonitis or suspicion of intestinal leak, plans to take the patient back to the operating room are made.

In the operating room, thorough exploration of the abdominal cavity is performed to rule out the presence of a septic focus or an anastomotic leak that may have predisposed to the dehiscence. Management of the infection is critical before attempting to close. Management of the incision is a function of the condition of the fascia. When technical mistakes are made and the fascia is strong and intact, primary closure is warranted. If the fascia is infected or necrotic, débridement is performed. The incision can be closed with retention sutures; however, to avoid tension, use of a prosthetic material may be preferred. Closure with an absorbable mesh (polyglactin or polyglycolic acid) may be preferable because the mesh is well tolerated in septic wounds and allows bridging the gap between the edges of the fascia without tension, prevents evisceration, and allows the underlying cause of the patient's dehiscence to resolve. After granulation of the wound has occurred, a skin graft is applied, and wound closure is achieved by advancing local tissue. This approach uniformly results in the development of a hernia, the repair of which requires the subsequent removal of the skin graft and use of a permanent prosthesis. An alternative method of closure is dermabrasion of the skin graft followed by fascial closure using the component separation technique. Attempts to close the fascia under tension guarantee a repeat dehiscence and, in some cases, result in intra-abdominal hypertension (IAH). The incision is left open (laparotomy), closed with a temporary closure device (open abdomen technique), closed with synthetic mesh or biologic graft (acellular dermal matrix), or closed by using negative-pressure wound therapy.

The open abdomen technique avoids IAH, preserves the fascia, and facilitates reaccess of the abdominal cavity. With laparotomy, the wound is allowed to heal with secondary intention or subsequently closed with a skin graft or local or regional tissue. This approach is associated with prolonged healing time, fluid loss, and risk of complex enterocutaneous fistula formation as a result of bowel exposure, desiccation, and traumatic injury. Furthermore, definitive surgical repair to restore the integrity of the abdominal wall is eventually required. A temporary closure device (vacuum pack closure) protects abdominal contents, keeps patients dry, can be quickly removed with increased IAP, and avoids secondary complications seen with laparotomy. A fenestrated, nonadherent, polyethylene sheet is applied on the bowel omentum, moist surgical towels or gauze with drains are placed on top, and an iodophor-impregnated adhesive dressing is placed. Continuous suction is then applied. If the fascia cannot be closed in 7 to 10 days, the wound is allowed to granulate and then covered with a skin graft.

Absorbable synthetic mesh provides wound stability and is resistant to infection. It is associated with fistula and hernia formation repair, which is difficult and may require reconstruction of the abdominal wall. Repair with nonabsorbable synthetic mesh such as polypropylene, polyester, or polytetrafluoroethylene is associated with complications that require removal of the mesh (e.g., abscess formation, dehiscence, wound sepsis, mesh extrusion, bowel fistulization). Although polytetrafluoroethylene is more desirable because it is nonadherent to underlying bowel, it is expensive, it does not allow skin grafting, and it is associated with chronic infections. An acellular dermal matrix (bioprosthesis) has the mechanical properties of a mesh for abdominal wall reconstruction and physiologic properties that make it resistant to contamination and infection. The bioprosthesis provides immediate coverage of the wound and serves as mechanical support in a single-stage reconstruction of compromised surgical wounds. It is bioactive because it functions as tissue replacement or scaffold for new tissue growth; it stimulates cellular attachment, migration, neovascularization, and repopulation of the implanted graft. A bioprosthesis also reduces long-term complications (e.g., erosion, infection, chronic pain). Available acellular materials are animal-derived (e.g., porcine intestinal submucosa, porcine dermis, cross-linked porcine dermal collagen) or human-derived (e.g., cadaveric human dermis). However, the rate of wound complications (e.g., superficial wound or graft infection, graft dehiscence, fistula formation, bleeding) and hernia formation or laxity of the abdominal wall is 25% to 50%.[2]

Negative-pressure wound therapy is based on the concept of wound suction. A vacuum-assisted closure device is most commonly used. The device consists of a vacuum pump, canister with connecting tubing, open-pore foam (e.g., polyurethane ether, polyvinyl alcohol foam) or gauze, and semiocclusive dressing. The device provides immediate coverage of the abdominal wound, acts as a temporary dressing, does not require suturing to the fascia, minimizes IAH, and prevents loss of domain. Applying suction of 125 mm Hg, the open-pore foam decreases in size and transmits the negative pressure to surrounding tissue, leading to contraction of the wound (macrodeformation); removal of extracellular fluid via decrease in bowel edema, evacuation of excess abdominal fluid, and decrease in wound size; stabilization of the wound environment; and microdeformation of the foam-wound interface, which induces cellular proliferation and angiogenesis. The secondary effects of the vacuum-assisted closure device include acceleration of wound healing, reduction and changes in bacterial burden, changes in biochemistry and systemic responses, and improvement in wound bed preparation—increase in local blood perfusion and induction healing response through microchemical forces.[3] This approach results in successful closure of the fascia in 85% of cases. However, the device is expensive and cumbersome to wear and may cause significant pain, cause bleeding (especially in patients on anticoagulant therapy), be associated with increased levels of certain bacteria, and be associated with evisceration and hernia formation. There is also an increased incidence of intestinal fistulization at enterotomy sites and enteric anastomoses and in the absence of anastomoses.

Surgical Site Infection (Wound Infection)

Causes

Surgical site infections (SSIs) are a significant problem for surgeons. Despite major improvements in antibiotics, better anesthesia, superior instruments, earlier diagnosis of surgical problems, and improved techniques for postoperative vigilance, wound infections continue to occur. Although some may view the problem as merely cosmetic, that view represents a shallow understanding of this problem, which causes significant patient suffering, morbidity, and mortality and is a financial burden to the health care system. Furthermore, SSIs represent a risk factor for the development of incisional hernia, which requires surgical repair. In the United States, SSIs account for almost 40% of hospital-acquired infections among surgical patients.

The surgical wound encompasses the area of the body, internally and externally, that involves the entire operative site. Wounds are generally categorized as follows:

1. Superficial, which includes the skin and subcutaneous tissue
2. Deep, which includes the fascia and muscle
3. Organ space, which includes the internal organs of the body if the operation includes that area

The U.S. Centers for Disease Control and Prevention proposed specific criteria for the diagnosis of SSIs (Box 12-2).[4]

BOX 12-2 Centers for Disease Control and Prevention Criteria for Defining a Surgical Site Infection

Superficial Incisional

Infection less than 30 days after surgery

Involves skin and subcutaneous tissue only, *plus* one of the following:

- Purulent drainage
- Diagnosis of superficial SSI by a surgeon
- Symptoms of erythema, pain, and local edema

Deep Incisional

Less than 30 days after surgery with no implant and soft tissue involvement

Infection less than 1 year after surgery with an implant; involves deep soft tissues (fascia and muscle), *plus* one of the following:

- Purulent drainage from the deep space but no extension into the organ space
- Abscess found in the deep space on direct or radiologic examination or on reoperation
- Diagnosis of a deep space SSI by the surgeon
- Symptoms of fever, pain, and tenderness leading to wound dehiscence or opening by a surgeon

Organ Space

Infection less than 30 days after surgery with no implant

Infection less than 1 year after surgery with an implant and infection; involves any part of the operation opened or manipulated, *plus* one of the following:

- Purulent drainage from a drain placed in the organ space
- Cultured organisms from material aspirated from the organ space
- Abscess found on direct or radiologic examination or during reoperation
- Diagnosis of organ space infection by a surgeon

Adapted from Mangram AJ, Horan TC, Pearson ML, et al: Guideline for prevention of surgical site infection. *Infect Control Hosp Epidemiol* 20:252, 1999.

SSI, surgical site infection.

SSIs develop as a result of contamination of the surgical site with microorganisms. The source of these microorganisms is mostly patients' flora (endogenous source) when integrity of the skin or wall of a hollow viscus is violated. Occasionally, the source is exogenous when a break in the surgical sterile technique occurs, allowing contamination from the surgical team, equipment, implant or gloves, or surrounding environment. The pathogens associated with SSI reflect the area that provided the inoculum for the infection to develop. However, the microbiology varies, depending on the types of procedures performed in individual practices. Gram-positive cocci account for half of the infections (Table 12-1)—*Staphylococcus aureus* (most common), coagulase-negative *Staphylococcus,* and *Enterococcus* spp. *S. aureus* infections normally occur in the nasal passages, mucous membranes, and skin of carriers. The organism that has acquired resistance to methicillin (methicillin-resistant *S. aureus* [MRSA]) consists of two subtypes, hospital-acquired and community-acquired MRSA. Hospital-acquired MRSA is associated with nosocomial infections and affects immunocompromised individuals. It also occurs in patients with chronic wounds, patients subjected to invasive procedures, and patients with prior antibiotic treatment. Community-acquired MRSA is associated with various skin and soft tissue infections in patients with and without risk factors for MRSA. Community-acquired MRSA (e.g., the USA300 clone) has also been noted to affect SSIs. Hospital-acquired MRSA isolates have a different antibiotic susceptibility profile—they are usually resistant to at least three β-lactam antibiotics and are usually susceptible to vancomycin, teicoplanin, and sulfamethoxazole. Community-acquired MRSA is usually susceptible to clindamycin, with variable susceptibility to erythromycin, vancomycin, and tetracycline. There is evidence to indicate that hospital-acquired MRSA is developing resistance to vancomycin (vancomycin-intermediate *S. aureus* and vancomycin-resistant *S. aureus*).[5] *Enterococcus* spp. are commensals in the adult gastrointestinal (GI) tract, have intrinsic resistance to various antibiotics (e.g., cephalosporins, clindamycin, aminoglycoside), and are the first to exhibit resistance to vancomycin.

TABLE 12-1 Pathogens Isolated from Postoperative Surgical Site Infections at a University Hospital

PATHOGEN	PERCENTAGE OF ISOLATES
Staphylococcus (coagulase-negative)	25.6
Enterococcus (group D)	11.5
Staphylococcus aureus	8.7
Candida albicans	6.5
Escherichia coli	6.3
Pseudomonas aeruginosa	6.0
Corynebacterium	4.0
Candida (non-*albicans*)	3.4
Alpha-hemolytic *Streptococcus*	3.0
Klebsiella pneumoniae	2.8
Vancomycin-resistant *Enterococcus*	2.4
Enterobacter cloacae	2.2
Citrobacter spp.	2.0

From Weiss CA, Statz CI, Dahms RA, et al: Six years of surgical wound surveillance at a tertiary care center. *Arch Surg* 134:1041–1048, 1999.

In approximately one third of SSI cases, gram-negative bacilli (*Escherichia coli, Pseudomonas aeruginosa,* and *Enterobacter* spp.) are isolated. However, the predominant bacterial species are the gram-negative bacilli at locations at which high volumes of GI operations are performed. Infrequent pathogens are group A beta-hemolytic streptococci and *Clostridium perfringens.* In recent years, involvement of resistant organisms in the genesis of SSIs has increased, most notably in MRSA.

A host of patient-related and operative procedure–related factors may contribute to the development of SSIs (Table 12-2).[6] The risk of infection is related to the specific surgical procedure performed, and surgical wounds are classified according to the relative risk of SSI occurring—clean, clean-contaminated, contaminated, and dirty (Table 12-3). In the National Nosocomial Infections Surveillance System, the risk of patients is stratified according to three important factors: (1) wound classification (contaminated or dirty); (2) longer duration operation, defined as duration that exceeds the 75th percentile for a given procedure; and (3) medical characteristics of patients as determined by American Society of Anesthesiology classification of III, IV, or V (presence of severe systemic disease that results in functional limitations, is life-threatening, or is expected to preclude survival from the operation) at the time of operation.[7]

Presentation

SSIs most commonly occur 5 to 6 days postoperatively but may develop sooner or later than that. Approximately 80% to 90% of all postoperative infections occur within 30 days after the

TABLE 12-2 Risk Factors for Postoperative Wound Infection

PATIENT FACTORS	ENVIRONMENTAL FACTORS	TREATMENT FACTORS
Ascites	Contaminated medications	Drains
Chronic inflammation	Inadequate disinfection/sterilization	Emergency procedure
Undernutrition	Inadequate skin antisepsis	Inadequate antibiotic coverage
Obesity		
Diabetes	Inadequate ventilation	Preoperative hospitalization
Extremes of age	Presence of foreign body	Prolonged operation
Hypercholesterolemia		
Hypoxemia		
Peripheral vascular disease		
Postoperative anemia		
Previous site of irradiation		
Recent operation		
Remote infection		
Skin carriage of staphylococci		
Skin disease in area of infection		
Immunosuppression		

Data from National Nosocomial Infections Surveillance Systems (NNIS) System Report: Data summary from January 1992–June 2001, issued August 2001. *Am J Infect Control* 29:404–421, 2001.

operative procedure. With the increased use of outpatient surgery and decreased length of stay in hospitals, 30% to 40% of all wound infections have been shown to occur after hospital discharge. Nevertheless, although less than 10% of surgical patients are hospitalized for 6 days or less, 70% of postdischarge infections occur in that group.

Superficial and deep SSIs are accompanied by erythema, tenderness, edema, and occasionally drainage. The wound is often soft or fluctuant at the site of infection, which is a departure from the firmness of the healing ridge present elsewhere in the wound. The patient may have leukocytosis and a low-grade fever. According to The Joint Commission, a surgical wound is considered infected if (1) grossly purulent material drains from the wound, (2) the wound spontaneously opens and drains purulent fluid, (3) the wound drains fluid that is culture-positive or Gram stain–positive for bacteria, and (4) the surgeon notes erythema or drainage and opens the wound after determining it to be infected.

TABLE 12-3 Classification of Surgical Wounds

CATEGORY	CRITERIA	INFECTION RATE (%)
Clean	No hollow viscus entered Primary wound closure No inflammation No breaks in aseptic technique Elective procedure	1-3
Clean-contaminated	Hollow viscus entered but controlled No inflammation Primary wound closure Minor break in aseptic technique Mechanical drain used Bowel preparation preoperatively	5-8
Contaminated	Uncontrolled spillage from viscus Inflammation apparent Open, traumatic wound Major break in aseptic technique	20-25
Dirty	Untreated, uncontrolled spillage from viscus Pus in operative wound Open suppurative wound Severe inflammation	30-40

Treatment

Prevention of SSIs relies on changing or dealing with modifiable risk factors that predispose to SSIs. However, many of these factors cannot be changed, such as age, complexity of the surgical procedure, and morbid obesity. Patients who are heavy smokers are encouraged to stop smoking at least 30 days before surgery, glucose levels in patients with diabetes must be treated appropriately, and severely malnourished patients should be given nutritional supplements for 7 to 14 days before surgery.[8] Obese patients must be encouraged to lose weight if the procedure is elective and there is time to achieve significant weight loss. Similarly, patients who are taking high doses of corticosteroids have lower infection rates if they are weaned off corticosteroids or are at least taking a lower dose. Patients undergoing major intra-abdominal surgery are administered a bowel preparation in the form of a lavage solution or strong cathartic, followed by an oral nonabsorbable antibiotic, particularly for surgery of the colon and small bowel. Bowel preparation reduces the patient's risk for infection from that of a contaminated case (25%) to a clean-contaminated case (5%). Hair is removed by clipping immediately before surgery, and the skin is prepared at the time of operation with an antiseptic agent (e.g., alcohol, chlorhexidine, iodine).

The role of preoperative decolonization in carriers of *S. aureus* undergoing general surgery is questionable, and the routine use of prophylactic vancomycin or teicoplanin (effective against MRSA) is not recommended. Although perioperative antibiotics are widely used, prophylaxis is generally recommended for clean-contaminated or contaminated procedures in which the risk of SSIs is high or in procedures in which vascular or orthopedic prostheses are used because the development of SSI would have grave consequences (Table 12-4). For dirty or contaminated wounds, the use of antibiotics is for therapeutic purposes rather than for prophylaxis. For clean cases, prophylaxis is controversial. For some surgical procedures, a first-generation or second-generation cephalosporin is the accepted agent of choice. A small but significant benefit may be achieved with prophylactic administration of a first-generation cephalosporin for certain types of

TABLE 12-4 Prophylactic Antimicrobial Agent for Selected Surgical Procedures

PROCEDURE	RECOMMENDED AGENT	POTENTIAL ALTERNATIVE
Cardiothoracic	Cefazolin or cefuroxime	Vancomycin, clindamycin
Vascular	Cefazolin or cefuroxime	Vancomycin, clindamycin
Gastroduodenal	Cefazolin	Cefoxitin, cefotetan, aminoglycoside, or fluoroquinolone + antianaerobe
Open biliary	Cefazolin	Cefoxitin, cefotetan, or fluoroquinolone + antianaerobe
Laparoscopic cholecystectomy	None	—
Nonperforated appendicitis	Cefoxitin, cefotetan, cefazolin + metronidazole	Ertapenem, aminoglycoside, or fluoroquinolone + antianaerobe
Colorectal	Cefoxitin, cefotetan, ampicillin-sulbactam, ertapenem, cefazolin + metronidazole	Aminoglycoside, or fluoroquinolone + antianaerobe, aztreonam + clindamycin
Hysterectomy	Cefazolin, cefuroxime, cefoxitin, cefotetan, ampicillin-sulbactam	Aminoglycoside, or fluoroquinolone + antianaerobe, aztreonam + clindamycin
Orthopedic implantation	Cefazolin, cefuroxime	Vancomycin, clindamycin
Head and neck	Cefazolin, clindamycin	—

From Kirby JP, Mazuski JE: Prevention of surgical site infection. *Surg Clin North Am* 89:365–389, 2009.

clean surgery (e.g., mastectomy, herniorrhaphy). For clean-contaminated procedures, administration of preoperative antibiotics is indicated. The appropriate preoperative antibiotic is a function of the most likely inoculum based on the area being operated. For example, when a prosthesis may be placed in a clean wound, preoperative antibiotics would include protection against *S. aureus* and streptococcal species. A first-generation cephalosporin, such as cefazolin, would be appropriate in this setting. For patients undergoing upper GI tract surgery, complex biliary tract operations, or elective colonic resection, administration of a second-generation cephalosporin such as cefoxitin or a penicillin derivative with a β-lactamase inhibitor is more suitable. Alternatively, ertapenem can be used for lower GI tract surgery. The surgeon gives a preoperative dose, intraoperative doses approximately 4 hours apart, and two postoperative doses appropriately spaced. The timing of administration of prophylactic antibiotics is critical. To be most effective, the antibiotic is administered intravenously within 30 minutes before the incision so that therapeutic tissue levels have developed when the wound is created and exposed to bacterial contamination. Usually, the period of anesthesia induction, preparation, and draping is adequate to allow tissue levels to build up to therapeutic levels before the incision is made. Of equal importance is ensuring that prophylactic antibiotics are not administered for extended periods postoperatively. Extensive antibiotic use in the prophylactic setting invites the development of drug-resistant organisms as well as serious complications, such as *Clostridium difficile*–associated colitis.

At the time of surgery, the operating surgeon plays a major role in reducing or minimizing the presence of postoperative wound infections. The surgeon must be attentive to his or her personal hygiene (hand scrubbing) as well as that of the entire team. In addition, the surgeon must ensure that the patient undergoes thorough skin preparation with appropriate antiseptic solutions and is draped in a sterile, careful fashion. During the operation, the following steps have a positive impact on outcome:

1. Careful handling of tissues
2. Meticulous dissection, hemostasis, and débridement of devitalized tissue
3. Compulsive control of all intraluminal contents
4. Preservation of blood supply of the operated organs
5. Elimination of any foreign body from the wound
6. Maintenance of strict asepsis by the operating team (e.g., no holes in gloves; avoidance of the use of contaminated instruments; avoidance of environmental contamination, such as debris falling from overhead)
7. Thorough drainage and irrigation with warm saline of any pockets of purulence in the wound
8. Ensuring that the patient is kept in a euthermic state, is well monitored, and is fluid-resuscitated
9. Expressing a decision about closing the skin or packing the wound at the end of the procedure

The use of drains for prevention of postoperative wound infections is controversial. In general, there is almost no indication for drains in this setting. However, placing closed suction drains in very deep, large wounds and wounds with large wound flaps to prevent the development of a seroma or hematoma is a worthwhile practice.

Treatment of SSIs depends on the depth of the infection. For superficial and deep SSIs, skin staples are removed over the area of the infection, and a cotton-tipped applicator may be easily passed into the wound, with efflux of purulent material and pus. The wound is gently explored with the cotton-tipped applicator or a finger to determine whether the fascia or muscle tissue is involved. If the fascia is intact, débridement of any nonviable tissue is performed; the wound is irrigated with normal saline solution and packed to its base with saline-moistened gauze to allow healing of the wound from the base anteriorly, preventing premature skin closure. If widespread cellulitis or significant signs of infection (e.g., fever, tachycardia) are noted, administration of IV antibiotics must be considered. Empirical therapy is started and tailored according to culture and sensitivity data. The choice of empirical antibiotics is based on the most likely culprit, including the possibility of MRSA. MRSA is treated with vancomycin, linezolid, or clindamycin. Cultures are not routinely performed except for patients who will be treated with antibiotics so that resistant organisms can be treated adequately. However, if the fascia has separated or purulent material appears to be coming from deep to the fascia, there is concern about dehiscence or an intra-abdominal abscess that may require drainage or possibly a reoperation.

Wound cultures are controversial. If the wound is small, superficial, and not associated with cellulitis or tissue necrosis, cultures may be unnecessary. However, if fascial dehiscence and a more complex infection are present, a culture is sent. A deep SSI associated with grayish, dishwater-colored fluid and frank necrosis of the fascial layer raise suspicion for the presence of a necrotizing type of infection. The presence of crepitus in any surgical wound or gram-positive rods (or both) suggests the possibility of infection with *C. perfringens*. Rapid and expeditious surgical débridement is indicated in these settings.

Most postoperative infections are treated with healing by secondary intention, allowing the wound to heal from the base anteriorly, with epithelialization being the final event. In some cases, when there is a question about the amount of contamination, delayed primary closure may be considered. In this setting, close observation of the wound for 5 days may be followed by closure of the skin or negative-pressure wound therapy if the wound looks clean and the patient is otherwise doing well.

COMPLICATIONS OF THERMAL REGULATION

Hypothermia

Causes

Optimal function of physiologic systems in the body occurs within a narrow range of core temperatures. A 2° C decrease in body temperature or a 3° C increase signifies a health emergency that is life-threatening and requires immediate intervention. Hypothermia can result from numerous mechanisms preoperatively, intraoperatively, or postoperatively. A trauma patient with injuries in a cold environment can experience significant hypothermia, and paralysis can lead to hypothermia because of loss of the shiver mechanism.

Hypothermia develops in patients undergoing rapid resuscitation with cool IV fluids, transfusions, or intracavitary irrigation with cold irrigant and in patients undergoing a prolonged surgical procedure with low ambient room temperature and a large, exposed operative area subjected to significant evaporative cooling. Almost all anesthetics impair thermoregulation and render the patient susceptible to hypothermia in the typically cool operating room environment.[9] Advanced age and opioid analgesia also reduce perioperative shivering. Propofol causes vasodilation and significant redistribution hypothermia. Postoperatively, hypothermia can result from cool ambient room temperature, rapid administration of IV fluids or blood, and failure to keep patients covered when they are only partially responsive. More than 80% of elective operative procedures are associated with a decrease in body temperature, and 50% of trauma patients are hypothermic on arrival in the operating suite.

Presentation

Hypothermia is uncomfortable because of the intense cold sensation and shivering. It may also be associated with profound effects on the cardiovascular system, coagulation, wound healing, and infection. A core temperature lower than 35° C after surgery triggers a significant peripheral sympathetic nervous system response, consisting of an increased norepinephrine level, vasoconstriction, and elevated arterial blood pressure. Patients in shock or with a severe illness often have associated vasoconstriction that results in poor perfusion of peripheral organs and tissues, an effect accentuated by hypothermia. In a high-risk patient, a core temperature lower than 35° C is associated with a twofold to threefold increase in the incidence of early postoperative ischemia and a similar increase in the incidence of ventricular tachyarrhythmia. Hypothermia also impairs platelet function and reduces the activity of coagulation factors, resulting in an increased risk for bleeding. Hypothermia results in impaired macrophage function, reduced tissue oxygen tension, and impaired collagen deposition, which predisposes wounds to poor healing and infection. Other complications of hypothermia include a relative diuresis, compromised hepatic function, and some neurologic manifestations. Similarly, the patient's ability to manage acid-base abnormalities is impaired. In severe cases, the patient can have significant cardiac slowing and may be comatose, with low blood pressure, bradycardia, and a very low respiratory rate.

Treatment

Prevention of hypothermia entails monitoring core temperature, especially in patients undergoing body cavity surgery or surgery lasting longer than 1 hour, children, older adults, and patients in whom general epidural anesthesia is being conducted.[9] Sites of monitoring include pulmonary artery blood, tympanic membrane, esophagus and pharynx, rectum, and urinary bladder. Significant evaporative cooling can occur while the patient is being anesthetized and during skin preparation; the patient is kept warm by increasing the ambient temperature and using heated humidifiers and warmed IV fluid. After the patient is draped, the room temperature can be lowered to a more comfortable setting. A forced-air warming device that provides active cutaneous warming is placed on the patient. Passive surface warming is ineffective in conserving heat. There is some evidence that a considerable amount of heat is lost through the head of the patient, so simply covering the patient's head during surgery may prevent significant heat loss.

In the perioperative period, mild hypothermia is common, and patients usually shiver because the anesthesia impairs thermoregulation. However, many patients who shiver after anesthesia are hypothermic. Treatment of hypothermia with forced-air warming systems and radiant heaters also reduces shivering.[9] In a severely hypothermic patient who does not require immediate operative intervention, attention must be directed toward rewarming by the following methods:

1. Immediate placement of warm blankets as well as currently available forced-air warming devices
2. Infusion of blood and IV fluids through a warming device
3. Heating and humidifying inhalational gases
4. Peritoneal lavage with warmed fluids
5. Rewarming infusion devices with an arteriovenous system
6. In rare cases, cardiopulmonary bypass

Special attention must be paid to cardiac monitoring during the rewarming process because cardiac irritability may be a significant problem. Similarly, acid-base disturbances must be aggressively corrected while the patient is being rewarmed. In the operating room, measures noted earlier to keep the patient warm are applied.

Malignant Hyperthermia

Causes

Malignant hyperthermia (MH) is a life-threatening hypermetabolic crisis manifested during or after exposure to a triggering general anesthetic in susceptible individuals. It is estimated that MH occurs in 1 in 30,000 to 50,000 adults. Mortality from MH has decreased to less than 10% in the last 15 years as a result of improved monitoring standards that allow early detection of MH, availability of dantrolene, and increased use of susceptibility testing.

Susceptibility to MH is inherited as an autosomal dominant disease with variable penetrance. To date, two MH susceptibility genes have been identified in humans, and four have been mapped to specific chromosomes but not definitely identified. The mutation results in altered calcium regulation in skeletal muscle in the form of enhanced efflux of calcium from the sarcoplasmic reticulum into the myoplasm. Halogenated inhalational anesthetic agents (e.g., halothane, enflurane, isoflurane, desflurane, and sevoflurane) and depolarizing muscle relaxants (e.g., succinylcholine, suxamethonium) cause an increase in the myoplasmic Ca^{2+} concentration. When an individual who is susceptible to MH is exposed to a triggering anesthetic, there is abnormal release of Ca^{2+}, which leads to prolonged activation of muscle filaments, culminating in rigidity and hypermetabolism. Uncontrolled glycolysis and aerobic metabolism give rise to cellular hypoxia, progressive lactic acidosis, and hypercapnia. The continuous muscle activation with adenosine triphosphate breakdown results in excessive generation of heat. If untreated, myocyte death and rhabdomyolysis result in hyperkalemia and myoglobulinuria. Eventually, disseminated coagulopathy, congestive heart failure (CHF), bowel ischemia, and compartment syndrome develop.

Presentation and Management

MH can be prevented by identifying at-risk individuals before surgery. MH susceptibility is suspected preoperatively in a patient with a family history of MH or a personal history of myalgia after exercise, a tendency for the development of fever, muscular disease, and intolerance to caffeine. In these cases, the creatine kinase level is checked, and a caffeine and halothane contraction test (or an in vitro contracture test developed in Europe) may be performed on a muscle biopsy specimen from the thigh.[10] Individuals with MH susceptibility confirmed by abnormal skeletal muscle biopsy findings or individuals with suspected MH susceptibility who decline a contracture test are given a trigger-free anesthetic (e.g., barbiturate, benzodiazepine, opioid, propofol, etomidate, ketamine, nitrous oxide, nondepolarizing neuromuscular blocker).

Individuals with unsuspected MH susceptibility may manifest MH for the first time during or immediately after the administration of a triggering general anesthetic. The clinical manifestations of MH are not uniform and vary in onset and severity. Some patients manifest the abortive form of MH (e.g., tachycardia, arrhythmia, increased temperature, acidosis). Other patients, after intubation with succinylcholine, demonstrate loss of twitches on neuromuscular stimulation and develop muscle rigidity. An inability to open the mouth as a result of masseter muscle spasm is a pathognomonic early sign and indicates susceptibility to MH. Other manifestations include tachypnea, hypercapnia, skin flushing, hypoxemia, hypotension, electrolyte abnormalities, rhabdomyolysis, and hyperthermia.

When MH is suspected or diagnosed, the steps outlined in Box 12-3 are followed. Dantrolene is a muscle relaxant. In the solution form, it is highly irritating to the vein and must be administered in a large vein. When given intravenously, dantrolene blocks up to 75% of skeletal muscle contraction and never causes paralysis. The plasma elimination half-life is 12 hours. Dantrolene is metabolized in the liver to 5-hydroxydantrolene, which also acts as a muscle relaxant. Side effects reported with dantrolene therapy include muscle weakness, phlebitis, respiratory failure, GI discomfort, hepatotoxicity, dizziness, confusion, and drowsiness. Another agent, azumolene, is 30 times more water-soluble than and equipotent to dantrolene in the treatment of MH; similar to dantrolene, it does not affect the heart. Its main side effect is marked pulmonary hypertension. However, azumolene is not in clinical use at this time.

Postoperative Fever

Causes

One of the most concerning clinical findings in a patient postoperatively is the development of fever. Fever is an increase in core temperature, the modulation of which is managed by the anterior hypothalamus. Fever may result from bacterial invasion or bacterial toxins, which stimulate the production of cytokines. Trauma (including surgery) and critical illness also invoke a cytokine response. Cytokines are low-molecular-weight proteins that act in an autocrine, paracrine, or endocrine fashion to influence a broad range of cellular functions and exhibit proinflammatory and anti-inflammatory effects. The inflammatory response results in the production of various mediators that induce a febrile inflammatory response, also known as systemic inflammatory response syndrome.[11] Fever in the postoperative period may be the result of an infection or caused by systemic inflammatory response syndrome. Fever after surgery is reported to occur in two thirds of patients, and infection is the cause of fever in approximately one third of cases. Numerous disease states can cause fever in the postoperative period (Table 12-5).

The most common infections are health care–associated infections—SSI, urinary tract infection (UTI), intravascular catheter–related bloodstream infection (CR-BSI), and pneumonia. UTI is a common postoperative event and a significant source of morbidity in postsurgical patients. A major predisposing factor is the presence of a urinary catheter; the risk increases with increased duration of catheterization (>2 days). Endogenous bacteria (colonic flora, most common *E. coli*) are the most common source of catheter-related UTI in patients with short-term catheterization. Additional bacteria are found with prolonged catheterization. In a critically ill surgical patient, candiduria accounts for approximately 10% of nosocomial UTIs. The presence of an indwelling catheter, diabetes mellitus, use of antibiotics, advanced age, and underlying anatomic urologic abnormalities are risk factors for candiduria.[12]

The use of central venous catheters carries a risk of CR-BSI that increases hospital stay and morbidity and mortality. The infections are preventable and are considered a "never" complication by the Centers of Medicare and Medicaid Services.[13] CR-BSI results from microorganisms that colonize the hubs or from

BOX 12-3 Management of Malignant Hyperthermia

Discontinue the triggering anesthetic.
Hyperventilate the patient with 100% oxygen.
Administer alternative anesthesia.
Terminate surgery.
Give dantrolene, 2.5 mg/kg, as a bolus and repeat every 5 minutes, then 1 to 2 mg/kg/hr until normalization or disappearance of symptoms.
Check and monitor arterial blood gas and creatine kinase, electrolyte, lactate, and myoglobin levels.
Monitor the ECG, vital signs, and urine output.
Adjunctive and supportive measures are carried out:

- Volatile vaporizers are removed from the anesthesia machine.
- Carbon dioxide canisters, bellows, and gas hoses are changed.
- Surface cooling is achieved with ice packs and core cooling with cool parenteral fluids.
- Acidosis is monitored and treated with sodium bicarbonate.
- Arrhythmias are controlled with beta blockers or lidocaine.
- Urine output more than 2 mL/kg/hr is promoted; furosemide (Lasix) or mannitol and an infusion of insulin and glucose (0.2 U/kg in a 50% glucose solution) are given for hyperkalemia, hypercalcemia, and myoglobulinuria.

The patient is transferred to the ICU to monitor for recurrence.

ECG, electrocardiogram; *ICU*, intensive care unit.

TABLE 12-5 Causes of Postoperative Fever

INFECTIOUS	NONINFECTIOUS
Abscess	Acute hepatic necrosis
Acalculous cholecystitis	Adrenal insufficiency
Bacteremia	Allergic reaction
Decubitus ulcers	Atelectasis
Device-related infections	Dehydration
Empyema	Drug reaction
Endocarditis	Head injury
Fungal sepsis	Hepatoma
Hepatitis	Hyperthyroidism
Meningitis	Lymphoma
Osteomyelitis	MI
Pseudomembranous colitis	Pancreatitis
Parotitis	Pheochromocytoma
Perineal infections	Pulmonary embolus
Peritonitis	Retroperitoneal hematoma
Pharyngitis	Solid organ hematoma
Pneumonia	Subarachnoid hemorrhage
Retained foreign body	Systemic inflammatory response syndrome
Sinusitis	Thrombophlebitis
Soft tissue infection	Transfusion reaction
Tracheobronchitis	Withdrawal syndromes
UTI	Wound infection

MI, myocardial infarction; *UTI*, urinary tract infection.

contamination of the injection site of the central venous catheter (intraluminal source) or skin surrounding the insertion site (extraluminal source). Coagulase-negative staphylococci, hospital-acquired bacteria (e.g., MRSA, multidrug-resistant gram-negative bacilli, fungal species *[Candida albicans]*) are the most common organisms responsible for CR-BSI. *S. aureus* bacteremia is associated with higher mortality and venous thrombosis. Metastatic infections (endocarditis) are uncommon but represent a serious complication of CR-BSI. Risk factors for bloodstream infection include the duration of central venous catheter placement, patient location (outpatient versus inpatient), type of catheter, number of lumens and manipulations daily, emergent placement, need for total parenteral nutrition (TPN), presence of unnecessary connectors, and whether best care practices are followed.[14]

Presentation and Management

In evaluating a patient with fever, one has to take into consideration the type of surgery performed, immune status of the patient, underlying primary disease process, duration of hospital stay, and epidemiology of hospital infections.

High fever that fluctuates or is sustained and that occurs 5 to 8 days after surgery is more worrisome than fever that occurs early postoperatively. In the first 48 to 72 hours after abdominal surgery, atelectasis is often believed to be the cause of the fever. Occasionally, clostridial or streptococcal SSIs can manifest as fever within the first 72 hours of surgery. Temperatures that are elevated 5 to 8 days postoperatively demand immediate attention and, at times, intervention. Evaluation involves studying the six "W's": wind (lungs), wound, water (urinary tract), waste (lower GI tract), wonder drug (e.g., antibiotics), and walker (e.g., thrombosis). The patient's symptoms usually indicate the organ system involved with infection; cough and productive sputum suggest pneumonia, and dysuria and frequency indicate UTI. Watery foul-smelling diarrhea develops as a result of infection with *C. difficile,* pain in the calf may be caused by deep vein thrombosis (DVT), and flank pain may be caused by pyelonephritis. Physical examination may show SSI; phlebitis; tenderness on palpation of the abdomen, flank, or calf; or cellulitis at the site of a central venous catheter.

Complete blood count, urinalysis and culture, radiograph of the chest, and blood culture are essential initial tests. A chest radiograph may show a progressive infiltrate suggestive of the presence of pneumonia. Urinalysis showing more than 10^5 colony-forming units (CFU)/mL in a noncatheterized patient and more than 10^3 CFU/mL in a catheterized patient indicates UTI. The diagnosis of CR-BSI is based on culture data because physical examination is usually unrevealing. There is no gold standard for how to use blood cultures. Two simultaneous blood cultures or paired blood cultures (i.e., simultaneous peripheral and central blood cultures) are commonly used. Peripheral blood cultures showing bacteremia and isolation of 15 CFUs or 10^2 CFUs from an IV catheter indicate the presence of CR-BSI. In tunneled catheters, a quantitative colony count that is 5-fold to 10-fold higher in cultures drawn through the central venous catheter is predictive of CR-BSI. If paired cultures are obtained, positive culture more than 2 hours before peripheral culture indicates the presence of CR-BSI. After removal of the catheter, the tip may be sent for quantitative culture. Serial blood cultures and a transesophageal echocardiogram are obtained in patients with *S. aureus* bacteremia and valvular heart disease, prosthetic valve, or new onset of heart murmur. Patients who continue to have fever, slow clinical progress, and no discernible external source may require computed tomography (CT) of the abdomen to look for an intra-abdominal source of infection.

Prevention of UTI starts with minimizing the duration of catheterization and maintenance of a closed drainage system. When prolonged catheterization is required, changing the catheter before blockage occurs is recommended because the catheter serves as a site for pathogens to create a biofilm. The efficacy of strategies to prevent or delay the formation of a biofilm, such as the use of silver alloy or impregnated catheters and the use of protamine sulfate and chlorhexidine, in reducing catheter-related UTIs has yet to be established.[15]

Most, if not all, CR-BSIs are preventable by adopting maximal barrier precautions and infection control practice during insertion. Educational programs that stress best practice that target the individuals placing the catheter and the individuals responsible for maintenance of the catheter are important. Removal of catheters when they are not needed is paramount. On placing the catheter, there must be strict adherence to aseptic technique, the same as in the operating room—hand hygiene, skin antisepsis, full barrier precaution, and stopping insertion when breaks in sterile technique occur. The subclavian vein is preferable to the jugular and femoral veins. Involvement of a catheter care team for proper catheter care after insertion has proven effective in reducing the incidence of CR-BSIs. Antiseptic-impregnated and antibiotic-impregnated catheters decrease catheter colonization and CR-BSIs, but their routine use is not recommended.

Treatment

Management of postoperative fevers is dictated by the results of a careful workup. Management of the elevated temperature itself is controversial. Although the fever may not be life-threatening, the patient is usually uncomfortable. Attempts to bring the temperature down with antipyretics are recommended. If pneumonia is suspected, empirical broad-spectrum antibiotic therapy is started and then altered according to culture results.

UTI is treated with removal or replacement of the catheter with a new one. In patients with systemic illness, broad-spectrum antibiotics are started because most offending organisms exhibit resistance to several antibiotics and then tailored according to culture and susceptibility results. In patients with asymptomatic bacteriuria, antibiotics are recommended for immunocompromised patients, patients undergoing urologic surgery, patients undergoing implantation of a prosthesis, or patients with infections caused by strains with a high incidence of bacteremia. Patients with candiduria are managed in a similar fashion. The availability of fluconazole, a less toxic antifungal than amphotericin B has encouraged clinicians to use it more frequently.

The treatment of CR-BSI entails removal of the catheter with adjunctive antibiotic therapy. A nontunneled catheter can be removed easily after establishing an alternative venous access. Single-agent therapy is sufficient and usually involves vancomycin, linezolid, or empirical coverage of gram-negative bacilli and *Candida* spp. in patients with severe sepsis or immunosuppression. Treatment is continued for 10 to 14 days. For patients with septic thrombosis or endocarditis, treatment is continued for 4 to 6 weeks. Catheter salvage is indicated in patients with tunneled catheters that are risky to remove or replace or in patients with coagulase-negative staphylococci who have no evidence of metastatic disease or severe sepsis, do not have tunnel infection, or do not have persistent bacteremia. Catheter salvage is achieved by antibiotic lock therapy whereby the catheter is filled with antibiotic solution for several hours.

RESPIRATORY COMPLICATIONS

General Considerations

Numerous factors contribute to abnormal pulmonary physiology after an operative procedure. First, loss of functional residual capacity is present in almost all patients. This loss may be the result of a multitude of problems, including abdominal distention, painful upper abdominal incision, obesity, strong smoking history with associated chronic obstructive pulmonary disease, prolonged supine positioning, and fluid overload leading to pulmonary edema. Almost all patients who undergo an abdominal or thoracic incision have a significant alteration in their breathing pattern. Vital capacity may be reduced 50% of normal for the first 2 days after surgery for reasons that are unclear. The use of narcotics substantially inhibits the respiratory drive, and anesthetics may take some time to wear off. Most patients who have respiratory problems postoperatively have mild to moderate problems that can be managed with aggressive pulmonary toilet. However, in some patients, severe postoperative respiratory failure develops; this may require intubation and ultimately may be life-threatening.

Two types of respiratory failure are commonly described. Type I, or hypoxic, failure results from abnormal gas exchange at the alveolar level. This type is characterized by a low partial arterial oxygen pressure (PaO_2) with a normal partial arterial carbon dioxide pressure ($PaCO_2$). Such hypoxemia is associated with ventilation-perfusion ($\dot{V}/\dot{Q}$) mismatching and shunting. Clinical conditions associated with type I failure include pulmonary edema and sepsis. Type II respiratory failure is associated with hypercapnia and is characterized by a low PaO_2 and high $PaCO_2$. These patients are unable to eliminate carbon dioxide adequately. This condition is often associated with excessive narcotic use, increased carbon dioxide production, altered respiratory dynamics, and adult respiratory distress syndrome (ARDS). The overall incidence of pulmonary complications exceeds 25% in surgical patients. Of all postoperative deaths, 25% are caused by pulmonary complications, and pulmonary complications are associated with 25% of the other lethal complications. It is of critical importance that the surgeon anticipate and prevent the occurrence of serious respiratory complications.

One of the most important elements of prophylaxis is careful preoperative screening of patients. Most patients have no pulmonary history and need no formal preoperative evaluation. However, all patients with a history of heavy smoking, maintenance on home oxygen, inability to walk one flight of stairs without severe respiratory compromise, or major lung resection and older patients who are malnourished must be carefully screened with pulmonary function tests. Similarly, patients managed by long-term bronchodilator therapy for asthma or other pulmonary conditions need to be assessed carefully. Although the value of perioperative assessment is controversial, most careful clinicians study a high-risk pulmonary patient before making an operative decision. The assessment may start with posteroanterior and lateral chest radiographs to evaluate the appearance of the lungs. This assessment serves as a baseline if the patient should have problems postoperatively.

Similarly, a patient with polycythemia or chronic respiratory acidosis warrants careful assessment. A room temperature arterial blood gas analysis is carried out in high-risk patients. Any patient with a PaO_2 less than 60 mm Hg is at increased risk. If $PaCO_2$ is more than 45 to 50 mm Hg, perioperative morbidity might be anticipated. Spirometry is a simple test that high-risk patients undergo before surgery. Probably the most important parameter in spirometry is the forced expiratory volume in 1 second (FEV_1). Studies have demonstrated that any patient with FEV_1 greater than 2 liters is unlikely to have serious pulmonary problems. Conversely, patients with FEV_1 less than 50% of the predicted value are likely to have exertional dyspnea. If bronchodilator therapy demonstrates an improvement in breathing patterns by 15% or more, bronchodilation is considered. Consultation with the patient includes a discussion about cessation of cigarette smoking 48 hours before the operative procedure and a careful discussion about the importance of pulmonary toilet after the operative procedure.

Atelectasis and Pneumonia

The most common postoperative respiratory complication is atelectasis. As a result of the anesthetic, abdominal incision, and postoperative narcotics, the alveoli in the periphery collapse, and a pulmonary shunt may occur. If appropriate attention is not directed to aggressive pulmonary toilet with the initial symptoms, the alveoli remain collapsed, and a buildup of secretions occurs and becomes secondarily infected with bacteria, resulting in pneumonia. The risk appears to be particularly high in patients who are heavy smokers, are obese, and have copious pulmonary secretions.

Pneumonia is the most common nosocomial infection occurring in hospitalized patients. Pneumonia occurring more than 48 hours after admission and without antecedent signs of infection is referred to as hospital-acquired pneumonia. Aspiration of oropharyngeal secretions is a significant contributing factor in development of hospital-acquired pneumonia. Extended intubation results in ventilator-associated pneumonia—pneumonia occurring 48 hours after but within 72 hours of the initiation of ventilation. Health care–associated pneumonia refers to pneumonia occurring in patients who were hospitalized in the last 90 days; patients in nursing facilities or frequenting a hemodialysis unit; and patients who have received recent antibiotics, chemotherapy, or wound care. Although some consider hospital-acquired pneumonia and health care–associated pneumonia to be the same disease process because both have the same prevalent organisms, the prognosis is different. Hospital-acquired pneumonia arising early (<5 days) has a better prognosis than hospital-acquired pneumonia arising late (>5 days). Numerous factors are associated with increased risk for pneumonia, including depressed immune status; concomitant disease; poor nutritional status; increased length of hospital stay; smoking; advanced age; uremia; alcohol consumption; prior antibiotic therapy; presence of an endotracheal, nasogastric (NG), or enteric tube; and proton pump inhibitor (PPI) therapy. Used to prevent stress ulceration, PPI therapy increases colonization of the stomach with pathogenic bacteria that can increase the risk of ventilator-associated pneumonia. Tubes traversing the aerodigestive tract serve as conduits for bacteria to migrate to the lower respiratory tract.[16]

The most common pathogens encountered in patients with hospital-acquired pneumonia depend on prior antibiotic therapy. In patients with early hospital-acquired pneumonia and no prior antibiotic therapy, the most common organisms are *Streptococcus pneumoniae* (colonizes upper airway), *Haemophilus influenzae,* Enterobacteriaceae spp. (*E. coli, Klebsiella* spp., and *Enterobacter* spp.), and *S. aureus* (mostly MRSA). Patients with early hospital-acquired pneumonia and recent antibiotic therapy and patients with late hospital-acquired pneumonia also have gram-negative bacilli involved. The bacteria are occasionally resistant to first-generation cephalosporins. The organisms in patients with late-onset hospital-acquired pneumonia and prior history of antibiotics exhibit multidrug resistance (*P. aeruginosa, Acinetobacter baumannii,* and MRSA).

Diagnosis

The most common cause of a postoperative fever in the first 48 hours after the procedure is atelectasis. Patients present with a low-grade fever, malaise, and diminished breath sounds in the lower lung fields. Frequently, the patient is uncomfortable from the fever but has no other overt pulmonary symptoms. Atelectasis is so common postoperatively that a formal workup is not usually required. With the use of incentive spirometry, deep breathing, and coughing, most cases of atelectasis resolve without any difficulty. However, if aggressive pulmonary toilet is not instituted or the patient refuses to participate, development of pneumonia is likely. A patient with pneumonia has a high fever and occasional mental confusion, produces a thick secretion with coughing, and shows leukocytosis; a chest radiograph reveals infiltrates. If the patient is not expeditiously diagnosed and treated, this condition may progress rapidly to respiratory failure and require intubation. Concurrently with the initiation of aggressive pulmonary toilet, induced sputum for culture and sensitivity should be sent immediately to the laboratory. Quantitative cultures of the lower airways obtained by blind tracheobronchial aspiration, bronchoscopically guided sampling (bronchoalveolar lavage), or protected specimen brush allow more targeted antibiotic therapy and, most importantly, decrease antibiotic use. Although pneumonia acquired in the hospital affects only 5% of all patients, the process may rapidly progress to frank respiratory failure requiring intubation, particularly in older patients.

Treatment

To prevent atelectasis and pneumonia, smokers are encouraged to stop smoking for at least 1 week before surgery, and the treatment of patients with chronic obstructive pulmonary disease, asthma, and CHF is optimized. Adequate pain control and proper pulmonary hygiene are important in the postoperative period. A patient-controlled analgesia device seems to be associated with better pulmonary toilet, as does the use of an epidural infusion catheter, particularly in patients with epigastric incisions. Encouraging the patient to use the incentive spirometer and cough while applying counterpressure with a pillow on the abdominal incision site is most helpful. Rarely, other modalities such as intermittent positive-pressure breathing and chest physiotherapy may be required. Patients on the ventilator are best kept in a semirecumbent position and subjected to proper oral hygiene. Chlorhexidine rinse or nasal gel has been shown to reduce the rate of ventilator-associated pneumonia. Treatment with sucralfate as opposed to a PPI for stress ulcer prophylaxis may be considered for patients not at high risk for GI bleeding. Proper endotracheal tube care, elimination of secretions pooling around the endotracheal cuff, frequent suctioning with a closed suction technique, and use of protocols designed to minimize mechanical ventilation can lead to decreased ventilator-associated pneumonia. After the diagnosis is made, while awaiting culture results, treatment with empirical antibiotic therapy is associated with decreased mortality. The choice of antimicrobial agent depends on the patient's risk factors, length of hospital stay, duration of mechanical ventilation, prior antibiotic therapy and culture results, and immunosuppression.

Aspiration Pneumonitis and Aspiration Pneumonia

Causes

Aspiration of oropharyngeal or gastric contents into the respiratory tract is a serious complication of surgery. Aspiration pneumonitis (Mendelson syndrome) is acute lung injury that results from the inhalation of regurgitated gastric contents, whereas aspiration pneumonia results from the inhalation of oropharyngeal secretions that are colonized by pathogenic bacteria. Although there is some overlap between the two disease entities with regard to predisposing factors, their clinicopathologic features are distinct.

Factors that predispose patients to regurgitation and aspiration include impairment of the esophageal sphincters (upper and lower) and laryngeal reflexes, altered GI motility, and absence of preoperative fasting. Many iatrogenic maneuvers place the patient at increased risk for aspiration in a hospital setting. In the perioperative period, aspiration is more likely in patients undergoing urgent surgery, in patients with altered levels of consciousness, and in patients with GI and airway problems. Trauma patients and patients with peritonitis and bowel obstruction may have a depressed level of consciousness and airway reflexes, a full stomach as a result of a recent meal or gastric stasis, or GI pathology that predisposes to retrograde emptying of intestinal contents into the stomach. Patients with depressed levels of consciousness as a result of high doses of narcotics and patients who have sustained cerebrovascular accidents are obtunded and have neurologic dysphagia and dysfunction of the gastroesophageal junction. Anesthetic drugs reduce esophageal sphincter tone and depress the patient's level of consciousness. Diabetics have gastroparesis and gastric stasis. Patients with an increased bacterial load in the oropharynx and depressed defense mechanisms as a result of an altered level of consciousness are at risk for aspiration pneumonia.

Older adults are particularly susceptible to oropharyngeal aspiration because of an increased incidence of dysphagia and poor oral hygiene. Patients with NG tubes or who are debilitated are also at risk for aspiration because they have difficulty swallowing and clearing their airway. The risk for aspiration pneumonia is similar in patients receiving feeding via NG, nasoenteric, and gastrostomy tubes; patients receiving nutrition via a gastrostomy tube frequently have scintigraphic evidence of aspiration of gastric contents. Critically ill patients are at an increased risk for aspiration and aspiration pneumonia because they are in a supine position, have an NG tube in place, exhibit gastroesophageal reflux even with the absence of an NG tube, and have altered GI motility. Prophylactic histamine 2 (H_2) receptor antagonists or PPIs that increase gastric pH and allow the gastric contents to become colonized by pathogenic organisms, tracheostomy, reintubation, and previous antibiotic exposure are other factors associated with an increased risk for health care–related pneumonia. The risk of aspiration is high after extubation because of the residual effect of sedation, NG tube, and oropharyngeal dysfunction.

The pathophysiology of aspiration pneumonitis is related to the pulmonary intake of gastric contents at a low pH associated with particulate matter. The severity of lung injury increases as the volume of aspirate increases and its pH decreases. The process often progresses rapidly, may require intubation soon after the injury occurs, and later sets the stage for bacterial infection. The infection is refractory to management because of the combination of infection occurring in an injured field. The pathophysiology of aspiration pneumonia is related to bacteria gaining access to the lungs.

Presentation and Diagnosis

A patient with aspiration pneumonitis often has associated vomiting and may have received general anesthesia or had an NG tube placed. The patient may be obtunded or have altered levels of consciousness. Initially, the patient may have associated wheezing and labored respiration. Many patients who aspirate gastric contents have a cough or a wheeze. However, some patients have silent aspiration suggested by an infiltrate on a chest radiograph or decreased PaO_2. Other patients have cough, shortness of breath, and wheezing that progress to pulmonary edema and ARDS. Among most patients with aspiration pneumonia, in a susceptible patient, the condition is diagnosed after a chest radiograph shows an infiltrate in the posterior segments of the upper lobes and the apical segments of the lower lobes.

Treatment

Prevention of aspiration in patients undergoing surgery is achieved by instituting measures that reduce gastric contents, minimize regurgitation, and protect the airway. For adults, a period of no oral intake, usually 6 hours after a night meal, 4 hours after clear liquids, and a longer period for diabetics, is necessary to reduce gastric contents before elective surgery.[17] Routine use of H_2 antagonists or PPIs to reduce gastric acidity and volume has not been shown to be effective in reducing the mortality and morbidity associated with aspiration and is not recommended. When a difficult airway is encountered, awake fiberoptic intubation is performed. In emergency situations in patients with a potentially full stomach, preoxygenation is accomplished without lung inflation, and intubation is performed after applying cricoid pressure during rapid-sequence induction. In the postoperative period, identification of an older or overly sedated patient or a patient whose condition is deteriorating mandates instituting maneuvers to protect the patient's airway. Postoperatively, it is important to avoid the overuse of narcotics, encourage the patient to ambulate, and feed cautiously a patient who is obtunded, older, or debilitated.

A patient who experiences aspiration of gastric contents needs to be placed on oxygen immediately and have a chest radiograph to confirm clinical suspicions. A diffuse interstitial pattern is usually seen bilaterally and is often described as bilateral, fluffy infiltrates. Close surveillance of the patient is essential. If the patient is maintaining oxygen saturation via a face mask without excessively high work of breathing, intubation may not be required. However, if the patient's oxygenation deteriorates or the patient is obtunded, and the work of breathing increases, as manifested by an increased respiratory rate, prompt intubation must be accomplished. After intubation for suspected aspiration, suctioning the bronchopulmonary tree confirms the diagnosis and removes any particulate matter. Administration of antibiotics shortly after aspiration is controversial except in patients with bowel obstruction or other conditions associated with colonization of gastric contents. Administration of empirical antibiotics is also indicated for a patient with aspiration pneumonitis that does not resolve or improve within 48 hours of aspiration. Corticosteroid administration does not provide any beneficial effects to patients with aspiration pneumonitis. Antibiotic therapy with activity against gram-negative organisms is indicated for patients with aspiration pneumonia.

Pulmonary Edema, Acute Lung Injury, and Adult Respiratory Distress Syndrome

Causes

A wide variety of injuries to the lungs or cardiovascular system, or both, may result in acute respiratory failure. Three of the most common manifestations of acute respiratory failure are pulmonary edema, acute lung injury, and ARDS. The clinician's ability to recognize and distinguish among these conditions is critical because clinical management of these three entities varies considerably.

Pulmonary edema is associated with accumulation of fluid in the alveoli. As a result of the fluid in the lumen of the alveoli, oxygenation cannot take place, and hypoxemia occurs. As a consequence, the patient must increase the work of breathing, including an increased respiratory rate and exaggerated use of the muscles of breathing. Pulmonary edema is usually caused by increased vascular hydrostatic pressure associated with CHF and acute myocardial infarction (MI). It is also commonly associated with fluid overload as a result of overly aggressive resuscitation (Box 12-4).

A consensus conference identified acute lung injury and ARDS as two separate grades of respiratory failure secondary to injury. In contrast to pulmonary edema, which is associated with increased pulmonary capillary wedge pressure (PCWP) and right-sided heart pressure, acute lung injury and ARDS are associated with hypo-oxygenation because of a pathophysiologic inflammatory response that leads to the accumulation of fluid in the alveoli as well as thickening in the space between the capillaries and the alveoli. Acute lung injury is associated with a PaO_2/fraction of inspired oxygen (FIO_2) ratio of less than 300, bilateral infiltrates on chest radiograph, and PCWP less than 18 mm Hg. It tends to be shorter in duration and not as severe. ARDS is associated

BOX 12-4 Conditions Leading to Pulmonary Edema, Acute Lung Injury, and Adult Respiratory Distress Syndrome

Increased Hydrostatic Pressure

Acute left ventricular failure
Chronic CHF
Obstruction of left ventricular outflow tract
Thoracic lymphatic insufficiency
Volume overload

Altered Permeability State

Acute radiation pneumonitis
Aspiration of gastric contents
Drug overdose
Near-drowning
Pancreatitis
Pneumonia
Pulmonary embolus
Shock states
Systemic inflammatory response syndrome and multiorgan failure
Sepsis
Transfusion
Trauma and burns

Mixed or Incompletely Understood Pathogenesis

Hanging injuries
High-altitude pulmonary edema
Narcotic overdose
Neurogenic pulmonary edema
Postextubation obstructive pulmonary edema
Reexpansion pulmonary edema
Tocolytic therapy
Uremia

CHF, congestive heart failure.

with a PaO_2/FIO_2 ratio of less than 200 and has bilateral infiltrates and PCWP less than 18 mm Hg.

Presentation and Management

Patients with pulmonary edema often have a corresponding cardiac history, recent history of massive fluid administration, or both. In the presence of a frankly abnormal chest radiograph, invasive monitoring in the form of a Swan-Ganz catheter for evaluation of PCWP may be indicated. Patients with an elevated PCWP are managed by fluid restriction and aggressive diuresis. Administration of oxygen via face mask in mild cases and intubation in more severe cases is also clinically indicated. In most cases, pulmonary edema resolves quickly after diuresis and fluid restriction.

Patients with acute lung injury and ARDS generally experience tachypnea, dyspnea, and increased work of breathing, as manifested by exaggerated use of the muscles of breathing. Cyanosis is associated with advanced hypoxia and is an emergency. Auscultation of the lung fields reveals poor breath sounds associated with crackles and occasionally with rales. Arterial blood gas analysis reveals the presence of a low PaO_2 and high $PaCO_2$. Administration of oxygen alone does not usually result in improvement of hypoxia.

In patients with impending respiratory failure, including tachypnea, dyspnea, and air hunger, management of acute lung injury and ARDS is initiated by immediate intubation plus careful administration of fluids; invasive monitoring with a Swan-Ganz catheter to assess PCWP and right-sided heart pressure is occasionally helpful. The strategy involves maintaining the patient on the ventilator with assisted breathing while the injured lung heals. A patient with severe acute lung injury or ARDS is initially placed on FIO_2 of 100% and then weaned to 60% as healing occurs. Positive end-expiratory pressure is a valuable addition to ventilator management of patients with this injury. Similarly, tidal volume needs to be 6 to 8 mL/kg, with peak pressure kept at 35 cm H_2O. Tidal volume is set at 10 to 12 mL/kg of body weight, and the respiratory rate is chosen to produce a $PaCO_2$ near 40 mm Hg. In addition, the inspiratory-to-expiratory ratio is set at 1 : 2. Most patients will require heavy sedation and pharmacologic paralysis during the early phases of recuperation.

Careful monitoring of oxygenation, improvement of the respiratory rate with intermittent mandatory ventilation, and general alertness will suggest when the patient is ready to be extubated. Criteria for extubation are listed in Table 12-6.

TABLE 12-6 Criteria for Weaning from the Ventilator

PARAMETER	WEANING CRITERIA
Respiratory rate	<25 breaths/min
PaO_2	>70 mm Hg (FIO_2 of 40%)
$PaCO_2$	<45 mm Hg
Minute ventilation	8-9 liters/min
Tidal volume	5-6 mL/kg
Negative inspiratory force	−25 cm H_2O

FIO_2, fraction of inspired oxygen; *$PaCO_2$*, partial arterial carbon dioxide pressure; *PaO_2*, partial arterial oxygen pressure.

Pulmonary Embolism and Venous Thromboembolism

Causes

VTE comprises DVT and pulmonary embolism (PE). PE is a serious postoperative complication that represents a source of preventable morbidity and mortality in the United States and is responsible for 5% to 10% of all in-hospital deaths. Undiagnosed PE has a hospital mortality rate of 30%, which decreases to 8% if diagnosed and treated appropriately. VTE is caused by a perturbation of the homeostatic coagulation system induced by intimal injury, stasis of blood flow, and a hypercoagulable state. Risk factors for the development of VTE are listed in Table 12-7.[18]

Thrombophilia describes hereditary and acquired biochemical states that predispose to VTE. One in four fatal PE cases occurs in surgical patients. Survivors of VTE are at increased risk for recurrence. The highest risk of VTE occurs in patients hospitalized for surgery. The prevalence of PE in patients with malignancy is 11%. The relative risk of DVT and PE in patients with inflammatory bowel disease is approximately 5% and 3%, respectively.

TABLE 12-7 Risk Factors for Venous Thromboembolism

CATEGORY	FACTORS
General factors	Advanced age
	Hospitalization or nursing home (with or without surgery)
	Indwelling venous catheters
	Neurologic disease (plegia and paresis)
	Cardiomyopathy, MI, or heart failure secondary to valve disease
	Acute pulmonary disease (ARDS and pneumonia)
	Chronic obstructive pulmonary disease
	Varicose veins
Inherited thrombophilia	Protein C deficiency
	Protein S deficiency
	Antithrombin III deficiency
	Dysfibrinogenemia
	Factor V Leiden mutation
	Prothrombin gene mutation
	Hyperhomocysteinemia
	Anticardiolipin antibody
	Paroxysmal nocturnal hemoglobinemia
Acquired thrombophilia	Malignancy
	Inflammatory bowel disease
	Heparin-induced thrombocytopenia
	Trauma
	Major surgery
	Pregnancy/postpartum
	Nephrotic syndrome
	Behçet syndrome
	Systemic lupus erythematosus
	History of VTE

ARDS, adult respiratory distress syndrome; *MI*, myocardial infarction; *VTE*, venous thromboembolism.

In victims of major trauma, the incidence of DVT exceeds 50%, with fatal emboli occurring in 0.4% to 2% of cases. Critically ill patients and patients in the intensive care unit (ICU) have multiple risk factors and are also at higher risk for VTE. Central venous catheter–related thromboses are more common with femoral placement. Thrombosis ranges from 4% to 28% after subclavian vein cannulation and 4% to 33% after internal jugular catheterization. Among patients with subclavian or axillary vein thrombosis, PE is reported in 9.4%.

Most pulmonary emboli originate from an existing DVT in the legs, and the iliofemoral venous system represents the site from which most clinically significant pulmonary emboli arise. Approximately 50% of patients with proximal DVT develop PE. Rare causes of PE include a fat embolus associated with fractures of long bones and air embolism, often related to operative procedures and the presence of central lines.

Presentation and Diagnosis

The physiologic response to PE depends on the size of the thrombus, coexisting cardiopulmonary disease, and various neurohormonal effects. More than 50% of DVTs are silent, and PE may be the first manifestation of the disease. Most symptoms and signs associated with symptomatic PE are nonspecific and may be encountered with other disease states, such as MI, pneumothorax, and pneumonia (Box 12-5). Chest radiograph has limited value in the diagnosis of PE and is mainly used to rule out other causes of a patient's symptoms. Approximately 5% to 10% of patients develop a massive PE that results in hemodynamic instability (hypotension, with or without shock) and death. The probability of an individual having PE (pretest probability) is assessed by the sum of points given to VTE risk factors: the patient's symptoms, signs, and laboratory results (e.g., electrocardiogram [ECG], chest radiograph, and arterial blood gas) most likely to be associated with PE. Using various scoring systems, patients are stratified into low-probability, moderate-probability, and high-probability categories.

Establishing the diagnosis of PE requires confirmatory tests (helical CT scan or pulmonary angiogram) and ancillary tests (venous duplex ultrasound [VUS] and D dimer assay). Helical CT, also known as spiral CT or CT pulmonary angiography, has high specificity (92%) and sensitivity (86%), especially for central PE (main pulmonary artery or subsegmental branches) and has replaced the $\dot{V}/\dot{Q}$ scan as the initial test of choice. In addition to the findings listed in Box 12-5, spiral CT also allows diagnosis of other pulmonary causes of a patient's symptoms. However, the test requires an IV contrast agent; may be unavailable after normal working hours; requires a cooperative patient to avoid artifacts; may miss emboli in subsegmental arteries, which account for 20% of all pulmonary emboli; and may be inconclusive in approximately 10% of cases. Pulmonary angiogram is the gold standard test because it visualizes the arterial tree directly and detects intravascular filling defects. However, it is used less commonly because it is invasive, it requires expertise, and after-hours availability is limited.

BOX 12-5 Symptoms and Signs of Pulmonary Embolism

Pleuritic chest pain*
Sudden dyspnea*
Tachypnea
Hemoptysis*
Tachycardia*
Leg swelling*
Pain on palpation of the leg*
Acute right ventricular dysfunction
Hypoxia
Fourth heart sound*
Loud second pulmonary sound*
Inspiratory crackles*

*More common with pulmonary embolism.

Echocardiography is a rapid, noninvasive, available bedside test that provides quick results in a critically ill or hemodynamically unstable patient. Transthoracic echocardiography shows the hemodynamic consequences of acute ventricular pressure overload—right ventricular dysfunction (hypokinesia and dilation), interventricular septal flattening and paradoxical motion, elevated tricuspid gradient, pulmonary hypertension, and patent foramen ovale.[19] Dysfunction of the right ventricle occurs in 30% to 50% of patients with PE who undergo echocardiography. Transesophageal echocardiography also shows secondary changes in cardiac chamber size and functions caused by hemodynamic effects of PE and may reveal a proximal intrapulmonary or free-floating intracardiac clot. Echocardiography also rules out other causes of shock, such as a pericardial tamponade. Transesophageal echocardiography is not always available and requires specialty training.

VUS of the extremities is used as an indirect test for diagnosing PE. Approximately one third of patients with PE demonstrate lower extremity findings consistent with DVT, and 80% of patients with PE have a DVT on the venogram. D dimer is a degradation product of a cross-linked fibrin blood clot. Levels are typically elevated in patients with acute thromboembolism. Of the many D dimer tests, enzyme-linked immunosorbent assay (ELISA) is the most sensitive, with quick results. A negative test excludes the diagnosis, but a positive test does not rule in the diagnosis.

Based on the pretest clinical probability, a patient suspected to have PE requires a chest radiograph, ECG, arterial blood gas analysis, and D dimer assay. If leg symptoms are present, VUS is performed. If VUS is positive, the patient is considered to have PE and receives anticoagulant medication because treatment is similar to that for PE. If leg symptoms are absent, the spiral CT approach may be used. If the findings on spiral CT are suboptimal or negative and there is a high clinical probability of PE, an angiogram is obtained. This approach is inappropriate for patients with iodinated dye allergy.

In critically ill patients in whom there is a high suspicion for PE and patients with suspected massive PE, the workup depends on their hemodynamic stability. In stable patients, anticoagulation is started if there are no contraindications, VUS is performed, and a spiral CT scan is obtained urgently. In unstable patients, anticoagulation is started, and VUS and echocardiography are performed. If the echocardiographic results are positive, thrombolytic therapy is started; if results are negative, a pulmonary angiogram is obtained.

Treatment

Medications used in the treatment of VTE include heparins, fondaparinux, VKAs, and thrombolytic agents. Heparin prevents the thrombin-mediated conversion of fibrinogen to fibrin and stops propagation of the thrombus. UFH is inexpensive and highly effective, enhances antithrombotic activity of antithrombin III and factor Xa, and has a short plasma half-life. LMWH primarily inactivates factor Xa and has a longer half-life and more predictable anticoagulant property. VKAs (e.g., warfarin) have a delayed onset of action and the potential to interact with other medications. Fondaparinux is a synthetic pentasaccharide that selectively inhibits factor Xa. Thrombolytic agents (e.g., streptokinase, urokinase, recombinant tissue plasminogen activator) are used in the treatment of massive PE.

Treatment of PE starts with prevention. Because most pulmonary emboli originate from existing clots in the deep venous system of the legs in at-risk patients, identifying patients at risk for DVT and applying preventive measures is the only way to decrease VTE-related morbidity and mortality. The intensity of prophylaxis must match the risk for VTE and potential complications of the medication (e.g., bleeding, heparin-induced thrombocytopenia). According to the American College of Chest Physicians, assessment of patients into low-risk, moderate-risk, and high-risk categories for VTE is based on the type of surgery performed, patient mobility, risk of bleeding, and VTE risk based on the presence of additional risk factors.[20] Age is a significant risk factor, with the risk doubling with each decade beyond age 40 years. Most hospitalized patients have at least one risk factor for VTE, and approximately 50% have more than three risk factors. Pharmacologic prophylaxis is an accepted and effective strategy.[21] In critically ill patients, heparin is first-line prophylaxis. Prophylaxis is achieved with the administration of low-dose UFH given subcutaneously every 8 hours or LMWH given as a daily dose. Studies have suggested that LMWH is more effective prophylaxis than low-dose UFH in critically ill patients and is associated with a reduced risk of major hemorrhage. Overt bleeding and thrombocytopenia are contraindications to chemical prophylaxis. In patients undergoing surgery, low-dose UFH is administered (5000 U, 3 to 4 hours preoperatively and then every 8 hours). Fondaparinux has emerged as an alternative prophylactic after major orthopedic surgery. Nonpharmacologic prophylaxis can be achieved with elastic stockings, graduated compression stockings, intermittent pneumatic compression devices, or venous foot pumps. Compression devices are not associated with bleeding. They produce a satisfactory reduction in risk for DVT in high-risk surgical patients. However, little is known about their efficacy as sole prophylaxis in critically ill patients, and they may be most beneficial in combination with pharmacologic prophylaxis in the subset of high-risk patients or solely in patients for whom the risk of bleeding is high. The presence of leg ulcers and peripheral vascular disease precludes the use of mechanical devices.

Anticoagulation is the standard of care treatment for VTE. It prevents clot propagation and allows endogenous fibrinolytic activity to dissolve existing thrombi, a process that occurs over weeks and months. Incomplete resolution is common and predisposes to recurrent VTE. The initial treatment is with LMWH, UFH, or fondaparinux, followed by VKA, which is administered on the same day as LMWH or UFH, with overlap for 5 days or longer until the target INR is achieved. In patients with VTE and active cancer, anticoagulation is continued indefinitely. Surgical patients within 24 hours of surgery may be considered for a retrievable inferior vena cava filter until anticoagulation is initiated. In patients with a contraindication to anticoagulation, placement of an inferior vena cava filter protects against PE.

UFH is given intravenously (a weight-adjusted bolus of 70 U/kg is followed by 1000 U/hr) to achieve a partial thromboplastin time 1.5 to 2 times the control value. Activated partial thromboplastin time is determined 6 hours after the loading dose and then on a daily basis, and the dose of heparin is adjusted accordingly. UFH is easily reversible and the agent of choice. LMWH is given subcutaneously once or twice daily (enoxaparin, 1.5 mg/kg/day, or dalteparin, 10,000 to 18,000 U/day, depending on weight). Monitoring of LMWH is unnecessary. UFH and LMWH may be associated with heparin-induced thrombocytopenia, and the platelet count is monitored between days 3 and 5. Warfarin is given orally, and this therapy is allowed to overlap with heparin therapy until the INR is therapeutic for 2 consecutive days before heparin is discontinued. Therapy is continued for more than 3 months, with the goal to reach an INR of 2.5.

In massive PE, the goal of therapy is to maintain hemodynamic stability, enhance coronary flow, and minimize right ventricular ischemia. When massive PE is suspected, resuscitation is initiated, oxygen is administered, and IV UFH therapy is started. In hemodynamically unstable patients, IV vasoactive medications are required. Thrombolytic therapy, if not contraindicated, has the advantage of dissolving the clot quickly, with rapid improvement in pulmonary perfusion, hemodynamic alterations, gas exchange, and right ventricular function. The role of surgical embolectomy is controversial. The transcatheter technique (with or without low-dose thrombolytic therapy) is another therapeutic approach. Placement of an inferior vena cava filter reduces the risk for recurrence of PE. Novel anticoagulants under investigation include factor Xa inhibitors (direct inhibitor [hypermethylated derivative of fondaparinux with a long half-life given intravenously or subcutaneously] or indirect inhibitor mediated by antithrombin [given orally or parenterally]) and direct thrombin inhibitors.

CARDIAC COMPLICATIONS

Postoperative Hypertension

Causes

Hypertension is a serious problem that can cause devastating complications in the preoperative, intraoperative, and postoperative periods. Perioperative hypertension (or hypotension) occurs in 25% of patients undergoing surgery. The risk of hypertension is related to the type of surgery performed and the presence of perioperative hypertension. Cardiovascular, thoracic, and intra-abdominal procedures are most commonly associated with hypertensive events. Preoperatively, most hypertension is essential hypertension; much less common are cases associated with renovascular causes and, even more rarely, vasoactive tumors. Intraoperatively, fluid overload and pharmacologic agents may cause hypertension. Postoperatively, numerous causative factors are associated with hypertension, including pain, hypothermia, hypoxia, fluid overload in the postanesthesia period caused by fluid mobilization from the extravascular compartment, and discontinuation of long-term antihypertensive therapy before surgery. Other causes of postoperative hypertension include intra-abdominal bleeding, head trauma, clonidine withdrawal syndrome, and pheochromocytoma crisis.

Presentation and Management

Most cases of hypertension are detected during the routine preoperative workup. An observant surgeon considers hypertension in the preoperative screening of patients, recognizing that failure to detect significant problems with hypertension can lead to needless hypertension-related complications. By definition, any patient who has a diastolic blood pressure greater than 110 mm Hg must be assessed and treated preoperatively if elective surgery is being contemplated. Patients taking long-term antihypertensive medications who are undergoing elective surgery are instructed to continue taking the medication up to the day of surgery. Patients receiving oral clonidine can be switched to a clonidine patch for at least 3 days before surgery. In emergency cases, the medications administered during induction and maintenance of anesthesia assist in lowering the blood pressure. Intraoperatively, the anesthesiologist must carefully monitor blood pressure; ensure that it stays within acceptable limits; and avoid fluid overload, hypoxia, and hypothermia. In the postoperative period, the patient is given adequate analgesia for pain control, and long-term antihypertensive medications are resumed. In patients who are unable to take oral medications, beta blockers, angiotensin-converting enzyme (ACE) inhibitors, calcium channel antagonists, or diuretics are given parenterally, or clonidine is administered as a transdermal patch.

Although hypertension in the postoperative period is common, a hypertensive crisis is uncommon, especially after noncardiac surgery. A hypertensive crisis is characterized by severe elevation of blood pressure associated with organ dysfunction—cerebral and subarachnoid hemorrhage and stroke, acute cardiac events, renal dysfunction, and bleeding from the operative wound. Hypertensive crisis appears to be particularly likely in carotid endarterectomy, aortic aneurysm surgery, and many head and neck procedures. Diastolic hypertension (>110 mm Hg) is significantly associated with cardiac complications, and systolic hypertension (>160 mm Hg) is associated with an increased risk for stroke and death. In patients with new-onset or severe perioperative hypertension and patients with a hypertensive emergency, treatment to lower blood pressure with agents that have a rapid onset of action, short half-life, and few autonomic side effects is essential. Medications most commonly used in this setting include nitroprusside and nitroglycerin (vasodilators), labetalol and esmolol (beta blockers), enalaprilat (useful for patients taking long-term ACE inhibitors), and nicardipine (calcium channel blocker). It is crucial in the acute setting not to decrease blood pressure more than 25% to avoid ischemic strokes and hypoperfusion injury to other organs.

Perioperative Ischemia and Infarction

Cause

Approximately 30% of all patients undergoing a surgical procedure have some degree of CAD. High risk for an acute coronary syndrome in the postoperative period is present in older patients, patients with peripheral artery disease, and patients undergoing vascular, thoracic, major orthopedic, or upper abdominal procedures. Major risk factors for developing CAD are smoking, family history, adverse lipid profiles, diabetes mellitus, and elevated blood pressure.[22] Although management of nonoperative MI has improved, the mortality associated with perioperative MI remains approximately 30%. Perioperative myocardial complications result in at least 10% of all perioperative deaths. In the 1970s, the risk for recurrence of MI within 3 months of a first MI was reported to be 30%, and if a patient underwent surgery within 3 to 6 months of infarction, the reinfarction rate was 15%; the reinfarction rate was only 5% 6 months postoperatively. However, improved preoperative assessment, advances in anesthesia and intraoperative monitoring, and the availability of more sophisticated ICU monitoring have resulted in improvement in the outcome of patients at risk for an acute cardiac event. Individuals undergoing an operation within 3 months of an infarction have an 8% to 15% reinfarction rate; between 3 and 6 months postoperatively, the reinfarction rate is only 3.5%. The general mortality associated with MI in patients without a surgical procedure is 12%.

Myocardial ischemia and MI result from the imbalance between myocardial oxygen supply and demand. Primary causes that reduce myocardial perfusion and oxygen supply include coronary artery narrowing caused by a thrombus that develops on a disrupted atherosclerotic plaque, dynamic obstruction caused by spasm of an epicardial coronary artery or diseased blood vessel, and severe narrowing caused by progressive atherosclerosis. Secondary causes that increase myocardial oxygen requirements, usually in the presence of a fixed restricted oxygen supply (limited myocardial perfusion), are extrinsic cardiac factors that include fever and tachycardia (increased myocardial oxygen demand), hypotension (reduced coronary blood flow), and anemia and hypoxemia (reduced myocardial oxygen delivery). The increased circulating catecholamines associated with surgical stress further increase myocardial oxygen demand.

Presentation and Diagnosis

Acute coronary syndrome comprises a constellation of clinical symptoms that are compatible with myocardial ischemia and encompasses MI: ST segment elevation myocardial infarction (STEMI) and depression (Q wave and non–Q wave), and unstable angina/non–ST segment elevation myocardial infarction (NSTEMI). Unstable angina/NSTEMI is defined as ST segment depression or prominent T wave inversion or positive biomarkers of myonecrosis in the absence of ST segment elevation and in an appropriate clinical setting. The risk for myocardial ischemia and MI is greatest in the first 48 hours after surgery, and it may be difficult to make the diagnosis. The classic manifestation—chest pain radiating into the jaw and left arm region—is often not present. Patients may have shortness of breath, increased heart rate, hypotension, or respiratory failure. Perioperative myocardial ischemia and MI are often silent and, when they occur, are marked by shortness of breath (heart failure, respiratory failure), increased heart rate (arrhythmias), change in mental status, or excessive hyperglycemia in patients with diabetes. Many perioperative MIs are non–Q wave NSTEMI. Periprocedural MI is associated with the release of biomarkers of necrosis, such as MB isoenzymes of creatine kinase (CK-MB) and troponins, into the circulation. The troponin complex consists of three subunits, T (TnT), I (TnI), and C (TnC). TnT and TnI are derived from heart-specific genes and are referred to as cardiac troponins. Cardiac troponins are not present in healthy individuals; their early release is attributable to the cytosolic pool, and late release is attributable to the structural pool.

Patients considered to have acute coronary syndrome should have a 12-lead ECG and be placed in an environment with continuous ECG monitoring and defibrillator capability. Biomarkers of myocardial necrosis are measured. CK-MB has a short half-life and is less sensitive and less specific than cardiac troponins. Troponins can be detected in blood by 2 to 4 hours, but elevation may be delayed for 8 to 12 hours. The timing of elevation of cardiac troponins is similar to CK-MB, but cardiac troponins persist longer, for up to 5 to 14 days. Elevated cardiac troponin levels above the 99th percentile of normal in two or more blood samples collected at least 6 hours apart indicate the presence of myocardial necrosis. Equivalent information is obtained with cTnI and cTnT except in patients with renal dysfunction, in whom cTnI has a specific role. Each patient should have a provisional diagnosis of acute coronary syndrome with unstable angina (changes on ECG of ischemia and no biomarkers in the circulation), STEMI, or NSTEMI. The distinction has therapeutic implications because patients with STEMI may be considered for immediate reperfusion therapy (fibrinolysis or percutaneous intervention).[22]

Treatment

Preventing coronary ischemia is a function of identifying patients likely at risk for a perioperative cardiac complication. Identification of such patients would allow improvement of the patient's condition, possibly reducing the risk; selection of the patient for invasive or noninvasive cardiac testing; and determining whether the patient would benefit from more intensive perioperative monitoring. Preoperative cardiac risk assessment includes adequate history taking, physical examination, and basic diagnostic tests. The history is important to identify patients with cardiac disease or patients at risk for cardiac disease, including patients with previous cardiac revascularization or history of MI or stroke, as well as patients with valvular heart disease, heart failure, arrhythmia, hypertension, diabetes, lung disease, and renal disease. Unstable chest pain, especially crescendo angina, warrants careful evaluation and probable postponing of an elective operation. Physical examination may reveal uncontrolled hypertension, evidence of peripheral artery disease, arrhythmia, or clinical stigmata of heart failure. Chest radiograph may show pulmonary edema, ECG may show an arrhythmia, blood gas analysis may reveal hypercapnia or a low PaO_2, and blood tests may show abnormal kidney function. A patient who is found to have heart failure on physical examination or by history must have the problem treated before consideration for an elective operative procedure. *Guidelines for Perioperative Cardiovascular Evaluation for Noncardiac Surgery,* published by the American College of Cardiology and American Heart Association, stratified clinical predictors of increased perioperative cardiovascular risk leading to MI, CHF, or death into major, intermediate, and minor risks (Table 12-8) and stratified cardiac risk into high, intermediate, and low (Table 12-9).[21]

The American College of Cardiology/American Heart Association guidelines permit more appropriate use of preoperative testing (echocardiography, dipyridamole myocardial stress perfusion imaging, traditional exercise stress test, or angiography) and beta blocker therapy, with probable cancellation of the elective operative procedure.[23] An algorithm for perioperative cardiovascular evaluation is presented in Figure 12-1. The role of preoperative coronary artery revascularization has yet to be determined. Percutaneous transluminal coronary angioplasty may be beneficial in reducing perioperative cardiac morbidity in a select group of patients.

Patients identified as being at high risk for myocardial events in the perioperative period are managed with beta blockers, careful intraoperative monitoring, maintenance of perioperative normothermia and vital signs, and continued postoperative pharmacologic management including the administration of adequate pain medication. Beta blockers (e.g., atenolol), given several days before surgery and continued for several days afterward, have been shown to reduce perioperative myocardial ischemia by 50% in patients with CAD or CAD risk factors.[24] Patients with chronic stable angina continue with their antianginal medications, and beta blockers are continued to the time of surgery and thereafter. An ECG is obtained before, immediately after, and for 2 days after surgery. Patients are monitored for 48 hours after surgery, high-risk patients are monitored for 5 days, and cardiac enzyme levels are also checked. Invasive hemodynamic monitoring is appropriate for patients with left ventricular dysfunction, fixed cardiac output (CO), and unstable angina or recent MI.

TABLE 12-8 Clinical Predictors of Increased Perioperative Cardiovascular Risk Leading to Myocardial Infarction, Heart Failure, or Death

LEVEL OF RISK	RISK FACTOR
Major	Unstable coronary syndromes
	Acute or recent MI with evidence of considerable ischemic risk as noted by clinical symptoms or noninvasive studies
	Unstable or severe angina (Canadian class III or IV)
	Decompensated heart failure
	Significant arrhythmias
	High-grade atrioventricular block
	Symptomatic ventricular arrhythmias in the presence of underlying heart disease
	Supraventricular arrhythmias with uncontrolled ventricular rate
	Severe valve disease
Intermediate	Mild angina pectoris (Canadian class I or II)
	Previous MI identified by history or pathologic evidence
	Q waves
	Compensated or previous heart failure
	Diabetes mellitus (particularly insulin dependent)
	Renal insufficiency
Minor	Advanced age
	Abnormal ECG (e.g., left ventricular hypertrophy, left bundle branch block, ST-T abnormalities)
	Rhythm other than sinus (e.g., atrial fibrillation)
	Low functional capacity (e.g., inability to climb 1 flight of stairs with a bag of groceries)
	History of stroke
	Uncontrolled systemic hypertension

ECG, electrocardiogram; *MI,* myocardial infarction.

TABLE 12-9 Cardiac Risk Stratification for Noncardiac Surgical Procedures

LEVEL OF RISK	RISK FACTOR
High (cardiac risk often >5%)	Emergency major operations, particularly in elderly patients
	Aortic and other major vascular surgery
	Peripheral vascular surgery
	Anticipated prolonged surgical procedures associated with large fluid shifts and blood loss
Intermediate (cardiac risk generally <5%)	Carotid endarterectomy
	Intraperitoneal and intrathoracic surgery
	Orthopedic surgery
	Prostate surgery
Low (cardiac risk generally <1%)	Endoscopic procedures
	Superficial procedures
	Cataract surgery
	Breast surgery

From Eagle KA, Berger PB, Calkins H, et al: ACC/AHA Guideline Update for Perioperative Cardiovascular Evaluation for Noncardiac Surgery—Executive Summary. A report of the American College of Cardiology/American Heart Association Task Force on Practice Guidelines (Committee to Update the 1996 Guidelines on Perioperative Cardiovascular Evaluation for Noncardiac Surgery). *Anesth Analg* 94:1052–1064, 2002.

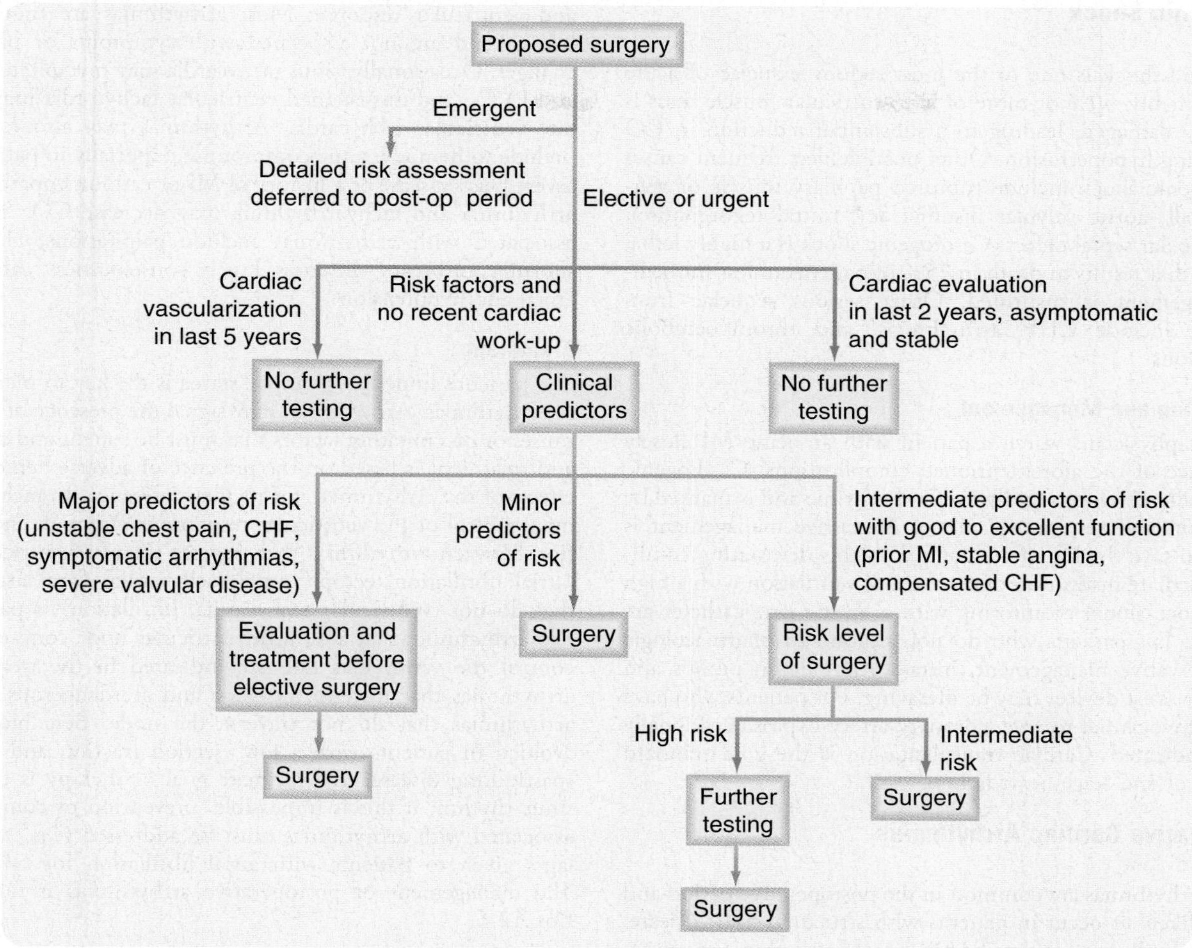

FIGURE 12-1 Algorithm for perioperative cardiovascular evaluation for noncardiac surgery. Patients with major predictors of risk and patients with intermediate predictors of risk and a planned high-risk procedure undergo additional testing and resultant indicated treatment before elective surgery. *CHF*, congestive heart failure; *MI*, myocardial infarction. (Adapted from Eagle KA, Brundage BH, Chaitman BR, et al: Guidelines for perioperative cardiovascular evaluation for noncardiac surgery. Report of the American College of Cardiology/American Heart Association Task Force on Practice Guidelines. *J Am Coll Cardiol* 27:910–945, 1996.)

Shortness of breath and chest pain are the two postoperative symptoms that must always be carefully evaluated and never written off as postoperative discomfort. Subtle changes in the ST segment and T wave suggest possible ischemia or MI. Evaluation of a patient suspected to have an intraoperative or postoperative MI includes immediate assessment by ECG and measurement of biomarkers of myocardial necrosis. Constant ECG monitoring is required so that any potentially lethal arrhythmia that develops can be treated immediately. If the level of cardiac function is a concern, echocardiography is considered. Cardiac troponin levels identify patients with myocardial necrosis but do not identify the cause of necrosis. Cardiac-specific troponin levels begin to increase by 3 hours after myocardial injury. A TnI level greater than 1 ng/mL is specific, and elevations persist for 7 to 10 days. TnT elevations persist for 10 to 14 days after MI. Medical management of myocardial ischemia and MI includes immediate administration of high-flow oxygen, transfer to the ICU, and early consultation with a cardiologist.

The goals of management of myocardial ischemia are to preserve the maximal amount of myocardial muscle possible, improve coronary blood flow, and decrease myocardial work. Immediate administration of beta blockers (oral or IV, dose-titrated to decrease heart rate to <70 beats/min) and aspirin (160 to 325 mg) is essential. Beta blockers are not indicated for patients with bradycardia, hypotension, severe left ventricular dysfunction, heart block, or severe bronchospastic disease. Nitroglycerin (given as a continuous IV infusion after a loading dose) alleviates pain and is beneficial for patients with MI complicated by heart failure or pulmonary edema. Systemic heparinization (or subcutaneous LMWH), if not contraindicated, is administered. In most cases, thrombolytic therapy is contraindicated in the postoperative period and can be used only in situations in which minor surgery is performed. Studies have shown that emergency stricture dilation and coronary artery stent placement may be more effective than thrombolytic therapy. ACE inhibitors may be given early after MI, especially anterior MI or with a low left ventricular ejection fraction, and is likely to be continued as a long-term therapy. Angiography must be strongly considered if the patient has ongoing myocardial ischemia that does not respond to pharmacologic therapy.

Cardiogenic Shock

Causes

Cardiogenic shock is one of the most serious sequelae of acute MI. Presumably, 50% or more of left ventricular muscle mass is irreversibly damaged, leading to a substantial reduction in CO and resulting hypoperfusion. Other possible, less frequent causes of cardiogenic shock include ruptured papillary muscle or ventricular wall, aortic valvular insufficiency, mitral regurgitation, and ventricular septal defect. Cardiogenic shock is a highly lethal condition that results in death in 75% of patients unless immediate management is instituted. Other serious sequelae from acute MI include CHF, arrhythmias, and thromboembolic complications.

Presentation and Management

Observant physicians watch a patient with an acute MI closely for evidence of the aforementioned complications. Cardiogenic shock usually develops rapidly over a short time and is marked by hypotension and respiratory failure. Aggressive management is required to save the life of a patient with this devastating condition. Immediate institution of mechanical ventilation with a high FIO_2 and occasional monitoring with a Swan-Ganz catheter are important. For patients who do not respond to pharmacologic and conservative management, intra-aortic balloon pumps and ventricular assist devices may be lifesaving. For patients who have adequate myocardial reserve, coronary artery bypass occasionally may be indicated. Cardiac transplantation is the gold standard treatment of end-stage heart failure.

Postoperative Cardiac Arrhythmias

Causes

Cardiac arrhythmias are common in the postoperative period and are more likely to occur in patients with structural heart disease. Cardiac arrhythmias are classified into tachyarrhythmia, bradyarrhythmia, and heart block. Tachyarrhythmia is further subdivided into supraventricular (sinus, atrial, nodal) and ventricular (premature ventricular contraction [PVC], ventricular tachycardia, ventricular fibrillation). Sustained supraventricular arrhythmia in patients undergoing major noncardiac surgery may be associated with an increased risk for a cardiac event (e.g., heart failure, MI, unstable angina) and cerebrovascular event.[24] Factors associated with increased risk for supraventricular arrhythmias are increasing age, history of heart failure, and type of surgery performed. Sinus tachycardia and atrial flutter or fibrillation are the most common types of tachyarrhythmia. Sinus tachycardia is caused by pain, fever, hypovolemia, anemia, and anxiety; less common causes are heart failure, MI, thyrotoxicosis, and pheochromocytoma. Atrial flutter or fibrillation occurs commonly in patients with electrolyte imbalance, history of atrial fibrillation, and chronic obstructive pulmonary disease.

Ventricular ectopy occurs in one third of patients after major noncardiac surgery. Factors associated with an increased risk for PVCs include the presence of preoperative PVCs, history of CHF, and cigarette smoking. Postoperative risk factors include hypoxia, acute hypokalemia, and hypercapnia. Ventricular arrhythmias consist of largely benign and sustained ventricular tachycardia and fibrillation. Nonsustained ventricular tachycardia commonly occurs during or after major vascular procedures.

Presentation

The physiologic impact of an arrhythmia depends on the type and duration of arrhythmia and the patient's underlying cardiac status and ventricular response. Most arrhythmias are transient and benign and are not associated with symptoms or physiologic changes. Occasionally, sinus tachycardia may precipitate ischemia and PVCs, and unsustained ventricular tachycardia may precipitate ventricular tachycardia. Arrhythmias may also represent a prelude to hemodynamic compromise, especially in patients with severe heart disease or a history of MI or cardiomyopathy. Bradyarrhythmia and tachyarrhythmia may decrease CO. Symptoms associated with arrhythmias include palpitations, chest pain, shortness of breath, dizziness, loss of consciousness, cardiac ischemia, and hypotension.

Treatment

The patient's underlying cardiac status is the key to management of arrhythmias. Arrhythmias may signal the presence of reversible causes or precipitating factors that must be sought and addressed, and treatment is based on the presence of adverse hemodynamic effects of the arrhythmia, not its mere presence. In tachyarrhythmia, control of the ventricular response is essential, and distinction between arrhythmias that traverse the atrioventricular node (atrial fibrillation, ectopic atrial tachycardia) from arrhythmias that do not (ventricular tachycardia, fibrillation) is paramount. Antiarrhythmics that alter atrioventricular node conduction and control the ventricular rate are indicated in the treatment of arrhythmias that traverse the node and are dangerous to use in arrhythmias that do not traverse the node. Beta blockers are avoided in patients with a low ejection fraction and bronchospastic lung disease. The ultimate goal of therapy is to achieve sinus rhythm; if this is impossible, prevention of complications associated with arrhythmias must be addressed (e.g., anticoagulants given to patients with atrial fibrillation for >48 hours). The management of postoperative arrhythmias is outlined in Box 12-6.

Postoperative Heart Failure

Causes

Heart failure is a clinical syndrome characterized by any structural or functional cardiac disorder that impairs the ability of the ventricle to fill with or eject blood.[25] Several risk factors predispose to the development of heart failure, the most significant of which are CAD, hypertension, and increasing age. Poorly controlled heart failure is one of the most serious cardiac risk factors for a preoperative patient, whereas patients with well-managed heart failure generally do well during an operation. Many factors can lead to new-onset heart failure or decompensation of preexisting heart failure in the perioperative period, including perioperative myocardial ischemia or MI, volume overload, hypertension, sepsis, occult cardiac valvular disease, PE, and new-onset atrial fibrillation. The risk for heart failure is greatest immediately after surgery and in the first 24 to 48 hours after surgery.

Presentation

Patients with poorly controlled heart failure or new-onset heart failure experience shortness of breath and wheezing. Physical examination often reveals tachycardia, a narrow pulse pressure, low pressure or orthostatic hypotension, jugular venous distention, peripheral edema, rales, and general evidence of poor peripheral perfusion. ECG may reveal MI, ventricular hypertrophy, atrial enlargement, or arrhythmias. A chest radiograph may indicate cardiomegaly, pulmonary edema, and pleural effusion. Echocardiography assesses ventricular function and provides information about regional wall motion and valve function.

BOX 12-6 Management of Postoperative Cardiac Arrhythmias

Cardiology consultation
Monitoring of patient on a telemetry floor or in ICU
12-lead ECG and long strip to differentiate between atrial and ventricular arrhythmia
Clinical assessment
- Vital signs
- Peripheral perfusion
- Cardiac ischemia and CHF
- Level of consciousness

Treatment of tachyarrhythmia
- Unstable: Cardioversion
- Stable
  - Supraventricular tachyarrhythmia: Beta blockers (esmolol), ibutilide, or alternatives (e.g., digoxin, calcium channel blockers, amiodarone)
  - Paroxysmal supraventricular tachyarrhythmia: Vagal stimulation or adenosine; digoxin, amiodarone, or calcium channel blocker if adenosine fails
  - Multifocal atrial tachycardia: Beta blocker, calcium channel blocker, or amiodarone
  - Ventricular tachycardia: Lidocaine, procainamide, or amiodarone

Treatment of bradyarrhythmia
- Sustained: Atropine or β-adrenergic agonist
- Transient: No therapy

Treatment of heart block
- Persistent high-grade second-degree or third-degree block: Insertion of permanent pacemaker

CHF, congestive heart failure; *ECG*, electrocardiogram; *ICU*, intensive care unit.

Treatment

Management of patients with heart failure is directed at optimizing preload, afterload, and myocardial contractility. Afterload reduction is accomplished by lowering the vascular resistance against which the heart must contract, and ACE inhibitors are a cornerstone of therapy for heart failure. Nitrates (venodilator) and hydralazine (vasodilator) reduce excessive preload and are used as an alternative in patients who cannot tolerate ACE inhibitors. β-Adrenergic blockade (selective or nonselective) for heart failure has proved effective in reducing mortality in patients with ischemic and nonischemic heart failure.[26] Digoxin (a sympatholytic agent) has traditionally been used for patients with heart failure in sinus rhythm. Its use has decreased given the superior and definitive beneficial effects of ACE inhibitors and beta blockers. Diuretics are necessary in all patients with heart failure for the management of volume overload and relief of symptoms of congestion. Calcium channel blockers are used only for the treatment of hypertension or angina not adequately controlled with other agents, such as ACE inhibitors or beta blockers. Inotropes increase cardiac contractility and are used in critically ill patients and patients with end-stage heart failure.

RENAL AND URINARY TRACT COMPLICATIONS

Urinary Retention

Causes

The inability to evacuate a urine-filled bladder is referred to as urinary retention. This is a common postoperative complication that is seen with particularly high frequency in patients undergoing perianal operations and hernia repair. Urinary retention may also occur after surgery for low rectal cancer when an injury to the nervous system affects bladder function. Most commonly, however, the complication is a reversible abnormality resulting from discoordination of the trigone and detrusor muscles as a result of increased pain and postoperative discomfort. Urinary retention is also occasionally seen after spinal procedures and may occur after overly vigorous IV administration of fluid. Benign prostatic hypertrophy and, rarely, a urethral stricture also may be causes of urinary retention.

Presentation and Management

Patients with postoperative urinary retention complain of a dull constant discomfort in the hypogastrium. Urgency and actual pain in this area occur as the retention worsens. Percussion just above the pubis reveals fullness and tenderness.

To prevent urinary retention in the population at greatest risk, older adults and patients who have undergone low anterior resection, these patients must be watched carefully. Adequate management of pain, including operative injection of local anesthetics, may also diminish the incidence of urinary retention. Judicious administration of IV fluids during the procedure and in the immediate postoperative period, especially in patients who have undergone anorectal surgery for benign disease, may similarly diminish the likelihood of postoperative urinary retention. Awareness of how much time has passed since the last voiding to the present time is crucial in preventing acute retention. Most patients should not go more than 6 to 7 hours without passing some urine, and an observant clinician ensures that no patient goes longer than that before undergoing straight catheterization.

General management principles for acute urinary retention include initial straight catheterization or placement of a Foley catheter, especially in older patients and patients who have undergone anterior resection because they may be unable to sense the fullness associated with retention. In high-risk patients, cystoscopy and cystometry may be required.

Acute Renal Failure

Causes

Acute renal failure (ARF) is characterized by a sudden reduction in renal output that results in the systemic accumulation of nitrogenous wastes. This hospital-acquired renal insufficiency is more prevalent after major vascular procedures (ruptured aneurysm), renal transplantation, cardiopulmonary bypass procedures, major abdominal cases associated with septic shock, and major urologic operations. It may also occur in patients undergoing procedures in which there is major blood loss, patients with transfusion reactions, patients with advanced diabetes undergoing operations, patients with life-threatening trauma, patients with major burn injuries, and patients with multiorgan system failure. Hospital-acquired renal insufficiency adversely affects surgical outcomes and is associated with significant mortality, especially when dialysis is required. Two types of ARF have been identified, oliguric and nonoliguric. Oliguric renal failure refers to urine in which volumes less than 480 mL are seen in a day. Nonoliguric renal failure involves output exceeding 2 liters/day and is associated with large amounts of isosthenuric urine that clears no toxins from the bloodstream. Factors leading to ARF can be inflow, parenchymal, or outflow—historically referred to as prerenal, renal, or postrenal (Table 12-10).

TABLE 12-10 Causes of Postoperative Acute Renal Failure

INFLOW OR PRERENAL	PARENCHYMAL OR RENAL	OUTFLOW OR POSTRENAL
Sepsis	Renal ischemia	Cellular debris (acute tubular necrosis)
Medications	Drugs (aminoglycosides, amphotericin)	Crystals
Nonsteroidal anti-inflammatory drugs	Iodinated contrast media	Uric acid
Angiotensin-converting enzyme inhibitors	Interstitial nephritis	Oxalate
Intravascular volume contraction		Pigment
Hypovolemia		Myoglobin
Hemorrhage		Hemoglobin
Dehydration		
Atherosclerotic emboli		
Third spacing		
Cardiac failure		

In normal kidneys, effective perfusion of the glomeruli is maintained by an autoregulatory mechanism involving the afferent and efferent arterioles. Any factor that interferes with or disrupts this mechanism results in ARF. Afferent constriction or efferent dilation decreases the glomerular filtration rate. Inflow, or prerenal, failure is secondary to hypotension, which causes afferent arteriolar constriction and efferent dilation; nonsteroidal anti-inflammatory drugs (NSAIDs), which inhibit afferent vasodilation; and gram-negative sepsis, which causes decreased peripheral vascular resistance while increasing renal vasoconstriction. Renal vascular stenosis and thrombosis can also be causes, although these are much less common. Outflow, or postrenal, ARF is caused by tubular obstruction from debris, crystals, or pigments; ureteric obstruction; or urinary bladder outflow obstruction. Ischemia, toxins, or nephritis cause parenchymal ARF.

The incidence of contrast-induced nephropathy has been increasing. Tubular damage can occur within 48 hours of contrast dye administration. Diabetic patients with vascular disease are at risk for major renal injury when contrast agents are administered. Administration of contrast agents to hypovolemic patients and patients with preexisting renal dysfunction guarantees some degree of renal injury. The tubular injury is generally self-limited and reversible. However, diabetic patients with creatinine clearance less than 50 mL/min who receive 100 mL of contrast dye can sustain severe tubular damage and may require dialysis. Blunt trauma with associated crush injuries places the patient at risk for ARF because of high serum levels of hematin and myoglobin, both of which are injurious to the renal tubules. ARF is a prominent feature in patients with acute compartment syndrome.[27] Growing awareness of this problem has led surgeons to intervene surgically, often resulting in dramatic improvement in renal function and preservation of renal filtering capacity.

Presentation and Management

Prevention of hospital-acquired renal insufficiency requires the following: identification of patients with preexisting renal dysfunction; avoidance of hypovolemia, hypotension, and medications that depress renal function; and judicious use of nephrotoxic drugs. In the presence of renal impairment, the dose of antibiotics given for serious infections must be adjusted. The risk for contrast-induced nephropathy is reduced by adequate hydration and premedication with a free radical scavenger (e.g., *N*-acetylcysteine) or the use of an alternative contrast agent (e.g., gadolinium). Renal hypoperfusion is avoided by optimizing CO and volume expansion. Administration of fluid must be particularly judicious in patients with a history of heart failure. Monitoring renal function in all surgical patients, sometimes including creatinine clearance, is a sound clinical practice. Early intervention in cases of postrenal obstruction and abdominal compartment syndrome can prevent the development of renal injury.

Anuria that suddenly develops postoperatively in an otherwise healthy individual with no preexisting renal disease is postrenal in nature until proven otherwise. A kink in the Foley catheter or obstruction must be cleared. In patients who have undergone major pelvic surgery, ligation of the ureters is suspect. If renal ultrasound or a CT scan shows hydronephrosis, immediate surgical treatment is indicated. Postrenal causes of ARF are the most dramatic and straightforward to diagnose and treat, with significant immediate improvement after treatment.

ARF is otherwise diagnosed when there is an increase in the serum creatinine level, decrease in creatinine clearance, and urine output less than 400 mL/day (<20 mL/hr). However, distinguishing between prerenal and renal azotemia is complicated. Careful history taking may identify patients with preexisting renal dysfunction. Patients with large fluid losses from the GI tract (e.g., diarrhea, vomiting, fistula, high ileostomy output) often have associated profound dehydration. In such cases, the increase in the blood urea nitrogen level is usually more than the increase in the creatinine level, and the ratio of blood urea nitrogen to creatinine is more than 20. Examination of the patient may reveal distended neck veins, rales in the lungs, and a cardiac gallop—all signs that a failing heart may be underperfusing the kidneys as the cause of the oliguria. Brown urine in the Foley bag in a trauma patient raises suspicion of myoglobinuria and requires rapid hydration, diuresis, and alkalinization of the urine. Evaluation of spun urine is helpful. The presence of hyaline casts indicates hypoperfusion, and the presence of coarse granular casts indicates acute tubular necrosis. Lipoid casts are found with NSAID-induced and contrast-induced nephropathy, and white and red cell casts are found with pyelonephritis. In patients with prerenal azotemia, the concentrating ability of the nephrons is normal, resulting in normal urine osmolality and fractional excretion of sodium (>500 mOsm/liter and FE_{Na} <1%, respectively). Conversely, with acute tubular necrosis, the concentrating ability of the kidney is lost, and the patient produces urine with an osmolality equal to serum and high urine sodium levels (350 mOsm and >50 mg/L, respectively) (Table 12-11). The best laboratory test for discriminating prerenal from renal azotemia is probably FE_{Na}. In patients with prerenal azotemia, FE_{Na} is 1% or less, whereas in patients with renal azotemia, it often exceeds 3%.

When ARF is diagnosed, one has to ascertain whether the hypoperfusion of the kidney is caused by hypovolemia or cardiac failure. Distinguishing the two is critical because giving patients with heart failure more fluid exacerbates an already failing system. Similarly, giving diuretics to a hypovolemic patient can worsen the renal failure. If a patient with prerenal azotemia has no history of cardiac disease, administration of isosmotic fluid (normal saline or lactated Ringer solution, or blood in patients who have hemorrhaged) is indicated. The IV fluid can be given rapidly (1 liter over a 20- to 30-minute period) in young patients with healthy hearts

TABLE 12-11 Diagnostic Evaluation of Acute Renal Failure

PARAMETER	PRERENAL	RENAL	POSTRENAL
Urine osmolality	>500 mOsm/liter	= Plasma	Variable
Urinary sodium	<20 mOsm/liter	>50 mOsm/liter	>50 mOsm/liter
Fractional excretion of sodium	<1%	>3%	Variable
Urine, plasma creatinine level	>40	<20	<20
Urine, plasma urea level	>8	<3	Variable
Urine, plasma osmolality	<1.5	>1.5	Variable

and a Foley catheter in place to measure hourly urine output and must be administered until the patient is producing a minimum of 30 to 40 mL/hr of urine. If fluid administration does not result in improvement of the oliguria, placement of a central venous pressure or Swan-Ganz catheter is indicated to measure left-sided or right-sided heart filling pressure. In the presence of CHF, diuretics, fluid restriction, and appropriate cardiac medications are indicated. Ultrasound may show renal atrophy, reflecting the presence of chronic metabolic disease.

Treatment of ARF includes the management of fluid and electrolyte imbalance, careful monitoring of fluid administration, avoidance of nephrotoxic agents, provision of adequate nutrition, and adjustment of doses of renally excreted medications until recovery of renal function. Treatment of hyperkalemia and fluid overload is most urgent in management of ARF. Hyperkalemia can be managed with a sodium-potassium exchange resin, insulin plus glucose, an aerosolized β_2-adrenergic agonist, and calcium gluconate. Insulin and β_2-adrenergic agonists shift potassium intracellularly. Hyperkalemia-associated cardiac irritability (prolonged P–R interval or peaked T waves) is treated urgently with the administration of a 10% calcium gluconate solution over a 15-minute period and simultaneous IV administration of insulin and glucose (10-U IV bolus with 50 mL of a 50% dextrose solution, followed by continuation of glucose to prevent hypoglycemia). A β_2-adrenergic agonist is given as a nebulizer containing 10 to 20 mg in 4 mL of saline over 10 minutes or as an IV infusion containing 0.5 mg. Calcium gluconate is given as 10 mL of a 10% solution over a 5-minute period to reduce arrhythmias. Refractory hyperkalemia associated with metabolic acidosis and rhabdomyolysis requires hemodialysis. In less severe hyperkalemia, an ion exchange resin (sodium polystyrene [Kayexalate]) in enema form helps lower potassium levels. Phosphate levels also require careful monitoring. Hypophosphatemia can induce rhabdomyolysis and respiratory failure and is treated with oral administration of Fleet Phospho-soda. Hyperphosphatemia with hypercalcemia increases the risk for calciphylaxis and is treated with administration of phosphorus binders (calcium carbonate) or dialysis. IV fluids are monitored with an emphasis on fluid restriction and occasional use of catheters to measure right-sided and left-sided heart filling pressure to avoid fluid overload.

When supportive measures fail, hemodialysis must be considered.[28] Indications for hemodialysis are listed in Box 12-7. Although some hemodynamic instability may occur during dialysis, it is usually transient and may be treated with fluids. Dialysis

BOX 12-7 Indications for Hemodialysis

Serum potassium >5.5 mEq/liter
Blood urea nitrogen >80 to 90 mg/dL
Persistent metabolic acidosis
Acute fluid overload
Uremic symptoms (pericarditis, encephalopathy, anorexia)
Removal of toxins
Platelet dysfunction causing bleeding
Hyperphosphatemia with hypercalcemia

may be continued on an intermittent basis until renal function has returned, which occurs in most cases.

ENDOCRINE GLAND DYSFUNCTION

Adrenal Insufficiency

Causes

Adrenal insufficiency is an uncommon but potentially lethal condition associated with failure of the adrenal glands to produce adequate glucocorticoids. Cortisol, the predominant corticosteroid secreted from the adrenal cortex, is under the influence of adrenocorticotropic hormone released from the pituitary gland, which is under the influence of hypothalamic corticotropin-releasing hormone; both hormones are subject to negative feedback by cortisol itself. Cortisol is a stress hormone.

Chronic adrenal insufficiency may result from primary destruction of the adrenal gland or be secondary to a disease state or disorder involving the hypothalamus or anterior pituitary gland. Primary adrenal insufficiency is most frequently caused by autoimmune adrenalitis (Addison disease), in which the adrenal cortex is destroyed by cytotoxic lymphocytes. Secondary adrenal insufficiency is most commonly caused by long-term administration of pharmacologic doses of glucocorticoids. Long-term use of glucocorticoids causes suppression of the hypothalamic-pituitary-adrenal axis, induces adrenal atrophy, and results in isolated adrenal insufficiency.

Acute adrenal insufficiency may occur as a result of abrupt cessation of pharmacologic doses of long-term glucocorticoid therapy, surgical excision or destruction of the adrenal gland (adrenal hemorrhage, necrosis, or thrombosis in patients with sepsis or antiphospholipid syndrome), or surgical excision or destruction (postpartum necrosis) of the pituitary gland. In addition, so-called functional or relative acute adrenal insufficiency may develop in critically ill and septic patients.

Presentation and Diagnosis

The clinical manifestations of adrenal insufficiency depend on the cause of the disease and associated endocrinopathies.[29] Symptoms and signs of chronic primary and secondary adrenal insufficiency are similar and nonspecific—fatigue, weakness, anorexia, weight loss, orthostatic dizziness, abdominal pain, diarrhea, depression, hyponatremia, hypoglycemia, eosinophilia, and decreased libido and potency. Patients with primary hypoadrenalism also show manifestations of elevated plasma levels of corticotropin and hyperpigmentation of the skin and mucous membranes. In contrast, patients with secondary disease initially have neurologic or ophthalmologic symptoms (headaches, visual disturbances) before showing signs of hypothalamic-pituitary-adrenal axis disease (hypopituitarism). Manifestations of hypothalamic-pituitary-adrenal axis suppression include hypoadrenalism, decreased levels of corticotropin, and manifestations of other hormone deficiencies (e.g., pallor, loss of hair in androgen-dependent areas, oligomenorrhea, diabetes insipidus, hypothyroidism).

Laboratory test abnormalities, including hyponatremia, hyperkalemia, acidosis, hypoglycemia or hyperglycemia, normocytic anemia, eosinophilia, and lymphocytosis, are present to a variable extent. The diagnosis is established by measuring the morning plasma cortisol concentration. A level greater than 19 μg/dL (525 nmol/liter) rules out adrenal insufficiency, and less than 3 μg/dL (83 nmol/liter) indicates the presence of adrenal insufficiency. A basal plasma corticotropin level greater than 100 pg/mL (22 nmol/liter), low or low-normal basal aldosterone level, and increased renin concentration are indicative of primary hypoadrenalism. When testing for primary adrenal insufficiency, the rapid corticotropin stimulation test to determine adrenal responsiveness is the diagnostic procedure of choice (Box 12-8).

The metyrapone test is performed to confirm the diagnosis of secondary adrenal insufficiency. An insufficient increase in plasma 11-deoxycortisol and a low plasma cortisol concentration (<8 μg/dL) after oral administration of metyrapone indicate the presence of secondary adrenal insufficiency. Magnetic resonance imaging (MRI) allows evaluation of the pituitary-hypothalamic region in patients with neurologic and ophthalmologic symptoms, and CT is used to evaluate the adrenal glands in patients with primary hypoadrenalism.

The diagnosis of acute adrenal insufficiency can be especially difficult to make in critically ill patients. The condition is suspected in patients exhibiting manifestations of preexisting or undiagnosed chronic adrenal insufficiency in whom unexplained hypotension or hemodynamic instability develops despite fluid resuscitation as well as ongoing evidence of inflammation without an obvious source of infection. Hyponatremia is usually present and does not respond to saline infusion. A sodium level less than 120 mmol/liter is dangerous and may lead to delirium, coma, and seizures. Hypoglycemia and azotemia may also be present. ECG occasionally reveals low voltage and peaked T waves. To diagnose the condition, cortisol and corticotropin concentrations are checked, and the short corticotropin stimulation test is performed.

Treatment

Prevention and avoidance of adrenal insufficiency are achieved by a thorough preoperative history, detailed instruction of patients receiving long-term corticosteroid therapy regarding the dangers of abrupt termination of the medication, and adequate perioperative corticosteroid administration. Specific patients with rheumatoid arthritis, inflammatory bowel disease, or autoimmune disease and recipients of organ transplants are targeted. In critically ill patients, a high index of suspicion can prevent a fatal outcome. A stress dose of hydrocortisone (100 mg) may be given with induction of anesthesia. For minor surgical procedures, the usual maintenance dose is continued postoperatively. For major surgical procedures, a stress dose (100 mg) is continued every 8 hours until the patient is stable or free of complications and then tapered to the usual maintenance dose.

Symptomatic patients are treated with hydrocortisone or cortisone. Fludrocortisone (substitute for aldosterone) is also administered to patients with primary disease. Patients who have received more than 20 mg of prednisone daily (or equivalent dose of another corticosteroid) (Table 12-12) for more than 3 weeks within the previous year and patients with Cushing syndrome who are undergoing surgery are presumed to have hypothalamic-pituitary-adrenal axis suppression and must be treated in a similar fashion.

Treatment of functional acute adrenal insufficiency involves immediate, rapid administration of high-dose hydrocortisone or methylprednisolone, with appropriate monitoring until clinical improvement is seen. Hypovolemia and hyponatremia are corrected with saline infusion.

Hyperthyroid Crisis

Causes

Hyperthyroidism refers to a sustained increase in the synthesis of thyroid hormones, and thyrotoxicosis is a clinical syndrome that results from an abnormal elevation of circulating levels of thyroid hormone, regardless of cause. Thyroid hormones are under the influence of pituitary gland thyroid-releasing hormone, which is under the influence of hypothalamic thyrotropin-releasing hormone; both are subject to negative feedback by the thyroid hormones. Thyroid hormones have physiologic effects on many organ systems, but the greatest effect is on the cardiovascular system.

Thyroid crisis is a medical emergency that occurs in thyrotoxic patients with toxic adenoma or toxic multinodular goiter but most often in patients with Graves disease. The crisis is frequently

BOX 12-8 Rapid Adrenocorticotropic Hormone Stimulation Test in Patients With Adrenal Insufficiency

Determine baseline serum cortisol level.

- Give IV (or IM) cosyntropin, 250 μg.
- Measure serum cortisol levels 30 to 60 minutes after cosyntropin is given.

Results

- Normal adrenal function: Basal or postcorticotropin plasma cortisol concentration is at least 18 μg/dL (500 nmol/liter) or preferably 20 μg/dL (550 nmol/liter).
- Primary adrenal insufficiency: Cortisol secretion is not increased.
- Severe secondary adrenal insufficiency: Cortisol levels increase a little or not at all because of adrenocortical atrophy.

TABLE 12-12 Relative Corticosteroid Potency Compared With Hydrocortisone

	GLUCOCORTICOID ACTIVITY	MINERALOCORTICOID ACTIVITY
Short-Acting		
Hydrocortisone	1	1
Cortisone	0.8	0.8
Intermediate-Acting		
Prednisone	4	0.25
Prednisolone	4	0.25
Methylprednisolone	5	Trace
Triamcinolone	5	Trace
Long-Acting		
Dexamethasone	20	Trace

Adapted from Druck P, Andersen DK: Diabetes mellitus and other endocrine problems. In Stillman RM, editor: Surgery: *Diagnosis and therapy,* New York, 1989, Lange, p 205.

precipitated by a stressful event and characterized by exacerbation of hyperthyroidism and decompensation of one or more organ systems. Mortality is high, ranging from 20% to 50% if the crisis is unrecognized and left untreated.

Presentation and Diagnosis

Clinical manifestations of hyperthyroidism include nervousness; fatigue; palpitations; heat intolerance; weight loss; atrial fibrillation (in older patients); and ophthalmopathy characterized by eyelid retraction or lag, periorbital edema, and proptosis. The onset of thyroid crisis is sudden and manifested by accentuation of the symptoms and signs of thyrotoxicosis and organ system dysfunction, including hyperpyrexia, tachycardia out of proportion to fever, dehydration and collapse, central nervous system dysfunction (delirium, psychosis, seizure, coma), cardiac manifestations, GI symptoms, and liver dysfunction.

The diagnosis of thyrotoxicosis requires demonstration of elevated levels of circulating thyroid hormone and suppressed thyroid-stimulating hormone (TSH) levels and identification of the cause of the thyrotoxicosis. Free thyroxine (T_4) and triiodothyronine (T_3) represent the small unbound fraction of total thyroxine that is biologically active and correlate directly with the presence and severity of thyroid dysfunction. Thyroid scintigraphy with technetium-99m pertechnetate or iodine-123 (^{123}I) provides information about the functional anatomy of the gland. In Graves disease, there is diffuse uptake; in Plummer disease (toxic multinodular goiter), there is an inhomogeneous pattern with hot, cold, and warm areas; and with Goetsch disease (toxic solitary nodule), there is intense activity in the area of the nodule, with suppression of paranodular tissue.

Treatment

In addition to the identification and treatment of the precipitating factors and supportive care, specific medications (e.g., iodine, propylthiouracil, β-adrenergic blockers, dexamethasone) that target hormonal synthesis and release and block peripheral effects of the hormone are administered (Box 12-9).[30] Steroids are required to block the peripheral conversion of T_4 to T_3 and as a supplement because there is increased steroid demand and turnover and decreased physiologic effectiveness. Cardioversion for supraventricular tachyarrhythmia is ineffective during the thyrotoxic storm.

Definitive therapy for Graves disease is accomplished with radioactive iodine (^{123}I) or surgery. Radioactive iodine has obvious advantages in older, high-risk patients but needs to be avoided in children, pregnant women, and patients with large toxic adenomas. Thyrotoxicosis can be successfully managed in 85% to 90% of patients with doses of ^{123}I in the range of 10 mCi (5 to 15 mCi) and subsequent levothyroxine. The main side effect of radioactive iodine is hypothyroidism. Surgery usually includes one of two operations: total thyroidectomy or a lobectomy on one side with a subtotal lobectomy on the other side. Total thyroidectomy is associated with a lower recurrence rate than subtotal thyroidectomy (4% to 15%) but requires lifelong T_4 replacement postoperatively. Excision of the lesion is indicated for toxic adenoma, whereas total thyroidectomy is indicated for toxic multinodular goiter. Before surgery, patients must be made euthyroid with antithyroid drugs, and iodine is given for 7 days before surgery.

BOX 12-9 Management of Thyroid Crisis

Identify and treat precipitating factor.
Supportive care
- Oxygen
- IV fluid therapy
- Sedation (chlorpromazine)
- VTE prophylaxis with heparin
- Dexamethasone

Fever: Antipyretics and cooling
Heart failure: Digoxin and diuretics
Atrial fibrillation: IV heparin
Beta blockers: Oral propranolol (or diltiazem), 60 to 80 mg every 4 hours, is given to reduce heart rate below 100 beats/min. In very sick patients, esmolol is given intravenously, and reserpine is given to patients refractory to large doses of propranolol.
Propylthiouracil or methimazole
Lugol solution is given 4 hours after propylthiouracil.
Plasmapheresis and charcoal plasma perfusion or exchange transfusion are reserved for recalcitrant cases if no response in 24 to 48 hours.
When euthyroidism is achieved, definitive therapy must be considered to prevent a second crisis.

VTE, venous thromboembolism.

Hypothyroidism

Causes

Hypothyroidism is characterized by low systemic levels of thyroid hormone and may be exacerbated in the postoperative period in patients with preexisting chronic hypothyroidism or as a result of severe stress. Severe illness, physiologic stress, and drugs may inhibit the peripheral conversion of T_4 to T_3 and induce a hypothyroid-like state. Hypothyroidism may be primary (e.g., surgical removal, ablation, disease of the thyroid gland), secondary (e.g., hypopituitarism), or tertiary (e.g., hypothalamic disease).

Presentation and Diagnosis

Patients with chronic hypothyroidism may be asymptomatic or, rarely, have the severe form (myxedema coma) characterized by coma, loss of deep tendon reflexes, cardiopulmonary collapse, and high mortality (≈40% to 50%). However, most patients exhibit symptoms of cold intolerance, constipation, brittle hair, dry skin, sluggishness, weight gain, and fatigue. The impact of hypothyroidism is greatest on the cardiovascular system, with effects such as bradycardia, hypotension, impaired cardiac function, conduction abnormalities, pericardial effusion, and increased risk for CAD. In critically ill patients (e.g., trauma or sepsis), hypothyroidism is associated with worsening of pulmonary function, a predisposition to pleural effusion, and susceptibility to hypothermia.

ECG usually shows bradycardia, low voltage, and prolonged P–R, QRS, and Q–T intervals. In patients with primary hypothyroidism, serum total T_4, free T_4, and free T_3 levels are low, whereas the TSH level is elevated. In secondary disease, the TSH level, free T_4 index, and free T_3 are low. Distinguishing the two is important because adrenal insufficiency is present in secondary disease, and administration of levothyroxine must be accompanied by cortisol or the disease could be exacerbated.

Treatment

Patients with known hypothyroidism who are receiving replacement hormonal therapy and are in the euthyroid state do not require any special treatment before surgery but are instructed to continue taking their medications. In patients with symptomatic chronic hypothyroidism, surgery is postponed until a euthyroid state has been achieved.

Patients with myxedema coma or patients showing clinical signs of significant hypothyroidism (e.g., severe postoperative hypothermia, hypotension, hypoventilation, psychosis, obtundation) are immediately treated with thyroid hormone, concomitant with IV administration of hydrocortisone, to avoid an addisonian crisis. IV levothyroxine or T_3 may be given until oral ingestion is possible.

Syndrome of Inappropriate Antidiuretic Hormone Secretion

Causes

The syndrome of inappropriate antidiuretic hormone secretion (SIADH) is the most common cause of chronic normovolemic hyponatremia. Hyponatremia is defined as a serum sodium concentration less than 135 mmol/liter. SIADH is diagnosed in any patient who remains hyponatremic despite all attempts to correct the imbalance in the presence of persistent antidiuretic activity from elevated arginine vasopressin levels. Vasopressin is a naturally occurring antidiuretic hormone that regulates free water excretion. It is synthesized in the hypothalamus, transported to the posterior pituitary, and stored until specific stimuli cause it to be secreted into the bloodstream. Thirst, hypovolemia, nausea, hypoglycemia, and drugs are among the many stimuli for vasopressin. Disorders and conditions that predispose to this relatively rare condition include trauma, stroke, antidiuretic hormone–producing tumors, drugs (ACE inhibitors, dopamine, NSAIDs), and pulmonary conditions.

Presentation

The clinical features of SIADH include anorexia, nausea, vomiting, obtundation, and lethargy. With more rapid onset, seizures, coma, and death can result. Clinical expression of SIADH is caused by hyponatremia and is a function of the degree of hyponatremia as well as the rapidity of its onset. The cardinal criteria of SIADH include hyponatremia with hypotonicity of plasma, urine osmolality in excess of plasma osmolality, increased renal sodium excretion, absence of edema or volume depletion, and normal renal function.

Treatment

Management of SIADH includes treatment of the underlying disease process and removal of excess water (i.e., treatment of hyponatremia). Fluid restriction is the mainstay of management of chronic SIADH. IV administration of normal saline is used only in significantly symptomatic patients with chronic SIADH or patients with symptomatic acute SIADH, with a duration of less than 3 days. Correction must occur at a rate of 0.5 mmol/liter/hr until the serum sodium concentration is 125 mg/dL or higher. Rapid correction leads to serious permanent neurologic damage. Diuretics such as furosemide occasionally help correct the imbalance. In some cases, IV administration of 3% saline solution may be required, but correction must be accomplished in a constant, sustained fashion because overly rapid correction can result in seizure activity.

GASTROINTESTINAL COMPLICATIONS

Ileus and Early Postoperative Bowel Obstruction

Causes

Early postoperative bowel obstruction denotes obstruction occurring within 30 days after surgery. The obstruction may be functional (i.e., ileus), caused by inhibition of propulsive bowel activity, or mechanical as a result of a barrier. Ileus that occurs immediately after surgery in the absence of precipitating factors and resolves within 2 to 4 days is termed *primary* or *postoperative ileus*. Ileus that occurs as a result of a precipitating factor and is associated with a delay in return of bowel function is termed *secondary, adynamic,* or *paralytic ileus*.[31] Mechanical bowel obstruction may be caused by a luminal, mural, or extraintestinal barrier.

The precise mechanism and cause of postoperative ileus are incompletely understood. Several events that occur during an abdominal surgical procedure and in the perioperative period may interfere with or alter the contractile activity of the small bowel, which is governed by a complex interaction among the enteric nervous system, central nervous system, hormones, and local molecular and cellular inflammatory factors. Surgical stress and manipulation of the bowel result in sustained inhibitory sympathetic activity, release of hormones and neurotransmitters, and activation of a local molecular inflammatory response that results in suppression of the neuromuscular apparatus.[32] In the immediate postoperative period, restricted oral intake and postoperative narcotic analgesia also contribute to altered small bowel motility. Opiates and opioid peptides in the enteric nervous system suppress neuronal excitability. After transection and reanastomosis of the small bowel, the distal part of the bowel does not react to the pacemaker (found in the duodenum), and the frequency of contractions decreases. Other conditions listed in Box 12-10 are associated with or result in adynamic ileus.

Mechanical early postoperative small bowel obstruction is commonly caused by adhesions (92%), a phlegmon or abscess, internal hernia, intestinal ischemia, or intussusception. Intussusception occurring in the postoperative period is uncommon and is a rare occurrence after colorectal surgery. A phlegmon or abscess may be caused by leakage of intestinal contents from a disrupted anastomosis or by iatrogenic injury to the bowel during enterolysis or closure of laparotomy incision. With mechanical obstruction, there is an increased incidence of discrete, clustered contractions proximal to the obstruction that propel the intestinal contents past the point of obstruction (in cases of partial obstruction) and result in cramps. In high-grade or complete obstruction, the contents do not move distally but accumulate in the proximal part of the bowel and initiate retrograde contractions that empty the small bowel contents into the stomach in preparation for expulsion during vomiting.

Presentation

Postoperative ileus affects the stomach and colon primarily. After laparotomy, small bowel motility returns within several hours; gastric motility, within 24 to 48 hours; and colonic motility, within 48 to 72 hours. Secretions and swallowed air are not emptied from the stomach, and gastric dilation and vomiting may

BOX 12-10 Causes of Intestinal Paralytic Ileus

- Pancreatitis
- Intra-abdominal infection (peritonitis or abscess)
- Retroperitoneal hemorrhage and inflammation
- Electrolyte abnormalities
- Lengthy surgical procedure and prolonged exposure of abdominal contents
- Medications (e.g., narcotics, psychotropic agents)
- Pneumonia
- Inflamed viscera

occur. The return of bowel activity is heralded by the presence of bowel sounds, flatus, and bowel movements.

Patients with early postoperative small bowel obstruction do not show manifestations of bowel activity or have temporary return of bowel function. In adynamic ileus, the stomach, small bowel, and colon are affected. In mechanical obstruction, the obstruction may be partial or complete, may occur in the proximal part of the small bowel (high obstruction) or in the distal part of the small bowel (low obstruction), and may be a closed-loop or open-ended obstruction.[33] There is stasis and progressive accumulation of gastric and intestinal secretions and gas; the bowel may lose its tone and dilate, resulting in abdominal distention, pain, nausea and vomiting, and obstipation. The extent of the clinical manifestations varies with the cause, degree, and level of obstruction. Patients with high mechanical small bowel obstruction vomit early in the course and usually have no or minimal distention. The vomitus is generally bilious. Patients with distal obstruction vomit later in the course and have more pronounced abdominal distention. The vomitus may initially be bilious and then becomes more feculent. Differentiation between adynamic ileus and mechanical obstruction can be difficult. With adynamic ileus, patients have diffuse discomfort but no sharp colicky pain and a distended abdomen. They often have a quiet abdomen, with few bowel sounds detected on auscultation with a stethoscope. With mechanical obstruction, high-pitched, tinkling sounds may be detected. Fever, tachycardia, manifestations of hypovolemia, and sepsis may also develop.

The diagnosis of bowel obstruction is usually based on clinical findings and plain radiographs of the abdomen.[33] However, in the postoperative period, differentiation between adynamic ileus and mechanical obstruction is imperative because the treatment is completely different. A CT scan, abdominal radiographs, and small bowel follow-through are variably used to establish the diagnosis and assist in treatment decision making. In adynamic ileus, abdominal radiographs reveal diffusely dilated bowel throughout the intestinal tract, with air in the colon and rectum. Air-fluid levels may be present, and the amount of dilated bowel varies greatly. With mechanical bowel obstruction, there is small bowel dilation with air-fluid levels and thickened valvulae conniventes in the bowel proximal to the point of obstruction and little or no gas in the bowel distal to the obstruction. A CT scan is more accurate for differentiating functional from mechanical obstruction by identifying the so-called transition point or cutoff at the obstruction site in cases of mechanical obstruction. It also determines the level (high or low) and degree of obstruction (partial versus high-grade or complete), differentiates between uncomplicated and complicated (compromised bowel, perforation) obstruction, and identifies specific types of obstruction (closed-loop obstruction, intussusception). In addition, CT may identify other associated disease states (e.g., bowel ischemia, phlegmon, abscess, pancreatitis). Small bowel follow-through is indicated if the clinical picture of postoperative small bowel obstruction is confusing, radiographs of the abdomen are not diagnostic, or the response to expectant management is inadequate. A standard battery of laboratory tests is also obtained, including complete blood cell count with differential; determination of amylase, lipase, electrolyte, magnesium, and calcium levels; and urinalysis.

Treatment

Preventive measures must be started intraoperatively and continued in the immediate postoperative period. A concerted effort must be made during any abdominal operation to minimize injury to the bowel and other peritoneal surfaces, the recognized source of adhesion formation. During the operation, the surgeon must handle the tissues gently and limit peritoneal dissection to only what is essential. The bowel must not be allowed to desiccate by prolonged exposure to air without protection. Moist laparotomy pads must be used to cover the bowel and must be moistened frequently if contact with the bowel is prolonged. Instrument injury to the bowel must be avoided. Given the importance of adhesion formation and the large magnitude of serious problems related to adhesions, adjunctive measures, such as antiadhesion barriers, may be considered. Numerous antiadhesion barriers are available, including an oxidized cellulose product and a product that is a combination of sodium hyaluronate and carboxymethyl cellulose. These agents may inhibit adhesions wherever they are placed. However, a decrease in the number of adhesions at the site of application does not translate into a decrease in the rate of small bowel obstruction.

In the postoperative period, electrolyte levels are monitored, and any imbalance is corrected. Alternative analgesia to narcotics, such as NSAIDs and placement of a thoracic epidural with local anesthetic, may be used when possible. Intubation of the stomach with an NG tube needs to be applied selectively. Routine intubation does not confer any appreciable effect and is associated with discomfort; inhibits ambulation; and predisposes to aspiration, sinusitis, otitis, esophageal injury, and electrolyte imbalance. The use of prokinetic agents does not alter the outcome after colorectal surgery, and other pharmacologic manipulations, such as parasympathetic agents, adrenergic blocking agents, and metoclopramide, have no impact on resolving postoperative ileus.[32] The role of early postoperative feeding is unclear.

When early postoperative obstruction is suspected or diagnosed, a three-step approach is essential to guarantee a favorable outcome—resuscitation, investigation, and surgical intervention.[33] Emergency repeat laparotomy is performed if there is a closed-loop, high-grade, or complicated small bowel obstruction, intussusception, or peritonitis. Adynamic ileus is treated by resolving some of the abnormalities listed in Box 12-10 and waiting expectantly for resolution, with surgery not usually being required. Partial mechanical small bowel obstruction is also initially managed expectantly and for a longer period, 7 to 14 days, if the patient is stable and clinical and radiologic improvement continues. During this time, nutritional support is initiated, and surgical intervention is performed if there are signs of deterioration or no improvement.

Acute Abdominal Compartment Syndrome

Cause

Abdominal compartment syndrome (ACS) comprises increasing organ dysfunction or failure as a result of IAH. IAH is present when there is consistent increased IAP greater than 12 mm Hg, determined by a minimum of three measurements conducted 4 to 6 hours apart, measured at the end of expiration in a relaxed patient. ACS may be primary or secondary and develops when IAP is 20 mm Hg or greater, with or without abdominal perfusion pressure less than 50 mm Hg (at least three measurements performed 1 to 3 hours apart); it is associated with failure of one or more organ systems that was not present previously.

Primary ACS develops as a result of pathologic IAH caused by intra-abdominal pathology, and secondary ACS develops in the absence of intra-abdominal primary pathology, injury, or intervention. Primary ACS is most commonly encountered in victims of multiple trauma, especially after damage control surgery, and develops as a result of ileus caused by bowel edema and contamination, continued bleeding, coagulopathy, packing used to control bleeding, capillary leak, and massive fluid resuscitation and transfusion. Closure of a noncompliant abdominal wall under tension in these situations is associated with IAH in 100% of cases. In nontrauma patients, IAH and possibly primary ACS have been reported to occur in patients with ascites, retroperitoneal hemorrhage, pancreatitis, or pneumoperitoneum and after reduction of chronic hernias that have lost their domain, repair of ruptured abdominal aortic aneurysm, complex abdominal procedures, and liver transplantation. Secondary ACS is in part iatrogenic and commonly encountered in patients with shock requiring aggressive fluid resuscitation with crystalloids, thermally injured and shock trauma victims, critically ill hypothermic and septic patients, and patients who have sustained cardiac arrest. Shock and ischemia increase capillary permeability; combined with excessive crystalloid resuscitation (leading to dilution of plasma) and gut reperfusion, which further increase microvascular permeability, exudation of fluid with resultant interstitial edema, bowel wall edema, and ascites occurs.

In healthy individuals, IAP ranges from subatmospheric to 5 mm Hg and fluctuates with respiration, body mass index, and activity. IAP ranges from 3 to 15 mm Hg after uncomplicated abdominal surgery. IAP reflects intra-abdominal volume and abdominal wall compliance. With increased volume, there is a decrease in compliance, and any further change in volume results in an increase in pressure, leading to IAH. In the early stages of IAH, changes in organ function are not detectable and of questionable clinical significance. With further increase in IAP, deleterious effects are observed in the intra-abdominal and extra-abdominal organs and abdominal wall.[27] Upward displacement of the diaphragm results in decreased thoracic volume and compliance and increased intrapleural pressure. An increase in peak airway pressure (PAP), ventilation-perfusion ($\dot{V}/\dot{Q}$) mismatch, hypoxia, hypercapnia, and acidosis result. When IAP reaches 25 mm Hg, there is an increase in end-respiratory pressure to achieve a fixed tidal volume. However, modest IAH can exacerbate acute lung injury, inhalation injury, or respiratory distress syndrome. Compression of the inferior vena cava and portal vein occurs and results in decreased venous return and a decrease in preload and pooling of blood in the splanchnic and lower extremity vascular beds and increased peripheral vascular resistance. Venous return decreases with IAP greater than 20 mm Hg. As a result, CO, cardiac index, and right atrial and pulmonary artery occlusion pressures decrease. Increased intrathoracic pressure also decreases left ventricular compliance, reducing contractility and further decreasing CO. Ventricular compliance is reduced when IAP is greater than 30 mm Hg. CO decreases, despite normovolemia or apparent high filling pressures and a normal ejection, when the IAP is 20 to 25 mm Hg. Systemic delivery of oxygen decreases and whole body oxygen consumption is significantly reduced at an IAP greater than 25 mm Hg.

Direct compression of the kidneys and obstruction of venous outflow, with resultant increase in prerenal vascular resistance and shunting of blood from the cortex to the medulla, results in a decrease in the glomerular filtration rate, renal plasma flow, glucose reabsorption, and urine output. In a postoperative patient admitted to the ICU with an IAP greater than 18 mm Hg, renal function is impaired by 30%, independent of prerenal circulation. Renal output decreases in 65% of patients with an IAP greater than 25 mm Hg and in 100% of patients with an IAP greater than 35 mm Hg. Compression of the mesenteric vasculature leads to a decrease in splanchnic perfusion, mesenteric venous hypertension, and decreased hepatic arterial flow. This results in severe intramucosal acidosis, intestinal edema, and visceral swelling; increased intestinal permeability; and possible bacterial translocation. Gastric intramucosal acidosis develops with IAP greater than 20 to 25 cm H_2O or 15 mm Hg. Elevated central venous pressure interferes with venous cerebral outflow, with consequent cerebral pooling and increase in intracerebral pressure. Also, with diminished CO and increasing intracerebral pressure, cerebral perfusion pressure decreases. Interleukin 6 (IL-6) and IL-1β levels increase in response to increased IAP. Blood flow to the abdominal wall decreases with a progressive increase in IAP; this may result in an increased rate of abdominal wound complications.

Diagnosis

The clinical manifestations of primary and secondary ACS are similar. However, the effects of secondary ACS are more subtle, so the diagnosis may be missed, and the clinical deterioration of the patient is usually attributed to severity of the primary illness or occurrence of irreversible shock. Secondary ACS often occurs during aggressive fluid resuscitation in patients with burns, extra-abdominal injury, or sepsis. Patients with ACS have difficulty breathing or are difficult to ventilate and exhibit increasing PAP, decreased volumes, hypoxia, worsening hypercapnia, and deteriorating compliance. Oliguria rarely occurs in the absence of respiratory dysfunction or failure. The CO is reduced, despite apparent high filling pressures, and vasopressor therapy is required. The abdomen becomes distended and tense, and neurologic deterioration may occur. The central venous pressure, PCWP, and PAP become elevated, and acidosis develops. Anuria, exacerbation of pulmonary failure, cardiac decompensation, and death ultimately occur.

Use of the urinary bladder catheter has been the gold standard and is the indirect method used to measure IAP.[28] IAP is measured in the following ways: (1) using a regular Foley catheter, disconnect from drainage tubing, directly inject 50 mL, clamp, insert needle, and measure; (2) using a three-way Foley catheter, inject saline into one port, and measure IAP through the other; or (3) serially connect a regular Foley catheter to a three-way stopcock and a transducer. Other measurement kits are commercially available. Once measured, the pressure is graded: GI (IAP <10 to 15 cm H_2O), GII (IAP <16 to 25 cm H_2O), GIII (IAP <26 to 35 cm H_2O), and GIV (IAP >36 cm H_2O).

Treatment

The prevention of primary ACS entails leaving the peritoneal cavity open in patients at risk for IAH and after high-risk surgical procedures. Patients at risk for secondary ACS receiving crystalloid resuscitation must be monitored closely, and IAP must be measured when patients are given more than 6 liters of crystalloid in a 6-hour period. In addition to blood pressure and urine output, monitoring abdominal perfusion pressure (abdominal perfusion pressure = mean arterial pressure − IAP) by continuously measuring IAP throughout resuscitation is a helpful indicator of the resuscitation end point. Routine measurement of IAP also must be considered in critically ill patients because IAH is the leading cause of chest wall impairment in ARDS. Monitoring gastric pH can detect cases of secondary ACS early after admission to the ICU. A high incidence of suspicion is paramount, especially in cases of secondary ACS, in which the onset is insidious and manifestations are subtle. Patients exhibiting the prodromal phase of ACS benefit from timely intervention to relieve IAH and prevent progression to ACS (Box 12-11). Conservative fluid resuscitation; administration of analgesia, sedatives, and pharmacologic paralysis; patient positioning; drainage of intra-abdominal fluid; escharotomy; renal placement therapy; and diuretics are measures that may prevent progression to ACS.

Optimizing treatment and identifying patients with IAH-ACS likely to benefit from decompression is a challenging task. The decision to intervene surgically is not based on IAH alone but rather on the presence of organ dysfunction in association with IAH. Few patients with a pressure of 12 mm Hg have any organ dysfunction, whereas IAP greater than 15 to 20 mm Hg is significant in every patient. With grade III IAH, decompression may be considered when the abdomen is tense and signs of extreme ventilatory dysfunction and oliguria develop. In grade IV IAH, with signs of ventilator and renal failure, decompression is indicated. In patients with severe head injury and IAP greater than 20 mm Hg, even without overt ACS, or intractable intracranial hypertension without obvious head injury, abdominal decompression must be considered. In contrast to primary ACS, in which reopening of the preexisting laparotomy incision for decompression can be easily done, there is usually reluctance to perform a formal laparotomy for decompression in cases of secondary ACS, especially in the absence of primary intra-abdominal pathology. If nonoperative measures (see earlier) prove ineffective, fascial release without exposing the peritoneal cavity using minimally invasive techniques has proven effective in lowering IAP in experimental animals.[34] Decompression (formal laparotomy) is an emergency and is performed in the operating room. Decompression leads to reduction of IAH, severe hypotension as a result of sudden decrease in systemic vascular resistance, and abrupt increase in the true tidal volume delivered to the patient, with washout of the byproducts of anaerobic metabolism from below the diaphragm. Respiratory alkalosis; decrease in effective preload; and a bolus of acid, potassium, and other byproducts delivered to the heart, where they cause arrhythmia or asystolic arrest, result. Decompression is performed after adequate preload with volume has been established. Most patients respond to decompression and survive. When stable, the patient may be returned to the operating room for definitive closure. If primary closure is impossible, closure may be effected with skin flaps only, composite mesh, bioprosthesis, bilateral medial advancement of rectus muscle and its fascia with lateral skin relaxation incisions, or tissue expanders and myocutaneous flaps.

BOX 12-11 Prevention of Abdominal Compartment Syndrome

Patients at risk for IAH and abdominal compartment syndrome are identified (e.g., major trauma, complex abdominal procedure).

Organ function is monitored and assessed:

- Lungs: Hypercapnia, hypoxia, difficult ventilation, elevated pulmonary artery pressure, decrease in PaO_2/FIO_2 ratio, decreased compliance, intrapulmonary shunt, increased dead space
- Heart: Decreased CO and cardiac index and need for vasopressors
- Kidneys: Oliguria unresponsive to fluid therapy
- Central nervous system: Glasgow Coma Scale score <10 or neurologic deterioration in the absence of neurotrauma
- Abdomen: Distention; CT scan to check for fluid collections, narrowing of inferior vena cava, compression of kidneys, and rounding of abdomen

Intra-abdominal pressure is measured and monitored with a urinary bladder or gastric catheter.

Other tests are done to check organ dysfunction:

- Gastric mucosal pH
- Near-infrared spectroscopy to measure muscle and gastric tissue oxygenation
- Abdominal perfusion pressure = mean arterial pressure − intra-abdominal pressure
- Renal filtration gradient = mean arterial pressure − 2 × intra-abdominal pressure
- CT scan

Measures to lower IAH are implemented:

- Drainage of intra-abdominal fluid collections
- Muscle relaxation

Avoid primary closure of the incision—laparotomy or mesh, Bogota bag, biologic mesh, or vacuum-assisted closure.

CO, cardiac output; *CT,* computed tomography; *FIO_2,* fraction of inspired oxygen; *IAH,* intra-abdominal hypertension; *PaO_2,* partial arterial oxygen pressure.

Postoperative Gastrointestinal Bleeding

Causes

Postoperative GI bleeding is one of the most worrisome complications encountered by general surgeons. Possible causes in the stomach include peptic ulcer disease, stress erosion, Mallory-Weiss tear, and gastric varices; possible causes in the small intestine include arteriovenous malformations and bleeding from an anastomosis; and possible causes in the large intestine include anastomotic hemorrhage, diverticulosis, arteriovenous malformations, and varices.

In critically ill patients, GI bleeding caused by stress ulceration is a serious complication. The incidence of bleeding from stress ulceration has decreased in the past 15 years, mainly because of improved supportive care, superior acid suppression, and enhanced resuscitative measures. Clinically significant bleeding that leads to hemodynamic instability, the need for transfusion of blood products, and occasionally operative intervention occurs in less than 5% of cases and is associated with significant mortality. Risk factors for stress ulceration are listed in Box 12-12.

Presentation and Diagnosis

When considering the source of the hemorrhage, a previous history is important when assessing the patient. A history of peptic ulcer disease and previous upper GI bleeding leads one to consider a duodenal ulcer. Severe trauma, major abdominal surgery, central nervous system injury, sepsis, or MI may be associated with stress ulceration. An antecedent history of violent emesis leads to consideration of Mallory-Weiss tear, and a history of portal hypertension or variceal bleeding is a clue regarding the

BOX 12-12 Risk Factors for Development of Stress Erosions

Multiple trauma
Head trauma
Major burns
Clotting abnormalities
Severe sepsis
Systemic inflammatory response syndrome
Cardiac bypass
Intracranial operations

presence of esophageal varices. A previous history of diverticulosis may indicate that the hemorrhage is diverticular in nature. With a recent surgical history of intestinal anastomosis, oozing from the suture or staple line may be the source of GI bleeding. In distal colorectal anastomoses, bleeding may be the first sign of anastomotic breakdown. A previous history of aortic aneurysm repair may indicate the presence of an aortoduodenal fistula. A history of intake of NSAIDs or anticoagulant or platelet inhibitor therapy identifies patients at high risk for postoperative bleeding.

In general, bright red blood is considered to come from a colonic or distal small bowel source. Melanotic stools suggest a gastric cause of bleeding. However, rapid bleeding at any site may result in bright red blood. Bleeding from the anastomosis may be a slow ooze or a rapid hemorrhage that can lead to hypotension. Patients who appear to have lost a significant amount of blood have associated tachycardia or hypotension or have a significant decrease in hematocrit level.

Treatment

To prevent stress ulceration and decrease the risk for bleeding, patients at risk must receive aggressive fluid resuscitation to improve oxygen delivery and prophylaxis that neutralizes or reduces gastric acid. Patients with respiratory failure and coagulopathy benefit the most from prophylaxis. Maintaining the gastric pH above 4 is essential to minimize gastric mucosal injury and propagation of injury by acid; this can be achieved with antacids, H_2 blockers, M_1 cholinoreceptor antagonists, sucralfate, or PPIs.

The basic principles of management of postoperative GI bleeding include the following:

1. Fluid resuscitation and restoration of intravascular volume
2. Checking and monitoring clotting parameters and correcting abnormalities, as needed
3. Identification and treatment of aggravating factors
4. Transfusion of blood products
5. Identification and treatment of the source of the bleeding

In general, management of GI bleeding is best conducted in the ICU. Fluid resuscitation with isosmotic crystalloids is begun after securing venous access. Blood samples are sent to assess the hematocrit, platelet count, prothrombin time, partial thromboplastin time, and INR. If the INR is elevated, vitamin K and fresh-frozen plasma are administered. Platelet transfusion is administered to patients with a prolonged bleeding time or patients who have been taking antiplatelet drugs; desmopressin acetate may also be given to patients with renal failure. Hypothermia, if present, is corrected.

Blood transfusion is recommended when tachycardia and hypotension refractory to volume expansion are present, with a hemoglobin concentration 6 to 10 g/dL and the extent of blood loss unknown, a hemoglobin concentration less than 6 g/dL, and rapid blood loss more than 30% as well as in patients at risk for ischemia or patients with an oxygen extraction ratio greater than 50%, with a decrease in VO_2.[35] An NG tube is placed, and the effluent is checked for the presence of blood. Nonbloody bilious drainage almost rules out a gastroduodenal source of the bleeding. If blood is present, lavage with saline at room temperature is performed.

Identification and treatment of the source of bleeding can be achieved with endoscopy, angiography, or, occasionally, laparotomy. Endoscopic control of bleeding can be achieved with an injection of epinephrine, electrocoagulation, laser coagulation, heater probe, argon plasma coagulator, clip application, banding, or any combination of these modalities, depending on the source of bleeding. Visceral angiography is indicated for patients who are actively bleeding or when endoscopy fails to control the bleeding. When an actively bleeding vessel is identified, embolization (e.g., with absorbable gelatin sponge [Gelfoam], autologous blood clot, coils) often controls the bleeding. Infusion of vasopressin may be used in patients with severe stress ulceration, diverticulosis, and ongoing bleeding. Bleeding from an intestinal anastomosis and stress ulceration usually cease with expectant management. Rarely, a patient with an anastomosis may require a reoperation to resect the anastomosis and reconnect the bowel. Similarly, surgery for stress ulceration is reserved for patients who fail medical management. Usually, a generous gastrotomy is performed to evacuate the blood clots and oversew sites of active bleeding; uncommonly, total or subtotal gastrectomy, with or without vagotomy, is performed. With both approaches, recurrence is prevented in 50% to 80% of cases.

Stomal Complications

Causes

Stomas are widely used in the treatment of colorectal, intestinal, and urologic diseases. An intestinal stoma can be an ileostomy, colostomy, or urostomy; end, loop, or end-loop; temporary or permanent; diverting or decompressing; or continent or incontinent. A tube cecostomy and a blowhole are considered temporary decompressing colostomies performed in emergencies. Several causative factors are associated with stomal complications. Technical factors are most important in minimizing the complication rate of stoma construction and are largely preventable. Stomal complications are numerous (Table 12-13) and range from a bothersome problem with fit of the stomal appliance to major skin erosion and bleeding. Complications that occur within 30 days after surgery are considered early complications.

Presentation and Diagnosis

Ischemic necrosis results from impaired perfusion to the terminal portion of the bowel as a result of a tight aperture, overzealous trimming of mesentery, or mesenteric tension. Stomal retraction occurs early as a result of tension on the bowel or ischemic necrosis of the stoma. Late retraction is caused by increased thickness of

TABLE 12-13 Stomal Complications

	COMPLICATION	
CATEGORY	EARLY	LATE
Stoma	Poor location Retraction* Ischemic necrosis Detachment Abscess formation* Opening wrong end	Prolapse Stenosis Parastomal hernia Fistula formation Gas Odor
Peristomal skin	Excoriation Dermatitis*	Parastomal varices Dermatoses Cancer Skin manifestations of inflammatory bowel disease
Systemic	High output*	Bowel obstruction Nonclosure

*May also develop as a late complication.

the abdominal wall with weight gain. Stenosis occurs as a result of a small aperture, so-called natural maturation, ischemia, recurrence of Crohn's disease, or development of carcinoma. Mucocutaneous separation develops as a result of ischemia, inadequate approximation of mucosa to the dermal layer of skin, excessive bowel tension, or peristomal infection.

Stomal prolapse is most alarming to the patient and can result in incomplete diversion of stool, interfere with the stoma appliance, lead to leakage of stool, or become associated with obstructive symptoms and incarceration. Parastomal hernia formation occurs to some degree in most patients. A peristomal fistula is often a sign of Crohn's disease, may result from a deep suture used to mature the stoma, or may be caused by trauma from an appliance.

Chemical dermatitis is caused by contact of the stoma effluent with peristomal skin as a result of a large opening in the faceplate or leakage from an ill-fitted faceplate. Chemical dermatitis is initially manifested as erythema, ulceration (ileostomy effluent), encrustation (urostomy effluent), or pseudoepitheliomatous hyperplasia. Infectious dermatitis may be caused by fungus, bacteria, tinea corporis, or *C. albicans*. Allergic dermatitis may be related to any of the stomal equipment (e.g., faceplate, tape, belt), with skin manifestations appearing at the site of contact. Traumatic dermatitis occurs during change of the stomal device, from stripping of adhesive, or as a result of friction or pressure from the stomal device or supportive belt. Traumatic dermatitis is manifested as erythema, erosion, and ulceration.

Patients with a stoma are at risk for diarrhea and dehydration. The risk for dehydration depends on the type of stoma, the underlying primary disease process, and any concomitant bowel resection. Dehydration commonly occurs in older patients, in hot weather, during strenuous exercise, and in association with short bowel syndrome.

Cutaneous manifestations of the disease may develop in the damaged peristomal skin in patients with certain skin conditions, such as psoriasis. Pyoderma gangrenosa may develop in patients with inflammatory bowel disease, and parastomal varices may develop in patients with liver disease.

Treatment

To prevent most stomal complications, adherence to sound surgical technique is imperative. Application of the technical points presented in Box 12-13 ensures the construction of a healthy and well-positioned stoma in patients undergoing surgery. In emergencies and difficult cases (e.g., obese patients, patients with distended bowel, and patients with shortened mesentery), to ensure delivery of a viable stoma free of tension, the fascial aperture may be made larger, the bowel may have to be extensively mobilized, the ileocolic artery and inferior mesenteric artery may have to be divided at their origin, windows may need to be created in the mesentery, the stoma may be brought out at a site with less subcutaneous fat (e.g., above the umbilicus), or alternative stomas may be selected.

After construction of a stoma, a dusky appearance indicates some degree of ischemia. The ischemia may be mucosal or full thickness, and the extent and depth of ischemia dictate the need for immediate revision of the stoma. Viability of the stoma is checked with a test tube and a flashlight or endoscopy. Necrosis extending to and beyond the fascia requires immediate reoperation. Ischemia limited to a few millimeters is observed and may not result in any long-term sequelae. Repair of stomal retraction often requires laparotomy.

BOX 12-13 Technical Aspects of Stoma Construction

Abdominal Wall Aperture

Excision of circular piece of skin (≈2 cm in size)
Preservation of subcutaneous fat to provide support for stoma
Transrectus muscle placement of stoma
Fascial aperture to admit two fingers

Stoma

Selection of normal bowel for stoma
Adequate mobilization of bowel to avoid tension on stoma
Preservation of blood supply to end of bowel (marginal artery of the colon and last vascular arcade of small bowel mesentery must be preserved)
Small bowel serosa must not be denuded of more than 5 cm of mesentery

Maturation

Primary maturation of end stoma or afferent limb of loop ileostomy
Avoidance of traversing skin with sutures during maturation

Other Maneuvers*

Tunneling of bowel through extraperitoneal space of abdominal wall
Mesenteric-peritoneal closure
Fixation of mesentery or bowel to fascial ring
Use of supportive rod with loop stomas

*May be performed but have not been proved to be effective in preventing postoperative complications.

Skin-level stenosis can be repaired locally, and stenoses from other causes can be repaired via laparotomy. Complete separation or detachment usually requires revision. Local repair of end stomal prolapse can be achieved with a circumferential incision at the mucocutaneous junction, excision of redundant bowel, and rematuration. Repair of loop stomal prolapse is achieved by local revision to an end stoma. Laparotomy may be required for the treatment of recurrent prolapse and prolapse associated with a parastomal hernia. Large permanent or complicated parastomal hernias are treated by relocating the stoma or reinforcing the fascia ring with mesh (synthetic or biomaterial). Treatment of a peristomal fistula entails resection of the diseased or involved segment of bowel and relocation of the stoma. Treatment of mucosal islands ranges from ablation with electrocautery to relocation of the stoma.

Treatment of chemical dermatitis entails cleaning the damaged skin, use of barriers, and a properly fitting stomal management system. *Candida* dermatitis is best treated with nystatin powder. Allergic dermatitis is treated by removal of the offending item; symptomatic relief is produced by oral antihistamine or topical or oral steroid therapy. Traumatic dermatitis is treated by patient education, and application of a skin barrier under the tape is used to secure the faceplate in place. Occasionally, in cases of severe dermatitis, the patient has to be admitted to the hospital and placed on TPN until the skin around the stoma heals enough to allow subsequent placement of an appliance.

Clostridium difficile Colitis

Causes

C. difficile colitis (CDC) is an inflammatory bowel disease caused by toxins produced by unopposed proliferation of the bacterium *C. difficile*. Several factors are associated with increased risk for CDC (Table 12-14). There has been an increased incidence and

TABLE 12-14 Factors Associated With Increased Risk for *Clostridium difficile* Colitis

CATEGORY	RISK FACTORS
Patient-related factors	Increasing age Preexisting renal disease Preexisting chronic obstructive pulmonary disease Impaired immune defense Underlying malignancy Underlying GI disease
Treatment-related factors	Preoperative bowel cleansing Antibiotic use Immunosuppressive therapy Surgery Prolonged hospital stay
Facility-related factors	ICUs Caregivers Long-term care facilities

GI, gastrointestinal; *ICU*, intensive care unit.

diagnosis rate of *C. difficile* infection (CDI) in hospitalized patients as well as an increase in severity, requiring admission to the ICU, treatment failure of the disease, colectomies, and 30-day mortality (4.7% in 1992 to 13.8% in 2003).[36,37] These changes are caused by increased awareness of the disease, advanced age and numerous comorbidities of inpatients, ubiquitous use of antibiotics, and emergence and spread of a hypervirulent strain. Historically, cephalosporins, clindamycin, and ampicillin-amoxicillin were most commonly associated with CDI. Fluoroquinolones have emerged as the class of antibiotics most prone and at increased risk to cause CDI, and the increased use of newer generation fluoroquinolones is implicated in outbreaks of a fluoroquinolone-resistant strain. Since 2000, a hypervirulent toxinotype III strain of *C. difficile* (designated BI/NAP1/027 strain) has been identified in Canada, the United States, and England. Virulence of the wild-type *C. difficile* bacteria is related to enterotoxin A and cytotoxin B encoded by the genes *tcdA* and *tcdB*. Polymorphisms or partial deletions (18-base pair deletion) in *tcdC* may lead to increased production of toxins A and B at levels 16 and 23 times higher than the wild-type bacteria.

Antibiotic use continues to precede almost all cases of infection. Of patients contracting CDC, 90% have received antibiotic therapy, and 70% have been treated with multiple antibiotics. Patients receiving prolonged courses of antibiotic therapy are particularly susceptible, and patients receiving prophylaxis are also at risk. Prolonged hospital stay allows exposure to contaminated environmental surfaces by more susceptible people. ICUs and long-term care facilities are sites of heavy environmental contamination as well as housing critically ill and vulnerable patients. Impaired host immune defense as a result of advanced age, surgery, immunosuppressive medications, HIV, and chemotherapy are major risk factors. In the past decade, the proportion of immunocompromised patients infected with *C. difficile* increased from 20% to 30%. Surgical patients account for 45% to 55% of cases of CDC, and the highest rates of infection are noted in patients undergoing general and vascular surgery. *C. difficile* is a gram-positive anaerobic spore-forming bacillus; approximately 5% to 35% of bacteria do not produce toxins and do not cause colitis. The organism produces a capsule that resists degradation by phagocytes. The spore is heat-resistant, persists in the environment for months and years in a dormant phase, and survives on inanimate objects. Approximately 3% to 5% of the general population has the organism in their stool; the percentage increases to 8.6% of patients with hematologic malignancies and 10% to 25% of adults during hospitalization.

Antibiotic use leads to a disturbance in the microflora of the colon and allows the nosocomial organism to grow, proliferate, and produce toxins. Toxin A, an enterotoxin, causes cell rounding, mucosal damage and inflammation, and release of inflammatory mediators. Toxin B is a potent cytotoxin that causes identical cell rounding and activates the release of cytokines from human monocytes. The toxins translocate to the portal circulation. Phagocytosis of toxins by macrophages in the liver results in the elaboration of several cytokines that act in the propagation of the systemic septic response.

Presentation and Diagnosis

Overgrowth of the toxigenic strain of *C. difficile* results in various disease states, with varied clinical courses. Watery diarrhea is the hallmark symptom and usually starts during or shortly after antibiotic use. One dose of antibiotic can result in the disease, but the incidence with prophylactic antibiotics increases with extended use of antibiotics beyond the recommended period. Approximately 25% to 40% of patients become symptomatic 10 weeks after completion of antibiotic therapy. The stools are foul smelling and may be positive for the presence of occult blood. In mild to moderate cases, systemic signs of infection are absent or present to a mild degree. In severe colitis, the diarrhea becomes associated with abdominal cramps and anorexia, abdominal tenderness, dehydration, tachycardia, increased leukocyte (white blood cell [WBC]) count, and bandemia (>10%). Pseudomembranous colitis is the more dramatic form of the disease and develops in 40% of patients who present with significant symptoms.

Cell cytotoxin assay in tissue culture is a highly sensitive and specific test for the detection of toxin B (rounding effect) and is the gold standard diagnostic test for CDC. ELISA that detects toxin A or B in stool is highly sensitive and specific. In contrast to the stool cytotoxic test, which requires 24 to 48 hours, results of ELISA are obtained within hours, the test is less expensive, and it does not require specific training. Endoscopy reveals nonspecific colitis in moderate disease (mucosal edema and patchy erythema) or pseudomembranes in severe disease. The presence of pseudomembranes may be limited to the proximal colon in 10% of cases, and the rectum may be spared in 60% of cases. Radiographs of the abdomen may be normal or show adynamic ileus, colonic dilation, thumbprinting, or haustral thickening. CT scans may show a thickened and edematous colon wall and free peritoneal fluid.

Despite timely medical therapy, approximately 2% to 5% of patients develop fulminant colitis and may experience cytokine-mediated cardiovascular collapse and die. Fulminant colitis frequently develops in hospitalized and postoperative patients but may occur outside the hospital setting. At-risk patients include immunocompromised patients or patients taking multiple antibiotics, patients with a previous diagnosis of CDI, patients with vasculopathy, older patients, patients with chronic obstructive pulmonary disease, and patients with renal failure. In fulminant colitis, abdominal cramps, distention, and tenderness become more prominent and are associated with systemic signs of toxicity. Diarrhea may be absent in 5% to 12% of cases; the WBC count may be depressed but is most commonly increased with a rapid elevation (>20,000 cells/mm^3) and bandemia (>30%). A leukemoid reaction is a prominent feature that may suggest CDC or herald the onset of fulminant disease. Frank peritoneal signs and toxic megacolon may develop and progress rapidly to shock. Toxic megacolon usually develops slowly and is characterized by obstipation, a dilated colon, and systemic toxicity. In fulminant disease, the toxin assay is negative in 12.5% of cases. CT scanning is diagnostic and typically shows a boggy, edematous, and thickened colon wall (>3 mm) in 88%, pancolitis in 50%, serous ascites in 35%, pericolic inflammation in 35%, a clover leaf or accordion sign in 20%, and megacolon (transverse colon >8 cm) in 25% of cases. Sigmoidoscopy shows pseudomembranes in 90% of cases versus 23% in mild cases.

Treatment

Treatment of CDC starts with prevention. However, prevention is difficult because disinfectants may eliminate *C. difficile,* but not the highly resistant spores; antibiotics are ineffective in clearing stools of carriers; and steam sterilization, although effective, is expensive. Judicious use of antibiotics, application of standard hygiene measures to hospital staff, use of disposable gloves and single-use disposable thermometers, and ward closure and decontamination in case of outbreaks are important for decreasing the mortality and morbidity associated with CDC.

When a diagnosis of CDC is made, medical therapy and timely surgical intervention improve recovery and reduce the mortality rate. Death is related to delay in diagnosis, reliance on negative toxin assay, subtotal abdominal colectomy, and additional patient-related factors. Infections with *C. difficile* usually follow a benign course. Although some patients respond to discontinuation of antibiotic therapy, others require treatment and respond within 3 to 4 days, and symptoms resolve in 95% to 98% within 10 days. Vancomycin (125 mg, four times/day) is given orally, via the NG tube, or as an enema, or metronidazole (Flagyl) is given orally (250 mg, four times/day) or intravenously (500 mg, three times/day) for 2 weeks. Antimotility agents and narcotics are avoided. IV fluid therapy is instituted to correct dehydration. Oral intake is allowed in the absence of ileus. Approximately 25% to 30% of patients develop recurrent disease as a result of reinfection with a second strain or reactivation of toxigenic spores that persist in the colon. Treatment of relapse is similar to treatment of the primary infection. In patients with recurrent attacks, pulsed vancomycin therapy, combination therapy with vancomycin and rifampicin, or administration of competitive organisms (e.g., *Lactobacillus acidophilus* and *Saccharomyces cerevisiae*) may be tried.

Most patients with CDI respond to medical treatment, but the disease occasionally progresses to a more severe form, such as fulminant colitis, despite appropriate and timely medical treatment. Fulminant colitis is characterized by severe systemic inflammatory response (fever, hypotension, tachycardia, leukocytosis, requirement for volume resuscitation), shock, multiorgan failure, and death caused by toxin-induced inflammatory mediators (e.g., IL-8, macrophage inflammatory protein-2, substance P, tumor necrosis factor-α) released locally in the colon. Alarming premortem signs include hypotension that requires vasopressor support despite adequate volume resuscitation, lactate level 5 mmol/liter or greater, respiratory failure and ventilator support, and an increase in organ dysfunction.[36,38]

Colectomy is indicated when medical treatment fails or when the patient develops hemodynamic instability, fulminant disease, toxic megacolon, or peritonitis. The timing of intervention is not well established. Although the end point of failure of medical therapy is unknown, a 24- to 48-hour trial is considered minimal. Early intervention commits the patient to a major surgical procedure and an ileostomy, and delayed intervention is associated with high mortality (35% to 75%).[36-38]

When the patient develops fulminant CDC, multiorgan failure, and hypotension, surgical intervention is less likely to be beneficial. Mortality is also increased with advanced age (>65 years), prolonged duration of CDI, length of medical treatment, and elevated serum lactate levels.[36-38] Consequently, to reduce mortality of severe CDI, patients at risk for fulminant disease are identified, and the clinical features of the disease must be recognized. Most importantly, surgical intervention must be considered during a critical window that precedes the onset of multiorgan failure and hemodynamic collapse from prolonged septic shock. Early surgical intervention noted in more recent years (2000-2006 versus 1995-1996) has changed the outcome, with a decrease in mortality from 65% to 32%.[36,37] The procedure of choice is total abdominal colectomy and ileostomy. Lesser procedures are less effective and associated with high mortality (70%) compared with 11% with abdominal colectomy.

Anastomotic Leak

Causes

Numerous factors can cause or are associated with an increased risk for anastomotic leak (Table 12-15). Mechanical bowel preparation has long been considered a critical factor in preventing infectious complications after elective colorectal surgery. In emergencies, surgeons have resorted to on-table colonic lavage to cleanse the colon and primary anastomosis, with good results. With decreased morbidity rates as a result of effective antibiotic prophylaxis, modern surgical techniques, and advances in patient care, the need for mechanical bowel preparation has been questioned. Studies have shown that mechanical bowel preparation results in adverse physiologic changes and structural alterations in the colonic mucosa and inflammatory changes in the bowel wall. Furthermore, some studies have suggested that its use in elective cases is not only unnecessary but also associated with increased anastomotic

TABLE 12-15 Risk Factors Associated With Anastomotic Leak

DEFINITIVE FACTORS	IMPLICATED FACTORS
Technical aspects	Mechanical bowel preparation
Blood supply	Drains
Tension on suture line	Advanced malignancy
Airtight and watertight anastomosis	Shock and coagulopathy
Location in GI tract	Emergency surgery
Pancreaticoenteric	Blood transfusion
Colorectal	Malnutrition
Above peritoneal reflection	Obesity
Below peritoneal reflection	Gender
Local factors	Smoking
Septic environment	Steroid therapy
Fluid collection	Neoadjuvant therapy
Bowel-related factors	Vitamin C, iron, zinc, and cysteine deficiency
Radiotherapy	Stapler-related factors
Compromised distal lumen	Forceful extraction of stapler
Crohn's disease	Tears caused by anvil or gun insertion
	Failure of stapler to close

GI, gastrointestinal.

leaks, intra-abdominal and wound infections, and reoperation.[39] Proponents of intraoperative lavage have also become content with simply decompressing the dilated colon and milking away fecal matter in the area of the anastomosis instead of aggressive cleansing. Although there is a trend toward elimination of cleansing of the colon in elective and emergent colon resection, one must be cautioned against abandoning the practice completely, especially for anterior resections, in which the presence of stool in the rectum poses a problem with the use of staplers.

The level of the anastomosis in the GI tract is important. Although small bowel, ileocolic, and ileorectal anastomoses are considered safe, esophageal, pancreaticoenteric, and colorectal anastomoses are considered high risk for leakage. In the esophagus, lack of serosa appears to be a significant contributing factor. In the pancreas, the texture of the gland and size of the pancreatic duct, the presence of pancreatic duct obstructive lesions, the experience of the operating surgeon, and probably the type of enteric anastomosis are implicated (see later). In the rectum, the highest leak rate is found in anastomoses in the distal rectum, 6 to 8 cm from the anal verge.

Adequate microcirculation at the resection margins is crucial for the healing of any anastomosis. Factors interfering with the perianastomotic microcirculation include smoking, hypertension, locally enhanced coagulation activity as a result of surgical trauma, perianastomotic hematoma, and presence of macrovascular disease. In colorectal anastomoses, relative ischemia in the rectal remnant is a factor because its blood supply is derived from the internal iliac artery via the inferior hemorrhoidal vessels; contribution from the middle hemorrhoidal artery is minimal and, at best, variable because the vessels are mostly absent and, when present, are unilateral. Total mesorectal excision, neoadjuvant therapy, and extended lymphadenectomy with high ligation of the inferior mesenteric artery are additional contributing factors.

Intraluminal distention is believed to be responsible for rupture of an anastomosis. The mechanical strength of the anastomosis is important and, in the early period, is dependent on sutures or staples, with endothelial cells and fibrin-fibrinonectin complex additionally contributing to the tension force. Construction of a watertight and airtight anastomosis is essential. Antiadhesive agents may predispose to leaks because they isolate the anastomosis from the peritoneum and omentum and, as found in animal studies, decrease anastomotic bursting pressure and hydroxyproline levels.[40]

Intra-abdominally placed open rubber drains are not helpful and are associated with an increased risk of infection if left for more than 24 to 48 hours. In the pelvis, drains have been shown in some studies to be associated with a higher leak rate. Conversely, drains may remove blood, cellular debris, and serum that act as good culture media for perianastomotic sepsis or abscess formation. Local sepsis affects the integrity of the anastomosis negatively as it reduces collagen synthesis and increases collagenase activity, which results in increased lysis of collagen at the anastomosis. Defunctioning or protective stomas do not decrease the overall leak rate, but rather minimize the severity and sequelae of perianastomotic contamination and decrease the reoperation rate. However, defunctioning stomas deprive the colon of short-chain fatty acids, resulting in exclusion colitis and delay in epithelialization of the anastomosis, and are associated with altered collagen metabolism observed in left-sided anastomoses.

Bevacizumab, an angiogenesis inhibitor, is associated with increased risk for surgical site complications. This agent is a humanized monoclonal antibody that targets vascular endothelial growth factor (VEGF). VEGF is a critical factor for the survival of endothelial cells and is selectively present in the neovasculature of growing tumors. Bevacizumab binds with high specificity and affinity to VEGF, inhibiting the binding of VEGF to its receptors and negatively affecting angiogenesis or the remodeling of the existing network of blood vessels. Bevacizumab is used in combination with standard chemotherapy (irinotecan, 5-fluorouracil, and leucovorin) in the treatment of patients with metastatic colorectal cancer. In animal studies, antiangiogenic cancer therapy inhibits dermal wound healing in a dose-related fashion and compromises healing of colonic anastomoses. In patients with metastatic colorectal cancer, it increases the risk of surgical site complications—spontaneous dehiscence of primary anastomosis and colocutaneous fistula formation from an anastomosis. Such complications may occur 2 years after surgery.[41] The mechanism is probably related to microthromboembolic disease leading to bowel ischemia, inhibition of angiogenesis in the microvascular bed of the new anastomosis, inhibition of neoangiogenesis in postradiated tissue, and reduction in the number of newly formed vessels in granulation tissue surrounding anastomotic sites. Risk factors for delayed anastomotic complications include a history of anastomotic complications, radiotherapy, and rectal location of anastomoses.

Emergency bowel surgery is associated with high morbidity and mortality, in part because of sepsis and anastomotic leakage; this is related to the poor nutritional status of the patient, presence of underlying malignancy, immunocompromised state, presence of intra-abdominal contamination or sepsis, and hemodynamic instability. Transfusion, on the one hand, causes impaired cell-mediated immunity and predisposes to infection and, on the other hand, alleviates anemia and improves the oxygen-carrying capacity of red blood cells that may have a positive impact on healing. Obesity increases the difficulty and complexity of the surgery; has been shown to be associated with increased postoperative complications; and is an independent risk factor for an increasing leakage rate, especially after a low colorectal anastomosis. Steroids affect healing by decreasing collagen synthesis, delaying the appearance of the inflammatory reaction, and reducing the production of transforming growth factor-β and insulin-like growth factor in wounds, which are essential for wound healing.

Presentation and Diagnosis

Anastomotic leak results in sepsis and enteric fistula formation, leads to reoperation and a possible permanent stoma, and is associated with decreased survival and increased local recurrence rate after curative resection of cancer and possibly leads to death.[42] The clinical manifestations are the result of a cascade of events that start with loss of integrity of the anastomosis and leakage of intestinal contents. The leakage may be diffuse throughout the peritoneal cavity (uncontrolled leak) or become walled off by omentum; abdominal wall; and contiguous loops of bowel, pelvic wall, or adhesions from prior operations. If a surgical drain is present, intestinal contents are discharged onto the skin. Intra-abdominal fluid collections may contain intestinal contents, frank pus, or pus mixed with intestinal contents. If the fluid collection is drained surgically or percutaneously, there is an initial discharge of purulent material followed by feculent material heralding the formation of an enterocutaneous fistula (controlled fistula). If allowed to drain through the surgical incision or abdominal wall, surgical wound infection and dehiscence with evisceration or an abdominal wall abscess may occur. If the fluid collection burrows into a contiguous structure such as the urinary bladder or vagina, spontaneous drainage occurs, with the formation of an enterovesical or enterovaginal fistula.

After the index surgery, a patient may have an initial normal postoperative course or may not have been progressing as expected. The early warning signs of anastomotic leak are malaise, fever, abdominal pain, ileus, localized erythema around the surgical incision, and leukocytosis. Patients may also develop bowel obstruction, induration and erythema in the abdominal wall, rectal bleeding, or suprapubic pain. There may be initial excessive drainage from the surgical wound or surgical wound dehiscence or evisceration or both. An intra-abdominal fluid collection or abdominal wall abscess may be identified and drained surgically or percutaneously. Patients may also experience pneumaturia, fecaluria, and pyuria. When a fistulous communication is established, problems related to the loss of intestinal contents, perifistula skin, surgical wound, and malnutrition soon ensue.

Sepsis is a prominent feature of anastomotic leakage and results from diffuse peritonitis or localized abscess, abdominal wall infection, or contamination of a sterile site with intestinal contents. Abdominal wall infection develops as a result of contact of purulent material with the muscle and subcutaneous tissue; tissue necrosis associated with fascial sutures; or contact of corrosive intestinal juices with the abdominal wall, resulting in chemical erosion and extension of the infectious process. Nonclostridial necrotizing infections of the abdominal wall occur, particularly with fistulas of the lower GI tract that contain high concentrations of Enterobacteriaceae, non–group A beta-hemolytic streptococci, and anaerobic cocci or penicillin-sensitive *Bacteroides* spp. Contamination of the urinary bladder with intestinal contents (enterovesical fistula) results in urosepsis.

Treatment

Treatment of anastomotic leakage starts with prevention. In elective cases, nutritional support for 5 to 7 days is appropriate for patients who are malnourished or have lost significant amounts of weight. Mechanical and chemical bowel preparations are still recommended by many surgeons before colorectal resection. In patients receiving or who have received bevacizumab, the appropriate interval between the last dose administered and the surgery is unknown. The terminal half-life of the medication is long—20 days—so wound-healing complications are documented 56 days after treatment. It is advisable to delay elective surgery for at least 4 to 8 weeks or, preferably, three half-lives (60 days) after treatment. In patients with newly constructed anastomoses who are candidates for bevacizumab therapy, evaluation of the anastomosis before initiation of therapy with fine-cut CT scanning, barium enema, and colonoscopy allows identification of patients at risk for anastomotic complications. In emergencies, especially in hemodynamically unstable, immunocompromised, and nutritionally depleted patients, in the presence of fecal peritonitis, significant bowel dilation, and edema, an anastomosis is best avoided because a leak may prove fatal.

Construction of an anastomosis that is at low risk for disruption requires the following:

1. Adequate exposure, gentle handling of tissues, aseptic precaution, and meticulous, careful dissection
2. Adequate mobilization so that the two attached organs have a tension-free anastomosis
3. Correct technical placement of sutures or staples with little variance
4. Matching of the lumens of the two organs to be connected, which can be done by various techniques
5. Preservation of the blood supply to the ends of structures to be anastomosed

Sufficient microcirculation is essential for healing of the anastomosis. In intestinal anastomoses, the marginal artery of the colon and last vascular arcade of small bowel mesentery must be preserved. The small bowel serosa must not be denuded of mesentery more than 3 to 4 cm for hand-sewn anastomoses. In the distal colon, the following maneuvers may be required to ensure a tension-free anastomosis: inferior mesenteric artery divided at its origin, windows created in the mesentery of the small bowel up to the third portion of the duodenum, and small branches interrupted between the arcades creating mesenteric windows and dividing the ileocolic vessels at their origin. For intestinal and colorectal anastomoses, there is no difference in the rate of anastomotic leakage between hand-sewn and stapled anastomoses and among various stapling techniques, provided that sound surgical technique is followed. The decision to construct a one-layer or two-layer intestinal anastomosis is a matter of preference. A colorectal anastomosis is easier to perform in one layer. However, since the advent of stapling devices, an anastomosis deep in the pelvis has most commonly been stapled. The technique is not only faster but also improves asepsis because the anastomosis is performed in a closed fashion compared with a hand-sewn anastomosis, which is considered an "open anastomosis" and allows for more contamination. In low anterior resection, the omentum may be advanced to the pelvis and placed around the colorectal anastomosis. This maneuver may reduce the rate of anastomotic leak or disruption but mostly appears to decrease the severity of the complication. Drainage of a colorectal anastomosis is advisable in difficult cases and when technical problems are encountered or when neoadjuvant therapy has been used. Defunctioning stomas are used for extraperitoneal anastomoses, when technical difficulties are encountered, or after neoadjuvant therapy.

When constructing a pancreaticoenteric anastomosis, a pancreaticojejunostomy is equivalent to pancreaticogastrostomy. An end to side–duct to mucosa pancreaticojejunostomy is associated with a lower leak rate compared with an end-to-end invaginating pancreaticojejunostomy; obliteration of the main pancreatic duct with protamine gel or human fibrin sealant, or suture closure of the remnant pancreas without an anastomosis, is associated with the highest leak rate.[43] The routine placement of drains in proximity to pancreatic anastomoses is controversial. Drains and octreotide can be used when an anastomosis is performed to a soft pancreas with a small duct and in centers with lower surgical volume or centers with a high leak rate (>10%). Pancreatic duct stents (placed intraoperatively) continue to be used, despite the lack of data to suggest that they decrease the leak rate.[43] A pancreatic stent placed before a distal pancreatectomy decompresses the pancreatic duct by abolishing the pressure gradient between the pancreatic duct and duodenum and may decrease the risk of fistula formation, allowing the site of a leak to seal.

When an anastomotic leak is suspected or diagnosed, resuscitation is started immediately because patients are in the postoperative period and have been without nutrition. Furthermore, they have a contracted intravascular volume because of third spacing and lost intestinal contents and may have an electrolyte imbalance. Intravascular volume is restored with crystalloid fluids and a blood transfusion if anemia is present, and electrolyte imbalances are corrected. Oral intake is stopped, and the bowel is put at rest to decrease luminal contents and GI stimulation and secretion. An NG tube is placed if obstructive symptoms are present. Infected surgical wounds are opened, and any abdominal wall abscesses are incised and drained. Reoperation is indicated if there is diffuse peritonitis, intra-abdominal hemorrhage, suspected intestinal ischemia, major wound disruption, or evisceration. Reoperation is a major undertaking and is associated with significant mortality and morbidity. The procedure is bloody and carries the risk of bowel injury. Primary closure of the leaking point only is avoided because failure is certain.

The management of duodenal and proximal jejunal leaks is challenging. In these situations, transgastric placement of a jejunal tube helps divert gastric and biliopancreatic secretions, and placement of drains in close proximity to the leak allows external drainage of the intestinal contents. Pyloric exclusion and gastrojejunostomy should be used judiciously in these situations. Management of jejunal, ileal, and colorectal leaking anastomoses depends on the severity and duration of contamination, condition of the bowel, and hemodynamic stability of the patient. In a critically ill and unstable patient, especially a patient with fecal peritonitis, a damage control type of procedure is performed—the anastomosis is taken down, the ends of the bowel are stapled, peritoneal lavage is performed, and the incision is left open. A second-look laparotomy with stomal formation is performed in 24 to 48 hours or when the patient is more stable. Otherwise, in the small bowel, an anastomosis may be performed or the ends of the bowel are delivered as stomas; in the colon, the proximal end of the colon is brought out as a colostomy, and the distal end is closed or brought out as a mucous fistula; and in the rectum, the distal end is closed, and the proximal end of the colon is delivered as a stoma. A proximal diverting stoma with drainage of the pelvis is inadequate treatment of leaking colorectal anastomoses associated with diffuse peritonitis. If the abdomen is left open, covering the bowel with the greater omentum (if available) or a biologic implant protects the bowel and prevents desiccation and spontaneous fistula formation. Negative-pressure wound therapy is best avoided when bowel is exposed, especially in the presence of unprotected suture or staple line.[44]

In the absence of diffuse peritonitis and evisceration, a CT scan may identify single or multiple abscesses, pneumoperitoneum, ascites, and sometimes extravasation of oral contrast agent into the peritoneal cavity. Multiple abscesses require open drainage, a single intra-abdominal abscess can be drained percutaneously, and a pelvic abscess can be drained transrectally or transvaginally. An external fistula may develop after drainage. The management of a controlled fistula is outlined in the next section. If percutaneous drainage fails to control sepsis, reoperation is indicated. At the time of open drainage of a pelvic abscess, if there is any doubt about the origin of the abscess (de novo abscess versus abscess secondary to a small anastomotic leak that has sealed), a defunctioning stoma is constructed, unless there is complete disruption of the anastomosis. In that case, the ends of the bowel are exteriorized as a stoma. A pancreaticojejunostomy leak, if small, can be treated by placing a drain next to the leak. However, for an anastomosis that has almost fallen apart, the patient would probably require completion pancreatectomy. A patient who has a bile duct leak requires drainage of the infection and placement of a drain next to the leak or, in the case of a large leak, may require bile duct reconstruction.

Intestinal Fistulas

Causes

A fistula represents an abnormal communication between two epithelialized surfaces, one of which is a hollow organ. In the GI tract, a fistula may develop between any two digestive organs or between a hollow organ and the skin and may be developmental or acquired. Acquired fistulas account for most GI fistulas and can be traumatic, spontaneous, or postoperative in nature.

GI fistulas are most commonly iatrogenic, develop after an operation, and may occur anywhere in the GI tract. Esophageal, aortoenteric, and rectal fistulas are not discussed in this section. In the past, acquired GI fistulas most commonly developed as a result of a difficult appendectomy. At the present time, they commonly occur as the result of anastomotic breakdown, dehiscence of a surgically closed segment of stomach or bowel, unrecognized iatrogenic bowel injury after adhesiolysis, or during closure of a laparotomy incision. Occasionally, they develop after instrumentation or drainage of a pancreatic, appendiceal, or diverticular fluid collection or abscess. Predisposing factors for fistula formation include the presence of intrinsic intestinal disease, such as Crohn's disease; radiation enteritis; distal obstruction, or a hostile abdominal environment, such as an abscess or peritonitis. The risk is also higher in emergencies when the patient may be malnourished or poorly prepared.

Gastric fistulas are uncommon and frequently occur after resection for cancer and less frequently after resection for peptic ulcer disease, resection for necrotizing pancreatitis, an antireflux procedure, or bariatric surgery. Pancreatic fistulas develop as a result of disruption of the main pancreatic duct or its branches secondary to trauma or postoperatively after pancreatic biopsy; distal pancreatectomy; pancreaticoduodenectomy; pancreatic necrosectomy; or surgery on the stomach, biliary tree, or spleen. Intestinal fistulas develop after resection for cancer, diverticular disease, inflammatory bowel disease, or closure of a stoma.

Presentation and Diagnosis

Enterocutaneous fistulas are usually associated with a triad of sepsis, fluid and electrolyte imbalance, and malnutrition. Patients are usually in the postoperative period and may not be progressing as expected or may have an initial normal postoperative course. They then start showing the manifestations of leakage of intestinal contents (see earlier). The seriousness and severity of these manifestations depend on the surgical anatomy and physiology of the fistula. Anatomically, the fistula may originate from the stomach, duodenum, small bowel (proximal or distal), or large bowel. The tract of the fistula may erode into another portion of the intestines (enteroenteric fistula) or another hollow organ (enterovesical), forming an internal fistula, or into the body surface (enterocutaneous and pancreatic fistula) or vagina (enterovaginal fistula), forming an external fistula. A mixed fistula describes an internal fistula associated with an external fistula. A superficial fistula drains on top of an open or granulating wound. In a deep fistula, the tract traverses the abdominal cavity and drains onto the skin. Physiologically, the fistula is classified as high output or low output on the basis of the volume of discharge in 24 hours. The exact definition of low output and high output varies from 200 to 500 mL/24 hr. However, three different categories are recognized—low output (<200 mL/24 hr), moderate output (200 to 500 mL/24 hr), and high output (>500 mL/24 hr). The ileum is the site of the fistula in 50% of high-output fistulas. The discussion in this section focuses mainly on external fistulas.

Sepsis is a prominent feature of postoperative intestinal fistulas and is present in 25% to 75% of cases. As noted earlier, sepsis is the result of diffuse peritonitis or localized abscess, abdominal wall or necrotizing infection, or contamination of a sterile hollow organ with intestinal contents.

Loss of intestinal contents through the fistula results in hypovolemia and dehydration, electrolyte and acid-base imbalance, loss of protein and trace elements, and malnutrition. In a high intestinal fistula, it also results in loss of the normal inhibitory effect on gastric secretion, resulting in a gastric hypersecretory state. With high-output enterocutaneous fistulas, there is also intrahepatic cholestasis related to the loss of bile salts, disruption of enterohepatic circulation, and bacterial overgrowth in the defunctionalized intestine. Malnutrition results from loss of protein-rich secretions, lack of nutrient intake, loss of absorption caused by bypass of the gut (e.g., gastrocolic, duodenocolic, high enterocutaneous fistulas), and sepsis that sets the stage for nutritional deficiency and rapid breakdown of body muscle mass. In gastroduodenal and proximal small bowel fistulas, the output is high, and the fluid loss, electrolyte imbalance, and malabsorption are profound. In distal small bowel and colonic fistulas, the output is low, and dehydration, acid-base imbalance, and malnutrition are uncommon. Significant electrolyte imbalance occurs in 45% of patients, and malnutrition occurs in 55% to 90%.

Skin and surgical wound complications develop as a result of contact of GI effluent with skin or the wound. Effluent dermatitis results from the corrosive effect of intestinal contents, which cause irritation, maceration, excoriation, ulceration, and infection of the skin. Fecal dermatitis is marked by erythema and desquamation and may lead to skin sepsis. Superficial and deep surgical wound and necrotizing infections also develop. Pain and itching caused by contact of effluent with unprotected skin is intolerable and affects the morale of the patient.

Treatment

Although postoperative intestinal fistulas are not a new problem, their etiogenesis has changed, and their management continues to evolve. In the past, the main focus of management involved suctioning of the intestinal effluent and early surgical intervention. This approach has proven ineffective and is associated with significant patient morbidity and mortality and a high reoperation rate. At the present time, management requires the involvement of a surgeon, nutritionist, enterostomal therapist, interventional radiologist, and gastroenterologist; it entails initial medical treatment to allow spontaneous healing of the fistula, early surgical intervention in a select group of patients, and planned definitive surgery for patients whose fistulas have failed to heal. External intestinal fistulas result in prolonged hospital stays and enormous cost to the hospital and are associated with significant patient disability, morbidity, and mortality (6% to 30%). Although spontaneous closure occurs in 40% to 80% of cases, operative intervention may be required in 30% to 60% of cases.

The first step in the management of a GI fistula is to prevent its occurrence. Reducing the likelihood of an anastomotic leak requires adherence to sound surgical principles and proper techniques (see earlier). If a fistula forms, management involves several phases that are applied systematically and simultaneously (Table 12-16).

When a leak is diagnosed or suspected, management involves resuscitation, TPN, correction of electrolyte imbalances, and transfusions, as appropriate. Oral intake is stopped, and the bowel is put at rest, decreasing luminal contents and reducing GI stimulation and secretion. An NG tube is placed if obstructive symptoms are present. Routine NG tube placement is not helpful and subjects the patient to complications, such as sinusitis and aspiration. Broad-spectrum IV antibiotic therapy is started and adjusted later according to cultures.

The indications for early surgical intervention were discussed earlier. Otherwise, resuscitation is continued. Treatment with H_2 antagonists or PPI helps decrease peptic ulceration and may decrease fistula output but does not aid in closure of the fistula. Accurate measurement of output from all orifices and the fistula is paramount in maintaining fluid balance. Effective control of all sources of sepsis is important because continued sepsis is a major source of mortality that results in a state of hypercatabolism and the failure of exogenous nutritional support to restore and maintain body mass and immune function; it is also associated with a decreased rate of healing of GI fistulas. Infected surgical wounds are opened and drained, abdominal wall abscesses are incised and drained, and intra-abdominal fluid collections are drained percutaneously or surgically. Percutaneous drainage is tolerated better and allows changing a complex fistula (fistula associated with an

TABLE 12-16 Factors Affecting Healing of External Intestinal Fistulas

FACTORS	FAVORABLE	UNFAVORABLE
Surgical anatomy of fistula	Long tract, >2 cm	Short tract, <2 cm
	Single tract	Multiple tracts
	No other fistulas	Associated internal fistulas
	Lateral fistula	End fistula
	Nonepithelialized tract	Epithelialized tract
	Origin (jejunum, colon, duodenal stump, and pancreaticobiliary)	Origin (lateral duodenum, stomach, and ileum)
	No adjacent large abscess	Adjacent large abscess
Status of bowel	No intestinal disease	Intrinsic intestinal disease (Crohn's disease, radiation enteritis, recurrent or incompletely resected cancer)
	No distal bowel obstruction	Distal bowel obstruction
	Small enteral defect, <1 cm	Large enteral defect, >1 cm
Condition of abdominal wall	Intact	Disrupted (fistula opens into base of disrupted incision)
	Not diseased	Infiltrated with malignancy or intestinal disease
	No foreign body	Foreign body (mesh)
Physiology of patient	No malnutrition	Malnutrition
	No sepsis	Sepsis
Output of fistula	No influence	Influence

abscess) to a simple fistula that has a better chance of spontaneous closure. A small pigtail catheter may be changed to a larger catheter that allows irrigation of the abscess cavity, later injection of contrast agent to assess resolution of the abscess, and study of the anatomy of the fistula.

Nutrition is one of the most important factors contributing to a successful outcome in the management of intestinal fistulas. TPN must be started early after the correction of electrolyte imbalance and repletion of volume. TPN allows bowel rest, which decreases output, eliminates negative nitrogen balance, improves the patient's nutritional status, allows better timing of the operation when needed, increases the rate of recovery, and may slightly improve the closure rate when sepsis is controlled. Trace elements, multivitamins, vitamin K, and medications such as octreotide may be added to the TPN. TPN is the initial nutritional support for any patient with a fistula and is continued in patients with high-output fistulas or patients who cannot tolerate oral intake. Somatostatin analogues (e.g., octreotide, with a long half-life) help in management of the fistula by reducing GI secretions and inhibiting GI motility, controlling and reducing its output. Their value in healing intestinal fistulas is yet to be proven, and routine use is limited because they are not without side effects. Somatostatin leads to cellular apoptosis, villous atrophy, and interruption of intestinal adaptation and may be associated with acute cholecystitis. Enteral nutrition (low-residue diet, elemental diet, liquid whole protein diet) is administered to patients with low-output small bowel and colonic external fistulas. Fistuloclysis (i.e., infusion of nutrition directly through the fistula into the bowel distal to the fistula) is another option to deliver enteral nutrition to patients whose fistula has not healed spontaneously, provided that there is more than 75 cm of healthy bowel distal that is in continuity with the fistula.[45] Fistuloclysis is safer and less expensive than TPN and prevents atrophy of the bowel distal to the fistula.

Early control of fistula output is essential to protect the perifistula skin from the corrosive effects of intestinal effluent, promote healing of damaged skin and surgical wounds, and facilitate nursing care of the patient. Early involvement by an enterostomal therapist and wound care team cannot be overemphasized. Protection of the skin is achieved with barriers, sealants, adhesives, and pouches. Negative-pressure wound therapy is another treatment strategy whereby the continuous suction of fistula output minimizes contact between intestinal contents and surrounding tissue. It protects perifistula skin, reduces the need for dressing changes, promotes wound healing, and accelerates fistula closure, especially in deep fistulas. Closure has been reported to occur in 46% to 84% of cases.[46]

When initial sepsis is controlled, nutrition is provided, and wound and fistula care is provided, studies are performed to define the surgical pathology of the fistula (origin, course, length of the fistula) and condition of the bowel (presence of intrinsic intestinal disease, presence of distal obstruction, continuity of the bowel) and to evaluate resolution of the intra-abdominal abscess. A fistulogram is performed by injecting a water-soluble contrast medium or barium through an existing drain or by inserting a 5 Fr pediatric feeding tube or a Foley catheter into the external opening of the fistula. A fistulogram delineates the anatomy of the fistula and identifies associated cavities, other fistulas, and distal obstructions. A contrast enema demonstrates the presence of a colocutaneous fistula in 90%, a colovesical fistula in 34%, and a coloenteric fistula in most cases. Enteroclysis allows evaluation for intrinsic intestinal disease. Cystoscopy identifies the fistula opening in 40% of enterovesical fistulas, but the findings of localized bullous edema, with erythema and possible ulceration, are suggestive of the diagnosis in most patients. GI endoscopy allows direct visualization of colonic, intestinal, and gastroduodenal mucosa. CT scan allows evaluation for the resolution of intra-abdominal abscesses and presence of intrinsic intestinal disease.

With such an orchestrated approach, most external fistulas heal spontaneously. Factors associated with spontaneous healing or failure to close are listed in Table 12-16. After control of sepsis, approximately 60% to 90% of external intestinal fistulas with favorable factors close spontaneously with medical management, 90% close within 4 to 6 weeks, and less than 10% close in 2 to 3 months. There are limited therapeutic options for enterocutaneous fistulas that fail to close—accept the fistula as a stoma awaiting optimal time for definitive closure or attempt direct closure.

Direct repair is applicable to a superficial bud fistula, whereby limited dissection is performed to identify and close the edges of the fistula extraperitoneally and protect the suture line with a biologic dressing, with or without tissue adhesive. Although several attempts may be required to achieve successful closure of the fistula, the surgery is a local low-risk procedure and can be repeated. Definitive repair requires careful planning and may be a daunting task. Definitive closure requires a waiting period of 8 to 12 weeks and requires that sepsis be controlled, nutrition provided, and the skin protected. The waiting period is crucial to allow recovery of immunologic competence, improvement of nutritional status, and resolution of the period of dense inflammatory reaction. There are no well-established guidelines to help in determining the timing of surgery. However, the experience of the surgeon, general condition of the patient, softness of the abdominal wall and abdominal cavity, and surgical anatomy of the fistula must be taken into consideration. A dense intra-abdominal inflammatory reaction occurs 10 to 21 days after surgery and lasts 6 to 8 weeks before starting to resolve. A 6-month period is required for a neoperitoneal cavity to develop in fistulas within a laparoscopy wound. A simple fistula—a single fistula with direct communication between the bowel and skin, a short tract and small enteral opening, and associated with other favorable factors—can be closed 12 weeks after the index surgery. A complex fistula—a fistula with a long tract and associated with other internal fistulas, large abscess cavity, fistula that opens into the base of a disrupted wound, or other unfavorable factors—is closed 6 to 12 months after the index surgery. Complex fistulas associated with intrinsic intestinal disease require definitive surgical intervention after the initial sepsis is controlled because spontaneous closure is highly unlikely, and extirpation of the diseased bowel is essential. In a select group of patients with Crohn's disease, infliximab (Remicade) may also be used to aid in closure of the fistula.

A controlled enterocutaneous fistula that opens into the base of an interrupted wound requires abdominal wall construction at the time of definitive repair of the fistula. The fistulizing segment must not be excluded or bypassed to avoid the risk of blind loop syndrome. The fistula is excised, continuity of the GI tract is reestablished, and the freshly constructed anastomosis is wrapped with omentum if available. Gastric, duodenal, and proximal jejunal fistulas that cannot be resected without a major surgical procedure are best managed with a Roux-en-Y intestinal anastomosis. The laparotomy incision is closed primarily with durable well-vascularized coverage. Autogenous tissue reduces the risk of infection. Pedicle or free flaps with microvascular reconstruction may be considered; however, component separation when the rectus muscle is intact, with or without augmentation with acellular dermal matrix or synthetic mesh, is the preferred procedure.[47] Postoperative morbidity, ventral hernia formation, and recurrent enterocutaneous fistulas develop in approximately 20% to 25% of cases. Biologic material (e.g., acellular human or porcine dermal matrix, porcine submucosa) used for visceral overlay protection or reconstruction is another viable option in this setting of compromised operative field because the implant resists infection, and when postoperative infection occurs, removal of the implant is unnecessary. However, biologic materials are expensive, and the procedure is associated with a high rate of hernia formation and abdominal wall laxity.[48] Occasionally the incision is closed in stages. The incision may be left open (laparotomy), an absorbable mesh (polyglactin or polyglycolic acid) may be used to bridge the fascial defect, or negative-pressure wound therapy can be instituted. After granulation tissue has formed, a split-thickness skin graft is applied.

New innovative approaches, such as transcatheter injection of diluted thrombin, endoscopic tissue sealant or clip application, and porcine small intestinal submucosa, have been used in recalcitrant cases or as adjunctive therapy to hasten healing of the intestinal fistula, with some success.

Pancreatic Fistulas

Overall, the physiologic classification, diagnosis, management, and outcome of postoperative external pancreatic fistulas are similar to external intestinal fistulas. However, pancreatic fistulas have additional distinctive features. After pancreaticoduodenectomy, texture of the pancreas, size of the pancreatic duct, blood supply to the stump, and volume of pancreatic juice produced are the most significant risk factors for fistula formation. Pulmonary problems, autodigestion, and erosion into adjacent organs are additional significant morbidities associated with pancreatic fistulas. Sepsis and hemorrhage are associated with significant mortality (20% to 40%) and result in prolonged hospitalization and increased hospital expense. Postoperative pancreatic fistula is diagnosed when there is drain output of any measurable volume of fluid after postoperative day 3 with an amylase content more than three times the serum amylase activity. More often, the fluid amylase content is in the tens of thousands units per liter. The fistula is demonstrated on a fistulogram or CT scan.

Efforts to decrease the morbidity and mortality of pancreatic fistulas after pancreaticoduodenectomy focus on preventing, decreasing, and controlling pancreatic leaks at the pancreatic-enteric reconstruction (see earlier, "Anastomotic Leak"). The benefit of perioperative somatostatin or its analogue was evaluated in a meta-analysis study.[49] One study noted that somatostatin and octreotide reduced the rate of biochemical fistula but not the incidence of clinical anastomotic dehiscence, whereas the other noted a significant reduction in pancreatic fistula rate but no significant difference in postoperative mortality. Intraoperatively, a modified side-to-end pancreaticojejunal anastomosis provides a tension-free anastomosis to a pancreatic stump, with adequate blood supply and unobstructed flow of pancreatic juice. This modified pancreaticojejunostomy commonly includes mobilization of the pancreatic stump to allow invagination of 3 to 4 cm of pancreatic stump into the jejunum, ablation of the jejunal mucosa in the area of the jejunum-pancreas interface, suturing of the capsular edge of the pancreatic stump to mucosa of the everted jejunum, or the use of traction sutures between the capsular edge and jejunum proximal edge to avoid slippage of the stump out of the jejunum.

When a pancreatic fistula has formed, medical treatment results in spontaneous closure in almost all fistulas after a pancreaticoduodenectomy and in 80% of all other cases of pancreatic fistulas. Octreotide therapy is beneficial because it significantly reduces fistula output and decreases the time to fistula closure. Endoscopic retrograde cholangiopancreatography (ERCP) is valuable because it defines the pancreatic duct anatomy and ductal obstruction and allows the placement of a stent that bypasses the high-resistance areas of the sphincter of Oddi, ductal strictures, and calculi, allowing pancreatic secretions to follow the path of least resistance. The stent may also block the ductal opening of the fistula. Operative treatment of a benign pancreaticocutaneous fistula depends on the location of the fistula (proximal versus distal portion of the pancreas) and status of the pancreatic duct (dilated versus stenotic duct). High excision of the fistula with fistuloenterostomy has been associated with the best results. Pseudocyst enterostomy is associated with an unacceptable recurrence and failure rate.

HEPATOBILIARY COMPLICATIONS

Bile Duct Injuries

Causes

The most dreaded complication of gallbladder surgery is injury to the extrahepatic bile duct system. Cholecystectomy accounts for most postoperative biliary injuries and strictures. The rate of major bile duct injury after laparoscopic cholecystectomy ranges from 0.4% to 0.7%, as opposed to 0.2% after open cholecystectomy.[50] Bile leak may be caused by a bile duct injury, cystic duct stump leak, divided accessory duct, or injury to the intestine. Acute cholecystitis, a foreshortened cystic duct, anomalies of the biliary tree, hemorrhage from injury to the cystic or hepatic artery, dissection with thermal instruments in the triangle of Calot, and failure to define the anatomy in the triangle of Calot clearly are among the most important factors associated with a higher frequency of duct injury after laparoscopic cholecystectomy.

The most common injury sustained during the laparoscopic procedure is complete transection at or below the hepatic duct bifurcation. Other, less complex injuries include occlusion of the duct with a clip, thermal injury, avulsion of the cystic duct, and partial laceration.

Presentation and Diagnosis

Most bile duct injuries are not identified at the time of surgery. Early in the postoperative period, patients may have manifestations related to a bile leak or have signs of a bile duct stricture later. Bile leaking from a lacerated divided duct may accumulate in the subhepatic space and form a biloma or seep into the peritoneal cavity and result in bile ascites. Patients in this situation have right upper quadrant pain, fever, nausea, abdominal distention, and malaise. The bile may drain through an intraoperatively placed drain and manifest as a bile leak. In this setting, patients may have leukocytosis and a slightly elevated bilirubin level. Patients with a clipped bile duct do not usually have symptoms but do have elevated liver enzyme levels. Bile duct strictures are usually accompanied by cholangitis, pain, fever, chills, and jaundice.

Diagnosis of bile duct injury requires the use of nuclear medicine imaging to demonstrate the presence of a leak or obstruction, CT scan to identify bile collections or ascites, and ERCP to define the type and level of injury accurately. Percutaneous transhepatic cholangiography is indicated in cases of complete transection to define the proximal anatomy and site of injury. Magnetic resonance cholangiopancreatography is becoming the test of choice to diagnose late strictures and define the bile duct anatomy.

Treatment

Prevention of bile duct injury starts with proper surgical technique and adequate identification of the anatomy. The anatomic variability associated with severe inflammation creates a low threshold for converting a laparoscopic to an open cholecystectomy. During laparoscopic cholecystectomy, the infundibulum of the gallbladder must be retracted laterally and inferiorly to expose the triangle and widen the cystic–common bile duct angle. Dissection of the cystic duct and artery must begin close to the infundibulum of the gallbladder. The cystic duct and artery are divided when the anatomy is clearly delineated. Excessive traction on the gallbladder must be avoided because it would result in tenting of the common duct. If there is bleeding in the area of the cystic duct, blind clipping and cautery must be avoided, and adequate exposure must be achieved, even if placement of another port is required. If there is an unexpected bile leak, unusual anatomy, or a second bile duct identified, or when technical difficulties and excessive bleeding are encountered, intraoperative cholangiography helps identify the anatomy and any injuries. Early conversion to an open procedure must also be considered.

When a leak is diagnosed intraoperatively, immediate repair must be performed. The procedure is converted to an open one, and the extent of duct injury is assessed. An accessory duct can be ligated, partial transection of the common duct can be repaired over a T tube, a divided duct or almost circumferential transection of the common duct can be repaired with an end-to-end anastomosis over a T tube, and a high injury can be repaired with a Roux-en-Y biliary enteric anastomosis. If repair of a high duct injury is difficult, drains are placed in the subhepatic space, and the patient is referred to a tertiary center.

A leak or injury identified early in the postoperative period is treated as follows. The biloma is drained percutaneously, and a sphincterotomy is performed or a stent is placed, or both can be done if ERCP demonstrates a leak or partial narrowing. Surgical intervention is indicated for patients with major obstruction of the bile duct, major injury, or suspicion of a bowel injury. After adequate resuscitation, administration of antibiotics, and adequate drainage, patients are watched for a few days to ensure that they are not septic at the time of the operation. If there is evidence of adequate control of the leak, the surgeon may wait 5 to 7 days for inflammation in the area to subside before undertaking operative repair. Meticulous and careful dissection is required in this area because there is usually loss of common bile duct substance. After identifying the source of the bile extravasation, dissection plus débridement of nonviable common bile duct is prudent. When it has been ascertained that there is tissue with good integrity, a Roux-en-Y limb can be anastomosed to the common bile duct. Multiple drains are left around the site of the repair.

NEUROLOGIC COMPLICATIONS

Delirium, Cognitive Disorder, and Psychosis

Cause

Delirium refers to a state of acute confusion and is a common complication of surgery. Numerous factors are implicated in causing delirium (Box 12-14). The presence of a structural brain disorder (infarct) increases the individual's susceptibility to delirium. Anticholinergic medications and conditions that decrease the production of acetylcholine can precipitate delirium. In addition, a planned operation with loss of the patient's routine schedule, stress of the disease process, fear of the operation, loss of personal control, placement in an unfamiliar environment, addition of mind-altering pain medications, and pain can lead to dramatic alterations in behavior in postoperative patients. Older patients, patients with a previous history of substance abuse or psychiatric disorders, and pediatric patients are at particularly high risk for behavioral disorders in the postoperative period.

BOX 12-14 Causes of Acute Delirium

Advanced age
Alcohol intoxication and withdrawal
Drugs (overdose or withdrawal)
- Anticholinergic drugs (tricyclic antidepressants, antihistamine)
- Oral hypoglycemic agents
- Antibiotics (cephalosporins)
- Histamine receptor blocking agents
- Anti-inflammatory drugs (e.g., steroidal, nonsteroidal)
- Anticonvulsant medications
- Anxiolytics (diazepam)
- Narcotics
- Cardiac medications (beta blockers, digoxin)

Structural brain abnormalities (e.g., edema, transient ischemic attack, neoplasm)
Metabolic and hemodynamic disturbances
- Electrolyte imbalance
- Hypoglycemia
- Hypoxemia
- Hypovolemia

Endocrine dysfunction
- Thyrotoxicosis
- Hypothyroidism
- Adrenocortical insufficiency

Sepsis and infections
Respiratory dysfunction (e.g., respiratory failure, PE, chronic obstructive pulmonary disease)
Liver, renal, and cardiac disease (e.g., CHF, renal failure)
Trauma (surgical or otherwise)
Critical illness and ICU stay

CHF, congestive heart failure; *ICU*, intensive care unit; *PE*, pulmonary embolism.

Presentation and Diagnosis

Early in the postoperative period, a patient may become acutely agitated, uncooperative, and confused. However, patients with a previous psychiatric disorder may become more withdrawn and depressed. Some patients may become noncommunicative and emotionally flat and may withdraw from any emotional exchange. Patients may also show an altered level of consciousness and changes in cognition. They may have reduced ability to focus, decreased levels of awareness, and difficulty with attention. In addition, they may have hallucinations and altered psychomotor activity and sleep-wake cycle. These changes have a tendency to fluctuate during the course of the day and are worse at night (sundowning). The severity of these manifestations depends on the underlying cause.

The incidence of postoperative delirium and cognitive disorders in geriatric patients varies with the type of surgery performed and preexisting dementia. Postoperative anemia (secondary to acute blood loss), electrolyte imbalance, sepsis, malnutrition, bladder catheterization, physical restraints, extended duration of anesthesia, infection, and respiratory complications are significant precipitating factors.

The most immediately threatening disorder encountered by physicians is delirium tremens, which may occur 48 hours to 14 days after acute alcohol withdrawal. In addition, delirium tremens is associated with extreme autonomic hyperactivity. Early signs of delirium tremens include fever, tremor, and tachycardia, and late signs include confusion, psychosis, agitation, and seizures. Because of the serious underlying nutritional and medical deficiencies, these patients have moderately high mortality, which approaches 20% in some series.

Treatment

Management of delirium and cognitive disorders in a postoperative patient is a frustrating and challenging clinical scenario. Prevention starts with the identification of high-risk individuals before surgery and careful follow-up thereafter. Minimizing the dose or eliminating medications that interrupt mental function must be considered. Optimizing fluid status, providing nutrition and adequate pain control, and removing restraints early, including the Foley catheter, are essential. Early ambulation and transfer from the ICU are encouraged.

Treatment of patients with acute confusion or a sudden change in behavior after surgery requires the following:

1. Recognition of the disorder
2. Close observation and monitoring
3. Identification and elimination of the precipitating factor
4. Treatment of any associated laboratory abnormalities
5. Selective use of imaging or other studies to rule out an organic brain lesion
6. Application of measures to protect the patient and staff
7. Treatment

A history of drug or alcohol abuse and of cardiac, pulmonary, renal, or liver disease or psychiatric illness must be sought. A list of medications used in the perioperative period must be checked. Clinical evaluation is performed to look for evidence of sepsis or a recent neurologic event. A thorough neurologic examination is performed while focusing on the level of consciousness and presence of focal neurologic deficits, ataxia, paresis, or paralysis. Cognitive tests are conducted. Blood samples are sent to check for evidence of infection and to identify metabolic, electrolyte, nutritional, and blood gas abnormalities. Chest radiograph and urinalysis are performed to look for a source of infection. An ECG is obtained to look for evidence of MI. CT or MRI and occasionally a spinal tap may be helpful in select cases.

Measures to protect the patient and staff may include the occasional use of physical restraints, reassurance by speaking to the patient, and allowing family members to be involved in patient care. Medical therapy includes haloperidol, a neuroleptic (0.5 to 2 mg, given intravenously or intramuscularly to achieve a rapid effect and then orally for maintenance therapy). Benzodiazepines are the drug of choice for acute alcohol withdrawal. Other medications, including haloperidol (to control psychosis), beta blockers (to control autonomic manifestations), and clonidine (to control hypertension) are given in addition to benzodiazepine to patients with acute alcohol withdrawal.

Seizure Disorders

Causes

Seizures are caused by paroxysmal electrical discharges from the cerebral cortex and may be primary or secondary. Primary causes include intracranial tumor, hemorrhage, trauma, and idiopathic seizure activity. Secondary causes include metabolic derangement, sepsis, systemic disease processes, and pharmacologic agents. Patients at particularly high risk for postoperative seizure include patients with a previous history of epilepsy and patients experiencing acute withdrawal from alcohol or medications or receiving other pharmacologic agents, including antidepressants, hypoglycemic agents, and lidocaine.

Presentation and Management

Seizures characterized by convulsions, rhythmic myoclonic activity, loss of consciousness, and change in mental status are often associated with fecal and urinary incontinence, lack of neurologic responsiveness, and postevent amnesia. On recognizing evidence of seizure activity, the patient must be carefully restrained so that injury is not sustained during convulsions and is carefully observed. Administration of IV benzodiazepines is essential to stop the seizure activity and is the standard for immediate care. Phenytoin (Dilantin) is the most commonly used anticonvulsant for new-onset generalized or focal seizures. It may be administered intravenously during acute convulsions or orally for maintenance. Side effects of phenytoin include rash and liver dysfunction. Occasionally, phenobarbital may be used, but because of sedation, it is not an agent of choice. The two most commonly used agents for maintenance after seizures or for someone with status epilepticus are carbamazepine (Tegretol) and valproic acid. Neither of these agents can be given intravenously and are used for maintenance only. Gabapentin can be administered when the patient's condition is refractory to other agents. After adequate control of the seizure, a diagnostic workup for its cause is initiated. Workup includes a detailed history and physical examination, history of previous medication and drug use, WBC count to rule out occult infection, and electrolyte and metabolic assessment. CT or MRI is indicated for a patient with new-onset seizure activity because tumors are often the cause. Similarly, an electroencephalogram is obtained at some point to look for abnormal waveform activity.

Stroke and Transient Ischemic Attacks

Causes

A stroke in the perioperative period is devastating and correlates with the type of operative procedure performed, age of the patient, and presence of risk factors for cardiovascular disease. Strokes are more commonly associated with cardiovascular procedures. Although older adults with cardiovascular disease are at a higher risk for stroke, younger individuals are not exempt, especially individuals with an underlying inherited thrombophilia.

Postoperative strokes may be ischemic or hemorrhagic in nature. Ischemic strokes most commonly result from perioperative hypotension or overzealous control of hypertension or from cardioemboli in patients with atrial fibrillation. Other sources of cardioemboli include MI and bacterial endocarditis. An embolus arising from DVT and traversing a patent foramen ovale (i.e., paradoxical embolization) may be responsible for strokes of unknown cause. Hemorrhagic strokes are less common and are mostly related to therapy with anticoagulants. Factors related to coagulation disorders, such as chronic abuse of alcohol, AIDS, cocaine use, bleeding diathesis, and preexisting cerebrovascular anomalies, are associated with an increased risk for hemorrhagic stroke.

Presentation and Management

In all cases of stroke, the neurologic changes represent a dramatic departure from normal patient function. A focal alteration in motor function, alteration in mental status, aphasia, or occasionally unresponsiveness may be noted. Hemorrhagic strokes are uncommon, and their effect can be more devastating than ischemic strokes that are transient (occurring for seconds to minutes) or reversible (occurring for minutes to hours). In truly irreversible injury, the impact on the patient's overall health is immeasurable, and the patient's ability to function and enjoy a good quality of life is severely compromised.

Prevention of a perioperative stroke starts with the identification of at-risk patients. Patients with hypertension must receive adequate treatment, and overzealous correction must be avoided. Patients with atrial fibrillation benefit from prophylaxis with anticoagulants. Patients with a carotid bruit must be evaluated with noninvasive vascular studies and treated accordingly. Patients undergoing a high-risk surgical procedure (e.g., carotid endarterectomy) may be monitored intraoperatively with transcranial Doppler and electroencephalography. Adequate hydration and monitoring in the perioperative period to avoid hypotension and fluctuations in blood pressure are essential to avoid ischemic strokes.

When the clinical signs and symptoms of a stroke are recognized, the patient must have an IV line placed and be monitored for cardiac arrhythmias. Coagulation parameters are assessed for the presence of a coagulopathy, and blood is sent for culture and determination of the sedimentation rate to check for bacteremia and bacterial endocarditis. A diagnostic workup is started immediately to distinguish between hemorrhagic and ischemic stroke with a CT scan or MRI of the brain. Further tests depend on the clinical scenario, such as echocardiography to assess the heart for structural disease, carotid duplex scanning to assess patency of the carotid artery, and cerebral angiography to evaluate for vascular anomalies. Therapy is dictated by the underlying mechanism of the stroke. A hypertensive hemorrhagic stroke is treated by aggressive control of the hypertension, an embolic stroke (cardiogenic or secondary to inherited thrombophilia) is treated by anticoagulation (in the absence of a contraindication) to prevent recurrence, and a hemorrhagic stroke is treated by reversal of the coagulopathy with protamine if secondary to heparin or platelet transfusion if secondary to antiplatelet therapy. Mannitol and dexamethasone are given to reduce cerebral swelling. Treatment of any underlying cardiac arrhythmia is imperative to prevent recurrent embolization. Surgical intervention is indicated for patients with a localized hematoma or vascular anomaly, depending on the location and size of the hematoma, status of the patient, and accessibility of the aneurysm. Thrombolytic therapy (recombinant tissue plasminogen activator) is effective in restoring cerebral blood flow and minimizing brain injury if instituted early after the onset of an embolic event. Otherwise, low-dose aspirin therapy is the standard for acute ischemic infarction; antiplatelet agents (e.g., clopidogrel bisulfate, ticlopidine hydrochloride) are added in patients who continue to have symptoms.

EAR, NOSE, AND THROAT COMPLICATIONS

Epistaxis

Epistaxis may be associated with primary blood dyscrasias such as leukemia and hemophilia, excessive anticoagulation, and hypertension. Epistaxis is divided into two general categories—anterior and posterior. Anterior trauma is often caused by contusion or laceration of the nasal septum or turbinates during insertion of an NG or endotracheal tube. Firm pressure applied between the thumb and index finger to the nasal ala and held for 3 to 5 minutes is generally successful in stopping most cases of anterior epistaxis. Occasionally, packing with strip gauze for 10 to 15 minutes aids in a particularly refractory case. If the bleeding fails to stop, packing for an extended period with petroleum jelly–covered strip gauze may be required. Removal of the packing in 1 to 3 days is usually associated with successful treatment of refractory epistaxis, along with treatment of the underlying condition or reversal of anticoagulation.

A more serious scenario is posterior nasal septal bleeding, which can be life-threatening. If all attempts to stop anterior nasal septal bleeding are unsuccessful, one may infer the probability of a posterior nasal hemorrhage, which may necessitate placement of a posterior pack of petroleum jelly–covered strip gauze. For particularly refractory cases, a Foley catheter with a 30-mL balloon can be passed through the nasal passages, and after the pack is placed, pressure can be applied to it by pulling on the Foley catheter. This type of epistaxis may require concomitant anterior nasal packing for successful treatment. For a difficult hemorrhage such as this, the packs may need to be left in place for 2 to 3 days. For epistaxis that defies all attempts at conservative management, ligation of the sphenopalatine artery or anterior ethmoidal artery may be required.

Acute Hearing Loss

Abrupt loss of hearing in the postoperative period is uncommon. An immediate physical examination is performed to ascertain the degree of hearing loss. Unilateral hearing loss is generally associated with obstruction or edema related to an NG or feeding tube. Bilateral hearing loss is more often neural in nature and is usually associated with pharmacologic agents, such as aminoglycosides and diuretics. Examination with an otoscope often reveals the presence of cerumen impaction or edema from a middle ear infection. If the otologic examination is completely normal, neural injury related to the agents just mentioned should be suspected. These drugs need to be discontinued immediately, and hearing needs to be monitored over the ensuing 2 to 3 days to see whether recovery occurs. For cerumen impaction, use of a delicate speculum under direct vision is indicated. If the hearing loss is associated with edema related to an NG tube, merely removing the NG tube results in resolution of the edema.

Nosocomial Sinusitis

Nosocomial sinusitis is a recognized complication in critically ill patients. Left untreated, sinusitis may be complicated by brain abscess formation, postorbital cellulitis, and nosocomial pneumonia. Patients receiving ventilatory support via a nasotracheal tube and patients with nasal colonization with gram-negative bacteria are at high risk for sinusitis. Patients with facial trauma, patients with an NG or feeding tube, and patients who have received antibiotic therapy are also at risk.

Most nosocomial sinusitis occurs in the second week of hospitalization, and the maxillary sinuses are the most commonly affected. The classic signs encountered with community-acquired sinusitis (e.g., facial pain, malaise, fever, purulent nasal discharge) may not be present because the patient is usually unconscious and intubated, has other sources of infection, and is receiving analgesics and antipyretics. The diagnosis is often made when CT is performed to look for a source of fever and the sinuses are included in the cuts. The CT scan generally shows thickened mucosa and the presence of an air-fluid level or opacification of the sinus.

When nosocomial sinusitis is diagnosed or suspected, nasal tubes are removed, decongestant is administered, and antibiotic therapy targeting the two most common organisms, *S. aureus* and *Pseudomonas* spp., is given. Other organisms that play a major role in nosocomial infections, such as MRSA and vancomycin-resistant *Enterococcus* and *Acinetobacter* spp., are also included in antibiotic coverage. With such treatment, a clinical response occurs in 48 hours, and a clinical and radiologic cure occurs in two thirds of patients. Failure of medical therapy leads to surgical drainage of the sinus involved. In rare cases, severe intractable sinusitis may require a drainage procedure via an operative technique.

Parotitis

Parotitis most commonly occurs in an older man with poor oral hygiene and poor oral intake, with an associated decrease in saliva production. The pathophysiology involves obstruction of the salivary ducts or an infection in a diabetic or immunocompromised patient. The patient is noted to have significant edema and focal tenderness surrounding the parotid gland, which eventually progresses to involve edema of the floor of the mouth. If left undiagnosed and untreated, parotitis can cause life-threatening sepsis. In the worst-case scenario, the infection can dissect into the mediastinum and cause stridor from partial airway obstruction. Patients with advanced parotitis have dysphagia and some respiratory occlusion. If the diagnosis of parotitis is being considered, the patient receives IV high-dose, broad-spectrum antibiotics with good coverage of *Staphylococcus,* the most common agent cultured from this disease. In the presence of a fluctuant area, incision plus drainage is indicated, with care taken to avoid the facial nerve. Rarely, advanced disease may require emergency tracheostomy. In most patients with parotitis, the condition arises 4 to 12 days after an initial operation. Because of the rapid progression of this disease, one must be aware of the diagnosis when present and institute immediate therapy, including occasional emergency surgery for patients with an obvious fluctuant area.

SELECTED REFERENCES

Almanaseer Y, Mukherjee D, Kline-Rogers EM, et al: Implementation of the ACC/AHA guidelines for preoperative risk assessment in a general medicine preoperative clinic: Improving efficiency and preserving outcomes. *Cardiology* 103:24–29, 2005.

This article describes the clinical predictors of increased cardiovascular risk leading to acute cardiac events in surgical patients. Implementation of these predictors also may allow better selection of patients who require more specific preoperative cardiac evaluation and beta blocker therapy.

Anderson DJ, Kaye KS, Classen D, et al: Strategies to prevent surgical site infections in acute care hospitals. *Infect Control Hosp Epidemiol* 29(Suppl 1):S51–S61, 2008.

Surgical site infections are a serious cause of significant postoperative morbidity, increased cost, and poor outcomes. A realistic strategy is provided for reducing or preventing surgical site infections in the acute care hospital setting.

Anderson JL, Adams CD, Antman EM, et al: ACC/AHA 2007 guidelines for the management of patients with unstable angina/non-ST-elevation myocardial infarction: A report of the American College of Cardiology/American Heart Association Task Force on Practice Guidelines (Writing Committee to Revise the 2002 Guidelines for the Management of Patients With Unstable Angina/Non-ST-Elevation Myocardial Infarction) developed in collaboration with the American College of Emergency Physicians, the Society for Cardiovascular Angiography and Interventions, and the Society of Thoracic Surgeons endorsed by the American Association of Cardiovascular and Pulmonary Rehabilitation and the Society for Academic Emergency Medicine. *J Am Coll Cardiol* 50:e1–e157, 2007.

Patients with angina, particularly unstable angina, represent a high-risk group for surgery. Practical guidelines are provided for management of this challenging group of patients.

Cooper MS, Stewart PM: Corticosteroid insufficiency in acutely ill patients. *N Engl J Med* 348:727–734, 2003.

This article discusses functional adrenal insufficiency in critically ill patients and outlines the workup and treatment strategies.

Dronge AS, Perkal MF, Kancir S, et al: Long-term glycemic control and postoperative infectious complications. *Arch Surg* 141:375–380, 2006.

This article addresses the importance of glycemic control as it relates to postoperative infections.

Eagle KA, Berger PB, Calkins H, et al: ACC/AHA Guideline Update for Perioperative Cardiovascular Evaluations for Noncardiac Surgery—Executive Summary. A report of the American College of Cardiology/American Heart Association Task Force on Practice Guidelines (Committee to Update the 1996 Guidelines on Perioperative Cardiovascular Evaluation for Noncardiac Surgery). *Anesth Analg* 94:1052–1064, 2002.

This important report from the American College of Cardiology and American Heart Association carefully outlines the management of patients with cardiac risk factors who undergo a noncardiac operation.

Geerts WH, Bergqvist D, Pineo GF, et al: Prevention of venous thromboembolism: American College of Chest Physicians Evidence-Based Clinical Practice Guidelines (8th Edition). *Chest* 133:381S–453S, 2008.

The American College of Chest Physicians offers evidence-based guidelines for preventing deep vein thrombosis in postoperative patients.

Heller L, Levin SL, Butler CE: Management of abdominal wound dehiscence using vacuum-assisted closure in patients with compromised healing. *Am J Surg* 191:165–172, 2006.

This article discusses the integration of vacuum-assisted closure systems in the management of wound dehiscence.

Lin HJ, Spoerke N, Deveney C, et al: Reconstruction of complex abdominal wall hernias using acellular human dermal matrix: A single institution experience. *Am J Surg* 197:599–603, 2009.

The development of a biologic prosthesis that can be placed in a contaminated field during hernia repair provided a new treatment paradigm for management of these complex patients. This article is a retrospective review of the experience of a single institution with one type of biologic prosthesis.

Migneco A, Ojetti V, Testa A, et al: Management of thyrotoxic crisis. *Eur Rev Med Pharmacol Sci* 9:69–74, 2005.

The manifestations and treatment of an uncommon but potentially devastating complication of thyrotoxicosis are outlined.

Moore AFK, Hargest R, Martin M, et al: Intra-abdominal hypertension and the abdominal compartment syndrome. *Br J Surg* 91:1102–1110, 2004.

This important article details the pathophysiology of intra-abdominal hypertension and abdominal compartment syndrome and provides guidelines for medical and surgical management of patients with these complications.

Perry SL, Ortel TL: Clinical and laboratory evaluation of thrombophilia. *Clin Chest Med* 24:153–170, 2003.

This review outlines the causes of a hypercoagulable state and the workup of patients with this complication and provides recommendations for testing these high-risk patients.

Sailhamer EA, Carson K, Chang Y, et al: Fulminant *Clostridium difficile* colitis: Patterns of care and predictors of mortality. *Arch Surg* 144:433–439, 2009.

This article is highly relevant because of its description of a more virulent, resistant, and aggressive form of Clostridium difficile.

Simon TL, Alverson DC, AuBuchon J, et al: Practice parameter for the use of red blood cell transfusions: Developed by the Red Blood Cell Administration Practice Guideline Development Task Force of the College of American Pathologists. *Arch Pathol Lab Med* 122:130–138, 1998.

This article is the result of a consensus conference held by the College of American Pathologists regarding blood transfusion and its usefulness for the treatment of surgical patients.

Slim K, Vicaut E, Panis Y, et al: Meta-analysis of randomized clinical trials of colorectal surgery with or without mechanical bowel preparation. *Br J Surg* 91:1125–1130, 2004.

This article sheds light on the usefulness of mechanical bowel preparation before colorectal surgery.

REFERENCES

1. Douketis JD, Berger PB, Dunn AS, et al: The perioperative management of antithrombotic therapy: American College of Chest Physicians Evidence-Based Clinical Practice Guidelines (8th Edition). *Chest* 133:299S–339S, 2008.
2. Diaz JJ, Jr, Conquest AM, Ferzoco SJ, et al: Multi-institutional experience using human acellular dermal matrix for ventral hernia repair in a compromised surgical field. *Arch Surg* 144:209–215, 2009.
3. Heller L, Levin SL, Butler CE: Management of abdominal wound dehiscence using vacuum-assisted closure in patients with compromised healing. *Am J Surg* 191:165–172, 2006.
4. Mangram AJ, Horan TC, Pearson ML, et al: Guideline for prevention of surgical site infection, 1999. Hospital Infection Control Practices Advisory Committee. *Infect Control Hosp Epidemiol* 20:250–278, 1999.
5. Awad SS, Elhabash SI, Lee L, et al: Increasing incidence of methicillin-resistant *Staphylococcus aureus* skin and soft-tissue infections: Reconsideration of empiric antimicrobial therapy. *Am J Surg* 194:606–610, 2007.
6. National Nosocomial Infections Surveillance (NNIS): System Report, Data Summary from January 1992–June 2001, issued August 2001. *Am J Infect Control* 29:404–421, 2001.
7. Culver DH, Horan TC, Gaynes RP, et al: Surgical wound infection rates by wound class, operative procedure, and patient risk index. National Nosocomial Infections Surveillance System. *Am J Med* 91:152S–157S, 1991.
8. Anderson DJ, Kaye KS, Classen D, et al: Strategies to prevent surgical site infections in acute care hospitals. *Infect Control Hosp Epidemiol* 29(Suppl 1):S51–S61, 2008.
9. Buggy DJ, Crossley AW: Thermoregulation, mild perioperative hypothermia and postanaesthetic shivering. *Br J Anaesth* 84:615–628, 2000.
10. Rosenberg H, Antognini JF, Muldoon S: Testing for malignant hyperthermia. *Anesthesiology* 96:232–237, 2002.
11. Jawa RS, Kulaylat MN, Baumann H, et al: What is new in cytokine research related to trauma/critical care? *J Intensive Care Med* 21:63–85, 2006.
12. Bukhary ZA: Candiduria: A review of clinical significance and management. *Saudi J Kidney Dis Transpl* 19:350–360, 2008.
13. Centers for Medicare and Medicaid Services (CMS), HHS: Medicare program; changes to the hospital inpatient prospective payment systems and fiscal year 2008 rates. *Fed Regist* 72:47129–48175, 2007.
14. Edwards JR, Peterson KD, Andrus ML, et al: National Healthcare Safety Network (NHSN) Report, data summary for 2006, issued June 2007. *Am J Infect Control* 35:290–301, 2007.
15. Ksycki MF, Namias N: Nosocomial urinary tract infection. *Surg Clin North Am* 89:475–481, 2009.
16. American Thoracic Society; Infectious Diseases Society of America: Guidelines for the management of adults with hospital-acquired, ventilator-associated, and healthcare-associated pneumonia. *Am J Respir Crit Care Med* 171:388–416, 2005.
17. Practice guidelines for preoperative fasting and the use of pharmacologic agents to reduce the risk of pulmonary aspiration: Application to healthy patients undergoing

elective procedures: A report by the American Society of Anesthesiologist Task Force on Preoperative Fasting. *Anesthesiology* 90:896–905, 1999.
18. Heit JA, Silverstein MD, Mohr DN, et al: Risk factors for deep vein thrombosis and pulmonary embolism: A population-based case-control study. *Arch Intern Med* 160:809–815, 2000.
19. Goldhaber SZ: Echocardiography in the management of pulmonary embolism. *Ann Intern Med* 136:691–700, 2002.
20. Geerts WH, Bergqvist D, Pineo GF, et al: Prevention of venous thromboembolism: American College of Chest Physicians Evidence-Based Clinical Practice Guidelines (8th Edition). *Chest* 133:381S–453S, 2008.
21. Eagle KA, Berger PB, Calkins H, et al: ACC/AHA Guideline Update for Perioperative Cardiovascular Evaluation for Noncardiac Surgery—Executive Summary. A report of the American College of Cardiology/American Heart Association Task Force on Practice Guidelines (Committee to Update the 1996 Guidelines on Perioperative Cardiovascular Evaluation for Noncardiac Surgery). *Anesth Analg* 94:1052–1064, 2002.
22. Anderson JL, Adams CD, Antman EM, et al: ACC/AHA 2007 guidelines for the management of patients with unstable angina/non-ST-elevation myocardial infarction: A report of the American College of Cardiology/American Heart Association Task Force on Practice Guidelines (Writing Committee to Revise the 2002 Guidelines for the Management of Patients With Unstable Angina/Non-ST-Elevation Myocardial Infarction) developed in collaboration with the American College of Emergency Physicians, the Society for Cardiovascular Angiography and Interventions, and the Society of Thoracic Surgeons endorsed by the American Association of Cardiovascular and Pulmonary Rehabilitation and the Society for Academic Emergency Medicine. *J Am Coll Cardiol* 50:e1–e157, 2007.
23. Almanaseer Y, Mukherjee D, Kline-Rogers EM, et al: Implementation of the ACC/AHA guidelines for preoperative cardiac risk assessment in a general medicine preoperative clinic: Improving efficiency and preserving outcomes. *Cardiology* 103:24–29, 2005.
24. Polanczyk CA, Goldman L, Marcantonio ER, et al: Supraventricular arrhythmia in patients having noncardiac surgery: Clinical correlates and effect on length of stay. *Ann Intern Med* 129:279–285, 1998.
25. Hunt SA, Baker DW, Chin MH, et al: ACC/AHA guidelines for the evaluation and management of chronic heart failure in the adult: Executive summary. *J Heart Lung Transplant* 21:189–203, 2002.
26. Bonet S, Agusti A, Arnau JM, et al: Beta-adrenergic blocking agents in heart failure: Benefits of vasodilating and non-vasodilating agents according to patients' characteristics: A meta-analysis of clinical trials. *Arch Intern Med* 160:621–627, 2000.
27. Moore AF, Hargest R, Martin M, et al: Intra-abdominal hypertension and the abdominal compartment syndrome. *Br J Surg* 91:1102–1110, 2004.
28. Karsou SA, Jaber BL, Pereira BJ: Impact of intermittent hemodialysis variables on clinical outcomes in acute renal failure. *Am J Kidney Dis* 35:980–991, 2000.
29. Cooper MS, Stewart PM: Corticosteroid insufficiency in acutely ill patients. *N Engl J Med* 348:727–734, 2003.
30. Migneco A, Ojetti V, Testa A, et al: Management of thyrotoxic crisis. *Eur Rev Med Pharmacol Sci* 9:69–74, 2005.
31. Postoperative Ileus Management Council: *Proceedings of consensus panel to define postoperative ileus. Colorectal surgery consensus report,* Atlanta, 2006, Thomson American Health Consultants.
32. Schwarz NT, Kalff JC, Turler A, et al: Selective jejunal manipulation causes postoperative pan-enteric inflammation and dysmotility. *Gastroenterology* 126:159–169, 2004.
33. Kulaylat MN, Doerr RJ: Small bowel obstruction. In Holzheimer RG, Mannick JA, editors: *Surgical treatment—evidence-based and problem-oriented,* New York, 2001, Zuckschwerdt, pp 102–113.
34. Kirkpatrick AW, Balogh Z, Ball CG, et al: The secondary abdominal compartment syndrome: Iatrogenic or unavoidable? *J Am Coll Surg* 202:668–679, 2006.
35. Simon TL, Alverson DC, AuBuchon J, et al: Practice parameter for the use of red blood cell transfusions: Developed by the Red Blood Cell Administration Practice Guideline Development Task Force of the College of American Pathologists. *Arch Pathol Lab Med* 122:130–138, 1998.
36. Seder CW, Villalba MR, Jr, Robbins J, et al: Early colectomy may be associated with improved survival in fulminant *Clostridium difficile* colitis: An 8-year experience. *Am J Surg* 197:302–307, 2009.
37. Sailhamer EA, Carson K, Chang Y, et al: Fulminant *Clostridium difficile* colitis: Patterns of care and predictors of mortality. *Arch Surg* 144:433–439, discussion 439–440, 2009.
38. Pepin J, Vo TT, Boutros M, et al: Risk factors for mortality following emergency colectomy for fulminant *Clostridium difficile* infection. *Dis Colon Rectum* 52:400–405, 2009.
39. Slim K, Vicaut E, Panis Y, et al: Meta-analysis of randomized clinical trials of colorectal surgery with or without mechanical bowel preparation. *Br J Surg* 91:1125–1130, 2004.
40. Uzunkoy A, Akinci OF, Coskun A, et al: Effects of antiadhesive agents on the healing of intestinal anastomosis. *Dis Colon Rectum* 43:370–375, 2000.
41. August DA, Serrano D, Poplin E: "Spontaneous," delayed colon and rectal anastomotic complications associated with bevacizumab therapy. *J Surg Oncol* 97:180–185, 2008.
42. Branagan G, Finnis D: Prognosis after anastomotic leakage in colorectal surgery. *Dis Colon Rectum* 48:1021–1026, 2005.
43. Stojadinovic A, Brooks A, Hoos A, et al: An evidence-based approach to the surgical management of resectable pancreatic adenocarcinoma. *J Am Coll Surg* 196:954–964, 2003.
44. Orgill DP, Manders EK, Sumpio BE, et al: The mechanisms of action of vacuum-assisted closure: More to learn. *Surgery* 146:40–51, 2009.
45. Teubner A, Morrison K, Ravishankar HR, et al: Fistuloclysis can successfully replace parenteral feeding in the nutritional support of patients with enterocutaneous fistula. *Br J Surg* 91:625–631, 2004.
46. Wainstein DE, Fernandez E, Gonzalez D, et al: Treatment of high-output enterocutaneous fistulas with a vacuum-compaction device. A ten-year experience. *World J Surg* 32:430–435, 2008.
47. Wind J, van Koperen PJ, Slors JF, et al: Single-stage closure of enterocutaneous fistula and stomas in the presence of large abdominal wall defects using the components separation technique. *Am J Surg* 197:24–29, 2009.

48. Lin HJ, Spoerke N, Deveney C, et al: Reconstruction of complex abdominal wall hernias using acellular human dermal matrix: A single institution experience. *Am J Surg* 197:599–603, 2009.
49. Alghamdi A, Jawas A, Hart R: Use of octreotide for the prevention of pancreatic fistula after elective pancreatic surgery: A systematic review and meta-analysis. *Can J Surg* 50:459–466, 2007.
50. Krahenbuhl L, Sclabas G, Wente MN, et al: Incidence, risk factors, and prevention of biliary tract injuries during laparoscopic cholecystectomy in Switzerland. *World J Surg* 25:1325–1330, 2001.

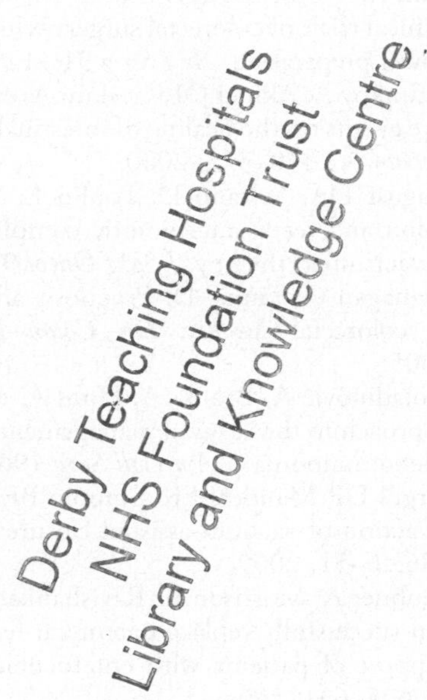

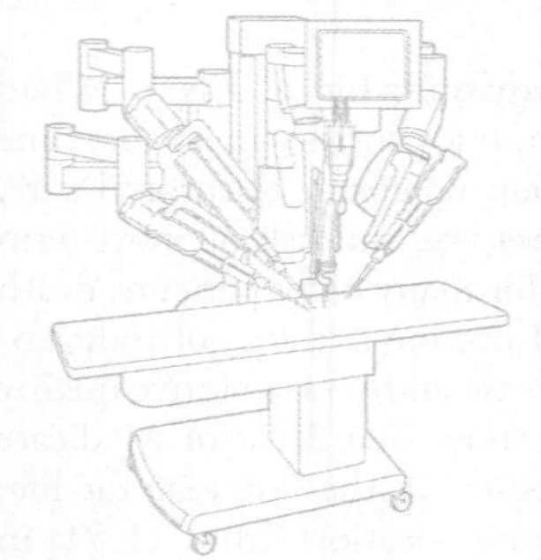

CHAPTER 13

Surgery in the Geriatric Patient

Heather Yeo, Jeffrey Indes, Ronnie A. Rosenthal

OUTLINE

In the last several decades, life expectancy has increased dramatically such that the average 65-year-old woman today can expect to live an additional 20 years, nearly twice as long as her counterpart in 1900. The average 80-year-old woman currently can expect to live nearly 10 years longer (Table 13-1).[1] With this increase in life expectancy comes an increase in the number of people living into old age with diseases and chronic conditions that would have caused death in earlier years. At the present time, more than 75% of people older than 65 years have at least one chronic condition, and 20% of Medicare patients have five or more chronic conditions.[2] Many of these diseases and chronic conditions, such as cancer, degenerative joint disease, coronary artery disease, and visual impairment, have a surgical option as part of the treatment algorithm.

As of 2012, nearly 10,000 Americans turn 65 every day. Over the next few decades, as the 78 million people in the Baby Boomer generation (born during the period 1946-1964) begin to reach age 65, there will be a rapid aging of the U.S. population (Fig. 13-1).[3] It is expected that by 2030, one in five people will be older than 65 years, and by 2050, almost 20 million people will be older than 85 years. In contrast to older persons in prior generations, members of the Baby Boomer generation expect to remain active and independent long after retirement. The demand for health care services is likely to overwhelm the system if new ways to increase supply and improve delivery are not developed.

In April 2008, in response to the impending crisis in providing health services to older adults, the Institute of Medicine issued a report in which the Institute of Medicine "charged the Committee on the Future Health Care Workforce for Older Americans with determining the health care needs of Americans over 65 years of age and analyzing the forces that shape the health care workforce for these individuals."[2] The committee determined that to meet these needs, a three-pronged approach was necessary:

1. Enhancing the competence in working with geriatric patients of the entire health care workforce
2. Increasing the recruitment and retention of geriatrics specialists
3. Improving the way health care is delivered

As a first step in the process of enhancing the competence of surgeons and surgical trainees in working with geriatric patients, the American Board of Surgery with the support of the American Geriatrics Society, the American Medical Association, and the John A. Hartford Foundation convened a meeting of seven surgical specialty boards to develop a series of competencies that could be used for certification purposes across disciplines. Although there was a general consensus that caring for older surgical patients requires specific competencies and a set of competencies was developed,[4] the adoption of these competencies by various boards has been variable. However, geriatric content has been added to training examinations, residency review committee requirements, and board examinations in most specialties (Fig. 13-2), and efforts continue to incorporate geriatric competencies into all certification processes.

The aim of this chapter is to enhance the knowledge of geriatrics for surgeons and surgical trainees by highlighting the issues that make surgical care of older patients different. We also present the physiologic background that underlies the differences, describe the current methods to assess the impact of decline and comorbidity, identify the important complications to anticipate and how to avoid them, and review the current status of the treatment of common surgical diseases of aging.

FOCUSING THINKING ABOUT SURGERY IN OLDER ADULTS

When planning surgery for a geriatric patient, two considerations are of utmost importance. First, surgical disease in older adults may not be identical to surgical disease in younger adults. The pattern, presentation, and natural history of disease are often different, and treatment options must take these differences into account. Second, the older surgical patient is different from a physiologic and psychosocial perspective. Surgical decision making must focus on what is best for the older adult patient based on the nature of the disease, the overall health status, and, most importantly, the treatment goals and preferences of the individual. Palliation of symptoms may be

TABLE 13-1 Life Expectancy of Older Persons at Various Ages

	ALL RACES	
AGE (YR)	MALE	FEMALE
65	17.9	20.5
70	14.4	16.6
75	11.2	12.9
80	8.3	9.7
85	5.9	7.0
90	4.1	4.8
95	2.8	3.3
100	2.0	2.3

From National Center for Health Statistics: Deaths: Final data for 2013. *Natl Vital Stat Rep* 64, 2013. Available at: <http://www.cdc.gov/nchs/data/nvsr/nvsr64/nvsr64_02.pdf>.

the primary concern rather than cure of disease with potentially longer, but less satisfactory, quality of life.

Pattern, Presentation, and Natural History of Disease

In many surgical disciplines, the landscape has changed dramatically over the past few decades as the population ages. For example, in the trauma bay of the emergency department, the number of older patients presenting with a fall has surpassed the number of younger patients presenting with more dramatic injuries. Falls are responsible for most injuries in people older than 65 years (Fig. 13-3).[5] Although the mechanism of injury may seem less significant, serious injuries and disability are common. A fall may also be the first manifestation, or a subsequent consequence, of a serious underlying condition. Awareness that a minor fall may have serious ramifications in an older individual has increased; however, algorithms that address the functional outcome and impact of a fall on quality of life and subsequent independence of the individual are often lacking.

The presentation of other surgical problems in older patients may also be misleading. The symptom pattern and natural history of common diseases are often different from that seen in younger patients. The absence of typical signs and symptoms often leads to errors in diagnosis and delays in treatment. As a result, it is not unusual for an acute complication to be the first indication of disease. For example, acute cholecystitis and common bile duct (CBD) stones are more common indications for cholecystectomy in patients older than 65 years, whereas biliary colic is more common in patients younger than 65 years. In addition, the extent of disease found at the time of surgery is often far more advanced in older patients compared with younger counterparts. Among patients requiring hospitalization for cholecystectomy, patients older than 65 years were found to have more complex diagnoses and a greater need for open and additional procedures than younger patients, with patients older than 80 years having the highest rates.[6] In patients with appendicitis, greater than 50% of patients older than 65 years have perforation at the time of appendectomy compared with less than 25% of patients younger than 65 years. A high index of suspicion is necessary to identify surgical disease early in older patients presenting with vague symptoms or unexplained changes in mental status.

Surgical Decision Making

For general and acute care surgeons, the presentation of an abdominal emergency in an older patient with multiple comorbidities presents a particularly difficult problem. When faced with the need to make a decision for surgery in a short time frame, for pathology that is potentially amenable to surgical cure, consideration is often focused entirely on the risk of short-term mortality and morbidity. However, for many older patients, death is less of a concern than functional decline and loss of independence. The patient's overall goals of care and postoperative quality of life are often overlooked. Data show that 33% of Medicare decedents received a surgical procedure in the last year for life; this rate varied widely with geographic location (from 11.5% in Hawaii to 34.5% in Indiana).[7] Other data indicate that patient preferences for life-sustaining treatments do not differ by location[8]; this indicates that factors other than what the patient wants control the treatment that is received.

Traditionally, surgeons have measured surgical success in terms of 30-day mortality and morbidity. However, for older patients, the definition of success is more complex. Although we are now able to perform even the most major surgery on the oldest patients with traditional surgical success, the quality of the outcome in the patient's view is more likely to depend on whether he or she can continue to function as before surgery. For some older patients, losing functional independence as a result of a major surgical intervention may be a far worse outcome than living with, or even dying of, the disease for which surgery is offered. In a study of older patients with limited life expectancy because of serious chronic disease, Fried and colleagues[9] examined the impact of treatment burden (low—minor interventions, such as intravenous [IV] antibiotics; high—major interventions, such as surgery) and expected outcome (desirable versus undesirable) on patient preferences for treatment. Results indicated that more than 70% of older patients would not want a low burden treatment if severe functional impairment or cognitive impairment was the expected outcome. The concern for functional and cognitive impairment was more dramatic than the concern for death (Fig. 13-4).

In another study of preferences for permanent nursing home placement in seriously ill hospitalized patients, 56% of patients were very unwilling or would rather die than live permanently in a nursing home. Correlation between the patient's wishes and the opinion of the surrogate and the physician of the patient's wishes was poor.[10] It is essential that an older patient be given a realistic estimate of the overall functional outcome of the proposed surgical treatment, in addition to the likelihood of control or cure of the particular disease. It is also essential that the surgeon understands the patient's preferences in the context of this broader view of surgical success.

Palliative Care

Honoring a patient's preferences for treatment at the end of life is a necessary component of quality health care. Studies have documented that the extent of burden plays a role in patients' decisions to choose aggressive care. If the risk and benefits are appropriately discussed, aging patients often may choose less aggressive treatment.[9]

For patients with a poor prognosis, discussion regarding palliative care should occur early in the treatment conversation. Palliative care does not preclude treatment of the disease or symptoms. Patients and their family members should be encouraged to complete and discuss advance directives, which have been shown to make decisions for care at the end of life easier for patients and their families and more in line with patients' wishes. Early palliative care has been shown to lead to substantial improvements in

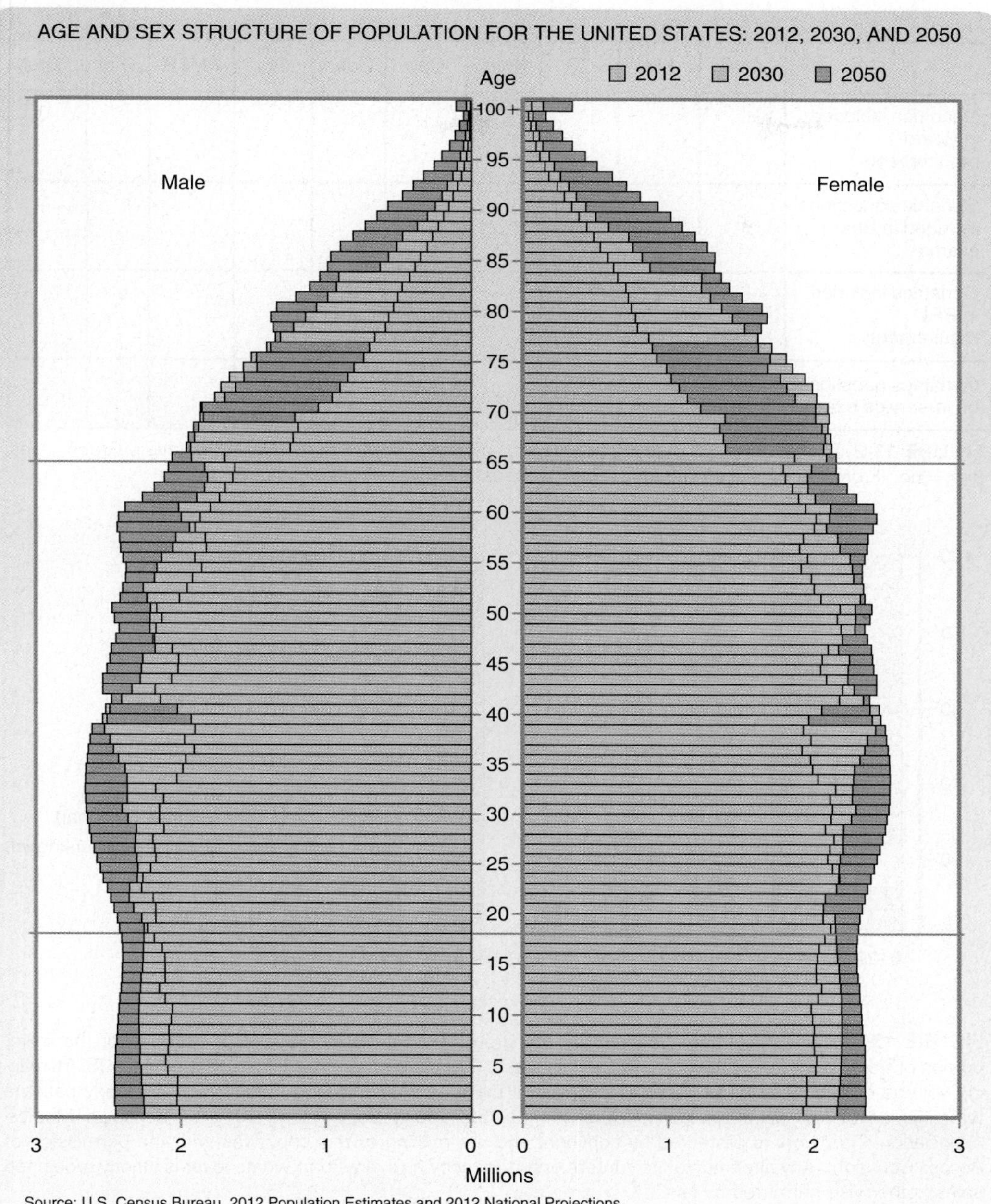

FIGURE 13-1 The aging of the Baby Boomer generation and their offspring in the United States in 2013, 2030, and 2050. (From Ortman JM, Velkoff VA, Hogan H: *An aging nation: The older population in the United States*, Current Populations Reports, P25–1140. Washington, DC, 2014, U.S. Census Bureau.)

quality of life and mood and was even shown to increase survival in some studies.[11] As there has been an increased focus on quality of care, physicians and surgeons have come to understand that treatment is not only about curing disease but also about quality of life and alleviating suffering in patients.

PHYSIOLOGIC DECLINE

With aging, there is a decline in physiologic function in all organ systems, but the magnitude of this decline is variable among organs and individuals. In the resting state, this decline usually has minimal functional consequence, although physiologic reserves may be used just to maintain homeostasis. However, when physiologic reserves are required to meet the additional challenges of surgery or acute illness, overall performance may deteriorate. This progressive age-related decline in organ system homeostatic reserves is termed *homeostenosis* and was first described by Cannon, a physiologist in the 1940s. Figure 13-5 is a graphic representation of the present concepts of homeostenosis.[12] In older age, there is increased use of physiologic reserves just to maintain normal homeostasis. When the body is stressed, fewer reserves are available to meet the challenge, and overall function may be pushed over the precipice of organ failure or death.

Over the past several decades, an enormous amount of research has been conducted to define the specific changes in organ

	Anes	EM	GS	Gyn	Oph	Ortho	Oto	PM&R	Thor	Urol
Geriatrics included in Board requirements										
Geriatrics questions included in Board exams										
Geriatrics included in RRC requirements										
Geriatrics questions on in-service exams										

FIGURE 13-2 The Solomon score card: adoption of geriatric content by surgical specialties. Green = yes; pink = no. (From the American Geriatrics Society Geriatrics-for-Specialists Initiative, 2013.)

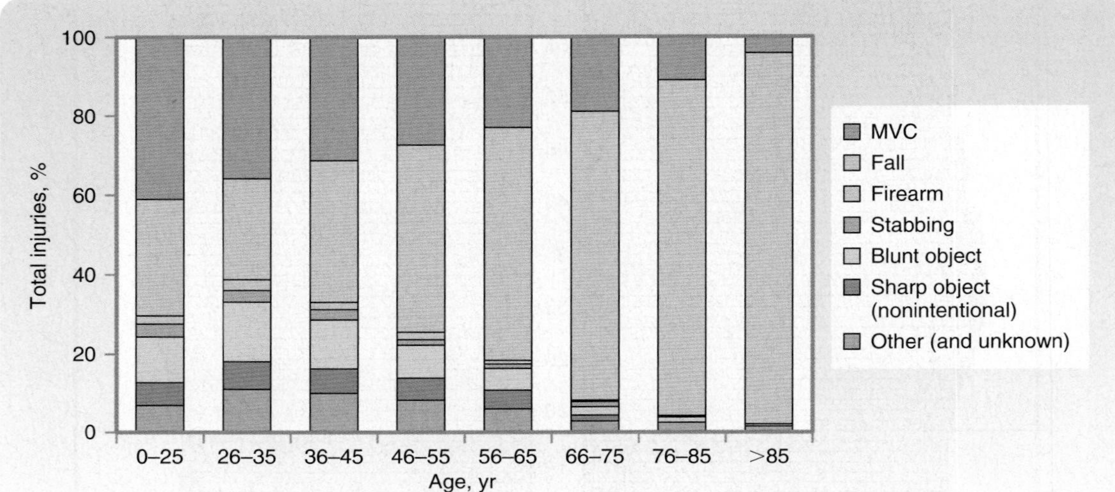

FIGURE 13-3 Etiology of traumatic injury by age group. With increasing age, falls account for the major portion of traumatic injuries. *MVC*, motor vehicle crash. (From Liberman M, Mulder DS, Sampalis JS: Increasing volume of patients at level I trauma centres: Is there a need for triage modification in elderly patients with injuries of low severity? *Can J Surg* 46:446–452, 2003.)

function that are directly attributable to aging. This task is inherently difficult because aging is also accompanied by increased vulnerability to disease. It is often difficult to determine whether an observed decline in function is secondary to aging per se or to disease associated with aging. However, the overall effect is still the same—a much smaller margin for error in the care of older patients. Understanding the changes in organ function can help minimize these errors.

Cardiovascular System

Cardiovascular disease is the leading cause of death in the United States in men and women. Of these deaths, 83% occur in persons older than 65 years. The prevalence of heart failure approaches 10 in 1000 persons in this age group. Congestive heart failure is a risk factor for several postoperative complications, including surgical site infections. Cardiac events are common in the postoperative period in older patients and are attributable to disease and to changes in the structure and function of the heart that accompany aging (Box 13-1).

Morphologic changes are found in the myocardium, conducting pathways, valves, and vasculature of the heart and great vessels with increasing age. The number of myocytes declines as the collagen and elastin content increases, resulting in fibrotic areas throughout the myocardium and an overall decline in ventricular compliance. Almost 90% of the autonomic tissue in the sinus node is replaced by fat and connective tissue, and fibrosis interferes with conduction in the intranodal tracts and bundle of His. These changes contribute to the high incidence of sick sinus syndrome, atrial arrhythmia, and bundle branch block. Sclerosis and calcification of the aortic valve are common but are usually of no functional significance. Progressive dilation of all four valvular annuli is probably responsible for the multivalvular regurgitation demonstrated in healthy older adults. Finally, there is a progressive increase in rigidity and decrease in distensibility of the coronary

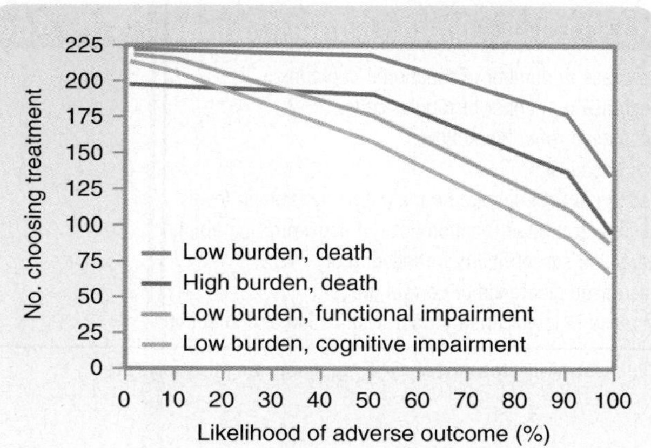

FIGURE 13-4 Many patients are willing to undertake high-burden or low-burden treatments, even if the risk of death is high (up to 50%). However, when there is a small risk of cognitive or functional decline, the number of patients willing to undergo even a low-burden treatment sharply declines. (From Fried TR, Bradley EH, Towle VR, et al: Understanding the treatment preferences of seriously ill patients. *N Engl J Med* 346:1061–1066, 2002.)

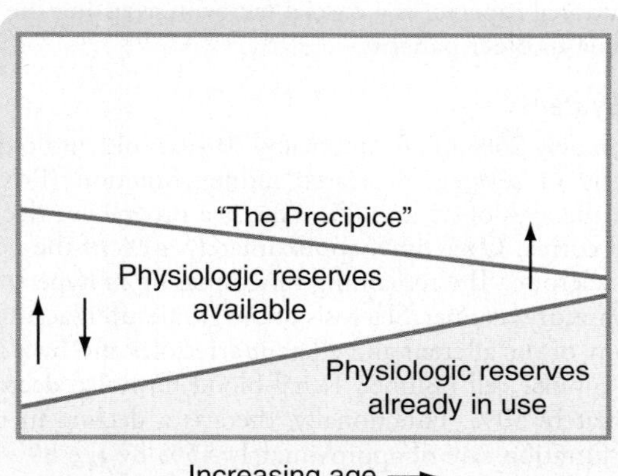

FIGURE 13-5 Graphic representation of homeostenosis. With advancing age, physiologic reserves are increasingly used to maintain homeostasis. *Vertical arrows* represent challenges such as surgical stress or acute illness. Because reserves are already used, there are fewer available to meet these challenges. As a result, the precipice is crossed by a stress that would be easily tolerated at a younger age. This precipice may be any relevant clinical marker, such as organ dysfunction or failure or death. (From Taffett GE: Physiology of aging. In Cassel CK, Leipzig RM, Cohen HJ, et al, editors: *Geriatric medicine: An evidence-based approach*, ed 4, New York, 2003, Springer-Verlag, pp 27–35.)

BOX 13-1 Major Cardiovascular Changes With Age

- Decreased number of myocytes
- Fibrosis of conducting pathways with increased arrhythmias
- Decreased ventricular and arterial compliance (increased afterload)
- Decreased β-adrenergic responsiveness
- Increased dependence on preload (including atrial kick)
- Increased diastolic dysfunction
- Increased silent ischemia

arteries and great vessels. Changes in the peripheral vasculature contribute to increased systolic blood pressure, increased resistance to ventricular emptying, and compensatory loss of myocytes, with ventricular hypertrophy.

The direct functional implications of these changes are difficult to assess accurately because age-related changes in body composition, metabolic rate, general state of fitness, and underlying disease all influence cardiac performance. It is now generally accepted that systolic function is well preserved with increasing age. Cardiac output and ejection fraction are maintained, despite the increase in afterload imposed by stiffening of the outflow tract. However, the mechanism whereby cardiac output is maintained during exercise is different. In younger persons, output is maintained by increasing the heart rate in response to β-adrenergic stimulation. With aging, there is a relative hyposympathetic state in which the heart becomes less responsive to catecholamines, possibly secondary to declining receptor function. The aging heart maintains cardiac output not by increasing rate, but by increasing ventricular filling (preload). Because of the dependence on preload, even minor hypovolemia can result in significant compromise in cardiac function.

Diastolic function, which depends on relaxation rather than contraction, is affected by aging.[13] Diastolic dysfunction is responsible for 50% of cases of heart failure in patients older than 80 years. Myocardial relaxation is more energy-dependent and requires more oxygen than contraction. With aging, there is a progressive decrease in the partial pressure of oxygen. Consequently, even mild hypoxemia can result in prolonged relaxation, higher diastolic pressure, and pulmonary congestion. Because early diastolic filling is impaired, maintenance of preload becomes even more reliant on atrial kick. Loss of the atrial contribution to preload can result in further impairment of cardiac function.

The manifestation of cardiac disease in older adults may be nonspecific and atypical. Although chest pain is still the most common symptom of myocardial infarction, atypical symptoms, such as shortness of breath, syncope, acute confusion, or stroke, occur in 40% of older patients.

Aging also impairs blood vessel function and leads to cardiovascular disease. Vascular dysfunction is caused by the following: (1) oxidative stress enhancement, (2) reduction of nitric oxide bioavailability by diminished nitric oxide synthesis or augmented nitric oxide scavenging or both, (3) production of vasoconstrictor/vasodilator factor imbalances, (4) low-grade proinflammatory environment, (5) impaired angiogenesis, and (6) endothelial cell senescence. The aging process in vascular smooth muscle is characterized by the following: (1) altered replicating potential, (2) change in cellular phenotype, (3) changes in responsiveness to contracting and relaxing mediators, and (4) changes in intracellular signaling functions. Systemic arterial hypertension is an age-dependent disorder; almost 50% of elderly adults are hypertensive. Treatment for hypertension is recommended in elderly patients. Lifestyle modifications, natural compounds, and hormone therapies are useful for initial stages and as supporting treatment with medication, but evidence from clinical trials in this population is needed. Because all antihypertensive agents can lower blood pressure in elderly patients, the choice of agent should be based on potential side effects and drug interactions.[14]

Respiratory System

Chronic lower respiratory disease is the fourth leading cause of death after heart disease, cancer, and stroke. Respiratory problems are the most common postoperative complications in older

BOX 13-2 Major Respiratory Changes With Age

Decreased chest wall compliance
Decline in maximum inspiratory and expiratory force
Decreased lung elasticity (small airway collapse)
Ventilation-perfusion mismatch
Decrease in PaO_2, no change in $PaCO_2$
Decreased FVC and FEV_1
Decline in ventilator responses to hypoxemia and hypercapnia
Decline in normal airway protective mechanisms (increased risk for aspiration)

FEV_1, forced expiratory volume in 1 second; *FVC,* forced vital capacity; *$PaCO_2$,* arterial carbon dioxide pressure; *PaO_2,* arterial oxygen pressure.

BOX 13-3 Major Renal Changes With Age

Decrease in number of functional nephrons
Decrease in number of tubular cells
Decreased renal blood flow
Decreased GFR
Decline in CrCl despite normal serum creatinine level
Decline in tubular function (loss of concentrating ability)
Increased susceptibility to dehydration
Decreased clearance of certain drugs
Increase in lower urinary tract dysfunction and infection

CrCl, creatinine clearance; *GFR,* glomerular filtration rate.

patients (Box 13-2). Disease-related and age-related changes in lung structure and function contribute to this vulnerability.[15]

There is a decline in respiratory function with aging that is attributable to changes in the chest wall and lungs. Chest wall compliance decreases secondary to changes in structure caused by kyphosis and is exaggerated by vertebral collapse. Calcification of the costal cartilage and contractures of the intercostal muscles result in a decline in rib mobility. Maximum inspiratory and expiratory forces can decrease by 50% as a result of a progressive decrease in the strength of the respiratory muscles.

In the lung, there is loss of elasticity, which leads to increased alveolar compliance with collapse of the small airways and subsequent uneven alveolar ventilation with air trapping. Uneven alveolar ventilation leads to ventilation-perfusion mismatches, which causes a decline in arterial oxygen tension of approximately 0.3 or 0.4 mm Hg/year. The partial pressure of carbon dioxide does not change, despite an increase in dead space; this may partly be the result of the decline in production of carbon dioxide that accompanies the falling basal metabolic rates. Air trapping is also responsible for an increase in residual volume, or the volume remaining after maximal expiration.

Loss of support of the small airways also leads to collapse during forced expiration, which limits dynamic lung volumes and flow rates. Forced vital capacity decreases by 14 to 30 mL/year and forced expiratory volume in 1 second decreases by 23 to 32 mL/year in men. The overall effect of loss of elastic inward recoil of the lung is balanced by the decline in chest wall outward force. Total lung capacity remains unchanged, and there is only a mild increase in resting lung volume, or functional residual capacity. Because total lung capacity remains unchanged, the increase in residual volume results in a decrease in vital capacity.

Control of ventilation is also affected by aging. Ventilatory responses to hypoxia and hypercapnia decrease by 50% and 40%, respectively. The exact mechanism of this decline has not been well defined, but it may be caused by declining chemoreceptor function at the peripheral or central nervous system level.

In addition to these intrinsic changes, pulmonary function is affected by alterations in the ability of the respiratory system to protect against environmental injury and infection. Clearance of particles from the lung through the mucociliary elevator is decreased and associated with ciliary dysfunction. Many complex changes in immunity with aging contribute to increased susceptibility to infections, including a less robust immune response from the innate and the adaptive immune systems (see later).[16]

There is also a decrease in several components of swallowing function. Loss of the cough reflex secondary to neurologic disorders, combined with swallowing dysfunction, may predispose to aspiration. The increased frequency and severity of pneumonia in older persons have been attributed to these factors and to an increased incidence of oropharyngeal colonization with gram-negative organisms. This colonization correlates closely with comorbidity and with the ability of older patients to perform activities of daily living (ADL). This fact lends support to the idea that functional capacity is a crucial factor in assessing the risk for pneumonia in older patients.

Renal System

Approximately 25% of all Americans 70 years old and older have moderately or severely decreased kidney function (Box 13-3). Between the ages of 25 and 85, there is a progressive decrease in the renal cortex. Over time, approximately 40% of the nephrons become sclerotic. The remaining functional units hypertrophy in a compensatory manner. Sclerosis of the glomeruli is accompanied by atrophy of the afferent and efferent arterioles and by a decrease in renal tubular cell number. Renal blood flow also decreases by approximately 50%. Functionally, there is a decline in the glomerular filtration rate of approximately 45% by age 80 years.

Renal tubular function also declines with advancing age. The ability to conserve sodium and excrete hydrogen ion decreases, resulting in a diminished capacity to regulate fluid and acid-base balance. Dehydration becomes a particular problem because losses of sodium and water from nonrenal causes are not compensated for by the usual mechanisms. The inability to retain sodium is believed to be caused by a decline in the activity of the renin-angiotensin system. The increasing inability to concentrate the urine is related to a decline in end-organ responsiveness to antidiuretic hormone. The marked decline in the subjective feeling of thirst is also well documented but not well understood. Alterations of osmoreceptor function in the hypothalamus may be responsible for the failure to recognize thirst despite significant elevations in serum osmolality.

Circulating levels of erythropoietin (EPO) are higher in healthy elderly adults compared with younger individuals. Increased EPO production in elderly adults is interpreted as a counterregulatory mechanism aimed at preserving normal red blood cell mass in response to a higher turnover as well as to EPO resistance. However, EPO levels are reduced in anemic elderly individuals, suggesting an impaired counterregulatory response to low hemoglobin levels. Elderly individuals may develop vitamin D deficiency as a result of the impaired capacity of the aging kidney to convert 25-hydroxyvitamin D to 1,25-dihydroxyvitamin D, but

Cockcroft-Gault equation

$$C_{cr} = [(140 - \text{Age in years}) \times \text{Weight in kilograms}]/(72 \times \text{Serum creatinine in mg/dL})$$

MDRD study equation

$$GFR = 175 \times (\text{Standardized serum creatinine in mg/dL})^{-1.154} \times (\text{Age in years})^{-0.203}$$

FIGURE 13-6 Equations for calculating creatinine clearance. *MDRD,* Modification of Diet in Renal Disease.

extrarenal factors (i.e., 25-hydroxyvitamin D availability) are at least equally responsible for vitamin D insufficiency in this age group.[17]

Because of the decline in renal function with aging, it is often important to measure glomerular filtration rate in older patients as part of preoperative risk assessment and in the hospital to provide accurate medication dosing. In older hospitalized patients, direct measurement of creatinine clearance (CrCl) is difficult because incontinence and cognitive impairment make 24-hour urine collection unreliable. Serum creatinine level may be an unreliable indicator of renal function status because this value may remain unchanged as a result of a concomitant decrease in lean body mass and a decrease in creatinine production. A serum creatinine level of 1.0 mg/dL may represent a CrCl of greater than 100 mL/min in a 30-year-old individual but less than 60 mL/min in an 85-year-old individual.

To overcome these problems, formulas have been developed to estimate CrCl from plasma creatinine and patient characteristics. The most commonly used formulas are the Cockcroft-Gault equation and the Modification of Diet in Renal Disease equation (Fig. 13-6). In a large study of older hospitalized patients, the Cockcroft-Gault equation was shown to correlate more closely with directly measured CrCl.[18]

Acute kidney injury (AKI) is defined as a 0.3-mg/dL or 50% or higher change in the serum creatinine level from baseline or a reduction in urine output of less than 0.5 mL/kg/hr over a 6-hour interval within a 48-hour period, following adequate volume resuscitation. AKI is a frequent occurrence after major surgery. AKI can develop in 7.5% of patients with a normal preoperative serum creatinine level. AKI is associated with increased short-term morbidity and mortality and increased long-term mortality. Age, emergency surgery, ischemic heart disease, and congestive heart failure are risk factors for the development of postoperative AKI. Furthermore, older patients with already compromised renal function are at increased risk of postoperative AKI. The key to avoiding postoperative AKI is to understand that older patients are at increased risk and to take steps to avoid unnecessary hypovolemia and ensure proper dosing of drugs that are cleared by the kidney and of drugs that are nephrotoxic.

The lower urinary tract also changes with increasing age. In the bladder, increased collagen content leads to limited distensibility and impaired emptying. Overactivity of the detrusor muscle secondary to neurologic disorders or idiopathic causes has also been identified. In women, decreased circulating levels of estrogen and decreased tissue responsiveness to this hormone cause changes in the urethral sphincter that predispose to urinary incontinence. In men, prostatic hypertrophy impairs bladder emptying. Together, these factors lead to urinary incontinence in 10% to 15% of older persons living in the community and 50% of older persons in nursing homes. There is also an increased prevalence of asymptomatic bacteriuria with age, which ranges from 10% to 50% depending on sex, level of activity, underlying disorders, and place of residence. Urinary tract infections alone are responsible for 30% to 50% of all cases of bacteremia in older patients. Alterations in the local environment and declining host defenses are thought to be responsible.

BOX 13-4 Major Hepatobiliary Changes With Age

- Decreased liver volume
- Increased hepatocyte size and ploidy
- Decrease in number of hepatocyte mitochondria
- Decreased hepatic blood flow
- Synthetic capacity unchanged
- Increased sensitivity to and decreased clearance of certain drugs
- Increased incidence of gallstones and gallstone-related diseases

Hepatobiliary System

Overall, hepatic function is well preserved with aging. However, liver disease and liver disease–related mortality are increased in persons between the ages of 45 and 85 years. Morphologic changes include a reduction in overall liver weight, size, and volume. Hepatocyte size and the number of binucleated cells increase, and the number of mitochondria decreases.[19] Functionally, hepatic blood flow decreases by 35% to 50%.

The synthetic capacity of the liver, as measured by standard tests of liver function, remains unchanged (Box 13-4). However, the metabolism of and sensitivity to certain types of drugs are altered. Drugs requiring microsomal oxidation (phase I reactions) before conjugation (phase II reactions) may be metabolized more slowly, whereas drugs requiring conjugation only may be cleared at a normal rate. Drugs that act directly on hepatocytes, such as warfarin (Coumadin), may produce the desired therapeutic effects at lower doses in older adults because of an increased sensitivity of cells to these agents. Some evidence has also suggested that aging may be associated with a decline in the ability of the liver to protect against the effects of oxidative stress.

The most significant correlate of altered hepatobiliary function in older adults is the increased incidence of gallstones and gallstone-related complications. Gallstone prevalence increases steadily with age, although there is variability in the absolute percentages, depending on the population. Stones have been demonstrated in 80% of nursing home residents older than 90 years. Biliary tract disease is the most common indication for abdominal surgery in older adults (see later).

BOX 13-5 Major Changes in Immune Function With Age

Involution of thymus gland
Decreased production and differentiation of naïve T cells
Decreased T cell mitogenic activity
Increase in inflammatory cytokines
Increase in autoantibodies

Immune Function

Immune competence, similar to other physiologic parameters, declines with advancing age (Box 13-5).[20] This immunosenescence is characterized by enhanced susceptibility to infections, an increase in autoantibodies and monoclonal immunoglobulins, and an increase in tumorigenesis. In addition, similar to other physiologic systems, this decline may not be apparent in the unchallenged state. For example, there is no decline in neutrophil count with age, but the ability of the bone marrow to increase neutrophil production in response to infection may be impaired. Older patients with major infections frequently have normal white blood cell (WBC) counts, but the differential count shows a profound shift to the left, with a large proportion of immature forms.

With aging, there is a decline in the hematopoietic stem cell pool in the bone marrow that leads to decreased production of naïve T cells from the thymus and of B cells from the bone marrow. Involution of the thymus gland, with a decline in thymic hormone levels, further impairs the production and differentiation of naïve T cells and leads to an increased proportion of memory T cells. This change in the population of T cells leaves older adult hosts less able to respond to new antigens.

Some B cell defects have been identified, although it is thought that the functional deficits in antibody production are related to altered T cell regulation rather than intrinsic B cell changes. In vitro, there is increased helper T cell activity for nonspecific antibody production as well as a decreased ability of suppressor T cells from old mice to recognize and suppress specific antigens from self. This is reflected in an increase in the prevalence of autoantibodies to more than 10% by 80 years of age. The mix of immunoglobulins also changes; immunoglobulin M (IgM) levels decrease, whereas IgG and IgA levels increase slightly.

Changes in the immune system with aging are similar to changes seen in chronic inflammation and cancer. In addition to the reduced mitogenic responses of T cells, there is an increase in the levels of acute-phase proteins. It is hypothesized that persistently elevated levels of inflammatory cytokines may be responsible for the downregulation of interleukin-2 production by chronically stimulated T cells. Markers of inflammation such as interleukin-6 have been shown to be increased in older patients. Chronic inflammation has been implicated in the syndrome of frailty, which is characterized by loss of muscle mass (sarcopenia), undernutrition, and impaired mobility. Inflammatory cytokines are also implicated in normocytic anemia that is common in frail older adults.

The clinical implications of these changes are difficult to determine. When superimposed on the known immunosuppression caused by the physical and psychological stresses of surgery, insufficient immunologic responses are to be expected in older adults. However, the increased susceptibility to many infectious agents in the postoperative period is more likely the result of a combination of stress and comorbid disease rather than physiologic decline alone.

Glucose Homeostasis

Data from the National Health and Nutrition Examination Survey have shown an increase in the prevalence of disorders of glucose homeostasis with age; more than 20% of persons older than 60 years have type 2 diabetes. An additional 20% have glucose intolerance characterized by normal fasting glucose and a postchallenge glucose level greater than 140 mg/dL but less than 200 mg/dL. Glucose intolerance may be the result of a decrease in insulin secretion, increase in insulin resistance, or both (Fig. 13-7).[21]

Beta cell function declines with age. This change is manifested by failure of the beta cell to adapt to the hyperglycemic milieu with an appropriate increase in insulin response. The question of insulin resistance is more controversial. Although insulin action has been shown to decrease in older adults, this change is thought to be more a function of changing body composition, with increased adipose tissue and decreased lean body mass, rather than age per se. Other authors believe that there is an increase in insulin resistance directly attributable to aging, as manifested by a decrease in insulin-mediated glucose uptake in muscle that is normally regulated by the glucose transporter GLUT-4. There is also an increase in intracellular lipid accumulation, which interferes with normal insulin signaling. These changes may be associated with the decline in mitochondrial function that also accompanies aging.[21]

These factors, combined with comorbid illness, medications, and genetic predisposition, come together to render older surgical patients at particularly high risk for uncontrolled hyperglycemia when subjected to the usual insulin resistance that accompanies the physiologic stress of surgery. The endogenous glucose response to traumatic stress and glycemic response to an exogenous glucose load are exaggerated in injured older patients.

Although most data on glucose control and surgical outcomes are in the cardiac surgery literature, more recent evidence has confirmed that uncontrolled hyperglycemia in the immediate perioperative period is associated with an increase in infections in almost all types of surgery. However, the optimum level of glucose control is still controversial. Earlier prospective studies indicated that tight control of blood sugar (80 to 110 mg/dL) achieved by continuous infusion of insulin improved some outcomes, including mortality in critically ill patients in the surgical intensive care unit, but more recent data have cast doubt on the benefits of such strict control. In general, maintenance of the blood glucose level less than 180 mg/dL in the perioperative period is now widely accepted as an appropriate target, even in older patients.

PREOPERATIVE ASSESSMENT

Increasing age appears to have a negative effect on the outcome of surgery. Previous small or single-institution studies demonstrated similar outcomes in older and younger patients for even the most complex procedures, such as Whipple resection for pancreatic cancer. These studies likely were limited by selection bias with only the fittest of older patients being offered surgery. More recent large database studies indicate that operative mortality of surgery for major gastrointestinal diseases increases with advancing age even after adjustment for comorbid conditions.[22]

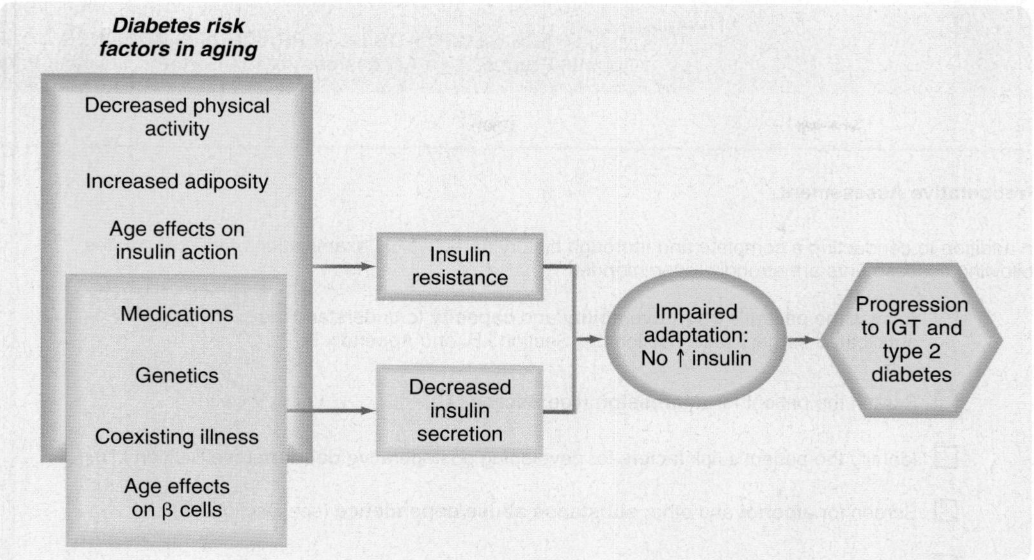

FIGURE 13-7 The normal response to hyperglycemia is for the beta cell to adapt and secrete sufficient insulin to restore euglycemia. In aging, there is a decrease in insulin secretion and a probable increase in insulin resistance, which, when combined with comorbid illness, genetic factors, and medications, leads to a failure of this glucoregulatory process. *IGT,* impaired glucose tolerance. (From Chang AM, Halter JB: Aging and insulin secretion. *Am J Physiol Endocrinol Metab* 284:E7–12, 2003.)

TABLE 13-2 Similarities Between Pediatrics and Geriatrics

PEDIATRIC	GERIATRIC
Congenital defects	Degenerative diseases
Unable to express symptoms	Atypical symptoms
Immature physiologically	Declining physiologically
Need for perioperative adjustments	Need for perioperative adjustments
Abuse/neglect/poverty	Abuse/neglect/poverty/isolation

Several risk calculation models have been developed to assess overall surgical risk in all preoperative surgical patients. Among these is the American College of Surgeons National Surgical Quality Improvement Programs model, which provides an online risk calculator available for use by all.[23] Although this model provides a useful tool for risk assessment, it is limited in elderly patients by the lack of variables specific to older patients, such as cognitive decline and frailty (see later).

Older adults are different from younger adults, much the way children are different. Although we have long accepted that pediatric surgical patients are a unique group, with specific childhood diseases and psychosocial concerns, we have been slower in recognizing the unique concerns of the geriatric surgical population (Table 13-2). We also recognize that there is a spectrum of vulnerability among pediatric patients, with older children at less risk than premature neonates. Similarly, there is a spectrum of vulnerability in older patients with adults who have aged in good health at lower risk than adults who have become frail. More recent literature suggests that frail older adults are at greatest risk for postoperative morbidity, mortality, and functional decline with loss of independence. In contrast to prematurity, frailty is not well defined and is often overlooked or underappreciated.[24]

To ensure the best surgical decision making and the best surgical outcome for the individual older patient, the preoperative assessment must be thorough and must address all of the relevant concerns. The American College of Surgeons and the American Geriatrics Society worked together to define a set of best practice guidelines for the preoperative assessment of the geriatric patient.[25] These guidelines include a 13-item checklist of cognitive, comorbid, functional, and psychosocial factors that have been shown to have an impact on the outcome of care for older surgical patients (Fig. 13-8).

Cognitive Assessment

Cognitive Decline and Dementia

Preoperative cognitive status as a risk factor for negative postoperative outcomes in older patients is often overlooked. Cognitive assessment is rarely a part of the preoperative history and physical examination. However, preoperative cognitive deficits are common; the prevalence of dementia is approximately 1.5% in adults 65 years old and approximately doubles with every 5 additional years of life. More than one third of persons older than 70 years have some cognitive impairment or dementia. Preexisting cognitive dysfunction can impair a patient's capacity to give informed consent and can have significant short-term and long-term consequences in the postoperative period. A history of dementia before surgery has been associated with increased rates of mortality and serious morbidity. Dementia is also the greatest risk factor for postoperative delirium.

Delirium is defined as an acute disorder of cognition and attention and is among the most common and potentially devastating complications seen in older surgical patients. The incidence of delirium in older surgical patients ranges from 5% to greater than 50%. Delirium is associated with longer hospital stays; increased rates of mortality, morbidity, and poor functional recovery; and more discharges to locations other than home (see later).

There are several methods to assess baseline cognitive status. The Mini-Cog[26] is an accurate test for cognitive impairment that is easy to perform in a busy clinic setting. The Mini-Cog

ACS NSQIP©/AGS BEST PRACTICE GUIDELINES:
Optimal Preoperative Assessment of the Geriatric Surgical Patient

Preoperative Assessment

In addition to conducting a complete and thorough history and physical examination of the patient, the following assessments are strongly recommended:

- ☐ Assess the patient's **cognitive ability** and **capacity** to understand the anticipated surgery (see Section I.A, Section I.B, and Appendix I).
- ☐ Screen the patient for **depression** (see Section I.C).
- ☐ Identify the patient's risk factors for developing postoperative **delirium** (see Section I.D).
- ☐ Screen for **alcohol** and other **substance abuse/dependence** (see Section I.E).
- ☐ Perform a preoperative **cardiac** evaluation according to the American College of Cardiology/American Heart Association (ACC/AHA) algorithm for patients undergoing noncardiac surgery (see Section II and Appendix II).
- ☐ Identify the patient's risk factors for postoperative **pulmonary** complications and implement appropriate strategies for prevention (see Section III).
- ☐ Document **functional status** and history of **falls** (see Section IV).
- ☐ Determine baseline **frailty** score (see Section V and Appendix III).
- ☐ Assess patient's **nutritional status** and consider preoperative interventions if the patient is at severe nutritional risk (see Section VI and Appendix IV).
- ☐ Take an accurate and detailed **medication history** and consider appropriate perioperative adjustments. Monitor for **polypharmacy** (see Section VII, Appendix V, Appendix VI, and Appendix VII).
- ☐ Determine the patient's **treatment goals** and **expectations** in the context of the possible treatment outcomes (see Section VIII).
- ☐ Determine patient's **family** and **social support system** (see Section VIII).
- ☐ Order appropriate preoperative **diagnostic tests** focused on elderly patients (see Section IX).

FIGURE 13-8 Best practice guidelines checklist for assessment of geriatric surgical patients. (From Chow WB, Rosenthal RA, Merkow RP, et al: Optimal preoperative assessment of the geriatric surgical patient: A best practices guideline from the American College of Surgeons National Surgical Quality Improvement Program and the American Geriatrics Society. *J Am Coll Surg* 215:453–466, 2012.)

comprises a three-item word learning and recall task (0 to 3 points; each correctly recalled word = 1 point) and a simple clock-drawing task (abnormal clock = 0 points; normal clock = 2 points) used as a distraction before word recall. Total possible Mini-Cog scores range from 0 to 5 points, with 0 to 2 suggesting a high likelihood of cognitive impairment and 3 to 5 suggesting a low likelihood of cognitive impairment.

Capacity

To give informed consent, a patient must have decision-making capacity. The essentials of decision-making capacity are well described.[27] In essence, a patient must be able to understand the nature of his or her illness, the risks and benefits of the treatment recommended, and the risks and benefits of the treatment alternatives. To be considered competent to give consent, the patient must be able to do the following:

1. Clearly indicate a treatment choice
2. Understand the relevant information given
3. Appreciate the medical condition and the consequences of treatments
4. Reason about the treatment options

Depression

Depression is present in approximately 11% of persons older than 71 years. Unrecognized depression in the postoperative period may explain poor oral intake, lack of participation in the postoperative treatment plan, and higher requirements for analgesics. Depression also has been associated with higher mortality and longer hospital stays in patients undergoing cardiac surgery. Screening for depression is easily accomplished using the Patient Health Questionnaire-2,[28] which requires the patient to answer the following two questions:

1. In the past 12 months, have you ever had a time when you felt sad, blue, depressed, or down for most of the time for at least 2 weeks?
2. In the past 12 months, have you ever had a time, lasting at least 2 weeks, when you did not care about the things that you usually care about or when you did not enjoy the things that you usually enjoy?

Delirium

Cognitive dysfunction and depression are risk factors for delirium; however, other factors also must be assessed. Risk factors for delirium are divided into two groups, preoperative or predisposing factors and precipitating factors, or factors that occur in the postoperative period (Table 13-3).[29] In addition to advanced age and cognitive dysfunction, predisposing factors include functional impairment, malnutrition, comorbid illness, sensory impairment, alcohol/substance abuse, psychotropic medications, severe illness, and type of surgery.

Comorbidity

Extensive testing for disease in every organ system is not cost-effective, practical, or necessary for most patients. A thorough history and physical examination provide information to direct further workup, if necessary. It is important to adjust the history and physical examination to look carefully for risk factors, signs, and symptoms of more common comorbid conditions.

Cardiovascular Disease

Of all comorbid conditions, cardiovascular disease is the most prevalent, and cardiovascular events are a leading cause of severe perioperative complications and death. The main thrust of preoperative evaluation in most patients, regardless of age, has focused on identifying patients at risk for cardiac complications. The American College of Cardiology and American Heart Association Task Force on Practice Guidelines first published an in-depth set of guidelines for preoperative cardiac evaluation in 1996, with the most recent update published in 2014.[30] These guidelines provide a stepwise Bayesian strategy for determining which patients need further testing to clarify risk or further treatment to minimize risk. Stratification is based on factors related to the patient and type of surgery. For older patients with known cardiac disease, rigorous workup may be necessary. For most patients, assessment of exercise tolerance and functional capacity is an accurate method of predicting the adequacy of cardiac and pulmonary reserves (see later).

Pulmonary Complications

Although the main focus of preoperative evaluation has been cardiac status, pulmonary complications in older patients are at least as common as cardiac complications, if not more common. Risk factors for pulmonary complications are not as well studied as risk factors for cardiac complications, although many of the same issues apply to both. Poor exercise capacity and poor general health predict pulmonary and cardiac complications. In a systematic review of the literature for risk factors for pulmonary complications after noncardiac surgery (not limited to older adults), patient and procedural factors were identified (Table 13-4).[31] Age older than 80 years was associated with the highest odds ratio of a pulmonary complication, even after adjusting for comorbidity. Indicators of impaired function, nutrition, and cognition, among others, were also important. Aortic aneurysm and thoracic and abdominal operations were the strongest procedure-related factors, but others, such as abdominal surgery, prolonged surgery, and emergency surgery, were also important.

In older patients, additional comorbid conditions, such as prior stroke, gastroesophageal reflux disease (GERD), and poor dentition, are risk factors for aspiration. Subtle changes in cognitive and swallowing function are also common and frequently unrecognized. Initial screening for aspiration risk can be accomplished easily with a simple 3-ounce water swallow test, which

TABLE 13-3 Risk Factors and Precipitating Factors for Delirium

RISK (PREDISPOSING) FACTORS	PRECIPITATING FACTORS
Advanced age	Infection
Cognitive impairment	Medications
Functional impairment	Hypoxemia
Poor nutrition	Electrolyte abnormalities
Comorbidity	Undertreated/overtreated pain
Alcohol abuse	Neurologic events
Psychotropic medications	Dehydration
Sensory impairment	Sensory deprivation
Type of surgery	Sleep disruption
Severe illness	Use of bladder catheters
	Unfamiliar environment
	Use of physical restraints

TABLE 13-4 Potential Risk Factors for Postoperative Pulmonary Complications

PATIENT-RELATED FACTORS	ODDS RATIO	PROCEDURE-RELATED FACTORS	ODDS RATIO
Age (yr)		Aortic aneurysm repair	6.90
70-79	3.90	Thoracic surgery	4.24
≥80	5.63	Abdominal surgery	3.01
ASA class II or higher	3.12-4.87	Upper abdominal surgery	2.91
Abnormal CXR	4.81	Neurosurgery	2.53
CHF	2.93	Prolonged surgery	2.26
Functionally dependent	1.62-2.51	Head and neck surgery	2.21
COPD	2.36	Emergency surgery	2.21
Weight loss	1.62	Vascular surgery	2.10
Medical comorbidity	1.48	General anesthesia	1.83
Cigarette use	1.40	Perioperative transfusion	1.47
Impaired sensorium	1.39		
Alcohol use	1.21		

Adapted from Smetana GW, Lawrence VA, Cornell JE: Preoperative pulmonary risk stratification for noncardiothoracic surgery: Systematic review for the American College of Physicians. *Ann Intern Med* 144:581–595, 2006.

ASA, American Society of Anesthesiologists; *CHF*, congestive heart failure; *COPD*, chronic obstructive pulmonary disease; *CXR*, chest radiograph.

has been shown to have high sensitivity and negative predictive value. This test is accomplished by asking the patient to swallow 90 mL of water without stopping. Choking, coughing, wet quality to the voice after swallowing, or failure to complete the test indicates that a more thorough swallowing examination may be in order. Passing this test indicates a low risk for aspiration; however, the false-positive rate is high. Aspiration precautions should be instituted for all older patients with any risk factors for aspiration.

Strategies to reduce postoperative pulmonary complications include preoperative use of incentive spirometry, smoking cessation regardless of timing, and optimization of pulmonary function for patients with underlying pulmonary comorbidity. Other strategies, such as the selective use of nasogastric decompression (rather than routine use), short-acting (as opposed to long-acting) intraoperative neuromuscular blockade, epidural anesthesia and analgesia, laparoscopic versus open approaches, and nutritional supplementation, have been suggested, but the evidence to support their use is mixed.

Function

Postoperative outcome in geriatric surgical patients is largely determined by the impact of physiologic decline and comorbidity on an individual's functional reserves. Limited preoperative functional reserves also contribute to postoperative immobility, which leads to complications such as atelectasis and pneumonia, venous stasis and pulmonary embolism, and multisystem deconditioning (see later). Function can be assessed in many ways.

American Society of Anesthesiologists Classification

For decades, the physical status classification of the American Society of Anesthesiologists (ASA) has been used successfully to stratify operative risk. This simple classification ranks patients according to the functional limitations imposed by coexisting disease. When curves for mortality versus ASA class are examined with regard to age, there is little difference between younger and older patients, which indicates that mortality is a function of coexisting disease rather than chronologic age. The ASA classification has been shown to predict postoperative mortality accurately even in patients older than 80 years.

Activities of Daily Living

The ability to perform ADL (e.g., feeding, continence, transferring, toileting, dressing, bathing) and instrumental ADL (e.g., telephone use, transportation, meal preparation, shopping, housework, medication management, managing finances) has also been shown to correlate with postoperative mortality and morbidity. In a study of patients older than 80 years, function (defined as independent, partially dependent, or totally dependent in ADL) was a better predictor of mortality than age.

Exercise Tolerance

Of all the methods of assessing overall functional capacity, exercise tolerance is the most sensitive predictor of postoperative cardiac and pulmonary complications in older adults. The metabolic requirements for many routine activities have been determined and are quantitated as metabolic equivalents (MET). The basal oxygen consumption of a 70-kg, 40-year-old man at rest is represented as 1 MET (defined as 3.5 mL/kg/min). Estimated energy requirements for various activities are shown in Figure 13-9. An inability to function above 4 METs has been associated with increased perioperative cardiac events and long-term risk. By asking appropriate questions about the level of activity, functional capacity can be accurately determined.

Gait, Mobility, and Fall Risk Assessment

Falls, considered one of the geriatric syndromes, are a leading cause of injury in older persons and are associated with declining overall health. A fall in the hospital is considered a never event. Evidence also suggests that a fall in the preoperative period may predict negative postoperative outcomes.[32] Every older patient should be asked about a history of falls and should be assessed for

ESTIMATED ENERGY REQUIREMENTS FOR VARIOUS ACTIVITIES*

1 MET	Can you take care of yourself? Eat, dress, or use the toilet? Walk indoors around the house? Walk a block or two on level ground at 2–3 mph or 3.2–4.8 km/h? Do light work around the house like dusting or washing dishes?
4 METs	
4 METs	Climb a flight of stairs or walk up hill? Walk on level ground at 4 mph or 6.4 km/h? Run a short distance? Do heavy work around the house like scrubbing floors or lifting or moving heavy furniture? Participate in moderate recreational activities like golf, bowling, dancing, doubles tennis, or throwing a baseball or football? Participate in strenuous sports like swimming, singles tennis, football, basketball, or skiing?
10 METs	

*MET, metabolic equivalent (see text).

FIGURE 13-9 Estimated energy requirements for various activities. With increasing activity, the number of METs increases. An inability to function above 4 METs has been associated with increased perioperative cardiac events and long-term risk. (From Eagle KA, Berger PB, Calkins H, et al: ACC/AHA guideline update for perioperative cardiovascular evaluation for noncardiac surgery—executive summary: A report of the American College of Cardiology/American Heart Association Task Force on Practice Guidelines [Committee to Update the 1996 Guidelines on Perioperative Cardiovascular Evaluation for Noncardiac Surgery]. *Circulation* 105:1257–1267, 2002.)

gait and mobility factors that may predispose to a fall. A simple way to assess gait and mobility impairment is the Timed Up and Go test,[33] which can be accomplished easily in the office setting. The patient is asked to rise from a chair without using the armrests, walk a measured 10 feet, turn, and return to the chair and sit back down. The inability to rise from the chair without the armrests and a test time of more than 15 seconds are considered indications of a high fall risk. Patients identified as high risk for fall should be considered for preoperative gait and balance training if time allows and should have a physical therapist assist with early mobilization in the postoperative period.

Frailty

Frailty is a geriatric syndrome in which declines in reserves across many organ systems leave the individual with decreased ability to respond to many stressors and increased vulnerability to poor outcomes. Similar to prematurity in neonates, frailty in older adults defines a population at increased risk for negative outcomes with any intervention. The study of frailty is complicated by the many different methods used to define the characteristics of a frail individual. However, loss of muscle mass (sarcopenia), chronic undernutrition, weakness, and decreased exercise tolerance are common to all methods. The presence of frailty is associated with many poor health outcomes, such as falls, disability, hospitalization, and death.

The Fried frailty phenotype[34] is the most widely used method to describe frailty. It defines the frail phenotype by five characteristics: weight loss, weak grip strength, self-reported exhaustion, slow walking speed, and low energy expenditure. Using this definition, frail patients undergoing elective surgery were found to have more postoperative complications, longer lengths of stay, and more frequent discharge to a location other than home.

Another method of describing frailty is the multidomain model, which includes measures of cognition and mood, function, malnutrition, chronic disease, and geriatric syndromes. Using elements of this model (cognition, ADL, low serum albumin, anemia, comorbidity, and falls), frail patients undergoing surgery that required an intensive care unit stay were found to have higher rates of mortality at 6 months after surgery.[35] Other surrogate measures of frailty that are simple to perform in the office setting include the Timed Up and Go test (>15 seconds), mentioned previously; measurement of gait speed (timed walk 15 feet in >6 seconds); and the simplified frailty index, which includes weight loss, low energy level, and the inability to rise from a chair five times in succession without using the arms.

Nutritional Status

The impact of poor nutrition as a risk factor for perioperative mortality and morbidity such as pneumonia and poor wound healing has long been appreciated. Various psychosocial issues and comorbid conditions common to older adults place them at high risk for nutritional deficits. Malnutrition is estimated to occur in approximately 0% to 15% of community-dwelling older persons, 35% to 65% of older patients in acute care hospitals, and 25% to 60% of institutionalized older adults. Factors that lead to inadequate intake and uptake of nutrients in older adults include the ability to obtain food (e.g., financial constraints, availability of food, limited mobility), desire to eat food (e.g., living situation, mental status, chronic illness), ability to eat and absorb food (e.g., poor dentition, chronic gastrointestinal disorders such as GERD or diarrhea), and medications that interfere with appetite or nutrient metabolism (Box 13-6).

BOX 13-6 Factors Associated With Increased Risk of Malnutrition

- Recent weight loss
- Limited ability to obtain food
  - Immobility
  - Poverty
- Disinterest in eating
  - Depression
  - Isolation
  - Cognitive impairment
  - Decreased appetite
  - Decreased taste
- Difficulty eating
  - Poor dentition
  - Swallowing disorder
  - GERD
- Increased gastrointestinal losses
  - Diarrhea
  - Malabsorption
- Systemic diseases
  - Chronic lung
  - Liver
  - Cardiac
  - Renal
  - Cancer
- Drugs and medication
  - Alcohol
  - Suppressed appetite
  - Block nutrient metabolism

GERD, gastroesophageal reflux disease.

In a frail older adult, numerous factors contribute to neuroendocrine dysregulation of the signals that control appetite and satiety and lead to what is termed the *anorexia of aging*. Although the anorexia of aging is a complex interaction of many interrelated events and systems, the result is chronic undernutrition and loss of muscle mass (sarcopenia). Malnutrition has also been associated with increased risk of falls and hospital admission.

Measurement of nutritional status in older adults is difficult. Standard anthropomorphic measures do not take into account the changes in body composition and structure that accompany aging. Immune measures of nutrition are influenced by age-related changes in the immune system in general. Furthermore, criteria for the interpretation of biochemical markers in this age group have not been well established. Complicated markers and indices of malnutrition exist but are unnecessary in the routine surgical setting. Subjective assessment by history and physical examination, in which risk factors and physical evidence of malnutrition are evaluated, has been shown to be as effective as objective measures of nutritional status.

Several screening tools may be used, including the Subjective Global Assessment (SGA) and Mini Nutritional Assessment (MNA). The SGA is a relatively simple, reproducible tool for assessing nutritional status from the history and physical examination. SGA ratings are most strongly influenced by loss of subcutaneous tissue, muscle wasting, and weight loss. The SGA has been validated in older and critically ill patients and has been related to the development of postoperative complications.[36] The MNA, which measures 18 factors, including body mass index (BMI), weight history, cognition, mobility, dietary history, and self-assessment, is also a reliable method for assessing nutritional status. Nutritional status, as determined by the SGA and MNA, has been shown to predict outcome in outpatient and hospitalized geriatric medical patients.

Severe nutritional deficits can be identified by measuring the BMI (weight in kilograms/height in meters^2) and serum albumin and inquiring about unintentional weight loss. BMI less than 18.5 kg/m^2, albumin less than 3.0 g/dL, and unintentional weight loss greater than 10% to 15% within 6 months identify patients at high risk for nutritional related complications. For these patients, a course of preoperative nutritional supplementation may be warranted, even if surgery needs to be delayed for several weeks.

Medication Management

Physiologic changes, such as decreased lean muscle mass and decline in renal function (see "Renal System," earlier), affect the distribution and elimination of many drugs. As a result, older patients are at increased risk for adverse events related to inappropriate drugs or inappropriate dosing of drugs. The Beers list is a comprehensive list of medications that should be avoided or used with caution in older adults.[37] The most common drugs to be avoided include all benzodiazepines, the analgesic meperidine (Demerol), and the antihistamine diphenhydramine (Benadryl).

Use of multiple medications also poses a risk to older patients in the perioperative period. In a random sample of older adults living in the community, more than 80% were found to take at least one prescription medication, with 68% taking an over-the-counter drug or supplement as well. Greater than 50% of adults older than 60 years take five or more medications and supplements, many of which are unnecessary or inappropriately prescribed.[25] A thorough review of all medications should be conducted before surgery. All nonessential medications should be stopped, including all supplements because the content of these is frequently unclear. Other medications, such as medications with potential for withdrawal including beta blockers, should be continued in the perioperative period. For patients with significant cardiac or vascular disease who are not currently receiving beta blockers or statin therapy, consideration should be given to starting these medications.

Patient Counseling

As mentioned earlier, older patients do not make decisions in same context as younger patients. Death may be less of a concern than an unacceptable quality of continuing life. Patients should be counseled about the likelihood of functional decline requiring nursing home placement as well as the likelihood of complications and death.

Advance Directives

Once the decision to operate has been made, it is essential that there is a clear understanding of the patient's desires for life-sustaining treatments. All patients should be encouraged to make a formal advance directive and identify a surrogate decision maker should the patient become unable to make his or her own decisions. Providers should discuss the patient's preferences directly with the patient because surrogate decisions may not always reflect the wishes of the patient. Providers should also ensure that advance directives are clearly documented in the patient's medical record.

Postoperative Discharge Planning

Postoperative planning should begin early in the surgical evaluation. It is important to discuss expectations of patients and their families regarding length of stay as well as likelihood of the need for rehabilitation or home services. In addition, expectations regarding functional outcomes should be discussed. For patients coming from a nursing home, there may be specific requirements for them to be able to keep their place in the home. In the emergency setting, meeting such requirements is not possible, but as soon as needs are realized, case management should be involved in the care.

Important factors in discharge planning include assessment of family involvement, home readiness (i.e., does the patient have stairs, what will the patient need to be able to do functionally to return home), a physical and occupational therapy evaluation, and an open discussion with the patient about the surgeon's and physician's expectations for return of function. Studies have shown that advanced discharge planning with involvement of case management can improve patient outcomes, improve patient satisfaction, and decrease readmission—improving cost of care.[38] Finally, although it may be resource-intensive, there is some evidence that a more intensive follow-up by nursing staff aimed at looking for early warning signs (e.g., dehydration) may promote earlier treatment and decrease rates of readmission in these high-risk patients.

SPECIFIC POSTOPERATIVE COMPLICATIONS

Although older surgical patients with comorbid disease are at higher risk for many of the same surgical complications that occur in patients of all ages, several serious complications are more specific to this age group. These likely reflect an overall decline in physiologic capacity and reserve.

Delirium

Delirium, a disturbance of consciousness and cognition that manifests over a short period of time, with a fluctuating course, is among the most common and potentially devastating postoperative complications seen in older patients. Postoperative delirium is associated with higher rates of morbidity (30 days) and mortality (6 months), longer intensive care unit length of stay, longer hospital length of stay, higher rates of institutionalization after discharge, and higher overall hospital costs.[39] The incidence of postoperative delirium in older patients varies with the type of procedure: less than 5% after cataract surgery, 35% after vascular surgery, and 40% to 60% after hip fracture repair. The incidence in older patients requiring treatment in an intensive care unit is greater than 50%.

Postoperative delirium is usually the result of an interaction between preexisting conditions (risk factors) and postoperative events or complications (precipitating factors) (see Table 13-3). The onset of delirium may be the first indication of a serious postoperative complication. The best strategy at the present time to prevent delirium is to identify risk factors preoperatively and minimize precipitating factors intraoperatively and postoperatively. The American Geriatrics Society has released a formal Guideline for Postoperative Delirium (available at: http://geriatricscareonline.org/ProductAbstract/postoperative_delirium/CL018/?param2=search).

Risk Factors

The most important risk factor for postoperative delirium in older patients is a preexisting cognitive deficit, so some form of cognitive assessment is an essential part of the preoperative workup. Other risk factors include poor functional status, undernutrition or malnutrition, serious coexisting illness, sensory deficits, depression, alcohol consumption, preoperative psychotropic drug use, severity of illness, and magnitude of surgical stress. In a large prospective study of patients older than 50 years undergoing elective noncardiac surgery, Marcantonio and coworkers[40] determined the relative importance of some of these factors in predicting delirium and developed a quantitative predictive rule to identify patients at risk.

Precipitating Factors

Precipitating factors for delirium in the postoperative setting include common postoperative complications (e.g., hypoxia, sepsis, metabolic disturbances), untreated or undertreated pain, medications (e.g., certain antibiotics, analgesics, antihypertensives, beta blockers, benzodiazepines), situational issues (e.g., unfamiliar environment, immobility, loss of sensory assist devices such as glasses and hearing aids), use of bladder catheters and other indwelling devices or restraints, and disruption of the normal sleep-wake cycle (e.g., medications and treatments given during usual sleep hours). No association has been found with the route of anesthesia (epidural versus general) or the occurrence of intraoperative hemodynamic complications. However, intraoperative blood loss, need for blood transfusion, and postoperative hematocrit level less than 30% are associated with a significantly increased risk for postoperative delirium.

Diagnosis and Treatment

Although delirium is common in older patients after surgery, the diagnosis is frequently not appreciated. Agitation and confusion are usually recognized, but depressed levels of consciousness may also be present. The Confusion Assessment Model developed by Wei and colleagues[41] is a simple, well-validated tool to diagnose delirium. A positive Confusion Assessment Model requires the following: (1) acute onset with waxing and waning course and (2) inattention, with (3) disordered thinking or (4) altered level of consciousness.

The best treatment for delirium is prevention. Strategies that focus on maintaining orientation (e.g., family at the bedside, sensory devices available), encouraging mobility, maintaining normal sleep-wake cycles (no medications during sleep hours), and avoiding dehydration and inappropriate medications have been shown to decrease the number and duration of episodes of delirium in hospitalized patients. Pharmacologic prevention trials have not yet shown consistently positive results.

After delirium is diagnosed, a thorough search for precipitating factors, such as infections, hypoxia, metabolic disturbances, inappropriate medications, and undertreated pain, should be conducted. Invasive devices and catheters should be removed as soon as possible, and restraints should be avoided. The history should be thoroughly reviewed, and the family should be queried about possible predisposing factors, such as unrecognized alcohol consumption.

Aspiration

Aspiration is a common cause of morbidity and mortality in older patients in the postoperative period. The incidence of postoperative aspiration pneumonia increases almost exponentially with increasing age, with patients older than 80 years having a 9-fold to 10-fold greater risk than patients 18 to 29 years old.[42]

Swallowing is a complex, coordinated interaction of many neuromuscular events. One third of independent functioning older persons report some difficulty with swallowing. There is a decline in several of the elements of normal swallowing with age that predispose to aspiration. These elements include loss of teeth, decrease in the strength of the muscles of mastication, slowing of the swallow time, decreased laryngopharyngeal sensation, and decreased cough strength. Poor oral hygiene and the edentulous state are also associated with an overgrowth of pathologic organisms, which predispose to pneumonia after aspiration.

In general, other risk factors for aspiration in older patients can be categorized as disease-related (e.g., stroke, dementia, neuromuscular disorders such as Parkinson's disease, GERD), medication-related (e.g., drugs that cause dry mouth or altered mental status), and iatrogenic factors. Iatrogenic factors are particularly relevant to surgical patients. The presence of devices crossing the oropharynx (e.g., nasogastric tubes, endotracheal tubes, esophageal thermometers, transesophageal echocardiography probes) has been shown to disrupt the swallowing mechanism further. The need for prolonged intubation is associated with swallowing dysfunction and aspiration, as is the use of enteral feeding tubes. The routine use of nasogastric tubes in patients undergoing colon resection has been correlated with an increased risk of aspiration pneumonia, as has the use of transesophageal echocardiography probes in patients undergoing cardiac surgery. The occurrence of postoperative ileus also predisposes to aspiration.

Aspiration risk should be assessed preoperatively in all older patients with risk factors for aspiration and in patients with any report of a swallowing abnormality (see "Preoperative Assessment," earlier). Aspiration precautions should be ordered for any patient thought to be at risk. These precautions include 30-degree to 45-degree upright positioning, careful evaluation of gastrointestinal function before starting feeding and frequently thereafter, careful monitoring of gastric residuals in patients with feeding tubes, and upright position during meals and for 30 to 45 minutes after meals in patients on an oral diet.

Deconditioning

In older patients, the prolonged period of immobility that follows hospitalization for a major surgical procedure often results in functional decline and overall deconditioning. Functional decline has been observed after 2 days of immobility. Deconditioning is a distinct clinical entity characterized by specific changes in function of many organ systems (Table 13-5).[43] Deconditioned individuals have ongoing functional limitations, despite improvement in the original acute illness. The period for functional recovery may be three times longer than the period of immobility. Prolonged bed rest also leads to other postoperative complications, such as pressure ulcers and falls.

A major risk factor for deconditioning during hospitalization is a preexisting functional limitation. For example, patients requiring ambulation assist devices such as canes or walkers before hospitalization are more likely to experience significant further functional decline. Other, less obvious functional limitations, such as the inability to perform activities such as walking up a flight of steps carrying a bag of groceries (4 METs), are also associated with higher rates of postoperative complications and greater chances of functional decline. Other risk factors include two or more comorbidities, five or more medications, and a hospitalization or emergency department visit in the preceding year. Patients who develop delirium while in the hospital are also at greater risk of developing serious functional decline and of requiring placement in short-term rehabilitation or long-term care facilities.

TABLE 13-5 Organ System Effects of Bed Rest

SYSTEM	EFFECT
Cardiovascular	↓ Stroke volume, ↓ cardiac output, orthostatic hypotension
Respiratory	↓ Respiratory excursion, ↓ oxygen uptake, ↑ potential for atelectasis
Muscles	↓ Muscle strength, ↓ muscle blood flow
Bone	↑ Bone loss, ↓ bone density
Gastrointestinal	Malnutrition, anorexia, constipation
Genitourinary	Incontinence
Skin	Sheering force, potential for skin breakdown
Psychological	Social isolation, anxiety, depression, disorientation

From Kleinpell RM, Fletcher K, Jennings BM: Reducing functional decline in hospitalized elderly. In Hughes RG, editor: *Patient safety and quality: An evidence-based handbook for nurses*, AHRQ Publication No. 08-0043, Rockville, MD, 2008, Agency for Healthcare Research and Quality, pp 251–265.

Assessment of functional capacity is an essential part of the preoperative assessment (see earlier). In patients identified to be at risk for functional decline, a plan for early directed methods to promote mobility, including early physical therapy consultation, should be established before surgery. The "out of bed" order may be the most important of all routine postoperative orders for older patients.

Structured models for in-hospital care have been developed for geriatric patients hospitalized for medical illnesses. Adaptation of these models for surgical patients could promote improvements in functional and cognitive status. Preoperative conditioning to improve function before surgery, termed *prehabilitation*, has theoretical merit, although evidence to support its usefulness is lacking.

SURGERY OF MAJOR ORGAN SYSTEMS

Endocrine Surgery

Thyroid Disease

Thyroid disease is common. Hypothyroidism occurs in 10% of women and 2% of men older than 60 years; hyperthyroidism occurs in 0.5% to 6% of persons older than 55. Hypothyroidism is caused by autoimmune disease, previous radioablation or surgery, and drugs that interfere with the synthesis of thyroid hormone, such as amiodarone. Hyperthyroidism is usually caused by toxic multinodular goiter, with Graves disease being less common than in younger persons. Medical treatment of hypothyroidism in older adults is similar to treatment in younger patients. Surgical treatment of hyperthyroidism may be necessary for large goiters compressing the trachea. As with disorders of many other organ systems, symptoms of hypothyroidism and hyperthyroidism in this age group are easily overlooked or attributed to other causes. Failure to recognize the presence of either condition can result in serious perioperative problems.

The incidence of thyroid nodules increases throughout life, with nodules detected by physical examination, ultrasound, or autopsy, although physical examination is less sensitive because of fibrosis of the soft tissues of the neck and the gland. The incidence of nodules in autopsy series is 50%. Thyroid nodules are four times more common in women, but the risk for cancer in a nodule is higher in men. In the United States, thyroid cancer is the fastest growing cancer; the incidence of thyroid cancer increased from 3.6 per 100,000 in 1973 to 8.7 in 2002; an estimated 62,980 new cases were expected to be diagnosed in 2014.[44]

Well-differentiated thyroid cancer is divided into papillary and follicular subtypes. Sporadic papillary thyroid cancer has an almost bell-shaped distribution of age at diagnosis, with a decreasing trend in patients older than 60 years. Age is a negative prognostic factor for survival and other outcomes; patients older than 60 years have an increased risk for local recurrence, and patients younger than 20 and older than 60 have a higher risk for the development of distant metastasis. Similar results have been noted for follicular cancer. Increasing patient age correlates with increased risk for death by approximately twofold over a span of 20 years. Guidelines for the management of thyroid nodules and well-differentiated cancers are in the 2009 report of the American Thyroid Association Guidelines Task Force.[45]

When thyroidectomy is indicated, it can usually be performed safely, even in patients much older than 80 years. However, older age confers a higher risk of complications, longer hospital stays, higher mean costs, more likely discharges to a location other than home, and higher rates of perioperative mortality. Surgical outcomes in older patients with multiple comorbidities have been shown to be better when the operative volume of the surgeon is more than 30 thyroidectomies per year.[46] For this population with complicated comorbidities, surgical risks and benefits must be carefully weighed.

Parathyroid Disease

The most common reason for the finding of hypercalcemia in an elderly patient in the outpatient setting is primary hyperparathyroidism. The incidence of primary hyperparathyroidism increases with age; it affects approximately 2% of older persons, with a 3 : 1 female preponderance (1 in 1000 postmenopausal women). The disease is characterized by elevated serum calcium levels, often within 1 mg of normal, in the presence of elevated parathyroid hormone to levels 1.5 to 2 times normal. Most cases in older adults are solitary adenomas.

Until the 1970s, parathyroid disease was often symptomatic with nephrolithiasis (stones), overt skeletal disease (bones), and neuropsychiatric symptoms (psychic groans) on presentation. With the advent of routine calcium testing as part of automated chemistry analysis, this pattern has changed, and now 80% of cases are asymptomatic. A careful history frequently reveals the presence of less obvious psychological and emotional symptoms. Other subtle symptoms in older persons include memory loss, personality changes, inability to concentrate, exercise fatigue, and back pain. Several studies have shown that only 5% to 8% of patients are truly asymptomatic.

In response to the controversy regarding treatment of asymptomatic hyperparathyroidism, the National Institutes of Health (NIH) consensus conference met in 1990 and again in 2002 to define parameters for care. In 2008, an international workshop on hyperparathyroidism reviewed the old guidelines and provided updated recommendations.[47] Surgery is recommended in otherwise asymptomatic patients if there are elevations in serum calcium more than 1 mg/dl above the normal range, increased 24-hour urine calcium excretion (>400 mg), decreased CrCl, reduction in bone density of more than 2.5 SDs below peak bone mass (T-score <2.5), follow-up is difficult because of other comorbidities, or the patient is younger than 50 years old. This definition still leaves uncertain whether weakness and depression indicate symptomatic disease, although approximately 40% of patients with hyperparathyroidism have one or both symptoms. Because the risk for morbidity and mortality associated with surgery is low, even in older patients, parathyroidectomy remains the treatment of choice unless other comorbid conditions preclude surgery.

Minimally invasive parathyroid surgery has gained acceptance with the adoption of sestamibi-directed surgery, intraoperative parathyroid hormone assay, and videoscopic surgery. Cure rates in patients older than 70 years at one center increased from 84% in the pre–minimally invasive surgery era (before 2001) to 98% after the introduction of radiologically guided minimally invasive surgery under regional anesthesia.[48]

Breast Disease

Epidemiology. Increasing age is a major risk factor for developing breast cancer. Worldwide, almost one third of breast cancer cases occur in patients older than 65 years. In the United States, more than 50% of new cases of breast cancer and approximately two thirds of breast cancer–related deaths occur in patients older than 65 years. Breast cancer incidence increases with age, peaking at age 75 and declining slightly thereafter. It is predicted that as life expectancy continues to improve in Western countries, the proportion and absolute numbers of elderly women with breast cancer will increase dramatically.

Presentation and screening. The presentation of breast cancer is similar in older and younger populations. The most common symptom of breast cancer is a painless mass. In older women, a new breast lump is likely to represent a malignancy. Breast pain, skin thickening, breast swelling, or nipple discharge or retraction should be vigorously pursued with biopsy in older women. Breasts become less dense with aging, making the clinical examination easier in older women. This difference also translates into an improved positive predictive value of an abnormal mammogram in women older than 65 years. The American Cancer Society recommends monthly breast self-examination, annual clinical breast examination, and annual mammography beginning at age 40, with no upper age limit as long as a woman remains in good health. If a woman has an estimated life expectancy of less than 3 to 5 years, has severe functional limitations, or has multiple comorbidities that are likely to impair survival, discontinuation of screening is appropriate. The American Geriatrics Society Position Statement recommends annual or at least biennial mammography to age 75 years. Beyond the age of 75, mammography should be biennial or at least every 3 years if life expectancy is more than 4 years.[49]

Pathology and treatment overview. Overall, breast cancers in older patients tend to be associated with more favorable pathologic prognostic factors. As patient age increases, breast tumors are associated with more favorable tumor biology, as indicated by increased hormone sensitivity, attenuated epidermal growth factor receptor 2 (*EGFR2*) overexpression, and lower grades and proliferative indices. However, older patients are more likely to present with larger and more advanced tumors, and reports have suggested that lymph node involvement increases with age. Data suggest that older women are less likely to be treated according to recommended guidelines; they are less likely to receive definitive surgery, breast-conserving surgery, postlumpectomy radiotherapy, adjuvant hormonal therapy, or adjuvant chemotherapy. In addition, some studies show that although there has been significant improvement in recurrence and mortality as a result of improvements in screening and treatment, this improvement has been smaller among older women.

Breast cancer trials in the United States have a disproportionately low enrollment of older women. Women 65 years old and older are less likely than stage-matched and physician-matched younger women to be offered participation in breast cancer trials. Most recommendations for the treatment of older women with breast cancer have been derived from studies done in women younger than 70 years. In contrast to treatment of younger women with breast cancer, life expectancy is a central concept in decision making in older women with breast cancer. Accurate predictions and knowledge of life expectancy are inherently important in decisions regarding screening older populations using mammography, treatment of the primary lesion, and use of systemic adjuvant therapy. Currently available treatment options often carry short-term risks and toxicities in older women that are not mitigated by long-term survival gains. Current recommendations from the Society of Geriatric Oncology strongly recommend involving a geriatrician to help manage comorbidities and provide a realistic understanding of life expectancy.[50]

Surgery. The gold standard for treating localized breast cancer at any age is surgery. Surgical mortality in elderly women in reasonably good health is low (<1%). Surgical resection of the primary tumor is recommended for all older patients unless they are poor surgical candidates, and breast-conserving therapy should be recommended when possible. Despite evidence that age is not a contraindication to breast-conserving surgery, older women have historically had lower rates of breast-conserving cancer surgery than younger women. More recent studies have indicated that the proportion of older women undergoing breast-conserving therapy is increasing. Omitting surgery exposes patients to a higher risk of local relapse and is considered a suboptimal option, even for unfit older women. Tamoxifen alone had been previously recommended for the treatment of patients unfit for surgery and with short life expectancies because tamoxifen antagonizes the estrogen receptor. In contrast to premenopausal women in whom the ovaries are responsible for estrogen production, the adrenal gland produces estrogen in postmenopausal women. Aromatase inhibitors, which block the synthesis of estrogen, are also associated with better response rates and fewer thromboembolic complications than tamoxifen; however, the use of aromatase inhibitors in patients with severe osteoporosis is cautioned (see later).

The role of axillary lymph node dissection in the management of women with breast cancer has evolved over the last 10 to 15 years. Axillary lymph node dissection should be used when there is clinical suspicion of axillary lymph node involvement or a high-risk tumor. Biopsy of sentinel lymph nodes is a safe alternative to axillary lymph node dissection in patients with clinically node-negative tumors. Older patients with tumor size smaller than 2 to 3 cm and no clinical evidence of axillary involvement should be offered a sentinel lymph node biopsy.[50]

Radiation therapy. For women 70 years old or older who have early, estrogen receptor–positive breast cancer, the addition of adjuvant radiation therapy to tamoxifen does not significantly decrease the rate of mastectomy for local recurrence, increase the survival rate, or increase the rate of freedom from distant metastases. Tamoxifen alone is a reasonable choice for adjuvant treatment in such women. For older women with small, node-negative tumors, the decision to include breast irradiation after lumpectomy should be made on a case-by-case basis after careful discussion of the risks of locoregional recurrence and the side effects of radiation therapy. Alternatively, partial breast irradiation with multicatheter interstitial brachytherapy, balloon catheter brachytherapy, three-dimensional conformal external-beam radiotherapy, and intraoperative radiotherapy can be an option in selected older patients. Older women treated with mastectomy should be offered chest wall irradiation if they have tumors larger than 5 cm or more than four involved axillary lymph nodes.[50]

Chemotherapy. Adjuvant endocrine therapy is generally recommended for older women with estrogen receptor–positive breast cancer. Tamoxifen and aromatase inhibitors, such as anastrozole, improve overall survival, reduce local recurrence, and reduce the risk of contralateral breast cancer for hormone-sensitive tumors in older women. Tamoxifen and anastrozole have side effects that can reduce their tolerance. Tamoxifen is associated with deep vein thrombosis, pulmonary emboli, cerebrovascular events, endometrial carcinoma, vaginal discharge and bleeding, and hot flashes. There are considerably more musculoskeletal symptoms, including arthralgias and fractures, with anastrozole. It is important to monitor bone density and treat patients who have bone density loss while on aromatase inhibitors.

Older women have generally been underrepresented in adjuvant chemotherapy trials; however, more recent data suggest that standard adjuvant chemotherapy has a role in the treatment of fit older women. The added value of chemotherapy in older women who receive endocrine therapy is influenced greatly by comorbidity and life expectancy. Models for estimating the benefits of chemotherapy in hormone receptor–positive older women have been developed and demonstrate that a high risk of recurrence is needed to achieve a small survival benefit with adjuvant chemotherapy. For example, to reduce mortality risk at 10 years by 1% with chemotherapy, the risk of breast recurrence at 10 years has to be at least 25% for a 75-year-old woman in average health. These data suggest that chemotherapy for older women with hormone receptor–positive breast cancer should be offered only to patients with node-positive disease who are in reasonably good health, with a high risk of recurrence, and with a life expectancy of more than 5 years. Older patients with node-negative disease are unlikely to benefit from chemotherapy unless they have large hormone receptor–positive tumors with adverse pathologic characteristics or hormone receptor–negative tumors larger than 2 cm. An Internet-based tool that incorporates age, health status, and tumor characteristics can help determine the potential benefit of adjuvant chemotherapy for breast cancer patients (available at: http://www.adjuvantonline.com).

Gastrointestinal Surgery

Esophagus

Motility disorders. The esophagus undergoes characteristic changes with aging. Dysfunction of the proximal aspects of swallowing is noted during normal aging. Resting upper esophageal sphincter pressure and relaxation are decreased in the older normal population compared with a younger control population. The duration of oropharyngeal swallowing and the sensory threshold for initiating a swallow are increased with advancing age. These factors increase the risk of pharyngeal stasis and potential for aspiration. Dysmotility of the cricopharyngeus (upper esophageal sphincter) with increasing age can result in Zenker diverticula (see Chapter 41). In normal healthy individuals, the physiologic function of the esophagus itself appears to be preserved until patients reach around 80 years of age. In this group, the amplitude of esophageal contractions is decreased.

Gastroesophageal reflux disease. It has been suggested that GERD is associated with the peristaltic dysfunction that occurs with aging. Although the lower esophageal sphincter resting pressure is normal and relaxes appropriately after deglutition, the sphincter fails to contract rapidly back to baseline, resulting in prolonged decreased tone. There is also an increased incidence of sliding hiatal hernia with aging that is due to laxity at the gastroesophageal junction. These conditions, along with delayed gastric emptying, predispose older patients to GERD. Also, many medications prescribed for older patients increase the relaxation of the lower esophageal sphincter.[51]

The complications of GERD, including erosive esophagitis, Barrett esophagus, and esophageal adenocarcinoma, are seen with an increased frequency in older patients. However, more recent studies have demonstrated that symptoms may be attenuated in older adults. Specifically, older patients with severe esophagitis are least likely to have severe heartburn. Instead, they present with more nonspecific symptoms, such as dysphagia, anorexia, anemia, weight loss, and vomiting. The absence of classic symptoms may be the result of an age-related decreased esophageal sensitivity to pain. More aggressive diagnosis or treatment of GERD may be warranted for older patients, regardless of their presenting symptoms.

Laparoscopic Nissen fundoplication for the correction of GERD in older patients provides a viable alternative to lifelong medications, which may be less effective in older patients. Relief of symptoms, particularly vomiting and aspiration, is reported by 90% of older patients after a Nissen procedure. Laparoscopic Nissen has been shown to be safe with comparable outcomes in elderly adults.

Paraesophageal hernias. Paraesophageal hernias also increase with advancing age and can reach an enormous size without symptoms (Fig. 13-10). In the past, the fear of gastric volvulus, with subsequent strangulation, mandated immediate repair of

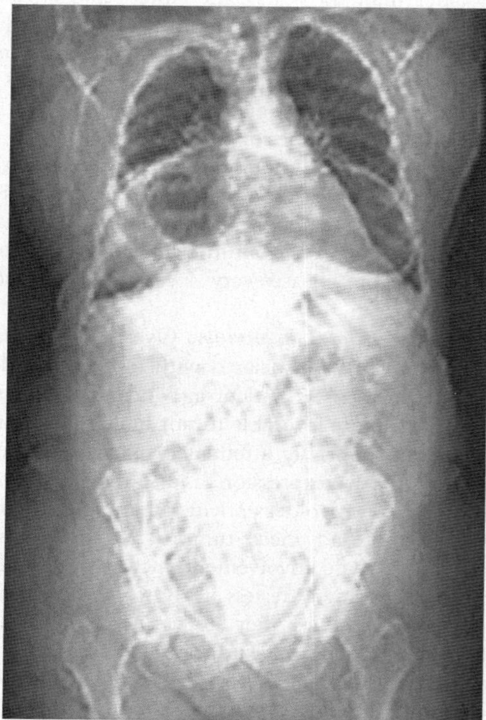

FIGURE 13-10 Scout film for a computed tomography scan showing a giant paraesophageal hernia with the entire stomach in the chest, rotated in an organoaxial direction.

paraesophageal hernias, even in the absence of symptoms. At the present time, watchful waiting is generally recommended rather than immediate surgery for asymptomatic hernia, which has been demonstrated to have a low (1.1%) annual probability of requiring an emergency operation.

Dysphagia. Dysphagia is a frequent symptom in older adults that can cause significant problems in the perioperative period. Dysphagia in older adults can be divided into two categories—abnormalities affecting the neuromuscular mechanisms controlling movement of the tongue, pharynx, and upper esophageal sphincter (oropharyngeal dysphagia) and disorders affecting the esophagus itself (esophageal dysphagia). Causes of oropharyngeal dysphagia include stroke, Parkinson disease, myasthenia gravis, diabetes, carcinomas, Zenker diverticulum, and osteophytes. Causes of esophageal dysphagia can be divided into problems with motility, such as achalasia, diffuse esophageal spasm, and scleroderma, and structural problems, such as carcinoma, benign stricture, webs, and vascular compression.

Esophageal cancer. Esophageal resection remains the only established curative treatment for cancer of the esophagus and gastric cardia. A major problem is that the surgery required is extensive, with a considerable risk of complications. Although the short-term mortality has decreased in recent years, the complication rate remains high. Studies have suggested that survival after resection of esophageal cancer is improving; however, this may be partly the result of detection and treatment of tumors at an earlier stage. There appears to be no difference in surgical complication rates between younger and older patients undergoing esophagectomy. However, there is an increase in operative and in-hospital mortality and a decreased 5-year survival in older patients; this is most likely because of an increase in cardiopulmonary complications and other major morbidities seen in the older age group undergoing esophageal resection. Some evidence indicates that laparoscopy and minimally invasive techniques have decreased length of stay and morbidity and comparable outcomes to open surgery in elderly patients.

Stomach

A progressive cephalad migration of the antral-fundic junction occurs with age. Studies have shown that 25% to 80% of older adults have fasting achlorhydria. This condition is caused by progressive loss of parietal cells and decreased antral and serum concentrations of gastrin. Achlorhydria results in derangements in folate, iron, and vitamin B_{12} absorption.[51]

Peptic ulcer. The incidence of peptic ulcer disease increases with age. Patients older than 65 years account for 80% of deaths related to peptic ulcer. Other factors that increase the risk of peptic ulcer disease in older adults are the use of nonsteroidal anti-inflammatory drugs (NSAIDs) and infection with *Helicobacter pylori*. NSAID use has increased markedly in recent years, especially in older adults. The use of NSAIDs increases the risk of developing complicated peptic ulcer disease in older patients compared with younger patients. Actual NSAID use is also a useful prognostic indicator; the mortality rate from peptic ulcer disease in older patients who take NSAIDs is twice that of older patients who do not take NSAIDs. Similarly, 80% of all ulcer-related deaths occur in patients taking NSAIDs. Despite this finding, NSAIDs are frequently prescribed to older patients, including patients with previous gastrointestinal problems. *H. pylori* infections are believed to occur at a rate of 1% per year, yielding a substantial percentage of older adults harboring infections.

Older patients typically present for surgical correction of peptic ulcer disease in a delayed fashion and with more advanced disease. This situation translates to statistically significant increases in operative mortality for older patients undergoing surgery for complicated peptic ulcer disease. Age alone has not been shown to be an independent predictor of surgical risk. Multivariate analysis reveals three risk factors for operative mortality in perforated ulcer—the presence of concomitant disease, preoperative shock, and more than 48 hours of perforation. Age, amount of peritoneal soilage, and length of history of ulcer disease do not appear to be significant risks.

Gastric cancer. The incidence of gastric cancer increases progressively with age, with most patients between the ages of 50 and 70 years at presentation. Risks include dietary (e.g., pickled vegetables, salted fish, nitrates, nitrites), occupational (e.g., metal, asbestos, rubber workers), and geographic (Asia versus Western Hemisphere) factors. Chronic atrophic gastritis, previous gastric surgery, and chronic *H. pylori* infection, more frequently found in older patients, are associated with an increased risk of gastric cancer. Chronic atrophic gastritis and *H. pylori* infection are also risk factors for gastric lymphoma and its precursor, mucosal-associated lymphoid tissue. These patients typically present in the sixth decade of life.

The presentation of gastric cancer is changing in older persons, leading to the need for more aggressive surgery. Older patients present with a predominance of intestinal-type tumors rather than the more aggressive diffuse type. There is also a progression of the location of the tumor to more proximal areas of the stomach. As a result, total gastrectomy for cure in this population is now required in 13% to 34% of cases. No difference in resectability or the rate of positive lymph nodes found at surgery (60% to 70%) has been noted between younger and older patients.[52] Early reports of minimally invasive gastrectomy have demonstrated decreased morbidity and cost because of decreased length of stay. Long-term outcomes are less clear.

Biliary Tract Disease

In almost all populations and both sexes, the prevalence of gallstones increases with advancing age, although the magnitude of this increase varies with the population. Biliary tract disease is the most common cause of acute abdominal symptoms in patients older than 65 years in the United States and accounts for approximately one third of all abdominal surgeries in this age group. In 2006, adults older than 65 years accounted for 50% of hospital discharges for a primary diagnosis of cholelithiasis and one third of the more than 400,000 inpatient cholecystectomies performed that year.

The increased frequency of gallstones in older adults is thought to result from changes in the composition of bile and impaired biliary motility. Alterations in the composition of bile with advancing age include an increase in the activity of 3-hydroxy-3-methylglutaryl coenzyme A (the rate-limiting enzyme in the synthesis of cholesterol) and a decrease in the activity of 7α-hydroxylase (the rate-limiting enzyme in the synthesis of bile salts from cholesterol). These changes result in the supersaturation of bile with cholesterol and a decrease in the primary bile salt pool. The ratio of secondary to primary bile salts also increases. It is postulated that these secondary bile salts promote cholesterol gallstone formation by enhancing cholesterol synthesis, increasing the protein content of bile, decreasing nucleation time, and increasing the production of specific phospholipids that are thought to affect the production of mucin. It has also been suggested that the increase in secondary bile salts in older adults may promote the recycling of bilirubin, which leads to the unconjugated bilirubin supersaturation necessary for pigment stone formation.

Alterations in gallbladder motility and bile duct motility are thought to be central to the development of cholesterol and brown pigment stones, respectively. The role of motility in black pigment stone formation is less clear. Biliary motility is a complex interaction of hormonal and neural factors, but the major stimulus for gallbladder emptying is cholecystokinin (CCK). In animal models, the sensitivity of the gallbladder wall to CCK has been shown to decrease with increasing age. In humans, gallbladder sensitivity to CCK is also decreased. However, there is a compensatory increase in the production of CCK in response to a stimulus that results in normal gallbladder contraction. The significance of this observation with regard to gallstone formation is unknown.

The indications for treatment of gallstone disease in older patients are the same as in younger patients, although complications of the disease, rather than biliary colic, are more common in older patients. Older patients admitted to the hospital for cholecystectomy are more likely to have multiple biliary diagnoses, carry a concomitant diagnosis of cholangitis, undergo open operation, and require additional procedures such as endoscopic retrograde cholangiopancreatography or CBD exploration.[53] The increased rate of complicated disease seen in older patients may be attributable to the increased severity of the disease, an increased prevalence of comorbid illnesses, or both. However, it is more likely to be a combination of factors, including delays in diagnosis and treatment caused by the frequent absence of typical biliary tract symptoms. Biliary colic, or episodic right upper quadrant pain radiating to the back, precedes the development of a complication only half as often in older patients as in younger patients. Even in the presence of acute cholecystitis, 25% of older patients may have no abdominal tenderness, one third have no elevation in temperature or WBC count, and 59% have no peritoneal signs in the right upper quadrant.

The outcome of biliary tract surgery in older patients hospitalized for treatment has not improved much over the past several decades. Older patients have more complicated disease at the time of surgery, longer lengths of stay, higher rates of in-hospital mortality, and much higher rates of discharge to sites other than home (Fig. 13-11).[53] Until predictors of impending complications other than symptoms are identified, improving the outcome of biliary tract disease in older adults will be difficult. Increased awareness of the atypical manifestations of gallstone-related illness in this age group is essential.

Treatment of acute cholecystitis in older adults is controversial. Although considerable evidence supports the safety and efficacy of early laparoscopic cholecystectomy for acute cholecystitis in general, some authors favor percutaneous drainage, followed by delayed cholecystectomy, in older adults. Evidence has suggested that 25% of older patients admitted to the hospital with a diagnosis of acute cholecystitis do not undergo cholecystectomy on the initial admission. However, readmission rates in this group are high, and 2-year survival is worse, even after adjustment for comorbidities and other patient risk factors.[54]

The presence of CBD stones increases the likelihood of postoperative complications and death. In the prelaparoscopic era, CBD stones were addressed at the time of cholecystectomy. Although open CBD exploration was extremely successful in clearing the bile duct of stones, it was associated with a significant increase in operative mortality and morbidity over simple cholecystectomy alone. Most clinicians now agree that if CBD stones are suspected from a dilated duct on ultrasound or from abnormal liver or pancreatic test results, a preoperative attempt at sphincterotomy and extraction via endoscopic retrograde cholangiopancreatography should be carried out. Successful duct clearance by this approach is reported in more than 90% of cases. However, recurrence of CBD stones after sphincterotomy, even with antecedent or subsequent cholecystectomy, is higher in older patients compared with younger patients (20% versus 4%). Risk factors

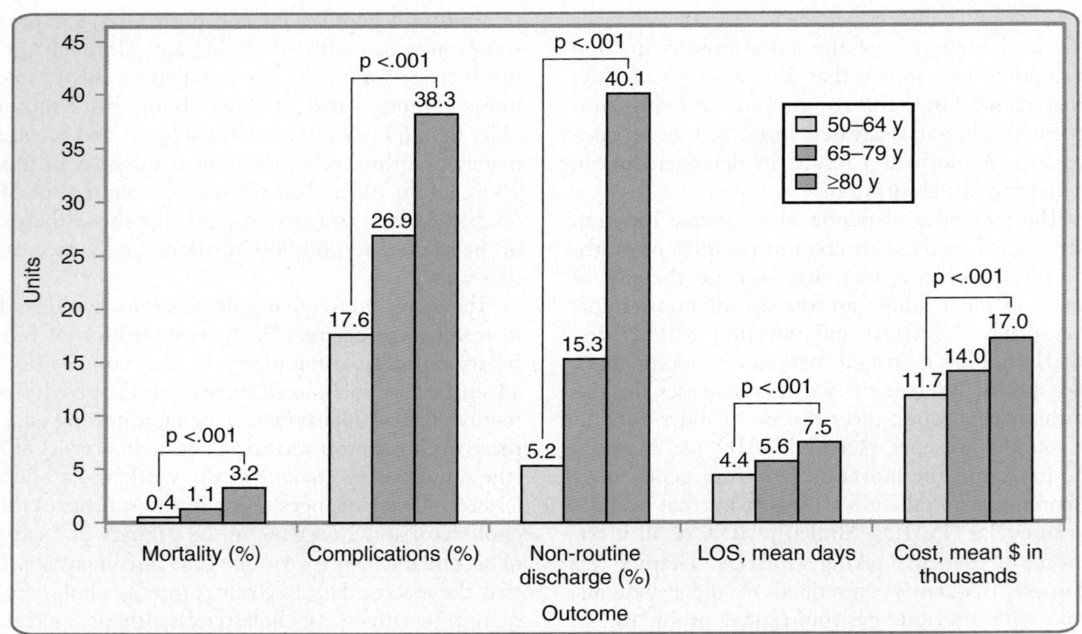

FIGURE 13-11 Outcomes of inpatient cholecystectomy with increasing age. *LOS*, length of stay. (From Kuy S, Sosa JA, Roman SA, et al: Age matters: A study of clinical and economic outcomes following cholecystectomy in elderly Americans. *Am J Surg* 201:789–796, 2011.)

for recurrence include a dilated CBD, duodenal diverticulum, angulation of the CBD, and previous cholecystectomy.

Management of the gallbladder after successful endoscopic treatment of CBD stones in patients without coincident acute cholecystitis is controversial. Several studies indicated that a complication related to the gallbladder eventually develops in 4% to 24% of patients managed by endoscopic sphincterotomy alone and that 5.8% to 18% require subsequent cholecystectomy. Because patients managed in this fashion are frequently the oldest and frailest patients, the mortality related to subsequent acute cholecystitis in these patients can be 25%.

Liver

Over the past 20 years, mortality associated with liver resection in patients older than 65 years has decreased. Advances in operative technique, anesthetic management, and intensive care have greatly reduced morbidity and mortality. Today, the rates in younger and older patients are comparable. Results are so similar that age alone is not a contraindication to simultaneous resection of colorectal malignancy and liver metastases. Previous studies on the safety of resection in elderly patients cited mortality and morbidity of approximately 4% to 5% and 30% to 40%, respectively. Postoperative liver function in well-selected elderly patients has proven comparable to their younger counterparts.

Tumors of the liver are 20 times more likely to arise from metastatic disease than from primary cancer. Metastatic tumors from gastrointestinal tract primaries are the most common type referred for resection. Patients with colon cancer have a 35% risk for recurrence in the liver, but only 10% to 20% of patients identified have resectable disease. Patients who undergo resection have more than a 30% 5-year survival rate versus 0% without resection. Resection of colon and rectal liver metastases has been shown to be safe and effective in a select group of elderly patients.

When determining appropriateness of resection, it is important to consider the higher prevalence of insulin resistance and nonalcoholic fatty liver disease in elderly patients. Although age itself is not a contraindication, careful consideration of comorbidities must be taken into account. For patients in whom commodities cause prohibitive risk, other options to treat hepatic cancer include radiologic embolization, cryotherapy, and radiofrequency ablation therapy, which can be performed operatively or transcutaneously.

Small Bowel Obstruction

Small bowel obstruction (SBO) is the most common and surgically relevant disorder of small intestinal function encountered in older patients. Although the exact incidence of SBO in older adults is difficult to ascertain, lysis of adhesions is the third most common gastrointestinal procedure after cholecystectomy and partial excision of the large bowel. Of the deaths associated with SBO, 50% occur in patients older than 70 years.

In Western countries, adhesions are responsible for most SBOs, followed by incarcerated hernias, neoplasms, and inflammatory bowel disease. Patients with incarcerated hernias are slightly older than patients with adhesive obstruction. In addition, certain types of hernias, such as hernias that occur through the obturator foramen, are found almost exclusively in older adults and are particularly difficult to diagnose. Luminal obstruction, other than from deliberately ingested objects, accounts for less than 5% of cases. However, most cases of this type of obstruction occur in older adults. The two most common objects obstructing the lumen in adults are phytobezoars and gallstones. Phytobezoars, or large concretions of poorly digested fruit and vegetable matter, form with increased frequency in the stomach of older patients with poor dentition, decreased gastric acid, impaired gastric motility, and previous gastrectomy. In the stomach, these masses can become enormous without any symptoms. However, when a portion breaks free and migrates into the small bowel, obstruction ensues. Gallstones enter the small bowel usually through a fistula between the gallbladder and duodenum. Obstruction of the small bowel lumen by an aberrantly located gallstone, incorrectly termed *gallstone ileus,* accounts for 1% to 3% of all SBOs but has been implicated in 25% of obstructions in patients older than 65 years with no abdominal wall hernia or history of previous surgery.

The pathophysiology, diagnosis, and treatment of SBO are discussed elsewhere in the text. However, two important issues that determine management strategy—distinguishing functional (ileus) from mechanical obstruction and distinguishing simple from strangulated obstruction—are even more complex in older patients. Many of the factors associated with ileus, such as systemic infections, intra-abdominal infections, metabolic abnormalities, and medications that affect motility, are more common in older adults. The relevance of these factors to the finding of abdominal distention is not always appreciated. Signs and symptoms of underlying infections, such as pneumonia, urinary tract infection, or appendicitis, may be subtle. Bowel distention may be erroneously considered the primary problem rather than a secondary event. Vomiting from various nonobstructive causes can rapidly lead to dehydration and subsequent electrolyte abnormalities in older adults. The constellation of vomiting and bowel distention can easily be mistaken for obstruction.

In patients of all ages suspected to have adhesive SBO, initial nonoperative management with nasogastric decompression and IV hydration is standard. Although rates vary, only approximately 30% of patients with adhesive SBO require surgery, usually for failure to progress or fear of strangulation. However, an accurate distinction between strangulated and simple mechanical SBO is difficult to make, particularly in older adults, because there are no objective markers that consistently identify which patient will require small bowel resection for ischemia at the time of surgery for SBO. Clinical findings of fever, tachycardia, elevated WBC count, and focal tenderness are notoriously misleading, particularly in older adults, in whom the risk for strangulation is the highest.

Several additional considerations are important in older adults. Although the natural reflex is to avoid unnecessary operations in sick older patients, prolonged conservative management can present new problems. Prolonged bed rest is associated with an increased incidence of venous stasis, pulmonary complications, and deconditioning. Prolonged nasogastric intubation is associated with an increased incidence of aspiration and pneumonia. Even a short period of nutritional deprivation may present a significant risk to an older patient with a baseline nutritional deficit. These factors together may result in a poor outcome if surgery becomes necessary after a prolonged attempt to avoid it.

In a review of more than 32,000 patients treated for SBO in California, 24% required surgery on the index admission.[55] Although length of stay was longer for patients who had surgery, mortality was lower, readmissions for SBO were fewer, and the time interval to readmission for SBO was longer. The authors specifically stated that further research is needed to determine the importance of time to surgery on outcomes for the oldest and sickest patients.

In older patients who have undergone previous abdominal operations for malignant disease, the decision about when to operate is even more difficult. Metastatic obstruction presents several technical and ethical problems. Obstructing lesions are frequently found at numerous points in the bowel, and resection may be impossible. Bypass of long, partially obstructed segments may be technically feasible but can leave the patient with a functionally short gut. For this form of obstruction, 30-day operative mortality rates in older patients exceed 35%, and most patients die within 6 months. This discouraging outcome has led some clinicians to advocate prolonged periods of nonoperative decompression. However, this approach produces only transient relief of obstructive symptoms. Furthermore, a previous history of malignancy is not an absolute indication that the obstruction is caused by metastatic disease. In 10% to 38% of patients with suspected malignant obstruction, a benign cause is found at the time of surgery.

Over the past decade, there has been increasing interest in using minimally invasive techniques to diagnose and treat SBO. At first glance, the laparoscopic approach in older adults has considerable appeal. Early intervention with minimal surgical stress would seem ideal. Numerous small series by experienced laparoscopic surgeons show diagnostic success in more than 90% of cases and total therapeutic success rates of 50% to 90%. However, laparoscopy in this setting can be technically challenging and not without complications. It is unclear at the present time how widely this option will be adopted as more surgeons become skilled in these advanced laparoscopic techniques.

Appendicitis

Although appendicitis typically occurs in the second and third decades of life, 5% to 10% of cases manifest in old age. Appendicitis in older adults has increased in recent decades, whereas the incidence in younger patients is declining. This increase is thought to be due in part to increasing life expectancy and a larger proportion of elderly adults. Inflammation of the appendix accounts for 2.5% to 5% of acute abdominal disease in patients older than 60 to 70 years. The overall mortality from appendicitis is only 0.8%, but most deaths occur in very young and very old patients. In adults, the mortality rate after appendectomy is strongly related to age, ranging from a minimum of 0.07/1000 appendectomies in patients 20 to 29 years old to a maximum of 164/1000 in nonagenarians.

The classic presentation of appendicitis—periumbilical pain that localizes over several hours to the right lower quadrant, fever, anorexia, and leukocytosis—occurs in less than 20% of older patients with appendicitis. Although almost all older patients with acute appendicitis present with abdominal pain, only 50% to 75% have pain localized to the right lower quadrant. Almost one third of patients have diffuse nonlocalizable abdominal pain. Because vague abdominal pain is a common symptom in older adults, its significance may be overlooked, leading to delays in treatment. Other signs of acute appendicitis are also unreliable in older adults. The WBC count and temperature are normal in 20% to 50% of older patients with appendicitis. Nausea, vomiting, and anorexia are also found less frequently in older patients.[56]

The indolent and nonspecific nature of the initial symptoms of appendicitis in older adults usually leads to delays of 48 to 72 hours before medical attention is sought. These delays are compounded by a delay in diagnosis when the patient reaches the hospital. Delays to operation longer than 24 hours are three times as likely to occur in older patients compared with younger patients. As a result of these delays, more than 50% of older patients have perforated appendicitis identified at operation.[56] Older patients undergoing appendectomy for perforated appendicitis have a higher risk of complications and death than older patients undergoing simple appendectomy for appendicitis without peritonitis.

The use of computed tomography (CT) scanning in the diagnosis of acute appendicitis has increased dramatically. Less than 20% of patients underwent preoperative CT before urgent appendectomy in 1998 compared with greater than 90% of patients in 2007. The negative appendectomy rate in older adults has not changed during this same time period. Because of the atypical presentation of appendicitis, the high rate of perforation at the time of presentation, and the expanded differential diagnosis in older adults, CT scanning has been advocated.[57] If an abscess is found, percutaneous drainage and IV antibiotics are often preferable to exploration in the presence of a large abscess. In younger patients, this approach is followed by interval appendectomy approximately 6 weeks after the abscess has resolved. In older adults, recurrent appendicitis after resolution of the abscess is uncommon, and interval appendectomy is not necessary in all cases. However, the possibility of perforated cancer in this age group mandates a thorough evaluation of the colon when the acute process is controlled. Older patients presenting with signs and symptoms of acute appendicitis, but with longer duration of symptoms and a lower hematocrit than expected, should raise the concern for colon or appendiceal cancer.

The use of laparoscopic surgery for the treatment of acute appendicitis has increased dramatically over the past decade. At laparoscopy, a significantly higher incidence of complicated appendicitis and other pathology is observed in older adults. These factors lead to a higher conversion rate to open surgery in older patients. There is no difference in infectious related morbidity between younger and older patients undergoing laparoscopic appendectomy; however, older patients experience a higher rate of cardiopulmonary complications. Laparoscopic appendectomy is associated with a higher likelihood of discharge home compared with discharge to a skilled or nonskilled nursing facility and reduced mortality rates compared with open appendectomy.

Despite improvement in diagnosis and management of appendicitis in elderly patients, morbidity and mortality for this group remain high—28% to 60% and 10%, respectively. A delay in diagnosis is thought to be the cause of high morbidity and mortality in many cases, so clinical suspicion should remain high.

Carcinoma of the Colon and Rectum

Colorectal cancer is the third most common type of cancer and second most common cause of cancer-related deaths in the United States. Colorectal cancer is predominantly a disease of aging and is a major cause of morbidity and mortality in the older population. Colorectal cancer incidence is directly associated with increasing age, with most cases affecting older adults; 71% of new cases occur in adults 65 years old and older, and 42% occur in adults 75 years old and older. The annual incidence of colon cancer is almost 40 times higher for individuals older than 85 years compared with individuals 40 to 44 years old. With the aging of the U.S. population, it is projected that the incidence of colorectal cancer will continue to increase.

Increasing age is a poor prognostic factor in colorectal cancer. Patients older than 75 years have a significantly decreased 5-year disease-free survival compared with younger patients. Although differences in colorectal cancer survival could be attributed in part to cancer biology and physiologic function specific to older adults, explicit differences in processes of care have been shown to be responsible for these outcome differences. Specifically, treatment disparities related to diagnosis, surgical care, and adjuvant and neoadjuvant therapies have been identified when comparing younger and older patients.[58]

The presenting signs and symptoms of colorectal cancer depend on the location of the tumor and do not vary substantially with age. Right-sided lesions tend to cause microcytic anemia from occult bleeding, and patients present with fatigue, weakness, syncope, or a fall. Patients with left-sided tumors tend to present with constipation, diarrhea, or a change in stool caliber. However, because fatigue, falls, constipation, and bowel dysfunction are accepted as common sequelae of aging, these symptoms are frequently ignored by the patient and physician, and the diagnosis is often not made until a complication occurs.

Older adults, regardless of the number of comorbidities they have, are less likely to receive screening for colorectal cancer. As a result, older patients are more likely to present with more advanced disease than younger patients. In addition, the proportion of unstaged cancers increases with advancing age. The U.S. Preventive Services Task Force recommends screening for colorectal cancer in adults beginning at age 50 years and continuing until age 75 years for individuals with average risk. Recommendations for screening include annual fecal occult blood testing and flexible sigmoidoscopy every 5 years, with full colonoscopy for positive occult blood or adenomatous polyps on flexible sigmoidoscopy, or colonoscopy every 5 to 10 years. Because older patients have an increased incidence of right-sided cancers and because more than 50% of patients with right-sided cancers have no lesions within reach of the flexible sigmoidoscope, colonoscopy may be a more effective screening tool in older patients. Colorectal cancer screening is not advised for older adults unlikely to live 5 years or for older adults who have significant comorbid medical conditions precluding treatment. Screening trials indicate that a difference in colorectal cancer mortality between screened and unscreened persons does not become noticeable until at least 5 years after screening. Therefore, persons with a life expectancy of 5 years or less are not likely to benefit from screening but are at risk for complications from procedures and the treatment of clinically unimportant disease.

Surgical resection is the only curative treatment for resectable colorectal cancer, regardless of the patient's age. For tumors of the abdominal colon, prohibitive anesthetic risk secondary to severe comorbidity and the presence of advanced metastatic disease are the only factors that should negatively influence the decision for surgery. There has been some concern about the ability of older patients to tolerate resection of low rectal cancers, including abdominoperineal resection, low anterior resection, and sphincter-saving coloanal anastomosis. Although technically more demanding than traditional abdominoperineal resection, coloanal anastomosis provides a sphincter-saving alternative that is well tolerated by older adults in terms of operative mortality and postoperative complications, and several studies have shown that the long-term results are comparable in highly selected patients. Both procedures are equally effective for cure provided that there is at least a 2-cm distal resection margin. Coloanal reconstruction can achieve continence in almost 80% of older individuals. Assessment of anal function is crucial in patient selection for low rectal anastomosis because many of these patients have poor functional results after sphincter-preserving surgery. Fecal incontinence may result in a worse quality of life than a well-controlled end-sigmoid colostomy, and it is important for physicians to talk about these risks with their patients.

Several randomized studies comparing laparoscopic colectomy with open colectomy have been completed; however, older patients are underrepresented. Available series data suggest that in elderly patients there is no significant difference between laparoscopic colectomy and open colectomy in perioperative mortality rates, need for blood transfusion, or incidence of reoperation and that elderly patients may benefit more from the minimally invasive approach than younger patients. Cardiopulmonary morbidity appears to be lower in older patients undergoing a minimally invasive approach to resection of colorectal cancer. Gastrointestinal and respiratory recovery are quicker after laparoscopic colectomy, and patients report less pain, require less narcotic analgesia, experience a shorter hospital stay, and are more likely to return to independent status after laparoscopic colectomy. Adequacy of oncologic clearance is equivalent in both treatment groups.

For patients with significant comorbidities and early-stage cancers, local excision of low-lying rectal cancers may be an option. Although the local recurrence rate is significantly higher for local excision, overall 5-year survival is similar. For frail older or high-risk patients, lesser procedures, including transanal excision and fulguration, can provide local control of the tumor without disrupting continence. Local control of rectal tumors with chemoradiation is also possible to control pain and bleeding in poor-risk patients with metastatic disease and a short life expectancy. The use of colonic stents to palliate poor surgical candidates with impending obstruction should be considered when technically feasible.

Operative mortality for colorectal cancer in older patients is determined by the same two factors that influence operative mortality in older adults in general—the presence of coexisting disease and the need for emergency surgery. In patients with few or no comorbidities, operative mortality is similar regardless of age. Even in patients older than 80 years, elective operative mortality rates are only approximately 2%. However, because of the issues described, older patients are more likely to require emergency surgery than younger patients. Patients with colorectal cancer who are 85 years old are twice as likely to need emergency surgery as patients 65 years old. In addition, with advancing age, a decreasing proportion of patients undergo curative resection at the time of surgery. When surgery is performed as an emergency, mortality increases threefold to fourfold over elective mortality for similar procedures. Length of hospital stays and hospital costs also increase. In addition, patients who survive emergent operations are only half as likely to return to independent living as patients after elective emergency surgery.

Long-term survival after a diagnosis of colorectal cancer in older adults is disproportionately poor compared with younger patients. Methodology taking into account competing causes of death established that older patients die more frequently from colorectal cancer, over and above expected age-related rates of death. In older patients with colon and rectal cancers, the 5-year mortality after surgical resection is 1.5 to 2.5 times greater than for younger patients. The poorer survival seen in older patients with colorectal cancer may be a result of the reduced use of adjuvant therapy in this group. Despite the fact that most patients with colorectal cancer are older than 70 years, only 20% of patients in randomized trials are older than 70 years. The efficacy and tolerance of adjuvant chemotherapy for colon cancer and neoadjuvant chemoradiotherapy for rectal cancer in older patients have been demonstrated; however, less than 30% of patients older

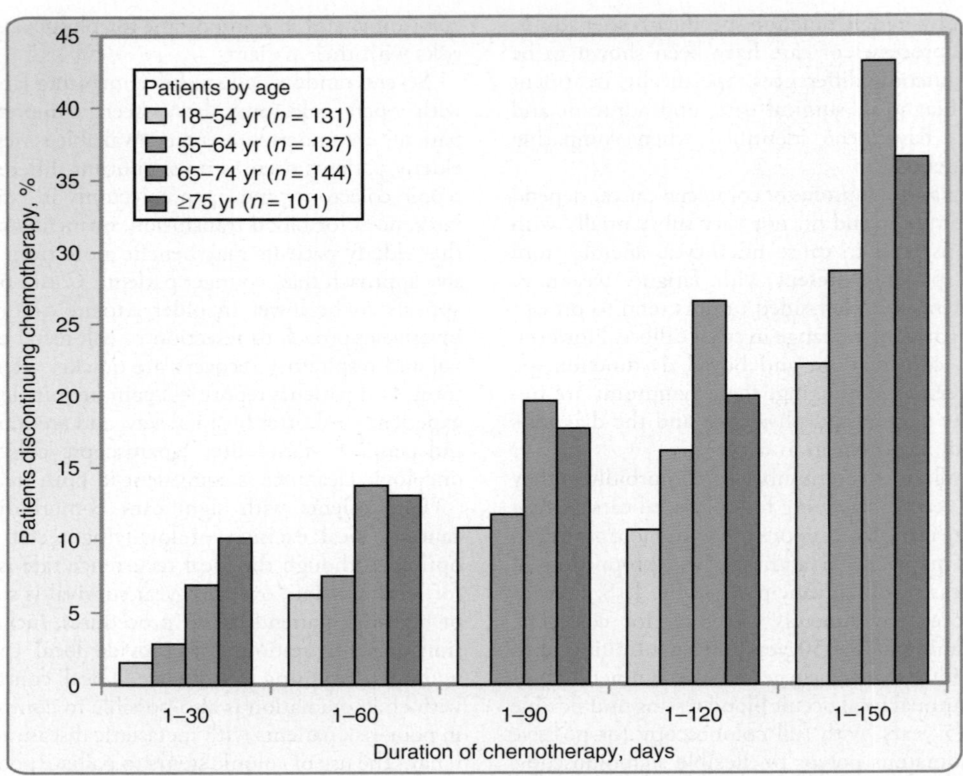

FIGURE 13-12 Cumulative proportion of patients discontinuing chemotherapy by age. (From Kahn KL, Adams JL, Weeks JC, et al: Adjuvant chemotherapy use and adverse events among older patients with stage III colon cancer. *JAMA* 303:1037–1045, 2010.)

than 75 receive adjuvant therapy. Moreover, of patients who do receive adjuvant therapy, more than 50% do not receive the appropriate therapy for the recommended duration (Fig. 13-12).[58]

Surgical therapy of colorectal liver metastasis is being used with increasing frequency. Resection of metastatic lesions is associated with improved survival and operative morbidity, and mortality has been declining; however, older patients are poorly represented in studies evaluating liver resection for colorectal cancer liver metastasis. Inaccurate provider perceptions of high postoperative mortality and concerns about lack of oncologic benefit may contribute to this pattern. Although there are some physiologic changes in liver function with increasing age, these changes are not usually sufficient to influence the outcome of liver resection. Mortality rates after liver resection in older adults are less than 5%. Older adults derive a significant benefit from a surgical approach to colorectal liver metastases and have reasonable morbidity and mortality. The 5-year survival after resection has been reported to be 32% compared with 10.5% in patients not undergoing hepatectomy.[59]

Abdominal Wall Hernia

Repair of abdominal wall hernia is the most common surgical procedure in the United States. The lifetime risk for inguinal hernia is 27% for men and 3% for women, with about 27% performed in adults older than 65 years. More than 750,000 inguinal hernias are repaired every year in the United States with a bimodal distribution. Most develop for the first time in patients younger than 1 year and in patients 55 to 85 years old. The estimated incidence of abdominal wall hernia in persons older than 65 years is 13/1000, with a fourfold to eightfold higher incidence in men than in women. In patients older than 70 years, 65% of all hernias are inguinal, 20% are femoral, 10% are ventral, 3% are umbilical, and 1% are esophageal hiatal. Although most groin hernias occur in men, 80% of femoral hernias occur in women. Older adults are also at risk for the more occult types of hernias, such as paraesophageal hernias and obturator hernias that do not become apparent until a complication has occurred.

Hernias pose some additional challenges in older adults. For example, they are often long-standing, and many have been present for more than 10 years. As a result of the chronic nature of these hernias, often the normal anatomy is distorted, and there is loss of tissue planes. In addition, loss of tissue strength many make an anatomic repair more difficult. Even with these challenges, symptomatic groin and umbilical hernias in older adults should preferentially be repaired electively. Open, tension-free mesh repair of inguinal, femoral, and umbilical hernias can be performed as an outpatient procedure under epidural or local anesthesia with IV sedation. Mortality rates are low, even in patients with concomitant medical disease, and many reports have demonstrated mortality rates of 0%. Laparoscopic repair requires a general anesthetic in most cases, takes more operative time to complete, and incurs greater hospital costs. In older adults, the decreased economic benefit to society of an earlier return to normal activities and work seems to obviate the overall cost benefit of the laparoscopic operation. The trend in most centers is for laparoscopic repair to be restricted to bilateral and recurrent inguinal hernias, for which the results are excellent.

The issue of watchful waiting instead of immediate repair of asymptomatic and mildly symptomatic hernia in older adults is controversial. Although authors of some randomized studies have favored watchful waiting, others have suggested that repair may improve general health and decrease possible serious morbidity. Most studies agree that the risk of incarceration of asymptomatic hernias is small. One consideration that is most important in the decision to choose watchful waiting over repair is how the presence of the hernia might limit the activities of the aging individual. Maintenance of function and mobility is an important predictor of long-term survival and quality of life in older persons. In a follow-up to one randomized trial that initially showed watchful waiting was safe, family members were surveyed about the ability of the hernia patient to perform four activities—normal activities around the home, normal work activities, social activities, and recreational activities.[60] Of family members in the watchful waiting group, 25% to 30% reported some level of concern about the patient's ability to perform these activities. It was suggested these results favor repair.

Approximately 15% to 30% of hernia repairs for older adults are performed on an emergent basis. Incarceration, if it occurs, can be catastrophic, particularly for frail older patients. This complication is mainly the result of the high incidence of strangulation found at the time of surgery. Intestinal resection is required in 12% to 20% of incarcerated inguinal hernias and 40% of incarcerated femoral hernias. The decision to operate for asymptomatic or mildly symptomatic hernias is made on an individual basis by balancing the possible consequences of watchful waiting with the risks of the surgery. It should be determined by seeking input from the family whether the patient has limited his or her activities to avoid mild discomfort. Decreased activity presents more of a risk to the overall health of most older persons than the operative risk associated with inguinal hernia repair.

Incisional hernias in older adults are common and may be challenging to repair. In contrast to laparoscopic inguinal hernia repair, there is a clear benefit to using this technique as long as preexisting comorbidities and technical difficulty do not preclude the use of laparoscopic techniques. Studies have shown decreased wound complications and length of stay in the laparoscopic groups.

Vascular Surgery

The most frequent peripheral vascular diseases seen in older patients are abdominal aortic aneurysms (AAAs), carotid artery disease, and peripheral arterial occlusive disease. Under elective conditions and in patients with well-managed concomitant disease, vascular surgery is safe and effective; in many cases, endovascular technology is changing patterns of intervention.

Abdominal Aortic Aneurysm

Mortality from elective AAA repair is generally considered to be less than 5% in patients 65 years old and older, despite the high incidence of comorbidities in this age group. However, more recent evidence has called into question the effects of age on the outcome of AAA repair. On the basis of several studies, it has been shown that there is a strong effect of age on mortality; men 85 years old and older have almost five times the perioperative mortality rate of younger men, and women 85 years old and older have greater than 10 times the mortality rate of younger women. Similarly, 5-year mortality after AAA repair in older men and women is approximately 80% to 90% compared with 25% to 30% in younger patients. Octogenarians are more difficult to treat by endovascular aneurysm repair (EVAR) than younger patients because of poorer anatomic suitability and a higher incidence of complications. Recovery of quality of life in octogenarians takes longer (>12 months) than expected.[61] As EVAR has become more prevalent, experience with open AAA repair is diminishing, with concomitant increased mortality and morbidity associated with open surgery. In older patients, complications occur in approximately one third of open AAA repairs with infrarenal clamping and in more than 50% of repairs with suprarenal clamping. Also, suprarenal clamping is associated with increases in 30-day mortality, renal insufficiency, intraoperative blood loss, hospital length of stay, and rate of discharge to a nursing home. These results suggest that open AAA repair is becoming even less appropriate for most older patients, especially as the mean age of "older" patients increases.

In a prospective randomized trial, the Veterans Affairs Cooperative Study Group compared EVAR with open repair in 881 patients with asymptomatic AAA. The previously reported reduction in perioperative mortality with EVAR was sustained at 2 years and at 3 years but not thereafter. There were 10 aneurysm-related deaths in the EVAR group (2.3%) versus 16 in the open repair group (3.7%) (P = .22). Six aneurysm ruptures were confirmed in the EVAR group versus none in the open repair group (P = .03). A significant interaction was observed between age and type of treatment (P = .006); survival was increased among patients younger than 70 years old in the EVAR group, but tended to be better among patients 70 years old or older in the open repair group (Fig. 13-13).[62] The true usefulness of EVAR may be with the repair of ruptured AAA. Emergency open repair for rupture is still associated with an operative mortality rate higher than 50% and an extremely high morbidity rate in patients who do survive. However, reports of EVAR for ruptured aneurysms with reduced mortality are encouraging. A more recent collective review of worldwide experience with more than 1700 patients with ruptured aneurysms showed in experienced centers a 30-day mortality rate of 19.7% in patients treated with EVAR compared with 36.3% in patients treated with open repair. In addition, the outcome of ruptured AAA might be improved by wider use of local anesthesia for EVAR.[63] It is probable that the durability of stent grafts will increase over time, suggesting that EVAR is likely to be appropriate for older patients with suitable anatomy for repair. Future directions involve fenestrated grafts for juxtarenal and pararenal aneurysms, which will extend the seal zone to include the superior mesenteric and celiac arteries.

Carotid Artery Disease

Treatment of carotid disease for the prevention of stroke is a common issue for older patients. In patients older than 65 to 80 years, the stroke rate from surgery is approximately 2.8%, and the mortality rate is 2.4%. Survival of patients older than 80 years after carotid endarterectomy is similar to the general population. The incidence of neurologic symptoms after endarterectomy is lower than in an unoperated patient (13% versus 33%), and the incidence of late stroke is much lower (2% versus 17%), confirming the efficacy of endarterectomy in older patients. Suitable indications in octogenarians are similar to indications in younger patients and include high-grade carotid lesions and hemispheric symptoms with well-controlled concomitant disease. The development of carotid artery angioplasty and stenting was originally thought to be a breakthrough, minimally invasive treatment for carotid disease with wide applicability.[64] Among elderly patients with symptomatic or asymptomatic carotid stenosis, the risk of the composite primary outcome of stroke, myocardial infarction, or death did not differ significantly in the group undergoing carotid artery angioplasty and stenting and the group undergoing

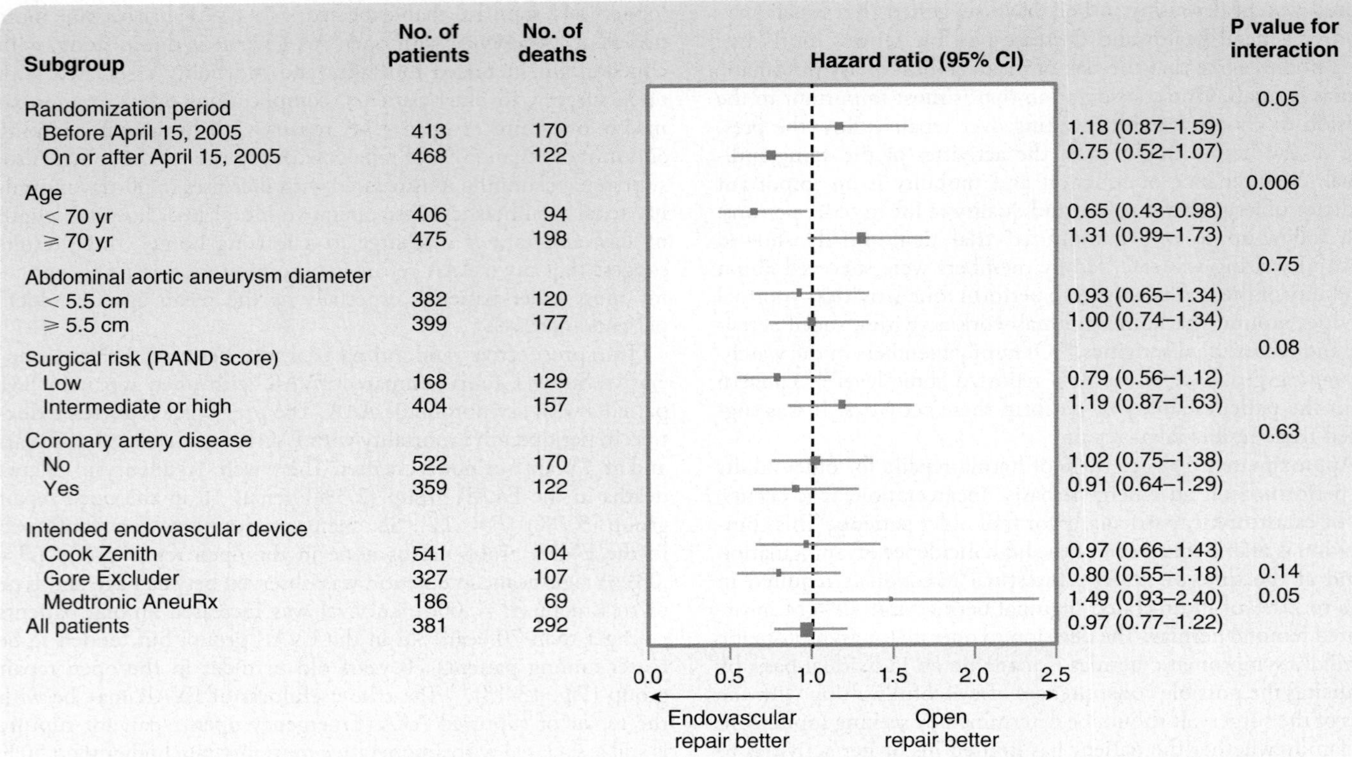

Subgroup
No. of patients
No. of deaths
Hazard ratio (95% CI)
P value for interaction
Randomization period
Before April 15, 2005 413 170 1.18 (0.87–1.59)
On or after April 15, 2005 468 122 0.75 (0.52–1.07)
0.05
Age
< 70 yr 406 94 0.65 (0.43–0.98)
⩾ 70 yr 475 198 1.31 (0.99–1.73)
0.006
Abdominal aortic aneurysm diameter
< 5.5 cm 382 120 0.93 (0.65–1.34)
⩾ 5.5 cm 399 177 1.00 (0.74–1.34)
0.75
Surgical risk (RAND score)
Low 168 129 0.79 (0.56–1.12)
Intermediate or high 404 157 1.19 (0.87–1.63)
0.08
Coronary artery disease
No 522 170 1.02 (0.75–1.38)
Yes 359 122 0.91 (0.64–1.29)
0.63
Intended endovascular device
Cook Zenith 541 104 0.97 (0.66–1.43)
Gore Excluder 327 107 0.80 (0.55–1.18) 0.14
Medtronic AneuRx 186 69 1.49 (0.93–2.40) 0.05
All patients 381 292 0.97 (0.77–1.22)
0.0 0.5 1.0 1.5 2.0 2.5
Endovascular repair better
Open repair better

FIGURE 13-13 Factors predictive of death in endovascular and open repair. (From Lederle FA, Freischlag JA, Kyriakides TC, et al: Long-term comparison of endovascular and open repair of abdominal aortic aneurysm. *N Engl J Med* 367:1988–1997, 2012.)

carotid endarterectomy (Fig. 13-14). During the periprocedural period, there was a higher risk of stroke with stenting and a higher risk of myocardial infarction with endarterectomy.[65] Patients older than 75 years have increased arch calcium deposits and increased arch tortuosity compared with younger patients, suggesting that increased stroke risk is inherent to standard femoral approaches generally used for carotid artery angioplasty and stenting. Age should be considered when planning a carotid intervention. Carotid stenting has an increased risk of adverse cerebrovascular events in elderly patients but mortality equivalent to younger patients. Carotid endarterectomy is associated with similar neurologic outcomes in elderly and young patients, at the expense of increased mortality.[66]

Peripheral Vascular Disease

Peripheral vascular surgery for limb salvage is indicated for ischemic pain at rest, nonhealing ulcers, or frank gangrene. Although reports show that age older than 80 years is a relative risk factor for increased perioperative mortality, surgery generally can be safely performed in older patients, especially when performed electively. In patients older than 80 years, the mortality rate associated with surgery is less than 5%, and limb salvage rates over a period of 3 to 5 years are 50% to almost 90%. The 5-year graft patency rates have been reported to be better in older patients compared with younger patients with prosthetic and autologous graft materials, although the small numbers of patients that have been studied suggests that larger series are needed to validate these single-center reports. Nevertheless, older patients do no worse than younger patients after infrageniculate bypass surgery. Treatment of graft infections in older patients is morbid, although aggressive wound care and muscle flap coverage is an option with good results (>50% graft salvage and 90% limb salvage). Endovascular approaches can also be used in the periphery in older patients, with reasonable durability in patients with limited life expectancy. Angioplasty of the superficial femoral artery has a 5-year cumulative primary patency rate greater than 50% and a secondary patency rate of up to 70% in older patients. It is unclear whether these results will lead to increased treatment of older patients with claudication, as it has in younger patients.[67] In a study of mostly elderly patients, endovascular-first and open-first revascularization strategies had equivalent limb salvage rates and amputation-free survival at 5 years in properly selected patients with critical limb ischemia.[68]

Quality of life and preservation or restoration of functional independence are most important considerations in older patients. Amputation can be performed safely in older patients, with rates of perioperative mortality less than 10%. However, long-term survival after amputation is poor, with 1-year survival rates of approximately 50%; independent risk factors for mortality include high-level amputation, congestive heart failure, and inability to ambulate in the community. These functionally poor results of amputation lead many surgeons to continue to offer an aggressive approach to limb salvage in older patients.

Cardiothoracic Disease

Cardiovascular disease has been the leading cause of death in the United States for almost 100 years. At the present time, approximately 64 million Americans, or 23% of the population, have cardiovascular disease. Most deaths attributable to cardiovascular disease occur in older patients.

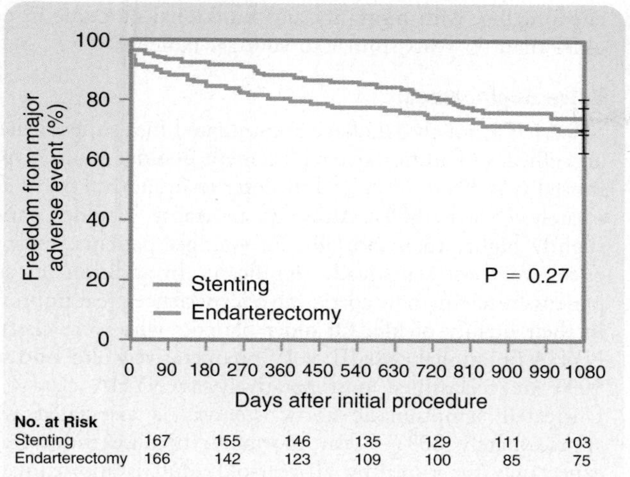

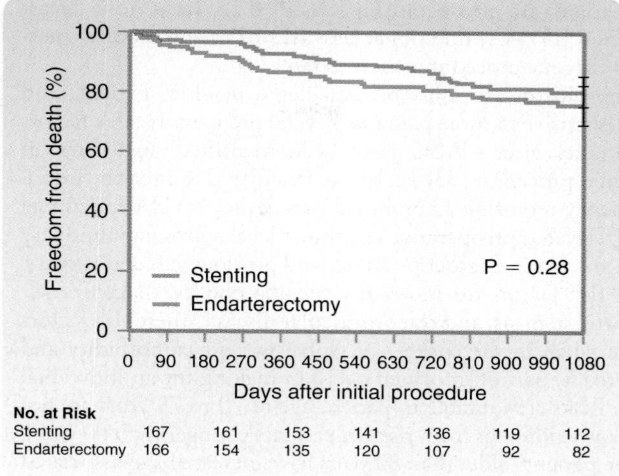

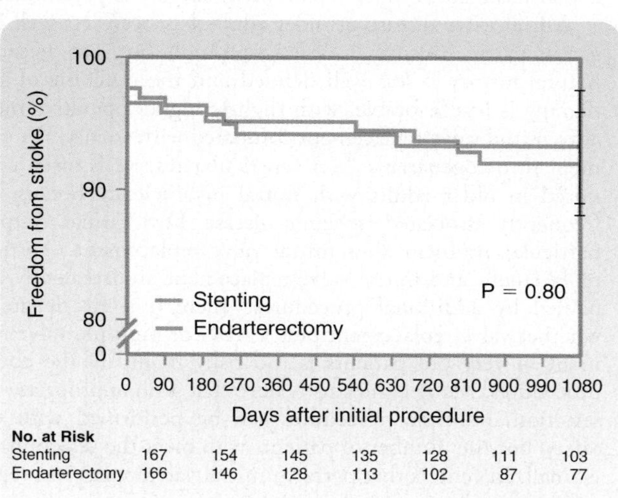

FIGURE 13-14 A-C, Kaplan-Meier curves depicting outcomes of major adverse events, stroke, and death in patients undergoing carotid endarterectomy and carotid stenting. (From Gurm HS, Yadav JS, Fayad P, et al: Long-term results of carotid stenting versus endarterectomy in high-risk patients. *N Engl J Med* 358:1572–1579, 2008.)

Cardiac surgery is usually a dramatic event for patients and is one of the most frequently studied surgical procedures. Older patients have excellent results after cardiac surgery; as minimally invasive treatment of cardiac atherosclerosis changes patterns of referral to cardiac surgeons, patients are becoming older, with more frequent and severe comorbid conditions. Nevertheless, the uniformly good results with coronary artery bypass grafting and valve replacement have encouraged the continued performance of cardiac surgery, even in marginal candidates. Mortality in nonagenarians is approximately 14%, but 5-year survival is approximately 59%.[69] Factors associated with excellent outcome in older patients include technically flawless surgery, meticulous hemostasis, excellent myocardial protection, and perfect anesthesia management.

Coronary Artery Disease

The number of CABG procedures performed on patients older than 65 years increased from 2.6 operations/1000 in 1980 to 13.0 operations/1000 in 1993. However, with the increasing use and success of percutaneous coronary artery interventions, the rate of CABG in persons older than 65 years decreased to 8.9/1000. This pattern is reflective of the performance of CABG in the general population, increasing from 7.2 cases/1000 discharges in 1988 to 12.2 cases in 1997, decreasing to 9.1 cases in 2003; nevertheless, overall mortality after CABG decreased from 5.4% in 1988 to approximately 3.3% in 2003.

Patients who are now referred for CABG usually have more complex disease or have failed alternative procedures. More than 50% of CABG procedures are now performed on patients older than 65 years. As the mortality and morbidity associated with cardiac surgical procedures have decreased, there has been a growing willingness to offer surgical therapy to older patients with reconstructible coronary artery disease. Older patients referred for cardiac surgery have a higher incidence of advanced disease (e.g., triple-vessel disease, left main or main equivalent disease, poor left ventricular function) and more symptomatic disease (90% of octogenarians are preoperatively classified as New York Heart Association [NYHA] functional class III or IV) and require emergency or urgent procedures more often.

Comorbid disease must be considered in older patients and may be extensive in some patients. Several preoperative risk factors for mortality after CABG have been identified, including an emergency procedure, severe left ventricular dysfunction, mitral insufficiency requiring a combined procedure, NYHA functional class IV, elevated preoperative creatinine level, chronic pulmonary disease, anemia (hematocrit <34%), and previous vascular surgery. Further risk factors for morbidity include obesity, diabetes mellitus, aortic stenosis, and cerebrovascular disease. These risk factors must be taken in the context of global patient comorbidity and considered as part of informed decision making for an individual patient. Risks attributable to patient age of 70 to 79 years are not significantly different from risks in patients younger than 60 years; however, patients older than 80 years have increased age-associated risk, equivalent to the presence of shock or acute (<6 hours) myocardial infarction.

In patients older than 80 years, CABG is associated with an acceptable overall mortality of 7% to 12%, with mortality after elective procedures less than 3%. Nonagenarians have a perioperative mortality of approximately 15% to 20% but a 5-year postoperative survival of approximately 50%, which represents a significant survival benefit associated with surgery. Early elective surgery is preferable to emergency surgery, which is associated with 2 to 10 times higher mortality. With persistent reluctance to offer elective operations to many older patients, some series report a significant percentage—40%—of older patients requiring urgent or emergency operations.

In elderly patients undergoing percutaneous coronary intervention (PCI), major adverse coronary event rates are relatively high, but successful revascularization is associated with a reduction in these outcomes at 5-year follow-up.[70] When examining the outcomes of elderly patients treated with drug-eluting stents, the rates of 1-year all-cause death were nearly four times higher in octogenarians than in nonoctogenarians. However, the rates of 1-year recurrent myocardial infarction, target vessel revascularization, and CABG are similar.[71]

Morbidity after coronary surgery in older patients is high in many series. Pulmonary failure requiring prolonged intubation, neurologic events such as cerebrovascular accidents and delirium, and sternal wound infections increase with age and are associated with postoperative mortality. Other complications, including reoperation for bleeding, need for pacemaker insertion, perioperative myocardial infarction, and superficial wound infections, occur with equal frequency in younger and older patients, although some studies have noted a slightly higher incidence of sternal wound infection in older patients.

In a study comparing CABG with PCI, 304 consecutive patients 80 years old or older with uncomplicated left main coronary artery stenosis treated with PCI or CABG were selected and analyzed in a large multinational registry. During hospitalization, a trend toward a higher mortality rate was reported in patients treated with PCI. The incidence of target vessel revascularization at follow-up was higher in patients treated with PCI. After adjustment with propensity score, the revascularization strategy was not significantly correlated to the rate of mortality.[72] Older patients with end-stage heart failure have traditionally been excluded from the option of cardiac transplantation because of the scarcity of donor hearts and an inability to tolerate pharmacologic immunosuppression easily. Reports of partial left ventriculectomy are encouraging, with mortality and functional outcome in patients older than 65 years similar to younger patients.

Valve Replacement

Since 1975, much data have accumulated that support the safety and efficacy of aortic valve replacement in older adults. Operative mortality is 3% to 10%, and the long-term survival rate is approximately 75% to 80%. Although mortality in older patients is slightly higher than mortality in younger patients, most differences were not statistically significant. In addition, most older patients receiving new aortic valves experience great improvement in their quality of life. Of older patients who were classified as NYHA functional class III or IV preoperatively and who survive, 90% are reclassified postoperatively as NYHA class I or II. Untreated symptomatic aortic stenosis is associated with an approximately 80% 4-year mortality; because the average life expectancy for a healthy 70-year-old adult is approximately 13 years and life expectancy for an 80-year-old adult is approximately 8 years, safe aortic valve replacement surgery is preferable.

Mitral valve disease in older adults has been less well investigated, partly because it is less common but also because the natural history is less well defined and the outcome of surgical therapy is less favorable, with slightly higher operative mortality after mitral valve replacement compared with aortic valve replacement in octogenarians. Left ventricular reserve is often compromised in older adults with mitral insufficiency because of the frequently associated ischemic disease. Low cardiac output is a particular problem after mitral valve replacement. Aortic valve replacement and mitral valve replacement are frequently accompanied by additional procedures. There is some debate about whether valve replacement plus CABG or multiple valve replacement in very old patients is too risky to justify the combined procedures. Many clinicians believe that with appropriate patient selection, multiple procedures can be performed with relative safety, but the number of patients who meet the selection criteria is small. In centers that perform mitral valvuloplasty to repair the valve in patients with low ejection fractions, results in older patients are similar to results in younger patients.

The choice of valve material is also an important consideration in older patients. Mechanical valves are extremely durable but require lifelong anticoagulation. In patients older than 75 years, the mortality from long-term anticoagulation alone is almost 10% per year. Bioprosthetic valves are less durable but do not require anticoagulation and may suffice for patients with a life expectancy of less than 10 years.

As experience with minimally invasive procedures increases, it is likely that these procedures will become safer and will be used with increased frequency in older patients. Early clinical trials confirm the safety and efficacy of percutaneous aortic valves, especially in elderly patients requiring aortic valve replacement.[73] In addition, percutaneous catheter–based methods for mitral valvular pathology for valve repair have been developed and have been proposed as an alternative measure in high-risk and elderly patients.

Lung Cancer

Lung cancer, usually adenocarcinoma or squamous cell carcinoma, is a leading cause of death in industrialized countries; more than 150,000 deaths are caused by lung cancer in the United States annually. Smoking is the most important risk factor for lung cancer, and smoking cessation is an appropriate preventive measure for all patients. Appropriate therapy depends on accurate staging, and CT and ^{18}F-fluorodeoxyglucose positron emission tomography play diagnostic roles.

The incidence of non–small cell lung cancer (NSCLC) increases with age. Thus, the more recent recommendations of the American Association of Thoracic Surgery Task Force for Lung Cancer Screening and Surveillance differed from recommendations of other professional societies in two particular areas: an increase in the age of the screened population to age 79 years and an annual scan schedule that extends beyond a 3-year start.[74] There is still bias that older patients with early-stage (I to III) NSCLC do poorly with surgical resection, and these patients are often referred for limited resection or radiation therapy. Aggressive chemotherapy, particularly platinum-based adjuvant therapy, is often poorly tolerated by older patients. Studies comprising elderly patients and patients with mainly stage IB to IIIA showed that preoperative chemotherapy significantly improves overall survival, time to distant recurrence, and recurrence-free survival in resectable NSCLC. The findings suggest this is a valid treatment option for most of these patients. Toxic effects could not be assessed in the study.[75] Many older patients have less than a full staging workup, incomplete histologic diagnoses, or undocumented performance status. Stage IV disease is initially diagnosed in most patients with NSCLC, and they may be treated with combined chemotherapy and radiation therapy. However, older patients are not often considered candidates for this therapy. The use of single-agent (oral etoposide) chemotherapy is not recommended in this population based on inferior survival compared with multidrug IV treatment. Likewise, dose attenuation of the standard cisplatin/etoposide regimen was associated with poorer outcome. There is a significant interaction of poor performance status with age, favoring cisplatin-based treatment in younger patients (≤70 years old) and carboplatin-based treatment in older patients. Neoadjuvant therapy is generally prescribed in older patients who are borderline candidates for surgery, would benefit from tumor downstaging, or would best be treated definitively by radiation therapy.

Evidence has suggested improved outcomes in older patients after surgical treatment of lung cancer.[76] Surgical resection for lung cancer is associated with an operative mortality rate of approximately 6%, although approximately 50% of patients still experience some postoperative morbidity, such as atrial fibrillation, pneumonia, or retained secretions requiring bronchoscopy. The 5-year survival in older patients after pulmonary resection for cancer is approximately 35%, with 40% survival in patients undergoing lobectomy only. Video-assisted thoracic surgery (VATS) is finding increased application, with some surgeons performing VATS for lung cancer resection. The potential for less operating time and blood loss as well as shorter hospital length of stay and improved recovery time, holds great promise for all patients, especially older adults. Perioperative mortality rate for octogenarians treated with VATS is 2%. VATS is associated with a similar 5-year survival rate compared with conventional open surgery. Advanced age is associated with more complications but only marginally worse survival. Results such as these suggest that VATS may increase the number of older patients who would be candidates for surgical therapy. In a review of retrospective series, lobectomy emerged as the surgical treatment of choice for carefully selected, operable octogenarians with early-stage lung cancer. The reported 5-year survival for stage I NSCLC was 56% and increased to 62% for stage Ia.

Future reports are likely to define combinations of adjuvant and neoadjuvant therapy as well as analyze oncologic genomic signatures to increase the number of older patients who would be surgical candidates and achieve disease-free survival. However, the outlook for older patients with preexisting pulmonary disease or other severe comorbid conditions remains poor.

Trauma

Trauma is currently the fifth leading cause of death in older adults. People older than 65 years account for one third of trauma cases and 30% to 40% of trauma deaths, with more recent rates being the highest. Older patients have increased mortality, longer hospital stays, increased morbidity, and worse functional outcomes than younger patients. Motor vehicle accidents are the most common form of fatal injury in patients younger than 80 years, and falls are the most frequent fatal injury after the age of 80. The incidence of death from motor vehicle accidents in older adults is the same whether they are passengers or pedestrians.

Older adults are at increased risk for blunt trauma and its complications. Age-associated central nervous system changes decrease coordination and mobility and increase the risk for accidents. Cerebral atrophy and decreased viscoelastic properties within the cranial vault make the brain more susceptible to blunt injury. Increased bone fragility results in an increased tendency for fracture. Decreased cardiac reserve and inability to increase cardiac output prevent avoidance of accidents. Concomitant use of drugs such as anticoagulants and antiplatelet agents increases the morbidity associated with traumatic events in older patients.

Significant injury can result from simple falls from a level surface to the ground. The incidence of fracture or serious injury from such a fall is 40% in an older adult. Significant morbidity is associated with a fall that results in injury. Of patients hospitalized after a fall, 50% need to be discharged from the hospital to a nursing facility, and only 50% are alive 1 year later. Elevator injuries in older patients are most commonly a slip, trip, or fall but are associated with hospital admission in 15% of cases; 40% of these admissions are for a fractured hip.

Older patients have increased morbidity and mortality after head trauma, particularly when taking anticoagulant medications. Older people have increased rates of traumatic brain injury after head trauma and have longer disability. They take much longer to recover from head trauma than younger people and require more intensive rehabilitation. Blunt head trauma in an older person carries a particularly high mortality. Mortality in older patients with a Glasgow Coma Scale score of 5 is more than twice that of patients 20 to 40 years old; only 2% of older patients have a favorable recovery compared with 38% of younger patients.

Injury from burns accounts for 8% of trauma in older patients. Older adults are at particular risk for burns because of impaired vision, decreased reaction time, depressed alertness, and decreased sensation of pain. In most older burn victims, injuries occur as a result of actions during ADL—scalding, cooking accidents with flame, and electrical burns. In all patients, survival from burns is directly related to the total body surface area affected, but this association is more pronounced in older adults. In general, burns involving more than 40% of the total body surface area in older persons have a poor prognosis. Reasons for increased mortality are concomitant medical disease, burn wound sepsis, and multisystem failure, including pneumonia. Among survivors of serious burns who are 59 years old or older, less than 50% are discharged to independent living, one third are discharged to assisted living at home, and 20% are discharged to nursing facilities.

Older patients, whether they live with relatives or are institutionalized, are at risk for trauma as a result of elder abuse. It is estimated that 5% of older adults living in the community are subject to this type of maltreatment. It has also been shown that only 1 in 13 or 14 cases of elder abuse is reported. Maltreatment of older people can take one or more of six basic forms: physical abuse, sexual abuse, neglect, psychological abuse, financial exploitation, and violation of rights. As the older adult population increases, surgeons treating older trauma victims must learn to detect and report signs of physical and sexual abuse in addition to providing physical care of the patient's injuries, much as they have been mandated to do with children.[77]

Transplantation

In 1946, the first successful renal transplantation was performed. Early results with cadaveric renal transplants in patients older than 45 years were poor. The introduction of cyclosporine in the 1980s led to dramatic improvements, particularly in high-risk patients. As experience at transplantation centers has grown and the population older than 60 years has increased, the number of older patients who could potentially benefit from transplantation has also increased. Over the past 2 decades, the number of persons older than 65 requiring renal replacement therapy in the United States has doubled and the number of persons older than 75 years has tripled.

There is proven benefit of renal transplantation for elderly patients; however, this benefit may be compromised because of difficulties in access to transplant. In one study of renal transplantation, patients older than 60 years had more delayed graft function and a longer initial hospital stay, but the incidence of acute rejection episodes was lower.[78] Patient survival, graft survival, and death-censored graft survival did not differ between older and younger patients, although follow-up of older patients was shorter (4.1 years versus 6.7 years). The main cause of organ loss in older patients was death with a functioning kidney. Other studies showed that 10-year allograft survival was higher in older patients than in patients younger than 60 years. However, the survival rate at 10 years in patients older than 60 was 44% versus 81% for younger patients. Given the shortage of organ donors, the ethics of transplantation in older individuals with a higher likelihood of dying with a functioning allograft is questioned, although many believe that the evidence does not justify denying transplantation on the basis of age alone. Consideration of factors such as physical and cognitive function and frailty in addition to comorbidity may enhance the process of evaluation for transplant in geriatric patients. Kidneys with high Kidney Donor Profile Index scores and living donor organs may become the most realistic transplant options for elderly patients in light of amended allocation policy.[78]

The number of older persons requiring liver transplantation has also increased. The percentage of liver recipients older than 65 years increased from 4.9% in 1991 to 6.8% in 2002. Although age has been identified as a risk factor for a poorer outcome after liver transplantation, when patients are in better health (e.g., living at home at the time of transplantation), age is not a factor. Many studies supported liver transplantation in low-risk, properly evaluated older adults.[78] As the number of older transplant patients has increased, one important factor has emerged: The rate of acute and chronic rejection is lower in older patients. The lower rate of rejection has been attributed to the overall decline in immunocompetence with age. However, this decline also renders older patients more susceptible to infection and malignancy. The high incidence of lymphoproliferative disorders in older transplant patients in general and the high rate of recurrent hepatitis C in older liver transplant patients in particular may be the result of excessive immunosuppression in these already compromised patients. Decreasing immunosuppression in older patients may improve long-term and short-term survival.

SELECTED REFERENCES

1. Fried TR, Bradley EH, Towle VR, et al: Understanding the treatment preferences of seriously ill patients. *N Engl J Med* 346:1061–1066, 2002.

Elderly patients were asked about their preferences for treatment based on the likelihood of and adverse outcome. The authors found that the burden of treatment, its outcomes and the likelihood of outcomes all influence patient treatment preferences. Most patients chose low burden therapy. If patients felt they had a risk of severe cognitive impairment, most would not want to receive the therapy. This work supports the importance of talking with patients about treatment options and outcomes.

2. Finlayson E, Wang L, Landefeld CS, et al: Major abdominal surgery in nursing home residents: A national study. *Ann Surg* 254:921–926, 2011.

Using national Medicare claims data and the nursing home Minimum Data Set nursing home patients were compared to non-nursing home patients. Results show that nursing home residents experience substantially higher rates of mortality and invasive interventions after surgery than other Medicare beneficiaries. These findings should be used to council patients and for physicians to consider in their discussion.

3. Chow W, Rosenthal RA, Merkow RP, et al: Optimal preoperative assessment of the geriatric surgery patient: a best practice guideline from the American College of Surgeons National Surgery Quality Improvement Program and the American Geriatrics Society. *J Am Coll Surg* 215:453–466, 2012.

With the support of the John a Hartford Foundation, the American College of Surgeons-National Surgical Quality Improvement Program (ACS-NSQIP) and the American Geriatrics Society assembled a 21 member expert panel to create a best practice guidelines for the optimal preoperative assessment of the geriatric patient. This guidelines is based on evidence where available and on consensus expert opinion where evidence is not available. It provides a comprehensive checklist and supporting tools to help clinicians perform a thorough evaluation of factors that impact the surgical outcomes of older adults.

4. Lederle FA, Freischlag JA, Kyriakides TC, et al: Long-term comparison of endovascular and open repair of abdominal aortic aneurysm. *N Engl J Med* 367:1988–1997, 2012.

This is a prospective randomized trial of 444 patients assigned to endovascular repair and 437 patients assigned to open repair for abdominal aortic aneurysms. Patients were selected from 42 Veteran Affairs medical centers and were all over 49 years of age. They found that endovascular repair and open repair resulted in similar long-term survival.

The perioperative survival advantage with endovascular repair was sustained for several years, but rupture after repair remained a concern. Endovascular repair led to increased long-term survival among younger patients but not among older patients, for whom a greater benefit from the endovascular approach had been expected.

5. Garg K, Kaszubski PA, Moridzadeh R, et al: Endovascular-first approach is not associated with worse amputation-free survival in appropriately selected patients with critical limb ischemia. *J Vasc Surg* 59:392–399, 2014.

This was a retrospective analysis of patients with critical limb ischemia that were initially revascularized with either an endovascular or open approach. The endo-first was performed in 187 (62%), open-first in 105 (35%), and 10 (3%) had hybrid procedures. The authors showed that at 5 years, the endo-first and open-first revascularization strategies had equivalent limb salvage rates and amputation free survival rates in patients with critical limb ischemia when properly selected. A patient-centered approach with close surveillance improves long-term outcomes for both open and endo approaches.

REFERENCES

1. National Center for Health Statistics: Deaths: Final data for 2013. *Natl Vital Stat Rep* 64:2013.
2. Rowe JW, Committee on the Future Health Care Workforce for Older Americans, Board on Health Care Services: Retooling for an aging America: Building the health care workforce. In Washington, DC, 2008, The National Academies Press, pp xi–xii.
3. Ortman JM, Velkoff VA, Hogan H: *An aging nation: The older population in the United States*, Current Populations Reports, P25–1140. Washington, DC, 2014, U.S. Census Bureau.
4. Bell RH, Jr, Drach GW, Rosenthal RA: Proposed competencies in geriatric patient care for use in assessment for initial and continued board certification of surgical specialists. *J Am Coll Surg* 213:683–690, 2011.
5. Liberman M, Mulder DS, Sampalis JS: Increasing volume of patients at level I trauma centres: Is there a need for triage modification in elderly patients with injuries of low severity? *Can J Surg* 46:446–452, 2003.
6. Kuy S, Sosa JA, Roman SA, et al: Age matters: A study of clinical and economic outcomes following cholecystectomy in elderly Americans. *Am J Surg* 201:789–796, 2011.
7. Kwok AC, Semel ME, Lipsitz SR, et al: The intensity and variation of surgical care at the end of life: A retrospective cohort study. *Lancet* 378:1408–1413, 2011.
8. Barnato AE, Herndon MB, Anthony DL, et al: Are regional variations in end-of-life care intensity explained by patient preferences? A study of the US Medicare population. *Med Care* 45:386–393, 2007.
9. Fried TR, Bradley EH, Towle VR, et al: Understanding the treatment preferences of seriously ill patients. *N Engl J Med* 346:1061–1066, 2002.
10. Mattimore TJ, Wenger NS, Desbiens NA, et al: Surrogate and physician understanding of patients' preferences for living permanently in a nursing home. *J Am Geriatr Soc* 45:818–824, 1997.
11. Detering KM, Hancock AD, Reade MC, et al: The impact of advance care planning on end of life care in elderly patients: Randomised controlled trial. *BMJ* 340:c1345, 2010.
12. Taffett GE: Physiology of aging. In Cassel CK, Leipzig RM, Cohen HJ, et al, editors: *Geriatric medicine: An evidence-based approach*, ed 4, New York, 2003, Springer-Verlag, pp 27–35.
13. Sanders D, Dudley M, Groban L: Diastolic dysfunction, cardiovascular aging, and the anesthesiologist. *Anesthesiol Clin* 27:497–517, 2009.
14. Rubio-Ruiz ME, Perez-Torres I, Soto ME, et al: Aging in blood vessels. Medicinal agents for systemic arterial hypertension in the elderly. *Ageing Res Rev* 18:132–147, 2014.
15. Sharma G, Goodwin J: Effect of aging on respiratory system physiology and immunology. *Clin Interv Aging* 1:253–260, 2006.
16. Lowery EM, Brubaker AL, Kuhlmann E, et al: The aging lung. *Clin Interv Aging* 8:1489–1496, 2013.
17. Bolignano D, Mattace-Raso F, Sijbrands EJ, et al: The aging kidney revisited: A systematic review. *Ageing Res Rev* 14:65–80, 2014.
18. Pequignot R, Belmin J, Chauvelier S, et al: Renal function in older hospital patients is more accurately estimated using the Cockcroft-Gault formula than the modification diet in renal disease formula. *J Am Geriatr Soc* 57:1638–1643, 2009.
19. Schmucker DL: Age-related changes in liver structure and function: Implications for disease? *Exp Gerontol* 40:650–659, 2005.
20. Gruver AL, Hudson LL, Sempowski GD: Immunosenescence of ageing. *J Pathol* 211:144–156, 2007.
21. Chang AM, Halter JB: Aging and insulin secretion. *Am J Physiol Endocrinol Metab* 284:E7–E12, 2003.
22. Finlayson E, Wang L, Landefeld CS, et al: Major abdominal surgery in nursing home residents: A national study. *Ann Surg* 254:921–926, 2011.
23. Bilimoria KY, Liu Y, Paruch JL, et al: Development and evaluation of the universal ACS NSQIP surgical risk calculator: A decision aid and informed consent tool for patients and surgeons. *J Am Coll Surg* 217:833–842.e3, 2013.
24. Anaya DA, Johanning J, Spector SA, et al: Summary of the panel session at the 38th Annual Surgical Symposium of the Association of VA Surgeons: What is the big deal about frailty? *JAMA Surg* 149:1191–1197, 2014.
25. Chow WB, Rosenthal RA, Merkow RP, et al: Optimal preoperative assessment of the geriatric surgical patient: A best practices guideline from the American College of Surgeons National Surgical Quality Improvement Program and the American Geriatrics Society. *J Am Coll Surg* 215:453–466, 2012.
26. Borson S, Scanlan J, Brush M, et al: The mini-cog: A cognitive "vital signs" measure for dementia screening in multilingual elderly. *Int J Geriatr Psychiatry* 15:1021–1027, 2000.
27. Appelbaum PS: Clinical practice. Assessment of patients' competence to consent to treatment. *N Engl J Med* 357:1834–1840, 2007.
28. Li C, Friedman B, Conwell Y, et al: Validity of the Patient Health Questionnaire 2 (PHQ-2) in identifying major depression in older people. *J Am Geriatr Soc* 55:596–602, 2007.
29. Lagoo-Deenadayalan SA, Newell MA, Pofahl WE: Common perioperative complications in older patients. In Rosenthal

RA, Zenilman ME, Katlic MR, editors: *Principles and practice of geriatric surgery*, ed 2, New York, 2011, Springer, pp 361–376.

30. Fleisher LA, Fleischmann KE, Auerbach AD, et al: 2014 ACC/AHA guideline on perioperative cardiovascular evaluation and management of patients undergoing noncardiac surgery: A report of the American College of Cardiology/American Heart Association Task Force on practice guidelines. *J Am Coll Cardiol* 64:e77–e137, 2014.
31. Smetana GW, Lawrence VA, Cornell JE, et al: Preoperative pulmonary risk stratification for noncardiothoracic surgery: Systematic review for the American College of Physicians. *Ann Intern Med* 144:581–595, 2006.
32. Jones TS, Dunn CL, Wu DS, et al: Relationship between asking an older adult about falls and surgical outcomes. *JAMA Surg* 148:1132–1138, 2013.
33. Podsiadlo D, Richardson S: The timed "Up & Go": A test of basic functional mobility for frail elderly persons. *J Am Geriatr Soc* 39:142–148, 1991.
34. Fried LP, Tangen CM, Walston J, et al: Frailty in older adults: Evidence for a phenotype. *J Gerontol A Biol Sci Med Sci* 56:M146–M156, 2001.
35. Robinson TN, Eiseman B, Wallace JI, et al: Redefining geriatric preoperative assessment using frailty, disability and co-morbidity. *Ann Surg* 250:449–455, 2009.
36. D'Alegria B, Cohen C, Medeiros F, et al: Nutritional diagnosis obtained by subjective global assessment in surgical patients and occurrence of postoperative complications. *Nutr Hosp* 23:621, 2008.
37. American Geriatrics Society Beers Criteria Update Expert Panel: American Geriatrics Society updated Beers Criteria for potentially inappropriate medication use in older adults. *J Am Geriatr Soc* 60:616–631, 2012.
38. Naylor MD, Brooten D, Campbell R, et al: Comprehensive discharge planning and home follow-up of hospitalized elders: A randomized clinical trial. *JAMA* 281:613–620, 1999.
39. Robinson TN, Raeburn CD, Tran ZV, et al: Postoperative delirium in the elderly: Risk factors and outcomes. *Ann Surg* 249:173–178, 2009.
40. Marcantonio ER, Goldman L, Mangione CM, et al: A clinical prediction rule for delirium after elective noncardiac surgery. *JAMA* 271:134–139, 1994.
41. Wei LA, Fearing MA, Sternberg EJ, et al: The Confusion Assessment Method: A systematic review of current usage. *J Am Geriatr Soc* 56:823–830, 2008.
42. Kozlow JH, Berenholtz SM, Garrett E, et al: Epidemiology and impact of aspiration pneumonia in patients undergoing surgery in Maryland, 1999-2000. *Crit Care Med* 31:1930–1937, 2003.
43. Kleinpell RM, Fletcher K, Jennings BM: Reducing functional decline in hospitalized elderly. In Hughes RG, editor: *Patient safety and quality: An evidence-based handbook for nurses*, AHRQ Publication No. 08-0043, Rockville, MD, 2008, Agency for Healthcare Research and Quality, pp 251–265.
44. Siegel R, Ma J, Zou Z, et al: Cancer statistics, 2014. *CA Cancer J Clin* 64:9–29, 2014.
45. American Thyroid Association (ATA) Guidelines Taskforce on Thyroid Nodules and Differentiated Thyroid Cancer, Cooper DS, Doherty GM, et al: Revised American Thyroid Association management guidelines for patients with thyroid nodules and differentiated thyroid cancer. *Thyroid* 19:1167–1214, 2009.
46. Sosa JA, Mehta PJ, Wang TS, et al: A population-based study of outcomes from thyroidectomy in aging Americans: At what cost? *J Am Coll Surg* 206:1097–1105, 2008.
47. Bilezikian JP, Khan AA, Potts JT, Jr, et al: Guidelines for the management of asymptomatic primary hyperparathyroidism: Summary statement from the third international workshop. *J Clin Endocrinol Metab* 94:335–339, 2009.
48. Morris LF, Zelada J, Wu B, et al: Parathyroid surgery in the elderly. *Oncologist* 15:1273–1284, 2010.
49. Schonberg MA, Hamel MB, Davis RB, et al: Development and evaluation of a decision aid on mammography screening for women 75 years and older. *JAMA Intern Med* 174:417–424, 2014.
50. Biganzoli L, Wildiers H, Oakman C, et al: Management of elderly patients with breast cancer: Updated recommendations of the International Society of Geriatric Oncology (SIOG) and European Society of Breast Cancer Specialists (EUSOMA). *Lancet Oncol* 13:e148–e160, 2012.
51. Salles N: Basic mechanisms of the aging gastrointestinal tract. *Dig Dis* 25:112–117, 2007.
52. Saif MW, Makrilia N, Zalonis A, et al: Gastric cancer in the elderly: An overview. *Eur J Surg Oncol* 36:709–717, 2010.
53. Kuy S, Sosa JA, Roman SA, et al: Age matters: A study of clinical and economic outcomes following cholecystectomy in elderly Americans. *Am J Surg* 201:789–796, 2011.
54. Riall TS, Zhang D, Townsend CM, Jr, et al: Failure to perform cholecystectomy for acute cholecystitis in elderly patients is associated with increased morbidity, mortality, and cost. *J Am Coll Surg* 210:668–669, 2010.
55. Foster NM, McGory ML, Zingmond DS, et al: Small bowel obstruction: A population-based appraisal. *J Am Coll Surg* 203:170–176, 2006.
56. Sheu BF, Chiu TF, Chen JC, et al: Risk factors associated with perforated appendicitis in elderly patients presenting with signs and symptoms of acute appendicitis. *Aust N Z J Surg* 77:662–666, 2007.
57. Pooler BD, Lawrence EM, Pickhardt PJ: MDCT for suspected appendicitis in the elderly: Diagnostic performance and patient outcome. *Emerg Radiol* 19:27–33, 2012.
58. Kahn KL, Adams JL, Weeks JC, et al: Adjuvant chemotherapy use and adverse events among older patients with stage III colon cancer. *JAMA* 303:1037–1045, 2010.
59. Anaya DA, Becker NS, Abraham NS: Global graying, colorectal cancer and liver metastasis: New implications for surgical management. *Crit Rev Oncol Hematol* 77:100–108, 2011.
60. Gibbs JO, Giobbie-Hurder A, Edelman P, et al: Does delay of hernia repair in minimally symptomatic men burden the patient's family? *J Am Coll Surg* 205:409–412, 2007.
61. Pol RA, Zeebregts CJ, van Sterkenburg SM, et al: Outcome and quality of life after endovascular abdominal aortic aneurysm repair in octogenarians. *J Vasc Surg* 60:308–317, 2014.
62. Lederle FA, Freischlag JA, Kyriakides TC, et al: Long-term comparison of endovascular and open repair of abdominal aortic aneurysm. *N Engl J Med* 367:1988–1997, 2012.
63. IMPROVE trial investigators, Powell JT, Hinchliffe RJ, et al: Observations from the IMPROVE trial concerning the clinical care of patients with ruptured abdominal aortic aneurysm. *Br J Surg* 101:216–224, discussion 224, 2014.

64. Gurm HS, Yadav JS, Fayad P, et al: Long-term results of carotid stenting versus endarterectomy in high-risk patients. *N Engl J Med* 358:1572–1579, 2008.
65. Brott TG, Hobson RW, 2nd, Howard G, et al: Stenting versus endarterectomy for treatment of carotid-artery stenosis. *N Engl J Med* 363:11–23, 2010.
66. Antoniou GA, Georgiadis GS, Georgakarakos EI, et al: Meta-analysis and meta-regression analysis of outcomes of carotid endarterectomy and stenting in the elderly. *JAMA Surg* 148:1140–1152, 2013.
67. Malas MB, Enwerem N, Qazi U, et al: Comparison of surgical bypass with angioplasty and stenting of superficial femoral artery disease. *J Vasc Surg* 59:129–135, 2014.
68. Garg K, Kaszubski PA, Moridzadeh R, et al: Endovascular-first approach is not associated with worse amputation-free survival in appropriately selected patients with critical limb ischemia. *J Vasc Surg* 59:392–399, 2014.
69. Speziale G, Nasso G, Barattoni MC, et al: Operative and middle-term results of cardiac surgery in nonagenarians: A bridge toward routine practice. *Circulation* 121:208–213, 2010.
70. Hoebers LP, Claessen BE, Dangas GD, et al: Long-term clinical outcomes after percutaneous coronary intervention for chronic total occlusions in elderly patients (≥75 years): Five-year outcomes from a 1,791 patient multi-national registry. *Catheter Cardiovasc Interv* 82:85–92, 2013.
71. Yamanaka F, Jeong MH, Saito S, et al: Comparison of clinical outcomes between octogenarians and non-octogenarians with acute myocardial infarction in the drug-eluting stent era: Analysis of the Korean Acute Myocardial Infarction Registry. *J Cardiol* 62:210–216, 2013.
72. Conrotto F, Scacciatella P, D'Ascenzo F, et al: Long-term outcomes of percutaneous coronary interventions or coronary artery bypass grafting for left main coronary artery disease in octogenarians (from a Drug-Eluting stent for LefT main Artery registry substudy). *Am J Cardiol* 113:2007–2012, 2014.
73. Shrestha M, Folliguet TA, Pfeiffer S, et al: Aortic valve replacement and concomitant procedures with the Perceval valve: Results of European trials. *Ann Thorac Surg* 98:1294–1300, 2014.
74. Jaklitsch MT, Jacobson FL: Age limits and frequency of negative scans: When should lung cancer screening end? *J Surg Oncol* 108:301–303, 2013.
75. NSCLC Meta-analysis Collaborative Group: Preoperative chemotherapy for non-small-cell lung cancer: A systematic review and meta-analysis of individual participant data. *Lancet* 383:1561–1571, 2014.
76. Dominguez-Ventura A, Allen MS, Cassivi SD, et al: Lung cancer in octogenarians: Factors affecting morbidity and mortality after pulmonary resection. *Ann Thorac Surg* 82:1175–1179, 2006.
77. Kwan E, Straus SE: Assessment and management of falls in older people. *Can Med Assoc J* 186:E610–E621, 2014.
78. Tso PL: Access to renal transplantation for the elderly in the face of new allocation policy: A review of contemporary perspectives on "older" issues. *Transplant Rev (Orlando)* 28:6–14, 2014.

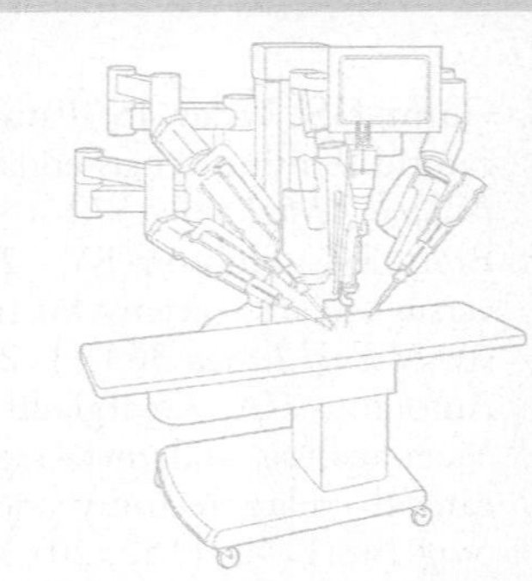

Anesthesiology Principles, Pain Management, and Conscious Sedation

Antonio Hernandez, Edward R. Sherwood

OUTLINE

The relatively brief history of anesthesiology began only a little more than 150 years ago with administration of the first ether anesthetic. Throughout much of the subsequent history, the risk of anesthesia-related mortality and morbidity was unacceptably high as a consequence of primitive equipment, complication-prone drugs, and lack of adequate monitors. However, during the past 4 decades, rapid technologic and pharmacologic progress has resulted in the ability to provide anesthesia safely for complex surgical procedures, even in patients with severe underlying disease.

The most notable advances in anesthesia equipment have been the development of anesthetic machines that reduce the possibility of providing hypoxic gas mixtures, vaporizers that provide accurate doses of potent inhalational agents, and intraoperative anesthesia ventilators that provide more precise and sophisticated respiratory support. Pharmacologic advances have generally consisted of shorter acting drugs with fewer important side effects. However, the greatest advances have been in monitoring devices. These include in-circuit oxygen analyzers, capnometers to assess the presence of exhaled carbon dioxide (CO_2), pulse oximeters, and anesthetic vapor–specific analyzers. Although these monitors do not guarantee a successful outcome, they markedly increase its probability. This chapter first sets the stage for discussing anesthetic management by reviewing the unique aspects of the anesthetic environment: the drugs, equipment, and monitors that are the basis for safe practice. Subsequent sections address preanesthetic assessment and preparation for anesthesia, selection of anesthetic techniques and drugs, airway management, conscious sedation, postanesthetic care, and management of acute postoperative pain.

PHARMACOLOGIC PRINCIPLES

The initial practice of anesthesiology used single drugs such as ether or chloroform to abolish consciousness, prevent movement during surgery, ensure amnesia, and provide analgesia. In contrast, current anesthesia practice combines multiple agents, often including regional techniques, to achieve specific end points. Although inhalational agents remain the core of modern anesthetic combinations, most anesthesiologists initiate anesthesia with intravenous (IV) induction agents and maintain anesthesia with inhalational agents supplemented by IV opioids and muscle relaxants. Benzodiazepines are often added to induce anxiolysis and amnesia. In many cases, total intravenous anesthesia (TIVA) is desirable and is executed through administration of anesthetics such as propofol in combination with opioids and other adjuncts.

Inhalational Agents

The original inhalational anesthetics—ether, nitrous oxide, and chloroform—had important limitations. Ether was characterized by notoriously slow induction and equally delayed emergence but could produce unconsciousness, amnesia, analgesia, and lack of movement without the addition of other agents. In contrast, induction and emergence were rapid with nitrous oxide, but the agent lacked sufficient potency to be used alone. Nevertheless, nitrous oxide is still used in combination with other agents in modern practice. Chloroform was associated with hepatic toxicity and occasionally fatal cardiac arrhythmias.

Subsequent drug development emphasized inhalational agents that facilitate rapid induction and emergence and are nontoxic; these agents include isoflurane, sevoflurane, and desflurane. Although halothane and enflurane were also commonly used in the past, the use of both agents has decreased dramatically more recently. The important aspects of each volatile anesthetic can be summarized in terms of key clinical attributes (Table 14-1). Two of the most important characteristics of inhalational anesthetics are the blood/gas (B/G) solubility coefficient and the minimum alveolar concentration (MAC). The B/G solubility coefficient is a measure of the uptake of an agent by blood. In general, less soluble agents (lower B/G solubility coefficients), such as nitrous oxide and desflurane, are associated with more rapid induction of and emergence from anesthesia, whereas induction and emergence are slower with agents having high solubility in blood, such as

TABLE 14-1 Important Characteristics of Inhalational Agents

ANESTHETIC	POTENCY	SPEED OF INDUCTION AND EMERGENCE	SUITABILITY FOR INHALATIONAL INDUCTION	SENSITIZATION TO CATECHOLAMINES	METABOLIZED (%)
Nitrous oxide	Weak	Fast	Insufficient alone	None	Minimal
Diethyl ether	Potent	Very slow	Suitable	None	10
Halothane	Potent	Medium	Suitable	High	≥20
Enflurane	Potent	Medium	Not suitable	Medium	<10
Isoflurane	Potent	Medium	Not suitable	Minimal	<2
Sevoflurane	Potent	Rapid	Suitable	Minimal	<5
Desflurane	Potent	Rapid	Not suitable	Minimal	0.02

halothane. Isoflurane and sevoflurane have intermediate rates of induction and emergence. MAC is the concentration of agent required to prevent movement in response to a skin incision in 50% of patients and is a way of describing the potency of a volatile anesthetic. A higher MAC represents a less potent volatile anesthetic. Among volatile agents, halothane is the most potent with a MAC of 0.75%; desflurane has a MAC of 6% and is the least potent of the hydrocarbon-based volatile agents. Nitrous oxide has a MAC of 104% at sea level, meaning that nitrous oxide alone is generally not suitable for maintenance of general anesthesia. The pungency of anesthetic agents also has practical implications. Agents with low pungency, such as halothane and sevoflurane, do not cause significant airway irritation when delivered at commonly used concentrations and are useful for inhalation induction of anesthesia. Desflurane is highly irritating to the airways and is not useful for inhalation induction under most conditions.

Nitrous Oxide

Nitrous oxide provides only partial anesthesia at atmospheric pressure because its MAC is 104% of inspired gas at sea level. Nitrous oxide minimally influences respiration and hemodynamics. In addition, it has low solubility in blood. Therefore, it is often combined with a potent volatile agent to permit a lower dose of the potent volatile agent, limiting side effects, reducing cost, and facilitating rapid induction and emergence. The most important clinical problem with nitrous oxide is that it is 30 times more soluble than nitrogen and diffuses into closed gas spaces faster than nitrogen diffuses out, increasing gas volume and pressure within the closed space. Because of this characteristic, nitrous oxide is contraindicated in the presence of closed gas spaces such as pneumothorax, small bowel obstruction, or middle ear surgery, as well as in retinal surgery, in which an intraocular gas bubble is created. Because nitrous oxide gradually accumulates in the pneumoperitoneum, some clinicians avoid its use during laparoscopic procedures. However, periodic venting can prevent gas accumulation.[1]

The ENIGMA trial, reported in 2007, indicated that patients having major surgical procedures lasting more than 2 hours had a higher incidence of postoperative complications and severe postoperative nausea and vomiting (PONV) if they received 70% nitrous oxide as part of their anesthetic regimen compared with patients randomly assigned to not receive nitrous oxide.[2] However, the more recent ENIGMA II trial, published in 2014, reported that use of nitrous oxide was not associated with an increased incidence of death, cardiovascular complications, or wound infection in high-risk surgical patients. Although the incidence of severe PONV was higher (15% versus 11%) in patients receiving nitrous oxide compared with controls, the occurrence of PONV in the nitrous oxide group was effectively controlled by antiemetic prophylaxis.[3]

Isoflurane

Approved by the U.S. Food and Drug Administration (FDA) in 1979, isoflurane rapidly replaced halothane as the most commonly used potent inhalational agent. Despite the subsequent release of sevoflurane and desflurane, isoflurane is commonly used in modern operating rooms, at least partly because the cost of the generic compound is much less than that of the newer agents. Isoflurane has several advantages over halothane, including less reduction in cardiac output, less sensitization to the arrhythmogenic effects of catecholamines, and minimal metabolism (Table 14-2; see Table 14-1). However, isoflurane-induced tachycardia, a variable response, can increase myocardial oxygen consumption. Careful observation of the heart rate is necessary when it is used in patients with coronary artery disease (CAD). In concentrations of 1.0 MAC or less, isoflurane causes little increase in cerebral blood flow and intracranial pressure (ICP) and depresses cerebral metabolic activity more than halothane or enflurane does. Its pungent odor virtually precludes its use for inhalational induction.

Sevoflurane

The relatively low blood solubility of sevoflurane facilitates rapid induction and relatively rapid emergence. Sevoflurane is associated with faster emergence than isoflurane, especially in longer cases, although its slightly faster emergence does not result in earlier discharge after outpatient surgery. Sevoflurane is associated with a lower incidence than isoflurane of postoperative somnolence and nausea in the postanesthesia care unit (PACU) and in the first 24 hours after discharge. In contrast to isoflurane, sevoflurane is pleasant to inhale, making it suitable for inhalational induction in children. However, the clinical differences between halothane and sevoflurane are subtle. In premedicated pediatric patients undergoing bilateral myringotomy and tube placement and randomly assigned to receive sevoflurane or halothane, anesthesiologists correctly identified the agent (to which they were blinded) in only 56.6% of cases.

Sevoflurane is clinically suitable for outpatient surgery, mask induction of patients with potentially difficult airways, and maintenance of patients with bronchospastic disease. When sevoflurane, halothane, and isoflurane were compared with thiopental/nitrous oxide anesthesia, all three of the potent agents decreased respiratory resistance in endotracheally intubated nonasthmatics; sevoflurane reduced airway resistance more than halothane or isoflurane.[4] Another advantage of sevoflurane is that cardiovascular side effects are minimal.

TABLE 14-2 Cardiopulmonary Effects of Inhalational Anesthetics

INHALATIONAL AGENT	BLOOD PRESSURE	HEART RATE	CARDIAC OUTPUT	SENSITIZATION TO CATECHOLAMINES	VENTILATORY DEPRESSION	BRONCHODILATION
Nitrous oxide	Little effect	Little effect	Little effect	No	Minimal	No
Halothane	Marked dose-dependent decrease	Moderate decrease	Marked dose-dependent decrease	Marked	Moderate dose-dependent effect	Moderate
Enflurane	Marked dose-dependent decrease	Moderate decrease	Moderate dose-dependent decrease	Moderate	Moderate dose-dependent effect	Minimal
Isoflurane	Moderate dose-dependent decrease	Variable increase	Minimal decrease	Minimal	Marked dose-dependent effect	Moderate
Sevoflurane	Moderate dose-dependent decrease	Little effect	Moderate dose-dependent decrease	Minimal	Moderate dose-dependent effect	Moderate
Desflurane	Minimal decrease	Variable; marked increase with rapid increase in concentration	Minimal decrease	Minimal	Marked dose-dependent effect	Moderate

Considerable metabolic transformation of sevoflurane takes place and results in increases in the serum fluoride ion concentration and, in the presence of soda lime or Baralyme, production of Compound A, a metabolite that is nephrotoxic in experimental animals. However, β-lyase, the enzyme responsible for the formation of Compound A, has 8 to 30 times greater activity in rat kidneys than in human kidney tissue. The toxicity of Compound A in humans appears to be theoretical and not clinically important.

Desflurane

Desflurane is rapidly taken up and eliminated. After anesthesia lasting more than 3 hours, desflurane was associated with more rapid recovery than isoflurane. The most volatile and least potent of the volatile anesthetics, desflurane must be administered through specialized electrically heated vaporizers. However, its pungent odor precludes inhalational induction. In addition, desflurane is associated with tachycardia and hypertension if the concentration is increased too rapidly.

When exposed to dry CO_2 absorbent, desflurane, isoflurane, and enflurane are partially converted to carbon monoxide. Desflurane, enflurane, and isoflurane produce more carbon monoxide than halothane or sevoflurane. Carbon monoxide production is greater with dry CO_2 absorbent, with Baralyme than with soda lime, at higher temperatures, and at higher anesthetic concentrations. Because continued gas flow in an unused machine desiccates the CO_2 absorbent, turning gas flow off in anesthesia machines when they are not in use can reduce carbon monoxide production.

Intravenous Agents

Since the introduction of thiopental, IV agents have become an indispensable component of modern anesthetic practice. IV agents are used primarily for induction of anesthesia and as part of a multidrug combination to produce TIVA.

Induction Agents

Most adult patients and many older children prefer IV induction to inhalational induction. IV induction is rapid, pleasant, and safe for most patients, although there are situations in which IV induction introduces hazards. Although several agents can be used for IV induction of anesthesia, propofol is the most widely used agent in the United States. Other agents include sodium thiopental, ketamine, methohexital, etomidate, and midazolam (Table 14-3).

Propofol is a short-acting induction agent that is associated with smooth, nausea-free emergence. Small doses are also useful for short-term sedation during brief procedures such as retrobulbar or peribulbar eye blocks, and propofol is commonly used as a continuous infusion during TIVA and for sedation during less invasive procedures such as gastrointestinal endoscopy. The primary limitations of propofol are pain on injection and blood pressure reduction. Propofol should be used with caution in patients who may be hypovolemic or who may tolerate hypotension poorly, such as patients with severe CAD.

Propofol produces excellent bronchodilation. In asthmatic patients, 0% of patients who received propofol wheezed at 2 or 5 minutes after intubation versus 45% of patients who received a thiobarbiturate and 26% of patients who received an oxybarbiturate.[5] In nonasthmatic patients, three quarters of whom smoked, airway resistance was less after induction with propofol than after induction with thiopental or etomidate. Evidence indicates that the bronchodilatory effects of propofol and ketamine are mediated through blockade of vagus nerve–mediated cholinergic bronchoconstriction.

Ketamine, which produces a dissociative state of anesthesia, is the only IV induction agent that increases blood pressure and heart rate and decreases bronchomotor tone. Usually associated with increased sympathetic tone, ketamine causes direct cardiac depression that may become evident if given to patients with high preanesthetic sympathetic tone, as in patients in hemorrhagic shock. In markedly reduced doses (15% to 20% of the usual induction dose), ketamine is an appropriate choice for IV induction of severely hypovolemic patients, in whom it causes the least decrease in blood pressure of any of the induction agents. Ketamine is an appropriate agent for IV induction of asthmatic patients because it reduces the increase in bronchomotor tone associated with endotracheal intubation. Among IV induction agents, ketamine also causes the least amount of ventilatory

TABLE 14-3 Clinical Characteristics of Intravenous Induction Agents

IV INDUCTION AGENT	DOSE (MG/KG)	COMMENTS	SIDE EFFECTS	SITUATIONS REQUIRING CAUTION	RELATIVE INDICATIONS
Thiopental	2-5	Inexpensive; slow emergence after high doses	Hypotension	Hypovolemia; compromised cardiac function	Suitable for induction in many patients
Ketamine	1-2	Psychotropic side effects controllable with benzodiazepines; good bronchodilator; potent analgesic at subinduction doses	Hypertension; tachycardia	Coronary disease; severe hypovolemia	Rapid-sequence induction of asthmatics; patients in shock (reduced doses)
Propofol	1-2	Burns on injection; good bronchodilator; associated with low incidence of postoperative nausea and vomiting	Hypotension	CAD; hypovolemia	Induction of outpatients; induction of asthmatics
Etomidate	0.1-0.3	Cardiovascularly stable; burns on injection; spontaneous movement during induction	Adrenal suppression (with continuous infusion)	Hypovolemia	Induction of patients with cardiac contractile dysfunction; induction of patients in shock (reduced doses)
Midazolam	0.15-0.3	Relatively stable hemodynamics; potent amnesia	Synergistic ventilatory depression with opioids	Hypovolemia	Induction of patients with cardiac contractile dysfunction (usually in combination with opioids)

CAD, coronary artery disease; *IV*, intravenous.

depression and loss of airway reflexes. However, because of the induction of copious oropharyngeal secretions, a drying agent such as glycopyrrolate is generally administered with ketamine.

Ketamine can be used as the sole anesthetic for brief, superficial procedures because it produces profound amnesia and somatic analgesia. However, it is less useful for abdominal cases or delicate surgery because it produces no muscular relaxation, does not control visceral pain, and may not completely control patient movement. The potent pain-relieving effects of ketamine have been exploited for preemptive analgesia. In patients in whom ketamine was infused continuously before incision and continued through wound closure, postoperative morphine consumption was significantly lower on postoperative days 1 and 2 compared with patients who did not receive ketamine.[6]

In patients with CAD, ketamine is usually avoided because tachycardia and increased blood pressure may cause myocardial ischemia. In patients with increased ICP (e.g., after traumatic brain injury), ketamine may increase ICP further because it is the only IV agent that increases cerebral blood flow. Another clinically important side effect of ketamine is emergence delirium. In adults and older children, supplemental benzodiazepines or volatile agents are generally effective in preventing emergence delirium.

Etomidate is an imidazole compound that produces minimal hemodynamic changes. Because it preserves blood pressure in most patients, etomidate is often chosen as an alternative for induction of patients with cardiovascular disease or severe hypovolemia. Major drawbacks include burning pain on injection, abnormal muscular movements (myoclonus), and adrenal suppression when given as a prolonged infusion for sedation of critically ill patients.

Induction with thiopental, the oldest IV induction agent, is rapid and pleasant. Although the drug is remarkably well tolerated by a wide variety of patients, it is not commonly used in modern anesthetic practice, and several clinical situations necessitate caution (see Table 14-3). In hypovolemic patients and patients with congestive heart failure, thiopental-induced vasodilation and cardiac depression can lead to severe hypotension unless doses are markedly reduced. In such patients, etomidate or ketamine is an alternative agent. Although thiopental does not directly precipitate bronchospasm, bronchospasm may develop in patients with reactive airway disease in response to the intense airway stimulation produced by endotracheal intubation. Consequently, propofol or ketamine is often chosen as an alternative for induction in patients with reactive airways disease. In the usual doses used for induction of anesthesia, thiopental is associated with rapid emergence because of redistribution of the agent from the brain to peripheral tissues, particularly fat. In higher doses, circulating blood levels increase, and the action of thiopental must be terminated by hepatic metabolism, which eliminates only about 10% per hour.

Midazolam is sometimes used for induction because it usually causes minimal cardiovascular side effects and has a much shorter duration of action than diazepam. Its onset of action is acceptably rapid; even in smaller doses, it induces profound amnesia for painful or anxiety-producing events. Midazolam is frequently selected for induction of patients for cardiovascular surgery. Because midazolam combines powerful anxiolytic and amnesic effects, smaller doses are also commonly used to premedicate anxious patients and as a component of a multidrug anesthetic.

Opioids

Opioids are used in most patients undergoing general anesthesia and are given systemically to a large proportion patients receiving regional or local anesthesia. As a component of a multifaceted anesthetic, opioids produce profound analgesia and minimal cardiac depression. Disadvantages include ventilatory depression and inconsistent hypnosis and amnesia, which usually must be provided by other agents.

There are several reasons for the universal popularity of opioids in anesthetic management. First, they reduce the MAC of potent inhalational agents. For example, fentanyl (3 ng/mL plasma concentration) decreased the MAC of sevoflurane by 59% and reduced MAC_{awake} (the alveolar concentration at which an emerging patient responds to commands) by 24%.[7] Second, they blunt the hypertension and tachycardia associated with manipulations such as endotracheal intubation and surgical incision. Third, they provide analgesia that extends through the early postemergence interval and facilitates smoother awakening from anesthesia. Fourth, in doses 10 to 20 times the analgesic dose, opioids act as complete anesthetics in a high proportion of patients by providing not only analgesia but also hypnosis and amnesia. This characteristic has prompted their use in patients undergoing cardiac surgery, sometimes as sole anesthetic agents and more often as a major component of a multimodal anesthetic. Finally, they are often added to local anesthetic solutions in epidural and intrathecal blocks to improve the quality of analgesia.

Morphine, hydromorphone, and meperidine are inexpensive, intermediate-acting agents that are less commonly used for maintenance of anesthesia than for postoperative analgesia. Fentanyl, a synthetic opioid that is 100 to 150 times more potent than morphine, is commonly used for maintenance of anesthesia because of its shorter duration of action and rapid onset. Newer synthetic, short-acting opioids, including sufentanil and alfentanil, are also used during anesthesia because they are quickly metabolized and excreted. Remifentanil, an opioid metabolized by serum esterases, is particularly short acting. Remifentanil does not accumulate during prolonged infusions and is often used as part of IV anesthetics.

Neuromuscular Blockers

Anesthesia 50 years ago was typically conducted with single potent inhalational agents that produced all the components of general anesthesia, including whatever degree of muscle relaxation was necessary for the conduct of surgery. Among the drawbacks of this approach was the fact that the depth of anesthesia necessary to produce profound muscle relaxation was much deeper than that necessary to provide hypnosis and amnesia. The addition of muscle relaxants afforded the opportunity to deliver only enough of the inhalational and IV agents to achieve hypnosis, amnesia, and analgesia, while still providing satisfactory operating conditions.

The two categories of neuromuscular blockers in clinical use are depolarizing (noncompetitive) and nondepolarizing (competitive) agents. The depolarizing agents exert agonistic effects at the cholinergic receptors of the neuromuscular junction, initially causing contractions evident as fasciculations, followed by an interval of profound relaxation. The nondepolarizing neuromuscular blockers compete for receptor sites with acetylcholine in the neuromuscular junction, with the magnitude of block dependent on the availability of acetylcholine, the concentration of neuromuscular blocker in the neuromuscular junction, and the affinity of the agent for the receptor.

Succinylcholine, the only depolarizing agent still in clinical use, remains popular for endotracheal intubation because of its rapid onset and short duration of action. However, it is associated with serious hazards, including hyperkalemia and malignant hyperthermia, in a small proportion of patients. The drug can be administered in a relatively high dose for intubation because it is rapidly metabolized by plasma pseudocholinesterase except in a small fraction of patients with atypical or absent pseudocholinesterase. Because its duration of action is only 5 minutes, a patient who cannot be successfully intubated can be ventilated by mask for a short time until spontaneous respiration resumes. However, a patient who cannot be ventilated by mask after succinylcholine administration is not likely to resume spontaneous breathing before the onset of life-threatening hypoxemia.[8]

Side effects of succinylcholine include bradycardia, especially in children, and severe, life-threatening hyperkalemia in patients with burns, paraplegia, quadriplegia, and massive trauma. Succinylcholine, alone or when combined with a volatile agent, is also implicated in triggering malignant hyperthermia in susceptible individuals. It is best avoided in patients at risk for malignant hyperthermia, including patients with muscular dystrophy or a family history of malignant hyperthermia. Some anesthesiologists avoid succinylcholine in children because masseter spasm is a common occurrence that may presage malignant hyperthermia, but it is usually a benign effect. Because succinylcholine is a depolarizing agent that causes visible muscle fasciculations, it has been implicated in postoperative muscle pain, which can be reduced by pretreatment with a small, precurarizing dose of a nondepolarizing agent. As a result of the multiple sporadic problems associated with the use of succinylcholine, some anesthesiologists reserve its use only for situations in which an airway must be rapidly secured (i.e., rapid-sequence induction). In other situations, nondepolarizing agents, chosen largely on the basis of their mode of excretion and duration of action, are preferable. For example, cisatracurium is largely metabolized in serum by Hofmann elimination and is suitable for patients with reduced renal function, in whom pancuronium and vecuronium would be unsuitable because they are partially eliminated by the kidneys.

Nondepolarizing relaxants are used when succinylcholine is contraindicated, as an alternative to succinylcholine for patients in whom easy endotracheal intubation is anticipated, and when intraoperative relaxation is required to facilitate surgical exposure. Knowledge of the side effects of individual agents (often related to vagolysis or release of histamine) and routes of metabolism plays a major role in the selection of specific agents for individual cases. Doses required to provide satisfactory operating conditions are summarized in Table 14-4. Dosing of nondepolarizing agents requires knowledge of several important characteristics. First, the use of neuromuscular blockers prevents movement in response to noxious stimuli. Chemical paralysis can mask the signs of inadequate anesthesia (or sedation or analgesia in postoperative patients). Medicolegal claims of intraoperative awareness during general anesthesia were more than twice as frequent in patients receiving intraoperative muscle relaxants.[9] Second, higher doses are required to provide satisfactory conditions for intubation than for surgical relaxation. If a nondepolarizer is used only after intubation, smaller doses are required. Third, other anesthetic drugs potentiate the actions of nondepolarizing agents. Succinylcholine used for intubation decreases subsequent requirements for nondepolarizers. Potent inhalational agents potentiate the effects of competitive neuromuscular blockers in a dose-dependent fashion. The newer inhalational agent desflurane potentiates the effects of vecuronium approximately 20% more than isoflurane. Fourth, individual responses to muscle relaxants vary widely, with patients demonstrating markedly increased and markedly decreased neuromuscular blockade compared with expected levels.

Finally, fifth and most important, subtle blockade can be difficult to detect and can be associated with postoperative complications. The importance of subtle residual paralysis has been quantified by using the train-of-four (TOF) fade ratio, a semiquantitative monitoring technique used to assess the adequacy of neuromuscular blockade and the adequacy of pharmacologic reversal. At the conclusion of anesthesia, a TOF ratio greater than 0.90 has been considered adequate return of neuromuscular function. This ratio means that the fourth of four muscle twitches in response to supramaximal stimuli delivered at 0.5-second intervals to the ulnar nerve is at least 90% of the magnitude of the first twitch. In a 2003 study, at TOF ratios less than 0.90, subjects had

TABLE 14-4 Dose-Response Relationships of Nondepolarizing Neuromuscular Blocking Drugs in Humans

DRUG	DURATION	ED_{50} (MG/KG)	ED_{95} (MG/KG)	INTUBATING DOSE (MG/KG)
Tubocurarine	Long	0.23 (0.16-0.26)	0.48 (0.34-0.56)	0.5-0.6
Pancuronium	Long	0.036 (0.022-0.042)	0.067 (0.059-0.080)	0.08-0.12
Vecuronium	Intermediate	0.027 (0.015-0.031)	0.043 (0.037-0.059)	0.1-0.2
Cisatracurium	Intermediate	0.026 (0.15-0.31)	0.04 (0.32-0.55)	0.15-0.2
Mivacurium	Short	0.039 (0.027-0.052)	0.067 (0.045-0.081)	0.15-0.2
Rocuronium	Intermediate	0.147 (0.069-0.220)	0.305 (0.257-0.521)	0.6-1.0

Modified from Naguib M, Lien CA: Pharmacology of muscle relaxants and their antagonists. In Miller RD, Fleisher LA, Johns RA, et al, editors: *Miller's anesthesia*, ed 6, Philadelphia, 2005, Churchill Livingstone, pp 481–572.
NOTE: ED50 and ED95 values are means (95% confidence limits). Larger doses are required to facilitate endotracheal intubation.
ED_{50}, effective dose for surgical relaxation in 50% of patients; *ED_{95}*, effective dose for surgical relaxation in 95% of patients.

diplopia and difficulty tracking objects in all directions. The ability to strongly oppose the incisors did not return until the TOF ratio was greater than 0.90. The authors concluded that satisfactory return of neuromuscular function requires return of the TOF ratio to greater than 0.90 and ideally to 1.0.[10] In patients who received the intermediate-acting neuromuscular blockers atracurium, vecuronium, or rocuronium only for endotracheal intubation, the TOF ratio was less than 0.9 in 37% of patients 2 hours after receiving the muscle relaxant. More recent studies showed that patients with TOF ratios less than 0.9 had an increased incidence of postoperative respiratory complications and delayed PACU discharge.[11] It is important to optimize return of neuromuscular function at the end of surgery through judicious use of muscle relaxants and reversal agents.

The use of neuromuscular blocking agents in general and nondepolarizing agents in particular necessitates a strategy to ensure adequate muscular function at the conclusion of anesthesia. Many of the complications associated with neuromuscular blockers relate to inadequate reversal at the conclusion of cases or inadequate assessment of reversal. Nondepolarizing relaxants are generally pharmacologically reversed with an anticholinesterase (neostigmine or edrophonium), accompanied by atropine or glycopyrrolate to counteract the muscarinic effects of the anticholinesterase. However, recovery depends on the intensity of neuromuscular blockade at the time that reversal is attempted and on the effects of the reversal agent. At the end of anesthesia, profound neuromuscular blockade may preclude reliable antagonism by an anticholinesterase within 5 to 10 minutes. For those reasons, pancuronium has been largely removed from modern anesthesia practice.

With the longer acting muscle relaxants, residual blockade can potentially complicate postoperative recovery. In a clinical trial of reversal of muscle relaxation, 691 patients undergoing abdominal, gynecologic, or orthopedic surgery under general anesthesia were randomly assigned to receive pancuronium, vecuronium, or atracurium. After reversal with neostigmine, a higher proportion (26%) of patients who had received pancuronium had residual neuromuscular blockade (TOF <70) than patients who had received vecuronium or atracurium (5.3% combined). Patients who received pancuronium and had a TOF ratio less than 0.70 had a higher incidence of atelectasis or pneumonia on postoperative chest radiographs (16.9% of 59 patients in that category). There was no association between postoperative pulmonary complications and residual blockade with the other two muscle relaxants.

One key factor determining recovery from neuromuscular blockade is the ability to metabolize and excrete the drugs. In patients with renal disease, the half-lives of tubocurarine, rocuronium, vecuronium, and pancuronium are prolonged. In such patients, alternative drugs such as cisatracurium, which is metabolized by Hofmann elimination and does not have a prolonged half-life in patients with renal dysfunction, should be considered.

ANESTHESIA EQUIPMENT

Anesthesia equipment has undergone rapid development over the past few decades. The central piece of equipment for delivery of anesthesia is the modern anesthesia machine. The anesthesia machine functions primarily to deliver oxygen and volatile anesthetics to the patient. In addition, modern anesthetic machines have sophisticated ventilators that allow for effective respiratory support and have integrated monitors that accurately measure oxygen delivery, inspired and end-tidal gas concentrations, airway pressures, minute ventilation, and fresh gas flows. Despite many years of improving designs, hazards of gas delivery systems must still be considered. The primary concern is inadvertent delivery of a hypoxic gas mixture. Adverse anesthetic outcomes were associated with gas delivery equipment in 72 of 3791 cases in the American Society of Anesthesiologists (ASA) closed claims database. Misuse of equipment occurred in 75% of incidents, and 78% could have been detected with monitoring of pulse oximetry or capnography. The essential elements of an anesthesia machine are gas sources (oxygen, nitrous oxide, and air), flowmeters, and a flow-proportioning device. In most cases, gases are delivered to the anesthesia machine from a bank of large H cylinders housed in a central area within the hospital. A backup system of E cylinders is attached directly to the anesthesia machine and provides a source of gases, particularly oxygen, if the central gas source becomes unavailable. The flowmeters allow independent administration of individual gases. To minimize the chance of delivering a hypoxic gas mixture, so-called fail-safe valves that require pressurization of the oxygen line before nitrous oxide can be delivered and flow-proportioning devices that automatically reduce the flow of nitrous oxide if the flow of oxygen is reduced below a safe concentration are present. The measurement of inspired oxygen concentration provides a further safeguard against delivering hypoxic gas mixtures.

In addition to the anesthesia machine, the other major components of anesthesia equipment are monitors. The use of monitors to assess changes in respiratory and cardiovascular function during anesthesia and surgery has been instrumental in improving overall safety (Box 14-1).

PATIENT MONITORING DURING AND AFTER ANESTHESIA

Effective monitoring is a crucial aspect of anesthesia care. The essential components of monitoring include observation and vigilance, instrumentation, data analysis, and institution of corrective measures, if indicated. The goal of patient monitoring is to provide optimal anesthetic management and detect abnormalities early in their course so that corrective measures can be instituted before serious or irreversible injury occurs. Although it is difficult to relate improved patient outcomes directly with specific monitors, the reduction in anesthesia-related morbidity and mortality has paralleled the institution of current monitoring practices.

The indications, risks, and benefits associated with the use of noninvasive and invasive electronic monitors must be assessed for each individual patient (see Box 14-1). These decisions are guided by the patient's medical condition, the type of surgery, and the potential complications associated with invasive monitoring. However, the proliferation of electronic monitoring devices does not circumvent the need for clinical skills, such as observation, inspection, auscultation, and palpation. The ASA has established standards for basic anesthetic monitoring that were most recently updated in 2011 (http://www.asahq.org/quality-and-practice-management/standards-and-guidelines). These standards are designed to integrate clinical skills and electronic monitoring with the goal of enhancing patient safety.

Standard I asserts that a qualified anesthesia care provider must be continuously present in the operating room during the administration of anesthesia. The practitioner must continuously monitor the status of the patient and alter anesthesia care based on the patient's response to the dynamic changes associated with anesthesia and surgery.

Standard II mandates continuous assessment of ventilation, oxygenation, circulation, and temperature during all anesthetics. Specific requirements include the following:

1. An oxygen analyzer with a low–oxygen concentration alarm must be used during general anesthesia.
2. Quantitative assessment of blood oxygenation such as by pulse oximetry must be performed.
3. The adequacy of ventilation must be continuously ensured by clinical evaluation. Quantitative monitoring of the CO_2 content in expired gas and the volume of expired gas is strongly recommended.
4. Clinical assessment and monitors to determine the presence of CO_2 in expired gases are required to ensure correct endotracheal tube placement after intubation. A device capable of detecting disconnection of breathing system components during mechanical ventilation must be in continuous use. This device must give an audible signal when its alarm threshold is exceeded.
5. Electrocardiography (ECG) must be continuously monitored during anesthesia, and blood pressure and heart rate must be evaluated at least every 5 minutes. In patients undergoing general anesthesia, adequacy of circulatory function must be continuously monitored by electronic means, palpation, or auscultation.

BOX 14-1 Routine and Specialized Electronic Monitors Used in Anesthetic Practice and Their Indications

Routine Monitors

Pulse oximetry
- Blood oxygen saturation
- Heart rate
- Tissue perfusion (via plethysmography)

Automated blood pressure cuff
- Blood pressure

ECG
- Heart rhythm
- Heart rate
- Monitor of myocardial ischemia

Capnography
- Adequacy of ventilation
- Intratracheal placement of endotracheal tube
- Pulmonary perfusion

Oxygen analyzer
- Monitoring of delivered oxygen concentration

Ventilator pressure monitor
- Ventilator disconnection during general anesthesia
- Monitoring of airway pressure

Temperature monitoring

Specialized Monitors

Monitoring of urine output (Foley catheter)
- Gross indicator of intravascular volume status and renal perfusion

Arterial catheter
- Continuous measurement of arterial blood pressure
- Sampling of arterial blood

Central venous catheter
- Continuous measurement of central venous pressure
- Delivery of centrally acting drugs
- Rapid administration of fluids and blood

Pulmonary artery catheter
- Measurement of pulmonary artery pressure
- Measurement of left ventricular pressure
- Measurement of cardiac output
- Measurement of mixed venous oxygenation

Precordial Doppler
- Detection of air embolism

Transesophageal echocardiography
- Evaluation of myocardial performance
- Assessment of heart valve function
- Assessment of intravascular volume
- Detection of air embolism

Esophageal Doppler
- Assessment of descending aortic blood flow
- Assessment of cardiac preload

Transpulmonary indicator dilution
- Measurement of cardiac output
- Measurement of preload

Esophageal and precordial stethoscope
- Auscultation of breathing and heart sounds

EEG/BIS
- Depth of anesthesia

BIS, bispectral index; *ECG*, electrocardiography; *EEG*, electroencephalography.

6. A means of temperature evaluation must be readily available in the operating room and is used during periods of intended or expected changes in body temperature.

Blood Pressure Monitoring

Blood pressure monitoring is required during all anesthetics. Noninvasive blood pressure monitoring is appropriate for most surgical cases, and most modern operating rooms are equipped with automated oscillometric blood pressure analyzers. Indications for invasive blood pressure monitoring include intraoperative use of deliberate hypotension; continuous blood pressure assessment in patients with significant end-organ damage or during high-risk surgical procedures; anticipation of wide perioperative blood pressure swings; need for multiple blood gas analyses; and inadequacy of noninvasive blood pressure measurements, such as in morbidly obese patients. Several sites for arterial cannulation are available, each with inherent advantages and potential for complications. The radial artery is most commonly cannulated because of its superficial location, relative ease of cannulation, and adequate collateral flow from the ulnar artery in most patients. Other potential sites for percutaneous arterial cannulation include the femoral, brachial, axillary, ulnar, dorsalis pedis, and posterior tibial arteries. Possible complications of intra-arterial monitoring include hematoma, neurologic injury, arterial embolization, limb ischemia, infection, and inadvertent intra-arterial injection of drugs. Intra-arterial catheters are not placed in extremities with potential vascular insufficiency. However, with proper patient selection, the complication rate associated with intra-arterial cannulation is low, and its benefits can be important.

Electrocardiography

ECG monitoring is a standard of care during the administration of anesthesia. Information regarding dysrhythmias and cardiac ischemia can be readily obtained from ECG data. Analysis of ECG tracings is the cornerstone of cardiopulmonary resuscitation protocols.

Ventilation Monitoring

Sedation and opioid administration and the induction of general or regional anesthesia can depress or abolish spontaneous ventilation and necessitate intraoperative ventilatory support. Several means are available to assess the adequacy of ventilation, including physical assessment of chest expansion, auscultation of breath sounds, and evaluation for evidence of upper airway obstruction and stridor. Precordial and esophageal stethoscopes provide continuous input regarding air movement and the development of wheezing. During mechanical ventilation, monitors of airway pressure and minute ventilation alert the anesthesiologist to conditions that can impair ventilation, such as disconnection of the ventilatory circuit, dislodgment of the endotracheal tube, obstruction of the gas delivery system, and changes in airway resistance or compliance or both.

The advent of end-tidal carbon dioxide ($ETCO_2$) monitoring has greatly enhanced the monitoring of ventilation and detection of esophageal intubation. In normal individuals, the difference between $ETCO_2$ and arterial carbon dioxide pressure ($PaCO_2$) is 2 to 5 mm Hg. The gradient between $ETCO_2$ and arterial CO_2 reflects dead space ventilation, which is increased in cases of decreased pulmonary blood flow, such as pulmonary air embolism or thromboembolism and decreased cardiac output. $ETCO_2$ monitoring can also provide important information regarding systemic perfusion. Specifically, $ETCO_2$ decreases during periods of decreased cardiac output and pulmonary perfusion.

Oxygenation Monitoring

Monitoring of fraction of inspired oxygen (FIO_2) and hemoglobin oxygen saturation is a standard of care during all general anesthetics. Modern anesthesia machines are equipped with oxygen analyzers that detect FIO_2. This monitor, in combination with fail-safe devices, low–oxygen delivery alarms, and oxygen ratio monitors, greatly decreases the chance of delivering a hypoxic gas mixture during anesthesia.

Temperature Monitoring

Temperature is monitored in all patients undergoing general anesthesia. The site of measurement depends on the surgical procedure and the physical characteristics of the patient. Esophageal temperature is most commonly measured during general anesthesia. Other sites of temperature monitoring include rectal, cutaneous, tympanic membrane, bladder, nasopharynx, and the pulmonary artery in patients with pulmonary artery catheters. Because of the potential morbidity associated with hypothermia and hyperthermia, it is important to monitor body temperature and institute measures to maintain temperature as close to normal as possible (Box 14-2).

Neuromuscular Blockade Monitoring

Because of variability in sensitivity to and metabolism of neuromuscular blockers among patients, it is essential to monitor neuromuscular function in patients receiving intermediate-acting and long-acting muscle relaxants. The most common sites of monitoring are at the ulnar or orbicularis oculi muscles. The basis of neuromuscular monitoring is assessment of muscle activity after proximal nerve stimulation (see Box 14-2). This evaluation

BOX 14-2 Techniques for Assessing Neuromuscular Blockade

Train-of-Four: Four Successive 200-μSec Stimuli in a 2-Sec Period

Twitch height progressively fades with increasing blockade

- Loss of the fourth twitch indicates 75% receptor blockade
- Loss of the third twitch indicates 80% blockade
- Loss of the second twitch indicates 90% blockade
- Loss of the first twitch indicates 100% blockade
- Clinical relaxation requires 75%-95% blockade

Presence of four twitches without fade suggests adequate reversal of neuromuscular blockade

Double-Burst Stimulation: Two Successive Sets of 50-Hz Bursts (Three Stimuli/Burst) Separated by 750 Msec (Appears as Two Twitches)

Easier to detect fade visually with this technique than with train-of-four

Loss of second twitch indicates 80% receptor blockade

Presence of two twitches without fade suggests adequate reversal of neuromuscular blockade

Tetany: Sustained 50-Hz or 100-Hz Burst

Duration of sustained contraction fades with increasing blockade

Sustained contraction for 5 sec suggests adequate reversal of neuromuscular blockade gives an indication of acetylcholine receptor blockade at the neuromuscular junction. The degree of neuromuscular blockade is indicated by a decreased evoked response to twitch stimulation. As noted earlier in this chapter, it is essential to monitor neuromuscular blockade and to ensure resolution of blockade at the end of anesthesia to minimize the incidence of postoperative complications related to residual neuromuscular blockade.

Central Nervous System Monitoring

Awareness during anesthesia is an uncommon but disturbing complication. Many years of experience with intraoperative electroencephalography signal processing resulted in development of the bispectral index (BIS), which is believed to monitor awareness during anesthesia. The monitor is essentially a modified electroencephalogram that assesses brain wave activity and reports numbers from 0 to 100, which correlate with the level of awareness. A value of 100 represents complete awareness, and 0 represents complete suppression of brain wave activity. Data suggest that BIS is an accurate indicator of the depth of anesthesia.[12] Monitoring the depth of anesthesia may allow for more precise titration of volatile and IV anesthetics and may improve time to awakening and discharge in the outpatient setting. Furthermore, some reports indicate that BIS values of less than 40 for more than 5 minutes during general anesthesia may be associated with increased perioperative morbidity including myocardial infarction and stroke in high-risk patients.[13] A meta-analysis concluded that BIS monitoring can reduce intraoperative awareness in high-risk patients, but it is unclear if the use of BIS monitoring provides advantages in that regard over monitoring end-tidal anesthetic gas concentration in most patients.[14] In addition to intraoperative use, BIS monitors are gaining acceptance as a means of assessing awareness in locations such as emergency departments and intensive care units.

PREOPERATIVE EVALUATION

The ASA has established basic standards for preanesthetic care in which an anesthesiologist is required to evaluate the medical status of the patient, derive a plan for anesthetic care, and discuss the plan with the patient (http://www.asahq.org/quality-and-practice-management/standards-and-guidelines). The Joint Commission requires that all patients receiving anesthesia undergo a preanesthetic evaluation. Because a decreasing percentage of patients are admitted to the hospital on the day before surgery, preoperative testing clinics have been developed to facilitate preoperative evaluation. The advent of preoperative clinics has facilitated efficient use of operating room resources. Ferschl and colleagues[15] reported that development of an anesthesia preoperative evaluation clinic in a teaching hospital reduced day-of-surgery cancellations and delays. Optimally, preoperative clinics need to be efficient, predictable, and thorough. In modern practice, many patients without complicated medical problems who are scheduled for elective, low-risk procedures are interviewed by telephone before surgery and given preoperative instructions.

The anesthesia preoperative evaluation serves multiple purposes. First, the patient has the opportunity to speak to an anesthesiologist and discuss the expected impact of anesthesia, including the patient's fears and concerns regarding anesthesia and postoperative pain management. Second, the preanesthetic interview focuses on the type of surgery, the underlying conditions necessitating surgery, any history of previous anesthetics, and the presence of coexisting diseases. The preoperative interview allows evaluation of the patient's medical status to determine whether additional medical evaluation or treatment is needed before surgery. This process requires a focused history, physical examination, and, if indicated, laboratory evaluation. Current medications must be reviewed to anticipate potential drug interactions and manage medical problems during the perioperative period. Instructions regarding oral intake, changes in medication use, and other important issues that need to be addressed before surgery are communicated to the patient during the preoperative interview.

A well-focused history allows the practitioner to perform targeted physical and laboratory examinations. Laboratory tests performed within 6 months of surgery generally do not need to be repeated unless a significant change in the patient's medical status has occurred. Healthy patients undergoing elective procedures may not need any preoperative laboratory testing. In the current climate of cost containment, preoperative testing must be minimized but effective. The use of routine preoperative testing is associated with significant costs, both in dollars and in potential harm. False-positive tests can cause needless delays in surgery and could require follow-up, which increases costs and could lead to harm or injury associated with further tests and procedures. Studies have shown that routine testing adds to costs but has little impact on patient care. However, targeted testing based on results of the history and physical examination can significantly improve overall patient care. Investigation of conditions associated with increased perioperative morbidity is important for reducing the risks related to anesthesia and surgery. Coexisting conditions that must be carefully evaluated include intravascular volume status; airway abnormalities; cardiovascular disease; pulmonary disease; neurologic disease; renal and hepatic disease; and disorders of nutrition, endocrinology, and metabolism. Preoperative pregnancy testing is controversial. The rationale for performing preoperative pregnancy testing is the potential for spontaneous abortion and birth anomalies associated with surgery and anesthesia. There is no clear evidence to demonstrate an association of anesthetic drugs with the development of fetal anomalies in humans, but animal studies have shown that some anesthetics, such as nitrous oxide, may cause developmental abnormalities. A clear sexual history and documentation of the last menstrual cycle is obtained in women of childbearing age. In ambiguous situations, a preoperative pregnancy test is indicated.

Airway Examination

Assessing the airway is a crucial step in developing an anesthetic plan. Even if regional anesthesia is planned, general anesthesia and the need to maintain a patent airway could be necessary in the event of failed block, surgical needs, or complications. The goal of the airway examination is to identify characteristics that could hinder assisted mask ventilation or tracheal intubation. A history of diseases or conditions that are associated with airway closure or difficult laryngoscopy alerts the practitioner to potential airway difficulties. Review of previous anesthetic records can provide invaluable information regarding previous airway management. The airway examination is completed by systematic inspection of the mouth opening, thyromental distance, neck mobility, and the size of the tongue in relation to the oral cavity (Box 14-3).

The patient is observed in frontal and profile views because many airway abnormalities, such as a receding mandible, are not evident from a frontal view. The size of the tongue in relation to

BOX 14-3 Important Factors in Performing an Airway Examination

Patient History

Previous anesthetic history
Medical history (e.g., history of oropharyngeal mass, pharyngeal disease)
Review of chart to assess prior airway management during previous anesthetics

Physical Examination

Mouth opening (should be 6-8 cm [3-4 fingerbreadths])
Cervical spine mobility
Mallampati classification
Thyromental distance (should be 6-8 cm [3-4 fingerbreadths])
Frontal and profile view
Assessment for disease-associated airway abnormalities
Presence of facial hair

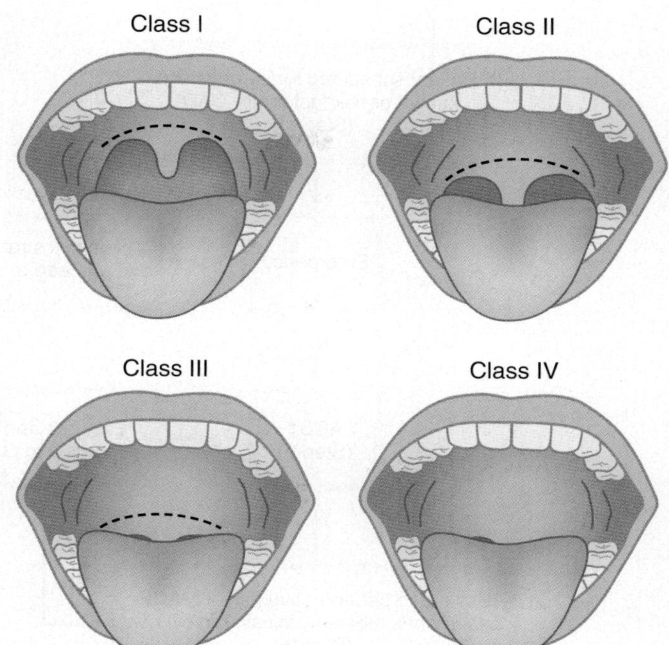

FIGURE 14-1 The Mallampati classification relates tongue size to pharyngeal size. This test is performed with the patient in the sitting position, the head held in a neutral position, the mouth wide open, and the tongue protruding to the maximum. The classification is assigned according to the pharyngeal structures that are visible: class I, visualization of the soft palate, fauces, uvula, anterior and posterior pillars; class II, visualization of the soft palate, fauces, and uvula; class III, visualization of the soft palate and the base of the uvula; and class IV, soft palate not visible at all. (From Mallampati SR, Gatt SP, Gugino LD, et al: A clinical sign to predict difficult tracheal intubation: A prospective study. *Can Anaesth Soc J* 32:429–434, 1985.)

the oral cavity can be graded by using the Mallampati classification (Fig. 14-1). The Mallampati examination is performed with the patient sitting and the head in a neutral position, the mouth opened as wide as possible, and the tongue protruded maximally. The observer views the oral and pharyngeal structures that are evident. In general, patients in whom the uvula, tonsillar pillars, and soft palate are visible (class I) are easy to mask ventilate and intubate. Patients in whom only the hard palate is visible, a class IV airway, have a higher likelihood of being difficult to mask ventilate and intubate. However, the Mallampati classification is only one component of the airway examination and must be used in conjunction with other aspects of the airway examination and the patient's history to provide a complete airway assessment. Other physical factors that are associated with uncomplicated airway management are adequate mouth opening, neck extension, and thyromental distance. In a meta-analysis examining more than 50,000 patients, Shiga and colleagues[16] reported that individual physical characteristics by themselves have poor predictive value for identifying airway difficulties. However, the combined presence of two or more physical characteristics that predict difficult airway management increasingly improves sensitivity and specificity.

Cardiovascular Disease

The risk for perioperative myocardial ischemia and infarction and the risk for cardiac death have become important issues as progressively more complex surgery has been offered to patients with increasingly severe systemic disease. The apparent incidence of perioperative myocardial ischemia depends on the perspective of the study (prospective or retrospective), the sensitivity of the markers used, and the type of surgical procedure. Based on review of the available literature, the American College of Cardiology (ACC) and American Heart Association (AHA) published guidelines for perioperative cardiovascular evaluation and management of patients undergoing noncardiac surgery.[17] The guidelines focus on the patient's history of cardiovascular disease, exercise tolerance, and the type of surgery proposed. A detailed history and physical examination are required to assess the presence of underlying cardiovascular disease. Assessment of functional status and the ability to perform common daily tasks is a critical part of the assessment. Patients with active major cardiovascular conditions require evaluation and treatment before undergoing elective noncardiac surgery. In the 2014 revision of the ACC/AHA guidelines, the committee developed a revised, algorithm-based approach for assessment of cardiovascular risk and determination of the need for perioperative cardiovascular testing.

Functional status is a reliable predictor of perioperative and long-term cardiovascular risk. Patients with poor functional status are at increased risk of cardiovascular events, whereas patients with good exercise tolerance are at lower risk. In the absence of recent exercise testing, a patient's functional status can be assessed based on determination of ability to perform common activities. Functional capacity is commonly expressed in terms of metabolic equivalents (METs), where 1 MET is the resting or basal oxygen consumption of a 40-year-old, 70-kg man. In the perioperative literature, functional capacity is classified as excellent (>10 METs), good (7 to 10 METs), moderate (4 to 6 METs), poor (<4 METs), or unknown. Perioperative cardiac and long-term risks are increased in patients unable to perform 4 METs of work during daily activities. Examples of activities requiring less than 4 METs are slow ballroom dancing, golfing with a cart, playing a musical instrument, and walking at approximately 2 to 3 mph. Examples of activities requiring more than 4 METs are climbing a flight of stairs or walking up a hill, walking on level ground at 4 mph, and performing heavy work around the house. Assessment tools such as the Duke Activity Status Index and the Specific Activity Scale allow for more detailed assessment of functional status. Figure 14-2 provides a framework for determining which patients are candidates for preoperative cardiac testing. The clinician must consider the urgency of surgery, the patient's functional capacity,

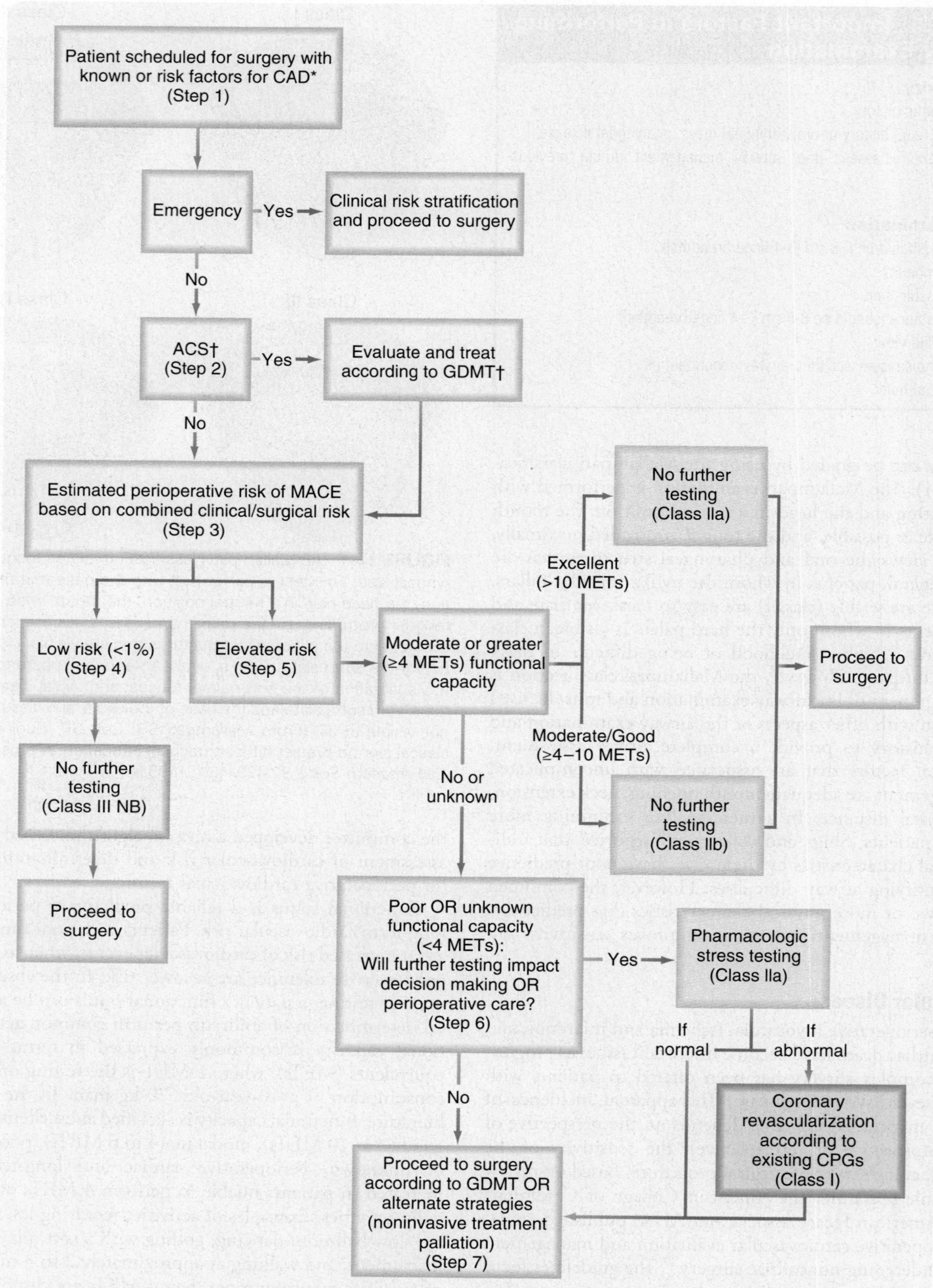

FIGURE 14-2 Stepwise approach to perioperative cardiovascular assessment for patients undergoing noncardiac surgery. The need for preoperative testing is based on the patient's functional status, type of surgery, and urgency of surgery. *ACS,* acute coronary syndrome; *CAD,* coronary artery disease; *CPG,* clinical practice guideline; *GDMT,* goal-directed medical therapy; *MACE,* major adverse cardiac event; *METs,* metabolic equivalents. (From Fleisher LA, Fleischmann KE, Auerbach AD, et al: 2014 ACC/AHA Guideline on Perioperative Cardiovascular Evaluation and Management of Patients Undergoing Noncardiac Surgery: A report of the American College of Cardiology/American Heart Association Task Force on Practice Guidelines. *J Am Coll Cardiol* 64:e77–137, 2014.)

and the type of surgery and give them appropriate weight. Since the publication of the perioperative cardiovascular evaluation guidelines in 2002 and revision in 2007, several new randomized trials and cohort studies have led to modification of the original algorithm. For a detailed overview of the current ACC/AHA Guidelines, clinicians should refer to the most recently published update. The following stepwise approach is recommended:[17]

Step 1: In patients scheduled for surgery with risk factors for or known CAD, heart failure, valvular heart disease, or arrhythmias, determine the urgency of surgery. If an emergency, determine the clinical risk factors that may influence perioperative management and proceed to surgery with appropriate monitoring and management strategies based on the clinical assessment.

Step 2: If the surgery is urgent or elective, determine if the patient has an active coronary syndrome. If yes, refer the patient for cardiology evaluation and management according to guideline-directed medical therapy.

Step 3: If the patient has risk factors for stable CAD, estimate the perioperative risk of a major adverse cardiac event (MACE) on the basis of the combined clinical and surgical risk. This estimate can be determined using the American College of Surgeons National Surgical Quality Improvement Program risk calculator (http://www.surgicalriskcalculator.com) or incorporating the Revised Cardiac Risk Index with an estimation of surgical risk. For example, a patient undergoing very low-risk surgery (e.g., ophthalmologic surgery), even with multiple risk factors, would have a low risk of MACE, whereas a patient undergoing major vascular surgery with few risk factors would have an elevated risk of MACE.

Step 4: If the patient has a low risk of MACE (<1%), no further testing is needed, and the patient may proceed to surgery.

Step 5: If the patient is at elevated risk of MACE, determine functional capacity with an objective measure or scale such as the Duke Activity Status Index. If the patient has moderate, good, or excellent functional capacity (≥4 METs), proceed to surgery without further evaluation.

Step 6: If the patient has poor (<4 METs) or unknown functional capacity, the clinician should consult with the patient and perioperative team to determine whether further testing will have an impact on patient decision making (e.g., decision to perform original surgery or willingness to undergo coronary artery bypass grafting or percutaneous coronary intervention, depending on the results of the test) or perioperative care. If yes, pharmacologic stress testing is appropriate. In patients with unknown functional capacity, exercise stress testing may be reasonable to perform. If the stress test is abnormal, consider coronary angiography and revascularization depending on the extent of the abnormal test. The patient can proceed to surgery with guideline-directed medical therapy, or consider alternative strategies, such as noninvasive treatment of the indication for surgery (e.g., radiation therapy for cancer) or palliation. If the test is normal, proceed to surgery according to guideline-directed medical therapy.

Step 7: If testing would not affect decision making or care, proceed to surgery according to guideline-directed medical therapy or consider alternative strategies, such as noninvasive treatment of the indication for surgery (e.g., radiation therapy for cancer) or palliation.

The need for specific testing depends on the patient's exercise tolerance, comorbidities, and the type of surgery proposed. Box 14-4 defines current recommendations on specific perioperative testing including preoperative ECG, echocardiography, stress testing, radionuclide perfusion scans, and coronary angiography. It is recommended that practitioners refer to the most recent ACC/AHA guidelines for detailed recommendations and level of evidence to support the guidelines.[17]

BOX 14-4 Recommendations for Supplemental Preoperative Evaluation

12-Lead ECG

Preoperative resting 12-lead ECG is reasonable for patients with known coronary heart disease or other significant structural heart disease except for low-risk surgery.

Preoperative resting 12-lead ECG may be considered for asymptomatic patients except for low-risk surgery.

Routine preoperative resting 12-lead ECG is not useful for asymptomatic patients undergoing low-risk surgical procedures.

Assessment of LV Function

It is reasonable for patients with dyspnea of unknown origin to undergo preoperative evaluation of LV function.

It is reasonable for patients with heart failure with worsening dyspnea or other change in clinical status to undergo preoperative evaluation of LV function.

Reassessment of LV function in clinically stable patients may be considered.

Routine preoperative evaluation of LV function is not recommended.

Exercise stress testing for myocardial ischemia and functional capacity.

For patients with elevated risk and excellent functional capacity, it is reasonable to forgo further exercise testing and proceed to surgery.

For patients with elevated risk and unknown functional capacity, it may be reasonable to perform exercise testing to assess for functional capacity if it would change management.

For patients with elevated risk and moderate to good functional capacity, it may be reasonable to forgo further exercise testing and proceed to surgery.

For patients with elevated risk and poor or unknown functional capacity, it may be reasonable to perform exercise testing with cardiac imaging to assess for myocardial ischemia.

Routine screening with noninvasive stress testing is not useful for low-risk noncardiac surgery.

Cardiopulmonary Exercise Testing

Cardiopulmonary exercise testing may be considered for patients undergoing high-risk procedures.

Noninvasive Pharmacologic Stress Testing Before Noncardiac Surgery

It is reasonable for patients at elevated risk for noncardiac surgery with poor functional capacity to undergo either DSE or MPI if it would change management.

Routine screening with noninvasive stress testing is not useful for low-risk noncardiac surgery.

Preoperative Coronary Angiography

Routine preoperative coronary angiography is not recommended.

Adapted from Fleisher LA, Fleischmann KE, Auerbach AD, et al: 2014 ACC/AHA Guideline on Perioperative Cardiovascular Evaluation and Management of Patients Undergoing Noncardiac Surgery: A report of the American College of Cardiology/American Heart Association Task Force on Practice Guidelines. *J Am Coll Cardiol* 64:e77–137, 2014.
DSE, dobutamine stress echocardiography; *ECG,* electrocardiography; *LV,* left ventricular; *MPI,* myocardial perfusion imaging.

Perioperative medical management is guided by the patient's cardiovascular status, the patient's current drug regimen, and the type of surgery proposed. The need for preoperative coronary revascularization is limited to patients who are candidates for emergency or urgent revascularization under any circumstances; this includes patients with unstable angina, active myocardial infarction, or arrhythmias caused by active ischemia. Current evidence does not support elective coronary revascularization to decrease perioperative cardiovascular complications in most patients undergoing noncardiac surgery. It is recommended that surgery be delayed a minimum of 14 days for patients who have undergone angioplasty and 30 days for patients receiving bare metal stents (BMS). In patients receiving drug-eluting stents (DES), current evidence indicates that the risk of stent thrombosis is stabilized at 6 months after DES placement. Although the risk of restenosis is higher with BMS compared with DES, thrombosis is generally not life-threatening in patients receiving BMS and can be treated with repeat angioplasty. In cases where the need for noncardiac surgery is time sensitive, insertion of BMS should be considered. If noncardiac surgery is urgent or an emergency and the risk of bleeding is high, the risks and benefits of coronary revascularization should be weighed, and coronary artery bypass grafting should be considered as a revascularization strategy. Recommendations for management of patients who have undergone recent coronary revascularization are shown in Figure 14-3.

Numerous investigators have assessed the efficacy and safety of beta blockers in the management of cardiovascular disease during the perioperative period. Current studies suggest that beta blockers reduce perioperative myocardial ischemia and may reduce the risk of myocardial infarction and cardiovascular death in high-risk patients. At the present time, the ACC/AHA recommends continuation of beta blocker therapy in patients who are on long-term beta blocker therapy.[17] The use of beta blockers should be considered based on risk stratification and titrated based on clinical

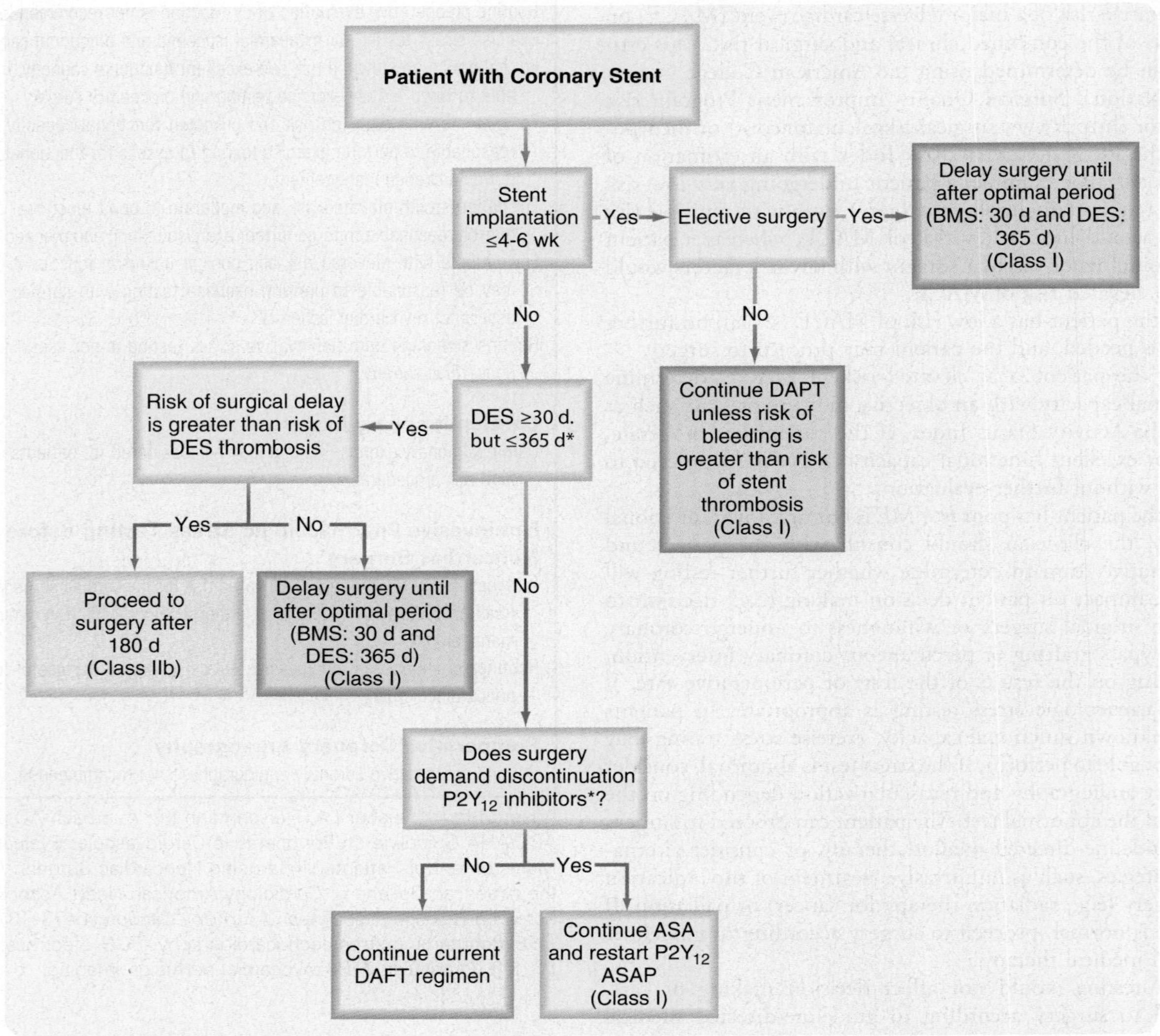

FIGURE 14-3 Stepwise approach to patients who have undergone recent coronary stent placement and present for surgery. *ASA,* acetylsalicylic acid; *ASAP,* as soon as possible; *BMS,* bare metal stent; *DAPT,* dual antiplatelet therapy; *DES,* drug-eluting stent. (From Fleisher LA, Fleischmann KE, Auerbach AD, et al: 2014 ACC/AHA Guideline on Perioperative Cardiovascular Evaluation and Management of Patients Undergoing Noncardiac Surgery: A report of the American College of Cardiology/American Heart Association Task Force on Practice Guidelines. *J Am Coll Cardiol* 64:e77–137, 2014).

circumstances. In beta blocker–naïve patients, perioperative beta blocker therapy should be initiated with caution and based on clinical judgment. Similarly, the perioperative use of calcium channel blockers should be based on patient comorbidities and clinical judgment. Statins should be continued in patients on long-term statin therapy. Perioperative initiation of statin therapy should be considered in patients undergoing vascular surgery and patients at risk for cardiovascular disease who are undergoing high-risk procedures. It is reasonable to continue treatment with angiotensin-converting enzyme inhibitors and angiotensin receptor antagonists during the perioperative period and to reinitiate these agents postoperatively in patients in whom the drugs were withheld preoperatively. The use of α_2 agonists for prevention of cardiac events is not recommended, based on the current literature. An overview of recommendations for perioperative medical management is provided in Box 14-5.[17]

Endocarditis Prophylaxis

Some patients with congenital or valvular heart disease are at increased risk for the development of infective endocarditis (IE). The AHA previously proposed long-standing guidelines that recommended antibiotic prophylaxis for patients at risk for the development of IE who underwent dental, urinary, gastrointestinal, or respiratory surgical procedures. However, the AHA guidelines for endocarditis prophylaxis were changed significantly in 2007.[18] The revised recommendations are based on research that indicates the chance of developing IE is much more likely to result from random bacteremias caused by daily activities such as chewing and toothbrushing rather than as a result of bacteremia generated by dental and surgical procedures. Therefore, antibiotic prophylaxis is not recommended based solely on an increased lifetime risk of developing IE and should be reserved for patients at highest risk (Box 14-6). The AHA panel recommends that antibiotic

BOX 14-5 Recommendations for Perioperative Medical Management

Coronary Revascularization Before Noncardiac Surgery

Revascularization before noncardiac surgery is recommended when indicated by existing clinical practice guidelines.

Coronary revascularization is not recommended before noncardiac surgery exclusively to reduce perioperative cardiac events.

Timing of Elective Noncardiac Surgery in Patients With Previous PCI

Noncardiac surgery should be delayed after PCI—14 days after balloon angioplasty, 30 days after BMS implantation.

Noncardiac surgery should be delayed 365 days after DES implantation.

A consensus decision regarding the relative risks of discontinuation or continuation of antiplatelet therapy can be useful.

Elective noncardiac surgery after DES implantation may be considered after 180 days.

Elective noncardiac surgery should not be performed in patients in whom DAPT would need to be discontinued perioperatively within 30 days after BMS implantation or within 12 mo after DES implantation.

Elective noncardiac surgery should not be performed within 14 days of balloon angioplasty in patients in whom aspirin would need to be discontinued perioperatively.

Perioperative Beta Blocker Therapy

Beta blockers should be continued in patients who are on long-term beta blocker therapy.

Management of beta blockers after surgery should be guided by clinical circumstances.

In patients with intermediate-risk or high-risk preoperative test results, it may be reasonable to begin beta blocker therapy.

In patients with three or more RCRI factors, it may be reasonable to begin beta blockers before surgery.

Initiating beta blockers in the perioperative setting as an approach to reduce perioperative risk is of uncertain benefit in patients with a long-term indication but no other RCRI risk factors.

It may be reasonable to begin perioperative beta blockers long enough in advance to assess safety and tolerability, preferably >1 day before surgery.

Beta blocker therapy should not be started on the day of surgery.

Perioperative Statin Therapy

Statins are continued in patients currently taking statins.

Perioperative initiation of statin use is reasonable in patients undergoing vascular surgery.

Perioperative initiation of statins may be considered in patients with a clinical risk factor who are undergoing elevated-risk procedures.

α_2 Agonists

α_2 Agonists are not recommended for prevention of cardiac events.

ACE Inhibitors

Continuation of ACE inhibitors or ARBs is reasonable perioperatively.

If ACE inhibitors or ARBs are held before surgery, it is reasonable to restart as soon as clinically feasible postoperatively.

Antiplatelet Agents

DAPT is continued in patients undergoing urgent noncardiac surgery during the first 4-6 wk after BMS or DES implantation, unless the risk of bleeding outweighs the benefit of stent thrombosis prevention.

In patients with stents undergoing surgery that requires discontinuation of $P2Y_{12}$ inhibitors, aspirin is continued, and the $P2Y_{12}$ platelet receptor-inhibitor is restarted as soon as possible after surgery.

Management of perioperative antiplatelet therapy should be determined by consensus of the treating clinicians and the patient.

In patients undergoing nonemergency/nonurgent noncardiac surgery without prior coronary stent placement, it may be reasonable to continue aspirin when the risk of increased cardiac events outweighs the risk of increased bleeding.

Initiation or continuation of aspirin is not beneficial in patients undergoing elective noncardiac noncarotid surgery who have not had a previous coronary stent.

Perioperative Management of Patients With CIEDs

Patients with ICDs should be on a cardiac monitor continuously during the entire period of inactivation, and external defibrillation equipment should be available. ICDs must be reprogrammed to active therapy.

Adapted from Fleisher LA, Fleischmann KE, Auerbach AD, et al: 2014 ACC/AHA Guideline on Perioperative Cardiovascular Evaluation and Management of Patients Undergoing Noncardiac Surgery: A report of the American College of Cardiology/American Heart Association Task Force on Practice Guidelines. *J Am Coll Cardiol* 64:e77–137, 2014.

ACE, angiotensin-converting enzyme; *ARB,* angiotensin receptor blocker; *BMS,* bare metal stent; *CIED,* cardiac implantable electronic device; *DAPT,* dual antiplatelet therapy; *DES,* drug-eluting stent; *ICD,* implantable cardioverter-defibrillator; *PCI,* percutaneous coronary intervention; *RCRI,* Revised Cardiac Risk Index.

prophylaxis is reasonable for dental procedures that involve manipulation of gingival tissues, the periapical region of teeth, or perforation of oral mucosa as well as respiratory tract procedures or procedures that manipulate infected skin or musculoskeletal structures in patients at highest risk. Antibiotic prophylaxis solely to prevent IE is not recommended for genitourinary or gastrointestinal tract procedures. For recommended procedures and indications, oral amoxicillin is the drug of choice. Alternative drugs and routes are recommended for patients who are unable to take oral medications or patients with penicillin allergy (Table 14-5).

Pulmonary Disease

Surgical patients often have obstructive or restrictive pulmonary disease. The preoperative history focuses on functional status, exercise tolerance, severity of the disease, and current medications. Recent worsening of symptoms needs to be closely evaluated. A thorough chest physical examination must be performed. Findings on the history and physical examination as well as an understanding of the planned surgical procedure suggest appropriate preoperative testing, which may include chest radiography, arterial blood gas analysis, and pulmonary function testing. The goal of preoperative evaluation is to detect and treat reversible pulmonary pathology, optimize medical management, and allow planning for postoperative ventilatory support, if indicated.

The perioperative risk associated with preexisting pulmonary disease has been extensively studied. Qaseem and coworkers,[19] reviewing preoperative pulmonary evaluation, identified patient-related risk factors; factors related to the surgical site; and other factors related to surgery, such as the duration of surgery, choice of general anesthesia, and intraoperative use of pancuronium (Table 14-6). Major patient-associated risk factors are ASA class greater than II, age older than 60 years, functional dependence, and the presence of chronic obstructive pulmonary disease (COPD) or congestive heart failure. A serum albumin concentration of less than 3.5 g/dL was also a strong predictor of pulmonary complications. Current smoking was a minor predictor of pulmonary complications. The presence of obesity or mild to moderate asthma was not significantly associated with perioperative pulmonary complications.

Obstructive sleep apnea (OSA) is an increasingly common condition in surgical patients that requires preoperative evaluation and optimization. Patients with OSA present significant challenges regarding perioperative decision making. OSA is characterized by periodic upper airway obstruction during sleep resulting in repetitive arousal from sleep to restore airway patency. The condition can result in daytime somnolence, episodic hypoxia and hypercarbia, and cardiovascular dysfunction. Perioperative complications include exaggerated respiratory depression from anesthetics and analgesics, postoperative pulmonary complications, cardiac dysrhythmias, and prolonged hospital stays.[20] The ASA has developed Practice Guidelines for the Perioperative Management of Patients with OSA.[21] The guidelines emphasize the importance of preoperative evaluation and development of protocols to optimize the perioperative care of patients with OSA.

Patients with asthma or COPD should be evaluated preoperatively and optimized before surgery. Assessment should include physical examination and history to assess bronchodilator and steroid use, number and severity of recent respiratory exacerbations, history of previous intubation, and precipitating factors.[22] The approach to preoperative optimization depends on the patient's history and current disease severity and includes use of inhaled β_2 agonists, anticholinergics, and steroids as well as treatment of other existing comorbidities. The choice of anesthetic

BOX 14-6 Cardiac Conditions Associated With Highest Risk of Adverse Outcome from Endocarditis for Which Prophylaxis With Dental Procedures is Reasonable

Prosthetic cardiac valve or prosthetic material used for cardiac valve repair

Previous IE

CHD*

- Unrepaired cyanotic CHD, including palliative shunts and conduits
- Completely repaired congenital heart defect with prosthetic material or device, whether placed by surgery or by catheter intervention, during the first 6 mo after the procedure†
- Repaired CHD with residual defects at the site or adjacent to the site of a prosthetic patch or prosthetic device (which inhibit endothelialization)

Cardiac transplantation recipients who develop cardiac valvulopathy

CHD, congenital heart disease; *IE,* infective endocarditis.
*Except for the conditions listed, antibiotic prophylaxis is no longer recommended for any other form of CHD.
†Prophylaxis is reasonable because endothelialization of prosthetic material occurs within 6 months after the procedure.

TABLE 14-5 Antibiotic Regimens for Dental Procedures

	REGIMEN (SINGLE DOSE ADMINISTERED 30 MIN TO 60 MIN BEFORE THE PROCEDURE)		
SITUATION	AGENT	ADULTS	CHILDREN
Able to take oral medication	Amoxicillin	2 g	50 mg/kg
Unable to take oral medication	Ampicillin	2 g IM or IV	50 mg/kg IM or IV
	Cefazolin or ceftriaxone	1 g IM or IV	50 mg/kg IM or IV
Allergic to penicillin or ampicillin	Cephalexin	2 g	50 mg/kg
	Clindamycin	600 mg	20 mg/kg
	Azithromycin or clarithromycin	500 mg	15 mg/kg
Allergic to penicillin or ampicillin and unable to take oral medication	Cefazolin or ceftriaxone	1 g IM or IV	50 mg/kg IM or IV
	Clindamycin	600 mg IM or IV	20 mg/kg IM or IV

Note: Cephalosporins should not be used in an individual with a history of anaphylaxis, angioedema, or uticaria with penicillins or ampicillin.
IM, Intramuscular; *IV,* intravenous.

TABLE 14-6 Risk Factors Associated With Postoperative Pulmonary Complications

PATIENT-ASSOCIATED RISK FACTORS	RELATIVE RISK ASSOCIATED WITH FACTOR	PROCEDURE-ASSOCIATED RISK FACTORS	RELATIVE RISK ASSOCIATED WITH FACTOR
Age >60 yr	2.1-3.0	Surgery >3 hr	2.1
Functional dependence	2.5	General anesthesia	1.8
ASA class >II	4.9	Emergency surgery	2.2
Congestive heart failure	2.9		
Smoking	1.3		
Obesity	1.3		
COPD	1.8		

ASA, American Society of Anesthesiologists; *COPD,* chronic obstructive pulmonary disease.
Modified from Qaseem A, Snow V, Fitterman N, et al: Risk assessment for strategies to reduce perioperative pulmonary complications for patients undergoing non-cardiovascular surgery: A guideline from the American College of Physicians. *Ann Intern Med* 144:575–580, 2006.

agents and technique depends on the patient's condition and the type of surgery. In patients with active disease, elective surgery should be postponed until the patient is adequately treated.

The other major factors predicting perioperative pulmonary complications are related to surgical and anesthetic interventions and include surgery lasting longer than 3 hours, emergency surgery, and the use of general anesthesia. Procedures with an increased risk for pulmonary complications include abdominal surgery, thoracic surgery, neurosurgery, head and neck surgery, and vascular surgery.

Pulmonary function testing is controversial, partly because of changing expectations regarding the ability of patients with chronic pulmonary disease to tolerate extensive surgery. Pulmonary function testing has variable predictive value, cannot define a threshold above which the risk associated with surgery is prohibitive, and identifies no group at high risk but without clinical evidence of pulmonary disease. Also, arterial blood gas analysis does not identify a group for whom the risk of surgery is prohibitive. Spirometry may be helpful in a patient who has unexplained cough, dyspnea, or exercise intolerance or if there is a question regarding optimal improvement of air flow obstruction. Warner and associates[23] compared 135 patients who had undergone spirometry, were scheduled to undergo abdominal surgery, and met objective criteria for obstructive pulmonary disease (mean forced expiratory volume in 1 second, 0.9 ± 0.2 liter) with 135 patients matched for sex, surgical site, smoking history, and age. Although there was a significantly greater incidence of bronchospasm, the incidence of prolonged endotracheal intubation, prolonged intensive care unit admission, or readmission was no different. These results are reiterated in the meta-analysis performed by Qaseem and coworkers.[19]

Renal and Hepatic Disease

Renal and hepatic dysfunctions alter the metabolism and disposition of many anesthetic agents and impair many systemic functions. Patients with acute renal or hepatic insufficiency do not undergo elective surgery until these conditions can be adequately stabilized. Chronic renal insufficiency provides many perioperative management challenges, including acid-base abnormalities, electrolyte disturbances, and coagulation disorders. A thorough history must include the cause of chronic renal insufficiency, the presence of systemic complications related to chronic renal insufficiency, and other systemic diseases. Current daily urinary output, the type and frequency of dialysis, and dialysis-related complications also must be evaluated. The physical examination focuses on identifying systemic complications of chronic renal insufficiency, including evidence of altered volume status, coagulopathy, anemia, pericardial effusion, and encephalopathy. Laboratory evaluation includes assessment of anemia, electrolyte abnormalities, coagulopathy, and cardiovascular disease. Dialysis is performed 18 to 24 hours before surgery to avoid the fluid and electrolyte shifts that occur immediately after dialysis.

A patient with chronic liver disease poses many perioperative challenges. The presence of liver disease alters anesthetic drug metabolism, and hypoalbuminemia increases the free fraction of many drugs, making these patients sensitive to the acute and the long-term effects of many anesthetics. The perioperative risks associated with anesthesia and surgery depend on the severity of hepatic dysfunction. The preoperative evaluation focuses on hepatic synthetic and metabolic function and the presence of coagulopathy, encephalopathy, and ascites as well as the nutritional status of the patient.

Nutrition, Endocrinology, and Metabolism

Diabetes mellitus warrants discussion because of its high prevalence and potential for comorbidity. Preanesthetic evaluation focuses on the duration and type of diabetes and the current medical regimen. Review of end-organ function with emphasis on autonomic dysfunction, cardiovascular disease, renal insufficiency, retinopathy, and neurologic complications is mandatory. Patients with diabetes are considered to have delayed gastric emptying and to be at risk for gastroesophageal reflux. Perioperative plasma glucose levels need to be well controlled, yet hypoglycemia must be prevented. Appropriate control of perioperative blood sugar in diabetics is difficult to define. There is compelling evidence of a correlation between hyperglycemia and long-term diabetic and perioperative complications.[24] It is much less clear whether blood sugar must be tightly controlled during the acute stress of surgery. However, there is a strong correlation between mortality and tight control of glucose in critically ill patients, including surgical patients.[25] Furthermore, given the heterogeneity of the diabetic population, it is unlikely that a single standard approach is appropriate for all patients.

In diabetic patients undergoing surgery, the following principles of management are generally accepted:

1. Insulin pumps should be continued at sleep basal rates.
2. On the morning of surgery, a reduced dose of intermediate-acting or long-acting insulin should be provided and short-acting insulin should be held.
3. When a diabetic patient who is NPO is given insulin, glucose should be provided in IV fluids or plasma glucose concentrations should be closely monitored.

4. Plasma glucose concentrations should be checked before surgery and before discharge as a minimum.
5. In patients with type 2 diabetes, most authors suggest holding oral antidiabetic medications and noninsulin injectable medications on the day of surgery.
6. Metformin is usually stopped because of a slight risk for perioperative drug-induced lactic acidosis. Perioperative insulin requirements vary depending on body weight, liver disease, steroid therapy, infection, and the use of cardiopulmonary bypass.

Patients who have received systemic glucocorticoids before surgery may be unable to respond adequately to surgical stress. Because of the remote risk for adrenal insufficiency during anesthesia, patients who are on long-term glucocorticoid therapy generally receive perioperative glucocorticoid coverage. Recommendations regarding identification of patients at risk and appropriate dosing are based on anecdotal evidence. Newer recommendations are based on the preoperative dosage of glucocorticoid, the duration of therapy, and the type of surgery. For minor surgical stress, the equivalent of 25 mg of hydrocortisone on the day of surgery is recommended; for moderate surgical stress, 50 to 75 mg equivalent for 1 to 2 days; and for major surgical stress, 100 to 150 mg/day for 2 to 3 days.

Fasting Before Surgery

Pulmonary aspiration of gastric contents during anesthesia is an uncommon but serious complication. To prevent aspiration, NPO guidelines have been developed for patients scheduled for anesthesia and surgery. Traditionally, orders for "NPO after midnight" forbade any intake of liquids and solids. However, applying the same guidelines for clear liquids (gastric emptying time, 1 to 2 hours) and solids (gastric emptying time, 6 hours) has been questioned. The ASA adopted guidelines in 1998 that recommended a minimum fasting period of 2 hours after the ingestion of clear liquids and 6 hours for solids and nonclear liquids such as milk or orange juice (Table 14-7). Clear liquids are defined as liquids that you can see through and do not contain solids or particulates. The routine use of gastrointestinal stimulants, gastric acid secretion blockers, antacids, and antiemetics is not recommended. However, many patients have medical conditions that cause decreased gastric emptying. In these patients, the use of agents to improve gastric emptying and neutralize gastric acid may be warranted. In addition, precautions are instituted to decrease the risk for aspiration during anesthesia in patients undergoing emergency procedures.

The reported incidence of aspiration during anesthesia in various studies has ranged from 1.4 to 11 per 10,000 anesthetics. A higher incidence has been noted during emergency surgery and in patients with underlying disease processes that cause decreased gastric emptying. Some reports suggest that aspiration is at least as common during emergence from anesthesia as during the induction phase. Of patients in whom aspiration is suspected, less than half exhibit evidence of pulmonary injury. In one study, approximately one third of patients with suspected aspiration during anesthesia required postoperative intubation and ventilation. Most of these patients were extubated within 6 hours of surgery. Approximately 10% of patients required intubation and ventilation for 24 hours or longer. Approximately half of the patients requiring ventilation for longer than 24 hours after aspiration of gastric contents died of pulmonary complications.

TABLE 14-7 Preoperative Fasting Recommendations to Reduce Risk of Pulmonary Aspiration*

INGESTED MATERIAL	MINIMUM FASTING PERIOD (HR)
Clear liquids†	2
Breast milk	4
Infant formula	6
Nonhuman milk	6
Solid food	6

Adapted from Practice guidelines for preoperative fasting and the use of pharmacologic agents to reduce the risk of pulmonary aspiration: A report of the ASA Task Force on Preoperative Fasting. *Anesthesiology* 90:896–905, 1999.

*Applies to healthy patients undergoing elective procedures.

†Examples of clear liquids are water, fruit juices without pulp, black coffee, clear tea, and carbonated beverages.

Assessment of Physical Status

The ASA has developed a graded, descriptive scale as a means of categorizing preoperative comorbidity. The classification is independent of operative procedure and serves as a standardized method of communicating patient physical status to anesthesiologists and other health care providers. Patients are categorized as follows:

ASA I: A patient with no organic, physiologic, biochemical, or psychiatric disturbance.

ASA II: A patient with mild systemic disease that results in no functional limitation. Examples are well-controlled hypertension and uncomplicated diabetes mellitus.

ASA III: A patient with severe systemic disease that results in functional impairment. Examples are diabetes mellitus with vascular complications, previous myocardial infarction, and uncontrolled hypertension.

ASA IV: A patient with severe systemic disease that is a constant threat to life. Examples are congestive heart failure and unstable angina pectoris.

ASA V: A moribund patient who is not expected to survive with or without the surgery. Examples are ruptured aortic aneurysm and intracranial hemorrhage with elevated ICP.

ASA VI: A patient who has been declared brain dead whose organs are being harvested for transplantation.

E: Emergency surgery is required. For example, ASA IE represents an otherwise healthy patient undergoing emergency appendectomy.

SELECTION OF ANESTHETIC TECHNIQUES AND DRUGS

The selection of anesthetic techniques and drugs begins with the preoperative anesthetic evaluation. Recognition of important preexisting conditions and long-term use of medications may suggest that certain approaches are preferable. Then the requirements of the surgical procedure and surgeon are considered. What is the operative site? How will the patient be positioned? What is the expected duration of surgery? Is the patient expected to return home after an ambulatory procedure or is hospital admission anticipated? Finally, in this era of cost constraints, are the costs of newer drugs justified by probable clinical benefit? Evidence of the increasing safety of anesthesia is the fact that multiple options can often be used safely and effectively for the same procedure and the same patient.

After completing the preanesthetic evaluation, the anesthesiologist discusses various options regarding anesthetic care with the patient. Together, sometimes with input from the patient's surgeon, the anesthesiologist and patient choose an anesthetic technique. Continued progress in the pharmacology of anesthetic drugs, improvements in the accuracy and applicability of monitoring devices, and parallel improvements in the management of chronic disease processes have resulted in the ability to customize the anesthetic management of individual patients extensively.

Risk of Anesthesia

Patients often desire information regarding the risk of death or major complications associated with anesthesia. However, because perioperative death and major complications have become rare, the risk associated with anesthesia is difficult to quantify. Each year, an estimated 234 million surgical cases are performed worldwide. In developed nations, surgical mortality is estimated to be 0.4% to 0.8% with morbidity rates of 3% to 17%.[26] The risk for cardiac arrest attributable to anesthesia appears to be less than 1 in 10,000 cases.[27,28] Schwilk and colleagues[29] prospectively studied preoperative risk factors as predictors of perioperative adverse events in 26,907 patients undergoing noncardiac surgery. There were 14 variables that proved to be independent risk factors, including sex, age, ASA status, functional status, nutritional state, coronary disease, airway and lung pathology, Mallampati classification, fluid and electrolyte balance, metabolic state, grade of urgency, operative site, duration of surgery, and anesthetic technique (lower risk with regional than with general anesthesia). With the use of a point system, patients could be reliably separated into low-risk and high-risk groups.

Because so many surgical procedures are now performed without admission to the hospital, the risk associated with ambulatory anesthesia is particularly important. To assess this risk, 38,598 patients who had undergone 45,090 consecutive ambulatory surgical procedures were contacted within 72 hours and 30 days of surgery (99.94% and 95.9% of patients, respectively). No patient died of a medical complication within 1 week of surgery.[30] The total death rate was 1 in 11,273 (4 deaths), and the total complication rate was 1 in 1366. A study by Fleisher and associates[31] reported similar findings with mortality rates of 0.025% to 0.05% for patients undergoing outpatient surgery in physician offices, ambulatory surgery centers, and outpatient hospital facilities. Patient and procedure selection are important factors in determining the safety of outpatient anesthesia and surgical procedures. The associated risk is a summation of surgery and anesthesia. The individual contributions of each component are difficult to determine.

Selection of a Specific Technique

The first step in selecting a specific anesthetic technique for an individual patient is to consider whether the procedure can be appropriately performed with monitored anesthesia care, regional anesthesia (including regional upper and lower extremity blocks, subarachnoid blocks, and epidural anesthesia), or general anesthesia. Monitored anesthesia care supplements local anesthesia performed by surgeons. Anesthesiologists usually participate because an individual patient or procedure requires higher doses of potent sedatives or opioids or because an acutely or chronically ill patient requires close monitoring and hemodynamic or respiratory support. Regional anesthesia (discussed in detail in a later section) is useful for operations on the upper and lower extremities, pelvis, and lower part of the abdomen. Certain other procedures, such as carotid endarterectomy and awake craniotomy, also can be successfully performed under a regional or field block. Patients receiving regional anesthesia can generally remain awake and, if needed, can receive IV sedation or analgesics. Although regional anesthesia avoids general anesthesia and intuitively appears to be safer, hazards specific to regional anesthesia must be considered. Such hazards include, among others, post–dural puncture headache, local anesthetic toxicity, high neuraxial block, and peripheral nerve injury. In addition, an inadequate regional anesthetic may require rapid transition to heavy sedation or general anesthesia.

General anesthesia is a reversible state of unconsciousness. Although the mechanism of general anesthetics remains speculative and controversial, the four components of general anesthesia (amnesia, analgesia, inhibition of noxious reflexes, and skeletal muscle relaxation) are usually achieved in modern anesthesia by a combination of IV anesthetics and analgesics, inhalational anesthetics, and frequently muscle relaxants. Because the drugs that produce these components cause desirable and undesirable physiologic changes, the pharmacologic effects of the agents must be matched to the pathophysiology of the patient's medical problems. The major adverse changes associated with anesthetic drugs are respiratory depression, cardiovascular depression, and loss of airway maintenance and protection. Important complications of general anesthesia include hypoxemia (with possible CNS damage), hypotension, cardiac arrest, and aspiration of acidic gastric contents (which can lead to severe pulmonary damage). Dental damage is more frequent but not life-threatening. General anesthesia can be maintained by inhalation of volatile agents or by infusion of IV agents. Both techniques can have advantages under certain conditions, and individual patient factors should be considered.

Regardless of the suitability of a particular technique for a specific surgical procedure, other factors, including the patient's preferences, must be considered. For example, regional anesthesia might not be chosen if a patient is extremely anxious or cannot communicate effectively because of a language barrier. Monitored anesthesia care might be inappropriate if a patient is unlikely to lie quietly during delicate or prolonged surgery. Any procedure planned under regional anesthesia or monitored anesthesia care can require conversion to general anesthesia if the original choice proves unsatisfactory.

AIRWAY MANAGEMENT

Airway management is perhaps the most critical skill in anesthesiology. As discussed earlier, the preoperative evaluation focuses on recognition of patients who may be difficult to mask ventilate or intubate. Knowledge of and skill with various techniques for establishment of a patent airway constitutes the central group of skills that are critical for the safe practice of anesthesiology. The incidence of difficult intubations is low. Difficult direct laryngoscopy occurs in 1.5% to 8.5% of general anesthetics, and failed intubation occurs in 0.13% to 0.3% of general anesthetics. The laryngeal mask airway, the lighted stylet, and an array of videolaryngoscopes are more recent developments that make ventilation and intubation possible in many patients who fail intubation with a conventional laryngoscope. The fiberoptic bronchoscope is an additional tool for the management of a difficult airway.

Because of the importance of a prompt, effective response to difficult intubation, the ASA has developed guidelines for managing difficult airways (Fig. 14-4). A key factor is the initial airway examination and recognition of a patient with a potentially difficult airway. If the practitioner suspects that mask ventilation and tracheal intubation will be difficult, it is recommended that spontaneous ventilation be preserved. Approaches to these patients include awake intubation or the use of anesthetic techniques that preserve spontaneous ventilation. In some cases, establishment of a surgical airway in an awake patient under local anesthesia may be indicated. However, some patients are found to have a difficult airway only after anesthesia and muscle relaxation have been induced. This is an emergency situation that must be rectified quickly to avoid hypoxemia, brain injury, or death. Various airway adjuncts are available to preserve ventilation and facilitate tracheal intubation under emergency conditions. The practitioner always must call for assistance in these situations to optimize patient care and consider re-establishment of spontaneous ventilation. It is essential to have alternative means for securing the airway available for all patients in the event of an unanticipated difficult airway.

REGIONAL ANESTHESIA

Regional anesthesia is an attractive anesthetic option for many types of operative procedures and can provide excellent postoperative pain management in selected patients. However, similar to any anesthetic technique, the risks and benefits associated with regional anesthesia must be assessed for each individual. Several regional techniques are in common use, including spinal, epidural, and peripheral nerve blocks. Each technique has specific benefits and risks, which depend in part on the choice of local anesthetic drugs.

Local Anesthetic Drugs

Local anesthetics have played a critical role in intraoperative anesthesia almost since they were first described. The two classes of local anesthetic drugs in common use are aminoesters and aminoamides (often described as *esters* and *amides*). The mechanism of action of local anesthetics is dose-dependent blockade of sodium currents in nerve fibers. Local anesthetic drugs differ in terms of their physicochemical characteristics. Of these characteristics, the most important are pK_a, protein binding, and the degree of hydrophobicity. pK_a refers to the pH at which half the drug exists in the basic uncharged form and half exists in the cationic form. In general, agents with a lower pK_a have a faster onset than agents with a higher pK_a, although some agents, such as chloroprocaine, can be given at much higher concentrations, offsetting the effects of a high pK_a. Because all commonly used local anesthetics have relatively high pK_a values, they are largely ineffective in acidotic (inflamed) environments, in which local anesthetics exist primarily in the ionized form, which does not penetrate nerves. In general, greater hydrophobicity is associated with greater potency, and increased protein binding correlates with a longer duration of action. The speed of onset, duration of action, and typical doses of agents commonly used for regional anesthesia or local anesthesia are summarized in Table 14-8.

In using local anesthetics clinically, the priority is to prevent local anesthetic toxicity. When used for regional anesthesia, the toxicity of local anesthetics depends on the site of injection and the speed of absorption. Inadvertent intravascular injection of local anesthetics produces toxicity with much smaller doses. The main symptoms of local anesthetic toxicity involve the CNS and cardiovascular system. The earliest signs of an overdose or inadvertent intravascular injection are numbness or tingling of the tongue or lips, a metallic taste, light-headedness, tinnitus, or visual disturbances. Signs of toxicity can progress to slurred speech, disorientation, and seizures. With higher doses of local anesthetics, cardiovascular collapse ensues.

The best defenses against local anesthetic toxicity are aspiration to detect unplanned vascular entry before injecting large doses of local anesthetics and knowledge of the maximal safe dose of the drug being injected. Adding epinephrine, which slows absorption, also decreases the likelihood of a toxic response secondary to rapid absorption. The primary treatments of local anesthetic toxicity are oxygen and airway support. If a seizure does not terminate spontaneously, a benzodiazepine (e.g., midazolam) or thiopental is given. Cardiovascular support may be needed.

Cardiovascular toxicity from bupivacaine may be particularly difficult to treat. One approach intended to reduce the cardiovascular toxicity of bupivacaine (a racemic mixture of the *levo* and *dextro* isomers) has been to produce a solution consisting of only the *levo* isomer. In healthy male volunteers, slow IV infusion of levobupivacaine reduced the mean stroke index, acceleration index, and ejection fraction less than racemic bupivacaine. Ropivacaine, a newer potent amide local anesthetic, was compared with bupivacaine and lidocaine in volunteers receiving a slow IV infusion until CNS symptoms first occurred. Echocardiography and ECG were used to quantify systolic, diastolic, and electrophysiologic effects. Bupivacaine increased QRS width during sinus rhythm compared with the other two treatments and reduced systolic and diastolic function, whereas ropivacaine reduced systolic function only. The anesthetic properties of ropivacaine are similar to bupivacaine, and based on its decreased toxicity profile, ropivacaine is commonly used as an alternative to bupivacaine by many practitioners. Many case reports and experimental studies have reported the efficacy of lipid emulsion infusion as a means of rescuing subjects from severe local anesthetic toxicity. Although the mechanisms of action of lipid emulsion therapy are not completely understood, the use of lipid emulsion

FIGURE 14-4 American Society of Anesthesiologists difficult airway algorithm. The likelihood and clinical impact of basic management problems, such as difficult intubation, difficult mask ventilation, and difficulty with patient cooperation or consent, should be assessed in all patients in whom airway management is being contemplated. The clinician should consider the relative merits and feasibility of basic management choices, including the use of awake intubation techniques, preservation of spontaneous ventilation, and the use of surgical approaches to establish a secure airway. Primary and alternative strategies should be considered: (a) other options include, but are not limited to, surgery under mask anesthesia, surgery under local infiltration or nerve block, and intubation attempts after induction of general anesthesia; (b) alternative approaches include the use of different laryngoscope blades, awake intubation, blind oral or nasal intubation, fiberoptic intubation, an intubating stylet or tube changer, light wand, retrograde intubation, and surgical airway access; (c) see awake intubation; (d) options for an emergency nonsurgical airway include transtracheal jet ventilation, laryngeal mask airway, and Combitube. (From American Society of Anesthesiologists: Practice guidelines for management of the difficult airway: A report by the American Society of Anesthesiologists task force on management of the difficult airway. *Anesthesiology* 78:597–602, 1993.)

DIFFICULT AIRWAY ALGORITHM

1. Access the likelihood and clinical impact of basic management problems:
   - A. Difficult ventilation
   - B. Difficult intubation
   - C. Difficulty with patient cooperation or consent
   - D. Difficult tracheostomy
2. Actively pursue opportunities to deliver supplemental oxygen throughout the process of difficult airway management
3. Consider the relative merits and feasibility of basic management choices:

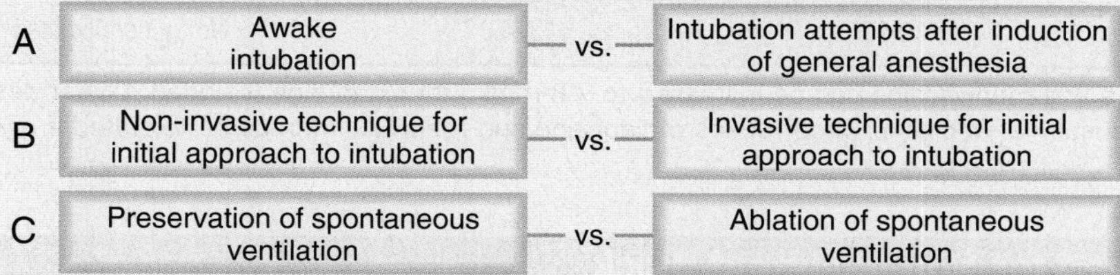

4. Develop primary and alternative strategies:

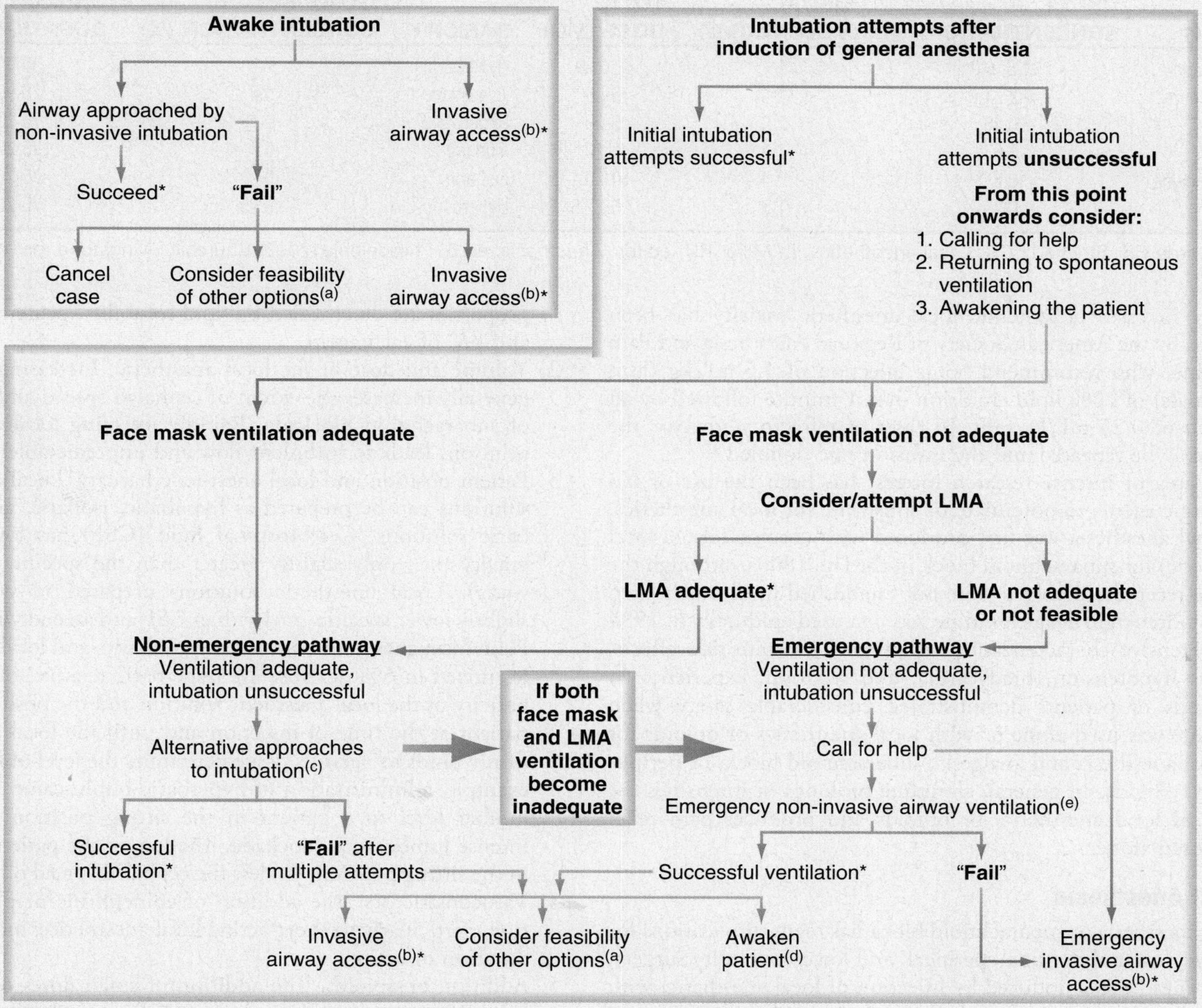

Awake intubation

Airway approached by non-invasive intubation

Invasive airway access(b)*

Succeed*

"Fail"

Cancel case

Consider feasibility of other options(a)

Invasive airway access(b)*

Intubation attempts after induction of general anesthesia

Initial intubation attempts successful*

Initial intubation attempts **unsuccessful**

From this point onwards consider:
1. Calling for help
2. Returning to spontaneous ventilation
3. Awakening the patient

Face mask ventilation adequate

Face mask ventilation not adequate

Consider/attempt LMA

LMA adequate*

LMA not adequate or not feasible

Non-emergency pathway
Ventilation adequate, intubation unsuccessful

Alternative approaches to intubation(c)

If both face mask and LMA ventilation become inadequate

Emergency pathway
Ventilation not adequate, intubation unsuccessful

Call for help

Emergency non-invasive airway ventilation(e)

Successful intubation*

"Fail" after multiple attempts

Successful ventilation*

"Fail"

Invasive airway access(b)*

Consider feasibility of other options(a)

Awaken patient(d)

Emergency invasive airway access(b)*

***Confirm ventilation, tracheal intubation, or LMA placement with exhaled CO_2**

a. Other options include (but are not limited to): surgery utilizing face mask or LMA anesthesia, local anesthesia infiltration or regional nerve blockade. Pursuit of these options usually implies that mask ventilation will not be problematic. Therefore, these options may be of limited value if this step in the algorithm has been reached via the Emergency Pathway.
b. Invasive airway access includes surgical or percutaneous tracheostomy or cricothyrotomy.
c. Alternative noninvasive approaches to difficult intubation include (but are not limited to): use of different laryngoscope blades, LMA as an intubation conduit (with or without fiberoptic guidance), fiberoptic intubation, intubating stylet or tube changer, light wand, retrograde intubation, and blind oral or nasal intubation.
d. Consider repreparation of the patient for awake intubation or canceling surgery.
e. Options for emergency non-invasive airway ventilation include (but are not limited to): rigid bronchoscope, esophageal-tracheal combitube ventilation, or transtracheal jet ventilation.

TABLE 14-8 Important Characteristics of Local Anesthetics Used for Major Nerve Blocks

LOCAL ANESTHETIC	AMINOAMIDE OR AMINOESTER	SPEED OF ONSET (MIN)	DURATION OF ACTION (MIN)	MAXIMAL DOSE* (AXILLARY BLOCK)
Lidocaine	Aminoamide	10-20	60-180	5 mg/kg
Mepivacaine	Aminoamide	10-20	60-180	5 mg/kg
Bupivacaine	Aminoamide	15-30	180-360	3 mg/kg
Ropivacaine	Aminoamide	15-30	180-360	3 mg/kg
Chloroprocaine	Aminoester	10-20	30-50	Not generally used

*Maximal dose without epinephrine; doses of lidocaine and mepivacaine can be increased to 7-8 mg/kg if epinephrine is added. Lower doses may be toxic if infiltrated subcutaneously, as for intercostal nerve blocks; larger doses of lidocaine and mepivacaine may be tolerated if given by epidural injection.

TABLE 14-9 Local Anesthetics Used for Subarachnoid Block

DRUG	USUAL CONCENTRATION (%)	USUAL VOLUME (ML)	TOTAL DOSE (MG)	BARICITY	GLUCOSE CONCENTRATION (%)	USUAL DURATION (MIN)
Lidocaine	1.5, 5.0	1-2	30-100	Hyperbaric	7.5	30-60
Tetracaine	0.25-1.0	1-4	5-20	Hyperbaric	5.0	75-200
	0.25	2-6	5-20	Hyperbaric	0	75-200
	1.0	1-2	5-20	Isobaric	0	75-200
Bupivacaine	0.5	2-4	10-20	Isobaric	0	75-200
	0.75	1-3	7.5-22.5	Hyperbaric	8.25	75-200

From Berde CB, Strichartz GR: Local anesthetics. In Miller RD, editor: *Anesthesia*, ed 5, Philadelphia, 2000, Churchill Livingstone, pp 491–522.

therapy in cases of systemic local anesthetic toxicity has been adopted by the American Society of Regional Anesthesia and Pain Medicine, who recommend bolus injection of 1.5 mL/kg (lean body mass) of 20% lipid emulsion over 1 minute followed by an infusion of 0.25 mL/kg/min. In cases of refractory toxicity, the bolus may be repeated and the infusion rate doubled.[32]

An area of intense research interest has been the use of α_2-adrenergic agents to potentiate or substitute for local anesthetics. Regional anesthesia was first produced with cocaine (also a local anesthetic) for subarachnoid block in the late 1800s, although the specific receptors involved were not established until much later. The α_2-adrenergic drug clonidine was first used epidurally in 1984 after extensive characterization in animals. Despite side effects, such as hypotension, bradycardia, and sedation, experience in thousands of patients demonstrated considerable safety when clonidine was used alone or with local anesthetics or opioids for epidural anesthesia and analgesia, subarachnoid block, or peripheral nerve block. In general, clonidine prolongs or intensifies the effects of local anesthetics or opioids and produces pain relief when used alone.

Spinal Anesthesia

Spinal anesthesia or subarachnoid block has many applications for urologic, lower abdominal, perineal, and lower extremity surgery. Spinal anesthesia is induced by injection of local anesthetic, with or without opiates, into the subarachnoid space. A well-performed subarachnoid block provides excellent sensory and motor blockade below the level of the block. The block generally has a relatively rapid and predictable onset. Several factors determine the level, speed of onset, and duration of spinal blockade, as follows:

1. Local anesthetic agent. Local anesthetics have varying potencies, durations of action, and speeds of onset after subarachnoid administration. Typical doses and durations of action are shown in Table 14-9. Bupivacaine and tetracaine have significantly longer durations of action than lidocaine. These properties are determined by lipid solubility, protein binding, and pK_a of each agent.
2. Volume and dose of the local anesthetic. Increasing the dose generally increases the extent of cephalad spread and duration of subarachnoid blockade. Rapidly injecting local anesthetic solutions leads to turbulent flow and unpredictable spread.
3. Patient position and local anesthetic baricity. Local anesthetic solutions can be prepared as hypobaric, isobaric, and hyperbaric solutions. Cerebrospinal fluid (CSF) has low specific gravity (i.e., only slightly greater than the specific gravity of water). Local anesthetic solutions prepared in water have slightly lower specific gravity than CSF and ascend within CSF. Plain local anesthetic solutions are isobaric, and local anesthetics mixed in 5% dextrose are hyperbaric relative to CSF. The baricity of the local anesthetic solution and the position of the patient at the time of injection and until the local anesthetic firmly binds to nervous tissue determine the level of block. For example, administration of hyperbaric bupivacaine at the low lumbar level to a patient in the sitting position results in intense lumbosacral blockade. The longer the patient remains in the sitting position, the less the cephalad spread of the block.
4. Vasoconstrictors. The addition of epinephrine or phenylephrine, particularly to short-acting local anesthetics, increases the duration of action.
5. Addition of opioids. The addition of small doses of fentanyl (e.g., 20 μg) or morphine (e.g., 0.25 mg) prolongs the duration of analgesia and increases the duration of analgesia and tolerance for tourniquet pain.
6. Anatomic and physiologic factors. A higher than expected level of spinal anesthesia can result from anatomic factors that decrease the relative volume of the subarachnoid space, such as obesity, pregnancy, increased intra-abdominal pressure, previous spine surgery, and abnormal spinal curvature. Elderly patients tend to be more sensitive to intrathecally injected local anesthetics.

Spinal anesthesia provides the advantage of avoiding manipulation of the airway and the potential complication of tracheal intubation as well as the potential side effects of general anesthetics, such as nausea, vomiting, and prolonged emergence or drowsiness. Spinal anesthesia also provides advantages for several types of surgery, including endoscopic urologic procedures, particularly transurethral resection of the prostate, in which an awake patient provides a valuable monitor for assessment of hyponatremia or bladder perforation. Less confusion and postoperative delirium have been reported in elderly patients after repair of hip fractures under spinal anesthesia. Intrathecal opiate administration can provide high-quality postoperative analgesia for patients undergoing abdominal, lower extremity, urologic, and gynecologic procedures.

In most cases, spinal anesthesia is administered as a single bolus injection. The block is of limited duration and is not suitable for prolonged procedures. The practice of continuous spinal anesthesia with the use of small-bore catheters has largely been abandoned because of neurologic complications associated with local anesthetic toxicity. However, continuous spinal anesthesia with relatively large-bore epidural catheters can provide the advantages of incremental titration and the ability to administer additional doses in selected elderly patients. This technique has a high likelihood of inducing a post–dural puncture headache in young patients.

Complications of subarachnoid block include hypotension (sometimes refractory), bradycardia, post–dural puncture headache, transient radicular neuropathy, backache, urinary retention, infection, epidural hematoma, and excessive cephalad spread resulting in cardiorespiratory compromise. Frank neurologic injury, although described with continuous techniques using small-bore catheters, is quite rare. Hypotension, which occurs as a consequence of sympathectomy, usually responds readily to fluids and small doses of pressors such as ephedrine. The efficacy of fluid preloading in providing prophylaxis against hypotension is controversial.

Post–dural puncture headache occurs after a small proportion of subarachnoid blocks. Factors that increase the incidence include female sex, younger age, and larger needles. Epidural analgesia would appear to avoid the complication, but if the dura mater is inadvertently punctured, it leaves a much larger dural rent. Compared with epidural anesthesia, spinal anesthesia has a quicker onset, is more predictably satisfactory for surgery, and is less frequently associated with backache. Transient radicular neuropathy, a painful but usually self-limited condition, became evident in association with an increase in enthusiasm for the use of lidocaine for subarachnoid block.

When cardiac arrest results from excessive cephalad spread of subarachnoid block or protracted hypotension, cardiopulmonary resuscitation is notoriously difficult. Patients who experience cardiac arrest during subarachnoid block have poor survival, possibly because the profound sympathectomy causes difficulty in generating adequate coronary perfusion pressure. Relatively large doses of epinephrine may be necessary to achieve adequate perfusion pressure during cardiopulmonary resuscitation after spinal anesthesia. Absolute contraindications to spinal anesthesia include sepsis, bacteremia, infection at the site of injection, severe hypovolemia, coagulopathy, therapeutic anticoagulation, increased ICP, and patient refusal.

Epidural Anesthesia

Epidural block, another form of neuraxial regional block, has application in a wide variety of abdominal, thoracic, and lower extremity procedures. Induction of epidural anesthesia or analgesia results from injection of local anesthetics, with or without opiates, into the lumbar or thoracic epidural space. Generally, a catheter is inserted after the epidural space has been located with a needle. The presence of the catheter provides several advantages. First, local anesthetic can be added in a controlled fashion so that the time to onset of the block can be well controlled. Second, the catheter can be used for repeated dosing so that anesthesia can be provided for the duration of lengthy procedures. Third, local anesthetics or opiates can be administered for several days to provide postoperative analgesia.

Epidural anesthesia has specific advantages for thoracic surgery, peripheral vascular surgery, and gastrointestinal surgery. Epidural anesthesia has also been shown to decrease blood loss and deep venous thrombosis during total joint arthroplasty. Postoperative epidural analgesia for thoracic surgery provides superior pain control, less sedation, and better pulmonary function than parenteral opiates.

In a Cochrane Database analysis, it was determined that the use of epidural anesthesia was associated with a significant decrease in 0- to 30-day mortality and a decreased incidence of pneumonia compared with the use of general anesthesia in a broad group of surgical procedures. The incidence of perioperative myocardial infarction was not different among groups. Similarly, the use of epidural analgesia after general anesthesia decreased the incidence of postoperative pneumonia compared with the use of general anesthesia alone but did not change 0- to 30-day mortality or incidence of myocardial infarction.[33]

The use of low concentrations of local anesthetics in conjunction with epidural opiates has been associated with earlier ambulation and less postoperative ileus after abdominal surgery. Thoracic epidural anesthesia, but not lumbar epidural anesthesia, appears to be associated with more rapid recovery of gastrointestinal function after major abdominal surgery. However, IV lidocaine also resulted in more rapid return of bowel function (flatus and bowel movement). Circulating systemic lidocaine may account for at least some of the effects of epidural anesthesia on postoperative bowel function. A study by Swenson and colleagues[34] did not show a significant difference in return to bowel function, hospital length of stay, or postoperative pain control when comparing epidural analgesia with continuous lidocaine infusion in patients undergoing colon resection. A continuing controversy relates to whether epidural or subarachnoid analgesia reduces subsequent analgesic requirements after the block has resolved (so-called preemptive analgesia).

The complications and contraindications associated with epidural anesthesia are similar to those associated with spinal anesthesia. However, a special cautionary note is indicated regarding epidural anesthesia and anticoagulation. Because of the risk of spinal hematoma, placement and removal of epidural catheters in patients receiving oral or parenteral anticoagulation is performed in conjunction with an anesthesiologist. The advent of low-molecular-weight heparin (LMWH) for prophylaxis of deep venous thrombosis resulted in an increase in the incidence of epidural hematomas associated with the removal or placement of epidural catheters. Although LMWH is effective as prophylaxis against venous thromboembolism, spinal hematomas have occurred in association with perioperative use of LMWH in patients given neuraxial analgesia. The timing of catheter placement and removal in the setting of LMWH use is critical to avoiding this rare but catastrophic complication. Although many of the guidelines are based on evidence provided by small clinical studies and case reports, a general consensus exists regarding the placement and removal of epidural catheters in patients receiving LMWH.[35] In general, an epidural catheter should not be placed earlier than 24 hours after treatment with LMWH, and LMWH should not be started before 6 hours after epidural catheter placement. An epidural catheter should not be removed earlier than 12 hours after the last dose of LMWH, and LMWH should not be restarted earlier than 2 hours after catheter removal. A high index of suspicion of epidural hematoma must be maintained in patients undergoing neuraxial blockade who have received or will receive LMWH. All persons involved in the care of patients receiving continuous epidural analgesia need to be aware of the signs of epidural hematoma, including back pain, lower extremity sensory and motor dysfunction, and bladder and bowel abnormalities. To reduce the risk, needle placement is not performed less than 10 to 12 hours after the last dose, and subsequent dosing is delayed at least 2 hours. Epidural catheters are withdrawn at least 10 to 12 hours after the last dose of LMWH. A final rare complication, epidural abscess, is considered in patients in whom back pain develops after epidural injection; magnetic resonance imaging is an effective diagnostic tool in such patients.

Peripheral Nerve Blocks

Blockade of the brachial plexus, lumbar plexus, and specific peripheral nerves is an effective means of providing surgical anesthesia and postoperative analgesia for many surgical procedures involving the upper and lower extremities. The advantage of peripheral nerve blocks is reduced physiologic stress compared with spinal or epidural anesthesia, avoidance of airway manipulation and the potential complications associated with endotracheal intubation, and avoidance of the potential side effects associated with general anesthesia. Successful nerve block anesthesia requires a cooperative patient, an anesthesiologist skilled in peripheral nerve blocks, and a surgeon who is accustomed to operating on awake patients. All patients undergoing peripheral nerve block receive full preoperative evaluation under the assumption that general anesthesia can be used if the block is inadequate.

Improvements in nerve block equipment and methodology and the availability of a wide range of local anesthetics have greatly improved the effectiveness and safety of peripheral nerve blocks. In addition to providing surgical anesthesia, peripheral nerve blocks and the placement of indwelling catheters for a prolonged nerve block provide excellent analgesia for many types of upper extremity surgery and trauma. An additional application of indwelling catheters is enhancement of blood flow after reattachment of amputated limbs and in patients with peripheral vascular disease. Each particular block has specific associated risks and benefits. General complications of peripheral nerve blocks include local anesthetic toxicity, neurologic injury, inadvertent neuraxial block, and intravascular injection of local anesthetics.

CONSCIOUS SEDATION

When anesthesiologists participate in the sedation of patients undergoing surgical procedures, the procedure is termed *monitored anesthesia care.* Monitored anesthesia care encompasses a wide range of depths of sedation ranging from minimal sedation to brief intervals of complete unconsciousness (e.g., during placement of a retrobulbar block by an ophthalmologist). When non-anesthesia personnel administer sedation for surgical procedures, the process is generally termed *conscious sedation,* although the term *moderate sedation* is preferable. Moderate sedation implies that the patient can respond purposefully to verbal or tactile stimulation, has a patent airway requiring no intervention, demonstrates adequate spontaneous ventilation, and has maintained cardiovascular function. There is a narrow margin between minimal sedation, which may be inadequate for surgery to continue, and deep sedation, which may result in airway compromise and cardiovascular and respiratory depression. Although relatively rare in this setting, a closed claim analysis showed that hypoventilation and hypoxemia were the most common major complications.[36] Because of the risks associated with moderate sedation, the Joint Commission requires that patients be managed with precautions similar to what they would receive if an anesthesiologist were managing the sedation. Important factors include the necessity for preprocedure evaluation, continuous presence of a trained monitoring assistant who has no other responsibilities throughout the procedure, immediate availability of airway and resuscitation equipment, monitoring after the procedure until the effects of sedation have resolved, and specific written postoperative instructions. Physicians who perform procedures under conscious sedation are granted privileges in line with their training and experience in the appropriate resuscitative procedures.

Drugs used for moderate sedation usually consist of opioids such as fentanyl or morphine, often combined with an anxiolytic such as midazolam. Titration of these agents requires careful assessment of a patient's level of pain or anxiety and the requirements for the surgical procedure. Induction agents such as propofol are becoming increasingly popular for induction of moderate sedation outside of the operating room. Although generally safe when used under the proper conditions, these agents introduce an added element of risk and increase the need for caution because of potentially rapid progression to deep sedation or even general anesthesia. Most hospitals now have specific policies and procedures governing moderate sedation. Clinicians who use moderate sedation outside hospitals (e.g., in office-based surgical practices) need to follow the same precautions as practiced in the hospital environment.

POSTANESTHESIA CARE

The PACU is the area designated for the care of patients recovering from the immediate physiologic and pharmacologic consequences associated with anesthesia and surgery. The PACU ideally is located close to the operating rooms. Monitors for the assessment of ventilation, oxygenation, and circulation must be available for all recovering patients. Care also includes periodic assessment of neuromuscular function, mental status, temperature, pain, fluid status, urine output, nausea and vomiting, and bleeding and drainage. The extent of monitoring depends on the condition of the patient. The ASA has established standards of postanesthesia care.[37] Recovery from anesthesia is usually uneventful and routine. Most patients stay in the PACU for 30 to 60 minutes until they are fully reactive and can move to a second-stage recovery area (for ambulatory patients who are returning home that day) or to a bed on a surgical floor. However, several criteria need to be met before the patient can be safely discharged from the PACU. All patients must be awake and oriented and have stable vital signs. Patients must be breathing without difficulty, able to protect their airways, and oxygenating appropriately. Pain, shivering, nausea, and vomiting must be adequately controlled. Patients receiving regional anesthesia must be observed for resolution of the block. There can be no evidence of surgical complications such as postoperative bleeding. Several types of anesthesia-related complications can be encountered in the PACU and must be promptly recognized and treated to prevent serious injury.

Postoperative Agitation, Delirium, and Cognitive Decline

Pain and anxiety are often manifested as postoperative agitation. However, agitation may also signal serious physiologic disturbances such as hypoxemia, hypercapnia, acidosis, hypotension, hypoglycemia, surgical complications, and adverse drug reactions. Serious underlying conditions must be excluded as the cause of agitation before empirically treating patients with pain medications, sedatives, or physical restraints.

Postoperative delirium is a common complication of surgery and anesthesia that occurs in 70% of patients older than age 60 who undergo major procedures requiring inpatient care. Development of postoperative delirium in elderly patients is associated with increased mortality, persistent cognitive decline, and prolongation of in-hospital care. Multiple factors contribute to postoperative delirium, including preoperative cognitive function, extent of surgery, and the need for postoperative intensive care. Approaches to minimize postoperative delirium are under investigation, but no definitive recommendations can be given at this time.

Respiratory Complications

Respiratory problems are the most frequently occurring major complications in the PACU. Airway obstruction is most commonly due to obstruction of the oropharynx by the tongue or oropharyngeal soft tissues as a result of the residual effects of general anesthetics, pain medications, or muscle relaxants. Other causes of airway obstruction include laryngospasm; blood, vomitus, or debris in the airway; glottic edema; vocal cord paralysis; and external compression of the airway by a hematoma, dressing, or cervical collar. Oxygen must be administered to a patient with airway obstruction as measures are taken to relieve the obstruction. The characteristic physical signs of airway obstruction are sonorous respiratory sounds and paradoxical chest movement.

Many obstructions can be relieved by applying a head-tilt and jaw-thrust maneuver with or without placement of an oral or nasopharyngeal airway. Suctioning the airway may also be beneficial, and the patient needs to be examined for evidence of external airway compression. In cases of laryngospasm, continuous positive airway pressure is applied, followed by the administration of 10 to 20 mg of succinylcholine if continuous positive airway pressure is ineffective. Patients may require mask ventilation and endotracheal intubation if the laryngospasm does not resolve promptly. In children, glottic edema or postextubation croup can result in airway obstruction. Mild cases are treated with humidified oxygen. Refractory obstruction may require the administration of systemic steroids and racemic epinephrine by nebulization. Reintubation may also be required.

Hypoxemia is a common problem; administration of supplemental oxygen during transportation to the PACU and during the immediate postoperative period decreases the incidence and severity of hypoxemia. The incidence of mild hypoxemia (oxygen saturation [SpO_2] of 86% to 90%) and severe hypoxemia (SpO_2 ≤85%) was 7% and 0.7%, respectively, in the PACU for patients undergoing superficial elective plastic surgery; 38% and 3%, respectively, for patients undergoing upper abdominal surgery; and 52% and 20%, respectively, for patients undergoing thoracoabdominal surgery.[38] Hypoxemia can result from hypoventilation, ventilation-perfusion mismatching, or right-to-left intrapulmonary shunting. Reluctance to inspire deeply after abdominal or thoracic surgery may also result in hypoxemia. Clinically, hypoxemia must be suspected as an underlying problem in patients exhibiting restlessness, tachycardia, or cardiac irritability. Bradycardia, hypotension, and cardiac arrest are late signs. Hypoxemia in the PACU may be secondary to atelectasis, which may respond to incentive spirometry or vigorous encouragement to inspire deeply and cough. Treatment of hypoxemia requires the administration of oxygen, assurance of adequate ventilation, and treatment of the underlying causes.

Hypoventilation (synonymous with hypercapnia) can result from airway obstruction; central respiratory depression caused by the residual effects of anesthetic agents; hypothermia; CNS injury; or restriction of ventilation secondary to muscle relaxants, abdominal distention, and electrolyte abnormalities. Signs include prolonged somnolence, a slow (or rapid) respiratory rate, airway obstruction, shallow breathing, tachycardia, and arrhythmias. Severe hypoventilation can result in hypoxemia, although augmented inspired oxygen limits the severity of hypoventilation-induced hypoxemia. Treatment is aimed at identification and treatment of the underlying problem. In all cases, ventilation must be supported until corrective measures are instituted. Obtundation, circulatory depression, and severe respiratory acidosis are indications for endotracheal intubation and ventilatory support.

Postoperative Nausea and Vomiting

Perhaps one of the most annoying problems for patients and personnel in the PACU is PONV. A wide variety of agents have varying degrees of effectiveness for prevention or treatment of PONV (Table 14-10). No single technique has yet proved to be uniformly therapeutic and cost-effective. The use of propofol for induction of anesthesia has also been shown to be effective in decreasing the incidence of PONV. One important complication related to the IV coadministration of ondansetron and metoclopramide has been the production of bradyarrhythmias, including a slow junctional escape rhythm and ventricular bigeminy. More recently, the FDA placed a black box warning on the use of droperidol in cases in which additional ECG monitoring is required before and after administration of the drug because of an alleged increase in serious cardiac arrhythmias caused by Q–T prolongation. The FDA warning has been controversial because of the good safety profile of droperidol for 30 years and relative lack of scientific evidence to support the recommendation.[39] A study comparing droperidol and saline did not show a significant effect of either intervention on the Q–T interval during or after anesthesia.[40] Nevertheless, the FDA recommendation has caused a significant reduction in the use of droperidol for the treatment of PONV.

The approach to the prophylaxis and treatment of PONV is guided by an understanding of the mechanisms causing nausea and vomiting. Areas in the brainstem that control nausea and vomiting reflexes, such as the chemoreceptor trigger zone, contain receptors for dopamine, acetylcholine, histamine, and serotonin. Binding of all of these receptors may precipitate nausea or vomiting or both. Effective pharmacologic approaches to the treatment of PONV include the use of anticholinergics, serotonin receptor antagonists, antidopaminergics, corticosteroids and antihistamines (see Table 14-10). The use of any particular agent is based

TABLE 14-10 Commonly Used Antiemetic Agents

DRUG CLASS	COMMON SIDE EFFECTS
Dopamine Receptor Antagonists (D_2)	
Phenothiazines	
Fluphenazine	
Chlorpromazine	
Prochlorperazine	Sedation
Butyrophenones	Dissociation
Droperidol	Extrapyramidal effects
Haloperidol	
Substituted benzamide	
Metoclopramide	
Antihistamines (H_1)	
Diphenhydramine	Sedation
Promethazine	Dry mouth
Anticholinergics	
Scopolamine	Sedation
Atropine	Dry mouth
	Tachycardia
Serotonin Receptor Antagonists	
Ondansetron	Headache
Dolasetron	
Corticosteroids	
Dexamethasone	Glucose intolerance
Methylprednisolone	Altered wound healing
Hydrocortisone	Immunosuppression
	Renal effects

on efficacy, potential side effects, and cost. In patients at high risk of PONV or in patients with a history of PONV, it is often effective to employ a multimodal approach.

Hypothermia

Hypothermia has been extensively studied as a perioperative complication. The most important issues related to perioperative hypothermia include the risk of increased oxygen consumption postoperatively as a result of shivering, alterations in drug metabolism, effects on blood coagulation, and the possibility that hypothermia could increase the rate of surgical infections. Increased oxygen consumption could be a particular problem in patients with CAD, in whom shivering could trigger myocardial ischemia. However, the risk associated with mild hypothermia has not been well defined in otherwise healthy patients. Nevertheless, the Center for Medicare and Medicaid Services has designated perioperative normothermia as a Pay for Performance issue. This means that hospitals and medical centers that report on and achieve perioperative normothermia (36° C within 30 minutes of arrival in the PACU for procedures lasting for >1 hour) receive financial incentives.

General anesthesia has profound effects on thermoregulatory mechanisms, and active intraoperative warming is required to maintain normothermia under most conditions. Forced air and circulating water warmers are the most effective techniques for providing active intraoperative warming, each having advantages under different conditions. IV fluid warmers and airway warming devices can also be useful for minimizing heat loss but do not allow for active warming. Because of the effects of anesthesia on heat redistribution to the skin and peripheral tissues, preoperative warming is required to minimize core hypothermia in patients undergoing procedures lasting less than 1 hour. Studies indicate that prophylactic warming decreases the incidence of postoperative hypothermia and need for intervention in the outpatient surgical setting. However, time to PACU discharge and patient satisfaction were not affected. The use of prophylactic warming is associated with a significant increase in cost. Guidelines for temperature management during short, outpatient surgical procedures remain to be fully implemented.

Circulatory Complications

Hypotension in the PACU is most commonly due to hypovolemia, left ventricular dysfunction, or arrhythmias. Other causes include anaphylaxis, transfusion reactions, cardiac tamponade, pulmonary emboli, adverse drug reactions, adrenal insufficiency, and hypoxemia. Treatment involves support of the circulation with fluids, administration of inotropic agents, use of the Trendelenburg position, and delivery of oxygen until the underlying cause is diagnosed and treated.

Hypertension is a common finding in the PACU. Common causes include pain, anxiety, and inadequately managed essential hypertension. Hypoxemia and hypercapnia always need to be ruled out. Other, less common causes include hypoglycemia; drug reactions; diseases such as hyperthyroidism, pheochromocytoma, or malignant hyperthermia; and bladder distention. The fundamental goal in control of postoperative hypertension is to identify and correct the underlying cause.

Postoperative Visual Loss

Postoperative visual loss is a rare but devastating complication that occurs most commonly in patients undergoing prolonged surgery in the prone position (spine surgery) or cardiac surgery. The overall incidence is reported as 0.02%. Causes include retinal artery occlusion, cortical blindness, and ischemic optic neuropathy. Risk factors for the development of postoperative visual loss are not completely understood, but more recent studies have identified obesity, prolonged length of surgery, high intraoperative blood loss, and lack of use of colloids for resuscitation as possible risk factors. Because of the seriousness of the complication, the ASA has released a practice advisory on postoperative visual loss.[41]

ACUTE PAIN MANAGEMENT

Pain, one of the most common symptoms experienced by surgical patients, has historically been poorly evaluated and frequently undertreated. There have been important changes in medical care with respect to pain management, with inclusion of pain management in medical school curricula, establishment of institutional protocols and procedures for pain management, development of the subspecialty of pain medicine, creation of organizations focused on pain, and increased interest on the part of governmental and third-party payers. These changes are expected to continue into the future, and medical personnel must continue to increase their knowledge of pain control and their commitment to provide optimal analgesia as a key component of patient care. Surveys demonstrate that continued improvement is necessary to reduce further the high incidence of moderate to severe acute postoperative pain.

Acute pain occurs frequently in the setting of surgery and trauma. The pain experience may be part of the symptom complex that prompts the patient to seek medical care, or it may be caused by tissue injury sustained as a result of surgery or trauma. Acute pain is pain that is expected to be of relatively short duration and that should resolve with tissue healing or withdrawal of the noxious stimulus. Acute pain generally resolves within minutes, hours, or days. Chronic pain, which can persist for years, is defined as pain that persists for at least 1 month beyond the usual course of an acute disease or beyond a reasonable time in which an injury would be expected to heal. The acute stress response associated with acute pain serves a useful function, although undertreatment may result in harmful pathophysiologic changes. Chronic pain serves no useful function and is now recognized not only as a part of certain disease processes such as cancer but also often as a disease itself.

Mechanisms of Acute Pain

The International Association for the Study of Pain defines pain as "an unpleasant sensory and emotional experience associated with actual or potential tissue damage or described in terms of such damage." This definition emphasizes not only the sensory experience but also the affective component of pain. The tissue injury that leads to the complaint of pain results in a process called *nociception,* which has four steps: transduction, transmission, modulation, and perception. With transduction, the noxious stimulus is converted into an electrical signal at free nerve endings, which are also known as nociceptors. Nociceptors are widely distributed throughout the body in somatic and visceral tissues.

With transmission, the electrical signal is sent via nerve pathways toward the CNS. Nerve pathways include primary sensory afferents (primarily Aδ and C fibers) that project to the spinal cord, ascending tracts (including the spinothalamic tract) to the brainstem and thalamus, and thalamocortical pathways to the cortex. Modulation, the process that either enhances or suppresses the pain signal, occurs primarily in the dorsal horn of the spinal cord, in particular, the substantia gelatinosa. Perception, the final step in the nociceptive process, occurs when the pain signal reaches the cerebral cortex. The first three steps in nociception are important for the sensory and discriminative aspects of pain. The fourth step, perception, is integral to the subjective and emotional experience.

Methods of Analgesia

Multiple agents, routes of administration, and modalities are available for effective management of acute pain (Fig. 14-5). Analgesic agents include opioids, nonsteroidal anti-inflammatory drugs (NSAIDs), acetaminophen, and local anesthetics. Less traditional agents that may be used more frequently in the future include clonidine, dexmedetomidine, guanfacine, dextromethorphan, and gabapentin. Routes of administration include oral, parenteral, epidural, and intrathecal routes. The oral route is the preferred route for analgesic delivery. Patients experiencing mild to moderate acute pain and who can receive agents orally can obtain effective analgesia. Parenteral administration is preferred for patients experiencing moderate to severe pain, patients who require rapid control of pain, and patients who cannot receive agents through the gastrointestinal tract. The IV route is preferred over intramuscular and subcutaneous injections when the parenteral route is indicated. Intramuscular injections are painful, result in erratic absorption, and lead to variable blood levels of the administered agent.

Opioids

Opioids are potent analgesic agents that are effective but frequently underused. By binding to opioid receptors in the CNS and probably also in peripheral tissues, opioids modulate the nociceptive process. The best-characterized opioid receptors are μ_1, μ_2, δ, κ, ε, and σ receptors. The μ_1 receptors are involved in supraspinal analgesia. The δ and κ receptors are involved in spinal analgesia. Opioids can be administered by multiple routes, including oral, parenteral, neuraxial, rectal, and transdermal.

Opioids have varying degrees of potency. Strong opioids are ideal for moderate to severe pain and for pain that is constant in frequency. Weak opioid agents are suitable for mild to moderate pain that is intermittent in frequency. Morphine, the prototype strong opioid, can be delivered by various routes and techniques. Other strong opioids include hydromorphone, fentanyl, and meperidine. Morphine is metabolized to morphine-3-glucuronide and morphine-6-glucuronide, which can accumulate in patients who have renal impairment. Fentanyl and hydromorphone are more suitable agents for moderate to severe pain in patients with renal dysfunction. Historically, meperidine has frequently been the preferred strong opioid. This practice has declined because meperidine is metabolized to normeperidine, a unique toxic metabolite that can accumulate and cause seizure-like activity. Elderly patients, patients who are dehydrated, and patients with renal impairment are particularly vulnerable to this side effect. Fentanyl is available in a transdermal preparation, but this route is not recommended for acute pain management.

Weak opioid agents, such as hydrocodone and codeine, are commonly combined with aspirin or acetaminophen. Tramadol is an analgesic that is a nonopioid but has some opioid-like effects. It is a centrally acting agent that is administered orally and can be used for mild to moderate pain. Common opioid-related side effects include nausea, pruritus, sedation, mental clouding, decreased gastric motility, urinary retention, and respiratory depression. Appropriate selection of agents, monitoring, and treatment can prevent or ameliorate these side effects.

One major barrier to the effective use of opioid agents by patients, physicians, and other health care providers is the fear of addiction, which can be manifested as underdosing, use of excessively wide dosing intervals, administration of weak opioids for moderate to severe pain, and underreporting of pain. In the setting of acute postoperative pain, the use of opioids has not been shown to be a risk factor for the development of an addiction disorder. Key terms to understand include *tolerance, addiction* (psychological dependence), and *physical dependence.* Tolerance occurs when a previously effective opioid dose fails to provide adequate analgesia. It is a normal physiologic effect and should not be confused with addiction. Tolerance develops not only to the analgesic effect of opioids but also to most opioid-related side effects. The duration of opioid exposure also plays a role in the development of tolerance. In patients manifesting tolerance, an increased dose is required to achieve effective analgesia. Addiction or psychological dependence is a compulsive disorder manifested by preoccupation with obtaining and inappropriate use of a substance, continued use despite harm, decreased quality of life, and denial. Psychological dependence should not be confused with physical dependence, which is a normal physiologic process. Physical dependence is manifested by the occurrence of a withdrawal syndrome when use of a drug is stopped suddenly or when an antagonist is given. The duration of opioid treatment is a factor in the development of physical dependence. The short-term use of opioids in the perioperative period rarely results in physical

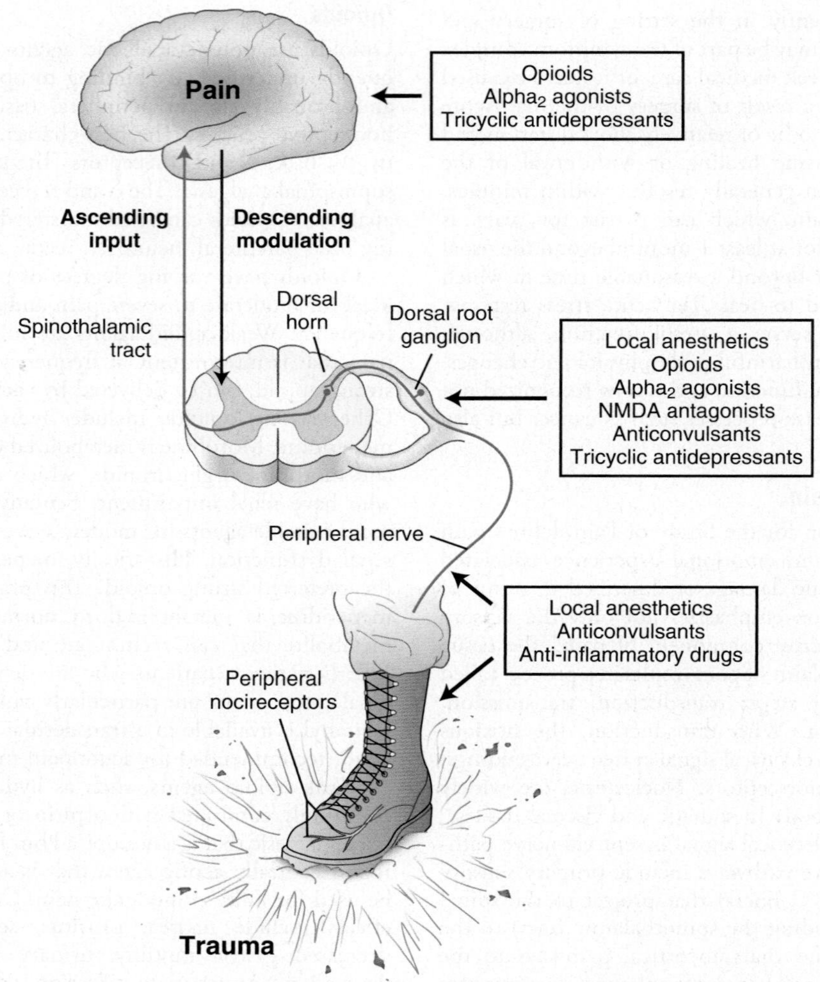

FIGURE 14-5 Schematic diagram outlining the nociceptive pathway for transmission of painful stimuli. Interventions that prevent nociceptive transmission are shown at the points in the pathway that are thought to be their sites of action. (From Buckenmaier CC, III, Bleckner LL, editors: *Military Advanced Regional Anesthesia and Analgesia*, Washington, DC, 2008, Borden Institute, Walter Reed Army Medical Center.)

dependence. Slow tapering of opioids generally prevents withdrawal symptoms.

Nonsteroidal Anti-Inflammatory Drugs

NSAIDs are an important component of perioperative analgesia that, when used as part of a multimodal analgesic approach, reduce pain and can decrease opioid consumption. Their mechanism of action is achieved through inhibition of cyclooxygenase (COX) enzyme activity, which results in decreased production of prostaglandins. Prostaglandins are potent mediators of pain that act directly at nociceptors and increase nociceptor sensitivity. Inhibition of prostaglandin production results in analgesia but can also lead to side effects such as gastric ulceration, bleeding, and renal injury. These side effects have limited the use of NSAIDs in the perioperative period. Contrary to previous evidence that NSAIDs act mainly in peripheral tissues, there is now evidence that NSAIDs also work in the CNS.

This analgesic class contains a wide range of compounds with differing chemical structures. Most of these agents are intended for oral administration, which limits their use perioperatively. Ketorolac is available for parenteral administration and has been shown to be effective for analgesia and safe with appropriate patient selection. Ketorolac is avoided in patients with a history of gastropathy, platelet dysfunction, or thrombocytopenia; in patients with a history of allergy to the agent; and in patients with renal impairment or hypovolemia. It is used with caution in elderly patients. A loading dose of 30 mg intravenously followed by 15 mg intravenously every 6 hours for a short course can provide effective analgesia for mild to moderate pain or can be a useful adjunct for moderate to severe pain when combined with opioids or other analgesic techniques. Moodie and colleagues[42] conducted a double-blinded, placebo-controlled trial in patients undergoing abdominal and orthopedic surgery. On recovering from anesthesia, subjects received intranasal 30 mg or 10 mg of ketorolac or placebo spray. Patient-controlled analgesia (PCA) morphine pump dose over 40 hours was lowest in the 30-mg ketorolac (37.8 mg) group compared with the 10-mg ketorolac (54.3 mg) and placebo (56.5 mg) groups. At 6 hours, the 30-mg dose of ketorolac was associated with lower pain, but the difference in either the pain level or the incidence of nausea or pruritus was not significant beyond this time point.[42]

The most recent advance in this analgesic category is the introduction of agents that are selective in their inhibition of subtypes of the COX enzyme. There are at least two subtypes of this enzyme: COX-1 (constitutive) and COX-2 (inducible). Traditional NSAIDs are nonselective inhibitors of COX. Newer agents (celecoxib, rofecoxib, valdecoxib) are selective COX-2 inhibitors. COX-2 inhibitors appear to offer similar analgesia with a reduced risk of causing gastrointestinal bleeding, bleeding diathesis, and renal compromise. They have mostly been studied and used clinically in the management of arthritis-related pain but are becoming more frequently used in the perioperative period. Currently available COX-2 inhibitors are for oral administration. In a study by Huang and colleagues,[43] the COX-2 selective inhibitor celecoxib was administered to patients undergoing total knee arthroplasty under subarachnoid blockade. A 200-mg dose of celecoxib was administered 1 hour before surgery and every 12 hours thereafter for 5 days. PCA morphine use was lower in the celecoxib (15.1 mg) group compared with the placebo (19.7 mg) group. Celecoxib use was associated with a lower pain score during the first postoperative 48 hours and increased knee range of motion during the first 3 postoperative days. Morphine-related adverse effects (nausea and vomiting) did not differ between groups.[43] Parecoxib is being studied for parenteral use. There are indications that COX-2 inhibitors are associated with a lower incidence of gastropathy. Concerns about the use of these selective NSAIDs include the risk for cardiovascular events and their effects on bone healing. Some of these agents (rofecoxib, valdecoxib) have been removed from the market because of the risk for cardiovascular complications. Valdecoxib was removed from commercial distribution because of the risk for severe skin reaction and cardiovascular complications.

N-methyl-D-aspartate antagonists. Ketamine has long been recognized as a powerful induction agent with strong analgesic properties, albeit at the expense of psychotropic adverse effects including dysphoria and psychosis at higher doses of the drug. Discovery of *N*-methyl-D-aspartate (NMDA) antagonists and their role in sensitizing the CNS has led to a re-emergence of this class of agents for use in management of acute pain in perioperative medicine. A prospective randomized, double-blinded, placebo-controlled study by Zakine and colleagues[44] compared two ketamine regimens against placebo. They used intraoperative ketamine (500 μg/kg load followed by 2 μg/kg/min) or intraoperative and postoperative ketamine (2 μg/kg/min) versus placebo in patients undergoing major abdominal surgery under general anesthesia. The authors noted lower morphine PCA use in the perioperative (intraoperative and postoperative) ketamine group (27 mg) compared with intraoperative ketamine (48 mg) and placebo (50 mg). Pain scores were lower in both ketamine groups compared with placebo and the incidence of nausea and vomiting was highest in the placebo group.[44] Similar results were noted in a study of patients undergoing total knee replacement surgery. Furthermore, a study by Remerand and colleagues[45] demonstrated perioperative ketamine to be associated with a 6-month reduction in chronic pain: 8% in the ketamine group compared with 21% in the placebo group. However, if ketamine is not administered via continuous infusion (i.e., PCA or intraoperative alone), it seems to be ineffective, as noted in a gynecologic surgery study (PCA) and pediatric scoliosis surgery study (intraoperative alone). Lastly in the NMDA group, magnesium has also been recognized to possess NMDA antagonist properties. However, it seems to be ineffective as an analgesic unless administered in high doses.

α_2-adrenergic agonists. There is a high density of α_2-adrenergic receptors in the substantia gelatinosa of the dorsal horn in humans, where it is believed that α_2-adrenergic agonists impair the transmission of pain signals. Clonidine, because of its potent antihypertensive properties, is of limited use in perioperative medicine. However, dexmedetomidine has been demonstrated to be effective in perioperative medicine with only transient effects on hemodynamics in exchange for improved analgesia and lower opiate use and lower related opiate side effects. In a study by Tufanogullari and colleagues,[46] which included patients undergoing laparoscopic bariatric surgery under general anesthesia, patients were randomly assigned into one of four groups: IV dexmedetomidine, 0.2 μg/kg/hour, 0.4 μg/kg/hour, or 0.8 μg/kg/hour, or placebo infusion therapy during the operation alone. The authors noted less PCA morphine use for up to 48 hours in the dexmedetomidine groups. The incidence of nausea and vomiting was lower and the PACU stay was shorter in the dexmedetomidine groups. However, pain scores were not different between groups, which the authors suggested may have been a result of not continuing the infusion in the postoperative period.[46] Aside from analgesic benefits, dexmedetomidine seems to have other preoperative advantages. Ji and coworkers[47] evaluated the association of dexmedetomidine in patients undergoing cardiac surgery beginning the infusion on weaning from cardiopulmonary bypass and continuing into the intensive care unit but for less than 24 hours. In their study, they noted reduction in hospital, 30-day, and 1-year mortality and reduction of complications including delirium. Pain scores were not described by the authors, and we cannot conclude if pain was lower with the administration of dexmedetomidine.[47] Guanfacine is another α_2-adrenergic agonist that is receiving attention as an agent to decrease postoperative delirium and serve as an adjunct for pain management. Guanfacine is delivered orally and has minimal cardiovascular side effects. Further study is needed to determine the efficacy of guanfacine as a perioperative adjunct.

Local Anesthetics for Management of Acute Pain

Local anesthetics work by blocking conduction in nerve fibers, the second step in the process of nociception. These agents are used to provide regional anesthesia for surgery, but their effects last into the postoperative period and contribute to preemptive analgesia. Local anesthetics used in lower doses than required for anesthesia can also provide analgesia by various application techniques, including local infiltration, topical application, epidural infusion, and peripheral nerve infusion. Local anesthetic infiltration was previously considered to aid postoperative analgesia, but emerging evidence suggests this therapy may lead to inconsistent results. In a study by Hariharan and colleagues,[48] patients undergoing abdominal hysterectomy were randomly assigned into one of four groups including local anesthetic (1% lidocaine with 0.25% bupivacaine, with 2 μg/mL epinephrine). Patients received local anesthetic infiltration under the skin preoperatively and postoperatively, preoperatively alone, or postoperatively alone or placebo. PCA morphine and pain scores were not different among all four groups suggesting these techniques are ineffective for perioperative analgesia in this patient population.[48] Topical application of local anesthetic includes the use of agents such as eutectic mixture of local anesthetics (EMLA cream), which contains prilocaine and lidocaine. This agent can be used for superficial procedures and can be placed before the surgical incision. Peripheral nerve catheters for local anesthetic infusion are frequently placed for postoperative pain management. The development of disposable and lightweight infusion pumps has led to increasing use of peripheral nerve infusion in the ambulatory setting.

Peripheral nerve infusion analgesia has been shown to provide improved postoperative pain control compared with opioid administration.

Combination Analgesic Therapy

Synergy may be obtained by combining agents from different analgesic classes. Synergy results in potentiation of effect and reduced dosage of each individual agent with fewer and less severe side effects from each agent. Common combinations include opioids and NSAIDs in an analgesic regimen or epidural administration of a local anesthetic with an opioid. The choice of agent and technique depends on factors such as the patient's medical history, the patient's preference, the extent of surgery, the expected degree of postoperative pain, the experience of the staff providing care for the patient, and the postoperative setting in which the patient will recover. Gabapentin, an anticonvulsant used for management of chronic neuropathic pain, has shown efficacy for analgesia in the acute postoperative period, including improved pain control and reduced opioid-related side effects. However, studies demonstrating benefit from gabapentin used doses of 900 mg or 1200 mg to demonstrate an analgesic benefit. In a study by Khan and associates[49] including patients undergoing lumbar laminectomy, patients received either 900 mg or 1200 mg of gabapentin in the preoperative or postoperative period. The authors found reduced morphine use in the first 24 hours postoperatively and lower pain scores with fewer side effects, regardless of the timing of (preoperative or postoperative) gabapentin administration.[49] In addition to acute pain benefits, gabapentin may play a role in chronic pain. Although pregabalin is not a new agent, its role in acute pain remains to be determined. There are a few negative trials, but emerging evidence may demonstrate an optimal strategy that will likely involve therapy beyond the hospitalization period.[50] In a study by Buvanendran and colleagues,[50] patients underwent a total knee arthroplasty under combined epidural-intrathecal anesthesia for postoperative epidural analgesia. Epidural analgesia was used until 32 to 42 hours postoperatively. Pregabalin 300 mg or placebo was administered preoperatively and tapered over 14 days. Epidural use was lower in the pregabalin group at the expense of increased sedation and confusion on postoperative day 0. However, there was an associated reduction in neuropathic pain at 3 months and 6 months in the pregabalin group. Other studies are ongoing.

Preemptive analgesia continues to be actively explored and used in the perioperative period. Induced by various agents and techniques, the goal of preemptive analgesia is to influence the analgesic process before initiation of the noxious stimulus (e.g., surgical incision). This analgesia minimizes sensitization of the nervous system and moderates the process of nociception described previously. Effective preemptive analgesia results in decreased postoperative pain, reduced postoperative analgesic requirement, decreased side effects from analgesics, increased compliance with postoperative rehabilitation, and decreased incidence of chronic postsurgical pain syndromes.

Neuraxial Analgesia

Neuraxial routes of administration include the epidural and intrathecal (subarachnoid) routes. These modes of administration require consultation from acute pain specialists, usually anesthesiologists who receive specialized training in use of the neuraxial route for the administration of anesthesia and analgesia. Neuraxial agents are delivered by a single injection into the epidural or subarachnoid space, by intermittent injections through an indwelling epidural catheter, by continuous infusion through an indwelling epidural catheter, or by patient-controlled epidural analgesia through an indwelling catheter. Indwelling subarachnoid catheters are rarely used for acute pain. An important consideration in selecting patients for neuraxial analgesia is the presence of abnormal coagulation, including concurrent use of antiplatelet and anticoagulant agents. Knowledge of such coagulation issues is important to minimize the risk for intraspinal bleeding and spinal hematoma formation, which can lead to severe neurologic injury. The neuraxial route requires education of the medical and nursing staff and the use of protocols and guidelines. In general, patients can be managed on surgical floors with these analgesic techniques. However, monitoring procedures need to be in place to minimize the development of side effects and enhance patient safety.

Agents such as opioids and local anesthetics are given via the neuraxial route to achieve analgesia. Other agents that have been used neuraxially include clonidine, neostigmine, and acetaminophen. Opioids, when delivered by the neuraxial route, provide analgesia by their action at opioid receptors located in the dorsal horn of the spinal cord. An important determinant of opioid action when delivered by the neuraxial route is the drug's degree of lipid solubility. Morphine is hydrophilic, which accounts for its slow onset of analgesia, long duration of action, ability to provide analgesia over a wide dermatomal distribution, and the risk for late respiratory depression. Fentanyl is lipophilic, which accounts for its fast onset and short duration of action, ability to provide segmental analgesia, and limited risk for late respiratory depression. A hydrophilic opioid such as morphine, when delivered into the epidural or subarachnoid space, remains in the CSF longer than a lipophilic opioid. The drug can travel rostrally to the brain and influence the respiratory centers hours after initial delivery.

Local anesthetics, when used for neuraxial analgesia, provide analgesia by blocking nerve conduction. To achieve neuraxial analgesia, local anesthetics are delivered in smaller doses and weaker concentrations than required to achieve surgical anesthesia. This resulting sensory blockade is sufficient to provide analgesia but not sufficiently profound to interfere with motor function and mask complications. Analgesic concentrations of local anesthetics also cause less impairment of sympathetic tone. Bupivacaine and ropivacaine are the most commonly used local anesthetics for epidural analgesia and peripheral nerve infusion analgesia. They affect sensory fibers more than motor fibers (differential blockade) and have a lower incidence of tachyphylaxis (tolerance to local anesthetic action). Neuraxial analgesia for acute pain commonly combines opioids and local anesthetics. Each agent has a different mechanism of action; combining these agents produces synergistic analgesia and results in reduced doses of each agent and a decreased incidence and severity of side effects. A meta-analysis of the efficacy of postoperative epidural analgesia concluded that epidural analgesia, regardless of agent, location of catheter placement, and type of pain assessment, provided analgesia superior to that of parenteral opioids.[51]

Intravenous Patient-Controlled Analgesia

An increasingly popular and effective modality using the parenteral route of administration is IV PCA. This modality minimizes the steps involved in the delivery of analgesia and increases patient autonomy and control. Opioids are the agent of choice for IV PCA. Comparing IV PCA with conventional intermittent nurse-administered opioid delivery, patients obtain prompt analgesia, receive smaller doses of opioids at more frequent intervals, can maintain blood concentration of drug in the analgesic range, and have a lower incidence of drug-related side effects. Candidates for IV PCA are patients who can understand the basic steps involved in use of the device, who are willing to assume control of their analgesia, and who are physically capable of activating the device. Such patients include children 4 years old and older and most adults, including geriatric patients.

The preferred agents for IV PCA are opioids, with morphine sulfate most commonly chosen. Other opioids used for IV PCA include hydromorphone, fentanyl, and meperidine. IV PCA with methadone has been described. Physicians' orders for IV PCA must specify the drug, drug concentration, loading dose, bolus dose, continuous infusion rate (basal rate), lockout interval, and dose limits. Selection of these parameters is based on the patient's age, medical status, and level of pain. The routine use of a continuous basal infusion rate with IV PCA is controversial. With a continuous infusion, drug is delivered to the patient regardless of demand, resulting in the potential for a higher incidence of drug-related side effects, including respiratory depression. It is safest to restrict the use of basal infusions to patients in special categories, including patients with severe pain from extensive surgery or trauma and patients who are tolerant because of long-term opioid use.

The use of structured protocols and guidelines is encouraged for facilities using IV PCA. The medical and nursing staff need to receive training in the care of patients using this modality. There is an increased risk for complications if staff members are not trained to understand the concept of IV PCA; to perform appropriate patient selection, education, and assessment; to use appropriate drug and dose selection; and to establish appropriate monitoring requirements and protocols for management of side effects.

Selection of Methods of Postoperative Analgesia

The choice of postoperative pain management strategies is a function of patient factors, surgeon preferences, the anesthesiologist's skills, and the availability of resources for postoperative care and monitoring.

Chronic Pain

In a subset of patients, pain persists after the expected healing time despite the lack of sufficient pathology to account for the pain. Pain that persists for 1 month beyond the expected time for recovery or initial onset is considered evidence of a chronic pain syndrome. Patients with persistent pain frequently use words such as "burning," "shooting," and "shocklike" to describe their pain, which is generally associated with a neuropathic pain syndrome. Neuropathic pain syndromes occur when there has been injury to the nervous system (central, peripheral, or both). Central sensitization is believed to underlie the development of neuropathic pain. Examples include patients with persistent pain after head and neck surgery, thoracotomy, mastectomy, hernia repair, and amputation. Certain factors that may increase the risk for chronic pain include infection at the surgical site, intraoperative trauma to nerves, diabetes mellitus, and nerve entrapment by cancer. There is some evidence that preemptive analgesia may help minimize the occurrence of these syndromes.

Because chronic pain syndromes can be difficult to diagnose in the early postoperative period, it is important for physicians to perform appropriate pain assessment during postoperative follow-up. For example, after amputation, patients might consider it strange to continue to feel sensation and pain in the location of an amputated limb and might be reluctant to volunteer information that they believe could suggest psychological instability. In such circumstances, appropriate questioning may elicit the complaint and result in patient reassurance and appropriate treatment. Referral to a pain medicine consultant is appropriate when the diagnosis of a chronic postoperative pain syndrome is made. Treatment modalities include the use of adjuvant medications such as antidepressants and anticonvulsants, nerve blocks, physical therapy, and psychological techniques.

Specific Types of Patients With Acute Pain

Patients With a History of Chronic Pain

Patients who have a history of chronic pain may experience acute pain as a result of surgery or trauma differently from patients who have no history of chronic pain. Their experience of pain is affected by their experience with chronic pain. Some of these patients may be receiving long-term opioid therapy as a part of their chronic pain management. It is likely that these patients will manifest tolerance to opioid therapy and have a decreased pain threshold, which may result in the patient reporting higher levels of pain and the physician increasing the opioid dose. Obtaining a pain history preoperatively, choosing anesthetic and surgical techniques to minimize tissue trauma and the response to trauma, and appropriate planning for postoperative analgesia can assist in achieving effective analgesia.

Patients With a History of Substance Abuse

Patients with a history of substance abuse are frequently undertreated for acute pain complaints. The stigma associated with drug abuse, misunderstanding on the part of health care providers, and inappropriate pain behavior contribute to undertreatment in this patient population. Effective analgesia can be obtained with strict guidelines, patient education, and appropriate use of consultants and modalities such as regional analgesia.

Pediatric Patients

Pediatric patients experience severity of acute postoperative and post-traumatic pain similar to adults. A major historical myth that has been refuted is the belief that neonates, infants, and children do not perceive pain as adults do. Effective analgesia for a pediatric patient experiencing acute pain can be achieved with pain assessment tools that are tailored for this population and modalities and agents similar to those used for adults. Dosage selection in a pediatric patient must be guided by calculations based on patient weight. With neonates, nurse-controlled analgesia is standard. Older children can use PCA effectively. Regional anesthesia is increasingly used for pediatric surgery, with the benefits of analgesia extending into the postoperative period and reduced opioid requirements. Epidural analgesia, usually via a caudally placed catheter or a single injection into the caudal canal, can provide effective analgesia. Placement of a peripheral catheter for infusion of local anesthetics can also be used. Topical anesthesia with local anesthetics such as the application of EMLA cream can likewise minimize pain from IV catheter placement and superficial procedures.

Elderly Patients

As the proportion of elderly adults in the general population increases, a growing percentage of geriatric patients are undergoing surgery or being treated for trauma. These patients require pain assessment and evaluation tailored to their mental status and cognitive abilities. The modalities and agents used to manage acute pain in this population must take into consideration underlying disease states and decreased organ function.

CONCLUSION

Largely because of important advances in anesthesia equipment, monitors, and drugs, modern anesthesia is safe and effective for most patients. With a wide variety of specific techniques available, selection of anesthetic and postoperative pain regimens for each patient can be based on the requirements of the surgical procedure, the patient's preferences, and the experience and expertise of the anesthesiologist. Patients with more significant comorbidities are receiving surgical care. Anesthesia practice is evolving to provide adequate risk assessment and risk adjustment and to optimize the care of the perioperative patient.

SELECTED REFERENCES

American Society of Anesthesiologists Task Force on Perioperative Management of Patients with Obstructive Sleep Apnea: Practice guidelines for the perioperative management of patients with obstructive sleep apnea: An updated report by the American Society of Anesthesiologists Task Force on Perioperative Management of Patients with Obstructive Sleep Apnea. *Anesthesiology* 120:268–286, 2014.

This report presents guidelines for preoperative assessment, perioperative management, and postoperative disposition of patients with obstructive sleep apnea.

Benumof JL, Dagg R, Benumof R: Critical hemoglobin desaturation will occur before return to an unparalyzed state following 1 mg/kg intravenous succinylcholine. *Anesthesiology* 87:979–982, 1997.

Using a combination of pharmacologic and physiologic information from the literature, the authors discuss in detail factors that influence the rate at which clinically important hypoxemia occurs in relation to the expected duration of succinylcholine. This article contributes an important counter to the common misconception that succinylcholine will be metabolized before hypoxemia-induced harm occurs.

Fleisher LA, Fleischmann KE, Auerbach AD, et al: 2014 ACC/AHA Guideline on Perioperative Cardiovascular Evaluation and Management of Patients Undergoing Noncardiac Surgery: A report of the American College of Cardiology/American Heart Association Task Force on Practice Guidelines. *J Am Coll Cardiol* 64:e77–e137, 2014.

In this extensive review, a joint task force of the American College of Cardiology and American Heart Association reports guidelines for evaluation of patients with cardiovascular disease who are scheduled for noncardiac surgery. The task force thoroughly examines the importance of the history, physical findings, functional status, and influence of various types of surgery as well as current recommendations on perioperative use of beta blockers, statins, and other medications. The value of preoperative testing is also evaluated. This report is a valuable update of a consensus approach to this topic.

Grosse-Sundrup M, Henneman JP, Sandberg WS, et al: Intermediate acting non-depolarizing neuromuscular blocking agents and risk of postoperative respiratory complications: Prospective propensity score matched cohort study. *BMJ* 345:e6329, 2012.

In a study of 18,579 surgical patients, the authors determined that the use of intermediate-acting neuromuscular blocking agents is associated with a higher incidence of respiratory complications during the postoperative period. The importance of ensuring adequate reversal of neuromuscular blockade at the end of surgery is emphasized.

Myles PS, Leslie K, Chan MT, et al: The safety of addition of nitrous oxide to general anaesthesia in at-risk patients having major non-cardiac surgery (ENIGMA-II): A randomised, single-blind trial. *Lancet* 384:1446–1454, 2014.

In contrast to previous trials, the ENIGMA II trial reported that use of nitrous oxide was not associated with an increased incidence of death, cardiovascular complications, or wound infection in high-risk surgical patients. Although the incidence of severe postoperative nausea and vomiting was higher (15% versus 11%) in patients receiving nitrous oxide compared with control subjects, the occurrence of postoperative nausea and vomiting in the nitrous oxide group was effectively controlled by antiemetic prophylaxis.

Punjasawadwong Y, Phongchiewboon A, Bunchungmongkol N: Bispectral index for improving anaesthetic delivery and postoperative recovery. *Cochrane Database Syst Rev* (6):CD003843, 2014.

The meta-analysis concluded that bispectral index monitoring can reduce intraoperative awareness in high-risk patients, but it is unclear if the use of bispectral index monitoring provides advantages in that regard over monitoring end-tidal anesthetic gas concentration in most patients.

Qaseem A, Snow V, Fitterman N, et al: Risk assessment for and strategies to reduce perioperative pulmonary complications for patients undergoing noncardiothoracic surgery: A guideline from the American College of Physicians. *Ann Intern Med* 144:575–580, 2006.

A consensus conference reviewed the topic of preoperative pulmonary evaluation. This group identified patient-related risk factors; factors related to the surgical site; and other factors related to surgery, such as the duration of surgery, choice of general anesthesia, and intraoperative use of muscle relaxants. Major patient-associated risk factors were American Society of Anesthesiologists class greater than II, age older than 60 years, functional dependence, and presence of chronic obstructive pulmonary disease or congestive heart failure. A serum albumin concentration of less than 3.5 g/dL was also a strong predictor of pulmonary complications.

Sprung J, Warner ME, Contreras MG, et al: Predictors of survival following cardiac arrest in patients undergoing noncardiac surgery: A study of 518,294 patients at a tertiary referral center. *Anesthesiology* 99:259–269, 2003.

Cardiac arrest occurred in 223 of 518,294 patients (4.3 per 10,000) undergoing noncardiac surgery between January 1, 1990, and December 31, 2000. The frequency of cardiac arrest in patients receiving general anesthesia decreased over time (7.8 per 10,000 during 1990-1992; 3.2 per 10,000 during 1998-2000). The immediate survival rate after cardiac arrest was 46.6%, and the hospital survival rate was 34.5%. In 24 patients (0.5 per 10,000), cardiac arrest was related primarily to anesthesia.

REFERENCES

1. Diemunsch PA, Van Dorsselaer T, Torp KD, et al: Calibrated pneumoperitoneal venting to prevent N2O accumulation in the CO2 pneumoperitoneum during laparoscopy with inhaled anesthesia: An experimental study in pigs. *Anesth Analg* 94:1014–1018, 2002.
2. Myles PS, Leslie K, Chan MT, et al: Avoidance of nitrous oxide for patients undergoing major surgery: A randomized controlled trial. *Anesthesiology* 107:221–231, 2007.
3. Myles PS, Leslie K, Chan MT, et al: The safety of addition of nitrous oxide to general anaesthesia in at-risk patients having major non-cardiac surgery (ENIGMA-II): A randomised, single-blind trial. *Lancet* 384:1446–1454, 2014.
4. Rooke GA, Choi JH, Bishop MJ: The effect of isoflurane, halothane, sevoflurane, and thiopental/nitrous oxide on respiratory system resistance after tracheal intubation. *Anesthesiology* 86:1294–1299, 1997.
5. Eames WO, Rooke GA, Wu RS, et al: Comparison of the effects of etomidate, propofol, and thiopental on respiratory resistance after tracheal intubation. *Anesthesiology* 84:1307–1311, 1996.
6. Fu ES, Miguel R, Scharf JE: Preemptive ketamine decreases postoperative narcotic requirements in patients undergoing abdominal surgery. *Anesth Analg* 84:1086–1090, 1997.
7. Katoh T, Ikeda K: The effects of fentanyl on sevoflurane requirements for loss of consciousness and skin incision. *Anesthesiology* 88:18–24, 1998.
8. Benumof JL, Dagg R, Benumof R: Critical hemoglobin desaturation will occur before return to an unparalyzed state following 1 mg/kg intravenous succinylcholine. *Anesthesiology* 87:979–982, 1997.
9. Domino KB, Posner KL, Caplan RA, et al: Awareness during anesthesia: A closed claims analysis. *Anesthesiology* 90:1053–1061, 1999.
10. Debaene B, Plaud B, Dilly MP, et al: Residual paralysis in the PACU after a single intubating dose of nondepolarizing muscle relaxant with an intermediate duration of action. *Anesthesiology* 98:1042–1048, 2003.
11. Grosse-Sundrup M, Henneman JP, Sandberg WS, et al: Intermediate acting non-depolarizing neuromuscular blocking agents and risk of postoperative respiratory complications: Prospective propensity score matched cohort study. *BMJ* 345:e6329, 2012.
12. Kreuer S, Bruhn J, Larsen R, et al: A-line, bispectral index, and estimated effect-site concentrations: A prediction of clinical end-points of anesthesia. *Anesth Analg* 102:1141–1146, 2006.
13. Leslie K, Myles PS, Forbes A, et al: The effect of bispectral index monitoring on long-term survival in the B-aware trial. *Anesth Analg* 110:816–822, 2010.
14. Punjasawadwong Y, Phongchiewboon A, Bunchungmongkol N: Bispectral index for improving anaesthetic delivery and postoperative recovery. *Cochrane Database Syst Rev* (6): CD003843, 2014.
15. Ferschl MB, Tung A, Sweitzer B, et al: Preoperative clinic visits reduce operating room cancellations and delays. *Anesthesiology* 103:855–859, 2005.
16. Shiga T, Wajima Z, Inoue T, et al: Predicting difficult intubation in apparently normal patients: A meta-analysis of bedside screening test performance. *Anesthesiology* 103:429–437, 2005.
17. Fleisher LA, Fleischmann KE, Auerbach AD, et al: 2014 ACC/AHA Guideline on Perioperative Cardiovascular Evaluation and Management of Patients Undergoing Noncardiac Surgery: A report of the American College of Cardiology/American Heart Association Task Force on Practice Guidelines. *J Am Coll Cardiol* 64:e77–e137, 2014.
18. Wilson W, Taubert KA, Gewitz M, et al: Prevention of infective endocarditis: Guidelines from the American Heart Association: A guideline from the American Heart Association Rheumatic Fever, Endocarditis and Kawasaki Disease Committee, Council on Cardiovascular Disease in the Young, and the Council on Clinical Cardiology, Council on Cardiovascular Surgery and Anesthesia, and the Quality of Care and Outcomes Research Interdisciplinary Working Group. *J Am Dent Assoc* 138:739–745, 747–760, 2007.
19. Qaseem A, Snow V, Fitterman N, et al: Risk assessment for and strategies to reduce perioperative pulmonary complications for patients undergoing noncardiothoracic surgery: A guideline from the American College of Physicians. *Ann Intern Med* 144:575–580, 2006.
20. Park JG, Ramar K, Olson EJ: Updates on definition, consequences, and management of obstructive sleep apnea. *Mayo Clin Proc* 86:549–554, quiz 554–555, 2011.
21. American Society of Anesthesiologists Task Force on Perioperative Management of Patients with Obstructive Sleep Apnea: Practice guidelines for the perioperative management of patients with obstructive sleep apnea: An updated report by the American Society of Anesthesiologists Task Force on Perioperative Management of Patients with Obstructive Sleep Apnea. *Anesthesiology* 120:268–286, 2014.
22. Yamakage M, Iwasaki S, Namiki A: Guideline-oriented perioperative management of patients with bronchial asthma and chronic obstructive pulmonary disease. *J Anesth* 22:412–428, 2008.
23. Warner DO, Warner MA, Barnes RD, et al: Perioperative respiratory complications in patients with asthma. *Anesthesiology* 85:460–467, 1996.
24. Sebranek JJ, Lugli AK, Coursin DB: Glycaemic control in the perioperative period. *Br J Anaesth* 111(Suppl 1):i18–i34, 2013.
25. van den Berghe G, Wouters P, Weekers F, et al: Intensive insulin therapy in critically ill patients. *N Engl J Med* 345:1359–1367, 2001.
26. Moonesinghe SR, Mythen MG, Grocott MP: High-risk surgery: Epidemiology and outcomes. *Anesth Analg* 112:891–901, 2011.
27. Newland MC, Ellis SJ, Lydiatt CA, et al: Anesthetic-related cardiac arrest and its mortality: A report covering 72,959 anesthetics over 10 years from a US teaching hospital. *Anesthesiology* 97:108–115, 2002.

28. Sprung J, Warner ME, Contreras MG, et al: Predictors of survival following cardiac arrest in patients undergoing noncardiac surgery: A study of 518,294 patients at a tertiary referral center. *Anesthesiology* 99:259–269, 2003.
29. Schwilk B, Muche R, Treiber H, et al: A cross-validated multifactorial index of perioperative risks in adults undergoing anaesthesia for non-cardiac surgery. Analysis of perioperative events in 26907 anaesthetic procedures. *J Clin Monit Comput* 14:283–294, 1998.
30. Warner MA, Shields SE, Chute CG: Major morbidity and mortality within 1 month of ambulatory surgery and anesthesia. *JAMA* 270:1437–1441, 1993.
31. Fleisher LA, Pasternak LR, Herbert R, et al: Inpatient hospital admission and death after outpatient surgery in elderly patients: Importance of patient and system characteristics and location of care. *Arch Surg* 139:67–72, 2004.
32. Neal JM, Mulroy MF, Weinberg GL, et al: American Society of Regional Anesthesia and Pain Medicine checklist for managing local anesthetic systemic toxicity: 2012 version. *Reg Anesth Pain Med* 37:16–18, 2012.
33. Guay J, Choi P, Suresh S, et al: Neuraxial blockade for the prevention of postoperative mortality and major morbidity: An overview of Cochrane Systematic Reviews. *Cochrane Database Syst Rev* (1):CD010108, 2014.
34. Swenson BR, Gottschalk A, Wells LT, et al: Intravenous lidocaine is as effective as epidural bupivacaine in reducing ileus duration, hospital stay, and pain after open colon resection: A randomized clinical trial. *Reg Anesth Pain Med* 35:370–376, 2010.
35. Horlocker TT, Wedel DJ, Benzon H, et al: Regional anesthesia in the anticoagulated patient: Defining the risks (the second ASRA Consensus Conference on Neuraxial Anesthesia and Anticoagulation). *Reg Anesth Pain Med* 28:172–197, 2003.
36. Metzner J, Domino KB: Risks of anesthesia or sedation outside the operating room: The role of the anesthesia care provider. *Curr Opin Anaesthesiol* 23:523–531, 2010.
37. Apfelbaum JL, Silverstein JH, Chung FF, et al: Practice guidelines for postanesthetic care: An updated report by the American Society of Anesthesiologists Task Force on Postanesthetic Care. *Anesthesiology* 118:291–307, 2013.
38. Xue FS, Li BW, Zhang GS, et al: The influence of surgical sites on early postoperative hypoxemia in adults undergoing elective surgery. *Anesth Analg* 88:213–219, 1999.
39. White PF: Droperidol: A cost-effective antiemetic for over thirty years. *Anesth Analg* 95:789–790, 2002.
40. White PF, Song D, Abrao J, et al: Effect of low-dose droperidol on the QT interval during and after general anesthesia: A placebo-controlled study. *Anesthesiology* 102:1101–1105, 2005.
41. American Society of Anesthesiologists Task Force on Perioperative Visual Loss: Practice advisory for perioperative visual loss associated with spine surgery: An updated report by the American Society of Anesthesiologists Task Force on Perioperative Visual Loss. *Anesthesiology* 116:274–285, 2012.
42. Moodie JE, Brown CR, Bisley EJ, et al: The safety and analgesic efficacy of intranasal ketorolac in patients with postoperative pain. *Anesth Analg* 107:2025–2031, 2008.
43. Huang YM, Wang CM, Wang CT, et al: Perioperative celecoxib administration for pain management after total knee arthroplasty—a randomized, controlled study. *BMC Musculoskelet Disord* 9:77, 2008.
44. Zakine J, Samarcq D, Lorne E, et al: Postoperative ketamine administration decreases morphine consumption in major abdominal surgery: A prospective, randomized, double-blind, controlled study. *Anesth Analg* 106:1856–1861, 2008.
45. Remerand F, Le Tendre C, Baud A, et al: The early and delayed analgesic effects of ketamine after total hip arthroplasty: A prospective, randomized, controlled, double-blind study. *Anesth Analg* 109:1963–1971, 2009.
46. Tufanogullari B, White PF, Peixoto MP, et al: Dexmedetomidine infusion during laparoscopic bariatric surgery: The effect on recovery outcome variables. *Anesth Analg* 106:1741–1748, 2008.
47. Ji F, Li Z, Nguyen H, et al: Perioperative dexmedetomidine improves outcomes of cardiac surgery. *Circulation* 127:1576–1584, 2013.
48. Hariharan S, Moseley H, Kumar A, et al: The effect of preemptive analgesia in postoperative pain relief—a prospective double-blind randomized study. *Pain Med* 10:49–53, 2009.
49. Khan ZH, Rahimi M, Makarem J, et al: Optimal dose of pre-incision/post-incision gabapentin for pain relief following lumbar laminectomy: A randomized study. *Acta Anaesthesiol Scand* 55:306–312, 2011.
50. Buvanendran A, Kroin JS, Della Valle CJ, et al: Perioperative oral pregabalin reduces chronic pain after total knee arthroplasty: A prospective, randomized, controlled trial. *Anesth Analg* 110:199–207, 2010.
51. Block BM, Liu SS, Rowlingson AJ, et al: Efficacy of postoperative epidural analgesia: A meta-analysis. *JAMA* 290:2455–2463, 2003.

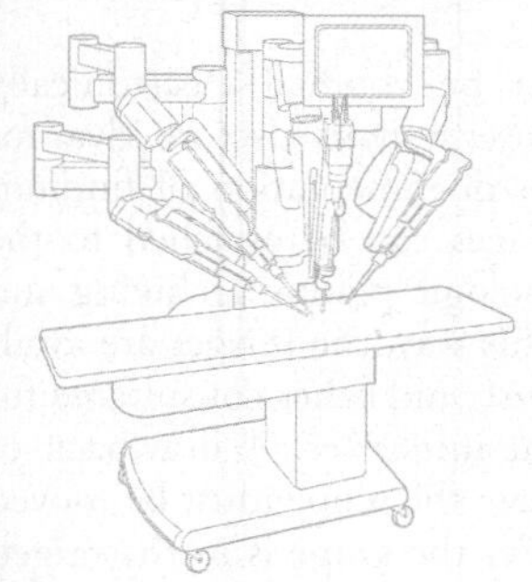

CHAPTER 15

Emerging Technology in Surgery: Informatics, Robotics, Electronics

Carmen L. Mueller, Gerald M. Fried

OUTLINE

 **Please access ExpertConsult.com to view the corresponding video for this chapter.**

There has been a dramatic change in surgical care over the past 25 years with the introduction of digitization, miniaturization, improved optics, novel imaging techniques, and computerized information systems in the operating room (OR) (Fig. 15-1). Surgery has traditionally required incisions sufficiently large to allow the surgeon to introduce his or her hands into the body and to allow sufficient light to see the structures being operated on; however, innovations have stimulated a radical change in the way surgical procedures are performed. Many surgical procedures have become image-guided. These procedures can be done by manipulating instruments from outside the patient, directing them by looking at displays of direct images of the target tissues (e.g., endoscopic or laparoscopic surgery) or at indirect images of the region of interest (e.g., endovascular catheter-based treatments, energy-focused ablation of tumors). Image-guided surgery has enabled the use of very small incisions or punctures to introduce surgical instruments. In other cases, the surgical instruments can be passed to the target tissue through anatomic conduits (e.g., arteries or veins) or natural orifices (e.g., mouth, anus, vagina, or urethra) without the need for any visible incision.

Although patients may benefit substantially from new technologies that minimize the invasiveness of surgical therapies, employment of novel techniques often requires an entirely novel skill set for surgeons. The concept of the procedure may be familiar to the surgeon, but the skills required to perform the surgery are different and must be learned and practiced to avoid the risk of complications during this learning or transition phase. Furthermore, "new" does not always mean better, and critical assessment of the utility, safety, and cost-effectiveness of new technology remains a cornerstone of the process of adopting innovations in surgery. This chapter describes more recent groundbreaking surgical innovations, highlights emerging technologies that are poised to change the OR significantly in the near future, and addresses approaches to training and establishing proficiency as new technologies emerge.

The authors gratefully acknowledge the contributions made by the authors of the previous editions of this chapter.

SIGNIFICANT ADVANCES IN SURGICAL TECHNOLOGY

Minimally Invasive Surgery

Accessing internal body cavities, such as the chest, abdomen, and pelvis, requires an incision. The size of the incision is determined by the need of the surgeon to see and to manipulate the target tissues. If resection is required, the incision size must take into account the dimensions of the tissues to be removed. In some cases, thorough histologic examination of the removed tissue is not critical (e.g., splenectomy for idiopathic thrombocytopenic purpura or hysterectomy for fibroids), and the resected organ may be pulverized or morcellated to ease its removal through a small incision. In other cases, such as colectomy for cancer, it is important to examine the removed tissues closely for the purposes of accurate staging and grading and to ensure that the resection margins are free of disease. In the latter cases, the incision must be sufficient to avoid compromising the accuracy of the pathologic examination. The goal of minimal access surgery is to diminish the trauma of access without compromising the overall goal of the surgical procedure (Fig. 15-2).

The "cost" to the patient of the access incision is multifactorial. Generally, larger incisions are associated with more postoperative pain, longer recovery periods, a period of physical disability, greater morbidity in cases of wound infection, more risk of incisional hernias, and a higher rate of symptomatic adhesive bowel obstruction in the future. It is estimated that approximately 20% to 30% of laparotomies result in incisional hernias. Because the success of incisional hernia repair is poor—approximately 30% of repairs fail—a large laparotomy incision in itself may lead to a second operation in 30% of patients and a third operation in a further 9% or more of patients to deal with complications of access.

The widespread adoption of minimally invasive surgery (MIS) has greatly diminished postoperative pain and the morbidity of wound infection as well as the longer term problems related to hernias and adhesions. However, the smaller incisions present some specific challenges to the operating surgeon.[1]

Laparoscopic surgery involves the placement of a small telescope into the body cavity. The scope provides illumination of the target tissues and conveys a bright, magnified, high-definition image to the surgeon through an attached or incorporated camera system. The view, particularly when using high-definition cameras, is startling in its clarity (Fig. 15-3). It eliminates shadows and affords all members of the operating team an identical view of the surgery. An important limitation of laparoscopic imaging is that it is generally monocular (compared with the binocular view we have in open surgery) because traditional scopes have a single lens system. With a monocular scope, the surgeon obtains a two-dimensional view of the body displayed on a video monitor. Other cues must be developed to appreciate the relative positions of the instruments and visualized tissues in three-dimensional view. This is a learned skill, and most surgeons are able to adjust to laparoscopic imaging with a little practice.

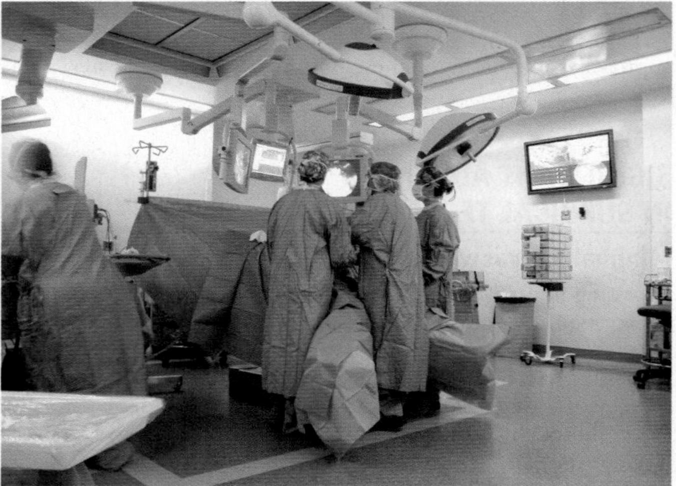

FIGURE 15-1 Integrated operating room (OR). The integrated OR provides digital information on multiple displays, controlled by the surgical team. The large flat-panel screen displays four images (endoscopic view, patient's vital signs, image of the abdomen captured by a camera in the OR light, and a room view). The central display in the surgical field is a touch screen allowing the surgeon to control the OR environment. The green lighting allows the surgical team to see well and do their work, while avoiding glare on the surgical displays.

Most scope-camera systems can be zoomed electronically and adjusted for light sensitivity. These systems also are ideal for recording static images or videos for documentation of findings or for teaching purposes. These images can be attached to the medical record and stored with radiologic picture archiving and communication system images. In this way, the images are available for the radiologist, the pathologist, and other consultants for patient care or quality improvement initiatives. A drawback of laparoscopy is the limited field of view; the scope must be moved to maintain an ideal image. The closer the scope is to the target, the better the illumination, magnification, and image detail, but the field of view is more limited. Constant communication between the surgeon doing the operation and the assistant managing the telescope is essential for safe surgery.

Laparoscopic images give the surgeon a view of the surface of tissues. In open surgery, the surgeon can palpate and compress tissues to gain a sense of the presence of pathology that lies deep to the surface. Because direct manual evaluation is unavailable during laparoscopy, the surgeon must adopt other methods to evaluate the tissues beneath the surface. Some of this information can be acquired before surgery by assessing the patient with cross-sectional imaging, such as ultrasound, computed tomography (CT) and magnetic resonance imaging (MRI). Digital images from CT and MRI scans can be displayed in the OR using surface markers to help the surgeon consolidate these findings with the visual display of the tissue surface during surgery. Advantages of ultrasound (Fig. 15-4) are that it is easy to use intraoperatively and it can be positioned to provide real-time information of the tissue being viewed through the scope. A surgeon proficient in intraoperative ultrasound can incorporate the surface and the cross-sectional information to evaluate the target tissues carefully.

Digitally Augmented Surgery

During MIS, the surgeon's eye is on the display monitor. One advantage presented by this setup is the display of multiple pieces of information on the imaging screen.[2] Most data required by the surgical team are available digitally and can be routed to any display device. Important hemodynamic data on the patient acquired by the anesthesiologist can be displayed on the surgeon's monitor. When operating on an unstable patient, this display provides valuable real-time data to the surgeon. Similarly, the surgeon can display real-time imaging information provided by intraoperative ultrasound, flexible endoscopy or fluoroscopy, or preoperatively acquired images (e.g., CT, MRI) simultaneously with the laparoscopic images using picture-in-picture, split-screen,

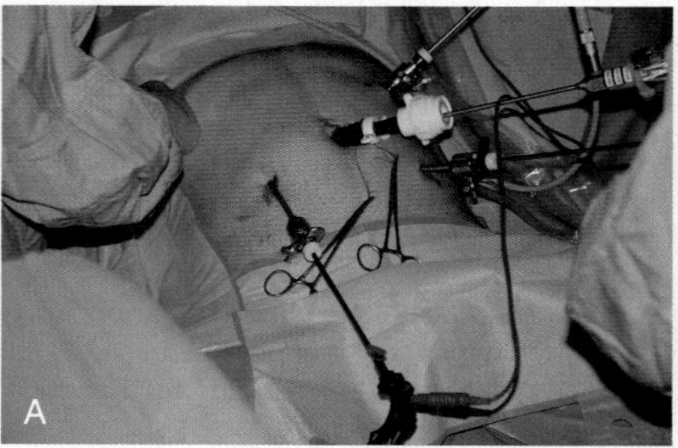

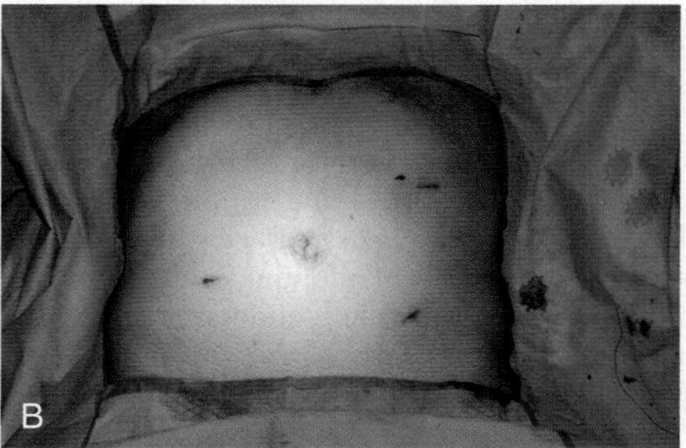

FIGURE 15-2 Surgical field for laparoscopic colectomy. **A,** The instruments are passed through trocars in the abdominal wall. **B,** The small incisions at the completion of the surgery. The largest incision at the umbilicus was to extract the specimen.

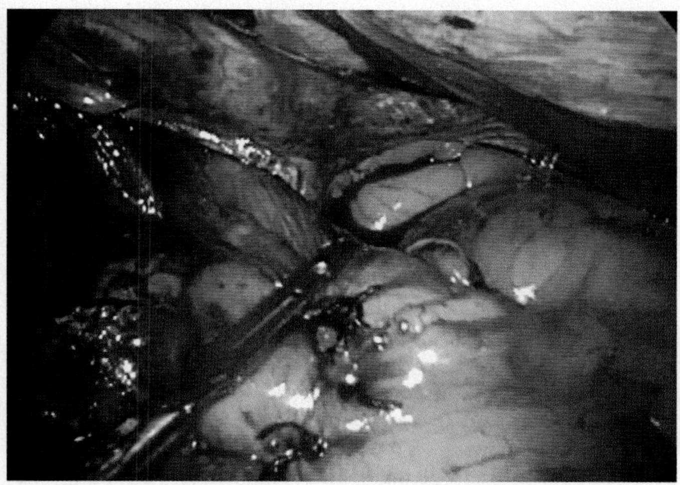

FIGURE 15-3 Laparoscopic image provides a magnified, high-resolution, and well-illuminated view for the entire surgical team.

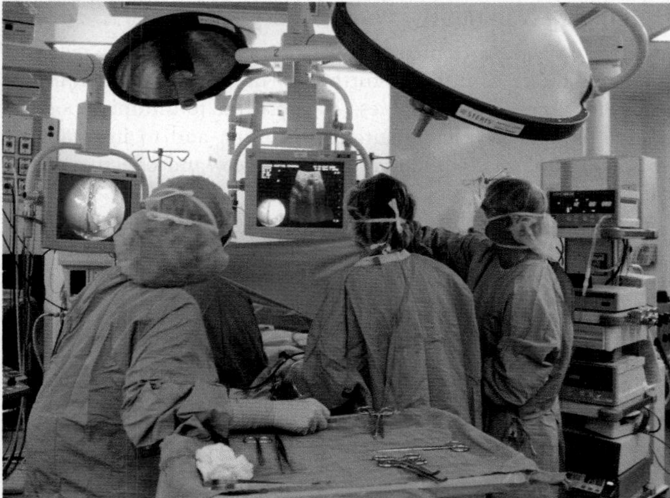

FIGURE 15-4 Laparoscopic ultrasound. Surface imaging by laparoscopy and cross-section imaging with ultrasound are complementary.

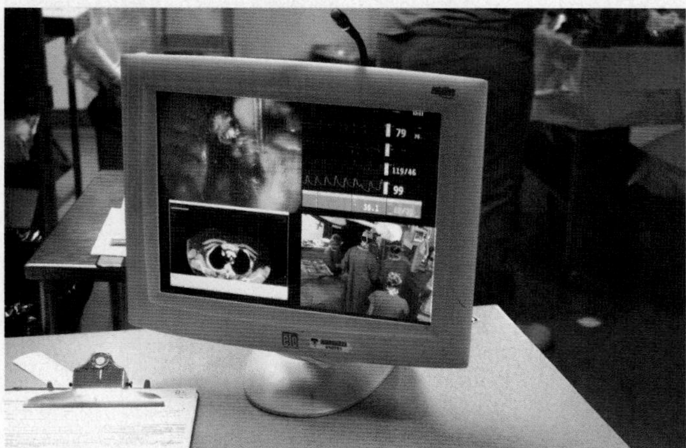

FIGURE 15-5 Quad-split screen display. The surgeon can select up to four images to be displayed simultaneously on a monitor. This display at the nursing station shows the endoscopic image, the preoperative computed tomography image, vital signs, and the room view.

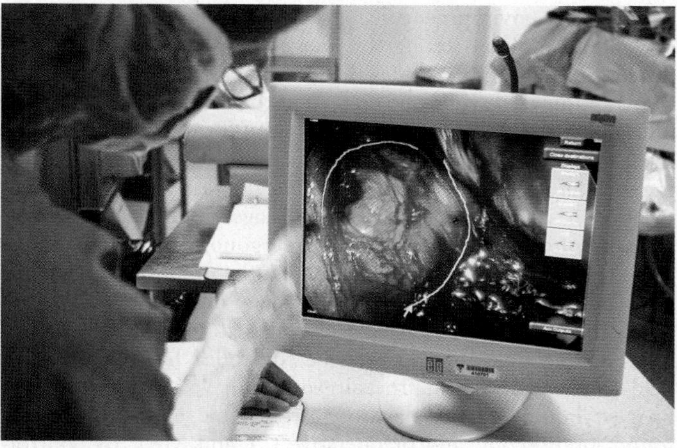

FIGURE 15-6 Telestration allows the surgeon to use the touch screen to annotate the image for documentation or teaching.

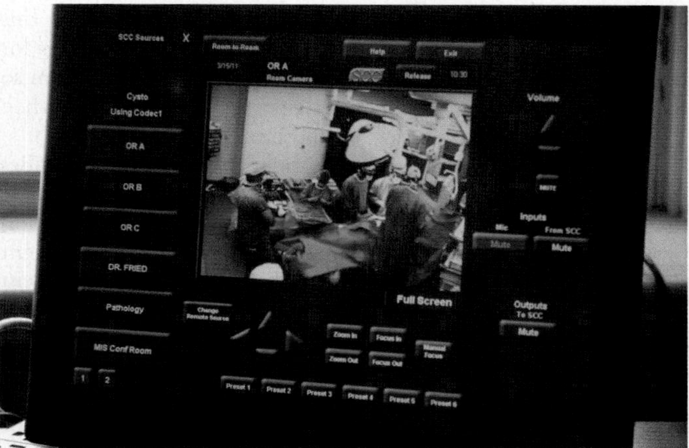

FIGURE 15-7 The touch interface in the surgeon's office allows him to select the image source and display this remotely.

or quad-split screen displays (Fig. 15-5). The surgeon can use telestration techniques (such as used to outline plays on television sports broadcasts) to communicate with the assistant or point out findings to students (Fig. 15-6).

Videoconferencing can be readily available and built into today's ORs, bringing consultant surgical specialists, pathologists, and radiologists into the previously closed surgical arena. Videoconferencing provides a useful context for intraoperative interpretation of findings from nonsurgical members of the patient care team. In digitally augmented surgery, the surgeon can have access to a whole dashboard of information and select the relevant data for heads-up display during the procedure. The routing of digital information to displays can be carried out using voice controls or touch screens in the surgical field. The OR images can also be accessed remotely in real time with appropriate security and privileges (Fig. 15-7). Furthermore, videoconferencing technology has allowed for remote training and mentoring through the processes of telementoring and teleproctoring in the OR and in surgical simulation. Video feeds of live surgical procedures can include audio commentating and allow large groups of surgeons to learn simultaneously from a single expert.[3] This technology also has been adapted for open surgery, with head-mounted camera systems able to project and record procedures the same way surgeons have been doing with laparoscopic procedures for years.

The OR environment has been completely redesigned to provide an optimal setting for image-guided surgery.[3] Ambient tinted room lighting provides the surgeon a glare-free view of the display monitors, while allowing the others in the OR sufficient illumination to move around the room and carry out their work safely. The surgical team has access to multiple monitors to display the surgical images and other digital information. It is not unusual to have six or seven monitors in an image-guided surgical suite. Each monitor can be moved into an ergonomically comfortable viewing position; it has been shown that the monitor position has an impact on the precision and efficiency of the surgical procedure. Integrated ORs have been designed so that all devices, lighting, and image routing can be controlled from the surgical field or a control station. The surgeon can have access to multiple images simultaneously—laparoscopy, flexible endoscopy, ultrasound, fluoroscopy, and preoperative CT and MRI. By controlling the interface, any digital image or combination of images can be routed to any monitor. Any image can be recorded to document the surgical findings. The images or video clips can be annotated by verbal recordings or by textual description. This provides very valuable documentation of the surgical findings for the medical record. Prompts can be embedded into the system so that a visual or auditory reminder can alert the surgical team when it is time for the next dose of antibiotics.

Despite the many advantages, minimal access surgery provides some very specific challenges. When operating through a large incision, there are relatively few constraints on the range of motion of surgical instruments. If a surgeon wants to move the instrument tip upward, he or she can move the whole hand and instrument upward. In laparoscopy, the abdomen is insufflated with gas to create a working space. Generally, 5 to 6 liters of carbon dioxide is pumped into the abdominal cavity, separating structures and allowing the lens to focus on the target tissue from a suitable distance. To avoid loss of this working space, instruments must be passed through airtight trocars or ports placed through the abdominal wall. These ports have gaskets that seal around the instruments, maintaining the positive pressure and working space. The design of these ports poses some limitations on instrument design, such as the geometry and curvature of the instrument shafts (Fig. 15-8). Because the handles of the instruments are outside the patient, the shafts are generally quite long. Interposing the laparoscopic instrument between the surgeon's hands and the target tissue dampens tactile feedback. Surgeons rely on their determination of texture and compressibility to evaluate tissue characteristics and pathology. In laparoscopic surgery, the surgeon must learn how to interpret these characteristics through the instrument. In robotic laparoscopic surgery, the surgeon operates a device at a console outside the patient, which controls instruments inside the patient. Using robotic technology without haptic feedback results in complete loss of the sense of touch to evaluate tissues. Prototype instruments are being developed that incorporate haptics or that can display force feedback (tissue resistance) optically or by sound feedback; however, they have not yet been widely incorporated into clinical care.

As surgeons have become more skilled in laparoscopy, the variety of surgical procedures to which MIS techniques have been applied has continued to grow, bolstered by evidence of effectiveness and safety, patient demand, and better instrumentation. Relative contraindications have continued to diminish. At the present time, most elective and many emergency abdominal surgical procedures are frequently done laparoscopically.

Optimizing Minimally Invasive Surgery

Having realized the tremendous benefit of laparoscopy to patients, there is a desire to improve further by diminishing the injury of access to internal body cavities. The goals are to diminish postoperative pain, to accelerate surgical recovery, and to improve the cosmetic outcome, while maintaining safety and effectiveness of the surgical treatment.

One approach is further miniaturization of the diameter of the surgical instruments and telescopes (Fig. 15-9). As camera light sensitivity and image quality improve, high-quality images can be obtained through progressively smaller scopes. Previously, a 10-mm-diameter telescope was needed to provide sufficient light and image quality to perform surgery; at the present time, 5-mm scopes can provide images that are hard to distinguish from images of 10-mm scopes. Progressive reduction in scope diameter allows

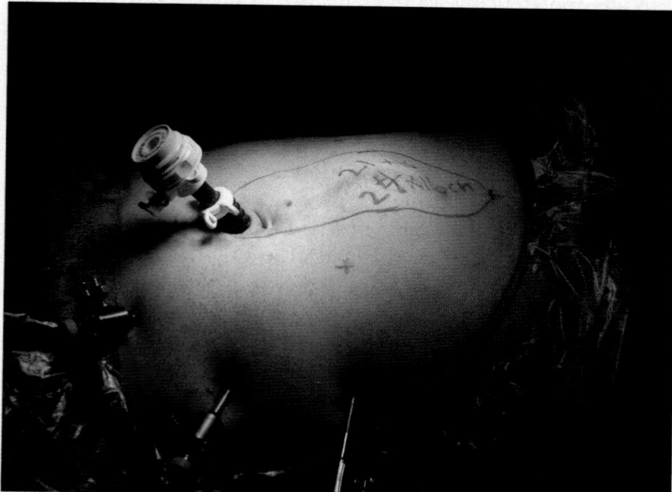

FIGURE 15-8 Surgeon working through trocars during incisional hernia repair.

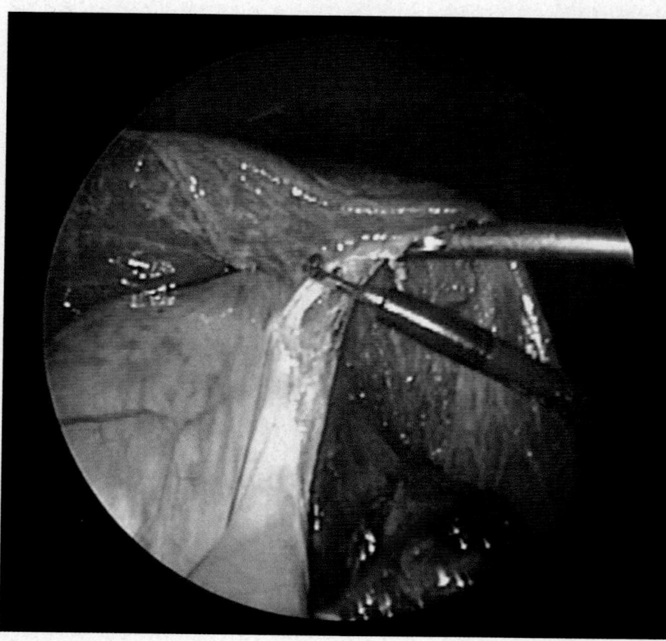

FIGURE 15-9 Laparoscopic cholecystectomy using 3-mm instruments and scope.

the surgeon to move the scope easily from port to port to provide different views of the surgical target and to minimize the cosmetic and functional problems related to these incisions.

Smaller surgical instruments with 2-mm diameters have also been designed, minimizing even further the incisions required for surgical access (minilaparoscopy) (Fig. 15-10), although these tend to be less robust and more limited in curvature than traditional laparoscopic instruments.[4] Single-incision laparoscopy was developed as a means to introduce all instruments through a single port, through an incision that can be hidden in most patients at the umbilicus and heal with virtually no scar. Although cosmetically appealing, single-incision laparoscopy has been fraught with limitations, including technical challenges in instrument design, interference between adjacent instruments and energy devices, a significant learning curve for the surgeon, and increased wound complications.[5]

Natural orifice transluminal endoscopic surgery (NOTES) is an evolving approach whereby access to a body cavity is achieved without any incision in the body wall. NOTES is truly scarless surgery, conducted by accessing the target organ through a natural orifice (mouth, rectum, vagina). After placing a flexible or rigid endoscope through a natural orifice, an organ (esophagus, stomach, colon, or vagina) is intentionally perforated, and the scope is advanced directly to the target tissue. One way this is accomplished is by passing a flexible endoscope through the mouth into the stomach and then through the stomach wall into the abdominal cavity. Other surgical instruments are advanced through or around the gastroscope and out this opening into the abdominal cavity. After the procedure is completed, the resected tissue is retrieved through the mouth, and the gastrotomy is closed. As might be imagined, this technique is fraught with challenges. Very long instruments are required, and they need to be directed by manipulating the visualization platform (endoscope) using specially designed elevators at the distal end of the scope; this makes it difficult to move the instruments without moving the view. The operating platform is flexible, and it is unstable for the surgeon to work. It also requires an iatrogenic perforation of a viscus to obtain access. Any failure of healing can result in peritonitis. Although access through the vagina is less risky than access through the stomach or colon, its potential use is limited to women, and the risk of postoperative dyspareunia remains to be determined.[6]

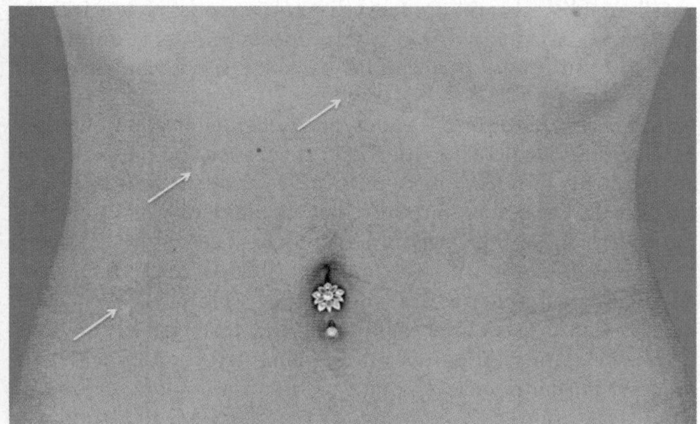
FIGURE 15-10 Incisions after minilaparoscopy cholecystectomy.

Clinical trials indicate that NOTES transvaginal cholecystectomy may be safe but requires significantly longer operative times and does not offer significant advantages over conventional laparoscopic cholecystectomy in terms of pain and recovery time.[7] NOTES techniques may be more applicable to procedures other than cholecystectomy, such as procedures that already require an opening in the digestive tract.

A new technique that is rapidly gaining popularity is treatment of achalasia by peroral endoscopic myotomy (POEM) (Fig. 15-11). The POEM procedure is a natural orifice technique that involves creation of a long esophageal myotomy using a flexible gastrointestinal endoscope. After incising the esophageal mucosa, a tunnel is created in the esophageal wall, the circular muscle is divided to a point distal to the lower esophageal sphincter, and the esophageal mucosal opening is closed with clips. Preliminary trials in skilled hands showed short-term effectiveness of the POEM procedure, equivalent to surgical myotomy in control of dysphagia, with low morbidity and rapid recovery; however, the procedure appears to be associated with a higher rate of gastroesophageal reflux compared with a Heller myotomy combined with an antireflux procedure.[8,9]

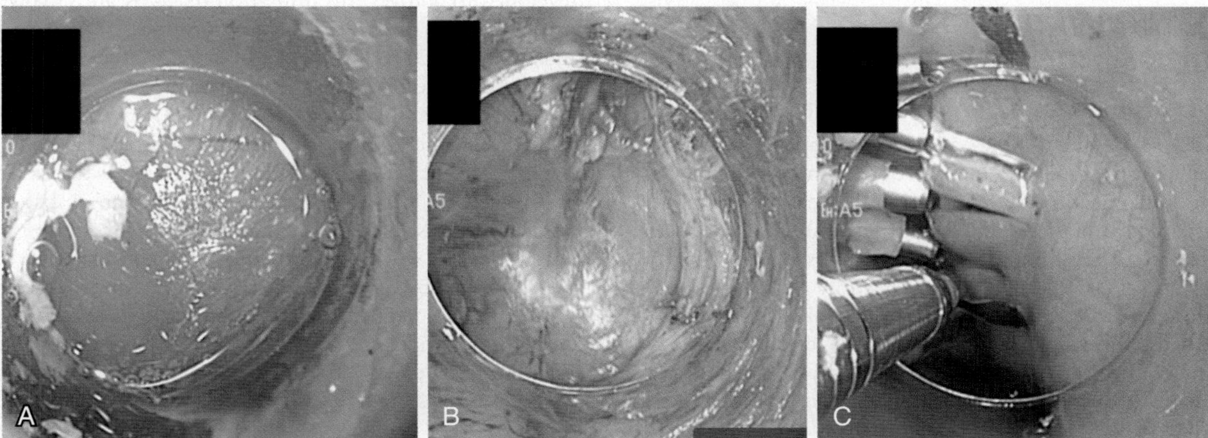
FIGURE 15-11 Peroral endoscopic myotomy. **A,** View of endoscopic submucosal tunnel. **B,** Almost complete myotomy with only a few circular muscle fibers remaining to be divided. **C,** Closure of mucosal incision with clips. (Courtesy Dr. Melina Vassiliou and Dr. Daniel von Renteln.)

Catheter-Based Therapies

Vascular surgery has traditionally involved replacing or bypassing occluded or aneurysmal vessels. Endovascular procedures have revolutionized vascular surgery in much the same way laparoscopy has impacted abdominal and thoracic surgery. Imaging is provided by fluoroscopy, and contrast solution is injected to outline the vascular anatomy. By accessing the vascular system by puncture or cut-down, instruments can be threaded along the vessel, narrow vessels can be dilated with balloons, and intraluminal stents can be threaded into position guided by real-time fluoroscopic imaging. Large incisions required for access in patients with serious comorbidity can be avoided entirely. Results of endovascular procedures are excellent, recovery is hastened, and the requirements for prolonged hospitalization and intensive care unit stays are reduced.[10,11]

In cardiac surgery, similar transcatheter endovascular approaches have been used to treat coronary artery disease, close septal defects, dilate stenotic valves, and replace cardiac valves. The idea of avoiding the stress and morbidity of a major incision is particularly appealing in these patients with serious underlying disease. Despite this appeal, the effectiveness and durability of these less invasive therapies must be compared with traditional surgical approaches.

Image-Guided Ablative Therapies

High-intensity focused ultrasound (HIFU) is a technique whereby ultrasound or MRI can be used to direct focused ultrasound energy to pathologic tissues. The acoustic energy absorbed by the targeted tissue causes rapid heating and destruction of the tissue. At the present time, applications are mostly for the ablation of uterine fibroids and benign prostatic hyperplasia. HIFU is an exciting example of image-guided surgery without any incision. The application of HIFU is growing; it is being evaluated for destruction of metastatic disease and treatment of arrhythmias.[12,13]

An analogous image-guided therapy is radiofrequency ablation (RFA). Using any of numerous imaging techniques (e.g., laparoscopy, ultrasound, CT, MRI), RFA energy is used to destroy pathologic tissues. Although HIFU can be delivered transcutaneously, RFA requires direct access to the target tissue for its effect. RFA has been shown to be an effective modality to treat tumors of lung, liver, bone, and kidney.[14]

EVOLVING INNOVATIVE TECHNOLOGIES IN SURGERY

Flexible Endoscope as a Surgical Platform

The development of the flexible endoscope has opened up a whole field of diagnostic and therapeutic opportunities. With only topical anesthesia or intravenous sedation, it is easy to pass a flexible endoscopic through the mouth or nose into the upper gastrointestinal tract or respiratory tree or a colonoscope through the rectum (Fig. 15-12). The scope is advanced by deflecting the tip of the endoscope using wheels at the handle, guided by the image provided by the miniature charge-coupled device chip at the end of the scope and displayed on a monitor. Channels in the scope provide access for instruments, and the lens can be irrigated and the field suctioned through the scope. Instruments that can be used with the flexible endoscope include specially developed instruments for punch biopsy, needles for injection and needle knives for incisions, snares to remove polyps or foreign bodies, balloons to stretch strictures, clips to occlude bleeding vessels or seal perforations, and stents for deployment across strictures or perforations. Energy can be delivered down the scope in the forms of monopolar or multipolar electrocautery, lasers, or heater probes to stop bleeding or ablate tumors. The flexible endoscope can provide high-definition images of the interior of the body and is a well-established and important diagnostic modality. It is increasingly being used for therapeutic purposes and is an important tool for surgeons performing gastrointestinal and thoracic procedures.

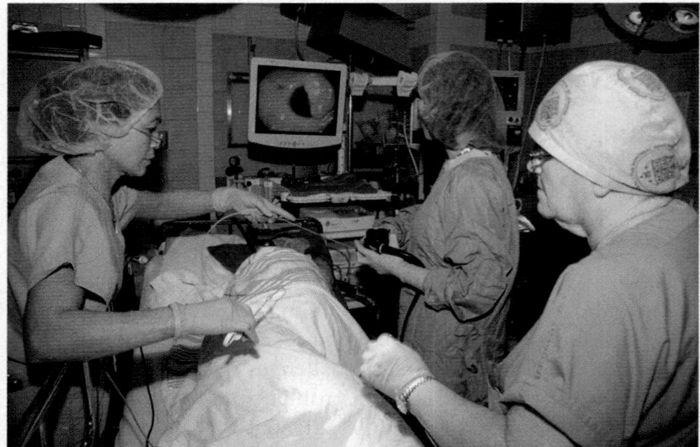

FIGURE 15-12 Flexible endoscopy is a platform for surgical therapy or an adjunct to open or laparoscopic surgery.

Surgical applications of endoscopes include resection of esophageal, gastric, and colonic mucosal tumors, sparing the patient an anatomic organ resection for early-stage cancers in which lymphadenectomy is not required or that would result in intolerable morbidity in a frail patient. Techniques currently employed include endoscopic mucosal resection (EMR) (Fig. 15-13) and endoscopic submucosal dissection (ESD) (Fig. 15-14), both of which require specialized equipment and technical skills. EMR involves elevating the tumor off the muscularis propria with submucosal injection, creating one or more tumor "polyps" through band application, and removing the lesion in a manner similar to polypectomy. This technique can effectively remove large mucosal lesions; however, piecemeal excisions create difficulty for the pathologist trying to assess lateral resection margins. ESD was developed to address this limitation of EMR and involves elevating the tumor off the muscularis propria through submucosal injection and dissecting beneath the tumor in the submucosal plane to remove it en bloc. The advantage of ESD over EMR is an intact and complete surgical specimen; however, this approach requires considerably more technical skill, particularly in areas that are difficult to reach endoscopically, such as the gastroesophageal junction. Highly specialized equipment is also required, including endoscopes with enhanced range of motion at the tip and additional working and water irrigation channels as well as specialized endoscopic dissection and hemostasis tools.

Despite the challenges associated with these techniques, the endoscope is increasingly being used to treat disease states that previously mandated a transabdominal surgical approach. Mainstream examples include gastrostomy tube insertion and common bile duct stone extraction; these two procedures are now almost exclusively performed endoscopically.

As surgeons have become increasingly comfortable with the flexible endoscope as a surgical platform, they have sought some

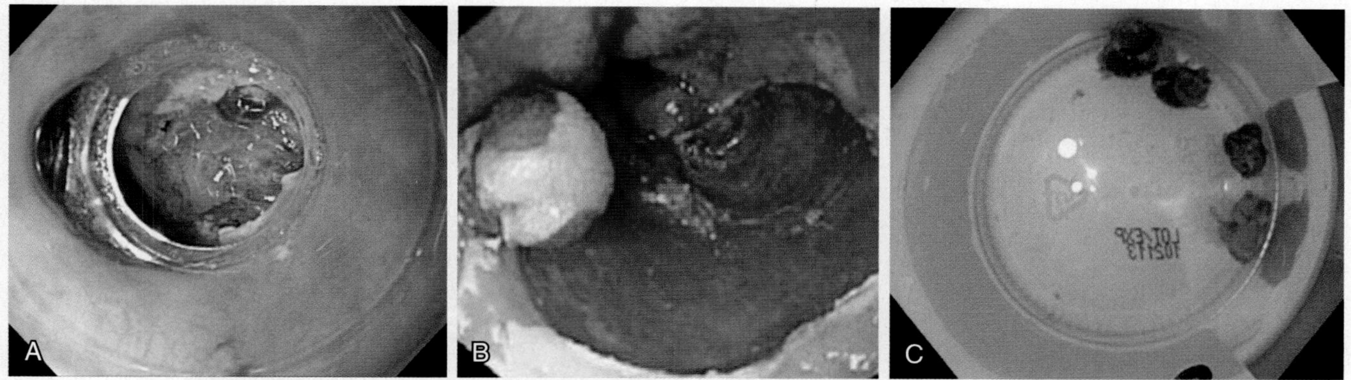

FIGURE 15-13 Endoscopic mucosal resection. **A,** View of target lesion through endoscopic cap. **B,** Target lesion is raised off underlying tissue by submucosal injection and banded to create a pseudopolyp, which is removed by a technique similar to snare polypectomy. **C,** Large lesions must be removed piecemeal using this technique. (Courtesy Dr. Lorenzo Ferri.)

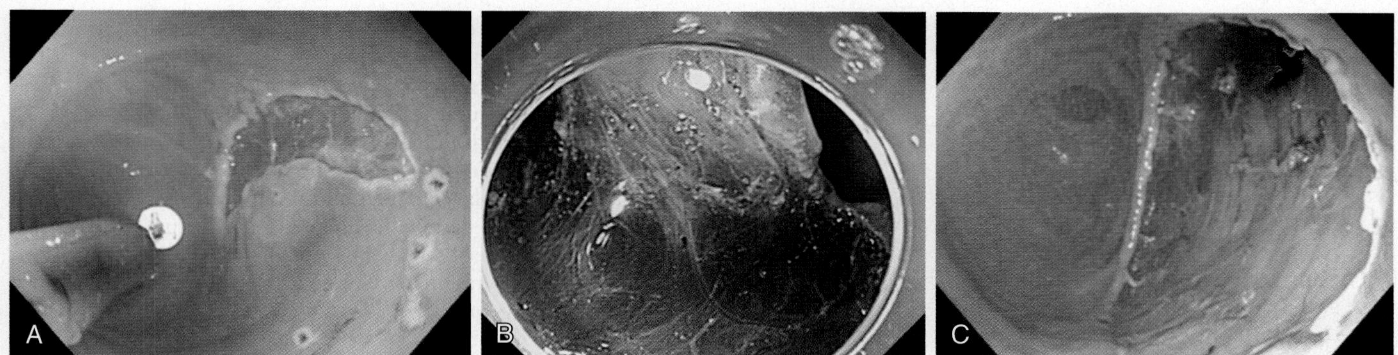

FIGURE 15-14 Endoscopic submucosal dissection. **A,** The target lesion is mapped out with radiofrequency energy and raised off the underlying tissue through submucosal injection. The mucosa is then circumferentially cut around the target lesion. **B,** The mucosal lesion is dissected from the submucosa. **C,** Resulting mucosal defect after en bloc removal of the target lesion. (Courtesy Dr. Lorenzo Ferri.)

of these capabilities for use in laparoscopic surgery. Thus, flexible tip laparoscopes have been developed that can provide effective visualization of hard-to-reach areas in the chest, abdomen, and pelvis.

Similar to other image-guided therapies, the flexible endoscope demands the surgeon be comfortable operating while viewing a monitor with a monocular optical system and be able to effect therapies using long instruments interposed between his or her hands and the target tissue. More recent advances have combined the outstanding imaging capability of the flexible endoscope with an ultrasound transducer at the distal end. Applications in the gastrointestinal tract (endoscopic ultrasound [EUS]) and bronchial tree (endobronchial ultrasound) extend the capability of the endoscope to visualize the complete thickness of the wall of the organ (for staging of tumors), adjacent lymph nodes (for biopsy), and adjacent structures (e.g., evaluation of the common bile duct or pancreas through the duodenum or stomach during EUS). Surgical procedures can be performed using EUS guidance, such as pancreatic pseudocyst drainage into the stomach.

Minimally Invasive Robotic Surgery

The concept of robotic surgery is to use the enabling characteristics of robots to improve the capabilities of the surgeon compared with working freehand.[15] In contrast to the use of robotics in industry, the robot does not work autonomously in most surgical applications, but rather acts as an interface between the operating surgeon and the patient. In this master-slave relationship, the surgeon (master) sits at a console, in an ergonomic and comfortable position, and uses movements of the hands and feet to control movement of the laparoscope and instruments (slave) in the patient. The commercially available robotic system in North America uses a proprietary laparoscope with two optical systems providing binocular (three-dimensional) vision. The surgical instruments are "wristed" near their distal tips, so the movements of the surgeon's hands can be reproduced by the instruments without the usual limitations of the fulcrum effect seen with traditional laparoscopic instruments. The degrees of freedom of the instrument are increased making it easier to do fine maneuvers than with traditional laparoscopic surgery. The surgeon can work from within the OR or remotely because there is no direct contact between the surgeon at the console and the instruments (Fig. 15-15). One consequence of this interface is that the surgeon has no tactile sense of the tissues and must adapt by using visual information.

Robotic surgery has opened up the concept of telesurgery. Theoretically, the surgeon can operate on patients at great distance[16]; however, trained personnel would still be required onsite to prepare the patient, insert the ports, dock the robot, change instruments, and intervene to treat complications or unexpected findings that cannot be controlled robotically. Before remote

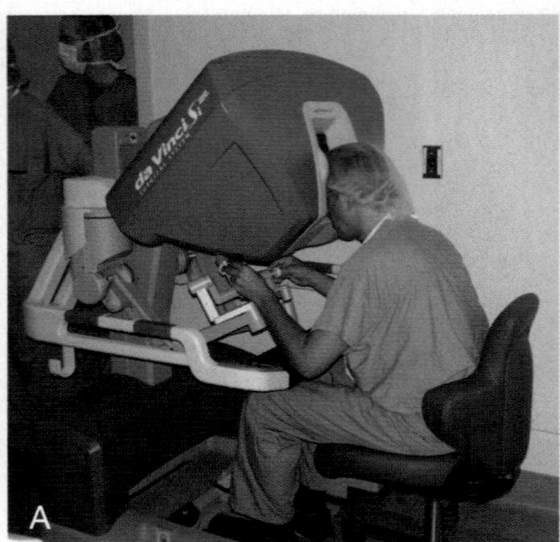

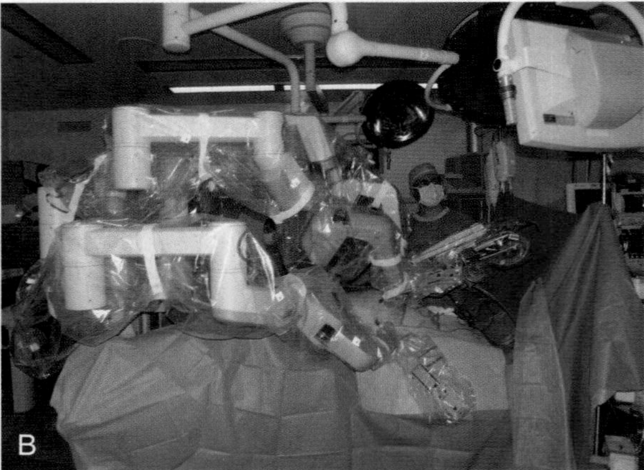

FIGURE 15-15 Robotic surgery. **A,** The surgeon at the console uses his hands and feet to control the robot arms. **B,** Robotic setup at the patient.

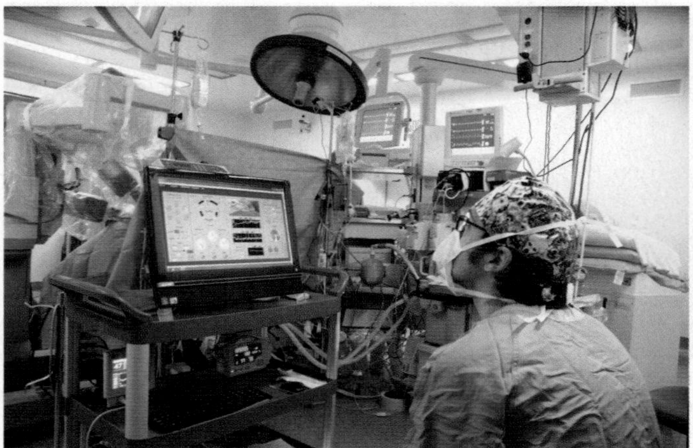

FIGURE 15-16 In this operation, robotic prostatectomy is being done with robotic-controlled anesthesia.

surgery can be applied practically, issues of licensing and liability must be addressed, and latent delays between the motion of the surgeon and the movement of the instrument must be resolved. The longer the distance that the data need to be transmitted from the console to the patient, the greater the latent delay. Delays of more than 250 msec can have a significant impact on the quality of the surgery.[17] Robotic surgical platforms are very appealing for support of injured soldiers and for support of patients in hostile environments, such as outer space missions, deep sea exploration, and polar expeditions.

Robotic surgery provides other exciting opportunities to enhance surgical performance. Because there is an interface between the surgeon and the effector instruments, it is possible to modulate the relationship between the surgeon's movement and the movement of the instrument electronically. The robot can adjust the gain or the scale of movement. In this way, the surgeon may make larger movements to effect very fine movements of the instrument tip; this can be very helpful for surgery that requires very fine and precise movements, such as suturing small vessels together. Algorithms can also be incorporated to dampen tremor using embedded filters. More recently, robotic surgery has been carried out in conjunction with robotic-assisted anesthesia (Fig. 15-16). Robotic-assisted anesthesia involves an automated platform where anesthesia agents are controlled using computer-assisted devices that calculate moment-to-moment anesthesia doses in a closed loop system to provide optimal dosing.[18] Similar systems have been used to enhance performance and safety in regional anesthesia.[19]

At the present time, MIS robotic systems are widely used in urologic surgery and gynecologic surgery and to a lesser extent in cardiac surgery, otolaryngology, and general surgery.[19-27] The main drawbacks are the costs, the bulkiness and setup time for the equipment, and the absence of compelling data to show superiority of robotic operations over operations done by well-trained laparoscopic surgeons.

Influence of Robotics on Other Domains in Surgery

Although conventional laparoscopy influenced much of robotic technology, innovation continues to flow in both directions between these domains, and lessons learned from robotic technology have been used to enhance conventional laparoscopic equipment. Traditional laparoscopic instruments are straight to allow them to pass through small-diameter working ports. However, this design presents significant challenges to the surgeon who often must move the tissues around the instruments rather than the other way around to complete a dissection. New articulating laparoscopic instruments address this problem by incorporating some of the range of motion traditionally offered by robotic platforms. Furthermore, three-dimensional laparoscopic imaging systems, originally available only for robotic surgery, have been developed for use in conventional laparoscopy as well. Evidence suggests three-dimensional camera technology shortens the learning curve for laparoscopic skills for novices and may enhance proficiency at complex tasks such as fine dissection and suturing for even experienced surgeons.[28,29] Limitations involve increased cost over traditional laparoscopes, the need for the surgeon to wear three-dimensional glasses to see the image properly, and reduced visualization when using energy devices as a result of the snowlike appearance of surgical smoke in three-dimensional view.

Perhaps the greatest influence robotics will have on surgery in the near future is the robotization of endoscopy. The execution of complex surgical tasks using endoscopes is conceivable, but currently available technology limits the practicality and feasibility of most endoscopic surgery today. Significant hurdles include lack of triangularization and instability of the flexible endoscope making lengthy and complex procedures difficult. In addition, the single-operator nature of contemporary endoscopes limits simultaneous operators working in the same surgical field to provide exposure and retraction. Robotic-assisted endoscopy could potentially address these issues. Although no commercially available robotic endoscope exists at the present time, numerous prototypes have emerged around the world, and this technology may be realized in the clinical setting in the near future.

Three-Dimensional Printing and Bioprinting

Three-dimensional printing technology emerged in the mid-1980s and was originally known as additive manufacturing. The process involves the deposition of materials other than ink from printer-like nozzles onto a moving platform according to computerized algorithms to create three-dimensional objects. Originally used in the manufacture of simple objects, such as objects containing glass, plastic, and metal, three-dimensional printing technology could conceivably be applied to create objects involving food, electronics, and even human tissue. The potential uses in medicine are vast, and this technology has only just begun to be explored for medical and surgical applications. At the present time, only approximately 2% of a 700 million USD industry is being directed toward medical applications, but this is projected to expand to a 1.9 billion USD industry for medical applications alone within the next 10 years.

In medicine, three-dimensional printing applications are being investigated for remote "printing" of prescription drugs, custom-fit prosthesis modeling, and preoperative fracture modeling for surgical planning and simulation training, among other applications. The use of three-dimensional printers to create human organs for transplantation (and other related forms of "bioprinting") may perhaps be realized in the not-so-distant future.[30,31]

Measuring and Predicting Innovation in Surgery

Keeping pace with changes in surgical technology and innovation can be daunting given the often rapid pace of technologic advancement and number of potential new technologies surfacing at any one time. A proposed mechanism to quantify and even predict emerging technologies in surgery is to track trends in the types of peer-reviewed publications and patent applications within surgical technology domains. It has been shown that new technologies that eventually become mainstream follow a sigmoidal pattern of prevalence of usage, with relatively little use at first (innovation phase), then increasing use (early adopter phase), then widespread acceptance (late adopter phase), and finally plateauing (maintenance phase). Literature publication and patent application numbers have been shown to follow this same pattern except that they precede the usage curve, meaning that such measures could serve as predictors of which technologies are likely to become adopted into the mainstream. Most recently, patent applications and peer-reviewed publications in surgical robotics and image guidance technology have emerged as front-runners, suggesting these domains may become the next fields from which the new technologies with the most impact develop.[32,33]

SIMULATION FOR SURGICAL TRAINING AND OPERATIVE PLANNING

Use of new technology in surgery, whether performed by laparoscopy, robotics, flexible endoscopy, transcatheter methods, or other techniques, generally requires a set of specific technical skills distinct from the skills required for traditional open surgical procedures. Each technique makes specific demands on the surgeon, requiring specific training programs. It cannot be assumed that a surgeon who is proficient at doing a splenectomy by laparotomy can smoothly adopt the laparoscopic technique for this operation without further training. Moreover, ensuring the adequate training of surgeons remains a critical step in the transition of a new technology from inception to a widely accepted practice norm.

There is a concept of the learning curve during which the surgeon acquires proficiency with a technique in the course of applying the technique in surgical practice. The evaluation of a new technology or techniques can be biased by evaluating the outcome of the procedure in the hands of a surgeon in the learning curve, and it may be unclear when the learning curve is completed. In this regard, outcomes measured at the introduction of a new technology may be more reflective of the surgeon's experience or proficiency with the technique than the merits of the procedure itself.

Learning a surgical technique in a simulation environment has many practical advantages. Specific learning objectives can be defined and modeled for learning, allowing the surgeon to practice repeatedly the specific skills that are required to make the transition to using a new technique. Practice on a simulator focuses the experience on the learner and not the patient. The learner can be allowed to progress at his or her own pace and go beyond his or her comfort level and experiment with different techniques or approaches. The surgeon can be allowed to make errors and to be required to correct them. Performance can be measured in a standardized and objective way and compared with an accepted performance standard (proficiency level).[34-36] We explore here the role of simulation-based education for the training of surgeons to do laparoscopic surgery. Many of the principles learned through this process have provided educational paradigms for teaching other innovative surgical techniques.

Simulation Training for Minimally Invasive Surgery

The advent of the laparoscopic era with the shift to image-based surgical technologies required abdominal surgeons to learn new skills. This was not a seamless transition, as evidenced by the increase in common bile duct injuries associated with the introduction of laparoscopic cholecystectomy in the early 1990s. Weekend courses simply did not adequately prepare experienced open surgeons to be proficient in the new image-based two-dimensional environment with the reduction in tactile feedback and increased hand-eye coordination required. Similarly, training programs struggled with how best to prepare residents for laparoscopic surgery. Coincident with the need to teach image-based surgery, other forces challenged the traditional apprenticeship model of surgical training, including an increased focus on patient safety, increasing OR costs, and limitations in resident work hours. These needs led to the development of models to allow the acquisition and assessment of fundamental laparoscopic skills outside the OR, through simulation.[37,38] This training paradigm shift was also occurring for open surgical skills[35,39] and in other technical specialties such as anesthesia, analogous to the use of flight simulators in the aviation industry.

Simulation allows for the acquisition of skills through learner-centered, deliberate practice in a safe environment, analogous to practicing an instrument. For example, instead of learning how to dissect the gallbladder from the liver bed during laparoscopic cholecystectomy in the OR, trainees acquire the fundamental psychomotor skills in a simulation center (Fig. 15-17), allowing them to focus on operative strategy, anatomy, and judgment with their clinical proctor in the OR. As such, simulation is best seen

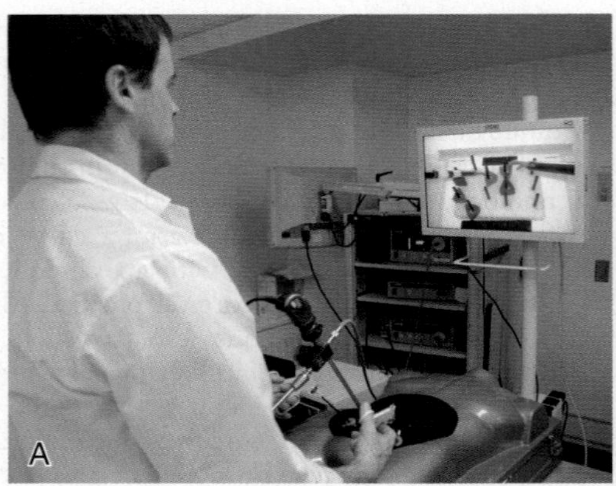

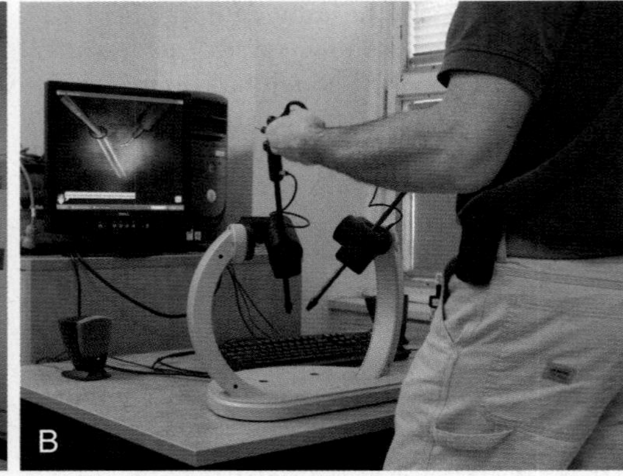

FIGURE 15-17 Surgical simulation. The learner is practicing fundamental laparoscopic skills in the simulation center on a physical box trainer (**A**) and a virtual reality simulator (**B**).

as a potentially important adjunct to clinical experience, especially during early training for a particular skill or procedure, and ideally within a developed curriculum. In laparoscopy, simulations include live animals, human cadavers, box trainers, and virtual reality (VR) trainers. Simulations may teach and assess fundamental skills (part task trainers) or entire procedures, teamwork, and interprofessional skills. Innovations such as the integration of trainers with actors to create human-simulator hybrids may enhance effectiveness. Simulation is often costly in terms of technologic and human resources. Objective assessment of performance is an important component of simulation-based training, to set practice goals, guide remediation, and judge the effectiveness of these new educational interventions. An overview of the role of simulation in surgical education is presented, focusing on its role in training and assessment for image-guided interventions and highlighting evidence supporting the transferability of skills from the simulated to clinical environments.

Teaching Fundamental Skills With Part Task Trainers

Part task simulators are used to teach and assess the component skills required to perform procedures and do not model entire operations. In laparoscopic surgery, these include box trainers and VR systems with tasks that develop depth perception, hand-eye coordination, and bimanual dexterity using various drills requiring the coordinated use of both hands in a two-dimensional space and more complex tasks such as suturing. The primary role of the simulators is to enable novice surgeons to acquire baseline psychomotor skills through deliberate practice outside of the OR.

A widely available part task box trainer system is the Fundamentals of Laparoscopic Surgery (FLS) program.[37] FLS incorporated the McGill Inanimate System for Training and Evaluation of Laparoscopic Skills box trainer to teach and certify fundamental technical skills in laparoscopy. Similar to other box trainers, FLS consists of a box covered with an opaque membrane through which trocars for instruments and a camera are placed. The trainee visualizes the interior of the box on a monitor, modeling image-guided surgery. Standard laparoscopic instruments, including curved dissectors, scissors, and needle drivers are used. FLS includes five tasks, scored for efficiency and accuracy in a standardized fashion, with error scores applied to penalize specific actions that should be discouraged. There is ample published evidence to support the validity and reliability of the performance metrics,[38] and FLS performance correlates with intraoperative performance as measured during gallbladder dissection from the liver bed in laparoscopic cholecystectomy. A proficiency-based curriculum has been developed based on FLS training to a specific performance goal. FLS training to proficiency results in greater improvements in OR performance compared with standard clinical training.[40] In other words, fundamental psychomotor skills acquired in a low-fidelity part task trainer such as FLS transfer to the OR environment. Simulation-based training is efficient and effective. The FLS program has established minimal standards of knowledge about laparoscopic surgery and the technical skill that must be demonstrated as the basis for practicing laparoscopy; the American Board of Surgery now requires FLS certification for general surgeons to qualify for the board examination. The requisite skills may be developed by practicing using simple box trainer simulations, or more complex VR systems.

After acquiring proficiency using part task trainer simulations, these skills can be applied to the performance of laparoscopic procedures. Using VR and physical training systems, entire procedures can be learned and performance assessed in the safety of a simulation environment. The advantage of this approach is that the learner can acquire skills rapidly, explore different approaches to performing an operation, assess specific enabling devices and instrumentation, and practice dealing with complications that are apt to occur in practice. Simulation is oriented around the learner, whereas patient safety is paramount in the clinical learning environment. When the procedure evolves (e.g., from multiport laparoscopy to single-port laparoscopy), the learner can upgrade his or her skills using simulation to decrease the learning curve (Fig. 15-18).

Based on the box trainer platform, numerous other laparoscopic skills tasks can and have been developed to facilitate training in specialized laparoscopic skills. Models can simulate partial advanced laparoscopic tasks, such as running a suture line or needle, or mimic complete operations, such as hernia repair and hiatal surgery.[41,42] The box trainer platform, a simple yet high-fidelity training model, allows motivated instructors and trainees to develop new training tasks to suit their individual needs locally, without incurring high equipment and development costs.

Reliable and valid rating scales have been developed for assessment of clinical performance during laparoscopic surgery. These tools provide specific assessment of performance during each critical phase of an operation and reflect specific skills fundamental to performance of that operation. Using this information as a "needs assessment," a specific curriculum can be developed for each individual learner, creating a highly efficient and effective personal learning program.[43-46]

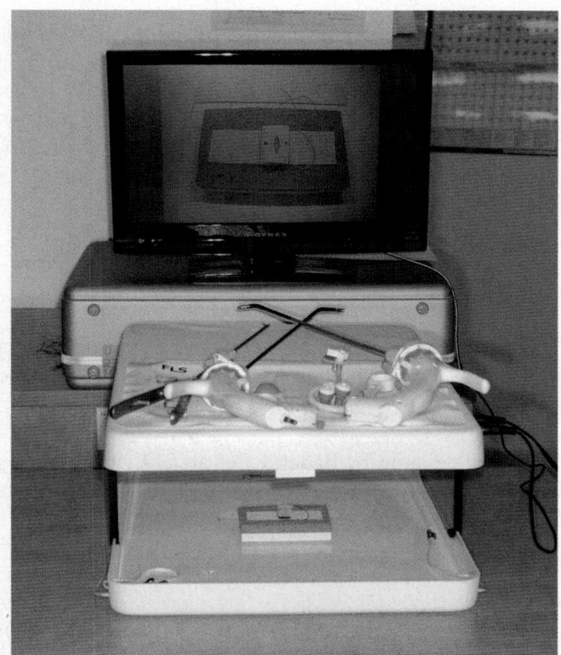

FIGURE 15-18 Part task trainer box used for the Fundamentals of Laparoscopic Study program can be readily modified to practice skills required for single-port laparoscopy.

Simulation for Endovascular Procedures

Endovascular procedures are ideally suited for simulation training. Numerous high-fidelity simulators are available to learn these procedures. VR displays provide images of the clinical problem; wires, balloons, and stents can be deployed to treat various pathologies in almost any anatomic location. This is a very effective platform to train in endovascular procedures for vascular surgeons, cardiac surgeons, radiologists, or cardiologists. A single simulator can provide educational opportunities to practice interventions on the carotids, cerebral aneurysms, coronary arteries, iliofemoral vessels, and aortic valve replacement.

Urology Simulators

Urology has a long history of application of image-guided or minimally invasive therapies. Transurethral approaches to the prostate, bladder, and urinary tract are well established. Advances in tissue ablation, such as the holmium laser, have enabled prostatectomy for benign disease to be done with very low morbidity. Most urinary stone disease can be treated by endoscopic or percutaneous methods or lithotripsy on an ambulatory basis without the need for general anesthesia. Because many of these procedures require specific skills unique to the procedure, simulation has proven to be a very useful platform to develop and practice these skills. Similar to endovascular procedures, commercially available VR systems are excellent platforms to practice a large variety of urologic procedures. Scenarios are available to challenge the learner with cases of varying difficulty, and performance can be easily evaluated.

Flexible Gastrointestinal and Respiratory Endoscopy Simulators

Although the flexible endoscope is an exciting platform for diagnosis and therapy, it requires substantial experience before its utility can be fully mastered. Numerous simulators have been developed for teaching gastrointestinal and respiratory endoscopy, including endoscopic therapeutic procedures, endoscopic ultrasound, and endoscopic retrograde cholangiopancreatography. These devices come with various clinical scenarios of different degrees of difficulty and complexity. The learner can become comfortable with the endoscope interface, can practice manipulating the scope to navigate the appropriate anatomic channel, can test his or her diagnostic acumen, and can experience various endoscopic therapies delivered through the scope. Metrics embedded in the simulator allows the learner to track performance over time and to compare his or her performance with that of a peer group or to a proficiency standard.

Until more recently, standardized ways to verify achievement of proficiency in flexible endoscopy were lacking, and competence historically was judged based on self-reported case numbers and clinical exposure. However, these measures are notoriously imprecise and give little objective information regarding an individual's endoscopy skills. To provide a more objective measure of basic endoscopy skills, the Society of American Gastrointestinal and Endoscopic Surgeons developed the Fundamentals of Endoscopic Surgery (FES) program. Similar to the FLS program, FES includes a didactic educational component, a knowledge test, and a hands-on skills assessment on a VR model. The VR hands-on component includes five tasks that test core skills needed to be proficient in flexible endoscopy: scope navigation, loop reduction, retroflexion, mucosal evaluation, and instrument targeting. The FES hands-on task scores have good internal consistency, and performance on these tasks has been shown to correlate highly with experience level and clinical performance.[47-49]

Simulation for Surgical Planning

The Holy Grail of surgical simulation is the concept of preoperative surgical rehearsal based on the anatomy and pathology of the specific patient being operated on. Because sophisticated imaging techniques provide anatomic and functional information in a digital format, three-dimensional VR models can be produced preoperatively that simulate the operative environment. Patient-specific imaging data can be modeled into a VR simulator with realistic haptic properties and with deformation with pressure and traction mimicking human tissue characteristics. The surgeon could then explore different approaches to performing a complex or high-risk surgical procedure, being able to interact with the patient's unique anatomy and pathology in the safety of the VR environment before actually undertaking the operation in the patient. Such modeling systems have been developed in neurosurgery, allowing surgeons to determine the optimal operative approach to challenging surgical problems such as arteriovenous malformations.[50] The application for neurosurgery is particularly attractive because the skull forms a rigid framework to the brain allowing accurate stereotactic representation.

Ongoing work in this area is also resulting in the development of applications of such technology to abdominal procedures, such as liver resection.[51] Preoperative imaging modalities such as CT and MRI can be used to render three-dimensional composite images that can be manipulated by the surgeon in VR preoperatively and intraoperatively. Information from these models can be used to guide the operative approach, predict the anatomy to be encountered at each operative step, and customize port placement to optimize operative ergonomics based on each patient's unique anatomy. In theory, an operation could be created similar to a movie, with editing of parts of the procedure that can be done better, recording all the movements, and playing back the perfect operation in the OR.

Measuring Surgical Performance During Simulation

The best incentive to improve technical skills is to measure them. Having a measure of performance skill allows the establishment of norms, proficiency target goals for training, comparison to peers, and an objective standard for certification. This measurement is possible only when performance can be assessed using metrics that have passed the standards of reliability and validity required to use these measures in a high-stakes environment. The parameters measured must reflect and predict clinical performance, must be practical to apply, must be meaningful to the learner, and must be generalizable to different learning environments. The attraction of measuring performance in a simulated environment is that the context for testing can be standardized, unaffected by patient differences in body habitus, anatomy, and pathology. The level of difficulty can be altered systematically and in a reproducible and standardized fashion. By providing a consistent test environment, the metrics can be evaluated scientifically, and improvement and learning curves can be tracked.

SUMMARY

Surgery is going through a rapid growth spurt as advancements in technology continue to be adapted to the OR. This is a stimulating time. The rate of innovation holds great promise for the rapid advancement of patient care. As previously distinct technologies such as surgery, endoscopy, and radiology continue to overlap in the ORs in the future, surgeons will be progressively challenged to embrace and master new techniques throughout their careers. In this landscape, simulation is predicted to feature prominently as a key training tool for surgeons of all disciplines.

SELECTED REFERENCES

Bhayani NH, Kurian AA, Dunst CM, et al: A comparative study on comprehensive, objective outcomes of laparoscopic Heller myotomy with per-oral endoscopic myotomy (POEM) for achalasia. *Ann Surg* 259:1098–1103, 2014.

Although a single-institution study, this article highlights the process of objective evaluation of new technology with reproducible, quantifiable, and clinically significant end points.

Faulkner H, Regehr G, Martin J, et al: Validation of an objective structured assessment of technical skill for surgical residents. *Acad Med* 71:1363–1365, 1996.

This article describes objective structured assessment of technical skill (OSATS), developed to evaluate surgical skill, and provides good validation data in support of its use. OSATS is one of the most widely used metrics for technical skill evaluation.

Fried GM, Feldman LS, Vassiliou MC, et al: Proving the value of simulation in laparoscopic surgery. *Ann Surg* 240:518–525, discussion 518–525, 2004.

An excellent summary is presented of the process of validation of simulation as a useful and effective way to assess technical skill in surgery. Using the hands-on component of the Fundamentals of Laparoscopic Study program as an example, the authors describe the way the metrics were validated and how the educational effectiveness was measured.

Krummel TM: Forecasting innovation in surgery. *Ann Surg* 260:212–213, 2014.

This article reports a novel and clever method of predicting innovations in surgery that are likely to become widely adopted and practice-changing technologies.

Mutter D, Dallemagne B, Bailey C, et al: 3D virtual reality and selective vascular control for laparoscopic left hepatic lobectomy. *Surg Endosc* 23:432–435, 2009.

This case report with associated videos demonstrates the integration of three-dimensional imaging and virtual reality simulation and the application of this technology to preoperative "rehearsal" of a complex laparoscopic procedure (in this case, left hepatic lobectomy).

Nagendran M, Gurusamy KS, Aggarwal R, et al: Virtual reality training for surgical trainees in laparoscopic surgery. *Cochrane Database Syst Rev* (8):CD006575, 2013.

This systematic review summarizes the literature regarding the impact of virtual reality simulation training on operating room performance. The article highlights knowledge gaps in the current literature regarding the impact of simulation training on clinical outcomes and provides direction for future studies.

Seol YJ, Kang HW, Lee SJ, et al: Bioprinting technology and its applications. *Eur J Cardiothorac Surg* 46:342–348, 2014.

The principles of three-dimensional printing technology and the current and soon-to-emerge applications of bioprinting in medicine are summarized.

REFERENCES

1. Himal HS: Minimally invasive (laparoscopic) surgery. *Surg Endosc* 16:2002, 1647–1652.
2. Bova F: Computer based guidance in the modern operating room: A historical perspective. *IEEE Rev Biomed Eng* 3:209–222, 2010.
3. Gambadauro P, Torrejon R: The "tele" factor in surgery today and tomorrow: Implications for surgical training and education. *Surg Today* 43:115–122, 2013.
4. Gurusamy KS, Vaughan J, Ramamoorthy R, et al: Miniports versus standard ports for laparoscopic cholecystectomy. *Cochrane Database Syst Rev* (8):CD006804, 2013.
5. Trastulli S, Cirocchi R, Desiderio J, et al: Systematic review and meta-analysis of randomized clinical trials comparing single-incision versus conventional laparoscopic cholecystectomy. *Br J Surg* 100:191–208, 2013.

6. Liu L, Chiu PW, Reddy N, et al: Natural orifice transluminal endoscopic surgery (NOTES) for clinical management of intra-abdominal diseases. *Dig Endosc* 25:565–577, 2013.
7. Noguera JF, Cuadrado A, Dolz C, et al: Prospective randomized clinical trial comparing laparoscopic cholecystectomy and hybrid natural orifice transluminal endoscopic surgery (NOTES) (NCT00835250). *Surg Endosc* 26:3435–3441, 2012.
8. Bhayani NH, Kurian AA, Dunst CM, et al: A comparative study on comprehensive, objective outcomes of laparoscopic Heller myotomy with per-oral endoscopic myotomy (POEM) for achalasia. *Ann Surg* 259:1098–1103, 2014.
9. Pescarus R, Shlomovitz E, Swanstrom LL: Per-oral endoscopic myotomy (POEM) for esophageal achalasia. *Curr Gastroenterol Rep* 16:369, 2014.
10. van Beek SC, Conijn AP, Koelemay MJ, et al: Editor's Choice: Endovascular aneurysm repair versus open repair for patients with a ruptured abdominal aortic aneurysm: A systematic review and meta-analysis of short-term survival. *Eur J Vasc Endovasc Surg* 47:593–602, 2014.
11. Malas MB, Freischlag JA: Interpretation of the results of OVER in the context of EVAR trial, DREAM, and the EUROSTAR registry. *Semin Vasc Surg* 23:165–169, 2010.
12. Rueff LE, Raman SS: Clinical and technical aspects of MR-guided high intensity focused ultrasound for treatment of symptomatic uterine fibroids. *Semin Intervent Radiol* 30:347–353, 2013.
13. Marien A, Gill I, Ukimura O, et al: Target ablation—image-guided therapy in prostate cancer. *Urol Oncol* 32:912–923, 2014.
14. Tatli S, Tapan U, Morrison PR, et al: Radiofrequency ablation: Technique and clinical applications. *Diagn Interv Radiol* 18:508–516, 2012.
15. Maeso S, Reza M, Mayol JA, et al: Efficacy of the da Vinci surgical system in abdominal surgery compared with that of laparoscopy: A systematic review and meta-analysis. *Ann Surg* 252:254–262, 2010.
16. Haidegger T, Sandor J, Benyo Z: Surgery in space: The future of robotic telesurgery. *Surg Endosc* 25:681–690, 2011.
17. Lum MJ, Rosen J, King H, et al: Teleoperation in surgical robotics—network latency effects on surgical performance. *Conf Proc IEEE Eng Med Biol Soc* 2009:6860–6863, 2009.
18. Hemmerling TM, Taddei R, Wehbe M, et al: Robotic anesthesia—a vision for the future of anesthesia. *Transl Med UniSa* 1:1–20, 2011.
19. Wehbe M, Giacalone M, Hemmerling TM: Robotics and regional anesthesia. *Curr Opin Anaesthesiol* 27:544–548, 2014.
20. Kang DC, Hardee MJ, Fesperman SF, et al: Low quality of evidence for robot-assisted laparoscopic prostatectomy: Results of a systematic review of the published literature. *Eur Urol* 57:930–937, 2010.
21. Ploussard G, de la Taille A, Moulin M, et al: Comparisons of the perioperative, functional, and oncologic outcomes after robot-assisted versus pure extraperitoneal laparoscopic radical prostatectomy. *Eur Urol* 65:610–619, 2014.
22. Tinelli R, Malzoni M, Cosentino F, et al: Robotics versus laparoscopic radical hysterectomy with lymphadenectomy in patients with early cervical cancer: A multicenter study. *Ann Surg Oncol* 18:2622–2628, 2011.
23. Gurusamy KS, Samraj K, Fusai G, et al: Robot assistant versus human or another robot assistant in patients undergoing laparoscopic cholecystectomy. *Cochrane Database Syst Rev* (9):CD006578, 2012.
24. Trastulli S, Farinella E, Cirocchi R, et al: Robotic resection compared with laparoscopic rectal resection for cancer: Systematic review and meta-analysis of short-term outcome. *Colorectal Dis* 14:e134–e156, 2012.
25. Aboumarzouk OM, Stein RJ, Eyraud R, et al: Robotic versus laparoscopic partial nephrectomy: A systematic review and meta-analysis. *Eur Urol* 62:1023–1033, 2012.
26. Hambraeus M, Arnbjornsson E, Anderberg M: A literature review of the outcomes after robot-assisted laparoscopic and conventional laparoscopic Nissen fundoplication for gastro-esophageal reflux disease in children. *Int J Med Robot* 9:428–432, 2013.
27. Wang F, Xu Y, Zhong H: Robot-assisted versus laparoscopic pyeloplasty for patients with ureteropelvic junction obstruction: An updated systematic review and meta-analysis. *Scand J Urol* 47:251–264, 2013.
28. Tanagho YS, Andriole GL, Paradis AG, et al: 2D versus 3D visualization: Impact on laparoscopic proficiency using the fundamentals of laparoscopic surgery skill set. *J Laparoendosc Adv Surg Tech A* 22:865–870, 2012.
29. Lusch A, Bucur PL, Menhadji AD, et al: Evaluation of the impact of three-dimensional vision on laparoscopic performance. *J Endourol* 28:261–266, 2014.
30. Seol YJ, Kang HW, Lee SJ, et al: Bioprinting technology and its applications. *Eur J Cardiothorac Surg* 46:342–348, 2014.
31. Schubert C, van Langeveld MC, Donoso LA: Innovations in 3D printing: A 3D overview from optics to organs. *Br J Ophthalmol* 98:159–161, 2014.
32. Hughes-Hallett A, Mayer EK, Marcus HJ, et al: Quantifying innovation in surgery. *Ann Surg* 260:205–211, 2014.
33. Krummel TM: Forecasting innovation in surgery. *Ann Surg* 260:212–213, 2014.
34. Nagendran M, Gurusamy KS, Aggarwal R, et al: Virtual reality training for surgical trainees in laparoscopic surgery. *Cochrane Database Syst Rev* (8):CD006575, 2013.
35. Faulkner H, Regehr G, Martin J, et al: Validation of an objective structured assessment of technical skill for surgical residents. *Acad Med* 71:1363–1365, 1996.
36. Dawe SR, Windsor JA, Broeders JA, et al: A systematic review of surgical skills transfer after simulation-based training: Laparoscopic cholecystectomy and endoscopy. *Ann Surg* 259:236–248, 2014.
37. Swanstrom LL, Fried GM, Hoffman KI, et al: Beta test results of a new system assessing competence in laparoscopic surgery. *J Am Coll Surg* 202:62–69, 2006.
38. Fried GM, Feldman LS, Vassiliou MC, et al: Proving the value of simulation in laparoscopic surgery. *Ann Surg* 240:518–525, discussion 518–525, 2004.
39. Grantcharov TP, Reznick RK: Teaching procedural skills. *BMJ* 336:1129–1131, 2008.
40. Sroka G, Feldman LS, Vassiliou MC, et al: Fundamentals of laparoscopic surgery simulator training to proficiency improves laparoscopic performance in the operating room—a randomized controlled trial. *Am J Surg* 199:115–120, 2010.
41. Kurashima Y, Feldman LS, Al-Sabah S, et al: A tool for training and evaluation of laparoscopic inguinal hernia repair: The Global Operative Assessment of Laparoscopic Skills–Groin Hernia (GOALS-GH). *Am J Surg* 201:54–61, 2011.

42. Kurashima Y, Feldman L, Al-Sabah S, et al: A novel low-cost simulator for laparoscopic inguinal hernia repair. *Surg Innov* 18:171–175, 2011.
43. Zevin B, Bonrath EM, Aggarwal R, et al: Development, feasibility, validity, and reliability of a scale for objective assessment of operative performance in laparoscopic gastric bypass surgery. *J Am Coll Surg* 216:955–965, e958; quiz 1029–1031, 1033, 2013.
44. Ghaderi I, Vaillancourt M, Sroka G, et al: Evaluation of surgical performance during laparoscopic incisional hernia repair: A multicenter study. *Surg Endosc* 25:2555–2563, 2011.
45. Vassiliou MC, Feldman LS, Andrew CG, et al: A global assessment tool for evaluation of intraoperative laparoscopic skills. *Am J Surg* 190:107–113, 2005.
46. Shanmugan S, Leblanc F, Senagore AJ, et al: Virtual reality simulator training for laparoscopic colectomy: What metrics have construct validity? *Dis Colon Rectum* 57:210–214, 2014.
47. Mueller CL, Kaneva P, Fried GM, et al: Colonoscopy performance correlates with scores on the FES manual skills test. *Surg Endosc* 28:3081–3085, 2014.
48. Vassiliou MC, Dunkin BJ, Fried GM, et al: Fundamentals of endoscopic surgery: Creation and validation of the hands-on test. *Surg Endosc* 28:704–711, 2014.
49. Poulose BK, Vassiliou MC, Dunkin BJ, et al: Fundamentals of endoscopic surgery cognitive examination: Development and validity evidence. *Surg Endosc* 28:631–638, 2014.
50. Ferroli P, Tringali G, Acerbi F, et al: Brain surgery in a stereoscopic virtual reality environment: A single institution's experience with 100 cases. *Neurosurgery* 67:ons79–ons84, discussion ons84, 2010.
51. Mutter D, Dallemagne B, Bailey C, et al: 3D virtual reality and selective vascular control for laparoscopic left hepatic lobectomy. *Surg Endosc* 23:432–435, 2009.

SECTION III

Trauma and Critical Care

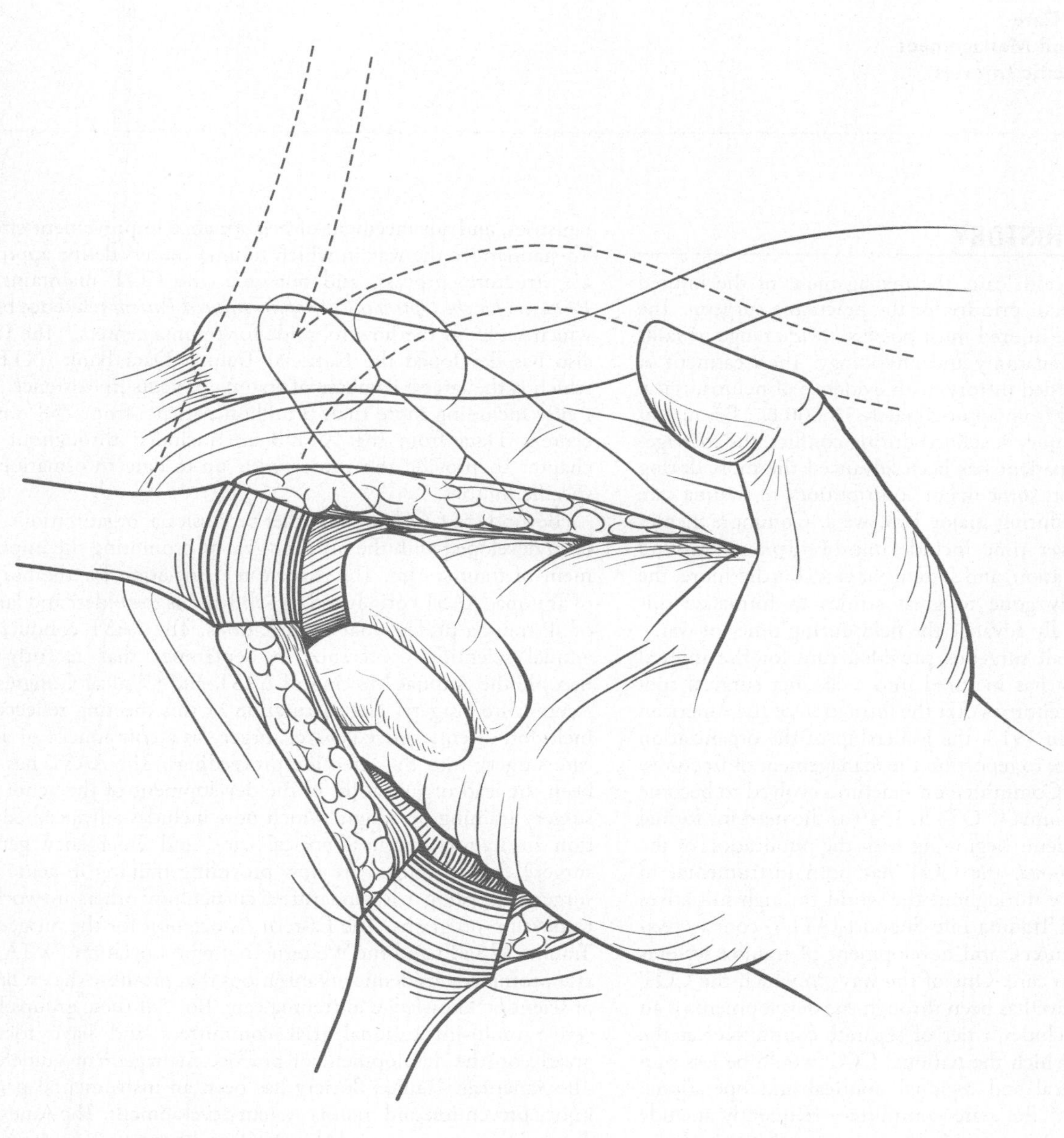

16 CHAPTER

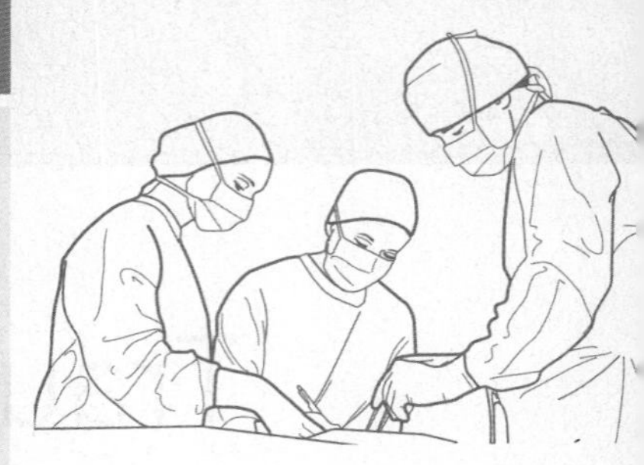

Management of Acute Trauma

R. Shayn Martin, J. Wayne Meredith

OUTLINE

OVERVIEW AND HISTORY

Since the dawn of health care, the management of the injured patient has been a major priority for the practicing surgeon. The surgeon managing the injured must possess a wide range of skills spanning all areas of anatomy and physiology. The treatment of injuries predates recorded history, with evidence of neurosurgical procedures discovered from approximately 10,000 BC. Because of the high burden on injury sustained during conflict, the management of the injured patient has been advanced the most during wartime. Box 16-1 lists some major contributions to trauma care that were developed during major U.S. wars. Common themes that have evolved over time include improvements in wound management, resuscitation, and systems of care. Furthermore, the military have recently gone to great strides to formalize this research to more rapidly advance the field during times of war.

Whereas initially all surgeons provided care for the injured patient, traumatology has matured into a distinct surgical specialty during the last century. After the formation of the American College of Surgeons in 1913, the leadership of the organization appointed a committee to report on the management of fractures. Created in 1922, the Committee on Fractures evolved to become the Committee on Trauma (COT) in 1949 as the need for formal oversight became evident. Beginning with the publication of the *Early Care of the Injured,* the COT has been instrumental in advancing trauma care throughout the world through initiatives such as the Advanced Trauma Life Support (ATLS) course, verification of trauma centers, and development of trauma systems that improve access to care. One of the ways in which the COT has been highly effective has been through the development of an infrastructure that includes a tier of separate committees at the state level, a level at which the national COT would be less successful because of local and regional political and operational structure. Activities of the state committees frequently include trauma system development with the creation of triage documents, maximizing the use of prehospital and hospital resources, injury prevention initiatives, maintenance of statewide trauma registries, and advancement of performance improvement efforts. To standardize the way in which trauma centers define appropriate structure, process, and outcome, the COT maintains the *Resources for the Optimal Care of the Injured Patient* reference book, which serves as the how-to guide for trauma centers.[1] The COT also has developed the National Trauma Data Bank (NTDB), which is the largest database of trauma patients in existence, currently including more than 6 million patients from 758 trauma centers. Data from the NTDB are included throughout this chapter to provide the reader with up-to-date information on specific injuries.

Beyond the COT, several other professional organizations have been developed with the primary goal of promoting the improvement of trauma care. The American Association for the Surgery of Trauma (AAST) originated in 1938 and is the oldest and largest of all trauma professional organizations. The AAST conducts an annual scientific conference in September that recently has become the Annual Meeting of AAST and Clinical Congress of Acute Care Surgery. The maturation of this meeting reflects the inclusion of emergency general surgery as a component of acute care surgery into the scientific proceedings. The AAST has also been the lead organization in the development of the acute care surgery training paradigm, which now includes advanced education in trauma, surgical critical care, and emergency general surgery. Several centers are now providing training in acute care surgery according to a standardized curriculum; others are working to develop programs. The Eastern Association for the Surgery of Trauma (EAST) and the Western Trauma Association (WTA) are also prominent academic organizations that promote the exchange of scientific knowledge in trauma care. Both of these groups have active multi-institutional trial committees and have focused greatly on the development of practice management guidelines. The American Trauma Society has been an instrumental part of injury prevention and trauma system development. The American Trauma Society was founded in 1968 and has been a leader at the national level by advocating for the injured patient and promoting trauma-related legislation. Finally, the Orthopaedic Trauma

BOX 16-1 Advances and Discoveries in Trauma Care During War

French and Indian War (1754-1763)
Wound contraction during healing
Primary and secondary healing
Description of granulation tissue and epithelialization

American Revolutionary War (1775-1783)
Exhaustive therapy (bleeding, diarrhea, vomiting, salivation, sweating)
Centralization of medical care
Establishment of first medical school

American Civil War (1861-1865)
Primary amputation (versus secondary)
Use of topical antiseptic agents
Whole blood infusion
Development of specialty hospitals (eye/ear, orthopedics, hernia)
Extremity traction splinting

World War I (1914-1918)
Laparotomy for penetrating abdominal trauma
Wound débridement and delayed closure
Early use of plasma and crystalloid
First blood bank

World War II (1939-1945)
Guillotine amputation and delayed primary closure
Exteriorization of colon injuries
Mobile surgical teams
Organ dysfunction after injury described

Korean War (1950-1953)
Vascular surgery for limb salvage
Hypovolemic shock recognition
Mobile surgical hospital units (MASH units)

Vietnam War (1955-1964)
Aeromedical transfer (helicopter)
Sulfamylon for burn care
Recognition of acute respiratory distress syndrome (Da Nang lung)

Operation Enduring Freedom (Iraq, 2003 to Present)
Damage control resuscitation
Highly efficient trauma systems
Re-emergence of tourniquet use

Association, American Association of Neurological Surgeons, and Society of Trauma Nurses represent three organizations whose members are part of the multidisciplinary team dedicated to improving the care of the injured patient.

TRAUMA SYSTEMS

The importance of trauma systems is best demonstrated by the following example. Interstate 40 runs 2550 miles from Wilmington, on the coast of North Carolina, to Barstow, California. If a car crash were to occur along this long stretch of road, the unfortunate reality is that even with similar injuries, a patient's outcome is highly dependent on where along the highway the crash occurs. This illogical finding is a reflection of the variability in a patient's

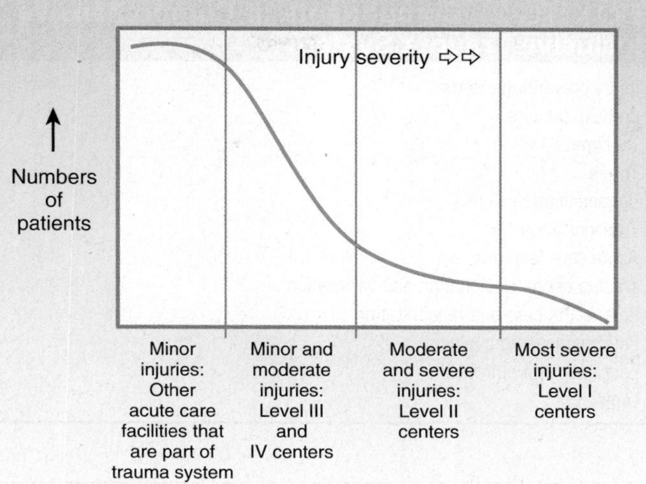

FIGURE 16-1 The inclusive trauma system including the relationship between number of patients and severity of injury with respect to trauma facilities. The system is designed to optimally match the level of injury with the capabilities of the medical center. (From American College of Surgeons Committee on Trauma: *Resources for the optimal care of the injured patient 2014*, ed 6, Chicago, 2014, American College of Surgeons.)

access to care from location to location. Regions that respond the best to injury have developed an organized approach to providing all of the elements that maximize the potential for meaningful recovery, called a trauma system. Trauma systems include the entire care continuum, starting at the time of the injury, with a patient's access to care, and extending through the rehabilitation process. At the most basic level, the goal of a trauma system is to get *the right patient to the right place at the right time.*

As our health care system developed, trauma care was initially centered around the large, academic hospitals. All patients were transported to the trauma center regardless of the degree of injury. Although this was found to be beneficial to the severely injured who were transported to the trauma center, this type of approach, now described as an exclusive trauma system, resulted in the movement of significant numbers of minimally injured patients who could have been cared for at the local hospital. Essentially, this type of system fails to capitalize on the resources available at the nontrauma centers. The solution was the development of trauma systems that are inclusive and thus involve all hospitals to address the needs of all injured patients, regardless of the severity of injury or geographic location (Fig. 16-1). Inclusive trauma systems capitalize on the resources of all hospitals from critical access facilities to the large level I and level II trauma centers. Guided by triage protocols, injured patients are transported to facilities that are appropriate to provide the necessary level of care based on the severity of the injuries. At times, this requires transfer of patients from smaller hospitals to trauma centers, although in this system, most patients can receive the appropriate treatment at the local hospital. Box 16-2 lists the common components of an inclusive trauma system that must be coordinated to maximize the efficiency of getting the injured patient to the care location needed most. The benefits of this approach include the efficient use of all available resources, reduction in potentially overwhelming trauma centers with patients of lower acuity, and allowing most patients to receive appropriate care within their own

BOX 16-2 Components of Comprehensive Inclusive Trauma System

Injury prevention efforts
Prehospital care
Tachypnea
Triage
Communication
Transportation
Acute care facilities
Trauma center designation and verification
Post–acute care and rehabilitation
Performance improvement
Education and outreach
Legislation

TABLE 16-1 Abbreviated Injury Scale (AIS) Body Regions

AIS FIRST DIGIT	BODY REGION
1	Head
2	Face
3	Neck
4	Thorax
5	Abdomen
6	Spine
7	Upper extremity
8	Lower extremity
9	Unspecified

community. Finally, the importance of legislative support cannot be overstated. Only through ongoing governmental support can trauma systems flourish and patients can be ensured access to high-quality trauma care.

The establishment of trauma systems is a relatively new development, with Illinois and Maryland first creating trauma systems approximately 40 years ago. Congress recognized the need for a coordinated approach to the management of the injured and passed the Trauma Care Systems Planning and Development Act of 1990, which formally addressed the need for trauma systems. Further advancement occurred in 1992 when the Health Resources and Services Administration released the Model Trauma Care System Plan.[2] Revised in 2006 and renamed the *Model Trauma System Planning and Evaluation* document, this work applied a public health approach to trauma and provided valuable direction for developing and evaluating trauma systems. Within the public health domain, trauma was identified as a disease, the impact of which can be prevented or decreased by applying already established systems that address other health-related issues, such as infectious diseases. As an added benefit, the American College of Surgeons COT established the Trauma Systems Consultation Program in 1996 to guide states or regions in the process of developing a systematic approach to trauma care.

The establishment of highly functional trauma systems saves lives as evidenced by several studies. In 2006, the National Study on Costs and Outcomes of Trauma (NSCOT) was performed to evaluate variations in the care provided between trauma centers and nontrauma center hospitals. Supported by the National Center for Injury Prevention and Control of the Centers for Disease Control and Prevention, NSCOT represents one of the largest epidemiologic studies ever to evaluate the care of the injured patient. Including more than 5000 patients from 69 hospitals, NSCOT established that patient outcomes are improved when care is provided at a trauma center versus a nontrauma center. After correction for injury severity, care at a trauma center was associated with a 20% in-hospital mortality reduction and a 25% reduction in 1-year mortality.[3] At the system level, Nathens and colleagues demonstrated the value of a coordinated response to injury after studying 400,000 patients during a 17-year period.[4] The study spanned a length of time during which trauma systems were established and optimized. After accounting for all possible contributors to improved outcomes, the development of a trauma system resulted in an 8% reduction in mortality during a 10-year period.[4] Whereas these studies represent the seminal work on this subject, others have also reported this effect, demonstrating an improvement in outcomes in areas that establish a systematic approach to injury management.

The development and maintenance of trauma systems are highly dependent on multidisciplinary teams that represent locations ranging from the smallest rural hospital to the largest academic medical center. Even in areas in which definitive trauma care is not provided, health care personnel play a vital role by establishing triage plans and providing initial stabilization and patient transfer. Highly functional trauma systems require the involvement of local leaders from hospitals, government, and prehospital agencies to develop the regional trauma system and to work with surrounding trauma centers to ensure appropriate care for patients with all levels of injury severity. It is valuable for the physician to learn about the structure of the local system and to identify his or her specific role to optimize the functionality of the system.

INJURY SCORING

The development of systems for comparing injuries has been extremely important and the subject of a great deal of work in the last 45 years. Scoring systems are typically based on either injury anatomy or the physiology demonstrated after one or more injuries are sustained. The Abbreviated Injury Scale (AIS) has been the most used anatomic system of injury classification since it was first released in 1971. Injuries are characterized by a six-digit taxonomy that describes the body region, type of anatomic structure, and specific anatomic detail of the injury. Table 16-1 demonstrates the body regions and the associated first digit code within the AIS lexicon that allow users of this system to clearly know the location of the injury. Perhaps of even more widespread use is the AIS severity code (frequently described as the post-dot code). This seventh digit describes the severity and potential risk of death for each injury in the AIS system. Post-dot codes range from 1 (minimal severity) to 6 (presumably fatal) and are frequently used to cohort injuries and to compare outcomes. The Association for the Advancement of Automotive Medicine frequently embarks on the rigorous process of refining the AIS to be sure that is stays current in its ability to accurately characterize injury.

The AIS represents the foundation for other scoring systems that are better able to account for the severity of multiple combined injuries. In 1974, Baker and colleagues presented the Injury Severity Score (ISS), calculated by summing the squares of the AIS severity codes for the three most severely injured body regions.[5] The ISS ranges from 1 to 75, with severity groupings being defined as minor injury (ISS less than 9), moderate injury (ISS between 9 and 16), serious injury (ISS between 16 and 15), and severe injury (ISS more than 25). The ISS has been commonly used throughout the literature to quantify the overall burden of injury sustained by a patient. As a further development in anatomic injury scoring, the Organ Injury Scale (OIS) released by the AAST has been incorporated into the more recent versions of the AIS.[6] By introducing the concept of injury grades, the OIS has added greater anatomic detail for specific organs and incorporated the ability to better delineate organ injury severity. This OIS severity has been validated with the NTDB to optimize the associated risk of morbidity and mortality.[6]

In addition to anatomic scoring systems, other scales have been developed that include the physiologic insult of the burden of injury. These physiologic scoring systems are more capable of identifying the patient's overall condition and can also better guide real-time decision making. One commonly used scale of this type is the Glasgow Coma Scale (GCS), which reflects a patient's level of consciousness. With scores ranging from 3 to 15, the GCS is composed of a measure of eye opening, verbal response, and motor function. The GCS and more specifically the motor score alone have been found to be reflective of a patient's outcome after traumatic brain injury.[7] The Revised Trauma Score (RTS) is another well-studied physiologic scoring system that characterizes the injured patient's condition by incorporating the GCS, systolic blood pressure, and respiratory rate. These scores have been of value for research purposes and have been successfully used to make triage decisions. To better demonstrate the way in which the GCS and RTS are designed, Tables 16-2 and 16-3 reflect how these scores are calculated.

PREHOSPITAL TRAUMA CARE

Immediately after a patient is injured, the trauma system engages the prehospital phase of care. The goal of the prehospital system is to move a patient to a location capable of providing definitive injury management as quickly as possible. The prehospital team plays an integral role in the management of the trauma patient because of the time-dependent nature of injury. The initial approach to the injured patient in the prehospital setting includes four key priorities:

1. Evaluate the scene.
2. Perform an initial assessment.
3. Make triage-transport decision.
4. Initiate critical interventions and transport the patient.

Despite being brief, this list of priorities is extremely effective because it is designed to expedite rapid hemorrhage control. As a rule, transport should be initiated as quickly as possible with the majority of interventions performed on the way to the definitive care facility.

After scene safety is ensured to protect our prehospital providers, the initial assessment should be rapidly completed. The initial assessment consists of a systematic approach to immediately identify life-threatening conditions that require urgent intervention. The ABC mnemonic guides the initial assessment, during which ***a***irway, ***b***reathing, and ***c***irculation are sequentially evaluated and addressed. While the spine is protected, the patient's airway is secured, and assisted ventilation is provided as necessary. External hemorrhage is identified and immediately controlled while fluid resuscitation is initiated.

Emergent interventions in the field can be immediately lifesaving, but optimal outcomes ultimately depend on quickly making an effective triage and transport decision. Using the "load and go" approach, all essential prehospital interventions can be provided while the patient is being transported. All prehospital teams know that immediate departure from the scene is paramount, but identifying where to go and how to get there can be more challenging. Well-defined protocols should guide the field triage process so that teams know immediately where to transport a patient. Figure 16-2 demonstrates the Field Triage Decision Scheme, which was developed by the Centers for Disease Control and Prevention and included in recent editions of the COT's *Resources for the Optimal Care of the Injured Patient* reference.[8] Using physiologic status, mechanism of injury details, and other indicators of a high-risk patient, this tool assists in determining which patients might benefit from care at a trauma center. Most prehospital agencies attempt to rapidly assess a patient and initiate the transport process while keeping the scene time to within 15 minutes.

The initial clinical concern that the prehospital team must assess is the injured patient's airway. The "gold standard" for

TABLE 16-2 Glasgow Coma Scale

Eye Opening	Spontaneous	4
	To voice	3
	To pain	2
	None	1
Verbal Response	Oriented	5
	Confused	4
	Inappropriate	3
	Incomprehensible	2
	None	1
Motor Response	Obeys commands	6
	Localizes pain	5
	Withdraws to pain	4
	Flexion	3
	Extension	2
	None	1
Total Glasgow Coma Scale Score		3-15

TABLE 16-3 Revised Trauma Score

Glasgow Coma Scale Score	13-15	4
	9-12	3
	6-8	2
	4-5	1
	3	0
Systolic Blood Pressure (mm Hg)	>89	4
	76-89	3
	50-75	2
	1-49	1
	0	0
Respiratory Rate (breaths/min)	10-29	4
	>29	3
	6-9	2
	1-5	1
	0	0
Total Revised Trauma Score		0-12

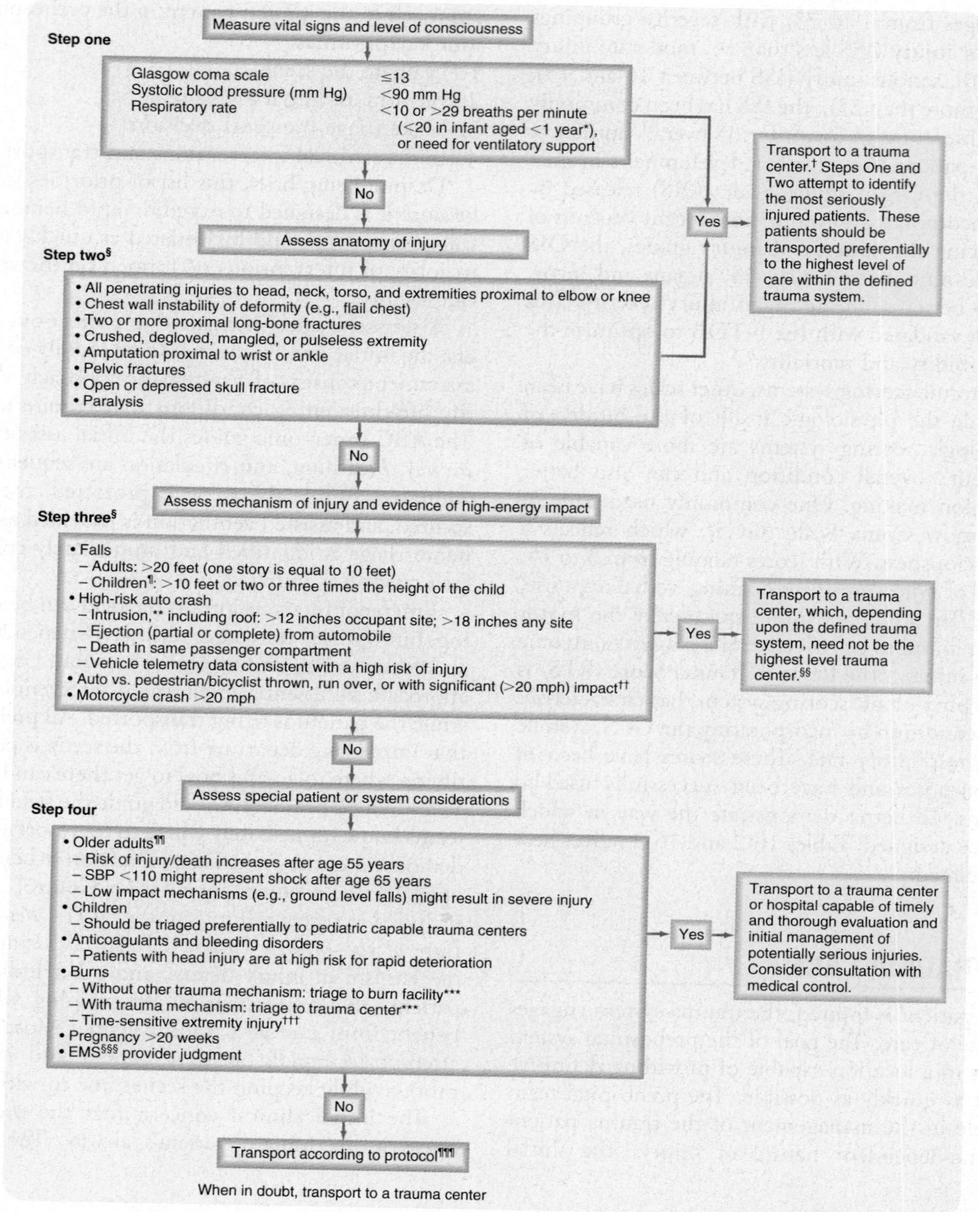

Step one
Measure vital signs and level of consciousness
Glasgow coma scale ≤13
Systolic blood pressure (mm Hg) <90 mm Hg
Respiratory rate <10 or >29 breaths per minute (<20 in infant aged <1 year*), or need for ventilatory support
Yes
Transport to a trauma center.[†] Steps One and Two attempt to identify the most seriously injured patients. These patients should be transported preferentially to the highest level of care within the defined trauma system.
No
Step two[§]
Assess anatomy of injury
• All penetrating injuries to head, neck, torso, and extremities proximal to elbow or knee
• Chest wall instability of deformity (e.g., flail chest)
• Two or more proximal long-bone fractures
• Crushed, degloved, mangled, or pulseless extremity
• Amputation proximal to wrist or ankle
• Pelvic fractures
• Open or depressed skull fracture
• Paralysis
No
Step three[§]
Assess mechanism of injury and evidence of high-energy impact
• Falls
– Adults: >20 feet (one story is equal to 10 feet)
– Children[¶]: >10 feet or two or three times the height of the child
• High-risk auto crash
– Intrusion,** including roof: >12 inches occupant site; >18 inches any site
– Ejection (partial or complete) from automobile
– Death in same passenger compartment
– Vehicle telemetry data consistent with a high risk of injury
• Auto vs. pedestrian/bicyclist thrown, run over, or with significant (>20 mph) impact[††]
• Motorcycle crash >20 mph
Yes
Transport to a trauma center, which, depending upon the defined trauma system, need not be the highest level trauma center.[§§]
No
Step four
Assess special patient or system considerations
• Older adults[¶¶]
– Risk of injury/death increases after age 55 years
– SBP <110 might represent shock after age 65 years
– Low impact mechanisms (e.g., ground level falls) might result in severe injury
• Children
– Should be triaged preferentially to pediatric capable trauma centers
• Anticoagulants and bleeding disorders
– Patients with head injury are at high risk for rapid deterioration
• Burns
– Without other trauma mechanism: triage to burn facility***
– With trauma mechanism: triage to trauma center***
– Time-sensitive extremity injury[†††]
• Pregnancy >20 weeks
• EMS[§§§] provider judgment
Yes
Transport to a trauma center or hospital capable of timely and thorough evaluation and initial management of potentially serious injuries. Consider consultation with medical control.
No
Transport according to protocol[¶¶¶]
When in doubt, transport to a trauma center

FIGURE 16-2 Guidelines for field triage of injured patients, which were created to guide the development of state and local EMS systems triage protocols. The guidelines use four decision steps (physiologic, anatomic, mechanism of injury, and special considerations) to direct triage decisions within the local trauma system. *SBP*, systolic blood pressure. (From Sasser SM, Hunt RC, Faul M, et al; Centers for Disease Control and Prevention: Guidelines for field triage of injured patients: Recommendations of the National Expert Panel on Field Triage, 2011. *MMWR Recomm Rep* 61:1–20, 2012.)

Source: Adapted from American College of Surgeons. Resources for the optimal care of the injured patient. Chicago, IL: American College of Surgeons; 2006. Footnotes have been added to enhance understanding of field triage by persons outside the acute injury care field.

*The upper limit of respiratory rate in infants is >29 breaths per minute to maintain a higher level of overtriage for infants.

†Trauma centers are designated Level I-IV, with Level I representing the highest level of trauma care available.

§Any injury noted in Steps Two and Three triggers a "yes" response.

¶Age <15 years.

**Intrusion refers to interior compartment intrusion, as opposed to deformation which refers to exterior damage.

††Includes pedestrians or bicyclists thrown or run over by a motor vehicle or those with estimated impact >20 mph with a motor vehicle.

§§Local or regional protocols should be used to determine the most appropriate level of trauma center; appropriate center need not be Level I.

¶¶Age >55 years.

***Patients with both burns and concomitant trauma for whom the burn injury poses the greatest risk for morbidity and mortality should be transferred to a burn center. If the nonburn trauma presents a greater immediate risk, the patient may be stabilized in a trauma center and then transferred to a burn center.

†††Injuries such as an open fracture or fracture with neurovascular compromise.

§§§Emergency medical services.

¶¶¶Patients who do not meet any of the triage criteria in Steps One through Four should be transported to the most appropriate medical facility as outlined in local EMS protocols.

airway maintenance in the severely injured patient remains oral endotracheal intubation, typically using a rapid-sequence technique. One must always assume that the patient has a spine injury and appropriately maintain spinal precautions. The utility of advanced airway management in the field has been questioned, with the literature providing conflicting recommendations. In a retrospective analysis of 496 injured patients, Eckstein and colleagues found that airway management with endotracheal intubation was associated with an increased mortality rate compared with bag valve mask ventilation.[9] Conversely, other studies have confirmed the benefit of advanced prehospital airway support, especially in the setting of severe traumatic brain injury.[10] To assist with securing the challenging airway, blind insertion airway devices have become common and add great value in providing a bridge to a more definitive solution. Regardless of the approach implemented by the prehospital agency, personnel need to have the ability to manage all levels of airway compromise while transporting the patient to definitive care.

External hemorrhage control and initiation of resuscitation are critical needs during the prehospital phase of care. Direct pressure remains the mainstay of hemorrhage control, although tourniquet use has become more common in the management of exsanguinating extremity trauma. For some time, tourniquets were infrequently used because of concern about causing unnecessary muscle and nerve injury. Driven by recent military experience and advances in device development, tourniquets have demonstrated benefit in select situations. Several series now have demonstrated improved outcomes related to the use of tourniquets in the military theater.[11] Prehospital agencies now commonly include tourniquets on their standard equipment lists so that they may be used when a patient with uncontrolled extremity bleeding is encountered. Many commercial devices are available, and Figure 16-3 illustrates an example of a tourniquet that can be used in the prehospital setting.

Patients in shock require initiation of resuscitation to correct intravascular volume depletion after hemorrhage control. The appropriate magnitude of crystalloid volume administration has been questioned recently, and the concept of a controlled resuscitation has become well accepted. The reason for this evolution is the belief that overresuscitation before management of bleeding could potentially increase the rate of blood loss by disrupting areas that had become hemostatic. This concept was best studied in a group of patients with penetrating torso trauma who were randomized to either standard crystalloid administration or the withholding of all resuscitation until a patient is at the trauma center and can be taken to the operation room.[12] The group of patients who had resuscitation withheld until reaching the hospital had a lower mortality than the standard, immediate resuscitation group.[12] In terms of widespread application of this approach, the study was limited by the inclusion of a unique cohort of penetrating trauma patients in an urban setting, with short transport times to definitive care. Despite this, most prehospital agencies have evaluated the traditional practices and worked toward providing a more controlled resuscitation that still provides adequate organ perfusion.

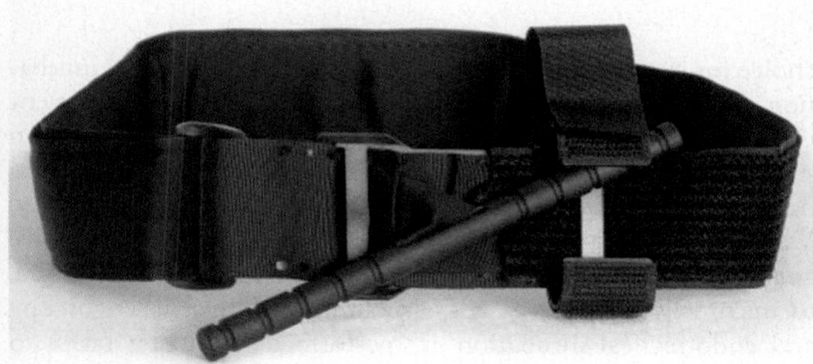

FIGURE 16-3 Example of a tourniquet. Tourniquets are commonly being used to prevent extremity exsanguination in military and civilian prehospital environments.

INITIAL ASSESSMENT AND MANAGEMENT

The mainstay of the initial approach to the injured patient is the ATLS course. Since its development in 1980, the ATLS course has provided a structured, standardized approach to the injured patient that is based on the concept of rapidly identifying and addressing life-threatening conditions during the initial assessment of the patient.[13] More specifically, ATLS conveys three important concepts that greatly enhance the ability to manage injured patients, regardless of where care is provided:

1. Treat the greatest threat to life first.
2. The lack of a definitive diagnosis should not delay the application of an indicated urgent treatment.
3. An initial, detailed history is not essential to begin the evaluation of a patient with acute injuries.

Following a defined order of assessment, life-threatening conditions are immediately addressed at the time of identification. This initial assessment, also termed the *primary survey*, follows the mnemonic ABCDE (Fig. 16-4):

Airway and cervical spine protection
Breathing
Circulation
Disability or neurologic condition
Exposure and environmental control

In addition, the primary survey can be repeated any time there is a change in the patient's condition. Despite being simple in design, the primary survey offers a tool that the surgeon can trust to identify what life-threatening condition exists and where to direct clinical effort. The following outlines the performance of the primary survey.

Airway

On the arrival of the patient in the trauma bay, the status of the injured patient's airway should be immediately assessed. Simply eliciting a verbal response provides the most meaningful information because the ability to speak usually indicates adequate airway protection. Patients who cannot speak have either mental status depression or some obstruction to air flow, both of which are indications for airway management. Further indicators of airway compromise include noisy breathing, severe facial trauma (specifically with oropharyngeal blood or foreign body), and agitation of the patient. A determination of the adequacy of the airway as well as a decision to obtain better airway control, if necessary, should be completed within seconds of the patient's arrival. After the initial assessment, frequent reassessment for deterioration and the development of airway compromise is paramount.

Until it is ruled out with an appropriate evaluation, all injured patients should be assumed to have an injury to the vertebral column and have the appropriate precautions maintained. This is

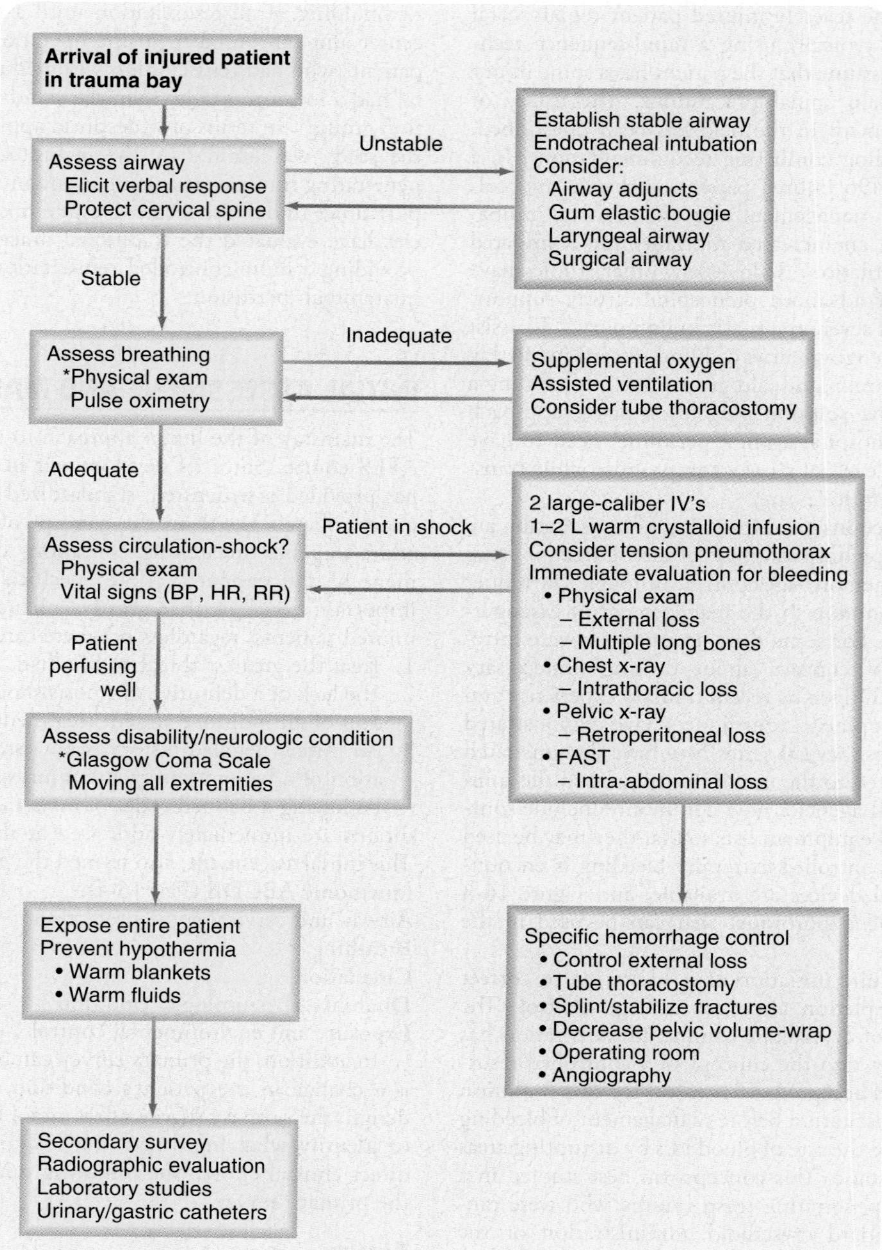

FIGURE 16-4 Algorithm for the initial assessment of the injured patient. *BP*, Blood pressure; *HR*, heart rate; *RR*, respiratory rate.

of significant importance during the manipulation of the head and neck while the airway is being managed. Cervical spine protection includes the use of a hard cervical collar and the maintenance of the log roll technique for all movement of the patient. During airway assessment and management, the anterior portion of the cervical collar can be removed to optimize exposure, but manual stabilization from an assistant should be provided when the collar is not securely in place. Rigid long spine boards may be of value during transport of the patient but should be removed as soon as possible to avoid pressure-related wounds that can occur within a short time.

When the injured patient's airway is deemed inadequate, a definitive airway must be established. The definitive airway of choice for most injured patients remains oral endotracheal intubation provided by a rapid-sequence technique. While the patient is being prepared for intubation, bag valve mask ventilation should be provided, and adjuncts such as oropharyngeal and nasopharyngeal airways may assist in maintaining airway patency. With cricoid pressure applied, the patient is provided a sedative and fast-acting neuromuscular blocker, such as succinylcholine, to maximally enhance glottic visualization. Direct laryngoscopy and endotracheal intubation are performed, with care taken to avoid cervical spine motion. The appropriate position of the tube in the trachea is confirmed by chest and abdomen auscultation, end-tidal carbon dioxide measurement, and ultimately a chest radiograph. The presence of experienced airway personnel is critical and in trauma centers is often an important component of the trauma alert system.

The trauma team must always be prepared to secure the difficult airway that cannot be adequately managed with direct laryngoscopy. The gum elastic bougie has been shown to improve the rate of successful intubation, especially in the setting of a challenging airway. When the normal view of the glottis is obscured, the bougie can be placed with a limited view of the vocal cords, resulting in an improved rate of appropriately placing an endotracheal tube. A recent advance in the area of advanced airway management has been the emergence of video-assisted laryngoscopy. Several devices are now available that provide the clinician a view of the upper airway anatomy that is displayed on a video monitor. By eliminating challenges related to the angle of the airway, video-assisted laryngoscopy has been shown to increase first attempt success and to decrease the incidence of esophageal intubation in the setting of the difficult airway.[14] The blind insertion airway device offers an additional tool to be applied when attempts at intubation are unsuccessful. Devices such as the laryngeal mask airway, multilumen esophageal airway (Combitube), and laryngeal tube airway (King LT-D) are placed blindly and function by occluding the esophagus and the posterior pharynx, allowing assisted ventilation to pass selectively down the trachea. Blind insertion airways have been found to be easy to place and are considered to be an effective salvage approach.[15]

As airway specialists are transitioning to advanced techniques, preparation for a surgical airway should begin. Before physiologic deterioration, a cricothyroidotomy should be performed when other approaches have failed. The inability to maintain oxygenation with a bag valve mask between intubation attempts is a reasonable indication for establishment of a surgical airway. A cricothyroidotomy (Fig. 16-5) is performed by making a transverse incision over the cricothyroid membrane, which can be palpated between the thyroid cartilage and cricoid ring. It is critical that the surgeon frequently palpate the underlying structures to guide the dissection and to avoid injury to more lateral structures of the neck. Spreading the overlying soft tissue reveals the cricothyroid membrane, which is then transversely incised. The cricothyroidotomy is spread longitudinally, and a tracheostomy or endotracheal tube is advanced through the incised membrane and down the trachea. Care must be taken to avoid advancing the tube past the carina, which is common in these situations. Tube position is immediately confirmed with lung auscultation and end-tidal carbon dioxide determination. Finally, patients suspected of having a laryngeal injury might have abnormal anatomy in the vicinity of the cricothyroid membrane and therefore may require a tracheostomy instead of a cricothyroidotomy.

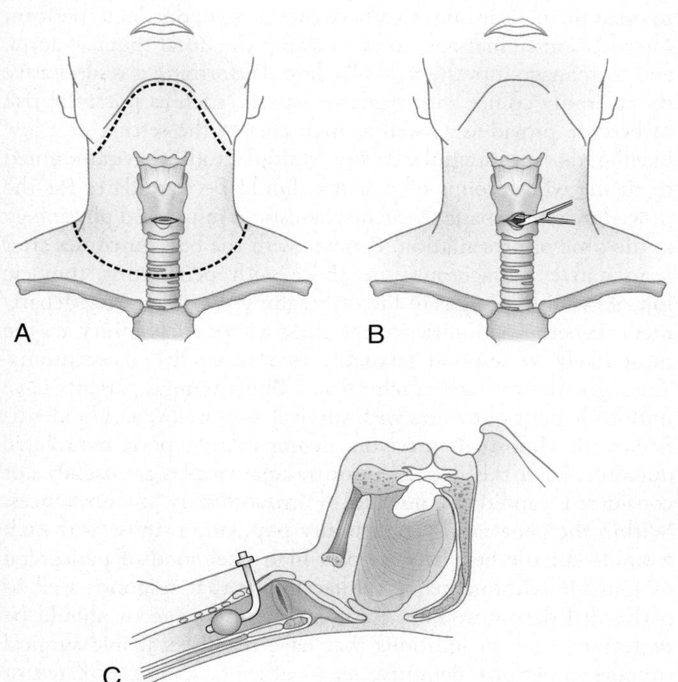

FIGURE 16-5 Technique of Cricothyroidotomy. The cricothyroid membrane is identified by palpation, and a transverse incision is made over the membrane **(A)**. The incision and dissection are continued through the cricothyroid membrane and the cricothyroidotomy is spread **(B)**, allowing the passage of a tracheal tube **(C)**.

Breathing

Following the management of the airway, breathing is evaluated by visualizing chest movement, auscultating breath sounds, and measuring oxygen saturation. Limited respiratory effort or dyspnea requires support of ventilation and further assessment of the chest. Ventilation problems may be secondary to tension pneumothorax, massive hemothorax, or flail chest with pulmonary contusion. Tension pneumothorax may cause respiratory deterioration but may also be in the form of cardiovascular collapse. It is a clinical diagnosis that should be recognized on the primary survey without need for radiographic confirmation before treatment. Deviation of the trachea in the sternal notch with unilaterally absent or diminished breath sounds and cardiopulmonary compromise should immediately suggest tension pneumothorax. Thoracic decompression should be rapidly performed with a large-bore needle or a tube thoracostomy, depending on the availability of equipment and supplies. Massive hemothorax also requires tube thoracostomy with evacuation of blood and re-expansion of the lung. Severe pulmonary contusion is managed with aggressive mechanical ventilation, often with elevated levels of positive end-expiratory pressure. To avoid the loss of positive end-expiratory pressure, one should resist continually disconnecting the ventilator to suction or bag valve to ventilate the patient when oxygenation will only improve with uninterrupted mechanical ventilation.

Circulation

An assessment of the cardiovascular system follows, with the primary goal of determining whether the patient is in shock. Patients must be rapidly evaluated for the clinical signs of shock as demonstrated in Box 16-3. Although hypotension clearly indicates cardiovascular decompensation, patients can be in shock well

BOX 16-3 Indicators of Shock in the Injured Patient

Agitation or confusion
Tachycardia
Tachypnea
Diaphoresis
Cool, mottled extremities
Weak distal pulses
Decreased pulse pressure
Decreased urine output
Hypotension

before the blood pressure decreases because of the body's ability to compensate. By far the most common cause of shock in the injured patient is hemorrhage. Blood loss must be ruled out before other causes of shock are deemed to be responsible. On recognizing the presence of shock, resuscitation is immediately initiated with 1 to 2 liters of warm crystalloid solution infused through two large-bore, short, peripheral intravenous (IV) catheters. The patient must next undergo a rapid screen to identify the cause of life-threatening blood loss. There are essentially five major locations through which exsanguination can occur, and therefore the subsequent evaluation focuses on identifying which of these locations is the cause of shock. Exsanguinating blood loss can occur by external blood loss and through the chest, abdomen, retroperitoneum (pelvic fracture), or multiple long bone fractures. The initial physical examination identifies sources of external blood loss and long bone fractures. These are managed immediately with direct pressure and fracture splinting, respectively. A chest radiograph can then evaluate for thoracic blood loss, and a pelvic radiograph will identify a pelvic fracture. To evaluate the abdomen, the focused abdominal sonography in trauma (FAST) scan is a rapidly obtainable ultrasound examination that assesses for intraperitoneal fluid. Specifically, the FAST scan assesses the hepatorenal, splenorenal, and pelvic spaces for fluid, which is presumed to be blood in the setting of trauma. The value of the FAST scan is that it can be performed quickly in the trauma bay by the surgeon and can be rapidly repeated if necessary. As an example, blood in the hepatorenal space on FAST scan is demonstrated by Figure 16-6.

After the initial administration of IV fluid, patients are assessed for ongoing signs of shock. Those who respond by demonstrating a normalizing physiologic state then undergo a comprehensive evaluation to identify all injuries. A common pitfall during this time is to continue administering IV fluids at a high rate that might mask ongoing blood loss. A failure to respond to the initial crystalloid bolus indicates continued blood loss that requires immediate intervention. External blood loss should be controlled and fractures reduced and splinted. A tube thoracostomy is required for thoracic blood loss when the chest radiograph demonstrates a hemothorax. Ongoing intrathoracic bleeding after chest tube placement may require thoracotomy. Intra-abdominal bleeding in the hemodynamically unstable patient warrants

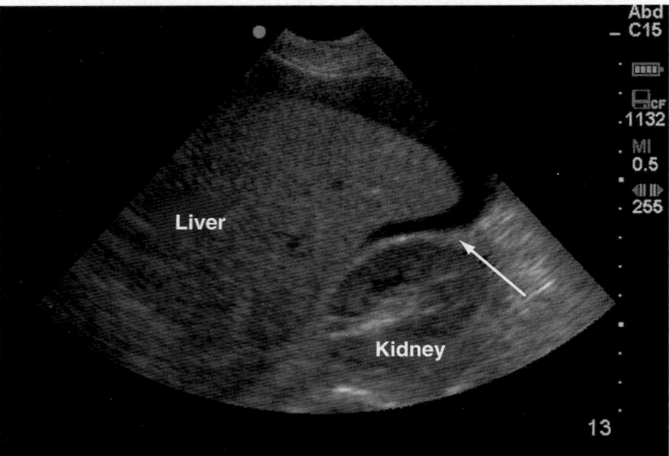

FIGURE 16-6 Focused abdominal sonography in trauma (FAST) scan demonstrating fluid in the hepatorenal space (Morison pouch). The *arrow* identifies fluid (blood) between the liver and the right kidney.

emergent laparotomy. Pelvic fractures require immediate management of any increased pelvic volume with a binder or sheet, followed by pelvic angiography with embolization for arterial hemorrhage. Simultaneous with the management of ongoing bleeding, blood products should be provided to maintain adequate intravascular volume.

Disability and Exposure

During the primary survey, it is valuable to make a rapid determination of neurologic function. Of particular importance is globally characterizing neurologic function to assess for traumatic brain injury and spinal cord injury. The GCS score should be determined to identify deficits in eye opening, verbal ability, and motor responses to potentially reflect the degree of neurologic injury. When sedating medications are required, noting the baseline level of neurologic function before administration can be beneficial. The spinal cord is grossly assessed by visualizing movement of the extremities. A lack of extremity movement may indicate a spinal cord injury that may ultimately be the source of shock after sources of blood loss have been ruled out. All clothing is removed at this time to allow an adequate examination and any required intervention. A core body temperature is obtained, and keeping the injured patient warm is important. Patients in shock have significant physiologic derangements that impede the ability to maintain body temperature. Therefore, environmental control should be maintained with warm blankets and increased room temperature as well as with other interventions, such as heated fluid administration and body warmers.

Resuscitative Thoracotomy

After critical injury, select patients who experience cardiac arrest may benefit from resuscitative thoracotomy in the emergency department. Resuscitative thoracotomy provides the opportunity to open the pericardium to relieve cardiac tamponade, to perform internal cardiac massage, to cross-clamp the distal thoracic aorta, and to manage intrathoracic bleeding. Performing a resuscitative thoracotomy comes with negative aspects, such as potential risk to bedside providers as well as high cost in the setting of a low likelihood of meaningful recovery. Multiple studies have attempted to define what groups of patients should be candidates for the procedure on the basis of the mechanism of injury and physiology at the time of presentation. Patients with the best outcomes after resuscitative thoracotomy are those with penetrating thoracic injuries who have signs of life on reaching the emergency department. Penetrating injuries to the chest with cardiac injury are the most likely to respond favorably to resuscitative thoracotomy, although survival rates reach 35%.[16] Blunt trauma patients have uniformly poor outcomes with survival rates as low as 1% identified, with almost all survivors demonstrating poor neurologic outcome.[16] For this reason, blunt trauma patients are usually not considered candidates outside of extraordinary circumstances. Within the penetrating chest injury population, those with stab wounds fair the best because of a high likelihood of pericardial tamponade without major cardiac injury that responds well to pericardial decompression. Resuscitative thoracotomy should be performed only in locations that have readily available surgical support to perform definitive repair of thoracic injuries if return of spontaneous circulation is achieved.

Endovascular occlusion of the aorta during the initial resuscitation has recently emerged as a promising method of obtaining temporary hemorrhage control in the agonal patient.[17] Resuscitative endovascular balloon occlusion of the aorta (REBOA) is commonly used in the setting of ruptured abdominal aortic aneurysms to essentially slow bleeding and to allow enough time for an adequate repair to be performed. Also driven by military needs, REBOA is now being used at select trauma centers to occlude the aorta in the trauma bay in the setting of advanced shock and imminent cardiac arrest. By essentially cross-clamping the aorta, REBOA shunts blood to the heart and brain while also slowing blood loss from abdominal and pelvic injuries. Although more work is required to better evaluate the procedure, REBOA may offer a quicker, less invasive method of achieving aortic occlusion during the initial resuscitation of the injured patient, thus providing another tool to combat early exsanguinating blood loss.[17]

Secondary Survey

A thorough head to toe examination is required to assist in identifying all potential injuries. This is often performed immediately after the primary survey in patients who are stable and not requiring emergent intervention. Findings identified during the secondary survey often prompt further evaluation with imaging or other diagnostic modalities. A more detailed neurologic evaluation can be completed at this time and abnormalities of the face and neck identified. Posterior surfaces that are more difficult to visualize because of the cervical collar are now better examined. The torso is evaluated to identify evidence of pulmonary dysfunction, and findings consistent with peritonitis must be recognized. Seat belt marks or other superficial injury to the neck and abdomen may prompt further evaluation. The pelvis is assessed for tenderness, with care taken to avoid excessive compression because this technique to identify stability may disrupt hemostasis. A rectal examination with a nonbloody glove to assess the position of the prostate and the presence of gross gastrointestinal blood should be included. The extremities are manipulated to identify open or closed deformities, and distal perfusion must be carefully assessed, especially in the presence of fractures or dislocations. Formal evaluation consisting of distal blood pressure measurements with comparison to uninjured extremities is valuable to identify vascular injuries. The patient is rolled to evaluate the spine for deformity or tenderness, and the long spine board should be removed if it is still present. In the setting of penetrating trauma, all possible areas of skin must be visualized, including those in hidden locations, such as the scalp, posterior neck, mouth, axilla, perineum, and back. Marking of penetrating injuries with radiopaque markers can be extremely helpful if subsequent imaging studies are obtained.

MANAGEMENT OF SPECIFIC INJURIES

Damage Control Principles

The concept of damage control evolved in contrast to the traditional approach of definitive repair of all injuries during the initial operation. Some patients would experience progressive physiologic derangement during these operations, often developing hypothermia, coagulopathy, and metabolic acidosis, a combination that has been labeled the deadly triad. Damage control emerged as a way of halting this rapid physiologic deterioration by quickly managing bleeding, providing aggressive resuscitation, and leaving more definitive reconstruction for a time when stability has been established. Rotondo and associates coined the term *damage control* to describe this approach to management of patients who were progressing rapidly toward death.[18] Surgical bleeding is quickly controlled, which may include intrathoracic or intra-abdominal packing to achieve hemostasis. Hollow visceral injury can be managed by primary repair or resection with temporary gastrointestinal discontinuity to expedite the operation. Temporary closure of the chest or abdomen is achieved, often with a vacuum-type closure method, to avoid the development of intracompartment hypertension and to manage large amounts of fluid drainage. Resuscitation in the intensive care unit follows, with return to the operating room on normalization of body temperature, coagulopathy, and metabolic acidosis. Damage control began as an approach to severe abdominal injuries but now is used in the chest, pelvis, and extremities. Many now advocate for a similar approach to orthopedic injuries based on the theory that rapid fracture stabilization may reduce the inflammatory response to injury.

Consistent with damage control surgery, an approach to resuscitation that includes the provision of equivalent amounts of all of the components within blood has recently emerged. Termed damage control resuscitation or massive transfusion, military experience has prompted an approach to resuscitation that replaces lost blood with equal amounts of packed red blood cells, plasma, platelets, and cryoprecipitate. The military experience and more recently some civilian centers have demonstrated the prevention of severe coagulopathy, which has been associated with less physiologic derangement after severe injury.[19] Others have reported data refuting these findings, although the majority of trauma centers have adopted this approach and now have a well-defined massive transfusion protocol.

Finally, the latest addition to the area of damage control principles and early resuscitation is tranexamic acid (TXA). TXA inhibits fibrinolysis and has been found to decrease blood loss on elective surgery. The CRASH-2 trial randomized 20,211 injured patients to either early administration of TXA (within 8 hours) or placebo.[20] Patients who received TXA demonstrated a decrease in all-cause mortality compared with placebo (14.5% versus 16%; $P = .0035$).[20] There have been some concerns about an increased risk of thromboembolic events secondary to administration of an antifibrinolytic agent, although TXA has become a part of the initial resuscitation within many prehospital systems and trauma centers.

Injuries to the Brain

Even in the setting of optimal care, traumatic brain injuries (TBIs) result in substantial morbidity and mortality. Those who survive often experience permanent disability that ranges from mild deficits to conditions requiring total care. The outcomes faced by patients who sustain multiple injuries are often dictated predominantly by the TBI. As injury epidemiology has evolved, falls now are the most common cause of brain injuries, with those at the extremes of age being the most vulnerable. At the tissue level, brain injuries are the result of either direct transmission of energy or the accumulation of blood within the cranium. Energy transmitted to the cranium and the underlying brain tissue can cause direct injury both at the location of contact and on the contralateral side. Further, the tearing of blood vessels at the time of injury can result in the accumulation of blood within the cranium. As is the case with most tissue, injured brain develops edema after injury that can be worsened by ongoing ischemia. According to the Monro-Kellie doctrine, any increase in the volume of intracranial contents (from blood or edema) results in an elevation of intracranial pressure (ICP) with an associated decrease in the volume of other tissues, such as the brain parenchyma and cerebrospinal fluid. As seen in Figure 16-7, an increase in intracranial volume results in an exponential increase in ICP once the volume

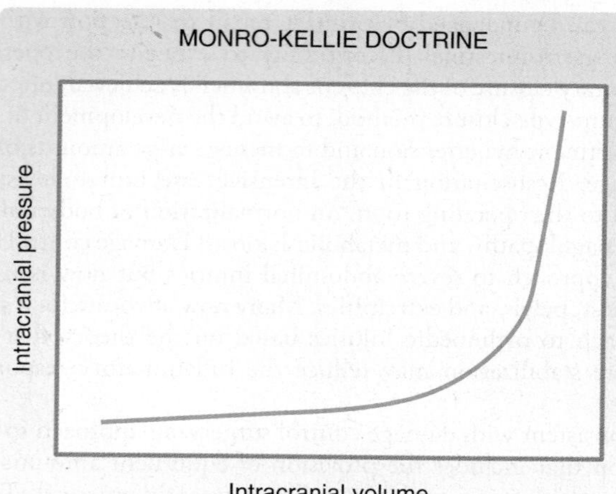

FIGURE 16-7 Monro-Kellie doctrine, which describes the increase in intracranial pressure as intracranial volume increases from hemorrhage or edema. This relationship of pressure to volume is a result of the rigid cranial vault that exhibits a fixed volume.

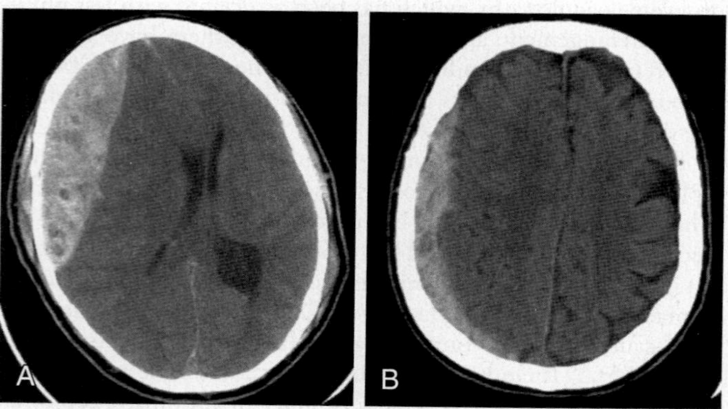

FIGURE 16-8 Cranial CT demonstrating **(A)** an epidural hematoma and **(B)** a subdural hematoma. Blood appears as high-density fluid *(white)* identified on the right side of both images. The epidural hematoma is associated with a significant midline shift. Note how the subdural hematoma follows the contour of the underlying brain.

exceeds that which is present within the rigid cranial vault. This significantly elevated ICP only worsens cerebral perfusion and oxygenation, which results in further edema.

In terms of specific TBIs, epidural hematomas (Fig. 16-8) typically result from a lateral fracture of the cranium causing bleeding from the middle meningeal artery or a nearby vessel. Classically, the clinical course consists of an initial loss of consciousness followed by a lucid interval, during which time the hematoma is expanding. On reaching a significant size, the epidural hematoma causes profound neurologic deterioration. Recognition of this clinical course early can result in treatment with decompression that leads to a favorable outcome. Fortunately, the underlying brain tissue is often not severely injured in the setting of an epidural hematoma. This is in distinction to subdural hematomas, which commonly are associated with severe underlying brain tissue injury (see Fig. 16-8). Subdural hematomas are commonly caused by tearing of the bridging veins between the dura mater and the cerebral cortex. Although the hematoma itself can be compressive, it is usually the underlying brain contusion and axonal injury that predict the outcome after these injuries. Bleeding within the subarachnoid space is indicative of diffuse bleeding from brain tissue and in itself is not deleterious. Despite this, subarachnoid hemorrhages are not benign, and surveillance is mandated to identify deterioration. Parenchymal contusions of brain tissue result from the direct transmission of energy to the cranium and underlying brain as well as from movement of the brain within the rigid cranial vault, resulting in injury on the opposite side (contrecoup injury). Secondary brain injury resulting from cerebral edema is the greatest cause of morbidity after intraparenchymal contusion. Finally, diffuse axonal injury describes the phenomenon of disruption of the axon from the neuronal body secondary to severe rotational forces that are believed to create a shearing effect. Imaging often underestimates the severity of diffuse axonal injury, with only punctate hemorrhages and possibly a loss of differentiation of gray and white matter being present. Commonly, diffuse axonal injury becomes evident when patients experience a poor neurologic outcome in the setting of underwhelming imaging studies.

Immediate Management

Secondary brain injury prevention is the primary goal of the management of TBI. The primary brain injury process cannot be reversed or corrected, and the outcome after TBI is dictated by how well secondary injury is prevented. As the pathophysiologic process suggests, the mainstay of preventing secondary brain injury consists of maintenance of acceptable cerebral perfusion and subsequent oxygenation. Airway control and ventilatory support are therefore critical immediately after TBI. Hemorrhage control and resuscitation should be initiated to prevent hypoperfusion, which can further worsen the ischemic insult to the brain. Quantifying the degree of neurologic deficit by determining the GCS score may be helpful in comparing the patient's neurologic function throughout the continuum of care. Because anticoagulant and antithrombotic medications can worsen intracranial bleeding, urgent reversal is indicated as soon as the presence of these agents becomes evident. Patients who require operative decompression should be immediately transferred to a facility capable of neurosurgical procedures. When necessary, transfer should be a high priority and not be delayed to obtain studies that will have no immediate impact on the care of the patient.

Evaluation

A brief neurologic assessment is first performed during the primary survey when the GCS score is determined. The motor function component of the GCS is the most predictive of future neurologic outcome, with the ability to localize stimulation or to follow commands being favorable. An assessment of the size and reactivity of the pupils is also included because this can be indicative of intracranial hypertension with impingement on the cranial nerves. When possible, a neurologic examination should be performed before the administration of any sedating or paralyzing agents so as not to obscure pertinent findings.

Following in priority the management of airway, breathing, and circulation, patients with TBI benefit from immediate imaging of the head to expedite decompression when it is needed. Cranial computed tomography (CT) without the IV administration of a contrast agent is the most important diagnostic study during the initial evaluation of TBI because it is highly sensitive for detecting intracranial hemorrhage. On cranial CT, acute blood appears as high-density fluid that may be identified in various locations within the head. Contusions within the brain parenchyma with associated edema can be visualized on CT; mass effect with lateral shifting of brain matter is also an important CT finding. Intracranial abnormalities found on CT may require emergent craniotomy, so promptly obtaining the study is paramount. Magnetic resonance imaging (MRI) may be able to provide better anatomic detail, but it has no role in the initial evaluation of the brain-injured patient.

Management

Immediate cranial CT will provide the information required to prompt operative therapy. Neurosurgical consultation should be obtained early to allow rapid transfer to the operating room when necessary. Most commonly, epidural and subdural hematomas with mass effect benefit from drainage and decompression in the operating room. Depressed skull fractures may require early operative intervention to manage hemorrhage and to elevate the displaced bone. Epidural and subdural hematomas are managed with craniotomy, followed by evacuation of hematoma and cessation of intracranial bleeding. After surgery, management includes ongoing surveillance of neurologic function and avoidance of intracranial hypertension. In the setting of severe intracranial hypertension, patients will occasionally benefit from decompressive craniectomy to remove a portion of the cranium and possibly to perform a parenchymal resection.

Patients with intracranial hemorrhage frequently require close neurologic monitoring, which is usually performed in a higher level of care, such as the intensive care unit. On occasion, less severe TBIs can be monitored in a lower level of care when the risk of ongoing bleeding is low and neurosurgical assistance is readily available. The Brain Trauma Foundation provides a comprehensive assessment of the available literature to arrive at evidence-based recommendations.[21] To limit secondary injury, support of cardiovascular and pulmonary function is of great importance. ICP is often measured, with the goal being to reduce brain tissue edema as much as possible. Cerebral perfusion pressure (CPP), which is the difference between the mean arterial pressure and the ICP, is also commonly used to guide severe TBI management. Although ICP and CPP are both frequently used to guide the management of patients with severe TBI, neither of these measurements has been found to be superior. Despite this, it has been recognized that the overaggressive treatment of CPP may in fact be deleterious. A suggested approach to the management of severe TBI is presented in Figure 16-9.

Ongoing intracranial hypertension may require various interventions to manage ICP. Head of bed elevation is a simple technique that can provide gravity-assisted reduction in ICP, but the

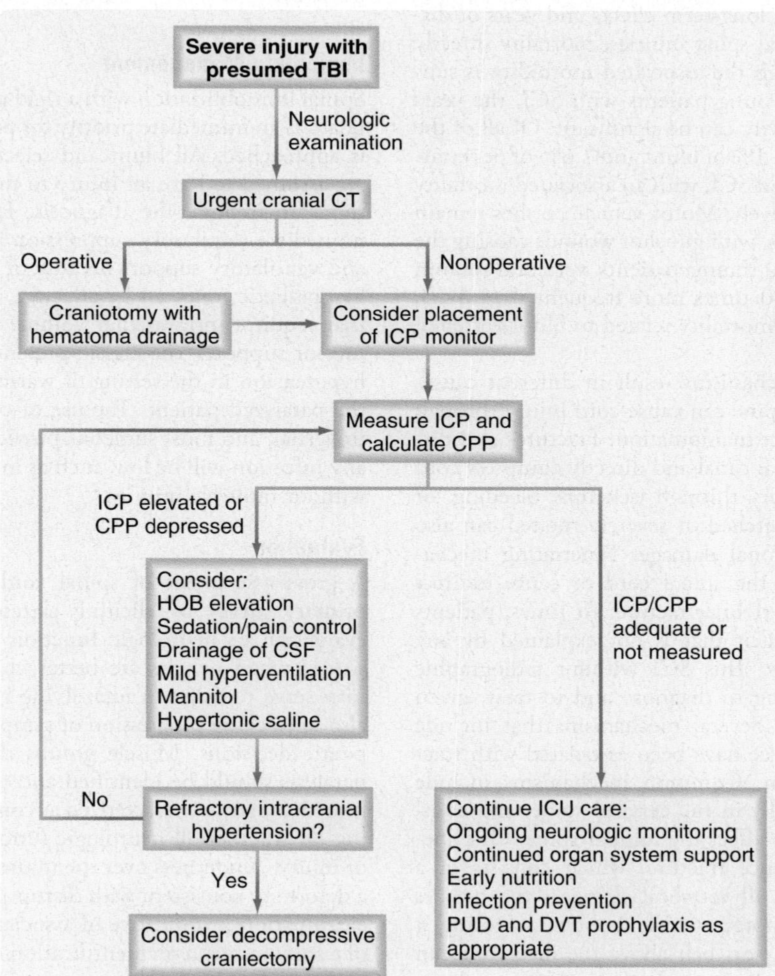

FIGURE 16-9 Algorithm for the management of traumatic brain injury. *CPP,* Cerebral perfusion pressure; *CSF,* cerebrospinal fluid; *CT,* computed tomography; *DVT,* deep venous thrombosis; *HOB,* head of bed; *ICP,* intracranial pressure; *ICU,* intensive care unit; *PUD,* peptic ulcer disease; *TBI,* traumatic brain injury.

thoracolumbar spine must be stable to be in the upright position. A ventriculostomy may be placed to drain cerebrospinal fluid, which may assist with intracranial hypertension. Although the use of significant hyperventilation has been found to be deleterious, increased ventilation resulting in a PCO_2 between 30 and 35 mm Hg results in an optimal amount of vasoconstriction to decrease intracranial hypertension while maintaining cerebral oxygen delivery. Sedation and pain control aimed at reduction of ICP is valuable, although the depth of neurologic suppression should be kept at a minimum to ensure a productive examination. Hyperosmolar therapy with mannitol or hypertonic saline that functions by reducing brain tissue edema is frequently useful. The administration of mannitol and hypertonic saline requires monitoring of serum osmolarity to prevent severe electrolyte derangement. When ICP remains refractory to these interventions, paralysis and barbiturate coma induction may be beneficial. All available evidence continues to demonstrate that corticosteroid administration has no role in the management of TBI. Patients who respond to the initial TBI management will experience a slow decrease in ICP as edema decreases and neurologic function improves.

Injuries to the Spinal Cord and the Vertebral Column

Although not a common cause of early mortality, spinal cord injuries (SCIs) result in severe long-term effects and years of disability. Except for high cervical spine injuries, mortality directly related to SCIs is low, although the associated morbidity is substantial and irreversible. For young patients with SCI, the years of disability and lost productivity can be significant. Of all of the injured patients in the NTDB, 1% of blunt and 1.6% of penetrating trauma patients sustained an SCI, with an associated mortality of 13.0% and 17.0%, respectively. Motor vehicle crashes remain the leading cause of blunt SCIs, with gunshot wounds causing the most penetrating SCIs. In blunt trauma patients, vertebral column fracture alone is more than 10 times more frequent than SCIs. Although it is more frequent, mortality related to blunt vertebral spine injuries is only 5.5%.

Blunt and penetrating mechanisms result in different causes of SCI. Blunt trauma to the spine can cause cord injury through direct impingement or indirect manipulation. Fractures and dislocations can collapse the spinal canal and directly compress cord tissue or cause secondary injury through ischemia, bleeding, or edema. Cord tissue that is stretched or severely rotated can also be injured, resulting in neuronal damage. Penetrating mechanisms either directly lacerate the spinal cord or cause indirect injury through ischemia or vertebral fracture. At times, patients present with a neurologic deficit that is not explained by any vertebral column abnormality. This SCI without radiographic abnormality can be challenging to diagnose and to treat, given the lack of bone irregularity. Several mechanisms that include different forms of physical force have been associated with fractures of the vertebral column. Common mechanisms include flexion and extension, especially in the cervical spine, and compressive forces that commonly affect the lumbar spine. One specific injury pattern is a Chance fracture, which consists of a transverse disruption through all vertebral elements that occurs most commonly during a motor vehicle accident. During a frontal crash, a malpositioned seat belt above the iliac crest can cause excessive flexion and distraction of lumbar vertebrae, resulting in this fracture pattern. Figure 16-10 exhibits a lumbar spine radiograph that demonstrates a lateral view of a Chance fracture.

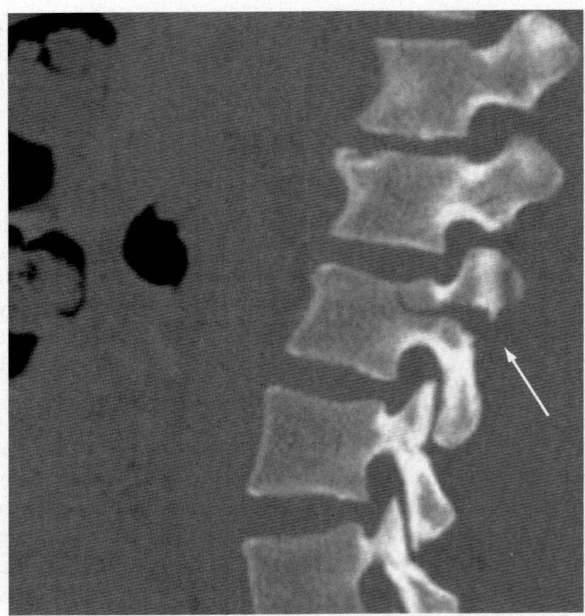

FIGURE 16-10 Chance fracture on lumbar spine CT in sagittal view. Note the fracture involvement of all posterior elements as identified by the *arrow*.

Immediate Management

Spinal immobilization with a rigid cervical collar and a long spine board is an immediate priority for prehospital personnel as a scene is approached. All blunt and select penetrating trauma patients are assumed to have an injury to the spine until a proper evaluation can exclude the diagnosis. High cervical SCIs may have immediate respiratory suppression requiring airway management and ventilatory support because of paresis of the phrenic nerves. Sympathetic tone can be affected, resulting in neurogenic shock that requires intravascular volume expansion and possible vasopressor support. The classic presentation of neurogenic shock is hypotension in the setting of warm, well-perfused extremities in the paralyzed patient. The use of corticosteroids for SCI is controversial, and most surgeons provide them only when the risk of any infection will be low, such as in the setting of an isolated SCI without multiple injuries.[22]

Evaluation

A gross assessment of spinal cord function occurs during the primary survey by eliciting extremity movement. A thorough evaluation of neurologic function occurs during the secondary survey when deficits are better characterized. This information may serve to assist in identifying the location of the injury but also in tracking progression of symptoms, which may affect therapeutic decisions. Muscle groups that demonstrate weakness or paralysis should be identified and the level of sensory loss determined. SCIs are characterized as complete or incomplete, depending on whether all neurologic function is absent below the level of injury. Tenderness over the injured vertebrae or the presence of a deformity consistent with disruption of the vertebral column on examination is indicative of associated fracture. The involvement of a spine surgeon on identification of an injury may guide further evaluation and expedite operative intervention when it is needed. Patients who have no findings on examination, demonstrate no decreased level of consciousness, and have no distracting injuries can undergo clearance of the spine by clinical means alone.

Imaging of the cervical, thoracic, and lumbar portions of the spine is commonly required to further evaluate for vertebral column injury. Although plain radiographs of the spine are acceptable, the high-quality images and rapid availability associated with CT have made this the modality of choice in most emergency departments. Because of the challenges of visualizing the cervicothoracic junction on plain radiography, a dedicated cervical spine CT scan is now often obtained during the initial imaging of the patient. Sagittal and coronal reconstruction of CT imaging of the spine provides better anatomic visualization. CT imaging offers excellent evaluation of bone injuries, but SCIs are poorly delineated because of limited soft tissue detail. Nevertheless, spinal canal compromise and soft tissue edema on CT are highly suggestive of injury to the spinal cord. Figure 16-11 demonstrates a severe cervical spine fracture with subluxation and anterior displacement of the vertebral body.

Although CT has supplanted plain radiography for imaging of the cervical spine, plain radiography remains more conducive to evaluation of the thoracic and lumbar vertebrae. These images provide an assessment of vertebral height and the alignment of the vertebral bodies. Many centers have now developed the ability to avoid obtaining these radiographs by using images obtained during CT examination of the chest, abdomen, and pelvis. These images can be reformatted to specifically visualize the thoracic and lumbar spines in the sagittal and coronal planes. The anatomic detail provided by these images is excellent, and they have been shown to be more sensitive than plain radiographs for bone injury. Many centers have now abandoned plain radiographs in exchange for these reformatted thoracic and lumbar spine CT images. Dedicated CT scans of the spine may still be necessary, particularly when there is significant injury that requires advanced operative planning. As previously described, CT is less effective in the evaluation of the spinal cord, and MRI is often needed to better characterize soft tissue injury. MRI of the spine may provide valuable information to guide early operative intervention. Obtaining these images, especially in the acute setting, must be carefully considered with respect to the patient's overall level of stability.

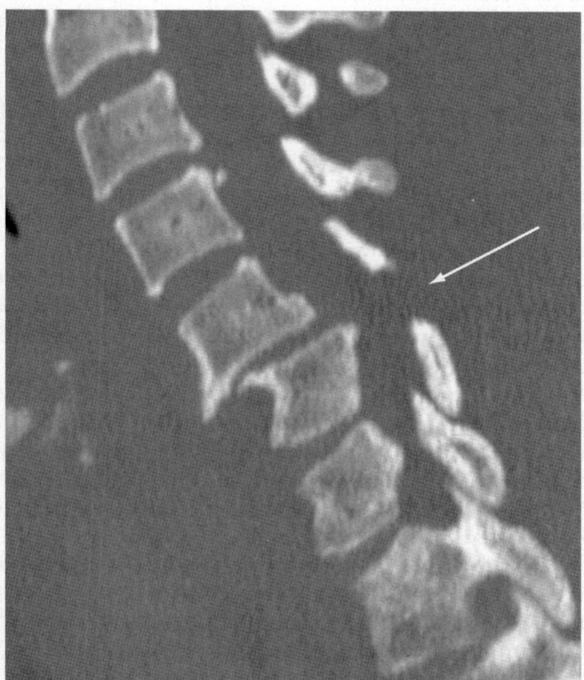

FIGURE 16-11 Cervical spine fracture with severe anterior subluxation and compromise of the spinal canal. The *arrow* identifies the severe narrowing of the spinal canal.

Management

Throughout the patient's entire evaluation, the spine should be protected from further injury by maintaining strict immobilization until injuries can be ruled out. Nevertheless, early removal of the long spine board to avoid the development of pressure wounds is extremely important. On recognition of an SCI, consultation with a spine surgeon should be obtained promptly. Immediate arrangements should be made for transfer when spine surgery services are not available. To avoid delays, subsequent imaging should be avoided unless the results will have an immediate impact on the care provided. Cervical SCIs with neurogenic shock require resuscitation because of a loss of sympathetic tone. Most patients with neurogenic shock respond to volume expansion with crystalloid solution, but some require vasopressor agents, such as dopamine or epinephrine. Cord ischemia and progression of the SCI may worsen in the setting of hypotension, so shock should be treated aggressively. Corticosteroid therapy for SCI has been well studied but remains controversial. Several large randomized trials have demonstrated small improvements in recovery after methylprednisolone administration, especially when it is initiated early after injury.[22] Other investigators have challenged these findings and demonstrated an increased incidence of steroid-related complications, such as infection. Therefore, most physicians agree that steroids remain an option that should be considered after consultation with a spine surgeon. When it is administered, methylprednisolone is provided as a bolus of 30 mg/kg body weight followed by an infusion of 5.4 mg/kg/hr for 23 hours if the bolus was given within 3 hours of injury. The infusion duration is extended to 48 hours if the bolus was administered between 3 and 8 hours after injury, whereas SCIs that occurred more than 8 hours prior should not be treated.

The management of spine injuries varies greatly, depending on the injury pattern and the associated vertebral column stability. Cervical fracture-dislocation injuries may benefit from the application of traction in the emergency department to restore vertebral column alignment. Some SCIs benefit from early operative decompression to reduce cord impingement, especially in the setting of incomplete lesions that demonstrate the ability to improve if further damage is avoided. Vertebral column injuries with instability often require operative fixation as soon as emergent issues are managed and the patient can undergo spine surgery. Fractures without instability may require only immobilization with a hard collar or brace until bone healing can occur. Table 16-4 lists commonly encountered vertebral column fractures with the associated management options. After treatment of injuries to the spine, the patient's neurologic status should be monitored closely for changes that might prompt urgent intervention.

Injury to the Maxillofacial Region

The face is commonly injured in the setting of blunt trauma, although these injuries are rarely life-threatening. Tissue damage that compromises the airway is the greatest concern with maxillofacial injuries, and bleeding can be a significant issue as well. Commonly, poor outcomes after facial injuries are due to a concomitant TBI. Facial injuries can result from direct impact during a blunt mechanism that results in the transmission of energy to

TABLE 16-4 Fractures of the Vertebral Column

FRACTURE	DESCRIPTION	TYPICAL MANAGEMENT
C1 Jefferson fracture	Disruption of C1 ring in multiple locations; blow-out of ring	Stable transverse ligament: hard collar Unstable transverse ligament: traction or surgery
Odontoid fractures	Type I: tip of odontoid Type II: through base Type III: involves C2 body	Type I: hard collar Type II: halo vest or surgery Type III: halo vest
C2 hangman fracture	Bilateral C2 pedicles with spondylolisthesis	Halo vest or surgery if displacement is severe
Cervical vertebral body fractures	Compression or burst of vertebral body with or without retropulsion into canal	Mild loss of height: hard collar Involvement of multiple columns or presence of retropulsion into canal: surgical stabilization
Thoracic vertebral body fractures	Compression or burst of vertebral body with or without retropulsion into canal	Anterior column only: TLSO Anterior and posterior columns: surgical stabilization
Lumbar vertebral body fractures	Compression or burst of vertebral body with or without retropulsion into canal	Anterior column only: TLSO Anterior and posterior columns: surgical stabilization
Chance fracture	Avulsion of posterior elements of lumbar vertebrae seen with high seat belt use	Surgical stabilization

TLSO, Thoracolumbosacral orthosis.

the structures of the face. As a result, facial bone fractures and soft tissue injuries are commonly identified. One specific injury pattern includes the Le Fort class of facial fractures, which consist of three variations of midface disruption from the surrounding facial bones. Penetrating mechanisms, such as gunshot and knife-related wounds, are relatively common and can result in large soft tissue injuries, especially with the passage of a bullet through the face. Significant morbidity can result from injuries to the face, particularly when there is associated sensory disruption from injury to the eyes, ears, nose, or mouth.

Immediate Management

Injury to the face requires prompt assessment and management of the patient's airway, especially when there is lower face soft tissue and bone involvement. Because edema can worsen rapidly, early intubation when there is a concern about airway stability can be lifesaving. Blood or debris in the oropharynx can greatly complicate intubation, and the application of backup airway options, including a surgical approach, may be necessary. Given the vascularity of the face, bleeding can be an immediate concern and should be managed with direct pressure and the initiation of resuscitation. Rapid closure of wounds may be required, although facial bleeding may be challenging to identify. Bleeding from deep vessels or fractured bone may require angioembolization for control to be obtained. Frequently, bleeding from the face is exacerbated by hypothermia and coagulopathy, which should be aggressively prevented or treated.

Evaluation

Facial injuries are first identified on physical examination, during which the extent of soft tissue involvement is determined. The eyes are grossly examined for diplopia and subjective changes in visual acuity. The condition of the globe and the surrounding orbit requires careful evaluation for rupture or extraocular muscle entrapment, which requires urgent treatment. The external ear is examined, and drainage from the ear canal is identified when it is present. Midface and mandibular stability and the condition and proper occlusion of the dentition and alveolar ridge are assessed. Forehead and midface deformities are indicative of underlying frontal and maxillary bone fractures, respectively. When fractures or soft tissue injuries are identified, the motor function of the face should be assessed to evaluate facial nerve function.

Injuries to the face often benefit from three-dimensional imaging with thin-cut CT to adequately visualize the facial bones. Sagittal and coronal as well as three-dimensional reconstructions can aid in the thorough assessment of the bones and deep soft tissue. CT is indicated when severe external injury is identified on secondary survey or when facial abnormality is identified on cranial CT. Imaging of the face should be performed only after life-threatening injuries have been addressed because management of facial injuries is not time sensitive in most cases.

Management

Facial fractures and severe soft tissue injuries often benefit from the involvement of a maxillofacial surgery specialist to assist in management. As previously described, airway management and bleeding are the most immediate priority. Direct pressure and wound closure are often effective in managing facial bleeding. In severe cases, angiography with embolization of bleeding facial blood vessels may be necessary. Before wound closure, jagged or nonviable skin edges should be débrided, followed by irrigation of the wound with sterile fluid. Lacerations can frequently be closed with local anesthesia using deep absorbable sutures followed by closure of the skin with 5-0 or 6-0 interrupted or running sutures. Lacerations to the lip, nose, ear, and orbit are more complex in nature, and closure requires special consideration to facilitate optimal wound healing.

The management of facial fractures is infrequently required in the acute setting and can be deferred until after other injuries are addressed. Severely depressed facial bone fractures are the exception because these may involve the underlying brain and require urgent reduction. Most facial fractures are repaired after time allows the associated edema to decrease. Large open wounds and fractures involving sinuses or the aerodigestive tract require antibiotics shortly after admission, but overextending this course should be avoided. When repair is appropriate, fractures often benefit from open reduction and internal fixation, typically with screws and plates. Reconstructive efforts are aimed at optimizing functional and cosmetic outcomes. This includes the preservation of normal extraocular motor function by addressing orbital fractures with rectus muscle involvement. Mandibular fractures can be treated with maxillary-mandibular fixation, although significant fracture displacement may require internal fixation with plating.

Injuries to the Neck

The neck contains multiple vital structures close to one another and therefore may be challenging and overwhelming to address when it is injured. Nevertheless, as with other areas of the body, managing neck injuries can be made reasonable by implementing an organized approach. Neck injuries are uncommon but result in the highest mortality rate of all body regions (20.0% mortality for AIS ≥3 injuries in the NTDB). Penetrating injuries from gunshot and stab wounds are the most common mechanism of injury. Penetrating injuries can directly lacerate vascular and aerodigestive structures, resulting in substantial bleeding or contamination, respectively. Although uncommon, blunt mechanisms can cause compression, with fracture of the larynx or trachea. Blunt pharyngeal or esophageal injuries are even less common but can result in leakage into the surrounding soft tissue, causing neck or mediastinal infection if they are not adequately managed. Blunt force to the neck can cause injury to the carotid or vertebral arteries. These blunt cerebrovascular injuries (BCVIs) result from seat belt compression or severe flexion-extension mechanisms. BCVI severity ranges from intimal tears, with or without thrombosis, to full-thickness injury with pseudoaneurysm formation. The morbidity associated with a BCVI predominantly includes stroke secondary to thromboembolism that is caused by the disrupted vessel wall.

Immediate Management

Neck injuries can often require rapid intervention because of the vulnerability of the contained vital structures. The highest priority concern is establishment of a secure airway, especially given the rapidity with which deterioration can occur in the setting of a neck injury. Direct injury to the larynx or trachea is the most common cause of airway compromise. Expanding neck hematomas can quickly compress the upper airway, leading to inadequate ventilation. Immediate intubation should occur in the setting of an expanding neck hematoma or if there is concern about impending airway compromise. Suspected laryngotracheal injury presents one of the most challenging airway management situations. Patients who are maintaining their own airway should have a planned approach to airway management that might include intubation or awake tracheostomy in the operating room. Attempted intubation could worsen a tenuous situation and should not be performed without a well-developed backup plan. A loss of airway requires emergent intervention that might include performing a surgical airway. The surgical airway of choice for an upper airway injury is a tracheostomy because injury to the larynx could make cricothyroidotomy ineffective.

In the immediate setting, hemorrhage is the other major concern that might occur after neck injury. Direct pressure effectively manages most bleeding from the neck, at least during transport to the operating room and initiation of neck exploration. Injury to the large vessels of the neck will often require control in the operating room. Bleeding should be immediately treated with digital pressure on the wound until operative exposure can be achieved. Large quantities of blood can be lost quickly, so resuscitation with blood products should be rapidly initiated. Patients with suspected injury should be rapidly transferred to the operating room for surgical management of ongoing bleeding.

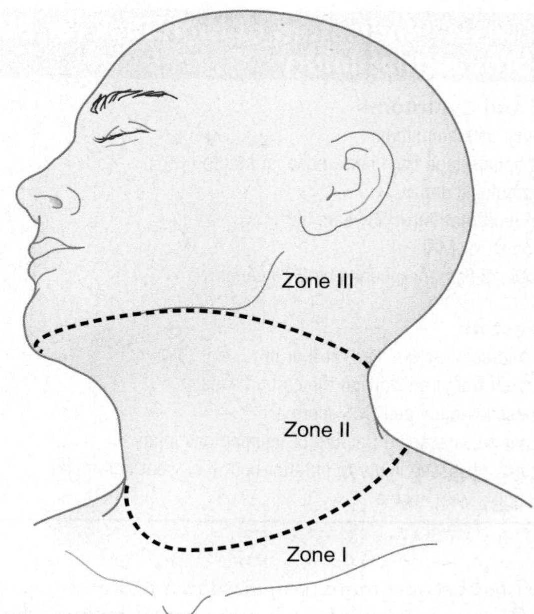

FIGURE 16-12 Zones of the Neck. Zone 1 extends from the thoracic inlet to the cricoid cartilage. Zone 2 is between the cricoid cartilage and the angle of the mandible. Zone 3 extends from the angle of the mandible to the skull base.

Evaluation

Unstable patients should be taken immediately to the operating room, and the structures of the neck will be evaluated with direct visualization. Stable patients require further evaluation for neck injury with physical examination and imaging. Penetrating injuries are characterized by anatomic location, which is demonstrated in Figure 16-12. Zone I extends from the thoracic inlet to the cricoid cartilage and contains large vascular structures as well as the trachea and esophagus. Stretching from the cricoid cartilage to the angle of the mandible, zone II is the most accessible surgically and contains the carotid and vertebral arteries, jugular veins, and structures of the aerodigestive tract. Zone III includes the neck between the angle of the mandible and the base of the skull. Structures within zone III include blood vessels that are difficult to expose surgically. Although zone II injuries traditionally mandated operative exploration, it has since been recognized that only those patients with evidence of active bleeding or an obvious aerodigestive injury require surgery. Regardless of anatomic location, stable neck injuries can be evaluated with selective diagnostic studies.[23]

Diagnostic studies evaluating the neck must assess for injury to the vascular structures. Commonly, this can be achieved with CT angiography, which delineates the vascular anatomy of the neck with great accuracy. CT angiography can be performed quickly in the emergency department and effectively reveals vascular injuries to the neck. Of secondary benefit is the identification of the track of penetrating objects, which may permit selective evaluation of other structures of the neck. Metallic missile debris causes image scatter and may limit the utility of CT angiography. Standard digital subtraction angiography does not suffer from this limitation and may provide added information in this setting. Duplex ultrasonography provides an additional adjunct that can evaluate the carotid and vertebral arteries for injury.

BOX 16-4 Indicators of High Risk for Blunt Cerebrovascular Injury

Signs and Symptoms

Expanding neck hematoma
Arterial hemorrhage from neck, nose, or mouth
Focal neurologic deficit
Cervical bruit (patient < 50 years old)
Stroke on CT or MRI
Neurologic deficit unexplained by CT findings

Risk Factors

Severe midface fracture, Le Fort II or III
Basilar skull fracture involving the carotid canal
Diffuse axonal injury and GCS score ≤ 6
Significant cervical spine fracture or ligamentous injury
Significant soft tissue injury to anterior neck (i.e., seat belt mark)
Near-hanging with anoxia

BCVI has become more recognized as a major source of morbidity after severe injury. Initially thought to be rare, the emergence of high-risk screening criteria and improved imaging technology have led to a significant increase in the diagnosis of BCVIs. Early studies identified criteria that accurately identified patients at high risk of having a BCVI.[24] Digital subtraction angiography subsequently confirmed BCVI in 30% of this high-risk cohort. Commonly referred to as the Denver criteria, these risk factors are used to screen patients and to prompt further evaluation (Box 16-4).[24] The emergence of CT angiography has now replaced digital subtraction angiography as the study of choice for diagnosis of BCVI. On occasion, standard angiography is still necessary, but the improved logistics of obtaining a CT scan and the more favorable associated risk profile have caused most centers to rely heavily on CT imaging for BCVI evaluation.

Neck injuries commonly require an evaluation of the aerodigestive tract. The trachea is best evaluated by performing bronchoscopy. More superior injuries require laryngoscopy, although laryngeal injuries can be challenging to identify. The evaluation of the esophagus is best achieved by performing both contrast esophagography and esophagoscopy. When performed in isolation, these studies can miss a significant number of injuries, although together the sensitivity is high. Often, when CT imaging has been previously performed, this information can be used to selectively obtain diagnostic studies when the involvement of a given structure has clearly been avoided. Figure 16-13 presents a coordinated approach to the evaluation of penetrating neck injuries as developed by the WTA.[25]

Management

Active bleeding, expanding neck hematoma, and obvious aerodigestive injuries require immediate neck exploration. Most commonly, structures of the neck are exposed by an incision along the anterior border of the sternocleidomastoid muscle on the side of the injury. A collar incision may be more versatile, especially if both sides of the neck need exploration. The platysma is divided, exposing the anterior border of the sternocleidomastoid muscle, which is dissected from the underlying tissue. The internal jugular vein is next identified and exposed. An injured internal jugular vein may require direct repair or ligation if closure is not possible. The facial vein is identified entering the anterior surface of the internal jugular vein. Ligation of the facial vein allows the deep structures of the neck to be exposed. With the internal jugular vein retracted laterally, the carotid sheath is identified and opened. If necessary, the carotid artery is controlled proximally and distally if an arterial injury is suspected. Care should be taken to avoid injury to the adjacent vagus nerve and the hypoglossal nerve, which crosses the internal carotid artery superiorly. Short-segment carotid artery injuries should be repaired with either simple closure or end-to-end anastomosis. More extensive injuries require reconstruction with a synthetic graft or autologous vein. In damage control situations, the carotid artery can be ligated if no other options exist, although cerebral blood flow may be compromised.

Exploration of the trachea and esophagus is achieved by retracting the carotid artery laterally. Dissection is continued medially and may be aided by the placement of a nasogastric tube to allow palpation of the esophagus. Injuries to the esophagus should be débrided to expose the entirety of the perforation, which is often larger than initially visualized. Closure of the esophageal wall can be in one or two layers, and wide drainage is important. Covering the esophageal repair with viable muscle may be highly beneficial, especially in the setting of adjacent tracheal or vascular repair. Massive tissue loss or delayed presentation poses a challenge and may require esophageal diversion with esophagostomy followed by delayed reconstruction. Tracheal lacerations can be primarily closed with absorbable suture if the injury is small and will approximate in a tension-free fashion. Large tracheal defects often require resection and anastomosis, although some anterior tracheal injuries can be managed by creating a tracheostomy through the injury. After the tracheostomy tract matures, the tube can be removed, and closure usually occurs spontaneously.

As the evaluation of BCVIs has evolved, treatment has also become more advanced. To decrease the risk of thromboembolic stroke, anticoagulation or antiplatelet therapy is required after the diagnosis of BCVI. Bleeding risk from associated injuries often limits the ability to begin immediate anticoagulation or antiplatelet therapy, but treatment should be initiated as soon as safely possible. Fortunately, a significant percentage of strokes occur days to weeks after injury and therefore still benefit from delayed initiation of therapy. Figure 16-14 presents an approach to the diagnosis and management of BCVIs published by the WTA.[26] Anticoagulation with heparin should be started with the goal of achieving a partial thromboplastin time between 40 and 50 seconds. Antiplatelet therapy is now believed to be as effective as full anticoagulation in most circumstances. CT angiography can be repeated at 7 days and therapy discontinued if complete healing has occurred. Persistent injury requires treatment for 3 months, followed by repeated imaging. Pseudoaneurysms may benefit from endovascular management with stent placement or embolization for vertebral artery injuries.

Injuries to the Chest

Injuries to the thorax are common, occurring in more than 20% of patients in the NTDB. The chest contains vital cardiopulmonary structures, and therefore these injuries can be life-threatening. Chest injuries result equally from blunt and penetrating mechanisms, with an overall mortality of 9.9%.[27] Falls and motor vehicle crashes cause the majority of blunt chest injuries by the transmission of energy to the chest wall and underlying structures. Direct compression and deceleration and rotational physical mechanisms are the causes of thoracic injuries at the tissue level. The prominence of the chest makes it vulnerable to penetrating mechanisms,

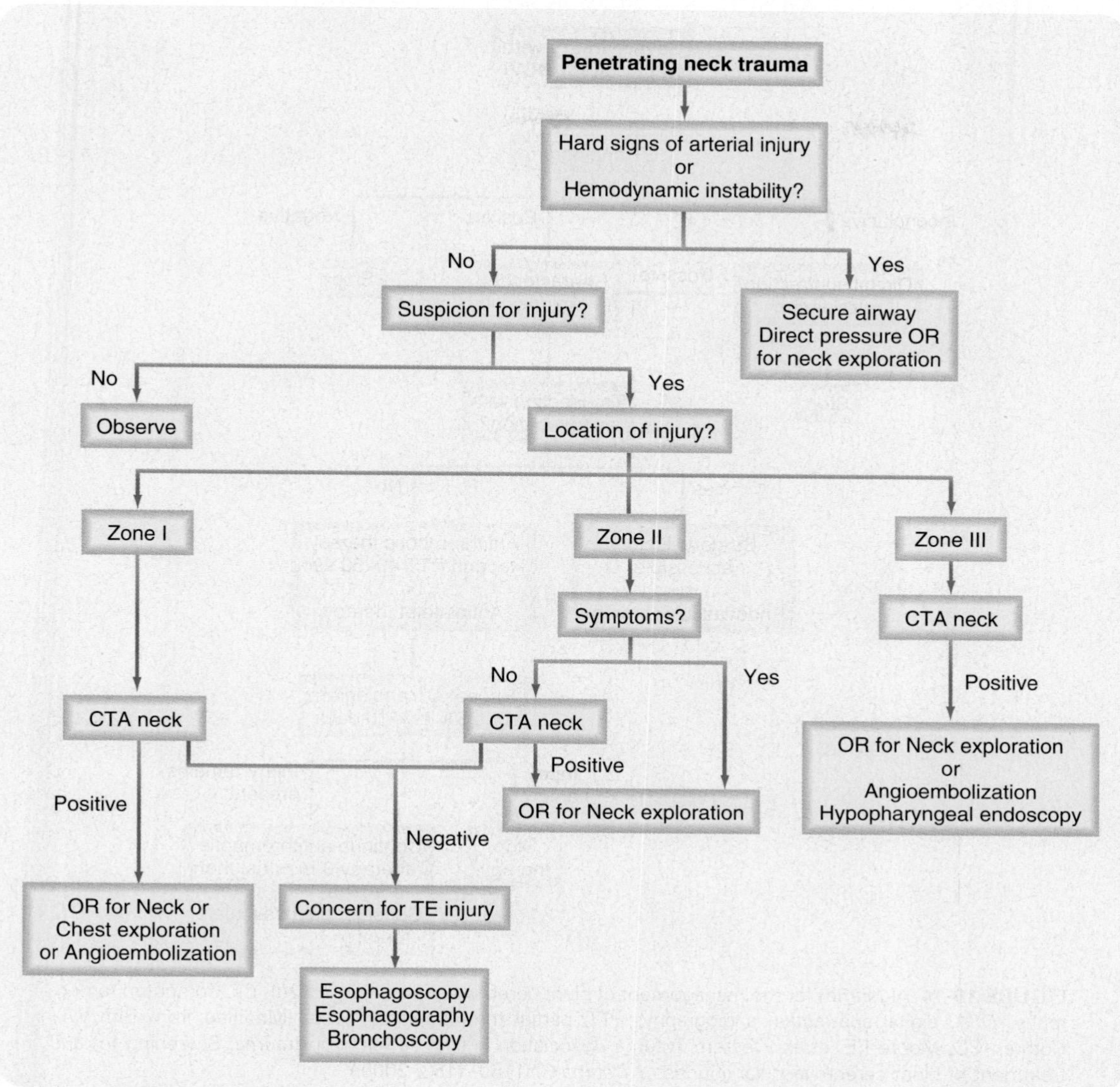

FIGURE 16-13 Algorithm for the management of penetrating neck injuries. Hard signs include active bleeding, expanding neck hematoma, air bubbling from wound, neurologic deficit, and hematemesis. *CTA,* Computed tomography angiography; *OR,* operating room; *TE,* tracheoesophageal. (Modified from Sperry JL, Moore EE, Coimbra R, et al: Western Trauma Association critical decisions in trauma: Penetrating neck trauma. *J Trauma Acute Care Surg* 75:936–940, 2013.)

such as gunshot and stab wounds. Penetrating mechanisms result in direct laceration of pulmonary and mediastinal structures. Gunshot wounds can also cause significant lung contusion to tissue adjacent to the track of the missile. Despite the serious nature of these injuries, most can be treated effectively with basic interventions.

Immediate Management

Thoracic injuries often require intervention during the primary survey because of the impact on cardiopulmonary function. Chest injuries with pulmonary compromise require immediate management of the airway with ventilatory assistance. Decreased breath sounds with poor pulmonary compliance are consistent with a tension pneumothorax and may require urgent placement of a tube thoracostomy. External bleeding should be controlled with direct pressure while resuscitation with crystalloid solution and blood products is initiated. Hemodynamic instability most commonly indicates hemorrhage that requires control of bleeding and resuscitation. In addition, hypotension may be due to a tension pneumothorax as well as cardiac dysfunction secondary to pericardial tamponade, cardiac contusion or myocardial infarction, or coronary air embolism. Following an assessment for sources of blood loss, a search for pericardial fluid with ultrasound or pericardial window is needed, especially after penetrating trauma. Patients in shock with ongoing blood loss from the chest or pericardium often require operative intervention. Cardiac arrest, especially in the setting of penetrating mechanisms, may benefit from resuscitative thoracotomy (see earlier section). Figure 16-15 demonstrates an approach to the initial evaluation and management of penetrating chest injuries.

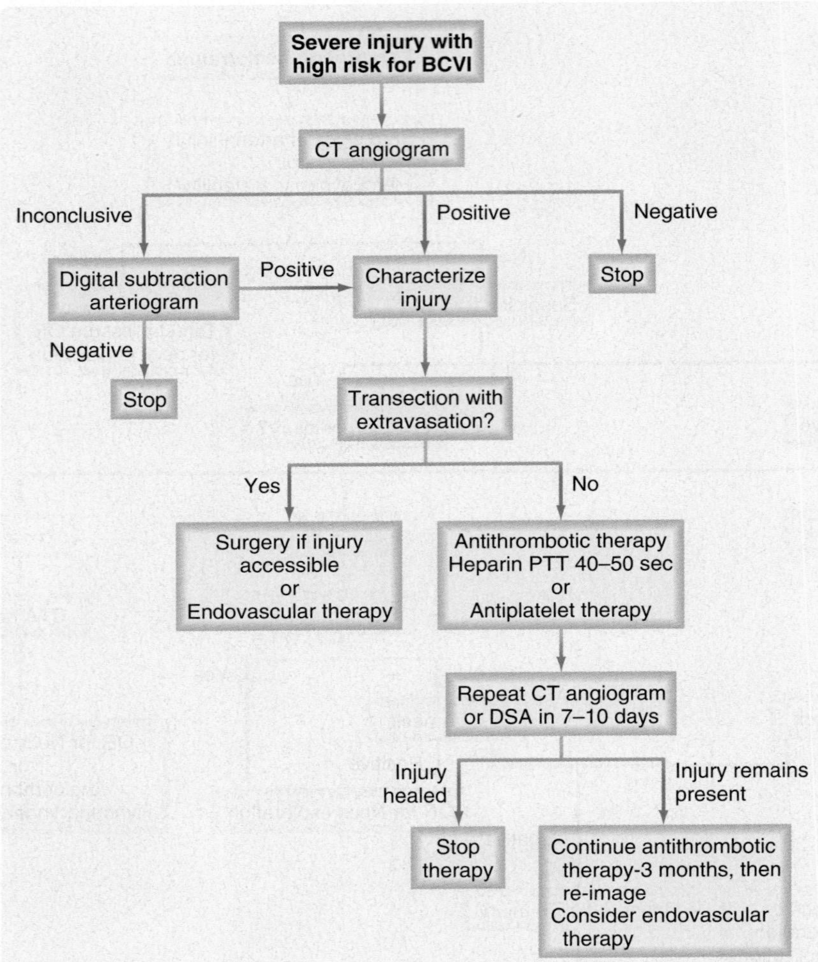

FIGURE 16-14 Algorithm for the management of blunt cerebrovascular injury (BCVI). *CT,* Computed tomography; *DSA,* digital subtraction angiography; *PTT,* partial thromboplastin time. (Modified from Biffl WL, Cothren CC, Moore EE, et al: Western Trauma Association critical decisions in trauma: Screening for and treatment of blunt cerebrovascular injuries. *J Trauma* 67:1150–1153, 2009.)

Evaluation

The majority of chest injuries can be diagnosed with physical examination and plain chest radiography. External injuries, such as chest wall defects and penetrating wounds, will be identified on physical examination. Chest wall tenderness and abnormal movement can be identified to reflect injuries to the ribs and sternum. Deviation of the trachea at the sternal notch may reveal intrathoracic tension on the side opposite the trachea. Chest radiography is performed on all significantly injured patients at risk for thoracic injuries. A chest radiograph can be obtained rapidly in the trauma bay during the initial assessment. Most important, the chest is evaluated for the presence of a pneumothorax or hemothorax that would require immediate tube thoracostomy. Whereas the chest radiograph may suggest aortic injury, thoracic CT angiography has become the standard approach to evaluation of the chest. CT provides visualization of the chest wall and hemithoraces, allowing identification of rib fractures, pneumothoraces, hemothoraces, and pulmonary contusion. Furthermore, chest CT angiography is able to identify transection of the aortic wall as well as lower grade injuries that involve only the aortic intima. CT angiography has become accepted as sufficient to guide operative intervention without the need for standard angiography of the chest.

Penetrating injuries that are believed to involve or to cross the mediastinum require further evaluation. Wounds within the area defined by the sternal notch superiorly, the costal margin inferiorly, and the nipples laterally constitute these high-risk injuries. Cardiovascular and aerodigestive structures within the mediastinum require assessment for bleeding or perforation. Immediate ultrasound is performed to evaluate the pericardium for effusion, although communication with one of the hemithoraces may yield false-negative results. The great vessels are evaluated for injury with CT angiography, although this can be impeded by the presence of retained missile fragments that cause scatter. This is one setting in which standard angiography may be valuable. Depending on the trajectory of the penetrating object, the trachea and proximal airways may require evaluation with bronchoscopy. To evaluate the esophagus, a combination of esophagoscopy and contrast esophagography is diagnostic. As described in the neck injury section, these studies have an approximate 20% false-negative rate in isolation, although their combined sensitivity approaches 100%.

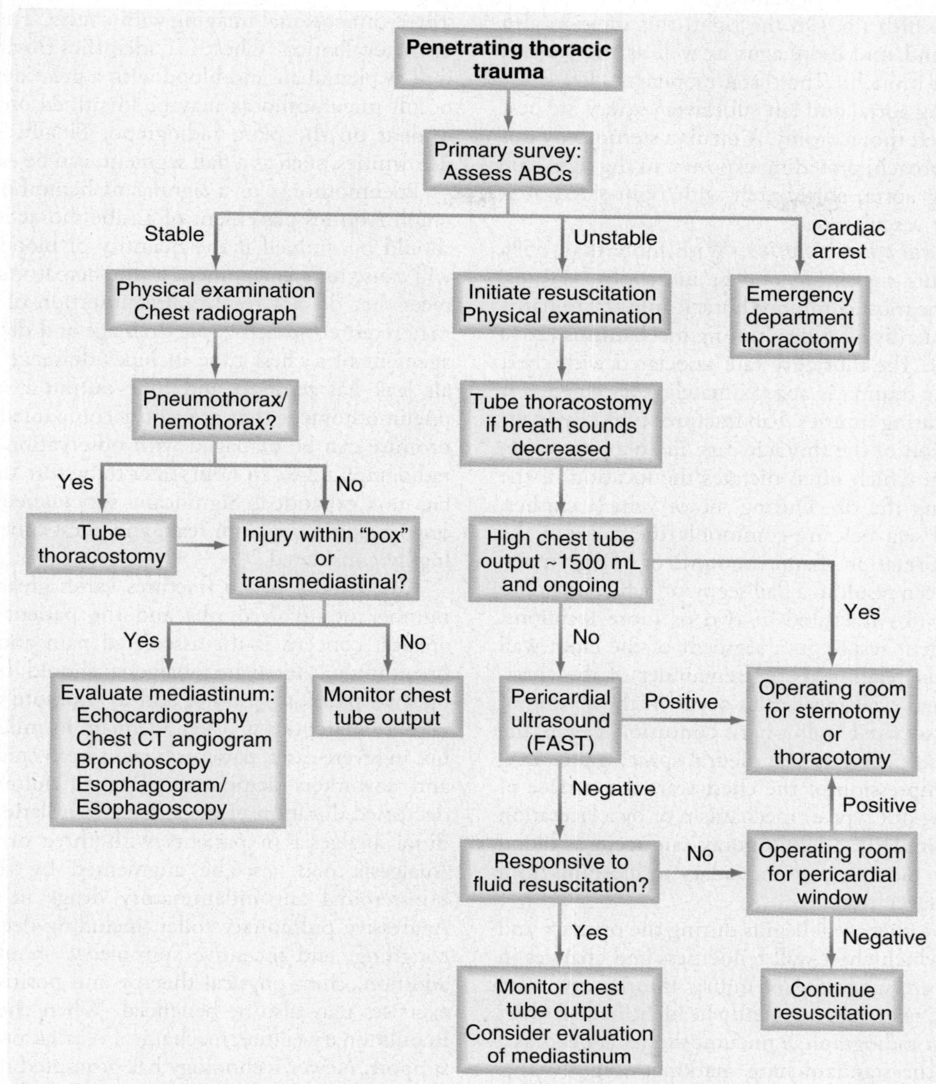

FIGURE 16-15 Algorithm for the management of penetrating thoracic injuries. *FAST,* Focused abdominal sonography in trauma.

Management

Thoracic injuries are often straightforward to manage, with up to 85% successfully treated with tube thoracostomy alone. Although chest tubes are often urgently required, placement may still be performed in a controlled manner to include strict sterile preparation and excellent surgical technique. To avoid the development of an empyema, the chest should be prepared appropriately by wide preparation with chlorhexidine (not just a splash of povidone-iodine) as well as full body draping to maintain the sterility of the field. After infusion of local anesthetic, the skin incision should be made at the level of the nipple to stay superior enough to avoid the highest reach of the diaphragm. A subcutaneous tunnel is created in a superior direction, and the chest is entered bluntly in an interspace above the skin incision. The lung is palpated to confirm chest entry and to evaluate for intrathoracic adhesions. A chest tube large enough to drain blood (typically 32 to 36 Fr) is then advanced through the incision and positioned posterior to the lung. If the tube is being placed only for a pneumothorax, the anterior hemithorax is a more appropriate position. To confirm that the tube is not kinked, it is helpful to be sure that the tube freely spins before completion of the procedure. The tube is then connected to an underwater drainage device providing 20 cm H_2O suction.

Tube thoracostomies that drain large amounts of blood on initial placement or demonstrate ongoing output indicate active intrathoracic bleeding requiring thoracotomy. The widely accepted indications for immediate thoracotomy include more than 1500 mL of blood drained on chest tube insertion or more than 300 mL/hr of drainage for 3 consecutive hours. Although these values may indicate intrathoracic bleeding, it is most important to determine if ongoing surgical bleeding is present. For example, chest tubes that initially drain 1500 mL but then have little ongoing output in the setting of hemodynamic stability may not require thoracotomy. Other indications for thoracotomy include a massive air leak with associated pneumothorax and drainage of esophageal or gastric contents from the chest tube. When thoracotomy is required, the choice of surgical approach depends on the suspected injury. Access to the lungs, pulmonary vasculature, and hemidiaphragm is achieved through a posterolateral thoracotomy that is best performed through the fifth interspace, with possible removal of the fifth rib. On the right, this incision also exposes the proximal and mid esophagus as well as the trachea and bilateral mainstem bronchi. The distal esophagus, left lung, left ventricle, descending aorta, and left subclavian artery are best approached through a left thoracotomy. A median sternotomy can be a highly versatile approach, providing exposure to the right side of the heart, ascending aorta, aortic arch with right-sided arch vessels, and pulmonary vasculature.

Chest wall and pleural space injuries. With more than 65% of blunt trauma patients sustaining one or more rib fractures, chest wall injuries are the most common thoracic injury. Similarly, rib fractures occur frequently after penetrating mechanisms (28% of cases in the NTDB). The mortality rate associated with chest wall injuries after blunt trauma is approximately 7%, whereas it exceeds 19% for penetrating injuries. Rib fractures typically occur secondary to compression of the thoracic cage in an anteroposterior or lateral direction, which often dictates the location of the cortical disruption along the rib. During motor vehicle crashes, the steering wheel and seat belt are commonly the cause of the inciting chest wall deformation. Large amounts of energy transferred to the chest wall can result in a flail segment, which includes two or more adjacent ribs fractured in two or more locations. Essentially, a flail segment results in a segment of the chest wall that moves separately in relation to the remainder of the chest. Although abnormal chest wall mechanics occur in the setting of a flail segment, the associated pulmonary contusion causes the greatest physiologic insult. Within the pleural space, a pneumothorax occurs after compression of the chest tears the surface of the lung through a blow-out type of mechanism or by a laceration from a fractured rib. Similarly, a hemothorax can occur as blood accumulates within the pleural space secondary to bleeding from the chest wall or lung laceration.

The evaluation of the chest wall begins during the primary and secondary surveys, in which chest wall tenderness and changes in pulmonary mechanics are suggestive of injury. Injuries involving the chest wall or pleural space can frequently be identified on chest radiographs. On a chest radiograph, a pneumothorax appears as a lucency peripheral to the standard lung markings (Fig. 16-16).

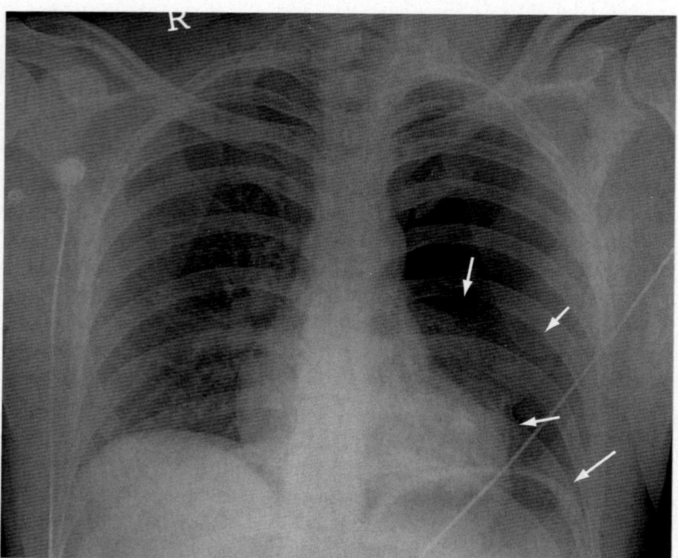

FIGURE 16-16 Large left-sided pneumothorax on plain chest radiograph. The *arrows* identify the lateral border of the collapsed lung.

Three-dimensional imaging with chest CT is often a valuable part of the evaluation. Chest CT identifies rib and sternal fractures as well as pleural air and blood with a great degree of sensitivity. An occult pneumothorax may be identified on chest CT that is not evident on the plain radiograph. Finally, significant chest wall deformities, such as a flail segment, can be easily identified on CT.

Pneumothorax or a significant hemothorax on a chest radiograph requires placement of a tube thoracostomy. Hemothoraces should be drained if the quantity of blood in the pleural space will cause lung entrapment as the hematoma matures. Hemothoraces that do not resolve after insertion of a tube thoracostomy may require thoracoscopic drainage and decortication. The management of a chest tube includes drainage until any pulmonary air leak has resolved and tube output is not excessive. Occult pneumothoraces that are not accompanied by respiratory compromise can be managed with observation and a repeated chest radiograph 12 to 24 hours later to be sure that the pneumothorax has not expanded. Significant subcutaneous air often suggests ongoing pulmonary air leak, and chest tube placement should be highly considered.

The severity of rib fractures varies greatly, depending on the number of involved ribs and the patient's characteristics. The greatest concern is the associated pain and the development of pneumonia. Adequate analgesia should be provided to allow optimal pulmonary toilet and to promote comfort. Pain control with IV narcotics is often adequate in mild and moderate cases, but in severe cases, patients benefit from epidural analgesia. Bulger and coworkers demonstrated fewer pulmonary infections and decreased duration of mechanical ventilation with the use of epidural analgesia in patients with three or more rib fractures.[28] Analgesia may also be augmented by the administration of nonsteroidal anti-inflammatory drugs in appropriate patients. Aggressive pulmonary toilet, including deep breathing, frequent coughing, and incentive spirometry, should be encouraged. In addition, chest physical therapy and positive expiratory pressure exercises may also be beneficial. When chest wall injuries result in pulmonary failure, mechanical ventilation is required to provide support. Newer technology has prompted renewed interest in the operative fixation of rib fractures, although the appropriate indications for these procedures and the associated benefit remain incompletely defined. Sternal fractures are often managed similarly to rib fractures with pulmonary toilet techniques and analgesia. The presence of an associated mediastinal hematoma with active bleeding from the adjacent internal mammary artery may require angioembolization or open ligation.

Pulmonary injuries. Lung injuries are common after chest trauma, with 31.9% of patients in the NTDB sustaining a pulmonary contusion. Mortality after pulmonary contusion is approximately 10%, predominantly as a result of respiratory failure from the acute respiratory distress syndrome or pneumonia. Pulmonary contusion is caused by energy transfer through the chest wall to the pulmonary parenchyma, resulting in tissue damage as well as hemorrhage into the alveolar and interstitial spaces. This tissue damage is manifested as physiologic shunt with hypoxemia. The majority of morbidity is secondary to a profound inflammatory response that can progress to multiple organ dysfunction or failure. Frequently, pulmonary contusion occurs with a flail segment and is often more clinically important than the rib fractures themselves. Lung injury can also be caused by penetrating mechanisms, with gunshot wounds being the most common. Typically, the missile directly lacerates the parenchyma and then can cause significant contusion of the surrounding tissue.

The drainage of large amounts of blood or air from a tube thoracostomy is often the first indication of a pulmonary injury. Chest radiographs obtained shortly after the patient's arrival may demonstrate pneumothorax or hemothorax, which may be suggestive of underlying pulmonary injury. Lung contusions may be present on the initial chest radiograph but typically require time to become visualized. Pulmonary contusions that are identified early on chest film are frequently severe and often rapidly progress to respiratory failure. Thoracic CT is valuable for the identification of pulmonary contusion, although at times it can be challenging to differentiate contusion from atelectasis. A valuable rule of thumb is that atelectasis does not cross pulmonary fissures, whereas contusions are not limited by ventilatory segments. Furthermore, injured pulmonary tissue in the vicinity of chest wall injuries, especially when it is not in dependent areas, is highly suggestive of pulmonary contusion. Injured lung tissue on CT appears as higher density, as can be seen on Figure 16-17.

Thoracotomy may be required for lung injury when large quantities of blood or air drain from a chest tube. Although there are classic guidelines for chest tube drainage (described earlier), the decision to operate needs to be based on the likelihood of ongoing bleeding. For this reason, ongoing drainage of blood from the chest tube is more important than the amount of initial output. In most cases, tube thoracostomy alone with lung expansion adequately manages low-pressure lung bleeding and small air leaks. Ongoing drainage of blood indicates a more central, high-pressure source, which should prompt thoracotomy and control of bleeding. Bleeding from the pulmonary parenchyma is controlled through suture ligation of bleeding vessels. Missile tracks can be opened by passing a stapler through the wound and performing a tractotomy, which then exposes the injured vessels. When larger segments of lung are injured, pulmonary resection is occasionally required through either an anatomic or nonanatomic approach. Damage control requires the control of surgical bleeding with sutures or staplers, followed by packing of the chest with laparotomy sponges and temporary closure. As opposed to abdominal packing, packs in the chest should occupy minimal space and be constructed to allow maximal lung expansion.

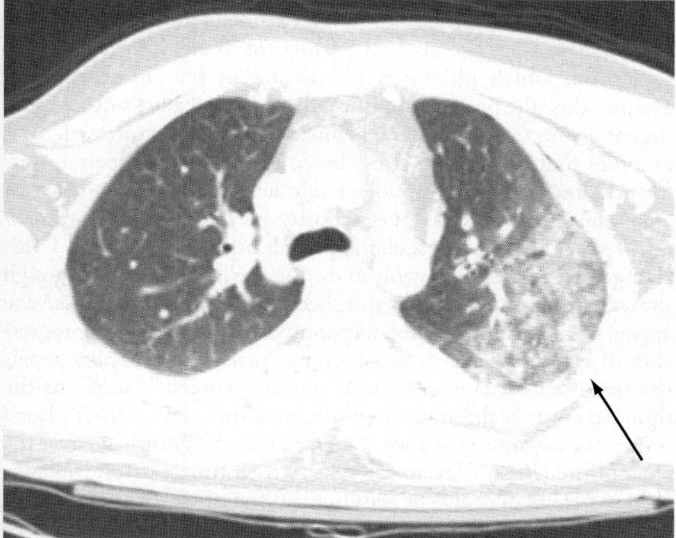

FIGURE 16-17 Left pulmonary contusion on thoracic CT. The *arrow* identifies contused lung, which appears as higher density tissue because of air space hemorrhage and associated edema.

Pulmonary contusion often requires little more than supportive care. Patients should be monitored for hypoxemia, increased work of breathing, and agitation, which indicate respiratory decompensation that often requires intubation and mechanical ventilation. Pulmonary contusions will resolve with time, although patients require support until adequate lung function returns. Efforts to prevent ventilator-associated pneumonia are required because of a significantly increased risk. Although mechanical ventilation is often required, intubation should be guided by the patient's observed respiratory function and should not be performed prophylactically. Similarly, the presence of a pulmonary contusion or flail chest does not require mandatory chest tube placement in the absence of a pneumothorax or hemothorax. A misconception is that pulmonary contusions should be managed with fluid restriction, although appropriate resuscitation to maintain acceptable whole-body perfusion should be provided as for other severely injured patients. When needed, a pulmonary artery catheter may guide fluid administration, especially when significant ventilatory support is required. Aggressive pulmonary toilet, as well as adequate pain control when chest wall injuries are also present, can be beneficial.

Cardiac injuries. Despite being uncommon, cardiac injuries are some of the most severe injuries sustained by patients after penetrating and blunt trauma. Penetrating injury to the heart occurred in 1.8% of patients with penetrating trauma in the NTDB and in 8.7% of the subset with penetrating chest trauma alone. These statistics likely underestimate the true incidence of penetrating cardiac injuries because most are immediately lethal and never present to a hospital. For those penetrating cardiac injuries that do present to the emergency department in the NTDB, the mortality rate is 72.9%.

The location of penetrating injury on initial examination will often be suggestive of cardiac injury. Patients may present in extremis with pericardial tamponade or bleeding into one of the hemithoraces. Those who need resuscitative thoracotomy may have a cardiac injury identified at that time. In others, indicators of pericardial tamponade may be present, including hypotension with distended neck veins and muffled heart sounds, although these signs may not always be evident. Ultrasound is a valuable tool for quickly assessing the pericardium for fluid and should be performed in all patients with hemodynamic instability. When the results of ultrasound are inconclusive, a subxiphoid pericardial window is required to evaluate for the presence of blood in the pericardium. On making of a small opening in the pericardium, the pericardial space can be directly visualized. The pericardial window can then be extended to perform a median sternotomy in the setting of visualized blood.

For cardiac injuries that cause cardiovascular collapse, a left anterolateral thoracotomy is performed in the emergency department as previously described. When time permits, most cardiac injuries are best approached through a median sternotomy. Injuries to the atria can be grasped in a side-biting fashion with a Satinsky clamp and then closed with running or interrupted permanent monofilament sutures. Ventricular injuries can be more challenging and usually are associated with significant bleeding. The laceration can be held together manually while the defect is closed with horizontal mattress sutures reinforced with pledgets. To gain temporary control and to allow transport to the operating room, skin staples may provide short-term closure of the cardiac laceration. Another option is the passage of a Foley catheter through the wound, followed by inflation of the balloon and maintenance of outward tension. This occludes the defect until definitive closure can be achieved.

Blunt injury to the heart occurs less commonly, being seen in only 2.2% of blunt chest trauma cases. Most of these cases represent a contusion of the myocardium that results in arrhythmias and are frequently self-limited. In rare cases, blunt cardiac injury results in heart failure with cardiogenic shock. The diagnosis of cardiac contusion has been well studied but remains controversial. Although several laboratory and radiographic studies have been found to be associated with cardiac contusion, treatment is driven by the presence of clinical sequelae, thus questioning the need for confirmatory testing. Arrhythmia on the electrocardiogram, most commonly tachyarrhythmia, and cardiogenic shock are the pertinent clinical sequelae that require intervention. Clinical findings of cardiac contusion that are absent on admission are unlikely to develop and, in their continued absence, require no further evaluation. Laboratory studies, such as elevated cardiac enzyme levels, and further imaging do not alter the treatment regimen dictated by clinical and electrocardiographic findings. The presence of hemodynamic instability with evidence of heart failure should prompt echocardiography to assess cardiac wall and septal motion as well as function of the valves, which in rare cases can be injured during blunt thoracic trauma.

Patients suspected of having a blunt cardiac injury should undergo electrocardiography at the time of initial evaluation. Patients with mild electrocardiographic changes, such as sinus tachycardia, should be monitored for 12 hours with telemetry. No further intervention is required if telemetry has revealed no arrhythmias and a follow-up electrocardiographic recording is normal. The presence of arrhythmias on admission requires telemetry for 24 to 48 hours and therapy initiated for the specific electrical abnormality. In most cases, arrhythmias that are identified during the initial assessment resolve quickly during the course of monitoring and do not require medical treatment. Cardiogenic shock may require treatment with inotropic support and right ventricular afterload reduction, given the frequent involvement of the right side of the heart. Patients who demonstrate structural abnormalities on echocardiography may require urgent operation to repair cardiac injuries, such as valvular failure.

Thoracic aortic injuries. Thoracic aortic injuries are fortunately uncommon but are associated with poor outcomes. In the NTDB, aortic injury was present in only 0.3% of patients sustaining blunt trauma, although the associated mortality exceeded 37%. As with other severe injuries, the described incidence of these injuries underestimates the actual frequency because aortic transection is a common cause of immediate death in blunt trauma patients who never present to the emergency department. Penetrating aortic injury is also uncommon, being present in only 2.9% of penetrating chest trauma, although the associated mortality is extensive, with 88% resulting in death. Blunt aortic injuries are believed to be a result of rapid deceleration, which tears the aortic wall in the vicinity of the ligamentum arteriosum, where it is fixed to the thorax. More recent theories suggest that lateral mechanisms also contribute, during which the aortic arch acts as a lever and causes torque to develop at the aortic isthmus. The result of these mechanisms can range from a tear in the aortic intima to full-thickness transection of the vessel wall. With full-thickness injuries, only those who experience containment of the rupture by the surrounding mediastinal tissue survive to hospital presentation.

A chest radiograph that demonstrates findings such as a widened mediastinum, apical capping, loss of the aortic knob, or deviation of the left mainstem bronchus suggests blunt aortic injury. Because of a high rate of missed injuries with use of chest radiography as a screening study, most patients involved in high-energy injury mechanisms undergo helical CT angiography of the chest to evaluate for aortic injury. On chest CT, an aortic injury ranges from a disruption in the intima to a pseudoaneurysm with a mediastinal hematoma, which appears as contrast material contained outside the aortic lumen. As CT technology has evolved, chest CT alone is usually sufficient to plan operative repair, and standard angiography is rarely necessary. Figure 16-18 reveals a chest CT image that demonstrates a contained pseudoaneurysm from an aortic transection. Similarly, aortic injury from penetrating injury may be identified on CT imaging or at the time of thoracotomy or sternotomy, often in the setting of a patient in extremis.

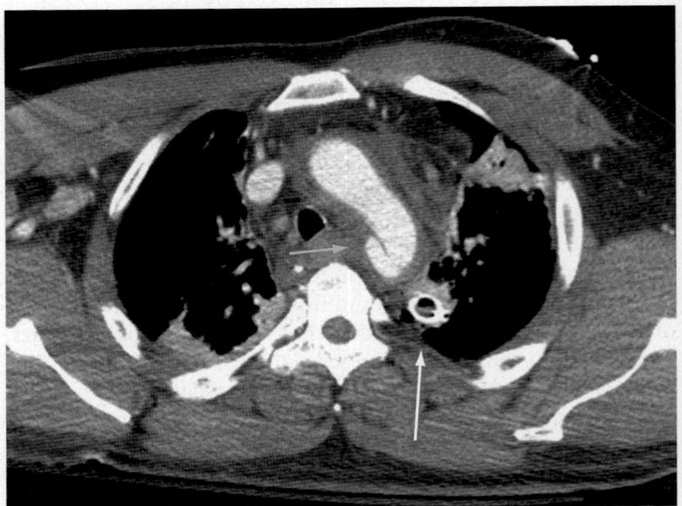

FIGURE 16-18 Aortic transection with pseudoaneurysm and associated hematoma on thoracic CT. This injury occurred at the typical location, just distal to the left subclavian artery at the aortic isthmus. The *yellow arrow* identifies a pseudoaneurysm; the *white arrow* identifies a left-sided tube thoracostomy.

Blunt thoracic aortic injury with pseudoaneurysm will require operative repair. The natural history of these injuries is slow expansion, which ultimately culminates in free aortic rupture. Despite this, the progression is usually slow and allows other more urgent issues, such as acute hemorrhage, to be addressed. It is essential that aortic wall stress be controlled until repair is performed, and this is usually adequately achieved with beta-receptor antagonist medications. The majority of these injuries are now repaired with an endovascular approach using a stent graft.[29] This change in treatment has evolved during the last 10 years, although the scientific support has not been robust. Nevertheless, the appeal of the minimally invasive approach with the rapid progression of catheter-based technology has made endovascular repair the treatment of choice at most trauma centers.[29] Access to the thoracic aorta is through the groin, and the stent graft is placed under fluoroscopic guidance. On occasion, the graft will cover the ostia of the left subclavian artery, at which time a carotid to subclavian bypass may also be required. When open surgical repair is required, the aorta is exposed through a left thoracotomy. Large penetrating injuries and blunt transection require replacement of a segment of the aorta with a prosthetic graft. This is most commonly performed with the assistance of cardiopulmonary bypass, with full bypass through a femoral-femoral approach or with a centrifugal pump and left-sided heart bypass. The use of cardiopulmonary bypass has been associated with a decreased incidence of paraplegia, which can result from cessation of aortic blood flow if a clamp and sew technique is used.

As the ability to visualize small intimal defects on CT has evolved, there are aortic injuries that may not require operative repair. Some patients with a small intimal tear only may be candidates for nonoperative management because many of these injuries will heal without intervention. Patients should be treated with beta-blocker therapy and undergo follow-up imaging to ensure the absence of expansion and ultimately the resolution of the injury.

Tracheobronchial injuries. Tracheobronchial tree injuries are uncommon but are associated with significant morbidity and mortality. Penetrating mechanisms are the most common cause, although these injuries still represent only 0.4% of all penetrating chest injuries in the NTDB. Despite this low incidence, the associated mortality was significant at 57.9%. Blunt injury to the tracheobronchial tree can occur but is extraordinarily rare, representing only 0.07% of blunt thoracic injuries. It is thought that these injuries result from the application of a large amount of energy to the anterior chest, which pulls the lungs laterally and avulses the bronchi from the fixed carina. Furthermore, a tracheal rupture may occur when lungs and airways are rapidly compressed against a closed glottis, which perforates the trachea along the membranous portion. Penetrating tracheobronchial injuries are predominantly a result of gunshot wounds that cause direct laceration of the tracheobronchial tree.

The location of the airway disruption will dictate the clinical presentation and the method of injury identification. Injuries that involve the thoracic trachea and proximal bronchi may result in large amounts of pneumomediastinum identified by chest radiography or CT imaging. More distal airway injuries will typically cause a pneumothorax requiring insertion of a tube thoracostomy. A continuous air leak with persistent pneumothorax is highly suggestive of an injury to a bronchus or large bronchiole. Significant subcutaneous air may also be present on physical examination. Diagnosis is made with either rigid or flexible bronchoscopy, depending on the location of the injury and the ability to manipulate the neck. Bronchoscopy allows the identification of the injury and a detailed characterization, such as the location and severity of the disruption.

The management of tracheobronchial injuries begins with careful assessment and control of the airway. With the placement of any airway, avoidance of further disruption is vital, and it may benefit from bronchoscopic guidance under direct visualization. Bronchial injuries that occupy less than one third of the luminal circumference may be considered for nonoperative management if lung expansion with a chest tube results in resolution of the pneumothorax and associated air leak. Management includes humidified oxygen, careful suctioning, and close observation to monitor for infectious sequelae that may develop. Operative management of the trachea, right-sided airways, and proximal left mainstem bronchus is best approached through a right posterolateral thoracotomy. Distal left-sided injuries are repaired through a left thoracotomy. A vascularized intercostal muscle flap should be mobilized and preserved during creation of the thoracotomy because placement of a retractor will prevent harvest of this valuable tissue coverage. Devitalized tissue should be débrided and injures closed with absorbable suture. Large injuries may require segmental resection with anastomosis. Coverage of the repair with a tissue pedicle, such as the previously created intercostal muscle flap, may improve healing. If possible, patients who require ongoing mechanical ventilation should have the endotracheal tube advanced so that the end of the tube is distal to the repair and protected from positive pressure. Other options include dual-lung ventilation and extracorporeal life support during the immediate postoperative period.

Esophageal injuries. Similar to the tracheobronchial tree, the thoracic esophagus is uncommonly injured by either blunt or penetrating mechanisms. Penetrating injury is more common, but only 1.6% of penetrating chest injuries in the NTDB had involvement of the esophagus. Most of these are caused by gunshot wounds, followed by stab wounds in less than 20% of cases. The mortality associated with penetrating esophageal injuries is substantial at 35.6% as a result of mediastinal sepsis and because of the adjacent vital structures that can also be injured along with the esophagus. Blunt esophageal injury is exceedingly rare, identified in only 0.02% of blunt trauma patients in the NTDB. Although these injuries are rare, the mortality is significant at 29.6%, often because of challenges with timely diagnosis and treatment. Whereas penetrating injury causes direct tissue laceration, blunt esophageal injury is likely to be caused by a rapid elevation in intraluminal pressure during compression of the chest or abdomen. An impact to the upper abdomen can compress the distended stomach, leading to transmission of air and fluid up the esophagus and resulting in a perforation of the wall, usually in the distal segment.

The location of penetrating injuries and the presumed trajectory are often suggestive of esophageal injury. Penetrating injuries in the vicinity of the mediastinum require consideration of possible esophageal injury. The esophagus is best evaluated through a combination of contrast esophagography and esophagoscopy. Together these two modalities result in a sensitivity of almost 100% for esophageal injury. Diagnostic studies may reveal extravasation of contrast material from the esophageal lumen or a disruption of the mucosa visualized during endoscopy. The location of the injury should be determined to assist in operative planning. A large amount of mediastinal air is suggestive of esophageal injury that may benefit from further evaluation. Often, chest CT reveals air adjacent to the esophagus but outside the lumen as well as surrounding soft tissue inflammation. High-resolution CT imaging may even demonstrate the esophageal wall defect. Low esophageal injuries at the gastroesophageal junction may result in abdominal pain and tenderness.

Esophageal injuries with associated mediastinal contamination require immediate identification and repair because delays are associated with worse outcomes. Esophageal injuries require operative repair to close the esophageal defect and to provide adequate mediastinal drainage. The upper and midthoracic esophagus is best approached through a right posterolateral thoracotomy through the fourth or fifth interspace, whereas the lower esophagus is exposed from the left through the sixth or seventh interspace. As with tracheobronchial injuries, creation of a vascularized intercostal muscle flap on entry into the chest will allow excellent coverage of the repair. When the location of the injury is at the gastroesophageal junction, it may best be approached through a laparotomy. The injury is entirely exposed, which usually requires opening of the muscle layer superiorly and inferiorly to reveal the extent of the mucosal defect, which is commonly larger than the muscle disruption. The esophageal injury is then closed in one or two layers, frequently with an absorbable mucosa suture followed by interrupted muscle sutures of a permanent material. Coverage of the repair with a muscle flap or adjacent tissue may help reduce the high rate of leak. Esophageal repairs at the gastroesophageal junction can be covered with a fundoplication of gastric tissue. Wide drainage of the mediastinum and chest is extremely important to control any leak that may develop. A gastrostomy and feeding jejunostomy are frequently performed to allow gastric decompression and early nutritional support. Inflammation within the mediastinum develops quickly, and primary repair of injuries that are identified late may not be possible. Esophagectomy may be the only option to allow recovery from the associated inflammatory insult, followed by planned elective reconstruction, when it is feasible.

Diaphragmatic injuries. Injuries to the diaphragm are common after penetrating injuries to the chest, occurring in 17.4% of cases in the NTDB. The associated mortality is significant at 26.3%, although almost all of these deaths are a result of injury to adjacent vital organs because diaphragmatic injuries themselves are usually of limited threat to life. Conversely, blunt diaphragmatic injuries occur in only 1.6% of blunt thoracic injuries and are believed to be a result of a rapid increase in intra-abdominal pressure during an anterior impact that causes a blow-out of the diaphragmatic tissue. The left side of the diaphragm is the injured location in approximately 75% of the cases because of the coverage of the right side with the liver. Despite the low incidence, the mortality is significant at 20.9%, probably because of the high energy required to create a blunt diaphragmatic rupture. The morbidity related to diaphragmatic injuries is occasionally identified months to years later when the perforation was not initially repaired. The natural history of these injuries includes progressive enlargement with herniation of abdominal viscera into the chest.

Injuries to the diaphragm can be a diagnostic challenge and require a high index of suspicion, even with the most subtle indicators. Penetrating diaphragmatic injuries are usually discovered on operative exploration of the chest or abdomen. During exploration, following the trajectory of the injury will usually allow identification of the diaphragmatic defect. Blunt injuries can be more elusive. The chest radiograph may demonstrate the presence of abdominal viscera, most commonly the stomach, within the chest, although this finding may be absent in a significant number of injuries (Fig. 16-19). Passage of a nasogastric tube can be of assistance if the tube is identified in the lower left hemithorax, and the injection of gastric contrast material may add to the detection. Chest and abdominal CT scans may demonstrate the presence of abdominal viscera in the chest or an abnormality of the diaphragm itself, such as thickening, elevation, or a defect. Given the challenge of diagnosis, operative exploration may be required when imaging is suggestive. In patients who have no other indication for laparotomy, video-assisted thoracoscopy or cautious laparoscopy conducted to avoid tension pneumothorax may offer less invasive means of visualizing the diaphragm.

Diaphragmatic injuries are typically repaired by débriding nonviable tissue and then closing the defect. The diaphragm exhibits enough redundancy for all but the largest defects to be closed primarily. Closure is performed with a single layer of nonabsorbable suture incorporating large full-thickness bites of healthy diaphragmatic tissue. It is important to obtain hemostasis because diaphragmatic injuries can bleed significantly from branches of the phrenic artery that can be exposed at the edges of the tear. Large areas of tissue loss are rare in traumatic rupture but, when present, may require reconstruction with a prosthetic. Nonabsorbable synthetic materials can be used to reconstruct the diaphragm in clean surgical fields but should be avoided in the setting of contamination. A peripheral detachment of the diaphragm from the wall of the torso can be repaired by reinserting the injured tissue one or two interspaces superior.

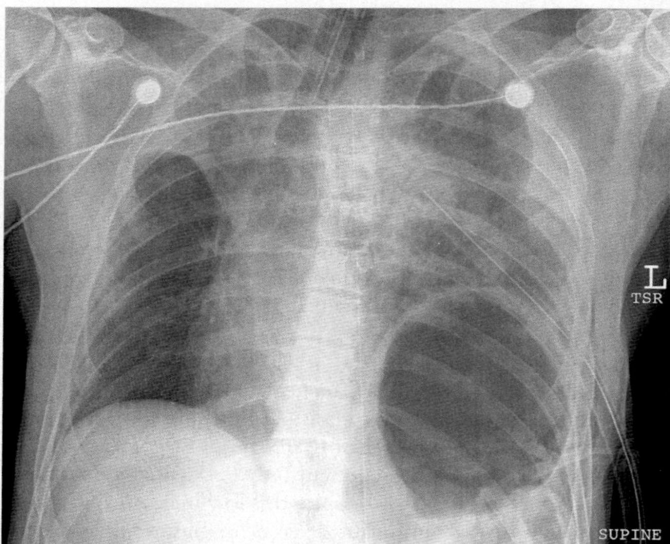

FIGURE 16-19 Left-sided diaphragmatic injury on plain chest radiograph. The gas-filled stomach can be visualized on the left side of the chest because of herniation through a large diaphragmatic laceration.

Injuries to the Abdomen

The abdomen is a commonly injured body region and frequently requires the care of a surgeon for definitive management. Within the 2012 NTDB, 14.8% of all patients sustained abdominal injuries, with penetrating mechanisms being proportionately greater than blunt (23.8% versus 12.1%). The vital nature of the organs contained within the abdomen makes evaluation and management a priority. The predominant sources of morbidity and mortality are bleeding and visceral perforation with associated sepsis. In the setting of blunt trauma, solid organs often sustain contusion or laceration, causing bleeding that may require surgical management. Furthermore, blunt forces can cause rupture of hollow viscera due to rapid compression of a segment of intestine containing fluid and air. Penetrating mechanisms directly lacerate solid and hollow viscera, resulting in bleeding and intra-abdominal contamination that often require surgical repair.

Immediate Management

The immediate management of abdominal injuries includes the initiation of resuscitation and a rapid assessment for sources of bleeding. Patients in shock require the administration of crystalloid solutions and blood products to support cardiovascular function as bleeding is controlled. Furthermore, a rapid survey for bleeding including assessment of the abdomen is completed to prompt transfer to the operating room when needed. Retained foreign bodies traversing the abdominal wall should be maintained throughout the initial evaluation and protected from excessive movement. These should then be removed only after defining a definitive plan, which almost always includes abdominal operation to manage associated injuries.

Blunt Abdominal Trauma Evaluation

The evaluation of the injured patient varies on the basis of blunt versus penetrating mechanisms. Blunt trauma patients who are

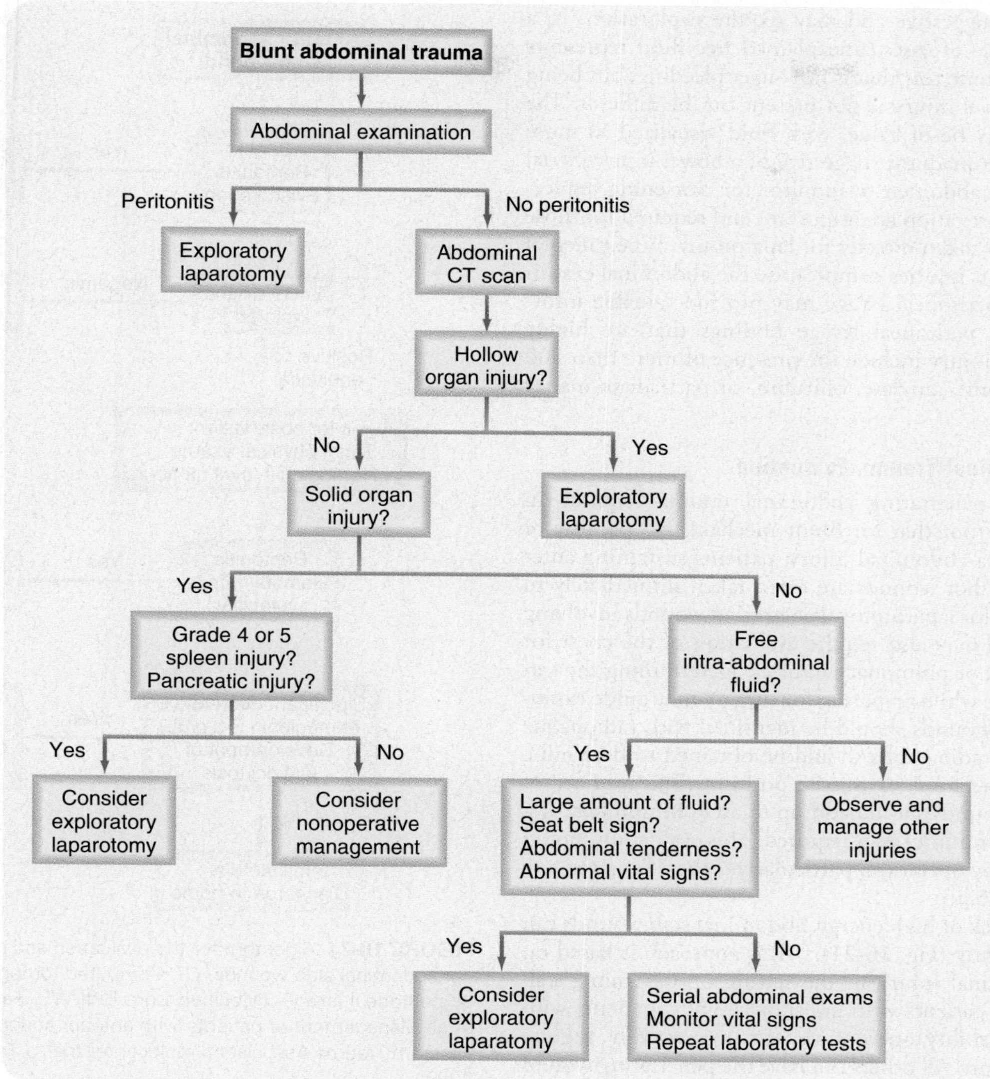

FIGURE 16-20 Algorithm for the evaluation and management of blunt abdominal trauma.

unstable and have intra-abdominal fluid identified on FAST require an emergent laparotomy to manage bleeding.[30] If FAST examination capabilities are unavailable, diagnostic peritoneal lavage revealing 10 mL or more of gross blood suggests an intra-abdominal source of shock requiring emergent operation. The presence of peritonitis is also an indication for immediate transfer to the operating room for laparotomy. All other patients will undergo an evaluation of the abdomen as depicted in Figure 16-20.

Abdominal CT is the primary method of imaging of the stable blunt trauma patient and has supported the evolution of the nonoperative management of many solid abdominal organ injuries. Abdominal CT is typically performed with IV administration of a contrast agent timed to capture the portal venous phase, which best demonstrates the perfusion of the solid abdominal organs. Abdominal CT provides the necessary visualization of the solid organs to allow the determination of injury severity, including the presence of active bleeding. These imaging findings prompt management decisions, such as the need for operative, nonoperative, or angiographic therapy. Historically, blood within the abdomen mandated a laparotomy, although commonly the bleeding from solid organs had stopped by the time of exploration. It was recognized that the patient's physiologic state was often more indicative of the need for laparotomy than the presence of the injury alone. The recognition that ongoing bleeding was uncommon in the setting of cardiovascular stability led to the management of many of these injuries nonoperatively. Three-dimensional imaging with CT also provides the ability to visualize the retroperitoneum, which cannot be evaluated with FAST or diagnostic peritoneal lavage.

Despite being sensitive for solid organ injury, CT is less capable of detecting injuries to the hollow viscera. This ability has improved as CT technology has evolved, but overall there are still significant limitations. Injury to the gastrointestinal tract is suggested by bowel wall thickening, inflammation in the surrounding adipose tissue seen as stranding, or the presence of free intraperitoneal fluid. Oral contrast material is uncommonly provided as it adds little to the value of the study. Unexplained free fluid must be carefully considered because of a high risk of associated bowel injury. The presence of an abdominal seat belt mark or tenderness on examination is suggestive and may require exploration. In a significant percentage of cases, unexplained free fluid represents blood from a mesenteric tear that is no longer bleeding, but being confident that a bowel injury is not present can be difficult. The amount of fluid may be of value, with fluid visualized in more than one abdominal quadrant suggestive of a bowel injury. Serial examinations of the abdomen to monitor for worsening tenderness and peritoneal irritation are important and required for those patients who are not taken directly for laparotomy. When mental status or concomitant injuries compromise the abdominal examination, diagnostic peritoneal lavage may provide valuable information. Diagnostic peritoneal lavage findings that are highly suggestive of bowel injury include the presence of more than 500 white blood cells/mm^3, amylase, bilirubin, or particulate matter in the lavage fluid.

Penetrating Abdominal Trauma Evaluation

The evaluation of penetrating abdominal trauma requires an approach different from that for blunt mechanisms. Because of the high rate of intra-abdominal injury, patients sustaining anterior abdominal gunshot wounds are often taken immediately to the operating room for laparotomy. Penetrating wounds involving the upper abdomen may also require evaluation of the chest for mediastinal, pleural, or pulmonary injuries. Determining the trajectory of the missile while preparing for surgery may guide exploration. Penetrating wounds should be identified with radiopaque markers, and plain radiographs should be obtained to determine their location and relation to missile position. The number of missiles and skin wounds should add up to an even number, or a more intense search for injuries is required. This evaluation should be brief and not delay operation, particularly if there has been any hemodynamic instability.

Because of the lack of high energy, abdominal stab wounds can be managed differently (Fig. 16-21).[31] This approach is based on a low risk of intestinal injury in the setting of abdominal stab wounds. Similar to patients with gunshot wounds, patients with hemodynamic instability, peritonitis, or evisceration require immediate laparotomy. All others can have the penetrating wound explored to determine whether the anterior or posterior abdominal fascia is violated. Patients without any fascial penetration can be considered for discharge. If the local wound exploration reveals any evidence of possible fascial penetration, patients should be monitored with serial abdominal examinations and laboratory studies. The development of peritonitis, hemodynamic instability, significant decreases in hemoglobin level, or leukocytosis should prompt further evaluation, usually with laparotomy. Patients without clinical change after 24 hours can have a diet instituted and be considered for discharge. Of note, this approach does require the presence of an infrastructure that allows close surveillance of these patients, which may not be available in all facilities. There remain some surgeons who think that penetration of the abdominal fascia warrants exploration immediately, with the understanding that this will result in a higher nontherapeutic laparotomy rate.

Laparoscopy provides an additional tool to use in the presence of an abdominal stab wound to evaluate for peritoneal penetration. It remains fairly well accepted that laparoscopy is not sufficient to explore the entire abdomen, but it can be used to identify violation of the parietal peritoneum, which can then prompt laparotomy to repair injuries. In the absence of other injuries, patients without peritoneal penetration can be discharged to home after recovery from anesthesia. Despite increasing the number of patients who may be candidates for immediate discharge, this approach carries a higher rate of nontherapeutic laparotomies.

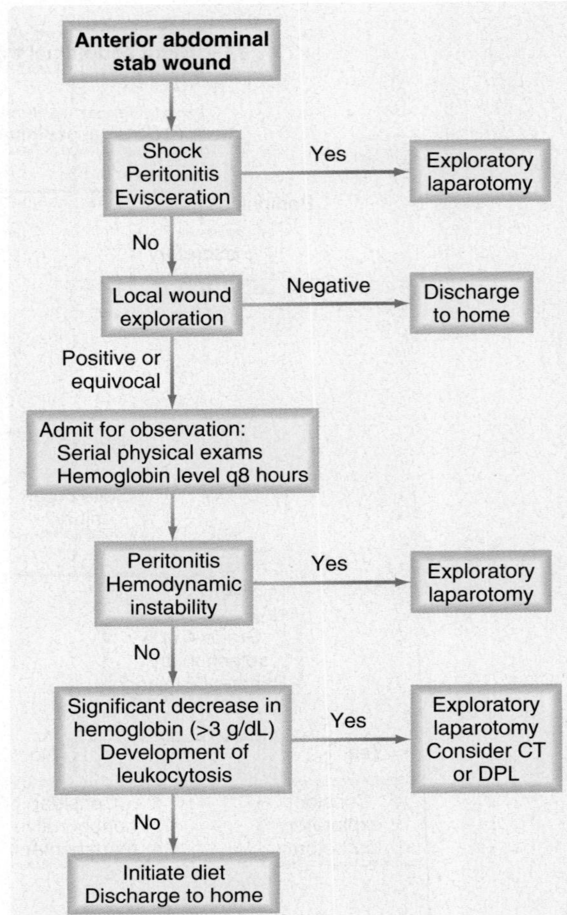

FIGURE 16-21 Algorithm for the evaluation and management of anterior abdominal stab wounds. *CT,* Computed tomography; *DPL,* diagnostic peritoneal lavage. (Modified from Biffl WL, Kaups KL, Cothren CC, et al: Management of patients with anterior abdominal stab wounds: A Western Trauma Association multicenter trial. *J Trauma* 66:1294–1301, 2009.)

Penetrating wounds that occur posterior to the midaxillary lines and throughout the back may benefit from three-dimensional imaging with CT. Patients with peritonitis or a wound that clearly enters the abdomen require abdominal exploration. Otherwise, significant structures are often avoided because of the thickness and density of the retroperitoneum. CT can often determine the track of the penetrating injury by aligning the external markers with internal missiles and locules of air within the tissues. Establishment of the injury track allows the proximity to vital structures to be determined, including the vertebral column, spinal cord, pelvis, and blood vessels. Penetrating injury tracks identified by CT that are close to intra-abdominal organs typically require abdominal exploration. The presence of retained metallic missiles can limit this approach by causing radiographic scatter, which may obscure findings on CT imaging.

Management

A laparotomy is performed to explore the abdomen and to repair injuries that are identified. It is important that the exploration of the abdomen be performed systematically to avoid missing injuries that may be subtle. As described in the setting of damage control, this approach may require abbreviation in the setting of deteriorating physiologic condition. As a standard technique, the abdomen is opened from the xiphoid process to the pubic symphysis to provide adequate exposure. The falciform ligament can be divided, separating the liver from the abdominal wall to improve retraction and to facilitate perihepatic packing. With use of a hand-held retractor, blood is quickly evacuated from all four quadrants of the abdomen, and laparotomy sponges are placed to provide temporary hemostasis. A fixed retractor can be placed to facilitate optimal exposure. Sponges placed in the four quadrants are removed to address bleeding but can be replaced as needed in the setting of damage control. The entire gastrointestinal tract is carefully evaluated, from the gastroesophageal junction to the proximal rectum at the peritoneal reflection. The lesser sac is also entered to visualize the posterior stomach and the pancreas. At times, the only evidence of injury may be blood staining beneath the peritoneum, and these areas should be explored to confirm the absence of serious injury. When injuries are identified, they are repaired, as detailed in subsequent sections. The development of physiologic compromise prompts the need to abbreviate the operation and to proceed with damage control methods. This recognition benefits greatly from effective two-way communication between the surgical and anesthesia teams. If the operation can be completed without conversion to damage control, the abdominal fascia is closed and the subcutaneous wound addressed as dictated by the level of intra-abdominal contamination.

Splenic injuries. The spleen is the most commonly injured abdominal organ in the NTDB, with 23.8% of patients with abdominal trauma demonstrating splenic injuries. The frequency of these injuries requires the surgeon to possess a sound understanding of the management of splenic injuries. Many splenic injuries are self-limited, demonstrating no evidence of ongoing bleeding; others require splenectomy, which in most cases is straightforward. Despite this, the mortality after blunt splenic injury in the NTDB is 9.3%. Many of these deaths are likely caused by associated injuries and prehospital delays because definitive management can be rapidly achieved. Direct compression of the spleen with parenchymal fracture is a common pathophysiologic mechanism at the tissue level, although injury can also be secondary to rapid deceleration that tears the splenic parenchyma or capsule where it is fixed to the retroperitoneum. This can cause a subcapsular hematoma, which is demonstrated in Figure 16-22 at the time of splenectomy. Hemorrhage from a splenic injury can be ongoing at the time of presentation or more commonly will have stopped, causing no more blood loss. Injuries that stop bleeding can often be managed without splenectomy, although patients can experience a delayed reinitiation of hemorrhage. This is the greatest concern for patients who undergo nonoperative management, and many studies have been devoted to identifying patients at high risk of delayed hemorrhage as well as to ways of mitigating these events. The rate of late bleeding was determined to be 10.6% in a large series, although this rate varies greatly with the grade of splenic injury. Penetrating splenic trauma is less common but is still present in 8.5% of all penetrating abdominal injuries in the NTDB. This is consistent with the rate reported in a large series from Grady Memorial Hospital and Ben Taub General Hospital during the 1980s and 1990s, in which 9.2% and 7.6%, respectively, of penetrating abdominal injuries involved the spleen.[32]

Unstable patients who are taken emergently to the operating room may have a splenic injury identified at the time of laparotomy. Unstable patients with intra-abdominal fluid on FAST

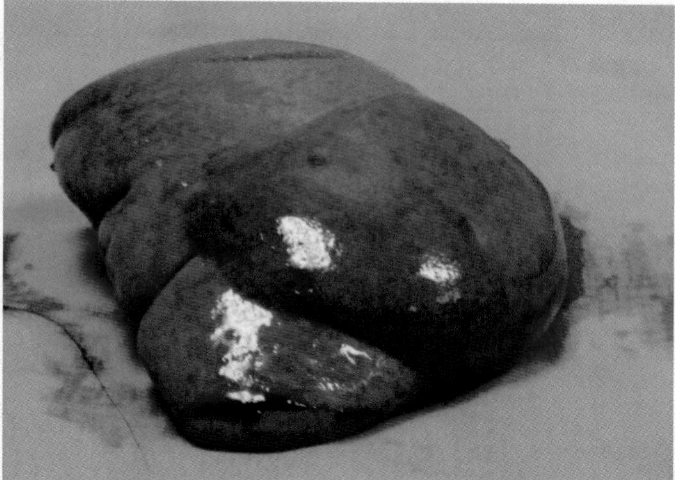

FIGURE 16-22 Splenic injury with subcapsular hematoma. Despite only a 1-cm capsular tear, this injury demonstrated ongoing hemorrhage.

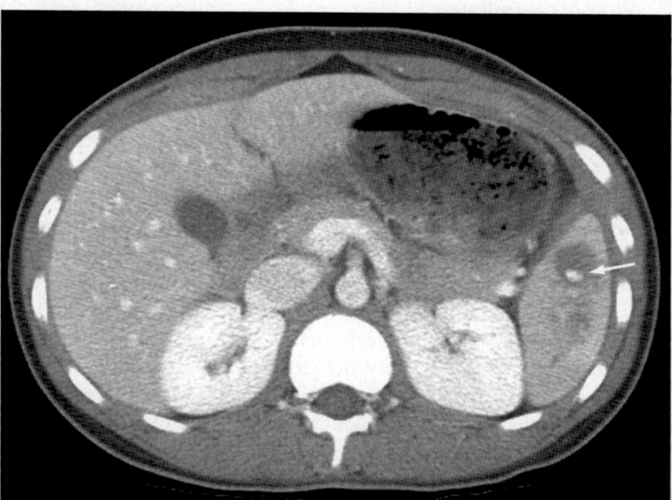

FIGURE 16-23 Grade III splenic laceration on abdominal CT. Note the focus of active extravasation of contrast material within the injured splenic parenchyma as identified by the *arrow*.

require exploration, with the spleen commonly being the bleeding intra-abdominal organ. In all other patients, abdominal CT with IV administration of a contrast agent is the most valuable study for identifying and characterizing splenic injuries. Splenic injuries appear as disruptions in the normal splenic parenchyma, frequently with surrounding hematoma and free intra-abdominal blood. On occasion, active bleeding can be identified by visualizing extravasation of contrast material that appears as a high-density blush or accumulation of contrast-laden blood. At times, this extravasation will be free into the peritoneal space; at other times, it will be contained within an intraparenchymal pseudoaneurysm. A splenic injury with active extravasation into a pseudoaneurysm is demonstrated in Figure 16-23. Other types of splenic injury can include a hematoma confined to the subcapsular space and even complete devascularization of the organ caused by injury of the hilar vessels. Spleen injuries are characterized by the AAST Injury Scoring Scale, which grades injuries on the basis of parenchymal or subcapsular abnormality and the presence of vascular involvement (Table 16-5).

TABLE 16-5 AAST Spleen Injury Scale

INJURY GRADE	INJURY TYPE	DESCRIPTION OF INJURY
I	Hematoma	Subcapsular, <10% surface area
	Laceration	Capsular tear, <1 cm parenchymal depth
II	Hematoma	Subcapsular, 10% to 50% surface area; intraparenchymal, <5 cm in diameter
	Laceration	Capsular tear, 1 to 3 cm parenchymal depth that does not involve a trabecular vessel
III	Hematoma	Subcapsular, >50% surface area or expanding; ruptured subcapsular or parenchymal hematoma; intraparenchymal hematoma ≥5 cm or expanding
	Laceration	>3 cm parenchymal depth or involving trabecular vessels
IV	Laceration	Laceration involving segmental or hilar vessels producing major devascularization (>25% of spleen)
V	Hematoma	Completely shattered spleen
	Laceration	Hilar vascular injury devascularizes spleen

The use of splenic angiography and embolization represents the most recent advance in the evaluation and management of spleen injuries. Commonly, centers use angiography to evaluate and often to treat stable patients who demonstrate active extravasation on CT imaging. The best way to use splenic angiography is still being elucidated, but it has become almost uniformly used in some capacity at most centers. One major benefit of angiography is the potential to obstruct sites of bleeding endovascularly by angioembolization. Stable patients who are found to have a pseudoaneurysm on CT may benefit from angioembolization to eliminate blood flow through the injured segment of spleen. Some centers have developed approaches that include mandatory angiography with embolization to reduce the risk of delayed hemorrhage. There is evidence suggesting that this intervention may increase the rate of splenic injuries that can be safely managed nonoperatively.[33] Nevertheless, only patients not in shock should be considered for angiographic evaluation and possible angioembolic treatment.

Many patients with blunt splenic trauma can be managed without splenectomy when careful selection of patients is applied. It is critical that only patients who are stable and have no evidence of ongoing blood loss be considered for nonoperative management. It should not be overlooked that the definitive management for splenic bleeding remains splenectomy, and this approach does not carry with it an overly significant risk profile, especially in comparison to the adverse outcomes related to ongoing hemorrhage. Therefore, no unstable bleeding patient should go without splenectomy, especially in an attempt to push the figurative nonoperative envelope. Nevertheless, the majority of patients are no longer bleeding at presentation and do benefit from avoiding an unnecessary operation. Based on the patient's physiologic state, it is usually possible to identify those who have a hemostatic splenic injury and are appropriate candidates for nonoperative management. Nonoperative management does not mean that there is a lack of intervention or care provided. In fact, nonoperative management of splenic injury can be more labor-intensive than operative therapy and require greater resources for a longer time. It is necessary to have the appropriate care model to provide the ongoing surveillance required to manage a spleen injury without surgery. To be considered for nonoperative management, patients must have no physiologic indication of ongoing bleeding. Hemodynamic stability is required without any ongoing intravascular volume support. Physiologic stability includes a normal blood pressure, lack of tachycardia, no physical examination findings indicating shock, and absence of metabolic acidosis. Care should be taken in interpreting the initial hemoglobin level as actual blood loss may not be recognized until intravascular equilibration occurs. Patients who stabilize after crystalloid infusion are still candidates for nonoperative management, although a lower threshold for operation should be maintained.

A great deal of work has been performed in an attempt to better identify which patients with spleen injuries can be safely managed nonoperatively. Age of the patient has been evaluated in two retrospective studies that compared nonoperative failure rates between groups older and younger than 55 years, although disparate results were obtained.[34,35] The larger of these studies demonstrated a significantly greater failure rate (19% versus 10%) of nonoperative management in patients older than 55 years.[35] Nevertheless, more than 80% of older patients who underwent attempted nonoperative management still succeeded, so most would agree that age alone is not a contraindication to management without surgery. The grade of injury at the time of presentation has also been extensively considered, although a consistent approach has not been agreed on. One multi-institutional retrospective study conducted by EAST identified failure rates of 33.3% in grade IV and 75% in grade V injuries, with 8% of failures occurring more than 9 days after injury.[36] In another multicenter study, these high-grade injuries were not as common, but all of them failed nonoperative management.[37] Surgeons have interpreted these data in different ways. Some believe that failure rates after high-grade splenic injuries are unacceptably high, especially given that almost one in 10 may occur after hospital discharge and that splenectomy does not carry a markedly high morbidity. Others interpret the significant number of patients with high-grade injuries who are ultimately managed with a successful nonoperative approach as support for more frequent attempts at avoiding surgery. The result is that this decision remains the surgeon's preference and is often guided by surgical intuition. Our preference is to reserve nonoperative management for stable grade I, II, and III injuries, with the assistance of angioembolization when the bleeding risk is more substantial.

Operative management of splenic injuries may be required in the setting of instability at the time of admission or after failed nonoperative management when the spleen rebleeds after a period of stability. Regardless, the best approach is through a midline incision, followed by the packing of all four quadrants when the patient is unstable. A fixed retractor can improve exposure, and the packs are removed to expose the injured spleen. To mobilize the spleen, the peritoneum is divided laterally by retracting the spleen posteromedially to expose the retroperitoneal attachments. This division of the peritoneum begins at the white line of Toldt (splenocolic ligament) and then continues superiorly until the short gastric vessels are encountered. After the peritoneum is opened laterally, a blunt plane is created posterior to the spleen in a medial direction, extending behind the tail of the pancreas. This maneuver mobilizes the entire spleen and distal pancreas, allowing the spleen to be delivered up into the wound. While avoiding the greater curve of the stomach, the short gastric vessels are ligated and divided. Finally, the spleen is removed after the hilar vessels are clamped and ligated, being sure not to injure the tail of the pancreas. A drain should be placed only if there is concern that the tail of the pancreas was injured. Postsplenectomy vaccines must be provided to ensure protection from encapsulated bacteria, including *Streptococcus pneumoniae, Neisseria meningitidis,* and *Haemophilus influenzae.* Whereas splenic salvage techniques are well described, their utility is limited in the era of highly effective nonoperative management and endovascular approaches to splenic trauma. Splenic injury secondary to penetrating abdominal trauma is usually identified during laparotomy and should be addressed on the basis of the presence or absence of ongoing bleeding.

Hepatic injuries. Liver injuries are extremely common after blunt trauma; only the spleen demonstrates a higher incidence. Within the NTDB, liver injuries occurred in 3.0% of all patients, whereas 22.2% of patients with blunt mechanisms sustained hepatic trauma. The outcomes after blunt liver injury have improved, with the associated mortality rate down to 12.5% in the latest version of the NTDB. The work of Richardson and colleagues, in which they reported their 25-year experience, remains the largest series of liver injuries.[38] During that time, the total number of liver injuries increased significantly, although the incidence of major hepatic trauma remained stable, ranging from 12% to 15%.[38] The death rate of all patients with hepatic trauma decreased from 19% to 9% during the study period, which the authors attributed to improved management of venous injuries. Mechanisms of blunt hepatic trauma include compression with direct parenchymal damage and shearing forces, which tear hepatic tissue and disrupt vascular and ligamentous attachments. The liver is partially protected by the thoracic cage, although even the rigid ribs provide little support during high-energy mechanisms. Because of the large amount of the abdomen occupied by the liver, penetrating injuries are common as well. Nicholas and coworkers described liver injury in 34.4% and 29.3% of cases of penetrating abdominal trauma reported from two busy trauma centers.[32] Similarly, the liver is the most commonly injured abdominal organ after penetrating trauma in the NTDB, present in 26.1% of cases. The mortality associated with these penetrating injuries is significant at 22.0%. Penetrating mechanisms directly lacerate the hepatic parenchyma while also causing adjacent tissue contusion. The associated morbidity can also be significantly greater when vascular or biliary tree structures are involved.

Similar to other abdominal organs, liver injuries are often first diagnosed on entering the abdomen in the unstable patient explored for free fluid on FAST examination. Those who do not require immediate operation should be imaged with abdominal CT enhanced with IV administration of a contrast agent. CT is capable of providing excellent anatomic detail that allows highly accurate characterization of injuries. Common findings on CT indicative of liver injury include disruption of the hepatic parenchyma with perihepatic blood or hematoma and hemoperitoneum. Bleeding from the liver can be seen on CT as extravasation of contrast material either within the liver parenchyma or into the peritoneal space as seen in Figure 16-24. The characteristics of the liver injury on CT can be used to categorize the injury with the AAST Injury Scoring Scale, which accounts for parenchymal involvement and the presence of vascular injury (Table 16-6).

Hemodynamic instability in the emergency department in the setting of free fluid on FAST examination requires immediate laparotomy. Even though there have been great advances in the nonoperative management of liver injuries, it should not be overlooked that unstable patients require operative management of bleeding. Operative management of hepatic injuries as developed by the WTA is presented in Figure 16-25.[39] Similar to spleen injuries, most injuries to the liver have stopped bleeding by the time of evaluation. Those patients who demonstrate hemodynamic stability benefit from a more conservative approach. Hemostatic injuries do not require operation but instead benefit from close surveillance for indicators of rebleeding or associated complications. Nonoperative management of liver injuries has been shown to demonstrate excellent results, with success achieved in 85% to 97% of cases.[40] In addition to avoiding unnecessary operation in a significant number of patients, the application of a nonoperative approach for select patients has resulted in a decrease in mortality for liver injuries, despite an increase in overall injury severity during the last 3 decades.[38] Candidates for nonoperative management must demonstrate evidence that all

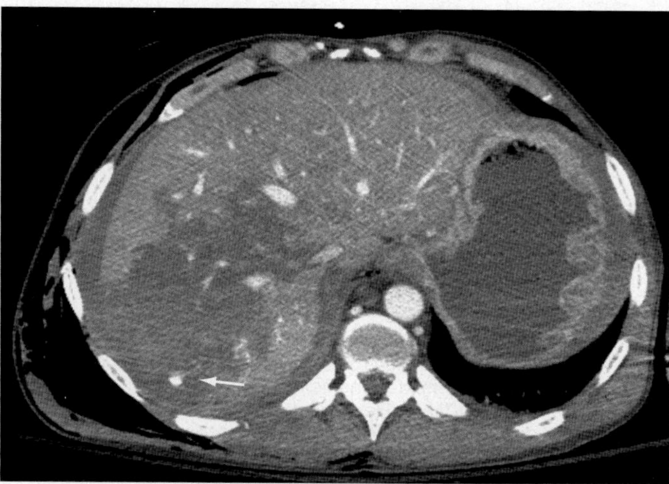

FIGURE 16-24 Grade IV liver laceration involving the right hepatic lobe on abdominal CT. Note the focus of active extravasation of contrast material within the injured liver parenchyma at the periphery of the injury as identified by the *arrow*.

TABLE 16-6 AAST Liver Injury Scale

INJURY GRADE	INJURY TYPE	DESCRIPTION OF INJURY
I	Hematoma	Subcapsular, <10% surface area
	Laceration	Capsular tear, <1 cm parenchymal depth
II	Hematoma	Subcapsular, 10% to 50% surface area; intraparenchymal, <10 cm in diameter
	Laceration	Capsular tear, 1 to 3 cm parenchymal depth, <10 cm in length
III	Hematoma	Subcapsular, >50% surface area of ruptured subcapsular or parenchymal hematoma; intraparenchymal hematoma >10 cm or expanding
	Laceration	>3 cm parenchymal depth
IV	Laceration	Parenchymal disruption involving 25% to 75% hepatic lobe or 1 to 3 Couinaud segments
V	Laceration	Parenchymal disruption involving >75% of hepatic lobe or >3 Couinaud segments within a single lobe
	Vascular	Juxtahepatic venous injuries (i.e., retrohepatic vena cava/central major hepatic veins)
VI	Vascular	Hepatic avulsion

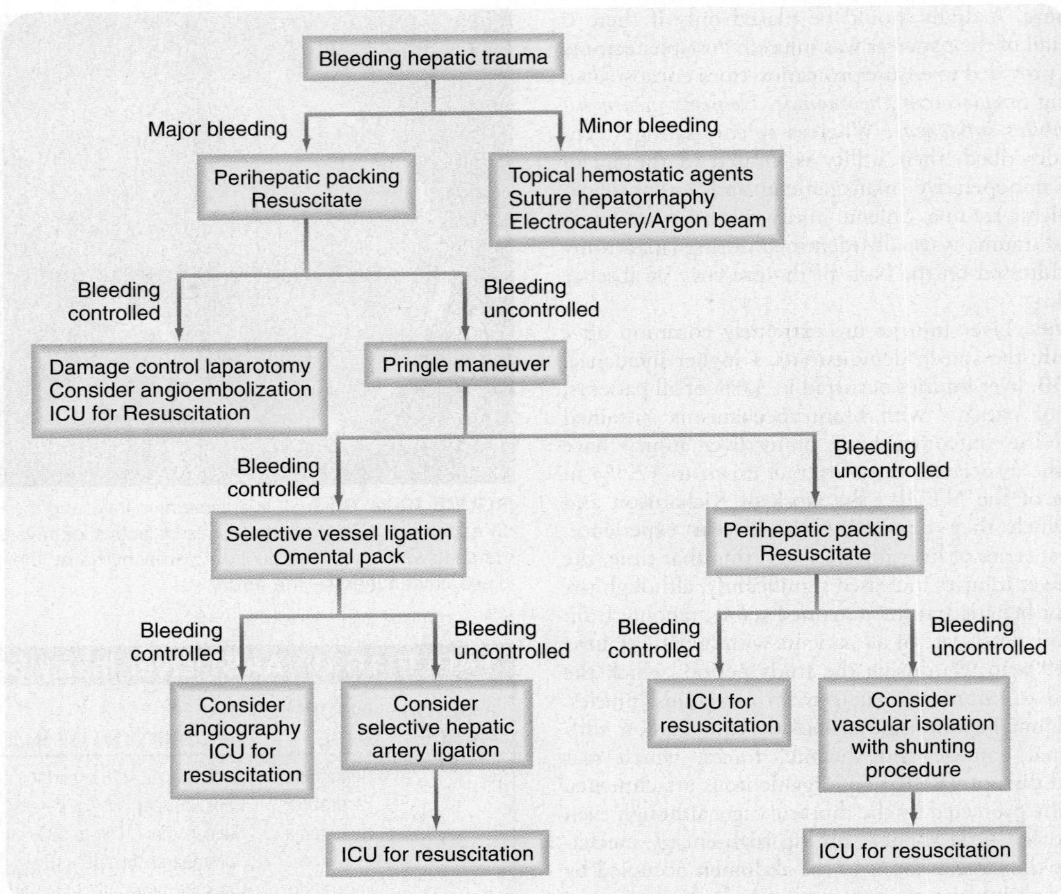

FIGURE 16-25 Algorithm for the operative management of hepatic injuries. *ICU*, Intensive care unit. (Modified from Kozar RA, Feliciano DV, Moore EE, et al: Western Trauma Association/critical decisions in trauma: Operative management of adult blunt hepatic trauma. *J Trauma* 71:1–5, 2011.)

bleeding from the liver has stopped. These patients have no tachycardia, hypotension, metabolic acidosis, or physical examination evidence of shock. In addition, they cannot be receiving ongoing fluid resuscitation that might mask cardiovascular compromise. To a greater degree than in splenic injuries, physiologic stability is the major predictor of successful nonoperative management of hepatic trauma. Even in the setting of high-grade injuries, nonoperative management can be attempted as long as the patient remains hemodynamically stable without evidence of bleeding.

As opposed to spleen injuries, the operative intervention for liver trauma is less definitive and can be challenging. Therefore, the surgeon needs to diligently determine whether the patient has liver bleeding that would benefit from surgery. For this reason, slow decreases in hemoglobin levels are at times tolerated and even occasionally treated with transfusion. This is especially true in the multiply injured patient who may have several sites of slow blood loss, and the decline in hemoglobin level may not represent ongoing hepatic bleeding. As with other solid organ injuries, it is possible that a hollow visceral injury could be present but overlooked if intra-abdominal fluid is attributed solely to the liver injury. For this reason, frequent abdominal examinations to detect evidence of intestinal injury are an important part of nonoperative management.

Extravasation of IV contrast material into the liver parenchyma on CT usually represents a pseudoaneurysm from a disrupted intrahepatic vascular structure. The natural history of hepatic pseudoaneurysms is not entirely elucidated, but it is believed that they may be associated with an increased risk of delayed bleeding, especially when they are associated with hepatic arterial branches. Hepatic angiography with embolization offers an attractive approach to eliminating the intraparenchymal pseudoaneurysm. After successful embolization, patients need standard surveillance required for all hepatic injuries managed nonoperatively. In appropriately selected patients, the use of angioembolization has improved the rate of successful nonoperative management with a reduction in conversion to surgical treatment.[41,42] Furthermore, many higher grade injuries that historically might have required operation become candidates for nonoperative management with the addition of angioembolization.

Even successful nonoperative management may require the treatment of complications, such as bile leaks with biloma formation, hemobilia, and development of liver abscesses. Frequently, these are suggested by the development of abdominal symptoms, with the addition of systemic infection or inflammation at times. CT or ultrasound imaging can be valuable in evaluating for abscess and biloma; these can usually be managed with percutaneous drainage guided by CT or ultrasound. Endoscopic retrograde cholangiopancreatography (ERCP) with stent placement is occasionally required to decompress the biliary tree and to promote healing of a bile leak. Biliary ascites not amenable to percutaneous drainage may require laparoscopy or laparotomy for adequate drainage to be obtained. Hemobilia is managed with angiography, which includes embolization of the hepatic vessel that is communicating with the biliary tree.

When operative management is required, a midline laparotomy is the most versatile approach for managing any liver injury that might be encountered. The falciform ligament is divided, and perihepatic sponges are placed to temporarily manage bleeding from the liver. A fixed retractor can be placed to improve exposure of the right upper quadrant structures. When needed, perihepatic packing and manual compression can temporize bleeding to provide the opportunity to catch up with the resuscitation. Once the patient is reasonably stable, the packs are removed and the injuries to the liver are evaluated. Mild injuries with minimal ongoing bleeding may be managed with further compression, topical hemostatic agents, or suture hepatorrhaphy. Management of liver injuries may be facilitated by dividing the triangular ligaments to mobilize the right or left hepatic lobes. This will allow injuries to be better exposed for repair but may also allow more effective packing by optimizing anterior to posterior compression. Any mobilization of the liver must be carefully considered if there is any chance that the attachments of the liver are providing lifesaving tamponade of retrohepatic bleeding. Most liver injuries will require only superficial techniques for hemostasis to be obtained.

When more severe bleeding from the liver is present, a Pringle maneuver is a valuable adjunct to slow blood flow enough to visualize the injury. The hepatoduodenal ligament is encircled with a vessel loop or vascular clamp to occlude hepatic blood flow from the hepatic artery and portal vein. This maneuver helps distinguish hepatic arterial and portal venous bleeding from hepatic vein bleeding, which will persist with the hepatoduodenal ligament clamped. In many cases, the liver laceration can then be explored and any actively bleeding vessels controlled with suture ligation. Hepatic parenchyma that appears to be devitalized should be débrided, and drains should be placed when injuries appear to be at risk for a bile leak. A vascularized pedicle of omentum may reduce parenchymal bleeding and promote healing of the laceration when it is packed within the liver injury.

Liver injuries in the vicinity of the retrohepatic vena cava that are not actively bleeding should be packed and not explored. There are many heroic techniques described in the literature that outline the repair of retrohepatic vena cava injuries, but the approach with the greatest likelihood of success is preserving the body's natural tamponade of this low-pressure region when feasible. An atriocaval (Shrock) shunt is one method that includes isolation of the retrohepatic vena cava by placing an intravascular shunt between the right atrium and infrahepatic vena cava. Isolation of the liver with an atriocaval shunt with the addition of a Pringle maneuver theoretically allows repair of the vena cava or hepatic veins with less ongoing blood loss. Damage control techniques may be required because many patients who require operative intervention for liver injuries have already deteriorated physiologically. Control of surgical bleeding is obtained and the liver is packed, followed by temporary abdominal closure. It is inappropriate to leave surgical bleeding and to hope that packing alone will provide adequate control. Conversely, diffuse liver bleeding due to coagulopathy will not respond to repeated attempts at placement of suture but instead requires reversal of physiologic derangements. Patients are then resuscitated in the intensive care unit until hypothermia, coagulopathy, and acidosis resolve, at which time the abdomen can be re-explored and packs removed. After damage control, angiography with embolization may provide additional assistance with management of ongoing bleeding from hepatic artery branches. Despite this, the mortality in this cohort of patients remains high.[41]

Gastric injuries. Penetrating mechanisms are the most common cause of injuries to the stomach, with these being present in 17.6% and 17.3% of cases from two busy urban trauma centers.[32] More recent data from the NTDB reflect a slightly lower incidence, with 11.3% of patients with penetrating abdominal trauma sustaining a gastric injury. Within this cohort of patients, the associated mortality is 21.5%. Frequently, penetrating gastric injuries cause full-thickness perforations with likely spillage of gastric contents into the abdomen. Conversely, blunt gastric injuries are rare, occurring in 0.05% of all blunt trauma patients and 4.3% of patients with any blunt hollow visceral injury.[43] The mortality associated with these injures is significant, reaching 28.2% in an EAST multi-institutional trial. When studied with regression analysis, gastric injury was independently associated with death (relative risk, 2.8; 95% confidence interval, 1.8 to 4.4).[43] The NTDB contains a similarly low incidence of blunt gastric injuries, with less than 1% of patients with blunt abdominal trauma injuring the stomach. The associated mortality for this cohort of patients is 13.8%. Blunt gastric rupture is caused by an acute increase in intraluminal pressure from external forces that result in bursting of the gastric wall. Because of the high-energy nature of this mechanism, associated injury to the liver, spleen, pancreas, and small bowel is common, and mortality is frequently attributed to these associated injuries.

Like other hollow visceral injuries, gastric injuries will often be identified on physical examination by the presence of peritonitis. Furthermore, the location of penetrating wounds may be suggestive of gastric injury. Some gastric injuries are evident on CT, but the overall sensitivity for hollow visceral injury is limited. Finally, the evaluation of gastric injuries follows the approach to that of other hollow abdominal viscera (see earlier).

The approach to repair of gastric injuries is based on the amount of tissue loss and the injury location. Hematomas within the gastric wall should be evacuated to ensure the absence of perforation, followed by control of bleeding and closure of the seromusculature with nonabsorbable suture. Injuries that are full thickness should have all nonviable tissue débrided; the gastric wall is then closed in one or two layers. A common approach is to close the perforation with absorbable suture and then to invert the suture line with nonabsorbable seromuscular stitches. A stapler can also be used to close a perforation because of the redundancy of the gastric tissue and the unlikelihood of overly decreasing the volume of the stomach lumen. Injuries involving the gastroesophageal junction, lesser curve, fundus, and posterior wall may be more challenging to approach and require better exposure of the upper abdomen. Rarely, highly destructive injuries that cause the loss of large portions of the stomach will require partial or even total gastrectomy. Reconstruction could require Billroth I or II gastroenterostomy or creation of a Roux-en-Y esophagojejunostomy, depending on the extent of the resection.

Duodenal injuries. Duodenal injuries are uncommon after blunt and penetrating trauma but can pose a diagnostic and therapeutic challenge. Because of the retroperitoneal location of the duodenum, most injuries are due to penetrating mechanisms, occurring in 4.0% of cases. Gunshot wounds are the predominant cause, and the associated mortality is significant at 24.5% in the NTDB. Blunt duodenal injuries are much less common, occurring in 0.1% of cases. Compared with other blunt injuries to the gastrointestinal tract, the duodenum sustains injury 12% of the time.[43] The associated mortality has been reported as 14.8%, which is similar to rates found in the NTDB.[43] Blunt injuries are caused by a blow to the epigastrium by a narrow object, resulting in contusion of the wall or a blow-out secondary to acute elevation of intraluminal pressure. The classic description includes the abdomen's being struck by a steering wheel or, in children, a bicycle handlebar.

Penetrating duodenal injuries are often first diagnosed at laparotomy that is initiated on the basis of the location of the penetrating wound. Blunt duodenal injuries can be more challenging to identify and therefore require a high index of suspicion to avoid missed injuries. Physical examination findings can be lacking because of the retroperitoneal location of the duodenum. Even full-thickness duodenal perforations may not demonstrate peritoneal signs unless the perforation involves an intraperitoneal segment. The most valuable tool for diagnosis is abdominal CT with a low threshold for operative exploration. Abdominal CT may demonstrate a thickened duodenal wall, air or fluid outside the bowel lumen, or extravasation of contrast material if an oral contrast agent was administered. Low-grade injuries, such as a duodenal hematoma, can be identified by CT, although it is important also to evaluate the pancreas because associated injury is common. Any evidence of duodenal perforation on examination or imaging requires immediate operative intervention. Findings can at times be subtle, but a low threshold for exploration must be maintained because of the potential for false-negative abdominal CT results. Upper gastrointestinal contrast studies, diagnostic peritoneal lavage, and laboratory studies such as serum amylase level determination may provide additional information but have a limited role in the evaluation of duodenal injuries.

The approach to management of duodenal injuries depends on the location of the injury and the amount of tissue destruction. Hematomas of the duodenal wall will often resolve without intervention and are an issue only if they cause a gastric outlet obstruction. Treatment of obstructing hematomas consists of gastric decompression and initiation of total parenteral nutrition, with re-evaluation of gastric emptying with a contrast study after 5 to 7 days. If the duodenal obstruction persists after approximately 2 weeks, operative exploration is warranted to evaluate for perforation, stricture, or associated pancreatic injury. Hematomas will frequently decompress spontaneously during mobilization of the duodenum, and the intestinal wall should then be evaluated for perforation. Duodenal hematomas identified incidentally during laparotomy should not be intentionally opened unless there is a concern for full-thickness injury.

Most duodenal wall perforations can be repaired primarily by a single- or double-layer approach after débridement of devitalized tissue. Complete mobilization of the duodenum with a wide Kocher maneuver is required to provide necessary exposure and to ensure a tension-free repair. Larger amounts of tissue loss or duodenal transection can be managed with resection and primary anastomosis as long as the ampulla is not involved and the injured segment is short. Longer segments of duodenal injury or areas adjacent to the ampulla may require enteric bypass with a Roux-en-Y reconstruction. If possible, a healthy piece of omentum should be placed over any repair, and protection from enteric contents can be achieved by performing a pyloric exclusion and creating a gastroenterostomy. In the damage control setting, the use of a duodenostomy tube or resection leaving the gastrointestinal tract in discontinuity is highly effective for temporarily controlling contamination.

Pancreatic injuries. Pancreatic injuries commonly occur in association with injury to the duodenum because of their proximity. A penetrating mechanism is more commonly the cause, with 4.4% of patients with penetrating abdominal trauma sustaining a pancreatic injury. Although infrequent, these injuries remain a serious problem, resulting in mortality rates of 15.3% and 29.8% for blunt and penetrating mechanisms, respectively. Delays in diagnosis and management are believed to contribute to these significant mortality rates. Pancreatic enzymes are caustic, making delays in management of the injuries a source of massive systemic inflammation and subsequent poor outcomes. Pancreas tissue injury can result from direct laceration of the organ or through the transmission of blunt force energy to the retroperitoneum. A common mechanism of blunt pancreatic injury involves the crushing of the body of the pancreas between a rigid structure, such as a steering wheel or seat belt, and the vertebral column. The impact to the pancreas causes injury that ranges from mild contusion to complete transection with ductal disruption.

The identification of pancreas injuries can be challenging, particularly because available imaging modalities are not highly effective. As with the duodenum, the retroperitoneal location of the pancreas makes physical examination findings less helpful for diagnosis. Three-dimensional imaging with IV contrast–enhanced abdominal CT provides the best view of the pancreas and associated injury. Despite this, the extent of parenchymal injury and the degree of ductal involvement remain poorly characterized, as identified in a large multicenter trial.[44] Based on the technology employed, the ability to detect parenchymal injury and pancreatic duct disruption remained below 60%. Peitzman and colleagues reported better performance by CT in a prospective study in which the sensitivity of CT was approximately 80%, likely reflecting the variations in radiologic interpretation between centers.[45] CT alone may not be satisfactory to rule out a clinically significant pancreatic injury, and a high index of suspicion must be maintained. On abdominal CT, findings suggestive of pancreatic injuries include malperfusion of the pancreatic parenchyma, surrounding fluid, or hematoma and stranding in the adjacent soft tissue. An injury involving the neck of the pancreas on CT is demonstrated in Figure 16-26.

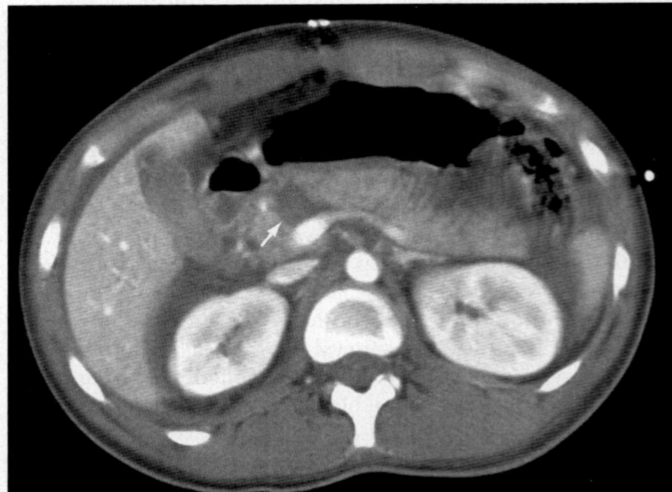

FIGURE 16-26 Pancreatic injury on abdominal CT. The injury involves the pancreatic neck and appears as a 2-cm segment of nonperfused pancreas tissue with surrounding edema as identified by the *arrow*.

The identification of clinically significant pancreatic injuries may require the use of other diagnostic studies. It is of great value to minimize the time to diagnosis of these injuries because delays in obtaining control can result in worse outcomes. Patients who are experiencing an unexpectedly poor response to their injuries require further evaluation for injuries to organs like the pancreas that may have been missed. Repeated CT imaging may suggest a pancreatic injury that required time to develop radiographically evident pancreatic inflammation. When it is obtained more than 3 hours after injury occurrence, an elevated serum amylase level may reflect pancreatic trauma. Used in this way, serum amylase levels are reasonably sensitive but are lacking in specificity and therefore are of limited value. Imaging of the pancreatic ducts with ERCP or magnetic resonance cholangiopancreatography may be helpful, especially for those patients who have a suggestion of pancreatic injury. These additional modalities continue to be studied and may occasionally be valuable in planning therapy and determining an operative approach.

Pancreatic injuries of any significance require surgical management. Exposure of the entire pancreas is required to evaluate for injury and to develop an effective surgical plan. This exposure includes mobilization of the hepatic flexure of the colon and division of the gastrocolic ligament to retract the transverse colon and mesocolon inferiorly. A Kocher maneuver will mobilize the pancreatic head and facilitate visualization. Assessment of the pancreas includes determining the amount of parenchymal involvement, location of the injury, and presence of ductal involvement. Pancreatic ductal injuries to the left of the superior mesenteric vessels are managed with a distal pancreatectomy. The proximal pancreatic stump can be managed by individually ligating the duct and oversewing the parenchyma or using a stapling device. Healing of the retained pancreas may be enhanced by coverage with a piece of healthy omentum, and a closed suction drain should be placed to manage any pancreatic enzyme leak. Managing injuries of the ductal system within the head of the pancreas can be more challenging. When tissue destruction is limited, managing these injuries with drainage alone often diverts the leakage of pancreatic fluid externally, creating a controlled fistula that frequently will close spontaneously. The closure of a fistula may be facilitated by biliary decompression through the placement of stents by ERCP. Massive destruction of the pancreatic head with devitalized parenchyma or combined pancreatic and duodenal injuries may require a pancreaticoduodenectomy (Whipple procedure). This presents the patient with a large surgical burden and is associated with a high postoperative complication rate. Only patients who are stable are candidates for pancreaticoduodenectomy; others undergo an abbreviated operation with later reconstruction. Damage control for pancreatic injury includes hemorrhage control, external drainage, and temporary abdominal closure with plans for re-exploration.

Effective external drainage is an important component in the management of pancreatic injuries, the value of which cannot be overstated. Pancreatic enzyme diversion is required to prevent retroperitoneal exposure to caustic enzymes, which will provoke a massive inflammatory response and progressive organ dysfunction. Less severe pancreatic injuries that do not involve the pancreatic duct, including hematomas, parenchymal contusions, and lacerations of the capsule or superficial parenchyma, should be managed with external drainage. Closed suction systems are associated with a reduced rate of abscess development compared with open-style drains.[46] Distal feeding access may be valuable to provide early enteral nutrition, depending on the overall clinical picture. Figure 16-27 demonstrates an approach to the operative management of pancreatic injuries.

Small bowel injuries. Likely secondary to the large percentage of the abdomen occupied, the small intestine is one of the more frequently injured organs after penetrating abdominal trauma. Series have reported the incidence to be as high as 60% in patients with penetrating abdominal trauma, although recent data from the NTDB demonstrated significantly lower presence of small intestinal injury (12.9%).[32] Mortality rates range from 15% to 20%, with most caused by associated vascular injuries.[43] Penetrating injuries can range from tiny perforations to large destructive injuries that devitalize circumferential segments of small bowel. Blunt injuries of the small bowel are less common, present in 1.7% of all blunt abdominal injuries in the NTDB, although these injuries are associated with a significant mortality rate of 14.0%. At the tissue level, injury can be secondary to crushing, rupture, and shearing mechanisms. Direct tissue injury can occur when the small bowel is crushed between the steering wheel or seat belt and a rigid structure, such as the vertebral column. Small bowel rupture occurs when the intraluminal pressure rapidly increases, causing a blow-out along the antimesenteric border. Deceleration mechanisms can result in a shearing of the serosa or muscularis throughout a segment of small bowel. Finally, injuries to the small bowel mesentery can result in devascularization and subsequent intestinal necrosis without direct tissue injury.

In the setting of penetrating mechanisms, small bowel injuries are often identified at the time of abdominal exploration. Patients may have peritonitis on examination at the time of presentation, or their abdominal examination findings may worsen in the hours after presentation. As with other hollow abdominal viscera, the evaluation can be challenging and is similar to the evaluation of the stomach and duodenum as described earlier. Abdominal CT imaging has significant limitations, and a high index of suspicion must exist to avoid a missed injury.

The repair of small bowel injuries depends on the amount of intestinal wall destruction in relation to the overall luminal circumference. Injuries to the intestinal serosa can be reinforced with interrupted nonabsorbable suture, which imbricates the injury. Small perforations can be repaired primarily with one or two layers after débridement of devitalized tissue. Care must be taken to avoid overly compromising the size of the intestinal lumen. In the setting of multiple perforations, primary repair can still be safely performed as long as the injuries are not so close as to result in narrowing of the bowel lumen when closed. Despite this, many surgeons choose to perform a resection with anastomosis when multiple perforations are present within a segment of bowel. When injuries involve more than 50% of the intestinal wall circumference, bowel resection with anastomosis should be performed. There has been no difference in leak rates demonstrated between stapled and hand-sewn anastomoses following resection. Selection of the anastomosis technique should be based on the preference of the surgeon and the amount of experience with the chosen technique. Hand-sewn anastomoses are frequently constructed in two layers, but single-layer methods are equally efficacious. Damage control for small bowel injuries includes rapid closure of perforations to control contamination with resection when large injuries are present. Patients in shock may benefit from resection without immediate anastomosis because of a higher risk of anastomotic dehiscence and the need for an abbreviated operation. The abdomen is temporarily closed, and the patient is resuscitated to correct physiologic derangements. After resuscitation,

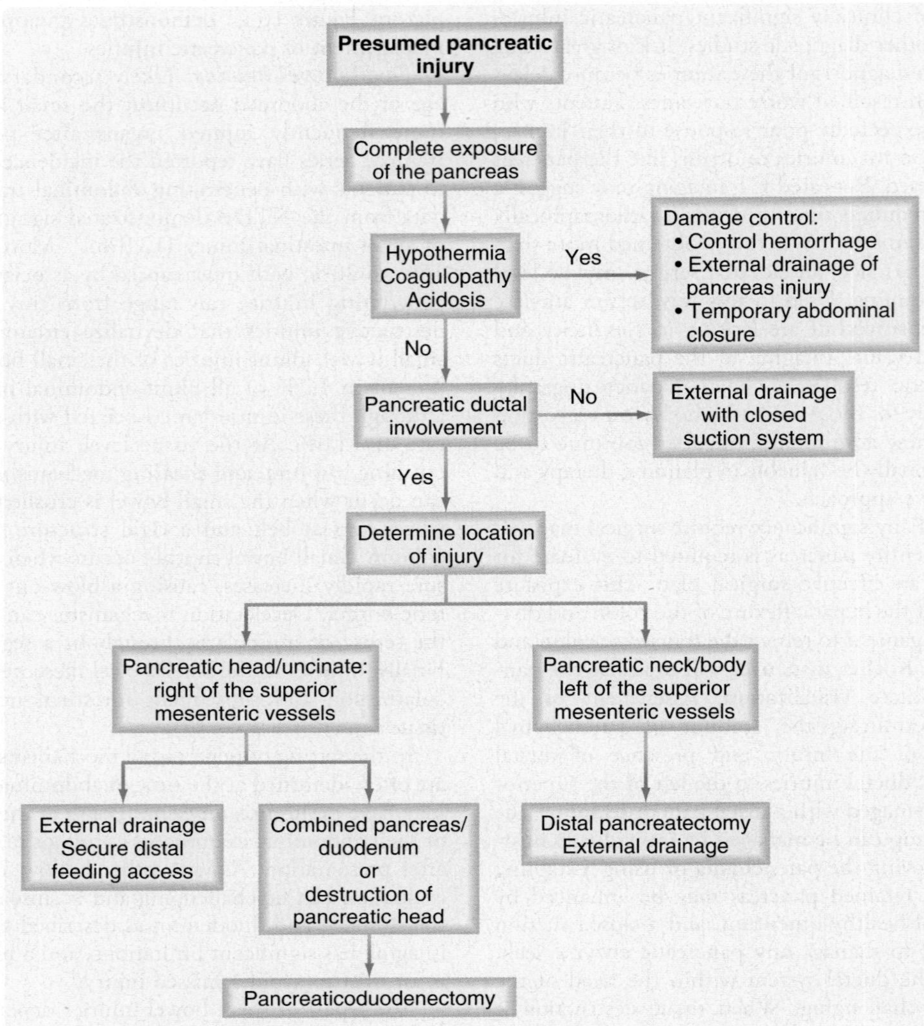

FIGURE 16-27 Algorithm for the operative management of pancreatic injury.

intestinal continuity can be re-established on return to the operating room.

Colon injuries. Colon and rectal injuries occur most commonly after penetrating abdominal trauma and rarely after blunt mechanisms. After penetrating abdominal trauma, injury to the colon is second only to small bowel trauma, occurring in 36.4% of patients in a series of 250 cases.[32] The incidence of colon injury in the NTDB also remains high at 24.6% in the most recent database. Despite this, the associated mortality for colon and rectal injuries is the lowest of all the abdominal viscera in the NTDB at 12.3%. Colonic tissue loss from penetrating injuries can range in severity, depending on the level of energy associated with the mechanism. From an examination standpoint, the retroperitoneal location of the right and left colon can obscure findings and injury identification. Colon and rectal injuries occur in less than 1% of all blunt trauma patients, demonstrating an associated mortality of 13%. When only patients with blunt hollow visceral injury are considered, the colon or rectum is involved in 30.2% of cases.[43] In a large series of blunt hollow visceral injuries, the mortality associated with colon and rectal injuries equaled 19.4%.[43] Injuries to the colon are caused by mechanisms similar to those that occur in the small bowel. The colonic wall can be directly crushed by physical forces or rupture when the rate of compression results in a rapid elevation in intraluminal pressure. Depending on the involved colonic segment, the colon injury and perforation can occur into the retroperitoneum. Most commonly seen in the retroperitoneal portions of the colon, shearing forces can cause a separation of the serosa or muscularis from the underlying mucosa over a long segment. The results of this injury mechanism are evident in Figure 16-28. Finally, injury to the rectum can also occur when severe pelvic fractures with sharp bone fragments cause a laceration.

Colonic injuries may first be identified at the time of laparotomy that was prompted by hemodynamic instability or a suggestive penetrating mechanism. The evaluation of the colon is similar to that of the small bowel. Abdominal CT is limited in capability, although it may demonstrate colonic wall thickening with surrounding stranding or fluid. Furthermore, imaging may identify the track of a penetrating mechanism, allowing the surgeon to assess proximity to the colon. Finally, care must be taken to adequately assess the segments of the colon that are retroperitoneal in location.

Evaluation of the rectum may require a different approach. Blood identified on rectal examination or a penetrating trajectory

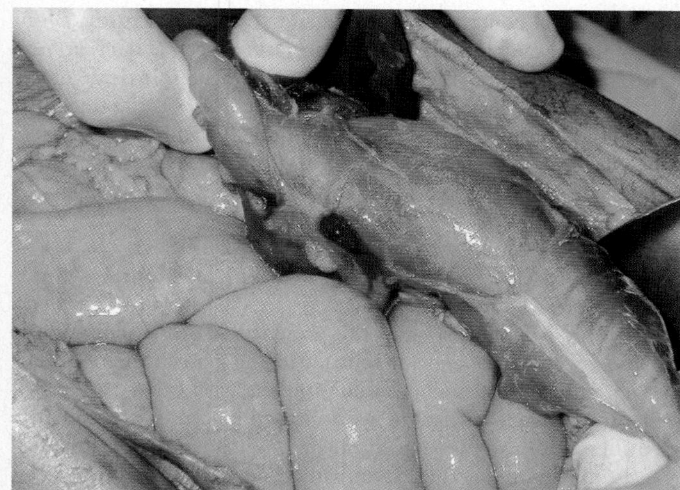

FIGURE 16-28 Blunt left-sided colon injury at the time of laparotomy. The injury mechanism resulted in a deserosalizing-type injury that involved a segment of colon several centimeters long.

that suggests rectal involvement requires further evaluation. Rigid proctosigmoidoscopy can be valuable to provide visualization of the rectum and distal sigmoid colon. In hemodynamically stable patients, this can assist with operative planning. Findings on endoscopy include a clear injury to the rectum or demonstrate only hematoma in the rectal wall or a large amount of blood in the rectal vault. Determination of the size of the injury and location on the rectal wall may be valuable for planning surgical management. Upper rectal injuries, especially those on the anterior or lateral surfaces, may be first identified during visualization of the pelvic structures at the time of laparotomy.

The approach to operative repair depends on the extent of the colonic wall injury and the patient's overall condition. Historically, the approach to all colon injuries included resection with the creation of a colostomy because anastomotic dehiscence was of great concern. Subsequent experience questioned the need for proximal fecal diversion to manage colonic perforations. Several randomized prospective trials have concluded that primary repair or resection with anastomosis is safe in select patients, resulting in a leak rate that is not significantly greater than with colonic diversion.[47,48] Therefore, injuries that involve less than 50% of the colonic wall circumference can be repaired with one or two layers, being sure to imbricate the mucosal edge. Destructive colon injuries that involve more than 50% of the colonic wall should be resected, and immediate anastomosis is possible in many cases. Injuries proximal to the middle colic artery are best managed with a right hemicolectomy and ileocolostomy anastomosis. Distal injuries require segmental resection with colocolostomy anastomosis. In the setting of shock, immediate anastomosis should be avoided because of an unacceptably high leak rate.

Colon injuries that are encountered in the unstable patient should be resected. Depending on the need to abbreviate the operation, colostomy can be created then or the gastrointestinal tract left in discontinuity until after the patient has been adequately resuscitated. Delayed primary anastomosis or creation of a colostomy can be performed on return to the operating room. Leak rates after delayed primary anastomosis have been found to be equivalent to those with immediate anastomosis performed in the setting of hemodynamic stability.[49] Significant associated injuries, underlying medical disease, or delayed injury recognition with the development of severe peritoneal inflammation may also suggest the need for colostomy.

Rectal injuries that result in perforation can cause significant contamination leading to pelvic sepsis. For this reason, operative management is often required. Rectal injuries are predominantly managed with fecal diversion and presacral drainage until healing has occurred, at which time the colostomy can be reversed. An end colostomy or a loop configuration can be used as long as complete fecal diversion is achieved. Drainage of the presacral space has traditionally been a component of managing rectal perforations as a result of experience gained in the military theater. More recent work has suggested that presacral drainage is unnecessary, especially in the setting of low-energy, nonmilitary types of penetrating rectal trauma.[50] Until more definitive studies emerge, one approach is to drain lower rectal injuries that occur posteriorly or laterally because these have likely entered the presacral space and are at greater risk of abscess formation. Other injuries sustained by the extraperitoneal rectum can be managed with fecal diversion alone. Rectal injuries that involve more than 50% of the luminal circumference may require resection of the rectum above the injury with the creation of an end colostomy.

Abdominal great vessel injuries. The major blood vessels of the abdomen are predominantly located within the retroperitoneum, with some larger vessels also in the intestinal mesenteries. Because of massive associated blood loss, visualization of the vessels can be compromised, making management of these injuries challenging. Most commonly, major abdominal vascular injuries are secondary to penetrating mechanisms. In the setting of blunt trauma, hematomas within the retroperitoneum are often secondary to pelvic fractures with bleeding from pelvic blood vessels that dissect superiorly. Abdominal vascular injuries are addressed elsewhere in this text (Section XII, Vascular), so only those concepts related to initial assessment and management are presented here.

Abdominal vascular injuries are often first recognized at the time of laparotomy being performed for penetrating abdominal trauma. These injuries are frequently associated with significant ongoing blood loss and hemodynamic instability. The specific vascular injury is better delineated after exploration and exposure of the retroperitoneal structures. Penetrating injuries to the back frequently benefit from three-dimensional imaging, given that most do not enter the peritoneal cavity. CT is often used to identify the path of the injury and therefore to suggest possible involvement of adjacent structures. Similarly, evaluation of the abdominal vasculature after blunt trauma is best achieved with contrast-enhanced CT. On occasion, retroperitoneal vascular injury is identified during urgently performed laparotomy, although further identification of specific injuries depends on the location of the hematoma.

Penetrating injuries to the retroperitoneum identified during laparotomy require exploration and repair. Although the details of these repairs are discussed elsewhere, a knowledge of the basic exposure of these structures is important. Hematomas of the infrarenal vasculature or the right renal hilum are exposed with a right medial visceral mobilization, also known as the Cattell-Braasch maneuver. A wide Kocher maneuver is performed, and the peritoneal dissection is continued inferiorly to mobilize the right colon. The dissection continues around the cecum and superiorly up the mesenteric root. Retraction of the abdominal viscera superior and to the left will expose the lower midline vascular structures. Basic tenets of vascular repair including proximal and distal control of the injured vessel are achieved when possible.

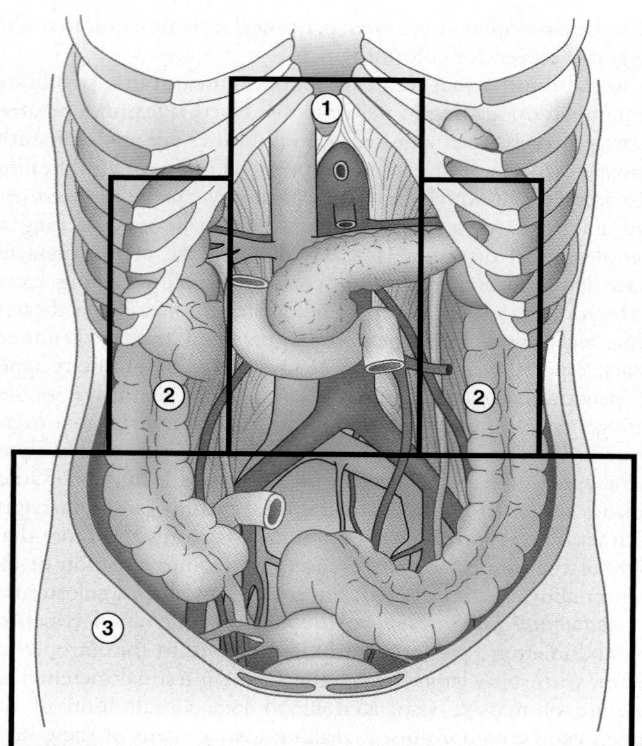

FIGURE 16-29 Zones of the retroperitoneum visualized at the time of laparotomy. Zone 1 includes the central vascular structures, such as the aorta and vena cava. Zone 2 includes the kidneys and adjacent adrenal glands. Zone 3 describes the retroperitoneum associated with the pelvic vasculature.

Injuries to the suprarenal great vessels or the left renal hilum are exposed by performing a left medial visceral mobilization (the Mattox maneuver). This is achieved by dividing the peritoneum along the entire left side of the abdomen, from above the spleen down to the distal left colon. The plane posterior to the colonic mesentery and the pancreas is developed, and the abdominal viscera are retracted to the right to expose the superior retroperitoneal vasculature.

Blunt abdominal vascular injuries that are not actively bleeding may require operative repair or may be considered for endovascular therapy, depending on the nature of the vascular disease. During laparotomy, the location of retroperitoneal hematoma guides surgical decision making. As seen in Figure 16-29, the retroperitoneum can conceptually be divided into three zones. Zone 1 hematomas require exploration because these frequently involve the aorta, proximal visceral vessels, or inferior vena cava, although an exception may be the dark hematoma behind the liver, which suggests a retrohepatic vena cava injury. Injuries to the retrohepatic vena cava are best served by not exposing the contained, low-pressure injury and by gently packing the surrounding area. A hematoma in the region of zone 2, which predominantly contains the kidneys, should be explored only if it appears that the hematoma is expanding and continuing to lose blood. Finally, a hematoma in zone 3 is usually secondary to pelvic fracture bleeding and should not be explored unless exsanguinating hemorrhage is obvious.

Genitourinary injuries. The genitourinary organs include the kidneys, ureters, bladder, and urethra, all of which are contained within the retroperitoneum. Bleeding and extravasation of urine are the major concern with injuries to these structures. Blunt mechanisms can result in renal laceration or bladder rupture, which can occur into the peritoneal space or the soft tissue of the pelvis. The typical mechanism for bladder injuries is the transmission of significant energy to the urine-filled bladder, resulting in wall rupture. This is almost universally associated with some amount of pelvic fracture. All genitourinary structures are vulnerable to penetrating mechanisms, many of which cause urine extravasation.

The approach to evaluating and managing genitourinary injuries is described elsewhere in this text (see Chapter 72) and therefore is only briefly outlined. The presence of gross hematuria is the most valuable screen for injuries to the genitourinary organs and should prompt further evaluation. As with other abdominal structures, imaging with IV contrast–enhanced CT frequently identifies injuries to the genitourinary organs. Abdominal CT reveals injuries to the kidneys and adjacent adrenal glands and can demonstrate findings suggestive of urine extravasation. When suspicion exists, injury to the bladder can be evaluated by obtaining a CT cystogram. In male patients, blood at the urethral meatus or a displaced prostate on rectal examination is suggestive of a urethral injury and requires evaluation. This is best achieved by performing retrograde urethrography, especially before placement of a urinary catheter. Penetrating genitourinary injuries may be first identified at the time of laparotomy or diagnosed with imaging studies. Penetrating injuries to the back benefit from CT, which can characterize the injury track and delineate adjacent organs.

During laparotomy, penetrating trauma to the retroperitoneum in the vicinity of the kidney should be explored to ensure hemostasis but also to assess for a urine leak. Although it is not always feasible, obtaining proximal control at the renal hilum is ideal and should be performed whenever possible. Many renal injuries are hemostatic at the time of exploration, whereas many will respond favorably to simple techniques. Conversely, devastating renal injuries, especially in the setting of shock with ongoing bleeding, may require nephrectomy. Assessment of the contralateral side for a kidney is valuable, but the potential for renal salvage should be dictated by the patient's physiologic condition. The repair of ureteral injuries can be achieved in several different ways ranging from primary repair to nephrectomy. Intraperitoneal bladder injuries can be repaired in two layers of absorbable suture and the bladder drained with a Foley catheter or suprapubic cystostomy tube. Extraperitoneal bladder ruptures require only decompression with a urinary catheter, followed by cystography to confirm healing after a period of recovery.

Blunt injury to genitourinary structures is commonly identified on imaging and can be managed nonoperatively in most cases. Bleeding from the kidneys and adrenal glands is often self-limited and requires no specific intervention. Injuries that demonstrate no evidence of ongoing bleeding are candidates for nonoperative management. Physiologic deterioration requires laparotomy with management of uncontrolled bleeding. Patients with hemodynamic stability but pseudoaneurysm from a renal injury on imaging may benefit from angioembolization. As described before, a renal hematoma after blunt trauma identified at laparotomy should be explored only if it appears that the hematoma is expanding.

Injuries to the Pelvis and Extremities

The majority of injuries sustained by trauma patients involve the musculoskeletal system. Orthopedic injuries to the pelvis and extremities are extremely common and described in depth elsewhere in this text. A basic approach to management as it relates to the general or trauma surgeon is presented here. Orthopedic injuries constituted the greatest number of cases in the 2014 NTDB report, with 29.5% of patients having upper extremity and 37.0% having lower extremity trauma. Although the mortality is low for each group, the long-term morbidity and functional implications can be significant. Pelvic fractures alone were seen in 6.9% of cases and had a greater mortality at approximately 7%. A variety of physical mechanisms are responsible for orthopedic injuries, with falls and motor vehicle crashes being the most common causes.

Evaluation for musculoskeletal injuries begins with a thorough physical examination, which easily identifies fractures that are open or demonstrate severe deformity. Plain radiography remains highly effective for diagnosis, although some fractures, such as complex pelvic fractures, benefit from CT. Pelvic fractures are typically identified on initial pelvic radiography and then better characterized on abdominal CT. In addition to evaluating the bone structures, CT can identify associated hematomas and the presence or absence of active extravasation of contrast medium, which appears as high-density material within the hematoma. Extremity examination must include a thorough vascular assessment and evaluation for compartment syndrome. Clinical evidence of vascular injury may require angiography to localize and to characterize the abnormality. CT angiography has evolved and now constitutes a major contributor to the evaluation of peripheral vascular trauma.

Bleeding from complex pelvic fractures presents a unique challenge and requires a coordinated approach. As depicted in Figure 16-30, unstable patients should have a pelvic radiograph quickly obtained and interpreted for pelvic fracture. An important point is that although some pelvic fracture patterns are higher risk, any fracture is capable of bleeding and should be addressed in the unstable patient. Pelvic fractures that demonstrate an increase in pelvic volume should be compressed with a pelvic binder or sheet wrapped around the hips to reduce the space available for hematoma formation. Pelvic compression will frequently address venous bleeding, but ongoing instability suggests an arterial source, which should be addressed with angiography and embolization. Some recent work has suggested that packing of the pelvis may be an alternative to embolization, especially when endovascular therapy is not immediately available. Stabilization of the pelvic ring with external fixation or definitive repair is then

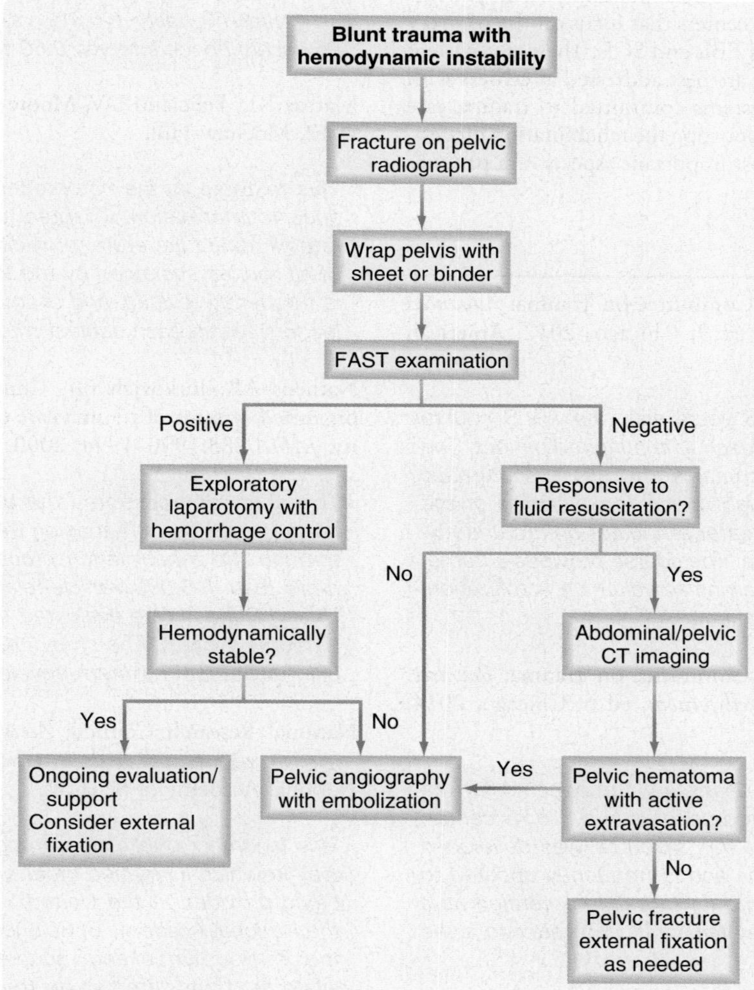

FIGURE 16-30 Algorithm for the evaluation and management of pelvic fractures with associated hemorrhage.

performed to maintain reduction of the pelvic volume and to limit ongoing venous bleeding.

REHABILITATION

Although the acute management of injuries plays the greatest role in the reduction of mortality, it is the process of rehabilitation that limits the long-term morbidity of injury. The rehabilitation process can be substantially longer than the hospital phase of care and is indispensable in restoring functionality and allowing patients to return to productive lives after injury. Despite a great deal of emphasis being placed on trauma-related fatalities, there were approximately 31 million nonfatal injuries in 2013, many of which required rehabilitative services.

The rehabilitation process begins immediately after the acute needs of the injured patient have been met. Early mobilization is extremely important to circumvent deconditioning. Physical and occupational therapists frequently begin the process by initiating therapy and determining what resources may be required when the patient leaves the hospital. With these recommendations available, case managers and social workers can begin the process of identifying the inpatient or outpatient resources required to address the unique rehabilitation needs of the patient. Early engagement by the rehabilitation team can expedite referrals and transfer to appropriate facilities. Select populations of patients may benefit from rehabilitation centers that focus on the recovery from specific conditions, such as TBIs and SCIs. These two patient cohorts have specific needs that are best addressed at centers with specialized expertise. Health systems committed to trauma care must place a high priority on supporting the rehabilitation process, given that this is one of the most important aspects of a patient's long-term recovery.

SELECTED REFERENCES

American College of Surgeons Committee on Trauma: *Advanced trauma life support for doctors*, ed 9, Chicago, 2012, American College of Surgeons.

First released more than 35 years ago, the ATLS course revolutionized the initial approach to the injured patient. The ninth edition of this text contains the same systematic approach that has been taught since the initiation of the course as well as an even greater emphasis on the underlying support from the literature. The course provides a framework to successfully perform an initial evaluation, stabilization, and transfer of the injured patient.

American College of Surgeons Committee on Trauma: *Resources for the optimal care of the injured patient*, ed 6, Chicago, 2014, American College of Surgeons.

This document outlines the necessary components for the optimal management of injured patients in a trauma center. Known as the Orange Book, this resource was developed by the Committee on Trauma and is frequently updated to remain current. The requirements to become verified as a trauma center and then to maintain verification are contained within this document.

Brain Trauma Foundation; American Association of Neurological Surgeons; Congress of Neurological Surgeons: Guidelines for the management of severe traumatic brain injury. *J Neurotrauma* 24(Suppl 1):S1–S106, 2007.

These guidelines represent the most comprehensive compilation of all literature related to traumatic brain injury. Evidence-based guidelines are provided on the basis of the strength of the associated studies. Application of the guidelines has been associated with improved outcomes after traumatic brain injury.

MacKenzie EJ, Rivara FP, Jurkovich GJ, et al: A national evaluation of the effect of trauma-center care on mortality. *N Engl J Med* 354:366–378, 2006.

The National Study on Costs and Outcomes of Trauma (NSCOT) is a large multicenter project supported by the Centers for Disease Control and Prevention that was initiated to define variations in injury care and outcomes between trauma centers and nontrauma centers. The project included more than 5000 patients from 69 hospitals spanning 12 states. This study demonstrated the benefit of care provided at a trauma center versus a nontrauma center. After correction for injury severity, trauma center care was associated with a reduction of in-hospital mortality (7.6% vs. 9.5%; relative risk, 0.80; 95% confidence interval, 0.66 to 0.98) as well as 1-year mortality (10.4% vs. 13.8%; relative risk, 0.75; 95% confidence interval, 0.60 to 0.95).

Mattox KL, Feliciano DV, Moore EE: *Trauma*, ed 7, New York, 2012, McGraw-Hill.

This textbook is the comprehensive resource for all injury-specific information. Chapters within the textbook incorporate all recent literature, providing an excellent presentation of all injuries sustained by the trauma patient. The textbook is frequently revised, and chapters are written by the world leaders within each subject matter.

Nathens AB, Jurkovich GJ, Cummings P, et al: The effect of organized systems of trauma care on motor vehicle crash mortality. *JAMA* 283:1990–1994, 2000.

This study demonstrated the benefit of establishing a systematic method of managing trauma from the time of injury through the rehabilitation process. During a 17-year span, more than 400,000 vehicle-related fatalities throughout the United States were evaluated for the effect of establishing a trauma system. The study identified a mortality benefit of 8% from trauma system development.

National Research Council: *Accidental death and disability: the neglected disease of modern society*, Washington, DC, 1966, National Academy of Sciences.

This landmark publication brought to light the substandard way in which injury and other emergency medical care was being provided in the United States. Published in 1966 by the National Academy of Sciences, this document prompted the development of and improvement in emergency medical systems. Considered to be the white paper of emergency care, this report provides valuable perspective regarding the maturation of modern-day emergency medical services.

Rotondo MF, Schwab CW, McGonigal MD, et al: 'Damage control': An approach for improved survival in exsanguinating penetrating abdominal injury. *J Trauma* 35:375–383, 1993.

This article was the first to present the concept of damage control, which has become the standard of care in managing multiple severe injuries. It was not until the development of this approach that surgeons employed the abbreviation of abdominal surgery to prevent the deadly cycle of worsening hypothermia, coagulopathy, and acidosis. Based on the success of this methodology, other areas of trauma management, such as orthopedics and resuscitation, have developed similar approaches.

U.S. Department of Health and Human Services, Health Resources and Services Administration: Model trauma systems planning and evaluation. 2006. Available at: <http://www.ncdhhs.gov/dhsr/ems/trauma/pdf/hrsatraumamodel.pdf>, Accessed June 10, 2015.

In response to studies that demonstrated a paucity of trauma systems in the United States, the Health Resources and Services Administration released this document, which outlines how systems for the management of injuries are developed and evaluated. The document emphasizes the value of a public health approach to trauma care. It has also been valuable in securing governmental funding for trauma system development.

REFERENCES

1. American College of Surgeons Committee on Trauma: *Resources for the optimal care of the injured patient*, ed 6, Chicago, 2014, American College of Surgeons.
2. U.S. Department of Health and Human Services, Health Resources and Services Administration: Model trauma systems planning and evaluation. Available at: <http://www.ncdhhs.gov/dhsr/ems/trauma/pdf/hrsatraumamodel.pdf>, 2015 (Accessed June 10).
3. MacKenzie EJ, Rivara FP, Jurkovich GJ, et al: A national evaluation of the effect of trauma-center care on mortality. *N Engl J Med* 354:366–378, 2006.
4. Nathens AB, Jurkovich GJ, Cummings P, et al: The effect of organized systems of trauma care on motor vehicle crash mortality. *JAMA* 283:1990–1994, 2000.
5. Baker SP, O'Neill B, Haddon W Jr, et al: The injury severity score: A method for describing patients with multiple injuries and evaluating emergency care. *J Trauma* 14:187–196, 1974.
6. Tinkoff G, Esposito TJ, Reed J, et al: American Association for the Surgery of Trauma Organ Injury Scale I: spleen, liver, and kidney, validation based on the National Trauma Data Bank. *J Am Coll Surg* 207:646–655, 2008.
7. Healey C, Osler TM, Rogers FB, et al: Improving the Glasgow Coma Scale score: Motor score alone is a better predictor. *J Trauma* 54:671–678, discussion 678–680, 2003.
8. Sasser SM, Hunt RC, Faul M, et al: Guidelines for field triage of injured patients: Recommendations of the National Expert Panel on Field Triage, 2011. *MMWR Recomm Rep* 61:1–20, 2012.
9. Eckstein M, Chan L, Schneir A, et al: Effect of prehospital advanced life support on outcomes of major trauma patients. *J Trauma* 48:643–648, 2000.
10. Winchell RJ, Hoyt DB: Endotracheal intubation in the field improves survival in patients with severe head injury. Trauma Research and Education Foundation of San Diego. *Arch Surg* 132:592–597, 1997.
11. Kragh JF Jr, Walters TJ, Baer DG, et al: Survival with emergency tourniquet use to stop bleeding in major limb trauma. *Ann Surg* 249:1–7, 2009.
12. Bickell WH, Wall MJ Jr, Pepe PE, et al: Immediate versus delayed fluid resuscitation for hypotensive patients with penetrating torso injuries. *N Engl J Med* 331:1105–1109, 1994.
13. American College of Surgeons Committee on Trauma: *Advanced trauma life support for doctors*, ed 9, Chicago, 2012, American College of Surgeons.
14. De Jong A, Molinari N, Conseil M, et al: Video laryngoscopy versus direct laryngoscopy for orotracheal intubation in the intensive care unit: A systematic review and meta-analysis. *Intensive Care Med* 40:629–639, 2014.
15. Parmet JL, Colonna-Romano P, Horrow JC, et al: The laryngeal mask airway reliably provides rescue ventilation in cases of unanticipated difficult tracheal intubation along with difficult mask ventilation. *Anesth Analg* 87:661–665, 1998.
16. Burlew CC, Moore EE, Moore FA, et al: Western Trauma Association critical decisions in trauma: Resuscitative thoracotomy. *J Trauma Acute Care Surg* 73:1359–1363, 2012.
17. Brenner ML, Moore LJ, DuBose JJ, et al: A clinical series of resuscitative endovascular balloon occlusion of the aorta for hemorrhage control and resuscitation. *J Trauma Acute Care Surg* 75:506–511, 2013.
18. Rotondo MF, Schwab CW, McGonigal MD, et al: 'Damage control': An approach for improved survival in exsanguinating penetrating abdominal injury. *J Trauma* 35:375–382, discussion 382–383, 1993.
19. Fox CJ, Gillespie DL, Cox ED, et al: The effectiveness of a damage control resuscitation strategy for vascular injury in a combat support hospital: Results of a case control study. *J Trauma* 64:S99–S106, discussion S106–S107, 2008.
20. CRASH-2 trial collaborators, Shakur H, Roberts I, Bautista R, et al: Effects of tranexamic acid on death, vascular occlusive events, and blood transfusion in trauma patients with significant haemorrhage (CRASH-2): A randomised, placebo-controlled trial. *Lancet* 376:23–32, 2010.
21. Brain Trauma Foundation; American Association of Neurological Surgeons; Congress of Neurological Surgeons: Guidelines for the management of severe traumatic brain injury. *J Neurotrauma* 24(Suppl 1):S1–S106, 2007.
22. Bracken MB, Holford TR: Neurological and functional status 1 year after acute spinal cord injury: Estimates of functional recovery in National Acute Spinal Cord Injury Study II from results modeled in National Acute Spinal Cord Injury Study III. *J Neurosurg* 96:259–266, 2002.
23. Golueke PJ, Goldstein AS, Sclafani SJ, et al: Routine versus selective exploration of penetrating neck injuries: A randomized prospective study. *J Trauma* 24:1010–1014, 1984.
24. Biffl WL, Moore EE, Offner PJ, et al: Optimizing screening for blunt cerebrovascular injuries. *Am J Surg* 178:517–522, 1999.
25. Sperry JL, Moore EE, Coimbra R, et al: Western Trauma Association critical decisions in trauma: Penetrating neck trauma. *J Trauma Acute Care Surg* 75:936–940, 2013.

26. Biffl WL, Cothren CC, Moore EE, et al: Western Trauma Association critical decisions in trauma: Screening for and treatment of blunt cerebrovascular injuries. *J Trauma* 67:1150–1153, 2009.
27. American College of Surgeons Committee on Trauma: *National Trauma Data Bank annual report 2014*, Chicago, 2014, American College of Surgeons.
28. Bulger EM, Edwards T, Klotz P, et al: Epidural analgesia improves outcome after multiple rib fractures. *Surgery* 136:426–430, 2004.
29. DuBose JJ, Leake SS, Brenner M, et al: Contemporary management and outcomes of blunt thoracic aortic injury: A multicenter retrospective study. *J Trauma Acute Care Surg* 78:360–369, 2015.
30. McKenney M, Lentz K, Nunez D, et al: Can ultrasound replace diagnostic peritoneal lavage in the assessment of blunt trauma? *J Trauma* 37:439–441, 1994.
31. Biffl WL, Kaups KL, Cothren CC, et al: Management of patients with anterior abdominal stab wounds: A Western Trauma Association multicenter trial. *J Trauma* 66:1294–1301, 2009.
32. Nicholas JM, Rix EP, Easley KA, et al: Changing patterns in the management of penetrating abdominal trauma: The more things change, the more they stay the same. *J Trauma* 55:1095–1108, discussion 1108–1110, 2003.
33. Haan JM, Bochicchio GV, Kramer N, et al: Nonoperative management of blunt splenic injury: A 5-year experience. *J Trauma* 58:492–498, 2005.
34. Cocanour CS, Moore FA, Ware DN, et al: Age should not be a consideration for nonoperative management of blunt splenic injury. *J Trauma* 48:606–610, discussion 610–612, 2000.
35. Harbrecht BG, Peitzman AB, Rivera L, et al: Contribution of age and gender to outcome of blunt splenic injury in adults: Multicenter study of the Eastern Association for the Surgery of Trauma. *J Trauma* 51:887–895, 2001.
36. Peitzman AB, Heil B, Rivera L, et al: Blunt splenic injury in adults: Multi-institutional Study of the Eastern Association for the Surgery of Trauma. *J Trauma* 49:177–187, discussion 187–189, 2000.
37. Cogbill TH, Moore EE, Jurkovich GJ, et al: Nonoperative management of blunt splenic trauma: A multicenter experience. *J Trauma* 29:1312–1317, 1989.
38. Richardson JD, Franklin GA, Lukan JK, et al: Evolution in the management of hepatic trauma: A 25-year perspective. *Ann Surg* 232:324–330, 2000.
39. Kozar RA, Feliciano DV, Moore EE, et al: Western Trauma Association/critical decisions in trauma: Operative management of adult blunt hepatic trauma. *J Trauma* 71:1–5, 2011.
40. Meredith JW, Young JS, Bowling J, et al: Nonoperative management of blunt hepatic trauma: The exception or the rule? *J Trauma* 36:529–534, discussion 534–535, 1994.
41. Duane TM, Como JJ, Bochicchio GV, et al: Reevaluating the management and outcomes of severe blunt liver injury. *J Trauma* 57:494–500, 2004.
42. Asensio JA, Roldan G, Petrone P, et al: Operative management and outcomes in 103 AAST-OIS grades IV and V complex hepatic injuries: Trauma surgeons still need to operate, but angioembolization helps. *J Trauma* 54:647–653, discussion 653–654, 2003.
43. Watts DD, Fakhry SM, EAST Multi-Institutional Hollow Viscus Injury Research Group: Incidence of hollow viscus injury in blunt trauma: An analysis from 275,557 trauma admissions from the East multi-institutional trial. *J Trauma* 54:289–294, 2003.
44. Phelan HA, Velmahos GC, Jurkovich GJ, et al: An evaluation of multidetector computed tomography in detecting pancreatic injury: Results of a multicenter AAST study. *J Trauma* 66:641–646, discussion 646–647, 2009.
45. Peitzman AB, Makaroun MS, Slasky BS, et al: Prospective study of computed tomography in initial management of blunt abdominal trauma. *J Trauma* 26:585–592, 1986.
46. Fabian TC, Kudsk KA, Croce MA, et al: Superiority of closed suction drainage for pancreatic trauma. A randomized, prospective study. *Ann Surg* 211:724–728, discussion 728–730, 1990.
47. Stone HH, Fabian TC: Management of perforating colon trauma: Randomization between primary closure and exteriorization. *Ann Surg* 190:430–436, 1979.
48. Demetriades D, Murray JA, Chan L, et al: Penetrating colon injuries requiring resection: Diversion or primary anastomosis? An AAST prospective multicenter study. *J Trauma* 50:765–775, 2001.
49. Miller PR, Chang MC, Hoth JJ, et al: Colonic resection in the setting of damage control laparotomy: Is delayed anastomosis safe? *Am Surg* 73:606–609, discussion 609–610, 2007.
50. Gonzalez RP, Falimirski ME, Holevar MR: The role of presacral drainage in the management of penetrating rectal injuries. *J Trauma* 45:656–661, 1998.

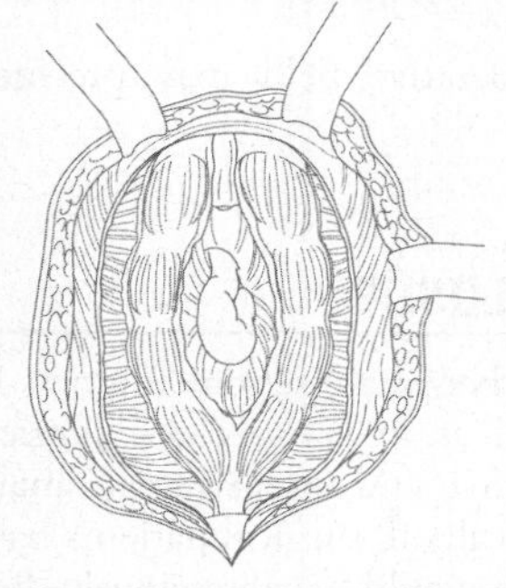

CHAPTER 17

The Difficult Abdominal Wall

Oliver L. Gunter, Richard Miller

OUTLINE

 **Please access ExpertConsult.com to view the corresponding video for this chapter.**

Despite the fact that the laparotomy incision is a common factor in any number of abdominal operations, there is little evidence to guide surgeons in optimal closure of the abdominal wall. The goal of this chapter is to illustrate techniques of permanent as well as temporary closure of the abdominal wall, with further attention given to situations that fall outside of normal conditions.

SUTURE MATERIAL

Abdominal wall closure has changed over time, in large part because of improvements in suture materials and characteristics. The ideal suture material for abdominal wall closure would be one that resists infection, provides adequate tensile strength to prevent abdominal wall disruption, minimizes tissue damage, and is absorbable. In current practice, a significant percentage of abdominal wall incisions are closed with slowly absorbing monofilament suture, such as polydioxanone (PDS; Ethicon, Johnson & Johnson), which is frequently used as a double-stranded suture to increase tensile strength. Polydioxanone has an advantage over polyglactin for abdominal closure, with a longer strength retention profile and absorption time, as well as being a monofilament that may resist infection to a greater degree than braided suture. Use of nonabsorbable sutures for abdominal closure (e.g., polypropylene) has been associated with increased pain and sinus track formation and has not shown any significant difference in the incidence of incisional hernia formation, wound dehiscence, or surgical site infection.[1,2]

CLOSURE TECHNIQUE

Principles of wound closure applied to the closure of the abdominal wall are essentially the same for closure of any surgical incision. Minimization of tissue damage is imperative, and this may be done by limiting the incorporation of the abdominal wall musculature in the closure. A 4 : 1 ratio of suture bites versus suture advancement has been advocated, although recent evidence suggests that smaller fascial bites may decrease the incidence of dehiscence and ventral hernia, likely a result of decreased tissue ischemia and damage.[3,4] Layered closure of the abdominal wall to include separate layered closure of the peritoneum and subcutaneous tissues in addition to the skin and fascia is discouraged, and mass closure is preferred.[3] A continuous suture of slowly absorbable suture material is the recommended method of closure in elective abdominal surgery, although there is little evidence to guide closure in the emergency setting.[5]

Although retention sutures are frequently employed, there is little evidence to suggest benefit to their use.[6] Whereas they are intended to prevent evisceration, there is no consensus on the ideal adjunct to standard techniques of abdominal wall closure. Retention sutures have been associated with increased pain, increased wound inflammation, wound complications and skin breakdown, and problems with ostomy appliance placement.[7] Thus, routine use of retention sutures, although theoretically advantageous, is not without potential complications. Patients at high risk of acute fascial dehiscence may benefit from some method of evisceration prophylaxis, and some have promoted the use of synthetic mesh in high-risk abdominal wall closures.[8-10] Identification of the patient who is at higher risk of abdominal wall dehiscence may alter surgical technique of abdominal wall closure and should be considered in any abdominal operation.

ABDOMINAL FASCIAL DEHISCENCE

The incidence of fascial dehiscence has been reported as high as 3.5% after major abdominal surgery and is associated with significant morbidity and mortality.[6] Acute fascial dehiscence may be heralded by increased serosanguineous drainage from the laparotomy wound and can be confirmed on physical examination. Predisposing risk factors to acute fascial dehiscence are illustrated in Box 17-1.[11] Wound infection has been found to be highly associated with fascial dehiscence in multiple studies.[12-14] The primary technical causes of acute fascial dehiscence are knot failure (rare), fascial damage (frequently related to tension, ischemia, or surgical site infection), and suture material damage and failure.

Surgical management of acute dehiscence relies on a number of factors. The cause of the dehiscence should be investigated either at the time of surgery or with preoperative imaging if indicated. Fascial dehiscence may be associated with either surgical site infection or intra-abdominal abscess, and this will vary by the type of index operation performed.[15,16] Although the risk of fascial dehiscence may persist beyond 3 weeks postoperatively, the usual time frame is within the first 7 days after primary closure.[17] Depending on the degree of intraperitoneal inflammatory process and formation of adhesions and peritoneal sclerosis, the abdomen may be inaccessible for repeated laparotomy, and fascial dehiscence would be managed as a planned ventral incisional hernia with reconstruction in a delayed fashion. If laparotomy is feasible, determination of the cause of fascial dehiscence followed by abdominal wall closure is considered standard management. Frequently, abdominal wall closure is made difficult by tissue edema and excessive tension, and patients may benefit from delayed closure once the acute physiologic process has normalized. Any associated bowel injury or anastomotic disruption creating an enterocutaneous fistula substantially increases the complexity of reoperation. The use of prophylactic mesh may be helpful to facilitate abdominal wall closure because the ventral incisional hernia rate is increased after dehiscence despite repair, although contamination of the operative field may preclude its use.

BOX 17-1 Risk Factors for Fascial Dehiscence

- Wound closure technique
- Type of incision
- Operative indication
- Increasing abdominal pressure
- Age >65 years
- Chronic obstructive pulmonary disease
- Hemodynamic instability
- Malnutrition
- Diabetes
- Obesity
- Ascites
- Jaundice
- Steroid use

TEMPORARY ABDOMINAL CLOSURE

Techniques in damage control have become essential adjuncts in trauma and general surgery as well as in subspecialty surgical procedures. Advancements in operative and intensive care management of severely injured and critically ill surgical patients have improved survival rates in those who would have previously died of their injury or disease processes. One such advanced technique is the application of serial abdominal operations before primary fascial closure and the creation of a temporary abdominal closure (TAC) (Box 17-2). Current options for TAC include a tension-free atraumatic abdominal visceral coverage and dynamic techniques in which the fascial edges are closed with serial plication (Table 17-1). In addition, multiple case reports describe a number of modifications to these tension-free and dynamic closure techniques.

In an attempt to reduce the time from a TAC to primary fascial closure and to help minimize management variability in patients with an open abdomen and loss of abdominal domain, we have proposed a five-stage management algorithm for this population of patients (Fig. 17-1). With current resuscitation strategies, the abdominal fascia can be successfully closed during stage 3 of this algorithm in the majority of patients.[18]

The goal of delayed primary fascial closure is to have the fascia closed as soon as possible, ideally within the first 8 days to minimize potential complications related to open abdomen management.[19] However, the risk for development of intra-abdominal hypertension and abdominal compartment syndrome from

BOX 17-2 Indications for Temporary Abdominal Closure

- Damage control
  - Severe hemorrhage
  - Hypothermia, coagulopathy, acidosis
  - Delayed definitive operation secondary to patient's physiologic state
- Intra-abdominal hypertension or compartment syndrome
- Questionable visceral viability
- Planned acute reoperation
- Severe intra-abdominal sepsis
- Triage

TABLE 17-1 Current Techniques of Temporary Abdominal Closure

TECHNIQUE	DESCRIPTION	EXAMPLE
Vacuum pack	Perforated polyethylene sheet placed under fascia, covering abdominal viscera Sterile surgical towels and suction drains placed in wound, covered with adhesive plastic drape; drains placed to continuous suction	Barker vacuum pack
Negative pressure wound therapy	Polyethylene encapsulated foam system placed under fascia with negative pressure sponge applied to vacuum device	KCI ABThera open abdomen negative pressure therapy
Artificial burr	Two opposing Velcro sheets with hooks and loops, sutured to fascial edges Velcro sheets connect in the midline	Wittman patch
Dynamic retention sutures	Sutures or elastomers placed transabdominally, just lateral to rectus fascia bilaterally	Canica ABRA silicone elastomer
Inlay patch	Impermeable prosthesis sutured to fascial edges	Bogota bag
Skin-only closure	Use of towel clips to reapproximate skin in the midline	Towel clip closure

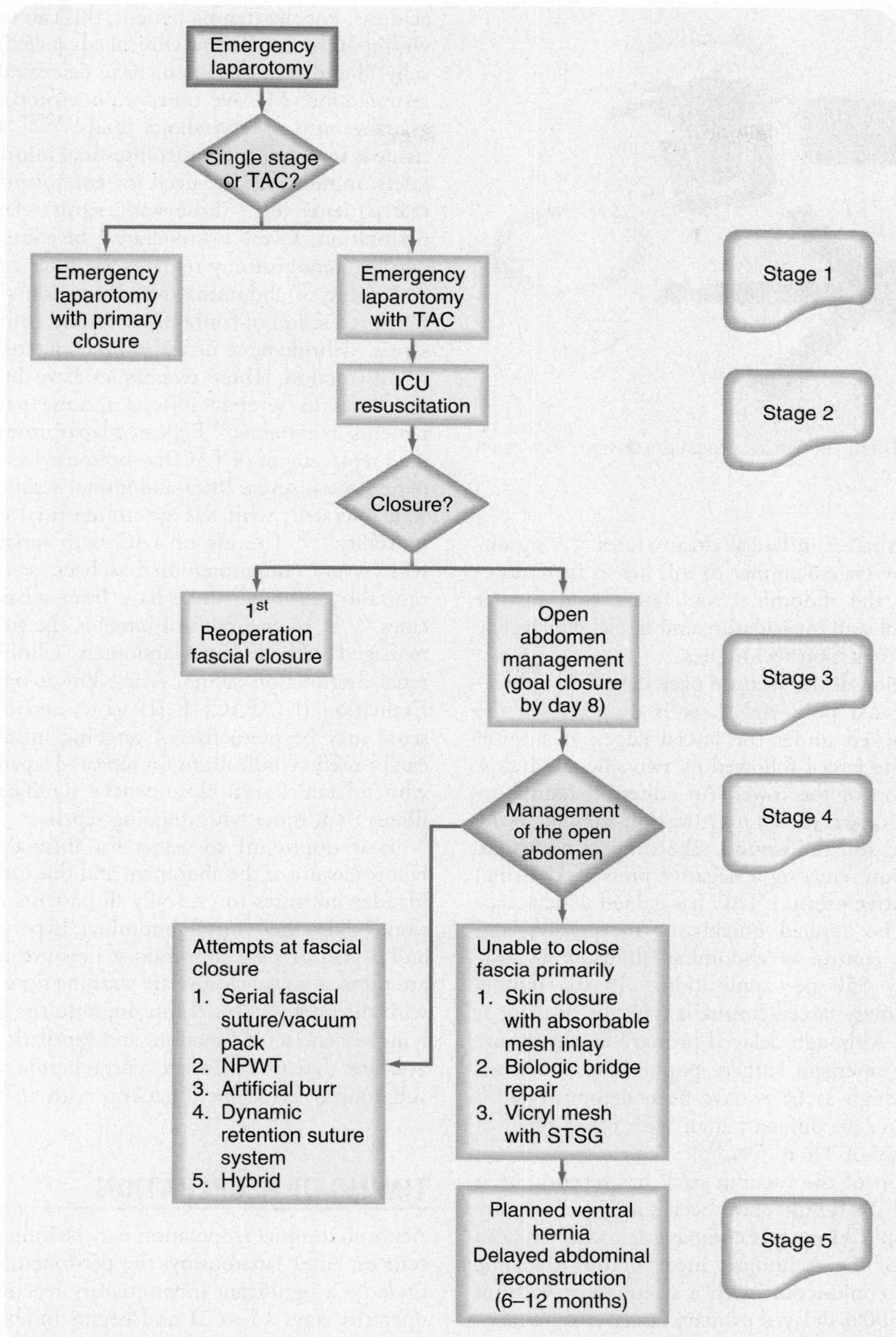

FIGURE 17-1 Five-stage proposed algorithm for management of the open abdomen. *ICU,* intensive care unit; *NPWT,* negative pressure wound therapy; *STSG,* split-thickness skin graft; *TAC,* temporary abdominal closure.

ongoing inflammatory response syndrome, visceral edema, and lack of source control and intra-abdominal abscess or enterocutaneous fistula may be reason to delay primary closure. In this setting, the surgeon may have to accept a planned delayed abdominal wall reconstruction and use alternative means of visceral coverage (stages 4 and 5).

Commonly used for TAC, the artificial burr system consists of two sheets of hook and burr material, similar to Velcro, that are sewn to the fascial edges after a plastic drape is placed over the viscera. The hook and burr are then overlapped with limited tension to provide a secure TAC. Gauze is used to pack the subcutaneous tissue.[20] Pulling the Velcro-like material apart easily allows reexploration of the abdomen. At the completion of the subsequent operations, the patch can be tightened to keep fascial tension. Repeated tightening allows a sequential approximation of the fascia until it can be closed without undue tension. There is some evidence that the artificial burr, along with dynamic retention sutures paired with a commercially available vacuum pack

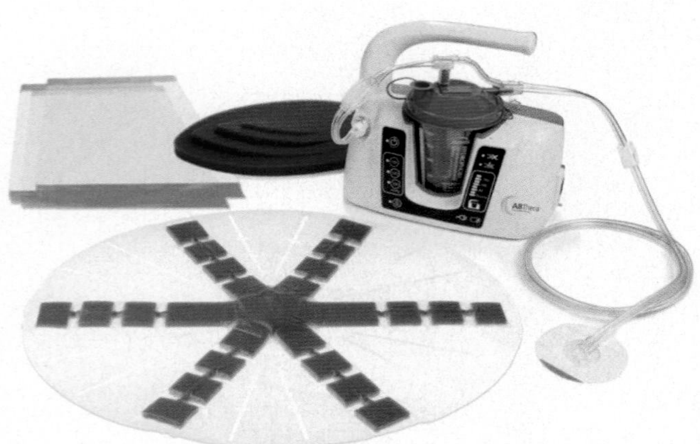

FIGURE 17-2 KCI ABThera negative pressure device for open abdomen management.

device, has the highest success in fascial closure rates.[21] A significant disadvantage of any system similar to this lies in its requirement to be sutured to the abdominal wall fascia, thus further damaging the abdominal wall musculature and fascia, which may complicate future reconstruction techniques.

The original description of the vacuum pack described a three-layer TAC.[22] A fenestrated polyvinyl sheet is draped over the exposed viscera and tucked under the fascial edges. A surgical towel is placed under the fascia, followed by two silicone drains, which are placed on top of the towel. An adhesive, iodophor-impregnated polyester drape is placed over the skin laterally to the anterior axillary lines to seal the wound. The surgical drains are connected to wall suction, creating a negative pressure dressing. The vacuum pack–negative pressure TAC has gained wide acceptance because it can be applied quickly, is inexpensive and atraumatic, and allows control of abdominal fluids. It is cost-effective, approximately $50 per application.[21] In the trauma population, delayed primary fascial closure is typically possible at the second laparotomy. Although delayed primary fascial closure is less common in the emergent surgery population, combined fascial closure rates as high as 68% have been demonstrated.[23] Fistula and leak rates are no different than with other types of TAC, with reported rates of 3% to 5%.[23,24]

A commercial version of the vacuum pack has recently been made available (Fig. 17-2). Results have been similar to primary fascial closure and complication rates comparable to the vacuum pack. A modification of the technique, incorporating dynamic serial fascial closure in conjunction with a commercial vacuum pack, has demonstrated 90% delayed primary fascial closure rates. This technique extends beyond the 8-day benchmark, with low complication rates in some series.[23-25] A review has suggested that the vacuum pack and artificial burr are associated with the highest closure rates as well as with the lowest mortality rates, although identification of the population of patients that would most benefit from this method of closure can be challenging.[21]

ASSESSING READINESS FOR ABDOMINAL CLOSURE

Patients are prepared to return for reconstruction of internal injuries once they have been adequately resuscitated.[26,27] The goal of resuscitation is correction of hypothermia, coagulopathy, and acidosis. For the trauma patient, this can usually be accomplished within 36 hours. Recent clinical advances in the care for the critically ill and trauma patient have decreased the time to adequate resuscitation. Massive transfusion protocols have minimized the excessive use of crystalloid fluids.[18,28,29] Injured or devitalized tissue is resected, and gastrointestinal injuries can be anastomosed safely, minimizing the need for enterostomy. However, for high-risk patients (e.g., those with sepsis related to gastrointestinal perforation, severe postoperative bleeding, intraoperative hypotension), enterostomy remains the most conservative approach.[30]

Staging of abdominal reconstruction serves three main functions: reduction of contamination and control of intra-abdominal sepsis, débridement of devitalized or contaminated tissue, and reconstruction. These techniques have been shown to improve outcomes in severely injured trauma patients, particularly for patients in extremis.[31] Repeated laparotomy with routinely scheduled replacement of TAC has been used as a means to manage the patient with severe intra-abdominal sepsis effectively. It has been well tolerated, with few gastrointestinal complications and low mortality.[32,33] The use of TAC with serial reoperations in cases with severe contamination has been associated with improved mortality, although there have been mixed results in less severe cases.[20,34,35] Source control remains the priority in most patients managed with an open abdomen. Clinical parameters such as renal dysfunction values, Acute Physiology and Chronic Health Evaluation II (APACHE II) score, and multiorgan dysfunction score may be predictive of ongoing intra-abdominal sepsis and can be used as indications for repeated laparotomy.[26,32,36,37] Patients who tolerate fascial closure have significantly lower severity of illness than those with ongoing sepsis.

It is important to assess for intra-abdominal hypertension before closure of the abdomen, and this can be done by measuring bladder pressures in critically ill patients on mechanical ventilation.[38] Sustained intra-abdominal hypertension (>20 mm Hg) and a rise of peak inspiratory pressure of 10 cm H_2O during attempts at fascial closure are warning signs of high fascial tension, with the potential for compromise to the abdominal wall, underlying viscera, renal function, and ventilation. Closure of the fascia at a later date or a planned ventral hernia may be prudent for this subgroup of critically ill patients with an open abdomen.[39,40]

TIMING OF REOPERATION

Acute abdominal reoperation may be indicated in specific circumstances. After laparotomy, the peritoneum and peritoneal cavity undergo a significant inflammatory reaction that builds by postoperative days 14 to 21 and begins to abate by approximately 6 weeks postoperatively. Thus, in the early postoperative period, there is a limited time frame for safe abdominal reoperation. The postoperative healing process creates a scenario that resembles temporary sclerosing peritonitis, making it difficult or impossible to mobilize the viscera and to explore the abdomen thoroughly. The risk of injury is not insignificant, and any need for operative intervention must take into account this risk versus potential benefit of the procedure. In the event that the abdomen cannot be safely entered, nonoperative or percutaneous techniques should be pursued.

With regard to timing of reoperative surgery, the extent and circumstances of the index operation must be taken into account. Laparoscopic procedures incur much less interruption of normal peritoneal physiology and anatomy, thus resulting in fewer

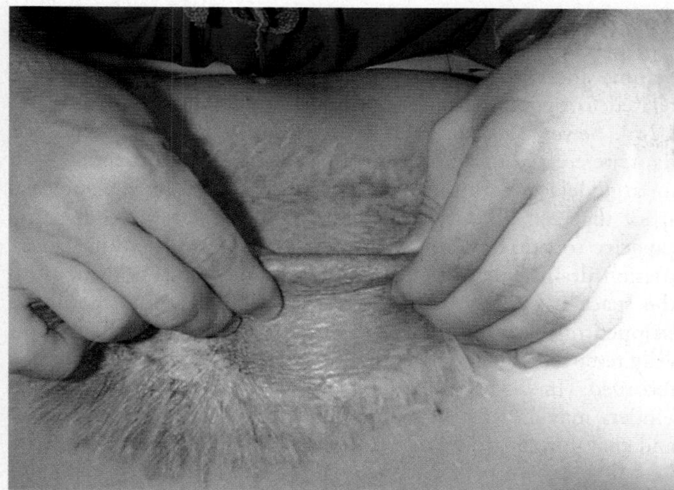

FIGURE 17-3 Pinch test after abdominal wall skin graft indicating release of the graft from underlying viscera.

postoperative adhesions. Patients managed with open abdomen and eventual skin graft typically require 6 to12 months before consideration of abdominal reconstruction. In the setting of trauma, this may require further delay as other injuries are addressed. After application of an abdominal wall skin graft over the open abdomen, the blood supply is derived from the underlying bowel. Ideal timing of reoperation in these patients occurs when the graft releases from the underlying viscera and the graft is able to pass the so-called pinch test (Fig. 17-3). With regard to timing of ostomy takedown, a longer time between ostomy creation and reversal has been associated with fewer complications, and adhesions appeared to diminish at about 15 weeks and beyond.[41] As adhesions may be associated with increased operative complexity, this time frame should be considered before elective reoperative surgery. After an open operation (e.g., Hartmann procedure), typical delays of 6 months or more should be expected before ostomy reversal.

SYNTHETIC MESH FAILURE

The use of synthetic prosthetic mesh is well established as the surgical treatment of choice for repair of ventral incisional hernias and in the majority of cases can provide a long-lasting repair with low recurrence rates. The development of synthetic mesh material was a major advancement in hernia surgery, and its advantages include decreased recurrence rates, ease of use, and relatively low cost compared with biologic mesh.[42] This has resulted in synthetic mesh being the most commonly used prosthetic for reinforcement for initial incisional and recurrent hernia repairs.

Although the application of synthetic mesh has resulted in a significant improvement in failure and recurrence rates, the use of these mesh materials may result in specific complications that range from minor to potentially life-threatening. Synthetic mesh may variably become infected, depending on the degree of contamination of the wound and the nature of the prosthetic material used.

Infections must be eradicated before any major repair is considered, and measures should be taken to heal open wounds as bacterial colonization may be significant even in the absence of a frank infection. In the setting of mesh infection, this requires

BOX 17-3 Challenges in Ventral Hernia Repair in a Contaminated Field

- Multiple previous attempts at hernia repair
- Significant disruption of tissue planes
- Enterocutaneous fistulas must be resected
- Accompanying prosthetic material must be removed
- Large fascial defect
- Replacing with permanent prosthetic mesh is relatively contraindicated in the acute phase
- Protein-calorie malnutrition
- Primary repair has high rate of failure

removal of the infected mesh material and anchoring sutures, drainage of any abscesses, and débridement of the wound. Studies of mesh infections after open ventral incisional hernia repairs recently revealed that the lighter weight, macroporous meshes carry a lower risk of infection compared with the heavier microporous meshes, such as expanded polytetrafluoroethylene.[43] Any mesh that is not incorporated should be excised completely from the edge of the wound to healthy tissues. If the wound has a large amount of contamination or requires major débridement, bowel resection, or enterocutaneous fistula takedown, for example, a multistage approach may be required to achieve a clean wound before definitive abdominal wall reconstruction is entertained. There are many challenges to hernia repair in an infected field (Box 17-3).

When there is insufficient autologous tissue for layered closure, often the case after emergent surgery in the setting of peritonitis, the surgeon is then faced with several challenges that must be addressed in a prioritized fashion. After the infection is eradicated, bowel resection performed, and necrotic tissue débrided, the visceral sac must then be contained. In this scenario, it is generally not advisable to create large skin flaps or to perform myofascial component separations during the acute phase of management. After source control and treatment of infections, preparation of the wound for definitive repair should not interfere with possible reconstruction options in the future. Tissue repair during this time is an anabolic process, and malnourished or actively catabolic patients may have significantly impaired wound healing. In addition, the open abdomen probably contributes to the systemic inflammatory response and catabolism state.

Although it is less than ideal, it may be necessary to rely on TAC and fascial bridge techniques first to reduce the bacterial burden and then to develop a clean wound for later definitive repair. Determining the proper way to deal with this residual defect is still a source of controversy. Negative pressure devices have been used to help in this situation, first to eradicate all infection and then to cover a biologic mesh bridged repair.

BIOLOGIC MESH

Biologic mesh material for abdominal wall reconstruction was introduced in the late 1990s. These materials provided additional flexibility in surgical options for the repair of complex abdominal wall defects. Biologic mesh was developed and promoted primarily for use in contaminated fields, in which synthetic mesh use was contraindicated. Since the introduction of these biosynthetic materials, there has been an ever-expanding market of new biologic materials that claim superiority, yet few of these materials have been subject to critical evaluation of their outcomes in humans for abdominal wall reconstruction.

Each of these biologic prosthetics has unique methods of processing that result in different handling characteristics and physiologic properties. Biologic mesh has the purported benefit of its ability to be used in a contaminated field, and explantation may not be necessary if the biologic mesh becomes infected. Compared with conventional mesh, biologic mesh has been shown to improve bacterial clearance and to harbor significantly less quantitative bacterial counts in animal models.[44] Non–cross-linked biologics have been shown to perform better in both categories compared with cross-linked biologics.

In the setting of sepsis with a large abdominal wound defect, local wound care is required until the bacterial burden is reduced, followed by a temporizing abdominal closure. The ideal closure is autologous tissue; however, this is not always feasible. If the skin cannot be closed over the abdominal wall defect, our current practice involves use of a non–cross-linked biologic mesh as an inlay bridge repair. Although this does not provide definitive hernia repair, the primary theoretical advantage of using biologic mesh is to prevent desiccation of underlying bowel, which may prevent fistula formation. Wound management systems that use topical antimicrobials and minimize desiccation are useful to keep the graft moist and to limit the bacterial burden.

The biologic mesh may desiccate and form an eschar, which may require local débridement, although this typically does not occur for weeks after mesh placement (Fig. 17-4). Once the wound bed appears healthy with adequate granulation tissue, it can either be allowed to granulate and heal by secondary intention or be covered with native skin or a skin graft. This biologic bridge technique is useful for patients with significant comorbidities, for the acutely ill, and in cases in which definitive reconstruction is a prohibitive risk. There is clear evidence that if the biologic mesh is used as a bridge repair, the result is a high recurrence rate because of stretching of the biologic over time, causing laxity, bulging, or actual recurrence within a year.[45] Thus, the bridge repair should be thought of not as a definitive reconstruction alternative but more as biologic cover of the peritoneal cavity that prevents desiccation and possible enterocutaneous fistula formation.

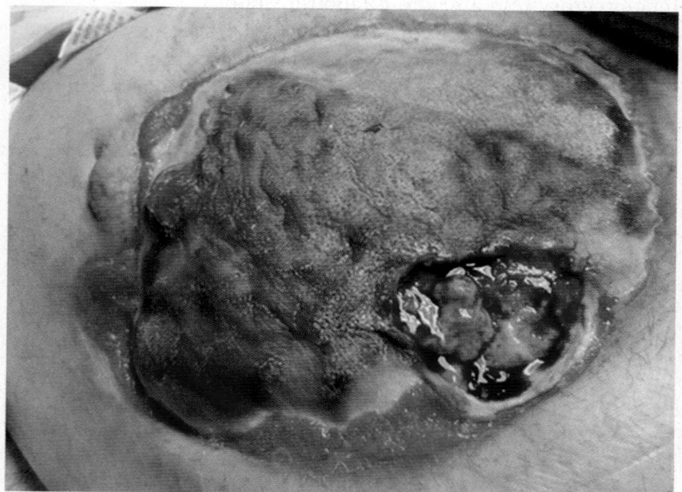

FIGURE 17-4 Desiccation of biologic mesh bridge repair.

SEROMA AND SKIN NECROSIS

Seroma and skin necrosis formation are frequent complications related to major abdominal wall reconstruction (Figs. 17-5 and 17-6). Seromas occur because large skin and subcutaneous fat flaps are created to release fascial planes or to reapproximate skin in large defects with previous skin grafts. This creates a potential space that can fill with exudate from the tissues, exceeding the capacity to be reabsorbed. To reduce seroma formation, closed suction drains should be placed in the subcutaneous tissue until the space is obliterated. These closed suction drains should be stripped regularly in the early postoperative period and are typically removed when less than 30 mL in a 24-hour period has been recorded. In addition, external compression with abdominal binders may aid in the abdominal wall and skin flap adherence and may hinder fluid collection formation. Care must be taken

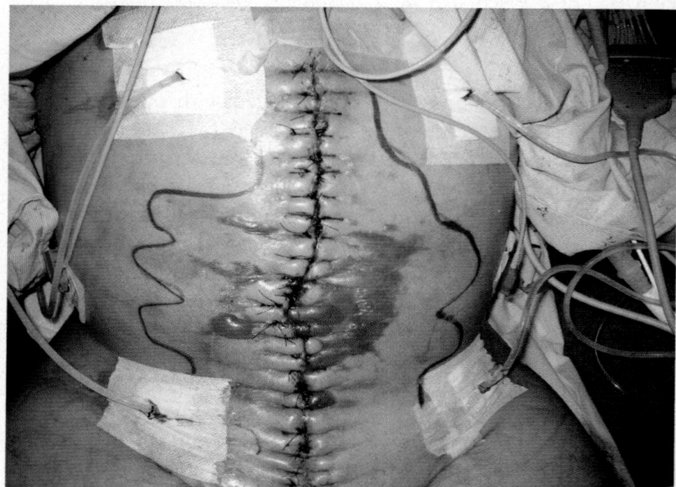

FIGURE 17-5 Skin necrosis complicating abdominal wall reconstruction.

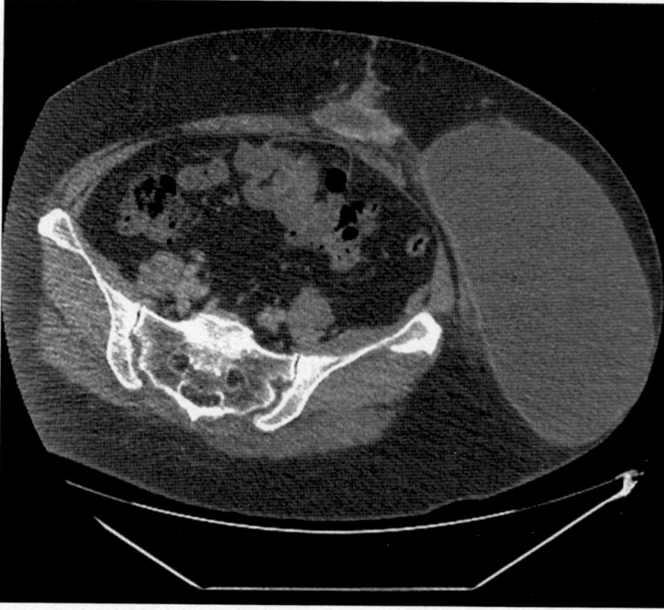

FIGURE 17-6 Postoperative seroma complicating ventral incisional hernia repair.

with leaving drains for an extended time as they may provide an entry point for skin organisms and contribute to infection. The use of prophylactic antibiotics while closed suction drains are in place to prevent infection should be discouraged as there is no evidence to support their use.

Other methods that have been described in the literature to decrease seroma formation include the use of quilting stitches, fibrin glue, and talc application under the skin flaps. However, there are no large studies to definitively show the benefit of these methods, and they should be considered on a case-by-case basis. If closed suction drains fail, reoperation may be indicated, particularly in the setting of infected seroma.

The blood supply to the skin is primarily distributed through the subcutaneous fat and perforators originating from the deep inferior epigastric artery. Intraoperative methods for optimizing and preserving the circulation to the skin and preventing postoperative skin necrosis are essential. Techniques to preserve the perforators are well described in the literature. The perforators' density is highest around the periumbilical area, and thus it is important to spare a circular distance of about 3 cm around the umbilicus during the dissection.

Impending skin necrosis can be manifested as duskiness, blistering, and blanching redness that can progress to definitive necrotic tissue. Management clearly varies by the depth and the total area of the necrosis. Superficial skin necrosis can be treated locally with hydrating gels or enzymatic débriding agents. These agents reduce the bacterial and necrotic tissue burden and maintain a moist environment for healing. Full-thickness wounds require skin and subcutaneous sharp débridement. Negative pressure wound management systems can aid in sterile wound coverage for this complication. Preliminary trials are under way in using a vacuum-assisted closure that cyclically infuses antibiotics or enzymatic débridement agents to treat infected wounds or infected hardware.

PREPARATION FOR ABDOMINAL WALL RECONSTRUCTION

The goal of definitive reconstruction is first to optimize the patient's condition and then to restore the structure and functional continuity of the musculofascial system and provide stable and durable wound coverage to minimize additional complications.

Once the decision has been made to operate, preoperative risk factors must be carefully evaluated and optimized before an elective complex abdominal wall reconstruction is performed. Figure 17-7 depicts the results of a recent survey of surgeons who were asked to list what they considered common contraindications to hernia repair.[46] Modifiable risk factors deserve special attention in this population of complex patients, and comorbidities must be optimized preoperatively. Every effort should be made to control diabetes and to maximize protein-calorie repletion and cardiopulmonary status. Mandatory cigarette smoking cessation is required for at least 4 to 6 weeks before repair. In patients with a previous methicillin-resistant *Staphylococcus aureus* (MRSA) infection, consideration should be given to decolonizing the patient or suppressing MRSA carriers preoperatively and using vancomycin prophylaxis perioperatively. Mesh infection is better prevented than treated (Table 17-2). Understanding of preoperative risk factors during the process of patient and procedure selection is essential to minimizing adverse postoperative occurrences (Table 17-3).[47]

DEFINITIVE REPAIR: CREATING A DYNAMIC ABDOMINAL WALL

Even with a great deal of preoperative planning, there is still no single approach that will solve all the needs for the reconstruction

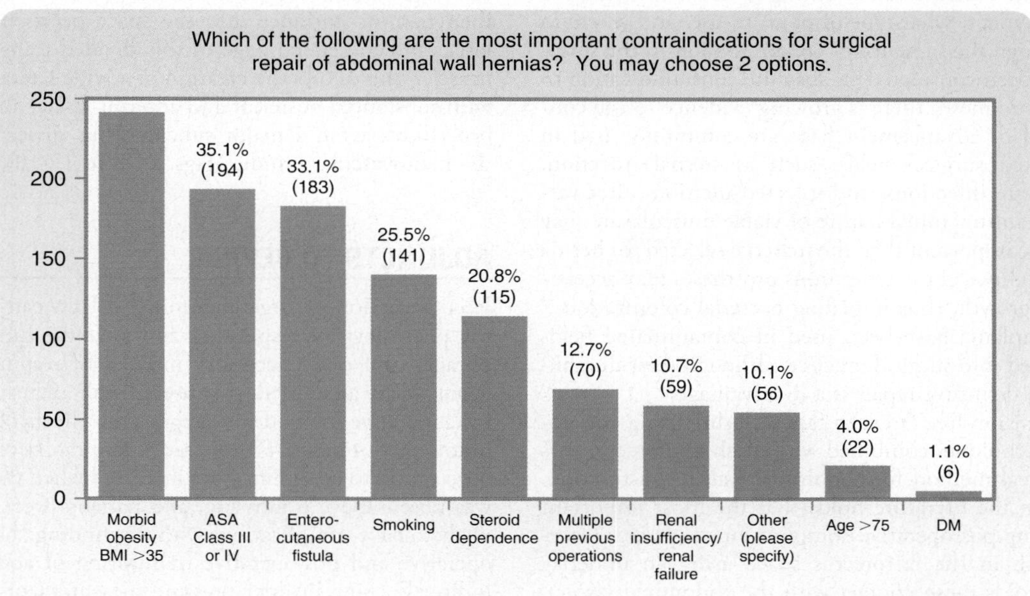

FIGURE 17-7 Survey data showing common contraindications to hernia repair. *ASA,* American Society of Anesthesiologists; *BMI,* body mass index; *DM,* diabetes mellitus.

TABLE 17-2 Prevention of Mesh Infection

Preoperative measures	Discontinuation of smoking Preoperative antibacterial shower Preoperative and intraoperative intravenous antibiotics Antiseptics at the surgical site Mechanical bowel preparation in chronically incarcerated hernia defects
Intraoperative measures	Iodine-impregnated polyurethane films Avoidance of wrinkles and redundant mesh Soaking of synthetic mesh in antibiotic solution Avoidance of contacting the mesh with the skin Judicious use of drains

TABLE 17-3 Modified Hernia Risk Stratification System

GRADE 1	GRADE 2	GRADE 3
Low Risk	**Comorbid**	**Contaminated**
Low risk of complications No history of wound infection	Smoker Obese COPD Diabetes mellitus History of wound infection	Clean-contaminated Contaminated Dirty
SSO = 14%	SSO = 27%	SSO = 46%

COPD, chronic obstructive pulmonary disease; *SSO*, surgical site occurrence.

of a complex abdominal wall defect. It is essential that the surgeon review all of the prior operative reports and have a clear understanding of what remains in the wound and in what location. A preoperative computed tomography scan of the abdominal wall is necessary before any consideration of major reconstruction.

In cases of previous contamination or infection, the surgeon is often faced with the difficult task of having to decide when to use mesh for reinforcement, what type of mesh to use, and where to position it. Although the presence of contamination in the surgical field has long been considered an absolute contraindication to the use of prosthetic mesh, there is growing evidence to the contrary.[48] Rotational or advancement flaps are commonly used in other contaminated surgical fields, such as sternal infection, orthopedic hardware infections, and infected incisions after vascular bypass. The antimicrobial nature of viable musculature may ultimately be more important than the material selected for hernia repair, although lightweight macroporous prostheses may accelerate local tissue ingrowth, thus impeding bacterial colonization.[43] Biologic mesh implants have been used in contaminated fields since being adopted into surgical practice, although their durability as a long-term definitive repair is a disadvantage.

Currently, a tension-free fascia to fascia closure using component separation techniques combined with mesh reinforcement is considered the ideal method for abdominal wall reconstruction. Expert opinion in the literature holds that the most important factor in preventing postoperative complications is proper placement of the mesh in the retrorectus space using an underlay technique that avoids mesh contact with the abdominal viscera. In general, the retrorectus repair and the underlay placement of mesh have resulted in the lowest complication rate, including less infection, seroma formation, and hernia recurrence, compared with the onlay or interposition techniques.

Various techniques for mobilization of the fascia medially with component separation provide a tension-free repair of the rectus fascia and subsequent protection from infection from the overlying subcutaneous fat and skin. The classically described Ramirez technique for component separation requires large subcutaneous flaps for access to be gained to the lateral abdominal wall to release the external oblique fascia.[49] This technique has high wound morbidity and is in general no longer recommended for high-risk patients. Recently developed endoscopic methods to perform component separation release of the external oblique aponeurosis by using an endoscopic camera and avoiding division of the perforators have now been described. However, the improved appreciation of abdominal wall function to create a dynamic abdominal wall unit has popularized two ideal reconstruction techniques: the modified Rives-Stoppa repair and the transversus abdominis release repair.[50,51] Both use a retromuscular sublay of mesh and have become the "gold standard" repair by the American Hernia Society. The retromuscular space has a rich vascularization, and these two techniques preserve the abdominal wall neurovascular bundle with favorable outcomes. Both of these techniques use a posterior component separation and the placement of lightweight macroporous synthetic mesh in the retrorectus space and outside of the peritoneal cavity. These techniques serve as optimal protection of the bowel from the mesh provided by the posterior rectus sheath, peritoneum, and omentum.

MODIFIED RIVES-STOPPA AND TRANSVERSUS ABDOMINIS RELEASE TECHNIQUES

In the modified Rives-Stoppa technique, the posterior rectus sheath is incised approximately 0.5 cm from the fascial edge of the defect. The retromuscular plane is then developed to the lateral extent of the dissection: the linea semilunaris. If this dissection is insufficient to close the posterior rectus fascia, an extension of this technique is the transversus abdominis release. In this technique, the transversus abdominis muscle is divided, which then permits entrance into the space between the transversalis fascia and the lateral edge of this divided transversus abdominis muscle. This allows the creation of a wide lateral dissection plane with substantial posterior and anterior fascial advancement. Both procedures avoid a major subcutaneous dissection and preserve the neurovascular bundle (Figs. 17-8 to 17-10).

ADJUNCTS TO REPAIR

Reconstruction of large abdominal defects can markedly change the physiology of respiration and alter the function of the diaphragm and other accessory muscles of respiration. Many surgeons have advocated the use of the plateau pressure as an intraoperative method for gauging the effects of hernia repair on pulmonary function. Postoperative respiratory complications have been found to be significantly increased when the plateau pressure was raised above 6 mm Hg, and patients were nine times more likely to have complications with this finding.[52] In addition, intraoperative and postoperative monitoring of abdominal pressures indirectly using bladder pressure measurements is routinely recommended when the abdominal wall defect is more than 600 cm^2.[52]

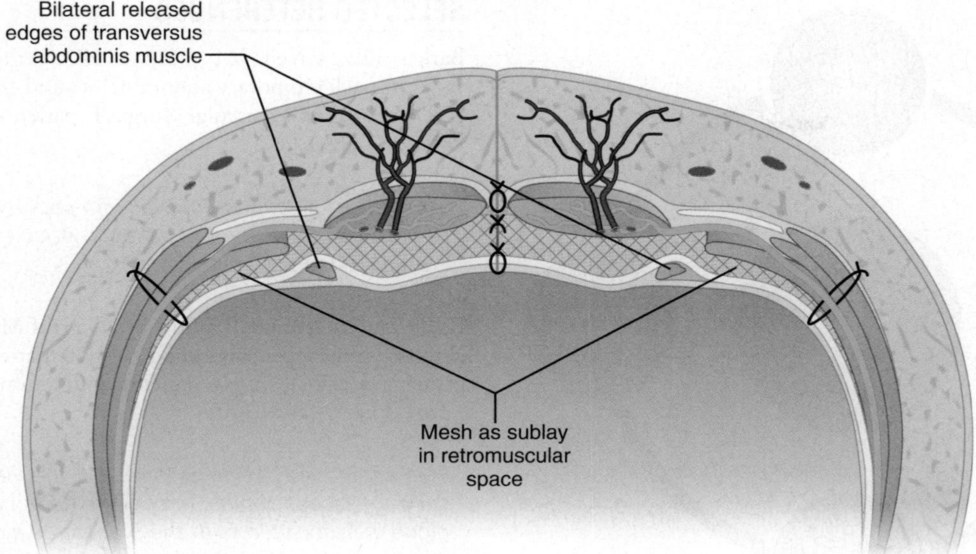

FIGURE 17-8 Anatomic depiction of retromuscular ventral incisional hernia repair with mesh with release of transversus abdominis muscle, positioning the mesh in a preperitoneal/retromuscular plane with wide overlap.

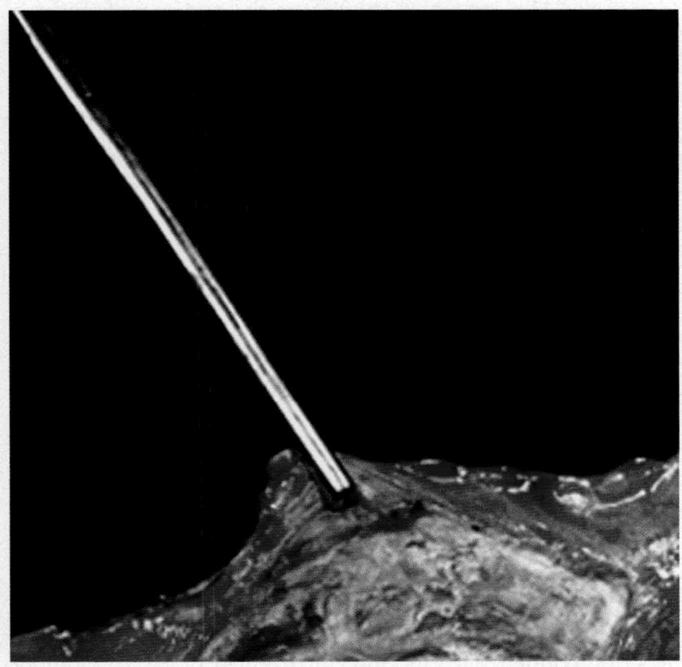

FIGURE 17-9 Development of the retrorectus plane after dividing the rectus sheath in the midline.

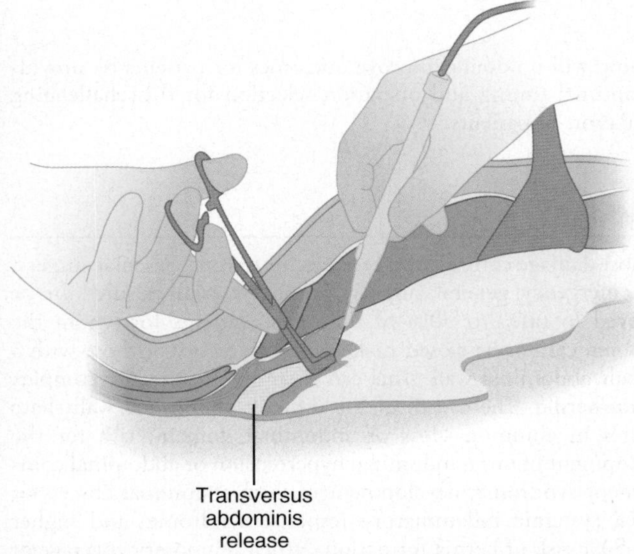

FIGURE 17-10 Transversus abdominis release in retromuscular hernia repair.

Pain management is essential in these patients, and epidural catheters and transversus abdominis plane blocks substantially improve pain relief and significantly reduce narcotic use within the postoperative phase as well as having beneficial effects on costs and postoperative morbidity.[53] Both techniques also increase early mobilization, thus reducing additional complications related to this extensive surgery. Long-acting injectable bupivacaine local anesthetic provides prolonged relief of pain and also reduces the use of narcotics. As mentioned previously, the use of abdominal binders also significantly improves the patient's ambulation, pain control, and comfort.

As previously stated, a thorough understanding of the determinants of outcomes may be the most important factor in reducing complications, and even death, in these patients (Fig. 17-11). Perhaps nonoperative close observation strategies for asymptomatic large incisional hernias may be prudent in certain populations of patients. Currently, there is no study evaluating patients with known incisional hernias who are managed nonoperatively.

Most recently, the American Hernia Society has developed a Quality Collaborative to improve the value of hernia care delivered to patients. It was formed in 2013 by hernia surgeons both in private practice and in academic centers. The goal of the Quality Collaborative is to use concepts of continuous quality improvement to improve outcomes and to optimize costs. Ongoing data collection, performance feedback, and collaborative

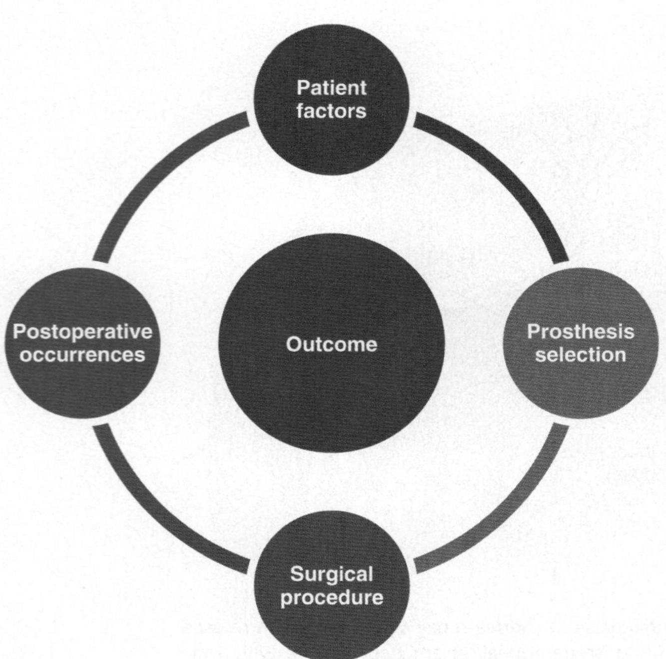

FIGURE 17-11 Factors determining outcome in abdominal wall reconstruction.

learning will no doubt improve outcomes for patients by providing optimal timing and operation selection for this challenging population of patients.

SUMMARY

In most damage control laparotomies for trauma, vascular surgery, and emergency general surgery, primary fascial closure can be achieved in 60% to 90% of the cases. Patients for whom the abdomen cannot be closed make up the category of those with a difficult abdominal wall. This can then give rise to the complex ventral hernia. The causes of the difficult abdominal wall share features in common—loss of abdominal domain, risk for the development of intra-abdominal hypertension or abdominal compartment syndrome, development of intra-abdominal abscess or fistula, systemic inflammatory response syndrome, and higher than 50% risk of hernia formation. When temporary coverage of the abdomen is necessary, the technique should be easy to apply, tension free, atraumatic, and inexpensive and allow a high rate of delayed primary fascial closure.

After normalization of the physiologic status, reexploration and a staged repair may be performed. It is not advisable to attempt delayed primary fascial closure if there is undue tension on the fascia or the peak inspiratory pressure rises more than 10 cm H_2O. However, the inability to close the open abdomen by 8 days is associated with a significant increase in complications, including enteroatmospheric fistulas.[19] For this reason, some surgeons have bridged an abdominal wall defect with biologic mesh to protect the abdominal viscera. However, this repair should be considered a temporizing measure because most bridging repairs will develop bulging or laxity within 1 year of closure. Delayed ventral hernia repair using component separation reinforced with biologic mesh has produced excellent results and is recommended for the closure of the complicated abdominal wall.

SELECTED REFERENCES

Barker DE, Green JM, Maxwell RA, et al: Experience with vacuum-pack temporary abdominal wound closure in 258 trauma and general and vascular surgical patients. *J Am Coll Surg* 204:784–792, 2007.

This study describes 717 vacuum-pack closures that were performed in 258 surgical patients. Abdominal complications are described in detail.

Boele van Hensbroek P, Wind J, Dijkgraaf MG, et al: Temporary closure of the open abdomen: A systematic review on delayed primary fascial closure in patients with an open abdomen. *World J Surg* 33:199–207, 2009.

This study was designed to review the literature systematically to assess which temporary abdominal closure technique is associated with the highest delayed primary fascial closure rate. The techniques described were vacuum-assisted closure, vacuum pack, artificial burr, mesh or sheet, zipper, silo, skin closure, dynamic retention sutures, and loose packing.

Carbonell AM, Criss CN, Cobb WS, et al: Outcomes of synthetic mesh in contaminated ventral hernia repairs. *J Am Coll Surg* 217:991–998, 2013.

Contamination of the surgical field has long been thought to be an absolute contraindication to the use of prosthetic mesh for hernia repair. There is growing evidence that synthetic materials may be safely used despite the presence of contamination, potentially resulting in improved long-term outcomes of hernia repair.

Connolly PT, Teubner A, Lees NP, et al: Outcome of reconstructive surgery for intestinal fistula in the open abdomen. *Ann Surg* 247:440–444, 2008.

This is a discussion of the factors that influence the outcome of surgical techniques to close enterocutaneous fistulas within the open abdomen. Simultaneous reconstruction of the intestinal tract and abdominal wall remains associated with a high complication rate, justifying the management of such patients in specialized units.

de Vries Reilingh TS, van Goor H, Rosman C, et al: "Components separation technique" for the repair of large abdominal wall hernias. *J Am Coll Surg* 196:32–37, 2003.

This study evaluates the use of the component separation technique as a method for abdominal wall reconstruction. Special attention is dedicated to the reconstruction of large abdominal wall hernias, especially under contaminated conditions, in which the use of prosthetic material is contraindicated.

Fabian TC, Croce MA, Pritchard FE, et al: Planned ventral hernia. Staged management for acute abdominal wall defects. *Ann Surg* 219:643–650, 1994.

An analysis of a staged management scheme for the initial and definitive management of acute abdominal wall defects is provided. A four-stage scheme for managing acute abdominal wall defects is described: stage I, prosthetic insertion; stage II, 2 to 3 weeks after prosthetic insertion and wound granulation, removal of prosthesis; stage III, 2 to 3 days later, planned ventral hernia (split-thickness skin graft or full-thickness skin and subcutaneous fat graft); stage IV, 6 to 12 months later, definitive reconstruction. Cases were evaluated retrospectively for the benefits and risks of the techniques used.

Miller RS, Morris JA, Jr, Diaz JJ, Jr, et al: Complications after 344 damage-control open celiotomies. *J Trauma* 59:1365–1371, 2005.

This study evaluated a large number of damage control abdomens. Morbidity is associated with the timing and method of wound closure and transfusion volume but is independent of injury severity. Best outcomes occurred with delayed primary fascial closure before 8 days.

Morris JA, Jr, Eddy VA, Blinman TA, et al: The staged celiotomy for trauma. Issues in unpacking and reconstruction. *Ann Surg* 217:576–584, 1993.

This article describes the important clinical events and decisions surrounding the reconstruction/unpacking portion of the staged celiotomy for trauma. The authors examined medical records to identify and to characterize indications and timing of reconstruction, criteria for emergency return to the operating room, complications after reconstruction, and abdominal compartment syndrome.

Novitsky YW, Elliott HL, Orenstein SB, et al: Transversus abdominis muscle release: A novel approach to posterior component separation during complex abdominal wall reconstruction. *Am J Surg* 204:709–716, 2012.

This is a landmark surgical anatomy description that expounds on the knowledge of the retrorectus space by describing a closed internal component separation method. The anatomical details of the transversus abdominis space are described that set the basis for the transversus abdominis release hernia repair.

Ramirez OM, Ruas E, Dellon AL: "Components separation" method for closure of abdominal-wall defects: An anatomic and clinical study. *Plast Reconstr Surg* 86:519–526, 1990.

This study suggests that large abdominal wall defects can be reconstructed with functional transfer of abdominal wall components without the need for the distant transposition of free muscle flaps. This demonstrated that the external oblique muscle can be separated from the internal oblique in a relatively avascular plane. The rectus muscle, with its overlying rectus fascia, can be elevated from the posterior rectus sheath. The compound flap of the rectus muscle, with its attached internal oblique transversus abdominis muscle, can be advanced 10 cm around the waistline.

Schecter WP, Hirshberg A, Chang DS, et al: Enteric fistulas: Principles of management. *J Am Coll Surg* 209:484–491, 2009.

The aim of this review is to present current principles in the management of enteric fistulas. Traditional management principles are evaluated to improve management and to better understand the physiology and natural history of enteric fistulas.

Stone HH, Strom PR, Mullins RJ: Management of the major coagulopathy with onset during laparotomy. *Ann Surg* 197:532–535, 1983.

This is a classic description of the technique of abbreviated laparotomy, abdominal packing, and correction of coagulopathy in 31 patients with an acceptable level of survival in previously nonsalvageable situations.

REFERENCES

1. Krukowski ZH, Cusick EL, Engeset J, et al: Polydioxanone or polypropylene for closure of midline abdominal incisions: A prospective comparative clinical trial. *Br J Surg* 74:828–830, 1987.
2. Corman ML, Veidenheimer MC, Coller JA: Controlled clinical trial of three suture materials for abdominal wall closure after bowel operations. *Am J Surg* 141:510–513, 1981.
3. Ceydeli A, Rucinski J, Wise L: Finding the best abdominal closure: An evidence-based review of the literature. *Curr Surg* 62:220–225, 2005.
4. Seiler CM, Bruckner T, Diener MK, et al: Interrupted or continuous slowly absorbable sutures for closure of primary elective midline abdominal incisions: A multicenter randomized trial (INSECT: ISRCTN24023541). *Ann Surg* 249: 576–582, 2009.
5. Diener MK, Voss S, Jensen K, et al: Elective midline laparotomy closure: The INLINE systematic review and meta-analysis. *Ann Surg* 251:843–856, 2010.
6. Khorgami Z, Shoar S, Laghaie B, et al: Prophylactic retention sutures in midline laparotomy in high-risk patients for wound dehiscence: A randomized controlled trial. *J Surg Res* 180:238–243, 2013.
7. Rink AD, Goldschmidt D, Dietrich J, et al: Negative side-effects of retention sutures for abdominal wound closure. A prospective randomised study. *Eur J Surg* 166:932–937, 2000.
8. Caro-Tarrago A, Olona-Casas C, Olona-Cabases M, et al: Impact on quality of life of using an onlay mesh to prevent incisional hernia in midline laparotomy: A randomized clinical trial. *J Am Coll Surg* 219:470–479, 2014.
9. Caro-Tarrago A, Olona Casas C, Jimenez Salido A, et al: Prevention of incisional hernia in midline laparotomy with an onlay mesh: A randomized clinical trial. *World J Surg* 38:2223–2230, 2014.
10. Argudo N, Pereira JA, Sancho JJ, et al: Prophylactic synthetic mesh can be safely used to close emergency laparotomies, even in peritonitis. *Surgery* 156:1238–1244, 2014.
11. Eke N, Jebbin NJ: Abdominal wound dehiscence: A review. *Int Surg* 91:276–287, 2006.
12. van Ramshorst GH, Nieuwenhuizen J, Hop WC, et al: Abdominal wound dehiscence in adults: Development and validation of a risk model. *World J Surg* 34:20–27, 2010.

13. Duttaroy DD, Jitendra J, Duttaroy B, et al: Management strategy for dirty abdominal incisions: Primary or delayed primary closure? A randomized trial. *Surg Infect (Larchmt)* 10:129–136, 2009.
14. Hendrix SL, Schimp V, Martin J, et al: The legendary superior strength of the Pfannenstiel incision: A myth? *Am J Obstet Gynecol* 182:1446–1451, 2000.
15. Tillou A, Weng J, Alkousakis T, et al: Fascial dehiscence after trauma laparotomy: A sign of intra-abdominal sepsis. *Am Surg* 69:927–929, 2003.
16. Graham DJ, Stevenson JT, McHenry CR: The association of intra-abdominal infection and abdominal wound dehiscence. *Am Surg* 64:660–665, 1998.
17. Carlson MA: Acute wound failure. *Surg Clin North Am* 77:607–636, 1997.
18. Cotton BA, Au BK, Nunez TC, et al: Predefined massive transfusion protocols are associated with a reduction in organ failure and postinjury complications. *J Trauma* 66:41–48, discussion 48–49, 2009.
19. Miller RS, Morris JA, Jr, Diaz JJ, Jr, et al: Complications after 344 damage-control open celiotomies. *J Trauma* 59:1365–1371, discussion 1371–1374, 2005.
20. Wittmann DH, Aprahamian C, Bergstein JM, et al: A burr-like device to facilitate temporary abdominal closure in planned multiple laparotomies. *Eur J Surg* 159:75–79, 1993.
21. Boele van Hensbroek P, Wind J, Dijkgraaf MG, et al: Temporary closure of the open abdomen: A systematic review on delayed primary fascial closure in patients with an open abdomen. *World J Surg* 33:199–207, 2009.
22. Brock WB, Barker DE, Burns RP: Temporary closure of open abdominal wounds: The vacuum pack. *Am Surg* 61:30–35, 1995.
23. Barker DE, Green JM, Maxwell RA, et al: Experience with vacuum-pack temporary abdominal wound closure in 258 trauma and general and vascular surgical patients. *J Am Coll Surg* 204:784–792, discussion 792–793, 2007.
24. Navsaria PH, Bunting M, Omoshoro-Jones J, et al: Temporary closure of open abdominal wounds by the modified sandwich-vacuum pack technique. *Br J Surg* 90:718–722, 2003.
25. Cipolla J, Stawicki SP, Hoff WS, et al: A proposed algorithm for managing the open abdomen. *Am Surg* 71:202–207, 2005.
26. Holzheimer RG, Gathof B: Re-operation for complicated secondary peritonitis—how to identify patients at risk for persistent sepsis. *Eur J Med Res* 8:125–134, 2003.
27. Morris JA, Jr, Eddy VA, Blinman TA, et al: The staged celiotomy for trauma. Issues in unpacking and reconstruction. *Ann Surg* 217:576–584, discussion 584–586, 1993.
28. Cotton BA, Gunter OL, Isbell J, et al: Damage control hematology: The impact of a trauma exsanguination protocol on survival and blood product utilization. *J Trauma* 64:1177–1182, discussion 1182–1183, 2008.
29. Duchesne JC, Hunt JP, Wahl G, et al: Review of current blood transfusions strategies in a mature level I trauma center: Were we wrong for the last 60 years? *J Trauma* 65:272–276, discussion 276–278, 2008.
30. Weinberg JA, Griffin RL, Vandromme MJ, et al: Management of colon wounds in the setting of damage control laparotomy: A cautionary tale. *J Trauma* 67:929–935, 2009.
31. Hirshberg A, Wall MJ, Jr, Mattox KL: Planned reoperation for trauma: A two year experience with 124 consecutive patients. *J Trauma* 37:365–369, 1994.
32. Stawicki SP, Brooks A, Bilski T, et al: The concept of damage control: Extending the paradigm to emergency general surgery. *Injury* 39:93–101, 2008.
33. Wittmann DH, Aprahamian C, Bergstein JM: Etappenlavage: Advanced diffuse peritonitis managed by planned multiple laparotomies utilizing zippers, slide fastener, and Velcro analogue for temporary abdominal closure. *World J Surg* 14:218–226, 1990.
34. Diaz JJ, Jr, Mejia V, Subhawong AP, et al: Protocol for bedside laparotomy in trauma and emergency general surgery: A low return to the operating room. *Am Surg* 71:986–991, 2005.
35. Mayberry JC, Burgess EA, Goldman RK, et al: Enterocutaneous fistula and ventral hernia after absorbable mesh prosthesis closure for trauma: The plain truth. *J Trauma* 57:157–162, discussion 163–163, 2004.
36. Goris RJ: Mediators of multiple organ failure. *Intensive Care Med* 16(Suppl 3):S192–S196, 1990.
37. Marshall JC: SIRS and MODS: What is their relevance to the science and practice of intensive care? *Shock* 14:586–589, 2000.
38. Malbrain ML, De Laet IE, De Waele JJ: IAH/ACS: The rationale for surveillance. *World J Surg* 33:1110–1115, 2009.
39. Cheatham ML: Nonoperative management of intraabdominal hypertension and abdominal compartment syndrome. *World J Surg* 33:1116–1122, 2009.
40. Malbrain ML, Cheatham ML, Kirkpatrick A, et al: Results from the International Conference of Experts on Intra-abdominal Hypertension and Abdominal Compartment Syndrome. I. Definitions. *Intensive Care Med* 32:1722–1732, 2006.
41. Keck JO, Collopy BT, Ryan PJ, et al: Reversal of Hartmann's procedure: Effect of timing and technique on ease and safety. *Dis Colon Rectum* 37:243–248, 1994.
42. Fischer JP, Basta MN, Mirzabeigi MN, et al: A comparison of outcomes and cost in VHWG grade II hernias between Rives-Stoppa synthetic mesh hernia repair versus underlay biologic mesh repair. *Hernia* 18:781–789, 2014.
43. Diaz-Godoy A, Garcia-Urena MA, Lopez-Monclus J, et al: Searching for the best polypropylene mesh to be used in bowel contamination. *Hernia* 15:173–179, 2011.
44. Harth KC, Broome AM, Jacobs MR, et al: Bacterial clearance of biologic grafts used in hernia repair: An experimental study. *Surg Endosc* 25:2224–2229, 2011.
45. Iacco A, Adeyemo A, Riggs T, et al: Single institutional experience using biological mesh for abdominal wall reconstruction. *Am J Surg* 208:480–484, discussion 483–484, 2014.
46. Evans KK, Chim H, Patel KM, et al: Survey on ventral hernias: Surgeon indications, contraindications, and management of large ventral hernias. *Am Surg* 78:388–397, 2012.
47. Kanters AE, Krpata DM, Blatnik JA, et al: Modified hernia grading scale to stratify surgical site occurrence after open ventral hernia repairs. *J Am Coll Surg* 215:787–793, 2012.
48. Carbonell AM, Criss CN, Cobb WS, et al: Outcomes of synthetic mesh in contaminated ventral hernia repairs. *J Am Coll Surg* 217:991–998, 2013.
49. Ramirez OM, Ruas E, Dellon AL: "Components separation" method for closure of abdominal-wall defects: An anatomic and clinical study. *Plast Reconstr Surg* 86:519–526, 1990.

50. Bauer JJ, Harris MT, Gorfine SR, et al: Rives-Stoppa procedure for repair of large incisional hernias: Experience with 57 patients. *Hernia* 6:120–123, 2002.
51. Novitsky YW, Elliott HL, Orenstein SB, et al: Transversus abdominis muscle release: A novel approach to posterior component separation during complex abdominal wall reconstruction. *Am J Surg* 204:709–716, 2012.
52. Blatnik JA, Krpata DM, Pesa NL, et al: Predicting severe postoperative respiratory complications following abdominal wall reconstruction. *Plast Reconstr Surg* 130:836–841, 2012.
53. Fischer JP, Nelson JA, Wes AM, et al: The use of epidurals in abdominal wall reconstruction: An analysis of outcomes and cost. *Plast Reconstr Surg* 133:687–699, 2014.

18 CHAPTER

Emergency Care of Musculoskeletal Injuries

Daniel K. Witmer, Silas T. Marshall, Bruce D. Browner

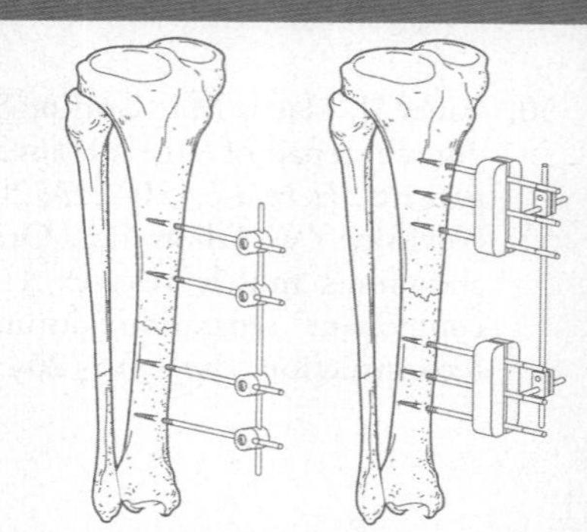

OUTLINE

EPIDEMIOLOGY OF ORTHOPEDIC INJURIES

Accidents continue to be a leading cause of death and disability throughout the world. Last year in the United States, trauma was the number one cause of death in the first five decades of life[1] and the third most common cause of death among all age groups. In general, the amount of energy absorbed by a multiply injured patient corresponds to the extent of the musculoskeletal injuries. Because high energy is frequently involved, fractures and soft tissue injuries are common. It has been estimated that 46% of patients sustaining a traumatic injury in the United States have an orthopedic injury, and between 13% and 25% of these patients require an orthopedic traumatologist.[2] The patients who suffer these injuries endure not just physical but financial hardships to recover. Trauma in the United States accounts for billions of dollars in lost productivity, medical costs, and property damage each year.

At the national and global levels, substantial improvements in transportation safety and delivery of medical care have helped address this growing pandemic. Seat belt and helmet laws, enforcement of drunk driving laws, mandates for improved safety features in automobiles, rapid deployment of emergency medical teams, and establishment of trauma centers have decreased the number of accident scene fatalities. With more victims now likely to survive accidents that might have been fatal in the past, caregivers will be challenged with managing more complex fractures and soft tissue wounds. These realities demand that trauma teams be aware of the frequency and consequences of musculoskeletal injuries in every trauma patient. An appreciation for the unique features of skeletal injury in patients who may also have severe head, thoracic, or intra-abdominal trauma is essential. In this way, a cohesive, integrated approach to the diagnosis and treatment of musculoskeletal injuries may be used in the care of the multiply injured patient.

TERMINOLOGY

Communication among collaborating specialists is central to patient care. Trauma and emergency department (ED) findings need to be relayed precisely to consulting specialists. This task is particularly challenging in view of the variety of anatomic locations, fracture patterns, and associated soft tissue injuries encountered in orthopedics. Although many injuries are identified by eponyms within the orthopedic community, the most practical and universally understood characterizations of injuries are those that adhere to basic anatomic and mechanical principles.

Fracture Types

A fracture is a disruption of the normal architecture of bone. Fractures can be acute, subacute, or chronic. Acute fractures have sharp, well-defined edges of the fragments. Subacute fractures have signs of healing present on radiography. The edges become blunted and less well defined as bone resorption and new bone formation occur. Chronic fractures have a rounded and sclerotic appearance after resorption and remodeling of bone have occurred at the fracture ends (Fig. 18-1). This distinction can usually be made on clinical examination. Chronic fractures are often termed *delayed unions* or *nonunions.* A delayed union is defined as a fracture that is taking longer to show progression toward healing than would normally be expected. The expected healing time varies, depending on the age of the patient and anatomic location of the fracture. For example, long bones in adults typically take 6 to 8 weeks to achieve full bone union, whereas pediatric fractures and metaphyseal fractures take less time. A nonunion is a fracture that has lost the potential to progress with healing. In general, nonunion of a long bone is a fracture that has failed to show evidence of healing during a 4- to 6-month period.[3] Chronic repetitive trauma can also cause microscopic disruptions when bone is stressed beyond its failure point. These injuries are termed *stress fractures* and are considered overuse injuries.

Because of increased plasticity, a more substantial periosteum, and the presence of growth plates, children's bones are at risk for a different set of fractures (Fig. 18-2). Plastic deformity of a long bone in a pediatric patient is deformation of the bone without actual disruption of the bone cortex. Diagnosis of the deformity often necessitates radiography of the contralateral extremity to confirm asymmetry. Axial loads of long bones in children can lead to buckling of the cortex without a visible fracture line,

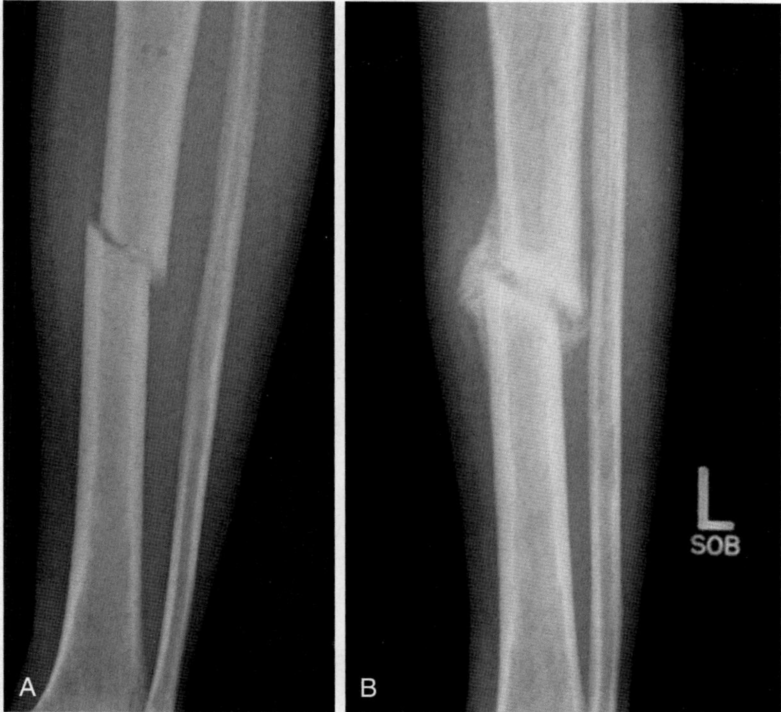

FIGURE 18-1 A, Acute fracture. Note the sharp, well-defined edges. **B,** Nonunion; 6 months later, the fracture line is still clearly visible, the edges of this fracture are blunted, and the bone ends are sclerotic. There was still motion at the fracture site on clinical examination. The patient had significant chronic pain.

appropriately termed a *buckle fracture.* Incomplete disruptions of the cortex are termed *greenstick fractures* in children or *infractions* in adults. A greenstick fracture consists of a cortical disruption on one side of the bone, with a buckle fracture or plastic deformation on the opposite side. The dense periosteal layer in children can contribute stability to many of these fractures if the layer remains intact. A fracture through the cartilaginous growth plate (physis) is another fracture type unique to children. Physeal fractures are described by the Salter-Harris classification (Fig. 18-3*A*). Types I and V, pure physeal injuries, may be difficult to identify with standard radiographs. A high level of clinical suspicion is necessary to diagnose these injuries.

When a bone fails through an area weakened by preexisting disease, it is termed a *pathologic fracture.* Causes may include weakness from primary bone tumors, metastatic lesions, infection, metabolic disease, and injury to an old fracture site. Although they are not commonly referred to in this way, fractures in osteoporotic bone are technically pathologic. However, the term *insufficiency* or *fragility fracture* is most frequently used to describe these injuries. In contradistinction to acute fractures in healthy bone, fragility fractures normally result from accidents with much lower energy, such as a fall from standing height. Hip fractures, compression fractures of the vertebral bodies, and distal radius fractures in older adults are common examples.

A fracture is considered open when an overlying wound produces communication between the fracture site and the outside environment. These fractures can range from an inside-to-outside poke hole in the skin to severe crush injuries or soft tissue degloving. High-energy fracture patterns indicate that the soft tissues as well as the bones have absorbed large forces. Although the skin laceration is the most obvious component, the energy of the fracture, degree of contamination, and soft tissue injury must all be taken into account in grading the severity of the injury. Final grading of open fractures occurs in the operating room, after a thorough débridement and evaluation of the soft tissue envelope. Contamination of bone can lead to the development of osteomyelitis and all its catastrophic consequences and thus necessitates emergency treatment.

An intra-articular fracture extends into a joint. When there is significant cartilage damage, late degenerative changes are likely. These injuries are normally caused by an axial load across the joint. Displaced intra-articular fractures require anatomic reduction and rigid fixation to minimize the risk of post-traumatic arthritis. Anatomic reduction can be achieved directly with open arthrotomy or by arthroscopic means. It can also be achieved indirectly with fluoroscopic guidance.

Long bone fractures are characterized by anatomic location (Fig. 18-3*B*). The epiphysis includes the area between the physis, or physeal scar, and articular surface. The metaphysis is located between the epiphysis and shaft and includes the growth plate. The diaphysis encompasses the shaft of the bone between the proximal and distal metaphyses. The diaphysis is made up of mostly dense cortical bone, which has less vascularity than the soft cancellous bone of the metaphysis. This difference in vascularity affects the rate at which the bone heals. Fractures can be described according to location within these three sections or according to the location in the bone—proximal, middle, and distal. In addition, fractures within the diaphysis are usually divided into thirds (i.e., proximal, middle, and distal thirds). Distally, the humerus and femur flare to form their articular surfaces. These flares are termed the *epicondyles,* and fractures in these areas are referred to as supracondylar or intracondylar. The articular surfaces distal to the epicondyles are known as condyles. Intracondylar fractures are intra-articular and may extend proximally. Such distinctions are

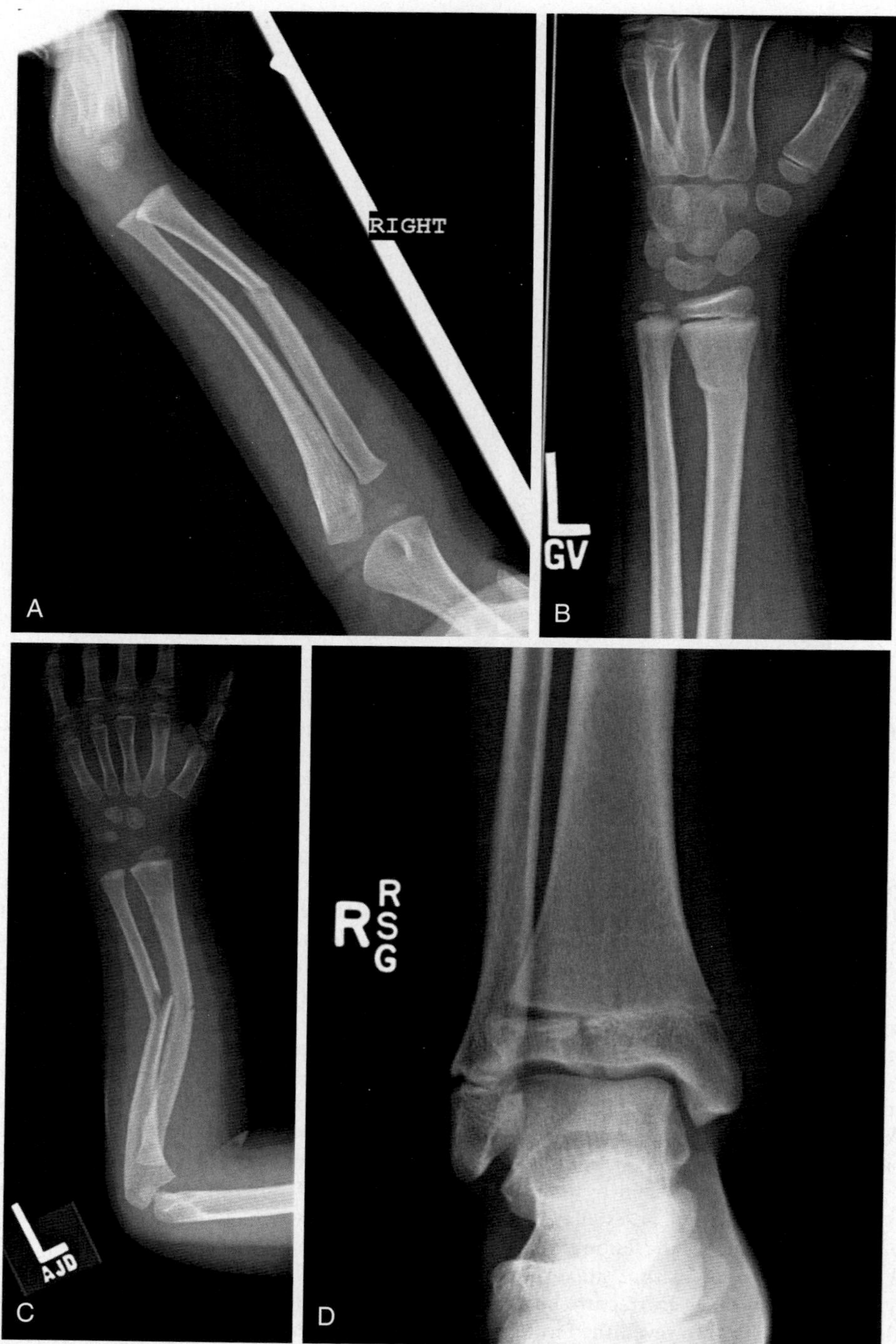

FIGURE 18-2 **A,** Plastic deformity. Note the bowing of the ulna. **B,** Buckle fracture. The cortex of the distal radius is deformed but intact. **C,** Greenstick fracture; disruption of radial cortices, without disruption of the ulnar cortices, in this forearm fracture in both bones. **D,** Physeal fracture. Note the gapping of the lateral tibial physis.

important because these injuries present difficult treatment challenges.

A fracture may also be described by the pattern of cortical disruption (Fig. 18-4). The orientation of the primary fracture line may be transverse, oblique, or spiral. Transverse and oblique fractures occur when a bending moment is applied. Oblique fractures can be further characterized as long or short oblique. Spiral fractures generally result from a rotational force about the long axis of the bone. Comminution refers to the presence of multiple fragments within an individual fracture site and usually indicates a higher energy injury or weakened bone in an older patient. A butterfly fragment is an area of comminution in one of the simple fracture patterns described earlier. Segmental fractures are fractures that occur at multiple levels in the same bone.

Displacement, if present, is described from a combination of principles. These deformities may occur in any plane. When

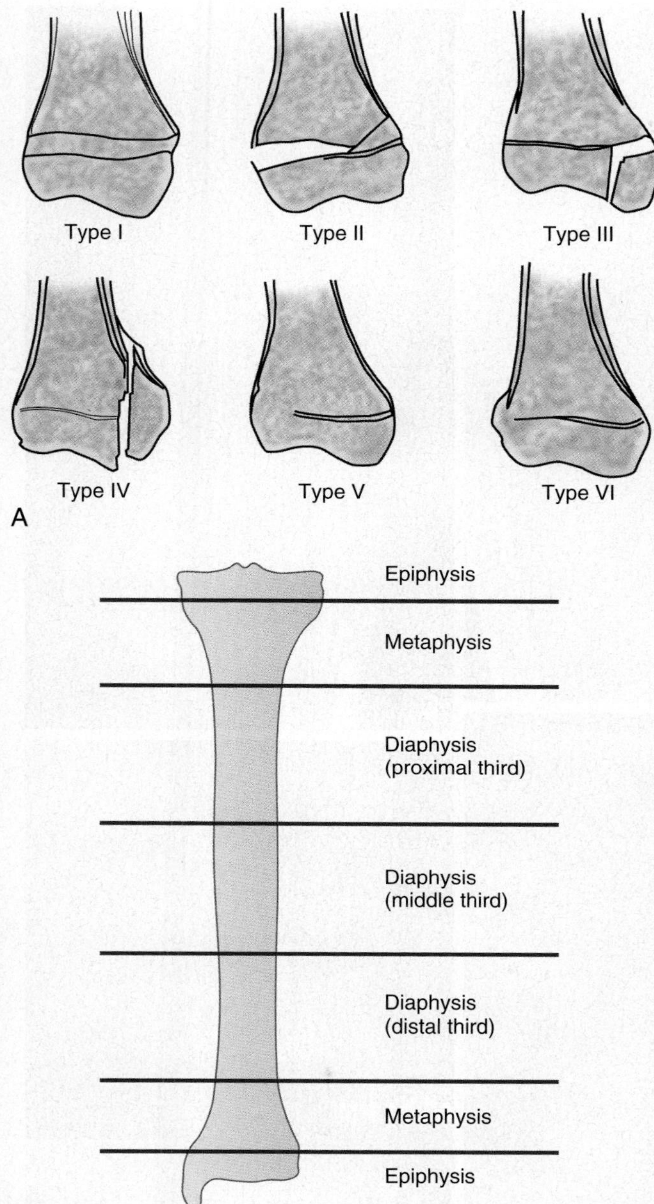

FIGURE 18-3 A, Salter-Harris classification of growth plate injuries. **B,** Anatomic regions of the tibia. (**A,** From Janicki JA: Salter-Harris fractures. In Miller M, Hart JF, MacNight JM, editors: *Essential orthopaedics*, Philadelphia, 2010, Saunders Elsevier, pp 939–943.)

viewed on plain radiographs, all injuries will be resolved into pure coronal or sagittal displacement. However, the true displacement usually occurs in a plane that is somewhere in between. Translation, angulation, rotation, and shortening are all components of fracture displacement. Translation is the relationship of the proximal fracture fragment to the distal one. It is described in terms of percentage of overlap. A fracture with 100% translation in any plane is completely displaced. Angulation is simply the angle created by the displaced fracture fragments. It is conventionally described in two ways. The first is by the direction of displacement of the distal fragment, and the second is by the direction of the apex of the fracture. For example, the fracture shown in Figure 18-5 may be described as dorsally angulated or apex volarly angulated. The final component is rotation. To describe rotation exactly, a full-length film of the limb segment involved, including the joints above and below, must be examined. Alternatively, rotational deformity may be assessed clinically by comparing the injured limb with the contralateral side.

Once a fracture has been identified, it must be described in a consistent, systematic manner. All descriptions begin with whether the fracture is open or closed. The amount of soft tissue involvement is described. A closed fracture is assumed if, after careful evaluation, there is no observed communication between the fracture and outside world. The presence of an intra-articular fracture is then communicated. The side of the body and injured bone are stated next. A description of the pattern, followed by its location in the bone, is indicated. The displacement of the fracture fragments is related. Finally, it is important to indicate any associated, nonorthopedic injuries that may alter the timing and type of initial orthopedic management. Adherence to this scheme allows complete understanding of the fracture.

Other Injuries

Ligamentous injuries are commonly encountered in association with traumatic injuries to bones and joints. When a ligament is damaged but is still in continuity, it is termed a *sprain.* Sprains can range in severity from minor injuries to significant instability about a joint. Grade I ligamentous injuries are caused by stretching of a ligament or ligament complex. They do not normally result in instability. A simple ankle sprain is a typical example of this type of injury. Partial ruptures of ligaments can result in minor instability and are considered grade II injuries. Complete ruptures, or grade III injuries, lead to significant instability at the associated joint. Avulsion fractures at the insertion of ligamentous structures also fall into this category. Ligamentous injuries cannot be overlooked because they can produce significant joint instability and endanger the surrounding soft tissue and neurovascular structures. This detail is critical in evaluating musculoskeletal injuries. A full neurovascular examination should be performed whenever there is suspicion of joint instability. Although most ligamentous injuries do not require urgent orthopedic management, stabilization or immobilization of the joint with a splint or brace is usually advisable.

A strain is an injury to a muscle or tendon. These injuries are most commonly of an overuse nature. Further loading of the already weakened structure can compound these injuries and lead to muscle or tendon rupture. Rest, ice, compression, and elevation are the mainstays of treatment for a strain; however, more urgent orthopedic management is necessary for a rupture. Although many tendon ruptures can be treated nonoperatively, proper positioning of the joint is important to ensure that the tendon scars down in a functional position. If operative management is pursued, it should occur fairly urgently. Scarring of the tendon tract and contracture of the muscle significantly complicate the operative procedure.

Joint injury without fracture is common in axial load injuries. Articular contusions, or bone bruises, usually heal with a period of rest and restricted weight bearing but can lead to late degenerative changes in the joint. A more significant osteochondral defect occurs when a piece of articular cartilage, along with its underlying subchondral bone, is separated from the surrounding joint surface. Small osteochondral defects can be asymptomatic; however, many of these lesions can lead to chronic pain and joint degeneration. In some cases, the osteochondral fragment is large

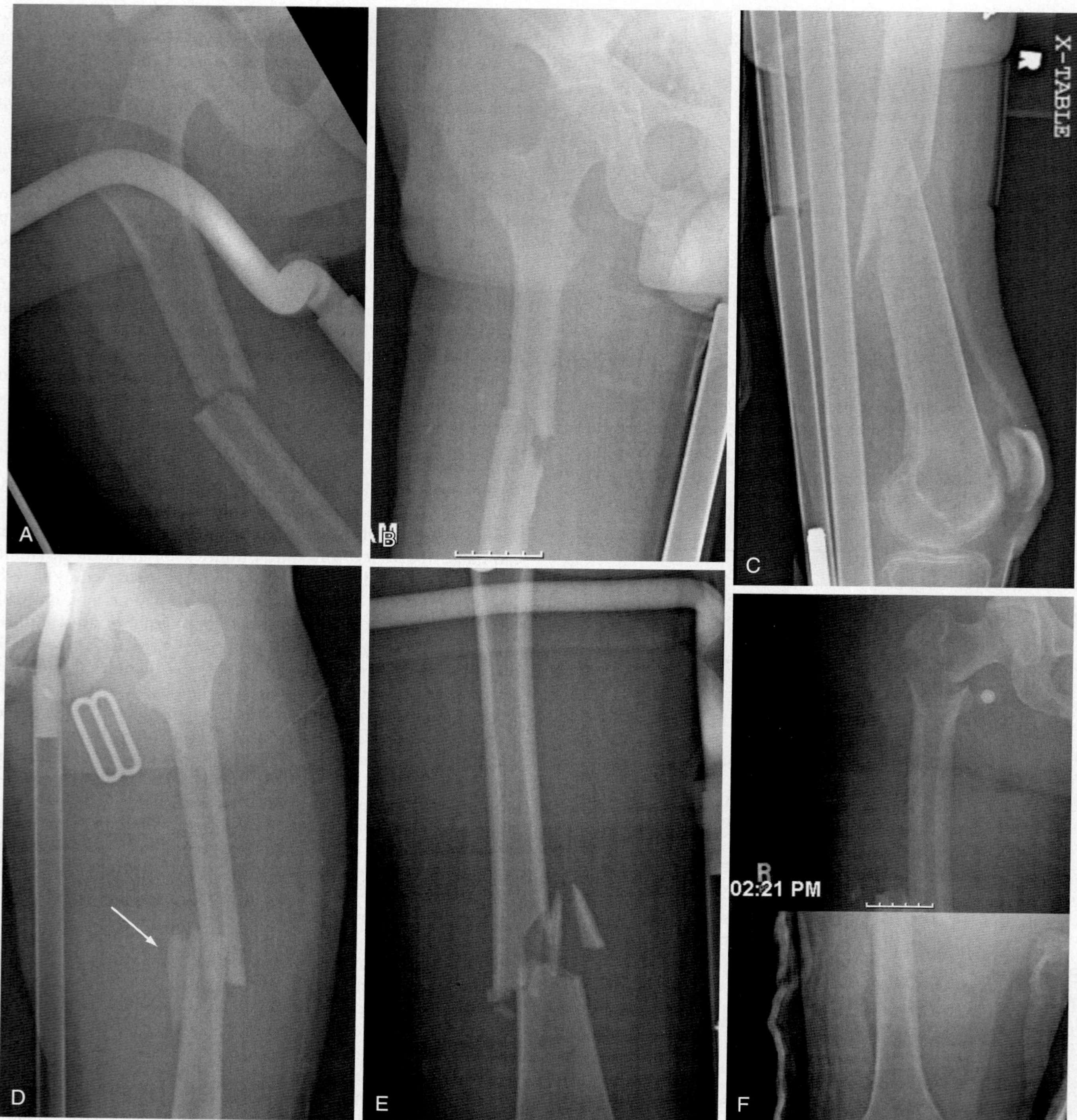

FIGURE 18-4 Femur Fracture Patterns. **A,** Transverse. **B,** Oblique. **C,** Spiral. **D,** Butterfly fragment *(arrow)*. **E,** Comminuted. **F,** Segmental.

enough to be seen on plain radiographs. In these cases, it is important to immobilize the joint to minimize joint damage from the free-floating bone fragment. Other commonly injured joints are the intervertebral discs in the spine. These discs are made up of a viscoelastic nucleus pulposus surrounded by a dense, fibrous anulus fibrosus. With a great enough axial load, the nucleus pulposus can herniate through the anulus, resulting in a disc herniation. This disc bulge can impinge on nerve roots, causing back and radicular pain. Disc herniations rarely need surgical intervention and often resolve with a course of physical therapy. Very rarely, severe disc bulge in the lumbar spine can cause significant impingement on the cauda equina, resulting in cauda equina syndrome. This is a surgical emergency and is discussed in more detail later in the chapter.

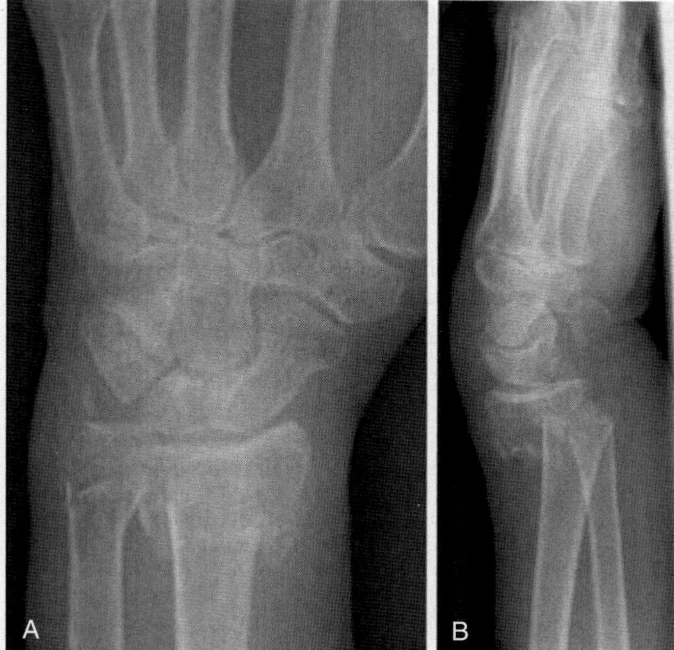

FIGURE 18-5 Posteroanterior **(A)** and lateral **(B)** left wrist radiographs of a 75-year-old woman who fell and sustained a displaced distal radius fracture and a comminuted displaced distal ulna fracture. The distal radius fracture was an open injury. The distal radius fracture was fixed with external fixation, and the distal ulna fracture was fixed with the intrafocal pin plate. (From Foster B, Bindra R: Intrafocal pin plate fixation of distal ulna fractures associated with distal radius fractures. *J Hand Surg* 137:356–350, 2012.)

FIXATION PRINCIPLES

External Fixation

External fixation provides stabilization of an injured limb segment through the use of pins or wires embedded in the bone. These pins are then connected to rods or rings by clamps. With the exception of the pins or wires, the rigid construct is external to the body, as the name implies. Newer designs are more complex but easier to apply and more stable than previous designs. The addition of modularity has added to their prospective uses and has led to more adaptable and adjustable constructs.

External fixation is used for the treatment of open fractures, fractures in unstable patients who cannot tolerate significant anesthesia times or blood loss, complex fractures in which open reduction with internal fixation (ORIF) is not warranted, and fractures with associated vascular injuries requiring stabilization and urgent vascular repair. Specialized external fixation devices are also used in limb reconstruction surgery. In fractures with soft tissue injuries, placement of percutaneously inserted pins that minimize further soft tissue damage and avoid the area of contamination helps decrease the incidence of infection and delayed union. External fixators may be used for temporary stabilization or for definitive treatment in select cases. In complex fractures around joints, fixation with implanted plates or screws may not provide adequate stability. In addition, overlying soft tissue damage makes operative exposure dangerous. In these cases, an external fixator, with the pins placed at a distance from the fracture and injured soft tissues, can provide the osseous stability necessary for fracture healing.

External frames are constructed from three components: pins, connectors, and rods or rings (Fig. 18-6). Pins are threaded or

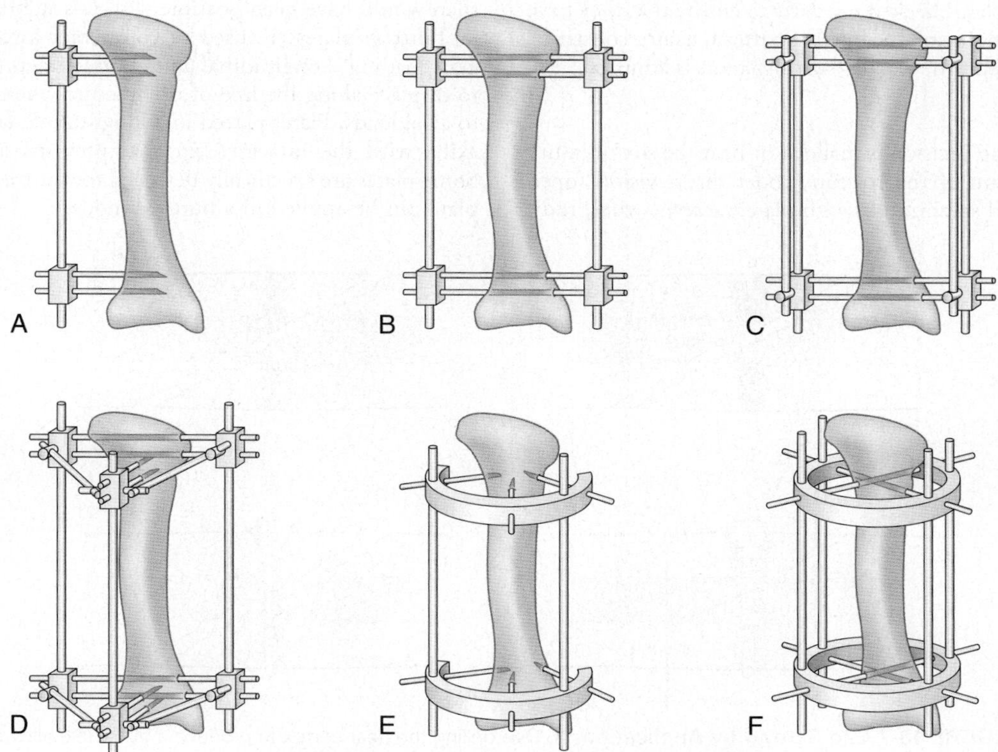

FIGURE 18-6 Basic Fixator Configurations. **A,** Unilateral. **B,** Bilateral. **C,** Multiplanar (quadrilateral). **D,** Multiplanar (delta configuration). **E,** Hybrid fixator. **F,** Ring fixator. (From Green SA: Principles and complications of external fixation. In Browner BD, Levine AM, Jupiter JB, et al, editors: *Skeletal trauma: Basic science, management, and reconstruction*, ed 4, Philadelphia, 2008, WB Saunders.)

smooth and vary in length and diameter. They serve to connect the bone to the rest of the device. Pin placement is chosen to stabilize the fracture best while not compromising the viability of the fragments. Pins are never placed through compromised or infected skin. A variety of different clamps serve as connectors and secure pins to the rods that form the external frames. Most are universal joints that allow multiple degrees of freedom. Connecting clamps have advanced to the point that they now snap in place onto the pins and rods. They may be combined with rings or hinged rods and allow infinite permutations of frame constructs. Stabilizing rods are almost universally radiolucent to allow radiographic examination after application. Threaded rods, bone transport rails, motorized lengthening devices, and dynamic struts represent a small sample of the types of rods that can be used to achieve specific results.

A number of factors affect the stiffness of the fixation construct. The stiffness of the pin material (usually stainless steel) and connecting bar material (titanium, stainless steel, or carbon fiber) as well as the diameter of the pins and bars contributes to the stiffness of the frame. However, the loss of stiffness seen with more flexible materials, such as carbon fiber, or smaller diameter pins can easily be overcome by the frame configuration chosen. Increasing stiffness is seen with an increasing number of pins, increasing pin spread (distance between pins), decreasing distance between the bar and bone, increasing number of bars, and use of multiplanar constructs.

Once applied, external fixators require regular care and monitoring. Pin care is begun immediately and consists of cleansing with normal saline or half-strength peroxide solution. Drainage from pin sites must be addressed with local care, antibiotics, curettage of pin tracks, pin removal and replacement, or a combination of these measures. Pins are checked regularly to ensure that they have not loosened. Depending on the fracture pattern, fixator construct, and goals of treatment, the weight-bearing status is adjusted.

Internal Fixation

ORIF implies that an incision is made at or near the site of injury to facilitate reduction of the fracture under direct vision (open reduction) and rigid stabilization with plates, screws, wires, rods, or combinations thereof (internal fixation). This technique allows anatomic reduction and the creation of constructs of varying levels of stability. Different types of implants can be used to achieve these results.

Pins and Screws

Pins and screws are the simplest implants. They can be introduced in a variety of areas and are often placed percutaneously through a poke hole in the skin. Kirschner wires may be used temporarily and frequently are used for the stabilization of small fragments. They can also be used provisionally to hold the fracture reduction while more stable fixation is applied. Screws can be used for interfragmentary compression when they are placed with a lag technique (Fig. 18-7). This technique involves the use of a gliding hole in one fragment to allow the screw to compress one fragment against another. Figure 18-7*B* shows a position screw. Without a gliding hole, a fully threaded screw will capture both fragments without compressing the far fragment to the near one, thus holding the position of the fragments.

Plates

Plates are used frequently for the internal fixation of fractures. They allow even distribution of force across their length and can serve various biomechanical functions. The biomechanical properties of a plate depend on the material used (usually titanium or stainless steel), dimensions of the plate (thickness, width, and length), and technique with which it is applied (Fig. 18-8).

A neutralization plate is used to protect another form of fixation from excessive force. Often used in combination with a lag screw, these plates add stability by preventing torsion and bending. The addition of a neutralization plate allows mobilization earlier than would have been possible with less stable fixation.

Buttress plates are used to counteract forces that occur with axial loading. Longitudinal and oblique fractures near joints tend to displace along the line of the fracture when they are subjected to axial loads. Plates placed in a longitudinal fashion can form an axilla with the intact cortex that prevents axial displacement. Some plates are specifically designed for buttressing; however, any plate can be applied in a buttress mode.

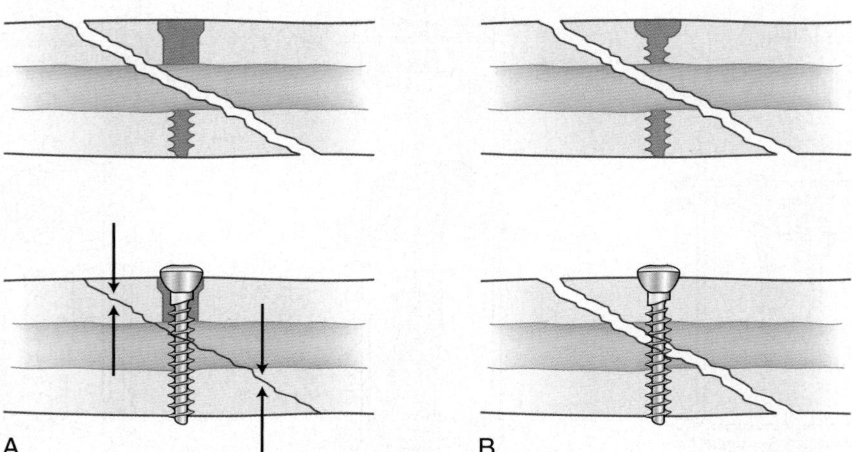

FIGURE 18-7 Lag Screws by Application. A, Overdrilling the near cortex to produce a glide hole allows a cortical screw to act as a lag screw, compressing the far cortex to the near cortex. **B,** In the absence of a glide hole, a cortical screw inserted across the fracture site will maintain fracture gapping. (From Mazzocca AD, DeAngelis JD, Caputo AE, et al: Principles of internal fixation. In Browner BD, Levine AM, Jupiter JB, et al, editors: *Skeletal trauma: Basic science, management, and reconstruction*, ed 4, Philadelphia, 2008, WB Saunders.)

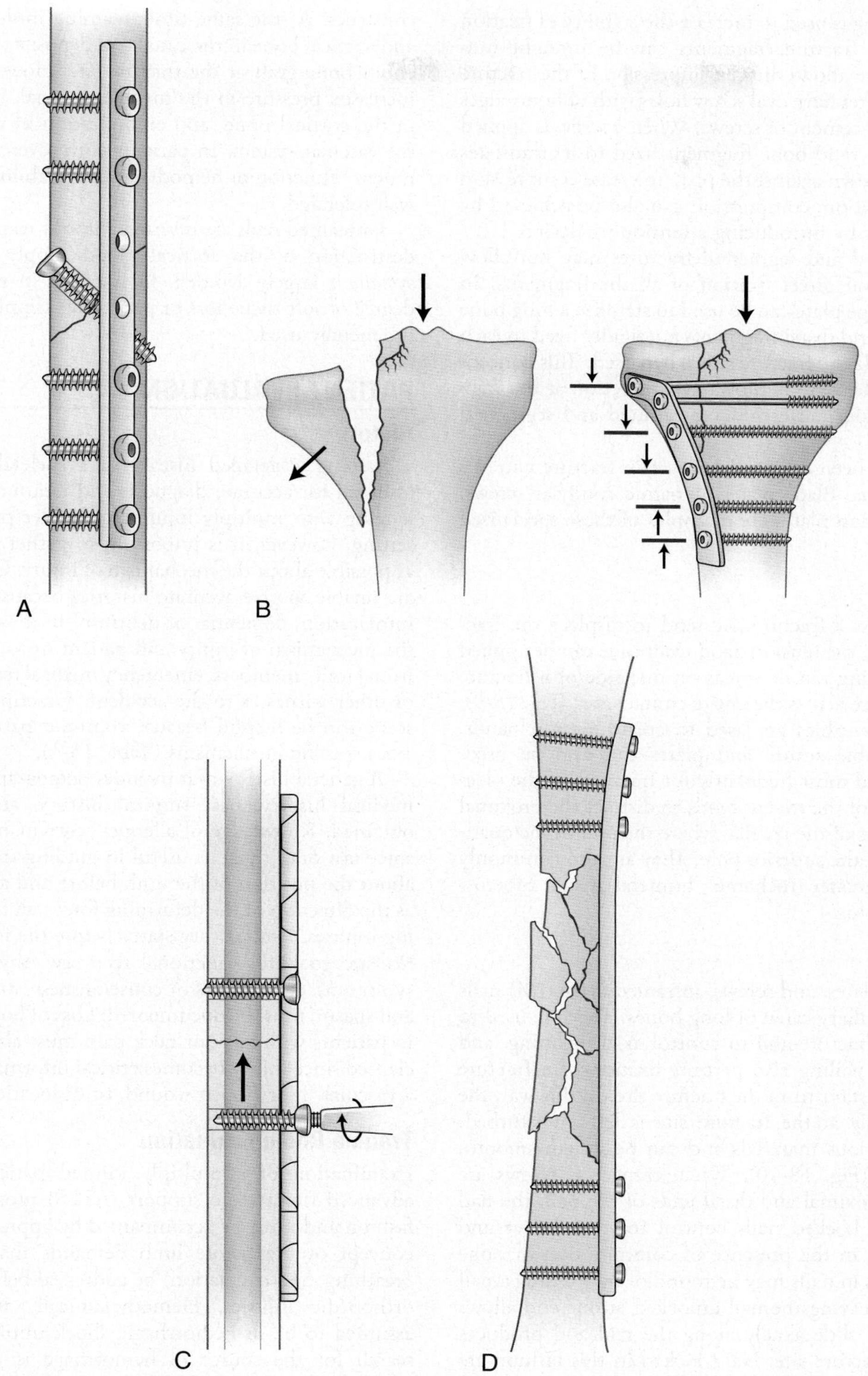

FIGURE 18-8 **A,** Interfragmentary screw fixation with a neutralization plate effectively resisting an external load. **B,** Buttress plate supporting the underlying cortex, effectively resisting displacement, which otherwise would result in angular deformity of the joint. The plate acts as a buttress or retaining wall. **C,** In the compression mode, the screw is inserted 1 mm eccentric to its final position in the hole on the side away from the fracture site. When the screw is tightened, its head slides down along the inclined plane, merging the eccentric circles and causing horizontal movement of the plate (1 mm). This results in fracture compression. **D,** The bridge plate maintains length and alignment by fixing to bone away from the comminution and preserving critical blood supply to that area by limiting surgical dissection. (From Mazzocca AD, DeAngelis JD, Caputo AE, et al: Principles of internal fixation. In Browner BD, Levine AM, Jupiter JB, et al, editors: *Skeletal trauma: Basic science, management, and reconstruction*, ed 4, Philadelphia, 2008, WB Saunders.)

Compression plating is used to increase the stability of fixation when the two major fracture fragments can be brought into contact. This technique allows direct compression of the fracture ends. Compression plates have oval screw holes with oblique edges that allow eccentric placement of screws. When a screw is applied eccentrically, the plate (and bone fragment fixed to it) translates as the screw tightens down against the plate to create compression at the fracture. In addition, compression can also be achieved by overbending a plate or by introducing a tensioning device.

Highly comminuted and segmental fractures may not allow anatomic reduction and direct fixation of all the fragments. In these situations, a bridge plate can be used to stabilize a long bone rigidly. The proximal and distal fragments are rigidly fixed to each other with a plate while the fracture site is bypassed. This concept has been popularized because it allows less dissection at the fracture site, which may devitalize the comminuted and segmental fragments.

Special plates have been designed for certain fracture patterns and anatomic locations. Blade plates, dynamic condylar screws, and pelvic reconstruction plates are examples of these specialized plates.

Tension Bands

When the forces across a fracture site tend to displace the fractured pieces in tension, the tension band technique can be applied to convert the displacing tensile forces on one side of a fracture into a compressive force across the entire contact area (Fig. 18-9). Traditionally, wires or cables are used to create tension bands. However, nonabsorbable suture and plates can also be used. Tension bands are used most frequently for fractures of the olecranon, where the pull of the triceps tends to distract the proximal fragment, and fractures of the patella, where the pull of the quadriceps tends to distract the superior pole. They are also commonly used for the femoral greater trochanter, humeral greater tuberosity, and medial malleolus.

Intramedullary Nails

In contrast to wires, plates, and screws, intramedullary (IM) nails are placed in the medullary canal of long bones. They are used to splint or to bridge a fracture and to control axial, bending, and rotational forces. IM nailing also permits fixation of a fracture through an incision distant from the fracture site. In this way, the periosteal blood supply at the fracture site is left undisturbed. Nails are made of various materials and can be fluted, smooth, solid, or cannulated (Fig. 18-10). When transverse screws are placed through the proximal and distal ends of the nail, the nail is said to be locked. Locked nails control rotation better and maintain bone length in the presence of comminution or bone loss. The locking holes in nails may be round or oval. Using a nail with an oval hole or leaving the nail unlocked at one end allows the bone fragment to slide axially along the nail and produces compression at the fracture site. Nails locked in this fashion are dynamically locked. When screws are inserted through round holes in both ends of the nail, no motion is allowed within the construct; they are statically locked (Fig. 18-11).

IM nails can be introduced in a proximal to distal or distal to proximal direction and are termed *antegrade* and *retrograde,* respectively. Nails may be inserted with or without canal preparation by reaming. Reaming involves passing a large drill down the medullary canal to remove the cancellous bone and effectively widen the canal. This increased width allows the insertion of a larger diameter nail to increase the strength and stiffness of the construct. At the same time, reaming morcellizes the cancellous and cortical bone in the canal and deposits this exceptional autogenous bone graft at the fracture site. However, reaming leads to increased pressure in the medullary canal, increased temperature in the cortical bone, and embolization of marrow contents into the vascular system. In patients with severe derangement of pulmonary function or hemodynamic instability, embolization is not well tolerated.

Unreamed nails are inserted without reaming of the canal, and destruction of the cortical blood supply from the medullary system is largely avoided. In fractures in which there is a large degree of soft tissue loss or periosteal stripping, an unreamed nail is generally used.

PATIENT EVALUATION

History

Obtaining a detailed history of a skeletally injured patient is essential for accurate diagnosis and treatment. This can be challenging with multiply injured and older patients in the trauma setting; however, it is important to gather as much information as possible about the mechanism of injury. Often, trauma patients are unable to give accurate histories because of unconsciousness, intoxication, dementia, or delirium. In these cases, an account of the mechanism of injury and patient history should be obtained from family members, emergency medical response crew members, or other witnesses to the accident. Descriptions from the injury scene can be helpful because common patterns of injury follow from specific mechanisms (Table 18-1).

A general history that includes demographic information, past medical history, past surgical history, and social history are obtained. Knowledge of allergies, current medications, and time since last oral intake is useful in guiding treatment. Information about the position of the limb before and after the injury as well as the direction of the deforming force can help predict the resulting injuries. Ambulatory status before the injury helps determine realistic goals for functional recovery. Any transient neurologic symptoms, such as loss of consciousness, numbness, paresthesias, and spasm, must be documented. Loss of bowel or bladder control in patients with back or neck pain must also be noted. The time elapsed since injury becomes critical information in a patient with a vascular injury, open wound, or dislocation.

Trauma Room Evaluation

Examination of a multiply injured patient must first follow advanced trauma life support (ATLS) protocols in a systematic fashion and must be accompanied by appropriate treatment. The concept of life before limb demands that the ABCs (*a*irway, *b*reathing, and *c*irculation) be addressed before evaluating for any orthopedic injuries. Hemodynamically unstable patients are assumed to be in hemorrhagic shock until proven otherwise. A search for the source of hemorrhage is undertaken and may include examination of the pleural cavities, abdomen, extremities, retroperitoneum, and pelvis. A plain chest radiograph may quickly reveal a hemothorax. Chest tubes are placed if necessary.

Pelvic instability and the need for rapid external pelvic fixation are addressed. A single examination of the pelvis for instability, performed by an experienced examiner, can be undertaken. There is debate about whether the anteroposterior (AP) pelvic film, which has traditionally been considered part of the standard trauma radiographic series, is justified with the advent of newer, ultrafast computed tomography (CT) scanners. Paydar and

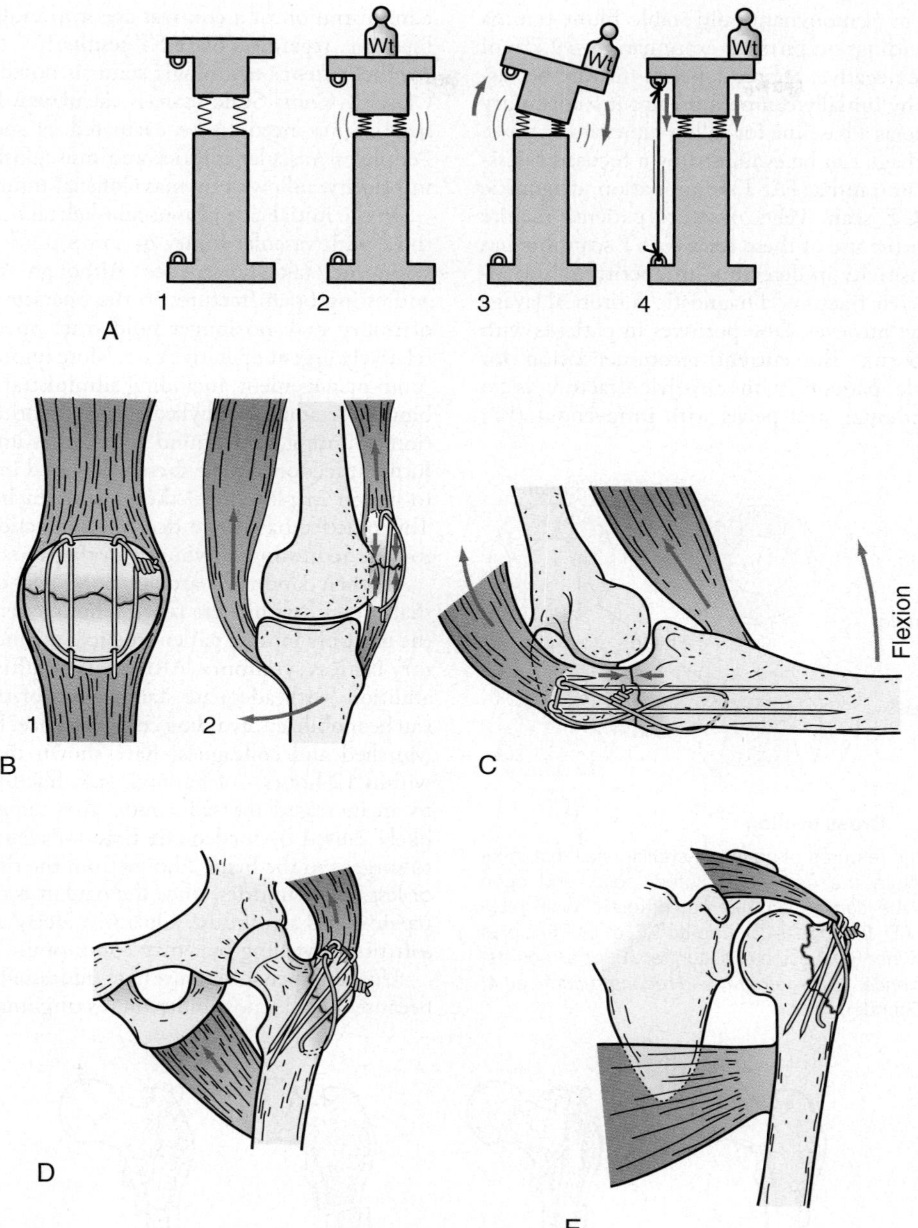

FIGURE 18-9 Tension Band Principles. **A,** (1) An interrupted I-beam connected by two springs. (2) The I-beam is loaded with a weight (Wt) placed over the central axis of the beam; there is uniform compression of both springs at the interruption. (3) When the I-beam is loaded eccentrically by placing the weight at a distance from the central axis of the beam, the spring on the same side compresses, whereas the spring on the opposite side is placed in tension and stretches. (4) If a tension band is applied before the eccentric loading, it resists the tension that would otherwise stretch the opposite spring, thus causing uniform compression of both springs. **B,** The tension band principle applied to fixation of a transverse patellar fracture. (1) The AP view shows placement of the parallel Kirschner wires and anterior tension band. (2) The lateral view demonstrates antagonistic pull of the hamstrings and quadriceps, causing a bending moment of the patella over the femoral trochlea. An anterior tension band transforms this eccentric loading into compression at the fracture site. **C,** The tension band principle applied to fixation of a fracture of the ulna. The antagonistic pull of the triceps and brachialis causes a bending moment of the ulna over the humeral trochlea. The dorsal tension band transforms this eccentric load into compression at the fracture site. **D,** The tension band principle applied to fixation of a fracture of the greater trochanter. With the hip as a fulcrum, the antagonistic pull of the adductors and abductors causes a bending moment in the femur. The lateral tension band transforms this eccentric load into compression at the greater trochanteric fracture site. **E,** The tension band principle applied to fixation of a fracture of the greater tuberosity of the humerus. Using the glenoid as a fulcrum, the antagonistic pull of the pectoralis major and supraspinatus causes a bending moment of the humerus. The lateral tension band transforms this eccentric load into compression at the greater tuberosity fracture site. (From Mazzocca AD, DeAngelis JD, Caputo AE, et al: Principles of internal fixation. In Browner BD, Levine AM, Jupiter JB, et al, editors: *Skeletal trauma: Basic science, management, and reconstruction*, ed 4, Philadelphia, 2008, WB Saunders.)

associates[4] found that in hemodynamically stable blunt trauma patients with normal findings on physical examination, 99.7% of pelvic radiographs were negative. Should a pelvic fracture be suspected, plain radiography initially can be done not just for injury characterization but also as a baseline for follow-up examinations. Intraperitoneal hemorrhage can be evaluated by a focused assessment with sonography in trauma (FAST) examination, diagnostic peritoneal lavage, or CT scan. Pelvic fracture patients require special consideration in the use of these tests. FAST scanning has been shown to lack sensitivity in detecting intraperitoneal bleeding in patients with a pelvic fracture.[5] Diagnostic peritoneal lavage has increased sensitivity; however, false positives in patients with pelvic fractures can occur. The current recommendation for hemodynamically stable patients with a pelvic fracture is to undergo CT of the abdomen and pelvis with intravenous (IV) administration of a contrast agent to evaluate for intraperitoneal bleeding, regardless of FAST results.[5]

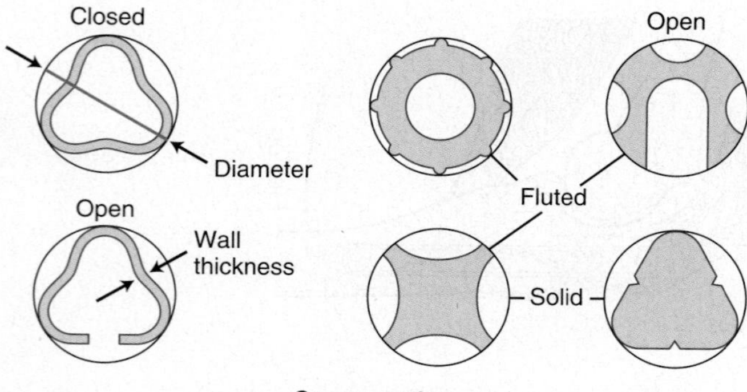

FIGURE 18-10 Geometric features of an intramedullary nail that influence its performance. Note the cloverleaf, fluted, solid, and open designs. All these have the same diameter but different wall thicknesses. (From Mazzocca AD, DeAngelis JD, Caputo AE, et al: Principles of internal fixation. In Browner BD, Levine AM, Jupiter JB, et al, editors: *Skeletal trauma: Basic science, management, and reconstruction*, ed 4, Philadelphia, 2008, WB Saunders.)

The patient's neurologic status is noted on admission, and the Glasgow Coma Scale score is calculated. Patients with suspected head injury need to be evaluated as soon as possible by CT. Peripheral vascular injuries and musculoskeletal injuries are next in priority, followed by maxillofacial injuries.

In the initial care of musculoskeletal injuries, open fractures or those with vascular injury or compromise, such as compartment syndrome, take precedence. Although the previous dictum of addressing open fractures in the operating room within 6 hours of injury may no longer hold true, open fractures still require relatively urgent operative care. More important, emergent trauma room management, including administration of appropriate antibiotics, tetanus prophylaxis, gross débridement, copious irrigation, splinting, and wound coverage, is imperative for preventing future infection. Sterile dressings placed in the trauma room need to be left in place until the patient reaches the operating room. This practice has led to decreased infection rates compared with routine redressing of wounds in the trauma area.

In their landmark article, Bone and coworkers[6] have shown that urgent (within the first 24 hours) versus late stabilization in the multiply injured patient reduces the incidence of adult respiratory distress syndrome (ARDS) and multisystem organ failure. In addition, with adequate stabilization of the fracture, the patient can be mobilized, avoiding convalescence. However, more recently, Morshed and colleagues[7] have shown that emergent fixation—within 12 hours—of femoral shaft fractures in polytrauma leads to an increased mortality rate. They suggest that this finding is likely caused by inadequate time for resuscitation in those taken to surgery in the first 12 hours from the time of injury. In isolated or less severe injuries, once the patient is stabilized, the timing of repair is less significant. Operative delay allows resolution of the soft tissue swelling that may compromise soft tissue closure.

Unstable pelvic fractures are addressed in the primary survey because of the possibility of exsanguination. Traumatic spine

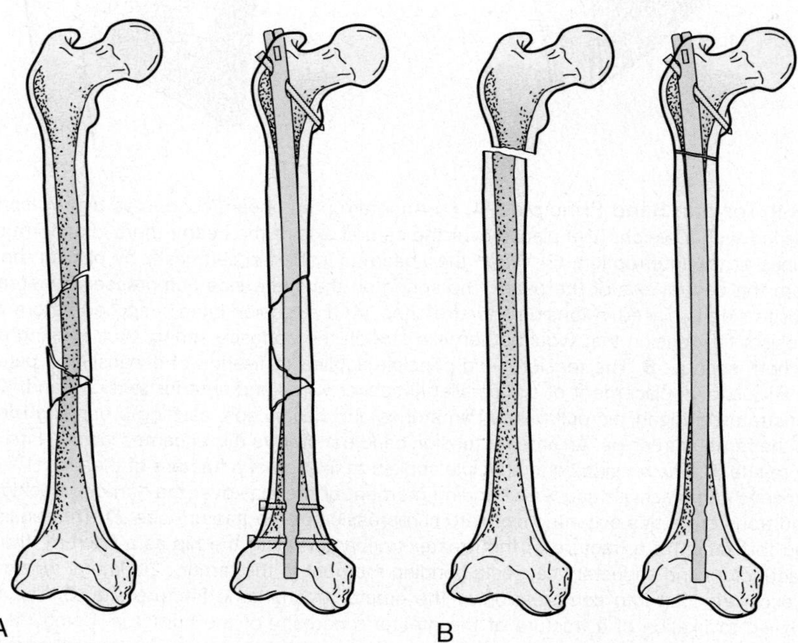

FIGURE 18-11 A, Static locked intramedullary nail fixed to both the proximal and distal fragments. **B,** Dynamic locked intramedullary nail fixed to the proximal (as shown) or distal fragment, but not to both.

TABLE 18-1 Common Patterns and Associated Injuries

INJURY PATTERN OR MECHANISM	ASSOCIATED INJURIES
Fall from a height	Calcaneus fracture Tibial plateau fracture Fractures around the hip (proximal femur, acetabulum) Vertebral burst fracture
Fall on outstretched hand	Distal radius fracture Posterior elbow dislocation Pediatric Both-bones forearm fracture Supracondylar humerus fracture
Ejection from a vehicle	Closed head injury Spine fractures
T-bone motor vehicle accident	Lateral compression–type pelvic fracture Closed head injury Thoracic injury
Head-on motor vehicle accident	Abdominal visceral injury Open-book pelvic fracture Retroperitoneal bleeding Injuries caused by floor board intrusion Calcaneal fracture Tibial plateau fracture Posterior hip dislocation
Posterior knee dislocation	Popliteal artery injury
Supracondylar humerus fracture	Brachial artery injury Nerve injury (median or radial)
Anterior shoulder dislocation	Axillary nerve injury
Posterior hip dislocation	Sciatic (peroneal division) nerve injury

injuries with associated neurologic compromise also deserve immediate attention. These exceptions aside, examination and management of the extremities are deferred to the secondary survey after the airway has been controlled and hemodynamic stability has been obtained. In a team approach, these examinations and treatments take place simultaneously. One caveat to this protocol is the conscious patient who is able to follow commands but will need intubation to protect the airway. In this case, a cursory neurologic examination of the extremities should be performed before sedation or intubation. Documentation of motor and sensory function in the upper and lower extremities is valuable information and takes only seconds to carry out. Throughout the resuscitation phase and during the remainder of the hospital course, reexamination in the form of the tertiary survey will ensure that no injury goes unrecognized.

Evidence of pelvic fractures is assessed early in the resuscitative effort. Massive flank or buttock contusions and swelling are indicative of significant bleeding. The Morel-Lavallée lesion is an ecchymotic lesion over the greater trochanter that represents a subcutaneous degloving injury. This lesion is frequently associated with acetabular fractures. Blood at the urethral meatus, signifying injury to the genitourinary tract, may be a sign of an underlying pelvic fracture. Palpation of the symphysis pubis and the sacroiliac joints can help determine the presence of disruption of these joints. Gentle rocking and lateral compression through the anterior iliac crests can provide helpful clues to the stability of the pelvic ring. Any opening or looseness signifies instability and may represent a source of hemorrhage. Rectal and vaginal examinations are performed, noting the presence of gross blood, lacerations, bone fragments, hematomas, or masses. Wounds and palpable bone fragments found on either of these examinations are diagnostic of an open pelvic fracture, which carries a poor prognosis. Rectal examination can also reveal a high-riding prostate gland, another indication of injury to the genitourinary tract.

The trauma team must always take steps to protect the patient from self-inflicted or iatrogenic spinal cord injury. Therefore, full spine precautions must be observed until it is confirmed that the patient's vertebral column is intact, either by physical examination and clinical findings or by radiologic confirmation, when warranted. Fitting the patient with a hard cervical collar stabilizes the cervical spine. Maintaining the patient in a supine flat position at all times protects the thoracic, lumbar, and sacral segments of the spine. If the patient is to be moved, a strict log roll technique is used. At times, a patient may have to be physically restrained to prevent potential self-inflicted injury by head or lower extremity movements that could impart rotational, translational, or bending moments to the vertebral column. Special care must be taken with combative patients or those with altered mental status who may have lost the ability to protect themselves from further injury. On examination of the back, the examiner notes the presence of deformity, edema, or ecchymosis. Tenderness elicited on palpation of the spine is recorded for each level at which the patient complains of pain. Distinction is made regarding whether the pain is midline or paraspinal. Perianal sensation and rectal sphincter tone should be evaluated to test sacral nerve root function. Deep tendon reflexes and pathologic reflexes, such as the bulbocavernosus and Babinski reflexes, are tested.

Plain radiographs of the cervical spine, including AP, lateral, and open-mouth odontoid views, were previously considered part of the standard trauma series of radiographs. Recently, however, Mathen and associates[8] have shown that the standard plain films fail to identify 55.5% of clinically relevant fractures identified by multislice CT and add no clinically relevant data. Similarly, CT of the thoracic, lumbar, and sacral spine is faster and more accurate than radiography at identifying traumatic injury. With most trauma patients undergoing CT of the chest, abdomen, and pelvis, reformatting of the data into spinal reconstructions adds neither time nor radiation exposure. With these data, plain films are no longer indicated.

Examination of the extremities in a patient with isolated injuries or in a multitrauma patient follows a simple, systematic, and reproducible pattern. Even when an isolated extremity injury is the primary reason for evaluation, the entire skeleton must be examined. The examiner must not be distracted from the task by obvious or severe injuries. Deformity, edema, ecchymosis, crepitus, tenderness, and pain with motion are the cardinal signs of an acute fracture. Each limb segment needs to be examined for lacerations and the signs of trauma described earlier. All joints are put through passive range of motion, at a minimum. Active range of motion is tested whenever possible. Joint effusions are evidence of intra-articular disease (e.g., ligament or cartilage damage or an intra-articular fracture). The joints are then manually stressed to assess the integrity of the ligamentous structures. A neurovascular examination is performed and documented. Pulses are recorded and compared with the opposite uninvolved extremity when possible. Doppler signals are obtained when palpable pulses are not present or are weak. Measuring the ankle-brachial index (ABI) is important when vascular injury is suspected. Motor function and sensation must be documented for the extremity dermatomes as

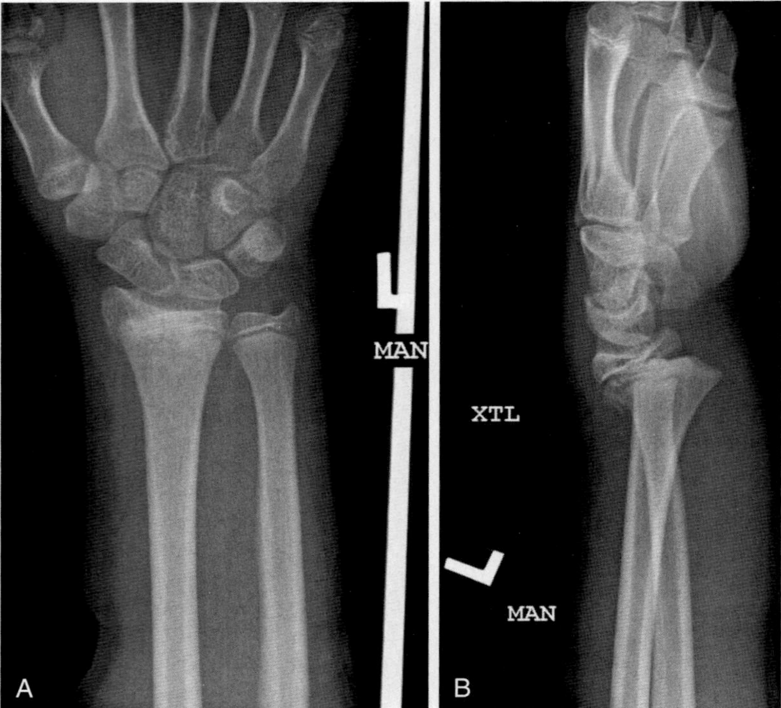

FIGURE 18-12 A, AP radiograph of the wrist showing disruption of the distal radial physis but adequate alignment. **B,** Lateral view showing complete physeal separation, with 50% dorsal displacement and significant angulation.

well as for the trunk in a patient with thoracic spine pain. To avoid the complications of a missed compartment syndrome, palpation of the involved compartments is performed. Any firm or tense compartments are checked for increased pressure if time and the patient's condition allow. Fasciotomies are performed urgently if pressures are elevated. Gross alignment and interim immobilization of long bone fractures are achieved before transportation of the patient from the trauma room. This helps prevent further damage to underlying soft tissues, reduces the patient's discomfort, facilitates transportation, and may help prevent further embolization of IM contents.[9] Traction splints or skeletal traction is applied when indicated.

Diagnostic Imaging

Radiographic examination is used to supplement and to enhance the information gathered during the primary survey, history, and physical examination. In a multiply injured patient, the ATLS protocol calls for a lateral cervical spine film and AP views of the pelvis and chest. However, as noted earlier for a stable, conscious patient with no physical examination findings of pelvic trauma, the pelvic film may be deferred for the pelvic CT scan. Cervical spine radiographs should be deferred for a CT scan of the cervical spine (if available). The secondary survey then dictates which extremity radiographs are necessary. In filming long bone injuries, it is important to verify the integrity of adjacent limb segments. Therefore, the joints above and below the level of injury are always included in the films. They are filmed separately if the cassette is not large enough to accommodate the entire view. Similarly, when pathologic change is suspected in a joint, the long bones above and below are also imaged. This practice helps identify commonly associated injuries to the adjacent limb segments that might otherwise be missed.

Because bone is a three-dimensional object, a single two-dimensional radiograph cannot describe a fracture. To understand the position and direction of the fracture fragments, orthogonal views (images taken at 90 degrees to one another) must be obtained. A bone may appear minimally displaced in one plane but in another view may be significantly displaced (Fig. 18-12). All extremities with deformity need to be rotated to the anatomic position before radiographs are taken to help decrease confusion in describing the fracture. When finer detail is necessary to evaluate a fracture pattern better or to confirm the findings of an equivocal radiograph, a CT scan should be ordered. Magnetic resonance imaging (MRI) has become a particularly useful imaging modality. It is used to evaluate soft tissue, acute fractures, stress fractures, spinal cord injuries, and intra-articular disease. Its role in the trauma setting has expanded as well, and it is particularly helpful in the setting of spinal cord injury. More frequently, MRI is used in the outpatient setting to evaluate soft tissue injuries and pathologic lesions. MRI is now commonly used for the diagnosis of acute fractures when plain films are negative.

Although AP and lateral views are generally adequate for most long bone fractures, there are a number of osseous structures that necessitate specific radiographs or routinely require more specialized studies, such as CT or MRI.

Shoulder

True AP and lateral views of the shoulder must be taken in relation to the scapula because of the orientation of the joint. The most useful lateral view is an axillary radiograph. The tube is angled cephalad, with the plate on the superior aspect of the abducted shoulder. This view is often difficult to obtain because of pain or instability at the proximal end of the humerus. The Velpeau view is a modified axillary view that provides orthogonally equivalent

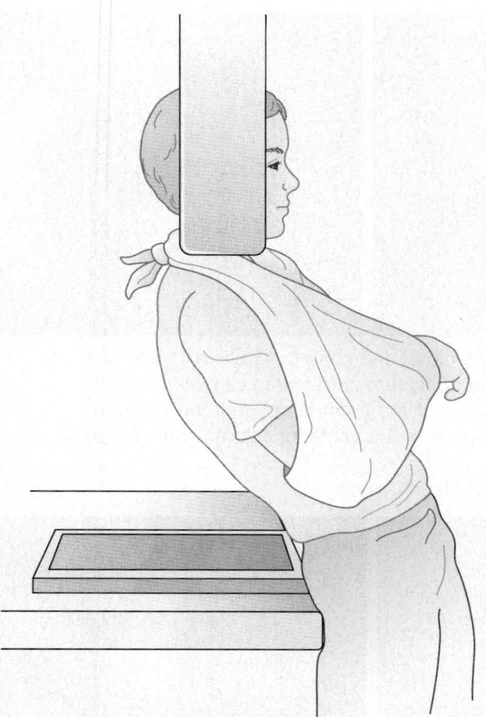

FIGURE 18-13 Velpeau or Bloom-Obata modified axillary view. (From Green A, Norris TR: Proximal humeral fractures and glenohumeral dislocations. In Browner BD, Levine AM, Jupiter JB, et al, editors: *Skeletal trauma: Basic science, management, and reconstruction*, ed 4, Philadelphia, 2008, WB Saunders.)

images. While wearing a sling, the patient leans backward 30 degrees over the cassette on the table. The x-ray tube is placed above the shoulder, and the beam is projected vertically down through the shoulder onto the cassette (Fig. 18-13). This allows the radiograph to be taken with the shoulder adducted and in a sling, allowing acquisition of the axillary images without the pain of shoulder abduction.

Elbow

AP and lateral views of the elbow provide visualization of most of the bone anatomy. Internal and external oblique views are included in a complete elbow series and allow better visualization of the medial and lateral epicondyles. On the lateral view, look for the fat pad sign or the sail sign for evidence of an occult fracture. The sail sign can be noted when hemiarthrosis from an intra-articular fracture forces the anterior and posterior fat pads out of the coronoid and olecranon fossae, respectively. On radiography, the visualized fat pads resemble a sail (Fig. 18-14). Although the anterior fat pad can be visualized in a normal elbow, the presence of a posterior fat pad sign is strongly suggestive of occult fracture and, if clinically appropriate, warrants a CT scan.

Pelvis and Acetabulum

The standard AP radiograph of the pelvis provides an overview to the structural integrity of the hips and pelvic ring. If pelvic disease is noted on this film or suspected from physical examination, further views are necessary. Judet views, or 45-degree oblique views of the pelvis, are used to evaluate the acetabuli (Fig. 18-15). Because of the spatial orientation of the acetabulum, these views represent orthogonal projections when the x-ray tube is canted toward or away from the affected side. Similarly, inlet and outlet views of the pelvis allow closer examination of the sacroiliac joints and the sacrum itself, as well as identifying AP disruption in the pelvic ring. The inlet view is taken with the beam angled 60 degrees caudad, thus making the beam perpendicular to the pelvic brim. The sacral ala, displacement of the sacroiliac joints, and displacement of the pubic symphysis in the AP plane are easily seen. The outlet view is a 30-degree oblique view, with the tube angled cephalad. The sacrum is pictured en face, and the neural foramina are easily evaluated. If it has not already been obtained as part of the trauma workup, pelvic CT should be ordered to evaluate fractures of the acetabuli and sacrum. This allows detailed evaluation of the amount of articular involvement or displacement and of the presence of bone fragments within the joint. It also provides information about sacral displacement or neural foraminal involvement. Finally, it allows evaluation for intrapelvic hematoma. MRI has little role in acute, traumatic pelvic ring injury; however, it is the imaging modality of choice for suspected osteomyelitis or pelvic abscess.

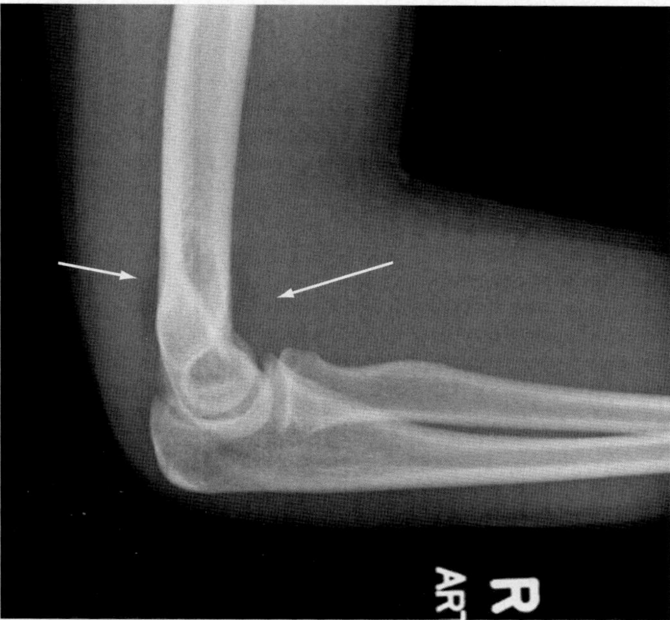

FIGURE 18-14 Positive fat pad or sail sign in a patient with a nondisplaced radial neck fracture. Note the anterior and posterior areas of radiolucency *(arrows)* representing the extruded fat pads.

Hip

A hip series consists of AP and cross-table lateral radiographs. In an adult patient with acute groin pain and inability to bear weight, an occult hip fracture should be ruled out with MRI or bone scan. In older patients with occult osteopenic hip fractures, bone scans, although accurate, are unreliable within 48 hours after injury. MRI has been shown to be at least as accurate as bone scans in the diagnosis of acute fractures. In addition, the sensitivity and specificity of MRI were the same within 24 hours of admission as later. Earlier diagnosis can potentially lead to shorter hospital stays and therefore, in theory, offset the additional cost of MRI. In patients with femoral shaft fractures, the incidence of ipsilateral femoral neck fracture is as high as 9%. A protocol of intraoperative live fluoroscopic rotation views can prevent this injury from being missed, as recent data have shown that preoperative

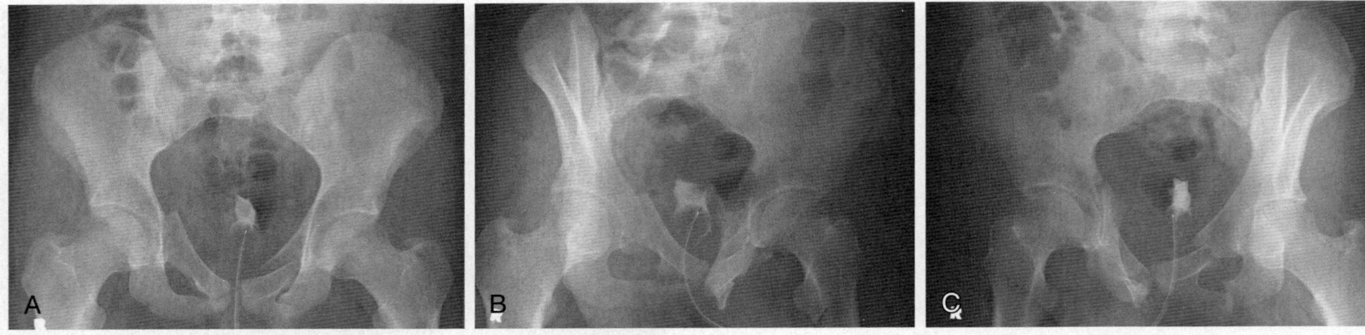

FIGURE 18-15 AP and Judet pelvic radiographs clearly show the anterior and posterior walls and columns of both acetabuli. **A,** AP view showing bilateral inferior and superior pubic ramus fractures as well as a right acetabular fracture. **B,** Right obturator oblique view shows disruption of the anterior column and posterior wall of the right acetabulum. **C,** Right iliac oblique view shows disruption of the posterior column and anterior wall of the right acetabulum.

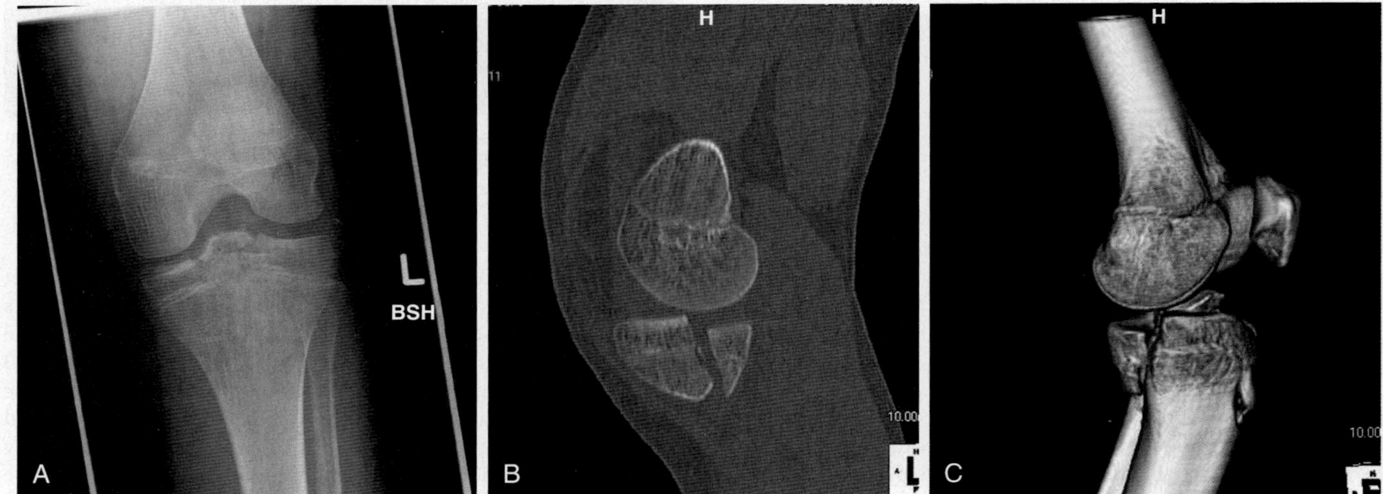

FIGURE 18-16 A, Minimally displaced fracture of the tibial eminence. **B,** CT scan of the knee shows a significant step-off of the posterior medial tibial plateau. **C,** Three-dimensional reconstruction.

radiographs and CT scans have poor sensitivity for diagnosis of these occult injuries.[10]

Knee

AP, lateral, and internal or external oblique plain films allow visualization of most traumatic osseous abnormalities of the knee. If possible, standing films are useful for evaluating knee alignment and joint space narrowing. The lateral film can show an effusion, patellar fracture, posterior tibial plateau fracture, or tibial tubercle injury. If there is any doubt as to the degree of articular involvement, displacement, or depression, a CT scan should be ordered (Fig. 18-16). Although MRI can be helpful in the acute setting, evaluation of ligamentous derangement is not urgent and can be deferred to the outpatient setting. In the setting of a knee dislocation, vascular injury should be assumed until proven otherwise. Serial measurements of the ABI are useful to monitor for vascular compromise, but vascular imaging in the form of CT angiography or MR angiography should be strongly considered in the setting of an acute knee dislocation.

Ankle

In the ankle, it is important to confirm maintenance of the mortise. The stability of the mortise depends on bone and ligamentous support. With AP, mortise, and lateral radiographs, disruptions in the bone anatomy can be visualized directly. Although the ligamentous structures cannot be visualized directly, assumptions about their continuity can be made by evaluating the spaces between the bones. Three main parameters commonly used are the tibia-fibula overlap, tibia-fibula clear space, and medial clear space (Fig. 18-17). All three parameters should be measured on the AP radiograph. The medial clear space is the distance between the medial border of the talus and lateral border of the medial malleolus. A normal value is less than 4 mm. The tibia-fibula clear space is the distance between the medial border of the fibula and floor of the incisura fibularis. A normal value is less than 5 mm. The tibia-fibula overlap is the amount of the lateral tibia overlapping the medial fibula. A normal value is more than 10 mm. In an adult ankle, there should be some degree of tibia-fibula overlap in all views. Both the tibia-fibula clear space and overlap are measured 10 mm proximally to the tibial plafond. Excluding a direct blow injury, sustaining an isolated medial malleolar fracture is exceedingly rare. Most ankle injuries are caused by a twisting moment imparted to the ankle. The energy that enters through the medial malleolus must exit at some point on the lateral ankle. This may result in a lateral collateral ligament tear (rare), lateral malleolar fracture, or more proximal fibula

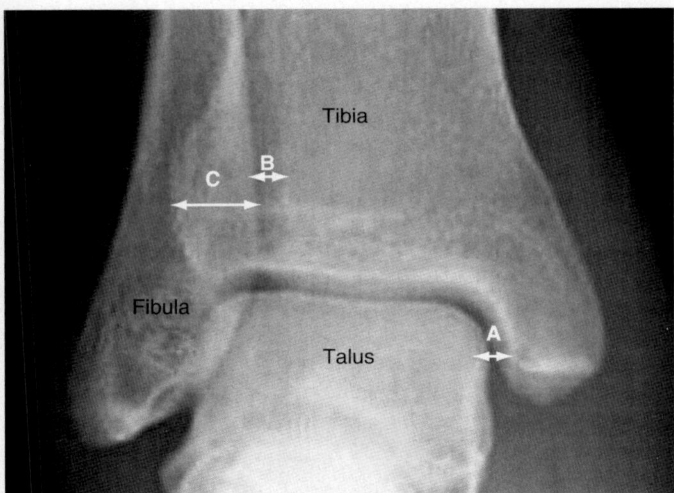

FIGURE 18-17 AP radiograph of the ankle showing medial clear space (A), tibia-fibula clear space (B), and tibia-fibula overlap (C).

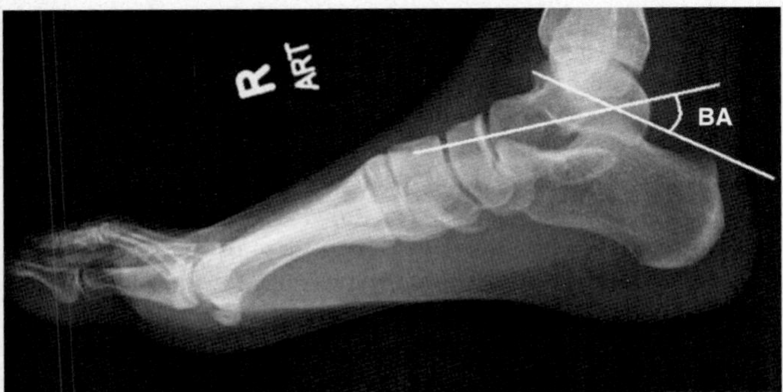

FIGURE 18-18 Lateral radiograph of the foot showing Bohler angle (BA).

fracture. In some cases, the energy passes through the syndesmosis and exits at the proximal fibula. This is known as a Maisonneuve fracture. The disruption results in an unstable ankle mortise, which influences the treatment plan. Because of this, any isolated medial malleolar fracture should always have full-length AP and lateral tibia-fibula radiographs. In the case of an intra-articular fracture of the weight-bearing surface of the tibia (pilon fracture), CT can be useful to evaluate the joint surface.

Foot

When an injury of the foot is suspected, the workup should start with a standard series of AP, lateral, and oblique radiographs. However, because of the complex three-dimensional structure of the foot, this standard series of films may not be adequate to visualize certain bones. In the case of a calcaneus fracture, a Harris axial view should be added to evaluate the varus-valgus alignment of the tuberosity as well as any sagittal splits in the bone. Bohler angle—an angle formed by the bisection of a line drawn from the superior aspect of the calcaneal tuberosity to the superior aspect of the posterior facet and a line drawn from the tip of the anterior process to the superior aspect of the posterior facet—should be evaluated in the lateral view (Fig. 18-18). A normal Bohler angle is between 20 and 40 degrees. A decrease in this angle usually indicates fracture, with depression of the posterior facet. When in doubt, films of the uninjured foot should be taken for

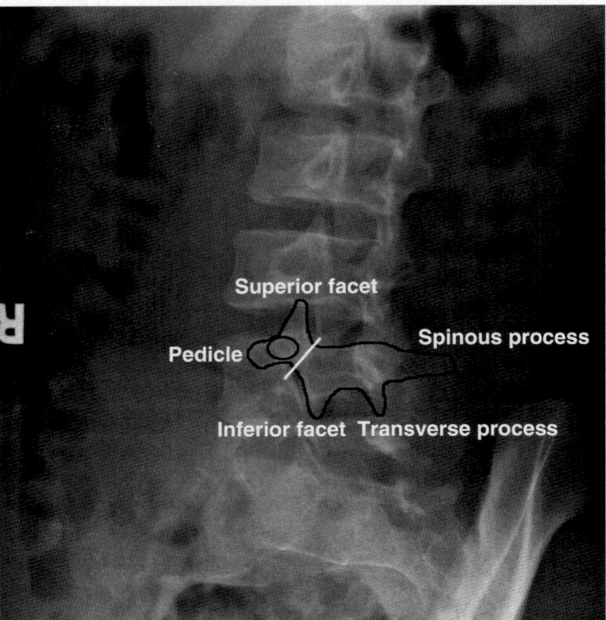

FIGURE 18-19 Oblique radiograph of the lumbar spine with the Scotty dog outlined. Back leg, transverse process; ear, superior articular facet; eye, pedicle; front leg, inferior articular facet; neck, pars interarticularis; tail, spinous process; *white line* (the collar) represents a fracture.

comparison. For fractures of the talus, the AP and lateral films should be evaluated for articular congruence at the tibiotalar, subtalar, and talonavicular joints. There are specialized views of the bone (e.g., Canale view for the talar neck and Broden view for evaluation of the subtalar joint); however, these views are radiology technician dependent. In many cases, if a fracture is seen on the AP or lateral view, a CT scan is a faster and more cost-effective way to evaluate the displacement pattern. If radiographs are negative or equivocal and the patient has evidence of fracture—ecchymosis, pain out of proportion to plain film findings, significant soft tissue swelling—a CT scan should be ordered. All but the most minimally displaced intra-articular fractures of the talus and calcaneus warrant a CT scan to define the fracture pattern and extent of articular displacement better. Except in the case of suspected osteomyelitis, MRI of the foot is of little use in the emergency setting.

Spine

In patients with acute back pain, AP and lateral radiographs of the spine can be useful to look for fractures, spondylolisthesis, malalignment, or congenital anomalies. Oblique views are sometimes necessary to evaluate the bone anatomy of the spine more completely. Figure 18-19 shows the outline of the so-called Scotty dog. Each body part of the "dog" represents a portion of the vertebral body anatomy. The bone link between the superior and inferior facets, the pars interarticularis, is visualized as the neck of the dog. A "collar" around the dog's neck represents disruption of this bone link, fracture or spondylolysis, which can represent an unstable injury. In most cases of traumatic injury presenting with a complaint of back pain, suggestive findings on plain films, back pain out of proportion to radiographic findings, or neurologic deficit, further imaging is needed. CT is useful for defining bone anatomy. If ligamentous injury or neurologic compromise is suspected, MRI should be performed. In patients for whom MRI is

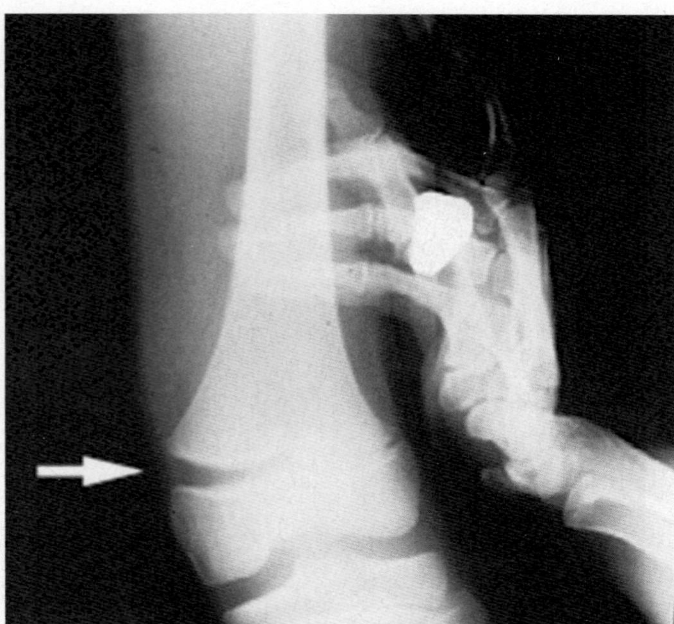

FIGURE 18-20 Stress radiograph of a physeal injury of the distal femur. An AP radiograph with valgus stress applied reveals unstable physeal disruption.

contraindicated, a bone scan can be considered if occult fracture is suspected, and CT myelography can be used to look for compromise of the spinal canal or intervertebral foramina.

Intra-Articular Fractures

The goal of radiographic assessment of intra-articular fractures is quantitation of articular incongruity and degree of malalignment. Orthogonal views of the joint and adjacent long bones are obtained. Radiographs made parallel to the articular surface best display any step-off that might be present. In complex intra-articular fractures, a CT scan is usually necessary to understand the position and displacement of all articular fragments fully. CT scans provide fine detail, help locate small fragments in the joint, and can further describe the extension of intra-articular fracture lines. They must not be used in lieu of acceptable plain radiographs, however. Plain radiographs are better suited to describe overall fracture characteristics and limb alignment accurately.

Stress Radiographs

Stress radiographs are taken when ligamentous or growth plate injuries are suspected after clinical examination but are not evident on plain films. Gapping of the joint or physis while stressing the structure in question is diagnostic (Fig. 18-20). Cervical spine ligamentous injuries are often diagnosed in this way with active flexion-extension radiographs. Passive flexion-extension must not be attempted.

Vascular Injuries

Angiography is another important modality used for the evaluation of extremity and pelvic injuries. It is indicated whenever signs of distal ischemia are noted in an extremity. In addition, it should be considered for a patient with pelvic fractures who is hemodynamically unstable. Knee dislocations are concerning because of the high incidence of associated vascular injury. There is a reported 18% to 30% rate of vascular injury after traumatic knee dislocation.[11] Current recommendations for evaluation of the leg after a knee injury include serial vascular examinations, using both manual palpation of pulses and the ABI, followed by selective arteriography of patients with abnormal examination findings.[12]

INITIAL MANAGEMENT

Care of musculoskeletal injuries begins in the prehospital phase of care. The extent of fracture and wound management differs with the level of training and experience of the first responders—laypeople, police, and emergency medical personnel. Therefore, it is essential that the initial treating physician perform a thorough assessment and begin initial management, including splinting and wound care.

Wound Management

After a thorough physical examination, treatment is begun immediately. All wound dressings and nontraction splints placed in the field should be removed by a single examiner to evaluate the degree of deformity and soft tissue injury. Superficial contamination by dirt, gravel, or grass may be removed. By sterile technique, wounds should be irrigated with sterile saline and mechanically débrided in the ED. Sterile saline solution or povidone-iodine–soaked dressings are then applied. After sterile dressings are placed over the wounds in the ED, they should remain in place until the time of operative irrigation and débridement. Careless wound management in the ED has been shown to increase the ultimate infection rate by 300% to 400%.[13] Tetanus prophylaxis and broad-spectrum IV antibiotics are administered. Immobilization is then undertaken in the same manner as for a closed injury. External bleeding in the extremities is controlled by direct manual pressure.

Reduction and Immobilization

All displaced fractures and dislocations are gently reduced to reestablish limb alignment provisionally. If the patient's condition allows, precise reductions are performed and the extremities are splinted formally to maintain the fracture reduction. With time, the difficulty of reduction increases because of edema and muscle spasm. Therefore, reduction needs to be attempted as soon as possible and with the patient as relaxed as possible. Often, narcotic analgesics and sedatives are necessary, particularly with large joint dislocations. Muscle spasm can obstruct atraumatic reduction of these injuries. If a joint is still dislocated after adequate sedation and relaxation, general anesthesia may be necessary.

Reduction maneuvers follow the same principles for all fracture and dislocation types. First, in-line traction is applied to the limb. If the soft tissue envelope surrounding the fracture fragments is intact, in-line traction alone may produce satisfactory alignment through ligamentotaxis. In most cases, the deformity must be re-created and exaggerated to unhook the fractured ends. While still pulling traction, the mechanism of injury is reversed and the fracture reduced. Neurovascular status is documented before and after any reduction maneuver or splint application. Once satisfactory reduction or alignment is achieved, it must be maintained by immobilization through casting, splinting, or continuous traction. The joints above and below the fracture must be included to prevent displacement. Postreduction radiographs are required to confirm alignment and rotation. Nondisplaced fractures are treated like displaced fractures, without reduction. Most nondisplaced fractures do not require surgical treatment. Splints are placed initially and then changed to circumferential casts after the swelling subsides.

Ligamentous injuries may also require immobilization. The joint is fully evaluated as described earlier, and a thorough neurovascular examination is performed on the limb. Frequently, pain, effusions, or hemarthroses occur; these represent intra-articular disease. Therapeutic aspiration of a traumatic hemarthrosis is not recommended because this can lead to iatrogenic infection. In addition, release of the pressure of the effusion can precipitate more bleeding. The limb is then immobilized and reevaluated after the acute pain and swelling decrease.

The rationale for immobilization is threefold. First, splinting, particularly with traction or compression devices, reduces bleeding by reducing the volume of the muscle compartments. Second, additional soft tissue injury may be averted, and the chance of converting a closed to an open fracture by sharp bone fragments is reduced. Third, immobilization of the fracture reduces the patient's discomfort and facilitates transportation and radiographic evaluation of the patient. All fractures and dislocations are splinted or immobilized in the ED. Splints are usually fashioned from padded plaster or fiberglass. Different splinting techniques are used to immobilize each type of fracture. A volar or ulnar gutter splint is used for fractures of the hand. A sugar tong splint (Fig. 18-21*A-D*) is used for wrist or forearm fractures. This splint prevents flexion and extension at the wrist and elbow as well as pronation and supination of the forearm. Fractures about the elbow are placed in a posterior long arm splint. For humeral shaft fractures, a coaptation or posterior splint is used. When there is minimal swelling present with a humeral shaft fracture, a functional fracture brace may be applied in the ED. A short leg splint consisting of a posterior slab and a U or stirrup component (Fig. 18-21*E-H*) is used for disease of the foot and ankle. With the addition of side slabs crossing the knee, this splint can be extended into a long leg splint for tibial fractures or knee dislocations (Fig. 18-21*I* and *J*). Splints can be secured with a bias-cut stockinette, elastic wraps, or gauze bandage, provided they are wrapped in a nonconstrictive fashion.

For fractures that require reduction, it is important to mold the initial splint or cast to maintain the reduction. The natural tendency of many fractures is to displace back into their injured position. Three-point molding of the splint is required to maintain the reduction in the proper position. Common examples of molding include a slight valgus mold for humeral shaft fractures and a volarly directed mold for dorsally displaced distal radius fractures (Fig. 18-22).

The role of circumferential casting in the acute setting is questionable. Because swelling of the injured extremity increases for 48 to 72 hours, a circular cast can be too constrictive and may lead to pressure necrosis or compartment syndrome. In select cases, in which a cast will be the definitive treatment (pediatric fractures or select nondisplaced fractures in adults), the initial circumferential cast can be applied and then cut longitudinally on two sides to allow swelling without splitting of the padding. This technique is called bivalving the cast; it maintains a reduction more effectively than an open splint while still allowing soft tissue swelling.

Traction

Traction is used to immobilize fractures or dislocations displaced by muscle forces that cannot be adequately controlled with simple splints. The most common indications are vertical shear injuries of the pelvis, hip dislocations, acetabular fractures, and fractures of the proximal femur or femoral shaft. Traction may be applied through the skin using a Buck traction boot or through the bone using a skeletal traction pin placed through the bone distal to the fracture (Fig. 18-23). Traction of more than 8 pounds through the skin for any extended period causes skin damage. Therefore, skin traction is practical only for geriatric hip fractures and pediatric injuries requiring limited distraction force. The Hare traction splint applies a distraction force through an ankle stirrup and can provide effective immobilization for femoral shaft fractures (Fig. 18-24). It can be applied in the field and helps facilitate transport and mobilization, but it should be used only temporarily because of the risk of skin breakdown from the stirrup.

Skeletal traction may be maintained for longer periods with more weight than that possible with skin traction. Up to 10% of body weight may be applied to a lower extremity skeletal traction pin. Radiographs of the anticipated pin site should be obtained before placement. Neurovascular structures must be avoided during placement of the pins. As a rule of thumb, pins should be placed from the side of the extremity containing the known structure at risk. This allows control over where the pin enters in relation to these structures. In the distal femur, the pin should be passed from medial to lateral to avoid the adductor hiatus containing the femoral artery and nerve. The pin should be placed parallel to the knee joint at the level of the superior pole of the patella and in the midpoint of the bone on the lateral radiograph. In the proximal tibia, the pin should be passed from lateral to medial to avoid the common peroneal nerve passing around the fibular head. The ideal pin placement is parallel to the joint, approximately 2 cm distal and 2 cm posterior to the top of the tibial tubercle. In the calcaneus, the pin should be passed medial to lateral to avoid the neurovascular bundle passing around the medial malleolus. The pin should be placed in the tuberosity, parallel to the ankle joint, as far posterior and inferior as possible while still passing through good bone. Once the pins are placed, the skin is checked for tension, which is relieved with incisions if necessary. The wounds are then dressed with povidone-iodine–soaked sponges. Pin track infections are a common complication and can lead to osteomyelitis in the worst cases. For this reason, all pin sites are cleaned with a half-strength hydrogen peroxide solution, and a sterile dressing is applied at least twice daily.

The availability of an operating room and expected time to surgery should be considered before applying skeletal traction. A study by Even and colleagues[14] prospectively evaluated 65 patients with diaphyseal femur fractures randomized to cutaneous (Buck) versus skeletal traction. All patients underwent fixation within 24 hours of hospitalization. There was no difference in preoperative pain control or intraoperative time to reduction between groups. For patients predicted to undergo operative fixation within 24 hours, application of cutaneous traction can avoid any unnecessary risks of ED traction pin placement. Multitrauma patients or those likely not to be taken in a timely manner to the operating room should have skeletal traction placed.

Prioritization of Surgical Care

After the secondary survey is completed and necessary diagnostic studies are obtained, a multiply injured patient may be moved to the operating room. Because operative decisions are made on a continuous basis as the patient's condition evolves, the trauma surgeon serves as the coordinator of care and prioritizes all surgical procedures after consulting with the anesthesiologist, neurosurgeon, and orthopedic surgeon. Critical procedures are carried out first, and each additional intervention is reviewed as the patient's

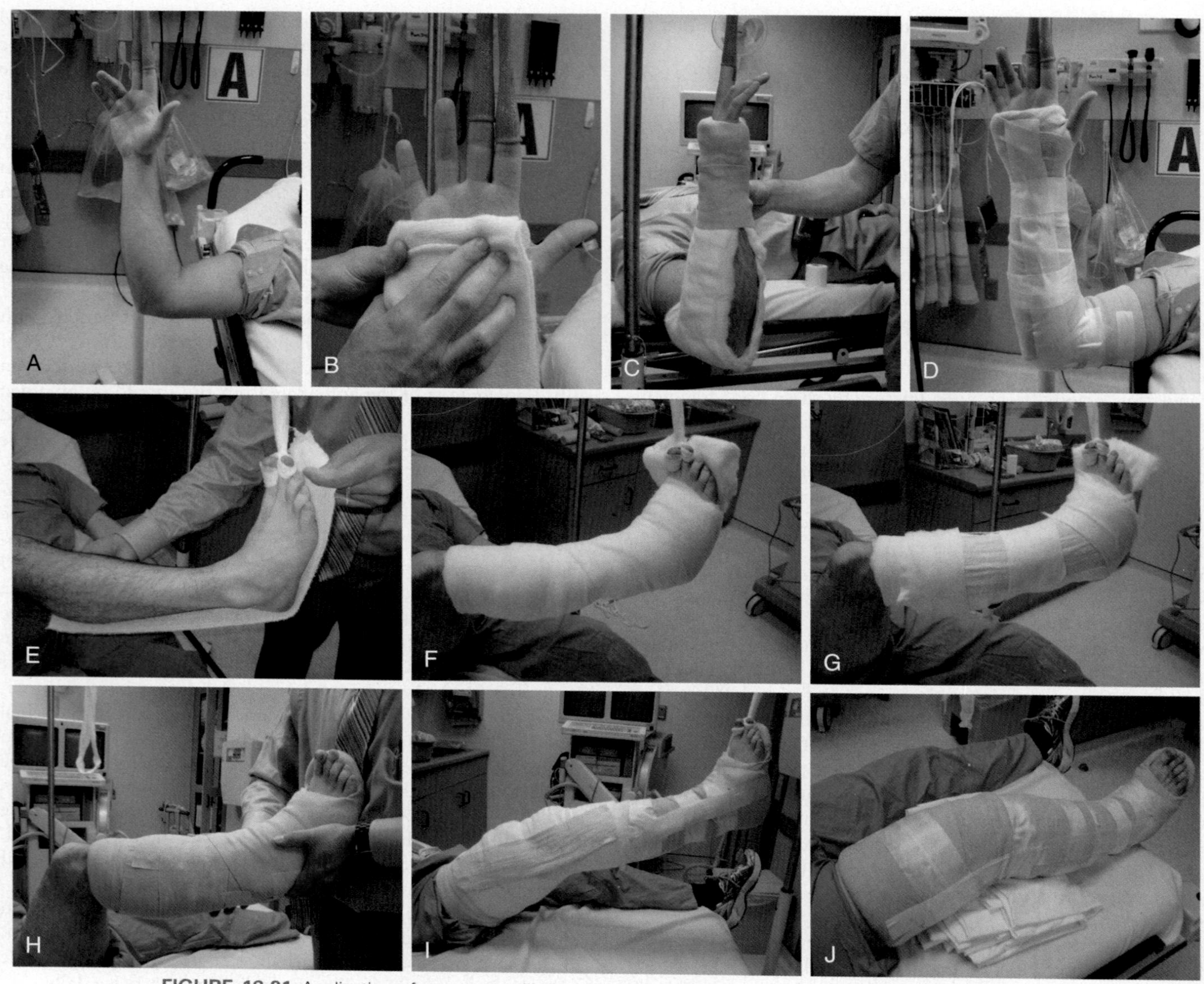

FIGURE 18-21 Application of sugar tong **(A-D)**, short leg **(E-H)**, and long leg **(I and J)** splints. **A,** Finger traps are used to apply gravity traction. **B** and **C,** A well-padded splint (plaster or fiberglass) is measured and applied to the limb. The splint should extend from the distal palmar crease volarly **(B)** to the metacarpophalangeal joints dorsally. This allows motion of the metacarpophalangeal joints. **D,** The compressive wrap (bias bandage or elastic wrap) is applied and secured with tape. **E,** Gravity traction is applied by hanging the limb by the toes in a figure-4 position across the bed. This serves two functions. First, flexion at the knee relaxes the pull of the gastrocnemius muscle across the ankle; second, the inversion produced by this position helps maintain fibular length and the reduction of the medial malleolus. Both a posterior slab and a U or stirrup component (plaster or fiberglass) are measured. **F,** The limb is protected with a soft dressing (circumferential Robert Jones cotton). **G,** The posterior followed by the stirrup splints are applied to the injured extremity and held in place with cast padding. **H,** The compressive wrap (bias bandage or elastic wrap) is applied and secured with tape. When possible, the knee is flexed and the ankle is placed in neutral position to prevent equinus contracture. **I,** The short leg splint may be extended into a long leg splint by protecting the remainder of the limb with a soft dressing and then applying medial and lateral side slabs overlapping the short leg splint and extending to the proximal thigh. **J,** Again, the compressive wrap (bias bandage or elastic wrap) is applied and secured with tape.

status evolves. Intra-abdominal, intrapelvic, thoracic, retroperitoneal, and intracranial hemorrhages are immediate surgical priorities. These injuries include acute visceral hemorrhage, aortic or caval injuries, injuries to the heart and pulmonary vessels, intracranial mass lesions, depressed skull fractures, and pelvic fractures with associated instability. In addition to hemorrhage, immediate surgery is indicated for the prevention of local and systemic infections from open or devitalized wounds and for limb salvage.

Stabilization of severe open and femoral shaft fractures may be performed simultaneously with or after hemodynamic stabilization of the surgical patient. Limb-threatening vascular injuries are managed on an emergency basis because limiting the warm ischemia time to 6 hours is essential for optimal recovery.[15] Decisions about limb viability, compartment syndrome, and the need for amputation of a mangled extremity are made in concert with all services involved. Consideration must also be given to emergency capsulotomy and ORIF of femoral head fractures as well as reduction of posterior hip dislocations to prevent avascular necrosis. Definitive care of complex upper extremity fractures or intra-articular fractures is undertaken if the patient's condition permits. Spine, acetabular, and upper extremity injuries are addressed next. The operative repair of maxillofacial injuries can usually be delayed for several days, depending on the status of the patient.

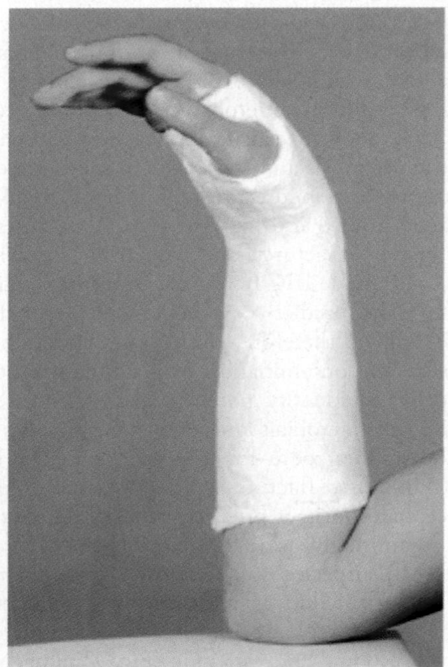

FIGURE 18-22 Distal radius mold. (© The Royal Children's Hospital, Melbourne, Australia. <http://www.rch.org.au/fracture-education/management_principles/Management_Principles/>.)

ORTHOPEDIC EMERGENCIES

Open Fractures

Until recently, open fractures were considered surgical emergencies. The 6-hour rule dictated that open fractures require immediate operative management, within 6 hours of injury. It was believed that delay beyond the 6-hour window significantly increased the risk of deep infection in this population of patients. The research behind this belief has been shown to be outdated. Currently, open fractures are treated as urgencies rather than emergencies. The majority of studies performed in the last decade have shown no difference in infection rate when surgery is delayed up to 24 hours.[16] Other trials have shown that higher grade fractures, those with gross contamination, and those in the lower extremity may have a higher rate of infection with delayed treatment.[17] Timely transfer to a definitive trauma center and early antibiotic administration (<1 hour after arrival) have been shown to be important factors in prevention of infection.[18,19] Overall, the current belief is that open fractures warrant emergent ED management (antibiotics, tetanus, irrigation, and débridement) followed by urgent operative débridement, within 24 hours, because the long-term complications of infection or nonunion may threaten the patient's limb and can, with systemic sepsis, threaten the patient's life. The difficulty of open fracture management has been recognized for centuries. Amputation was the mainstay of treatment until the mid-1800s, when antiseptic technique came into use. Antisepsis, combined with débridement of all contaminated

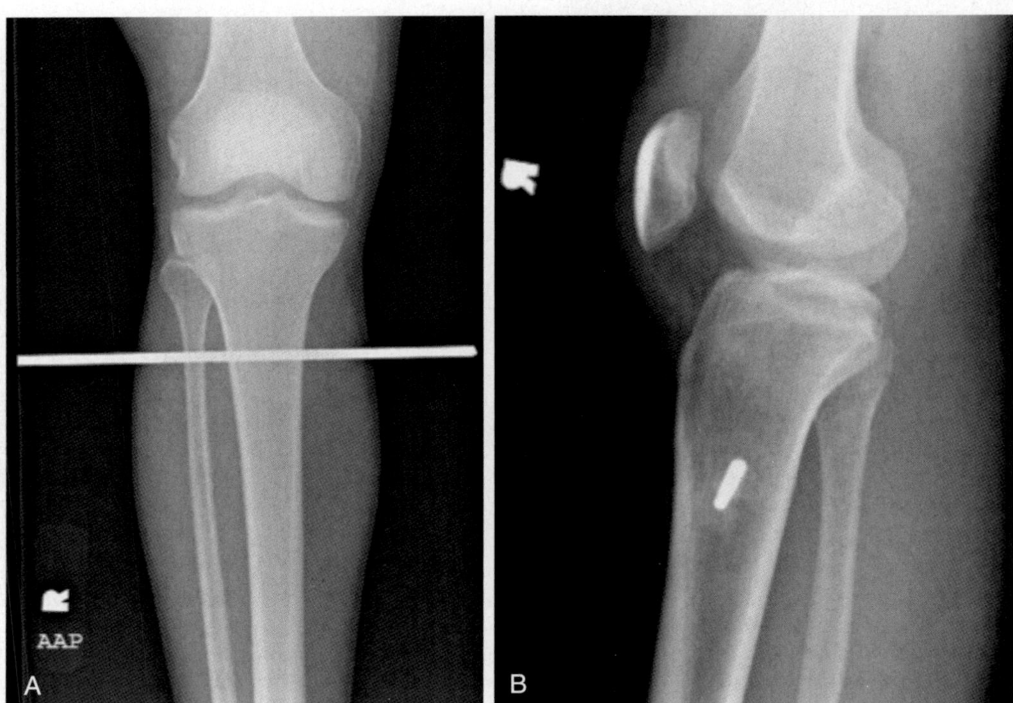

FIGURE 18-23 A and **B,** Proximal tibial traction pin.

and devitalized tissue, provided the first reduction in open fracture–related mortality. Contemporaneous advances in antibiotic prophylaxis, aggressive débridement, open wound management, rotational muscle flaps, free tissue transfer, and bone grafting techniques have dramatically enhanced our capacity to treat severe open fractures resulting from high-energy trauma.

Classification

A fracture is considered open when the fracture site communicates with the environment. Although the laceration or skin avulsion is the most obvious component, the entire zone of injury must be fully appreciated at the time of surgical exploration to assign an adequate severity grade (Fig. 18-25*A*). Gustilo and Anderson have devised the most commonly cited classification of fractures with soft tissue injury.[20] They divided fractures into three grades based on the length of the skin opening, degree of comminution, soft tissue injury, and contamination (Table 18-2). Grade III fractures are further divided into three subtypes, depending on the degree of soft tissue stripping and presence or absence of vascular injury. This classification scheme represents a continuum. Sharp divisions between groups are difficult to discern, particularly among the intermediate grades; thus, interobserver variation occurs.

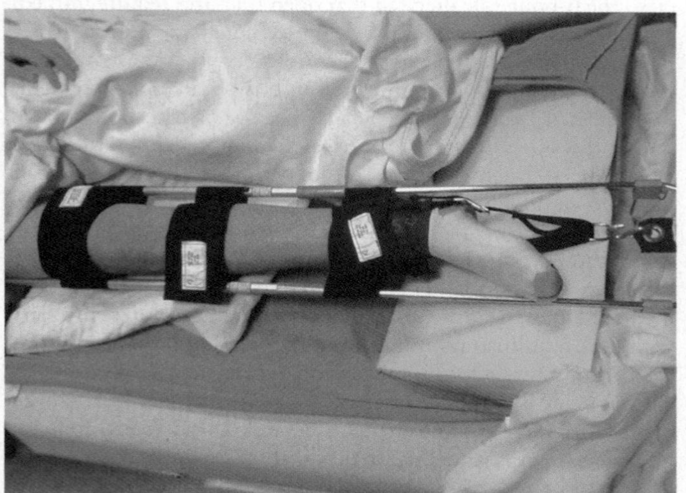

FIGURE 18-24 Hare traction splint placed at the scene of the accident to stabilize a femoral shaft fracture.

The Gustilo-Anderson classification provides useful information about the prognosis and treatment of the injured extremity. Infection rates tend to increase from grades I through III. Infection rates range from 0% to 2% for grade I fractures, from 2% to 10% for grade II fractures, and from 10% to 50% for grade III fractures, with grade IIIC fractures exhibiting the highest rates of infection.[19] The predictive value of cultures before formal débridement is low. Therefore, the recommendation is to treat presumed bacterial contamination by a standard protocol rather than attempting to identify potential pathogens. Regardless of fracture grade, antimicrobials and tetanus prophylaxis are administered in the trauma room for any open fracture. In all open fractures and in closed fractures with soft tissue injuries, a first-generation cephalosporin is preferred. Most authors recommend addition of an aminoglycoside for grades II and III fractures. For any fracture with suspected soil contamination ("barnyard" injuries), high-dose penicillin is added to the regimen to cover *Clostridium* spp (see Table 18-2). Current recommendations for duration of antibiotic therapy include 48 to72 hours of treatment

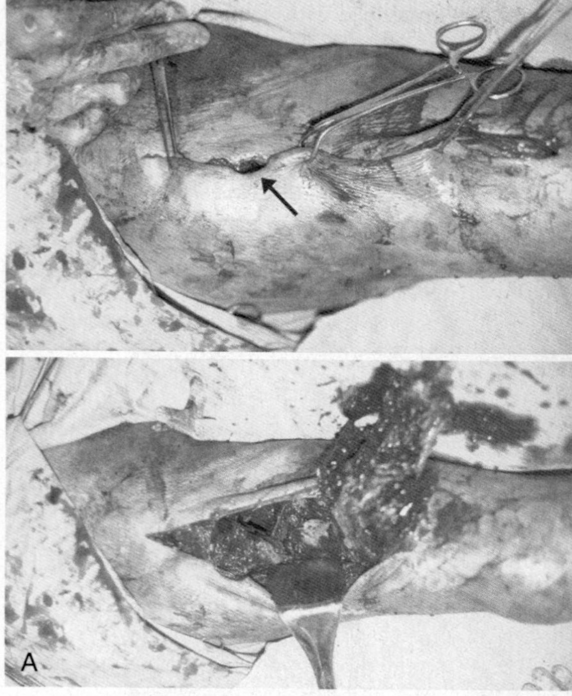

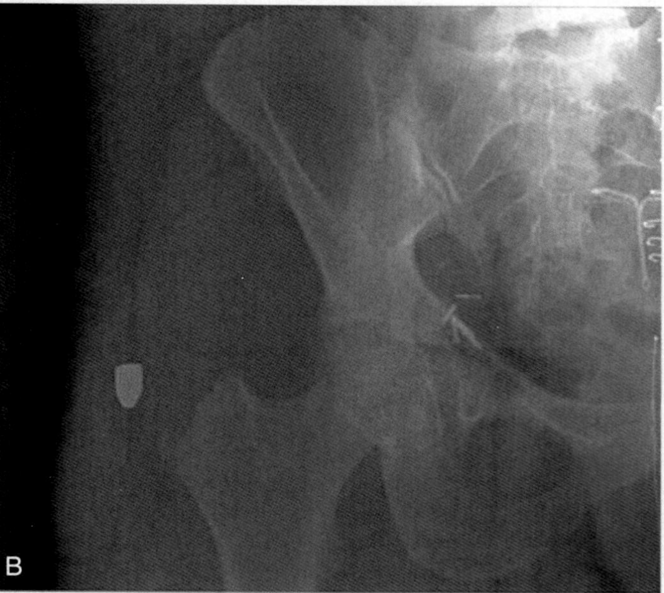

FIGURE 18-25 A, Débridement of an open wound. The small original skin wound *(arrow)* is shown in the center of a surgical incision. The full extent of underlying soft tissue damage cannot be appreciated until after exploration. **B,** Transabdominal gunshot wound involving an acetabular fracture and hip joint violation. (**B,** From Miller A, Carrol E, Tyler-Paris Pilson H: Transabdominal gunshot wounds of the hip and pelvis. *J Am Acad Orthop Surg* 21:286–292, 2013.)

TABLE 18-2 Gustilo-Anderson Classification of Open Fractures

FRACTURE TYPE	DESCRIPTION	ANTIBIOTICS
I	Skin opening <1 cm, clean; most likely inside-to-outside lesion; minimal muscle contusion; simple transverse or oblique fracture	First-generation cephalosporin
II	Laceration >1 cm with extensive soft tissue damage, flaps, or avulsion; minimal to moderate crushing; simple transverse or short oblique fracture with minimal comminution	First-generation cephalosporin ± aminoglycoside
III	Extensive soft tissue damage, including muscle, skin, and neurovascular structures; often a high-velocity injury with a severe crushing component (barnyard injuries)	First-generation cephalosporin + aminoglycoside + penicillin G
IIIA	Extensive laceration, adequate bone coverage; segmental fracture; gunshot injuries	
IIIB	Extensive soft tissue damage with periosteal stripping and bone exposure necessitating formal soft tissue coverage; usually associated with massive contamination	
IIIC	Any open fracture with a vascular injury requiring repair	

From Gustilo R, Mendoza R, Williams DN: Problems in the management of type III (severe) open fractures. *J Trauma* 24:742–746, 1984.

initially and another 48 to 72 hours of therapy after each trip to the operating room for surgical débridement or closure.

The soft tissue destruction in a closed injury can be worse than that in comparable open injuries. Tscherne and Gotzen[13] have classified closed fractures by creating a spectrum similar to what was recognized in open fractures (Table 18-3). Although this system has not been critically validated with outcome measures, it provides a means to gauge the significance of associated soft tissue injury. When these tissues become necrotic or if a surgical approach is carried out through them, infection rates could potentially increase.

TABLE 18-3 Tscherne Classification of Fractures With Soft Tissue Injuries

FRACTURE TYPE	DESCRIPTION
0	Minimal soft tissue damage; indirect violence; simple fracture patterns (e.g., torsion fracture of the tibia in skiers)
I	Superficial abrasion or contusion caused by pressure from within; mild to moderately severe fracture configuration (e.g., pronation fracture-dislocation of the ankle joint with a soft tissue lesion over the medial malleolus)
II	Deep contaminated abrasion associated with localized skin or muscle contusion; impending compartment syndrome; severe fracture configuration (e.g., segmental bumper fracture of the tibia)
III	Extensive skin contusion or crushing injury; underlying muscle damage may be severe; subcutaneous avulsion; decompensated compartment syndrome; associated major vascular injury; severe or comminuted fracture configuration

From Tscherne H, Oestern H: Die Klassifizierung des Weichteilschadens bei offenen und geschlossenen Frakturen. *Unfallheikunde* 85:111–115, 1982.

Initial Management

Early irrigation and débridement are the mainstays of treatment. Once the patient is in the operating room, dressings can be removed, along with all loose debris. Débridement requires meticulous removal and resection of all foreign and nonviable material from the wound and should proceed in a systematic fashion. The goal is reduction of the bacterial count by leaving only clearly viable tissue behind. Separate drapes and instruments should be used if the initial irrigation and débridement are to be followed by internal fixation. The wound is typically extended proximally and distally because the zone of injury is always larger than initially evident. Areas in which the extent of injury is commonly misjudged include the thigh and posterior leg because of their considerable muscle bulk. The fascial compartments are not completely decompressed by open fractures, and therefore fasciotomies are liberally performed during débridement to prevent compartment syndrome. Irrigation with copious amounts of sterile saline solution is then done. Grade I, II, and III fractures are typically irrigated with 3, 6, and 9 L of saline, respectively. This is done using either low-flow irrigation or pulsatile lavage. Recent research has shown that low-flow irrigation systems may decrease the rate of reoperation for infection, wound healing problems, and nonunion compared with pulsatile lavage.[21] Repeated débridement is performed 48 to 72 hours later because the tissue may demarcate and necrose. Surgical incisions used to enlarge the wound for exploration are closed primarily. The original wound created by the injury is usually left open, although it may be closed in select clean grade I and grade II injuries. Open wounds are now commonly managed with wound vacuum therapy, which has been shown to decrease the rate of deep infection after open fractures compared with conventional dressings.[22]

Planning for wound coverage begins with the initial débridement. Early plastic surgery consultation may be helpful. If skin grafting or muscle flap coverage is necessary, it should be performed within the first 72 hours before secondary colonization and wound fibrosis develop. The desire to avoid nosocomial infection has promoted a trend toward immediate coverage of open fracture wounds. If there is a large soft tissue or bone void present after débridement, local antibiotic delivery may be beneficial while waiting for definitive soft tissue coverage. By using an antibiotic bead pouch (antibiotic-impregnated polymethyl methacrylate beads under an impermeable surgical dressing), high levels of local antibiotics can be delivered without the toxic effects that the same systemic dose would have on the patient.

Limb Salvage versus Primary Amputation

The choice between primary amputation and salvage of a severely injured extremity is a difficult one. Successful salvage depends on a number of factors, including vascular status, extent of soft tissue injury, degree of comminution, bone loss, and neurologic function. In addition to these local factors, ultimate success depends on systemic and psychological elements. Patients with poor nutrition, multisystem injuries, or psychoses and those unable to cooperate with a lengthy reconstructive process may not be candidates for limb salvage. Several scoring systems have been devised to help assess the need for primary amputation objectively. These systems were developed retrospectively in reference to injuries involving the lower part of the leg. Severely injured upper extremities have a far greater impact on the overall functioning status of the patient, and thus indications for upper extremity amputation are significantly more limited.

The Mangled Extremity Severity Score (MESS) is the most widely validated classification system. It is the product of a retrospective review of 25 charts of patients with severe open fractures of the lower extremity (Table 18-4).[15] Investigators found that limb salvage was related to vascular status, age of the patient, duration of ischemia, and absorbed energy. A score of 7 or higher consistently predicted the need for amputation, whereas all limbs with initial scores of 6 or less remained viable in the long term. This system has been validated prospectively, and subsequent studies have almost uniformly supported the specificity of MESS in evaluating a severely injured lower leg. Subsequent studies have confirmed the high specificity (i.e., a low score reliability predicts limb salvage); however, these studies have also shown the sensitivity of the MESS to be low (i.e., a high score does not necessarily predict the need for amputation).[23] Other scoring systems have been shown to be equally poor predictors of the need for amputation.

The combined experiences of the U.S. military dealing with combat-related blast injuries and the Lower Extremity Assessment Project (LEAP) have shaped the current trends in dealing with the mangled extremity. The LEAP study was a prospective, multicenter trial conducted to study patients with severe lower extremity injuries.[24] This study represents the highest evidence available on management of the mangled lower extremity, and several key findings were noted in this group's 7-year follow-up. The first finding was that functional outcomes were similar in patients 2 and 7 years after limb salvage or amputation. Similar rates of pain, return to work, and disability were also found. The lifetime cost to the patient was noted to be higher in the amputation group, mostly because of the cost of prosthetics. The study also raised questions about a previously held absolute indication for amputation, which was lack of plantar foot sensation on arrival indicating disruption of the tibial nerve. A subgroup study showed that many patients with this finding managed with limb salvage had sensation return within 2 years from the index injury, and outcomes for these patients were no different from those of patients with intact sensation on presentation.[25] The MESS, the Limb Salvage Index, and many other scoring systems were also found in this study to have poor utility in predicting which limbs required amputation.

The military conflicts of the last decade resulted in an increased experience with combat-related blast injuries. Lower extremity amputations versus limb salvage in this population were studied in the Military Extremity Trauma Amputation/Limb Salvage (METALS) study.[26] This was a retrospective cohort of 324 patients who underwent limb salvage versus amputation after a wartime injury. The study found similar rates of depression and return to any activity (work and school) as in the LEAP study; however, functional outcomes were notably higher in the amputation group. It is thought that the lower average age as well as the ability immediately to begin structured rehabilitation in the military may have contributed to this finding.

These studies have influenced our current management of the mangled extremity. Absolute indications for amputation are few and include a severe crush injury, a mangled stump or distal tissue not amenable to repair, and a missing extremity. An extremity with warm ischemia time of more than 6 hours should be strongly considered for amputation as well. Finally, if possible, a discussion with the patient should be undertaken to determine the patient's wishes. This may take place after an initial limb salvage procedure if the patient is obtunded on presentation. Should primary amputation be indicated, thorough documentation must take place. It is important to document all pertinent local and systemic factors accurately. A MESS should be calculated for each patient but should be used with caution as a guideline to supplement the clinical findings. Whenever possible, pictures should be taken and added to the permanent medical record. When the indications are not absolute, it is essential that several surgeons evaluate the patient independently and document their opinions in the medical record.

After amputation, multidisciplinary management is critical. Patients should be screened for symptoms of depression and posttraumatic stress disorder and referred appropriately. Physical therapy and orthotics providers should be involved with the patient as soon as the condition permits. Future expectations, including possible repeated surgeries for infection, neuroma, heterotopic ossification, and stump revision, should be discussed with the patient early in the course of treatment.

TABLE 18-4 Mangled Extremity Severity Score

COMPONENT	POINTS
Skeletal and Soft Tissue Injury	
Low energy (stab, simple fracture, civilian gunshot wound)	1
Medium energy (open or multiplex fractures, dislocation)	2
High energy (close-range shotgun or military gunshot wound; crush injury)	3
Very high energy (same as above plus gross contamination, soft tissue avulsion)	4
Limb Ischemia (Doubled If >6 Hours)	
Pulse reduced or absent but perfusion normal	1
Pulseless, paresthesias, diminished capillary refill	2
Cool, paralyzed, insensate, numb	3
Shock	
Systolic blood pressure always >90 mm Hg	0
Hypotensive transiently	1
Persistent hypotension	2
Age (Years)	
<30	0
30-50	1
>50	2

From Johansen K, Daines M, Howey T, et al: Objective criteria accurately predict amputation following lower extremity trauma. *J Trauma* 30:568–573, 1990.

Fractures Secondary to Firearm Injury

Firearm injuries are common in the United States and frequently can involve injury to the musculoskeletal system. Fractures secondary to firearm injury are typically classified according to whether a high-energy (>2000 ft/s projectile velocity) or low-energy (<2000 ft/s) weapon was involved. Most handguns have low muzzle velocity, whereas most hunting and military rifles have a high muzzle velocity. The velocity of the weapon translates into the energy imparted and thus the damage caused to the soft tissues of the body.

Fractures caused by low-velocity weapons are typically treated as sterile, closed fractures. Irrigation and débridement in the ED, tetanus prophylaxis, and a short course of oral antibiotics are the typical treatment for these fractures. Fracture stabilization is dictated by the fracture pattern, as if it was a closed injury. Entrance and exit wounds are usually left open to allow drainage.

Fractures caused by high-velocity weapons are treated per an open fracture protocol. Aggressive débridement, tetanus prophylaxis, and IV antibiotics are the standard of care for these injuries. Temporary stabilization with external fixation is employed to allow soft tissue management until definitive fixation can occur. Most fractures caused by close-range shotguns, despite that they are lower energy weapons, are typically treated in this manner, given the concomitant soft tissue injury.

Intra-articular gunshot injuries deserve special attention. Bullets or fragments that remain lodged in a joint can lead to plumbism or systemic lead toxicity. They can also lead to a breakdown of articular cartilage and the development of early osteoarthritis from third-body wear. These risks as well as the possibility of septic arthritis warrant urgent exploration and removal of intra-articular bullets. This can be performed with formal open arthrotomy or with arthroscopic assistance.

Bullets traversing the intra-abdominal cavity are associated with fractures of the hip, pelvis, and spine (Fig. 18-25*B*). A review has noted that even in injuries that involve a hollow viscus perforation, retained bullet fragments in nonoperative fractures to the pelvis or spine may be managed with a simple course of IV antibiotics for the prevention of osteomyelitis.[27] Broad-spectrum coverage for gram-positive and gram-negative organisms is required. For periarticular gunshots, a CT scan can be a useful adjunct to determine if any fragments remain in the joint. Air seen in the joint space is an indicator that a bullet has violated the joint capsule, in which case irrigation and débridement are indicated. Any involvement of the hip joint and fragments that cause incomplete spinal cord injury warrant consideration for removal.

Skeletal Stabilization

Skeletal stabilization has been shown to be crucial for soft tissue healing. Compared with cast and splints, internal or external fixation permits greater access for wound care and is more effective in controlling pain during mobilization. At the cellular level, the inflammatory response is shortened and the spread of bacteria is diminished. The decision to use one mode of fixation over another is dependent on the fracture pattern, the degree of contamination, and the surgeon's preference.

One of the most widely accepted methods of fixation has been external fixation. In unstable patients or grossly contaminated wounds, standard or ringed external fixation can be used for temporary stabilization or for definitive fixation. External fixation minimizes dissection and avoids the insertion of large metallic implants. It is easily removed, replaced, and adjusted and can be combined with other means of fixation. However, external fixators are not without their problems. Although pin track osteomyelitis has become rare with changes in design and the technique of pin insertion, superficial infection with drainage occurs in approximately 30% of all patients. Because of their size and location, further débridement and coverage can be cumbersome. In the tibia, for example, pin insertion through the subcutaneous anteromedial border reduces pin track infection but often results in obstructed access for plastic and reconstructive surgery. In other cases, more extensive fracture patterns may require more complex frame constructs that further limit access. Although effective in providing skeletal stabilization during soft tissue reconstruction, external fixation is not ideal for achieving fracture union. Additional surgery, including bone grafting or conversion to internal fixation, is often necessary.

For these reasons, IM nailing appears to be an attractive option. Definitive fracture care can usually be accomplished in a single operation. Without bulky exposed hardware, mobilization and daily wound care are facilitated. Concerns about infection have been raised since these methods have been in use, particularly with reamed IM nails. Originally, the increased infection rate was believed to be caused by destruction of cortical blood flow by reaming. The injury itself causes periosteal stripping and significant soft tissue loss. The loss of the medullary blood supply potentially further weakens the bone's healing potential and resistance to infection. However, studies in animals have shown that the endosteal blood supply is reconstituted during a relatively short time. Reaming the IM canal before insertion of the nail allows placement of a larger diameter nail and forces bone marrow in between the fractured bone ends, which facilitates healing. However, studies have shown a higher risk of reoperation when reamed IM nails are used, with higher energy mechanisms of injury, and when a fracture gap is left over the nail.[28] Previous meta-analyses, however, have shown no difference specifically in infection rate between reamed and unreamed nails. Although there is still controversy about reamed versus unreamed nailing, the general consensus is that in a stable patient, IM nailing is the fixation of choice for open tibial fractures. High rates of infection have been shown when delayed conversion from external fixation to IM nailing is performed; however, the infection rate is significantly reduced when the conversion happens within 2 weeks. Open periarticular fractures and fractures of the upper extremity should be treated with plate fixation if the patient's condition warrants. Many fractures that in isolation are treated conservatively (clavicle fractures, humeral shaft fractures) are operatively stabilized in the multitrauma patient to allow earlier weight bearing in those limbs for physical therapy.

Acute Compartment Syndrome

Compartment syndrome can occur in any closed fascial space. Usually, this occurs in a myofascial space secondary to trauma. The causes of compartment syndrome are numerous and include but are not limited to open and closed fractures, arterial injury, gunshot wounds, snake bites, extravasation at venous and arterial access sites, limb crush injuries, burns, constrictive dressings, and tight casts. Rapid diagnosis and management of compartment syndrome is paramount to achieve a successful clinical outcome. This section addresses the pathogenesis, diagnosis, and management of acute compartment syndrome, specifically in the forearm and lower part of the leg.

Early recognition and treatment of compartment syndrome are critical in a trauma patient to avoid limb dysfunction, limb amputation, and even death. Volkmann was the first to describe the sequelae of postischemic contracture more than a century ago. He attributed permanent muscle contracture to trauma, swelling, and tight bandaging. As the late complications of compartment syndrome of the upper and lower extremities have been elucidated, the importance of early recognition and fasciotomy have become apparent. Failure to diagnose and to treat this complication has resulted in numerous cases of preventable morbidity, rare cases of mortality, and litigation. Missed or delayed diagnosis of compartment syndrome is one of the most common causes of malpractice litigation for orthopedic surgeons.

Pathogenesis

Compartment syndrome occurs secondary to increased pressure in the enclosed fascial space. The most common cause of compartment syndrome in an orthopedic patient is muscle edema from direct trauma to the extremity or reperfusion after vascular injury. This edema causes an increase in compartment pressure, which prevents venous outflow from the affected extremity. The backflow congestion furthers the cycle of increasing pressure and muscle ischemia. In the case of an orthopedic trauma patient with a long bone fracture, bleeding from the fracture produces a space-occupying hematoma that exacerbates the situation. On reduction of the fracture, compartment pressures increase secondary to a decrease in the compartmental volume. External compressive casts or bandages further reduce the ability of the compartment to expand.

Controversy exists about the level of compartment pressure for which surgical intervention is required. Mubarak and Hargens[29] have determined that an absolute tissue pressure of 30 mm Hg is the critical value at which fasciotomy should be performed. They concluded that because normal capillary pressure is 30 mm Hg, higher pressure would result in tissue necrosis. Other authors have argued that the absolute pressure may be less important than the pressure in relation to the diastolic pressure (ΔP). McQueen and Court-Brown[30] have shown that in patients who had sustained intracompartmental pressure difference of 30 mm Hg or more relative to the diastolic blood pressure, there was no residual muscle damage at follow-up. They recommended this ΔP as an indication for fasciotomy. Current recommendations vary, but most authors agree that a ΔP of 30 mm Hg or less is an absolute indication for compartment release.

Although there is controversy about when a fasciotomy should be performed, there is little debate about the effect of prolonged ischemia on skeletal muscle and nerve tissue. Investigators have determined that peripheral nerves and muscles can survive for as long as 4 hours under ischemic conditions without irreversible damage. An ischemia time of 6 hours results in a variable return of function in muscle and nerve tissue, and a total ischemia time longer than 8 hours leads to irreversible nerve and muscle injury.[31]

Diagnosis

The diagnosis of acute compartment syndrome requires a high degree of clinical suspicion, a full understanding of the mechanism of injury, and careful serial physical examinations (Fig. 18-26). Tscherne and Gotzen[13] have stated that the more severe the initial soft tissue injury, the greater the probability that soft tissue complications, including compartment syndrome, will develop. The diagnosis of compartment syndrome relies on an understanding of high-risk injury patterns, the subjective complaints of the patients, and an appreciation of early and late physical and clinical findings.

The classic signs of compartment syndrome are taught as the six *p*'s: pain out of proportion to injury, pallor, paralysis, paresthesias, pulselessness, and poikilothermia. In clinical practice, all of these findings except pain are either unreliable or not

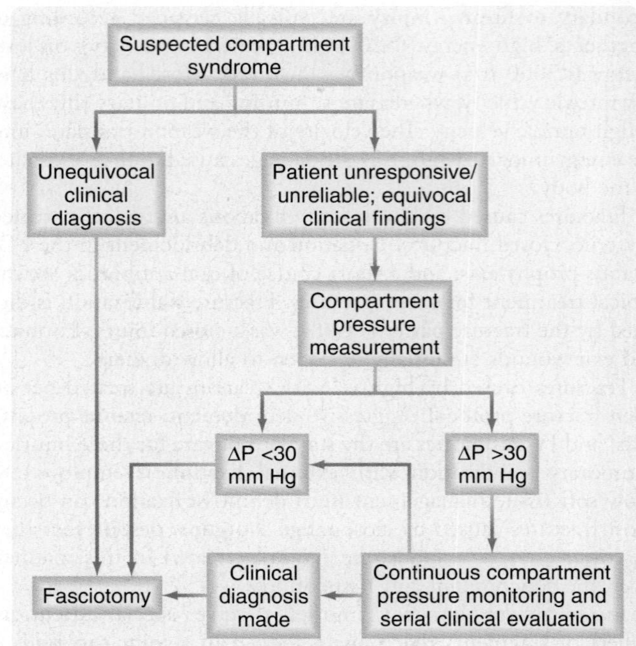

FIGURE 18-26 Algorithm for the management of a patient with suspected compartment syndrome.

manifested until permanent injury has occurred. Patients who are thought to have compartment syndrome should undergo either immediate fasciotomies or serial clinical examinations if the diagnosis is unclear. Compartment pressure measurements should be avoided in the awake patient who is able to give a good examination. In this type of patient, findings concerning for compartment syndrome (pain with passive stretch, tight compartments to palpation, increased narcotic requirements) should be treated as such and managed operatively.

Awake patients with a truly equivocal examination should undergo serial examinations and compartment measurement at the discretion of the attending physician. The trend away from spot compartment measurements in these patients is due to the recent evidence showing a lack of reliability and a high false-positive rate with one-time compartment measurements.[32] New research by McQueen and coworkers[33] documenting a 10-year experience with continuous intracompartmental monitoring of 850 patients with tibial fractures has shown this to be a safe, sensitive, and specific method for diagnosis. This method, however, has not been shown to make a difference in time to fasciotomy in previous trials and requires intensive care unit (ICU) care and equipment to perform. Obtunded patients are treated separately, with a reliance on the methods of compartment measurement as they cannot provide an accurate physical examination. Overall, compartment measurements remain controversial in their application and what pressure constitutes an indication for release, yet they remain a valuable tool for the obtunded patient or the patient with an equivocal serial examination.

Tissue Pressure Measurement Technique

Many methods have been described for evaluation of compartment pressures. The two most common techniques include the wick catheter and side port needle. The wick catheter has the benefit of continuous pressure monitoring by using a continuous, low-volume infusion technique. This may be used as an indwelling device for recording compartment pressures at multiple time

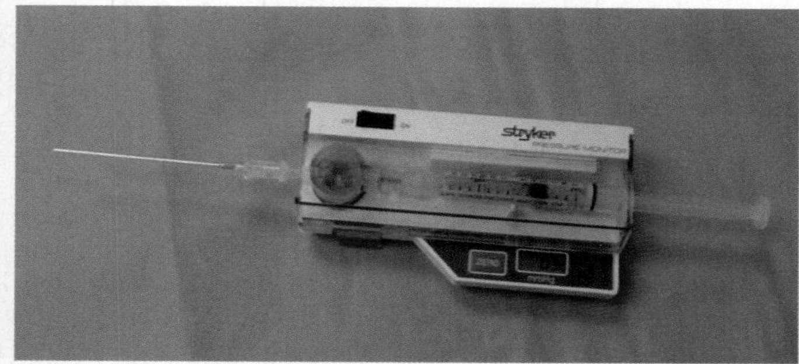

FIGURE 18-27 Stryker STIC catheter.

points. The most common method of measurement is the Stryker Intra-Compartmental Pressure Monitor System (STIC; Stryker, Mahwah, NJ), which uses the side port needle technique (Fig. 18-27). This hand-held electronic device is easily calibrated and used. Pressures are obtained by inserting the needle into each compartment and infusing a low volume of fluid until pressure equilibrium is reached. It is generally used to make measurements at one point in time and is not an indwelling device.

In place of invasive methods of measuring compartment pressure, fiberoptic devices are available in which near-infrared spectroscopy is used to measure tissue perfusion as a function of hemoglobin saturation. These devices allow continuous transcutaneous monitoring and are becoming more widely available. By using the absorptive wavelength of venous muscle oxyhemoglobin, near-infrared spectroscopy can evaluate the viability of a compartment at risk. Increased application of this technology in the diagnosis of chronic compartment syndrome has led to its more routine use in the acute and subacute setting.

Surgical Treatment

The two-incision approach to fasciotomy (Fig. 18-28) of the lower part of the leg is a reliable and straightforward procedure, given that the anatomy is well understood (Table 18-5). This approach involves making an anterolateral incision over the anterior and lateral compartments and a medial incision just posterior to the medial aspect of the tibia. The anterolateral incision is centered halfway between the fibular shaft and tibia. Once the fascia is identified, a small transverse incision is made to identify the anterior and lateral compartments as well as the superficial peroneal nerve traveling in the lateral compartment. It is important to release the entire compartment, including the most proximal and distal aspects. The posteromedial incision is used to decompress the superficial and deep posterior compartments. The incision is made approximately 2 cm posterior to the tibial shaft. Care must be taken to preserve the saphenous nerve and vein. Once the fascia is identified, a transverse incision is made to delineate the superficial and deep compartments. The superficial posterior compartment is released first, proximal and distal to the medial malleolus. In similar fashion, the deep posterior compartment is released. To decompress the deep compartment completely, the soleus muscle must be taken down off the medial side of the tibia.

The skin incisions should not be closed primarily after fasciotomy (although closing one incision may be appropriate if a tension-free closure is possible). Even though the fascia has been released, closing the skin can lead to a dangerous increase in intramuscular pressures. Secondary closure may be attempted when limb swelling has been reduced (3 to 5 days). Wound management before closure consists of wet to dry dressing changes or placement of a negative pressure dressing. Negative pressure

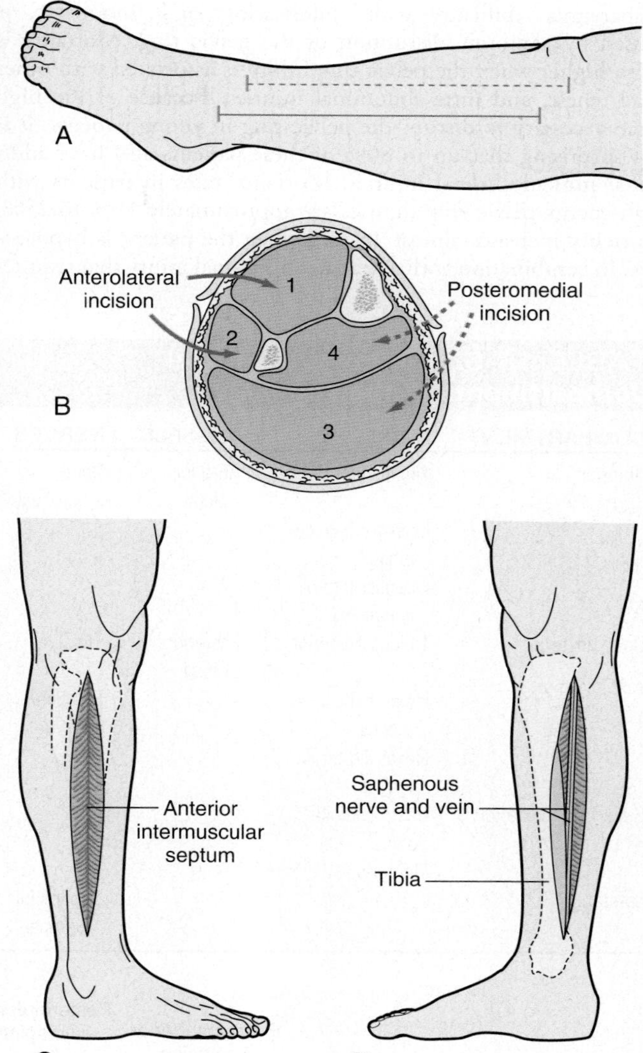

FIGURE 18-28 **A,** Double-incision technique for performing fasciotomies of all four compartments of the lower extremity. **B,** Cross section of the lower extremity showing positions of anterolateral and posteromedial incisions that allow access to the anterior and lateral compartments (*1* and *2*) and the superficial and deep posterior compartments (*3* and *4*). **C,** The anterior intramuscular septum should be identified in the lateral incision as it marks the division of the anterior and lateral leg compartments. **D,** The saphenous nerve and vein are identified in the medial incision and should be protected during compartment release.

dressings help reduce swelling and may help bring the skin edges together without undue tension. Skin closure of the fasciotomy can also be facilitated with vessel loops laced through staples placed along the skin edges. The vessel loops can be tightened daily at the bedside as the soft tissue swelling diminishes, which may eliminate the need for skin grafting. If a tension-free closure is not possible, the exposed muscle can be covered with a split-thickness skin graft.

Pelvic Ring Disruption

Pelvic ring disruption is a major cause of morbidity and mortality in multiply injured patients. Fatalities result from uncontrolled retroperitoneal hemorrhage and other associated injuries. Long-term disability, such as low back pain, leg length discrepancies, dyspareunia, difficulty with childbearing, and impotence, is caused by anatomic disruption of the pelvic ring. Mortality is often higher when the pelvic ring injury is associated with other head, chest, and intra-abdominal injuries. Because of the high force necessary to disrupt the pelvic ring in young patients, it is not surprising that up to 80% of these patients also have additional musculoskeletal injuries. Mortality rates in patients with high-energy pelvic ring injuries are approximately 15% to 25%. Mortality increases almost 13-fold when the patient is hypotensive. In combination with a head or abdominal injury that requires surgical intervention, mortality increases to 50%. When both procedures are necessary, mortality approaches 90%.[7]

Classification

Pelvic ring disruption can be broadly classified into two major groups, stable and unstable. A stable pelvis is defined as one that can withstand normal physiologic forces without being displaced. This stability depends on the integrity of the osseous and ligamentous structures (Fig. 18-29). Instability can be divided into rotational and vertical components (Fig. 18-30). Stable injuries include nondisplaced fractures of the pelvic ring and fractures resulting in less than 2.5 cm of displacement of anterior structures, the pubic rami or pubic symphysis. Rotational instability is characterized by widening of the symphysis pubis or displacement of pubic ramus fractures by more than 2.5 cm. Superior translation of a hemipelvis through fractures of the sacrum or ilium and vertical disruption of the sacroiliac joint by more than 1 cm constitute vertical instability. Serial sectioning studies have revealed that division of the symphyseal ligaments alone leads to an anterior diastasis of 2.5 cm or less and maintenance of stability.[34] Further sectioning of the anterior sacroiliac ligaments and sacrospinous and sacrotuberous ligaments (pelvic floor) imparts rotational instability. Vertical instability results only after the posterior sacroiliac ligaments are sectioned. Transverse process fractures of the L5 vertebrae should raise suspicion for pelvic instability secondary to disruption of the iliolumbar ligament. Displaced fractures (e.g., superior and inferior pubic ramus fractures, sacral or iliac wing fracture) can result in similar instability patterns. Because the pelvis is a true ring structure, significant anterior displacement must be accompanied by posterior disruption. Disruptions in the pelvic ring are usually a combination of osseous and ligamentous injury.

Early recognition of an unstable pelvic ring is essential because pelvic instability is associated with potentially fatal hemorrhage.

TABLE 18-5 Contents of Fascial Compartments in the Leg

COMPARTMENT	MUSCLES	VESSELS	NERVES
Anterior	Tibialis anterior	Anterior tibial	Deep peroneal
	Extensor hallucis longus		
	Extensor digitorum communis		
Deep posterior	Tibialis posterior	Posterior tibial	Tibial
	Flexor hallucis longus		Peroneal
	Flexor digitorum longus		
Superficial posterior	Gastrocnemius		
	Soleus		
	Plantaris		
Lateral			Superficial peroneal

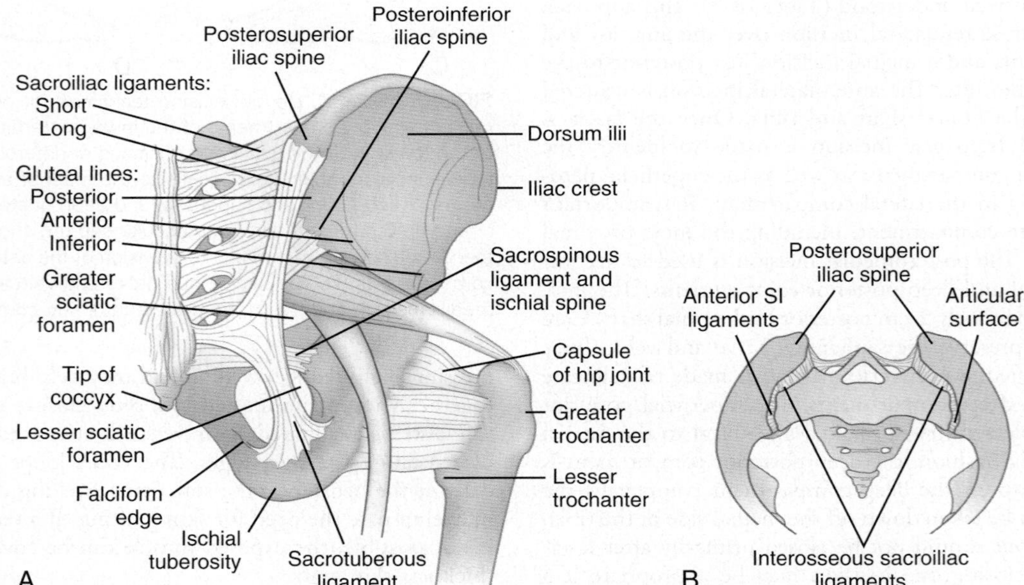

FIGURE 18-29 Ligamentous Complexes of the Pelvis. A, Posteriorly, the major ligaments noted in the region of the sacroiliac (SI) joint are the posterior SI ligaments, both long and short. The long ligaments blend with the sacrospinous and sacrotuberous ligaments. **B,** In cross section, the orientation of the very thick posterior interosseous SI ligaments is noted. (From Stover MD, Mayo KA, Kellam JF: Pelvic ring disruptions. In Browner BD, Levine AM, Jupiter JB, et al, editors: *Skeletal trauma: Basic science, management, and reconstruction*, ed 4, Philadelphia, 2008, WB Saunders.)

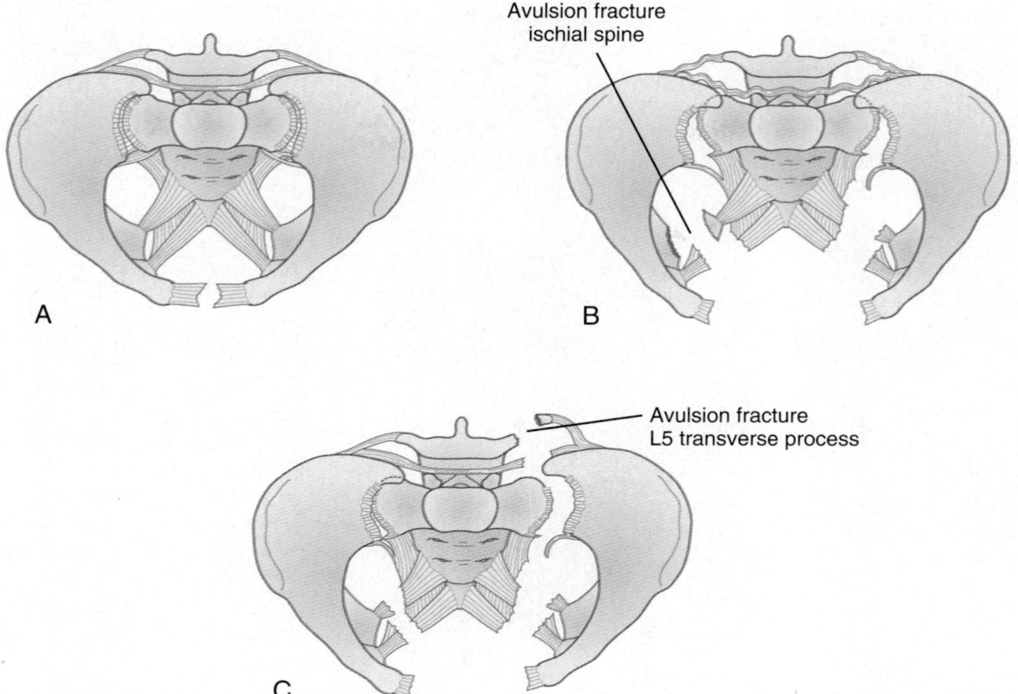

FIGURE 18-30 A, Division of the symphysis pubis allows the pelvis to open to approximately 2.5 cm with no damage to any posterior ligamentous structures. **B,** Division of the anterior sacroiliac and sacrospinous ligaments, either by direct division of their fibers *(right)* or by avulsion of the tip of the ischial spine *(left)*, allows the pelvis to rotate externally until the posterior superior iliac spines abut the sacrum. Note, however, that the posterior ligamentous structures (e.g., the posterior sacroiliac and iliolumbar ligaments) remain intact. Therefore, no displacement in the vertical plane is possible. **C,** Division of the posterior band ligaments, that is, the posterior sacroiliac as well as the iliolumbar, causes complete instability of the hemipelvis. Note that global displacement is now possible. (From Stover MD, Mayo KA, Kellam JF: Pelvic ring disruptions. In Browner BD, Levine AM, Jupiter JB, et al, editors: *Skeletal trauma: Basic science, management, and reconstruction*, ed 4, Philadelphia, 2008, WB Saunders.)

In addition, these injuries require intervention to reestablish the pelvic ring anatomy and to minimize late disability. Determination of the stability of the injured hemipelvis must be established through a combination of physical examination and review of the imaging studies. An anterior defect can sometimes be detected by palpation at the symphysis pubis. Rotational instability can be appreciated with lateral compression of the pelvis through the anterior iliac spines. Because repeated manipulation can cause iatrogenic injury, such handling needs to be done only once. Vertical instability may be appreciated with push-pull radiographs. These are obtained by taking two separate AP pelvic radiographs, one view with lower extremity traction and one with an axial load applied to the leg on the affected side. In 90% of cases, the physical examination and AP pelvic radiograph are sufficient to assess stability and to guide initial treatment. Anterior injuries are easily identified on this projection, and most unstable posterior injuries can also be appreciated.

Detailed classification systems have been developed on the basis of the direction of force, stability of the pelvis, location of the fracture, and whether it is an open or closed injury. The Young and Burgess classification characterizes pelvic ring fractures on the basis of the mechanism of injury (Fig. 18-31).[7] Fracture patterns are divided into three types (A, B, C), depending on the direction of the deforming force. Type A results from a lateral compression (LC) force, type B results from an AP compression (APC) force, and type C results from a vertical shear force. Type A and type B fractures are further subdivided into types I, II, and III patterns, depending on the amount of ligamentous or osseous disruption. In both cases, type I fractures are stable, type II are rotationally unstable, and type III are rotationally and vertically unstable. APC injuries have the greatest risk for retroperitoneal hemorrhage. The APC III, also known as an open-book pelvis, significantly increases the volume of the pelvis, allowing massive blood loss in a short time (Fig. 18-32). Intrapelvic visceral injuries are also more common with the AP patterns. Mortality in APC injuries is related to a combination of retroperitoneal bleeding and visceral injuries. LC and vertical shear fractures are associated with intra-abdominal and head injuries. Whereas intrapelvic hemorrhage occurs in LC fractures, the most common cause of death in a patient with this injury pattern is associated closed head trauma.[7]

Management

Pelvic stabilization and control of hemorrhage are the goals of initial management of unstable pelvic ring injuries. In most pelvic fractures, hemorrhage results from disruption of the pelvic venous plexus posteriorly and bleeding cancellous bone. Most bleeding resulting from pelvic fracture comes from the presacral venous plexus (Fig. 18-33). As a result, initial treatment of hemorrhage must focus on control of venous bleeding by reduction and stabilization of the pelvic ring. Reduction leads to a decrease in pelvic volume and tamponade of the bleeding vessels through compression of the viscera and pelvic hematoma. Stabilization maintains

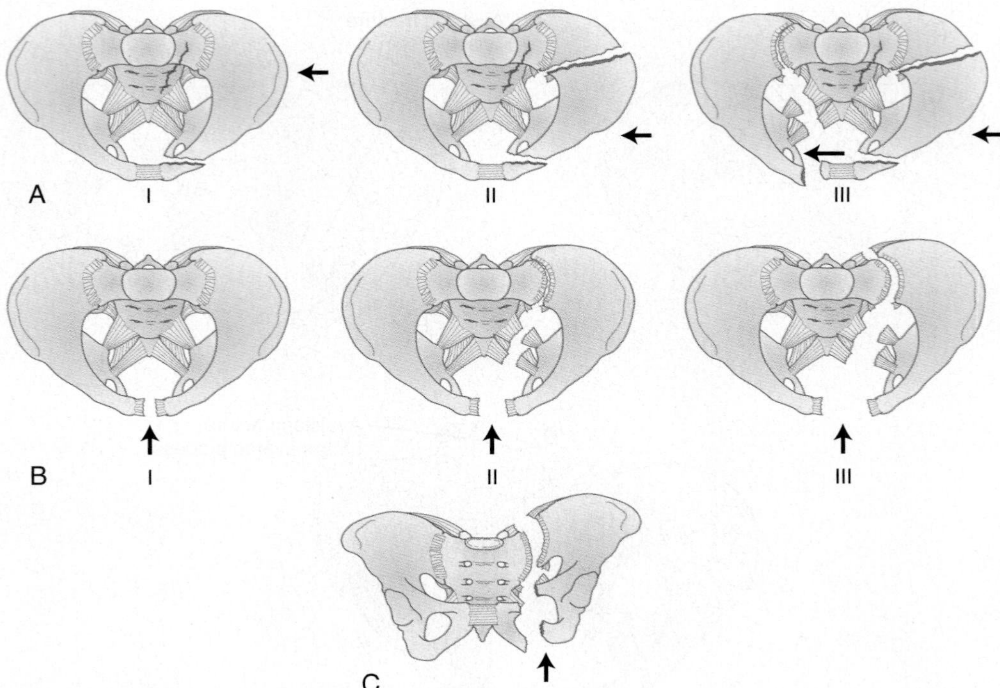

FIGURE 18-31 **Young and Burgess Classification. A,** Lateral compression force. Type I, a posteriorly directed force causing a sacral crushing injury and horizontal pubic ramus fractures ipsilaterally. This injury is stable. Type II, a more anteriorly directed force causing horizontal pubic ramus fractures with an anterior sacral crushing injury and either disruption of the posterior sacroiliac joints or fractures through the iliac wing. This injury is ipsilateral. Type III, an anteriorly directed force that is continued and leads to a type I or type II ipsilateral fracture with an external rotation component to the contralateral side; the sacroiliac joint is opened posteriorly, and the sacrotuberous and spinous ligaments are disrupted. **B,** AP compression fractures. Type I, an AP-directed force opening the pelvis but with the posterior ligamentous structures intact. This injury is stable. Type II, continuation of a type I fracture with disruption of the sacrospinous and potentially the sacrotuberous ligaments and an anterior sacroiliac joint opening. This fracture is rotationally unstable. Type III, a completely unstable or vertical instability pattern with complete disruption of all ligamentous supporting structures. **C,** A vertically directed force at right angles to the supporting structures of the pelvis leading to vertical fractures in the rami and disruption of all the ligamentous structures. This injury is equivalent to an AP type III or a completely unstable and rotationally unstable fracture. (Adapted from Young JWR, Burgess AR: *Radiologic management of pelvic ring fractures*, Baltimore, 1987, Urban and Schwarzenberg.)

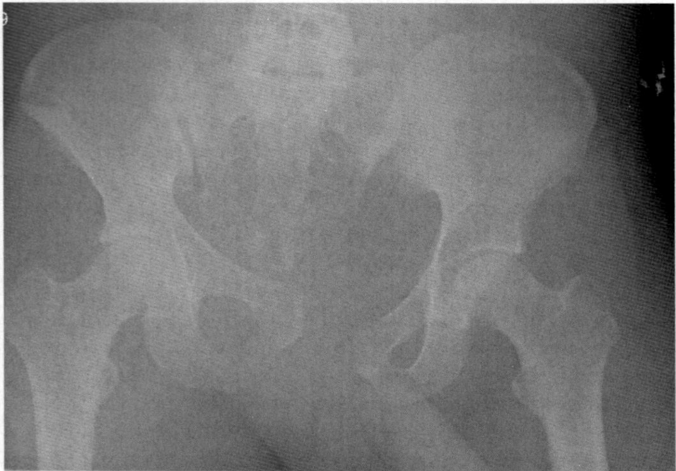

FIGURE 18-32 AP pelvic radiograph showing the so-called open-book pelvis. Complete disruption of the anterior and posterior ligamentous structures leaves this pelvis rotationally and vertically unstable.

the reduction and avoids movement of the hemipelvis, thereby reducing pain and limiting disruption of any organizing thrombus. In patients who remain hemodynamically unstable after initial resuscitation and stabilization, a source of arterial bleeding must be considered. A prospective study of 143 high-energy pelvic fracture patients showed that 10% had arterial injury.[35] Factors predicting arterial bleeding included a base deficit of 6 mmol/L, a systolic blood pressure below 104 mm Hg, and the need for transfusion in the ED.[35] CT angiography is another useful tool to evaluate patients who may benefit from angiographic or open control of pelvic bleeding. The significance of a "pelvic blush" finding on CT, however, remains controversial. A study by Verbeek and coworkers[36] demonstrated that of 42% of patients with pelvic ring injuries who had a pelvic blush on CT, only 47% of them required pelvic hemorrhage control. The negative predictive value of CT angiography is much higher, typically above 90%.

Stabilization of pelvic ring injuries accomplishes more than simply control of hemorrhage. Patients with a stabilized pelvis may more easily be transferred in bed, be repositioned, and have the head of the bed elevated. This facilitates the care of these

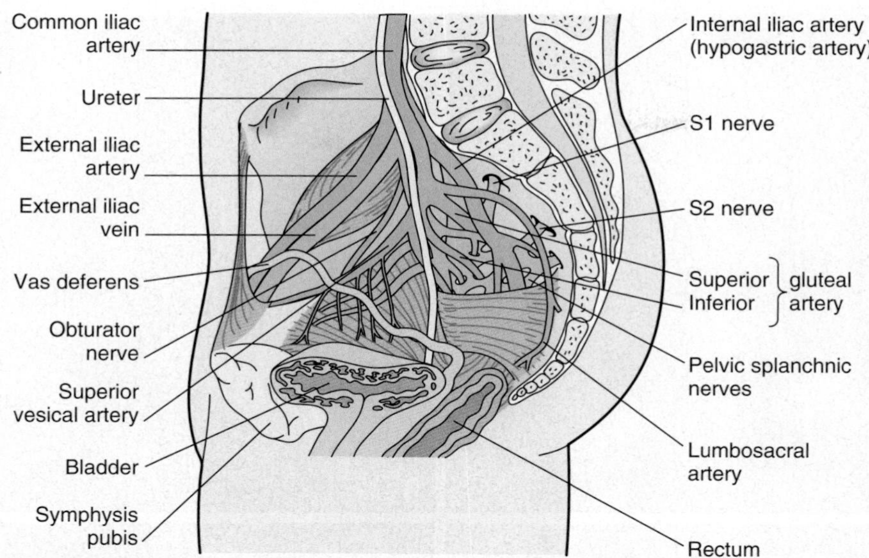

FIGURE 18-33 Internal aspect of the pelvis showing the great vessels and lumbosacral plexus as well as the pelvic floor, bladder, and rectum. (From Stover MD, Mayo KA, Kellam JF: Pelvic ring disruptions. In Browner BD, Levine AM, Jupiter JB, et al, editors: *Skeletal trauma: Basic science, management, and reconstruction*, ed 4, Philadelphia, 2008, WB Saunders.)

usually multiply injured patients in the ICU. Pain management and the decrease in the inflammatory cascade associated with an unstable, mobile fracture site are also benefits.

Initial stabilization. The initial stabilization of a patient with a pelvic ring injury occurs in the prehospital setting. When field personnel detect unstable pelvic ring disruptions on physical examination, they can begin treatment by binding the pelvis with a rolled sheet or applying pneumatic antishock garments (PASGs). Like air splints applied to the extremities, the garment functions by compressing the pelvis. If they are applied in the field, PASGs should not be deflated until the patient is being resuscitated in the trauma room. A PASG has the advantage of ease of use, application in the field, and reusability. However, it blocks access to the patient and restricts excursion of the diaphragm, and there have been reports of gluteal and thigh compartment syndromes developing after extended use of PASGs in hypotensive patients. Because of this, the use of the pelvic binder has become more common. These devices have been shown through biomechanical studies and clinical experience to effectively reduce pelvic volume.[37] Binders or sheets are properly applied by centering them over the greater trochanters and applying pressure. The more proximal part of the construct may be cut away to allow access to the lower abdomen if necessary. Internally rotating both legs and holding this position with tape across the ankles or knees also assists in pelvic reduction. These devices should be removed from the patient as soon as possible as skin breakdown can begin to occur quickly. In LC-type pelvic injuries, the binder may over-reduce the fracture by applying the same force on the pelvis as the initial injury, and it is not recommended in these patterns.

The standard method for controlling pelvic hemorrhage after sheet or binder removal has been the application of an anterior external fixation frame. When it is applied properly, an anterior pelvic external fixator should provide stability to the pelvis and hematoma while allowing access to the abdomen for surgical procedures. Although these devices can be applied in the ED, placement is frequently deferred until the patient is brought to the operating suite. In these cases, the pelvis can remain displaced for many hours, with venous bleeding continuing uncontrolled.

If an external fixator cannot be applied expeditiously, another method of provisional stabilization must be used. Devices called pelvic C-clamps have been developed that can be applied rapidly to reduce and provisionally stabilize the pelvis in the ED. Their design allows compression of the pelvis through percutaneous pins applied to the outer surface of the ilium, and they permit easy access to the abdomen or extremities (Fig. 18-34). The C-clamps can remain in place throughout the resuscitation phase and then be replaced by definitive stabilization methods when appropriate. Binders and sheets remain the preferred method of stabilization before external fixation because serious complications can result with C-clamp use from misplacement of the pins without fluoroscopic control.

Definitive management. Long-term definitive care of pelvic ring disruption is dependent on the pattern of injury and its severity. Stable fracture patterns usually require no more than restricted weight bearing. Frequently, an external fixator can provide definitive stabilization of unstable injuries if it is applied effectively and reduction is maintained. In cases in which the fixator may be obstructing access to the abdomen or an interim binder has been applied, ORIF or closed reduction and percutaneous fixation may be indicated. When rotational or vertical instability is present, the anterior and posterior pelvis must be stabilized. Anteriorly, the symphysis is often secured with a plate and screws. Posteriorly, more options exist. The sacroiliac joint or sacral fractures can be secured with plates, bars, or percutaneously inserted cannulated screws (Fig. 18-35). When only rotational instability is present, the posterior ligaments are usually only partially disrupted. After the anterior pelvis is secured, pelvic ring stability should be reexamined. Often, no posterior fixation is necessary.

Spinal Injuries

Evaluation

The initial evaluation of the trauma patient for spinal injuries follows the ATLS protocol as described earlier in this chapter. All

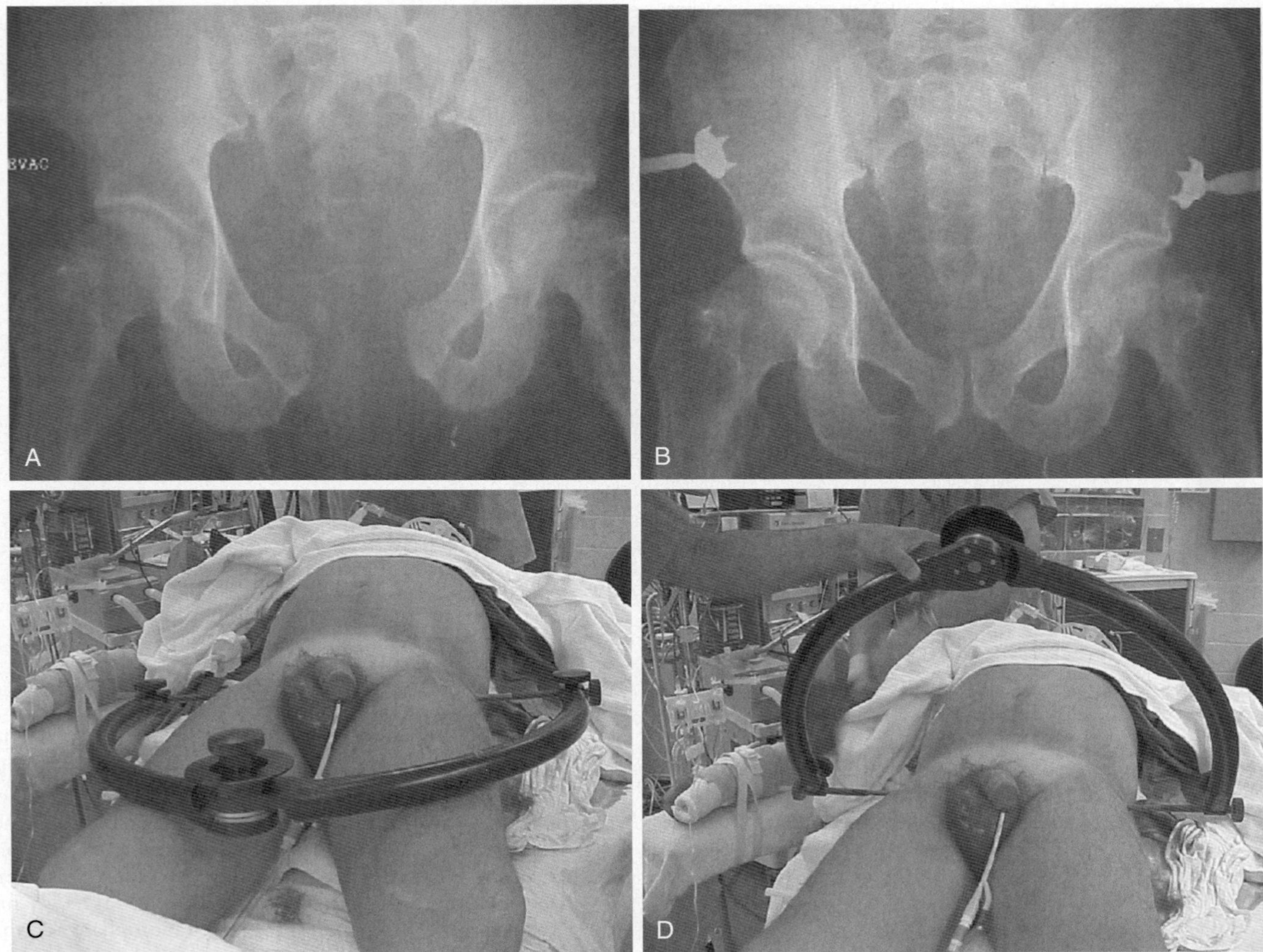

FIGURE 18-34 **Pelvic Ring Disruption with Massive Hemorrhage.** **A,** AP radiograph of the pelvis showing disruption of the symphysis pubis and sacroiliac joint. **B,** AP view of the pelvis after reduction by the application of a pelvic stabilizer. **C** and **D,** Patient with the pelvic stabilizer in the standard position and elevated to allow access to the perineum or to permit flexion of the hips for change to the lithotomy position.

trauma patients are typically placed in a cervical collar in the prehospital or ED phase of care, especially if neck pain is present or the patient has a distracting injury. Level 1 evidence suggests that the awake, sober, neurologically intact patient without distracting injury should have the collar removed as soon as possible if certain criteria are met.[38] To have the collar removed, these patients must have no tenderness to palpation in the cervical spine and must have full pain-free active range of motion. If midline neck pain or tenderness is present, CT evaluation is indicated. Likewise, the intoxicated patient or those with multiple distracting injuries should also have a CT evaluation. MRI may be used to identify injury to the posterior ligamentous structures.

Acute compression of the spinal cord can lead to spinal shock, which is detectable by physical examination. For diagnosis of spinal shock, the bulbocavernosus reflex is tested by tugging on the Foley catheter and looking for an anal wink. An absent reflex indicates spinal shock if the spinal column injury is above the lumbar spine. As spinal shock resolves, usually during 48 hours, this reflex returns. Examination at this point will provide a more accurate indication of neurologic deficits. The presence of sacral sparing (intact perianal sensation, rectal tone, or great toe flexion) represents at least partial continuity of the white matter long tracts. After a full neuromotor examination, an ASIA classification may be assigned to the spine-injured patient (Fig. 18-36).

Management

The spinal cord is divided into three columns (Fig. 18-37). The anterior column consists of the anterior two thirds of the vertebral body as well as the anterior longitudinal ligament. The middle column includes the posterior third of the vertebral body and the posterior longitudinal ligament. The posterior column includes all bone and ligamentous structures posterior to the posterior longitudinal ligament. In general, injury to one column results in a stable injury. Injury to two or three columns results in an unstable spinal segment. Instability in the spinal column puts the spinal cord at risk. Burst fractures, by definition, involve injury to the anterior and middle columns. These fractures are to be differentiated from compression fractures, which involve the anterior column only and are rarely associated with spinal cord injury. Burst fractures commonly occur after a fall from a height in which

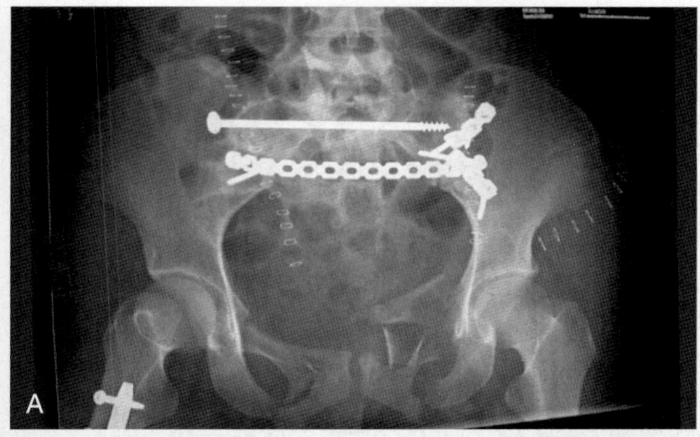

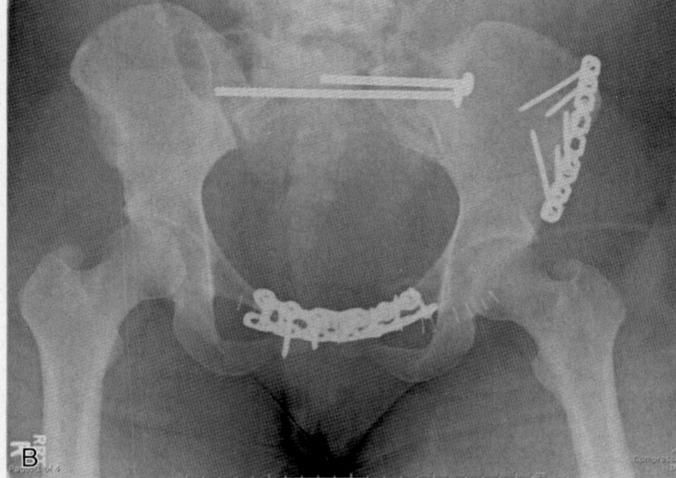

FIGURE 18-35 **Fixation of Unstable Pelvic Fractures. A,** One transiliac screw, one transiliac plate, and two left sacroiliac plates were used to stabilize the posterior elements in this fracture. **B,** One transiliac screw and one sacroiliac screw were used to stabilize the posterior elements of this fracture. Plates were used to stabilize the pubic symphysis. An iliac crest plate was used to fix the left iliac wing fracture.

an axial load is transmitted to the upper axial skeleton when the feet strike the ground first. This mechanism results in a common pattern of fractures, including calcaneus, tibial plateau, proximal femur, and lumbar burst fractures (see Table 18-1). Depending on the fracture pattern, treatment of spine injuries may range from observation to bracing, surgical fixation, or external halo fixation. However, treatment of all injuries begins with strict immobilization and spine precautions.

Cervical spine injuries can occur by several mechanisms, which can be divided into three main categories. The first involves direct trauma to the neck itself. The second mechanism involves motion of the head relative to the axial skeleton. This injury can occur by direct trauma to the head or continued movement of the head relative to the fixed body (whiplash), as often occurs in blunt trauma such as motor vehicle accidents, when the body is restrained. In attempting to tether the head against motion, the cervical spine endures a large bending or twisting moment that results in flexion-extension injuries or rotational injuries, respectively. A third mechanism of cervical spine injury involves a direct axial load imparted on the cranium that causes axial compression forces across the cervical vertebrae. This may result in a burst fracture and potential spinal cord injury. This pattern of injury is more commonly seen in the lumbar spine. An algorithm for diagnosis of cervical spine injuries is presented in Figure 18-38.

Thoracolumbar injuries are typically divided into compression (simple or burst), rotation/translation, or distraction mechanisms. The Thoracolumbar Injury Classification and Severity (TLICS) score is used to describe these injuries and to guide their management (Table 18-6).[39] The classification system has shown good reliability and validity and helps guide management. Compression fractures are typically managed nonoperatively if there is not a significant (>25%) loss of height. Bracing or kyphoplasty may be offered if pain limits a patient's recovery.

Burst fractures are manifested with varying levels of bone deformity. The three radiographic measures used to determine the severity of the injury are body height loss, focal kyphosis, and retropulsion of bone fragments into the canal (Fig. 18-39). In general, indications for surgical decompression and stabilization of a lumbar burst fracture include retropulsion of more than 50% of the spinal canal, 50% body height loss, and 25 degrees of focal kyphosis.[3] Retropulsion and focal kyphosis can lead to spinal canal compromise and acute cord or cauda equina compression. Translational or distracting injuries are managed on the basis of the fracture pattern and neurologic status of the patient. MRI can be used to determine the stability of the posterior ligamentous complex. Spinal stabilization with or without fusion and removal of fragments causing canal compromise can be offered for surgical treatment.

Cauda equina syndrome may be caused by space-occupying lesions such as fractures, herniated discs, tumor, and hematoma. The classic symptoms of cauda equina syndrome include varying degrees of back pain, bladder dysfunction (characterized early by urinary retention, followed later by overflow incontinence), saddle anesthesia, lower extremity numbness, and weakness and reduced rectal tone (a late finding). If cauda equina syndrome is suspected, MRI should be ordered immediately to look for canal compromise. If MRI is not available or the patient cannot undergo MRI, CT myelography can be performed. When a diagnosis of cauda equina syndrome is confirmed, surgical exploration and decompression should be performed.

Dislocations

Dislocation of any joint is considered an orthopedic emergency. Prolonged dislocation can lead to cartilage cell death, post-traumatic arthritis, ankylosis, and avascular necrosis. Dislocations of major joints (e.g., shoulder, elbow, hip, knee, or ankle) are particularly concerning because of the high risk of neurovascular injury. These injuries, which are more likely to occur in young active patients, can have devastating consequences.

Patient Evaluation

Most dislocations have characteristic physical findings. After a dislocation, muscles around the joint typically become spasmodic, thereby limiting range of motion as the limb assumes a distinctive position. In posterior hip dislocations, the thigh is held flexed and internally rotated. The affected limb is often shortened and cannot be passively extended. An anterior shoulder dislocation causes an externally rotated and adducted arm position. Elbow and knee dislocations (most commonly posterior) result in an extremity locked in extension (Fig. 18-40). As with all extremity injuries, a meticulous neurovascular examination must be performed and documented before and after manipulation.

Hip and knee dislocations require special discussion because of the extreme consequences of failure to recognize and to address

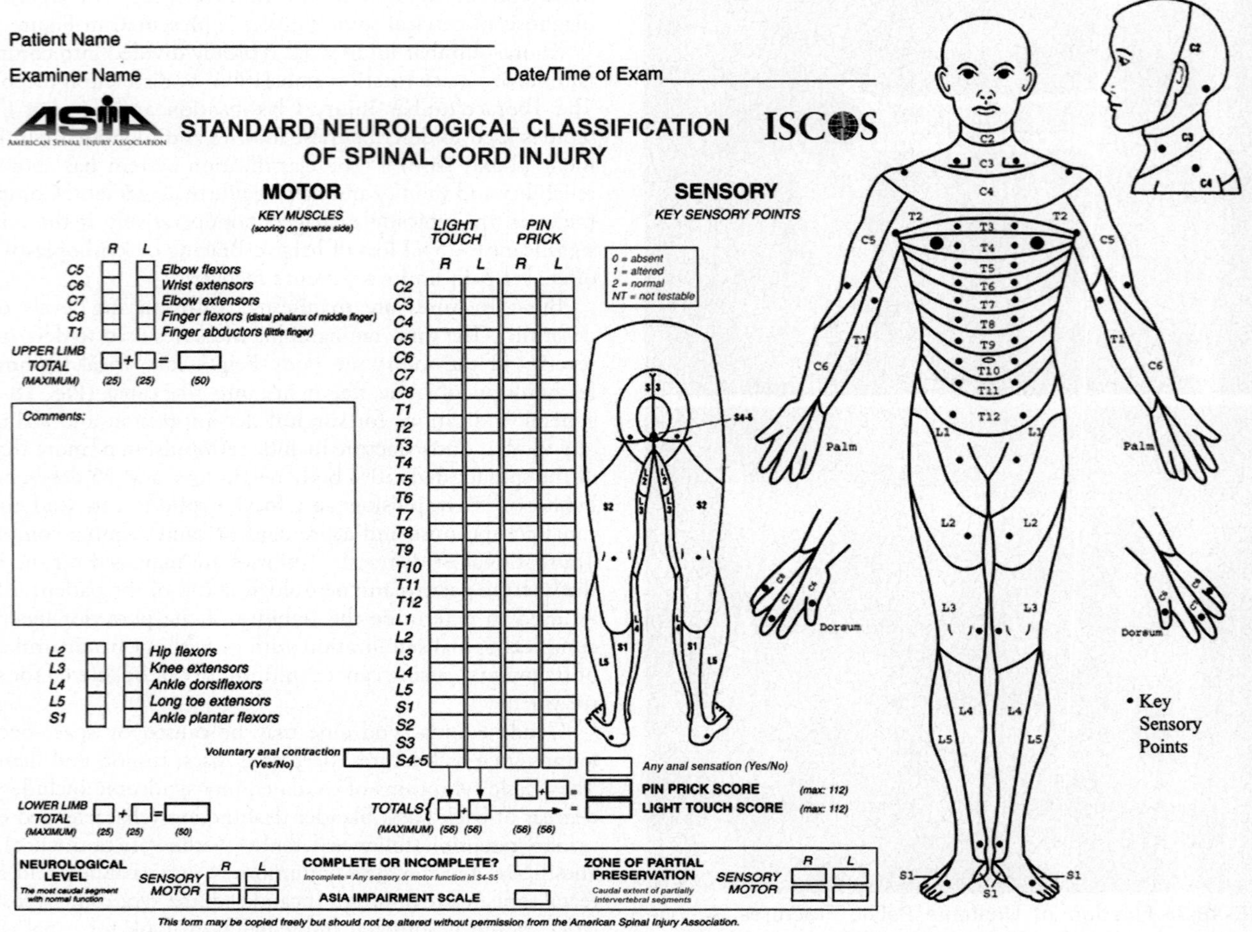

Patient Name ______________________

Examiner Name ______________________ Date/Time of Exam ______________________

ASIA — American Spinal Injury Association

STANDARD NEUROLOGICAL CLASSIFICATION OF SPINAL CORD INJURY ISCOS

MOTOR

KEY MUSCLES (scoring on reverse side)

	R	L	
C5			Elbow flexors
C6			Wrist extensors
C7			Elbow extensors
C8			Finger flexors (distal phalanx of middle finger)
T1			Finger abductors (little finger)

UPPER LIMB TOTAL (MAXIMUM) ☐ + ☐ = ☐ (25) (25) (50)

Comments:

	R	L	
L2			Hip flexors
L3			Knee extensors
L4			Ankle dorsiflexors
L5			Long toe extensors
S1			Ankle plantar flexors

Voluntary anal contraction (Yes/No) ☐

LOWER LIMB TOTAL (MAXIMUM) ☐ + ☐ = ☐ (25) (25) (50)

LIGHT TOUCH R L — PIN PRICK R L

C2, C3, C4, C5, C6, C7, C8, T1, T2, T3, T4, T5, T6, T7, T8, T9, T10, T11, T12, L1, L2, L3, L4, L5, S1, S2, S3, S4-5

TOTALS (MAXIMUM) (56) (56) (56) (56)

0 = absent
1 = altered
2 = normal
NT = not testable

Any anal sensation (Yes/No)

PIN PRICK SCORE (max: 112)

LIGHT TOUCH SCORE (max: 112)

SENSORY

KEY SENSORY POINTS

• Key Sensory Points

NEUROLOGICAL LEVEL (The most caudal segment with normal function) — SENSORY R L / MOTOR R L

COMPLETE OR INCOMPLETE? (Incomplete = Any sensory or motor function in S4-S5)

ASIA IMPAIRMENT SCALE

ZONE OF PARTIAL PRESERVATION (Caudal extent of partially innervated segments) — SENSORY R L / MOTOR R L

This form may be copied freely but should not be altered without permission from the American Spinal Injury Association.

FIGURE 18-36 ASIA classification. (©American Spinal Injury Association. <http://www.asia-spinalinjury.org/elearning/ISNCSCI.php>.)

them in timely fashion. In the case of a hip dislocation, sciatic nerve injury, cartilage cell death, and avascular necrosis can result from delay in treatment. Of these complications, avascular necrosis is the most devastating because of its propensity to cause collapse of the femoral head and the subsequent development of degenerative joint disease. This problem can lead to the need for total hip replacement or hip fusion at a young age. Avascular necrosis usually develops in a time-dependent fashion. In the dislocated position, tension on the capsular blood vessels restricts blood flow to the femoral head. If the hip remains dislocated for 24 hours, avascular necrosis will ensue in 100% of cases. Although irreversible damage to the blood supply may occur at the time of injury, reduction within 6 hours is generally believed to reduce the incidence of ischemic changes.

Knee dislocations are a common cause of arterial injury secondary to the proximity of the popliteal vessels. The vessels are tethered proximally at the adductor hiatus and distally as they exit the popliteal fossa and are subjected to a great deal of force when a knee dislocation occurs. Prompt reduction of these injuries is mandatory, followed by reevaluation of vascular status. Some authors have suggested that any patient with an acute knee dislocation should have angiography. However, this study is a costly procedure, with potential complications. Therefore, there has been a shift toward selective angiography. Database studies have estimated the rate of vascular injury after knee dislocation at 1% to 3%, with as many as 13% of patients requiring operative repair.[40] Rates as high as 64% have been reported in the literature, although most of these studies are small, given the rarity of the injury. Many have suggested that arteriography should be performed only in patients with abnormal vascular examination results, including decrease in pedal pulses, decrease in color or temperature, expanding hematoma about the knee, and history of abnormal examination findings before presentation in the ED.[13] The ABI should be included as part of the vascular evaluation. CT angiography has been shown to be effective in the diagnosis of vascular injury after knee dislocation and can also be considered. An algorithm for diagnosis of vascular injury after knee dislocation is shown in Figure 18-41.

Treatment

Reduction of dislocations often requires IV sedation to reduce the muscle spasm at the joint. In general, proper reduction technique of any dislocation includes re-creating the injury, gentle traction, and reversal of the injury. For example, in a posterior hip dislocation, the position of the hip at the time of dislocation was most likely flexed and internally rotated. When the hip dislocates, the femoral head usually hinges on the posterior wall of the acetabulum, which inhibits reduction. To reduce the joint, it should first

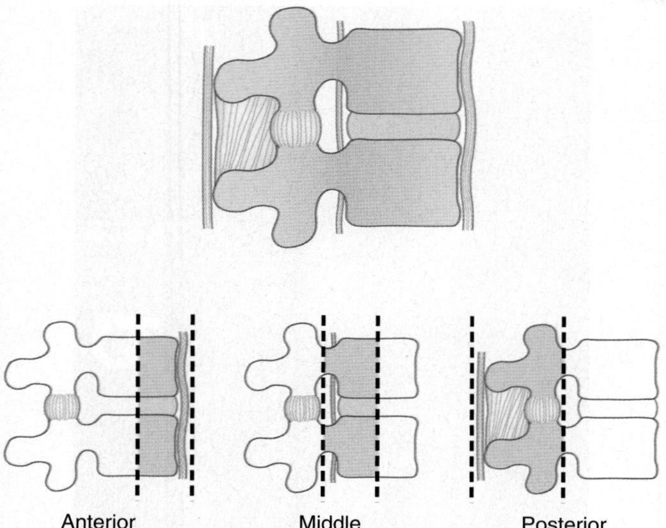

FIGURE 18-37 Denis' three-column model of the spine. The anterior column consists of the anterior two thirds of the vertebral body and anterior longitudinal ligament. The middle column includes the posterior third of the vertebral body and posterior longitudinal ligament. The posterior column includes all bone and ligamentous structures posterior to the posterior longitudinal ligament. (From Lee Y, Templin C, Eismont F, et al: Thoracic and upper lumbar spine injuries. In Browner BD, Levine AM, Jupiter JB, et al, editors: *Skeletal trauma: Basic science, management, and reconstruction*, ed 4, Philadelphia, 2008, WB Saunders.)

be flexed and internally rotated, unhinging it from the posterior wall. Next, traction will help pull the head back into the acetabulum. Finally, extension and external rotation will ensure that the joint remains reduced. It is important to use gentle constant traction rather than forceful pulling, which allows muscle spasm relaxation and improves the patient's comfort. If a joint cannot be reduced by closed methods with adequate sedation, general anesthesia is required. Attempts are made to reduce the joint by closed techniques in the operating room, with staff and instruments available for open reduction if this fails.

Vascular Injuries

Incidence

Although the rate of vascular injuries associated with blunt and penetrating extremity trauma is relatively low, the morbidity and limb loss associated with these injuries are significant. Distal ischemia is the most frequent manifestation of vascular injury in this setting; overt hemorrhage is less common. The orthopedic injuries most frequently associated with vascular insults include posterior knee dislocations, supracondylar humerus fractures, elbow dislocations, and unstable pelvic fractures. Other fractures that are less frequently associated with vascular injury include supracondylar femur fractures, tibial plateau fractures, and combined tibial-fibular fractures.

Although upper extremity injuries account for almost 30% of all peripheral vascular injuries, lower extremity vascular trauma carries a poorer prognosis and is potentially more serious. In

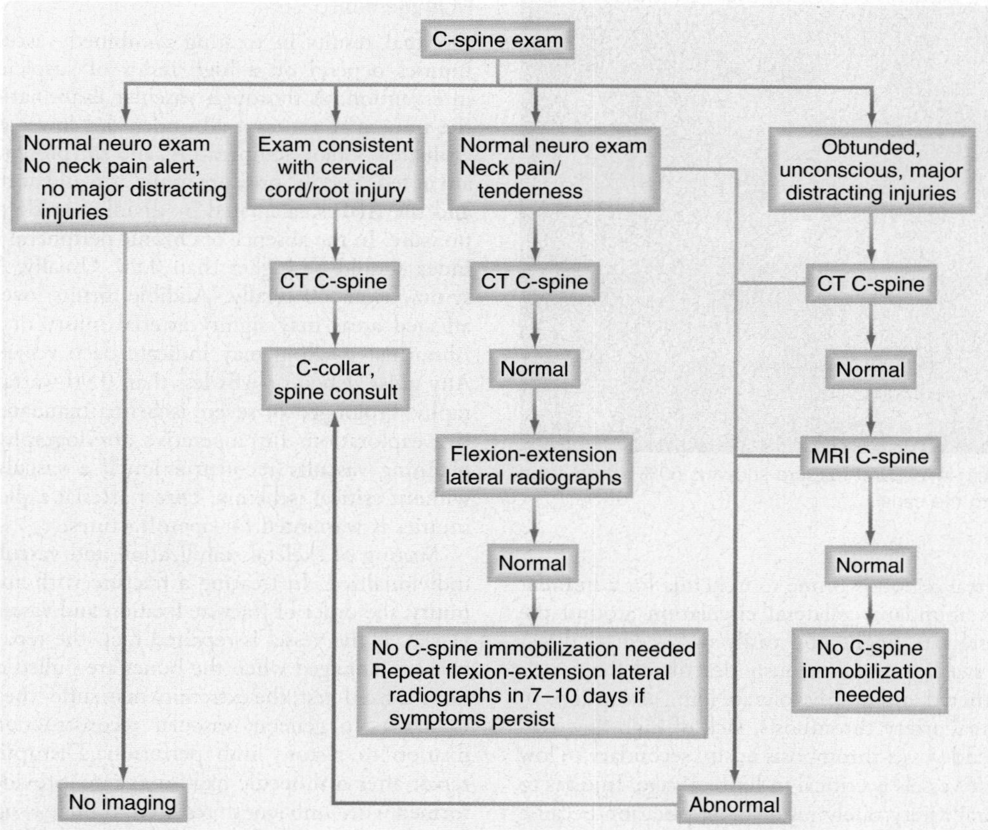

FIGURE 18-38 Algorithm for imaging diagnosis of cervical spine (C-spine) injury. (Adapted from Lee Y, Templin C, Eismont F, et al: Thoracic and upper lumbar spine injuries. In Browner BD, Levine AM, Jupiter JB, et al, editors: *Skeletal trauma: Basic science, management, and reconstruction*, ed 4, Philadelphia, 2008, WB Saunders.)

TABLE 18-6 Point System for TLICS Score

	POINTS
Type	
Compression	1
Burst	2
Translational/rotational	3
Distraction	4
Integrity of Posterior Ligamentous Complex	
Intact	0
Suspected/indeterminate	2
Injured	3
Neurologic Status	
Intact	0
Nerve root	2
Cord, conus medullaris, complete	2
Cord, conus medullaris, incomplete	3
Cauda equina	3

Clinical qualifiers: extreme kyphosis, marked collapse, lateral angulation, open fractures, soft tissue compromise, adjacent rib fractures, inability to brace, multisystem trauma, severe head injury, sternum fracture.

From Patel AA, Vaccaro AR: Thoracolumbar spine trauma classification. *J Am Acad Orthop Surg* 18:63–71, 2010.

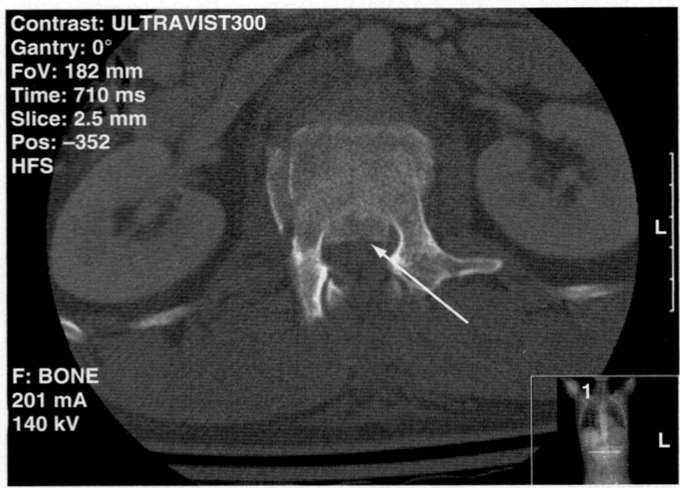

FIGURE 18-39 Lumbar-level burst fracture showing 50% retropulsion of bone fragments into the canal.

particular, the popliteal region is prone to ischemia for a number of reasons. There is abundant collateral circulation around the knee, but these vessels are fragile and easily damaged by direct trauma or adjacent swelling. As previously described, the vessels in this region are tethered and poorly tolerate joint disruption. In the setting of popliteal artery thrombosis, lack of high-flow collaterals may lead to end-vessel thrombosis in situ secondary to low flow. Patency of these vessels is critical in limb salvage. Injuries to the superficial femoral artery rarely result in amputation because of the rich collateral circulation with the profunda femoris artery. Although it is rarely injured, injury to the profunda femoris may be clinically silent, and the diagnosis must be made by angiography.

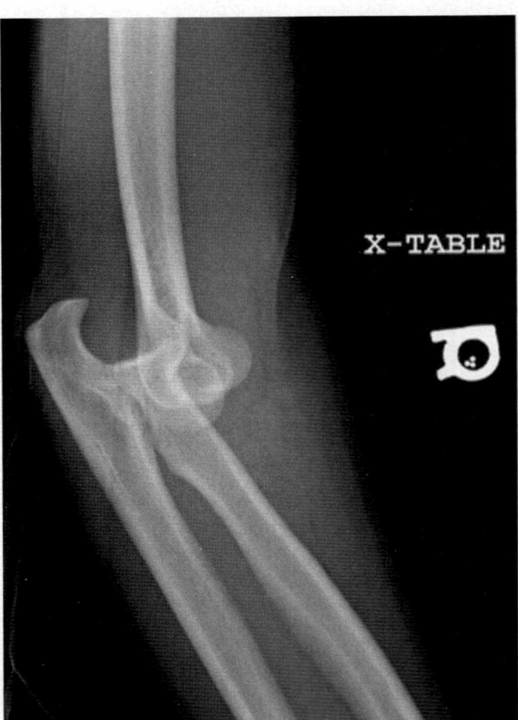

FIGURE 18-40 Posterior elbow dislocation characteristically locked in extension.

Management

Optimal results in treating combined vascular and orthopedic injuries depend on a high index of suspicion and expeditious intervention. A thorough vascular examination is performed in the trauma room, and all upper and lower extremity pulses are evaluated. Color, temperature, and the presence of pain or paresis are noted. Systolic pressure in the arm and at the ankle is recorded, and the ABI is calculated by dividing ankle pressure by brachial pressure. In the absence of chronic peripheral vascular disease, the index should be higher than 0.90. Usually, ABIs and pulses are symmetrical bilaterally. Audible bruits over blood vessels at affected areas may signify arterial injury or a traumatic fistula. Abnormal swelling may indicate deep vessel injury or rupture. Any pulse deficit or ABI less than 0.90 warrants formal arteriography. Prolonged or severe ischemia mandates immediate operative exploration. Intraoperative arteriography may be useful in planning vascular reconstruction if a vascular injury is present without critical ischemia. Direct arterial exploration of suspected injuries is warranted for open fractures.

Staging of skeletal stabilization and vascular repair should be individualized. In treating a fracture with an associated vascular injury, the order of fracture fixation and vascular repair is controversial. If the vessel is repaired first, the repair may be stretched or even damaged when the bones are pulled out to length. If the bone is fixed first, the extremity may suffer the effects of prolonged ischemia. In general, vascular reconstruction precedes fracture fixation to restore limb perfusion. Disruption of the vascular repair after orthopedic fixation is rare, provided the repair is performed with limb length restored. If there is significant shortening accompanying the fracture, placement of a temporary external fixator or femoral distracter is a fast and effective way to obtain appropriate limb length during vascular repair. The ipsilateral and contralateral limbs are prepared widely to allow access to the distal

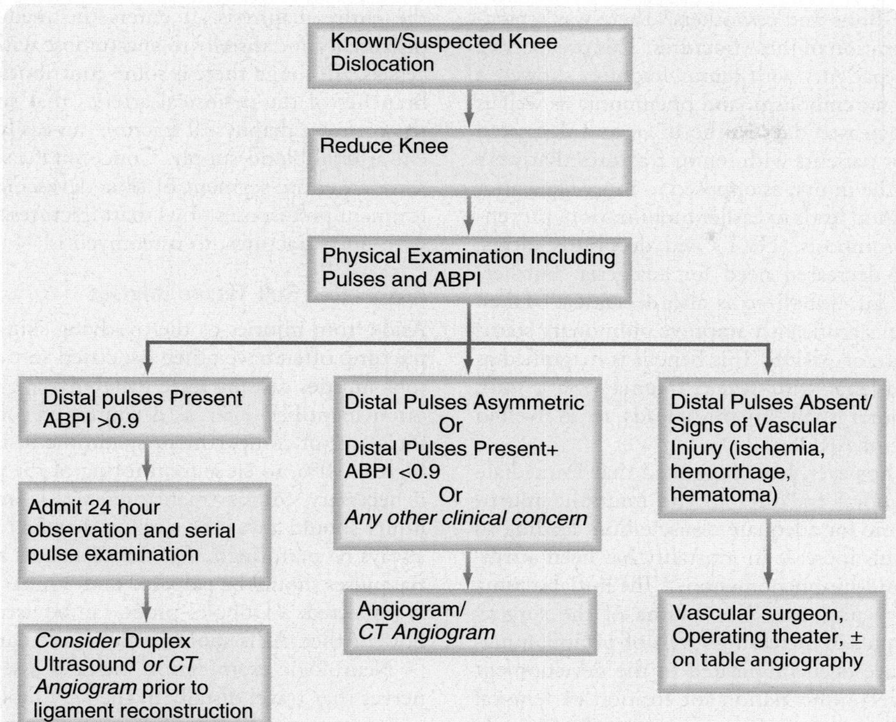

FIGURE 18-41 An algorithm for diagnosis of vascular injury after knee dislocation. *ABPI,* ankle-brachial pressure index. (From Howells NR, Brunton LR, Robinson J, et al: Acute knee dislocation: An evidence based approach to the management of the multiligament injured knee. *Injury* 42:1198–1204, 2011.)

vessels and contralateral saphenous vein. Fasciotomy is performed before vascular repair if compartment syndrome is suspected. In knee dislocations, it is advisable to release the compartments of the lower part of the leg because of the chance of reperfusion injury and the development of compartment syndrome. Proximal and distal control is obtained before exploration of the hematoma. The artery and vein are carefully inspected, and the injury is assessed.

In unstable fractures with vascular disruption, an external fixator is typically applied away from the zone of vascular injury to maintain length and to stabilize the area before vascular repair. Repair typically involves shunt or graft placement to provide a bypass over the injured area. Resection of the damaged proximal and distal vessel injury is performed. A completion arteriogram is routinely obtained because limb salvage depends on arterial patency. All major vein injuries are repaired to increase the patency rate of the arterial repair and to prevent the sequelae of chronic venous congestion.

COMMON LONG BONE FRACTURES

Femur Fractures

Epidemiology and Significance

Femur fractures occur at a rate of 1 per 10,000 people per year. A closed femoral shaft fracture is considered a major injury in calculating the Injury Severity Score (ISS). Therefore, another major injury in any other organ system qualifies the patient as multiply injured. With the exception of pathologic or insufficiency fractures in older patients, these fractures are the result of a high-energy injury. Frequently, these injuries lead to significant bleeding. Because of the geometry of the thigh, several units of blood can be lost into the tissues, with little external evidence of bleeding. Transfusion with packed red blood cells is often necessary. In addition to concerns about bleeding, the treating team should have a high suspicion of concomitant femoral neck fractures for all patients with femoral shaft fractures. As noted, there is almost a 10% incidence of these associated injuries.

Initial Management

All femur fractures must be immobilized before the patient is transported from the scene of the accident. Without immobilization, displaced femoral shaft fractures can cause increased edema, bleeding, and further damage to the surrounding soft tissues. Continued motion at the fracture site also results in increased fat embolization and contributes to the development of ARDS. Proper immobilization begins with in-line traction, which decreases the diameter of the thigh compartment, reducing its volume. The soft tissues are then under tension and can tamponade bleeding at the fracture site. As noted earlier, in-line traction in the field can be accomplished with a Hare traction splint (see Fig. 18-24).[41] For patients in extremis, a posterior splint alone will suffice until formal traction or immobilization can be achieved. As previously discussed, a traction pin can be placed through the proximal tibia to provide skeletal traction and to allow access to the distal femur (see Fig. 18-23). Up to 10% of a patient's body weight can be applied to a properly placed skeletal traction.

Definitive Stabilization

Timing of definitive fixation of femoral shaft fractures is controversial. Until the end of the 20th century, delayed fixation of femoral fractures, sometimes up to 2 weeks after the initial injury, was the standard of care. However, in the early 1990s, thanks in large part to the work of Bone and coworkers,[6] there was a paradigm shift toward early fixation of these fractures. This prospective randomized trial of 178 patients with femur fractures showed a decreased rate of ARDS, fat embolism, and pneumonia as well as shorter hospital stays, decreased days in the ICU, and decreased cost of hospitalization for patients with femur fractures that were fixed within 24 hours of the injury, as opposed to those fixed after 48 hours. Immediate fixation leads to earlier mobilization, prevention of deep venous thrombosis (DVT) and decubitus ulcers, easier nursing care, and decreased need for analgesia. Furthermore, the magnitude of fat embolized is also decreased.[6] Taken together, these factors can significantly improve pulmonary status and decrease the incidence of ARDS. This benefit is magnified as the ISS increases. In patients with severe trauma (ISS > 40), delayed fixation of femoral shaft fractures leads to a fivefold increase in the incidence of ARDS.

More recent studies, however, have suggested that immediate definitive fixation of femoral fractures in the multiply injured patient may not allow time for adequate resuscitation, leading to higher mortality rates. This increase in mortality has been attributed to the so-called second-hit phenomenon.[42] The initial trauma leads to an inflammatory response. The trauma of the surgery further increases this response, increasing levels of proinflammatory cytokines, which have been implicated in the development of ARDS. The current recommendation for fixation of femoral shaft fractures in the polytrauma patient is to proceed with early fixation if the patient is hemodynamically stable, not hypothermic, and oxygenating well.[43] Markers of resuscitation should be evaluated, with patients achieving a lactate level of less than 2.2 mmol/L, a mean arterial pressure above 60 mm Hg, and a base deficit of between −2 and +2 before definitive fixation. This protocol can reduce the patient's time in the ICU, time on the ventilator, and secondary procedures.[43]

The fixation of femoral shaft fractures has become fairly uniform. The treatment of choice for closed fractures and types I through IIIA open fractures is closed, locked IM nailing. In contrast to open reduction methods, closed IM nailing reduces bleeding and soft tissue disruption at the fracture site. These minimally invasive techniques reduce perioperative stress and decrease the incidence of infection and nonunion. Treatment of types IIIB and IIIC open femoral shaft fractures is usually staged, with immediate irrigation and débridement and external fixation, followed by IM nailing or plating when there is sufficient soft tissue coverage of the bone.

Tibial Shaft Fractures

Epidemiology and Significance

Almost 26 tibia fractures occur per 100,000 people per year. The incidence has increased to approximately 500,000 cases in the United States annually. Fractures of the diaphysis of the tibia occur by direct and indirect mechanisms. Common mechanisms are bumper injuries, gunshot wounds, and bending or torsional injuries with a firmly planted foot. Because of the anatomy of the blood supply in the lower leg and the high energy involved in these injuries, treatment of tibial shaft fractures can present many difficulties. Further complicating matters, approximately 24% of all tibial shaft fractures are open injuries.[9]

Blood Supply

Tibial shaft fractures tend to be slow healing as a result of their tenuous blood supply and limited soft tissue envelope. A single nutrient artery that branches from the posterior tibial artery serves the entire diaphysis. It enters the medullary canal and travels proximally and distally to anastomose with metaphyseal endosteal vessels. Although there is some contribution from the penetrating branches of the periosteal arteries that supply the outer third of the cortex, a diaphyseal fracture can easily compromise the nutrient arterial blood supply. Concomitant soft tissue stripping may leave an entire segment of tibia devascularized. This fragile environment predisposes tibial shaft fractures to impaired healing and, with open fractures, to osteomyelitis.

Associated Soft Tissue Injuries

Aside from injuries to the overlying skin and muscle, tibial shaft fractures often have other associated soft tissue injuries. Ligamentous injuries causing knee instability are not uncommon and are often identified later as a source of continued morbidity. The incidence of compartment syndrome in tibial shaft fractures is as high as 10%, so close monitoring of the patient's symptoms and, if necessary, compartment pressures is important. Neurovascular injury should always be suspected and a careful examination must always be performed. The dorsalis pedis and posterior tibial arterial pulses should be palpated and capillary refill assessed. If injury is suspected, a Doppler probe can be used to assess arterial blood flow further. ABIs should also be calculated.

Neurologic examination includes assessment of all five major nerves that travel distally in the leg (Table 18-7). The deep peroneal nerve, traveling in the anterior compartment, can be evaluated by testing first dorsal web space sensation and foot and toe dorsiflexion. Testing of sensation along the dorsum of the foot and eversion strength can assess the superficial peroneal nerve, which travels in the lateral compartment. The tibial nerve travels in the deep posterior compartment and provides sensation to the sole of the foot and motor function to the foot and toe plantar flexors. The sural and saphenous nerves travel superficially to the muscle compartments. They are both pure sensory nerves. The sural nerve supplies sensation to the lateral aspect of the heel, and the saphenous nerve supplies sensation to the medial malleolus.

Management and Treatment

Management and treatment of tibial shaft fractures have evolved over the years. A closed fracture with minimal displacement can be treated by cast immobilization and functional bracing. However, most fractures are now treated surgically to allow early weight bearing and rehabilitation. Reamed IM nailing is the technique of choice, when appropriate.

Plate fixation has fallen out of favor for diaphyseal fractures because of the high risk for wound healing complications. However, it remains a valuable treatment option for diaphyseal fractures that extend proximally or distally into the metaphysis, which are less amenable to IM stabilization. Minimally invasive percutaneous plating techniques have improved the results of plate fixation by limiting surgical dissection in the zone of injury. External fixation is an option for a patient who is unstable or when soft tissue injury precludes definitive fixation. Although it is generally reserved for temporary stabilization, with a good reduction, an external fixator can be used as definitive fixation. For complex fractures, a ringed external fixator is a powerful tool for correcting significant deformity or bone defects.

Humeral Shaft Fractures

Epidemiology and Significance

Humeral shaft fractures represent 3% to 5% of all fractures in adults. There is a bimodal distribution of incidence, with a small

TABLE 18-7 Nerves to the Foot

NERVE	SENSORY	MOTOR
Deep peroneal	First dorsal web space	Great toe dorsiflexion (extensor hallucis longus)
Superficial peroneal	Dorsum of foot	Eversion (peroneals)
Tibial	Plantar surface of foot	Great toe plantar flexion (flexor hallucis longus)
Sural	Lateral heel	None
Saphenous	Medial malleolus	None

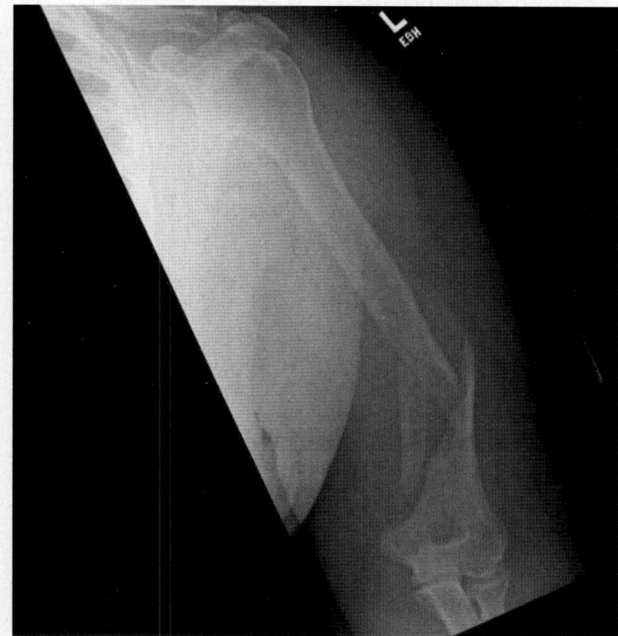

FIGURE 18-42 Holstein-Lewis fracture of the humeral shaft. This patient had no radial nerve function at presentation. At the time of surgery, the nerve was found to be intact but interposed between two fracture fragments. Full radial nerve function returned by 6 months.

peak in the third decade for young men and a larger peak in the seventh decade for women. In younger patients, the injury is the result of high-energy trauma, whereas in older patients, these fractures tend to be the result of osteoporosis. Most humeral shaft fractures can be treated nonoperatively. Studies have shown more than 95% union in those fractures treated without surgery.[43] In addition, the mobility of the shoulder and elbow joints will tolerate up to 15 degrees of malrotation, 20 degrees of flexion-extension deformity, 30 degrees of varus-valgus deformity, and 3 cm of shortening, without significant compromise in function or appearance.

A thorough neurovascular examination is imperative for patients with humeral fractures. There is an up to 18% incidence of radial nerve injury in humeral shaft fractures. With distal-third spiral fractures (the so-called Holstein-Lewis fracture), the incidence is even higher because the radial nerve is at risk as it courses distally in the spiral groove (Fig. 18-42). In the trauma setting, right-sided humeral shaft fractures can be predictive of concomitant injury to the liver and other intra-abdominal organs.

Treatment

Various nonoperative options exist for treating humeral shaft fractures; hanging arm casts, coaptation splints, sling and swathe, and functional bracing are all still used in the treatment of these fractures. Typically, a coaptation splint is applied in the acute setting and subsequently replaced by a functional fracture brace after the initial painful fracture period has passed (3 to 7 days). Patients are then allowed free elbow flexion-extension and arm abduction to 60 degrees. Gravity serves to correct alignment and to pull the bones out to length. Motion is encouraged to stimulate fracture healing because the hydraulic compression created by muscle contraction helps achieve fracture union.[43]

In certain circumstances, operative intervention is indicated. Failed closed reduction, intra-articular fractures, ipsilateral forearm or elbow fractures (floating elbow), segmental fractures, open fractures, and polytrauma patients all benefit from surgical management. Morbid obesity is a relative indication for operative treatment of these fractures. Obesity reduces the effectiveness of a functional fracture brace, and the relatively abducted resting position of the arm in an obese patient leads to a high incidence of varus malunion. Of patients with radial nerve palsies, 70% to 90% are neurapraxias and recover spontaneously during 3 to 6 months. Surgical intervention for patients with radial nerve palsy after humeral shaft fractures is controversial. An algorithm for treatment of this problem is presented in Figure 18-43. Operative options include IM nailing, plate and screw fixation, and external fixation.

CHALLENGES AND COMPLICATIONS

Missed Injuries

Missed musculoskeletal injuries account for a large proportion of delays in diagnosis within the first few days of care of a critically injured patient. Severely injured patients, especially those with a high ISS and a Glasgow Coma Scale score below 8, are more likely to have missed injuries.[44] Clinical reassessment of trauma patients within 24 hours has reduced the incidence of missed injuries by almost 40%. Patients should be reexamined as they regain consciousness and resume activity. Repeated assessments should be routinely performed in all patients, especially unstable and neurologically impaired patients. The tertiary trauma survey includes a comprehensive examination and review of laboratory results and radiographs within 24 hours of initial evaluation. Specific injury patterns should be reviewed closely, especially in patients with multiple injuries and severe disability. External soft tissue trauma may be indicative of a more severe underlying injury. Formal radiology rounds can facilitate increased recognition of occult injuries.

Drug and Alcohol Use

The incidence of drug and alcohol use in patients with musculoskeletal injuries has been reported to be as high as 50%. Prescription opiate use and abuse has also become more common in recent years. A study showed that among patients presenting with orthopedic trauma, 15.5% had filled an opiate prescription in the 3 months before injury compared with 9.2% of the general population.[45] Alcohol and drug use result in more severe orthopedic injuries and more frequent injuries requiring longer hospitalization. Associated complications include those from cocaine use, such as fever, hypertension, acute myocardial ischemia, arrhythmias, and stroke. Cocaine can also facilitate cardiac arrhythmias when it is combined with halothane, nitrous oxide, or ketamine. Furthermore, the use of alcohol or drugs can adversely affect the administration of premedicating drugs. Prophylaxis for delirium tremens in postoperative patients should be performed when

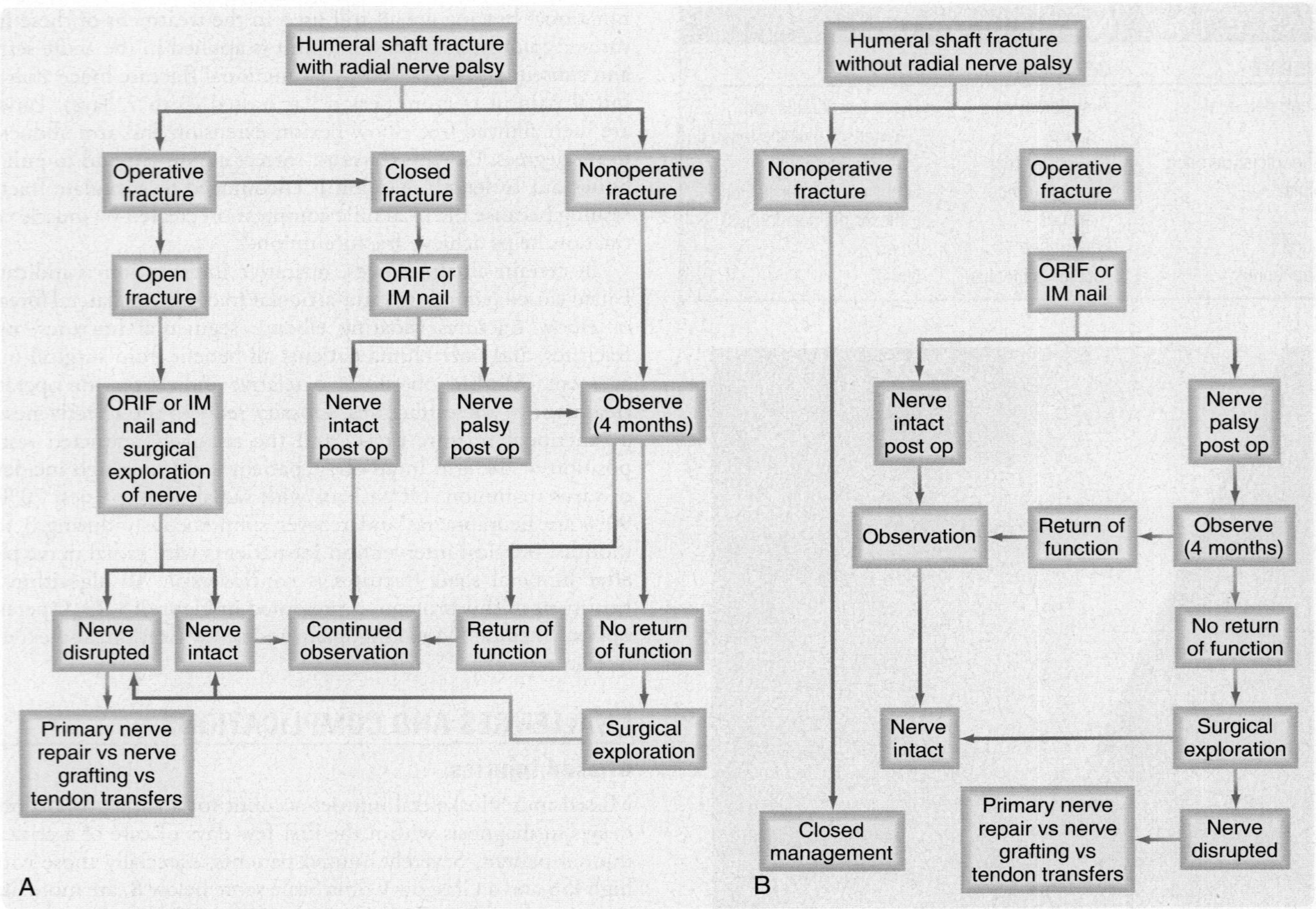

FIGURE 18-43 Algorithms for management of a patient presenting with a humeral shaft fracture with **(A)** and without **(B)** radial nerve palsy.

indicated. Inpatient detoxification consultation should be obtained before discharge.

Thromboembolic Complications

Compared with patients with isolated injuries, multiply injured patients have an increased incidence of thromboembolic complications, including DVT and pulmonary embolism (Fig. 18-44). Pulmonary embolism remains a leading cause of mortality in hospitalized trauma patients. In their study of venous thromboembolism (VTE) in trauma patients, Geerts and associates[46] have shown an overall incidence of 58%, with an 18% incidence of proximal clots. In addition to multiply injured trauma patients, patients undergoing elective neurosurgical, orthopedic, and oncologic surgery are also at increased risk for VTE. Long bone fractures, pelvic fractures, advanced age, spinal cord injuries, and surgical procedures are associated with an increased risk for VTE in trauma patients. The most common forms of pharmacologic prophylaxis include adjusted-dose unfractionated heparin, low-molecular-weight heparin (LMWH), warfarin, and aspirin. In addition, newer direct factor Xa inhibitors such as rivaroxaban (Xaltero) have been used for prophylaxis in elective hip and knee arthroplasty. Other forms of prophylaxis include mechanical devices, such as foot pumps and sequential calf compression pumps, and barrier devices, such as inferior vena cava filters.

It is generally agreed that prophylaxis is critical for a high-risk trauma patient. Two controversial issues in the prevention of VTE in a trauma patient are currently being debated. The first is the role of venous surveillance. Some physicians recommend routine duplex surveillance to detect thromboembolic events because the incidence of proximal DVT reported in some studies is higher than previously suspected. More recent literature, however, suggests that this is not necessary and that routine screening should be performed only for patients who are at high risk for VTE (e.g., in the presence of a spinal cord injury, lower extremity or pelvic fracture, or major head injury) and who have not received adequate thromboprophylaxis.[47] The second issue is appropriate prophylaxis. Adjusted-dose heparin and LMWH are currently the most common forms of prophylaxis. However, in a randomized study comparing low-dose unfractionated heparin with LMWH, Geerts and coworkers[46] documented an overall 44% incidence of DVT in trauma patients receiving low-dose unfractionated heparin versus 31% in those receiving enoxaparin. There was a slight increase in major bleeding in the enoxaparin-treated group; however, in none of the patients did the hemoglobin level drop by more than 2 g/dL.

In the most recent edition of the evidence-based recommendations for prevention of VTE, the American College of Chest Physicians recommended the use of routine prophylaxis with LMWH while the patient is in the hospital. In patients with

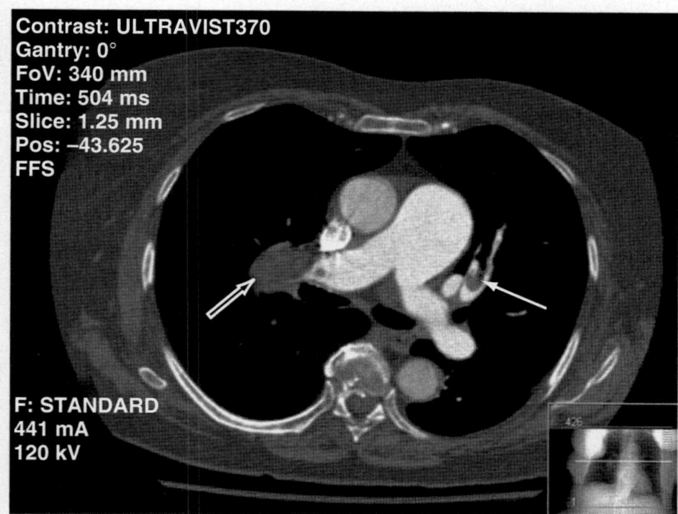

FIGURE 18-44 CT angiogram showing a large pulmonary embolism completely occluding the right pulmonary artery *(solid arrowhead)* and a smaller pulmonary embolism occluding one of the segmental branches of the left pulmonary artery *(open arrowhead)*.

impaired mobility or those going to an inpatient rehabilitation facility, they recommended discharge with LMWH or warfarin (with an international normalized ratio goal of 2.0 to 3.0). In patients with a contraindication to anticoagulation, they recommended the use of intermittent pneumatic compression devices. These devices deliver sequential rhythmic compression to the calf or thigh and can help reduce the rate of DVT in trauma patients. In patients with lower extremity fractures or wounds, foot pumps should be used. Finally, the American College of Chest Physicians recommended against the routine use of inferior vena cava filters for patients at high risk of VTE. Because of the potential complications of filter placement, including migration of the filter, bleeding during or after placement, and filter thrombosis, these devices should be reserved for patients with known proximal DVT and either an absolute contraindication to chemical anticoagulation or impending major surgery. In either case, they recommended starting therapeutic anticoagulation as soon as the contraindication resolves.[47] Further research in this area is needed to determine the efficacy and safety of some of the newer agents for trauma patients with orthopedic injuries.

Pulmonary Failure: Fat Emboli Syndrome and Adult Respiratory Distress Syndrome

Fat emboli syndrome (FES) is a condition characterized by respiratory distress, altered mental status, and skin petechiae. First described in humans in 1862, it occurs in multiply injured patients, especially those with orthopedic injuries. Clinical signs are evident hours to days after an injury involving long bone or pelvic fractures. Recent literature has suggested a higher rate of fat embolism found at autopsy in trauma patients compared with nontrauma patients (82% versus 63%).[48] In patients with isolated long bone fractures, the incidence is between 2% and 5%. In a multiply injured patient with long bone or pelvic fractures, the incidence of FES is as high as 19%. Marrow fat from the fracture site is believed to enter the pulmonary circulation, where it causes activation of the coagulation cascade, platelet dysfunction, release of vasoactive substances and inflammatory cytokines, and subsequent neutrophil infiltration.[49] The treatment of FES is mostly supportive, but a meta-analysis by Bederman and colleagues[50] has shown that the use of corticosteroids in patients with multiple long bone fractures reduces the rate of FES by 78% without significantly increasing the risk of complications related to treatment of the fractures. Before the advent of modern ICU care, mortality rates in patients with FES were reported to be as high as 20%.

FES may represent a subset of ARDS. ARDS is a pulmonary failure state defined as a PaO_2/FIO_2 ratio lower than 200 regardless of the level of positive end-expiratory pressure, a pulmonary artery occlusion pressure of 18 mm Hg or less, or bilateral diffuse infiltrates on chest radiographs in the absence of congestive heart failure.[51] Early fixation of fractures has been shown to reduce the incidence of FES and ARDS in trauma patients; however, there has been some debate about whether the method of fixation affects the incidence of FES. In theory, IM nailing causes an increased embolic load, which could lead to an increased incidence of FES, but clinical and experimental studies have suggested that the presence of chest injury, not the method of fracture fixation, is responsible for ARDS.[42] Therefore, in patients with an acute chest injury with concomitant long bone fractures, it may be advisable to delay definitive fixation of the fracture until the patient's pulmonary status has stabilized.

POSTOPERATIVE MOBILIZATION

The benefits of early fixation and mobilization of multiply injured patients have been discussed. However, a distinction between mobilization and weight bearing is essential. Mobilization is transfer of the patient from the supine position, either under the patient's own power or with the help of nurses or therapists. This includes turning the patient every shift by the nurse, sitting the patient up in bed, or transferring the patient to a chair. All patients should be mobilized by the first or second postoperative day if their general condition permits. Mobilization helps prevent the development of pulmonary and septic complications.

Weight bearing, in contrast, is transmission of a load through an extremity. For a patient to be allowed to bear weight on an injured extremity, the following three conditions must be met:

1. There must be bone to bone contact at the fracture site as demonstrated intraoperatively or on postreduction radiographs. Without contact of the fracture ends, the fixation devices will be subjected to all the stresses applied to the extremity, which will frequently result in failure of the fixation.
2. Stable fixation of the fracture must be achieved. By definition, stable fixation is not disrupted when it is subjected to normal physiologic loads. Stable fixation is dependent on a number of factors. Fixation may be less than ideal in patients with osteopenic bone or severely comminuted fractures. When excessive loads are anticipated, such as with heavy or obese patients, the typical fixation may not be adequate.
3. The patient must be able to comply with the weight-bearing status. Frequently, reliability of the patient is a significant consideration in the determination of weight-bearing status. Social, psychological, or emotional circumstances can affect a patient's ability to comply with weight-bearing restrictions.

Unless all three criteria are met, the fixation will need to be protected with restricted weight-bearing status. Touch-down weight bearing (TDWB) allows the patient to place the foot of the affected extremity flat on the floor, without bearing any of the patient's body weight. TDWB is often permitted in patients with injuries around the hip and allows extension of the hip and knee and dorsiflexion at the ankle. This natural position relaxes the hip musculature and minimizes joint reactive forces. Crutch walking with the foot off the floor (non–weight bearing) leads to a significant increase in force across the hip joint because of contraction of the muscles about the hip. Toe-touch weight bearing, a phrase often used synonymously with TDWB, is an unfortunate use of terminology. Most patients attempt to walk while touching only the toe of the injured extremity to the ground. In this position, the hip and knee are flexed and the ankle is held in equinus. When this status is maintained for any significant amount of time, contractures at the hip, knee, and ankle are common. For this reason, use of this terminology is discouraged.

Partial weight bearing is defined in terms of the percentage of body weight applied to an injured extremity. It is gradually increased as the fracture gains stability through healing. With the use of a scale, the patient can learn what different amounts of body weight feel like. When a fracture and the patient are stable enough to withstand normal loads, weight bearing as tolerated is instituted. It is believed that reliable patients limit their own weight bearing according to their pain.

Even when weight bearing is not allowed, mobilization of affected and adjacent joints is typically performed within a few days. After surgical treatment, joints are typically immobilized briefly and then allowed passive or active range of motion in bed if weight bearing is not prudent. Early joint mobilization decreases the likelihood of fibrosis and therefore increases early mobility. Furthermore, joint motion is necessary for the good health of articular cartilage. Cartilage is nourished from synovial fluid most efficiently when the joint is moving. Early joint mobilization has become a basic tenet of orthopedic care and has led to a decrease in the morbidity associated with musculoskeletal injuries.

SUMMARY

In the setting of acute trauma, preservation of a patient's life takes precedence over preservation of a limb. However, injuries to the extremities and axial skeleton may be life-threatening in rare circumstances (e.g., hemorrhage secondary to vascular injury from pelvic or long bone fractures). These must be recognized early and managed appropriately. Once the critical period has passed, musculoskeletal injuries are a major cause of post-traumatic morbidity, as demonstrated by increased health care costs, lost work days, physical disability, emotional distress, and diminished quality of life. Accordingly, it is essential that a detailed and complete extremity and axial musculoskeletal survey be performed on every patient, that injuries be identified early, and that the consulting orthopedic surgical team be notified of the specifics of these injuries in a timely fashion. It is essential that the trauma team have a high index of suspicion for the orthopedic emergencies discussed for any patient who has experienced high-energy trauma. Moreover, the patient should not be transported from the trauma room, unless necessary for lifesaving interventions, until the orthopedic team has evaluated and stabilized the involved extremity to protect it against further injury and morbidity. Finally, appropriate treatment of musculoskeletal injuries is a multidisciplinary undertaking. With cooperation and collaboration of all treating teams—general surgery, vascular surgery, neurosurgery, plastic surgery, internal medicine, and physical therapy—we will be able to ensure the best possible outcome for our patients.

SELECTED REFERENCES

Bone LB, Johnson KD, Weigelt J, et al: Early versus delayed stabilization of femoral shaft fractures: A prospective randomized study. *J Bone Joint Surg Am* 71:336–340, 1989.

This classic article has shaped the treatment of multiply injured patients. It was the first clearly to define the benefits of early stabilization of femoral shaft fractures prospectively.

Browner BD, Levine AM, Jupiter JB, et al, editors: *Skeletal trauma: Basic science, management and reconstruction*, ed 4, Philadelphia, 2008, WB Saunders.

This is one of the premiere comprehensive texts covering traumatic musculoskeletal injuries, and this two-volume set is now in its fourth edition. It is clearly written and visually appealing. The chapter authors are the elite orthopedic trauma surgeons in the world. It is an excellent reference for any physician dealing with a multiply injured patient.

Egol KA, Koval KJ, Zuckerma JD: *Handbook of fractures*, ed 4, Philadelphia, 2010, Lippincott Williams & Wilkins.

This conveniently sized handbook is the ideal reference for physicians managing musculoskeletal injuries in the emergency setting. Comprehensive but concise, this guide discusses epidemiology, anatomy, mechanism of injury, clinical evaluation, radiologic evaluation, classification, treatment, and management of complications of most acute musculoskeletal injuries.

Gustilo R, Anderson J: Prevention of infection in the treatment of 1025 open fractures of long bones: Retrospective and prospective analyses. *J Bone Joint Surg Am* 58:453–458, 1976.

This classic article defined the classification and proposed management guidelines in patients with open fractures. It includes more than 300 cases reviewed retrospectively and another 600 prospective cases in which the new classification was applied.

Lieberman J: *AAOS comprehensive orthopaedic review*, Rosemont, Ill, 2009, American Academy of Orthopaedic Surgeons.

This text is a comprehensive review of all orthopedic subspecialties. Its bulleted format and well-organized layout allow convenient referencing of a multitude of topics. It is an excellent reference for managing orthopedic patients.

Tscherne H, Gotzen L: *Fractures with soft tissue injuries*, Berlin, 1984, Springer-Verlag.

This fracture textbook is comprehensive in its coverage of open and closed fractures with soft tissue injuries. It covers all classifications, immediate management, fracture care, and wound care of these injuries. It uses the team approach to dealing with these complicated injuries.

REFERENCES

1. Centers for Disease Control and Prevention, National Center for Injury Prevention and Control: *Web-based Injury Statistics Query and Reporting System (WISQARS)*. Available at: <http://www.cdc.gov/injury/wisqars/>. Accessed February 19, 2015.
2. Clement RC, Carr BG, Kallan MJ, et al: Who needs an orthopedic trauma surgeon? An analysis of US national injury patterns. *J Trauma Acute Care Surg* 75:687–692, 2013.
3. Lieberman J: *AAOS comprehensive orthopaedic review*, Rosemont, Ill, 2009, American Academy of Orthopaedic Surgeons.
4. Paydar S, Ghaffarpasand F, Foroughi M, et al: Role of routine pelvic radiography in initial evaluation of stable, high-energy, blunt trauma patients. *Emerg Med J* 30:724–727, 2013.
5. Deunk J, Brink M, Dekker HM, et al: Predictors for the selection of patients for abdominal CT after blunt trauma: A proposal for a diagnostic algorithm. *Ann Surg* 251:512–520, 2010.
6. Bone LB, Johnson KD, Weigelt J, et al: Early versus delayed stabilization of femoral fractures. A prospective randomized study. *J Bone Joint Surg Am* 71:336–340, 1989.
7. Morshed S, Miclau T, 3rd, Bembom O, et al: Delayed internal fixation of femoral shaft fracture reduces mortality among patients with multisystem trauma. *J Bone Joint Surg Am* 91:3–13, 2009.
8. Mathen R, Inaba K, Munera F, et al: Prospective evaluation of multislice computed tomography versus plain radiographic cervical spine clearance in trauma patients. *J Trauma* 62:1427–1431, 2007.
9. Browner BD, Levine AM, Jupiter JB, et al, editors: *Skeletal trauma: Basic science, management, and reconstruction*, ed 4, Philadelphia, 2008, WB Saunders.
10. O'Toole RV, Dancy L, Dietz AR, et al: Diagnosis of femoral neck fracture associated with femoral shaft fracture: Blinded comparison of computed tomography and plain radiography. *J Orthop Trauma* 27:325–330, 2013.
11. Medina O, Arom GA, Yeranosian MG, et al: Vascular and nerve injury after knee dislocation: A systematic review. *Clin Orthop Relat Res* 472:2621–2629, 2014.
12. Levy BA, Fanelli GC, Whelan DB, et al: Controversies in the treatment of knee dislocations and multiligament reconstruction. *J Am Acad Orthop Surg* 17:197–206, 2009.
13. Tscherne H, Gotzen L: *Fractures with soft tissue injuries*, Berlin, 1984, Springer-Verlag.
14. Even JL, Richards JE, Crosby CG, et al: Preoperative skeletal versus cutaneous traction for femoral shaft fractures treated within 24 hours. *J Orthop Trauma* 26:e177–e182, 2012.
15. Johansen K, Daines M, Howey T, et al: Objective criteria accurately predict amputation following lower extremity trauma. *J Trauma* 30:568–572, 1990.
16. Crist BD, Ferguson T, Murtha YM, et al: Surgical timing of treating injured extremities: An evolving concept of urgency. *Instr Course Lect* 62:17–28, 2013.
17. Malhotra AK, Goldberg S, Graham J, et al: Open extremity fractures: Impact of delay in operative debridement and irrigation. *J Trauma Acute Care Surg* 76:1201–1207, 2014.
18. Pollak AN, Jones AL, Castillo RC, et al: The relationship between time to surgical debridement and incidence of infection after open high-energy lower extremity trauma. *J Bone Joint Surg Am* 92:7–15, 2010.
19. Obremsky WT, Molina C, Collins C, et al: Current practice in the initial management of open fractures among orthopaedic trauma surgeons. *J Orthop Trauma* 28:198–202, 2014.
20. Gustilo RB, Anderson JT: Prevention of infection in the treatment of one thousand and twenty-five open fractures of long bones: Retrospective and prospective analyses. *J Bone Joint Surg Am* 58:453–458, 1976.
21. Petrisor B, Sun X, Bhandari M, et al: Fluid lavage of open wounds (FLOW): A multicenter, blinded, factorial pilot trial comparing alternative irrigating solutions and pressures in patients with open fractures. *J Trauma* 71:596–606, 2011.
22. Blum ML, Esser M, Richardson M, et al: Negative pressure wound therapy reduces deep infection rate in open tibial fractures. *J Orthop Trauma* 26:499–505, 2012.
23. Ly TV, Travison TG, Castillo RC, et al: Ability of lower-extremity injury severity scores to predict functional outcome after limb salvage. *J Bone Joint Surg Am* 90:1738–1743, 2008.
24. Higgins TF, Klatt JB, Beals TC: Lower Extremity Assessment Project (LEAP)—the best available evidence on limb-threatening lower extremity trauma. *Orthop Clin North Am* 41:233–239, 2010.
25. Bosse MJ, McCarthy ML, Jones AL, et al: The insensate foot following severe lower extremity trauma: An indication for amputation? *J Bone Joint Surg Am* 87:2601–2608, 2005.
26. Doukas WC, Hayda RA, Frisch HM, et al: The Military Extremity Trauma Amputation/Limb Salvage (METALS) study: Outcomes of amputation versus limb salvage following major lower-extremity trauma. *J Bone Joint Surg Am* 95:138–145, 2013.
27. Miller A, Carrol E, Tyler-Paris Pilson H: Transabdominal gunshot wounds of the hip and pelvis. *J Am Acad Orthop Surg* 21:286–292, 2013.
28. Schemitsch EH, Bhandari M, Guyatt G, et al: Prognostic factors for predicting outcomes after intramedullary nailing of the tibia. *J Bone Joint Surg Am* 94:1786–1793, 2012.
29. Mubarak S, Hargens A: *Compartment syndromes and Volkmann's contracture*, Philadelphia, 1981, WB Saunders.
30. McQueen MM, Court-Brown CM: Compartment monitoring in tibial fractures. The pressure threshold for decompression. *J Bone Joint Surg Br* 78:99–104, 1996.
31. Whitesides TE, Heckman MM: Acute compartment syndrome: Update on diagnosis and treatment. *J Am Acad Orthop Surg* 4:209–218, 1996.
32. Whitney A, O'Toole RV, Hui E, et al: Do one-time intracompartmental pressure measurements have a high false-positive rate in diagnosing compartment syndrome? *J Trauma Acute Care Surg* 76:479–483, 2014.
33. McQueen MM, Duckworth AD, Aitken SA, et al: The estimated sensitivity and specificity of compartment pressure monitoring for acute compartment syndrome. *J Bone Joint Surg Am* 95:673–677, 2013.
34. Tile M: Pelvic ring fractures: Should they be fixed? *J Bone Joint Surg Br* 70:1–12, 1988.
35. Toth L, King KL, McGrath B, et al: Factors associated with pelvic fracture–related arterial bleeding during trauma resuscitation: A prospective clinical study. *J Orthop Trauma* 28:489–495, 2014.
36. Verbeek DO, Ponsen KJ, van Delden OM, et al: The need for pelvic angiographic embolisation in stable pelvic fracture patients with a "blush" on computed tomography. *Injury* 45:2111, 2014.

37. Knops SP, Schep NW, Spoor CW, et al: Comparison of three different pelvic circumferential compression devices: A biomechanical cadaver study. *J Bone Joint Surg Am* 93:230–240, 2011.
38. Anderson PA, Gugala Z, Lindsey RW, et al: Clearing the cervical spine in the blunt trauma patient. *J Am Acad Orthop Surg* 18:149–159, 2010.
39. Patel AA, Vaccaro AR: Thoracolumbar spine trauma classification. *J Am Acad Orthop Surg* 18:63–71, 2010.
40. Natsuhara KM, Yeranosian MG, Cohen JR, et al: What is the frequency of vascular injury after knee dislocation? *Clin Orthop Relat Res* 472:2615–2620, 2014.
41. Tornetta P, 3rd, Kain MS, Creevy WR: Diagnosis of femoral neck fractures in patients with a femoral shaft fracture. Improvement with a standard protocol. *J Bone Joint Surg Am* 89:39–43, 2007.
42. Morley JR, Smith RM, Pape HC, et al: Stimulation of the local femoral inflammatory response to fracture and intramedullary reaming: A preliminary study of the source of the second hit phenomenon. *J Bone Joint Surg Br* 90:393–399, 2008.
43. Bone LB, Giannoudis P: Femoral shaft fracture fixation and chest injury after polytrauma. *J Bone Joint Surg Am* 93:311–317, 2011.
44. Pfeifer R, Pape HC: Missed injuries in trauma patients: A literature review. *Patient Saf Surg* 2:20, 2008.
45. Holman JE, Stoddard GJ, Higgins TF: Rates of prescription opiate use before and after injury in patients with orthopaedic trauma and the risk factors for prolonged opiate use. *J Bone Joint Surg Am* 95:1075–1080, 2013.
46. Geerts WH, Code KI, Jay RM, et al: A prospective study of venous thromboembolism after major trauma. *N Engl J Med* 331:1601–1606, 1994.
47. Geerts WH, Bergqvist D, Pineo GF, et al: Prevention of venous thromboembolism: American College of Chest Physicians Evidence-Based Clinical Practice Guidelines (8th Edition). *Chest* 133:381S–453S, 2008.
48. Eriksson EA, Rickey J, Leon SM, et al: Fat embolism in pediatric patients: An autopsy evaluation of incidence and Etiology. *J Crit Care* 30:221.e1–221.e5, 2015.
49. Blankstein M, Byrick RJ, Nakane M, et al: Amplified inflammatory response to sequential hemorrhage, resuscitation, and pulmonary fat embolism: An animal study. *J Bone Joint Surg Am* 92:149–161, 2010.
50. Bederman SS, Bhandari M, McKee MD, et al: Do corticosteroids reduce the risk of fat embolism syndrome in patients with long-bone fractures? A meta-analysis. *Can J Surg* 52:386–393, 2009.
51. Irwin R, Rippe J: *Manual of intensive care medicine*, ed 5, Philadelphia, 2010, Lippincott, Williams & Wilkins.

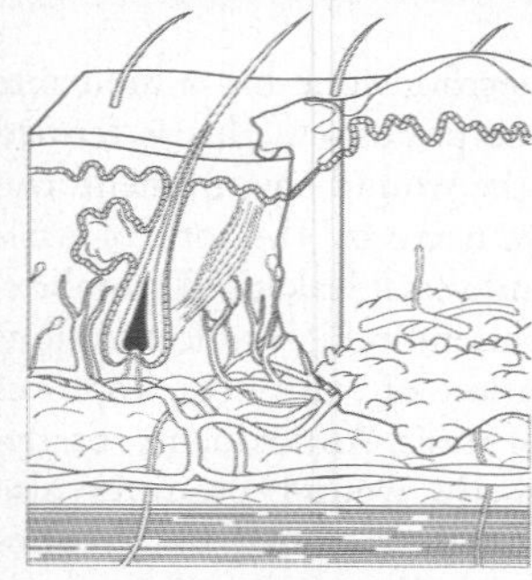

CHAPTER 19

Burns

Marc G. Jeschke, David N. Herndon

OUTLINE

More than 500,000 burn injuries occur annually in the United States.[1] Although most of these burn injuries are minor, approximately 40,000 to 60,000 burn patients require admission to a hospital or major burn center for appropriate treatment. The devastating consequences of burns have been recognized by the medical community and significant amounts of resources and research have been dedicated, successfully improving these dismal statistics.[2] Specialized burn centers (Box 19-1) and advances in therapy strategies, based on improved understanding of resuscitation, enhanced wound coverage, more appropriate infection control, improved treatment of inhalation injury, and better support of the hypermetabolic response to injury, have further improved the clinical outcome of this unique population of patients during the past years.[3,4] However, severe burns remain a devastating injury affecting nearly every organ system and leading to significant morbidity and mortality.[5,6]

ETIOLOGY OF BURN INJURY

There is no greater trauma than major burn injury, which can be classified according to different burn causes and different depths (Box 19-2). Of all cases, nearly 4000 people die of complications related to thermal injury.[7] As in all trauma-related deaths, burn deaths generally occur either immediately after the injury or weeks later as a result of multisystem organ failure. Sixty-six percent of all burns occur at home, and fatalities are predominant in the extremes of age—the very young and the elderly. The most common causes of burn are flame and scald burns.[8] Scald burns are most common in children up to 5 years of age.[8] There is a significant percentage of burns in children that are due to child abuse. A number of risk factors have been linked to burn injury, specifically age, location, demographics, and low economic status.[9] These risk factors underscore the fact that most burn injuries and fatalities are preventable and mandate intervention and prevention strategies. Overall, no single group is immune to the public health debt caused by burns.

Location plays a major role in the risk for and treatment of a burn. The available resources in a given community greatly influence morbidity and mortality. A lack of adequate resources affects the education, rehabilitation, and survival rates for burn victims. An individual with a severe burn in a resource-rich environment can receive care within minutes, whereas a burned person in an austere environment may suffer for an extended time waiting for care. Ideal treatment of burns requires the collaboration of surgeons, anesthesiologists, occupational therapists and physiotherapists, nurses, nutritionists, rehabilitation therapists, and social workers just to accommodate the very basic needs of a major burn survivor.[10] Any delay in reaching these resources compounds a delay in resuscitation and thus adds to the mortality risk.[11] For those who have access to adequate burn care, survival from a major burn is the rule, no longer the exception. In fact, the survival rate for all burns is 94.6%, but for at-risk populations, in communities lacking medical, legal, and public health resources, survival can be nearly impossible.[8]

PATHOPHYSIOLOGY OF BURN INJURY

Local Changes

Locally, thermal injury causes coagulative necrosis of the epidermis and underlying tissues; the depth of injury depends on the temperature to which the skin is exposed, the specific heat of the causative agent, and the duration of exposure. Burns are classified into five different causal categories and depths of injury. The causes include injury from flame (fire), hot liquids (scald), contact with hot or cold objects, chemical exposure, and conduction of electricity (Box 19-2). The first three induce cellular damage by the transfer of energy, which induces coagulation necrosis. Chemical burns and electrical burns cause direct injury to cellular membranes in addition to the transfer of heat and can cause a coagulation or colliquation necrosis.

The skin, which is the largest organ of the human body, provides a staunch barrier in the transfer of energy to deeper tissues, thus confining much of the injury to this layer. Once the inciting focus is removed, however, the response of local tissues can lead to injury in the deeper layers. The area of cutaneous or superficial injury has been divided into three zones: zone of coagulation, zone of stasis, and zone of hyperemia (Fig. 19-1). The necrotic area of burn where cells have been disrupted is termed the *zone of coagulation*. This tissue is irreversibly damaged at the time of injury. The area immediately surrounding the necrotic zone has a moderate degree of insult with decreased tissue perfusion. This is termed the *zone of stasis* and, depending on the wound environment, can either survive or go on to coagulative necrosis. The zone of stasis is associated with vascular damage and vessel leakage. Thromboxane A2, a potent vasoconstrictor, is present in high concentrations in burn wounds, and local application of inhibitors improves blood flow and decreases the zone of stasis. Antioxidants, bradykinin antagonists, and subatmospheric wound pressures also improve blood flow and affect the depth of injury. Local endothelial interactions with neutrophils mediate some of the local inflammatory responses associated with the zone of stasis. Treatment directed at the control of local inflammation immediately after injury may spare the zone of stasis, indicated by studies demonstrating the blockage of leukocyte adherence with anti-CD18 or anti-intercellular adhesion molecules; monoclonal antibodies improve tissue perfusion and tissue survival in animal models. The last area is the *zone of hyperemia,* which is characterized by vasodilation from inflammation surrounding the burn wound. This region contains the clearly viable tissue from which the healing process begins and is generally not at risk for further necrosis.

BOX 19-1 Burn Unit Organization and Personnel

Experienced burn surgeons (burn unit director and qualified surgeons)
Dedicated nursing personnel
Physical and occupational therapists
Social workers
Dietitians
Pharmacists
Respiratory therapists
Psychiatrists and clinical psychologists
Prosthetists

BOX 19-2 Burn Classifications

Causes

Flame: damage from superheated, oxidized air
Scald: damage from contact with hot liquids
Contact: damage from contact with hot or cold solid materials
Chemicals: contact with noxious chemicals
Electricity: conduction of electrical current through tissues

Depths

First degree: injury localized to the epidermis
Superficial second degree: injury to the epidermis and superficial dermis
Deep second degree: injury through the epidermis and deep into the dermis
Third degree: full-thickness injury through the epidermis and dermis into subcutaneous fat
Fourth degree: injury through the skin and subcutaneous fat into underlying muscle or bone

Burn Depth

The depth of burn varies by the degree of tissue damage. Burn depth is classified into degree of injury in the epidermis, dermis, subcutaneous fat, and underlying structures (Fig. 19-2).

First-degree burns are, by definition, injuries confined to the epidermis. First-degree burns are painful and erythematous and blanch to the touch with an intact epidermal barrier. Examples include sunburn or a minor scald from a kitchen accident. These burns do not result in scarring, and treatment is aimed at comfort with the use of topical soothing salves with or without aloe and oral nonsteroidal anti-inflammatory agents.

Second-degree burns are divided into two types: superficial and deep. All second-degree burns have some degree of dermal damage, by definition, and the division is based on the depth of injury into the dermis. Superficial dermal burns are erythematous and painful, blanch to touch, and often blister. Examples include scald injuries from overheated bathtub water and flash flame burns. These wounds spontaneously re-epithelialize from retained epidermal structures in the rete ridges, hair follicles, and sweat glands in 1 to 2 weeks. After healing, these burns may have some slight skin discoloration in the long term. Deep dermal burns into the

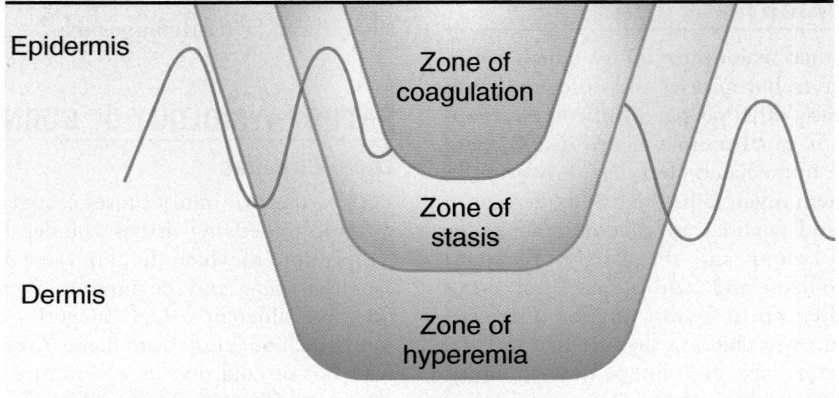

FIGURE 19-1 Zones of Injury after a Burn. The zone of coagulation is the portion irreversibly injured. The zones of stasis and hyperemia are defined in response to the injury.

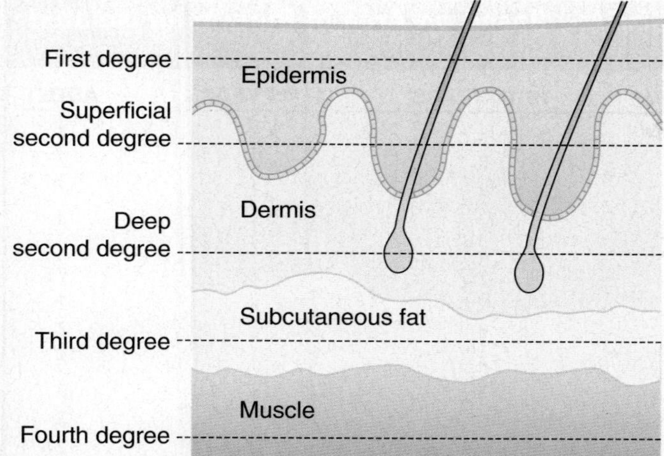

FIGURE 19-2 Depths of a Burn. First-degree burns are confined to the epidermis. Second-degree burns extend into the dermis (dermal burns). Third-degree burns are "full thickness" through the epidermis and dermis. Fourth-degree burns involve injury to underlying tissue structures, such as muscle, tendons, and bone.

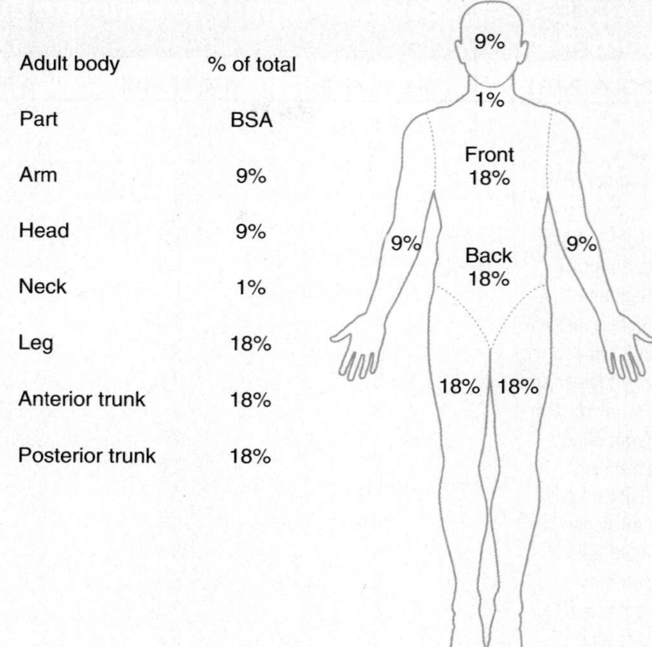

Adult body Part	% of total BSA
Arm	9%
Head	9%
Neck	1%
Leg	18%
Anterior trunk	18%
Posterior trunk	18%

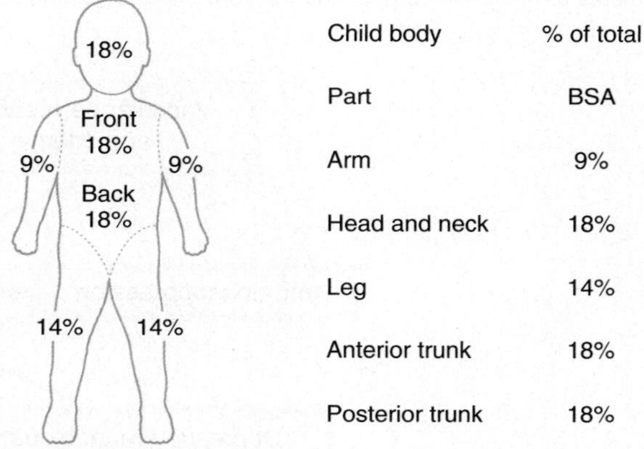

Child body Part	% of total BSA
Arm	9%
Head and neck	18%
Leg	14%
Anterior trunk	18%
Posterior trunk	18%

FIGURE 19-3 Estimation of burn size using the rule of nines. *BSA*, body surface area. (From Advanced Burn Life Support Provider Manual, Chicago, IL, 2005, American Burn Association.)

reticular dermis appear more pale and mottled, do not blanch to touch, but remain painful to pinprick. These burns heal in 2 to 5 weeks by re-epithelialization from hair follicles and sweat gland keratinocytes, often with severe scarring as a result of the loss of dermis.

Third-degree burns are full thickness through the epidermis and dermis and are characterized by a hard, leathery eschar that is painless and black, white, or cherry red. No epidermal or dermal appendages remain; thus, these wounds must heal by re-epithelialization from the wound edges. Deep dermal and full-thickness burns require excision with skin grafting from the patient to heal the wounds in a timely fashion.

Fourth-degree burns involve other organs beneath the skin, such as muscle, bone, and brain.

Currently, burn depth is most accurately assessed by judgment of experienced practitioners. Accurate depth determination is critical to wound healing as wounds that will heal with local treatment are treated differently from those requiring operative intervention. Examination of the entire wound by the physicians ultimately responsible for their management then is the "gold standard" used to guide further treatment decisions. New technologies, such as the multisensor laser Doppler flowmeter, hold promise for quantitative determination of burn depth. Several reports claim superiority of this method over clinical judgment in the determination of wounds requiring skin grafting for timely healing, which may lead to a change in the standard of care in the near future.

Burn Size

Determination of burn size estimates the extent of injury. Burn size is generally assessed by the "rule of nines" (Fig. 19-3). In adults, each upper extremity and the head and neck are 9% of the total body surface area (TBSA), the lower extremities and the anterior and posterior trunk are 18% each, and the perineum and genitalia are assumed to be 1% of the TBSA. Another method of estimating smaller burns is to equate the area of the open hand (including the palm and the extended fingers) of the patient to be approximately 1% TBSA and then to transpose that measurement visually onto the wound for a determination of its size. This method is crucial in evaluating burns of mixed distribution.

Children have a relatively larger portion of the body surface area in the head and neck, which is compensated for by a relatively smaller surface area in the lower extremities. Infants have 21% of the TBSA in the head and neck and 13% in each leg, which incrementally approaches the adult proportions with increasing age. The Berkow formula is used to accurately determine burn size in children (Table 19-1).

Systemic Changes

Severe burns covering more than 20% TBSA in adults and 40% TBSA in pediatric patients are typically followed by a period of stress, inflammation, and hypermetabolism, characterized by a hyperdynamic circulatory response with increased body temperature, glycolysis, proteolysis, lipolysis, and futile substrate cycling (Fig. 19-4). These responses are present in all trauma, surgical, and critically ill patients, but the severity, length, and magnitude are unique for burn patients.[5]

TABLE 19-1 Berkow Formula to Estimate Burn Size (%) Based on Area of Burn in an Isolated Body Part*

BODY PART	0-1 YEARS	1-4 YEARS	5-9 YEARS	10-14 YEARS	15-18 YEARS	ADULT
Head	19	17	13	11	9	7
Neck	2	2	2	2	2	2
Anterior trunk	13	13	13	13	13	13
Posterior trunk	13	13	13	13	13	13
Right buttock	2.5	2.5	2.5	2.5	2.5	2.5
Left buttock	2.5	2.5	2.5	2.5	2.5	2.5
Genitalia	1	1	1	1	1	1
Right upper arm	4	4	4	4	4	4
Left upper arm	4	4	4	4	4	4
Right lower arm	3	3	3	3	3	3
Left lower arm	3	3	3	3	3	3
Right hand	2.5	2.5	2.5	2.5	2.5	2.5
Left hand	2.5	2.5	2.5	2.5	2.5	2.5
Right thigh	5.5	6.5	8	8.5	9	9.5
Left thigh	5.5	6.5	8	8.5	9	9.5
Right leg	5	5	5.5	6	6.5	7
Left leg	5	5	5.5	6	6.5	7
Right foot	3.5	3.5	3.5	3.5	3.5	3.5
Left foot	3.5	3.5	3.5	3.5	3.5	3.5

*Estimates are made, recorded, and then summed to gain an accurate estimate of the body surface area burned.

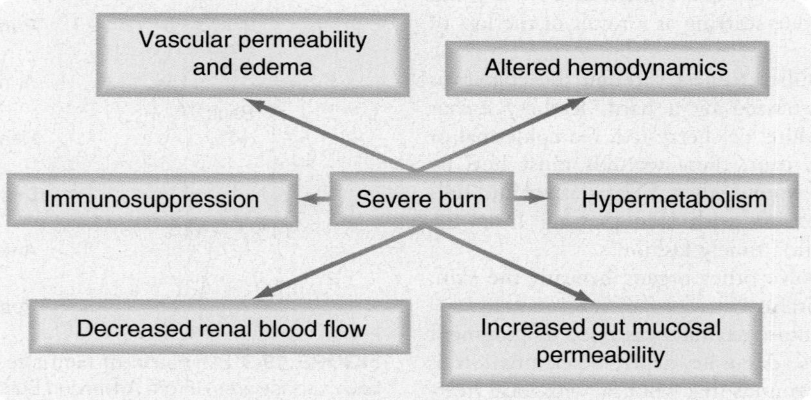

FIGURE 19-4 Systemic effects of a severe burn.

Hypermetabolic Response to Burn Injury

Marked and sustained increases in catecholamine, glucocorticoid, glucagon, and dopamine secretion are thought to initiate the cascade of events leading to the acute hypermetabolic response with its ensuing catabolic state.[12] The cause of this complex response is not well understood. However, interleukins 1 and 6, platelet-activating factor, tumor necrosis factor, endotoxin, neutrophil adherence complexes, reactive oxygen species, nitric oxide, and coagulation as well as complement cascades have also been implicated in regulating this response to burn injury.[13] Once these cascades are initiated, their mediators and byproducts appear to stimulate the persistent and increased metabolic rate associated with altered glucose metabolism seen after severe burn injury.[13]

The postburn metabolic phenomena occur in a timely manner, suggesting two distinct patterns of metabolic regulation after injury. The first phase occurs within the first 48 hours of injury and has classically been called the ebb phase, characterized by decreases in cardiac output, oxygen consumption, and metabolic rate as well as impaired glucose tolerance associated with its hyperglycemic state. These metabolic variables gradually increase within the first 5 days after injury to a plateau phase (called the flow phase), characteristically associated with hyperdynamic circulation and the hypermetabolic state.[12,14] Insulin release during this time was found to be twice that of controls in response to glucose load,[15] and plasma glucose levels are markedly elevated, indicating the development of an insulin resistance.[15] Current understanding has been that these metabolic alterations resolve soon after complete wound closure. However, studies found that the hypermetabolic response to burn injury may last for more than 12 months after the initial event.[16] We found that sustained hypermetabolic alterations after a burn, indicated by persistent elevations of total urine cortisol levels, serum cytokines, catecholamines, and basal energy requirements, were accompanied by impaired glucose metabolism and insulin sensitivity that persisted for up to 3 years after the initial burn injury.[16]

A 10-fold to 50-fold elevation of plasma catecholamines and corticosteroid levels occurs in major burns that persists up to 3 years after injury.[5,14,16] Cytokine levels peak immediately after burn injury, approaching normal levels only after 1 month. Constitutive and acute-phase proteins are altered beginning 5 to 7 days after burn injury and remain abnormal throughout the acute hospital stay. Serum insulin-like growth factor I (IGF-I), IGF-binding protein 3 (IGFBP-3), parathyroid hormone, and osteocalcin drop immediately after the burn injury 10-fold and remain significantly decreased up to 6 months compared with normal levels.[14] Sex hormones and endogenous growth hormone levels decrease around 3 weeks after a burn injury (Fig. 19-5).[14]

For severely burned patients, the resting metabolic rate at thermal neutral temperature (30° C) exceeds 140% of normal at admission and is reduced to 130% once the wounds are fully healed, then to 120% at 6 months and 110% at 12 months after burn injury.[14] Increases in catabolism result in loss of total body protein, decreased immune defenses, and decreased wound healing.[5,14]

Immediately after a burn injury, patients have low cardiac output characteristic of early shock. However, 3 to 4 days after the burn injury, cardiac output is more than 1.5 times that of nonburned, healthy volunteers.[14] The heart rate of pediatric burn patients approaches 1.6 times that of nonburned, healthy volunteers.[12] After a burn injury, patients have increased cardiac work.[5] Myocardial oxygen consumption surpasses that of marathon runners and is sustained well into the rehabilitative period.

There is profound hepatomegaly after injury. The liver increases its size by 225% of normal by 2 weeks after burn injury and remains enlarged at discharge by 200% of normal.[14]

After burn injury, muscle protein is degraded much faster than it is synthesized.[17] Net protein loss leads to loss of lean body mass and severe muscle wasting, leading to decreased strength and failure to fully rehabilitate. Significant decreases in lean body mass related to chronic illness or hypermetabolism can have dire consequences. A 10% loss of lean body mass is associated with immune dysfunction. A 20% loss of lean body mass positively correlates with decreased wound healing. A loss of 30% of lean body mass leads to increased risk for pneumonia and pressure sores. A 40% loss of lean body mass can lead to death. Uncomplicated severely burned patients can lose up to 25% of total body mass after acute burn injury.[14] Protein degradation persists up to nearly 1 year after severe burn injury, resulting in significant negative whole body and cross-leg nitrogen balance (Fig. 19-6).[5] Protein catabolism has a positive correlation with increases in metabolic rates. Severely burned patients have a daily nitrogen loss of 20 to 25 g/m^2 of burned skin.[5] At this rate, a lethal cachexia can be reached in less than 1 month. The protein loss of burned pediatric patients leads to significant growth retardation for up to 24 months after injury.[16]

Elevated circulating levels of catecholamines, glucagon, and cortisol after severe thermal injury stimulate free fatty acids and glycerol from fat, glucose production by the liver, and amino acids from muscle (Fig. 19-7).[5,12] Specifically, glycolytic-gluconeogenetic cycling is increased 250% during the postburn hypermetabolic response coupled with an increase of 450% in triglyceride–fatty acid cycling.[5] These changes lead to hyperglycemia and impaired insulin sensitivity related to postreceptor insulin resistance demonstrated by elevated levels of insulin and fasting glucose and significant reductions in glucose clearance. Whereas glucose delivery to peripheral tissues is increased up to threefold, glucose oxidation is restricted. Increased glucose production is directed, in part, to the burn wound to support the relatively inefficient anaerobic metabolism of fibroblasts and endothelial and inflammatory cells. The end product of anaerobic glucose oxidation—lactate—is recycled to the liver to produce more glucose through gluconeogenic pathways.[5] Serum glucose and serum insulin increase after burn injury and remain significantly increased through the acute hospital stay. Insulin resistance appears during the first week after burn injury and persists significantly after discharge up to 3 years.[14,16]

Septic patients have a profound increase in metabolic rates and protein catabolism up to 40% more compared with those with like-size burns who do not develop sepsis.[18,19] A vicious circle develops, as patients who are catabolic are more susceptible to sepsis because of changes in immune function and immune response. The emergence of multidrug-resistant organisms has led to increases in sepsis, catabolism, and mortality (Fig. 19-8). Modulation of the hypermetabolic, hypercatabolic response, thus preventing secondary injury, is paramount in the restoration of structure and function of severely burned patients.

Inflammation and Edema

Significant burns are associated with massive release of inflammatory mediators, both in the wound and in other tissues. These mediators produce vasoconstriction and vasodilation, increased capillary permeability, and edema locally and in distant organs. The generalized edema is in response to changes in Starling forces in both burned and unburned skin. Initially, the interstitial hydrostatic pressures in the burned skin decrease, and there is an associated increase in nonburned skin interstitial pressures. As the plasma oncotic pressures decrease and interstitial oncotic pressures increase as a result of increased capillary permeability–induced protein loss, edema forms in the burned and nonburned tissues. The edema is greater in the burned tissues because of lower interstitial pressures.

Many mediators have been proposed to account for the changes in permeability after burn injury, including histamine, bradykinin, vasoactive amines, prostaglandins, leukotrienes, activated complement, and catecholamines, among others. Mast cells in the burned skin release histamine in large quantities immediately after injury, which elicits a characteristic response in venules by increasing intercellular junction space formation. The use of antihistamines in the treatment of burn edema, however, has had limited success. In addition, aggregated platelets release serotonin to play a major role in edema formation. This agent acts directly to increase pulmonary vascular resistance, and it indirectly aggravates the vasoconstrictive effects of various vasoactive amines. Serotonin blockade improves cardiac index, decreases pulmonary artery pressure, and decreases oxygen consumption after burn injury. When the antiserotonin methysergide was given to animals after scald injury, wound edema formation decreased as a result of local effects.

Another mediator likely to play a role in changes in permeability and fluid shifts is thromboxane A2. Thromboxane increases dramatically in the plasma and wounds of burned patients. This potent vasoconstrictor leads to vasoconstriction and platelet aggregation in the wound, contributing to expansion of the zone of stasis. It also caused prominent mesenteric vasoconstriction and decreased gut blood flow in animal models that compromised gut mucosal integrity and decreased gut immune function.

Effects on Cardiovascular System

Microvascular changes induce cardiopulmonary alterations characterized by loss of plasma volume, increased peripheral vascular

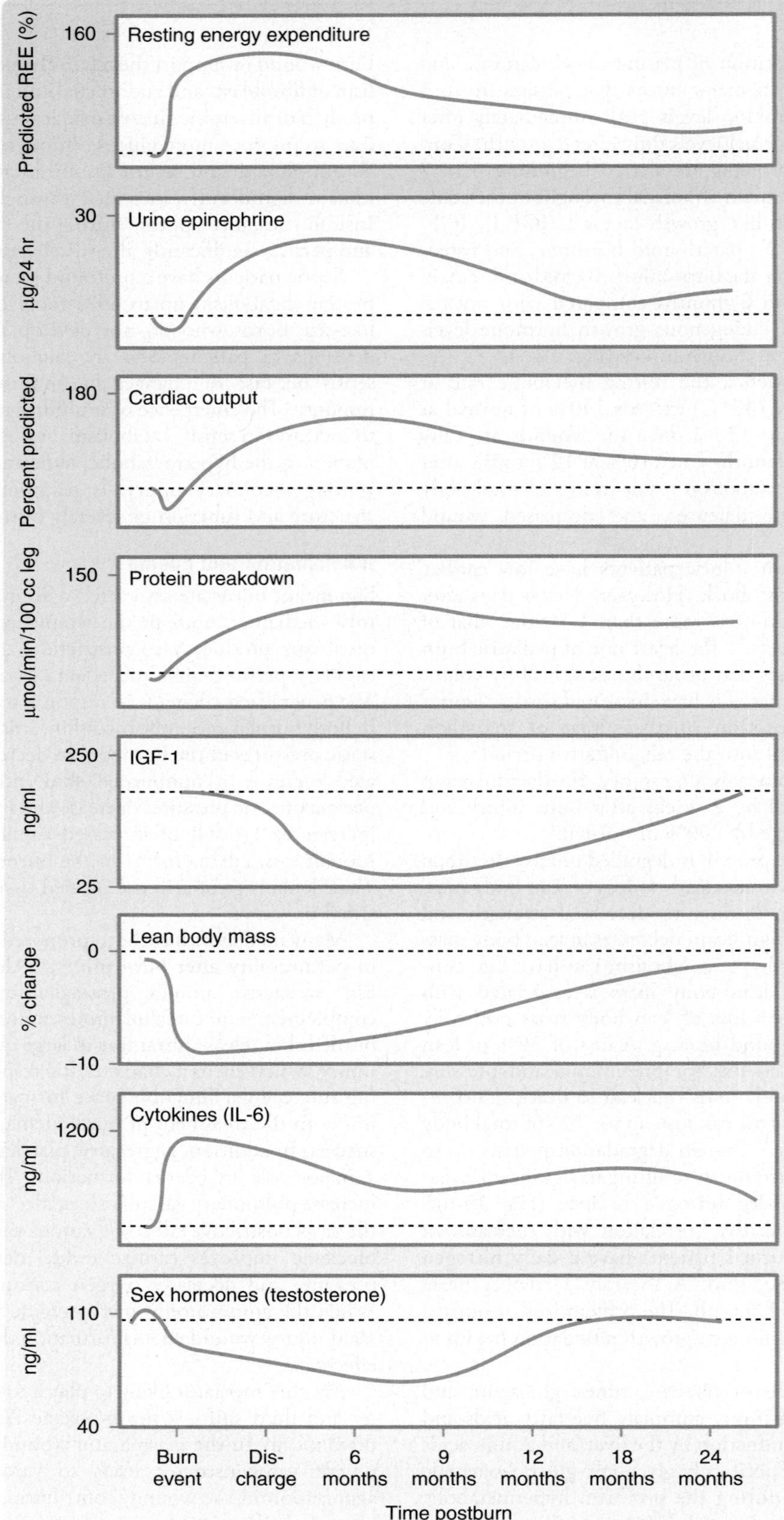

FIGURE 19-5 Physiologic and metabolic changes after severe burn injury. Changes are demonstrated in resting energy expenditure (REE), stress hormones (epinephrine), cardiac function (cardiac output), gender hormones (testosterone), cytokines (interleukin-6), and body composition (lean body mass). Data were summarized from published works from our institution. Averages for burn patients are represented by *solid curves*. Values from nonburned, normal patients are represented by *dashed lines*. (From Williams FN, Jeschke MG, Chinkes DL, et al: Modulation of the hypermetabolic response to trauma: Temperature, nutrition, and drugs. *J Am Coll Surg* 208:489–502, 2009.)

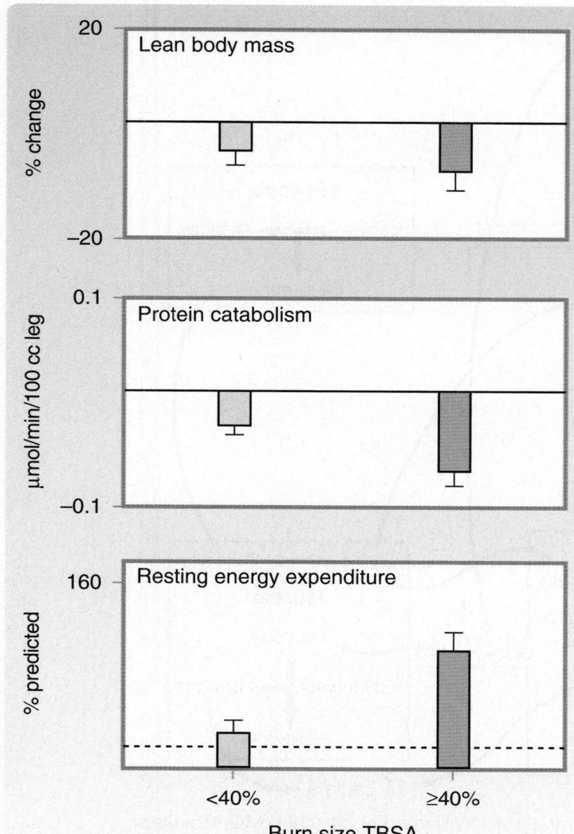

FIGURE 19-6 Effect of burn size on body mass, resting energy expenditure, and protein degradation. Changes in net protein balance of muscle protein synthesis and breakdown induced by burn injury were measured by stable isotope studies using d5-phenylalanine infusion. Graphs are averages ± standard error of the mean. The *yellow bars* represent patients with burns <40% total body surface area (TBSA). The *blue bars* represent patients with burns ≥40% TBSA. Values from nonburned, normal patients are represented by *dashed lines*. (From Williams FN, Jeschke MG, Chinkes DL, et al: Modulation of the hypermetabolic response to trauma: Temperature, nutrition, and drugs. *J Am Coll Surg* 208:489–502, 2009.)

resistance, and subsequent decreased cardiac output immediately after injury. Cardiac output remains depressed from decreased blood volume and increased blood viscosity as well as decreased cardiac contractility. Ventricular dysfunction in this period is attributed to a circulating myocardial depressant factor present in lymphatic fluid, although the specific factor has never been isolated. Burn patients with burns over 40% of their TBSA demonstrated an increased cardiac output that significantly decreased over time. This was accompanied by an increase in heart rate. Severely burned pediatric patients had a marked tachycardia of 160% to 170% predicted, which remained high at discharge from the intensive care unit (ICU) at around 150%. Cardiac output at admission was 150% and remained high at discharge at around 130% predicted. There is some evidence that heart rate remains elevated up to 2 years after burn injury.[14] Increased cardiac stress after burn injury is associated with myocardial depression, which was shown in several studies.[20] The hypothesis that one of the main contributors to mortality in large burns may be cardiac stress and myocardial dysfunction was confirmed in a retrospective autopsy study, implying the therapeutic need to improve cardiac stress and function.[21]

Effects on the Renal System

Diminished blood volume and cardiac output result in decreased renal blood flow and glomerular filtration rate. Other stress-induced hormones and mediators, such as angiotensin, aldosterone, and vasopressin, further reduce renal blood flow immediately after the injury. These effects result in oliguria, which, if left untreated, will cause acute tubular necrosis and renal failure. Twenty years ago, acute renal failure in burn injuries was almost always fatal. Today, newer techniques in dialysis became widely used to support the kidneys during recovery. The latest reports indicate an 88% mortality rate for severely burned adults and a 56% mortality rate for severely burned children in whom renal failure develops in the postburn period. Early resuscitation decreases risks of renal failure and improves the associated morbidity and mortality.[11]

Effects on the Gastrointestinal System

The gastrointestinal response to burn is highlighted by mucosal atrophy, changes in digestive absorption, and increased intestinal permeability. Atrophy of the small bowel mucosa occurs within 12 hours of injury in proportion to the burn size and is related to increased epithelial cell death by apoptosis. The cytoskeleton of the mucosal brush border undergoes atrophic changes associated with vesiculation of microvilli and disruption of the terminal web actin filaments. These findings were most pronounced 18 hours after injury, which suggests that changes in the cytoskeleton, such as those associated with cell death by apoptosis, are processes involved in the changed gut mucosa. Burn also causes reduced uptake of glucose and amino acids, decreased absorption of fatty acids, and reduction in brush border lipase activity. These changes peak in the first several hours after burn injury and return to normal at 48 to 72 hours, a timing that parallels mucosal atrophy.

Intestinal permeability to macromolecules, which are normally repelled by an intact mucosal barrier, increases after burn injury. Intestinal permeability to polyethylene glycol 3350, lactulose, and mannitol increases after injury, correlating to the extent of the burn. Gut permeability increases even further when burn wounds become infected. A study using fluorescent dextrans showed that larger molecules appeared to cross the mucosa between the cells, whereas the smaller molecules traversed the mucosa through the epithelial cells, presumably by pinocytosis and vesiculation. Mucosal permeability also paralleled increases in gut epithelial apoptosis.

Changes in gut blood flow are related to changes in permeability. Intestinal blood flow was shown to decrease in animals, a change that was associated with increased gut permeability at 5 hours after burn injury. This effect was abolished at 24 hours. Systolic hypotension has been shown to occur in the hours immediately after burn injury in animals with a 40% TBSA full-thickness injury. These animals showed an inverse correlation between blood flow and permeability to intact *Candida*.

Effects on the Immune System

Burns cause a global depression in immune function, which is shown by prolonged allograft skin survival on burn wounds. Burned patients are then at great risk for a number of infectious complications, including bacterial wound infection, pneumonia, and fungal and viral infections. These susceptibilities and

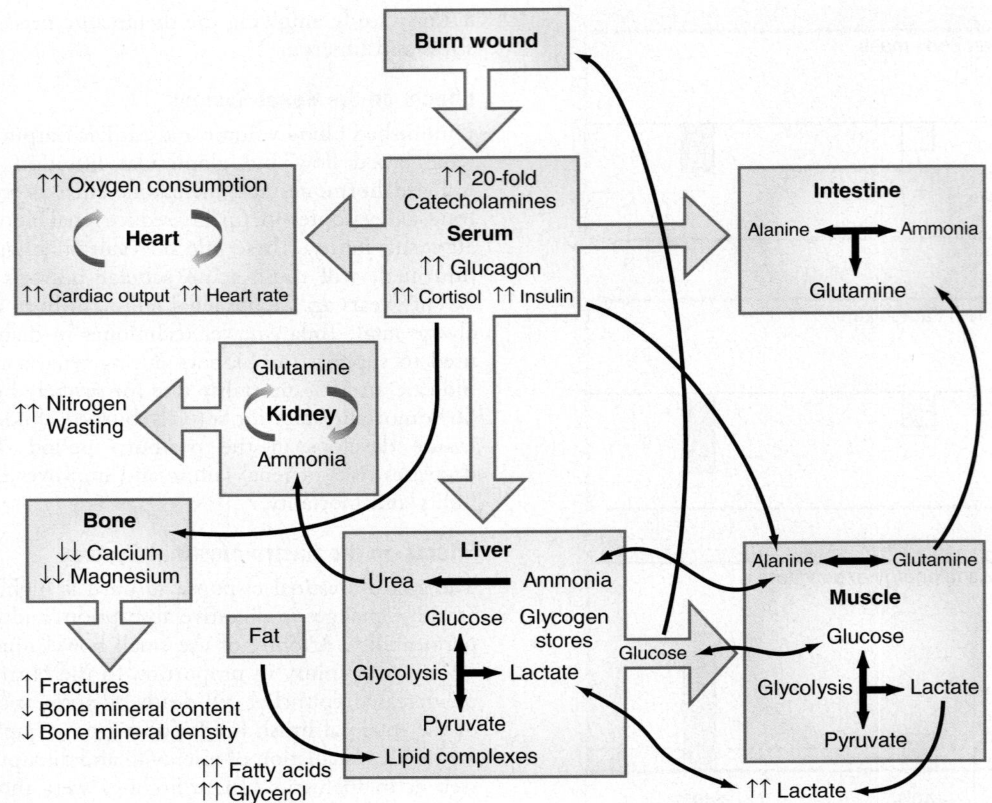

FIGURE 19-7 Effects of metabolic dysfunction after burn injury. (From Williams FN, Jeschke MG, Chinkes DL, et al: Modulation of the hypermetabolic response to trauma: Temperature, nutrition, and drugs. *J Am Coll Surg* 208:489–502, 2009.)

conditions are based on depressed cellular function in all parts of the immune system, including activation and activity of neutrophils, macrophages, T lymphocytes, and B lymphocytes. With burns of more than 20% TBSA, impairment of these immune functions is proportional to burn size.

Macrophage production after burn injury is diminished, which is related to the spontaneous elaboration of negative regulators of myeloid growth. This effect is enhanced by the presence of endotoxin and can be partially reversed with granulocyte colony-stimulating factor (G-CSF) treatment or inhibition of prostaglandin E2. Investigators have shown that G-CSF levels actually increase after severe burn. However, bone marrow G-CSF receptor expression is decreased, which may in part account for the immunodeficiency seen in burns. Total neutrophil counts are initially increased after burn injury, a phenomenon that is related to a decrease in cell death by apoptosis. However, neutrophils that are present are dysfunctional in terms of diapedesis, chemotaxis, and phagocytosis. These effects are explained, in part, by a deficiency in CD11b/CD18 expression after inflammatory stimuli, decreased respiratory burst activity associated with a deficiency in $p47^{phox}$ activity, and impaired actin mechanics related to neutrophil motile responses. After 48 to 72 hours, neutrophil counts decrease somewhat, like macrophages, with similar causes.

T-helper cell function is depressed after a severe burn that is associated with polarization from the interleukin-2 and interferon-γ cytokine-based T-helper 1 (Th1) response toward the Th2 response. The Th2 response is characterized by the production of interleukin-4 and interleukin-10. The Th1 response is important in cell-mediated immune defense, whereas the Th2 response is important in antibody responses to infection. As this polarization increases, so does the mortality rate. Administration of interleukin-10 antibodies and growth hormone has partially reversed this response and improved mortality rate after burn injury in animals. Burn also impairs cytotoxic T-lymphocyte activity as a function of burn size, thus increasing the risk of infection, particularly from fungi and viruses. Early burn wound excision improves cytotoxic T-cell activity.

BASIC TREATMENT OF BURN INJURY

Prehospital Management

Before undergoing any specific treatment, burned patients must be removed from the source of injury and the burning process stopped. Inhalation injury should always be suspected, and 100% oxygen should be given by face mask. While the patient is being removed from the source of injury, care must be taken so that the rescuer does not become another victim. All caregivers should be aware that they might be injured by contact with the patient or the patient's clothing. Universal precautions, including wearing of gloves, gowns, mask, and protective eyewear, should be used whenever there is likely to be contact with blood or body fluids. Burning clothing should be extinguished and removed as soon as possible to prevent further injury. All rings, watches, jewelry, and belts should be removed because they retain heat and can produce a tourniquet-like effect. Room temperature water can be poured on the wound within 15 minutes of injury to decrease the depth of the wound, but any subsequent measures to cool the wound should be avoided to prevent hypothermia during resuscitation.

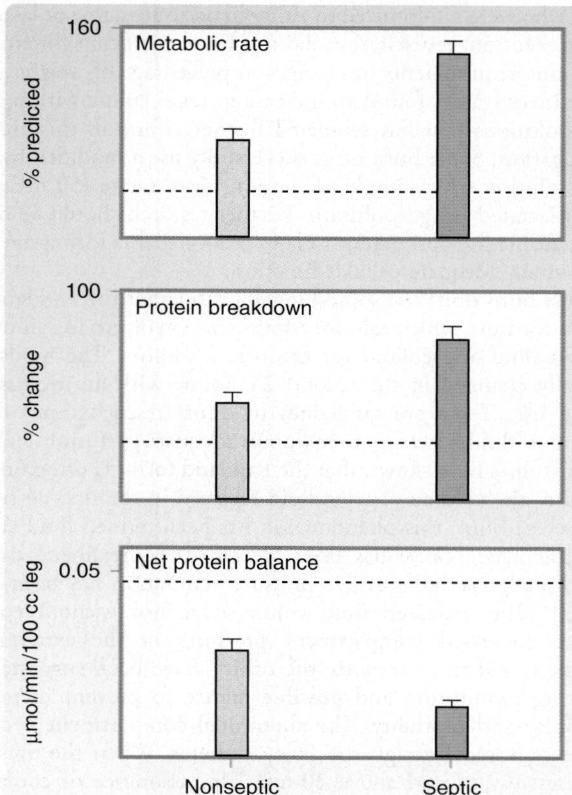

FIGURE 19-8 Effect of sepsis on resting energy expenditure, muscle protein breakdown, and fractional synthetic rate of muscle protein synthesis compared with like-sized burns. Changes in net protein balance of muscle protein synthesis and breakdown induced by burn injury were measured by stable isotope studies using d5-phenylalanine infusion. Graphs are averages ± standard error of the mean. The *yellow bars* represent nonseptic patients with burns ≥40% total body surface area (TBSA). The *blue bars* represent septic patients with burns ≥40% TBSA. Values from nonburned, normal patients are represented by *dashed lines.* (From Williams FN, Jeschke MG, Chinkes DL, et al: Modulation of the hypermetabolic response to trauma: Temperature, nutrition, and drugs. *J Am Coll Surg* 208:489–502, 2009.)

Initial Assessment

As with any trauma patient, the initial assessment of a burned patient is divided into a primary and secondary survey. In the primary survey, immediate life-threatening conditions are quickly identified and treated. In the secondary survey, a more thorough head-to-toe evaluation of the patient is undertaken.

Exposure to heated gases and smoke results in damage to the upper respiratory tract. Direct injury to the upper airway results in edema, which, in combination with generalized whole body edema associated with severe burn, may obstruct the airway. Airway injury must be suspected with facial burns, singed nasal hairs, carbonaceous sputum, and tachypnea. Upper airway obstruction may develop rapidly, and respiratory status must be continually monitored to assess the need for airway control and ventilatory support. Progressive hoarseness is a sign of impending airway obstruction, and endotracheal intubation should be instituted early before edema distorts the upper airway anatomy. This is especially important in patients with massive burns, who may appear to breathe without problems early in the resuscitation period until several liters of volume are given to maintain homeostasis, resulting in significant airway edema.

The chest should be exposed to assess breathing; airway patency alone does not ensure adequate ventilation. Chest expansion and equal breath sounds with CO_2 return from the endotracheal tube ensure adequate air exchange.

Blood pressure may be difficult to obtain in burned patients with edematous or charred extremities. Pulse rate can be used as an indirect measure of circulation; however, most burned patients remain tachycardic even with adequate resuscitation. For the primary survey of burned patients, the presence of pulses or Doppler signals in the distal extremities may be adequate to determine adequate circulation of blood until better monitors, such as arterial pressure measurements and urine output, can be established.

In those patients who have been in an explosion or deceleration accident, a possibility exists for spinal cord injury. Appropriate cervical spine stabilization must be accomplished by whatever means necessary, including use of cervical collars to keep the head immobilized until the condition can be evaluated.

Initial Wound Care

Prehospital care of the burn wound is basic and simple because it requires only protection from the environment with application of a clean dry dressing or sheet to cover the involved part. Damp dressings should not be used. The patient should be wrapped in a blanket to minimize heat loss and for temperature control during transport. The first step in diminishing pain is to cover the wounds to prevent contact to exposed nerve endings. Intramuscular or subcutaneous narcotic injections for pain should never be used because drug absorption is decreased as a result of the peripheral vasoconstriction. This might become a problem later when the patient is resuscitated, and vasodilation increases absorption of the narcotic depot with resulting apnea. Small doses of intravenous morphine may be given after complete assessment of the patient and after it is determined to be safe by an experienced practitioner.

Although prehospital management is simple, it is often difficult to enact, particularly in at-risk populations. A study in New Zealand showed that initial burn first aid treatment was inadequate in 60% of patients interviewed. These authors also showed that inadequate first aid care was clearly associated with poorer outcomes. They suggested that defined education programs targeted on at-risk populations might improve these outcomes.[22]

Transport

Rapid, uncontrolled transport of the burn victim is not a priority, except when other life-threatening conditions coexist. In most incidents involving major burns, ground transportation of victims to the receiving hospital is appropriate. Helicopter transport is of greatest use when the distance between the accident and the hospital is 30 to 150 miles. For distances of more than 150 miles, transport by fixed-wing aircraft is most appropriate. Whatever the mode of transport, it should be of appropriate size and have emergency equipment available, with trained personnel on board, such as nurses, physicians, paramedics, or respiratory therapists who are familiar with multiply injured trauma patients.

Resuscitation

Adequate resuscitation of the burned patient depends on the establishment and maintenance of reliable intravenous access. Increased times to beginning resuscitation of burned patients result in poorer outcomes, and delays should be minimized. Venous access is best attained through short peripheral catheters in unburned skin; however, veins in burned skin can be used and are preferable to no intravenous access. Superficial veins are often thrombosed in full-thickness injuries and therefore are not suitable for cannulation. Saphenous vein cutdowns are useful in cases of difficult access and are used in preference to central vein cannulation because of lower complication rates. In children younger than 6 years, experienced practitioners can use intraosseous access in the proximal tibia until intravenous access is accomplished. Lactated Ringer solution without dextrose is the fluid of choice except in children younger than 2 years, who should receive 5% dextrose in lactated Ringer solution. The initial rate can be rapidly estimated by multiplying the TBSA burned by the patient's weight in kilograms and then dividing by 8. Thus, the rate of infusion for an 80-kg man with a 40% TBSA burn would be

$$80\ \text{kg} \times 40\%\ \text{TBSA}/8 = 400\ \text{mL/hr}$$

This rate should be continued until a formal calculation of resuscitation needs is performed.

Many formulas have been devised to determine the proper amount of fluid to give a burned patient, all originating from experimental studies on the pathophysiology of burn shock. These experimental studies established the basis for modern fluid resuscitation protocols. They showed that edema fluid in burn wounds is isotonic and contains the same amount of protein as plasma and that the greatest loss of fluid is into the interstitium.[23] They used various volumes of intravascular fluid to determine the optimal amount in terms of cardiac output and extracellular volume in a canine burn model, and this was applied to the clinical realm in the Parkland formula. Plasma volume changes were not related to the type of resuscitation fluid in the first 24 hours, but thereafter colloid solutions could increase plasma volume by the amount infused. From these findings, it was concluded that colloid solutions should not be used in the first 24 hours until capillary permeability returned closer to normal. Others have argued that normal capillary permeability is restored somewhat earlier after burn injury (6 to 8 hours), and therefore colloids could be used earlier.

Concurrently, researchers showed the hemodynamic effects of fluid resuscitation in burns, which culminated in the Brooke formula. They found that fluid resuscitation caused an obligatory 20% decrease in both extracellular fluid and plasma volume that concluded after 24 hours. In the second 24 hours, plasma volume returned to normal with the administration of colloid. Cardiac output was low in the first day despite resuscitation, but it subsequently increased to supernormal levels as the flow phase of hypermetabolism was established. Since these studies, it has been found that much of the fluid needs are due to "leaky" capillaries that permit passage of large molecules into the interstitial space to increase extravascular colloid osmotic pressure. Intravascular volume follows the gradient to tissues, into both the burn wound and the nonburned tissues. Approximately 50% of fluid resuscitation needs are sequestered in nonburned tissues in 50% TBSA burns.

Hypertonic saline solutions have theoretical advantages in burn resuscitation. These solutions decrease net fluid intake, decrease edema, and increase lymph flow, probably by the transfer of volume from the intracellular space to the interstitium. When these solutions are used, hypernatremia must be avoided, and it is recommended that serum sodium concentrations not exceed 160 mEq/dL. However, for patients with more than 20% TBSA burns who were randomized to either hypertonic saline or lactated Ringer solution, resuscitation did not have significant differences in volume requirements or changes in percentage of weight gain. Other investigators found an increase in renal failure with hypertonic solutions that has tempered further efforts in this area of investigation. Some burn units successfully use a modified hypertonic solution of 1 ampule of sodium bicarbonate (50 mEq) in 1 L of lactated Ringer solution. Further research should be done to determine the optimal formula to reduce edema formation and to maintain adequate cellular function.

Most burn units use something akin to either the Parkland or Brooke formula, which calls for administration of varying amounts of crystalloid and colloid for the first 24 hours. The fluids are generally changed in the second 24 hours, with an increase in colloid use. These are guidelines to direct resuscitation of the amount of fluid necessary to maintain adequate perfusion. In fact, recent studies have shown that the Parkland formula often underestimates the volume of crystalloid received in the first 24 hours after severe burn; this phenomenon has been termed fluid creep. No clear single cause has been identified. More liberal use of opioid analgesia and positive pressure ventilation has been suggested.[24] The increased fluid volumes are not without consequence; increased compartment pressures in the extremities, abdomen, and most recently the orbit[25] have been suggested as requiring monitoring and possible release to prevent increased morbidity and mortality. The abdominal compartment is clinically monitored through the Foley catheter. When the pressure increases toward and above 30 mm Hg, assurance of complete abdominal escharotomy is made, and paralytics are considered. If the increased abdominal pressure persists (>30 mm Hg), an improved outcome rests in the performance of a decompressive laparotomy. However, the patients who require this procedure have mortality rates of 60% to nearly 100%, depending on the series. Therefore, monitoring of the resuscitation is crucial to ensure acceptable outcome. This is easily monitored in burned patients with normal renal function by following the volume of urine output, which should be at 0.5 mL/hr in adults and 1.0 mL/kg/hr in children. Changes in intravenous fluid infusion rates should be made on an hourly basis determined by the response of the patient to the particular fluid volume administered. The exact formulas are shown in Table 19-2.

For burned children, formulas are commonly used that are modified to account for changes in surface area to mass ratios. These changes are necessary because a child with a comparable burn to that of an adult requires more resuscitation fluid per kilogram. The Galveston formula uses 5000 mL/TBSA burned

TABLE 19-2 Resuscitation Formulas

FORMULA	CRYSTALLOID VOLUME	COLLOID VOLUME	FREE WATER
Parkland	4 mL/kg per % TBSA burn	None	None
Brooke	1.5 mL/kg per % TBSA burn	0.5 mL/kg per % TBSA burn	2.0 L
Galveston (pediatric)	5000 mL/m^2 burned area + 1500 mL/m^2 total area	None	None

These guidelines are used for the initial fluid management after a burn injury. The response to fluid resuscitation should be continuously monitored, and adjustments in the rate of fluid administration should be made accordingly. *TBSA,* total body surface area.

(in m^2) + 1500 mL/m^2 total for maintenance in the first 24 hours. This formula accounts for both maintenance needs and the increased fluid requirements of a child with a burn. All of the formulas listed in Table 19-2 calculate the amount of volume given in the first 24 hours, half of which is given in the first 8 hours.

The use of albumin during intravenous resuscitation has recently come under criticism. The Cochrane group showed in a meta-analysis of 31 trials that the risk of death was higher in burned patients receiving albumin compared with those receiving crystalloid, with a relative risk of death at 2.40 (95% confidence interval, 1.11 to 5.19). Another meta-analysis of all critically ill patients refuted this finding, showing no differences in relative risk between albumin-treated and crystalloid-treated groups. In fact, as quality of the trials improved, the relative risks were reduced. Additional recent evidence suggests that albumin supplementation even after resuscitation does not affect the distribution of fluid among the intracellular and extracellular compartments. What we can conclude from these trials and meta-analyses is that albumin used during resuscitation is at best equal to crystalloid and at worst detrimental to the outcome of burned patients. For these reasons, we cannot recommend the use of albumin during resuscitation.

To combat any regurgitation with an intestinal ileus, a nasogastric tube should be inserted in all patients with major burns to decompress the stomach. This is especially important for all patients being transported in aircraft at high altitudes. In addition, all patients should be restricted from taking anything by mouth until the transfer has been completed. Decompression of the stomach is usually necessary because the apprehensive patient will swallow considerable amounts of air and distend the stomach. In addition, a Dobhoff tube should be placed into the first part of the duodenum to continuously feed the severely burned.

Recommendations for tetanus prophylaxis are based on the condition of the wound and the patient's immunization history. All patients with burns of more than 10% TBSA should receive 0.5 mL of tetanus toxoid. If prior immunization is absent or unclear or the last booster dose was more than 10 years ago, 250 units of tetanus immune globulin are also given.

Escharotomies

When deep second- and third-degree burn wounds encompass the circumference of an extremity, peripheral circulation to the limb can be compromised. Development of generalized edema beneath a nonyielding eschar impedes venous outflow and eventually affects arterial inflow to the distal beds. This can be recognized by numbness and tingling in the limb and increased pain in the digits. Arterial flow can be assessed by determination of Doppler signals in the digital arteries and the palmar and plantar arches in affected extremities. Capillary refill can also be assessed. Extremities at risk are identified either on clinical examination or on measurement of tissue pressures higher than 40 mm Hg. These extremities require escharotomies, which are releases of the burn eschar performed at the bedside by incision of the lateral and medial aspects of the extremity with a scalpel or electrocautery unit. The entire constricting eschar must be incised longitudinally to completely relieve the impediment to blood flow (Fig. 19-9). The incisions are carried down onto the thenar and hypothenar eminences and along the dorsolateral sides of the digits to completely open the hand, if it is involved. If it is clear that the wound will require excision and grafting because of its depth, escharotomies are safest to restore perfusion to the underlying nonburned

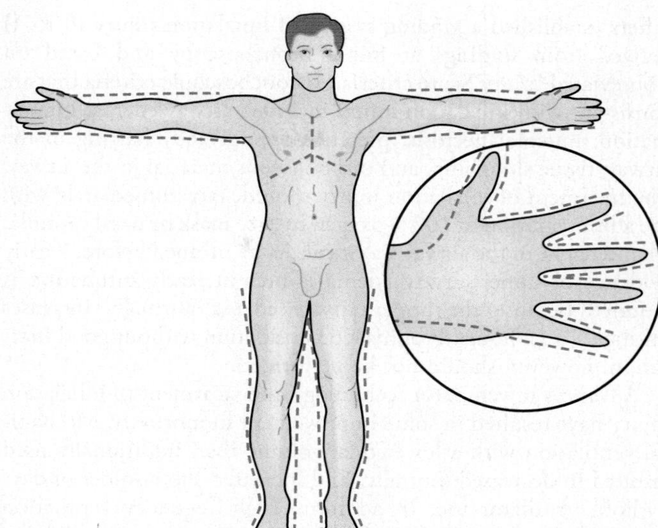

FIGURE 19-9 Recommended escharotomies. In limbs requiring escharotomies, the incisions are made on the medial and lateral sides of the extremity through the eschar. In the case of the hand, incisions are made on the medial and lateral digits and on the dorsum of the hand.

tissues until formal excision. If vascular compromise has been prolonged, reperfusion after an escharotomy may cause reactive hyperemia and further edema formation in the muscle, making continued surveillance of the distal extremities necessary. Increased muscle compartment pressures may necessitate fasciotomies. The most common complications associated with these procedures are blood loss and the release of anaerobic metabolites, causing transient hypotension. If distal perfusion does not improve with these measures, central hypotension from hypovolemia should be suspected and treated.

A constricting truncal eschar can cause a similar phenomenon, except the effect is to decrease ventilation by limiting chest excursion. Any decrease in ventilation of a burned patient should produce inspection of the chest with appropriate escharotomies to relieve the constriction and to allow adequate tidal volumes. This need becomes evident in a patient on a volume-control ventilator whose peak airway pressures increase.

SPECIFIC TREATMENT OF BURNS

Inhalation Injury

Even though mortality from major burns has significantly decreased during the past 20 years, inhalation injury still constitutes one of the most critical concomitant injuries following thermal insult. Approximately 80% of fire-related deaths result not from burns but from inhalation of the toxic products of combustion, and inhalation injury has remained associated with an overall mortality rate of 25% to 50% when patients require ventilator support for more than 1 week after injury.[11,26] Early diagnosis of bronchopulmonary injury is thus critical for survival and is conducted primarily clinically, based on a history of closed-space exposure, facial burns, and carbonaceous debris in mouth, pharynx, or sputum. Evidence-based experience on diagnosis of inhalation injury, however, is rare. Chest radiographs are routinely normal until complications, such as infections, have developed. The standard diagnostic method should therefore be bronchoscopy of the upper airway of every burn patient. Gamelli and others established a grading system of inhalation injury (0 to 4) derived from findings at initial bronchoscopy and based on Abbreviated Injury Score criteria.[27] Bronchoscopic criteria that are consistent with inhalation injury included airway edema, inflammation, mucosal necrosis, presence of soot and charring in the airway, tissue sloughing, and carbonaceous material in the airway. The treatment of inhalation injury should start immediately with the administration of 100% oxygen by face mask or nasal cannula. Maintenance of the airway is critical. As mentioned before, if early evidence of upper airway edema is present, early intubation is required because the upper airway edema normally increases during 9 to 12 hours. Prophylactic intubation without good indication, however, should not be performed.

Advances in ventilator technology and treatment of inhalation injury have resulted in some improvement in mortality. Mechanical ventilation with a lower tidal volume than traditionally used resulted in decreased mortality and increased the number of days without ventilator use. In addition, high-frequency ventilation decreased mortality to 29% from 41%. Management of inhalation injury consists of ventilatory support, aggressive pulmonary toilet (Table 19-3), bronchoscopic removal of casts, and nebulization therapy. Nebulization therapy can consist of heparin, alpha mimetics, or polymyxin B and is applied between two and six times a day. Pressure-control ventilation with permissive hypercapnia is a useful strategy in the management of these patients, and $PaCO_2$ levels of as much as 60 mm Hg can be well tolerated if they are arrived at gradually. Prophylactic antibiotics are not indicated but are imperative with documented lung infections. Clinical diagnosis of pneumonia includes two of the following[18]: chest radiograph revealing a new and persistent infiltrate, consolidation, or cavitation; sepsis, as defined in Table 19-4; or a recent change in sputum or purulence in the sputum as well as quantitative culture. Clinical diagnosis can be modified after using microbiologic data of three categories according to the American Burn Association Consensus Conference to Define Sepsis and Infection in Burns.[18] Empirical choices for the treatment of pneumonia before culture results are available should include coverage of methicillin-resistant *Staphylococcus aureus* and gram-negative organisms such as *Pseudomonas* and *Klebsiella*.[28]

TABLE 19-3 Inhalation Treatments of Smoke Inhalation Injury

TREATMENT	TIME, DOSAGE, AND METHOD
Bronchodilators (Albuterol)	q2h
Nebulized heparin	5000-10,000 units with 3 mL normal saline q4h
Nebulized acetylcysteine	20%, 3 mL q4h
Hypertonic saline	Induces effective coughing
Racemic epinephrine	Reduces mucosal edema

TABLE 19-4 Clinical Indications for Intubation

CRITERIA	VALUE
PaO_2	<60 mm Hg
$PaCO_2$	>50 mm Hg (acutely)
PaO_2/FIO_2 ratio	<200
Respiratory or ventilatory failure	Impending
Upper airway edema	Severe

Wound Care

After the airway is assessed and resuscitation is under way, attention must be turned to the burn wound. Treatment depends on the characteristics and size of the wound. All treatments are aimed at rapid and painless healing. Current therapy directed specifically toward burn wounds can be divided into three stages: assessment, management, and rehabilitation. Once the extent and depth of the wounds have been assessed and the wounds have been thoroughly cleaned and débrided, the management phase begins. Each wound should be dressed with an appropriate covering that serves several functions. First, it should protect the damaged epithelium, minimize bacterial and fungal colonization, and provide splinting action to maintain the desired position of function. Second, the dressing should be occlusive to reduce evaporative heat loss and to minimize cold stress. Third, the dressing should provide comfort over the painful wound.

The choice of dressing is based on the characteristics of the treated wound (Table 19-5). First-degree wounds are minor with minimal loss of barrier function. These wounds require no dressing and are treated with topical salves to decrease pain and to keep the skin moist. Systemic nonsteroidal anti-inflammatory agents given by mouth assist in pain control. Second-degree wounds can be treated with daily dressing changes with topical antibiotics, cotton gauze, and elastic wraps. Alternatively, the wounds can be treated with a temporary biologic or synthetic covering to close the wound. Deep second-degree and third-degree wounds require excision and grafting for sizable burns, and the choice of initial dressing should be aimed at holding bacterial proliferation in check and providing occlusion until the operation is performed.

Antimicrobials

The timely and effective use of antimicrobials has revolutionized burn care by decreasing invasive wound infections. The untreated burn wound rapidly becomes colonized with bacteria and fungi because of the loss of normal skin barrier mechanisms. As the organisms proliferate to high wound counts ($>10^5$ organisms per gram of tissue), they may penetrate into viable tissue. Organisms then invade blood vessels, causing a systemic infection that often leads to the death of the patient. This scenario has become uncommon in most burn units because of the effective use of antibiotics and wound care techniques. The antimicrobials that are used can be divided into those given topically and those given systemically.

Available topical antibiotics can be divided into two classes: salves and soaks. Salves are generally applied directly to the wound with cotton dressings placed over them, and soaks are generally poured into cotton dressings on the wound. Each of these classes of antimicrobials has advantages and disadvantages. Salves may be applied once or twice a day but may lose their effectiveness between dressing changes. Frequent dressing changes can result in shearing with loss of grafts or underlying healing cells. Soaks remain effective because antibiotic solution can be added without removal of the dressing; however, the underlying skin can become macerated.

Topical antibiotic salves include 11% mafenide acetate (Sulfamylon), 1% silver sulfadiazine (Silvadene), polymyxin B, neomycin, bacitracin, mupirocin, and the antifungal agent nystatin. No single agent is completely effective, and each has advantages and disadvantages. Silver sulfadiazine is the most commonly used. It

TABLE 19-5 Burn Wound Dressings

DRESSINGS	ADVANTAGES AND DISADVANTAGES
Antimicrobial Salves	
Silver sulfadiazine (Silvadene)	Broad-spectrum antimicrobial; painless and easy to use; does not penetrate eschar; may leave black tattoos from silver ion; mild inhibition of epithelialization
Mafenide acetate (Sulfamylon)	Broad-spectrum antimicrobial; penetrates eschar; may cause pain in sensate skin; wide application may cause metabolic acidosis; mild inhibition of epithelialization
Bacitracin	Ease of application; painless; antimicrobial spectrum not as wide as above agents
Neomycin	Ease of application; painless; antimicrobial spectrum not as wide
Polymyxin B	Ease of application; painless; antimicrobial spectrum not as wide
Nystatin (Mycostatin)	Effective in inhibiting most fungal growth; cannot be used in combination with mafenide acetate
Mupirocin (Bactroban)	More effective staphylococcal coverage; does not inhibit epithelialization; expensive
Antimicrobial Soaks	
0.5% Silver nitrate	Effective against all microorganisms; stains contacted areas; leaches sodium from wounds; may cause methemoglobinemia
5% Mafenide acetate	Wide antibacterial coverage; no fungal coverage; painful on application to sensate wound; wide application associated with metabolic acidosis
0.025% Sodium hypochlorite (Dakin solution)	Effective against almost all microbes, particularly gram-positive organisms; mildly inhibits epithelialization
0.25% Acetic acid	Effective against most organisms, particularly gram-negative ones; mildly inhibits epithelialization
Synthetic Coverings	
OpSite	Provides a moisture barrier; inexpensive; decreased wound pain; use complicated by transudate and exudate requiring removal; no antimicrobial properties
Biobrane	Provides a wound barrier; associated with decreased pain; use complicated by accumulation of exudate, risking invasive wound infection; no antimicrobial properties
TransCyte	Provides a wound barrier; decreased pain; accelerated wound healing; use complicated by accumulation of exudate; no antimicrobial properties
Integra	Provides complete wound closure and leaves a dermal equivalent; sporadic take rates; antimicrobial properties
Biologic Coverings	
Xenograft (pig skin)	Completely closes the wound; provides some immunologic benefits; must be removed or allowed to slough
Allograft (homograft, cadaver skin)	Provides all the normal functions of skin; can leave a dermal equivalent; epithelium must be removed or allowed to slough

has a broad spectrum of activity because its silver and sulfa moieties cover gram-positive, most gram-negative, and some fungal forms. Some *Pseudomonas* species possess plasmid-mediated resistance. Silver sulfadiazine is relatively painless on application, has a high patient acceptance, and is easy to use. On occasion, patients complain of a burning sensation after it is applied, and, in a few patients, a transient leukopenia develops 3 to 5 days after its continued use. This leukopenia is generally harmless and resolves with or without treatment cessation.

Mafenide acetate is another topical agent with a broad spectrum of activity because of its sulfa moiety. It is particularly useful against resistant *Pseudomonas* and *Enterococcus* species. It also can penetrate eschar, which silver sulfadiazine cannot. Disadvantages include painful application on skin, such as in second-degree wounds. It also can cause an allergic rash, and it has carbonic anhydrase inhibitory characteristics that can result in a metabolic acidosis when it is applied over large surfaces. For these reasons, mafenide sulfate is typically reserved for small full-thickness injuries.

Petroleum-based antimicrobial ointments with polymyxin B, neomycin, and bacitracin are clear on application, are painless, and allow easy wound observation. These agents are commonly used for treatment of facial burns, graft sites, healing donor sites, and small partial-thickness burns. Mupirocin is a relatively new petroleum-based ointment that has improved activity against gram-positive bacteria, particularly methicillin-resistant *S. aureus* and selected gram-negative bacteria. Nystatin, in either a salve or powder form, can be applied to wounds to control fungal growth. Nystatin-containing ointments can be combined with other topical agents to decrease colonization of both bacteria and fungus. The exception is the combination of nystatin and mafenide acetate; each inactivates the other.

Available agents for application as a soak include 0.5% silver nitrate solution, 0.025% sodium hypochlorite (Dakin solution), 0.25% acetic acid, and mafenide acetate as a 5% solution. Silver nitrate has the advantage of being painless on application and having complete antimicrobial effectiveness. The disadvantages include its staining of surfaces to a dull gray or black when the solution dries. This can become a problem in deciphering wound depth during burn excisions and in keeping the patient and his or her surroundings clean of the black staining. The solution is hypotonic as well, and continuous use can cause electrolyte leaching, with rare methemoglobinemia as another complication. A new commercial dressing containing biologically potent silver ions (Acticoat) that are activated in the presence of moisture is available. This dressing holds the promise of retaining the effectiveness of silver nitrate without the problems of silver nitrate soaks.

Dakin solution (0.25% sodium hypochlorite) has effectiveness against most microbes; however, it also has cytotoxic effects on the healing cells of patients' wounds. Low concentrations of sodium hypochlorite (0.025%) have fewer cytotoxic effects while maintaining most of the antimicrobial effects. Hypochlorite ion is inactivated by contact with protein, so the solution must be continually changed. The same is true for acetic acid solutions, which may be more effective against *Pseudomonas*. Mafenide acetate soaks have the same characteristics of the mafenide acetate salve, except in liquid form.

The use of perioperative systemic antimicrobials also has a role in decreasing burn wound sepsis until the burn wound is closed. Common organisms that must be considered in choosing a perioperative regimen include *S. aureus* and *Pseudomonas* species, which are prevalent in burn wounds.

Burn Wound Excision

Methods for handling burn wounds have changed in recent decades and are similar in adults and children. Increasingly aggressive early tangential excision of the burn tissue and early wound closure primarily by skin grafts have led to significant improvement of mortality rates and substantially lower costs in this particular population of patients. Early wound closure has furthermore been found to be associated with decreased severity of hypertrophic scarring, joint contractures, and stiffness, and it promotes quicker rehabilitation. Techniques of burn wound excision have evolved substantially during the past decade. In general, most areas are excised with a hand skin graft knife or powered dermatome. Sharp excision with a knife or electrocautery is reserved for areas of functional cosmetic importance, such as the hand and face. In partial-thickness wounds, an attempt is being made to preserve viable dermis, whereas in full-thickness injury, all necrotic and infected tissue must be removed, leaving a viable wound bed of fascia, fat, or muscle. The following techniques are mainly used.

Tangential excision. This technique, first described by Janzekovic in the 1970s, requires repeated shaving of deep dermal partial-thickness burns using a Braithwaite, Watson, or Goulian knife or dermatome set at a depth 0.005 to 0.010 inch until a viable dermal bed is reached, which is manifested clinically by punctate bleeding from the dermal wound bed.

Full-thickness excision. A hand knife such as the Watson or powered dermatome is set at 0.015 to 0.030 inch, and serial passes are made excising the full-thickness wound. Excision is aided by traction on the excised eschar as it passes through the knife or dermatome. Adequate excision is signaled by a viable bleeding wound bed, which is usually fat.

Fascial excision. This technique is reserved for burn extending down through the fat into muscle, when the patient presents late with large infected wounds and life-threatening invasive fungal infections. It involves surgical excision of the full thickness of the integument including the subcutaneous fat down to the fascia using Goulian knives and No. 11 blades. Unfortunately, fascial excision is mutilating and leaves a permanent contour defect, which is nearly impossible to reconstruct. Lymphatic channels are excised in this technique, and peripheral lymphedema may develop.

Most patients can be managed with layered excisions that optimize later appearance and function. Published estimates of the amount of bleeding associated with these operations range within 3.5% to 5% of the blood volume for every 1% of the body surface excised. The control of blood loss is one of the main determinants for outcome.[29] Therefore, several techniques should be applied to control blood loss. Local application of fibrin or thrombin spray, topical application of epinephrine 1:10000 to 1:20000, epinephrine-soaked laboratory pads (1:40000), and immediate electrocautery of the blood vessel can control blood loss.[30] The use of a sterilized tourniquet can also limit blood loss. Last, pre-excisional tumescence with epinephrine saline can be used on the trunk, back, and extremities but not on the fingers.

Burn Wound Coverage

After burn wound excision, it is vital to obtain wound closure. Various biologic and synthetic substrates have been employed to replace the injured skin after a burn. Autografts from uninjured skin remain the mainstay of treatment for many patients. Because early wound closure using autograft may be difficult when full-thickness burns exceed 40% TBSA, allografts (cadaver skin) frequently serve as skin substitute in severely burned patients (Fig. 19-10). Although this approach is still commonly used in burn centers throughout the world, it bears considerable risks, including antigenicity and cross-infection as well as limited availability. Xenografts have been used for hundreds of years as temporary replacement for skin loss. Even though these grafts provide a

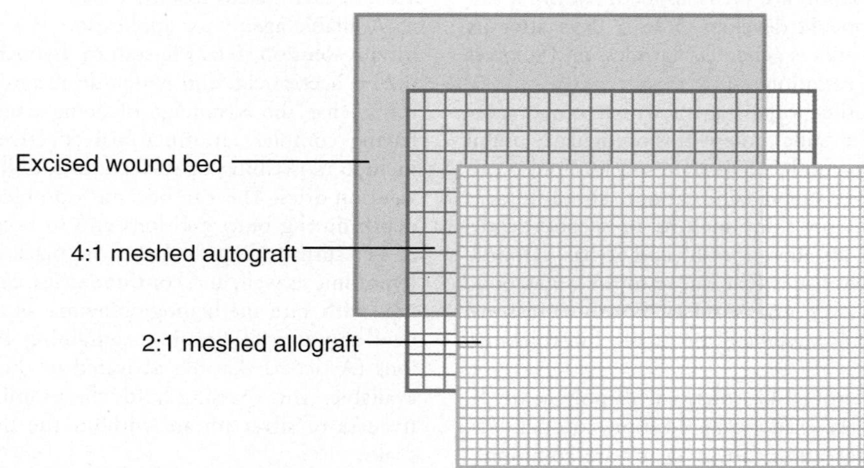

FIGURE 19-10 Diagram of skin closure using widely meshed autografts. A widely meshed autograft is placed on a freshly excised viable wound bed. The remaining open wound between the interstices of the autograft is closed with an overlying layer of allograft, which can also be meshed to allow transudate, exudate, and hematoma to escape.

biologically active dermal matrix, the immunologic disparities prevent engraftment and predetermine rejection over time. However, both xenografts and allografts are a means of only temporary burn wound cover. True closure can be achieved only with living autografts or isografts. Autologous epithelial cells grown from a single full-thickness skin biopsy specimen have been available for nearly 2 decades. These cultured epithelial autografts have been shown to decrease mortality in massively burned patients in a prospective, controlled trial. Our institution found cultured epithelial autografts used in combination with wide mesh autograft and allograft overlay in a population of pediatric patients with burns of 90% or more TBSA to be associated with improved cosmetic results. However, widespread use of cultured autografts has been primarily hampered by poor long-term clinical results, exorbitant costs, and fragility and difficult handling of these grafts; these problems have been consistently reported by different burn units treating deep burns, even when cells were applied on properly prepared wound beds. Alternatively, dermal analogues have been made available for clinical use in recent years. Integra was approved by the U.S. Food and Drug Administration for use in life-threatening burns and has been successfully used in immediate and delayed closure of full-thickness burns, leading to reduction in length of hospital stay, favorable cosmetics, and improved functional outcome in a prospective and controlled clinical study. Our group conducted a randomized clinical trial using Integra in the management of severe full-thickness burns of 50% TBSA or more in a population of pediatric patients, comparing it with standard autograft-allograft technique, and found Integra to be associated with attenuated hepatic dysfunction, improved resting energy expenditure, and improved aesthetic outcome.[31] AlloDerm, an acellular human dermal allograft, has been advocated for the management of acute burns. Small clinical series and case reports suggest that AlloDerm may be useful in the treatment of acute burns. Tissue engineering technology is advancing rapidly. Fetal constructs have been successfully trialed by Hohlfeld and colleagues,[32] and the bilaminar skin substitute of Boyce (cultured skin substitute)[33] is in clinical use and is very promising.[30] Advances in stem cell culture technology may represent another promising therapeutic approach to deliver cosmetic restoration for burn patients.

Multiorgan Failure

Early, aggressive resuscitation regimens have improved survival rates dramatically. With the advent of vigorous fluid resuscitation, irreversible burn shock has been replaced by sepsis and subsequent multiorgan failure as the leading cause of death associated with burns. In our pediatric burn population with burns of more than 80% TBSA, sepsis defined by bacteremia developed in 17.5% of the children.[11] The mortality rate in the whole group was 33%; most of these deaths were attributable to multiorgan failure. Some of the patients who died were bacteremic and "septic," but most were not. These findings highlight the observation that development of multiorgan failure is often associated with infectious sepsis, but infection is by no means required for development of multiorgan failure. What is required is an inflammatory focus, which in severe burns is the massive skin injury that requires inflammation to heal. It has been postulated that the progression to multiorgan failure exists in a continuum with the systemic inflammatory response syndrome. Nearly all burned patients meet the criteria for systemic inflammatory response syndrome as defined by the consensus conference of the American College of Chest Physicians and the Society of Critical Care Medicine. It is therefore not surprising that multiorgan failure is common in burned patients.

Etiology and Pathophysiology

The progression from the systemic inflammatory response syndrome to multiorgan failure is not well explained, although some of the responsible mechanisms are recognized. Most of these are found in patients with inflammation from infectious sources. In the burned patient, these infectious sources most likely emanate from invasive wound infection or from lung infections (pneumonia). As organisms proliferate out of control, endotoxins are liberated from gram-negative bacterial walls and exotoxins from gram-positive and gram-negative bacteria. Their release causes the initiation of a cascade of inflammatory mediators that can result, if unchecked, in organ damage and progression to organ failure. On occasion, failure of the gut barrier with penetration of organisms into the systemic circulation may incite a similar reaction. However, this phenomenon has been demonstrated only in animal models, and it remains to be seen whether this is a cause of human disease.

Inflammation from the presence of necrotic tissue and open wounds can incite an inflammatory mediator response similar to that seen with endotoxin. The mechanism by which this occurs, however, is not well understood. Regardless, it is known that a cascade of systemic events is set in motion, either by invasive organisms or from open wounds, that initiates the systemic inflammatory syndrome, which may progress to multiorgan failure. Evidence from animal studies and clinical trials suggests that these events converge to a common pathway, which results in activation of several cascade systems. Those circulating mediators can, if secreted in excessive amounts, damage organs distal from their site of origin. Among these mediators are endotoxin, arachidonic acid metabolites, cytokines, neutrophils and their adherence molecules, nitric oxide, complement components, and oxygen free radicals.

Prevention

Because different cascade systems are involved in the pathogenesis of burn-induced multiorgan failure, it is so far impossible to pinpoint a single mediator that initiates the event. Thus, because the mechanisms of progression are not well known, prevention is currently the best solution. The current recommendations are to prevent the development of organ dysfunction and to provide optimal support to avoid conditions that promote the onset.

The great reduction of mortality from large burns was observed with early excision and an aggressive surgical approach to deep wounds. Early removal of devitalized tissue prevents wound infections and decreases inflammation associated with the wound. In addition, it eliminates small, colonized foci, which are a frequent source of transient bacteremia. Those transient bacteremias during surgical manipulations may prime immune cells to react in an exaggerated fashion to subsequent insults, leading to whole body inflammation and remote organ damage. We recommend complete early excision of clearly full-thickness wounds within 48 hours of the injury or as early as possible.

Oxidative damage from reperfusion after low-flow states makes early, aggressive fluid resuscitation imperative. This is particularly important during the initial phases of treatment and operative excision with its attendant blood losses. Furthermore, the volume of fluid may not be as important as the timeliness with which it is given. In the study of children with more than 80% TBSA burns, it was found that one of the most important contributors to survival was the time required to start intravenous resuscitation, regardless of the initial volume given.

Topical and systemic antimicrobial therapy has significantly diminished the incidence of invasive burn wound sepsis. Perioperative antibiotics clearly benefit patients with burn injuries of more than 30% TBSA. Vigilant and scheduled replacement of intravascular devices minimizes the incidence of catheter-related sepsis. We recommend changes of indwelling catheters every 5 days. The first can be done over a wire using sterile Seldinger technique, but the second change requires a new site. This protocol should be kept as long as intravenous access is required. When possible, peripheral veins should be used for cannulation, even through burned tissue. The saphenous vein, however, should be avoided because of the high risk of thrombophlebitis.

Pneumonia, which contributes significantly to death in burned patients, should be vigilantly anticipated and aggressively treated. Every attempt should be made to wean patients as early as possible from the ventilator to reduce the risk of ventilator-associated nosocomial pneumonia. Furthermore, early ambulation is an effective means of preventing respiratory complications. With sufficient analgesics, even patients on continuous ventilatory support can be out of bed and in a chair.

The most common sources of sepsis are the wounds and the tracheobronchial tree; efforts to identify causative agents should be concentrated there. Another potential source, however, is the gastrointestinal tract, which is a natural reservoir for bacteria. Starvation and hypovolemia shunt blood from the splanchnic bed and promote mucosal atrophy and failure of the gut barrier. Early enteral feeding reduces septic morbidity and prevents failure of the gut barrier. At our institution, patients are fed immediately through a nasogastric tube. Early enteral feedings are tolerated in burned patients, preserve the mucosal integrity, and may reduce the magnitude of the hypermetabolic response to injury. Support of the gut goes along with carefully monitored hemodynamics.

Organ Failure

Even with the best efforts at prevention, the presence of the systemic inflammatory syndrome that is ubiquitous in burned patients may progress to organ failure. It was recently found that approximately 28% of patients with more than 30% TBSA burns will develop severe multiorgan dysfunction, of which 14% will also develop severe sepsis and septic shock. The general development begins in either the renal or pulmonary system and can progress through the liver, gut, hematologic system, and central nervous system. Whereas the development of multiorgan failure does not predict mortality, a study found a greater than 50% prevalence of multiorgan failure among nonsurvivors of burn injury.[19]

Renal Failure

With the advent of early aggressive resuscitation, the incidence of renal failure coincident with the initial phases of recovery has diminished significantly in severely burned patients. However, a second period of risk for the development of renal failure 2 to 14 days after resuscitation is still present. Renal failure is hallmarked by decreasing urine output, fluid overload, electrolyte abnormalities including metabolic acidosis and hyperkalemia, development of azotemia, and increased serum creatinine level. Treatment is aimed at averting complications associated with these conditions.

Urine output of more than 1 mL/kg is an adequate measure of renal perfusion in the absence of underlying renal disease. Decreasing the volume of fluid being given can alleviate volume overload in burned patients. These patients have increased insensible losses from the wounds, which can be roughly calculated at 1500 mL/m^2 TBSA + 3750 mL/m^2 TBSA burned. Further losses are accrued on air beds (1 L/day in an adult). Decreasing the infused volume of intravenous fluids and enteral feedings to less than the expected insensate losses alleviates fluid overload problems. Electrolyte abnormalities can be minimized by decreasing potassium administration in the enteral feedings and giving oral bicarbonate solutions. Almost invariably, severely burned patients require exogenous potassium because of the heightened aldosterone response that results in potassium wasting.

If the problems listed earlier overwhelm the conservative measures, some form of dialysis may be necessary. The indications for dialysis are volume overload and electrolyte abnormalities not amenable to other treatments. Peritoneal dialysis is effective in burned pediatric patients to remove volume and to correct electrolyte abnormalities. In adults, hemofiltration is an effective approach. Continuous venous-venous hemodialysis is sometimes indicated because of the fluid shifts that occur. All hemodialysis techniques should be done in conjunction with experienced nephrologists who are well versed in these techniques.

After dialysis is begun, renal function may return, especially in pediatric patients and adult patients who maintain some urine output. Therefore, patients requiring such treatment may not require lifelong dialysis. It is a clinical observation that whatever urine output was present will decrease once dialysis is begun, but it may return in several days to weeks once the acute process of closing the burn wound nears completion.

Pulmonary Failure

Many burned patients require mechanical ventilation to protect the airway in the initial phases of their injury. We recommend that these patients be extubated as soon as possible after the risk is diminished. A trial of extubation is often warranted in the first few days after injury, and reintubation in this setting is not a failure. To perform this technique safely, however, requires the involvement of experts in obtaining an airway. The goal is extubation as soon as possible to allow the patients to clear their own airways because they can perform their own pulmonary toilet better than through an endotracheal tube or tracheostomy. The first sign of impending pulmonary failure is a decline in oxygenation. This is best followed up with continuous oximetry, and a decrease in saturation to less than 92% is indicative of failure. Increasing concentrations of inspired oxygen are necessary, and when ventilation begins to fail, denoted by increasing respiratory rate and hypercapnia, intubation is needed.

Some have stated that early tracheostomy (within the first week) might be indicated in those with significant burn who are likely to require long-term ventilation. In one study, it was found in severely burned children who underwent early tracheostomy that the peak inspiratory pressures were lower after tracheostomy, with higher ventilatory volumes and pulmonary compliance and higher PaO_2/FIO_2 ratios. No instances of tracheostomy site infections or tracheal stenoses were identified in the 28 patients studied. Another randomized study comparing those severely burned patients who underwent early tracheostomy with those who did not found similar improvements in oxygenation; however, no significant differences could be found in outcome measures such as ventilator days, length of stay, incidence of pneumonia, or survival. In fact, 26% of those not undergoing tracheostomy were successfully extubated within 2 weeks of admission, implying that they would not have required tracheostomy at all. It seems that although tracheostomy may be required in some severely burned patients on ventilatory support, the advantages of early tracheostomy do not outweigh the disadvantages. Further data from other centers may change this conclusion in the future.

Hepatic Failure

The development of hepatic failure in burned patients is a challenging problem without many solutions. The liver synthesizes circulating proteins, detoxifies the plasma, produces bile, and provides immunologic support. After severe burn injury, the liver increases in size to more than 200% of normal.[14] When the liver begins to fail, protein concentrations of the coagulation cascade decrease to critical levels and the patient becomes coagulopathic. Toxins are not cleared from the bloodstream, and concentrations of bilirubin increase. Complete hepatic failure is not compatible with life, but a gradation of liver failure with some decline of the function is common. Efforts to prevent hepatic failure are the only effective methods of treatment.

With the development of coagulopathies, treatment should be directed at replacement of factors II, VII, IX, and X until the liver recovers. Albumin replacement may also be required. Attention to obstructive causes of hyperbilirubinemia, such as acalculous cholecystitis, should be considered as well. Initial treatment of this condition should be gallbladder drainage, which can be done percutaneously.

Hematologic Failure

Burned patients may become coagulopathic through two mechanisms: (1) depletion and impaired synthesis of coagulation factors and (2) thrombocytopenia. Factors associated with factor depletion are through disseminated intravascular coagulation associated with sepsis. This process is also common with coincident head injury. With breakdown of the blood-brain barrier, brain lipids are exposed to the plasma, which activates the coagulation cascade. Varying penetrance of this problem results in differing degrees of coagulopathy. Treatment of disseminated intravascular coagulation should include infusion of fresh-frozen plasma and cryoprecipitate to maintain plasma levels of coagulation factors. For disseminated intravascular coagulation induced by brain injury, the concentration of fibrinogen and levels with cryoprecipitate are the most specific indicators. Impaired synthesis of factors from liver failure is treated as alluded to earlier.

Thrombocytopenia is common in severe burns from depletion during burn wound excision. Platelet counts lower than 50,000 are common and do not require treatment. Only when the bleeding is diffuse and is noted to occur from intravenous sites should administration of exogenous platelets of considered.

Paradoxically, it was found that severely burned patients are also at risk for thrombotic and embolic complications likely related to immobilization. It was found that complications of deep venous thrombosis were associated with increasing age, weight, and TBSA burned. These data intimate that deep venous thrombosis prophylaxis would be prudent for adult patients in the absence of bleeding complications.

Central Nervous System Failure

Obtundation is one of the hallmarks of sepsis, and burn patients are no exception. A new onset of mental status changes not attributed to sedative medications in a severely burned patient should incite a search for a septic source. Treatment is supportive.

ATTENUATION OF THE HYPERMETABOLIC RESPONSE

Nonpharmacologic Modalities

Nutritional Support

The response to injury known as hypermetabolism occurs dramatically after severe burn. Increases in oxygen consumption, metabolic rate, urinary nitrogen excretion, lipolysis, and weight loss are directly proportional to the size of the burn. This response can be as high as 200% of the normal metabolic rate and returns to normal only with the complete closure of the wound. Because the metabolic rate is so high, energy requirements are immense. These requirements are met by mobilization of carbohydrate, fat, and protein stores. Because the demands are prolonged, these energy stores are quickly depleted, leading to loss of active muscle tissue and malnutrition. This malnutrition is associated with functional impairment of many organs, delayed and abnormal wound healing, decreased immunocompetence, and altered cellular membrane active transport functions. Malnutrition in burns can be subverted to some extent by delivery of adequate exogenous nutritional support. The goals of nutrition support are to maintain and to improve organ function and to prevent protein-calorie malnutrition.

Several formulas are used to calculate calorie requirements in burned patients. One formula multiplies the basal energy expenditure determined by the Harris-Benedict formula by 2 in burns of 40% TBSA, assuming a 100% increase in total energy expenditure. When total energy expenditure was measured by the doubly labeled water method, actual expenditures were found to be 1.33 times the predicted basal energy expenditure for pediatric patients with burns of more than 40% TBSA. To meet the minimal needs of all the patients in this study, 1.55 times the predicted basal energy expenditure would be required; however, giving calorie loads in excess of this probably leads to fat accumulation without affecting lean mass accretion. This correlated to 1.4 times the measured resting energy expenditure by indirect calorimetry. These studies indicate that the calculation of 2 times the predicted basal energy expenditure might be too high.

Other commonly used calculations include the Curreri formula, which calls for 25 kcal/kg/day plus 40 kcal per percentage of TBSA burned per day. This formula provides for maintenance needs plus the additional calorie needs related to the burn wounds. This formula was devised as a regression from nitrogen balance data in severely burned adults. In children, formulas based on body surface area are more appropriate because of the greater body surface area per kilogram of weight. We recommend the formulas depending on the child's age (Table 19-6). These

TABLE 19-6 Formulas to Predict Calorie Needs in Severely Burned Children

AGE GROUP	MAINTENANCE NEEDS	BURN WOUND NEEDS
Infants (0-12 months)	2100 kcal/% TBSA burned/24 hours	1000 kcal/% TBSA burned/24 hours
Children (1-12 years)	1800 kcal/% TBSA burned/24 hours	1300 kcal/% TBSA burned/24 hours
Adolescents (12-18 years)	1500 kcal/% TBSA burned/24 hours	1500 kcal/% TBSA burned/24 hours

TBSA, total body surface area.

formulas were determined to maintain body weight in severely burned children. The formulas change with age on the basis of the body surface area alterations that occur with growth.

The composition of the nutritional supplement is also important. The optimal dietary composition contains 1 to 2 g/kg/day of protein, which provides a calorie to nitrogen ratio at around 100:1 with the earlier suggested calorie intakes. This amount of protein provides for the synthetic needs of the patient, thus sparing to some extent the proteolysis occurring in the active muscle tissue. Nonprotein calories can be given either as carbohydrate or as fat. Carbohydrates have the advantage of stimulating endogenous insulin production, which may have beneficial effects on muscle and burn wounds as an anabolic hormone. In addition, it was recently shown that almost all of the fat transported in very-low-density lipoprotein after severe burn is derived from peripheral lipolysis and not from de novo synthesis of fatty acids in the liver from dietary carbohydrates. As fat transporters are markedly decreased, we suggest use of a low-fat diet because additional fat to deliver noncarbohydrate calories has little support.

The diet may be delivered in two forms: either enterally through enteric tubes or parenterally through intravenous catheters. Parenteral nutrition may be given in isotonic solutions through peripheral catheters or with hypertonic solutions in central catheters. In general, the calorie demands of burned patients prohibit the use of peripheral parenteral nutrition. Total parenteral nutrition delivered centrally in burned patients has been associated with increased complications and mortality rate compared with enteral feedings. Total parenteral nutrition is reserved only for those patients who cannot tolerate enteral feedings. Enteral feeding has been associated with some complications, which include mechanical complications, enteral feeding intolerance, and diarrhea.

Interest in nutritional adjunctive treatment with anabolic agents has recently received attention as a means to decrease lean mass losses after severe injury. Agents used include growth hormone, insulin-like growth factor, insulin, oxandrolone, testosterone, and propranolol. Each of these agents has different actions to stimulate protein synthesis through an increase in protein synthetic efficiency. Put simply, the free amino acids available in the cytoplasm from stimulated protein breakdown with severe injury or illness are preferentially shunted toward protein synthesis rather than export out of the cell. Some of these agents, such as insulin and oxandrolone, have shown efficacy not only in improving protein kinetics but also in improving lean mass after severe burn. Further research will reveal whether these biochemical and physiologic measures translate to improved function.

Environmental Support

Burn patients can lose as much as 4000 mL/m^2 burned skin per day of body water through evaporative loss from extensive burn wounds that have not definitively healed. The altered physiologic state resulting from the hypermetabolic response attempts to at least partly generate sufficient energy to offset heat losses associated with this inevitable water loss. The body attempts to raise skin and core temperatures to 2° C above normal. Raising the ambient temperature from 25° C to 33° C can diminish the magnitude of this obligatory response from 2.0 to 1.4 resting energy expenditure in patients exceeding 40% TBSA (Fig. 19-11).[12] This simple environmental modulation is an important primary treatment goal that frequently is not realized.

Exercise and Adjunctive Measures

A balanced physical therapy program is essential to restore metabolic variables and to prevent burn wound contracture. Progressive resistance exercises in convalescent burn patients can maintain and improve body mass, augment incorporation of amino acids into muscle proteins, and increase muscle strength and the ability to walk distances by approximately 50%. It has been demonstrated that resistance exercising can be safely accomplished in pediatric burn patients without exercise-related hyperpyrexia as the result of an inability to dissipate the generated heat. Although the initial burn injury and sepsis-related complications principally determine the extent of the metabolic response in burn victims, obligatory activity, background and procedure-related pain, and anxiety also greatly increase metabolic rates. Judicious maximal narcotic support, appropriate sedation, and supportive psychotherapy are mandatory to minimize their effects.

Pharmacologic Modalities

Recombinant Human Growth Hormone

Daily intramuscular administration of recombinant human growth hormone (rhGH) at doses of 0.2 mg/kg as a daily injection during acute burn care has favorably influenced the hepatic acute-phase response, increased serum concentrations of its secondary mediator IGF-I, improved muscle protein kinetics, maintained muscle growth, decreased donor site healing time by 1.5 days, improved resting energy expenditure, and decreased cardiac output.[34] These beneficial effects of rhGH are mediated by IGF-I, and patients receiving treatment demonstrated 100% increases in serum IGF-I and IGFBP-3 relative to healthy individuals. However, in a prospective, multicenter, double-blind, randomized, placebo-controlled trial involving 247 patients and 285 critically ill nonburned patients, Branski and coworkers[34] found that high doses of rhGH (0.10 ± 0.02 mg/kg body weight) were associated with increased morbidity and mortality. Others demonstrated growth hormone treatment to be associated with hyperglycemia and insulin resistance. However, neither short-term nor long-term administration of rhGH was associated with an increase in mortality in severely burned children.

Insulin-like Growth Factor

Because IGF-I mediates the effects of growth hormone, the infusion of equimolar doses of recombinant human IGF-I and IGFBP-3 to burned patients has been demonstrated to effectively improve protein metabolism in catabolic pediatric subjects and adults with significantly less hypoglycemia than with rhGH itself. It attenuates muscle catabolism and improves gut mucosal integrity in children with serious burns. Immune function is effectively improved by attenuation of the type 1 and type 2 hepatic acute-phase responses, increased serum concentrations of constitutive proteins, and vulnerary modulation of the hypercatabolic use of body protein.[12] However, studies by Langouche and Van den Berghe[35] indicate that the use of IGF-I alone is not effective in critically ill patients without burns.

Oxandrolone

Treatment with anabolic agents such as oxandrolone, a testosterone analogue that possesses only 5% of its virilizing androgenic effects, improves muscle protein catabolism through enhanced protein synthesis efficiency, reduces weight loss, and increases donor site wound healing. In a prospective randomized study, Wolf and colleagues[36] demonstrated that administration of 10 mg of oxandrolone every 12 hours decreased hospital stay. In a large

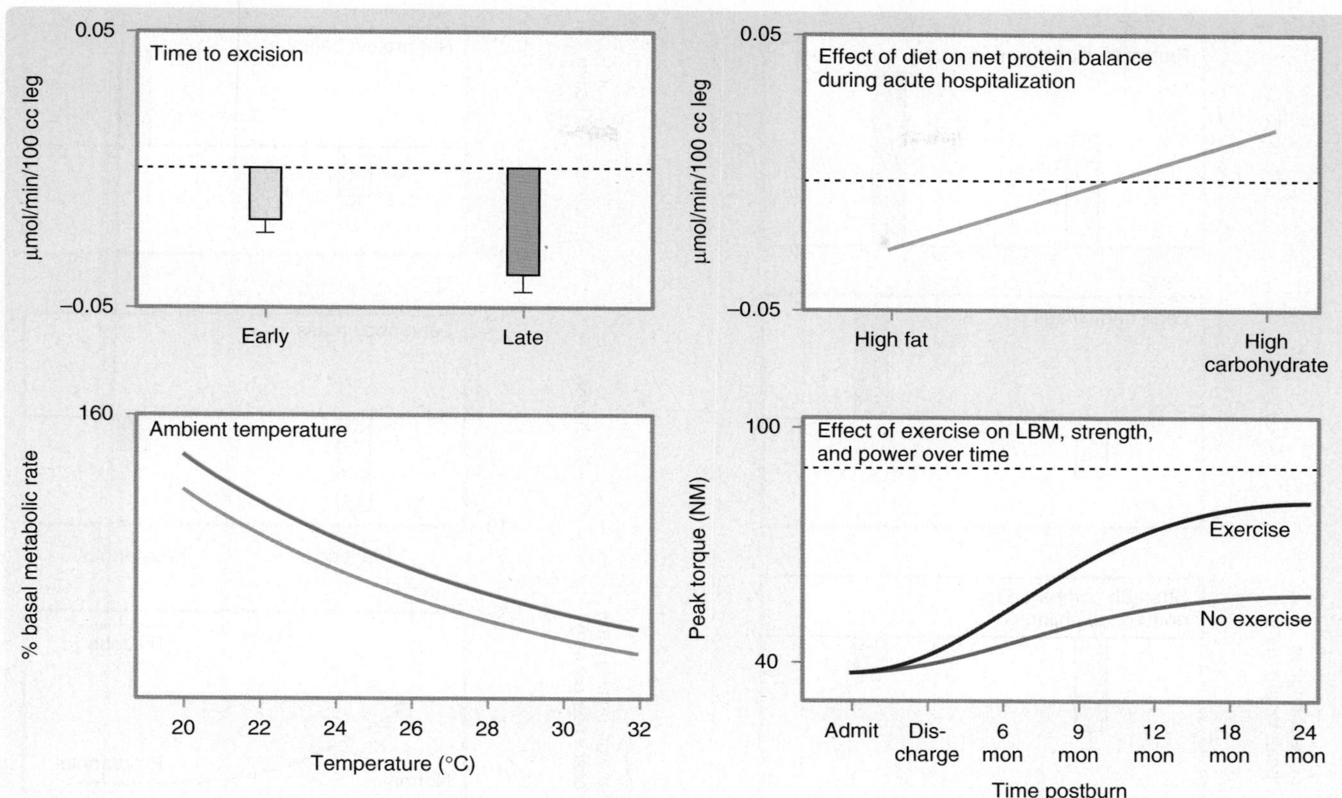

FIGURE 19-11 Nonpharmacologic modulations of the hypermetabolic response after burn injury. The effect is demonstrated of early excision and grafting, environmental thermoregulation, high-carbohydrate diet, and exercise on physiologic derangements after burn injury. Graphs are averages ± standard error of the mean. The *yellow bars* represent patients with burns ≥40% total body surface area (TBSA) who had early excision. The *blue bars* represent patients with burns ≥40% TBSA who had late excision of burn eschar. Averages for burn patients are represented by *solid curves*. Values from nonburned, normal patients are represented by *dashed lines*. *LBM,* lean body mass. (From Williams FN, Jeschke MG, Chinkes DL, et al: Modulation of the hypermetabolic response to trauma: Temperature, nutrition, and drugs. *J Am Coll Surg* 208:489–502, 2009.)

prospective, double-blinded, randomized single-center study, oxandrolone given at a dose of 0.1 mg/kg every 12 hours shortened length of acute hospital stay, maintained lean body mass, and improved body composition and hepatic protein synthesis (Fig. 19-12).[37] The effects were independent of age. Long-term treatment with this oral anabolic during rehabilitation in the outpatient setting is more favorably regarded than parenteral anabolic agents by pediatric subjects. Oxandrolone successfully abates the effects of burn-associated hypermetabolism on body tissues and significantly increases body mass over time, lean body mass (at 6, 9, and 12 months after burn injury), and bone mineral content by 12 months after injury versus unburned controls.[38] Patients treated with oxandrolone show few complications relative to those treated with rhGH. However, although anabolic agents can increase lean body mass, exercise is essential to development of strength.

Propranolol

β-Adrenergic blockade with propranolol represents probably the most efficacious anticatabolic therapy in the treatment of burns. Long-term use of propranolol during acute care in burn patients, at a dose titrated to reduce heart rate by 15% to 20%, was noted to diminish cardiac work (Fig. 19-13). It also reduced fatty infiltration of the liver, which typically occurs in these patients as the result of enhanced peripheral lipolysis and altered substrate handling. Reduction of hepatic fat results from decreased peripheral lipolysis and reduced palmitate delivery and uptake by the liver, producing smaller livers that adversely affect diaphragmatic function less frequently. Stable isotope and serial body composition studies showed that administration of propranolol reduces skeletal muscle wasting and increases lean body mass after burn injury.[12] The underlying mechanism of action of propranolol is still unclear; however, its effect appears to be due to an increased protein synthesis in the face of a persistent protein breakdown and reduced peripheral lipolysis.[39] Data suggest that administration of propranolol given at 4 mg/kg body weight every 24 hours also markedly decreases the amount of insulin necessary to decrease elevated glucose level after burn injury (unpublished data). Propranolol may thus constitute a promising approach to overcome postburn insulin resistance.

Attenuation of Hyperglycemia after Burn Injury

Insulin

Insulin represents probably one of the most extensively studied therapeutic agents, and novel therapeutic applications are constantly being found. Besides its ability to decrease blood glucose

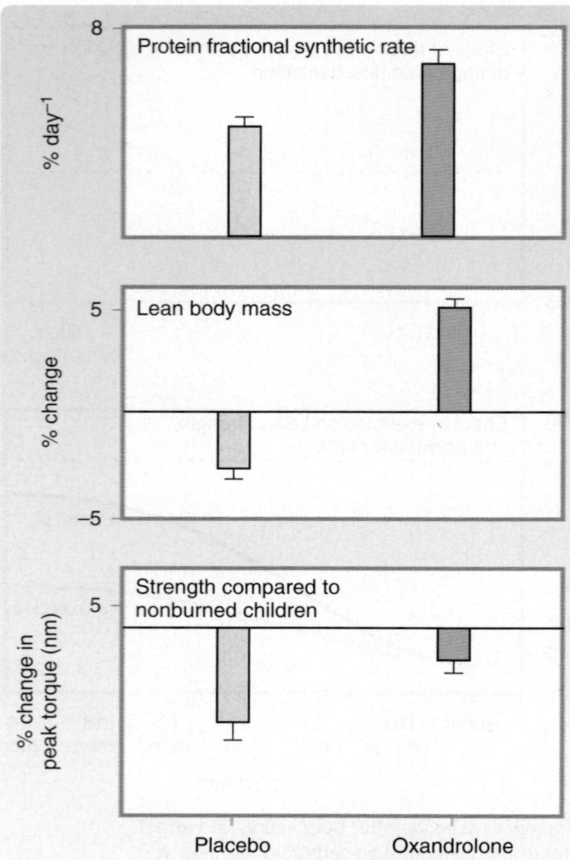

FIGURE 19-12 Effect of oxandrolone treatment on the fractional synthetic rate of muscle protein synthesis, lean body mass, and strength. Changes in net protein balance of muscle protein synthesis and breakdown induced by burn injury were measured by stable isotope studies using d5-phenylalanine infusion. Graphs are averages ± standard error of the mean. The *yellow bars* represent patients with burns ≥40% total body surface area (TBSA) who received no anabolic agents. The *blue bars* represent patients with burns ≥40% TBSA who were randomized to receive oxandrolone. (From Williams FN, Jeschke MG, Chinkes DL, et al: Modulation of the hypermetabolic response to trauma: Temperature, nutrition, and drugs. *J Am Coll Surg* 208:489–502, 2009.)

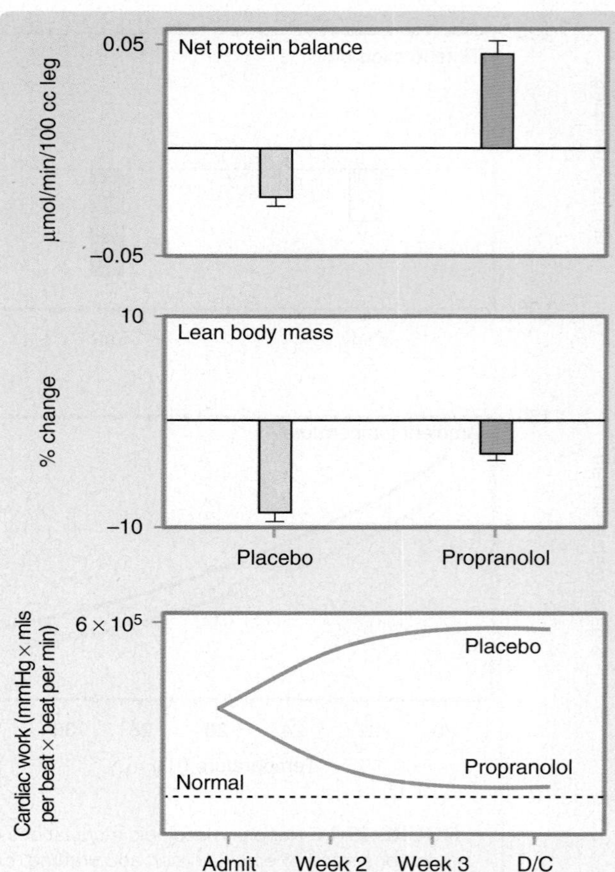

FIGURE 19-13 Effect of propranolol treatment on the fractional synthetic rate of muscle protein synthesis, lean body mass, and cardiac work. Changes in net protein balance of muscle protein synthesis and breakdown induced by burn injury were measured by stable isotope studies using d5-phenylalanine infusion. Graphs are averages ± standard error of the mean. The *yellow bars* represent patients with burns ≥40% total body surface area (TBSA) who received no anabolic agents. The *blue bars* represent patients with burns ≥40% TBSA who were randomized to receive propranolol. Values from nonburned, normal patients are represented by *dashed lines.* (From Williams FN, Jeschke MG, Chinkes DL, et al: Modulation of the hypermetabolic response to trauma: Temperature, nutrition, and drugs. *J Am Coll Surg* 208:489–502, 2009.)

concentration by mediating peripheral glucose uptake into skeletal muscle and adipose tissue and suppressing hepatic gluconeogenesis, insulin is known to increase DNA replication and protein synthesis through control of amino acid uptake, to increase fatty acid synthesis, and to decrease proteinolysis.[13] The last makes insulin particularly attractive for the treatment of hyperglycemia in severely burned patients because insulin given during acute hospitalization has been shown to improve muscle protein synthesis, to accelerate donor site healing time, and to attenuate lean body mass loss and the acute-phase response (Fig. 19-14).[13] In addition to its anabolic actions, insulin was shown to exert totally unexpected anti-inflammatory effects potentially neutralizing the proinflammatory actions of glucose.[40,41] These results suggest a dual benefit of insulin administration: reduction of proinflammatory effects of glucose by restoration of euglycemia and a proposed additional insulin-mediated anti-inflammatory effect.[42] Insulin administered to maintain glucose at levels below 110 mg/dL decreased mortality, incidence of infections, sepsis, and sepsis-associated multiorgan failure in surgically critically ill patients. It was also found to significantly reduce newly acquired kidney injury, to accelerate weaning from mechanical ventilation, and to accelerate discharge from the ICU and the hospital.[43] When given during the acute phase, it not only improved acute hospital outcomes but also improved long-term rehabilitation and social reintegration of critically ill patients during a period of 1 year, indicating the advantage of insulin therapy.[44,45] However, because strict blood glucose control to maintain normoglycemia was required to obtain the most clinical benefit, a dialogue has emerged between those who believe that tight glucose control is beneficial for patient outcome and others who fear that high doses of insulin may lead to increased risk for hypoglycemic events and its associated consequences in these patients. In fact, a multicenter trial in Europe, Efficacy of Volume Substitution and Insulin Therapy in Severe Sepsis (VISEP), investigated the effects of insulin administration on morbidity and mortality in patients with severe infections and sepsis.[46] The authors found that insulin administration

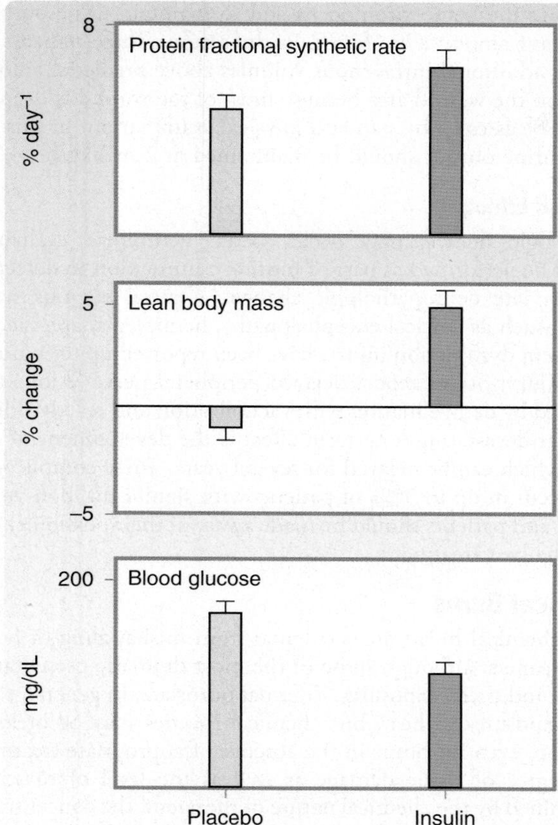

FIGURE 19-14 Effect of insulin therapy on the fractional synthetic rate of muscle protein synthesis, lean body mass, and average blood glucose levels. Changes in net protein balance of muscle protein synthesis and breakdown induced by burn injury were measured by stable isotope studies using d5-phenylalanine infusion. Graphs are averages ± standard error of the mean. The *yellow bars* represent patients with burns ≥40% total body surface area (TBSA) who received no anabolic agents or insulin. The *blue bars* represent patients with burns ≥40% TBSA who were randomized to receive insulin. (From Williams FN, Jeschke MG, Chinkes DL, et al: Modulation of the hypermetabolic response to trauma: Temperature, nutrition, and drugs. *J Am Coll Surg* 208:489–502, 2009.)

did not affect mortality, but the rate of severe hypoglycemia was fourfold higher in patients receiving intensive insulin therapy compared with the conventional therapy group.[46] Another large multicenter study examined the use of a continuous hyperinsulinemic, euglycemic clamp throughout ICU stay and found a dramatic increase in serious hypoglycemic episodes.[47] The ideal target glucose range therefore has not been found, and several groups are currently undertaking clinical trials to define ideal glucose levels for the treatment of ICU and burned patients. Currently, the Surviving Sepsis Campaign recommendation is to maintain glucose levels below 150 mg/dL.[48] However, maintaining a continuous hyperinsulinemic, euglycemic clamp in burn patients is particularly difficult because these patients are being continuously fed large calorie loads through enteral feeding tubes in an attempt to maintain euglycemia. Because burn patients require weekly operations and daily dressing changes, enteral nutrition needs occasionally to be stopped, which may lead to disruption of gastrointestinal motility and increased risk of hypoglycemia.[5]

Metformin

Metformin (Glucophage), a biguanide, can be used as an alternative means to correct hyperglycemia in severely injured patients. By inhibiting gluconeogenesis and augmenting peripheral insulin sensitivity, metformin directly counters the two main metabolic processes that underlie injury-induced hyperglycemia. In addition, metformin has been rarely associated with hypoglycemic events, thus possibly eliminating this concern associated with the use of exogenous insulin. In a small randomized study reported by Gore and colleagues,[49] metformin reduced plasma glucose concentration, decreased endogenous glucose production, and accelerated glucose clearance in severely burned patients. A follow-up study looking at the effects of metformin on muscle protein synthesis confirmed these observations and demonstrated an increased fractional synthetic rate of muscle protein and improvement in net muscle protein balance in metformin-treated patients.[49] Thus, analogous to insulin, metformin may have efficacy in critically injured patients as both an antihyperglycemic and a muscle protein anabolic agent. Despite the advantages and potential therapeutic uses, treatment with metformin or other biguanides has been associated with lactic acidosis. To avoid metformin-associated lactic acidosis, the use of this medication is contraindicated in certain diseases or illnesses in which there is a potential for impaired lactate elimination (hepatic or renal failure) or tissue hypoxia, and it should be used with caution in subacute burn patients.

Novel Therapeutic Options

Other ongoing trials to decrease postburn hyperglycemia include the use of glucagon-like peptide 1 and peroxisome proliferator-activated receptor gamma (PPAR-γ) agonists (e.g., pioglitazone, thioglitazones) or the combination of various antidiabetic drugs. PPAR-γ agonists, such as fenofibrate, have been shown to improve insulin sensitivity in patients with diabetes. Cree and colleagues[50] found in a double-blind, prospective, placebo-controlled randomized trial that fenofibrate treatment significantly decreased plasma glucose concentrations by improving insulin sensitivity and mitochondrial glucose oxidation. Fenofibrate also led to significantly increased tyrosine phosphorylation of the insulin receptor and insulin receptor-substrate 1 in muscle tissue after hyperinsulinemic-euglycemic clamp compared with placebo-treated patients, indicating improved insulin receptor signaling.[50]

SPECIAL CONSIDERATIONS: ELECTRICAL AND CHEMICAL BURNS

Electrical Burns

Initial Treatment

Three percent to 5% of all admitted burned patients are injured from electrical contact. Electrical injury is unlike other burn injuries in that the visible areas of tissue necrosis represent only a small portion of the destroyed tissue. Electrical current enters a part of the body, such as the fingers or hand, and proceeds through tissues with the lowest resistance to current, generally the nerves, blood vessels, and muscles. The skin has a relatively high resistance to electrical current and is therefore mostly spared. The current then leaves the body at a "grounded" area, typically the foot. Heat generated by the transfer of electrical current and passage of the current itself then injures the tissues. During this exchange, the muscle is the major tissue through which the current flows, and thus it sustains the most damage. Most muscle is close to bones.

Blood vessels transmitting much of the electricity initially remain patent, but they may proceed to progressive thrombosis as the cells either die or repair themselves, thus resulting in further tissue loss from ischemia.

Injuries are divided into high- and low-voltage injuries. Low-voltage injury is similar to thermal burns without transmission to the deeper tissues; zones of injury from the surface extend into the tissue. Most household currents (110 to 220 V) produce this type of injury, which causes only local damage. The worst of these injuries are those involving the edge of the mouth (oral commissure) sustained when children gnaw on household electrical cords.

The syndrome of high-voltage injury consists of varying degrees of cutaneous burn at the entry and exit sites combined with hidden destruction of deep tissue. Often, these patients also have cutaneous burns associated with ignition of clothing from the discharge of electrical current. Initial evaluation consists of cardiopulmonary resuscitation if ventricular fibrillation is induced. Thereafter, if the initial electrocardiogram findings are abnormal or there is a history of cardiac arrest associated with the injury, continued cardiac monitoring is necessary along with pharmacologic treatment for any dysrhythmias. The most serious derangements occur in the first 24 hours after injury. If patients with electrical injuries have no cardiac dysrhythmias on initial electrocardiogram or recent history of cardiac arrest, no further monitoring is necessary.

Patients with electrical injuries are at risk for other injuries, such as being thrown from the electrical jolt or falling from heights after disengaging from the electrical current. In addition, the violent tetanic muscle contractions that result from alternating current sources may cause a variety of fractures and dislocations. These patients should be assessed in the same manner as any other patient with blunt traumatic injuries.

The key to managing patients with an electrical injury lies in the treatment of the wound. The most significant injury is within the deep tissue, and subsequent edema formation can cause vascular compromise to any area distal to the injury. Assessment should include circulation to distal vascular beds because immediate escharotomy and fasciotomy may be required. If the muscle compartment is extensively injured and necrotic, such that the prospects for eventual function are dismal, early amputation may be necessary. We advocate early exploration of affected muscle beds and débridement of devitalized tissues, with attention given to the deeper periosteal planes because this is the area with the most muscle tissue. Fasciotomies should be complete and may require nerve decompressions, such as carpal tunnel and Guyon canal releases. Tissue that has questionable viability should be left in place, with planned reexploration in 48 hours. Many such reexplorations may be required until the wound is completely débrided. Electrical damage to vessels may be delayed, and the extent of necrosis may extend after the initial débridements. After the devitalized tissues are removed, closure of the wound becomes paramount. Although skin grafts suffice as closure for most wounds, flaps may offer a better alternative, particularly with exposed bones and tendons. Even exposed and superficially infected bones and tendons can be salvaged with coverage by vascularized tissue. Early involvement by reconstructive surgeons versed in the various methods of wound closure is optimal.

Muscle damage results in release of hemochromogens (myoglobin), which are filtered in the glomeruli and may result in obstructive nephropathy. Therefore, vigorous hydration and infusion of intravenous sodium bicarbonate (5% continuous infusion) and mannitol (25 g every 6 hours for adults) are indicated to solubilize the hemochromogens and to maintain urine output if significant amounts are found in the serum. These patients also require additional intravenous volumes above predicted amounts based on the wound area because most of the wound is deep and cannot be assessed by standard physical examination. In this situation, urine output should be maintained at 2 mL/kg/hr.

Delayed Effects

Neurologic deficits may occur. Serial neurologic evaluations should be performed as part of routine examination to detect any early or late neuropathologic changes. Central nervous system effects, such as cortical encephalopathy, hemiplegia, aphasia, and brainstem dysfunction injury, have been reported up to 9 months after injury; others report delayed peripheral nerve lesions characterized by demyelination with vacuolization and reactive gliosis. Another devastating long-term effect is the development of cataracts, which can be delayed for several years. These complications may occur in up to 30% of patients with significant high-voltage injury, and patients should be made aware of their possibility even with the best treatment.

Chemical Burns

Most chemical burns are accidental from mishandling of household cleaners, although some of the most dramatic presentations involve industrial exposures. Thermal burns are, in general, short-term exposures to heat, but chemical injuries may be of longer duration, even for hours in the absence of appropriate treatment. The degree of tissue damage as well as the level of toxicity is determined by the chemical nature of the agent, the concentration of the agent, and the duration of skin contact. Chemicals cause their injury by protein destruction, with denaturation, oxidation, formation of protein esters, or desiccation of the tissue. In the United States, the composition of most household and industrial chemicals can be obtained from the Poison Control Center in the area, which can give suggestions for treatment.

Speed is essential in the management of chemical burns. For all chemicals, lavage with copious quantities of clean water should be done immediately after removal of all clothing. Dry powders should be brushed from the affected areas before irrigation. Early irrigation dilutes the chemical, which is already in contact with the skin, and timeliness increases effectiveness. Several liters of irrigant may be required. For example, 10 mL of 98% sulfuric acid dissolved in 12 L of water decreases the pH to 5.0, a range that can still cause injury. If the chemical composition is known (acid or base), monitoring of the spent lavage solution pH gives a good indication of lavage effectiveness and completion. A good rule of thumb is to lavage with 15 to 20 L of tap water or more for significant chemical injuries. The lavage site should be kept drained to remove the earlier, more concentrated effluent. Care should be taken to drain away from uninjured areas to avoid further exposure.

All patients must be monitored according to the severity of their injuries. They may have metabolic disturbances, usually from pH abnormalities, because of exposure to strong acids or caustics. If respiratory difficulty is apparent, oxygen therapy and mechanical ventilation must be instituted. Resuscitation should be guided by the body surface area involved (burn formulas); however, the total fluid needs may be dramatically different from the calculated volumes. Some of these injuries may be more superficial than they appear, particularly in the case of acids, and therefore require less resuscitation volume. Injuries from bases, however, may penetrate beyond that which is apparent on examination and therefore

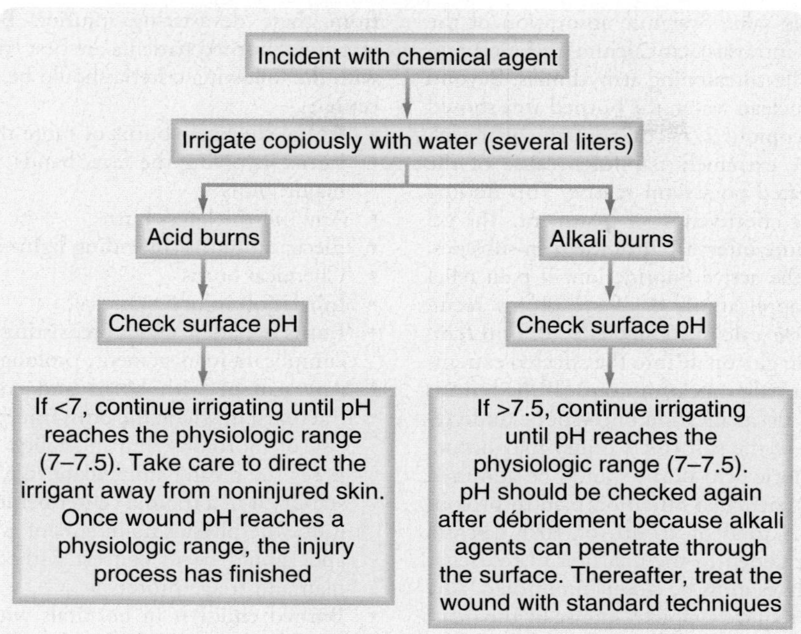

FIGURE 19-15 Treatment of acid and alkali burns.

require more volume. For this reason, patients with chemical injuries should be observed closely for signs of adequate perfusion, such as urine output. All patients with significant chemical injuries should be monitored with indwelling bladder catheters to accurately measure outputs.

Operative débridement, if indicated, should take place as soon as a patient is stable and resuscitated (Fig. 19-15). After adequate lavage and débridement, burn wounds are covered with antimicrobial agents or skin substitutes. Once the wounds have stabilized with the indicated treatment, they are taken care of as with any loss of soft tissue. Skin grafting or flap coverage is performed as needed.

Alkali

Alkalis, such as lime, potassium hydroxide, bleach, and sodium hydroxide, are among the most common agents involved in chemical injury. Accidental injury frequently occurs in infants and toddlers exploring cleaning cabinets. There are three factors involved in the mechanism of alkali burns: (1) saponification of fat causes the loss of insulation of heat formed in the chemical reaction with tissue; (2) massive extraction of water from cells causes damage because of the hygroscopic nature of alkali; and (3) alkalis dissolve and unite with the proteins of the tissues to form alkaline proteinates, which are soluble and contain hydroxide ions. These ions induce further chemical reactions, penetrating deeper into the tissue. Treatment involves immediate removal of the causative agent with lavage of large volumes of fluid, usually water. Attempts to neutralize alkali agents with weak acids are not recommended because the heat released by neutralization reactions induces further injury. Particularly strong bases should be treated with lavage and consideration for the addition of wound débridement in the operating room. Tangential removal of affected areas is performed until the tissues removed are at a normal pH.

Cement (calcium oxide) burns are alkali in nature, occur commonly, and are usually work-related injuries. The critical substance responsible for the skin damage is the hydroxyl ion. Often, the agent has been in contact with the skin for prolonged periods, such as underneath the boots of a cement worker who seeks treatment hours after the exposure or after the cement penetrates clothing and, when combined with perspiration, induces an exothermic reaction. Treatment consists of removal of all clothing and irrigation of the affected area with water and soap until all the cement is removed and the effluent has a pH of less than 8. Injuries tend to be deep because of exposure times, and surgical excision and grafting of the resultant eschar may be required.

Acids

Acid injuries are treated initially like any other chemical injury, with removal of all chemicals by disrobing the affected area and copious irrigation. Acids induce protein breakdown by hydrolysis, which results in a hard eschar that does not penetrate as deeply as that caused by the alkalis. These agents also induce thermal injury by heat generation with contact of the skin, further causing soft tissue damage. Some acids have added effects, which are discussed here.

Formic acid injuries are relatively rare, usually involving an organic acid used for industrial descaling and as a hay preservative. Electrolyte abnormalities are of great concern for patients who have sustained extensive formic acid injuries, with metabolic acidosis, renal failure, intravascular hemolysis, and pulmonary complications (acute respiratory distress syndrome) being common. Acidemia detected by a metabolic acidosis on arterial blood gas analysis should be corrected with intravenous sodium bicarbonate. Hemodialysis may be required when extensive absorption of formic acid has occurred. Mannitol diuresis is required if severe hemolysis occurs after deep injury. A formic acid wound typically has a greenish appearance and is deeper than what it initially appears to be; it is best treated by surgical excision.

Hydrofluoric acid is a toxic substance used widely in both industrial and domestic settings and is the strongest inorganic acid known. Management of these burns differs from that of other acid burns in general. Hydrofluoric acid produces dehydration and corrosion of tissue with free hydrogen ions. In addition, the fluoride ion complexes with bivalent cations such as calcium and magnesium to form insoluble salts. Systemic absorption of the fluoride ion then can induce intravascular calcium chelation and hypocalcemia, which causes life-threatening arrhythmias. Beyond initial copious irrigation with clean water, the burned area should be treated immediately with copious 2.5% calcium gluconate gel. These wounds in general are extremely painful because of the calcium chelation and associated potassium release. This finding can be used to determine the effectiveness of treatment. The gel should be changed at 15-minute intervals until the pain subsides, an indication of removal of the active fluoride ion. If pain relief is incomplete after several applications or if symptoms recur, intradermal injections of 10% calcium gluconate (0.5 mL/cm^2 affected), intra-arterial calcium gluconate into the affected extremity, or both may be required to alleviate symptoms. If the burn is not treated in such a fashion, decalcification of the bone underlying the injury and extension of the soft tissue injury may occur.

All patients with hydrofluoric acid burns should be admitted for cardiac monitoring, with particular attention paid to prolongation of the QT interval. A total of 20 mL of 10% calcium gluconate solution should be added to the first liter of resuscitation fluid, and serum electrolytes must be closely monitored. Any electrocardiographic changes require a rapid response by the treatment team with intravenous calcium chloride to maintain heart function. Several grams of calcium may be required in the end until the chemical response has run its course. Serum magnesium and potassium also should be closely monitored and replaced. Speed is the key to effective treatment.

Hydrocarbons

The organic solvent properties of hydrocarbons promote cell membrane dissolution and skin necrosis. Symptoms include erythema and blistering, and the burns are typically superficial and heal spontaneously. If they are absorbed systemically, toxicity can produce respiratory depression and eventual hepatic injury thought to be associated with benzenes. Ignition of the hydrocarbons on the skin induces a deep full-thickness injury.

OUTCOMES

Many of the treatments for burn are directed at improving functional, psychological, and work outcomes, which are only now being systematically studied. Authors are now reporting new methods to evaluate outcomes through burn-specific health scales and measures of adjustment. Authors found that severely burned adult patients adjust relatively well, although some develop clinically significant psychological disturbances, such as somatization and phobic anxiety. Children with severe burns were found to have similar somatization problems as well as sleep disturbances but in general were well adjusted. Time off work in adult patients was found to be associated with increasing percentage TBSA burned, psychiatric history, and extremity burns with considerable job disruption. In general, major burns can lead to significant disturbances in psychiatric health and outcomes, but they can be overcome.

BURN UNITS

Improvements in burn care originated in specialized units specifically dedicated to the care of burned patients. These units consist of experienced personnel with resources to maximize outcome from these devastating injuries. Because of these specialized resources, burned patients are best treated in such places. Patients with the following criteria should be referred to a designated burn center:

- Partial-thickness burns of more than 10% TBSA
- Burns involving the face, hands, feet, genitalia, perineum, or major joints
- Any full-thickness burn
- Electrical burns, including lightning injury
- Chemical burns
- Inhalation injury
- Burns in patients with preexisting medical disorders that could complicate management, prolong recovery, or affect outcome
- Any patient with burns and concomitant trauma (such as fractures) in which the burn injury poses the greater immediate risk of morbidity and mortality. In such cases, if the trauma poses the greater immediate risk, the patient may be initially stabilized in a trauma center before being transferred to a burn unit. The physician's judgment is necessary in such situations and should be in concert with the regional medical control plan and triage protocols.
- Burned children in hospitals without qualified personnel or equipment to care for children
- Burns in patients who will require special social, emotional, or long-term rehabilitative intervention

Specialized care for severely burned patients in burn centers has contributed to the significant improvements in morbidity and mortality. Today, the overall LD_{50} for all burns is a 70% TBSA, meaning that today, a 70% TBSA burn has a 50% mortality for all ages.[8] Twenty years ago, the LD_{50} was a 50% TBSA.

SUMMARY

The treatment of burns is complex. Minor injuries can be treated in the community by knowledgeable physicians. Moderate and severe injuries, however, require treatment in dedicated facilities with resources to maximize the outcomes from these often devastating events.

Novel concepts and techniques have been proposed and significantly improved during the past 30 years, resulting in a considerable decline in burn-related deaths and hospital admissions in the United States. The single greatest advancement in treating patients with severe thermal injuries during the last 20 years has probably been early excision and closure of the burn wound, leading to substantially reduced resting energy requirements and subsequent improvement of mortality rates in this particular population of patients. The adequate and rapid institution of fluid resuscitation maintains tissue perfusion and prevents organ system failure. Sepsis is successfully controlled by early excision of burn wounds and topical antimicrobial agents. Patients suffering from sustained inhalation injury require additional fluid resuscitation, humidified oxygen, and, occasionally, ventilatory support. Enteral tube feeding is commenced early to control stress ulceration, to maintain intestinal mucosal integrity, and to provide fuel for the resulting hypermetabolic state. Therapeutic approaches to overcome this persistent hypermetabolism and associated hyperglycemia have remained challenging. At present, β-adrenergic blockade with propranolol represents probably the most efficacious anticatabolic therapy in the treatment of burns. Other pharmacologic strategies that have been successfully used to attenuate the hypermetabolic response to burn injury include growth hormone,

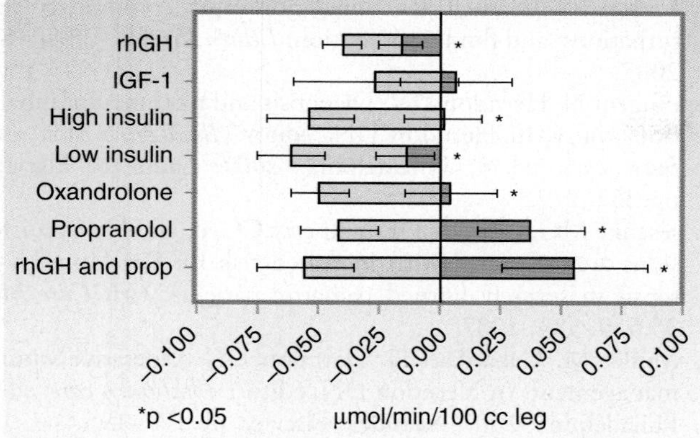

FIGURE 19-16 Relative efficacy of the different anabolic agents to improve muscle protein synthesis compared with standard of care alone. Changes in net protein balance of muscle protein synthesis and breakdown induced by burn injury were measured by stable isotope studies using d5-phenylalanine infusion. $*P < .05$. Graphs are averages ± standard error of the mean. The *yellow bars* represent patients with burns ≥40% total body surface area (TBSA) who received no anabolic agents. The *blue bars* represent patients with burns ≥40% TBSA who were randomized to receive drug. (From Williams FN, Jeschke MG, Chinkes DL, et al: Modulation of the hypermetabolic response to trauma: Temperature, nutrition, and drugs. *J Am Coll Surg* 208:489–502, 2009.)

insulin-like growth factor, and oxandrolone (Fig. 19-16). Maintaining blood glucose at levels below 110 mg/dL with intensive insulin therapy has been shown to reduce mortality and morbidity in critically ill patients; however, associated hypoglycemic events have led to the investigation of alternative strategies, including the use of metformin and the PPAR-γ agonist fenofibrate.

Further studies are needed to address the primary determinants of death, inhalation injury complications, and pneumonia as well as to ameliorate pain and scar formation, which are the persistent sequelae of this thermal injury. Better understanding of the basic mechanisms underlying the metabolic alterations after burn injury may lead to the development of novel therapeutic options. Centralized care in burn units and multidisciplinary team approaches will advance and extend current therapeutic strategies, thus further improving the prognosis of these unique patients.

SELECTED REFERENCES

Baxter CR: Fluid volume and electrolyte changes of the early postburn period. *Clin Plast Surg* 1:693–703, 1974.

This article defined the development and use of the Parkland formula for the resuscitation of burned patients.

Bull JP, Squire JR: A study of mortality in a burns unit: Standards for the evaluation of alternative methods of treatment. *Ann Surg* 130:160–173, 1949.

This landmark article was one of the first to describe the incidence of burn mortality.

Herndon DN, Hart DW, Wolf SE, et al: Reversal of catabolism by beta-blockade after severe burns. *N Engl J Med* 345:1223–1229, 2001.

This landmark clinical trial showed that propranolol, a nonselective beta receptor antagonist, attenuates the profound hypermetabolic response and the muscle-protein catabolism after severe burn injury.

Herndon DN, Tompkins RG: Support of the metabolic response to burn injury. *Lancet* 363:1895–1902, 2004.

This review was one of the premier articles to highlight the many methods to attenuate the hypermetabolic response and to thoroughly describe the physiologic and metabolic derangements postburn.

Jeschke MG, Chinkes DL, Finnerty CC, et al: Pathophysiologic response to severe burn injury. *Ann Surg* 248:387–401, 2008.

This landmark clinical trial delineated the complexity of the hypermetabolic, hypercatabolic response to severe burn injury.

Williams FN, Jeschke MG, Chinkes DL, et al: Modulation of the hypermetabolic response to trauma: Temperature, nutrition, and drugs. *J Am Coll Surg* 208:489–502, 2009.

This review highlights the significant pharmacologic and nonpharmacologic modulators of the postburn hypermetabolic response that have been shown to improve morbidity and mortality.

Wolf SE, Rose JK, Desai MH, et al: Mortality determinants in massive pediatric burns. An analysis of 103 children with > or = 80% TBSA burns (> or = 70% full-thickness). *Ann Surg* 225:554–565, 1997.

The treatment of severely burned pediatric patients and the major determinants of mortality are described in this article. A formula was also devised to predict those who will survive or succumb to their injuries.

REFERENCES

1. Guidelines for the operation of burn centers. *J Burn Care Res* 28:134–141, 2007.
2. Wolf SE: Critical care in the severely burned: Organ support and management of complications. In Herndon DN, editor: *Total burn care*, ed 3, Philadelphia, 2007, Saunders Elsevier, pp 454–476.
3. Herndon DN: *Total burn care*, ed 3, Philadelphia, 2007, Saunders Elsevier.
4. Klein MB, Goverman J, Hayden DL, et al: Benchmarking outcomes in the critically injured burn patient. *Ann Surg* 259:833–841, 2014.
5. Jeschke MG, Herndon DN: Burns in children: Standard and new treatments. *Lancet* 383:1168–1178, 2014.
6. Bull JP, Squire JR: A study of mortality in a burns unit: Standards for the evaluation of alternative methods of treatment. *Ann Surg* 130:160–173, 1949.
7. Flynn JD, National Fire Protection Association: Children playing with fire. Available at: <http://www.nfpa.org/assets/files/PDF/ChildrenPlayingExSummary.pdf>. Accessed February 18, 2015.

8. Centers for Disease Control and Prevention. Fire deaths and injuries: Fact sheet. Available at: <http://www.cdc.gov/HomeandRecreationalSafety/Fire-Prevention/fires-factsheet.html>.
9. National Burn Repository: Report of data from 1999-2008. American Burn Association. Available at: <http://www.ameriburn.org/>. Accessed February 18, 2015.
10. Herndon DN, Blakeney PE: Teamwork for total burn care: Achievements, directions, and hopes. In Herndon DN, editor: *Total burn care*, ed 3, Philadelphia, 2007, Saunders Elsevier, pp 9–13.
11. Wolf SE, Rose JK, Desai MH, et al: Mortality determinants in massive pediatric burns. An analysis of 103 children with > or = 80% TBSA burns (> or = 70% full-thickness). *Ann Surg* 225:554–565, 1997.
12. Williams FN, Jeschke MG, Chinkes DL, et al: Modulation of the hypermetabolic response to trauma: Temperature, nutrition, and drugs. *J Am Coll Surg* 208:489–502, 2009.
13. Gauglitz GG, Herndon DN, Jeschke MG: Insulin resistance postburn: Underlying mechanisms and current therapeutic strategies. *J Burn Care Res* 29:683–694, 2008.
14. Jeschke MG, Chinkes DL, Finnerty CC, et al: Pathophysiologic response to severe burn injury. *Ann Surg* 248:387–401, 2008.
15. Cree MG, Aarsland A, Herndon DN, et al: Role of fat metabolism in burn trauma–induced skeletal muscle insulin resistance. *Crit Care Med* 35:S476–S483, 2007.
16. Gauglitz GG, Herndon DN, Kulp GA, et al: Abnormal insulin sensitivity persists up to three years in pediatric patients post-burn. *J Clin Endocrinol Metab* 94:1656–1664, 2009.
17. Herndon DN, Hart DW, Wolf SE, et al: Reversal of catabolism by beta-blockade after severe burns. *N Engl J Med* 345:1223–1229, 2001.
18. Greenhalgh DG, Saffle JR, Holmes JH, 4th, et al: American Burn Association consensus conference to define sepsis and infection in burns. *J Burn Care Res* 28:776–790, 2007.
19. Williams FN, Herndon DN, Hawkins HK, et al: The leading causes of death after burn injury in a single pediatric burn center. *Crit Care* 13:R183, 2009.
20. Willis MS, Carlson DL, Dimaio JM, et al: Macrophage migration inhibitory factor mediates late cardiac dysfunction after burn injury. *Am J Physiol Heart Circ Physiol* 288:H795–H804, 2005.
21. Pereira C, Murphy K, Herndon D: Outcome measures in burn care. Is mortality dead? *Burns* 30:761–771, 2004.
22. Sagraves SG, Phade SV, Spain T, et al: A collaborative systems approach to rural burn care. *J Burn Care Res* 28:111–114, 2007.
23. Baxter CR: Fluid volume and electrolyte changes of the early postburn period. *Clin Plast Surg* 1:693–703, 1974.
24. Sullivan SR, Friedrich JB, Engrav LH, et al: "Opioid creep" is real and may be the cause of "fluid creep". *Burns* 30:583–590, 2004.
25. Sullivan SR, Ahmadi AJ, Singh CN, et al: Elevated orbital pressure: Another untoward effect of massive resuscitation after burn injury. *J Trauma* 60:72–76, 2006.
26. Finnerty CC, Herndon DN, Jeschke MG: Inhalation injury in severely burned children does not augment the systemic inflammatory response. *Crit Care* 11:R22, 2007.
27. Endorf FW, Gamelli RL: Inhalation injury, pulmonary perturbations, and fluid resuscitation. *J Burn Care Res* 28:80–83, 2007.
28. Nugent N, Herndon DN: Diagnosis and treatment of inhalation injury. In Herndon DN, editor: *Total burn care, total burn care*, ed 3, Philadelphia, 2007, Saunders Elsevier, pp 262–272.
29. Jeschke MG, Chinkes DL, Finnerty CC, et al: Blood transfusions are associated with increased risk for development of sepsis in severely burned pediatric patients. *Crit Care Med* 35:579–583, 2007.
30. Muller M, Gahankari D, Herndon DN: Operative wound management. In Herndon DN, editor: *Total burn care*, ed 3, Philadelphia, 2007, Saunders Elsevier, pp 177–195.
31. Branski LK, Herndon DN, Pereira C, et al: Longitudinal assessment of Integra in primary burn management: A randomized pediatric clinical trial. *Crit Care Med* 35:2615–2623, 2007.
32. Hohlfeld J, de Buys Roessingh A, Hirt-Burri N, et al: Tissue engineered fetal skin constructs for paediatric burns. *Lancet* 366:840–842, 2005.
33. Jeschke MG, Finnerty CC, Shahrokhi S, et al: Wound coverage technologies in burn care: Novel techniques. *J Burn Care Res* 34:612–620, 2013.
34. Branski LK, Herndon DN, Barrow RE, et al: Randomized controlled trial to determine the efficacy of long-term growth hormone treatment in severely burned children. *Ann Surg* 250:514–523, 2009.
35. Langouche L, Van den Berghe G: Glucose metabolism and insulin therapy. *Crit Care Clin* 22:119–129, vii, 2006.
36. Wolf SE, Edelman LS, Kemalyan N, et al: Effects of oxandrolone on outcome measures in the severely burned: A multicenter prospective randomized double-blind trial. *J Burn Care Res* 27:131–139, 2006.
37. Jeschke MG, Finnerty CC, Suman OE, et al: The effect of oxandrolone on the endocrinologic, inflammatory, and hypermetabolic responses during the acute phase postburn. *Ann Surg* 246:351–360, 2007.
38. Przkora R, Jeschke MG, Barrow RE, et al: Metabolic and hormonal changes of severely burned children receiving long-term oxandrolone treatment. *Ann Surg* 242:384–389, 2005.
39. Pereira CT, Jeschke MG, Herndon DN: Beta-blockade in burns. *Novartis Found Symp* 280:238–251, 2007.
40. Jeschke MG, Klein D, Bolder U, et al: Insulin attenuates the systemic inflammatory response in endotoxemic rats. *Endocrinology* 145:4084–4093, 2004.
41. Jeschke MG, Kulp GA, Kraft R, et al: Intensive insulin therapy in severely burned pediatric patients: A prospective randomized trial. *Am J Respir Crit Care Med* 182:351–359, 2010.
42. Dandona P, Chaudhuri A, Mohanty P, et al: Anti-inflammatory effects of insulin. *Curr Opin Clin Nutr Metab Care* 10:511–517, 2007.
43. Van den Berghe G, Wilmer A, Hermans G, et al: Intensive insulin therapy in the medical ICU. *N Engl J Med* 354:449–461, 2006.
44. Ellger B, Debaveye Y, Vanhorebeek I, et al: Survival benefits of intensive insulin therapy in critical illness: Impact of maintaining normoglycemia versus glycemia-independent actions of insulin. *Diabetes* 55:1096–1105, 2006.
45. Ingels C, Debaveye Y, Milants I, et al: Strict blood glucose control with insulin during intensive care after cardiac

surgery: Impact on 4-years survival, dependency on medical care, and quality-of-life. *Eur Heart J* 27:2716–2724, 2006.

46. Brunkhorst FM, Engel C, Bloos F, et al: Intensive insulin therapy and pentastarch resuscitation in severe sepsis. *N Engl J Med* 358:125–139, 2008.
47. Jeschke MG, Pinto R, Herndon DN, et al: Hypoglycemia is associated with increased postburn morbidity and mortality in pediatric patients. *Crit Care Med* 42:1221–1231, 2014.
48. Dellinger RP, Levy MM, Carlet JM, et al: Surviving Sepsis Campaign: International guidelines for management of severe sepsis and septic shock: 2008. *Crit Care Med* 36:296–327, 2008.
49. Gore DC, Herndon DN, Wolfe RR: Comparison of peripheral metabolic effects of insulin and metformin following severe burn injury. *J Trauma* 59:316–322, 2005.
50. Cree MG, Zwetsloot JJ, Herndon DN, et al: Insulin sensitivity and mitochondrial function are improved in children with burn injury during a randomized controlled trial of fenofibrate. *Ann Surg* 245:214–221, 2007.

20 CHAPTER

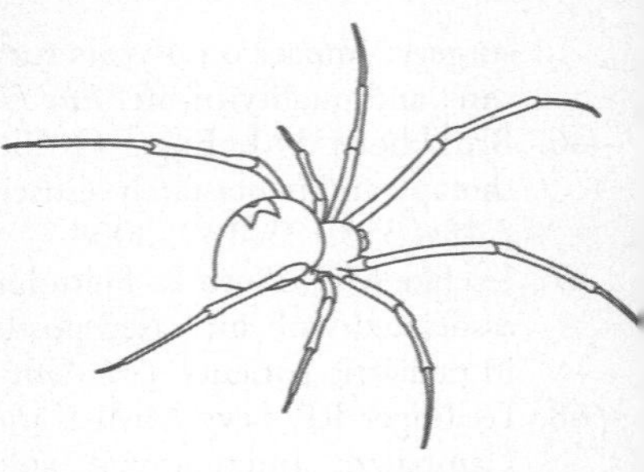

Bites and Stings

Lillian F. Liao, Robert L. Norris, Paul S. Auerbach, Elaine E. Nelson, Ronald M. Stewart

OUTLINE

SNAKEBITES

Epidemiology

Snakebites are a public health problem primarily in warm areas across the globe. The burden of injury is greatest in the tropical and subtropical regions of the world, primarily affecting Southeast Asia, India, Australia, South America, and parts of Africa. The World Health Organization reports approximately 5 million snakebites worldwide with 2.5 million venomous snakebites each year and 125,000 deaths worldwide.[1] The actual number of bites may be underreported. In the United States, approximately 7000 to 8000 venomous bites occur annually with approximately five deaths in the reported population. It is estimated that more deaths would occur if injured individuals did not seek medical care. Long-term morbidity from snakebites is unknown because extended long-term follow-up of these patients is not usually conducted.[1,2]

Venomous Species Indigenous to United States

Clinically important venomous snakes that inhabit the United States can be divided into two broad classes, Crotalinae and Elapidae. Crotalinae are a subfamily of Viperidae, more commonly known as pit vipers, named for their infrared sensing facial pit. Crotalinae species are numerous and occupy a broad range of habitats, present throughout all of the contiguous United States with the exception of Maine. Crotalinae include rattlesnakes (Fig. 20-1), copperheads (Fig. 20-2), and cottonmouths/water moccasins. Several characteristics distinguish Crotalinae from nonvenomous snakes. Crotalinae tend to have relatively triangular heads, elliptical pupils, heat-sensing facial pits, and large, retractable anterior fangs (Figs. 20-3 and 20-4). All but one species of rattlesnakes have a terminal rattle as a typical distinguishing feature (see Fig. 20-1). Non-Crotalinae, which with the exception of coral snakes are nonvenomous, have more rounded heads, circular pupils, and no fangs. The only indigenous Elapidae of the United States is the coral snake (Fig. 20-5), which encompasses three distinct species: the eastern coral snake (*Micrurus fulvius*), Texas coral snake (*Micrurus tener*), and Sonoran coral snake (*Micruroides euryxanthus*). North American coral snakes have distinctly colored stripes arranged in a typical pattern on their skin, perhaps remembered best through folk rhymes as "red on yellow, kill a fellow; red on black, venom lack."

Lower extremity bites are more common when the victim is not intentionally handling the snake. Upper extremity bites predominate in victims intentionally handling venomous snakes. Most patients with Crotalinae envenomations present with swelling and pain to the site of injury.[3-5] Coral snake envenomations may have minimal or no local findings.

Pathophysiology

Clinical findings of envenomation from the two subfamilies of snakes differ. Snakes in the Crotalinae family cause 95% of venomous snakebites in the United States. Crotalinae envenomation is typically deposited into the subcutaneous tissue by the fangs of the viper. Less commonly, it is deposited into intramuscular compartments and causes major local effects of tissue necrosis and sometimes severe systemic effects with hematologic abnormalities as a result of its hemotoxic affects.[4,5] Envenomation, which leads to diffuse capillary leakage, can result in pulmonary edema, hypotension, and shock. In addition to primary hemotoxins, a consumptive coagulopathy may follow the severe tissue injury.[6,7] Envenomation can result in diffuse bleeding within 1 hour of envenomation. Although intravenous (IV) envenomation is exceedingly rare, it produces profound shock and organ dysfunction with onset of these symptoms within minutes.

Crotalinae venom contains a wide array of complex components, including peptides and various enzymes. The venom typically contains zinc-dependent metalloproteinases. These enzymes cause damage at the basement membrane level, disrupting the endothelial cell connections, causing hemorrhage and fluid extravasation.[5] Bite severity in each case is related to the volume deposited and the concentrations of toxin produced by the species of Crotalinae. Rattlesnake envenomations are typically more severe and more likely to require antivenin therapy.

Elapidae venom contains alpha neurotoxin, which results in a direct neurotoxic effect. Toxins affect presynaptic and postsynaptic receptors. The venom can result in respiratory depression with progression to neurogenic shock. Patients with these symptoms

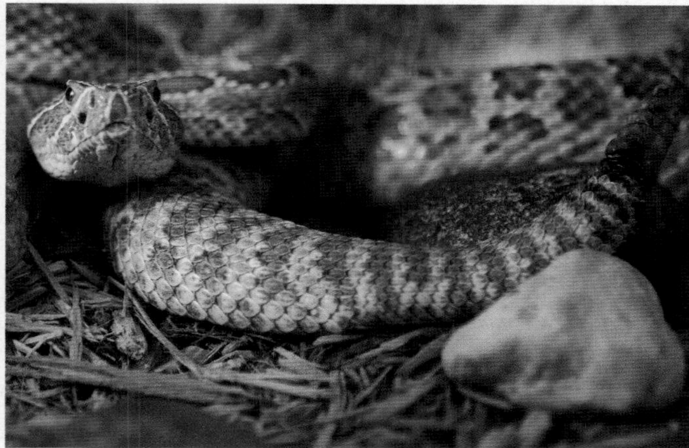

FIGURE 20-1 A typical rattlesnake of the Crotalinae subfamily. There are 32 different species in North America, and all but one species has the terminal rattle. (Courtesy Ronald M. Stewart.)

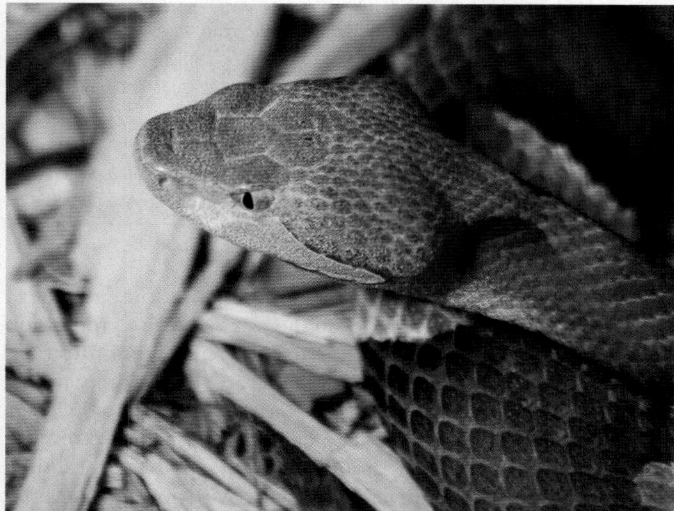

FIGURE 20-2 Typical features of a North American copperhead. Many, if not most, copperhead and water moccasin envenomations are less severe than the related rattlesnake species. (Courtesy Ronald M. Stewart.)

have a high risk of mortality, and immediate medical attention is required.[8]

Clinical Manifestations

Local signs and symptoms of Crotalinae snakebites include swelling, pain, and ecchymosis. Swelling may progress to bullae formation and typically progresses along the path of the lymphatic drainage of the region bitten (Fig. 20-6). Pain is reported as a burning that starts within minutes of envenomation. Swelling, if progressive, can develop into compartment syndrome of the extremity. Tissue necrosis can also occur, with delays in treatment resulting in loss of function from Crotalinae bites. Systemic signs are due to diffuse circulatory collapse as a result of envenomation. Patients report initial nausea, perioral paresthesias, metallic taste, and muscle twitching. Laboratory derangements include increased partial thromboplastin time, prothrombin time, fibrin split products, elevated creatinine, creatine phosphokinase, proteinuria, hematuria, and anemia.[9]

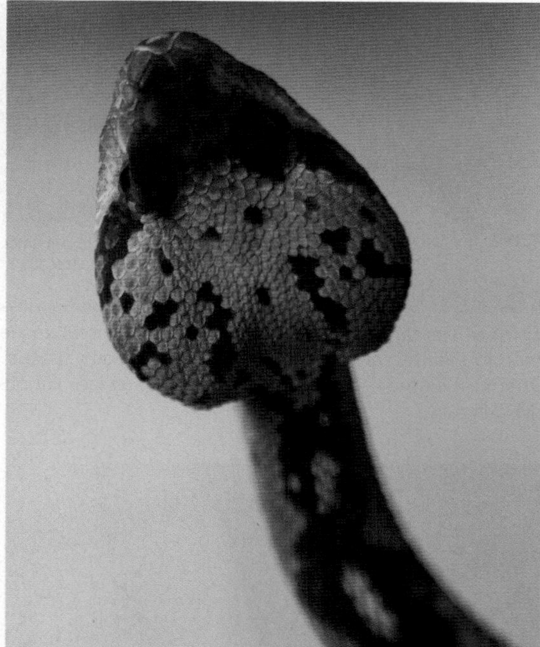

FIGURE 20-3 This rattlesnake displays the typical broad, triangular head characteristic of Crotalinae species. (Courtesy Ronald M. Stewart.)

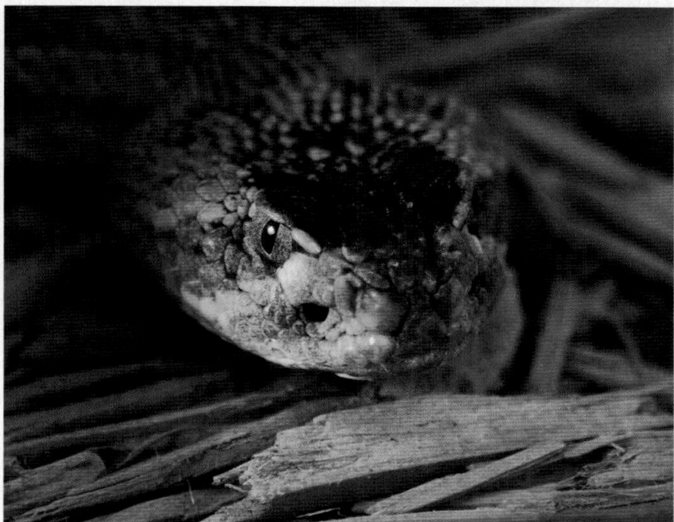

FIGURE 20-4 Crotaline species have characteristic facial pits that are extremely sensitive to infrared radiation and elliptical pupils. (Courtesy Ronald M. Stewart.)

In contrast, patients with coral snake envenomation, which primarily causes neurotoxicity, may present with respiratory failure or neurologic symptoms with minimal local findings. Systemic signs of coral snakebites, including cranial nerve dysfunction and loss of deep tendon reflexes, may progress to respiratory depression and paralysis over several hours. Differences in therapy make it important to distinguish between coral snake and pit viper bites.[7-9]

Management

Initial management of a snakebite victim is to remove the victim from the area of danger. The wound should be cleaned locally, the

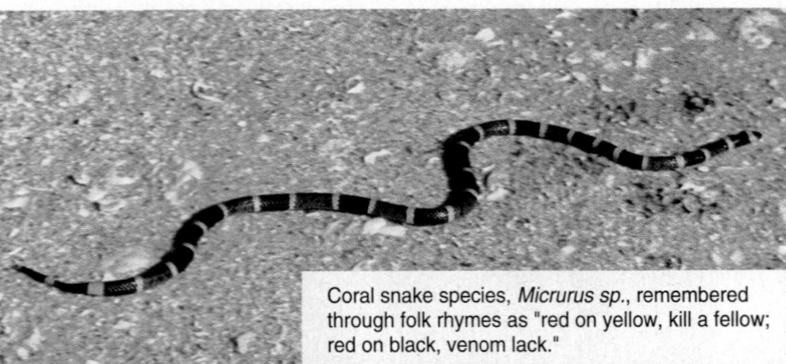

Coral snake species, *Micrurus sp.*, remembered through folk rhymes as "red on yellow, kill a fellow; red on black, venom lack."

FIGURE 20-5 Typical markings of North American coral snakes. It is uncommon to see the furtive coral snake in broad open spaces. (Courtesy Luther C. Goldman, U.S. Fish and Wildlife Service, annotated by Ronald M. Stewart.)

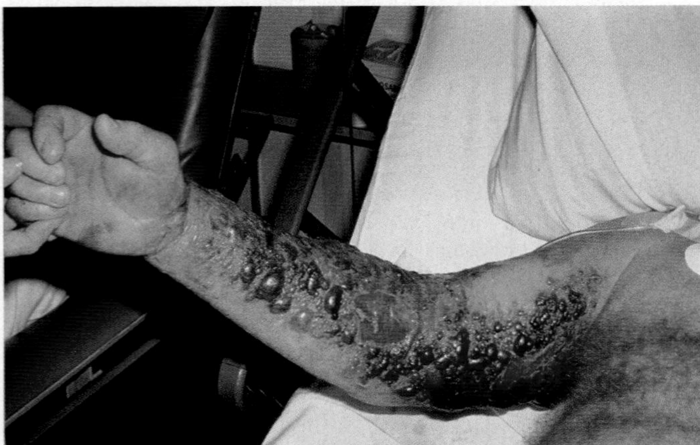

FIGURE 20-6 Signs of a severe envenomation (grade 3) with extensive bullae formation after a rattlesnake bite to the hand. This appearance is now uncommon in patients treated early with antivenin.

affected area should be elevated to the level of the heart if possible, and the patient should be transported to a nearby hospital for determination of need for antivenin administration. Historical recommendations of x-cut aspiration, freshly killed bird, cryotherapy, suction, tourniquets, and electrical shock therapy are harmful and should not be adopted (Table 20-1).

Initial hospital evaluation should follow the protocols and guidelines according to the Advanced Trauma Life Support Course.[10] A detailed history should be obtained from the patient or field health care provider regarding the timing of injury, type of snake involved, and prior history of envenomation. Patients or their family members often bring in the snake (alive or dead); however, these animals should not be handled because bite reflex can occur for up to 1 hour after the snake has been dead. The area of the bite should be marked, and the affected area should be assessed every 15 minutes for progression until the progression has stabilized.[7-9]

Complete laboratory evaluation is needed for patients with Crotalinae bites. Patients with Elapidae bites also need respiratory monitoring. A chest radiograph and electrocardiogram is needed for older patients or patients with systemic symptoms. All patients with signs of envenomation should be observed for at least 24 hours in the hospital. Patients with Crotalinae bites without signs of envenomation or laboratory abnormalities can be discharged after 6 to 8 hours of observation. Potential coral snake envenomations should be observed for a longer time, typically 24 hours.

TABLE 20-1 Outdated or Disproven Treatment Modalities for Snakebites

X-CUT ASPIRATION	CONSTRICTOR BAND
Freshly killed bird dressing	Partial or radical excision of wounds
Electrical stimulation	Steroids
Ice—ligature cryotherapy	Heat
Fasciotomy (prophylactic)	Tourniquet

TABLE 20-2 Snakebite Severity Grading Scale

0	Fang mark; local swelling, ecchymosis <2.5 cm; minimal pain and tenderness; no systemic symptoms
1	Fang mark; history of immediate pain with bite; swelling and erythema 5-15 cm; no systemic symptoms
2	Fang mark; history of immediate severe pain; swelling and erythema 15-40 cm; mild systemic symptoms or abnormal laboratory findings or both
3	Fang mark; history of immediate severe pain; swelling and erythema >40 cm; petechiae and bullae; moderate systemic symptoms; bleeding or disseminated intravascular coagulopathy or both; abnormal laboratory values
4	Fang mark; signs of multiple envenomation sites; history of immediate severe pain; severe systemic signs—coma, shock, bleeding, disseminated intravascular coagulation, and paralysis

A grading scale has been used for estimating the severity of Crotalinae bites.[11] The grading tool helps to evaluate progression of injury and determine the need for antivenin administration. This is an important tool because CroFab (BTG International Inc., West Conshohocken, PA) is expensive, and, although generally safe, it can have adverse side effects. The snakebite severity grading scale (Table 20-2) should be used as part of the initial assessment for use of antivenin. Patients with minimal severity without progression would likely not benefit from antivenin. Conversely, patients with moderate to severe bites would likely benefit from antivenin administration (Fig. 20-7).[8-12]

Antivenin Therapy

Antivenin therapy is the mainstay of treatment for significant envenomations from Crotalinae and Elapidae species.[13] A decision to use antivenin therapy requires clinical judgment, and consultation with experienced clinicians is recommended. Administration of antivenin is time-sensitive in both categories of envenomation: The earlier antivenin is administered, the more effective the therapy. CroFab is a commercially available polyvalent antivenin effective against a wide range of Crotalinae species in the United States. The antibodies used for this product are derived from sheep, and clinical experience has demonstrated the product to be significantly safer than the polyvalent antivenom used before 2000. Antivenin therapy is mediated by antibody to antigen binding. CroFab, as its name implies, consists of fragment antigen-binding segments of the antibodies (Fab). Because there must be enough antibody to neutralize a given amount of antigen, antivenin dosing is determined by the amount of venom injected by the snake rather than the mass or size of the patient. The initial standard dosing is 4 to 6 vials in pediatric and adult patients. The bolus is repeated until the signs and symptoms are stabilized, after

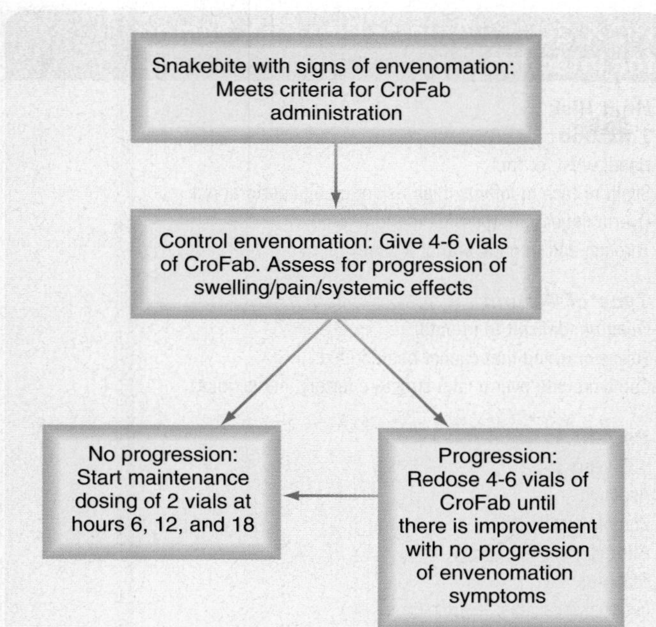

FIGURE 20-7 Straightforward algorithm for management of patients with significant envenomation. Dosing is based on an estimate of the degree of envenomation, not on weight.

which 2 vials of CroFab are given every 6 hours for three additional doses. Pregnancy is not a contraindication to CroFab.[11-13]

Coral snake *(Micrurus fulvius)* antivenin was produced by Pfizer (New York, NY) and is available in limited quantities for coral snakebites. The antivenin is not currently being produced, and the expiration dates of available antivenin supply have been extended since 2011. The U.S. Food and Drug Administration, in partnership with Pfizer, has been trying to secure more coral snake antivenin. However, at the present time, the supply is highly uncertain, and contacting hospital pharmacies and the regional poison control center is mandatory to assess treatment options. Antivenin treatment should be started early for patients who definitively sustained coral snakebites, as signs and symptoms initially can be minimal. The antivenin carries a risk of anaphylaxis, so administration in a facility where ready availability of treatment for anaphylaxis (epinephrine, steroids, antihistamine, and airway control) is mandatory. For envenomations from nonindigenous species in the United States, poison control centers and zoos can provide important information regarding the procurement of antivenin and management. The American Association of Poison Control Centers (800-222-1222) is a useful source of information for physicians needing help in managing venomous snakebites. Given the shortage of some antivenin products, the poison control center contacts are particularly important.[12]

Coagulopathy of Envenomation

Crotalinae envenomation can result in a cascade of systemic coagulopathy.[14] Blood product is required only if the coagulation defect is not reversed by antivenin, or if there is active, significant hemorrhage. Serious bleeding requires the administration of appropriate blood product components based on laboratory values. However, antivenin should begin before replacement of any blood products because treating the primary cause of bleeding is of utmost importance. Coagulopathy can last 2 weeks after injury, and elective surgery must be avoided during this time.[5,9,12]

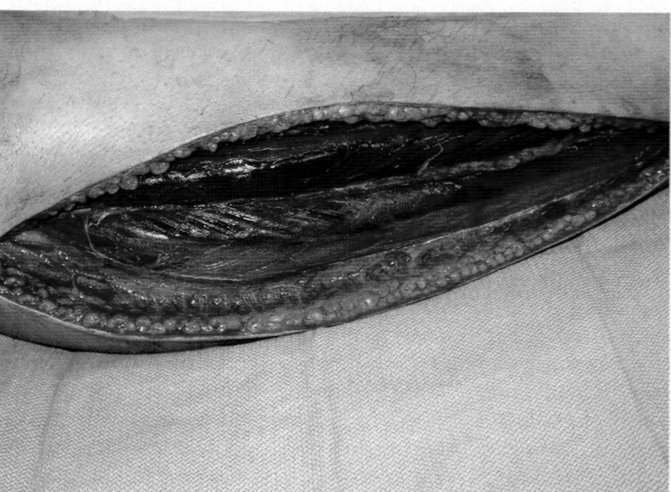

FIGURE 20-8 Fasciotomy of the lower extremity in a victim of a severe rattlesnake bite on the lower leg. Intracompartmental pressures were documented to be exceedingly elevated in this patient, despite limb elevation and large doses of antivenom. (Courtesy Ronald M. Stewart.)

Fasciotomy

Based on probability, most venom is injected into the subcutaneous space, so fasciotomy is very rarely required; however, venom occasionally is injected into muscle compartments (Fig. 20-8). Children and patients with bites to the hands or fingers are most likely to sustain intramuscular injection of venom. In cases of intramuscular injection, compartment syndrome may develop, and evaluation must be done serially. There is no role for prophylactic fasciotomy.[15] Animal data demonstrate that fasciotomy may increase the severity of local myonecrosis, and antivenin is effective in reducing compartment syndrome[16,17]; however, if adequate antivenin has been administered and a compartment syndrome is highly likely or demonstrated by increased compartmental pressures, fasciotomy may be required. One must refrain from débridement of injured muscle groups because the usual evaluation of muscle viability (contraction, coloration, general appearance) is unreliable in the setting of intramuscular envenomation, as this may be a sign of venom injury rather than muscle necrosis. Premature débridement can result in unnecessary morbidity.[15] Antivenin administration is the primary treatment for these patients. Additionally, negative pressure wound therapy is appropriate for coverage of fasciotomy sites.

MAMMALIAN BITES

Epidemiology

The incidence of mammalian bite injuries is unknown because most patients with minor wounds never seek medical care. Although death from animal bites is uncommon in the United States, thousands of people are killed around the world each year, primarily by large animals such as lions and tigers. Dogs are responsible for 80% to 90% of animal bites in the United States, followed by cats and humans; an estimated 4.7 million dog bites occur annually in the United States and account for 1% of emergency department visits.[18] Most of these bites are from a family pet or a neighborhood dog. Pit bulls and Rottweilers account for most fatal dog bites in the United States.[18] Animal bites occur most frequently on the extremities of adults and on the head, face, and neck of children, which increases the risk for death and serious morbidity in children. More than 60% of reported bites occur in children, especially boys 5 to 9 years old.

Treatment

Evaluation

Humans attacked by animals are at risk for blunt and penetrating trauma. Animals produce blunt injuries by striking with their extremities, biting with their powerful jaws, and crushing with their body weight. Teeth and claws can puncture body cavities, including the cranium, and amputate extremities. Patients with serious injuries are managed in a similar fashion as other potentially seriously injured victims, with special attention given to wound management. Useful laboratory tests include a hematocrit when blood loss is of concern and cultures when an infection is present. Radiographs are obtained to diagnose potential fractures, joint penetration, severe infections, and retained foreign bodies, such as teeth. The patient's tetanus immunization status needs to be updated as necessary.

Wound Care

Local wound management reduces the risk for infection and maximizes functional and esthetic outcomes. Early wound cleaning is the most important therapy for preventing infection and zoonotic diseases such as rabies. Intact skin surrounding dirty wounds is scrubbed with a sponge and 1% povidone-iodine or 2% chlorhexidine gluconate solution. Alternatively, a dilute povidone-iodine solution can be used for irrigation, as long as the wound is flushed afterward with normal saline or water. Wounds that are dirty or contain devitalized tissue are cleaned lightly with gauze or a porous sponge and sharply débrided. Optimal wound management may require treatment in the operating room under general or regional anesthesia.

Options for wound repair include primary, delayed primary, and secondary closure. The anatomic location of the bite, source of the bite, and type of injury determine the most appropriate method. Primary closure is appropriate for head and neck wounds that are initially seen within 24 hours of the bite and for which esthetic results are important and infection rates are low.[19,20] Primary closure can also be used for low-risk wounds to the arms, legs, and trunk if seen within 6 to 12 hours of the bite. Severe human bites and avulsion injuries of the face that require flaps have been successfully repaired by primary closure; however, this technique is controversial. Wounds prone to the development of infection (Box 20-1), such as wounds initially seen longer than 24 hours after the bite (or >6 hours if ear or nose cartilage is involved), are covered with moist dressings and undergo delayed primary closure after 3 to 5 days. Puncture wounds have an increased incidence of infection and are not sutured. Deep irrigation of small puncture wounds and wide excision have not proved beneficial. However, larger puncture wounds usually benefit from irrigation and débridement. Healing by secondary intention generally produces unacceptable scars in cosmetically sensitive areas. The clinician should be alert to the fact that significant dog bites may have extensive undermined areas created by the large canine teeth. These wounds require operative intervention under general or regional anesthesia.

Bites involving the hands or feet have a much greater chance of becoming infected and are left open.[20] The primary goal in repairing bite wounds on the hand is to maximize functional outcome. Even with adequate therapy, approximately one third of dog bites on the hand become infected.[20] Healing by secondary intention is recommended for most hand lacerations. After thorough exploration, irrigation, and débridement, the hand is immobilized, wrapped in a bulky dressing, and elevated. Although high-quality data are limited, preventive, empirical antibiotics in these settings may be warranted.[21]

A common human bite wound associated with high morbidity is a clenched fist injury (fight bite) resulting from striking the tooth of another person's mouth. Regardless of the history obtained, injuries over the dorsum of the metacarpophalangeal joints are treated as clenched fist injuries. Although these wounds appear minor, they often result in serious injury to the extensor tendon or joint capsule and have significant oral bacterial contamination. The extensor tendon retracts when the hand is opened, so evaluation needs to be carried out with the hand in the open and clenched positions. Minor injuries are irrigated, débrided, and left open. Potentially deeper injuries and infected bites require exploration and débridement in the operating room and administration of IV antibiotics.[22] All bite injuries are reevaluated in 1 or 2 days to rule out secondary infection.

BOX 20-1 Animal Bite Risk Factors for Infection

High Risk

Location

Hand, wrist, or foot
Scalp or face in infants (high risk of cranial perforation)
Over a major joint (possible perforation)
Through-and-through bite of a cheek

Type of Wound

Puncture (difficult to irrigate)
Tissue crushing that cannot be débrided
Carnivore bite over a vital structure (artery, nerve, joint)

Patient

>50 years old
Asplenic
Chronic alcoholism
Altered immune status
Diabetes
Peripheral vascular insufficiency
Long-term corticosteroid therapy
Prosthetic or diseased heart valve or joint

Species

Domestic cat
Large cat (deep punctures)
Human (hand bites)
Primates
Pigs

Low Risk

Location

Face, scalp, or mouth

Type of Wound

Large, clean lacerations that can be thoroughly irrigated

Adapted from Keogh S, Callaham ML: Bites and injuries inflicted by domestic animals. In Auerbach PS, editor: *Wilderness medicine: Management of wilderness and environmental emergencies*, ed 4, St Louis, 2001, Mosby, pp 961–978.

Microbiology

Given the large variety and concentration of bacteria in mouths, it is not surprising that wound infection is the main complication of bites, with 3% to 18% of dog bite wounds and approximately 50% of cat bite wounds becoming infected. Infected wounds contain aerobic and anaerobic bacteria and yield an average of five isolates/culture (Box 20-2). Although many wounds are infected by *Staphylococcus* and *Streptococcus* spp. and anaerobes, *Pasteurella* spp. are the most common bacterial pathogen, found in 50% of dog bites and 75% of cat bites. Human bite wounds, as in other bite wounds, are related to the oral flora of the biting offender. These wounds are typically contaminated with *Eikenella corrodens* in addition to the microorganisms found after dog and cat bites.[22,23]

Systemic diseases such as rabies, cat-scratch disease, cowpox, tularemia, leptospirosis, and brucellosis can be acquired through animal bites. Human bites can transmit hepatitis B and C, tuberculosis, syphilis, and HIV.[24] Although HIV transmission from human bites is rare, seroconversion is possible when a person with an open wound, either from a bite or a preexisting injury, is exposed to saliva containing HIV-positive blood.[24] In this scenario, baseline and 6-month postexposure HIV testing is performed, and prophylactic treatment with anti-HIV drugs is considered.

BOX 20-2 Common Bacteria Found in Mouths of Animals

Acinetobacter spp.
Actinobacillus spp.
Aeromonas hydrophila
Bacillus spp.
Bacteroides spp.
Bordetella spp.
Brucella canis
Capnocytophaga canimorsus
Clostridium perfringens
Corynebacterium spp.
Eikenella corrodens
Enterobacter spp.
Escherichia coli
Eubacterium spp.
Fusobacterium spp.
Haemophilus aphrophilus
Haemophilus haemolyticus
Klebsiella spp.
Leptotrichia buccalis
Micrococcus spp.
Moraxella spp.
Neisseria spp.
Pasteurella aerogenes
Pasteurella canis
Pasteurella dagmatis
Pasteurella multocida
Peptococcus spp.
Peptostreptococcus spp.
Propionibacterium spp.
Proteus mirabilis
Pseudomonas spp.
Serratia marcescens
Staphylococcus aureus
Staphylococcus epidermidis
Streptococcus spp.
Veillonella parvula

Adapted from Keogh S, Callaham ML: Bites and injuries inflicted by domestic animals. In Auerbach PS, editor: *Wilderness medicine: Management of wilderness and environmental emergencies*, ed 4, St Louis, 2001, Mosby, pp 961–978.

Antibiotics

Although data are limited, preventive antibiotics are recommended for patients with high-risk bites.[21] The initial antibiotic choice and route are based on the type of animal and severity and location of the bite. Cat bites often cause puncture wounds that require antibiotics. Patients with low-risk dog and human bites do not benefit from prophylactic antibiotics unless the hand or foot is involved.[23] Patients seen 24 hours after a bite without signs of infection do not usually need prophylactic antibiotics. Routine cultures of uninfected wounds have not proved useful and are reserved for infected wounds.

Initial antibiotic selection needs to cover *Staphylococcus* and *Streptococcus* spp., anaerobes, *Pasteurella* spp. for dog and cat bites, and *E. corrodens* for human bites. Amoxicillin-clavulanate is an acceptable first-line antibiotic for most bites. Alternatives include second-generation cephalosporins, such as cefoxitin, or a combination of penicillin and a first-generation cephalosporin. Patients who are allergic to penicillin can receive clindamycin combined with ciprofloxacin (or combined with trimethoprim-sulfamethoxazole if the patient is pregnant or a child).[18] Moxifloxacin has also been suggested as monotherapy. Infections developing within 24 hours of the bite are generally caused by *Pasteurella* spp. and are treated by antibiotics with appropriate coverage. Patients with serious infections require hospital admission and parenteral antibiotics such as piperacillin-tazobactam, ampicillin-sulbactam, and ticarcillin-clavulanate. For penicillin-allergic patients, options include clindamycin combined with either a fluoroquinolone or trimethoprim-sulfamethoxazole and or doxycycline.

Rabies

Annually, thousands of people die of rabies worldwide, with dog bites or scratches being the major source.[25] In the United States, rabies is primarily found in wildlife, with raccoons being the primary source, followed by skunks, bats, and foxes.[26] Cats and dogs account for less than 5% of cases since the establishment of rabies control programs. Although the number of infected animals in the United States continues to increase, with the total approaching 8000/year, human infection rates remain constant at one to three cases annually. Bats have been the main source of human rabies reported in the United States during the past 20 years, although a history of bat contact is absent in most victims.

Rabies is caused by a rhabdovirus found in the saliva of animals and is transmitted through bites or scratches. Acute encephalitis develops, and patients almost invariably die. The disease usually begins with a prodromal phase of nonspecific complaints and paresthesias, with itching or burning at the bite site spreading to the entire bitten extremity. The disease progresses to an acute neurologic phase. This phase generally takes one of two forms. The more common encephalitic or furious form is typified by fever and hyperactivity that can be stimulated by internal or external factors such as thirst, fear, light, or noise, followed by fluctuating levels of consciousness, aerophobia or hydrophobia, inspiratory spasm, and abnormalities of the autonomic nervous system. The paralytic form of rabies is manifested by fever, progressive weakness, loss of deep tendon reflexes, and urinary incontinence. Both forms progress to paralysis, coma, circulatory collapse, and death.

Adequate wound care and postexposure prophylaxis can prevent the development of rabies.[27] Wounds are washed with soap and water and irrigated with a virucidal agent such as povidone-iodine solution. If rabies exposure is strongly suspected, consider leaving the wound open. The decision to administer rabies prophylaxis after an animal bite or scratch depends on the offending species and nature of the event. Guidelines for administering rabies prophylaxis can be obtained from local public health agencies or from the Advisory Committee on Immunization Practices and the U.S. Centers for Disease Control and Prevention.[27] Research indicates that rabies prophylaxis is not being administered according to guidelines, which results in costly overtreatment or potentially life-threatening undertreatment.

Worldwide, almost 1 million people receive rabies prophylaxis each year; this includes 40,000 people from the United States.[25] Unprovoked attacks are more likely to occur by rabid animals. All wild carnivores must be considered rabid, but birds and reptiles do not contract or transmit rabies. In cases of bites by domestic animals, rodents, or lagomorphs, the local health department needs to be consulted before beginning rabies prophylaxis. A bite from a healthy-appearing domestic animal does not require prophylaxis if the animal can be observed for 10 days (see Boxes 20-1 and 20-2).

Rabies prophylaxis involves passive (with rabies immune globulin) and active (with rabies vaccine) immunization. Passive immunization consists of administering 20 IU/kg body weight of rabies immune globulin. As much of the dose as possible is infiltrated into and around the wound. The rest is given intramuscularly at a site remote from where the vaccine was administered. If the human rabies immune globulin is not given immediately, it can still be administered for up to 7 days. Active immunization for healthy patients consists of administering 1 mL of human diploid cell vaccine or 1 mL of purified chick embryo cell vaccine intramuscularly into the deltoid of adults and into the anterolateral aspect of the thigh in children on days 0, 3, 7, and 14. For immunocompromised patients, a five-dose schedule is recommended on days 0, 3, 7, 14, and 28.[27] Patients with preexposure immunization do not require passive immunization and need active immunization only on days 0 and 3.[27]

ARTHROPOD BITES AND STINGS

Although mammalian and reptilian bites inflict more serious injuries and are generally more dramatic in their presentations, many more people in the United States die from insect bites and stings, most often caused by anaphylaxis. Also, even more people contract vector-related infectious diseases from the bites of insects.

Black Widow Spiders

Widow spiders (genus *Latrodectus*) are found throughout the world. At least one of five species inhabits all areas of the United States except Alaska. The best-known widow spider is the black widow *(Latrodectus mactans)*. The female has a leg span of 1 to 4 cm and a shiny black body with a distinctive red ventral marking (often hourglass-shaped) (Fig. 20-9). Variations in color occur among other species, with some appearing brown or red and some without the ventral marking. The nonaggressive female widow spider bites in defense. Males are too small to bite through human skin.

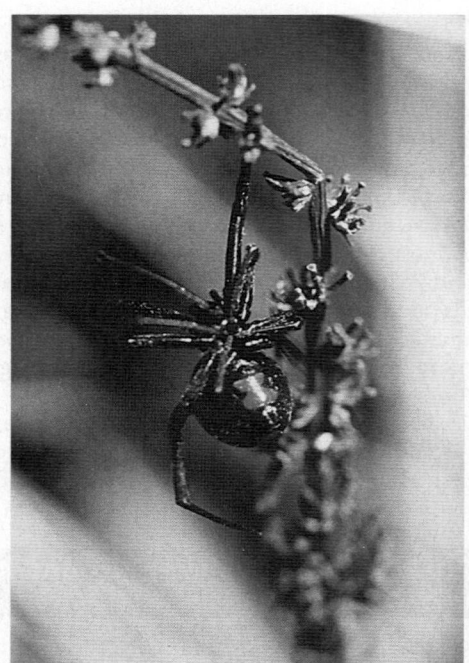

FIGURE 20-9 Female black widow spider *(Latrodectus mactans)* with the characteristic hourglass marking. (Courtesy Paul Auerbach.)

Toxicology

Widow spiders produce neurotoxic venom with minimal local effects. The major component is alpha-latrotoxin, which acts at presynaptic terminals by enhancing the release of neurotransmitters. The ensuing clinical picture results from excess stimulation of neuromuscular junctions as well as the sympathetic and parasympathetic nervous systems.

Clinical Manifestations

The bite itself may be painless or felt as a pinprick. Local findings are minimal. The patient may have systemic complaints and no history of a spider bite, making the diagnosis challenging. Neuromuscular symptoms may occur 30 minutes after the bite and include severe pain and spasms of large muscle groups. Abdominal cramps and rigidity could mimic a surgical abdomen, but rebound is absent. Dyspnea can result from chest wall muscle tightness. Autonomic stimulation produces hypertension, diaphoresis, and tachycardia. Other symptoms include muscle twitching, nausea and vomiting, headache, and paresthesias.

Treatment

Mild bites are managed with local wound care—cleansing, intermittent application of ice, and tetanus prophylaxis as needed. The possibility of delayed severe symptoms makes an observation period of several hours prudent. The optimal therapy for severe envenomation is controversial. IV calcium gluconate, previously recommended as a first-line drug to relieve muscle spasms after widow spider bites, has no significant efficacy. Narcotics and benzodiazepines are more effective agents to relieve muscular pain. Antivenin has been shown to reduce or eliminate symptoms of latrodectism.[28]

In the United States, antivenom derived from horse serum is available (Black Widow Spider Antivenin; Merck, West Point,

PA). Because this antivenom can cause anaphylactoid reactions or serum sickness, it must be reserved for serious cases. Antivenom is currently recommended for pregnant women, children younger than 16 years, adults older than 60 years, and patients with severe envenomation and uncontrolled hypertension or respiratory distress. Skin testing for possible allergy to the U.S. antivenom is recommended by the manufacturer and is outlined in the package insert, although the reliability of such testing is low. Patients about to receive antivenom may be pretreated with antihistamines to reduce the likelihood or severity of a systemic reaction to the serum. The initial recommended dose is 1 vial intravenously or intramuscularly, repeated as necessary, although it is exceedingly rare for more than 2 vials to be required. Studies have demonstrated that antivenom can decrease a patient's hospital stay, with discharge several hours after administration.[28] A high-quality antivenom is also available in Australia for *Latrodectus* bites, and a new purified Fab fragment *Latrodectus mactans* antivenom (Analatro) is currently undergoing clinical trials (ClinicalTrials.gov Identifier: NCT00657540). Manufacturer: Instituto Bioclon S.A. de C.V., Mexico City, Mexico.

Brown Recluse Spiders

Envenomation by brown spiders of the genus *Loxosceles* is termed *necrotic arachnidism* or *loxoscelism*. These arthropods primarily inhabit North and South America, Africa, and Europe. Several species of *Loxosceles* are found throughout the United States, with the greatest concentration in the Midwest. Most significant bites in the United States are by *Loxosceles reclusa*, the brown recluse. The brown spiders are varying shades of brownish gray, with a characteristic dark brown, violin-shaped marking over the cephalothorax—hence, the name *violin spider* (Fig. 20-10). Although most spiders have four pairs of eyes, brown spiders have only three pairs. Male and female spiders can bite and may do so when threatened.

Toxicology

Although several enzymes have been isolated from the venom, the major deleterious factor is sphingomyelinase D, which causes dermonecrosis and hemolysis. It is a phospholipase that interacts with the cell membranes of erythrocytes, platelets, and endothelial cells and causes hemolysis, coagulation, and platelet aggregation.

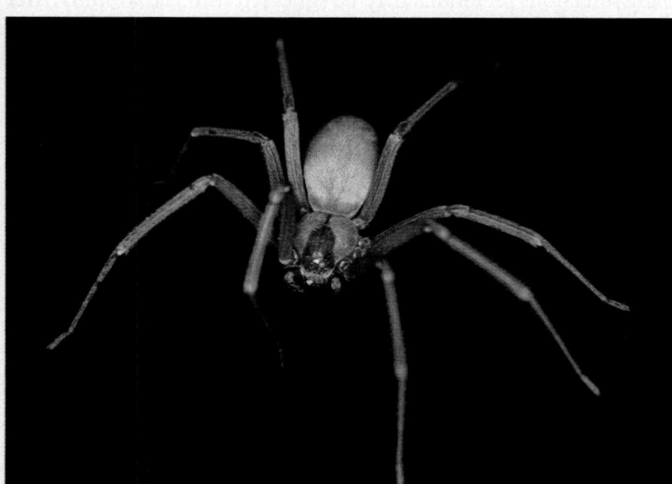

FIGURE 20-10 Brown recluse spider *(Loxosceles reclusa)* with a typical violin-shaped marking on the cephalothorax. (Courtesy Rose Pineda, www.rosapineda.com.)

Host responses have some significance in determining the severity of envenomation because functioning polymorphonuclear leukocytes and complement are necessary for the venom to have maximal effect.

Clinical Manifestations

Local findings at the bite site range from mild irritation to severe necrosis with ulceration.[29] The patient is often completely unaware of the bite or may have felt a slight stinging. It is unusual for the victim to see or capture the spider. This can make the diagnosis very challenging because similar skin lesions can represent bites by other arthropods, skin infections (including methicillin-resistant *S. aureus*), herpes zoster, dermatologic manifestation of a systemic illness, or other causes of dermatitis and vasculitis.[30] Within several hours of a *Loxosceles* bite, local tissue ischemia develops in some patients, with resulting pain, itching, swelling, and erythema. A blister may form at the site. In more severe bites, the central area turns purple as a result of microvascular thrombosis. Peripheral vasoconstriction can also create a pale border surrounding the central region of necrosis. Over the next several days, an eschar develops over the widening necrotic area. The eschar separates and leaves an ulcer that usually heals over a period of many weeks to months, but occasionally skin grafting is required. Necrosis is most severe in fatty areas such as the abdomen and thigh.

Systemic features include headache, nausea and vomiting, fever, malaise, arthralgia, and maculopapular rash. Additional findings may include thrombocytopenia, disseminated intravascular coagulation, hemolytic anemia, coma, and possibly death. Renal failure can result from intravascular hemolysis.

In patients with lesions consistent with brown spider bites, a search for evidence of systemic involvement (viscerocutaneous or systemic loxoscelism) is initiated, particularly if the victim has any systemic complaints. Appropriate laboratory tests include a complete blood count with platelet count and a bedside urine test for blood. If the results of any of these tests are abnormal, electrolyte, liver function, and coagulation studies are in order, but no truly diagnostic studies are available. Systemic loxoscelism is more common in children and can occur with minimal local findings.

Treatment

All recommended management is controversial, and recommendations should be viewed with a measure of healthy skepticism, especially when the etiology is uncertain. The bite site is splinted, elevated, and treated with cold compresses. Cold therapy inhibits venom activity and has been reported to reduce inflammation and necrosis. Heat application, in contrast, enhances tissue damage and ulcer development. Although controversial, a lipophilic prophylactic antibiotic such as erythromycin or cephalexin can be administered in standard doses for a few days. Tetanus status is updated as needed. Brown spider bites in which necrosis does not develop within 72 hours generally heal well and require no additional therapy. No commercial antivenom is available in the United States.

Some research has suggested that more severe lesions may benefit from dapsone if administered within the first few days after the bite, even though the drug is not approved for this indication.[31] Dapsone may reduce local inflammation and necrosis by inhibiting neutrophil function. The suggested adult dosage is 100 mg/day. Dapsone can cause methemoglobinemia and is contraindicated in patients with glucose-6-phosphate dehydrogenase deficiency. Levels of this enzyme are checked as therapy begins, and dapsone is discontinued if the enzyme level is found to be deficient. Dapsone is not approved for use in children. Given the conflicting data on efficacy and the side-effect profile, dapsone use is of questionable benefit.

Early surgical intervention, other than simple conservative débridement of obviously necrotic tissue, is avoided. It is difficult or impossible to predict with any certainty the extent of eventual necrosis, and early surgery is apt to be overaggressive and needlessly disfiguring. Pyoderma gangrenosum, manifested as nonhealing ulcers and failure of skin grafts, occurs more often in patients undergoing early excision and débridement, possibly as a result of the rapid spread of venom.[28] After 1 to 2 weeks, when eschar margins are defined, débridement can be performed as necessary. In severe cases, wide excision and split-thickness skin grafting are necessary while dapsone therapy is continued.

The efficacy of using hyperbaric oxygen therapy for *Loxosceles* bites is extremely controversial.[32] Steroid administration, by any route, has never been proved to be beneficial in limiting dermonecrosis.

Patients with rapidly expanding necrotic lesions or a clinical picture suggesting systemic loxoscelism are admitted for close observation and management. Primary staphylococcal soft tissue infections are much more prevalent than brown recluse spider bites and are often attributed to "spider bites"; alternative diagnoses that may cause rapid expanding tissue necrosis should also be strongly considered in this situation, including serious soft tissue infection. Patients with less serious lesions can be monitored on an outpatient basis with frequent wound checks. Visits during the first 72 hours include reassessment for any evidence of systemic involvement based on symptoms and signs and possibly a bedside urine test for blood.

Scorpions

Significant scorpion envenomation occurs worldwide by species belonging to the family Buthidae. In this group, the bark scorpion *(Centruroides sculpturatus)* is the only potentially dangerous species in the United States. It is found throughout northern Mexico, Arizona, and southern California. Numerous other *Centruroides* species exist throughout the southern United States extending as far north as Nebraska. The bark scorpion is a yellow-to-brown crablike arthropod up to 5 cm in length. Approximately 15,000 scorpion stings were reported during 2004 in the United States, and this is almost certainly a significant underestimate of the total number of stings that occurred. Scorpions tend to be nocturnal and sting when threatened.

Toxicology

Neurotoxic scorpion venoms, such as that produced by the bark scorpion, contain multiple low-molecular-weight basic proteins but possess very little enzymatic activity. The neurotoxins target excitable tissues and work primarily on ion channels, particularly sodium and potassium channels. They cause massive release of multiple neurotransmitters throughout the autonomic nervous system and the adrenal medulla.[33] Almost any organ system can be adversely affected, either by direct toxin effects or by the flood of autonomic neurotransmitters. Because of the speed of their systemic absorption, these neurotoxic scorpion venoms can cause rapid systemic toxicity and potentially death.

Clinical Manifestations

Most scorpion stings in the United States cause short-lived, searing pain and mild, local irritation with slight swelling. Stings by the bark scorpion typically produce local paresthesias and burning pain. Systemic manifestations may include cranial nerve and neuromuscular hyperactivity and respiratory distress.[33] Signs of adrenergic stimulation, accompanied by nausea and vomiting, may also develop. Young children are at greatest risk for severe stings from the bark scorpion. Death can occur from bark scorpion stings, but this is very rare in the United States. As with spider bites, the clinician is advised to consider other common conditions when the etiology is uncertain, as methamphetamine overdose has been misdiagnosed as scorpion envenomation.

Treatment

All patients receive tetanus prophylaxis if indicated, application of cold compresses to the sting site, and analgesics for pain. Victims of bark scorpion stings with signs of systemic envenomation require supportive care, with close monitoring of cardiovascular and respiratory status in an intensive care setting. If systemic signs are present, an equine-derived Fab antivenin approved by the Food and Drug Administration is available for use, Centruroides Immune F(ab′)2 (Anascorp) is manufactured by Rare Disease Therapeutics Inc (Franklin, TN). This antivenin was studied in a very small randomized clinical trial and found to be effective in reducing systemic symptoms.[34]

Ticks

Several potentially serious diseases occur from tick bites, including Rocky Mountain spotted fever, ehrlichiosis, tularemia, babesiosis, Colorado tick fever, relapsing fever, and Lyme disease. Timely and adequate removal of the tick is important to prevent disease. Common lay recommendations for tick removal, such as the application of local heat, gasoline, methylated spirits, and fingernail polish, are ineffective. Proper removal involves grasping the tick by the body as close to the skin surface as possible with an instrument and applying gradual, gentle axial traction, without twisting. Commercial tick removal devices are superior to standard tweezers for this purpose.[35] An alternative removal method involves looping a length of suture material in a simple overhand knot around the body of the tick. The loop is slipped down as close to the patient's skin surface as possible. The knot is tightened, and the tick is pulled backward and out, over its head in a somersault action. Crushing the tick is avoided because potentially infectious secretions may be squeezed into the wound. After extraction, the wound is cleansed with alcohol or povidone-iodine. Any retained mouthparts of the tick are removed with the tip of a needle. If the tick was embedded for less than 24 hours, the risk of transmitting infection is very low. Tetanus immunization needs to be current. Occasionally, a granulomatous lesion requiring steroid injection or surgical excision may develop at the tick bite site a few weeks after the incident.[36] Patients in whom a local rash or systemic symptoms develop within 4 weeks of exposure to tick-infested areas, even in the absence of a known bite, need to be evaluated for infectious complications such as Lyme disease, the most common vector-borne disease in the United States.

Lyme disease is caused by the spirochete *Borrelia burgdorferi* and may initially be seen in any of three stages—early localized (stage 1), early disseminated (stage 2), or late-persistent (stage 3). Stage 1 findings of limited infection include a rash in at least 80% of patients that develops after an incubation period of approximately 3 to 30 days.[37,38] The rash, termed *erythema migrans,* is typically a round or oval erythematous lesion that begins at the bite site and expands at a relatively rapid rate, up to 1 cm/day, to a median size of 15 cm in diameter.[39] As the rash expands, there may be evidence of central clearing and, less commonly, a central vesicle or necrotic eschar. Fatigue, myalgia, headache, fever, nausea, vomiting, regional lymphadenopathy, sore throat, photophobia, anorexia, and arthralgia may accompany the rash. Without treatment, the rash fades in approximately 4 weeks. If untreated, the infection may disseminate, and multiple erythema migrans lesions (generally smaller than the primary lesion) and neurologic, cardiac, or joint abnormalities may develop 30 to 120 days later. Neuroborreliosis occurs in approximately 15% of untreated patients and is characterized by central or peripheral findings such as lymphocytic meningitis, subtle encephalitis, cranial neuritis (especially facial nerve palsy, which may be unilateral or bilateral), cerebellar ataxia, and motor neuropathies.[40] Cardiac findings occur in approximately 5% of untreated patients and are usually manifested as atrioventricular nodal block or myocarditis. Oligoarticular arthritis is a common finding in early disseminated Lyme disease and occurs in approximately 60% of untreated victims. There is a particular propensity for larger joints such as the knee, which becomes recurrently and intermittently swollen and painful. Findings of early disseminated Lyme disease eventually disappear with or without treatment. Over time, up to 1 year after the initial tick bite, Lyme disease can progress to its chronic form, manifested by chronic arthritis, chronic synovitis, neurocognitive disorders, chronic fatigue, or any combination of these findings.

The diagnosis of Lyme disease is based largely on the presence of classic erythema migrans in a patient with a history of possible tick exposure in an endemic area or the presence of one or more findings of disseminated infection (e.g., nervous system, cardiovascular system, or joint involvement) and positive serology. Serologic testing is done in two stages. The first test is an enzyme-linked immunosorbent assay for IgM and IgG antibodies to *B. burgdorferi*. If this test is reactive or indeterminate, it needs to be confirmed with a second test, a Western blot. If the patient has been ill for longer than 1 month, only IgG is assayed because an isolated positive IgM antibody level is probably a false-positive finding at this stage. Patients from highly endemic areas with the classic findings of stage 1 disease, including erythema migrans, can be treated without serologic confirmation because testing may be falsely negative at this early stage.[41]

First-line treatment of early or disseminated Lyme disease, in the absence of neurologic involvement, is oral doxycycline for 14 to 21 days. The second-line agent for use in children 8 years of age or younger and pregnant women is amoxicillin. An equally effective third choice is cefuroxime axetil. Each of these oral agents provides a cure in more than 90% of patients.[38] In more complex management situations, including the possibility of neuroborreliosis or patients with cardiac manifestations, treatment consists of daily IV ceftriaxone for 14 to 28 days with consultation with appropriate infectious disease physicians.[39,42] Treatment of persistent arthritis after antibiotic therapy consists of anti-inflammatory agents or arthroscopic synovectomy.

Decisions to treat a victim of a tick bite prophylactically to prevent Lyme disease are controversial. Some authors condemn such an approach given the low (approximately 1.4%) risk for transmission after a tick bite, even in an endemic area.[39] However, research has shown that a single dose of doxycycline 200 mg orally given within 72 hours of a tick bite can further reduce the already low risk of disease transmission.[38,43] A vaccine against Lyme disease has been withdrawn from the market. The best prevention for tick-borne diseases such as Lyme disease is the use of insect repellent and frequent body checks for ticks when traveling through their habitat.

Hymenoptera

Most arthropod envenomation occurs by species belonging to the order Hymenoptera, which includes bees, wasps, yellow jackets, hornets, and stinging ants. In the United States, Hymenoptera account for most human fatalities, more than snake and mammalian bites combined. The winged Hymenoptera are located throughout the United States, whereas so-called fire ants are currently limited to the southeastern and southwestern regions. The Africanized honeybee, which characteristically attacks in massive numbers, has migrated into the southwestern United States.

Toxicology

Hymenoptera sting humans defensively, especially if their nests are disturbed. The stingers of most Hymenoptera are attached to venom sacs located on the abdomen and can be used repeatedly. However, some bees have barb-shaped stingers that prevent detachment from the victim and render the bees capable of only a single sting. Hymenoptera venom contains vasoactive compounds such as histamine and serotonin, which are responsible for the local reaction and pain. The venom also contains peptides, such as melittin, and enzymes, primarily phospholipases and hyaluronidases, which are highly allergenic and elicit an IgE-mediated response in some victims.[44] Fire ant venom consists primarily of nonallergenic alkaloids that release histamine and cause a mild local necrosis. Allergenic proteins constitute only 0.1% of fire ant venom.

Clinical Reactions

A Hymenoptera sting in a nonallergic individual produces immediate pain followed by a wheal and flare reaction. Stings from fire ants characteristically produce multiple pustules from repetitive stings at the same site. Multiple Hymenoptera stings can produce a toxic reaction characterized by vomiting, diarrhea, generalized edema, cardiovascular collapse, and hemolysis, which can be difficult to distinguish from an acute anaphylactic reaction.

Large exaggerated local reactions develop in approximately 17% of envenomed subjects.[44] These reactions are manifested as erythematous, edematous, painful, and pruritic areas larger than 10 cm in diameter and may last 2 to 5 days. The precise pathophysiology of such reactions is unclear, although they may be partly IgE-mediated.[45] Patients in whom large local reactions develop are at risk for similar episodes with future stings but do not appear to be at increased risk for systemic allergic reactions.

Bee sting anaphylaxis develops in 0.3% to 3% of the general population and is responsible for approximately 40 reported deaths annually in the United States.[44] Fatalities occur most often in adults, usually within 1 hour of the sting. Symptoms generally occur within minutes and range from mild urticaria and angioedema to respiratory arrest secondary to airway edema and bronchospasm and finally cardiovascular collapse. A positive IgE-mediated skin test to Hymenoptera extract helps predict an allergic sting reaction. Unusual reactions to Hymenoptera stings include late-onset allergic reactions (>5 hours after the sting), serum sickness, renal disease, neurologic disorders such as Guillain-Barré syndrome, and vasculitis. The cause of these reactions is thought to be immune-mediated.

Treatment

If an offending bee has left behind a stinger, it is removed as quickly as possible to prevent continued injection of venom.[46] The sting site is cleaned and locally cooled. Topical or injected lidocaine can help decrease pain from the sting. Antihistamines administered orally or topically can decrease pruritus. Blisters and pustules (typically sterile) from fire ant stings are left intact. Tetanus status is updated as needed.

Treatment of an exaggerated, local envenomation includes the aforementioned therapy in addition to elevation of the extremity and analgesics. A 5-day course of oral prednisone (1 mg/kg/day) is also recommended.[44] Isolated local reactions, typical or exaggerated, do not require epinephrine or referral for immunotherapy.

Mild anaphylaxis can be treated with 0.01 mg/kg (up to 0.5 mg) of 1:1000 (1 mg/mL, or 0.1%) intramuscular (mid-anterolateral thigh) epinephrine and an oral or parenteral antihistamine. More severe cases are also treated with steroids and may require oxygen, endotracheal intubation, IV epinephrine infusion, bronchodilators, IV fluids, or vasopressors. These patients are observed for approximately 24 hours in a monitored environment for any recurrence of severe symptoms.

Venom immunotherapy effectively prevents recurrent anaphylaxis from subsequent stings in patients with positive skin tests.[47] Patients with previous severe, systemic allergic reactions to Hymenoptera stings or in whom serum sickness develops are referred to an allergist for possible immunotherapy. Referral is also recommended for adults with purely generalized dermal reactions, such as diffuse hives. Children with skin manifestations alone appear to be at relatively low risk for more serious anaphylaxis after subsequent stings and do not need referral. Patients with a history of systemic reactions resulting from Hymenoptera stings need to carry injectable epinephrine with them at all times; they also need to wear an identification medallion identifying their medical condition.[47]

MARINE BITES AND STINGS

Of all living creatures, 80% reside underwater. Humans primarily in temperate or tropical seas encounter hazardous marine animals. Exposure to marine life through recreation, research, and industry leads to frequent encounters with aquatic organisms. Injuries generally occur through bites, stings, or punctures and infrequently through electrical shock from creatures such as the torpedo ray.

Initial Assessment

Injuries from marine organisms can range from mild local irritant skin reactions to systemic collapse from major trauma or severe envenomation. Several environmental aspects unique to marine trauma may make treatment of these patients challenging. Immersion in cold water predisposes patients to hypothermia and near-drowning. Rapid ascent after an encounter with a marine organism can cause air embolism or decompression illness in a scuba diver. Anaphylactic reaction to venom may further complicate an envenomation. Late complications include unique infections caused by a wide variety of aquatic microorganisms and immune-mediated phenomena.

Microbiology

Most marine isolates are gram-negative rods.[48] *Vibrio* spp. are of primary concern, particularly in immunocompromised hosts and patients with cirrhosis. In fresh water, the related vibrio-like organisms *Aeromonas* spp. can be particularly aggressive pathogens. *Staphylococcus* and *Streptococcus* spp. are also frequently cultured from infections. The laboratory is notified that cultures are being requested for aquatic-acquired infections to alert them of the need for appropriate culture media and conditions.

General Management

Initial management is focused on the airway, breathing, and circulation. Anaphylaxis needs to be anticipated and the victim treated accordingly. Patients with extensive blunt and penetrating injuries are managed as major trauma victims. Patients who have been envenomed receive specific intervention directed against a toxin (discussed separately, according to the marine animal), in addition to general supportive care. Contact of the regional poison control center is highly advised. Antivenom can be administered, if available, and should be directed by experienced clinicians or the poison control center. Antitetanus immunization is updated after a bite, cut, or sting. Radiographs are obtained to locate foreign bodies and fractures. Magnetic resonance imaging is more useful than ultrasound or computed tomography to identify small spine fragments.

Selection of antibiotics is tailored to marine bacteriology. Third-generation cephalosporins provide adequate coverage for gram-positive and gram-negative microorganisms found in ocean water, including *Vibrio* spp.[48] Ciprofloxacin, cefoperazone, gentamicin, and trimethoprim-sulfamethoxazole are acceptable antibiotics. Outpatient regimens include ciprofloxacin, trimethoprim-sulfamethoxazole, or doxycycline. Patients with large abrasions, lacerations, puncture wounds, or hand injuries and immunocompromised patients receive prophylactic antibiotics. Infected wounds are cultured. If a wound, commonly on the hand after a minor scrape or puncture, appears erysipeloid in nature, infection by *Erysipelothrix rhusiopathiae* is suspected. A suitable initial antibiotic based on this presumptive diagnosis would be penicillin, cephalexin, or ciprofloxacin.

Wound Care

Meticulous wound care is necessary to reduce the risk for infection and optimize the esthetic and functional outcomes.[49] Wounds are irrigated with normal saline. Débridement of devitalized tissue can decrease infection and promote healing. Large or complex wounds require exploration and management in the operating room. As noted with other bite wounds, the decision to close a wound primarily must balance the cosmetic result against the risk for infection.[50] Wounds are loosely closed and drainage allowed. Primary closure is avoided with distal extremity wounds, punctures, and crush injuries. For large shark wounds, postoperative management may be prolonged, and common complications and sequelae of shock, massive blood transfusion, myoglobinuria, and respiratory failure may occur. Rehabilitation may include the creation of prosthetic devices.[51]

Antivenom

Antivenom is available for several types of envenomation, including from the box jellyfish, sea snake, and stonefish.[52] Patients demonstrating severe reactions to such envenomation benefit from antivenom. Skin testing to determine which patients might benefit from pretreatment with diphenhydramine or epinephrine can be performed before antivenom is administered, but it is not an absolute predictor of severe reactions. Ovine-derived antivenom (Commonwealth Serum Laboratories, King of Prussia, PA) to treat severe *Chironex fleckeri* (box jellyfish) envenomation has been administered intramuscularly by field rescuers for many years without reports of a serious adverse reaction. Serum sickness is a complication of antivenom therapy and can be treated with corticosteroids. In the case of managing one of these envenomations in the United States, the regional poison control center is contacted, or major marine aquariums or zoos may be helpful.

Injuries from Nonvenomous Aquatic Animals

Sharks

Approximately 50 to 100 shark attacks are reported annually. However, these attacks cause fewer than 10 deaths/year.[49,51] Tiger, great white, gray reef, and bull sharks are responsible for most attacks. Most incidents occur at the surface of shallow water within 100 feet of the shore.[40] Sharks locate prey by detecting motion, electrical fields, and sounds and by sensing body fluids through smell and taste. Most sharks bite the victim once and then leave. Most injuries occur to the lower extremities.

Powerful jaws and sharp teeth produce crushing, tearing injuries. Hypovolemic shock and near-drowning are life-threatening consequences of an attack.[49] Other complications include soft tissue and neurovascular damage, bone fractures, and infection.[51] Most wounds require exploration and repair in the operating room (see Chapter 6). Radiographs may reveal one or more shark teeth in the wound. Occasionally, bumping by sharks can produce abrasions, which are treated as second-degree burns.

Moray Eels

Morays are bottom dwellers that reside in holes or crevices. Eels bite defensively and produce multiple small puncture wounds and, rarely, gaping lacerations. The hand is most frequently bitten. Occasionally, the eel remains attached to the victim, with decapitation of the animal required for release. Puncture wounds and bites on the hand from all animals, including eels, are at high risk for infection and must not be closed primarily if the capability exists for delayed primary closure.

Alligators and Crocodiles

Crocodiles can attain a length of more than 20 feet and travel at speeds of 20 mph in water and on land. Similar to sharks, alligators and crocodiles attack primarily in shallow water. These animals can produce severe injuries by grasping victims with their powerful jaws and dragging them underwater, where they roll while crushing their prey. Injuries from alligator and crocodile attacks are treated similarly to shark bites.

Miscellaneous

Other nonvenomous animals capable of attacking include the barracuda, giant grouper, sea lion, mantis shrimp, triggerfish, needlefish, and freshwater piranha. Except for the needlefish, which spears a human victim with its elongated snout, these animals bite. Barracuda are attracted to shiny objects and have bitten fingers, wrists, scalps, or dangling legs adorned with reflective jewelry.

Envenomation by Invertebrates

Coelenterates

The phylum Cnidaria (formerly Coelenterata) consists of hydrozoans, which include fire coral, hydroids, and Portuguese man-of-war; scyphozoans, which include jellyfish and sea nettles; and anthozoans, which include sea anemones. Coelenterates carry specialized living stinging cells called cnidocytes that encapsulate intracytoplasmic stinging organelles called cnidae, which include nematocysts.[52,53]

Mild envenomation, typically inflicted by fire coral, hydroids, and anemones, produces skin irritation.[52] The victim notices immediate stinging followed by pruritus, paresthesias, and throbbing pain with proximal radiation. Edema and erythema develop in the involved area, followed by blisters and petechiae. This can progress to local infection and ulceration.

Severe envenomation is caused by anemones, sea nettles, and jellyfish.[50] Patients have systemic symptoms in addition to the local manifestations. An anaphylactic reaction to the venom may contribute to the pathophysiology of envenomation. Fever, nausea, vomiting, and malaise can develop. Any organ system can be involved, and death is attributed to shock and cardiorespiratory arrest. One of the most venomous creatures on earth, found primarily off the coast of northern Australia, is the box jellyfish *Chironex fleckeri* (sea wasp). In the United States, *Physalia physalis, Chiropsalmus quadrigatus,* and *Cyanea capillata* are substantial stingers.

Therapy consists of detoxification of nematocysts and systemic support. Dilute (5%) acetic acid (vinegar) can inactivate most coelenterate toxins and is applied for 30 minutes or until the pain is relieved.[52] This treatment is critical with the box jellyfish. If a detoxicant is unavailable, the wound may be rinsed in seawater and gently dried.[52] Fresh water and vigorous rubbing can cause nematocysts to discharge. For a sting from the box jellyfish, Australian authorities previously recommended the pressure immobilization technique, but this is no longer recommended. Instead, the envenomed limb is kept as motionless as possible, and the victim is promptly taken to a setting in which antivenom and advanced life support are available.

To decontaminate other jellyfish stings, isopropyl alcohol is used only if vinegar is ineffective. Baking soda may be more effective than acetic acid for inactivating the toxin of U.S. eastern coastal Chesapeake Bay sea nettles.[52] Baking soda must not be applied after vinegar without a brisk saline or water rinse in between application of the two substances to avoid an exothermic reaction. Powdered or solubilized papain (meat tenderizer) may be more effective than other remedies for sea bather's eruption (often misnamed sea lice) caused by thimble jellyfishes or larval forms of certain sea anemones. Fresh lime or lemon juice, household ammonia, olive oil, or sugar may be effective, depending on the species of stinging creature.

After the skin surface has been treated, any remaining nematocysts must be removed. One method is to apply shaving cream or a flour paste and shave the area with a razor. The affected area again is irrigated, dressed, and elevated. Medical care providers need to wear gloves for self-protection. Cryotherapy, local anesthetics, antihistamines, and steroids can relieve pain after the toxin is inactivated. Prophylactic antibiotics are not usually necessary. Safe Sea jellyfish-safe sun block (Nidaria Technology, Jordan Valley, Israel) has been shown to reduce the risk of being stung and may be recommended as a preventive measure before entering the water.[54]

Sponges

Two syndromes occur after contact with sponges.[50] The first is an allergic plant–like contact dermatitis characterized by itching and burning within hours of contact. This dermatitis can progress to soft tissue edema, vesicle development, and joint swelling. Large areas of involvement can cause systemic toxicity with fever, nausea, and muscle cramps. The second syndrome is an irritant dermatitis after penetration of the skin with small spicules. Sponge diver's disease is caused by anemones that colonize the sponges rather than by the sponges themselves.

Treatment consists of gently washing and drying the affected area. Dilute (5%) acetic acid (vinegar) is applied for 30 minutes three times daily.[50] Any remaining spicules can be removed with adhesive tape. A steroid cream can be applied to the skin after decontamination. Occasionally, a systemic glucocorticoid and an antihistamine are required.

Echinodermata

Starfish, sea urchins, and sea cucumbers are members of the phylum Echinodermata. Starfish and sea cucumbers produce venom that can cause contact dermatitis.[52] Sea cucumbers occasionally feed on coelenterates and secrete nematocysts, so local therapy for coelenterates also needs to be considered. Sea urchins are covered with venomous spines capable of causing local and systemic reactions similar to those from coelenterates. First aid consists of soaking the wound in warm, but tolerable water. Residual spines can be located with soft tissue radiographs or magnetic resonance imaging. Purple skin discoloration at the site of entrance wounds may be indicative of dye leached from the surface of an extracted urchin spine. This temporary tattoo disappears in 48 hours, which often confirms the absence of a retained foreign body. A spine is removed only if it is easily accessible or closely aligned to a joint or critical neurovascular structure. Reactive fusiform digit swelling attributed to a spine near a metacarpal bone or flexor tendon sheath may be alleviated by a high-dose glucocorticoid administered in an oral 14-day tapering schedule. Retained spines may cause the formation of granulomas that are amenable to excision or intralesional injection with triamcinolone hexacetonide, 5 mg/mL.

Mollusks

Octopuses and cone snails are the primary envenoming species in the phylum Mollusca. Most harmful cone snails are found in Indo-Pacific waters. Envenomation occurs from a detachable harpoon-like dart injected via an extensible proboscis into the victim.[50,52] Blue-ringed octopuses can bite and inject tetrodotoxin, a paralytic agent. Both species can produce local symptoms such as burning and paresthesias. Systemic manifestations are primarily neurologic and include bulbar dysfunction and systemic muscular paralysis. Management of the bite site is best achieved by pressure and immobilization to contain the venom. Immediate transport to a medical facility is mandatory to assess the bandage and for supportive care.

Annelid Worms (Bristleworms)

Annelid worms (bristleworms) carry rows of soft, easily detached fiberglass-like spines capable of inflicting painful stings and irritant dermatitis. Inflammation may persist for 1 week. Visible bristles are removed with forceps and adhesive tape or a commercial facial peel. Alternatively, a thin layer of rubber cement may be used to trap the spines and then peel them away. Household vinegar, rubbing alcohol, or dilute household ammonia may provide additional relief. Local inflammation is treated with a topical or systemic glucocorticoid.

Envenomation by Vertebrates

Stingrays

Rays are bottom dwellers ranging from a few inches to 12 feet long (tip to tail). Venom is stored in whiplike caudal appendages. Stingrays react defensively by thrusting their spines into a victim, causing puncture wounds and lacerations. The most common site of injury is the lower part of the leg and top of the foot. Local damage can be severe, with occasional penetration of body cavities; this is worsened by the vasoconstrictive properties of the venom, which produce cyanotic-appearing wounds. The venom is often myonecrotic. Systemic complaints include weakness, nausea, diarrhea, headache, and muscle cramps. The venom can cause vasoconstriction, cardiac dysrhythmias, respiratory arrest, and seizures.[53]

If an experienced medical provider is present, the wound is irrigated and soaked in nonscalding hot water (up to 45° C [113° F]) for 1 hour.[53] Caution with hot water is warranted. Débridement, exploration, and removal of spines are carried out during or after hot water soaking. Immersion cryotherapy is thought to be detrimental. The wound is not closed primarily. Lacerations heal by secondary intention or are repaired by delayed closure. The wound is dressed and elevated. Pain is relieved locally or systemically. Radiography is performed to locate any remaining spines. Acute infection with aggressive pathogens is anticipated.[50] In the event of a nonhealing draining wound, retention of a foreign body is suspected.

Miscellaneous Fish

Other fish with spines that can produce injuries similar to those of stingrays include lionfish, scorpionfish, stonefish, catfish, and weeverfish. Each can cause envenomation, puncture wounds, and lacerations, with spines transmitting venom. Clinical manifestations and therapy are similar to those pertaining to stingrays. In the case of lionfish, vesiculations are sometimes noted. An equine-derived antivenom (Commonwealth Serum Laboratories) is available for administration in case of significant stonefish envenomation.

Sea Snakes

Sea snakes of the family Hydrophiidae appear similar to land snakes. They inhabit the Pacific and Indian Oceans. The venom produces neurologic signs and symptoms, with possible death from paralysis and respiratory arrest. Local manifestations can be minimal or absent. Therapy is similar to that for coral snake (Elapidae) bites. The pressure immobilization technique is recommended in the field. Polyvalent sea snake antivenom is administered if any signs of envenomation develop.[53] The initial dose is one ampule, repeated as needed. Consultation with an experienced clinician, toxicologist, or poison control center is recommended.

SELECTED REFERENCES

Auerbach PS, editor: *Wilderness medicine*, ed 6, Philadelphia, 2012, Mosby.

This textbook is an authoritative, in-depth review of wilderness medicine. Bites and stings by many organisms are discussed in detail by experts from each field. Many pertinent studies are reviewed.

Casale TB, Burks AW: Clinical practice. Hymenoptera-sting hypersensitivity. *N Engl J Med* 370:1432–1439, 2014.

The reactions to Hymenoptera stings are well organized in this practical monograph. The natural history of stinging insect allergy is reviewed, and therapeutic considerations regarding acute management, immunotherapy to prevent recurrent anaphylaxis, and who should receive immunotherapy are discussed.

Gold BS, Dart RC, Barish RA: Bites of venomous snakes. *N Engl J Med* 347:347–356, 2002.

This article is a concise, practical review of snake venom poisoning in the United States. Proper use of North American antivenom is well summarized.

Isbister GK, Graudins A, White J, et al: Antivenom treatment in arachnidism. *J Toxicol Clin Toxicol* 41:291–300, 2003.

This article provides an excellent review of the use of antivenom in spider bites around the world.

Mebs D: *Venomous and poisonous animals*, Boca Raton, FL, 2002, CRC Press.

This book is a superbly illustrated collection of fascinating, detailed information about venoms and poisons in the animal kingdom, including marine and terrestrial animals.

Shapiro ED: Clinical practice. Lyme disease. *N Engl J Med* 370:1724–1731, 2014.

This article provides a thorough review of the current understanding of Lyme borreliosis and outlines diagnosis and treatment.

Swanson DL, Vetter RS: Bites of brown recluse spiders and suspected necrotic arachnidism. *N Engl J Med* 352:700–707, 2005.

This excellent review of necrotic arachnidism includes the approach to diagnosis and management.

Williamson JA, Fenner PJ, Burnett JW, editors: *Venomous and poisonous marine animals*, Sydney, Australia, 1996, University of New South Wales Press.

This book discusses all common and uncommon toxic marine animals.

REFERENCES

1. Chippaux JP: Snake-bites: Appraisal of the global situation. *Bull World Health Organ* 76:515–524, 1998.
2. Kasturiratne A, Wickremasinghe AR, de Silva N, et al: The global burden of snakebite: A literature analysis and modelling based on regional estimates of envenoming and deaths. *PLoS Med* 5:e218, 2008.
3. Spano S, Macias F, Snowden B, et al: Snakebite Survivors Club: Retrospective review of rattlesnake bites in Central California. *Toxicon* 69:38–41, 2013.
4. Corneille MG, Larson S, Stewart RM, et al: A large single-center experience with treatment of patients with crotalid envenomations: Outcomes with and evolution of antivenin therapy. *Am J Surg* 192:848–852, 2006.
5. Moss ST, Bogdan G, Dart RC, et al: Association of rattlesnake bite location with severity of clinical manifestations. *Ann Emerg Med* 30:58–61, 1997.
6. Hall EL: Role of surgical intervention in the management of crotaline snake envenomation. *Ann Emerg Med* 37:175–180, 2001.
7. Correa JA, Fallon SC, Cruz AT, et al: Management of pediatric snake bites: Are we doing too much? *J Pediatr Surg* 49:1009–1015, 2014.
8. Balde MC, Chippaux JP, Boiro MY, et al: Use of antivenoms for the treatment of envenomation by Elapidae snakes in Guinea, Sub-Saharan Africa. *J Venom Anim Toxins Incl Trop Dis* 19:6, 2013.
9. Walker JP, Morrison RL: Current management of copperhead snakebite. *J Am Coll Surg* 212:470–474, discussion 474–475, 2011.
10. *Advanced Trauma Life Support Course (ATLS), 9*, Chicago, September 1, 2012, American College of Surgeons.
11. Dart RC, Hurlbut KM, Garcia R, et al: Validation of a severity score for the assessment of crotalid snakebite. *Ann Emerg Med* 27:321–326, 1996.
12. Cribari C: *Management of Poisonous Snakebites*, Chicago, 2004, American College of Surgeons Committee on Trauma.
13. Chippaux JP, Lang J, Eddine SA, et al: Clinical safety of a polyvalent F(ab′)2 equine antivenom in 223 African snake envenomations: A field trial in Cameroon. VAO (Venin Afrique de l'Ouest) Investigators. *Trans R Soc Trop Med Hyg* 92:657–662, 1998.
14. Budzynski AZ, Pandya BV, Rubin RN, et al: Fibrinogenolytic afibrinogenemia after envenomation by western diamondback rattlesnake *(Crotalus atrox)*. *Blood* 63:1–14, 1984.
15. Stewart RM, Page CP, Schwesinger WH, et al: Antivenin and fasciotomy/debridement in the treatment of the severe rattlesnake bite. *Am J Surg* 158:543–547, 1989.
16. Tanen DA, Danish DC, Clark RF: Crotalidae polyvalent immune Fab antivenom limits the decrease in perfusion pressure of the anterior leg compartment in a porcine crotaline envenomation model. *Ann Emerg Med* 41:384–390, 2003.
17. Tanen DA, Danish DC, Grice GA, et al: Fasciotomy worsens the amount of myonecrosis in a porcine model of crotaline envenomation. *Ann Emerg Med* 44:99–104, 2004.
18. Centers for Disease Control and Prevention (CDC): Nonfatal dog bite-related injuries treated in hospital emergency departments—United States, 2001. *MMWR Morb Mortal Wkly Rep* 52:605–610, 2003.
19. Paschos NK, Makris EA, Gantsos A, et al: Primary closure versus non-closure of dog bite wounds: A randomised controlled trial. *Injury* 45:237–240, 2014.
20. Maimaris C, Quinton DN: Dog-bite lacerations: A controlled trial of primary wound closure. *Arch Emerg Med* 5:156–161, 1988.
21. Callaham M: Prophylactic antibiotics in common dog bite wounds: A controlled study. *Ann Emerg Med* 9:410–414, 1980.
22. Perron AD, Miller MD, Brady WJ: Orthopedic pitfalls in the ED: Fight bite. *Am J Emerg Med* 20:114–117, 2002.
23. Broder J, Jerrard D, Olshaker J, et al: Low risk of infection in selected human bites treated without antibiotics. *Am J Emerg Med* 22:10–13, 2004.
24. Vidmar L, Poljak M, Tomazic J, et al: Transmission of HIV-1 by human bite. *Lancet* 347:1762, 1996.
25. World Health Organization: Rabies surveillance and control: The world survey of rabies. No. 35 for the year 1999. <http://www.who.int/rabies/resources/wsr1999/en>, 2002.
26. Krebs JW, Wheeling JT, Childs JE: Rabies surveillance in the United States during 2002. *J Am Vet Med Assoc* 223:1736–1748, 2003.
27. Department of Health and Human Services, Centers for Disease Control and Prevention: Use of a reduced (4-dose) vaccine schedule for postexposure prophylaxis to prevent human rabies: Recommendations of the Advisory Committee on Immunization Practices. <http://www.cdc.gov/mmwr/pdf/rr/rr5902.pdf>, 2010.

28. Offerman SR, Daubert GP, Clark RF: The treatment of black widow spider envenomation with antivenin *Latrodectus mactans:* A case series. *Perm J* 15:76–81, 2011.
29. Sams HH, Dunnick CA, Smith ML, et al: Necrotic arachnidism. *J Am Acad Dermatol* 44:561–573, quiz 573–566, 2001.
30. Swanson DL, Vetter RS: Bites of brown recluse spiders and suspected necrotic arachnidism. *N Engl J Med* 352:700–707, 2005.
31. King LE, Jr, Rees RS: Dapsone treatment of a brown recluse bite. *JAMA* 250:648, 1983.
32. Tutrone WD, Green KM, Norris T, et al: Brown recluse spider envenomation: Dermatologic application of hyperbaric oxygen therapy. *J Drugs Dermatol* 4:424–428, 2005.
33. LoVecchio F, McBride C: Scorpion envenomations in young children in central Arizona. *J Toxicol Clin Toxicol* 41:937–940, 2003.
34. Boyer LV, Theodorou AA, Berg RA, et al: Antivenom for critically ill children with neurotoxicity from scorpion stings. *N Engl J Med* 360:2090–2098, 2009.
35. Stewart RL, Burgdorfer W, Needham GR: Evaluation of three commercial tick removal tools. *Wilderness Environ Med* 9:137–142, 1998.
36. Metry DW, Hebert AA: Insect and arachnid stings, bites, infestations, and repellents. *Pediatr Ann* 29:39–48, 2000.
37. Montiel NJ, Baumgarten JM, Sinha AA: Lyme disease—part II: Clinical features and treatment. *Cutis* 69:443–448, 2002.
38. Shapiro ED: Clinical practice. Lyme disease. *N Engl J Med* 370:1724–1731, 2014.
39. Shapiro ED, Gerber MA: Lyme disease. *Clin Infect Dis* 31:533–542, 2000.
40. Steere AC: A 58-year-old man with a diagnosis of chronic Lyme disease. *JAMA* 288:1002–1010, 2002.
41. DePietropaolo DL, Powers JH, Gill JM, et al: Diagnosis of Lyme disease. *Am Fam Physician* 72:297–304, 2005.
42. Dinser R, Jendro MC, Schnarr S, et al: Antibiotic treatment of Lyme borreliosis: What is the evidence? *Ann Rheum Dis* 64:519–523, 2005.
43. Nadelman RB, Nowakowski J, Fish D, et al: Prophylaxis with single-dose doxycycline for the prevention of Lyme disease after an *Ixodes scapularis* tick bite. *N Engl J Med* 345:79–84, 2001.
44. Wright DN, Lockey RF: Local reactions to stinging insects (Hymenoptera). *Allergy Proc* 11:23–28, 1990.
45. Reisman RE: Insect stings. *N Engl J Med* 331:523–527, 1994.
46. Visscher PK, Vetter RS, Camazine S: Removing bee stings. *Lancet* 348:301–302, 1996.
47. Casale TB, Burks AW: Clinical practice. Hymenoptera-sting hypersensitivity. *N Engl J Med* 370:1432–1439, 2014.
48. Williamson JA, Fenner PJ, Burnett JW: *Venomous and poisonous marine animals*, Sydney, 1996, University of New South Wales Press.
49. Howard RJ, Burgess GH: Surgical hazards posed by marine and freshwater animals in Florida. *Am J Surg* 166:563–567, 1993.
50. Barber GR, Swygert JS: Necrotizing fasciitis due to *Photobacterium damsela* in a man lashed by a stingray. *N Engl J Med* 342:824, 2000.
51. Guidera KJ, Ogden JA, Highhouse K, et al: Shark attack. *J Orthop Trauma* 5:204–208, 1991.
52. McGoldrick J, Marx JA: Marine envenomations. Part 2: Invertebrates. *J Emerg Med* 10:71–77, 1992.
53. McGoldrick J, Marx JA: Marine envenomations. Part 1: Vertebrates. *J Emerg Med* 9:497–502, 1991.
54. Boulware DR: A randomized, controlled field trial for the prevention of jellyfish stings with a topical sting inhibitor. *J Travel Med* 13:166–171, 2006.

CHAPTER 21

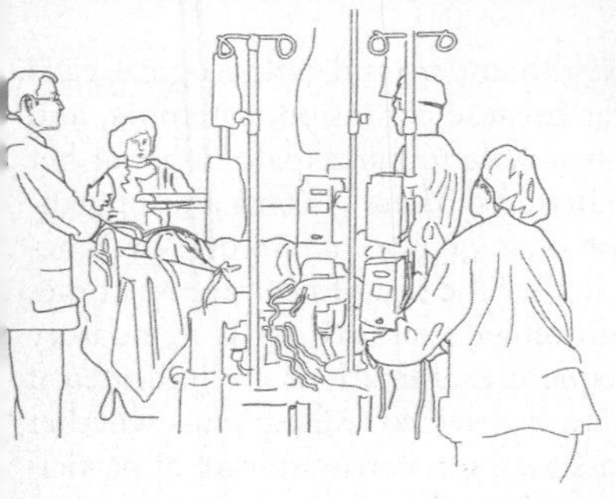

Surgical Critical Care

Andrew H. Stephen, Charles A. Adams, Jr., William G. Cioffi

OUTLINE

The demand for quality surgical critical care is expected to increase as the population of the United States ages, and care of these patients will be increasingly more complex because of their more numerous comorbidities. Surgical intensivists will need to stay abreast of advances in medical treatments across multiple disciplines to continue to deliver quality critical care. Approximately half of patients who require general surgical operations are taking medications unrelated to the surgical condition, and this rate is typically higher in patients destined for the intensive care unit (ICU). Although many tertiary care facilities treat surgical critical care patients in closed model ICUs, where care is directed by specially trained teams led by specialty boarded surgical intensivists, it is imperative that surgeons understand the concepts and thought processes involved in caring for these patients, particularly for patients cared for in open model or mixed ICUs lead by nonsurgical intensivists.

One of the greatest challenges for a critical care provider is to be cognizant of and to integrate fully advances in technology into clinical care for maximal benefit to critically ill patients. Each year brings an array of new devices, diagnostic tools, and complex therapies that pose a challenge to the intensivist. However, perhaps the greatest challenge of all is to deliver quality, cost-efficient care, especially in the present atmosphere of health care reform and dwindling financial resources. As a corollary of the so-called quality movement, awareness is increasing among health care providers of the long-term ramifications of critical illness and its devastating effects on quality of life after ICU discharge. With the advent of each new technology or therapy, one must remember that "more" in terms of volume, intensity, or complexity of care does not always translate into better results and that a critically ill surgical patient requires a measured and thoughtful systems-based approach that optimizes outcomes in the most efficient and cost-effective way. Surgical intensivists are critical care specialists, but in contrast to their medical colleagues, they have the unique ability to understand the impact of surgical disease and operative procedures on physiology in the ICU, and this distinctive knowledge base is thought to lead to better outcomes for critically ill surgical patients.

NEUROLOGIC SYSTEM

Dysfunction

Alterations in mental status in a critically ill surgical patient are commonplace. For example, in a review of mechanically ventilated ICU patients, delirium was identified in 60% to 80%; evidence has shown this increases costs, length of stay, risk of infections, and mortality.[1] It is unclear whether delirium causes these worsened outcomes or is a general marker of critical illness, but its impact on poor outcomes and complications is not debatable. The surgical ICU, with its goal to provide continuous care around-the-clock, does not afford patients a calming environment and rapidly disrupts circadian rhythms, particularly in elderly patients. The level of heightened stimulation in the ICU is due to many factors, including the need for frequent monitoring, procedures, and bedside care; patient spacing issues; and a multitude of tubes, lines, drains, and machinery typically required in care of a critically ill surgical patient. However, the diagnosis of "ICU delirium" is one of exclusion, and any alteration in mental status should lead the clinician to seek out organic causes, such as cerebrovascular accident (stroke), changes in intracranial pressure, medications, hypoxia or hypercapnia, sepsis, and metabolic causes.

The term *altered mental status* in the ICU encompasses a broad number of clinical entities on the continuum from confusion to delirium to encephalopathy and brain death. *Confusion* is one of the typical terms used to describe neurologic function in an ICU patient. Confusion is one of the least severe yet most common disturbances of neurologic function. It is defined by any type of disorientation to person, time, or place; inability to follow simple commands; or excess drowsiness. Confusion often exists before progression to more dangerous and difficult-to-treat alterations such as delirium, so any episode of confusion should prompt evaluation for possible organic causes. *Delirium* refers to a disturbance of attention, focus, or awareness to one's environment that occurs over a short time and is disparate from the patient's baseline level of function. Cognitive deficits such as memory loss and difficulty with language or visuospatial skills and a fluctuating course are the hallmarks of delirium. Active delirium, which is denoted by agitation, is often detected by critical care providers. However, negative delirium, which is denoted by lethargy and quiet inattentiveness, is often not recognized, and defined assessment measures for delirium have been advocated by the Society of Critical Care Medicine and the American Psychiatric Association to increase recognition of this entity.[2] The two most commonly used and well-known delirium assessment tools are the Confusion Assessment Method for the ICU (CAM-ICU) and the Intensive Care Delirium Screening Checklist. These tools are highly sensitive and specific for delirium in the ICU, and both have been validated in patients on ventilation and patients without ventilation assistance. Regardless of which tool is employed, it is important to use a regularly scheduled, objective measure for detection of delirium in the ICU. Elderly patients are particularly susceptible to hypoactive delirium, and detecting this condition can be difficult despite the application of tools such as CAM-ICU.

The term *encephalopathy* broadly describes any global brain dysfunction. It can result from organic and nonorganic causes and is often the result of direct effects on the brain, such as trauma, ischemia, or toxins. Encephalopathy also may be caused by things far removed from the central nervous system, as illustrated by the classic example of hepatic encephalopathy, which is caused by liver dysfunction resulting from impaired clearance of gut-derived compounds. The grading system for encephalopathy ranges from confusion to obtundation, stupor, and coma. Obtundation is a mental blunting or reduced interest in the surrounding environment, slowed response to stimuli, and increased periods of sleep even during the daytime. Stupor is one step further on the continuum and implies a severe lack of cognitive function in which one is almost unconscious and responds only to the most noxious stimuli. Coma is a state where the patient no longer is capable of responding to verbal or physical stimuli and has no understanding or awareness of his or her surroundings. Comatose patients have such an advanced state of neurologic dysfunction that they cannot protect their airway and should be intubated and placed on mechanical ventilation.

Catatonia, which is often associated with schizophrenia, is increasingly being recognized as a state of neurologic dysfunction in critically ill patients.[3] Classically, catatonia includes psychomotor disturbances such as mutism, rigidity, hyperactivity, and combativeness; it is actually more common in patients with medical and surgical illnesses than in patients with psychiatric disorders, and the ICU is one of the most common settings for its occurrence. Similar to delirium, there are excited and withdrawn subtypes of catatonia; also, similar to hypoactive delirium in elderly patients, the withdrawn subtype is typically under-recognized in ICU patients. Risk factors for catatonia include the use of dopamine antagonists for agitation (e.g., haloperidol), atypical antipsychotics (e.g., risperidone, quetiapine), and antiemetics (e.g., metaclopramide, promethazine). Again similar to delirium, catatonia is associated with negative outcomes, including myocardial infarction, pneumonia, venous thrombosis and pulmonary embolism, pressure ulceration, prolonged catheterization, infections, deconditioning, contractures, and death. Scales and measuring systems are available to grade catatonia; however, they are beyond the scope of this chapter. Basic treatment includes withholding the offending agents and judicious use of small doses of benzodiazepines. To distinguish catatonia from sedation or delirium, the clinician must look for the more subtle signs, such as active but motiveless resistance to movement, mimicking, mutism, and excessive continuation or cooperation to a command from the examiner.

It is crucial for the intensivist to understand and recognize each of the entities described so far because confusion, catatonia, and delirium all render the patient unable to participate in his or her care and contribute to bad outcomes. There is often an opportunity early on in the progression of any type of neurologic dysfunction to recognize and treat it so that the risk of negative outcomes can be mitigated. A daily neurologic examination is mandatory for all patients, and more frequent examinations are indicated if a change in neurologic function is detected. All patients, whether intubated or not, should be assessed for alertness; level of participation with the examination; orientation to person, time, and place; and motor strength in all four extremities. Any deficits in this examination should prompt a more thorough and detailed examination searching for subtle lateralizing findings such as asymmetry of sensation or strength. The physical examination findings should be coupled with a comprehensive review of vital signs, laboratory values, and medication adjustments or additions as well as a search for infectious sources. Any lateralizing signs warrant urgent computed tomography (CT) scan of the head, but scans performed for global (nonlateralizing) findings are often unrevealing. CT scans done in patients with obvious metabolic, infectious, or recent medication adjustments have an even lower yield.

The decision to send an ICU patient on a "diagnostic journey" should not be made lightly because there are numerous risks associated with transporting critically ill patients. The literature is replete with examples of significant mishaps, such as endotracheal tube dislodgment, worsening hypoxia, or hemodynamic compromise, during transport of ICU patients; a careful risk-benefit analysis must be performed before transport. Lastly, one of the most important aspects of the neurologic examination and assessment that is overlooked is discussion with the bedside nurse. Because of frequent bedside interactions with the patient and charting of objective data such as CAM-ICU, Glasgow Coma Scale, or Richmond Agitation and Sedation Scores (RASS), the bedside nurse is a crucial source of information and can facilitate early diagnosis of the patient's neurologic decline.

Specific treatment for the neurologic dysfunctions discussed so far is too broad to review, but the principles are to determine the underlying cause of the alteration, correct the problem in cases of encephalopathy, and withdraw the agent contributing to delirium or confusion whenever possible. In general, benzodiazepines should be avoided in the ICU, particularly in elderly patients, because they contribute to the development of delirium. However, once delirium manifests, it is typically treated with haloperidol or other antipsychotic agents. Providers should engage family members in reorienting patients, physical therapy should continue for mobilization and exercise, and restoration of normal sleep-wake cycles should be attempted. Daily routines, providing the patient with his or her eyeglasses or hearing aid or both, daytime stimulation, and nighttime quiet all are effective nonpharmacologic methods of preventing and treating delirium.

Analgesia, Sedation, and Neuromuscular Blockade

Pain and discomfort in ICU patients is a constant problem because of intubation and mechanical ventilation, invasive procedures and equipment, wounds, burns, and surgical incisions. In addition, the ICU environment is often hectic, unpredictable, and very stimulating, leading to increased anxiety, which itself is often a manifestation of inadequately treated pain. Nurse-driven analgesia and sedation protocols have grown in popularity as a means to facilitate early extubation for ventilated ICU patients, and although they have been successful in this regard, there is some concern because a large percentage of these patients recall feeling pain, anxiety, and fear when surveyed shortly after ICU discharge. The long-term consequences of these noxious memories is unknown, but inadequately treated pain and anxiety can lead to unplanned extubation and removal of important devices, increased physiologic demand from high sympathetic output states, cardiac decompensation, and prolonged pulmonary recovery. However, excessive use of analgesia and sedation agents is associated with many problems, including respiratory depression, hypotension, prolonged mechanical ventilation, increased rates of ventilator-associated events and pneumonia, prolonged lengths of stay, venous thrombosis, and increased costs. Accumulation of analgesic and sedative agents and their metabolites in adipose tissue is especially problematic when continuous infusions are used. The proper balance of analgesics and sedatives in ICU patients is critical if good outcomes are to be maximized and complications are to be minimized. In recent years, numerous randomized investigations have shown improved outcomes in mechanically ventilated patients through use of analgesia and sedation protocols.[4] Typically, these protocols are nurse-driven and incorporate daily awakening, which encourages spontaneous breathing trials (SBTs) and early liberation from mechanical ventilation. Additional benefits are shorter ICU and hospital stays, reduced pneumonia rates, less venous thromboembolism (VTE), and presumed reductions in overall health care costs.

Pain should be monitored and charted on an hourly basis in the ICU using one of numerous scoring systems and scales to measure pain; the most notable scales are the visual analog scale and Numeric Rating Scale. Awake patients who are able to self-report their pain level are the most easily treated; however, most critically ill patients cannot self-report because of intubation and other obstacles to communication, neurologic dysfunction, and medication effects. These patients are best assessed using objective assessments via the Critical Care Pain Observation Tool or RASS, and their pain is treated according to these objective measures.

Opioids are first-line agents for treating pain in the ICU because they have a rapid onset of action, are easily titrated, are inexpensive, and generally lack an accumulation of parent drug or active metabolites. The most commonly used opiates are morphine, fentanyl, and hydromorphone. Fentanyl has a rapid onset of action, has a short half-life, generates no active metabolites, and creates minimal cardiovascular depression. It is highly lipophilic, so continuous infusions are associated with accumulation in lipid stores resulting in a prolonged effect, and large doses have been associated with muscle rigidity syndromes. Morphine has a slower onset of action and longer half-life and is not suitable for hemodynamically unstable patients because of its potential to cause histamine release and vasodilation, which is also the reason for associated pruritus. Morphine is contraindicated in renal failure because an active metabolite, morphine-6-glucuronide, can accumulate and lead to undesirable long-term effects. Hydromorphone is a synthetic opioid that has a half-life similar to morphine but generates no active metabolites and does not cause histamine release. It seems to be better tolerated in some patients who experience nausea with morphine, but all opioid analgesics are associated to some extent with varying degrees of respiratory depression, hypotension, ileus, and nausea.

Pain may be treated with nonopioid agents such as nonsteroidal anti-inflammatory drugs (NSAIDs) including intravenous ketorolac or oral ibuprofen. NSAIDs, which block the production of prostaglandins, do not cause any adverse effects on hemodynamics or gut motility and work synergistically with opioid agents to treat pain effectively with lower opioid doses. NSAIDs have many undesirable effects, and their greatest toxicities are gastrointestinal bleeding and renal failure. Care should be exercised in elderly patients and patients with marginal creatinine clearance because these drugs may precipitate renal failure. All patients receiving these drugs are at risk for gastrointestinal bleeding. The mechanism of renal toxicity of NSAIDs is thought to be due to direct injury to renal tubular cells by vasoconstriction caused by decreased vasodilatory prostaglandins.

Acetaminophen is another pain reliever that can be used in conjunction with opioid agents or alone in elderly patients or patients with mild to moderate pain. In 2010, the U.S. Food and Drug Administration approved intravenous acetaminophen, and its use in ICU patients has expanded greatly. Some research has shown an opioid-sparing effect with intravenous acetaminophen, but evidence that it reduces opioid-related complications such as nausea and emesis is limited. Intravenous acetaminophen is theorized to be more efficacious than oral acetaminophen as a result of avoidance of the first-pass effect, but the cost of intravenous acetaminophen is many times that of the oral or rectal forms. It also requires delivery in 100 mL of fluid over 15 minutes, so administration can be cumbersome. However, in contrast to intravenous NSAIDs, the side-effect profile is very favorable, particularly in elderly patients.

Pain medication can be delivered in many ways, but in general continuous infusions should be avoided whenever possible. If the patient's gastrointestinal tract is functioning, oral agents can be used, but this route can be problematic in the setting of ileus, hemodynamic instability, or bowel discontinuity. Awake patients may be able to administer their own agents via patient-controlled analgesia devices. These devices deliver narcotics in a more timely fashion, provide better patient satisfaction, and diminish anxiety because the patient has some control over his or her medication administration; however, some studies suggest that patients using patient-controlled analgesia receive greater total doses than patients on intermittent or scheduled regimens. Epidural analgesia given through a catheter in the epidural space has been shown to provide many benefits in patients who undergo major thoracic or abdominal surgery. Patient-controlled epidural analgesia is becoming more prevalent and incorporates many of the benefits of patient-controlled analgesia compared with continuous epidural infusions. A meta-analysis of randomized trials found that patients who received epidural analgesia had lower rates of mortality, atrial arrhythmias, deep venous thrombosis (DVT), respiratory depression, and postoperative nausea and vomiting compared with patients who received systemic analgesics. Patients who received epidural analgesia also had earlier return of bowel function but more episodes of hypotension owing to sympatholytic activity.[5]

Similar to administration of pain and analgesic agents, nurse-driven protocols may be applied to the management of sedation. Much of the more recent literature regarding pain and sedation protocols overlaps, and there is good evidence that nurses can use such protocols to assess and manage patients' sedation needs when they are properly trained and educated on protocol use. Most of these protocols aim to keep patients calm but arousable, which corresponds to a level of −1 to −2 on the RASS. Benzodiazepines and propofol have long been the key agents used for sedation, but they provide no analgesia, so narcotics are still necessary. More recently, the concept of separate sedative-hypnotic approaches has been replaced at many institutions by an analgosedation approach where pain is treated first with the added benefit that the analgesic medication provides some sedation effect. Treating pain and discomfort first and using this concept of an analgesia-based sedation strategy has been shown to result in less time on mechanical ventilation, to shorten ICU length of stay, and to reduce dosing of benzodiazepines and other hypnotics.[6]

Midazolam and lorazepam are the most commonly used benzodiazepines for sedation in the ICU. Diazepam is a longer acting agent that is rarely used in this setting, but it may be beneficial in treating severe muscle spasms, especially muscle spasms associated with fractures. Benzodiazepines, which are γ-aminobutyric acid (GABA) agonists, induce a calming mood and can potentiate opioids, but, as mentioned previously, they may cause or worsen delirium. Midazolam is an agent with a short half-life that has significant amnestic properties and is often given by continuous infusion. It is metabolized by the liver but cleared renally, and so its active metabolites, hydroxymidazolams, can cause continued sedation in patients with renal failure. Lorazepam is a longer acting agent, which makes it useful for intermittent dosing. Propofol, also a GABA agonist, has rapid onset and clearance making it ideal for frequent neurologic examinations as required in patients with traumatic brain injury, but it can cause marked cardiovascular suppression and hypotension and unmask hypovolemia. Propofol is lipid based and can lead to hypertriglyceridemia, pancreatitis, and the rare propofol infusion syndrome. The propofol infusion syndrome must be recognized early because it has a very high mortality; patients typically present with severe metabolic derangements, including rhabdomyolysis, acute kidney injury (AKI), metabolic acidosis, and shock. The α_2-adrenergic agent dexmedetomidine has increased in popularity in recent years; its major advantage is that it does not cause respiratory depression or delirium. It is approved by the Food and Drug Administration to facilitate weaning ventilated patients, and it has been shown to result in reduced ventilator times compared with benzodiazepines. There is some evidence showing decreased opioid requirements with dexmedetomidine as well as decreased need for benzodiazepines in patients being treated for alcohol withdrawal, but these data are limited.

Although neuromuscular blocking agents were used extensively in ICU patients needing mechanical ventilation, most patients do not need neuromuscular blockade to tolerate mechanical ventilation. Indications for neuromuscular blockade include managing difficult-to-control intracranial pressure, ventilator dyssynchrony, profound hypoxemia, and reduction of oxygen consumption in certain patient populations. In cases of ventilator dyssynchrony, attempts should first be made to sedate patients adequately, and neuromuscular blockade should be viewed as an agent of last choice. Paralytics are useful adjuncts and provide enhanced safety for certain procedures, especially procedures involving the airway, such as intubation, tracheostomy, bronchoscopy, or endotracheal tube exchange. Because neuromuscular blocking agents provide no sedation or analgesia, it is crucial that providers ensure that paralyzed patients are well sedated and that adequate analgesia has been provided. Paralysis without analgesia and sedation is cruel and is associated with debilitating memories of the event and may contribute to post-traumatic stress disorder. There are two classes of neuromuscular blocking agents—depolarizing and nondepolarizing agents. Depolarizing agents are similar in structure to acetylcholine and bind to their receptors at the motor end plates, initially causing depolarization of the muscle while blocking repolarization. Nondepolarizing agents competitively block the acetylcholine binding sites in an antagonist fashion. Succinylcholine, the only depolarizing neuromuscular blocking agent, has a rapid onset of action, has a short half-life of about 15 seconds, and is often the paralytic used for rapid-sequence intubation and short invasive procedures but never as a continuous infusion. Succinylcholine is degraded by plasma pseudocholinesterases, and prolonged action may occur in patients with a genetic deficiency of this enzyme. Because succinylcholine causes intracellular potassium release, patients can develop transient hyperkalemia, which can be significant in patients with AKI, burns, crush injury, rhabdomyolysis, and spinal cord injury or prolonged immobility.

The nondepolarizing neuromuscular blocking agents are the steroidal agents pancuronium, vecuronium, and rocuronium in decreasing order of half-life, and they are metabolized and cleared by the liver and kidneys. The duration of action of pancuronium is approximately 90 minutes, and it has a significant vagolytic effect and so should not be used in patients with coronary artery disease or atrial fibrillation with rapid ventricular response because it causes marked tachycardia. Vecuronium and rocuronium are used as infusions or for short procedures but can accumulate in patients with renal dysfunction. Atracurium and cisatracurium cause minimal cardiovascular effects and have an almost immediate onset of action. Cisatracurium causes less histamine release than atracurium, and both agents are eliminated by plasma ester hydrolysis, known as Hoffmann elimination. Atracurium and cisatracurium are preferred in patients with renal or hepatic failure.

Patients receiving paralytic agents should be monitored for depth of neuromuscular blockade with train-of-four testing, and the goal should be to maintain a patient with one to two twitches. If patients are paralyzed too deeply, this may indicate a drug accumulation, which can be associated with increased risk of complications such as critical illness myopathy and critical illness polyneuropathy. Critical illness myopathy and critical illness polyneuropathy are now more recognized entities, and their occurrence should be minimized by stopping neuromuscular blocking agents as early as possible or by observing occasional periods off neuromuscular blockade, or "paralysis holidays." Corticosteroid use, prolonged mechanical ventilation, sepsis, and aminoglycoside use all have been identified as contributors to development of critical illness myopathy and critical illness polyneuropathy; both conditions dramatically extend a patient's recovery and are associated with long-term disabilities.

Alcohol Withdrawal and Opioid Dependence

An increasing number of patients who require critical care in the perioperative period have a history of alcohol or opioid abuse or opioid dependency. A history of alcohol abuse is present in 40% of admitted patients, and a significant number of these patients subsequently develop alcohol withdrawal syndrome. Alcohol withdrawal syndrome causes autonomic instability and increased metabolic demand resulting from tachycardia, hypertension, tremors, and agitation. Patients progressing to delirium tremens or alcohol-related seizures have a significantly increased risk of dying. The goal in caring for patients with a history of alcohol abuse should be to treat them early to prevent symptoms of withdrawal. Benzodiazepines are the mainstay for prevention and treatment of alcohol withdrawal syndrome, and they have been shown to reduce seizure risk markedly in these patients compared with neuroleptics such as haloperidol. Benzodiazepines calm patients and control the autonomic instability associated with alcohol withdrawal syndrome through GABAergic effects. The main drawback of benzodiazepines is their tendency to cause respiratory and cardiovascular depression. Propofol and barbiturates are also GABAergic, but these agents cause more severe respiratory and cardiovascular suppression, which greatly limits their use in the treatment of alcohol withdrawal syndrome. A few small studies examined dexmedetomidine, an α_2-adrenergic agonist, as an adjunct for treating alcohol withdrawal syndrome, and although there have been some encouraging results, it lacks GABA activity and is ineffective at preventing seizures. This agent is given as an infusion and leads to minimal respiratory depression but can cause bradycardia and hypotension. Dexmedetomidine is not approved for treating alcohol withdrawal syndrome; because this is considered an off-label use, it is associated with much higher medication costs. However, dexmedetomidine is effective as an adjunct to treat alcohol withdrawal syndrome effectively with much smaller amounts of benzodiazepines.

Alcohol withdrawal syndrome encompasses many subjective findings, and objective scoring systems such as the Clinical Institute Withdrawal Assessment (CIWA) are helpful in guiding the treatment of alcohol withdrawal syndrome. Use of CIWA results in reduced benzodiazepine dosing compared with fixed dosing. Although CIWA is an effective tool for managing alcohol withdrawal syndrome, its role in the ICU must be viewed with caution because the differential diagnosis of agitation and restlessness is broad and includes life-threatening entities such as hypoxia, sepsis, shock, and stroke. Agents such as clonidine and beta blockers blunt autonomic hyperactivity in alcohol withdrawal syndrome, whereas atypical antipsychotics such as olanzapine and quetiapine may control agitation but must be combined with benzodiazepines because they often lower the seizure threshold.

Opioid dependency is a burgeoning problem in the United States, and an increasing number of patients with opioid dependency present to surgical ICUs. Opioid dependency and treatment of this condition with methadone taper or mixed receptor agonists such as buprenorphine add layers of complexity to treating acute pain. Buprenorphine is commonly used to taper patients from opioid addiction or to treat chronic pain, and ICU providers should be familiar with its mechanism and use, as it is anticipated that the number of patients receiving this agent will increase. There are very few protocols and little randomized evidence to guide the administration of analgesics in this patient population, but key themes have emerged. Patients with opioid dependency who have undergone major surgery or have sustained significant traumatic injury require narcotic quantities in excess of their baseline dosing. If these patients are able to take oral medications, starting them on their baseline doses of buprenorphine or methadone will result in inadequate pain control, and they will require additional shorter acting agents for optimal pain control. Mixed agents such as buprenorphine limit the effectiveness of other opioids with the resultant need for escalating doses of opioids, so providers need to be on guard for respiratory depression, ileus, and other narcotic-related complications. It may be advisable to suspend use of this agent in the acute setting and reinitiate it after the patient's acute pain has lessened. Patients who are dependent on narcotics should have their pain addressed via a multifaceted approach, including the use of nonsteroidal agents and epidural and regional blocks as well as the added input of pain management specialists, clinical pharmacists, and social workers.

CARDIOVASCULAR SYSTEM

Comorbidities, Events, and Risk Mitigation

Elderly adults (≥65 years old) comprise the fastest growing segment of the U.S. population; by 2030, this subgroup will comprise almost 20% of the population. This age group tends to have more complex medical comorbidities, but if these chronic health conditions are managed effectively, older adults are able to live longer and more productive lives. Although previously elderly patients were denied open surgical care because of concerns of excess mortality, newer treatment options such as stent placement and endovascular surgery and minimally invasive techniques have allowed more elderly patients to have their health conditions addressed surgically. As a result, more elderly patients with complex cardiovascular issues undergo noncardiac surgery. In the past, these types of patients were often admitted to the ICU or surgical ward preoperatively to optimize their hemodynamic and fluid volume status, but a lack of evidence to support this in terms of better outcomes coupled with prohibitive costs of such an approach rendered this an unsustainable approach. At the present time, these patients are often admitted to the ICU with little or no advance warning, and the opportunity for approaches to minimize cardiovascular risk is extremely limited.

The most common perioperative events are arrhythmias, myocardial infarction, and nonfatal and fatal cardiac arrest. These events typically occur in the first 3 days after surgery and are likely due to the convergence of the patient's high sympathetic output and myocardial metabolic demand in the midst of the greatest intravascular volume shifts. Patient complaints of cardiac ischemia during this time are frequently lost in the background of postoperative complaints of pain and nausea, and intubated patients are extremely limited in their ability to relay cardiac distress. Cardiac events in the noncardiac surgery perioperative period are associated with an in-hospital mortality of 15% to 25% and increased risk of another myocardial infarction or cardiac death extending 6 months into the postoperative period. In a large review of patients at a tertiary care center, nonfatal cardiac arrest was associated with in-hospital mortality of 65%, and increased risk of cardiac death extended 5 years after the event. Historically, major cardiac events occur in 1% to 2% of patients older than age 50 undergoing elective noncardiac surgery; however, most of these retrospective reviews were conducted in the past, and it is likely that the present rate is much higher given the aging population. The rate of adverse cardiac events is even higher in emergency operations.

The combination of events in the perioperative period including intubation and extubation, bleeding and anemia, and immune-inflammatory activation is analogous to one long cardiac stress test. On ICU admission, the patient's cardiovascular comorbidities, such as coronary stents or bypasses, peripheral vascular disease, arrhythmias, valvular abnormalities (e.g., aortic stenosis), hypertension, and ischemic stroke, should be thoroughly explored so that risks of further cardiac events might be mitigated. The patient's medication history should be considered, and a plan should be made for continuing or reintroducing critical agents during the postoperative period, particularly if the patient will be NPO. Generally, anticoagulants and antiplatelet agents are held during the perioperative period because of concerns for bleeding. Most antihypertensives and diuretics can be held until the patient resumes oral intake and their volume status and hemodynamic abnormalities have normalized. Beta blockers and clonidine should not be abruptly discontinued because significant rebound effects may occur with disastrous consequences. The decision to start or stop antiplatelet agents in patients with coronary stents is a highly nuanced decision; although it is too complex to be discussed here in depth, the type of stent and duration it has been indwelling are critical components of this decision. The highest rates of stent thrombosis occur when antiplatelet agents are discontinued within 6 months of stent placement or with drug-eluting stents.

Surgery and traumatic injury cause immune-inflammatory activation marked by endothelial injury, capillary leak, hypercoagulability, and hormonal alterations that dramatically increase myocardial oxygen demand and place the coronary arteries and plaques under sheer stress. This is fertile ground for myocardial oxygen demand and supply imbalances leading to non–ST-segment elevation myocardial infarction (NSTEMI) and plaque rupture and thrombosis (ST-segment elevation myocardial infarction [STEMI]). Patients who have preexisting coronary artery stenosis are at greatest risk for perioperative coronary events. In these patients, beta blockers and 3-hydroxy-3-methylglutaryl-coenzyme A (HMG-CoA) reductase inhibitors are indicated and can reduce the risk of cardiac events in this stressful perioperative period. Beta blockers decrease heart rate, sympathetic output, and myocardial contraction leading to reduced metabolic and oxygen demand of the body and the myocardium, and there is some evidence to suggest that they reduce levels of inflammatory cytokines and may have an anti-inflammatory effect. Several investigations of beta blockers in noncardiac surgery showed improved outcomes from a cardiac viewpoint, but this is controversial because other studies showed that these benefits are offset by increased complications such as stroke. A randomized investigation exploring the benefit of beta blockers and HMG-CoA reductase inhibitors in patients undergoing noncardiac surgery showed that this group had a lower rate of myocardial infarction and cardiac death.[7] There was a trend toward improved outcomes in patients given fluvastatin versus the control group, but these results did not reach statistical significance. Many older trials showed a protective benefit of perioperative beta blockers, and evidence is mounting that HMG-CoA reductase inhibitors (statins) have a favorable effect on outcomes after trauma, sepsis, and other inflammatory conditions because of their global anti-inflammatory effects. Statins were shown to lower the risk of postoperative atrial fibrillation risk, an important and costly cardiac event that results in increased length of stay and health care expenses.[8]

The role of beta blockers in the ICU for patients who have not been on them previously is controversial. The only Class I recommendation the American Heart Association and American College of Cardiology have been able to make is that beta blockers should be resumed in patients who have been on them as early as possible because failure to do so results in increased mortality. The Cardiac Risk Index (CRI) system was designed to guide clinicians through the clinical decision process regarding beta blocker use in the perioperative period. The CRI is composed of six components: high-risk surgery, ischemic coronary disease, congestive heart failure, diabetes, cerebrovascular disease, and renal insufficiency (Box 21-1). Patients with two or more of these CRI components should be started on beta blocker therapy because 30-day mortality has been shown to be reduced in these patients with this approach.[9] The use and benefit of beta blockers in the perioperative period, particularly in the ICU, remain controversial, and the controversy is likely to persist until there are more randomized investigations. Patients with cardiac risk factors who are undergoing emergency surgery often have contraindications to beta blockers, such as shock or hypotension, but it may be prudent to use small doses of an intravenous agent such as metoprolol as soon as feasible in the postoperative period.

BOX 21-1 Cardiac Risk Factor Indicators for Beta Blocker Therapy

Consider beta blocker therapy if two or more of the following are present:
High-risk surgery (chest, abdomen, major vascular)
History of ischemic coronary disease (myocardial infarction, nitrate therapy, positive exercise stress test, Q waves)
Congestive heart failure (pulmonary congestion, S_3 gallop, bilateral rales)
Cerebrovascular disease (prior transient ischemic attack or stroke)
Diabetes
Renal insufficiency (baseline creatinine >2 mg/dL)

TABLE 21-1 Benefits of Early Postoperative Beta Blockers and 3-Hydroxy-3-Methylglutaryl-Coenzyme A Inhibitors

BETA BLOCKERS	HMG-CoA INHIBITORS
Decrease global and cardiac oxygen demand	Stabilize coronary plaques
Reduce shear stress on coronary plaque	Reduce incidence of atrial fibrillation
Anti-inflammatory	Anti-inflammatory

HMG-CoA, 3-hydroxy-3-methylglutaryl-coenzyme A.

Dysfunction: Ischemic Disease, Non–ST-Segment Elevation Myocardial Infarction, and Arrhythmias

Cardiac risk factor assessment in the preoperative period is controversial, but there are certain straightforward approaches that should be taken with these patients when they arrive in the surgical ICU. If the patient is to undergo acute emergency surgery, the cardiac risk assessment is limited to vital signs, estimations of volume status, and electrocardiogram (ECG). The ECG should be examined for ST-segment elevations or depressions, T-wave inversions, P–R interval, and rhythm. Awake patients should be queried about chest pain or pressure, jaw pain, and nausea, while recognizing that some of these complaints may be attributable to a laparotomy. ST-segment changes or ischemic symptoms should trigger assessment of troponin biomarkers looking for confirmation of myocardial infarction. A perioperative myocardial infarction has significant prognostic value in predicting 30-day postoperative mortality and mandates treatment to minimize further myocardial damage. A newer entity, myocardial injury after noncardiac surgery (MINS), likely represents a new understanding of NSTEMI.[10] MINS results in injury to the myocardium from ischemia that does not result in necrosis and typically occurs in the first 30 days postoperatively. Elevation of troponin, a biomarker of myocardial injury, is a predictor of postoperative mortality, but it is unclear if this is a cause-and-effect relationship or a marker of global illness because troponin may be elevated in nonischemic entities such as sepsis, pulmonary embolism, and cardioversion. Patients with MINS benefit from many of the same treatments that benefit patients with actual myocardial infarction—beta blockers, aspirin, and statins (Table 21-1). Patients who have ST-segment elevations or depressions (i.e., STEMI) that are persistent and accompanied by symptoms may benefit from attempts at revascularization by percutaneous techniques or by coronary artery bypass grafting. Percutaneous techniques usually mandate powerful platelet inhibitors, and this may not be feasible or safe in the immediate postoperative period. Alternatively, heparin infusion is typically started for STEMI to arrest propagation of coronary clots.

Dysrhythmias are common in the ICU because of increased levels of catecholamines and other circulating inflammatory mediators, but cardiac arrest is rare. The initial goal in the management of cardiac arrest is to deliver quality cardiopulmonary resuscitation (CPR) with a rate of 100 chest compressions per minute to maintain cerebral perfusion. The patient should be promptly attached to a monitor and the rhythm analyzed. Pulseless electrical activity and asystole are not amenable to cardioversion, but cardioversion is indicated in ventricular fibrillation and pulseless ventricular tachycardia. A definitive airway should be obtained, and 40 U of vasopressin can be given one time while CPR is underway; alternatively, 1 mg of epinephrine repeated every 3 to 5 minutes may be given. Throughout the resuscitative efforts, a search for the underlying cause (e.g., hemorrhage, hyperkalemia, hypovolemia, tension pneumothorax) of the arrest should be sought and treated if found. CPR should be stopped every 2 minutes to assess the patient's rhythm and pulse, and if a pulse has returned, more standard ICU resuscitation plans should continue, and the antiarrhythmic amiodarone should be given. Amiodarone is also indicated for all unstable tachyarrhythmias including ventricular tachycardia with and without a pulse. Calcium chloride is used in an attempt to stabilize the myocardium, especially if a hyperkalemic arrest is suspected, whereas magnesium sulfate is indicated in cases of torsades de pointes. Advanced cardiac life support guidelines stress the importance of maintaining adequate CPR throughout resuscitation efforts with as few interruptions for therapeutic interventions as possible.

Bradycardia, defined as a heart rate less than 60 beats/min, is evaluated first with an ECG, but if the patient has symptoms such as shortness of breath, chest pain, or dizziness or is hypotensive, atropine 0.5 or 1 mg should be given. Other β_2 agonists (e.g., epinephrine or dopamine) may be required to increase the heart rate and blood pressure while a workup for the cause of the bradycardia is sought. If these approaches fail, percutaneous pacing may be needed, but this modality is ineffective for long-term use, and transvenous methods may be required. Bradycardia may be a sign of profound myocardial ischemia, especially in patients with advanced coronary artery disease, so efforts to increase myocardial oxygen delivery should be started. Patients with wide QRS complexes and tachycardia should be given amiodarone and undergo cardioversion because this dysrhythmia is most likely ventricular in origin; however, the ECG should be evaluated to rule out aberrant conduction as a cause of the wide QRS complexes. If the QRS complex is narrow, and the patient is hemodynamically unstable from tachycardia, synchronized cardioversion is warranted. Sinus tachycardia is the most common tachycardia in the ICU. It is often an appropriate response to fever, pain, sympathetic stimulation, bleeding, hypotension, sepsis, or inflammation, and therapies should be directed at the underlying cause. If the width of the QRS complex is unclear, intravenous adenosine (6 mg, repeated once) may be administered and typically facilitates identification of the underlying rhythm. If the rate does not slow, it should be treated as a wide-complex tachycardia; if it slows, it should be treated as a narrow-complex tachycardia. The differential diagnosis includes supraventricular tachycardias, atrial fibrillation, atrial flutter, multifocal atrial tachycardia, and uncertain tachycardias, all of which require different treatments. A detailed discussion of the management of these rhythm abnormalities is beyond the scope of this chapter, and expert consultation may be necessary. Atrial fibrillation is the most common sustained dysrhythmia in the ICU and its occurrence is an indicator of the stresses and overall status of a patient. Etiologies of atrial fibrillation abound and include any condition associated with catecholamine release, increased sympathetic tone, or generalized inflammation. New-onset postoperative atrial fibrillation develops in 7% to 8% of patients undergoing noncardiac surgery and is associated with increased mortality and length of stay and other cardiac events such as stroke and myocardial infarction. Greater than 80% of patients with new-onset atrial fibrillation are able to be discharged in sinus rhythm without the need for anticoagulation or advanced antiarrhythmic agents. The most successful initial pharmacologic approach is to attempt rate control with beta blockers or calcium channel blockers to block the atrioventricular node and promote conversion back to sinus rhythm. Beta blockers have been shown to result in higher rates of conversion to sinus rhythm than calcium channel blockers at 2 and 12 hours after onset of atrial fibrillation. Amiodarone is also an effective therapy in atrial fibrillation and is preferred in patients with systolic heart failure. Patients who fail to convert to sinus rhythm within 48 hours of onset of atrial fibrillation typically require therapeutic anticoagulation, which is a challenging decision in the newly postoperative patient.

Shock and Hemodynamic Monitoring

The definition of shock has evolved significantly from the descriptions more than 100 years ago of a "peculiar effect on the animal system produced by violent injuries" to our current understanding that it is a condition in which tissue perfusion is inadequate to meet oxygen needs. This simple definition overcomes some of the disagreement about whether a patient is in shock resulting from the multitude of available definitions and avoids the pitfalls associated with embracing absolute values. There is no set blood pressure that defines the shock state, and patients can be hypotensive or hypertensive and be in shock. The etiologies of shock are numerous and include hypovolemia and hemorrhage, sepsis, cardiac pump failure, neurologic injury, and obstructive entities, but regardless of the cause, all shock states should begin with restoration of an adequate circulating volume. Even cardiac pump failure initially responds to crystalloid administration, but the challenge in resuscitation from shock lies in gauging when the ideal amount of fluid has been given. The process of administering intravenous crystalloids, blood, and blood products to restore an effective circulating volume is referred to as resuscitation and after resuscitation; vasopressor and inotropic agents are given based on data obtained from invasive means of hemodynamic monitoring.

Hypovolemic shock is the most common form of shock and results from loss of plasma volume as seen in gastrointestinal losses from diarrhea, fistulas, and vomiting; inadequate intake from short gut syndrome, malnutrition, and dehydration; or conditions such as epidermolysis and burns. The most dramatic form of hypovolemic shock is hemorrhagic shock, which typically has a more sudden onset and is due to surgery, trauma, or losses from gastrointestinal sources. Patients in hemorrhagic shock should initially be given blood and blood products instead of crystalloid. Patients in hypovolemic or hemorrhagic shock initially compensate for loss of intravascular volume with increased sympathetic output, which increases systemic vascular resistance and heart rate. Initially, such compensation may maintain blood pressure, but as the circulating volume decreases and the systemic vascular resistance reaches its maximum, end organ perfusion becomes inadequate, and the patient enters a shock state. Inadequate end organ perfusion is the basis for the physical findings of shock, such as tachycardia, dry mucous membranes, mottled skin, decreased mental status, and oliguria.

Cardiogenic shock is due to significantly decreased cardiac output as a result of diminished myocardial contractility or profound bradycardia. In the ICU, the most common etiologies are acute myocardial infarction, massive pulmonary embolism, or advanced heart block. Patients in cardiogenic shock develop increased ventricular filling pressures and significantly decreased cardiac output, and, similar to patients with hypovolemic shock, they compensate with increased systemic vascular resistance setting the stage for a cycle of cardiac decompensation, volume overload, and decreased coronary perfusion causing further myocardial injury. The key aspect of treating cardiogenic shock is inotropic and chronotropic support and for severe cases advanced modalities such as intra-aortic balloon pumps or ventricular assist devices. The physical findings of cardiogenic shock that help differentiate it from hypovolemic shock are the presence of pulmonary congestion, jugular venous distention, and other signs of marked volume overload.

Septic shock is often placed into a broader category known as distributive shock and is a result of loss of vasomotor tone and decreased systemic vascular resistance along with hypovolemia. Neurogenic shock is a form of distributive shock caused by interruption of the sympathetic nervous system, typically secondary to trauma, with a striking reduction of systemic vascular resistance. Septic shock is a far more common entity in the ICU and represents a host of physiologic derangements resulting from whole body immune-inflammatory activation. Bacterial endotoxin, cytokines, and nitric oxide result in loss of capillary gap junction and endothelial integrity, which promotes fluid loss from the intravascular space—hence septic shock always involves a degree of hypovolemia. Compounding the hypovolemia is a disruption in vasomotor tone decreasing the systemic vascular resistance and myocardial suppression, which diminishes the cardiac output. Although many clinicians associate sepsis with a hyperdynamic cardiac response, most patients subsequently develop ventricular systolic and diastolic dysfunction from mediators such as tumor necrosis factor and interleukin-1; however, most patients recover pump function when sepsis resolves.

Following the diagnosis of a shock state, it is desirable to obtain some type of hemodynamic monitoring keeping in mind that there is no single vital sign, physiologic variable, laboratory marker, or measurement that can tell a provider what is occurring at the tissue or organ level. An arterial catheter should be placed in the radial artery using full barrier sterile precautions because the risk of infection with arterial catheters is similar to the risk with central venous catheters. Femoral placement is the next preferred location for arterial cannulation, and this may be facilitated through the use of bedside ultrasound. The most reliable data obtained from an arterial line is the mean arterial pressure (MAP) because the MAP is not affected by systems issues such as stiffness and resistance of the catheter or the measuring system, which can result in overdamping or underdamping of the pressure tracing.

Laboratory markers may be helpful in monitoring resuscitation from the shock state and offer additional data to supplement invasive parameters. Lactic acid, arterial blood gases (ABG), and base deficit are global indicators of end organ perfusion and can help guide responses to therapy because early normalization of elevated lactic acid levels has been linked to increased survival in injured and critically ill patients. These laboratory measurements are static in nature, and although following their trends can yield valuable data, the quest to obtain minute-to-minute guidance inspired cardiologists in the 1960s to seek a more advanced means of monitoring. The landmark article by Swan and Ganz describing the pulmonary artery catheter (PAC) in 1970 started an era of more invasive and complex hemodynamic monitoring that has continued to the present day. There are several invasive means for guiding fluid resuscitation and gauging intravascular volume status; however, no one device or modality has emerged superior, and at best almost all claim equivalency to the PAC.

Central venous catheters have dual utility in that they provide intravenous access while measuring central venous pressure (CVP). CVP is a surrogate for end-diastolic pressure and volume in the right ventricle, but this is dependent on right ventricular compliance, cardiac valvular function, intrathoracic pressure, and several other variables. CVP is an even poorer and more unreliable marker for left-sided filling pressures because any pulmonary or valvular abnormalities significantly degrade the assumption that CVP correlates with the end-diastolic filling pressure of the left ventricle. Measuring central venous oxygen saturation ($ScvO_2$) in addition to CVP yields better detection of tissue and organ hypoperfusion and allows clinicians to estimate global oxygen parameters better. These catheters, coined "sepsis catheters," have been associated with improved outcomes in patients with sepsis, injury, and certain high-risk surgical procedures.

Central venous catheters are associated with two types of morbidity: immediate technical complications and long-term complications. Immediate complications are usually related to procedural mishaps and include pneumothorax, hemothorax, arteriovenous fistula, air embolus, dysrhythmia, and death. Pneumothorax occurs in about 1% to 5% of cases of subclavian vein cannulation, whereas arterial injury is more common when the internal jugular or femoral approach is used, but this risk has been significantly reduced with the advent of real-time bedside ultrasound. Long-term complications of central catheters are venous thrombosis and infection. Subclavian catheters are the least likely to become infected, and femoral catheters have the highest thrombosis and infectious risk as a result of their contaminated local environment. The femoral access site should be used as a last resort or in emergency situations when other venous access cannot be established. Patients admitted to the ICU from the emergency department or the field should have their venous access changed because breaks in sterile technique tend to occur when venous access is placed in a patient in extremis. Patients undergoing tracheostomy should have their internal jugular central access converted to the subclavian site because tracheal secretions have been shown to increase line infection rates significantly.

Although use of the PAC has declined significantly over the last 2 decades, it is still a valuable tool and should not be overlooked in critically ill patients. The PAC yields direct measurements of CVP, right atrial pressure, pulmonary arterial pressure, pulmonary artery wedge pressure, and mixed venous oxygen saturation (SvO_2) and calculations of cardiac output, oxygen consumption, and other parameters such as systemic vascular resistance and left ventricular stroke work. In contrast to the older devices that relied on one-time injections of chilled saline, newer PACs allow for continuous cardiac output. In more than 40 years, very few studies have clearly shown a mortality benefit when PACs are used in the management of critically ill patients; some data indicate that PACs may contribute to worse outcomes. However, in the right hands, the PAC is extremely useful in guiding fluid resuscitation and vasopressor and inotropic support. Some literature suggests that the ability of critical care providers to interpret the data yielded by the PAC accurately may be the true issue and not the catheters—that is, there is a knowledge gap of clinicians interpreting PAC data. The newest PACs monitor right ventricular end-diastolic pressure and calculate a right ventricular ejection fraction on a continuous basis, which may circumvent some of the problems presented by pulmonary and valvular abnormalities.

As stated previously, there is no single vital sign, physiologic variable, laboratory marker, or measurement that can tell a provider what is occurring at the tissue or organ level, but the trends and responses to management interventions are significant. The more derivations and calculations involved in modifying PAC data, the more likely that data might be skewed by unseen variables. Thus, systemic vascular resistance, which is expressed as dyne • sec/cm^5 is more contrived and less helpful to managing ICU patients than SvO_2, which is directly measured and is expressed as a percent (%). To some degree, PACs have been slighted as a hemodynamic monitoring tool because study designs evaluating their use have often been flawed, especially in terms of patient selection and the rationale behind PAC data guiding interventions. In a large National Trauma Data Bank review by Friese and colleagues,[11] outcomes, including mortality, were shown to be improved in severely injured elderly patients who received a PAC as part of their ICU management.

Complications associated with PAC use should not be underestimated. In addition to those attributable to central venous access, complications specific to PAC use such as heart block, ventricular tachycardia, valvular damage, pulmonary infarction, and the uniformly fatal event of pulmonary artery rupture have been described. Left bundle branch block is a relatively strong contraindication to PAC placement because complete heart block may result. It is crucial that all clinicians caring for patients with a PAC understand the waveforms, interpretations, and pitfalls associated with their use, but a detailed review of all the data is beyond the scope of this chapter.

There has been a focus more recently on bedside echocardiography performed by trained intensivists as a rapid, noninvasive, repeatable way to assess intravascular volume status and cardiac performance in critically ill surgical patients. Echocardiography is finally being recognized as a valuable tool in surgical ICU patients after being used for decades to assess high-risk surgical patients in the preoperative and intraoperative settings. Echocardiography can rapidly assess cardiac function and hemodynamics by looking at right ventricular and left ventricular systolic and diastolic function, valvular function, cardiac wall motion, and volume status by assessing inferior vena cava changes in response to fluid challenge. Additional information, such as the presence of pericardial fluid or collapse of the right ventricle signifying cardiac tamponade, are among the many other uses of this modality. Evidence suggests that echocardiography may be more accurate in determining left ventricular volume status than a PAC, but further study is necessary. As is the case with any new technology, there is skepticism regarding the true benefit of echocardiography because there is a paucity of randomized evidence showing that it leads to better outcomes. Over time and as evidence mounts, it is likely that echocardiography in surgical ICUs will become the norm, and the PAC may become a thing of the past.

Many less invasive hemodynamic monitoring tools, such as cardiac contour output analysis, lithium dilution, and peripheral catheter transpulmonary thermodilution, have emerged, but there are no significant data demonstrating superior outcomes with these new technologies compared with the PAC. Although it is hoped that these modalities will afford the ICU clinician additional, less invasive options for hemodynamic monitoring, many of these modalities require specialized proprietary equipment that render them not cost-effective. Techniques such as thenar eminence and gastric mucosal monitoring, near-infrared spectroscopy, and other technologies extrapolate regional tissue bed data into global indices of oxygen delivery and consumption with varying degrees of success. As technology progresses, miniaturization advances, and artificial intelligence emerges, it is likely that revolutionary improvements in critical care will continue to unfold, but at the present time, echocardiography, PACs, and a dedicated and thoughtful clinician still represent the most effective options for optimizing hemodynamics and improving outcomes for surgical ICU patients.

Resuscitation

Most patients in shock, regardless of the cause, benefit from a trial of fluid resuscitation given in the form of a crystalloid bolus. Interpretation of the response to this initial bolus can offer insight into the cause of the patient's shock and should be used to guide the fluid resuscitation strategy. A patient in hypovolemic shock should begin to show improvements in mentation, skin turgor and color, heart rate, blood pressure, and urine output after one or two boluses of crystalloid fluid, but it can be confusing because similar initial improvements are seen in cases of septic and hemorrhagic shock. Although the initial response to fluid is typically favorable in cardiogenic shock, this positive response is quickly lost as filling pressures rise even higher and cardiac output falls further on the Starling curve. Hemorrhagic shock responds favorably to fluid as well; although there are some improvements in hemodynamic parameters, markers of oxygen delivery worsen. Despite a growing body of literature confirming the benefits of restrictive transfusion strategies, none of these benefits apply to actively bleeding patients, and blood and blood products should remain the first-line therapy in resuscitating bleeding patients.

Recognizing when volume resuscitation is adequate is one of the most complex and challenging decisions in critical care, and this has remained controversial for decades. Over this time, a host of parameters, known as end points of resuscitation, have been touted as the ideal marker of volume resuscitation, and many patients have paid the price for clinicians wedded to one number instead of considering all the available data. The days of supranormal resuscitation originally promulgated by Shoemaker are long behind us, having been disproven by subsequent trials. For example, resuscitating burn patients with lower rates of fluid, as denoted by the Brooke formula, has decreased the rate of abdominal compartment syndrome (ACS) compared with the Parkland formula, which mandates more aggressive resuscitation, without incurring more renal failure.[12] Hyper-resuscitation, intra-abdominal hemorrhage, and catastrophes can lead to the development of ACS, which occurs when blood, ascetic edema fluid, or tissue swelling drives intra-abdominal pressure up as the limit of abdominal fascial compliance is exceeded. ACS progresses from intra-abdominal hypertension to the full-blown syndrome, which is marked by multisystem organ failure (MSOF). Treatment of this condition includes neuromuscular blockade and drainage of ascites as temporizing maneuvers, but decompressive laparotomy and temporary abdominal closure is usually required. Inadequate resuscitation leads to persistence of end organ ischemia and the shock state, which causes irreparable harm to the patient. The

Fluid and Catheter Treatment Trial (FACTT) in 2006 showed that surgical patients with lung injury and acute respiratory distress syndrome (ARDS) managed with a conservative fluid strategy guided by lower CVP and pulmonary capillary wedge pressure had significantly fewer days of mechanical ventilation compared with patients managed with liberal fluid practices without any increase in mortality or renal failure.[13]

Akin to the controversy surrounding how much fluid to give, debates centered on which fluid to give have raged on for more than a century. Lactated Ringer solution and normal saline are the two crystalloid fluids most commonly used, and each has its own subtle advantages and disadvantages. In large volumes, normal saline can cause a hyperchloremic metabolic acidosis, whereas lactated Ringer solution has been implicated as a cause of metabolic alkalosis when used for prolonged periods. Because lactate exists as a racemic mixture in solution, and the D-isomer of lactate is a known neurotoxin, there are some concerns that large volumes of lactated Ringer solution may result in encephalopathy; however, clear-cut proof of this concern is lacking. Because only one third of each liter of crystalloid remains in the intravascular space, whereas the rest occupies the interstitial or intracellular spaces, clinicians have sought colloids as resuscitative fluids under the premise that they would be more inclined to stay intravascularly. This notion fails to recognize that shock is associated with capillary leak and expansion of the intercellular compartment and that the breakdown of tight junctions results in pores far larger than the size of most colloids. Albumin, which can be given as a human derived colloid, normally provides 80% of intravascular oncotic pressure, and it has been used extensively as a resuscitative fluid. The debate about the ideal resuscitative fluid, crystalloid versus colloids, continues at the present time, and colloids have swung in and out of favor repeatedly.

The Saline Albumin Fluid Evaluation (SAFE) trial showed no significant differences in mortality, ICU length of stay, need for renal replacement therapy (RRT), or organ failure when patients were resuscitated with 4% albumin compared with normal saline, although albumin is much more expensive.[14] The SAFE trial looked at a very heterogeneous group of patients, whereas subsequent studies focused more on the role of albumin in resuscitating patients with severe sepsis or septic shock. Although albumin administration can reduce overall fluid requirements, there has been no short-term or long-term benefit compared with crystalloids alone. Synthetic colloids such as hydroxyethyl starch initially generated a lot of enthusiasm as a resuscitative fluid, but this has waned. Because these agents cause renal failure in septic patients and contribute to bleeding via platelet dysfunction, they have largely been abandoned as a resuscitative fluid. An area of avid investigation is centered on hemoglobin-based oxygen carriers, particularly for military and field usage, but after some initially encouraging results, these agents have not lived up to that enthusiasm.

Hemodynamic Support

After the initiation of fluid resuscitation, subsequent therapies designed to improve hemodynamics are largely pharmacologic and involve the use of vasopressor or inotropic agents. Vasopressors augment MAP and systemic perfusion by a direct constrictive action on blood vessels, but this does not lead to improved perfusion at the tissue level. Vasopressors may be harmful to tissue perfusion and may lead to a false sense of security because an elevated MAP generally implies good tissue perfusion. Vasopressor therapy should be guided by MAP and other physiologic parameters, such as mental status, urine output, lactate clearance, and resolution of acidosis. Ideally, clinicians should seek to actively wean patients off vasopressors, but this should not be done at the expense of excessive fluid administration. In cases of septic or distributive shock in which increased intravascular capacitance plays a significant role in the shock state, the goals should be first to restore an effective circulating volume and then to add vasopressors to augment alpha-adrenergic mediated vasomotor tone.

The terms *catecholamines* and *sympathomimetics* are synonymous and denote endogenous and synthetically derived agents that act directly on alpha- and beta-adrenergic receptors enhancing the sympathetic response of the individual. Phenylephrine is a selective α_1 agonist that works on receptors in the smooth muscle cells of vessels rendering it a potent vasoconstrictor. It is most useful in shock states in which intravascular volume is deemed to be adequate but systemic vascular resistance is exceedingly low, such as in neurogenic shock, epidural anesthesia–induced hypotension, or transient hypotension associated with inhaled anesthetics. Pure α_1 agonists have little role in treating septic or other forms of distributive shock because they lack any direct effect on the heart. Norepinephrine, by virtue of its alpha and beta effects, causes increased cardiac output by chronotropic and inotropic activities as well as vasoconstriction via a potent α_1 effect. Norepinephrine is the predominant agent used in septic shock because of its favorable mix of alpha and beta actions, and there is some evidence that it may attenuate the systemic inflammatory response. Although norepinephrine is the preferred pressor for septic shock because of its lack of adverse effects compared with dopamine, two large randomized controlled trials failed to show benefits related to mortality and organ failure when norepinephrine was compared with dopamine or vasopressin. Epinephrine is an endogenous catecholamine that has far more beta activity than alpha activity, rendering it the preferred agent for cardiac arrest, anaphylaxis, and cardiogenic shock and a second-line agent for septic shock. Similar to dopamine, epinephrine is associated with severe arrhythmias, and this is theorized to be due to increasing myocardial workload and oxygen demand. Vasopressin is an endogenous peptide, not an adrenergic agent, and its mechanism of action is different from the previously mentioned catecholamines. It works via a G protein–coupled receptor that appears to be less denatured by acidemia, increasing its effectiveness in severe septic shock. In many shock states, endogenous vasopressin may be depleted, and so it is usually administered at physiologic replacement doses. To date, no study has shown a benefit to monitoring vasopressin levels, and dosing this drug based on serum levels is not indicated; pharmacologic doses are associated with splanchnic vasoconstriction and bowel ischemia. The synthetic catecholamine dopamine is no longer a preferred agent in the ICU because it is an unpredictable agent with numerous negative side effects.

The management of acute heart failure and cardiogenic shock in the ICU is very challenging because these patients typically have a wide range of comorbidities as well as the usual confounding perioperative factors. The goals of managing acute heart failure are to optimize preload and intravascular volume, maximize contractility, and decrease myocardial demand and oxygen consumption. The synthetic catecholamine dobutamine is a useful to augment heart rate and contractility via its β_1 actions, while decreasing left ventricular preload through its β_2 vasodilatory effects. Owing to its β_2 effect, dobutamine should be avoided in hypovolemic states and septic shock because it can cause profound hypotension. Phosphodiesterase inhibitors milrinone and amrinone act via intracellular second messengers to prevent the breakdown of cyclic adenosine monophosphate, which essentially extends the time period of contraction and contractility of the myocardium. Although these agents are not adrenergic agonists, they behave similarly to dubutamine and increase contractility but also promote vasodilation resulting in hypotension and significant arrythymias. Afterload reducers and diuretics may have a role in management of heart failure and cardiogenic shock, but their use is too complex to be adequately discussed here. Similarly, mechanical assist devices, such as left ventricular assist devices, biventricular assist devices, and right ventricular assist devices, have become much more effective and portable allowing some patients to be discharged with them in place. Intra-aortic balloon pumps are useful tools as a bridge to cardiac recovery in patients with heart failure or cardiogenic shock refractory to pharmacologic therapy, patients awaiting cardiac transplant, and patients with post–coronary bypass heart failure.

RESPIRATORY SYSTEM

Respiratory Failure

Respiratory failure is one of the most frequent reasons surgical patients require ICU admission and may be due to diverse causes, such as blunt chest trauma, altered mental status, cardiothoracic surgery, sepsis, medical comorbidities, and shock. Even simple abdominal operations may cause splinting, hypoventilation, atelectasis, and hypoxemia leading to respiratory failure. Hypoxemia is the hallmark of type I respiratory failure, and hypercapnia and hypoxemia are associated with type II respiratory failure. Hypoventilation from pain, narcotics, and mental status changes can result in respiratory acidosis, whereas inadequate pulmonary toilet can lead to pooling of secretions, atelectasis, and pneumonia. Most surgical patients have type II respiratory failure because of multiple overlapping factors. Ideally, patients at high risk for respiratory failure are identified before they worsen to the point where they require intubation to allow for measures to treat or mitigate the underlying cause of the respiratory failure. Examples of these measures are adequately treating pain to avoid splinting and atelectasis, inducing diuresis in patients with volume overload, or adjusting narcotics and sedatives in overmedicated patients.

Assessing a patient with respiratory failure is an urgent and challenging endeavor for all clinicians, and a structured and systematic approach is indicated. Similar to the primary survey of the Advanced Trauma Life Support course, asking the patient a question and assessing his or her phonation, degree of breathlessness, and comfort in responding gives clues to airway patency, pulmonary reserve, work of breathing, and mental status. Stridor, or high-pitched upper airway obstructive sounds, is ominous, and arrangements should be made for prompt intubation of the patient. Prompt intubation is also indicated for unresponsive or comatose patients. If the patient's condition allows, supplemental oxygen should be delivered by a high-flow face mask, and a thorough chest examination should be done assessing chest rise, accessory muscle use, and retractions followed by careful auscultation of the type and quality of breath sounds. Physical examination findings and a brief history are critical in rapidly working through the vast differential diagnosis of acute respiratory failure. If the cause of the respiratory distress is not found after assessing the airway, breathing, and circulation, a more in-depth review of the patient's recent ICU course should be done with the patient's nurse. Clues to the patient's distress (e.g., aspiration, recent medications, procedures) likely can be learned from this discussion.

Chest x-ray (CXR) and ABG analysis are sensible components of the workup of a patient in respiratory distress. The CXR should be reviewed for pathology paying special attention to the location of the endotracheal tube in intubated patients. An ABG analysis is key to assessing oxygenation and ventilation as well as data about the patient's acid-base balance. Analysis of the ABGs can determine the alveolar-arterial (A-a) oxygen gradient, which is a comparison of the fractional inspired oxygen (FIO_2) to partial pressure of oxygen in the ABGs. A large A-a gradient without signs of abnormality on the CXR should raise suspicion for pulmonary embolism. Although CXR and ABGs are useful adjuncts, they are not necessary to make the decision to intubate a patient struggling to breathe. In less critical situations, the SOAP mnemonic can be used to guide the decision whether to intubate patients:

*S*ecretions that are excessive and cannot be cleared by the patient
*O*xygenation that is inadequate
*A*irway compromise or obstruction
*P*ulmonary function not meeting ventilatory needs

Intubation in the ICU is generally a risky undertaking because most patients have cardiopulmonary disturbances that do not allow for adequate preoxygenation coupled with a hyperdynamic state of very high oxygen consumption. There is little margin for error, and only one attempt is possible before cardiac arrest in many patients. For these reasons, clinicians in the ICU should have extensive training in intubating these patients; otherwise, it is imperative to seek assistance from someone more skilled. If time allows, the anesthesia record of postoperative patients should be reviewed to learn the airway findings, type of laryngoscope blade used, and any other difficulties previously encountered. Given the high degree of intra-abdominal processes in the surgical ICU, all patients should be treated as if they are at high risk for aspiration, and rapid-sequence intubation (RSI) should be considered the norm. The key principles of RSI are preoxygenation with 100% oxygen via a face mask, avoidance of bag-mask ventilation to reduce gastric distention, brisk induction with hypnotic agents, and short-onset paralytic agents followed by placement of an oral endotracheal tube by direct laryngoscopy. Patients who are in extremis and cannot be intubated or ventilated by bag-mask ventilation should undergo emergent cricothyroidotomy.

Although there are many pharmacologic options for RSI, a few standout as uniquely suited to for this purpose. Benzodiazepines, narcotics, and sedative-hypnotics all are suitable induction agents. Etomidate is a quick-onset and ultra-short-acting sedative-hypnotic agent that has minimal adverse effects on hemodynamics, which is a problem associated with many other sedating agents. Propofol, another ultra-short-acting hypnotic agent, and midazolam, a short-acting benzodiazepine, can be used for intubation but cause more hypotension, which is an undesirable complicating factor in urgent intubations. Ketamine is a dissociative agent that is chemically related to the street drug PCP (phenylcyclohexyl piperidine) and is a useful agent for RSI because it can provide sedation and hypnosis without causing hemodynamic compromise. Compared with etomidate, ketamine was shown to result in lower rates of adrenal insufficiency in a randomized trial of critically ill patients requiring intubation because etomidate directly inhibits cortisol production by blocking 11β-hydroxylase in the adrenal cortex. The anticortisol effect of etomidate is worth considering in patients with distributive shock of unclear cause because this effect may persist 12 to 24 hours after administration. Paralytics are part of the RSI algorithm, and the two most commonly used drugs are succinylcholine and rocuronium. As previously mentioned, succinylcholine is a short-acting depolarizing paralytic agent with a half-life of approximately 15 seconds that is useful in RSI because it wears off fairly quickly, which may be lifesaving in patients who cannot be intubated. Rocuronium is the most rapidly acting of all the nondepolarizing paralytic agents and is indicated in cases where succinylcholine is contraindicated (see "Analgesia, Sedation, and Neuromuscular Blockade" for these contraindications). Few clinical trials comparing the safety and effectiveness of paralytic agents have been performed in the ICU setting, but a randomized investigation did not show any difference in intubation failure rates, desaturation events, or intubation conditions when succinylcholine was compared with rocuronium.

Noninvasive and Mechanical Ventilation

In some special circumstances, it may be possible to avoid intubation and full mechanical ventilation, particularly if the cause of the respiratory failure is identified and can be readily reversed. Patients with hypoxemia and increased work of breathing may be temporarily supported with noninvasive means until intravenous diuretics can treat their volume overload. Similarly, hypoventilating patients who are overnarcotized may be supported with these devices while they are given narcotic reversal agents such as naloxone or their epidural infusion is turned down. Noninvasive ventilatory support is a bridging therapy and should not be considered as a definitive treatment; if the underlying cause of hypoxia or inadequate ventilation cannot be treated in a timely fashion, formal intubation is mandatory. Options for noninvasive ventilation include continuous positive airway pressure (CPAP), bilevel positive airway pressure (BiPAP), and high-flow humidified oxygen systems. CPAP acts by providing a continuous level of positive pressure through a tight-fitting mask maintaining a patient's functional residual capacity (FRC) and is more effective for treating type I respiratory failure. CPAP does not aid ventilation and should be used with caution in patients with an altered sensorium because they may vomit into the mask and aspirate and die. BiPAP, similar to CPAP, provides a continuous level of positive airway pressure to augment FRC but also adds a driving pressure when patients initiate a breath, which can augment ventilation. Through its support of oxygenation and ventilation, BiPAP is effective in treating type II respiratory failure. Patients on CPAP and BiPAP require careful monitoring, and plans should always be in place denoting the duration of the noninvasive trial, end points of therapy, and action plans should the respiratory failure worsen. High-flow oxygen humidification systems are a more recent addition to the respiratory support armamentarium and are effective in augmenting a patient's oxygenation without desiccating the upper airways and nasal passages. Literature has shown that postoperative surgical patients who develop recurrent respiratory failure after extubation should be promptly intubated except in certain rare circumstances, the most notable exception being antecedent chronic obstructive respiratory disease, where BiPAP may be effective in overcoming recurrent respiratory failure.

Many terms and management concepts are similar whether a patient is on CPAP, BiPAP, or standard mechanical ventilation. The FIO_2 is the concentration of oxygen in the inspiratory flow delivered to the patient. Positive end expiratory pressure (PEEP) is delivered at the end of exhalation and prevents small airway closure, which maintains or increases the FRC. PEEP and FIO_2 are the main determinants of oxygenation, but there are limits to how much they may be increased before the patient starts experiencing negative sequelae. High PEEP may adversely affect hemodynamics by decreasing venous return to the heart, where high FIO_2 can lead to the generation of oxygen free radicals, which may damage many cell types in the lungs. It is often easier to conceptualize oxygenation and ventilation as two separate and unrelated entities, each affected by different parameters. Although this conceptualization is helpful, it is not accurate because there is significant overlap and interplay between the determinants of each. Ventilation is governed by the minute volume, which is a product of the respiratory rate and tidal volume. Increasing the driving pressure increases the tidal volume but may result in barotrauma as pressures rise, whereas increasing the respiratory rate also increases the minute volume, but at higher rates the lungs may become hyperinflated because there is inadequate time for complete exhalation.

In general, the more ill the patient, the more controlled his or her ventilatory support should be. The clinician should set the ventilator so that most components of the respiratory cycle are governed by the machine, so the patient will get the desired minute and tidal volumes to ensure ventilation and oxygenation. Assist or support modes augment patient-initiated breaths by adding defined amounts of positive pressure to each breath and adding PEEP to maintain FRC. Patients placed on controlled modes of ventilation are usually cycled according to preset tidal volume and peak airway pressure goals; these are termed *volume control ventilation* and *pressure control ventilation*, respectively. When volume control ventilation is employed, decreases in airway, lung, or chest wall compliance alter the delivered tidal volume, and the ventilator's processors alter the pressure until the desired volume is delivered, but this mode may result in barotrauma. Most modern ventilators have a setting termed *pressure regulated volume control*, where a targeted tidal volume is delivered but the delineated peak pressure is not exceeded. Older modes such as assist control have limited utility and should be used only in patients who are deeply sedated or receiving neuromuscular blockade. Spontaneously breathing patients should not be on assist control because this typically results in overventilation and severe respiratory alkalosis.

Pressure control modes are best suited to situations in which the clinician is concerned about changing airway and lung compliance. In these modes, the driving pressure, respiratory rate, PEEP, and FIO_2 are set by the clinician, but the tidal volume delivered depends on the patient's thoracic compliance. Pressure control modes are more labor intensive because minute ventilation can vary as compliance changes. Investigations are often necessary to identify the causes of the changing compliance, but these modes may protect against barotrauma. In this mode, decreasing tidal volumes should prompt an evaluation for causes of decreased compliance, such as pneumothorax, mucous plugging, endotracheal tube obstruction, bronchospasm, worsening abdominal distention, and ACS. Pressure control modes can also be mandatory, assisted, or entirely patient initiated. The pressure control mode where all breaths are patient initiated is termed *pressure support ventilation* (PSV). In PSV modes, the driving pressure, PEEP, and FIO_2 are set, but the respiratory rate and tidal volume are determined by the patient, and it is generally more comfortable for patients. PSV typically results in less need for sedation, which renders it an excellent choice for weaning from mechanical ventilation.

Weaning and Extubation

From the very first moments an intubated patient arrives in the surgical ICU or shortly after an ICU patient is intubated, providers should be considering the possible duration of ventilation and formulating a plan to wean and extubate the patient. Prolonged mechanical ventilation is associated with ventilator-induced lung injury, pneumonia, deconditioning, and other adverse outcomes. Although there are several important benefits from liberation from mechanical ventilation, inappropriate or overzealous attempts at weaning should be avoided because they can result in extubation failure and the need for emergent reintubation with its attendant risks. Generally, one of the first questions that must be answered when considering extubating a patient is: Has the process that created the initial conditions requiring mechanical ventilation still present? When this question is answered, the clinician should review the response to daily awakening and SBTs, the patient's mental status and hemodynamics, anticipated procedures, and impending travel out of the ICU for diagnostic or therapeutic interventions. Despite large numbers of investigations over the last 2 decades, there is no one set of criteria or objective measures that can guide patient selection for weaning and extubation, and the decision-making process must combine objective elements with clinical judgment.

The decision to extubate an awake and oriented patient is far easier than deciding to extubate a patient with encephalopathy, traumatic brain injury (TBI), delirium, or other causes of altered mental status. An adequate mental status is an important determinant not only of a patient's ability to protect his or her airway but also whether they will participate in pulmonary toileting measures that are critical to staving off the need for reintubation. Information gathered during "sedation holidays" can greatly simplify this determination. After assessing the patient's mental status, focus should shift to an assessment of the patient's oxygenation, and the most recent ABG analysis should be reviewed. The partial pressure of oxygen from the ABG analysis can be divided by the FIO_2 to calculate a P : F ratio, which is an objective measure of the patient's oxygenation and is used in the Berlin definition of ARDS. Patients who have acute lung injury (P : F <300) or ARDS (P : F <200) are rarely successfully extubated, and efforts should be focused instead on optimizing their oxygenation rather than extubation. Another useful calculation is the rapid shallow breathing index (RSBI), which was developed in the early 1990s as a measure to predict suitability for extubation and has been successfully validated in several large clinical trials. RSBI is defined as the ratio of respiratory rate (breaths per minute) to tidal volume (liters) while a patient is on zero driving pressure and PEEP. Patients with an RSBI of 105 or greater are highly unlikely to be successfully extubated; patients scoring lower have higher chances of a successful extubation.[15] As stated earlier, SBTs are useful in predicting successful extubation, but there is no uniform definition of the technique for a SBT. Some techniques described include low-level PEEP (5 cm H_2O) without additional driving pressure, PSV with low-level settings of PEEP, and driving pressure or T-piece trials in which the patient is removed from positive pressure and is given supplemental oxygen only but remains intubated. It is likely that the lack of positive pressure and PEEP coupled with the airway resistance of the endotracheal tube is the real test of the patient's reserve and is the reason behind the predictive value of the SBT. Randomized studies comparing SBT strategies of PSV versus T-tube have not shown significant differences in percentages of patients who have remained extubated after 48 hours, but both of these measures are useful in formulating a decision to extubate a patient.

Pneumonia, Acute Respiratory Distress Syndrome, Salvage Modes of Ventilation, and Extracorporeal Membrane Oxygenation

Although pneumonia is not thought of as a surgical disease, the highest rates of ventilator-associated pneumonia (VAP) are observed in surgical critical care units, with the top rates of VAP occurring in trauma and neurosurgical ICUs. It is important to make this distinction because understanding the processes that increase the risk of patients developing VAP allows providers to embrace strategies to lessen its occurrence. Factors such as poor postoperative pain control, inadequate pulmonary toilet, immobilization, and prolonged mechanical ventilation all should be addressed to reduce the risk of VAP. Upper midline abdominal and thoracic incisions result in significant pain causing splinting, shallow respirations, atelectasis, and poor clearance of secretions; it is theorized that advancements in minimally invasive techniques such as video-assisted thoracic surgery, laparoscopic surgical approaches, and endovascular surgical approaches will lead to lower pneumonia rates. VAP is one of the leading nosocomial infections causing death in surgical ICUs. Although it may be an oversimplification, it is impossible to get VAP without a ventilator, and so the most effective preventive measure is timely extubation. The concept of combining several associated interventions to reduce VAP led to the development of the "VAP bundle," which seeks to improve the care of ventilated patients and to reduce the occurrence of VAP. The components of this bundle are head of bed elevation to 30 degrees, oral care with chlorhexidine solution, sedation interruption, and SBTs. Additional elements such as venous thromboembolic prophylaxis and preventive agents for stress ulcer bleeding have been added to this bundle as well, which is ironic because more recent evidence shows that proton pump inhibitors (PPIs) are associated with an increased risk of VAP. Many ICUs have adopted "VAP prevention" teams that make rounds multiple times a week with checklists to follow bundle compliance and have resulted in lower VAP rates.

Despite the severity of the problem, there is still no universally accepted definition of VAP. The U.S. Centers for Disease Control and Prevention (CDC) has introduced the concept of ventilator-associated events to include other conditions contributing to prolonged mechanical ventilation. The diagnosis of ventilator-associated events according to the CDC criteria is objective and systematic, but this is not the case with VAP, the diagnosis of which remains highly controversial. CXR findings have been shown to be highly subjective rendering them ill-suited for the diagnosis of VAP. Scoring systems such as the Clinical Pulmonary Infection Score may not be valid in certain patient populations as it has limited utility in surgical patients because of the presence of many factors consistent with the systemic inflammatory response syndrome (SIRS). In particular, the Clinical Pulmonary Infection Score is not helpful in diagnosing VAP in trauma patients because these patients tend to have the most pronounced SIRS response mimicking infections.[16] The most consistent finding in patients with VAP is hypoxemia, worsening oxygenation, and the inability to wean, so VAP should be high on the differential diagnosis list anytime these problems arise.

It has been well documented that ineffective or delayed therapy for VAP leads to higher mortality, and clinicians treating ICU patients with suspected VAP face the dual challenge of diagnosing this entity and initiating the correct therapy. The most effective strategy for treating patients with suspected VAP may center around the use of either blind or bronchoscopically directed quantitative cultures followed by administration of empirical antibiotics. The choice of the antibiotic is determined by several factors, including the antibiogram of the ICU, the time from hospital admission, and previous antibiotic therapy. Quantitative cultures do not increase the sensitivity of detecting pneumonia, but they dramatically increase diagnostic specificity, which allows de-escalation from broad-spectrum empirical agents to narrow-spectrum agents. Sputum culture is an inaccurate diagnostic modality that typically results in the growth of multiple organisms, which severely limits de-escalation.

Significant progress has been made in treating and preventing ARDS since Ashbaugh's first descriptions in the *Lancet* of a heterogeneous group of patients including patients with severe injuries, pneumonia, pancreatitis, burns, ventilator-induced injury, blood product transfusions, and infections who all manifested ARDS. The mortality of ARDS remains quite high; the cause of death is rarely profound hypoxia and more commonly multiorgan failure or infection. Terms such as "shock lung" or "white lung" are no longer used, and the Berlin definition is replacing the criteria put forth in 1994 by the American European Consensus Conference (AECC) that defined and categorized ARDS. The AECC criteria for ARDS stated that the following elements were required for a diagnosis: P : F 200 or less, bilateral and diffuse CXR infiltrates, and noncardiogenic pulmonary edema with pulmonary artery wedge pressure less than 18 if available. Acute lung injury was a precursor of ARDS and was defined as a P : F between 200 and 300. The main criticisms of the AECC criteria have been that they underestimate the prevalence of ARDS, have limited prognostic value, and are misleading because higher levels of PEEP may raise the P : F above 200. In 2012, the European Society of Intensive Care Medicine put forth the Berlin definition to broaden the hypoxemic categorization of ARDS to capture more patients with the syndrome. A P : F of 201 to 300 was consistent with mild ARDS, 101 to 200 was consistent with moderate ARDS, and less than 100 was consistent with severe life-threatening ARDS.[17]

The classic pathologic findings of ARDS are generalized lung inflammation and neutrophil infiltration caused by parenchymal cytokine release leading to diffuse alveolar and capillary damage. Endothelial injury results in leakage of protein-rich edema fluid into the alveoli and the formation of hyaline membranes. Efforts to modify the disease process using corticosteroids, dietary supplements, antioxidants, and surfactants have met with limited success; thus, prevention of ARDS is paramount. A landmark multicenter randomized trial found that ventilation using low tidal volumes (6 mL/kg of ideal body weight) compared with traditional tidal volumes (12 mL/kg) in patients with ARDS was associated with lower plateau pressures, more ventilator-free days, and overall reduced mortality.[18] No other investigation of ARDS has affected outcomes, management, and prevention of ARDS more than this one, and it ushered in a new era recognizing that excessive tidal volumes and airway pressures result in alveolar stretch, shear stresses, and damage to the pulmonary epithelium and endothelium. Patients ventilated with lower tidal volumes were found to have lower levels of interleukin-6 suggesting that this strategy causes less lung and systemic inflammation. The lower tidal volume group required higher levels of PEEP comparable to the higher tidal volume group, and it is theorized that higher mean and plateau pressures reduced alveolar shear and stretch, forces termed *volutrauma*. This appreciation of volutrauma led to ventilator management strategies that have lessened the incidence of ARDS and reduced systemic inflammation.

When patients develop hypoxemia that is refractory to maneuvers such as increasing FIO_2, PEEP, and driving pressure, salvage modes of mechanical ventilation should be considered. Two of these modes are airway pressure release ventilation (APRV) and high-frequency percussive ventilation (HFPV) via a volumetric diffusive respirator (VDR). The goals of APRV are to minimize alveolar phasic opening and closing, limiting shear stresses and maintaining a high mean airway pressure. In APRV, the patient is maintained at a pressure high (P-high) for a period of time (T-high) during which the patient can take spontaneous breaths followed by a brief period of release of pressure (T-low), at which time the airway pressure decreases down to a baseline level (P-low) that is akin to PEEP. The amount of time spent at T-low is less than the time it takes for the small airway to close; APRV maintains a high MAP and promotes oxygenation. It is typical for the ratio of time at P-high to P-low to be in the range of 4 or 5 seconds to 1 second, and this is probably why this mode was initially called "continuous positive airway pressure with an intermittent release phase." APRV mainly improves oxygenation but can cause problems in patients with chronic obstructive pulmonary disease because of the short pressure release times and air trapping.

HFPV is essentially a pressure-controlled mode of ventilation that requires a specialized machine, the VDR, to deliver subphysiologic tidal volumes at high frequencies superimposed on typical ventilator flow. The VDR uses lower peak pressures and PEEP than conventional settings because it maintains a higher mean airway pressure. It can mobilize secretions in patients with inhalation injury or pneumonia owing to eddy currents that form around the aliquots of air as the subphysiologic tidal volumes are delivered in a percussive fashion. Numerous investigations involving patients with inhalation injury and ARDS have shown improved P : F ratios and lower peak pressures with HFPV compared with conventional modes, but there are no significant randomized data to show mortality benefit with HFPV. APRV and HFPV are similar in that both use higher mean airway pressures and smaller tidal volumes; this likely minimizes volutrauma, although comparative studies are lacking.

The H1N1 influenza outbreak resulted in an increase in interest in extracorporeal membrane oxygenation (ECMO) as a salvage therapy for patients with florid ARDS. ECMO facilitates lung rest and healing and can break the cycle of ongoing lung injury because it can take over most of the patient's ventilation and oxygenation needs and avoids the high airway pressures and volutrauma that occur as part of ventilator management for patients with ARDS. The CESAR study in 2009 was one of the first randomized trials that assessed the benefits of ECMO for ARDS in 180 patients with severe respiratory failure.[19] These patients were randomly assigned to conventional ventilator versus ECMO, and the study found less disability and fatalities in the ECMO group 6 months after ICU discharge. The CESAR study demonstrated that ECMO therapy was approximately twice as expensive as conventional therapy, but that this cost was offset in gained quality-adjusted life-years.[19] The CESAR study findings have been echoed in more recent observational studies, and the concept of transferring patients with ARDS to ECMO centers is gaining popularity, even if it requires a mobile ECMO treatment team to transport these critically ill patients.

Prone positioning is useful for treating patients with severe ARDS. Similar to ECMO, there is some resistance to embrace this therapy because of the logistical challenges it presents. Prone positioning results in improved ventilation and perfusion matching as well as alveolar recruitment to improve oxygenation and reduce volutrauma. Multiple randomized trials have shown improved oxygenation with prone positioning, but until more recently few have shown a survival benefit. Although most ICU providers view prone positioning as a salvage therapy for patients with severe ARDS, emerging data show that this modality is an effective adjunct for treating ARDS, especially if used early in the disease process. Caring for patients in the prone position requires significant nursing resources, and there is always a concern about endotracheal or other tube dislodgments, skin breakdown, and limited access to the patient in emergent situations. Surgical patients in particular have unique challenges to prone positioning because of abdominal incisions, open abdomens, and unstable spine injuries.[20]

Special Issues: Tracheostomy and Obesity

Tracheostomy often conjures up negative images for patients, families, and providers, who sometimes equate it with signs of futility; however, numerous studies have shown it to be beneficial in critically ill patients. Placement of a tracheostomy can facilitate ventilator weaning in patients with chronic obstructive pulmonary disease or cardiomyopathy because of its ability to reduce dead space ventilation and work of breathing. It can improve clearance of secretions in patients with altered mental status, TBI, or neuromuscular weakness and provides a stable airway for comatose patients. Discontinuing an endotracheal tube results in a marked reduction in the patient's sedation requirements, which promotes wakefulness, spontaneous respiration, and ventilator weaning and increases liberation from mechanical ventilation. Tracheostomy can prevent airway narrowing and obstruction, which often plagues patients with long-term endotracheal intubation secondary to buildup of biofilm and debris on the inner wall of the tube because the inner cannula of the tracheostomy is easily changed.

The timing of tracheostomy in patients with prolonged respiratory failure is controversial; previously, patients commonly remained orally intubated for 14 or more days before the procedure was considered. More recent data show decreased ICU lengths of stay and duration of mechanical ventilation, without increased complication rates, when tracheostomy is performed within 7 days of the institution of mechanical ventilation. The benefits of early tracheostomy has been further supported by investigations showing similar results in a mixed population of medical, surgical, and trauma patients who underwent tracheostomy within 3 days of the initiation of mechanical ventilation. Bedside bronchoscopic-guided percutaneous tracheostomy in the ICU has become standard in most institutions and is associated with lower costs and less transport complications, delays, postoperative hemorrhage, and infections compared with open tracheostomy done in the operating room.[21] There are relatively few contraindications to percutaneous tracheostomy, and many of the previously identified contraindications, such as coagulopathy and obesity, have been disproven as evidence and experience with the procedure mount.

Obesity is a growing epidemic in the United States and the developed world and presents significant challenges to the entire critical care team. One in three Americans and one in four ICU patients has a body mass index greater than 30, which is the defining number for class I obesity. Almost every aspect of the respiratory system in an obese patient is more difficult, including bag-mask ventilations, intubation, emergency surgical airway placement, ventilator management and weaning, and tracheostomy. The anatomic effects of obesity on pulmonary physiology are too many to list but include increased airway resistance from parapharyngeal fat, collapsible airways from tracheomalacia, and decreased compliance from weight of the chest wall and pressure from abdominal girth. The most significant pulmonary problem from obesity is a consistent decrease in FRC, especially in dependent lung areas, that causes a marked ventilation/perfusion mismatch. At rest, obese patients have been shown to have a 60% increase in oxygen consumption compared with nonobese patients, and half of this extra oxygen consumption in the obese is energy required for the act of breathing.[22] These patients can have obesity hypoventilation syndrome, which has a neurally mediated mechanism that decreases respiratory drive leading to hypoxia and hypercarbia. Obstructive sleep apnea is much more common as body mass index increases, and this can be a particularly dangerous problem in a postoperative patient who has residual anesthetic and narcotics in his or her system. It is important for surgeons to consider obstructive sleep apnea as they formulate their postoperative care plans not only for patients with known obstructive sleep apnea but also for patients with obesity.

Obese patients are particularly subject to becoming hypoxemic during intubation because of their limited pulmonary reserve, increased oxygen demand, and anatomic obstacles such as a short stout neck and airway abnormalities. Once intubated, obese patients should be ventilated with tidal volumes based on their ideal body weight and not their actual body weight because the latter would lead to potentially injurious barotrauma. Ideal body weight for men is calculated as 50 ± 2.3 kg for each inch over 5 feet and for women is calculated as 45.5 ± 2.3 kg for each inch over 5 feet. Obese patients have diminished FRC, and slightly increased levels of PEEP may be helpful in reducing alveolar collapse and improving lung and chest wall compliance.

GASTROINTESTINAL SYSTEM

Background, Malnutrition, and Catabolism of Critical Illness

Major surgery, injury, and critical illness all induce a stress response that quickly leads to loss of lean body mass and an ongoing catabolic state; this remains an area of prime focus for many researchers interested in inflammation. Several converging factors align to contribute to this catabolic state, including decreased oral intake because of NPO states, anorexia secondary to injury and inflammation, and anatomic obstacles to enteral nutrition such as intestinal surgery. Many surgical diseases are treated with bowel rest including ileus, pancreatitis, intestinal ischemia, and intra-abdominal infections, which greatly limits the intake of substrate at a time of elevated catabolism. For most clinicians, nutritional issues are often secondary in terms of acuity or urgency compared with problems affecting the cardiovascular or respiratory systems, leading to the insidious nature of malnutrition and catabolism. The important contribution of nutrition and metabolism to outcomes has been recognized only more recently by many ICU providers. Although nutrition in the ICU is usually thought to be a way of preserving lean body mass to promote mobilization, weaning from mechanical ventilation, and overall recovery, it is now recognized that nutrition has a direct effect on infectious outcomes and complications.[23]

The catabolism associated with critically ill surgical patients appears to be multifactorial and is likely the result of a complex interplay among direct tissue injury, pain, immune-inflammatory activation, and ischemia-reperfusion injury leading to negative nitrogen balance and increased energy consumption. As part of the normal stress response, relative insulin resistance develops, and glucose is not as readily used by tissues leading to increased breakdown of protein and fat stores. The so-called protein-sparing effect of intravenous glucose solutions in critically ill patients is inconsequential, and this should never be thought of as addressing nutritional needs for the sickest patients. Not only are protein stores broken down during critical illness, but also there is a shift in protein synthesis to proteins necessary for creating and maintaining the inflammatory state; this is illustrated by the classic concept that serum albumin falls in response to illness because it is a "negative acute phase reactant," whereas C-reactive protein and other inflammatory mediators are greatly increased. In addition to protein and fat stores, the body's stores of vitamins and trace elements are consumed rapidly during this time. Many of these vitamins and trace elements have critical roles in organ function, immune competence, and wound healing, and deficiencies in these contribute to complications.

Muscle weakness and functional limitations may persist for years after ICU discharge. Although this prolonged period of weakness commences during the catabolic phase, the exact mechanisms have not been elucidated. It is known that for muscle stores to become depleted, the consumption of amino acids, especially the branched chain varieties—leucine, isoleucine, and valine—must exceed their intake because these are essential amino acids. A study from the United Kingdom looked at acute skeletal muscle wasting in critically ill patients who were in the ICU more than 7 days and on mechanical ventilation for at least 2 days and found that there were significant declines in the cross-sectional area of the quadriceps muscle, measured by ultrasound, and increased muscle breakdown. These negative effects were seen day 1 to day 7 of study enrollment and were greater in patients with multiorgan failure compared with patients with single-system failure, which suggests that the catabolic effects of critical illness are proportional to the "dose" of the illness. Furthermore, the degree of muscle loss correlated with increases in C-reactive protein levels and decreases in oxygenation, supporting the concept that muscle wasting is a product of critical illness and organ failure.[24] Although muscle loss and functional deficits are known to occur in healthy, well-fed individuals when placed on bed rest, these declines occur surprisingly quickly in critically ill patients, despite adequate delivery of calories and protein.

Assessment of Malnutrition and Energy Requirements

Regardless of the high prevalence of malnutrition and catabolism in the surgical ICU and years of research focusing on this problem, there is no uniform assessment method, laboratory value, or metric to identify the patients at greatest risk for nutrition-related poor outcomes. In the past, weight loss of a certain percentage of body weight coupled with physical examination findings in the setting of decreased caloric intake defined malnutrition. Although weight loss of greater than 10% to 15% of body weight before ICU admission has been shown to be associated with increased mortality in surgical patients, this is a very crude assessment of malnutrition. In 2010, the American Society for Parenteral and Enteral Nutrition (ASPEN) and the European Society for Clinical Nutrition and Metabolism proposed three distinct types of malnutrition: chronic starvation without inflammation, chronic disease-related malnutrition with mild to moderate chronic inflammation, and acute disease-related malnutrition with acute and severe inflammation. The incorporation of inflammation takes into consideration the "dose" of critical illness and alerts providers to patients, such as obese patients, who are more likely to develop malnutrition despite the perception of them being "overfed."[25]

ASPEN and the Academy of Nutrition and Dietetics modified the 2010 definitions by including the presence of two or more of the following: inadequate energy intake, unintentional weight loss, wasting on physical examination, and decreased grip strength or functional loss.[26] The Subjective Global Assessment and the Malnutrition Universal Screening Tool look at similar factors as the ASPEN screening guidelines, but both of these tools are limited in their ability to assess malnutrition in different hospital acuity levels, particularly the ICU. Obese patients are very difficult to assess because their body habitus often masks some of the physical examination findings on which many of these tools focus. Laboratory values are equally limited in their ability to define malnutrition. The often cited serum markers (e.g., albumin, prealbumin, retinol binding protein) are more indicative of inflammation or illness rather than a measure of how well the patient's nutritional needs are being met. Indirect calorimetry is a preferred modality that determines a patient's oxygen consumption and carbon dioxide production to provide accurate and objective guidance for nutritional delivery; however, it is expensive, not readily available in all institutions, and impractical in patients on high FIO_2. Indirect calorimetry is a static measurement, and its utility in identifying the nutritional needs of metabolic active and ever-changing ICU patients is limited. In the absence of good objective measurements or in difficult-to-assess patients, the standard recommendations of 25 kcal/kg/day and 1 to 2 g/kg of protein are a good fallback option; however, "one size does not fit all," and adjustments should be made based on premorbid nutritional status, functional status, medications, comorbidities, and the degree of injury or inflammation.

Body weight, physical examination, and to a lesser degree laboratory markers are subject to significant fluctuations in ICU patients as a result of fluid shifts between intravascular and extravascular compartments, which masks loss of muscle or adipose mass. Tissue imaging techniques to estimate lean body mass and nutritional status and body composition analysis have progressed rapidly from anthropometric measurements to x-ray absorptiometric techniques to present-day CT scan–dependent methods. CT is now recognized as the most accurate means of body composition analysis. With CT scanning, tissue densities and cross-sectional area of muscle groups can be assessed. The third lumbar vertebra has been identified as the conventional CT landmark where cross-sectional analysis of tissue best reflects total body muscle volume and lean body mass. Alternatively, psoas muscle cross-sectional area can be used as a marker of cachexia and malnutrition and may have some prognostic value based on more recent data. The shortcomings of using CT to assess nutritional status are cost, ionizing radiation, and need for transport; bedside tools such as ultrasound are gaining popularity and may become the standard way we monitor how effectively we are delivering nutrition to critically ill patients.

Enteral Feeding

Critically ill patients have multiple factors adversely affecting their ability to eat or take in substrate to meet their nutritional needs, but there is often hesitancy among providers to address this problem. Analogous to the prior discussion about a plan for ventilator weaning being established immediately after the initiation of mechanical ventilation, so too should a complete, individualized nutritional plan be established for ICU patients on admission. All intubated patients should have an oral or nasogastric tube placed for administration of medications and liquid food or "tube feeds," and the position of these tubes must be confirmed radiographically before anything is given through them. Patients who are not intubated and who are unable to eat because of an altered sensorium, sedatives, narcotics, or anorexia should have a small-bore nasogastric tube placed as well. These tubes are readily tolerated and are not as prone to clogging as pure feeding tubes; they also allow for gastric suctioning and decompression should that be required. The nutritional plan should never be "the patient will start eating tomorrow" because more often than not tomorrow never comes, and the patient's nutritional deficits become even greater. The advantages of enteral nutrition continue to accrue in the literature and include maintaining gut integrity, trophic effects on the liver, increased intestinal immunoglobulin production, decreased infection rates, and more stable glycemic profiles. In some patients, such as patients with burn injuries and patients with TBI, enteral nutrition has been shown not only to reduce the rates of ileus and gastroparesis but also to reduce septic complications and promote better neurologic outcomes.

Several barriers to the effective delivery of enteral nutrition exist, but one of the most common and troubling reasons that patient's needs are not met is frequent interruptions for various reasons, such as turning the patient for care, washing or bedding changes, diagnostic imaging studies, bedside procedures, and ill-conceived NPO orders. Patients undergoing elective surgery are kept NPO for 8 hours before intubation for fear of gastric aspiration; however, this reason does not make sense in an ICU patient with a critical need for nutrition who has a cuffed tube in the airway as well as a gastric tube for decompression. These patients should have their tube feeding stopped immediately before leaving the ICU for the operating room, their nasogastric tube or feeding tube flushed, and the stomach decompressed via suctioning. Perhaps the most vexing reason tube feedings are stopped centers around gastric residual volume (GRV) measurements. Trials have shown that GRV measurements of 500 mL should be tolerated so that the patient's nutritional needs are met, without fear of increased aspiration events.[27] Most clinicians picture the pylorus as a patent drain that allows unfettered egress of tube feeding from the stomach into the duodenum, but this is in direct opposition to gastric physiology, which mandates that receptive relaxation of the stomach must occur before gastric emptying ensues. Although feeding intolerance can result from gastroparesis and ileus, which are common entities in ICU patients, clinicians should have a higher tolerance for GRV without undue fear of aspiration. Patients with ongoing elevated GRV and feeding intolerance require a thoughtful evaluation because new-onset feeding intolerance is often a harbinger of impending sepsis or infectious complications. The medical record and bedside nurse should be queried to determine when the patient last had a bowel movement, and a digital rectal examination should be performed looking for fecal impaction. The feeding tube should be checked for patency and proper location on radiographs, which may also yield data on the presence of ileus, pseudo-obstruction, or suspected pneumonia, all of which are associated with feeding intolerance. Some patients, especially patients with extensive intra-abdominal surgery or injury, may require a CT scan to rule out intra-abdominal abscess as a cause of the intolerance. Patients who continue to fail attempts at gastric feeding can be treated with prokinetic agents such as erythromycin or metoclopramide or receive a postpyloric feeding tube. Postpyloric tubes are effective in circumventing gastroparesis but offer no advantage to patients with ileus and are not associated with lower rates of aspiration or pneumonia. Lastly, patients on moderate to high doses of vasopressors should not receive enteral nutrition because of the rare complication of bowel necrosis from the increased intestinal oxygen demand induced by feeding in the setting of splanchnic ischemia.

The concept of feeding to meet a 24-hour total nutritional goal has emerged more recently and shows promise in overcoming some of the previously discussed challenges to delivering enteral nutrition. Because any interruption in tube feeding hinders the delivery of the patient's required calories and yet some interruptions in tube feeding are unavoidable, the new strategy empowers the bedside nurse to alter the rate of continuous tube feeding drips or intervals between bolus tube feedings to compensate for any interruptions so that the patient's total caloric goal is met. Although this strategy has resulted in better and more complete delivery of enteral nutrition, it remains to be shown whether this has any direct effect on outcomes. Similarly, bolus tube feeding may be more effective in delivering nutrition because it is more physiologic and mirrors how patients eat normally. Bolus tube feeding has been shown to be a more effective method of delivering tube feeding in some patient populations, such as adult and pediatric burn patients, but experience in broader ICU populations is limited.

Parenteral Nutrition

One of the oldest adages in the ICU is "if the patient has a gut, use it," which reinforces the importance of good nutrition in critically ill patients and the benefits associated with enteral nutrition, but circumstances arise where patients cannot be fed enterally or the delivery of enteral nutrition has been inadequate despite aggressive measures. Bowel obstruction, enterocutaneous fistula, peritonitis, and active gastrointestinal bleeding all are contraindications to enteral nutrition, and in patients with these problems parenteral nutrition is an effective way to meet nutritional needs. The more difficult questions are: When will the patient regain gastrointestinal function? When should parenteral nutrition begin? How long can nutrition be withheld? In the United States, the typical approach is to wait 1 week for a patient who was previously well nourished to recover gastrointestinal function before starting parenteral nutrition. The Society for Critical Care Medicine and ASPEN support this approach in their guidelines because of concerns about complications of parenteral nutrition, including hypertriglyceridemia, hyperglycemia, cholestasis, and central line–associated bloodstream infections (CLABSI). Subsequent to these guidelines, randomized trials evaluated the effect of starting parenteral nutrition on the first day of ICU admission, but results of these studies have been mixed, and the only reproducible benefit has been reduced costs of enteral nutrition compared with parenteral nutrition. Some trials have shown decreased ICU length of stay and infections when patients received no nutrition compared with patients who received early parenteral nutrition; the optimal time to wait before starting parenteral nutrition remains unclear.

The risks and benefits of enteral nutrition and parenteral nutrition remain contentious and confusing because parenteral nutrition has received overly negative attention, and it is likely that the obstacles to delivering enteral nutrition have been understated. A randomized trial comparing enteral nutrition and parenteral nutrition within 36 hours of ICU admission demonstrated no differences in 90-day mortality, infectious complications, or several other secondary issues including the adequacy of caloric delivery between the two groups.[28] Previous investigations that demonstrated advantages of enteral nutrition over parenteral nutrition, especially in infectious outcomes, were limited by small sample sizes and confounding variables such as poor glycemic control. Parenteral nutrition tends to be far more reliable in its ability to meet nutritional needs because there are far fewer interruptions compared with enteral nutrition, and these needs are typically met sooner as well. Parenteral nutrition is usually ordered in a customized fashion with caloric needs established by weight-based calculations or indirect calorimetry. Amino acids, lipids, and dextrose are the key components along with electrolytes, vitamins, and trace elements. It is thought that the catabolism of critical illness that results in loss of lean body mass may be curtailed by increasing the protein content of parenteral formulas, but this is unsupported by evidence. Glutamine, the main fuel for enterocytes and leukocytes, has been added to parenteral nutrition in the hopes of maintaining immune competency as well as intestinal function, but insufficient evidence supports this practice. Customizing lipid preparations such that there are greater amounts of anti-inflammatory omega-3 fatty acids instead of proinflammatory omega-6 fatty acids has shown encouraging results, particularly in patients with ARDS. Patients on parenteral nutrition should receive balanced electrolytes in their formulas, and these should be adjusted daily as abnormalities emerge. Delivering nutrition after a prolonged period of starvation can result in life-threatening electrolyte imbalances termed *refeeding syndrome*, which is due to intracellular shift of potassium, magnesium, and phosphate leading to arrhythmias, respiratory failure, neurologic dysfunction, and possibly death, so permissive underfeeding is reasonable in these patients.

RENAL SYSTEM

AKI, one of the most common forms of organ failure, affects about one third of patients admitted to the surgical ICU within 24 hours of admission and is associated with increased mortality and a markedly diminished quality of life in patients requiring long-term RRT. AKI occurring in the ICU tends to recur more often than AKI occurring in other settings and greatly complicates the ICU management of patients because of its effects on fluid balance, acid-base status, electrolytes, arrhythmias, clearance of toxins and drug metabolites, encephalopathy, platelet function, and erythropoiesis. Because all organ systems are inter-related, AKI sometimes serves as the trigger in a cascade of organ systems leading to MSOF. AKI results in tremendous resource utilization and significantly increases ICU costs.

The Second International Consensus Conference of the Acute Dialysis Quality Initiative Group met and developed the AKI definition and subclassifications we know as the RIFLE criteria. RIFLE criteria consist of *r*isk, *i*njury, *f*ailure, *l*oss, and *e*nd-stage renal disease. In the past, the definition of renal dysfunction was not uniform, and at one point there were more than 30 definitions of this condition. RIFLE has been shown to be the most sensitive method for detecting AKI early in its course and is useful for prognostic purposes (Table 21-2).[29] The first sign of impending renal failure is oliguria, defined in adults as less than 0.5 mL/kg/hr or less than 400 mL per day or, less commonly, a sudden increase in serum creatinine. Oliguria is a common occurrence in the ICU and should prompt a thorough review of the patient's fluid balance, intake and output, and hemodynamics as well as a physical examination to assess the patient's volume status. Patients who have recently undergone a procedure should be carefully examined to ensure that bleeding is not the cause of oliguria, and a discussion with the bedside nurse should occur to determine if any new or recent medications have been administered. The causes of AKI fall broadly into three categories: prerenal causes secondary to diminished renal perfusion, intrinsic or parenchymal causes, and postrenal obstructive causes. Prerenal causes of AKI predominate in surgical patients, and the factors contributing to this are too numerous to list here. Often an initial appropriate first step is to administer a small bolus of isotonic crystalloid and observe the response while a diligent evaluation of the patient is undertaken. From the viewpoint of the kidney, systolic heart failure will appear to be a prerenal cause of oliguria because renal perfusion is diminished, but congestive failure ought to be easily discerned from dehydration on physical examination. A quick and relatively inexpensive way to confirm prerenal causes of oliguria involves checking urine electrolytes and calculating a fractional excretion of sodium (FeNa). A FeNa less than 1% is usually indicative of a prerenal cause, whereas FeNa greater than 3% indicates an intrinsic problem such as acute tubular necrosis (ATN). As already mentioned, there are caveats to a FeNa less than 1% because other conditions such as hepatorenal syndrome or congestive failure manifest this way, and recent diuretic administration tends to invalidate interpretation of the FeNa. Simple urinalysis contains a wealth of information to guide the workup of AKI because a high urine specific gravity and low pH are consistent with prerenal causes of AKI, whereas the presence of tubular or muddy brown casts is indicative of renal parenchymal disease such as ATN. The presence of eosinophils is associated with interstitial nephritis, whereas "large blood" with no red blood cells is indicative of muscle breakdown or intravascular hemolysis. ATN in the surgical ICU is often a progression from a prerenal condition that results from oxidative or ischemic injury to renal tubular cells, but similar to AKI itself, the causes of ATN are legion.

Restoring an effective circulating volume usually treats AKI resulting from prerenal hypovolemia, but there is no role for supranormal fluid resuscitation to encourage renal recovery. Once AKI is established, there are no interventions clinicians can employ to promote renal recovery, and the goals of management are to avoid further injury from nephrotoxins and recurrent hypoperfusion from hypovolemia and to adjust the dosing of renally cleared agents. Failure to adjust dosages of medications can have disastrous consequences, which is borne out by the example of enoxaparin, which can result in severe bleeding if administration

TABLE 21-2 RIFLE Criteria (Creatinine and Urine Output Indicators)

Risk	Increased serum creatinine × 1.5 or GFR decrease >25%	UOP <0.5 mL/kg/hr × 6 hr
Injury	Increased serum creatinine × 2 or GFR decrease >50%	UOP <0.5 mL/kg/hr × 12 hr
Failure	Increased serum creatinine × 3 or GFR decrease >75%	UOP <0.3 mL/kg/hr × 24 hr or anuria × 12 hr
Loss	Persistent ARF, complete loss of kidney function >4 wk	
ESRD	ESRD, complete loss of kidney function >3 mo	

ARF, acute renal failure; *ESRD*, end-stage renal disease; *GFR*, glomerular filtration rate; *UOP*, urine output.

is not adjusted for a decreasing creatinine clearance (C_{Cr}). The medications that require dosing adjustments or discontinuation are too numerous to list but include antibiotics, NSAIDs, antihypertensives, narcotics, and many others; it is a good idea to confer with a clinical pharmacist if available. An estimated C_{Cr} can be calculated by collecting a 24-hour urine collection and using the formula $C_{Cr} = (U_{Cr} \times V)/P_{Cr}$, where U_{Cr} = urine creatinine concentration (mg/dL), V = urine volume (mL/min), and P_{Cr} = plasma creatinine concentration (mg/dL), which yields the Cockcroft-Gault formula, $C_{Cr} = [(140 - \text{age}) \times \text{weight}]/(P_{Cr} \times 72)$. Weight is measured in kilograms, and in women the final value is multiplied by 0.85; normal C_{Cr} is about 95 mL/min in women and 120 mL/min in men. Because 24-hour urine collection is a lengthy process, many clinicians collect urine for shorter time periods and adjust the equation accordingly to extrapolate C_{Cr}. Lastly, diuretics should be held in patients with worsening AKI, and attempts to convert oliguric AKI to nonoliguric AKI do not affect the need for RRT or mortality.

One of the most common electrolyte disturbances in patients with AKI is hyperkalemia, which may result in arrhythmia and sudden cardiac death. New-onset hyperkalemia in the ICU should prompt a quick response from providers; the initial step is to repeat the laboratory test to confirm the first value. A plasma potassium level may be helpful in avoiding pseudohyperkalemia, which is common in postsplenectomy states and other thrombocytotic states. An ECG should also be assessed looking for peaked T waves and widening of the QRS complex, but literature shows that the detection of these findings in hyperkalemia is poor, even by trained cardiologists, so treatment should not be deferred in true cases of hyperkalemia based on ECG interpretation. Insulin, dextrose, sodium bicarbonate, and β_2 agonists all are effective at shifting potassium intracellularly and are effective temporizing measures, as is intravenous calcium, which stabilizes myocyte membranes. At higher levels of hyperkalemia, urgent hemodialysis should also be considered because it is the only effective way to reduce total body potassium. Diuretics and resins such as sodium polystyrene that pull electrolytes from the gastrointestinal tract have a limited role in the treatment of hyperkalemia because diuretics may worsen AKI, whereas resins with sorbitol have been associated with colonic ischemia and necrosis.

The need for RRT is often a critical branch point in the care of critically ill patients, and it is incumbent on providers to discuss goals of care with the patient's family and if possible the patient. Long-term outcomes for patients requiring RRT during critical illness are not favorable, and this needs to be discussed as part of a goal of therapy discussion. Indications for RRT are hyperkalemia, metabolic acidosis, severe volume overload, uremia causing encephalopathy or platelet-related bleeding, and some drug overdoses. Options for RRT included intermittent hemodialysis or continuous RRT. Hemodialysis works via a countercurrent exchange mechanism to remove solutes and ultrafiltration to remove volume and uses high flow rates, approaching 350 mL/min, which often results in tachycardia and hypotension. Hemodynamic instability and need for vasopressor support are relative contraindications for hemodialysis. Continuous venous hemofiltration, continuous venovenous hemodialysis, and continuous venovenous hemodiafiltration are the three most common forms of continuous RRT in the ICU, with the last-mentioned being the predominant mode. These continuous modes use low flow rates, which are better tolerated in hemodynamically unstable patients but at the expense of efficiency mandating their continuous usage. This slow rate is also associated with blood clotting in the dialysis circuit, so anticoagulants, heparin or citrates, are typically required, which may present problems for many patients in the surgical ICU. It remains to be seen whether the timing of RRT or the type of RRT (hemodialysis versus continuous RRT) improves outcomes such as mortality and renal recovery. A trial comparing hemodialysis with continuous RRT failed to show any appreciable differences in critically ill patients.[30]

HEPATIC SYSTEM

Cirrhosis and Perioperative Liver Decompensation

Few comorbidities present as daunting a challenge to intensivists as the management of cirrhosis in a surgical ICU patient. Similar to renal failure, liver failure is a complex and far-reaching condition because it entails management of diverse problems such as fluid shifts, coagulopathy, portal hypertension, hepatic encephalopathy, and hepatorenal syndrome, but in contrast to renal failure, there is no "liver dialysis" to support the patient. More patients with liver failure will present to the ICU in the future because the prevalence of infectious hepatitides and obesity-related nonalcoholic hepatic steatosis is expected to rise. More than 30 years ago, a landmark article examining the relationship between cirrhosis, abdominal surgery, and outcomes demonstrated mortality rates approaching 80% in patients with cirrhosis and a prothrombin time more than 2.5 seconds longer than in control subjects who underwent cholecystectomy. These fatalities were attributable to intra-abdominal hemorrhage, progressive hepatic and renal failure, and upper gastrointestinal hemorrhage resulting from portal hypertension. Prothrombin time was identified as a better marker of hepatocellular function than albumin because prothrombin more accurately estimates biosynthetic function of the liver. More recently, the Model for End-Stage Liver Disease score has been used to guide patient selection and prognosticate morbidity and mortality in patients with chronic liver disease undergoing major operations. The score is determined through calculations incorporating serum bilirubin, prothrombin time/international normalized ratio, and creatinine and has been predictive in several studies looking at outcomes. The Model for End-Stage Liver Disease has largely supplanted older subjective predictive models of outcomes such as Child-Pugh. However in contrast to renal failure, which is well defined by the RIFLE criteria, there is no true formal definition or grading of postoperative liver failure.

Multiple factors contribute to postoperative liver failure, but the basic physiology is driven by ischemia of the hepatocytes. Hypotension secondary to hypovolemia, hemorrhage, and vasodilation all result in a decreased MAP, which diminishes nutritive hepatic artery and portal vein flow. This mechanism is also involved in some cases of liver failure observed after general anesthesia or laparoscopic procedures in which hepatocyte hypoperfusion may not be as readily evident. Because the cirrhotic liver already has significantly reduced numbers of hepatocytes, the ischemic injury to the remaining hepatocytes is manifested in decreased synthetic function with insufficient generation of critical proteins such as clotting factors and albumin. In addition, the decrease in hepatocytes limits the ability of the liver to perform normal metabolic functions, and toxins such as ammonia and drug metabolites may build up. Many of the complications of liver failure (e.g., bleeding, encephalopathy, ascites) are in some way attributable to hepatocyte death. Patients with liver failure also have generalized immune dysfunction caused by loss of Kupffer cells as well as decreased production of critical elements of the inflammatory response, such as C-reactive protein, interleukins, complement, and many other cytokines.

Perioperative fluid management in patients with liver disease requires special attention to minimize delivery of sodium-containing solutions, which in the setting of a low intravascular oncotic pressure cause increased ascites and interstitial edema. Patients with cirrhosis have activation of the renin-angiotensin axis and can be intravascularly contracted, even though they have total body fluid overload. In addition, dysregulation in nitric oxide and many other vasoactive substances can lead to differing degrees of vasoconstriction or dilation at the level of the tissue. In extreme cases of liver failure, portal hypertension can inexplicably result in splanchnic vasodilation, which may activate the juxtaglomerular apparatus of the kidney resulting in significant afferent arteriole vasoconstriction and may lead to the development of hepatorenal syndrome. This condition is difficult to treat, and it is irreversible in most cases unless the patient undergoes liver transplantation. The mortality of patients with cirrhosis who develop AKI (with creatinine >2 mg/dL) in the ICU was shown to be more than 80%.[31] The classic finding in hepatorenal syndrome is FeNa less than 1% and very low urine sodium, indicating the kidney senses hypovolemia and attempts to conserve sodium. Albumin-containing solutions, which are low in sodium, are characteristically used to volume resuscitate patients with cirrhosis because they tend to minimize ascites and peripheral edema. Patients who have suffered significant blood loss should be resuscitated with blood and blood products and a minimal amount of crystalloid solutions—so-called all product resuscitation. Even albumin and other blood product colloids will leak from the intravascular space, especially in sepsis, and the cycle of ascites continues particularly if liver failure worsens. Patients who are not critically ill and taking oral nutrition should be on sodium and free water restriction as part of the management of ascites. Decompensated liver failure and worsening ascites can lead to respiratory failure as a result of increased intra-abdominal pressure, and diuresis, paracentesis, and transjugular intrahepatic portosystemic shunt may be required in extreme cases.

Hepatic encephalopathy is another manifestation of advanced liver failure and is due to impaired hepatic clearance of gut-derived substances such as mercaptans and ammonia. These compounds, which are normally produced by intestinal flora, have sedating effects mediated by GABA receptors in the brain. Ammonia, produced by the breakdown of urea in the gut, is a neurotoxin that readily crosses the blood-brain barrier and is normally metabolized by the liver to urea by a series of enzymes. Hepatic encephalopathy is the result of numerous hepatic insults (e.g., dehydration, infections, gastrointestinal bleeding, hepatically metabolized medications) and may be seen in chronic and acute liver failure. The degree of hepatic encephalopathy can be graded by the West Haven scale (Table 21-3). Management of hepatic encephalopathy centers on addressing the underlying cause of the hepatic decompensation and reducing excess intake of dietary protein and aromatic amino acids, but care must be taken to avoid malnutrition. Lactulose, a nonabsorbable disaccharide, creates an osmotic and cathartic effect that promotes the elimination of ammonia and mercaptans from the gut. It is usually given in 15- to 30-mL aliquots until the patient has three soft bowel movements a day; overzealous titration should be avoided because this can cause voluminous diarrhea, dehydration, and worsening liver failure. Rifaximin and other enteral antibiotics can treat hepatic encephalopathy by reducing the gut flora and the production of the compounds that cause hepatic encephalopathy. Studies have shown comparable results in terms of mental status improvements in patients with hepatic encephalopathy treated with lactulose versus rifaximin, and some literature suggests that osmotic laxatives alone may be equally effective. Special enteral formulas with varying amounts of aliphatic and branched chain amino acids have been evaluated in liver and hepatic encephalopathy with disappointing results.

TABLE 21-3 West Haven Criteria of Hepatic Encephalopathy

GRADE	LEVEL OF CONSCIOUSNESS	SYMPTOMS
0	Normal	None
1	Minor mental slowing	Diminished fine motor skills
2	Lethargic or apathetic	Slurred speech, ataxia
3	Somnolent	Clonus, asterixis
4	Coma	Signs of intracranial hypertension

HEMATOLOGIC SYSTEM

Review of Clotting Mechanisms and Thromboembolism

ICU patients are affected with coagulopathies and thrombophilias, and both conditions may occur in the same patient during the span of their ICU care. Coagulopathy tends to be more common and can be the result of nutritional deficiencies, liver dysfunction, congenital diseases such as hemophilia and von Willebrand disease, hemodilution, consumption, and many other surgical causes. Sepsis, trauma, and almost every medication given to ICU patients has been associated at some point with thrombocytopenia. Hypothermia, the scourge of trauma care, can magnify coagulopathy through its negative effects on clotting factors. Critical illness and inflammation cause activation of the coagulation cascade leading to microvascular clotting and organ dysfunction and is one theory behind the development of MSOF. Even after major injury with bleeding and coagulopathy, patients develop an increased risk of thrombosis as a result of endothelial injury, venous stasis, and immobility. On the surface, these dichotomies seem confusing, but when one considers that normal homeostasis is maintained by simultaneous activation of the clotting and fibrinolytic system, these conflicting conditions make more sense. Scant evidence exists on the relationships between coagulation abnormalities in the ICU and patient outcomes, and good data to guide the management of the complex interplay between these two competing systems are lacking.

The process of clotting is initiated when there is endothelial injury, which exposes vascular wall elements that activate platelets. Platelet activation draws in and activates more platelets leading to the creation of a platelet plug, which is known as primary hemostasis. Circulating clotting factors undergo a cascading activation that eventually leads to the activation of thrombin that converts fibrinogen to fibrin. Cross linking of fibrin monomers forms a strengthening lattice, reinforcing the platelet plug. Thrombin is one of the most important proteins in the coagulation cascade because it activates numerous other clotting factors; increases platelet activation and aggregation; and activates protein C, which is a modulating inhibitor of the cascade. There are two coagulation pathways, intrinsic and extrinsic, that coalesce into a common pathway where factor X is activated and converts prothrombin to thrombin and ultimately to deposition of fibrin. The effectiveness of the intrinsic pathway is typically measured by the partial thromboplastin time, and the extrinsic pathway, initiated by tissue injury and release of tissue factor, is measured by the prothrombin time. Prothrombin time and partial thromboplastin time are not functional tests of clotting and are limited in assessing clot strength, durability, or the quality of the clot formed by the interplay of platelets, von Willebrand factor, and fibrin. As previously stated, activation of clotting factors is coupled to the simultaneous activation of clotting inhibitors so that clotting is carefully countered by fibrinolysis. Disturbances in this delicate balance can lead to uncontrolled thrombosis, as is seen in disseminated intravascular coagulation, a complication of sepsis, major surgery, severe trauma, obstetric procedures, transfusion reactions, and malignancies. Hyperfibrinolysis, as seen in liver failure, may result in profound coagulopathy. The major regulators of clotting are protein C, which breaks down factors Va and VIIIa; antithrombin, which inactivates thrombin and factors Xa and IXa; and plasmin, which cleaves fibrin. Recombinant plasminogen activators are widely available and are used to treat myocardial infarction, ischemic stroke, and pulmonary embolism.

The most frequently used tests of the clotting system, such as prothrombin time, partial thromboplastin time, and the international normalized ratio (which is a standardized modification of the prothrombin time), are not functional assays of clotting. The addition of data from checking bleeding time, platelet counts, fibrinogen, or the concentration of individual clotting factors does little to improve the assessment of this important system. Thromboelastometry is based on an assay that was initially used more than 60 years ago and is a functional assay of clotting and clot lysis. This test is performed with a small amount of sampled blood (300 μL) to which a rotational force is applied, and a filament yields real-time data such as time to clot formation, clot strength, and clot breakdown. The first component of the thromboelastography tracing is the reaction or "R" time, which is analogous to the data gleaned from checking partial thromboplastin time and prothrombin time. The kinetic time measures the time it takes for clot strength amplitude to increase from 2 mm to 20 mm and is a measure of fibrin and platelet function. Maximum amplitude assesses the maximum strength of clot, and the lysis index measures the dissolution of clot over time with a low lysis index indicating hyperfibrinolysis.[32] The clinical benefits of functional clotting assays, especially from point-of-care testing in the ICU, are numerous and may lead to more effective use of blood, blood products, and other agents, which, it is hoped, will lead to fewer complications, lower costs, and better outcomes.

As previously stated, ICU patients have multiple factors that leave them susceptible to clotting complications such as DVT, pulmonary embolism, and heparin-induced thrombocytopenia (HIT). ICU patients do not present with typical symptoms of DVT, such as thigh or calf pain, and physical findings are often obscured by anasarca, but they are at high risk because of the presence of Virchow triad: endothelial injury, venous stasis, and a hypercoagulable state. Surveillance ultrasonography and venography studies in ICUs have shown rates approaching 40%, and of cases that extend to the thigh, approximately 50% result in pulmonary embolism. Ultrasound is the diagnostic study of choice to detect DVT because it is portable, quick, and relatively inexpensive. Because of the high rate of DVT in the ICU, prophylaxis is crucial, and all patients should have sequential compression devices, stockings, and a pharmacologic agent such as heparin or low-molecular-weight heparin unless otherwise contraindicated. Risk for DVT is highest in patients with major thoracic or abdominal operations lasting 30 minutes or longer, neurosurgical procedures, coronary artery bypass grafting, severe trauma, hip fracture, spinal cord injury, surgery or chemotherapy for malignancy, and congestive heart or respiratory failure. In high-risk patients with an absolute contraindication for pharmacologic DVT prophylaxis, an inferior vena cava filter is indicated, and most of these are now removable. Pulmonary embolisms can range from clinically insignificant subsegmental clots found incidentally on a CT scan to a main pulmonary trunk embolus that causes hypoxia, hemodynamic instability, and death. With increasing resolution of CT scans, more incidental subsegmental emboli are being found, but it appears that anticoagulation is not indicated for these patients. Patients with larger pulmonary embolisms should receive systemic anticoagulation with subsequent conversion to oral agents. Patients with marked hypoxia or hemodynamic instability typically require systemic thrombolytic therapy with tissue plasminogen activator unless otherwise contraindicated. Large symptomatic pulmonary embolisms also may be treated by interventional radiologic procedures and in rare cases surgical thrombectomy. The decision to use systemic anticoagulation or tissue plasminogen activator should not be made lightly because of bleeding risks. A careful appraisal of risks and benefits and a discussion with consultants and the surgeon of record should be undertaken and documented in the medical record.

Heparin-Induced Thrombocytopenia

HIT is a serious complication that can result from exposure to heparin products with unfractionated heparin having the highest risk and low-molecular-weight heparins having the least risk. There are two types of HIT. Type 1 HIT is a less serious, non–immune-mediated form that causes clumping of platelets, but the effects appear to be more transient and self-limited. Type 2 HIT involves the development of heparin-associated antiplatelet antibodies and occurs within a few days of heparin exposure or sooner if the patient has been sensitized from prior exposure. The manifestations of type 2 HIT can be severe and include venous and arterial thromboembolism. Because thrombocytopenia is common in the ICU but may portend dangerous type 2 HIT, many clinicians use the 4T score, which combines the timing and severity of the thrombocytopenia, occurrence of new thrombosis, and the presence of alternative explanations for thrombocytopenia to guide the workup and management of HIT. In one review, despite use of the 4T score, the diagnosis of HIT was considered in 15% of ICU patients but confirmed in less than 1%. Patients with a platelet count less than 50,000 μL or whose platelet count decreases 50% or more of baseline are usually evaluated for HIT with an enzyme-linked immunosorbent assay (ELISA) or serotonin release assay (SRA). ELISA testing is usually immediately available, but the confirmatory SRA typically requires reference laboratory testing; thus, for most patients, an ELISA screen can be performed as a screening test. If the ELISA is positive and the patient's pretest probability of HIT is high, a direct thrombin inhibitor such as argatroban should be started until results from the SRA are available. In one of the largest reviews to date, a positive ELISA was not confirmed by the SRA 86% of the time. It is prudent to withhold all heparinoids while the diagnosis of HIT is being ruled out, unless the patient's probability of HIT before testing is exceedingly low.

Critical Illness Anemia and Transfusion

Anemia in the ICU is common and is the result of decreased erythrocyte production, daily phlebotomy, hemodilution, and bleeding events. Evidence shows that greater than 25% of patients in a surgical ICU on any given day receive a transfusion, most often of packed red blood cells, and that 85% of patients who are in the ICU for more than 1 week receive a transfusion. Most critically ill patients with anemia do not have active blood loss, and the issue is more often one of inadequate erythrocyte production in the face of phlebotomy and dilution. Inflammatory conditions upregulate hepcidin, which results in iron sequestration in the liver and macrophages, diminishing erythropoiesis by the bone marrow. Anemia in the ICU is assumed to result in decreased oxygen carrying capacity and is theorized to contribute to poorer outcomes, but evidence to support this contention is lacking; however, there is a wealth of data showing that liberal transfusions contribute to many complications and poor outcomes. In light of these data, restrictive transfusion practices are the norm in most ICUs at the present time, although some clinicians still adhere to liberal transfusion strategies based on tradition. The exception to restrictive transfusion is an actively bleeding patient in whom transfusions need to replace not only what is lost but also what will be shortly lost.

Blood therapy remains a challenging and sometimes controversial topic in the ICU, despite a markedly decreased risk of blood-borne infectious complications compared with the past. Long gone are the days when blood was considered a "tonic" to perk up patients, and most clinicians now recognize that the oxygen carrying capacity of banked blood is limited because of depletion of 2,3-diphosphoglycerate and adenosine triphosphate, two factors critical to oxygen delivery at the cellular level. Additionally, many of the adverse effects of blood are being recognized (e.g., transfusion-related acute lung injury and immunosuppression). Transfusion-related acute lung injury appears to be mediated by soluble factors derived from the donor that cause pronounced immune activation in the recipient that may lead to ARDS and MSOF. In 1999, the TRICC trial, a landmark randomized trial that examined transfusion requirements in critical care, showed decreased mortality when a restrictive transfusion practice was compared with a liberal transfusion practice. This study established hemoglobin less than 7 mg/dL as a "transfusion trigger" for most patients, and the mortality benefit was still observed in patients with preexisting cardiac disease.[33] Additional research confirmed that hemoglobin levels of 7 mg/dL are well tolerated by ICU patients, and the only patients who benefit from more liberal transfusion are patients who are actively bleeding or manifesting acute coronary ischemia.

Massive Transfusion Strategies and Anticoagulation Reversal

Massive transfusion, defined as administration of 10 U of packed red blood cells given over a 24-hour period, is occasionally required for patients with severe trauma, gastrointestinal hemorrhage, or ruptured abdominal aneurysms. In these patients, large-volume resuscitation with crystalloid fluids must be avoided because this leads to worsening coagulopathy and death. Exsanguination is still the leading cause of death of trauma patients and is often the result of the deadly triad of coagulopathy, acidosis, and hypothermia; these conditions should be avoided and corrected at all costs. Once surgical control of bleeding is obtained, massive transfusion protocols can be lifesaving and aim to resuscitate patients with a balance of packed red blood cells, fresh-frozen plasma (FFP), and platelets, while minimizing the administration of crystalloid. This resuscitation strategy has been termed *hemostatic resuscitation*. Although the exact ratio of these products is still being defined and verified, it appears that patients approaching a 1 : 1 : 1 ratio have favorable outcomes. A retrospective review of more than 400 patients with trauma-induced coagulopathy confirmed that patients given a 1 : 1 ratio of FFP to red blood cells had markedly lower mortality (28% versus 51%) than patients given a 1 : 4 ratio. Concerns have arisen about the increased administration of FFP because of its pooled nature and potential to promote inflammatory responses such as transfusion-related acute lung injury and ARDS, and these concerns have been corroborated by a study that found elevated risk of ARDS and MSOF with increasing amounts of FFP but decreased risk when cryoprecipitate was used. Cryoprecipitate is a blood product that contains high amounts of fibrinogen, von Willebrand factor, and factor VIII. Many centers have added this product to their massive transfusion protocols to decrease the use of plasma and to avoid depletion of the factors in cryoprecipitate that are almost absent in FFP.

Factor VIIa, prothrombin complex concentrates (PCC), and tranexamic acid are massive transfusion protocol adjuncts that decrease the use of blood products and help to control hemorrhage. Activated recombinant factor VII promotes clotting by initiating a thrombin burst on the surface of activated platelets; it showed great promise as the "universal hemostat," but some of this enthusiasm has waned because of the drug's high cost and limited evidence that it reduces mortality in patients with severe traumatic injury. PCC is derived from human blood and contains varying amounts of the vitamin K–dependent factors II, VII, IX, and X and protein C and S. PCC is growing in popularity as a reversal agent for patients taking anticoagulants, especially the so-called novel anticoagulants. PCC was intended to counteract the coagulopathy induced by warfarin, which is mediated through inhibition of the terminal carboxylation of the vitamin K–dependent clotting factors. Three PCCs are composed of factors II, VII, and X, and four factor agents have those plus added factor VII. The emergence of innovative anticoagulants such as dabigatran and rivaroxaban, direct thrombin and factor Xa inhibitors, respectively, has expanded the role of PCC. Previously, warfarin was reversed through the administration of vitamin K or FFP if urgent reversal was indicated. PCCs are stored in powder form and can be quickly reconstituted for reversal of warfarin without the concerns for volume overload associated with large quantities of FFP administration. Tranexamic acid inhibits fibrinolysis by blocking a binding site on plasminogen and has been shown to reduce the risk of hemorrhage and death significantly in a study of more than 20,000 bleeding trauma patients. This trial, the CRASH-2 trial, demonstrated its mortality benefit without a significant increase in vascular occlusive events; however, the role of tranexamic acid outside of trauma is still being investigated.[34]

ENDOCRINE SYSTEM

Glucose Control

Hyperglycemia is common in the ICU and can be the result of many different conditions, but the two main causes are increased glucose production and peripheral insulin resistance. These conditions can occur in the same patient and even at the same time; thus, hyperglycemia is thought to be a marker of systemic inflammation. Multivariate analysis has shown that hyperglycemia is an independent risk factor for adverse outcomes after trauma, sepsis, and TBI because it contributes to infections, neuropathy, immunosuppression, and organ dysfunction. Many aspects of granulocyte function are adversely affected by glycosylation, including chemotaxis, phagocytosis, and the efficacy of the respiratory burst, so bacterial infections are more prevalent in hyperglycemic individuals. Previously, most of the evidence concerning the effect of hyperglycemia on outcomes was derived from patients undergoing open heart surgery and patients with myocardial infarction, but more recent data from diverse patient populations of critically ill patients have clarified some of the controversy.

The term *tight glucose control* was derived from the experience of patients undergoing open heart surgery and the finding that hyperglycemia led to increased rates of sternal dehiscence or mediastinitis after coronary bypass operations. Several years later, van den Berghe's group published a landmark article showing that patients with mechanical ventilation who had their glucose controlled in a very narrow range of 80 to 110 mg/dL had lower incidences of bloodstream infection, sepsis, need for renal replacement, ICU neuropathy, and mortality.[35] This single trial ushered in the era of tight glucose control for all ICU patients, and most quality organizations embraced this as "standard of care" drowning out the voices of some providers who questioned the reproducibility of the results. Later, the Normoglycaemia in Intensive Care Evaluation Survival Using Glucose Algorithm Regulation (NICE-SUGAR) study revealed that tight glucose control led to more episodes of hypoglycemia, which significantly increased mortality.[36] Subsequent trials confirmed this finding, and hypoglycemia was recognized as an independent predictor of mortality. At the present time, glucose values of most ICU patients are maintained in the range of 150 to 180 mg/dL, which was the range of the patients undergoing open heart surgery who had the better outcomes decades before. The experience with tight glucose control in the ICU is an excellent cautionary tale of what can happen when major shifts in care are driven by a single randomized controlled trial, no matter how well designed it is.

Adrenal Insufficiency

The hypothalamic-pituitary-adrenal axis is central to the "fight-or-flight" state and has served humans well in this capacity, but in times of severe critical illness it can soon become exhausted. Endogenous vasopressin and corticosteroids are often depleted in shock states with profound adverse effects on hemodynamics. The finding that supplementation of glucocorticoids and mineralocorticoids to patients in septic shock decreased short-term mortality began an era of widespread use of corticosteroids for shock, and similar to the experience following the article by van den Berghe and colleagues, steroid therapy became standard therapy based on this single publication despite concerns about immunosuppression, wound healing, and glucose control. In this study, patients were given a synthetic adrenocorticotropic hormone to identify the patients who had relative adrenal insufficiency requiring steroid supplementation; although steroids reduced pressor requirements and 28-day mortality, mortality at 1 year was unaffected.[37] In 2008, the Corticosteroid Therapy of Septic Shock (CORTICUS) randomized trial confirmed what many clinicians had anecdotally observed—that steroids might reduce vasopressor requirements, but mortality was not reduced.[38] Adrenocorticotropic hormone stimulation testing has fallen out of favor since CORTICUS confirmed that the results of this test are unimportant to guide therapy, and steroid supplementation is reserved for patients with shock refractory to fluids and vasopressors. ICU patients who are on long-term steroids for medical comorbidities should be given bioequivalent doses of intravenous hydrocortisone and converted to their long-term dose when they resume oral intake.

INFECTION IN THE INTENSIVE CARE UNIT

Fever and Approach to Infections

Critical illness increases the incidence of infections for a multitude of reasons, but surgical patients have an even greater risk because of factors unique to this patient population. Hemorrhagic shock, trauma, wounds and incisions, drains, catheters, tubes, devitalized tissue, hematomas, immunosuppressants, and malnutrition are just some of the many reasons why surgical ICU patients have the greatest risk of infection among all critical care settings. To complicate matters further, surgical ICU patients often have manifestations of SIRS, which limits the predictive value of the classic signs of infection, such as fever and leukocytosis. In light of these manifestations of SIRS, fever in surgical ICUs is typically defined as 101.5° F and much higher in patient with burns or a heavy burden of necrotic tissue.

The evaluation of fever should begin with consideration of all potential sources of infection in the patient followed by a focused physical examination that explores every one of those possibilities. All dressings, wounds, and devices should be evaluated. The saying "look for the hand of man" can help pinpoint the likely source of infection, and operative reports and the medical record should not be overlooked, keeping in mind that less than 20% of fever in the first 2 days after elective surgery is due to an infection.[39] Analogous to the secondary survey of trauma, the ICU patient should be examined from head to toe looking for the infectious source. Alterations in mental status, craniectomy, or monitoring devices render meningitis a possibility, whereas nasogastric or feeding tubes make sinusitis more likely. Intubation, aspiration, pulmonary contusion, and altered mental status all increase the risk of pneumonia, and chest tubes, surgery, and trauma make empyema a distinct possibility. All indwelling tubes and devices should be considered a breach in the normal host defense mechanisms and are potential points of ingress for bacteria and infection. As is the case in blunt trauma, the evaluation of the abdomen is most challenging because the potential sources here are almost too numerous to list; in addition to infections resulting from recent operations or injury, the patient may be at risk for common intra-abdominal processes such as appendicitis. Anastomotic breakdown, intra-abdominal abscess, infectious colitis, and acalculous cholecystitis are some of the more common causes of intra-abdominal infection, and patients should be approached the same methodical way as ICU patients with fever—a thorough consideration of potential sources, followed by a focused examination. If the source of the fever or infection is not found or if the provider is unsure, the decision to seek imaging studies or laboratory evaluation needs to be made.

For most patients, including patients on the ward, fever and leukocytosis are usually indicative of infection, but as noted previously, this is not the case in the ICU. Other signs of infection should be sought, including changes in vital signs such as tachycardia, oliguria, hyperglycemia, and new-onset hypoxemia. Feeding intolerance is often an early, subtle sign of an impending infection, and ileus usually accompanies any intra-abdominal process. Worsening liver dysfunction, increasing creatinine, new-onset lactic acidosis, and a left shift on the differential are worrisome findings and may be associated with infection. Any degradation in a previously stable organ system may be a manifestation of sepsis, as illustrated by worsening oxygenation despite stable ventilator settings in the case of VAP or peritonitis. In contrast to medical intensivists, surgical intensivists have the ability to obtain "source control." Complete compliance with all elements of the sepsis bundle do the patient little good unless perforated diverticulitis, fecal peritonitis, or necrotizing soft tissue infection is not addressed first. Keeping this in mind should alter how surgeons view antibiotics—that is to say, drainage of abscesses, resection of necrotic or infected tissue, or removal of infected devices should be undertaken without delay if possible, and antibiotics are adjuncts to this, the primary therapy. Occasionally, antibiotics are not needed once source control has been obtained, as is borne out by the treatment of a simple abscess, which is primarily incision and drainage. In regard to antibiotic therapy in ICU patients, less is often more, and the focus should be on detecting and treating the source, with antibiotics used in a rational fashion rather than indiscriminately starting or adding them haphazardly.

Central venous catheters are common in the ICU and are useful for medication or fluid administration, vasopressor agents, TPN, and hemodynamic monitoring. CLABSI is a serious, iatrogenic complication of ICU care that carries distinct morbidity and mortality risks as well as increased length of stay and hospital charges. Advances (e.g., antibiotic-impregnated catheters, antiseptic dressings and hubs) have had some positive effect on CLABSI rates, but the most important way to reduce the risk of CLABSI is remove the catheter. It is a good practice on ICU rounds to evaluate the need for each tube, catheter, or device every day so that the devices may be removed as soon as possible. Obviously infected lines, indicated by draining purulence or erythema, should be removed immediately, whereas catheters suspected of being infected may be wire changed and the tip sent for culture. Catheters must be removed if the tip culture returns with more than 15 colonies of bacteria. If there are positive blood cultures and a central line was present for more than 2 days including the day before or the day the cultures were drawn, the CDC criteria for a CLABSI have been met. Common pathogens are *Staphylococcus* species; gram-negative and fungal pathogens may infect lines placed in the femoral position. Central lines should be inserted following a standard protocol or bundle that includes hand washing, chlorhexidine skin preparation, maximal barrier precautions, and a bedside nurse monitor looking for breaks in sterility. Similar to many aspects of ICU patient care at the present time, central line insertion, maintenance, and access are governed by standardized protocols and bundles of care to reduce rates of CLABSI.

Pneumonia, discussed extensively in the Respiratory System, is the most common cause of death in patients with infections acquired in the ICU, and most of these cases are associated with mechanical ventilation. Ideally, VAP is diagnosed using quantitative cultures because this allows for the most effective de-escalation of antibiotics. Empirical antibiotics against the most likely organism should be started and then tailored as culture results become available. Methicillin-resistant *Staphylococcus aureus* and the non–lactose fermenting gram-negative rods termed *SPACE* organisms (*Serratia*, *Pseudomonas*, *Acinetobacter*, *Citrobacter*, and *Enterobacter*) should receive 14 days of therapy, whereas all other pathogens can be treated for 1 week. Lung penetration of many antibiotics is poor, and the pharmacokinetics of dosing antibiotics in critically ill patients can be challenging so input from a clinical pharmacist should be sought out if available.

Catheter-associated urinary tract infection (CAUTI) in the ICU is a common problem and typically due to the frequent use of bladder catheters. Similar to central venous catheters, the risk of developing an infection coincides with the duration the catheter is indwelling. Coverage of the catheter with a biofilm facilitates bacterial colonization and migration, and this process affects almost every indwelling foreign body over time. Workup for CAUTI involves sending a urinalysis and urine culture; however, the urinalysis can be unreliable because pyuria and leukocyte esterase are often absent in ICU patients with documented infections, whereas nitrates indicate only *Escherichia coli* or *Enterobacter* infection. In contrast to outpatient populations, ICU CAUTI is often due to multidrug-resistant gram-negative rods or fungal organisms, so duration of antibiotic treatment is typically 7 days because of the "complicated" nature of CAUTI in this setting. The presence of *Candida* organisms in the urine of ICU patients is termed *candiduria* and generally reflects colonization rather than true infection. Candiduria is more common in patients with poor glucose control and in patients who recently received broad-spectrum antibiotics. Antifungal agents are indicated when *Candida* organisms are recovered on culture from two different sites; however, it is prudent to initiate coverage in patients who have had recent genitourinary procedures, renal transplantation, or marked neutropenia. Most *Candida* species are susceptible to azole agents, such as fluconazole, but *Candida glabrata* and other strains of yeast exhibit resistance to this agent and may require treatment with an echinocandin such as caspofungin. For highly resistant organisms, amphotericin may be required and should be given as a bladder irrigant to avoid systemic toxicity. Similar to CLABSI and VAP, it is difficult to get a CAUTI if the Foley catheter is removed as soon as possible, so most institutions have embraced this philosophy, including in ICU patients.

Clostridium difficile infection is not as common as VAP or CAUTI, but it can follow a virulent course progressing rapidly to florid septic shock, renal failure, acidosis, and death. *C. difficile* infection is associated with dysbiosis or imbalances in colonic flora caused by exposure to antibiotics, with agents having a broad spectrum against anaerobes causing the greatest degree of dysbiosis. Treatment of *C. difficile* with metronidazole further disrupts the normal colonic flora, which sets the stage for recurrent episodes and carrier states. Although *C. difficile* is the most common cause of nosocomial diarrhea, it sometimes manifests as ileus and constipation, so providers should not equate this disease only with diarrhea. Most cases of diarrhea in the ICU are not due to *C. difficile* but rather medications such as sorbitol-containing elixirs, enteral tube feeds, and malabsorption. The diagnosis of *C. difficile* is accomplished through polymerase chain reaction, which is more sensitive than prior toxin assays, and standing orders for nurses to send stool specimens as they see fit have been shown to reduce time to diagnosis. The new NAP-1 strain of *C. difficile* often progresses to megacolon, shock, and need for emergent colectomy. Patients should initially be treated with metronidazole, but it is acceptable to add oral vancomycin in areas where NAP-1 predominates. Fidaxomicin, which has activity against *C. difficile* but causes less disturbance to normal colonic flora, has been shown to be an effective therapy and is associated with lower recurrence rates. *C. difficile* colitis that progresses to septic shock or renal failure is best treated by emergent colectomy because it is unlikely that antibiotics would be a successful therapy at that point. Initial reports of less invasive approaches for toxic colitis, such as loop ileostomy and colonic lavage with osmotic laxatives and antibiotics, have shown promising results, as has fecal transplant, but further investigation is necessary.

Sepsis Strategies

Approximately 40% of all ICU patients have sepsis on admission or manifest it at some point during their ICU stay, and the resource utilization and costs of treatment for it are staggering. The term *sepsis* is derived from the Greek word meaning "to rot or decay," and sepsis lies on a continuum of illness progressing from SIRS to severe sepsis and septic shock. These conditions were defined more than 2 decades ago, and this common language has helped guide therapy and the ability of clinicians to offer a prognosis for critically ill patients.[40] SIRS is defined by the presence of two or more of the following criteria: temperature less than 36° C or greater than 38° C, heart rate greater than 90 beats/min, white blood cell count less than $4000/mm^3$ or greater than $12,000/mm^3$ or band neutrophils greater than 10%, and respiratory rate greater than 20 or arterial carbon dioxide pressure less than 32 mm Hg. As previously noted, many surgical patients meet SIRS criteria on ICU admission, which can make the diagnosis of sepsis a challenge. Sepsis is defined by the presence of SIRS with an infection, whereas severe sepsis is sepsis with signs of end organ failure (e.g., oliguria, altered mental status, acidosis). Finally, septic shock is at the end of the spectrum and is present when patients with sepsis develop hypotension despite adequate fluid resuscitation and require vasopressor support.

The Surviving Sepsis Campaign (www.survivingsepsis.org), initially launched in 2002 and revised several times since, is a notable example of a strategy designed by clinicians and investigators to improve outcomes. The original concept was driven by a strategy that stressed early targeted physiologic goals of resuscitation that changed the management of critically ill medical patients far more than surgical patients. The campaign consists of two sets of bundled elements to be fulfilled in the first 3 and 6 hours from the time the patient is diagnosed with sepsis—the so-called time zero. The 3-hour bundle calls for measurement of lactic acid level, blood cultures to be drawn before initiating antibiotics, administration of broad-spectrum antibiotics, and boluses of 30 mL/kg of crystalloid fluid for hypotension or lactic acid greater than 4 mmol/liter. The later bundle suggests the use of vasopressors to maintain MAP greater than 65 mm Hg, measurement of CVP and $ScvO_2$, and rechecking lactic acid level levels. The targeted physiologic goals are a CVP 8 mm Hg or greater, $ScvO_2$ greater than 70%, and correction of lactic acidosis. The initial bundle elements of corticosteroids, tight glucose control, and activated protein C were modified as new evidence emerged about their use as noted in previous sections. Although activated protein C was initially promising, this drug was withdrawn from the market in 2011 after failing to improve outcomes, although many surgical patients could not receive this drug because of concerns over postoperative hemorrhage. The treatment of sepsis and septic shock continues to focus on meeting the bundled care goals in a timely fashion because high bundle compliance rates have been shown to reduce mortality. Although the bundled care elements of the Surviving Sepsis Campaign have benefited patients with sepsis syndromes, the importance of surgical source control cannot be overstated. Also, evidence regarding the long-term sequelae of surviving sepsis is often unfavorable because these patients have been shown to have significant and lasting functional and cognitive impairments that adversely affect quality of life.[41] There is a great need for high-quality, risk-stratified data on long-term outcomes of sepsis and critical illness, as emerging data show that many of these patients have significant issues regarding adverse quality of life.

Antibiotic Stewardship

It has been repeatedly shown that infected patients who receive the right empirical antibiotic at the right time have better outcomes because delays in effective antibiotic therapy lead to higher mortality. It has also been noted that unnecessary or extended antibiotic use exposes the patient and other patients to immediate and long-term hazards. These two conflicting truths highlight the predicament that clinicians face when dealing with a patient with a potential infection, and although most opt to start empirical antibiotic therapy, this decision is often questioned when faced with a patient in fulminant septic shock caused by unnecessary antibiotic-induced *C. difficile* colitis. Unnecessary overuse of antibiotics led the World Health Organization to publish a statement sounding the alarm as resistant pathogens are emerging at far faster rates than novel antimicrobials are being developed, which threatens to become a danger to the health of people worldwide. In addition to concerns over the development of resistance and *C. difficile* colitis, inappropriate antibiotic therapy exposes patients to nephrotoxicity, allergic reactions, opportunistic fungal infections, and volume overload, there are global issues of costs, waste, and drug shortages (Box 21-2). The concept of antibiotic stewardship is important in health care but more so in the ICUs because the highest rates of antibiotic use occur here. The components of this stewardship include a critical appraisal of the need for antibiotics on daily rounds, a review of culture results to eliminate unnecessary agents, de-escalation from broad-spectrum to narrow-spectrum agents whenever possible, and establishing a stop date for the antimicrobial therapy. Multidisciplinary stewardship programs have been shown to reduce inappropriate antibiotic use, decrease the development of resistance, and lessen hospital costs without worsening patient outcomes.

BOX 21-2 Benefits of Antibiotic Stewardship in the Intensive Care Unit

- Decreased development of resistant organisms
- Reduced nephrotoxicity and acute kidney injury
- Decreased *Clostridium difficile* risk
- Decreased opportunistic fungal infections
- Reduced costs and resource consumption

PROPHYLAXIS IN THE INTENSIVE CARE UNIT

Stress Ulcer Prophylaxis

Critically ill patients have factors (e.g., decreased mucosal bicarbonate and mucus production and splanchnic ischemia) that result in weakening of the gastric mucosal defenses setting the stage for gastritis and bleeding. Although these events are rare, occurring in less than 2% of ICU patients, bleeding may be heavy resulting in the need for transfusions and emergency surgery. Most critically ill patients have a reduction in their gastric acid secretion, and bleeding episodes are due entirely to loss of mucosal defenses. Stress ulcer bleeding is an ominous development because these patients have been shown to have markedly higher mortality rates. The classic finding on upper endoscopy is multiple areas of ulceration or petechial erosions, particularly in the gastric fundus; this entity cannot be treated endoscopically because diffuse bleeding arises from superficial mucosal capillaries. The primary prevention of stress ulcer bleeding centers around decreasing acid production despite the fact that the pathophysiology suggests the mucosal changes drive this process. In many ICU patients, prophylaxis is likely overused, and some data suggest that this predisposes the patient to pneumonia and *C. difficile* infections as well as increasing health care costs. Retrospective reviews have identified patients at high risk for stress ulcer bleeding, and patients with the following conditions should receive prophylaxis: respiratory failure and mechanical ventilation, hemodynamic instability requiring vasopressors, liver failure, coagulopathy, TBI, spinal cord injury, organ transplantation, and burns.

Various medications have been tried over the years to prevent stress ulcer bleeding, including anticholinergics and antacids, which had unwanted side effects and limited efficacy. The introduction of cimetidine, the first histamine 2 (H_2) receptor antagonist, ushered in a new era in medicine that saw a dramatic reduction not only in stress ulcer bleeding but also in peptic ulcer disease. The addition of sucralfate, an aluminum sulfate compound that functioned as a direct mucosal protection, offered additional therapeutic options, but this agent was cumbersome to use because medications and enteral feeding had to be held around its dosing several times a day. At the present time, sucralfate and cimetidine have been replaced entirely by more modern H_2 receptor antagonists and PPIs. The literature comparing the efficacy and costs of these two agents is conflicting, and although PPIs are far more potent than H_2 receptor antagonists, this potency has not been proven to offer superior efficacy against stress ulceration. A meta-analysis suggested that PPIs may be marginally more effective than H_2 receptor antagonists at reducing stress ulcer bleeding, but these benefits are likely offset by their significantly higher cost. At the present time, PPIs and H_2 receptor antagonists both appear to be effective agents against stress ulceration, and the choice boils down to costs and drug availability until more randomized data become available.

Venous Thromboembolism Prophylaxis

As mentioned in the Hematologic System, critically ill patients are at high risk for VTE because almost all of them have the factors comprising Virchow triad. Patients who have experienced total joint replacement surgery, multisystem trauma, severe orthopedic injuries, or recent spinal cord injury are at the highest risk for VTE, although any patients with prolonged immobility should be considered at risk. In contrast to stress ulcer bleeding events, VTEs are a frequent occurrence in the ICU, and surveillance studies of trauma patients found DVT rates of 50%.[42] The most significant consequence of VTE is pulmonary embolism (discussed in detail in the Respiratory System), which can be fatal. All ICU patients should receive mechanical VTE prophylaxis in the form of compression stockings and sequential pneumatic devices, which are thought to activate tissue plasminogen and promote local fibrinolysis. Patients with lower extremity fractures or ischemic peripheral vascular disease may not be candidates for these devices. For most ICU patients, mechanical VTE prophylaxis is inadequate, and pharmacologic prophylaxis is indicated.

Pharmacologic prophylaxis has been shown to reduce VTE and pulmonary embolism compared with mechanical devices or no prophylaxis at all. In the past, the most commonly used pharmacologic agent was unfractionated heparin given subcutaneously, but there has been a move away from heparin as newer agents have become available. Enoxaparin, a low-molecular-weight heparin, was found to reduce the risk of DVT by 30% compared with unfractionated heparin in a group of high-risk trauma patients, without a difference in adverse events. This trial and subsequent ones have established enoxaparin as preferred VTE prophylaxis for high-risk patients. In contrast to enoxaparin, only a small amount of unfractionated heparin is metabolized by the kidneys, and it is often used in patients with AKI.

With the increasing obesity epidemic, it is likely that many patients are receiving inadequate prophylactic doses of VTE prophylaxis. Enoxaparin was approved with fixed dosing, but the advent of an assay for activated factor X along with treatment failures in obese patients led to the interest in weight-based dosing. Enoxaparin dosed 0.5 mg/kg twice daily based on actual body weight, targeted for anti–factor Xa levels of 0.2 to 0.5 IU/mL has been shown to be an appropriate and safe strategy for obese ICU patients. Most of the data on dosing obese patients have come from the bariatric literature, and few data on critically ill obese patients are available. ICU patients who are at high risk for VTE but cannot be anticoagulated for an extended period, such as patients with hemorrhagic stroke, should receive an inferior vena cava filter. These filters do not prevent DVTs; they prevent large pulmonary embolisms, although small pulmonary embolisms may make it through to the lungs. Inferior vena cava filters are typically placed in the operating room, but bedside placement using intravascular ultrasound or fluoroscopic guidance is gaining interest. Bedside placement has realized savings in cost, operative time, and need for transport, while increasing timeliness of placement without problems of malpositioning.

SPECIAL ISSUES

Long-Term Intensive Care Unit Outcomes

Since the days of Semmelweiss and Codman, surgeons have been at the forefront of advancing quality in health care, a concept that has only more recently taken hold in the rest of health care as governmental and other organizations have embraced the "quality movement." Modern ICU care has made significant progress as technology and medications have improved, but some of the most dramatic advancements in the quality of care have been driven by the embrace of evidence-based practice. These changes coupled with an aging population who are living longer with more comorbidities has called into question some of the purpose of critical care as the focus turns from quantity of life to quality of life. Until more recently, most research in the ICU was based on short-term outcomes, such as 30-day mortality or survival to discharge, but as the amount of organ failure that can be supported has grown along with increasingly complex care, patients, families, and providers are questioning the outcomes of ICU survival. Research into the long-term physical, cognitive, and emotional outcomes of ICU discharge is in its infancy, and much remains to be learned, but this begs the difficult question: What will be the application of these outcomes data once known?

Some of the initial studies of long-term ICU care are becoming available, and some of the revelations are disconcerting. "Surviving intensive care: a report from the 2002 Brussels Roundtable" was a landmark article in *Intensive Care Medicine* that suggested that short-term outcomes such as in-hospital mortality were poor measures of "patient-centered outcomes." The authors also introduced the concept that the health and well-being of families of ICU patients should also be included in research looking at outcomes of critical care. Most importantly, the concept of health-related quality of life (HRQOL) arose from this gathering in Brussels as an outcomes measure to affirm focus on the patient beyond what transpires in the ICU.[43] Surgeons need to know about the long-term outcomes of critical illness so that they can better counsel patients and families during the perioperative period because care is "beginning and ending outside the ICU box."[43]

Most long-term ICU outcomes research has involved heterogeneous patient populations with far more medical ICU patients than surgical patients, and although this limits the applicability of these data to surgical patients, it does not completely invalidate the data. In a 2011 prospective longitudinal study, Khouli and associates[44] showed that one third of patients admitted to the ICU died within 6 months and that the oldest survivors had the poorest results on HRQOL questionnaires. In that study, chronic obstructive pulmonary disease present before ICU admission was the most significant predictor of mortality at 6 months. Mortality at 1 year after ICU discharge for septic patients was shown to be surprisingly high, as was the presence of lasting cognitive impairment. Compared with age-matched healthy control subjects, ICU patients who survive to 6 months after discharge demonstrated worse physical function, general health, and social functioning, and their HRQOL outcomes remained poor compared with baseline.[45] The need for RRT after ICU discharge has been associated with dismal results with almost uniform mortality at 3 months in nonsurgical patients older than 75 years. Patients with ARDS during their ICU stay have been shown to have lasting difficulties with muscle weakness, depression, and significant physical limitations but surprisingly few pulmonary limitations. Although long-term data after traumatic injury are limited, it appears that many of these patients return to their previous level of health and employment as long as they do not have significant TBI. Based on what little data we have about post-ICU outcomes, it appears that outcomes after ICU discharge for patients with traumatic injury and patients with ARDS are not as dismal as outcomes for patients with sepsis and oncologic patients.

TABLE 21-4 Adverse Long-Term Outcomes for Intensive Care Unit Survivors

PHYSICAL LIMITATIONS	COGNITIVE LIMITATIONS	EMOTIONAL ISSUES
Inability to do ADL	Inability to do ADL	Decreased social functioning
Loss of independence	Inability to concentrate	Depression
Poor exercise tolerance	Memory deficits	Sleep disturbances
Neuromyopathies	Poor problem solving	PTSD
Unsteadiness	Disorganization	Anxiety

ADL, activities of daily living; *PTSD*, post-traumatic stress disorder.

End-of-Life Care

One of the most difficult discussions that a physician can have with a patient centers around goals of care, particularly as the patient becomes elderly or develops a serious illness. Because this discussion is so difficult, many patients arrive in the ICU with their wishes regarding end-of-life care ill-defined. Similarly, less than 50% of Americans have a "living will" establishing what level of support they want if they are critically ill or if treatment is medically futile or what their long-term goals after discharge from the ICU would be. Patients with intra-abdominal catastrophes, shock, altered mental status, major trauma, or burns are not in any condition to have such a discussion. It is imperative that the ICU team remain in close contact with family members and health care representatives of critically ill patients at all times. Soon after a critically ill patient is admitted to the ICU and after the intensivist has had time to review the medical record, laboratory results, and other diagnostic studies, a meeting should be held with the patient's representatives to establish goals of care. At that time, the provider needs to offer a frank assessment of the patient's status and a reasonable prognosis based on a synthesis of all available data. It is equally important that the provider understand what the patient's wishes for outcomes after ICU discharge are, what restrictions or limitations the patient would be willing to accept, and how much the patient would be willing to endure to achieve those goals (Table 21-4). If the patient is unable to communicate the answers to these questions, the patient's representatives must provide answers. The amalgamation of all this information is how the goals of therapy are established, and a determination of an advance directive (i.e., code status) commonly is made at this time. Periodic meetings are needed as more information becomes available and the clinical picture becomes clearer. Open and nonadversarial communication becomes even more important when a patient in the ICU experiences a decline or has a complication of care, or there is an increased chance of death. These discussions are best held in a quiet, private location, rather than as an impromptu meeting in a hallway or the patient's room. Ideally, these meetings should be attended by representatives from the ICU care team, family members, and the primary surgeon if applicable. Small-scale meetings such as this typically occur on a daily basis, and larger extended meetings are typically held in response to significant developments, such as the need for mechanical ventilation or RRT in response to major complications or if there has been a significant event such that previously established goals are no longer possible. In the case of the latter, this may open the door to a discussion of futility, not in terms of medical futility, but rather futility that is patient defined.

Over the last 2 decades, there has been a major shift in how end-of-life care is approached in the ICU. Previously, such approaches used a paternalistic system where the physician was in a dominant role establishing the plan; at the present time, patient autonomy is foremost, and the physician serves more as an advisor and facilitator of the patient's wishes. Some authors call this "self-determination," which began in the early 1990s as more patients were noted to seek "do not resuscitate," "do not intubate," and "do not hospitalize" orders. Health care proxies were also more often officially named as surrogate decision makers in cases where patients lost mental capacity to make decisions. These trends have helped guide the ICU team and have reduced the number of futile situations in the ICU. Another change is a better understanding of the relationship between advances in ICU care, quality of life, and a patient's identity. With the vast technologic advances in critical care, including salvage ventilation modes for ARDS, ECMO, parenteral nutrition, and support devices such as left ventricular assist devices, there is increasing ability to support patients and stave off death for extended periods. End-of-life care has become complicated because these therapies can make it difficult for family members of patients to recognize just how ill or tenuous the patient is. When communicating with families, it is important that the ICU team convey the degree of illness and support the patient requires to shift the discussion from meanings of biologic or physiologic life to a different set of meanings. Walker and Lovat[46] defined a second level of life as a "sense of personhood and the essence or meaningfulness of human life." In essence, they were describing the paramount importance of quality of life from the point of view of the patient and the individuals who are meaningful to the patient's personhood. Thus, the discussion regarding end-of-life care has morphed from "can we?" to "should we?"

When care has become medically futile or obtaining the patient's long-term goals is impossible, care shifts to alternative strategies such as hospice care or withdrawal of support. Hospice care aims to provide physical and emotional support to patients and family members and may be rendered at home or in a facility. A wide range of services are possible, including analgesia and anxiolysis, oxygen, various medical devices, chaplain services, and counselors. For the sickest patients or patients on the highest levels of organ support, it is impossible to leave the ICU because any interruption of support would result in the patient's death. Hospice services can be arranged in an inpatient fashion, or the patient can be made "comfort measures only" or "no escalation of care" such that all potentially painful or invasive measures are withheld. A "comfort measures only" patient per The Joint Commission definition should receive only therapies that provide maximum comfort during the natural process of dying, and all other therapies should be avoided or discontinued. Mechanical ventilation is often discontinued, and the patient's air hunger is treated with morphine, which is an example of the principle of double effect. All attempts should be made to allow the patient's family to be at the bedside if the patient desires, and the patient should be offered privacy as well as medical social work and chaplain support services so that the patient may die with dignity and comfort in the presence of his or her extended family.

SELECTED REFERENCES

Caironi P, Tognoni G, Gattinoni L: Albumin replacement in severe sepsis or septic shock. *N Engl J Med* 371:84, 2014.

This randomized trial comparing fluid resuscitation strategies of albumin with crystalloid versus crystalloid alone in patients with severe sepsis or septic shock showed that albumin led to a higher mean arterial pressure in the first 7 days and lower net fluid balance, but there were no significant differences in mortality or secondary outcomes.

Casaer MP, Mesotten D, Hermans G, et al: Early versus late parenteral nutrition in critically ill adults. *N Engl J Med* 365:506–517, 2011.

In a randomized study of initiation of total parenteral nutrition (TPN) within 48 hours of intensive care unit (ICU) admission compared with initiation after 8 days in the ICU, mortality rates and functional outcomes were similar, but the late TPN group had fewer infections.

Dunkelgrun M, Boersma E, Schouten O, et al: Bisoprolol and fluvastatin for the reduction of perioperative cardiac mortality and myocardial infarction in intermediate-risk patients undergoing noncardiovascular surgery: A randomized controlled trial (DECREASE-IV). *Ann Surg* 249:921–926, 2009.

In a randomized trial of more than 1000 adults of intermediate cardiac risk undergoing noncardiac surgery, low-dose beta blocker therapy was associated with a significant reduction in 30-day cardiac death and nonfatal myocardial infarction. Fluvastatin improved outcomes as well, but this was not statistically significant.

Guerin C, Reignier J, Richard JC, et al: Prone positioning in severe acute respiratory distress syndrome. *N Engl J Med* 368: 2159–2168, 2013.

In a multicenter randomized trial of 466 adult patients with severe acute respiratory distress syndrome, one group was positioned prone for at least 16 hours per day, and the other group remained supine. The prone group had significantly lower 28-day and 90-day mortality.

Iwashyna TJ, Ely EW, Smith DM, et al: Long-term cognitive impairment and functional disability among survivors of severe sepsis. *JAMA* 304:1787–1794, 2010.

This prospective cohort study showed significant cognitive and physical limitations after discharge from the intensive care unit in patients admitted with severe sepsis who were 75 years old or older.

Kress JP, Pohlman AS, O'Connor MF, et al: Daily interruption of sedative infusions in critically ill patients undergoing mechanical ventilation. *N Engl J Med* 342:1471–1477, 2000.

This is an important randomized controlled trial of mechanically ventilated adults that showed sedation holidays result in shorter duration of mechanical ventilation and intensive care unit length of stay.

Peek GJ, Mugford M, Tiruvoipati R, et al: Efficacy and economic assessment of conventional ventilatory support versus extracorporeal membrane oxygenation for severe adult respiratory failure (CESAR): A multicentre randomised controlled trial. *Lancet* 374: 1351–1363, 2009.

In a randomized trial of 180 adults with severe respiratory failure comparing conventional ventilator management with extracorporeal membrane oxygenation (ECMO) therapy, ECMO resulted in improved rates of 6-month survival with lasting disability.

Sprung CL, Annane D, Keh D, et al: Hydrocortisone therapy for patients with septic shock. *N Engl J Med* 358:111–124, 2008.

A large, randomized trial comparing hydrocortisone with placebo in patients with severe sepsis or septic shock showed no mortality benefit and slightly increased rates of infection in the group receiving steroids.

Ventilation with lower tidal volumes as compared with traditional tidal volumes for acute lung injury and the acute respiratory distress syndrome. The Acute Respiratory Distress Syndrome Network. *N Engl J Med* 342:1301–1308, 2000.

This seminal article established the survival benefit of lung protective ventilation low tidal volumes in patients with acute respiratory distress syndrome. This study led to worldwide changes in ventilator management.

Vincent JL, Baron JF, Reinhart K, et al: Anemia and blood transfusion in critically ill patients. *JAMA* 288:1499–1507, 2002.

This prospective observational study detailed the prevalence of anemia in intensive care unit patients, the significant frequency of transfusions, and the increased mortality associated with transfusions. The authors also described the effect of transfusion on organ function.

REFERENCES

1. Morandi A, Brummel NE, Ely EW: Sedation, delirium and mechanical ventilation: The "ABCDE" approach. *Curr Opin Crit Care* 17:43–49, 2011.

2. van Eijk MM, van Marum RJ, Klijn IA, et al: Comparison of delirium assessment tools in a mixed intensive care unit. *Crit Care Med* 37:1881–1885, 2009.
3. Saddawi-Konefka D, Berg SM, Nejad SH, et al: Catatonia in the ICU: An important and underdiagnosed cause of altered mental status. A case series and review of the literature. *Crit Care Med* 42:e234–e241, 2014.
4. Kress JP, Pohlman AS, O'Connor MF, et al: Daily interruption of sedative infusions in critically ill patients undergoing mechanical ventilation. *N Engl J Med* 342:1471–1477, 2000.
5. Popping DM, Elia N, Van Aken HK, et al: Impact of epidural analgesia on mortality and morbidity after surgery: Systematic review and meta-analysis of randomized controlled trials. *Ann Surg* 259:1056–1067, 2014.
6. Devabhakthuni S, Armahizer MJ, Dasta JF, et al: Analgosedation: A paradigm shift in intensive care unit sedation practice. *Ann Pharmacother* 46:530–540, 2012.
7. Dunkelgrun M, Boersma E, Schouten O, et al: Bisoprolol and fluvastatin for the reduction of perioperative cardiac mortality and myocardial infarction in intermediate-risk patients undergoing noncardiovascular surgery: a randomized controlled trial (DECREASE-IV). *Ann Surg* 249:921–926, 2009.
8. Bhave PD, Goldman LE, Vittinghoff E, et al: Statin use and postoperative atrial fibrillation after major noncardiac surgery. *Heart Rhythm* 9:163–169, 2012.
9. London MJ, Hur K, Schwartz GG, et al: Association of perioperative beta-blockade with mortality and cardiovascular morbidity following major noncardiac surgery. *JAMA* 309: 1704–1713, 2013.
10. Botto F, Alonso-Coello P, Chan MT, et al: Myocardial injury after noncardiac surgery: A large, international, prospective cohort study establishing diagnostic criteria, characteristics, predictors, and 30-day outcomes. *Anesthesiology* 120:564–578, 2014.
11. Friese RS, Shafi S, Gentilello LM: Pulmonary artery catheter use is associated with reduced mortality in severely injured patients: A National Trauma Data Bank analysis of 53,312 patients. *Crit Care Med* 34:1597–1601, 2006.
12. Chung KK, Wolf SE, Cancio LC, et al: Resuscitation of severely burned military casualties: Fluid begets more fluid. *J Trauma* 67:231–237, discussion 237, 2009.
13. Wiedemann HP: A perspective on the fluids and catheters treatment trial (FACTT). Fluid restriction is superior in acute lung injury and ARDS. *Cleve Clin J Med* 75:42–48, 2008.
14. Finfer S, Bellomo R, Boyce N, et al: A comparison of albumin and saline for fluid resuscitation in the intensive care unit. *N Engl J Med* 350:2247–2256, 2004.
15. Yang KL, Tobin MJ: A prospective study of indexes predicting the outcome of trials of weaning from mechanical ventilation. *N Engl J Med* 324:1445–1450, 1991.
16. Croce MA, Swanson JM, Magnotti LJ, et al: The futility of the clinical pulmonary infection score in trauma patients. *J Trauma* 60:523–527, discussion 527–528, 2006.
17. ARDS Definition Task Force, Ranieri VM, Rubenfeld GD, et al: Acute respiratory distress syndrome: The Berlin Definition. *JAMA* 307:2526–2533, 2012.
18. Ventilation with lower tidal volumes as compared with traditional tidal volumes for acute lung injury and the acute respiratory distress syndrome. The Acute Respiratory Distress Syndrome Network. *N Engl J Med* 342:1301–1308, 2000.
19. Peek GJ, Mugford M, Tiruvoipati R, et al: Efficacy and economic assessment of conventional ventilatory support versus extracorporeal membrane oxygenation for severe adult respiratory failure (CESAR): A multicentre randomised controlled trial. *Lancet* 374:1351–1363, 2009.
20. Guerin C, Reignier J, Richard JC, et al: Prone positioning in severe acute respiratory distress syndrome. *N Engl J Med* 368:2159–2168, 2013.
21. Zagli G, Linden M, Spina R, et al: Early tracheostomy in intensive care unit: A retrospective study of 506 cases of video-guided Ciaglia Blue Rhino tracheostomies. *J Trauma* 68:367–372, 2010.
22. Kress JP, Pohlman AS, Alverdy J, et al: The impact of morbid obesity on oxygen cost of breathing (VO(2RESP)) at rest. *Am J Respir Crit Care Med* 160:883–886, 1999.
23. Mahanna E, Crimi E, White P, et al: Nutrition and metabolic support for critically ill patients. *Curr Opin Anaesthesiol* 28:131–138, 2015.
24. Puthucheary ZA, Rawal J, McPhail M, et al: Acute skeletal muscle wasting in critical illness. *JAMA* 310:1591–1600, 2013.
25. Jensen GL, Compher C, Sullivan DH, et al: Recognizing malnutrition in adults: Definitions and characteristics, screening, assessment, and team approach. *JPEN J Parenter Enteral Nutr* 37:802–807, 2013.
26. White JV, Guenter P, Jensen G, et al: Consensus statement: Academy of Nutrition and Dietetics and American Society for Parenteral and Enteral Nutrition: characteristics recommended for the identification and documentation of adult malnutrition (undernutrition). *JPEN J Parenter Enteral Nutr* 36:275–283, 2012.
27. Casaer MP, Mesotten D, Hermans G, et al: Early versus late parenteral nutrition in critically ill adults. *N Engl J Med* 365:506–517, 2011.
28. Harvey SE, Parrott F, Harrison DA, et al: Trial of the route of early nutritional support in critically ill adults. *N Engl J Med* 371:1673–1684, 2014.
29. Joannidis M, Metnitz B, Bauer P, et al: Acute kidney injury in critically ill patients classified by AKIN versus RIFLE using the SAPS 3 database. *Intensive Care Med* 35:1692–1702, 2009.
30. Schefold JC, Haehling S, Pschowski R, et al: The effect of continuous versus intermittent renal replacement therapy on the outcome of critically ill patients with acute renal failure (CONVINT): A prospective randomized controlled trial. *Crit Care* 18:R11, 2014.
31. Arabi Y, Ahmed QA, Haddad S, et al: Outcome predictors of cirrhosis patients admitted to the intensive care unit. *Eur J Gastroenterol Hepatol* 16:333–339, 2004.
32. Whiting D, DiNardo JA: TEG and ROTEM: Technology and clinical applications. *Am J Hematol* 89:228–232, 2014.
33. Hebert PC, Wells G, Blajchman MA, et al: A multicenter, randomized, controlled clinical trial of transfusion requirements in critical care. Transfusion Requirements in Critical Care Investigators, Canadian Critical Care Trials Group. *N Engl J Med* 340:409–417, 1999.
34. Shakur H, Roberts I, Bautista R, et al: Effects of tranexamic acid on death, vascular occlusive events, and blood transfusion in trauma patients with significant haemorrhage (CRASH-2): A randomised, placebo-controlled trial. *Lancet* 376:23–32, 2010.
35. van den Berghe G, Wouters P, Weekers F, et al: Intensive insulin therapy in critically ill patients. *N Engl J Med* 345:1359–1367, 2001.

36. Finfer S, Chittock DR, Su SY, et al: Intensive versus conventional glucose control in critically ill patients. *N Engl J Med* 360:1283–1297, 2009.
37. Annane D, Sebille V, Charpentier C, et al: Effect of treatment with low doses of hydrocortisone and fludrocortisone on mortality in patients with septic shock. *JAMA* 288:862–871, 2002.
38. Sprung CL, Annane D, Keh D, et al: Hydrocortisone therapy for patients with septic shock. *N Engl J Med* 358:111–124, 2008.
39. Barie PS, Hydo LJ, Eachempati SR: Causes and consequences of fever complicating critical surgical illness. *Surg Infect (Larchmt)* 5:145–159, 2004.
40. Bone RC, Balk RA, Cerra FB, et al: Definitions for sepsis and organ failure and guidelines for the use of innovative therapies in sepsis. The ACCP/SCCM Consensus Conference Committee. American College of Chest Physicians/Society of Critical Care Medicine. *Chest* 101:1644–1655, 1992.
41. Iwashyna TJ, Ely EW, Smith DM, et al: Long-term cognitive impairment and functional disability among survivors of severe sepsis. *JAMA* 304:1787–1794, 2010.
42. Geerts WH, Jay RM, Code KI, et al: A comparison of low-dose heparin with low-molecular-weight heparin as prophylaxis against venous thromboembolism after major trauma. *N Engl J Med* 335:701–707, 1996.
43. Angus DC, Carlet J, 2002 Brussels Roundtable Participants: Surviving intensive care: A report from the 2002 Brussels Roundtable. *Intensive Care Med* 29:368–377, 2003.
44. Khouli H, Astua A, Dombrowski W, et al: Changes in health-related quality of life and factors predicting long-term outcomes in older adults admitted to intensive care units. *Crit Care Med* 39:731–737, 2011.
45. Hofhuis JG, Spronk PE, van Stel HF, et al: The impact of critical illness on perceived health-related quality of life during ICU treatment, hospital stay, and after hospital discharge: A long-term follow-up study. *Chest* 133:377–385, 2008.
46. Walker P, Lovat T: Concepts of personhood and autonomy as they apply to end-of-life decisions in intensive care. *Med Health Care Philos* 18:309–315, 2015.

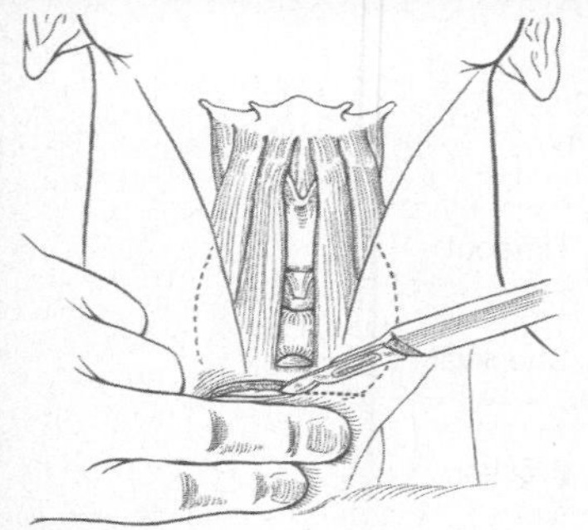

CHAPTER 22

Bedside Surgical Procedures

Addison K. May, Bradley M. Dennis, Oliver L. Gunter, Jose J. Diaz

OUTLINE

Bedside surgical procedures have become standard in many intensive care units (ICUs), replacing the operating room (OR) as the preferred location for select procedures in critically ill patients.[1] Performance of appropriately selected procedures within the ICU limits the risk of transporting critically ill patients, facilitates flexibility in timing and scheduling, and reduces cost.[2-12] The ability to perform some operations at the bedside may be lifesaving in critically ill patients too unstable to transport safely to the OR. Advancements in monitoring and sedation, in endoscopic and percutaneous techniques, and in bedside imaging have enabled the transition of several procedures traditionally performed in the OR and endoscopy and interventional radiology suites to the ICU. Some procedures now regularly performed in the ICU include bedside laparotomy, tracheostomy, percutaneous endoscopic feeding access, percutaneous drainage procedures, and the placement of inferior vena cava filters. For example, between 2006 and 2014, greater than 2800 percutaneous tracheostomies, 900 percutaneous endoscopic gastrostomy (PEG) or gastrojejunostomy tube placements, 450 exploration and irrigation of open abdomens, and 50 exploratory laparotomies were performed at the bedside in the ICUs at Vanderbilt University Medical Center. In unstable patients, other procedures also may be performed at the bedside, including irrigation and débridement of wounds, orthopedic stabilization with external fixation, fasciotomies, amputations, and diagnostic laparoscopy.

Although bedside operative procedures can be performed safely with complication rates equal to in the OR, doing so mandates that cases are appropriately selected and that appropriate safety practices are consistently implemented. The ICU represents a complex environment in which to perform complex processes and procedures. Recognition of the numerous potentials for error and adverse events in such settings is important. Based on the experience of industry and other high-reliability organizations, prevention of error and adverse events requires standardization of processes and elimination of variability.[13] Protocols and safety practices specifically for bedside operative procedures should be in place to ensure the ability to perform these procedures safely, with low infection rates, and with the assurance of comfort and amnesia. In this chapter, we discuss the following topics:

1. The rationale for bedside surgical procedures
2. Process of bringing the OR to the bedside
3. Systematic safety methodologies and practices to ensure safe performance of bedside procedures
4. Selection of patients for bedside surgical procedures
5. Specific considerations for common bedside procedures
   a. Bedside laparotomy
   b. Percutaneous tracheostomy
   c. Percutaneous endoscopic feeding tubes
   d. Bronchoscopy

RATIONALE FOR BEDSIDE SURGICAL PROCEDURES

For good reasons, most surgical procedures are performed in the OR. The centralization of resources, including anesthesia personnel and equipment, surgical equipment, radiology, specialized nursing and procedural support staff, and safety policies and principles, make the modern surgical suite an ideal venue for most operations (Fig. 22-1). However, OR demand may exceed available resources, complicating timely access to the OR and scheduling of unplanned, urgent, or emergent cases. Competition for OR space may delay or prevent timely operative procedures for critically ill patients. Additionally, performance of procedures in the OR mandate transportation of critically ill patients from the ICU and back and requires substantial resource utilization and costs. As the complexity and severity of illness of critical care patients have increased, so too has the risk related to their transport. The transport of critically ill patients frequently requires multiple personnel, including nursing staff, transport staff, respiratory care, and anesthesia staff. Furthermore, the change of venue and personnel caring for the patient necessitates detailed communication for handoff and represents a potential source of medical error.[2]

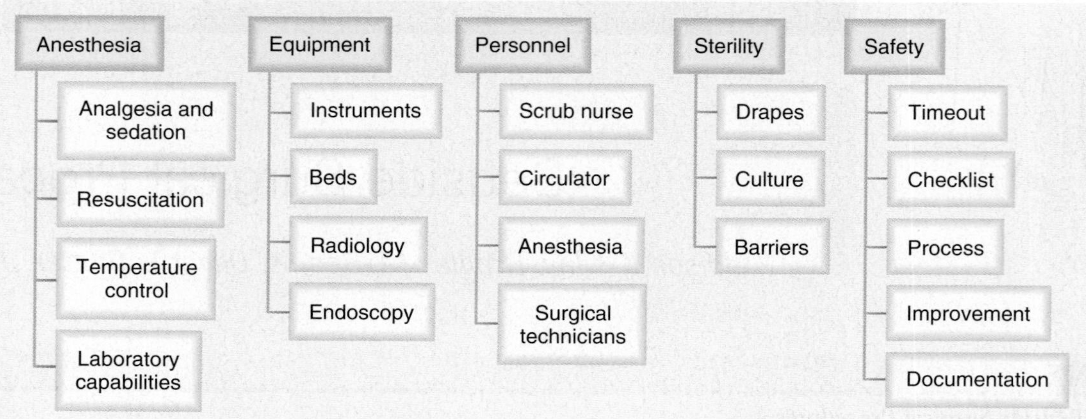

FIGURE 22-1 Resources available in the operating room.

The transport of a patient from the ICU to the OR is a resource sink, adds cost, and increases risk. Consideration of transport to the OR should be evaluated in the same manner as other treatments by assessing risk versus benefit for the individual patient.

TAKING THE OPERATING ROOM TO THE BEDSIDE

By creating and applying a well-constructed system, the major benefits of the OR can be reproduced at the bedside (Fig. 22-2). As Figure 22-2 infers, multiple factors are required to create and maintain a successful system for performing bedside procedures. Management guidelines may include standard operating procedures, preprocedure checklists including time-out procedures, and sedation protocols. Dedicated procedure support personnel not only decrease the variability in how an individual procedure is performed but also play important roles in compliance to guidelines, both of which are significant factors in reducing error. Appropriate access to supplies may require temporary storage of core equipment in an individual ICU with standardized restocking mechanisms, streamlining the supply chain. Finally, a facilitative mindset among staff is vital to the success of such a system.

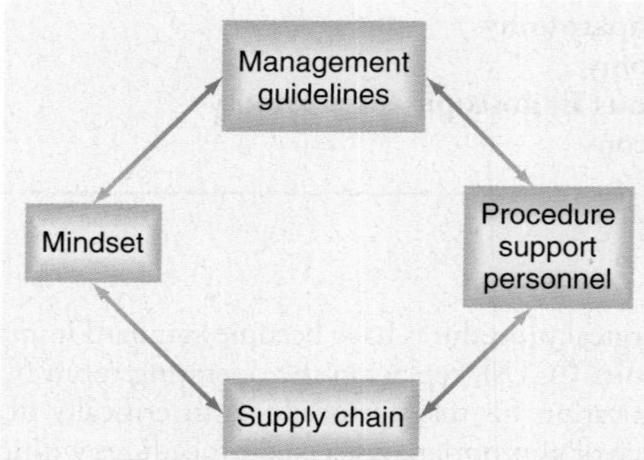

FIGURE 22-2 Fundamentals vital to the success of bedside surgical procedures.

SAFETY PRACTICES FOR BEDSIDE SURGICAL PROCEDURES

To ensure the safety of operative procedures performed at the bedside in the ICU, systematic measures should be in place for appropriate patient selection; adequate expertise of supporting personnel; limited procedural variability; adequate monitoring and anesthesia; and facilitation of concise, accurate, and specific intrateam communication. Measures shown to increase safety in the OR are also appropriate for procedures performed at bedside in the ICU. Implementation of the Safe Surgery Saves Lives program developed by the World Health Organization (WHO) has been associated with a significant global reduction in perioperative morbidity and mortality.[14] The 10 safety objectives outlined in the WHO Guidelines for Safe Surgery 2009 are as follows[15]:

1. The team will operate on the correct patient at the correct site.
2. The team will use methods known to prevent harm from administration of anesthetics, while protecting the patient from pain.
3. The team will recognize and effectively prepare for life-threatening loss of airway or respiratory function.
4. The team will recognize and effectively prepare for risk of high blood loss.
5. The team will avoid inducing an allergic or adverse drug reaction for which the patient is known to be at significant risk.
6. The team will consistently use methods known to minimize the risk for surgical site infection.
7. The team will prevent inadvertent retention of instruments and sponges in surgical wounds.
8. The team will secure and accurately identify all surgical specimens.
9. The team will effectively communicate and exchange critical information for the safe conduct of the operation.
10. Hospitals and public health systems will establish routine surveillance of surgical capacity, volume, and results.

The use of specifically trained procedure support personnel to support bedside operative procedures within the ICU greatly facilitates reduction in variability, compliance with standard operative procedures, reduction of communication errors, and maintenance of appropriate skill sets. Depending on the volume of procedures to be supported, these personnel can be dedicated to a specific unit or service or used to support bedside procedures on numerous services in multiple ICUs. Limiting this procedure support role to a small number of personnel allows greater degree of expertise to be developed and, in our experience, has been extremely valuable in maintaining procedural safety; this is particularly true with handling of the airway and endotracheal tube during percutaneous tracheostomies. Additionally, these personnel are charged with development and monitoring of safety practices and ensure their application during all procedures.

Management guidelines, protocols, and standard operating procedures should be in place before the routine performance of bedside operative procedures. They should be in line with procedures developed for the OR and be easily accessible, and compliance should be monitored. Because of variations in specific personnel and practice patterns in various ICUs, documents may be customized to each location to ensure their appropriate application during bedside operative procedures. These documents should address the selection of appropriate cases, mandatory personnel, equipment, medications, and monitoring. An example of a bedside operative guideline is provided in Box 22-1.[7] All patients should have blood pressure, electrocardiography, pulse oximetry, and ventilation routinely monitored throughout the procedures. Adequate personnel must be present to allow performance of the procedure, monitoring of sedation and anesthesia, medication administration, manipulation of ventilation if required, and documentation. The actual number of personnel required varies depending on the procedure and expertise of particular personnel. Analgesia and sedation must be ensured with appropriate medications under the direction of the adequately credentialed personnel. Additionally, guidelines and protocols should include standards for adequate preparation, equipment, and instrument accounting.

The use of preprocedure time-out and procedural checklists aids in ensuring appropriate safety practices. Use of these tools helps limit communication errors, facilitates compliance with standard operating procedures, and can be used to aid in documentation and compliance monitoring. These tools should be consistent with practices employed in the OR to reduce variability where appropriate. Figure 22-3 provides an example of such a procedural checklist. Ideally, these tools can be combined with forms required for documentation, and information can be captured for quality and performance analysis.

Ensuring a high degree of safety of bedside operative procedures and providing documentation of such when required mandate that mechanisms for tracking procedure performance, compliance monitoring, and adverse event review and reporting are developed. These mechanisms must be applicable locally to facilitate consistent, nonvariable performance and interface with global hospital safety mechanisms and initiatives. Development of process mapping flow charts and diagrams facilitates the integration of unit-specific, departmental, and hospital-wide processes and helps delineate lines of communication and authority.

BOX 22-1 Bedside Surgery Protocol

Indications

Decompressive celiotomy for abdominal compartment syndrome

Exploratory celiotomy for intra-abdominal hemorrhage after damage control and packing

Reexploration of a previously open abdomen for washout or closure

Exploratory celiotomy to rule out intra-abdominal sepsis in a patient with ventilatory requirements that prohibit safe transport to the OR

Protocol

ICU attending physician and operating surgeon will be present for the entire surgical procedure.

Informed consent will be obtained (if possible).

Preprocedure checklist will be reviewed by the bedside nurse.

Bedside nurse and a respiratory therapist will monitor patient and record procedure (conscious sedation sheet).

Indications to proceed to OR (level 1):

- Surgical bleeding
- Dead bowel
- Need to open another body cavity
- Surgeon preference

For laparotomies:

- A sterile perimeter will be set up in the patient's room. All individuals must wear a surgical head covering and mask.
- The ICU attending physician will oversee anesthetic management of the patient.
- General anesthesia will include narcotics, benzodiazepines, propofol, paralytics, and ventilator management.
- A sterile hand wash will be performed by the operating team.
- Preoperative antibiotics are indicated only if a new surgical wound is to be made (e.g., cefazolin [Ancef], 1-2 g intravenously).
- A povidone-iodine (Betadine)–chlorhexidine abdominal preparation will be used.
- A standard Bovie will be set up (when indicated).
- Wall suction canisters will be set up.
- A 4-liter warm irrigation with normal saline will be used.
- A standard bedside celiotomy tray will be set up with suture on a sterile field.

Adapted from Vanderbilt University Medical Center, Division of Trauma and Surgical Critical Care: Emergency general surgery protocols: Bedside surgery protocol, 2005 (https://medschool.vanderbilt.edu/trauma-and-scc/files/trauma-and-scc/public_files/Protocols/Bedside%20Surgery%20.pdf).

SELECTION OF PATIENTS FOR BEDSIDE SURGICAL PROCEDURES

As noted previously, if selected appropriately, bedside operative procedures can be performed with similar risk of complications as when performed in the OR, at lower cost, and without transportation risks.[2,6-10,12] However, there are no randomized studies and few retrospective reviews that evaluate the safety of bedside operative procedures or help delineate what the appropriate patient populations and operative procedures are. The safety and efficacy of bedside procedures vary depending on the local experience and application of safety practices. As experience is gained, indications may broaden, and frequency may increase. The decision to perform an operative procedure at the bedside considers the balance between the difficulty and risk of transport; the complexity of the operation; the ability to achieve timely OR space; and the safety, ease, and cost savings of performing the procedure at the bedside. Most major operative procedures should be performed in the OR. In general, the indications for bedside operative procedures fall into two categories: (1) the patient is too unstable for transport to the OR and the procedure is a required, lifesaving intervention, or (2) the procedure is modest enough that the risk of transport, difficulties of OR scheduling, and cost and resource utilization of the OR favor a bedside procedure.[16] Factors that generally favor performance of procedures in the OR include complex procedures, bleeding risk from major vascular structures, need for insertion of prosthetic materials, significant lighting requirements, and lengthy procedures. Commonly performed bedside procedures include percutaneous and open tracheostomy, PEG or percutaneous endoscopic gastrojejunostomy (PEGJ) tube placement, bronchoscopy, soft tissue débridement,

SICU Procedure "TIME-OUT" Check List			
Complete this form (a) just prior to beginning the procedure and (b) at the location where the procedure is to be performed			
Patient's Name: Medical record number:			
Procedure Type: ☐ Planned non-emergent ☐ Not planned non-emergent ☐ Emergent			
VERIFICATION			
1. Invasive procedure to be performed:			
		Circle one	
2. H&P completed if patient admitted within past 24 hours		Yes	No
3. Informed consent obtained? (Verified by Bedside RN and Procedure RN)		Yes	No
4. Correct patient identity? ☐ Arm Band ☐ MRN ☐ Consent If procedure is emergent, Bedside RN, Procedure RN, and Physician performing procedure need to verify patient ID and initial this form.		Yes	No
5. Agreement on procedure (Agreement b/w Physician performing procedure and Procedure RN)		Yes	No
6. Correct side/site verified and marked? ☐ NA ☐ Right ☐ Left ☐ Site: (Verified and marked by Physician performing procedure and Procedure RN)		Yes	No
7. Correct equipment available? (Verified by Physician performing procedure and Procedure RN)		Yes	No
8. Required resources available? (Verified by Physician performing procedure and Procedure RN)		Yes	No
9. Ready to setup procedure? (Verified by Procedure RN)		Yes	No
9. Ready to proceed with procedure? (Verified by Procedure RN)		Yes	No
TIME-OUT: All individuals performing and assisting with the procedure are to review the checklist and sign below.			
Physician performing procedure:			
Procedure RN name:			
Bedside RN name:			
Other:	Other:	Other:	
Staff calling "TIME-OUT": (Title and signature)			

FIGURE 22-3 Surgical intensive care unit procedure time-out checklist.

decompressive laparotomy for abdominal hypertension, washout and packing removal after a damage control laparotomy, placement of inferior vena cava filters, and damage control orthopedic procedures. Occasionally, the condition of extremely critically ill patients can be temporized at the bedside by the performance of a bedside operative procedure with subsequent performance of the definitive operation in the OR.

BEDSIDE LAPAROTOMY

Bedside laparotomy was initially a procedure of last resort in patients too sick to proceed to the OR—a heroic attempt to identify reversible intra-abdominal pathology as the patient was near death.[7] However, the recognition of abdominal compartment syndrome (ACS) as a frequent complication of resuscitation of acutely ill patients and the acceptance of the "damage control" approach to the management of acutely ill patients with intra-abdominal pathology has resulted in a dramatic increase in the application of bedside laparotomy in more controlled settings.[6,7,16-18] Damage control and management of ACS use an open abdomen approach in which the fascia remains open and necessitates the use of various temporary abdominal closure techniques. Indications for bedside laparotomy can be classified as emergent or semielective. Common emergent indications include (1) decompressive laparotomy for ACS, (2) control and packing for recurrent bleeding after a previous damage control laparotomy, and (3) suspicion of intra-abdominal infection in patients too critically ill to be transported to the OR. Common semielective indications include (1) pack removal after damage control laparotomy, (2) irrigation and débridement of the open abdomen, (3) source control for sepsis resulting from intra-abdominal pathology, and (4) management of traumatic abdominal defects.

Historically, the most common emergent indication for bedside laparotomy was for decompression of abdominal hypertension. Recognition and understanding of the pathophysiology of increased intra-abdominal pressure leading to organ system dysfunction—ACS—has increased significantly since Kron and associates first described the measurement of intra-abdominal pressure as an indication for abdominal reexploration.[17,19-21] ACS can be classified as primary, resulting from intra-abdominal processes, or secondary, resulting from bowel edema and intra-abdominal fluid secondary to the treatment and resuscitation of extra-abdominal pathology. Increasing intra-abdominal pressure leads to alterations in abdominal perfusion pressure, restricted venous return, and reduction of pulmonary compliance. These alterations can lead to cardiac failure, pulmonary decompensation, and oliguria. Severe elevations in abdominal pressure can lead to organ hypoperfusion and ischemia, although the pressure at which this occurs may vary depending on mean arterial pressure. Grading systems for the degree of abdominal hypertension have been proposed with grades III (21 to 25 mm Hg) and IV (>25 mm Hg) considered to be significantly elevated, defining ACS.[22] Management of ACS may involve only measures to ensure adequate abdominal perfusion pressures at lower pressures, but as intra-abdominal pressure increases, abdominal decompression by laparotomy is indicated. Appropriate treatment requires recognition of development of this syndrome. Routine monitoring of bladder pressures of patients requiring significant resuscitation after abdominal procedures and patients being resuscitated from a significant shock (base deficit >10) who receive 6 liters or more of crystalloid or 6 units or more of packed red blood cells in a 6-hour period is indicated.[17] With changes in resuscitation strategies in critically unstable patients, the incidence of ACS may be declining.

The acceptance of damage control, an abbreviated laparotomy to salvage trauma patients with exsanguination, has led to an increased application of bedside laparotomy for control of recurrent bleeding within the abdomen before correction of the patient's systemic physiology and for removal of abdominal packs, irrigation, and débridement.[23] Bedside laparotomy is common in most level I trauma centers where damage control and temporary abdominal closure for patients in extremis are frequently used. Numerous methods of temporary abdominal closure have been described and continue to evolve. We prefer to use negative pressure systems, and facility with the applications of these systems is required for patient management.

The open abdominal approach is also applied to the general surgery population, most commonly for the management of necrotizing pancreatitis, necrotizing soft tissue infection of the abdominal wall, diffuse peritonitis in patients at high risk of failure of source control, and mesenteric ischemia.[7,16] Damage control techniques with staged gastrointestinal reconstruction, serial abdominal washouts for source control, and delayed abdominal wall closure can be used in the management of these very complex patients. Controlled trials of these techniques are limited, and the indications and settings in which the open abdominal approach is most appropriate are not fully determined.

TRACHEOSTOMY

Tracheostomy is the most common surgical procedure in critically ill patients requiring prolonged mechanical ventilation.[24] Open and percutaneous dilatational tracheostomy (PDT) can be performed safely at the bedside in the ICU.[5,8,9,25,26] The ease and convenience of bedside tracheostomy in critically ill patients has made performance at the bedside the standard in many institutions.[27] Indications for tracheostomy in critically ill patients include the following:

- Presence of pathologic conditions predicting prolonged mechanical intubation, inability to protect airway, or both
- Airway edema and high-risk airway after maxillofacial and surgery and trauma
- High-risk airway resulting from cervical immobilization for fracture fixation
- Need for a surgical airway because of inability to intubate the patient

Identification of these indications is not always straightforward, and clinical decision making remains difficult. Perioperative mortality related to PDT in randomized studies appears to be less than 0.2%.[3,5,8,9,25,28] The safety of bedside PDT was confirmed in a retrospective analysis of more than 3000 consecutive procedures.[5] This analysis revealed a periprocedural major complication rate of 0.15% and a periprocedural mortality rate of less than 0.1% within this population of critically ill patients. Additionally, this review demonstrated the safety of bedside PDT in obese and superobese patients. These data are useful for decisions regarding the indications for tracheostomy in critically ill patients; patients in whom the risks of failure of extubation or airway loss are estimated to result in fatal outcome are greater than 1 in 1000 should be considered for tracheostomy. Timing of tracheostomy is controversial in patients with predicted prolonged mechanical ventilation. Studies have supported early tracheostomy (up to 7 days) versus delayed tracheostomy (after 7 days) with shorter ICU stays and less mechanical ventilation but with no difference in mortality in trauma and nontrauma populations.[28,29] However, a randomized study of medical ICU patients demonstrated a significant reduction in mortality (32% versus 62%), pneumonia (5% versus 25%), and accidental extubation (0 versus 6) when early tracheostomy (48 hours) was compared with delayed tracheostomy (14 to 16 days) for patients predicted to require 14 days of mechanical ventilation.[30] The early group also had significantly decreased ICU length of stay and ventilator days.

PDT has become widely used for elective tracheostomy in critically ill adult patients. Ciaglia and colleagues[31] first described elective PDT in 1985, and since that time, numerous modifications to the technique have been made. When comparing PDT with standard surgical tracheostomy performed in the OR, PDT demonstrated decreased wound infection, clinically relevant bleeding, and mortality.[8,25] Percutaneous tracheostomy has also been demonstrated to be more cost-effective in critically ill ICU patients.[3,9,26] Long-term complications have not been adequately studied in randomized trials to draw conclusions.

Reported perioperative complications of percutaneous tracheostomy include the following:

- Peristomal bleeding from injury to the anterior jugular veins or thyroid isthmus
- Injury of the trachea or esophagus or both by laceration through the back wall of the trachea
- Extraluminal placement by creating a false tract during placement of the tracheostomy tube
- Loss of airway

Major perioperative complications can be minimized by employing safety measures outlined in the previous sections. We find that specifically trained support personnel managing the airway is particularly helpful in limiting airway mishaps. Additionally, one of two techniques should be used to ensure proper positioning of the tracheostomy tube and to minimize risk of loss of airway by inadvertent extubation during the procedure: bronchoscopic guidance or semiopen technique with blunt dissection to the anterior trachea.[32,33] However, bronchoscopic guidance does not eliminate severe tracheal injuries, and involvement of experienced personnel is important to prevent these complications. PDT tracheostomies can be performed safely in morbidly obese patients; however, care must be taken in selecting the size and length of the tracheostomy tube.[5] There are no studies that appropriately describe methods to select the appropriate length of tracheostomy tubes in morbidly obese patients. However, our analysis of tracheostomy dislodgments within our institution suggested that inadequate tracheostomy length with a standard tube in morbidly obese patients was a major contributing factor. The routine use of proximally extended tracheostomy tubes rather than standard length tubes in patients with body mass index greater than 35 or in patients with severe anasarca eliminated this issue.

Long-term, the incidence of serious tracheal stenosis after percutaneous tracheostomy is low with reports of 6%,[34] and tracheal stenosis usually occurs early in the subglottic position. Subclinical tracheal stenosis is found in 40% of patients.[35] Follow-up of patients discharged from the ICU with tracheostomies is important to minimize and identify complications. Dedicated multidisciplinary tracheostomy teams have been shown to reduce time to decannulation, length of stay, and adverse events.[36]

PERCUTANEOUS ENDOSCOPIC GASTROSTOMY

Gauderer and coworkers[37] first described the PEG in 1980 for access into the stomach for enteral feedings using a "pull" technique. Various other techniques have since been described. The principle of a sutureless approximation of the stomach to the anterior abdominal wall has allowed the pull technique to become the most popular method used. The other two most commonly used techniques are the "push" and introducer techniques, both of which require the use of stay sutures to approximate the stomach to the anterior abdominal wall. Newer PEGJ tubes combine gastric and jejunal ports to allow distal feeding and proximal decompression.

Accepted primary indications for a PEG or PEGJ include inability to swallow, high risk of aspiration, severe facial trauma, and indications for mechanical ventilation for longer than 4 weeks.[4,38] Other indications include nutritional access for debilitated patients and patients with dementia with severe malnutrition. PEG tubes have been associated with reducing overall hospital cost.[39]

Numerous gastrostomy and gastrojejunostomy tubes are commercially available. Most allow simple gastrostomy assess with or without a valve. Some are flush with the skin and require a tube to be attached only during feeding. For critically ill patients with increased risk of aspiration, multilumen percutaneous endoscopic transgastric jejunostomy tubes are available. These tubes allow drainage of the stomach while feeding the proximal jejunum. A third lumen connects to a balloon that maintains apposition of the gastric and abdominal walls.[40] Although feeding can be started on the same day as the PEG is placed, most critically ill patients are not started on feedings for 24 hours.[41] Contraindications for PEG placement include the following:

- No endoscopic access
- Severe coagulopathy
- Gastric outlet obstruction
- Survival less than 4 weeks
- Inability to bring the gastric wall in approximation to the abdominal wall

There are a few relative contraindications, such as an inability to transilluminate through the anterior abdominal wall, gastric varices, and diffuse gastric cancer. Anterior wall inflammation or infection should be treated before the procedure. Ascites can be drained before the procedure and is not an absolute contraindication.[42] PEG tubes may be placed in the presence of a ventriculoperitoneal shunt or a dialysis catheter; however, placement should be separated by 1 to 2 weeks or more.[43,44] History of a previous or recent laparotomy is not a contraindication for PEG; however, a discrete indentation of the stomach when palpating the anterior abdominal wall and adequate transillumination should be ensured.[45]

PEG is thought to be a safe procedure whether it is performed in the gastrointestinal laboratory, the OR, or at bedside in the ICU. However, because PEG tube placement is frequently performed in debilitated or critically ill patients, complications are associated with a higher mortality than would be expected for most elective procedures.[46] Free intraperitoneal air after PEG is common and can persist for 4 weeks.[47] Abdominal wall infection can occur as an early complication of PEG placement; an ample skin incision that prevents creation of a closed space around the feeding tube and administration of antibiotics before the procedure have been demonstrated to decrease PEG site infections.[48] Dislodgment of the PEG from the stomach can occur and may be life-threatening. Dislodgment may occur acutely through the application of traction on the gastrostomy tube, pulling it partially or completely through the abdominal wall. Alternatively, the tube may necrose through the stomach wall if the PEG flange or balloon applies too much pressure on the gastric wall. If this complication occurs before development of a fibrous tract during the initial 10 to 14 days, it should be considered a surgical emergency because gastric contents would spill into the abdominal cavity. Operative closure of the gastrostomy is required. To minimize the risk of this complication, methods that prevent inadvertent movement of the gastrostomy tube should be used and meticulously followed. These methods include ensuring adequate fixation of the tube to the external abdominal wall, recording of the position of the gastrostomy tube at the skin surface immediately after the procedure with routine verification, and application of binders or other devices that limit the inadvertent application of traction of the tube.

BRONCHOSCOPY

Fiberoptic bronchoscopy of surgical patients is indicated for diagnostic and therapeutic indications. Therapeutic indications include insertion of an endotracheal tube, removal of foreign bodies inadvertently aspirated, removal of mucous plugs, reversal of atelectasis in mechanically ventilated patients, suctioning of thick tenacious secretions, and diagnosis of obstructive pneumonia.[49]

Diagnostic bronchoscopy is most commonly used for obtaining pulmonary specimens for diagnosis and management of pneumonia.[50] Quantitative cultures obtained via fiberoptic bronchoscopy have been shown to eliminate the diagnosis of pneumonia in nearly 50% of patients with clinical signs of pneumonia, to decrease inappropriate antibiotic use, and to improve mortality compared with nonquantitative techniques. Standardization of culture techniques should be undertaken.

The risk associated with bronchoscopy is related more to the need for conscious sedation and the required medications if performed in a nonintubated patient. Medication use could possibly result in depressed mental status progressing to hypoventilation, airway vulnerability, and the risk of aspiration. The risks of the procedure itself are pneumothorax, hypoxia, airway hyperreactivity, pulmonary hemorrhage, and systemic hypotension or hypertension.

SELECTED REFERENCES

Delaney A, Bagshaw SM, Nalos M: Percutaneous dilatational tracheostomy versus surgical tracheostomy in critically ill patients: A systematic review and meta-analysis. *Crit Care* 10:R55, 2006.

This meta-analysis of percutaneous dilatational tracheostomy (PDT) versus standard open surgical tracheostomy supports the benefits of PDT.

Dennis BM, Eckert MJ, Gunter OL, et al: Safety of bedside percutaneous tracheostomy in the critically ill: Evaluation of more than 3,000 procedures. *J Am Coll Surg* 216:858–865, discussion 865–867, 2013.

This article, which is the largest review of the safety of bedside percutaneous dilatational tracheostomy, documents safety across body mass index distribution.

Diaz JJ, Jr, Mejia V, Subhawong AP, et al: Protocol for bedside laparotomy in trauma and emergency general surgery: A low return to the operating room. *Am Surg* 71:986–991, 2005.

This primary article examines outcomes of bedside laparotomy with a protocol for indications and support.

Fagon JY: Diagnosis and treatment of ventilator-associated pneumonia: Fiberoptic bronchoscopy with bronchoalveolar lavage is essential. *Semin Respir Crit Care Med* 27:34–44, 2006.

The indications, benefits, and performance of bronchoscopy for the diagnosis of pneumonia are reviewed.

Griffiths J, Barber VS, Morgan L, et al: Systematic review and meta-analysis of studies of the timing of tracheostomy in adult patients undergoing artificial ventilation. *BMJ* 330:1243, 2005.

In this meta-analysis of studies evaluating the timing of tracheostomy, early tracheostomy was defined as less than 7 days.

Moore AF, Hargest R, Martin M, et al: Intra-abdominal hypertension and the abdominal compartment syndrome. *Br J Surg* 91:1102–1110, 2004.

This article provides a review of the pathophysiology and treatment of abdominal compartment syndrome.

Rumbak MJ, Newton M, Truncale T, et al: A prospective, randomized, study comparing early percutaneous dilational tracheotomy to prolonged translaryngeal intubation (delayed tracheotomy) in critically ill medical patients. *Crit Care Med* 32:1689–1694, 2004.

This primary article examining the benefit of tracheostomy at 48 hours versus 14 days demonstrated a significant reduction in complications and mortality when tracheostomy is performed early.

Shapiro MB, Jenkins DH, Schwab CW, et al: Damage control: Collective review. *J Trauma* 49:969–978, 2000.

This article is a collective review of the history, indications, and performance of damage control laparotomy.

Van Natta TL, Morris JA, Jr, Eddy VA, et al: Elective bedside surgery in critically injured patients is safe and cost-effective. *Ann Surg* 227:618–624, 1998.

This article is the first report of the safety and effectiveness of bedside surgical procedures.

REFERENCES

1. Barba CA: The intensive care unit as an operating room. *Surg Clin North Am* 80:957–973, 2000.
2. Beckmann U, Gillies DM, Berenholtz SM, et al: Incidents relating to the intra-hospital transfer of critically ill patients. An analysis of the reports submitted to the Australian

Incident Monitoring Study in Intensive Care. *Intensive Care Med* 30:1579–1585, 2004.
3. Bowen CP, Whitney LR, Truwit JD, et al: Comparison of safety and cost of percutaneous versus surgical tracheostomy. *Am Surg* 67:54–60, 2001.
4. Carrillo EH, Heniford BT, Osborne DL, et al: Bedside percutaneous endoscopic gastrostomy. A safe alternative for early nutritional support in critically ill trauma patients. *Surg Endosc* 11:1068–1071, 1997.
5. Dennis BM, Eckert MJ, Gunter OL, et al: Safety of bedside percutaneous tracheostomy in the critically ill: Evaluation of more than 3,000 procedures. *J Am Coll Surg* 216:858–865, discussion 865–867, 2013.
6. Diaz JJ, Jr, Mauer A, May AK, et al: Bedside laparotomy for trauma: Are there risks? *Surg Infect (Larchmt)* 5:15–20, 2004.
7. Diaz JJ, Jr, Mejia V, Subhawong AP, et al: Protocol for bedside laparotomy in trauma and emergency general surgery: A low return to the operating room. *Am Surg* 71:986–991, 2005.
8. Freeman BD, Isabella K, Lin N, et al: A meta-analysis of prospective trials comparing percutaneous and surgical tracheostomy in critically ill patients. *Chest* 118:1412–1418, 2000.
9. Freeman BD, Isabella K, Cobb JP, et al: A prospective, randomized study comparing percutaneous with surgical tracheostomy in critically ill patients. *Crit Care Med* 29:926–930, 2001.
10. Porter JM, Ivatury RR, Kavarana M, et al: The surgical intensive care unit as a cost-efficient substitute for an operating room at a Level I trauma center. *Am Surg* 65:328–330, 1999.
11. Porter JM, Ivatury RR: Preferred route of tracheostomy—percutaneous versus open at the bedside: A randomized, prospective study in the surgical intensive care unit. *Am Surg* 65:142–146, 1999.
12. Van Natta TL, Morris JA, Jr, Eddy VA, et al: Elective bedside surgery in critically injured patients is safe and cost-effective. *Ann Surg* 227:618–624, discussion 624–626, 1998.
13. Pronovost PJ, Thompson DA: Reducing defects in the use of interventions. *Intensive Care Med* 30:1505–1507, 2004.
14. Haynes AB, Weiser TG, Berry WR, et al: A surgical safety checklist to reduce morbidity and mortality in a global population. *N Engl J Med* 360:491–499, 2009.
15. WHO Guidelines for Safe Surgery 2009: *Safe Surgery Saves Lives*, Geneva, Switzerland, 2009, WHO Press.
16. Mayberry JC: Bedside open abdominal surgery. Utility and wound management. *Crit Care Clin* 16:151–172, 2000.
17. Biffl WL, Moore EE, Burch JM, et al: Secondary abdominal compartment syndrome is a highly lethal event. *Am J Surg* 182:645–648, 2001.
18. Miller RS, Morris JA, Jr, Diaz JJ, Jr, et al: Complications after 344 damage-control open celiotomies. *J Trauma* 59:1365–1371, discussion 1371–1374, 2005.
19. Kirkpatrick AW, Balogh Z, Ball CG, et al: The secondary abdominal compartment syndrome: Iatrogenic or unavoidable? *J Am Coll Surg* 202:668–679, 2006.
20. Leppaniemi A, Kemppainen E: Recent advances in the surgical management of necrotizing pancreatitis. *Curr Opin Crit Care* 11:349–352, 2005.
21. Moore AF, Hargest R, Martin M, et al: Intra-abdominal hypertension and the abdominal compartment syndrome. *Br J Surg* 91:1102–1110, 2004.
22. Sugrue M: Abdominal compartment syndrome. *Curr Opin Crit Care* 11:333–338, 2005.
23. Shapiro MB, Jenkins DH, Schwab CW, et al: Damage control: Collective review. *J Trauma* 49:969–978, 2000.
24. Cools-Lartigue J, Aboalsaud A, Gill H, et al: Evolution of percutaneous dilatational tracheostomy—a review of current techniques and their pitfalls. *World J Surg* 37:1633–1646, 2013.
25. Delaney A, Bagshaw SM, Nalos M: Percutaneous dilatational tracheostomy versus surgical tracheostomy in critically ill patients: A systematic review and meta-analysis. *Crit Care* 10:R55, 2006.
26. Heikkinen M, Aarnio P, Hannukainen J: Percutaneous dilational tracheostomy or conventional surgical tracheostomy? *Crit Care Med* 28:1399–1402, 2000.
27. Bittner EA, Schmidt UH: The ventilator liberation process: Update on technique, timing, and termination of tracheostomy. *Respir Care* 57:1626–1634, 2012.
28. Griffiths J, Barber VS, Morgan L, et al: Systematic review and meta-analysis of studies of the timing of tracheostomy in adult patients undergoing artificial ventilation. *BMJ* 330:1243, 2005.
29. Arabi Y, Haddad S, Shirawi N, et al: Early tracheostomy in intensive care trauma patients improves resource utilization: A cohort study and literature review. *Crit Care* 8:R347–R352, 2004.
30. Rumbak MJ, Newton M, Truncale T, et al: A prospective, randomized, study comparing early percutaneous dilational tracheotomy to prolonged translaryngeal intubation (delayed tracheotomy) in critically ill medical patients. *Crit Care Med* 32:1689–1694, 2004.
31. Ciaglia P, Firsching R, Syniec C: Elective percutaneous dilatational tracheostomy. A new simple bedside procedure: Preliminary report. *Chest* 87:715–719, 1985.
32. Paran H, Butnaru G, Hass I, et al: Evaluation of a modified percutaneous tracheostomy technique without bronchoscopic guidance. *Chest* 126:868–871, 2004.
33. Polderman KH, Spijkstra JJ, de Bree R, et al: Percutaneous dilatational tracheostomy in the ICU: Optimal organization, low complication rates, and description of a new complication. *Chest* 123:1595–1602, 2003.
34. Norwood S, Vallina VL, Short K, et al: Incidence of tracheal stenosis and other late complications after percutaneous tracheostomy. *Ann Surg* 232:233–241, 2000.
35. Walz MK, Peitgen K, Thurauf N, et al: Percutaneous dilatational tracheostomy—early results and long-term outcome of 326 critically ill patients. *Intensive Care Med* 24:685–690, 1998.
36. Garrubba M, Turner T, Grieveson C: Multidisciplinary care for tracheostomy patients: A systematic review. *Crit Care* 13:R177, 2009.
37. Gauderer MW, Ponsky JL, Izant RJ, Jr: Gastrostomy without laparotomy: A percutaneous endoscopic technique. *J Pediatr Surg* 15:872–875, 1980.
38. Adams GF, Guest DP, Ciraulo DL, et al: Maximizing tolerance of enteral nutrition in severely injured trauma patients: A comparison of enteral feedings by means of percutaneous endoscopic gastrostomy versus percutaneous endoscopic gastrojejunostomy. *J Trauma* 48:459–464, discussion 464–465, 2000.
39. Harbrecht BG, Moraca RJ, Saul M, et al: Percutaneous endoscopic gastrostomy reduces total hospital costs in head-injured patients. *Am J Surg* 176:311–314, 1998.

40. Shang E, Kahler G, Meier-Hellmann A, et al: Advantages of endoscopic therapy of gastrojejunal dissociation in critical care patients. *Intensive Care Med* 25:162–165, 1999.
41. Stein J, Schulte-Bockholt A, Sabin M, et al: A randomized prospective trial of immediate vs. next-day feeding after percutaneous endoscopic gastrostomy in intensive care patients. *Intensive Care Med* 28:1656–1660, 2002.
42. Wejda BU, Deppe H, Huchzermeyer H, et al: PEG placement in patients with ascites: A new approach. *Gastrointest Endosc* 61:178–180, 2005.
43. Schulman AS, Sawyer RG: The safety of percutaneous endoscopic gastrostomy tube placement in patients with existing ventriculoperitoneal shunts. *JPEN J Parenter Enteral Nutr* 29:442–444, 2005.
44. Taylor AL, Carroll TA, Jakubowski J, et al: Percutaneous endoscopic gastrostomy in patients with ventriculoperitoneal shunts. *Br J Surg* 88:724–727, 2001.
45. Eleftheriadis E, Kotzampassi K: Percutaneous endoscopic gastrostomy after abdominal surgery. *Surg Endosc* 15:213–216, 2001.
46. Lockett MA, Templeton ML, Byrne TK, et al: Percutaneous endoscopic gastrostomy complications in a tertiary-care center. *Am Surg* 68:117–120, 2002.
47. Dulabon GR, Abrams JE, Rutherford EJ: The incidence and significance of free air after percutaneous endoscopic gastrostomy. *Am Surg* 68:590–593, 2002.
48. Sharma VK, Howden CW: Meta-analysis of randomized, controlled trials of antibiotic prophylaxis before percutaneous endoscopic gastrostomy. *Am J Gastroenterol* 95:3133–3136, 2000.
49. Labbe A, Meyer F, Albertini M: Bronchoscopy in intensive care units. *Paediatr Respir Rev* 5(Suppl A):S15–S19, 2004.
50. Fagon JY: Diagnosis and treatment of ventilator-associated pneumonia: Fiberoptic bronchoscopy with bronchoalveolar lavage is essential. *Semin Respir Crit Care Med* 27:34–44, 2006.

23 CHAPTER

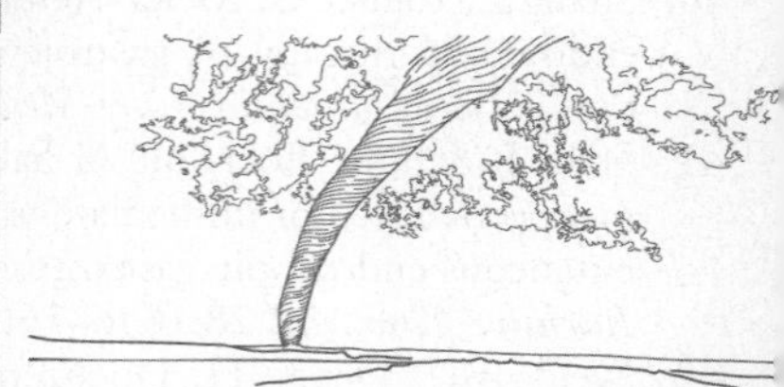

The Surgeon's Role in Mass Casualty Incidents

Michael Stein, Asher Hirshberg

OUTLINE

Surgeons are traditionally focused on trauma care of the individual critically injured patient. However, ongoing challenges across the globe ranging from urban terrorism to extreme weather events emphasize the growing importance of large-scale incidents and the selective public attention they command. For example, in July 2011, an urban bombing and mass shooting in Oslo, Norway, captured headlines worldwide, whereas a train derailment in Fatehpur, India, only 12 days earlier was barely mentioned in the media despite a larger number of casualties than the Oslo incident.

As surgeons become involved in the disaster response of their communities and institutions, many view trauma care in disasters as similar in principle to normal daily practice, only more of the same. Hence, disaster preparedness training is not a high priority for general surgery residents.[1] This view of disaster preparedness as a primarily logistical issue is a dangerous misconception because large numbers of casualties have a profound effect on trauma care inside and outside the hospital. Furthermore, such large-scale events confront surgeons with unusual injury patterns and unique clinical problems not seen in daily practice. Preparing for these challenges requires not only special planning and training but, most importantly, a different way of thinking about trauma care.

Across the wide array of large-scale scenarios, there is a single common denominator: a discrepancy between a sudden surge in wounded patients and the limited resources available to treat them. The wars in Iraq and Afghanistan and medical care for casualties of armed conflicts in remote regions have exposed surgeons (in the military and on humanitarian missions) to the brutal realities of these challenges and for a need for a special mindset. On the home front, incidents such as the Boston Marathon bombings in April 2013 demonstrated how a modern and prepared large metropolitan trauma system can deal very effectively with a major urban terror incident.[2] The aim of this chapter is to provide a concise overview of the medical response to large-scale events mostly from the perspective of the clinical surgeon practicing in a hospital that is part of a modern trauma system.

KEY CONCEPTS

Classification of Disasters and Implications for Trauma Care

In a mass casualty incident (MCI), a medical system is suddenly confronted by a large influx of casualties needing care within a short period of time. This unexpected surge creates a discrepancy between the number of injured patients and the resources available to treat them. MCIs can be classified by cause (natural or man-made), duration, location, and several other characteristics. From the clinical perspective of trauma care, scenarios usually conform to one of three traditional classes, each with different implications for trauma care (Table 23-1).[3,4]

Multiple Casualty Incidents

In multiple casualty incidents, arriving casualties strain the hospital resources beyond normal daily operations but do not overwhelm them. Such incidents (e.g., bus accident, school shooting) may involve dozens of casualties but are effectively handled using local hospital resources. As a rough guide, a hospital is facing a multiple casualty incident when the number of arriving casualties is less than the number of beds or gurneys in the emergency department (ED).

Mass Casualty Incidents

With mass casualty incidents, the surge of casualties exceeds the capacity of the ED, despite an effective disaster response. This situation results in significant delays in trauma care or a suboptimal level of care for some casualties. The term *mass casualty* implies some degree of failure to provide optimal timely trauma care to all severely injured patients.

Major Medical Disasters

Disasters typically result in many thousands of casualties and destruction of organized community support systems and infrastructure. In major medical disasters, the resources to treat severely injured patients have been largely destroyed. External medical

TABLE 23-1 Classification of Disasters and Implications for Trauma Care

DISASTER CLASS	TOTAL NUMBER OF CASUALTIES	IMPLICATIONS FOR TRAUMA CARE
Multiple casualty	Less than ED capacity	Standards of care maintained for all severe casualties
Mass casualty	More than ED capacity	Care of some severe casualties delayed or suboptimal
Major disaster	ED and hospital overwhelmed	Most severely injured patients die or survive without any medical care

ED, emergency department.

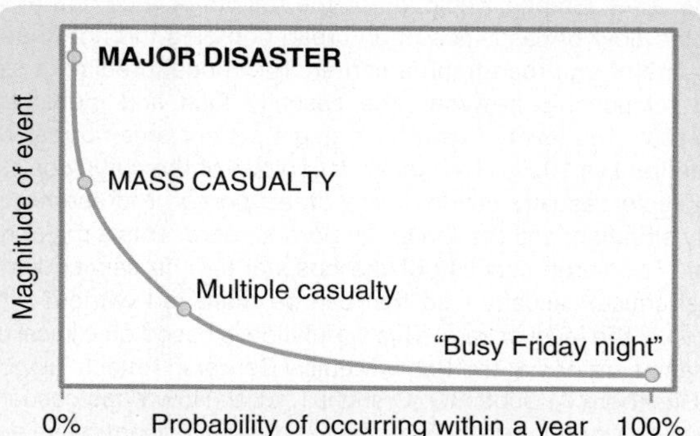

FIGURE 23-1 Graphic depiction of the inverse relationship between the magnitude of disaster scenarios and their frequency. Although most surgeons will not encounter a major natural disaster during their careers, busy Friday nights are a regular feature in most urban trauma centers.

teams with appropriate logistic support can make a difference in the management of some survivors, although help typically arrives late and deals primarily with delayed complications.

In this chapter, *MCI* is used as a generic term describing a large-scale event. When referring to a specific disaster class or scenario (e.g., multiple casualty incident), the term is fully spelled out. The magnitude of a MCI is inversely related to its frequency (Fig. 23-1). Most practicing surgeons will never encounter a major medical disaster during their careers. At the other end of the MCI spectrum are "busy Friday nights"—a trauma team on call coping with a cluster of severely injured patients that arrived within a short period of time and put a temporary strain on available resources. This situation, a frequent occurrence in inner-city hospitals, represents the lowermost end of a spectrum of MCI. A major earthquake or a devastating tsunami is at the other extreme. The paradox of disaster preparedness is that the most time and effort are spent on preparing for the largest and least likely doomsday scenarios instead of paying attention to the lessons from "busy Fridays" and improving the response to limited but much more imminent threats.

Injury Severity Distribution

A key feature of every MCI is the injury severity distribution. Regardless of the cause or magnitude of the event, only about 10% to 15% of survivors presenting to the hospital are severely wounded, of whom roughly one third have immediately

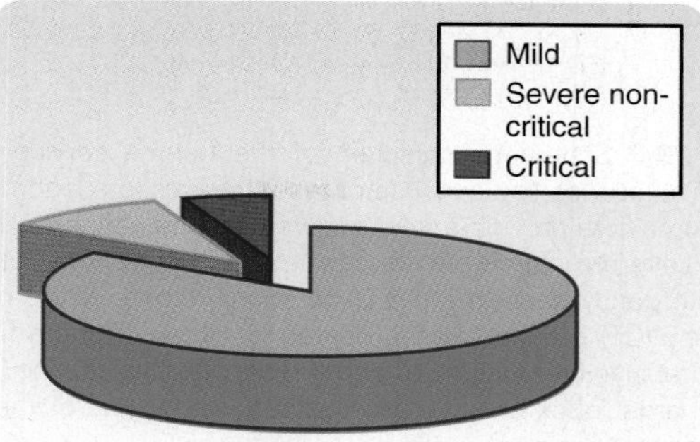

FIGURE 23-2 Generic injury severity distribution for disaster scenarios. Of all survivors arriving in the hospital, most (85%) will have only minor injuries. Of severely injured (Injury Severity Score >9) patients, only one third, or 1 in 20 arrivals, will have life-threatening injuries. This injury severity distribution forms the basis for planning the hospital disaster response.

life-threatening injuries (Fig. 23-2). Most survivors sustain minor or nonurgent injuries.[3] For example, during the London subway bombings in July 2005, the Royal London Hospital received 194 casualties within 3 hours, but only 27 (14%) were severely injured. Of these, only eight casualties (4% of the total) were critically wounded.[5]

Although the death toll at the scene depends on the cause of the MCI and may be very high when structural collapse occurs, the injury severity distribution remains roughly the same across a wide range of MCIs. In other words, although the total number of casualties may be vast, most do not require a high level of trauma care and are not urgent. These considerations form the rationale behind an effective medical response.[6]

MODERN TRAUMA CARE IN MASS CASUALTY

Goal of the Hospital Disaster Response

A well-known principle of medical disaster response is to do the greatest good for the greatest number of casualties. Surgeons and other trauma care providers must understand the clinical implications of this principle. From the trauma care perspective, a MCI is "a needle in a haystack" situation where a small number of severely injured patients who require immediate high-level trauma care is immersed within a much larger group of patients with minor injuries who can tolerate delays and even suboptimal care without adversely affecting outcome.[3] The ultimate goal of the entire hospital disaster response is to provide this small group of critically injured patients with a level of care that approximates the care provided to similarly injured patients on a normal working day. This goal has never been formally declared by the American College of Surgeons or any other professional organization but has always been implicitly understood by surgeons and is an expectation of the public. In a multiple casualty incident, this goal can be achieved through effective triage and priority-driven trauma care. In a mass casualty situation, it can still be achieved by diverting trauma resources from the less severely injured casualties to the critically wounded casualties, but this comes at a cost. Contrary to popular belief, the casualties whose management is delayed or compromised in a mass casualty scenario are not the patients with minor injuries, but rather the seriously injured patients with non–life-threatening injuries (e.g., major open fracture).

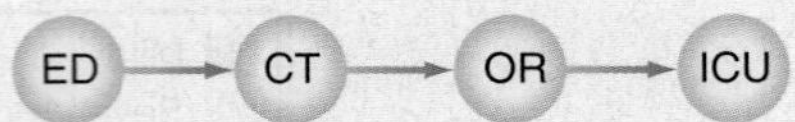

FIGURE 23-3 Schematic depiction of the trauma service line of a hospital. The service line consists of resources, assets, and facilities in which trauma care providers treat severely injured patients. The typical flow of a severely injured patient is from the trauma resuscitation bay of the emergency department (ED) to imaging, usually the computed tomography (CT) scanner, to the operating room (OR), and finally to a surgical intensive care unit (ICU) bed. Preserving this service line in the face of a large influx of severe casualties is the goal of the hospital disaster response.

Understanding the Trauma Service Line in Disasters

There is a strange dissociation between the dramatic advances in trauma systems in the past 30 years and disaster planning. Most hospital disaster plans (including those of Level 1 trauma centers) do not refer specifically to the hospital trauma service, even though any effective disaster response must rely on it. Simply put, hospitals with 21st century trauma services and facilities have disaster plans that are still based on concepts of trauma care from the 1970s.

Every modern trauma center maintains a dedicated *trauma service line* for severely injured patients during normal daily operations (Fig. 23-3). This service line includes trauma teams, assets, and facilities (e.g., resuscitation bays and operating rooms [ORs]), all readily available to treat seriously injured patients. The trauma service line has limited capabilities to treat multiple badly injured patients simultaneously. The goal of an effective disaster response is to preserve the hospital trauma service line in the face of an unusually large influx of casualties. From the trauma care perspective, success in dealing with a MCI is not streamlining the flow of 40 or 60 casualties through the ED, but rather preserving the capability to identify the 3 or 4 critically injured (but salvageable) patients and provide them with optimal trauma care.[6]

Casualty Load and Surge Capacity

Many hospital administrators have an exaggerated view of the ability of their institution to deal with large numbers of casualties, especially when the hospital is a trauma center. This exaggerated view is due to the fact that hospital disaster planning is typically based on counting ED gurneys and hospital beds, rather than on the rate at which casualties are processed through the hospital trauma service line. In reality, as the MCI unfolds and progressively more casualties arrive, finding an available resuscitation bay and staffing it with experienced trauma teams becomes increasingly difficult.

From the trauma care perspective, the arrival rate of severe casualties is a more meaningful metric of the burden on a trauma system than the total number of casualties. The casualty load can be defined by their arrival rate (number of casualties arriving per hour), and an increasing casualty load eventually leads to degradation of trauma care as more and more severely injured patients compete for limited assets and resources. An intact trauma service line provides each severe casualty with a trauma team, resuscitation bay, and other resources, such as a time slot in the computed tomography (CT) scanner, an available OR, and a vacant bed in the intensive care unit (ICU). The point beyond which this level of care cannot be maintained for new arrivals is the surge capacity of the trauma service line of the hospital.[7] Surge capacity is a dynamic measure of the processing capacity of the trauma service line.

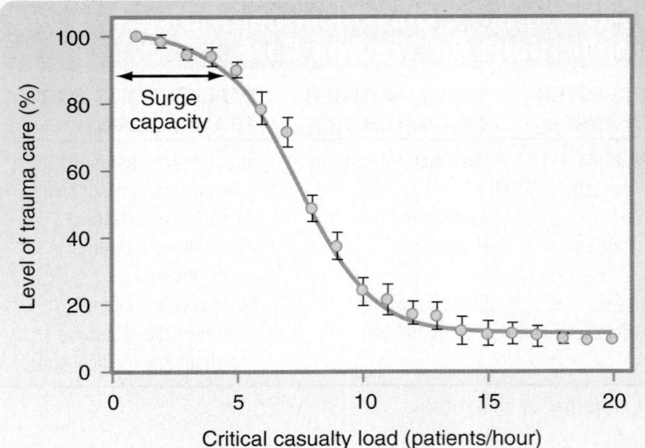

FIGURE 23-4 Graphic depiction of the results of a computer simulation of the flow of casualties of an urban bombing through the trauma service line of an urban trauma center. The model predicts a sigmoid-shaped relationship between the casualty load and global level of trauma care. The level of care for a single patient on a normal working day is defined as 100%. The *upper flat portion* of the curve corresponds to a multiple casualty incident, the *steep portion* represents a mass casualty situation, and the *lower flat portion* represents a major medical disaster. The surge capacity of the hospital trauma service line is the maximal critical casualty load that can be managed without a precipitous drop in the level of care. This simulation is based on clinical profiles of casualties treated at the Rabin Medical Center in Petach Tikva, Israel. (From Hirshberg A, Scott BG, Granchi T, et al: How does casualty load affect trauma care in urban bombing incidents? A quantitative analysis. *J Trauma* 58:686–693, 2005.)

Trauma surgeons know from experience that an increasing casualty load adversely affects the quality of trauma care because many casualties compete for the same limited trauma assets and resources, not least of which is the attention of a trauma team. Analysis using a computer model[7] described this relationship as a sigmoid-shaped curve (Fig. 23-4). The upper flat portion of the curve represents a multiple casualty incident handled by an intact trauma service line. Here the level of care for severe casualties approximates the care given to a single wounded patient on a normal working day. The steep portion represents a gradually failing trauma service line, corresponding to a mass casualty scenario. The lower flat portion represents a failed (or nonexistent) service line overwhelmed by a major medical disaster.

The surge capacity of the trauma service line is the point beyond which the level of care begins to drop, the shoulder of the sigmoid curve. An effective disaster response shifts the curve to the right, extending the surge capacity and resulting in a more gradual decline of the level of care. A traditional empirical estimate[8] puts the surge capacity of a hospital at one severely injured patient per hour for every 100 hospital beds. This rough estimate is in line with the results of computer simulations of hospitals coping with MCIs and can serve as a practical yardstick that can be used in planning the medical response.

Mass Casualty and Modern Trauma Systems

Most large-scale incidents in the urban setting are multiple casualty incidents that do not exceed the surge capacity of individual hospitals. Despite deliberate attempts by terrorist groups, from Madrid in 2004 to the Boston Marathon in 2013, to coordinate multiple simultaneous bombings designed to overwhelm the organized response, Western trauma systems have proven very resilient.

The best documented examples so far have been the Madrid trains bombing (March 2004),[9] the London subway bombing (July 2005),[5] and the Oslo bombing and mass shooting (July 2011).[10] These incidents clearly showed that modern emergency medical services (EMS) in large metropolitan areas serve as effective buffers that mitigate the impact of a large-scale event by distributing casualties among hospitals. With 2253 casualties in Madrid and more than 700 in London, rapid distribution of casualties among several hospitals resulted in each participating hospital facing only a multiple casualty incident with a handful of critically injured patients. However, this strong buffering mechanism was conspicuously absent in the U.S. Embassy bombing in Nairobi, Kenya, in 1998, where thousands of casualties flooded the Kenyatta National Hospital; this mass casualty incident was not adequately documented and reported in the trauma or disaster literature. This is a crucial fact that is worth re-emphasizing: No hospital that is served by a functioning metropolitan EMS system has ever been overwhelmed by a MCI. A highly effective buffering mechanism was evident during the Oslo bombing and shooting incident in July 2011, where a large number of mild casualties were diverted to an outpatient facility away from the trauma center, offloading the trauma center.[10] It was also a key element of the successful response to the Boston Marathon bombings,[11] although a definitive medical report is yet to be published. School shootings in the United States, such as the Virginia Tech shooting in 2007[12] or the Sandy Hook Elementary School shooting in 2012, were multiple casualty incidents involving dozens of casualties. These and other school shootings demonstrate that existing emergency planning and regional trauma systems can effectively deal with such incidents.

A major difficulty in trying to learn useful lessons from past incidents is the paucity of clinical data. Most published reports provide only global statistics, such as the total number of casualties and the mortality among the critically injured (critical mortality), with few clinical details about trauma care of individual patients. Difficulties and problems in trauma care must be inferred between the lines. One example is the alarmingly high number of negative laparotomies as a result of false-positive bedside sonography (focused abdominal sonography for trauma) examinations. This fact was hidden within the data of the main reports from Madrid[9] and London.[5] As a result, trauma teams in Oslo faced the same problem in 2011 but again omitted it from their formal report.[10,12] In the entire body of literature on disaster medicine, no hospital has ever reported having preventable morbidity and mortality. In view of the high public profile of such incidents and the tendency toward self-congratulatory reporting,[11] crucial details of adverse outcomes or difficulties in trauma care during MCIs are unlikely to be accurately reported.

The foundations of an effective medical response to any MCI are robust trauma systems and well-functioning trauma centers. The general public does not associate the financial health of trauma centers with the medical response to disasters. In the United States, while the national grid of functioning trauma centers is being eroded by lack of public funding, huge resources have been allocated to preparations for "all-hazard" scenarios including a major chemical or biological attack in rural states. Expensive preparations for such "all-hazard" scenarios have become a top priority despite their extremely small likelihood because of their huge commercial potential. The public does not realize this dangerous paradox. Without a strong national grid of trauma centers and robust EMS systems, no effective disaster response will be possible for either doomsday scenarios or plain civilian MCIs.

TABLE 23-2 Typical Timeline of Urban Mass Casualty Incident

SCENE PHASE	CHARACTERISTICS	IMPLICATIONS FOR ED
Chaotic	No organized medical care; mild casualties go to nearest hospital	First wave: A few walking wounded
Organized effort	Key is effective triage; priority-driven transport of casualties	Second wave: Main body of casualties
Site clearing	Remaining casualties transported	
Late	Sporadic mild casualties	Third wave: Slow trickle of mild casualties

ED, emergency department.

Medical Response at the Scene

Urban MCIs follow a typical timeline that can be divided into four distinct phases (Table 23-2).[13] The initial chaotic phase begins immediately after the inciting event, as many minor casualties run from the scene and find their way to the nearest hospital. The organized effort phase begins when a prehospital provider takes charge at the scene and initiates a systematic medical response, while also ensuring the safety and security of the medical teams. The most important aspect of this phase is effective field triage, which allows rapid distribution of casualties among several hospitals. This phase is followed by the site-clearing phase. It ends when the last live casualty is transported from the scene. The late phase is a poorly defined period during which minor casualties decide to seek medical attention, often after being persuaded by family and friends.

From the hospital perspective, this timeline translates into a characteristic three-wave casualty arrival pattern (see Table 23-2). The first wave is often a small cluster of minor casualties arriving on their own. After a variable interval, the main body of casualties begins to pour in, presenting with a wide variety of injury severities. Finally, a slow trickle of late arrivals with minor injuries or acute stress reaction continues over many hours.[2,13]

Because the time from injury to definitive care is a key determinant of mortality, the approach of most prehospital teams in an urban setting is to "scoop and run." The emphasis is on field triage and rapid transport; interventions are largely restricted to airway management and control of external hemorrhage. However, in a rural or remote setting, there may be a bottleneck because of limited means of transport or long distances from the scene to the hospital. This situation may require some form of trauma care at the scene for casualties awaiting transport.

Field triage schemes are based on a rapid assessment of clinical and physiologic parameters. One prominent algorithm in the United States is the SALT triage scheme (*s*ort, *a*ssess, *l*ifesaving interventions, *t*reatment/*t*ransport), which combines global assessment of the casualties (e.g., walking versus laying still) with a more detailed yet brief assessment of vital signs.[14] SALT has been endorsed by the American College of Surgeons and other professional organizations dealing with mass casualty triage. Although it has been promoted as a universal triage scheme for MCIs, its main usefulness is at the scene rather than for hospital triage at the ED door.

TRAUMA ASPECTS OF HOSPITAL DISASTER PLANS

Hospital Disaster Response

The goal of the hospital disaster plan is to augment rapidly the surge capacity of the trauma service line (including support elements such as the blood bank and laboratory). Each service or facility within the hospital response envelope activates a facility-specific disaster protocol designed to increase the processing capacity of the facility rapidly to accommodate a sudden large influx of casualties. The underlying principle of these protocols is suspension of normal daily activities while rapidly mobilizing staff reinforcements. An emergency operations center is the executive tool of the hospital leadership in coordinating the institutional effort.

Activation of the full disaster response of a large hospital takes time, disrupts normal daily activities, and is expensive. It is also usually unnecessary because most MCIs that the hospital is likely to face are limited events that can be successfully addressed by activating a more limited response. It makes sense to plan for a tiered response.[15] The plan for a limited MCI refers to a mass casualty incident. It centers primarily on the ED and relies on in-house staff and resources. The response to a large-scale MCI involves the entire hospital staff (including off-site personnel) and uses facilities outside the ED area.

From the perspective of trauma care, the hospital response consists of two distinct phases.[6,13] During the initial phase, the incident is still evolving, casualties are arriving, and their ultimate number is unknown. The central consideration is to preserve the assets and resources of the trauma service line in anticipation of additional casualties. The definitive phase begins when casualties are no longer arriving, the overall number of casualties is known, and the hospital response envelope has been fully deployed. The clinical focus shifts to providing definitive care to all casualties in a graded, priority-oriented fashion.

Preparing to Receive Casualties

The characteristic lag between notification and arrival of the first casualty provides a window of opportunity to initiate an effective response. Actions taken during this brief interval often shape the subsequent response. Nowhere is this window more crucial than in the ED, where a rapid evacuation plan is activated to create empty gurneys and physical space for a large influx of casualties. Based on their medical condition, patients in the ED can be discharged, rapidly admitted to the floor, or transferred to a designated "surge" facility within the hospital. Other priorities are positioning a triage officer outside the ED and improvising additional trauma bays close to the trauma resuscitation area. The command chain in the ED must be clear to all, and the staff must be briefed and assigned specific roles. For example, in the trauma resuscitation area, staff members are assigned to specific teams and told explicitly who will take the first, second, and subsequent critical arrivals. Emergency carts containing additional medical supplies are deployed in designated areas.

Incident Command and Clinical Decision Making

Hospital disaster plans are traditionally based on a top-down organizational hierarchy stemming from the incident command structure developed in the 1970s to streamline the field management of large-scale incidents. This organizational structure is based on a top-down military command hierarchy first introduced in the Franco-Prussian War in the second half of the 19th century. The implementation of these top-down command structures during a real incident is problematic because most MCIs are brief incidents. The rapid dynamics of a typical urban MCI far outpace the deployment of a typical top-down hospital disaster plan. By the time the hospital has an incident command center up and running, the incident is long over. More importantly, the top-down hierarchical tree means that problems are always escalated upward in anticipation of a solution from "someone in authority," which inevitably results in delays. In a real incident, communication systems (including cell phones) very often fail as they did during the Boston Marathon bombings in 2013,[2] and local managers communicate among themselves using text messaging.

The shortcomings of the rigid top-down command structure became obvious during the response to Hurricane Katrina in New Orleans in 2005[16] and stood in sharp contrast to many small-scale successes led by resourceful local managers who effectively collaborated with their peers in professional or organizational networks in and outside the hospital. An effective disaster response at any level must be based on such collaborative networks rather than on rigid top-down chains of command.[17] In real life, the effective response of the trauma service line to a sudden large casualty load always boils down to a small group of experienced trauma providers and local managers whose decisions drive the entire effort. In the ED, these individuals are the surgeon in charge, attending emergency physician, charge nurse, and triage officer. These decision makers understand the overarching goals of the hospital plan and should be empowered to address problems independently instead of merely reporting them upward. They should be trained to improvise and communicate horizontally with other local managers. Such collaborative network architectures provide flexibility, adaptability, and resiliency when parts of the system suddenly fail.[17]

During an MCI, there is a fundamental change in the medical decision making process.[18] In everyday clinical practice, trauma team leaders enjoy full autonomy in their clinical decisions regarding treatment priorities and the use of resources and facilities. The trauma team leader does not have to ask permission to take a patient to CT scan or to the OR. In a MCI, a large number of severely injured patients compete for the same resources and facilities. Key clinical decisions must be made by the surgeon in charge, who knows the "big picture" of the institutional situation. The autonomy of the individual team leader no longer exists. For example, the decision to take a patient with a penetrating abdominal injury and intra-abdominal bleeding to the OR is not automatic, and it cannot be made by the trauma team leader alone because it depends on the needs of other critical casualties and on the situation in the OR. The surgeon in charge is not merely a coordinator or supervisor but actually makes key clinical decisions about individual patients.

Hospital Triage

Triage is the central element of the hospital disaster response with implications far beyond the ED door.[19] There is a wide discrepancy between the theory of triage and the harsh reality of sorting bleeding casualties on the ambulance dock. Most hospital plans call for an experienced trauma surgeon to stand at the ED entrance and sort arriving casualties based on a brief assessment of physiologic parameters (e.g., palpable peripheral pulse or respiratory

TABLE 23-3 Traditional and Realistic Hospital Triage Categories

	TRIAGE MODE	
TRADITIONAL CATEGORIES	**SINGLE-STEP**	**SEQUENTIAL**
Immediate	Severe (to shock room)	Critical (to shock room)
Expectant		
Dead		
Delayed	All others (to ED holding)	Delayed (to ED holding)
Minimal		Minimal (treated outside ED)

ED, emergency department.

distress). Popular schemes divide casualties into five categories—immediate (life-threatening injuries), delayed (severe injuries that can wait for definitive care), minimal (walking wounded), expectant, and dead (Table 23-3).

Experience from real MCIs has shown that the triage officer has time for only a rapid cursory glance at each arrival. The triage decision must rely on a global impression of the patient's clinical condition rather than on physiologic measurements.[18] Furthermore, it is often impossible to distinguish immediate from delayed casualties based on this rapid cursory glance, and pronouncing death on the ambulance dock without a thorough examination and cardiac monitor is also an unrealistic expectation. Most problematic is the hopeless (or expectant) category because such determinations often depend on available resources; the same critical casualty may be deemed salvageable when the casualty load is light or hopeless when the ED is overwhelmed.[3] For all these reasons, realistic triage on the ambulance dock should be viewed as rapid and crude screening for severe casualties who require immediate access to the hospital trauma service line.

The quality of triage is traditionally expressed in terms of overtriage and undertriage rates.[20] The former is the erroneous assignment of nonsevere casualties to the trauma resuscitation area, whereas the latter is the erroneous assignment of severe casualties to a regular ED gurney. Overtriage is a system problem because these patients may compete with severe casualties for limited trauma resources. Undertriage is a medical error that may adversely affect the care of individual patients and lead to preventable morbidity and mortality. It has been suggested that hospital triage should be viewed as any other diagnostic screening test, using specificity and sensitivity rates as measures of triage accuracy.[20]

The major goal of effective triage is to facilitate better use of limited trauma resources. The key resource here is the specific attention of a trauma team. The cost of inaccurate triage can be quantified in terms of trauma team workload. A computer model showed that increasing triage accuracy reduces this workload.[20]

Triage does not end on the ambulance dock.[21] It is a reiterative process whereby each casualty is sequentially and repeatedly assessed as he or she progresses along the trauma service line. Each reevaluation increases the accuracy of the overall process and increases the likelihood that the patient will be triaged correctly and allocated the appropriate resources for the best possible clinical outcome.

Trauma Care in the Initial Phase

During the initial phase of a MCI (Box 23-1), the hospital operates two parallel (but separate) service lines for incoming casualties. The first one is a high-priority line reserved for severe casualties that includes the staff and resources to treat severely wounded patients during normal daily operations (see Fig. 23-3). This service line is staffed by experienced trauma care providers who deal with severely injured patients daily.

BOX 23-1 Goals and Principles of Trauma Care in the Initial Phase

Goals
Optimal trauma care for critical casualties
Minimal acceptable care for all others

Principles
Two parallel but separate service lines
Conservation of trauma assets and resources
Centralized clinical decision making
Loss of continuity of care

The second service line is designated for casualties with minor injuries, who require mostly treatment of trivial wounds and ruling out occult trauma. The service line is staffed by reinforcement staff who are not trauma care providers in their normal day jobs but are called up to help as part of the disaster plan. They are guided and supervised by a few experienced trauma care providers.

The roles of the trauma surgeon and trauma-trained nurse in MCIs have never been formally defined in published guidelines and are conspicuously absent from most templates for hospital disaster protocols. Depending on the structure and size of the trauma service at a specific institution, surgeons and nurses with trauma experience may be assigned to perform triage,[2] be in charge of the trauma resuscitation area,[18] or have medical control of other parts of the hospital response envelope. The underlying principle is that trauma surgeons and nurses should be positioned where they can have the most impact on the overall clinical result. Their roles should be defined well in advance and incorporated into the institutional disaster plan.

Critical casualties who enter the trauma service line are treated in a fashion similar to that of everyday care, with an emphasis on expediency, rapid turnover times, and smaller trauma teams. The crucial difference is that all major clinical decisions are referred to the surgeon in charge who roams in the trauma resuscitation area and acts as coordinator and ultimate clinical decision maker.[18] Clinical and administrative control is maintained through frequent rounds on all casualties in the ED made by the surgeon in charge, charge nurse, and ED attending physician. The product of these rounds is a list of casualties, their diagnoses, and their disposition (or plan). Knowing the total number of casualties and their injuries and dispositions as well as the situation at each trauma service point allows the surgeon in charge to consider clinical priorities against available resources and determine a feasible solution for each casualty.[22]

"MINIMAL ACCEPTABLE CARE"

The guiding principle for the care of noncritical casualties during the initial phase of a mass casualty incident is "minimal acceptable care."[13,22] This is empirical trauma care along the line of first aid in the field. The aim is to buy time, conserve trauma resources, and delay definitive care of nonurgent injuries to offload the trauma service line. The concept of minimal acceptable care is based on experience with civilian casualties of war, in which approximately two thirds of casualties survive for 1 week after injury without any medical care, and nonoperative management buys time and improves survival.[23] According to the principles of minimal acceptable care, clinical suspicion of a long bone fracture is treated by empirical splinting and analgesia, and the patient is rapidly admitted to a floor bed without imaging. Even penetrating abdominal trauma with peritoneal signs but no hemodynamic compromise (i.e., no intra-abdominal hemorrhage) can be initially managed with intravenous fluids, antibiotics, nasogastric suction, analgesia, and admission to a floor bed until an OR becomes available in the definitive care phase. One of the hallmarks of this temporizing philosophy is to limit access to the CT scanner only to patients for whom the scan is essential or potentially lifesaving (e.g., a head injury with lateralizing signs or a deteriorating level of consciousness); this approach was used during the Oslo bombing and shooting spree in 2012.[10,24]

Although "minimal acceptable care" is a key principle in the disaster response, surgeons practicing in Western hospitals that are part of a metropolitan EMS system will practically never use it because their hospitals are unlikely to be overwhelmed by a sudden influx of casualties even in a large-scale event. The metropolitan EMS system effectively distributes casualties between hospitals, reducing the impact on each. Minimal acceptable trauma care remains relevant only in exceptional circumstances, mostly in remote or austere environments. Western surgeons may encounter it on humanitarian missions or in field surgery in combat areas where resources are very limited and distribution of casualties to other facilities is not an option.

Other Aspects of Hospital Response

Another distinguishing feature of trauma care in disasters is discontinuity of care because in most real-life events, teams are assigned to service points rather than to individual critical patients. A critical casualty may be resuscitated in the shock room by one team, the imaging studies may be reviewed by a second team, and the operation may be performed by a third team. Few hospital disaster plans currently address this crucial issue and incorporate solutions (e.g., case managers) to mitigate the potential adverse effects of this loss of continuity of care.[25]

Although the CT scanner is a classic bottleneck in the flow of casualties, OR availability is not a major concern because only a very few casualties require emergency surgery during the initial phase.[26] Even in large-scale MCIs, such as the simultaneous terrorist bombings in Madrid and London, there were delays of more than an hour between activation of the disaster response and the first operative procedure, giving the OR time to prepare.

Contrary to the situation in the OR, the availability of ICU beds is always a source of grave concern.[27] In particular in urban bombing incidents, approximately one of every four admitted casualties will need to be admitted to the ICU. The surge in demand comes against a background of chronic surgical ICU bed shortage in many urban trauma centers. The hospital disaster response must include protocols for rapidly generating a substantial reserve of vacant ICU beds to be made available for incoming casualties. Such protocols typically involve transferring nonventilated patients to floor beds or using nonsurgical intensive care facilities within the hospital. The postanesthesia care unit is often the first to accommodate an overflow of ventilated patients simply because the ventilators and the nurses with critical care skills are already in place. Severely injured nonoperated patients from an urban bombing will need a surgical ICU bed 4 to 5 hours after arrival; there is a longer time span before operated casualties need an ICU bed.[5] These long delays allow the hospital to prepare beds, transfer patients, and mobilize staff reinforcements to achieve a substantial surge in ICU capacity.

Definitive Care Phase

During the definitive care phase, casualties are no longer arriving, their ultimate number is known, and the disaster response envelope of the hospital has been fully deployed. It is now possible to take stock and proceed with definitive care for all admitted casualties in an orderly and systematic fashion.[13,28] Care in this phase is based on rounds by members of the trauma service on all admitted casualties. These rounds derive prioritized lists of patients in need of imaging, consultations, operative procedures, and transfer to other institutions.

The definitive care phase consumes considerable time and resources,[28] so even limited multiple casualty incidents may disrupt the normal daily activities of the trauma service line and related facilities for several days or longer. Return to normal daily activities is gradual, and the investment of time and effort in providing care to complex trauma cases by multiple teams is often underestimated.[29] Although the ED may return to normal relatively quickly, the surgical ICU and OR will require additional staffing and support for several days to weeks after the incident. The Israeli experience with urban bombings contains useful descriptions of a general ICU coping with multiple casualty incidents, the importance of planning to relieve staff at regular intervals, and the use of staff reinforcements, nursing students, and volunteers.[29]

During the definitive care phase, consideration should be given to the secondary distribution of casualties by transferring some of them to other institutions. Interhospital transfer of burn patients to appropriate centers is an example. Such transfers are more problematic when the indication is logistic (e.g., shorter wait times for orthopedic procedures). Financial and administrative issues as well as considerations of institutional prestige create barriers to secondary distribution—often to the detriment of patients.

An urban bombing is an example of a short MCI, in which the main body of casualties arrives within a few hours of the explosion. However, in some types of MCIs, such as natural disasters or trauma care in areas of civilian strife and armed conflict, a continuous stream of casualties blurs the distinction between the initial phase and the definitive care phase. The hospital staff faces a seemingly endless stream of casualties that goes on and on for many days, weeks, or longer, without a formal ending. Such a "rolling MCI" poses a special kind of logistical and operational challenge and is typically not included in most hospital disaster plans.[30] In a "rolling MCI," a top priority is maintenance of capabilities and preservation of resources over time. The focus of the trauma teams must shift from the casualties at the door to the casualties presenting tomorrow—and the next day and the next week. Strict rationing of staff working hours, maintaining a robust supply chain for critical items such as blood products, and preparing accommodations for hospital staff to reside in-house for many days are elements of such a plan.

A crucial final step before return to normal is a formal debriefing as soon as possible after the incident. Ideally, all staff who took part in the effort should participate. The debriefing should be carefully structured to cover all key areas of clinical and administrative activity, while allowing free input from any participant who wishes to make a point. The aim is to learn lessons and identify barriers to the hospital response that can be incorporated into the hospital disaster plan.

SURGEON'S ROLE IN NATURAL DISASTERS

The medical aid stampede during the first few weeks after the Haiti earthquake in January 2010 demonstrated how little surgeons know about their role in natural disasters, as many volunteers with good intentions rushed to the stricken country in improvised teams, only to discover how little good intentions and surgical skills alone can achieve. Natural disasters vary in scope, magnitude, and number of casualties. Their consequences and cost in human lives are much higher in third-world countries compared with countries with resilient infrastructure and well-developed medical systems. For example, the earthquake that devastated Haiti in 2010 resulted in hundreds of thousands deaths. By comparison, the Northridge earthquake in California in 1994, an event of roughly the same magnitude, resulted in 33 immediate fatalities.

There are fundamental differences between the medical response to an urban MCI and organizing medical aid to a major natural disaster.[31] In the former, a functioning trauma system is coping with an unusually large casualty load over a brief period. In the latter, the catastrophic event compromises or destroys infrastructure and community support systems in the affected area (including trauma and health care facilities). External medical assets and resources must be imported into the disaster area to reinforce, support, or replace compromised local assets over a period of many weeks, months, and sometimes years.[31] Climate change increases the likelihood of extreme weather events and other climate-related disasters, bringing large-scale natural disasters closer to home for surgeons in the Western world[32] and posing entirely new challenges to health care providers worldwide.[33]

Injury Patterns in Natural Disasters

Natural disasters are associated with specific injury patterns. For example, in a major earthquake, the most important wounding mechanisms are falling debris and entrapment underneath collapsed buildings. Immediate search and rescue efforts by survivors in their immediate vicinity save more lives than the organized (but delayed) rescue efforts of external agencies.[34] During the first few hours after an earthquake, survivors present with a wide variety of extremity and visceral injuries; later, the prevailing patterns are extremity injuries and a high incidence of crush injuries. Only a small fraction of the total number of casualties are still alive after 48 hours underneath the rubble. Delayed extrication translates into a high incidence of crush syndrome and acute renal failure, as reported after the Marmara earthquake in Turkey in 1999.[35] The incidence of pediatric orthopedic trauma is higher than expected.[36]

The 2004 tsunami in Southeast Asia caused twice as many dead as injured survivors. The main injury patterns in survivors involved extremity fractures and soft tissue wounds.[37] In a volcanic eruption, injuries are caused by falling rocks, exposure to ash (a strong respiratory irritant), and inhalation injury from volcanic gases. The leading cause of death is suffocation. Knowing the characteristic injury patterns for each type of natural disaster is a prerequisite for planning an effective medical response.

Initiating the Medical Relief Effort

Contrary to the popular notion of the heroic medical volunteer racing to the rescue, there is a formal methodology underlying an effective international effort to provide support after a natural disaster in a remote region. The crucial first step is a rapid needs assessment, a formal task that is carried out as soon as possible after the catastrophe.[38] A United Nations Disaster Assessment and Coordination team, typically comprising two to six trained experts, is rapidly deployed to the disaster area to assess the immediate needs and report back to the international community. The rapid needs assessment, conducted in close collaboration with local authorities and facilities, not only defines the extent of the damage to infrastructure and medical resources but also estimates the numbers of casualties, types of injuries, and key priorities for disaster relief. Medical needs are often assigned a lower priority than essentials such as water, food, and shelter. Without an expert needs assessment and subsequent careful planning of a mission tailored to the specific circumstances of the disaster, the humanitarian effort will not be effective.

Trauma Care in the Disaster Area

The medical response to a major natural disaster consists of two distinct phases.[31] During the immediate phase, the first days and weeks after the catastrophe, the main goal is to provide trauma care to the injured survivors. In the late phase, in the subsequent months or years, the focus is on supporting the reconstruction of local medical services and facilities in the stricken area.

During the immediate phase, by the time outside medical help arrives, casualties with severe visceral injuries either have been treated already or have not survived. The clinical focus is on the management of extremity and soft tissue injuries (that may be neglected or infected) and complications such as renal failure from crush syndrome. Another important component of the work of outside medical teams is to provide solutions to ongoing surgical emergencies in the afflicted population. In the absence of functioning surgical facilities in the disaster area, even simple emergencies such as an incarcerated hernia or an obstetric condition requiring an urgent cesarean section may lead to preventable mortality.

In the immediate phase, the surgical management of extremity injuries follows the well-established principles of the management of war wounds. The focus is on straightforward procedures rather than complex reconstructions that are not feasible in the austere circumstances. Muscle compartments should be decompressed liberally and early, nonviable or heavily contaminated tissue should be excised while carefully preserving intact skin and viable soft tissue. Wounds are left open for delayed primary closure or for reexcision if needed. Unsalvageable or mangled extremities should be amputated early, with the stump left open for delayed primary closure.[31]

The composition and surgical capabilities of a team deployed to a disaster area must be carefully considered to fit the clinical needs. A typical team consists of general and orthopedic surgeons with trauma experience. More important than specific surgical skills is the ability to work in an austere environment in a spirit of collaboration with local and other external medical teams. A trained professional team with disaster relief experience, supported by a robust logistic, security, and communications envelope, has a much better chance of rendering effective medical care than an ad hoc team of enthusiastic volunteers. An effective intervention is limited in scope and duration and has well-defined realistic goals. A critical view of the most common errors and pitfalls in humanitarian relief efforts was published in 2010[39] in the wake of the Haiti earthquake, giving voice to grave concerns in the international community about the effectiveness of these efforts.

BLAST TRAUMA: CLINICAL PATTERNS AND SYSTEM IMPLICATIONS

Blast injury is an uncommon but devastating form of trauma, where one third of casualties admitted to the hospital have an Injury Severity Score higher than 15, a rate three times higher than seen in a typical civilian trauma practice. The overall number of casualties and rate of immediate on-scene mortality are determined by the size of the explosive charge, structural failure of the building, and indoor detonation, which results in a greatly amplified blast wave. Suicide bombers are particularly devastating weapons of urban terror because they specifically target crowded indoor locations or large open space gatherings to maximize the effect of the explosion.[22]

Blast trauma is viewed by trauma surgeons as a multidimensional injury because it often combines blast, penetrating, blunt, and burn mechanisms. The results are injury patterns of high severity and complexity and an unusually heavy burden on the trauma service line of the hospital. The classification of blast injuries is presented in Table 23-4.

Primary Blast Injury

The most common clinical sign of blast injury is eardrum perforation.[40] These perforations usually heal spontaneously but may result in various degrees of hearing loss in 25% of patients. Eardrum perforation is a useful marker of the proximity of the patient to the detonation, so arriving casualties should be screened for tympanic membrane rupture in the ED; individuals with a perforation should undergo an audiometric assessment for hearing loss. Although it is customary to admit otherwise asymptomatic patients with eardrum perforation for overnight observation because of their proximity to the detonation and concerns over the insidious onset of a blast lung injury, this practice is not evidence-based.

The blast wave from the detonation disrupts the alveolar-capillary interface of the lung, resulting in a spectrum of blast lung injury ranging from mild pulmonary contusion with intra-alveolar hemorrhage to severe and rapidly evolving acute respiratory distress syndrome.[41,42] Blast lung injury is uncommon, occurring in only 5% to 8% of live casualties in urban bombings, but the severity of this injury is the key determinant of mortality among early survivors. Patients with mild blast lung injury present with localized infiltrates on chest x-ray. Management is similar to management of a mild lung contusion, and the outcome is favorable. Patients with severe lung injury typically present with rapidly worsening hypoxia, develop bilateral diffuse infiltrates, and require early aggressive respiratory support.[41] Pneumothorax should be actively sought in these patients and immediately decompressed. Mortality may exceed 60% in these severe cases.

TABLE 23-4 Classification of Blast Trauma

CLASS OF BLAST INJURY	MECHANISM
Primary	Wounding of air-filled viscera as direct result of blast wave
Secondary	Penetrating trauma from bomb fragments and other projectiles of varying mass and velocity
Tertiary	Casualties propelled by blast wind, resulting in standard patterns of blunt trauma
Quaternary	Burns, crush, and all other trauma mechanisms not included above

Blast lung injury in the setting of an urban bombing poses a unique burden on the surgical ICU.[27,29] The trauma teams are facing several patients with severe and rapidly worsening hypoxia who arrive in the same wave of casualties. Each patient requires not only emergency endotracheal intubation but also advanced ventilatory support and the undivided attention of a team of critical care providers.[43] This logistic nightmare scenario is almost unique to urban bombing incidents and translates into a substantial medical, organizational, and staffing challenge centered around the ICU. The presence of associated injuries (e.g., burns or penetrating trauma) adds to the complexity of an already difficult situation.

Intestinal blast trauma ranges in severity from subserosal hemorrhage to full-thickness perforation.[44] Clinically important bowel blast injury is rare in urban bombings but is the most common form of trauma in an immersion blast from an underwater explosion. The clinical pitfall with these injuries is a delayed presentation, with some casualties developing peritoneal signs 48 hours or more after the explosion. The injury may occur in any portion of the bowel, but the terminal ileum and cecum are the most commonly affected organs.[44]

Secondary Blast Injury

Penetrating trauma from fragments of the bomb casing or from metal projectiles added to an improvised explosive device can cause a wide array of injuries, ranging from superficial skin lacerations to lethal visceral wounds. From the perspective of the trauma service line, the key consideration is the need for extensive imaging to locate penetrating fragments and define their trajectories because a physical examination is a poor predictor of the depth of penetration. The most expedient method is to use a helical CT scan to locate multiple projectiles rapidly and delineate their trajectories.[45] However, this method may create a bottleneck for patient flow and requires setting priorities and rationing access to the scanner during the initial phase of the hospital response.

Penetrating trauma by multiple projectiles may result in deep soft tissue wounds that bleed profusely. Because these wounds are typically located on the posterior aspect of the torso and extremities, the associated blood loss is often underestimated. When a patient is taken to the OR for emergency surgery, it is advisable to logroll the patient and rapidly pack the wounds with gauze before the main surgical procedure.[46]

Although classic management principles for traumatic wounds call for débridement of each wound and removal of embedded foreign bodies, this is often not a realistic option in casualties with multiple (sometimes dozens) asymptomatic penetrating wounds. A common-sense approach is to address only symptomatic or infected projectiles and projectiles in problematic locations (e.g., intra-articular).

Tertiary and Quaternary Blast Injuries

When casualties are propelled by the explosion against stationary objects, the results are standard patterns of blunt trauma. However, these tertiary blast injuries are typically combined with other types of trauma caused by the blast; this complicates the clinical picture and presents unusual dilemmas in terms of treatment priorities and resource allocation.

Quaternary blast trauma refers mostly to burns and crush injuries. Superficial flash burns, typically involving large body areas, are markers of proximity to the blast. They are common among casualties found dead at the scene and have been shown to be predictors of blast lung injury.[43] The ignition of flammable materials and clothes causes deep burns of variable extent, sometimes in conjunction with inhalation injury. A large number of burn casualties, many of them brought initially to hospitals that do not have a dedicated burn service, place an extraordinary burden on regional burn systems that generally have a limited surge capacity during normal daily operations. Secondary distribution of these patients to other burn centers outside the immediate vicinity of the bombing site is a key feature of MCIs involving a large number of burned casualties, such as the Bali nightclub bombing in Indonesia in 2002.[47]

CONCLUSION

The central message of this chapter is that amidst the wailing sirens of approaching ambulances, the terrible sights on television, the hectic activity of medical teams, and the emotional outrage of the public, surgeons must not forget their core mission: to preserve the trauma service line of their hospital and maintain the ability to provide the best possible trauma care to the next critical casualty. Contrary to the prevailing practice among disaster planners and hospital administrators to prepare for nightmare "mega-scenarios" that practicing surgeons are unlikely to encounter, the emphasis should be on preparing for realistic MCIs that happen in every community from time to time.

The ultimate goal of the entire hospital disaster plan is to provide a small number of critically injured casualties with a level of trauma care comparable to the care given to similarly injured patients on a normal working day. The many mildly injured patients are the "noise"—the casualties that are seen and heard on the evening news. The surgeon's role is to focus on the few casualties who are silent—the patients whose battle for survival unfolds away from the cameras, in the shock room, the OR, and the ICU. These very few critically injured patients are the crux of the entire effort.

SELECTED REFERENCES

Aylwin CJ, Konig TC, Brennan NW, et al: Reduction in critical mortality in urban mass casualty incidents: Analysis of triage, surge, and resource use after the London bombings on July 7, 2005. *Lancet* 368:2219–2225, 2006.

This report paints a detailed picture of the hospital response to the London subway bombings, including individual timelines for severe casualties. Although it shows how a modern trauma center copes with a large-scale event, it does not provide details on preventable morbidity and mortality.

Cushman JG, Pachter HL, Beaton HL: Two New York City hospitals' surgical response to the September 11, 2001, terrorist attack in New York City. *J Trauma* 54:147–154, 2003.

This is a classic report of the main hospital response to the World Trade Center destruction on September 11, 2001, with a discussion of the tiered hospital response plan.

Frykberg ER: Medical management of disasters and mass casualties from terrorist bombings: How can we cope? *J Trauma* 53:201–212, 2002.

This is the first overview of the medical response to urban terrorism that emphasizes the role of effective triage and looks at the medical response in quantitative terms. Frykberg was a pioneer in bringing the importance of disaster preparedness to the attention of surgeons.

Hirshberg A, Scott BG, Granchi T, et al: How does casualty load affect trauma care in urban bombing incidents? A quantitative analysis. *J Trauma* 58:686–693, 2005.

A computer model was used to simulate the response of a major U.S. trauma center to an urban bombing using casualty profiles from an Israeli hospital. The model predicts the now classic sigmoid-shaped relationship between the level of trauma care and increasing casualty load and defines the surge capacity of the hospital trauma service line.

Welling DR, Ryan JM, Burris DG, et al: Seven sins of humanitarian medicine. *World J Surg* 34:466–470, 2010.

A must-read for any surgeon contemplating participation in a humanitarian disaster relief effort, this editorial explains how good intentions can end up causing more damage than good.

REFERENCES

1. Dennis AJ, Brandt MM, Steinberg J, et al: Are general surgeons behind the curve when it comes to disaster preparedness training? A survey of general surgery and emergency medicine trainees in the United States by the Eastern Association for the Surgery for Trauma Committee on Disaster Preparedness. *J Trauma Acute Care Surg* 73:612–617, 2012.
2. Boston Trauma Center Chiefs' Consortium: Boston marathon bombings: An after-action review. *J Trauma Acute Care Surg* 77:501–503, 2014.
3. Hirshberg A, Holcomb JB, Mattox KL: Hospital trauma care in multiple-casualty incidents: A critical view. *Ann Emerg Med* 37:647–652, 2001.
4. O'Neill PA: The ABC's of disaster response. *Scand J Surg* 94:259–266, 2005.
5. Aylwin CJ, Konig TC, Brennan NW, et al: Reduction in critical mortality in urban mass casualty incidents: Analysis of triage, surge, and resource use after the London bombings on July 7, 2005. *Lancet* 368:2219–2225, 2006.
6. Hirshberg A: Multiple casualty incidents: Lessons from the front line. *Ann Surg* 239:322–324, 2004.
7. Hirshberg A, Scott BG, Granchi T, et al: How does casualty load affect trauma care in urban bombing incidents? A quantitative analysis. *J Trauma* 58:686–693, discussion 694–695, 2005.
8. De Boer J: Order in chaos: Modelling medical management in disasters. *Eur J Emerg Med* 6:141–148, 1999.
9. Gutierrez de Ceballos JP, Turegano Fuentes F, Perez Diaz D, et al: Casualties treated at the closest hospital in the Madrid, March 11, terrorist bombings. *Crit Care Med* 33:S107–S112, 2005.
10. Gaarder C, Jorgensen J, Kolstadbraaten KM, et al: The twin terrorist attacks in Norway on July 22, 2011: The trauma center response. *J Trauma Acute Care Surg* 73:269–275, 2012.

11. Walls RM, Zinner MJ: The Boston Marathon response: Why did it work so well? *JAMA* 309:2441–2442, 2013.
12. Kaplowitz L, Reece M, Hershey JH, et al: Regional health system response to the Virginia Tech mass casualty incident. *Disaster Med Public Health Prep* 1:S9–S13, 2007.
13. Stein M, Hirshberg A: Medical consequences of terrorism. The conventional weapon threat. *Surg Clin North Am* 79:1537–1552, 1999.
14. SALT mass casualty triage: Concept endorsed by the American College of Emergency Physicians, American College of Surgeons Committee on Trauma, American Trauma Society, National Association of EMS Physicians, National Disaster Life Support Education Consortium, and State and Territorial Injury Prevention Directors Association. *Disaster Med Public Health Prep* 2:245–246, 2008.
15. Cushman JG, Pachter HL, Beaton HL: Two New York City hospitals' surgical response to the September 11, 2001, terrorist attack in New York City. *J Trauma* 54:147–154, discussion 154–155, 2003.
16. McSwain N, Jr: Disaster preparedness perspective from 90.05.32w, 29.57.18n. *Crit Care* 10:108, 2006.
17. Mattox K, McSwain N, Frykberg E, et al: Position statement from the steering committee of the Atlantic-Gulf States Disaster Medical Coalition: Integrated collaborative networks will facilitate mass casualty medical response. *J Am Coll Surg* 205:612–616, 2007.
18. Almogy G, Belzberg H, Mintz Y, et al: Suicide bombing attacks: Update and modifications to the protocol. *Ann Surg* 239:295–303, 2004.
19. Frykberg ER: Triage: Principles and practice. *Scand J Surg* 94:272–278, 2005.
20. Hirshberg A, Frykberg ER, Mattox KL, et al: Triage and trauma workload in mass casualty: A computer model. *J Trauma* 69:1074–1081, discussion 1081–1082, 2010.
21. Kleber C, Cwojdzinski D, Strehl M, et al: Results of in-hospital triage in 17 mass casualty trainings: Underestimation of life-threatening injuries and need for re-triage. *Am J Disaster Med* 8:5–11, 2013.
22. Stein M: Urban bombing: A trauma surgeon's perspective. *Scand J Surg* 94:286–292, 2005.
23. Coupland RM: Epidemiological approach to surgical management of the casualties of war. *BMJ* 308:1693–1697, 1994.
24. Pillgram-Larsen J: A bomb in the city and an Island shooting spree: Lessons from Oslo. In Mattox KL, Allen MK, editors: *Medical Disaster Response Syllabus*, Las Vegas, March 2012, pp 59–68.
25. Einav S, Schecter WP, Matot I, et al: Case managers in mass casualty incidents. *Ann Surg* 249:496–501, 2009.
26. Hirshberg A, Stein M, Walden R: Surgical resource utilization in urban terrorist bombing: A computer simulation. *J Trauma* 47:545–550, 1999.
27. Shamir MY, Rivkind A, Weissman C, et al: Conventional terrorist bomb incidents and the intensive care unit. *Curr Opin Crit Care* 11:580–584, 2005.
28. Einav S, Aharonson-Daniel L, Weissman C, et al: In-hospital resource utilization during multiple casualty incidents. *Ann Surg* 243:533–540, 2006.
29. Aschkenasy-Steuer G, Shamir M, Rivkind A, et al: Clinical review: The Israeli experience: Conventional terrorism and critical care. *Crit Care* 9:490–499, 2005.
30. Ozoilo KN, Pam IC, Yiltok SJ, et al: Challenges of the management of mass casualty: Lessons learned from the Jos crisis of 2001. *World J Emerg Surg* 8:44, 2013.
31. Ryan JM: Natural disasters: The surgeon's role. *Scand J Surg* 94:311–318, 2005.
32. Butler CD, Harley D: Primary, secondary and tertiary effects of eco-climatic change: The medical response. *Postgrad Med J* 86:230–234, 2010.
33. Fink S: *Five days at Memorial: Life and death in a storm-ravaged hospital*, New York, 2013, Crown Publishers.
34. Redmond AD: Natural disasters. *BMJ* 330:1259–1261, 2005.
35. Erek E, Sever MS, Serdengecti K, et al: An overview of morbidity and mortality in patients with acute renal failure due to crush syndrome: The Marmara earthquake experience. *Nephrol Dial Transplant* 17:33–40, 2002.
36. Bar-On E, Lebel E, Blumberg N, et al: Pediatric orthopedic injuries following an earthquake: Experience in an acute-phase field hospital. *J Trauma Acute Care Surg* 74:617–621, 2013.
37. Dries D, Perry JF, Jr: Tsunami disaster: A report from the front. *Crit Care Med* 33:1178–1179, 2005.
38. Redmond AD, WHO: Needs assessment of humanitarian crises. *BMJ* 330:1320–1322, 2005.
39. Welling DR, Ryan JM, Burris DG, et al: Seven sins of humanitarian medicine. *World J Surg* 34:466–470, 2010.
40. Okpala N: Management of blast ear injuries in mass casualty environments. *Mil Med* 176:1306–1310, 2011.
41. Ritenour AE, Baskin TW: Primary blast injury: Update on diagnosis and treatment. *Crit Care Med* 36:S311–S317, 2008.
42. Wolf SJ, Bebarta VS, Bonnett CJ, et al: Blast injuries. *Lancet* 374:405–415, 2009.
43. Pizov R, Oppenheim-Eden A, Matot I, et al: Blast lung injury from an explosion on a civilian bus. *Chest* 115:165–172, 1999.
44. Owers C, Morgan JL, Garner JP: Abdominal trauma in primary blast injury. *Br J Surg* 98:168–179, 2011.
45. Sosna J, Sella T, Shaham D, et al: Facing the new threats of terrorism: Radiologists' perspectives based on experience in Israel. *Radiology* 237:28–36, 2005.
46. Bala M, Rivkind AI, Zamir G, et al: Abdominal trauma after terrorist bombing attacks exhibits a unique pattern of injury. *Ann Surg* 248:303–309, 2008.
47. Fisher D, Burrow J: The Bali bombings of 12 October, 2002: Lessons in disaster management for physicians. *Intern Med J* 33:125–126, 2003.

SECTION IV

Transplantation and Immunology

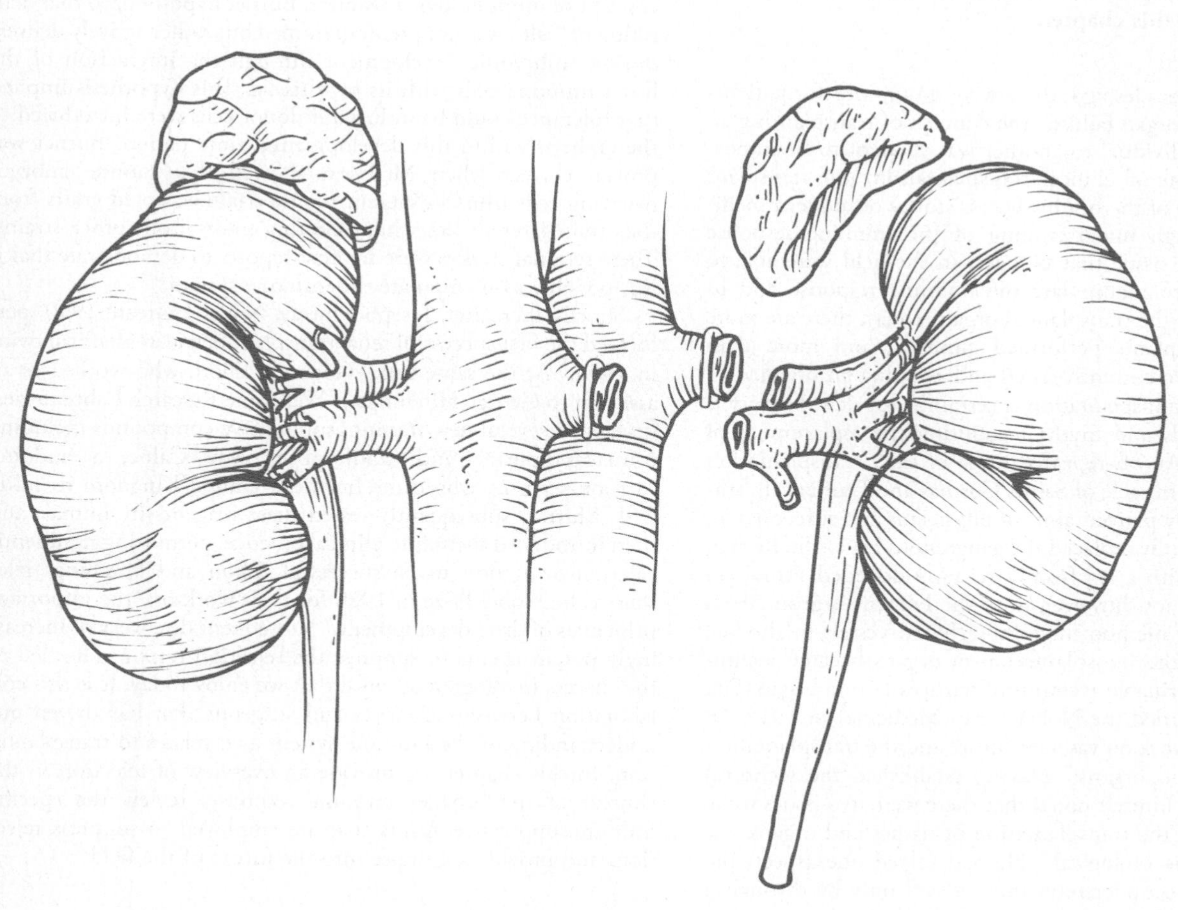

24 CHAPTER

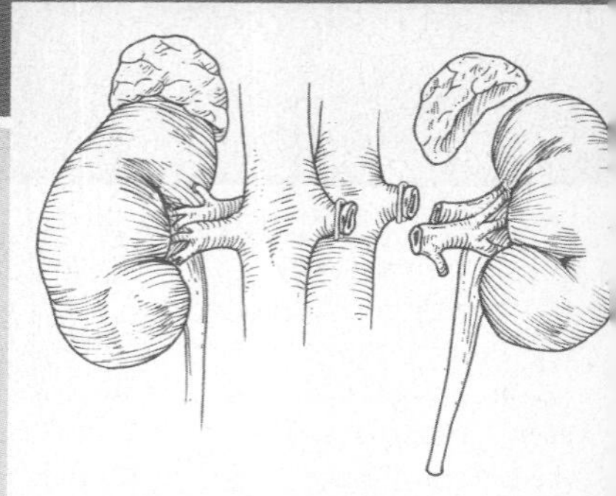

Transplantation Immunobiology and Immunosuppression

Andrew B. Adams, Mandy Ford, Christian P. Larsen

OUTLINE

 **Please access ExpertConsult.com to view the corresponding video for this chapter.**

Only a few short decades ago, there were no options for patients dying of end-stage organ failure. The concept of transplanting an organ from one individual to another was thought to be impossible. The evolution of clinical transplantation and transplant immunology is one of the bright success stories of modern medicine. It was through understanding of the immune response to the transplanted tissue that pioneers in the field were able to develop therapies to manipulate the immune response and to prevent rejection of the transplanted organ. Today, there are more than 25,000 transplants performed annually, and more than 100,000 patients are currently listed and awaiting an organ.

The concept of transplantation is certainly not new. History is replete with legends and myths recounting the replacement of limbs and organs. An oft-repeated myth of early transplantation is derived from the miracle of Saints Cosmas and Damian (brothers and subsequently patron saints of physicians and surgeons), in which they successfully replaced the gangrenous leg of the Roman deacon Justinian with a leg from a recently deceased Ethiopian (Fig. 24-1). It was not, however, until the French surgeon Alexis Carrel developed a method for joining blood vessels in the late 19th century that the transplantation of organs became technically feasible and verifiable accounts of transplantation began (Fig. 24-2). He was awarded the Nobel Prize (Medicine) in 1912 "in recognition of his work on vascular suture and the transplantation of blood vessels and organs." Having established the technical component, Carrel himself noted that there were two issues to be resolved regarding "the transplantation of tissues and organs . . . the surgical and the biological." He had solved one aspect, the surgical, but he also understood that "it will only be through a more fundamental study of the biological relationships existing between living tissues" that the more difficult problem of the biology would come to be solved.[1]

Forty years would pass before another set of eventual Nobel Prize winners, Peter Medawar and Frank Macfarlane Burnet, would begin to define the process by which one individual rejects another's tissue (Fig. 24-3).[2] Medawar and Burnet had developed an overall theory on the immunologic nature of self and the concept of immunologic tolerance. Burnet hypothesized that definition of "self" was not preprogrammed but rather actively defined during embryonic development through the interaction of the host's immune cells with its own tissue. This hypothesis implied that tolerance could be induced if donor cells were introduced to the embryo within this developmental time period. Burnet was proven correct when Medawar showed that mouse embryos receiving cells from a different mouse strain accepted grafts from the strain later in life while rejecting grafts from other strains. These seminal studies were the first reports to demonstrate that it was possible to manipulate the immune system.[3]

Shortly thereafter, Joseph Murray, Nobel Laureate 1990, performed the first successful renal transplant between identical twins in 1954.[4] At the same time, Gertrude Elion, who worked as an assistant to George Hitchings at Wellcome Research Laboratories, developed several new immunosuppressive compounds including 6-mercaptopurine and azathioprine. Roy Calne, a budding surgeon-scientist who came from the United Kingdom to study with Murray, subsequently tested these reagents in animals and then introduced them into clinical practice, permitting nonidentical transplantation to be successful. Elion and Hitchings later shared the Nobel Prize in 1988 for their work on "the important principles of drug development." Subsequent discovery of increasingly potent agents to suppress the rejection response has led to the success in allograft survival that we enjoy today. It is this collaboration between scientists and surgeons that has driven our understanding of the immune system as it relates to transplantation. In this chapter, we provide an overview of rejection in the context of the broader immune response, review the specific immunosuppressive agents that are employed to suppress rejection, and provide a glimpse into the future of the field.

THE IMMUNE RESPONSE

The immune system, of course, did not evolve to prevent the transplantation of another individual's tissue or organs; rejection, rather, is a consequence of a system that has developed over thousands of years to protect against invasion by pathogens and to prevent subsequent disease. To understand the rejection process and in particular to appreciate the consequences of pharmacologic suppression of rejection, a general understanding of immune response as it functions in a physiologic setting is required.

The immune system has evolved to include two complementary divisions to respond to disease: the innate and acquired immune systems. Broadly speaking, the innate immune system recognizes general characteristics that have, through selective pressure, come to represent universal pathologic challenges to our species (ischemia, necrosis, trauma, and certain nonhuman cell surfaces).[5] The acquired arm, on the other hand, recognizes specific structural aspects of foreign substances, usually peptide or carbohydrate moieties, recognized by receptors generated randomly and selected to avoid self-recognition. Although the two systems differ in their specific responsibilities, they act in concert to influence each other to achieve an optimal overall response.

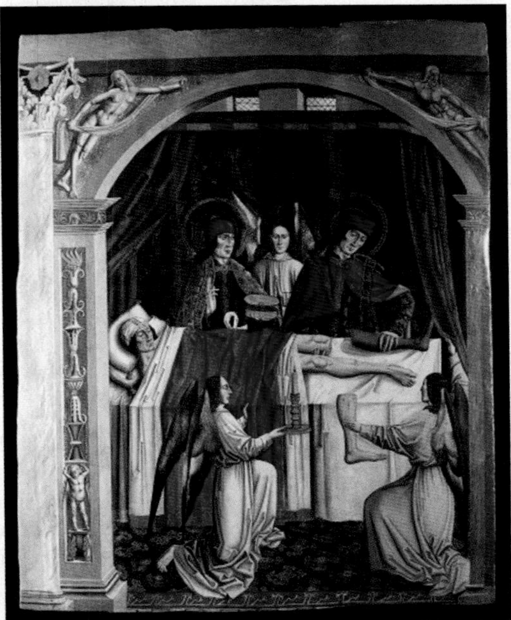

FIGURE 24-1 A 15th century painting of Cosmas and Damian, patron saints of physicians and surgeons. The legend of the Miracle of the Black Leg depicts the removal of the diseased leg of Roman Justinian and replacement with the leg of a recently deceased Ethiopian man.

INNATE IMMUNITY

The innate immune system is thought to be a holdover from an evolutionarily distant response to foreign pathogens. In contrast to the acquired immune system, which employs an innumerable host of specificities to identify any possible antigen, the innate system uses a select number of protein receptors to identify specific motifs consistent with foreign or altered and damaged tissues. These receptors can exist on cells, such as macrophages, neutrophils, and natural killer (NK) cells, or free in the circulation, as is the case for complement. Whereas they fail to exhibit the specificity of the T cell receptor (TCR) or antibody, they are broadly reactive against common components of pathogenic organisms,

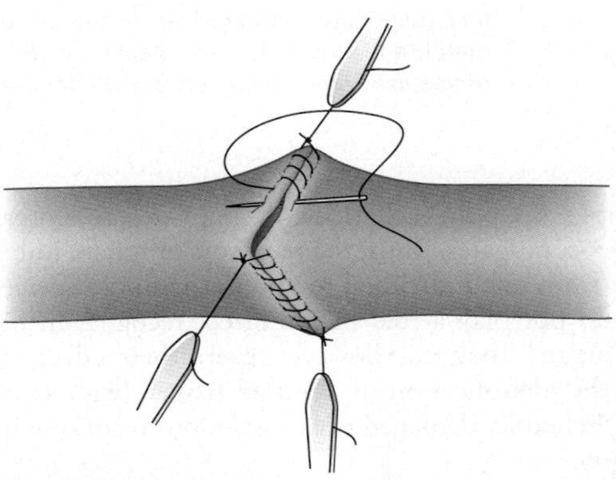

FIGURE 24-2 Triangulation technique of vascular anastomosis by Alexis Carrel. (Reprinted from Edwards WS, Edwards PD: *Alexis Carrel: Visionary surgeon*, Springfield, Ill, 1974, Charles C Thomas.)

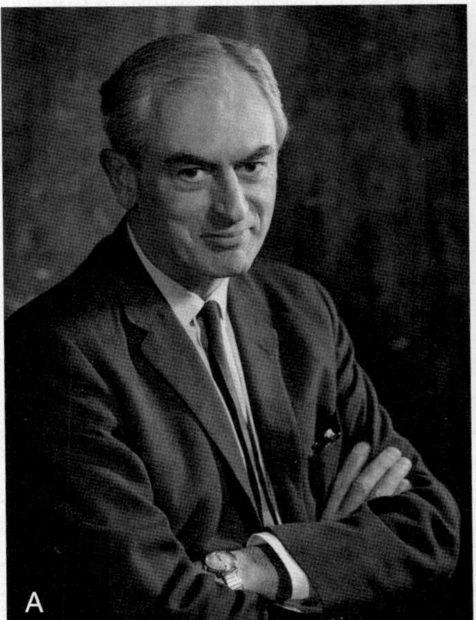

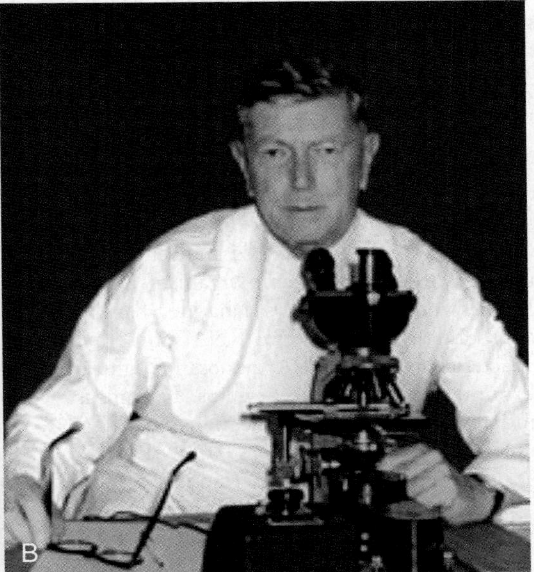

FIGURE 24-3 **A,** Sir Peter Medawar. (Courtesy Bern Schwartz Collection, National Portrait Gallery, London.) **B,** Sir Frank Macfarlane Burnet. (Courtesy Walter and Eliza Hall Institute of Medical Research.)

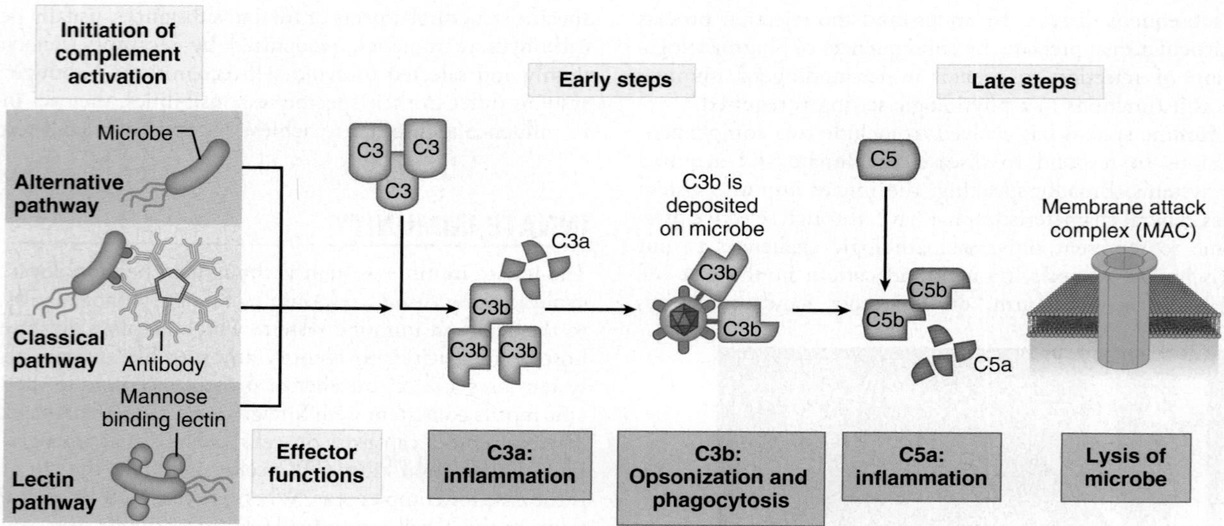

FIGURE 24-4 Complement Activation. There are three distinct pathways that lead to complement activation. All three pathways lead to production of C3b, which initiates the late steps of complement activation. C3b binds to the microbe and promotes opsonization and phagocytosis. C5a stimulates the local inflammatory response and catalyzes formation of the membrane attack complex, which results in microbial cell membrane disruption and death by lysis. (Adapted from Abbas AK, Lichtman AH, Pillai S: *Cellular and molecular immunology*, ed 8, Philadelphia, 2015, Saunders Elsevier.)

for example, lipopolysaccharides on gram-negative organisms or other glycoconjugates. Thus, the receptors of innate immunity are the same from one individual to another within a species and, in general, do not play a role in the direct recognition of a transplanted organ. They do, however, exert their effects indirectly through the identification of "injured tissue" (e.g., as is the case when an ischemic, damaged organ is moved from one individual to another).

Once activated, the innate system performs two vital functions. It initiates cytolytic pathways for the destruction of the offending organism, primarily through the complement cascade (Fig. 24-4). In addition, the innate system can convey the encounter to the acquired immune system for a more specific response through byproducts of complement activation by activation of antigen-presenting cells (APCs). Macrophages and dendritic cells not only engulf foreign organisms that have been bound by complement, but they can also distinguish pathogens as they can be identified through receptors for foreign carbohydrates (e.g., mannose receptors). Recently, a highly evolutionarily conserved family of proteins known as Toll-like receptors (TLRs) has been described to play an important role as activation molecules for innate APCs. They bind to pathogen-associated molecular patterns (PAMPs), motifs common to pathogenic organisms. Some examples of TLR ligands include lipopolysaccharide, flagellin (from bacterial flagella), double-stranded viral RNA, unmethylated CpG islands of bacterial and viral DNA, zymosan (β-glucan found in fungi), and numerous heat shock proteins. In contrast to PAMPs, which initiate a response to an infectious challenge, danger-associated molecular pattern molecules (DAMPs) also called alarmins, trigger the innate inflammatory response to noninfectious cell death and injury. Many DAMPs are nuclear or cytosolic proteins or even DNA that is released or exposed in the setting of cell injury. These signals alert the innate immune system that injury has occurred and a response is required. DAMP receptors include some of the TLRs, including TLR2 and TLR4, but also a variety of other proteins, such as RAGE (receptor for advanced glycation end products) and TREM-1 (triggering receptor expressed on myeloid cells 1). In the setting of a transplant surgery where an organ is cut out of one individual with a period of obligatory ischemia, cooled to near freezing, and then replaced in another individual, DAMPs play an active role in stimulating the innate inflammatory response. Once an injury or infectious insult has been identified, the cellular components of the innate system begin to initiate a response.

Monocytes

Mononuclear phagocytes are bone marrow–derived cells that initially emerge as monocytes within peripheral blood. In the setting of certain inflammatory signals, they home to sites of injury or inflammation, where they mature and become macrophages. Their function is to acquire, process, and present antigen as well as to serve as effector cells in certain situations. Once activated, they elaborate various cytokines that regulate the local immune response. They play a significant role in facilitating the acquired T cell response through antigen presentation, and their cytokines induce substantial tissue dysfunction in sites of inflammation. Thus, their recruitment to sites of injury and cell death can subsequently provoke T cell activation and rejection.

Dendritic Cells

Dendritic cells are specialized macrophages that are regarded as professional APCs. They are the most potent cells that present antigen and are distributed throughout the lymphoid and nonlymphoid tissues of the body. Immature dendritic cells can be found along the gut mucosa, within the skin, and in other sites of antigen entry. Once they have encountered antigen in sites of injury, they undergo a process of maturation, including the upregulation of both major histocompatibility complex (MHC) molecules, class I and class II, as well as various costimulatory molecules. They also begin to migrate toward peripheral lymphoid tissue (i.e., lymph nodes), where they can interact with antigen-specific T cells and potentiate their activation. The dendritic cell is involved in the licensing of $CD8^+$ T cells for cytotoxic function, stimulates T cell clonal expansion, and provides signals for helper T cell (Th) differentiation. There are also subsets of dendritic cells that serve distinct functions in inducing and regulating the cellular response. For example, myeloid dendritic cells are more immunogenic, whereas plasmacytoid dendritic cells are more tolerogenic and may work to suppress the immune response.

Natural Killer Cells

NK cells are large granular lymphocytes with potent cytolytic function that constitute a critical component of innate immunity. They were initially discovered during studies focused on tumor immunology. There was a small subset of lymphocytes that exhibited the ability to lyse tumor cells in the absence of prior sensitization, described as "naturally" reactive. These "natural killer" cells exhibited rapid cytolytic activity and existed in a relatively mature state (i.e., morphology characteristic of activated cytotoxic lymphocytes—large size, high protein synthesis activity with abundant endoplasmic reticulum, and rapid killing activity). Further studies have indicated that NK cells lyse cell targets that lack expression of self MHC class I, termed the missing self hypothesis, a situation that could arise as a result of viral infection with suppression of self class I molecules or in tumors under strong selection pressure of killer T cells. Since those initial studies, NK cells have been found to express cell surface inhibitory receptors, which include KIRs (killer inhibitory receptors). These molecules function to deliver inhibitory signals when they bind class I MHC molecules, thus preventing NK-mediated cytolysis on otherwise healthy host cells. NK cells produce various cytokines, including interferon-γ (IFN-γ), which may function to activate macrophages, which can in turn eliminate host cells infected by intracellular microbes. Similar to macrophages, NK cells express cell surface Fc receptors, which bind antibody and participate in antibody-dependent cellular cytotoxicity. NK cells also play an important role in the immune response after bone marrow transplantation and xenotransplantation. Their role in solid organ transplantation is less well defined.

ACQUIRED IMMUNITY

The distinguishing feature of the acquired immune system is specific recognition and disposition of foreign elements as well as the ability to recall prior challenges and to respond appropriately. Highly specific receptors, discussed later, have evolved to distinguish foreign from normal tissue through antigen binding. The term *antigen* is used to describe a molecule that can be recognized by the acquired immune system. An epitope is the portion of the antigen, generally a carbohydrate or peptide moiety, that actually serves as the binding site for the immune system receptor and is the base unit of antigen recognition. Thus, there may be one or many epitopes on any given antigen. The acquired response is divided into two distinct arms: cellular and humoral. The predominant effector cell in each arm is the T cell and B cell, respectively. Accordingly, the two main types of receptors that the immune system employs to recognize any given epitope are the TCR and B cell receptor or antibody. In general, individual T or B lymphocytes express identical receptors, each of which binds only to a single epitope. This mechanism establishes the specificity of the acquired immune response. The antigenic encounter alters the immune system such that future challenges with the same antigen provoke a more rapid and vigorous response, a phenomenon known as immunologic memory. There are vast differences in the way each division of the acquired immune response identifies an antigen. The B cell receptor or antibody can identify its epitope directly without preparation of the antigen, either on an invading pathogen itself or as a free-floating molecule in the extracellular fluid. T cells, however, recognize only their specific epitope after it has been processed and bound to a set of proteins, unique to the individual, which are responsible for presentation of the antigen. This set of proteins, crucial to antigen presentation, are termed histocompatibility proteins and, as their name suggests, were defined through studies examining tissue transplantation. The case of the immune response in tissue transplantation is unique and is discussed in its own section.

Major Histocompatibility Locus: Transplant Antigens

The major histocompatibility complex (MHC) refers to a cluster of highly conserved polymorphic genes on the sixth human chromosome. Much of what we know about the details of the immune response grew from initial studies defining the immunogenetics of the MHC. Studies began in mice, in which the MHC gene complex, termed H-2, was described by Gorer and Snell as a genetic locus that segregated with transplanted tumor survival. Subsequent serologic studies identified a similar genetic locus in humans called the HLA (human leukocyte antigen) locus. The products of these genes are expressed on a wide variety of cell types and play a pivotal role in the immune response. They are also the antigens primarily responsible for human transplant rejection, and their clinical implications are discussed later.

MHC molecules play a role in both the innate and acquired immune systems. Their predominant role, however, lies in antigen presentation within the acquired response. As mentioned earlier, the TCR does not recognize its specific antigen directly; rather, it binds to the processed antigen that is bound to cell surface proteins. It is the MHC molecule that binds the peptide antigen and interacts with the TCR, a process called antigen presentation. Thus, all T cells are restricted to an MHC for their response. There are two classes of MHC molecules, class I and class II. In general, $CD8^+$ T cells bind to antigen within class I MHC, and $CD4^+$ T cells bind to antigen within class II MHC.

Human Histocompatibility Complex

The antigens primarily responsible for human allograft rejection are those encoded by the HLA region of chromosome 6 (Fig. 24-5). The polymorphic proteins encoded by this locus include class I molecules (HLA-A, B, and C) and class II molecules (HLA-DP, DQ, and DR). There are additional class I genes with limited polymorphism (E, F, G, H, and J), but they are not currently used in tissue typing for transplantation and are not considered here. There are class III genes as well, but they are not cell surface proteins involved in antigen presentation directly but rather include molecules that are pertinent to the immune response by various mechanisms: tumor necrosis factor-α, lymphotoxin β, components of the complement cascade, nuclear transcription factor-β, and heat shock protein 70. Other conserved genes within the HLA include genes necessary for class I and class II presentation of peptides, such as the peptide transporter proteins TAP1 and TAP2 and proteasome proteases LMP2 and LMP7.[6] Although other polymorphic genes, referred to as minor histocompatibility antigens, exist in the genome outside of the HLA locus, they play a more limited role in transplant rejection and are not covered

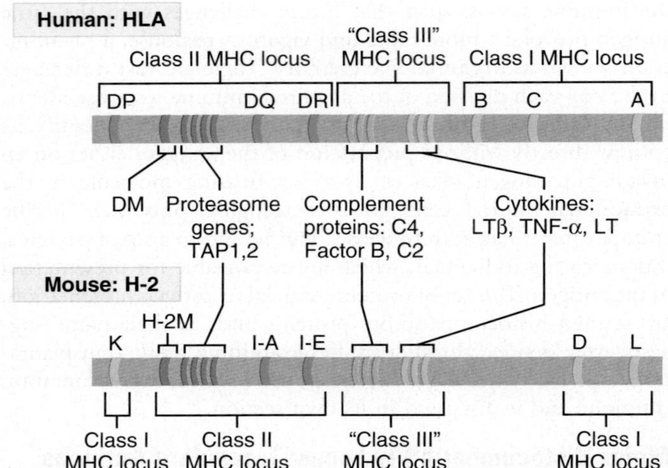

FIGURE 24-5 Location and organization of the HLA complex on human chromosome 6 and H-2 complex on murine chromosome 17. The complex is conventionally divided into three regions: I, II, and III. Class III genes are not related to class I and class II genes, structurally or functionally. (Adapted from Abbas AK, Lichtman AH, Pillai S: *Cellular and molecular immunology*, ed 8, Philadelphia, 2015, Saunders Elsevier.)

here. It is, however, important to point out that even HLA-identical individuals are subject to rejection on the basis of these minor differences. The blood group antigens of the ABO system must also be considered transplant antigens, and their biology is critical to humoral rejection.

Although initially identified as transplant antigens, class I and class II MHC molecules actually play vital roles in all immune responses, not just those to transplanted tissue. HLA class I molecules are present on all nucleated cells. In contrast, class II molecules are found almost exclusively on cells associated with the immune system (macrophages, dendritic cells, B cells, and activated T cells) but can be upregulated and appear on other parenchymal cells in the setting of cytokine release due to an immune response or injury.

The importance to transplantation of MHC gene products stems from their polymorphism. Unlike most genes, which are identical within a given species, polymorphic gene products differ in detail while still conforming to the same basic structure. Thus, polymorphic MHC proteins from one individual are foreign alloantigens to another individual. Recombination within the HLA locus is uncommon, occurring in approximately 1% of molecules. Consequently, the HLA type of the offspring is predictable. The unit of inheritance is the haplotype, which consists of one chromosome 6 and therefore one copy of each class I and class II locus (HLA-A, B, C, DP, DQ, and DR). Thus, donor-recipient pairings that are matched at all HLA loci are referred to as HLA-identical allografts, and those matched at half of the HLA loci are termed haploidentical. Note that HLA-identical allografts still differ genetically at other genetic loci and are distinct from isografts. Isografts are organs transplanted between identical twins and are immunologically indistinguishable and thus are not rejected. The genetics of HLA is particularly important in understanding clinical living related donor transplantation. Each child inherits one haplotype from each parent; therefore, the chance of siblings being HLA identical is 25%. Haploidentical siblings occur 50% of the time, and completely nonidentical or HLA-distinct siblings occur 25% of the time. Biologic parents are haploidentical with their children unless there has been a rare recombination event. The degree of HLA match can also improve if the parents are homozygous for a given allele, thus giving the same allele to all children. Likewise, if the parents share the same allele, the likelihood of that allele being inherited improves to 50%. This is even more important in the field of bone marrow transplantation, in which the risks of donor-mediated cytotoxicity and resultant graft-versus-host disease become a more relevant issue.

Each class I molecule is encoded by a single polymorphic gene that is combined with the nonpolymorphic protein β_2-microglobulin (chromosome 15) for expression. The polymorphism of each class I molecule is extreme, with 30 to 50 alleles per locus. Class II molecules are made up of two chains, α and β, and individuals differ not only in the alleles represented at each locus but also in the number of loci present in the HLA class II region. The polymorphism of class II is thus increased by combinations of α and β chains as well as by hybrid assembly of chains from one class II locus to another. As the HLA sequence varies, the ability of various peptides to bind to the molecule and to be presented for T cell recognition changes. Teleologically, this extreme diversity is thought to improve the likelihood that a given pathogenic peptide will fit into the binding site of these antigen-presenting molecules, thus preventing a single viral agent from evading detection by T cells of an entire population.[7]

Class I Major Histocompatibility Complex

The three-dimensional structure of class I molecules (HLA-A, B, and C) was first elucidated in 1987.[8] The class I molecule is composed of a 44-kDa transmembrane glycoprotein (α chain) in a noncovalent complex with a nonpolymorphic 12-kDa polypeptide called β_2-microglobulin. The α chain has three domains, α_1, α_2, and α_3. The critical structural feature of class I molecules is the presence of a groove formed by two α helices mounted on a β pleated sheet in the α_1 and α_2 domains (Fig. 24-6). Within this groove, a 9–amino acid peptide, formed from fragments of proteins being synthesized in the cell's endoplasmic reticulum, is mounted for presentation to T cells. Almost all the significant sequence polymorphism of class I is located in the region of the peptide-binding groove and in areas of direct T cell contact. The assembly of class I is dependent on association of the α chain with β_2-microglobulin and native peptide within the groove. Incomplete molecules are not expressed. In general, all peptides made by a cell are candidates for presentation, although sequence alterations in this region favor certain sequences over others. The α_3 immunoglobulin-like domain, which is the domain closest to the membrane and interacts with the CD8 molecule on the T cell, demonstrates limited polymorphism and is conserved to preserve interactions with $CD8^+$ T cells.

Human class I presentation occurs on all nucleated cells, and expression can be increased by certain cytokines, thus allowing the immune system to inspect and to approve of ongoing protein synthesis. Interferons (IFN-α, IFN-β, and IFN-γ) induce an increase in the expression of class I molecules on a given cell by increasing levels of gene expression. T cell activation occurs when a given T cell encounters a class I MHC molecule carrying a peptide from a nonself protein presented in the proper context (e.g., viral protein is processed in an infected cell and the peptide fragments are presented on class I molecules for T cell recognition). So-called cross presentation may also occur in which certain APCs, namely, a subset of dendritic cells, have the ability to take up and process exogenous antigen and present it on class I molecules to $CD8^+$ T cells.[9] In the case of transplantation, this

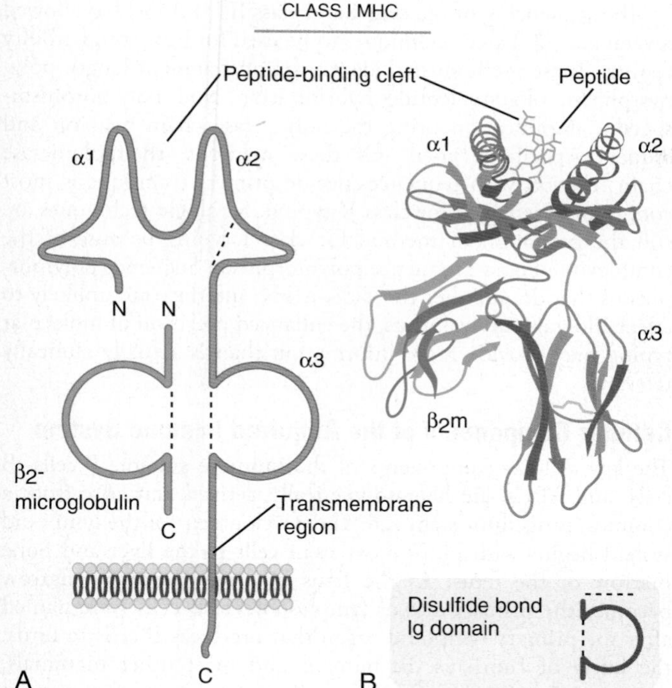

FIGURE 24-6 Structure of the MHC class I molecule. Class I molecules are composed of polymorphic α chain noncovalently attached to the nonpolymorphic β_2-microglobulin (β_2m). **A,** Schematic diagram. **B,** The ribbon diagram shows the extracellular structure of a class I molecule with a bound peptide. (Adapted from Abbas AK, Lichtman AH, Pillai S: *Cellular and molecular immunology*, ed 6, Philadelphia, 2010, Saunders Elsevier.)

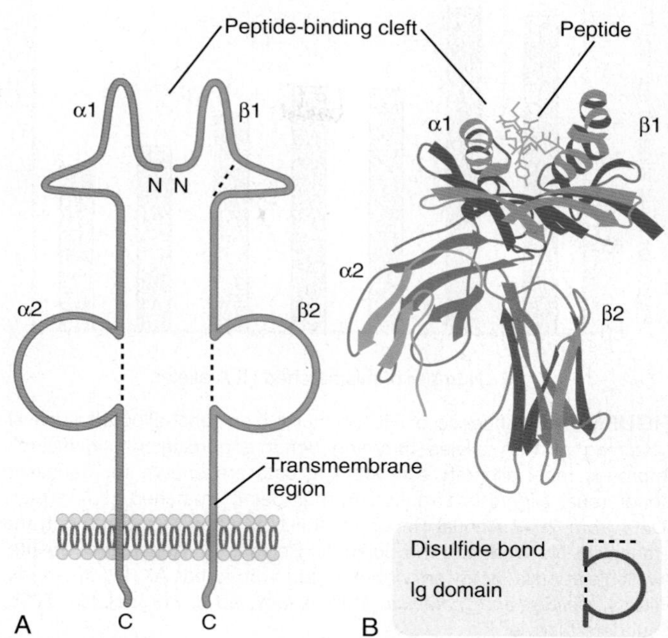

FIGURE 24-7 Structure of the MHC class II molecule. Class II molecules are composed of a polymorphic α chain noncovalently attached to a polymorphic β chain. **A,** Schematic diagram. **B,** The ribbon diagram shows the extracellular structure of a class II molecule with a bound peptide. (Adapted from Abbas AK, Lichtman AH, Pillai S: *Cellular and molecular immunology*, ed 6, Philadelphia, 2010, Saunders Elsevier.)

activation is not only possible when foreign peptide is identified after the donor MHC has been processed and presented on recipient APCs but more commonly occurs when a T cell interacts directly with the nonself class I MHC, the so-called direct alloresponse.

Class II MHC

The class II molecules are products of the, HLA-DP, HLA-DQ, and HLA-DR genes. The structural features of class II molecules are strikingly similar to those of class I molecules. The three-dimensional structure of class II molecules was inferred by sequence homology to class I in 1988 and eventually proven by x-ray crystallography in 1993 (Fig. 24-7).[10] The class II molecules contain two polymorphic chains, one approximately 32 kDa and the other approximately 30 kDa. The peptide-binding region is composed of the α_1 and β_1 domains. The immunoglobulin-like domain is composed of the α_2 and β_2 segments. Similar to the class I immunoglobulin-like α_3 domain, there is limited polymorphism in these segments, and the β_2 domain, in particular, is involved in the binding of the CD4 molecule, helping to restrict class II interactions to CD4$^+$ T cells. Class II molecule assembly requires association of both the α chain and β chain in combination with a temporary protein called the invariant chain.[11] This third protein covers the peptide-binding groove until the class II molecule is out of the endoplasmic reticulum and is sequestered in an endosome. Proteins that are engulfed by a phagocytic cell are degraded at the same time as the invariant chain is removed, allowing peptides of external sources to be associated with and presented by class II. In this way, the acquired immune system can inspect and approve of proteins that are present in circulation or that have been liberated from foreign cells or pathogens through the phagocytic process. Accordingly, class II molecules, in contrast to class I molecules, are confined to cells related to the immune response, particularly APCs (macrophages, dendritic cells, B cells, and monocytes). Class II expression can also be induced on other cells, including endothelial cells, under the appropriate conditions. After binding class II molecules, CD4$^+$ T cells participate in APC-mediated activation of CD8$^+$ T cells and antibody-producing B cells. In the case of transplanted organs, ischemic injury at the time of transplantation accentuates the potential for T cell activation by upregulation of both class I and class II molecules locally on the recipient. The trauma of surgery and ischemia also upregulate class II on all cells of the allograft, making nonself MHC more abundant. Host CD4$^+$ T cells may then recognize donor MHC directly (direct alloresponse) or after antigen processing (indirect alloresponse) and then proceed to participate in rejection.

HLA Typing: Implications for Transplantation

For the reasons already discussed, closely matched transplants are less likely to be recognized and rejected than are similar grafts differing by multiple alleles at the MHC. HLA matching has clear influence on the prolongation of graft survival. Humans have two different HLA-A, B, and DR alleles (one from each parent, six in total). Although clearly important, the HLA-C, DP, and DQ loci have previously been administratively dismissed in general organ allocation. More recently, there is an effort to expand genetic typing of donors to include HLA-DP and HLA-DQ so that these HLA molecules may be considered as well. Whereas current

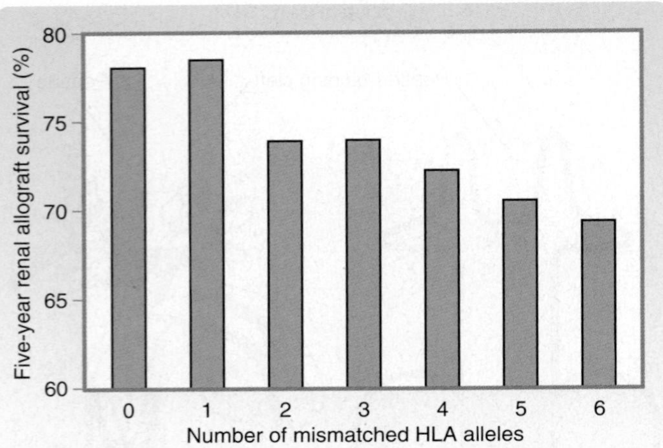

FIGURE 24-8 Influence of HLA matching on renal allograft survival. Matching of HLA alleles between donor and recipient significantly improves renal allograft survival. The data are shown for deceased donor renal allografts stratified by number of matched HLA alleles. (Data from 2012 Annual Report of the U.S. Organ Procurement and Transplant Network and the Scientific Registry of Transplant Patients. Available at *http://www.srtr.org*. Adapted from Abbas AK, Lichtman AH, Pillai S: *Cellular and molecular immunology*, ed 8, Philadelphia, 2015, Saunders Elsevier.)

immunosuppressive regimens negate much of the impact of matching, several studies have demonstrated improvements in renal allograft survival when the six primary alleles are matched between donor and recipient, a so-called six-antigen match (Fig. 24-8). Historically, MHC match has been defined using two cellular assays: the lymphocytotoxicity assay and the mixed lymphocyte reaction. Both assays define MHC epitopes but do not comprehensively define the entire antigen or the exact genetic disparity involved. Techniques now exist for precise genotyping by molecular techniques that distinguish the nucleotide sequence of an individual's MHC.

The mixed lymphocyte reaction is performed by incubating recipient T cells with irradiated donor cells in the presence of ^{3}H-thymidine (the irradiation treatment ensures that the assay measures only proliferation of recipient T cells). If the cells differ at the class II MHC locus, recipient $CD4^+$ T cells produce interleukin-2 (IL-2), which stimulates proliferation. Proliferating cells incorporate the labeled nucleotide into their newly manufactured DNA, which can be detected and quantified. Whereas class II polymorphism is detected by this assay, it takes several days to complete one assay. Thus, use of the mixed lymphocyte reaction as a prospective typing assay is limited to living related donors. The specific MHC alleles are not identified with this assay; instead, they are inferred from a series of reactions. Although this assay has been extremely valuable historically, it has now been largely supplanted by more modern molecular techniques. The lymphocytotoxicity assay involves taking serum from individuals with anti-MHC antibodies of known specificity and mixing it with lymphocytes from the individual in question. Exogenous complement is added, as is a vital dye, which is not taken up by intact cells. If the antibody binds to MHC, it activates the complement and leads to cell membrane disruption, and the cell takes up the vital stain. Microscopic examination of the cells can then determine if the MHC antigen was present on the cells. This, too, has been supplanted by more modern methods of MHC-specific antibody detection.

The sequencing of the class I and class II HLA loci has allowed several genetic-based techniques to be used for histocompatibility testing. These methods include restriction fragment length polymorphism, oligonucleotide hybridization, and polymorphism-specific amplification using the polymerase chain reaction and sequence-specific primers. Of these methods, the polymerase chain reaction with sequence-specific primers technique is most commonly employed for class II typing. Serologic techniques are still the predominant method for class I typing because of the complexity of class I sequence polymorphism. Sequence polymorphisms that do not alter the TCR-MHC interface are unlikely to affect allograft survival; thus, the enhanced precision of molecular typing may provide more information than is actually clinically relevant.

Cellular Components of the Acquired Immune System

The key cellular components of the immune system, T cells, B cells, and APCs, are hematopoietically derived and arise from a common progenitor stem cell. The development of the lymphoid system begins with pluripotent stem cells in the liver and bone marrow of the fetus. As the fetus matures, the bone marrow becomes the primary site of lymphopoiesis. B cells were named after the primary lymphoid organ that produces B cells in birds, the bursa of Fabricius. In humans and most other mammals, precursor B cells remain within the bone marrow as they mature and fully develop. Although precursor T cells also originate in the bone marrow, they soon migrate to the thymus, the primary site of T cell maturation, where they become "educated" to self and acquire their specific cell surface receptors and the ability to generate effector function. Mature lymphocytes are then released from the primary lymphoid organs, the bone marrow and thymus, to populate the secondary lymphoid organs, including lymph nodes, spleen, and gut, as well as peripheral tissues. Each of these cells has a unique role in establishing the immune response. The highly coordinated network is regulated in part through the use of cytokines (Table 24-1).

Both B and T cells are integral components of a highly specific response that must be prepared to recognize a seemingly endless array of pathogens. This is accomplished through a unique method that allows random generation of almost unlimited receptor specificity yet controls the ultimate product by eliminating or suppressing those that might react against self and perpetuate an autoimmune response. There are fundamental differences in the manner in which T and B cells recognize antigen. B cells are structured to respond to whole antigen and in response synthesize and secrete antibody that can interact with antigen at distant sites. T cells, on the other hand, are responsible for cell-mediated immunity and of necessity must interact with cells in the periphery to neutralize and to eliminate foreign antigens. From the peripheral blood, T cells enter the lymph nodes or spleen through highly specialized regions in the postcapillary venules. Within the secondary lymphoid organ, T cells interact with specific APCs, where they receive the appropriate signals that in effect license them for effector function. They then exit the lymphoid tissues through the efferent lymph, eventually percolating through the thoracic duct and returning to the bloodstream. From there, they can return to the site of the immune response, where they encounter their specific antigen and carry out their predefined functions.

T Cell Receptor

Considerable progress has been made in defining the mechanisms of T cell maturation and the development of a functional TCR.

TABLE 24-1 Summary of Cytokines

CYTOKINE	SOURCE	PRINCIPAL CELLULAR TARGETS AND BIOLOGIC EFFECTS
Interleukin-1	Macrophages, endothelial cells, some epithelial cells	Endothelial cell: activation (inflammation, coagulation) Hypothalamus: fever Liver: synthesis of acute-phase proteins
Interleukin-2	T cells	T cells: proliferation, ↑ cytokine synthesis, survival, potentiates Fas-mediated apoptosis, promotes regulatory T cell development NK cells: proliferation, activation B cells: proliferation, antibody synthesis (in vitro)
Interleukin-3	T cells	Immature hematopoietic progenitor cells: stimulates differentiation into myeloid lineage, proliferation of myeloid lineage cells
Interleukin-4	CD4⁺ T cells (Th2), Mast cells	B cells: isotype switching to IgE T cells: Th2 differentiation, proliferation Macrophages: inhibition of IFN-γ–mediated activation Mast cells: stimulates proliferation
Interleukin-5	CD4⁺ T cells (Th2)	Eosinophils: activation, ↑ production B cells: proliferation, IgA production
Interleukin-6	Macrophages, endothelial cells, T cells	Liver: ↑ synthesis of acute-phase proteins B cells: proliferation of antibody-producing cells
Interleukin-7	Fibroblasts, bone marrow stromal cells	Immature hematopoietic progenitor cells: stimulates differentiation into lymphoid lineage T and B cells: important for survival during development as well as for T cell memory
Tumor necrosis factor	Macrophages, T cells	Endothelial cells: activation (inflammation, coagulation) Neutrophils: activation Hypothalamus: fever Liver: ↑ synthesis of acute-phase proteins Muscle, fat: catabolism (cachexia) Many cell types: apoptosis
Interferon-γ	T cells (Th1, CD8⁺ T cells), NK cells	Macrophages: activation (increased microbicidal functions) B cells: isotype switching to IgG subclasses that facilitate complement fixation and opsonization T cells: Th1 differentiation Various cells: ↑ expression of class I and class II MHC, ↑ antigen processing and presentation to T cells
Type I interferons (IFN-α, IFN-β)	Macrophages: IFN-α Fibroblasts: IFN-β	All cells: stimulates antiviral activity including ↑ class I MHC expression NK cells: activation
Transforming growth factor-β	T cells, macrophages, other cell types	T cells: inhibition of proliferation and effector functions B cells: inhibition of proliferation, ↑ IgA production Macrophages: inhibits activation, stimulates angiogenic factors Fibroblasts: increased collagen synthesis
Lymphotoxin	T cells	Lymphoid organogenesis Neutrophils: increased recruitment and activation
BAFF (CD257)	Follicular dendritic cells, monocytes, B cells	B cells: survival and proliferation
APRIL (CD256)	T cells, follicular dendritic cells, monocytes	B cells: survival and proliferation
Interleukin-8	Lymphocytes, monocytes	Stimulates granulocyte activity Chemotactic activity
Interleukin-9	Activated Th2 lymphocytes	Enhances proliferation of T cells, mast cells
Interleukin-10	Macrophages, T cells (mainly regulatory T cells)	Macrophages and dendritic cells: inhibition of IL-12 production, stimulates expression of costimulatory molecules and class II MHC
Interleukin-11	Bone marrow stromal cells	Megakaryocytes: thrombopoiesis Liver: induces acute-phase proteins B cells: stimulates T-dependent antibody production
Interleukin-12	Macrophages, dendritic cells	T cells: Th1 differentiation NK and T cells: IFN-γ synthesis, increased cytotoxic activity
Interleukin-13	CD4⁺ T cells (Th2), NKT cells, mast cells	B cells: isotype switching to IgE Epithelial cells: increased mucus production Fibroblasts and macrophages: increased collagen synthesis
Interleukin-14	T cells, some B cell tumors	B cells: enhances proliferation of activated B cells, stimulates immunoglobulin production
Interleukin-15	Macrophages, others	NK cells: proliferation T cells: proliferation (memory CD8⁺ T cells)

Continued

TABLE 24-1 Summary of Cytokines—cont'd

CYTOKINE	SOURCE	PRINCIPAL CELLULAR TARGETS AND BIOLOGIC EFFECTS
Interleukin-17	T cells	Endothelial cells: increased chemokine production Macrophages: increased chemokine/cytokine production Epithelial cells: GM-CSF and G-CSF production
Interleukin-18	Macrophages	NK and T cells: IFN-γ synthesis
Interleukin-21	Th2, Th17, Tfh	Drives development of Th17 and Tfh B cells: activation, proliferation, differentiation NK cells: functional maturation
Interleukin-22	Th17	Epithelial cells: production of defensins, increased barrier functions Promotes hepatocyte survival
Interleukin-23	Macrophages, dendritic cells	T cells: maintenance of IL-17–producing T cells
Interleukin-27	Macrophages, dendritic cells	T cells: inhibits production of IL-17/Th17 cells, promotes Th1 differentiation NK cells: IFN-γ synthesis
Interleukin-33	Endothelial cells, smooth muscle cells, keratinocytes, fibroblasts	Th2 development and cytokine production

Adapted from Abbas AK, Lichtman AH, Pillai S: *Cellular and molecular immunology*, ed 8, Philadelphia, 2015, Saunders Elsevier.
G-CSF, granulocyte-colony stimulating factor; *GM-CSF*, granulocyte-macrophage colony-stimulating factor.

The formation of the TCR is fundamental to the understanding of its function.[12] When precursor T cells migrate from the fetal liver and bone marrow to the thymus, they have yet to obtain their specialized TCR or accessory molecules. On arrival to the thymus, T cells undergo a remarkable rearrangement of the DNA that encodes the various chains of the TCR (α, β, γ, and δ) (Fig. 24-9). The order of genetic rearrangement recapitulates the evolution of the TCR. T cells first attempt to recombine the γ and δ TCR genes and then, if recombination fails to yield a properly formed receptor, resort to the more diverse α and β TCR genes. The γδ configuration is typically not successful, and thus most T cells are αβ T cells. T cells expressing the γδ TCR have more primitive functions, including recognition of heat shock proteins and activity similar to NK cells as well as MHC recognition, whereas αβ T cells are more typically limited to recognition of MHC complexed with processed peptide.

Regardless of the genes used, individual cells recombine to express a TCR with only a single specificity. The rearrangements occur randomly, resulting in a population of T cells capable of binding 10^9 different specificities, essentially all combinations of MHC and peptide. As a result, the frequency of naïve T cells available to respond to any given pathogen is relatively small, between 1 in 200,000 and 1 in 500,000. These developing T cells also express both CD4 and CD8, accessory molecules that strengthen the TCR binding to MHC. These accessory molecules further increase the binding repertoire of the population to include either class I or class II MHC molecules. If the process of T cell maturation ended at this stage, there would be a host of T cells that could recognize self MHC–peptide complexes, resulting in an uncontrolled, global autoimmune response. To avoid the release of autoreactive T cells, developing cells undergo a process following recombination known as thymic selection (Fig. 24-10).[13] Cells initially interact with the MHC-expressing cortical thymic epithelium, which produces hormones (thymopoietin and thymosin) as well as cytokines (e.g., IL-7) that are critical to T cell development. If binding does not occur to self MHC, those cells are useless to the individual (e.g., they cannot bind self cells to assess for infection), and they are permitted to die by neglect through apoptosis, a process called positive selection. Thus, positive selection ensures that T cells are restricted to self MHC. Cells surviving positive selection then move to the thymic medulla and normally eventually lose either CD4 or CD8. If binding to self MHC in the medulla occurs with an unacceptably high affinity, there is an active process whereby death-promoting signals are delivered and programmed cell death is initiated, a process termed negative selection. Negative selection stands in contrast to the death that occurs by neglect when immature lymphocytes are not positively selected. Another possible although less common outcome of a high-affinity interaction with self peptide–MHC is the development of a regulatory T cell (Treg) phenotype. The precise nature of this affinity threshold remains a matter of intense investigation and involves interaction with hematopoietic cells that reside in the thymus as well as medullary thymic epithelial cells. These thymically derived "natural" Tregs emerge from the thymus and are involved in the suppression of autoreactive T cells in the periphery, which is discussed later.

The only cells released into the periphery are those that can both bind self MHC and avoid activation. Whereas T cells are restricted to bind self MHC–peptide complexes without activation, the selection process does not consider foreign MHC. Thus, by random chance, some cells with appropriate affinity for self MHC survive and have inappropriately high affinity for the MHC molecules of other individuals. In the setting of transplantation, these recipient T cells are able to recognize donor MHC–peptide complexes because there are sufficient conserved motifs shared between donor and self MHC molecules. However, because donor MHC was not present during the thymic education process, the binding of donor MHC by an "alloreactive" T cell leads to activation, and rejection ensues. The precursor frequency or the number of alloreactive T cells is much higher than the 1 in 200,000 or 1 in 500,000 T cells available to react toward any given antigen. Because T cells are selected to bind self MHC, the frequency specific for a similar, nonself MHC (i.e., alloreactive) is between 1% and 10% of all T cells.

In addition to thymic selection, it is now clear that mechanisms exist for peripheral modification of the T cell repertoire. Many of these mechanisms are in place for removal of T cells after an immune response and downregulation of activated clones. CD95, a molecule known as Fas, is a member of the tumor necrosis factor (TNF) receptor superfamily and is expressed on

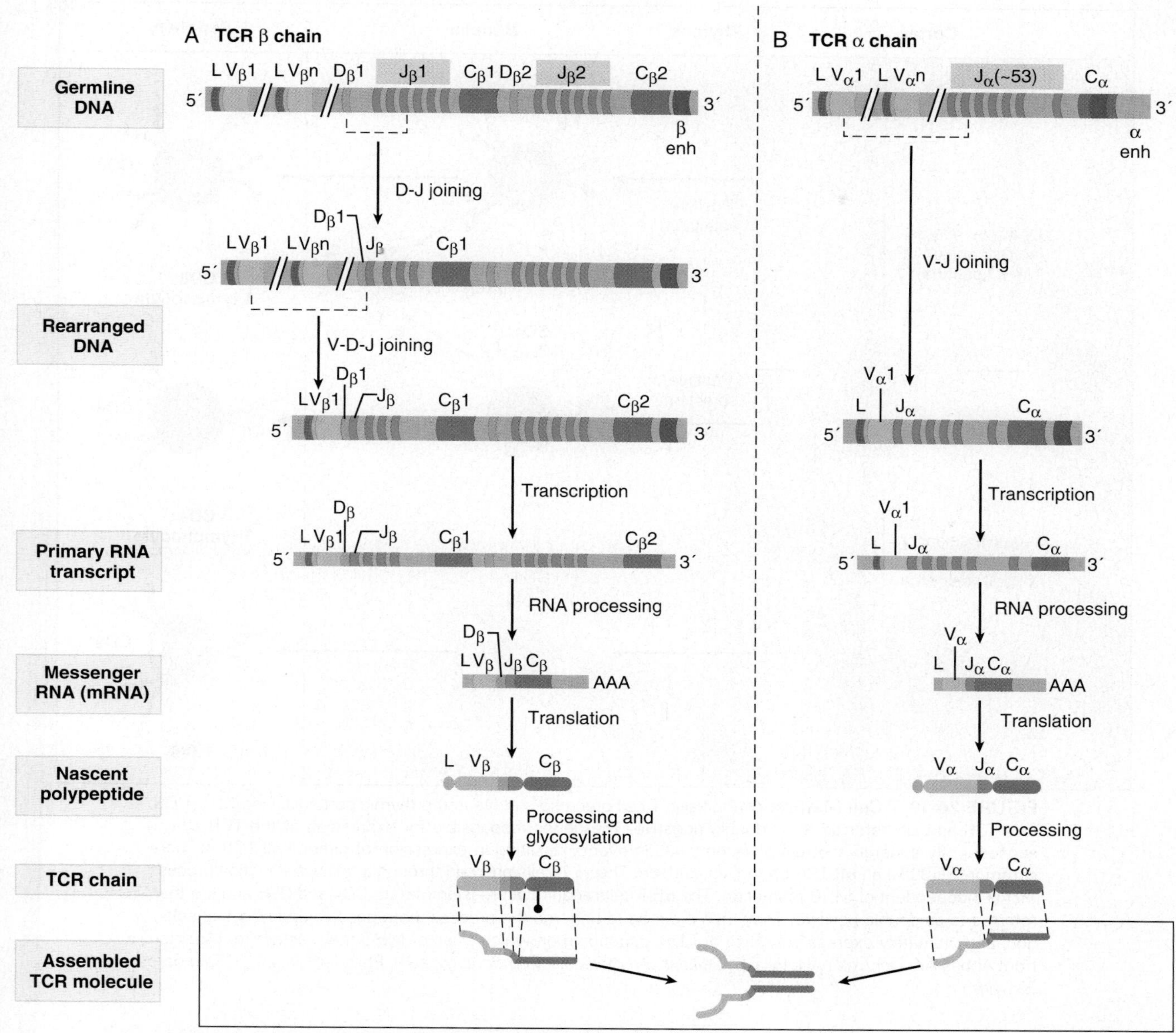

FIGURE 24-9 TCR recombination and expression (α and β loci shown here). There is an elaborate genetic rearrangement that leads to the formation of a diverse repertoire of T cell receptors. Genomic DNA is spliced under the direction of specific enzymes active during T cell development within the thymus. Random segments from regions termed variable (V), joining (J), diversity (D), and constant (C) are brought together to form a unique gene responsible for a unique TCR chain. The γ and δ loci recombine first, and if successful, a γδ TCR is formed. If unsuccessful, then α and β regions recombine to form an αβ TCR. Approximately 95% of T cells progress to express an αβ TCR. (Adapted from Abbas AK, Lichtman AH, Pillai S: *Cellular and molecular immunology*, ed 8, Philadelphia, 2015, Saunders Elsevier.)

activated T cells. Under appropriate conditions, binding of this molecule to its ligand, CD178, promotes programmed cell death of a cohort of activated T cells. This method is dependent on TCR binding and the activation state of the T cell. Complementing this deletional method to TCR repertoire control are nondeletional mechanisms that selectively anergize (make unreactive) specific T cell clones. In addition to signaling through the TCR complex, T cells require additional costimulatory signals (described in detail later). TCR binding leads to T cell activation only if the costimulatory signals are present, generally delivered by APCs. In the absence of costimulation, the cell remains unable to proceed toward activation and in some circumstances becomes refractory to activation even with the appropriate signals. Thus, TCR binding that occurs to self in the absence of appropriate antigen presentation or active inflammation results in an aborted activation and prevents self-reactivity.

T Cell Activation

T cell activation is a sophisticated series of events that have only recently been more fully described. The TCR, unlike antibody, recognizes its ligand only in the context of MHC. By requiring that T cells respond only to antigen encountered when it is

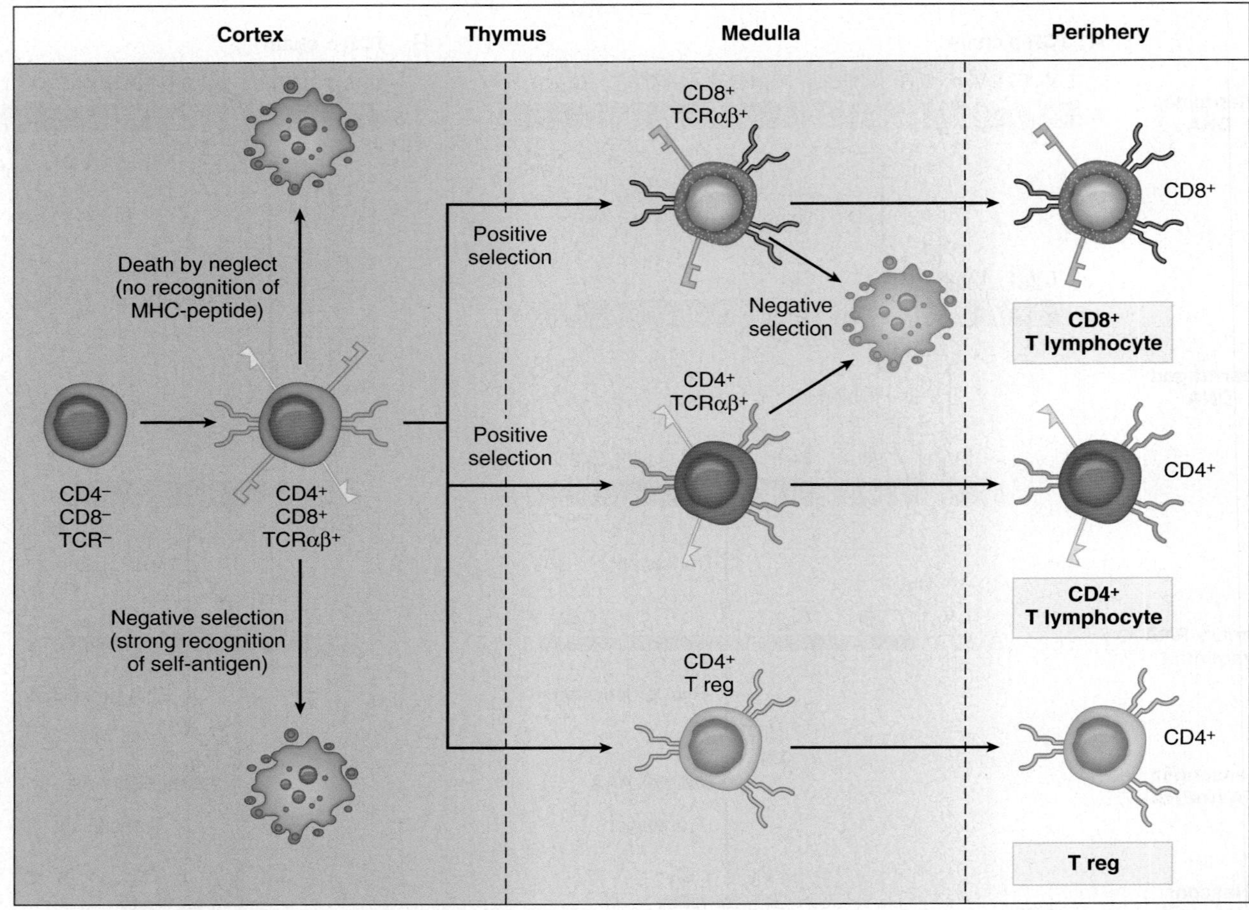

FIGURE 24-10 T Cell Maturation. Initially, T cell precursors arrive in the thymic cortex lacking CD4, CD8, or a TCR and are referred to as double negative. The genes responsible for expression of the TCR chains subsequently undergo a series of recombination events resulting in expression of either a γδ TCR or more commonly (>90%) an αβ TCR on the cell surface. The γδ T cells proceed through a distinct selection process that is independent of MHC restriction. The αβ T cells acquire expression of both CD4 and CD8 and are then referred to as double positive. They then proceed to undergo the process, both positive and negative selection, and ultimately express only CD4 or CD8, depending on which class of MHC they restrict to. (Adapted from Abbas AK, Lichtman AH, Pillai S: *Cellular and molecular immunology*, ed 8, Philadelphia, 2015, Saunders Elsevier.)

physically embedded on self cells, the system avoids constant activation by soluble molecules.

T cells can then specifically recognize and destroy cells that make peptide products of mutation or viral infection. Because the number of potential antigens is high and the likelihood is that self-antigens vary minimally from foreign antigens, the nature of the TCR-binding event has evolved such that a single interaction with an MHC molecule is not sufficient to cause activation. In fact, a T cell must register a signal from approximately 8000 TCR-ligand interactions with the same antigen before a threshold of activation is reached.[14] Each event results in the internalization of the TCR. Because resting T cells have low TCR density, sequential binding and internalization during several hours is required. Transient encounters are not sufficient. This threshold is reduced considerably by appropriate costimulation signals (detailed later).

Most TCRs are heterodimers composed of two transmembrane polypeptide chains, α and β. The αβ-TCR is noncovalently associated with several other transmembrane signaling proteins, including CD3 (composed of three separate chains, γ, δ, and ε) and ζ chain molecules as well as the appropriate accessory molecule from the T cell, either CD4 or CD8, which associates with its respective MHC molecule. Together these proteins are known as the TCR complex. When the TCR is bound to an MHC molecule and the proper configuration of accessory molecules stabilizes its binding, a signal is initiated by intracytoplasmic protein tyrosine kinases. These protein tyrosine kinases include p56lck (on CD4 or CD8), p59Fyn, and ZAP-70, the last two of which are associated with CD3. Repetitive binding signals combined with the appropriate costimulation eventually activate phospholipase-γ1, which in turn hydrolyzes the membrane lipid phosphatidylinositol bisphosphate, thereby releasing inositol trisphosphate and diacylglycerol. Inositol trisphosphate binds to the endoplasmic reticulum, causing a release of calcium that induces calmodulin to bind to and activate calcineurin. Calcineurin dephosphorylates the critical cytokine transcription factor nuclear factor of activated T cells (NFAT), prompting it, with the transcription factor nuclear factor κB (NF-κB), to initiate transcription of cytokines

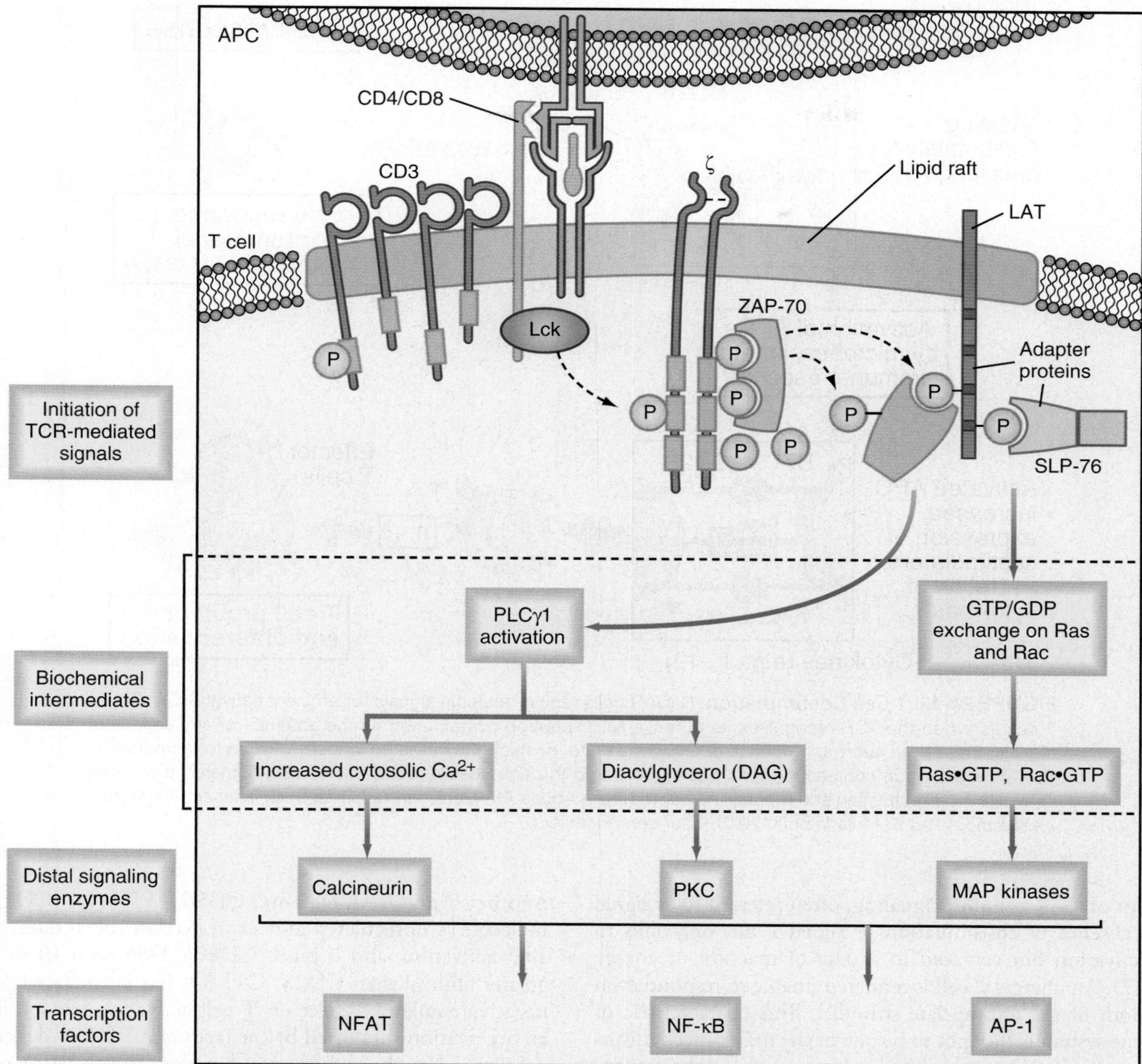

FIGURE 24-11 T Cell Activation. On antigen recognition, there is a clustering of TCR complexes and coreceptors that initiates a cascade of signaling events within the T cell. Tyrosine kinases associated with the coreceptors (e.g., Lck) phosphorylate CD3 and the ζ chain. The ζ chain association protein kinase (ZAP-70) subsequently associates with these regions and becomes activated. ZAP-70 phosphorylates various adaptor and coreceptor proteins, ultimately activating numerous cellular enzymes including calcineurin, PKC, and several MAP kinases. These enzymes then activate transcription factors that promote expression of various genes involved in proliferation and T cell responses. (Adapted from Abbas AK, Lichtman AH, Pillai S: *Cellular and molecular immunology*, ed 6, Philadelphia, 2010, Saunders Elsevier.)

including IL-2 and its receptor (Fig. 24-11). Resting T cells express only low levels of the IL-2 receptor (CD25), but with activation, IL-2R expression is increased. As the activated T cell begins to produce IL-2 secondary to events initiated by TCR activation, the cytokine begins to work in both autocrine and paracrine fashions, potentiating diacylglycerol activation of protein kinase C (PKC). PKC is important in activating many gene regulatory steps critical for cell division. This effect, however, is restricted only to T cells that have undergone activation after encountering their specific antigen leading to IL-2R expression. Thus, the process limits proliferation and expansion to only those clones specific for the offending antigen. As the antigenic stimulus is removed, IL-2R density decreases and the TCR complex is re-expressed on the cell surface. There is a negative feedback system between the TCR and the IL-2R resulting in a highly regulated and efficient system that is reactive only in the presence of antigen and ceases to function once antigen in removed. Many of these steps in T cell activation have been targeted in the development of immunosuppressive agents. These are discussed in detail in a subsequent section of this chapter.

Costimulation

Recognition of the antigenic peptide–MHC complex through TCR binding is usually not sufficient alone to generate a response in a naïve T cell. Additional signals through so-called costimulatory pathways are required for optimal T cell activation.[15,16] In

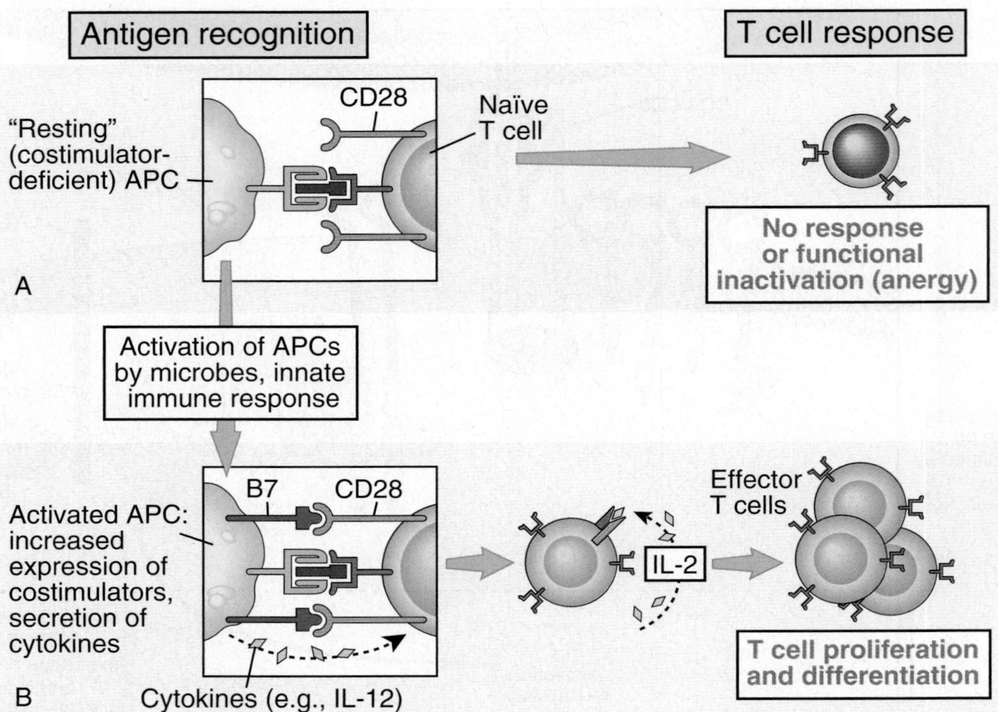

FIGURE 24-12 T Cell Costimulation. Naïve T cells require multiple signals for efficient activation. **A,** Signal 1 occurs when the TCR recognizes its putative MHC-peptide combination. In the absence of any additional signals, there is an aborted response or anergy, a state in which the cell is no longer available for stimulation. **B,** TCR signaling in conjunction with signals received through costimulatory molecules, signal 2, promotes effective T cell activation and function. (Adapted from Abbas AK, Lichtman AH, Pillai S: *Cellular and molecular immunology*, ed 6, Philadelphia, 2010, Saunders Elsevier.)

fact, receipt of TCR complex signaling, often referred to as signal 1, in the absence of costimulation or signal 2 not only fails to achieve activation but can lead to a state of inaction or anergy (Fig. 24-12). An anergic T cell is rendered unable to respond even if given both of the appropriate stimuli.[17] This characteristic of the immune system is thought to be one of the major mechanisms in tolerance to self-antigens in the periphery, crucial in the prevention of autoimmunity. Researchers have exploited this discovery using antibodies or receptor fusion proteins designed to block interactions between key costimulatory molecules at the time of antigen exposure. Much of the research to date has focused on the interactions of two costimulatory pathways, the CD28/B7 pathway (immunoglobulin-like superfamily members) and CD40/CD154 pathway (TNF/TNFR superfamily members). There have been, however, many additional pairings within these same families and others that have been found to have distinct roles in costimulatory function (Table 24-2).

CD28, present on T cells, and the B7 molecules CD80 and CD86 on APCs were among the first costimulatory molecules to be described. Ligation of CD28 is necessary for optimal IL-2 production and can lead to the production of additional cytokines, such as IL-4 and IL-8, and chemokines, such as RANTES, as well as protect T cells from activation-induced apoptosis through the upregulation of antiapoptotic factors such as Bcl-X_L and Bcl-2. CD28 is expressed constitutively on most T cells, whereas the expression of CD80 and CD86 is largely restricted to professional APCs, such as dendritic cells, monocytes, and macrophages. The kinetics of CD80/CD86 expression is complex, but they are typically increased with the induction of the immune response. Another ligand for CD80 and CD86 is CTLA-4 (CD152). This molecule is upregulated and expressed on the surface of T cells after activation, and it binds CD80/CD86 with 10 to 20 times greater affinity than CD28. CTLA-4 has been shown to have a negative regulatory effect on T cell activation and proliferation, an observation supported by the fact that CTLA-4–deficient mice develop a lymphoproliferative disorder. The negative regulatory effect of CTLA-4 is mediated through both cell intrinsic activation of intracellular phosphatases and a recently identified cell extrinsic mechanism in which CTLA-4 binding actually removes CD80/CD86 from the surface of the APC, thereby limiting the availability of ligands for CD28 costimulation. The therapeutic potential of costimulation blockade was first made apparent through the use of an engineered fusion protein composed of the extracellular portion of the CTLA-4 molecule and a portion of the human immunoglobulin (Ig) molecule. This compound binds CD80 and CD86 and prevents costimulation through CD28. Several clinical trials in autoimmunity have demonstrated the efficacy of CTLA-4–Ig (abatacept). More recently, a higher affinity, second-generation version, LEA29Y (belatacept), has been tested with success as a replacement for calcineurin inhibitors and was approved in 2011 for kidney transplant recipients.[18]

Closely related to the CD28/B7 pathway is the CD40/CD154 (CD40L) pathway. Evidence for the crucial role of the CD40/CD154 pathway in the immune response came to light after the observation that hyper-IgM syndrome results from a mutational defect in the gene encoding CD154. In addition to defects in the generation of T cell–dependent antibody responses, patients with hyper-IgM syndrome also have defects in T cell–mediated immune

TABLE 24-2 Costimulatory Molecules

RECEPTOR	DISTRIBUTION	LIGAND	DISTRIBUTION	PRINCIPAL EFFECTS AND FUNCTIONS
CD28	T cells	CD80/CD86	Activated APCs	Lowers the threshold for T cell activation Promotes survival, ↑ antiapoptotic factors Promotes Th1 phenotype
CD40	Dendritic cells, B cells, macrophages, endothelial cells	CD154	T cells, soluble platelets	Induces CD80/CD86 expression on APCs
CD27	T cells, NK cells, B cells	CD70	Thymic epithelium, activated T cells, activated B cells, mature dendritic cells	Enhances T cell proliferation and survival Acts after CD28 to sustain effector T cell survival Influences secondary responses more than primary Promotes B cell differentiation and memory formation
CD30	Activated T cells, activated B cells	CD153	B cells, activated T cells	Maintains survival of primed and memory T cells Promotes Th2 > Th1
CD95 (Fas)	T cells, B cells, APCs, stromal cells	CD178 (FasL)	T cells, APCs, stromal cells	Involved in peripheral T cell homeostasis through "fratricide," may deliver costimulatory signal
CD134 (OX40)	Activated T cells $CD4^+ > CD8^+$	CD252 (OX40L)	Activated T cells, mature dendritic cells, activated B cells	Important for $CD4^+$ T cell expansion and survival ↑ Antiapoptotic factors Functions after CD28 to sustain $CD4^+$ T cell survival Enhances cytokine production Augments effector and memory $CD4^+$ T cell function Promotes Th2 > Th1
CD137 (4-1BB)	Activated T cells $CD8^+ > CD4^+$ Monocytes, follicular dendritic cells, NK cells	4-1BBL	Mature dendritic cells, activated B cells, activated macrophages	Sustains rather than initiates $CD8^+$ T cell responses Functions after CD28 to sustain T cell survival Important in antiviral immunity Promotes $CD8^+$ effector function and cell survival
CD152 (CTLA-4)	Activated T cells	CD80/CD86	Activated APCs	Higher affinity for CD80/CD86 than CD28, inhibits T cell response
HVEM	T cells, monocytes, immature dendritic cells	CD258 (LIGHT)	Activated lymphocytes, immature dendritic cells, NK cells	Augments T cell responses, $CD8^+ > CD4^+$ Promotes dendritic cell maturation
		CD272 (BTLA)	Activated T cells, B cells, dendritic cells	Negative costimulator, inhibits IL-2 production BTLA remains expressed on Th1 but not Th2
		CD160	NK cells, cytolytic $CD8^+$ T cells, γδ T cells	Negative regulator of $CD4^+$ T cell activation Inhibits proliferation and cytokine production
CD265 (RANK)	Dendritic cells	CD254 (TRANCE)	Activated T cells $CD4^+ > CD8^+$	Enhances dendritic cell survival, upregulates Bcl-xl, (?) enhances IFN-γ production
CD279 (PD-1)	T cells	CD274 (PD-L1)	T cells, B cells, APCs, some parenchymal cells	Inhibits activation, proliferation, and acquisition of effector cell function Th1 > Th2
		CD273 (PD-L2)	Dendritic cells, macrophages	Inhibits activation, proliferation, and acquisition of effector cell function Th2 > Th1
CD278 (ICOS)	Activated T cells, memory T cells	CD275 (ICOSL)	Dendritic cells, B cells, macrophages	Promotes survival and expansion of effector T cells, (?) promotes Th2 responses
GITR	Treg cells, $CD8^+$ T cells, B cells, macrophages	GITRL	B cells, dendritic cells, macrophages, endothelial cells	Marker for Treg cells, allows proliferation of Tregs Promotes T cell proliferation and cytokine production Negative regulator for NK function

responses. CD40 is a cell surface molecule expressed on endothelium, B cells, dendritic cells, and other APCs. Its ligand, CD154, is primarily found on activated T cells. Upregulation of CD154 after TCR signaling allows signals to be sent to the APC through CD40; in particular, it is a critical signal for B cell activation and proliferation. CD40 binding is required for APCs to stimulate a cytotoxic T cell response. It leads to the release of activating cytokines, particularly IL-12, and the upregulation of B7 molecules. It also initiates innate functions of APCs, including nitric oxide synthesis and phagocytosis. Interestingly, CD154 is also released in soluble form by activated platelets. Thus, sites of trauma that attract activated platelets simultaneously recruit the ligand required to activate tissue-based APCs, providing a link between innate and acquired immunity. Antibody preparations to CD154 have shown great promise in experimental models, but clinical trials were halted because of concern for unexpected thrombotic complications. There continues to be hope that anti-CD154 antibodies that bind distinct epitopes or antibodies directed toward CD40 may circumvent this issue.

Since earlier investigations, multiple other pairings of molecules have been characterized and shown to demonstrate costimulatory or coinhibitory activity. It is the sum of these positive costimulatory and negative coinhibitory signals that shapes the character and magnitude of the T cell response.[19] CD278 (inducible costimulator or ICOS) is a CD28 superfamily expressed on activated T cells, and its ligand, CD275 (ICOSL or B7-H2), is expressed on APCs. Unlike CD28, ICOS is not present on naïve T cells, but instead expression is upregulated after T cell activation and persists on memory T cells. ICOS can function to boost activation of effector T cells in general but in particular plays a critical role in the function of follicular helper T cells (Tfh), a specialized CD4$^+$ T cell subset involved in the germinal center reaction and generation of class-switched antibody. Another member of the CD28 superfamily, PD-1 (CD279), and its ligands PD-L1 (CD274) and PD-L2 (CD273), both B7 family members, have been shown to be involved in negative regulation of cellular immunity. More recently, coinhibitory molecules PD-1H (also known as VISTA) and BTLA have joined this list. Several members of the TNF/TNFR superfamily have been shown to play important roles in T cell costimulation. These include CD134/CD252 (OX40/OX40L), CD137/CD137L (4-1BB/4-1BBL), CD27/CD70, CD95/CD178 (Fas/FasL), CD30/CD153, RANK/TRANCE, and others. Furthermore, members of the CD2 family function in both costimulatory (i.e., CD2) and coinhibitory (i.e., 2B4) roles during the execution of an alloimmune response. Finally, the T cell–immunoglobulin mucin-like (TIM) family of molecules have been shown to play important coinhibitory roles during alloimmunity, both on effector cells and on Tregs.

In addition to the multitude of costimulatory molecules, many other adhesion molecules expressed on the cell surface (intercellular adhesion molecule, selectins, integrins) control the movement of immune cells through the body, regulate their trafficking to specific areas of inflammation, and nonspecifically strengthen the TCR-MHC binding interaction. They differ from costimulation molecules in that they enhance the interaction of the T cell with its antigen without influencing the quality of the TCR response. There are two main families of cellular adhesion molecules within the immune system: the selectins and the integrins. The selectin family of adhesion molecules is responsible for "rolling," the initial attachment of leukocytes to vascular endothelial cells at sites of tissue injury and inflammation before their firm adhesion (mediated by integrin binding). The selectin family of proteins is composed of three closely related molecules, each having differential expression on immune cells: L-selectin is expressed on leukocytes, P-selectin is expressed on platelets, and E-selectin is expressed on endothelium. Structurally, all selectins share an amino-terminal lectin domain that interacts with a carbohydrate ligand, an epidermal growth factor–like domain, and two to nine short repeating units that share homology with sequences found in some complement-binding proteins. In contrast to most other adhesion molecules that also possess some signaling or costimulatory functionality, selectins function solely to facilitate leukocyte binding to vascular endothelium. This selectin-mediated loose binding is converted into tight adhesion after activation of leukocyte integrins. Integrins are transmembrane receptors that serve as bridges for cell-cell as well as for cell–extracellular matrix interactions. Many are expressed constitutively on cells of the immune system (i.e., leukocyte function antigen 1) but on sensing inflammatory cytokine or chemokine signals, such as IL-8, are induced to change conformation that results in higher avidity interaction with integrin ligands, resulting in leukocyte extravasation into inflamed tissue. Both selectins and integrins are potential therapeutic targets to inhibit access of donor-reactive T cells into the allograft.

T Cell Effector Functions

During thymic education, most T cells initially express both CD4 and CD8 molecules, but subsequently T cells become either CD4$^+$ or CD8$^+$, depending on which MHC class they restrict to. Thus, these accessory molecules govern which type of MHC and by extension which types of cells a given T cell can interact with and evaluate. Because there is nearly ubiquitous expression of class I MHC, all cell types are surveyed. These class I molecules display peptides that are generated within the cell (e.g., peptides from normal cellular processes or from internal viral replication). T cells responsible for inspecting all cells express the accessory molecule CD8, which in turn binds to class I and specifically stabilizes a TCR interaction with a class I–presented antigen. Thus, CD8$^+$ T cells evaluate most cell types and mediate destruction of altered cells. Appropriately, they have been termed cytotoxic T cells.

APCs are the predominant cell type that expresses class II MHC molecules in addition to class I. Class II molecules display peptides that have been sampled from surrounding extracellular spaces through phagocytosis and thus usually represent the presentation of newly acquired antigen. Cells initiating an immune response need to have access to this newly processed antigen. CD4 binds class II MHC and stabilizes the interaction of the TCR with the class II–peptide complex. Thus, under physiologic conditions, CD4$^+$ T cells are first alerted to an invasion of the body by hematopoietically derived APCs that present their newly acquired antigen in the form of processed peptide in a class II molecule. As a consequence of their MHC restriction, these subpopulations of T cells have several different functions. CD4$^+$ T cells typically contribute to the response in a helper or regulatory role, whereas CD8$^+$ T cells are much more likely to play a part in cell elimination through cytotoxic functions.

After activation, CD4$^+$ T cells initially play a critical role in the expansion of the immune response. After encountering an APC that expresses the specific antigenic peptide–MHC II pairing, the CD4$^+$ T cell can then signal back to the APC to promote factors that allow CD8$^+$ T cell activation. This process is accomplished by expression of specific costimulatory molecules and the release of certain cytokines. This licensing of CD8$^+$ T cells for cytotoxic function is a key step within the immune response. This describes in part how CD4$^+$ T cells become helper cells. More recently, there has been further elucidation of their cellular differentiation into several well-defined T helper (Th) subsets, including Th1, Th2, Th17, and Tfh cells, which are largely defined on the basis of the distinct transcription factors they express and the cytokines they elaborate (Fig. 24-13). The main cytokine driving the differentiation of Th1 cells is IL-12, and mature Th1 cells mediate effector function through the release of IFN-γ and TNF. The predominant role of IFN-γ is to enhance macrophage function and activity as well as to promote cell-mediated immunity. Activated macrophages then proceed to ingest and to kill invading microbes, and at the same time the acquired immune system is directed to produce antibodies that promote opsonization, thereby enhancing the overall process. Th2 cell differentiation, in contrast, is driven by the presence of IL-4 and results in release of IL-4, IL-5, IL-10, and IL-13, which ultimately inhibit macrophage activation and promote IgE production and eosinophil activation. Th17 cells are an inflammatory CD4$^+$ subset that plays a major role in the protective immune response against fungal pathogens and extracellular bacteria. Th17 cells are generated in the presence of transforming growth factor-β (TGF-β) and IL-6 and are potent secretors of the inflammatory cytokines IL-17 and IL-23. Interestingly, in

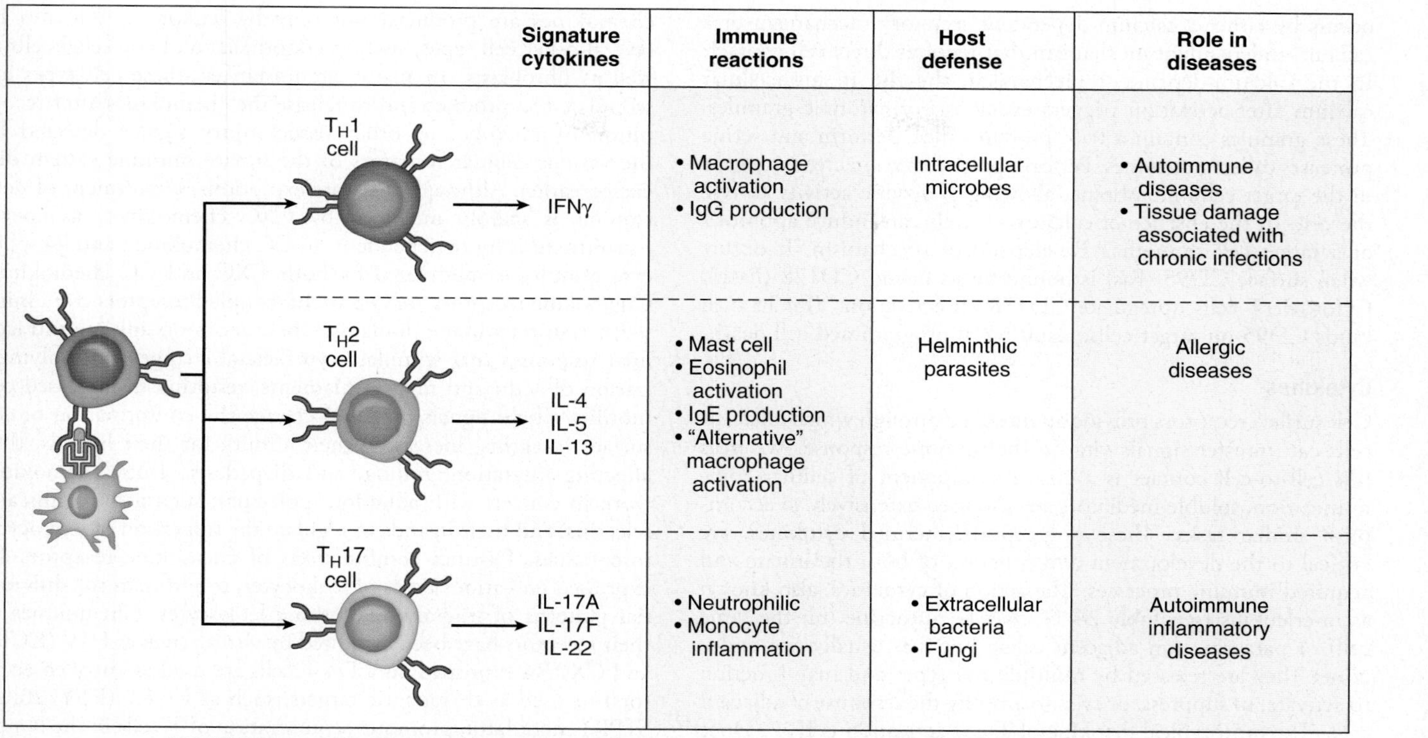

	Signature cytokines	Immune reactions	Host defense	Role in diseases
T_H1 cell	IFNγ	• Macrophage activation • IgG production	Intracellular microbes	• Autoimmune diseases • Tissue damage associated with chronic infections
T_H2 cell	IL-4 IL-5 IL-13	• Mast cell • Eosinophil activation • IgE production • "Alternative" macrophage activation	Helminthic parasites	Allergic diseases
T_H17 cell	IL-17A IL-17F IL-22	• Neutrophilic • Monocyte inflammation	• Extracellular bacteria • Fungi	Autoimmune inflammatory diseases

FIGURE 24-13 T Cell Subsets. Naïve CD4$^+$ T cells may differentiate into distinct subsets of effector cells in response to antigen, costimulatory or coinhibitory signals, and cytokines. Th1 cells produce IFN-γ, which activates macrophages to kill intracellular microbes. Th2 cells produce cytokines (IL-4, IL-5, and others) that stimulate IgE production and activate eosinophils in response to parasitic infection. Th17 cells secrete IL-17 and IL-22; they play an important role in responses to fungi and contribute to several autoimmune inflammatory diseases. (Adapted from Abbas AK, Lichtman AH, Pillai S: *Cellular and molecular immunology*, ed 8, Philadelphia, 2015, Saunders Elsevier.)

addition to their role in protective immunity, Th17 cells have been associated with several autoimmune diseases, including multiple sclerosis, rheumatoid arthritis, and psoriasis, and several immunomodulatory therapies are being developed to impair their activity in these patients. Finally, Tfh cells are ICOS$^+$ PD-1$^+$ cells that home to lymphoid germinal centers by virtue of their expression of the chemokine receptor CXCR5, where they provide help for the generation of class-switched, high-affinity IgG responses. Tfh cells provide this help in the form of CD154 expression and the secretion of IL-21.

An important feature of these CD4$^+$ Th cells is the ability of one subset to regulate the activity of the other. For example, IL-10 produced by Th2 cells and Tregs negatively regulates transcription of IFN-γ mRNA. Thus, the initial steps in differentiation depend greatly on the surrounding immunologic milieu, which ultimately influences the character of the immune response. Furthermore, more recent fate mapping studies have revealed a high degree of plasticity between Th subsets, demonstrating that cells of one Th subset can under certain conditions transdifferentiate into another Th subset.

Another subset of CD4$^+$ T cells that has been described to play a critical role in the ability of the immune system to temper its response is the Treg population. Tregs suppress immune responses either through direct cell-cell contact with effector cells or indirectly through their interaction with APCs. These cells not only have the ability to suppress cytokines, adhesion molecules, and costimulatory signals but are also able to focus this response by expression of integrins, which allow Tregs to home to the location of immune engagement. The most extensively studied population of Tregs are those CD4$^+$ T cells that express CD25 (the high-affinity α chain of the IL-2 receptor).[20] CD4$^+$CD25$^+$ cells express the transcription factor Foxp3, a protein that has been shown to be both necessary and sufficient for the differentiation of CD4$^+$ T cells into Tregs. Indeed, both mice and humans that lack functional Foxp3 molecule develop severe systemic autoimmunity. Thus, CD4$^+$CD25$^+$ Foxp3$^+$ T cells have been the target of numerous attempts to alter immune function and are being tested in clinical trials of cellular immunotherapy to control graft rejection after transplantation and to mitigate autoimmunity. Foxp3$^+$ Tregs develop during T cell thymic development after recognition of self-antigen in the thymus (with signal strength that is not sufficient to induce negative selection). These so-called natural Tregs (also termed thymic Tregs) express a TCR repertoire distinct from that of conventional T cells and are important for maintaining immune homeostasis and preventing autoimmunity. However, Foxp3$^+$ Tregs can also develop extrathymically during the course of an immune response, and studies have shown that these cells are elicited by stimulation with low-dose antigen or under conditions of limited CD154 costimulation. These so-called induced Tregs (also termed peripheral Tregs) are highly specific for the antigen by which they were elicited and thus may be more potent suppressors of autoimmunity and transplant rejection when used as cellular immunotherapy.

Unlike CD4$^+$ T cells, CD8$^+$ T cells function primarily to eliminate infected or defective cells. As mentioned before, licensing occurs through APC interactions, and subsequent cell killing occurs by either a calcium-dependent secretory mechanism or a calcium-independent mechanism that requires direct cell contact. In the calcium-dependent mechanism, the rise in intracellular calcium after activation triggers exocytosis of cytolytic granules. These granules contain a lytic protein called perforin and serine proteases called granzymes. Perforin polymerization creates defects in the target cell's membrane, allowing granzyme activity to lyse the cell. In the absence of calcium, T cells can induce apoptosis of a target cell through a Fas-dependent mechanism. It occurs when surface CD95 (Fas) is bound by its ligand CD178 (FasL). Cytotoxic T cells upregulate CD178 on activation. This in turn binds CD95 on target cells, resulting in programmed cell death.

Cytokines

Cell surface receptors provide an interface through which adjacent cells can transfer signals vital to the immune response. Whereas this cell-to-cell contact is a critical component of cellular communication, soluble mediators are also used extensively to accomplish similar tasks. These polypeptides, termed cytokines, are critical to the development and function of both the innate and acquired immune processes. The action of cytokines, also known as interleukins (see Table 24-1), may be autocrine (on the same cell) or paracrine (on adjacent cells), but it is usually not endocrine. They are released by multiple cell types and may function to activate, to suppress, or even to amplify the response of adjacent cells. The prototypical cytokine of T cell activation is IL-2. Once a given T cell encounters its specific antigen in the setting of appropriate costimulation, it will subsequently produce and release IL-2 as well as other cytokines that will influence any cell within its vicinity. As mentioned before, Th cellular subsets are differentiated on the basis of the pattern of cytokine expression. Th1 cells, which mediate cytotoxic responses such as delayed-type hypersensitivity, express IL-2, IL-12, IL-15, and IFN-γ. Th2 cells support the development of humoral or eosinophilic responses and consequently express IL-4, IL-5, IL-10, and IL-13. Th17 cells, a more recently described subset, are distinguished by their production of IL-17, IL-21, and IL-22.

Cytokine receptors are now known to function through Janus kinase (JAK) signal transduction proteins. They convey signals to signal transducers and activators of transcriptions (STATs), DNA-binding proteins that translocate to the nucleus to influence gene transcription. As is the case with most of the immune response, this pathway is tightly regulated. For example, suppressors of cytokine signaling (SOCS) proteins act in a negative feedback loop to inhibit STAT phosphorylation by binding and inhibiting JAKs or competing with STATs for phosphotyrosine-binding sites on cytokine receptors. There is evidence emerging for the involvement of SOCS proteins in human disease, which raises the possibility that therapeutic strategies based on the manipulation of SOCS activity might be of clinical benefit.

One particular subset of cytokines are termed chemokines for their ability to influence movement of leukocytes and to regulate their migration to and from secondary lymphoid organs, blood, and tissues. Chemokines, or chemotactic cytokines, are a unique set of cytokines that are structurally homologous, 8- to 10-kDa polypeptides that have a varying number of cysteine residues in conserved locations that are key to forming their three-dimensional shape. The two major families are CC chemokines (also called β), in which the two defining cysteine residues are adjacent, and the CXC (or α) family, in which these residues are separated by one amino acid. There are numerous CC (1-28) and CXC (1-16) chemokines with various targets and functions. The CC and CXC chemokines are produced not only by leukocytes but also by several other cell types, such as endothelial and epithelial cells as well as fibroblasts. In many circumstances, these cell types are stimulated to produce and to release the chemokines after recognition of microbes or other tissue injury signals detected by the various cellular receptors of the innate immune system discussed earlier. Although there are exceptions, recruitment of neutrophils is mainly mediated by CXC chemokines, monocyte recruitment is more dependent on CC chemokines, and lymphocyte homing is modulated by both CXC and CC chemokines. Chemokine receptors are G protein–coupled receptors containing seven transmembrane domains. These receptors initiate intracellular responses that stimulate cytoskeletal changes and polymerization of actin and myosin filaments, resulting in increased cell motility. These signals may also change the conformation of cell surface integrins, increasing their affinity for their ligands, thus affecting migration, rolling, and diapedesis. Thus, chemokines work in concert with adhesion molecules, such as integrins and selectins, and their ligands to regulate the migration of leukocytes into tissues. Distinct combinations of chemokine receptors are expressed on various types of leukocytes, resulting in the differential patterns of migrations of those leukocytes. Chemokines or their receptors have been exploited by viruses such as HIV (CCR5 and CXCR4 expressed on CD4 T cells are used as entry coreceptors) or used as therapeutic targets, such as CCR7 (FTY720, an S1PR1 modulator, promotes sequestration of T cells in the lymph node through a CCR7-dependent mechanism; see later). In addition to cytokines, there are a host of other soluble, small-molecule mediators that are released during an immune response or with other types of inflammation. These function to increase blood flow to the area and to improve the exposure of the area to lymphocytes and the innate immune system.

B Cells

The primary lymphoid organ responsible for B cell differentiation is the bone marrow. Similar to all other cells in the immune system, B cells are derived from pluripotent bone marrow stem cells. IL-7, produced by bone marrow stromal cells, is a growth factor for pre-B cells. IL-4, IL-5, and IL-6 are cytokines that stimulate the maturation and proliferation of mature primed B cells. The principal function of B cells is to produce antibodies against foreign antigens (i.e., the humoral immune response) as well as to be involved in antigen presentation. B cell development occurs through several stages, each stage representing a change in the genomic content at the antibody loci. During the differentiation process, there is an elegant series of nucleotide rearrangements that results in a nearly unlimited array of specificities, allowing a diverse recognition repertoire.

B cell receptor or antibody. Similar to the T cell and its receptor, each B cell has a unique membrane-bound receptor through which it recognizes specific antigen. In the case of the B cell, this immunoglobulin molecule may also be produced in a secreted form that can interact with the extracellular environment far from its cellular origin. Each mature B cell produces antibody of a single specificity.

Each antibody is composed of two heavy chains and two light chains. Five different heavy chain loci (μ, γ,α, ε, and δ) are found on chromosome 14 and two light chain loci (κand λ) are located on chromosome 2. Each chain is composed of V, D, J, and C regions, which are brought together randomly by the RAG1 and RAG2 complex to form a functional antigen receptor. Immunoglobulin has a basic structure of four chains, two of which are

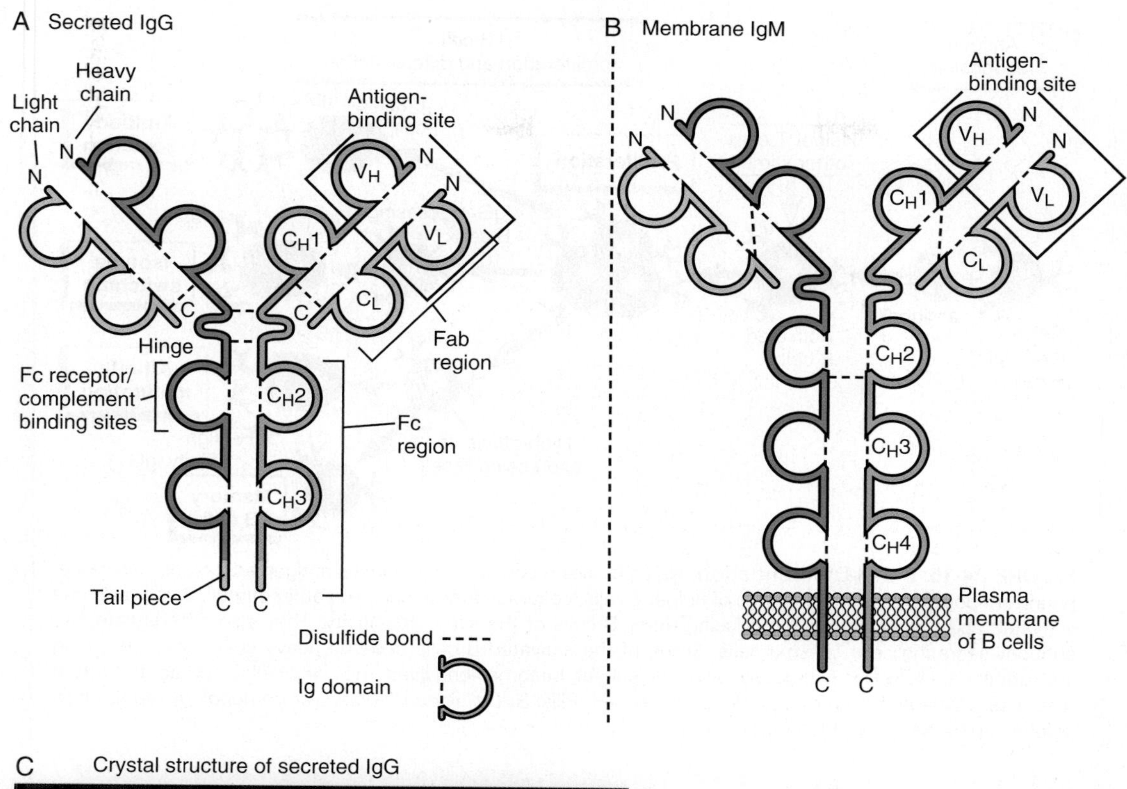

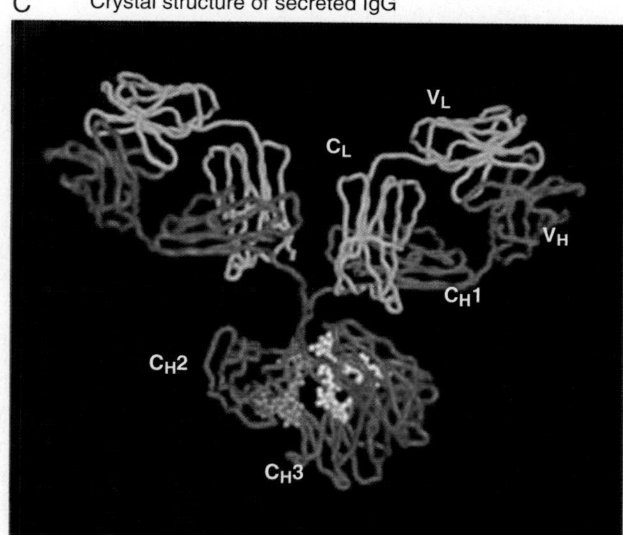

FIGURE 24-14 Structure of Immunoglobulin. A, Representation of secreted IgG molecule. The antigen-binding regions are formed by the variable regions of both light (V_L) and heavy (V_H) chains. The constant region of the heavy chain (C_H) is responsible for the Fc receptor and complement-binding sites. **B,** Schematic diagram of membrane-bound IgM. The membrane form of the antibody has C-terminal transmembrane and cytoplasmic portions that anchor the molecule in the plasma membrane. **C,** X-ray crystallography representation of IgG molecule. Heavy chains are colored *blue* and *red*, light chains are colored *green*, and carbohydrates are shown in *gray*. (Adapted from Abbas AK, Lichtman AH, Pillai S: *Cellular and molecular immunology*, ed 6, Philadelphia, 2010, Saunders Elsevier.)

identical heavy chains and two of which are identical light chains (Fig. 24-14). Both heavy and light chains have a constant region as well as a variable, antigen-binding region. The antigen-binding site is composed of both the heavy and light chain variable regions. The ability of antibody to neutralize microbes is entirely a function of this antigen-binding region.

In humans, there are nine different immunoglobulin subclasses or isotypes: IgM, IgD, IgG1, IgG2, IgG3, IgG4, IgA1, IgA2, and IgE. Heavy chain use defines the subtype of any given antibody. Whereas the variable regions are involved in antigen binding, the constant regions have functionality as well. The fragment crystallizable region or Fc region is in the tail portion composed of the

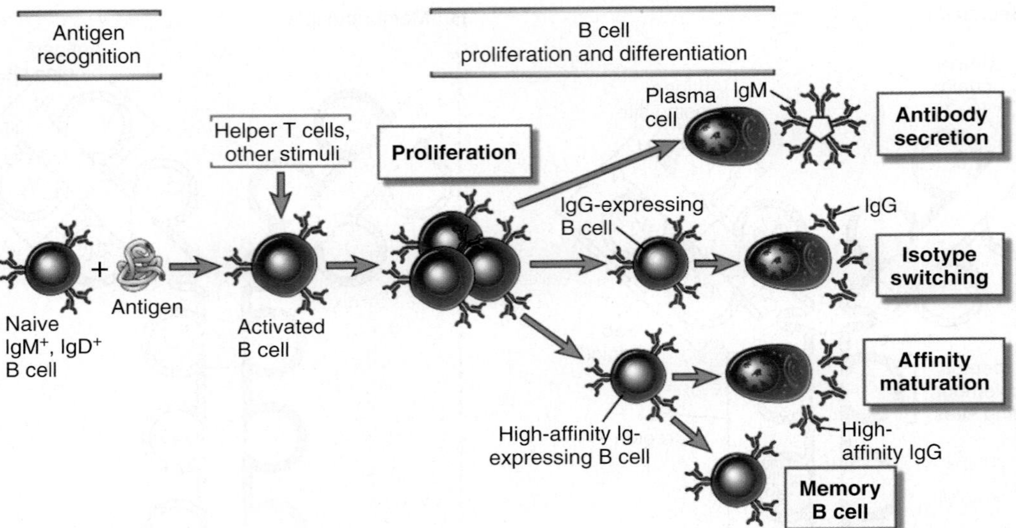

FIGURE 24-15 **B Cell Differentiation.** Naïve B cells recognize their specific antigen as it binds to surface-bound antibody. Under the influence of helper T cells, costimulatory signals, and other stimuli, B cells become activated and clonally expand, producing many B cells of the same specificity. They also differentiate into antibody-secreting cells, plasma cells. Some of the activated B cells undergo heavy chain class switching and affinity maturation. Ultimately, a small subset become long-lived memory cells, primed for future responses. (Adapted from Abbas AK, Lichtman AH, Pillai S: *Cellular and molecular immunology*, ed 8, Philadelphia, 2015, Saunders Elsevier.)

two heavy chain constant regions. It interacts with Fc receptors on phagocytic cells of the innate immune system to facilitate opsonization and subsequent destruction of the antigen to which the antibody is bound as well as facilitating antigenic peptide processing. The Fc portion of IgM and some classes of IgG also serves to activate complement. Distinct immune effector functions are assigned to each isotype. IgM and IgG antibodies provide a pivotal role in the endogenous or intravascular immune response. IgA is primarily responsible for mucosal immunity and is largely confined to the gastrointestinal and respiratory tracts. Resting B cells that have not yet been exposed to antigen express IgD and IgM on their cell surface. After interaction with antigen, the first isotype produced is IgM, which is efficient at binding complement to facilitate phagocytosis or cell lysis. Further activation and differentiation of the B cell occur after interactions with $CD4^+$ T cells. B cells undergo isotype switching, which results in a decrease in IgM titer with a concomitant rise in IgG titer. Unlike the TCR, the immunoglobulin loci undergo continued alteration after B cell stimulation to improve the affinity and functionality of the secreted antibody. A primed B cell may undergo further mutation within the variable regions that leads to increased affinity of antibody, termed somatic hypermutation. Such B cells are retained to provide the ability to generate a more vigorous response if the antigen happens to be re-encountered (Fig. 24-15).

B cell activation. When antigen is bound by two surface antibodies (or a multimeric form of antibody), the antibodies are brought together on the cell surface in a process known as cross linking. This is the event that stimulates B cell activation, proliferation, and differentiation into a plasma cell (antibody-producing cell). As for the T cell, the threshold for B cell activation is high. This can be lowered 100-fold by costimulatory signals received by the transmembrane complex CD19-CD21. B cells can also internalize antigens bound to surface antibodies and process them for presentation to T cells, thus participating in antigen presentation.

As discussed earlier, B cells may provide and receive certain costimulatory signals. For example, B cells express CD40 and when bound by CD154 expressed on activated T cells, the result is upregulation of B7 molecules on the B cell and delivery of important costimulatory signals to T cells as well.

Plasma cells (activated B cells) are distinguished histologically by their hypertrophied Golgi apparatus. They secrete large amounts of monoclonal (single specificity) antibody.

In addition to being secreted after exposure to an antigen, antibody can be present as part of a natural repertoire in circulation for initial response to common pathogens. Antigen exposure generally leads to B cell affinity maturation and isotype switching and produces high-affinity IgG antibodies. Naturally occurring antibodies, however, are generally IgM antibodies with low affinity and are generally thought to respond to a broad array of carbohydrate epitopes found on many common bacterial pathogens. Natural antibody is responsible for ABO blood group antigen responses and discordant xenograft rejection (see "Xenotransplantation").

This portion of the chapter has summarized the general response of the immune system to an infectious challenge. The next sections address the unique situation of the immune response to transplanted tissue and organs.

TRANSPLANT IMMUNITY

The study of modern transplant immunology is traditionally attributed to the experiments of Sir Peter Medawar, fueled by attempts to use skin transplantation as a treatment for burned aviators during World War II. While monitoring the victims with autologous (syngeneic) and homologous (allogeneic) skin grafts, he noted that not only did all allogeneic grafts universally fail promptly, but also secondary grafts from the same donor were rejected even more vigorously, suggesting immune involvement. He pursued this hypothesis with extensive experiments in rabbits, wherein he confirmed his previous observation and noted the presence of a heavy lymphocyte infiltrate in the rejecting graft. It was N. A. Mitchison, working in the early 1950s, who definitively identified a role for lymphocytes in the rejection of foreign tissue. Subsequent studies in tumor immunology as well as work by Snell using strains of genetically identical mice identified the genetic basis for graft rejection as the MHC, known in humans as HLA and in mice as the H-2 locus. These series of experiments during a short period of several years demonstrated that rejection of transplanted tissue was an immunologic process, implicated lymphocytes as the principal effector cells, and identified the MHC as the primary source of antigen in the rejection response. These pivotal studies laid the groundwork for the transition of transplantation from the experimental to the clinical realm.

Whereas the technical skill for the transplantation of skin and other organs had been available for some time, the vigorous rejection of allografts had prevented its widespread use for many years. It was not until 1954, after Medawar's critical studies had been published, that the first successful organ transplantation was performed. Despite Medawar's claim that the "biological force" responsible for rejection would "forever inhibit transplantation from one individual to another," Joseph Murray, a surgeon-scientist, persevered in his pursuit of making clinical transplantation a reality. At the time, there was evidence to suggest that the overall immunologic barrier was lacking between identical twins, and coincidentally Murray was busily perfecting a surgical technique for kidney transplantation in dogs. In 1954, the opportunity presented itself to test the hypothesis. Richard Herrick, who had incurable kidney damage, was the first candidate, and his identical sibling, Ronald, was willing to donate a kidney for transplantation to his brother. Murray confirmed the lack of immunologic reactivity between the two brothers by first placing skin grafts from each twin onto the other. Once he confirmed the lack of a response, he used the technique that he had perfected in the canine model, performing the first successful kidney transplant between identical twins in December 1954.[4] The operation proceeded without complication, and the kidney functioned well without the need for immunosuppression. Despite this landmark advance in transplantation, the majority of individuals in need of a transplant did not have an identical twin to donate an organ. Thereafter, the focus of the field was appropriately directed toward the development of methods to control the rejection response.

During the 1950s and 1960s, several discoveries were made that were of the utmost importance for future successes in transplantation. Following Gorer and Snell's description of the murine MHC system, Jean Dausset described the equivalent in humans using antibodies developed against HLA. This led to the first serologically based typing system for human transplant antigens. Snell and Dausset shared the Nobel Prize in 1980 for their observations.

In the late 1960s, Paul Terasaki reported on the significance of preformed antibody directed against donor MHC molecules and its impact on kidney graft survival. He developed the microlymphocyte cytotoxicity test, allowing pretransplantation detection of recipient-derived antidonor antibody. This formed the basis for the crossmatch assay that is used today to screen potential donor-recipient pairings. These techniques along with the development of new immunosuppressive compounds including 6-mercaptopurine and azathioprine led to the first successful kidney transplantation between relatives who were not identical twins and also to the first successful transplant using a kidney from a deceased donor.

Although early attempts at immunosuppression permitted extended allograft survival in selected patients, both the reproducibility and durability of results were far from adequate. In the 1970s, investigators sought novel treatments to improve the success rate for transplantation; these modalities included thoracic duct drainage and the use of antilymphocyte serum. Despite these efforts, the results for kidney transplantation remained poor, with the best centers achieving 1-year survival rates of 70% for living related kidney grafts and 50% for deceased donor kidney transplants. Then, a chance discovery of a promising agent from a fungal isolate dramatically changed the outlook for kidney and other types of transplantation. Jean-François Borel identified an active metabolite, cyclosporine (CsA), that showed selective in vitro inhibition of lymphocyte cultures but no significant myelotoxic effects. Promising results in dogs eventually led to clinical trials in humans, and the modern era of transplantation had begun.

The introduction of CsA ushered in the most dramatic improvement in the field of transplantation. Liver and heart transplant survival rates doubled, and the improved immunosuppression encouraged transplant teams around the world to begin broader investigational use, transplanting lung, small bowel, and pancreas. Now, with the use of CsA and newer agents, 1-year graft survival has exceeded 90% for virtually all organs except the small intestine. Despite the discovery and clinical introduction of ever increasingly potent immunosuppressants, the field of transplantation has many areas in need of improvement. Drug-related side effects and the intractable problem of chronic rejection still plague practitioners. The focus of the current research is the development of a clinically applicable strategy to promote "transplantation tolerance," thereby eliminating the pitfalls and shortcomings of current immunosuppressive therapy.

REJECTION

There are three classic histopathologic definitions of allograft rejection that are based on not only the predominant mediator but also the timing of the process (Fig. 24-16).

1. Hyperacute rejection occurs within minutes to days after transplantation and is primarily mediated by preformed antibody.
2. Acute rejection is a process mediated by T cells (although it is often accompanied by an acquired antibody response) and generally occurs within the first few weeks to months of transplantation but can occur at any time.
3. Chronic rejection is the most common cause of long-term allograft loss and is an indolent fibrotic process that occurs during months to years. It is thought to be secondary to both T and B cell processes including donor-specific antibody but is difficult to completely separate from nonimmune mechanisms of chronic organ damage (e.g., drug toxicity and cardiovascular comorbid diseases).

Hyperacute Rejection

Although essentially untreatable, hyperacute rejection is nearly universally preventable with the proper use of the lymphocytotoxic crossmatch or other means of detecting donor-specific antibodies before transplantation. This form of rejection occurs when donor-specific antibodies are present in the recipient's system before transplantation. These antibodies may be the result of

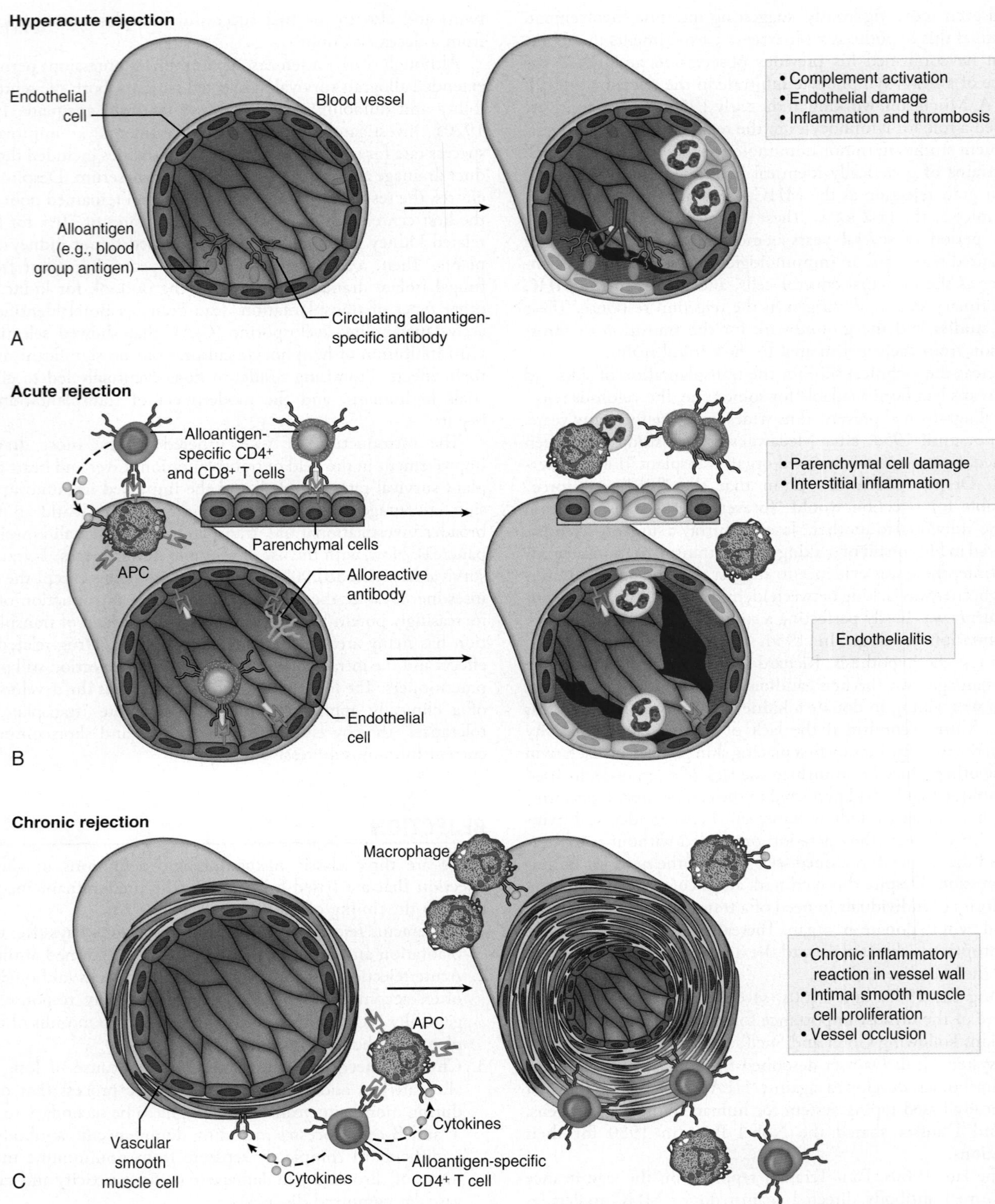

FIGURE 24-16 Mechanisms of Rejection. A, Hyperacute rejection occurs when preformed antibodies react with donor antigens on the vascular endothelium of the graft. Subsequent complement activation triggers rapid intravascular thrombosis and graft necrosis. **B,** Acute rejection is predominantly mediated by a cellular infiltrate of alloreactive T cells that attack donor cells both in the endothelium and in the parenchyma. Alloreactive antibodies also develop and contribute to acute humoral or vascular rejection. **C,** Chronic rejection is characterized by graft arteriosclerosis and fibrosis. Immune- and nonimmune-mediated mechanisms are responsible for abnormal proliferation of cells within the intima and media of the vessels of the graft, eventually leading to luminal occlusion. (Adapted from Abbas AK, Lichtman AH, Pillai S: *Cellular and molecular immunology*, ed 8, Philadelphia, 2015, Saunders Elsevier.)

"natural processes," such as the formation of antibody to blood group antigens, or the product of prior exposure to antigens with similar enough specificities as those expressed by the donor that cross-reactivity can occur. In the latter, sensitization is usually the result of a prior transplantation, transfusion, or pregnancy, but it may also be the result of prior environmental antigen exposure. As expected, hyperacute rejection can occur within the first minutes to hours after graft reperfusion. Antibodies bind to the donor tissue or endothelium and initiate complement-mediated lysis and endothelial cell activation, resulting in a procoagulant state and immediate graft thrombosis. On histologic evaluation, there may be platelet and thrombin thrombi, early neutrophil infiltration, and positive staining for the complement product C4d on the endothelial lining of small blood vessels (Fig. 24-17). Thankfully, this type of rejection is largely avoidable with pretransplantation testing by the crossmatch assay.

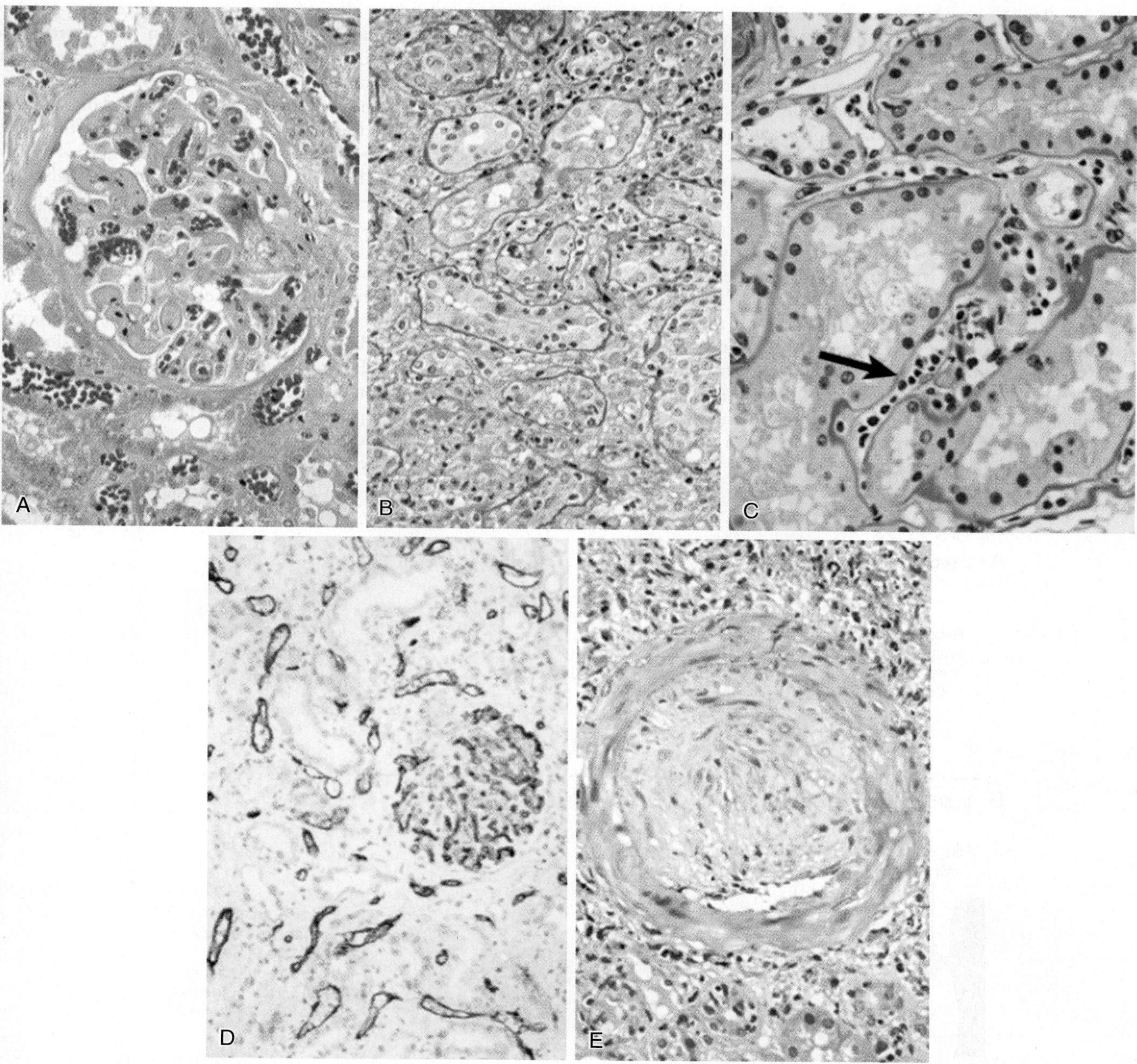

FIGURE 24-17 Histology of Rejection. A, Hyperacute rejection of a kidney allograft with characteristic endothelial damage, thrombus, and early neutrophil infiltrates. **B,** Acute cellular rejection of kidney with inflammatory cells within the connective tissue around the tubules and between tubular epithelial cells. **C,** Acute antibody-mediated rejection of kidney allograft with inflammatory reaction within a graft vessel resulting in endothelial disruption. **D,** C4d deposition in the small vessels of the transplanted kidney. **E,** Chronic rejection in a transplanted kidney with graft arteriosclerosis. The vascular lumen has been replaced with smooth muscle cells and fibrotic response. (Adapted from Abbas AK, Lichtman AH, Pillai S: *Cellular and molecular immunology*, ed 8, Philadelphia, 2015, Saunders Elsevier.)

Similar to the lymphocytotoxicity assay described previously that is used for MHC class I typing, the crossmatch is performed by mixing cells from the donor with serum from the recipient and the addition of complement if needed. Lysis of the donor cells indicates that antibodies directed against the donor are present in the recipient's serum; this is called a positive crossmatch. Thus, a negative crossmatch assay coupled with proper ABO matching will effectively prevent hyperacute rejection in 99.5% of transplants. Newer crossmatch techniques have become increasingly sophisticated, including those directed at both class I and class II antibodies, flow cytometric techniques, and bead-based screening assays to exclude non-HLA antibodies. As a given patient's sensitivity status may change over time, a more common technique for screening a patient's sensitization status is to screen a potential recipient's serum against a panel of random donor cells representing the likely regional donor pool. Known as the panel reactive antibody (PRA) assay, the results are expressed as a percentage of the panel within the randomly selected cell set that lyses when recipient serum is added. Thus, a nonsensitized patient would be given a score of 0%, and a highly sensitized patient might have a PRA score up to 100%. These screens can now be performed without the need for cells by using polystyrene beads coated with HLA antigens. In this situation, the laboratory detects all anti-HLA antibodies and calculates a PRA score on the basis of the expected frequency of the HLA types in the donor pool. There are now clinical protocols to attempt desensitization that use plasmapheresis or intravenous immune globulin (IVIG) to reduce circulating antibody.[21] A more promising method is to avoid crossmatch-positive donor-recipient pairs with paired donor exchange.

Acute Rejection

Of the three types of rejection, only acute rejection can be successfully reversed once it is established. T cells constitute the core element responsible for acute rejection, often termed T cell–mediated rejection. There is also a form of acute rejection that is particularly aggressive and involves vascular invasion by T cells known as acute vascular rejection. Finally, a more recently recognized form of acute rejection mediated by the humoral immune system, known as antibody-mediated rejection (AMR), is discussed briefly later. With the advent of increasingly effective immunosuppression, allograft loss from acute cellular rejection has become increasingly rare. Acute rejection can occur at any time after the first few postoperative days, the time needed to mount an acquired immune response; it most commonly occurs within the first 6 months after transplantation. Without adequate immunosuppression, the cellular response will progress during the course of days to a few weeks, ultimately destroying the allograft. As described earlier, there are two main pathways through which rejection can proceed, the direct and indirect alloresponses (Fig. 24-18). In either case, allospecific T cells encounter their appropriate antigen (either processed donor MHC peptides presented on self MHC or directly recognized donor MHC), undergo activation, and promote similar responses. The precursor frequency of T cells specific for either direct allorecognition or indirect allorecognition differs. Indirect allorecognition is similar to any given pathogen. Donor MHC protein is processed into peptides and presented on self MHC. The number of T cells specific for this antigen is approximately 1 in 200,000 to 1 in 500,000. Direct allorecognition, however, has a much higher precursor frequency. These T cells recognize donor MHC directly without

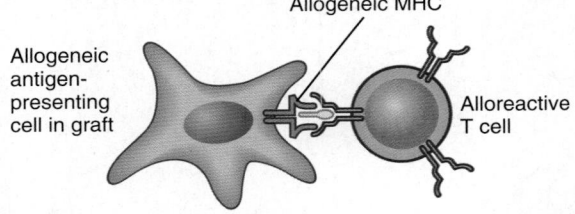

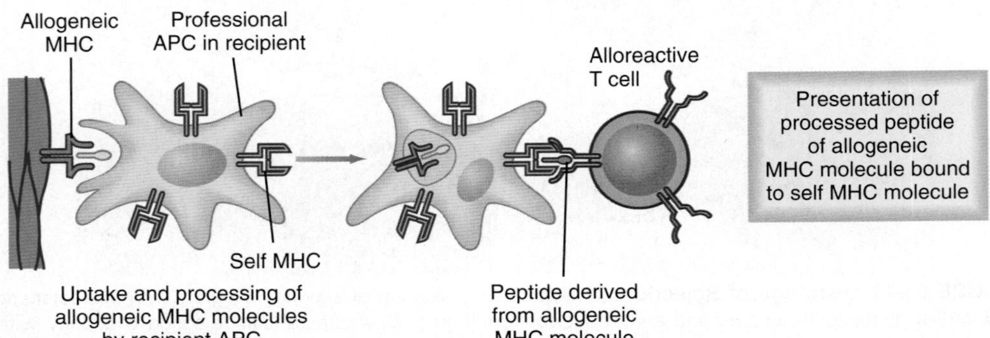

FIGURE 24-18 Direct versus Indirect Allorecognition. A, Direct allorecognition occurs when recipient T cells bind directly to donor MHC molecules on graft cells. **B,** Indirect allorecognition results when recipient antigen-presenting cells take up donor MHC and process the alloantigen. Allopeptides are then presented on recipient (self) MHC molecules in standard fashion to alloreactive T cells. (Adapted from Abbas AK, Lichtman AH, Pillai S: *Cellular and molecular immunology*, ed 6, Philadelphia, 2010, Saunders Elsevier.)

processing (Fig. 24-19). Given that T cells are selected to recognize self MHC molecules and that there are similarities between donor and recipient MHC, it is no surprise that a substantial number of T cells are alloreactive. Some estimates suggest that somewhere between 1% and 10% of all T cells are directly alloreactive. This high precursor frequency likely overwhelms many of the regulatory processes in place to control the much lower cell frequencies involved in physiologic immune responses. These alloreactive T cells, once activated, move to destroy the graft. Subsequently, there is massive infiltration of T cells and monocytes into the allograft, resulting in destruction of the organ through direct cytolysis and a general inflammatory milieu that leads to generalized parenchymal dysfunction and endothelial injury resulting in thrombosis (see Fig. 24-17).

The bulk of current immunosuppressive agents are directed toward the T cells themselves or interruption of pathways essential to their activation or effector functions. In an effort to prevent acute cellular rejection, induction therapy may be used during the initial stages after transplantation. These agents are discussed in the subsequent section but many times will be antibody therapies that serve to deplete or to inactive T cells globally during the immediate postoperative period of engraftment when ischemia-reperfusion injury is most likely to promote immune recognition. Immunosuppressive regimens are frequently scheduled to favor an intense regimen initially in the immediate postoperative period and then are tapered to lower, less toxic levels over time.

T cell–specific treatments lead to prevention of acute rejection in approximately 70% of transplants, and when it does occur, it can be reversed in most cases. Similar to hyperacute rejection resulting from preformed antibody responses, T cell presensitization will result in an accelerated form of cellular rejection mediated by memory T cells. It generally occurs within the first 2 or 3 days after transplantation and is often accompanied by a significant humoral response.

The humoral equivalent to acute cellular rejection is AMR. This occurs when offending antibodies specific for alloantigen exist in the circulation at levels undetectable by the crossmatch assay or, alternatively, B cell clones capable of producing donor-specific antibody are activated and stimulated to produce de novo alloantibodies. The former scenario is often seen in patients with a high PRA score that has decreased over time. Transplantation leads to restimulation of memory B cells responsible for the donor-specific antibodies. The result is initial graft function, followed by rapid deterioration within the first few postoperative days. Implementation of a more aggressive immunosuppressive regimen, including higher doses of steroids combined with nonspecific antibody depletion by plasmapheresis or IVIG (nonspecific immunoglobulin), is occasionally successful in reversing AMR.

Prompt recognition of acute rejection is essential to ensure prolonged graft survival. Untreated rejection leads to expansion of the immune response to involve multiple pathways, some of which are less sensitive to T cell–specific therapies. In addition, damage to the allograft, particularly for kidney, pancreas, and heart, is generally accompanied by a permanent loss of function that is proportional to the magnitude of involvement. Most acute rejection episodes are initially asymptomatic until the secondary effects of organ dysfunction occur. By this point, the rejection process has proceeded to a point that it is often more difficult to reverse. Accordingly, monitoring for acute rejection is usually intense initially, particularly during the first year after transplantation. In general, any unexplained graft dysfunction should prompt biopsy and evaluation for the lymphocytic

A Normal

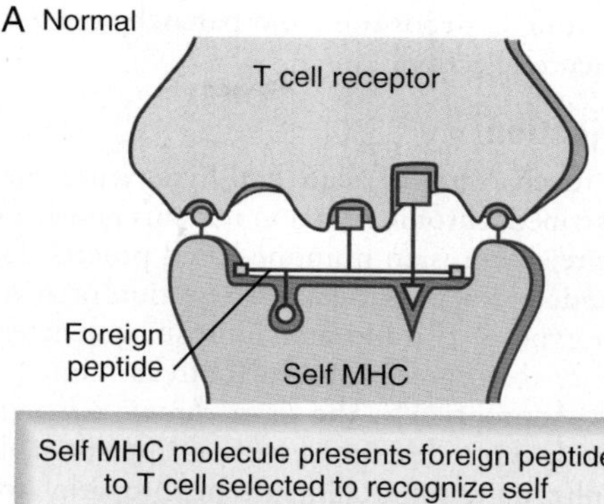

Self MHC molecule presents foreign peptide to T cell selected to recognize self MHC weakly, but may recognize self MHC-foreign peptide complexes well

B Allorecognition

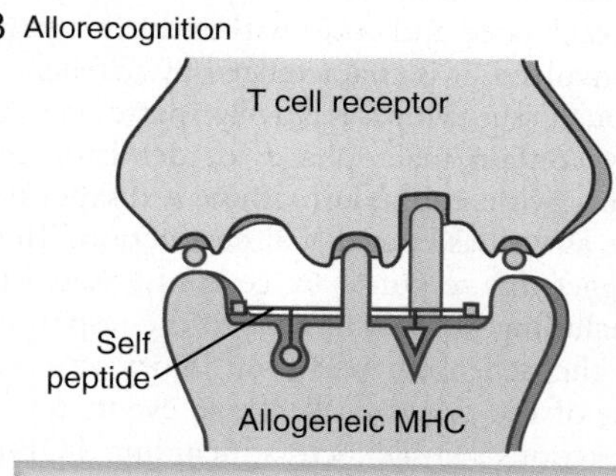

The self MHC-restricted T cell recognizes the allogeneic MHC molecule whose structure resembles a self MHC-foreign peptide complex

C Allorecognition

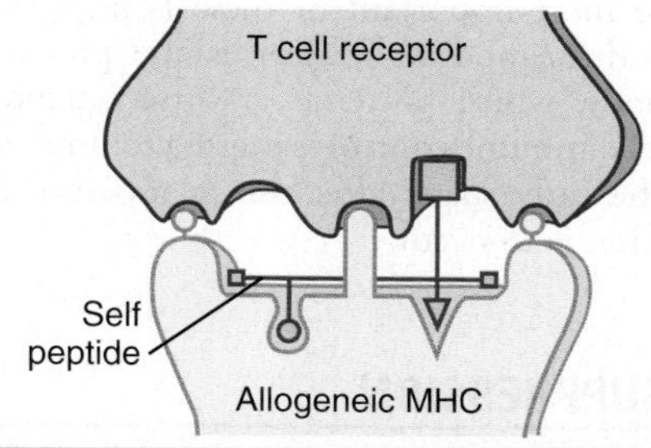

The self MHC-restricted T cell recognizes a structure formed by both the allogeneic MHC molecule and the bound peptide

FIGURE 24-19 Molecular Basis for Direct Allorecognition. Recipient T cells may recognize donor MHC molecules directly because of the similarities between MHC alleles but become activated because only T cells strongly reactive to self MHC were deleted in the thymus through negative selection. **A,** Normally, T cells encounter self MHC complexed with foreign peptide and become activated in the appropriate situation. **B,** T cells may encounter allogeneic MHC complexed with endogenous peptide and mistakenly react as the structure of the foreign MHC molecule itself resembles self MHC bound with foreign peptide. **C,** Alternatively, the combination of self peptide and allogeneic MHC may promote activation. (Adapted from Abbas AK, Lichtman AH, Pillai S: *Cellular and molecular immunology*, ed 6, Philadelphia, 2010, Saunders Elsevier.)

infiltration, antibody deposition, and parenchymal necrosis characteristic of acute rejection.

Chronic Rejection

Whereas the mechanisms of acute and hyperacute rejection have been well described, chronic rejection remains poorly understood. True chronic rejection is an immune-based process derived from repeated or indolent T cell–mediated rejection or AMR, but the clinical phenotype of chronic graft fibrosis and deterioration is often secondary to a combination of both immune and nonimmune effects. Appropriately, the term *chronic rejection* has been substituted with more descriptive terms: interstitial fibrosis and tubular atrophy or chronic allograft nephropathy for kidneys, chronic coronary vasculopathy for hearts, vanishing bile duct syndrome for livers, and bronchiolitis obliterans for lungs.[22] The process is insidious, usually occurring during a period of years, but it can be accelerated and occur within the first year. Regardless of the organ involved, it is characterized by parenchymal replacement by fibrous tissue with a relatively sparse lymphocytic infiltrate but may contain macrophages or dendritic cells (see Fig. 24-17). Organs with epithelium show a disappearance of the epithelial cells as well as endothelial destruction. The events that ultimately trigger this response are certainly related to the transplantation, including but not limited to the response to alloantigen as well as the ischemia-reperfusion injury associated with the actual transfer of the organ itself. These events set the stage for expression of various soluble factors including TGF-β leading to a remodeling of the parenchyma and ensuing fibrous replacement. Chronic inflammatory insults can also evoke a process of epithelial to mesenchymal dedifferentiation, leading to epithelial cells that regress into fibrocytes. Although to date these processes remain essentially untreatable once identified, several factors have been identified that predispose toward the development of chronic rejection. The most important of these is prior acute rejection episodes. Another important factor is the presence of donor-specific antibody, which portends a worse outcome. Thus, the more effectively immune control is exerted to limit acute rejection episodes in the early stages after transplantation, the less likely chronic rejection is to occur.

IMMUNOSUPPRESSION

Current immunosuppressive therapies in transplantation achieve excellent results, especially in terms of relatively short-term patient and allograft survival rates. Despite tremendous progress during the past 50 years, all agents designed to prevent rejection remain nonspecific to the alloimmune response. Given the redundancy of the immune system, recipients almost always need multiple agents to adequately control the normal immune response. In addition, none of these therapies specifically inhibits the response to the allograft; instead, most immunosuppressants target the immune response globally. In other words, all drugs that prevent rejection do so at the cost of preventing the normal host response to bacterial and viral infections as well as tumor surveillance. Whereas some of the newer therapies are more precise in their mechanisms, many target not only the mediators of the immune response but also any cells undergoing maturation or division. Consequently, there are many nonimmune side effects associated with immunosuppressive therapy that can directly or indirectly contribute to graft dysfunction. In addition, the societal costs are not trivial, considering that transplant recipients may take dozens of pills a day at an annual cost of $10,000 to $15,000.

The most critical time for immunoprotection is the first few days to months after transplantation. The graft is fresh, and there is a heightened state of inflammation secondary to inevitable graft injury from ischemia-reperfusion as well as the physical transfer of the organ itself. In addition, this is the time of initial antigen exposure, which will play a large role in establishing a lasting state of immune unresponsiveness. For this reason, immunosuppression is extremely intense in the early postoperative period and normally tapered thereafter. This initial conditioning of the recipient's immune system is known as induction immunosuppression. It usually involves complete deletion or at least aggressive reduction of the T cell response and consequently is tolerated only for a short time without lethal consequences. After this initial period, the agents used to prevent acute rejection for the remainder of the life of the patient are called maintenance immunosuppressants. These medications still carry with them a host of immune and nonimmune side effects that may also ultimately contribute to long-term graft failure. Immunosuppressants used to reverse an acute rejection episode are called rescue agents. They are generally the same as those agents used for induction therapy. The mechanisms of the various immunosuppressants are described here and detailed in Table 24-3.

Corticosteroids

Steroids, in particular glucocorticoids, remain one of the most commonly employed medications to prevent rejection. They are almost exclusively used in combination with other agents with which they seem to act synergistically to improve graft survival. They may also be used in higher doses as rescue therapy for acute rejection episodes. Although steroids possess potent immunosuppressive properties, they can contribute significantly to the morbidity of transplantation by their effects on wound healing and propensity to cause diabetes, hypertension, and osteoporosis. More recently, because of these side effects, there has been an emphasis on developing steroid-minimization or steroid-sparing protocols.

Although the Nobel Prize was awarded more than 50 years ago for work on the hormones of the adrenal cortex, the mechanism of the immunosuppressive effect of glucocorticoids was only recently elucidated.[23] Similar to other steroid hormones, glucocorticoids bind to an intracellular receptor after passing into the cytoplasm through nonspecific mechanisms. The receptor-steroid complex then enters the nucleus, where it acts as a transcription factor. One of the most important genes upregulated is the gene encoding IκB. This protein binds to and inhibits the function of NF-κB, a key activator of proinflammatory cytokines and an important transcription factor involved in T cell activation. Through this mechanism, steroids also act to diminish transcription of IL-1 and TNF-α by APCs as well as to prevent upregulation of MHC expression. Phospholipase A2, and consequently the entire arachidonic acid cascade, is also inhibited. They decrease the leukocyte response to various chemokines and chemotactins and by inhibiting vasodilators, such as histamine and prostacyclin, thus dampen the inflammatory response globally. This broad anti-inflammatory response quickly mollifies the intragraft environment and thus substantially improves graft function long before the offending cells have actually left the graft. The most commonly used oral glucocorticoid formulation is prednisone; its intravenous equivalent is methylprednisolone.

TABLE 24-3 **Summary of Immunosuppressive Drugs**

DRUG	DESCRIPTION	MECHANISM	NONIMMUNE TOXICITY AND COMMENTS
Prednisone	Corticosteroid	Binds nuclear receptor and enhances transcription of IκB, which inhibits NF-κB and T cell activation	Diabetes, weight gain, psychological disturbances, osteoporosis, ulcers, wound healing, adrenal suppression
Cyclosporine	11–Amino acid cyclic peptide from *Tolypocladium inflatum*	Binds to cyclophilin; complex inhibits calcineurin phosphatase and T cell activation	Nephrotoxicity, hemolytic uremic syndrome, hypertension, neurotoxicity, gingival hyperplasia, skin changes, hirsutism, post-transplantation diabetes, hyperlipidemia
Tacrolimus (Prograf)	Macrolide antibiotic from *Streptomyces tsukubaensis*	Binds to FKBP12; complex inhibits calcineurin phosphatase and T cell activation	Effects similar to cyclosporine but with lower incidence of hypertension, hyperlipidemia, skin changes, hirsutism, and gingival hyperplasia but higher incidence of post-transplantation diabetes and neurotoxicity
Sirolimus (rapamycin)	Triene macrolide antibiotic from *Streptomyces hygroscopicus* from Easter Island (Rapa Nui)	Binds to FKBP12; complex inhibits target of rapamycin and IL-2–dependent T cell proliferation	Hyperlipidemia, increased toxicity of calcineurin inhibitors, thrombocytopenia, delayed wound healing, delayed graft function, mouth ulcers, pneumonitis, interstitial lung disease
Everolimus (Zortress)	Derivative of sirolimus, similar mechanism and toxicities		
Mycophenolate mofetil (CellCept)	Mycophenolic acid from *Penicillium stoloniferum*	Inhibits synthesis of guanosine monophosphate nucleotides; blocks purine synthesis, preventing proliferation of T and B cells	Gastrointestinal symptoms (mainly diarrhea), neutropenia, mild anemia
Azathioprine (Imuran)	Prodrug that undergoes hepatic metabolism to form 6-mercaptopurine	Converts 6-mercaptopurine to 6-thioinosine-5′-monophosphate, which is converted to thioguanine nucleotides that interfere with DNA and purine synthesis	Leukopenia, bone marrow depression, liver toxicity (uncommon)
Antithymocyte globulin	Polyclonal IgG from rabbits or horses immunized with human thymocytes	Blocks T cell membrane proteins (CD2, CD3, CD45), causing altered function, lysis, and prolonged T cell depletion	Cytokine release syndrome, thrombocytopenia, leukopenia, serum sickness
OKT3 (muromonab-CD3)	Anti-CD3 murine monoclonal antibody	Binds CD3 associated with the TCR, leading to initial activation and cytokine release, followed by blockade of function, lysis, and T cell depletion	Severe cytokine release syndrome, pulmonary edema, acute renal failure, central nervous system changes
Basiliximab	Anti-CD25 chimeric monoclonal antibody	Binds to high-affinity chain of IL-2R (CD25) on activated T cells, causing depletion and preventing IL-2–mediated activation	Hypersensitivity reaction, uncommon
Daclizumab	Anti-CD25 humanized monoclonal antibody	Similar to that of basiliximab	Hypersensitivity reaction, uncommon
Rituximab	Anti-CD20 chimeric monoclonal antibody	Binds to CD20 on B cells and causes depletion	Infusion and hypersensitivity reactions, uncommon
Alemtuzumab	Anti-CD52 humanized monoclonal antibody	Binds to CD52 expressed on most T and B cells, monocytes, macrophages, and NK cells, causing lysis and prolonged depletion	Mild cytokine release syndrome, neutropenia, anemia, autoimmune thrombocytopenia, thyroid disease
FTY720	Sphingosine-like derivative of myricin from the fungus *Isaria sinclairii*	Functions as an antagonist for sphingosine-1-phosphate receptors on lymphocytes, enhancing homing to lymphoid tissues and preventing egress, causing lymphopenia	Reversible first-dose bradycardia, potentiated by general anesthetics and beta blockers, nausea, vomiting, diarrhea, increased liver enzyme levels
Belatacept (LEA29Y)	High-affinity homologue of CTLA-4–Ig	Binds to CD80/CD86 and prevents costimulation through CD28	In clinical trials, preliminary results suggest equal efficacy to CsA but improved glomerular filtration rate

Adapted from Halloran PF: Immunosuppressive drugs for kidney transplantation. *N Engl J Med* 351:2715–2729, 2004.

Antiproliferative Agents

Azathioprine

The purine analogue azathioprine was first described in the 1960s and remained a mainstay of immunosuppression for the next 30 years.[24] It is still used today in organ transplantation and in the treatment of some autoimmune diseases, such as autoimmune hepatitis. Similar to other antiproliferative agents, it is a nucleotide analogue that targets cells undergoing rapid division; in the case of an immune response, its goal is to limit the clonal expansion of T and B cells. Azathioprine undergoes hepatic conversion to several active metabolites, including 6-mercaptopurine and 6-thioinosine monophosphate. These derivatives inhibit DNA synthesis by alkylating DNA precursors and interfering with DNA repair mechanisms. In addition, they inhibit the enzymatic conversion of thioinosine monophosphate to adenosine monophosphate and guanosine monophosphate, effectively depleting the cell of adenosine. The effects of azathioprine are relatively nonspecific, and like other antiproliferative agents, it acts on all rapidly dividing cells requiring nucleotide synthesis. Consequently, its predominant toxicities are seen in the bone marrow, gut mucosa, and liver. It is primarily used as a maintenance agent in combination with other medications, such as a corticosteroid and calcineurin inhibitor.

Mycophenolate Mofetil

Mycophenolate mofetil (MMF) is an immunosuppressive agent with a similar mechanism of action to azathioprine. It is derived from the fungus *Penicillium stoloniferum*. Once ingested, it is metabolized in the liver to the active moiety mycophenolic acid. The active compound inhibits inosine monophosphate dehydrogenase, the enzyme that controls the rate of synthesis of guanosine monophosphate in the de novo pathway of purine synthesis, a critical step in RNA and DNA synthesis. Importantly, however, is the presence of a "salvage pathway" for guanosine monophosphate production in most cells except lymphocytes (hypoxanthine-guanine phosphoribosyltransferase–catalyzed guanosine monophosphate production directly from guanosine). Thus, MMF exploits a critical difference between lymphocytes and other body tissues, resulting in relatively lymphocyte-specific immunosuppressive effects. MMF blocks the proliferative response of both T and B cells, inhibits antibody formation, and prevents the clonal expansion of cytotoxic T cells.

There have been numerous clinical trials to evaluate MMF. Specifically, MMF has been shown to decrease the rate of biopsy-proven rejection and the need for rescue therapy compared with azathioprine.[25] Appropriately, MMF has replaced azathioprine in most immunosuppressive protocols as the third in the standard three-drug regimen, although recent evidence suggests that its therapeutic difference is less pronounced when it is used with more modern immunosuppressive regimens. It has also been used in combination with either a calcineurin inhibitor or sirolimus by many centers in steroid-sparing protocols. MMF is not, however, effective enough to use without either steroids or calcineurin inhibitors. The major clinical side effects include leukopenia and diarrhea.

Calcineurin Inhibitors

Cyclosporine

Jean-François Borel is credited with the discovery of CsA in 1972 while working as a microbiologist for Sandoz Laboratories (now Novartis). He apparently was vacationing in Norway and while there had collected soil samples for analysis in search of new antibiotics. Although the samples failed to show any significant antimicrobial activity, they did show potent immunosuppressive characteristics. Further studies demonstrated that the active component is a cyclic, nonribosomal peptide of 11 amino acids produced by the fungus *Tolypocladium inflatum*.[26] The mechanism of action of CsA is mediated primarily through its ability to bind the cytoplasmic protein cyclophilin. The CsA-cyclophilin complex binds to the calcineurin-calmodulin complex within the cytoplasm and blocks calcium-dependent phosphorylation and activation of NFAT, a critical transcription factor involved in T cell activation including upregulation of the IL-2 transcript (Fig. 24-20). The result is blockade of IL-2 production. Thus, CsA is used as a maintenance agent, blocking the initiation of an immune response, but it is ineffective as a rescue agent once IL-2 has already been produced. In addition, CsA acts to increase transcription of TGF-β, a cytokine involved in the normal processes that limit the immune response by inhibiting T cell activation, reducing regional blood flow, and stimulating tissue remodeling and wound repair. As discussed later, the toxicity and side effects of CsA may be in large part related to the effects of TGF-β.

CsA has poor water solubility and consequently must be given in a suspension or emulsion. This becomes a particular concern in liver transplantation because the oral absorption of CsA is dependent on bile flow; fortunately, this was addressed through the development of a microemulsion form that is less bile dependent. CsA is metabolized by the hepatic cytochrome P450 enzymes, and blood levels are therefore influenced by agents that affect the P450 system. P450 inhibitors, which include ketoconazole, erythromycin, calcium channel blockers, and grapefruit juice, result in higher CsA levels; inducers of P450, including rifampin, phenobarbital, and phenytoin, result in lower CsA levels.

The discovery of CsA and its subsequent development as an immunosuppressant contributed enormously to the advancement of organ transplantation. It was first approved for clinical use in 1983 and led to substantial improvement in the outcome of deceased donor renal transplantation and permitted the widespread practice of heart and liver transplantation. Whereas its potent immunosuppressive activity was welcomed, its attendant toxicities were less than ideal. CsA induces the expression of TGF-β, and much of CsA toxicity can be linked to increased TGF-β activity. One of the most important side effects of CsA is renal toxicity. CsA has a significant vasoconstrictor effect on proximal renal arterioles, resulting in a 30% decrease in renal blood flow. This action is most likely mediated through increased TGF-β levels that act to increase the transcription of endothelin, a potent vasoconstrictor, resulting in activation of the renin-angiotensin pathway and resultant hypertension.[27] The remodeling effects of TGF-β also induce fibrin deposition, which is thought to play a role in the fibrosis typically seen during chronic allograft nephropathy. CsA frequently causes neurologic side effects consisting of tremors, paresthesias, headache, depression, confusion, somnolence, and, rarely, seizures. Hypertrichosis (increased hair growth) is another frequent side effect, predominantly occurring on the face, arms, and back in up to 50% of patients. Gingival hyperplasia may also occur. The use of CsA in combination with corticosteroids has permitted a lowering of the CsA dose, resulting in decreased toxicity, particularly nephrotoxicity.

Tacrolimus

Tacrolimus was isolated from Japanese soil samples in 1984 as part of an effort to discover novel immunosuppressants. A

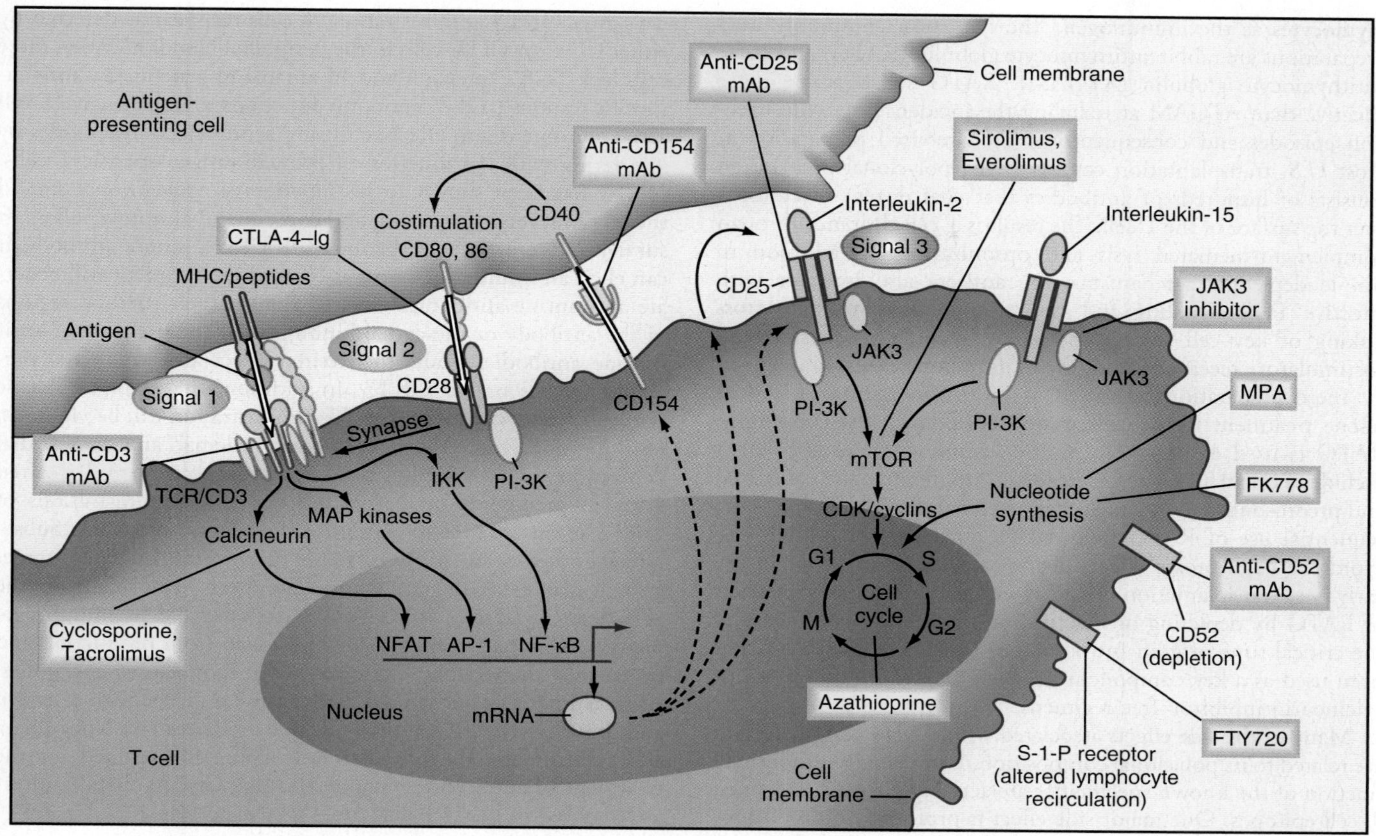

FIGURE 24-20 Molecular Mechanisms of Immunosuppression. Immunosuppressants may be small molecules, antibodies, or fusion proteins that block various pathways critical for T cell activation. TCR binding facilitates kinase activity by CD3 and the coreceptors (CD4 or CD8). The costimulatory molecules CD28, CD154, and others determine the relative potency of these signals. TCR signal transduction proceeds through a calcineurin-dependent pathway, resulting in dephosphorylation of NFAT, which subsequently enters the nucleus and acts in concert with NF-κB to facilitate cytokine gene expression. IL-2 functions in an autocrine fashion, binding to the IL-2R once the high-affinity chain (CD25) is expressed, to promote cell division. Cyclosporine and tacrolimus block TCR signal transduction by inhibiting calcineurin. Sirolimus and everolimus target mTOR to effectively block IL-2R signaling. Azathioprine and MMF/MPA interrupt the cell cycle by interfering with nucleic acid metabolism. Monoclonal antibodies (OKT3, anti–IL-2 receptor, alemtuzumab, anti-CD154, and others) or fusion proteins (CTLA-4–Ig, belatacept) function to deplete T cells or to interrupt key surface interactions required for T cell function. (From Halloran PF: Immunosuppressive drugs for kidney transplantation. *N Engl J Med* 351:2715–2729, 2004.)

macrolide, produced by the fungus *Streptomyces tsukubaensis*, tacrolimus was found to possess potent immunosuppressive properties.[28] Similar to CsA, it blocks the effects of NFAT, prevents cytokine transcription, and arrests T cell activation.[29] The intracellular target is an immunophilin protein distinct from cyclophilin known as FK-binding protein (FK-BP). In vitro, tacrolimus was found to be 100 times more potent in blocking IL-2 and IFN-γ production than CsA. Tacrolimus, like CsA, also increases TGF-β transcription, leading to both the beneficial and toxic effects of this cytokine. The side-effect profile for tacrolimus is similar to that of CsA with regard to renal toxicity, but the cosmetic side effects, such as abnormal hair growth and gingival hyperplasia, are substantially reduced. Neurotoxicity, including tremors and mental status changes, is more pronounced with tacrolimus, as is its diabetogenic effect. Tacrolimus has been shown to be extremely effective for liver transplantation and has become the drug of choice for most centers.

Lymphocyte Depletion Preparations

Most of the current induction regimens involve the use of some antilymphocyte antibody preparation. Their mechanism of action is probably not fully understood but involves some combination of either selective or nonselective depletion and inactivation. They cause profound immunosuppression, placing the recipient at increased risk for opportunistic infections or lymphoma, and are consequently generally limited to short-term use on the order of days to weeks.

Antilymphocyte Globulin

Antilymphocyte globulin preparations are produced by immunizing another species with an inoculum of human lymphocytes, followed by collection of the sera and purification of the gamma globulin fraction. The result is a polyclonal antibody preparation that contains antibodies directed at a multitude of antigens on lymphocytes. More recently, preparations have used human thymocytes as the immunogen. The two most commonly used preparations are rabbit antithymocyte globulin (RATG) and horse antithymocyte globulin (ATGAM). RATG seems to be more effective than ATGAM at reducing the incidence of acute rejection episodes and consequently is the preferred preparation at most U.S. transplantation centers.[30] The polyclonal preparation consists of hundreds of antibodies that coat dozens of epitopes over the surface of the T cell. The result is T cell clearance through complement-mediated lysis and opsonization. In addition to simple depletion mechanisms, the antisera also interfere with effective TCR signaling and can promote inappropriate cross linking of key cell surface molecules, including adhesion and costimulatory receptors, resulting in unresponsiveness or anergy.[31]

These preparations are used as induction agents as well as rescue treatment for acute rejection episodes. Most commonly, RATG is used as part of a multidrug induction protocol that includes a calcineurin inhibitor, an antiproliferative such as MMF, and prednisone. A frequent strategy in renal transplantation is the sequential use of RATG followed by a calcineurin inhibitor to avoid the nephrotoxic effects of the calcineurin inhibitor in the early post-transplantation period as well as to maximize the effects of RATG by depleting or inactivating the majority of T cells at the critical time of graft introduction. More recently, RATG has been used as a key component of newer steroid-minimization or calcineurin inhibitor–free regimens.[32,33]

Many of the side effects associated with RATG administration are related to its polyclonal composition. Surprisingly, only a small fraction of the known specificities are actually directed at defined T cell epitopes. One major side effect is profound thrombocytopenia secondary to platelet-specific antibodies within the polyclonal preparation. In addition to T cell depletion, leukopenia and anemia may also result. Overimmunosuppression is also a concern; given that these preparations are extremely effective at T cell depletion, there is an increase in viral reactivation and primary viral infections, including cytomegalovirus (CMV), Epstein-Barr virus (EBV), herpes simplex virus, and varicella-zoster virus. The effect on EBV-specific T cells also predisposes treated patients to a higher incidence of EBV-associated lymphoid malignant neoplasms. Overall, however, the drug is well tolerated by most transplant recipients. The most common symptoms are the result of transient cytokine release after antibody binding. Chills and fevers occur in up to 20% of patients, but this cytokine release syndrome is usually treatable with antipyretics and antihistamines. In addition, this response is often tempered in patients receiving corticosteroids as part of the induction regimen.

OKT3

Muromonab-CD3 (OKT3), a murine monoclonal antibody directed against the human CD3 ε chain (a component of the TCR signaling complex; see Fig. 24-11), was approved by the Food and Drug Administration for use in patients in 1986. It was the first commercially available monoclonal antibody preparation for use in organ transplantation. Similar to the polyclonal preparations, there are several proposed mechanisms of action for OKT3. On binding to CD3, OKT3 triggers internalization of the TCR complex, preventing antigen recognition and subsequent signal transduction. In addition, it also labels cells for elimination through opsonization and phagocytosis. Adequate dosing is usually monitored by flow cytometry and staining for $CD3^+$ T cells in recipients' blood samples; depletion to less than 10% of baseline is considered an adequate response. Interestingly, several days after OKT3 administration, T cells reappear as detected by either $CD4^+$ or $CD8^+$ cells in the peripheral blood; however, these cells lack TCR expression and are unable to generate an antigen-specific response. OKT3 not only functions to impair naïve T cell activation but is also effective during acute rejection episodes by interfering with the function of primed antigen-specific T cells. OKT3 has been shown to be superior to conventional steroid therapy in reversing rejection and consequently improves allograft survival.[34] Unfortunately, because OKT3 is a mouse antibody, it can elicit an immune response itself, and the recipient will generate antimurine antibodies directed against the structural regions of the antibody or the actual binding site. The presence of antimurine antibodies limits the desired effect and eventually precludes further use of OKT3. In addition, the cytokine release syndrome associated with OKT3 administration can be vigorous, resulting in hypotension, pulmonary edema, and myocardial depression. In fact, a high dose of intravenous steroid is often given as premedication before the first few administrations of OKT3 in an attempt to minimize the adverse reactions. Subsequent dosing is less likely to result in symptoms as most target cells available for degranulation have been removed from the periphery. Because of this vigorous response and its immunogenicity, OKT3 has recently been withdrawn from production and is generally unavailable. There are newer monoclonal antibodies, either chimeric or humanized, with a similar mechanism of action and specificity as OKT3; these include otelixizumab, teplizumab, and visilizumab. They are currently being investigated for the treatment of autoimmune conditions like Crohn's disease, ulcerative colitis, and type 1 diabetes.

Anti–IL-2 Receptor Antibodies

The cytokine IL-2 plays a critical role in T cell activation and function. After antigen recognition and signal transduction through the TCR complex, expression of IL-2 and its receptor is markedly upregulated. The receptor consists of three chains: α (CD25), β (CD122), and the common cytokine receptor γ chain (CD132). These chains associate in a noncovalent manner to form the IL-2 receptor complex. The α chain, CD25, is a type I transmembrane protein that is responsible for the high-affinity binding of IL-2 on activated T cells and is critical for T cell clonal expansion (see Fig. 24-20). Given its importance in the cellular response, two monoclonal antibodies were developed and approved for use in transplantation: daclizumab and basiliximab.[35,36] The two antibodies differ in their composition in that daclizumab is humanized and basiliximab is a mouse-human chimeric antibody. Both are directed against CD25 and function to block IL-2 binding. Because CD25 is preferentially expressed on recently activated T cells, the antibodies are semiselective in their effects, presumably affecting only T cells specific for the allograft that have been activated at the time of graft implantation. Once the T cell response is well under way, effector T cells are much less dependent on CD25 expression, and these antibodies are much less effective. For this reason, both anti-CD25 antibodies are used during the induction phase only. Much like antithymocyte globulin, they have been shown to prevent or to reduce the frequency of acute rejection when they are used in combination with the standard three-drug regimen. More recently, they have been employed as part of regimens to reduce or to eliminate calcineurin inhibitors or within steroid-minimization protocols. Both antibodies are very well tolerated clinically as they do not precipitate the same side effects seen with OKT3 or even with antithymocyte globulin, such as the cytokine release syndrome. Unlike OKT3, both daclizumab and basiliximab are the products of genetic engineering, with the structural components of the mouse antibody having been replaced with human IgG, and thus they are much less likely to invoke a neutralizing antibody response themselves. Daclizumab has since been discontinued as a result of diminished demand, leaving basiliximab as the sole option.

Other Immunoglobulin Therapies

Rituximab

Rituximab is a murine antihuman CD20 chimeric antibody that was initially developed for the treatment of B cell lymphoma and has since been used in the treatment of post-transplantation lymphoproliferative disorder (PTLD). CD20 is a cell surface protein expressed on all mature B cells but not on plasma cells. Rituximab binds to CD20 and facilitates antibody-dependent cellular cytotoxicity and complement-dependent cytotoxicity of B cells as well as promoting programmed cell death. More recently, rituximab has been used in a wide variety of autoimmune disorders and as a component in some investigational strategies designed as induction therapy in highly sensitized transplant recipients undergoing kidney transplantation or even in ABO-incompatible pairings. CD20 is not expressed on antibody-producing plasma cells; as such, its role in limiting aggressive forms of rejection may relate to the role of B cells in antigen presentation.

Alemtuzumab

Similar to rituximab, alemtuzumab was originally developed in the oncology field for the treatment of lymphoma. It is a humanized antibody against human CD52, a cell surface protein expressed on most mature lymphocytes and monocytes but not on their stem cell precursors. It has been used not only in patients with lymphoma but also in autoimmune processes, such as multiple sclerosis and rheumatoid arthritis. Administration of alemtuzumab is extremely effective at reducing the number of T cells both in the peripheral blood and in secondary lymphoid organs. In addition, it depletes, to a lesser extent, both B cells and monocytes. Unlike other strategies, this depletion may last for weeks to months after dosing. Investigational studies in transplantation employing alemtuzumab as an induction agent have allowed minimization of immunosuppression, particularly when it is combined with a calcineurin inhibitor.[37,38] Its optimal use in transplantation remains to be established.

Intravenous Immune Globulin

IVIG is composed of pooled plasma fractions from thousands of donors and essentially contains a representative sample of all antibodies found within that population. It is used frequently in the treatment of several autoimmune diseases, such as idiopathic thrombocytopenic purpura, Guillain-Barré syndrome, and myasthenia gravis, as well as in patients with severe immune deficiencies featuring low or absent antibody levels. IVIG is also used in organ transplantation, specifically in the treatment of humoral rejection or before transplantation in a highly sensitized recipient in an attempt to reduce the PRA score and potential positive crossmatch. More recently, it has also been used as part of ABO-incompatible protocols. IVIG probably works through several mechanisms to alter the immune response, including neutralization of circulating autoantibodies and alloantibodies through anti-idiotypic antibodies and selective downregulation of antibody production through Fc-mediated mechanisms.[39]

Mammalian Target of Rapamycin Inhibitors

Sirolimus (rapamycin) was isolated from a soil sample taken from Easter Island, a Polynesian island in the southeastern Pacific ocean also known as Rapa Nui, hence the name rapamycin. It is a macrolide derived from the bacterium *Streptomyces hygroscopicus* with potent immunosuppressive properties. Everolimus is a derivative of rapamycin that possesses similar properties. Both are similar in structure to tacrolimus and bind to the same intracellular target, FK-BP, but neither agent affects calcineurin activity and consequently does not inhibit expression of NFAT or IL-2 expression. Instead, the sirolimus–FK-BP complex inhibits the mammalian target of rapamycin (mTOR), specifically the mTOR complex 1 (see Fig. 24-20). mTOR is also called FRAP (FK-BP–rapamycin-associated protein) or RAFT (rapamycin and FK-BP target). RAFT-1 is a critical kinase involved in the IL-2 receptor signaling pathway. The result is inhibition of p70 S6 kinase activity, an enzyme essential for ribosomal phosphorylation, and arrest of cell cycle progression.[40] Other receptors are also affected, including those for IL-4, IL-6, and platelet-derived growth factor.

Both sirolimus and everolimus are potent inhibitors of rejection in experimental models. Sirolimus and tacrolimus can act synergistically to impair rejection, but the combination results in intolerable toxicity, specifically calcineurin inhibitor–mediated nephrotoxicity. More often, sirolimus is used as an alternative to calcineurin inhibitors in a multidrug regimen or combined with other agents, allowing a reduction in the dose and minimization of side effects, including calcineurin inhibitor–related nephrotoxicity or steroid-specific side effects. In addition to immunosuppressive properties, mTOR inhibitors have been shown to have promising antitumor effects as well. For example, sirolimus has been shown to promote programmed cell death in B cell lymphomas, and everolimus has demonstrated activity against EBV. Thus, both agents may play an important role in the prevention of PTLD. Sirolimus and everolimus have also been used in the development of drug-eluting coronary stents to limit the rate of in-stent restenosis because of their antiproliferative properties. There is an increased incidence of hypercholesterolemia and hypertriglyceridemia with both agents that often requires treatment with cholesterol-lowering agents or discontinuation of the drug. Oral ulcers, wound healing complications (in particular an increased incidence of lymphoceles), elevated levels of proteinuria, and thrombocytopenia remain frequent problems and limit universal application.

Newer Immunosuppressive Agents

Belatacept

Costimulation is a critical component of naïve T cell activation and has been extensively studied as a potential target for manipulation in organ transplantation. One of the most important pathways is the interaction between CD28 and CD80/CD86. Signaling through CD28 allows effective IL-2 production and promotes cell survival through upregulation of antiapoptotic molecules. CD152 (CTLA-4) is another cell surface molecule expressed on activated T cells that is more effective in binding CD80 and CD86 than CD28. Once activated, T cells begin to express CD152, which interacts with CD80 and CD86 with a higher affinity and effectively blocks CD28 binding. CD152 then delivers an inhibitory signal to the T cell as part of a downregulatory mechanism for the immune response. A fusion protein consisting of the extracellular component of CTLA-4 and the heavy chain of human IgG1 was developed to block CD28-CD80/

CD86 interactions and consequently to impair costimulation and T cell activation (see Fig. 24-20). CTLA-4–Ig (abatacept) is used clinically in several autoimmune indications, including rheumatoid arthritis and psoriasis.[41,42] Further efforts to improve the efficacy of CTLA-4–Ig resulted in a novel mutant form, LEA29Y (belatacept). LEA29Y is a second-generation CTLA-4–Ig molecule that differs by two amino acid residues within the binding domain, resulting in increased affinity for CD80 and CD86. The resultant improvement in binding affinity led to more potent immunosuppressive properties in vitro and in vivo.[43] Belatacept has since been used in both preclinical, nonhuman primate studies and phase 3 clinical trials in human renal transplantation. It has demonstrated efficacy equivalent to CsA in renal transplant recipients receiving MMF and steroids and appears to promote superior renal function as a calcineurin inhibitor–free regimen.[44] One potential drawback is that it must be administered parenterally. Instead of a few pills every day, the patient must come into the clinic or an infusion center every month for maintenance therapy. This need to receive the drug in a health care environment may improve drug adherence.

Fingolimod (FTY720)

Fingolimod, also known as FTY720, has a unique mechanism of action that results in sequestration of lymphocytes within lymph nodes, thereby preventing them from participating in allograft rejection or autoimmunity. It is derived from the fungus *Isaria sinclairii* and is an analogue of sphingosine. FTY720 requires phosphorylation by sphingosine kinase 2 to become active, after which it binds to a sphingosine-1-phosphate receptor, specifically S1PR1 (see Fig. 24-20). Binding of S1PR1 by FTY70-P results in aberrant internalization of the receptor. Lack of the receptor on the cell surface deprives lymphocytes of the signals necessary for egress from secondary lymphoid organs and functionally traps them within lymph nodes. Unfortunately, despite promising experimental data, FTY720 failed to show an improvement in efficacy in the prevention of renal allograft rejection in two large phase 3 studies. A common side effect was self-limited bradycardia, which had been documented in earlier safety trials. The phase 3 trials, however, revealed a surprising decrease in renal function within the FTY720 treatment arm. In addition, a worrisome number of patients developed macular edema. Given that there was no documented benefit in efficacy and new, unexpected side effects had appeared, clinical trials were halted in renal transplantation. Trials have continued in autoimmune conditions, such as multiple sclerosis. After a recent phase 3 clinical trial demonstrated that FTY720 was superior to interferon beta-1a in the treatment of multiple sclerosis, it was subsequently approved by the Food and Drug Administration as the first oral disease-modifying drug that reduces relapses and delays disease progression in patients with relapsing forms of multiple sclerosis.[45]

Eculizumab

The complement system is one of the main components of the innate immune response but also plays a significant role in regulating the adaptive immune system as well. Complement activation with formation of the membrane attack complex is the end point of a number of inflammatory processes that can cause damage to the transplanted organ. In particular, the role of complement in AMR or other processes that lead to immune complex deposition within the allograft or xenograft has recently been recognized as a potential target of therapeutic intervention. Eculizumab is a humanized monoclonal antibody targeting the complement component C5. Its binding to C5 inhibits formation of complement components downstream, including the split product C5a and membrane attack complex (see Fig. 24-4). It is approved to treat patients with paroxysmal nocturnal hemoglobinuria and atypical hemolytic uremic syndrome. More recently, there have been several reports employing eculizumab in solid organ transplantation as a means to treat or even to prevent AMR. It does appear to be effective when it is given prophylactically in combination with plasma exchange and IVIG in highly sensitized recipients, who are at higher risk for development of AMR. Unfortunately, it is not universally effective as a significant number of highly sensitized patients proceed to experience AMR despite treatment. This likely reflects the complexity of the processes leading to AMR, suggesting that additional mechanisms may be at play. Additional ongoing studies have shown promising early results with other reagents, such as an inhibitor of C1, but further trials are needed.

JAK3 Kinase Inhibition

Given the side-effect profile of calcineurin inhibitor therapy, in particular the nephrotoxic effects, there has been an intense effort to develop other therapeutic targets by exploiting the other pathways that are critical for T cell activation and effector function. Cytokines are critical signals and growth factors that influence T cell proliferation and differentiation. The cytokine receptors found on the T cell surface transduce their signal through the use of the JAK/STAT pathways. Given that this pathway is key for T cell activation and effector function, several JAK inhibitors have been developed. One in particular, tofacitinib, a JAK3 inhibitor, has been tested in kidney transplantation. JAK3, unlike other subtypes, is restricted in its expression to primarily hematopoietic cells and associates with the common γ chain, a shared component of the receptor for IL-2, IL-4, IL-7, IL-9, IL-15, and IL-21. JAK3 inhibition has been an effective treatment for various autoimmune conditions in clinical trials, ultimately leading to the approval of tofacitinib for the treatment of rheumatoid arthritis. In a phase 2b clinical trial, tofacitinib was found to be equally effective at preventing rejection as CsA in renal transplant recipients. In addition, patients treated with tofacitinib had better renal function (higher glomerular filtration rate), less chronic damage on kidney biopsy, and lower rates of post-transplantation diabetes than those patients who received CsA. Unfortunately, treatment with tofacitinib was associated with more anemia and neutropenia and a trend toward more infections, including BK virus and CMV infections, and cases of PTLD, likely accounting for the current reduced interest in transplantation.

Protein Kinase C Inhibition

Similar to JAK3 inhibition, PKC is an attractive target for immunosuppression as it mediates signaling downstream of the TCR. There are many different isoforms of PKC, but a few in particular play key roles in T and B cell signaling. Sotrastaurin is a small-molecular-weight immunosuppressant that blocks early T cell activation through selective inhibition of PKC-θ and PKC-α, isoforms that are critical for IL-2 and IFN-γ production, respectively. In a phase 2 study, sotrastaurin was evaluated as a replacement for tacrolimus as part of a standard immunosuppression protocol in renal transplant recipients. Although patients treated with sotrastaurin had superior renal function, there was an unacceptably high rate of acute rejection compared with the tacrolimus-treated controls, and the study was stopped because of lack of efficacy. It remains to be seen whether optimal dosing and drug combinations will be evaluated in future studies.

Complications of Immunosuppression

The development of immunosuppressive agents was the key step in the advancement of the field of transplantation. Unfortunately, these same agents are responsible for much of the morbidity associated with organ transplantation as well. All current immunosuppressants function to a greater or lesser degree in a nonspecific fashion (i.e., global immunosuppression instead of donor-specific or allospecific immunosuppression). The consequence is occasional overzealous suppression of the immune system, resulting in infectious complications, primarily viral infections, as well as an increased risk of malignant disease. In addition, many of these agents modify the function of proteins and pathways required for normal cell function, and consequently their inhibition results in undesired, nonimmune side effects, including direct organ injury.

Risk of Infection

There is a fine balance between sufficient immunosuppression to prevent rejection and preservation of the host response to nontransplant antigens and pathogens. Introduction of tissue from one individual to another always allows the potential transfer of a new organism. Currently, an extensive battery of testing is performed on both the donor and recipient before transplantation. These examinations have greatly decreased the potential exposure to the recipient, but no test is perfect, and testing can be limited by available technology and the time interval between explantation and implantation. Some infections may still be transferred unknowingly for various reasons, including early infection and lack of seropositivity. Infections may be donor derived, such as a CMV^+ organ placed into a CMV^- recipient, or may arise from less commonly transferred viruses, resulting in primary infections of HIV, hepatitis C virus, hepatitis B virus, tuberculosis, *Trypanosoma cruzi*, West Nile virus, lymphocytic choriomeningitis virus, or rabies.[46]

The threat comes not only from new pathogens but, more important, from those to which the recipient has likely already been exposed and harbors in a state of dormancy. Normally, these pathogens are controlled after the initial infection and remain quiescent. After the immune system is rendered impotent by pharmacologic suppression, these pathogens can spring to life and quickly become uncontrollable. Recipient-derived infections are much more common after transplantation than donor-derived infections. One common example is CMV reactivation. The majority of the population has been exposed to CMV at some point in their lives. On transplantation and induction immunosuppressive therapy, CMV reactivation can occur, resulting in pneumonitis, hepatitis, pancreatitis, or colitis. CMV has also been implicated in the lesions of heart transplant recipients with chronic rejection, highlighting the interplay between the immune response and chronic viral infections or the inflammation they may induce. Other recipient-derived infections include tuberculosis, certain parasites *(Strongyloides stercoralis, Trypanosoma cruzi)*, viruses (e.g., CMV, EBV, herpes simplex, varicella-zoster, hepatitis B, hepatitis C, and HIV), and endemic fungi (e.g., *Pneumocystis jiroveci, Histoplasma capsulatum, Coccidioides immitis*, and *Paracoccidioides brasiliensis*).

Fortunately, patterns of opportunistic infections after transplantation have been altered by the use of routine antimicrobial prophylaxis. The risk for reactivation is highest approximately 6 to 12 weeks after transplantation and again after periods of increased immunosuppression for acute rejection episodes. Transplant programs use various prophylactic regimens, depending on the organs transplanted. Many regimens include pneumococcal vaccine, hepatitis B vaccine, trimethoprim-sulfamethoxazole for *Pneumocystis* pneumonia and urinary tract infections, ganciclovir or valganciclovir for CMV infections, and clotrimazole troche or nystatin for oral and esophageal fungal infections. As immunosuppressive strategies have evolved, resulting in increases in both allograft and patient survival, the specific pathogens as well as the pattern of infection have also evolved. For example, the polyomaviruses BK and JC have recently been recognized to play a more important role in transplantation than previously understood. Infection with the polyomavirus BK has been found in association with a progressive nephropathy and ureteral obstruction, and the JC virus has been associated with progressive multifocal leukoencephalopathy. Detection of BK viral DNA in blood and urine has been useful for monitoring response to therapy, which includes minimizing immunosuppression and treatment with antiviral therapies.

Risk for Malignant Disease

The immune system not only plays a critical role in defending the host against attack from pathogens, it also plays an important role in the surveillance and detection of cancer, particularly those cancers driven by viral infection. The consequence is a nearly 10-fold increase in rates of malignant disease. Skin cancers, particularly squamous cell cancers, are the most common malignant conditions in transplant recipients and account for substantial morbidity and mortality.[47] As expected, virally mediated tumors tend to occur much more frequently in transplant recipients. For example, human papillomavirus is associated with cancer of the cervix, hepatitis B and C viruses with hepatocellular carcinoma, and human herpesvirus 8 with Kaposi sarcoma. EBV, in particular, can be associated with the development of PTLD, a broad term used to describe EBV-associated lymphomas that occur in transplant recipients. PTLD varies from asymptomatic to life-threatening, and accordingly treatment varies from simple reduction or withdrawal of immunosuppression to vigorous chemotherapeutic regimens. More recently, patients have been treated with antiviral agents targeting EBV or even chemotherapy including antibody therapy against the tumor cells, such as rituximab.

Nonimmune Side Effects

Although current immunosuppressants have become increasingly more specific, in general, they are still directed at pathways that play an important role in multiple systems other than immunity. Thus, inhibition of a pathway for the sake of immunosuppression can also lead to unintended consequences if the target is critical to other processes. For example, calcineurin inhibitors are potent suppressors of T cell activation, but their activity not only decreases IL-2 transcription, it also increases TGF-β expression. Elevated levels of TGF-β result in an increase in endothelin expression and eventually lead to hypertension. In addition, TGF-β is thought to play a critical role in the development of chronic allograft nephropathy, previously thought to be immune mediated but now likely to be, at least partly, secondary to nonimmune side effects secondary to calcineurin inhibitor use.

Histologic evidence of calcineurin inhibitor–associated nephrotoxicity is essentially universal in renal transplants by 10 years. Furthermore, these deleterious effects are not limited to only renal transplant recipients. The incidence of chronic renal failure in nonrenal transplant recipients is an astonishing 16.5%.[48] New-onset diabetes after transplantation is also an important problem, particularly in individuals receiving tacrolimus or steroids. The incidence of new-onset immunosuppressive-related diabetes mellitus approaches 30% in the first 2 years after renal transplantation, conferring a significantly higher risk of death. In addition to renal failure, hypertension, and diabetes, immunosuppressive therapy can also lead to hyperlipidemia, anemia, and accelerated cardiovascular disease, which is a leading cause of death in long-term transplant survivors. Thus, it appears that the very reagents that ushered in a new era of success in organ transplantation have proven to be major contributors in the demise of the transplanted organ or recipient. Clearly, there is a pressing clinical need to develop novel immunosuppressive agents that are more specific yet less toxic or to devise strategies to induce immune tolerance so that long-term immunosuppression may eventually be eliminated altogether.

TOLERANCE

Immunologic tolerance has been thought of as the "holy grail" of transplantation biology. Self-tolerance as discussed before involves regulation of the immune response to prevent undesired effects toward host tissues or proteins. This is established and maintained through both central (i.e., thymic selection and deletion) and peripheral mechanisms. The ability to selectively inactive the host response toward only the transplanted donor antigens while maintaining immunocompetence would be highly desirable. This would avoid the need for lifelong immunosuppression with its associated toxicities as well as eliminate chronic rejection, the major cause of late graft failure.

It has been more than 50 years since the first reports of acquired tolerance. The discovery of neonatal transplantation tolerance has been credited to Ray Owen, a geneticist who studied the inheritance of red blood cell antigens in cattle. He reported in 1945 that dizygotic twins had mixtures of their own cells and their twin partner's cells. Earlier observations had demonstrated that bovine dizygotic twins develop a fusion of their placentas during embryonic life. This results in a common intrauterine circulation and the unabated passage of sex hormones, explaining the phenomenon of freemartin cattle. Owen also recognized that this common circulation allows the exchange of hematopoietic cells during embryonic life and the establishment of a chimeric state. Interestingly, these calves did not develop isoantibodies to their twin, suggesting a state of immunologic tolerance.

Peter Medawar acknowledged the importance of Owen's observation and predicted that an exchange of skin grafts between dizygotic calves could verify the tolerance hypothesis, and together with his postdoctoral fellow, Rupert Billingham, he performed a series of grafting experiments that provided direct support for the concept of neonatally acquired transplantation tolerance. Subsequent experiments by Billingham, Leslie Brent, and Medawar demonstrated that neonatally acquired transplantation tolerance could be achieved in mice by inoculation of embryos or intravenous injection of newborn mice with allogeneic cells. Medawar shared the Nobel Prize in 1960 for the discovery of acquired immunologic tolerance.

Just as there are multiple methods to provide for self-tolerance in any given individual, there have been many proposed strategies to induce transplantation tolerance exploiting these pathways. Some of these include clonal deletion or elimination of donor-reactive cells, clonal anergy or functional inactivation of donor-reactive cells, and regulation or suppression of donor-reactive cells. There are rare reports of patients who have discontinued immunosuppression for various reasons and have not experienced rejection. Ongoing studies within this small population of patients seek to determine what mechanisms are responsible for graft maintenance in the absence of immunosuppression. One such study suggests that those kidney transplant patients who discontinue their immunosuppressive treatments for whatever reason and continue to enjoy stable allograft function also have elevated numbers of naïve and transitional B cells in their peripheral blood compared with those patients who remain on immunosuppression, suggesting a role for this cell population in the tolerant state.[49]

There are numerous reports of tolerance in experimental models, but most of these are not effective when translated to higher animal models such as nonhuman primates. Although there are several exciting avenues of research and even clinical trials in humans, currently there is no proven regimen to induce transplantation tolerance that would be widely applicable. Here are a few strategies of particular interest that are currently under investigation.[50]

T Cell Ablation

Most currently employed immunosuppressive regimens involve the use of induction therapy. Many rely on some form of antilymphocyte preparation, most commonly RATG, to eliminate or to inactive recipient cells at the time of transplantation. They are used in the very early post-transplantation period, which corresponds to the time when ischemia and reperfusion of the graft accompanied by the surgical trauma significantly increase immune recognition. These preparations successfully remove T cells from the circulation for several days, and those that are present remain anergic for some period. Use of these agents has significantly reduced the rate of acute rejection and allowed minimization of immunosuppression in several different protocols. A number of groups have undertaken clinical trials using early recipient T cell depletion in combination with various other immunosuppressive strategies to induce tolerance. The prevailing concept is one of T cell clone reduction in an effort to allow existing tolerance mechanisms to be effective. Several studies have used alemtuzumab to induce profound T cell depletion. Despite achieving depletion that was similar to promising preclinical studies with respect to kinetics, magnitude, and effectiveness within the secondary lymphoid tissues, treatment with alemtuzumab alone or in combination with deoxyspergualin was not sufficient to induce tolerance in adult humans.[38] Newer studies have combined alemtuzumab with belatacept and rapamycin with promising results, although tolerance was not achieved.[51] The failure of these T cell–centric approaches suggests that other components of the immune system, such as B cells, NK cells, or monocytes, may need to be specifically targeted to achieve tolerance. Whereas depletion alone has not been able to establish tolerance, it has allowed minimization of immunosuppression to a single agent in some cases and likely facilitates other protolerant approaches.

Costimulation Blockade

T cell activation requires not only interaction between the TCR complex and MHC-bound peptide but also sufficient costimulatory signals to promote a successful response. TCR ligation in the absence of appropriate costimulation results in T cell inactivation or anergy. This mechanism is used presumably as a mechanism of peripheral tolerance to control any aberrant, self-reactive T cell that may have escaped the thymic selection process. Researchers have tried to exploit this through the development of antibodies or fusion proteins designed to block these costimulatory interactions. Interruption of costimulatory pathways at the time of transplantation should thus selectively inactivate or anergize only those cells specific for donor antigen, leaving nonreactive cells unaffected. Preexisting immunity and innate responses should be unaffected by this approach. There are multiple animal models of transplantation in which this has proved to be the case, particularly with simultaneous blockade of the CD28 and CD40 pathways. This approach in both rodents and primates has resulted in prolonged survival of cardiac and renal allografts without the need for any subsequent immunosuppression and without any infectious or malignant side effects. The extrapolation of these results to clinical practice has been thus far disappointing. In the only human tolerance trial of costimulation blockade, hu5C8, a humanized anti-CD154 monoclonal antibody, demonstrated limited efficacy and was associated with potential thromboembolic toxicity. Newly developed agents that block the CD28 pathway are now being tested as maintenance agents, which may pave the way for their use in future tolerance trials. In addition, there are numerous other therapeutic reagents that have been or are in development (such as antibodies to CD40, CD134 [OX40L], ICOS, and many other costimulatory pathways). It remains to be seen which of these will make it through the gauntlet of drug development, but there are exciting possibilities for tolerance regimens in the future.[19]

Mixed Chimerism

Mixed hematopoietic chimerism is associated with a particularly robust form of donor-specific tolerance. This approach involves both central and peripheral mechanisms for induction and maintenance of tolerance. Mixed chimerism refers to a recipient who possesses both self and donor-derived hematopoietic cells after bone marrow transplantation. Similar to the normal physiologic process, donor marrow elements migrate to the thymus and participate in thymic selection, resulting in central deletion of potentially donor-reactive T cells. Presumably similar events occur within the bone marrow for B cell selection. The peripheral compartment can be pharmacologically deleted in a nonspecific fashion at the time of transplantation, or alternatively, donor antigen delivered at the time of bone marrow infusion engages donor-reactive cells in the absence of appropriate costimulation, causing peripheral deletion, anergy, or regulation and resulting in donor-specific nonresponsiveness.

In humans, successful bone marrow transplantation allows the acceptance of subsequent organ allografts from the same donor in the absence of immunosuppression. Conventional bone marrow transplantation regimens, however, are typically myeloablative in nature, and the associated toxicities are too great for them to be employed as part of a solid organ tolerance trial. Newer advances in nonmyeloablative techniques with less toxicity have since paved the way for the clinical application and testing of mixed chimerism–based strategies. An initial trial to test the efficacy of a mixed chimerism strategy to induce tolerance was performed in highly selected patients suffering from both end-stage renal failure and multiple myeloma. These patients simultaneously received bone marrow and a kidney from an HLA-identical sibling. The regimen lead to chimerism in all six patients; four had transient chimerism, and the remaining two progressed into full chimeras. Three patients remain operationally tolerant without any immunosuppression after a reported follow-up of up to 7 years. Recently, the same group of investigators reported on a similar protocol in haploidentical living related donor-recipient pairs that resulted in the successful induction of transient chimerism and tolerance. None of these patients possessed concomitant indications for bone marrow transplantation, such as multiple myeloma, as was the case in the first trial. One allograft was lost to irreversible humoral rejection, but remarkably the other four recipients have sustained stable renal allograft function for up to 5 years after complete withdrawal of immunosuppressive drugs.[52] The conditioning regimen required resulted in profound T, B, and NK cell depletion and substantial myelosuppression, leading to severe leukopenia and capillary leak syndrome. Interestingly, the biologic phenomenon that inspired the protocol, mixed chimerism, was not achieved in any patient, suggesting that the predominant effect is one of intensive induction. Although there is still a significant need to develop regimens to induce transplantation tolerance, this effort will have to be balanced with the exceptional patient and allograft outcomes presently available with current immunosuppressive therapies.[53]

XENOTRANSPLANTATION

The most pressing problem in clinical transplantation is the shortage of available organs. More than 100,000 individuals are currently listed and awaiting organ transplantation. Many more individuals could benefit from transplantation but, given the shortage of organs, are not currently considered. Those who are placed on the list for transplantation must often wait a significant amount of time before an organ becomes available, during which time their clinical status can deteriorate, diminishing their ability to survive and to recover from surgery. An alternative source of organs could potentially come from another species, xenotransplantation. In addition to increasing the supply of available organs, xenotransplantation also offers some of the same benefits realized with living donors, such as decreased ischemic time and injury as well as optimization of the recipient's health status. There are potential novel disadvantages with xenotransplantation, such as zoonotic viral transmission. Xenografts may be concordant and discordant, depending on the proximity in evolution of the given species to humans. This proximity markedly influences the immune response, and the implications are discussed here.

Concordant Xenografts

Concordant xenografts refer to transplants between closely related species; for humans, these include Old World monkeys and apes. The critical element defining an animal as concordant is the assembly of carbohydrate antigens on the cell surface. Similar to humans, concordant species lack galactosyltransferase, and as a result, their carbohydrates are the typical blood group antigens and they lack the N-linked disaccharide galactose-α(1-3)-galactose (α-Gal). Thus, the natural antibodies present in the circulation of potential human recipients can be predicted by straightforward blood group typing, thereby avoiding the problem of hyperacute rejection. Even though hyperacute rejection is not a threat, the typical mechanisms of graft rejection remain, including acute cellular rejection, acute vascular rejection, and, presumably, chronic rejection. Surprisingly, most of the critical molecular elements responsible for antigen presentation and T cell–mediated rejection are evolutionarily conserved in mammals. That is to say, MHC molecules, adhesion proteins, and costimulatory molecules are similar across species and are adequate for immune function. Consequently, concordant xenografts undergo cellular and humoral rejection in a similar fashion as would a totally MHC-mismatched allograft in the absence of immunosuppression.

Several experimental models of concordant xenograft transplantation as well as occasional ventures into the clinical arena have clearly demonstrated that concordant xenotransplantation is feasible. The most famous case occurred almost 25 years ago when clinicians at Loma Linda transplanted a baboon heart into an infant born with hypoplastic heart syndrome. The child survived for 20 days after the transplantation before eventually succumbing to primarily humoral-mediated rejection.[54] This foray into the realm of clinical xenotransplantation highlighted the ethical issues associated with primate to human transplantation. Widespread application of concordant xenografts would quickly deplete the supply of nonhuman primates, particularly when a loss rate extrapolated from poorly matched allografts is taken into consideration. In addition, there is significant concern that zoonotic transfer of disease, in particular retroviral transmission, will put the patient and the public at undue risk. Given these factors, it is unlikely that concordant xenotransplantation will ever gain widespread application.

Discordant Xenografts

Transplant concordance among species is predominantly determined on the basis of the expression of the enzyme galactosyltransferase. This enzyme is responsible for differential expression of carbohydrate moieties on the cell surface of discordant species, primarily α-Gal expression. In considering human recipients, discordant xenograft donors would include New World monkeys and other mammals, but for physiologic concerns (e.g., organ size, availability), pigs would be the preferred animal donor. When organs from discordant species are transplanted into humans, they rapidly undergo hyperacute rejection. The primary mechanism relies on the presence of preformed IgM antibodies against cell surface carbohydrate moieties, particularly α-Gal. These so-called natural antibodies are similar to those antibodies that define the blood group antigens. On transplantation, they bind to the endothelial cells on the donor organ and in concert with complement precipitate an irreversible reaction of cell damage, thrombosis, and immediate graft failure. As with concordant xenografts, the remainder of the acquired and innate immune responses may also play an important role in the rejection process.

Despite the aggressive immune response elicited by discordant xenograft transplantation, enthusiasm and research continue toward establishing a xenogeneic source of donor organs. Several groups have now developed transgenic pigs that express various human complement regulator proteins, such as CD59, CD55 (decay-accelerating factor), and membrane cofactor protein. Other groups have developed α(1-3)-galactosyltransferase knockout animals, which would eliminate the expression of α-Gal, removing the major target of complement activation (Fig. 24-21). In fact, baboons transplanted with hearts from decay-accelerating factor transgenic pigs enjoy prolonged survival compared with control pig donors. More recently, there have been exciting reports of prolonged xenograft survival (in some cases >1 year) in preclinical nonhuman primate models of heart, islet, and kidney transplantation.[55-57] Whereas there are significant barriers before clinical application, genetic engineering may conceivably allow an endless supply of made-to-order organs.

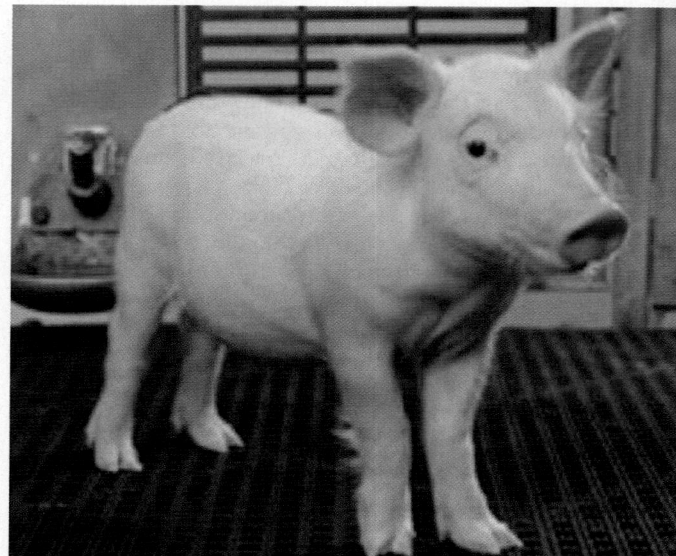

FIGURE 24-21 Xenotransplantation using genetically engineered porcine donors. Example of an α-galactosyltransferase knockout, human decay-accelerating factor (hDAF) transgenic donor pig. (Courtesy National Swine Resource and Research Center [NSRRC]; http://www.nsrrc.missouri.edu/NSRRC0009info.asp.)

NEW AREAS OF TRANSPLANTATION

Islet Cell Transplantation

The concept of islet cell transplantation to treat diabetes is not novel, but reliable reversal of diabetes after islet transplantation is a relatively recent accomplishment. Techniques for islet isolation have undergone refinement for most of the latter half of the last century. Clinical application of this technique, however, was largely hampered by both the lack of efficient isolation techniques and the lack of effective immunosuppressive regimens, many of which included diabetogenic drugs such as steroids, which promoted diabetes themselves, resulting in poor outcomes (~10% of recipients became insulin independent after transplantation). In 2000, a group from Edmonton, Alberta, demonstrated successful, consistent insulin independence after islet transplantation. The principal change was the development of a steroid-free immunosuppressive protocol composed of low-dose tacrolimus, sirolimus, and daclizumab. The initial report ignited incredible enthusiasm within the diabetes community, but the optimism has since been tempered by less promising long-term results. In a subsequent multicenter trial, less than half of the 36 patients achieved insulin independence 1 year after transplantation, and those who initially did achieve independence lost it over time. In addition to the questions of long-term efficacy, islet transplantation is associated with substantial costs, and there are questions about its safety and ultimate utility. Given these more recent results, the number of clinical islet transplantations performed worldwide has dramatically decreased in the last few years. Despite these setbacks, there is tremendous promise for the field of islet transplantation, including research focusing on ex vivo islet expansion and the use of stem cells, newer more effective yet less toxic immunosuppressive protocols, tolerance regimens, and xenotransplantation.

Vascularized Composite Tissue Transplantation

Vascularized composite tissue transplantation involves the transfer of multiple tissue types, including skin, fat, muscle, nerves, blood vessels, tendon, and bone, within one functional unit, such as a hand or face. Annually, there are millions of patients with lost limbs or extensive soft tissue injuries who could potentially benefit from reconstruction with composite tissue transfer. Several of these cases have been highlighted within the media in the last few years, and the ethical debate over non-lifesaving transplantation has generated extensive discussion. The first successful hand transplantation was performed in Lyon, France, in 1998, and since that time, more than 50 patients have undergone single- or double-hand transplants. Many have recovered remarkable levels of function, including tying shoes, dialing a cell phone, turning door knobs, and throwing a ball, as well as sensitivity to hot and cold. Unfortunately, some patients have required amputation of the transplanted hand after uncontrolled rejection, most of which has been attributed to noncompliance. Shortly after the early reports of hand transplantation, there have been numerous descriptions of other successful composite tissue allografts, including larynx, trachea,[58] and more recently face.[59]

The first successful face composite allograft was reported by a group of surgeons from France in 2005. Not long after, the first near-total human face transplantation in the United States was performed in 2008 on a patient with severe midface trauma after a gunshot wound. Many patients regain the ability to perform many normal daily activities, such as breathing through the nose, recovering a sense of smell and taste, speaking intelligibly, and using the mouth to eat solid foods and to drink from a cup (Fig. 24-22).[59] Unlike traditional solid organ transplantation, many of the cases of composite tissue transplantation provoke ethical, economic, and clinical dilemmas. Some may argue that subjecting recipients to the risks of surgery and lifelong immunosuppression for a non–life-sustaining transplant may not be appropriate. Nevertheless, these transplants can totally transform the life of a severely disabled or disfigured patient, improving both form and function. With the advent of increasingly less toxic immunosuppressants and possible tolerance strategies, composite tissue transplantation will become an ever-increasing part of standard clinical treatment.

CONCLUSION

More than a half-century has passed since the first successful solid organ transplantation. Today, thousands of patients with end-stage diseases undergo lifesaving transplantation each year.

That which was once considered impossible is now an everyday occurrence, and those transplant recipients are leading healthy, productive lives with an organ from another individual functioning inside of them. The concept of replacing a diseased organ with a healthy one is simple in concept, yet the details of managing the rejection response can become complex. The immune system typically generates a highly organized yet regulated response when challenged. Many of the principal details of the normal immune response were described by researchers examining the mechanisms of allograft rejection. In fact, surgeons garnered multiple Noble Prizes in Medicine for their significant contributions to the field. Whereas short-term allograft survival rates have steadily improved, there are still many issues on which to improve. The availability of adequate donor organs remains the most pressing issue restricting the majority of potential recipients from receiving a life-sustaining transplant. There continues to be progress in xenotransplantation and tissue engineering, and they may yet provide for an unlimited supply of safe, transplantable organs. There are significant drawbacks to nonselective immunosuppressive therapy, such as increased risks of infections and malignant disease, economic constraints, and long-term effects, including renal insufficiency, diabetes, hyperlipidemia, and cardiovascular disease. Increasingly targeted immunosuppressive agents continue to be developed and tested. Ultimately, the goal would be risk-free, donor-specific immunosuppression. The development of a safe, widely applicable regimen that reliably produces transplantation tolerance would eliminate many of the problems currently associated with organ transplantation. Indeed, one of the medical miracles of the last century is the infancy and growth of organ transplantation. Although challenges remain, transplant surgeons and scientists will undoubtedly be at the forefront of discovery and innovation as we move forward.

SELECTED REFERENCES

Abbas AK, Lichtman AH, Pillai S: *Cellular and molecular immunology*, ed 8, Philadelphia, 2014, Saunders Elsevier.

Concise, well-developed textbook of immunology.

Brent L: *A history of transplantation immunology*, San Diego, 1997, Academic Press.

An interesting historical perspective on the development of transplantation immunology.

Chong AS, Alegre ML: The impact of infection and tissue damage in solid-organ transplantation. *Nat Rev Immunol* 12:459–471, 2012.

An excellent review on the importance of the innate immune response in the rejection process.

Fishman JA: Infection in solid-organ transplant recipients. *N Engl J Med* 357:2601–2614, 2007.

Insightful review of infection in transplantation.

Halloran PF: Immunosuppressive drugs for kidney transplantation. *N Engl J Med* 351:2715–2729, 2004.

Excellent overview of clinical transplantation and immunosuppression.

Wood KJ, Bushell A, Hester J: Regulatory immune cells in transplantation. *Nat Rev Immunol* 12:417–430, 2012.

A well-written review of regulatory cell populations and their importance in transplantation.

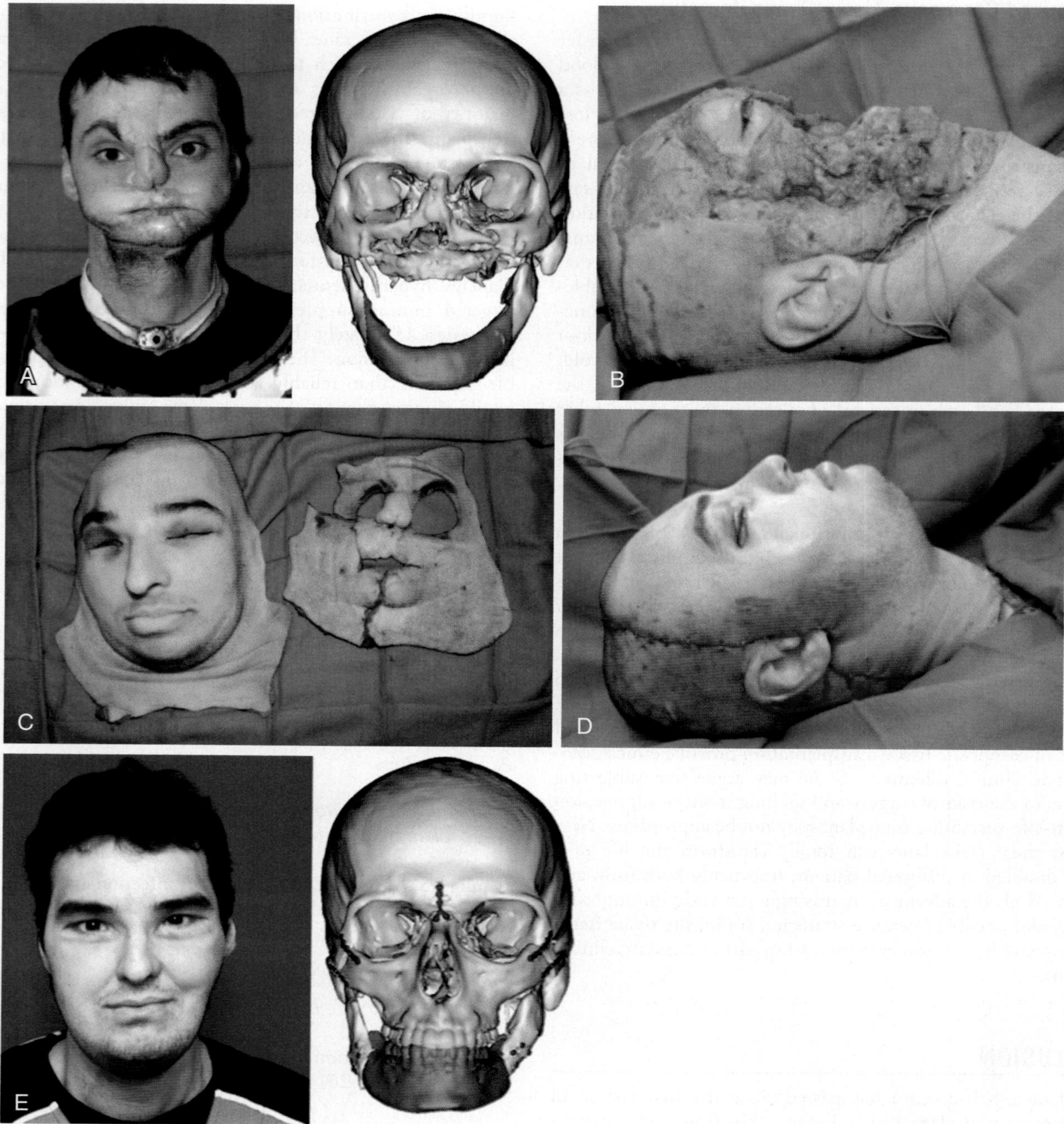

FIGURE 24-22 **A,** Frontal view and computed tomography scan reconstruction of patient before transplantation. **B,** Intraoperative photograph after removal of disfigured tissue, hardware, and bone. **C,** Side-by-side comparison of the donor face attached to its underlying skeletal architecture on the left and the recipient's face on the right. **D,** Intraoperative photograph of final facial reconstruction. **E,** Frontal view and computed tomography scan reconstruction 16 months after transplantation. (From Dorafshar A, Branko, B, Christy, M, et al: Total face, double jaw, and tongue transplantation: An evolutionary concept. *Plast Reconstr Surg* 131:241–251, 2013; Khalifian A, Brazio P, Mohan R, et al: Facial transplantation: The first 9 years. *Lancet* 384:2153–2163, 2014. Courtesy Eduardo D. Rodriguez, MD, DDS.)

REFERENCES

1. Carrel A: Landmark article, Nov 14, 1908: Results of the transplantation of blood vessels, organs and limbs. By Alexis Carrel. *JAMA* 250:944–953, 1983.
2. Billingham RE, Brent L, Medawar PB: Actively acquired tolerance of foreign cells. *Nature* 172:603–606, 1953.
3. Billingham RE, Brent L, Medawar PB: 'Actively acquired tolerance' of foreign cells. 1953. *Transplantation* 76:1409–1412, 2003.
4. Murray JE, Lang S, Miller BF: Observations on the natural history of renal homotransplants in dogs. *Surg Forum* 5:241–244, 1955.
5. Dempsey PW, Allison ME, Akkaraju S, et al: C3d of complement as a molecular adjuvant: Bridging innate and acquired immunity. *Science* 271:348–350, 1996.
6. Campbell RD, Trowsdale J: Map of the human MHC. *Immunol Today* 14:349–352, 1993.
7. Parham P, Ohta T: Population biology of antigen presentation by MHC class I molecules. *Science* 272:67–74, 1996.
8. Bjorkman PJ, Saper MA, Samraoui B, et al: Structure of the human class I histocompatibility antigen, HLA-A2. *Nature* 329:506–512, 1987.
9. Bevan MJ: Cross-priming. *Nat Immunol* 7:363–365, 2006.
10. Brown JH, Jardetzky TS, Gorga JC, et al: Three-dimensional structure of the human class II histocompatibility antigen HLA-DR1. *Nature* 364:33–39, 1993.
11. Teyton L, O'Sullivan D, Dickson PW, et al: Invariant chain distinguishes between the exogenous and endogenous antigen presentation pathways. *Nature* 348:39–44, 1990.
12. Davis MM, Bjorkman PJ: T-cell antigen receptor genes and T-cell recognition. *Nature* 334:395–402, 1988.
13. Kappler JW, Roehm N, Marrack P: T cell tolerance by clonal elimination in the thymus. *Cell* 49:273–280, 1987.
14. Viola A, Lanzavecchia A: T cell activation determined by T cell receptor number and tunable thresholds. *Science* 273:104–106, 1996.
15. Chambers CA, Allison JP: Co-stimulation in T cell responses. *Curr Opin Immunol* 9:396–404, 1997.
16. Larsen CP, Pearson TC: The CD40 pathway in allograft rejection, acceptance, and tolerance. *Curr Opin Immunol* 9:641–647, 1997.
17. Schwartz RH: A cell culture model for T lymphocyte clonal anergy. *Science* 248:1349–1356, 1990.
18. Rostaing L, Vincenti F, Grinyo J, et al: Long-term belatacept exposure maintains efficacy and safety at 5 years: Results from the long-term extension of the BENEFIT study. *Am J Transplant* 13:2875–2883, 2013.
19. Ford ML, Adams AB, Pearson TC: Targeting co-stimulatory pathways: Transplantation and autoimmunity. *Nat Rev Nephrol* 10:14–24, 2014.
20. Wood KJ, Sakaguchi S: Regulatory T cells in transplantation tolerance. *Nat Rev Immunol* 3:199–210, 2003.
21. Gloor JM, DeGoey SR, Pineda AA, et al: Overcoming a positive crossmatch in living-donor kidney transplantation. *Am J Transplant* 3:1017–1023, 2003.
22. Gourishankar S, Halloran PF: Late deterioration of organ transplants: A problem in injury and homeostasis. *Curr Opin Immunol* 14:576–583, 2002.
23. Rhen T, Cidlowski JA: Antiinflammatory action of glucocorticoids—new mechanisms for old drugs. *N Engl J Med* 353:1711–1723, 2005.
24. Calne RY, Murray JE: Inhibition of the rejection of renal homografts in dogs by Burroughs Wellcome 57-322. *Surg Forum* 12:118–120, 1961.
25. Sollinger HW: Mycophenolate mofetil for the prevention of acute rejection in primary cadaveric renal allograft recipients. U.S. Renal Transplant Mycophenolate Mofetil Study Group. *Transplantation* 60:225–232, 1995.
26. Borel JF, Feurer C, Gubler HU, et al: Biological effects of cyclosporin A: A new antilymphocytic agent. *Agents Actions* 6:468–475, 1976.
27. Kirk AD, Jacobson LM, Heisey DM, et al: Posttransplant diastolic hypertension: Associations with intragraft transforming growth factor-beta, endothelin, and renin transcription. *Transplantation* 64:1716–1720, 1997.
28. Kino T, Hatanaka H, Miyata S, et al: FK-506, a novel immunosuppressant isolated from a Streptomyces. II. Immunosuppressive effect of FK-506 in vitro. *J Antibiot (Tokyo)* 40:1256–1265, 1987.
29. Fruman DA, Klee CB, Bierer BE, et al: Calcineurin phosphatase activity in T lymphocytes is inhibited by FK 506 and cyclosporin A. *Proc Natl Acad Sci U S A* 89:3686–3690, 1992.
30. Hardinger KL, Rhee S, Buchanan P, et al: A prospective, randomized, double-blinded comparison of thymoglobulin versus Atgam for induction immunosuppressive therapy: 10-year results. *Transplantation* 86:947–952, 2008.
31. Merion RM, Howell T, Bromberg JS: Partial T-cell activation and anergy induction by polyclonal antithymocyte globulin. *Transplantation* 65:1481–1489, 1998.
32. Swanson SJ, Hale DA, Mannon RB, et al: Kidney transplantation with rabbit antithymocyte globulin induction and sirolimus monotherapy. *Lancet* 360:1662–1664, 2002.
33. Matas AJ, Kandaswamy R, Gillingham KJ, et al: Prednisone-free maintenance immunosuppression—a 5-year experience. *Am J Transplant* 5:2473–2478, 2005.
34. A randomized clinical trial of OKT3 monoclonal antibody for acute rejection of cadaveric renal transplants. Ortho Multicenter Transplant Study Group. *N Engl J Med* 313:337–342, 1985.
35. Vincenti F, Kirkman R, Light S, et al: Interleukin-2-receptor blockade with daclizumab to prevent acute rejection in renal transplantation. Daclizumab Triple Therapy Study Group. *N Engl J Med* 338:161–165, 1998.
36. Nashan B, Moore R, Amlot P, et al: Randomised trial of basiliximab versus placebo for control of acute cellular rejection in renal allograft recipients. CHIB 201 International Study Group. *Lancet* 350:1193–1198, 1997.
37. Calne R, Friend P, Moffatt S, et al: Prope tolerance, perioperative campath 1H, and low-dose cyclosporin monotherapy in renal allograft recipients. *Lancet* 351:1701–1702, 1998.
38. Kirk AD, Hale DA, Mannon RB, et al: Results from a human renal allograft tolerance trial evaluating the humanized CD52-specific monoclonal antibody alemtuzumab (CAMPATH-1H). *Transplantation* 76:120–129, 2003.
39. Samuelsson A, Towers TL, Ravetch JV: Anti-inflammatory activity of IVIG mediated through the inhibitory Fc receptor. *Science* 291:484–486, 2001.
40. Kuo CJ, Chung J, Fiorentino DF, et al: Rapamycin selectively inhibits interleukin-2 activation of p70 S6 kinase. *Nature* 358:70–73, 1992.

41. Kremer JM, Westhovens R, Leon M, et al: Treatment of rheumatoid arthritis by selective inhibition of T-cell activation with fusion protein CTLA4Ig. *N Engl J Med* 349:1907–1915, 2003.
42. Abrams JR, Lebwohl MG, Guzzo CA, et al: CTLA4Ig-mediated blockade of T-cell costimulation in patients with psoriasis vulgaris. *J Clin Invest* 103:1243–1252, 1999.
43. Larsen CP, Pearson TC, Adams AB, et al: Rational development of LEA29Y (belatacept), a high-affinity variant of CTLA-4–Ig with potent immunosuppressive properties. *Am J Transplant* 5:443–453, 2005.
44. Vincenti F, Larsen C, Durrbach A, et al: Costimulation blockade with belatacept in renal transplantation. *N Engl J Med* 353:770–781, 2005.
45. Cohen JA, Barkhof F, Comi G, et al: Oral fingolimod or intramuscular interferon for relapsing multiple sclerosis. *N Engl J Med* 362:402–415, 2010.
46. Fishman JA: Infection in solid-organ transplant recipients. *N Engl J Med* 357:2601–2614, 2007.
47. Euvrard S, Kanitakis J, Claudy A: Skin cancers after organ transplantation. *N Engl J Med* 348:1681–1691, 2003.
48. Ojo AO, Held PJ, Port FK, et al: Chronic renal failure after transplantation of a nonrenal organ. *N Engl J Med* 349:931–940, 2003.
49. Newell KA, Turka LA: Tolerance signatures in transplant recipients. *Curr Opin Organ Transplant* 20:400–405, 2015.
50. Newell KA, Larsen CP, Kirk AD: Transplant tolerance: Converging on a moving target. *Transplantation* 81:1–6, 2006.
51. Kirk AD, Guasch A, Xu H, et al: Renal transplantation using belatacept without maintenance steroids or calcineurin inhibitors. *Am J Transplant* 14:1142–1151, 2014.
52. Kawai T, Sachs DH, Sprangers B, et al: Long-term results in recipients of combined HLA-mismatched kidney and bone marrow transplantation without maintenance immunosuppression. *Am J Transplant* 14:1599–1611, 2014.
53. Sachs DH, Kawai T, Sykes M: Induction of tolerance through mixed chimerism. *Cold Spring Harb Perspect Med* 4:a015529, 2014.
54. Bailey LL, Nehlsen-Cannarella SL, Concepcion W, et al: Baboon-to-human cardiac xenotransplantation in a neonate. *JAMA* 254:3321–3329, 1985.
55. Iwase H, Liu H, Wijkstrom M, et al: Pig kidney graft survival in a baboon for 136 days: Longest life-supporting organ graft survival to date. *Xenotransplantation* 22:302–309, 2015.
56. Higginbotham L, Mathews D, Breeden CA, et al: Pre-transplant antibody screening and anti-CD154 costimulation blockade promote long-term xenograft survival in a pig-to-primate kidney transplant model. *Xenotransplantation* 22:221–230, 2015.
57. Mohiuddin MM, Singh AK, Corcoran PC, et al: Genetically engineered pigs and target-specific immunomodulation provide significant graft survival and hope for clinical cardiac xenotransplantation. *J Thorac Cardiovasc Surg* 148:1106–1113, discussion 1113-1114, 2014.
58. Delaere P, Vranckx J, Verleden G, et al: Tracheal allotransplantation after withdrawal of immunosuppressive therapy. *N Engl J Med* 362:138–145, 2010.
59. Siemionow M, Papay F, Alam D, et al: Near-total human face transplantation for a severely disfigured patient in the USA. *Lancet* 374:203–209, 2009.

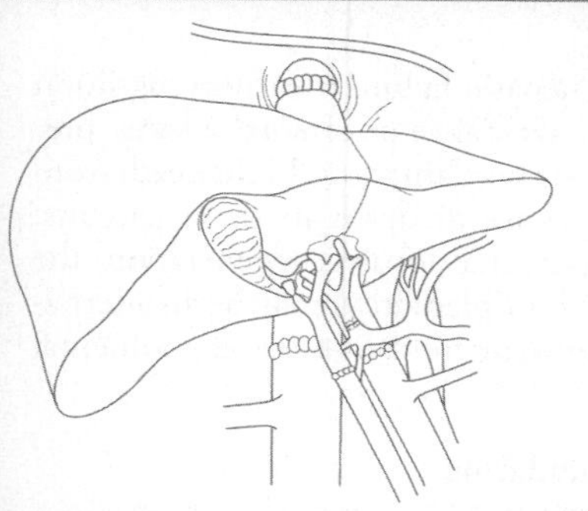

CHAPTER 25

Liver Transplantation

Nancy Ascher

OUTLINE

HISTORY

The ability to replace the human liver successfully reflects the rich history of transplantation. Transplantation moved beyond the exchange of skin and tissue with the development of vascular techniques. Sewing blood vessels together, as described by Alexis Carrel at the outset of the 20th century, made it possible for researchers to implant whole organs for the first time. This development set the stage for the implantation of organs into humans.

The kidney was the first organ for which transplantation was attempted. The procedure is straightforward with anastomosis of the vein, artery, and ureter, and the production of urine is an immediate visible marker of transplantation success. Work was undertaken for the other solid organs, but the technical aspects were more challenging than for kidney transplantation. Although progress in kidney transplantation was related to its technical ease, immunologic problems hampered progress until the development of the immunosuppressive agent azathioprine. The first successful human kidney transplantation was in 1954.[1] It avoided the need for immunosuppression because it was a live donor kidney transplant exchanged between identical twins; this case was proof of concept that solid organ transplantation could successfully be achieved. The field of kidney transplantation was further fueled by the U.S. government underwriting the support of patients with end-stage renal disease, which fostered advances in kidney transplantation and hemodialysis. The parallel development of the concept of brain death[2] resulted in a potential source of donor organs for the nascent filed of transplantation. The first human liver transplantation was performed in 1963 by Thomas Starzl. The patient suffered from biliary atresia, had coagulopathy, and did not survive the surgery.[3] Additional attempts in Berlin, Boston, and Paris were also unsuccessful. Subsequent initial successes in orthotopic liver transplantation were in patients with liver cancer. These patients had less portal hypertension and less complicated surgery but were not long-term survivors secondary to recurrent disease, technical problems, and lack of adequate immunosuppression.

In the early 1980s, liver transplantation in the United States was limited to a handful of programs; initial results were poor, with less than 30% 1-year survival. A major advance came with the clinical introduction of cyclosporine for immunosuppression in solid organ transplantation.[4] Its use and tacrolimus in liver transplant recipients allowed further developments in this field.

As success in liver transplantation increased, more centers initiated programs, and increasing numbers of patients availed themselves of this therapy. In attempts to provide timely transplantation to patients with the greatest need, local, regional, and national distribution schemes were developed and allocation to patients on the waiting list became based on need rather than on time on the list (see later, "Organ Shortage, Mode for End-Stage Liver Disease, and Liver Distribution").

The increasing disparity between available livers from brain dead deceased donors and potential recipients has led to a number of advances that serve to increase the donor pool. These include split liver transplantation, live donor liver transplantation, the use of donors after cardiac death, and the use of extended criteria donors. These topics are covered in detail.

INDICATIONS AND CONTRAINDICATIONS

Indications

As the outcome of liver transplantation has improved, the indications have expanded to include any compromise of life from chronic liver insufficiency, chronic liver disease with acute decompensation, acute liver failure, and enzyme deficiencies (Table 25-1). Liver transplantation is also indicated for a limited number of patients with primary liver tumors. Rarely, metastatic disease has been an indication for transplantation; whereas a metastatic neuroendocrine tumor is an accepted indication, metastatic gastrointestinal cancer is controversial.

The first issue in determining candidacy for transplantation is whether a given patient would benefit from liver replacement. The second issue that must be addressed is whether the patient can withstand the challenge of a liver transplantation surgery.

TABLE 25-1 Indications for Liver Transplantation

ADULTS	%	CHILDREN	%
Noncholestatic cirrhosis	65	Biliary atresia	58
Viral hepatitis B and C		Inborn errors of metabolism	11
Alcoholic*		Cholestatic	9
Cryptogenic		Primary sclerosing cholangitis	
Cholestatic	14	Alagille syndrome	
Primary biliary cirrhosis		Autoimmune	4
Primary sclerosing cholangitis		Viral hepatitis	2
Autoimmune	5	Miscellaneous	16
Malignant neoplasm	2		
Miscellaneous	14		

*Most alcoholic patients are coinfected with the hepatitis C virus.

Compromise in cardiac or pulmonary function may prohibit the patient as a candidate. In some cases, failure of an additional organ system may dictate combination transplantations. Although kidney-liver transplantations are relatively common, heart-liver and lung-liver transplantations are rarely performed.[5]

Regardless of the specific cause of liver disease, patients with chronic liver disease who have deteriorated tend to present with common signs and symptoms. These include coagulopathy, thrombocytopenia, muscle wasting, gynecomastia, ascites, varices, encephalopathy, and renal insufficiency. These physiologic perturbations may lead to life-threatening complications; patients with ascites are susceptible to spontaneous bacterial peritonitis, leading to sepsis or the development of a peritoneal-pleural fistula with respiratory compromise. Gastrointestinal bleeding is the potential complication of varices. An acute exacerbation of chronic liver disease can be triggered by sepsis, gastrointestinal bleeding, or progressive renal insufficiency. Some diseases, such as Wilson disease or autoimmune hepatitis, may be manifested with an acute decompensation without a prior diagnosis of liver disease.

The production of many essential proteins originates in the liver. The inborn errors of metabolism reflect failure of production of crucial enzymes in the liver. Liver transplantation cures the disease by replacing the liver cells with competent metabolic pathways; it is recommended for those diseases in which there is no central nervous system compromise.

Fulminant Hepatic Failure

Fulminant hepatic failure refers to the acute onset of liver failure with the absence of previous liver disease. The entity is defined as the presence of encephalopathy within 8 weeks of jaundice.

In addition to encephalopathy, the disease is characterized by jaundice, coagulopathy, metabolic acidosis, and renal insufficiency. Encephalopathy may progress to coma. Once a patient reaches stage 4 encephalopathy, the rate of successful treatment without transplantation ranges from 5% to 20%, depending on the cause.[6] The most common cause in the United States and England is acetaminophen overdose,[7] either accidental or intentional. In Asia, acute hepatitis from hepatitis B viral infection is the most common cause.[8] In a significant number of cases, the specific cause is unknown. Acetaminophen overdose carries a relatively good prognosis without transplantation if the metabolic functions related to the liver are maintained. Medication has been largely unsuccessful, as have liver support devices. Hypothermia may prove useful in younger patients.[9] The key to successful liver transplantation for fulminant hepatic failure is early recognition and listing for transplantation, avoidance of cerebral edema, prevention of infection, and timely transplantation. Brain death from cerebral edema is a common cause of death in these patients. Depending on the cause and potential for liver regeneration, the liver assist device or hepatocyte transplantation may be an alternative to liver transplantation, but these modalities are experimental at this time.

Hepatitis C and Liver Transplantation

Chronic hepatitis C virus (HCV) infection is the most common indication for transplantation in the West at present. In the United States, it is estimated that 5 million individuals are infected with HCV. In approximately 20% of these patients, a chronic injury state develops in the liver, with progression to cirrhosis and liver insufficiency. HCV can be subdivided into five groups or serotypes. The most common U.S. serotype is genotype 1, which is less responsive than genotype 2 or 3 to antiviral medication.

HCV infection recurs after transplantation because the virus resides in tissues other than the liver. The aggressiveness of the recurrent hepatitis C after liver transplantation cannot be predicted; risk factors include donor age, treatment for acute rejection, and level of hepatitis C viremia at the time of transplantation.[10] Another factor that predicts HCV reinfection severity after transplantation is the treatment for rejection after transplantation (with additional steroids or antilymphocyte preparations).[11] In the past, transplantation of a liver from a donor older than 40 years was associated with a greater risk of recurrent cirrhosis than in transplantation from a younger donor. Hepatitis C treatment with interferon and ribavirin is effective in approximately 50% of patients before transplantation.[12] These medications are poorly tolerated in patients with end-stage liver disease; renal insufficiency limits the dose of ribavirin, and hypersplenism with low white blood cell count limits the dose of interferon.

Recent developments in the treatment of hepatitis C with sofosbuvir and ribavirin have vastly changed the therapeutic landscape.[13] Marked reduction in viral load may be demonstrated shortly after initiation of the oral agents; the treatment is shorter than with the previous agents, and side effects are minimal. This class of direct-acting antiviral agents will likely decrease the need for retransplantation for recurrent hepatitis C. The cost of these agents is currently high, and the proposed use before versus after transplantation has been questioned.[14] It is easier to achieve a significant decrement in viral load in recipients of liver donor transplants compared with recipients of cadaveric grafts as the timing of transplantation is known. It is hoped that the direct-acting antiviral agents will decrease the need for transplantation in patients with hepatitis C from lack of progression to decompensation or the development of hepatocellular carcinoma (HCC).[15]

Hepatitis B

Chronic hepatitis B virus infection is the most common cause of chronic liver disease in endemic regions of Asia and Africa and the most common cause of death from hepatitis worldwide.[16]

The hepatitis B vaccine is effective in inducing the formation of antibodies that will protect against hepatitis B exposure. As the use of hepatitis B vaccine spreads worldwide, one can look forward to an overall decrease in the incidence of hepatitis B virus infection over time.

In the past, hepatitis B was a major problem after transplantation, with rapid reinfection of the graft. Effective therapy with antiviral agents and hyperimmune globulin has largely eradicated disease recurrence after transplantation.

Primary Biliary Cirrhosis

Primary biliary cirrhosis is a form of autoimmune cholestatic liver disease, with inflammatory injury to the bile ducts. It is a chronic cause of hepatic insufficiency and is characterized by autoimmune markers and some response to immunosuppressants.[17] This disease is more common in women. The disease may recur yeas after transplantation, but its recurrence is unlikely to progress to the need for retransplantation.

Primary Sclerosing Cholangitis

Primary sclerosing cholangitis is an autoimmune disease that is more frequent in men. It progresses over the years to a cholestatic picture associated with scarring of the intrahepatic and extrahepatic bile ducts. The disease is associated with ulcerative colitis in approximately 90% of patients. In a small number of patients (<10%), the process is associated with cholangiocarcinoma.[18] The bile duct involvement in primary sclerosing cholangitis dictates the use of choledochojejunostomy in patients undergoing liver transplantation. Primary sclerosing cholangitis may rarely recur after transplantation.

Alcoholic Liver Disease

Chronic alcohol abuse may cause scarring in the liver, leading to cirrhosis with decompensation. Patients who stop the use of alcohol can prevent progression of the disease. Alcoholic liver disease may be seen in association with other chronic insults to the liver, such as chronic hepatitis C, and in this setting is more likely to progress to decompensation. Most transplantation centers require abstinence from alcohol after transplantation and a period of abstinence (usually 6 months) before transplantation to demonstrate the patient's understanding of the contribution of alcohol to the disease and a commitment to abstinence. Acute alcoholic hepatitis has recently been suggested as an appropriate indication for liver transplantation in a select subset of patients.[19] As the disease has a dismal prognosis otherwise,[20] larger studies are necessary to determine the utility of this approach.

Nonalcoholic Steatohepatitis

Nonalcoholic steatohepatitis[21] reflects a pending epidemic of liver disease associated with the progression of obesity and metabolic syndrome throughout the world. Fatty infiltration of the liver with inflammation and subsequent injury and fibrosis are the histologic features. The associated metabolic syndrome and diabetes dictate evaluation of the coronary arteries of these potential recipients. Nonalcoholic steatohepatitis may recur after transplantation.

Biliary Atresia

Biliary atresia is the most common indication for liver transplantation in the pediatric patient and is a major concern in the infant with persistent jaundice after birth. Its diagnosis is made with liver biopsy and the finding of an absent extrahepatic bile duct at the time of laparotomy. Its cause is unclear.

Affected infants are treated with hepaticojejunostomy (Kasai procedure). The success of this procedure is dictated by surgery soon after birth and the size of the bile ducts in the bile duct plate. Post-Kasai cholangitis may hasten the need for transplantation. An early indication for transplantation in children is a failure to grow. Intervention with transplantation at this stage may allow catch-up growth. At transplantation, the Roux-en-Y procedure is required for biliary drainage of the transplanted organ.

Contraindications

Patients with liver disease are extensively evaluated to determine their candidacy for transplantation. Cardiac, pulmonary, and renal functions are assessed. Patients are also seen by a social worker or other mental health professional for psychosocial evaluation. Each patient is individually evaluated to determine the risk-benefit ratio of undertaking transplantation. There are generally accepted absolute and relative contraindications to transplantation. In general, contraindications reflect the expectation of a poor outcome.

Systemic infections are considered relative contraindications to transplantation, and uncontrolled bacterial and fungal infections are absolute contraindications to transplantation. Infections in the liver, such as cholangitis, may be an exception to this rule. HIV infection is considered by some groups to be a contraindication, but several studies have shown outcomes comparable to those of matched control patients if the virus is controlled.[22]

Failure of another organ may be a contraindication to transplantation if that organ cannot be replaced or expected to recover. Kidney transplantation accompanies liver transplantation in 5% of cases. On occasion, liver-heart transplantation is performed for diseases such as amyloidosis; combined liver-lung transplantation for diseases such as cystic fibrosis has been performed in rare circumstances.[5]

Patients with chronic liver disease can develop pulmonary manifestations of their liver disease. Portopulmonary hypertension is considered a contraindication with persistent pulmonary artery pressures higher than 50 mm Hg in the presence of elevated pulmonary vascular resistance.[23] Hepatopulmonary syndrome becomes a contraindication to transplantation when the PaO_2 does not demonstrate marked improvement with administration of 100% oxygen.[24] Inability to care for the transplanted organ adequately because of continued drug or alcohol abuse or lack of commitment to immunosuppressive drugs is considered a contraindication to transplantation. Continued commitment to immunosuppressive drugs is difficult to assess before transplantation; in some series, noncompliance after transplantation has been reported to be up to 35%.[25]

Anatomic considerations may be relative contraindications to liver transplantation. The presence of portal vein thrombosis may be overcome by removal of the thrombosis or a jump graft from the host superior mesenteric vein. With complete thrombosis of the portal system, portal inflow from the infrahepatic vena cava has been used, although use of this procedure is rare and morbidity is high.

Metastatic HCC is considered an absolute contraindication to transplantation, related to poor outcome. The risk of metastatic disease after liver transplantation is dependent on the size and number of HCC nodules in the liver. The Milan criteria for liver transplantation for HCC (single nodule <5 cm or less than three nodules, the largest of which is <3 cm) are used to predict the risk of recurrent disease after transplantation. Patients who meet these criteria have a risk of recurrence that is less than 20%, whereas patients outside the criteria have a recurrence rate of approximately 60%.[26] The Milan criteria are currently used to define acceptable candidates for transplantation in the United States; patients who meet the Milan criteria are given extra priority for transplantation. There is a controversy about transplantation for patients outside the Milan criteria, and there is an interest in finding other methods of identifying those patients who have a low recurrence risk after transplantation. Molecular biomarkers may prove reliable for selecting patients who will benefit from transplantation.[27-29]

Organ Shortage, Model for End-Stage Liver Disease, and Liver Distribution

The decision of whether a patient is a candidate for transplantation and what priority a given patient should have is dictated in part by the relative shortage of deceased donor livers. Despite substantial governmental and community efforts, the needs of the nearly 16,000 patients awaiting transplantation are not met by the approximately 5000 or so donors.[30] Tumors outside the Milan criteria may be treated by locoregional therapy with transarterial chemoembolization or radiofrequency ablation to decrease the tumor to the size prescribed by the Milan criteria; these patients enjoy nearly the same 5-year survival as patients with tumors within the Milan criteria.[31]

With recognition of the improved outcomes of liver transplantation in the 1980s, the transplantation programs proliferated. Livers were allocated to programs and teams rather than to patients, with the transplantation center selecting the most appropriate recipient for a given donor. Because of the concept that the organs should be allocated to patients rather than to centers, lists of patients were created and ordered according to the patient's time waiting on the list, and the organs were offered to the patients as they moved to the top of the list.

The current system of liver distribution in the United States is first on the level of the local organ procurement organization, then to the 11 United Network for Organ Sharing (UNOS) regions, and then shared on a national basis. A patient's priority on the waiting list is based on his or her medical status as determined by the model for end-stage liver disease (MELD) score, which reflects the likelihood of death within 3 months. The MELD score assigns points that reflect the severity of liver disease. The score is based on a formula that considers bilirubin and creatinine levels and the international normalized ratio (INR).[32]

Model for End-Stage Liver Disease Formula

$$\text{MELD score} = (0.957 \times \log_e \text{creatinine [mg/dL]}) + (0.378 \times \log_e \text{bilirubin [mg/dL]}) + (1.120 \times \log_e \text{INR}) + 0.643$$

The components of the MELD score were chosen because they represent objective criteria that can be reviewed and verified compared with ascites and encephalopathy, which were used previously (as part of the Childs-Pugh score) but are subjective and cannot be readily verified. The use of the MELD score to determine liver distribution has led to a significant decrease in the rate of death of potential recipients on the waiting list because it allows livers to be directed to the sickest patients. Patients with a high MELD score at the time of transplantation have slightly poorer survival after transplantation (Table 25-2). Recently, a change toward wider sharing of livers was instituted. The "Share 35" rule dictates that regional rather than local distribution of livers be done for patients with the greatest need (MELD score > 35). The hope is to further decrease death on the waiting list.

For patients with low MELD scores (<15), the risk of death while waiting for transplantation is less than the risk of death after transplantation.[33] The current allocation system therefore discourages transplantation of patients with MELD scores of less than 15 by allocating a liver to all the higher MELD score patients in the region before allowing local use in patients with scores of less than 15. These last two concepts, that sicker patients have a slightly higher risk of poor outcome after liver transplantation and that relatively healthy patients (MELD score < 15) have worse outcomes with transplantation than if they remained on the waiting list, suggest that both pretransplantation and post-transplantation outcomes should be considered in the allocation of livers. Currently, the MELD score weighs only the pretransplantation outcomes, and death on the waiting list has been reduced since the initiation of the MELD score. It has been proposed that the MELD score be replaced as a means to distribute organs with a system that determines potential survival benefit after transplantation or a combination of survival benefit before and after transplantation for patients with chronic liver disease.[34] For some patients, the risk of death or dropout from the list may not be reflected in the laboratory values in the MELD score. For example, patients with HCC benefit from transplantation, even when their laboratory test results are normal. To allow transplantation, an exception is made and additional MELD points are assigned to these patients.[35] This approach is used to transplant these patients before their tumors become so extensive that patients fall outside the limits of criteria for liver transplantation. "MELD exceptions" have also been also used for diseases such as amyloidosis, portopulmonary hypertension, and hepatopulmonary syndrome. MELD exceptions dictate petition to a local review board for access.

TABLE 25-2 Concordance With 3-Month Mortality

SCORE	CONCORDANCE (%)	95% CONFIDENCE INTERVAL
Model for end-stage liver disease (MELD)	0.88	0.85-0.90
Childs-Turcotte-Pugh	0.79	0.75-0.83

Pediatric donor livers are distributed to pediatric patients preferentially. The scoring used in pediatric patients is referred to as the pediatric end-stage liver disease (PELD) score.[36]

Patients with acute liver failure, such as fulminant hepatic failure, are given the highest priority (status 1) for donor organs to avoid the development of cerebral edema and other fatal outcomes. Status 1 supersedes the MELD score in the organ allocation process.

LIVE DONOR LIVER TRANSPLANTATION

Regardless of the distribution scheme used for deceased donor transplants, the need of potential liver transplant recipients far exceeds the supply. As a consequence of this disparity, a number of alternatives have been used to increase the supply, including live donor liver transplantation. The basis for this approach includes the work of Otte and colleagues,[37] who pared down adult-sized livers for use in pediatric patients, as well as the observation that the liver can regenerate after major liver resection for cancer.

Subsequently, Broelsch's team at the University of Chicago thoughtfully raised the medical and ethical issues of pediatric patients dying while awaiting liver transplantation as the foundation for the development of a live donor transplant program.[38]

This program yielded outstanding patient survival, greatly reduced death on the waiting list for the pediatric patients, and led the way for the development of adult-to-adult live donor liver transplantation. The development was further fueled in Asia by the absence of brain death legislation and the cultural and religious reluctance to embrace the brain death concept. Asia, India, and South America represent regions with the most active live donor liver transplant programs, far exceeding the use of cadaveric transplants.

The long history of live donor kidney transplantation has provided the cultural, ethical, and medical framework on which to build live donor liver transplantation, but the issues regarding live donor liver transplantation have been more complex. Long-term studies of kidney transplant donors showed low operative mortality and the same long-term morbidity as for age-matched controls, with no higher incidence of the need for dialysis over time in most patients.[39] To date, there are no longer term evaluations of live liver donors, but concern exists about their long-term course in terms of hepatic reserve and bile duct problems.

It rapidly became clear that operative mortality for live donor liver transplantation was significant, with early death from pulmonary emboli in those who donated the lateral segment of the liver to pediatric recipients and the highly publicized death of a right lobe donor in the United States in 2002. Subsequent deaths throughout the world have underscored the concern for the risks of the procedure. Current estimates are that the risk of death from liver donation is 1 in 500 to 1000; the risk of death from kidney donation is 1 in 3000.[40] The community awaits the effect of liver donation on long-term morbidity and mortality.

The balance between adequate liver mass for the recipient and risk to the donor underscores the challenges for progress in this field. The other major factor is that the perceived need for live donor liver transplantation varies across the United States because there are regional inequities in the availability of cadaver organs.[30] In the United States, live donor liver transplantation for adult patients decreased significantly after the institution of the MELD system and has remained low, constituting less than 5% of liver transplantations carried out.[30] In Asia, without the alternative of deceased donor transplantation, an increasing number of live donor transplantations are performed, with expanding recipient indications, and centers have experience with large numbers of live donor liver transplantations.[41]

A number of groups have been rethinking the use of left lobe grafts, largely because of concern for donor safety. The physiologic strains on the donor of the left lobe appear to be less; there have been no reports of a left lobe donor's requiring liver transplantation after donation compared with right lobe donation, for which the need for emergent liver transplantation has been reported.[41] The reservation about using the smaller piece of liver from left lobe donation is that the high portal flow generated by the enlarged spleen and other vascular manifestations of portal hypertension result in injury to the graft from hyperperfusion and endothelial damage. It has been estimated that the weight of the graft should be more than 0.8% of the recipient's body weight to prevent injury from hyperperfusion. The small left lobe grafts (generally, 30% to 40% of the total liver mass) may be protected from harm through decreasing portal vein blood flow by performing portacaval shunts, ligating the splenic artery, or performing splenectomy. Another strategy has been to use two left lobe donors for a single recipient, a strategy that attempts to minimize risk to the donor by using the left lobe from two donors while maximizing liver mass in the recipient.[42] The potential risk to two donors is the major concern to this approach. However, excellent outcomes have been reported with low live donor morbidity.

Of live liver donors, 30% to 40% suffer one or more postoperative complications.[43] The most serious include pulmonary emboli, portal vein thrombosis, bile duct injury, and liver insufficiency secondary to a resection that is too extensive.

The potential for death among live liver donors has led to a more clearly delineated informed consent process in the transplant community, the use of a donor advocate to ensure that the concern for donor safety is paramount, and the clear separation of donor and recipient teams to ensure that the donor is treated without ulterior motives, which might occur if the same team cared for both the donor and the recipient. Long-term follow-up will be necessary to determine whether the long-term sequelae for live donors are as benign as for living kidney donors.

The recent application of hand-assisted laparoscopic techniques for living donor right hepatic lobectomy may have a similar impact as laparoscopic donor nephrectomy in increasing live liver donation. This technique, using a midline incision for the hand port, needs wider application to realize its potential impact.[44]

There appears to be a learning curve with live donor liver transplantation. Centers with extensive experience note decreased rates of complications compared with inexperienced centers. In addition, groups in Asia with extensive experience have outstanding records of low complications in their live donor experience.[45]

The recipient outcomes from live liver donors are superior to those for patients awaiting transplantation and those receiving deceased donor transplants.[46] These differences are primarily explained by the opportunity to perform live donor liver transplantation when the recipient is in relatively good health, rather than relying on the MELD system, which distributes deceased donor livers to the most gravely ill hosts. Controlling for recipient condition and comparing recipients of live donor versus deceased donor transplants also favors outcomes in the recipients of live donor grafts; this may reflect the same factors that are operative in live donor kidney transplantation—the use of an organ that is free of preservation insult, the avoidance of the negative effects of brain death on organ viability, and the immunologic advantage of a live donor graft (most often immunologically related). In the early days of adult-to-adult live liver donation, high MELD score recipients were found to have poor outcomes, and many centers limited live donor transplantation with partial grafts to recipients with a MELD score of less than 25. More recently, excellent outcomes have been reported in high MELD score recipients of live liver donors.[47] This is likely to result in increased live liver donor transplantation in this group of patients.

Living donor transplantation, however, does suffer from the increased complications in the recipient related to the bile duct anastomosis. Because the branch of the bile duct is used in live donor transplantation rather than the trunk, as in deceased donor transplantation, the rate of biliary complications is roughly twice as high.

TECHNICAL ASPECTS OF LIVER TRANSPLANTATION

Unlike the kidney transplant (placed in a heterotopic position in the iliac fossa), the liver is placed orthotopically, in its native position within the abdomen. The procedure involves removal of the host liver and replacement with a whole or partial graft.

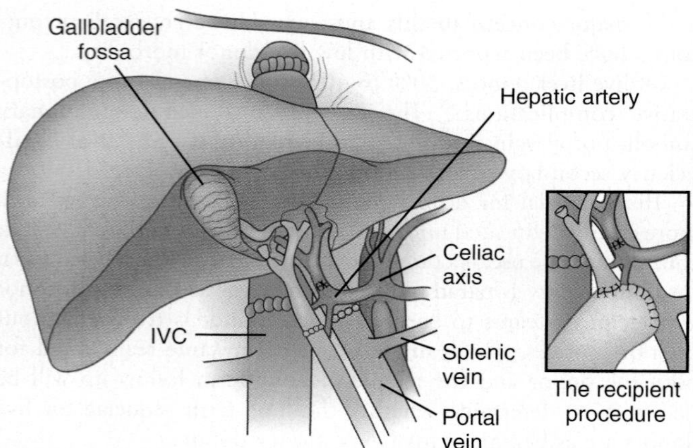

FIGURE 25-1 A choledochocholedochostomy (duct to duct) anastomosis in orthotopic liver transplantation. *IVC*, inferior vena cava. *Inset*, A choledochojejunostomy.

Figure 25-1 demonstrates a completed orthotopic liver transplantation using the bicaval approach. Alternatively, the donor liver may be placed by the piggyback technique.

Removal of the host liver is often challenging because of the portal hypertension and coagulopathy that frequently accompany chronic liver disease. After mobilization of the liver, the bile ducts are divided, and vascular clamps are placed on the suprahepatic vena cava, infrahepatic vena cava, portal vein, and hepatic artery. The anhepatic phase of the surgery relates to the period during which the new liver is sewn in and the patient is without a liver. In the conventional implantation technique, the suprahepatic vena cava, infrahepatic vena cava, portal vein, and hepatic artery are sewn in sequence. The alternative piggyback technique leaves the host vena cava intact and involves an anastomosis between the donor suprahepatic cava and the confluence of the hepatic veins. In this technique, the donor infrahepatic cava is oversewn. The piggyback method may shorten the anhepatic phase and has the potential for improved cardiovascular stability because it leaves the venacaval flow intact during the anhepatic phase.

Some centers use venovenous bypass, in which shunt tubing is placed in the host portal vein and infrahepatic cava and returned to the central venous circulation to maintain vascular stability during the anhepatic phase. Centers that do not use the bypass technique rely more on anesthesia support of the blood pressure through volume administration and pressors.

The piggyback technique is necessary for patients undergoing live donor liver or split liver transplantation when a donor vena cava is not available. In the case of a right lobe graft (segments 5 to 8), the venous drainage is the right hepatic vein; the inflow is the right hepatic artery and right portal vein.

The anhepatic phase ends with reperfusion of the graft, with inflow from the portal vein and outflow through the vena cava. Subsequently, arterial inflow is reestablished, and biliary drainage is accomplished through a choledochocholedochostomy or choledochojejunostomy (usually in the case of biliary atresia or sclerosing cholangitis, in which the host duct is unsuitable).

Split Liver Transplant

The identification of separate units within the liver with unique blood supply, venous drainage, and biliary drainage makes possible the use of a single deceased donor liver applicable for two recipients. Figure 25-2 demonstrates the segments of liver (1 to 8) that can be defined by their separate venous and arterial inflow, venous outflow, and biliary drainage.

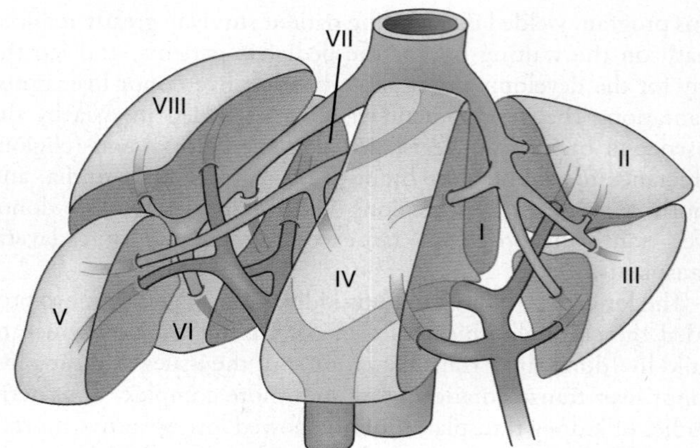

FIGURE 25-2 Anatomic segments of the liver.

The split is usually done between a child (receiving segments 2 and 3 or segments 2, 3, and 4) and an adult (receiving segments 1, 4, 5, 6, 7, and 8 or segments 1, 5, 6, 7, and 8). The right lobe graft most commonly includes the donor vena cava and right hepatic artery; the pediatric graft is based on the celiac trunk, providing the left hepatic artery, left portal vein, and left hepatic vein.

The splitting of a deceased donor liver for use in two adult patients has been infrequent. Inadequate left lobe mass may be a problem.

LIVE DONOR OPERATION

Figure 25-3 depicts the line of resection for a segment 2-3 hepatectomy (line A) in the setting of an adult-to-child live donor liver operation or for a cadaveric split for an adult and child (line A).

The use of segments 2 and 3 is most appropriate for infants and small children (up to 5 years of age). The donor operation can be performed through a midline incision. The round ligament is divided, retracted, and mobilized. The left triangular ligament is taken down. The left hepatic artery and left portal vein are mobilized. Numerous branches from the left portal vein to segments 1 and 4 are ligated and divided. The left hepatic vein is mobilized. A resection line is drawn from the right edge of the left hepatic vein, coursing approximately 1 cm to the right of the falciform ligament to the bile duct plate, which sits superiorly above the left portal vein as it enters segments 2 and 3. The liver parenchyma is carefully divided, with clipping or ligature of large vessels and ducts. The plane just to the right of the falciform ligament is usually used because it usually yields a single 2-3 bile duct for reimplantation. After the parenchymal dissection medially, the segment 2-3 is lifted superiorly and dissected free from segment 1. This results in an isolated segment 2-3 with left hepatic artery, left portal vein, and left hepatic vein along with the segment 2-3 duct. The segment 2-3 is flushed through the left portal vein and left hepatic artery.

Right Lobe Dissection for Live Donor Liver Transplantation

The right lobe (segments 5 to 8) is most commonly used for adult-to-adult live donor liver transplantation. The right lobe

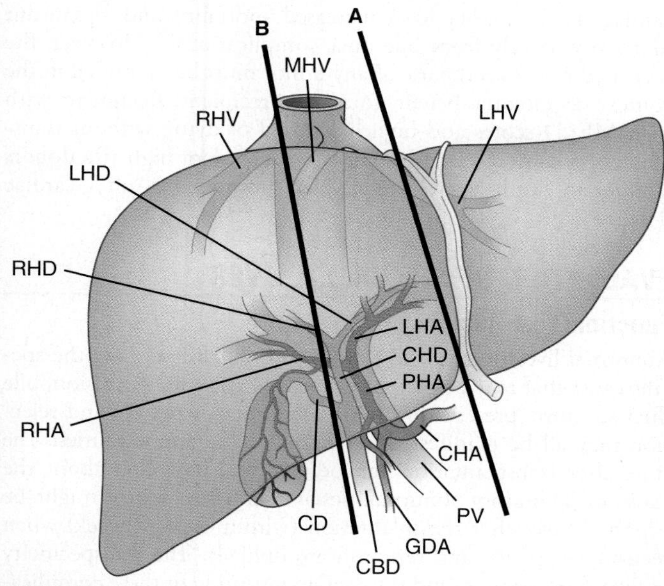

FIGURE 25-3 Planes of dissection for the 2-3 hepatectomy *(line A)* and for a right-left lobe split *(line B)*. *LHV*, left hepatic vein; *MHV*, middle hepatic vein; *RHV*, right hepatic vein; *LHD*, left hepatic duct; *RHD*, right hepatic duct; *RHA*, right hepatic artery; *CD*, cystic duct; *CBD*, common bile duct; *GDA*, gastroduodenal artery; *LHA*, left hepatic artery; *CHD*, common hepatic duct; *PHA*, proper hepatic artery; *CHA*, common hepatic artery; *PV*, portal vein.

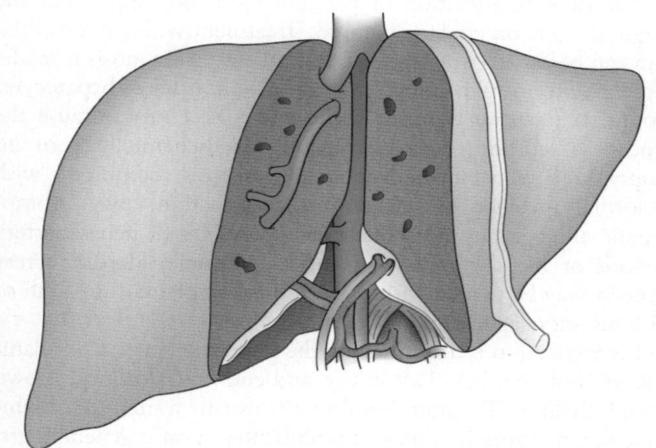

FIGURE 25-4 Plane of donor dissection for right or left live donor liver transplantation and for split liver transplantation.

represents 60% to 80% of the liver mass. A bilateral subcostal or trap door incision is made, or midline incision is done if laparoscopic mobilization of the right triangular ligaments is used. A cholecystectomy is performed. The right hepatic artery and right portal vein are isolated and temporarily occluded to establish the line of demarcation, which is used to plan the plane of resection (Fig. 25-4; also see Fig. 25-3, resection line B). This line typically runs at the left edge of the gallbladder fossa to the medial aspect of the right hepatic vein. The right lobe is mobilized by division of the right triangular ligaments and suture ligation of the perforating veins between the right lobe and infrahepatic vena cava. The right hepatic vein and accessory right hepatic veins (>5 mm) are isolated. The right hepatic duct is mobilized; it may be divided before or after the parenchymal dissection.

Various techniques may be used to divide the parenchyma; the preferred technique is dissection with the Cavitron ultrasonic surgical aspirator (Cooper Medical, Santa Clara, Calif), which allows the identification of vessels and ducts for ligation. Venous branches from segments 5 and 8 may be preserved for reimplantation; there is controversy as to whether this is necessary to prevent venous outflow obstruction and congestion of the graft. In centers with extensive experience, these veins are generally preserved and reimplanted.[45] Once the parenchymal dissection is complete and the right duct divided, vascular clamps are placed on the right hepatic artery, right portal vein, and right hepatic vein for resection of the right lobe.

Left Lobe Dissection for Live Donor Liver Transplantation

The left lobe graft is based on segments 1, 2, 3, and 4 with inflow from the left hepatic artery and left portal vein and outflow from the middle and left hepatic veins. The middle and left hepatic veins frequently have a confluent trunk as they enter the vena cava (see Fig. 25-3, resection line B). The operation includes parenchymal dissection along Cantlie's line, the same line as for the right hepatic lobectomy. The middle and left hepatic veins may need to be taken separately or as a single trunk, depending on the level of confluence of these vessels. The parenchymal dissection is done in the same manner as for right hepatic lobectomy, with care to clip or to suture ligate large vessels and bile ducts. At our center, the left lobe graft includes segment 1, adding a small amount of additional liver mass.

Implantation of Partial Liver Graft

The piggyback technique is the basis for implantation of a split liver graft or a graft from a live donor. If the split liver comes intact with a vena cava, a conventional transplantation procedure may be done.

The piggyback technique involves ligation and division of the perforating veins from the right lobe of the host liver to the vena cava. Accessory right hepatic veins are also sacrificed. The venous anastomosis is usually created between the graft hepatic vein and a wide cavotomy, typically using the orifices of the recipient hepatic veins. Depending on whether the donor graft is the right or left lobe, either the right or left hepatic artery branches from the recipient may be used for inflow. Similarly, inflow may be from the right or left portal vein branch. If a left lobe graft is used and a portacaval shunt is planned to decompress the portal system to prevent portal hyperperfusion, the right portal vein branch may be used to create the shunt to the vena cava and the left portal vein branch used for inflow into the donor portal vein branch. Biliary drainage is achieved through a duct-to-duct anastomosis or a Roux-en-Y anastomosis to the donor duct, depending on the duct sizes. Care must be taken to avoid tension on this anastomosis.

EARLY COMPLICATIONS OF LIVER TRANSPLANTATION

Early signs that a newly implanted liver is functioning are acid clearance, normalization of clotting parameters, and bile production; these signs may be apparent within a few minutes after reperfusion. Primary nonfunction refers to a condition in which the transplanted liver does not work. It is rare (<2%) and fatal without retransplantation. Ultrasonography with Doppler evaluation may be useful to eliminate vascular thrombosis as a cause. Hepatic artery thrombosis occurs in 2% to 4% of adult transplantation procedures[48] but has a threefold to fourfold higher incidence in children. Although early thrombectomy of the hepatic artery may prevent retransplantation in some patients, most patients require retransplantation. Portal venous thrombosis may be unnoticed but may be manifested with gastrointestinal bleeding or coagulopathy and may require therapy for new or persistent portal hypertension. Other complications include bleeding, inadequate production of clotting factors (poor initial function), and inadequate replacement of factors at the time of transplantation (e.g., platelet or fresh-frozen plasma replacement). The need to reoperate on a given patient is dictated by cardiovascular stability, liver function, presence of abdominal compartment syndrome (which may be manifested by acute or progressive renal failure), and total blood products used. Bile duct stricture or leak is a complication that may be seen early after transplantation or later; its cause likely reflects compromised blood supply of the donor or recipient duct. Early strictures likely represent inflammation or edema at the anastomosis and frequently are self-limited. The first line of therapy for an anastomotic stricture is dilation and stent placement performed through endoscopic retrograde cholangiopancreatography or a transhepatic route. Strictures that persist or recur after dilation or stenting are treated surgically, with conversion to a choledochojejunostomy.

Outcome

Progress in the technical and immunologic aspects of liver transplantation has led to excellent graft and patient survival, with 1- and 5-year patient survival rates of 88% and 75%, respectively.[30] Results depend on the specific disease for which the transplantation is performed.

EXTENDED CRITERIA DONORS

Although liver transplantation is successful with both live and deceased donors, it is increasingly difficult to find a perfect deceased donor. The ideal liver donor (young and otherwise completely healthy) is increasingly rare because the cause of death for most donors has shifted from trauma to cerebrovascular accidents. Using UNOS data, Feng and coworkers[49] have defined the donor factors increasing the risk of failure after liver transplantation into a formula called the donor risk index. Factors contributing to risk with use of livers from donation after brain death include advanced donor age, fatty infiltration, and use of split livers from these donors. The donor risk issues must be taken in context of the recipient for whom it is used. In the past, the use of an older donor was particularly hazardous in the HCV-positive recipient. With current antiviral agents for HCV, this risk appears to be mitigated. Many transplantation programs balance the recipient's risk of death on the basis of the MELD score with the risk of recurrent cirrhosis in HCV-positive patients.

Another donor source, the use of which has increased significantly during the past 5 years, is the donor after cardiac death. These are donors who do not meet brain death criteria and become donors after they are removed from life support and experience cessation of cardiac function. Most centers use a 30-minute cutoff from the time of withdrawal of life support to the perfusion of the organ as a criterion for accepting such donors, but there is variability. Even with these criteria, the recipients of livers from cardiac death donors have increased mortality and significant morbidity, largely from bile duct complications.[50] However, the increased risk from the use of any donor must be examined in the context of potential benefit to a given recipient. Recipients with high MELD scores and high likelihood of dying without transplantation show survival benefit from the use of high-risk donors after brain death as well as of livers from donors after cardiac death.

EVALUATION OF ABNORMAL LIVER

Function Test Results

Abnormal liver function test results do not differentiate the specific cause that may be present in the liver; vascular occlusion, bile duct stricture, preservation injury, recurrent hepatitis, and rejection may all be manifested with nonspecific abnormalities. The time after transplantation can be an important clue about the cause of laboratory abnormalities. Preservation injury might be expected early after transplantation (within the first week) when recurrent hepatitis and rejection are unlikely. The nonspecificity of liver function tests and the overlap in timing of these complications dictate an organized approach to the patient with perturbation in laboratory test results. Doppler ultrasonography is recommended to evaluate hepatic artery and portal vein flow and bile duct caliber. If the ultrasound study reveals intact inflow and absent bile duct dilation, a percutaneous liver biopsy is performed and used to make the diagnosis of acute rejection, recurrent hepatitis, or preservation injury. Biliary obstruction may be manifested by bile duct proliferation or pericholangitis on biopsy, but the diagnosis rests on cholangiography. Treatment with stent or dilation can be carried out at the same time as the diagnosis is made. Preservation injury is manifested by vacuolization of hepatocytes around the central vein; no treatment is necessary because the process is self-limited and reversible. An ischemic pattern on biopsy with hepatocyte dropout or necrosis, combined with abnormal findings on ultrasound examination, may prompt hepatic angiography to evaluate the possibility of hepatic artery stenosis or median arcuate ligament syndrome. Hepatic artery stenosis may be treated with balloon dilation or stenting, with or without anticoagulation.

Liver rejection is diagnosed by the presence of a portal inflammatory infiltrate, bile duct injury, and endothelial injury, known as endotheliitis. The portal infiltrate is usually a mixture of lymphocytes, neutrophils, and eosinophils. Rejection is generally first treated with increased steroids or change in immunosuppressive therapy. In patients with underlying hepatitis C, increased steroids are avoided in favor of increasing immunosuppression to avoid enhanced viral replication induced by steroids. Typically, the increased immunosuppression would be an increase in the tacrolimus or mycophenolate dose or the addition of a mammalian target of rapamycin (mTOR) inhibitor.

Recurrent hepatitis C generally occurs later than the complications noted but may be seen within a few weeks of transplantation. Distinguishing recurrent hepatitis C from rejection by liver biopsy can be difficult. The time after transplantation can be an important clue to deciding whether it is rejection or recurrent hepatitis C; recurrent hepatitis C usually occurs within 6 weeks of transplantation. Recurrent hepatitis C may be treated with direct antiviral agents.

Hepatic artery occlusion is an indication for retransplantation if it occurs in the early postoperative period. It is associated with progressive saccular dilation of the biliary tree secondary to bile duct ischemia and the development of liver abscesses. If the hepatic artery occludes slowly over time, adequate collaterals may develop and obviate the need for retransplantation.

IMMUNOSUPPRESSION AFTER LIVER TRANSPLANTATION

The liver has been referred to as a privileged organ because, in general, the need for immunosuppression decreases over time, and unlike the situation in kidney and heart transplantation, chronic rejection is uncommon.

The mainstay of immunosuppression after liver transplantation is the use of a combination of a calcineurin inhibitor (tacrolimus or cyclosporine), steroids (methylprednisolone), and antiproliferative agent (e.g., mycophenolate mofetil). The calcineurin inhibitors are used in 95% of transplantation centers, despite their known nephrotoxicity. These agents are also associated with hypertension, diabetes, and neurologic effects, including seizures.[51] The major advantages of the mycophenolate derivatives are their lack of renal toxicity, although their toxicities include gastrointestinal irritation[52] and bone marrow suppression. Steroid-free protocols may be useful to minimize de novo diabetes mellitus, cytomegalovirus infection, hypercholesterolemia, and, in HCV-infected patients, the recurrence of hepatitis C.[53]

The mTOR inhibitors have a place in preventing and treating rejection; they effectively decrease interleukin-2 production by a mechanism distinct from that of the calcineurin inhibitors. The antineoplastic effect makes their use attractive in patients with HCC as an indication for transplantation.[54,55] The mTOR inhibitors are associated with hyperlipidemia and inhibition of wound healing. Some groups avoid their use in the immediate postoperative period.

RETRANSPLANTATION AND RECURRENT DISEASE

Rejection, although frequent early after transplantation, is rarely the cause of graft failure. This is in contradistinction to other types of solid organ transplantation in which chronic rejection is a common cause of the need for retransplantation. Recurrent disease is most frequently the cause of graft failure in patients with chronic hepatitis C, although this is likely to change with new antivirals. Recurrent disease may, rarely, be the cause of graft failure in patients with chronic hepatitis B, primary biliary cirrhosis, sclerosing cholangitis, nonalcoholic steatohepatitis, and autoimmune liver disease. Alcoholic liver disease may recur if the patient returns to alcohol. HCC may also recur, but its recurrence rarely causes graft failure and is not always limited solely to the graft.

ROLE OF LIVER TRANSPLANTATION FOR HEPATOCELLULAR CARCINOMA

There is considerable controversy as to whether patients with HCC are better served with liver transplantation versus liver resection. In the early days of liver transplantation, a number of first transplantations were done in patients with cancer. The immediate postoperative success likely reflected less severe liver disease and absent portal hypertension. Although the operation and early post-transplantation course could be judged a success in these patients, they succumbed with recurrent cancer. As a consequence, liver transplantation for HCC was not pursued on a large scale for many years. Mazzaferro and colleagues[26] clearly defined those patients with HCC who were likely to have survival that matched survival with other indications for transplantation. This group defined the Milan criteria, which selected candidates with good short- and long-term outcomes and a low rate of tumor recurrence. The Milan criteria dictate that transplantation be limited to patients with a single tumor smaller than 5 cm or more than three tumors, the largest of which must be less than 3 cm. These criteria have been applied throughout the world and adapted by the central agency distributing livers in the United States (UNOS) to provide the basis for additional points to modify the MELD score. The Milan criteria, based on the disease of the explanted organ, have been challenged because preoperative imaging may be inaccurate in as many as 30% of patients, both in overestimating and in underestimating the number and size of cancers. In addition, the criteria have been challenged as being too restrictive by a number of groups who have demonstrated excellent short- and long-term survival; they expanded the criteria to include bigger solitary tumors and an increase in the number of tumors.[56,57]

HCC most commonly develops on the background of chronic scarring of the liver—cirrhosis. In the setting of cirrhosis, the issue of hepatic reserve and potential for decompensation limit the suitability of resection as a first-line approach to patients with cirrhosis and HCC. The other limitation of resection as definitive treatment for HCC is the potential for recurrence in the remaining liver. Because HCC occurs on the background of chronic liver disease, its occurrence reflects a field effect and therefore the potential evolution to HCC in other portions of the liver.

Data from patients observed after resection or radiofrequency ablation have demonstrated that 40% to 50% of patients will have recurrence by 3 years.[58] Although outcomes from resection have improved significantly during the past 20 years, with 1-year patient survival that matches the outcomes of liver transplantation, the 5-year disease-free survival for resection is far lower than the outcomes for transplantation when tumors of the same size are treated.[59]

The major limitation in the use of transplantation as treatment for HCC is the limited number of donors. The disparity between the number of potential deceased donors and patients listed for transplantation is significant; HCC is increasingly the indication for transplantation, accounting for 25% of transplantations done in 2012.[30] The use of live donors or extended criteria deceased donors has not met the continued need. Use of transplantation in a patient with HCC removes from the donor pool a lifesaving organ for a patient who may not have an alternative therapy, such as resection. It is hoped that better selection of patients using biologic markers of the tumor or of the remnant liver may predict those patients at highest risk of recurrence after resection and funnel those patients toward transplantation, and the remaining patients, at low risk for recurrence, would undergo resection.

It has been suggested that liver resection be used as first-line therapy for HCC, with salvage transplantation if the cancer recurs.[60] One could consider this a "poor man's" biologic marker using the remnant liver's biology over time to delineate those patients at risk for recurrence. This approach would avoid unnecessary transplantation and unwarranted immunosuppression in patients in whom the tumor does not recur. However, this is hampered by the fact that many recurrences are outside the criteria for transplantation, with multiple intrahepatic tumors, and transplantation after resection may be more difficult.

The recurrence after resection may be more aggressive and likely to be outside of transplantation criteria because of extensive tumor within the liver or as the result of metastatic disease. There are conflicting data in the literature in this regard.[61,62]

ROLE OF CELLULAR TRANSPLANTATION IN LIVER REPLACEMENT

The replacement of the liver involves a major surgical procedure, with complex technical and immunologic aspects. The notion, therefore, of using cells instead of the entire organ is an attractive alternative.

Hepatocyte transplantation makes the most logical sense for replacing missing enzymes, in which only a small number of cells would be needed to correct deficiencies. Examples of such defects include urea cycle defects such as ornithine transcarbamylase deficiency and the defect in bilirubin conjugation, Crigler-Najjar syndrome. Animal models have demonstrated the possibility of at least temporary correction of enzyme deficits using hepatocyte transplantation.[63]

Hepatocytes could also be used in fulminant hepatic failure in which the hepatic scaffolding is left intact, and a few case reports have suggested its usefulness. Hepatocyte transplantation has also been used in chronic liver disease, but the results have not been convincing. When advanced liver disease is associated with portal hypertension, it is unlikely to be of benefit.

The potential role for the use of hepatocytes or stem cells from the host has expanded with the reintroduction of these cells and is the hope for the future. This approach may avoid the need for liver replacement and may also obviate the need for immunosuppression.[64]

SELECTED REFERENCES

Baker TB, Jay CL, Ladner DP, et al: Laparoscopy-assisted and open living donor right hepatectomy: A comparative study of outcomes. *Surgery* 146:817–823, 2009.

The use of minimally invasive surgery for live donor kidney transplantation markedly increased the donor pool. This article reports results of the application of minimally invasive surgery for live donor liver transplantation.

Feng S, Goodrich NP, Bragg-Gresham JL, et al: Characteristics associated with liver graft failure: The concept of a donor risk index. *Am J Transplant* 6:783–790, 2006.

It is recognized that the outcome after liver transplantation must take into account comorbid conditions in the recipient. This article articulates the donor factors that also influence post-transplantation survival.

Kamath PS, Wiesner RH, Malinchoc M, et al: A model to predict survival in patients with end-stage liver disease. *Hepatology* 33:464–470, 2001.

This article describes the scoring system currently used to distribute livers in the United States. It also predicts for chance of death without liver replacement.

Mazzaferro V, Regalia E, Doci R, et al: Liver transplantation for the treatment of small hepatocellular carcinomas in patients with cirrhosis. *N Engl J Med* 334:693–699, 1996.

This landmark article demonstrates for the first time that patients with small hepatocellular carcinomas undergoing liver transplantation have comparable results to patients with other diagnoses.

Pillai AA, Levitsky J: Overview of immunosuppression in liver transplantation. *World J Gastroenterol* 15:4225–4233, 2009.

This article provides a broad overview of the drugs used for immunosuppression in liver transplantation.

Schaubel DE, Guidinger MK, Biggins SW, et al: Survival benefit–based deceased-donor liver allocation. *Am J Transplant* 9:970–981, 2009.

Avoidance of death before transplantation and survival benefit after transplantation are blended together to dictate a new potential distribution of livers for transplantation.

Yao FY: Liver transplantation for hepatocellular carcinoma: Beyond the Milan criteria. *Am J Transplant* 8:1982–1989, 2008.

The outcomes after liver transplantation using the Milan criteria represent excellent results but exclude a large number of patients. Expanding the criteria serves more patients without sacrificing outcome.

REFERENCES

1. Murray G, Holden R: Transplantation of kidneys, experimentally and in human cases. *Am J Surg* 87:508–515, 1954.
2. A definition of irreversible coma. Report of the Ad Hoc Committee of the Harvard Medical School to Examine the Definition of Brain Death. *JAMA* 205:337–340, 1968.
3. Starzl TE, Groth CG, Brettschneider L, et al: Orthotopic homotransplantation of the human liver. *Ann Surg* 168:392–415, 1968.
4. Borel JF, Feurer C, Gubler HU, et al: Biological effects of cyclosporin A: A new antilymphocytic agent. *Agents Actions* 6:468–475, 1976.
5. Kotru A, Sheperd R, Nadler M, et al: Combined lung and liver transplantation: The United States experience. *Transplantation* 82:144–145, author reply 145, 2006.
6. Ostapowicz G, Fontana RJ, Schiodt FV, et al: Results of a prospective study of acute liver failure at 17 tertiary care centers in the United States. *Ann Intern Med* 137:947–954, 2002.
7. Marudanayagam R, Shanmugam V, Gunson B, et al: Aetiology and outcome of acute liver failure. *HPB (Oxford)* 11: 429–434, 2009.
8. Lee WM: Etiologies of acute liver failure. *Semin Liver Dis* 28:142–152, 2008.
9. Karvellas CJ, Stravitz R, Battenhouse H, et al: US Acute Liver Failure Study Group: Therapeutic hypothermia in acute liver failure: A multicenter retrospective cohort analysis. *Liver Transpl* 21:4–12, 2015.

10. Roche B, Samuel D: Risk factors for hepatitis C recurrence after liver transplantation. *J Viral Hepat* 14(Suppl 1):89–96, 2007.
11. Everson GT: Impact of immunosuppressive therapy on recurrence of hepatitis C. *Liver Transpl* 8:S19–S27, 2002.
12. Berenguer M: Systematic review of the treatment of established recurrent hepatitis C with pegylated interferon in combination with ribavirin. *J Hepatol* 49:274–287, 2008.
13. Meissner EG, Nelson A, Marti M, et al: Sustained virologic response for chronic hepatitis C infection after 27 days of treatment with sofosbuvir and ribavirin. *Open Forum Infect Dis* 1:013, 2014.
14. Gallegos-Orozco JF, Charlton M: Treatment of HCV prior to liver transplantation to prevent HCV recurrence—wise or wasteful? *Liver Int* 35:9–11, 2015.
15. Kutala BK, Guedy J, Asselah T, et al: Impact of treatment against hepatitis C virus on overall survival of naive patients with advanced liver disease. *Antimicrob Agents Chemother* 59:803–810, 2015.
16. Beasley RP: Hepatitis B virus. The major etiology of hepatocellular carcinoma. *Cancer* 61:1942–1956, 1988.
17. Liermann Garcia RF, Evangelista Garcia C, McMaster P, et al: Transplantation for primary biliary cirrhosis: Retrospective analysis of 400 patients in a single center. *Hepatology* 33:22–27, 2001.
18. Gow PJ, Chapman RW: Liver transplantation for primary sclerosing cholangitis. *Liver* 20:97–103, 2000.
19. Mathurin P, Moreno C, Samuel D, et al: Early liver transplantation for severe alcoholic hepatitis. *N Engl J Med* 365:1790–1800, 2011.
20. Kim W, Kim DJ: Severe alcoholic hepatitis—current concepts, diagnosis and treatment options. *World J Hepatol* 6:688–695, 2014.
21. Younossi ZM: Review article: Current management of non-alcoholic fatty liver disease and non-alcoholic steatohepatitis. *Aliment Pharmacol Ther* 28:2–12, 2008.
22. Tan-Tam CC, Frassetto LA, Stock PG: Liver and kidney transplantation in HIV-infected patients. *AIDS Rev* 11:190–204, 2009.
23. Saner FH, Nadalin S, Pavlakovic G, et al: Portopulmonary hypertension in the early phase following liver transplantation. *Transplantation* 82:887–891, 2006.
24. Martinez-Palli G, Taura P, Balust J, et al: Liver transplantation in high-risk patients: Hepatopulmonary syndrome and portopulmonary hypertension. *Transplant Proc* 37:3861–3864, 2005.
25. Dew MA, DiMartini AF, De Vito Dabbs A, et al: Rates and risk factors for nonadherence to the medical regimen after adult solid organ transplantation. *Transplantation* 83:858–873, 2007.
26. Mazzaferro V, Regalia E, Doci R, et al: Liver transplantation for the treatment of small hepatocellular carcinomas in patients with cirrhosis. *N Engl J Med* 334:693–699, 1996.
27. Silva MF, Sherman M: Criteria for liver transplantation for HCC: What should the limits be? *J Hepatol* 55:1137–1147, 2011.
28. Kakodkar R, Soin AS: Liver transplantation for HCC: A review. *Indian J Surg* 74:100–117, 2012.
29. Raza A, Sood GK: Hepatocellular carcinoma review: Current treatment, and evidence-based medicine. *World J Gastroenterol* 20:4115–4127, 2014.
30. Health Resources Services Administration, U.S. Department of Health & Human Services: Organ Procurement and Transplantation Network. <http://optn.transplant.hrsa.gov>, 2012.
31. Yao FY, Mehta N, Flemming JA, et al: Downstaging of hepatocellular cancer before liver transplant: Long-term outcome compared to tumors within Milan Criteria. *Hepatology* 61:1968–1977, 2015.
32. Kamath PS, Wiesner RH, Malinchoc M, et al: A model to predict survival in patients with end-stage liver disease. *Hepatology* 33:464–470, 2001.
33. Martin AP, Bartels M, Hauss J, et al: Overview of the MELD score and the UNOS adult liver allocation system. *Transplant Proc* 39:3169–3174, 2007.
34. Schaubel DE, Guidinger MK, Biggins SW, et al: Survival benefit–based deceased-donor liver allocation. *Am J Transplant* 9:970–981, 2009.
35. Ioannou GN, Perkins JD, Carithers RL, Jr: Liver transplantation for hepatocellular carcinoma: Impact of the MELD allocation system and predictors of survival. *Gastroenterology* 134:1342–1351, 2008.
36. Barshes NR, Lee TC, Udell IW, et al: The pediatric end-stage liver disease (PELD) model as a predictor of survival benefit and post-transplant survival in pediatric liver transplant recipients. *Liver Transpl* 12:475–480, 2006.
37. Otte JB, de Ville de Goyet J, Alberti D, et al: The concept and technique of the split liver in clinical transplantation. *Surgery* 107:605–612, 1990.
38. Millis JM, Cronin DC, Brady LM, et al: Primary living-donor liver transplantation at the University of Chicago: Technical aspects of the first 104 recipients. *Ann Surg* 232:104–111, 2000.
39. Segev DL, Muzaale AD, Caffo BS, et al: Perioperative mortality and long-term survival following live kidney donation. *JAMA* 303:959–966, 2010.
40. Trotter JF, Adam R, Lo CM, et al: Documented deaths of hepatic lobe donors for living donor liver transplantation. *Liver Transpl* 12:1485–1488, 2006.
41. Hwang S, Lee SG, Lee YJ, et al: Lessons learned from 1,000 living donor liver transplantations in a single center: How to make living donations safe. *Liver Transpl* 12:920–927, 2006.
42. Song GW, Lee SG, Hwang S, et al: Dual living donor liver transplantation with ABO-incompatible and ABO-compatible grafts to overcome small-for-size graft and ABO blood group barrier. *Liver Transpl* 16:491–498, 2010.
43. Ghobrial RM, Freise CE, Trotter JF, et al: Donor morbidity after living donation for liver transplantation. *Gastroenterology* 135:468–476, 2008.
44. Baker TB, Jay CL, Ladner DP, et al: Laparoscopy-assisted and open living donor right hepatectomy: A comparative study of outcomes. *Surgery* 146:817–823, 2009.
45. Lee SG: A complete treatment of adult living donor liver transplantation: A review of surgical technique and current challenges to expand indication of patients. *Am J Transplant* 15:17–38, 2015.
46. Berg CL, Gillespie BW, Merion RM, et al: Improvement in survival associated with adult-to-adult living donor liver transplantation. *Gastroenterology* 133:1806–1813, 2007.
47. Selzner M, Kashfi A, Cattral MS, et al: Live donor liver transplantation in high MELD score recipients. *Ann Surg* 251:153–157, 2010.

48. Stewart ZA, Locke JE, Segev DL, et al: Increased risk of graft loss from hepatic artery thrombosis after liver transplantation with older donors. *Liver Transpl* 15:1688–1695, 2009.
49. Feng S, Goodrich NP, Bragg-Gresham JL, et al: Characteristics associated with liver graft failure: The concept of a donor risk index. *Am J Transplant* 6:783–790, 2006.
50. Skaro AI, Jay CL, Baker TB, et al: The impact of ischemic cholangiopathy in liver transplantation using donors after cardiac death: The untold story. *Surgery* 146:543–552, discussion 552–543, 2009.
51. Pillai AA, Levitsky J: Overview of immunosuppression in liver transplantation. *World J Gastroenterol* 15:4225–4233, 2009.
52. Sollinger HW: Mycophenolates in transplantation. *Clin Transplant* 18:485–492, 2004.
53. Sgourakis G, Radtke A, Fouzas I, et al: Corticosteroid-free immunosuppression in liver transplantation: A meta-analysis and meta-regression of outcomes. *Transpl Int* 22:892–905, 2009.
54. Watson CJ, Friend PJ, Jamieson NV, et al: Sirolimus: A potent new immunosuppressant for liver transplantation. *Transplantation* 67:505–509, 1999.
55. Klintmalm GB, Nashan B: The role of mTOR inhibitors in liver transplantation: Reviewing the evidence. *J Transplant* 2014:845438, 2014.
56. Yao FY: Liver transplantation for hepatocellular carcinoma: Beyond the Milan criteria. *Am J Transplant* 8:1982–1989, 2008.
57. Marsh JW, Schmidt C: The Milan criteria: No room on the metro for the king? *Liver Transpl* 16:252–255, 2010.
58. Ng KK, Poon RT, Lo CM, et al: Analysis of recurrence pattern and its influence on survival outcome after radiofrequency ablation of hepatocellular carcinoma. *J Gastrointest Surg* 12:183–191, 2008.
59. Morris-Stiff G, Gomez D, de Liguori Carino N, et al: Surgical management of hepatocellular carcinoma: Is the jury still out? *Surg Oncol* 18:298–321, 2009.
60. Poon RT, Fan ST, Lo CM, et al: Long-term survival and pattern of recurrence after resection of small hepatocellular carcinoma in patients with preserved liver function: Implications for a strategy of salvage transplantation. *Ann Surg* 235:373–382, 2002.
61. Hu RH, Ho MC, Wu YM, et al: Feasibility of salvage liver transplantation for patients with recurrent hepatocellular carcinoma. *Clin Transplant* 19:175–180, 2005.
62. Cucchetti A, Vitale A, Gaudio MD, et al: Harm and benefits of primary liver resection and salvage transplantation for hepatocellular carcinoma. *Am J Transplant* 10:619–627, 2010.
63. Fitzpatrick E, Mitry RR, Dhawan A: Human hepatocyte transplantation: State of the art. *J Intern Med* 266:339–357, 2009.
64. Locke JE, Shamblott MJ, Cameron AM: Stem cells and the liver: Clinical applications in transplantation. *Adv Surg* 43:35–51, 2009.

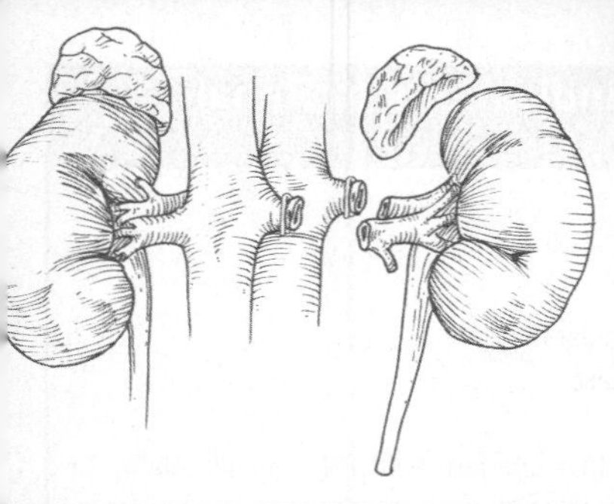

CHAPTER 26

Kidney and Pancreas Transplantation

Yolanda Becker, Piotr Witkowski

OUTLINE

HISTORICAL PERSPECTIVE

Interest in transplanting organs into humans dates to the early 1900s, when Floresco described anastomosis of the renal graft to the iliac fossa in 1905. In 1906, Jaboulay attempted to use a pig kidney to cure a patient with acute nephritis. He anastomosed the renal xenograft to the brachial arteries of the patient, and urine was noted for 1 hour after reperfusion. Alexis Carrel was developing techniques of triangulation of vascular anastomoses by performing various organ transplants in animals and received the Nobel Prize in 1912. Organ function was minimal, and further attempts at organ transplantation were abandoned. However, in the early 1950s, Medawar and colleagues described the prevention of rejection in mice, and human organ transplantation was again attempted. Joseph Murray performed the first successful renal transplantation in 1954 between identical twins. He received the Nobel Prize in 1990 for his groundbreaking work. Other major milestones in transplantation have included the discovery of cyclosporine and other effective immunosuppressive medications, the description of the histocompatibility antigens, and the perfecting of preservation solutions (Box 26-1).

The history of the discovery of diabetes and insulin is fascinating and well documented. Pancreas transplantation has also developed as a durable way to provide constant insulin to the type 1 diabetic. Hedon performed the first pancreas transplantation in an animal in 1913. He attempted placement of a pancreas allograft in the neck of pancreatectomized dogs. William Kelly and Richard Lillehei at the University of Minnesota performed the first successful human pancreas transplantation. They transplanted a duct-ligated segmental pancreas graft simultaneously with a kidney graft from the same deceased donor. The pancreas failed because of thrombosis and was removed on the seventh postoperative day. Management of the exocrine pancreas secretions has remained a problem; many revisions over the years have been a donor duodenal button technique, bladder drainage, duct ablation by injection, and finally enteric drainage. Much progress has been achieved recently in clinical islet transplantation, and this procedure has been recognized as an approved alternative to whole organ pancreas transplantation in Canada, Australia, and much of Europe. This chapter describes key clinical considerations in kidney, pancreas, and islet transplantation. Recipient and donor factors as well as long-term outcomes are discussed.

KIDNEY TRANSPLANTATION

Indications

Kidney transplantation offers patients a better long-term outcome than dialysis. The patient's quality of life is improved, and survival is projected to be 10 years longer than if the patient remains on dialysis.[1] During the past decade, the kidney waiting list has grown and the death of candidates who die while waiting has doubled. This reflects a change in demographics in the recipient waiting list; patients are listed at older ages, and an increasing number of patients are inactive on the waitlist.[2]

The most common causes of renal disease have evolved during the last 10 years. Overall, the percentage of patients with diabetes and hypertension as the cause of failure has increased from 24% to 28%, and the percentage of glomerular disease has declined from 42% to 21%.[2] In addition, the incidence of chronic kidney disease had also rapidly increased from 209,000 patients in 1991 to 472,000 in 2004.[3] Coresh and colleagues noted that the higher prevalence of diabetes, hypertension, and higher body mass index (BMI) explain this trend. The current prevalence of end-stage renal disease (ESRD) has risen rapidly, and at the end of the fourth quarter of 2012, there were more than 640,000 prevalent cases (www.USRDS.org). Similarly, the waitlist for kidney transplantation continues to grow every year. Potential recipients are also older than in past decades, with the group aged 50 to 64 years seeing the greatest increase (Fig. 26-1). This change in demographics has certainly presented challenges in preparation of these patients for transplantation and immunosuppression. It is also estimated that by 2015, there will be 136,000 patients with incident ESRD per year and 712,000 with prevalent disease (www.USRDS.org).

Patient Selection

The evaluation of patients as appropriate candidates for transplantation can be an arduous process. Patients with ESRD have significant comorbidities, and these must be taken into account in evaluating for transplantation. Guidelines for evaluation of these

BOX 26-1 Major Milestones in the History of Transplantation

1954	Joseph Murray performs the first successful kidney transplantation between identical twins
1966	Kelly and Lillehei perform the first pancreas transplantation
1967	First simultaneous kidney and pancreas transplantation
1970's	Borel, Stahelin, Calne, and White initiate trials of use of cyclosporine in transplantation
1980's	Belzer and Southard develop University of Wisconsin Solution (ViaSpan)
1990	Murray receives the Nobel Prize in Medicine
1990	Scharp and Lacy report the first successful human clinical islet transplantation

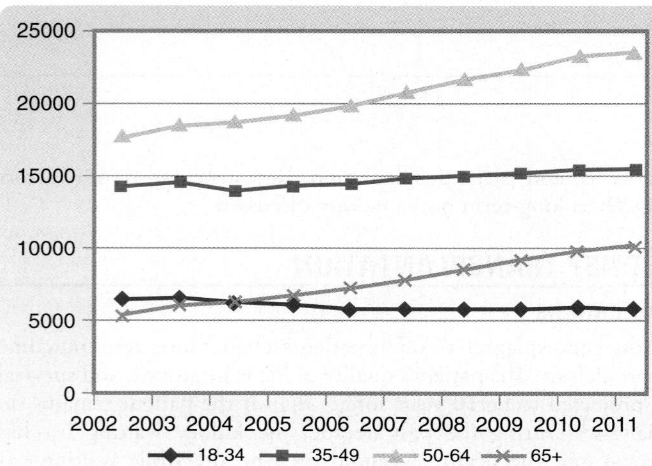

FIGURE 26-1 Additions to the United Network for Organ Sharing/Organ Procurement and Transplantation Network kidney waiting list by age. (From Annual Data Report of the US Organ Procurement and Transplantation Network. Preface. *Am J Transplant* 14[Suppl 1]:5–7, 2014.)

patients have been established.[4] Emphasis should be placed on obtaining the original cause of renal disease so the patient can be given reasonable expectations for graft survival. A graded association has been reported between reduced glomerular filtration rate (GFR) and risk of death and cardiovascular events.[5] Mortality rates are above 20% per year with dialysis. Long-term follow-up of kidney transplant recipients has shown a clear survival advantage over remaining on dialysis.[6] Studies have also shown significant improvements in quality of life and participation measures.[7]

The first step in the evaluation process is referral to a transplant center. Many factors may affect the ability of the patient to come for evaluation. Furth and colleagues[8] showed that lower socioeconomic status, female gender, and lower level of education resulted in fewer referrals. There has been concern that geographic distance to a transplant center might negatively influence access to care. However, a study of rural populations showed that remote or rural residence was not associated with a longer waitlist time.

Recipients must be carefully evaluated for surgical risk as well as for their ability to tolerate long-term immunosuppression. With improvements in perioperative management, the indications for kidney transplantation have increased. The absolute and relative contraindications for transplantation are shown in Box 26-2. According to the Kidney Disease Outcomes Quality Initiative guidelines, patients with a GFR of 30 mL/min/1.72 m^2 or lower and stage 3 or 4 chronic kidney disease should be referred to a nephrologist (http://www.kidney.org/professionals/kdoqi/index.cfm). Patients whose GFR falls below 20 mL/min/1.72 m^2 should be evaluated as possible kidney transplant patients if they do not have an absolute contraindication.

BOX 26-2 Contraindications to Renal Transplantation

Absolute

Active malignant disease
Active infection
Unreconstructable peripheral vascular disease
Severe cardiac or pulmonary disease
Active IV drug abuse
Significant psychosocial barriers that interfere with the patient's ability to comply with a complex medical regimen

Relative

Limited life expectancy
History of nonadherence to medication regimen
History of noncompliance with dialysis
Financial barriers
Psychiatric issues
Renal disease with high recurrence rate (active lupus, autoimmune disease)
Morbid obesity (BMI is center dependent)
Frailty

HIV infection was once a contraindication to transplantation; however, select patients with appropriate cell counts ($CD4^+$ above 400 cells/mm^3) and an undetectable viral load have good results with transplantation as a treatment modality for HIV-associated nephropathy. There has been an increase in transplantation as a treatment modality for HIV-associated nephropathy since 2006.[9]

Common causes of renal failure leading to the need for replacement therapy include diabetes, hypertension, glomerular diseases, interstitial diseases, cystic diseases, and chronic allograft nephropathy with subsequent failure of a transplanted kidney. Kidney diseases can recur in the allograft with varying frequency. Some diseases may lead to transplant failure with an inability to retransplant, such as aggressive focal sclerosing glomerulonephritis (recurrence of 20% to 30%). Common primary renal diseases and their probability of recurrence are listed in Table 26-1.[10-15]

Screening of potential recipients should begin with a detailed history, with particular attention paid to the original cause of disease. The length of time on dialysis has been noted to be an independent risk factor for poorer outcomes.[1] Gathering of the past medical history should include exposures to infectious diseases (especially tuberculosis, cytomegalovirus [CMV], Epstein-Barr virus, hepatitis) as well as malignant disease. Cardiac risk factors should be evaluated. Family history of renal disease or other systemic illnesses should be documented. Routine age-appropriate screening examinations, such as Papanicolaou smears, mammograms, colonoscopy, dental prophylaxis, and bone density, should be obtained as recommended by clinical practice guidelines.[4] Prostate-specific antigen levels should be checked in men older than 50 years. In addition, the patient should be questioned about thrombotic events, such as miscarriages, multiple dialysis access events, deep venous thrombosis, and pulmonary embolism,

TABLE 26-1 Primary Renal Diseases and Recurrence Rates

DISEASE	RECURRENCE RATE (%)	GRAFT LOSS (%)
Diabetes	100	Low until 10 years after transplantation
Focal segmental glomerulonephritis	20-30, first transplant; 80, second transplant	40-50
MPGN type 1	20-30	20-60
MPGN type 2	50-100	10
IgA nephropathy	40-50	30
Membranous nephropathy	40	Up to 50
Hemolytic uremic syndrome	30	20-30
Systemic lupus	30	Rare
Polycystic kidney disease	0	0

MPGN, membranoproliferative glomerulonephritis.

so a hypercoagulable profile can be obtained. The ability of the patient to tolerate immunosuppression should be evaluated. This involves consideration not only of the medical conditions but also of the ability to comply with a complex medical regimen and the financial ability to obtain the medications.

Patients with ESRD are at increased risk for cardiovascular disease.[5] Hence, a careful preoperative cardiac screening must be completed. There is little consensus as to the optimal screening algorithm; however, dobutamine stress echocardiography has been shown to have superiority in accuracy and predictability for perioperative cardiac events.[16] Patients should have a baseline electrocardiogram, recognizing that nearly 75% will have evidence of left ventricular hypertrophy. The patient's risk profile should be assessed to determine whether any risk factors can be modified (diet, weight management). Low-risk patients include those who have good functional capacity and no cardiac disease previously identified. These are typically patients with isolated renal disease, such as IgA nephropathy or polycystic kidney disease, and have little comorbidity. Moderate-risk patients should undergo stress testing. It is important to ensure that the stress is diagnostic and a reasonable heart rate was achieved. Moderate-risk patients include those without cardiac symptoms but who have diabetes, a prior history of heart disease, or two or more other risk factors for coronary disease (smoking, strong family history, hyperlipidemia, hypercholesterolemia). High-risk patients include those with a positive result on noninvasive testing, long-standing diabetes, or history of severe congestive heart failure. These patients require cardiac catheterization before being accepted for the transplant list. Cardiac revascularization should occur before transplantation. Patients are required by national policy to be reevaluated on a yearly basis. At any reevaluation, the cardiac status should be routinely reviewed and updated.

A full physical examination should be completed. Renal failure patients are at increased risk for cerebrovascular events, and the stroke risk is 10 times higher than that of the general population.[17] Therefore, if carotid bruits are discovered, patients should be screened for significant carotid stenosis. Atrial fibrillation can also be discovered on physical examination. The femoral, dorsalis pedis, and posterior tibial arteries should be palpated and any

TABLE 26-2 Kidney Donor Profile Index (KDPI) Score Components

Age	Height
Weight	Ethnicity
Brain death or circulatory death	Creatinine level
Stroke	Hypertension
Diabetes	Hepatitis C

bruits documented. If the pulses are abnormal or the patient has undergone previous amputation for vascular disease, a noncontrast abdominal and pelvic computed tomography (CT) scan should be obtained to assess the level of peripheral vascular disease. It may be that iliac inflow is significantly compromised, which would prevent the patient from having a successful outcome. If inflow is compromised, one can consider whether a revascularization with conduits is warranted before or at the time of transplantation.[18]

Kidney organs can be obtained from living or deceased donors. The demand for kidney transplant and appropriate organs has continually increased, given the increase in the burden of ESRD. Whereas living donation and living unrelated donation have increased in recent years, expanding the deceased donor pool is crucial. In 2003, the national Organ Donation Breakthrough Collaborative was launched. The intent of this national effort was to increase the conversion rate (number of families consenting to donation in appropriate potential donors) to 75%. An update in 2005 sought to further increase donor organs by increasing the average organs transplanted per donor to 3.75.[19] Deceased donor kidneys have traditionally been placed in three broad categories: extended criteria donor (ECD), standard criteria donor (SCD), and donor after cardiac death (DCD). ECD kidneys are obtained from donors older than 60 years or from donors aged 50 to 59 years with at least two of the following: cerebrovascular accident as cause of death, terminal creatinine concentration above 15 mg/dL, or history of hypertension. Kidneys from donors meeting criteria for ECD have a 1.7 relative risk of graft loss compared with kidneys from other donors.[20] However, recipients of ECD kidneys clearly have a survival benefit compared with those remaining on the waitlist. In donation after cardiac death, the care team has determined that the patient is unlikely to make a reasonable recovery and the patient is being maintained on mechanical ventilation. If the family is interested in organ donation, a request is made to consider donation after cardiac death. If the family consents, the ventilator is disconnected in either the operating room or intensive care unit. If the heart stops within a designated time frame (depends on the organ to be procured), the team waits several minutes to ensure cardiac standstill. The patient is then declared dead by the care team (not a member of the organ recovery team), and the organs are procured en bloc.

There has been a recent significant change in the kidney allocation system. Effective December 4, 2014, all kidney organs will receive a score, the Kidney Donor Profile Index (KDPI). This profile is based on 10 clinical factors (Table 26-2). Patients will be required to sign an informed consent for kidneys whose score is greater than 85% because of the decreased long-term outcome. Details of the new allocation system are noted later.

Living Donor Selection

The first successful living kidney donation was performed in 1954. Since that time, data continue to show that living kidney donation provides the best graft and patient survival results in recipients. Donors may or may not be genetically related to their intended recipient. In some cases, living donors are anonymous. There are several reports of extended altruistic donor chains. In these cases, an initial donor-recipient pair cannot go forward with transplantation, usually because of ABO incompatibility or sensitization of the recipient. A reciprocal exchange with another incompatible pair allows a "domino transplant" with multiple exchanges, with centers across the country participating. There has been no difference in outcomes of kidneys requiring shipping in paired donation versus traditional living kidney donation.[21] The 5-year survival of an unrelated kidney transplant is the same as that of a kidney transplant from a related donor. The underlying premise of living donation is that the donor will not suffer any medical consequences from the donation and has minimal surgical risk.

Currently accepted eligibility criteria include the following: age, 18 to 70 years; BMI below 35; no cancer or active infection; and adequate renal function. ABO compatibility is also a consideration. However, recipients can undergo desensitization protocols, and transplantation can be performed across ABO barriers. The donor should be informed in these circumstances of an increased risk of rejection of the kidney by the recipient. There is some individual variation among transplant centers concerning acceptable GFR or BMI. Relative contraindications include renal stones, impaired glucose tolerance with a family history of type 2 diabetes, GFR of 70 to 80 mL/min/1.72 m^2, hypertension, and BMI above 35. Absolute contraindications are listed in Box 26-3. For screening, all donors should have a thorough history and physical examination completed. Potential donors should be asked about nonsteroidal use in addition to questions about any medical illnesses. Potential donors should be made aware of the need to be away from work for a time, and their willingness to donate free of coercion should be ascertained. An electrocardiogram and chest radiograph should be obtained. Routine laboratory work should include urinalysis, complete blood count, liver function testing, creatinine concentration (with estimated GFR), chemistries, lipid profile, microalbumin level, and oral glucose tolerance test. Prostate-specific antigen levels should be obtained in men. Mammograms and Papanicolaou smears should be completed in women of appropriate age. Radiographic evaluation of the anatomy of the renal arteries, veins, and collecting system should be performed and can be done by CT angiography, magnetic resonance imaging, or arteriography on the basis of local expertise. In addition, all donors must be evaluated by an independent donor advocate. The independent donor advocate is not influenced by a relationship with the intended recipient or the

BOX 26-3 Contraindications to Living Kidney Donation

BMI > 40
Diabetes
Active malignant disease
HIV positive
GFR < 70 mL/min/1.72 m^2
Significant albuminuria
Hypertension requiring multiple medications
Pelvic or horseshoe kidney
Significant psychiatric impairment
Nephrolithiasis with a high chance of recurrence (cystine, struvite)

transplant center. The donor and recipient pair must also adhere to the National Organ Transplant Act of 1984, which states, "It is unlawful for any person to knowingly acquire, receive, or otherwise transfer any human organ for valuable consideration for use in human transplantation." Many transplant centers ask potential donors to undergo a psychological or psychiatric evaluation.

Potential donors should be informed that the risk of perioperative mortality regardless of surgical technique is approximately 0.03%. Matas and colleagues[22] surveyed 234 United Network for Organ Sharing (UNOS)–listed kidney transplant programs and found that reoperation was required in 0.4% of patients undergoing open nephrectomy, in 1.0% of hand-assisted laparoscopic nephrectomy, and in 0.9% of total laparoscopic nephrectomy.

Donor nephrectomy may be performed by open or laparoscopic techniques. The open technique is performed through a flank incision. There are variations in the technique of laparoscopic donor nephrectomy. Some centers use a hand-assisted approach; others perform the procedure entirely laparoscopically and make a Pfannenstiel incision to retrieve the kidney. Some centers perform a single-incision donor nephrectomy and dissect the renal hilum using instruments placed through a GelPort system, which is ultimately the site of kidney retrieval. If unexpected anatomy or bleeding is encountered, it is important to promptly convert to open techniques to prevent any donor complications or prolonged surgery.

Laparoscopic Surgical Technique

Either the right or left kidney can be procured laparoscopically. The left renal anatomy is generally preferred as the renal vein is longer. Many studies have shown that the right kidney can be procured safely.[23] A left kidney dissection is described here as it is far more common. A 5-mm entry site is placed in the left lower quadrant, and a Veress needle is used to insufflate the abdomen to a pressure of 10 to 15 mm Hg. A 12-mm port is placed at the umbilicus. Two additional 5-mm ports are placed, one at the left costal margin and the last in the midaxillary line to retract the kidney.

The left colon and splenic flexure are taken down at the line of Toldt with the harmonic scalpel. The ureter and gonadal vein complex are identified at the pelvic brim and isolated from surrounding tissue. The renal vein is identified by following the gonadal vein to its entry point. The artery is identified, and lymphatic tissue overlying the artery and vein is divided with the harmonic scalpel.

The adrenal gland is visualized at the upper pole of the kidney and divided from the upper pole of the kidney. The adrenal vein is dissected free from surrounding tissue and transected. The kidney is retracted medially, and the posterior and lateral attachments outside of Gerota fascia are divided with the harmonic scalpel. A Pfannenstiel incision is made approximately 3 fingerbreadths above the pubis. The rectus abdominis muscles are split at the midline, and a purse-string suture with 0 Vicryl suture is made in the peritoneum. Electrocautery is used to enter the peritoneum, and an Endo Catch bag is introduced for retrieval of the kidney. The ureter and gonadal vein are transected with the linear Endo GIA white load stapler at the pelvic brim. The artery is isolated and divided with an Endo GIA white load linear cutting stapler. The vein is also divided with the Endo GIA stapler. The kidney is placed in the Endo Catch bag and brought out through the Pfannenstiel incision and given to the recipient surgeon for flushing.

Open Surgical Technique

The patient is placed in the lateral decubitus position. A subcostal incision is made from the tip of the twelfth rib anteriorly extending approximately 10 to 12 cm. The latissimus dorsi and posterior serratus are divided. The external and internal oblique muscles are divided starting at the posterior border. The retroperitoneal space is exposed, and Gerota fascia is identified. The twelfth rib may need to be resected to allow better exposure. However, this will increase the risk of a postoperative pneumothorax (0.09%).[22] Gerota fascia is then incised. The ureter is identified and dissected down to the iliac vessels, at which point it is clipped and divided, preserving an appropriate length for subsequent transplantation. Tissue overlying the renal artery and vein is identified and divided. At this point, the kidney is isolated on its vascular pedicle. When the recipient team is ready, a right-angle clamp is placed on the renal artery and the artery is divided. A Satinsky clamp is placed around the inferior vena cava for a right nephrectomy or on the renal vein for a left nephrectomy. The renal vein is divided, and the kidney is given to the recipient team. The renal artery stump is then suture ligated. The renal vein stump is oversewn with a 5-0 Prolene suture in a running fashion.

Postoperative Care and Follow-up

Postoperatively, the patient should be kept well hydrated and careful attention paid to urine output. The diet can be advanced quickly in either open or laparoscopic cases. The most common complications are urinary retention and ileus. Other less common complications are bleeding, deep venous thrombosis or pulmonary embolism, rhabdomyolysis, injury to the bowel or bladder, and injury to the spleen. Patients who undergo laparoscopic donor nephrectomy tend to have shorter hospital stays (2 to 4 days) compared with patients who undergo open nephrectomy (3 to 7 days). The long-term consequences of kidney donation have been carefully reviewed. However, a long-term donor registry is still not a reality. Survival and the development of ESRD do not appear to be affected by living donation. In a study of 3698 kidney donors from 1963 to 2007 at a single center, it was shown that ESRD developed in 180 cases per million persons per year in donors compared with 268 cases per million persons per year in the general population.[24] Scores of physical and mental health in the living kidney donor population were significantly better than those of the general U.S. population.

Concerns have been raised recently about the long-term consequences of decreased GFR seen in living kidney donors and the risk of subsequent renal failure.[25] At issue has been whether original control groups were appropriate in comparing living donors with an unscreened population. In the current study, the authors compare donors to the third National Health and Nutrition Examination Survey (NHANES III). They found that kidney donors had a higher risk for development of ESRD throughout their life (90 per 10,000) compared with a healthy population (14 per 10,000), but the risk was still much lower than in the general population (326 per 10,000). There was increased risk noted in African American, older, and related donors. A follow-up editorial by Gill and Tonelli noted that ESRD in the NHANES III control group may have been underestimated, and there were different methods used to ascertain ESRD in donors, resulting in exaggerating the risk in donors.[26]

Deceased Donors

Procurement occurs after declaration of death, either brain death (Box 26-4) or cardiac death. The University of Wisconsin created

BOX 26-4 Confirmatory Testing for a Determination of Brain Death

Cerebral Angiography

The contrast medium should be injected under high pressure in both anterior and posterior circulation.

No intracerebral filling should be detected at the level of entry of the carotid or vertebral artery to the skull.

The external carotid circulation should be patent.

The filling of the superior longitudinal sinus may be delayed.

Electroencephalography

A minimum of eight scalp electrodes should be used.

Interelectrode impedance should be between 100 and 10,000 Ω.

The integrity of the entire recording system should be tested.

The distance between electrodes should be at least 10 cm.

The sensitivity should be increased to at least 2 μV for 30 minutes with inclusion of appropriate calibrations.

The high-frequency filter setting should not be set below 30 Hz, and the low-frequency setting should not be above 1 Hz.

Electroencephalography should demonstrate a lack of reactivity to intense somatosensory or audiovisual stimuli.

Transcranial Doppler Ultrasonography

There should be bilateral insonation. The probe should be placed at the temporal bone above the zygomatic arch or the vertebrobasilar arteries through the suboccipital transcranial window.

The abnormalities should include a lack of diastolic or reverberating flow and documentation of small systolic peaks in early systole. A finding of a complete absence of flow may not be reliable because of inadequate transtemporal windows for insonation.

Cerebral Scintigraphy (Technetium Tc 99m Hexametazime)

The isotope should be injected within 30 minutes after its reconstitution.

A static image of 500,000 counts should be obtained at several time points: immediately, between 30 and 60 minutes later, and at 2 hours.

A correct intravenous injection may be confirmed with additional images of the liver demonstrating uptake (optional).

From Wijdicks EF: The diagnosis of brain death. *N Engl J Med* 344:1215–1221, 2001.

a tool to determine the likelihood of progression to cardiac death to allow centers to better inform families (Table 26-3).[27] The criteria for establishing brain death were published in the *New England Journal of Medicine* in 2001. A complete neurologic examination must first be completed when the patient has a core temperature above 32° C and there is no evidence of drug intoxication, poisoning, or neuromuscular blocking agents. There can be no other medical conditions that can confound the clinical assessment, such as severe electrolyte, acid-base, or endocrine disturbances or hypotension. A complete clinical neurologic examination includes documentation of coma, the absence of brainstem reflexes, and apnea. Confirmatory testing is also completed as outlined in Box 26-4.

A careful medical and social history is obtained from the medical record and the family. Potential donors are excluded if there is active infection or malignant disease. Renal function and urine output are assessed. If a donor has increased risk behavior as defined by the Centers for Disease Control and Prevention (CDC) for transmission of HIV infection or hepatitis C, the intended recipient must be informed that the donor is high risk,

TABLE 26-3 Tool for Predicting Progression to Cardiac Death

DCD Tool Score

POINTS	EXPIRATION IN <60 MINUTES (%)	EXPIRATION IN <120 MINUTES (%)
7-11	4-24	10-40
12-17	34-87	51-91
18-23	92-98	94-98

University of Wisconsin DCD Evaluation Tool

CRITERIA	ASSIGNED POINTS	POINT SCORE
Spontaneous Respirations after 10 minutes		
Rate >12	1	
Rate <12	3	
TV >200 mL	1	
TV <200 mL	3	
NIF >20	1	
NIF <20	3	
No Spontaneous Respirations	**9**	
BMI		
<25	1	
25-29	2	
>30	3	
Vasopressors		
No vasopressors	1	
Single vasopressor	2	
Multiple vasopressors	3	
Patient Age		
0-30	1	
31-50	2	
51+	3	
Intubation		
Endotracheal tube	3	
Tracheostomy	1	
Oxygenation after 10 minutes		
O_2 Sat >90%	1	
O_2 Sat 80%-89%	2	
O_2 Sat <79%	3	
Final score		
Date of extubation	Time of extubation	
Date of expiration	Time of expiration	
Total time		

DCD, donor after cardiac death; *TV,* tidal volume; *NIF,* negative inspiratory force.
From Lewis J, Peltier J, Nelson H, et al: Development of the University of Wisconsin Donation After Cardiac Death Evaluation Tool. *Prog Transplant* 13:265–273, 2003.

and a written consent for transplantation with an increased risk CDC donor must be obtained (Box 26-5). In managing a donor, it is important to monitor urine output carefully. Vasopressin may need to be given if diabetes insipidus develops. Many organ procurement specialists administer hormonal therapy to stabilize the donor after the catecholamine release that is common in acute brain death.[28] This catecholamine release can result in significant decreases in thyroid hormone, cortisol, and insulin levels.

Kidney Procurement and Preparation

The retroperitoneum is fully exposed. The ureters are identified and divided as close to the bladder as possible. In procuring the

BOX 26-5 Increased Risk CDC Donor: 2013 Update

Donors meeting one or more of the following 11 criteria should be identified as being at increased risk for recent HIV, hepatitis B virus (HBV), and hepatitis C virus (HCV) infection

1. Men who have had sex with another man (MSM) in the preceding 12 months
2. Women who have had sex with a man with a history of MSM behavior in the preceding 12 months
3. People who have had sex with a person who has injected drugs by intravenous, intramuscular, or subcutaneous route for nonmedical reasons in the preceding 12 months
4. People who have injected drugs by intravenous, intramuscular, or subcutaneous route for nonmedical reasons in the preceding 12 months
5. People who have engaged in sex in exchange for money or drugs in the preceding 12 months
6. Persons who have had sex in the preceding 12 months with a person known or suspected to have HIV, HBV, or HCV infection
7. Persons who have had sex with a person who has sex in exchange for money or drugs in the preceding 12 months
8. People who have been in lockup, jail, prison, or a juvenile correctional facility for more than 72 hours in the preceding 12 months
9. A child who is ≤18 months of age and born to a mother known to be infected with or at increased risk for HIV, HBV, or HCV infections
10. A child who has been breastfed within the preceding 12 months and the mother is known to be infected with or at increased risk for HIV infection
11. People who have been newly diagnosed with or have been treated for syphilis, gonorrhea, chlamydia, or genital ulcers in the preceding 12 months

right kidney, it is important to preserve the vena cava cuff so that the renal vein can be lengthened if needed to facilitate the recipient operation.

On the back table, Gerota fascia is removed. The renal artery and vein are identified. The ureter is identified, and the periureteric tissue as well as the tissue along the lower pole of the kidney is preserved to prevent ureter ischemia. If any lower pole renal arteries are identified, these must be reconstructed to ensure adequate blood supply to the ureter.

Preservation and Storage

Once the kidneys are procured, they must be transported to the respective transplant centers by the organ procurement organization. During this time, the kidneys experience changes from cold ischemia. The goal of preservation is to extend the period of organ viability. Delayed graft function significantly increases at 24 hours. Various preservation solutions have been developed over the years. The predominant storage solution currently used in the United States is ViaSpan (Dupont). The contents of ViaSpan are noted in Table 26-4.

Kidneys may be stored in static cold solution. However, there is increasing evidence supporting the use of pulsatile machine perfusion in the preservation of kidneys. With use of this technology, flow is maintained throughout the kidney and vasoconstriction can be minimized. A study by Ploeg and colleagues[29] showed that machine perfusion significantly decreased the risk of delayed graft function, and recipient creatinine concentration was significantly lower for the first 2 weeks after transplantation. Interestingly, there was no difference seen when a subgroup analysis of

TABLE 26-4 Contents of University of Wisconsin Preservation Solution (ViaSpan)

Lactobionic acid	100 mmol/L
KOH (5 M)	20 mL
NaOH (5 M)	5 mL
Adenosine	5 mmol/L
Allopurinol	3 mmol/L
KH_2PO_4	25 mmol/L
HES	5 g%
Glutathione	3 mmol/L
Raffinose	30 mmol/L
$MgSO_4$	5 mmol/L
Insulin	40 U/L
Dexamethasone	8 mg/L
Bactrim	2 mL/L

DCD, ECD, and SCD kidneys was completed. However, if delayed graft function did develop, the duration was 3 days shorter in machine-perfused kidneys (10 versus 13 days; $P = .04$).

Recipient Operation

The kidney is usually placed in a retroperitoneal position in the recipient. The donor renal vein is anastomosed to the common iliac vein, and the donor artery is anastomosed to the recipient common or external iliac artery. It should be noted if the recipient has significant upstream iliac atherosclerotic disease as this may affect transplant outcomes. The ureter is then spatulated, and an end-to-side anastomosis is completed to the bladder mucosa. A ureteral stent is placed that is then removed 4 to 6 weeks postoperatively.

Postoperative Surgical Complications

The overall rate of technical complications in kidney transplantation is low (5% to 10%). Most complications are manifested as a sudden drop in urine output. However, some recipients experience delayed graft function, so urine output is not a reliable marker of a surgical complication. Daily monitoring of serum creatinine and hemoglobin levels is crucial in the first days after kidney transplantation. Other parameters, such as β_2-microglobulin, can also be helpful to differentiate early rejection from a surgical complication. The most common surgical complications are outlined here.

Hemorrhage

If the kidney transplant was placed in the retroperitoneal space and no window was created to the peritoneal cavity, bleeding will be limited. Patients will commonly present with the acute onset of flank pain, and there may be a palpable mass at the incision site. An acute decrease in hematocrit or hemoglobin may also be seen. Because of compression of the kidney parenchyma, patients will sometimes present with hypertension rather than with the expected hypotension. Many patients are receiving beta blockers, so tachycardia is also not a reliable sign. The patient must be examined, and a high clinical suspicion should be maintained. Risk factors include obesity, antiplatelet agents, and anticoagulation.[30] An ultrasound examination can be helpful if time permits. Often, the bleeding site cannot be identified, and evacuation of a large hematoma is completed. Biopsy of the kidney should be performed as hyperacute rejection can lead to kidney swelling and disruption of the parenchyma as the cause of the bleed (Fig. 26-2).

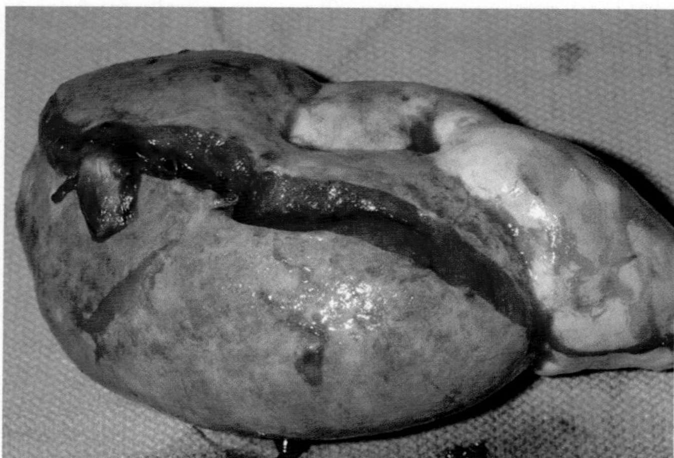

FIGURE 26-2 Acute rejection causing kidney parenchymal disruption and hemorrhage.

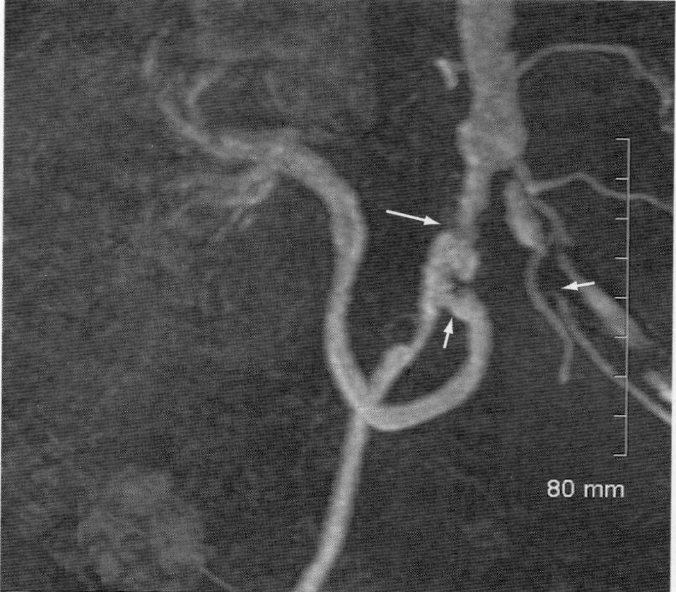

FIGURE 26-3 Angiogram demonstrating native iliac disease limiting arterial inflow to the transplant kidney.

Venous Thrombosis

Venous thrombosis occurs in 0.5% to 4% of cases and usually is manifested within the first week postoperatively.[31] The patient may develop sudden hematuria or decrease in urine output. Ultrasound examination confirms the diagnosis. The transplanted renal vein might be kinked at the time of the original transplantation because of compression in the retroperitoneal position or possibly external compression for a lymphocele or hematoma. Dialysis patients also have a high incidence of hypercoagulable states. A preoperative hypercoagulable workup should be completed if the patient reports multiple dialysis access thrombosis events (especially of native fistulas), a history of deep venous thrombosis or pulmonary embolism, or a high incidence of miscarriages. The graft is usually unable to be salvaged after renal vein thrombosis. There are case reports of salvage if the patient is able to be taken to the operating room within the hour after the diagnosis.[32] However, this is rare, and a transplant nephrectomy is usually required.

Arterial Thrombosis

Arterial thrombosis occurs in less than 1% of cases. The patient may have sudden cessation of urine output, or the failure of the β_2-microglobulin levels to fall after transplantation may herald the problem. Ultrasound is diagnostic. If there is normal anatomy and a single renal artery, the chance of salvage is minimal. The kidney will not tolerate warm ischemia, and a transplant nephrectomy is warranted. In rare cases, if a segmental artery or upper pole branch is affected, the remaining renal mass may be able to sustain the patient for a time. However, if a lower pole artery is thrombosed, the ureter becomes ischemic, and a urine leak may develop from ureteral necrosis.

Arterial Stenosis

Stenosis of the renal artery is a late complication. The incidence varies from 1% to 23%. Patients usually present with an asymptomatic rise in creatinine concentration. Some may have bilateral lower extremity edema and worsening hypertension. Magnetic resonance imaging or CT angiography can be performed to confirm the diagnosis. Patients may have upstream iliac disease, which will mimic transplant renal artery stenosis as the transplant is still ischemic. Many modalities can be used to treat the stenosis. If the native iliac artery is diseased, balloon angioplasty has been successful. Figure 26-3 demonstrates native iliac artery atherosclerotic disease. In this case, the renal artery was anastomosed to the recipient's hypogastric artery at the initial operation because of native atherosclerotic disease. Balloon angioplasty of transplant renal artery stenosis has success rates varying between 20% and 80%. Another alternative is to use ABO-compatible deceased donor iliac artery as a bypass graft from the native iliac artery to a point beyond the renal artery stenosis.[33]

Urologic Complications

The blood supply to the ureter comes from multiple sources including the gonadal artery, superior and inferior vesicular arteries, and common iliac and hypogastric arteries. During procurement of the donor kidney, it is important to avoid injury to the periureteric tissue in the "golden triangle," an anatomic area defined by the renal artery, the lower pole of the kidney, and the ureter. Approximately 15% to 20% of donors have a lower pole renal artery that is a major source of arterial inflow to the ureter. Complications of the ureter include leak, obstruction, and stenosis. Use of a stent at the time of implantation has been associated with fewer mechanical urologic complications. However, there is an increased incidence of urinary tract infections when stents are used. Stenosis may occur early or late and occurs in 2% to 15% of recipients.[34] Early in the course of transplantation, stenosis may be caused by extrinsic compression from a lymphocele or acute ischemia. Polyoma (BK) virus is a cause of late multiple strictures. Patients usually present with an asymptomatic rise in creatinine concentration. If a leak is present, patients may report significant pelvic pain. If the diagnosis is obstruction or stenosis, an ultrasound examination will demonstrate hydronephrosis (Fig. 26-4) and may also show a lymphocele obstructing the ureter. The acute obstruction can be relieved by placing a percutaneous nephrostomy tube. A more definitive study can then be performed to demonstrate the exact location of the obstruction. A short, very distal obstruction or stenosis can be repaired by reimplanting the ureter. A long stricture or very proximal stricture will need to be repaired by performing a ureteropyelostomy and using the native

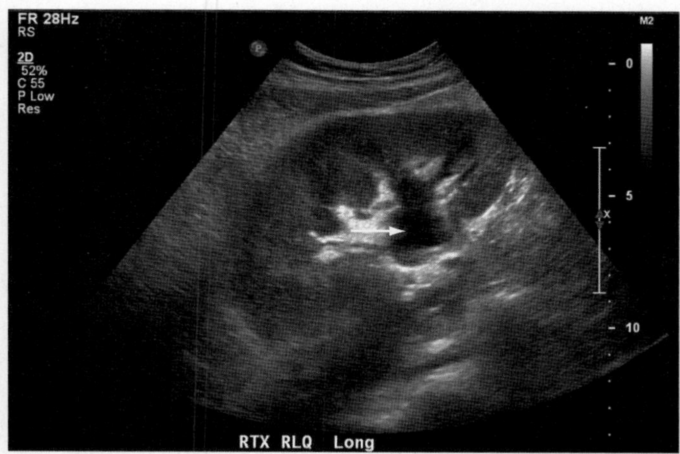

FIGURE 26-4 Ultrasound image demonstrating hydronephrosis.

ureter. It is important to determine that the patient has a normal native ureter before this reconstruction.

Urine leak can also develop. This occurs in 1% of cases overall but accounts for 25% of all urologic complications.[34] Patients present with pain as well as swelling at the transplant site, usually within the first week after transplantation. The creatinine concentration is also elevated. The diagnosis can be made by aspirating the perinephric fluid and checking the creatinine level. A nuclear medicine scan can also be performed. Delayed images will reveal the urine leak when the contrast material is seen outside of the bladder. Placement of a double-J stent at the time of transplantation may decrease the risk of this complication.[34] Graft loss is rare with urologic complications.

Lymphocele

During the routine recipient operation, the lymphatics overlying the iliac vessels are divided. Approximately 1% to 18% of recipients can develop a lymphocele when these lymphatics leak.[30] Careful ligation at the time of transplantation can help decrease the incidence of this complication, but it does not completely eliminate the risk. Many lymphoceles are asymptomatic. However, some patients may present with a swollen leg and increased creatinine concentration because of compression on the iliac vein or transplanted ureter. Ultrasound is diagnostic (Fig. 26-5). The treatment of symptomatic lymphoceles is surgical, with a peritoneal communication being established either by open techniques or laparoscopically. Percutaneous aspiration has poor results with a high rate or recurrence and also carries the risk of infecting the fluid collection. A systematic analysis of management of lymphoceles revealed a slightly lower recurrence rate with laparoscopic fenestration versus open techniques (16% versus 8%).[35] With the open technique, a large peritoneal window can be created. Laparoscopic techniques are successful and are associated with less postoperative pain and a slight decrease in hospital stay. Care must be taken not to injure the transplanted ureter in creating a window by either technique. The lymphocele fluid should be sent for creatinine levels at the time of surgery to ensure that there is no occult urine leak.

Infections

Infectious complications are common after transplantation in large part because of the use of immunosuppression. Up to 80% of recipients experience a urinary tract infection. There is a 1% to 10% chance of wound infections immediately after surgery. As expected, diabetes, obesity, and the use of steroids increase the risk. Viral infections are also common in the first 3 months after transplantation as this is the time that the patient is receiving the highest levels of maintenance immunosuppression and the effects of induction therapy are the most pronounced. Common viral infections include CMV, Epstein-Barr virus, and polyomavirus (BK-type). For this reason, many transplant centers will treat patients in the early post-transplantation phase with antivirals including ganciclovir, acyclovir, and valganciclovir. Another common opportunistic infection is *Pneumocystis jiroveci,* and trimethoprim-sulfamethoxazole (Bactrim) or pentamidine is used as prophylaxis.

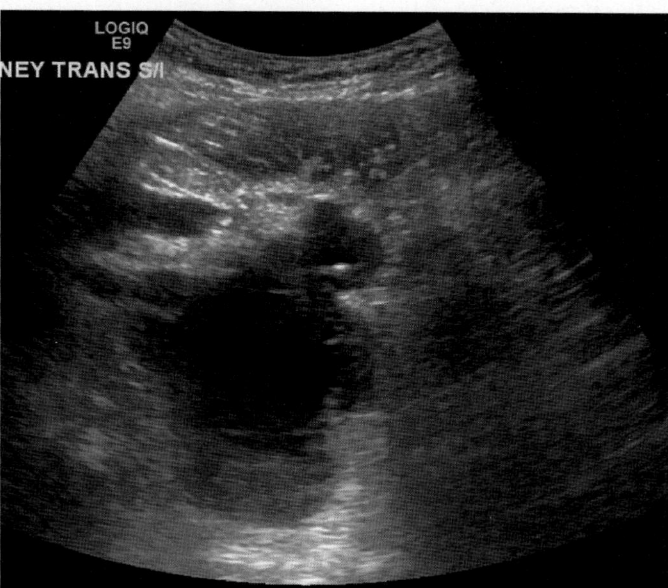

FIGURE 26-5 Ultrasound image demonstrating a lymphocele.

TABLE 26-5 Adult Kidney Graft Survival

	1 YEAR	5 YEARS	10 YEARS
Deceased donor, non-ECD	93.7%	75.6%	49.7%
Deceased donor, ECD	88.3%	60.7%	28.6%
Living donor	97.0%	84.7%	61.1%

ECD, extended criteria donor.
From Scientific Registry of Transplant Recipients annual report. <http://www.srtr.org/>, (Accessed December 10, 2014).

Outcomes

Transplantation offers patients a better quality of life compared with dialysis. It is also a cost-effective form of kidney replacement therapy associated with improved survival, especially if the patient can be transplanted before initiation of dialysis. Patient survival is excellent at 1 year; the survival rate is 98% for living donation recipients and 95% for recipients of deceased donor kidneys. At 5 years, recipients of living donation/living unrelated donation kidneys have a survival of 90%, and it exceeds that of non-ECD recipients, whose survival is 83%. Recipients of ECD kidneys have a 5-year survival of 69%. Graft survival at 1 year, 2 years, 5 years, and 10 years has steadily improved, probably because of decreased donor graft loss.[36] These percentages can certainly be affected by recipient selection.[19] Current 1-, 5-, and 10-year graft survival is shown in Table 26-5. The most common cause of graft loss is progressive interstitial fibrosis that ultimately leads to kidney failure.

Kidney Allocation

Significant concerns were raised that the kidney allocation system that had been in place for nearly 3 decades before 2013 was outdated and did not allow the best use of kidney allografts from deceased donors. In 2003, work began to diminish the system limitations that resulted in higher discard rates, variability in access, and unrealized graft survival years. In June 2013, the Organ Procurement and Transplantation Network Board of Directors approved sweeping changes to the current kidney allocation system. In the new system, recipients will receive an Estimated Post Transplant Survival (EPTS) score, which is calculated on the basis of four variables: recipient age, diabetic status, time on dialysis, and number of prior solid organ transplants. Those candidates with the longest potential survival will preferentially receive kidney allografts that are also estimated to have long survival times.

Deceased donor kidneys will also receive a score, the Kidney Donor Profile Index (KDPI), which is based on 10 variables (see Table 26-2). Kidneys will no longer be classified as ECD or DCD but will receive a score. Kidneys with the top 20% KDPI are preferentially allocated to the top 20% EPTS candidates. Those kidneys with a KDPI greater than 85% will be an "opt in" system that will require recipients to sign prior consent for these kidneys. Kidneys with a KDPI greater than 85% will be allocated on the basis of waiting time and local or regional area.[37]

It is estimated that this new system of allocation will gain more than 8000 years of graft longevity, and it is the hope that this will decrease the need for retransplantation, thereby effectively increasing the pool of donor organs available.[37]

PANCREAS TRANSPLANTATION

Diabetes is a major health concern in the United States and is the single leading cause of ESRD. Diabetic retinopathy is a leading cause of blindness. In 1999, the American Diabetes Association clinical guidelines advocated whole organ pancreas transplantation as a viable treatment option for type 1 diabetes. The guidelines state, "Pancreas transplantation should be considered an acceptable therapeutic alternative to continued insulin therapy in diabetic patients with imminent or established end-stage renal disease who have had or plan to have a kidney transplant, because the successful addition of a pancreas does not jeopardize patient survival, may improve kidney survival, and will restore normal glycemia" (www.guideline.gov). According to the International Pancreas Transplant Registry, as of December 2010, more than 35,000 pancreas transplants have been performed worldwide, with more than 24,000 in the United States alone.[38] Successful pancreas transplantation can improve the quality of life of patients with type 1 diabetes by eliminating the need for frequent glucose monitoring and decreasing the need for strict dietary monitoring. In addition, patients and their families no longer need to monitor for hypoglycemic events that are life-threatening.

The history of pancreas transplantation has been marked by the limitations of surgical complications and rejection. In the early era of pancreas transplantation, 25% of grafts were lost because of technical issues. With improvements in technique and immunosuppression, the current report of the Scientific Registry of Transplant Recipients reveals that 1-year patient survival for both pancreas transplantation alone (PTA) and simultaneous pancreas and kidney transplantation (SPK) is more than 95%. The 1-year pancreas graft survival is 85% for SPK, 76% for PTA, and 82% for pancreas after kidney (PAK) transplantation nationally.[39] Patients who undergo SPK have better renal graft function compared with patients receiving a kidney alone, without an increase in surgical complications.[40]

Patient Selection

Patients requiring pancreas transplantation are usually type 1 diabetics with a clear C-peptide deficiency. Given that insulin therapy can mitigate the complications of hyperglycemia, patients who are accepted as transplant recipients must balance the effects of lifelong immunosuppression and potential surgical risk with the opportunity to improve their quality of life and perhaps decrease the progression of microvascular complications. Patients may undergo SPK, PTA, or PAK transplantation from a different donor. For patients choosing PTA, there should be clear documentation of significant hypoglycemic events as well as of stable renal function. Because the patients will require calcineurin inhibitor therapy after PTA, a GFR of more than 70 to 80 mL/min/1.72 m^2 and proteinuria of less than 1 g are required in our program. In addition, these patients should be informed that PTA has been shown to be an independent risk factor for renal failure.[41] In PAK candidates, a GFR of more than 50 mL/min/1.72 m^2 is required to maintain renal function with a temporary increase in immunosuppression. Patients with minimal secondary complications are the best candidates for pancreas transplantation. However, it has been shown that many of the secondary complications of diabetes are ameliorated by a constant euglycemic state.

Diabetes is a major risk factor for atherosclerosis, so careful screening for cardiac disease and peripheral vascular disease is necessary. Cardiovascular disease is the leading cause of death among type 1 diabetics.[42] The evaluation of the cardiac reserve of a pancreas transplant candidate is controversial. Algorithms that differentiate patients at high and low risk for perioperative cardiac events have been shown to be effective in decreasing mortality.[42] Whereas concerns about preserving renal function are important, correction of cardiac lesions before transplantation is paramount to a successful outcome. Given the burden of disease in this population, cardiac catheterization is recommended for evaluation. A careful physical examination, with particular attention paid to the peripheral dorsalis pedis and posterior tibial pulses as well as the presence of carotid bruits, can help determine if further screening studies are required.

SPK has recently been offered to a growing number of patients with type 2 diabetes. The overall rate increased from 2% in 1995 to 7% in 2010. According to the same database, approximately 8% of SPK, 5% of PAK, and 1% of PTA transplantations were performed in patients with type 2 diabetes in 2010. UNOS has defined the following criteria for SPK: (1) insulin therapy and C-peptide level below 2 ng/mL; or (2) insulin therapy with C-peptide level above 2 ng/mL and BMI below 28. However, current results from all single-center and database studies do not provide a clear message about the pros and cons of SPK in type 2 diabetes with chronic kidney disease, and many physicians remain skeptical about its definite role as it carries significant surgical challenges, and it is not an immediately lifesaving procedure.[43]

Pancreas Donor

There are no reliable scoring systems to determine the suitability of a pancreas donor. A clinical judgment must be made at the

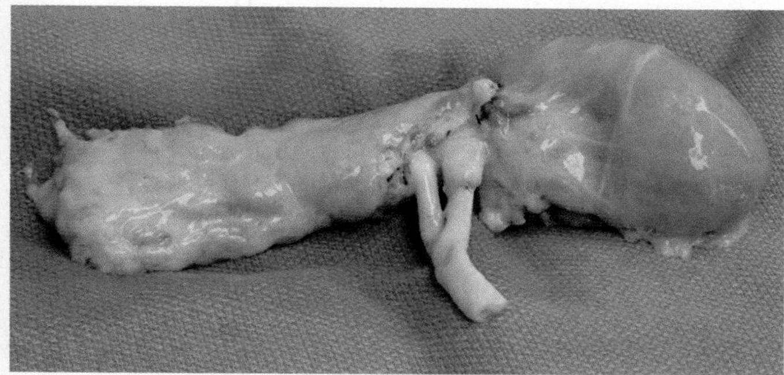

FIGURE 26-6 Photograph of the "ideal pancreas."

TABLE 26-6 Pancreas Graft Outcomes

	AGE	
OUTCOME	<18 YEARS (*N* = 63)	>18 YEARS (*N* = 237)
Glomerular filtration rate	65.6 ± 16	58.3 ± 17*
5-year glucose	85.3 ± 13	95.2 ± 29*
5-year hemoglobin A1c	5.47 ± 0.98	5.86 ± 3.5†
5-year kidney	85.0%	83.2%
5-year pancreas	85.3%	79.8%

*P ≤ .002.
†P = .013.

time of procurement to determine the quality of a pancreas.[44] The ideal pancreas is neither fatty nor edematous (Fig. 26-6). Pancreas organs can be safely procured from DCD with outcomes similar to donation after brain death.[45] In DCD, we recommend warm ischemia times of less than 45 minutes. The ideal age range is 10 to 45 years. Pediatric donors can be safely used. In a study at the University of Wisconsin, there were 142 pancreas donors younger than 18 years. The average donor weight was 24.5 ± 5 kg. The aggregate outcomes in the pediatric donors are compared with those in adult donors in Table 26-6. The lower limit of age in this study was 3 years, and the lower weight limit was 25 kg.[46]

Pancreas Procurement, Preparation, and Transplantation

During the procurement, minimal handling of the pancreas is optimal. A generous midline incision is made and a median sternotomy is accomplished. It is most common to procure the liver and pancreas en bloc and then to separate the organs in ice to minimize warm ischemia time. The right and left colon are mobilized, and a Kocher maneuver is accomplished to free the duodenum and head of the pancreas. The gastrohepatic ligament is carefully inspected to identify a replaced left hepatic artery. The gastrohepatic ligament is divided as well as the omentum along the greater curvature of the stomach. The pancreas is visualized and inspected for fibrosis or masses. The splenic attachments are freed, and the tail of the pancreas is mobilized from its attachments, with care taken to stay away from the pancreatic parenchyma. The left gastric artery is ligated and divided. The pancreas is mobilized to the level of the vena cava. The bowel mesentery is ligated and divided. The mesenteric vessels may be ligated with ties before flushing, or a vascular stapling device may be used after flushing. If a stapling device is used, the mesentery should be carefully oversewn as the pancreas is prepared for transplantation to prevent any mesenteric vessels from retracting and causing a significant hematoma at the head of the pancreas after organ reperfusion. The stomach is divided at the level of the pylorus with a TA stapler, and the small bowel is divided with a GIA 55 or 75 stapler just distal to the ligament of Treitz. The superior mesenteric artery (SMA) root is identified. The aorta is cross-clamped, and 2 liters of University of Wisconsin solution (ViaSpan) is flushed through the organs. University of Wisconsin solution remains the preferred solution as histidine-tryptophan-ketoglutarate preservation solution was associated with increased risk of thrombosis.[44] The pancreas and liver block is removed.

On the back table, the SMA is identified, and care is taken to preserve a replaced right hepatic artery if it is present. The splenic artery is identified, and a small 6-0 Prolene suture is used to mark the splenic artery as it enters the pancreatic body. The splenic artery is then divided. Division of the portal vein must be done carefully to ensure adequate length for both the liver and pancreas transplant recipients. At least 1 cm of portal vein should be preserved for the pancreas anastomosis. Extension of the portal vein for pancreas transplantation results in an unacceptable risk of transplant thrombosis.

Once the pancreas and liver are separated, the pancreas is bathed in University of Wisconsin solution and further back table preparation ensues. The spleen is removed from the tail of the pancreas. A probe is placed in the splenic artery and SMA to check patency. The duodenal segment is then prepared. The segment is stapled with a GIA 55 stapler just distal to the pylorus, with care taken to preserve the pancreatic duct drainage. The excess distal small bowel is also shortened with a GIA stapler. Both staple lines are oversewn with 3-0 silk in a Lembert fashion. The portal vein is then dissected. There is usually one small peripancreatic venous branch that can be safely ligated and divided, thereby lengthening the portal vein. The splenic artery and SMA are clearly identified. The excess celiac plexus tissue between the arteries is carefully ligated and divided. Extreme care must be taken to prevent injury to the pancreas at this point. Several figure-of-eight silk sutures are placed in this area to prevent bleeding after reperfusion.

The vascular reconstruction is then completed. The iliac artery is used as a Y-graft, and an end-to-end anastomosis of the external and internal iliac arteries to the pancreas splenic artery and SMA, respectively, is completed with 6-0 Prolene sutures in a running fashion.

The recipient is then prepared. A midline incision is made, and the iliac arteries are exposed for systemic drainage. The pancreas transplant is usually placed on the right side to prevent undue stretching of the venous anastomosis. For systemic venous drainage, the portal vein is anastomosed to the distal vena cava in an end-to-side fashion. The iliac artery graft is sutured to the common iliac artery of the recipient. For portal drainage, the donor portal vein is anastomosed to the recipient proximal superior mesenteric vein. A path is created in the small bowel mesentery so that the arterial Y-graft can be anastomosed to the iliac artery (usually the right). The vascular clamps are then removed. Slow, sequential removal of the clamps is essential to prevent hematoma formation. The venous clamp is slowly removed, and venous bleeding is controlled. The distal arterial clamp is removed, and hemorrhage is controlled. The proximal arterial clamp is then removed. For enteric drainage of exocrine secretions, the bowel anastomosis is then completed from the duodenal transplant stump side to side to the recipient mid jejunum. If necessary, a Roux-en-Y drainage may also be performed to prevent tension on the transplant duodenal stump. We prefer a hand-sewn double-layer anastomosis as stapled anastomoses are associated with an increased risk of bleeding. The exocrine secretions may also be drained to the bladder. A 4- to 5-cm cystostomy is made on the anterior dome of the bladder. A two-layer anastomosis is completed; the outer layer is created with nonabsorbable 3-0 or 4-0 suture and the inner layer with absorbable 4-0 to 5-0 suture.

After completion of the exocrine drainage anastomosis, another careful inspection of the graft should be accomplished to identify any delayed bleeding that may have developed after warming of the transplant.

Drainage Techniques: Endocrine and Exocrine Secretions

Enteric Drainage or Bladder Drainage

Managing the exocrine secretions of the pancreas transplant remains a challenge. A multitude of techniques have been used over the years, including duct exclusion by injection, duct ligation, and even open drainage to the peritoneal cavity. In the past, the duodenal stump was thought to be a cause for rejection and the size was minimized by a "button technique" or the stump was eliminated altogether and a direct duct anastomosis was completed. However, all these techniques were complicated by significant leak rates. The duodenal stump is now left intact and anastomosed to either the bladder or bowel as described in the previous section.

Bladder drainage offers the advantages of decreasing the risk of enteric content contamination from the native enterotomy and allowing monitoring of urinary amylase level as an early diagnostic tool for dysfunction or rejection of the transplant. However, significant metabolic acidosis as well as urinary tract complications may develop. There is a high incidence of urinary tract infections, dysuria, urethritis, and even urethral disruption. Leaks can occur in the early postoperative course, and patients may present with abdominal discomfort or there may be an asymptomatic rise in amylase or lipase. Urinary anastomotic leaks can be diagnosed with a bladder contrast-enhanced CT scan with delayed images. If the CT scan does not show a significant amount of intra-abdominal fluid, a Foley catheter can be placed for 7 to 10 days. A normal amylase level with normoglycemia represents clinical resolution of the leak, and no further imaging studies are required in our experience. However, if a large amount of fluid is seen, the patient will require prompt laparotomy with consideration of transplant pancreatectomy if there is significant compromise of the duodenal stump.

Evidence of better outcomes has emerged after conversion of bladder drainage to enteric drainage in a subset of patients.[47] Given the good outcomes in patients who underwent conversion of bladder to enteric drainage and the fact that enteric drainage is more physiologic, interest was renewed in enteric drainage beginning in early 2000. Follow-up studies have shown that enteric drainage is not associated with significant increases in infection, and by use of this technique, the complications of bladder drainage can be avoided. Currently, the majority of pancreas transplants are performed with enteric drainage of the exocrine secretions, with only 20% of programs reporting the use of bladder drainage to the International Pancreas and Islet Transplant Association database.

Systemic Drainage versus Portal Drainage

Hyperinsulinemia has been noted in pancreas transplant recipients who have systemic drainage, probably because of the loss of the first-pass effect of hepatic degradation. Stratta and colleagues[48] began to champion portal drainage, which was proposed to be more physiologic and would not result in a proatherosclerotic state due to hyperinsulinemia. In long-term studies comparing systemic drainage and portal drainage, there has been no clear advantage seen in portal drainage. Whereas theoretical concern exists about atherosclerosis, no clear metabolic advantages of portal drainage have been proved. At this point, the choice of systemic drainage or portal drainage lies with the surgeon.[49]

Surgical Complications

Leak

Leak from the enteric anastomosis was the Achilles heel of early attempts at pancreas transplantation. The incidence varies from 2% to 10%. Enteric leak presents with signs and symptoms similar to intestinal perforation, including abdominal pain, nausea and vomiting, fever, and tachycardia. Patients may have an elevated white blood cell count, but this is often nonspecific as patients are receiving steroids. The amylase levels are not always affected. However, serum creatinine levels are often elevated and can signal ongoing infection. As a consequence of immunosuppression, transplant patients may not display overt signs of infection or leak, and a high index of suspicion is critical to timely diagnosis and treatment. Clinical suspicion may be sufficient to mandate reoperation, but radiographic imaging can often provide confirmatory evidence in equivocal cases. The most useful imaging test in this setting is CT with oral administration of a contrast agent. CT is especially useful for identifying the duodenal stump and recipient small bowel because ultrasound may be hampered by overlying bowel.[50] Findings include free or loculated intraperitoneal fluid, extraluminal air, and extravasation of contrast material.

Enteric leak almost always requires reoperation. Early leaks are most often anastomotic, and treatment depends on the size of the leak and the condition of the donor duodenum. Simple oversewing may be sufficient for small leaks. If part of the duodenum is compromised, that portion may be resected and the remaining duodenum shortened. If the original anastomosis was performed in a side-to-side fashion, a Roux-en-Y limb may be created to divert the intestinal stream away from the graft. In the case of significant leak with sepsis or advanced peritonitis or in the setting of devitalized tissue, graft pancreatectomy is the procedure of choice.

Most leaks occur in the first several weeks after transplantation. However, there is a subset of patients who experience leaks late in their transplant course. Predisposing factors included biopsy-proven rejection, CMV infection, blunt abdominal trauma, and obstructive uropathy. In a series of patients with bladder drainage, 9 of 25 cases of leaks resolved with Foley catheter treatment only. In the remainder, direct suture repair or conversion to enteric drainage was successful.[51] When leaks from the bladder anastomosis occur after 10 years, the duodenal stump can be thin walled, and conversion is associated with a higher rate of anastomotic leak from the newly created enteric anastomosis. For this reason, we recommend that enteric conversion in a transplant after 10 years be created with a Roux-en-Y anastomosis to divert the intestinal stream. We also place perianastomotic drains at the time of the conversion.

Vascular Complications

Thrombosis. Graft thrombosis represents the most common nonimmunologic cause of pancreas transplant failure. An analysis of UNOS data through June 2004 demonstrated graft loss rates due to thrombosis ranging from 2.7% in bladder-drained SPK to 8% in enteric-drained PTA. The choice of exocrine drainage affected graft thrombosis rates only in SPK (2.7% for bladder drained versus 5.4% for enteric drained).[52] Whereas thrombosis rates have improved considerably compared with previous eras of analysis, thrombosis remains the most common cause of early technical graft loss.

A number of risk factors have been identified for graft thrombosis. In the donor, advanced age, cerebrovascular cause of death, hemodynamic instability, and massive resuscitation confer a high risk.[52] Use of a venous interposition graft to extend the portal vein may also increase the risk for thrombosis. Recipient factors likely also play a part in graft thrombosis. Coagulopathy related to uremia may confer protection from thrombosis in recipients of SPK transplants, whereas the diabetic state is known to be associated with hypercoagulability. Results from a study of 152 patients indicate that low-dose heparin (200 to 400 units/hr or 5 units/kg/hr) for 48 hours postoperatively may provide a protective benefit in prevention of early graft loss resulting from thrombosis without an increased risk of bleeding.[53]

The majority of graft thromboses occur early after transplantation and are suspected in the setting of graft tenderness, hyperglycemia, elevation in serum amylase and lipase, or decrease in urinary amylase for bladder-drained pancreas transplants. Patients with arterial thrombosis may have an acute rise in glucose concentration without pain as the graft is not swollen after arterial thrombosis. Graft thrombosis leads to a rapid decline in the patient's clinical status, with hypotension and tachycardia developing soon after the rise in glucose. Emergent exploratory laparotomy with transplant pancreatectomy is often necessary. In the case of partial arterial thrombosis, the graft may occasionally be rescued with a combination of mechanical or pharmacologic thrombolysis and resection. The appearance of the graft on reexploration is critical. It is usually obvious whether there is sufficient viable pancreas to save.

Pancreas transplant ultrasound is the initial diagnostic test of choice. Doppler flow imaging can provide an overall view of parenchymal vascularity, and flow signals should be identified in both the arterial and venous systems. Limitations of ultrasonography include operator dependence and interference from surrounding structures and overlying bowel.

Percutaneous thrombolysis or thrombectomy may be of benefit in selected patients, especially those with partial venous thrombosis. In one report, catheter-directed thrombolysis and percutaneous mechanical thrombectomy achieved graft salvage in three of four patients.[54]

Bleeding. Immediate post-transplantation bleeding can occur from the pancreatic parenchyma, particularly near the SMA or splenic arteries. The patient presents with hypotension, tachycardia, and abdominal distention. It is our practice to place several figure-of-eight superficial silk sutures in the peripancreatic tissue lying between the SMA and splenic arteries to prevent bleeding in this difficult to approach area.

Delayed gastrointestinal bleeding can also occur from the enteric anastomosis. This usually is manifested from postoperative days 6 to 10 and is self-limited. Patients present with a sudden drop in hemoglobin and are usually hemodynamically stable. It is important to correct any coagulopathy that may be preexisting. Single doses of vasopressin at 0.3 μg/kg as well as initiation of an octreotide infusion at 25 μg/hr are also helpful in limiting blood loss. Endoscopy or radiographic studies are usually not diagnostic in this instance. However, if the patient becomes hemodynamically unstable, another diagnosis, such as duodenal ulcer, should be considered.

Late gastrointestinal bleeding can ensue as a result CMV infection, duodenal ulcers of the duodenal stump from ischemia, or rejection. Massive late gastrointestinal bleeding might be fatal if the diagnosis of aortoenteric fistula is not taken into consideration as a source of the hemorrhage in the differential diagnosis.[55] In such cases, the source of bleeding is not identified on upper and lower endoscopy. Findings on angiography of the celiac trunk and superior and inferior mesenteric arteries are also normal, which may prompt the physician to engage in desperate surgical exploration and resection of the bowel or pancreas, leading to uncontrolled bleeding from the iliac artery and the patient's death. The proper approach requires immediate diagnostic iliac artery angiography instead and therapeutic placement of a covered stent if aortoenteric fistula or pseudoaneurysm is identified.[55] The same approach should be considered in case of sudden intraperitoneal bleeding while draining a collection in proximity to the pancreas graft. Both aortoenteric fistula and pseudoaneurysms are prone to develop in cases of chronic rejection or in proximity to already failed organs.[55]

Other Considerations

Infections, bowel obstruction, and pancreatitis can also occur after transplantation. Most often, these do not require open surgical therapy but must be considered in the differential diagnosis of transplant dysfunction.

Infection. After pancreas transplantation, infection may develop in the superficial or deep wound spaces. The appropriate use of perioperative antibiotics can limit this complication. Pancreas transplant recipients should be treated with 48 hours of gram-positive, gram-negative, and fungal coverage.

Surgical site infection, most commonly from gram-positive organisms, may occur in up to 50% of patients. Superficial wound infections are generally treated with local wound care and additional antibiotics. Deep space or intra-abdominal infections are less common but carry a significantly greater morbidity. Signs and symptoms of intra-abdominal infection are similar to those for enteric leak. Ultrasound and CT are the mainstays of diagnosis.

The stable patient with a localized abscess can generally be treated with percutaneous abscess drainage. Patients with widespread infection or hemodynamic instability should be reexplored. Culture specimens should be obtained to focus antimicrobial therapy. Intra-abdominal infection, especially when it is close to the vascular anastomosis, may predispose to pseudoaneurysm formation. Unexplained intra-abdominal bleeding in a patient with a history of abdominal abscess should raise the possibility of anastomotic pseudoaneurysm as described before.

Pancreatitis. Graft pancreatitis is common after transplantation, occurring in as many as 35% of patients. Early pancreatitis is likely to be related to reperfusion injury to the graft. The diagnosis is made in the setting of abdominal pain and hyperamylasemia. It is important to rule out the possibility of acute rejection, although abdominal pain is less likely with rejection. CT imaging of the graft reveals a swollen, hypervascular organ, often with a significant amount of surrounding fluid. Our treatment of graft pancreatitis includes aggressive fluid resuscitation, withholding of enteral nutrition with institution of total parenteral nutrition as required, treatment of superimposed or concurrent infection, and supportive management. Most cases of pancreatitis are self-limited.

Bowel obstruction. Significant intra-abdominal dissection is required in pancreas transplantation. In contrast to the retroperitoneal kidney transplantation alone, the intraperitoneal nature of the pancreas operation increases the risk of bowel complications. Small bowel obstruction may be caused by postsurgical adhesions or by internal hernia formation.

Patients typically present with nausea, vomiting, obstipation, and abdominal pain. Plain radiographs demonstrate air-fluid levels, and CT confirms the diagnosis. In the stable patient, resuscitation and nasogastric tube decompression may be sufficient. Unstable patients or those with peritonitis should be explored in the operating room.

Outcomes

Pancreas transplantation is a safe and reliable treatment for type 1 diabetes. There is a significant survival benefit, with a waitlist mortality of 30% compared with 9% after transplantation.[56] Normoglycemia is restored, and patients demonstrate normal hemoglobin A1c levels. Importantly, patients do not suffer from hypoglycemic unawareness. Early efforts at pancreas transplantation were hindered by surgical complications and difficulty with the diagnosis and treatment of rejection. However, with improvements in surgical technique, immunosuppression, and tissue typing, outcomes have significantly improved in the current decade. Graft survival is comparable to that of other transplants, with a 1-year patient survival above 95% and survival at 3 years above 90%.[57] We have shown that patient survival at 1 year, 10 years, and 20 years is 97%, 80%, and 58%, respectively, with pancreas graft survival of 88%, 63%, and 36% during the same time frame. Acute rejection rates have fallen to below 10% in the current era of immunosuppression with prednisone, mycophenolate mofetil, and tacrolimus. A major consideration for pancreas transplantation is the potential for prevention of the secondary complications of diabetes. However, there are no randomized clinical trials comparing the efficacy of pancreas transplantation to tight glycemic control with insulin therapy. It has become increasingly apparent that benefits may not be seen until 5 to 10 years after transplantation.[56] Peripheral neuropathy improved after 1 year as shown by increased nerve conduction velocity. In addition, in a comparison of neuropathy in patients 10 years after transplantation, those with functioning pancreas grafts had stable nerve action amplitudes, whereas those patients with failed grafts showed steady decline.[58] There has been debate about the effect of consistent normoglycemia on diabetic retinopathy. The grade of disease before transplantation may affect the response. Those with severe disease before transplantation may still progress to blindness. However, in long-term follow-up, retinopathy stabilizes and conjunctival microcirculation improves in patients with successful transplantation.[59]

Successful pancreas transplantation normalizing glucose control for at least 1 year significantly improves kidney graft survival not only when the pancreas is implanted simultaneously but also, to a lesser extent, when pancreas transplantation follows deceased or living donor kidney transplantation. Survival of the patient is also improved in such a scenario.[60]

The major cause of death in pancreas transplant recipients is cardiovascular disease. A careful preoperative screening is necessary in these patients to treat any silent cardiac disease before transplantation. From 2005 to 2007, 72% of University of Wisconsin pretransplant patients were screened with coronary angiography. In addition to normalization of hemoglobin A1c levels and nearly normal fasting glucose levels, patients enjoy freedom from hypoglycemic events, which significantly improves the quality of life for both the patients and their families.

ISLET TRANSPLANTATION

Because the main goal of pancreas transplantation is to replace beta cell function, endocrine tissue only (islet) transplantation has the potential to provide the same therapeutic effect. Moreover, islet transplantation is a minimally invasive procedure, thereby avoiding complex intra-abdominal surgery and related surgical complications as well as those related to exocrine secretions of the pancreas. In patients with severe peripheral vascular disease, islet injection may offer the only chance for improved glucose control and an insulin-free life without fear of hypoglycemic unawareness. Transplanting only the islets also obviates the need to manage the complications secondary to the exocrine secretions of the pancreas. The patient and physician must consider the balance between the secondary complications of diabetes and the side effects of immunosuppression.

Isolation Techniques

Islet Transplantation Technique

For islet transplantation, the pancreas is procured and preserved from a deceased donor in the same fashion as for whole organ transplantation, with special attention paid to proper cooling of the organ during the entire procedure and not injuring the capsule of the organ. Because blood vessels are not used during islet isolation, in case of replaced right hepatic artery, the SMA might be easily dissected and sent with the liver and the pancreas used for islet transplantation. In most countries, the best-quality donor pancreata are first allocated for whole organ transplantation; if rejected, they are then offered for islets. However, fatty organs from donors with a BMI above 32 might go directly to islet centers with high isolation yields. High- and low-quality donors might be differentiated on the basis of the donor scoring system developed in Edmonton.[61]

Choosing donors carefully allows centers to save time and money by minimizing the risk of a low yield or failed isolation. Islet cell processing takes place in clinical-grade facilities meeting Good Manufacture Practice requirements. First, the pancreas is dissociated during enzymatic digestion with collagenase, and then the islets are separated from acinar tissue during gradient purification. Next, islets can be cultured for up to 72 hours, allowing an elective procedure and preparation of the patient. Islets are infused into the portal vein by an interventional radiologist. The entire procedure can be performed under local anesthesia with minimal sedation. Intra-abdominal bleeding occurs in 3% to 15% of cases and is the main risk related to the procedure. However, less than 1% of patients who have a bleeding episode require surgery. The initial cohorts reported a small chance of portal vein thrombosis. In the current era, use of heparin and modern purification techniques that result in low pellet volume minimizes this risk. There is no long-term risk described to the liver, even after several sequential islet infusions.[62]

Outcomes

In a landmark study, Shapiro and colleagues[63] reported the outcomes of seven patients who were insulin free 1 year after islet transplantation on a steroid-free protocol of immunosuppression. During the last 14 years, new islet isolation and transplantation techniques have been optimized. New immunosuppressive protocols have been tested. Recent analysis of the Collaborative Islet Transplant Registry data from more than 600 patients indicates that islet transplantation may lead to a 50% insulin independence rate at 5 years, when induction with a T-cell depletion agent in combination with tumor necrosis factor-α blocker is used at the time of transplantation.[64] These results are replicable and were reported by seven independent centers.[62] Such an outcome is comparable to that of PTA. Results from Edmonton also indicate that subsequent sequential islet infusions (fourth and fifth) may safely extend the insulin-free period.[64] It should be highlighted that 90% of patients maintained islet function more than 5 years after the procedure, expressing normal levels of C-peptide in the bloodstream. This protects them from severe hypoglycemia and allows good glucose control with or without supporting insulin and a much improved quality of life. Nephrotoxicity of the immunosuppressive agents has been one of the major concerns of islet transplantation compared with remaining on insulin. Results from a crossover study indicated that the progression of kidney disease is faster in "brittle" type 1 diabetics remaining on the waiting list on optimal insulin therapy compared with patients who received islet transplants and maintained a therapeutic dose of tacrolimus.[65] In addition, inhibition of progression in neuropathy and angiopathy has been reported in islet transplant recipients.[65] Risk of sensitization and development of high panel reactive antibodies increased in those with suboptimal immunosuppression, especially in those who stopped completely.[62]

For highly selected patients, those with the brittle form of type 1 diabetes and hypoglycemic unawareness, islet transplantation offers a vital minimally invasive therapeutic option with durable long-term results. Because of the high cost and limited funding, further progress in the field in the United States requires approval and reimbursement of the procedure by the insurance payers. There is a guarded optimism that approval will take place soon because a multicenter U.S. trial sponsored by the National Institutes of Health and supervised by the Food and Drug Administration has been completed, and promising 1-year follow-up data have been collected.[66]

SELECTED REFERENCES

Friedewald JJ, Samana CJ, Kasiske BL, et al: The kidney allocation system. *Surg Clin North Am* 93:1395–1406, 2013.

This article succinctly outlines the challenges of creating new policies for kidney allocation. The new Kidney Donor Profile Index (KDPI) and the Estimated Post Transplant Survival (EPTS) score are explained as they relate to the allocation of deceased donor kidneys.

Gill JS, Tonelli M: Understanding rare adverse outcomes following living kidney donation. *JAMA* 311:577–579, 2014.

Muzaale AD, Massie AB, Wang MC, et al: Risk of end-stage renal disease following live kidney donation. *JAMA* 311:579–586, 2014.

These companion papers review outcomes after kidney donation and provide an analysis of populations at risk. It is crucial to review the data in Muzaale's paper with potential recipients and to understand the partner paper by Gill and Tonelli.

Shapiro AM, Lakey JR, Ryan EA, et al: Islet transplantation in seven patients with type 1 diabetes mellitus using a glucocorticoid-free immunosuppressive regimen. *N Engl J Med* 343:230–238, 2000.

This classic article launched a reinvigoration of the field of pancreas islet transplantation.

REFERENCES

1. Wolfe RA, Ashby VB, Milford EL, et al: Comparison of mortality in all patients on dialysis, patients on dialysis awaiting transplantation, and recipients of a first cadaveric transplant. *N Engl J Med* 341:1725–1730, 1999.
2. Leichtman AB, Cohen D, Keith D, et al: Kidney and pancreas transplantation in the United States, 1997-2006: The HRSA Breakthrough Collaboratives and the 58 DSA Challenge. *Am J Transplant* 8:946–957, 2008.
3. Coresh J, Selvin E, Stevens LA, et al: Prevalence of chronic kidney disease in the United States. *JAMA* 298:2038–2047, 2007.
4. Abramowicz D, Cochat P, Claas FH, et al: European Renal Best Practice Guideline on kidney donor and recipient evaluation and perioperative care. *Nephrol Dial Transplant* 2014. [Epub ahead of print].
5. Go AS, Chertow GM, Fan D, et al: Chronic kidney disease and the risks of death, cardiovascular events, and hospitalization. *N Engl J Med* 351:1296–1305, 2004.
6. Meier-Kriesche HU, Ojo AO, Port FK, et al: Survival improvement among patients with end-stage renal disease: Trends over time for transplant recipients and wait-listed patients. *J Am Soc Nephrol* 12:1293–1296, 2001.
7. Purnell TS, Auguste P, Crews DC, et al: Comparison of life participation activities among adults treated by hemodialysis, peritoneal dialysis, and kidney transplantation: a systematic review. *Am J Kidney Dis* 62:953–973, 2013.
8. Furth SL, Hwang W, Neu AM, et al: Effects of patient compliance, parental education and race on nephrologists' recommendations for kidney transplantation in children. *Am J Transplant* 3:28–34, 2003.
9. Yoon SC, Hurst FP, Jindal RM, et al: Trends in renal transplantation in patients with human immunodeficiency virus infection: An analysis of the United States Renal Data System. *Transplantation* 91:864–868, 2011.
10. Ponticelli C: Recurrence of focal segmental glomerular sclerosis (FSGS) after renal transplantation. *Nephrol Dial Transplant* 25:25–31, 2010.
11. Cochat P, Fargue S, Mestrallet G, et al: Disease recurrence in paediatric renal transplantation. *Pediatr Nephrol* 24:2097–2108, 2009.
12. Chadban S: Glomerulonephritis recurrence in the renal graft. *J Am Soc Nephrol* 12:394–402, 2001.
13. Dabade TS, Grande JP, Norby SM, et al: Recurrent idiopathic membranous nephropathy after kidney transplantation: A surveillance biopsy study. *Am J Transplant* 8: 1318–1322, 2008.
14. Zuber J, Le Quintrec M, Morris H, et al: Targeted strategies in the prevention and management of atypical HUS recurrence after kidney transplantation. *Transplant Rev (Orlando)* 27:117–125, 2013.

15. Goral S, Ynares C, Shappell SB, et al: Recurrent lupus nephritis in renal transplant recipients revisited: It is not rare. *Transplantation* 75:651–656, 2003.
16. Wang LW, Fahim MA, Hayen A, et al: Cardiac testing for coronary artery disease in potential kidney transplant recipients: A systematic review of test accuracy studies. *Am J Kidney Dis* 57:476–487, 2011.
17. Power A, Chan K, Singh SK, et al: Appraising stroke risk in maintenance hemodialysis patients: A large single-center cohort study. *Am J Kidney Dis* 59:249–257, 2012.
18. Coleman S, Kerr H, Goldfarb D, et al: Utilization of vascular conduits to facilitate renal transplantation in patients with significant aortoiliac calcification. *Urology* 84:967–970, 2014.
19. Womer KL, Kaplan B: Recent developments in kidney transplantation—a critical assessment. *Am J Transplant* 9:1265–1271, 2009.
20. Sung RS, Christensen LL, Leichtman AB, et al: Determinants of discard of expanded criteria donor kidneys: Impact of biopsy and machine perfusion. *Am J Transplant* 8:783–792, 2008.
21. Treat EG, Miller ET, Kwan L, et al: Outcomes of shipped live donor kidney transplants compared with traditional living donor kidney transplants. *Transpl Int* 27:1175–1182, 2014.
22. Matas AJ, Bartlett ST, Leichtman AB, et al: Morbidity and mortality after living kidney donation, 1999–2001: Survey of United States transplant centers. *Am J Transplant* 3:830–834, 2003.
23. Ko EY, Castle EP, Desai PJ, et al: Utility of the endovascular stapler for right-sided laparoscopic donor nephrectomy: A 7-year experience at Mayo Clinic. *J Am Coll Surg* 207:896–903, 2008.
24. Ibrahim HN, Foley R, Tan L, et al: Long-term consequences of kidney donation. *N Engl J Med* 360:459–469, 2009.
25. Muzaale AD, Massie AB, Wang MC, et al: Risk of end-stage renal disease following live kidney donation. *JAMA* 311:579–586, 2014.
26. Gill JS, Tonelli M: Understanding rare adverse outcomes following living kidney donation. *JAMA* 311:577–579, 2014.
27. Lewis J, Peltier J, Nelson H, et al: Development of the University of Wisconsin Donation After Cardiac Death Evaluation Tool. *Prog Transplant* 13:265–273, 2003.
28. Wijdicks EF: The diagnosis of brain death. *N Engl J Med* 344:1215–1221, 2001.
29. Moers C, Smits JM, Maathuis MH, et al: Machine perfusion or cold storage in deceased-donor kidney transplantation. *N Engl J Med* 360:7–19, 2009.
30. Humar A, Matas AJ: Surgical complications after kidney transplantation. *Semin Dial* 18:505–510, 2005.
31. Sadej P, Feld RI, Frank A: Transplant renal vein thrombosis: Role of preoperative and intraoperative Doppler sonography. *Am J Kidney Dis* 54:1167–1170, 2009.
32. Harraz AM, Shokeir AA, Soliman SA, et al: Salvage of grafts with vascular thrombosis during live donor renal allotransplantation: A critical analysis of successful outcome. *Int J Urol* 21:999–1004, 2014.
33. Shames BD, Odorico JS, D'Alessandro AM, et al: Surgical repair of transplant renal artery stenosis with preserved cadaveric iliac artery grafts. *Ann Surg* 237:116–122, 2003.
34. Wilson CH, Rix DA, Manas DM: Routine intraoperative ureteric stenting for kidney transplant recipients. *Cochrane Database Syst Rev* 6:CD004925, 2013.
35. Lucewicz A, Wong G, Lam VW, et al: Management of primary symptomatic lymphocele after kidney transplantation: A systematic review. *Transplantation* 92:663–673, 2011.
36. Matas AJ, Smith JM, Skeans MA, et al: OPTN/SRTR 2011 Annual Data Report: Kidney. *Am J Transplant* 13(Suppl 1):11–46, 2013.
37. Friedewald JJ, Samana CJ, Kasiske BL, et al: The kidney allocation system. *Surg Clin North Am* 93:1395–1406, 2013.
38. Gruessner AC: 2011 Update on pancreas transplantation: Comprehensive trend analysis of 25,000 cases followed up over the course of twenty-four years at the International Pancreas Transplant Registry (IPTR). *Rev Diabet Stud* 8:6–16, 2011.
39. Israni AK, Skeans MA, Gustafson SK, et al: OPTN/SRTR 2012 Annual Data Report: Pancreas. *Am J Transplant* 14(Suppl 1):45–68, 2014.
40. Gutierrez P, Marrero D, Hernandez D, et al: Surgical complications and renal function after kidney alone or simultaneous pancreas-kidney transplantation: A matched comparative study. *Nephrol Dial Transplant* 22:1451–1455, 2007.
41. Scalea JR, Butler CC, Munivenkatappa RB, et al: Pancreas transplant alone as an independent risk factor for the development of renal failure: A retrospective study. *Transplantation* 86:1789–1794, 2008.
42. Ma IW, Valantine HA, Shibata A, et al: Validation of a screening protocol for identifying low-risk candidates with type 1 diabetes mellitus for kidney with or without pancreas transplantation. *Clin Transplant* 20:139–146, 2006.
43. Fourtounas C: Transplant options for patients with type 2 diabetes and chronic kidney disease. *World J Transplant* 4:102–110, 2014.
44. Maglione M, Ploeg RJ, Friend PJ: Donor risk factors, retrieval technique, preservation and ischemia/reperfusion injury in pancreas transplantation. *Curr Opin Organ Transplant* 18:83–88, 2013.
45. Siskind E, Akerman M, Maloney C, et al: Pancreas transplantation from donors after cardiac death: An update of the UNOS database. *Pancreas* 43:544–547, 2014.
46. Fernandez LA, Turgeon NA, Odorico JS, et al: Superior long-term results of simultaneous pancreas-kidney transplantation from pediatric donors. *Am J Transplant* 4:2093–2101, 2004.
47. van de Linde P, van der Boog PJ, Baranski AG, et al: Pancreas transplantation: Advantages of both enteric and bladder drainage combined in a two-step approach. *Clin Transplant* 20:253–257, 2006.
48. Stratta RJ, Gaber AO, Shokouh-Amiri MH, et al: A prospective comparison of systemic-bladder versus portal-enteric drainage in vascularized pancreas transplantation. *Surgery* 127:217–226, 2000.
49. Bazerbachi F, Selzner M, Marquez MA, et al: Portal venous versus systemic venous drainage of pancreas grafts: Impact on long-term results. *Am J Transplant* 12:226–232, 2012.
50. Vandermeer FQ, Manning MA, Frazier AA, et al: Imaging of whole-organ pancreas transplants. *Radiographics* 32:411–435, 2012.
51. Nath DS, Gruessner A, Kandaswamy R, et al: Late anastomotic leaks in pancreas transplant recipients—clinical characteristics and predisposing factors. *Clin Transplant* 19: 220–224, 2005.

52. Gruessner AC, Sutherland DE: Pancreas transplant outcomes for United States (US) cases as reported to the United Network for Organ Sharing (UNOS) and the International Pancreas Transplant Registry (IPTR). *Clin Transpl* 45–56, 2008.
53. Scheffert JL, Taber DJ, Pilch NA, et al: Clinical outcomes associated with the early postoperative use of heparin in pancreas transplantation. *Transplantation* 97:681–685, 2014.
54. Gilabert R, Fernandez-Cruz L, Real MI, et al: Treatment and outcome of pancreatic venous graft thrombosis after kidney-pancreas transplantation. *Br J Surg* 89:355–360, 2002.
55. Fridell JA, Johnson MS, Goggins WC, et al: Vascular catastrophes following pancreas transplantation: An evolution in strategy at a single center. *Clin Transplant* 26:164–172, 2012.
56. van Dellen D, Worthington J, Mitu-Pretorian OM, et al: Mortality in diabetes: Pancreas transplantation is associated with significant survival benefit. *Nephrol Dial Transplant* 28:1315–1322, 2013.
57. Gruessner AC, Sutherland DE, Gruessner RW: Pancreas transplantation in the United States: A review. *Curr Opin Organ Transplant* 15:93–101, 2010.
58. Sutherland DE, Gruessner RW, Dunn DL, et al: Lessons learned from more than 1,000 pancreas transplants at a single institution. *Ann Surg* 233:463–501, 2001.
59. Shipman KE, Patel CK: The effect of combined renal and pancreatic transplantation on diabetic retinopathy. *Clin Ophthalmol* 3:531–535, 2009.
60. Luan FL, Kommareddi M, Cibrik DM, et al: The time interval between kidney and pancreas transplantation and the clinical outcomes of pancreas after kidney transplantation. *Clin Transplant* 26:403–410, 2012.
61. O'Gorman D, Kin T, Murdoch T, et al: The standardization of pancreatic donors for islet isolations. *Transplantation* 80:801–806, 2005.
62. Bruni A, Gala-Lopez B, Pepper AR, et al: Islet cell transplantation for the treatment of type 1 diabetes: Recent advances and future challenges. *Diabetes Metab Syndr Obes* 7:211–223, 2014.
63. Shapiro AM, Lakey JR, Ryan EA, et al: Islet transplantation in seven patients with type 1 diabetes mellitus using a glucocorticoid-free immunosuppressive regimen. *N Engl J Med* 343:230–238, 2000.
64. Barton FB, Rickels MR, Alejandro R, et al: Improvement in outcomes of clinical islet transplantation: 1999-2010. *Diabetes Care* 35:1436–1445, 2012.
65. Thompson DM, Meloche M, Ao Z, et al: Reduced progression of diabetic microvascular complications with islet cell transplantation compared with intensive medical therapy. *Transplantation* 91:373–378, 2011.
66. Ricordi C, Hering B, Bridges N, et al: Completion of the first FDA phase 3 multicenter trial of islet transplantation in type 1 diabetes by the NIH CIT consortium. *Cytotherapy* 16:S14, 2014.

27 CHAPTER

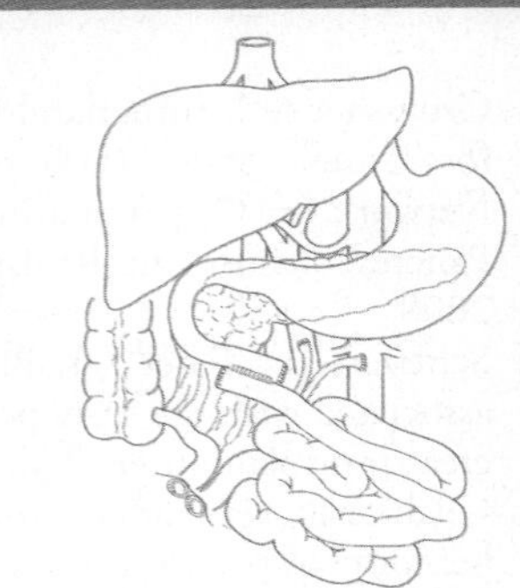

Small Bowel Transplantation

Aparna Rege, Debra L. Sudan

OUTLINE

HISTORY

Intestine transplantation has become a lifesaving treatment option for patients with intestinal failure. The term *intestinal failure* encompasses multiple disorders of inadequate intestinal length or function that prevent adequate nutrient absorption. In contrast, *enteral autonomy* is a term describing the ability of an individual to absorb all nutrient needs from the gastrointestinal tract. For the subset of patients who have intestinal failure because of loss of bowel length, the terms *short gut syndrome* and *short bowel syndrome* are used interchangeably. The causes of short bowel syndrome include congenital malformations, traumatic injury, and ischemia. The absolute length of remnant bowel required to sustain nutrient absorption varies among individuals and on the basis of age. As a rule of thumb, however, short bowel syndrome and lack of enteral autonomy are the norm after resection of more than 75% of the native intestine. Furthermore, in children who undergo surgical bowel resection of more than 75% of normal bowel length, more than 35% die in the first 18 months of life.[1]

Intestinal failure may also describe a subset of patients with normal or nearly normal intestinal length but with abnormal function as a result of Crohn's disease, motility disorders (such as intestinal pseudo-obstruction and long-segment Hirschsprung's disease), or diseases of the enterocytes (such as intestinal epithelial dysplasia). Disorders of intestinal function are less common than short bowel syndrome but share the same devastating consequences, leaving patients unable to absorb nutrients from the gut. In fact, before the 1960s, any cause of intestinal failure was nearly always fatal.

The first investigation of intestine transplantation as therapy for intestinal failure is attributed to Alexis Carrel in 1905.[2] Given the lack of understanding of transplant immunology at that time, it was not surprising that these early efforts were unsuccessful. Approximately 50 years later, in 1959 (after the first reports of successful kidney transplantation), Lillehei and colleagues[3] at the University of Minnesota published their successful experimental work transplanting intestines in a canine model. In 1962, Starzl (also working in a dog model) described transplantation of multiple abdominal organs, including the liver and entire gastrointestinal tract (from stomach through colon), termed homotransplantation of multiple visceral organs.[4] Human intestinal transplantation was subsequently attempted by Lillehei and coworkers in 1967.[5] Like Carrel's work, this effort and several additional attempts during the next 2 decades were unsuccessful in achieving complete enteral autonomy, although several intestine recipients survived for several months after transplantation.[6] The primary reasons for failure were early technical complications and the inability to control rejection, leading to development of overwhelming infections or post-transplantation lymphoma.

The clinical course of intestinal failure was dramatically altered when Dudrick and associates[7] described hyperalimentation, which is arguably one of the most significant medical breakthroughs of the century. Their work demonstrated that puppies could achieve nearly normal growth patterns while exclusively sustained by hyperalimentation, more commonly referred to currently as total parenteral nutrition (TPN). The clinical introduction of long-term TPN increased survival in individuals with intestinal failure.[8] Contemporary studies of the natural history of intestinal failure have reported overall 1- and 5-year survival of parenteral nutrition–dependent patients from 60% to 75% in children and 75% to 85% in adults.[9,10] Given the success of parenteral nutritional support in the early 1970s and the abysmal results after early attempts at intestine transplantation, there was diminished enthusiasm for further clinical trials of intestine transplantation.

Over time, potentially fatal complications associated with TPN administration were identified. These included severe catheter-associated bloodstream infections; technical difficulties in maintaining venous access because of catheter-associated venous thrombosis; and cholestasis leading to liver failure, also referred to as parenteral nutrition–associated liver disease (PNALD) or intestinal failure–associated liver disease (IFALD). IFALD develops in 40% to 60% of infants and is closely related to birth weight

(<1000 g) and duration of TPN (>3 months).[11] Risk of IFALD-induced steatosis in adults receiving home parenteral nutrition is lower, with reported rates of 15% to 40%. Once IFALD develops, however, it is associated with a 43% 5-year mortality in patients with remnant jejunum and ileum length of less than 50 cm.[12]

Concurrent with reports of severe TPN-associated complications, cyclosporine immunosuppression was introduced, resulting in marked improvements in kidney and liver allograft survival. With advances in immunosuppression, there was renewed interest in the field of intestine transplantation. The first successful human isolated intestine allograft (with the achievement of enteral autonomy) was reportedly performed by Deltz and colleagues[13] in 1988 with a living donor allograft procured from the sister of the 42-year-old recipient. Although rejection episodes recurred, these episodes were controlled with the use of cyclosporine, bolus steroids, and antilymphocyte treatments, eventually achieving enteral autonomy. A few months later, Grant and coworkers[14] performed the first cadaveric combined liver-intestine transplant to achieve complete enteral autonomy and more than 1-year patient and graft survival using cyclosporine. Despite these individual successes, 1-year expected patient survival after intestine transplantation using cyclosporine immunosuppression was approximately 25%, and failure to achieve enteral autonomy and risk for early death persisted.[6] In the early 1990s, the introduction of tacrolimus immunosuppression improved control of intestine allograft rejection, resulting in improved patient and graft survival after intestine transplantation.[15,16] Whereas this led to a mild increase in volume, the overall volume and experience with intestine transplantation have been dramatically less than with transplantation of other solid organ allografts. In the United States, the United Network for Organ Sharing (UNOS) has reported that only 2400 intestine transplants have been performed through June 30, 2014 (http://optn.transplant.hrsa.gov).

INDICATIONS FOR INTESTINE TRANSPLANTATION

Dependence on parenteral nutrition alone is not considered an indication for intestine transplantation in light of the excellent survival of most patients receiving parenteral nutrition. Indications for transplantation of the intestine were proposed by experts in the field at the Sixth International Small Bowel Transplant Symposium, including irreversible intestinal failure and one or more of the following:[17] (1) overt or impending liver failure caused by PNALD; (2) multiple thromboses of central veins limiting central venous access; (3) more than two episodes of catheter-related infection requiring hospitalization in any year; (4) single episode of fungal line infection; and (5) frequent and severe episodes of dehydration, despite intravenous (IV) fluid supplementation and TPN. Additional indications for intestine transplantation have subsequently been added, including intestinal failure that typically results in early death despite TPN (e.g., unreconstructible gastrointestinal tract) and diseases for which no alternative therapy is available (such as complete splanchnic venous thrombosis and unresectable benign or slow-growing mesenteric tumors).[18-20] Other potential indications include patients with high morbidity, poor quality of life, and severe fluid or electrolyte abnormalities that require frequent hospitalization, although these are not uniformly accepted.

The international Intestinal Transplant Registry (ITR) has collected demographic and outcome data on nearly all intestine transplants worldwide since the first successful cases in the late 1980s (Table 27-1). The most common primary underlying disease states reported by the ITR in pediatric recipients of an intestine allograft are gastroschisis (22%), volvulus (16%), and necrotizing enterocolitis (14%). In adult intestine transplant recipients, the most common underlying intestine diseases reported are ischemia (24%), Crohn's disease (11%), volvulus (8%), and trauma (7%).[21]

TABLE 27-1 Underlying Indications for Intestine Transplantation

PEDIATRIC	INCIDENCE (%)	ADULT	INCIDENCE (%)
Gastroschisis	22	Ischemia	24
Volvulus	16	Crohn's disease	11
Necrotizing enterocolitis	14	Trauma	7
Pseudo-obstruction	9	Desmoid tumors	9
Intestinal atresia	8	Motility disorders	8
Retransplantation	8	Volvulus	7
Hirschsprung's disease	7	Short gut, other	7
Microvillous inclusion disease	6	Retransplantation	6
Malabsorption, other	4	Miscellaneous	5
Short gut, other	4	Other tumors	4
Motility	2	Gardner syndrome	3
Tumor	1		

From Intestinal Transplant Association: Intestine transplant registry: 25 years of follow-up results. <http://intestinaltransplantassociation.com>. Accessed June 10, 2015.

EVALUATION

Recipient Evaluation

Timely referral to an intestine transplantation center (before or soon after the development of complications of parenteral nutrition administration) is the first step for the potential intestine transplant candidate. Evaluation for transplantation includes determination of residual intestine length, anatomy and function, extent of complications of intestinal failure, and presence and extent of comorbid conditions. Although each center develops its own protocols, diagnostic studies frequently performed during the evaluation are listed in Table 27-2.[22] After the evaluation, a multidisciplinary team (including transplant surgery, gastroenterology, anesthesia, social work, finance, nutrition, pharmacy, finance, and medical psychology) determines if a patient is an appropriate candidate on the basis of center-specific inclusion and exclusion criteria. If the patient is deemed a candidate, the center places the patient on the waiting list within the donor service area of UNOS. UNOS has developed allocation strategies for available cadaveric donor organs, which are publicly available (http://www.unos.org).

Donor Evaluation

An appropriate cadaveric donor is selected on the basis of compatible blood type and size of the donor compared with the recipient. Size is a significant consideration for the intestine donor because substantial loss of abdominal domain is common in the recipient after extensive resection. To address this problem of loss of domain, some centers have advocated that an ideal donor should have a body weight 50% to 75% that of the recipient.[23] Another

TABLE 27-2 Diagnostic Studies for Evaluation of the Intestine Transplant Candidate

DIAGNOSTIC STUDIES	TESTS AND PROCEDURES
Laboratory evaluation	Serum chemistries, liver function tests, complete blood count, prothrombin time–international normalized ratio, partial thromboplastin time, platelet count, albumin
Serologic tests for infectious diseases	CMV immunoglobulin G/immunoglobulin M, EBV antibodies, hepatitis B virus, hepatitis C virus, HIV
Endoscopy	Upper gastrointestinal endoscopy, colonoscopy with biopsy
Pathology	Percutaneous liver biopsy
Radiographic evaluation	Upper gastrointestinal series with small bowel follow-through, barium enema
	Computed tomography of abdomen and pelvis, liver ultrasound
	Doppler ultrasonography of jugular and subclavian veins (or magnetic resonance venography) to assess patency
	Gastric emptying study, motility testing
	Two-dimensional echocardiography
Other	Nutrition, psychosocial, cardiopulmonary, and anesthesia assessment

important aspect of donor selection is cold ischemia time. Prolonged cold ischemia time of the intestine allograft may lead to loss of mucosal integrity and bacterial translocation or intestinal perforation early after the transplant surgery. Transplant programs consider factors such as travel time between the recipient and donor medical centers and a history of extensive prior abdominal surgery in the recipient when selecting the intestine donor. Because of the sensitivity of the bowel graft to injury, most intestine donors are typically stable hemodynamically, require minimal vasopressor support, and are geographically close to the recipient transplant center.[24]

In children, viral serologic testing of the cadaveric donor for Epstein-Barr virus (EBV) and cytomegalovirus (CMV) is important because of the associated risk for primary viral transmission, leading to post-transplantation lymphoproliferative disorder and severe enteritis, respectively.[25,26]

Donor and Recipient Surgical and Technical Considerations

Isolated Intestine Transplantation

Isolated intestine (or small bowel) allografts typically include the entire jejunum and ileum with the associated vasculature, that is, the superior mesenteric artery (SMA) and vein (SMV) (Fig. 27-1). The most common variable in this type of allograft is the site of vascular transection (above or below the pancreas), which primarily depends on whether the pancreas from the intestine donor is allocated independent of the intestine allograft. In the neonatal donor or in any donor for whom the isolated pancreas has not been allocated separately for transplantation, the SMA is divided at the level of the aorta and the portal vein is divided at the superior border of the pancreas to provide maximum lengths of vessels to the intestine allograft. The donor jejunum is divided with a surgical stapler just distal to the ligament of Treitz, and the ileum is transected proximal to the ileocecal valve. In contrast, in adult and older pediatric donors without significant aberrations in anatomy, isolated intestine can be safely procured while still allowing use of the liver and pancreas from the same donor for other recipients.[27] In these circumstances, the donor operation requires additional careful dissection of the mesentery from the retroperitoneal organs, and the SMA and SMV are divided at the mesenteric root at the inferior border of the pancreas. Carotid or iliac arteries and iliac or jugular veins are also procured from the cadaveric donor to allow vascular reconstruction in the recipient.

During the recipient operation, arterial inflow is established by direct anastomosis of the donor SMA to the recipient infrarenal aorta or by interposition of a donor arterial conduit. Venous outflow from the allograft is provided by anastomosis of the donor SMV to the recipient portal vein or inferior vena cava, with or without an interposition of donor venous conduit. The continuity of the bowel is established proximally and distally by standard techniques for enteric anastomoses. Finally, a distal ileostomy is created to allow routine monitoring of the graft (Fig. 27-1).

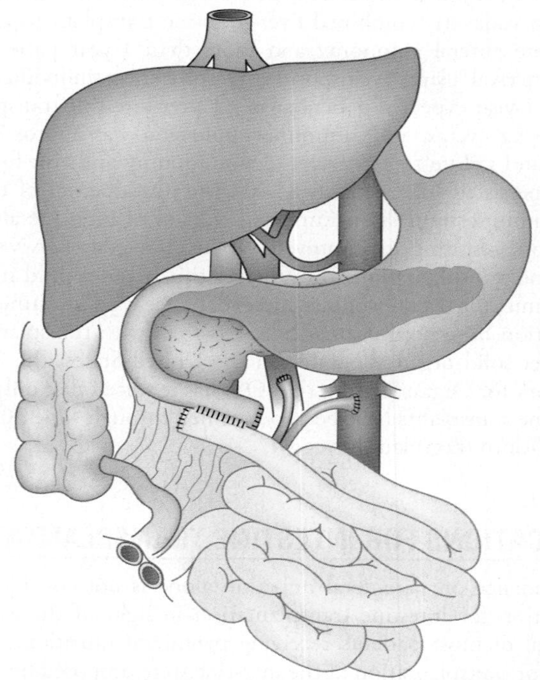

FIGURE 27-1 Isolated Intestine Transplant. Arterial inflow is established through anastomosis of the donor superior mesenteric artery with the recipient infrarenal aorta. Venous drainage is achieved by anastomosis of the donor superior mesenteric vein to the native portal vein or inferior vena cava. Bowel continuity is established through anastomosis of the proximal graft jejunum to the recipient duodenum, and the distal ileum is brought out as an ileostomy.

Intestine Allograft in Combination With Other Abdominal Organs

The nomenclature of grafts that include additional abdominal organs along with the intestine is less consistent than the isolated intestine graft and has varied over time and among various centers.

A liver–small bowel graft as described by Grant and colleagues[14] refers to the individual liver and intestine grafts procured from the same cadaveric donor, but each implanted separately. The technical aspects of donor procurement for grafts planned to be implanted separately are the same as those described for isolated intestine transplantation and in standard liver procurement. This composite graft requires a loop of defunctionalized (Roux-en-Y) allograft small bowel for biliary drainage. In this situation, the pancreas allograft could potentially be allocated to a different recipient. The second variant of the liver and intestine allograft is the en bloc version, in which the liver and intestine along with the duodenum and pancreas (or head of the pancreas) are procured and transplanted in continuity, thus preserving the extrahepatic biliary system[28,29] (Fig. 27-2). However, when the liver–small bowel graft is planned to be implanted en bloc, after complete mobilization of the abdominal organs along the avascular planes, the cadaveric donor procurement differs from that described before in that (1) no hilar dissection is performed (leaving the hepatic hilum, donor duodenum, and donor pancreas undisturbed), (2) the donor thoracic aorta is excised in continuity with the abdominal aorta (including the orifices of both the celiac axis and SMA), and (3) the donor spleen is typically removed from the tail of the pancreas on the back table. The sites for division of the bowel (just distal to the pylorus and proximal to the ileocecal valve) and division of the inferior vena cava (above and below the liver) are the same as in isolated liver or isolated intestine transplantation.

During the recipient operation, the native liver is excised along with most (or all) of the remnant small bowel to make room for the intestine allograft. The extent of native visceral resection may include the distal native stomach, native duodenum, pancreas, and spleen. Conditions that may affect the extent of native visceral resection include the extent or location of hilar or mesenteric root tumors, presence of enterocutaneous fistulas or anatomic abnormalities in any of these structures, and loss of abdominal domain that precludes placement of the graft because of size discrepancy. The suprahepatic inferior vena cava anastomosis is performed first as in a liver-only transplantation procedure. Reconstruction of the vena cava can be performed in either caval replacement or piggyback fashion (largely dependent on the presence or absence of size discrepancy between donor and recipient or preference of the center or surgeon). The caval anastomosis allows venous drainage

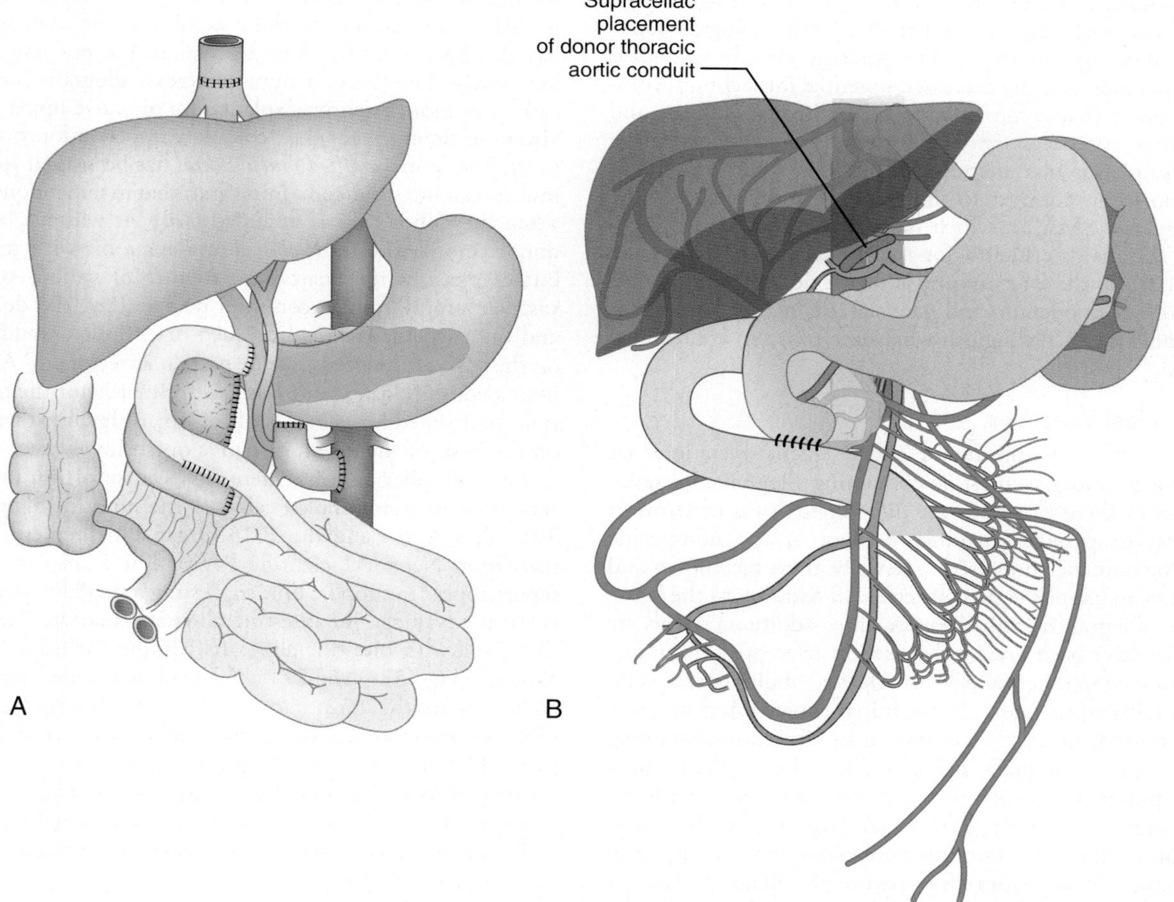

FIGURE 27-2 Liver-Intestine-Pancreas Transplant. A, The donor celiac axis and superior mesenteric arteries are left on an aortic conduit, which is anastomosed to the recipient aorta infrarenally. Venous outflow is through the anastomosis between the donor hepatic veins and the recipient suprahepatic inferior vena cava. The donor duodenum and the head of the pancreas (shown) or the entire donor pancreas are left intact to preserve the donor common bile duct. The donor jejunum is anastomosed to the native stomach, duodenum (shown), or proximal jejunum, depending on the native remnant anatomy. **B,** Supraceliac placement of donor thoracic aortic conduit.

of the composite organs because the donor portal system remains intact. Next, the arterial inflow is reestablished. Figure 27-2*A* demonstrates use of the donor thoracic aorta as a conduit for arterial inflow to the donor celiac trunk and SMA. This donor aortic conduit may be anastomosed to the recipient's infrarenal aorta or supraceliac aorta as shown in Figure 27-2*B*. Once the graft is revascularized, bowel continuity is restored proximally and distally; however, the site of anastomosis depends on the recipient's anatomy and the extent to which native viscera have been removed. In Figure 27-2*A*, the proximal bowel reconstruction is shown at the level of the native duodenum and allograft proximal jejunum, and the distal reconstruction is at the level of the allograft distal ileum and remnant native transverse colon.

When the recipient foregut is retained, a portacaval (or splenorenal) shunt must be performed to allow venous drainage of the native foregut (stomach, pancreas, spleen, and duodenum) to prevent formation of esophagogastric varices or refractory ascites from venous outflow obstruction. In this instance, the proximal bowel reconstruction is performed between the proximal native remnant jejunum and the donor allograft proximal jejunum.

The strategic advantage of individual implantation is the potential to explant a failed intestine allograft without disrupting the liver allograft if discordant injury occurs after transplantation, which was clearly a concern in the early experience in light of the high incidence and recurrent nature of intestine allograft rejection. The advantages of the en bloc strategy are the simplified recipient operation and the decreased potential for technical complications, given that reconstruction of the biliary drainage and portal vein is not necessary. In addition, the en bloc strategy requires a single vascular anastomosis to either a cuff or conduit of donor aorta, in contrast to individual reconstruction of the celiac artery and SMA, in which the grafts are implanted separately.[28,29] The major criticism for the nomenclature liver–small bowel for both of these techniques is that it does not distinguish when the donor duodenum and pancreas are included as part of the graft, nor does it distinguish what native viscera are retained or removed.[30]

Other Technical Variations

Technical variations in the donor and recipient operations are common for multiorgan intestine-containing allografts; however, the nuances of these variations are difficult to assess in terms of contribution to patient outcomes because of the nonspecific nature of the nomenclature used to describe these techniques and inconsistency in use of the various terms. In addition to the liver–small bowel allograft described earlier, three additional terms are presently (or have been previously) used in reference to multiorgan intestine-containing allografts: cluster, multivisceral, and modified multivisceral grafts. In the initial papers using the term *multivisceral* in the description of multiorgan intestine-containing allografts in dogs, the graft included the entire gastrointestinal tract from proximal stomach to transverse colon along with the liver.[4] As more commonly used today, *multivisceral* has been reserved for a multiorgan intestine-containing allograft that specifically contains donor stomach as part of the allograft, whether or not the colon is included as part of the graft.[31] Historically, the right and transverse colon, which receive their arterial supply based on the SMA, were included as part of the intestine transplant. The colon was placed orthotopically and anastomosed to the recipient colon or brought out as an end colostomy. An early series from Pittsburgh[32] described increased risk of graft loss with inclusion of the colon, and inclusion of the colon in multivisceral

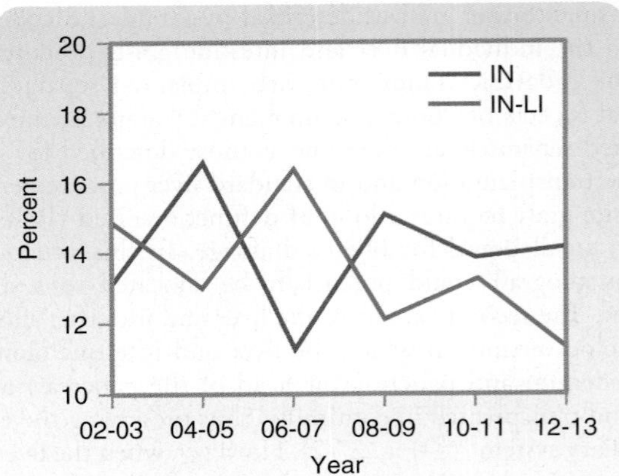

FIGURE 27-3 Graft failure within the first 90 days after transplantation among intestine transplant recipients. *IN*, intestine; *IN-LI*, intestine-liver.

grafts was largely abandoned for many years thereafter. More recent reports have refuted this perceived negative impact, and centers are increasingly including the colon with intestine allografts of all types.[33-35] The ITR report presented in 2013 showed that the rate of colon inclusion has increased from 4% in 2000 to 30% in 2012.[21] In addition to these variations, the term *multivisceral* has also been used by some to refer to the multiorgan en bloc liver–small bowel–duodenum–pancreas allograft (as described earlier) or more extensive explantation of native upper abdominal viscera in the recipient (i.e., complete upper abdominal exenteration). The term *modified multivisceral* has been used to describe a multiorgan intestine-containing graft that includes donor stomach when the donor liver is excluded (with or without inclusion of donor colon). The term *cluster* overlaps a bit with multivisceral but emphasizes the anatomic structure of various organs with vascular supply from a common pedicle (i.e., the donor aorta), and the particular organs included or excluded could be altered on the basis of the needs for the particular recipient.[8] As originally described, the cluster graft was used primarily for the transplantations performed for tumor, and the organs included were selected on the basis of the extent of native organ involvement.[36]

For a number of years, there has been suspicion that the liver was protective immunologically for the intestine allograft.[37] The 2013 ITR report and the 2013 Organ Procurement and Transplantation Network/Scientific Registry of Transplant Recipients report appear to support this, suggesting a small long-term patient survival advantage for intestine allografts that are liver inclusive compared with intestine allografts without inclusion of the liver allograft (Figs. 27-3 and 27-4).[38] The more detailed anatomic data collection in the most recent ITR report compared with the UNOS data set has allowed preliminary analysis of factors that may affect outcome, including the various organ combinations. Further studies are required to identify the advantages and disadvantages of the various techniques of donor organ implantation and the contribution to outcome based on the extent of recipient native organ removal.

IMMUNOSUPPRESSION

The increased immunogenicity of the intestine requires more potent immunosuppression regimens than are typically used with other solid organs. The introduction of cyclosporine was the key

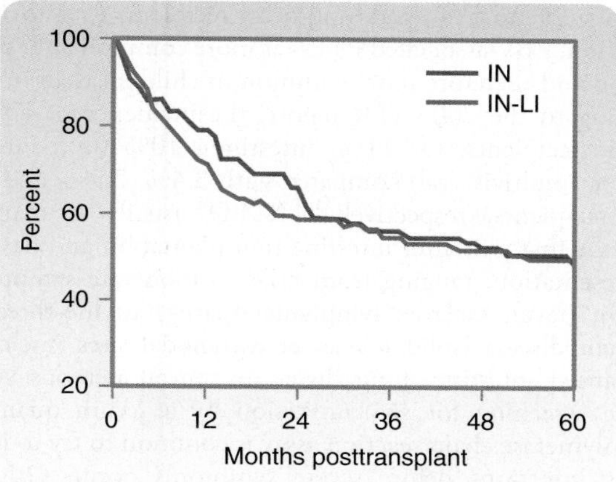

FIGURE 27-4 Five-year graft survival among intestine transplant recipients, 2008. *IN,* intestine; *IN-LI,* intestine-liver.

to the successful introduction of intestine transplantation. However, it was not until the introduction of tacrolimus (FK-506, Prograf), which forms the basis for most maintenance immunotherapy regimens today, that successful intestine transplantation reached acceptable rates. Steroids are also widely used, although the use of a steroid avoidance protocol has been reported with apparent success.[39] Most centers use induction immunosuppression intraoperatively with a monoclonal antibody (e.g., alemtuzumab [Campath] or basiliximab [Simulect]) or polyclonal antibody (e.g., antithymocyte globulin [Thymoglobulin]) preparation. Induction therapy has been associated with a substantial decrease in the incidence of early rejection, and the recent review by the ITR suggests an advantage for depletional induction therapy. Use of other immunosuppressive agents (including mycophenolate mofetil [CellCept] and sirolimus [Rapamune]) has been reported at various centers either routinely or when side effects of the standard immunosuppressive regimens are encountered.[40] Similar to the anatomic considerations in surgical techniques and choice of induction agent, no specific maintenance regimen has proved to be superior to another, and centers continue to use regimens based on preference of the physician, experience, and needs of the individual patient.

COMPLICATIONS

Surgical and Perioperative Complications

Despite the advances in intestine transplantation, it remains a surgical procedure with high morbidity, and reported complication rates approach 50%. The most common types of technical complications are bowel anastomotic leaks, intestine perforations, and wound complications. These can be catastrophic and require a high index of suspicion because of the extensive immunosuppression and at times lack of typical signs and symptoms. The management of these surgical complications in the intestine allograft recipient uses standard surgical principles to provide coverage to the bowel loops, to drain or to débride infectious material or tissue, and to close enteric defects. Vascular complications are rare but include both bleeding and thrombosis. Postoperative hemorrhage may result from recipient coagulopathy (especially in the case of native or allograft hepatic dysfunction) and be amplified by the extensive dissection usually required as a result of multiple adhesions from previous surgeries. Thrombosis of arterial inflow or venous outflow conduits is typically associated with devastating sudden graft necrosis and results in patient or graft loss. Biliary complications can be largely avoided in liver-intestine transplantations by including the duodenum and pancreas, thus avoiding any hilar dissection as noted before. Rare instances of intrahepatic biliary strictures due to preservation injury, prolonged cold ischemia, or late immunologic injury have been observed.

MONITORING AND REJECTION

Historically, rejection was frequent and often severe in intestine transplant recipients, with incidence as high as 70% to 80%.[14] More recently, with the evolution of various immunosuppressive strategies, a decrease in the incidence of rejection has been observed that correlates with improved patient survival.[39] Acute cellular rejection usually occurs within the first year after transplantation but can occur at any time. The most frequent clinical signs and symptoms of rejection may mimic those of viral gastroenteritis, including unexplained fever, abdominal pain or cramping, and increased stoma or stool output. Because of the insidious onset, lack of distinctive features, and absence of specific biomarkers, diagnosis may potentially be delayed. For this reason, rejection remains closely associated with rates of graft failure and mortality. Unlike in hepatic or renal transplantation, no convenient serochemical marker exists to monitor intestinal function. Stool calprotectin and serum citrulline levels have been examined as potential markers of intestinal function, but because of limited access and prolonged times to test results, neither of these tests is widely used at this time.[41,42] A measure of immune reaction to the donor HLA antigens has recently been approved by the Food and Drug Administration and shows significant promise for monitoring of children after intestine transplantation.

Ileoscopy through the ostomy provides a method of visualizing the mucosa and obtaining tissue for pathologic examination. Routine ileoscopy and biopsy typically begin between postoperative days 5 and 7, and most centers will obtain biopsy specimens once or twice weekly for the first 1 to 3 months and as needed for symptoms thereafter.

Acute cellular rejection is characterized histologically in mild forms by an inflammatory response that is localized to the lamina propria and the crypts, with increased numbers of apoptotic bodies seen in the crypts but with maintenance of an intact mucosal lining and normal or nearly normal villous height. Moderate acute cellular rejection is defined by markedly increased inflammation within the lamina propria, increased apoptotic bodies within the crypts, and blunting or distortion of the villous architecture. In severe acute cellular rejection, the damage to crypts is so marked that the intestinal architecture may be lost and severe mucosal ulceration or exfoliation is identified.[43] Although the mechanism is presently unclear, the liver appears to have a protective effect for rejection of the intestine, with some centers reporting a higher incidence or severity of acute cellular rejection in isolated intestine transplants compared with intestine transplants in combination with the liver.[44]

Once rejection has been established, treatment usually consists of large steroid doses and an increase in the target levels of maintenance immunosuppression. Resistant cases may be treated with more potent immunosuppression, such as rabbit antithymocyte globulin with or without additional immunosuppressive medications (e.g., sirolimus, mycophenolate mofetil) or rarely infliximab (a murine monoclonal antibody to tumor necrosis factor-α;

Remicade).[45] During treatment for rejection, the combination of increased immunosuppression and potential compromise of the gut mucosal barrier can lead to secondary infections, requiring close follow-up and a high index of suspicion for infections.

Infection

Infection is a serious risk in the short and long term and can lead to significant morbidity and mortality. Bacterial infections are prevalent, with incidence as high as 70% to 90% after intestine transplantation.[46] A number of preoperative and intraoperative factors contribute to a high rate of bacterial infection, including prolonged operative time, multiple blood transfusions, potential contamination from enteric spillage, preexisting liver disease, preexisting infections, and frequent need for prolonged central venous access. Ischemia-reperfusion injury may also lead to loss of the gut mucosal barrier and bacterial translocation or intestinal anastomotic leak in the immediate postoperative period. Rejection leads to a similar impairment of the gut mucosal barrier, but later in the postoperative course. Bacterial infections can be manifested as intra-abdominal infection, catheter-related infections, pneumonia, or wound infections, with central line infections being the most common. Organisms include typical gut flora such as *Escherichia coli, Klebsiella, Enterobacter,* enterococci, and polymicrobial infections. Special consideration should also be given to fungal infections; most centers use antifungals as part of their routine perioperative antimicrobial prophylaxis regimens.

Viral infections (particularly with members of the herpesvirus family) are common in patients receiving intestine transplants, with approximately two thirds of patients developing such infections. CMV is a common pathogen after intestine transplantation that often affects the allograft. The reported incidence of CMV infection ranges from 18% to 25%, with a 7% incidence of invasive CMV disease.[47]

Donor and recipient CMV serologic status is an important predictor of post-transplantation CMV infection. Transplanting bowel from the CMV-positive donor to a CMV-negative recipient facilitates transmission and may increase the risk for tissue-invasive CMV, recurrent CMV, and ganciclovir-resistant CMV infection.[48]

Similar to rejection, the presentation of CMV infection may be insidious and ranges from mild symptoms (fever, increased stoma or stool output, cramping, and abdominal pain) to severe symptoms (intestinal ulceration, bleeding, perforation, or frank ischemia). The potential severity of primary CMV infections has led some to propose the restriction of transplantation from a CMV-positive donor intestine into a CMV-negative recipient. Because the symptoms of CMV infection may mimic those of intestine allograft rejection, biopsy of the allograft may be needed to differentiate the two causes of graft injury. The presence of CMV inclusion bodies on hematoxylin and eosin stain or identification of CMV by immunohistochemistry or stool electron microscopy confirms the diagnosis of CMV enteritis. Fortunately, with appropriate antimicrobial treatment, typically IV ganciclovir (Cytovene) alone or in combination with CMV immune globulin (CytoGam), and reduction in immunosuppression, graft loss can be avoided in most cases.[49]

EBV, another member of the herpesvirus family, presents a unique challenge to intestine transplant recipients because of the association with development of post-transplantation lymphoproliferative disorder (PTLD). In intestine transplant recipients, the reported incidence of PTLD is 10% to 20%, which is considerably higher compared with kidney recipients (1% to 2%), liver recipients (2% to 5%), and lung-heart recipients (5% to 10%).[50] In addition, EBV-associated PTLD is more common after primary infection and therefore more common in children than in adults. According to the 2003 ITR report, the incidence of PTLD in pediatric recipients was 11% (intestine), 10% (liver-intestine), and 19% (multivisceral) compared with 3.4%, 2.9%, and 6% in adults recipients, respectively.[31] PTLD usually is manifested within the first year after intestine transplantation and has a variable presentation, ranging from mild to moderate symptoms of infection (fever, malaise, lymphadenopathy) to life-threatening malignant disease (solid masses at extranodal sites, such as the transplanted intestine, lung, liver, or central nervous system). Routine screening for seroconversion by a serum quantitative EBV polymerase chain reaction assay is common to try to identify primary infections before severe symptoms occur. Other risk factors for the development of PTLD include transplantation of organs from an EBV-positive donor to an EBV-negative recipient and the use of potent immunosuppressive agents for induction therapy or for treatment of rejection.[51] Reduction of immunotherapy (with or without antiviral medication) is the first line of treatment with a high response rate (45%). More severe cases and patients who develop Burkitt or T-cell lymphoma may require chemotherapy. Anti-CD20 monoclonal antibodies (e.g., rituximab) may also be useful in the treatment of PTLD when the EBV infection appears to be leading to B-cell tumors or proliferation. Surgical excision of localized disease, if possible (e.g., tonsillectomy, splenectomy, lobectomy, or enterectomy), is highly effective. Despite these treatments, EBV-associated PTLD has a mortality rate of 25% to 60%.[52]

Graft-versus-host disease occurs when donor lymphoid cells begin to target recipient tissues, most notably the epithelial cells in the skin and intestine. Because of the large amount of lymphoid tissue present in the intestine, it was predicted that an intestine recipient might be at higher risk for graft-versus-host disease, but surprisingly, it has been relatively uncommon. The reported incidence ranges from 0% to 14% and is most frequently associated with patients with concomitant severe combined immunodeficiency.[53,54] Increasing immunosuppression, mainly through the increase or addition of steroids or antithymocyte globulin, has been the mainstay of treatment, but the outcome varies according to severity, with a high rate of mortality in the most severe cases.

OUTCOMES

Patient and Graft Survival

Patient and graft survival rates have improved with time. One-year adjusted patient survival improved from 60.4% in 1997 to 78.4% by 2006 and has remained relatively stable since then (Table 27-3).[21,55] The most common reason for mortality after intestine transplantation is infection with sepsis, accounting for 50% of deaths. Similarly, 1-year adjusted graft survival has improved from 55.6% to 69.6%, although 5-year graft survival remains approximately 50%. Sepsis is the leading cause of graft loss (50%), followed by rejection (13%), cardiovascular events (8%), PTLD (6.8% to 9.9%), and technical complications (6.1%).[21] Age appears to influence the cause of graft loss. Children younger than 18 years are more likely than adults to lose their grafts as a result of rejection (62.4% versus 47.8%) and lymphoma (2.2% versus 0%).[21] In general, graft function after transplantation is good in survivors. According to the 2013 ITR report, of the patients surviving more than 6 months after transplantation, 67% are free from TPN and 25% require either partial supplementation or full

TABLE 27-3 Graft and Patient Survival (%) in Two Different Eras*

TRANSPLANT	SURVIVAL	1 YEAR (2005-2006)†	5 YEARS (2001-2006)†	1 YEAR (2011-2012)	5 YEARS (2008-2013)
Intestine	Graft survival	68.3	36.3	78.6	48
	Patient survival	81.4	56.2	80	50
Intestine-liver	Graft survival	73.1	50.6	70.6	48.9
	Patient survival	73.4	54.8	70	50
Liver (deceased donor)	Graft survival	82.4	67.6	89.3	78.1
	Patient survival	87.1	73.3		

*For intestine, intestine-liver, and liver transplants at 1 and 5 years after transplantation.

†Years in parentheses represent years of treatment. Data from U.S. Organ Procurement and Transplantation Network and the Scientific Registry of Transplant Recipients: 2013 OPTN/SRTR annual report: Transplant data 1999-2007. <http://optn.transplant.hrsa.gov/ar2013>. Accessed June 10, 2015.

TPN or IV hydration. In patients receiving a colon segment with their intestine graft, there is a 5% higher rate of freedom from parenteral nutrition or IV fluid support.

Costs and Quality of Life

Estimates of the annual cost for home TPN range from $100,000 to $250,000, including costs of supplies and infusion solutions (ranging from $75,000 to $122,000) and costs of hospitalizations for parenteral nutrition–related complications (ranging from $10,000 to $196,000).[56] Despite the high initial cost of the intestine transplantation procedure and hospitalization, when average costs of immunosuppressive medications and subsequent hospitalizations are considered, transplantation becomes cost-effective compared with home TPN, usually between 1 and 3 years after transplantation.[32] In addition to the assessment of cost-effectiveness, studies have attempted to evaluate potential improvements in quality of life after intestine transplantation, but these are limited. The ITR has reported that of patients who survive longer than 6 months after transplantation, 85% have a Karnofsky score higher than 90%, implying a good to excellent quality of life, with minimal symptoms. DiMartini and colleagues[57] have reported that adult intestine transplant recipients perceive an equal or better quality of life after transplantation compared with remaining on home TPN. Studies in pediatric intestine recipients are more difficult to perform because of the young age of most recipients with intestinal failure and the lack of appropriate and reliable tools for assessing this age group. Previous studies have reported that parents of intestine recipients perceive a slightly worse quality of life compared with the patients themselves, but the children rate their quality of life similar to that of normal age-matched children.[58] Results of neurodevelopmental assessments of infant multivisceral transplant recipients are concerning because of findings of significant cognitive and motor delays that continue for a substantial time after transplantation. Although these studies are small, they suggest the need for close monitoring for nutritional deficiencies both before and after transplantation as well as for physical therapy and speech and language services to maximize appropriate development in these children.[59]

One additional concern is the limited number of centers that have established expertise in management of the patient with intestinal failure or intestine transplantation worldwide. This has led to differential access to multidisciplinary management of intestinal failure based on location. The substantial costs of intestinal failure management (especially with parenteral nutrition) have contributed to a substantial number who rely on government payers (state Medicaid or Medicare). Given financial constraints of many patients with intestinal failure, access to experienced centers can be a challenge.

Other challenges in the field of intestine transplantation include the following:

1. The limited data available for recipients in existing registries
2. The need for multi-institutional studies (because of small numbers of recipients at individual centers) to identify
   - The most effective induction and maintenance immunosuppression strategies to minimize rejection and infectious complications
   - Biomarkers that can replace ileoscopy and biopsy for routine monitoring of the intestine allograft
   - The significance of and optimal treatment (if any) for patients developing donor-specific antibody
3. Development of clear indications for and risks associated with inclusion or exclusion of other organs along with the intestine allograft (e.g., stomach, colon, spleen)

CONCLUSIONS

The field of intestine transplantation has expanded slowly at least in part because of the successful widespread use of home TPN. PNALD and catheter-related complications (infections or venous thrombosis) remain the most frequent indications for intestine transplantation, although the incidence of PNALD appears to have decreased or to have been delayed by the introduction of recent parenteral nutrition management strategies. Intestine transplantation is no longer considered experimental and is offered to patients with life-threatening complications of parenteral nutrition administration or complete portomesenteric thrombosis. The transplant operation is frequently challenging and complex because of the frequency of prior surgery, altered anatomy, and presence of portal hypertension. Furthermore, the postoperative course is frequently complicated. Readmission to the hospital is often required for treatment of diarrhea, dehydration, infection, or rejection; however, after initial recovery, independence from TPN is the norm. Patient and graft survival has been increasing and approaching results of other solid organ transplants and is similar to patient survival on TPN. The improvements in morbidity and mortality have led to acceptance of intestine transplantation as a standard treatment for intestinal failure.

SELECTED REFERENCES

Deltz E, Schroeder P, Gebhardt H, et al: Successful clinical small bowel transplantation—report of a case. *Clin Transplant* 3:89–91, 1988.

A case report of what is considered the first successful living donor small intestine transplant.

Dudrick SJ, Rhoads JE, Vars HM: Growth of puppies receiving all nutritional requirements by vein. *Fortschr Parenteral Ernahrung* 2:16–18, 1967.

This is the landmark paper in which prolonged survival was demonstrated to be feasible in puppies using only hyperalimentation (intravenous nutrition, more commonly referred to today as parenteral nutrition).

Fryer J: Intestinal transplantation: Current status. *Gastroenterol Clin North Am* 36:145–159, 2007.

A review of intestinal transplantation and its current practices.

Grant D, Abu-Elmagd K, Mazariegos G, et al: Intestinal transplant registry report: Global activity and trends. *Am J Transplant* 15:210–219, 2015.

This is a summary of data from the Intestinal Transplant Registry database that includes statistics compiled from intestinal transplant recipients at transplant centers from 21 countries.

REFERENCES

1. Wales PW, De Silva N, Kim JH, et al: Neonatal short bowel syndrome—a cohort study. *J Pediatr Surg* 40:755–762, 2005.
2. Carrel A: Landmark article, Nov 14, 1908: Results of the transplantation of blood vessels, organs and limbs. *JAMA* 250:944–953, 1905.
3. Lillehei R, Goott B, Miller F: The physiological response of the small bowel of the dog to ischemia, including prolonged in vitro preservation of the bowel with successful replacement of survival. *Ann Surg* 150:543–560, 1959.
4. Starzl T, Kaupp H, Jr, Brock D, et al: Homotransplantation of multiple visceral organs. *Am J Surg* 103:219–229, 1962.
5. Lillehei RC, Idezuki Y, Feemster JA, et al: Transplantation of stomach, intestine, and pancreas: Experimental and clinical observations. *Surgery* 62:721–741, 1967.
6. Starzl T, Rowe M, Todo S, et al: Transplantation of multiple abdominal viscera. *JAMA* 261:1449–1457, 1989.
7. Dudrick SJ, Rhoads JE, Vars HM: Growth of puppies receiving all nutritional requirements by vein. *Fortschr Parenteral Ernahrung* 2:16–18, 1967.
8. Dudrick SJ, Wilmore DW, Vars HM, et al: Long-term total parenteral nutrition with growth, development, and positive nitrogen balance. *Surgery* 64:134–142, 1968.
9. Squires RH, Duggan C, Teitelbaum DH, et al: Pediatric Intestinal Failure Consortium: Natural history of pediatric intestinal failure: Initial report from the Pediatric Intestinal Failure Consortium. *J Pediatr* 161:723–728, 2012.
10. Howard L, Heaphey L, Fleming CR, et al: Four years of North American registry home parenteral nutrition outcome data and their implications for patient management. *JPEN J Parenter Enteral Nutr* 15:384–393, 1991.
11. Beale EF, Nelson RM, Bucciarelli RL, et al: Intrahepatic cholestasis associated with parenteral nutrition in premature infants. *Pediatrics* 64:342–347, 1979.
12. Messing B, Crenn P, Beau P, et al: Long-term survival and parenteral nutrition dependence in adult patients with the short bowel syndrome. *Gastroenterology* 117:1043–1050, 1999.
13. Deltz E, Schroeder P, Gebhardt H: Successful clinical small bowel transplantation—report of a case. *Clin Transplant* 3:89–91, 1988.
14. Grant D, Wall W, Mimeault R, et al: Successful small-bowel/liver transplantation. *Lancet* 335:181–184, 1990.
15. Todo S, Reyes J, Furukawa H, et al: Outcome analysis of 71 clinical intestinal transplantations. *Ann Surg* 222:270–282, 1995.
16. Abu-Elmagd KM, Reyes J, Fung JJ, et al: Evolution of clinical intestinal transplantation: Improved outcome and cost effectiveness. *Transplant Proc* 31:582–584, 1999.
17. Kaufman SS, Atkinson JB, Bianchi A, et al: American Society of Transplantation: Indications for pediatric intestinal transplantation: A position paper of the American Society of Transplantation. *Pediatr Transplant* 5:80–87, 2001.
18. Abu-Elmaqd KM: Intestinal transplantation for short bowel syndrome and gastrointestinal failure: Current consensus, rewarding outcomes, and practical guidelines. *Gastroenterology* 130(Suppl 1):S132–S137, 2006.
19. Fishbein TM, Matsumoto CS: Intestinal replacement therapy: Timing and indications for referral of patients to an intestinal rehabilitation and transplant program. *Gastroenterology* 130 (Suppl):S147–S151, 2006.
20. Vianna RM, Mangus RS: Present prospects and future perspectives of intestinal and multivisceral transplantation. *Curr Opin Clin Nutr Metab Care* 12:281–286, 2009.
21. Grant D, Abu-Elmagd K, Mazariegos G, et al: Intestinal Transplant Association: Intestinal transplant registry report: Global activity and trends. *Am J Transplant* 15:210–219, 2015.
22. Beneditti E, Panaro F, Holterman M, et al: Surgical approaches and intestinal transplantation. *Best Pract Res Clin Gastroenterol* 17:1017–1040, 2003.
23. Fryer JP: Intestinal transplantation: Current status. *Gastroenterol Clin North Am* 36:145–159, 2007.
24. Matsumoto CS, Kaufman SS, Girlanda R, et al: Utilization of donors who have suffered cardiopulmonary arrest and resuscitation in intestinal transplantation. *Transplantation* 86:941, 2008.
25. Reyes J, Green M, Bueno J, et al: Epstein Barr virus associated posttransplant lymphoproliferative disease after intestinal transplantation. *Transplant Proc* 28:2768–2769, 1996.
26. Kusne S, Mañez R, Frye BL, et al: Use of DNA amplification for diagnosis of cytomegalovirus enteritis after intestinal transplantation. *Gastroenterology* 112:1121, 1997.
27. Abu-Elmagd K, Fung J, Bueno J, et al: Logistics and technique for procurement of intestinal, pancreatic, and hepatic grafts from the same donor. *Ann Surg* 232:680–687, 2000.
28. Bueno J, Abu-Elmagd K, Mazariegos G, et al: Composite liver–small bowel allografts with preservation of donor duodenum and hepatic biliary system in children. *J Pediatr Surg* 35:291–296, 2000.
29. Sudan DL, Iyer KR, Deroover A, et al: A new technique for combined liver/small intestinal transplantation. *Transplantation* 72:1846–1848, 2002.

30. Kato T, Ruiz P, Thompson JF, et al: Intestinal and multivisceral transplantation. *World J Surg* 26:226–237, 2002.
31. Grant D, Abu-Elmagd K, Reyes J, et al, Intestine Transplant Registry: 2003 Report of the intestine transplant registry: A new era has dawned. *Ann Surg* 241:604–613, 2005.
32. Todo S, Reyes J, Furukawa H, et al: Outcome analysis of 71 clinical intestinal transplantations. *Ann Surg* 222:270–280, 1995.
33. Goulet O, Auber F, Fourcade L, et al: Intestinal transplantation including the colon in children. *Transplant Proc* 34:1885–1886, 2002.
34. Matsumoto CS, Kaufman SS, Fishbein TM: Inclusion of the colon in intestinal transplantation. *Curr Opin Organ Transplant* 16:312–315, 2011.
35. Kato T, Selvaggi G, Gaynor JJ, et al: Inclusion of donor colon and ileocecal valve in intestinal transplantation. *Transplantation* 86:293–297, 2008.
36. Starzl TE, Todo S, Tzakis A, et al: Abdominal organ cluster transplantation for the treatment of upper abdominal malignancies. *Ann Surg* 210:374, 1989.
37. Abu-Elmagd KM, Costa G, Bond GJ, et al: Five hundred intestinal and multivisceral transplantations at a single center: Major advances with new challenges. *Ann Surg* 250:567–581, 2009.
38. Smith JM, Skeans MA, Horslen SP, et al: OPTN/SRTR 2013 Annual Data Report: Intestine. *Am J Transplant* 15(Suppl 2):1–16, 2015.
39. Abu-Elmagd KM, Costa G, Bond GJ, et al: Evolution of the immunosuppressive strategies for the intestinal and multivisceral recipients with special reference to allograft immunity and achievement of partial tolerance. *Transpl Int* 22:96–109, 2009.
40. Reyes J, Mazariegos GV, Abu-Elmagd K, et al: Intestinal transplantation under tacrolimus monotherapy after perioperative lymphoid depletion with rabbit anti-thymocyte globulin (Thymoglobulin). *Am J Transplant* 5:1430, 2005.
41. Hibi T, Nishida S, Garcia J, et al: Citrulline level is a potent indicator of acute rejection in the long term following pediatric intestinal/multivisceral transplantation. *Am J Transplant* 12:S27–S32, 2012.
42. Sudan D, Vargas L, Sun Y, et al: Calprotectin: A novel noninvasive marker for intestinal allograft monitoring. *Ann Surg* 246:311–315, 2007.
43. Remotti H, Subramanian S, Martinez M, et al: Small-bowel allograft biopsies in the management of small-intestinal and multivisceral transplant recipients: Histopathologic review and clinical correlations. *Arch Pathol Lab Med* 136:761–771, 2012.
44. Abu-Elmagd KM, Wu G, Costa G, et al: Preformed and de novo donor specific antibodies in visceral transplantation: Long-term outcome with special reference to the liver. *Am J Transplant* 12:3047–3060, 2012.
45. Berger M, Zeevi A, Farmer DG, et al: Immunologic challenges in small bowel transplantation. *Am J Transplant* 12(Suppl 4):S2–S8, 2012.
46. Guaraldi G, Cocchi S, Codeluppi M, et al: Outcome, incidence, and timing of infectious complications in small bowel and multivisceral organ transplantation patients. *Transplantation* 80:1742–1748, 2005.
47. Florescu DF, Langnas AN, Grant W, et al: Incidence, risk factors, and outcomes associated with cytomegalovirus disease in small bowel transplant recipients. *Pediatr Transplant* 16:294–301, 2012.
48. Kotton CN, Kumar D, Caliendo AM, et al, Transplantation Society International CMV Consensus Group: Updated international consensus guidelines on the management of cytomegalovirus in solid organ transplantation. *Transplantation* 96:333–360, 2013.
49. Florescu DF, Abu-Elmagd K, Mercer DF, et al: An international survey of cytomegalovirus prevention and treatment practices in intestinal transplantation. *Transplantation* 97:78–82, 2014.
50. Allen U, Preiksaitis J, AST Infectious Diseases Community of Practice: Epstein-Barr virus and posttransplant lymphoproliferative disorder in solid organ transplant recipients. *Am J Transplant* 13:107–120, 2013.
51. Quintini C, Kato T, Gaynor JJ: Analysis of risk factors for the development of post-transplant lymphoproliferative disorder among 119 children who received primary intestinal transplants at a single center. *Transplant Proc* 38:1755–1758, 2006.
52. Ramos E, Hernández F, Andres A, et al: Post-transplant lymphoproliferative disorders and other malignancies after pediatric intestinal transplantation: Incidence, clinical features and outcome. *Pediatr Transplant* 17:472–478, 2013.
53. Mazariegos GV, Abu-Elmagd K, Jaffe R, et al: Graft versus host disease in intestinal transplantation. *Am J Transplant* 4:1459–1465, 2004.
54. Gilroy RK, Coccia PF, Talmadge JE, et al: Donor immune reconstitution after liver–small bowel transplantation for multiple intestinal atresia with immunodeficiency. *Blood* 103:1171–1174, 2004.
55. Grant D: Intestinal transplantation: 1997 report of the international registry. Intestinal Transplant Registry. *Transplantation* 67:1061–1064, 1999.
56. Hofstetter S, Stern L, Willet J: Key issues in addressing the clinical and humanistic burden of short bowel syndrome in the US. *Curr Med Res Opin* 29:495–504, 2013.
57. DiMartini A, Rovera G, Graham T, et al: Quality of life after small intestinal transplantation and among home parenteral nutrition patients. *JPEN J Parenter Enteral Nutr* 22:357–362, 1998.
58. Ngo KD, Farmer DG, McDiarmid SV, et al: Pediatric health-related quality of life after intestinal transplantation. *Pediatr Transplant* 15:849–854, 2011.
59. Thevenin DM, Baker A, Kato T, et al: Neurodevelopmental outcomes of infant multivisceral transplant recipients: A longitudinal study. *Transplant Proc* 38:1694–1695, 2006.

SECTION V

Surgical Oncology

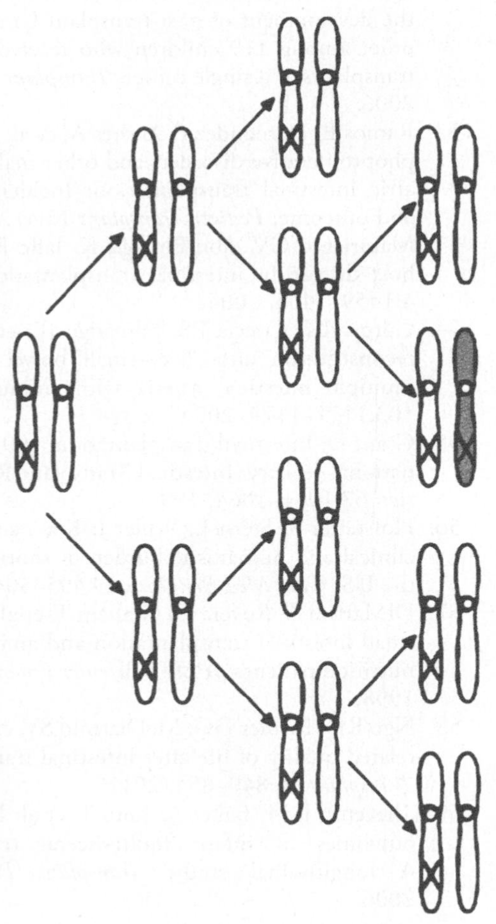

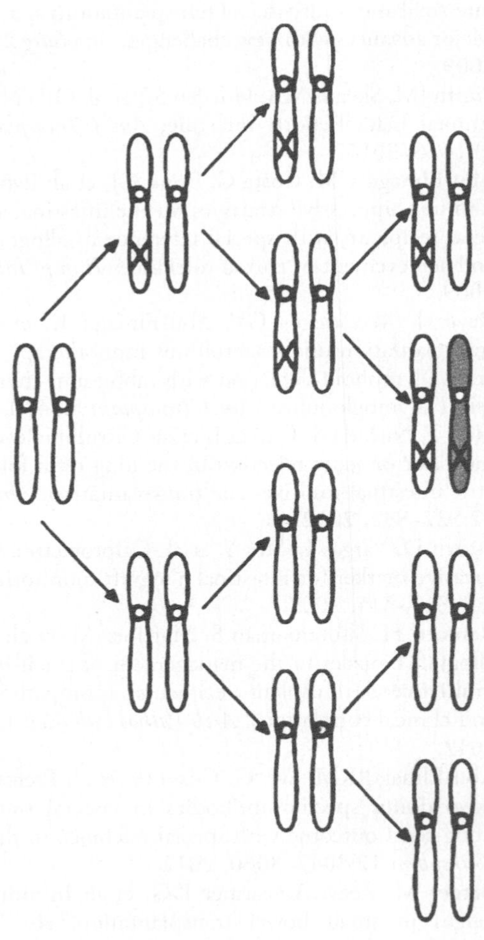

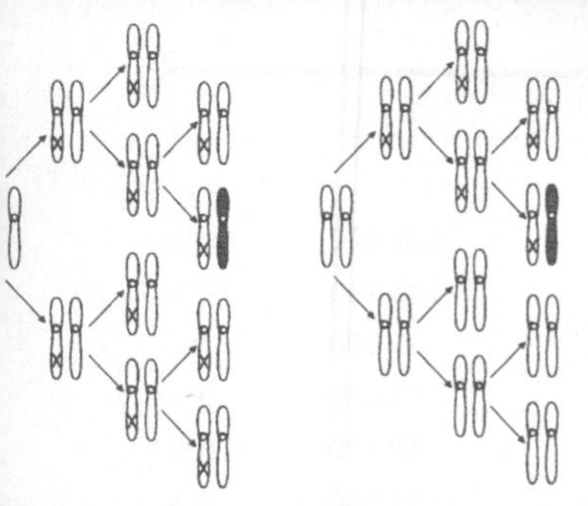

CHAPTER 28

Tumor Biology and Tumor Markers

Dominic E. Sanford, S. Peter Goedegebuure, Timothy J. Eberlein

OUTLINE

Neoplasia (literally meaning "new growth") is the uncontrolled proliferation of cells. The term *tumor*, which was originally used to describe the swelling caused by inflammation, is now used interchangeably with neoplasm. Transformation is the multistep process in which normal cells acquire malignant characteristics, such as the ability to invade tissues and to spread to distant sites (metastasize). Each step in transformation reflects one or more genetic alterations that confer a growth advantage over normal cells. Cancers are simply malignant tumors. There are a number of essential characteristics expressed by neoplastic cells that enable cancer progression.[1] These characteristics are shared by most if not all human cancers.

EPIDEMIOLOGY

Incidence is the number of new cases within a specified time frame, usually expressed as cases per 100,000 people per year. Prevalence is the number of patients with a disease in the population at a given point in time. A person's risk of developing or dying of cancer is usually expressed in terms of lifetime risk (risk during the course of a lifetime) or, in describing the relationship of specific risk factors with a particular cancer, the relative risk (comparing those with a certain exposure or trait with those who do not have it).

About 1.7 million new cases of cancer are expected to be diagnosed in 2014, excluding the more than 1 million new cases of basal and squamous cell cancers (Fig. 28-1). In men, the most common cancers are of the prostate, lung, colorectum, and urinary bladder. In women, the most common cancers are of the breast, lung, colorectum, and uterus. Cancer is the second most common cause of death in the United States, accounting for one of every four deaths, and is the most common cause of death in men and women between the ages of 40 and 79 years. In 2014, more than 580,000 Americans will die of cancer, corresponding to roughly 1600 deaths per day.[2] The national trends in incidence and death rates for select cancers are shown in Figures 28-2 and 28-3.

Global Burden of Cancer

Worldwide, cancer is responsible for one in eight deaths. The distribution and types of cancer that occur continue to change, being affected primarily by (1) the growth and aging of populations, (2) the increasing encroachment of modifiable risk factors (cigarette smoking, Western diet, and physical inactivity) in developing countries, and (3) the relatively slower decrease in infection-related cancers.[3] By 2020, 70% of all cancer-related deaths will be in developing countries, where survival rate (20% to 30%) is half that of developed countries.[4] Indeed, 80% to 90% of people diagnosed with cancer in developing countries present with late-stage, terminal cancer.[4] In the United States alone, cancer-associated medical costs were more than $120 billion in 2010 and are projected to reach $150 billion by 2020. Therefore, the majority of cancer deaths will occur in the countries least equipped to handle the burden.

Aging and Cancer

The incidence of cancer increases with age; thus, cancer disproportionately affects people aged 65 years and older.[5] In the United States, this age group composes 56% of all newly diagnosed cancer patients and 71% of all cancer deaths. The median ages of death for cancers common to both men and women (including lung, colorectal, pancreas, stomach, and urinary bladder) range from 71 to 77 years. The proportion of the U.S. population aged 65 years and older is growing rapidly. From 2010 to 2050, this segment of the U.S. population is expected to more than double in size, which is a recognized trend throughout the developed world. With an expanding older population, the incidence of cancer will increase, thereby raising the overall cancer burden on society. In addition, cancer care will also be of increasingly greater complexity in this population; reasons for this include more comorbidities of greater severity in the setting of declining physiologic reserve, difficulties with access to care, and lack of social support.

Cancer treatment in the elderly is less well studied, and it has been shown that the elderly population is underrepresented in clinical trials.[6-8] Clearly, surgeons must more carefully weigh individuals' operative risk in the context of the morbidity of the procedure, with greater consideration for quality of life and functional status, beyond just postoperative mortality and mortality, and long-term survival. Furthermore, there have been a number of reports regarding the underuse of adjuvant therapy in the aging

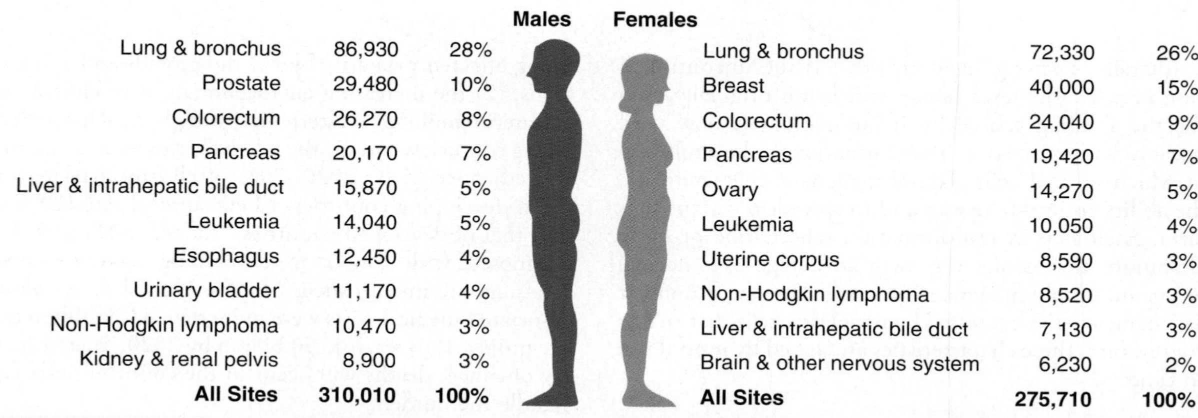

Estimated New Cases*

Males			Females		
Prostate	233,000	27%	Breast	232,670	29%
Lung & bronchus	116,000	14%	Lung & bronchus	108,210	13%
Colorectum	71,830	8%	Colorectum	65,000	8%
Urinary bladder	56.390	7%	Uterine corpus	52,630	6%
Melanoma of the skin	43,890	5%	Thyroid	47,790	6%
Kidney & renal pelvis	39,140	5%	Non-Hodgkin lymphoma	32,530	4%
Non-Hodgkin lymphoma	38,270	4%	Melanoma of the skin	32,210	4%
Oral cavity & pharynx	30,220	4%	Kidney & renal pelvis	24,780	3%
Leukemia	30,100	4%	Pancreas	22,890	3%
Liver & intrahepatic bile duct	24,600	3%	Leukemia	22,280	3%
All Sites	**855,220**	**100%**	**All Sites**	**810,320**	**100%**

Estimated Deaths

Males			Females		
Lung & bronchus	86,930	28%	Lung & bronchus	72,330	26%
Prostate	29,480	10%	Breast	40,000	15%
Colorectum	26,270	8%	Colorectum	24,040	9%
Pancreas	20,170	7%	Pancreas	19,420	7%
Liver & intrahepatic bile duct	15,870	5%	Ovary	14,270	5%
Leukemia	14,040	5%	Leukemia	10,050	4%
Esophagus	12,450	4%	Uterine corpus	8,590	3%
Urinary bladder	11,170	4%	Non-Hodgkin lymphoma	8,520	3%
Non-Hodgkin lymphoma	10,470	3%	Liver & intrahepatic bile duct	7,130	3%
Kidney & renal pelvis	8,900	3%	Brain & other nervous system	6,230	2%
All Sites	**310,010**	**100%**	**All Sites**	**275,710**	**100%**

FIGURE 28-1 Top 10 cancer types for estimated new cancer cases and deaths by sex in 2014 for the United States. *Estimates are rounded to the nearest 10 and exclude basal cell and squamous cell skin cancers and in situ carcinoma except urinary bladder. (From Siegel R, Ma J, Zou Z, et al: Cancer statistics, 2014. *CA Cancer J Clin* 64:9–29, 2014.)

population despite evidence that adjuvant therapies have a similar relative effectiveness and safety in the elderly.[9,10]

Obesity and Cancer

The prevalence of overweight (body mass index of 25 to 30 kg/m^2) and obesity (body mass index ≥30 kg/m^2) in most developed countries (and in urban areas of many less developed countries) has increased markedly during the past 2 decades. In the United States, more than one third of the population is now classified as obese. Although obesity has long been recognized as an important cause of diabetes and cardiovascular disease, the relationship between obesity and cancer has received less attention. Epidemiologic studies indicate that adiposity contributes to the increased incidence of and death from cancers of the colon, breast (in postmenopausal women), endometrium, kidney (renal cell), esophagus (adenocarcinoma), gastric cardia, pancreas, gallbladder, and liver (hepatocellular carcinoma). It has been estimated that 15% to 20% of all cancer deaths in the United States can be attributed to overweight and obesity.[11]

The mechanisms by which obesity increases cancer risk appear to involve the metabolic and endocrine effects of obesity through their alterations in levels of peptide and steroid hormones. For example, greater amounts of adipose tissue lead to increased circulating levels of free fatty acids. This in turn causes liver, muscle, and other tissues to increase their use of fats for energy production, thereby reducing their need for uptake and metabolism of glucose and eventually leading to hyperglycemia. This functional insulin resistance forces an increase in pancreatic insulin secretion. Epidemiologic and experimental evidence suggests that chronic hyperinsulinemia increases the risk of cancers of the colon and endometrium and probably other tumors (e.g., those of the pancreas and kidney).

Circulating levels of estrogens are strongly related to adiposity. For cancers of the breast (in postmenopausal women) and endometrium, the effects of overweight and obesity on cancer risk are largely mediated by increased estrogen levels. For patients with breast cancer, adiposity has been associated with both poorer survival and increased likelihood of recurrence, an effect that

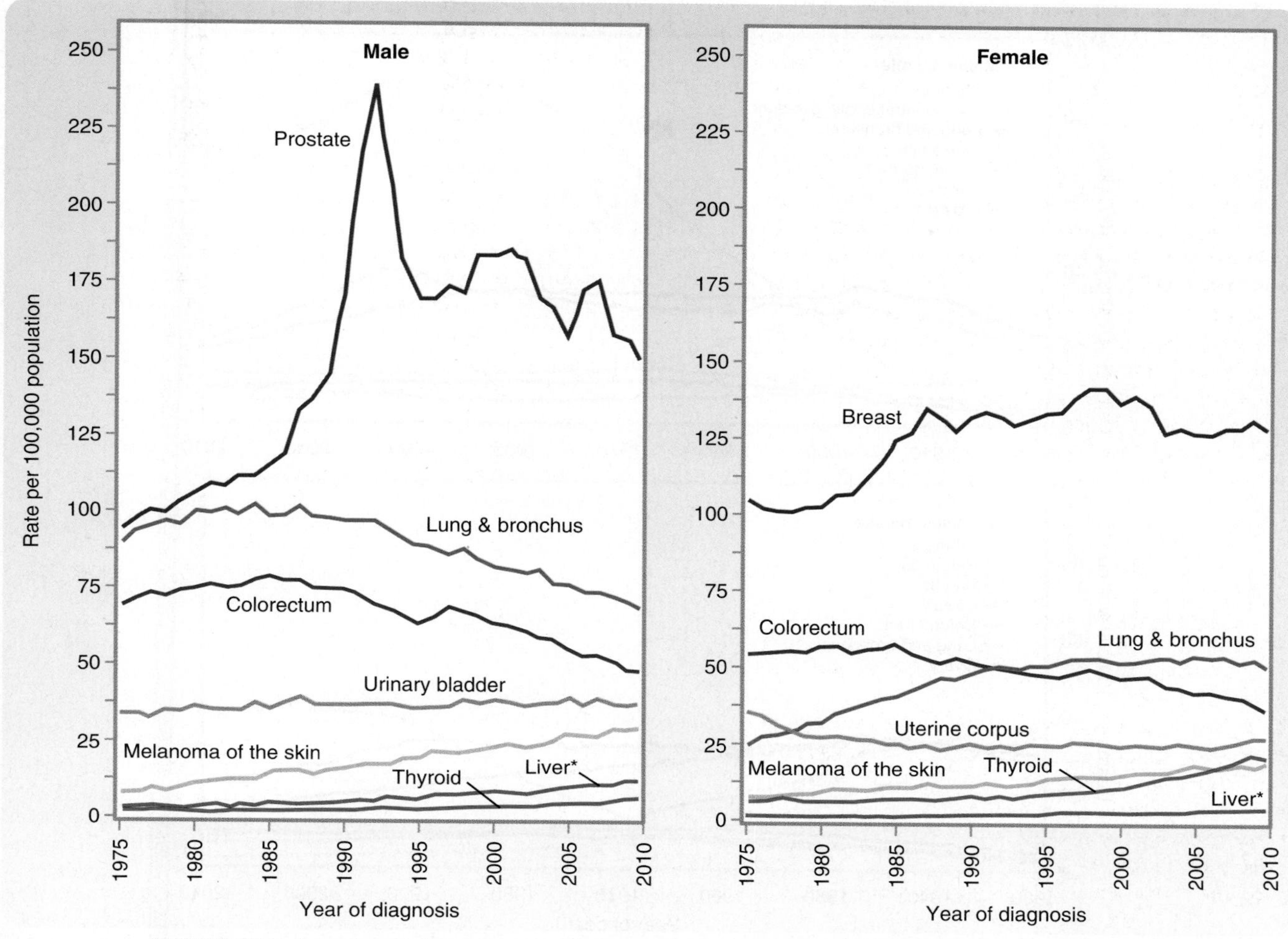

FIGURE 28-2 Annual age-adjusted cancer incidence rates for males and females for selected cancers in the United States, 1975-2010. *Includes intrahepatic bile duct. (From Siegel R, Ma J, Zou Z, et al: Cancer statistics, 2014. *CA Cancer J Clin* 64:9–29, 2014.)

persisted after adjustment for tumor stage and grade, hormone receptor status, and adjuvant therapy.

TUMOR BIOLOGY

Solid tumors are composed of neoplastic cells and stroma. It has become clear that these two compartments are interdependent and function as a unit to promote tumor growth, therapeutic resistance, invasion, and metastasis. Much has been learned about the multistep process of tumorigenesis. For example, the transformation of melanocytes into malignant melanoma can be divided histopathologically and clinically into five major identifiable steps (Table 28-1). Successive genetic changes confer a physiologic growth advantage leading to progressive conversion of normal cells into cancer cells. In addition to changes in tumor cells, the cells of the nearby stroma undergo phenotypic changes that further perpetuate tumor progression. A number of distinct physiologic changes are essential to tumorigenesis (discussed later), many of which are therapeutic targets (Fig. 28-4).

Sustaining Proliferative Signaling

Cells within normal tissues are largely instructed to grow by neighboring cells (paracrine signals) or through systemic (endocrine) signals. Likewise, cell-to-cell growth signaling occurs in the majority of tumors as well. The immediate tumor cell environment (the stroma) contains residing nonmalignant cells, such as parenchymal cells, epithelial cells, fibroblasts, and endothelial cells. In addition, most tumors are characterized by infiltrating immune cells, such as lymphocytes, polymorphonuclear cells, mast cells, and macrophages. In some tumors, these cooperating cells may eventually transform themselves, coevolving with the tumor cells to sustain the growth of the tumor cells. Finally, basement membranes form the extracellular matrix (ECM) that provides a scaffold for proliferation of fibroblast and endothelial cells. Together, tumor cells and stroma produce factors (autocrine and paracrine factors) that, in cell-bound, matrix-bound, or soluble form, directly or indirectly influence tumor development. Autocrine factors secreted by tumor cells promote growth of tumor cells but may also stimulate neighboring cells. In addition, tumor cells secrete paracrine factors that act on host cells or ECMs, generating a supportive microenvironment. For example, transforming growth factor-β (TGF-β) may induce angiogenesis, production of ECM molecules, and production of other cytokines by fibroblasts and endothelial cells. Simplified, tumor growth is dependent on the response of tumor cells to paracrine and autocrine factors (Fig. 28-5). These factors include angiogenesis factors, growth factors, chemokines (polypeptide signaling

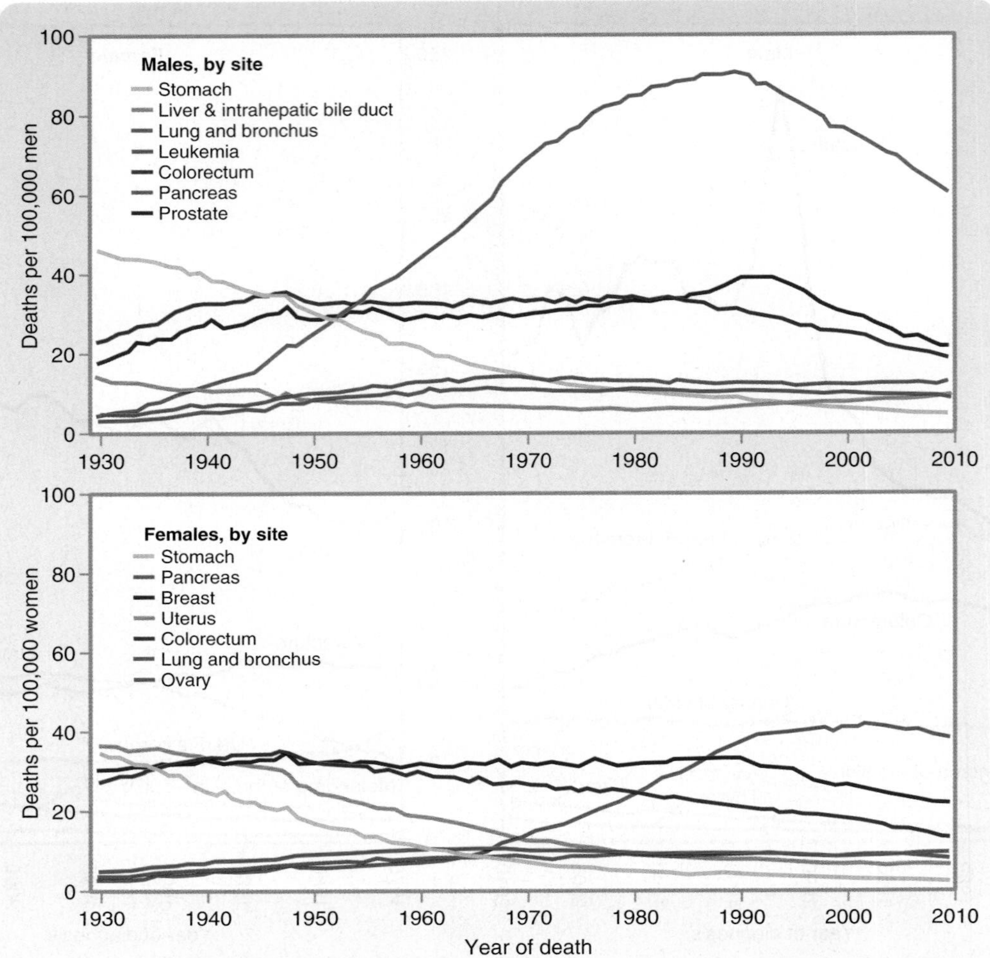

FIGURE 28-3 Trends in death rates for selected sites by sex, United States, 1930 to 2010. (From Siegel R, Ma J, Zou Z, et al: Cancer statistics, 2014. *CA Cancer J Clin* 64:9–29, 2014.)

TABLE 28-1 Stepwise Progression from Melanocyte to Metastatic Melanoma

STEP*	CHARACTERISTICS
1	Common melanocytic nevus
2	Dysplastic nevus
3	Radial growth phase of melanoma
4	Vertical growth phase of melanoma
5	Metastatic melanoma

Adapted from Clark WH, Jr, Elder DE, Guerry D, 4th, et al: A study of tumor progression: The precursor lesions of superficial spreading and nodular melanoma. *Hum Pathol* 15:1147–1165, 1984.

*Common acquired and congenital nevi without cytologic atypia (step 1) may progress into dysplastic nevi with clear atypical histologic and cytologic features (step 2). Most of these lesions are stable, but a few may progress to a malignant melanoma that tends to grow outward along the radius of the plaque (step 3). Within the plaque, a nodule develops of fast-growing cells that expand in a vertical direction, invading the dermis and elevating the epidermis (step 4). Finally, the tumor metastasizes (step 5).

molecules originally characterized by their ability to induce chemotaxis), cytokines, hormones, enzymes, and cytolytic factors that may promote or reduce tumor growth (Table 28-2).

During the evolution of a tumor, its responsiveness to growth signals changes. Paracrine growth mechanisms are dominant during the early development of tumor. Tumors become resistant to paracrine growth inhibitors and gain responsiveness to paracrine growth promoters. However, autocrine growth mechanisms become more prominent as tumors further develop. The observation that metastatic tumor cells tend to spread more randomly through the body in late-stage tumors suggests that autocrine growth mechanisms may be more dominant than paracrine growth mechanisms. Advanced breast cancers, for example, lose hormone responsiveness. It is even possible for a tumor to grow completely autonomously (acrine state) and to be independent of growth factors and inhibitors (Fig. 28-6).

To achieve growth self-sufficiency, growth signaling pathways are altered. This involves alteration of extracellular growth signals, of transmembrane transducers of those signals, or of intracellular signaling pathways that translate those signals into action. Growth factor receptors are overexpressed in many cancers. Receptor overexpression may enable the cancer cell to respond to low levels of

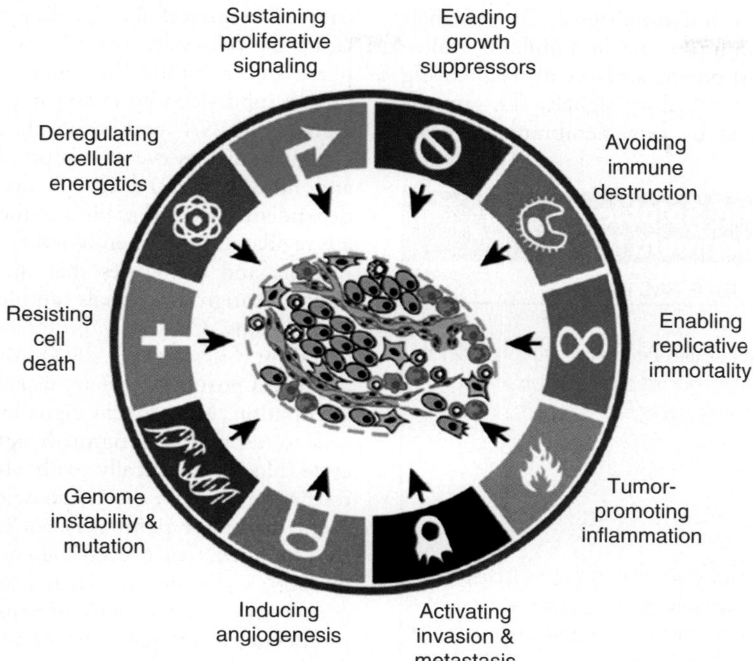

FIGURE 28-4 Key physiologic changes associated with progressive conversion of normal cells into malignant tumor cells. The indicated traits are common to the majority of human cancers, together conferring cell survival or tumor expansion. (Adapted from Hanahan D, Weinberg RA: The hallmarks of cancer. *Cell* 144:646–674, 2011.)

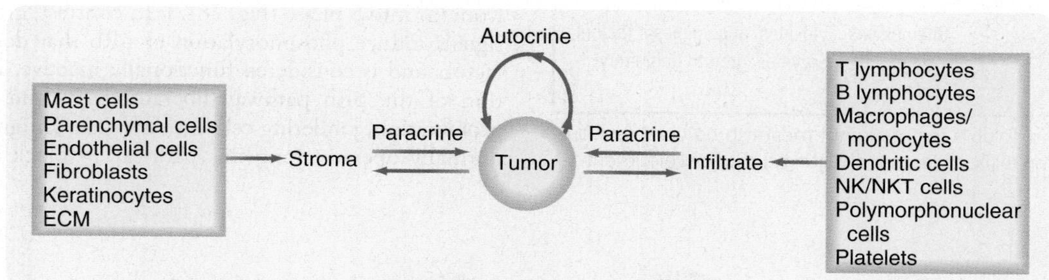

FIGURE 28-5 Paracrine and Autocrine Growth Mechanisms. Both stromal cells and infiltrating cells secrete paracrine factors that affect tumor development. In addition, tumor cells secrete autocrine as well as paracrine factors that in turn act on stromal cells and infiltrating cells. *ECM,* extracellular matrix; *NK,* natural killer.

growth factor that normally would not trigger proliferation. For example, the epidermal growth factor receptor (EGFR) and the HER2/neu receptor are overexpressed in breast and other epithelial cancers. In addition, gross overexpression of growth factor receptors can elicit growth factor–independent signaling. This can also be achieved through structural alteration of receptors, such as truncated versions of EGFR that lack much of its cytoplasmic domain and are constitutively activated.

Cancer cells can also modulate their stromal environment, including the ECM, through secretion of factors such as basic fibroblast growth factor, platelet-derived growth factor, TGF-β, and others. ECM components, such as collagens, fibronectins, laminins, and vitronectins, may bind to two or more receptors and may also bind other ECM molecules. The matrix molecule–receptor interaction induces signals that influence cell behavior, including entrance into the active cell cycle. Cancer cells can switch the types of ECM receptors (integrins and heparan sulfate proteoglycans) they express, favoring ones that transmit pro-growth signals.

A more complex mechanism for acquisition of self-sufficiency in growth signals stems from changes in intracellular signaling pathways, some of which actively engage in crosstalk. Many of the oncogenes (e.g., activating mutations in *KRAS*) mimic normal growth signaling and induce mitogenic signals without stimulation from upstream regulators. This results in autonomous cell proliferation independent of external signals. Last, negative-feedback mechanisms that help regulate normal signaling pathways can be disrupted and thereby enhance proliferative signaling.

Evading Growth Suppressors

Cell division is an ordered, tightly regulated process involving both stimulatory and inhibitory signals. Thus, in addition to acquiring stimulatory growth signals, tumor cells need to overcome or to neutralize growth-inhibitory signals. These signals include both soluble growth inhibitors and immobilized inhibitors embedded in the ECM and on the surfaces of neighboring cells. Similar to many of the stimulatory signals, the growth-inhibitory signals are transduced by transmembrane receptors coupled to intracellular signaling pathways that target genes regulating the cell cycle. The cell cycle can be divided into an interphase and a mitotic (M) phase (Fig. 28-7).[12] The interphase is further subdivided into two gap phases (G_1 and G_2), separated by a phase of DNA synthesis (S phase). The two gap phases involve crucial regulatory events that prepare the cell for DNA replication and mitosis. Central to cell cycle progression are the cyclin-dependent kinases that bind to the cyclin proteins. These proteins are regulated by numerous other proteins including tumor suppressors and oncogenes that induce stimulatory or inhibitory signals. Antigrowth signals can block cell division by two distinct mechanisms. Cells may be forced to exit the cell cycle into a quiescent (G_0) state (Fig. 28-7). Alternatively, cells may be induced to enter a postmitotic state, usually associated with terminal differentiation. Many of the signaling pathways that enable normal cells to respond to antigrowth signals are associated with the cell cycle block, specifically with the components governing the restriction point in the G_1 phase of the cell cycle. The restriction point marks the point between early and late G_1 phase passage that represents an irreversible commitment to undergo one cell division. Cells monitor their external environment during this period and, on the basis of sensed signals, decide whether to proliferate, to be quiescent, or to enter into a postmitotic state. At the molecular level, many and perhaps all antiproliferative signals involve the retinoblastoma protein (pRb) and its two family members, p107 and p130.[12] pRb is a key negative regulator at the restriction point. In quiescent cells, pRb is hypophosphorylated and blocks cell division by binding E2F transcription factors that control the expression of many genes essential for progression from G_1 into S phase (Fig. 28-7). In contrast, growth-stimulatory signals induce phosphorylation of pRb that does not bind E2F factors and is considered functionally inactive. Likewise, disruption of the pRb pathway liberates E2Fs and thus allows cell proliferation, rendering cells insensitive to antigrowth factors that normally operate along this pathway to block advance through

TABLE 28-2 Cells and Soluble Factors Affecting Tumor Development*

CELLS	SOLUBLE FACTORS
Stroma	
Parenchymal cells Endothelial cells Fibroblasts Mast cells Extracellular matrix Keratinocytes	Growth factors, growth inhibitors, nutritional factors, hormones, degradative enzymes, cytokines, angiogenesis factors
Infiltrate	
T lymphocytes B lymphocytes Natural killer cells Natural killer T cells Macrophages-monocytes Dendritic cells Polymorphonuclear cells Platelets	Cytokines, chemokines, cytolytic factors, angiogenesis factors, growth (inhibitory) factors, degradative enzymes, cytostatic factors, antibodies
Tumor	Chemokines, cytokines, angiogenesis factors, degradative enzymes, growth (inhibitory) factors

*The list of cells and soluble factors is not meant to be complete but to illustrate the complexity of factors affecting tumor development.

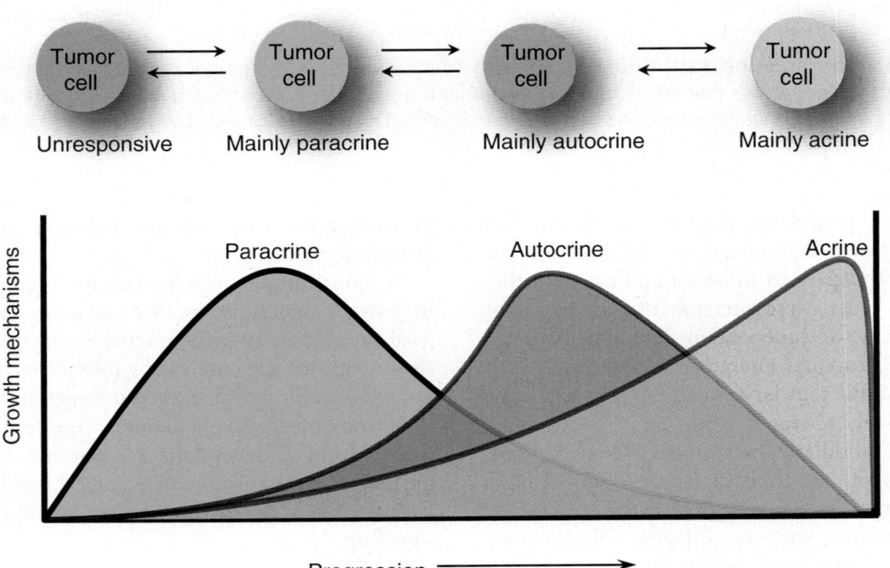

FIGURE 28-6 Changes in Contribution of Growth Mechanisms to Tumor Development. During tumor progression, the contribution of paracrine growth mechanisms decreases, and the tumor becomes more dependent on autocrine growth mechanisms. At later stages, the tumor may even become independent of growth mechanisms (acrine state).

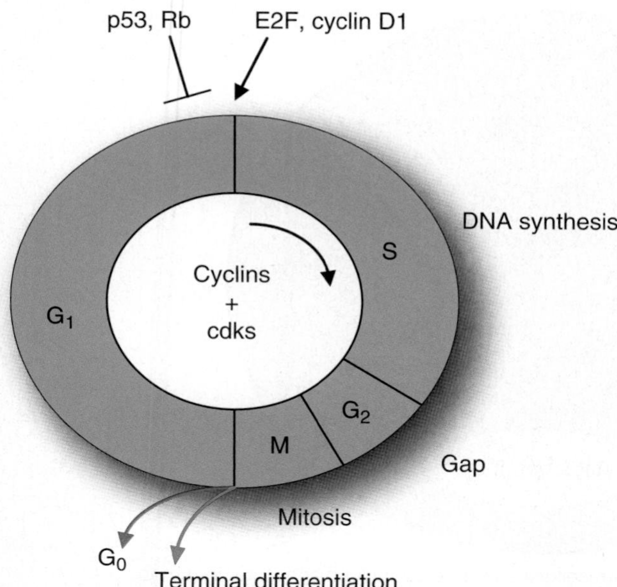

FIGURE 28-7 Schematic Overview of the Cell Cycle. Cell division is governed by cyclin proteins and cyclin-dependent kinases (cdks). After mitosis, a cell can terminally differentiate, enter a quiescent state, or re-enter the cell cycle. A critical point in the cell cycle control is the transition from G_1 to S. After passing this checkpoint, the cell is committed to division. Tumor suppressor genes such as the retinoblastoma *(Rb)* gene and *p53* block G_1 to S transition, whereas oncogenes such as cyclin D1 and E2F promote transition.

the G_1 phase of the cell cycle. For example, TGF-β prevents the phosphorylation of pRb that inactivates pRb and thereby blocks advance through G_1. In some tumors, such as breast, colon, liver, and pancreatic cancers, TGF-β responsiveness is lost through downregulation of TGF-β receptors or through expression of mutant, dysfunctional receptors. In others, such as colon, lung, and liver cancers, the cytoplasmic Smad4 protein, which transduces signals from ligand-activated TGF-β receptors to downstream targets, may be eliminated through mutation of its encoding gene. Alternatively, in cervical carcinomas induced by human papillomavirus, the viral oncoprotein E7 binds pRb and thereby induces dissociation of E2F and subsequent transcription of genes necessary for cell cycle progression. In addition, cancer cells can also turn off expression of integrins and other cell adhesion molecules (CAMs) that send antigrowth signals. In summary, the antigrowth signaling pathways converging onto Rb and the cell cycle are disrupted in a majority of human cancers. Cyclin–cyclin-dependent kinase complexes, essential for cell cycle progression, are regulated by two families of cyclin–cyclin-dependent kinase inhibitors in normal cells. However, in tumor cells, these regulatory proteins, such as the p16 member of the INK4 family, are frequently deleted, allowing tumor cells to bypass cell cycle arrest.

In addition to avoiding antigrowth signals, tumor cells may also avoid terminal differentiation, for example, through overexpression of the oncogene c-*myc*, which encodes a transcription factor regulating expression of cyclins and cyclin-dependent kinases, or through upregulation of Id (short for inhibitor of DNA-binding/differentiation) family members. Likewise, during human colon carcinogenesis, mutations of *APC*, a negative regulator of β-catenin, lead to the constitutive activation of Wnt/β-catenin signaling, which serves to block the terminal differentiation of enterocytes in colonic crypts.

Resisting Cell Death

The growth of tumors is determined by the ability of tumor cells to proliferate, offset by cell death. Most if not all types of tumors are characterized by defects in cell death signaling pathways and are resistant to cell death. Cell death in tumors is caused primarily by programmed cell death, or apoptosis, which is the most common and well defined form of cell death.[13] Apoptosis is a physiologic cell suicide program essential for embryonic development, functioning of the immune system, and maintenance of tissue homeostasis. Apoptosis is characterized by disruption of membranes and chromosomal degradation in a matter of hours. The general apoptosis signaling pathway involves the release of cytochrome *c* from mitochondria that activates various caspases (a family of at least 10 proteases) in sequence (Fig. 28-8).

Activation of caspase cascades leads to DNA fragmentation and apoptosis. Induction of apoptosis is either death receptor dependent (extrinsic pathway) or independent (intrinsic pathway). The two best understood death receptor pathways are the Fas receptor and death receptor 5 that bind the extracellular Fas ligand and TRAIL, respectively. Binding of the ligands triggers activation of caspase 8 and promotes the cascade of procaspase activation leading to release of cytochrome *c* from mitochondria and eventually apoptosis. The intrinsic pathway is triggered by various extracellular and intracellular stresses, such as growth factor withdrawal, hypoxia, DNA damage, and oncogene induction. Receptor-independent pathways involve translocation of proapoptotic molecules from the cytoplasm to the mitochondria, causing mitochondrial damage and release of cytochrome *c*. Cytochrome *c* is directly involved in the activation of caspase 9, which activates caspase 3, which then leads to apoptosis.

The idea that apoptosis forms a constraint to cancer was first raised in 1972 when massive apoptosis was observed in the cells populating rapidly growing, hormone-dependent tumors after hormone withdrawal.[14] The discovery of *bcl-2* oncogene as having antiapoptotic activity opened up the investigation of apoptosis in cancer at the molecular level.[15] Bcl-2 promotes formation of B cell lymphomas through a chromosomal translocation linking the *bcl-2* gene to an immunoglobulin locus, which results in constitutive activation of *bcl-2*, driving lymphocyte survival. Further research has demonstrated that altering components of the apoptotic machinery allows a cell to resist death signals, providing it with a selective growth advantage. For example, functional inactivation of the tumor suppressor p53 is observed in more than 50% of human cancers. p53 is a key regulator of apoptosis by sensing DNA damage that cannot be repaired and subsequent activation of the apoptotic pathway. Other abnormalities, such as hypoxia and oncogene overexpression, are also channeled in part through p53 to the apoptotic machinery and fail to elicit apoptosis when p53 function is lost. In addition, alterations in cell survival pathways can suppress or alter apoptosis. For example, the phosphatidylinositol 3-kinase/AKT pathway, which transmits antiapoptotic survival signals, is likely involved in inhibiting apoptosis in many human tumors. This signaling pathway can be activated by extracellular factors such as insulin-like growth factors I and II or interleukin-3 (IL-3), by intracellular signals from Ras, or by loss of the pTEN tumor suppressor that negatively regulates the phosphatidylinositol 3-kinase/AKT pathway. A final example is the discovery of a nonsignaling decoy receptor for FAS ligand

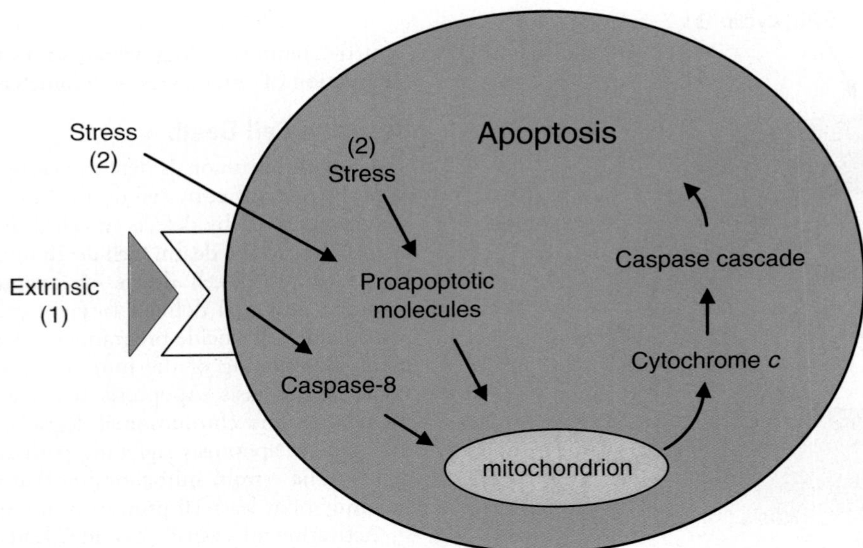

FIGURE 28-8 Apoptotic Pathways. Extracellular and intracellular stresses can induce apoptosis in tumor cells. Extracellular triggering can occur through a receptor-dependent (1) or receptor-independent (2) pathway. Both pathways induce release of cytochrome *c* from mitochondria, which triggers activation of various caspases in sequence, ultimately leading to apoptosis.

in a high fraction of lung and colon carcinoma cell lines. Expression of this decoy receptor dilutes the death signal mediated through FAS.

Nonapoptotic types of cell death that can promote tumor growth include necrosis, autophagy, and mitotic catastrophe. Necrosis is normally induced by pathophysiologic conditions such as infection, inflammation, and ischemia. Necrosis is characterized by unregulated cell destruction associated with the release of proinflammatory signals. Inflammatory cells, in particular those of myeloid origin that are recruited to the tumor environment, actively promote tumor growth through induction of angiogenesis, immune suppression, tumor invasiveness, and metastasis formation. Autophagy is triggered by growth factor withdrawal, hypoxia, DNA damage, and differentiation and developmental triggers.[13,16] Degraded intracellular organelles give rise to metabolites that allow survival of tumor cells in stressed, nutrient-limited environments. Finally, aberrant mitosis caused by failure of the G_2 checkpoint to block mitosis when DNA is damaged can lead to cell death, known as mitotic catastrophe. The signaling pathways involved in these types of nonapoptotic cell death are less well defined compared with those that regulate apoptosis, but it is clear that defects in nonapoptotic cell death pathways have been linked to cancer. For example, amplification of the MDM2 oncogene, which negatively regulates expression of p53, results in inadequate expression of p53 and thereby loss of tumor suppressor function. Another example is the deletion of the autophagy-regulating gene *becklin-1* in high percentages of ovarian, breast, and prostate cancers. In addition to cell death, cells can undergo permanent growth arrest, called senescence, when repair of damaged DNA fails. Senescent cells lose their clonogenicity, but defects in the senescent program contribute to tumor development.

Enabling Replicative Immortality

Acquired disruption of cell-to-cell signaling by itself does not ensure expansive tumor growth on its own. This is due to the intrinsic programmed decline in replication potential that limits multiplication of normal somatic cells. This program must be disrupted for a clone of cells to develop into a macroscopic tumor. Normal cells have a finite replicative potential. Once a cell population has progressed through a certain number of doublings, they stop growing but remain viable, a process termed senescence.

With the exception of stem cells, activated lymphocytes, and germline cells, normal cells have a limited replicative potential. Stem cells give rise to progenitor cells that can progress through a certain number of doublings with an increasing degree of differentiation. Fully differentiated cells do not have replicative potential. The number of doublings is controlled by telomeres, the ends of chromosomes that are composed of several thousand repeats of a short 6–base pair sequence element.[17] Telomeres prevent end-to-end chromosomal fusion. However, each DNA replication is associated with a loss of 50 to 100 base pairs of telomeric DNA from the ends of every chromosome. The progressive shortening of telomeres through successive cycles of replication eventually causes them to lose their ability to protect the ends of chromosomal DNA. When the critical length is bridged, the unprotected chromosomal ends participate in end-to-end chromosomal fusions, yielding a karyotype disarray that almost inevitably results in the death of the affected cell.[17] Telomeric attrition is negated by the enzyme telomerase that elongates telomeric DNA. Telomerase activity is high during embryonic development and in certain cell populations, such as stem cells in adults. However, many tumors are characterized by elevated telomerase activity. Alternatively, telomeres are maintained through recombination-based interchromosomal exchanges of sequence information. Thus, by maintaining a telomere length above a critical threshold, the tumor cells have unlimited proliferative potential and are considered immortal.

Evidence has recently been obtained for the existence of cancer stem cells (CSCs), or cancer-initiating cells, that give rise to tissue-specific progenitor cells and phenotypically diverse cancer cells with limited replicative potential.[18] The definition of CSCs is still a subject of some debate, but a CSC subclass has now been described in most types of cancer. Characteristic of CSCs is the exponentially enhanced ability to seed new tumors, relative to the non-CSC population, in immunodeficient mice. These cells are extraordinarily rare within the tumor and usually make up less than 10% of neoplastic cells and often less than 5%. CSCs may generate tumors through self-renewal as well as through differentiation into multiple cell types. Various cell surface markers have been used to define CSCs, such as CD44, CD133, and CXCR4. Interestingly, CSCs possess similar transcriptional profiles with normal tissue stem cells, further supporting their designation as stem-like. Furthermore, evidence suggests that CSCs are more resistant to traditional therapeutic modalities, such as chemotherapy and radiation.

Inducing Angiogenesis

Based on the observation that many individuals who died of non–cancer-related causes had in situ tumors at the time of autopsy, physicians and scientists concluded that these microscopic tumors are in a dormant state. The reason for tumor dormancy is that the body blocks the tumor from recruiting its own blood supply to provide tumor cells with the required oxygen and nutrients. The growth of new blood vessels, angiogenesis, is a highly regulated process to ensure supply to all cells within an organ. Surprisingly, the microscopic tumors lack the ability to induce angiogenesis, and only an estimated 1 in 600 acquire angiogenic activity. Research pioneered by Judah Folkman has demonstrated that naturally occurring endogenous angiogenesis inhibitors prevent tumors from expanding.[19] The angiogenesis inhibitors keep the tumors in check by counterbalancing the angiogenic signals. These signals are mediated by soluble factors and their receptors on endothelial cells as well as by integrins and adhesion molecules mediating cell-matrix and cell-cell interactions. Angiogenic activity is induced by growth factors such as vascular endothelial growth factor (VEGF), basic and acidic fibroblast growth factor, and platelet-derived growth factor. Each binds to transmembrane tyrosine kinase receptors displayed primarily by endothelial cells that are connected to intracellular signaling pathways. Angiogenesis inhibitors are associated with specific tissues or circulate in the blood. The first inhibitor, interferon-α, was reported in 1980, and additional endogenous inhibitors have been identified since then.[19] These include thrombospondin, tumstatin, canstatin, endostatin, and angiostatin. Evidence for the importance of inducing and sustaining angiogenesis in tumors is overwhelming. For example, the switch of dormant human tumors into fast-growing tumors in immune-compromised mice is associated with an angiogenesis gene signature. Most telling are the results of clinical studies with the anti-VEGF antibody bevacizumab (Avastin), the first angiogenesis inhibitor approved by the Food and Drug Administration for treatment of colon cancer. Bevacizumab significantly prolongs the survival of patients with advanced cancer. Similarly, a dominant-interfering version of the VEGF receptor 2 proved to impair neovascularization and growth of subcutaneous tumors in mice.

The ability to induce and to sustain angiogenesis seems to be acquired in a discrete step (or steps) during tumor development through a switch to the angiogenic phenotype.[19,20] Tumors appear to activate the angiogenic switch by changing the balance between the total angiogenic stimulation and the total angiogenic inhibition.[21] This occurs in most cases when the angiogenesis stimulators overwhelm the angiogenesis inhibitors. In some tumors, these changes may be linked. It is likely that such disruption in the angiogenic balance is under control of the genetic makeup of the individual tumor cell and its microenvironment. Angiogenesis inducers and inhibitors may be genetically controlled by tumor suppressor genes such as *p53*, whereas oncogenes (e.g., *ras*) may downregulate transcription of endogenous inhibitors or activate inducers. For example, *bcl-2* activation leads to significantly increased expression of VEGF and angiogenesis. Another dimension of regulation is through proteases, which can control the bioavailability of angiogenic activators and inhibitors. Thus, a variety of proteases can release basic fibroblast growth factor stored in the ECM, whereas plasmin, a proangiogenic component of the clotting system, can cleave itself into an angiogenesis inhibitor form called angiostatin. Another angiogenesis inhibitor, endostatin, is an internal fragment of the basement membrane collagen XVIII. Finally, hypoxia and other metabolic stressors, mechanical stress from proliferating cells, or inflammatory immune responses can trigger angiogenesis. The coordinated expression of proangiogenic and antiangiogenic signaling molecules and their modulation by proteolysis appear to reflect the complex homeostatic regulation of normal tissue angiogenesis and of vascular integrity. Different types of tumors use distinct molecular strategies to activate the angiogenic switch.

Endothelial cells are key in the formation of new blood vessels through production or expression of angiogenesis-promoting factors. These factors include proinflammatory cytokines such as IL-6, VEGF, and hematopoietic growth factors such as colony-stimulating factors that recruit and activate bone marrow–derived progenitor cells. Among the progenitor cells are myeloid precursors that further promote the proinflammatory responses at the tumor and actively contribute to angiogenesis by producing matrix metalloprotease-9, a critical regulator of tumor angiogenesis through the induced release of VEGF. Bone marrow–derived endothelial precursors foster tumor blood vessel assembly.

Activating Invasion and Metastasis

Progressing tumors give rise to distant metastases that are the cause of 90% of human cancer deaths. Invasion and metastatic growth of tumor cells do not appear to be random processes. Paget observed in 1889 that breast carcinoma often metastasized to the liver, lungs, bone, adrenals, or brain. He hypothesized that tumor cells (the "seed") would grow only in selective environments (the "soil"), where conditions supported tumor growth, hence the so-called seed-and-soil hypothesis. Since then, additional studies have confirmed this hypothesis. For example, malignant melanoma metastasizes to the brain, but ocular malignant melanoma frequently metastasizes to the liver. Prostate cancer metastasizes to the bone and colon carcinoma to the liver.

Whereas metastatic spread is in part determined by circulation patterns, the retention of disseminated tumor cells in distant organs and successful development suggest the existence of specific molecular interactions. Molecular analysis has provided several theories to explain preferential outgrowth of tumor cells. One theory, the growth factor theory, proposes that tumor cells in the blood or lymphatics invade organs at similar frequency, but only those that find favorable growth factors multiply. Transferrins, for example, are iron-transferring ferroproteins required for cell growth that have additional mitogenic properties beyond their iron-transporting function. Increased concentrations of transferrin are found in lung, bone, and the brain and are associated with elevated levels of transferrin receptors on metastasizing tumor cells. Another theory, the adhesion theory, proposes that endothelial cells lining the blood vessels in certain organs express adhesion molecules that bind tumor cells and permit extravasation. A third theory is that chemokines secreted by the target organ can enter the circulation and selectively attract tumor cells that express receptors for the chemokines. Evidence for the importance of chemokines in tumor progression was recently obtained for breast cancer cells preferentially metastasizing in bone marrow, liver, lymph nodes, and lung.[22] These organs were found to secrete CXCL12, which is the ligand for the chemokine receptor CXCR4, enriched on breast cancer cells compared with normal breast epithelial cells. A similar phenomenon was observed for melanoma cells that were found to express elevated levels of the receptors CXCR4, CCR7, and CCR10 compared with normal melanocytes.[22] Lymph nodes, lung, liver, bone marrow, and skin express the highest levels of the ligands for these receptors and are the preferred sites for metastatic spread of melanomas. Because chemokines are now known to affect angiogenesis and expression of cytokines, adhesion molecules, and proteases in addition to inducing migration, it appears that chemokines and their receptors play an essential role in the successful outgrowth of tumors at preferential sites.

Detailed analysis of primary tumors indicates that gene functions mediating metastatic activities are present early in the disease. These functions result from genetic or epigenetic alterations. The genes can be grouped into classes, such as metastasis-initiating genes that control invasion, angiogenesis, circulation, and bone marrow mobilization. Similarly, metastasis progression genes control extravasation, survival, and reinitiation, whereas metastasis virulence genes regulate organ-specific colonization. These intrinsic properties of the tumor together with its cellular origin determine the organ specificity and temporal course of metastasis formation.

The formation of tumor metastases is characterized by detachment of some tumor cells from the primary tumor and infiltration into the bloodstream or lymphatics (intravasation). The reciprocal process occurs at other locations in the body (extravasation). Both intravasation and extravasation are characterized by changes in ECMs and their interactions with tumor cells. The cell-cell and cell-matrix interactions are mediated through CAMs, primarily by members of the immunoglobulin and calcium-dependent cadherin families,[23] the hyaluronan receptor CD44, selectins, and integrins,[24] which link cells to ECM substrates. Studies have shown that the molecules mediating adhesion are also capable of signal transduction. As such, changes in expression of adhesion molecules will alter signaling pathways, and conversely, signaling molecules can directly affect the function of adhesion molecules in tumor cells.

Epithelial (E)–cadherin is the prototype cadherin responsible for cell polarity and organization of epithelium. E-cadherin function is lost in most epithelial tumors during progression to tumor malignancy and may in fact be a prerequisite for tumor cell invasion and metastasis formation. In normal cells, extracellular domains of E-cadherin on opposing cells couple and form cell-cell junctions (Fig. 28-9). The cytoplasmic cell adhesion complex is linked to the actin cytoskeleton through catenins (α, β, and γ). Mechanisms that include mutational inactivation of the E-cadherin or β-catenin genes, transcriptional repression, or proteases of the extracellular cadherin domain induce loss of E-cadherin function.[23] This prevents catenins from binding and leads to their accumulation in the cytoplasm. Inactivation of nonsequestered β- and γ-catenin is dependent on the presence of the tumor suppressor gene *APC* and an inactive Wnt signaling pathway (Fig. 28-9). However, when *APC* function is lost, as is the case in many colon cancers or in the case of Wnt activation, β-catenin is not degraded but instead translocates to the nucleus, where transcription is activated of genes involved in cell proliferation and tumor progression, such as *c-myc*, cyclin D1, CD44, and others.

Changes in expression of CAMs in the immunoglobulin superfamily also appear to play critical roles in the processes of invasion and metastasis.[23,25] Neuronal (N)–CAM, for example, undergoes a switch in expression from a highly adhesive isoform to poorly

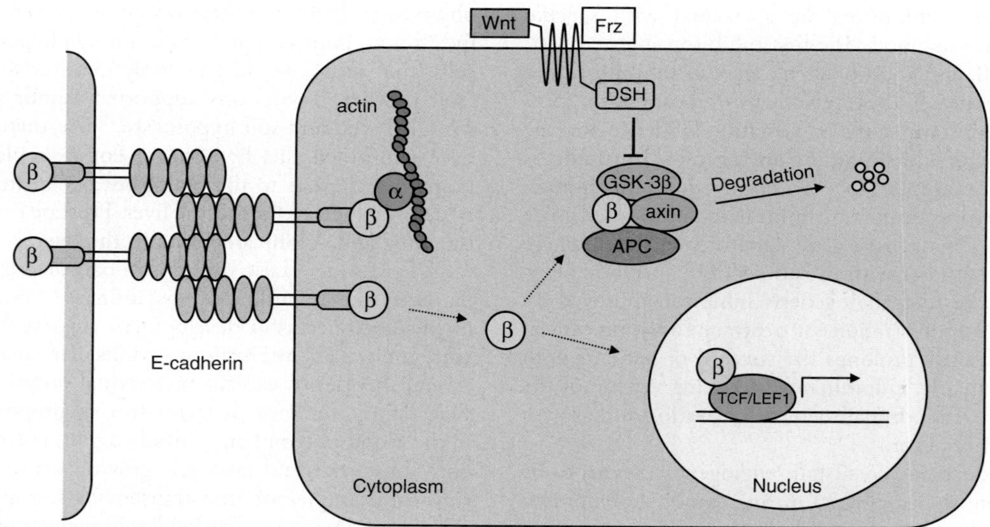

FIGURE 28-9 Loss of E-Cadherin Permits Tumor Progression. Functional loss of E-cadherin to sequester β-catenin leads to accumulation of β-catenin in the cytoplasm. Likewise, Wnt signaling inactivates GSK-3β, which leads to stabilization of β-catenin instead of its degradation. Also, loss of *APC* function may result in accumulation of β-catenin in the cytoplasm. This leads to translocation of β-catenin to the nucleus, where it binds the T cell–specific transcription factor/lymphoid enhancer factor-1 (TCF/LEF-1), inducing a genetic program that leads to tumor progression. *α*, α-catenin; *APC*, adenomatous polyposis coli; *β*, β-catenin; *Frz*, frizzled (transmembrane receptor for Wnt growth factors); *DSH*, disheveled; *GSK-3β*, glycogen synthase kinase 3β.

adhesive (or even repulsive) forms in Wilms tumor, neuroblastoma, and small cell lung cancer. In invasive pancreatic cancer and colorectal cancers, the overall expression of N-CAM is reduced.

Selectins are a family of transmembrane molecules consisting of E (endothelial), L (leukocyte), and P (platelet) selectins that normally mediate blood cell–endothelial cell interactions. However, alterations in the expression level of selectins or their ligands, such as the E- and L-selectin ligand CD44, have been associated with increased invasiveness and poor survival in several malignant neoplasms, such as breast cancer and colorectal cancer.

Changes in integrin expression are also evident in invasive and metastatic cells. For invading and metastasizing cells to be successful, they need to adapt to changing tissue microenvironments. This is accomplished through shifts in the spectrum of integrin α and β subunits displayed on the cell surface by the migrating cells. The large extracellular domain of integrins can bind to ECM molecules (such as collagens, laminin, and fibronectin), to ligands associated with vascular and coagulation physiology (such as thrombospondin and factor X), or with other CAMs. Each integrin molecule consists of an α subunit and a β subunit, but a particular β subunit can dimerize with several different α subunits. These novel permutations result in different integrin subtypes (currently 24 combinations have been described) having distinct substrate preferences. In addition, integrins may exhibit different specificities when expressed on different cell types. Thus, carcinoma cells facilitate invasion by shifting their expression of integrins from those that favor ECM present in normal epithelium to other integrins that preferentially bind the degraded stromal components produced by extracellular proteases.[25] For example, expression of $\alpha_4\beta_1$, which binds fibronectin, correlates with progression of melanoma. The changes are incompletely understood because of the large number of distinct integrin genes, the even larger number of heterodimeric receptors resulting from combinatorial expression of various α and β receptor subunits, and the increasing evidence of complex signals emitted by the cytoplasmic domains of these receptors. Changes in integrin expression may also be essential for expansion of the tumor stem cell compartment by inhibiting differentiation or apoptosis.[26]

The second general parameter of the invasive and metastatic capability involves extracellular proteases that regulate ECM turnover. It has become clear that tumor progression may involve an increased expression of proteases, decreased expression of protease inhibitors, and inactive zymogen forms of proteases that are converted into active enzymes. Expression of the protease tenascin, which neutralizes adhesion to fibronectin, is increased 10-fold in invasive breast carcinoma compared with normal breast tissue. Matrix metalloproteases are overexpressed in melanoma, invasive breast carcinoma, and invasive squamous cell carcinoma. Matrix-degrading proteases are characteristically associated with the cell surface by synthesis with a transmembrane domain, binding to specific protease receptors, or association with integrins. One imagines that docking of active proteases on the cell surface can facilitate invasion by cancer cells into nearby stroma, across blood vessel walls, and through normal epithelium cell layers. That notion notwithstanding, it is difficult to unambiguously ascribe the functions of particular proteases solely to this capability, given their evident roles in other hallmark capabilities, including angiogenesis and growth signaling, which in turn contribute directly or indirectly to the invasive and metastatic capability. A further complexity derives from the multiple cell types involved in protease expression and display, including stromal and inflammatory cells such as neutrophils and macrophages.

The activation of extracellular proteases and the altered binding specificities of cadherins, CAMs, selectins, and integrins are clearly central to the acquisition of invasiveness and metastatic potential. The clonal and genetic diversity of tumors permits adhesion and detachment from the same matrix. Some tumor cells within a primary tumor may have the correct genotype and phenotype to permit both detachment from the surrounding tissue and entry into blood vessels or lymphatic vessels. Likewise, extravasation may be mediated by a few tumor cells that express the required receptors for certain ECM molecules. In general, those mutations that confer escape from homeostatic control mechanisms in the host or that give the tumor cell a growth advantage over others are favorably selected. Thus, tumor clones that best complement the environment with expression of particular ECM receptors may thrive because this provides an advantage over other clones. However, the regulatory pathways and molecular mechanisms that govern these changes are incompletely understood and appear to differ from one tissue environment to another.

It has recently been demonstrated that epithelial cancer cells can acquire a mesenchymal phenotype. This cellular program, known as epithelial-mesenchymal transition (EMT), is an essential phenomenon during normal embryogenesis. However, cancer cells use EMT to become invasive and to metastasize. During EMT, cancer cells downregulate the expression of cellular adhesion molecules, such as E-cadherin, and become spindle shaped, thus allowing them to invade surrounding tissues, to intravasate into the bloodstream, and to metastasize. Once cells in EMT arrive at distant sites of metastasis, they extravasate and undergo a process of mesenchymal-epithelial transition, whereby these cells revert back to their original epithelial phenotype for clonal expansion and establishment of metastasis. Recent work suggests that cells in EMT acquire similar stem-like properties to CSCs, and thus EMT could give rise to CSCs.[18]

Avoiding Immune Destruction

In the early 1900s, it was proposed by Paul Ehrlich that the frequency of cancerous transformations would be very high if it were not for the defense system of the host. This concept was later substantiated in the 1950s and 1960s. Burnet hypothesized that the development of T lymphocyte–mediated immunity during evolution was specific for elimination of transformed cells. He further proposed that there is a continuous surveillance of the body for transformed cells, hence the term *immunosurveillance*. Extensive studies on immune infiltrate in primary human cancers have established that memory T cells, particularly of the T helper ($CD4^+$) type 1 subtype, and cytotoxic ($CD8^+$) T cells are prognostic factors for disease-free and overall survival at all stages of clinical disease.[27] Alternatively, tumors infiltrated with abundant myeloid cells, particularly macrophages, correlate with worse prognosis in many types of cancers, such as pancreas and breast. Data from mouse and human studies combined suggest that immune surveillance of cancer does exist, mediated through immune cells and soluble factors. Whereas the immune system may eliminate most transformed cells, some cells manage to escape and may develop into tumors.

The continuous pressure of the immune system in an immunocompetent host determines to a great degree if and how tumors evolve, a process called *immunoediting* (Fig. 28-10).[28] In this process, the immune system plays a dual role in the interactions between tumor and the host. On one hand, the immune system effectively eliminates highly immunogenic tumor cells. At the same time, however, the immune system fails to eliminate tumor

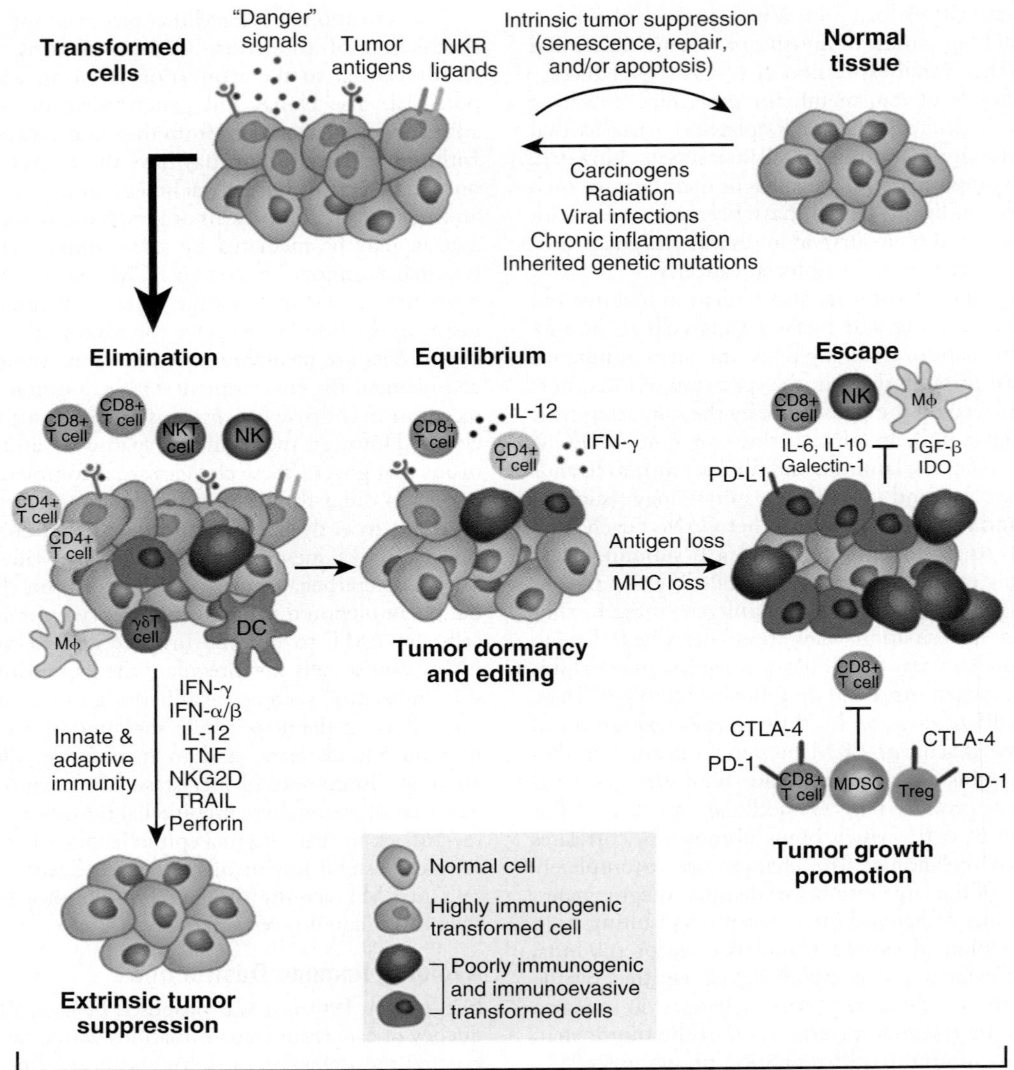

FIGURE 28-10 Schematic Overview of Immunoediting. When developing tumors disrupt local tissue structures, proinflammatory cytokines are released and together with secreted chemokines attract innate immune cells, such as macrophages, natural killer (NK) cells, NKT cells, and γ/δ cells. Innate immune cells can directly recognize and lyse tumor cells but also induce an adaptive immune response mediated by $CD8^+$ and $CD4^+$ lymphocytes. Whereas most tumor cells are eliminated (elimination phase), tumor cell variants may survive and expand. However, the activated immune system keeps the tumor in check by eliminating those tumor cells that are sufficiently immunogenic (equilibrium phase). The immunologic pressure may cause selection toward tumor cell variants with reduced immunogenicity that are capable of escaping from immune recognition (escape phase). These variants can expand in an immunologically intact environment. (From Schreiber RD, Old LJ, Smyth MJ: Cancer immunoediting: Integrating immunity's roles in cancer suppression and promotion. *Science* 331:1565–1570, 2011.)

cells with reduced immunogenicity, thereby selecting for tumor variants that have acquired immune evasion mechanisms. Over time, this selection leads to outgrowth of tumor cells that fail to induce an effective immune response. As such, the interactions between an intact immune system and tumor cells evolve through three phases, referred to as the elimination phase, the equilibrium phase, and the escape phase. The recognition and elimination of transformed cells is a concerted effort between innate and adaptive immunity, representing the two arms of the immune system. Local disruption of tissue that occurs as a result of expansion of transformed cells is associated with release of chemokines and proinflammatory cytokines such as interferons, IL-1, IL-6, and tumor necrosis factor-α that trigger innate immunity.

The innate immune system represents the first line of defense against transformed cells (and microorganisms). The most important outcome of these initial events is the production of interferon-γ by activated innate immune cells. Interferon-γ has direct antitumor effects and further boosts tumor cell lysis by innate immune cells. The resulting availability of tumor antigen triggers an adaptive immune response. Key in this process is the uptake of tumor antigen by antigen-presenting cells, primarily dendritic cells. The dendritic cells migrate to tumor-draining lymph nodes and stimulate T and B lymphocytes. The development of adaptive immunity represents the second line of defense against tumors and, together with innate immunity, could completely eliminate the tumor. However, this does not always occur and may lead to what is referred to as the equilibrium phase. This phase is characterized by a balance between tumor growth and tumor elimination, as the name suggests. Antitumor immunity leads to destruction of immunogenic tumor cells, whereas tumor cells with reduced immunity go unnoticed.

Over time, genetic instability and heterogeneity of the tumor cells may give rise to tumor variants better able to withstand the immunologic pressure. Contributing to the failure of the immune system are tumor-induced immune suppressor mechanisms. Once this point has been reached, referred to as the escape phase, the immune system can no longer contain the tumor, and the tumor grows progressively. During the last decade, multiple mechanisms have been identified through which tumors escape from elimination by the immune system. These mechanisms include host-related factors, tumor-related factors, and a combination of both. Among host-related factors are treatment-related immunosuppression, acquired or inherited immunodeficiency, and aging. The list of tumor-related escape mechanisms includes loss of major histocompatibility complex alleles, reduced antigen processing or presentation, decreased expression of costimulatory molecules required for T cell recognition, secretion of immunosuppressive factors (TGF-β, IL-10), stimulation of suppressor cells, and mechanisms that actively induce tolerance or apoptosis in activated immune cells. A thorough discussion of tumor immunology and immunotherapy is discussed elsewhere in this textbook.

Deregulating Cellular Energetics

Otto Warburg first described the anomalous predilection of cancer cells to limit their energy metabolism to glycolysis, even in the presence of oxygen (aerobic glycolysis), an observation termed the Warburg effect. Because glycolysis has a roughly 18-fold lower energy yield compared with aerobic metabolism through mitochondrial oxidative phosphorylation, cancer cells must dramatically upregulate the rate of glycolysis (up to 200-fold higher than normal cells) to keep up with the rapid metabolism of rapidly dividing neoplastic cells. One mechanism used by tumor cells to increase the rate of glycolysis is to upregulate the expression of glucose transporters, such as GLUT1. Clinically, the Warburg effect is used to diagnose or to stage cancers, such as visualizing glucose uptake by positron emission tomography with ^{18}F-fluorodeoxyglucose. In addition, clinical trials of glycolytic inhibitors in cancer are currently ongoing.

Genomic Instability and Mutation

Genomic alteration is emerging as a key enabling characteristic to many of the traits outlined before. Under normal physiologic conditions, the genome is maintained under extraordinary fidelity by important caretaker genes. Alterations of this important cellular machinery can result in loss of the ability to detect DNA damage, loss of the ability to directly repair damaged DNA, and inability to inactivate or to intercept mutagenic molecules before DNA damage can occur. Mutant copies of some caretaker genes can predictably result in an increased incidence of certain types of cancer. *TP53* is an important tumor suppressor gene, and it plays a key role in orchestrating the detection and resolution of mutations; hence, it is often referred to as the guardian of the genome. However, *TP53* is the most commonly mutated tumor suppressor gene in cancer. Once proper maintenance of the genome is lost, cells are free to accumulate multiple genetic alterations, any of which can convey the key characteristics for tumor progression discussed previously.

Tumor-Promoting Inflammation

Tumor-promoting inflammation is also emerging as a key enabling characteristic of many types of cancer. As previously described, immune cells may play an important role in antitumor defense. However, paradoxically, these same immune cells can also enhance tumor progression. It has long been recognized that many tumors are densely infiltrated by various immune cells. Similar to a chronic wound, leukocytes in the tumor produce various growth factors, which can promote tumor growth, angiogenesis, and therapeutic resistance. Often, inflammation is an early event in tumorigenesis and can incite the conversion of a premalignant lesion into a full-blown cancer. For example, leukocytes can elaborate various reactive oxygen species that can cause damage to the DNA of nearby cells, thus fostering the progression to malignancy.

In addition, it has recently become evident that tumors can alter the functionality of infiltrating immune cells, causing functional leukocytes to become anergic or even immunosuppressive. For example, macrophages isolated from tumors, such as pancreatic cancer, are potently immunosuppressive and prevent antitumor immune responses by T cells; however, monocytes from the blood of these same cancer patients are capable of promoting immune responses, suggesting that the tumor environment can alter the functionality of infiltrating leukocytes to escape immune-mediated elimination.

CARCINOGENESIS

Cancer Genetics

Malignant transformation is the process by which a clonal population of cells acquires alterations that confer a growth advantage over normal cells. Many of these alterations occur at the genetic level, involving the gain of function by oncogenes or the loss of function by tumor suppressor genes. A multistep model for colorectal tumorigenesis has been described (Fig. 28-11). Designation as an oncogene or tumor suppressor gene relates to the directionality of effect, without implications about molecular detail. Indeed, the original name for what came to be known as tumor suppressor genes was in fact antioncogenes.

Genetic mutations that are inherited from one's parents and are present in all cells of the body are called *germline* (or constitutional) mutations; in contrast, *somatic* mutations are acquired during an individual's lifetime and cannot be passed on to one's children. Somatic mutations, which account for most mutations in cancer, may be caused by exposure to carcinogens in the form of radiation, chemicals, or chronic inflammation (see later).

A tumor that arises in an individual may be classified as either hereditary or sporadic. In hereditary cases, a germline mutation is responsible for the predisposition to neoplasia. The index case or *proband* is the individual who is first diagnosed as having the syndrome, even if earlier generations are later recognized as also having the syndrome. If the patient with a tumor does not have an inherited predisposition and the tumor's genetic mutations are all somatic, the tumor is classified as sporadic. In some hereditary cancer syndromes, the germline mutation causes a tendency for the cell to accumulate somatic mutations.

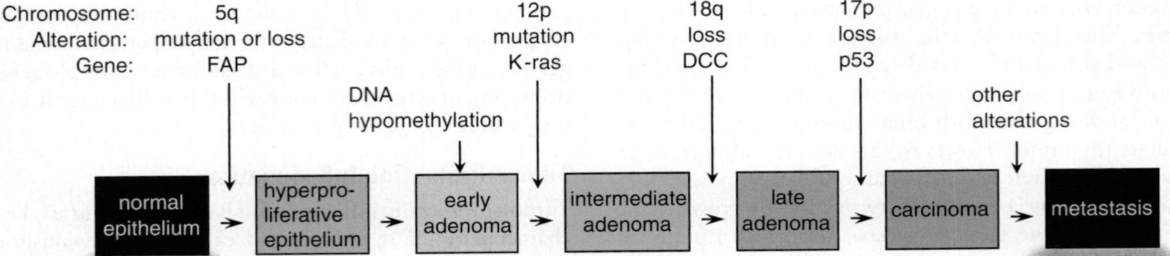

FIGURE 28-11 A Genetic Model for Colorectal Tumorigenesis. Tumorigenesis proceeds through a series of genetic alterations involving oncogenes *(ras)* and tumor suppressor genes (particularly those on chromosomes 5q, 12p, 17p, and 18q). The three stages of adenomas in general represent tumors of increasing size, dysplasia, and villous content. In patients with familial adenomatous polyposis (FAP), a mutation on chromosome 5q (*APC* gene) is inherited. This alteration may be responsible for the hyperproliferative epithelium present in these patients. Hypomethylation is present in very small adenomas in patients with or without polyposis, and this alteration may lead to aneuploidy, resulting in the loss of suppressor gene alleles. The *ras* gene mutation appears to occur in one cell of a preexisting small adenoma and, through clonal expansion, produces a larger and more dysplastic tumor. Allelic deletions of chromosome 17p and 18q usually occur at a later stage of tumorigenesis than do deletions of chromosome 5q or *ras* gene mutations. The order of these changes is not invariant, however, and accumulation of these changes, rather than their order with respect to one another, seems most important. Tumors continue to progress once carcinomas have formed, and the accumulated loss of suppressor genes on additional chromosomes correlates with the ability of the carcinomas to metastasize and cause death. (From Fearon ER: A genetic model for colorectal tumorigenesis. *Cell* 61:759, 1990.)

Although hereditary cancer syndromes are rare, their study has provided powerful insights into more common forms of cancer (Table 28-3). Key germline mutations in hereditary cancers are often the same as somatic mutations present in sporadic cancers. *TP53* gene mutations, if inherited, cause Li-Fraumeni syndrome. Familial adenomatous polyposis (FAP) is caused by a germline mutation in the adenomatous polyposis coli *(APC)* gene. More than 80% of sporadic colorectal cancers also have a somatic mutation of this same gene. Similarly, mutation in the *RET* proto-oncogene is responsible for the predisposition to development of the familial form of medullary thyroid cancer (MTC). Somatic mutations of *RET* are found in about 50% of sporadic MTCs.

Predisposition in familial cancer syndromes is generally inherited in an autosomal dominant fashion. Exceptions include ataxia-telangiectasia and xeroderma pigmentosa, which are transmitted in an autosomal recessive manner. Not all inherited genetic mutations have complete penetrance. There is almost complete penetrance of colorectal cancer in FAP and of MTC in multiple endocrine neoplasia type 2 (MEN2). In contrast, penetrance is less than 50% for pheochromocytoma in neurofibromatosis. Penetrance can also vary considerably for different characteristics of the same syndrome. However, the factors determining penetrance remain largely unknown.

There are a number of features of hereditary cancers that distinguish them phenotypically from their sporadic counterparts. The former tend to cause the development of multifocal, bilateral cancer at an early age, whereas in the latter, cancer occurs later and is usually unilateral. Hereditary cancers will display clustering of the same cancer type in relatives and may be associated with other conditions, such as mental retardation and pathognomonic skin lesions.

Selected Familial Cancer Syndromes

Retinoblastoma

Retinoblastoma is a pediatric retinal tumor that holds an important place in the history of cancer genetics because the causative gene, *RB1*, was the first tumor suppressor gene to be cloned. Most cases are detected by the age of 7 years, but bilateral disease is manifested earlier, usually within the first year of life. It is associated with extraocular malignant neoplasms including sarcomas, melanomas, and tumors of the central nervous system. Distinct sporadic and hereditary forms of retinoblastoma have long been recognized, with predisposition conferred by a germline mutation in approximately 40% of cases. Knudson reasoned that the germline mutation is necessary but not by itself sufficient for tumorigenesis because some children with an affected parent do not develop a tumor but later produce an affected child, indicating that they are carriers of the germline mutation. Most affected children with an affected parent develop tumors bilaterally. He further hypothesized that hereditary retinoblastoma requires two mutations, one of which is germline and the other somatic. In children with unilateral disease and no family history, both mutations are somatic. The hereditary and nonhereditary forms of the tumor require the same number of events—the "two-hit" hypothesis (Fig. 28-12). The *RB1* protein product is a key regulator of the cell cycle, and its loss results in failure of retinoblasts to differentiate properly.

Li-Fraumeni Syndrome

In 1969, Li and Fraumeni reported a new familial syndrome involving sarcomas (of both soft tissue and bone), breast cancers (the most common malignant neoplasm in this syndrome), brain tumors, leukemias, adrenocortical carcinomas, and a variety of other cancers. The syndrome that now bears their name has been defined as (1) a proband diagnosed with sarcoma before the age of 45 years, with (2) a first-degree relative with any cancer diagnosed before the age of 45 years, plus (3) an additional first- or second-degree relative with either a sarcoma at any age or any cancer before the age of 45 years. Half of Li-Fraumeni kindreds have mutations in *TP53* gene, which produces the protein p53. Inheritance is in an autosomal dominant fashion. Penetrance is 50% by the age of 40 years and 90% by the age of 60 years.

TABLE 28-3 **Familial Cancer Syndromes**

SYNDROME	GENES	LOCATIONS	CANCER SITES AND ASSOCIATED TRAITS
Breast/ovarian syndrome	*BRCA1*	17q21	Cancers of the breast, ovary, colon, prostate
	BRCA2	13q12.3	Cancers of the breast, ovary, colon, prostate, gallbladder and biliary tree, pancreas, stomach; melanoma
Cowden disease	*PTEN*	10q23.3	Cancer of the breast, endometrium, and thyroid
Familial adenomatous polyposis	*APC*	5q21	Colorectal carcinoma, duodenal and gastric neoplasms, medulloblastomas, osteomas
Familial melanoma	*p16; CDK4*	9p21; 12q14	Melanoma, pancreatic cancer, dysplastic nevi, atypical moles
Hereditary diffuse gastric cancer	*CDH1*	16q22	Gastric cancer
Hereditary nonpolyposis colorectal cancer	*hMLH1; hMSH2; hMSH6; hPMS1; hPMS2*	3p21; 2p22-21; 2p16; 2q31.1; 7p22.2	Colorectal cancer; endometrial cancer; transitional cell carcinoma of the ureter and renal pelvis; and carcinomas of the stomach, small bowel, pancreas, and ovary
Hereditary papillary renal cell carcinoma	*MET*	7q31	Renal cell cancer
Hereditary paraganglioma and pheochromocytoma	*SDHB; SDHC; SDHD*	1p36.1-p35; 1q21; 11q23	Paraganglioma, pheochromocytoma
Juvenile polyposis coli	*BMPRIA*	10q21-q22	Juvenile polyps of the gastrointestinal tract, gastrointestinal malignant neoplasms
	SMAD4/DPC4	18q21.1	
Li-Fraumeni	*p53*	17p13	Breast cancer, soft tissue sarcoma, osteosarcoma, brain tumors, adrenocortical carcinoma, Wilms tumor, phyllodes tumor (breast), pancreatic cancer, leukemia, neuroblastoma
	hCHK2	22q12.1	
Multiple endocrine neoplasia type 1	*MEN1*	11q13	Pancreatic islet cell tumors, parathyroid hyperplasia, pituitary adenomas
Multiple endocrine neoplasia type 2	*RET*	10q11.2	Medullary thyroid cancer, pheochromocytoma, parathyroid hyperplasia
MYH-associated adenomatous polyposis	*MYH*	1p34.3-p32.1	Cancer of the colon, rectum, breast, stomach
Neurofibromatosis type 1	*NF1*	17q11	Neurofibromas, neurofibrosarcoma, acute myelogenous leukemia, brain tumors
Neurofibromatosis type 2	*NF2*	22q12	Acoustic neuromas, meningiomas, gliomas, ependymomas
Nevoid basal cell carcinoma	*PTC*	9q22.3	Basal cell carcinoma
Peutz-Jeghers syndrome	*STK11*	19p13.3	Gastrointestinal carcinomas, breast cancer, testicular cancer, pancreatic cancer, benign pigmentation of the skin and mucosa
Retinoblastoma	*RB*	13q14	Retinoblastoma, sarcomas, melanoma, malignant neoplasms of the brain and meninges
Tuberous sclerosis	*TSC1; TSC2*	9q34; 16p13	Multiple hamartomas, renal cell carcinoma, astrocytoma
von Hippel–Lindau syndrome	*VHL*	3p25	Renal cell carcinoma, hemangioblastomas of the retina and central nervous system, pheochromocytoma
Wilms tumor	*WT*	11p13	Wilms tumor, aniridia, genitourinary abnormalities, mental retardation

From Marsh D, Zori R: Genetic insights into familial cancers—update and recent discoveries. *Cancer Lett* 181:125–164, 2002.

Patients exhibit increased sensitivity to radiation; the irradiated field is susceptible to the development of new malignant neoplasms. For those kindreds who lack germline *TP53* mutations, a number of candidate genes have been proposed, including the cell cycle checkpoint kinases *CHK1* and *CHK2*, which directly phosphorylate p53. It is likely that other such causative genes serve similar tumor suppressive functions to p53 or are involved in the regulation of p53.

Familial Adenomatous Polyposis

FAP accounts for 1% of the total colorectal cancer burden. It is an autosomal dominant condition caused by mutation in the *APC* gene, located on chromosome 5q21. Penetrance is extremely high, with more than 90% of affected individuals developing colorectal cancer. It is characterized clinically by the development of several hundred to more than a thousand adenomatous polyps that carpet the colon. The first clear FAP kindreds were described in 1925 by the surgeon Lockhart-Mummery. The phenotype usually emerges during the second and third decades of life. The polyps are indistinguishable (macroscopically and microscopically) from sporadic adenomatous polyps, and each individual polyp does not have a greater propensity to undergo malignant degeneration than sporadic polyps. Rather, it is the sheer number of polyps that makes the collective risk of malignancy so high. Untreated individuals typically present with colorectal cancer at 35 to 40 years of age, around 30 years earlier than the median age for sporadic colorectal cancer. Extracolonic manifestations of FAP include upper gastrointestinal polyps, desmoid tumors (15%), and thyroid cancer (1% to 2%; usually papillary). Polyps of the stomach and duodenum are present in more than 90% of patients by the age of 70 years, with two thirds of duodenal polyps located in the periampullary region. Indeed, duodenal adenocarcinoma is the third leading cause of death in FAP, after metastatic colorectal carcinoma and desmoid tumors. Desmoid tumors are locally invasive fibromatoses that occur within the abdomen or abdominal wall. Patients with FAP have a relative risk for development of desmoid disease 850 times that of the general population.

The *APC* gene was first localized in 1987, then cloned in 1991, after mutation analyses of FAP kindreds. It encodes a 300-kDa protein, expressed in a variety of cell types, whose major function

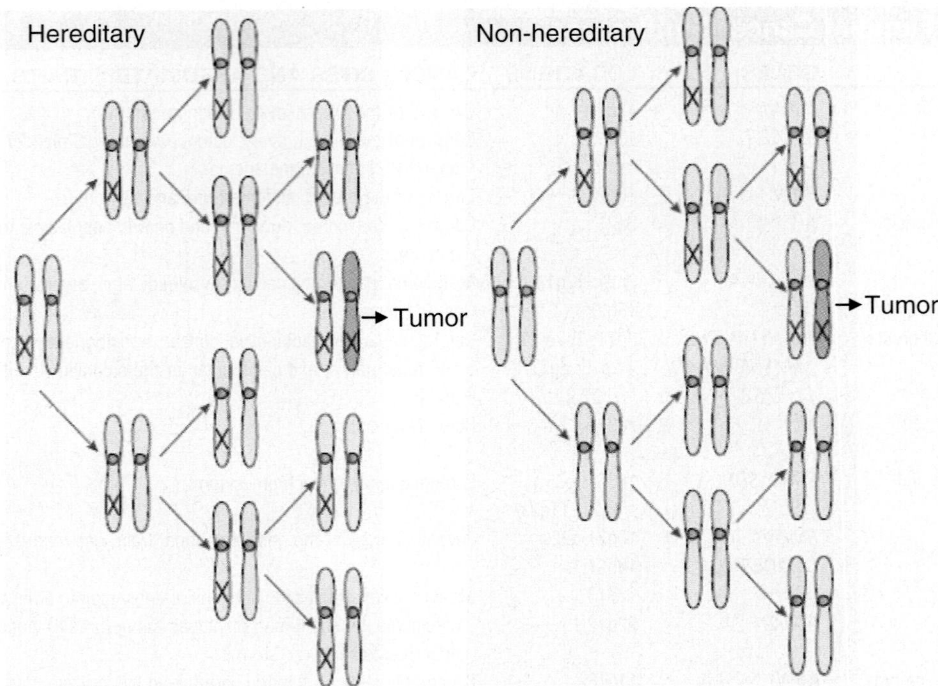

FIGURE 28-12 Two Genetic Hits to Cancer. In hereditary retinoblastoma, all retinoblasts are heterozygous for the mutant allele (indicated by X); they all have already sustained "one hit." In contrast, the preneoplastic clone in nonhereditary retinoblastoma must acquire this mutation before sustaining the "second hit" to complete malignant transformation. (Modified from Knudson AG: Two genetic hits [more or less] to cancer. *Nat Rev Cancer* 1:157–162, 2001.)

is as a scaffolding protein, affecting cell adhesion and migration. It is part of a protein complex, modulated by the Wnt signaling pathway, that regulates the phosphorylation and degradation of β-catenin. When *APC* is mutated, β-catenin is not phosphorylated and accumulates in the cytoplasm, where it binds to the TCF family of transcription factors, altering the expression of various genes involved in cell proliferation, migration, differentiation, and apoptosis. More than 700 disease-causing mutations in the *APC* gene have been reported. The most common of these involve a frameshift mutation (68%), a nonsense mutation (30%), or a large deletion (2%). Most of these mutations are located in what is referred to as the *mutation cluster region*, at the 5′ end of exon 15.

The location of the mutation plays a role in determining the phenotype. Mutations between 976 and 1067 are associated with a threefold to fourfold increased risk for development of duodenal adenomas. Congenital hypertrophy of the retinal pigment epithelium is associated with mutations between codons 463 and 1387. Gardner syndrome is associated with mutations between codons 1403 and 1578[29] and, in addition to colorectal cancer, manifests osteomas of the mandible or skull, epidermal cysts, and multiple skin and soft tissue tumors, especially desmoids and thyroid tumors. Attenuated FAP is a phenotypically distinct variant of FAP in which (1) affected individuals have fewer than 100 adenomas, (2) the polyps are more proximally distributed in the colon, and (3) the onset of colorectal cancer is about 15 years later than in patients with FAP. Mutations responsible for this variant occur in the extreme upstream or downstream portions of the *APC* gene.

MYH-associated polyposis (MAP) is a syndrome caused by mutations in the human *MutY homologue (MYH)* gene. It accounts for about a third of patients who have attenuated polyposis but who test negative for *APC* mutations. Unlike FAP, MAP is inherited in an autosomal *recessive* manner. Phenotypically, MAP-associated colorectal cancer is indistinguishable from attenuated FAP, although it is manifested later, around the age of 50 years. The polyps are distributed throughout the colon, although there are conflicting data about right- and left-sided tumor predominance. Extracolonic manifestations include breast cancer (18%) and upper gastrointestinal polyps (one third).[30] The *MYH* gene encodes a DNA glycosylase involved in the base excision repair pathway, important in preventing mutations due to oxidative damage. Y165C and G382D mutations account for more than 80% of all mutations discovered thus far. Penetrance is estimated at 50%.[30] Homozygotes or compound heterozygotes for germline mutations of the *MYH* gene have a 93-fold increased risk of colorectal cancer.[31] Mutation leads to chromosomal instability in which there is an accelerated rate of chromosomal misaggregation during cell division. This leads to aneuploidy, which has been recognized as an early genetic change in the stepwise carcinogenesis of both FAP and MAP tumors. Polyps bearing *MYH* mutations have twice the overall incidence of aneuploidy compared with those in patients with FAP. Current evidence suggests that carriers of single mutated alleles are unlikely to have more than a 50% increased risk of colorectal cancer.

Hereditary Nonpolyposis Colorectal Cancer

Also known as Lynch syndrome, hereditary nonpolyposis colorectal cancer (HNPCC) accounts for 2% of all colorectal cancers. It is an autosomal dominant condition caused by mutations in DNA mismatch repair genes. When originally described by Lynch, kindreds were subclassified into types I and II on the basis of whether only colorectal cancer developed (type I) or extracolonic cancers were present (type II). Penetrance is high. The broad phenotype of HNPCC is of right-sided predominance of colonic cancers (70% proximal to the splenic flexure) that appear at an earlier age (median age of diagnosis is 45 years), with increased likelihood of synchronous and metachronous cancers. Extracolonic malignant neoplasms occur, especially of the endometrium and ovary. Whereas the actual incidence of adenomatous polyps is the same as for those who develop sporadic colorectal cancer, once a tumor develops, there is an increased rate of tumor progression (accelerated carcinogenesis). This is due to the fact that the rate of genetic mutation in HNPCC tumors is two to three times higher than in normal cells. A colonic adenoma may progress to carcinoma within 2 to 3 years, in contrast to the 8 to 10 years typical of sporadic cases.

Mutations in DNA mismatch repair genes cause microsatellite instability. Microsatellites are genomic regions in which short DNA sequences are repeated. During replication of these sequences, slippage of the DNA polymerase complex can occur, resulting in the formation of daughter strands that contain too many or too few copies of these sequences. Mutations may occur when these microsatellites are misaligned. The mutations then persist when the DNA mismatch repair proteins fail to correct the errors. This causes inactivation of tumor suppressor genes, such as *TGFBR2*, *IGFR2*, and *BAX*. Mutations in a number of DNA mismatch repair genes have been identified in patients with HNPCC. Mutations in *MSH2* and *MLH1* account for about two thirds of cases. *MSH6* mutations account for a further 10% of cases. Other mismatch repair genes in which mutations lead to HNPCC include *PMS1* and *PMS2*. It should be noted that 15% of sporadic colorectal cancers have microsatellite instability, but it occurs through methylation silencing of the *hMLH1* gene rather than through mutation as in HNPCC.

BRCA1 and *BRCA2*

About 5% to 10% of all breast cancers are hereditary and attributable to mutations in high-penetrance susceptibility genes. However, only two of these have been identified: *BRCA1* and *BRCA2*. One quarter of high-risk kindreds have mutations in either of these genes. Although the estimated risk of breast cancer for a 70-year-old woman with a germline mutation in *BRCA1* or *BRCA2* is 80%, different mutations vary in their risk of malignancy.

Carriers are at risk for other cancers, especially of the ovary. Risk of ovarian cancer in a patient who is a carrier for *BRCA1* or *BRCA2* is 60% and 27%, respectively. Approximately 5% of all ovarian cancers are attributed to *BRCA1* germline mutations. The risk of ovarian cancer for those patients with *BRCA2* mutations is lower, around 15% to 20%. Male carriers are at greater risk for prostate cancer. *BRCA2* mutation is also associated with increased risk of melanoma and cancers of the pancreas, stomach, gallbladder, and biliary system.

The *BRCA1* gene is located on the long arm of chromosome 17. It is a large gene of some 100,000 nucleic acids, and more than 250 different mutations have been reported. The sheer number of mutations makes the task of identifying the specific mutation in a new kindred very difficult. The *BRCA2* gene is even larger than *BRCA1*, and about 100 mutations have been reported. As for *BRCA1*, the majority of alterations are frameshift or nonsense mutations, which produce a truncated protein. Both *BRCA1* and *BRCA2* are tumor suppressor genes; they are nonfunctional in malignant cells as a result of combined germline mutation followed by inactivation of the second allele in the tumor (the Knudson two-hit hypothesis). These genes have key roles in DNA damage repair, regulation of gene expression, and cell cycle control.

Multiple Endocrine Neoplasia Type 1

MEN1 is an autosomal dominant condition characterized phenotypically by tumors of the parathyroid gland (leading to hyperparathyroidism), pancreatic islet cells, and the pituitary gland. Affected individuals can also develop lipomas, adenomas of the adrenal and thyroid glands, cutaneous angiofibromas, and carcinoid tumors.

Mutations in the tumor suppressor gene, called *MEN1*, located on chromosome 11q13, are responsible for this syndrome; 80% of mutations identified result in the loss of function of the gene product, called menin. Menin is a 67-kDa protein predominantly found in the nucleus. It binds with a variety of proteins with roles in the regulation of transcription, DNA repair, and organization of the cytoskeleton. None of these menin pathways has yet been found to be critical in *MEN1* tumorigenesis, although a number of candidates, such as JunD, have been proposed.

Multiple Endocrine Neoplasia Type 2

All affected individuals with MEN2 develop MTC. It is subclassified into type A and type B. MEN2A is characterized by pheochromocytoma (50%) and hyperparathyroidism (25%). In addition to MTC and pheochromocytoma, MEN2B is characterized by mucosal neuromas on the tongue and lips and subconjunctival areas, intestinal ganglioneuromatosis, and a marfanoid body habitus. The majority of cases of MEN2B are the result of spontaneous new *RET* mutations.

Both types are caused by germline mutations in the *RET* (REarranged during Transfection) proto-oncogene, located on chromosome 10q11. It encodes a transmembrane tyrosine kinase receptor, which is expressed on a wide variety of neuroendocrine and neural cells, including thyroid C cells, adrenal medullary cells, and autonomic ganglion cells. Once mutated, the receptor constitutively activates various signaling pathways, including p38/MAPK and JNK pathways.

Von Hippel–Lindau Syndrome

Von Hippel–Lindau is a rare, autosomal dominant syndrome characterized by the development of highly vascularized tumors in multiple organs. These include hemangioblastomas of the retina and central nervous system, renal cysts that develop into clear cell renal cell cancer, and pheochromocytomas. It is caused by mutations in the *VHL* gene. Penetrance is 90% by the age of 65 years, with the mean age at diagnosis being 26 years. Since the discovery of the role of the *VHL* gene in this syndrome, mutations of this same gene have been found in the majority of sporadic clear cell renal cell carcinomas. That loss of *VHL* function is a critical event during renal cell carcinogenesis is supported by experiments in which introduction of wild-type *VHL* into *VHL*-deficient renal cancer cell lines resulted in suppression of tumor growth.

The protein product of the *VHL* gene, pVHL, functions as a tumor suppressor and is part of the cell's response mechanism to hypoxia. Under conditions of low cellular oxygen tension, hypoxia-inducible factors (HIFs) 1 and 2 regulate genes involved in metabolism, angiogenesis, erythropoiesis, and cell proliferation. pVHL targets the α subunit of HIF for oxygen-dependent proteolysis. Therefore, lack of pVHL results in persistence of the HIF complex, with increased HIF transcriptional activity and upregulation of HIF target genes, including *VEGF*, *GLUT1*, and erythropoietin, independent of cellular oxygen levels. pVHL also has roles in regulating ECM turnover and microtubule stability.

Cancer Epigenetics

Epigenetic inheritance is defined as cellular information, other than the nucleotide sequence, that is heritable during cell division. There are three main interrelated forms: DNA methylation, genomic imprinting, and histone modification. These epigenetic templates control gene expression and can be transmitted to daughter cells independently of the DNA sequence.

One of the best studied types of epigenetic change is the cytosine methylation at CpG dinucleotides. CpG islands (CGIs) are approximately 1-kilobase stretches of DNA containing clusters of CpG dinucleotides that are usually unmethylated in normal cells and are often located near the 5′ ends of genes. Methylation of promoter CGIs is associated with a closed chromatin structure and transcriptional silencing of the associated gene. This has been shown to be a common event in carcinogenesis. Tumor suppressor genes such as *CDKN2A*, *RB*, *VHL*, and *BRCA1* are inactivated by hypermethylation of their promoter CGIs.

Conversely, genes that are hypomethylated, leading to increased transcription, have been identified. For example, promoter CpG demethylation has been shown to lead to overexpression of cyclin D2 and maspin in gastric cancer.[32] DNA hypomethylation has also been associated with genomic instability. Loss of methylation is particularly severe in pericentromeric satellite sequences, and cancers of the ovary and breast frequently contain unbalanced chromosomal translocations with breakpoints in the pericentromeric regions of chromosomes 1 and 16. The demethylation of these satellite sequences may predispose to their breakage and recombination.

Genomic imprinting refers to the conditioning of the maternal and paternal genomes during gametogenesis, such that a specific parental allele is more abundantly (or exclusively) expressed in the offspring. In Wilms tumors, loss of imprinting has been demonstrated to lead to pathologic biallelic expression of *IGF2*. This appears to occur in combination with hypermethylation of regions of the reciprocally imprinted *H19* gene. These two phenomena are the earliest detectable genetic changes in this cancer, strongly suggesting a gatekeeper role for epigenetic alterations in cancer.

CGI methylation is associated with a condensed chromatin structure that blocks the access of transcription factors to DNA promoter sites, leading to transcriptional silencing. The modification of histones (e.g., by acetylation, methylation, or phosphorylation) is important in the compaction of chromatin structure. Recent work in colorectal cancer suggests that the combination of DNA hypermethylation together with histone modifications plays a critical role in the maintenance of gene silencing.[33] This is an emerging area of research.

Carcinogens

Any agent that can contribute to tumor formation is referred to as a carcinogen, which can be chemical, physical, or biologic. The International Agency for Research on Cancer (IARC) maintains a registry of human carcinogens that is available on the Internet (www.iarc.fr). The compounds are categorized into five groups based on epidemiologic studies, animal models, and short-term mutagenesis tests. Group 1 contains what are considered to be proven human carcinogens. Group 2A agents are probable human carcinogens, for which there is limited evidence of carcinogenicity in humans but sufficient evidence to prove carcinogenicity in experimental animals. The group 2B category includes agents that are possibly carcinogenic to humans, for which there is limited evidence of carcinogenicity in humans and less than sufficient evidence of carcinogenicity in experimental animals. There is inadequate evidence for carcinogenicity in humans or experimental animals for agents included in group 3. Group 4 agents are probably not carcinogenic to humans.

Chemical Carcinogens

Chemicals that initiate carcinogenesis are extremely diverse in structure and function and include both natural and synthetic products (Tables 28-4 and 28-5). They fall into one of two categories: direct-acting compounds, which do not require chemical transformation for their carcinogenicity; and indirect-acting compounds, or procarcinogens, which require metabolic conversion in vivo for their carcinogenic effects. All these compounds, or their active metabolites in the latter category, share the essential property of being highly reactive electrophiles (have electron-deficient atoms) that can react with nucleophilic (electron-rich) sites in the cell. These reactions are nonenzymatic and result in the formation of covalent adducts between the chemical carcinogens and (almost always) DNA.

The majority of chemical carcinogens require metabolic activation for their carcinogenic effects. The metabolic pathway that produces the active metabolite may be just one of a number of metabolic pathways required for the degradation of the parent compound. Thus, the carcinogenic potency of the carcinogen is determined not just by the reactivity of the electrophilic derivatives but also by the balance between the metabolic activation and inactivation reactions. Most of the known carcinogens are metabolized by cytochrome P450–dependent mono-oxygenases. Because these enzymes are essential for the activation of procarcinogens, individual susceptibility to carcinogenesis is regulated in part by polymorphisms in the genes that encode these enzymes. For example, the product of the P450 gene *CYP1A1* metabolizes polycyclic aromatic hydrocarbons such as benzo(a)pyrene. About 10% of the white population has a highly inducible form of this enzyme that is associated with an increased risk of lung cancer in smokers. Light smokers with the susceptible genotype of *CYP1A1* have a sevenfold higher risk for development of lung cancer compared with smokers without the permissive genotype. Age, sex, and nutritional status also have an effect on the metabolism of carcinogens and thus their probability of inducing malignancy.

DNA is the primary target of chemical carcinogens. The ability of these compounds to induce mutations is termed mutagenic potential. The Ames test is the most common method for evaluating mutagenic potential and measures the ability of a chemical to induce mutations in the bacterium *Salmonella typhimurium*. The majority of known chemical carcinogens score positive on the Ames test, so it is useful for screening. However, not all compounds with mutagenic potential in vitro also have in vivo effects. Whereas there is no one mutation unique to all chemical carcinogens, individual compounds have been found to induce characteristic changes in DNA. For example, aflatoxin B1 induces a G:C → T:A transconversion in codon 249 of the *TP53* gene (249^{ser} *p53* mutation). Individuals from areas where there is a high level of exposure to aflatoxin B1 develop hepatocellular carcinoma (HCC) with this characteristic mutation. This mutation is an otherwise uncommon occurrence in HCC caused by other agents, such as the hepatitis B virus.

The carcinogenicity of some chemicals is augmented by subsequent administration of other agents, called promoters, which are

TABLE 28-4 Selected IARC Group 1 Chemical Carcinogens

CHEMICAL CARCINOGEN	MEANS OF EXPOSURE	PREDOMINANT TUMOR TYPE
Aflatoxins	Ingestion of contaminated maize and peanuts grown in hot, humid climates	Hepatocellular carcinoma
Arsenic	Ingestion; also inhalation by smelter workers	Skin cancer
Asbestos	Inhalation	Mesothelioma, lung cancer
Benzene	Inhalation, especially in gasoline-related industries or in the production of other chemicals from benzene	Leukemia
Benzidine	Inhalation by workers in the dye industry	Cancer of the urinary bladder
Beryllium	Inhalation by workers in the refining of the metal and production of beryllium-containing products; also those in the aircraft, aerospace, electronics, and nuclear industries	Lung cancer
Cadmium	Inhalation by workers in cadmium production and refining, nickel-cadmium battery manufacturing, other cadmium-related industries	Lung cancer
Chromium compounds	Inhalation during chromium plating, chromate production, welding	Lung cancer
Ethylene oxide	Inhalation during production of various industrial chemicals (e.g., ethylene glycol)	Leukemia, lymphoma
Nickel	Inhalation, ingestion, or skin contact in nickel or nickel alloy production plants, welding, or electroplating operations	Lung cancer, nasal cancer
Radon	Inhalation in underground mines	Lung cancer
Vinyl chloride	Inhalation during production of polyvinyl chloride	Hepatic angiosarcoma, hepatocellular carcinoma, brain tumors, lung cancer, hematopoietic malignant neoplasms
Coal tars	Inhalation, transcutaneous absorption in a variety of industrial settings	Skin cancer, scrotal cancer
Tobacco smoke	Inhalation	Lung cancer, oral cancer, pharyngeal cancer, laryngeal cancer, esophageal cancer

Based on information from IARC Monographs on the Evaluation of Carcinogenic Risks to Humans: International Agency for Research on Cancer (IARC), 2014. <http://monographs.iarc.fr/ENG/Classification/ClassificationsGroupOrder.pdf>.

TABLE 28-5 Selected IARC Group 1 Pharmaceutical Carcinogens

PHARMACEUTICAL CARCINOGEN	PREDOMINANT TUMOR TYPE
Azathioprine	Non-Hodgkin lymphoma, squamous cell cancer of the skin, hepatocellular carcinoma, cholangiocarcinoma
Cyclophosphamide	Cancer of the urinary bladder, leukemia
Chlorambucil	Leukemia
Tamoxifen	Endometrial cancer
Estrogens (OCP, HRT)	Cancer of the breast and endometrium

Based on information from IARC Monographs on the Evaluation of Carcinogenic Risks to Humans: International Agency for Research on Cancer (IARC), 2014. <http://monographs.iarc.fr/ENG/Classification/ClassificationsGroupOrder.pdf>.
HRT, hormone replacement therapy; *OCP*, oral contraceptive pill.

by themselves nontumorigenic. Such chemicals include phorbol esters, hormones, and phenols. Their fundamental characteristic is their ability to induce cell proliferation. Promotion may involve multiple compounds acting as promoters acting on different regulatory pathways. The end result is the clonal expansion of initiated cells.

Radiation Carcinogenesis

The two most important forms of radiation causing malignant change in humans are ultraviolet (UV) radiation and ionizing radiation (IR). Whereas IR has been found to cause a variety of cancers, UV radiation is principally implicated in the causation of skin cancers. There is typically a long latency period between radiant exposure and clinical development of cancer.

UV radiation is a known risk factor for squamous cell carcinoma, basal cell carcinoma, and possibly malignant melanoma. The degree of risk depends on the type of UV rays, the intensity of exposure, and the quantity of melanin present in the individual's skin. The UV portion of the electromagnetic spectrum can be divided into three wavelength ranges: UVA (320-400 nm), UVB (280-320 nm), and UVC (200-280 nm). Of these, UVB is the most important. UVC, also a potent mutagen, is filtered out by the planetary ozone layer. The carcinogenicity of UVB is due to its formation of pyrimidine dimers in DNA. This damage may be repaired by the nucleotide excision repair pathway. This is a multistep process involving recognition of the damaged DNA strands, their incision and removal, and synthesis of a patch containing the correct nucleotide sequence, which is then annealed to the DNA structure. With excessive sun exposure, it is postulated that the capacity of this pathway is overwhelmed, and some DNA damage remains unrepaired. Xeroderma pigmentosa, a family of autosomal recessive disorders characterized by extreme photosensitivity and a 2000-fold increased risk of skin cancer, is caused by mutations in the genes involved in nucleotide excision repair. Mutations in the *ras* and *p53* genes occur early in skin cancers, mainly at dipyrimidine sequences.

IR includes both electromagnetic (x-rays, gamma rays) and particulate (alpha particles, beta particles, protons, neutrons) forms. IR is both a carcinogen and a therapeutic agent; low-dose exposure can increase an individual's risk for development of cancer, but when given at high doses, it can slow or stop tumor growth. IR has a multitude of effects on tissues, affecting both cells and their microenvironment. IR leads to a rapid, global, and persistent activation of the microenvironment. Inflammation leads to the production of reactive oxygen species or reactive nitrogen species by tissue macrophages or neutrophils. Long-term sublethal exposure to these inflammatory products may cause genomic instability in parenchymal cells, eventually leading to chromosomal abnormalities or gene mutations. In addition, it is becoming apparent that irradiated stroma has a persistent "activated" phenotype. Irradiated stroma has been shown to contribute to the selection and proliferation of malignant clones in animal models.

Survivors of the atomic bombs dropped on Hiroshima and Nagasaki developed leukemias after an average latency period of 7 years but have also suffered an increased incidence of solid organ tumors (e.g., breast, colon, thyroid, and lung). Irradiation of the head and neck in childhood has been associated with a high incidence of thyroid cancer in adulthood.

There is a defined vulnerability of different tissues to radiation-induced carcinogenesis. Most vulnerable is the hematopoietic cell line, causing leukemias (except chronic lymphocytic leukemia), followed by the thyroid gland. In the intermediate category are breast, lung, and salivary glands. The skin, bone, and gastrointestinal tract are relatively radioresistant.

Infectious Carcinogens

One of the first observations that cancer may be caused by transmissible agents was by Peyton Rous in 1911, when he demonstrated that cell-free extracts from sarcomas in chickens could transmit sarcomas to other animals injected with these extracts. This was subsequently discovered to represent viral transmission of cancer by the Rous sarcoma virus. Infectious agents (Table 28-6) may cause or increase the risk of malignancy by a number of mechanisms, including direct transformation, expression of oncogenes that interfere with cell cycle checkpoints or DNA repair, expression of cytokines or other growth factors, and alteration of the immune system.

Viral carcinogenesis. Approximately 15% of all human tumors worldwide are caused by viruses. This number reflects predominantly two malignant neoplasms: cervical cancer caused by human papillomavirus, and hepatocellular cancer caused by hepatitis B virus (HBV) and hepatitis C virus (HCV).

TABLE 28-6 Selected IARC Group 1 Infectious Carcinogens

INFECTIOUS CARCINOGEN	PREDOMINANT TUMOR TYPE
Epstein-Barr virus	Burkitt lymphoma, Hodgkin disease, immunosuppression-related lymphoma, nasopharyngeal carcinoma
Hepatitis B	Hepatocellular carcinoma
Hepatitis C	Hepatocellular carcinoma
Human immunodeficiency virus type 1	Kaposi sarcoma
Human papillomavirus types 16 and 18	Cervical cancer, anal cancer
Human T cell lymphotropic virus type 1	Adult T cell leukemia
Helicobacter pylori	Gastric adenocarcinoma
Opisthorchis viverrini	Cholangiocarcinoma, hepatocellular carcinoma
Schistosoma haematobium	Cancer of the urinary bladder

Based on information from IARC Monographs on the Evaluation of Carcinogenic Risks to Humans: International Agency for Research on Cancer (IARC), 2014. <http://monographs.iarc.fr/ENG/Classification/ClassificationsGroupOrder.pdf>.

Tenets of viral carcinogenesis (Box 28-1). Human tumor viruses display different mechanisms of cell transformation and fall into both direct- and indirect-acting categories. Direct-acting viruses carry one or more oncogenes, whereas the indirect-acting agents appear not to possess an oncogene. Both types establish long-term persistent infections in their target cell types.

Small DNA tumor viruses. Because of their limited genetic content, small DNA tumor viruses (e.g., human papillomaviruses) are dependent on the host cell machinery to replicate the viral genome. Virus-encoded nonstructural proteins stimulate resting cells to enter S phase to provide the enzymes and environment conducive to viral DNA replication. Because of this ability to usurp cell cycle control, such proteins are also responsible for cell transformation. The binding of viral oncoproteins to cellular tumor suppressor proteins p53 and pRb is fundamental to the effects of the small DNA tumor viruses on host cells. For example, the E6 oncoprotein of human papillomavirus forms a complex with p53, targeting it for ubiquitin-mediated degradation.

Hepatitis B virus. The development of HCC after HBV infection probably involves a combination of indirect and direct mechanisms. Chronic liver injury secondary to persistent viral infection leads to necrosis, inflammation, and hepatocyte regeneration. The constitutive induction of liver cell progression into the cell cycle overwhelms DNA repair mechanisms in the presence of mutational events. This may induce fixed DNA mutations and chromosomal rearrangements, which are major determinants of cell transformation; concurrently, fibrosis disrupts the normal lobular structure and modifies cell-cell and cell-ECM interactions, with further loss of control over cell growth. Integration of HBV DNA into the host genome occurs in 90% of HBV-related HCC and has been postulated as an early event in chronic viral infection. Thus far, no specific genes have been identified to be the preferential target for HBV insertion. However, the insertion itself may induce general genomic instability. Dysregulation of cellular genes controlling immortalization (*hTERT*), proliferation (*MAPK1*, cyclin A), and viability (tumor necrosis factor receptor–associated protein 1) has been observed.[34] The HBV cell surface proteins have been shown to increase hepatocyte proliferation and may contribute to carcinogenesis by accumulating in the endoplasmic reticulum, thereby inducing endoplasmic reticulum stress. The HBV X protein (HBx) may also act as a potential viral oncoprotein. It is a potent transcriptional activator, acting on a number

BOX 28-1 Tenets of Viral Carcinogenesis

- Viruses can cause neoplasia in animals and humans.
- Tumor viruses frequently establish persistent infections in natural hosts.
- Viral infections are more common than virus-related tumor formation.
- Long latent periods usually elapse between initial viral infection and tumor appearance.
- Host factors are important determinants of virus-induced tumorigenesis.
- Viruses may be either direct- or indirect-acting carcinogenic agents.
- Viruses are seldom complete carcinogens.
- Viral strains may differ in oncogenic potential.
- Oncogenic viruses modulate growth control pathways in cells.
- In tumors affected by viral carcinogenesis, viral markers are usually present in neoplastic cells.
- One virus may be associated with more than one type of neoplasia.

Adapted from Butel JS: Viral carcinogenesis: Revelation of molecular mechanisms and etiology of human disease. *Carcinogenesis* 21:405–426, 2000.

of viral and cellular promoters. It influences signal transduction pathways both in the cytoplasm and in the mitochondrion. HBx also binds p53 and inhibits several critical p53-mediated processes, including DNA sequence-specific binding, transcriptional transactivation, and apoptosis.

RNA viruses. After viral infection, the single-stranded RNA viral genome is transcribed into a double-stranded DNA copy, which is then integrated into the chromosomal DNA of the cell. Retroviral infection is permanent. Oncogenic retroviruses carry oncogenes derived from cellular genes, which, for the most part, are involved in mitogenic signaling and growth control. Examples of such proto-oncogenes are protein kinases, G proteins, growth factors, and transcription factors. Alternatively, retroviruses that do not possess oncogenes may cause tumors during integration into the cellular genome. If this occurs near normal cellular proto-oncogenes, the strong promoter and enhancer sequences of the provirus (which allow viral replication) will also affect the expression of proto-oncogenes. This mechanism is termed proviral insertional mutagenesis.

Hepatitis C virus. Unlike retroviruses, HCV does not appear to cause integration of its DNA into the cellular genome.[35] The predominant mechanism of HCV in the development of HCC appears to be indirect, that is, by the induction of chronic hepatocellular injury, coupled with inflammation and liver cell regeneration. However, a number of HCV proteins have been implicated in its carcinogenic activity.[36] Both the HCV core protein and NS3 protein modulate the expression of the cyclin-dependent inhibitor $p21^{WAF1}$ and affect the activity of p53. The E2 protein interacts with CD82, inhibiting T and NK cells. The NS5A protein acts as a transcription factor and interacts with cellular signaling pathways and various cell cycle regulatory kinases to block the apoptotic cellular response to persistent HCV infection.

Helicobacter pylori. *H. pylori* infection is the most important risk factor for the development of gastric cancer. It was the first bacterium linked to human cancer and was classified as a group 1 carcinogen by the IARC in 1996. The mechanisms by which *H. pylori* causes cancer remain largely unknown but are thought to involve both host and bacterial characteristics. The chronic inflammatory response to the infection elicited by *H. pylori* is considered an important mechanism by which infection may eventually lead to neoplasia. However, it is unknown why and how the infection and resulting inflammation select certain individuals but not others to enter the neoplastic cascade. The gastric microenvironment, such as acid secretion, may play a key role. IL-1β is a potent inhibitor of acid secretion. Polymorphisms of the gene encoding this cytokine and also the gene encoding the IL-1β receptor antagonist gene, part of the same gene cluster, have been associated with increased risk for gastric cancer.

Infection with strains of *H. pylori* that carry the cytotoxin-associated antigen A *(cagA)* gene is associated with gastric carcinoma. The *cagA* gene product, CagA, is delivered into gastric epithelial cells by the bacterial type IV secretion system—in essence, a molecular syringe. Once it is intracellular, CagA is tyrosine phosphorylated by SRC family kinases and then is able to specifically bind and activate the cellular oncoprotein SHP2. Thus, it can be seen that CagA deregulation of SHP2 mimics a situation in which SHP2 acquires a gain-of-function mutation. CagA is thought to be important during early phases of gastric carcinogenesis, in particular, the progression from superficial gastritis to atrophic gastritis to intestinal metaplasia. However, the presence of CagA alone is not sufficient for transformation of gastric epithelial cells into a malignant phenotype.

Chronic Inflammation

Chronic inflammation in the absence of infection has long been linked with the development of cancer. Examples include the development of squamous cell carcinoma of the skin in areas of chronic ulceration (Marjolin ulcer) and the high risk for colorectal cancer in patients with ulcerative colitis. However, the exact mechanistic changes that occur during chronic inflammation that lead to malignant transformation are just beginning to be elucidated. For example, in ulcerative colitis–associated colorectal cancer, a dual mechanism has been proposed. Ulceration of the epithelium exposes underlying cell layers to the contents of the bowel lumen. The intestinal flora triggers the nuclear factor κB pathway in macrophages, causing them to release proinflammatory agents such as prostaglandins, chemokines, and interleukins that indirectly promote survival of transformed epithelial cells.

TUMOR MARKERS

Tumor markers are indicators of cellular, biochemical, molecular, or genetic alterations by which neoplasia can be recognized. They are surrogate measures of the biology of the cancer, providing insight into the clinical behavior of the tumor. This is particularly useful when the cancer is not clinically detectable. The information provided may be diagnostic, distinguishing benign from malignant disease; it may correlate with the amount of tumor present ("tumor burden"); it may allow subtype classification to more accurately stage patients; it may be prognostic, either by the presence or absence of the marker or by its concentration; and it may guide choice of therapy and predict response to therapy.

The ideal tumor marker has three defining characteristics. First, the marker should be expressed exclusively by the particular tumor. Second, collection of the specimen for the tumor marker assay should be easy. Third, the assay itself should be reproducible, rapid, and inexpensive. Currently, there is no one marker that fulfils all these criteria for any cancer, nor is there any specific cancer for which there are biomarkers that completely describe its behavior.

Tumor markers fall into three broad categories: proteins, genetic mutations, and epigenetic changes (Box 28-2). All three may be found in the tumor tissue itself. Tumor markers found in body fluids, particularly blood and urine, have the greatest potential for clinical application because of the ease of access to these fluids for analysis and because repeated sampling allows in vivo monitoring of the malignant disease for such things as progression or recurrence, metastasis, and response to therapy.

BOX 28-2 Potential Nonprotein Tumor Markers

RNA-Based Markers

Overexpressed or underexpressed transcripts
Regulatory RNAs (e.g., micro-RNAs)

DNA-Based Markers

Single-nucleotide polymorphisms
Chromosomal translocations: *bcr-abl* (Philadelphia)
Changes in DNA copy number
Microsatellite instability
Epigenetic changes (e.g., differential promoter-region methylation)

From Ludwig JA, Weinstein JN: Biomarkers in cancer staging, prognosis and treatment selection. *Nat Rev Cancer* 5:845–856, 2005.

Rather than provide an exhaustive review of all tumor markers, this section outlines the major categories of tumor markers and focuses on the evidence for the tumor markers currently in clinical use.

Protein Tumor Markers

Proteins were the first type of tumor marker identified and hence are considered the "classic" tumor markers. However, despite decades of research, few are in clinical use. Those routinely used are in general limited by poor sensitivity and specificity. Their concentrations in serum or plasma generally correlate with tumor burden as they are shed from the expanding neoplasm.

Carcinoembryonic Antigen

Carcinoembryonic antigen (CEA) is probably the most studied cancer tumor marker and is predominantly used clinically in patients with cancer of the colon and rectum. It is an oncofetal protein that is normally present during fetal life but can be present in low concentrations in healthy adults. Structurally, it is a glycoprotein with a molecular mass of 200 kDa and is a component of the glycocalyx, located on the luminal side of the cell membrane of normal epithelial intestinal cells. CEA is a member of a large family of proteins that are related to the immunoglobulin gene superfamily. The molecule itself is secreted into the circulation and is also found in the mucous secretions of the stomach, small intestine, and biliary tree. Although its exact function is unknown, CEA has been shown to be involved in cell adhesion and is able to inhibit apoptosis induced by loss of anchorage to the ECM.

Testing. Immunoassay kits allow determination of serum CEA levels accurately, reproducibly, and relatively inexpensively. Serum levels of less than 2.5 ng/mL are normal; 2.5 to 5.0 ng/mL, borderline; and greater than 5.0 ng/mL, elevated. Borderline levels occur with benign disorders such as inflammatory bowel disease, pancreatitis, cirrhosis, and chronic obstructive pulmonary disease. Smoking can also increase CEA; the upper limit of normal in smokers should be considered 5 ng/mL.

Screening. CEA is not useful as a screening test because of its low sensitivity in early-stage disease. Elevated CEA levels occur in only 5% to 40% of patients with localized disease.

Prognosis. Elevated CEA levels reflect the burden of tumor present. The degree of CEA elevation correlates with increasing stage of disease, and therefore CEA levels have prognostic value. Preoperative serum CEA is an independent predictor of survival; the higher the preoperative serum level, the poorer the prognosis. This effect persists even after patients are stratified for resectability and extent of local tumor invasion. The 5-year survival is significantly worse in patients with elevated preoperative CEA levels compared with those with a normal preoperative CEA level. Furthermore, 5-year survival is higher in those patients whose elevated preoperative CEA level normalized postoperatively. Finally, patients with elevated preoperative CEA levels have higher recurrence rates compared with those with normal CEA levels.

Monitoring. The most common application of CEA is in monitoring of patients for recurrent disease. CEA is most sensitive for hepatic or retroperitoneal metastasis and relatively insensitive for local, pulmonary, or peritoneal involvement. About 75% of patients with recurrent colorectal cancer have an elevated serum CEA level before development of symptoms. The pattern or magnitude of the rise in the CEA level is of no value in distinguishing localized recurrence from distant disease. However, because elevations of CEA may be transient, repeated measurement should be performed as confirmation of the trend. A confirmed rising trend in CEA should prompt evaluation for recurrent disease.

Because CEA reflects tumor burden, it is useful in monitoring response to chemotherapy in patients with metastatic cancer. An elevated CEA level is an independent factor associated with poor survival and progression on 5-fluorouracil chemotherapy in patients with metastatic colorectal cancer. Patients with advanced cancer whose CEA levels fall during chemotherapy survive significantly longer than those patients whose CEA levels do not change or increase.

α-Fetoprotein

α-Fetoprotein (AFP) is used in the detection and management of HCC. It is an oncofetal antigen, consisting of a single-chain polypeptide with molecular mass of 700 kDa. Levels are elevated in the fetus, fall to low levels after birth, and are elevated during pregnancy. It is synthesized by hepatocytes and endodermally derived gastrointestinal tissues.

Testing. AFP is measured with immunoassay kits, either enzyme-linked immunoassays or radioimmunoassays. The upper limit of normal for a healthy, nonpregnant adult is less than 25 ng/mL;10% to 20% of HCCs do not have detectable levels of AFP. Levels are also raised in nonseminomatous testicular cancer, for which it is a valuable tumor marker (see discussion later). Twenty percent of patients with gastric or pancreatic cancer and 5% of patients with colorectal or lung cancer have significant elevations (>5 ng/mL) of serum AFP levels. Elevated levels are also seen in hepatitis, inflammatory bowel disease, and cirrhosis.

Screening. AFP has an estimated sensitivity of 25% to 75%, a specificity of 76% to 94%, and a positive predictive value of 9% to 50%. However, the sensitivity and specificity vary with the cutoff value chosen. If the cutoff value is set at 20 ng/mL, the sensitivity and specificity are 30% and 87%, respectively; but if the cutoff value is raised to 100 ng/mL and 400 ng/mL, sensitivity and specificity vary from 72% and 56% to 70% and 94%, respectively.

The combination of AFP and ultrasound improves efficacy of screening. One surveillance study of 1125 patients with HCV reported a sensitivity of 100% with a combination of AFP and ultrasound compared with a sensitivity of 75% for AFP alone and 87% for ultrasound alone.[37] Cost-effectiveness analysis calculates the costs of each additional life year gained in terms of quality-adjusted life years (QALYs). A QALY less than $50,000 is considered cost-effective. In the United States, studies suggest that surveillance of patients with HCV-related cirrhosis with a combination of AFP and an imaging modality (either ultrasound or computed tomography) would gain QALYs at acceptable cost.[38-40]

Prognosis. AFP concentration reflects tumor size, with levels above 400 ng/mL associated with larger tumors. As a result, it has been shown that AFP correlates with stage and prognosis. The rate of increase, expressed as AFP doubling time, has also been associated with poorer prognosis.

Monitoring. AFP has been shown to decline after resection or ablation. After complete resection, AFP levels should drop and remain less than 10 ng/mL. Shirabe and colleagues[41] found that in patients with HCC whose preoperative AFP level was higher than 100 ng/mL and in whom the postoperative AFP level did not fall below 20 ng/mL, early recurrence within the first postoperative year should be strongly suspected. For those patients whose AFP levels do normalize postoperatively, a subsequent rise in AFP during the course of serial serum measurements has been found to be the best indicator of recurrent disease. It was the first measured abnormality in 34% of these patients. However, in some patients who had elevated serum levels of AFP with their original HCC, postoperative levels of AFP were unreliable in detecting recurrence. Five (12%) patients did not have elevated serum levels despite the presence of recurrent disease.

Tumor regrowth after treatment with chemoembolization does not correlate with rate of AFP rise or tumor burden.

AFP levels usually decline in response to effective chemotherapy. Monitoring of AFP therefore avoids prolonged use of ineffective and potentially toxic chemotherapy.

Carbohydrate Antigen 19-9

Carbohydrate antigen 19-9 (CA 19-9) is widely used as a serum marker of pancreatic cancer, but its use is limited to monitoring responses to therapy, not as a diagnostic marker. It is a mucin-type glycoprotein expressed on the surface of pancreatic cancer cells and was initially detected by monoclonal antibodies raised against colon cancer cell lines in a mouse model. The CA 19-9 epitope is normally present within the biliary tree. Biliary tract disease, both acute and chronic, can elevate serum CA 19-9 levels.

Testing. CA 19-9 is detected by an immunoassay, with the upper limit of normal for a healthy adult being 37 U/mL. Sensitivities of CA 19-9 in the diagnosis of pancreatic cancer range from 67% to 92%, with specificities ranging from 68% to 92%. The utility of CA 19-9 as a diagnostic marker is limited in a number of ways. First, patients with negative Lewis[a] blood group antigen cannot synthesize CA 19-9, and therefore it should not be used as a serologic marker in these individuals, who make up about 10% of the population. Second, patients with benign biliary tract disease can have levels of up to 400 U/mL, with 87% having concentrations above 70 U/mL. Significant numbers of patients with pancreatitis, either acute or chronic, also have elevated levels. Third, besides pancreas cancer, CA 19-9 levels are also elevated in patients with other cancers, including those of the biliary tree (95%), stomach (5%), colon (15%), liver (HCC, 7%), and lung (13%). For lung cancer, CA 19-9 levels add little clinically useful information to determination of CEA levels.

Screening. CA 19-9 is not useful as a screening modality because of its low sensitivity in early-stage disease. With increasing levels of CA 19-9, the diagnosis of pancreatic cancer becomes more accurate. When a cutoff level of 100 U/mL is used, a number of studies have demonstrated that whereas sensitivity ranges from 60% to 84%, specificity for pancreas cancer is 95% or greater. Levels above 1000 U/mL are almost diagnostic of pancreatic cancer. Because of its frequent elevation in benign biliary tract disease, CA 19-9 is not useful in distinguishing benign from malignant distal common bile duct strictures.

Prognosis. In those patients with pancreas cancer who have CA 19-9 detectable in their serum, the level has been shown to correlate with tumor burden. For example, higher CA 19-9 levels typically correlate with higher tumor stage, and more than 95% of patients with unresectable disease have levels above 1000 U/mL. Of patients who undergo curative resection, those whose CA 19-9 levels returned to normal survived longer than those whose levels fell but never normalized.

Monitoring. Serial measurement of CA 19-9 is used to monitor response to therapy. A rise in CA 19-9 level after curative resection has been shown to precede clinical or computed tomography evidence of recurrence by 2 to 9 months. In patients with unresectable or metastatic disease, failure of CA 19-9 levels to fall with chemotherapy reflects poor tumor response. However, in both settings, the lack of alternative effective therapies limits the utility of serial monitoring of CA 19-9.

Prostate-Specific Antigen

Prostate-specific antigen (PSA) is a serine protease that is formed in the prostatic epithelium and secreted into the prostatic ducts. Its function is to digest the gel that is formed in seminal fluid after ejaculation. Under normal circumstances, only small amounts of PSA leak into the circulation. With enlargement of the gland (e.g., in patients with benign prostatic hyperplasia) or distortion of its architecture, serum PSA levels increase. Thus, PSA is considered a tissue-specific rather than a prostate cancer–specific marker; patients who have undergone curative radical prostatectomy as well as women have no detectable PSA.

Testing. PSA is detected with an immunoassay. Besides benign prostatic hyperplasia, other instances in which serum PSA levels may be elevated include prostatitis, prostatic massage, prostatic biopsy, and digital rectal examination. Initial studies set the upper limit of normal for PSA at 4 ng/mL, with levels greater than 10 ng/mL suggestive of malignancy and levels of 4 to 10 ng/mL being indeterminate. Since then, it has been found that the upper limit of the normal range of PSA increases with age. The limit is 2.5 ng/mL for those aged 40 to 49 years, 3.5 ng/mL for those 50 to 59 years, 4.5 ng/mL for those 60 to 69 years, and 6.5 ng/mL for those 70 years and older. The rate of increase of PSA in a normal 60-year-old is 0.04 ng/mL per year.

Expressing PSA relative to prostatic volume and time has also helped discriminate cancer from benign conditions when the PSA level is less than 10 ng/mL but greater than the upper limit of normal for the patient's age. PSA density is defined as the ratio of PSA to prostatic volume, as measured by transrectal ultrasound or magnetic resonance imaging. Higher PSA densities are more suggestive of malignancy compared with benign prostatic hyperplasia because the amount of PSA released per gram of prostate cancer is significantly greater than that released from normal prostatic tissue.

The ratio of free to total PSA has also been found to improve the specificity of prostate cancer diagnosis in the PSA range of 4 to 10 ng/mL. PSA slope (also known as PSA velocity) is the rate of change of the concentration of PSA over time. For individuals with initial levels below 4.0 ng/mL, a PSA slope of greater than 0.75 ng/mL per year is considered significant; for patients whose baseline level is above 4.0 ng/mL, a slope of more than 0.4 ng/mL is considered significant.

Screening. PSA is widely used as a screening tool for prostate cancer, enabling early detection and diagnosis of this disease. However, its use has recently been called into question by the results of two recent trials. The European Randomized Study of Screening for Prostate Cancer (ERSPC) randomized 162,387 men to either screening with PSA or no screening. With a median follow-up of 9 years, there were 214 prostate cancer deaths in the screening group and 326 in the control group, resulting in an adjusted rate ratio for death of 0.8 for the screening group. In other words, to prevent one death from prostate cancer, more than 1400 men need to be screened and 48 men treated. In the Prostate, Lung, Colorectal and Ovary Cancer (PLCO) trial, 76,693 U.S. men were randomized, and with an average of 7 years of follow-up, mortality between the screened and control groups did not differ (rate ratio for death of 1.1). These data have added to concerns about overdiagnosis and overtreatment of this disease, with the associated effects on the patient's quality of life.[42] Autopsy studies have found that prostate cancer can be found in 55% of men in their fifth decade of life and 64% in their seventh decade, indicating that a significant proportion of these cancers are not lethal. Only one in eight screen-detected cancers is likely to kill its host if left untreated.

Monitoring response to therapy. After operative resection, the PSA level is expected to normalize after 2 to 3 weeks. Patients whose PSA level remained elevated 6 months after radical prostatectomy eventually developed recurrent disease. In contrast, it takes 3 to 5 months for the PSA level to normalize after radiotherapy. However, failure of the PSA level to normalize after radiotherapy also predicts relapse. Rise in serum PSA level is usually the first sign of either local recurrence or metastatic progression. In patients with advanced disease, PSA levels are also used to monitor response to systemic therapy.

Carbohydrate Antigen 125

Carbohydrate antigen 125 (CA 125) is a carbohydrate epitope on a glycoprotein carcinoma antigen. It is present in the fetus and in derivatives of the coelomic epithelium, including peritoneum, pleura, pericardium, and amnion. In healthy adults, CA 125 has been detected by immunohistochemistry in the epithelium of the fallopian tubes, endometrium, and endocervix. However, neither adult nor fetal ovarian epithelium expresses CA 125.

Testing. CA 125 levels are measured by an immunoassay, with the upper limit of normal set at 35 U/mL. Elevated levels are detected in 80% of patients with ovarian cancer. In patients with ovarian masses, an elevated CA 125 level has a sensitivity of 75% and a specificity of approximately 90% for malignancy. It is also detectable in a high percentage of patients with cancer of fallopian tube, endometrium, and cervix as well as in nongynecologic malignant neoplasms of the pancreas, colon, lung, and liver. Benign conditions in which CA 125 is elevated include endometriosis, adenomyosis, uterine fibroids, pelvic inflammatory disease, cirrhosis, and ascites. Like CA 19-9 in patients with pancreas cancer, CA 125 is an adjunct to diagnosis rather than being diagnostic of itself.

Screening. By itself, CA 125 is not useful as a screening tool for ovarian cancer because of its poor specificity. However, the United Kingdom Collaborative Trial of Ovarian Cancer Screening is evaluating the effectiveness of CA 125 in postmenopausal women. In this study, those women classified as high risk according to their CA 125 level are further screened with transvaginal ultrasound. Final results from this trial are highly anticipated, and are expected to be released in the near future.

Prognosis. Patients with elevated CA 125 levels at the time of diagnosis have a worse prognosis compared with those patients with normal levels. Absolute levels of CA 125 do not clearly correlate with tumor stage, although with increasing stage, greater percentages of patients have elevated CA 125 levels: 50% of stage I patients, 70% of stage II patients, 90% of stage III patients, and 98% of stage IV patients.

Monitoring response to therapy. CA 125 is of value in monitoring disease course. Partial or complete response to therapy is associated with a decrease in the CA 125 level in more than 95% of patients. Increasing levels of CA 125 correlate with disease recurrence and precede clinical or imaging evidence of recurrence by a median time of 3 months. When rising CA 125 levels are used as an indication for second-look laparotomies, recurrent disease is found approximately 90% of the time.

CA 125 levels in peritoneal fluid may be more sensitive than serum levels. Thus, in those patients whose serum CA 125 level normalizes during therapy, peritoneal fluid CA 125 levels may better be able to distinguish those patients with residual disease from those without. The upper limit of normal for peritoneal fluid CA 125 is 200 U/mL.

AFP and Human Chorionic Gonadotropin in Testicular Germ Cell Tumors

Nonseminomatous testicular cancers comprise several different histologic types, including embryonal carcinoma, syncytiotrophoblasts (choriocarcinoma), yolk sac tumors, and teratomas. Marker expression can be predicted on the basis of the predominant histologic type. Human chorionic gonadotropin (HCG) is detected in more than 90% of choriocarcinomas, whereas AFP is expressed by 90% to 95% of yolk sac tumors, 20% of teratomas, and 10% of embryonal carcinomas.

Diagnosis. Of patients with proven nonseminomatous testicular germ cell tumors, about 50% will have elevated serum levels of HCG and 60% of AFP; either marker is elevated in 90% of cases. The determination of both marker levels is important because nearly half of these tumors secrete only one of these substances. In addition to the high rate of marker positivity, there have been few cases of spuriously elevated serum levels of HCG or AFP in patients without testicular cancer. The presence of a testicular tumor in combination with an elevated level of AFP or HCG is suggestive of testicular cancer without being diagnostic. Elevated levels of these markers in a man younger than 40 years without signs of a testicular tumor may indicate extratesticular germ cell cancer.

Prognosis. An absolute AFP concentration of more than 500 ng/mL or HCG level of more than 1000 ng/mL predicts poor prognosis. These tumor markers are useful in identifying biologically distinct categories of morphologically similar tumors. In one study considering pretreatment levels of AFP and HCG, 92% of patients with normal levels of both markers achieved complete remission, compared with just 26% of those with elevated AFP only, 46% of those with elevated HCG only, and 35% of those with elevations of both. Similarly, in comparing groups of patients with similar disease burdens, those with elevated marker levels have a worse prognosis compared with those with normal marker levels.

Monitoring. In the majority of patients with nonseminomatous germ cell tumors, tumor marker levels correlate with response to chemotherapy. The rate of marker decline (half-life), calculated from weekly determinations after initiation of chemotherapy, can be used to identify early those patients who respond poorly to chemotherapy. Half-lives of more than 3.5 days for HCG or more than 7 days for AFP suggest patients requiring aggressive therapy, such as high-dose chemotherapy in combination with stem cell transplantation. However, there is a significant percentage of patients whose levels of tumor markers fall despite failure of their tumors to regress with therapy.

After completion of primary therapy, increasing marker concentrations, even in the absence of other features of recurrence, may lead to salvage chemotherapy. Therefore, it is important to exclude false-positive results. The level of HCG should be measured in the urine, where the concentration should be similar to that of serum. In contrast, interfering substances are not excreted into the urine. Intensive chemotherapy may induce hypogonadism with associated HCG levels of up to 5 to 10 IU/liter. It can be differentiated from relapse by measurement of luteinizing hormone and follicle-stimulating hormone; like the postmenopausal state in women, levels above 30 to 50 IU/liter indicate that HCG is derived from the pituitary.

DNA-Based Markers

Specific mutations in oncogenes, tumor suppressor genes, and mismatch repair genes can serve as biomarkers. These mutations may be germline, such as the *RET* proto-oncogene of MEN2 and the *APC* gene of FAP, or somatic mutations, such as the occurrence of *p53* mutations in a wide variety of tumors. Chromosomal abnormalities such as the 9 : 22 translocation that creates the *bcr-abl* oncogene are also useful biomarkers. Specific single-nucleotide polymorphisms have been identified that are associated with increased risk for specific cancers, and haplotype assessment has been shown to predict susceptibility to several cancers, including prostate, breast, lung, and colon.

DNA-based markers are beginning to have a profound influence on clinical practice. For example, HER2/neu amplification status is now being routinely used to guide treatment with trastuzumab in patients with breast cancer. The American Society of Clinical Oncology recommends that all patients with metastatic colorectal carcinoma who are candidates for anti-EGFR antibody therapy should have their tumor tested for *KRAS* mutation. If *KRAS* mutation in codon 12 or 13 is detected, these patients should not receive anti-EGFR antibody therapy as part of their treatment. This represents the first major step toward individualized treatment for patients with metastatic colorectal cancer.

Somatic *EGFR* mutations have been found to represent an important mechanism of resistance to tyrosine kinase inhibitors in non–small cell lung cancer. Deletions in exon 19 and L858R are associated with response of non–small cell lung cancer to gefitinib or erlotinib monotherapy, whereas mutations in exon 20 (particularly the T790M point mutation) confer resistance to erlotinib and gefitinib. As a result, *EGFR* mutation analysis is being used to identify patients who are likely to respond to monotherapy with tyrosine kinase inhibitors. Similarly, 40% to 60% of melanomas harbor a mutation of the serine/threonine kinase BRAF, which is involved in the activation of the MAP kinase/ERK signaling pathway. More than 90% of the mutations are due to a substitution of glutamic acid for valine at the amino acid 600 position (V600E). A recent phase 3 clinical trial (BRIM-III) demonstrated that treatment with a BRAF kinase inhibitor, vemurafenib, was associated with significantly increased response rates as well as with improved progression-free and overall survival compared with dacarbazine.[43] Targeting of therapies to specific mutations expressed by tumors represents an area of active clinical investigation and could hold significant promise.

Epigenetic Changes

Testing for epigenetic changes is still at an early discovery stage and has not yet reached the clinic. However, it has great potential for a number of reasons. First, DNA assays for aberrant methylation are easier and more sensitive than those for point mutations. Second, cancer-specific DNA methylation patterns can be detected in tumor-derived free DNA in the bloodstream and in epithelial tumor cells shed into the lumen. This ease of access to sample medium may facilitate efforts at detection and monitoring of cancer. Third, DNA methylation profiles are more chemically and biologically stable than RNA or most proteins. As a result, they may be more reliably detected in diverse biologic fluids. Methylation biomarker studies have been performed in a variety of cancers, including breast, esophageal, gastric, colorectal, and prostate. The sources of the DNA have included plasma or serum, urine, sputum, and saliva. A number of general observations have been made. Targeted biologic fluid sources of DNA, such as urine for bladder cancer, tended to give higher clinical sensitivities than serum or plasma analysis. In contrast, the specificity of plasma or serum detection of tumor-specific markers was found to be extremely high—approximately 100%. Combining DNA methylation assays may complement existing screening methods of high sensitivity but low specificity, such as PSA in prostate cancer. Use of panels of methylation targets in these studies improved the clinical sensitivity of the assay.

Potential Applications

Early detection. Although abnormal epigenetic silencing of genes can occur at any time during carcinogenesis, it appears to occur most frequently early in the transformation process. Aberrant crypt foci, which contain preneoplastic hyperplastic colonic epithelial cells, have been found to contain abnormal methylation in promoter regions of genes involved in the abnormal activation of the Wnt signaling pathway.[44] Abnormal methylation patterns in histologically normal cells may emerge as useful markers for cancer risk assessment.

Prediction of response to therapy. Methylation of specific genes can be linked to the biologic behavior of the tumor. A number of studies have reported associations between DNA methylation markers and response to chemotherapy. The most extensive work has been done on CpG hypermethylation of the O^6-methylguanine DNA methyltransferase (MGMT) gene, which appears to confer sensitivity to various alkylating chemotherapeutic agents. MGMT methylation was associated with prolonged survival in glioma patients treated with carmustine and in patients with large diffuse B cell lymphoma who were treated with cyclophosphamide as part of multidrug regimens.[45] In addition, methylation of the *ESR1* gene and the *PGR* gene predicts estrogen and progesterone receptor status, respectively, and response to tamoxifen. Individual methylation markers, such as of the E-cadherin promoter, have also been linked to breast cancer metastasis.

Prognostication. Abnormal methylation of combinations of genes has been associated with poor outcome.

On an opposite note, loss of methylation is being increasingly recognized as an important event in carcinogenesis. Hypomethylated CGIs have been associated with the activation of nearby genes. For example, hypomethylation of the promoter for the cancer/testis antigen CAGE correlates with the gene's increased expression and is found in premalignant lesions of the stomach.[46] Similar instances of demethylated promoters activating their downstream genes have been found in numerous other cancers, including those of the colon, pancreas, liver, uterus, lung, and cervix.[32] In a study of ovarian carcinogenesis, hypomethylation of centromeric and juxtacentromeric satellite DNA was found to be increased in tumors of advanced stage or high grade, and this strong hypomethylation was an independent marker of poor prognosis.[47] Furthermore, genome-wide hypomethylation has also been detected in cancer cells and may contribute to genomic instability.

DNA methylation profiles, examining both hypermethylation and hypomethylation, may provide greater insights into tumor behavior than either profile alone.

RNA-Based Markers

RNA-based markers have been identified in the context of global mRNA expression using high-throughput technologies. These microarrays ("gene chips") provide a means to measure the expression of 30,000 to 40,000 human genes in a single experiment.

Statistical modeling then allows selection of groups of genes, "fingerprints," that best distinguish disease states.

In 2004, Paik and colleagues described an algorithm to predict likelihood of distant recurrence in patients with node-negative, tamoxifen-treated breast cancer based on the expression of 21 genes in tumor tissue.[48] This multigene assay, known as Oncotype DX, includes 16 tumor-associated genes and 5 reference genes, with the result expressed as a recurrence score (RS). Higher expression levels of "favorable" genes result in a lower RS, whereas higher expression of "unfavorable" genes results in a higher RS. Validation studies have demonstrated that this assay is more accurate in predicting clinical outcome in estrogen receptor–positive, lymph node–negative breast cancer patients treated with tamoxifen than traditional clinicopathologic characteristics. Several studies have found that use of this test has altered treatment choice in approximately 25% of patients.[49]

The MammaPrint assay is another multigene assay, using 70 genes, designed to individualize treatment for patients with either estrogen receptor–positive or estrogen receptor–negative, lymph node–negative breast cancer. Its accuracy to select early-stage breast cancer patients who are highly likely to develop distant metastases and therefore may benefit most from adjuvant chemotherapy is being tested prospectively in the MINDACT (Microarray In Node-negative Disease may Avoid ChemoTherapy) clinical trial. Preliminary results from this trial support the notion that gene expression testing and standard assessment methods often produce different risk stratification (31% of patients), but final results from the trial are still pending.

Proteomic Profiling

Proteomics is the study of all the proteins expressed by the genome. Ultimately, genetic mutations are manifested at the protein level, involving derangements of protein function and communication within diseased cells and with their microenvironment. Execution of the disease process occurs through altered protein function. Protein tumor biomarkers are thought to be low abundance proteins (of concentrations in the nanomolar range), shed from tumor cells or from the tumor-host interface into the circulation.[50] Detection and measurement of these proteins provide information about the clinical behavior of the cancer. Proteomic profiling using mass spectrometry technologies generates complex fingerprints of ion peaks corresponding to protein concentrations that can be correlated with disease states. Numerous studies, using samples from blood (plasma or serum), urine, and pancreatic juice, have demonstrated the feasibility of this technology for biomarker discovery and for the early detection of ovarian, breast, prostate, and pancreas cancer. Identification of reproducible protein signatures of specific diseases has the potential to achieve much higher diagnostic sensitivity and specificity than of currently available biomarkers. Proteomic profiling lacks a standardized methodology and remains time and labor intensive. For the moment, these technologies are not ready for routine clinical use. Their principal role is in protein biomarker discovery. Candidate biomarkers discovered through this process can be validated by standard immunometric techniques after the development of specific antibodies.

The role of biomarkers in cancer is expanding rapidly. Clearly, the future holds great promise for the use of biomarkers in the clinical management of patients with cancer (Table 28-7). It is likely that biomarkers will play an increasingly important role in cancer prognosis and therapeutic selection as well as, perhaps, in early detection.

TABLE 28-7 Biomarkers and Biologically Targeted Therapies

CANCER	BIOMARKER	THERAPY
Breast	Estrogen receptor, progesterone receptor	Tamoxifen/aromatase inhibitors
Lymphoma	CD20	Rituximab
Chronic myelogenous leukemia	*bcr-abl*	Imatinib
Gastrointestinal stromal tumor	c-*kit*	Imatinib
Non–small cell lung cancer	*EGFR* mutation	Gefitinib
Breast	*HER2/neu*	Trastuzumab
Melanoma	*BRAF* V600E mutation	Vemurafenib

From Ludwig JA, Weinstein JN: Biomarkers in cancer staging, prognosis and treatment selection. *Nat Rev Cancer* 5:845–856, 2005. Biomarker expression is being increasingly used, independent of formal staging criteria, to decide which patients receive biologically targeted therapies.

SELECTED REFERENCES

Allegra CJ, Jessup JM, Somerfield MR, et al: American Society of Clinical Oncology provisional clinical opinion: Testing for KRAS gene mutations in patients with metastatic colorectal carcinoma to predict response to anti–epidermal growth factor receptor monoclonal antibody therapy. *J Clin Oncol* 27:2091–2096, 2009.

This paper summarizes the role and rationale for KRAS mutation testing to determine treatment in patients with metastatic colorectal cancer.

Beck B, Blanpain C: Unravelling cancer stem cell potential. *Nat Rev Cancer* 13:727–738, 2013.

A review of the latest scientific evidence for cancer stem cells.

Clark WH, Jr, Elder DE, Guerry D, 4th, et al: A study of tumor progression: The precursor lesions of superficial spreading and nodular melanoma. *Hum Pathol* 15:1147–1165, 1984.

This paper summarizes observations of tumor progression and defines the series of proliferative lesions that constitute the progression from melanocytic neoplasia to malignant melanoma. Based on their observations, the authors provide a paradigm for the development of neoplasia in general and provide a list of six lesional steps.

Dawson MA, Kouzarides T: Cancer epigenetics: From mechanism to therapy. *Cell* 150:12–27, 2012.

Excellent overview of developments and progress in the field of cancer epigenetics.

Fang H, Declerck YA: Targeting the tumor microenvironment: From understanding pathways to effective clinical trials. *Cancer Res* 73:4965–4977, 2013.

Review of tumor cell–stroma interactions and clinical implications for therapies.

Fearon ER, Vogelstein B: A genetic model for colorectal tumorigenesis. *Cell* 61:759–767, 1990.

This is the classic paper detailing the first genetic model for tumorigenesis involving a series of genetic mutations, including mutational activation of oncogenes and inactivation of tumor suppressor genes.

Hanahan D, Weinberg RA: The hallmarks of cancer: The next generation. *Cell* 144:646–674, 2011.

The authors provide an update to their landmark paper from 10 years prior, in which they detail the current understanding of common physiologic and molecular characteristics of cancer.

Knudson AG: Two genetic hits (more or less) to cancer. *Nat Rev Cancer* 1:157–162, 2001.

This paper provides a perspective on the number of genetic mutations that lead to cancer by using retinoblastoma as a model.

Schreiber RD, Old LJ, Smyth MJ: Cancer immunoediting: Integrating immunity's roles in cancer suppression and promotion. *Immunity* 21:137–148, 2004.

This paper reviews the evidence and theory behind immunoediting in cancer.

Sparano JA, Paik S: Development of the 21-gene assay and its application in clinical practice and clinical trials. *J Clin Oncol* 26:721–728, 2008.

This paper reviews the use of the Oncotype DX assay in the clinical decision making for patients with node-negative, tamoxifen-treated breast cancer.

REFERENCES

1. Hanahan D, Weinberg RA: Hallmarks of cancer: The next generation. *Cell* 144:646–674, 2011.
2. Siegel R, Ma J, Zou Z, et al: Cancer statistics, 2014. *CA Cancer J Clin* 64:9–29, 2014.
3. Thun MJ, DeLancey JO, Center MM, et al: The global burden of cancer: Priorities for prevention. *Carcinogenesis* 31:100–110, 2010.
4. Sener SF, Grey N: The global burden of cancer. *J Surg Oncol* 92:1–3, 2005.
5. Thakkar JP, McCarthy BJ, Villano JL: Age-specific cancer incidence rates increase through the oldest age groups. *Am J Med Sci* 348:65–70, 2014.
6. Hutchins LF, Unger JM, Crowley JJ, et al: Underrepresentation of patients 65 years of age or older in cancer-treatment trials. *N Engl J Med* 341:2061–2067, 1999.
7. Lewis JH, Kilgore ML, Goldman DP, et al: Participation of patients 65 years of age or older in cancer clinical trials. *J Clin Oncol* 21:1383–1389, 2003.
8. Trimble EL, Carter CL, Cain D, et al: Representation of older patients in cancer treatment trials. *Cancer* 74:2208–2214, 1994.
9. Hung A, Mullins CD: Relative effectiveness and safety of chemotherapy in elderly and nonelderly patients with stage III colon cancer: A systematic review. *Oncologist* 18:54–63, 2012.
10. Jin Y, Qiu MZ, Wang DS, et al: Adjuvant chemotherapy for elderly patients with gastric cancer after D2 gastrectomy. *PLoS ONE* 8:e53149, 2013.
11. Calle EE, Rodriguez C, Walker-Thurmond K, et al: Overweight, obesity, and mortality from cancer in a prospectively studied cohort of U.S. adults. *N Engl J Med* 348:1625–1638, 2003.
12. Burkhart DL, Sage J: Cellular mechanisms of tumour suppression by the retinoblastoma gene. *Nat Rev Cancer* 8:671–682, 2008.
13. Okada H, Mak TW: Pathways of apoptotic and non-apoptotic death in tumour cells. *Nat Rev Cancer* 4:592–603, 2004.
14. Kerr JF, Wyllie AH, Currie AR: Apoptosis: A basic biological phenomenon with wide-ranging implications in tissue kinetics. *Br J Cancer* 26:239–257, 1972.
15. Korsmeyer SJ: Chromosomal translocations in lymphoid malignancies reveal novel proto-oncogenes. *Annu Rev Immunol* 10:785–807, 1992.
16. Kelekar A: Autophagy. *Ann N Y Acad Sci* 1066:259–271, 2005.
17. Shin JS, Hong A, Solomon MJ, et al: The role of telomeres and telomerase in the pathology of human cancer and aging. *Pathology* 38:103–113, 2006.
18. Beck B, Blanpain C: Unravelling cancer stem cell potential. *Nat Rev Cancer* 13:727–738, 2013.
19. Folkman J: Angiogenesis. *Annu Rev Med* 57:1–18, 2006.
20. Naumov GN, Folkman J, Straume O: Tumor dormancy due to failure of angiogenesis: Role of the microenvironment. *Clin Exp Metastasis* 26:51–60, 2009.
21. Hanahan D, Folkman J: Patterns and emerging mechanisms of the angiogenic switch during tumorigenesis. *Cell* 86:353–364, 1996.
22. Zlotnik A: Chemokines and cancer. *Int J Cancer* 119:2026–2029, 2006.
23. Cavallaro U, Christofori G: Cell adhesion and signalling by cadherins and Ig-CAMs in cancer. *Nat Rev Cancer* 4:118–132, 2004.
24. Makrilia N, Kollias A, Manolopoulos L, et al: Cell adhesion molecules: Role and clinical significance in cancer. *Cancer Invest* 27:1023–1037, 2009.
25. Hanahan D, Weinberg RA: The hallmarks of cancer. *Cell* 100:57–70, 2000.
26. Janes SM, Watt FM: New roles for integrins in squamous-cell carcinoma. *Nat Rev Cancer* 6:175–183, 2006.
27. Pages F, Galon J, Dieu-Nosjean MC, et al: Immune infiltration in human tumors: A prognostic factor that should not be ignored. *Oncogene* 29:1093–1102, 2010.
28. Schreiber RD, Old LJ, Smyth MJ: Cancer immunoediting: Integrating immunity's roles in cancer suppression and promotion. *Science* 331:1565–1570, 2011.
29. Fearon ER: Human cancer syndromes: Clues to the origin and nature of cancer. *Science* 278:1043–1050, 1997.
30. Nielsen M, Franken PF, Reinards TH, et al: Multiplicity in polyp count and extracolonic manifestations in 40 Dutch patients with MYH associated polyposis coli (MAP). *J Med Genet* 42:e54, 2005.

31. Galiatsatos P, Foulkes WD: Familial adenomatous polyposis. *Am J Gastroenterol* 101:385–398, 2006.
32. Feinberg AP, Tycko B: The history of cancer epigenetics. *Nat Rev Cancer* 4:143–153, 2004.
33. Kondo Y, Shen L, Issa JP: Critical role of histone methylation in tumor suppressor gene silencing in colorectal cancer. *Mol Cell Biol* 23:206–215, 2003.
34. Chemin I, Zoulim F: Hepatitis B virus induced hepatocellular carcinoma. *Cancer Lett* 286:52–59, 2009.
35. Butel JS: Viral carcinogenesis: Revelation of molecular mechanisms and etiology of human disease. *Carcinogenesis* 21:405–426, 2000.
36. Anzola M: Hepatocellular carcinoma: Role of hepatitis B and hepatitis C viruses proteins in hepatocarcinogenesis. *J Viral Hepat* 11:383–393, 2004.
37. Izzo F, Cremona F, Ruffolo F, et al: Outcome of 67 patients with hepatocellular cancer detected during screening of 1125 patients with chronic hepatitis. *Ann Surg* 227:513–518, 1998.
38. Arguedas MR, Chen VK, Eloubeidi MA, et al: Screening for hepatocellular carcinoma in patients with hepatitis C cirrhosis: A cost-utility analysis. *Am J Gastroenterol* 98:679–690, 2003.
39. Lin OS, Keeffe EB, Sanders GD, et al: Cost-effectiveness of screening for hepatocellular carcinoma in patients with cirrhosis due to chronic hepatitis C. *Aliment Pharmacol Ther* 19:1159–1172, 2004.
40. Saab S, Ly D, Nieto J, et al: Hepatocellular carcinoma screening in patients waiting for liver transplantation: A decision analytic model. *Liver Transpl* 9:672–681, 2003.
41. Shirabe K, Takenaka K, Gion T, et al: Significance of alpha-fetoprotein levels for detection of early recurrence of hepatocellular carcinoma after hepatic resection. *J Surg Oncol* 64:143–146, 1997.
42. Eckersberger E, Finkelstein J, Sadri H, et al: Screening for prostate cancer: A review of the ERSPC and PLCO trials. *Rev Urol* 11:127–133, 2009.
43. Chapman PB, Hauschild A, Robert C, et al: Improved survival with vemurafenib in melanoma with BRAF V600E mutation. *N Engl J Med* 364:2507–2516, 2011.
44. Baylin SB, Ohm JE: Epigenetic gene silencing in cancer—a mechanism for early oncogenic pathway addiction? *Nat Rev Cancer* 6:107–116, 2006.
45. Laird PW: The power and the promise of DNA methylation markers. *Nat Rev Cancer* 3:253–266, 2003.
46. Cho B, Lee H, Jeong S, et al: Promoter hypomethylation of a novel cancer/testis antigen gene CAGE is correlated with its aberrant expression and is seen in premalignant stage of gastric carcinoma. *Biochem Biophys Res Commun* 307:52–63, 2003.
47. Widschwendter M, Jiang G, Woods C, et al: DNA hypomethylation and ovarian cancer biology. *Cancer Res* 64:4472–4480, 2004.
48. Paik S, Shak S, Tang G, et al: A multigene assay to predict recurrence of tamoxifen-treated, node-negative breast cancer. *N Engl J Med* 351:2817–2826, 2004.
49. Sparano JA, Paik S: Development of the 21-gene assay and its application in clinical practice and clinical trials. *J Clin Oncol* 26:721–728, 2008.
50. Hanash SM, Pitteri SJ, Faca VM: Mining the plasma proteome for cancer biomarkers. *Nature* 452:571–579, 2008.

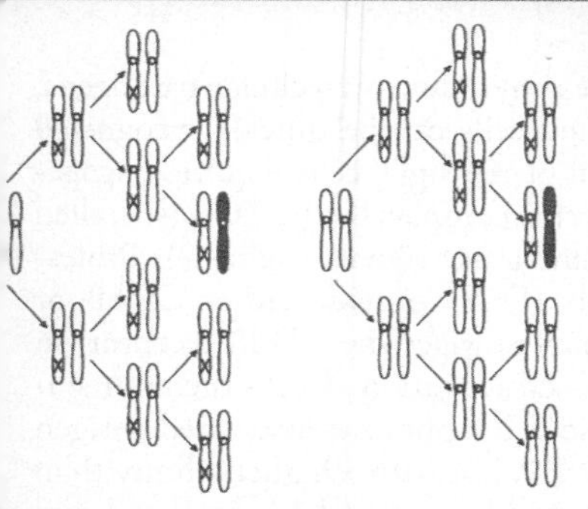

CHAPTER 29

Tumor Immunology and Immunotherapy

James S. Economou, James C. Yang, James S. Tomlinson

OUTLINE

The immune system is our most powerful defense against infectious disease[1] and the mediator of rejection in transplantation. For an increasing larger subset of patients, modern immune-based therapies can also effect dramatic and durable rejection of bulky systemic disease in several solid and hematopoietic malignant neoplasms. This attests to the capacity of the adaptive and perhaps of the innate immune system to recognize and to destroy malignant neoplasms. These complete responses are generally durable, which is even more remarkable. The adaptive arm of the human immune system recognizes peptide epitopes expressed in the context of the major histocompatibility complex (MHC) on the cell surface; we now know that these may be either self-antigens or acquired tumor-specific mutations that are presented to the immune system through this MHC restricting element. The immune system has evolved mechanisms of immunologic tolerance that allows discrimination between self and nonself. Almost half of the human T cell repertoire is self-reactive—generally of low affinity, having escaped thymic deletion—which explains how some antitumor immune responses are in fact autoimmune in nature. There are likely many potential immune targets associated with solid and hematopoietic malignant neoplasms, both normal self-proteins and tumor-specific mutations, against which human cytotoxic T cells can be activated and expanded. Genome-based advances as well have provided promising recombinant immunomodulatory molecules, such as cytokines and checkpoint inhibitors.[2] Thus, there is broad potential in human cancer immunotherapy as we are beginning to have better understanding of the biologic rules.

OVERVIEW OF TUMOR IMMUNOLOGY

T Lymphocytes and Natural Killer Cells

Bone marrow–derived progenitor cells enter the thymus, from which T cells eventually emerge. In the thymus, an enormous repertoire of T cell receptors (TCRs) is randomly generated by recombinations and mutations in their α and β chains. Progenitors with TCRs of high affinity for self-antigens undergo deletion (negative selection). Some of those with low affinity for self-antigens survive and are positively selected, so that a significant percentage of self-reactive T cells emerge from the thymus. Only a very small percentage of the cells entering and proliferating within the thymus survive this education process. Several types of T cells emerge into the periphery. $CD8^+$ T cells recognize antigen in the context of MHC class I molecules, express αβ TCRs, are commonly referred to as cytotoxic T cells, and produce a number of cytokines. $CD4^+$ T cells recognize antigen in the context of MHC class II molecules. There are several subsets of $CD4^+$ T cells (Fig. 29-1). Among the better recognized are Th1 cells (helper type 1 T cells) that secrete interleukin-2 (IL-2), tumor necrosis factor-α (TNF-α), and interferon-γ (IFN-γ) and Th2 cells that produce IL-4, IL-5, IL-6, IL-10, and IL-13. Th1 cells promote cytotoxicity and inflammation, whereas Th2 cells assist in the stimulation of B cells to produce antibody. T helper cells will favor Th1 (cell-mediated) or Th2 (humoral) immune responses, but a subset of regulatory cells (Treg cells) plays a critical role in dampening autoimmunity. These Treg cells constitute 5% to 10% of $CD4^+$ cells and express the transcription factor Foxp3 and dominantly suppress autoimmune responses; mutation of the Foxp3 gene in humans and mice leads to multiorgan autoimmune disease. A fourth type of T cell subtype is the so-called Th17 cell, which preferentially produces IL-17, IL-21, and IL-22 and is important in the pathogenesis of autoimmune diseases.

$CD4^+$ T cells also play an important role in the initiation and maintenance of $CD8^+$ T cell responses.[2] They may do this through a variety of mechanisms. Activated $CD4^+$ T cells can interact with dendritic cells (DCs), professional antigen-presenting cells, through an interaction between the CD40 receptor and its ligand, CD40L. This activation or "licensing" of DCs allows these antigen-presenting cells to promote the differentiation of $CD8^+$ T cells and to establish a durable memory T cell response. $CD4^+$ T cells also produce IL-2 and IFN-γ, which could potentially support CD8 function. Thus, the importance of $CD4^+$ T cells in shaping a productive antitumor response has been incorporated into many tumor immunotherapy strategies.

Another T cell subset (γδ) represents a minor population (1% to 10%) of $CD3^+$ T cells that is even more enriched in mucosal epithelium and expresses TCRs that recognize bacterial and viral antigens. Natural killer T (NKT) cells express phenotypic markers of T and NK cells and express a specific family of TCRs that recognize glycolipid antigens presented by CD1d molecules. These NKT cells are thought to help initiate T cell responses through the production of large amounts of the cytokines IFN-γ and IL-4.

Mature T cells have a broad repertoire of αβ TCRs with diverse antigen specificity. This diversity is generated during T cell differentiation by a process of gene rearrangement of variable (V), joining (J), and diversity (D) gene segments. TCRs are composed of α and β chains; it is estimated that recombination events could potentially yield a repertoire exceeding 10^{12} unique TCRs. These TCRs recognize antigen in the context of MHC proteins found on the surface of cells. Proteins within the cell are digested in the proteasome complex into short peptide fragments (8 to 12 amino acid residues), which are transported to the cell surface bound in the groove of MHC class molecules; the specific peptide sequence presented is determined by the MHC (in humans, also called HLA [human leukocyte antigen]) allele. These class I–restricted peptides are recognized by $CD8^+$ T cells. This provides the immune system with a continuous surveillance system for intracellular pathogens, such as viruses, so that infected cells can be quickly recognized and eliminated. The activation of resting T cells requires engagement of the correct MHC-peptide complex by the TCR (so-called signal 1) and additional costimulatory signals (signal 2). Professional antigen-presenting cells (DCs) provide either CD80 or CD86 (B7 family genes), which engages the CD28 receptor on the T cell, a requirement for T cell activation. T cells then upregulate another receptor, cytotoxic T lymphocyte–associated antigen 4 (CTLA-4), which also binds B7, but with a higher affinity than CD28. Engagement of CTLA-4 induces an inhibitory signal that downregulates T cell activation.[3] This is a natural immunomodulatory mechanism for dampening immune responses. Monoclonal antibodies that bind to CTLA-4 can block this interaction and inhibit the negative regulatory signaling (Fig. 29-2). Studies in human subjects have demonstrated that CTLA-4 blockade can break peripheral tolerance to self-antigens and induce antitumor and antiself autoimmune responses.

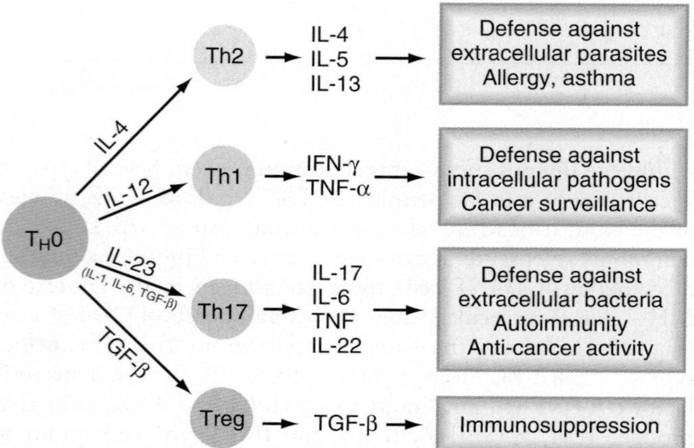

FIGURE 29-1 CD4 T Cell Subsets and Their Properties. A T_H0 cell is a naïve T cell that has differentiated successfully and undergone positive and negative selection in the thymus. Naïve helper T cells ($CD4^+$) can differentiate into several subsets whose general properties and predominant cytokine production are shown.

Another important pathway is the PD-1/PD-L1 axis in which the inhibitory ligand (PD-L1) commonly expressed in many cancers, when it engages T cell PD-1, abrogates lymphocyte activation (Fig. 29-2).[4] Interruption of this negative signaling benefits a significant proportion of patients with several solid tumors.

Although much emphasis in antitumor immunity has been focused on adaptive responses (T lymphocytes and antibodies), effector cells of the innate immune system, specifically NK cells, can act alone or in concert with adaptive immunity.[5,6] NK cells can recognize and kill target cells without prior sensitization. These cells express activating and inhibitory cell surface receptors and, when their activating receptors are engaged without concomitant ligation of their inhibitory receptors, can kill targets directly. NK cells have been traditionally viewed as providing a first line of defense against virally infected cells. NK cells can also interact with the adaptive immune system. They can modulate the function of professional antigen-presenting cells (e.g., DCs), promote the generation of Th1 responses, and potentially dampen

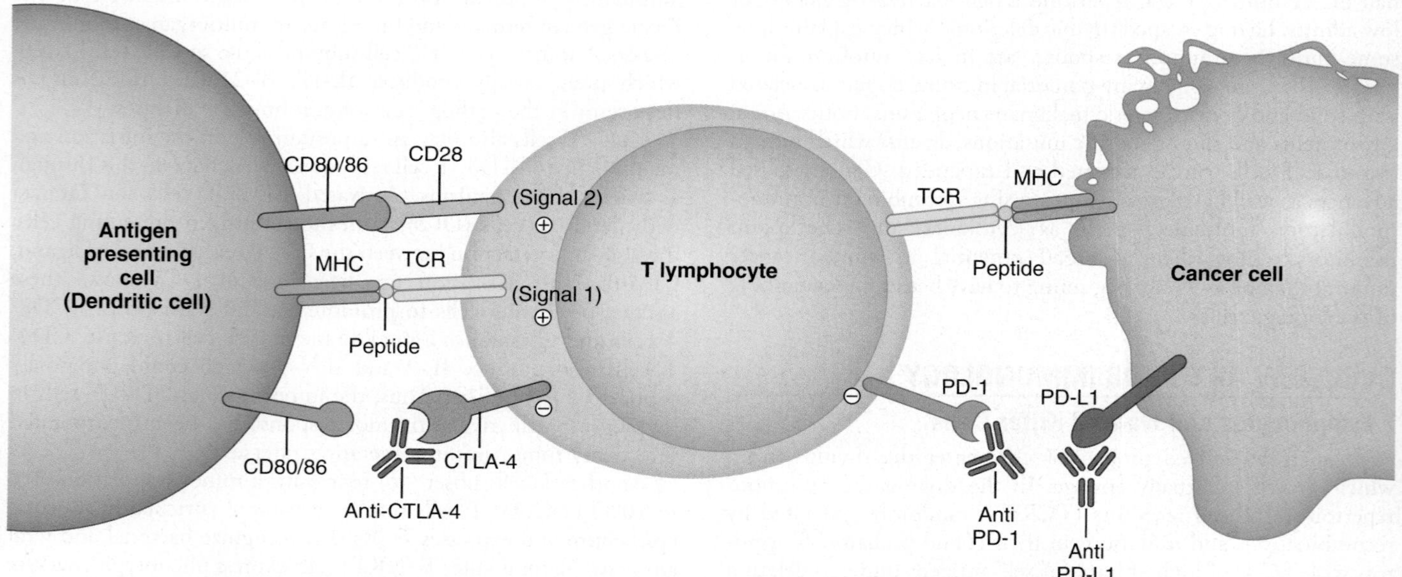

FIGURE 29-2 Important activation and inhibitory signaling in T lymphocytes and modern therapeutic interventions. Activation of T cells requires TCR engagement of antigen in the context of MHC and a second costimulatory signal, CD80/86 and CD28. Inhibitory signaling by CTLA-4 or PD-1/PD-L1 can be blocked with monoclonal antibodies.

autoimmune immunopathologic changes. Because their inhibitory receptors engage MHC molecules, NK cells specifically recognize cells that have lost MHC class I molecules, which can occur during viral infections or malignant transformation. NK cells are strongly activated by exogenous cytokines such as IL-2 and have been termed lymphokine-activated killer cells (LAK cells). LAK cells have greatly enhanced cytotoxicity for a much broader range of target cells.

The cytotoxic pathways initiated by the activation of cytotoxic T lymphocytes and NK cells include the granule-exocytosis pathway, which results in the release of membrane-destructive perforin and granzymes, and the death receptor pathways mediated by TNF-α, TRAIL, and FasL binding their cognate receptors on the target cell surface (Fig. 29-3).[7] These receptors activate the caspase cascade involving caspase 8 autoprocessing, activation of caspase 3, and cleavage of death substrates (e.g., poly[ADP-ribose] polymerase), with subsequent induction of apoptosis. Another mechanism for inducing apoptosis, which is more typical for some chemotherapeutic drugs, uses a mitochondrial pathway involving permeabilization of the mitochondrial membrane and mitochondrial collapse. Mitochondrial integrity is preserved by a balance between antiapoptotic (e.g., Bcl-2, Bcl-xL, Bfl-1/A1, Mcl-1) and proapoptotic Bcl-2 family members (e.g., Bax, Bid, Bad, Bik, Bcl-xS). Mitochondrial destabilization will facilitate the cytosolic release of apoptogenic molecules, which expedites caspase 9 activation and in turn activates caspase 3, leading to apoptosis. The expression of these gene products is tightly regulated by the activity of survival signaling pathways (nuclear factor κB, AKT/PI3K, ERK1/2, p38, and JNK).

Antigen-Presenting Cells

DCs are professional antigen-presenting cells whose role is to take up, process, and present antigen to the immune system[8]; they are essential during the initial activation of resting T cells. There are different subtypes of DCs with specialized functions that depend on their anatomic location. DCs are found in lymphoid tissues, in the skin, and on the mucosal surfaces of many organs. DCs in the gastrointestinal tract can sample bacteria in the intestinal lumen and initiate secretory immunoglobulin A (IgA) responses. In the lung, DCs help maintain tolerance to inhaled allergens. In the peripheral blood, DC precursors can migrate to sites of inflammation and initiate immune responses. DC function is powerfully modulated by a variety of receptors including Toll-like receptors (TLRs) and surface C-type lectin receptors. DCs at different stages of differentiation vary in their ability to migrate, to take up antigen by phagocytosis, and to effectively stimulate T cells. Immature DCs patrol their environment, sampling by pinocytosis and receptor-mediated endocytosis. Extracellular antigens are taken up into endosomes, which fuse with protease-containing lysosomes, and within these compartments, antigens are cleaved into peptides that can bind to MHC class II molecules and be delivered to the cell surface. Proteins in the cytoplasmic compartment of antigen-presenting cells are degraded by the proteosome and actively transported into the endoplasmic reticulum, where they are loaded onto MHC class I molecules and delivered to the cell surface. Some exogenous or environmental antigens can also find their way into the MHC class I antigen presentation pathway; this is termed *cross-presentation* and is an important mechanism for generating $CD8^+$ class I–restricted T cell responses. DCs can

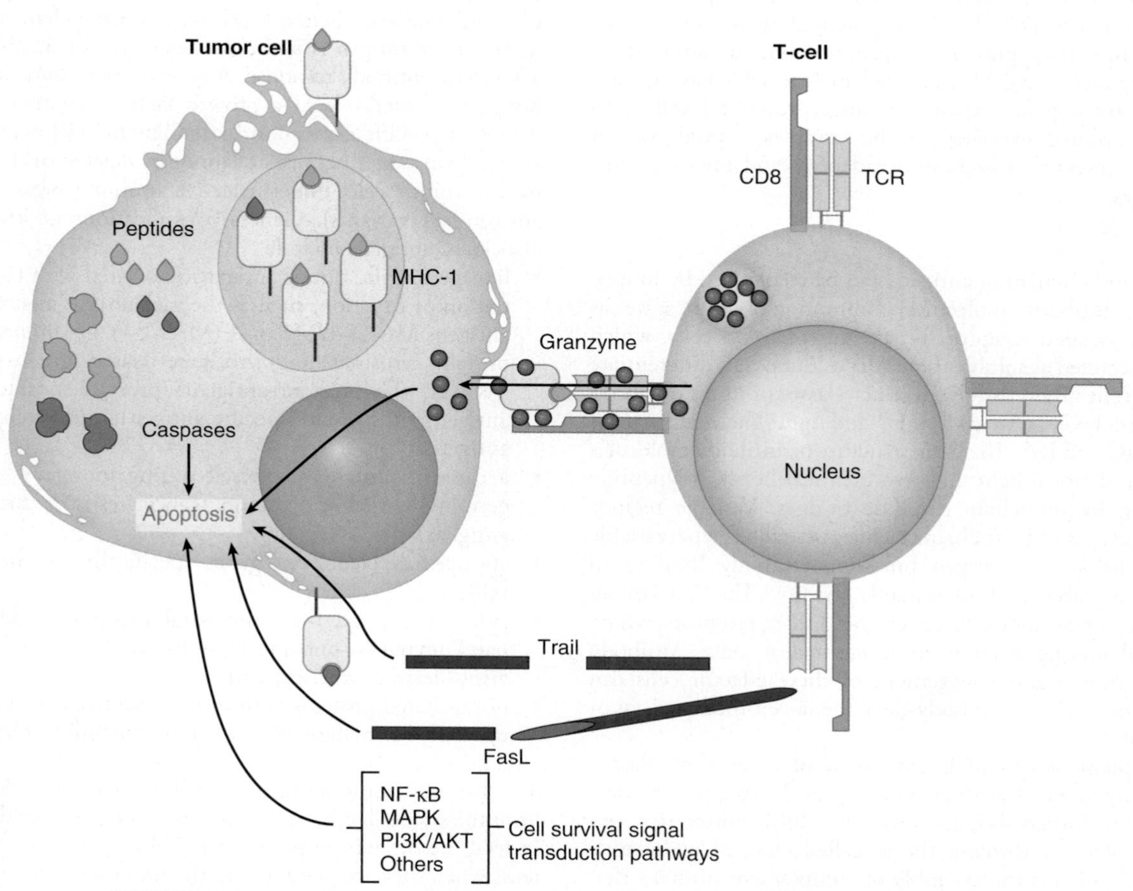

FIGURE 29-3 Mechanisms of target cell killing by cytotoxic lymphocytes (see text for details).

acquire antigen in the periphery and travel to lymph nodes, where they interact with T cells and present antigen. DCs originate from pluripotent stem cells from bone marrow, enter the blood, and localize to almost all tissues and lymphoid organs. Myeloid DCs (these include DCs found in deep epithelial tissues and Langerhans cells present in the epidermis) and plasmacytoid DCs are a major source of type I interferon.

DCs have cell surface receptors termed *pattern recognition receptors* that screen the environment for pathogens. The TLR family is the best characterized; these can recognize bacterial products (e.g., lipopolysaccharide, flagellin), viral products such as double-stranded RNA, and specific CpG-rich DNA motifs, more common in microbial genomes. These signals, along with various proinflammatory cytokines, can deliver a danger signal to DCs that establishes the context within which they see and present antigens. TLR signaling drives immature DCs into a more mature phenotype with much higher expression of MHC, costimulatory molecules, and DC-derived cytokines (such as IL-12). Immature DCs are migratory and highly efficient in antigen capture, whereas mature DCs are less mobile but more efficient in processing and presenting antigen in an immunostimulatory context.

Distinct sets of molecules govern migration of DCs to and from the periphery and to lymph nodes. Prominent among these signals are a variety of chemokines and their receptors (e.g., CCR7, CCL19, CCL21). Signals that induce maturation of immature DCs include CD40 ligand delivered by T cells as well as signals by NK cells, a variety of proinflammatory cytokines (e.g., IL-1, TNF, IL-6), and engagement of TLR and C-type lectins. The context of antigen presentation and the maturational phenotype of DCs will determine and shape the type of T cell response. Immature DCs have the potential to be tolerogenic, perhaps because they present antigen without an appropriate costimulatory second signal. Activated mature DCs have greater potency in activating and expanding antigen-reactive T cells. This is an oversimplified overview of the complex central role of various DC subsets that orchestrate adaptive and innate antitumor responses.

Antibody

Cell surface and circulating antigens can be recognized by immunoglobulins (antibody molecules). Immunoglobulins serve as membrane-associated receptors on the surface of B cells, which can then be secreted as soluble molecules as these cells differentiate into plasma cells. There are five distinct classes of immunoglobulin molecules: IgG, IgA, IgM, IgD, and IgE. There are several isotypes of IgG and IgA. The basic structure of antibody molecules includes two identical light and two identical heavy polypeptide chains linked by interchain disulfide bridges. Variable regions within the heavy and light chains create a so-called hypervariable region responsible for antigen binding. Antibody binding to antigen is reversible and of variable avidity. The C-terminal portion of certain antibody classes can bind to Fc receptors, which are expressed among a range of mononuclear cells. Antibody binding to antigen and engagement of these effector cells can trigger phagocytosis or antibody-dependent cell-mediated cytotoxicity (ADCC).

The complement system is composed of a series of plasma proteins, many of which exist as proenzymes that require cleavage for activation. Surface-bound IgG and IgM antibodies can activate complement through the so-called classical pathway, a byproduct of which is the assembly of complement proteins that effect transmembrane pore formation in target cells. Complement byproducts can also promote chemotaxis of mononuclear cells that release cytokines. Thus, complement activation not only can kill targets but can label them as pathogens for elimination. The alternative pathway allows complement activation without antibody.

Tumor Antigens

A molecular understanding of tumor recognition has been achieved only recently. The first molecularly defined antigen recognized by a tumor-reactive T cell was only discovered in 1991.[9] This advance first required elucidation of the biology of antigen processing and presentation and its interaction with MHC molecules, which occurred in the late 1980s. These discoveries demonstrated that antigens presented by MHC class I molecules were largely derived from intrinsic cytoplasmic proteins whose proteasome-degraded peptides are expressed on the cell surface in the context of MHC class I molecules, whereas antigens presented by class II MHC molecules are often environmental proteins. Mature T cells express the CD8 or CD4 coreceptor, which binds to invariant portions on all class I or class II MHC molecules, respectively. This additional ligation increases the affinity of the T cell interaction with the antigen-presenting cell. Therefore, T cells expressing CD4 typically recognize antigens presented by MHC class II molecules, and $CD8^+$ T cells usually recognize class I–presented antigens.

Cancer cells can overexpress or abnormally express a variety of normal cellular proteins. Because the human T cell repertoire can recognize self-proteins, some of these self-proteins could potentially serve as targets for immune-based therapies. As discussed in detail later, gene products resulting from tumor-specific mutations may be even better T cell targets. One characteristic of an ideal cancer antigen is its immunogenicity, or its ability to elicit a T cell or antibody response. A gene product associated with the neoplastic process (e.g., a growth factor receptor) with a high degree of specific expression by malignant cells may prove to be an excellent target because it cannot be deleted or downregulated by the tumor cells under selective immune pressure (so-called antigen-loss variants). General classifications of known tumor-associated antigens include

- lineage-specific tumor antigens associated with tissue differentiation or function, such as the melanocyte-melanoma lineage antigens MART-1/Melan-A (MART-1), gp100 protein, mda-7 protein, tyrosinase and tyrosinase-related protein (TRP-1 and TRP-2), the prostate antigens (prostate-specific membrane antigen and prostate-specific antigen), and carcinoembryonic antigen;
- a class of proteins expressed during ontogeny and in adult germline tissues and tumors (cancer-testis or cancer-germline antigens);
- epitopes derived from genes specifically mutated in tumor cells;
- epitopes derived from oncoviral processes, such as human papillomavirus oncoproteins E6 and E7 or Epstein-Barr virus–derived proteins; and
- nonmutated proteins with tumor-selective expression contributing to the malignant phenotype, including HER2/neu and hTERT.

The list of tumor antigens continues to grow. Although the immune system has been widely exposed to some of these epitopes in fetal life or later, responses can still be generated to these proteins when they are presented to the immune system in an immunostimulatory context (Box 29-1). A cytotoxic response to any

BOX 29-1 Tumor Antigens Recognized by T Cells

Tissue differentiation antigens: Specialized proteins with a functional role in the tumor's tissue of origin
- Melanoma and melanocytes, proteins involved in pigment production (e.g., tyrosinase, gp100, and MART-1)

Tumor-testis antigens: Family of proteins expressed by tumors and germline tissues but not other normal tissues
- Some identified by cloning antigens using native T cells with tumor reactivity
- Others found by serologic expression cloning using high-affinity IgGs in serum of some cancer patients (leading to discovery of T cell epitopes in these proteins)
- Examples: the MAGE family of proteins and NY-ESO-1

Proteins overexpressed after transformation: Often contribute to malignant transformation or growth but are also normal proteins with conventional functions
- Examples: normal p53 molecule (overexpressed when a mutant allele is present), erbB-2, and hTERT (from telomerase)

Tumor-specific mutations
- Mutation occurs in normal protein within a peptide naturally processed and presented from that protein
- Mutations contributing to transformation or tumor growth most significant (immune evasion by mutation loss less likely)
- Examples: CDK4, β-catenin, HLA-A*1101 (all in melanoma)

BOX 29-2 Cancer Cell Defense Mechanisms

T regulatory (Treg) cells: $CD4^+$-$CD25^+$ T cell population, which inhibits T cell function and proliferation
- In mice, deletion of these cells can induce autoimmunity
- In mice, adversely affects antitumor immunity
- Circumstantial evidence for a role in humans

CTLA-4 (CD152): Inhibitory receptor induced by T cell activation that binds to CD80 and CD86 ligands
- Blockade can induce tumor regression in some patients

PD-1 (CD279; programmed death 1): Another inhibitory receptor on T cells, prevalent on lymphocytes in the tumor microenvironment
- Binds to ligand PD-L1 (CD274); also present on some human tumors

SOCS (suppressors of cytokine signaling): Family of proteins that bind and inhibit kinases in the JAK/STAT pathway through which a number of cytokines signal

Myeloid suppressor cells: Cells of myeloid lineage that inhibit T cells
- Inhibited by a variety of putative mechanisms, including effects on dendritic cells and modulation of arginine and nitric oxide metabolism
- Accumulate in tumor-bearing state

TGF-β: Multifunctional and complex cytokine with many effects on the immune response, some of which are inhibitory

nonmutated self-protein has a risk of causing autoimmune toxicity. Directing immune responses to tumor-specific mutated antigens avoids this risk, but the patient-specific nature of such mutations hampers the generation of reagents of use in multiple patients.

The identification of the specific molecular targets on tumor cells that provoke immune responses opened the door to new approaches to the age-old concept of vaccinating patients against cancer. The concept is to generate new T cell or antibody responses to these defined targets that would induce the regression or rejection of antigen-expressing tumors. Some investigators have tried targeting known epitopes on proven antigens (identified by cloning the antigen recognized by an empirically procured tumor-reactive T cell clone), whereas others have explored generating T cells against unproven candidate antigens chosen by a favorable pattern of differential expression on tumors and normal tissues. As noted, TCRs engage small, cleaved, processed peptides bound to specific MHC molecules. From the thousands of potential antigenic proteins and millions of possible amino acid fragments within these proteins, very few are actually liberated enzymatically, are transported into the correct MHC loading compartment within the cell, and successfully bind with adequate affinity to an MHC molecule to be exported and displayed on the cell surface.

Immunosuppressive Tumor Microenvironment

There is abundant evidence that cancer cells have acquired an array of defense mechanisms to thwart their destruction by the immune system.[10] These are summarized in Box 29-2. Most human cancers present peptide epitopes in the context of MHC molecules that can be recognized by antigen-reactive T cells, but tumor cells themselves do not present antigen in an immunostimulatory context. Human T cells require additional signaling through costimulatory molecules, such as CD80/86 (B7 family), for optimal T cell activation and expansion. Without these other signals, T cells can become anergic. Tumor cells can also downregulate antigen expression by a variety of mechanisms, such as epigenetic silencing, loss of MHC expression, and loss of function of the intracellular machinery that processes and transports peptides to the cell surface.

The immune system also has complex and generally fine-tuned downregulatory signaling to modulate responses.[11] Contraction of an acute immune response after 1 to 2 weeks may be appropriate for a viral infection but will be counterproductive to rejecting a large mass of malignant tissue. Autoimmune and allograft immune responses represent the types of chronic ongoing processes that would favor antitumor immune responses and underscore the need for a better understanding of the basic biology of immune regulation.

In addition to CTLA-4 signaling (see earlier), negative signaling can also be transduced through programmed death receptor 1 (PD-1). DCs express the programmed death receptor ligand PD-L1 (or B7-H1); its expression by DCs can skew T cells toward an unresponsive phenotype.[3,12] DCs found within the tumor microenvironment have been shown to express high levels of PD-L1, which contribute to decreased local T cell function. Some tumor cells themselves can present this inhibitory ligand, and expression of PD-L1, as with renal cancer, is associated with a poorer clinical outcome. Blockade of this PD-L1/PD-1 interaction using decoy receptors or antibodies is effective in improving immune therapies in animal models and when translated into human cancer immunotherapy trials has yielded impressive antitumor responses (see later).

A small subpopulation of $CD4^+$ T cells (5% to 10%) constitutively express the α chain of the IL-2 receptor CD25; most of these cells also express transcription factor Foxp3 (a forkhead-winged helix family member) and GITR (glucocorticoid-induced tumor necrosis factor receptor) as well as CTLA-4. These cells, Treg cells, produce immunosuppressive cytokines such as IL-10 and transforming growth factor-β (TGF-β) and can also inhibit through cell contact–dependent mechanisms. Mice or humans with a genetic mutation in Foxp3 lack Treg cells and develop a fulminant and lethal autoimmune disorder. Animal studies have clearly shown that Treg cells are responsible for suppressing the self-reactive T cell repertoire, and the clinical manifestations from genetic loss of Foxp3 suggest that this may also be true in humans. Human Treg cells are enriched in tumor specimens and in draining lymph nodes of many solid tumors, and there is emerging evidence supporting a dominant role in suppressing self-reactive antitumor immune responses. Moderating Treg cell function could potentially favor antitumor immune responses. The use of lymphodepleting strategies before adoptive cell therapy (described later), which clearly enhances the antitumor biology of adoptively transferred T cells, may be caused in part by the depletion of host resident Treg cells.

Myeloid-derived suppressor cells (MDSCs) and tumor-associated macrophages are found in increased numbers in the bone marrow, blood, and lymphoid organs of tumor-bearing mice. These MDSCs include granulocytes and immature myelomonocytic precursors. They clearly suppress T cell function through a variety of mechanisms. Although not as well studied in human solid tumors, MDSCs have been isolated and have an immunosuppressive phenotype.

Tumors themselves, and at times tumor stroma, can produce immunosuppressive substances; a prominent factor is TGF-β. TGF-β directly inhibits cytotoxic T cell activation, cytokine production, helper T cell responses, and activation of DCs and can promote the differentiation of Treg cells. Inhibition of TGF-β can have a salutary effect on antitumor immunity. T cells rendered insensitive to TGF-β signaling using a dominant-negative receptor have enhanced function in vivo. Neutralizing antibodies, small molecule inhibitors, and engineered T cells are currently under study in clinical trials. Vascular endothelial growth factor (VEGF) is important in angiogenesis but can also inhibit the function of DCs. Thus, anti-VEGF therapy could also function through an immune mechanism. An isoform of the enzyme cyclooxygenase 2 is overexpressed in many tumors and catalyzes the synthesis of prostaglandin E2. Prostaglandin E2 has a generally adverse impact on the immune system, particularly on DC and T cell function.

Amino acid metabolism can profoundly affect immune cell function; two key amino acids in this respect are arginine and tryptophan. Indoleamine 2,3-dioxygenase (IDO) metabolizes the essential amino acid L-tryptophan and arginase metabolizes arginine. High levels of either enzyme are associated with functional inhibition of T cells and other cell populations, such as DCs. IDO overexpression has been observed in a variety of human cancers and can be an independent adverse prognostic factor. IDO can also be induced in DCs and macrophages in the tumor microenvironment by Treg cells. A specific small molecule inhibitor of IDO, 1-methyl-tryptophan, and a similar inhibitor for arginase, *N*-methylarginine, are being studied preclinically and clinically.

IMMUNOTHERAPY

Cytokine Therapy

The cellular immune system often communicates among its component cells and exerts its effector functions using secreted proteins that bind to specific receptors. These secreted proteins are referred to as cytokines, and most often, they act in a paracrine fashion, exerting their action on cells in their local environment. The family of interleukins (which currently includes more than 35 members) has a protean scope of interactions. In the clinical use, several cytokines have been demonstrated to be of value, typically administered in pharmacologic doses as systemic agents.

Although the interferons (type I interferons, consisting of the many species of IFN-α and IFN-β; and type II interferon, which consists only of IFN-γ) have important and diverse roles in immunity, they have limited clinical utility. Systemically administered IFN-α has some activity against renal cancer, hairy cell leukemia, chronic myeloid leukemia, and HIV-associated Kaposi sarcoma, but interferon for all these diseases has largely been superseded by other more effective biologicals.

IL-2 was the first cytokine to demonstrate reproducibly curative outcomes in patients with several types of widely metastatic cancer. Multiorgan toxicity is observed with high-dose IL-2 administration, including hypotension, capillary leak, transient hepatic and renal insufficiency, and mental status changes, which are in many ways reminiscent of events in sepsis. Toxicity is managed by judicious limitations on IL-2 dosing, fluid management, and supportive care because these toxicities are almost always self-limited and fully reversible. In an experienced clinical environment, the treatment-related mortality of high-dose IL-2 should be no more than 1%, with some centers reporting more than 800 consecutive courses administered without death.[13] Initial studies of IL-2 included patients with tumors of many histologic types, but it soon became apparent that the two most consistently responsive cancers are melanoma and renal cell cancer (RCC). For patients with metastatic disease, the objective response rates (partial and complete) for melanoma and RCC were approximately 15% and 20%, respectively.[14,15] Whereas the response rate was not remarkable, some of these patients (4% to 7%) achieved complete regression of widespread disease, responses that have proved durable more than 20 years (Fig. 29-4).[16,17] The ability to cure widely metastatic solid tumors with any systemic treatment is rare. However, for patients with RCC and melanoma, those achieving a complete response rarely relapsed. Considerable efforts have failed to provide predictors of which patients will respond to IL-2. For patients with metastatic clear cell renal cancer, two randomized studies have suggested that high-dose IL-2 regimens produce higher response rates (22% partial and complete responses with high-dose treatments versus 12% with lower dose regimens) as well as more durable responses than with low-dose regimens, but they were underpowered to evaluate differences in overall survival.[18]

There have been numerous clinical efforts to combine cytokines with other agents, particularly chemotherapy, to improve efficacy. Biochemotherapy using combinations of cisplatin, vinblastine, and dacarbazine (DTIC) with IL-2 and IFN-α, in general, have failed to show any survival benefit and had increased toxicity. Combinations of IL-2 and IFN-α had a similar clinical trials history: no improvement in response but increased toxicity. Use of biologic therapies in the adjuvant setting after complete resection of high-risk local regional melanoma remains controversial. The U.S. Food and Drug Administration (FDA) has approved the use of high-dose IFN-α (1 month of maximal-dose intravenous therapy followed by 11 months of lower dose subcutaneous treatment) after resection of node-positive melanoma on the basis of a randomized prospective study showing a delay in time to progression and borderline improved overall survival. In subsequent follow-up, the survival benefit in the original study was no longer significant, and a larger randomized study showed delayed time to progression, with no survival benefit.[19] Underpowered attempts to demonstrate a benefit of adjuvant IL-2 administration for high-risk melanoma have never suggested a benefit. This

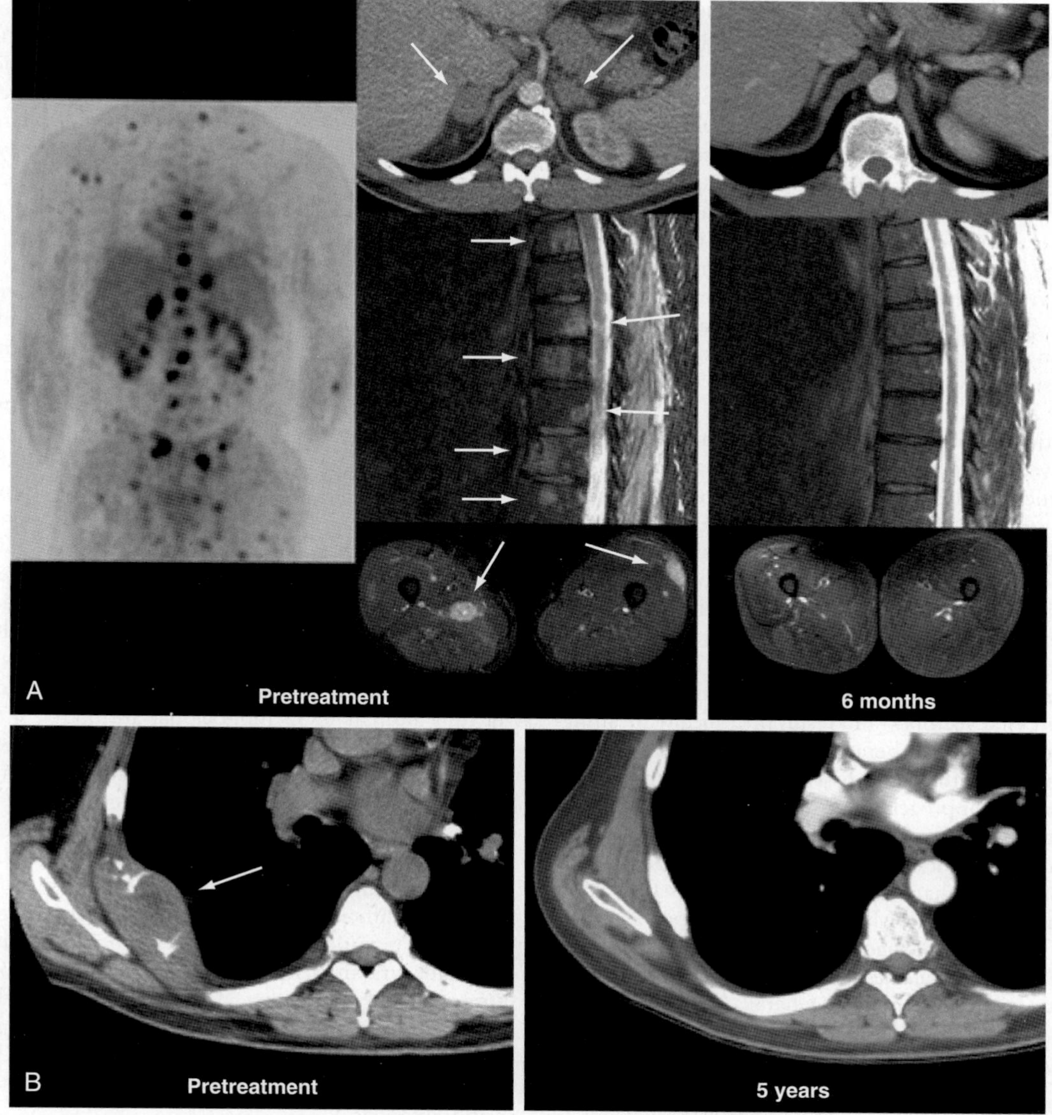

FIGURE 29-4 Complete responses to high-dose IL-2. **A,** Patient with diffuse metastatic melanoma by computed tomography and positron emission tomography scanning who received high-dose IL-2 therapy and had complete regression of all measurable disease, which is still ongoing 2 years later. **B,** Patient with multiple bone metastases from RCC, with a complete response sustained 5 years later.

should not be surprising because a drug that achieves responses in a small minority of patients in a metastatic setting may require enormously powered studies to evaluate it properly in the adjuvant setting.

Several other cytokines have been studied. IL-15 is a T cell and NK cell growth factor that also inhibits antigen-induced T cell death, in contrast to IL-2. IL-7 is another T cell growth factor with a role in homeostatic T cell expansion in response to lymphopenia; it causes dramatic increases in total body $CD4^+$ and $CD8^+$ T cells when it is administered to human subjects. IL-21 is another T cell growth factor that has been reported to cause tumor regressions in one early clinical study. Yet the systemic use of these agents as monotherapy for the treatment of cancer has not progressed beyond these early studies. Ultimately, their role may be in combination with other more potent immunotherapeutic agents.

Vaccines

Successful presentation of a peptide epitope on an MHC molecule does not automatically result in a brisk T cell response (see Fig. 29-2). To initiate a good T cell response, an antigen must be presented to the immune system along with appropriate costimulatory molecules (signal 2, where the peptide MHC complex is signal 1), or it may be rendered anergic instead of reactive. The CD28 receptor usually serves this coreceptor function, although other mechanisms exist. Another important principle is that even well-presented normal self-proteins are general weak immunogens; the most avid self-reactive T cell clones have been in the thymus.

Early cancer vaccine strategies used autologous or allogeneic cell-based vaccines. These efforts were based on half-century-old studies with carcinogen-induced murine tumor models. Whole cell vaccines contain multiple antigens that could be cross-presented by host antigen-presenting cells (DCs) and whose function could be further enhanced with an adjuvant. Initial crude adjuvants such as alum and the tuberculosis vaccine bacille Calmette-Guérin (BCG) have been replaced by molecules such as imiquimod or unmethylated CG dinucleotides, which stimulate antigen-presenting cells through TLRs. The results of whole tumor cell vaccine trials have been disappointing. The largest randomized study of an allogeneic cancer vaccine used three carefully selected melanoma cell lines with BCG (Canvaxin) in patients with stage III or resected stage IV melanoma and showed no impact on survival. Even when whole cell tumor vaccines were genetically engineered to produce cytokines such as granulocyte-macrophage colony-stimulating factor with adjuvant activities, no improvement in survival was observed in recently conducted randomized trials.

The identification of tumor rejection antigens and their specific epitopes has allowed new molecularly driven approaches to tumor vaccines. These include the use of synthetic peptides instead of whole cells or proteins (thus bypassing inefficient antigen-processing pathways) and incorporation of genes encoding these antigens into recombinant viral vectors to allow specific antigens to be more effectively targeted. Cell-based vaccines have employed in vitro–generated DCs. These DC-based vaccines have incorporated a variety of strategies—pulsing DCs with immunogenic peptide, genetically engineering with defined tumor antigens using recombinant viral vectors—and result in clinically meaningful tumor responses in a small percentage of patients with melanoma and perhaps a few other cancers (Fig. 29-5). The application of multiple vaccination approaches against cancer-associated antigens has not led to consistent success in causing cancer regression. Dozens of vaccine approaches against dozens of target antigens in hundreds of clinical trials have largely been unsuccessful against measurable metastatic disease. Many trials have reported infrequent anecdotal responses, primarily in patients with melanoma confined to the skin and nodal sites, which appear to be somewhat more amenable to immunotherapy in general. A review of more than 1200 patients vaccinated for cancer reported an overall objective response rate of 3.6%.[20] Analyses of these trials have shown that there is little evidence for the generation of significant numbers of new tumor-reactive T cells by most vaccines. Whereas there is clear evidence that many vaccine formulations can activate and expand tumor antigen–reactive T cells, they are still inadequate as stand-alone treatments and may need to be used in combination, perhaps with immunomodulation reagents.

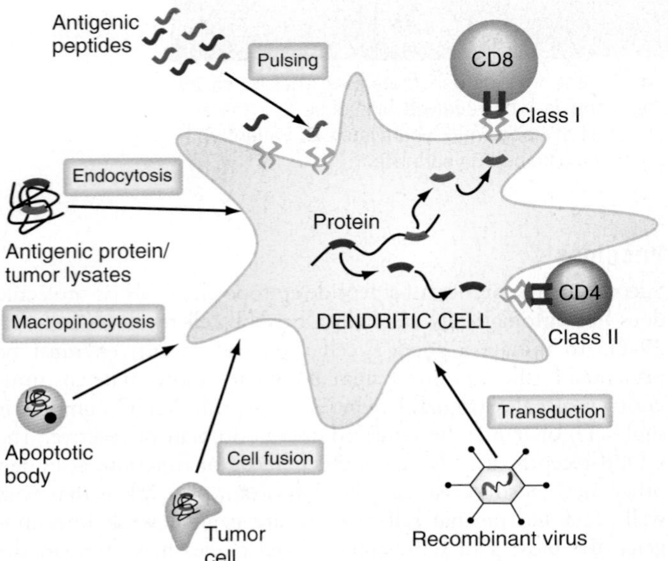

FIGURE 29-5 Tumor Antigen Acquisition by Dendritic Cells. These professional antigen-presenting cells can acquire and process antigen through endocytosis or pinocytosis or be manipulated ex vivo with peptide loading or genetic engineering to produce a cell-based vaccine.

Targeting Immunomodulatory Pathways

Although the two-signal model (TCR engagement plus costimulatory signal) has been largely validated, the adaptive immune response is modulated by additional costimulatory and coinhibitory signals as it orchestrates an appropriate antigen-reactive response. With respect to antitumor immunity, preclinical animal studies that have been translated into human cancer trials have shown, in particular, that the blockade of coinhibitory molecules such as CTLA-4 and PD-1/PDL-1 can yield dramatic and durable tumor regressions in several types of solid tumors (Fig. 29-6). CTLA-4, through engagement with its ligands CD80 and CD86, attenuates activation and expansion of antigen-reactive T cells; it can be thought of as one of the "breaking" mechanisms of the immune system. Monoclonal antibodies that block CTLA-4 in humans have been developed: ipilimumab, now FDA approved (a fully human IgG1k monoclonal antibody); and tremelimumab (a fully human IgG2 monoclonal antibody). CTLA-4 blockade has demonstrated a significant survival advantage and long-term benefit in a minority of melanoma patients (approximately 10%) but has only rare activity against other tumors.[21] The significant toxicities of CTLA-4 blockade are autoimmune in nature and directed toward skin (rash, vitiligo), bowel (diarrhea, colitis), liver (hepatitis), and endocrine tissues (hypophysitis, hypothyroidism, adrenal insufficiency) with a resultant mortality of approximately 1%. The remarkable antitumor responses initiated by CTLA-4 blockade are mediated by the dense infiltration of metastatic tumor by T lymphocytes. These antitumor T cells as well as the anti–self-reactive T cells mediating the autoimmune side effects presumably preexisted in these patients and were held in check by CTLA-4 inhibition until this was released with this blocking antibody.

A second coinhibitory receptor expressed on T cells is PD-1, which is engaged by its ligands PD-L1 and PD-L2. PD-L1 and to a lesser extent PD-L2 are expressed by a broad range of human malignant neoplasms—melanoma, non–small cell lung cancer, colon, breast, urothelial, ovarian, and pancreatic as well as hematologic cancers. Engagement of PD-1 by these tumor-expressed ligands now appears to be an important mechanism by which some human cancers evade an otherwise effective antitumor immune response. Monoclonal antibodies directed against PD-1 or PD-L1, with the goal of interrupting this inhibitory signaling, are undergoing extensive testing in human cancer trials.[22] Anti–PD-1 monoclonal antibodies produced clinical responses in patients with melanoma, renal cancer, bladder cancer, and non–small cell lung cancer ranging from 15% to 30% (Fig. 29-7). In some trials, the response rate in melanoma approached 50%, with a significant minority being complete responses. PD-L1–specific monoclonal antibodies likewise have shown activity in phase 1 clinical trials for patients with melanoma, renal cancer, and non–small cell lung cancer. CTLA-4 and PD-1/PD-L1 coinhibitory signaling plays a nonredundant role in immune regulation; blockade of CTLA-4 acts on activated naïve and memory T cells, whereas blockade of PD-1/PD-L1 interrupts negative signaling in

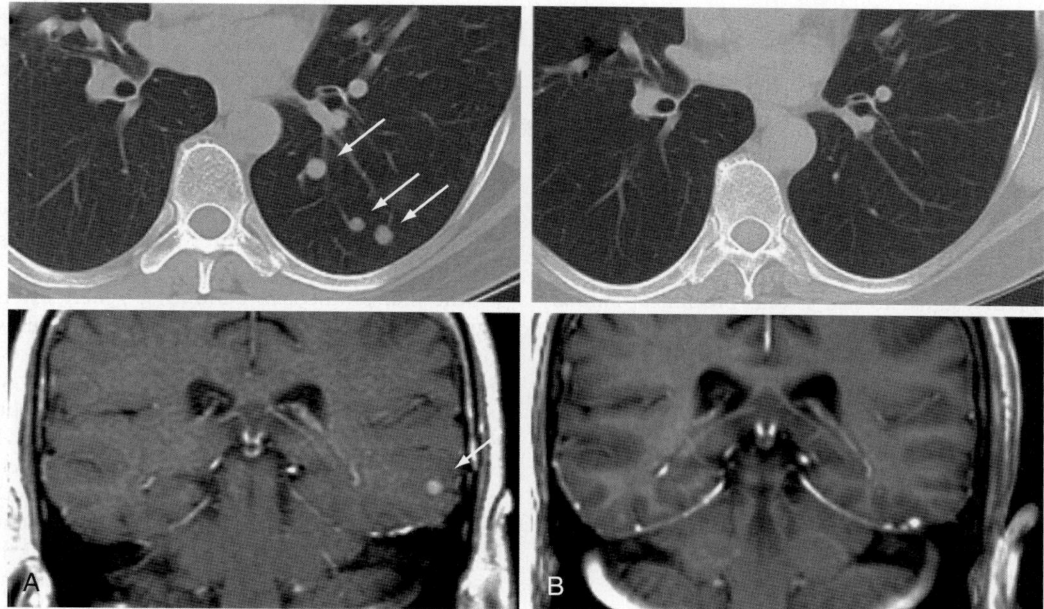

FIGURE 29-6 Regression of lung and brain metastases from melanoma in a patient treated with ipilimumab (anti–CTLA-4 antibody). **A,** Patient with lung, subcutaneous, and brain metastases received ipilimumab. **B,** He then developed immune-mediated hypopituitarism but achieved a complete regression of all disease, which is ongoing 7 years later.

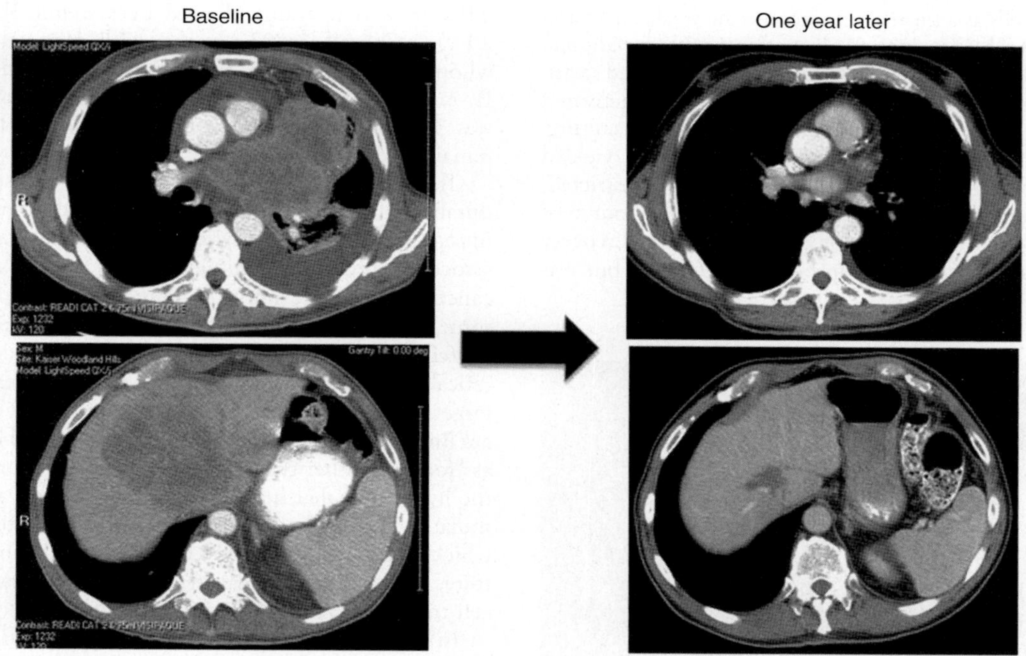

FIGURE 29-7 Response of bulky metastatic melanoma to PD-1–blocking antibody. A dramatic response during a period of a year in a patient who failed to respond to biochemotherapy, high-dose IL-2, and CTLA-4–blocking antibody.

the tumor microenvironment. Based on these mechanisms and sites of action, PD-1/PD-L1–directed therapies predictably have far fewer side effects and can produce antitumor responses in patients who fail to respond to CTLA-4 blockade. One anti–PD-1 antibody, pembrolizumab, has recently been approved by the FDA for patients with treatment-refractory metastatic melanoma.

Our improved understanding of human tumor immune biology afforded by these clinically active checkpoint inhibitors provides many opportunities for their use in combination, with modern cancer vaccines and with T cell–based therapies (see later).

The objective response criteria for immune therapies cannot be accommodated by the response criteria in use for many decades with cytotoxic chemotherapies. For these immunomodulatory therapies, the kinetics of response may be very slow and the achievement of a complete response may evolve during 1 to 2 years, making overall survival the most significant objective response criterion. These observations underscore the need for better biomarkers to predict and to confirm responses.

Immune modulation can also be positively driven by stimulation of coreceptors, which enhances immunity. A receptor-like protein expressed on $CD4^+$ and $CD8^+$ T cells after activation is 4-1BB (CD137); cross-linking of 4-1BB with a ligand or antibody delivers a costimulatory signal to the T cell. Preclinical animal studies have demonstrated enhanced tumor rejection in established tumor models. This strategy for immunomodulation using an agonist anti-CD137 human monoclonal antibody is undergoing trials in human subjects. Another early clinical trial using an agonist antibody to CD40, an activating receptor on DCs, showed objective tumor regressions, again all in patients with melanoma. Combining such activating strategies with blocking of inhibitory receptors and perhaps vaccines may be needed to achieve more impressive and consistent clinical responses.

T Cell Adoptive Therapy

With the recognition that T lymphocytes are the effectors of tumor rejection and immunologic memory in animal models, early human studies focused on tumor-reactive lymphocytes isolated from patients with IL-2–responsive cancers, largely in melanoma. The basic approach was to isolate, expand, and readminister tumor-reactive T cells as a means to overcome the weak expansion of such cells in vivo by vaccination. In patients with melanoma, more than 80% of metastatic lesions were enriched with such resident tumor-reactive T cells, which could be activated and expanded in vitro simply by adding IL-2 to cell culture. These tumor-infiltrating lymphocyte (TIL) cultures yielded large numbers of oligoclonal populations of MHC-restricted, melanoma-reactive effector cells (Fig. 29-8). This rich source of polyclonal tumor-reactive T cells not only served as a discovery tool for numerous shared antigens in human melanoma but was

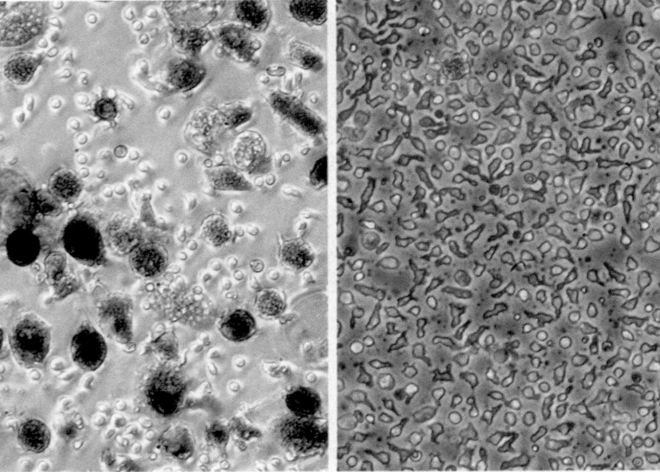

FIGURE 29-8 Expansion of TILs from resected metastatic melanoma in culture with IL-2. Photomicrograph of fresh melanoma after enzymatic dispersal *(left)* shows tumor cells and small numbers of infiltrating lymphocytes. After several weeks of culture in IL-2, there is T cell outgrowth and lysis of all tumor cells *(right)*, with most cultures then demonstrating immunologic recognition of tumor.

critical in demonstrating that the transfer of ex vivo expanded autologous tumor-reactive T cells could cause complete and durable regressions of metastatic cancer. The initial attempt at such an approach used huge numbers of cells grown in vitro (a median of 2×10^{11} cells were administered to patients), supported with high-dose systemic IL-2 to enhance TIL survival and in vivo function.[23] An overall objective response rate of 33% was seen and was not influenced by prior IL-2 failure. However, the major shortcoming of this study was that most responses were of short duration (median, 7 months).

The first protocol to administer genetically modified cells to humans was used to track TILs after administration using a marker gene and showed that almost all infused TILs had disappeared from the circulation within days.[24,25] A chemotherapy-induced lymphodepletion regimen before adoptive transfer was found to enhance lymphocyte survival and to improve T cell persistence. Murine models suggest that the mechanisms were (1) removal of suppressive Treg cells; (2) stimulation of T cell growth factors in the host in response to lymphodepletion (homeostatic proliferation); (3) reduction in competition for these homeostatic cytokines from endogenous T cells or NK cells; and (4) increased immunostimulatory microbial factors, such as lipopolysaccharide. In clinical protocols, several immunosuppressive regimens have been used to deplete host lymphocytes. The basic regimen consisted of high-dose cyclophosphamide and fludarabine, with some patients also receiving total body irradiation. When peripheral leukocyte counts are essentially zero, a median of 5×10^{10} cultured TILs are given, again followed by systemic IL-2 support (Fig. 29-9).[26] Overall, in 93 patients with metastatic melanoma, of whom 86% had visceral tumor involvement and 84% had prior IL-2, the objective response rate was 56% and the 5-year survival was 30%; 19 of the 20 patients achieving complete regressions remain free of disease 5 to 10 years later.

There is emerging evidence that the TILs mediating these durable regressions may in fact be directed not toward the shared lineage-specific melanocytic antigens but rather to tumor-associated mutations unique to each patient's tumor. Human cancers accumulate multiple mutations in their gene products, some driving the cancer process and many other "bystander" proteins resulting from carcinogens and genetic instability. Theoretically, such mutated proteins would be the ideal tumor rejection targets; the amino acid changes may not affect protein function, are limited to the tumor, and may be seen by the immune system as "foreign" rather than "self." These observations have generated the hypothesis that human cancers with larger numbers of accumulated mutations may present more mutated "neoepitopes," which in turn provides for a more robust antitumor T cell repertoire, a repertoire that can be exploited clinically with adoptive cell transfer or release of inhibitory signaling.[27]

In the field of adoptive T cell therapy, the advent of efficient gene engineering methods for human T cells has enabled novel approaches to generate tumor-reactive T cells. Recombinant gamma retroviruses and lentiviruses can introduce new genes into mature human peripheral blood T cells with high efficiency. These techniques have been applied to introduce genes encoding a variety of receptors that can recognize targets on tumors and trigger a T cell response. There are several types of such receptors in clinical trials. The traditional two-chain TCR consists of α and β chains that engage the peptide-MHC complex of a tumor antigen and transduce a signal by noncovalent association with the CD3 complex in the T cell. Another receptor, termed chimeric antigen receptor (CAR), uses an antigen-binding extracellular

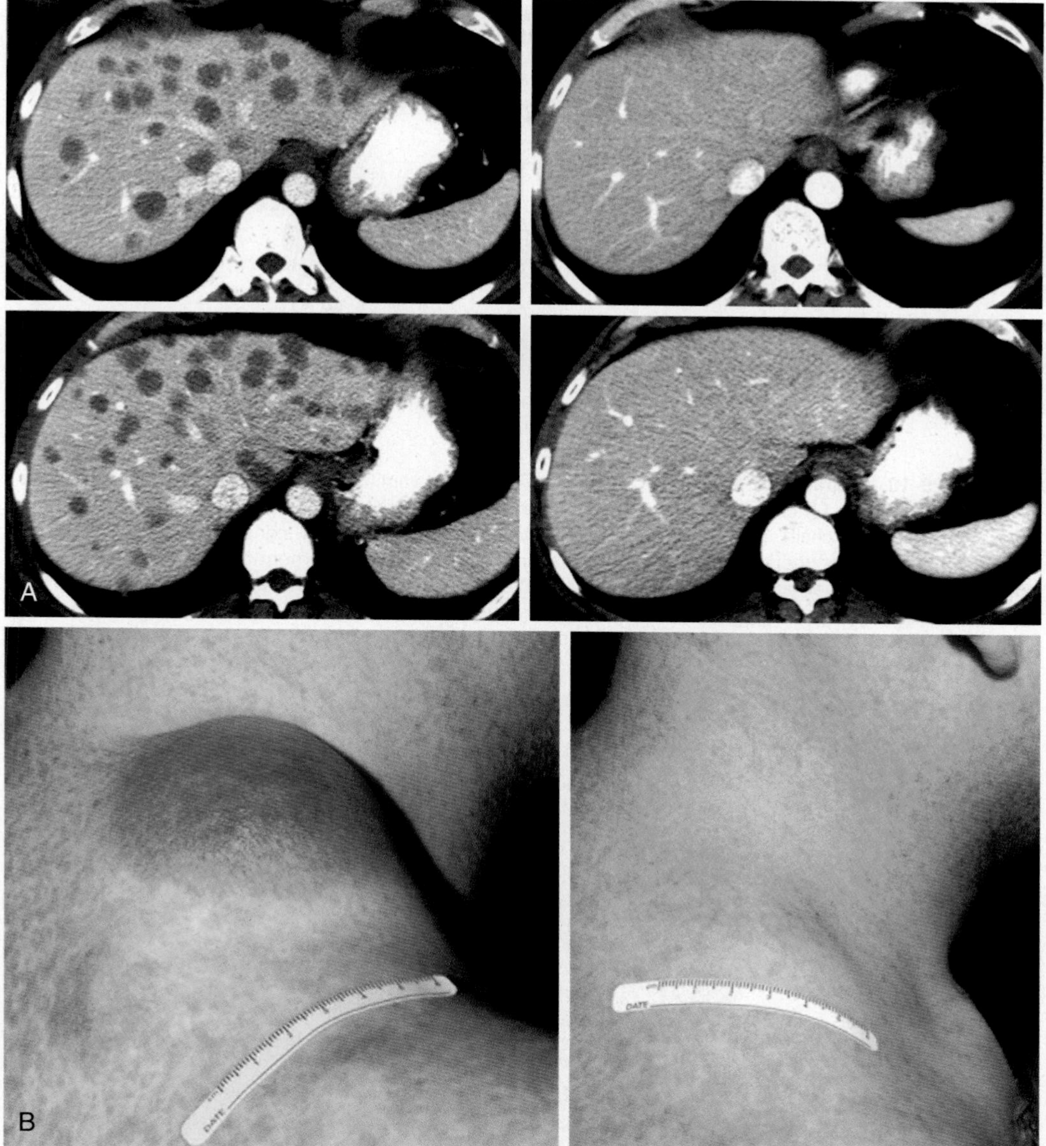

FIGURE 29-9 Clinical responses in patients with metastatic melanoma to adoptive transfer of in vitro expanded TILs with systemic IL-2, following preparative lymphodepletion. Responses can be durable and rapid. **A,** Patient with extensive liver disease remains free of disease more than 5 years after one T cell transfer. **B,** Another patient showed rapid regression of bulky subcutaneous disease only 12 days after cell transfer, achieving a complete response, durable at 4 years.

domain (often a single-chain version of the Fab fragment of a monoclonal antibody) covalently linked in tandem to a transmembrane domain and the CD3 ζ molecule for signal transduction (Fig. 29-10). Several generations of CAR receptors employ different intracellular signaling moieties, such as CD28 or CD137 (4-1BB). These antibody-based CARs bind to a target molecule expressed on the external surface of the cell membrane and therefore have the advantage of not being MHC restricted. Traditional two-chain TCRs (encoded in a bicistronic retroviral vector) have been used to successfully target pigment-related antigens in melanoma, such as MART-1 and gp100, and to achieve tumor regressions (Fig. 29-11). Expression of the same target molecules by melanocytes of the skin, anterior eye, and inner ear resulted in "on-target, off-tumor" toxicities that can be limiting (rash, uveitis, and hearing loss). These sometimes dramatic clinical events underscore the remarkable potency of adoptive cell transfer to find and to kill antigen-positive cells throughout the body. Similar results have been observed when carcinoembryonic antigen was targeted; while producing some evidence of tumor regression, this therapy was accompanied by severe colitis. The use of a TCR against the NY-ESO-1 protein, a more tumor-specific cancer-germline antigen, has been shown to induce high rates of regressions of melanoma and synovial sarcoma without apparent normal tissue toxicity. These impressive clinical responses and off-target toxicities further emphasize the importance of identifying tumor-restricted antigen targets.

CARs use the Fab portion of the antibody molecule as the recognition unit of surface antigens. The most successful effort to

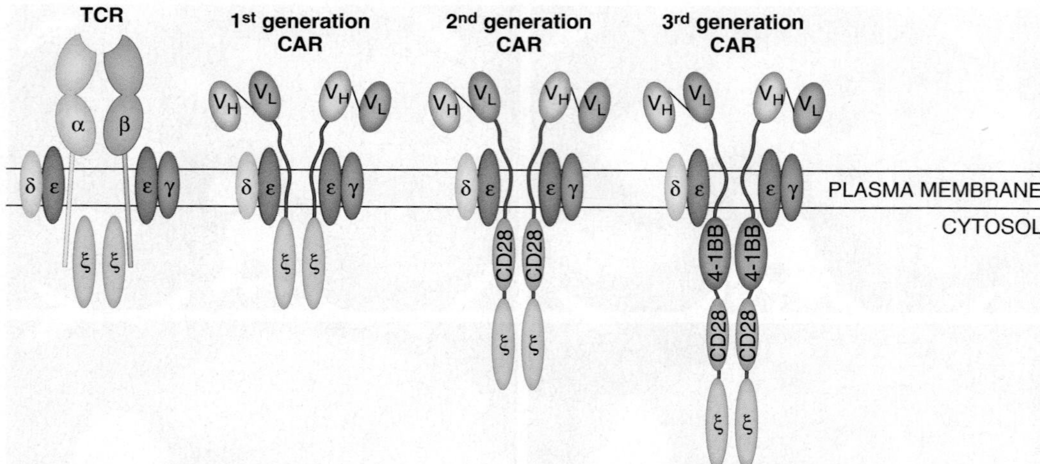

FIGURE 29-10 Illustration of a native T cell receptor (TCR) and various chimeric antigen receptors (CARs). The native TCR α and β chains noncovalently associate with the CD3 complex consisting of two ζ chains, two ε chains, one γ chain, and one δ chain to transduce a T cell activation signal. First-generation CARs covalently attach an antigen-binding domain from a single-chain variable fragment of a monoclonal antibody to the ζ chain of CD3, which then associates with the remainder of the CD3 complex to signal. Second- and third-generation CARs add one or two interposed costimulation domains (respectively) from a variety of T cell costimulators to enhance activation (here illustrated with CD28 and 4-1BB).

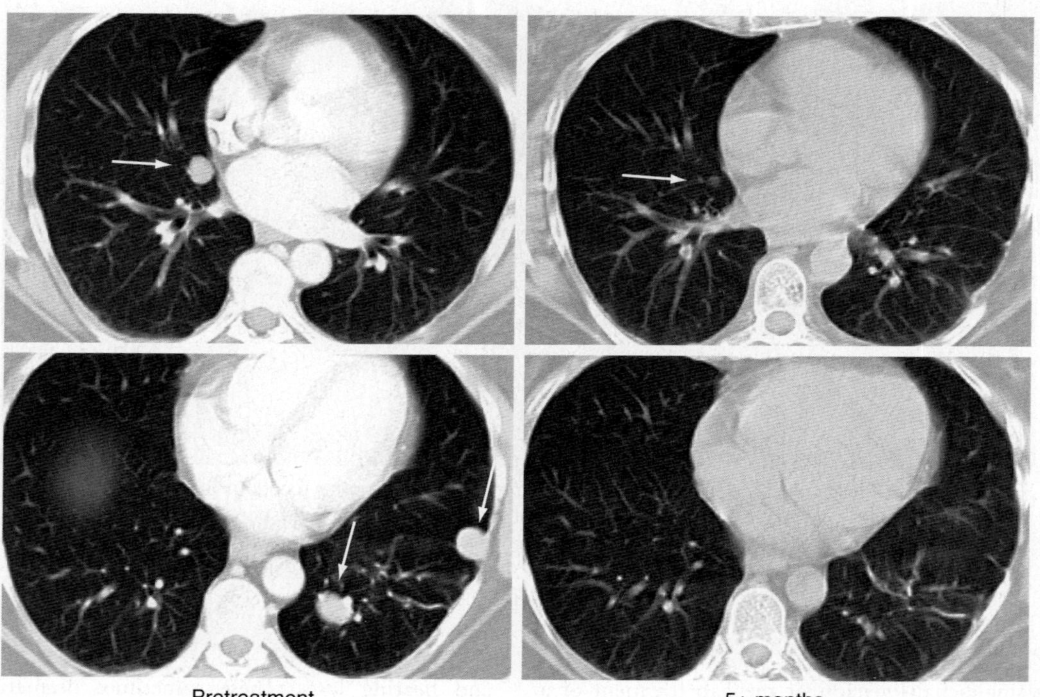

FIGURE 29-11 Patient with metastatic melanoma responding to MART melanoma antigen TCR-engineered T cell adoptive immunotherapy.

date has been in targeting the CD19 molecule on B cell malignant neoplasms (Fig. 29-12). Several versions of an anti-CD19 CAR have moved into clinical trials, in which they have shown dramatic effects against chemotherapy-refractory chronic lymphocytic leukemia, diffuse large B cell lymphoma, and acute lymphocytic leukemia.[28] Patients undergoing CD19 CAR treatment also generally develop B cell aplasia because CD19 is expressed by normal B cells; this can be successfully managed with immunoglobulin infusion and infection control and is considered an acceptable toxicity. The response rate in early phase 1/2 trials with patients has been high. Overall, these various T cell adoptive therapy trials have demonstrated that the infusion of tumor-reactive T cells can be a potent new therapeutic modality but will require target antigens of the highest specificity to be administered safely.

Monoclonal Antibody Therapy

The concept of the immune system's providing targeted therapy in the treatment of disease has its origins in experiments

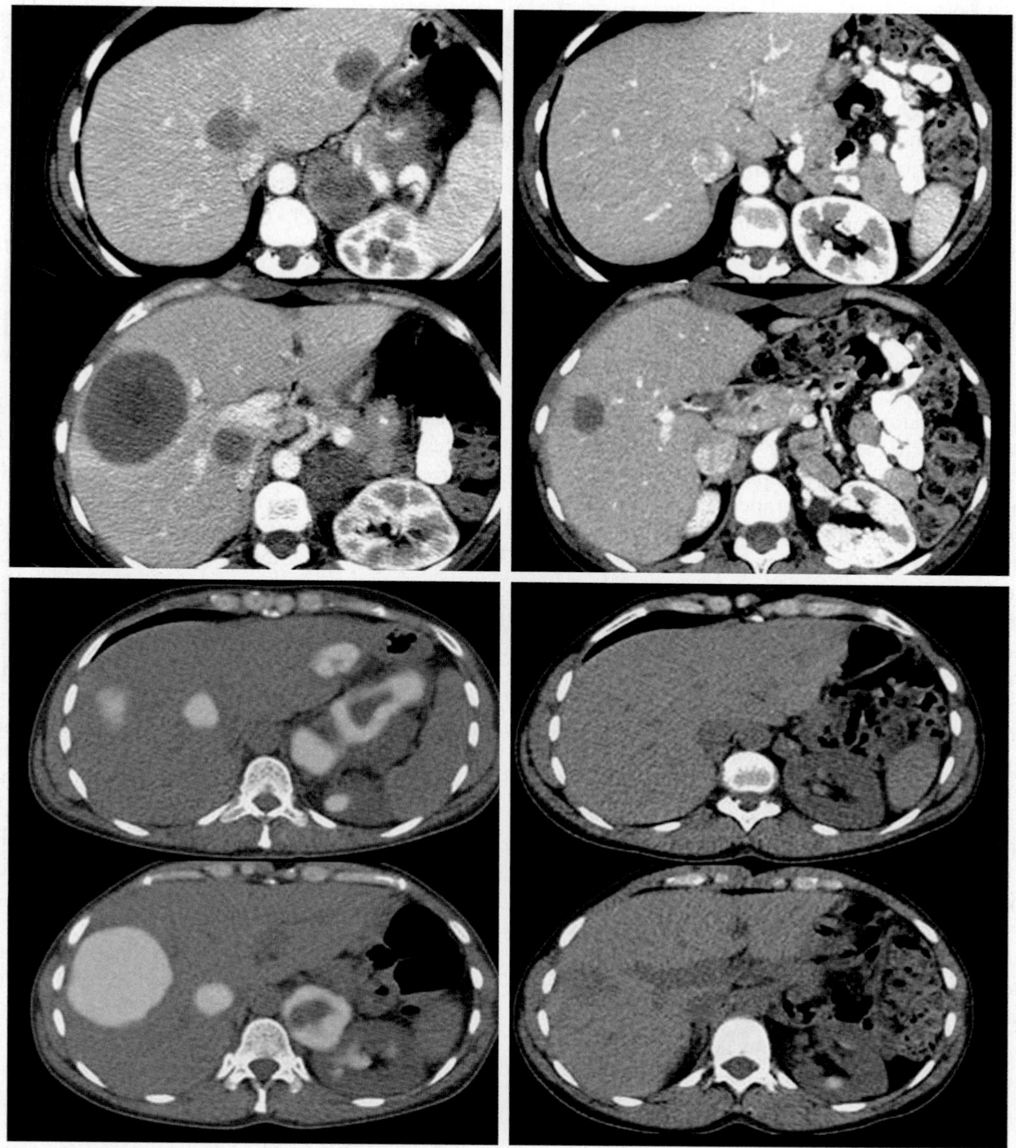

FIGURE 29-12 Positron emission tomography/computed tomography scan of a patient with chemotherapy-resistant diffuse large B cell lymphoma. Pretreatment scan on the left demonstrates liver, gastric, and retroperitoneal lymph node involvement. The patient received CD19 CAR adoptive cell therapy and achieved complete response. Scan on right taken at 13 months of follow-up (liver residual metabolically inactive).

performed in 1890 by von Behring and Kitasato. They determined that immunity to infectious diseases could be transferred from one rat to the next through a serum transfusion; they coined the term *passive serotherapy.* The first application of passive serotherapy in the treatment of cancer was performed in 1895 by Hericourt and Richet, when they immunized dogs with human sarcoma and transferred the serum to patients in an attempt to provide cancer immunity. After almost 100 years since the first cancer immunotherapy trial, the FDA approved the first monoclonal antibody to be used in the treatment of cancer. Today, therapeutic monoclonal antibodies are considered to be the fastest growing class of new therapeutic agents. Although many had predicted the therapeutic potential of monoclonal antibodies during the past century, it was not until mouse hybridoma technology was developed by Kohler and Milstein in 1975 that the ability to produce monoclonal antibodies directed against a specific target antigen became a reality.[29,30]

Unfortunately, monoclonal antibodies created from mouse hybridoma technology were specific but limited in their therapeutic potential secondary to xenogeneic reasons. First, they are recognized by the immune system as foreign and stimulate the production of human anti-mouse antibodies, commonly referred to as the HAMA response. This immunogenic response usually limits murine monoclonal antibodies to a single dose. Second, murine monoclonal antibodies are unable to activate other effector functions (e.g., complement, NK cells, phagocytes) of the human immune system. Finally, murine monoclonal antibodies suffer from a much reduced serum half-life compared with human antibodies, resulting in decreased time of exposure to the target antigen. To overcome many of these limitations, molecular engineering techniques were developed to generate antibodies in which the murine sequences were partially or fully replaced by human protein sequences. A chimeric monoclonal antibody refers to a murine antibody in which the variable regions responsible for the antigen specificity remain murine and the constant region (Fc) is replaced by human sequences. A humanized monoclonal antibody refers to a monoclonal antibody created by engrafting murine complementarity-determining regions onto a human monoclonal antibody variable region. Most recently, fully human antibodies have been produced through human hybridomas and transgenic mice expressing human immunoglobulin genes.[31] Also, engineered monoclonal antibody fragments have been developed and characterized that have unique pharmacokinetic and therapeutic properties (Fig. 29-13).[32,33]

It is estimated that monoclonal antibodies account for approximately 30% of new biotech (genetically engineered) drugs in development. To date, the FDA has approved more than 35 monoclonal antibody/antibody-based therapeutics to treat various diseases, such as cancer, autoimmune diseases, and transplant rejection, with many more currently in clinical trials (Table 29-1). Currently, there are more than 750 clinical trials open to evaluate antibody therapeutics. Given the rapid introduction and development of monoclonal antibody therapeutics, the U.S. Adopted Names Council, in collaboration with the World Health Organization International Nonproprietary Names Committee, has established guidelines for the naming of new monoclonal antibodies. Each name is composed of four syllables, with each syllable providing information. The first syllable is a unique prefix. The second syllable describes the indication; for example, all monoclonal antibodies intended to treat tumors will have the second syllable of *-tu* for tumor. The third syllable identifies the source of the antibody (murine, *-o*; chimeric, *-xi*; human, *-u*). The last syllable is always *-mab*, identifying the therapeutic agent as a monoclonal antibody.

To highlight the clinical potential of and challenges to monoclonal antibody therapeutics, the remaining portion of this section describes monoclonal antibody therapy as it pertains to cancer.[34,35] The mechanism of action used by monoclonal antibodies in the fight against cancer can be divided into two types. The first results from the physical binding of the monoclonal antibody to the specific tumor antigen. Many antigenic targets are cell surface receptors connected to signaling pathways, which are important in cancer progression. The best example of this is trastuzumab (Herceptin), which blocks signaling through an overexpressed growth factor receptor (HER2/neu) in a subset of breast cancers. Second, and perhaps more important, a monoclonal antibody directed against a tumor antigen can activate the patient's own immune system to attack the tumor tissue. This mechanism is mediated through interactions of the Fc region of the antibody and effector cells of the immune system bearing the Fcγ receptor, such as NK cells, phagocytes, and neutrophils. Activation of these professional phagocytes leads to tumor cell destruction and is referred to as ADCC.[36] Also, the Fc domain of the antibody can activate the complement system through interactions with complement-activating protein (C1q), resulting in the formation of the membrane attack complex, which causes cell lysis. This is referred to as complement-dependent cytotoxicity (CDC). Furthermore, there is mounting evidence that monoclonal antibodies are likely to enhance tumor antigen presentation by professional antigen-presenting cells such as DCs, which may ultimately lead to the induction of tumor antigen–specific cytotoxic T cell responses and result in lasting immunity. Amplification of the immune response to other tumor antigens may also occur because it is likely after ADCC or CDC that many tumor peptides have the opportunity to undergo professional antigen presentation, with the potential of also inciting a cytotoxic T cell response.[37,38]

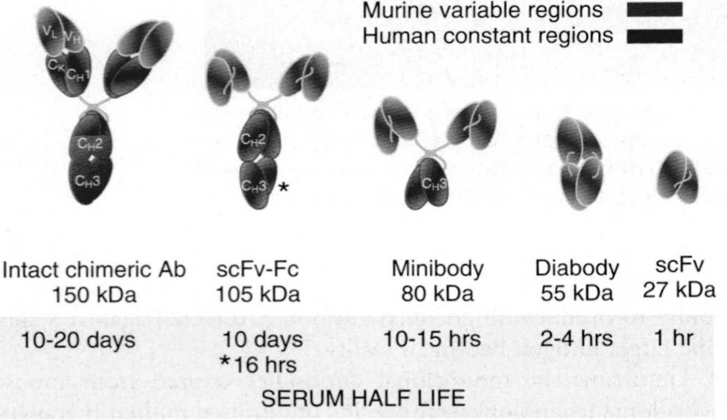

FIGURE 29-13 Chimeric monoclonal antibody (Ab) and engineered antibody fragments. A chimeric intact monoclonal antibody is depicted, showing the retained murine domains *(green)* and human domains *(red)*. Engineered antibody fragments are depicted to the right of the intact chimeric antibody. These fragments are listed in decreasing size from right to left, with their corresponding serum half-life. Note that the 105-kDa fragment (scFv-Fc) normally has a half-life of 10 days. However, when a point mutation is introduced *(star)*, the fragment has a half-life of 16 hours, comparable to the much smaller 80-kDa minibody fragment. This is the result of a point mutation introduced into the FcRn-binding region in the C_H3 domain, which decreases the fragment's affinity for the FcRn, resulting in a much decreased serum half-life.

Factors Governing the Therapeutic Potential of Monoclonal Antibodies

Endogenous IgG has a half-life of approximately 3 weeks. This relatively long serum persistence is a result of its interaction with the FcRn (neonatal or Brambell receptor) on endothelial cells. Most serum proteins undergo pinocytosis, followed by progressive acidification of the endosome, which eventually fuses with a lysosome and results in the destruction of entrapped proteins. IgG, however, binds the FcRn of the endosomal membrane under acidic conditions and is thus protected from lysosomal degradation; it is shuttled back to the serum and released from FcRn under a physiologic pH (7.4). Site-specific mutagenesis has identified the specific amino acid residues responsible for the Fc-FcRn interaction that leads to the long serum half-life of IgG antibodies. Thus, by introducing specific amino acid changes into the Fc region of an engineered antibody, one can tailor the pharmacokinetic properties to fit the clinical or therapeutic indication.[39] For example, by substitution of one amino acid (H310A), the serum half-life of an engineered chimeric monoclonal antibody fragment was reduced by 90%, from 10 days to 16 hours. One can imagine therapeutic applications in which a shorter serum half-life would be beneficial, such as a conjugated monoclonal antibody with toxin or radionuclide in which rapid clearance would serve to decrease the exposure of the normal tissues of the body to the toxin.

Monoclonal antibodies of the IgG subtype are large (150-kDa) proteins. Their relatively large size may limit their ability to penetrate tissues to bind the targeted tumor antigen. It is estimated that the average intervessel distance in tumors is approximately 40 to 100 μM. Obviously, in hypoxic areas of a tumor, this distance is probably increased. Therefore, a smaller molecule will be

TABLE 29-1 **FDA-Approved Monoclonal Antibody–Based Therapeutics**

WORLD HEALTH ORGANIZATION'S INTERNATIONAL NONPROPRIETARY NAMES (INN)	TRADE NAME	ANTIBODY TARGET; TYPE	CLINICAL INDICATION	FDA APPROVAL
Muromonab-CD3	Orthoclone Okt3	Anti-CD3; murine IgG2a	Kidney transplant rejection; T cell depletion	1986
Abciximab	ReoPro	Anti-GPIIb/IIIa; chimeric IgG1 Fab	Prevention of thrombosis/clotting after angioplasty	1994
Rituximab	MabThera, Rituxan	Anti-CD20; chimeric IgG1	Non-Hodgkin lymphoma	1997
Basiliximab	Simulect	Anti–IL-2R; chimeric IgG1	Kidney transplant rejection	1998
Daclizumab	Zenapax	Anti–IL-2R; humanized IgG1	Kidney transplant rejection	1997
Palivizumab	Synagis	Anti-RSV; humanized IgG1	Respiratory syncytial virus	1998
Infliximab	Remicade	Anti-TNF; chimeric IgG1	Crohn's disease	1998
Trastuzumab	Herceptin	Anti-HER2; humanized IgG1	Breast cancer	1998
Gemtuzumab ozogamicin	Mylotarg	Anti-CD33; humanized IgG4; conjugated immunotoxin	Acute myeloid leukemia	2000
Alemtuzumab	MabCampath, Campath-1H	Anti-CD52; humanized IgG1	Chronic myeloid leukemia	2001
Adalimumab	Humira	Anti-TNF; human IgG1	Rheumatoid arthritis	2002
Ibritumomab tiuxetan	Zevalin	Anti-CD20; murine IgG1; conjugated to radionuclide (yttrium-90)	Non-Hodgkin lymphoma	2002
Efalizumab	Raptiva	Anti-CD11a; humanized IgG1	Psoriasis	2003
Tositumomab-I131	Bexxar	Anti-CD20; murine IgG2a; conjugated to radionuclide (iodine-131)	Non-Hodgkin lymphoma	2003
Omalizumab	Xolair	Anti-IgE; humanized IgG1	Asthma	2003
Cetuximab	Erbitux	Anti-EGFR; chimeric IgG1	Colorectal cancer	2004
Bevacizumab	Avastin	Anti-VEGF; humanized IgG1	Colorectal cancer	2004
Natalizumab	Tysabri	Anti-α_4 integrin; humanized IgG4	Multiple sclerosis	2004
Ranibizumab	Lucentis	Anti-VEGF; humanized IgG1 Fab	Macular degeneration	2006
Panitumumab	Vectibix	Anti-EGFR; human IgG2	Colorectal cancer	2006
Eculizumab	Soliris	Anti-C5; humanized IgG2/4	Paroxysmal nocturnal hemoglobinuria	2007
Certolizumab pegol	Cimzia	Anti-TNF; humanized Fab, pegylated	Crohn's disease	2008
Golimumab	Simponi	Anti-TNF; human IgG1	Rheumatoid and psoriatic arthritis, ankylosing spondylitis	2009
Canakinumab	Ilaris	Anti–IL-1β; human IgG1	Muckle-Wells syndrome	2009
Ofatumumab	Arzerra	Anti-CD20; human IgG1	Chronic lymphocytic leukemia	2009
Ustekinumab	Stelara	Anti–IL-12/23; human IgG1	Psoriasis	2009
Tocilizumab	RoActemra, Actemra	Anti–IL-6R; humanized IgG1	Rheumatoid arthritis	2010
Denosumab	Prolia	Anti–RANK-L; human IgG2	Bone loss	2010
Belimumab	Benlysta	Anti-BLyS; human IgG1	Systemic lupus erythematosus	2011
Ipilimumab	Yervoy	Anti–CTLA-4; human IgG1	Metastatic melanoma	2011
Brentuximab vedotin	Adcetris	Anti-CD30; chimeric IgG1; immunoconjugate	Hodgkin lymphoma	2011
Pertuzumab	Perjeta	Anti-HER2; humanized IgG1	Breast cancer	2012
Raxibacumab	Raxibacumab	Anti-*B. anthracis* PA; human IgG1	Anthrax infection	2012
Trastuzumab emtansine	Kadcyla	Anti-HER2; humanized IgG1; immunoconjugate	Breast cancer	2013
Vedolizumab	Entyvio	Anti-$\alpha_4\beta_7$ integrin; humanized IgG1	Inflammatory bowel disease	2014
Obinutuzumab	Gazyva	Anti-CD20; humanized IgG1; glycoengineered	Chronic lymphocytic leukemia	2014
Ramucirumab	Cyramza	Anti-VEGFR2; human IgG1	Gastric cancer	2014
Siltuximab	Sylvant	Anti–IL-6; chimeric IgG1	Castleman disease	2014
Secukinumab	Cosentyx	Anti–IL-17A; human IgG1	Immunosuppression	2015
Nivolumab	Opdivo	Anti–PD-1; human IgG4	Melanoma	2015
Pembrolizumab	Keytruda	Anti–PD-1; humanized IgG4	Melanoma	2015
BMS-936559	(undecided)	Anti–PD-L1; human IgG4; inhibits the binding of PD-L1 to both PD- and CD80	Solid cancers	Investigational (2015)

able to diffuse or to penetrate farther and more quickly. Also, small molecules have different clearance mechanisms. It is generally accepted that molecules smaller than 80 kDa are below the renal threshold and are able to be cleared solely through the kidney. To this end, protein engineers have been able to create very small antibody fragments that retain the antigen-binding specificity but no longer retain the ability to bind the FcRn. The smallest of these entities is the single-chain Fv, with a molecular mass of 27 kDa. Many of these fragments, with ultrashort half-lives, are being tested in mouse models for the ability to target tumors for imaging, diagnostics, and potential transport of larger toxic molecules and chemotherapeutic agents to the tumor.

Compared with traditional chemotherapy, the side-effect profile of nonconjugated monoclonal antibody immunotherapy is rather mild. Most of the toxicity is related to hypersensitivity reactions caused by the protein sequences of mouse origin present in chimeric and humanized monoclonal antibodies. Although fatal infusion reactions are rare, they have been reported. These reactions usually occur during or just after the first dose of the monoclonal antibody. Other side effects may occur as a result of the binding of the monoclonal antibody to its cognate antigen. For example, cetuximab, a chimeric monoclonal antibody that binds the epidermal growth factor receptor (EGFR), is associated with skin eruptions secondary to the blockade of EGFR signaling. Also, bevacizumab (Avastin), a monoclonal antibody that binds VEGF, is associated with hemorrhagic and thrombotic events associated with the decreased signaling through the VEGF receptor (VEGFR).

Unconjugated Antibodies

As noted, the treatment of disease with unconjugated monoclonal antibodies became popular in the 1980s, after murine monoclonal antibodies became available secondary to hybridoma technology. These early therapeutic monoclonal antibodies suffered from poor clinical efficacy and immunogenicity secondary to the HAMA response, leading to the termination of most clinical monoclonal antibody studies. It was not until the development of chimeric, humanized, and fully human therapeutic monoclonal antibodies that clinical efficacy was routinely witnessed in monoclonal antibody studies. Although many therapeutic monoclonal antibodies start as murine monoclonal antibodies, much of the murine antibody is replaced by human IgG protein sequences. For example, a chimeric IgG molecule is approximately 75% human and 25% murine. A humanized murine monoclonal antibody is approximately 95% human, with only the complementarity-determining regions of the variable region remaining murine.

Rituximab is an excellent example of the development of a monoclonal antibody clinically effective against a cancer after transitioning to the chimeric form of the antibody from the parent murine monoclonal antibody. Rituximab, but not its parent murine monoclonal antibody, has demonstrated cytotoxicity in experimental systems. Rituximab is a chimeric monoclonal antibody directed against a cell surface antigen found on mature B cells of non-Hodgkin lymphoma (NHL) and was the first monoclonal antibody to be approved by the FDA, in 1997, for use in the treatment of a human malignant neoplasm. Initially, rituximab was used as single-agent therapy for recurrent or refractory low-grade B cell lymphomas and demonstrated an overall response rate of 48% and a complete response rate of 10%.[40] The cytotoxic activity of rituximab is thought to be a combination of CDC and ADCC; this clarifies the inactivity of the parent murine monoclonal antibody, which lacks the human Fc region to interact with the serum complement protein (C1q) and the Fcγ receptor of the professional phagocytes to elicit ADCC. Evidence in support of ADCC as the mechanism of action was the finding that Fcγ receptor polymorphisms predict response rates in patients with follicular lymphoma treated with rituximab. With high response rates and limited toxicity in the setting of recurrent or refractory NHL, studies were undertaken to investigate rituximab as a first-line therapy. Initially, rituximab was shown to increase the sensitivity of chemotherapy-resistant cell lines, which spawned a trial of rituximab added to a first-line chemotherapy regimen of cyclophosphamide, doxorubicin, vincristine, and prednisolone (CHOP). The addition of rituximab to CHOP, commonly referred to as R-CHOP, resulted in a 95% overall response rate, including a 55% complete response rate. Long-term follow-up revealed a statistically improved survival without significant differences in toxicity.

Trastuzumab is a humanized antibody derived from a murine monoclonal antibody directed against HER2/neu. This receptor tyrosine kinase is a member of the EGFR family, which was noted to be overexpressed because of gene amplification in approximately 25% of breast cancers. Therefore, the strategy was undertaken to target this overexpressed cell surface receptor that was associated with a more aggressive biology in an attempt to disrupt the cancer-promoting mitogenic signaling through antibody blockade of this receptor. Initial phase 2 trials, conducted in the setting of metastatic HER2/neu-positive breast cancers, demonstrated modest objective response rates of 12% to 16%. Given the evidence for single-agent activity, further trials were conducted with trastuzumab in combination with standard chemotherapy regimens, which demonstrated a doubling of the response rates (25% to 57%) compared with chemotherapy alone. In addition, in the adjuvant setting, trastuzumab has been associated with a 50% reduction in 1-year recurrence rates in phase 3 trials.[41,42] The mechanism of action responsible for the response rates of trastuzumab in the treatment of breast cancer has not been fully elucidated. Although some studies have provided evidence that the interruption of intracellular signaling by HER2/neu plays a major role in its antitumor activity, others consider ADCC to be a major component of the antitumor activity of trastuzumab. Cardiomyopathy is the major side effect of trastuzumab therapy, especially when it is combined with taxanes and anthracyclines.

Cetuximab (Erbitux) also targets a receptor tyrosine kinase, EGFR. This chimeric monoclonal antibody binds to the receptor in a nonactivating manner with a much higher affinity than the natural ligands. This causes receptor blockade and eventual internalization of the receptor, leading to an overall decrease in receptor signaling. Cetuximab was approved for use in the treatment of colorectal cancer in 2004 on the basis of a trial that compared cetuximab with cetuximab plus irinotecan in patients with metastatic disease. The addition of cetuximab to irinotecan demonstrated superior activity. Interestingly, cetuximab demonstrated moderate response rates in previously chemoresistant patients and appeared to be synergistic when combined with chemotherapy.[43] Recently, cetuximab has been approved for use in squamous cell head and neck cancers in combination with radiotherapy.[44] The addition of cetuximab to radiotherapy has decreased local regional recurrence by 32% and significantly improved overall survival. Toxicity associated with cetuximab therapy is an acneiform rash. There is some evidence that the severity of the rash is associated with improved antitumor activity. Moreover, some medical oncologists are proposing that dosing should be escalated until a rash forms.

Bevacizumab (Avastin) is a humanized monoclonal antibody that targets VEGF, the soluble ligand of the VEGFR expressed on endothelial cells. Signaling through VEGFR is thought to play a major role in the development of new vessels or angiogenesis. Many tumors are known to be associated with increased production of VEGF, leading to increased tumor angiogenesis, which is thought to play an important role in cancer progression and metastases. Bevacizumab has been approved for use in the treatment of metastatic colorectal cancer.[45] Currently, it is combined with fluorouracil and oxaliplatin or irinotecan as first-line therapy for metastatic colorectal cancer. A proposed mechanism of action is actually to normalize tumor vasculature, which helps in the delivery of cytotoxic chemotherapy. Also, bevacizumab has received FDA approval for use in some patients with other cancers, such as RCC (combined with IFN-α), non–small cell lung cancer, breast cancer, and glioblastoma. Associated toxicities reported are delayed wound healing and hemorrhagic events. It is customary to delay elective surgical procedures until 6 weeks after the last dose of bevacizumab.

Immunoconjugates

Antibodies conjugated to radionuclides were among the first immunoconjugates. External beam radiation delivers focused high-dose radiation during several weeks to treat local areas of disease. Targeted radioimmunotherapy such as that provided by an immunoconjugate could be delivered intravenously as a systemic therapy to treat tumor deposits throughout the body. Another important difference with external beam radiation is that the radiation source is delivered to the site of the tumor; thus, the tumor is continually exposed to the radiation. Radionuclides can be categorized with respect to the characteristics of the energy emitted on nuclear decay. Some radionuclides are considered high-energy beta emitters (yttrium-90 and rhenium-188), and the path length of cytotoxic radiation can penetrate a tumor up to a distance of 1 cm. This relatively long path length of cytotoxic radiation could overcome some of the limitations of radioimmunoconjugates, such as poor tumor penetration and heterogeneous antigen expression, by achieving a large bystander effect. Radionuclides such as lutetium-177 and iodine-131 are considered medium-energy beta emitters whose energy can traverse approximately 1 mm. If one considers the diameter of a cell to be approximately 20 μm, the bystander effect should encompass approximately 50 cells in all directions. One could imagine that radioimmunoconjugates transporting medium-energy beta emitters could be used in the treatment of micrometastatic disease. Using these radionuclides may limit the radiation dose to the normal tissue surrounding the small tumor deposits.

Two anti-CD20 IgG radioimmunoconjugates are currently FDA approved for the treatment of NHL. Ibritumomab (Zevalin) is conjugated to yttrium-90, and tositumomab (Bexxar) is conjugated to iodine-131. Interestingly, both are murine monoclonal antibodies, yet the feared HAMA response rarely occurs. The lack of this immunogenic response is thought to be related to the destruction of the CD20-positive B cell population, which would elicit the HAMA response. Both of these radioimmunoconjugates are associated with high response rates. Patients treated with tositumomab had an overall response rate of 67%, and patients with bulky disease also demonstrated a significant clinical response. Also, in a head-to-head comparison of tositumomab conjugated to ^{131}I versus the unconjugated antibody, the addition of the radionuclide improved overall response rates, and importantly, complete response rates were tripled.[46] Moreover, these complete responses proved to be durable compared with responses achieved by rituximab, an unconjugated anti-CD20 monoclonal antibody. The primary toxicity associated with radioimmunotherapy is the exposure of the highly sensitive bone marrow to radioactivity, resulting in dose-limiting myelosuppression.

CONCLUSION

Future work in human tumor immunotherapy will need to define and then address the underlying mechanisms that limit a productive antitumor response. These include strategies to optimize the delivery of defined tumor antigens to professional antigen-presenting cells, such as DCs, and in an immunostimulatory context to initiate a robust CD8$^+$ and CD4$^+$ T cell response. Provision of adequate precursors, through genetic engineering of T cells or hematopoietic stem cells, may also be needed. T cell activation and expansion can be promoted in vivo through a variety of strategies that include blocking of negative regulatory signaling and provision of cytokines. As antigen-reactive effector T cells enter a tumor, they encounter a hostile immunosuppressive microenvironment. Tumor cell targets have also frequently acquired constitutively active survival pathways. However, there are promising strategies being developed to address each of these limiting steps, as evidenced by the progressive improvement in clinical tumor immunotherapy occasioned by our better understanding of the underlying basic science.

Financial disclosure: JSE is a scientific cofounder of Kite Pharma, a cancer immunotherapy company.

SELECTED REFERENCES

Cheever MA: Twelve immunotherapy drugs that could cure cancers. *Immunol Rev* 222:357–368, 2008.

An overview of the most promising strategies to enhance antitumor immunity.

Dudley ME, Wunderlich JR, Yang JC, et al: Adoptive cell transfer therapy following nonmyeloablative but lymphodepleting chemotherapy for the treatment of patients with refractory metastatic melanoma. *J Clin Oncol* 23:2346–2357, 2005.

A phase II study showing the effectiveness of adoptively transferring cultured melanoma-reactive T cells to a patient after preparative lymphodepletion. The response rate of 51% and the achievement of durable complete responses in some patients illustrate the potential of this approach to immunotherapy.

Jakobovits A, Amado RG, Yang X, et al: From XenoMouse technology to panitumumab, the first fully human antibody product from transgenic mice. *Nat Biotechnol* 25:1134–1143, 2007.

One of the major drawbacks to therapeutic monoclonal antibody development and efficacy is the immunogenicity of murine protein sequences. This review summarizes the powerful development of a transgenic mouse (XenoMouse), in which the mouse antibody production genes were replaced by human immunoglobulin heavy- and light-chain loci. Panitumumab was the first fully human monoclonal antibody developed by immunizing the XenoMouse against a cancer cell line that overexpresses EGFR.

Rosenberg SA, Lotze MT, Yang JC, et al: Experience with the use of high-dose interleukin-2 in the treatment of 652 cancer patients. *Ann Surg* 210:474–484, 1989.

A broad experience in the use of interleukin-2 to treat melanoma and renal cancer, documenting its ability to cause regressions and some apparent cures of metastatic disease.

van der Bruggen P, Traversari C, Chomez P, et al: A gene encoding an antigen recognized by cytolytic T lymphocytes on a human melanoma. *Science* 254:1643–1647, 1991.

A groundbreaking description of the first molecular characterization of a tumor-associated antigen recognized by a T cell. This was an impressive accomplishment, following so quickly after the first understanding of how antigens are processed, presented by MHC, and recognized by T cells. It proved to be the MAGE-1 antigen on a melanoma, presented by HLA-A1.

REFERENCES

1. Loose D, Van de Wiele C: The immune system and cancer. *Cancer Biother Radiopharm* 24:369–376, 2009.
2. Zhang S, Zhang H, Zhao J: The role of CD4 T cell help for CD8 CTL activation. *Biochem Biophys Res Commun* 384:405–408, 2009.
3. Yao S, Zhu Y, Chen L: Advances in targeting cell surface signalling molecules for immune modulation. *Nat Rev Drug Discov* 12:130–146, 2013.
4. Ribas A: Tumor immunotherapy directed at PD-1. *N Engl J Med* 366:2517–2519, 2012.
5. Cheever MA: Twelve immunotherapy drugs that could cure cancers. *Immunol Rev* 222:357–368, 2008.
6. Topham NJ, Hewitt EW: Natural killer cell cytotoxicity: How do they pull the trigger? *Immunology* 128:7–15, 2009.
7. Chavez-Galan L, Arenas-Del Angel MC, Zenteno E, et al: Cell death mechanisms induced by cytotoxic lymphocytes. *Cell Mol Immunol* 6:15–25, 2009.
8. Ferrantini M, Capone I, Belardelli F: Dendritic cells and cytokines in immune rejection of cancer. *Cytokine Growth Factor Rev* 19:93–107, 2008.
9. van der Bruggen P, Traversari C, Chomez P, et al: A gene encoding an antigen recognized by cytolytic T lymphocytes on a human melanoma. *Science* 254:1643–1647, 1991.
10. Pittet MJ: Behavior of immune players in the tumor microenvironment. *Curr Opin Oncol* 21:53–59, 2009.
11. Peggs KS, Quezada SA, Allison JP: Cancer immunotherapy: Co-stimulatory agonists and co-inhibitory antagonists. *Clin Exp Immunol* 157:9–19, 2009.
12. Merelli B, Massi D, Cattaneo L, et al: Targeting the PD1/PD-L1 axis in melanoma: Biological rationale, clinical challenges and opportunities. *Crit Rev Oncol Hematol* 89:140–165, 2014.
13. Kammula US, White DE, Rosenberg SA: Trends in the safety of high dose bolus interleukin-2 administration in patients with metastatic cancer. *Cancer* 83:797–805, 1998.
14. Smith FO, Downey SG, Klapper JA, et al: Treatment of metastatic melanoma using interleukin-2 alone or in conjunction with vaccines. *Clin Cancer Res* 14:5610–5618, 2008.
15. Klapper JA, Downey SG, Smith FO, et al: High-dose interleukin-2 for the treatment of metastatic renal cell carcinoma: A retrospective analysis of response and survival in patients treated in the surgery branch at the National Cancer Institute between 1986 and 2006. *Cancer* 113:293–301, 2008.
16. Rosenberg SA, Yang JC, White DE, et al: Durability of complete responses in patients with metastatic cancer treated with high-dose interleukin-2: Identification of the antigens mediating response. *Ann Surg* 228:307–319, 1998.
17. Rosenberg SA, Lotze MT, Yang JC, et al: Experience with the use of high-dose interleukin-2 in the treatment of 652 cancer patients. *Ann Surg* 210:474–484, 1989.
18. Yang JC, Sherry RM, Steinberg SM, et al: Randomized study of high-dose and low-dose interleukin-2 in patients with metastatic renal cancer. *J Clin Oncol* 21:3127–3132, 2003.
19. Kirkwood JM, Ibrahim JG, Sondak VK, et al: High- and low-dose interferon alfa-2b in high-risk melanoma: First analysis of intergroup trial E1690/S9111/C9190. *J Clin Oncol* 18:2444–2458, 2000.
20. Rosenberg SA, Yang JC, Restifo NP: Cancer immunotherapy: Moving beyond current vaccines. *Nat Med* 10:909–915, 2004.
21. Pardoll DM: The blockade of immune checkpoints in cancer immunotherapy. *Nat Rev Cancer* 12:252–264, 2012.
22. Topalian SL, Hodi FS, Brahmer JR, et al: Safety, activity, and immune correlates of anti-PD-1 antibody in cancer. *N Engl J Med* 366:2443–2454, 2012.
23. Rosenberg SA, Yannelli JR, Yang JC, et al: Treatment of patients with metastatic melanoma with autologous tumor-infiltrating lymphocytes and interleukin 2. *J Natl Cancer Inst* 86:1159–1166, 1994.
24. Rosenberg SA, Aebersold P, Cornetta K, et al: Gene transfer into humans—immunotherapy of patients with advanced melanoma, using tumor-infiltrating lymphocytes modified by retroviral gene transduction. *N Engl J Med* 323:570–578, 1990.
25. Dubinett SM, Patrone L, Huang M, et al: Interleukin-2-responsive wound-infiltrating lymphocytes in surgical adjuvant cancer immunotherapy. *Immunol Invest* 22:13–23, 1993.
26. Dudley ME, Yang JC, Sherry R, et al: Adoptive cell therapy for patients with metastatic melanoma: Evaluation of intensive myeloablative chemoradiation preparative regimens. *J Clin Oncol* 26:5233–5239, 2008.
27. Tran E, Turcotte S, Gros A, et al: Cancer immunotherapy based on mutation-specific $CD4^+$ T cells in a patient with epithelial cancer. *Science* 344:641–645, 2014.
28. Kochenderfer JN, Dudley ME, Kassim SH, et al: Chemotherapy-refractory diffuse large B-cell lymphoma and indolent B-cell malignancies can be effectively treated with autologous T cells expressing an anti-CD19 chimeric antigen receptor. *J Clin Oncol* 33:540–549, 2015.
29. Kohler G, Milstein C: Continuous cultures of fused cells secreting antibody of predefined specificity. *Nature* 256:495–497, 1975.
30. Jakobovits A, Amado RG, Yang X, et al: From XenoMouse technology to panitumumab, the first fully human antibody product from transgenic mice. *Nat Biotechnol* 25:1134–1143, 2007.
31. Lonberg N: Human antibodies from transgenic animals. *Nat Biotechnol* 23:1117–1125, 2005.

32. Beckman RA, Weiner LM, Davis HM: Antibody constructs in cancer therapy: Protein engineering strategies to improve exposure in solid tumors. *Cancer* 109:170–179, 2007.
33. Wu AM, Senter PD: Arming antibodies: Prospects and challenges for immunoconjugates. *Nat Biotechnol* 23:1137–1146, 2005.
34. Griggs J, Zinkewich-Peotti K: The state of the art: Immune-mediated mechanisms of monoclonal antibodies in cancer therapy. *Br J Cancer* 101:1807–1812, 2009.
35. Campoli M, Ferris R, Ferrone S, et al: Immunotherapy of malignant disease with tumor antigen-specific monoclonal antibodies. *Clin Cancer Res* 16:11–20, 2010.
36. Steplewski Z, Lubeck MD, Koprowski H: Human macrophages armed with murine immunoglobulin G2a antibodies to tumors destroy human cancer cells. *Science* 221:865–867, 1983.
37. Weiner LM, Dhodapkar MV, Ferrone S: Monoclonal antibodies for cancer immunotherapy. *Lancet* 373:1033–1040, 2009.
38. Selenko N, Majdic O, Jager U, et al: Cross-priming of cytotoxic T cells promoted by apoptosis-inducing tumor cell reactive antibodies? *J Clin Immunol* 22:124–130, 2002.
39. Olafsen T, Kenanova VE, Wu AM: Tunable pharmacokinetics: Modifying the in vivo half-life of antibodies by directed mutagenesis of the Fc fragment. *Nat Protoc* 1:2048–2060, 2006.
40. McLaughlin P, Grillo-Lopez AJ, Link BK, et al: Rituximab chimeric anti-CD20 monoclonal antibody therapy for relapsed indolent lymphoma: Half of patients respond to a four-dose treatment program. *J Clin Oncol* 16:2825–2833, 1998.
41. Piccart-Gebhart MJ, Procter M, Leyland-Jones B, et al: Trastuzumab after adjuvant chemotherapy in HER2-positive breast cancer. *N Engl J Med* 353:1659–1672, 2005.
42. Romond EH, Perez EA, Bryant J, et al: Trastuzumab plus adjuvant chemotherapy for operable HER2-positive breast cancer. *N Engl J Med* 353:1673–1684, 2005.
43. Jonker DJ, O'Callaghan CJ, Karapetis CS, et al: Cetuximab for the treatment of colorectal cancer. *N Engl J Med* 357:2040–2048, 2007.
44. Bonner JA, Harari PM, Giralt J, et al: Radiotherapy plus cetuximab for squamous-cell carcinoma of the head and neck. *N Engl J Med* 354:567–578, 2006.
45. Hurwitz H, Fehrenbacher L, Novotny W, et al: Bevacizumab plus irinotecan, fluorouracil, and leucovorin for metastatic colorectal cancer. *N Engl J Med* 350:2335–2342, 2004.
46. Davis TA, Kaminski MS, Leonard JP, et al: The radioisotope contributes significantly to the activity of radioimmunotherapy. *Clin Cancer Res* 10:7792–7798, 2004.

30 CHAPTER

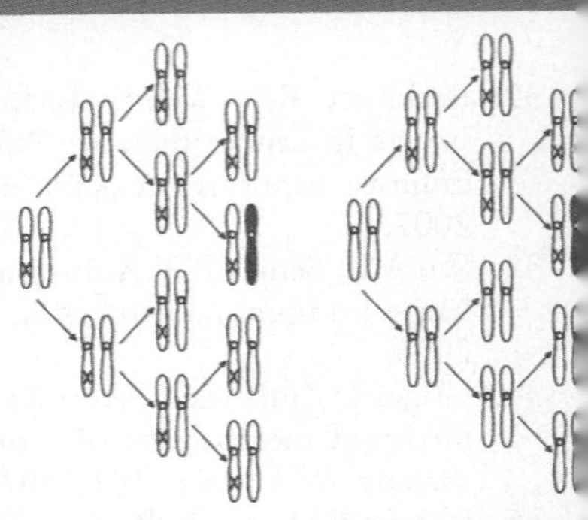

Melanoma and Cutaneous Malignant Neoplasms

Charles W. Kimbrough, Marshall M. Urist, Kelly M. McMasters

OUTLINE

Skin cancer is the most common form of cancer, accounting for at least half of all malignant neoplasms. Almost one in five Americans will be diagnosed with skin cancer in their lifetime. The high incidence of skin cancer is largely attributable to environmental exposures, particularly sunlight. Squamous cell carcinoma and basal cell carcinoma compose the bulk of all skin cancers, although melanoma represents the most common cause of skin cancer–related death. This chapter focuses primarily on these three malignant neoplasms as well as on a few less common cutaneous neoplasms that are encountered by surgeons.

CUTANEOUS MELANOMA

John Hunter is attributed with the first published account of melanoma, a nodal metastasis described in 1787. René Laennec, who identified metastatic melanoma deposits in distant viscera, described it as "cancer noire." He subsequently named the disease melanosis in 1812.[1] Since these early descriptions, our understanding of melanoma has seen incredible progress. Building on a steady accumulation of research, recent insights into the molecular and genetic mechanisms of this disease have ushered in an exciting new era of advances in melanoma therapy.

Epidemiology

Even though melanoma accounts for less than 2% of skin cancer cases, it is currently the fifth most common cancer in men and the seventh most common cancer among women in the United States. Melanoma also causes the majority of skin cancer–related deaths.[2] For 2014, the American Cancer Society estimated 76,100 new cases of melanoma in the United States, with approximately 9170 deaths. These numbers may continue to climb; melanoma incidence has steadily increased worldwide during the last 50 years. Overall, incidence rates have been greatest in Australia, New Zealand, North America, and northern Europe. The steady rise in incidence has been attributed to lifestyle changes leading to increased sun exposure as well as to improved surveillance and detection of early lesions. In the United States, incidence has increased roughly 2.8% annually since the 1980s.[3] Although recent trends demonstrate a stabilization of incidence rates in high-risk countries including the United States (Fig. 30-1), some reports suggest an underlying shift toward a higher incidence in young women.

The degree of pigmentation in the skin is a relative protective factor against cutaneous melanoma, and those with lighter skin tones are at increased risk. As a result, cutaneous melanoma is predominantly a disease of whites. In particular, patients with a fair complexion, blond or red hair, and blue eyes are at increased risk, as are those who sunburn easily, have a tendency to develop freckles, or have an inability to tan. In the United States, the average annual age-adjusted melanoma incidence per 100,000 persons is 21.9 for whites compared with 4.7 for Hispanics, 4.5 for Native Americans (including Alaska Natives), 1.5 for Asians/Pacific Islanders, and 1.0 for African Americans.[4] Melanoma is slightly more common in males than in females, although the prognosis is slightly better in females.

Although the median age of melanoma patients is about 60 years, it occurs in a wide age distribution and affects patients at all stages of life (Fig. 30-2). The incidence is greatest in older patients, but it is one of the most common cancers in young adults and adolescents. Because of the relatively young median age of melanoma patients, the average melanoma mortality results in more than 20 years of potential life lost. Genetic risk factors for melanoma include high-risk skin types (Fitzpatrick types I and II), family history of melanoma, and xeroderma pigmentosum. Patients with a prior history of melanoma or other skin cancers as well as those with a large number of melanocytic nevi, dysplastic nevi, or giant congenital nevi are also at increased risk. Environmental risk factors include episodes of intense intermittent sun exposure associated with severe blistering sunburns, immunosuppression, and upper socioeconomic status.

Whereas the causes of melanoma are not completely defined, there is a clear association with ultraviolet (UV) radiation. Compared with some nonmelanoma skin cancers, which appear to be related to chronic sun exposure, melanoma may result more from intermittent episodes of intense UV radiation. UV light can be classified as either UVA or UVB; UVA has a longer wavelength and penetrates more deeply into the skin than UVB. Although UVA radiation has long been known to play a major role in skin aging and wrinkling, growing evidence has implicated UVA radiation as a cause of melanoma and nonmelanoma skin cancers alike. UVA is the predominant wavelength in tanning beds, and in

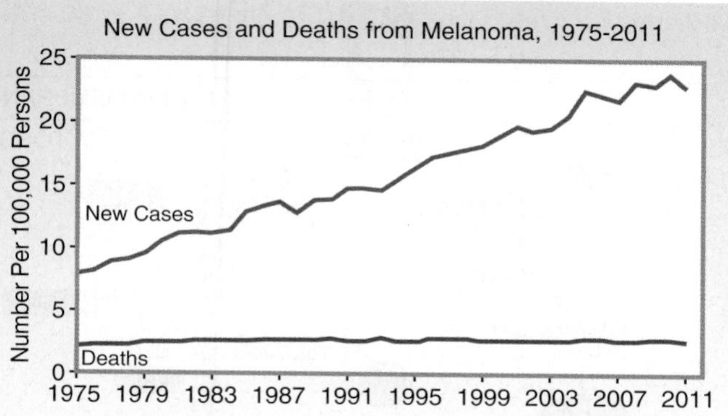

FIGURE 30-1 New cases and deaths from melanoma, 1975-2011. Source: SEER 9 incidence and U.S. mortality 1975-2011, all races, both sexes. Rates are age adjusted. (From SEER Fact Sheets: Melanoma of the skin. http://seer.cancer.gov/statfacts/html/melan.html.)

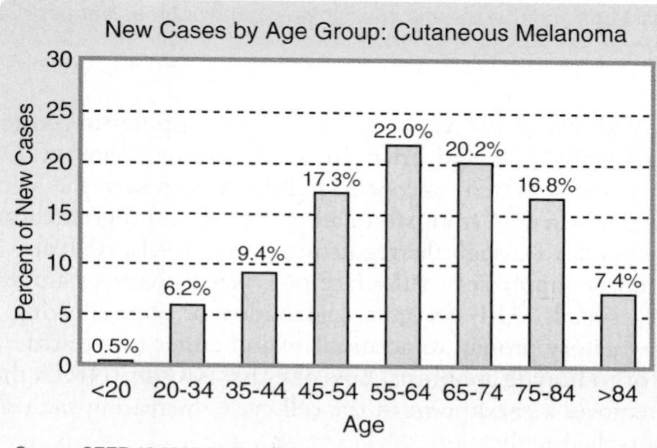

FIGURE 30-2 New cutaneous melanoma cases by age group, 2007-2011. Source: SEER 18 2007-2011, all races, both sexes. (From SEER Fact Sheets: Melanoma of the skin. http://seer.cancer.gov/statfacts/html/melan.html.)

melanoma centers around the country, teenagers and young adults who frequent tanning beds are increasingly found with melanoma. Another major risk factor is UVB exposure from natural sunlight, especially among those with fair skin. UVB damages the skin's more superficial epidermal layers and is the chief cause of sunburn. It has long been implicated in the development of melanoma, and recent findings suggest a direct link between UVB and specific mutations that drive oncogenesis.[5]

Much of the excessive exposure to UV radiation is intentional and completely preventable, particularly sunbathing and tanning bed use. Recommendations for reducing melanoma risk include avoidance of these activities, use of protective clothing, and use of sunscreens. Although at least one randomized controlled trial demonstrated a decreased incidence of melanoma with adequate sunscreen use, sunscreen alone should not be substituted for additional protective measures.

Precursor Lesions

Although melanomas frequently arise de novo, up to 40% may arise within preexisting lesions, including dysplastic nevi, congenital nevi, and Spitz nevi. In addition, up to 5% to 10% of melanoma patients will have a family history of the disease.

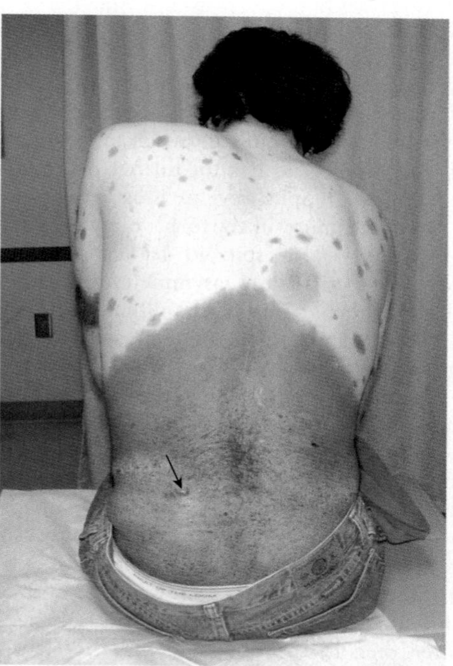

FIGURE 30-3 Giant congenital nevus of the trunk with a melanoma *(arrow)*.

Variously termed dysplastic nevus syndrome, familial atypical multiple mole–melanoma syndrome, and B-K mole syndrome, these syndromes include patients with melanoma in one or more first- or second-degree relatives and large numbers of melanocytic nevi (often >100). On close clinical or histologic examination, some of these nevi will appear atypical or dysplastic. There may also be a family history of other malignant diseases, especially pancreatic cancer. These patients require detailed dermatologic evaluation several times annually, with periodic biopsies of the most suspicious lesions.

In general, a dysplastic nevus is a 6- to 15-mm macular (flat) pigmented skin lesion with indistinct margins and variable color. The clinical distinction between a nevus with dysplasia and a nevus without dysplasia is often difficult, and therefore, these lesions require careful monitoring over time to evaluate for progression. Most nevi are benign, but some may reflect early atypia associated with increased intracellular growth signaling and can progress to invasive disease with the accumulation of additional mutations.[6] Although most dysplastic nevi do not progress to melanoma, suspicious lesions require biopsy. Dysplastic nevi are typically described as having mild, moderate, or severe dysplasia on histologic examination. Those with moderate or severe dysplasia should be excised with negative margins; wide local excision (WLE) is unnecessary. Those with mild dysplasia usually do not require excision with negative margins but should be closely observed over time.

The risk to those with congenital nevi is proportional to the size and number of nevi (Fig. 30-3). Small- or medium-sized congenital nevi represent a low risk and are therefore observed unless they change in appearance. Giant congenital nevi (>20 cm in diameter) are rare and estimated to occur in anywhere from 1 in 20,000 to 1 in 500,000 newborns, but they carry an increased lifetime risk for the development of melanoma. These patients are also at increased risk for other tumors, particularly sarcomas. Complete excision should be considered when possible. At a minimum, these patients should undergo regular dermatologic evaluation.[7]

Spitzoid melanocytic lesions constitute a wide range of histopathology, from the typical benign Spitz nevus to spitzoid melanoma. A Spitz nevus is a rapidly growing, pink or brown, benign skin lesion with little or no risk for further progression to melanoma. Whereas benign Spitz nevi are most common in children, lesions in adults are more likely to have atypical features or to represent melanoma with spitzoid features. Atypical features include size larger than 10 mm, asymmetry, ulceration, and poor circumscription; these lesions can be difficult to distinguish histologically from melanoma. Consultation with an expert dermatopathologist is recommended; however, even the best pathologists may have difficulty in determining the malignant potential of spitzoid tumors. Although complete excision with negative margins is adequate for an unequivocal Spitz nevus, the diagnosis is often not so clear-cut. If there is any concern that the lesion may be melanoma, WLE with margins appropriate for melanoma is performed. Sentinel lymph node (SLN) biopsy is appropriate for invasive spitzoid melanomas and can be used as a prognostic measure in indeterminate cases.[8] However, use of SLN biopsy routinely for atypical Spitz tumors is controversial as atypical cells are often seen in the SLN and may not have prognostic significance.[9]

Pathogenesis

During the last few decades, the molecular mechanisms that underlie melanoma progression have been an exciting area of research and discovery. In general, there are several hallmark steps in the development of cancer: self-sufficient growth signaling, evasion of tumor suppressor signals, downregulation of apoptosis, unlimited replication, sustained angiogenesis, and progression to invasion or metastasis.[10] Whereas many of the mechanisms behind melanoma remain unknown, several genes and molecular pathways have been identified as key steps in melanoma development.[6] With the introduction of novel agents to treat melanoma, understanding of these pathways has become increasingly important.

One of the canonical pathways involved in the development of tumors is the mitogen-activated protein kinase (MAPK) signaling pathway (Fig. 30-4). Normally, signals generated at extracellular receptors initiate a signaling cascade that passes down the MAPK pathway to modulate gene expression in the nucleus. Gain-of-function mutations affecting any of the constituent steps along this cascade can result in oncogenes that continuously drive cell proliferation. Not surprisingly, several mutations in this pathway have been identified that contribute to the development of invasive melanoma. Activating mutations in *BRAF* have been reported in approximately 50% of melanomas, most commonly the result of the substitution of glutamic acid for valine at codon 600 (V600E). Upstream of *BRAF*, mutations associated with *NRAS* affect about 15% of melanomas. Mutations in the tyrosine kinase extracellular receptor *KIT* may affect up to 20% of melanomas, depending on the subtype.[11] The development of targeted therapies specifically directed against these overactive signaling molecules is a promising area of research.

Gain-of-function mutations alone are likely not enough to generate melanoma; *BRAF* mutations are observed at a similar frequency in some benign nevi and malignant disease. In addition, the loss of key tumor suppressor genes is necessary for further neoplastic development. For instance, an inactivating mutation in the gene *CDKN2A* occurs in 25% to 40% of familial melanomas. A well-characterized gene with key roles in cell cycle control,

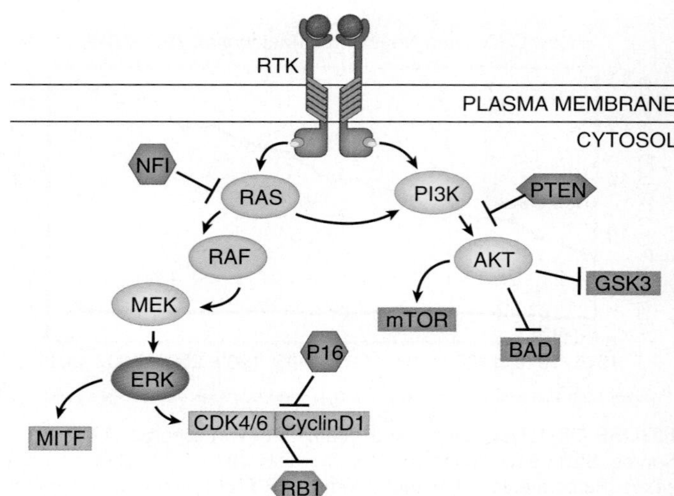

FIGURE 30-4 Core signaling pathways involved in the pathogenesis of melanoma. (From Chen G, Davies MA: Targeted therapy resistance mechanisms and therapeutic implications in melanoma. *Hematol Oncol Clin North Am* 28:523–536, 2014.)

CDKN2A codes for two separate tumor suppressor proteins, INK4A ($p16^{INK4A}$) and ARF ($p14^{ARF}$). In the event of DNA damage or activated oncogenes, INK4A prevents the cyclin-dependent kinase 4 from stimulating the cell to progress through the cell cycle. Through the regulation of p53 levels, ARF also acts as a tumor suppressor in the face of DNA damage or amplified growth signals. ARF prevents degradation of p53, allowing this key regulatory protein to accumulate and either to arrest the cell cycle or to initiate apoptosis. Loss of either ARF or INK4A therefore removes a checkpoint in the cell cycle, increasing the risk of uncontrolled replication.

An additional tumor suppressor frequently affected in melanoma is *PTEN* on chromosome 10. *PTEN* inhibits signaling through phosphatidylinositol 3,4,5-trisphosphate (PIP_3), which represents the second major signaling pathway in melanoma (in addition to MAPK). PIP_3 acts downstream through protein kinase B, also called AKT. AKT not only increases cellular proliferation but also inactivates the proapoptotic protein BCL-2 antagonist of cell death (BAD). Loss of *PTEN* occurs in approximately 25% to 50% of nonfamilial melanomas and may represent one pathway involved in the development of resistance to targeted therapies.

Initial Evaluation

Melanoma commonly is manifested as an irregular pigmented skin lesion that has grown or changed over time. The ABCDEs of melanoma are used to guide diagnosis and the decision to perform a biopsy: *a*symmetry, irregular *b*orders, *c*olor changes, *d*iameter greater than 6 mm, and *e*volution or change over time (Fig. 30-5).

The first and most important step in the evaluation of a patient diagnosed with melanoma is a thorough history and physical examination. The history should elicit factors related to the primary melanoma, including duration, change over time, and symptoms such as itching and bleeding. In addition, other factors, such as sun exposure, tanning bed use, immunosuppression, prior history of cancer, and family history, should be investigated. A detailed physical examination should specifically include a complete skin examination, with inspection and palpation of the skin to detect any other suspicious skin lesions, including in-transit

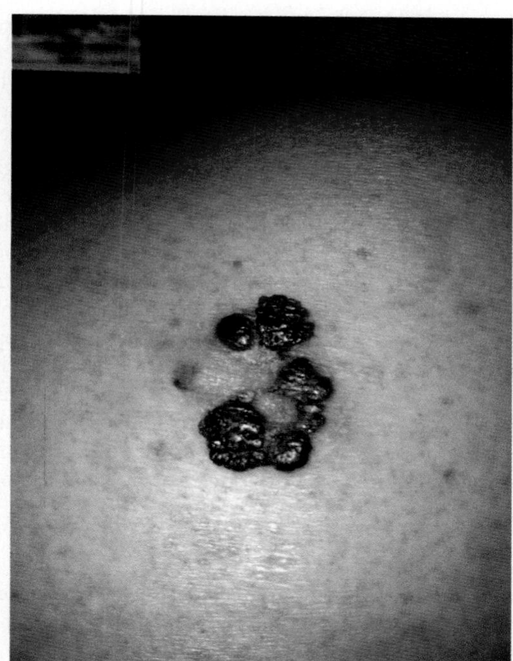

FIGURE 30-5 The ABCDE characteristics of melanoma include *a*symmetry, irregular *b*orders, variegated *c*olors, large *d*iameters, and *e*volution or change over time.

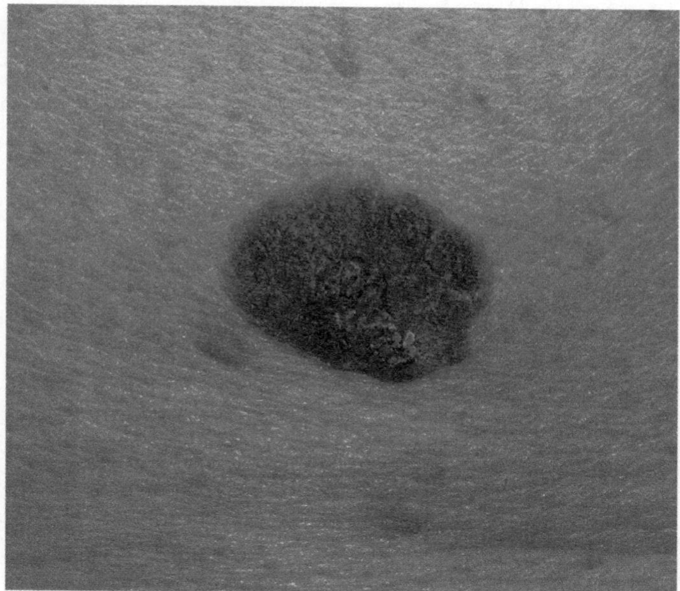

FIGURE 30-6 Seborrheic keratosis.

disease. Palpation of the cervical, axillary, and inguinal lymph nodes should always be performed, with palpation of the epitrochlear or popliteal nodes as appropriate for distal upper or lower extremity melanomas. Although it is widely recognized that a skin examination should be part of the routine physical examination by primary care physicians and others, it is rarely performed. A full skin examination requires only that the patient undress, and it may take only 1 minute to perform a complete survey. Many lives have been saved by early detection of melanomas by physicians who took the time to evaluate the skin.

The majority of melanomas occur de novo, but they can arise within a congenital or acquired nevus. Even for experienced clinicians, the distinction between a benign nevus and an early melanoma can be difficult. Benign pigmented lesions are so prevalent that it is challenging to detect an early melanoma among many benign lesions. The most common benign pigmented skin lesions are seborrheic keratoses (Fig. 30-6). Known for their propensity to accumulate over time in elderly patients, these are typically scaly, waxy, raised lesions with a stuck-on look that makes them appear as if they could easily be scraped off with a fingernail. The characteristic appearance usually is completely diagnostic, and these lesions do not need to be removed. However, even the most experienced dermatologists have been fooled by what appeared to be an irritated seborrheic keratosis that turned out to be melanoma.

An additional atypical presentation is amelanotic melanoma; it is not pigmented and is manifested as a raised pink or flesh-colored skin lesion. A high index of clinical suspicion is needed, and particular attention should be paid to any history of change in a lesion. If a patient presents with a skin lesion that has changed in size, color, or shape and is itching or bleeding, there should be a low threshold for biopsy. Telling a patient "let's keep an eye on it" simply means that it will be ignored.

Fortunately, given the increased awareness of this disease, locally advanced melanomas are infrequently encountered (Fig. 30-7). Nonetheless, roughly 10% of patients will present with regional disease; up to 5% may present with distant metastases. Regional disease refers to the lymphatic spread of tumor to the regional nodal basin, which is the set of lymph nodes that receives the first drainage from the site of the primary tumor. In-transit melanoma is a form of regional lymphatic metastasis in which the tumor spreads within the draining lymphatic channels and becomes evident as cutaneous or subcutaneous nodules between the site of the primary tumor and regional lymph nodes (Fig. 30-8). Distant metastasis refers to the hematogenous spread of melanoma to distant organs. Although it is uncommon at the time of initial diagnosis, it is important to elicit symptoms of metastatic disease, such as any masses, neurologic symptoms or headaches, anorexia, weight loss, bone pain, or respiratory symptoms.

Biopsy

Primary care physicians as well as dermatologists and surgeons should be trained to perform a skin biopsy. There are three basic types of skin biopsy: excisional, incisional (including punch biopsy), and shave biopsy. In the majority of cases, an excisional biopsy is the most appropriate method to diagnose and completely remove a pigmented skin lesion, particularly small lesions. Most patients who have a suspicious-appearing pigmented lesion will prefer to have it completely removed anyway. With use of local anesthesia, a narrow-margin excision is performed, with the subsequent defect closed by sutures. The depth of excision should extend to subcutaneous fat to ensure a full-thickness biopsy specimen. Attention should be paid to the orientation; a fusiform excision should be oriented in such a way as to easily allow subsequent wide excision if that becomes necessary. In particular, a longitudinal orientation on the extremities is best. In other areas, consideration should be given to an orientation that would allow closure with the least tension and best cosmetic outcome in the event that wider excision is needed.

For larger lesions, it may be appropriate to obtain a tissue diagnosis with a full-thickness incisional biopsy before performing complete excision. The simplest incisional biopsy is a punch biopsy, in which a disposable instrument is twisted into the anesthetized skin to remove a 2- to 8-mm cylinder of skin and subcutaneous tissue, followed by closure of the defect with one or two simple sutures. Punch biopsies of at least 4 mm should be performed because smaller tissue samples often do not provide adequate tissue for pathologic evaluation. The punch biopsy should be performed through the thickest area of the lesion, not on the edge of the lesion, and multiple punch biopsies can be performed to sample larger lesions.

Shave biopsies are frequently performed by dermatologists and are appropriate for many nonpigmented skin lesions. This is a good way to diagnose squamous cell and basal cell carcinoma. A shave biopsy is performed by elevating the skin lesion with forceps or inserting a small needle beneath the lesion, followed by shaving of the lesion with a razor blade or scalpel. Hemostasis is achieved with topical agents or by electrocautery. The patient then treats the area with topical antibiotic ointment, and the wound heals by secondary intention. Because a shave biopsy is easy to perform and does not require sutures, it is a popular method of biopsy. However, shave biopsy should not be performed for pigmented lesions and certainly not if melanoma is suspected. If melanoma is actually diagnosed through a shave biopsy, the procedure can easily transect the lesion and forfeit any real assessment of tumor thickness. To circumvent this problem, dermatologists often perform deep shave or saucerization biopsies, which completely remove the lesion down to subcutaneous fat. In the hands of experienced clinicians, this can be an effective biopsy technique.

All pigmented lesions should be sent for pathologic evaluation using fixation and permanent section. Ablation of pigmented skin lesions by cryotherapy, cautery, or lasers is specifically discouraged; there are many examples of prolonged delays in diagnosis as a result of these practices.

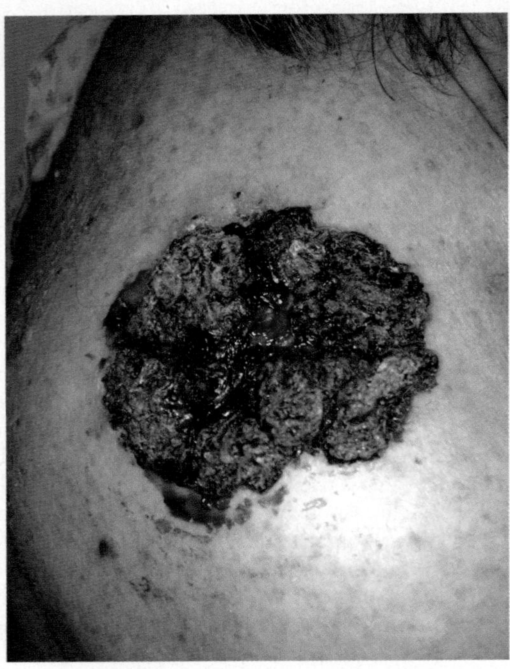

FIGURE 30-7 Locally advanced melanoma.

Pathology

Unequivocal designation of pigmented lesions as benign or malignant can be challenging. Given the consequences of a missed diagnosis, pathologists often have a low threshold to classify equivocal lesions as malignant melanoma. It is now common for a pathology report to contain a long description essentially stating that the lesion may be anything from a severely dysplastic nevus to melanoma in situ to early invasive melanoma. In such cases, the prudent decision is to treat such lesions as an early invasive melanoma by WLE with a 1-cm margin. Although melanoma in situ does not invade beyond the basement membrane into blood vessels and lymphatics, it can be considered a premalignant lesion, given that there remains a significant likelihood of progression to invasive melanoma. Partly for this reason, excision with a 0.5- to 1-cm margin is recommended (see "Wide Local Excision").

On histologic evaluation, invasive cutaneous melanoma is divided into four major types based on growth pattern and location. These include lentigo maligna, superficial spreading, acral lentiginous, and nodular melanoma. All melanomas initially proliferate in the basal layer of the skin. As they multiply, these cells expand radially in the epidermis and superficial dermal layer, termed the radial growth phase. With time, growth begins in a vertical direction and the skin lesion may become palpable, known as the vertical growth phase. The vertical growth phase allows

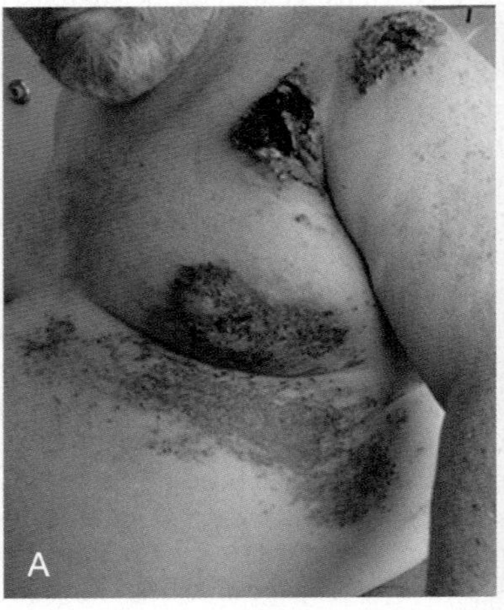

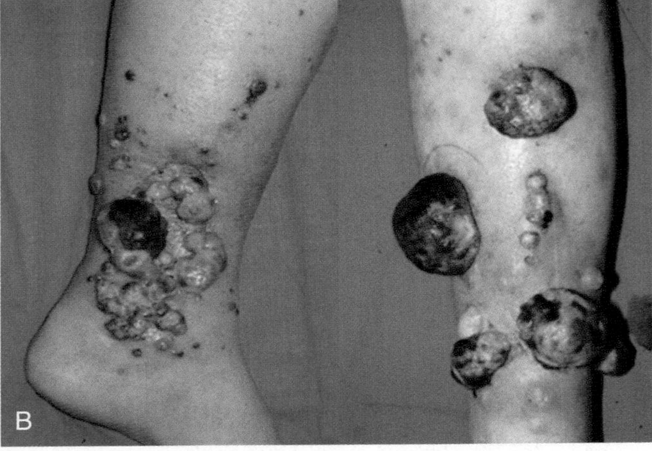

FIGURE 30-8 In-transit melanoma.

invasion into the deeper layers of the skin, where the tumor may ultimately achieve metastatic potential by invasion of blood vessels and lymphatic channels. Whereas the histologic subtype is not in general a major factor in prognosis, some histologic subtypes progress to the vertical growth phase earlier in tumor development and therefore are more likely to be manifested at an advanced stage.

The most common histologic type is superficial spreading melanoma (Fig. 30-9). It is not necessarily associated with sun-exposed skin, and it most commonly appears on the trunk and proximal extremities. As the name suggests, superficial spreading melanoma initially appears as a flat pigmented lesion growing in the radial dimension. These lesions are often asymmetrical with irregular borders and can display a wide variety of pigments. If they are allowed to progress, these melanomas will subsequently develop a vertical growth phase, invade more deeply into the skin, and possibly ulcerate.

Lentigo maligna melanoma occurs most commonly on the sun-exposed areas of older individuals and is manifested as a flat, dark, variably pigmented lesion, with irregular borders and a history of slow development (Fig. 30-10). Lentigo maligna

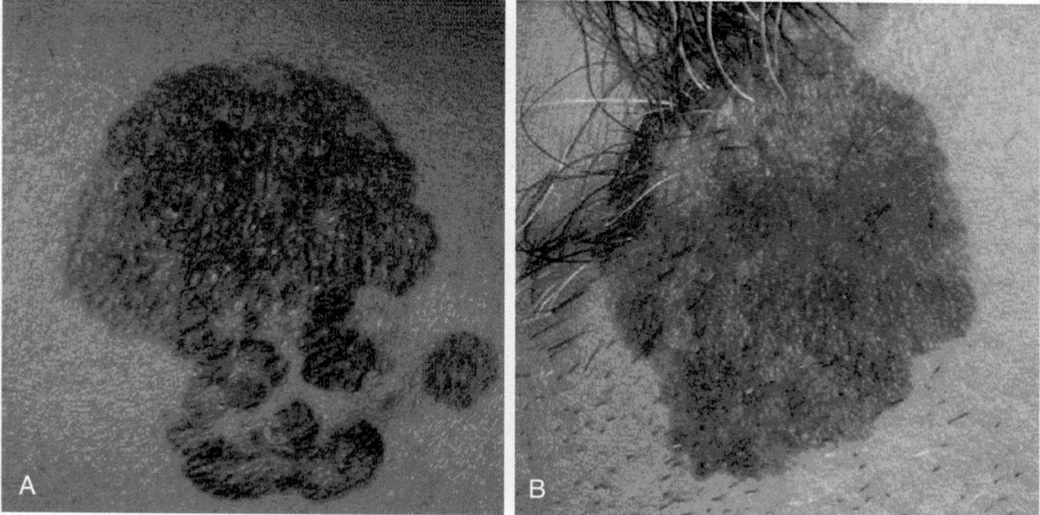

FIGURE 30-9 Superficial spreading melanoma.

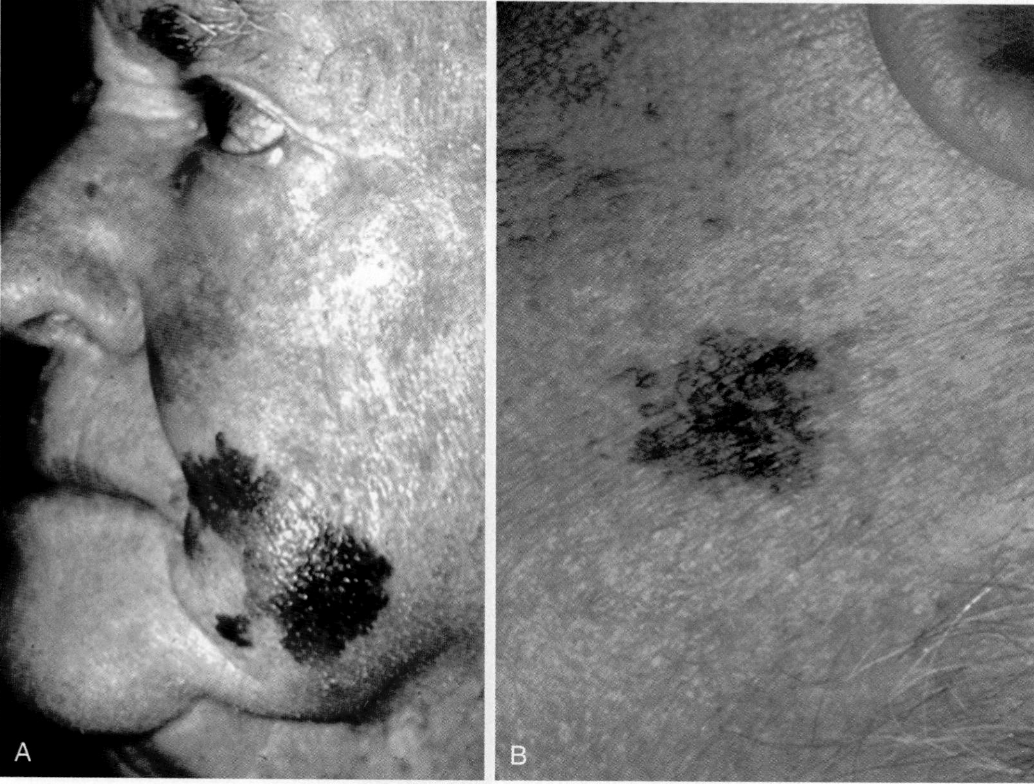

FIGURE 30-10 Lentigo maligna melanoma.

melanomas may become relatively large before diagnosis as the slow progression can escape the patient's notice. Overall, the prognosis of lentigo maligna melanoma is better than for the other subtypes, given the superficial nature of these tumors. Nonetheless, lentigo maligna melanomas can pose management problems because of their propensity to develop in cosmetically challenging areas, such as the face. Furthermore, the histologic extent of the lesion may extend well beyond the clinically apparent borders of the pigmented lesion. Thus, achieving negative margins may be difficult. Before proceeding with complex tissue flaps for closure, it is prudent to ensure negative margins. This may necessitate delaying the closure until the final pathology report indicates negative margins of excision.

Acral lentiginous melanoma is classified by its anatomic site of origin. These tumors develop in the subungual areas beneath fingernails and toenails as well as on the palms of the hand and soles of the feet (Fig. 30-11). This is the most common type of melanoma in black patients. The histologic appearance of acral lentiginous melanoma is similar to that of mucosal melanoma. The diagnosis is often made at an advanced stage, which accounts for the poor prognosis of these tumors in general. Subungual acral lentiginous melanomas are often mistaken for subungual hematomas, leading to a delay in diagnosis. However, whereas pigment from a hematoma should migrate distally with growth of the nail, subungual melanomas will remain in place and sometimes cause a streak in the nail. Biopsy of subungual melanomas can be accomplished by performing a digital block with local anesthesia and removing the nail or by performing a punch biopsy through the nail itself.

Nodular melanomas are raised papular lesions that can occur anywhere on the body and that tend to develop a vertical growth pattern early in their course (Fig. 30-12). These melanomas can have atypical presentations that do not always conform to ABCDE criteria, including a higher rate of amelanotic lesions compared with the other subtypes. As a result, nodular melanomas often have a poor prognosis because of greater average tumor thickness and frequent ulceration at initial presentation.

Desmoplastic melanoma has an atypical presentation characterized by the combination of melanoma cells with a prominent stromal fibrosis. Often amelanotic, diagnosis can be challenging and presentation will often be delayed. There are two main types, classified as pure or mixed, depending on the degree of desmoplasia present. Desmoplastic melanomas have a greater propensity for local recurrence and often exhibit neurotropism. Whereas it was generally held that desmoplastic melanoma had a lower risk for nodal spread, recent findings suggest that the incidence of nodal metastasis may be higher than previously thought, and the rate of nodal disease among mixed lesions is similar to that seen in other melanoma subtypes.[12]

Prognostic Factors and Staging

Although most melanoma patients are ultimately cured, the reputation of melanoma as a deadly cancer will rightfully generate anxiety in most patients. Given the poor survival that accompanies advanced disease, often measured in months, this is certainly to be expected. However, most patients present with early, localized disease, and the overall 5-year survival among all patients approaches 91%.[13] It is therefore of substantial importance to accurately risk stratify these patients to predict prognosis and appropriately guide management decisions.

Wallace Clark first described a classification system for melanoma that correlated with survival in 1969.[14] Known as Clark's level of invasion, this scheme was based on the extent of invasion into the anatomic layers of the skin (Fig. 30-13). Shortly after Clark introduced his levels of invasion, Alexander Breslow described a simpler system based on a measurement of the vertical thickness of the melanoma in 1970. Now known as Breslow thickness, this is the distance from the top of the granular layer down to the lowest tumor cell.[15] Over time, Breslow thickness has largely supplanted Clark level as it has been shown to be a more accurate method of predicting prognosis. Melanomas are commonly referred to as thin (≤1 mm Breslow thickness),

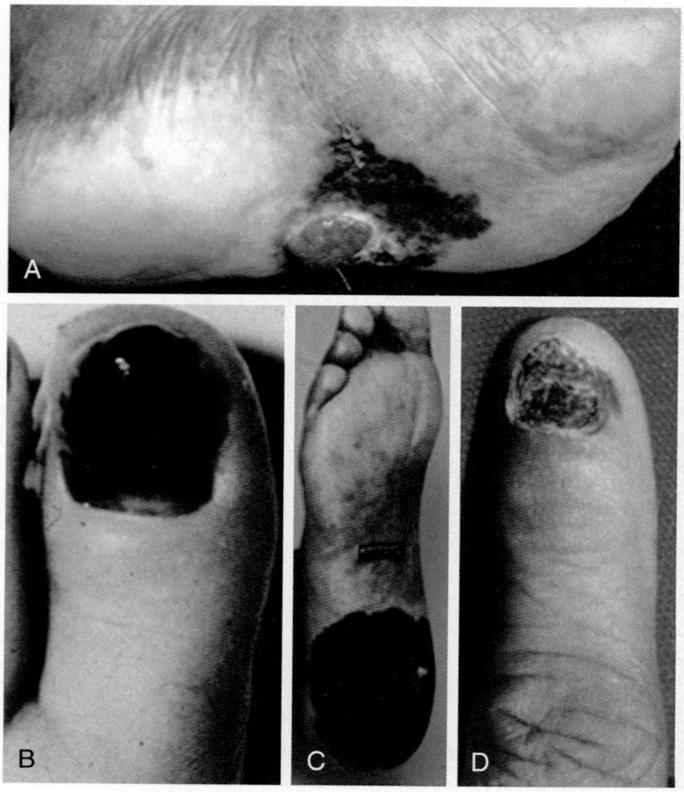

A B C D

FIGURE 30-11 Acral lentiginous melanoma.

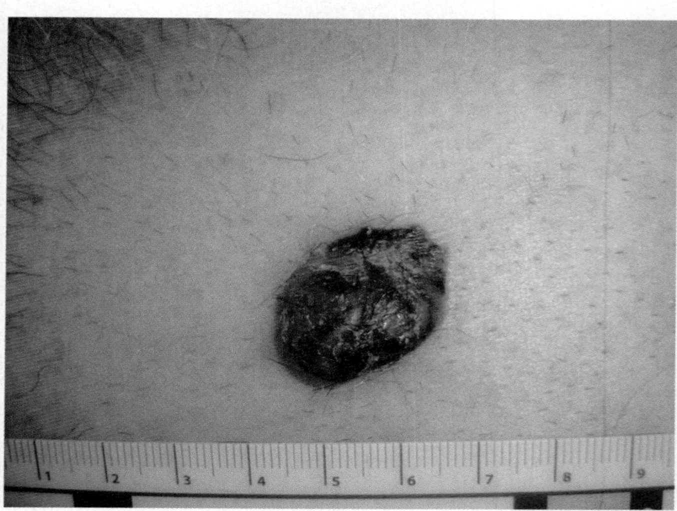

FIGURE 30-12 Nodular melanoma.

intermediate thickness (>1 to 4 mm), and thick (>4 mm). As the thickness of the melanoma increases, the prognosis worsens.

Since the pioneering work of Clark and Breslow, additional factors associated with melanoma survival have been identified. The status of the regional lymph nodes is the single most important prognostic factor predicting survival; Gershenwald demonstrated that metastasis to the sentinel nodes increases the chances of death from melanoma substantially to more than 6.5 times that of patients without nodal disease.[16] Other major prognostic factors, in order of impact on survival, include Breslow thickness, ulceration, age, anatomic location of the primary tumor, and gender.[17] More recently, mitotic rate has emerged as an independent predictor for survival, particularly in thin melanomas.

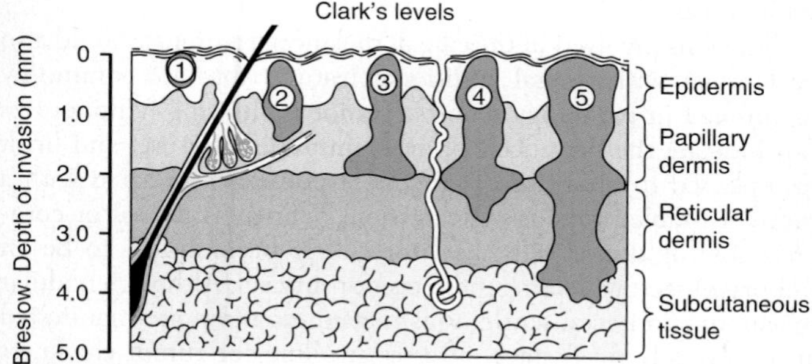

FIGURE 30-13 Clark's levels of invasion: (1) epidermis, (2) extension to papillary dermis, (3) filling the papillary dermis, (4) reticular dermis, and (5) subcutaneous fat.

AJCC Staging

In a continual effort to improve risk stratification, the American Joint Committee on Cancer (AJCC) Melanoma Staging Committee has analyzed data including outcomes and major prognostic factors from centers across North America, Europe, and Australia to develop a staging system for melanoma. Currently, the AJCC staging system for cutaneous melanoma uses a tumor, node, and metastasis (TNM) classification (Tables 30-1 and 30-2). For the seventh edition (published in 2009), 38,918 patients with cutaneous melanoma, including 7972 with metastatic disease, were analyzed. Important prognostic factors in the staging system include Breslow thickness, ulceration, nodal status, and other manifestations of lymphatic spread (e.g., satellite lesions, in-transit disease) as well as the presence of distant metastatic disease. Taking all these factors into consideration, the system provides good discrimination of survival among patients as classified by stage (Fig. 30-14).

T stage. Current AJCC staging classifies all primary melanomas as T1 to T4 on the basis of Breslow thickness (Table 30-1). In addition to thickness, all lesions are further categorized by ulceration status. Ulceration, defined histologically as the absence of an intact epithelium over the melanoma, appears to be a phenotypic marker for worse tumor biology and has emerged as a robust predictor of prognosis (Fig. 30-15). Patients with ulcerated melanomas have a worse prognosis than those with nonulcerated melanomas, even among patients with regional nodal metastasis. The most recent AJCC staging system introduced mitotic rate as an additional criterion for T1 lesions, replacing Clark level. As a marker of cellular proliferation, a cutoff of at least 1 mitosis/mm^2 has been correlated with decreased survival.

TABLE 30-1 TNM Staging Categories for Cutaneous Melanoma

T CLASSIFICATION	THICKNESS	ULCERATION STATUS/MITOSES
T1	≤1.0 mm	a: Without ulceration and mitosis <1/mm^2 b: With ulceration or mitoses ≥1/mm^2
T2	1.01-2.0 mm	a: Without ulceration b: With ulceration
T3	2.01-4.0 mm	a: Without ulceration b: With ulceration
T4	>4.0 mm	a: Without ulceration b: With ulceration
N CLASSIFICATION	**NO. OF METASTATIC NODES**	**NODAL METASTATIC MASS**
N1	1 node	a: Micrometastasis* b: Macrometastasis†
N2	2-3 nodes	a: Micrometastasis* b: Macrometastasis† c: In transit metastases/satellites without metastatic nodes
N3	4 or more metastatic nodes, or matted nodes, or in transit metastases/satellites with metastatic nodes	
M CLASSIFICATION	**SITE**	**SERUM LDH**
M1a	Distant skin, subcutaneous, or nodal metastases	Normal
M1b	Lung metastases	Normal
M1c	All other visceral metastases	Normal
	Any distant metastasis	Elevated

From Balch CM, Gershenwald JE, Soong SJ, et al: Final version of 2009 AJCC melanoma staging and classification. *J Clin Oncol* 27:6199–6206, 2009.

LDH, lactate dehydrogenase.

*Micrometastases are diagnosed after sentinel lymph node biopsy and completion lymphadenectomy (if performed).

†Macrometastases are defined as clinically detectable nodal metastases confirmed by therapeutic lymphadenectomy or when nodal metastasis exhibits gross extracapsular extension.

TABLE 30-2 Stage Groupings for Cutaneous Melanoma

CLINICAL STAGING*				PATHOLOGIC STAGING†			
	T	N	M		T	N	M
0	Tis	N0	M0	0	Tis	N0	M0
IA	T1a	N0	M0	IA	T1a	N0	M0
IB	T1b	N0	M0	IB	T1b	N0	M0
	T2a	N0	M0		T2a	N0	M0
IIA	T2b	N0	M0	IIA	T2b	N0	M0
	T3a	N0	M0		T3a	N0	M0
IIB	T3b	N0	M0	IIB	T3b	N0	M0
	T4a	N0	M0		T4a	N0	M0
IIC	T4b	N0	M0	IIC	T4b	N0	M0
III	Any T	Any N	M0	IIIA	T1-4a	N1a	M0
					T1-4a	N2a	M0
				IIIB	T1-4b	N1a	M0
					T1-4b	N2a	M0
					T1-4a	N1b	M0
					T1-4a	N2b	M0
					T1-4a	N2c	M0
				IIIC	T1-4b	N1b	M0
					T1-4b	N2b	M0
					T1-4b	N2c	M0
					Any T	N3	M0
IV	Any T	Any N	Any M	IV	Any T	Any N	Any M

From Balch CM, Gershenwald JE, Soong SJ, et al: Final version of 2009 AJCC melanoma staging and classification. *J Clin Oncol* 27:6199–6206, 2009.

*Clinical staging includes microstaging of the primary melanoma and clinical/radiologic evaluation for metastases. By convention, it should be used after complete excision of the primary melanoma with clinical assessment for regional and distant metastases.

†Pathologic staging includes microstaging of the primary melanoma and pathologic information about the regional lymph nodes after partial or complete lymphadenectomy. Pathologic stage 0 or stage IA patients are the exception; they do not require pathologic evaluation of their lymph nodes.

N stage. For patients with regional lymph node disease, independent prognostic factors include the number of involved nodes and nodal tumor burden at the time of staging in addition to the thickness and ulceration status of the primary tumor. Tumor burden is characterized as either microscopic disease detected by SLN biopsy or clinically apparent macroscopic disease that is subsequently confirmed on pathologic examination. In-transit or satellite metastases found between the primary lesion and the draining nodal basin are considered N2c or N3, depending on the status of the regional nodes (see Table 30-1).

M stage. Melanoma is notorious in its ability to spread to diverse distant sites, although metastases to the skin, lung, brain, liver, and small bowel are most common. Stratifying overall survival by location of metastasis has generated three classifications for the AJCC M stage: distant skin, subcutaneous tissue, or lymph nodes (M1a); lung metastasis (M1b); and all other visceral metastases or distant sites (M1c). In addition, survival is significantly reduced in patients with elevated serum lactate dehydrogenase at the time of stage IV diagnosis. The source and mechanism behind elevated lactate dehydrogenase levels in these patients are not well understood.

Additional Factors

Several factors that have consistently been shown to have an impact on survival are not incorporated into the current AJCC staging system. Older patients have a greater risk of melanoma mortality than younger patients, despite the fact that younger patients are more likely to have nodal metastasis. Patients with axial (trunk, head, and neck) melanomas have a worse prognosis than those with extremity tumors. Women have a better prognosis than men, for reasons that are unclear. Although advancements in staging have diminished the role that Clark level plays as a prognostic factor, it continues to be reported routinely. Patients and physicians alike will frequently confuse Clark level with the overall AJCC stage, even though there is obviously a large difference between a Clark level 4 melanoma, which may have a very good prognosis, and stage IV melanoma, indicating distant metastatic disease.

Surgeons involved in the care of melanoma patients should also be familiar with several additional features that are commonly mentioned in pathology reports. Tumor infiltrating lymphocytes can indicate the presence of a host immune response, and brisk (as opposed to nonbrisk or absent) response is associated with a more favorable prognosis. Regression, defined as partial or complete loss of tumor cells, has not clearly been shown to be an important factor affecting metastasis or survival. Although nodular melanoma and acral lentiginous melanoma often are manifested at a more advanced stage, after controlling for tumor thickness and other factors, there is no survival difference based on histologic subtype.[18]

Staging Beyond TNM

Given that not all prognostic factors are accounted for within the current AJCC staging system, additional tools that may further refine patient risk stratification have been developed. Using the same database that generated the current TNM guidelines, the AJCC has also developed an electronic predictive tool *(www.melanomaprognosis.org)* that takes into consideration patient-specific demographic and pathologic information. After patient information is entered according to simple prompts, 1-, 2-, 5-, and 10-year survival estimates are displayed with 95% confidence intervals. An even more robust prognostic tool, specifically for patients 18 to 70 years old with melanoma of 1 mm in thickness or more undergoing SLN biopsy, is available online at *www.melanomacalculator.com* and as a free app for iPhone and Android devices.[19] Ultimately, tools such as these may give a more accurate prognosis than simple stage designation and are useful for counseling patients about their risk of recurrence and suitability for clinical trials of novel adjuvant therapy.

Future efforts will likely move beyond models like the TNM system, which is based largely on clinical and pathologic features, and incorporate gene signatures and molecular profiles. Improvements in our understanding of melanoma biology on a genetic and molecular basis have led to the identification of multiple new biomarkers that may aid in both diagnosis and prognosis.[20] Cutaneous melanoma was one of the cancers selected by the National Cancer Institute for The Cancer Genome Atlas, whereby hundreds of melanoma samples were sequenced to identify the genetic alterations that occur in these tumors. Sequencing results are available online to researchers and, it is hoped, will lead to advances in our understanding of melanoma biology. Genetic profiling projects have also attracted the private sector, and during the last few years, commercial tests based on gene signatures have been developed for multiple cancers, including melanoma.

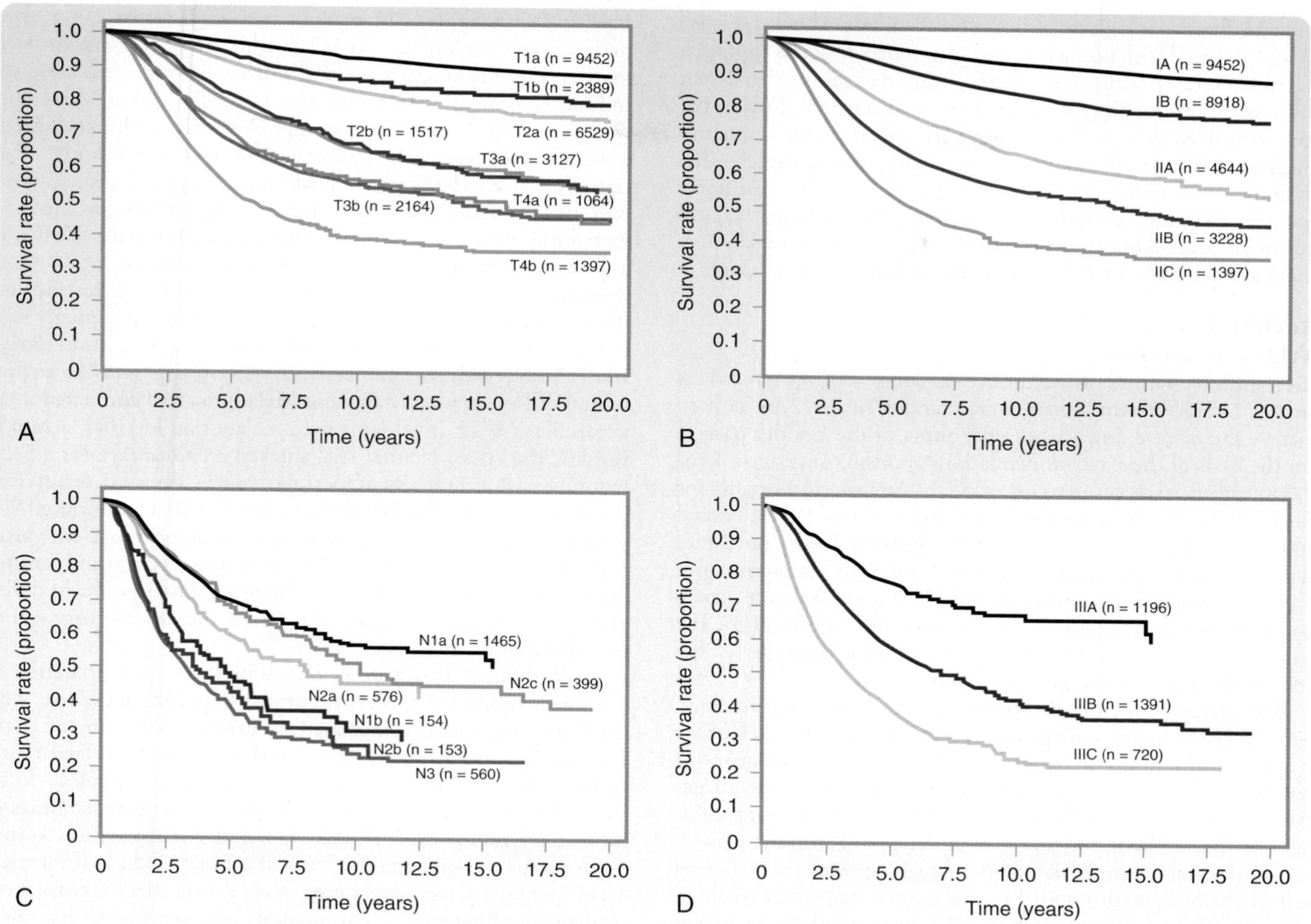

FIGURE 30-14 Survival curves from the AJCC Melanoma Staging Database by T stage **(A)** as well as by the AJCC classifications for stage I and stage II melanoma **(B)**. For stage III melanoma, survival by N stage **(C)** and AJCC stage III groupings **(D)** is shown. (From Balch CM, Gershenwald JE, Soong SJ, et al: Final version of 2009 AJCC melanoma staging and classification. *J Clin Oncol* 27:6199–6206, 2009.)

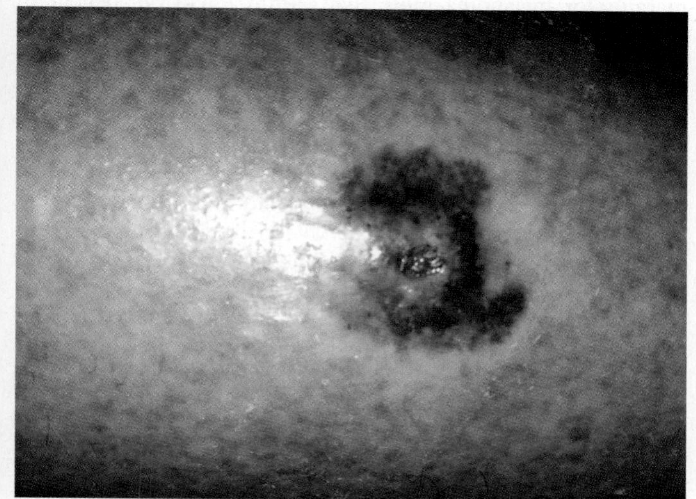

FIGURE 30-15 Ulcerated melanoma.

Additional Workup and Imaging

Most melanoma patients who seek surgical consultation will have already been diagnosed with melanoma. Patients clinically staged with localized stage I or stage II disease do not require any further tests unless they are symptomatic. Formerly, liver function tests or serum lactate dehydrogenase levels were commonly assessed; however, there is no evidence that blood tests are helpful for detecting metastatic disease in patients with localized melanoma. Similarly, additional imaging studies are unnecessary for most patients with localized disease, although patients with thick primary tumors (stage IIC) can be considered for further workup. In patients with stage III disease detected by sentinel node biopsy, additional imaging workup is controversial. The probability of detecting real disease in patients with microscopic nodal metastasis by radiographic studies such as positron emission tomography (PET) and computed tomography (CT) scanning is surprisingly low, with an estimated 11 false positives for every true metastasis in one study.[21] Patients with advanced stage III disease who have clinically detectable nodal metastasis or patients in earlier disease stages who present with symptoms suggestive of metastasis should undergo further imaging studies. The distinction between stage III and stage IV melanoma is important in deciding the appropriate treatment options, and imaging can determine the extent and resectability of any metastatic lesions in stage IV disease. For these advanced presentations, PET, CT, and magnetic resonance imaging (MRI) of the brain are generally recommended. The National Comprehensive Cancer Network (NCCN) routinely updates guidelines including the appropriate workup, surgical treatment, and adjuvant therapy for patients with melanoma. These are available for reference online at *http://www.nccn.org*.

Treatment

Wide Local Excision

The aggressive nature of melanoma has long been recognized; as early as 1857, William Norris recommended surgery "not only to remove the disease, but to cut away some of the healthy parts."[1] On the basis of these recommendations and the concern for lymphatic spread, excision margins of 5 cm were surgical dogma for much of the previous century. Beginning in the 1970s, several surgeons (including Breslow) began to report no adverse outcomes in patients who underwent excision with a narrower margin. Since that time, multiple randomized controlled trials evaluating excision margins have established current guidelines (Table 30-3). The principal determinant for appropriate excision margins is the Breslow thickness of the primary tumor.

Based largely on clinical experience and consensus guidelines, 5-mm excision margins are generally recommended for melanoma in situ. However, several papers have questioned the adequacy of narrower margins; one study of 1072 patients demonstrated negative margins in only 86% of patients with 6-mm margins compared with 98.9% of patients who underwent 9-mm excisions.[22] In addition, close reanalysis of pathologic specimens including both melanoma in situ and thin melanomas can often result in upstaging of these lesions, such that 5-mm margins are no longer adequate.[23] With this in mind, it is prudent to attempt 1-cm margins for lesions in anatomic areas that will permit easy primary closure. Although no randomized controlled trials have specifically addressed excision margins for thin invasive melanoma, the general consensus is that 1-cm margins are sufficient.

Several key randomized controlled trials have evaluated the margins needed for intermediate-thickness melanoma.[24-29] None of these studies has demonstrated an advantage in overall survival, disease-free survival, or local recurrence with wider excision margins (3 to 5 cm). In the first trial, conducted by the World Health Organization, 612 patients with melanomas 2-mm thick or less were randomized to WLE with either a 1-cm or 3-cm margin. Local recurrence as a site of first recurrence was observed in four patients, all with melanomas larger than 1- to 2-mm thick that were in the 1-cm margin group. Nonetheless, this small trend toward increased local recurrence did not significantly affect overall survival. The Intergroup Melanoma Surgical Trial randomized 462 patients with melanomas of the trunk or proximal extremities between 1-mm and 4-mm thick to receive WLE with a 2-cm or 4-cm margin. After a median follow-up of 10 years, there was no significant difference in overall survival. In addition, the incidence of local recurrence was the same for patients with either 2-cm or 4-cm margins (2.1% versus 2.6%, respectively). Both the Swedish Melanoma Study Group trial and the French Group of Research on Malignant Melanoma trial compared 2-cm versus 5-cm WLE in patients with melanomas less than 2 mm in Breslow thickness. Neither trial showed an advantage for a 5-cm margin excision in terms of local recurrence, disease-free survival, or overall survival. The British Collaborative Trial randomized 900 patients with melanomas 2-mm thick or larger to a 1-cm versus 3-cm margin excision; elective lymph node dissection and sentinel node biopsy were not permitted. There were no significant differences in local and in-transit recurrence, disease-free survival, or overall survival.

TABLE 30-3 Recommended Margins of Wide Local Excision

THICKNESS	MARGIN*
In situ	0.5 cm
<1 mm	1 cm
1-2 mm	1-2 cm†
>2-4 mm	2 cm
>4 mm	2 cm‡

*Lesser margins may be justified in specific cases to achieve better functional or cosmetic outcome.

†A 1-cm margin may be associated with a slightly greater risk of local recurrence in this Breslow thickness category.

‡There is no evidence that margins >2 cm are beneficial; however, greater margins may be considered for advanced melanomas when local recurrence risk is high.

Even though these studies established the appropriateness of narrow margins for most patients with melanoma, there were findings suggestive of increased recurrence with use of 1-cm margins in some patients. The British Collaborative Trial found significantly greater locoregional recurrence (pooled local, in-transit, and nodal recurrence) in patients with melanomas of more than 2 mm in thickness who underwent excision with a 1-cm versus a 3-cm margin.[28] On the basis of these findings, a 1-cm margin for melanoma more than 2-mm thick is considered inadequate. However, 2-cm margins are acceptable for these lesions.[29] In the World Health Organization trial, a nonsignificant increase in local recurrence for melanomas 1- to 2-mm thick was observed in patients with 1-cm compared with 3-cm margins (4.2% versus 1.5%, respectively).[24] Given this trend, it is thought that 1-cm margins may increase the risk of local recurrence in lesions 1- to 2-mm thick.

As a result of these trials, current guidelines recommend 2-cm margins for melanoma more than 2-mm thick. No benefit in overall survival, disease-free survival, or local recurrence has been demonstrated with margins larger than 2 cm. Whereas 1- to 2-cm margins are sufficient for tumors 1- to 2-mm thick, 1-cm excision margins in these patients may increase locoregional recurrence. When it is feasible, 2-cm margins should be attempted for these patients. Limited trial data exist for melanomas more than 4-mm thick, although retrospective studies indicate that a 2-cm margin is likely to be adequate. Nevertheless, wider excision may be appropriate for thicker lesions with a high risk of local recurrence.

Technique. WLE can be performed under local anesthesia in most cases, although general anesthesia is preferred for patients who will also undergo sentinel node biopsy or lymphadenectomy. The appropriate margins of excision are measured from the edge of the lesion or previous biopsy scar. This usually represents a fusiform incision that encompasses the margins of excision to allow primary closure (Fig. 30-16). WLE is performed to remove the skin and subcutaneous tissue down to the muscle fascia. Excision of the fascia is not necessary in most cases but may be performed for patients with thick primary tumors. The specimen is

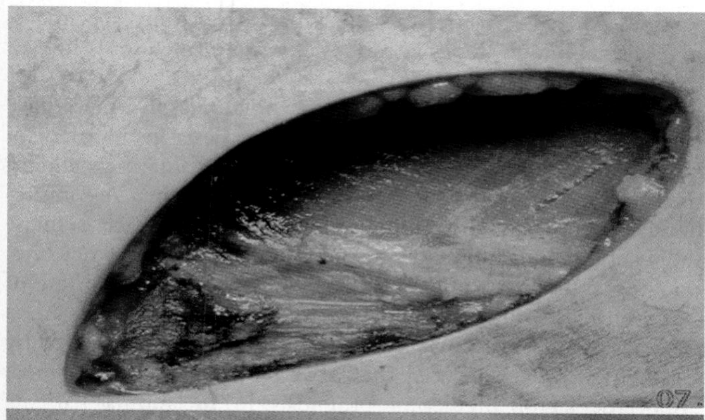

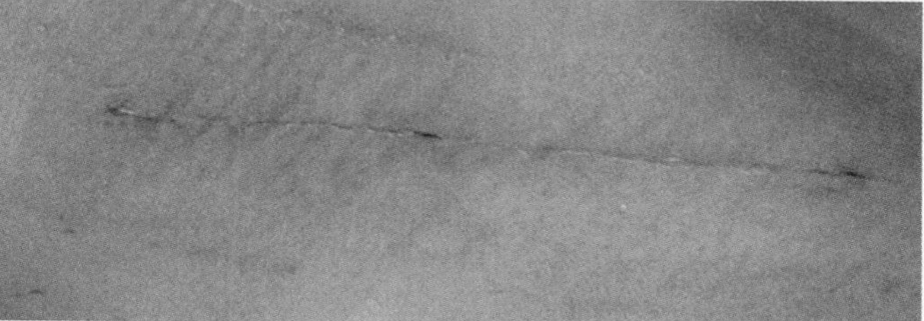

FIGURE 30-16 Fusiform incision and closure.

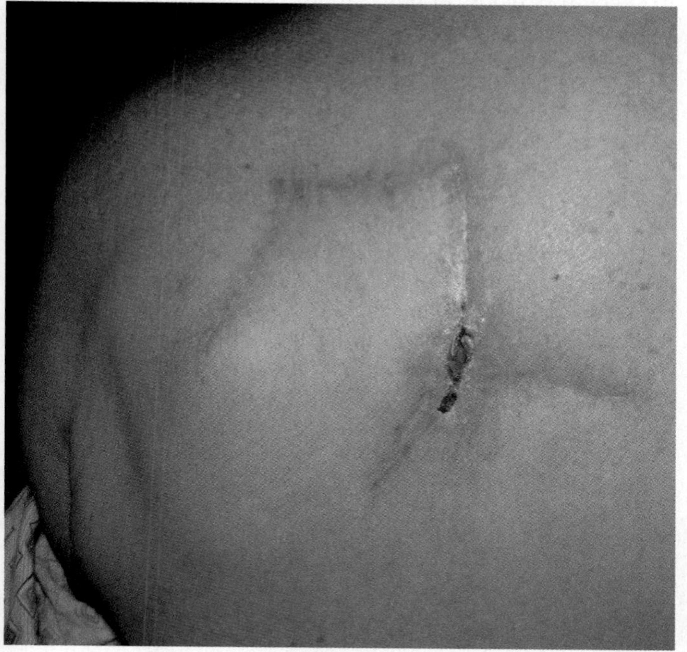

FIGURE 30-17 Unnecessarily complex closure.

submitted for permanent section pathology; frozen section analysis of margins is not performed. In most cases, the incision is closed by mobilizing the skin without the need for complex tissue rearrangement or skin grafting (Fig. 30-17). Complex tissue flaps or skin grafts are rarely necessary, except for melanomas of the head and neck and distal extremities. Tumors arising in proximity to structures such as the nose, eye, and ear may require compromise of conventional margins to avoid deformities or disabilities. Subungual melanomas are treated with amputation of the distal digit to provide a 1-cm margin from the tumor. For fingers, ray amputations are unnecessary because the melanoma commonly involves only the distal phalanx, and amputation at the distal interphalangeal joint is sufficient. In all cases, resection should achieve histologically negative margins. The recommended margins of excision are the clinically measured margins; it is unnecessary to re-excise the melanoma if the final pathology report indicates that the measured distance from the melanoma to the edge of the excised skin is less than the recommended margin unless the margin is involved or almost involved by tumor.

Mohs' micrographic surgery (MMS) involves the sequential tangential excision of skin cancers with immediate pathologic margin assessment. It is used most often for nonmelanoma skin cancers such as squamous cell and basal cell carcinomas, with good results. In melanoma, MMS is used primarily for in situ lesions, although some centers have begun to use MMS for invasive melanoma. MMS is preferred for cosmetically sensitive areas such as the face, where it may minimize the skin defect while still achieving negative margins of excision. Success can be highly operator dependent and requires full pathologic examination of the excised margins. Although there have been several single-institution reports indicating that MMS results in low local recurrence rates for melanoma, it remains controversial.

Management of the Regional Lymph Nodes

Similar to WLE, management of the regional lymph nodes has been refined over the years from earlier aggressive strategies. To understand these developments, first it is important to understand the proper terminology regarding the operations performed for regional lymph nodes. Elective lymph node dissection (ELND) is performed for patients without clinical evidence of nodal metastasis, that is, those without palpable nodes or imaging studies to suggest regional nodal disease. Therapeutic lymph node dissection (TLND) refers to lymphadenectomy performed for nodal disease detected by palpation or imaging studies. Completion lymph node dissection (CLND) is the operation performed after finding nodal metastasis by SLN biopsy.

Elective lymph node dissection. Herbert Snow recognized the propensity for melanoma to metastasize to the regional lymph nodes, and in 1892, advocated that treatment for melanoma include WLE combined with an ELND.[1] Snow realized that melanoma first spread to regional lymph nodes before metastasizing to distant sites. He, therefore, recommended elective nodal dissection both as a curative measure and to improve regional control. These recommendations remained controversial for more than a century, with opponents countering that ELND exposed patients to unnecessary morbidity.

The controversy about elective lymphadenectomy led to several randomized controlled trials. None has demonstrated an overall survival benefit for ELND, although two trials warrant mention for findings on subgroup analysis. In the Intergroup Melanoma Surgical Trial, 740 patients with melanoma 1 to 4 mm thick were randomized to ELND or nodal observation.[27] Although there was no survival difference between the groups overall, subgroup analysis suggested a survival benefit for patients younger than 60 years, those without ulcerated melanomas, those with melanomas 1 to 2-mm thick, and those with extremity melanomas. In 1998, a World Health Organization study randomized 240 patients with truncal melanomas of 1.5 mm or more in thickness to ELND or nodal observation and found no survival advantage for ELND.[30] However, subgroup analysis revealed a significant 5-year survival advantage for patients with occult nodal metastasis found by ELND compared with those who developed nodal disease while under observation and subsequently required TLND (48% versus 27%, respectively; $P = .04$). This provided some support for the notion that early removal of nodal metastasis is more efficacious than waiting for the patients to progress to large palpable nodes.

One reason that these studies failed to show any overall survival benefit is that only approximately 20% of patients with melanomas of 1 mm or more in thickness have nodal metastases at the time of presentation. Therefore, the 80% of patients without nodal metastases cannot possibly benefit from lymphadenectomy. Because the morbidity of lymph node dissection can be substantial, including wound complications, chronic pain, and lymphedema, there has been little enthusiasm for ELND in the absence of a demonstrable survival benefit. On the other hand, the rationale for ELND stemmed from the concept that regional nodal metastases might, in turn, metastasize to distant sites, and that the greater the tumor burden in the regional nodes, the greater the chance for distant metastasis. In this sense, Snow's observations were prescient in that patients rarely develop distant metastases without first developing nodal disease. Early removal of microscopic nodal metastases was therefore thought to improve survival. Retrospective studies have provided support for this concept.

Sentinel lymph node biopsy. The entire controversy about ELND resolved with the development of techniques for SLN biopsy. In 1977, Robinson and colleagues[31] published a study on the use of cutaneous lymphoscintigraphy to identify the nodes that drained truncal melanomas with ambiguous drainage patterns. Because truncal melanomas can potentially drain to cervical, axillary, or inguinal lymph nodes, the decision about which nodal basin should undergo ELND was based on Sappey's anatomic studies from the 19th century. With lymphoscintigraphy, radioactive tracer is injected into the skin around the melanoma, and tracer particles are then allowed to drain through the lymphatic channels into the regional lymph nodes. Nuclear imaging can then identify the location of the draining nodal basin (Fig. 30-18).

Although it now seems obvious that the first nodes in the nodal basin to receive radioactive tracer would also be the first nodes to receive metastatic tumor cells, the concept of a sentinel node was not actually established until the pioneering work of Donald Morton. In 1992, Morton and coworkers[32] published the first report of SLN biopsy for melanoma and found that the sentinel node accurately determined the presence or absence of microscopic nodal metastasis. The study proved the theory of the sentinel node; in a series of 187 lymphadenectomy specimens, nonsentinel lymph nodes were the only site of metastasis in 2 of the 3079 nodes examined.[32]

Since Morton's initial publication, thousands of articles have been published to validate the SLN hypothesis in a variety of malignant neoplasms, and SLN biopsy has become the standard method for staging the regional nodes in melanoma. A comprehensive meta-analysis combined 71 of these studies to evaluate the reliability and validity of SLN biopsy as a staging procedure. Looking at results from more than 25,000 patients, the rate of successful SLN identification was found to be 98.1%, with a false-negative rate of 12.5%.[33] Furthermore, a landmark study by Gershenwald demonstrated that SLN biopsy is the single most important factor predicting prognosis in melanoma patients without clinical evidence of nodal metastasis.[34] Because SLN biopsy is a minimally invasive procedure, this prognostic information comes with fewer associated complications than in a complete lymph node dissection.

Multicenter Selective Lymphadenectomy Trial. The only randomized controlled trial to compare outcomes between SLN biopsy and nodal observation is the first Multicenter Selective Lymphadenectomy Trial (MSLT-I). Overall, 1347 patients with intermediate-thickness melanoma (1.2 to 3.5 mm thick) and 314 patients with thick melanoma (>3.5 mm thick) were randomized to either SLN biopsy or observation. Patients with disease identified by SLN biopsy underwent immediate completion lymphadenectomy. The frequency of nodal metastasis across all groups was 20.8% and was similar within each treatment arm. No difference in 10-year melanoma-specific survival was found between SLN biopsy and observation in either the intermediate-thickness (81.4% versus 78.3%; $P = .18$) or thick melanoma groups (58.9% versus 64.4%; $P = .56$).[35] However, improved 10-year disease-free survival was observed with SLN biopsy in both intermediate and thick melanomas. The status of the sentinel node was the strongest predictor of recurrence or death from melanoma; in patients with intermediate-thickness melanoma, 10-year survival was 85.1% with a negative SLN biopsy compared with 62.1% for positive nodes (hazard ratio [HR], 3.09; 95% confidence interval [CI], 2.12-4.49; $P < .001$).[35] Interestingly, on subgroup analysis limited only to patients with nodal metastasis (disease identified on SLN biopsy or that developed while under observation), improved

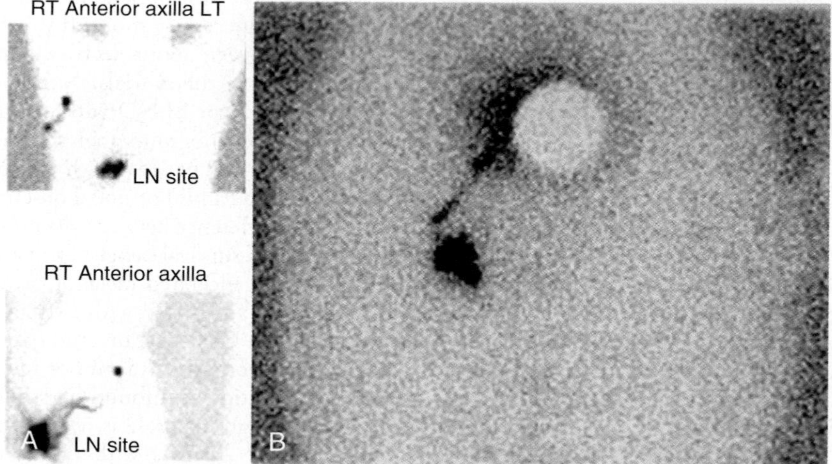

FIGURE 30-18 Preoperative lymphoscintigraphy can aid in the identification of sentinel nodes. **A,** Melanoma of the back with drainage to the axilla. *LN,* lymph node. **B,** Periumbilical lesion with draining sentinel nodes located in the left groin.

melanoma-specific survival, disease-free survival, and distant disease-free survival was observed in the SLN biopsy arm among patients with intermediate-thickness lesions.

Indications. Although SLN biopsy is a minimally invasive procedure, it is not without morbidity and certainly not without cost. Like other staging tests, it should not be overused in low-risk patients and requires careful balancing of risk and benefit. However, given the results from MSLT-I and other studies suggesting that approximately 20% of lesions more than 1-mm thick will have nodal metastasis, there is general consensus that SLN biopsy is appropriate for patients with intermediate-thickness melanoma. However, the role of SLN biopsy in either thin or thick melanoma has been the source of some controversy.

Thin melanoma. In the United States, upwards of 70% of melanomas are less than 1-mm thick. The overall risk of nodal metastasis in these patients is estimated at 5% or less; however, subsets of this population can have rates of nodal disease that approach those seen with thicker lesions. Whereas routine use of SLN biopsy is not recommended for thin melanoma, if these lesions have any features that are associated with an increased risk for nodal spread, SLN biopsy may be indicated.[36] Features of the primary lesion that have been linked to an increased risk of nodal metastasis include ulceration and mitotic rate (≥1 mitosis/mm^2), and as a result, these factors have been incorporated into current AJCC staging. Presence of either ulceration or a mitotic rate of more than 1 mitosis/mm^2 discriminates a T1a from a T1b melanoma and upstages these lesions from stage IA to stage IB. It is, therefore, recommended that patients with T1b melanomas be considered for SLN biopsy.

The thickness of the primary lesion represents another consideration for SLN biopsy. Whereas lesions less than 0.75-mm thick have an SLN metastasis rate of 2.7%, this rises to 6.2% for lesions more than 0.75 mm.[36] Given the low risk of nodal disease, routine SLN biopsy for melanoma less than 0.75 mm is not recommended. The yield of positive SLN for patients with melanomas less than 0.75-mm thick, even if classified as T1b, is low; reasonable clinicians could conclude that SLN biopsy is not warranted for most such patients. On the other hand, some recommend SLN biopsy for all lesions more than 0.75 mm.[37] Certainly, patients with melanomas of more than 0.75 mm that are associated with ulceration or a mitotic rate of 1 mitosis/mm^2 or more should be considered for SLN biopsy. Additional risk factors, such as Clark level, age, and gender, may also inform the decision for SLN biopsy. Whereas Clark level alone may not be sufficient, Clark level 4 or level 5 lesions in combination with other high-risk features may warrant SLN biopsy.[36,38] Similarly, SLN biopsy may be reasonable in patients younger than 40 years if other high-risk factors are present, but no clear age cutoff has been established.[36,39] Male gender may indicate increased risk in the presence of other high-risk factors; in one study, men with thin melanomas more than 0.75-mm thick and a mitotic rate greater than zero had an estimated SLN metastasis rate of 16.1%.[40]

Thick melanoma. As thick primary melanoma (>4 mm) places patients at an increased risk for distant metastatic disease, prior dogma held that SLN biopsy or lymph node dissection was not beneficial for these patients. However, a number of studies have shown that thick melanoma patients with tumor-negative SLN have a better prognosis than those with tumor-positive SLN. One review of 240 patients with melanomas more than 4-mm thick found that 58% of patients had a negative SLN biopsy, and compared with patients with a positive node, a negative biopsy was associated with both improved distant disease-free survival and overall survival.[41] Because there is a continuum of risk that does not abruptly end at 4 mm Breslow thickness, SLN biopsy for thick melanomas may provide improved regional disease control and possibly cure for these patients. Similarly, although the benefit remains unproven, there are reports detailing SLN biopsy for some patients with locally recurrent or in-transit melanoma.

Technical details. The technical details of proper SLN biopsy are worthy of attention. First, all patients should undergo preoperative lymphoscintigraphy, typically performed on the same day as the operation to perform SLN biopsy and WLE. Technetium Tc 99m sulfur colloid (0.5 mCi) should be injected into the dermis, raising a wheal, in four aliquots around the melanoma or biopsy site. It is important to inject the tracer into the normal skin approximately 0.5 cm away from the melanoma or scar from the biopsy and not into the melanoma or biopsy scar itself. A common mistake is to inject the radioactive tracer too deeply into the subcutaneous tissue, which will result in failure to detect a sentinel node. If no sentinel nodes are identified after the initial injection, repeated injection should be performed with the proper technique by an experienced clinician. In almost all cases, this will result in identification of sentinel nodes. Imaging is performed with a gamma camera, with dynamic and static images that allow identification of lymphatic channels and sentinel nodes. Although patterns of lymphatic drainage can be predictable at times, lymphoscintigraphy often identifies lymph nodes in locations that are not anticipated. This is especially true for melanomas in ambiguous lymphatic drainage areas, such as the trunk, head, or neck, where anatomic predictions of nodal spread are unreliable. In such cases, lymphoscintigraphy may identify sentinel nodes in more than one nodal basin. Furthermore, it is not uncommon to identify sentinel nodes outside the traditional cervical, axillary, and inguinal nodal basins. So-called interval, intercalated, or in-transit nodes may be found in subcutaneous locations or between muscle groups. For distal upper or lower extremity melanomas, it is important to assess the presence of epitrochlear or popliteal sentinel nodes, respectively (Fig. 30-19). These interval nodes have the same risk of harboring melanoma cells as sentinel nodes in traditional nodal basins; therefore, it is recommended that they be removed at the time of sentinel node biopsy. In addition, 85% of the time, the interval lymph node is the only positive node, even for those patients with other SLNs identified in traditional

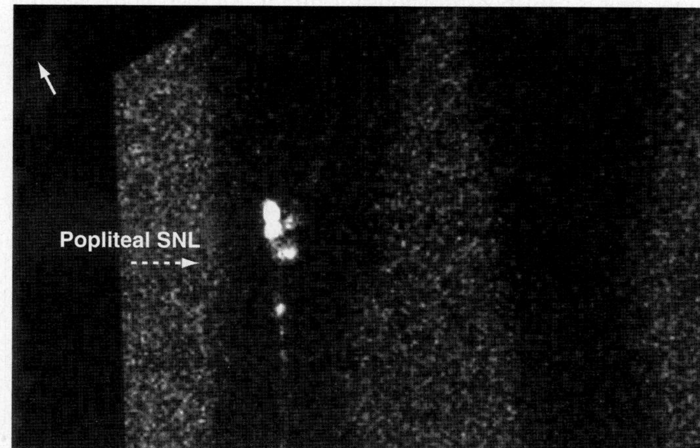

FIGURE 30-19 Popliteal sentinel lymph nodes identified by lymphoscintigraphy.

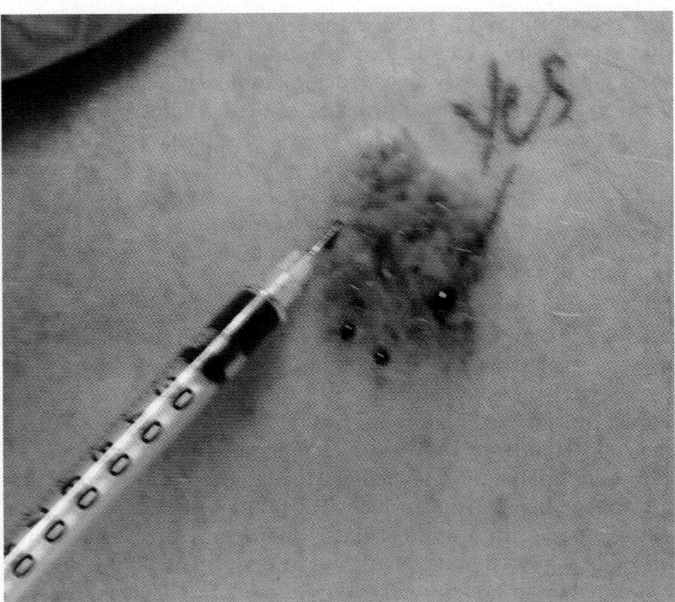

FIGURE 30-20 Raising a wheal with an intradermal injection of vital blue dye.

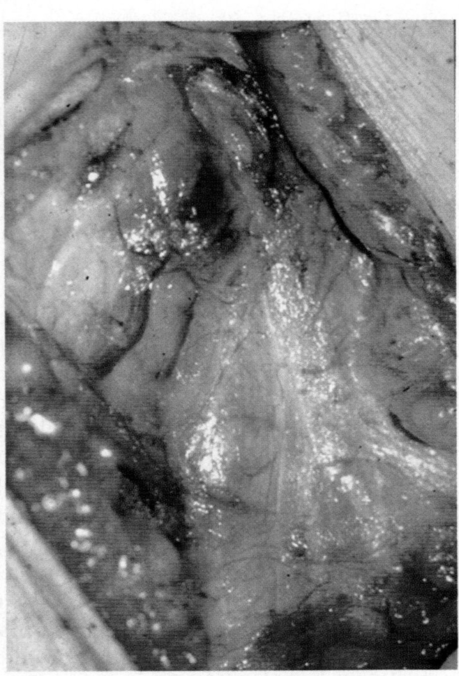

FIGURE 30-21 Blue lymphatic channels leading to a blue node during sentinel lymph node biopsy.

basins. Therefore, sentinel nodes should be removed in all nodal basins identified by preoperative lymphoscintigraphy.

At operation, which is generally performed under general anesthesia, a vital blue dye (e.g., isosulfan blue) is injected into the dermis around the melanoma site in a manner similar to that for injection of the radioactive tracer (Fig. 30-20). This combined lymphatic mapping technique allows the identification of the sentinel nodes in 99% of patients. Because the blue dye will not persist in the sentinel nodes for prolonged periods, it is injected just before the operation. One to 5 mL is used, depending on the size of the melanoma site. Because blue dye will persist in the skin for many months after injection, it is best to inject it within the margins of the planned WLE. A hand-held gamma probe is used to identify the location of the sentinel nodes, and dissection is performed to identify blue lymphatic channels entering into any blue lymph nodes (Fig. 30-21). A sentinel node is defined as any lymph node that is the most radioactive node in the nodal basin, any node that is blue, any node that has a radioactive count of 10% or higher of the most radioactive node in that basin, or any node that is palpably suspicious for tumor. All such nodes require resection, and following these guidelines minimizes the false-negative rate of SLN biopsy. Although multiple radioactive lymph nodes may be evident within a nodal basin on lymphoscintigraphy, many of these represent second-echelon nodes that do not need to be removed; there is often a poor correlation between the number of nodes visualized on the lymphoscintigram and the number of sentinel nodes identified. In general, the average number of sentinel nodes identified is two per nodal basin. Tissue should be sent for permanent section histopathology with immunohistochemical stains for melanoma markers (e.g., S-100, HMB-45, and Melan-1). Immediate frozen section histology should be avoided because even expert pathologists have difficulty in diagnosing micrometastatic melanoma in the SLN on frozen sections.

SLN biopsy is more challenging in the head and neck than for other regions, probably because of the rich lymphatic drainage network in this location. Correspondingly, the false-negative rate for SLN biopsy is generally higher for melanomas in these locations. Precise knowledge of the anatomy in this region is essential to avoid inadvertent neurologic or other injury. Parotid sentinel nodes can be identified and removed, usually without the need for superficial parotidectomy. However, if there is any concern for facial nerve injury, superficial parotidectomy may be a safer option. A common site for cervical SLN is directly adjacent to the spinal accessory nerve, which should be visualized and preserved.

Lymph Node Dissection

Completion lymphadenectomy. Although the status of the regional nodal basin is the most important prognostic factor in cutaneous melanoma, the prognosis of patients with a positive sentinel node varies widely. Depending on the presence of other risk factors, overall 5-year survival can range from 15% to 85% with stage III disease. The presence of disease in nonsentinel nodes is an independent predictor of decreased survival in stage III patients, and most patients with a positive sentinel node are offered completion lymphadenectomy to improve disease control. Nonetheless, despite current recommendations that call for completion lymphadenectomy in the setting of positive lymph nodes, some have questioned the need for CLND, given that nodal metastasis is often not found beyond the SLN. However, in two large prospective randomized trials (MSLT-I and the Sunbelt Melanoma Trial), the rate of tumor-positive nonsentinel nodes among patients who underwent CLND for tumor-positive sentinel nodes was 16%. Similarly, a retrospective multi-institutional study by Wong and colleagues found that regional nodal recurrence developed in 15% of 134 patients with positive sentinel node metastases who did not undergo CLND. From these studies, it can be estimated that the risk of nodal recurrence after SLN biopsy is at least 15% if CLND is not performed.

Several studies have tried to identify subgroups of sentinel node–positive patients who may be at a lower risk of nonsentinel

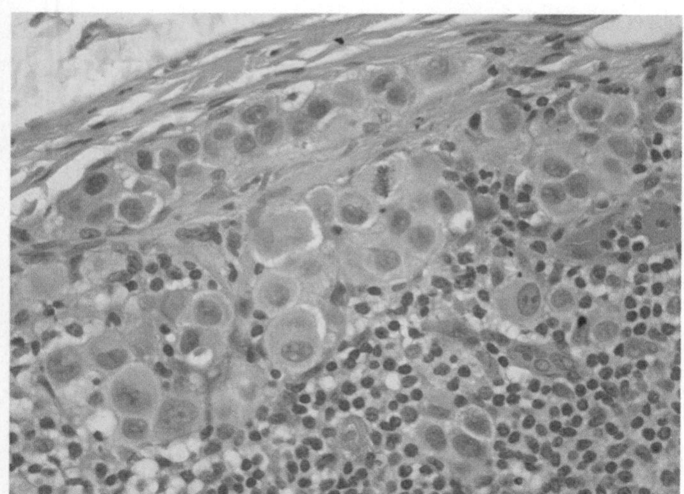

FIGURE 30-22 Subcapsular micrometastatic melanoma deposits within the lymph node.

node metastasis. Multiple different scoring systems evaluating the burden of micrometastatic disease within the lymph node have been developed, with criteria including location of tumor deposits, tumor cross-sectional area, tumor diameter (either summed across all foci or only within the largest focus), and depth of invasion into the lymph node (Fig. 30-22). One study comparing different classifications for tumor burden with the sentinel node found that the maximum diameter of the largest focus of micrometastatic disease was the most powerful predictor of nonsentinel node status, overall survival, and disease-free survival.[42] Nonetheless, tumor deposits within the lymph node may reflect a continuum of disease, and there is currently no consensus regarding which patients may safely avoid completion lymphadenectomy.

Regional disease control and cure are the two principal goals of completion lymphadenectomy. Even if cure is unlikely, regional disease control remains an important goal of therapy; allowing patients to progress can result in significant pain and suffering from advanced nodal metastases (Fig. 30-23). In MSLT-I, the rate of regional nodal recurrence after CLND was 4.2%; in the Sunbelt Melanoma Trial, it was 4.9%. Therefore, although it remains uncertain whether CLND cures more patients or improves overall survival, it does appear to provide excellent regional disease control. Currently, the MSLT-II is under way to determine if CLND offers a survival benefit over SLN alone. Until the results of MSLT-II are available, it is recommended that patients with metastatic disease in the SLN undergo completion lymphadenectomy. For patients with SLNs identified in more than one nodal basin, CLND should be performed only for the basins with positive sentinel nodes.

Therapeutic lymph node dissection. Patients with nodal metastasis suspected by palpation or imaging studies should undergo confirmation with fine-needle aspiration biopsy in most cases. In some cases, palpable nodes may be benign, and dissection for patients who have benign lymphadenopathy should be avoided. In equivocal cases, excisional biopsy may confirm the diagnosis. In the absence of metastatic disease, lymph node dissection can result in long-term survival and potentially cure for a significant fraction of patients. Prognosis depends on the extent of the nodal disease. There is a wide range of overall survival, depending on such factors as the number of positive nodes and

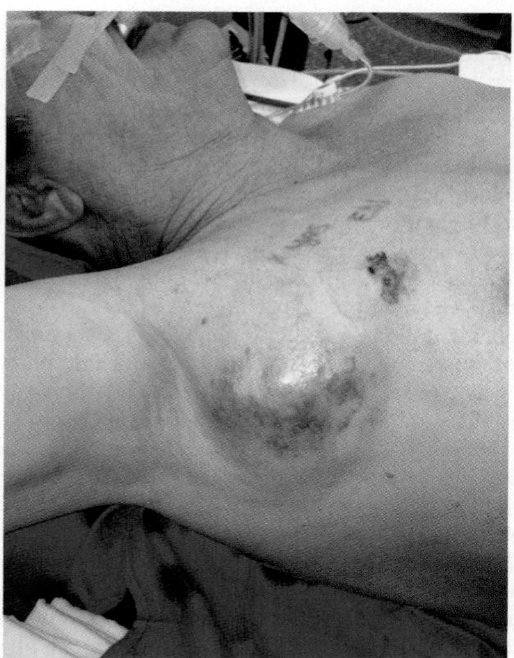

FIGURE 30-23 Advanced axillary nodal disease.

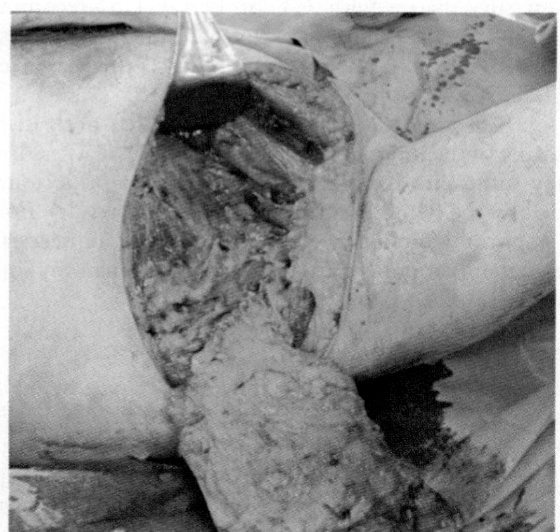

FIGURE 30-24 Complete en bloc excision of axillary lymph nodes for advanced disease.

the disease burden within the lymph node (e.g., microscopic versus macroscopic disease).

Extent. Because of the lack of effective adjuvant therapy agents, lymphadenectomy should be as complete as possible. There is a marked difference, for example, in the axillary lymph node dissection performed for breast cancer compared with surgery for melanoma. In breast cancer, a level I or II lymph node dissection is performed to gain important staging information while hormonal therapy, chemotherapy, and radiation provide effective regional control. In melanoma patients, effective regional control results from a thorough level I, II, and III axillary dissection (Fig. 30-24). For instance, in breast cancer, conventional wisdom dictates minimizing attempts to clear level II nodes cephalad to the axillary vein and not clearing level III nodes at all in an effort to decrease the risk of lymphedema. However, failure to completely clear these level II and III nodes can be a frequent cause of nodal recurrence in melanoma patients after axillary lymphadenectomy. Therefore, complete removal of all fibrofatty tissue around the axillary vein, thoracodorsal and medial pectoral neurovascular bundles, and long thoracic nerve should be performed. To clear bulky level II and III nodes, the pectoralis minor muscle may need to be divided near its insertion on the coracoid process. On rare occasions, the pectoralis major muscle may need to be divided as well. The axillary vein may be ligated and divided if it becomes involved with tumor, often with less consequence in terms of edema than one might anticipate.

Inguinal lymph node dissection includes the superficial inguinal (femoral) lymph nodes and may also include dissection of deep or pelvic (internal iliac, external iliac, and obturator) nodes. For most cases of lower extremity melanoma metastatic to inguinal sentinel nodes, a superficial inguinal lymph node dissection is sufficient. There is no consensus as to when adding a pelvic dissection is necessary. For patients with palpable nodal disease or with imaging suggestive of involved pelvic lymph nodes, the deep nodes should be dissected in most cases. Metastasis to Cloquet's node, which links the femoral and iliac nodal chains underneath the inguinal ligament, has traditionally been a common indication for a deep dissection. Similarly, gross involvement of multiple nodes on superficial dissection is another traditional indication for pelvic dissection. For patients with inguinal nodal disease, follow-up surveillance with CT or PET/CT is recommended because pelvic nodal recurrence may be difficult to detect clinically until it is bulky and extensive. Once this has occurred, regional disease control may be lost.

For cervical lymphadenectomy, a functional neck dissection with sparing of the internal jugular vein and spinal accessory nerve is usually sufficient. The need for superficial parotidectomy may be guided by the lymphoscintigraphy and SLN results. Epitrochlear or popliteal lymphadenectomy is frequently unnecessary but requires careful attention to the particular anatomy in these regions (Fig. 30-25).

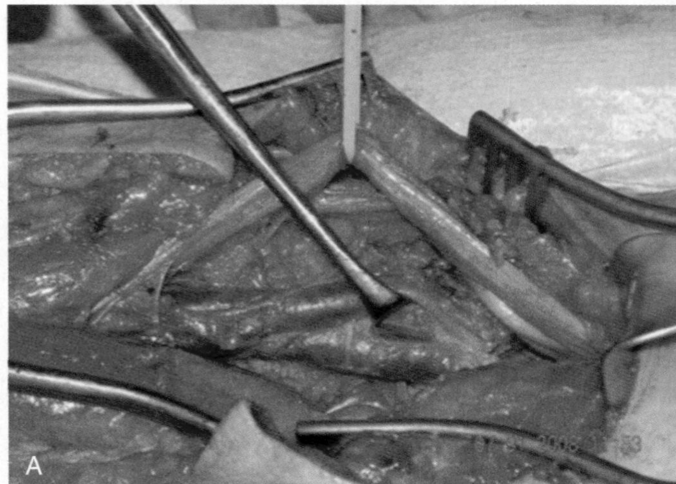

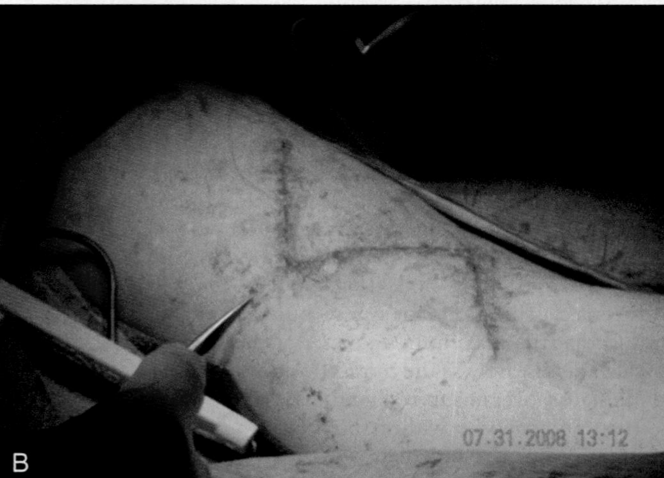

FIGURE 30-25 Popliteal lymphadenectomy with closure.

Adjuvant Therapy

The development of successful adjuvant therapies in melanoma has been hindered by a lack of effective systemic therapies. At least 25 randomized trials in stage II to stage III melanoma have evaluated a variety of adjuvant therapies, including chemotherapy and immune stimulants, without any clear survival advantage shown. Outside of clinical trials, current NCCN guidelines recommend interferon and radiotherapy as the two principal options for adjuvant therapy in select patients with stage II or stage III melanoma, although there are good reasons to remain skeptical about these options. Given the recent development of new targeted therapies and immunotherapies for stage IV disease (see "Treatment of Metastatic Disease"), effective adjuvant treatment for melanoma may be on the horizon. This underscores the need to encourage participation in clinical trials to evaluate novel agents in the setting of adjuvant therapy.

Interferon alfa-2b. The only systemic adjuvant therapy approved by the U.S. Food and Drug Administration (FDA) is high-dose interferon alfa-2b. Interferon alfa-2b is administered at nearly the maximum tolerated dose, with 1 month of intravenous therapy followed by 11 months of subcutaneous injections three times weekly. The therapeutic index is relatively low, and there are substantial associated adverse effects. These include influenza-like symptoms, fatigue, malaise, anorexia, neuropsychiatric side effects, and potential hepatic toxicity.

The clinical efficacy of high-dose interferon alfa-2b has been evaluated in several prospective randomized trials. In 1984, the Eastern Cooperative Oncology Group conducted the first trial, E1684. Most of the 287 high-risk melanoma patients enrolled in this study had palpable nodal disease, and an advantage in both disease-free and overall survival was observed with interferon at a median follow-up of 6.9 years. On the basis of these findings, the FDA approved high-dose interferon alfa-2b for high-risk patients. However, with longer follow-up (median, 12.6 years), only disease-free survival remained significant. Similar results were seen in the larger follow-up study, E1690, which demonstrated a marginal improvement in disease-free survival but no difference in overall survival. A third study, E1694, randomized patients to high-dose interferon versus a ganglioside vaccine (G_{M2}). This study was stopped early because of the clear superiority of interferon compared with the vaccine in terms of disease-free and overall survival. Initially interpreted as evidence of the beneficial effect of interferon, considerable doubt was placed on E1694 after follow-up studies demonstrated a significant detrimental effect once the G_{M2} vaccine was compared with placebo. The European Organization for Research and Treatment of Cancer (EORTC) evaluated 5 years of pegylated interferon alfa-2b versus observation. In this trial (EORTC 18991), an improvement in disease-free survival was seen, but there was no benefit in distant metastasis-free interval or overall survival. Finally, the Sunbelt Melanoma Trial randomized patients with a single positive sentinel node (all of whom underwent CLND) to observation versus high-dose interferon alfa-2b. Although it was somewhat underpowered to detect small differences in disease-free or overall survival, this study showed neither trends nor significant differences to suggest a benefit from high-dose interferon in this population.

Because of the toxicity of high-dose interferon, multiple studies have evaluated alternative dosing schedules. In the largest such trial, EORTC trial 18952, intermediate doses of interferon were evaluated in patients with stage IIB or stage III disease. Although there was demonstrable improvement in disease-free survival, no improvement in distant metastasis-free interval or overall survival was seen. Additional studies have largely had similar results, suggesting that lower doses may provide a disease-free survival advantage similar to that of high-dose interferon.

Altogether, these studies suggest that adjuvant interferon may prolong disease-free survival, but there is likely no survival benefit for most patients. Given the cost and toxicity of high-dose interferon alfa-2b, it has not gained widespread acceptance. Interestingly, in the Sunbelt Melanoma Trial, the 5-year survival for sentinel node–positive patients who did not receive interferon was 67% after CLND, suggesting that clinically occult nodal disease has an intermediate mortality risk. Therefore, observation in these patients is likely a reasonable option.

Radiation Therapy

Melanoma is relatively resistant to irradiation, and adjuvant radiation therapy is not used routinely. However, there may be a role in select patients after lymphadenectomy to limit nodal recurrence. In one randomized controlled trial, 250 patients considered to be at high risk for nodal recurrence were allocated to either adjuvant radiotherapy (48 Gy in 20 fractions) or observation. High risk was defined as one or more involved parotid nodes, two or more cervical or axillary nodes, three or more involved inguinal nodes, presence of extranodal extension, or maximum diameter of the largest lymph node greater than 4 cm (3 cm for cervical nodes). With a median follow-up of 40 months, risk of nodal relapse was lower in the radiotherapy group (HR, 0.56; 95% CI, 0.32-0.98), although there were no differences observed in disease-free or overall survival between the two groups.[43] In addition to patients who fit the high-risk criteria outlined before, radiotherapy may also be considered in patients who present with palpable nodal disease or in select patients with desmoplastic neurotropic melanoma who have inadequate margins of excision.

Follow-Up after Treatment of Melanoma

Whereas there are no clear guidelines on appropriate follow-up for patients after they have been treated for melanoma, some general principles should be considered. Follow-up is dictated largely by each patient's risk of recurrence, which takes into consideration disease stage as well as any other patient-specific risk factors. In addition to the risk of recurrence related to the initial melanoma, patients are at an estimated 8% to 10% increased risk for development of a second primary melanoma, not to mention other skin cancers. For this reason, the most important component of surveillance is a thorough history and physical examination, performed at least annually for life. Most recurrences will be detected within the first 5 years after treatment of the primary melanoma, although it is possible to detect metastatic disease decades afterward. In general, most recurrences are detected by the patient or on history and physical examination, and relatively few are found with laboratory or imaging tests. There are no data to suggest that routine screening with imaging affects overall survival. Similarly, routine laboratory tests are generally not needed.

With this is mind, a general follow-up strategy can be based on an individual patient's risk of metastasis. Stage 0, I, and IIA patients are at low risk of recurrence and should be observed by history and physical examination at least every 6 months for the first 3 years and at least annually thereafter. A careful history is necessary to elicit symptoms such as new skin lesions, nodal masses, pain, headaches, neurologic changes, weight loss, and gastrointestinal and pulmonary symptoms. Patients should be educated about common symptoms and signs of recurrence so that they can report any important changes that arise between scheduled visits. Physical examination should include a complete skin inspection, including palpation to detect regional nodal or in-transit recurrence. For stage IIB, IIC, and III melanoma patients, a reasonable follow-up schedule would be a history and physical examination every 3 or 4 months for the first 3 years, every 6 months for the next 2 years, and annually thereafter. The use of laboratory tests and imaging tests such as CT, MRI, or PET/CT is controversial but not unreasonable for these patients. Patients with stage IV melanoma will have regular clinical, laboratory, and radiologic evaluations to monitor the response to treatment.

Treatment of Recurrent Disease

Local recurrence. Recurrent tumors within 2 cm of the WLE scar or skin graft are considered local recurrences and represent aggressive tumor biology associated with a poor overall survival. Recurrence risk increases with tumor thickness and has been estimated as 0.2%, 2%, 6%, and 13% for melanomas less than 0.75 mm, 0.75 to 1.5 mm, 1.5 to 4 mm, and larger than 4 mm, respectively. Treatment for local recurrence is surgical resection to histologically negative margins. Although WLE guidelines for primary tumors do not apply, at least a 1-cm margin should be attempted with complete resection of the prior WLE scar. SLN biopsy of local recurrences may detect positive regional nodes, but its role in this situation is unclear, and it is considered on a case-by-case basis.

In-transit disease. In-transit recurrences arise from tumor deposits within lymphatic channels draining the primary tumor and are manifested as either subcutaneous or cutaneous tumor nodules located between the primary tumor site and regional nodal basin. They are frequently not pigmented or clearly visible, and the only sign on examination may be a palpable nodule. If in-transit disease is suspected, patients may require fine-needle aspiration or biopsy to confirm the diagnosis and should have an imaging evaluation to detect distant metastatic disease. Limited in-transit disease amenable to resection is adequately treated by excision to negative margins. SLN biopsy is of unclear value but may be considered. Only approximately 20% of patients will have no progression of disease after resection, but those with recurrent in-transit disease can be managed with repeated excision and maintain a good quality of life for years. To treat in-transit lesions that are not amenable to wide excision, intralesional injections have been used. Available agents (none of which are FDA approved for this indication) include bacille Calmette-Guérin, interleukin-2, interferon alfa, PV-10 (a red dye with antitumoral activity likely by the immune response), and talimogene laherparepvec (an oncolytic virus encoded with the gene for granulocyte-macrophage colony-stimulating factor). Whereas most of these therapies have been evaluated only with small studies, both partial and complete responses have been reported. Additional options include topical therapy with imiquimod for superficial lesions and the use of radiation, although radiotherapy is usually ineffective for in-transit disease.

Extensive or recurrent in-transit disease confined to the upper or lower extremity may be treated by hyperthermic isolated limb perfusion (HILP). With HILP, either the femoral or axillary vessels are cannulated and connected to a pump oxygenator that circulates heated chemotherapy while a tourniquet isolates the extremity to limit systemic toxicity. Concentrations of chemotherapy that are 15 to 25 times higher than systemic delivery methods can be reached, and drug is delivered at temperatures up to 42°C. In the United States, melphalan (L-phenylalanine mustard) is the most common agent used; in Europe, tumor necrosis factor-α (TNF-α) is commonly added to melphalan. The American College of Surgeons Oncology Group evaluated the addition of TNF-α to melphalan in a large randomized controlled trial but found no significant advantage in overall or complete response rates. In addition, the use of TNF-α was associated with a significantly higher rate of toxicity and adverse events.

Since Creech and colleagues first performed HILP at Tulane University in the 1950s, several single-institution studies have demonstrated overall response rates of approximately 80% (Fig. 30-26). Complete response rates vary and may be as high as 60%. Unfortunately, durable complete responses are less common, as many patients will have recurrence within 1 year. Many recurrences can be managed with local therapies, such as excision and intratumoral injection, although repeated perfusion can be performed in patients who initially responded to HILP. Despite the likelihood of recurrence, an initial complete response still may predict a better prognosis. Ten-year survival in patients with a complete response approaches 50%. Given the success of HILP in patients with in-transit disease, it was hypothesized that HILP could serve as an adjuvant therapy to help decrease the risk of recurrence after excision of high-risk primary melanoma (>1.5 mm Breslow thickness). More than 800 patients were randomized to WLE alone or WLE with HILP, with no benefit seen in overall survival or disease-free survival at more than a 6-year median follow-up. Based on this, HILP is recommended only for patients with established in-transit disease.[44]

The toxicity of HILP can be substantial, and long-term morbidity is seen in more than 40% of patients. Common complications include compartment syndrome, neuropathy, skin reaction, blistering, and lymphedema; amputation may become necessary in 1% to 3% of patients (Fig. 30-27). To limit regional and systemic toxicity, Kroon and Thompson[45] introduced isolated limb infusion (ILI), a less invasive method of delivering regional chemotherapy. Vascular access with ILI is accomplished by insertion of percutaneous catheters, with pneumatic tourniquet isolation of the involved extremity. Perfusion is performed through manual circulation with a syringe and is therefore less resource intensive than HILP. Without the pump oxygenator, ILI is a hypoxic procedure with lower flow rates that HILP. Studies have demonstrated comparable results to HILP with less limb toxicity, although response rates for ILI are on the lower end of what is reported for HILP. ILI is especially appealing for treatment of patients with in-transit disease who do not require regional lymphadenectomy or who have undergone prior HILP. In patients with extensive in-transit disease refractory to therapy, amputation is seldom if ever indicated. These patients carry a high risk of having distant metastases, and long-term survival is not achieved by amputation.

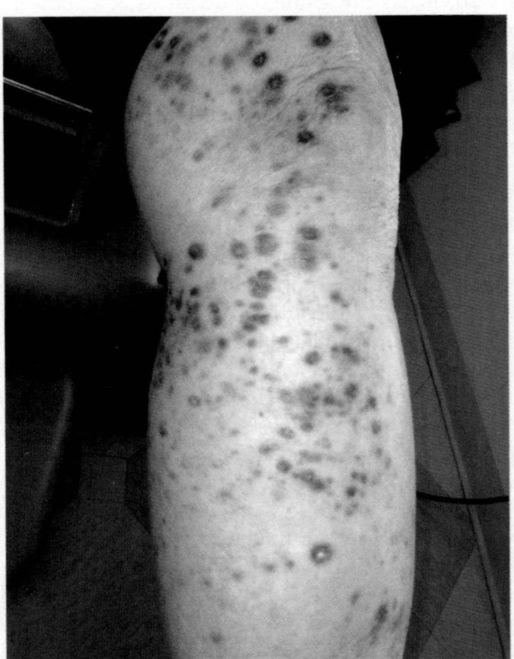

FIGURE 30-26 Response of in-transit disease after HILP. Note that the skin can remain pigmented after therapy.

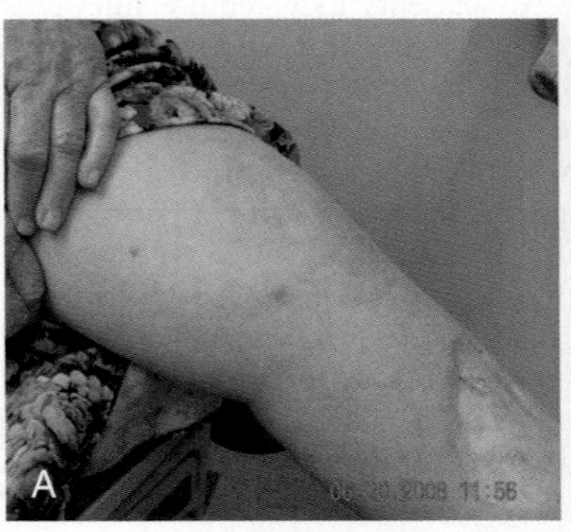

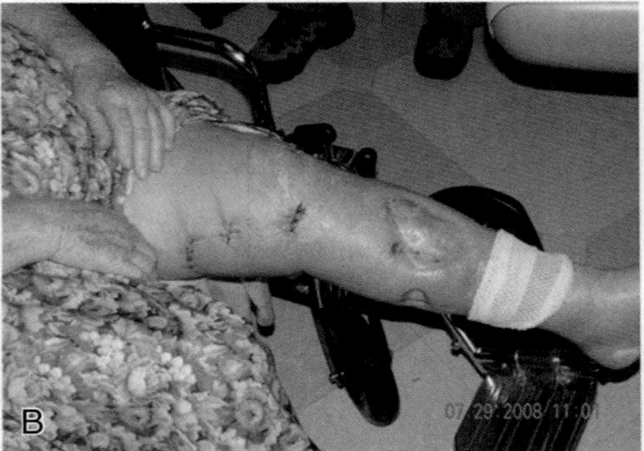

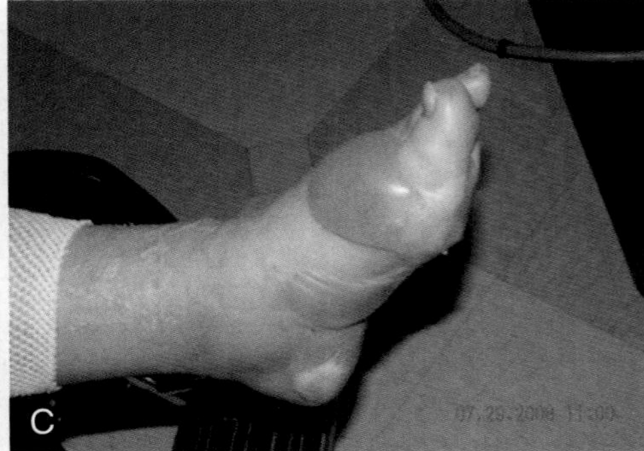

FIGURE 30-27 **A,** Recurrent in-transit melanoma. **B,** Erythema after HILP. **C,** Lower extremity blisters after HILP.

Regional nodal recurrence. Regional nodal recurrence is treated by lymphadenectomy in patients who previously have not had a complete lymph node dissection. If a patient has a recurrence within a previously resected nodal basin, excision of the recurrence to negative margins is recommended. Left untreated, advanced regional nodal disease can develop with subsequent loss of regional disease control. These recurrences can encase neurovascular structures and ulcerate through the skin, resulting in pain, bleeding, infection, and decreased quality of life. Adjuvant systemic or radiation therapy can be considered, depending on the extent of disease, including enrollment in clinical trials.

Treatment of Metastatic Disease

Systemic therapy. For all intents and purposes, there has not been effective systemic therapy for advanced metastatic melanoma since Hunter's initial description of the disease in the 18th century. To this day, disseminated melanoma has one of the worst survival rates among all cancers, with a median overall survival of 6 to 10 months. Historically, the only two approved therapies for metastatic melanoma were dacarbazine (DTIC) and high-dose interleukin-2. Whereas these agents demonstrated modest response rates, no benefit in overall survival was ever found. Biochemotherapy, an approach combining three chemotherapeutic agents (cisplatin, vinblastine, and dacarbazine) with interleukin-2 and interferon, similarly showed no overall survival benefit despite some limited success in achieving overall and complete response rates. Essentially, although individual patients would occasionally respond well to therapy, these events were too infrequent to demonstrate any benefit to the overall population. On top of that, these therapies were accompanied by significant toxicity and side effects.

The landscape has changed drastically during the last several years after the introduction of several novel agents that have demonstrated an overall survival benefit in metastatic melanoma.[46] As a result of our greatly improved understanding of the genetic and molecular mechanisms behind melanoma, two separate approaches have emerged: immunotherapy and targeted therapy. These strategies depend, in part, on identifying the specific mutations that are active in particular melanomas, allowing therapies to be tailored to individual patients.[11]

Immunotherapy. Immunotherapy has long been a strategy for melanoma; prior treatment with interleukin-2, interferon alfa, and granulocyte-macrophage colony-stimulating factor as well as multiple vaccine trials attempted to boost inherent immunity to fight cancer cells. Through a better understanding of immune checkpoints, newer strategies focus on blocking negative feedback systems that suppress T cell activity.

Ipilimumab is a monoclonal anti–CTLA-4 antibody that was the first systemic agent to demonstrate improved overall survival in patients with metastatic melanoma. In activated T cells, the CTLA-4 receptor traffics to the extracellular membrane, where it inhibits costimulatory ligands on antigen-presenting cells and thereby prevents continued antigen-presenting cell stimulation of the T cell. By blocking CTLA-4, ipilimumab effectively prolongs the T cell response (Fig. 30-28). In one study that randomized 502 patients to either ipilimumab plus DTIC or DTIC and placebo, the ipilimumab group demonstrated significantly prolonged overall survival (11.2 months versus 9.1 months; $P <$ .001), with the survival benefit extending out to 3 years (20.8% versus 12.2%).[47] Grade 3 or 4 complications occurred in 56.3% of those treated with ipilimumab, including colitis, hepatitis, and rashes. Whereas there were no bowel perforations, surgeons should know that this is a known complication to ipilimumab therapy. Occasional autoimmune-related treatment-induced deaths have also been reported. Ipilimumab is FDA approved for treatment of metastatic melanoma.

The programmed death 1 (PD-1) inhibitors represent a newer family of immune checkpoint regulators. Similar to CTLA-4, interaction of the PD-1 receptor with its ligands PD-L1 and PD-L2 promotes T cell anergy and apoptosis (Fig. 30-29). Some tumors even express PD-L1, and in effect, will turn off the T cells with which they come into contact. In several phase 1 trials, use of PD-1–blocking antibodies led to durable, objective responses observed across several types of solid tumors. Concurrent use of PD-1 inhibitors with ipilimumab in 53 patients with unresectable stage III or stage IV melanoma led to an objective response in 53% of patients, all with a tumor reduction greater than 80%.[48] Further studies are under way, but PD-1 inhibitors have the potential to be a first-line therapy for melanoma. In fact, pembrolizumab was approved in 2014 for the treatment of patients with unresectable or metastatic melanoma and disease progression after therapy with ipilimumab and, if *BRAF* V600 mutation positive, a BRAF inhibitor.

Targeted therapy. The development of targeted therapies has resulted from the identification of driver mutations such as *BRAF* (see "Pathogenesis") in malignant melanoma. Understanding of these mutations has allowed the development of drugs that specifically inhibit overactive signaling molecules (Fig. 30-30). The first of these agents was vemurafenib, a small-molecule kinase inhibitor effective against the V600E mutated version of *BRAF*. In a phase 3 randomized controlled trial comparing vemurafenib with DTIC in the treatment of 675 patients with metastatic melanoma, vemurafenib demonstrated both a significant survival benefit (HR, 0.37; 95% CI, 0.26-0.55) and a prolonged median progression-free survival (5.3 months versus 1.6 months; $P <$ .001).[49] Common side effects included arthralgias, fatigue, rash, and photosensitivity. As a result, the FDA approved vemurafenib for use in metastatic melanoma. At the most recent follow-up, vemurafenib demonstrated increased median overall survival (13.6 months versus 9.7 months; $P = .0008$), and maintained a prolonged median progression-free survival (6.9 months versus 1.6 months; $P < .0001$).[50] Additional BRAF inhibitors have demonstrated comparable success. Dabrafenib, another selective BRAF inhibitor that targets the V600E mutation, demonstrated a similar increase in progression-free survival compared with DTIC (5.1 months versus 2.7 months; $P < .0001$).[51]

A major concern for BRAF inhibitors is that most patients become resistant to therapy and can relapse within 6 months. For instance, with prolonged follow-up, the survival benefit seen with vemurafenib begins to narrow; whereas there was an HR of 0.37 at 3.8 months, the HR increases to 0.70 at 1 year.[49,50] There are multiple reports describing patterns of resistance to vemurafenib, most of which describe the increased use of alternative signaling pathways or upregulation of the MAPK pathway downstream through increased MEK activity. For this reason, combination therapy using BRAF and MEK inhibitors has been evaluated. In one study, combination therapy using the MEK inhibitor trametinib with dabrafenib prolonged progression-free survival compared with dabrafenib alone (9.3 months versus 8.8 months; $P =$ .03); this combination is now FDA approved for the treatment of unresectable or metastatic melanoma.[52]

Moving forward, combinations of immunotherapy and targeted therapy as well as other systemic options may further improve survival in metastatic melanoma. During the next several

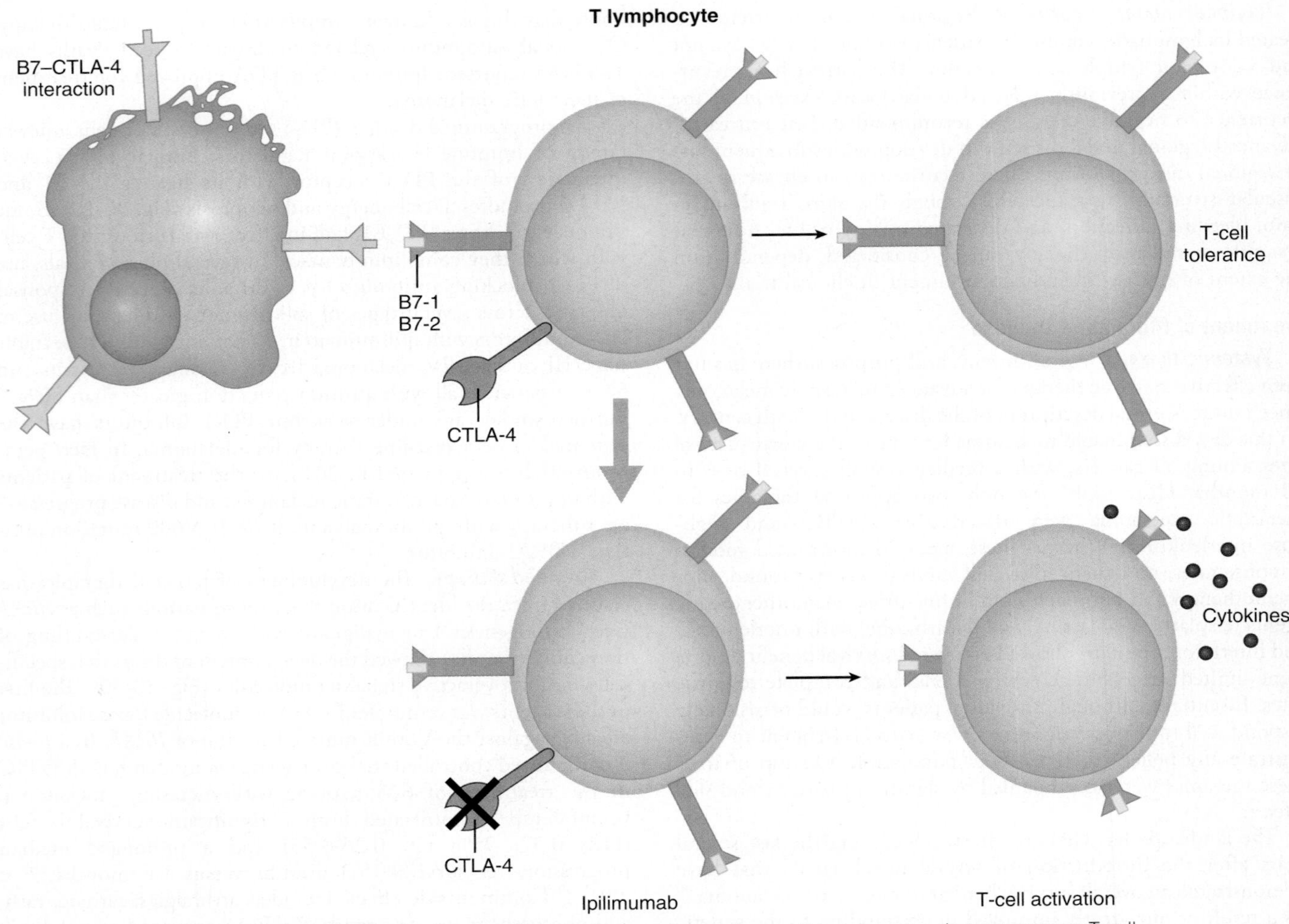

FIGURE 30-28 CTLA-4 is a key negative regulator on the surface of T lymphocytes that suppresses T cell function. Blockade of CTLA-4 with ipilimumab permits T cells to continue with antitumor activity. (From Srivastava N, McDermott D: Update on benefit of immunotherapy and targeted therapy in melanoma: The changing landscape. *Cancer Manag Res* 6:279–289, 2014.)

years, the landscape will continue to evolve as multiple randomized controlled trials determine the optimal treatment strategies. Engaging patients in clinical trials not only will give them the best chance for a clinical response but will also continue to drive this exciting development of new therapies.

Metastasectomy. Although most patients with stage IV melanoma will present with disseminated lesions that are not amenable to resection, patients with limited metastatic disease should undergo resection when it is feasible. Not only does resection offer palliation, but for some stage IV patients, resection provides a survival advantage similar to that seen after lymphadenectomy for advanced stage III patients. Whereas overall the median survival of patients with stage IV melanoma is approximately 6 to 10 months, in well-selected patients, resection of metastatic disease can lead to 5-year survival rates ranging from 15% to 40%. Even patients with brain metastases may benefit from complete resection, further emphasizing that complete extirpation of all disease may be the best treatment, even for advanced disease. Careful selection of patients is paramount; important things to consider in evaluating a patient for resection of metastatic disease include the patient's underlying functional status and comorbidities, the location and number of metastatic lesions, and the features reflective of the underlying tumor behavior, such as the disease-free interval from the time of primary resection. An emerging consideration is the role of novel systemic therapies, which may provide an effective neoadjuvant option that, up to this time, has been absent in melanoma care. With the introduction of these agents, the indications for and timing of resection for stage IV will be an area of active research.

Special Situations and Noncutaneous Melanoma

Unknown Primary Melanoma

In rare cases, patients will present with stage III or stage IV melanoma and no preceding diagnosis of cutaneous melanoma. This occurs in less than 2% of melanoma cases overall and in less than 5% of all cases involving metastatic disease. A diagnosis of unknown primary melanoma should prompt a thorough skin examination, including the perianal area, external genitalia, nail beds, scalp, and external auditory canal. Endoscopic evaluation of the oral cavity and nasopharynx as well as of the anus and rectum can identify mucosal melanoma. Women should undergo a thorough pelvic examination, and an ophthalmology examination may be required to rule out ocular melanomas. PET/CT and MRI of the brain are warranted to assess the extent of disease.

Some hypothesize that unknown primary melanomas arise from benign nevus cells already trapped within lymph nodes.

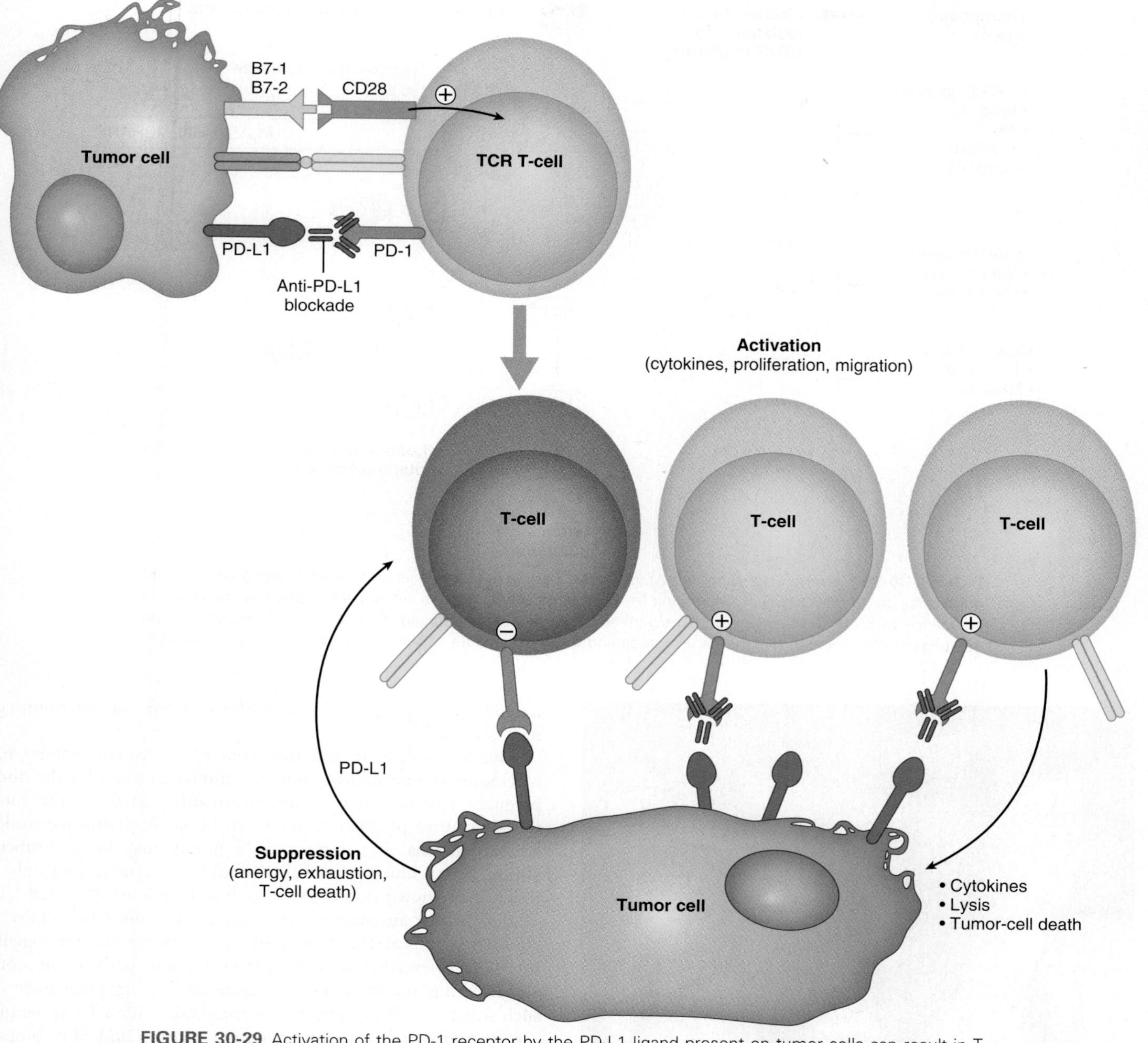

FIGURE 30-29 Activation of the PD-1 receptor by the PD-L1 ligand present on tumor cells can result in T cell anergy and death. Receptor blockade with anti–PD-1 prevents suppression of T cell activity, allowing an improved antitumor response. *TCR,* T cell receptor. (From Srivastava N, McDermott D: Update on benefit of immunotherapy and targeted therapy in melanoma: The changing landscape. *Cancer Manag Res* 6:279–289, 2014.)

Alternatively, cutaneous melanoma is known to undergo spontaneous regression in rare cases, presumably as a result of an immune response to the primary tumor. Therefore, a history of a prior pigmented skin lesion that has disappeared or clinical evidence of vitiligo should be closely scrutinized (Fig. 30-31). Not infrequently, patients will provide a history of pigmented skin lesions that have been excised, cauterized, or treated with lasers. Pathology review of any previously excised skin lesions should be performed.

In the setting of lymph node metastasis without a primary lesion, TLND is performed with the assumption that it represents stage III disease. Interestingly, patients with unknown primary melanomas who present with lymph node involvement have equivalent or possibly better overall survival compared with patients with a known primary lesion. This may suggest a stronger immune response in these patients that resulted in regression of the primary melanoma.

Melanoma and Pregnancy

Close to one third of all women diagnosed with melanoma are of childbearing age, and lesions that arise during pregnancy can raise difficult clinical questions. Whether there is a link between

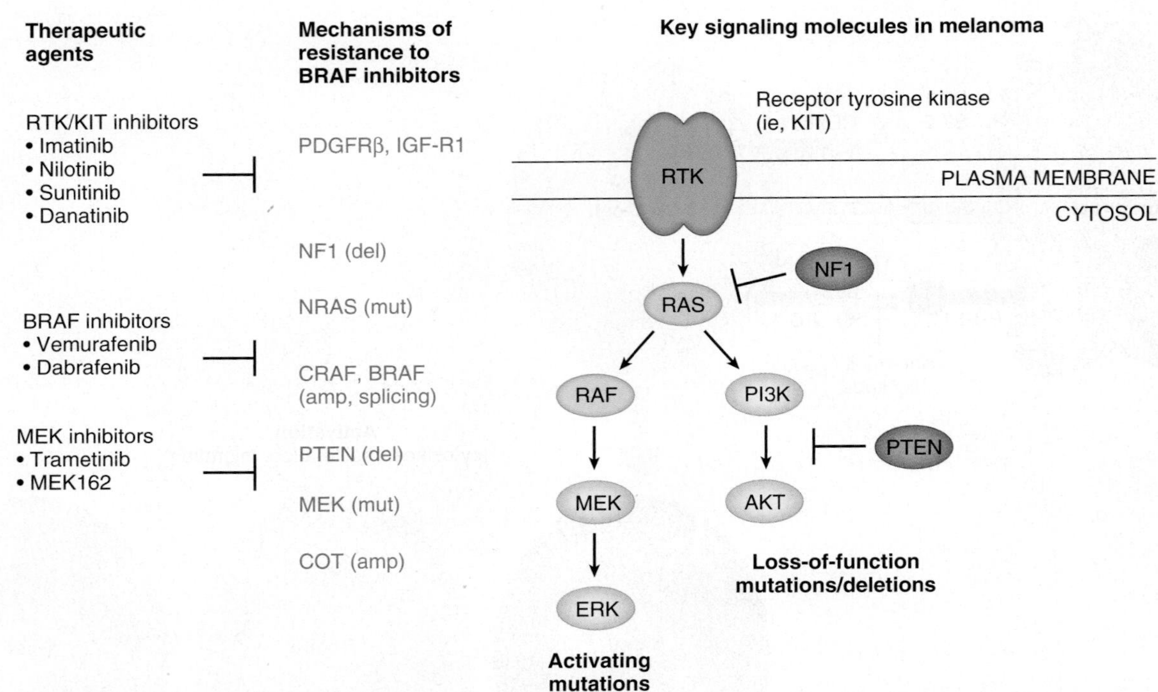

FIGURE 30-30 Common signaling pathways involved in the pathogenesis of melanoma along with current options for targeted therapies. Alterations to multiple different steps in the signaling cascade can result in resistance to BRAF inhibitors. (From Griewank KG, Scolyer RA, Thompson JF, et al: Genetic alterations and personalized medicine in melanoma: Progress and future prospects. *J Natl Cancer Inst* 106:djt435, 2014.)

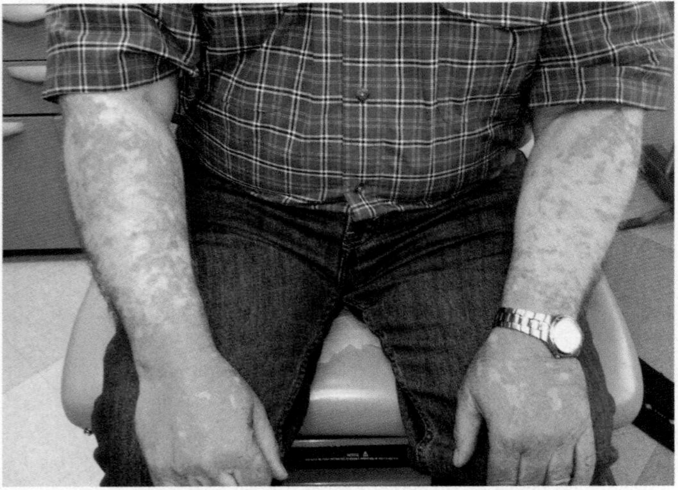

FIGURE 30-31 Vitiligo after immunotherapy. On occasion, patients with an unknown primary melanoma will present with similar findings.

pregnancy and the overall risk for development of melanoma is not well understood. Whereas early studies suggested that hormonal changes during pregnancy led to increasing pigmentation and an environment conducive to melanoma development, current evidence does not support these theories. Therefore, any nevus or pigmented lesion with suspicious changes during pregnancy should not be attributed to hormones or the expected physiology of pregnancy, and appropriate workup is required. In addition, although early studies may have suggested worse outcomes for melanoma in pregnancy, once controlling for tumor-related factors, it has become clear that the prognosis for patients treated during pregnancy is no different from that for nonpregnant patients.[53]

Overall, evaluation and treatment of a pregnant patient for melanoma should follow guidelines similar to those for the nonpregnant patient. There is no therapeutic benefit to the early termination of pregnancy. WLE can be safely performed under local anesthesia. If necessary, SLN biopsy may be performed, although vital blue dye probably should not be used. Not only is there an unknown risk to the fetus, but there is an estimated 1 in 10,000 risk of an anaphylactic reaction. Lymphoscintigraphy is considered safe as the dose used is well below the teratogenic threshold. Nevertheless, some physicians and patients are concerned about use of radioactive materials during pregnancy; in such situations, WLE under local anesthesia with a 1-cm margin can be performed, with wider margin excision and SLN biopsy reserved until after the baby is delivered. For patients who have tumors with poor prognostic factors, it may be advisable to wait 2 to 3 years before the next pregnancy as this represents the time during which recurrence is most likely.

Noncutaneous Melanomas

Although the neural crest cells that ultimately yield melanocytes migrate predominantly to the skin during fetal development, they will also localize to several other organs and tissues. As a result, melanomas may arise in other locations, including on mucosal surfaces, within the eye, or in the leptomeninges.

Within the eye, melanocytes are found in the retina and uveal tract (iris, ciliary body, and choroids). In the United States, ocular melanoma is the most common intraocular malignant neoplasm in adults. Primary treatment consists of enucleation or iodine-125 brachytherapy, although other options include photocoagulation and partial resection. Unlike cutaneous melanoma, given the lack of lymphatic vessels in the uveal tract, metastatic spread of ocular melanoma occurs hematogenously. Metastasis occurs almost exclusively in the liver, but resection of liver metastases from ocular melanoma is rarely possible. Although CT scans may suggest a solitary liver metastasis, more sensitive modalities such as MRI may display hundreds of small lesions. There are no accepted effective treatments for ocular melanoma metastatic to the liver, and patients can be encouraged to participate in clinical trials.

The most common sites for mucosal melanomas are the head and neck (oral cavity, oropharynx, nasopharynx, and paranasal sinuses), anal canal, rectum, and female genitalia. Because of the occult location of many of these lesions, patients tend to present with more advanced disease and have a poor prognosis. When possible, these tumors should be excised to negative margins. Given the high risk of metastatic disease, extensive local resections, such as abdominoperineal resection or pelvic exenteration, do not improve overall survival. However, these procedures may decrease the risk of local recurrence. In general, a role for SLN biopsy has not been established, and lymph node dissection is not indicated unless patients have clinically evident lymphadenopathy. The majority of mucosal melanomas may be associated with *KIT* amplifications, whereas *BRAF* or *NRAS* mutations are rare. Clinical trials in mucosal melanoma have, therefore, focused on targeted therapies with KIT inhibitors.

CUTANEOUS MALIGNANT NEOPLASMS: NONMELANOMA SKIN CANCER

Squamous Cell Carcinoma and Basal Cell Carcinoma

Nonmelanoma skin cancer (NMSC) represents the most common type of malignant neoplasm in the world. In the United States, it is estimated that almost one in five Americans will develop NMSC during their lifetime. Approximately 80% are basal cell carcinoma (BCC), with squamous cell carcinoma (SCC) representing nearly 20%. Much rarer types of NMSC make up the remainder of cases. Sun exposure is the predominant risk factor, and similar to melanoma, the overall incidence of NMSC is increasing. Accurate estimates of NMSC incidence are difficult to ascertain as many are treated without obtaining a histologic diagnosis, and most cases are not reported within national registries. The American Cancer Society reports more than 2 million cases of BCC and SCC per year in the United States. After an initial diagnosis of BCC or SCC, there is an increased risk for the development of additional cancers, including a second NMSC, melanoma, or even some nonskin cancers. For this reason, patients with a prior diagnosis of skin cancer require long-term periodic surveillance. Fortunately, as a result of early detection and effective therapy, mortality rates for NMSC are declining.

Squamous Cell Carcinoma

Risk factors for development of SCC include exposure to sunlight, susceptible skin types, compromised immunity, environmental exposures, and underlying genetic disorders. Most SCCs occur on sun-exposed surfaces, particularly the head and neck. In susceptible individuals (those with fair skin, blond hair, and blue eyes), prolonged sun exposure correlates directly to an increased risk for SCC. In contrast to melanoma or BCC, the cumulative effect of chronic UV radiation likely plays a larger role in SCC than intermittent, intense exposures. As with melanoma, individuals with dark complexions have a lower risk, even with prolonged sun exposure. The risk for NMSC increases with occupational or recreational sun exposure, advancing age, and proximity to the equator. The amount of sun exposure is also proportional to the incidence of known precursor lesions for SCC, including actinic keratosis.

It is thought that UV radiation, and UVB in particular, increases the risk of SCC through several mechanisms. First, there is the direct carcinogenic effect of UV light on the frequently dividing keratinocytes within the basilar layer of the epidermis. Unrepaired mutations from UV light damage can drive tumor proliferation and growth. Second, UVB-induced silencing of the *p53* tumor suppressor gene occurs in more than 90% of SCCs.[54] With loss of p53, keratinocytes are unable to arrest the cell cycle or to initiate apoptosis in the face of cellular damage from UV radiation. With subsequent mutations, cells can then progress from dysplasia to in situ or invasive disease.

Occupational and environmental carcinogens, including arsenic, organic hydrocarbons, ionizing radiation, and cigarette smoke have also been associated with an increased risk for SCC. Genetic disorders, including xeroderma pigmentosum and albinism, are associated with increased risk for many types of skin cancer. A history of chronic inflammation from burn scars (Marjolin ulcer), draining sinuses, infections (including osteomyelitis), and nonhealing ulcers can precede the development of SCCs. In the setting of chronic nonhealing wounds, or even with previously healed wounds that subsequently break down, biopsy may be prudent to rule out SCC.

Immunosuppression is a well-established cause of SCCs of the skin, particularly with the suppression of cell-mediated immunity after solid organ transplantation. Skin cancer is the most frequent malignant neoplasm in organ transplant recipients, with SCC and BCC representing 95% of these cancers. Whereas the risk of BCC increases 10-fold after transplantation, these patients have an incidence of SCC that is 65 times that of the normal population (Fig. 30-32). Not only is there an increased risk for development of

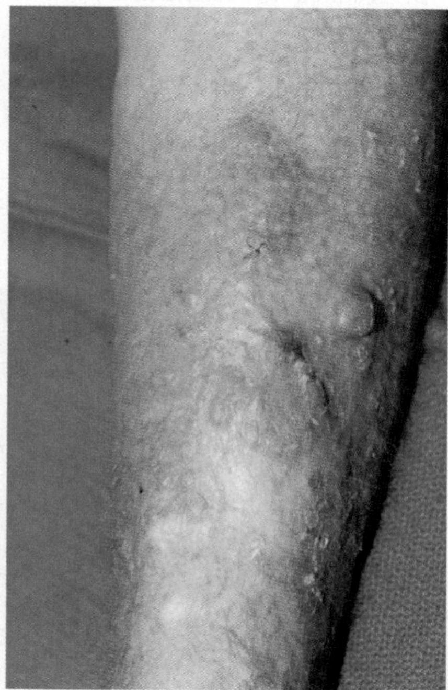

FIGURE 30-32 Multiple squamous cell carcinomas on the forearm of a patient after kidney transplantation.

cancers, but the tumors that develop appear more aggressive with an increased rate of metastases. The intensity of immunosuppression and the duration of therapy both correlate with the risk of malignancy. Whereas malignant neoplasms develop in 10% to 27% of patients after 10 years of immunosuppression, this number increases to 40% to 60% after 20 years. Patients with transplants such as heart or lung that require stronger immunosuppression regimens are at increased risk compared with those who require less medication.[55] In addition to pharmacologic immunosuppression, conditions associated with acquired impairments of cell-mediated immunity (lymphomas, leukemias, and autoimmune diseases) have an increased risk for SCC. Human papillomavirus, an infection associated with immunosuppression, is proposed as a causative factor for the development of SCCs. BRAF inhibition is also associated with the development of SCC.

Most SCCs begin with a proliferation of keratin cells in the basal layer of the epidermis that appear as red or pink areas, clinically termed actinic keratoses (solar keratoses). Local symptoms may wax and wane for a period of many months. Lesions are scaling, with an uneven surface and an erythematous base (Fig. 30-33). Individual lesions are usually smaller than 1 cm in diameter and appear in chronically sun-damaged skin. The diagnosis is both clinical and histologic as actinic keratoses share many microscopic features with SCC in situ. The overall risk for malignant conversion to invasive SCC is low and estimated to be in the range of 1 in 1000 lesions/year. Bowen disease, which appears histologically as SCC in situ, initially is manifested with a reddened area that progresses to thickened plaques and may vary from small lesions (<1 cm) to large areas. When it is confined to the glans penis or vulva, Bowen disease is sometimes referred to as erythroplasia of Queyrat.

Invasive SCCs are palpable scaling lesions that become ulcerated centrally and have elevated, firm edges. In addition to spreading horizontally, these lesions may grow vertically and become fixed to underlying tissue. They may be confused with keratoacanthoma, a benign lesion that can also thicken and ulcerate. Biopsy may be required to differentiate between these two conditions.

Most SCCs can be treated locally with excellent results (see "Treatment Options for Squamous and Basal Cell Carcinoma"). Recurrence is associated with tumor size, degree of differentiation, depth of invasion, perineural involvement, immune status of the patient, and anatomic site. Local recurrence is associated with an increased risk for regional and distant metastases. High-risk areas for development of metastasis include tumors originating from the dorsal hands, lips, ears, and penis. The first site of metastasis is usually the regional lymph nodes.

Basal Cell Carcinoma

BCC is the most common NMSC, and lesions are most commonly found on the sun-exposed areas of the head and neck. Risk factors for development of BCC are similar to those for SCC, although basal cell lesions may result more from intense, intermittent exposure to UV radiation. On a molecular level, 90% of BCCs have been linked to mutations in the hedgehog signaling pathway.[54] A key signaling pathway in embryonic development, it is largely inactive in adult tissues. In the presence of hedgehog (Hh) signaling peptides, the Patched (PTCH) receptor releases the transmembrane Smoothened (SMO) protein, allowing SMO to initiate a signaling cascade that activates the expression of several target genes. Normally, PTCH will inhibit SMO in the absence of Hh signals. Both activating mutations in SMO and inactivating mutations in PTCH have been linked to BCC, ultimately leading to unrestricted growth signaling.

In contrast to SCCs and actinic keratoses, there is no precursor skin lesion for BCCs. These lesions may have an appearance that varies from nodules in the skin to a large nonhealing sore, with drainage and crusting. In comparison to SCCs, they have a slow growth rate, which can lead to a delay in diagnosis. BCCs commonly infiltrate locally but rarely metastasize. Metastases are associated with advanced age of the patient and neglected large lesions. The primary site will often undergo resection multiple times before metastases appear. Once metastatic disease appears, the median survival drops to less than 1 year.

BCCs grow in multiple distinctive patterns, and although there is not a universally accepted classification system, there are several common subtypes. The nodular growth pattern is characterized by a well-defined, elevated lesion with a waxy appearance (Fig. 30-34). As the lesion grows, pearly opalescent nodules develop along the margins. A central depression with umbilication or ulceration and rolled edges is a classic sign. Distinct blood vessels (telangiectasia) may be seen across the surface or along the edges of the mass. Although most BCCs are pink or skin colored, they may also have shades of brown or black pigmentation, thereby mimicking a benign mole or melanoma. Cystic BCCs are less common but have a distinctive appearance. Their surface is translucent, and they may appear blue or gray and be confused with a

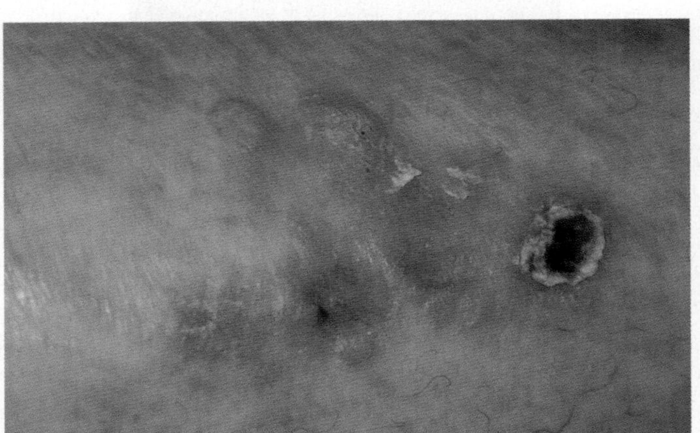

FIGURE 30-33 Squamous cell carcinoma with red, scaling skin.

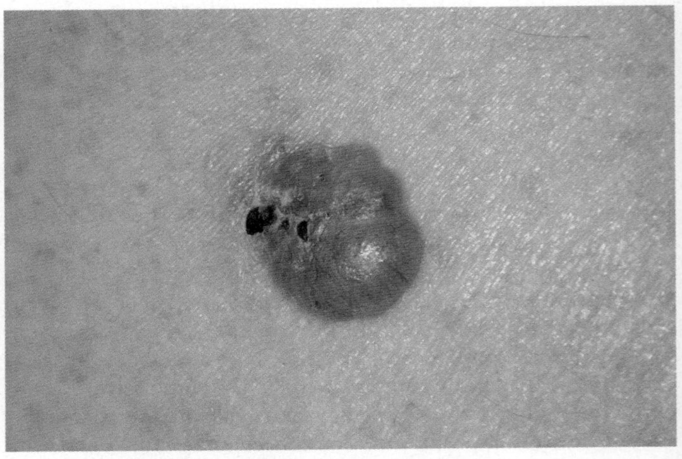

FIGURE 30-34 Nodular basal cell carcinoma.

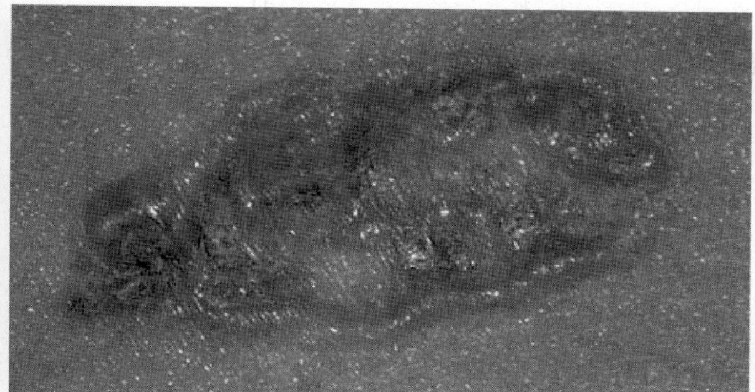

FIGURE 30-35 Morpheaform basal cell carcinoma.

blue nevus. Superficial BCCs are more macular than other growth patterns and may extend over the surface of the skin in a multicentric pattern. The center can ulcerate, and the margins are often irregular and ill-defined. These lesions may appear similar to those of psoriasis, tinea, or eczema. In micronodular lesions, there may be several mildly elevated pink or red lesions that pepper the skin. Associated with a more aggressive growth pattern, there is often extension well beyond visible changes in the skin surface. The white scarring varieties of this growth pattern are termed morpheaform BCC; these lesions are among the most locally invasive subtypes and can penetrate deep into the underlying subdermis (Fig. 30-35).

Treatment Options for Squamous and Basal Cell Carcinoma

NMSC is staged by different criteria than melanoma. The overall favorable prognosis and low risk of metastasis in NMSC have limited the applicability of a formal staging system, although recent evidence-based updates that incorporate known high-risk features may improve risk stratification for affected patients.[56] In the seventh edition of the AJCC staging manual, these updates were based primarily on high-risk features for SCC, although the staging system can continue to be applied to other NMSCs, such as BCCs. The T stage is determined by the largest diameter of the lesion on the skin surface and by invasion of extradermal structures and incorporates high-risk features such as perineural invasion, Clark level 4 or higher, location (ear or nonglabrous lip), and differentiation.

Evaluation for surgical treatment of SCCs and BCCs begins with an assessment for high-risk factors as this will help guide selection from the multiple treatment modalities that are available (Table 30-4). In assessing high-risk factors, appropriate considerations include size, location, histology, and individual patient factors. Treatment options include surgical excision as well as any number of field therapies. Whereas surgical resection techniques include histopathologic analysis to define the margins of resection, field therapies treat a generalized area but do not define the status of margins. Field therapy approaches include radiation therapy, cryosurgery, photodynamic therapy, electrodessication and curettage, and topical agents like imiquimod. In addition, as in melanoma, several targeted therapies have been developed for use in NMSC. Vismodegib was recently approved for use in advanced or metastatic BCC and works by targeting SMO gain-of-function mutations within the hedgehog pathway. In SCC, both epidermal growth factor receptor antagonists and tyrosine kinase inhibitors may have some benefit.[54]

Standard surgical excision is the preferred treatment for most SCCs and BCCs. This procedure is usually performed under local

TABLE 30-4 Basal Cell and Squamous Cell Skin Cancer: Risk Factors for Local Recurrence Based on Characteristics of the Primary Tumor

FACTOR	LOW RISK	HIGH RISK
Location		
Trunk and extremities	<20 mm	≥20 mm
Forehead and neck	<10 mm	≥10 mm
Central part of the face	<6 mm	≥6 mm
Borders	Well defined	Poorly defined
Incidence	Primary	Recurrent
Immunosuppression	Negative	Positive
Previous radiation therapy/ chronic inflammation	Negative	Positive
Rapid growth rate	Negative	Positive
Neurologic symptoms	Negative	Positive
Differentiation	Well	Moderate or poorly
Perineural/vascular invasion	Negative	Positive

Adapted with permission from the NCCN clinical practice guidelines in oncology (NCCN Guidelines) for basal cell skin cancer version 1.2015.

anesthesia. According to the most recent NCCN Clinical Practice Guidelines in Oncology (NCCN Guidelines), a 4- to 6-mm margin is adequate for low-risk tumors, whereas 10-mm margins should be sought for high-risk lesions. The risk for local recurrence is less when wider margins are obtained, especially in the presence of micronodular, infiltrative, and morpheaform histologic patterns. After excision, the local cure rate is greater than 90%. An alternative surgical approach is MMS, which attains a high rate of local tumor control through the use of horizontal frozen sections. The high success rate of MMS is attributed to closer examination of a greater proportion of the excision margins in addition to identification of the precise location of any positive margins. Along positive margins, excision continues until clear margins are obtained. MMS may be preferred for recurrent or high-risk tumors, those with irregular margins, and tumors in anatomic areas such as the eye, nose, mouth, and ear, where tissue preservation is important.

Although field therapy techniques do not define the margins of treatment histologically, they may still be effective for local tumor control. Cryotherapy is best suited for small superficial lesions and can be expected to achieve local control rates greater than 90%. Treated areas are allowed to heal slowly by secondary intention, often resulting in pale scars. Curettage may be used for patients with superficial lesions less than 2 cm in size. Radiation therapy is highly effective for the treatment of BCC and SCC, especially for preserving wide areas of skin in the head and neck region. In areas at high risk for recurrence after extensive surgical excision, radiation may also serve as a useful adjunctive therapy. Radiation should be avoided in SCCs that arise within chronic ulcers or scars; these often will require surgical excision.

In precursor lesions of SCC, such as actinic keratosis, cryotherapy is a commonly performed therapy. Alternative treatments include topical 5-fluorouracil, electrodessication and curettage, carbon dioxide laser, dermabrasion, and chemical peel. Tissue biopsy is indicated when the actinic keratosis is raised or recurrent after topical therapy.

Uncommon Cutaneous Malignant Neoplasms

Among the myriad lesser-known skin conditions and tumors, several uncommon skin malignant neoplasms are important for the general surgeon to understand and to know how to manage. Cutaneous angiosarcoma is a rare, aggressive, soft tissue sarcoma derived from blood or lymphatic vessel endothelium. Cutaneous angiosarcoma predominantly occurs in elderly whites and most commonly arises on the head and neck. In addition, angiosarcoma has been observed to follow chronic lymphedema after axillary dissection for breast cancer (Stewart-Treves syndrome) and may arise in irradiated tissues after prolonged intervals. The typical finding is a smooth, firm or spongy subcutaneous growth that develops a violaceous erythema similar to a bruise. Left alone, it may subsequently develop into an ulcerated mass up to 10 cm or more in size. On histologic evaluation, angiosarcomas are high grade and often multifocal, with skip areas of normal-appearing skin. Abnormal, pleomorphic, malignant-appearing endothelial cells are pathognomonic. Although principal spread is hematogenous, compared with other sarcomas, there is a high incidence of lymph node metastasis. Treatment consists of complete resection with histologically negative margins and irradiation of the involved field. Lymph node dissection is indicated if lymphadenopathy appears before distant metastases are identified. There is no consensus about the role of adjuvant chemotherapy. Overall, 5-year survival rate is approximately 35%.[57]

Dermatofibrosarcoma protuberans (DFSP) is a low-grade sarcoma arising from dermal fibroblasts. Lesions appear as smooth, flesh-colored nodules in or immediately beneath the skin and generally are manifested in patients between 20 and 50 years of age. Most appear on the trunk (50%), with the remainder on the proximal extremities (20% to 35%) or on the head and neck (10% to 15%). Because of their slow growth, lesions are commonly 1 to 5 cm at diagnosis. Their external appearance belies their true character as tumor cells will frequently invade the underlying soft tissues and contribute to incomplete excision and local recurrence. Treatment consists of WLE with a 2- to 4-cm margin. Specimen orientation and pathologic analysis of margins are required. Distant metastases are uncommon and are preceded by two or more local recurrences. A variant of DFSP is associated with fibrosarcomatous change on pathologic examination; these lesions may have a more aggressive course with a higher risk for distant disease. Adjuvant radiation therapy has been used effectively after resection for recurrences. Interestingly, the translocation t(17:22) has been found in approximately 90% of DFSP lesions. This has led to the use of imatinib in patients with locally advanced or metastatic disease and sometimes as neoadjuvant therapy.[58]

Extramammary Paget disease (EMPD) is a rare form of adenocarcinoma that arises from apocrine glands of the skin, most commonly in the perianal area, vulva, and scrotum. The clinical appearance is that of an erythematous plaque, but white or depigmented areas with crusts and scaling may also be present. The size is variable, from smaller than 1 cm to an entire area in the anogenital region. Because EMPD can have many clinical characteristics in common with eczema, bacterial and fungal infections, and nonspecific dermatitis, the diagnosis is often made by biopsy of lesions not responding to standard therapies. In most cases, EMPD is confined to the epidermis and is well controlled with excision. When invasion of the deeper structures occurs, the disease becomes increasingly difficult to control, and the mortality rate increases to about 50%. Because EMPD is also associated with an increased risk for simultaneous internal malignant neoplasms in the genitourinary and gastrointestinal tracts, a complete workup includes a survey of these locations. Standard treatment is surgical resection extending to histologically negative margins, which may require a number of procedures because the histologic changes are best seen on permanent section. Patients require close clinical follow-up because local recurrences are common. Radiation therapy has been reported to reduce the incidence of local recurrence after excision.

Kaposi sarcoma, a low-grade soft tissue malignant neoplasm, arises from lymphatic vascular endothelial cells in the skin. The incidence is increasing because it is most often seen in patients with acquired immunodeficiency syndrome (AIDS) and other immunosuppressed states, such as organ transplantation. In patients infected with human immunodeficiency virus (HIV), human herpesvirus 8 has been identified as the causative agent of Kaposi sarcoma. There is also a classic variant seen on the lower extremities of older men of eastern European and Mediterranean descent. The clinical picture is variable; asymptomatic purple to brown bruises develop and progress to spots, plaques, or nodules on both lower extremities. Local symptoms appear late as the tumors become advanced. In AIDS patients, skin changes respond best to aggressive antiretroviral therapy. Symptomatic skin lesions can be treated with radiation therapy, intralesional injection of chemotherapeutic agents, cryotherapy, or excision.

Although rare, Merkel cell carcinoma (MCC) is an aggressive and often fatal malignant neoplasm. There is debate as to whether Merkel cells arise from epidermal or neural crest progenitors, but on histologic evaluation, MCC may be indistinguishable from small cell carcinoma and other small round blue cell tumors. There is emerging evidence to suggest that the transformation of Merkel cells into MCC is the result of a novel virus, the Merkel cell polyomavirus.[59] The diagnosis is confirmed by biopsy, and initial workup may require additional tests and imaging, such as chest radiograph to rule out other tumors. Partly because of the poor overall survival in these patients compared with other NMSCs, the AJCC developed an MCC-specific staging system in 2010. The primary treatment is WLE (2- to 3-cm margins), although MMS has been used for some lesions where tissue conservation is necessary. SLN biopsy is generally recommended to identify patients with occult regional lymphatic metastases, which may occur in up to one third of cases. Nodal status affects prognosis, and patients with nodal disease have a significantly decreased overall survival. MCC is a relatively radiosensitive tumor, and adjuvant radiation has been shown to reduce the local recurrence rate at the primary tumor site. If the SLN is positive, adjuvant radiation to the nodal basin after CLND may decrease the rate of regional recurrence and improve overall survival. Although metastases may be responsive to chemotherapy, there is currently little evidence to support adjuvant systemic therapy.[59]

Many other cutaneous lesions and conditions are associated with malignancy but are beyond the scope of this chapter. However, the important principles in the management of these entities are the same as those reviewed earlier:

- Clinicians must have a low threshold for biopsy of new or changing skin lesions.
- The diagnosis is made by biopsy and histologic analysis.
- If appropriate, surgical excision is performed, with the goal of obtaining histologically negative margins.
- Further treatment and follow-up schedule will be dictated by the specific diagnosis.

SELECTED REFERENCES

Balch CM, Gershenwald JE, Soong SJ, et al: Final version of 2009 AJCC melanoma staging and classification. *J Clin Oncol* 27:6199–6206, 2009.

A detailed explanation of the most recent updates to the AJCC staging system for melanoma.

Breslow A: Thickness, cross-sectional areas and depth of invasion in the prognosis of cutaneous melanoma. *Ann Surg* 172:902–908, 1970.

The original paper describing the Breslow thickness classification for primary melanoma.

Chapman PB, Hauschild A, Robert C, et al: Improved survival with vemurafenib in melanoma with BRAF V600E mutation. *N Engl J Med* 364:2507–2516, 2011.

The initial trial demonstrating a survival benefit for the BRAF inhibitor vemurafenib.

Clark WH, Jr, From L, Bernardino EA, et al: The histogenesis and biologic behavior of primary human malignant melanomas of the skin. *Cancer Res* 29:705–727, 1969.

Clark's original description of the Clark level classification for melanoma.

Eggermont AM, Spatz A, Robert C: Cutaneous melanoma. *Lancet* 383:816–827, 2014.

Excellent overview of the advances in our understanding of melanoma and the emergence of novel therapies during the last decade.

Gershenwald JE, Thompson W, Mansfield PF, et al: Multi-institutional melanoma lymphatic mapping experience: The prognostic value of sentinel lymph node status in 612 stage I or II melanoma patients. *J Clin Oncol* 17:976–983, 1999.

Landmark paper describing the prognostic significance of the sentinel node for melanoma.

Griewank KG, Scolyer RA, Thompson JF, et al: Genetic alterations and personalized medicine in melanoma: Progress and future prospects. *J Natl Cancer Inst* 106:djt435, 2014.

Excellent review of the molecular and genetic pathways involved in melanoma and the development of targeted therapies.

Hanahan D, Weinberg RA: Hallmarks of cancer: The next generation. *Cell* 144:646–674, 2011.

Outstanding overview of the cellular biology that drives the development of cancer.

Morton DL, Wen DR, Wong JH, et al: Technical details of intraoperative lymphatic mapping for early stage melanoma. *Arch Surg* 127:392–399, 1992.

Initial description of the technique for sentinel lymph node biopsy in melanoma.

Morton DL, Thompson JF, Cochran AJ, et al: Final trial report of sentinel-node biopsy versus nodal observation in melanoma. *N Engl J Med* 370:599–609, 2014.

Final trial results of the Multicenter Selective Lymphadenectomy Trial from the late Dr. Morton.

Nieweg OE, Kroon BB: Isolated limb perfusion with melphalan for melanoma. *J Surg Oncol* 109:332–337, 2014.

Detailed overview of the development and current status of hyperthermic isolated limb perfusion.

Robert C, Thomas L, Bondarenko I, et al: Ipilimumab plus dacarbazine for previously untreated metastatic melanoma. *N Engl J Med* 364:2517–2526, 2011.

Initial trial report for ipilimumab, the first systemic therapy to affect overall survival.

REFERENCES

1. Neuhaus SJ, Clark MA, Thomas JM: Dr. Herbert Lumley Snow, MD, MRCS (1847-1930): The original champion of elective lymph node dissection in melanoma. *Ann Surg Oncol* 11:875–878, 2004.
2. American Cancer Society: *Cancer facts and figures, 2014*, Atlanta, 2014, American Cancer Society.
3. Little EG, Eide MJ: Update on the current state of melanoma incidence. *Dermatol Clin* 30:355–361, 2012.
4. Wu XC, Eide MJ, King J, et al: Racial and ethnic variations in incidence and survival of cutaneous melanoma in the United States, 1999-2006. *J Am Acad Dermatol* 65:S26–S37, 2011.
5. Hodis E, Watson IR, Kryukov GV, et al: A landscape of driver mutations in melanoma. *Cell* 150:251–263, 2012.
6. Miller AJ, Mihm MC, Jr: Melanoma. *N Engl J Med* 355:51–65, 2006.
7. Alikhan A, Ibrahimi OA, Eisen DB: Congenital melanocytic nevi: Where are we now? Part I. Clinical presentation, epidemiology, pathogenesis, histology, malignant transformation, and neurocutaneous melanosis. *J Am Acad Dermatol* 67:495.e1–495.e7, 2012.
8. Hill SJ, Delman KA: Pediatric melanomas and the atypical spitzoid melanocytic neoplasms. *Am J Surg* 203:761–767, 2012.
9. Lallas A, Kyrgidis A, Ferrara G, et al: Atypical Spitz tumours and sentinel lymph node biopsy: A systematic review. *Lancet Oncol* 15:e178–e183, 2014.
10. Hanahan D, Weinberg RA: Hallmarks of cancer: The next generation. *Cell* 144:646–674, 2011.
11. Griewank KG, Scolyer RA, Thompson JF, et al: Genetic alterations and personalized medicine in melanoma: Progress and future prospects. *J Natl Cancer Inst* 106:djt435, 2014.
12. Chen LL, Jaimes N, Barker CA, et al: Desmoplastic melanoma: A review. *J Am Acad Dermatol* 68:825–833, 2013.

13. Balch CM, Gershenwald JE, Soong SJ, et al: Final version of 2009 AJCC melanoma staging and classification. *J Clin Oncol* 27:6199–6206, 2009.
14. Clark WH, Jr, From L, Bernardino EA, et al: The histogenesis and biologic behavior of primary human malignant melanomas of the skin. *Cancer Res* 29:705–727, 1969.
15. Breslow A: Thickness, cross-sectional areas and depth of invasion in the prognosis of cutaneous melanoma. *Ann Surg* 172:902–908, 1970.
16. Gershenwald JE, Thompson W, Mansfield PF, et al: Multi-institutional melanoma lymphatic mapping experience: The prognostic value of sentinel lymph node status in 612 stage I or II melanoma patients. *J Clin Oncol* 17:976–983, 1999.
17. Balch CM, Soong SJ, Gershenwald JE, et al: Prognostic factors analysis of 17,600 melanoma patients: Validation of the American Joint Committee on Cancer melanoma staging system. *J Clin Oncol* 19:3622–3634, 2001.
18. Payette MJ, Katz M, 3rd, Grant-Kels JM: Melanoma prognostic factors found in the dermatopathology report. *Clin Dermatol* 27:53–74, 2009.
19. Callender GG, Gershenwald JE, Egger ME, et al: A novel and accurate computer model of melanoma prognosis for patients staged by sentinel lymph node biopsy: Comparison with the American Joint Committee on Cancer model. *J Am Coll Surg* 214:608–617, discussion 617–609, 2012.
20. Weinstein D, Leininger J, Hamby C, et al: Diagnostic and prognostic biomarkers in melanoma. *J Clin Aesthet Dermatol* 7:13–24, 2014.
21. Pandalai PK, Dominguez FJ, Michaelson J, et al: Clinical value of radiographic staging in patients diagnosed with AJCC stage III melanoma. *Ann Surg Oncol* 18:506–513, 2011.
22. Kunishige JH, Brodland DG, Zitelli JA: Margins for standard excision of melanoma in situ. *J Am Acad Dermatol* 69:164, 2013.
23. Santillan AA, Messina JL, Marzban SS, et al: Pathology review of thin melanoma and melanoma in situ in a multidisciplinary melanoma clinic: Impact on treatment decisions. *J Clin Oncol* 28:481–486, 2010.
24. Cascinelli N: Margin of resection in the management of primary melanoma. *Semin Surg Oncol* 14:272–275, 1998.
25. Cohn-Cedermark G, Rutqvist LE, Andersson R, et al: Long term results of a randomized study by the Swedish Melanoma Study Group on 2-cm versus 5-cm resection margins for patients with cutaneous melanoma with a tumor thickness of 0.8-2.0 mm. *Cancer* 89:1495–1501, 2000.
26. Khayat D, Rixe O, Martin G, et al: Surgical margins in cutaneous melanoma (2 cm versus 5 cm for lesions measuring less than 2.1-mm thick). *Cancer* 97:1941–1946, 2003.
27. Balch CM, Soong SJ, Smith T, et al: Long-term results of a prospective surgical trial comparing 2 cm vs. 4 cm excision margins for 740 patients with 1-4 mm melanomas. *Ann Surg Oncol* 8:101–108, 2001.
28. Thomas JM, Newton-Bishop J, A'Hern R, et al: Excision margins in high-risk malignant melanoma. *N Engl J Med* 350:757–766, 2004.
29. Gillgren P, Drzewiecki KT, Niin M, et al: 2-cm versus 4-cm surgical excision margins for primary cutaneous melanoma thicker than 2 mm: A randomised, multicentre trial. *Lancet* 378:1635–1642, 2011.
30. Cascinelli N, Morabito A, Santinami M, et al: Immediate or delayed dissection of regional nodes in patients with melanoma of the trunk: A randomised trial. WHO Melanoma Programme. *Lancet* 351:793–796, 1998.
31. Robinson DS, Sample WF, Fee HJ, et al: Regional lymphatic drainage in primary malignant melanoma of the trunk determined by colloidal gold scanning. *Surg Forum* 28:147–148, 1977.
32. Morton DL, Wen DR, Wong JH, et al: Technical details of intraoperative lymphatic mapping for early stage melanoma. *Arch Surg* 127:392–399, 1992.
33. Valsecchi ME, Silbermins D, de Rosa N, et al: Lymphatic mapping and sentinel lymph node biopsy in patients with melanoma: A meta-analysis. *J Clin Oncol* 29:1479–1487, 2011.
34. Gershenwald JE, Tseng CH, Thompson W, et al: Improved sentinel lymph node localization in patients with primary melanoma with the use of radiolabeled colloid. *Surgery* 124:203–210, 1998.
35. Morton DL, Thompson JF, Cochran AJ, et al: Final trial report of sentinel-node biopsy versus nodal observation in melanoma. *N Engl J Med* 370:599–609, 2014.
36. Andtbacka RH, Gershenwald JE: Role of sentinel lymph node biopsy in patients with thin melanoma. *J Natl Compr Canc Netw* 7:308–317, 2009.
37. Han D, Zager JS, Shyr Y, et al: Clinicopathologic predictors of sentinel lymph node metastasis in thin melanoma. *J Clin Oncol* 31:4387–4393, 2013.
38. Balch CM, Gershenwald JE, Soong SJ, et al: Update on the melanoma staging system: The importance of sentinel node staging and primary tumor mitotic rate. *J Surg Oncol* 104:379–385, 2011.
39. Sondak VK, Wong SL, Gershenwald JE, et al: Evidence-based clinical practice guidelines on the use of sentinel lymph node biopsy in melanoma. *Am Soc Clin Oncol Educ Book* 320–325, 2013.
40. Kesmodel SB, Karakousis GC, Botbyl JD, et al: Mitotic rate as a predictor of sentinel lymph node positivity in patients with thin melanomas. *Ann Surg Oncol* 12:449–458, 2005.
41. Scoggins CR, Bowen AL, Martin RC, 2nd, et al: Prognostic information from sentinel lymph node biopsy in patients with thick melanoma. *Arch Surg* 145:622–627, 2010.
42. Egger ME, Bower MR, Czyszczon IA, et al: Comparison of sentinel lymph node micrometastatic tumor burden measurements in melanoma. *J Am Coll Surg* 218:519–528, 2014.
43. Burmeister BH, Henderson MA, Ainslie J, et al: Adjuvant radiotherapy versus observation alone for patients at risk of lymph-node field relapse after therapeutic lymphadenectomy for melanoma: A randomised trial. *Lancet Oncol* 13:589–597, 2012.
44. Nieweg OE, Kroon BB: Isolated limb perfusion with melphalan for melanoma. *J Surg Oncol* 109:332–337, 2014.
45. Kroon HM, Thompson JF: Isolated limb infusion: A review. *J Surg Oncol* 100:169–177, 2009.
46. Eggermont AM, Spatz A, Robert C: Cutaneous melanoma. *Lancet* 383:816–827, 2014.
47. Robert C, Thomas L, Bondarenko I, et al: Ipilimumab plus dacarbazine for previously untreated metastatic melanoma. *N Engl J Med* 364:2517–2526, 2011.
48. Wolchok JD, Kluger H, Callahan MK, et al: Nivolumab plus ipilimumab in advanced melanoma. *N Engl J Med* 369:122–133, 2013.

49. Chapman PB, Hauschild A, Robert C, et al: Improved survival with vemurafenib in melanoma with BRAF V600E mutation. *N Engl J Med* 364:2507–2516, 2011.
50. McArthur GA, Chapman PB, Robert C, et al: Safety and efficacy of vemurafenib in BRAF(V600E) and BRAF(V600K) mutation-positive melanoma (BRIM-3): Extended follow-up of a phase 3, randomised, open-label study. *Lancet Oncol* 15:323–332, 2014.
51. Hauschild A, Grob JJ, Demidov LV, et al: Dabrafenib in BRAF-mutated metastatic melanoma: A multicentre, open-label, phase 3 randomised controlled trial. *Lancet* 380:358–365, 2012.
52. Long GV, Stroyakovskiy D, Gogas H, et al: Combined BRAF and MEK inhibition versus BRAF inhibition alone in melanoma. *N Engl J Med* 371:1877–1888, 2014.
53. Jhaveri MB, Driscoll MS, Grant-Kels JM: Melanoma in pregnancy. *Clin Obstet Gynecol* 54:537–545, 2011.
54. Dubas LE, Ingraffea A: Nonmelanoma skin cancer. *Facial Plast Surg Clin North Am* 21:43–53, 2013.
55. Zwald FO, Brown M: Skin cancer in solid organ transplant recipients: Advances in therapy and management: Part I. Epidemiology of skin cancer in solid organ transplant recipients. *J Am Acad Dermatol* 65:253–261, 2011.
56. Farasat S, Yu SS, Neel VA, et al: A new American Joint Committee on Cancer staging system for cutaneous squamous cell carcinoma: Creation and rationale for inclusion of tumor (T) characteristics. *J Am Acad Dermatol* 64:1051–1059, 2011.
57. Young RJ, Brown NJ, Reed MW, et al: Angiosarcoma. *Lancet Oncol* 11:983–991, 2010.
58. Bogucki B, Neuhaus I, Hurst EA: Dermatofibrosarcoma protuberans: A review of the literature. *Dermatol Surg* 38:537–551, 2012.
59. Wang TS, Byrne PJ, Jacobs LK, et al: Merkel cell carcinoma: Update and review. *Semin Cutan Med Surg* 30:48–56, 2011.

31 CHAPTER

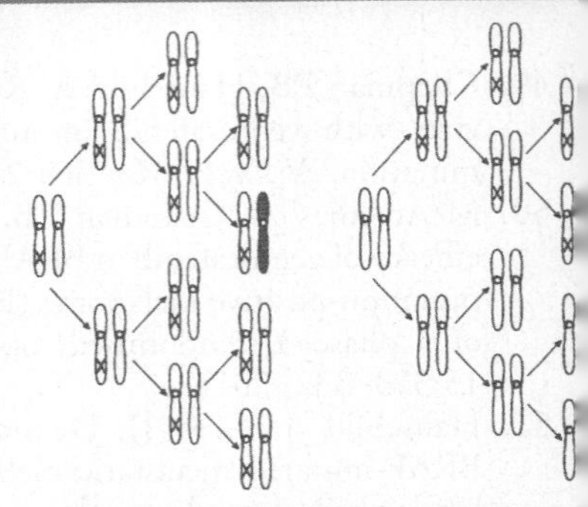

Soft Tissue Sarcoma

Carlo M. Contreras, Martin J. Heslin

OUTLINE

EPIDEMIOLOGY

Soft tissue sarcoma (STS) is a diverse group of more than 60 neoplasms that can arise from virtually any anatomic site and can affect the very young as well as the elderly. The tissue types of STS origin include skeletal muscle, adipose cells, blood and lymphatic vessels, and connective tissue or those cells with a common mesoderm origin (Fig. 31-1 and Table 31-1). Also included are peripheral nerves derived from the neuroectoderm. Its clinical behavior occupies a wide spectrum, from indolent low-grade neoplasms, such as benign lipomas, to tumors with aggressive tumor biology, such as metastatic angiosarcoma. STS is relatively rare, with 12,020 estimated new cases and an estimated 4740 deaths for the year 2014. Whereas this accounts for 1% of cancer incidence in the United States, it accounts for 2% of cancer-related deaths. The diagnosis of patients with STS is challenging because although it is rare in the general population, a number of common, nonneoplastic conditions can mimic STS (see Box 31-1).

Although there is a great deal of overlap between the various STS subtypes, the most traditional categorization separates trunk and extremity STS from retroperitoneal sarcomas. Before these varieties are discussed in detail, this chapter first reviews core concepts that are relevant to all STS. These core concepts include STS etiology, STS staging, consideration of the lipomatous tumor spectrum, and the STS category previously referred to as malignant fibrous histiocytoma (MFH). A more detailed discussion of trunk and extremity STS and retroperitoneal sarcoma follows. Other specific and relevant STS subtypes are addressed in more detail throughout the chapter as well.

Large published series demonstrate that extremity and trunk STS is more common than intraperitoneal and retroperitoneal STS.[1] Among extremity STS, the proximal limb is more commonly affected than the distal portion, with the thigh the most common location, accounting for 44% of patients. The age at diagnosis and the histologic STS subtype are often closely linked. Rhabdomyosarcoma, hemangioma, neurofibroma, and alveolar sarcoma tend to disproportionately affect children and young adults. Most STS occurs sporadically, but other well-documented causes include germline mutations, radiation exposure, and environmental exposure.

CORE CONCEPTS

Germline Mutations

Neurofibromatosis Type 1

Neurofibromatosis type 1 (NF1) is an autosomal dominant condition caused by mutations of the *NF1* gene, which is located at chromosome 17q11.2. *NF1* codes for a protein called neurofibromin, which acts as a tumor suppressor of the *ras* oncogene signaling pathway. In addition to the ubiquitous development of multiple cutaneous neurofibromas, these patients have a 10% risk for development of a malignant peripheral nerve sheath tumor (MPNST, which is covered in more detail later in this chapter). NF1 is also related to a variety of other tumors, including schwannomas and gliomas.

Li-Fraumeni Syndrome

The Li-Fraumeni syndrome is a rare autosomal dominant disorder caused by mutations of the *TP53* gene, which is located at chromosome 17p13.1. The *TP53* gene codes for p53, a protein that acts as a tumor suppressor. Wild-type p53 functions to facilitate the clearance of damaged cellular DNA and to prevent the clonal propagation of these mutated sequences. *TP53* mutations therefore contribute to an increased risk of various malignant neoplasms. In order of decreasing prevalence, these include breast cancer, STS (especially rhabdomyosarcoma, undifferentiated pleomorphic sarcoma, and pleomorphic sarcoma), adrenocortical carcinoma, brain cancer, osteosarcoma, and hematologic malignant neoplasm. Patients affected by the Li-Fraumeni syndrome exhibit a range of phenotypes, depending on the types of mutations involved, with some patients developing rhabdomyosarcoma before 4 years of age.

Familial Adenomatous Polyposis and Gardner Syndrome

The familial adenomatous polyposis (FAP) syndrome is an autosomal dominant disorder caused by mutation of the *APC* gene,

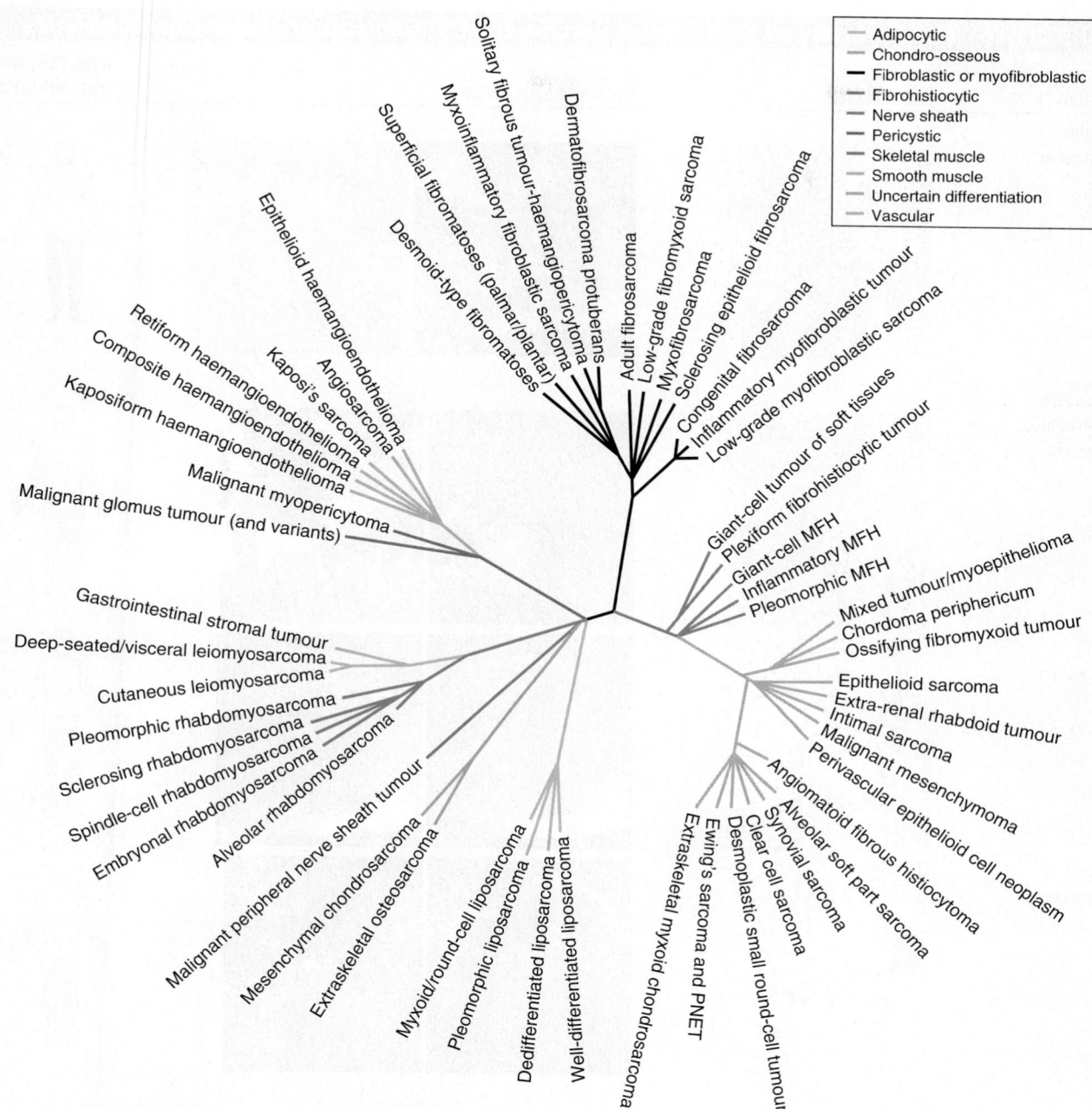

FIGURE 31-1 Taxonomy of Soft Tissue Sarcoma. This unrooted phylogeny shows about 60 sarcoma subtypes, as originally defined by the World Health Organization International Agency for Research on Cancer, amended and updated on the basis of current knowledge. The classification reflects relationships among lineage, prognosis (malignant, intermediate or locally aggressive, intermediate or rarely metastasizing), driver alterations, and additional parameters. Branch lengths are determined by nearest neighbor joining of a discretized distance matrix based on the aforementioned variables. Initial branching reflects differences in lineage, with associated lineages appearing closer in distance (such as skeletal and smooth muscle). Subsequent branching denotes similarity in prognosis, whether they are translocation associated, and if so, the genes shared among distinct fusions (in this order). Although incomplete, as many subtypes lack sufficient global molecular profiling data on which to base a phylogeny, this initial formulation minimally reflects the relationships among lineage and major molecular lesions in the subtypes. The illustration excludes 52 benign types of tumor. *MFH,* undifferentiated pleomorphic sarcoma; *PNET,* primitive neuroectodermal tumor. (From Taylor BS, Barretina J, Maki RG, et al: Advances in sarcoma genomics and new therapeutic targets. *Nat Rev Cancer* 11:541–557, 2011.)

TABLE 31-1 The Diversity of Soft Tissue Sarcoma (STS) Clinicopathologic Characteristics

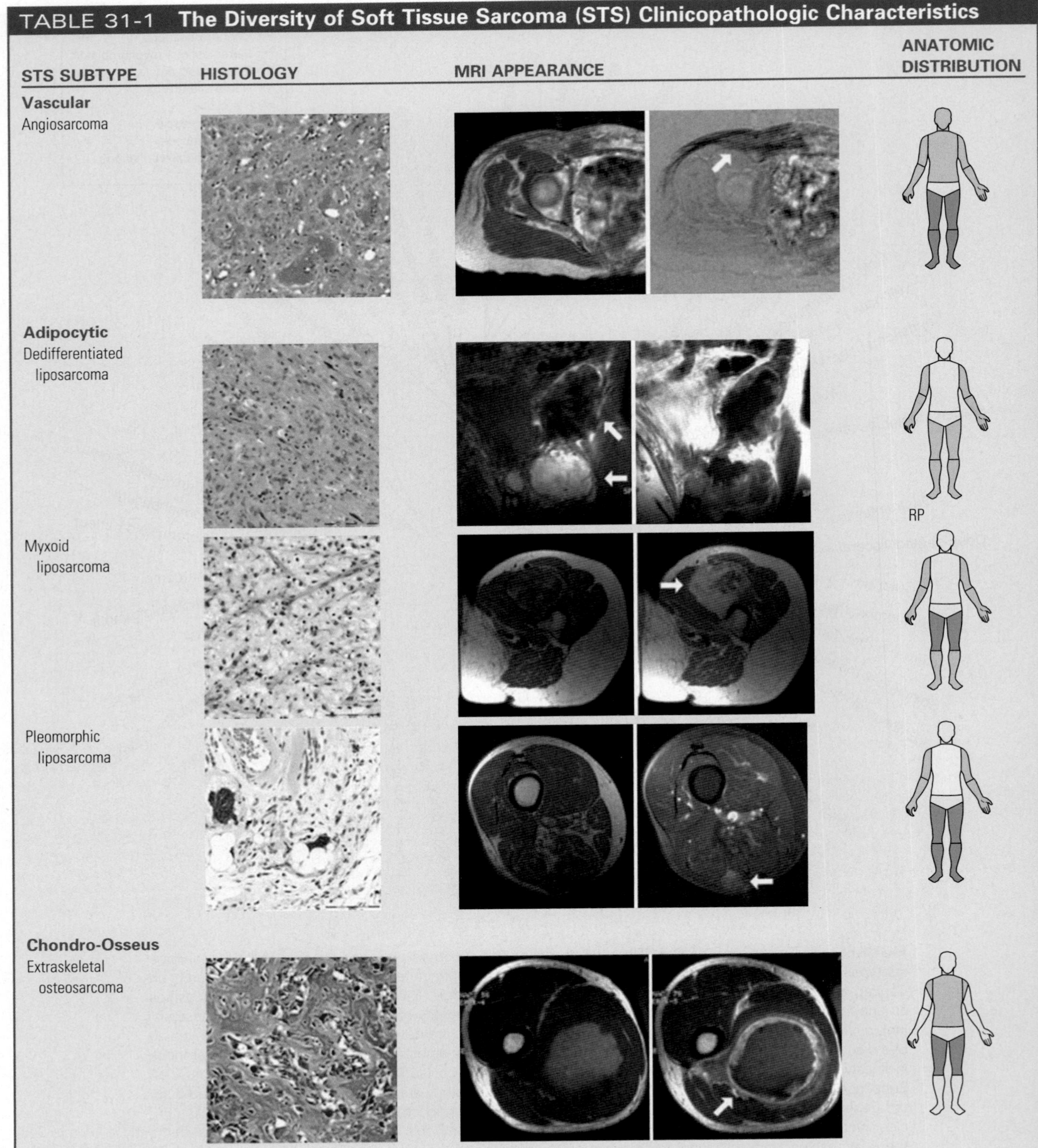

STS SUBTYPE	HISTOLOGY	MRI APPEARANCE	ANATOMIC DISTRIBUTION
Vascular			
Angiosarcoma			
Adipocytic			
Dedifferentiated liposarcoma			RP
Myxoid liposarcoma			
Pleomorphic liposarcoma			
Chondro-Osseus			
Extraskeletal osteosarcoma			

TABLE 31-1 The Diversity of Soft Tissue Sarcoma (STS) Clinicopathologic Characteristics—cont'd

STS SUBTYPE	HISTOLOGY	MRI APPEARANCE	ANATOMIC DISTRIBUTION
Myofibroblastic			
Myxofibrosarcoma	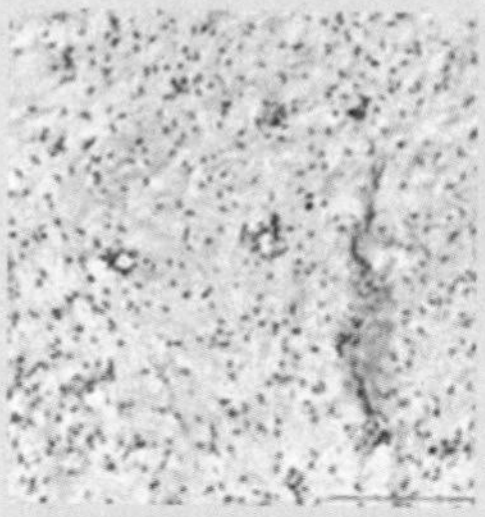	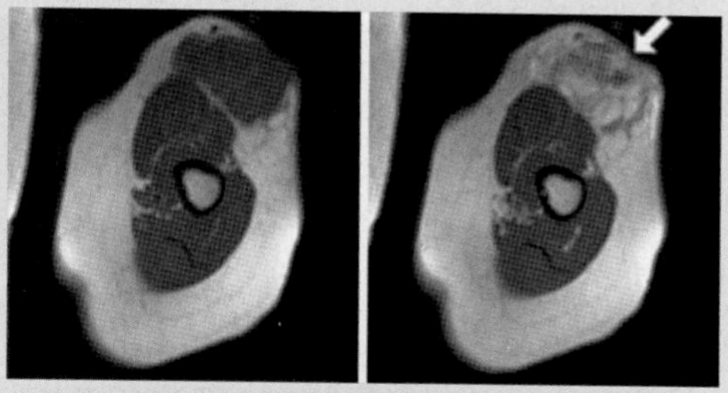	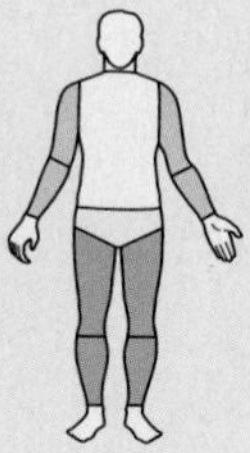
Low-grade fibromyxoid sarcoma	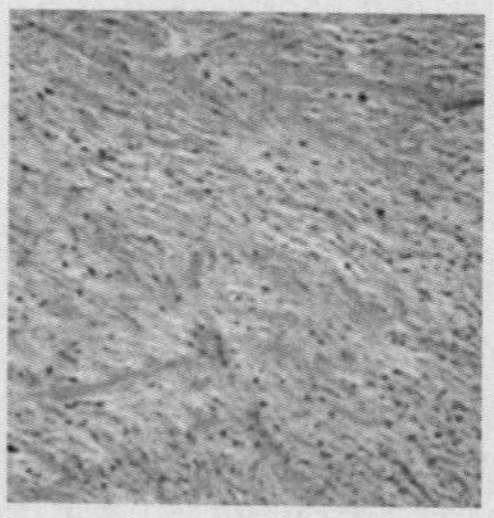	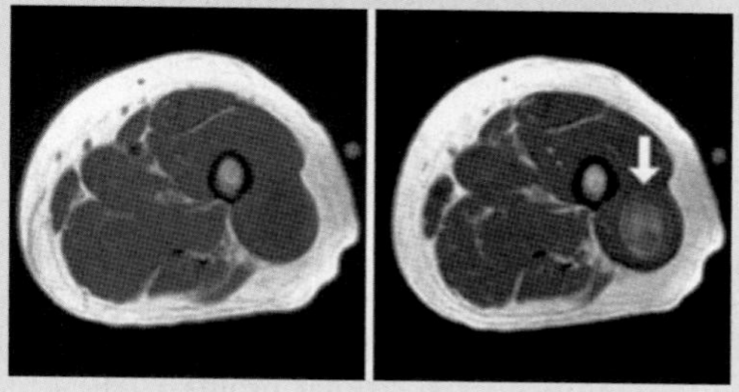	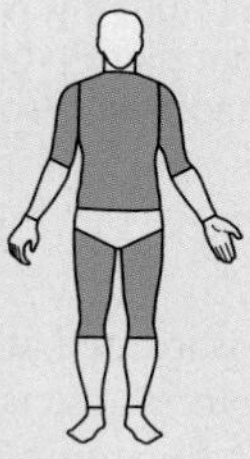 RP
Smooth Muscle			
Leiomyosarcoma	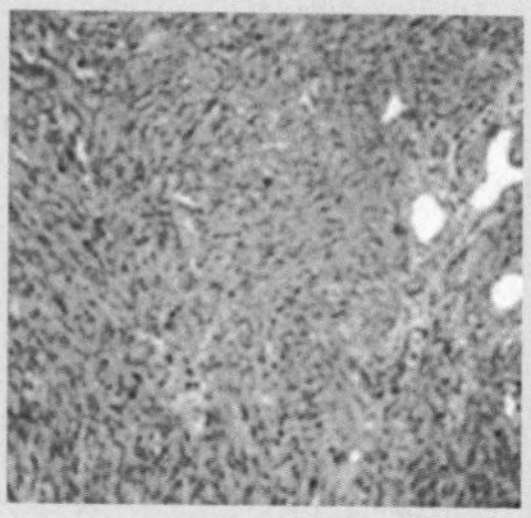	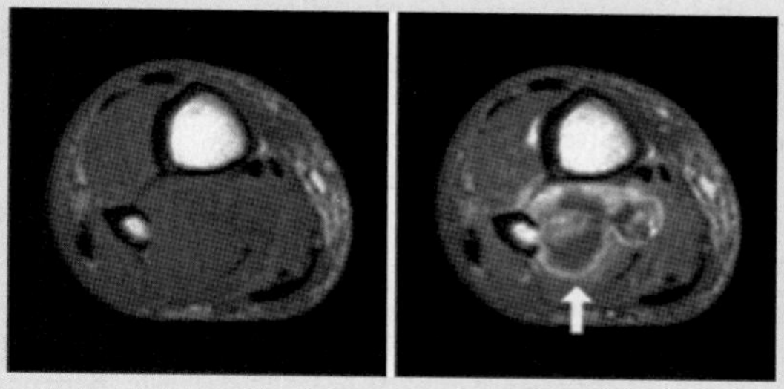	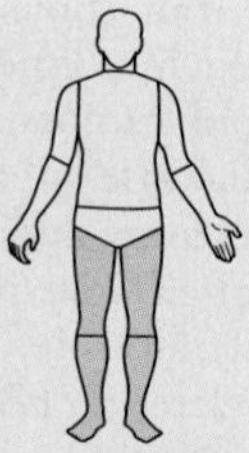 RP, pelvis, vascular
Uncertain Differentiation			
Synovial sarcoma	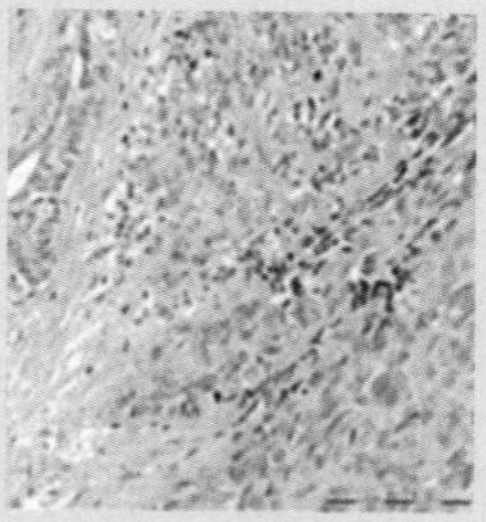	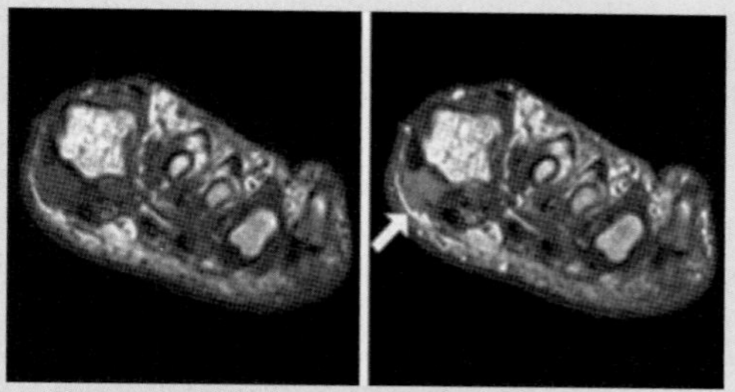	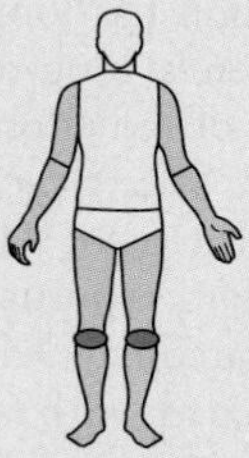 Joints, tendons
Undifferentiated pleomorphic sarcoma	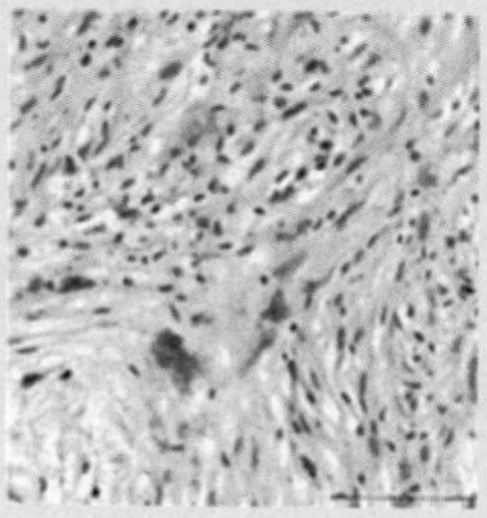	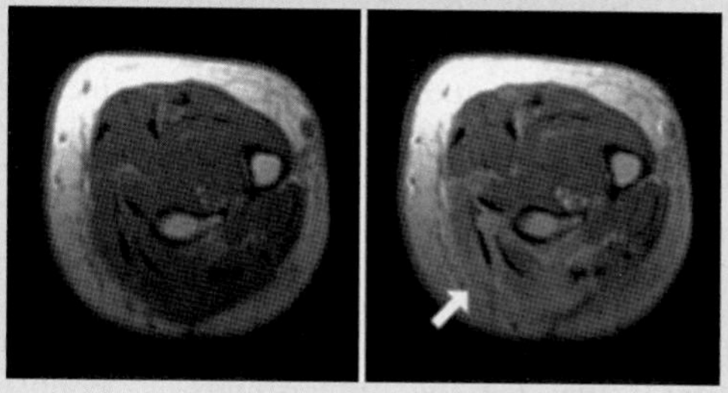	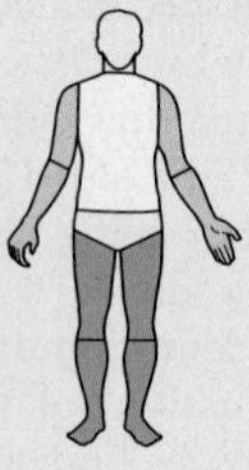

Continued

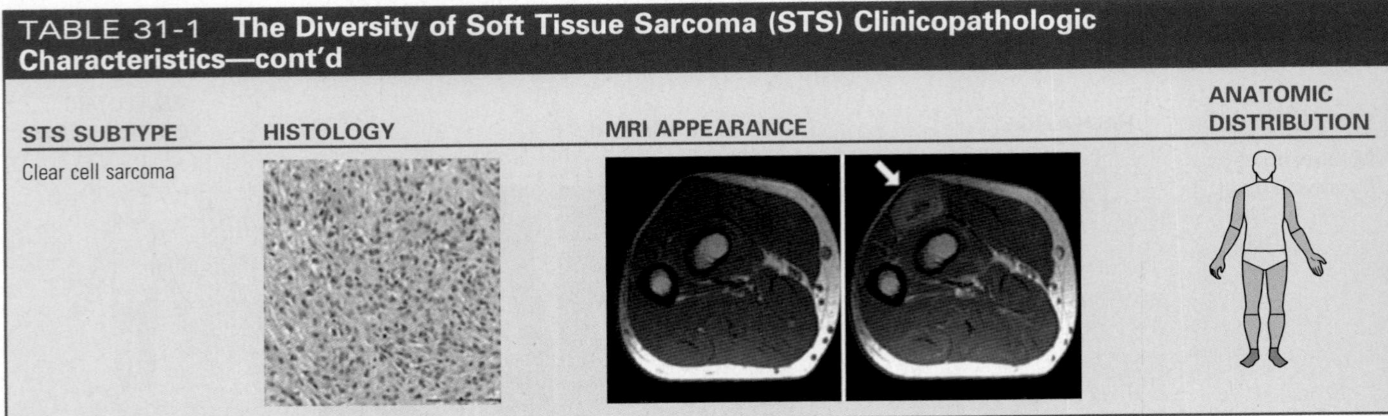

TABLE 31-1 The Diversity of Soft Tissue Sarcoma (STS) Clinicopathologic Characteristics—cont'd

STS SUBTYPE	HISTOLOGY	MRI APPEARANCE	ANATOMIC DISTRIBUTION
Clear cell sarcoma			

Adapted from van Vliet M, Kliffen M, Krestin G, et al: Soft tissue sarcomas at a glance: Clinical, histological, and MR imaging features of malignant extremity soft tissue tumors. *Eur Radiol* 19:1499–1511, 2009.
MRI, magnetic resonance imaging; *RP,* retroperitoneum.

which is located at chromosome 5q21-q22. This gene also encodes a protein that acts as a tumor suppressor, inhibiting the localization of β-catenin to the nucleus. The truncated mutant protein fails to regulate β-catenin, resulting in unchecked cellular proliferation. The cardinal clinical feature is innumerable colonic polyps, but some patients also develop extracolonic manifestations, such as epidermoid cysts, osteomas, and desmoid tumors. Desmoid tumors, covered in more detail later in this chapter, typically arise approximately 5 years after FAP-related prophylactic colectomy and are a major source of morbidity and mortality. They often arise in prior surgical sites but can be manifested at virtually any site. Intra-abdominal tumors are much more likely to be related to FAP, whereas desmoids of the extremities are typically sporadic.

Radiation

Radiation has long been suspected to significantly contribute to a patient's long-term risk of STS development. Whereas the effects of radiation are thought to be dose dependent, radiation-related STS typically occurs at the periphery of the radiation field. The main STS subtypes thought to be associated with prior radiation exposure include unclassified pleomorphic sarcoma, angiosarcoma, leiomyosarcoma, fibrosarcoma, and MPNST.[2] Compared with sporadic forms of these same STS subtypes, those arising after radiation exposure tend to have a shorter disease-specific survival. In the setting of adjuvant radiation therapy for breast cancer, a large cohort of 122,991 women demonstrated that radiation contributes to an absolute increase in the risk of STS of 0.13% during 10 years.[3] Patients who later develop STS after being treated as children for cancers requiring radiation therapy do so a median of 11.8 years later, also in a dose-dependent fashion. The development of angiosarcoma after a combination of postmastectomy lymphedema and radiation therapy is known as Stewart-Treves syndrome; it also has a latency of about 10 years after initial therapy. Interestingly, Stewart-Treves syndrome–related angiosarcoma usually occurs outside the previous radiation field but within the zone of lymphedema. An increased risk of STS not only is attributable to therapeutic doses of radiation but also has been linked to lower doses encountered by pediatric patients undergoing routine computed tomography (CT) scan.

Carcinogens

Hepatic angiosarcoma is related to several carcinogenic substances including Thorotrast, polyvinyl chloride, and arsenic. Thorotrast is a thorium-based intravenous contrast agent that was used between the years 1930 and 1955. In affected patients, hepatic angiosarcoma is diagnosed 20 to 30 years after exposure. Polyvinyl chloride is an extremely common form of plastic, but prolonged and unprotected exposures have been linked to the development of hepatic angiosarcoma.

Staging

Tumor Grade

Because of the inclusion of tumor grade, the American Joint Committee on Cancer (AJCC) staging system for STS is unique compared with most other types of cancer. Internationally, the two most widely applied grading systems are the French Fédération Nationale des Centres de Lutte Contre le Cancer (FNCLCC) system and the National Cancer Institute (NCI) system. The FNCLCC is a score based on the sum of three categories: tumor differentiation, rate of mitoses, and amount of tumor necrosis. The NCI system is similar but for certain STS subtypes requires that the pathologist state the degree of tumor cellularity and pleomorphism, which can limit its reproducibility. The FNCLCC and the NCI systems were compared, and the FNCLCC was found to be superior in estimating the risk of distant metastasis and survival.[4]

Beyond tumor grade, the other important staging parameters include tumor size, depth of tumor, nodal involvement, and involvement of distant sites. The schema for the AJCC staging system, seventh edition, is shown in Tables 31-2 and 31-3. The AJCC staging system states that either the FNCLCC or the NCI may be used for STS staging.

The performance of the STS AJCC seventh edition staging system has been challenged. A degree of generalization across a population of tumors is inherent to any staging system. Currently, multiple histologic STS subtypes are considered together in the AJCC STS staging system. As cancer staging systems have evolved, it has become apparent that grouping of these heterogeneous tumors decreases the prognostic power compared with a schema in which separate subtypes are individually considered. This realization has driven the creation of a separate AJCC staging system

TABLE 31-2 AJCC Staging for Soft Tissue Sarcomas

Primary Tumor (T)	
Primary tumor cannot be assessed	TX
No evidence of primary tumor	T0
Tumor 5 cm or less in greatest dimension	T1
Superficial tumor	T1a
Deep tumor	T1b
Tumor more than 5 cm in greatest dimension	T2
Superficial tumor	T2a
Deep tumor	T2b
Regional Lymph Nodes (N)	
Regional lymph nodes cannot be assessed	NX
No regional lymph node metastasis	N0
Regional lymph node metastasis	N1
Distant Metastasis (M)	
No distant metastasis	M0
Distant metastasis	M1

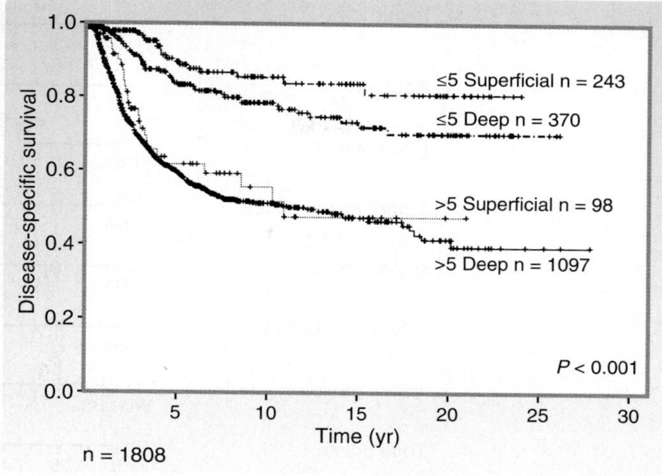

FIGURE 31-2 Importance of size and depth among primary high-grade STS tumors. (From Brennan MF, Antonescu CR, Moraco N, et al: Lessons learned from the study of 10,000 patients with soft tissue sarcoma. *Ann Surg* 260:416–422, 2014.)

TABLE 31-3 Anatomic Stage and Prognostic Groups for Soft Tissue Sarcomas

GROUP	T	N	M	GRADE
Stage IA	T1a	N0	M0	G1
	T1b	N0	M0	G1
Stage IB	T2a	N0	M0	G1
	T2b	N0	M0	G1
Stage IIA	T1a	N0	M0	G2, G3
	T1b	N0	M0	G2, G3
Stage IIB	T2a	N0	M0	G2
	T2b	N0	M0	G2
Stage III	T2b	N0	M0	G3
	Any T	N1	M0	Any grade
Stage IV	Any T	Any N	M1	Any grade

for gastrointestinal stromal tumor (GIST), bone sarcoma, uterine sarcoma, Kaposi sarcoma, and dermatofibrosarcoma protuberans (DFSP). Additional modifications may continue to improve future AJCC editions. The AJCC seventh edition STS staging criteria do not differentiate between extremity and retroperitoneal STS. Compared with extremity STS, visceral and retroperitoneal STS appears to have a lower disease-specific survival. In the case of visceral STS, this decreased disease-specific survival is driven by the likelihood for distant metastasis; but for retroperitoneal STS, the low disease-specific survival is driven by the risk of local recurrence.[1]

The importance of the size of the primary STS to prognosis is well described (Fig. 31-2), but the current 5-cm size threshold specified by the AJCC seventh edition has been challenged.[1] Greater prognostic discrimination may be possible with use of four size categories (≤5 cm, >5 to 10 cm, >10 to 15 cm, and >15 cm), while multiple authors have demonstrated that the size of retroperitoneal sarcoma does not affect survival. Tumor depth is also included in the AJCC seventh edition staging, although this criterion is not relevant to visceral or retroperitoneal sarcoma. In patients with trunk or extremity sarcoma, the T stage is subdivided into T*x*a and T*x*b on the basis of whether the STS is located superficial or deep to the investing fascia of the trunk or limb. For extremity STS of 5 cm or smaller, stratification based on tumor depth confers a measurable difference in the disease-specific survival; there is little difference in comparing superficial and deep extremity STS of more than 5 cm.[1] The limitations of AJCC staging for retroperitoneal sarcoma were also highlighted in a single-institution retrospective review of 343 patients treated during 10 years.[5] Because of the nature of retroperitoneal sarcoma, most patients with retroperitoneal sarcoma segregate into either AJCC stage I disease or stage III disease. Representing only 4% of patients in this series, AJCC stage II disease was infrequently observed because all retroperitoneal sarcomas are T*x*b by definition, retroperitoneal sarcoma of 5 cm or less at diagnosis is extremely rare, and retroperitoneal sarcomas of more than 5 cm are likely to be high grade. In practical terms, the only retroperitoneal sarcomas that fall under AJCC stage II criteria are low- to intermediate-grade tumors larger than 5 cm. Because of the few patients with stage II disease, the survival curves are reduced to a binary distribution, stage I patients or stage II/III patients. Anaya and colleagues demonstrated that a more descriptive and clinically relevant method of estimating prognosis involves segregating patients into three histologic groups: well-differentiated liposarcoma, dedifferentiated or pleomorphic liposarcoma, and all other retroperitoneal sarcoma histologic types.

Overall, regional lymph node involvement for STS is uncommon (2% to 10%). The most common STS subtypes undergoing lymphadenectomy for nodal metastases are angiosarcoma, rhabdomyosarcoma, MFH (recently reclassified as undifferentiated pleomorphic sarcoma), epithelioid sarcoma, clear cell sarcoma, and liposarcoma.[6] Although regional nodal involvement is an important prognosticator of survival, patients with multiple positive nodes, a single lymph node, and distant metastatic disease all have similar survival.[1,6] Some groups have proposed the use of sentinel lymph node dissection for epithelioid sarcoma, clear cell sarcoma, and rhabdomyosarcoma in the pediatric population, but the accuracy is generally unacceptable, and the technique has never been successfully applied to STS in a well-designed clinical trial.

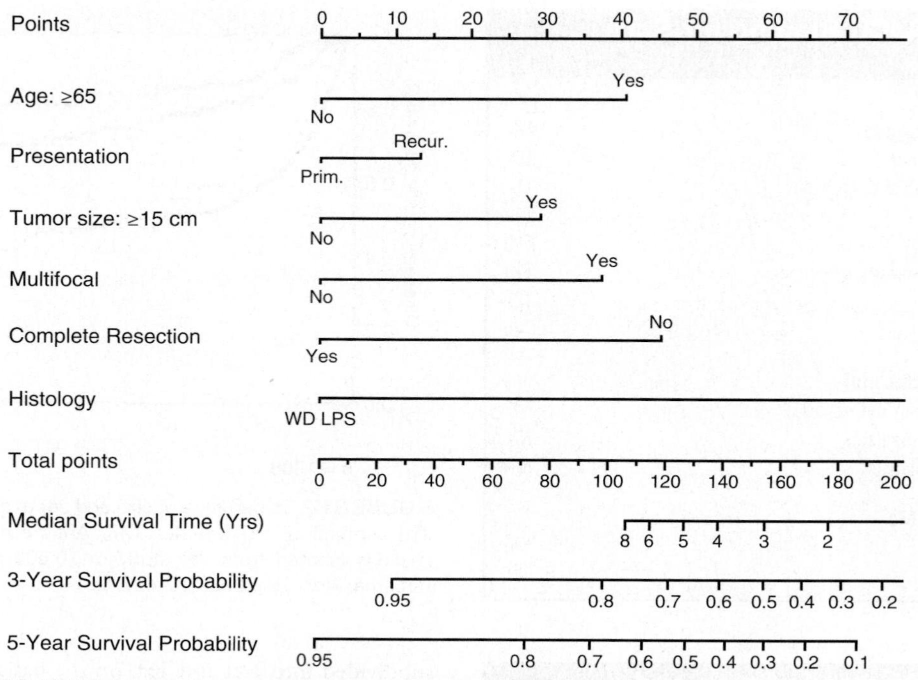

FIGURE 31-3 Postoperative nomogram for median, 3- and 5-year overall survival prediction in patients with nonmetastatic, resectable, retroperitoneal sarcoma. *DD lipo,* dedifferentiated/pleomorphic liposarcoma; *OS,* overall survival; *WD lipo,* well-differentiated liposarcoma. (From Anaya, DA, Lahat G, Wang X, et al: Postoperative nomogram for survival of patients with retroperitoneal sarcoma treated with curative intent. *Ann Oncol* 21:397–402, 2010. Oxford University Press, European Society of Medical Oncology.)

Nomograms have recently been developed in response to the fact that standard staging systems, like the AJCC, do not adequately consider the relevant parameters and therefore cannot accurately estimate prognosis of patients with STS. No fewer than 13 different nomograms have been published for STS alone. The nomograms were developed to address a number of oncologic outcomes but most typically predict local recurrence or overall survival (Fig. 31-3). In general, the nomograms are reported to more accurately prognosticate outcome than traditional staging systems, but few have been validated in a data set beyond that which was used to generate the nomogram. Nonetheless, they can provide meaningful information that, when used appropriately, can have an impact on the care of patients with STS. It remains to be seen how the proliferation of these nomograms will affect future editions of traditional staging systems.

Clinical Evaluation

There are dozens of STS subtypes that affect the trunk and extremities. The most common clinical presentation is of a patient with a painless mass without prior evaluation. If STS is included in the differential diagnosis, appropriate oncologic staging should be undertaken. This staging starts by performing a detailed history and physical examination. These are important in determining the likelihood of STS versus other more common mimicking diagnoses, such as hypertrophic scar, myositis ossificans, hematoma, or cyst (Box 31-1). Small, superficial and mobile masses highly suggestive of STS that are separate from skeletal or neurovascular structures may be taken to the operating room for resection with wide gross margins, depending on the location relative to vital structures. Tumors close to vital structures may be referred to a center with expertise treating STS. In these patients, a preoperative biopsy is unnecessary. Undesirable consequences of an unnecessary preoperative biopsy include a pathology report that provides the incorrect non-STS diagnosis because of an insufficient specimen, a nonideal placement of the biopsy site leading to a larger incision than otherwise necessary, and delay in therapy.

BOX 31-1 Entities That May Mimic Soft Tissue Sarcoma

- Hypertrophic scar
- Retroperitoneal lymphadenopathy: lymphoma, germ cell tumor, or metastasis from gastrointestinal primary
- Hematoma
- Myositis ossificans
- Benign lipoma
- Cyst
- Abscess
- Cutaneous malignant neoplasms, including melanoma

Larger or otherwise more complicated lesions require additional oncologic staging. The extent of staging is highly individualized and adapted to each patient. In general, the indications for preoperative imaging and biopsy include the following:

- Inability to determine the extent of the mass on physical examination
- Suspected neurovascular involvement
- Suspicion for regional or distant metastasis
- Need for operation that would likely result in significant functional deficits
- Suspicion that the mass is unresectable or resectable with questionable surgical margins at presentation

Rigorous studies evaluating the utility of magnetic resonance imaging (MRI) versus CT are dated. Whereas MRI is generally considered the most informative imaging modality for trunk and extremity STS, there are important roles for the use of contrast-enhanced CT and ultrasound. In addition to imaging of the primary STS site, a chest CT should generally be obtained as this is the most frequent site of metastasis. When they are available, the biopsy results may prompt consideration of additional imaging. For example, CT of the abdomen and pelvis should be considered for patients with more aggressive histologic types, such as myxoid or round cell liposarcoma, epithelioid sarcoma, angiosarcoma, and leiomyosarcoma. Brain imaging may be considered to exclude metastasis from alveolar soft part sarcoma, clear cell sarcoma, and angiosarcoma.

The surgeon may choose from a variety of biopsy methods. Given the rarity of STS and the scant amount of tissue procured, a fine-needle aspirate is generally unsatisfactory except in the diagnosis of a local recurrence. An image-guided core needle biopsy is more likely to provide a reliable diagnosis, but when it is applied to large cystic lesions or lesions with a considerable myxoid component, a core needle biopsy may still be nondiagnostic. To decrease the risk of local recurrence, the core biopsy approach should be planned so that the entire needle trajectory can be easily incorporated into the forthcoming surgical resection volume. If the core needle biopsy attempts are still nondiagnostic, an incisional biopsy may be necessary. Here, again, it is critical to plan the incision so that the entire biopsy trajectory is ultimately included within the resection volume.

Armed with radiographic and pathologic information, a multidisciplinary team at a high-volume STS center, with representatives from surgical oncology, medical oncology, diagnostic radiology, pathology, and radiation oncology in attendance, ideally discusses the case. The goal of this discussion is to assess which treatment modalities are most appropriate for each patient and in what sequence each modality should be implemented (Fig. 31-4). Up to 74% of patients who undergo an unplanned trunk or extremity sarcoma resection have residual disease at the time of re-resection. Thirty-day mortality, rates of limb preservation,

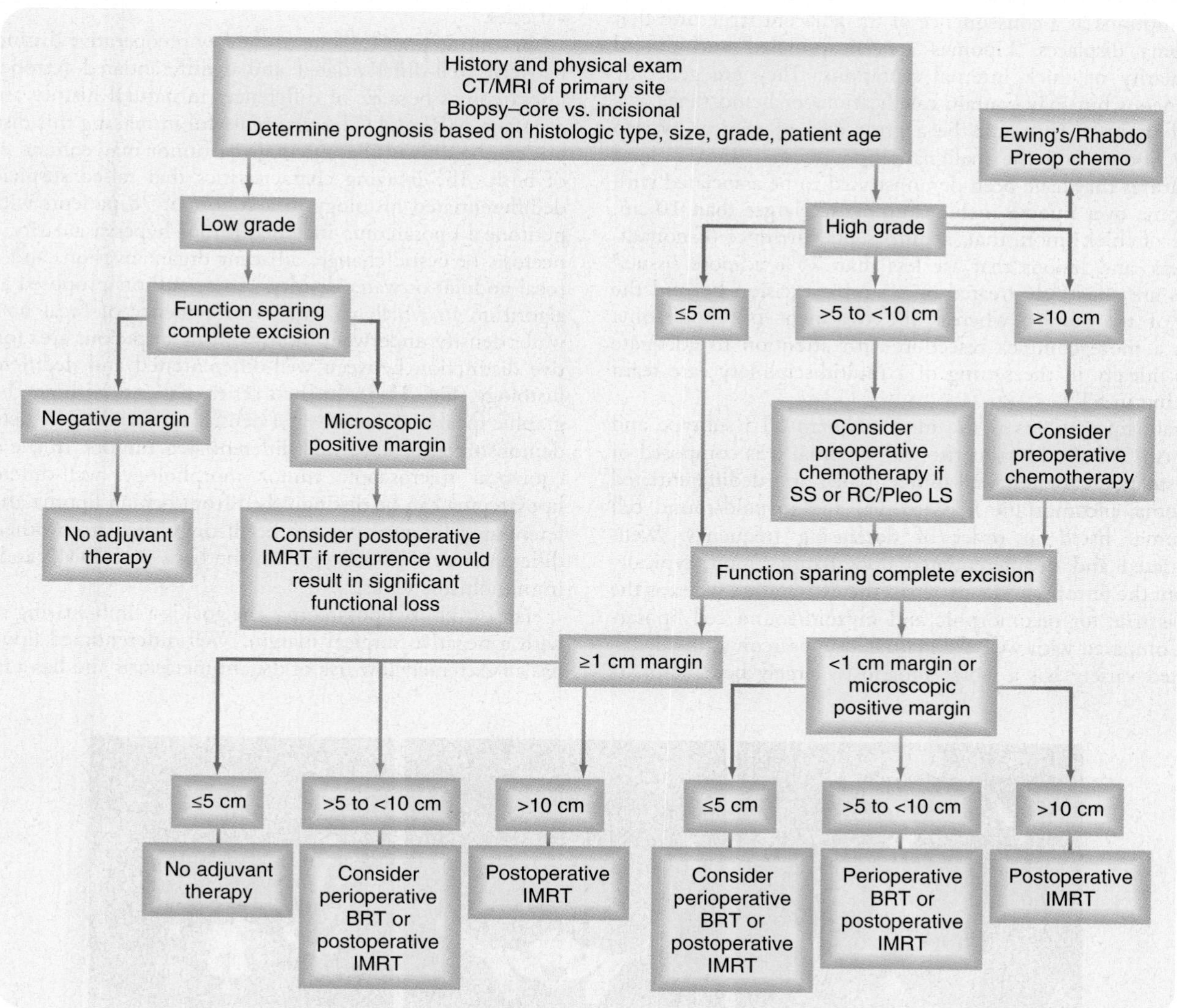

FIGURE 31-4 Algorithm for the management of primary (with no metastases) extremity or trunk soft tissue sarcoma, using a biologic rationale (i.e., size and grade of tumor). *BRT,* brachytherapy; *EBRT,* external beam radiation therapy; *IMRT,* intensity-modulated radiation therapy; *RC/Pleo LS,* round cell–pleomorphic liposarcoma; *SS,* synovial sarcoma.

and overall survival have been linked to care delivered at high-volume STS centers.[7]

Because of the considerable risk for recurrence, close postoperative surveillance is important for STS patients. In general, these patients should undergo a physical examination every 3 to 6 months for 2 or 3 years, then every 6 months for the next 2 years, and then annually. Radiographic surveillance of the chest, abdomen, and pelvis should also be undertaken at regular intervals. The modality (CT versus MRI) and the frequency should be individualized to the patient and the tumor characteristics. The most informative preoperative imaging modality is favored, but consideration should also be given to avoiding unnecessary radiation exposure by ultrasound or MRI. The imaging frequency for STS patients has not been rigorously studied, but a shorter imaging frequency may be appropriate for a patient with close surgical margins or a patient with a particularly ominous histologic type.

Lipomatous Tumors

Lipomas are adipocytic tumors that can arise from any part of the body. By definition, they are benign neoplasms, but they can cause symptoms as a consequence of the adjacent structures that the lipoma displaces. Lipomas are encapsulated and devoid of nodularity or thick internal septations. They are generally homogeneous but may contain calcifications or hemorrhage as a result of trauma. There can be a great deal of clinical overlap between lipoma and the malignant liposarcoma. The CT and MRI features that have been demonstrated to be associated with liposarcoma over lipoma include tumor size larger than 10 cm, presence of thick (more than 2 mm) septa, presence of nonadipose areas, and lesions that are less than 75% adipose tissue.[8] Lipomas are effectively treated by a simple excision beyond the capsule of the tumor, whereas the treatment of liposarcoma involves a more complex resection with attention to adequate margins, ideally in the setting of a multidisciplinary care team specializing in STS.

Overall, liposarcoma is the most frequent STS subtype and represents 45% of all retroperitoneal sarcoma; it is composed of three histologic varieties: well-differentiated and dedifferentiated liposarcoma, pleomorphic liposarcoma, and myxoid/round cell liposarcoma, listed in order of decreasing frequency. Well-differentiated and dedifferentiated liposarcomas more typically arise from the retroperitoneum versus the extremities, whereas the inverse is true for pleomorphic and myxoid/round cell liposarcoma. Compared with well-differentiated liposarcoma, the dedifferentiated variety has a worse prognosis, largely because of its much greater risk of distant metastasis compared with well-differentiated liposarcoma. Local recurrence is common in both types. The malignant behavior of well-differentiated and dedifferentiated liposarcomas is attributable to the amplification of chromosome 12q13-15, which accounts for the upregulation of MDM2 and CDK4. Both well-differentiated and dedifferentiated retroperitoneal liposarcomas are often multifocal. Myxoid and round cells are descriptive terms based on their histologic appearance. These liposarcoma varieties are characterized by distinct translocations, t(12;16)(q13;p11) and more rarely t(12;22)(q13;q12). Multiple tumor-promoting pathways including MET, RET, and PI3K/Akt are activated as a result of these translocations. Myxoid liposarcoma is unusual in its relative sensitivity to radiation and chemotherapy, resulting in a 10-year disease-specific survival of 87%. Considered a poorly differentiated form of the myxoid variety, the round cell variety has a worse outcome than myxoid liposarcoma, with metastasis developing in 21% of patients in one large series. Pleomorphic liposarcoma is another example of a poorly differentiated liposarcoma with a poor outcome. It displays a variety of genetic abnormalities, none as reliable as those described for the preceding liposarcoma varieties.

In routine practice, one of the key preoperative distinctions is between well-differentiated and dedifferentiated retroperitoneal liposarcomas because of differences in natural history and management. MRI and CT scan are useful in making this distinction but can be difficult because a given tumor may contain elements of both. The imaging characteristics that raised suspicion of a dedifferentiated histology in a cohort of 78 patients with retroperitoneal liposarcoma included tumor hypervascularity, areas of necrosis or cystic change, adjacent organ invasion, and areas of focal nodular or water density.[9] These authors proposed a clinical algorithm in which patients with evidence of focal nodular or water density underwent biopsy of this suspicious area for definitive distinction between well-differentiated and dedifferentiated histology (Fig. 31-5). In their series, patients without the radiographic focal nodular or water density uniformly were definitively demonstrated to have well-differentiated tumors. In the event of equivocal microscopic tumor morphology, well-differentiated liposarcoma can be distinguished from benign lipoma and dedifferentiated liposarcoma can be distinguished from other poorly differentiated STS subtypes on the basis of MDM2 and CDK4 immunohistochemistry.

For extremity liposarcoma, the goal is a limb-sparing resection with a negative surgical margin. Well-differentiated liposarcoma has an extremely low risk of distant metastasis and has a favorable

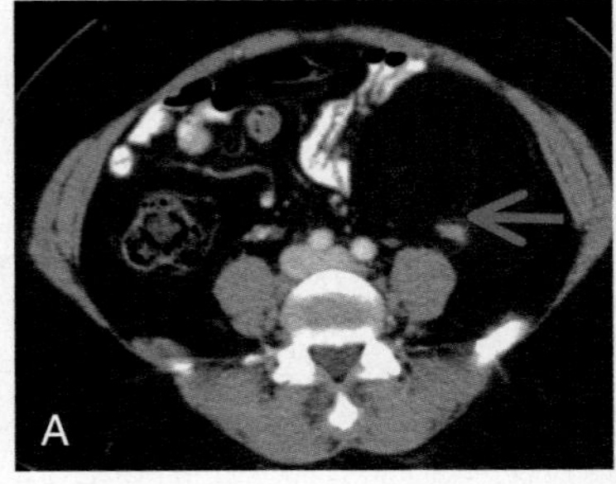

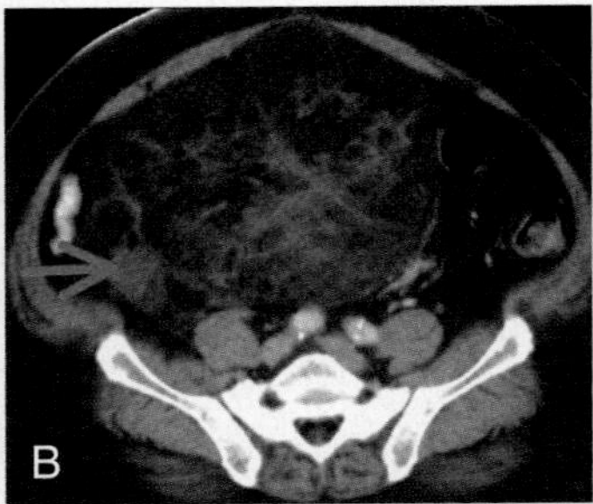

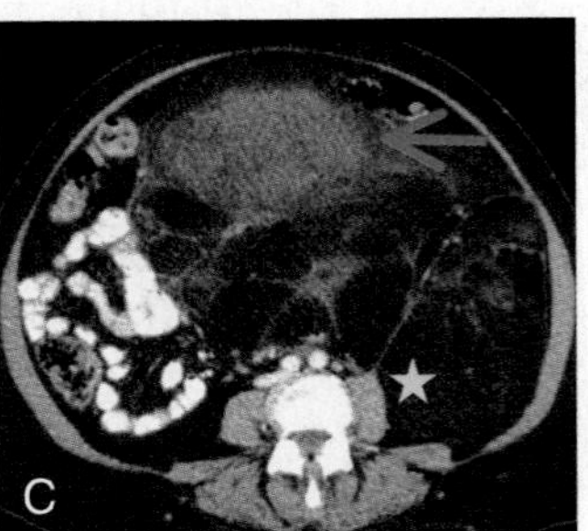

FIGURE 31-5 Variability in CT appearance of retroperitoneal liposarcoma. **A,** Simple, predominantly fatty, well-differentiated tumor; the *arrow* marks the inferior mesenteric vein. Thin septa are appreciable within the tumor. **B,** A hypercellular well-differentiated tumor with a focal nodular or water density area *(arrow)*. **C,** This tumor contains well-differentiated areas *(star)* as well as dedifferentiated elements *(arrow)*.

overall survival. This, combined with its resistance to radiation therapy and most chemotherapy agents, essentially eliminates the need for adjuvant therapy. On the other hand, patients with dedifferentiated extremity liposarcoma should be referred for consideration of adjuvant radiation therapy.

The treatment of patients with retroperitoneal liposarcoma is more complex. The principal goal is a gross complete resection as incomplete gross resection is associated with an increased risk of mortality.[10] Traditionally, retroperitoneal sarcoma has been treated by resection with a generous gross margin, with resection of organs and structures that are contiguous with or invading the tumor when feasible. More recently, some have advocated for a "complete compartmental resection," which mandates the resection of adjacent organs, even if they are not directly involved with the tumor.[11] Although it is controversial, the concept that "the resection is only as good as the closest margin" is an important one. This takes into account the relationships between vital structures on one side of the tumor and not resecting contiguous but uninvolved organs. Understanding of the patterns of retroperitoneal liposarcoma recurrence is important in planning the optimal approach. For patients with well-differentiated retroperitoneal liposarcoma, a unifocal versus multifocal presentation does not appear to confer an adverse prognosis, but patients with dedifferentiated disease multifocality have a worse overall survival.[12] Patients who develop recurrence after initial resection are likely to develop multifocal disease. This appears to be reflective of the tumor biology because an initial resection with positive margins does not appear to affect whether a patient develops a unifocal versus multifocal recurrence. The complete compartmental resection approach results in frequent multivisceral resections, with the following organs resected in more than 50% of cases: spleen, pancreas, diaphragm, adrenal gland, and kidney.[11] Proponents of a more traditional approach in which only tumor-contiguous organs are removed point out that 15% of patients who have recurrence after undergoing standard resection do so beyond the compartmental bounds of their initial tumor.[12] These out-of-field recurrences are unlikely to have been prevented with an aggressive complete compartmental resection strategy, and patients who may eventually benefit from nephrotoxic systemic chemotherapy are adversely affected by a potentially unnecessary complete compartmental resection–related nephrectomy.

Although grossly incomplete resections are to be avoided, a margin-negative resection is not possible in some situations. At times, this can be predicted on the basis of the preoperative imaging, but at other times, the difficulty of the resection is not appreciated until during the operation. A single-institution retrospective study compared the outcome of patients with retroperitoneal liposarcoma who underwent an incomplete resection versus patients who underwent exploration and biopsy without tumor resection. Even incomplete resection provides a statistically significant improvement in survival compared with no resection, 26 versus 4 months. In addition, 75% of patients undergoing incomplete resection reported palliation of their presenting symptoms.[13] In the setting of recurrent retroperitoneal liposarcoma, the rate of recurrent tumor growth is associated with prognosis. Patients whose recurrence grows less than 0.9 cm per month benefitted from complete resection of the recurrence, whereas recurrent tumor growth of more than 0.9 cm per month was associated with poor outcome.[14] Together these observations contribute to the complexity of developing an individualized treatment plan for retroperitoneal liposarcoma.

MFH Reclassification

In past decades, MFH was considered the most common STS in adults. Improvements and innovations in the pathologic review of STS have drastically altered the definition of MFH. Various authors have retrospectively reevaluated tumors originally classified as MFH and found that the majority merited reclassification. In one seminal manuscript, 63% were reclassified, and only 13% truly met pathologic criteria for MFH. These data shifted the diagnosis of MFH to one of exclusion, and this movement culminated in the 2013 World Health Organization classification of soft tissue tumors that completely eliminated the term. Tumors that still meet pathologic criteria for MFH are now referred to as unclassified or undifferentiated pleomorphic sarcoma. Careful histologic and immunohistochemical review by a pathologist with STS expertise is crucial in the accurate diagnosis and treatment of these patients. With precise pathologic review, patients with tumors originally classified as MFH have demonstrably different prognoses based on the actual line of STS differentiation.[15]

TRUNK AND EXTREMITY SARCOMA

Extremity STS poses a particular challenge with respect to balancing the degree of limb function with tumor control. Historically, surgeons had a much lower threshold to recommend extremity amputation for STS. Data from clinical trials have prompted a shift toward limb preservation in these patients. The ability to offer limb preservation is a result of improvements in the multidisciplinary care of these patients. One of the seminal trials conducted at the NCI proposed that extremity STS resection might be addressed by a limb-sparing approach instead of amputation.[16] Forty-three patients with high-grade extremity STS were randomized to undergo a limb-sparing operation followed by adjuvant radiation therapy versus amputation alone; both groups received adjuvant chemotherapy. This approach resulted in a slightly higher but nonstatistically significant difference in local recurrence in the limb-sparing group. Despite this, disease-free and overall survival rates were equivalent between the two groups. These results were supported by a similar contemporary trial that compared 126 patients who were randomized to limb-sparing STS resection with or without adjuvant brachytherapy in the absence of chemotherapy.[17] In this trial, only the patients with high-grade STS had a statistically significant decrease in local recurrence. In a later NCI study, patients demonstrated a decrease in local recurrence regardless of tumor grade with the addition of external beam radiation therapy. The STS literature lacks a randomized trial to identify in which patients adjuvant radiation therapy can be safely omitted because of the large sample size required to satisfy the accompanying power calculation.[18] Retrospective data indicate that adjuvant radiation therapy may be omitted for T1 extremity STS that is resected with negative surgical margins, even considering that 58% of these patients had high-grade tumors.[19] A large retrospective Scandinavian study of 1093 patients found that whereas a narrow or involved surgical margin does increase the risk of local recurrence, adjuvant radiation therapy improved local control independent of tumor grade, tumor depth (superficial or deep), or margin status. In the event that adjuvant radiation therapy is indicated, the surgeon should consider two technical maneuvers. The first is placement of a few metallic clips at the boundaries of the resection bed in the event that adjuvant radiation therapy is indicated; the second is that when a surgical drain is necessary, the skin exit site should be placed near the incision as the entire surgical drain track is usually included in the radiation field. Metallic clips within the resection bed will assist with radiation planning, and careful drain placement reduces an otherwise unnecessary augmentation of the radiation field.

Above and beyond the established local control benefits of adjuvant radiation, delivery of neoadjuvant radiation for STS offers a number of conceptual advantages. Before surgical resection, the target tissue oxygenation is superior, which facilitates the generation of intratumoral free radicals and ultimately tumor cell destruction. When radiation is administered neoadjuvantly, the radiation field includes a smaller volume of adjacent nontumor tissue compared with the radiation field after surgical resection.[20] When radiation is delivered with the tumor in situ, a lower preoperative dose is required versus in the postoperative setting. If radiation is delivered preoperatively, patients would be predicted to complete all components of their therapy more promptly as delayed wound healing can delay initiation of postoperative radiation therapy.[21] In contrast to other tumors, administration of neoadjuvant radiation therapy rarely results in measurable tumor shrinkage but may cause varying degrees of histologic tumor necrosis.[22] A complete pathologic response after neoadjuvant therapy is an important prognostic factor in a variety of malignant neoplasms including breast cancer, esophageal cancer, and rectal cancer. Unfortunately, this relationship does not appear to hold true for STS. When most of the resected tumor is nonviable after neoadjuvant radiation therapy or chemoradiotherapy, patients with STS do not have improvements in overall survival or local recurrence.[23] Patients with a positive surgical margin after undergoing preoperative radiation therapy do not appear to derive a significant reduction in local recurrence by administration of a postoperative radiation boost.

Only one clinical trial has randomized patients with extremity STS to receive either neoadjuvant or postoperative radiation therapy. In this trial, neoadjuvant external beam radiation therapy was associated with an increased risk of wound complications.[20] Although the authors reported a statistically significant difference in overall survival favoring the neoadjuvant arm, survival was a secondary end point, and the trial was not properly powered to evaluate this parameter. One would expect that another conceptual advantage of choosing a neoadjuvant approach would be to decrease the incidence and consequences of positive surgical margins by delivering tumoricidal doses preoperatively to the areas most at risk. In actuality, the existing randomized trial showed equivalent rates of negative surgical margins in patients receiving preoperative versus postoperative radiation therapy (83% and 85%, respectively).[20] Using the existing retrospective data to explore this question is problematic as there are clear selection biases in which patients receive neoadjuvant therapy and their subsequent risk for positive surgical margins. Finally, the definition of a positive or negative surgical margin differs among manuscripts, which contributes to the difficulty in interpreting the reported data. The long-term implications of a positive margin are independent of whether radiation therapy is delivered preoperatively or postoperatively; positive margins are associated with an increased risk for local recurrence, whereas overall survival is generally unchanged.

Preoperative regimens combining chemotherapy and radiation therapy have also been investigated. A retrospective review of 112 patients undergoing either neoadjuvant chemoradiation or neoadjuvant radiation versus surgery alone found equivalent oncologic outcomes among the three approaches. When stratified by size, the overall survival of patients with tumors larger than 5 cm was improved in treatment with either neoadjuvant chemoradiation or neoadjuvant radiation therapy compared with surgery alone.[24] Preoperative chemoradiation therapy followed by surgical resection and additional chemotherapy was shown to be associated with an increased overall survival. This was suggested in a retrospective study of 48 patients whose chemotherapy included combination of doxorubicin, ifosfamide, and dacarbazine. All 48 patients had high-grade extremity STS measuring at least 8 cm, and additional postoperative radiation therapy was delivered in the event of positive surgical margins.[25] Patients undergoing this intensive preoperative and postoperative chemotherapy regimen were matched to historical controls. In this study, the resection margin status was similar between the two groups. The outcomes of this preoperative and postoperative chemoradiation treatment schema were verified in RTOG 9514, a single-arm, multi-institutional phase 2 trial.[26]

The use of chemotherapy in the adjuvant setting for STS is controversial. EORTC 62931 was a randomized multi-institutional trial that randomized 351 patients to receive adjuvant chemotherapy (doxorubicin, ifosfamide, and the hematopoietic growth factor lenograstim) versus no chemotherapy. The overall and relapse-free survivals were equivalent in both groups. A meta-analysis of 1953 patients who had participated in 18 trials showed that those patients who received adjuvant doxorubicin had statistically significant improvements in local, distant, and overall recurrence. A randomized phase 2 study of 150 patients showed that neoadjuvant chemotherapy (doxorubicin and ifosfamide) was not associated with improvements in disease-free or overall survival. Because of the abundance of conflicting data, consensus guidelines such as those of the National Comprehensive Cancer Network and the European Society for Medical Oncology remain guarded in their recommendation for adjuvant chemotherapy.

Another treatment strategy that has been employed in patients with locally advanced extremity STS is regional chemotherapy, namely, limb perfusion. More commonly used in the treatment of locally advanced melanoma, this involves placement of both intravenous and intra-arterial catheters that are positioned within the affected limb proximal to the tumor. The combination of the limb vasculature and the intravascular catheters completes a circuit through which hyperthermic chemotherapy is circulated. A tourniquet proximal to the tips of the catheters separates the limb circulation from the systemic circulation to minimize systemic chemotherapy toxicity. The most common perfusion agents used are melphalan, tumor necrosis factor-α, and interferon-γ. Isolated limb perfusion is often combined with other modalities, namely, surgical resection. The technical demands and potential for local toxicities limit the application of this therapy. Currently, only one randomized trial has compared regional chemotherapy with other standard STS therapies. Overall, there is insufficient published data to conclusively establish the role of regional chemotherapy in the care of extremity STS.

The question as to what constitutes an adequate STS resection margin is complex, but the following is clear: the volume of tissue that is resected has clear implications as to the postoperative function of the limb, and a quantitative definition of an adequate surgical margin has never been defined in a randomized, prospective format. Whereas advances in rehabilitation medicine and prosthetic construction have significantly improved the functional capacity of patients who undergo extremity STS resection, the aforementioned data demonstrate that the goal of effective tumor extirpation with the smallest functional deficit is possible. Unlike in the melanoma literature, patients with extremity STS have never been randomized to compare surgical margin widths. Retrospectively, the local recurrence rate after resection of extremity STS with a microscopic margin of 1 cm or more is superior to when the margin is less than 1 cm.[27] However, in a different retrospective study, the only factor associated with an increased risk of local recurrence was tumor at the margin of resection.[28]

Because re-resection has been associated with improvements in local recurrence, patients with positive margins should be offered re-resection to achieve margins of 1 cm.[29] In difficult anatomic situations, pursuit of clear surgical margins should be weighed against the natural history of extremity STS and the risk of an increased functional deficit. Even in the setting of multimodality therapy, the risk of distant metastasis consistently outweighs the risk of local recurrence in high-grade tumors.

The gross morphology of STS is such that during resection, the plane of least resistance is usually along a tumor pseudocapsule. The pseudocapsule is a characteristic plane of thickened tissue that radiographically and during intraoperative palpation gives the impression of representing the interface between tumor and normal tissue. Resections that proceed along the pseudocapsule plane are generally enucleations with involved margins. Traditionally, a 1- to 2-cm grossly negative margin beyond the pseudocapsule is recommended, but this may be difficult or impossible to achieve in certain anatomic sites and may be unnecessary in dealing with low-grade tumors. Neoadjuvant therapy may be associated with formation of a more robust tumor pseudocapsule populated by fewer tumor cells.[30,31] Ultimately, as discussed in the section on retroperitoneal sarcoma, any resection margin is only as good as the closest margin in any region of the tumor, so that extending resections to increase morbidity in one region is not necessary if a closer margin exists in another region.

STS tends to metastasize hematogenously principally to the lungs but also to the liver and bone. Tumor grade is the most important predictor of metastasis, with a 43% rate of metastasis-free survival in patients with high-grade tumors.[32] Other important predictors of metastasis include tumor size, bone or neurovascular involvement, and tumor depth (superficial versus deep). The prevalence of pulmonary metastases among patients previously treated for extremity STS is approximately 19%. Isolated pulmonary metastases should be resected whenever feasible.[33] A prolonged disease-free interval between initial STS treatment and development of lung metastasis is generally a favorable prognostic factor. In the absence of effective systemic therapies, repeated pulmonary metastasectomy is also a consideration. Patients who are not candidates for metastasectomy should be evaluated for ablative or systemic therapies. Many types of STS are relatively chemoresistant; notable exceptions include angiosarcoma and synovial sarcoma. Typical agents for metastatic STS include doxorubicin, dacarbazine, ifosfamide, gemcitabine, and docetaxel. To date, no adequately powered randomized controlled trial has been able to show a statistically significant improvement in overall survival of patients with metastatic STS. Agents under investigation that show early promise in metastatic STS include DNA minor groove inhibitors (trabectedin), tyrosine kinase inhibitors (sorafenib, pazopanib), MDM2 antagonists, and modified ifosfamide compounds (palifosfamide, TH-302).

Malignant Peripheral Nerve Sheath Tumors

MPNSTs occur in roughly equal frequency sporadically and as part of NF1. These tumors are the malignant form of the benign schwannoma. Although they arise from a peripheral nerve or the nerve sheath, they are often painless on presentation. The most common age at presentation is 20 to 50 years. Historically, other names have been applied to MPNST, such as malignant schwannoma, neurogenic sarcoma, and neurofibrosarcoma. The term *malignant schwannoma* is avoided because not all MPNSTs actually arise from Schwann cells. These are generally aggressive tumors; recent large series have shown a local recurrence rate of about 20% and a 10-year disease-specific survival of more than 40%. The key prognostic factors include tumor size at presentation and tumor grade. There is no consensus in the literature as to whether MPNST in the setting of NF1 carries a worse prognosis than spontaneous cases. Treatment of these tumors is similar to that of other STS subtypes, with a focus on margin-negative resection. Although it has not been studied prospectively in the MPNST population, most retrospective reports agree that adjuvant radiation therapy is indicated to decrease the rate of local recurrence in extremity and superficial trunk lesions.

Desmoid Tumor

Desmoid tumors, also known as aggressive fibromatosis, are an uncommon group of fibroblastic tumors that have a curious natural history in that distant metastases are extremely rare. Approximately 75% to 85% of cases arise sporadically; the others are related to FAP. Among the sporadic cases, recent pregnancy and antecedent trauma are recognized associations. These tumors are two to three times more common in women than in men and are most commonly diagnosed in patients aged 30 to 40 years. Approximately 20% of FAP patients develop desmoid tumors, and a common presentation involves a desmoid at the prior colectomy scar.[34] Desmoid tumors are usually preceded by colonic polyposis in FAP patients and represent the second leading cause of death in FAP patients.[35] A detailed family history should be obtained from patients presenting with desmoid tumors to rule out unappreciated FAP, and consideration should also be given to screening colonoscopy.

The molecular underpinnings of desmoids, regardless of sporadic or syndromic association, are related to the WNT signaling pathway. In sporadic cases, *CTNNB1* mutations result in the expression of a stabilized form of β-catenin, which ultimately accumulates and is transported to the nucleus, where it exerts its proliferative effects through activation of transcription factors. In the setting of FAP, *APC* mutations also cause β-catenin stabilization, which also activates nuclear transcription and cellular proliferation. Specific *APC* codon mutations appear to confer a higher desmoid risk than other codon mutations.[34]

Clinically, the most common areas of origin include the extremity, intraperitoneal, abdominal wall, and chest wall. Affected patients may present with a painful versus asymptomatic firm mass, bowel obstruction, or bowel ischemia. Desmoid tumors are usually slow-growing but on occasion do grow aggressively. On radiographic evaluation, these tumors are generally homogeneous and solid in appearance. They may have either a distinct or an infiltrating boundary. CT scan and MRI are both useful imaging modalities. Especially in sporadic cases, desmoid tumors are indistinguishable from a variety of other STS subtypes based on imaging alone. Core needle biopsy is indicated in situations in which treatment recommendations will be altered on the basis of tumor histology.

Treatment of these tumors can be challenging. When tumors are large or infiltrating crucial anatomic structures, surgical resection with widely negative margins may not be possible. Even when the tumors are adequately resected, especially in the FAP population, desmoid tumors show a high likelihood of local recurrence.

These observations have prompted various recommendations for consideration of active surveillance for desmoid tumors rather than reflexive resection on diagnosis. In addition, the role of radiation may be appropriate, especially in recurrent extremity tumors. When considering that many desmoids are indolent and show very little growth after presentation and that resection may mandate significant functional deficits, an active surveillance strategy may be appropriate for selected patients.

Angiosarcoma

Angiosarcoma is a malignant tumor that arises from the endothelial lining of blood vessels and therefore can arise from almost any site. Overall, it accounts for 2% of all STS, but approximately 40% of all angiosarcomas are radiation associated.[2] In decreasing order of frequency, the most important primary sites are the trunk, head, and neck (particularly the scalp) and the viscera. Within the head and neck, the scalp is often the site of angiosarcoma origin. Angiosarcoma typically is diagnosed in the seventh and eighth decades. Although most angiosarcoma is sporadic, risk factors include previous therapeutic radiation exposure and lymphedema (see previous section). Angiosarcoma, in contrast to other STS, does have a higher frequency of involved regional lymph nodes. Approximately 20% of patients present with metastasis, most frequently to the lung.[36] On histologic evaluation, these tumors range from extremely well differentiated, mimicking hemangioma, to very poorly differentiated. Consistent with this, there is a wide variety of cytogenetic changes. On immunohistochemical examination, CD31 and FLI-1 are the most consistent markers.

The primary therapy for these lesions is surgical resection with negative margins. On microscopic examination, these tumors often infiltrate well beyond the area of gross involvement. For patients with head and neck angiosarcoma, this can present a reconstructive challenge. Angiosarcoma that arises within the breast after breast-conserving therapy is managed with mastectomy. Even after surgical resection, the outcome is poor, with a 5-year disease-specific survival of 53%.[36] In the cohort with resectable disease, tumor size larger than 5 cm and histologic evidence of an epithelioid component are indicators of poor prognosis.[36] After resection, distant failure predominates over local failure, although both are common. These tumors are often locally advanced and unresectable at presentation; fortunately, these tumors are responsive to chemotherapy and radiation therapy, and a neoadjuvant approach may be feasible.

The median survival of stage IV angiosarcoma is 8 to 12 months. Unlike other STS, metastatic angiosarcoma may be manifested with hemopneumothorax. Breast angiosarcoma may metastasize to the liver. The most typical agents employed in the unresectable or metastatic setting include paclitaxel and doxorubicin, followed by radiation therapy, except perhaps in patients whose tumor was incited by previous radiation therapy. A host of ongoing trials including angiosarcoma patients are underway that are exploring the utility of a range of agents including tyrosine kinase inhibitors and combination therapy of antiangiogenesis inhibitors together with cytotoxic agents *(clinicaltrials.gov).*

Dermatofibrosarcoma Protuberans

DFSP is an uncommon STS that affects approximately one in 4.2 million patients in the United States. This tumor affects men and women equally and appears to be more common in African American patients than in whites. The typical range of presentation is between the fourth and seventh decades. The trunk, upper extremity, and lower extremity are equally frequent sites of DFSP, followed by the head and neck. On physical examination, these are firm, indurated nodules that are reddish or brown in appearance. On histologic evaluation, DFSP is a dermal or subdermal tumor without penetration into the epidermis. Cytogenetically, the majority of DFSP displays the t(17;22)(q22;q13) translocation, which fuses the *COL1A1* and platelet-derived growth factor B *(PDGFB)* genes and accounts for its PDGFB overexpression. In difficult cases, this gene fusion can be detected by fluorescence in situ hybridization. Because of its somewhat bland visual appearance and the lack of associated pain, it can often be large at presentation, having been mistaken for a hypertrophic scar or a keloid.

DFSP frequently recurs locally, and consequently the treatment is surgical resection with wide margins. As is true with most STS, there are no well-designed clinical trials to define an adequate margin. Recurrence can be successfully treated with resection. The 5-year survival is 99.2%.[37] DFSP rarely metastasizes, but when it does, it often implies degeneration to fibrosarcoma. Because of the PDGFB upregulation, patients with unresectable disease may be treated with neoadjuvant imatinib.

RETROPERITONEAL AND VISCERAL SARCOMA

Retroperitoneal sarcoma represents approximately 15% of all STS. The sequestered location of the retroperitoneum probably accounts for the fact that the average tumor size at presentation is 15 cm.[38] The most frequent retroperitoneal sarcoma subtypes are liposarcoma, leiomyosarcoma, and MFH (see discussion earlier in this chapter).[38] The predominant intraperitoneal STS subtypes are GIST and leiomyosarcoma, which are discussed separately. The average age at presentation is 54 years, and there is an equal male to female distribution. In most series, the overall survival of patients presenting with retroperitoneal sarcoma is 33% to 39%. Even after optimal surgical resection, at least 70% of patients will relapse. In one large retrospective series, approximately 12% of patients presented with metastatic disease, predominantly pulmonary or hepatic.

The presentation of retroperitoneal sarcoma is variable, depending on the size and location of the tumor. Some are asymptomatic and incidentally discovered. Symptomatic tumors may be manifested with abdominal pain, weight loss, early satiety, nausea, emesis, back or flank pain, paresthesias, and weakness. CT and MRI are widely used for the evaluation of retroperitoneal sarcoma because of their excellent spatial resolution and reproducible axial image acquisition. The advantages of CT scan include rapid image acquisition, nearly universal availability, and a concise image set that can be more intuitive for the nonradiologist to interpret. The advantages of MRI include a wider range of soft tissue differentiation, but the disadvantages include an increased susceptibility to claustrophobia and motion artifact, the more limited availability, and a greater number of implant-related contraindications compared with CT scan. These modalities can be complementary, and at times both provide useful information. The patient must be carefully evaluated along with the imaging studies to verify that the retroperitoneal mass does not represent an unappreciated lymphoma, germ cell tumor, or metastasis from another primary tumor as the management of these tumors is quite different from that of retroperitoneal sarcoma.

A number of consensus guidelines strongly recommend performing a preoperative biopsy, but as previously discussed with extremity STS, biopsy for retroperitoneal sarcoma is not mandatory and has drawbacks in certain situations. By definition, a surgical biopsy ruptures the tumor, seeding the operative field and potentially reducing the possibility of a margin-negative resection. Preoperative biopsy can be particularly misleading in patients with large tumors as the biopsy is susceptible to a significant degree of sampling bias. This sampling bias can provide inappropriately reassuring information. The preoperative CT scan often contains enough information to proceed with treatment without a preoperative biopsy as long as the other basic considerations in the differential diagnosis are considered excluded. This includes lymphoma, germ cell tumors, and other metastatic disease (see Box 31-1). In a retrospective study from a large, single, tertiary care institution, the initial staging CT was sufficient in assessing the need for preoperative biopsy and assigning a treatment approach for those tumors for which biopsy is not indicated; this approach is discussed in greater detail in the lipomatous tumor section.[9] For this reason, if preoperative biopsy is obtained from a heterogeneous mass, the specimen should be obtained from the most concerning region under image guidance.

When possible, treatment should proceed with a complete gross resection. In the retroperitoneal sarcoma literature, the concept of margin status is different from that for extremity STS. Because extremity STS tumors are usually smaller than retroperitoneal sarcoma tumors, microscopic evaluation of the entire surgical specimen margin is often feasible. Given the much larger tumor dimensions of most retroperitoneal sarcomas, it is not practical and often impossible to microscopically evaluate 100% of the surgical specimen margin surface area. Consequently, most of the retroperitoneal sarcoma literature refers to complete gross resection. In one large series, complete gross resection was achieved in 80% of initial sarcoma resections, 57% of operations for first recurrence, 33% of operations at second recurrence, and 14% of operations at third recurrence. In 75% of patients, achieving complete gross resection may mean resecting contiguous or inseparable adjacent organs, such as the kidney, bowel, or pancreas and vascular structures. Predicting histologic invasion on the basis of gross intraoperative findings can be inaccurate. Before the era of modern CT technology, patients who underwent nephrectomy because of intraoperative evidence of suspected involvement during retroperitoneal sarcoma resection were further evaluated for histologic evidence of sarcoma invasion. In 73% of cases, the nephrectomy specimen did not contain STS. Improvements in the quality of preoperative imaging probably decrease the rate of adjacent organ resection based solely on intraoperative suspicion. As expected, predictors of poor prognosis include gross residual disease after resection, unresectable disease (either metastatic or locally advanced), and high tumor grade. Patients with a complete gross resection have a median survival of 103 months compared with 18 months for patients with incomplete resections. Even with optimal chemotherapy and radiation therapy, the median survival of patients with unresectable disease is 10 months.[39]

In contradistinction to extremity sarcoma, the role of multimodality therapy is more controversial in retroperitoneal sarcoma. Given the success of adjuvant radiation in extremity STS, this approach has been applied to retroperitoneal sarcoma, but with fewer randomized data to support its efficacy. The 60- to 70-Gy dose that is considered sarcoma lethal and typically used for extremity STS is not feasible in the adjuvant setting for retroperitoneal sarcoma because of bowel toxicity. Even dose reduction to 50 to 55 Gy results in significant enteritis. These tolerability issues prompted consideration of neoadjuvant radiation for retroperitoneal sarcoma. An advantage of neoadjuvant radiation is that the in situ tumor displaces the bowel anteriorly, thus facilitating the delivery of a higher radiation dose posteriorly, which is the most likely site of a positive histologic margin (Fig. 31-6). This approach delivers 45 Gy to the planned target volume, and the projected at-risk margins are boosted up to 65 Gy. Two separate studies have demonstrated that the neoadjuvant approach is well tolerated and that long- and short-term oncologic outcomes are favorable compared with historical cohorts treated with resection alone.[40,41]

For patients with metastatic retroperitoneal sarcoma, there are few effective chemotherapeutic options. Single or combination therapy with anthracyclines can be used as first-line therapy. A second-line regimen is gemcitabine and docetaxel. Novel agents undergoing further study include trabectedin, tyrosine kinase inhibitors, MDM2 antagonists, peroxisome proliferator-activated receptor gamma agonists, and CDK4 antagonists.

Gastrointestinal Stromal Tumor

GIST is the most common variety of visceral STS. These tumors are believed to originate from the interstitial cells of Cajal within the gastrointestinal myenteric plexus and emanate from nearly any part of the alimentary tract, from esophagus to anus. The most prevalent GIST sites are the stomach, the small bowel, and the rectum. Cajal cells are thought to function as pacemaker cells in

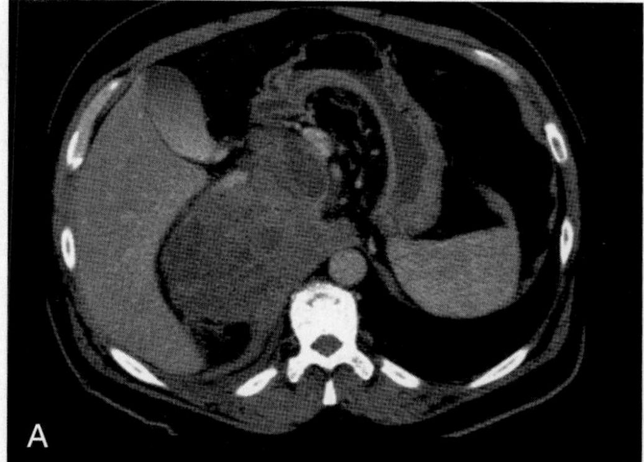

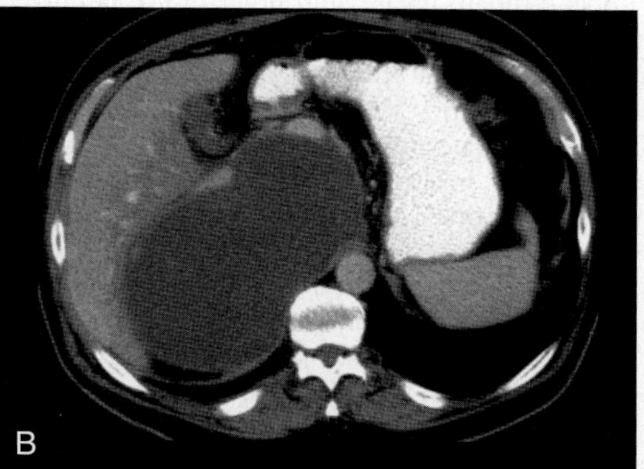

FIGURE 31-6 Liquefaction of a high-grade retroperitoneal sarcoma before **(A)** and after **(B)** administration of 60-Gy preoperative radiation therapy. The tumor was subsequently resected with negative surgical margins, and no viable tumor was histologically identifiable.

the viscera, mediating contractions. Cajal cells and GIST share common markers for CD117 and a calcium-activated chloride channel called DOG1. CD117 is another name for the *KIT* gene, which codes for a tyrosine kinase transmembrane receptor called c-kit. These molecular descriptions led to dramatic refinements in the diagnosis and treatment of patients with GIST. In morphologic appearance, GIST is classically a spindle cell neoplasm of smooth muscle origin. Although these tumors were previously described as leiomyoma or leiomyosarcoma, GISTs are differentiated on the basis of CD34, CD117, and DOG1 expression and the lack of smooth muscle staining.

The c-kit receptor is a proto-oncogene that belongs to the platelet-derived growth factor receptor (PDGFR) superfamily. The natural c-kit ligand is a stem cell factor, and its binding causes tyrosine kinase receptor homodimerization, autophosphorylation, and activation of multiple pathways, including RAS, RAF, MAPK, AKT, and STAT3. Certain mutations of the c-kit receptor confer constitutive activation of the receptor, which ultimately results in cellular proliferation. The other relevant gene, also found on chromosome 4, that bears striking similarity to c-kit is the platelet-derived growth factor receptor alpha (PDGFRA) receptor. Overall, about 70% of GIST tumors have *KIT* gene mutations, approximately 7% have *PDGFRA* mutations, and 15% have wild-type *KIT* and *PDGFRA* genotypes. These GIST tumors are characterized by a number of other mutations affecting succinate dehydrogenase (*SDH*), *BRAF*, *KRAS*, and *NF1*. *SDH* mutations are related to GIST in patients affected by the Carney-Stratakis syndrome, and *NF1* mutations drive GIST formation in patients with type 1 neurofibromatosis.

The clinical presentation of these tumors is variable, ranging from incidental to symptomatic with respect to pain, nausea, vomiting, or, more rarely, gastrointestinal blood loss. On endoscopic examination, GIST usually appears as a smooth submucosal tumor that extrinsically impinges on the visceral lumen as opposed to an ulcerated mucosal mass. The endoscopic differential diagnosis of an intramural visceral mass includes GIST, neuroendocrine tumor, intramural lipoma, and lymphoma. Some GIST tumors are serosally pedunculated and do not contribute to intestinal obstruction. On CT, these tumors are well encapsulated and generally have heterogeneous contrast enhancement because of regions of necrosis within the tumor. Metastasis is not rare, but affected sites include the liver and peritoneal surface. The majority of GIST tumors are sporadic, but there are notable examples of syndromic involvement. These include NF1, germline succinate dehydrogenase mutations, the Carney-Stratakis syndrome, von Hippel–Lindau disease, and other minor familial GIST syndromes.

Because these are submucosal tumors, endoscopic forceps biopsies are often nondiagnostic. Tumors situated between the ligament of Treitz and the ileocecal valve can be localized by double-balloon enteroscopy or capsule endoscopy. Blood loss related to GIST may indicate that the tumor has ulcerated through the mucosa. An endoscopic ultrasound-guided needle biopsy generally shows a spindle cell neoplasm; if sufficient tissue is available, this can be submitted for CD117 evaluation. Preoperative biopsy for suspected GIST is not mandatory, but preoperative histologic verification of GIST obviates the need for empirical lymphadenectomy at the time of resection, which would be crucial for neuroendocrine tumor or intestinal adenocarcinoma. Appropriate preoperative staging for GIST includes contrast-enhanced CT of the chest, abdomen, and pelvis. Localized lesions are taken to the operating room for resection with grossly negative surgical margins. Obtaining wide surgical margins has not been demonstrated to improve local recurrence rates or overall survival. Given the rarity of lymph node involvement, lymphadenectomy is not mandatory for GIST. Care should be taken not to compromise the capsule of the tumor as rupture can seed the exposed tissues and adversely affect the prognosis of the patient. As long as the risk of tumor rupture is not elevated, consideration of minimally invasive surgical resection techniques is appropriate and may accelerate the recovery. The operative note should clearly document the integrity of the tumor capsule as it can profoundly affect recommendations for adjuvant therapy.

Ideally, the pathology report follows a synoptic guideline to ensure that all relevant parameters are communicated to the multidisciplinary team. The key parameters include the tumor site organ of origin, tumor size, tumor focality, mitotic rate, immunohistochemical CD117 status, margin status, and results of molecular genetic studies, if performed. The mitotic rate is defined as the total count of mitoses per 5 mm^2 on the glass slide section and is reported in the most proliferative area of the tumor. In GIST tumors, the mitotic rate parameter is synonymous with the tumor grade that is included with most other STS subtypes. Entities that can mimic GIST microscopically include melanoma, paraganglioma, neuroendocrine tumors, and nerve sheath tumors.

Distinct from other STS subtypes, the AJCC seventh edition staging system has a schema for GIST tumors that separates gastric and omental GIST from nongastric GIST (Tables 31-4 to 31-6). A number of tools available to predict prognosis after resection can then be used on the basis of these pathologic and clinical parameters. The Memorial Sloan Kettering Cancer Center (MSKCC) group developed a nomogram based on the size of the resected GIST, the mitotic rate, and the anatomic site of origin, which is validated to predict the probabilities of 2- and 5-year recurrence-free survival.[42] The nomogram was developed using data from 127 patients treated at MSKCC and then validated in

TABLE 31-4 AJCC Staging for GIST

Primary Tumor (T)	
TX	Primary tumor cannot be assessed
T0	No evidence for primary tumor
T1	Tumor 2 cm or less
T2	Tumor >2 cm, ≤5 cm
T3	Tumor >5 cm, ≤10 cm
T4	Tumor >10 cm
Regional Lymph Nodes (N)	
N0	No regional lymph node metastasis
N1	Regional lymph node metastasis
Distant Metastasis (M)	
M0	No distant metastasis
M1	Distant metastasis
M1a	Lung
M1b	Other distant site
Histologic Grade (G)	
GX	Grade cannot be assessed
G1	Low grade; mitotic rate ≤5 per 50 high-power fields
G2	High grade; mitotic rate >5 per 50 high-power fields

From Edge SB, American Joint Committee on Cancer: *AJCC cancer staging manual*, ed 7, New York, 2010, Springer.

TABLE 31-5 Anatomic Stage and Prognostic Groups for Gastric and Omental GIST

GROUP	T	N	M	GRADE
Stage IA	T1 or T2	N0	M0	Low
Stage IB	T3	N0	M0	Low
Stage II	T1	N0	M0	High
	T2	N0	M0	High
	T4	N0	M0	Low
Stage IIIA	T3	N0	M0	High
Stage IIIB	T4	N0	M0	High
Stage IV	Any T	N1	M0	Any rate
	Any T	Any N	M1	Any rate

From Edge SB, American Joint Committee on Cancer: *AJCC cancer staging manual*, ed 7, New York, 2010, Springer.

TABLE 31-6 Anatomic Stage and Prognostic Groups for Nongastric* GIST

GROUP	T	N	M	GRADE
Stage IA	T1 or T2	N0	M0	Low
Stage II	T3	N0	M0	Low
Stage IIIA	T1	N0	M0	High
	T4	N0	M0	Low
Stage IIIB	T2	N0	M0	High
	T3	N0	M0	High
	T4	N0	M0	High
Stage IV	Any T	N1	M0	Any rate
	Any T	Any N	M1	Any rate

From Edge SB, American Joint Committee on Cancer: *AJCC cancer staging manual*, ed 7, New York, 2010, Springer.

*Nongastric includes small bowel, colorectal, esophageal, mesentery, and peritoneal.

TABLE 31-7 National Institutes of Health Consensus Criteria for GIST Estimated Risk of Recurrence

ESTIMATION OF RISK	LARGEST TUMOR DIMENSION (cm)	MITOSES, PER 50 HIGH-POWER FIELDS
Very low risk	<2	<5
Low risk	2-5	<5
Intermediate risk	<5	6-10
	5-10	<5
High risk	>5	>5
	>10	Any mitotic rate
	Any size	> 10

Adapted from Fletcher CDM, Berman JJ, Corless C, et al: Diagnosis of gastrointestinal stromal tumors: A consensus approach. *Hum Pathol* 33:459–465, 2002.

two independent GIST populations from other institutions. The target population of this nomogram is patients undergoing complete GIST resection who did not receive adjuvant therapy. Another prognostic tool is the Armed Forces Institute of Pathology criteria, designed to predict the risk of progressive disease after resection and based on data from more than 1900 patients with resected GIST who also did not receive adjuvant therapy. Inputs into this schema include mitotic rate, size, and anatomic site of origin. This series has not been validated to the same degree as the MSKCC nomogram but was developed using a more robust sample size. The modified National Institutes of Health criteria were established on the basis of several data sets, including the Armed Forces Institute of Pathology criteria, and have subsequently been validated (Table 31-7).[43,44]

As predictors of outcome after surgical resection, these risk assessment tools are routinely used to also assess the need for adjuvant therapy. Although none of these risk assessment tools includes it as an input parameter, the success of adjuvant therapy is dependent on the GIST molecular phenotype. Specific *KIT* mutations differentially affect long-term prognosis and response to therapy. The specific *KIT* exon in which the GIST mutation resides affects the molecular and clinical phenotype. For example, a *KIT* mutation in exon 13 resides within the tyrosine kinase domain and confers susceptibility to imatinib therapy. Exon 9 mutations correspond to the extracellular domain of the c-kit receptor, are observed principally in small bowel or colon GIST, and are less sensitive to imatinib. Routine genetic analysis to determine the precise mutated exon is not currently recommended by consensus guidelines, but this information may alter treatment recommendations.

Systemic therapy is indicated for adjuvant therapy after GIST resection, for the treatment of metastatic GIST, and for the neoadjuvant therapy of unresectable or locally advanced tumors. Imatinib, the best studied of these systemic agents, is an oral tyrosine kinase inhibitor of c-kit. In general, the presence of a *KIT* mutation is highly associated with response to this oral medication. Again, because of the similarities to the c-kit and *PDGFRA* receptors, some patients with wild-type *KIT* are sensitive to imatinib. Other available agents capable of GIST-related tyrosine kinase inhibition include sunitinib and regorafenib. The third major molecular GIST group is characterized by *SDH* mutations. Patients with these mutations are generally younger, have multiple gastric GISTs, and have a poor response to imatinib. Although it is not universally accepted as standard of care, advanced molecular analysis should be considered for all patients. This may affect the choice and dose of tyrosine kinase inhibitor for patients with *KIT* or *PDGFRA* mutations, and in patients with wild-type *KIT* and *PDGFRA* GISTs, further molecular evaluation may identify clinically relevant *SDH* or *BRAF* mutations.

Imatinib was first developed to treat Philadelphia chromosome–positive chronic myelogenous leukemia. Soon after, its efficacy was demonstrated in the setting of metastatic GIST, adjuvant therapy for resected GIST, and neoadjuvant therapy for unresectable GIST. Imatinib was demonstrated to be associated with a dramatic improvement in the median overall survival of metastatic GIST from 20 months to 57 months.[45] In the adjuvant setting after complete surgical resection, two randomized studies have demonstrated improved disease-free recurrence.[46,47] Because these trials vary in their clinicopathologic inclusion criteria and study design, there remains debate as to which patients should receive imatinib and for what duration.

The ACOSOG Z9001 was a double-blind trial that randomized patients with a grossly negative GIST resection to receive imatinib versus placebo for 1 year. All tumors were larger than 3 cm, and all were c-kit positive by immunohistochemistry. One year of adjuvant imatinib was associated with a statistically significant improvement in the recurrence-free survival versus placebo (98% versus 83%, respectively).[46] A subsequent Z9001 follow-up study demonstrated a persistent improvement in recurrence-free survival but did not demonstrate any improvement in overall survival.[48] In a separate trial, patients were randomized to 1 versus 3 years of adjuvant imatinib after resection of c-kit–positive GIST. This trial stipulated that patients must have high-risk disease per the National Institutes of Health consensus criteria. The 3-year duration of therapy was associated with improvements not only in recurrence-free survival but also in overall survival.

Joensuu and colleagues[49] recently published the first data describing the parameters associated with tumor recurrence after resection in patients already treated with adjuvant imatinib. Data sets from two of the aforementioned three randomized trials were used to construct and to validate a risk stratification score. Two such scores were developed. The five-parameter score includes mitotic count, organ of origin, size, tumor rupture, and duration of imatinib therapy; the two-parameter score includes mitotic count and organ of origin. These data support a 3-year duration of imatinib therapy and indicate that nongastric organ of origin and a high mitotic count adversely affect recurrence-free survival. Because the previous risk assessment schemas were developed using patient cohorts who had never been treated with adjuvant imatinib, this stratification score may prove to be clinically relevant.

Leiomyosarcoma

Leiomyosarcoma is a malignant smooth muscle tumor that can originate from virtually any part of the body. The most common sites affected are the retroperitoneum and the peritoneal cavity, namely, the uterus; about 25% rise from the trunk and extremities. Overall, after liposarcoma, leiomyosarcoma is the second most frequent STS subtype.[1] The peak incidence of leiomyosarcoma is in the sixth and seventh decades. Retroperitoneal and uterine leiomyosarcoma is more common in women, but there is a male predominance in other leiomyosarcoma sites. Predisposing risk factors for leiomyosarcoma include prior radiation exposure and immunosuppression combined with Epstein-Barr virus–related tumor promotion. Leiomyosarcoma does not arise from a degenerated leiomyoma, a common benign soft tissue tumor.

Leiomyosarcoma is generally a heterogeneous, well-circumscribed tumor with an often cystic or necrotic central area. This tumor stains positive for desmin and smooth muscle actin. It has a wide variety of cytogenetic aberrations but no reliable or pathognomonic markers. Before the description of *KIT* mutations, tumors that are now appreciated to represent GIST were described as leiomyosarcoma.

First-line therapy for leiomyosarcoma is surgical resection with negative margins. For uterine leiomyosarcoma, a total abdominal hysterectomy and bilateral oophorectomy is indicated. Resection of tumors that invade or are intimately associated with the inferior vena cava (IVC) require special planning. Depending on the size and position of the tumor, an approach including neoadjuvant radiation therapy may be a consideration. The intraoperative options include tumor resection with IVC ligation, patching of the IVC, and interposition graft of the IVC. Tumors involving the IVC typically have a great deal of collateralization already in place. For a tumor that requires segmental resection of the infrahepatic IVC, if the collaterals can be preserved, ligation without reconstruction may be an acceptable maneuver as postoperative lower extremity edema is well tolerated. Because of the rarity of IVC leiomyosarcoma, a future randomized trial further evaluating these maneuvers is unlikely.

Regardless of the organ of origin, adjuvant therapy is not currently recommended, although this is the subject of ongoing trials, especially for uterine leiomyosarcoma. Affecting 44% of patients, metastasis is usually hematogenous in nature, mainly to the lung and liver. Doxorubicin, ifosfamide, docetaxel, and gemcitabine are used in the metastatic setting, although leiomyosarcoma responds more poorly to chemotherapy than liposarcoma and synovial sarcoma do.

SUMMARY

STS is a fascinating aspect of surgical oncology that requires an understanding of multiple tumor types. To effectively treat STS patients, the surgeon must have a strong understanding of tumor biology, the physiologic consequences of various resection strategies, and the ability to effectively work within the context of a multidisciplinary oncology team. Recent discoveries relating to the molecular and genetic underpinnings demonstrate that although they are rare, these tumors may offer opportunities in the development of novel targeted therapies.

SELECTED REFERENCES

Anya DA, Lahat G, Wang X, et al: Postoperative nomogram for survival of patients with retroperitoneal sarcoma treated with curative intent. *Ann Oncol* 21:397–402, 2010.

A thoughtful, pragmatic, and easily applicable approach to the management of retroperitoneal sarcomas.

Brennan MF, Antonescu CR, Moraco N, et al: Lessons learned from the study of 10,000 patients with soft tissue sarcoma. *Ann Surg* 260:416–421, discussion 421–422, 2014.

The largest surgical series of soft tissue sarcoma demonstrates a number of key concepts that relate to natural history and management of patients with this disease.

Fletcher CD, Gustafson P, Rydholm A, et al: Clinicopathologic re-evaluation of 100 malignant fibrous histiocytomas: Prognostic relevance of subclassification. *J Clin Oncol* 19:3045–3050, 2001.

This illustrates the concept that the historical term malignant fibrous histiocytoma *is pathologically imprecise and fails to accurately predict outcome.*

Heslin MJ, Lewis JJ, Nadler E, et al: Prognostic factors associated with long-term survival for retroperitoneal sarcoma: Implications for management. *J Clin Oncol* 15:2832–2839, 1997.

An important manuscript demonstrating the natural history of patients undergoing resection for retroperitoneal sarcoma.

Joensuu H, Eriksson M, Hall KS, et al: Risk factors for gastrointestinal stromal tumor recurrence in patients treated with adjuvant imatinib. *Cancer* 120:2325–2333, 2014.

Whereas most retrospective reviews focus on GIST prognosis after resection alone, this paper describes a methodology to stratify the risk of GIST recurrence in patients treated with adjuvant imatinib.

Joensuu H, Vehtari A, Riihimaki J, et al: Risk of recurrence of gastrointestinal stromal tumour after surgery: An analysis of pooled population-based cohorts. *Lancet Oncol* 13:265–274, 2012.

Data from 10 published series regarding the risk for GIST recurrence after resection are used to help define which patients are likely to be cured by surgery alone.

O'Sullivan B, Davis AM, Turcotte R, et al: Preoperative versus postoperative radiotherapy in soft-tissue sarcoma of the limbs: A randomised trial. *Lancet* 359:2235–2241, 2002.

The NCI of Canada/Canadian Sarcoma Group SR2 clinical trial represents the only prospective randomized comparison of preoperative versus postoperative radiation therapy for extremity sarcoma.

Pisters PW, Pollock RE, Lewis VO, et al: Long-term results of prospective trial of surgery alone with selective use of radiation for patients with T1 extremity and trunk soft tissue sarcomas. *Ann Surg* 246:675–681, 2007.

Compelling data supporting the selective use of adjuvant radiation for early-stage soft tissue sarcoma.

Rosenberg SA, Tepper J, Glatstein E, et al: The treatment of soft-tissue sarcomas of the extremities: Prospective randomized evaluations of (1) limb-sparing surgery plus radiation therapy compared with amputation and (2) the role of adjuvant chemotherapy. *Ann Surg* 196:305–315, 1982.

This phase 3 NCI study paved the way for a generation of studies examining the role for limb-sparing surgery in the setting of multimodal therapy.

Taylor BS, Barretina J, Maki RG, et al: Advances in sarcoma genomics and new therapeutic targets. *Nat Rev Cancer* 11:541–557, 2011.

A unique perspective on the taxonomy and classification of soft tissue sarcoma, driven by the molecular genetics of this diverse tumor family.

van Vliet M, Kliffen M, Krestin GP, et al: Soft tissue sarcomas at a glance: Clinical, histological, and MR imaging features of malignant extremity soft tissue tumors. *Eur Radiol* 19:1499–1511, 2009.

This manuscript is a concise atlas of soft tissue sarcoma that correlates the natural history of the disease to the imaging and histologic characteristics.

REFERENCES

1. Brennan MF, Antonescu CR, Moraco N, et al: Lessons learned from the study of 10,000 patients with soft tissue sarcoma. *Ann Surg* 260:416–422, 2014.
2. Gladdy RA, Qin LX, Moraco N, et al: Do radiation-associated soft tissue sarcomas have the same prognosis as sporadic soft tissue sarcomas? *J Clin Oncol* 28:2064–2069, 2010.
3. Karlsson P, Holmberg E, Samuelsson A, et al: Soft tissue sarcoma after treatment for breast cancer—a Swedish population-based study. *Eur J Cancer* 34:2068–2075, 1998.
4. Guillou L, Coindre JM, Bonichon F, et al: Comparative study of the National Cancer Institute and French Federation of Cancer Centers Sarcoma Group grading systems in a population of 410 adult patients with soft tissue sarcoma. *J Clin Oncol* 15:350–362, 1997.
5. Anaya DA, Lahat G, Wang X, et al: Establishing prognosis in retroperitoneal sarcoma: A new histology-based paradigm. *Ann Surg Oncol* 16:667–675, 2009.
6. Johannesmeyer D, Smith V, Cole DJ, et al: The impact of lymph node disease in extremity soft-tissue sarcomas: A population-based analysis. *Am J Surg* 206:289–295, 2013.
7. Gutierrez JC, Perez EA, Moffat FL, et al: Should soft tissue sarcomas be treated at high-volume centers? An analysis of 4205 patients. *Ann Surg* 245:952–958, 2007.
8. Kransdorf MJ, Bancroft LW, Peterson JJ, et al: Imaging of fatty tumors: Distinction of lipoma and well-differentiated liposarcoma 1. *Radiology* 224:99–104, 2002.
9. Lahat G, Madewell JE, Anaya DA, et al: Computed tomography scan-driven selection of treatment for retroperitoneal liposarcoma histologic subtypes. *Cancer* 115:1081–1090, 2009.
10. Heslin MJ, Lewis JJ, Nadler E, et al: Prognostic factors associated with long-term survival for retroperitoneal sarcoma: Implications for management. *J Clin Oncol* 15:2832–2839, 1997.
11. Bonvalot S, Rivoire M, Castaing M, et al: Primary retroperitoneal sarcomas: A multivariate analysis of surgical factors associated with local control. *J Clin Oncol* 27:31–37, 2009.
12. Tseng WW, Madewell JE, Wei W, et al: Locoregional disease patterns in well-differentiated and dedifferentiated retroperitoneal liposarcoma: Implications for the extent of resection? *Ann Surg Oncol* 21:2136–2143, 2014.
13. Shibata D, Lewis JJ, Leung DH, et al: Is there a role for incomplete resection in the management of retroperitoneal liposarcomas? *J Am Coll Surg* 193:373–379, 2001.
14. Park JO, Qin LX, Prete FP, et al: Predicting outcome by growth rate of locally recurrent retroperitoneal liposarcoma: The one centimeter per month rule. *Ann Surg* 250:977–982, 2009.
15. Fletcher CDM, Gustafson P, Rydholm A, et al: Clinicopathologic re-evaluation of 100 malignant fibrous histiocytomas: Prognostic relevance of subclassification. *J Clin Oncol* 19:3045–3050, 2001.
16. Rosenberg SA, Tepper J, Glatstein E, et al: The treatment of soft-tissue sarcomas of the extremities. Prospective randomized evaluations of (1) limb-sparing surgery plus radiation therapy compared with amputation and (2) the role of adjuvant chemotherapy. *Ann Surg* 196:305–315, 1982.
17. Brennan MF, Casper ES, Harrison LB, et al: The role of multimodality therapy in soft-tissue sarcoma. *Ann Surg* 214:328, 1991.
18. Pisters PW, O'Sullivan B, Maki RG: Evidence-based recommendations for local therapy for soft tissue sarcomas. *J Clin Oncol* 25:1003–1008, 2007.
19. Pisters PWT, Pollock RE, Lewis VO, et al: Long-term results of prospective trial of surgery alone with selective use of radiation for patients with T1 extremity and trunk soft tissue sarcomas. *Ann Surg* 246:675–681, 2007.

20. O'Sullivan B, Davis AM, Turcotte R, et al: Preoperative versus postoperative radiotherapy in soft-tissue sarcoma of the limbs: A randomised trial. *Lancet* 359:2235–2241, 2002.
21. Hong NJ, Hornicek FJ, Harmon DC, et al: Neoadjuvant chemoradiotherapy for patients with high-risk extremity and truncal sarcomas: A 10-year single institution retrospective study. *Eur J Cancer* 49:875–883, 2013.
22. Canter RJ, Martinez SR, Tamurian RM, et al: Radiographic and histologic response to neoadjuvant radiotherapy in patients with soft tissue sarcoma. *Ann Surg Oncol* 17:2578–2584, 2010.
23. Mullen JT, Hornicek FJ, Harmon DC, et al: Prognostic significance of treatment-induced pathologic necrosis in extremity and truncal soft tissue sarcoma after neoadjuvant chemoradiotherapy. *Cancer* 120:3676–3682, 2014.
24. Curtis KK, Ashman JB, Beauchamp CP, et al: Neoadjuvant chemoradiation compared to neoadjuvant radiation alone and surgery alone for stage II and III soft tissue sarcoma of the extremities. *Radiat Oncol* 6:91, 2011.
25. Mullen JT, Kobayashi W, Wang JJ, et al: Long-term follow-up of patients treated with neoadjuvant chemotherapy and radiotherapy for large, extremity soft tissue sarcomas. *Cancer* 118:3758–3765, 2012.
26. Kraybill WG, Harris J, Spiro IJ, et al: Phase II study of neoadjuvant chemotherapy and radiation therapy in the management of high-risk, high-grade, soft tissue sarcomas of the extremities and body wall: Radiation Therapy Oncology Group Trial 9514. *J Clin Oncol* 24:619–625, 2006.
27. Baldini EH, Goldberg J, Jenner C, et al: Long-term outcomes after function-sparing surgery without radiotherapy for soft tissue sarcoma of the extremities and trunk. *J Clin Oncol* 17:3252–3259, 1999.
28. Heslin MJ, Woodruff J, Brennan MF: Prognostic significance of a positive microscopic margin in high-risk extremity soft tissue sarcoma: Implications for management. *J Clin Oncol* 14:473–478, 1996.
29. Zagars GK, Ballo MT, Pisters PWT, et al: Surgical margins and reresection in the management of patients with soft tissue sarcoma using conservative surgery and radiation therapy. *Cancer* 97:2544–2553, 2003.
30. Grabellus F, Podleska LE, Sheu SY, et al: Neoadjuvant treatment improves capsular integrity and the width of the fibrous capsule of high-grade soft-tissue sarcomas. *Eur J Surg Oncol* 39:61–67, 2013.
31. O'Donnell PW, Manivel JC, Cheng EY, et al: Chemotherapy influences the pseudocapsule composition in soft tissue sarcomas. *Clin Orthop Relat Res* 472:849–855, 2014.
32. Coindre JM, Terrier P, Guillou L, et al: Predictive value of grade for metastasis development in the main histologic types of adult soft tissue sarcomas: A study of 1240 patients from the French Federation of Cancer Centers sarcoma group. *Cancer* 91:1914–1926, 2001.
33. Blackmon SH, Shah N, Roth JA, et al: Resection of pulmonary and extrapulmonary sarcomatous metastases is associated with long-term survival. *Ann Thorac Surg* 88:877–885, 2009.
34. Bertario L, Russo A, Sala P, et al: Genotype and phenotype factors as determinants of desmoid tumors in patients with familial adenomatous polyposis. *Int J Cancer* 95:102–107, 2001.
35. Arvanitis ML, Jagelman DG, Fazio VW, et al: Mortality in patients with familial adenomatous polyposis. *Dis Colon Rectum* 33:639–642, 1990.
36. Lahat G, Dhuka AR, Hallevi H, et al: Angiosarcoma: Clinical and molecular insights. *Ann Surg* 251:1098–1106, 2010.
37. Criscione VD, Weinstock MA: Descriptive epidemiology of dermatofibrosarcoma protuberans in the United States, 1973 to 2002. *J Am Acad Dermatol* 56:968–973, 2007.
38. Stoeckle E, Coindre JM, Bonvalot S, et al: Prognostic factors in retroperitoneal sarcoma: A multivariate analysis of a series of 165 patients of the French Cancer Center Federation Sarcoma Group. *Cancer* 92:359–368, 2001.
39. Lewis JJ, Leung D, Woodruff JM, et al: Retroperitoneal soft-tissue sarcoma: Analysis of 500 patients treated and followed at a single institution. *Ann Surg* 228:355–365, 1998.
40. Pawlik TM, Pisters PW, Mikula L, et al: Long-term results of two prospective trials of preoperative external beam radiotherapy for localized intermediate- or high-grade retroperitoneal soft tissue sarcoma. *Ann Surg Oncol* 13:508–517, 2006.
41. Tzeng CWD, Fiveash JB, Popple RA, et al: Preoperative radiation therapy with selective dose escalation to the margin at risk for retroperitoneal sarcoma. *Cancer* 107:371–379, 2006.
42. Gold JS, Gönen M, Gutiérrez A, et al: Development and validation of a prognostic nomogram for recurrence-free survival after complete surgical resection of localised primary gastrointestinal stromal tumour: A retrospective analysis. *Lancet Oncol* 10:1045–1052, 2009.
43. Rutkowski P, Bylina E, Wozniak A, et al: Validation of the Joensuu risk criteria for primary resectable gastrointestinal stromal tumour—the impact of tumour rupture on patient outcomes. *Eur J Surg Oncol* 37:890–896, 2011.
44. Joensuu H, Vehtari A, Riihimäki J, et al: Risk of recurrence of gastrointestinal stromal tumour after surgery: An analysis of pooled population-based cohorts. *Lancet Oncol* 13:265–274, 2012.
45. Blanke CD, Demetri GD, von Mehren M, et al: Long-term results from a randomized phase II trial of standard- versus higher-dose imatinib mesylate for patients with unresectable or metastatic gastrointestinal stromal tumors expressing KIT. *J Clin Oncol* 26:620–625, 2008.
46. DeMatteo RP, Ballman KV, Antonescu CR, et al: Adjuvant imatinib mesylate after resection of localised, primary gastrointestinal stromal tumour: A randomised, double-blind, placebo-controlled trial. *Lancet* 373:1097–1104, 2009.
47. Joensuu H, Eriksson M, Sundby Hall K, et al: One vs three years of adjuvant imatinib for operable gastrointestinal stromal tumor: A randomized trial. *JAMA* 307:1265–1272, 2012.
48. Corless CL, Ballman KV, Antonescu CR, et al: Pathologic and molecular features correlate with long-term outcome after adjuvant therapy of resected primary GI stromal tumor: The ACOSOG Z9001 Trial. *J Clin Oncol* 32:1563–1570, 2014.
49. Joensuu H, Eriksson M, Hall KS, et al: Risk factors for gastrointestinal stromal tumor recurrence in patients treated with adjuvant imatinib. *Cancer* 120:2325–2333, 2014.

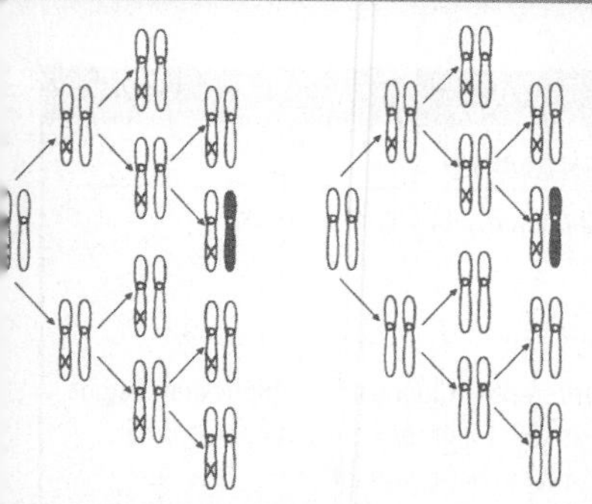

CHAPTER 32

Bone Tumors

Herbert S. Schwartz, Ginger E. Holt, Jennifer L. Halpern

OUTLINE

OVERVIEW

Orthopedic oncology is a complex surgical discipline that involves the diagnosis, management, and surveillance of primary mesenchymal malignant neoplasms (sarcomas), benign bone and soft tissue masses, and secondary neoplasms of bone and soft tissue. The unique structural qualities of bone along with its complex microenvironment must be considered in formulating strategies for management of bone tumors. This chapter reviews the complex biology of the bone microenvironment as it relates to tumor progression, skeletal stability, and potential treatment options. It also presents a general approach to the diagnosis, management, and appropriate triage of primary and secondary bone tumors, both benign and malignant. Although making a diagnosis is paramount, the restoration of function in the setting of skeletal compromise or instability is also critical in the management of bone tumors. Therefore, a complex understanding of what the tumor is doing to the bone, what the bone is doing to the tumor, where the lesion is, and what the lesion is making affects how bone tumors are managed (Table 32-1).

BONE MICROENVIRONMENT

An understanding of the bone microenvironment affects the macroscopic management of skeletal tumors. In the absence of tumor, bone is a dynamic and symbiotic organ, actively maintained by cells that respond to stimuli such as injury, stress, and metabolic need. Osteoblasts represent a terminal differentiation of a mesenchymal stem cell. They generate a collagen matrix that is then mineralized. When osteoblasts become surrounded by the matrix they create, they are deemed osteocytes and serve to maintain the bone environment. Osteoclasts are multinucleated cells derived from a hematopoietic lineage (macrophages) that resorb bone. The constant interplay of those cells (osteoblast, osteocyte, osteoclast) is necessary to maintain bone health. The marrow space is also home to other significant cell populations, such as mesenchymal stem cells. The active and ongoing homeostasis of bone and its intramedullary inhabitants generates a microenvironment rich in growth factors and signaling molecules, making it an ideal soil for osteophilic tumors.

In the setting of metastatic to bone neoplasms, intravascular tumor cells are attracted to the microenvironment of bone; it is preconditioned for tumor cell arrival by circulating factors, and it is inherently attractive because of the proteins, signaling molecules, and cells that it contains (Fig. 32-1). That concept was first coined the "seed and soil" theory by Stephen Paget in 1889.[1] For example, mesenchymal stem cells return (in part) to the bone marrow because of a signaling pathway involving the CXCL12 chemokine and the CXCR4 receptor. Intramedullary mesenchymal stem cells secrete CXCL12, and circulating stem cells that express the correlating CXCR4 receptor are recruited to the marrow space. Similarly, in the setting of metastatic breast cancer, as an example, tumor cells express CXCR4 receptor and therefore can also be recruited to the marrow space through the chemokine CXCL12.[2] In general, cell signaling molecules produced in the marrow space are recognized by tumor-based receptors and represent one example of how the bone microenvironment influences tumor deposition. Other players involved in homing of tumor cells to bone include but are not limited to exosomes and oncosomes, adhesion molecules, platelets, and circulating stem cells.[3]

Once in the bone microenvironment, in what is deemed the vicious cycle, tumor cells hijack the endogenous cells of bone to create an environment that fosters their own growth. Normally, the balance of lysis and bone formation in bone is maintained through the strategic production of signaling proteins. For example, nuclear factor κB ligand (RANKL) is generated by osteoblasts and recognized by its osteoclast receptor (RANK). When bound, RANKL stimulates osteoclastogenesis.[4] Osteoprotegerin, a decoy receptor secreted by osteoblasts, inhibits RANKL binding and therefore inhibits osteoclastogenesis.[5] Tumor cells can disturb bone homeostasis in a variety of ways. Tumor cells can directly stimulate osteoblasts to generate RANKL, which is the most prominent cytokine inducer of osteoclastogenesis.[6,7] Alternatively, tumor-secreted matrix metalloproteinase 7 can cleave extracellular matrix where bound and inactive RANKL resides,

TABLE 32-1 **Four Questions Asked to Evaluate Bone Tumors**

	QUESTION	ANSWER	CLINICAL SIGNIFICANCE	EXAMPLE
1	Where is the lesion—which bone and what part of that bone?	Which bone? (e.g., femur)	Some lesions occur most often in a specific bone.	Chondromyxoid fibroma—tibia
		Where is the bone? (e.g., epiphyseal, metaphyseal, diaphyseal)	There is a specific differential for lesions that occur in specific regions of the bone.	Differential diagnosis of epiphyseal lesions is giant cell tumor, chondroblastoma, infection, and ganglion.
2	What is the lesion doing to the bone?	Destructive	If a lesion essentially erases the bone, it implies that the lesion is aggressive and therefore likely to be malignant.	Metastatic lung carcinoma essentially erases the cortex, destabilizing the bone.
		No change in overall morphology	If the lesion does not deform, distort, or destroy the bone, it suggests that the lesion is benign.	An enchondroma is an eccentric cartilage deposit within the intramedullary canal. If covered up, the bone would look normal.
3	What is the bone doing to the lesion?	Failing to contain it	If the bone cannot respond to the assault of a tumor, the tumor is aggressive.	Osteosarcoma breaks out of the bone and elevates periosteum.
		Expanding and thinning	If the lesion is growing but the bone is trying to contain it, the bone may appear expanded and thinned. It may fall into the benign aggressive differential.	Aneurysmal bone cysts, giant cell tumors
		Creating a sclerotic border around the lesion	When the bone forms a sclerotic rim around a lesion, the lesion is typically benign.	Nonossifying fibroma, intraosseous ganglion
4	What is the lesion making?	Matrix-cartilage, bone, fibrous tissue	The matrix a tumor produces is part of its inherent classification.	Bone forming—osteoid osteoma, osteoblastoma, osteosarcoma

thereby releasing the active form of RANKL.[8] Once overactive osteoclastogenesis is initiated, tumor growth is fueled by this aggressive bone degradation, which frees an abundance of growth factors that can drive tumor proliferation.

This chapter is not intended to cover all aspects of the microenvironment tumor–native bone interplay. However, an appreciation of those complex relationships is important. Medical therapies can target not only tumor cells (the seed) but also the soil, essentially preventing tumor growth by making the environment less favorable. In patients with bone metastases and even in the setting of benign but locally aggressive lytic or osteoclast-filled tumors, systemic medications designed to limit osteoclast function are now used. The goal of those medicines is to reduce the number of skeletally related events (SREs), which include hypercalcemia of malignancy, bone pain, pathologic fracture, spinal cord compression, and the need for palliative radiation.

Bisphosphonates are a class of drugs that inhibit bone resorption and can decrease the number of SREs.[9] Nitrogen-containing bisphosphonates bind to and inhibit key enzymes of the intracellular mevalonate pathway, thereby preventing the prenylation and activation of small GTPases that are essential for the bone-resorbing activity and survival of osteoclasts. Bisphosphonates are taken up only by active osteoclasts. Zoledronic acid (Zometa) is commonly used for oncology patients as a means of preventing SREs.[10]

Denosumab (Xgeva) is a monoclonal antibody generated against RANKL. This drug mimics the natural action of osteoprotegerin, which prevents RANKL binding to RANK, thereby preventing osteoclast maturation. However, it does not also block the tumor necrosis factor–related apoptosis-inducing ligand (TRAIL), which is the principal mediator of tumor cell death by the human host cells.[11] Denosumab inhibits osteoclast recruitment, maturation, and function and ultimately induces apoptosis of activated osteoclasts and therefore stops bone resorption.[12] Examination of denosumab-treated bone shows an absence of osteoclasts.[13] Denosumab has been compared with zoledronic acid through a randomized double-blind trial in men with metastatic prostate cancer and shown to be more effective in preventing SREs than zoledronic acid.[14] Denosumab was also found to be superior to zoledronic acid in delaying time to SREs in patients with metastatic breast cancer.[15] Although these studies suggest that denosumab is superior to zoledronic acid in treatment of metastatic bone lesions in the case of breast and prostate cancer, denosumab is not universally used at this time for treatment of bone metastases. That fact likely relates to economic and availability issues as well as the need for studies to assess longer term follow-up and ideal dosing protocols.[13]

BONE MACROENVIRONMENT

Primary tumors of bone, both benign and malignant, tend to form in specific geographic regions of bone (Fig. 32-2). The primary differential diagnosis of epiphyseal tumors includes giant cell tumor, chondroblastoma, infection, and intraosseous ganglion. Clear cell chondrosarcoma is a less common epiphyseal lesion. Common diaphyseal lesions include adamantinoma, Ewing sarcoma, infection, osteoid osteoma or osteoblastoma, and fibrous dysplasia. Osteosarcoma most commonly forms in metaphyseal bone of the distal femur, proximal tibia, and proximal humerus. Metastatic bone disease can occur in all regions of the bone, although certain sites are considered more typical for specific cancers. Acral metastases and intracortical metastases are typically lung carcinomas. The common locations of tumors and the structural integrity and demands of the bone in those locations are important facts to consider in formulating plans for

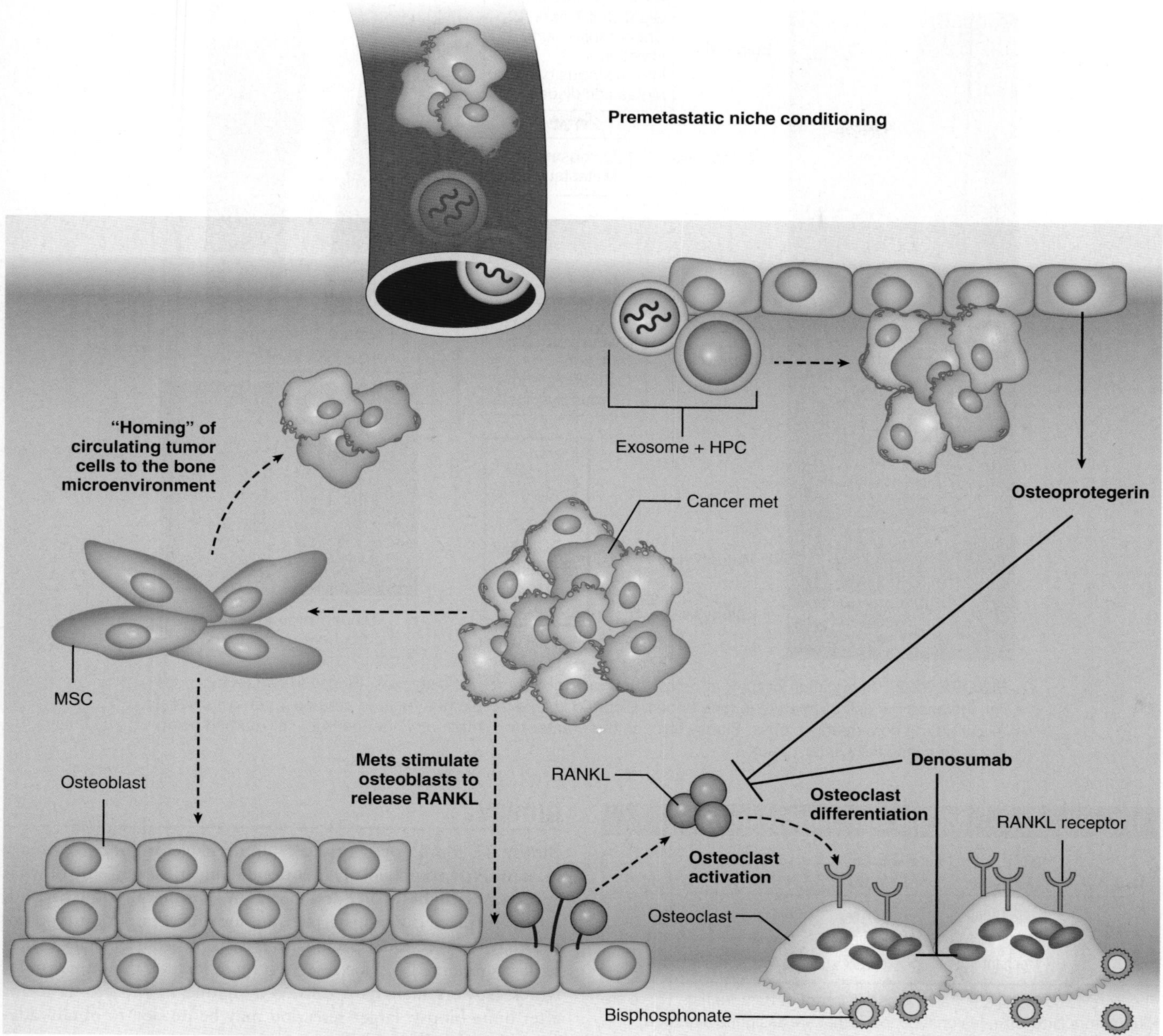

FIGURE 32-1 Circulating metastatic cancer cells find the bone microenvironment through a complex series of steps. Before their arrival, circulating factors optimize the bone (premetastatic niche conditioning). Cells are then recruited to the bone by signaling molecules called chemokines (homing). Once in the bone, tumor cells hijack normal bone metabolism (the vicious cycle). Medical therapies used in the treatment of metastatic bone cancers exploit the understanding of the vicious cycle. Denosumab is a human monoclonal antibody that binds RANKL and directly inhibits osteoclastogenesis. Zoledronic acid is a bisphosphonate that is taken up by and then inhibits activated osteoclasts. *HPC,* hematopoietic progenitor cell; *MSC,* mesenchymal stem cell. (Adapted from Cook LM, Shay G, Aruajo A, et al: Integrating new discoveries into the "vicious cycle" paradigm of prostate to bone metastases. *Cancer Metastasis Rev* 33:511–525, 2014.)

biopsy and reconstruction. For example, biopsy of an intraosseous, diaphyseal femoral lesion through a transcortical approach, even with a large-bore needle (core biopsy), can increase the risk of fracture at the site of biopsy (see Fig. 32-2). An alternative, depending on the proximity of the lesion to the greater trochanter, is to perform an intramedullary biopsy through a greater trochanteric starting point, using pituitary rongeurs to grab intramedullary bone at a predetermined location (see Fig. 32-2). That biopsy entrance site does not destabilize the bone, and it still can be resected as part of a wide tumor resection if needed. Alternatively, lesions at the metaphyseal flare can often be biopsied directly because the biomechanical stress in that area places it at much lower risk for fracture, even if a small bone window is created to obtain tissue.

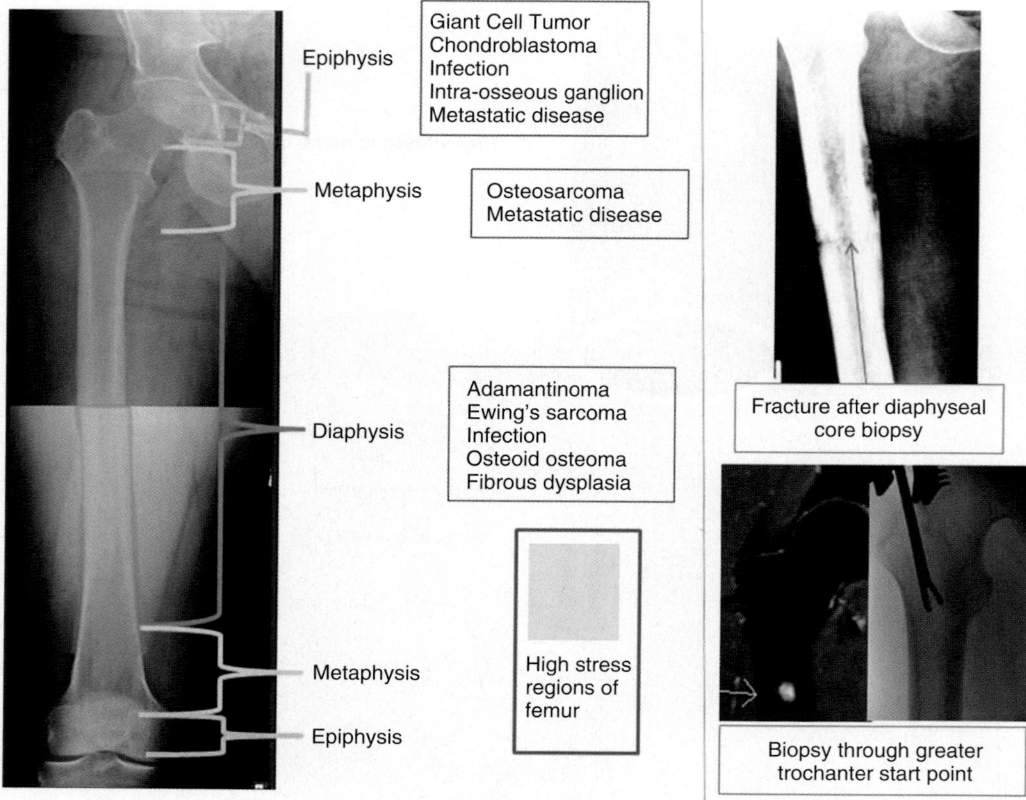

FIGURE 32-2 The location of tumors helps to narrow the differential diagnosis. Biopsy in certain locations can increase the risk of fracture in long bones. Pictured is an example of a fracture created in the diaphyseal femur after a core needle biopsy. Biopsy through the greater trochanter, an intramedullary nail starting point, is a biomechanically safer option.

TABLE 32-2 Mirels Scoring System

SCORE	SITE OF LESION	SIZE OF LESION	LESION TYPE	PAIN
1	Upper limb	>⅓ cortex	Blastic	Mild
2	Lower limb	⅓-⅔ cortex	Mixed	Moderate
3	Trochanteric	>⅔ cortex	Lytic	Functional

The Mirels scoring system allows assessment of fracture risk. There are four factors (site, size, lesion type, pain) that are assigned a numeric score of 1 to 3. The four scores are added together. If the overall score is more than 9, prophylactic fixation is indicated. A score of less than 7 can often be treated with radiation and medical therapies. Despite the utility of the scoring system, clinical judgment must always be taken into consideration regarding a specific patient.[16]

The relevance of tumor location is reflected in the Mirels criteria, which allow a more objective assessment of pathologic fracture risk in patients with bone tumors (Table 32-2). In that system, a numeric score is assigned to observed metastatic lesions in bone.[16] Lesions are categorized by location, size, and nature (lytic versus blastic). Based on a total score, recommendations can be made for operative prophylaxis. This classification/scoring system is designed to assist with decision making but in no way replaces clinical judgments made in consideration of each patient. However, it does capture the fact that lesions in high-stress, weight-bearing areas of the skeleton, such as the trochanteric femur, are at highest risk of fracture.

BIOPSY

Biopsy is a complex cognitive skill in the skeleton for two primary reasons. First, as previously mentioned, one must be aware of what approaches might further destabilize the bone in question. Second, one must place the biopsy tract in a location that accommodates future wide resection. Specifically, if a diagnosis of primary malignancy is rendered, a wide resection must include the biopsy tract, which harbors malignant cells. If a significant hematoma forms after bone biopsy, larger resection may be needed to obtain adequate margins (Fig. 32-3).

There are different modalities of bone biopsy. Fine-needle aspiration is rarely used unless there is a significant extraosseous soft tissue component that is accessible or significant bone lysis. Core biopsy, often performed with computed tomography (CT) guidance, can be performed through intact cortices (with adjunct use of a combined biopsy/drill system) or through areas of soft tissue extension. Incisional biopsy is a surgical procedure during which a carefully planned small incision is made in line with the tumor, with respect to neurovascular structures and bone biomechanics. Open biopsy allows acquisition of the most tissue compared with other techniques. If the cortex is intact, a high-speed burr is often used to create a less than dime-sized window into the bone. Meticulous hemostasis must be obtained to prevent contamination of surrounding tissues. Often, Surgicel and Gelfoam are packed into defects created in the soft tissue extraosseous component of the tumor, and then the tumor capsule and superficial layers are closed meticulously. If the cortex has been violated, bone

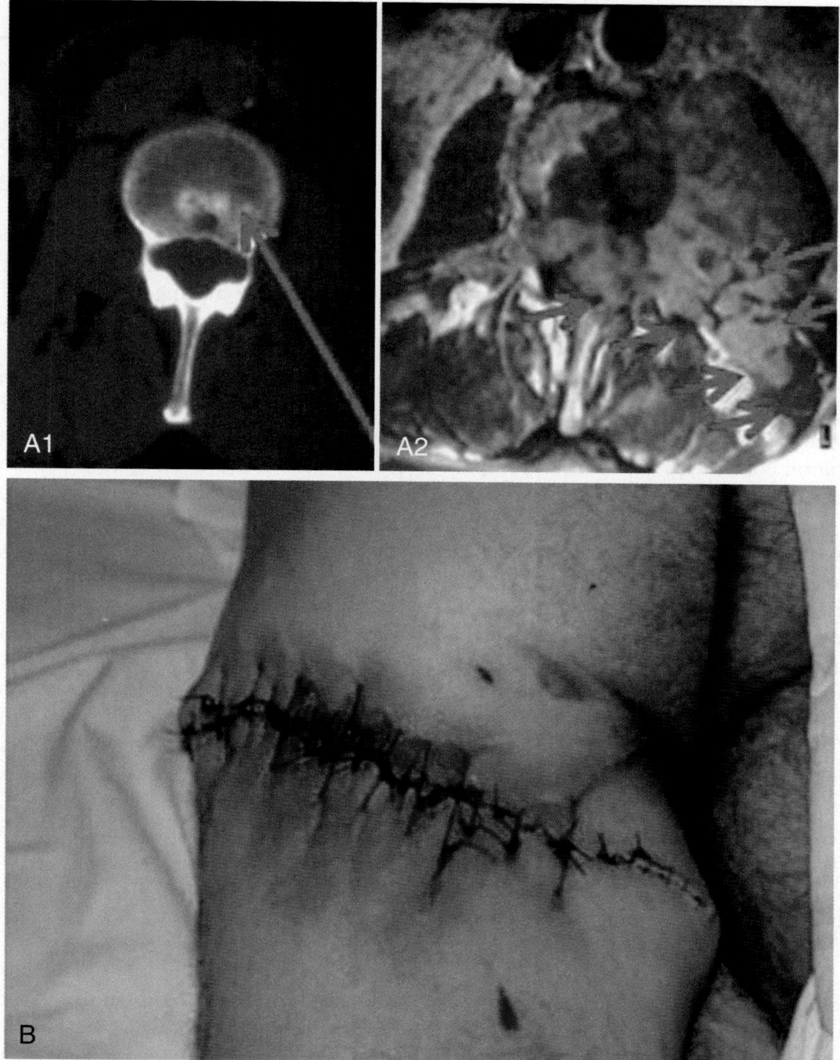

FIGURE 32-3 When planning a biopsy location, one must consider that the biopsy tract will be contaminated and in the case of malignant tumors will require resection. **A1,** A CT-guided biopsy tract into the vertebral body is demonstrated by the *arrow.* **A2,** The *arrows* indicate the extent of biopsy tract recurrence. **B,** An excellent example of an inappropriate biopsy, which mandated an otherwise unnecessary amputation in the patient. Biopsies must be performed in line with the incision that will eventually be required to resect a tumor. The entire biopsy tract must be resected. Therefore, a biopsy incision is typically small and strategically placed.

wax or a small plug of bone cement is often used to prevent intramedullary extravasation of blood and tumor into the biopsy tract.

Inappropriately placed biopsy tracts can change the nature of surgery required, even changing a potential limb salvage candidate into a patient requiring an amputation. Biopsy placement and execution are critical. It has been conclusively shown in several studies that surgeons inexperienced in musculoskeletal oncology principles have a three to four times increased rate of complication from a poorly placed biopsy site.[17-19]

STAGING

A critical part of biopsy planning includes a global understanding of the nature of a tumor—whether it is localized or part of a more systemic process. The patient's history and physical examination are vital parts of evaluation. Physical examination must include chaperoned breast examination or prostate examination in patients who potentially may have a metastatic to bone process. A series of radiologic studies are then performed to characterize the scope of the disease process. When a patient presents with an isolated bone lesion that may represent a malignant neoplasm, especially without antecedent history of cancer, the following studies or laboratory tests are typically obtained:

- Magnetic resonance imaging (MRI) of the entire affected bone with contrast enhancement identifies a soft tissue component of the tumor that, if present, may be easier to sample and also helps identify skip metastases.
- CT scan of the chest, abdomen, and pelvis with and without intravenous and oral administration of contrast material screens for common osteophilic carcinomas, including breast,

lung, renal, thyroid, and prostate, and also helps establish whether solid organ metastases are present.

- CT with two-dimensional reconstructions of the affected bone allows a better three-dimensional understanding of how the tumor has affected the bone.
- Whole body bone scan identifies other possible osseous sites and metastases.
- Plain radiographs of the affected bone show where in the bone the tumor is located (epiphyseal, metaphyseal, diaphyseal), show what the tumor is doing to the bone (lytic, blastic), show what the bone is doing to the tumor (containment versus failure to contain), and show the matrix of the lesion (e.g., bone, cartilage, fibrous) (see Table 32-1).
- Laboratory evaluation includes prostate-specific antigen, serum electrophoresis, calcium concentration to rule out hypercalcemia of malignancy, lactate dehydrogenase, alkaline phosphatase, complete blood count with differential, comprehensive metabolic panel, sedimentation rate, and C-reactive protein.

Two primary staging systems are used to describe skeletal sarcoma. In the Musculoskeletal Tumor Society staging system or Enneking system,[20] I refers to a low-grade skeletal sarcoma, II refers to a high-grade skeletal sarcoma, and III represents metastatic disease, either regional or distant. The letter A refers to intracompartmental tumor localization, whereas the letter B refers to extracompartmental extension. An example of extracompartmental extension is an osteosarcoma with extraosseous soft tissue mass or a pathologic fracture through an osteosarcoma, resulting in hematoma contamination. The American Joint Committee on Cancer staging system has been updated[21]; tumors are described by grade (I, low; II, high; III, tumor of any grade with skip metastases; IV, tumor of any grade with distant metastases) and size (<8 cm, A; >8 cm, B). Staging systems in general are designed to reflect prognosis and therefore to guide treatment algorithms.

Enneking also developed a staging system for benign bone tumors.[22] In the Enneking system, tumors are characterized as latent (1), active (2), or aggressive (3). Aggressive benign tumors often have a higher risk of local recurrence. Although aggressive benign tumors still can be technically resected in an intralesional fashion, resection must be meticulous, often using high-speed burrs and other adjuvants. The most important factor in preventing recurrence is likely to be adequacy of resection.[23]

ONCOLOGIC RESECTION

There are four types of surgical resection: intralesional, marginal, wide, and radical. The type of margin reflects the surgical dissection plane relative to the tumor or capsule of the tumor. Intralesional resections involve an incision made into the substance of tumor. Intralesional resections in bone are typically exemplified by curettage or debulking. They are used in the setting of benign bone tumors and metastatic to bone tumors. Marginal resections theoretically involve resection of the tumor around its capsule and by definition leave microscopic disease behind. Wide resections involve resection of the tumor with a surrounding rim of normal tissue, designed to remove the entirety of a tumor. Radical resections include not only the tumor and a rim of normal tissue but also the entirety of the compartment in which the tumor resides. Wide resections are more commonly used in the treatment of skeletal sarcomas as opposed to radical resections.

SKELETAL RECONSTRUCTION

The type of reconstruction needed often depends on the type of resection that is indicated. It also depends greatly on the reparative potential of the bone. For example, children can regenerate bone at a higher rate than adults, and therefore in the setting of benign tumors like aneurysmal bone cyst, bone graft might be used in a child, whereas bone cement might be used in an adult. Another important factor is the post-treatment impact of a tumor on bone. For example, a lytic lesion caused by multiple myeloma has a better chance of healing after medical therapies than a lytic lesion caused by lung cancer. The potential for bone regeneration at the site of tumor relates in many ways to the stromal content of the tumor. Lymphoma of bone is predominantly cellular, whereas lung carcinoma in bone has a significant stromal component. The footprint of the tumor cannot be erased in stromal-heavy tumors.

Skeletal stabilization or reconstruction comes in many forms. Plates and screws that span defects can be used after curettage of lesions. Bone strength can be augmented through the insertion of polymethyl methacrylate (bone cement) into skeletal defects along with plates and screws (rebar) (Fig. 32-4). Intramedullary nail fixation is a common strategy for prophylaxis of diaphyseal lesions, especially in the femur (Fig. 32-5). In the setting of metastatic disease with palliation as a goal, the reconstruction strategy selected should impart immediate stability and immediate full weight-bearing potential whenever possible.

In the case of wide resection (skeletal sarcomas), large segments of bone are resected. In those cases, reconstruction often involves the use of intercalary allografts (Fig. 32-6) or metal components, osteoarticular allografts, allograft-prosthetic composites, arthroplasty with megaprosthesis, or arthrodesis. Autologous vascularized free tissue transfer, such as vascularized free fibulas, can also be an option. Amputation is also always an alternative in select cases.

When a patient is identified who will require a large bulk allograft, templated radiographs of the bone needed (or the contralateral bone if there is too much deformity) are obtained. Approved tissue banks harvest materials with meticulous sterility and then can assess whether any in-stock cadaveric allografts match the bone being requested.[24] Allografts can be harvested with soft tissue attachments, and in that case the host tendons can be sewn into the allograft attachment sites. Allografts can be fortified with cement augmentation, if possible, and then secured to the native bone by plates and screws. Allografts are obviously nonviable scaffolds, and therefore ultimate healing at the native bone–allograft interface depends on the native bone use of the allograft as a scaffold through which new bridging bone is formed. Intercalary allografts are essentially bone place holders and can often be secured in situ through the use of intramedullary stabilization. Osteoarticular allografts include implantation of a new joint surface. In weight-bearing joints, osteoarticular allograft fracture and collapse over time are common. However, especially in the growing child, they allow delay of arthroplasty and generation of additional bone stock.

Arthroplasty is a common reconstruction strategy used after tumor resections that include portions of a joint (Fig. 32-7). The so-called megaprosthesis is named such because large modular metal implants are combined to restore length to the limb and to replace large bone defects. Those metal replacements are either potted into the bone with bone cement or press-fit into the long bone canal. Bone cement offers immediate stability but increased chance of aseptic loosening over time.[25] Press-fit stems require

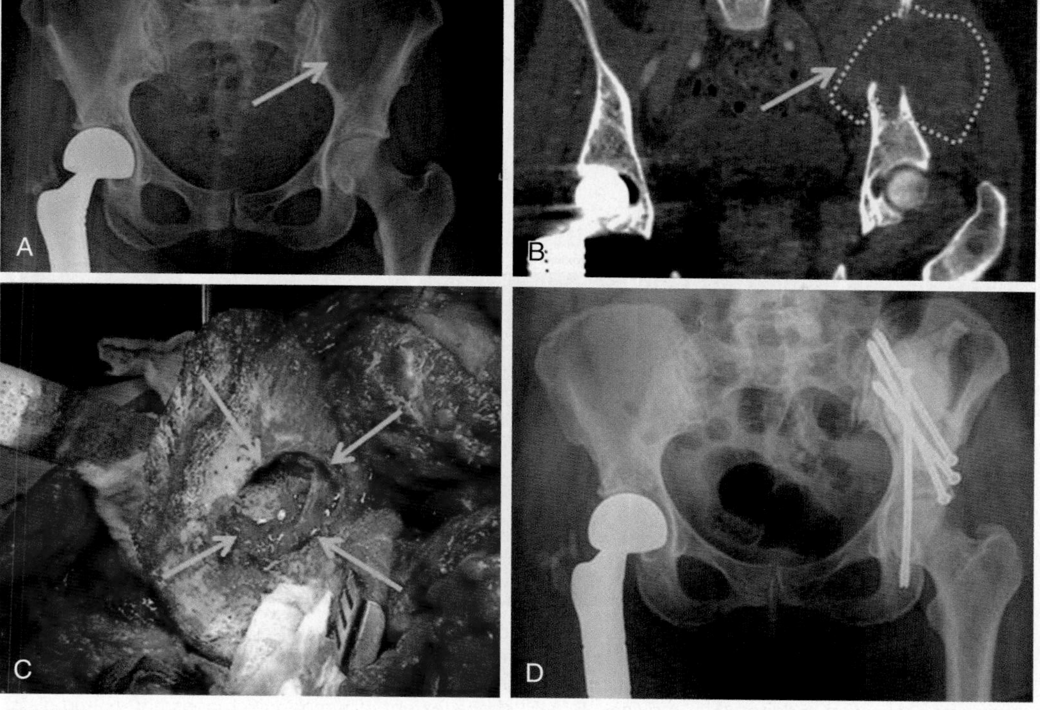

FIGURE 32-4 The patient had a prior right proximal femur metastatic lesion treated with proximal femur resection and megaprosthesis. She then developed a large, lytic, painful left iliac wing lesion that required intralesional resection and reconstruction with cement and 7.3-mm cannulated screws. **A,** Anteroposterior pelvis radiograph shows the lytic defect *(arrow)*. **B,** CT scan two-dimensional coronal reconstruction shows not only the bone defect but also the associated soft tissue mass (*arrow* and *dotted line*). **C,** Intraoperative view of the bone defect *(arrows)*. **D,** Postoperative anteroposterior view of pelvis.

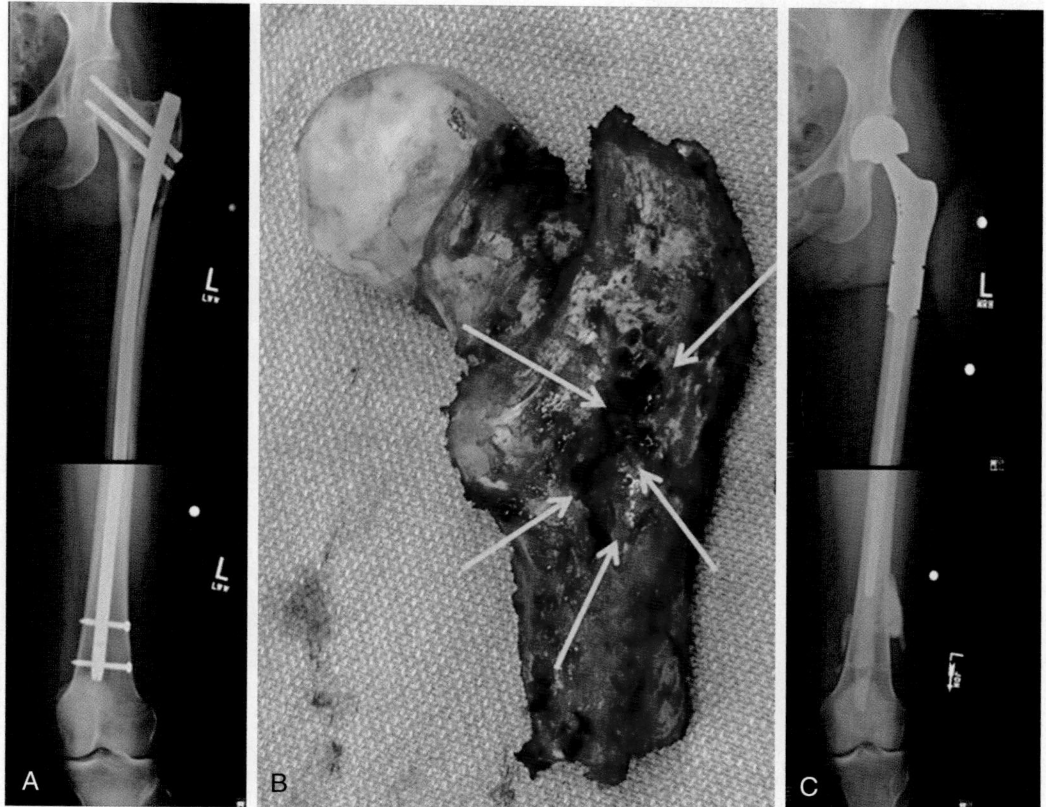

FIGURE 32-5 This patient had intramedullary nail stabilization and palliative radiation of the left femur for treatment of a peritrochanteric metastatic renal cell carcinoma lesion. **A,** Despite an appropriate attempt at stabilization and adjuvant therapies, she had persistent pain. **B,** Gross specimen revealed persistent lysis of the bone *(arrows)*. **C,** Reconstruction was subsequently performed with a long cemented stem proximal femur endoprosthesis.

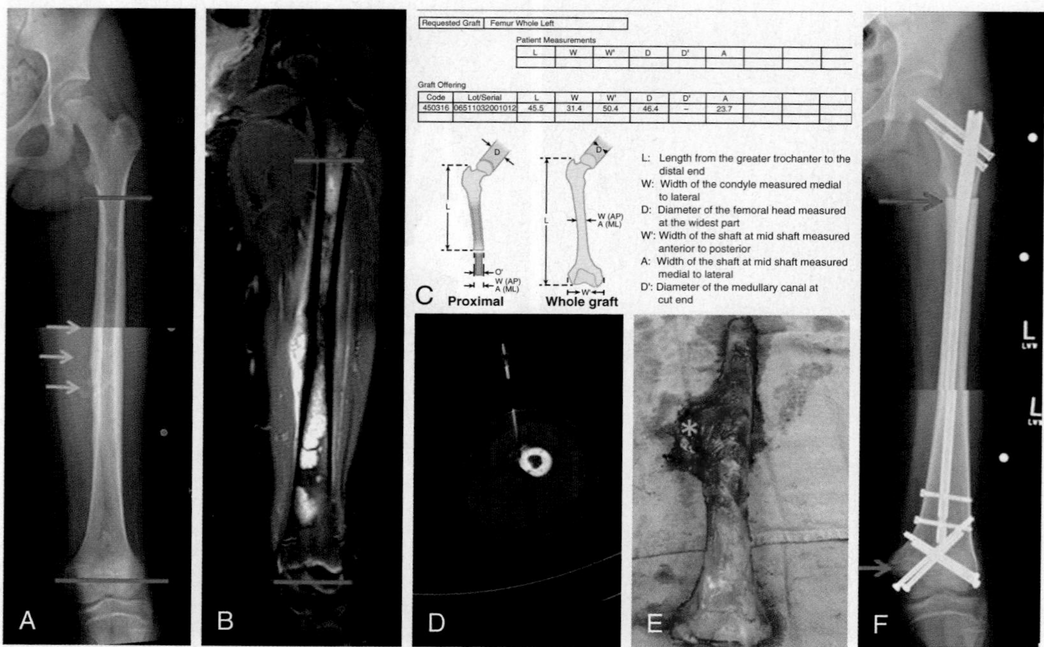

FIGURE 32-6 Allograft reconstruction can be used in osteoarticular, intercalary, or allograft-prosthetic composite reconstructions. This 11-year-old child had an extensive left femoral diaphyseal osteosarcoma with multiple skip metastases. **A,** Anteroposterior femur radiograph demonstrates periosteal reaction *(arrows)*. Anticipated resection is denoted by *red lines*. **B,** MRI shows extent of tumor, which does not extend distal to the physis. Proximal extent of tumor extends to the inferior aspect of lesser trochanter. MRI allows planning of intercalary femoral resection. **C,** Allograft matched. **D,** Biopsy tract. **E,** Resection performed with negative margins and includes the medial biopsy tract *(asterisk)*. **F,** Anteroposterior femur radiograph after resection. The *arrows* indicate allograft–native bone interfaces.

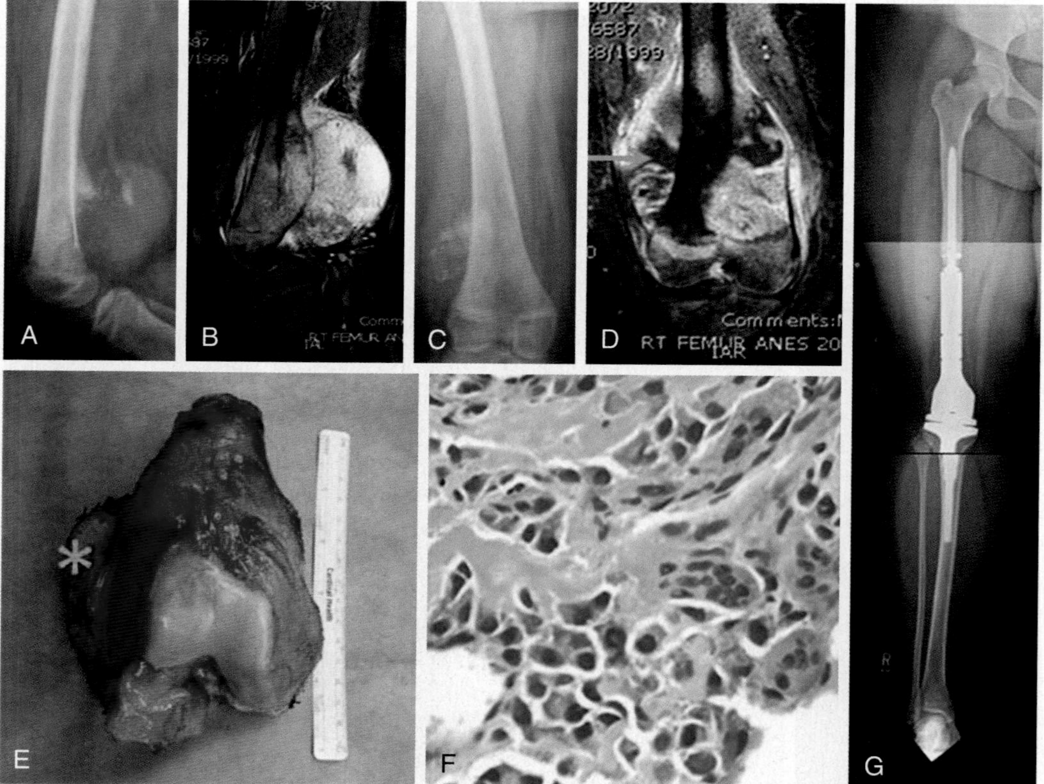

FIGURE 32-7 Endoprostheses are used to reconstruct periarticular malignant tumors. **A,** Lateral radiograph of distal femur shows aggressive bone tumor with large soft tissue extension. **B,** MRI T2 sagittal view shows true extent of bone involvement and soft tissue mass. **C,** Anteroposterior distal femur radiograph demonstrates osteoblastic matrix. **D,** MRI T2 coronal view shows planned biopsy trajectory to access soft tissue mass *(arrow)*. **E,** Resection specimen with biopsy tract *(asterisk)*. **F,** Histology analysis shows malignant cells with lace-like osteoid matrix. **G,** Right distal femur endoprosthesis using press-fit fixation into the femoral canal.

ingrowth or ongrowth of host bone over time around the stem periphery. In the case of the proximal humerus and proximal femur, no additional resurfacing of the acetabulum or glenoid is typically done. For distal femur or proximal tibia tumors, the tumor-unaffected side of the joint requires resurfacing to accommodate a hinge mechanism.

The means of reconstruction is often dictated by the weight-bearing demands of the bone in question. For example, an osteoarticular allograft is a good option for the proximal humerus, a technically non–weight-bearing limb. An allograft with soft tissue attachments allows the rotator cuff tendons to be sewn to the implant, thereby potentiating some overhead mobility. An osteoarticular allograft in the distal femur may be more of a problem because of weight-bearing demands. Therefore, arthroplasty may be preferred.

Amputation is indicated in the setting of primary tumors, when an adequate margin cannot be obtained through the use of limb salvage, or when the functional result achieved through limb salvage is worse than that achieved by amputation. Amputation may be indicated in the setting of metastatic or advanced cancers for the purposes of palliation.

BENIGN BONE TUMORS

The incidence of benign bone tumors far exceeds that of skeletal sarcomas. In the authors' clinical experience, there are at least five benign bone tumors for every primary malignant bone neoplasm; 54% of benign bone tumors are chondrogenic (enchondroma or osteochondroma).[26] The true prevalence of these tumors is unknown because many go undetected and unreported. Aggressive benign bone tumors, such as giant cell tumor and aneurysmal bone cysts, have a local recurrence rate as high as 30% and require meticulous intralesional resection with high-speed burr resection and other adjuvants.[27]

Enchondroma

Enchondromas are benign proliferations of hyaline cartilage typically found in the appendicular skeleton, less likely detected in the axial skeleton, and are centered in the metaphysis. They typically are incidental findings discovered during radiographic evaluations for other symptoms, except in the phalanges, where they can cause pathologic fracture. Enchondromas represent lobular cartilage islands that retain chondroid features and continue to grow until skeletal maturity, at which time they begin to undergo calcification. Their long-term physiologic activity is the reason that they remain scintigraphically active decades later on a bone scan. Isolated lesions do not cause progressive deformity of the bone. Malignant transformation is rare.

However, in patients with multiple enchondromas, such as Ollier disease or Maffucci syndrome (Ollier disease with subcutaneous hemangiomas), the risk of progressive bone deformity is higher, as is the risk of malignant transformation into a secondary chondrosarcoma. Interestingly, individuals with Maffucci syndrome also have a higher risk for development of occult carcinomas.[28]

Treatment of enchondromas remains conservative, and serial radiographic evaluation is the primary means of punctuated surveillance. Surgical intervention is required only if there is a question of malignant transformation. In that setting, albeit rare, the entire lesion is often curetted and submitted to surgical pathology. Cartilage lesions have areas of heterogeneity; therefore, in the case of malignant transformation, often only a small portion of the lesion appears malignant. The histopathologic interpretation of cartilage lesions depends on radiographic information and clinical information. For example, an enchondroma biopsied from the finger will look hypercellular, but because of its location, it will be called an enchondroma. The same material, however, if biopsied from the pelvis, would be called a higher grade chondrosarcoma. Clinical context is vital for proper evaluation of cartilage lesions (Fig. 32-8). If there is a question surrounding the diagnosis of enchondroma and open biopsy is performed, the biopsy entrance site, along with the lesion, is often packed with bone cement, and the bone is stabilized with a plate and screws. Bone grafting of the resected lesion is also an option. If lesions are called chondrosarcoma, then depending on the grade of the tumor, further resection or wide resection may be indicated.

Osteochondroma

Although discussed as a benign bone tumor, osteochondroma is better described as a hamartoma of bone. It develops from aberrant growth cartilage and radiographically is a cartilage-capped bone projection on the external surface of the bone according to the World Health Organization (Fig. 32-9). It is typically detected in the second decade of life. It is manifested as a painless mass or a mass associated with pain due to mechanical symptoms. There are two distinct radiographic types of osteochondroma, pedunculated and sessile. On three-dimensional imaging analysis, the intramedullary component of an osteochondroma should be confluent with the intramedullary canal of the affected bone. The lesion itself is capped by cartilage, and therefore the lesion grows through skeletal development and stops growing at skeletal maturity. If a lesion continues to grow after skeletal maturity or if radiographically a cartilage cap exceeds 2 cm in thickness after skeletal maturity, there is concern for potential malignant transformation. The majority of osteochondromas are solitary, and in those cases, the chance of malignant transformation is less than 1%.

However, osteochondromas can develop in a polyostotic fashion, as in hereditary multiple osteochondral exostosis or osteochondromatosis. Hereditary multiple osteochondral exostosis is an autosomal dominant condition. Three separate loci are implicated in its development: *EXT1* (8q24.1), *EXT2* (11p11-12), and *EXT3* (19p).[29,30] Affected children present with mass lesions and skeletal growth anomalies, including short stature, limb length discrepancies, angular deformity of knees and ankles, radial bowing and wrist deviation, and subluxation of the radiocapitellar joint.[31] The risk over time of malignant transformation of an osteochondroma in this scenario ranges from 10% to 30%. Osteochondromas that transform are called secondary chondrosarcomas.

Osteoid Osteoma

Osteoid osteoma is a benign osteoblastic tumor (Fig. 32-10). Although it is self-limited, the symptoms generated by this lesion that is less than 1 cm in diameter can be debilitating. Osteoid osteomas typically occur in the diaphysis of long bones but can occur anywhere, such as the posterior elements of the spine. Osteoblastomas are essentially giant osteoid osteomas that occur primarily in the spine. Both conditions can lead to scoliosis in the spine (related to pain and muscle spasm) or joint pain and sympathetic effusion in the proximity of a joint. On radiographic examination, these lesions show a radiolucent nidus, surrounded by an area of thickened cortical bone and sclerosis. On MRI, there is often extensive edema surrounding the lesions. The patient's

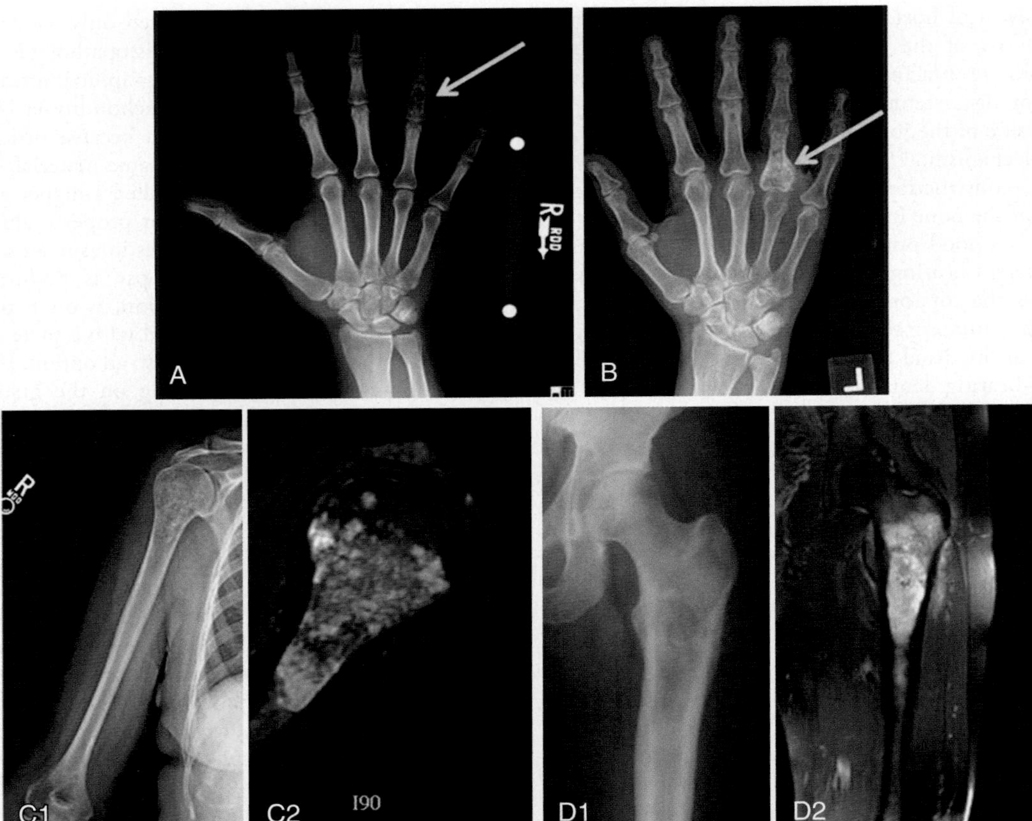

FIGURE 32-8 The differential diagnosis of cartilage lesions depends on clinical and radiographic information. **A,** Middle phalanx expansile lesion with internal calcification manifesting as pathologic fracture is a typical presentation for enchondroma. **B,** Although the more distal a cartilage lesion is, the less likely it is to be malignant, another patient presented with an aggressive proximal phalanx lesion, marked by pain, periosteal reaction, and internal calcification, and she was diagnosed with chondrosarcoma. **C,** On a radiograph of the proximal humerus, the patient has a cartilage lesion with expected calcification without destruction of surrounding cortex (**C1**). The lesion is lobular in nature, as apparent on MRI (**C2**). The patient is being observed radiographically. **D,** In comparison, another patient had an aggressive-appearing lesion in the left proximal femur, causing bone distortion (**D1**), which on MRI was associated with surrounding bone edema (**D2**). The patient was diagnosed with a high-grade chondrosarcoma and treated with proximal femoral resection and megaprosthesis.

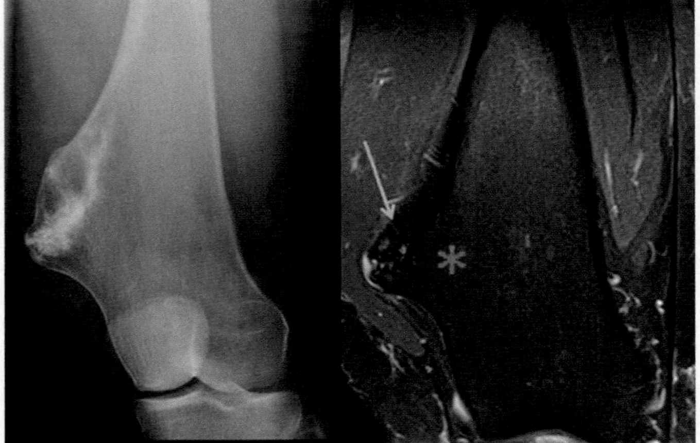

FIGURE 32-9 Osteochondromas are considered more a growth aberrancy than a tumor. Typical features in a skeletally mature individual are small cartilage cap less than 2 cm *(arrow)* and intramedullary canal of lesion confluent with intramedullary canal of the affected bone *(asterisk)*.

history elicited is classic in that pain is worse at night and relieved with nonsteroidal anti-inflammatory drugs. Although these self-limited lesions can be managed for a period of years with nonsteroidal anti-inflammatory drug therapy, watchful waiting, given the profound associated symptoms, is unacceptable to most patients. Osteoid osteoma can be treated with radiofrequency ablation by CT-guided percutaneous techniques. In that scenario, a lesion can be localized in three dimensions, biopsied to obtain definitive tissue for diagnosis, and then ablated with high-frequency radio waves that essentially heat the surrounding tissue around the probe. In areas not amenable to radiofrequency ablation, such as those that are too subcutaneous or near vital structures like the spinal cord, surgical resection of the lesion including the nidus is still performed.

Giant Cell Tumor

Giant cell tumor, which represents approximately 20% of benign bone tumors, is the most aggressive benign bone tumor (Fig. 32-11). Giant cell tumor occurs in the epiphyseal portion of a long bone or flat bones like the pelvis and sacrum in individuals

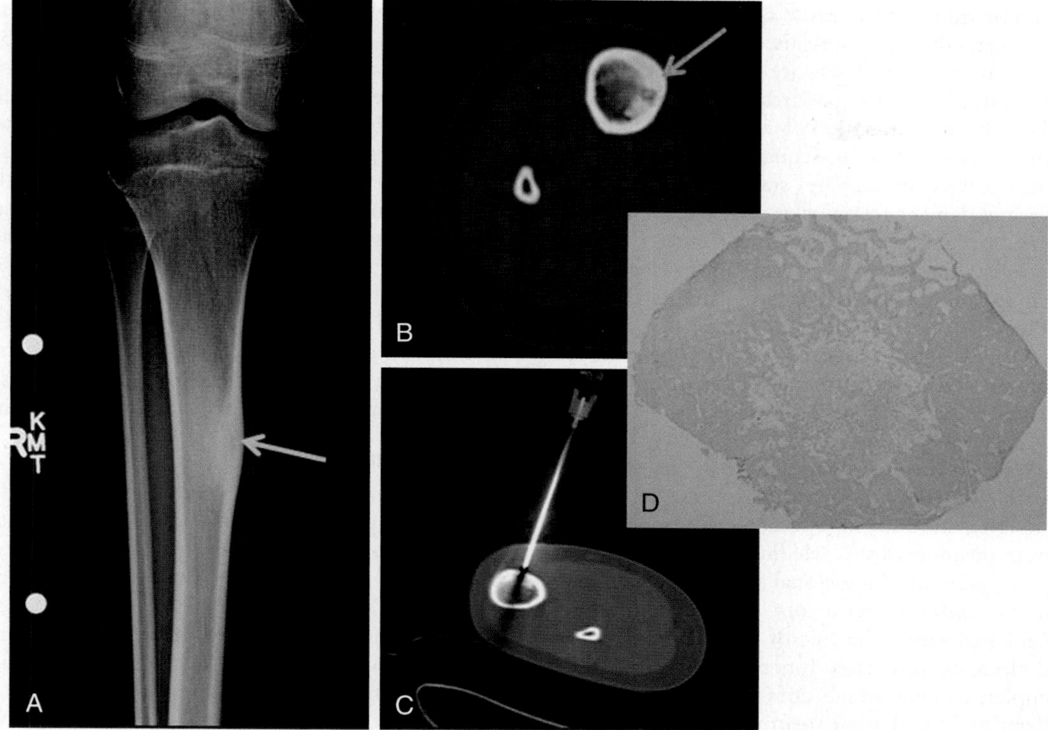

FIGURE 32-10 Osteoid osteomas are benign bone-forming lesions that despite their small size can cause significant pain. **A,** Anteroposterior tibia radiograph shows new bone formation and cortical thickening *(arrow).* **B,** Axial CT shows thickened cortex with a central nidus *(arrow).* **C,** In appropriate lesions, CT-guided biopsy for diagnosis can be followed by radiofrequency ablation for definitive treatment. **D,** An excised osteoid osteoma with a cherry-red nidus and surrounding bone.

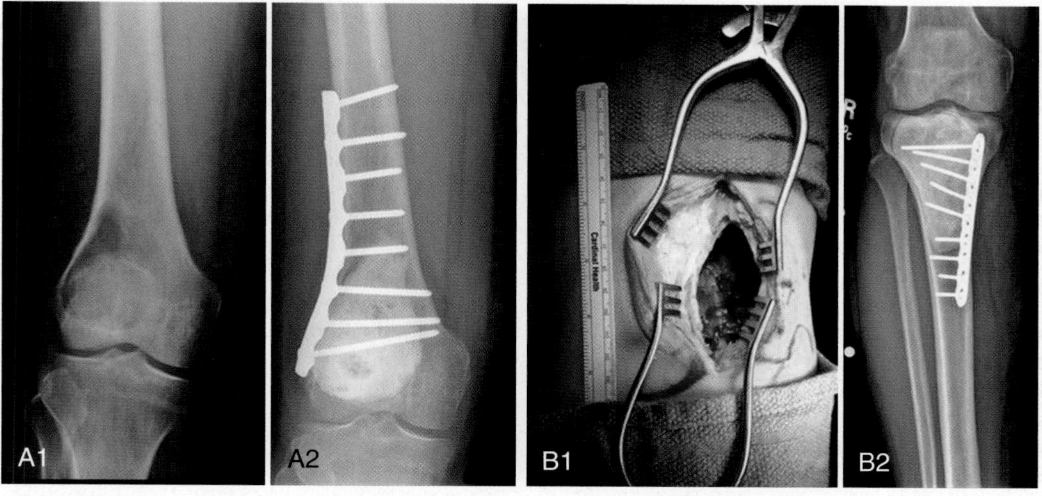

FIGURE 32-11 Giant cell tumors are destructive epiphyseal lesions that can cause articular surface compromise. **A1,** They are manifested as lytic lesions in the epiphyseal bone, as on this distal femur radiograph. **A2,** Intralesional resection and adjuvant treatment are performed, followed by cement and plate and screw reconstruction. **B1,** Although adjuvants are used, the most important part of limiting recurrence is meticulous resection. To accomplish that goal, a bone window often as large as the lesion itself must be created so that all aspects of the lesion can be addressed. **B2,** Cement reconstruction allows immediate stability as well as a means of radiographic monitoring for signs of recurrence.

between 20 and 40 years of age. Patients present with pain, which usually results from periarticular subchondral pathologic fractures. Along with eventual biopsy to rule out malignancy, preoperative evaluation also includes chest imaging and local site imaging. Surgical management requires exposure of the affected bone and creation of a large bone window allowing access to the entirety of the tumor cavity. Local recurrence rates after treatment of giant cell tumor in a bone can be as high as 40%, and therefore resection must be meticulous and often includes the use of adjuvants. After gross resection through curettage, a high-speed burr is used to resect tumor from characteristic bone pits. Additional adjuvants, such as polymethyl methacrylate bone cement, liquid nitrogen, phenol, or argon beam laser, are then used to try to decrease recurrence rates.[27] Finally, periarticular stabilization is performed, typically with a combination of cement and hardware. Bone grafting in those cases is often inadequate to restore stability. Periarticular cement offers immediate stability but may be associated with thermal damage to articular cartilage.[32] Giant cell tumors in the spine, sacrum, and pelvis present greater surgical challenges. Oftentimes, preoperative embolization is required because intraoperative tumor hemorrhage can be significant if the tumor has an aneurysmal bone cyst component.

Despite its benign description, there are instances of giant cell tumor lung metastases, which occur in approximately 1% to 2% of cases.[33] In those cases, the metastatic focus in the lung does not histopathologically meet the criterion for malignancy and is identical in appearance to the benign bone tumor in the skeleton. Survival rates are approximately 80% with aggressive treatment. Patients require long-term follow-up because recurrences may develop several years postoperatively. Medical therapies, such as bisphosphonates and human monoclonal RANKL antibodies (denosumab), can be useful in refractory giant cell tumor as well.[34,35] Those medicines target the role of osteoclasts in tumor development and decrease osteoclast function. However, their efficacy is not complete as denosumab does not affect neoplastic stromal cell proliferation.[36] Radiation treatment may have a role in primary giant cell tumors of the axial skeleton or in recurrent refractory giant cell tumors in a long bone. There is strong evidence, however, that irradiation of giant cell tumors increases the chance for malignant transformation to a frank giant cell sarcoma decades later.[37]

SKELETAL SARCOMAS

The American Cancer Society estimates that 3020 new cases of primary bone cancers will be diagnosed in 2014.[38] In adults, 40% of primary bone cancers are chondrosarcomas, 28% are osteosarcomas, 10% are chordomas, 8% are Ewing sarcomas, and 4% are skeletal sarcomas of bone not otherwise specified. In children, osteosarcoma is the most common primary bone tumor (56%), followed by Ewing sarcoma (28%) and chondrosarcoma (6%). The incidence of skeletal sarcomas is approximately equal in the pediatric and adult populations.

The modern-day algorithm for treatment of bone sarcomas was a serendipitous discovery in the 1970s.[39] During that time, intensive chemotherapy was administered to many teenagers with nonmetastatic osteosarcoma of the extremities after biopsy while they awaited fabrication of a custom endoprosthesis. After several months, the tumor was surgically removed and the implant inserted to preserve the limb. The resected bone was then examined histopathologically for evidence of chemotherapy effect. A survival benefit was noted in children who had received chemotherapy. That observation evolved into the modern-day treatment algorithm for skeletal sarcoma, which includes neoadjuvant chemotherapy, wide surgical resection, and subsequent adjuvant chemotherapy.

Wide surgical resections are mandated for skeletal sarcomas. The surgical goal is a local recurrence rate of less than 7%. Early studies by Simon[40] and Link[41] and their colleagues documented equivalent local recurrence and survival rates between limb salvage and amputation for distal femoral osteosarcoma. Cure rates are approximately 67% for extremity sarcomas, whereas axial tumors in the pelvis or spine have a worse prognosis (33%) for a similar tissue type.[42,43]

It has been demonstrated that limb salvage is more cost-effective during a period of decades than immediate amputation in the teenage population.[44] Implant survival is complicated in the short term by infection (allografts) and in the long term by aseptic loosening (metal).[45] Ten-year implant survival rates for metallic prostheses range from 50% to 80% in the proximal tibia, distal femur, and proximal femur.[46] Wound healing, especially while chemotherapy is being administered, is enhanced with healthy local flaps. Rotational flaps are often used around the knee to improve prosthetic coverage. For example, in proximal tibia resections, a medial gastrocnemius flap is needed to cover the prosthesis and to reconstruct the extensor mechanism.

Osteosarcoma

Osteosarcoma or osteogenic sarcoma is defined as a malignant tumor that produces neoplastic osteoid. Neoplastic cartilage or fibrous tissue may be present. There are many types of osteosarcoma, and they vary by location (intraosseous, surface, or extraskeletal), grade, or etiology. Spontaneous osteosarcomas are most common, but some osteosarcomas occur in the genetic syndromes of Li-Fraumeni and hereditary retinoblastoma and in postradiation scenarios. There is a bimodal age of tumor occurrence. Conventional osteosarcomas occur in the first 2 decades of life, whereas post-treatment or secondary (malignant transformation) osteosarcomas occur much later. Survival is best predicted by the degree of chemotherapy-induced necrosis.[47] Nonmetastatic extremity osteosarcoma with more than 90% chemotherapy-induced necrosis has survival rates of 80% at 5 years. Pelvic osteosarcoma with less than 90% chemotherapy-induced necrosis has a survival rate of approximately 30%.[42,43]

Ewing Sarcoma

Ewing sarcoma and primitive neuroectodermal tumor are small blue cell (microscopic appearance) malignant neoplasms of bone that cytogenetically represent the same entity. They share a common translocation, t(11;22)(q24;q12), in 85% of cases. Molecular cloning of the translocation reveals fusion between the 5′ end of the *EWS* gene from the 22q12 chromosome and the 3′ end of the 11q24 *FLI1* gene.[48-50] This tumor is exquisitely sensitive to chemotherapy and radiation treatment. Neither modality alone or in combination is sufficient to maximize the cure rate, however. Surgical extirpation in conjunction with chemotherapy is the preferred treatment. Reconstruction options follow those of other skeletal sarcomas.

Chondrosarcoma

Chondrosarcoma is a malignant skeletal neoplasm that produces hyaline cartilage. Several pathologic subtypes exist in which the neoplastic cells produce unusual matrices. Histopathology alone does not predict biologic behavior. Rather, a combination of histopathology, age, location, and radiographic appearance yields the best predictor of tumor aggressiveness. A low-grade cartilage tumor of the phalanx may have the same microscopic appearance as a pelvic chondrosarcoma. It would be exceedingly rare to die of a phalanx cartilage tumor. However, local control is notoriously difficult to achieve in pelvic chondrosarcomas, and long-term cure rates require massive resection. Secondary chondrosarcomas occur after malignant transformation of benign cartilage tumors, such as enchondroma or osteochondroma.

BONE METASTASES

Skeletal metastases are approximately 500 times more common than skeletal sarcomas.[51] Each year in the United States, 1.2 million new cases of carcinoma are diagnosed. The most common osteophilic carcinomas are prostate, thyroid, breast, lung, bladder, and renal carcinomas.

As cancer therapeutics improve, the prevalence of patients living with metastatic cancer also increases. Displaced pathologic fractures and impending pathologic fractures represent common problems for the orthopedic oncologist. The workup for a metastatic skeletal carcinoma of unknown primary origin includes a detailed physical examination, including breast and prostate examination. The radiographic studies ordered include a CT scan of the chest, abdomen, and pelvis; a whole body bone scan; serum protein electrophoresis; and assay for prostate-specific antigen.[52] If a diagnosis of metastatic to bone carcinoma is established, there are certain medical therapies that can be used to decrease the number of SREs in a patient (or clinically significant bone metastases).

Intralesional resection after tissue confirmation of the diagnosis and stabilization of bone lesions can provide excellent palliation of symptoms and improvements in quality of life. In considering surgical stabilization, whole bone prophylaxis is often performed with metal implants and cement augmentation. Postoperative radiation therapy must include delivery to the entire bone from joint to joint. A surgical goal of a local recurrence rate of less than 15% is preferred. Isolated metastases, such as from renal cell carcinoma or melanoma, can be treated aggressively if they are indeed isolated and occur after a long hiatus (several years) from initial diagnosis. Cures, in such instances, are not rare.

Reconstructive goals consist of choosing an implant durable enough to outlive the patient and understanding what if any healing capacity the bone may have. A variety of surgical techniques are used to reconstruct the skeleton (see Figs. 32-5 and 32-6). Palliative relief of pain and maximization of function are the goals of surgery.

CONCLUSION

The management of bone tumors requires an expertise and understanding of the bone microenvironment combined with a knowledge of macroscopic bone biomechanics. Tumor resections in the skeleton mandate concurrent plans for stable skeletal reconstruction. In the case of primary malignant bone tumors, studies demonstrate that patients have better outcomes when they are treated in a tertiary care facility with orthopedic oncology expertise. With regard to the management of secondary malignant neoplasms of bone, multiple factors—the nature of the tumor, the location of the lesion, and the demands of specific bone locations—may affect decisions about resection and reconstruction. Benign bone tumors often do not require surgical intervention, only surveillance. Aggressive benign tumors can be resected in an intralesional fashion, but that resection must be meticulous, and those patients must be observed for evidence of recurrence. Skeletal sarcomas are treated with wide excision and appropriate reconstruction. An evolving understanding of the bone microenvironment has translated into better pharmaceutical options for the treatment of bone tumor lesions and a better understanding of the bone-specific and tumor-specific demands in tumor reconstruction.

SELECTED REFERENCES

Enneking WF, Spanier SS, Goodman MA: A system for the staging of musculoskeletal sarcoma. *Clin Orthop Relat Res* 153:106–120, 1980.

This surgical staging system for musculoskeletal sarcomas stratifies bone and soft tissue tumors by the grade of biologic aggressiveness, by the anatomic setting, and by the presence of metastasis. It consists of three stages: I, low grade; II, high grade; and III, presence of metastases. These stages are subdivided by whether the lesion is anatomically confined within a compartment or beyond a compartment in ill-defined fascial planes and spaces. It has proved to be the most correlative system for predicting sarcoma outcomes.

Fizazi K, Carducci M, Smith M, et al: Denosumab versus zoledronic acid for treatment of bone metastases in men with castration-resistant prostate cancer: A randomised, double-blind study. *Lancet* 377:813–822, 2011.

In this phase 3, randomized controlled trial, denosumab was shown to be better than zoledronic acid in the prevention of skeletally related events. The results reflect the importance of understanding the bone microenvironment in which tumors proliferate. Denosumab is a human monoclonal antibody targeted against RANKL. Zoledronic acid is a bisphosphonate that inhibits the activated osteoclasts.

Mankin HJ, Mankin CJ, Simon MA: The methods of biopsy revisited. *J Bone Joint Surg Am* 78:656–663, 1996.

This investigation reviewed the hazards associated with biopsy of primary malignant musculoskeletal sarcomas and demonstrated that there were troubling rates in errors in diagnosis and technique, which adversely affected patient care. In addition, it was noted that patients had a decreased incidence of biopsy-related complications or adverse change in outcome when biopsy was performed in a sarcoma care center. On the basis of those observations, whenever possible, musculoskeletal tumor biopsies should be performed in a tertiary-type sarcoma center by an orthopedic oncologist or collaborating musculoskeletal radiologist.

Rougraff BT, Kneisl JS, Simon MA: Skeletal metastasis of unknown origin: A prospective study of a diagnosis strategy. *J Bone Joint Surg Am* 75:1276–1281, 1993.

In 85% of patients, the primary site of metastatic origin was identified by CT scan of the chest, abdomen, and pelvis. This diagnostic strategy was simple and highly successful for the identification of the site of an occult malignant tumor before biopsy in patients who had skeletal metastases of unknown origin. In a patient presenting with a skeletal lesion suggestive of a metastatic lesion with an unknown primary, CT scan is the test of choice to identify the primary lesion. In an era in which insurance approval of such tests is increasingly more difficult, it is important to advocate for patients to receive this standard of care examination.

Simon MA, Aschliman MA, Thomas N, et al: Limb-salvage treatment versus amputation for osteosarcoma of the distal end of the femur. *J Bone Joint Surg Am* 68:1331–1337, 1986.

This study compared three groups of patients who had a limb-sparing procedure, an above-the-knee amputation, or disarticulation of the hip for osteosarcoma of the distal femur. The use of a limb salvage procedure for osteosarcoma of the distal end of the femur did not shorten the disease-free interval or compromise long-term survival.

REFERENCES

1. Paget S: The distribution of secondary growths in cancer of the breast. *Lancet* 1:571–573, 1889.
2. Kang Y, Siegel PM, Shu W, et al: A multigenic program mediating breast cancer metastasis to bone. *Cancer Cell* 3:537–549, 2003.
3. Cook LM, Shay G, Aruajo A, et al: Integrating new discoveries into the "vicious cycle" paradigm of prostate to bone metastases. *Cancer Metastasis Rev* 33:511–525, 2014.
4. Boyle WJ, Simonet WS, Lacey DL: Osteoclast differentiation and activation. *Nature* 423:337–342, 2003.
5. Morony S, Capparelli C, Sarosi I, et al: Osteoprotegerin inhibits osteolysis and decreases skeletal tumor burden in syngeneic and nude mouse models of experimental bone metastasis. *Cancer Res* 61:4432–4436, 2001.
6. Mundy GR: Metastasis to bone: Causes, consequences and therapeutic opportunities. *Nat Rev Cancer* 2:584–593, 2002.
7. Weilbaecher KN, Guise TA, McCauley LK: Cancer to bone: A fatal attraction. *Nat Rev Cancer* 11:411–425, 2011.
8. Lynch CC, Hikosaka A, Acuff HB, et al: MMP-7 promotes prostate cancer–induced osteolysis via the solubilization of RANKL. *Cancer Cell* 7:485–496, 2005.
9. Pavlakis N, Schmidt R, Stockler M: Bisphosphonates for breast cancer. *Cochrane Database Syst Rev* (3):CD003474, 2005.
10. Aapro M, Abrahamsson PA, Body JJ, et al: Guidance on the use of bisphosphonates in solid tumours: Recommendations of an international expert panel. *Ann Oncol* 19:420–432, 2008.
11. Sheridan JP, Marsters SA, Pitti RM, et al: Control of TRAIL-induced apoptosis by a family of signaling and decoy receptors. *Science* 277:818–821, 1997.
12. Body JJ, Facon T, Coleman RE, et al: A study of the biological receptor activator of nuclear factor-κB ligand inhibitor, denosumab, in patients with multiple myeloma or bone metastases from breast cancer. *Clin Cancer Res* 12:1221–1228, 2006.
13. Rordorf T, Hassan AA, Azim H, et al: Bone health in breast cancer patients: A comprehensive statement by CECOG/SAKK Intergroup. *Breast* 23:511–525, 2014.
14. Fizazi K, Carducci M, Smith M, et al: Denosumab versus zoledronic acid for treatment of bone metastases in men with castration-resistant prostate cancer: A randomised, double-blind study. *Lancet* 377:813–822, 2011.
15. Stopeck AT, Lipton A, Body JJ, et al: Denosumab compared with zoledronic acid for the treatment of bone metastases in patients with advanced breast cancer: A randomized, double-blind study. *J Clin Oncol* 28:5132–5139, 2010.
16. Mirels H: Metastatic disease in long bones. A proposed scoring system for diagnosing impending pathologic fractures. *Clin Orthop Relat Res* 256–264, 1989.
17. Mankin HJ, Mankin CJ, Simon MA: The hazards of the biopsy, revisited. Members of the Musculoskeletal Tumor Society. *J Bone Joint Surg Am* 78:656–663, 1996.
18. Randall RL, Bruckner JD, Papenhausen MD, et al: Errors in diagnosis and margin determination of soft-tissue sarcomas initially treated at non-tertiary centers. *Orthopedics* 27:209–212, 2004.
19. Trovik CS: Scanadinavian Sarcoma Group Project: Local recurrence of soft tissue sarcoma. A Scandinavian Sarcoma Group Project. *Acta Orthop Scand Suppl* 72:1–31, 2001.
20. Enneking WF, Spanier SS, Goodman MA: A system for the surgical staging of musculoskeletal sarcoma. *Clin Orthop Relat Res* 106–120, 1980.
21. Bone. In Edge S, Byrd DR, Compton CC, et al, editors: *AJCC cancer staging manual*, ed 7, New York, 2010, Springer, pp 281–290.
22. Enneking WF: *Staging musculoskeletal tumors. Musculoskeletal Tumor Surgery*, New York, 1983, Churchill Livingstone, pp 87–88.
23. Blackley HR, Wunder JS, Davis AM, et al: Treatment of giant-cell tumors of long bones with curettage and bone-grafting. *J Bone Joint Surg Am* 81:811–820, 1999.
24. Joyce MJ: Safety and FDA regulations for musculoskeletal allografts: Perspective of an orthopaedic surgeon. *Clin Orthop Relat Res* 22–30, 2005.
25. Myers GJ, Abudu AT, Carter SR, et al: The long-term results of endoprosthetic replacement of the proximal tibia for bone tumours. *J Bone Joint Surg Br* 89:1632–1637, 2007.
26. Unni KK: *Dahlin's bone tumors: General aspects and data on 11,087 cases*, ed 5, Philadelphia, 1996, Lippincott-Raven.
27. Turcotte RE, Wunder JS, Isler MH, et al: Giant cell tumor of long bone: A Canadian Sarcoma Group study. *Clin Orthop Relat Res* 248–258, 2002.
28. Altay M, Bayrakci K, Yildiz Y, et al: Secondary chondrosarcoma in cartilage bone tumors: Report of 32 patients. *J Orthop Sci* 12:415–423, 2007.
29. Wuyts W, Van Hul W: Molecular basis of multiple exostoses: Mutations in the EXT1 and EXT2 genes. *Hum Mutat* 15:220–227, 2000.
30. Le Merrer M, Legeai-Mallet L, Jeannin PM, et al: A gene for hereditary multiple exostoses maps to chromosome 19p. *Hum Mol Genet* 3:717–722, 1994.
31. Vanhoenacker FM, Van Hul W, Wuyts W, et al: Hereditary multiple exostoses: From genetics to clinical syndrome and complications. *Eur J Radiol* 40:208–217, 2001.
32. Radev BR, Kase JA, Askew MJ, et al: Potential for thermal damage to articular cartilage by PMMA reconstruction of a bone cavity following tumor excision: A finite element study. *J Biomech* 42:1120–1126, 2009.
33. Dominkus M, Ruggieri P, Bertoni F, et al: Histologically verified lung metastases in benign giant cell tumours—14 cases from a single institution. *Int Orthop* 30:499–504, 2006.
34. Chawla S, Henshaw R, Seeger L, et al: Safety and efficacy of denosumab for adults and skeletally mature adolescents with giant cell tumour of bone: Interim analysis of an open-label, parallel-group, phase 2 study. *Lancet Oncol* 14:901–908, 2013.
35. Balke M, Campanacci L, Gebert C, et al: Bisphosphonate treatment of aggressive primary, recurrent and metastatic giant cell tumour of bone. *BMC Cancer* 10:462, 2010.
36. Mak IW, Evaniew N, Popovic S, et al: A translational study of the neoplastic cells of giant cell tumor of bone following

neoadjuvant denosumab. *J Bone Joint Surg Am* 96:e127, 2014.
37. Rock MG, Sim FH, Unni KK, et al: Secondary malignant giant-cell tumor of bone. Clinicopathological assessment of nineteen patients. *J Bone Joint Surg Am* 68:1073–1079, 1986.
38. Cancer facts and figures 2014. American Cancer Society. <http://www.cancer.org/acs/groups/content/@research/documents/webcontent/acspc-042151.pdf>.
39. Rosen G, Marcove RC, Caparros B, et al: Primary osteogenic sarcoma: The rationale for preoperative chemotherapy and delayed surgery. *Cancer* 43:2163–2177, 1979.
40. Simon MA, Aschliman MA, Thomas N, et al: Limb-salvage treatment versus amputation for osteosarcoma of the distal end of the femur. *J Bone Joint Surg Am* 68:1331–1337, 1986.
41. Link MP, Goorin AM, Miser AW, et al: The effect of adjuvant chemotherapy on relapse-free survival in patients with osteosarcoma of the extremity. *N Engl J Med* 314:1600–1606, 1986.
42. Pakos EE, Nearchou AD, Grimer RJ, et al: Prognostic factors and outcomes for osteosarcoma: An international collaboration. *Eur J Cancer* 45:2367–2375, 2009.
43. Goorin AM, Schwartzentruber DJ, Devidas M, et al: Presurgical chemotherapy compared with immediate surgery and adjuvant chemotherapy for nonmetastatic osteosarcoma: Pediatric Oncology Group Study POG-8651. *J Clin Oncol* 21:1574–1580, 2003.
44. Grimer RJ, Carter SR, Pynsent PB: The cost-effectiveness of limb salvage for bone tumours. *J Bone Joint Surg Br* 79:558–561, 1997.
45. Mankin HJ, Hornicek FJ, Raskin KA: Infection in massive bone allografts. *Clin Orthop Relat Res* 210–216, 2005.
46. Jeys LM, Kulkarni A, Grimer RJ, et al: Endoprosthetic reconstruction for the treatment of musculoskeletal tumors of the appendicular skeleton and pelvis. *J Bone Joint Surg Am* 90:1265–1271, 2008.
47. Picci P, Bacci G, Campanacci M, et al: Histologic evaluation of necrosis in osteosarcoma induced by chemotherapy. Regional mapping of viable and nonviable tumor. *Cancer* 56:1515–1521, 1985.
48. Aurias A, Rimbaut C, Buffe D, et al: Chromosomal translocations in Ewing's sarcoma. *N Engl J Med* 309:496–498, 1983.
49. de Alava E, Gerald WL: Molecular biology of the Ewing's sarcoma/primitive neuroectodermal tumor family. *J Clin Oncol* 18:204–213, 2000.
50. Hu-Lieskovan S, Zhang J, Wu L, et al: EWS-FLI1 fusion protein up-regulates critical genes in neural crest development and is responsible for the observed phenotype of Ewing's family of tumors. *Cancer Res* 65:4633–4644, 2005.
51. Jemal A, Siegel R, Ward E, et al: Cancer statistics, 2009. *CA Cancer J Clin* 59:225–249, 2009.
52. Rougraff BT, Kneisl JS, Simon MA: Skeletal metastases of unknown origin. A prospective study of a diagnostic strategy. *J Bone Joint Surg Am* 75:1276–1281, 1993.

SECTION VI

Head and Neck

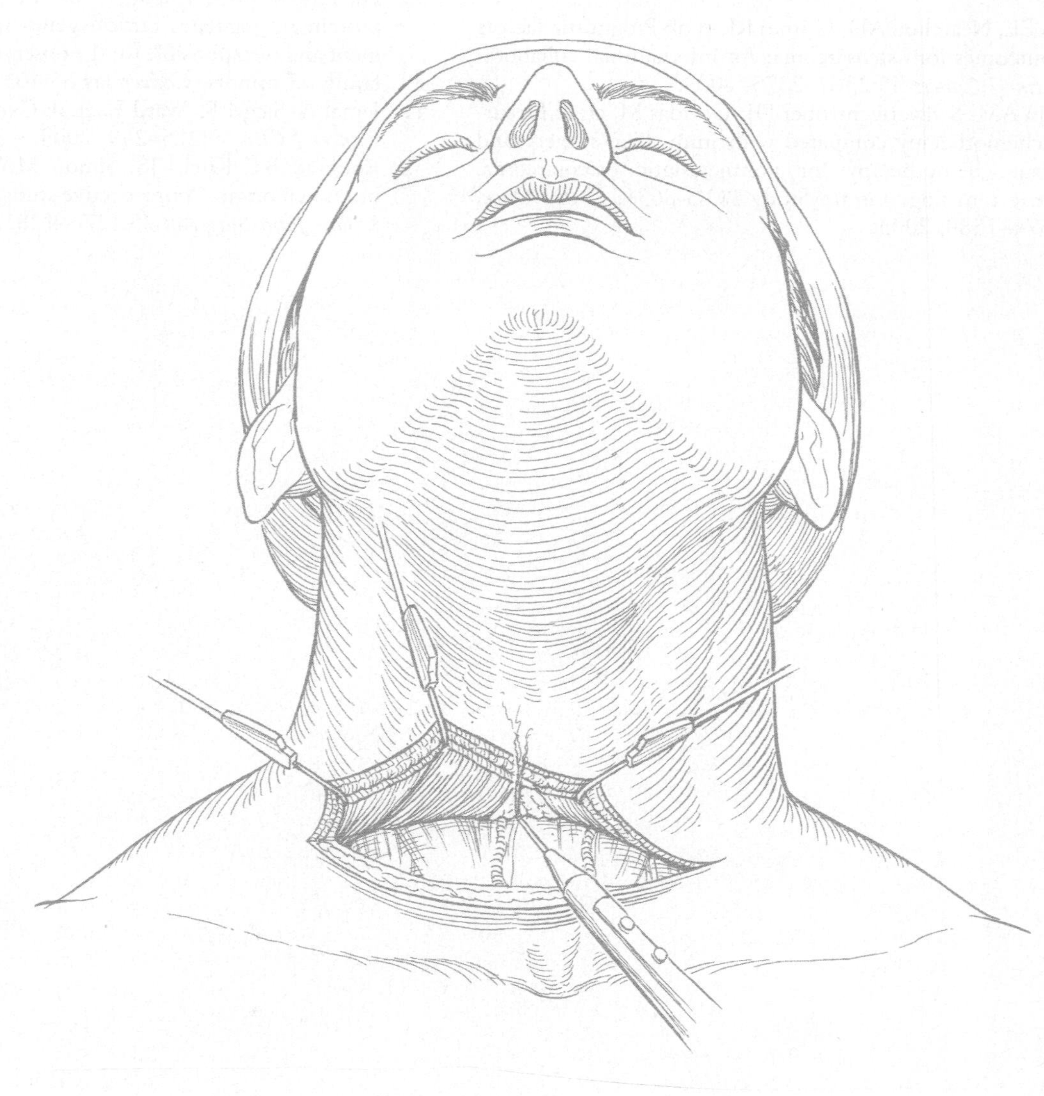

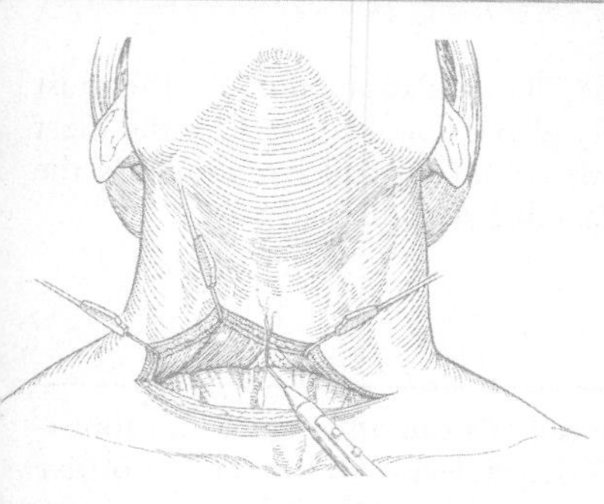

CHAPTER 33

Head and Neck

Robert R. Lorenz, Marion E. Couch, Brian B. Burkey

OUTLINE

NORMAL HISTOLOGY

The normal histology of the upper aerodigestive tract varies in each site. A complete review of the thyroid and parathyroid glands is beyond the scope of this chapter. The nasal vestibule is considered a cutaneous structure and is lined by keratinizing squamous epithelium. The limen nasi, or mucocutaneous junction, is where the epithelium changes to a ciliated pseudostratified columnar (respiratory) epithelium to line the nasal cavities. The exception is the olfactory epithelium at the roof of the nasal cavity, which is composed of bipolar, spindle-shaped olfactory neural cells with surrounding supporting cells. The paranasal sinuses are also lined by respiratory epithelium, but it tends to be thinner and less vascular than that of the nasal cavity. The nasopharyngeal lining varies from squamous to respiratory epithelium in an inconsistent manner. The adenoidal pad is composed of lymphoid tissue containing germinal centers without capsules or sinusoids. The oral cavity is lined by nonkeratinized stratified squamous epithelium with minor salivary glands throughout the submucosa and within the muscular tissue of the tongue. Although the oropharynx is lined by squamous epithelium, Waldeyer's ring is formed by lymphoid tissues of the palatine tonsils, adenoids, lingual tonsils, and adjacent submucosal lymphatics. The tonsils contain germinal centers without capsules or sinusoids, but, in contrast to the adenoids, the tonsils have crypts lined by stratified squamous epithelium.

The hypopharynx is lined by nonkeratinizing, stratified squamous epithelium. Seromucous glands are found throughout the submucosa of the hypopharynx, in the lower two thirds of the epiglottis, and in the potential space between the true and false vocal folds known as the ventricle. Nonkeratinizing stratified squamous epithelium lines the epiglottis and true vocal fold. Pseudostratified, ciliated respiratory epithelium lines the false vocal fold, ventricle, and subglottis. The thyroid, cricoid, and arytenoid cartilages are composed of hyaline cartilage, whereas the epiglottis, cuneiform, and corniculate cartilages are composed of elastic-type cartilage. The external ear is a cutaneous structure lined with keratinizing squamous epithelium and associated adnexal structures. The external third of the external auditory canal is unique in that it contains modified apocrine glands that produce cerumen. The middle ear is lined with respiratory epithelium.

Numerous noncancerous changes in squamous epithelium can be seen in the upper aerodigestive tract. *Leukoplakia*, which describes any white mucosal lesion, and *erythroplasia*, which describes any red mucosal lesion, are clinical descriptions and should not be used as diagnostic terms (Fig. 33-1). *Erythroplakia* is more often indicative of an underlying malignant lesion. *Hyperplasia* refers to thickening of the epithelium secondary to an increase in the total number of cells. *Parakeratosis* is an abnormal presence of nuclei in the keratin layers, whereas *dyskeratosis* refers to any abnormal keratinization of epithelial cells and is found in dysplastic lesions. *Koilocytosis* is a descriptive term for the vacuolization of squamous cells and is suggestive of viral infection, especially human papillomavirus (HPV).

EPIDEMIOLOGY

The American Joint Committee on Cancer (AJCC) staging system divides sites of malignancy originating in the head and neck into six major groups: lip and oral cavity, pharynx, larynx, nasal cavity and paranasal sinuses, major salivary glands, and thyroid.[1] Of the sites arising from the aerodigestive tract, laryngeal cancer is the most common cause of death (Table 33-1), whereas pharyngeal cancer has emerged as exhibiting the highest incidence over the past several years. Although there remains a male preponderance in aerodigestive tract malignancies, the male-to-female ratio has been steadily decreasing because of the direct association between tobacco as a causative agent and the increased incidence of female smokers. Tobacco abuse increases the odds ratio for the development of laryngeal cancer by 15 : 1, whereas alcohol abuse carries an odds ratio of 2 : 1. Combined abuse of alcohol and tobacco is not additive in terms of the odds ratio but multiplicative. More recent studies suggested that the epidemiology of head and neck cancer is shifting to mirror a change in the cause.[2] In the United States, during the period 1973-2003, the incidence rate for cancer sites causally related to HPV infection significantly increased (tongue base and tonsil subsites of the oropharynx), whereas significant declines in incidence were observed for oral cancers not causally related to HPV. In addition, HPV-associated cancers tended to affect younger (by 3 to 5 years) individuals and were less likely to be associated with alcohol or tobacco use. Worldwide, the highest incidence rates in men exceeded 30/100,000 in areas of France, Hong Kong, India, Spain, Italy, and Brazil as well as in black men in the United States, with dramatic increases in oral cancer being seen in Central and Eastern Europe, most notably Hungary, Poland, Slovakia, and Romania.[3] The highest female rates exceed 10/100,000 and are found in India, where chewing of betel quid and tobacco is common. Although aggregate rates are slowly declining in certain areas, such as India, Hong Kong, and Brazil as well as the United States among white individuals, rates are increasing in most other regions of the world. In addition to alcohol and tobacco consumption as causative factors, other risk factors include HPV and Epstein-Barr virus infection, Plummer-Vinson syndrome, metabolic polymorphisms, malnutrition, and occupational exposure to mutagenic agents. According to the National Cancer Database, squamous cell carcinoma (SCC) is the most common head and neck tumor of the major head and neck sites (88.9%), adenocarcinoma is the most common of the major salivary glands (56.4%), SCC is the most common of the sinonasal tract (43.6%), and lymphoma is the most common of the sites classified as "other" (82.5%).[4]

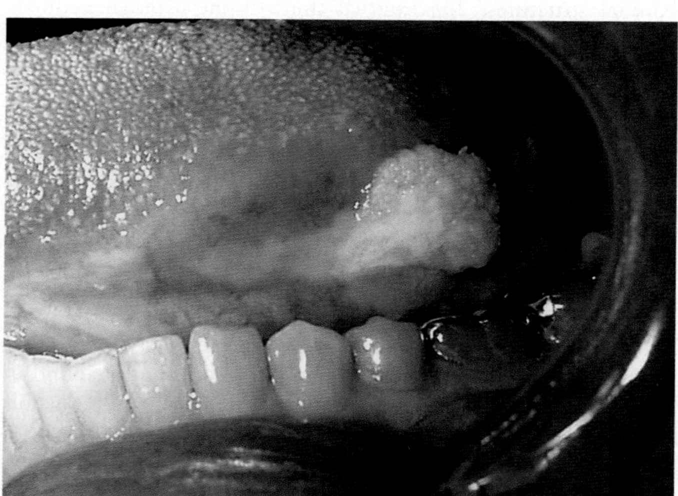

FIGURE 33-1 Leukoplakic lesion on the left mobile tongue. On biopsy, this lesion was determined to be hyperkeratosis without invasive cancer.

CARCINOGENESIS

HPV infection is now recognized as a causative agent for oropharyngeal carcinoma. Based on the molecular cause, HPV-positive and HPV-negative head and neck SCCs (HNSCCs) may be considered as two distinct cancers.[5] High-risk HPV strains (subtypes 16 and 18) suppress apoptosis and activate cell growth when the HPV E6 and E7 proteins disrupt regulatory cell cycle and DNA repair pathways. Malignant transformation begins with inactivation of the p53 tumor suppressor gene by E6, whereas E7 inactivates the retinoblastoma tumor suppressor protein (Rb). E6 targets the cellular ubiquitin-protein ligase E6-AP, which then targets p53 for ubiquitination and degradation; this results in unregulated cell growth. E7 associates with Rb and p21 by blocking the interaction of Rb with E2F, which initiates uncontrolled cell proliferation.[5] Viruses such as HPV can usurp cellular processes, but often the development of carcinoma is the result of a stepwise accumulation of genetic alterations.[6] Tobacco, a well-known risk factor, was one of the first carcinogens to be linked with p53 mutations. One tobacco carcinogen, benzo[α]pyrene diol epoxide, induces genetic damage by forming covalently bound DNA adducts throughout the genome, including p53. Damage induced by benzo[α]pyrene diol epoxide and other carcinogens is repaired with the nucleotide excision repair system. Several studies demonstrated that sequence variations in nucleotide excision repair genes contribute to HNSCC susceptibility.[7]

Many years after Slaughter proposed field cancerization, Califano and colleagues[8] described the molecular basis for histopathologic changes in HNSCC. Samples of dysplastic mucosa and benign hyperplastic lesions displayed loss of heterozygosity at specific loci (9p21, 3p21, 17p13). In particular, loss of heterozygosity at 9p21 or 3p21 is one of the earliest detectable events leading to dysplasia in this tumor progression model. From dysplasia, further genetic alteration in 11q, 13q, and 14q results in carcinoma in situ. The high rate of recurrence of HNSCC is believed to result from histopathologically benign squamous cell epithelium harboring a clonal population with genetic alterations.[8] Studies using microsatellite analysis and X chromosome inactivation verified that metachronous and synchronous lesions from distinct anatomic sites in HNSCC often originate from a common clone. This evidence confirms that genetically altered mucosa is difficult to cure in a patient with HNSCC because it is on the path to tumorigenesis, as predicted by this model.

TABLE 33-1 Head and Neck Cancer, 2009 Statistics: Upper Aerodigestive Tract

	ESTIMATED INCIDENCE			ESTIMATED DEATHS		
SITE	BOTH GENDERS	MALE	FEMALE	BOTH GENDERS	MALE	FEMALE
Tongue	10,530	7470	3060	1910	1240	670
Mouth	10,750	6450	4300	1810	1110	700
Pharynx	12,610	10,020	2590	2230	1640	590
Other oral cavity	1830	1300	530	1650	1250	400
Larynx	12,290	9920	2370	3660	2900	760

From Jemal A, Siegel R, Ward E, et al: Cancer statistics, 2009. *CA Cancer J Clin* 59:225–249, 2009.

Patients with HNSCC have a 3% to 7% annual incidence of secondary lesions in the upper aerodigestive tract, esophagus, or lung. A synchronous second primary lesion is defined as a tumor detected within 6 months of the index tumor. The occurrence of a second primary lesion more than 6 months after the initial lesion is referred to as metachronous. A second primary develops in the aerodigestive tract of 14% of patients with HNSCC over the course of their lifetime, with more than half of these lesions occurring within the first 2 years of the index tumor.

Evidence also suggests that changes in the programming of cells, including stem cells, may be involved in tumorigenesis in HNSCC because of the epithelial to mesenchymal transition.[9] Abnormalities in cadherins, tight junctions, and desmosomes lead to a decrease in cell-cell adherence and loss of polarity, increasing the mobility of these cells. As epithelial cells disassemble their junctional structures, undergo extracellular matrix remodeling, and begin expressing proteins of mesenchymal origin, they become migratory. When the process of epithelial to mesenchymal transition becomes pathologic, regulatory checkpoints are deficient. In the carcinogenic process, epithelial to mesenchymal transition may cause changes that contribute to tumor invasion and metastasis, enabling cancer cell dissemination.[9]

Epidermal growth factor receptor (EGFR) signaling has been strongly implicated in tumor progression in HNSCC. The ErbB family comprises four structurally related receptor tyrosine kinases. EGFR messenger RNA and protein are preferentially expressed in HNSCC compared with surrounding normal tissues, suggesting a significant role in carcinogenesis. EGFR is overexpressed in 80% to 100% of HNSCC tumors, with advanced-stage and poorly differentiated carcinomas more frequently demonstrating overexpression.[10] The most common mutation, *EGFRvIII*, occurs in 40% of HNSCCs. This mutant receptor is found only in cancer cells and has an in-frame deletion of exons 2 to 7, which results in a constitutively active receptor. The fact that *EGFRvIII* is not found in normal tissues makes this an attractive target for therapy. The two classes of therapies are monoclonal antibodies to EGFR receptor subunits and small-molecule EGFR tyrosine kinase inhibitors. When ligands bind to one of the ErbB receptors, a dimer forms, and the receptor's intracellular tyrosine residue then undergoes adenosine triphosphate–dependent autophosphorylation. Once phosphorylated, the receptor has the potential to trigger many different intracellular downstream pathways. The Janus kinase–signal transducers and activators of transcription (JAK-STAT), along with the phospholipase-Cγ–protein kinase C (PLCγ-PKC) pathways are activated in association with EGFR phosphorylation.

An emerging potential target for molecular-based cancer therapy is the insulin-like growth factor I receptor and its ligands, insulin growth factor I and insulin growth factor II.[11] With activation of the receptor, downstream signaling events include phosphorylation of insulin receptor substrate-1, activation of mitogen-activated protein kinases (MAPKs), and stimulation of the phosphatidylinositol-3 kinase (PI3K) pathway. This activation of both the Ras-MAPK-ERK and the PI3K-Akt pathways is similar to the downstream signaling seen with EGFR autophosphorylation.

With the advent of increasingly sophisticated molecular detection techniques, such as DNA microarrays, large numbers of genetic markers can now be tested with greater ease. Most single molecular markers studied to date have failed to demonstrate sufficient predictive potential in terms of incidence or prognosis. However, although single markers may not prove to have enough clinical applicability, panels of different molecular markers may offer more promising diagnostic and prognostic value.

STAGING

Staging of head and neck cancer follows the TNM classification established by the AJCC.[1] The T classification refers to the extent of the primary tumor and is specific to each of the six sites of origin, with subclassifications within each site. The N classification refers to the pattern of lymphatic spread within the neck nodes and is the same for most head and neck sites except thyroid, nasopharynx, mucosal melanoma, and skin (Table 33-2). In the seventh edition of the *AJCC Cancer Staging Manual*,[1] a descriptor has been added as ECS+ or ECS−, depending on the presence or absence of nodal extracapsular spread (ECS). Clinical staging of the neck is based primarily on palpation, although radiographic studies, including computed tomography (CT) and magnetic resonance imaging (MRI), have been shown to be accurate in detecting positive nodes. If the CT criteria of nodes with central necrosis or size larger than 1.0 cm are used to determine positivity, only 7% of pathologically positive lymph nodes would be missed, and these smaller nodes are most often found in necks with more extensive disease. Metastatic disease is reported simply as Mx (cannot be assessed), M0 (no distant metastases are present), or M1 (metastases present). The most common sites of distant spread are the lungs and bones, whereas hepatic and brain metastases occur less frequently. The risk for distant metastases depends more on nodal staging than on primary tumor size.

After complete resection of the primary and nodal disease, pathologic staging may be reported. This is designated by a preceding "p," as in pTNM. When measuring a pathologic mucosal specimen, tumor size may decrease up to 30% after resection.

TABLE 33-2 Metastatic Staging of Regional Lymph Nodes (N)

STAGE	DESCRIPTION
NX	Regional lymph nodes cannot be assessed
N0	No regional lymph node metastasis
N1*	Metastasis in a single ipsilateral lymph node, ≤3 cm in greatest dimension
N2*	Metastasis in a single ipsilateral lymph node, >3 cm but not >6 cm in greatest dimension, or in multiple ipsilateral lymph nodes, none >6 cm in greatest dimension, or in bilateral or contralateral lymph nodes, none >6 cm in greatest dimension
N2a*	Metastasis in single ipsilateral lymph node >3 cm but not >6 cm in greatest dimension
N2b*	Metastasis in multiple ipsilateral lymph nodes, none >6 cm in greatest dimension
N2c*	Metastasis in bilateral or contralateral lymph nodes, none >6 cm in greatest dimension
N3*	Metastasis in a lymph node >6 cm in greatest dimension

From Edge SB, Byrd DR, Compton CC, et al (editors): *AJCC cancer staging manual,* ed 7, New York, 2010, Springer-Verlag.

*A designation of U or L may be used for any N stage to indicate metastasis above the lower border of the cricoid (U) or below the lower border of the cricoid (L). Similarly, clinical or radiologic extracapsular spread (ECS) should be recorded as E− or E+, and histopathologic ECS should be designated as En (none), Em (microscopic), or Eg (gross).

Although clinical T staging is of primary concern, pathologic N staging allows detection of occult microscopic disease and is useful in determining prognosis. Site-specific staging systems are discussed according to the primary site. The major change in the 2010 edition of the AJCC staging system for HNSCC sites, in addition to the ECS+ or ECS− descriptor, is the addition of a separate classification for mucosal melanoma of the head and neck, a very rare tumor.[1]

CLINICAL OVERVIEW

Evaluation

Proper treatment of HNSCC requires careful evaluation and accurate clinical and radiographic staging. Patients with HNSCC are initially evaluated in a similar manner, regardless of the site of tumor. Patient histories focus on symptoms of the tumor, including the duration of symptoms, detection of masses, location of pain, and presence of referred pain. Special attention is paid to numbness, cranial nerve weakness, dysphagia, odynophagia, hoarseness, disarticulation, airway compromise, trismus, nasal obstruction, epistaxis, and hemoptysis. Alcohol and tobacco use histories are elicited. Office examination includes nasopharyngeal and laryngeal visualization with a mirror or fiberoptic endoscope. The examiner should be especially vigilant for second primary tumors and should not be preoccupied by the obvious primary lesion. Contrast-enhanced CT and MRI of the head and neck may be performed for evaluation of the tumor and detection of occult lymphadenopathy. CT scanning is best at evaluating bony destruction, whereas MRI can determine soft tissue involvement and is excellent at evaluating parotid and parapharyngeal space tumors. Chest radiography or chest CT is performed to rule out synchronous lung lesions. Levels of serum tumor markers such as alkaline phosphatase and calcium may be determined, but such tests are not standard.

Direct laryngoscopy and examination under anesthesia are commonly performed as part of the evaluation of HNSCC. These procedures allow the physician to evaluate tumors without patient discomfort and with muscle paralysis as well as evaluate the oropharynx, hypopharynx, and larynx and obtain biopsy samples. Pathologic confirmation of cancer is mandatory before initiating treatment. Concurrent bronchoscopy and esophagoscopy have historically been recommended for the detection of synchronous second primaries of the aerodigestive tract, which occur in 4% to 8% of patients who have one head and neck malignancy. With a normal chest radiograph or CT scan, bronchoscopy has a low yield for discovering bronchial tree second primaries. A barium esophagogram may substitute for esophagoscopy in patients at low risk for the development of esophageal tumors.

Positron Emission Tomography

^{18}F-fluorodeoxyglucose is a glucose analogue that is preferentially absorbed by neoplastic cells and can be detected by positron emission tomography (PET). The role of PET has been investigated in the initial evaluation of patients with HNSCC.[12] PET is more sensitive than CT in identifying the primary lesion but cannot detect unknown primary tumors with more than 50% sensitivity. More than one third of patients have a change in their TNM score based on PET findings, and 14% of patients are assigned a different stage when PET is added to the diagnostic workup. PET evaluates neck metastases with sensitivity equal to CT but with fewer false-positive results. PET can detect a higher percentage of lung metastases than chest radiography, bronchoscopy, or CT, but the specificity ranges from 50% to 80%, and how to treat a patient with a positive PET and an otherwise negative lung workup is still in question. In approximately 10% of patients, a synchronous second primary cancer is detected in various sites, including the stomach, pancreas, colon, and thyroid. Patients with tumors that demonstrate high uptake on PET have a worse prognosis than patients with less avid tumors and have less response to radiation therapy. The exact role of PET in the initial evaluation of HNSCC is still under investigation. Its use is becoming more routine, but it is not within the current standard of care.

Lymphatic Spread

The cervical lymphatic nodal basins contain 50 to 70 lymph nodes per side and are divided into seven levels (Figs. 33-2 and 33-3). Level I is subdivided:

- Level IA is bounded by the anterior belly of the digastric muscle, hyoid bone, and midline.
- Level IB is bounded by the anterior and posterior bellies of the digastric muscle and the inferior border of the mandible. Level IB contains the submandibular gland.

Level II is bounded superiorly by the skull base, anteriorly by the stylohyoid muscle, inferiorly by a horizontal plane extending posteriorly from the hyoid bone, and posteriorly by the posterior edge of the sternocleidomastoid muscle. Level II is further subdivided:

- Level IIA is anterior to the spinal accessory nerve.
- Level IIB, or the so-called submuscular triangle, is posterior to the nerve.

Level III begins at the inferior edge of level II and is bounded by the laryngeal strap muscles anteriorly, by the posterior border of the sternocleidomastoid muscle posteriorly, and by a horizontal plane extending posteriorly from the inferior border of the cricoid cartilage.

Level IV begins at the inferior border of level III and is bounded anteriorly by the strap muscles, posteriorly by the posterior edge of the sternocleidomastoid muscle, and inferiorly by the clavicle.

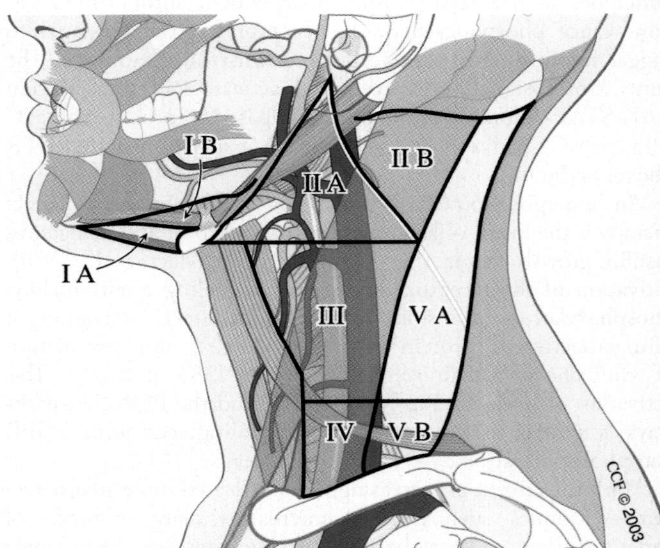

FIGURE 33-2 Diagram of cervical lymph node levels I through V. Level II is divided into regions A and B by the spinal accessory nerve. (Courtesy Cleveland Clinic Foundation, 2003.)

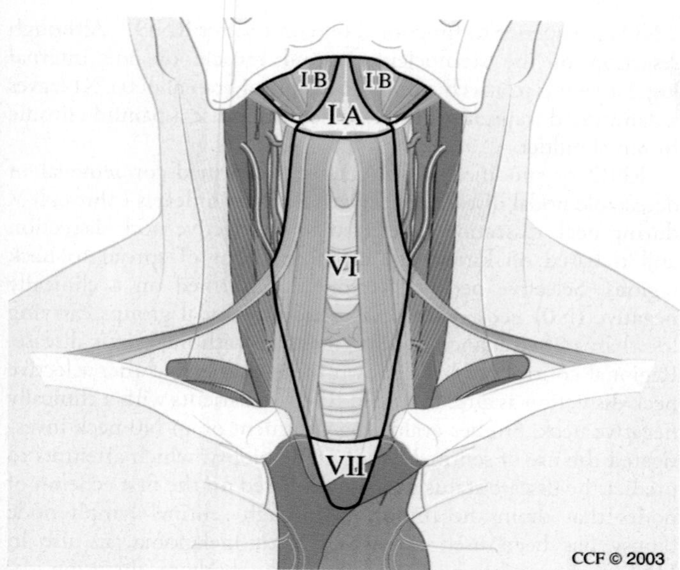

FIGURE 33-3 Diagram of anterior lymph node levels I, VI, and VII. Although large in area, most level VI lymph nodes are confined to the paratracheal region. (Courtesy Cleveland Clinic Foundation, 2003.)

Level V is posterior to the posterior edge of the sternocleidomastoid muscle, anterior to the trapezius muscle, superior to the clavicle, and inferior to the base of the skull.

Level VI is bounded by the hyoid bone superiorly, the common carotid arteries laterally, and the sternum inferiorly. Although level VI is large in area, the few lymph nodes that it contains are mostly in the paratracheal regions near the thyroid gland.

Level VII (superior mediastinum) lies between the common carotid arteries and is superior to the aortic arch and inferior to the upper border of the sternum.

Lymphatic drainage usually occurs in a superior to inferior direction and follows predictable patterns based on the primary site. Primary tumors of the lip and oral cavity generally metastasize to nodes in levels I, II, and III, although skip metastases may occur in lower levels. The upper lip primarily metastasizes ipsilaterally, whereas the lower lip has ipsilateral and contralateral drainage. Tumors in the oropharynx, hypopharynx, and larynx usually metastasize to levels II, III, and IV. Tumors of the nasopharynx spread to the retropharyngeal and parapharyngeal lymph nodes as well as to levels II through V. Other sites that metastasize to the retropharyngeal lymph nodes are the soft palate, posterior and lateral oropharynx, and hypopharynx. Tumors of the subglottis, thyroid, hypopharynx, and cervical esophagus spread to levels VI and VII. In addition to the lower lip, the supraglottis, base of the tongue, and soft palate have a high incidence of bilateral metastases.

Therapeutic Options

Therapeutic options for patients with HNSCC include surgery, radiation therapy, chemotherapy, and combination regimens. In general, early-stage disease (stage I or II) is treated by surgery or radiation therapy. Late-stage disease (stage III or IV) is best treated by a combination of surgery and radiation therapy or chemotherapy and radiation therapy, or all three modalities, depending on the site of the primary. Because surgery was the first therapeutic option available to physicians, it has the longest track record of the three and established the head and neck surgeon as the leader of the treatment team for HNSCC. Photon irradiation is superior to surgery for eradicating microscopic disease and is an excellent alternative to surgery for early lesions. Tonsil, tongue base, and nasopharyngeal primary tumors are especially responsive to photon irradiation. Neutron and proton irradiation are used much less often in the head and neck, although experience has grown with their role in salivary gland malignancies (neutron irradiation) and skull base cancers (proton irradiation). Electrons are not commonly used in the head and neck for noncutaneous tumors. With the advent of intensity-modulated radiation therapy, which can reduce the photon dosage to surrounding normal tissue through computer three-dimensional planning, the dogma that patients may not receive more than 7200 cGy to tissue of the head and neck has been called into question. Hyperfractionation is the practice of administering radiation more than once daily, and results of the European Organization for Research and Treatment of Cancer determined that hyperfractionation for HNSCC produces greater locoregional control than conventional once-daily regimens.[13] Radiation therapy is not as effective in treating large-volume, low-grade neoplasms or tumors in close proximity to the mandible because of the risk for osteoradionecrosis. The loss of salivary function with irradiation of the oral and oropharyngeal cavity can be disabling to patients, and its impact should not be minimized in the decision-making process.

A landmark chemotherapy trial for HNSCC was the Department of Veterans Affairs larynx trial, published in 1991.[14] Although chemotherapy alone is not curative in HNSCC, its role as a radiation sensitizer was established in this study. Two thirds of patients treated with radiation therapy and chemotherapy were able to keep their larynx, and survival was equal to patients treated with laryngectomy and radiation therapy. Recurrences after radiation therapy were shown to be multifocal in the bed of the original tumor, and the salvage surgeon should be familiar with the original tumor location and volume. Chemotherapy is commonly used in the treatment of incurable HNSCC, such as unresectable and metastatic disease, and can provide excellent symptom control in these patients.

Data from two large-scale, independent trials examined the benefit of adding chemotherapy to postoperative irradiation for HNSCC.[15,16] The European Organization for Research and Treatment of Cancer Trial and the Radiation Therapy Oncology Group 9501/Intergroup treated advanced-stage, high-risk patients with cisplatin concurrently with postoperative radiation therapy and compared the outcomes with patients undergoing postoperative irradiation alone. In the Radiation Therapy Oncology Group, the 2-year locoregional control rate was 82% for the group receiving chemoradiation therapy versus 72% for the radiation therapy–alone group. Disease-free survival was significantly longer in the chemoradiation therapy patients, although overall survival was not significantly different between the groups. Significantly more toxicity and treatment morbidity were seen in the combined-treatment group, and further prognostic indicators to determine which patients are at high risk for failure are needed to predict which groups warrant this more intensive adjuvant therapy.

The neck should be treated when there are clinically positive nodes or the risk for occult disease is more than 20%, based on the location and stage of the primary lesion. The decision to perform neck dissection or irradiate the neck is related to treatment of the primary lesion. If the index tumor is being treated with radiation, and the neck is N0 (no clinically detectable disease) or N1, the nodes are usually treated with irradiation. For surgically treated primary lesions, N0 or N1 neck disease may also be treated surgically. Negative prognostic factors such as extracapsular spread of tumor, perineural invasion, vascular invasion, fixation to surrounding structures, and multiple positive nodes are indicators for postoperative adjuvant radiation therapy. For N2 or N3 neck disease, neck dissection with planned postoperative radiation therapy is performed. When chemoradiation therapy protocols are used in treating the primary lesion and there is a complete response in the primary tumor and an N2 or N3 neck, planned neck dissection 8 weeks after chemoradiation therapy can contain cancer in one third of specimens.[17] If the neck mass persists, the percentage of residual disease increases to two thirds. When patients have advanced neck disease that involves the carotid artery or deep neck musculature, radiation or chemoradiation therapy is administered preoperatively in the hope that the tumor will reduce in size and become resectable. CT scans carry a high false-positive rate for determining carotid encasement. When carotid resection is necessary, the associated morbidity is high (major neurologic injury in 17%), with a 22% 2-year survival rate, and the decision to resect should be weighed carefully.

Radical neck dissection (RND) was attributed to Crile in 1906 and was considered the gold standard for the removal of nodal metastases (Fig. 33-4). Through a subsequent close reading of Crile's surgical notes, it was found that he had begun to modify his surgical technique to remove only selected regions of the neck, depending on the site of the primary tumor; this has become common surgical practice for HNSCC at the present time. All modifications of neck dissection are described in relation to the standard RND, which removes nodal levels I through V and the sternocleidomastoid muscle, internal jugular vein, cranial nerve XI, cervical plexus, and submandibular gland. Preservation of the sternocleidomastoid muscle, internal jugular vein, or cranial nerve XI in any combination is referred to as a modified RND, and the structures preserved are specified for nomenclature. A modified neck dissection may also be referred to as a Bocca neck dissection, named after the surgeon who demonstrated that not only is modified RND equally as effective in controlling neck disease as RND when structures are preserved that are not directly involved in tumor, but also the functional outcomes of patients after modified RND are superior to functional outcomes after RND.[18] Although resection of the sternocleidomastoid muscle or one internal jugular vein is relatively nonmorbid, loss of cranial nerve XI leaves a denervated trapezius muscle, which can cause a painful chronic frozen shoulder.

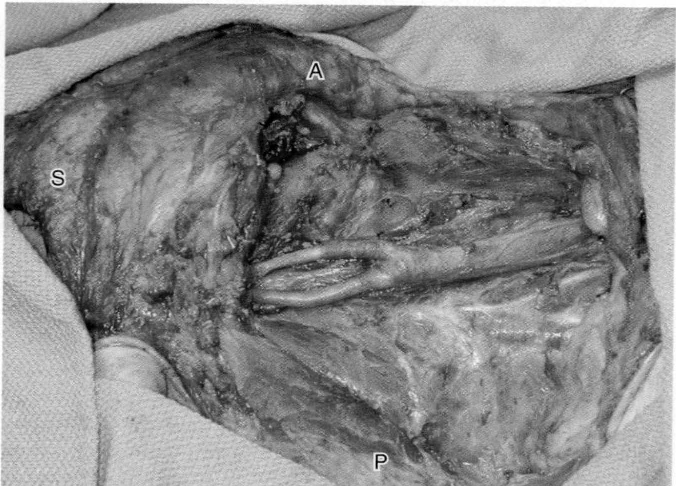

FIGURE 33-4 Proper appearance of the right neck after a radical neck dissection. In addition to all lymphatic tissue, the three structures of the internal jugular vein, sternocleidomastoid muscle, and spinal accessory nerve have been resected. *A*, anterior; *P*, posterior; *S*, superior.

RND or modified RND can be performed for removal of detectable nodal disease. Preservation of any of levels I through V during neck dissection is referred to as selective neck dissection and is based on knowledge of the patterns of spread to neck regions. Selective neck dissection is performed on a clinically negative (N0) neck, with preservation of nodal groups carrying less than a 20% chance of being involved with metastatic disease. Regional control has been shown to be as effective after selective neck dissection as after modified RND in patients with a clinically negative neck. Studies evaluating treatment of an N0 neck investigated the use of sentinel lymph node biopsy, which attempts to predict the disease status of the neck based on the first echelon of nodes that drain the tumor.[19] Although sentinel lymph node biopsy has been used extensively with melanoma, its use in HNSCC has come about more gradually. Early results using isosulfan blue dye alone suggested that this technique cannot consistently identify the sentinel node in HNSCC. More recent results using a gamma probe were more encouraging, although the isolated node should be serial step–sectioned at a thickness of 150 nm and be examined through permanent processing. Recommendations at the present time are that the technique should be restricted to early-stage (T1 or T2) oral and oropharyngeal cancers, with clinically N0 necks; the gamma probe continues to be an investigational tool pending validation by large randomized clinical trials.

ANATOMIC SITES

Lip

Anatomically, the lip is considered a subsite of the oral cavity. The lip begins at the junction of the vermilion border and skin and is composed of the vermilion surface, which refers to the mucosa that contacts the opposing lip. It is divided into the upper lip, lower lip, and oral commissures. Most lip cancers occur on the lower lip (90% to 95%), and cancers occur less often on the upper lip (2% to 7%) and commissures (1%). Lip cancer develops most commonly in white men 50 to 80 years old. Sun exposure and pipe smoking are associated with lip cancer. Although SCC is the most common lip cancer (90%), the most common cancer of the upper lip is basal cell carcinoma. Other lip cancers include variants of SCC (e.g., spindle cell and adenoid squamous carcinoma), mucosal melanoma, and minor salivary gland cancers.

The most common clinical manifestation of lip cancer is an ulcerative lesion on the vermilion or skin surface. Palpation is necessary to determine the submucosal extent of the lesion and possible fixation to underlying bone. Sensation of the chin should be tested to determine involvement of the mental nerve. Poor prognostic indicators include nerve involvement, fixation to the maxilla or mandible, cancer arising on the upper lip or commissure, positive nodal disease, and age younger than 40 years at diagnosis. The most frequently involved nodal basins are the submental and submandibular levels. A depth of tumor invasion of 4 mm has been shown to be a cutoff above which the incidence of cervical nodal disease is significantly increased.[20]

Similar to the rest of the oral cavity, lip cancer staging is based on size at initial evaluation. Early-stage disease may be treated by surgery or radiation therapy with equal success. Local surgery (wide local excision) with negative margin control of at least 3 mm is the preferred treatment, with supraomohyoid neck dissection performed for tumors with clinically negative necks but deeper primary invasion or size larger than 3 cm. Neck dissection with postoperative radiation therapy for patients with clinically evident neck disease has an acceptable 91% regional control rate in the neck.[21] The overall 5-year cure rate of 90% decreases to 50% in the presence of neck metastases. Postoperative irradiation is also indicated for advanced-stage primary disease, tumors with perineural involvement, or close or positive margins at the time of resection.

Goals of lip reconstruction include reinstitution of oral competence, cosmesis, and maintenance of dynamic function, while allowing adequate access for oral hygiene. The surgeon can remove up to half of the lip and still close the defect primarily, particularly defects in the lower lip, which contains more excess tissue than the upper lip. A lower lip wedge excision should not be carried below the mental crease unless the tumor dictates its excision. Care is taken to achieve close approximation of the white line on either side of the defect at the vermilion border because the eye is drawn to any mismatch that exists at this critical esthetic location.

Defects encompassing between one half and two thirds of the lip require augmentation. The Estlander and Abbé flaps are lip switch flaps based on the sublabial or superior labial artery. The Estlander flap is used when the defect involves the commissure, whereas the Abbé flap is used for more midline defects and requires second-stage division of the pedicle (Fig. 33-5). The Karapandzic flap consists of circumoral incisions with circular rotation of the skin flaps, while maintaining innervation of the orbicularis oris musculature. This one-stage procedure is used for defects involving more than two thirds of the lip. Microstomia is a potential complication from these types of flap reconstructions, and denture use may be impossible. For defects larger than two thirds, the Webster, Gillies, or Bernard types of repairs may also be used.

Oral Cavity

Because the oral cavity begins at the skin-vermilion junction, the lips are considered part of the oral cavity for staging purposes. Other subsites in the oral cavity include the buccal mucosa, upper and lower alveolar ridges, retromolar trigone, floor of the mouth, hard palate, and oral tongue. The tongue is divided into the oral tongue (two thirds of the tongue volume), anterior to the circumvallate papillae, and the base of tongue, which is not considered part of the oral cavity but rather the oropharynx. Staging of the oral cavity is based on size: T1, 0 to 2 cm; T2, 2 to 4 cm; T3, 4 to 6 cm; and T4, tumors larger than 6 cm or invading adjacent structures, including bone (cortical bone of the mandible or maxilla, not superficial erosion or tooth sockets), deep tongue musculature, or facial skin. SCC accounts for 90% of tumors located in these subsites, with a male preponderance in the fifth and sixth decades of life. There is a close association with alcohol and tobacco abuse.

Oral Tongue

The oral tongue begins at the junction between the tongue and floor of mouth and extends posteriorly to the circumvallate papillae. Tumors appear as exophytic, ulcerative, or submucosal masses that may be associated with tenderness or irritation with

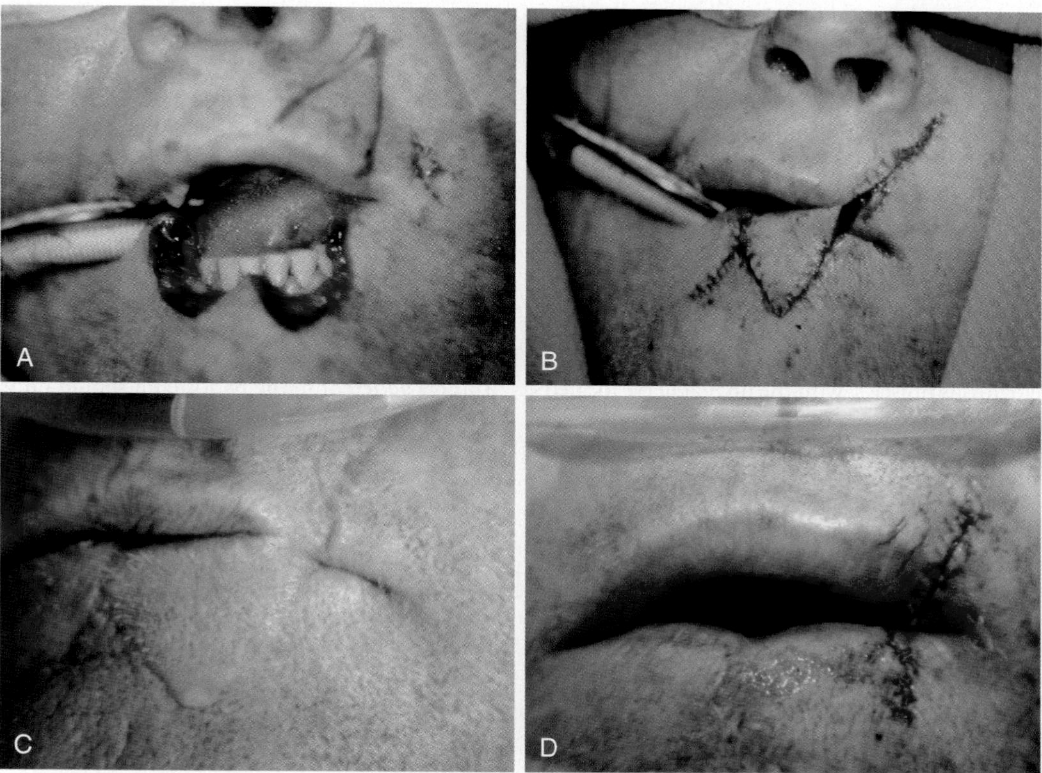

FIGURE 33-5 A, Squamous cell carcinoma resected from the lower lip, leaving approximately 25% of normal tissue. **B,** Abbé flap uses upper lip tissue pedicled on the labial artery. **C,** Before division of the flap after 6 weeks of healing. **D,** Appearance after pedicle division.

mastication. Benign tumors tend to be submucosal and include leiomyomas, neurofibromas, and granular cell tumors. Although granular cell tumors can arise in the larynx, they occur more frequently in the tongue and can be confused with SCC because of overlying pseudoepitheliomatous hyperplasia. Complete excision is curative, but histologic borders are notorious for extending beyond gross disease, and negative intraoperative margins are mandatory.

SCC is the most common type of malignancy, but leiomyosarcomas and rhabdomyosarcomas are also encountered (rarely). Neurotropic malignancies may involve the lingual or hypoglossal nerves, so tongue deviation or loss of sensation should be examined closely. Treatment of oral tongue cancer is primarily surgical, with wide local excision and negative margin control. The development of cervical metastases is related to the depth of invasion, perineural spread, advanced T stage, and tumor differentiation. Infiltration of more than 4 to 5 mm into the tongue musculature increases the incidence of occult cervical metastases. Metastases from the anterior of the tongue most frequently spread to the submental and submandibular regions. Tumors located more posteriorly often metastasize to levels II and III. Indications for postoperative radiation therapy include evidence of perineural or angiolymphatic spread or positive nodal disease.

Small tumors may be removed by wide local excision and primary closure or closure by secondary intention. Excision of larger tumors requires partial glossectomy or hemiglossectomy. Extirpation may result in significant dysfunction in terms of disarticulation and dysphagia from an inability to contact the palate, sense oral contents, or manipulate the tongue against the alveolus or lips. Reconstructive efforts should focus on maintaining tongue mobility without excess bulk. Split-thickness skin grafts, primary closure, or healing by secondary intention of larger tongue defects often results in tongue tethering. Thin, pliable fasciocutaneous flaps (e.g., the radial forearm free flap) are the preferred reconstructive technique for such defects. A palatal augmentation prosthesis may assist in maintaining palatal contact, which is important for speech and posterior propulsion of food boluses.

Floor of the Mouth

The floor of the mouth extends from the inner surface of the mandible medially to the ventral surface of the tongue and from the anteriormost frenulum posteriorly to the anterior tonsillar pillars. The mucosa of the floor of the mouth contains the openings of the sublingual gland and submandibular gland (via Wharton's ducts). The muscular floor comprises the genioglossus, mylohyoid, and hyoglossus muscles, with the lingual nerve located immediately submucosally.

Bimanual palpation can often determine fixation of tumors of the floor of the mouth to the mandible. CT demonstrates the depth of mandibular bony invasion, and widening of the cranial neural foramen, such as the foramen ovale, suggests neurotropic intracranial spread in advanced tumors. Determining mandibular invasion is of utmost importance for preoperative planning (Fig. 33-6). Invasion into the tongue musculature necessitates partial glossectomy concurrently with removal of the lesion on the floor of the mouth.

Treatment of lesions on the floor of the mouth is primarily surgical, with excision of the involved tongue or mandible as necessary to obtain negative margins. Removal of bone with soft tissue in continuity is commonly referred to as a commando or composite resection. Involvement of the neck may occur by direct extension of tumor through the floor of the mouth musculature or by lymphatic spread. The primary lesion and neck specimen should be taken in continuity so that accompanying lymphatic channels are resected. Adjuvant radiation therapy has similar indications as in oral tongue cancers. The primary goal of reconstruction is separation of the oral cavity from the neck by creating a watertight oral closure. This prevents orocutaneous salivary fistula formation. Secondary goals are maintaining tongue mobility, creating a lingual-alveolar sulcus, and preserving mandibular continuity. Local flaps for soft tissue reconstruction include the platysmal and submental myocutaneous pedicled flaps. Larger defects, including mandibular resection, require complex reconstruction, which is most often performed with free flaps.

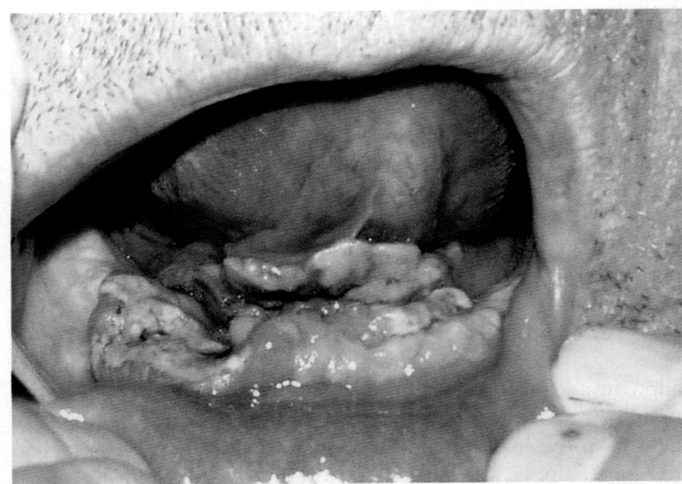

FIGURE 33-6 A 62-year-old man with squamous cell carcinoma of the anterior floor of the mouth invading the mandible.

Alveolus

The alveolus and its accompanying gingiva constitute the dental surfaces of the maxilla and mandible and extend from the gingivobuccal sulcus laterally to the floor of the mouth and hard palate medially. Posteriorly, the alveolus extends to the pterygopalatine arch and ascending ramus of the mandible, also referred to as the retromolar trigone. Because of the tight attachment between the mucosa and the underlying bone, treatment of alveolar SCC often involves treatment of the maxilla or mandible. Of gingival carcinomas, 70% occur on the lower gum. The periosteum of the mandible is a strong tumor barrier, and tumors that abut the bone often may be resected along with the adjacent periosteum only. Tumors adherent to the periosteum should undergo excision with marginal mandibulectomy, which involves resection of the superior or inner cortical portions of the mandible, with preservation of a continuous rim. Even superficial tumors that invade the outermost part of the mandible may be resected with a marginal mandibulectomy, although this is not oncologically sound if the tumor is a recurrence after radiation therapy. Segmental mandibulectomy entails excision of the full thickness of the mandible, interrupting mandibular continuity, and is indicated for patients with gross bone invasion by tumor. Primary radiation therapy for mandibular tumors is not a viable treatment option because of the high likelihood of osteoradionecrosis and poor response of involved bone to radiation therapy.

Buccal Mucosa

The buccal mucosa extends from the inner surface of the opposing surfaces of the lips to the alveolar ridges and pterygomandibular raphe. Buccal cancer is uncommon and represents 5% of all oral cavity carcinomas. Causative factors associated with buccal cancer include smoking, alcohol abuse, lichen planus, dental trauma, snuff dipping, and tobacco chewing. Approximately 65% of patients with buccal cancer are initially found to have extension beyond the cheek mucosa. Lymphatic drainage is to the submandibular lymph nodes; however, tumors in the posterior aspect of the cheek may spread to level II initially. Stage I cancers historically were treated by surgery and did not involve elective neck dissection because of the low rate of occult metastases. However, more recent studies suggested high rates of local recurrence for lesions treated by surgery alone, and adjuvant radiation therapy has been suggested even for early-stage lesions.[22] Deep invasion may require through and through excision of cheek skin, necessitating internal and external linings, usually with a fasciocutaneous free flap.

Palate

The hard palate is defined as the area medial to the maxillary alveolar ridges and extending posterior to the edge of the palatine bone. Chronic inflammatory lesions such as viral lesions, zoster, and pemphigoid can mimic neoplasms, and biopsy is indicated for persistent lesions. Necrotizing sialometaplasia is a benign, self-limited process of the minor salivary glands that has a predilection for the palate and can clinically mimic malignancy. The most common intraoral site for Kaposi sarcoma is the palate in immunosuppressed patients. Torus palatinus is a benign exostosis of the midline hard palate and may require surgery if it interferes with denture wearing.

Minor salivary gland tumors, along with SCC, make up most hard palate tumors. Adenoid cystic carcinoma, mucoepidermoid carcinoma, adenocarcinoma, and polymorphous low-grade adenocarcinoma are common malignancies of salivary gland origin that tend to arise at the junction of the hard and soft palate. Malignancies of the hard palate are treated by local excision, if found early, but most commonly require resection of bone because of close adherence of the mucosa to the palate. Inferior maxillectomy, subtotal maxillectomy, or total maxillectomy is indicated for progressively destructive tumors extending into the maxillary antrum. Adjuvant radiation therapy is given for advanced lesions. Reconstruction may be accomplished with soft tissue flaps for small defects, obturation with a dental prosthesis for defects with some remaining hard palate, or bony free tissue transfer for extensive palatal resections.

Oropharynx

The borders of the oropharynx include the circumvallate papillae anteriorly, plane of the superior surface of the soft palate superiorly, plane of the hyoid bone inferiorly, pharyngeal constrictors laterally and posteriorly, and medial aspect of the mandible laterally. The oropharynx includes the base of the tongue, inferior surface of the soft palate and uvula, anterior and posterior tonsillar pillars, glossotonsillar sulci, pharyngeal tonsils, and lateral and posterior pharyngeal walls. Similar to the oral cavity, T staging in the oropharynx depends on size. T4 tumors may extend out of the oropharynx posteriorly into the parapharyngeal space, inferiorly into the larynx, or laterally into the mandible.

Of tumors of the oropharynx, 90% are SCCs. Other tumors include lymphoma of the tonsils or tongue base or salivary gland neoplasms arising from minor salivary glands in the soft palate or tongue base. Initial symptoms include sore throat, bleeding, dysphagia and odynophagia, referred otalgia, and voice changes including a muffled quality or "hot potato" voice. Trismus suggests involvement of the pterygoid musculature. Imaging studies should focus on invasion through the pharyngeal constrictors, bony involvement of the pterygoid plates or mandible, invasion of the parapharyngeal space or carotid artery, involvement of the prevertebral fascia, and extension into the larynx. Lymph node metastases generally occur in the upper jugular chain (levels II to IV), although lesions may skip to lower levels and spread to level V; such lesions are more common with oropharyngeal tumors than with tumors of the oral cavity. Bilateral metastases are more common with tongue base and soft palate lesions, especially those with midline lesions.

Treatment of oropharyngeal SCC has focused increasingly on conservation therapy with chemotherapy and radiation therapy. Many tumors of the oropharynx are poorly differentiated and respond well to radiation. Chemotherapy has been used as a radiation sensitizer in numerous studies, and the local control rate achieved has been 90%, even in stage IV disease, although overall survival has not improved over more traditional surgery and radiation therapy.[23] A study of the cause of tonsil and tongue base cancers suggested that when the disease is associated with HPV infection, the prognosis is significantly improved over non-HPV tumors. In a phase II trial of investigational therapy in patients with oropharyngeal and laryngeal cancers (Eastern Cooperative Oncology Group study 2399), patients with HPV-positive tumors had a 73% reduction in risk of progression and a 64% reduction in risk of death compared with HPV-negative patients.[24] This landmark study was the first to demonstrate that tumor HPV status is a strong and favorable prognostic marker in uniform patient populations with similar treatment protocols. Many physicians have advised that tumor HPV status should be incorporated as a stratification factor in patients with oropharyngeal cancer, although basing treatment protocols on HPV status has yet to be definitively investigated.

Surgery is necessary for primary disease that involves the mandible and for resectable recurrent disease, and it has a role in very early superficial tumors that do not justify a full course of radiation therapy. Extensive surgery of the tongue base significantly alters a patient's ability to swallow. Reconstruction of the tongue with preservation of the larynx requires surgical techniques that maintain tongue mobility and suspend the larynx and neotongue to prevent aspiration.

Resection or contracture after irradiation of the soft palate may result in velopharyngeal insufficiency, which is manifested clinically as nasal regurgitation of liquids and solids and hypernasal speech. Augmentation of the soft palate may be performed surgically or via palatal obturation. Although a palatal obturator requires cleaning and is not permanent, patients can remove it for sleep. With surgical augmentation of the palate, a balance between reducing velopharyngeal insufficiency and causing obstructive sleep apnea is difficult to achieve. After tongue base resection, an inferiorly directed palatal obturator assists in achieving the contact at the tongue base that is necessary for the projection of food posteriorly during the oral and pharyngeal phases of swallowing.

Hypopharynx

The hypopharynx is the portion of the pharynx that extends inferiorly from the horizontal plane of the top of the hyoid bone to a horizontal plane extending posteriorly from the inferior border of the cricoid cartilage. The hypopharynx includes both piriform sinuses, lateral and posterior hypopharyngeal walls, and the postcricoid region. The postcricoid area extends inferiorly from the two arytenoid cartilages to the inferior border of the cricoid cartilage, connecting the piriform sinuses and forming the anterior hypopharyngeal wall. The piriform sinuses are inverted, pyramid-shaped potential spaces medial to the thyroid lamina; they begin at the pharyngoepiglottic folds and extend to the cervical esophagus at the inferior border of the cricoid cartilage.

Hypopharyngeal cancer is more common in men 55 to 70 years old with a history of alcohol abuse and smoking. The exception is in the postcricoid area, in which cancers are more common worldwide in women; this is directly related to Plummer-Vinson syndrome, a combination of dysphagia, hypopharyngeal and esophageal webs, weight loss, and iron deficiency anemia, usually occurring in middle-aged women. In patients who fail to undergo treatment consisting of dilation, iron replacement, and vitamin therapy, postcricoid carcinoma may develop just proximal to the web.

Hypopharyngeal tumors manifest as a chronic sore throat, dysphagia, referred otalgia, and a foreign body sensation in the throat. A high index of suspicion should be maintained because similar symptoms may be seen with the more common gastroesophageal reflux disease. In advanced disease, hoarseness may develop from direct involvement of the arytenoid, recurrent laryngeal nerve, or paraglottic space. The rich lymphatics that drain the hypopharyngeal region contribute to the fact that 70% of patients with hypopharyngeal cancer are initially seen with palpable lymphadenopathy. Patients with hypopharyngeal cancer have the highest rate of synchronous malignancies and the highest rate of development of second HNSCC primaries of any of the head and neck sites. Staging for hypopharyngeal cancer is based on the number of involved subsites or size of the tumor.

Physical examination for hypopharyngeal lesions includes fiberoptic endoscopy. Having the patient blow against closed lips and pinching the nose closed inflates the potential spaces of the piriformis and assists in visualization of the tumor. Palpation of the larynx may demonstrate a loss of laryngeal crepitus. A fixed larynx suggests posterior extension into the prevertebral fascia and unresectability. Barium swallow may demonstrate mucosal abnormalities associated with an exophytic tumor and is useful for determining the extent of involvement of the cervical esophagus. It also assists in determining the presence and amount of aspiration present. CT can be used to determine the presence of thyroid cartilage invasion, direct extension into the neck, and pathologic lymphadenopathy. Biopsy of the hypopharynx usually requires direct laryngoscopy under general anesthesia.

The most common area for lymphatic spread is the upper jugular nodes, even with inferior tumors. Other regions include the paratracheal and retropharyngeal nodes. The presence of contralateral cervical metastases or level V involvement is a grave prognostic indicator. Treatment of hypopharyngeal cancer yields poor results compared with other sites in the head and neck, presumably because of the late stage of the disease at diagnosis. For early lesions confined to the medial wall of the piriform or posterior pharyngeal wall, radiation or chemoradiation therapy is effective as a primary treatment modality. Seldom is laryngeal-sparing partial pharyngectomy possible. Small tumors of the medial piriform wall or pharyngoepiglottic fold may be amenable to conservation surgery, but they must not involve the piriform apex, and the patient must have mobile vocal cords and adequate pulmonary reserve.

The most common treatment of hypopharyngeal cancer is laryngopharyngectomy and bilateral neck dissection, including the paratracheal compartments, along with adjuvant radiation therapy. Trials of neoadjuvant chemotherapy followed by concomitant chemotherapy and radiation therapy have shown promise in organ preservation in hypopharyngeal cancer.[25] The estimated 5-year laryngeal preservation rate is 35%, and induction chemotherapy appears to decrease the rate of death from distant metastases.

After total laryngectomy and partial pharyngectomy, primary closure may be possible if at least 4 cm of viable pharyngeal mucosa remains. Primary closure using less than 4 cm of mucosa generally leads to stricture and an inability to swallow effectively. A pedicled cutaneous flap such as a pectoralis myocutaneous flap can be used to augment any remaining mucosa in these cases. When total laryngopharyngectomy with esophagectomy has been performed, a gastric pull-up may be used for reconstruction. More recently, free flap reconstruction with enteric flaps or tubed cutaneous flaps, such as radial forearm or anterolateral thigh flaps, has been used to reconstruct the total pharyngectomy defect.

Larynx

The three-dimensional boundaries of the larynx are complex, and exact definitions are necessary before understanding the pathologic conditions affecting this organ system. The anterior border of the larynx is composed of the lingual surface of the epiglottis, thyrohyoid membrane, anterior commissure, and anterior wall of the subglottis, which consists of the thyroid cartilage, cricothyroid membrane, and anterior arch of the cricoid cartilage. The posterior and lateral limits of the larynx are the arytenoids and interarytenoid region, aryepiglottic folds, and posterior wall of the subglottis, which is composed of the mucosa covering the cricoid cartilage. The superior limits are the tip and lateral borders of the epiglottis. The inferior limit is made up of the plane passing through the inferior edge of the cricoid cartilage.

For staging purposes, the larynx is divided into three regions—supraglottis, glottis, and subglottis. The supraglottis is composed of the epiglottis, laryngeal surfaces of the aryepiglottic folds, arytenoids, and false vocal folds. In addition to these supraglottic subsites, the epiglottis is divided into the suprahyoid and infrahyoid epiglottis, for a total of five supraglottic subsites. The inferior limit of the supraglottis is a horizontal plane through the ventricles, which is the lateral recess between the true and false vocal folds. This plane is also the superior border of the glottis; this is composed of the superior and inferior surfaces of the true vocal folds, extends inferiorly from the true vocal folds, and is 1 cm thick. Also included in the glottis are the anterior and posterior commissures. The subglottis extends from the lower border of the glottis to the lower margin of the cricoid cartilage.

Innervation of the larynx includes the superior laryngeal nerve, which supplies the cricothyroid and inferior constrictor muscles and contains afferent sensory fibers from the mucosa of the false vocal folds and piriform sinuses. The recurrent laryngeal nerve supplies motor innervation to all the intrinsic muscles of the larynx and sensation to the mucosa of the true vocal folds, subglottic region, and adjacent esophageal mucosa. The normal functions of the larynx are to provide airway patency, protect the tracheobronchial tree from aspiration, provide resistance for Valsalva maneuvers and coughing, and facilitate phonation. Tumors that involve the larynx impair these functions to a variable degree, depending on location, size, and depth of invasion.

Glottic tumors are often manifested early as hoarseness because the vibratory edge of the true vocal fold is normally responsible for the quality of the voice and is sensitive to even small lesions. Signs of airway compromise occur later in disease progression,

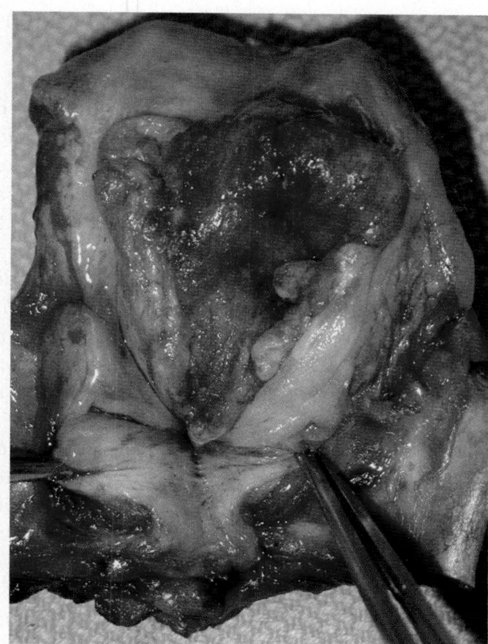

FIGURE 33-7 Pathologic specimen from a supracricoid laryngectomy for squamous cell carcinoma. The tumor involves almost the entire laryngeal surface of the epiglottis as well as the anterior commissure of the true vocal folds. Both vocal folds have been resected back to the vocal processes of the arytenoids, which are preserved to continue phonation and protect the airway from aspiration.

when tumor bulk obstructs the glottic opening. Impaired movement of the vocal fold may cause hoarseness, aspiration, impaired cough, or obstructive symptoms. Impaired movement is caused by tumor bulk, direct invasion of the thyroarytenoid muscle, invasion of the cricoarytenoid joint, or invasion of the recurrent nerve. Hemoptysis occurs with hemorrhagic lesions.

Compared with glottic tumors, supraglottic lesions are relatively indolent and are initially seen at a later stage of disease (Fig. 33-7). Patients often complain of a sore throat or odynophagia. Referred otalgia is caused by Arnold's nerve, the vagal branch that supplies part of the ear sensation. Bulky tumors of the epiglottis are often associated with a "hot potato" or muffled voice quality because of airway compromise. Dysphagia may cause weight loss and malnutrition. Subglottic tumors are rare and most often manifest as airway obstruction, vocal fold immobility, or pain.

The respiratory and squamous epithelia of the larynx are most often the cause of benign and malignant laryngeal neoplasms. Laryngeal papillomatosis is a benign exophytic growth of squamous epithelium with a tendency to recur, despite surgical excision. It has a bimodal distribution, referred to as the juvenile type and adult type. Granular cell tumors are also benign but may be confused with SCC because of a characteristic pseudoepitheliomatous hyperplasia that overlies this subepithelial lesion. Less frequent benign lesions include chondromas and rhabdomyomas. Non-neoplastic lesions of the larynx include vocal fold nodules and polyps, contact ulcers, subglottic stenosis, amyloidosis, and sarcoidosis. Finally, with exposure to carcinogens (e.g., tobacco), the epithelium of the larynx may undergo a series of precancerous changes, clinically referred to as leukoplakia (any white lesion of the mucosa) or erythroplakia (a red lesion), that consist of hyperplasia, metaplasia, or variable degrees of dysplasia.

The most common malignant lesion of the larynx is SCC, which is often classified as SCC in situ, microinvasive SCC, or invasive SCC. Spindle cell carcinoma and basaloid SCC are rare and represent more aggressive variants of SCC. Verrucous carcinoma is a highly differentiated variant of SCC that is locally destructive but does not metastasize and should respond to complete surgical excision. The nonepithelial components of the larynx may also undergo malignant transformation, leading to tumors of salivary origin such as adenocarcinoma, adenoid cystic carcinoma, and mucoepidermoid carcinoma. Other tumors include neuroendocrine carcinoma, adenosquamous carcinoma, chondrosarcoma, synovial sarcoma, and distant metastases from other organ systems.

The staging system for laryngeal cancers is based on subsite involvement and vocal fold mobility. The office examination includes flexible laryngoscopy to assess the location and functional impairment. Stroboscopic laryngoscopy can detect subtle impairment of true fold mucosal waves that suggest significant tumor penetration. Direct laryngoscopy under anesthesia allows examination of all laryngeal subsites, along with the ability to perform biopsy. Specific sites that are important to examine in supraglottic tumors include the ventricle, anterior commissure, vallecula, base of the tongue, piriform sinus, and preepiglottic space. Key areas of glottic involvement include the false vocal fold, ventricle, anterior commissure, arytenoids, subglottis, and posterior commissure or postcricoid mucosa. Under general anesthesia, paralysis of the vocal fold is differentiated from arytenoid fixation by palpation of the vocal process portion of the arytenoid.

CT is routinely performed for laryngeal lesions and images the preepiglottic and paraglottic regions and extent of cartilage involvement as well as determining direct extension into the deep neck structures. For the natural barriers and pathways of direct tumor spread, see the landmark histopathologic work of Kirchner.[26] CT scan should be performed with contrast agents and thin (1.5-mm) cuts through the larynx. Lymph node metastases are also identified by CT. The lymphatic drainage of the larynx differs in the supraglottic and glottic regions. Supraglottic epidermoid cancers metastasize early, with 50% of lesions having positive nodes. Contralateral and bilateral nodal metastases are common with supraglottic lesions because of the embryologic development of the supraglottis as a midline structure. Lymphatic drainage exits along the course of the superior laryngeal neurovascular pedicle and pierces the thyrohyoid membrane to drain to the subdigastric and superior jugular groups of nodes (levels II and III). Lymphatic drainage of tumors in the glottic and subglottic areas exits via the cricothyroid ligament and drains to the prelaryngeal (delphian) node, paratracheal nodes, and deep cervical nodes in the region of the inferior thyroid artery. Tumors confined to the glottis are only rarely associated with regional disease (4%), and positive nodes, when present, are most often ipsilateral.

Decision making in the treatment of laryngeal cancer is governed by tumor location, characteristics of tumor aggressiveness, and the patient's overall constitution and lifestyle. Poor prognostic factors include size, nodal metastasis, perineural invasion, and extracapsular spread. Low-grade epidermoid lesions of the larynx, such as dysplasia and carcinoma in situ, can be managed with local excision, such as microscopic excision of the mucosa. Concurrent denuding of the mucosa of both vocal folds near the anterior commissure can lead to the formation of an anterior web, which reduces voice quality and is a difficult complication to correct. Successful treatment of low-grade lesions includes close follow-up, with repeat office or operative laryngoscopy, and strict smoking cessation. For invasive disease, multiple treatment options are available, including conservation surgery and aggressive surgery, radiation therapy, and chemoradiation therapy. In general, conservation of the larynx in early-stage disease is key and can be accomplished with laryngeal preservation surgery or radiation therapy. Later stage disease that is still confined to the larynx is generally treated by chemoradiation therapy, with total laryngectomy used for salvage.

Laryngeal preservation surgery includes endoscopic surgery with cold steel, endoscopic laser resection, and open surgery, with preservation of some portion of the larynx to maintain the ability to talk. Transoral laser microsurgery, promoted by Ambrosch and colleagues[27] in Germany, has been used to treat not only all stages of laryngeal cancer but also oropharyngeal and hypopharyngeal tumors. Challenging the dogma that non–en bloc resection of tumors promotes locoregional recurrence, these authors demonstrated comparable cancer survival, while decreasing perioperative morbidity. In supraglottic cancers, this group reported 100% 5-year control rates for T1 tumors and 89% 5-year control rates for T2 tumors, with excellent functional outcomes, including minimal aspiration and short recovery periods.[27]

In recurrent glottic tumors after failure of radiation therapy, transoral laser microsurgery demonstrated an overall 3-year survival rate of 74%, comparable to that of total laryngectomy.[28] Although laser microsurgery requires significant technical expertise, acceptance of this oncologic technique has been increasing, changing the approach to upper aerodigestive tract malignancies.

Open conservation laryngeal surgery entails maintaining a conduit for air flow through the remnant of the larynx to permit the ability to talk without aspiration. When deciding whether a patient is a candidate for laryngeal preservation surgery, factors such as pulmonary function and cardiovascular status must be examined because these patients often have to tolerate some amount of aspiration or airway compromise.

Pulmonary function testing, such as spirometry and arterial blood gas analysis, is performed preoperatively. An excellent functional test is to have the patient climb two flights of stairs successively without becoming short of breath. The least invasive of the open procedures is open cordectomy, which is indicated for small midfold lesions and for which 100% 5-year control rates for T1 lesions and 97% 5-year control rates for T2 lesions have been reported.[29] Reconstruction is performed with a false vocal fold flap. For lesions involving the anterior commissure with less than 10 mm of inferior extension, an anterior frontal partial laryngectomy may be performed.

Conservation surgery options for more extensive tumors include vertical partial laryngectomy, supracricoid laryngectomy, and supraglottic laryngectomy. For T1 or T2 glottic lesions, vertical partial laryngectomy plus reconstruction with a false vocal cord pull-down or local muscle flap is indicated, as long as the cartilage is not involved. For T3 lesions not involving the preepiglottic space or arytenoid cartilage, supracricoid laryngectomy with cricohyoidopexy or cricohyoidoepiglottopexy is possible (Fig. 33-8). Excellent disease control has been achieved with this technique, largely because of removal of the paraglottic space and thyroid cartilage. Naudo and coworkers[30] showed that removal of feeding tubes and respiration without a tracheotomy can be achieved in 98% of patients. Standard supraglottic laryngectomy preserves both true vocal folds, both arytenoids, the tongue base, and the hyoid bone (Fig. 33-9). Because there are numerous extensions of this operation, in which more than the standard structures are resected, cure rates are difficult to compare, but, in general, T1 and T2 local control rates range from 85% to 100%, with decreased control for higher stage lesions.

If a decision has been made to undergo nonsurgical therapy, the patient must be able to complete the full course of radiation therapy, which usually includes 5 to 7 weeks of continuous daily therapy visits. Previous irradiation is a contraindication to further radiation therapy. Finally, the patient must be reliable in adhering to follow-up for years after treatment because recurrences may be indolent and difficult to detect.

For neoadjuvant or concurrent chemotherapy, the patient must have sufficient constitutional health to withstand the chemotherapeutic agents. For early laryngeal cancer (T1 or T2), irradiation provides excellent disease control, with good to excellent voice quality after therapy. For professional voice users with early lesions, irradiation is usually the choice of therapy.

The combination of chemotherapy and radiation therapy for advanced-stage disease (stages III and IV) was first brought into the mainstream with the Department of Veterans Affairs larynx trial in 1991.[14] Induction chemotherapy followed by radiation therapy was found to provide 2-year survival equal to that after total laryngectomy with postoperative radiation therapy, in addition to being able to preserve the larynx in 64% of patients. More recent trials with concurrent chemotherapy and radiation therapy demonstrated even better local control of advanced laryngeal cancers. Pretreatment vocal cord fixation does not preclude conservative nonsurgical therapy, but persistent immobility after treatment is a poor prognostic sign, and early surgical intervention should be considered.[31]

In patients who have disease extending outside the larynx, who fail conservative therapy (although some failures may still be amenable to conservation surgery), or who are not otherwise candidates for organ-preserving strategies, total laryngectomy is still commonly performed. It involves a permanent tracheostoma and loss of the voice, with permanent separation of the upper respiratory and digestive tracts.

Patients may experience a period of depression or social withdrawal after becoming aphonic. Speech and swallowing rehabilitation have become an integral part of laryngeal cancer treatment and should begin preoperatively. Speech rehabilitation options include speech with an electrolarynx, esophageal speech, and tracheoesophageal puncture. The electrolarynx is considered the easiest of the three methods to use and consists of a vibratory sound wave generator that is usually placed directly on the submandibular area or cheek. The patient mouths words to produce a monotone, electronic-sounding speech. Becoming understandable can take considerable time and patience.

Esophageal speech is produced by swallowing air into the esophagus and expulsing the air back through the pharynx, which vibrates as the air passes. The ability to master esophageal speech takes a motivated patient to be able to control the release of air through the upper esophageal sphincter, which occurs in only 20% of patients after laryngectomy.

Finally, tracheoesophageal puncture is a surgically created conduit between the tracheal stoma and pharynx that is made at the time of laryngectomy or secondarily. This conduit is fitted with a one-way valve that allows passage of air posteriorly from the trachea to the pharynx but prevents food and liquid from entering anteriorly into the airway. By occluding the stomal opening with the thumb during exhalation, the patient can pass air into the pharynx, which vibrates and allows remarkable clarity of speech. Patients who are good candidates for tracheoesophageal puncture have an 80% success rate of achieving fluent speech.

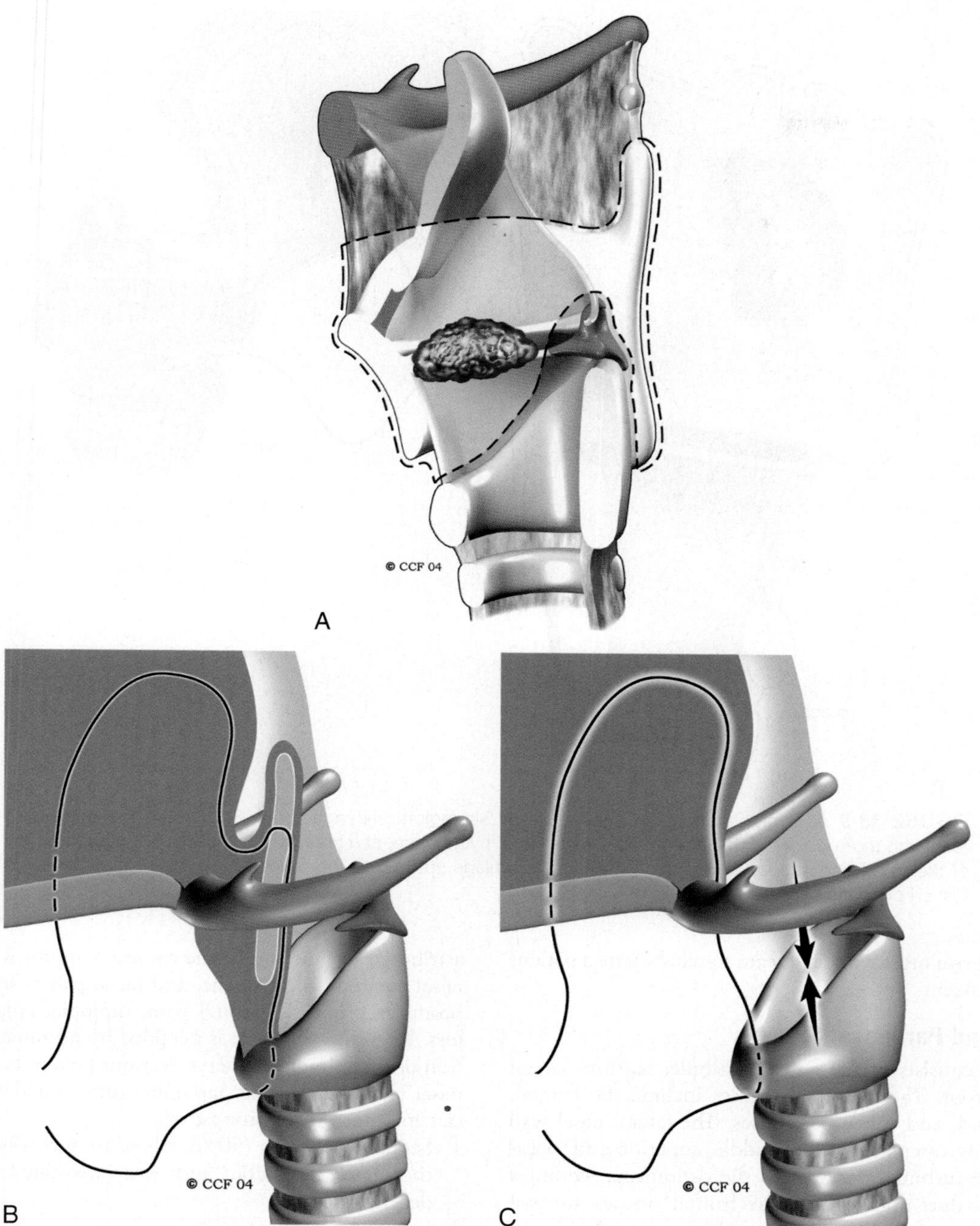

FIGURE 33-8 A, Lesion of the glottis deemed removable by supracricoid laryngectomy. The *dotted line* demonstrates resection of the true vocal fold to the arytenoid cartilages, including the entire laryngeal cartilage and paraglottic spaces laterally. **B,** Reconstruction by cricohyoidoepiglottopexy, with the cricoid cartilage sutured directly to the epiglottic remnant and hyoid bone. **C,** Reconstruction by cricohyoidopexy, with the cricoid sutured to the hyoid bone and tongue base directly. (Courtesy Cleveland Clinic Foundation, 2004.)

Swallowing rehabilitation is a second role of the speech therapist when rehabilitating a patient with laryngeal cancer, whether treated surgically or nonsurgically. Patients who undergo partial laryngectomy may have impaired pharyngeal movement and sensation, impaired vocal fold movement, decreased laryngeal elevation, and decreased subglottic pressure with poor cough, all contributing to possible aspiration.

Specially designed swallowing maneuvers and training in regard to food consistency are offered by the speech therapist to maintain an oral diet, although some patients may require gastric feeding or conversion to total laryngectomy if aspiration persists. Even patients after laryngectomy have difficulty relearning the act of swallowing. Radiation therapy and chemotherapy, although organ-preserving therapies, cause fibrosis, decreased sensation and movement, and decreased lubrication, which have a negative impact on swallowing. Furthermore, because of the exposed circumferential ulcerated mucosa of the pharynx that occurs with chemoradiation therapy, pharyngeal stenosis may develop during the recovery phase and necessitate dilation and pharyngeal augmentation surgery with healthy nonirradiated tissue. The speech

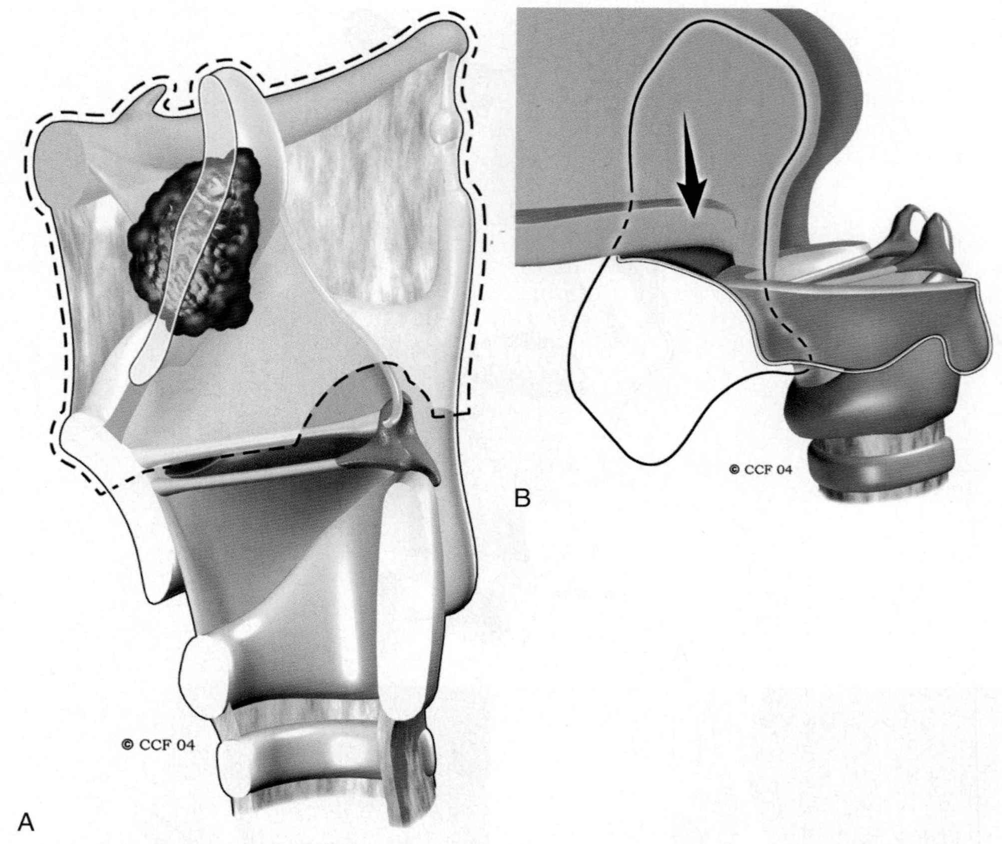

FIGURE 33-9 **A,** Supraglottic lesion, resectable by supraglottic laryngectomy. Shown are the borders of resection *(dotted line)*, including the false vocal folds, hyoid bone, and preepiglottic space. **B,** Reconstruction of the remaining inferior segment of the thyroid cartilage sutured to the tongue base. (Courtesy Cleveland Clinic Foundation, 2004.)

therapist and surgeon must work as a team to rehabilitate a patient with laryngeal cancer.

Nasal Cavity and Paranasal Sinuses

The nasal cavity consists of the nares, vestibule, septum, lateral nasal wall, and roof. The paranasal sinuses include the frontal, maxillary, ethmoid, and sphenoid sinuses. The lateral nasal wall includes the highly vascular inferior, middle, superior, and, occasionally, supreme turbinates as well as the ostiomeatal complex and nasolacrimal duct and orifice. The frontal sinuses are two asymmetrical air cavities within the frontal bone that drain into the nasal cavity via the frontal recesses. The ethmoid sinuses are a complex bony labyrinth directly beneath the anterior cranial fossa. The lamina papyracea is the paper-thin lateral wall of the ethmoid sinus that constitutes the medial wall of the orbit. The anterior ethmoids drain into the middle meatus (inferior to the middle turbinate), whereas the posterior ethmoids drain via the sphenoethmoidal recess. The sphenoid sinus lies in the middle of the sphenoid bone and drains via the sphenoethmoidal recess. The vital structures of the optic nerves, carotid arteries, and cavernous sinuses are contained within the lateral walls of the sphenoid sinus, whereas the sella turcica and optic chiasm lie superiorly within the roof. The maxillary sinuses drain into the middle meatus and are bound posteriorly by the pterygopalatine and infratemporal fossae.

Tumors of the nasal cavity and paranasal sinuses tend to be seen initially at a late stage because their symptoms are often attributed to more mundane causes. Symptoms include epistaxis, nasal congestion, headache, and facial pain. Orbital involvement produces proptosis, orbital pain, diplopia, epiphora, and vision loss. Nerve involvement is heralded by numbness in the distribution of the infraorbital nerve. Various benign tumors occur in the nasal region. Sinonasal papilloma (or schneiderian papilloma) is classified into three groups:

1. Septal papillomas (50%). These tumors arise on the septum; they are exophytic and not associated with malignant degeneration.
2. Inverted papilloma (47%).
3. Cylindrical cell papillomas (3%). These lesions arise on the lateral nasal wall or from the paranasal sinuses and are associated with malignant degeneration (10% to 15%), usually into SCC.

Although previously believed to require radical extirpation, sinonasal papillomas require only local surgical excision with negative margins.

Other benign nasal lesions include hemangioma, benign fibrous histiocytoma, fibromatosis, leiomyoma, ameloblastoma, myxoma, hemangiopericytoma (a benign, aggressive lesion with a tendency to metastasize), fibromyxoma, and fibro-osseous and osseous lesions, such as fibrous dysplasia, ossifying fibroma, and osteoma. Intracranial tissues may extend into the nasal area and give rise to encephaloceles, meningoceles, and pituitary tumors. CT and MRI demonstrate the intracranial connection, and biopsy without previous imaging is unwarranted because of the risk for cerebrospinal fluid (CSF) leakage or uncontrollable bleeding from vascular tumors.

Malignancies of the sinonasal tract represent only 1% of all cancers and 3% of upper respiratory tract malignancies and have a 2 : 1 male-to-female ratio. Because respiratory epithelium can differentiate into squamous or glandular histology, SCC and adenocarcinoma represent two of the most common sinonasal cancers.[4] Sinonasal carcinoma is related to exposure to nickel, Thorotrast (used as a radiographic contrast agent in the United States from about 1930 to the mid-1950s), and softwood dust. Chronic exposure to hardwood dust or leatherworking has been associated with adenocarcinoma of the sinonasal tract. Other malignancies include olfactory neuroblastoma, malignant fibrous histiocytoma, midline malignant reticulosis (also known as lethal midline granuloma or polymorphic reticulosis), osteosarcoma, chondrosarcoma, mucosal melanoma, lymphoma, fibrosarcoma, leiomyosarcoma, angiosarcoma, teratocarcinoma, and metastases from other organ systems (especially renal cell carcinoma).

Since the publication of the 2002 AJCC staging manual, the nasal cavity and ethmoid sinuses have been considered as separate primary sites, in addition to the maxillary sinus.[1] The staging system is only for carcinomatous malignancies and does not include the frontal or sphenoid sinuses as separate sites because of the rarity of tumors arising in these sites. Staging partly depends on local spread of the tumor. Ohngren's line extends from the medial canthus to the mandibular angle. Maxillary tumors superior to Ohngren's line have a poorer prognosis than tumors inferior to the line because of the proximity to the orbit and cranial cavity. Local spread of tumors may occur along nerves or vessels or directly through bone. Advanced tumors of the maxillary sinuses commonly involve the pterygopalatine and infratemporal fossae. Widening of the foramen rotundum (V2) or foramen ovale (V3) on imaging suggests neural spread with intracranial involvement (Fig. 33-10). Because olfactory neuroblastomas are believed to arise from the olfactory neuroepithelium, these tumors commonly involve the cribriform plate and spread intracranially toward the frontal lobes. Sphenoidal tumors may include extension to the cavernous sinuses, carotid arteries, optic nerves, or ophthalmic or maxillary branches of the trigeminal nerves. Lymph node metastases are generally uncommon (15%), and elective neck dissection or irradiation in the case of a clinically negative workup is most often unwarranted. Involved nodal groups include the retropharyngeal, parapharyngeal, submental, and upper jugulodigastric nodes.

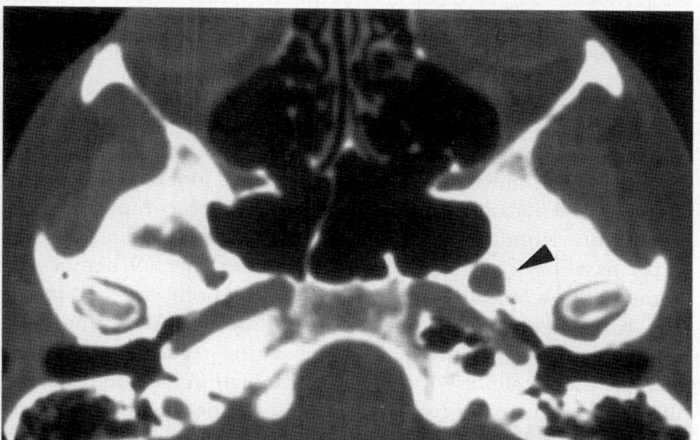

FIGURE 33-10 Computed tomography scan of a 38-year-old woman with adenoid cystic carcinoma demonstrating perineural spread along V3 and widening of the foramen ovale *(arrowhead)*. (Courtesy Dr. J. Netterville.)

The standard treatment of sinonasal malignancies is surgical resection, with postoperative radiation or chemoradiation therapy used for high-grade histology or advanced local disease. Because these cancers can involve the dentition, orbits, or brain, treatment requires a multidisciplinary team, including a head and neck surgeon, neurosurgeon, ophthalmologist, prosthodontist, oral surgeon, and reconstructive surgeon. After a preoperative workup consisting of imaging, endoscopy, and biopsy, a tumor map and operative plan are formulated. Vascular tumors are treated by embolization performed by an interventional radiologist, preferably within 24 hours of surgery. Patients with tumors requiring skull base exploration may need a lumbar drain to decompress the dura from the cranium and reduce the risk for postoperative CSF leakage. Routine prophylactic use of a tracheotomy for craniofacial surgery to reduce the risk for postoperative pneumocephalus is controversial.

Low-grade tumors limited to the lateral nasal wall, ethmoid sinuses, or septum have increasingly been removed with endoscopic techniques. A lateral rhinotomy incision is the classic open approach for a medial maxillectomy and entails removal of the lateral nasal wall. If the tumor involves the inferior maxilla, an inferior maxillectomy, including removal of the hard palate and the medial, lateral, and posterior maxillary sinus walls, is performed. For tumors more superior in the maxillary sinus, a total maxillectomy, including excision of the roof, is performed. If the bone of the floor of the orbit is involved, removal with postoperative reconstruction is indicated. If the orbital periosteum is involved with tumor, it may be resected with preservation of the orbit, although more extensive involvement of fat or muscle necessitates orbital exenteration (Fig. 33-11).[32]

If the anterior cranial floor is involved with tumor, as it often is in olfactory neuroblastomas, craniofacial resection is indicated. This procedure combines a craniotomy approach with a transfacial approach. Surgical disruption of the cribriform region causes postoperative anosmia. Reconstruction of the anterior cranial fossa requires separation of the cranial vault from the nasal cavity with a pericranial flap, temporoparietal fascial flap, fascia lata free graft, or, when extensive resection has been performed, a microvascular free flap. Unresectable lesions include lesions with brain involvement, carotid artery encasement, or bilateral optic nerve involvement.

Radiation therapy and chemotherapy for sinonasal malignancies are being used with increasing frequency. Sinonasal undifferentiated carcinoma, rhabdomyosarcoma, and midline reticulocytosis are examples of aggressive cancers in which neoadjuvant chemotherapy and radiation therapy play an integral role. Combining chemotherapy with radiation therapy and surgery for treatment of advanced sinonasal SCC has met with variable success.

Nasopharynx

The nasopharynx begins at the posterior nasal choana and ends at the horizontal plane between the posterior edge of the hard palate and posterior pharyngeal wall. The nasopharynx includes the vault; lateral walls, which contain the eustachian tube orifices and the fossae of Rosenmüller; roof, which is made up of the sphenoid rostrum; and posterior wall, which consists of the basiocciput or clivus. Malignant and benign tumors of the nasopharynx are usually related to the normal histology, which includes

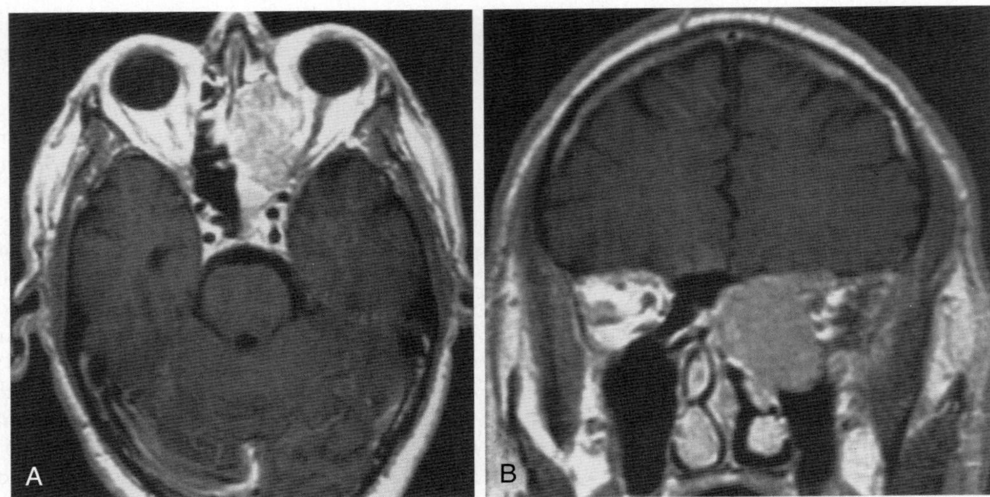

FIGURE 33-11 **A,** Axial magnetic resonance imaging (MRI) scan of a patient with adenosquamous carcinoma of the ethmoids involving the orbital fat. Orbital exenteration was necessary. **B,** Coronal MRI scan of the same patient demonstrating tumor extension to the floor of the anterior cranial fossa. (Courtesy Dr. J. Netterville.)

squamous and respiratory epithelium; the lymphoid tissues of the adenoids; and deeper tissues, including fascia, cartilage, bone, and muscle. Benign tumors of the nasopharynx are rare and include fibromyxomatous polyps, papillomas, teratomas, and pedunculated fibromas. Angiofibroma, a benign tumor that affects young male patients, is the most common benign tumor of the nasopharynx. Rathke's pouch cysts arise high in the nasopharynx at the sphenovomerian junction. The cyst develops from a remnant of ectoderm that normally invaginates to form the anterior pituitary and may become infected later in life. Thornwaldt's bursa is located more inferiorly and arises from a remnant of the caudal notochord; it can contain a jelly-like material. Thornwaldt's bursa may also become infected in later life, and marsupialization is most often all that is required to treat it and Rathke's pouch cysts. Craniopharyngiomas, extracranial meningiomas, encephaloceles, hemangiomas, paragangliomas, chordomas (which can cause extensive destruction), and antral-choanal polyps can also be seen in the nasopharynx.

The clinical findings in patients with nasopharyngeal tumors include symptoms of nasal obstruction, serous otitis with effusion and associated conductive hearing loss, epistaxis, and nasal drainage. Findings such as a cervical mass, headache, otalgia, trismus, and cranial nerve involvement suggest malignancy. Examination of the nasopharynx was historically performed with a mirror and has been greatly improved with the use of a rigid or flexible nasopharyngoscope in the office. CT is excellent for determining bony destruction and widening of foramina. MRI is used to assess soft tissue involvement and intracranial extension as well as nerve, cavernous sinus, and carotid involvement.

Angiofibromas are vascular lesions found exclusively in male patients, usually develop during puberty, and are commonly referred to as juvenile nasopharyngeal angiofibromas. Although they are benign tumors, angiofibromas often erode bone and cause significant structural and functional dysfunction as well as bleeding. CT findings of a nasopharyngeal mass, anterior bowing of the posterior wall of the antrum, erosion of the sphenoid bone, erosion of the hard palate, erosion of the medial wall of the maxillary sinus, and displacement of the nasal septum in an adolescent boy are highly suggestive of angiofibroma (Fig. 33-12). Surgery after embolization is the primary treatment modality, and understanding the location of origin is critical for complete tumor extirpation. Tumors originate at the posterolateral wall of the roof of the nasal cavity, at the sphenopalatine foramen. Whether performed endoscopically or via an open approach, such as lateral rhinotomy or the Caldwell-Luc operation, complete removal of all tumor and bone in the sphenopalatine region is crucial to decrease the possibility of recurrence. Radiation has been successfully used as treatment for these tumors, but because of the young age of patients at diagnosis and the lifelong risks associated with radiation exposure, it is usually reserved for unresectable angiofibromas and recurrences.

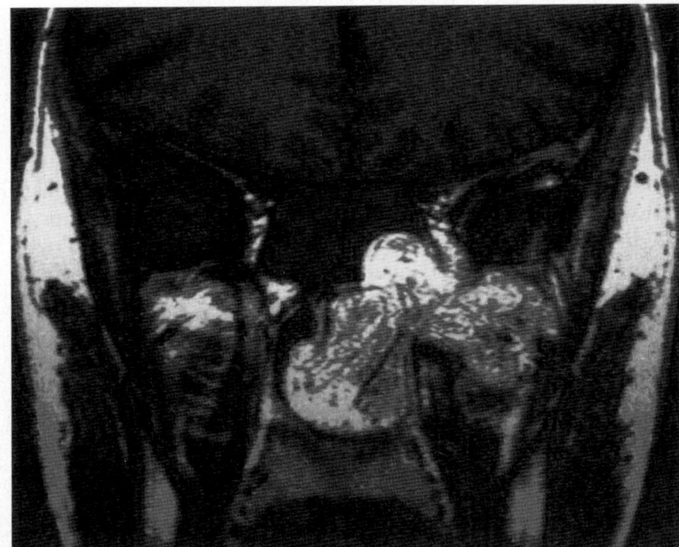

FIGURE 33-12 Magnetic resonance imaging scan of a 16-year-old boy with a left-sided juvenile angiofibroma. The tumor arose in the pterygomaxillary region and extended into the nasopharynx and infratemporal fossa. (Courtesy Dr. J. Netterville.)

Possible malignancies include nasopharyngeal carcinoma, low-grade nasopharyngeal papillary adenocarcinoma, lymphoma,

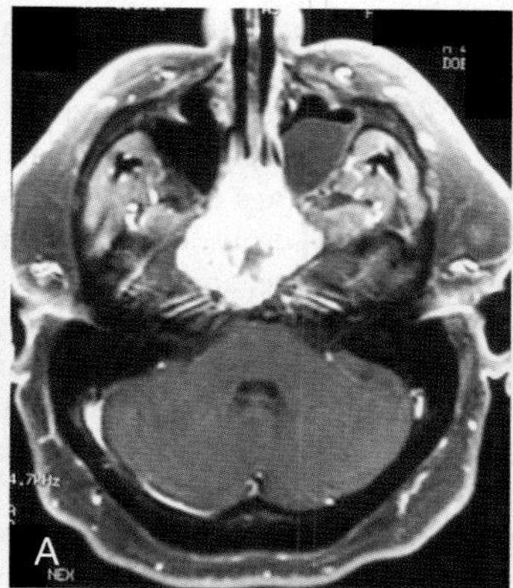

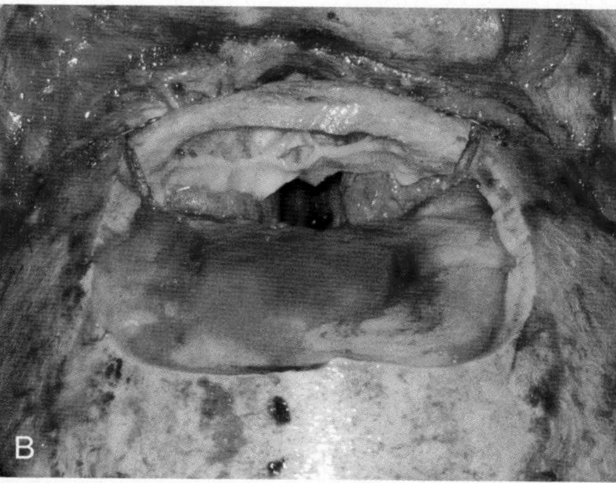

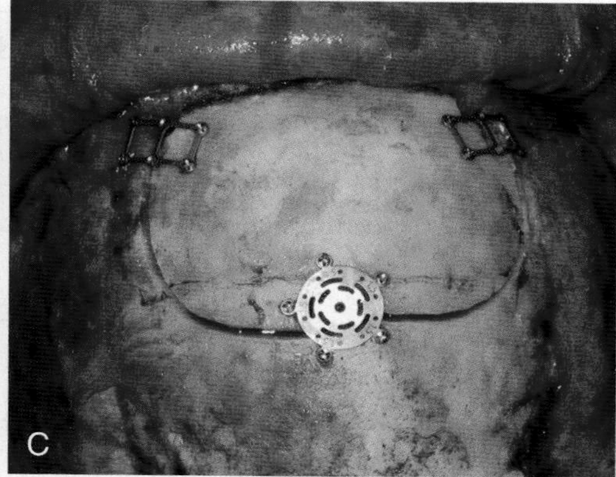

FIGURE 33-13 **A,** Magnetic resonance imaging scan of a 42-year-old man with a midline fibromyxoid sarcoma. **B,** Bicoronal incision with a combined subfrontal bar and craniotomy, allowing full access to the central anterior skull base. **C,** Replacement of the cranial bone along with a pericranial flap harvested from the deep surface of the flap for reconstruction of the skull base.

rhabdomyosarcoma, malignant schwannoma, liposarcoma, and aggressive chordoma. The staging system of malignant tumors of the nasopharynx is for epithelial tumors only and is based on confinement to the nasopharynx or spread to surrounding structures. Although nasopharyngeal carcinoma accounts for only 0.25% of all cancers in North America, it represents approximately 18% of all malignancies in China.[33] There is a strong correlation with Epstein-Barr virus, which has been demonstrated in all histologic subtypes of nasopharyngeal carcinoma. The World Health Organization divided nasopharyngeal carcinoma into three histologic variants: keratinizing (25%), nonkeratinizing (15%), and undifferentiated (60%). More recent classifications combine nonkeratinizing and undifferentiated tumors.[33] The most common initial sign is neck node metastases, especially to the posterior cervical triangle, and inferiorly positioned positive nodes predict poor outcomes. Treatment is based on radiation therapy to the primary site and bilaterally in the neck. With the addition of cisplatin and 5-fluorouracil, the rate of distant metastases decreases, and disease-free survival and overall survival increase.[34] Intracavitary irradiation is used to provide a boost at the primary site for advanced tumors and is used in cases of repeat irradiation. Surgery is reserved for persistent neck disease or for selected cases of local recurrence. Unique to these tumors is that the risk for recurrence with nonkeratinizing and undifferentiated carcinoma appears to be chronic and does not level off at 5 years, as it does with most other cancers. Rhabdomyosarcoma is the most frequent soft tissue sarcoma in pediatric patients and is the most common sarcoma occurring in the head and neck. Excluding the orbit, the most common site in the head and neck is the nasopharynx. Treatment is based on multimodality therapy consisting of nonradical surgery and radiotherapy plus multiagent chemotherapy.

Although surgery of the nasopharynx is performed primarily for benign pathologies, numerous approaches have been described, including endoscopic and open approaches, for the surrounding skull base region. Endoscopic skull base tumor resection has gained significantly in popularity, although the limits of the technique have not yet been clearly defined.[35] Endoscopic techniques not only avoid facial incisions but also allow shorter hospital stays. The most commonly described tumor removed via transnasal techniques is an inverting papilloma, which is excised in piecemeal fashion. Success has also been reported with endoscopic removal of mucoceles. Numerous open surgical approaches have been described to obtain access to the central skull base. For tumors of the nasopharynx, the transpalatal approach offers excellent visualization. The transfacial approach of lateral rhinotomy with unilateral or bilateral medial maxillectomy creates a facial incision but offers greater lateral exposure. The midfacial degloving procedure allows excellent bilateral exposure of the maxillae, paranasal sinuses, and nasopharynx without facial incisions. The posterior wall of the maxillary sinus may be removed to allow access to the pterygomaxillary fossa and deeper infratemporal fossa. For disease located more laterally, the transmastoid, transcochlear, and translabyrinthine approaches described by Fisch are used alone or in combination with more anterior approaches. More extensive approaches include the lateral facial split and mandibular swing, frontal-orbital or frontal-orbital-zygomatic approach, and maxillary swing; for disease of the high nasopharynx, the subfrontal approach affords excellent medial exposure (Fig. 33-13).

Pituitary Surgery

Although neurosurgery is the discipline responsible for comprehensive management of hypophyseal disease, a collaboration between otolaryngologists with endoscopic sinus surgery skills and neurosurgeons has resulted in the development of minimally invasive pituitary surgery.[35] The endoscopic transnasal transsphenoidal approach provides excellent visualization of the operative field and avoids intraoral or anterior nasal incisions, nasal packing, and postoperative complications such as septal deviation and lip anesthesia. Length of hospital stay, use of lumbar drains, and need for nasal packing have been demonstrated to be significantly reduced with minimally invasive pituitary surgery compared with open traditional approaches. Reconstruction of the sella by minimally invasive endoscopic repair has demonstrated that normal sphenoidal function can be maintained, while obtaining excellent results in terms of a low incidence of CSF leakage and harvest site morbidity (Fig. 33-14).[36]

Ear and Temporal Bone

When referring to tumors of the ear, the structures commonly involved include the external ear, middle ear, and inner ear. The external ear consists of the auricle or pinna and the external auditory canal to the tympanic membrane. The middle ear contains the tympanic cavity proper, ossicles, eustachian tube, epitympanic recess, and mastoid cavity. The borders of the middle ear include the tympanic membrane and squamous portion of the temporal bone laterally, petrous temporal bone medially, tegmen tympani or roof superiorly, carotid canal anteriorly, mastoid posteriorly, and floor of the tympanic bone inferiorly. The inner ear is contained within the petrous portion of the temporal bone and consists of the membranous and osseous labyrinth and internal auditory canal.

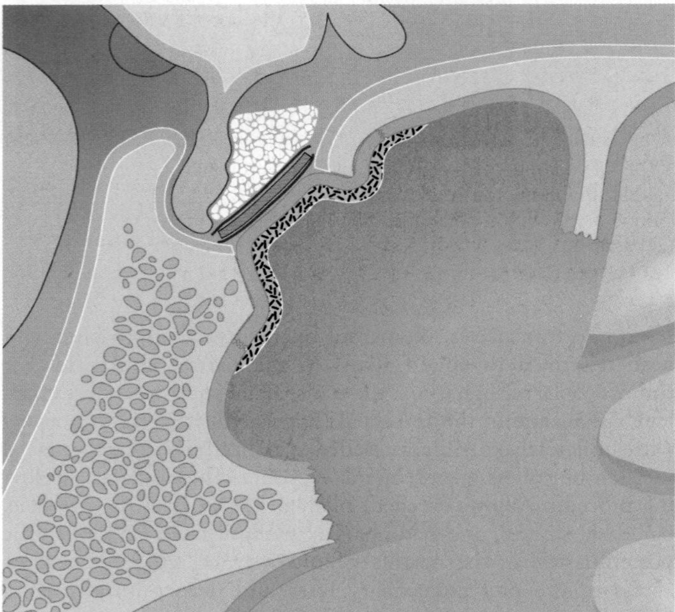

FIGURE 33-14 After endoscopically opening the sphenoid sinus in the minimally invasive hypophysectomy technique and resecting the pituitary tumor, sellar reconstruction is performed in a layered fashion. The sellar defect is partially filled with Gelfoam or fat, followed by layers of acellular human dermis, cartilage, acellular human dermis, mucosa, and fibrin glue. (From Lorenz RR, Dean RL, Chuang J, et al: Endoscopic reconstruction of anterior and middle cranial fossa defects using acellular dermal allograft. *Laryngoscope* 113:496–501, 2003.)

Evaluation of ear and temporal bone neoplasms requires appropriate physical examination and audiologic and vestibular testing, as well as radiologic assessment. Findings of hearing loss, vertigo, eustachian tube dysfunction with serous otitis media, cranial nerve deficits, pulsatile tinnitus, drainage, and deep boring pain are often associated with tumors and must be thoroughly evaluated. CT plays a crucial role in evaluating the temporal bone because of the complex anatomy contained within bony confines. MRI with gadolinium contrast agent is complementary and is used to define soft tissue anatomy (Fig. 33-15).

Neoplasms of the pinna are most often related to sun exposure and include basal cell carcinoma and SCC. Keratoacanthoma is a benign tumor characterized by rapid growth and spontaneous involution and may be confused with SCC. In the external auditory canal, ceruminous gland adenocarcinomas, adenoid cystic carcinoma, and atypical fibroxanthomas may arise. Within the temporal bone, benign neoplasms include adenoma, paraganglioma (at the tympanic membrane and at the jugular bulb), acoustic neuroma, and meningioma. SCC is the most common cancer of the temporal bone; others include adenocarcinoma of the middle ear or endolymphatic sac origin. In pediatric patients, soft tissue sarcomas such as rhabdomyosarcoma predominate. Metastases are an underrecognized cause of petrous bone tumors.

Malignancies of the pinna are treated similarly to skin cancers elsewhere on the face. Mohs microsurgery with frozen section control of margins minimizes the amount of normal tissue resected with the cutaneous malignancy. Involvement of underlying cartilage leads to more disseminated growth, necessitating partial or total auriculectomy. If the extent of disease is great, lateral temporal bone resection may be indicated, with attempted preservation of the facial nerve and inner ear. When the facial nerve or parotid gland is involved, lateral temporal bone resection with parotidectomy is performed. Radiation therapy may be used uncommonly for primary treatment or, more commonly, for adjuvant treatment in the case of perineural spread or poorly differentiated tumors.

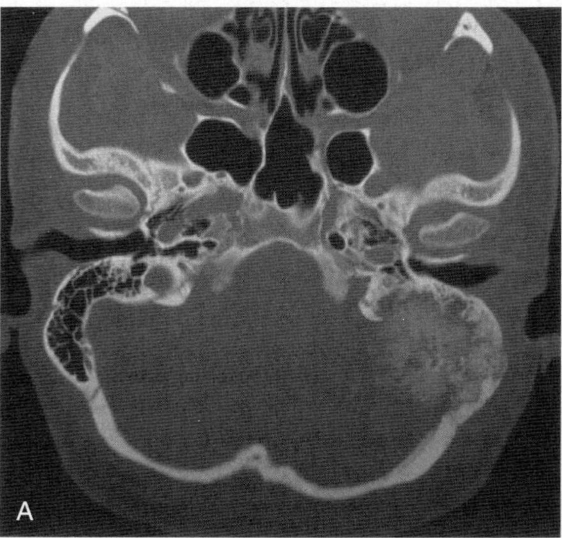

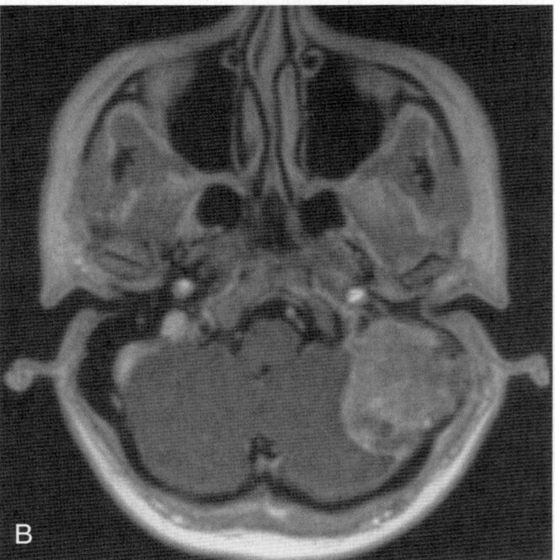

FIGURE 33-15 A, Computed tomography scan of a 19-year-old woman with osteosarcoma of the left temporal bone and bony destruction of the mastoid. **B,** Magnetic resonance imaging is useful for determining the extent of the tumor and the lack of brain invasion. (Courtesy Dr. J. Netterville.)

Treatment of tumors involving the middle ear and bony canal consists of en bloc resection of structures at risk for involvement. Rarely, when the tumor involves only the external canal without bony destruction, sleeve resection of the canal can be performed. Lateral temporal bone resection removes the bony and cartilaginous canal, tympanic membrane, and ossicles. Subtotal temporal bone resection involves removal of the ear canal, middle ear, petrous bone, temporomandibular joint, and facial nerve. Involvement of the petrous apex necessitates total temporal bone resection, with removal of the carotid artery. SCC within the petrous apex is considered incurable, although adenoid cystic carcinoma and select low-grade sarcomas may be excised with total temporal bone resection. The goals of reconstruction of temporal bone defects are protection from CSF leaks and coverage of vital structures and remaining bone to prepare for postoperative radiation therapy. Techniques for facial nerve rehabilitation are discussed next in "Salivary Gland Neoplasms." A prosthetic ear provides acceptable rehabilitation when a total auriculectomy has been performed.

Salivary Gland Neoplasms

The major salivary glands include the parotid glands, submandibular glands, and sublingual glands. There are also approximately 750 minor salivary glands scattered throughout the submucosa of the oral cavity, oropharynx, hypopharynx, larynx, parapharyngeal space, and nasopharynx. Salivary gland neoplasms are rare and constitute 3% to 4% of head and neck neoplasms. Most neoplasms arise in the parotid gland (70%), whereas tumors of the submandibular gland (22%) and sublingual and minor salivary glands (8%) are less common. The ratio of malignant to benign tumors varies by site as well—parotid gland, 80% benign and 20% malignant; submandibular gland and sublingual gland, 50% benign and 50% malignant; and minor salivary glands, 25% benign and 75% malignant.

The parotid gland is the largest salivary gland and is divided into the superficial lobe and deep lobe by the facial nerve. On imaging, the lobes can be differentiated by the retromandibular vein, which is commonly found at the division of the lobes. Deep lobe tumors lie within the parapharyngeal space. Stensen's duct is approximately 5 cm long; it pierces the buccal fat pad and opens in the oral cavity, opposite the second maxillary molar. The submandibular glands are closely associated with the lingual nerve in the submandibular triangle and empty via Wharton's duct into the papilla, just lateral to the frenulum. The sublingual gland lies on the inner table of the mandible and secretes via tiny openings (ducts of Rivinus) directly into the floor of the mouth or via several ducts that unite to form the common sublingual duct (Bartholin), which then merges with Wharton's duct.

Numerous non-neoplastic diseases commonly affect the salivary glands. Sialadenitis is an acute, subacute, or chronic inflammation of a salivary gland. Acute sialadenitis commonly affects the parotid and submandibular glands and can be caused by bacterial (usually *Staphylococcus aureus*) or viral (mumps) infection. Chronic sialadenitis results from granulomatous inflammation of the glands and is commonly associated with sarcoidosis, actinomycosis, tuberculosis, and cat-scratch disease. Sialolithiasis is the accumulation of obstructive calcifications within the glandular ductal system, more common in the submandibular gland (90%) than in the parotid (10%). When the calculi become obstructive, stasis of saliva may cause infection and create a painful, acutely swollen gland. Benign lymphoepithelial lesions of the salivary glands are non-neoplastic glandular enlargements associated with autoimmune diseases, such as Sjögren syndrome.

Salivary gland neoplasms most often manifest as slow-growing, well-circumscribed masses. Symptoms such as pain, rapid growth, nerve weakness, and paresthesias and signs of cervical lymphadenopathy and fixation to skin or underlying muscles suggest malignancy. When the initial symptom is complete unilateral facial paralysis, Bell palsy may be misdiagnosed as the cause; all patients with Bell palsy show some improvement in facial movement within 6 months of the onset of weakness. Trismus is associated with involvement of the pterygoid musculature by deep parotid lobe malignancies. Bimanual palpation of submandibular masses assists in determining fixation to surrounding structures. With deep parotid lobe cancers, CT and MRI tend to show irregular tumor borders and obliteration of fat planes in the parapharyngeal space. The accuracy of fine-needle aspiration cytology of the salivary glands has been well established. The sensitivity, specificity, and accuracy of parotid gland aspirates in one series were 92%, 100%, and 98%.[37] Excision of the gland is used to confirm the final diagnosis.

Benign tumors of the salivary glands include pleomorphic adenomas, various monomorphic adenomas (e.g., Warthin tumor, oncocytomas, basal cell adenomas, canalicular adenomas, and myoepitheliomas), various ductal papillomas, and capillary hemangiomas. Pleomorphic adenomas account for 40% to 70% of all tumors of the salivary glands and usually occur in the tail of the parotid. Similar to all benign parotid tumors, the treatment of choice is surgical excision with a margin of normal tissue (e.g., superficial parotidectomy). In the parotid gland, if excision is possible without complete removal of the affected lobe, the postoperative cosmetic appearance is superior to that in patients in whom a complete lobe is removed. Shelling out of pleomorphic adenomas should be avoided because it has been shown to correlate with increased rates of recurrence.[38] The facial nerve should not be sacrificed when removing a benign lesion (Fig. 33-16). Warthin tumor, or papillary cystadenoma lymphomatosum, is the second most common benign parotid tumor and occurs most often in older white men. Because of the high mitochondrial content within oncocytes, the oncocyte-rich Warthin tumor and oncocytomas incorporate technetium-99m and appear as hot spots on radionuclide scans. If fine-needle aspiration suggests a slow-growing Warthin tumor with confirmatory technetium scanning in a patient with contraindications to surgery, the tumor may be closely monitored because it has no malignant potential.

Malignant salivary tumors are staged according to size; T1 is smaller than 2 cm, T2 is 2 to 4 cm, T3 is larger than 4 cm (or any tumor with macroscopic extraparenchymal extension), and T4 involves invasion of surrounding tissues. Malignant salivary tumors are listed in Box 33-1. Mucoepidermoid carcinoma is the most common malignant tumor of the parotid gland and can be divided into low-grade and high-grade tumors. High-grade lesions have a propensity for regional and distant metastases and corresponding shorter survival rates than low-grade mucoepidermoid carcinomas. Adenoid cystic carcinoma constitutes 10% of all salivary neoplasms, with two thirds occurring in the minor salivary glands. The histologic types of adenoid cystic carcinoma are tubular, cribriform, and solid, listed in order from best to worst prognosis. An indolent growth pattern and a relentless propensity for perineural invasion characterize adenoid cystic carcinoma. Regional lymphatic spread is uncommon, although distant metastases occur within the first 5 years after diagnosis and may remain asymptomatic for decades. Malignant mixed tumors include cancers originating from pleomorphic adenomas, termed *carcinoma ex pleomorphic adenoma*, and de novo malignant mixed

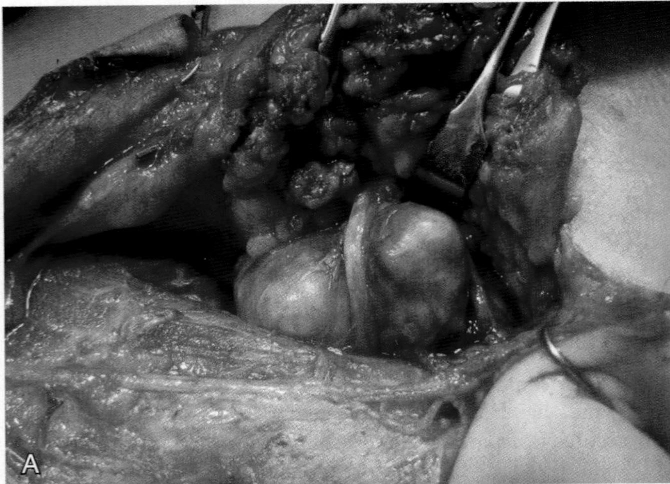

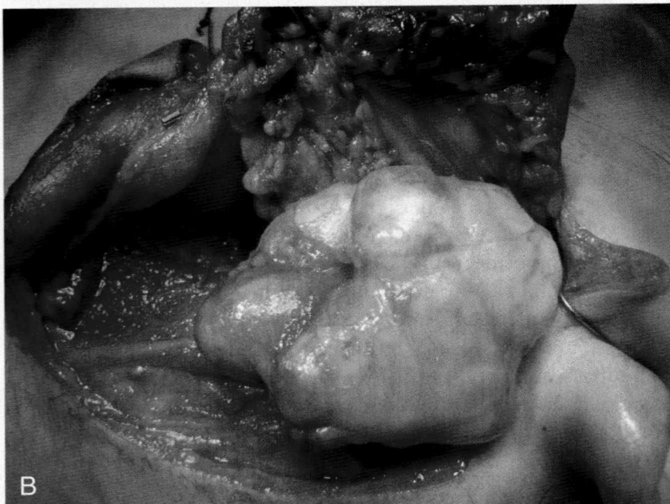

FIGURE 33-16 **A,** A 32-year-old woman with a deep parotid lobe pleomorphic adenoma. The facial nerve is displaced laterally. **B,** Once the mass is separated from the prestyloid space, it is delivered around the facial nerve, emptying the compressed parapharyngeal space and avoiding facial nerve injury.

BOX 33-1 Tumors of the Major and Minor Salivary Glands

Benign

Pleomorphic adenoma
Warthin tumor
Capillary hemangioma
Oncocytoma
Basal cell adenoma
Canalicular adenoma
Myoepithelioma
Sialadenoma papilliferum
Intraductal papilloma
Inverted ductal papilloma

Malignant

Acinic cell carcinoma
Mucoepidermoid carcinoma
Adenoid cystic carcinoma
Polymorphous low-grade adenocarcinoma
Epithelial-myoepithelial carcinoma
Basal cell adenocarcinoma
Sebaceous carcinoma
Papillary cystadenocarcinoma
Mucinous adenocarcinoma
Oncocytic carcinoma
Salivary duct carcinoma
Adenocarcinoma
Myoepithelial carcinoma
Malignant mixed tumor
Squamous cell carcinoma
Small cell carcinoma
Lymphoma
Metastatic carcinoma
Carcinoma ex pleomorphic adeno

tumors. The risk for malignant transformation of benign pleomorphic adenomas is 1.5% within the first 5 years, but risk increases to 9.5% when the benign tumor has been present for more than 15 years.[39] Most salivary gland lymphomas are of the non-Hodgkin variety (85%). The risk for malignant lymphoma in patients with Sjögren syndrome is 44-fold higher than in the normal population. Metastatic tumors are most often derived from cutaneous carcinomas and melanomas from the scalp, temporal area, and ear. Distant metastatic tumors are rare but may arise from the lung, kidneys, and breasts.

Treatment of salivary gland malignancies is en bloc surgical excision. Radiation therapy is administered postoperatively for high-grade malignancies demonstrating extraglandular disease, perineural invasion, direct invasion of surrounding tissue, or regional metastases. For tumors confined to the superficial lobe of the parotid gland, lateral lobectomy with preservation of the facial nerve may be performed. Gross tumor should not be left in situ, but if the facial nerve can be preserved by peeling tumor off the nerve, the nerve should be preserved, and radiation therapy should be used for microscopic residual disease. For cancers of the deep lobe, total parotidectomy is performed. Elective neck dissections are performed for high-grade malignancies, such as high-grade mucoepidermoid carcinoma. In patients with gross facial nerve involvement, temporal bone resection is performed, and the nerve is sacrificed proximally to obtain a negative margin. When the facial nerve is removed, rehabilitation with a simultaneous nerve graft may be performed in the hope of producing facial muscular tone. Although the primary goal of facial nerve rehabilitation is protection of the cornea from chronic exposure, other concerns include oral competency, nasal valve maintenance, and cosmesis. Upper lid gold weights, lateral tarsorrhaphies, static fascial slings, dynamic muscular slings, and delayed reinnervation procedures are also used for facial rehabilitation. Submandibular gland and minor salivary gland malignancies are treated similarly to parotid gland cancers by en bloc resection. Submandibular gland malignancies are removed with level I contents and accompanying modified RND. Gross involvement of the hypoglossal or lingual nerves requires sacrificing them and obtaining a negative margin by following the nerves toward the skull base. Adenoid cystic cancers are highly neurotropic; treatment consists of removal of gross tumor with radiation therapy for the microscopic disease that is assumed to exist at the periphery of the tumor.

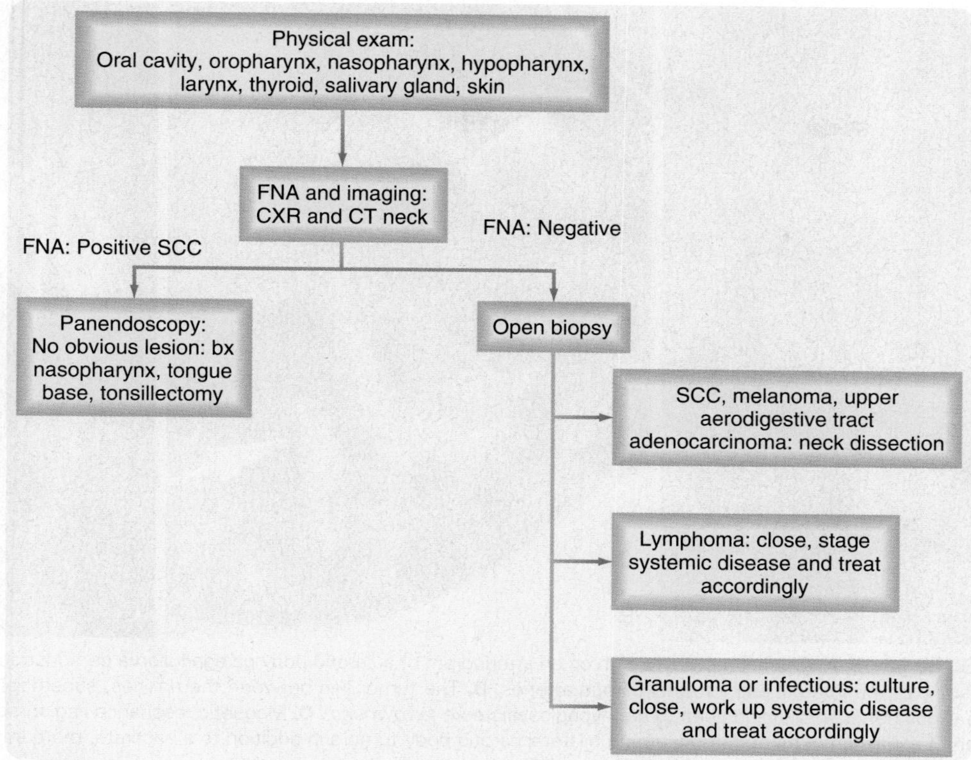

FIGURE 33-17 Workup of an asymptomatic unilateral neck mass in adults. *bx,* biopsy; *CT,* computed tomography; *CXR,* chest x-ray; *FNA,* fine-needle aspiration; *SCC,* squamous cell carcinoma.

Neck and Unknown Primary

The workup of a neck mass is different in children than in adults because of differing causes. Cervical masses are common in children and most often represent inflammatory processes or congenital abnormalities. Of pediatric neck masses that are persistent, 2% to 15% that are removed are malignant. Pediatric evaluation requires thorough head and neck examination, including endoscopy of the nasopharynx and larynx. The most common cause of cervical adenopathy is viral upper respiratory tract infections. The associated lymphadenopathy generally subsides within 2 weeks, although mononucleosis-related lymphadenopathy may persist for 4 to 6 weeks. The location of the mass as well as its character most often leads to the diagnosis. Lymphadenopathy not attributable to viral infections may represent a less common infectious process. Bacterial cervical adenitis is most often caused by group A β-hemolytic streptococci or *S. aureus.* Scrofula is cervical adenitis secondary to tuberculosis and is relatively uncommon in industrialized countries, although atypical mycobacteria may also cause cervical adenitis. Cat-scratch disease should be suspected if there is a history of cat contact, and indirect fluorescence antibody testing for *Bartonella henselae* should be performed. Midline masses include thyroglossal duct cysts, enlarged lymph nodes, dermoid cysts, hemangiomas, and pyramidal lobes of the thyroid. Nonlymphoid masses anterior to the sternocleidomastoid muscle are usually branchial cleft cysts. A soft compressible mass of the posterior triangle may represent a lymphangioma (or cystic hygroma), which usually develops before age 2 years. Cervical teratomas are present at birth and may involve compression of the airway or esophagus. Malignancies most commonly encountered in pediatric neck masses include sarcomas, lymphomas, and metastatic thyroid carcinoma.

Neck masses in adults represent malignancies more often than neck masses in children. Persistent masses larger than 2 cm represent cancer in 80% of cases. In addition to head and neck examination, CT assists in evaluating not only the masses but also potential primary sites. Fine-needle aspiration (<22-gauge needle) is performed as one of the initial steps in the workup of neck masses; it has an overall accuracy of 95% for benign neck masses and 87% for malignant masses (Fig. 33-17).[40] As in children, the location of the mass has a bearing on the likelihood of diagnosis: Midline masses may represent thyroglossal duct cysts, dermoid tumors, delphian nodes, thyroid masses, lipomas, or sebaceous cysts. Thyroglossal duct cysts represent the vestigial tract of descent that the thyroid followed from the foramen cecum to its normal location below the cricoid. The cyst may become enlarged later in life concurrent with an upper respiratory tract infection. Surgical excision should include the central portion of the hyoid bone (Sistrunk procedure), or recurrence is more likely.

Persistent lateral neck masses in adults may represent enlarged benign or malignant lymph nodes, neuromas or neurofibromas, carotid body tumors, branchial cleft cysts, lipomas, sebaceous cysts, parathyroid cysts, or a primary soft tissue tumor. Enlarged lymph nodes may have an infectious cause, similar to in the pediatric population, or be due to lymphoma, regional metastases from SCC, melanoma, thyroid carcinoma, salivary gland tumors, or distant metastases. Usually, lymphadenopathy in an adult is indicative of metastatic HNSCC, with lymphoma being less likely. Metastatic SCC is most frequently from the nasopharynx, oropharynx, or hypopharynx, and its presence is a negative prognostic indicator. In all cases of metastases to the neck, lymphadenectomy as treatment is valuable only in cases of SCC, salivary gland tumors, melanoma, and thyroid carcinoma. Otherwise,

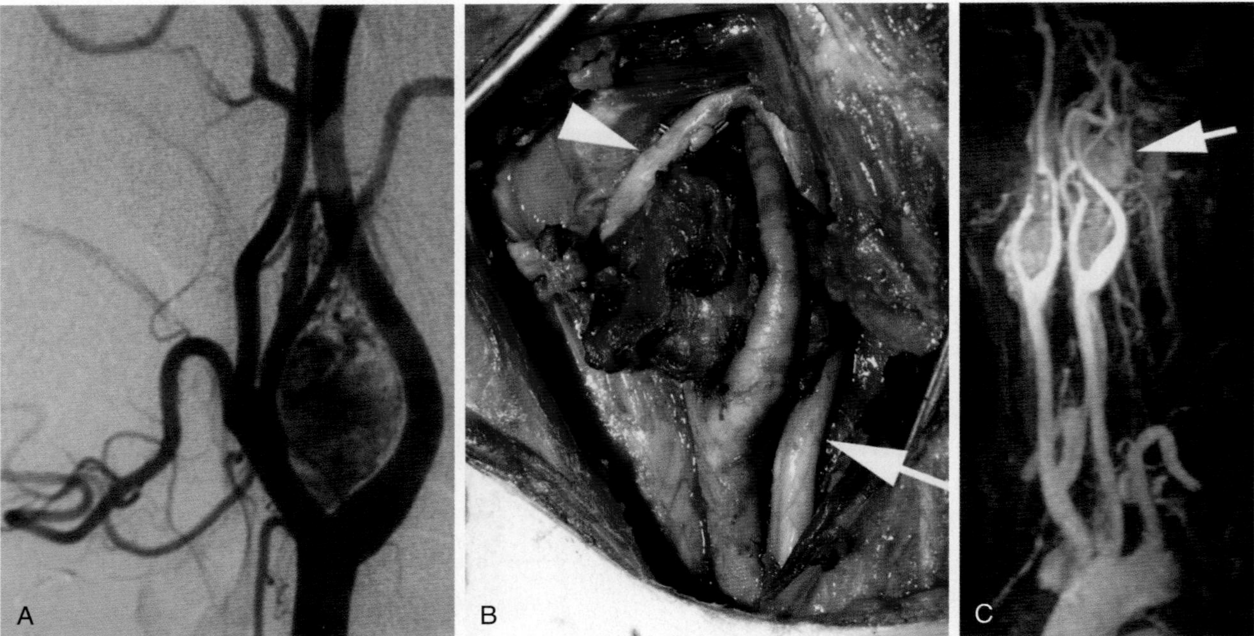

FIGURE 33-18 A, Characteristic lyre sign on an arteriogram of a carotid body paraganglioma demonstrating splaying of the internal and external carotid arteries. **B,** The tumor lies between the arteries, superficial to the vagus nerve *(arrow)* and deep to the hypoglossal nerve *(arrowhead)*. **C,** Magnetic resonance angiography scan of a different patient demonstrating bilateral carotid body tumors in addition to a separate, more superior, left vagal paraganglioma *(arrow)*. (Courtesy Dr. J. Netterville.)

removal of metastatic lymph nodes is indicated for diagnosis only, and systemic treatment must be initiated. In cases of multiple lymph node enlargement, a diagnosis of HIV infection, toxoplasmosis, or fungal infection should be investigated.

Less frequently, benign neck masses can develop in adults. The branchial cleft apparatus that persists after birth may give rise to many neck masses. First branchial cleft cysts develop in the preauricular or submandibular area, are intimately associated with the external auditory canal and parotid gland, and may require dissection of the facial nerve during excision. Second and third branchial cleft cysts and tracts develop anterior to the sternocleidomastoid muscle and often become symptomatic after upper respiratory tract infections. Although the second branchial cleft communicates with the ipsilateral tonsillar fossa, the third branchial cleft communicates with the piriform sinus. Removal of the cyst and tract necessitates dissection along the course of embryologic descent. Second branchial cleft tracts course between the internal and external carotid arteries. Third branchial cleft tracts course posterior to both branches of the carotid artery. Occasionally, a carcinoma may be found within the cyst. Debate continues about whether the carcinoma represents a cystic metastasis from the tongue base or tonsil or whether cancer may occur de novo within a branchial cleft cyst.[41]

Carotid body tumors or chemodectomas are more properly referred to as paragangliomas and arise from the branchiomeric paraganglia at the carotid body. These tumors are usually benign, unifocal, and nonhereditary; they are manifested as a nonpainful mass at the carotid bifurcation and have a characteristic lyre sign on carotid arteriography (Fig. 33-18). Because of their highly vascular nature, biopsy is contraindicated. Preoperative embolization is performed for tumors larger than 3 cm. The most frequent sequela from resection is cranial nerve injury, most commonly of the superior laryngeal nerve, but also the vagal nerve or hypoglossal nerve with large tumors.[42] Tumors larger than 5 cm are associated with a need for concurrent carotid artery replacement. The term *first-bite syndrome* was coined to describe the phenomenon of pain with the initiation of mastication; it is believed to be caused by removal of the sympathetic nerves surrounding the carotid bifurcation and reinnervation of the parotid secretory glands by parasympathetic fibers. Excision of bilateral carotid body tumors may lead to baroreceptor failure, with wide fluctuations in blood pressure.

Tumors of the parapharyngeal space are distinguished by their location; they are prestyloid, usually of salivary gland origin, or poststyloid, usually vascular or neurogenic in origin. Initial symptoms may consist of a superior neck mass, fullness of the parotid gland or tonsillar fossa, trismus, dysphagia, Horner syndrome, or cranial nerve impairment. Tumors include paraganglioma, salivary gland neoplasms, schwannoma or neurilemoma, lipoma, sarcoma, and lymphadenopathy. Access to these tumors is usually performed transcervically, and care must be taken to preserve uninvolved structures, such as the carotid artery and major cranial nerves (Fig. 33-19). A mandibulotomy approach is rarely required.

TRACHEOTOMY

Tracheotomy is generally used for patients requiring prolonged mechanical ventilation to reduce the risk of damage to the larynx, assist ventilation and pulmonary hygiene, and improve patient comfort and oral care. There is no hard rule about how long a translaryngeal endotracheal tube can be left in place. Some laryngologists recommend conversion to a tracheotomy after 3 days of intubation, although most use 2 to 3 weeks as a limit. Other

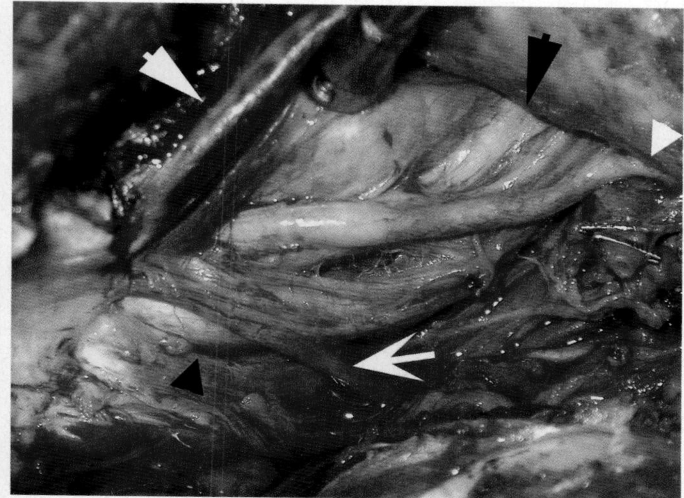

FIGURE 33-19 Left poststyloid space after removal of a parapharyngeal space tumor and lateral temporal bone resection. The carotid is seen anteriorly *(black arrowhead)* where it enters the skull base, whereas the internal jugular vein *(large white arrowhead)* is retracted posteriorly. The vagus nerve *(large black arrowhead)* is intimately associated with the hypoglossal nerve *(small white arrowhead)*, and separation of the two nerves at this level often leads to vocal cord paralysis. The glossopharyngeal nerve is seen anteriorly *(large white arrow)*.

common reasons for tracheotomy include chronic aspiration, acute airway obstruction secondary to facial or laryngeal trauma or oral or deep neck space infections, or perioperatively during radical cancer ablation.

The term *tracheotomy* implies formation of an opening that will close spontaneously once the tracheotomy tube has been decannulated. Closure via secondary intention generally occurs over a period of 5 to 7 days; the healing process should not be hastened by suturing the overlying skin closed, or an abscess may form in this highly contaminated wound. The term *tracheostomy* implies the formation of a permanent opening that remains open after removal of the tube. The surgeon can form a tracheostomy by suturing an inferiorly based tracheal ring flap to the skin at the time of surgery. Although this flap allows safer replacement of the tracheal tube should it become accidentally decannulated, once the mucocutaneous junction forms, a surgical procedure with rotational skin flaps is required to close the tracheostomy. A permanent tracheostomy should be considered for patients with extended mechanical ventilation, chronic aspiration, obstructive sleep apnea, or uncorrectable upper airway obstruction.

Preoperative assessment should include a history of previous tracheotomy or neck surgery, laryngeal pathology, bleeding difficulties, or cervical spine injuries. Perioperative complications of tracheotomy include bleeding, aspiration, pneumothorax and pneumomediastinum, recurrent laryngeal nerve injury, and hypoxia. Long-term problems include the formation of granulation tissue at the skin and within the trachea, collapse of tracheal cartilage and airway obstruction, and tracheoinnominate artery and tracheoesophageal fistulas.

Although the traditional open tracheotomy technique is still primarily used and preferred, percutaneous tracheotomy is being done more often. There have been reports of increased and decreased complication rates with the percutaneous technique versus the open technique.[43,44] Although one might suspect that the trauma from dilating the tracheal rings in the percutaneous technique might be associated with a substantial increase in long-term tracheal stenosis, this does not always seem to be the case; percutaneous tracheotomies have become common in many intensive care units in patients with favorable anatomy and supportive clinical settings.

VOCAL CORD PARALYSIS

More appropriately termed *vocal fold immobility*, loss of vocal cord function is a common occurrence. The recurrent laryngeal nerve supplies all the laryngeal musculature except for the cricothyroid muscle, which is supplied by the superior laryngeal nerve. Paralysis of the laryngeal muscles may occur from a lesion in the central nervous system or, usually, with peripheral nerve involvement (90%). Once the vagus nerve exits the jugular foramen, the superior laryngeal nerve divides superiorly in the parapharyngeal space and passes deep to the carotid artery. On the left side, the recurrent laryngeal nerve separates from the vagus nerve in the thorax, passes around the aortic arch at the ductus arteriosus, and travels superiorly in the tracheoesophageal groove to the cricothyroid joint. Probably as a result of the longer course of the left recurrent nerve, left vocal cord paralysis is more common than on right vocal cord paralysis. The right recurrent nerve separates from the vagus and passes around the right subclavian artery and back to the larynx (Fig. 33-20). A nonrecurrent recurrent laryngeal nerve is a rare finding (0.5% to 1.0%) on the right side; when present, the nerve separates from the vagus before descending into the chest, passes directly to the larynx, and is associated with a retroesophageal right subclavian artery. Approaches to the cervical spine should generally be performed from the left to reduce traction injury on the recurrent nerve because right-sided approaches have been associated with a higher rate of laryngeal nerve injury.[45]

Dysfunction of the superior laryngeal nerve usually occurs after thyroidectomy because the nerve is in close proximity to the superior thyroid vascular pedicle, and affected patients may have difficulty achieving precision in pitch, noticeable usually in professional voice users. Injury to the recurrent laryngeal nerve results in vocal fold paresis or paralysis. Patients with unilateral vocal cord immobility may have hoarseness, ineffective cough, dysphagia, aspiration, or airway compromise or may be completely asymptomatic because of their ability to compensate. Definitive diagnosis is made via laryngoscopy, and subtle weakness may require stroboscopic examination. Causes of paralysis include surgical trauma (usually thyroidectomy); malignancies of the thyroid, mediastinum, esophagus, or larynx; mediastinal compression; viral neuropathy; collagen vascular disease; sarcoidosis; diabetic neuropathy; and other reported factors. The cause is unknown in 20% of patients. Because recreating volitional abduction and adduction of the vocal cord is not currently feasible, the goal of treatment entails creating sufficient medialization of the involved vocal cord to allow efficient voicing and cough as well as reduce hoarseness and aspiration. Medialization may be accomplished with intracordal injection of various substances, including fat, absorbable gelatin sponge (Gelfoam), and human cadaveric collagen preparations. Because of the risk for granuloma formation, polytetrafluoroethylene (Teflon) injection is rarely used today. Medialization thyroplasty, with or without concurrent arytenoid adduction, consists of a surgically created window in the thyroid cartilage with the insertion of polymeric silicone substance (Silastic), hydroxyapatite, or Gore-Tex material and has shown excellent results. Laryngeal reinnervation via an ansa cervicalis–recurrent

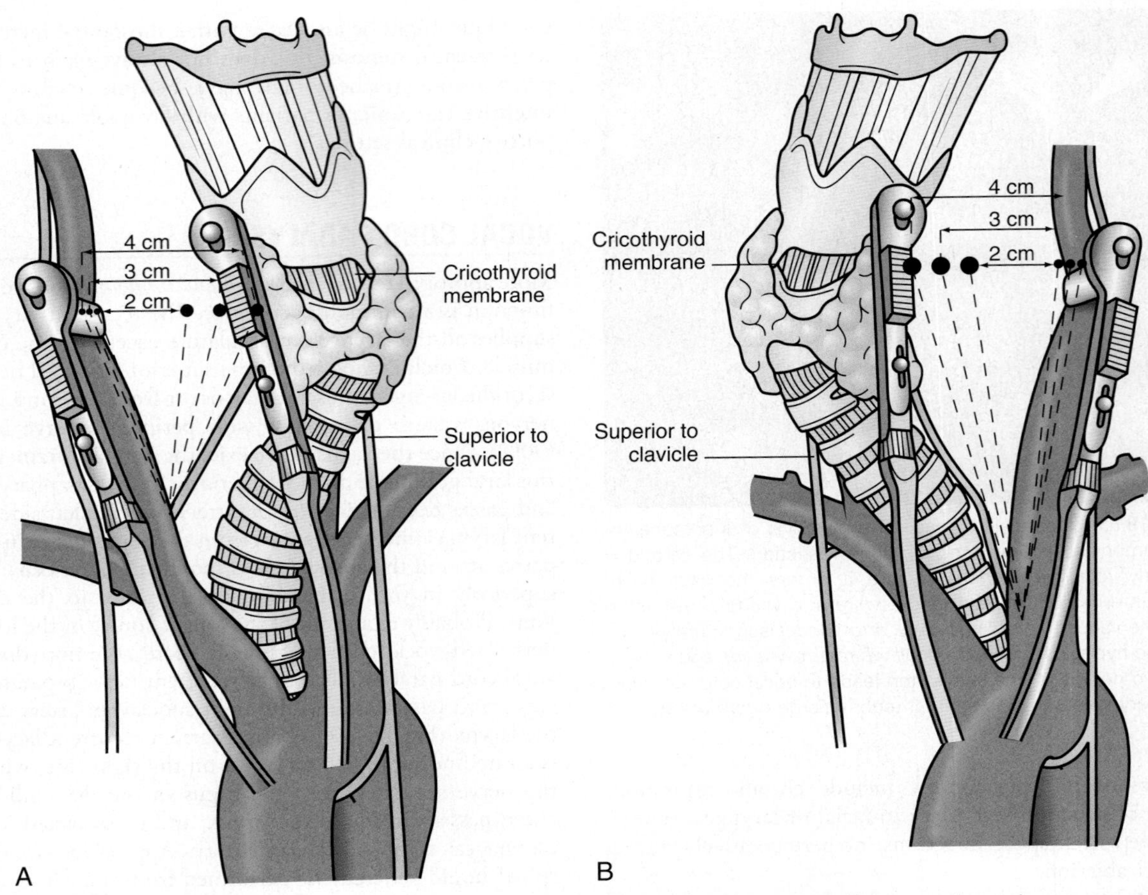

FIGURE 33-20 Anatomy of the right **(A)** and left **(B)** recurrent laryngeal nerves. The more diagonal course on the right side predisposes patients to traction injury during anterior cervical neck surgery. (From Netterville JL, Koriwchak MJ, Winkle M, et al: Vocal fold paralysis following the anterior approach to the cervical spine. *Ann Otol Rhinol Laryngol* 105:85–91, 1996.)

laryngeal nerve anastomosis provides medialization with tone to the paralyzed cord but takes several months to become effective.[46] Bilateral vocal fold paralysis is an uncommon scenario manifested by both vocal folds remaining near the midline position. Patients maintain a strong voice because the vocal folds continue to vibrate, but they might experience life-threatening airway obstruction and stridor and require immediate reintubation or tracheotomy.

RECONSTRUCTION

Perhaps the area of head and neck surgery that has undergone the most advancement in the past 25 years is reconstruction, fueled largely by the advent of microvascular free flaps. At the present time, there is almost no defect that cannot be repaired, which has afforded the ablative surgeon more leeway in obtaining tumor-free margins. The head and neck region is unique in the intricacy of its form and function, and careful reconstruction is needed to return patients back to their premorbid condition. Focus is usually on speech, swallowing, and cosmesis when considering rehabilitative goals. Swallowing may be impaired by resection of local tissues of the oral cavity, oropharynx, hypopharynx, larynx, and cervical esophagus. Loss of innervation—sensory or motor, locally or at the skull base—can severely impair swallowing. Irradiation leads to fibrosis of local tissues as well as loss of saliva and taste and may cause stenosis years after treatment is completed. Speech rehabilitation was discussed earlier (see "Larynx"). Because of the proximity and complexity of the airway and digestive tracts at the oral cavity, oropharynx, larynx, and hypopharynx, the ability to maintain the two functions is closely related. Frequently, aspiration occurs when the swallowing process is impeded. Although a tracheotomy tube helps protect the airway from aspiration and allows increased pulmonary suctioning, it also tethers the larynx to the skin and often exacerbates dysphagia. Once dysfunction has occurred, the physician is hampered by trying to maintain balance among airway, speech, and swallowing, and one function may have to be further impaired to improve another. In a severely dysfunctional upper airway, total sacrifice of one function may have to be accepted, and laryngectomy or a permanent gastric tube may be required.

Cosmetic deformities are most obvious in the head and neck area. Functional deficits not only occur in speech and swallowing but also affect eyelid function, oral competence, and maintenance of a nasal and oral airway. General principles of facial restoration include reconstructing the underlying bony framework, replacing skin with skin of matching quality, minimizing scar visibility and contracture, and reconstructing in zones of facial units. Skin should be matched by color, thickness, and hair-bearing units, when possible. The esthetic facial units include the forehead, eyes and periorbital area, midface, nose (which itself contains several subunits), and lips and mentum. A spectrum of reconstructive options exists, with healing by secondary intention and primary closure at one end and extensive reconstruction such as microvascular free flaps at the other. The option that is selected depends on the location and severity of the defect, overall health of the patient, available donor sites for flaps, status of the tissue adjacent to the defect (irradiated, infected, previously operated), and functionality of the area to be reconstructed. Not only must the reconstructive surgeon choose which option is best for a given defect, but also secondary and tertiary options should be planned in case of flap failure or recurrent disease.

Healing by secondary intention is an excellent option in several clinical scenarios. Mucosal defects with an underlying layer of vascularized muscle or bone that will not contract to the point of impeding function may be left to close by secondary intention. Examples include small tonsillectomy defects, tongue resections, and some laryngeal mucosal defects. Primary closure is likely to be the most commonly used option for closure of cutaneous defects. Attempts should be made to keep incisions within the lines of relaxed skin tension. These lines are caused by muscular insertion into the skin and form when there is mimetic motion. Incisions that parallel the lines of relaxed skin tension not only respect the esthetic units of the face but also have the least amount of tension along them, which decreases scarring. A Z-plasty may be used to reorient an unfavorable line of closure into a relaxed skin tension line.

Skin grafts are generally used for oral cavity, ear, or maxillectomy defects and for coverage of donor sites, such as the radial forearm and fibular free flaps and deltopectoral flap. Skin grafts are completely dependent for nutrition on the tissue over which they are placed and can heal well over muscle, perichondrium, and periosteum. They do not take well over bone or cartilage or on tissue that has been irradiated or infected or is hypovascular. Split-thickness skin grafts contain the epidermis and a portion of the dermis and are harvested with a dermatome at approximately 0.012-inch to 0.018-inch thickness. Thinner grafts require fewer nutrients to remain viable but also contract more when healing. Grafts may be meshed to allow greater surface coverage, but these types of grafts are generally restricted to the scalp or over muscle because of a less cosmetic result. A nonadherent antibiotic-impregnated bolster is commonly used to maintain stability between the split-thickness skin graft and recipient bed for 5 days to allow transmission of nutrients and capillary ingrowth while healing. Harvest sites include the anterior and lateral aspects of the thighs and buttocks.

Full-thickness skin grafts are characterized by a better color match, texture, and contour and less contracture, but success rates are lower than with split-thickness skin grafts. Commonly used donor sites include the postauricular, upper eyelid, and supraclavicular fossa skin. Composite grafts are occasionally needed for cartilage and skin reconstruction of the nasal ala and may be harvested from the conchal bowl without significantly affecting the appearance of the pinna. Acellular cadaveric human dermis that has been prepared by removing immunogenic cells while leaving the collagen matrix intact has grown in popularity as a skin graft substitute and avoids the need for a donor site.

Local skin flaps have an excellent tissue match because of their proximity to the defect. Commonly used designs include advancement, rotation, transposition, rhomboid, and bilobed flaps. Similar to primary closure, local flaps should be designed to be incorporated into the lines of relaxed skin tension. Although local flaps depend on the subdermal plexus of capillaries, regional flaps have an axial blood supply. This latter vascular pedicle is necessary for flap viability because greater distances are spanned by the flap and it is contained within the subcutaneous fascia, as in a fasciocutaneous flap, or within an underlying muscle, as in a myocutaneous flap. The deltopectoral, or Bakamjian, flap was one of the early regional flaps and was used extensively in head and neck reconstruction. Based on the intercostal perforating branches from the internal mammary artery, the flap is based medially and is designed over the upper pectoralis and deltoid regions. Because of the pliability of the transferred skin, it can be swung upward for skin defects or pharyngeal reconstruction.

Perhaps the development with the most significant impact on head and neck reconstruction was introduction of the pectoralis myocutaneous flap in 1978. Based on the pectoral branch of the thoracoacromial artery, the artery pierces the pectoralis muscle from the deep surface. A skin paddle designed over the muscle, or simply the muscle itself, may be transferred to reconstruct defects up to the nasopharynx. Historically, the pectoralis muscle was tunneled under the intervening skin to preserve the ipsilateral deltopectoral flap in case it was needed for future coverage. Division of the pectoral nerve branches ensures atrophy of the muscle and reduces the bulge over the clavicle. In addition to reconstruction of mucosal defects with the vascularized skin, coverage of an exposed carotid artery is an excellent use of the myogenous flap. The trapezius muscle offers multiple soft tissue flaps that may be rotated into head and neck defects. The lower trapezius myocutaneous flap, based on the dorsal scapular artery, has already been referred to as an excellent choice for lateral temporal bone defects. Finally, the submental and platysmal flaps are based on the facial artery and provide excellent local flap coverage for oral and oropharyngeal defects.

A free flap entails removal of composite tissue from a distant site, along with its blood supply, and reimplantation of the vasculature in the reconstructive field. The first successful human microvasculature transfer was a jejunal interposition flap in 1959; however, the modern era of microvasculature reconstruction did not arise until the 1970s, with improvements in instrumentation and technique. The current selection of donor sites allows the benefit of choosing among sites with large-caliber, long vascular pedicles that are anatomically consistent. In addition to favorable vascularity, optimal donor sites allow a simultaneous two-team approach of ablation and harvesting, possibility of a sensate flap, composite transfer of bone stock capable of accepting osseointegrated implants, transfer of secretory mucosa, or any combinations of these options. Patient selection for free flap reconstruction is of critical importance. Advanced age is not a contraindication to microvascular reconstruction, although previous recipient bed irradiation, contraction of tissues after secondary reconstruction, or previous free flap failure should raise concern in the reconstructive surgeon. Complete loss of a free tissue transfer should occur in less than 5% of cases.

The radial aspect of the forearm has emerged as the workhorse of soft tissue free flaps in head and neck reconstruction. A fasciocutaneous flap with sensate capabilities, the radial forearm flap is based on the radial artery and its venae comitantes, cephalic vein, or both for drainage. Variations of the flap include harvest of partial radius bone for bony reconstruction and palmaris longus tendon for suspensory reconstruction. The main advantage of the radial forearm flap is the thinness and pliability of the harvested skin, which makes it ideal not only for external cutaneous defects but also for reconstruction of the floor of the mouth or tongue (Fig. 33-21), soft palate and oropharyngeal wall, and pharynx as

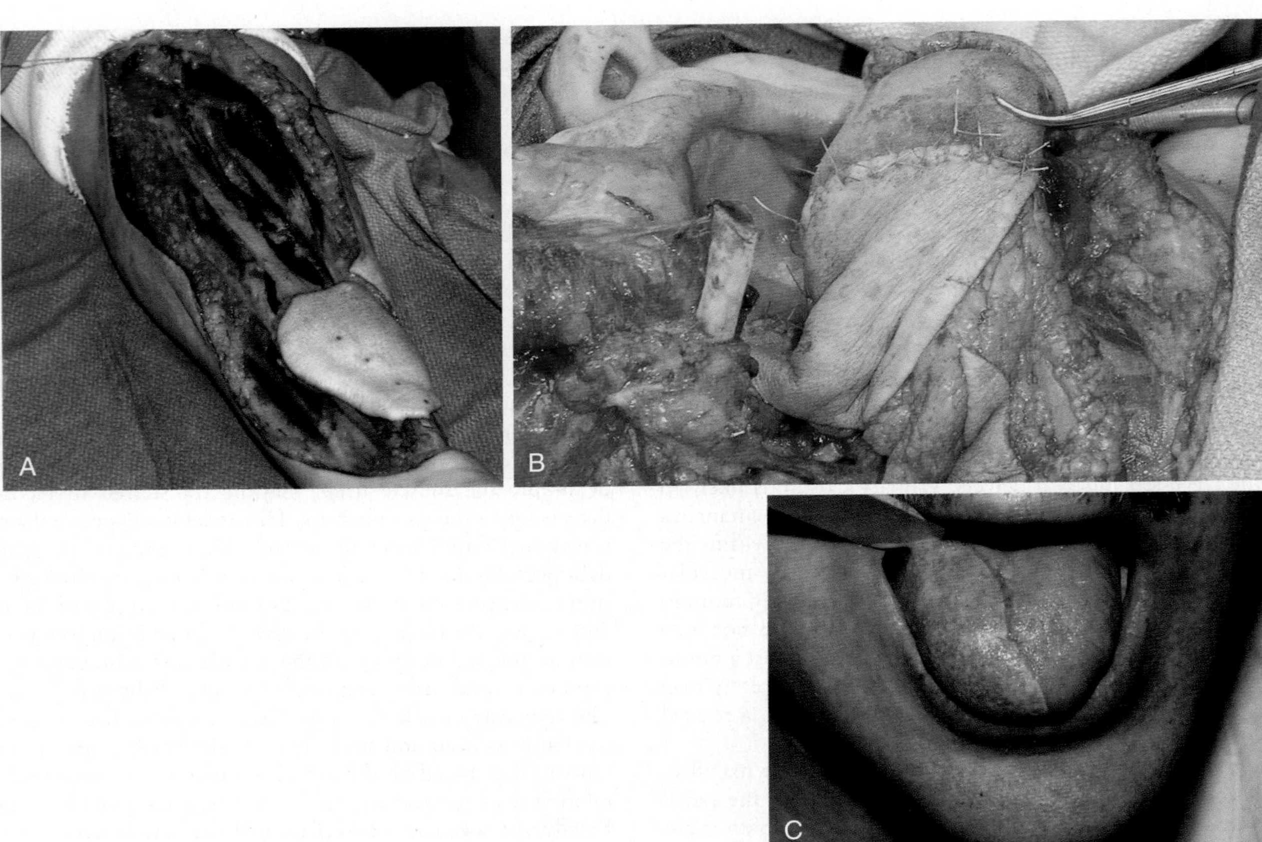

FIGURE 33-21 **A,** Harvest of a radial forearm fasciocutaneous free flap based on the radial artery. **B,** Right hemiglossectomy for squamous cell carcinoma of the right mobile tongue reconstructed with a radial forearm flap. **C,** Postoperative result 1 year later demonstrating excellent contour and tongue mobility.

well as skull base reconstruction. Although the donor site is more cosmetically obvious than other donor sites, long-term morbidity of the harvest is minimal. Other soft tissue flaps include the lateral arm flap, anterolateral thigh and lateral thigh flaps, latissimus dorsi flap, and rectus abdominis flap. The lateral arm flap is an excellent alternative to the radial forearm flap when the patient exhibits a dominant radial artery supply to the hand, which is a contraindication to use of the forearm site. The lateral arm flap is based on the posterior branches of the radial collateral vessels. It offers slightly more bulk than the radial forearm flap but is compromised to some extent by vessels that are smaller in caliber. Experience with thigh flaps has shown excellent results in tubed reconstruction of the pharynx. Latissimus dorsi and rectus abdominis flaps can be transferred as myogenous or myocutaneous flaps. Although skin match is not ideal, these flaps are best suited to large defects, including skull base repair or maxillectomy defects with orbital exenteration (Fig. 33-22). Harvest of the rectus abdominis may lead to the complication of postoperative hernia formation.

Enteric flaps include the gastro-omental flap and the jejunal flap. Disadvantages of these donor sites include the need for a laparotomy, which may preclude a two-team approach. In addition, the acceptable ischemia time is shortest with the enteric flaps because of their high tissue oxygen and nutrient demand. In contrast to other donor sites, the pedicle of these flaps cannot be divided even years postoperatively because the flap tissues do not incorporate blood supply from the surrounding tissue bed. The main advantages of enteric flaps are their pliability and ability to continue secreting mucus. In a patient who underwent radiation and has xerostomia, enteric reconstruction of recurrent oral or oropharyngeal tumors affords the opportunity to improve his or her quality of life significantly. The omentum of the gastro-omental flap may be draped into the neck to provide contour and bulk to a neck that has previously been dissected.

The most commonly used osseous free flaps include the fibula, scapula, and iliac crest. The fibular free flap is based on the peroneal artery and vein, and the blood supply to the foot should be investigated before harvesting this flap.[47] For mandibular or maxillary reconstruction with an osseous or osteocutaneous graft, 25 cm of fibula may be harvested, and donor site morbidity is minimal (Fig. 33-23). The bone stock of the fibula is sufficient to allow osseointegrated implantation for dentition or prosthetic anchors. The iliac crest osteocutaneous free flap allows even greater bone stock and is already naturally shaped in the form of a mandibular angle. Similar to the rectus abdominis flap, the iliac crest is hampered by the potential for postoperative hernias and has a relatively short vascular pedicle. Although the scapular free flap has the least bone stock of the three osseous flaps, it offers the advantage of simultaneous muscular, cutaneous, and bony reconstruction based on separate pedicles, allowing tremendous versatility in flap orientation. The megaflap includes the lateral border of the scapula based on the angular artery or the periosteal branch of the circumflex scapular artery, scapular or parascapular skin paddle based on cutaneous branches of the circumflex scapular artery, and latissimus dorsi and serratus anterior muscles supplied

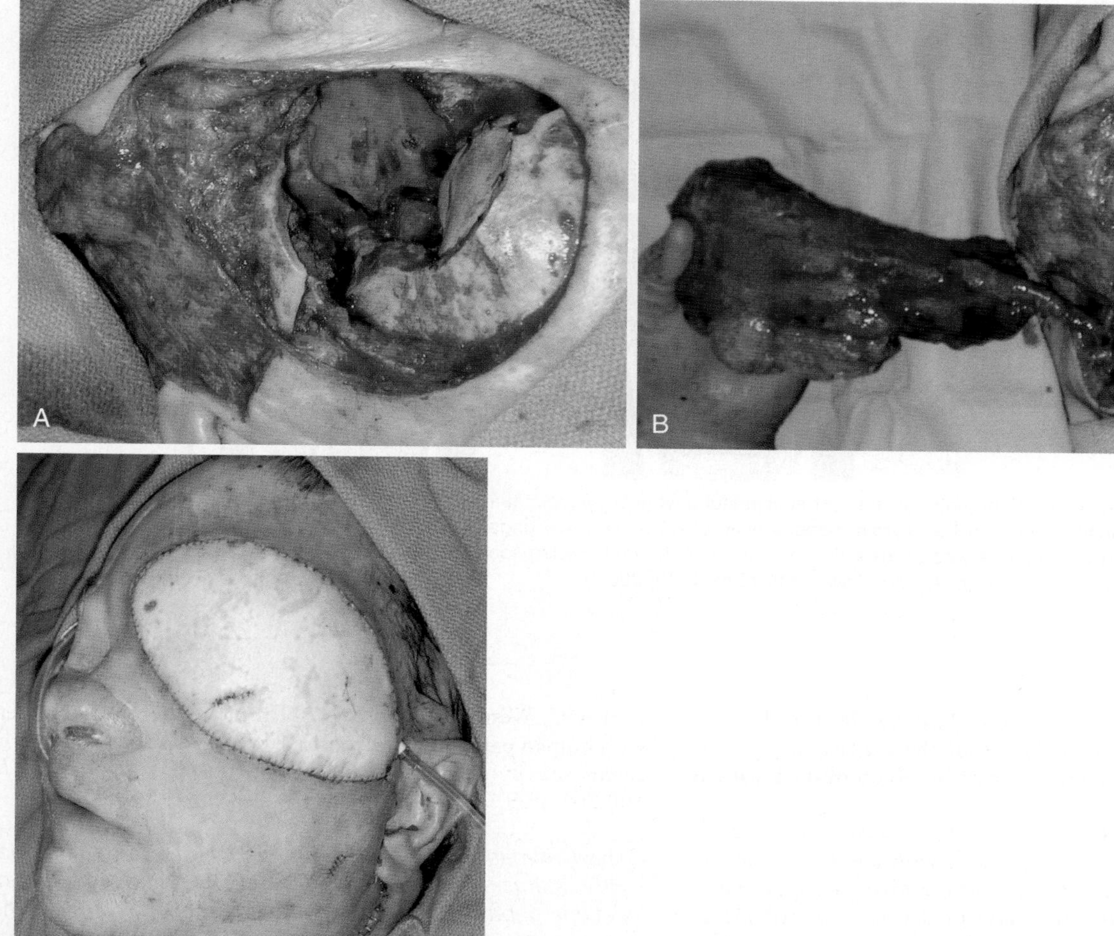

FIGURE 33-22 **A,** Resection of a recurrent skin squamous cell carcinoma invading the left orbit, paranasal sinuses, and frontal lobe dura. **B,** A rectus abdominis myocutaneous free flap has been revascularized with microvascular techniques into the recipient vessels of the neck, with the flap inset into place **(C)** for cutaneous and skull base reconstruction.

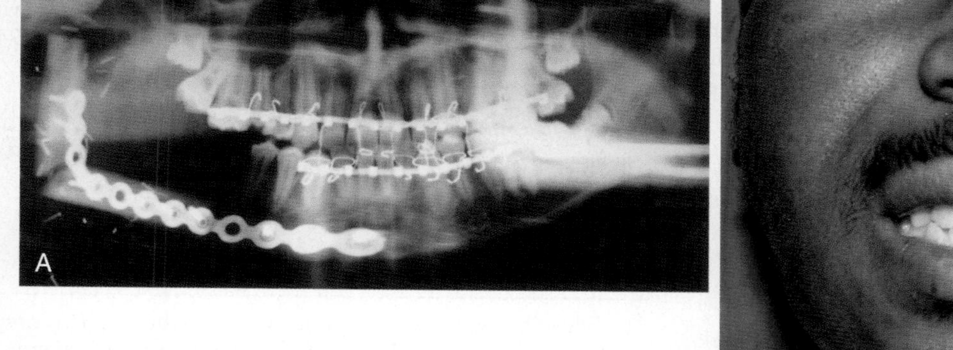

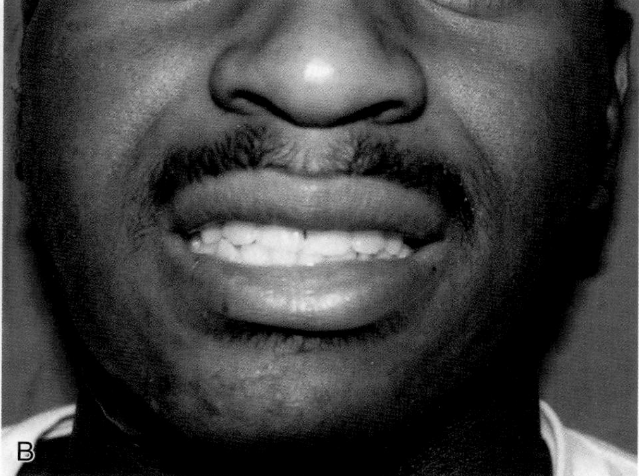

FIGURE 33-23 **A,** Immediate postoperative radiograph of a 35-year-old man after resection of an osteosarcoma of the mandibular ramus and reconstruction with a fibular osseocutaneous free flap. **B,** At 6 months postoperatively, the patient's dental occlusion has been preserved, along with excellent facial contour.

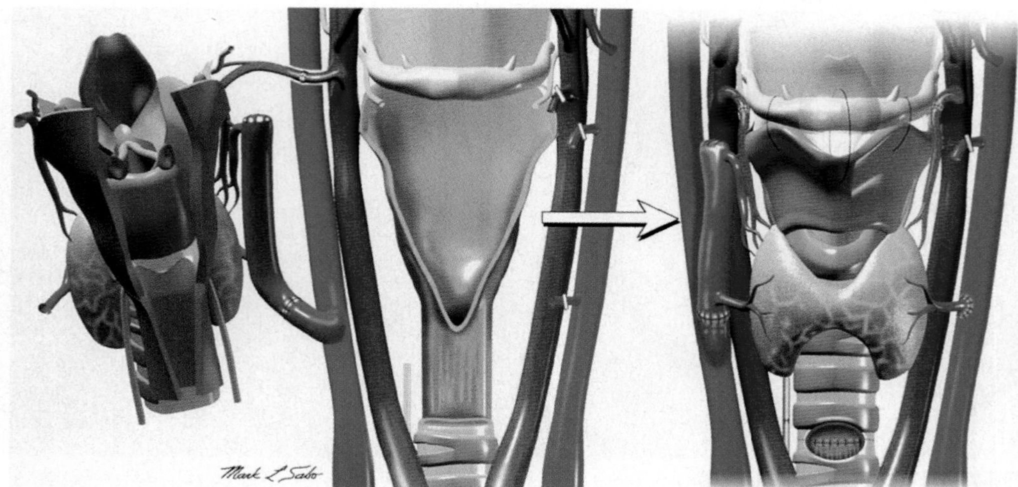

FIGURE 33-24 Schematic of the first successful laryngeal transplantation, performed in 1998. The larynx was transplanted with the thyroid, parathyroids, pharynx, and five rings of the trachea accompanying the vascularized and innervated organ. (From Strome M, Stein J, Esclamado R, et al: Laryngeal transplantation and 48-month follow-up. *N Engl J Med* 344:1676–1679, 2001.)

by the thoracodorsal artery. All arterial branches lead to the subscapular artery where it branches from the axillary artery, and revascularization of all segments may be accomplished with a single arterial anastomosis.

Perhaps the ultimate in head and neck reconstruction lies in the possibility of replacing ablated tissue with identical cadaveric donor tissue. In 1998, the first successful human laryngeal transplantation was performed with microvascular reconstruction (Fig. 33-24).[48] The larynx, pharynx, thyroid, parathyroids, and trachea were transplanted. Since the initial laryngeal transplant, further transplants of the larynx and the trachea have been performed successfully, but until nontoxic immunosuppressive drugs and protection against fostering tumor recurrence have been developed, nonvital organ transplantations are unlikely to become commonplace.

SELECTED REFERENCES

Induction chemotherapy plus radiation compared with surgery plus radiation in patients with advanced laryngeal cancer. The Department of Veterans Affairs Laryngeal Cancer Study Group. *N Engl J Med* 324:1685–1690, 1991.

This multi-institutional randomized trial demonstrated equal success between chemoradiation therapy and surgery with irradiation for laryngeal carcinoma while allowing patients who responded to the conservation treatment to keep their larynx.

Bocca E, Pignataro O: A conservation technique in radical neck dissection. *Ann Otol Rhinol Laryngol* 76:975–987, 1967.

This landmark article demonstrates equal control of metastatic neck disease with radical neck dissection and modified radical neck dissection, while avoiding the morbidity of unnecessary removal of neck structures.

Fakhry C, Westra WH, Li S, et al: Improved survival of patients with human papillomavirus-positive head and neck squamous cell carcinoma in a prospective clinical trial. *J Natl Cancer Inst* 100:261–269, 2008.

This landmark study was the first to demonstrate that tumor HPV status is a favorable prognostic marker in uniform patient populations with similar treatment protocols. The phase II trial suggested that when head and neck squamous cell carcinoma is associated with human papillomavirus (HPV) infection, the prognosis is significantly improved over non-HPV tumors. Many physicians advise that tumor HPV status should be incorporated as a stratification factor in patients with oropharyngeal cancer, although basing treatment protocols on HPV status has yet to be definitively investigated.

Naudo P, Laccourreye O, Weinstein G, et al: Complications and functional outcome after supracricoid partial laryngectomy with cricohyoidoepiglottopexy. *Otolaryngol Head Neck Surg* 118:124–129, 1998.

This article describes the outstanding functional results of supracricoid laryngectomy in terms of speech and swallowing while obtaining excellent local control of disease.

REFERENCES

1. Edge SB, Byrd DR, Compton CC, et al, editors: *AJCC cancer staging manual*, ed 7, New York, 2010, Springer-Verlag.
2. Chaturvedi AK, Engels EA, Anderson WF, et al: Incidence trends for human papillomavirus–related and unrelated oral squamous cell carcinomas in the United States. *J Clin Oncol* 26:612–619, 2008.
3. Johnson N: Tobacco use and oral cancer: A global perspective. *J Dent Educ* 65:328–339, 2001.

4. Cooper JS, Porter K, Mallin K, et al: The National Cancer Database report on cancer of the head and neck: 10-year update. *Head Neck* 31:748–758, 2009.
5. Gillison ML: Current topics in the epidemiology of oral cavity and oropharyngeal cancers. *Head Neck* 29:779–792, 2007.
6. Stadler M, Patel M, Couch M, et al: Molecular biology of head and neck cancer. *Hemat Oncol Clin N Am* 22:1099–1124, 2008.
7. Li C, Hu Z, Lu J, et al: Genetic polymorphisms in DNA base-excision repair genes ADPRT, XRCC1, and APE1 and the risk of squamous cell carcinoma of the head and neck. *Cancer* 110:867–875, 2007.
8. Califano J, van der Riet P, Westra W, et al: Genetic progression model for head and neck cancer: Implications for field cancerization. *Cancer Res* 56:2488–2492, 1996.
9. Hugo H, Ackland ML, Blick T, et al: Epithelial-mesenchymal and mesenchymal-epithelial transitions in carcinoma progression. *J Cell Physiol* 213:374–383, 2007.
10. Kalyankrishna S, Grandis JR: Epidermal growth factor receptor biology in head and neck cancer. *J Clin Oncol* 24:2666–2672, 2006.
11. Pollak MN, Schernhammer ES, Hankinson SE: Insulin-like growth factors and neoplasia. *Nat Rev Cancer* 4:505–518, 2004.
12. Kutler DI, Wong RJ, Kraus DH: Functional imaging in head and neck cancer. *Curr Oncol Rep* 7:137–144, 2005.
13. Bourhis J, Wibault P, Lusinchi A, et al: Status of accelerated fractionation radiotherapy in head and neck squamous cell carcinomas. *Curr Opin Oncol* 9:262–266, 1997.
14. Induction chemotherapy plus radiation compared with surgery plus radiation in patients with advanced laryngeal cancer. The Department of Veterans Affairs Laryngeal Cancer Study Group. *N Engl J Med* 324:1685–1690, 1991.
15. Bernier J, Domenge C, Ozashin M, et al: Postoperative irradiation with or without concurrent chemotherapy for locally advanced head and neck cancer. *N Engl J Med* 350:1945–1952, 2004.
16. Cooper JS, Pajak TF, Forastiere AA, et al: Postoperative concurrent radiotherapy and chemotherapy for high-risk squamous cell carcinoma of the head and neck. *N Engl J Med* 350:1937–1944, 2004.
17. Roy S, Tibesar RJ, Daly K, et al: Role of planned neck dissection for advanced metastatic disease in tongue base or tonsil squamous cell carcinoma treated with radiotherapy. *Head Neck* 24:474–481, 2002.
18. Bocca E, Pignataro O: A conservation technique in radical neck dissection. *Ann Otol Rhinol Laryngol* 76:975–987, 1967.
19. Kuriakose MA, Trivedi NP: Sentinel node biopsy in head and neck squamous cell carcinoma. *Curr Opin Otolaryngol Head Neck Surg* 17:100–110, 2009.
20. O'Brien CJ, Lauer CS, Fredricks S, et al: Tumor thickness influences prognosis of T1 and T2 oral cavity cancer—but what thickness? *Head Neck* 25:937–945, 2003.
21. Gooris PJ, Vermey A, de Visscher JG, et al: Supraomohyoid neck dissection in the management of cervical lymph node metastases of squamous cell carcinoma of the lower lip. *Head Neck* 24:678–683, 2002.
22. Strome SE, To W, Strawderman M, et al: Squamous cell carcinoma of the buccal mucosa. *Otolaryngol Head Neck Surg* 120:375–379, 1999.
23. Adelstein DJ, Saxton JP, Rybicki LA, et al: Multiagent concurrent chemoradiotherapy for locoregionally advanced squamous cell head and neck cancer: Mature results from a single institution. *J Clin Oncol* 24:1064–1071, 2006.
24. Fakhry C, Westra WH, Li S, et al: Improved survival of patients with human papillomavirus–positive head and neck squamous cell carcinoma in a prospective clinical trial. *J Natl Cancer Inst* 100:261–269, 2008.
25. Lefebvre JL, Chevalier D, Luboinski B, et al: Larynx preservation in piriform sinus cancer: Preliminary results of a European Organization for Research and Treatment of Cancer phase III trial. EORTC Head and Neck Cancer Cooperative Group. *J Natl Cancer Inst* 88:890–899, 1996.
26. Kirchner JA: *Vocal fold histopathology: A symposium*, San Diego, CA, 1986, College-Hill Press.
27. Ambrosch P, Kron M, Steiner W: Carbon dioxide laser microsurgery for early supraglottic carcinoma. *Ann Otol Rhinol Laryngol* 107:680–688, 1998.
28. Steiner W, Vogt P, Ambrosch P, et al: Transoral carbon dioxide laser microsurgery for recurrent glottic carcinoma after radiotherapy. *Head Neck* 26:477–484, 2004.
29. Muscatello L, Laccourreye O, Biacabe B, et al: Laryngofissure and cordectomy for glottic carcinoma limited to the mid third of the mobile true vocal cord. *Laryngoscope* 107:1507–1510, 1997.
30. Naudo P, Laccourreye O, Weinstein G, et al: Complications and functional outcome after supracricoid partial laryngectomy with cricohyoidoepiglottopexy. *Otolaryngol Head Neck Surg* 118:124–129, 1998.
31. Solares CA, Wood B, Rodriguez CP, et al: Does vocal cord fixation preclude nonsurgical management of laryngeal cancer? *Laryngoscope* 119:1130–1134, 2009.
32. Imola MJ, Schramm VL: Orbital preservation in surgical management of sinonasal malignancy. *Laryngoscope* 112:1357–1365, 2002.
33. Vasef MA, Ferlito A, Weiss LM: Clinicopathological consultation: Nasopharyngeal carcinoma, with emphasis on its relationship to Epstein-Barr virus. *Ann Otol Rhinol Laryngol* 106:348–356, 1997.
34. Al-Sarraf M, LeBlanc M, Giri PB, et al: Chemoradiotherapy versus radiotherapy in patients with advanced nasopharyngeal cancer: Phase III randomized Intergroup Study 0099. *J Clin Oncol* 16:1310–1317, 1998.
35. Jia WH, Huang QH, Liao J, et al: Trends in incidence and mortality of nasopharyngeal carcinoma over a 20–25 year period (1978/1983–2002) in Sihui and Cangwu counties in southern China. *BMC Cancer* 6:178, 2006.
36. Lorenz RR, Dean RL, Chuang J, et al: Endoscopic reconstruction of anterior and middle cranial fossa defects using acellular dermal allograft. *Laryngoscope* 113:496–501, 2003.
37. Stewart CJ, MacKenzie K, McGarry GW, et al: Fine-needle aspiration cytology of salivary gland: A review of 341 cases. *Diagn Cytopathol* 22:139–146, 2000.
38. Witt RL: The significance of the margin in parotid surgery for pleomorphic adenoma. *Laryngoscope* 112:2141–2154, 2002.
39. Seifert G: Histopathology of malignant salivary gland tumours. *Eur J Cancer B Oral Oncol* 28B:49–52, 1992.
40. Amedee RG, Dhurandhar NR: Fine-needle aspiration biopsy. *Laryngoscope* 111:1551–1557, 2001.

41. Zimmermann CE, von Domarus H, Moubayed P: Carcinoma in situ in a lateral cervical cyst. *Head Neck* 24:965–969, 2002.
42. Cohen SM, Burkey BB, Netterville JL: Surgical management of parapharyngeal space masses. *Head Neck* 27:669–675, 2005.
43. van Heurn LW, Goei R, de Ploeg I, et al: Late complications of percutaneous dilatational tracheotomy. *Chest* 110:1572–1576, 1996.
44. Kost KM: Endoscopic percutaneous dilatational tracheotomy: A prospective evaluation of 500 consecutive cases. *Laryngoscope* 115:1–30, 2005.
45. Netterville JL, Koriwchak MJ, Winkle M, et al: Vocal fold paralysis following the anterior approach to the cervical spine. *Ann Otol Rhinol Laryngol* 105:85–91, 1996.
46. Lorenz RR, Teker AM, Strome M, et al: Ansa cervicalis-to-recurrent laryngeal nerve anastomosis for unilateral vocal fold paralysis: A single institutional experience. *Ann Otol Rhinol Laryngol* 117:40–45, 2008.
47. Lorenz RR, Esclamado R: Preoperative magnetic resonance angiography in fibular free flap reconstruction of head and neck defects. *Head Neck* 23:844–850, 2001.
48. Strome M, Stein J, Esclamado R, et al: Laryngeal transplantation and 40-month follow-up. *N Engl J Med* 344:1676–1679, 2001.

SECTION VII

Breast

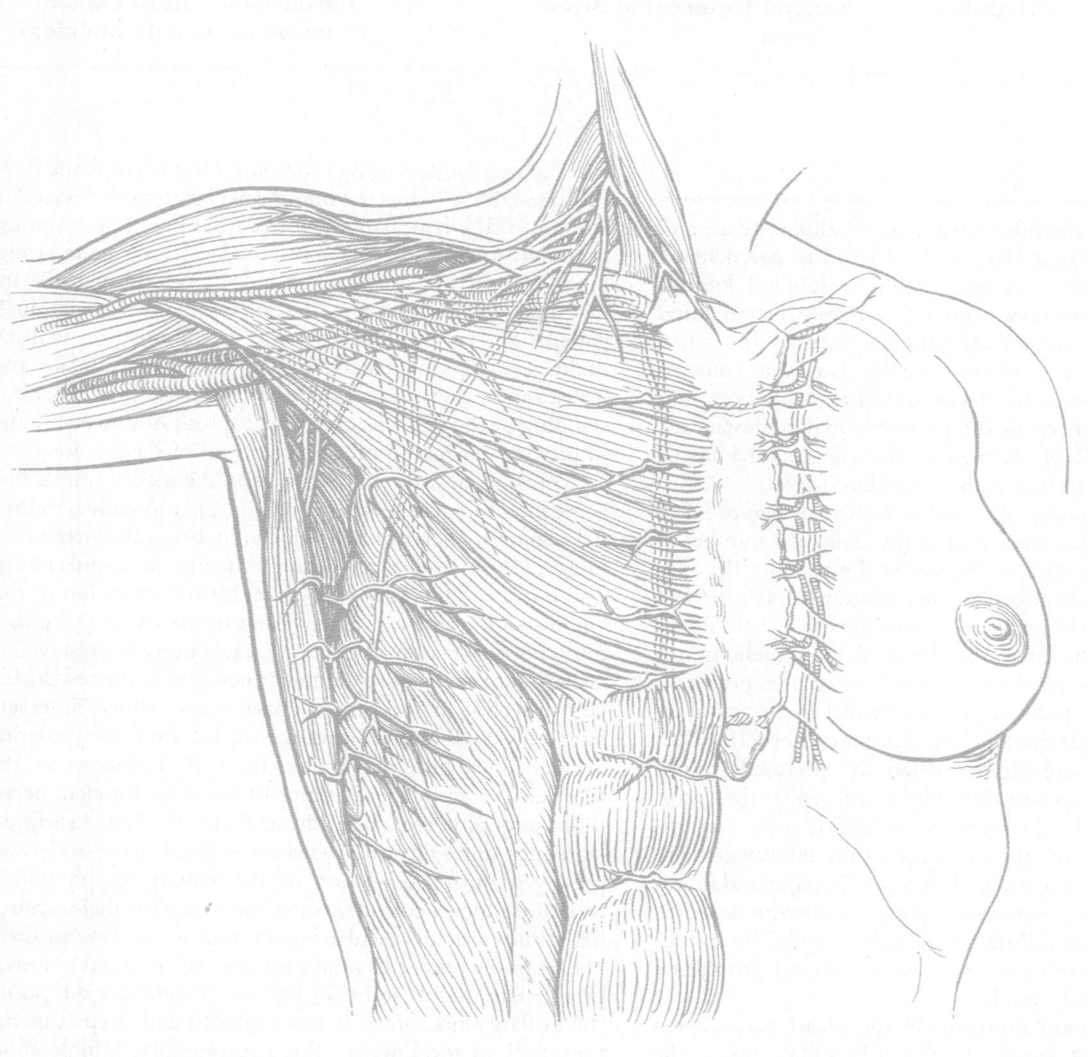

34 CHAPTER

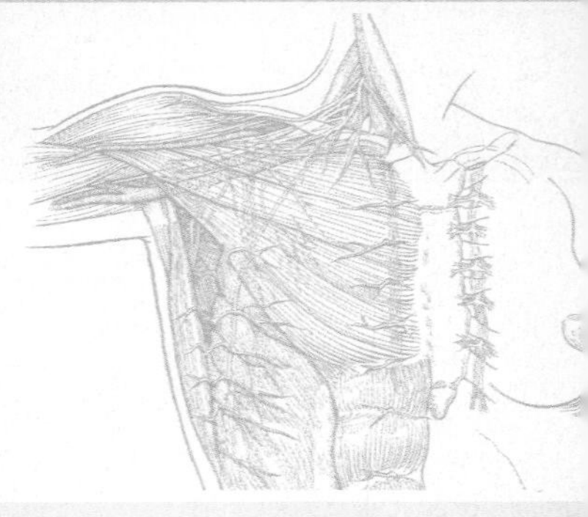

Diseases of the Breast

Kelly K. Hunt, Elizabeth A. Mittendorf

OUTLINE

ANATOMY

The breast lies between the subdermal layer of adipose tissue and the superficial pectoral fascia (Fig. 34-1). The breast parenchyma is composed of lobes that comprise multiple lobules. Fibrous bands termed the *suspensory ligaments of Cooper* provide structural support and insert perpendicularly into the dermis. The retromammary space, a thin layer of loose areolar tissue that contains lymphatics and small vessels, lies between the breast and pectoralis major muscle. Located deep to the pectoralis major muscle, the pectoralis minor muscle is enclosed in the clavipectoral fascia, which extends laterally to fuse with the axillary fascia.

The axillary lymph nodes, grouped as shown in Figure 34-2, are found within the loose areolar fat of the axilla; the number of lymph nodes varies according to the size of the patient. The axillary nodes are typically described as three anatomic levels defined by their relationship to the pectoralis minor muscle. Level I nodes are located lateral to the lateral border of the pectoralis minor muscle. Level II nodes are located posterior to the pectoralis minor muscle. Level III nodes are located medial to the pectoralis minor muscle and include the subclavicular nodes. Level III nodes are easier to visualize and remove when the pectoralis minor muscle is divided. The apex of the axilla is defined by the costoclavicular ligament (Halsted's ligament), at which point the axillary vein passes into the thorax and becomes the subclavian vein. Lymph nodes in the space between the pectoralis major and minor muscles are termed the *interpectoral group* or *Rotter's nodes*, as described by Grossman and Rotter. Unless these nodes are specifically exposed, they are not encompassed in surgical procedures that preserve the pectoral muscles.

Lymphatic channels are abundant in the breast parenchyma and dermis. Specialized lymphatic channels collect under the nipple and areola and form Sappey's plexus, named for the anatomist who described them in 1885. Lymph flows from the skin to the subareolar plexus and then into the interlobular lymphatics of the breast parenchyma. Appreciation of lymphatic flow is important for performing successful sentinel lymph node surgery (see "Lymph Node Staging" later on). Of the lymphatic flow from the breast, 75% is directed into the axillary lymph nodes. A minor amount of the lymphatic flow from the breast goes through the pectoralis muscle and into more medial lymph node groups (see Fig. 34-2). Lymphatic drainage also occurs through the internal mammary lymph nodes as the predominant drainage in 5% of patients and as a secondary route in combination with axillary drainage in approximately 20% of patients. A major route of breast cancer metastasis is through lymphatic channels; an understanding of the patterns of regional spread of cancer is important to provide optimal locoregional control of the disease.

Coursing close to the chest wall on the medial side of the axilla is the long thoracic nerve (see Fig. 34-2), also known as the external respiratory nerve of Bell, which innervates the serratus anterior muscle. This muscle is important for fixing the scapula to the chest wall during adduction of the shoulder and extension of the arm, and division of the nerve may result in the winged scapula deformity. For this reason, the long thoracic nerve is preserved during axillary surgery. The second major nerve encountered during axillary dissection is the thoracodorsal nerve, which innervates the latissimus dorsi muscle. This nerve arises from the posterior cord of the brachial plexus and enters the axillary space under the axillary vein, close to the entrance of the long thoracic nerve. The thoracodorsal nerve crosses the axilla to the medial surface of the latissimus dorsi muscle. The thoracodorsal nerve and vessels are preserved during dissection of the axillary lymph nodes. The medial pectoral nerve innervates the pectoralis major muscle and lies within a neurovascular bundle that wraps around the lateral border of the pectoralis minor muscle. The pectoral neurovascular bundle is a useful landmark because it indicates the position of the axillary vein, which is just cephalad and deep (superior and posterior) to the bundle. This neurovascular bundle should be preserved during standard axillary dissection.

The large sensory intercostal brachial or brachial cutaneous nerves span the axillary space and supply sensation to the undersurface of the upper part of the arm and skin of the chest wall along the posterior margin of the axilla. Dividing these nerves

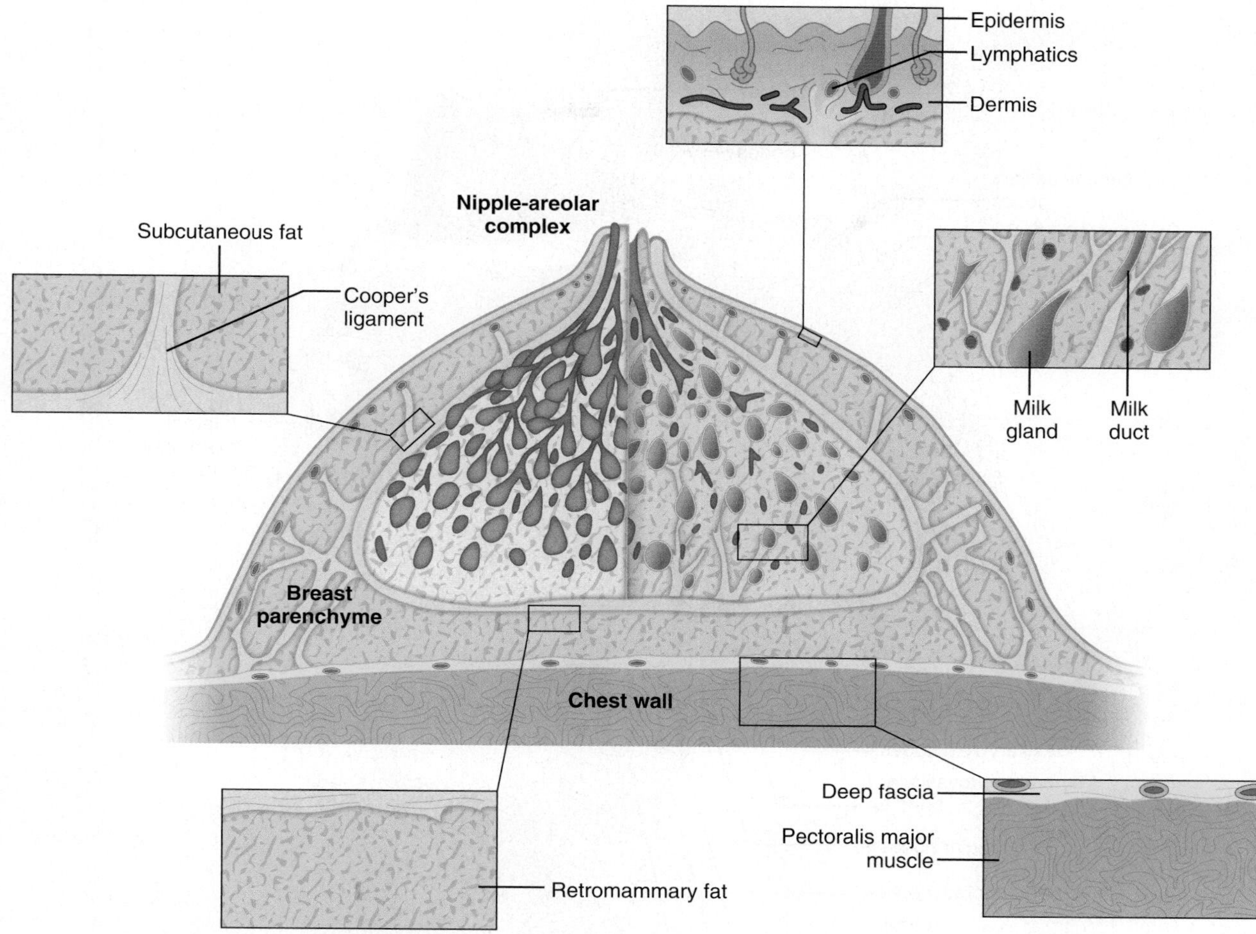

FIGURE 34-1 Cut-away diagram of a mature resting breast. The breast lies cushioned in fat between the overlying skin and pectoralis major muscle. The skin and the retromammary space under the breast are rich with lymphatic channels. Cooper's ligaments, the suspensory ligaments of the breast, fuse with the overlying superficial fascia just under the dermis, coalesce as the interlobular fascia in the breast parenchyma, and then join with the deep fascia of breast over the pectoralis muscle. The system of ducts in the breast is configured like an inverted tree, with the largest ducts just under the nipple and successively smaller ducts in the periphery. After several branching generations, small ducts at the periphery enter the breast lobule, which is the milk-forming glandular unit of the breast.

results in cutaneous anesthesia in these areas, and the possibility of this outcome should be explained to patients before axillary dissection. Denervation of the areas supplied by these sensory nerves causes chronic and uncomfortable pain syndromes in a small percentage of patients. Preservation of the most superior nerve maintains sensation to the posterior aspect of the upper part of the arm without compromising the axillary dissection in most patients.

MICROSCOPIC ANATOMY

The mature breast is composed of three principal tissue types: (1) glandular epithelium, (2) fibrous stroma and supporting structures, and (3) adipose tissue. The breast also contains lymphocytes and macrophages. In adolescents, the predominant tissues are epithelium and stroma. In postmenopausal women, the glandular structures involute and are largely replaced by adipose tissue. Cooper's ligaments provide shape and structure to the breast as they course from the overlying skin to the underlying deep fascia. Because these ligaments are anchored into the skin, infiltration of these ligaments by carcinoma commonly produces tethering, which can cause dimpling or subtle deformities on the otherwise smooth surface of the breast.

The glandular apparatus of the breast is composed of a branching system of ducts, organized in a radial pattern spreading outward and downward from the nipple-areolar complex (see Fig. 34-1). It is possible to cannulate individual ducts and visualize the lactiferous ducts with contrast agents. Figure 34-3 shows the arborization of branching ducts, which end in terminal lobules. The contrast dye opacifies only a single ductal system and does not enter adjacent and intertwined branches from functionally independent ductal branches. Each major duct has a dilated portion (lactiferous sinus) below the nipple-areolar complex. These ducts converge through a constricted orifice into the ampulla of the nipple.

Each of the major ducts has progressive generations of branching and ultimately ends in the terminal ductules or acini (Fig. 34-4). The acini are the milk-forming glands of the lactating breast and, together with their small efferent ducts or ductules,

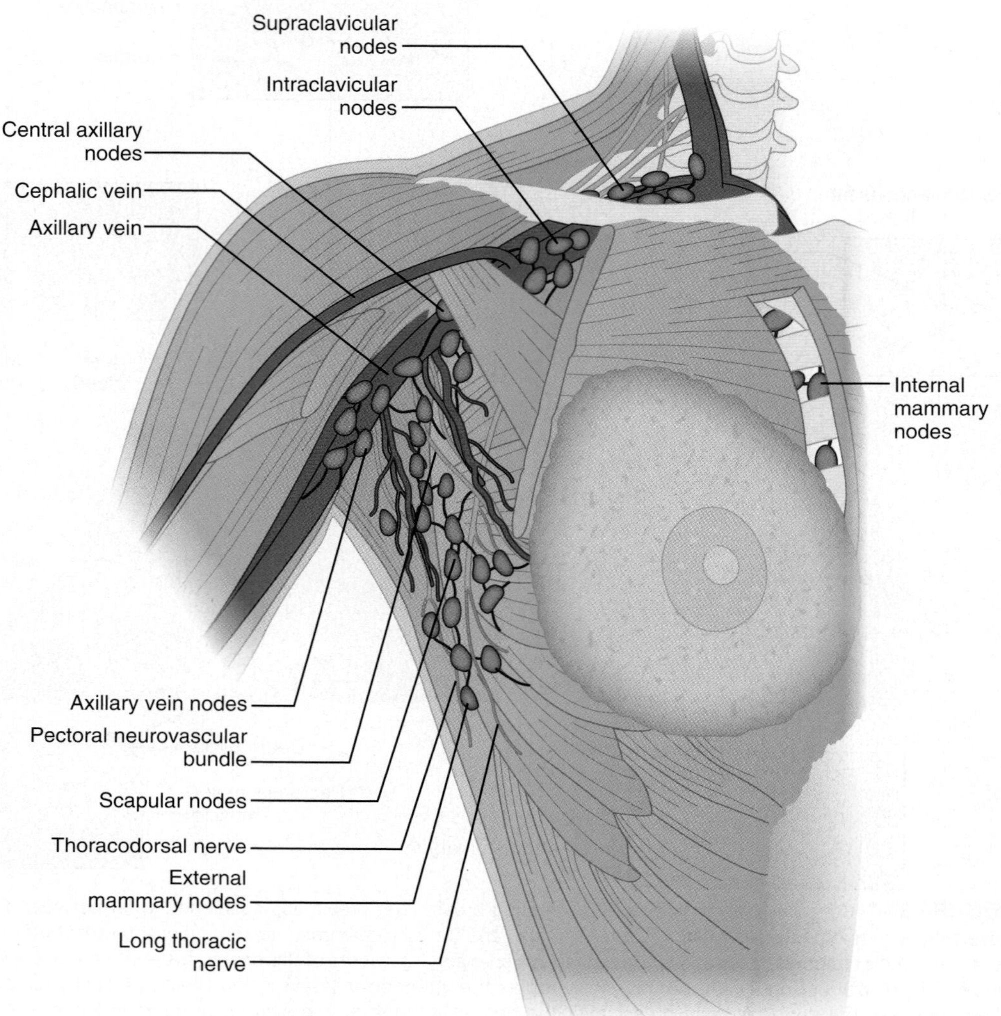

FIGURE 34-2 Contents of the axilla. In this diagram, there are five named and contiguous groupings of lymph nodes in the full axilla. Complete axillary dissection, as done in the historical radical mastectomy, removes all these nodes. However, the subclavicular nodes in the axilla are continuous with the supraclavicular nodes in the neck and nodes between the pectoralis major and minor muscles, called the *interpectoral nodes* in this diagram (also known as *Rotter's lymph nodes*). The sentinel lymph node is functionally the first node in the axillary chain and anatomically is usually found in the external mammary group. The relative positions of the long thoracic, thoracodorsal, and medial pectoral nerves are shown. These major nerves along with the pectoral neurovascular bundle should be preserved during surgery.

are known as *lobular units* or *lobules*. As shown in Figure 34-4, the terminal ductules are invested in a specialized loose connective tissue that contains capillaries, lymphocytes, and other migratory mononuclear cells. This intralobular stroma is clearly distinguished from the denser and less cellular interlobular stroma and from the adipose tissue within the breast.

The entire ductal system is lined by epithelial cells, which are surrounded by specialized myoepithelial cells that have contractile properties and serve to propel milk formed in the lobules toward the nipple. Outside the epithelial and myoepithelial layers, the ducts of the breast are surrounded by a continuous basement membrane containing laminin, type IV collagen, and proteoglycans. The basement membrane layer is an important boundary in differentiating in situ from invasive breast cancer. Continuity of this layer is maintained in ductal carcinoma in situ (DCIS), also termed *noninvasive breast cancer* (see "Pathology" later on). Invasive breast cancer is defined by penetration of the basement membrane by malignant cells invading the stroma.

BREAST DEVELOPMENT AND PHYSIOLOGY

Normal Development and Physiology

Before puberty, the breast is composed primarily of dense fibrous stroma and scattered ducts lined with epithelium. In the United States, puberty, as measured by breast development and the growth of pubic hair, begins between the ages of 9 and 12 years, and menarche (onset of menstrual cycles) begins at approximately 12 to 13 years of age. These events are initiated by low-amplitude pulses of pituitary gonadotropins, which increase serum estradiol concentrations. In the breast, this hormone-dependent maturation (thelarche) entails increased deposition of fat, the formation of new ducts by branching and elongation, and the first appearance of lobular units. This process of growth and cell division is under the control of estrogen, progesterone, adrenal hormones, pituitary hormones, and the trophic effects of insulin and thyroid hormone. There is evidence that local growth factor networks are also important. The exact timing of these events and the coordinated development of both breast buds may vary from the average in individual patients. The term *prepubertal gynecomastia* refers to symmetrical enlargement and projection of the breast bud in a girl before the average age of 12 years, unaccompanied by the other changes of puberty. This process, which may be unilateral, should not be confused with neoplastic growth and is not an indication for biopsy.[1]

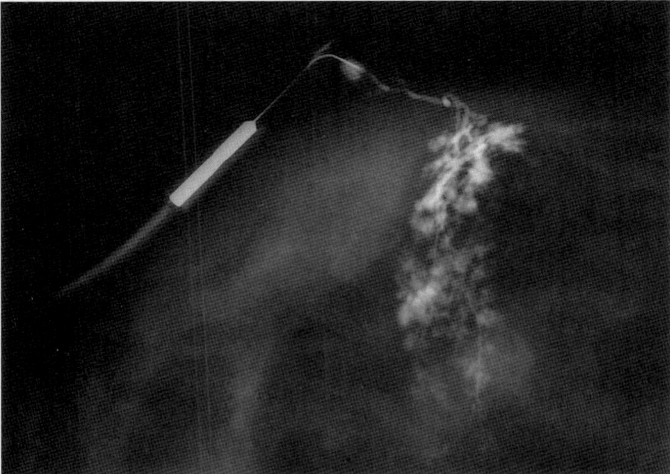

FIGURE 34-3 Injection of contrast material into a single ductal system (ductogram). Occasionally used to evaluate surgically significant nipple discharge, ductography is performed by cannulation of an individual duct orifice and injection of contrast material. This ductogram opacifies the entire ductal tree, from the retroareolar duct to the lobules at the end of the tree. It also demonstrates the functional independence of each duct system; there is no cross-communication between independent systems.

The postpubertal mature or resting breast contains fat, stroma, lactiferous ducts, and lobular units. During phases of the menstrual cycle or in response to exogenous hormones, the breast epithelium and lobular stroma undergo cyclic stimulation. The dominant process appears to be hypertrophy and alteration of morphology rather than hyperplasia. In the late luteal (premenstrual) phase, there is an accumulation of fluid and intralobular edema. This edema can produce pain and breast engorgement.

These physiologic changes can lead to increased nodularity and may be mistaken for a malignant tumor. Ill-defined masses in premenopausal women are generally observed through the course of the menstrual cycle before any intervention is undertaken. With pregnancy, there is diminution of the fibrous stroma and the formation of new acini or lobules, termed *adenosis of pregnancy.* After birth, there is a sudden loss of placental hormones, which, combined with continued high levels of prolactin, is the principal trigger for lactation. The actual expulsion of milk is under hormonal control and is caused by contraction of the myoepithelial cells that surround the breast ducts and terminal ductules. There is no evidence for innervation of these myoepithelial cells; their contraction appears to occur in response to the pituitary-derived peptide oxytocin. Stimulation of the nipple appears to be the physiologic signal for continued pituitary secretion of prolactin and acute release of oxytocin. When breastfeeding ceases, the prolactin level decreases and there is no stimulus for release of oxytocin. The breast returns to a resting state and to the cyclic changes induced when menstruation resumes.

Menopause is defined by cessation in menstrual flow for at least 1 year; in the United States, it usually occurs between the ages of 40 and 55 years, with a median age of 51 years. Menopause may be accompanied by symptoms such as vasomotor disturbances (hot flashes), vaginal dryness, urinary tract infections, and cognitive impairment (possibly secondary to interruption of sleep by hot flashes). Menopause results in involution and a general decrease in the epithelial elements of the resting breast.

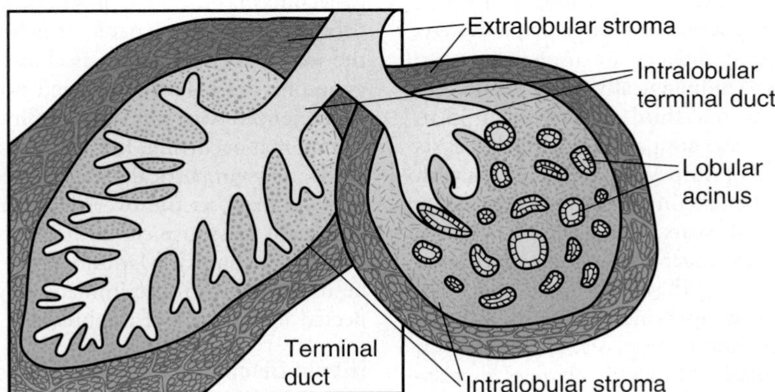

FIGURE 34-4 Mature resting lobular unit. At the distal end of the ductal system is the lobule, which is formed by multiple branching events at the end of terminal ducts, each ending in a blind sac or acini, and is invested with specialized stroma. The lobule is a three-dimensional structure but is seen in two dimensions in a histologic thin section, shown in the *lower right.* The intralobular terminal ductule and acini are invested in loose connective tissue containing a modest number of infiltrating lymphocytes and plasma cells. The lobule is distinct from the denser interlobular stroma, which contains larger breast ducts, blood vessels, and fat.

These changes include increased fat deposition, diminished connective tissue, and the disappearance of lobular units. The persistence of lobules, hyperplasia of the ductal epithelium, and cyst formation all can occur under the influence of exogenous ovarian hormones, usually in the form of postmenopausal hormone replacement therapy (HRT). Physicians should inquire about the menstrual history, age at onset of menses, and cessation of menses and record the use of HRT because all of these factors can influence a woman's risk of developing breast cancer. HRT can lead to increased breast density, which may decrease the sensitivity of mammography.

Fibrocystic Changes and Breast Pain

The condition previously referred to as *fibrocystic disease* represents a spectrum of clinical, mammographic, and histologic findings and is common during the fourth and fifth decades of life, generally lasting until menopause. An exaggerated response of breast stroma and epithelium to various circulating and locally produced hormones and growth factors is frequently characterized by the constellation of breast pain, tenderness, and nodularity. Symptomatically, the condition manifests as premenstrual cyclic mastalgia, with pain and tenderness to touch. This mastalgia can be worrisome to many women; however, breast pain is not usually a symptom of breast cancer. Pain without other signs or symptoms of breast cancer is uncommon, occurring in only approximately 5% of patients with breast cancer. In women with breast pain and an associated palpable mass, the presence of the mass is the focus of evaluation and treatment. Normal ovarian hormonal influences on breast glandular elements frequently produce cyclic mastalgia, pain generally in phase with the menstrual cycle. Noncyclic mastalgia is more likely idiopathic and difficult to treat. Women 30 years and older with noncyclic mastalgia should undergo breast imaging with mammography and ultrasonography in addition to a physical examination. If examination reveals a mass, this should become the focus of subsequent evaluation (see "Biopsy" later on). Occasionally, a simple cyst may cause noncyclic breast pain, and aspiration of the cyst usually resolves the pain. Most patients with simple cysts do not require further evaluation. Patients with complex cysts with solid intracystic components require additional evaluation including biopsy of the solid components.

Patients with fibrocystic changes have clinical breast findings that range from mild alterations in texture to dense, firm breast tissue with palpable masses. The appearance of large palpable cysts completes the picture. Fibrocystic changes are usually seen on mammography as diffuse or focal radiologically dense tissue. On ultrasonography, cysts are seen in one third of all women 35 to 50 years old; most of these cysts are nonpalpable. Palpable cysts or multiple small cysts are typical of fibrocystic disease. Cysts with or without fibrocystic disease are uncommon in women older than 60 years and younger than 30 years.

Histologically, in addition to macrocysts and microcysts, women with fibrocystic changes may have identified solid elements, including adenosis, sclerosis, apocrine metaplasia, stromal fibrosis, and epithelial metaplasia and hyperplasia. Depending on the presence of epithelial hyperplasia, fibrocystic changes are classified as nonproliferative, proliferative without atypia, or proliferative with atypia. All three types of changes can occur alone or in combination and to a variable degree, and in the absence of epithelial atypia, these changes represent the histologic spectrum of normal breast tissue. However, epithelial atypia (atypical ductal hyperplasia [ADH]) is a risk factor for the development of breast cancer. Atypical proliferations of ductal epithelial cells confer increased risk for breast cancer; however, fibrocystic change is not itself a risk factor for the development of breast malignancy.

Abnormal Development and Physiology

Absent or Accessory Breast Tissue

Absence of breast tissue (amastia) and absence of the nipple (athelia) are rare anomalies. Unilateral rudimentary breast development is more common, as is adolescent hypertrophy of one breast with lesser development of the other. Accessory breast tissue (polymastia) and accessory nipples (supernumerary nipples) are common. Supernumerary nipples are usually rudimentary and occur along the milk line from the axilla to the pubis in males and females. They may be mistaken for a small mole. Accessory nipples are usually removed only for cosmetic reasons. True polythelia refers to more than one nipple serving a single breast, which is rare. Accessory breast tissue is commonly located above the breast in the axilla. Rudimentary nipple development may be present, and lactation is possible with more complete development. Accessory breast tissue may be seen as an enlarging mass in the axilla during pregnancy and persists as excess tissue in the axilla after lactation is complete. The accessory mammary tissue may be removed surgically if it is large or cosmetically deforming or to prevent enlargement during future pregnancy.

Gynecomastia

Hypertrophy of breast tissue in men is a clinical entity for which there is frequently no identifiable cause. Pubertal hypertrophy occurs in boys between age 13 years and early adulthood, and senescent hypertrophy is diagnosed in men older than 50 years. Gynecomastia in teenage boys is common and may be bilateral or unilateral. Unless it is unilateral or painful, it may pass unnoticed and regress with adulthood. Pubertal hypertrophy is generally treated by observation without surgery. Surgical excision may be discussed if the enlargement is unilateral, fails to regress, or is cosmetically unacceptable. Hypertrophy in older men is also common. The enlargement is frequently unilateral, although the contralateral breast may enlarge with time. Many commonly used medications, such as digoxin, thiazides, estrogens, phenothiazines, and theophylline, may exacerbate senescent gynecomastia. In addition, gynecomastia may be a systemic manifestation of hepatic cirrhosis, renal failure, or malnutrition. In pubertal and senescent gynecomastia, the mass is smooth, firm, and symmetrically distributed beneath the areola. It is frequently tender, which is often the reason for seeking medical attention. Pubertal and senescent gynecomastia may be managed nonoperatively and can be fully characterized with ultrasonography. There is little confusion with carcinoma occurring in the breast. Carcinoma is not usually tender, is asymmetrically located beneath or beside the areola, and may be fixed to the overlying dermis or to the deep fascia. A dominant mass suspicious for carcinoma should be examined with core needle biopsy. Mammography and ultrasonography can also be useful tools to discriminate between gynecomastia and a suspected malignancy of the breast in older men.

Nipple Discharge

The appearance of discharge from the nipple (Fig. 34-5*A*) of a nonlactating woman is a common condition and is rarely associated with an underlying carcinoma. In one review of 270 subareolar biopsies for discharge from one identifiable duct and without an associated breast mass, carcinoma was found in only 16 patients (5.9%). In these cases, the fluid was bloody or tested strongly positive for occult hemoglobin. In another series of 249 patients

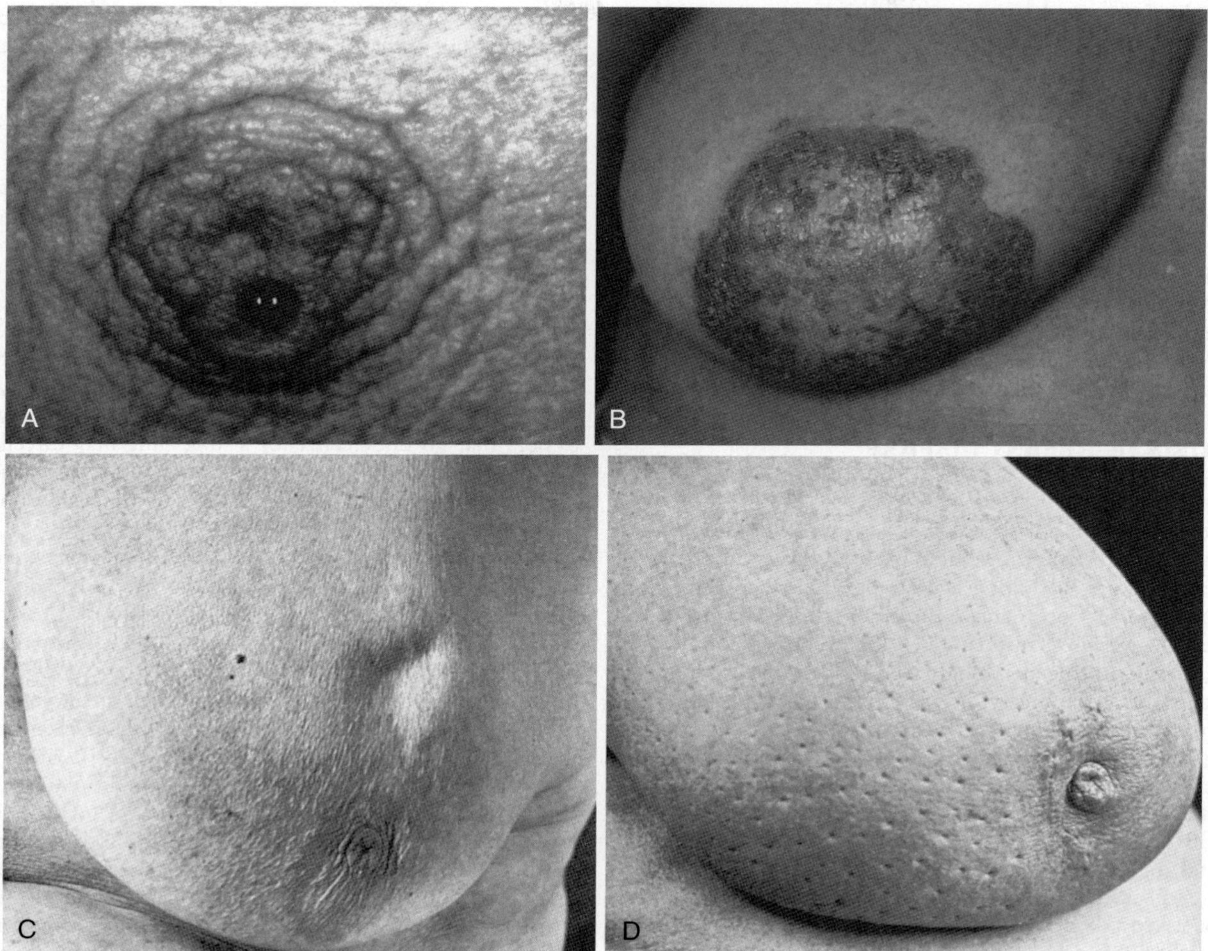

FIGURE 34-5 Common physical findings during breast examination. **A,** Nipple discharge. Discharge from multiple ducts or bilateral discharge is a common finding in healthy breasts. In the case shown, the discharge is from a single duct orifice and may signify underlying disease in the discharging duct. In this patient, a papilloma was the source of her symptoms. **B,** Paget disease of the nipple. Malignant ductal cells invade the epidermis without traversing the basement membrane of the subareolar duct or epidermis. The disease appears as a psoriatic rash that begins on the nipple and spreads off onto the areola and into the skin of the breast. **C,** Skin dimpling. Traction on Cooper's ligaments by a scirrhous tumor is distorting the surface of the breast and producing a dimple best seen with angled indirect lighting during abduction of the arms upward. **D,** Peau d'orange (skin of the orange) or edema of the skin of the breast. This finding may be caused by dependency of the breast, lymphatic blockage (from surgery or radiation), or mastitis. The most feared cause is inflammatory carcinoma, in which malignant cells plug the dermal lymphatics—the pathologic hallmark of the disease.

with discharge from a single identifiable duct, breast carcinoma was found in 10 patients (4%). In eight of these patients, a mass lesion was identified in addition to the discharge. In the absence of a palpable mass or suspicious findings on mammography, discharge is rarely associated with cancer.

It is important to establish whether the discharge comes from one breast or from both breasts, whether it comes from multiple duct orifices or from just one, and whether the discharge is grossly bloody or contains blood. A milky discharge from both breasts is termed *galactorrhea*. In the absence of lactation or a history of recent lactation, galactorrhea may be associated with increased production of prolactin. Radioimmunoassay for serum prolactin is diagnostic. However, true galactorrhea is rare and is diagnosed only when the discharge is milky (contains lactose, fat, and milk-specific proteins). Unilateral discharge from one duct orifice is often treated surgically when there is a significant amount of discharge. However, the underlying cause is rarely a breast malignancy.

The most common cause of spontaneous nipple discharge from a single duct is a solitary intraductal papilloma in one of the large subareolar ducts under the nipple. Subareolar duct ectasia producing inflammation and dilation of large collecting ducts under the nipple is common and usually involves discharge from multiple ducts. Cancer is a very unusual cause of discharge in the absence of other signs.

Nipple discharge that is bilateral and comes from multiple ducts is not usually a cause for surgery. Bloody discharge from a single duct often requires surgical excision to establish a diagnosis and control the discharge. A diagnosis of intraductal papilloma is found in most of these cases.

Galactocele

A galactocele is a milk-filled cyst that is round, well circumscribed, and easily movable within the breast. A galactocele generally occurs after the cessation of lactation or when feeding frequency has declined significantly, although galactoceles may occur 6 to 10 months after breastfeeding has ceased. The pathogenesis of galactocele is unknown, but inspissated milk within ducts is thought to be responsible. The cyst is usually located in the central portion of the breast or under the nipple. Needle aspiration produces thick, creamy material that may be tinged dark green or brown. Although it appears purulent, the fluid is sterile. Treatment is needle aspiration, and withdrawal of thick milky secretion confirms the diagnosis; surgery is reserved for cysts that cannot be aspirated or that become infected.

DIAGNOSIS OF BREAST DISEASE

Patient History

In a woman in whom breast disease is suspected, it is important for the examiner to determine the patient's age and to obtain a reproductive history, including age at menarche, age at menopause, and history of pregnancies including age at first full-term pregnancy. A previous history of breast biopsies should be obtained, including the pathologic findings, especially findings regarding proliferative breast disease. If the patient has had a hysterectomy, it is important to determine whether the ovaries were removed. In premenopausal women, a recent history of pregnancy and lactation should be noted. The history should include any use of HRT or use of hormones for contraception. The family history should detail any cancer of the breast and ovaries and the menopausal status of any affected relatives.

With respect to the specific breast complaint, the patient should be asked about history of a mass, breast pain, nipple discharge, and any skin changes. If a mass is present, the patient should be asked how long it has been present and whether it changes with the menstrual cycle. If a cancer diagnosis is suspected, inquiry about constitutional symptoms, bone pain, weight loss, respiratory changes, and similar clinical indications can direct investigations that could reveal evidence of metastatic disease.

Physical Examination

The physical examination begins with the patient in the upright sitting position. The breasts are carefully visually inspected for obvious masses, asymmetries, and skin changes. The nipples are inspected and compared for the presence of retraction, nipple inversion, or excoriation of the superficial epidermis such as that seen with Paget disease (Fig. 34-5*B*). The use of indirect lighting can unmask subtle dimpling of the skin or nipple caused by a carcinoma that places Cooper's ligaments under tension (Fig. 34-5*C*). Simple maneuvers such as stretching the arms high above the head or tensing the pectoralis muscles may accentuate asymmetries and dimpling. If carefully sought, dimpling of the skin or nipple retraction is a sensitive and specific sign of underlying cancer.

Edema of the skin produces a clinical sign known as *peau d'orange* (Fig. 34-5*D*). Peau d'orange and tenderness, warmth, and swelling of the breast are the hallmarks of inflammatory carcinoma but may be mistaken for acute mastitis. The inflammatory changes and edema are caused by obstruction of dermal lymphatic channels by emboli of carcinoma cells. Occasionally, a bulky tumor may produce obstruction of lymph channels that results in overlying skin edema. This is not typically the case with inflammatory carcinoma, where there is usually no discrete palpable mass but diffuse changes throughout the breast parenchyma. In 40 patients with inflammatory carcinoma described by Haagensen,[1] erythema and edema of the skin were present in all cases, a palpable mass or localized induration was noted in 19 patients, and no localized tumor was present in 21 patients.

Involvement of the nipple and areola can occur with carcinoma of the breast, especially when the primary tumor is located in the subareolar position. Direct involvement may result in retraction of the nipple. Flattening or inversion of the nipple can be caused by fibrosis in certain benign conditions, especially subareolar duct ectasia. In these cases, the finding is frequently bilateral, and the history confirms that the condition has been present for many years. Unilateral retraction or retraction that develops over weeks or months is more suggestive of carcinoma. Centrally located tumors that go undetected for a long time may directly invade and ulcerate the skin of the areola or nipple. Peripheral tumors may distort the normal symmetry of the nipples by traction on Cooper's ligaments.

Paget disease is a condition of the nipple that is commonly associated with an underlying breast cancer. First described by Paget in 1874, Paget disease produces histologically distinct changes within the dermis of the nipple. There is often an underlying intraductal carcinoma in the large sinuses just under the nipple (see Fig. 34-5*B*). Carcinoma cells invade across the junction of epidermal and ductal epithelial cells and enter the epidermal layer of the skin of the nipple. Clinically, dermatitis occurs that may appear eczematoid and moist or dry and psoriatic. It begins in the nipple, although it can spread to the skin of the areola. Many benign skin conditions affecting the breast, such as eczema, frequently begin on the areola, whereas Paget disease originates on the nipple and secondarily involves the areola.

Visual inspection should be followed by palpation of the regional lymph nodes and breast tissue. While the patient is still in the sitting position, the examiner supports the patient's arm and palpates each axilla to detect the presence of enlarged axillary lymph nodes. The supraclavicular and infraclavicular spaces are similarly palpated for enlarged nodes. Then the patient lies down, and the breast is palpated. Palpation of the breast is always done with the patient lying supine on a solid examining surface, with the arm stretched above the head. Palpation of the breast while the patient is sitting often leads to inaccurate interpretation because the overlapping breast tissue may feel like a mass or a mass may go undetected within the breast tissue. The breast is best examined with compression of the tissue toward the chest wall, with palpation of each quadrant and the tissue under the nipple-areolar complex. Palpable masses are characterized according to their size, shape, consistency, and location and whether they are fixed to the skin or underlying musculature. Benign tumors, such as fibroadenomas and cysts, can be as firm as carcinomas; usually, these benign entities are distinct, well circumscribed, and movable. Carcinoma is typically firm but less circumscribed, and moving a carcinoma produces a drag of adjacent tissue. Cysts and fibrocystic changes can be tender with palpation of the breast; however, tenderness is rarely a helpful diagnostic sign. Most palpable masses are self-discovered by patients during casual or intentional self-examination.

Biopsy

Fine-Needle Aspiration Biopsy

Historically, fine-needle aspiration biopsy (FNAB) was a common tool used in the diagnosis of breast masses. FNAB can be done with a 22-gauge needle, an appropriately sized syringe, and an alcohol preparation pad. The needle is repeatedly inserted into the mass while constant negative pressure is applied to the syringe. Suction is released, and the needle is withdrawn. The scanty fluid and cellular material within the needle are submitted in physiologically buffered saline or fixed immediately on slides in 95% ethyl alcohol. The slides are submitted for cytologic evaluation of the aspirated material. A limitation of FNAB in evaluating solid masses is that cytologic evaluation does not differentiate noninvasive lesions from invasive lesions if malignant cells are identified. If FNAB demonstrates malignancy, a core needle biopsy (see next) is still required for definitive histologic diagnosis before surgical intervention.

One clinical scenario in which FNAB still has utility is in the evaluation of a second suspicious lesion in the ipsilateral breast of a patient with a known malignancy. In this case, FNAB can be used to determine if the second lesion is malignant and confirm a diagnosis of multifocal breast cancer. This information can aid in determining the appropriate surgical plan. A second clinical scenario in which FNAB is commonly used is in the evaluation of lymph nodes that are suspicious on either physical examination or imaging, particularly high-resolution ultrasonography of the regional nodal basins. Suspicious lymph nodes can be evaluated by FNAB to determine whether metastatic disease is present. In this situation, FNAB has a reported sensitivity of approximately 90% and a specificity of up to 100%. Determining whether the tumor has spread to the lymph nodes is an important step in the initial staging of breast cancer that provides prognostic information and helps determine appropriate management strategies.

Core Needle Biopsy

Core needle biopsy is the method of choice to sample breast lesions. Core needle biopsy can be performed under mammographic (stereotactic), ultrasound, or magnetic resonance imaging (MRI) guidance. Mass lesions that are visualized on ultrasonography can be sampled under ultrasound guidance; calcifications and densities that are best seen on mammography are sampled under stereotactic guidance. During stereotactic core needle biopsy, the breast is compressed, most often with the patient lying prone on the stereotactic core needle biopsy table. A robotic arm and biopsy device are positioned by computed analysis of triangulated mammographic images. After local anesthetic is injected, a small skin incision is made, and a core biopsy needle is inserted into the lesion to obtain the tissue sample with vacuum assistance. There are standards for the appropriate number of core samples to be obtained for each type of abnormality being sampled. A clip should be placed to mark the site of the lesion, particularly for small lesions that may be difficult to find after extensive sampling. The specimens should be imaged to confirm that the targeted lesion has been adequately sampled. A similar approach is used for ultrasound-guided and MRI-guided biopsy of lesions.

Specimen radiography of excised cores is performed to confirm that the targeted lesion has been sampled and to direct pathologic assessment of the tissue. A mammogram obtained after biopsy confirms that a defect has been created within the target lesion and that the marking clip is in the correct position. Image-guided localization with either a wire or iodine-125 (^{125}I) radioactive seed and surgical excision are required if the lesion cannot be adequately sampled by core needle biopsy or if there is discordance between the imaging abnormality and pathologic findings.

The small samples obtained by core needle biopsy necessitate proper interpretation of the pathology results. Most patients undergoing core needle biopsy have benign findings and may return to routine screening with no other intervention required. If a malignancy is detected, histologic subtype, grade, and receptor status should be determined from the core needle biopsy sample. The patient may proceed to definitive treatment of the cancer if it is an early-stage breast cancer. Patients with locally advanced or inflammatory breast cancer should be treated with systemic chemotherapy before surgical intervention. Depending on the size of the imaging abnormality, approximately 10% to 20% of patients with a diagnosis of DCIS on core needle biopsy are found to have some invasive carcinoma at definitive surgery.

Excisional Biopsy

Use of a minimally invasive procedure, such as core needle biopsy, is the preferred approach for diagnosis of breast lesions. The use of excisional breast biopsy as a diagnostic procedure increases costs and results in delays of definitive surgery for patients with cancer.[2] Less than 10% of patients who undergo core needle biopsy have inconclusive results and require surgical biopsy for definitive diagnosis. Biopsy results that are not concordant with the targeted lesion (e.g., a spiculated mass on imaging and normal breast tissue on core needle biopsy) necessitate surgical excision. When ADH is found on core needle biopsy, surgical excision reveals DCIS or invasive carcinoma in 20% of cases because of the difficulty of distinguishing ADH and DCIS in a limited tissue sample. A finding of a cellular fibroadenoma on core needle biopsy requires excision to rule out a phyllodes tumor.

BREAST IMAGING

Breast imaging techniques are used to detect small, nonpalpable breast abnormalities, evaluate clinical findings, and guide diagnostic procedures. The primary imaging modality for screening asymptomatic women is mammography. During mammography, the breast is compressed between plates to reduce the thickness of the tissue through which the radiation must pass, separate adjacent structures, and improve resolution. On screening mammography, two views of each breast are obtained, mediolateral oblique and craniocaudal. For further evaluation of abnormalities identified on a screening mammogram or of clinical findings or symptoms, diagnostic mammography is indicated. Magnification views are obtained to evaluate calcifications, and compression views are used to provide additional detail when a mass lesion is suspected.

Sensitivity of mammography is limited by breast density, and 10% to 15% of clinically evident breast cancers have no associated abnormality on mammography. Digital mammography acquires digital images and stores them electronically, allowing manipulation and enhancement of images to facilitate interpretation. Digital mammography appears to be superior to traditional film-screen mammography for detecting cancer in younger women and women with dense breasts. Mammography in women younger than 30 years, whose breast tissue is dense with stroma and epithelium, may produce an image without much definition. As women age, the breast tissue involutes and is replaced by fatty tissue. On mammography, fat absorbs relatively little radiation and provides a contrasting background that favors detection of small lesions. Computer-assisted diagnosis has been shown to increase the sensitivity and specificity of mammography and ultrasonography over review by the radiologist alone.

Screening Mammography

Screening mammography is performed in asymptomatic women with the goal of detecting breast cancer that is not yet clinically evident. This approach assumes that breast cancers identified through screening will be smaller, have a better prognosis, and require less aggressive treatment than cancers identified by palpation. The potential benefits of screening are weighed against the cost of screening and the number of false-positive studies that prompt additional workup, biopsies, and patient anxiety.

Eight prospective randomized trials of screening mammography have been performed, with almost 500,000 women participating. In these trials, among women 39 to 49 years old, screening mammography reduced the risk for breast cancer death by 15% (relative risk [RR], 0.85; credible interval [CrI], 0.75 to 0.96). In the six trials that included women 50 to 59 years old, screening mammography reduced the risk for breast cancer death in this age group by 14% (RR, 0.86; CrI, 0.75 to 0.99). Two trials included women 60 to 69 years old, and screening mammography reduced the risk for breast cancer death in this age group by 32% (RR, 0.68; CrI, 0.54 to 0.87). Only one trial included women older than 70 years, and data were insufficient to recommend routine screening in this age group. On the basis of these results, the most recent U.S. Preventive Services Task Force report recommended biennial screening mammography for women 50 to 74 years old and recommended against screening for women 40 to 49 years old or older than 75 years.[2] The recommendations were based on the risk reduction, number of women needed to invite for screening to prevent one breast cancer death, and potential for harm from additional testing and biopsies (Table 34-1).

At the present time, the American Cancer Society continues to recommend annual screening mammography for women older than 40 years and suggests that this practice should continue as long as the woman is in good health. Younger women with a previous breast cancer, significant family history of breast cancer, or histologic risk factors for breast cancer may also benefit from screening with MRI. Although the randomized trials of screening mammography did not enroll women older than 74 years, breast cancer risk increases with age, and the sensitivity and specificity of mammography are highest in older women, whose breast tissue has usually been replaced by fat. It is reasonable to continue mammographic screening in older women who are in good general health who would be considered appropriate candidates for surgery.

Ultrasonography

Ultrasonography is useful in determining whether a lesion detected by mammography is solid or cystic. Ultrasonography can also be useful for discriminating lesions in patients with dense breasts. However, it has not been found to be a useful breast cancer screening tool because it is highly dependent on the operator performing the freehand screening and there are no standardized screening protocols. The American College of Radiology Imaging Network (ACRIN) performed a trial (ACRIN 6666) in high-risk women in whom mammography and ultrasonography were performed in randomized order to compare the sensitivity, specificity, and diagnostic yield of ultrasonography plus mammography compared with mammography alone.[3] The investigators found that the combination of mammography plus ultrasonography resulted in detection of an additional 4.2 cancers per 1000 women. However, the use of ultrasonography resulted in more false-positive events and required more call-backs and biopsies. There are no data available showing that the use of screening ultrasonography can reduce mortality caused by breast cancer.

Magnetic Resonance Imaging

MRI is increasingly being used for the evaluation of breast abnormalities. It is useful for identifying the primary tumor in the breast in patients who present with axillary lymph node metastases without mammographic evidence of a primary breast tumor (unknown primary tumor) or in patients with Paget disease of the nipple without radiographic evidence of a primary tumor. MRI may also be useful for assessing the extent of the primary tumor, particularly in young women with dense breast tissue; for evaluating for the presence of multifocal or multicentric cancer; for screening of the contralateral breast; and for evaluating invasive lobular cancers. Some surgeons use MRI preoperatively to determine eligibility for breast conservation; however, there are no high-level data showing that use of MRI to guide decision making about local therapy improves local recurrence rates or survival.

The sensitivity of MRI is greater than 90% for the detection of invasive cancer but only 60% or less for the detection of DCIS. The specificity of MRI is only moderate; there is significant overlap in the appearance on MRI of benign and malignant lesions. A meta-analysis of 22 studies reporting the detection of contralateral breast cancer by MRI revealed a mean incremental cancer detection rate of 4.1% and a positive predictive value of 47.9%. This high rate of detection may result partly from selection bias; however, it is of significant concern that more than 50% of the abnormalities detected on MRI represented false-positive findings, resulting in the need for additional imaging studies and biopsies.

The COMICE (Comparative Effectiveness of MRI in Breast Cancer) trial was a multicenter trial that recruited 1623 women

TABLE 34-1 Effect on Breast Cancer Mortality and False-Positive Mammograms by Age Group in Breast Cancer Screening Trials

AGE GROUP (YR)	NO. TRIALS	BREAST CANCER MORTALITY, RR (95% CRI)	NO. NEEDED TO INVITE FOR SCREENING TO PREVENT ONE BREAST CANCER DEATH (95% CRI)	FALSE-POSITIVE MAMMOGRAMS/ SCREENING ROUND*
39-49	8	0.85 (0.75-0.96)	1904 (929-6378)	97.8
50-59	6	0.86 (0.75-0.99)	1339 (322-7455)	86.6
60-69	2	0.68 (0.54-0.87)	377 (230-1050)	79.0
70-74	1	1.12 (0.73-1.72)	NA	68.8

Adapted from Nelson HD, Tyne K, Naik A, et al: U.S. Preventive Services Task Force: Screening for breast cancer: Systematic evidence review update for the U.S. Preventive Services Task Force. *Ann Intern Med* 151:727, 2009.

CRI, credible interval; *NA,* not available; *RR,* relative risk.

*Per 1000 screened.

BOX 34-1 American Cancer Society Risk Criteria for Breast Magnetic Resonance Imaging Screening

Women at high lifetime risk (≈20%-25% or greater) of breast cancer

- Known *BRCA1* or *BRCA2* gene mutation
- First-degree relative with *BRCA1* or *BRCA2* gene mutation, but have not had genetic testing themselves
- Lifetime risk of breast cancer of ≈20%-25% or greater
- Radiation therapy to the chest between the ages of 10 and 30
- Li-Fraumeni syndrome or Cowden syndrome or a first-degree relative with one of these syndromes

Women at moderately increased (15%-20%) lifetime risk

- Lifetime risk of breast cancer of 15%-20% according to risk assessment tools based mainly on family history
- Personal history of breast cancer, ductal carcinoma in situ, lobular carcinoma in situ, atypical ductal hyperplasia, or atypical lobular hyperplasia
- Extremely dense breasts or unevenly dense breasts when viewed by mammograms

aged 18 years or older with newly diagnosed breast cancer to assess the clinical efficacy of contrast-enhanced MRI.[4] Patients had standard clinical and radiologic examinations and were randomly assigned to undergo MRI or no further imaging. The primary end point was the proportion of patients undergoing another surgical procedure (reexcision or mastectomy) within 6 months. There was no statistically significant difference in reoperation rates between patients who did or did not undergo MRI. The contralateral breast cancer detection rate in the COMICE trial was 1.6%, significantly lower than that reported in other trials. This trial was criticized because MRI-guided biopsy was not available at all centers to assess suspicious findings identified on MRI. This situation led to numerous mastectomies without pathologic verification that the additional findings were malignancy.

With respect to using MRI for routine screening, the American Cancer Society has recommended annual MRI screening beginning at age 30 years for women at high lifetime risk for breast cancer development (approximately 20% to 25% or greater) (Box 34-1). Women at moderately increased lifetime risk (15% to 20%) are advised to discuss with their physicians the benefits and limitations of adding MRI screening. MRI is not recommended for women with a lifetime risk of developing breast cancer of less than 15%. When MRI is used for screening, it should be used in addition to screening mammography. Although MRI is more sensitive than mammography, it may still miss some malignancies that a mammogram would detect.

Nonpalpable Mammographic Abnormalities

Mammographic abnormalities that cannot be detected by physical examination include clustered microcalcifications and areas of abnormal density (e.g., masses, architectural distortions, asymmetries) that have not produced a palpable finding (Fig. 34-6). The Breast Imaging Reporting and Data System (BI-RADS) is used to categorize the degree of suspicion of malignancy for a mammographic abnormality (Table 34-2). To avoid unnecessary biopsies for low-suspicion mammographic findings, probably benign lesions are designated BI-RADS 3 and are monitored with short-interval mammograms over a 2-year period. Biopsy is performed only for lesions that progress during follow-up. Because 75% to 80% of patients for whom diagnostic biopsy of a nonpalpable mammographic lesion is recommended have benign findings, the less invasive and less costly image-guided core needle biopsy approach is preferred whenever feasible.

Image-Localized Surgical Excision of Nonpalpable Breast Lesions

Nonpalpable breast lesions should be assessed with image-guided core needle biopsy, as appropriate, according to the type of abnormality. If the diagnosis is not concordant with imaging findings or there is ADH in a field of microcalcifications that may represent DCIS, most patients should proceed to excisional biopsy for definitive diagnosis.

To ensure that the abnormality is completely excised, it should be localized with either a localizing wire or an ^{125}I radioactive seed that can be placed adjacent to the lesion under mammographic or ultrasound guidance. If a wire is used, it is placed through an introducer needle and has a hook that engages within the breast parenchyma at or near the abnormality to hold it in position after the introducer is withdrawn. Images with the wire in place are made available in the operating room to guide the surgeon. It is generally recommended that the surgical incision be placed directly over the lesion that is marked by the hook of the localizing wire and not where the wire enters the skin. Depending on the size of the breast and length of the localization wire, the hook may be a long distance from the skin entry site. Placing the surgical incision over the site of the hook wire minimizes the amount of normal breast tissue excised during the biopsy procedure. Depending on the size of the lesion and the degree of suspicion of malignancy, it is generally wise to excise a border of normal tissue around the lesion to ensure complete removal with a negative margin. After excision, the specimen is sent for specimen radiography to confirm that the targeted lesion has been excised. Patients who have a diagnosis of benign findings on excision should undergo new baseline mammography 4 to 6 months after the surgical procedure.

Although wire localization is the most common technique used to localize nonpalpable lesions to facilitate surgical resection, the technique has limitations, including patient discomfort, risk of wire displacement, and a negative impact on operating room efficiency because the wire must be placed on the day of surgery. Other techniques have been developed to facilitate resection of nonpalpable lesions, including radioactive seed localization, which involves positioning a 4.5-mm ^{125}I seed in the breast tissue. Radioactive seeds are preloaded into needles that are advanced under mammographic or ultrasound guidance into the lesion of interest, after which the seeds are deployed. Images with the seed in place are made available in the operating room to guide the surgeon. In the operating room, a gamma probe, which detects technetium-99m (^{99m}Tc), commonly used for sentinel lymph node dissection (SLND), and ^{125}I, can be used to guide the resection. After excision, the specimen is sent for specimen radiography to confirm that the targeted lesion and radioactive seed have been excised. In a single-institution report of an initial experience using radioactive seed localization, it was reported that compared with use of localizing wires, use of seeds improved operating room efficiency, and the volume of tissue excised and rates of negative margins were comparable for wire and seed localization.[5]

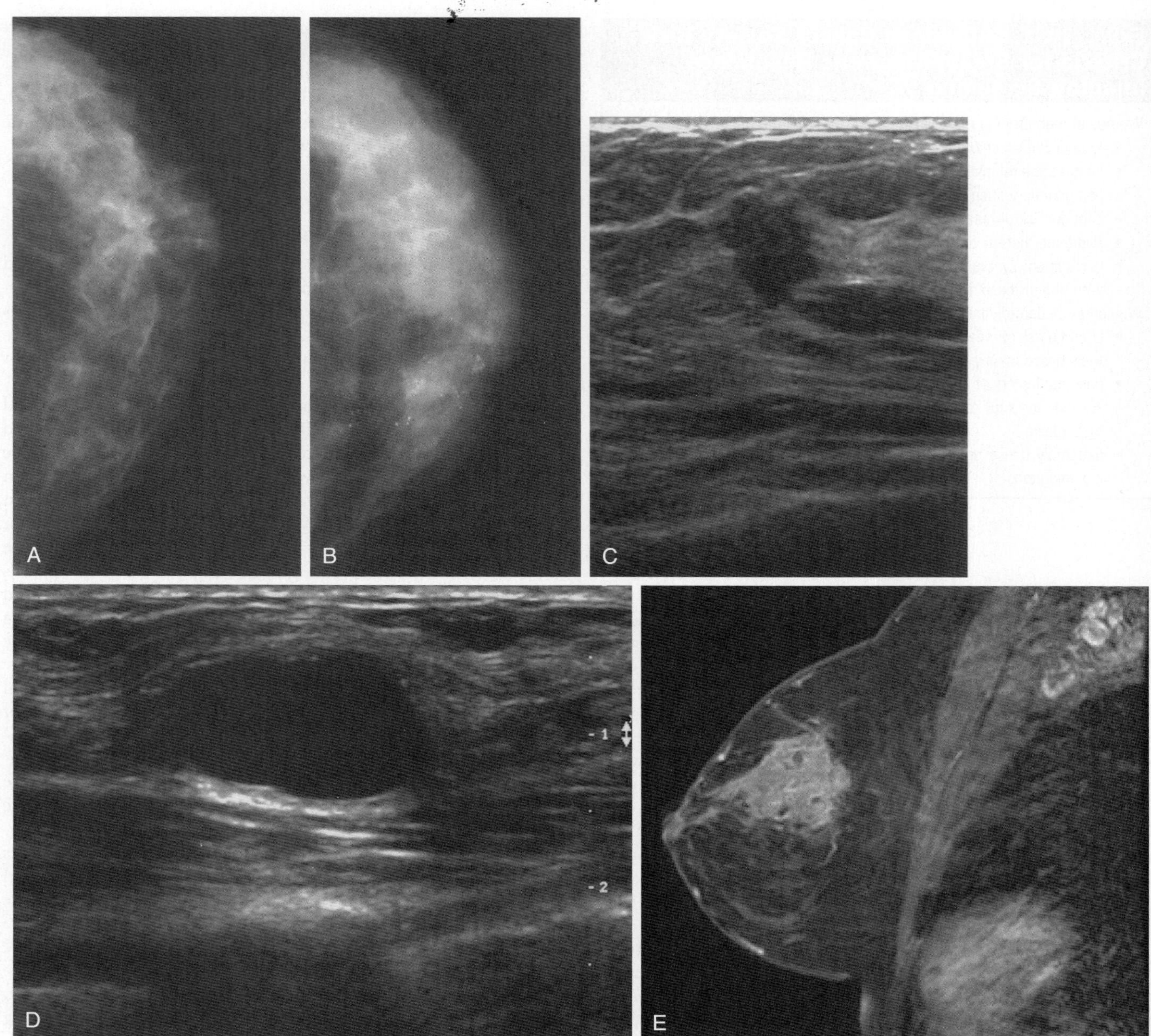

FIGURE 34-6 Mammography, ultrasound, and MRI findings in breast disease. **A,** Stellate mass in the breast. The combination of density with spiculated borders and distortion of surrounding breast architecture suggests a malignancy. **B,** Clustered microcalcifications. Fine, pleomorphic, and linear calcifications that cluster together suggest the diagnosis of ductal carcinoma in situ. **C,** Ultrasound image of breast cancer. The mass is solid, contains internal echoes, and displays an irregular border. Most malignant lesions are taller than they are wide. **D,** Ultrasound image of a simple cyst. On ultrasound, the cyst is round with smooth borders, there is a paucity of internal sound echoes, and there is increased through-transmission of sound with enhanced posterior echoes. **E,** Breast MRI showing gadolinium enhancement of a breast cancer. Rapid and intense gadolinium enhancement reflects increased tumor vascularity. Lesion contour and size may also be assessed by MRI.

IDENTIFICATION AND CARE OF HIGH-RISK PATIENTS

Risk Factors for Breast Cancer

Identification of factors associated with an increased incidence of breast cancer development is important in general health screening for women (Box 34-2). Risk factors for breast cancer can be divided into seven broad categories—age and sex, personal history of breast cancer, histologic risk factors, family history of breast cancer and genetic risk factors, reproductive risk factors, and exogenous hormone use.

Age and Sex

Age is probably the most important risk factor for breast cancer development. The age-adjusted incidence of breast cancer continues to increase with advancing age of the female population.

TABLE 34-2 Breast Imaging Reporting and Data System Final Assessment Category

CATEGORY	DEFINITION
0	Incomplete assessment—need additional imaging evaluation or prior mammograms for comparison
1	Negative—nothing to comment on; usually recommend annual screening
2	Benign finding—usually recommend annual screening
3	Probably benign finding (<2% malignant)—initial short-interval follow-up suggested
4	Suspicious abnormality (2%-95% malignant)—biopsy should be considered
5	Highly suggestive of malignancy (>95% malignant)—appropriate action should be taken
6	Known biopsy—proven malignancy

Adapted from Liberman L, Abramson AF, Squires FB, et al: The Breast Imaging Reporting and Data System: Positive predictive values of mammographic feature and final assessment categories. *AJR Am J Roentgenol* 171:35, 1998; and Liberman L, Menell JH: Breast Imaging Reporting and Data System (BI-RADS). *Radiol Clin North Am* 40:409, 2002.

BOX 34-2 Risk Factors for Breast Cancer

Risk Factors That Cannot be Modified

Increasing age
Female sex
Menstrual factors
Early age at menarche (onset of menses before age 12 yr)
Older age at menopause (onset beyond age 55 yr)
Nulliparity
Family history of breast cancer
Genetic predisposition (*BRCA1* and *BRCA2* mutation carriers)
Personal history of breast cancer
Race, ethnicity (white women have increased risk compared with women of other races)
History of radiation exposure

Risk Factors That Can Be Modified

Reproductive factors
Age at first live birth (full-term pregnancy after age 30 yr)
Parity
Lack of breastfeeding
Obesity
Alcohol consumption
Tobacco smoking
Use of hormone replacement therapy
Decreased physical activity
Shift work (night shifts)

Histologic Risk Factors

Proliferative breast disease
Atypical ductal hyperplasia
Atypical lobular hyperplasia
Lobular carcinoma in situ

Breast cancer is rare in women younger than 20 years and constitutes less than 2% of the total cases. Thereafter, the incidence increases to 1 in 233 from ages 30 to 39 years, 1 in 69 from ages 40 to 49, 1 in 42 from ages 50 to 59, 1 in 29 from ages 60 to 69, and 1 in 8 by age 80 years. Stated another way, women now have an average risk of 12.2% of being diagnosed with breast cancer at some time during their lives.

Sex is also an important risk factor because most breast cancers occur in women. Breast cancer does occur in men; however, the incidence in men is less than 1% of the incidence in women. Of 235,030 cases of invasive breast cancer anticipated in 2014, 2360 cases were expected to occur in men. Lumps in the breast in men are more likely to be benign and the result of gynecomastia (see earlier) or other noncancerous tumors rather than breast cancer.

Personal History of Breast Cancer

A history of cancer in one breast increases the likelihood of a second primary cancer in the contralateral breast. The magnitude of risk depends on the age at diagnosis of the first primary cancer, estrogen receptor (ER) status of the first primary cancer, and use of adjuvant systemic chemotherapy and endocrine therapy. In absolute terms, the actual risk varies from 0.5% to 1% per year in younger patients to 0.2% per year in older patients.[1,6]

Histologic Risk Factors

Histologic abnormalities diagnosed by breast biopsy constitute an important category of breast cancer risk factors. These abnormalities include lobular carcinoma in situ (LCIS) and proliferative changes with atypia. LCIS is an uncommon condition that is observed predominantly in younger premenopausal women. It is typically an incidental finding at biopsy for another condition and does not manifest as a palpable mass or suspicious microcalcifications on mammography. In a report on more than 5000 biopsies performed for benign disease, LCIS was found in 3.6% of cases.[1] In a review of 297 patients with LCIS treated by biopsy and careful observation, it was determined that the actuarial probability of carcinoma developing at the end of 35 years was 21.4%. Using data from the Connecticut Tumor Registry, it was determined that the risk ratio for patients with LCIS (ratio of observed to expected cases of invasive breast cancer) was 7:1. Significantly, 40% of the carcinomas that subsequently developed in patients with LCIS were purely in situ lesions, the invasive carcinomas that developed were predominantly ductal and not lobular in histology, and 50% of the carcinomas occurred in the contralateral breast. LCIS is not considered a breast cancer but rather a histologic marker for increased breast cancer risk, which is estimated at slightly less than 1% per year longitudinally.

For most patients with a diagnosis of LCIS, a conservative approach is favored. The three options that can be discussed with the patient are close observation, chemoprevention with tamoxifen or raloxifene, and bilateral mastectomy. LCIS predisposes to subsequent carcinoma, and the risk is lifelong and equal for both breasts. A 5-year course of tamoxifen provides a 56% reduction in breast cancer risk.[7] For patients who elect surgery rather than observation, bilateral total mastectomy is the procedure of choice.

Benign breast disease produces a spectrum of histologic lesions that are broadly divided into nonproliferative and proliferative epithelial changes. Nonproliferative changes include mild to moderate hyperplasia of luminal cells within breast ducts; these changes do not significantly increase a woman's lifetime risk for development of breast cancer. Proliferative changes within the breast ductal system are associated with an increased risk of developing breast cancer. Dupont and Page divided proliferative lesions into lesions with atypia and lesions without atypia; proliferative lesions without atypia sometimes are termed *severe hyperplasia*.

TABLE 34-3 Histologic Risk Factors for Development of Breast Cancer

HISTOLOGIC DIAGNOSIS	ESTIMATES, RR*
Nonproliferative disease†	1.0
Proliferative disease without atypia‡	1.3-1.9
Proliferative disease with atypia§	3.7-4.2
and strong family history	4-9
LCIS	>7

LCIS, lobular carcinoma in situ; *RR,* relative risk.
*Ratio of observed incidence over the incidence in women without proliferative disease.
†Fibrocystic change with no, usual, or mild hyperplasia.
‡Fibrocystic change with hyperplasia greater than mild or usual, papilloma, papillomatosis, sclerosing adenosis, radial scar, and other findings.
§Any diagnosis of atypical ductal or lobular hyperplasia, or both.
Data from Hartmann LC, Sellers TA, Frost MH, et al: Benign breast disease and the risk of breast cancer. *N Engl J Med* 353:229, 2005; London SJ, Connolly JL, Schnitt SJ, et al: A prospective study of benign breast disease and the risk of breast cancer. *JAMA* 267:1780, 1992; and Dupont WD, Parl FF, Hartmann WH, et al: Breast cancer risk associated with proliferative breast disease and atypical hyperplasia. *Cancer* 71:1258, 1993.

Subsequent studies adopted this classification scheme—nonproliferative lesions, proliferative changes without atypia (severe hyperplasia), and proliferative changes with atypia. ADH and atypical lobular hyperplasia (ALH) are categorized as proliferative changes with atypia. The risk for development of breast cancer in women with ADH or ALH is approximately four to five times the risk in the general population. A family history of breast cancer and atypical hyperplasia increases the risk to almost nine times that of the general population. The annual risk for development of breast cancer in a woman with ADH or ALH is 0.5% to 1% per year. The estimates of breast cancer risk according to histologic risk factors are influenced by age at diagnosis, menopausal status, and family history. Histologic risk factors are listed in Table 34-3.[8]

Family History of Breast Cancer and Genetic Risk Factors

Many studies have examined the relationship between family history of breast cancer and the risk for breast cancer. First-degree relatives (mothers, sisters, and daughters) of patients with breast cancer have a twofold to threefold excess risk for development of the disease. Risk is much higher if affected first-degree relatives had premenopausal onset and bilateral breast cancer. Risk is not significantly increased in women with distant relatives (cousins, aunts, grandmothers) with breast cancer, although breast cancer in paternal aunts may be associated with a genetic predisposition. In families with multiple affected members, particularly with bilateral and early-onset cancer, the absolute risk in first-degree relatives approaches 50%, consistent with an autosomal dominant mode of inheritance in these families.

Genetic factors are estimated to be responsible for 5% to 10% of all breast cancer cases, but they may account for 25% of cases in women younger than 30 years. In 1990, King and colleagues identified a region on the long arm of chromosome 17 (17q21) that contained a cancer susceptibility gene. The *BRCA1* gene was discovered in 1994; it is now known that mutations in *BRCA1* account for up to 40% of familial breast cancers. A second susceptibility gene, *BRCA2,* was discovered in 1995. In addition to being at increased risk for breast cancer, women with mutations in *BRCA1* or *BRCA2* are at increased risk for ovarian cancer (45% lifetime risk for *BRCA1* carriers).

Deleterious mutations in *BRCA1* or *BRCA2* are rare in the general population. The frequency of mutations is approximately 1 in 1000 (0.1%) in the U.S. population. Certain relatively closed populations may have higher prevalence rates and show preference for certain mutations, termed *founder mutations,* including the 185delAG and 5382insC mutations in *BRCA1,* which are found in 1.0% of the Ashkenazi Jewish population (Jews of Eastern European descent), and the C4446T mutation found in French Canadian families. *BRCA1* is a large gene with 22 coding exons and more than 500 mutations; many of these are unique and limited to a given family, which makes genetic testing technically difficult. *BRCA1* is a tumor suppressor gene with disease susceptibility inherited in an autosomal dominant fashion. Germline mutations inactivate a single inherited allele of *BRCA1* in every cell, and this precedes a somatic event in breast epithelial cells that eliminates the remaining allele and causes the cancer. The gene product may provide negative regulation of cell growth and is involved in recognition and repair of genetic damage.

The *BRCA2* gene is located on chromosome 13 and accounts for 30% of familial breast cancers; in contrast to *BRCA1*, *BRCA2* is associated with increased breast cancer risk in men. Women with a mutation in *BRCA2* also have a 20% to 30% lifetime risk for ovarian cancer. Founder mutations of *BRCA2* include the 617delT mutation, present in 1.4% of the Ashkenazi population; 8765delAG mutation, present in the French Canadian population, and 999del15 mutation, found in the Icelandic population. In Iceland, 7% of unselected women with breast cancer and 0.6% of individuals in the general population carry the 999del15 mutation.

The penetrance of a gene refers to the chance that carriers of mutations in the gene will actually develop breast cancer. The initial estimates of the penetrance of *BRCA1* and *BRCA2* mutations were high, but the penetrance of *BRCA1* and *BRCA2* mutations more recently has been estimated to be 56% (95% confidence interval [CI], 40% to 73%). It is reasonable to quote lifetime rates of breast cancer between 50% and 70% for carriers of *BRCA1* or *BRCA2* mutations.

The histopathology of *BRCA1*-associated breast cancer is unfavorable compared with *BRCA2*-associated cancer and includes tumors that are high grade, hormone receptor–negative, and aneuploid, with an increased S phase fraction. There is a strong association between the basal-like breast cancer subtype and *BRCA1* mutations. Women who carry a *BRCA1* mutation and develop breast cancer are highly likely to have basal-like breast cancer, and 10% of basal-like tumors arise in women with a *BRCA1* mutation. The same is not true for *BRCA2*-associated cancers, which are more commonly hormone receptor–positive. Overall mortality rates in patients with *BRCA1*-associated or *BRCA2*-associated breast cancer are similar to mortality rates in women with sporadic breast cancer. Because the risk for development of breast cancer is high in carriers of a *BRCA* gene mutation, prophylactic surgery is considered to be the most rational approach. MRI is encouraged for women who prefer intensive screening rather than prophylactic surgery. The efficacy of chemoprevention in *BRCA* mutation carriers is unclear, especially in women with *BRCA1* mutations, who tend to develop ER-negative breast cancers.

Reproductive Risk Factors

Reproductive milestones that increase a woman's lifetime estrogen exposure are thought to increase her breast cancer risk. These include onset of menarche before 12 years of age, first live childbirth after age 30 years, nulliparity, and menopause after age 55 years. There is a 10% reduction in breast cancer risk for each 2-year delay in menarche; the risk doubles with menopause after age 55. A first full-term pregnancy before age 18 years is associated with half the risk for development of breast cancer of a first full-term pregnancy after age 30 years. Induced abortion is not associated with increased breast cancer risk. Breastfeeding has been reported to reduce breast cancer risk, and this effect may be secondary to a decrease in the number of lifetime menstrual cycles. Compared with sex, age, histologic risk factors, and genetics, reproductive risk factors are relatively mild in terms of their contribution to risk (RR, 0.5 to 2.0). However, in contrast to family history or histologic factors, reproductive risk factors have a large influence on breast cancer prevalence in populations.[8]

Exogenous Hormone Use

Therapeutic or supplemental estrogen and progesterone are taken for various conditions, with the two most common scenarios being contraception in premenopausal women and HRT in postmenopausal women. Other indications for use of exogenous hormones include menstrual irregularities, polycystic ovaries, fertility treatment, and hormone insufficiency states. Studies have suggested that breast cancer risk is increased in current or past users of oral contraceptives but that the risk decreases as the interval after cessation of use increases.[9,10]

The use of HRT was studied in the Women's Health Initiative,[9] a prospective, randomized controlled trial in which healthy postmenopausal women 50 to 79 years old received various dietary and vitamin supplements and postmenopausal HRT. The study assessed the benefits and risks associated with HRT, a low-fat diet, and calcium and vitamin D supplementation and their effects on rates of cancer, cardiovascular disease, and osteoporosis-related fractures. During the period 1993-1998 at 40 centers in the United States, 16,608 women were randomly assigned to receive combined conjugated equine estrogens (e.g., Premarin, 0.625 mg/day) plus medroxyprogesterone acetate (2.5 mg/day) or placebo. Screening mammography and clinical breast examinations were performed at baseline and yearly thereafter. The study reached a stopping rule at 5.2 years of follow-up, at which time there were 245 cases of breast cancer (invasive and noninvasive) in the combined HRT group versus 185 cases in the placebo group. Compared with placebo, the combination of estrogen and progesterone, specifically Prempro, increased the risk of developing breast cancer in postmenopausal women with an intact uterus. Of greater concern was that breast cancer was more likely to be diagnosed at a more advanced stage in women receiving estrogen plus progesterone, and these women were substantially more likely to have abnormal mammograms.

Also in the Women's Health Initiative, 10,739 women who had had a hysterectomy were randomly assigned to conjugated equine estrogens (e.g., Premarin) at a dose of 0.625 mg daily or a placebo. After 7 years of follow-up, the two groups had equivalent rates of breast cancer (RR for the estrogen group, 0.80; 95% CI, 0.62 to 1.04).[10] There was a statistically significant difference between the treatment and control groups in the need for short-interval mammographic follow-up examinations, which was higher in the group that received Premarin (36.2% versus 28.1%).

These data show that women receiving combination HRT with estrogen and progesterone for 5 years have approximately a 20% increased risk for the development of breast cancer. Women who take estrogen-only formulations (because of previous hysterectomy) do not appear to be at increased risk for breast cancer.

Risk Assessment

A model for assessing breast cancer risk, known as the *Gail model*, was developed from case-control data in the Breast Cancer Detection Demonstration Project. (This model is available for clinical use at http://www.cancer.gov/bcrisktool.) In developing the model, factors influencing the risk for breast cancer were identified as age, race, age at menarche, age at first live birth, number of previous breast biopsies, presence of proliferative disease with atypia, and number of first-degree female relatives with breast cancer. The model does not include detailed information about genetic factors and may underestimate the risk for *BRCA1* or *BRCA2* mutation carriers and overestimate the risk for noncarriers. The model should not be used in women with a diagnosis of LCIS or DCIS. The Gail model for breast cancer risk was used in the design of the Breast Cancer Prevention Trial, which randomly assigned women at high risk (>1.67%) to receive tamoxifen or a placebo, and in the design of STAR (Study of Tamoxifen and Raloxifene),[11] which randomly assigned women at high risk to receive tamoxifen or raloxifene.

The Gail model assesses population risk using nongenetic factors, whereas hereditary and familial models assess genetic and familial factors of breast cancer. The Claus model is based on assumptions about the prevalence of high-penetrance breast cancer susceptibility genes. The Claus model provides individual estimates of breast cancer risk according to decade of life based on knowledge of first-degree and second-degree relatives with breast cancer and their ages at diagnosis.

Several models have been designed to assess the risk for harboring a mutation in *BRCA1* or *BRCA2*. These models can be useful in determining whether genetic testing is needed. The Couch model predicts risk for a mutation in the *BRCA1* gene. The BRCAPro model, developed by Myriad Genetics Laboratories, estimates the risk of *BRCA1* and *BRCA2* mutations. The Tyrer model incorporates personal risk factors and genetic analysis to give a more comprehensive and individual risk assessment. Such models have estimated that the incidence of clinically significant *BRCA1* or *BRCA2* mutations in the general population is approximately 1 in 300 to 500. Indications for consideration of genetic testing include breast cancer diagnosed before age 50, bilateral breast cancer, breast and ovarian cancer in the same individual, and breast cancer in men. Other factors that may be indications for testing are a family history (maternal or paternal) of two or more individuals with breast and ovarian cancer, a close male relative with breast cancer, a close relative with early-onset (<50 years) breast or ovarian cancer, and known *BRCA1* or *BRCA2* mutation in the family.

Care of High-Risk Patients

In practice, clinicians assess risk factors and consider the factors that are important to individual patients in making recommendations about breast cancer screening and intervention. Increased risk for breast cancer is defined as a 5-year calculated risk of 1.7% or higher using the National Cancer Institute (NCI) risk calculator, which is based on the Gail model. This is the average risk for a woman who is 60 years old; it has been used in the design of the U.S. prevention trials. This risk calculator is not applicable to women with a history of invasive breast cancer, DCIS, or LCIS. The model does not make adjustments for a first-degree relative with premenopausal or bilateral breast cancer and does not consider genetic mutations. The clinician must understand that risk may be significantly underestimated if these factors are present, and risk should be calculated within the context of the patient's overall personal and family history. However, even with these limitations, the Gail model provides a valuable starting point for the evaluation of breast cancer risk assessment. This risk assessment can provide a context for recommendations for primary prevention strategies and screening appropriate to the individual's risk level. For women found to be at high risk for the development of breast cancer, options include close surveillance with clinical breast examination, mammography, and breast MRI (depending on the lifetime risk) and interventions to reduce risk, such as chemoprevention or a bilateral prophylactic mastectomy or salpingo-oophorectomy.

Close Surveillance

Surveillance guidelines for individuals at high risk for breast cancer were established in 2002 by the National Comprehensive Cancer Network and the Cancer Genetics Studies Consortium. These guidelines are based primarily on expert opinion; screening guidelines for high-risk individuals are not established by prospective trials. Recommendations for women in a family with a breast and ovarian cancer syndrome include monthly breast self-examination beginning at age 18 to 20 years, semiannual clinical breast examination beginning at age 25 years, and annual mammography beginning at age 25 years or 10 years before the earliest age at onset of breast cancer in a family member. Nonetheless, studies of women with known *BRCA1* or *BRCA2* mutations found that 50% of the detected breast cancers were diagnosed as interval cancers; that is, they occurred between screening episodes and not during the course of routine screening. This observation prompted many groups to add annual screening MRI to screening mammography, with some groups recommending doing the two examinations simultaneously and others recommending staggering the two examinations. For women with a strong family history of early-onset breast and ovarian cancer who have not undergone genetic counseling, genetic counseling is offered; this includes a discussion of genetic testing for *BRCA1* and *BRCA2* mutations.

Chemoprevention for Breast Cancer

Drugs currently approved for reducing breast cancer risk are the selective ER modulators tamoxifen and raloxifene. Tamoxifen has proven beneficial for the treatment of ER-positive breast cancer (see "Endocrine Therapy" later on). Tamoxifen has been used as adjuvant treatment for breast cancer for several decades and is known to reduce the incidence of a second primary breast cancer in the contralateral breast of women who receive the drug as adjuvant therapy for a first primary breast cancer. The largest comprehensive analysis of the benefits of tamoxifen was done by the Early Breast Cancer Trialists' Collaborative Group (EBCTCG). This group meets every 5 years to review outcome data from breast cancer trials conducted worldwide. Findings from the EBCTCG overview analysis demonstrated that adjuvant tamoxifen reduces the risk for a second breast cancer in the unaffected breast by 47%. Four prospective randomized trials were completed that evaluated tamoxifen for chemoprevention in healthy women at increased risk for breast cancer.

In the NSABP (National Surgical Adjuvant Breast and Bowel Project) P-1 trial, 13,388 women who were 35 to 59 years old and had a diagnosis of LCIS, who had a moderately increased risk for breast cancer (RR, 1.66 over a 5-year period), or who were 60 years old or older were randomly assigned to tamoxifen or placebo. The risk estimates were based on the Gail model of risk (see earlier). In this study, tamoxifen reduced the risk for invasive breast cancer by 49% through 69 months of follow-up; the risk reduction was 59% in women with LCIS and 86% in women with ADH or ALH. The reduction in risk was noted only for ER-positive cancers. Tamoxifen treatment for 5 years was not without side effects and complications. In the tamoxifen treatment arm, endometrial cancers resulting from estrogen-like effects of the drug on the endometrium were increased by a factor of approximately 2.5. Pulmonary embolism (RR, 3) and deep venous thrombosis (RR, 1.7) were also more common in women who received tamoxifen. Data on the efficacy of tamoxifen for reduction of breast cancer risk in *BRCA1* and *BRCA2* mutation carriers were limited because mutation testing was not routinely performed on P-1 study participants. Tamoxifen is most effective at reducing the incidence of ER-positive breast cancers, so its role in *BRCA1* mutation carriers (who more often develop ER-negative breast cancers) is questionable.

Three other tamoxifen prevention trials were conducted approximately the same time as the NSABP P-1 trial, including the Italian Tamoxifen Prevention Study, Royal Marsden Hospital Pilot Tamoxifen Chemoprevention Trial, and IBIS-I (International Breast Cancer Intervention Study I). The Italian and Royal Marsden studies did not show any benefit of tamoxifen over placebo in terms of reduced incidence of breast cancer. There were some differences in the study populations and trial designs, which may explain the negative results compared with the P-1 trial. The IBIS-I trial showed a 33% reduction in the incidence of breast cancer with tamoxifen, slightly lower than the risk reduction in P-1 but confirming the risk reduction benefit of tamoxifen. Subsequently, a meta-analysis of all the tamoxifen prevention trials found that tamoxifen reduced the risk of breast cancer by 38%.[12] This analysis also confirmed the increased risks of endometrial cancer and venous thromboembolic events seen with tamoxifen use.

The NSABP P-2 trial (STAR trial)[11] compared tamoxifen with raloxifene in postmenopausal women. This comparison was based on the findings from the MORE trial, which included more than 10,000 women who received placebo versus raloxifene for the prevention and treatment of osteoporosis. In the MORE trial, at an average of 3 years of follow-up, there was a 54% reduction in the incidence of breast cancer and no increase in uterine cancer. The STAR trial enrolled 19,747 women at increased risk for breast cancer and demonstrated that tamoxifen and raloxifene each reduced the risk for invasive breast cancer by approximately 50%. Raloxifene had a more favorable toxicity profile: The number of uterine cancers was reduced by 36% in the raloxifene group compared with the tamoxifen group, and women taking raloxifene had 29% fewer episodes of venous thrombosis and a reduced incidence of pulmonary embolism compared with the tamoxifen group.

Because studies showed that aromatase inhibitors (AIs) prevent more contralateral breast cancers than tamoxifen in postmenopausal women with early-stage breast cancer, AIs have been evaluated for chemoprevention. The National Cancer Institute of Canada Clinical Trials Group completed the MAP.3 (Mammary Prevention 3) trial investigating the AI exemestane.[13] In this study, 4560 postmenopausal women who had at least one of several breast cancer risk factors (≥60 years old; Gail model 5-year risk score >1.66%; prior ADH, ALH, or LCIS; or prior DCIS with mastectomy) were randomly assigned to exemestane or placebo. After a median follow-up of 35 months, exemestane was associated with a 65% relative reduction in the annual incidence of invasive breast cancer, with 11 invasive cancers detected in the exemestane group and 32 detected in the placebo group. Adverse events occurred in 88% of subjects in the exemestane group and 85% of subjects in the placebo group ($P = .003$), with significant differences noted in the development of endocrine, gastrointestinal, and musculoskeletal symptoms. Exemestane has not been approved by the U.S. Food and Drug Administration as a chemopreventive agent; however, it has a category 1 recommendation for breast cancer prevention in the National Comprehensive Cancer Network clinical practice guidelines.

Prophylactic Mastectomy

Prophylactic mastectomy has been shown to reduce the chance of breast cancer development in high-risk women by 90%. Hartmann and colleagues[14] performed a retrospective review of 639 women with a family history of breast cancer who underwent prophylactic mastectomy. The women were divided into high-risk ($n = 214$) and moderate-risk ($n = 425$) groups, with women at high risk defined as women with a family history suggestive of an autosomal dominant predisposition to breast cancer. For women at moderate risk, the number of expected breast cancers was calculated according to the Gail model. On the basis of this model, 37.4 breast cancers were expected to develop, but only 4 cancers occurred, for an incidence risk reduction of 89%. For women in the high-risk cohort, the Gail model would underestimate the risk for development of breast cancer. The expected number of breast cancers was calculated by using three different statistical models from a control study of the high-risk probands (sisters). Three breast cancers developed after prophylactic mastectomy, for an incident risk reduction of at least 90%.

Several groups reported on prospective studies in *BRCA1* and *BRCA2* mutation carriers treated with prophylactic mastectomy versus surveillance and showed that mastectomy is highly effective in preventing breast cancers. More recently, results of risk-reducing mastectomy and risk-reducing salpingo-oophorectomy were reported in *BRCA1* and *BRCA2* mutation carriers followed in 22 centers as part of the PROSE consortium.[15] None of the participants who underwent risk-reducing mastectomy developed a subsequent breast cancer compared with 7% of the women who did not undergo this surgery. The use of risk-reducing salpingo-oophorectomy reduced the incidence of ovarian cancers from 5.8% to 1.1% and the incidence of breast cancers from 19.2% to 11.4%. Risk-reducing salpingo-oophorectomy was associated with a significant reduction in breast cancer–specific mortality, ovarian cancer–specific mortality, and all-cause mortality. The available data suggest that *BRCA* mutation carriers should be counseled to consider risk-reducing surgeries as a strategy to reduce cancer incidence and improve survival.

Women who undergo annual mammographic screening have an overall 80% chance of surviving breast cancer after it has been detected. Given the penetrance in the range of 50% to 60% for *BRCA1* or *BRCA2* mutation carriers, the chance of a *BRCA1* or *BRCA2* mutation carrier dying of breast cancer is approximately 10% if she chooses not to undergo risk-reducing surgery.[14]

The use of risk-reducing surgery in women who are not known to have deleterious mutations in *BRCA1* or *BRCA2* is controversial. Trends have suggested that more women with newly diagnosed breast cancer are choosing to undergo contralateral prophylactic mastectomy as a strategy for reducing the risk of contralateral breast cancer. Determining which patients may benefit from this approach has been challenging. Bedrosian and colleagues[16] used the Surveillance, Epidemiology, and End Results (SEER) database to study this issue and found that women with stage I or II breast cancer with ER-negative disease who underwent contralateral prophylactic mastectomy had an improvement in breast cancer–specific mortality of 4.8% at 5 years. Among women who did not undergo prophylactic mastectomy, the incidence of contralateral breast cancer was lower in women with ER-positive disease than in women with ER-negative disease.

Summary: Risk Assessment and Management

Understanding risk factors for the development of disease provides clues to pathogenesis and identifies patients likely to benefit from risk-reducing strategies. Although breast cancer can develop in both sexes, the risk of breast cancer development is much higher in women; breast cancer in men is uncommon. Age is a strong determinant of risk and is part of the NCI risk assessment tool. Family history is most significant when breast cancer affects first-degree relatives (mothers, sisters, and daughters) at a young age and when cases of ovarian cancer are found on the same side of the family. This type of family history may preclude the use of the NCI tool for accurate risk assessment. The most significant histologic risk factors for the development of breast cancer are LCIS, ADH, and ALH. A personal history of breast cancer predisposes to contralateral breast cancer.

BENIGN BREAST TUMORS AND RELATED DISEASES

Breast Cysts

Cysts within the breast parenchyma are fluid-filled, epithelial-lined cavities that vary in size from microscopic to large palpable masses containing 20 to 30 mL of fluid. A palpable cyst develops in at least 1 in every 14 women, and 50% of cysts are multiple or recurrent. The pathogenesis of cyst formation is not well understood; however, cysts appear to arise from destruction and dilation of lobules and terminal ductules. Microscopic studies showed that fibrosis at or near the lobule, combined with continued secretion, results in unfolding of the lobule and expansion of an epithelial-lined cavity containing fluid.[1,6]

Cysts are influenced by ovarian hormones, a fact that explains their variation with the menstrual cycle. Most cysts occur in women older than 35 years; the incidence steadily increases until menopause and sharply declines thereafter. New cyst formation in older women is generally associated with exogenous HRT.

Intracystic carcinoma is exceedingly rare. Rosemond reported that only three cancers were identified in more than 3000 cyst aspirations (0.1%). Other investigators confirmed this low incidence. There is no evidence of increased risk for breast cancer associated with cyst formation.

A palpable mass can be confirmed to be a cyst by direct aspiration or ultrasonography. Cyst fluid can be straw-colored, opaque, or dark green and may contain debris. Given the low risk for malignancy within a cyst, if the mass resolves after aspiration and the cyst contents are not grossly bloody, the fluid does not need to be sent for cytologic analysis. If the cyst recurs multiple times (more than twice is a reasonable rule), pneumocystography should be performed to evaluate for a solid component, and core needle biopsy should be performed to evaluate any solid elements. Surgical removal of a cyst is usually not indicated but may be required if the cyst recurs multiple times or if needle biopsy reveals findings of atypia.

Fibroadenomas and Other Benign Tumors

Fibroadenomas are benign solid tumors composed of stromal and epithelial elements. Fibroadenoma is the second most common tumor in the breast (after carcinoma) and is the most common tumor in women younger than 30 years. In contrast to cysts, fibroadenomas most often arise during the late teens and early reproductive years. Fibroadenomas are rarely seen as new masses in women after age 40 or 45 years. Clinically, fibroadenomas manifest as firm masses that are easily movable and may increase in size over several months. They slide easily under the examining fingers and may be lobulated or smooth. On excision, fibroadenomas are well-encapsulated masses that may detach easily from surrounding breast tissue. Mammography is of little help in discriminating between cysts and fibroadenomas; however, ultrasonography can readily distinguish between them because each has specific characteristics.

Fibroadenomas are benign tumors, although neoplasia may develop in the epithelial elements within them. Cancer in a newly discovered fibroadenoma is exceedingly rare; 50% of neoplasias that involve fibroadenomas are LCIS, 35% are invasive carcinomas, and 15% are intraductal carcinoma. When a tissue diagnosis confirms that the breast mass is a fibroadenoma, the patient can be reassured, and surgical excision is not needed. If the patient is bothered by the mass or it continues to grow, the mass can be excised.

Two subtypes of fibroadenoma are recognized. *Giant fibroadenoma* is a descriptive term applied to a fibroadenoma that attains an unusually large size (typically >5 cm). The term *juvenile fibroadenoma* refers to a large fibroadenoma that occasionally occurs in adolescents and young adults and histologically is more cellular than the usual fibroadenoma. Although these lesions may display remarkably rapid growth, surgical removal is curative.

Hamartomas and Adenomas

Hamartomas and adenomas are benign proliferations of variable amounts of epithelium and stromal supporting tissue. A hamartoma is a discrete nodule that contains closely packed lobules and prominent, ectatic extralobular ducts. On physical examination, mammography, and gross inspection, a hamartoma is indistinguishable from a fibroadenoma. Page and Anderson described an adenoma or tubular adenoma as a benign cellular neoplasm of ductules packed closely together so that they form a sheet of tiny glands without supporting stroma. During pregnancy and lactation, adenomas may increase in size, and histologic examination shows secretory differentiation. Biopsy is required to establish the diagnosis.

Breast Infections and Abscess

There are two general categories of infections of the breast: lactational infections and chronic subareolar infections associated with duct ectasia. Lactational infections are thought to arise from entry of bacteria through the nipple into the duct system and are characterized by fever, leukocytosis, erythema, and tenderness. Infections of the breast are most often caused by *Staphylococcus aureus* and may manifest as cellulitis with breast parenchymal inflammation and swelling, termed *mastitis*, or as abscesses. Treatment requires antibiotics and frequent emptying of the breast. True abscesses require drainage. Initial attempts at drainage should include needle aspiration; surgical incision and drainage should be reserved for abscesses that do not resolve after aspiration and treatment with antibiotics. In such cases, abscesses are generally multiloculated. Ultrasound evaluation can assist in characterizing a breast abscess and help to guide management.

In women who are not lactating, a chronic relapsing form of infection may develop in the subareolar ducts of the breast that is variously known as *periductal mastitis* or *duct ectasia*. This condition appears to be associated with smoking and diabetes. The infections are most often mixed infections that include aerobic and anaerobic skin flora. A series of infections with resulting inflammatory changes and scarring may lead to retraction or inversion of the nipple, masses in the subareolar area, and occasionally a chronic fistula from the subareolar ducts to the periareolar skin. Palpable masses and mammographic changes may result from the infection and scarring; these can make surveillance for breast cancer more challenging.

Subareolar infections may initially manifest as subareolar pain and mild erythema. Warm soaks and oral antibiotics may be effective treatment at this stage. Antibiotic treatment generally requires coverage for aerobic and anaerobic organisms. If an abscess has developed, needle aspiration is required in addition to antibiotics. Surgical incision and drainage is reserved for abscesses that do not resolve with these more conservative measures. Repeated infections are treated by excision of the entire subareolar duct complex after the acute infection has resolved completely, together with intravenous antibiotic coverage. Rarely, patients have recurrent infections requiring excision of the nipple and areola.

A presumed infection of the breast generally clears promptly and completely with antibiotic therapy. If erythema or edema persists, a diagnosis of inflammatory carcinoma should be considered.

Papillomas and Papillomatosis

Solitary intraductal papillomas are true polyps of epithelial-lined breast ducts. Solitary papillomas are most often located close to the areola but may be present in peripheral locations. Most papillomas are smaller than 1 cm but can grow to 4 or 5 cm. Larger papillomas may appear to arise within a cystic structure, probably representing a greatly expanded duct. Papillomas are not associated with an increased risk for breast cancer.

Papillomas located close to the nipple are often accompanied by bloody nipple discharge. Less frequently, they are discovered as a palpable mass under the areola or as a density seen on a mammogram. Treatment is excision through a circumareolar incision. For peripheral papillomas, the differential diagnosis is between papilloma and invasive papillary carcinoma.

It is important to distinguish papillomatosis from solitary or multiple papillomas. Papillomatosis refers to epithelial hyperplasia, which commonly occurs in younger women or is associated with fibrocystic change. Papillomatosis is not composed of true papillomas but rather consists of hyperplastic epithelium that may fill individual ducts similar to a true polyp but has no stalk of fibrovascular tissue.

Sclerosing Adenosis

Adenosis refers to an increased number of small terminal ductules or acini. Adenosis is frequently associated with a proliferation of stromal tissue that produces a histologic lesion, sclerosing adenosis, which can be confused with carcinoma grossly and histologically. Sclerosing adenosis can be associated with deposition of calcium, which can be seen on a mammogram in a pattern indistinguishable from the microcalcifications of intraductal carcinoma. In many series, sclerosing adenosis is the most common pathologic diagnosis in patients undergoing needle-directed biopsy of microcalcifications. Sclerosing adenosis is frequently listed as one of the component lesions of fibrocystic disease; it is common and is not believed to have significant malignant potential.

Radial Scars

Radial scars belong to a group of abnormalities known as *complex sclerosing lesions*. Radial scars can appear similar to carcinomas mammographically because they create irregular spiculations in the surrounding stroma. Radial scars contain microcysts, epithelial hyperplasia, and adenosis and have a prominent display of central sclerosis. The gross abnormality is rarely more than 1 cm in diameter. Larger lesions may form palpable tumors and appear as spiculated masses with prominent architectural distortion on a mammogram. These tumors can cause skin dimpling by producing traction on surrounding tissues. Radial scars generally require excision to rule out an underlying carcinoma. Radial scars are associated with a modestly increased risk for breast cancer.

Fat Necrosis

Fat necrosis can mimic cancer on mammography by producing a palpable mass or density that may contain calcifications. Fat necrosis may follow an episode of trauma to the breast or be related to a prior surgical procedure or radiation therapy. Calcifications are characteristic of fat necrosis and can often be visualized on ultrasonography as well. Histologically, fat necrosis is composed of lipid-laden macrophages, scar tissue, and chronic inflammatory cells. This lesion has no malignant potential.

EPIDEMIOLOGY AND PATHOLOGY OF BREAST CANCER

Epidemiology

It was estimated that 234,190 cases of invasive breast cancer and 60,290 cases of in situ breast cancer would be diagnosed in 2015 in the United States. Breast cancer is the second leading cause of cancer-related deaths, second to lung cancer, with approximately 40,000 deaths caused by breast cancer annually. Breast cancer is also a global health problem, with more than 1 million cases of breast cancer diagnosed worldwide each year. The overall incidence of breast cancer was increasing until approximately 1999 because of increases in the average life span, lifestyle changes that increase the risk for breast cancer, and improved survival rates for other diseases. Breast cancer incidence decreased from 1999 to 2006 by approximately 2% per year. This decrease was attributed to a reduction in the use of HRT after the initial results of the Women's Health Initiative were published but may also be the result of a reduction in the use of screening mammography (70.1% of women ≥40 years old were screened in 2000 versus 66.4% in 2005). During the years 2006-2010, breast cancer incidence rates were stable.

Survival rates in women with breast cancer have steadily improved over the last several decades, with 5-year survival rates of 63% in the early 1960s, 75% during the years 1975-1977, 79% during 1984-1986, and 90% during 1995-2005. The largest decreases in death rates from breast cancer have been in women younger than 50 years (decreases of 3.2% per year), although breast cancer death rates have also decreased in women older than 50 years (by 2% per year). The decreased mortality from breast cancer is thought to be the result of earlier detection via mammographic screening, a decreased incidence of breast cancer, and improvements in therapy. The current treatment of breast cancer is guided by pathology, staging, and more recent insights into breast cancer biology. There is an increased emphasis on defining disease biology and status in individual patients, with the subsequent tailoring of therapies.

Pathology

Noninvasive Breast Cancer

Noninvasive neoplasms of the breast are broadly divided into two major types, LCIS and DCIS (Box 34-3). LCIS is regarded as a risk factor for the development of breast cancer. LCIS is recognized by its conformity to the outline of the normal lobule, with expanded and filled acini (Fig. 34-7*A*). One variant of LCIS, pleomorphic LCIS, has been recognized more recently as a distinct, more aggressive histopathologic subtype. Pleomorphic LCIS shows marked nuclear pleomorphism compared with classic LCIS. One or more lobules are distended by discohesive cells with irregularly shaped, high-grade nuclei. Pleomorphic LCIS may or may not be associated with comedo necrosis and calcifications. If pleomorphic LCIS is associated with calcifications, it may be detected mammographically. The natural history of pleomorphic LCIS is unknown, and there is debate regarding treatment; many experts suggest that pleomorphic LCIS be treated with surgical excision similar to DCIS.

DCIS is more morphologically heterogeneous than LCIS, and pathologists recognize four broad types of DCIS: papillary, cribriform, solid, and comedo. The latter three types are shown in Figure 34-7. DCIS is recognized as discrete spaces filled with malignant cells, usually with a recognizable basal cell layer composed of presumably normal myoepithelial cells. The four morphologic types of DCIS are rarely seen as pure lesions; DCIS lesions are usually of mixed morphologic types. The papillary and cribriform types of DCIS are generally lower grade lesions and may take longer to transform to invasive cancer. The solid and comedo types of DCIS are generally higher grade lesions.

BOX 34-3 Classification of Primary Breast Cancer

Noninvasive Epithelial Cancers

Lobular carcinoma in situ

Ductal carcinoma in situ or intraductal carcinoma

- Papillary, cribriform, solid, and comedo types

Invasive Epithelial Cancers (Percentage of Total)

Invasive lobular carcinoma (10%)

Invasive ductal carcinoma

- Invasive ductal carcinoma, not otherwise specified (50%-70%)
- Tubular carcinoma (2%-3%)
- Mucinous or colloid carcinoma (2%-3%)
- Medullary carcinoma (5%)
- Invasive cribriform carcinoma (1%-3%)
- Invasive papillary carcinoma (1%-2%)
- Adenoid cystic carcinoma (1%)
- Metaplastic carcinoma (1%)

Mixed Connective and Epithelial Tumors

Phyllodes tumors, benign and malignant

Carcinosarcoma

Angiosarcoma

Adenocarcinoma

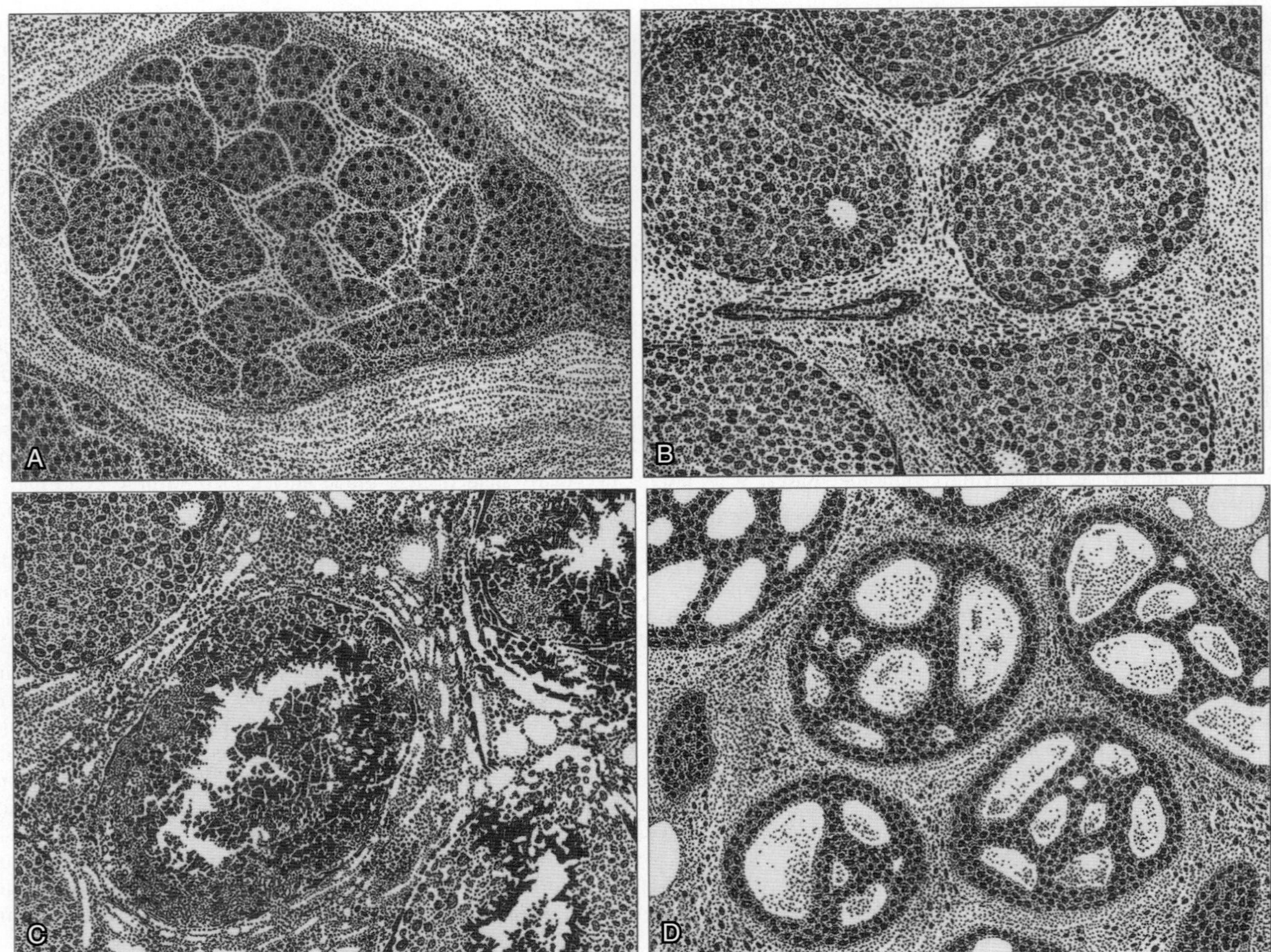

FIGURE 34-7 Noninvasive breast cancer. **A,** Lobular carcinoma in situ (LCIS). The neoplastic cells are small with compact, bland nuclei and are distending the acini but preserving the cross-sectional architecture of the lobular unit. **B,** Ductal carcinoma in situ (DCIS), solid type. The cells are larger than in LCIS and are filling the ductal rather than the lobular spaces. However, the cells are contained within the basement membrane of the duct and do not invade the breast stroma. **C,** DCIS, comedo type. In comedo DCIS, the malignant cells in the center undergo necrosis, coagulation, and calcification. **D,** DCIS, cribriform type. In this type, bridges of tumor cells span the ductal space and leave round, punched-out spaces.

As the cells inside the ductal membrane grow, they have a tendency to undergo central necrosis, perhaps because the blood supply to these cells is located outside the basement membrane. The necrotic debris in the center of the duct undergoes coagulation and finally calcifies, leading to the tiny, pleomorphic, and frequently linear forms of microcalcifications seen on mammograms. In some patients, an entire ductal tree may be involved in the malignancy, and the mammogram shows typical calcifications from the nipple extending posteriorly into the interior of the breast (termed *segmental calcifications*). For reasons that are not completely understood, DCIS, if not treated, usually transforms into an invasive cancer, usually recapitulating the morphology of the cells inside the duct. In other words, low-grade cribriform DCIS tends to be associated with low-grade invasive lesions that retain some cribriform features. There is no tendency for the grade to advance with invasion. DCIS frequently coexists with invasive cancers, and when this is the case, the two phases of the malignancy are usually morphologically similar.

Invasive Breast Cancer

Invasive breast cancers are recognized by their lack of overall architecture, infiltration of cells haphazardly into a variable amount of stroma, or formation of sheets of continuous and monotonous cells without respect for form and function of a glandular organ. Pathologists broadly divide invasive breast cancer into ductal and lobular histologic types, which probably do not reflect histogenesis and imperfectly predict clinical behavior. Invasive ductal cancer tends to grow as a cohesive mass; it appears as discrete abnormalities on mammograms and is often palpable as a discrete lump in the breast smaller than lobular cancers. Invasive lobular cancer tends to permeate the breast in a single-file nature, which explains why it remains clinically occult and often escapes detection on mammography or physical examination until the disease is extensive. The growth patterns of invasive ductal and lobular carcinomas are shown in Figure 34-8.

Invasive ductal cancer, also known as *infiltrating ductal carcinoma*, is the most common form of breast cancer; it accounts for

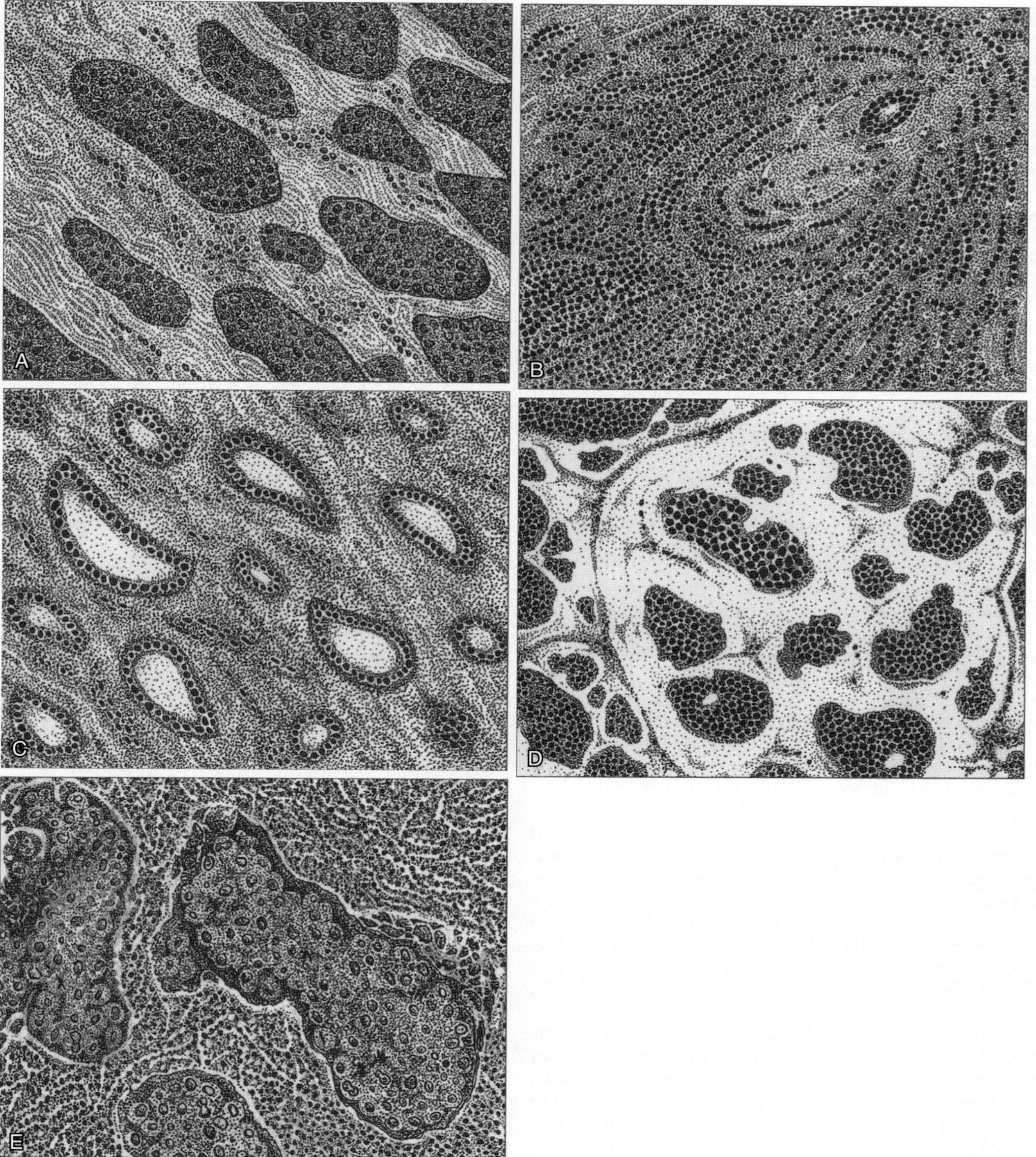

FIGURE 34-8 Invasive breast cancer. **A,** Invasive ductal carcinoma, not otherwise specified. The malignant cells invade in haphazard groups and singly into the stroma. **B,** Invasive lobular carcinoma. The malignant cells invade the stroma in a characteristic single-file pattern and may form concentric circles of single-file cells around normal ducts (targetoid pattern). **C,** Invasive tubular carcinoma. The cancer invades as small tubules, lined by a single layer of well-differentiated cells. **D,** Mucinous or colloid carcinoma. The bland tumor cells float like islands in lakes of mucin. **E,** Medullary carcinoma. The tumor cells are large and very undifferentiated, with pleomorphic nuclei. The distinctive features of this tumor are the infiltrate of lymphocytes and the syncytium-appearing sheets of tumor cells.

50% to 70% of invasive breast cancers. Invasive lobular carcinoma accounts for 10% of breast cancers, and mixed ductal and lobular cancers have been increasingly recognized and described in pathology reports. When invasive ductal carcinomas take on differentiated features, they are named according to the features that they display. If the infiltrating cells form small glands lined by a single row of bland epithelium, they are called *infiltrating tubular carcinoma* (see Fig. 34-8*C*). The infiltrating cells may secrete copious amounts of mucin and appear to float in this material. These lesions are called *mucinous* or *colloid tumors* (see Fig. 34-8*D*). Tubular and mucinous tumors are usually low-grade (grade I) lesions; these tumors each account for approximately 2% to 3% of invasive breast carcinomas.

Medullary cancer is characterized by bizarre invasive cells with high-grade nuclear features, many mitoses, and lack of an in situ component (see Fig. 34-8*E*). The malignancy forms sheets of cells in an almost syncytial fashion, surrounded by an infiltrate of small mononuclear lymphocytes. The borders of the tumor push into the surrounding breast rather than infiltrate or permeate the stroma. In its pure form, medullary cancer accounts for only approximately 5% of breast cancers; however, some pathologists have described a so-called *medullary variant* that has some features of the pure form of the cancer. These tumors are uniformly high grade, ER and progesterone receptor (PR) negative, and negative for the human epidermal growth factor receptor 2 (HER-2/neu; HER-2) cell surface receptor.

Another rare subtype of breast cancer that is typically high grade and negative for ER, PR, and HER-2 is metaplastic carcinoma. Most metaplastic carcinomas are node negative, but they have high potential for metastatic spread, and 10% of patients present with de novo metastatic disease. Even patients presenting with localized metaplastic carcinoma have a poor prognosis: Approximately 50% experience local or distant relapse.

Tumors that lack expression of ER, PR, and HER-2 are often called *triple-negative breast cancers*. Gene expression profiling and microarray analysis of breast cancers have revealed that triple-negative breast cancers are distinctly different from other ductal breast cancers and may also express molecular markers found in basal or myoepithelial cells. There may be some overlap between triple-negative breast cancer and *basal-like breast cancer,* but these categories were developed using differing technologies, and the two categories do not exactly overlap. The term *basal-like breast cancer* describes a specific subtype of breast cancer defined by microarray analysis, whereas triple-negative breast cancer is defined by lack of immunohistochemical detection of ER, PR, and HER-2.

The different histologic subtypes of breast cancer have some relationship with prognosis, although this is influenced by tumor size, histologic grade, hormone receptor status, HER-2 status, lymph node status, and other prognostic variables. The prognosis of invasive ductal carcinoma, not otherwise specified, is variable, modified by histologic grade and expression of molecular markers. Basal-like breast cancer is commonly aggressive, and because it is triple receptor negative, there are no targeted treatments for this form of cancer. Invasive lobular breast cancers carry an intermediate prognosis, and tubular and mucinous cancers have the best overall prognosis. These generalizations about the prognosis associated with different histologic subtypes are useful only in the context of tumor size, grade, and receptor status. Modern classification schemes based on determination of molecular markers and breast cancer subtype by microarray analysis are replacing these older morphologic descriptions.

Molecular Markers and Breast Cancer Subtypes

Numerous molecular markers have been reported to affect breast cancer outcomes, including molecules in the steroid hormone receptor pathway (ER and PR), molecules in the human epidermal growth factor receptor pathway (HER family), angiogenesis-related molecules, cell cycle–related molecules (e.g., cyclin-dependent kinases), apoptosis modulators, proteasomes, cyclooxygenase-2, peroxisome-proliferator-activated receptor γ, insulin-like growth factors (insulin-like growth factor family), transforming growth factor-γ, platelet-derived growth factor, and *p53*. Most of these markers are not routinely tested on breast cancer specimens at the time of diagnosis; such testing would not be feasible. Categorizing breast cancer according to the expression of molecular targets of treatments is practical, and the resulting classifications appear to agree with nonbiased classifications based on gene expression. Classification schemes reflect biology and predict treatment efficacy.

Incorporating predictive markers into the routine testing of breast cancers can help predict which patients would be most likely to benefit from therapies directed at those markers. The best example of this is testing for ER. Before the discovery of ER, all breast cancers were considered potentially sensitive to endocrine therapy. Pathologic assessment of ER is now performed on all primary tumors and predicts which patients should receive endocrine therapy. Patients whose tumors are ER negative can be spared endocrine therapy.

A second important predictive factor in breast cancer, discovered in 1985, is HER-2. This protein is the product of the *erb-B2* gene and is amplified in approximately 20% of human breast cancers. The extracellular domain of the receptor is present on the surface of breast cancer cells, and an intracellular tyrosine kinase enzyme links the receptor to the internal machinery of the cell. HER-2 is a member of the epidermal growth factor receptor family of receptor tyrosine kinases. The tyrosine kinase of HER-2 is activated when the HER-2 receptor heterodimerizes with other members of the family that have been bound by growth factors or when the HER-2 receptor homodimerizes. There is no known ligand that binds to the HER-2 receptor. HER-2 protein overexpression is measured clinically by immunohistochemistry and scored on a scale from 0 to 3+. Alternatively, fluorescent in situ hybridization, which directly detects the number of HER-2 gene copies, can be used to detect gene amplification. Inhibiting the function of the HER-2 receptor slows the growth of HER-2-amplified tumors in laboratory models and in clinical trials. Trastuzumab is a humanized monoclonal antibody directed against the extracellular domain of the HER-2 surface receptor and is effective treatment for HER-2-positive breast cancer (see "Trastuzumab-Based Targeted Therapy" later on). HER-2 testing is now a standard part of pathologic reporting on the primary tumor and is a predictive marker for HER-2-directed therapies.

A logical classification scheme for invasive breast cancer is based on the expression of ER status and HER-2 protein. This classification has the advantage of directing treatment choices. Patients with ER-positive tumors receive endocrine therapies, and patients with HER-2-positive tumors receive HER-2-targeted therapy. However, breast cancer is a heterogeneous disease, and different breast cancers behave in different ways. For example, some ER-positive tumors are indolent and not life-threatening, whereas other ER-positive tumors are very aggressive. In an attempt to subclassify the disease further, investigators are turning to global assessment of gene expression using microarrays; these are composed of oligonucleotide probes to almost every known

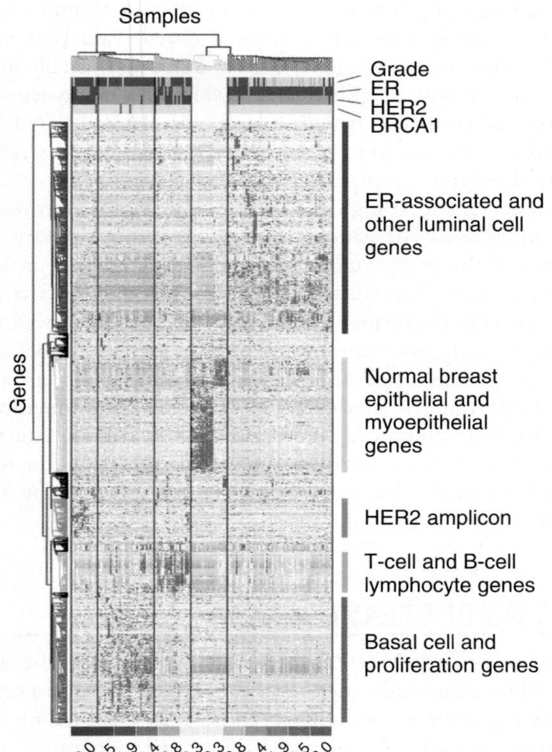

FIGURE 34-9 Microarray representation of human breast cancer. This portrayal of global gene expression is called a *heat map,* with shades of red indicating high gene expression and shades of blue indicating low gene expression relative to a mean across tissue samples. Tissue samples are present across the top in columns, and individual genes are in rows down the side; the intersection is an individual gene in a particular sample. A computer-clustering algorithm aligns samples with similar gene expression and genes with similar expression patterns in the samples (two-way clustering). This illustration provides an unbiased look at breast cancer according to gene expression. The dendrogram at the top depicts the degree of similarity of the tissue samples: *yellow,* normal breast epithelium; *blue,* predominantly ER-positive cancers; *red,* basal-like or triple-negative cancers; and *green,* HER-2-positive cancers (in two clusters defined by the degree of lymphocytic infiltrate). The *stripes* at the top indicate grade (shades of darker purple are higher grades), ER expression (purple is positive; green is negative), and HER-2 (purple is positive; green is negative). *BRCA1* mutation was determined for other reasons in this experiment. (Courtesy Dr. Andrea Richardson, Department of Pathology, Brigham and Women's Hospital, Boston, MA.)

expressed sequence of DNA in the human genome. Similar technologies based on single-nucleotide polymorphisms in the cancer DNA and profiles of expressed proteins are being developed to subclassify cancers and direct treatment.

A typical microarray experiment, commonly known as a *heat map,* is shown in Figure 34-9; the colors indicate levels of gene expression. Such a portrayal of the disease shows how different ER-positive tumors are from ER-negative tumors and underscores the modern concept that subclassification needs not only to define different groups of breast cancer but also to guide treatment.[17] In Figure 34-9, HER-2-positive tumors form two clusters (*in green at the top*), although these clusters are fused together in many depictions. HER-2-positive tumors cluster similarly and are responsive to inhibitors of the HER-2 receptor (e.g., trastuzumab). An unexpected finding is the uniqueness of tumors that are both ER negative and HER-2 negative. These tumors, also negative for PR, are called *triple-negative cancers.* They express proteins in common with myoepithelial cells at the base of mammary ducts and are also called *basal-like cancers* (see earlier). Women who carry a deleterious mutation in *BRCA1* (but not *BRCA2*) are much more likely to contract a basal-like cancer (triple-negative) than another subtype.

In addition to being used to classify breast cancer subtypes, molecular markers are used to select patients for systemic treatment (e.g., chemotherapy, endocrine therapy) and to predict the response of patients to these pharmacologic treatments. The simplest example is the use of ER or HER-2 status to predict the response to endocrine treatment or trastuzumab. Multiple gene products may be used in combination for these determinations. Microarray experiments use thousands of gene transcripts (messenger RNAs) to provide a snapshot of the molecular phenotype of an individual cancer. To adapt this technology for clinical application, investigators selected critical assemblies of gene products that provide the same predictive ability as a nonbiased, genome-wide analysis. The most advanced is a 21-gene test that can be used on paraffin-embedded tumor material from breast surgical specimens (Oncotype DX assay, a 21-gene recurrence score assay).[18] Originally designed to predict the recurrence of ER-positive, node-negative breast cancer treated with adjuvant endocrine therapy, the 21-gene recurrence score assay provides a recurrence score for ER-positive breast cancer that is used clinically to determine whether women with high-risk ER-positive breast cancer should receive adjuvant chemotherapy in addition to tamoxifen, an endocrine therapy (see "Endocrine Therapy" later on). Another multigene assay for determining prognosis is the MammaPrint assay. The MammaPrint assay analyzes data from 70 genes to develop a risk profile. The test provides a simple readout of low-risk or high-risk disease. This tool can be used for risk assessment in patients with ER-positive or ER-negative tumors. Tests based on critical combinations of genes will likely increasingly be used to guide clinical decision making regarding breast cancer treatment.

Other Tumors of the Breast

Phyllodes tumors. Tumors of mixed connective tissue and epithelium constitute an important group of unusual primary breast tumors. On one end of the spectrum are benign fibroadenomas, which are characterized by a proliferation of connective tissue and a variable component of ductal elements that may appear compressed by the swirls of fibroblastic growth. Clinically more challenging are phyllodes tumors, which contain a biphasic proliferation of stroma and mammary epithelium. First called *cystosarcoma phyllodes,* these tumors are now called *phyllodes tumors* in recognition of their usually benign course. However, with increasing cellularity, an invasive margin, and sarcomatous appearance, these tumors may be classified as malignant phyllodes tumors. Benign phyllodes tumors are firm lobulated masses that can range in size, with an average size of approximately 5 cm (larger than average fibroadenomas). Histologically, benign phyllodes tumors are similar to fibroadenomas, but the whorled stroma forms larger clefts lined by epithelium that resemble clusters of leaflike structures. The stroma is more cellular than in a fibroadenoma, but the fibroblastic cells are bland, and mitoses are infrequent.

Phyllodes tumors are seen on mammography as round densities with smooth borders and are indistinguishable from fibroadenomas. Ultrasonography may reveal a discrete structure with cystic spaces. The diagnosis is suggested by the larger size, history of rapid growth, and occurrence in older patients. Cytologic analysis is unreliable in differentiating a low-grade phyllodes tumor from a fibroadenoma. Core needle biopsy is preferred, although it is difficult to classify phyllodes tumors with benign or intermediate malignant potential on the basis of a limited sampling. The final diagnosis is best made by excisional biopsy followed by careful pathologic review.

Local excision of a benign phyllodes tumor, similar to local excision of a fibroadenoma, is curative. Intermediate tumors, also called *borderline phyllodes tumors,* are tumors to which it is difficult to assign a benign label. These tumors are treated by excision with margins of at least 1 cm to prevent local recurrence. Affected patients are at some risk for local recurrence, most often within the first 2 years after excision. Close follow-up with examination and imaging allows early detection of recurrence.

At the other end of the spectrum of tumors of mixed connective tissue and epithelium are frankly malignant stromal sarcomas. Malignant phyllodes tumors are characterized by features such as stromal overgrowth, cellular atypia, and high number of mitoses. These tumors are treated similarly to soft tissue sarcomas that occur on the trunk or extremities. Complete surgical excision of the entire tumor with a margin of normal tissue is advised. When the tumor is large with respect to the size of the breast, total mastectomy may be required. If mastectomy is performed and the margins are negative, radiation therapy is not recommended. If the margins are concerning or close, if the tumor involves the fascia or chest wall, or if the tumor is very large (>5 cm), irradiation of the chest wall is considered. If only wide local excision is performed, adjuvant radiation therapy is recommended. As with other soft tissue sarcomas, regional lymph node dissection is not required for staging or locoregional control. Metastases from malignant phyllodes tumors occur via hematogenous spread; common sites of metastasis include lung, bone, abdominal viscera, and mediastinum. The optimal palliative treatment of patients with metastatic phyllodes tumors has not been determined. Systemic therapeutic agents used for sarcomas have resulted in minimal success.

Angiosarcoma. Angiosarcoma, a vascular tumor, may occur de novo in the breast or within the dermis of the breast after irradiation for breast cancer. Angiosarcoma has also been seen to develop in the upper extremity of patients with lymphedema, historically after radical mastectomy. Angiosarcomas arising in the absence of previous radiation therapy or surgery generally form an ill-defined mass within the parenchyma of the breast. In contrast, angiosarcomas caused by prior radiation therapy arise in the irradiated skin as purplish vascular proliferations that may go unrecognized for a period of time. The differential diagnosis is frequently between malignant angiosarcoma and atypical vascular proliferations in irradiated skin. Histologically, angiosarcoma is composed of an anastomosing tangle of blood vessels in the dermis and superficial subcutaneous fat. The atypical and crowded vessels invade through the dermis and into subcutaneous fat. These tumors are graded by the appearance and behavior of the associated endothelial cells. Pleomorphic nuclei, frequent mitoses, and stacking of the endothelial cells lining neoplastic vessels are features seen in higher grade lesions. Necrosis, rarely seen in hemangiomas, is common in high-grade angiosarcomas. Clinically, radiation-induced angiosarcoma is identified as a reddish brown to purple raised rash within the radiation portals and on the skin of the breast. As the disease progresses, tumors protruding from the surface of the skin may predominate.

Mammography is unrevealing in most cases of angiosarcoma. In the absence of metastatic disease at initial evaluation, surgery is performed to secure negative skin margins and usually involves a total mastectomy. A split-thickness skin graft or myocutaneous flap may be needed to replace a large skin defect created by the resection. Metastasis to regional nodes is extraordinarily rare, and axillary dissection is not required.

Patients remain at high risk for local recurrence after resection of angiosarcoma. For patients who present with primary angiosarcoma of the breast, radiation therapy is beneficial in locoregional treatment. Patients with radiation-related angiosarcoma are not candidates for further radiotherapy. Metastatic spread occurs hematogenously, most commonly to the lungs and bone and less frequently to the abdominal viscera, brain, and contralateral breast. Adjuvant chemotherapy is generally recommended and may improve outcomes of patients with angiosarcoma. For patients free of metastatic disease at initial evaluation, the median time to recurrence after mastectomy is 8 months, and the median survival time is 2 years.

STAGING OF BREAST CANCER

Breast cancer stage is determined clinically by physical examination and imaging studies before treatment, and breast cancer stage is determined pathologically by pathologic examination of the primary tumor and regional lymph nodes after definitive surgical treatment. Staging is performed to group patients into risk categories that define prognosis and guide treatment recommendations for patients with a similar prognosis. Breast cancer is classified with the TNM classification system, which groups patients into four stage groupings based on the size of the primary tumor (T), status of the regional lymph nodes (N), and presence or absence of distant metastasis (M). The most widely used system is that of the American Joint Committee on Cancer. This system is updated every 6 to 8 years to reflect current understanding of tumor behavior. Some of the most significant changes in the most recent update (seventh edition) include a more stringent classification of isolated tumor cells based on the number of cells and whether the cells are almost confluent or nonconfluent. Stage I breast cancers are subdivided into IA and IB, with IB including T1 tumors associated with micrometastasis (N1mi) in the lymph nodes; a new category of M0(i+) includes patients with circulating tumor cells, disseminated tumor cells (bone marrow micrometastases), or cells found incidentally in other tissues that do not exceed 0.2 mm. The TNM classification is shown in Table 34-4; stage groupings are shown in Table 34-5.

Metastasis to ipsilateral axillary nodes predicts outcome after surgical treatment more powerfully than tumor size. Before the incorporation of systemic therapies in the management of breast cancer, when treatment was with surgery alone, the survival rate decreased almost linearly with increasing nodal involvement.

Although staging is an important part of the initial assessment of breast cancer patients, it is based on anatomic variables and does not incorporate other important prognostic factors. The new staging form has a place to record other variables, including tumor grade, ER status, PR status, HER-2 status, circulating tumor cells, disseminated tumor cells (in bone marrow), multigene recurrence score, and response to chemotherapy. These variables are not currently part of the staging system, but it is anticipated that future versions will incorporate important biologic variables for the stage groupings to reflect expected outcomes more accurately.

TABLE 34-4 TNM Classification for Breast Cancer (Pathologic Staging)

Primary Tumor (T)	
TX	Primary tumor cannot be assessed
T0	No evidence of primary tumor
Tis	Carcinoma in situ
Tis (DCIS)	DCIS
Tis (LCIS)	LCIS
Tis (Paget)	Paget disease of the nipple not associated with invasive carcinoma or carcinoma in situ (DCIS and/or LCIS) in underlying breast parenchyma
T1	Tumor ≤20 mm in greatest dimension
T1mi	Tumor ≤1 mm in greatest dimension
T1a	Tumor >1 mm but ≤5 mm in greatest dimension
T1b	Tumor >5 mm but ≤10 mm in greatest dimension
T1c	Tumor >10 mm but ≤20 mm in greatest dimension
T2	Tumor >20 mm but ≤50 mm in greatest dimension
T3	Tumor >50 mm in greatest dimension
T4	Tumor of any size with direct extension to the chest wall and/or to the skin
T4a	Extension to the chest wall, not including only pectoralis muscle adherence or invasion
T4b	Ulceration and/or ipsilateral satellite nodules and/or edema of the skin
T4c	Both T4a and T4b
T4d	Inflammatory carcinoma
Regional Lymph Nodes (N)	
pNX	Regional lymph nodes cannot be assessed
pN0	No regional lymph node metastasis
pN0(i–)	No regional lymph node metastasis histologically, negative IHC
pN0(i+)	Malignant cells in regional lymph nodes no greater than 0.2 mm
pN0(mol–)	No regional lymph node metastasis histologically, negative molecular findings (IHC)
pN0(mol+)	Positive molecular findings (RT-PCR), but no metastasis detected by histology or IHC
pN1	Micrometastases; or metastases in 1-3 axillary nodes and/or in internal mammary nodes with metastases detected by sentinel lymph node biopsy but not clinically detected
pN1mi	Micrometastases (>0.2 mm and/or >200 cells but none >2.0 mm)
pN1a	Metastases in 1-3 axillary nodes; at least one metastasis >2.0 mm
pN1b	Metastases in internal mammary nodes with micrometastasis or macrometastases detected by sentinel lymph node biopsy (not clinically detected)
pN1c	Metastases in 1-3 axillary nodes and in internal mammary nodes with micrometastases or macrometastases detected by sentinel lymph node biopsy but not clinically detected
pN2	Metastases in 4-9 axillary nodes or in clinically detected internal mammary lymph nodes in the absence of axillary lymph node metastases
pN2a	Metastases in 4-9 axillary nodes (at least one tumor deposit >2.0 mm)
pN2b	Metastases in clinically detected internal mammary lymph nodes in the absence of axillary lymph node metastases
pN3	Metastases in ≥10 axillary nodes; or in infraclavicular (level III axillary nodes) or in clinically detected ipsilateral internal mammary lymph nodes in the presence of one or more positive level I, II axillary nodes; or in >3 axillary lymph nodes and internal mammary lymph nodes, with micrometastases or macrometastases detected by sentinel lymph node biopsy but not clinically detected; or in ipsilateral supraclavicular lymph nodes
Distant Metastases (M)	
M0	No clinical or radiographic evidence of distant metastases
cM0(i+)	No clinical or radiographic evidence of distant metastases, but deposits of molecularly or microscopically detected tumor cells in circulating blood, bone marrow, or other nonregional nodal tissue that are no larger than 0.2 mm in a patient without symptoms or signs of metastases
M1	Distant detectable metastases as determined by classic clinical and radiographic means and/or histologically proven larger than 0.2 mm

From Edge SB, Byrd DR, Compton CC, et al, editors: *AJCC cancer staging manual*, ed 7, New York, 2010, Springer-Verlag.
DCIS, ductal carcinoma in situ; *IHC,* immunohistochemistry; *LCIS,* lobular carcinoma in situ; *RT-PCR,* reverse transcriptase polymerase chain reaction.

Some prefixes and suffixes are used with the cTNM (clinical) and pTNM (pathologic) staging systems to designate special cases. These do not affect the stage group but indicate that they must be analyzed separately. These prefixes and suffixes include the "m" suffix, which signifies multiple primary tumors, pT(m)NM; the "y" prefix, which denotes patients who have received systemic therapy, ypTNM; and the "r" prefix, which indicates a recurrent tumor, rTNM. In clinical practice, physicians use the anatomic stage grouping in addition to important biologic factors to determine risk and guide treatment recommendations.

SURGICAL TREATMENT OF BREAST CANCER

Historical Perspective

Through the mid-20th century, breast cancer was thought to arise in the breast and progress to other sites largely via centrifugal

TABLE 34-5 Stage Groupings for Breast Cancer

ANATOMIC STAGE	PROGNOSTIC GROUP		
0	Tis	N0	M0
IA	T1	N0	M0
IB	T0	N1mi	M0
	T1	N1mi	M0
IIA	T0	N1	M0
	T1	N1	M0
	T2	N0	M0
IIB	T2	N1	M0
	T3	N0	M0
IIIA	T0	N2	M0
	T1	N2	M0
	T2	N2	M0
	T3	N1	M0
	T3	N2	M0
IIIB	T4	N0	M0
	T4	N1	M0
	T4	N2	M0
IIIC	Any T	N3	M0
IV	Any T	Any N	M1

spread. In this model, more extensive surgical procedures were expected to reduce mortality by resecting locoregional disease before it could spread to distant sites. This model was supported, in part, by the results of the Halsted radical mastectomy, which was the first procedure that demonstrated improvements in breast cancer survival relative to the local excision of tumors. Introduced in the 1890s, the radical mastectomy included removal of the breast, overlying skin, and underlying pectoralis muscles in continuity with the regional lymph nodes along the axillary vein to the costoclavicular ligament. The procedure often required a skin graft to cover the large skin defect that was created. This approach was well suited to breast cancer biology of the time, when most tumors were locally advanced, frequently with chest wall or skin involvement and extensive axillary nodal disease. Radical mastectomy provided improved local control and led to an increasing population of long-term survivors. Radical mastectomy continued to be the mainstay of surgical therapy into the 1970s.

Numerous women continued to die of metastatic breast cancer after radical mastectomy and even after more extensive surgical procedures, including radical mastectomy with en bloc resection of the internal mammary and supraclavicular nodes. This situation eventually led to a shift in the theory of primary centrifugal spread to the more modern theory that breast cancer spreads centrifugally to adjacent structures and embolically via lymphatics and blood vessels to distant sites.

In the modern era, breast cancer treatment includes local and regional approaches (surgery and radiation therapy) in addition to medical therapies designed to treat systemic disease. Multimodality treatment approaches were the first to show significant improvements in locoregional control and survival. As breast cancer was being recognized at earlier stages, the radical mastectomy was abandoned in favor of more conservative surgical approaches in combination with radiation therapy. The result was dramatic reductions in the extent of surgery required for local control of breast cancer and decreases in treatment-related morbidity. Breast cancer is a heterogeneous disease, and current treatment is guided by properties of the individual patient's tumor as well as the size and location of the tumor.

Surgical Trials of Local Therapy for Operable Breast Cancer

Radical Mastectomy versus Total Mastectomy, With or Without Radiation Therapy

In the NSABP B-04 trial, patients with clinically negative nodes were randomly assigned to radical mastectomy, total mastectomy with irradiation of the chest wall and regional nodes, or total mastectomy alone with delayed axillary dissection if nodes became clinically enlarged. Patients with clinically positive nodes were randomly assigned to radical mastectomy or total mastectomy with irradiation of the chest wall and regional lymphatics. At 25 years of follow-up, overall survival (OS) and disease-free survival (DFS) were equivalent in all treatment arms within the node-positive and node-negative groups.[19] Of the patients with clinically node-negative disease who underwent radical mastectomy, 38% were found to have nodal metastases at surgery, yet only 18% of patients undergoing total mastectomy without axillary dissection or radiation therapy developed axillary recurrence requiring delayed dissection. Despite the differences in the timing of their treatment, patients with delayed axillary dissection had survival equivalent to patients who underwent radical mastectomy and patients who underwent mastectomy with irradiation of the axillary nodes. The results of this trial led to the conclusion that the mode and timing of treatment of axillary nodes does not alter DFS or OS. Immediate removal, delayed removal, and irradiation produced equivalent clinical results.

Mastectomy versus Breast-Conserving Therapy

Six prospective clinical trials that included more than 4500 patients compared mastectomy versus breast-conserving therapy (Table 34-6). In all these trials, there was no survival advantage for the use of mastectomy over breast preservation. The largest of these trials was NSABP B-06, which enrolled 1851 patients with tumors up to 4 cm in diameter and clinically negative lymph nodes. Patients were randomly assigned to undergo modified radical mastectomy, lumpectomy alone, or lumpectomy with postoperative irradiation of the breast without an extra boost to the lumpectomy site.[20] All patients with histologically positive axillary nodes received chemotherapy. At 20 years of follow-up, OS and DFS were the same in all three treatment groups.

NSABP B-06 provided valuable information about rates of ipsilateral breast cancer recurrence after lumpectomy, with or without breast irradiation. At 20 years of follow-up, local recurrence rates were 14.3% in women treated with lumpectomy and radiation therapy and 39.2% in women treated with lumpectomy alone ($P < .001$). For patients with positive nodes who received chemotherapy, the local recurrence rate was 44.2% for lumpectomy alone and 8.8% for lumpectomy plus radiation therapy.

Another important trial that evaluated breast-conserving therapy was the Milan I trial. This trial enrolled patients with smaller tumors and used more extensive surgery and radiation therapy than the NSABP B-06 trial. There were 701 women with tumors up to 2 cm and clinically negative nodes randomly assigned to undergo radical mastectomy or quadrantectomy with axillary dissection and postoperative irradiation. Patients with pathologically positive nodes received chemotherapy. OS at 20 years did not differ between the two groups. Locoregional failure

TABLE 34-6 Randomized Trials Comparing Breast Conservation versus Mastectomy

TRIAL	NO. PATIENTS	MAXIMUM TUMOR SIZE (CM)	SYSTEMIC THERAPY	FOLLOW-UP (YR)	% SURVIVAL LUMPECTOMY + XRT	% SURVIVAL MASTECTOMY	LOCAL RECURRENCE (BCT) (%)
NSABP B-06[a]	1851	4	Yes	20	47	46	14*
Milan Cancer Institute[b]	701	2	Yes	20	44	43	8.8*
Institute Gustave-Roussy[c]	179	2	No	14	73	65	13
National Cancer Institute[d]	237	5	Yes	10	77	75	16
EORTC[e]	868	5	Yes	10	65	66	17.6
Danish Breast Cancer Group[f]	905	None	Yes	6	79	82	3

BCT, breast-conserving therapy; *EORTC,* European Organization for Research and Treatment of Cancer; *NSABP,* National Surgical Adjuvant Breast and Bowel Project; *XRT,* radiation therapy.
*Includes only women whose excision margins were negative.
[a]Fisher B, Anderson S, Bryant J, et al: Twenty-year follow-up of a randomized trial comparing total mastectomy, lumpectomy, and lumpectomy plus irradiation for the treatment of invasive breast cancer. *N Engl J Med* 347:1233, 2002.
[b]Veronesi U, Cascinelli N, Mariani L, et al: Twenty-year follow-up of a randomized study comparing breast-conserving surgery with radical mastectomy for early breast cancer. *N Engl J Med* 347:1227, 2002.
[c]Arriagada R, Le M, Rochard F, et al: Conservative treatment versus mastectomy in early breast cancer: Patterns of failure with 15 years of follow-up data. *J Clin Oncol* 14:1558, 1996.
[d]Jacobson J, Danforth D, Cowan K, et al: Ten-year results of a comparison of conservation with mastectomy in the treatment of stage I and II breast cancer. *N Engl J Med* 332:907, 1995.
[e]van Dongen J, Voogd A, Fentiman I, et al: Long-term results of a randomized trial comparing breast-conserving therapy with mastectomy: European Organization for Research and Treatment of Cancer 10801 Trial. *J Natl Cancer Inst* 92:1143, 2000.
[f]Blichert-Toft M, Rose C, Andersen J, et al: Danish randomized trial comparing breast conservation therapy with mastectomy: Six years of life-table analysis. Danish Breast Cancer Cooperative Group. *J Natl Cancer Inst Monogr* 11:19, 1992.

rates differed between the groups: Chest wall recurrence occurred in 2.3% of women who underwent radical mastectomy, and ipsilateral breast tumor recurrence occurred in 8.8% of women who underwent quadrantectomy and radiation therapy (20-year follow-up). Contralateral breast cancer rates were identical, approximately 0.66% per year for all women, refuting the hypothesis that irradiation increases the incidence of contralateral breast cancers. After quadrantectomy, local failure rates were higher in younger women, with rates of 1% per year in women younger than 45 years and 0.5% per year in older women.

Three other randomized trials in patients with operable breast cancer found no survival benefit of mastectomy over breast-conserving therapy. In the EORTC (European Organization for Research and Treatment of Cancer) Trial 10801, in which 868 women were randomly assigned to modified radical mastectomy or lumpectomy and irradiation, there was no difference in survival at 10 years. This trial included patients with tumors up to 5 cm, and 80% of women enrolled had tumors larger than 2.0 cm. Positive margins were allowed, and the results showed lower rates of local recurrence with clear versus involved margins.

In the Institut Gustave-Roussy trial, 179 women with tumors smaller than 2 cm were randomly assigned to modified radical mastectomy or lumpectomy with a 2-cm margin of normal tissue around the cancer. No differences were observed between the two surgical groups in risk for death, metastases, contralateral breast cancer, or locoregional recurrence at 15 years of follow-up.

In the U.S. NCI trial, 237 women with tumors 5 cm or smaller were randomly assigned to lumpectomy with axillary dissection and radiation therapy or modified radical mastectomy. No differences were seen in OS or DFS rates at 10 years.

Planning Surgical Treatments

It is critical to establish the diagnosis of breast cancer firmly before initiation of definitive surgical treatment. Core needle biopsy of a palpable or image-detected lesion is the preferred approach for diagnosis. Open surgical biopsy is reserved for lesions not amenable to core needle biopsy and cases in which core needle biopsy has proved nondiagnostic. Examination of biopsy material should provide information about tumor histologic type and grade, ER and PR status, and HER-2 status.

A history and physical examination, in addition to appropriate imaging studies, are important to establish the extent of disease and assign a clinical stage. The most common sites of distant metastases from breast cancer are the liver, lungs, and bones. The National Comprehensive Cancer Network provides guidelines regarding the use of laboratory and radiologic testing in patients at initial diagnosis based on clinical stage. Computed tomography scans, bone scans, and other imaging studies are generally reserved for patients with abnormalities on blood chemistry tests or chest radiographs and for patients with locally advanced or inflammatory breast cancer. Thorough imaging of the ipsilateral and contralateral breast is performed to look for areas of concern other than the index lesion. Breast MRI may be used in selected cases to define the extent of tumor and look for additional breast lesions; however, there is no high-level evidence demonstrating that use of MRI to guide decisions regarding local therapy improves local recurrence rates or survival.

In the absence of metastatic disease, the first intervention for patients with early-stage breast cancer is surgery for excision of the tumor and surgical staging of the regional lymph nodes. Assessment of the primary tumor size and regional lymph nodes defines the pathologic stage and provides an estimate of the prognosis to inform decisions about systemic therapy. Patients with locally advanced and inflammatory breast cancers should receive systemic therapy before surgery (see "Neoadjuvant Systemic Therapy for Operable Breast Cancer" later on).

The selection of surgical procedures takes into account patient characteristics and other clinical and pathologic variables. Patient characteristics, including age, family history, menopausal status, and overall health, are assessed. Some patients may undergo genetic testing for *BRCA* gene mutations at the time of diagnosis. Patients with a known mutation are generally counseled toward bilateral mastectomy for treatment of the index breast and reduction of the risk of contralateral breast cancer. The location of the tumor within the breast and tumor size relative to breast size are evaluated. Patient preferences for breast preservation versus mastectomy are determined. For patients considering mastectomy, options for immediate reconstruction are discussed.

Selection of Surgical Therapy

Mastectomy and breast-conserving therapy have been shown to be equivalent in terms of patient survival, and the choice of surgical treatment is individualized. Patients who desire breast-conserving surgery must be willing to attend postoperative radiation therapy sessions and to undergo postoperative surveillance of the treated breast. Consultation with a radiation oncologist should be arranged before the planned surgery. Patients are advised about the risks and long-term sequelae of radiation therapy. A mastectomy is generally recommended for patients who have contraindications to radiation therapy (Box 34-4). Although pregnancy is an absolute contraindication to radiation therapy, many patients pregnant at diagnosis can complete their pregnancy and receive radiation therapy after delivery.

A significant factor in determining whether breast-conserving therapy is feasible is the relationship between tumor size and breast size. In general, the tumor must be small enough in relation to the breast size so that the tumor can be resected with adequate margins and acceptable cosmesis. In patients with large tumors for whom adjuvant (postoperative) systemic chemotherapy will likely be recommended, the use of preoperative chemotherapy may be considered. Chemotherapy administered before surgery may decrease the tumor size sufficiently to permit breast-conserving surgery in patients who would not otherwise appear to be good candidates. Another strategy is to consider local tissue rearrangement or pedicled myocutaneous flaps (latissimus dorsi) to fill the defect resulting from breast-conserving surgery. Patients with multicentric tumors are usually served best by mastectomy because it is difficult to perform more than one breast-conserving surgery in the same breast with acceptable cosmesis. Although high nuclear grade, presence of lymphovascular invasion, and negative steroid hormone receptor status all have been linked to increased local recurrence rates, none of these factors are considered contraindications to breast conservation.

BOX 34-4 Contraindications to Radiation

Absolute
- Pregnancy

Relative
- Systemic scleroderma*
- Active systemic lupus erythematosus*
- Prior radiation to breast or chest wall
- Severe pulmonary disease
- Severe cardiac disease (if tumor is left-sided)
- Inability to lie supine
- Inability to abduct arm on affected side
- *p53* mutation†

*Other collagen vascular diseases are not contraindications to radiation, although patients should not be taking immunosuppressants such as methotrexate because they are radiosensitizers.
†Patients with *p53* mutations are highly susceptible to radiation-induced cancers.

Factors Influencing Eligibility for Breast Conservation

Randomized trials have demonstrated the efficacy of breast-conserving therapy for a wide variety of breast cancers and have defined eligibility criteria for breast conservation. With these criteria and current surgical and radiation therapy approaches, local recurrence rates after lumpectomy and radiation therapy are less than 5% at 10 years at many large centers.

Tumor Size

Tumors 5 cm in size, tumors with clinically positive nodes, and tumors with lobular and ductal histology were included in the randomized trials of mastectomy versus breast-conserving therapy. In current practice, lumpectomy is considered when the tumor, regardless of size, can be excised with clear margins and an acceptable cosmetic result.

Margins

The appropriate margin width for lumpectomy specimens has been debated. Although the NSABP B-06 trial defined a negative margin as "no ink on tumor," other trials evaluating breast-conserving therapy did not specify a required margin width or did not evaluate microscopic margins. The optimal margin width has been open to interpretation, resulting in substantial variability in treatment and recommendations regarding the need for reexcision for wider margins. The Society of Surgical Oncology and American Society for Radiation Oncology convened a multidisciplinary panel to address the question of what margin width is required to minimize the risk of ipsilateral breast tumor recurrence.[21] The panel used a meta-analysis of margin width and ipsilateral breast tumor recurrence from a systematic review of 33 studies including 28,162 patients. They found that positive margins, defined as ink on invasive carcinoma or DCIS, were associated with a twofold increase in ipsilateral breast tumor recurrence risk compared with negative margins. The risk was not affected by any specific clinicopathologic features, including favorable biology, use of endocrine therapy, or administration of a radiation boost. In addition, more widely clear margins than no ink on tumor did not significantly decrease the ipsilateral breast tumor recurrence risk, including in patients with unfavorable biology, lobular cancers, or cancers with an extensive intraductal component. The panel concluded that "no ink on tumor" should be used as the standard for an adequate margin in invasive breast cancer.

Histology

Invasive lobular cancers and cancers with an extensive intraductal component can be treated with lumpectomy if clear margins can be achieved. Atypical hyperplasia (ductal and lobular) and LCIS at resection margins do not increase local recurrence rates.

Patient Age

Local recurrence rates after breast-conserving surgery are higher for younger women than for older women. Local recurrence rates are reduced in patients of all ages with the use of radiation therapy. A radiation boost to the tumor bed has been shown to reduce local failures after lumpectomy, particularly in younger women.

Breast-Conserving Surgery

Technical Aspects

Excision of the primary tumor with preservation of the breast has been referred to by many terms, including *lumpectomy*, *partial mastectomy*, *segmental mastectomy*, *segmentectomy*, *tylectomy*, and

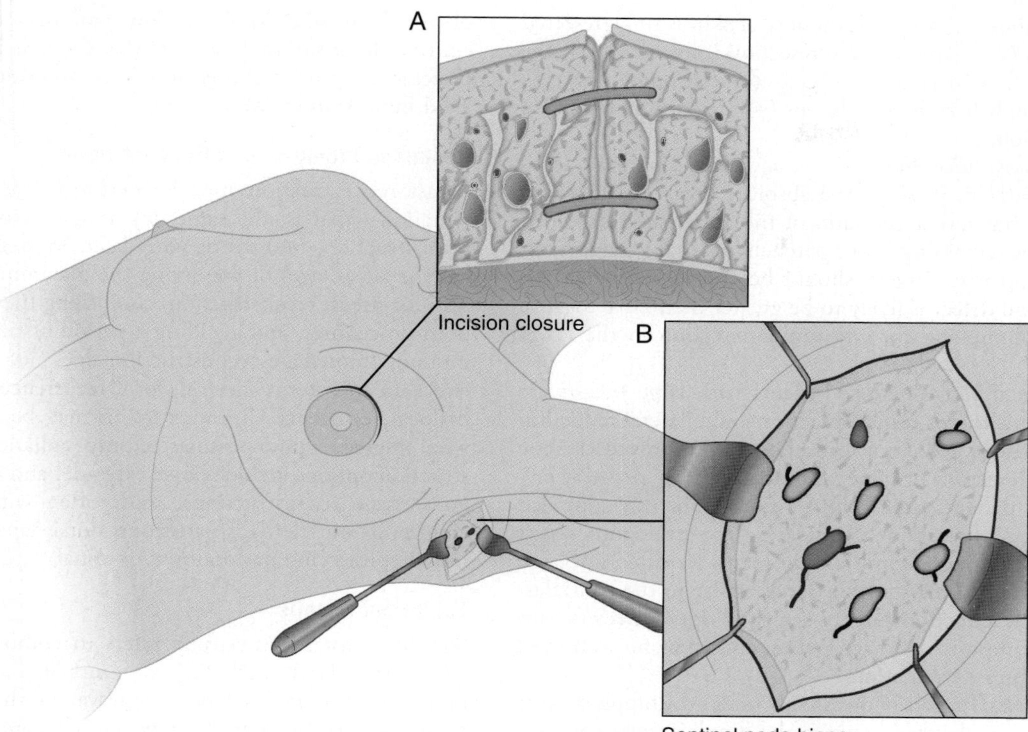

FIGURE 34-10 Breast-conserving surgery. **A,** Incisions to remove malignant tumors are placed directly over the tumor or around the areola. After the partial mastectomy has been completed, the parenchymal defect is closed *(inset)* to prevent a cosmetic deformity. **B,** A transverse incision below the axillary hairline is used for sentinel node biopsy or axillary dissection. The boundaries of the axillary dissection are the axillary vein superiorly, the latissimus dorsi muscle laterally, and the chest wall medially. The inferior dissection enters the tail of Spence (the axillary tail of the breast). In sentinel node biopsy, a similar transverse incision is made, which may be located by percutaneous mapping with the gamma probe to detect a hot spot from the radiolabeled colloid. It is extended through the clavipectoral fascia, and the true axilla is entered. The sentinel node is located by staining with blue dye *(inset)*, radioactivity, or both, and dissected free as a single specimen.

wide local excision. Breast-conserving surgery removes the malignancy with a surrounding rim of grossly normal breast parenchyma. This procedure is depicted in Figure 34-10, which shows the completed lumpectomy and skin incision for the axillary component of the procedure.

The breast specimen that is removed is oriented and its edges are inked before sectioning. Specimen radiography should be performed for all nonpalpable lesions or if there are microcalcifications associated with the palpable tumor. If a margin appears to be close or is positive histologically on intraoperative assessment, reexcision to remove more tissue frequently achieves a clear margin and allows conservation of the breast. Orientation of the surgical specimen allows focal reexcision of involved margins rather than global reexcision and improves the cosmetic result by reducing the amount of normal breast parenchyma that is excised.

The surgical defect created after lumpectomy is closed in cosmetic fashion. There is increasing interest in the use of advancement flap closure and other oncoplastic surgical techniques to maximize the cosmetic result.

Surgical staging of the axilla is performed through a separate incision in most patients undergoing breast conservation. SLND (see Fig. 34-10) has replaced anatomic axillary node dissection in patients with clinically negative axillary nodes. For patients who require axillary dissection, the extent of the dissection is identical to the axillary component of the modified radical mastectomy (see Fig. 34-10).

Cosmetic Challenges

The term *oncoplastic surgery* has been popularized to stress the importance of achieving the best possible esthetic result in the context of resecting the tumor with adequate oncologic margins. The goal is to retain as much of the natural breast size and contour as possible to provide optimal cosmesis and symmetry with the opposite breast. When the primary tumor is resected using an incision directly over the tumor and closure of the skin without reapproximation of any breast tissue, several deformities can occur, including volumetric deformity from a large parenchymal resection (retraction deformity when the seroma resorbs at the operative site); skin–pectoral muscle adherence deformity, in which the skin adheres to the underlying pectoral muscle; and lower pole deformity with downward turning of the nipple caused by excision of a tumor in the lower hemisphere of the breast. These deformities can make it difficult for patients to wear athletic clothing or bathing suits because significant asymmetry may be evident. It is important to correct these deformities before radiation therapy because the irradiation may further accentuate any asymmetry and make it more challenging to correct the defect in the future. The surgeon should consider oncoplastic techniques in the following situations: (1) a significant area of skin is to be resected with the tumor, (2) a large-volume resection is expected, (3) the tumor is in an area associated with poor cosmetic outcomes (e.g., lower hemisphere below the nipple), or (4) resection may lead to nipple malposition.

Extent of breast resection. When oncoplastic surgery techniques are considered, it is not the absolute breast volume that will be resected but rather the ratio of the anticipated defect to the volume of the remaining breast parenchyma that is important. In general, oncoplastic surgery should be considered when the size of the surgical defect is likely to be greater than 20% to 30% of the breast volume and for any tumor resection in the lower breast.

Breast size and body habitus. Patients with large breasts are often good candidates for tumor resection and bilateral reduction mammaplasty. Breast reduction can allow for improved esthetic outcomes after resection of large volumes of breast tissue at any location. Obese patients should be considered for this approach because they are often poor candidates for autologous tissue reconstruction after mastectomy, and implants are often not large enough to re-create a breast proportional in size to the contralateral breast. Breast reduction surgery is a good option because this can relieve the symptoms of macromastia and allow for improved outcomes after breast irradiation.

Tumor location. Tumors lying directly under the nipple-areolar complex and tumors located between the nipple-areolar complex and inframammary fold require special attention to avoid nipple-areolar complex distortion and contour deformity. In general, the skin and well-vascularized breast parenchyma must be adjusted to correct for the removal of breast tissue in these areas. As noted, deformities in the contour will be exacerbated by radiation and may be more challenging to correct at a later date.

Timing of Oncoplastic Surgery

Immediate repair of a partial mastectomy defect is almost always preferred to a delayed approach. Oncoplastic techniques such as tissue advancement and local tissue rearrangement at the time of the initial surgical procedure tend to provide the optimal solution. This approach has not been associated with delay in delivery of adjuvant systemic therapy or radiation. In general, local tissue transfer and breast reduction surgery cannot be performed on the irradiated breast; it is preferable to perform the procedure before radiation therapy. Tissue expanders and implants are not recommended to fill partial mastectomy defects because radiation may lead to capsular contracture, distortion, and infection.

If a cosmetic defect occurs after breast-conserving surgery and radiation therapy, reconstruction of the treated breast is generally not recommended for 1 to 2 years after radiation therapy has been completed. In irradiated tissue, there is a higher rate of tissue necrosis, seroma formation, and infection. The use of vascularized tissue from outside the radiation field is the favored approach. If the main deformity is caused by asymmetry with the contralateral breast, a mastopexy of the contralateral breast can be considered. In general, surgical procedures on the irradiated breast should be minimized because healing and recovery are impaired even when the skin appears healthy.

Mastectomy

Indications

Certain tumors still require mastectomy, including tumors that are large relative to breast size, tumors with extensive calcifications on mammography, tumors for which clear margins cannot be obtained on wide local excision, and tumors in patients with contraindications to breast irradiation (see Box 34-4). Patient preference for mastectomy or a desire to avoid radiation is also a valid indication for mastectomy.

Postmastectomy Breast Reconstruction

Breast reconstruction may be performed as immediate reconstruction—that is, the same day as mastectomy—or as delayed reconstruction, months or years later. Immediate reconstruction has the advantages of preserving the maximum amount of breast skin for use in reconstruction, combining the recovery period for both procedures, and avoiding a period of time without a breast mound. Immediate reconstruction does not have a detrimental effect on long-term survival, local recurrence rates, or detection of local recurrence. Reconstruction may be delayed in patients who might require postmastectomy radiation therapy. Reconstruction options include tissue expander and implant and autologous tissue reconstructions, most often with transverse rectus abdominis muscle flaps, latissimus dorsi flaps, or, more recently, muscle-preserving perforator abdominal flaps.

Technical Details

Simple or total mastectomy refers to complete removal of the mammary gland, including the nipple and areola. Modified radical mastectomy refers to removal of the mammary gland, nipple, and areola, with the addition of a complete axillary lymph node dissection (ALND) (Fig. 34-11). For either a total mastectomy or a modified radical mastectomy, an elliptical skin incision is planned to include the nipple and areola and usually any previous excisional biopsy scars (see Fig. 34-11). Skin flaps are raised to separate the underlying gland from the overlying skin along the subdermal plexus (see Fig. 34-11). If immediate reconstruction is not planned, sufficient skin is taken to allow smooth closure of skin flaps without redundant skin folds; this facilitates comfortable use of a breast prosthesis.

If immediate reconstruction is planned, a skin-sparing mastectomy may be performed in which only the nipple-areola complex is removed and the maximum amount of skin is left for use in the reconstruction. Nipple-areola–sparing mastectomy has been used with increasing frequency for selected patients with breast cancer. Multiple studies have shown the safety and feasibility of this approach, with many series showing no differences in recurrence rates or survival between patients undergoing nipple-areola–sparing mastectomy and patients undergoing skin-sparing mastectomy or standard total mastectomy.[22] Nipple-areola–sparing mastectomy has also been demonstrated to be safe in patients undergoing prophylactic mastectomy for risk reduction, including *BRCA1* and *BRCA2* gene mutation carriers.

Breast tissue is separated from the underlying pectoralis muscle, and the pectoral fascia is generally taken with the breast specimen. In a total mastectomy (see Fig. 34-11), breast tissue is separated from the axillary contents, and all breast tissue superficial to the fascia of the axilla is removed. In a modified radical mastectomy, the level I and II axillary lymph nodes are taken with the axillary breast tissue (see Fig. 34-11). Level I nodes are nodes inferior to the axillary vein and lateral to the pectoralis minor muscle, and level II nodes are nodes posterior to the pectoralis minor.

Lymph Node Staging

The pathologic status of the axillary lymph nodes is one of the most important prognostic factors in patients with breast cancer. Identification of metastatic tumor deposits in the axillary nodes

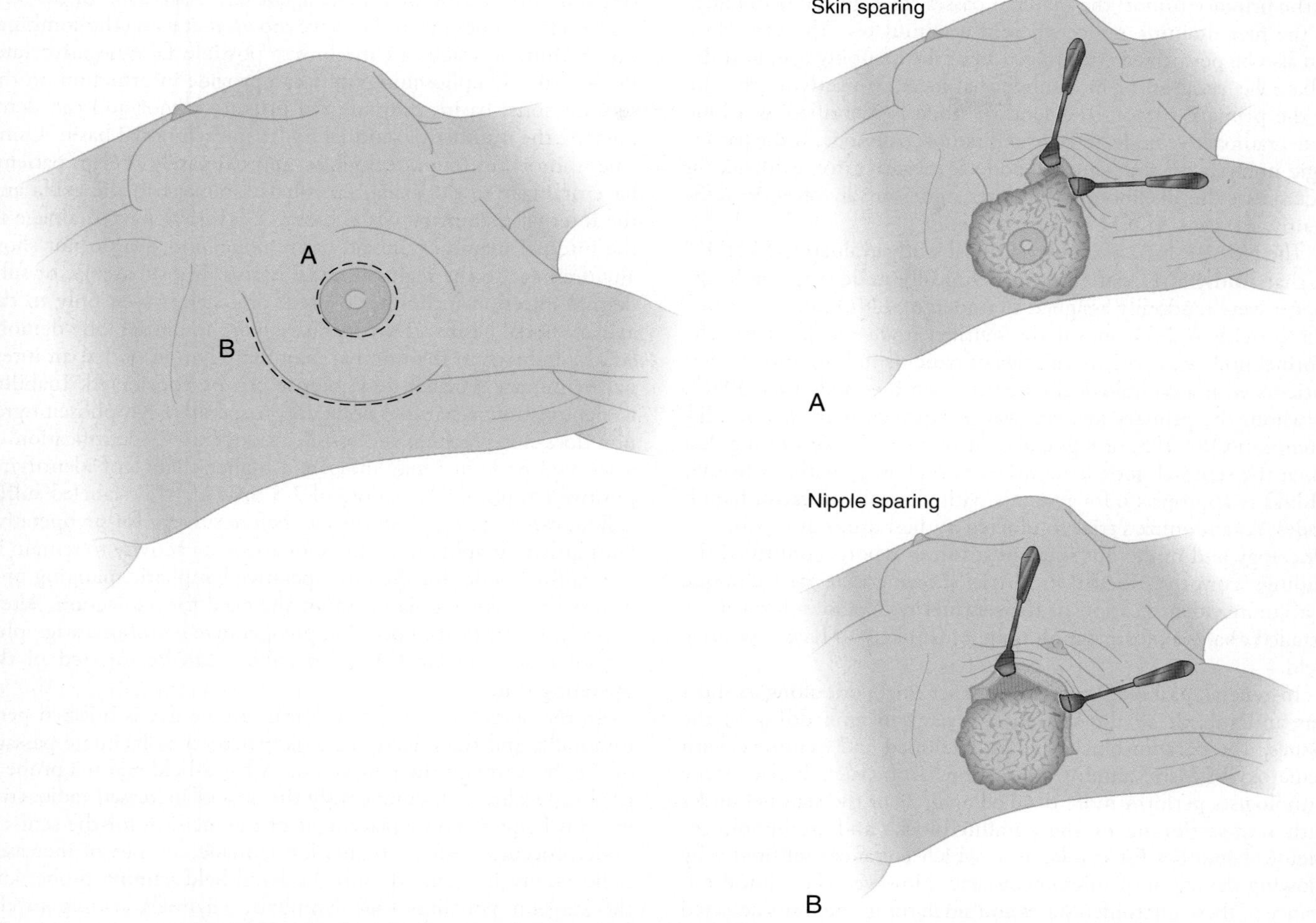

FIGURE 34-11 Total mastectomy with and without axillary dissection. For patients undergoing mastectomy without reconstruction, skin incisions are generally transverse and surround the central breast and nipple-areolar complex. **A,** Circumareolar incisions are most common for patients undergoing skin-sparing mastectomy with immediate reconstruction. Skin flaps are raised to separate the gland from the overlying skin and then the gland from the underlying muscle. Simple mastectomy divides the breast from the axillary contents and stops at the clavipectoral fascia. If axillary staging is planned, this is generally performed through a separate transverse axillary incision. **B,** An inframammary incision is shown for nipple-areolar–sparing mastectomy.

indicates a poorer prognosis and often prompts a recommendation for more aggressive systemic and locoregional therapies.

Historical Perspective

Historically, ALND was a routine component of the surgical management of breast cancer. It provides prognostic information about axillary nodal status and plays a therapeutic role in removing axillary disease in patients with positive nodes. The surgical procedure includes clearance of node-bearing tissue between the pectoralis major and latissimus dorsi muscles from the edge of the breast tissue in the low axillary region to the axillary vein and removal of the nodes posterior to the pectoralis minor muscle. Axillary dissection is the main source of morbidity in patients with early-stage breast cancer. The immediate problems include acute pain and paresthesias, need for hospitalization, reduced range of motion at the shoulder joint, and need for a drain in the surgical bed for 2 weeks or more. Long-term problems resulting from axillary dissection include lymphedema of the ipsilateral arm, numbness, chronic pain, and reduced range of motion at the shoulder joint.

Sentinel Lymph Node Dissection

The technique of SLND was developed to reduce the morbidity associated with axillary surgery, while still providing accurate staging information. Many patients now present with clinically node-negative disease, and SLND can identify patients with proven node-positive disease who may benefit from completion ALND. Patients with negative sentinel lymph nodes can avoid the morbidity of axillary dissection. Identification of the first, or sentinel, node draining the area of the primary tumor in the breast allows for this more selective approach to the axilla. The sentinel node is the most likely node to contain metastatic disease, if present, and the pathologist can focus the examination on the sentinel node without the added cost and time required to examine the full axillary contents. In sentinel node surgery, radiolabeled colloid, blue dye, or both are injected into breast tissue at the site of the primary tumor; the material passes through the lymphatics to the first draining node, where it accumulates. The procedure can also be performed with injection of the mapping agents at the subareolar position or in a subdermal location overlying the site of the primary tumor. The sentinel node is identified as a blue node, radioactive node, or blue and radioactive node. If the pathologic analysis of the sentinel node is negative for evidence of metastasis, the likelihood that other nodes are involved is sufficiently low that ALND is not required.

The NSABP B-32 trial was a critical study evaluating SLND.[23] In that study, 5611 patients with clinically node-negative breast cancer were randomly assigned to undergo SLND plus ALND or SLND with ALND only if the sentinel node was positive. The sentinel node was positive in 26% of patients in both groups. For patients with a pathologically negative sentinel node ($n = 3986$), in whom the primary analysis was performed, there was no difference in OS, DFS, or regional control rates, demonstrating that when the sentinel node is negative, SLND alone without further ALND is appropriate for patients with clinically negative lymph nodes. A randomized trial conducted at the European Institute of Oncology and numerous single-institution reports confirmed the findings from the NSABP B-32 trial showing that the technique is accurate. Identification of the sentinel node allows for a more detailed analysis of the lymph node most likely to have a positive yield.

In general, pathologists section the sentinel node along its short axis and submit all the sections for paraffin embedding of the tissues. The paraffin blocks can be sectioned and examined with hematoxylin-eosin staining of sections from each block. Some pathologists perform more detailed analysis of the sentinel nodes with step-sectioning of the paraffin blocks and immunohistochemical staining for cytokeratin, which enhances sensitivity by allowing detection of micrometastases. However, the clinical relevance of these micrometastases and small tumor deposits detected by immunohistochemical techniques has been questioned.[24] The NSABP B-32 trial provided an opportunity to investigate the clinical significance of occult metastatic disease.[24] For patients with negative sentinel nodes by hematoxylin-eosin staining, additional sections were evaluated by immunohistochemistry to identify occult metastases. The 5-year DFS rate was 86.4% for patients with occult metastases compared with 89.2% for patients without occult metastases (absolute difference = 2.8%), and the 5-year OS rate was 94.6% for patients with occult metastases compared with 95.8% for patients without occult metastases (absolute difference = 1.2%). These differences were statistically significant given the large number of patients enrolled in the study; however, because the absolute differences were small, the NSABP investigators concluded that the presence of occult metastases was not clinically significant. This conclusion was confirmed by the ACOSOG (American College of Surgeons Oncology Group) Z0010 trial, which was designed to evaluate the significance of sentinel node and bone marrow micrometastases in patients with early-stage breast cancer undergoing breast-conserving therapy.[25] In that study, the 5-year DFS rates for patients with immunohistochemistry-positive and immunohistochemistry-negative sentinel nodes were 90% and 92%, respectively ($P = .82$), whereas the 5-year OS rates were 95% and 96%, respectively ($P = .64$).

Lymphatic Mapping Technique and Selection of Patients for Sentinel Lymph Node Dissection

Lymphatic mapping can be performed with a combination of ^{99m}Tc-labeled sulfur colloid and a vital blue dye, isosulfan blue (Lymphazurin), or with a single agent for localization of the sentinel node. Numerous studies have shown that using the combination technique results in the lowest possible false-negative rate. Preoperative lymphoscintigraphy can provide information on the specific nodal basins draining the primary tumor and can demonstrate the number of sentinel nodes in each nodal basin. Using a peritumoral injection technique, approximately 70% of patients have drainage to the axilla, 20% have drainage to the axilla and the internal mammary nodal basin, 2% to 3% have drainage to the internal mammary nodal basin alone, and 8% do not show any drainage to the regional nodal basins. If a subareolar or subdermal injection technique is used, drainage is seen only to the axillary nodal basins. If preoperative lymphoscintigraphy demonstrates drainage to the internal mammary lymph nodes, an internal mammary sentinel node biopsy can be considered. Inability to demonstrate a sentinel node on preoperative lymphoscintigraphy does not preclude successful intraoperative identification of a sentinel node but may indicate a higher chance of identifying positive lymph nodes. A dose of 2.5 mCi of ^{99m}Tc-labeled sulfur colloid can be injected on the day before surgery for preoperative lymphoscintigraphy; this allows for adequate activity to remain in the sentinel nodes for the intraoperative lymphatic mapping procedure the following day without the need for reinjection. Alternatively, for surgeons not using preoperative lymphoscintigraphy, 0.5 mCi of ^{99m}Tc-labeled sulfur colloid can be injected in the operating suite.

In the operating suite, 3 to 5 mL of blue dye is injected peritumorally, and the injection site is massaged to facilitate passage of the dye through the lymphatics. A hand-held gamma probe is used to localize transcutaneously the area of increased radioactivity; this helps to guide placement of the incision for the sentinel node procedure. After the incision is made, an area of increased radioactivity is localized with the hand-held gamma probe, and the surgeon visualizes blue lymphatic channels leading to the sentinel node. Dissection is performed to avoid prematurely disrupting the afferent lymphatics. If a blue-stained lymphatic channel or a specific area of radioactivity ("hot spot") cannot be identified, the primary tumor can be resected to remove the site of injection, decreasing the background shine-through radioactivity. The sentinel node may be identified and removed, after which the nodal basin is checked again to confirm that the level of radioactivity has decreased. If the level of radioactivity remains high, additional sentinel nodes may remain in the nodal basin, and additional dissection should be completed to remove all sentinel nodes. Published studies have demonstrated an average of two or three sentinel nodes per patient.

Surgeons experienced in SLND can identify a sentinel node in more than 95% of patients. The false-negative rate for sentinel node surgery ranges from 0% to 10%, as reported in the NSABP B-32 trial.[23] Surgeons should be trained in SLND before using this procedure as a staging tool. Patients who present with clinically palpable lymph nodes should be evaluated with axillary ultrasonography and FNAB of the nodes. If axillary metastasis is confirmed, patients can proceed directly to standard axillary node dissection or be considered for preoperative chemotherapy. If axillary metastasis is not confirmed by FNAB, patients can proceed to sentinel node surgery for staging.

Some studies have shown that patients who have undergone previous excisional biopsy of the primary tumor are more likely to have a false-negative sentinel node.[23] The lymphatics may be disrupted by the biopsy, which can affect drainage patterns of the area surrounding the excisional biopsy site. To avoid this scenario, core needle biopsy is the preferred diagnostic approach in patients suspected to have breast cancer.

In older studies, SLND was reported to be less accurate in patients treated with preoperative chemotherapy. A meta-analysis of the published studies on sentinel node surgery after chemotherapy suggested that this technique is accurate; a more recent comparison showed that false-negative rates after chemotherapy compared favorably with false-negative rates observed in patients who undergo surgery first.[26] Patients with documented metastasis before the initiation of chemotherapy should undergo standard ALND on completion of chemotherapy.

Outcomes of Sentinel Lymph Node Dissection

Morbidity rates are substantially lower with SLND than with ALND. Another advantage is that SLND can be performed as an outpatient procedure and does not require a drain. Patients have more rapid return to full mobility and are able to return to work and other activities weeks sooner than after axillary dissection. Long-term morbidity, including lymphedema, numbness, and chronic pain, is greatly reduced.

SLND has been shown to provide reliable pathologic staging of the axilla, with false-negative rates generally less than 5% in experienced hands. Axillary recurrence rates have been shown to be extremely low after a negative sentinel node biopsy without axillary dissection. A negative sentinel node is now widely accepted as sufficient to establish node-negative disease in a patient, with no further axillary treatment required.[23]

When the sentinel node contains metastatic disease, the likelihood of additional involved nodes is directly proportional to the size of the primary breast tumor, presence of lymphatic vascular invasion, and size of the lymph node metastasis. In approximately 50% of patients with positive sentinel nodes, the sentinel node is the only positive node. In the presence of a positive sentinel node, treatment guidelines have dictated completion ALND as the standard; this is most commonly achieved with a completion level I and II axillary dissection. Although ALND has been standard practice for patients with positive sentinel nodes, the need for ALND in all patients with a positive sentinel node has been called into question because many patients have small-volume metastases, and the sentinel node is often the only positive node. A meta-analysis of studies evaluating patients with positive sentinel nodes showed that 53% of patients have additional positive nodes at ALND.[27] In the case of micrometastatic disease in the sentinel nodes, the rate of nonsentinel node involvement is 20%, and for patients with isolated tumor cells, it is less than 12%. These findings led to a trend of omitting ALND in selected patients with positive sentinel nodes. An analysis of SEER data from the years 1998-2004 revealed that 16% of patients with sentinel node–positive disease did not undergo ALND. These patients were more commonly older patients with low-grade, ER-positive tumors. During this time period, the proportion of patients with micrometastasis in the sentinel node who did not undergo ALND increased from 21% to 38%. A review of the National Cancer Data Base data from the years 1998-2005 revealed similar findings, with 20.8% of patients with sentinel node–positive disease avoiding ALND. There were no differences in axillary recurrence rates or survival between patients who had sentinel node surgery only and patients who underwent ALND.

One factor that may have contributed to the decrease in ALND for patients with positive sentinel nodes is the emergence of the use of nomograms that can predict the probability of disease burden in the undissected nonsentinel nodes. For patients with micrometastasis in one of several sentinel nodes or patients with disease detected by immunohistochemistry only, the estimated risk of additional positive nodes remaining in the axilla is low. The first nomogram developed was published by researchers from Memorial Sloan Kettering Cancer Center and is available to clinicians on the Internet (http://nomograms.mskcc.org/Breast/index.aspx; accessed August 20, 2015). A more recent tool, developed at the University of Texas MD Anderson Cancer Center, includes the important variable of sentinel node metastasis size. This nomogram is also available on the Internet (http://www3.mdanderson.org/app/medcalc/bc_nomogram2/index.cfm?pagename=nsln). Both nomograms have been validated to estimate the degree of additional nodal involvement on the basis of patient characteristics, primary tumor characteristics, number of sentinel nodes, and other factors. These and other nomograms can be used by the surgeon, in combination with clinical judgment and other available information, to estimate the risk of additional positive nonsentinel nodes in an individual patient.

The ACOSOG initiated a prospective randomized trial in 1999 designed specifically to evaluate the impact of ALND on locoregional recurrence and survival in patients with early-stage breast cancer.[28] The trial, ACOSOG Z0011, enrolled patients with clinical T1 or T2 breast cancer with one or two positive sentinel nodes who were planning to undergo breast-conserving surgery and whole breast irradiation. Patients were randomly assigned to undergo completion ALND or no further surgery (sentinel node surgery alone). The primary end point of the Z0011 study was OS; a secondary end point was locoregional recurrence. Patients enrolled in the Z0011 study had relatively favorable disease characteristics: The median age was 55 years, 70% of patients had T1 tumors, 82% had ER-positive tumors, 71% had only one positive sentinel node, and 44% had micrometastases. At a median follow-up of 6.3 years, local recurrence was seen in 3.6% (n = 29) of the ALND group versus 1.8% (n = 8) of the SLND-only group. Axillary recurrences were reported in 0.5% (n = 2) of patients in the ALND group versus 0.9% (n = 4) of patients in the SLND-only group. There were no differences in OS (91.9% after ALND versus 92.5% after SLND only; P = .24) or DFS (82.2% after ALND versus 83.8% after SLND only) at 5 years. The Z0011 study investigators concluded that the routine use of ALND was not justified in all patients with early-stage breast cancer with a positive sentinel node.

The results of the ACOSOG Z0011 study have changed treatment practices. It is now widely believed that ALND may be safely omitted in selected patients with clinically node-negative disease who have a positive sentinel node and are similar to the participants in the Z0011 trial—women with T1 or T2, clinically node-negative breast cancer who undergo breast-conserving surgery and whole breast irradiation and who have one or two positive sentinel nodes and are scheduled to undergo adjuvant systemic therapy. ALND remains the standard of care for patients with locally advanced breast cancer or inflammatory breast cancer, patients with a positive sentinel node who are scheduled for mastectomy, patients with a positive sentinel node who are scheduled for accelerated partial breast irradiation, and patients with a positive sentinel node after neoadjuvant chemotherapy.

TREATMENT OF DUCTAL CARCINOMA IN SITU

DCIS, or intraductal cancer, accounts for approximately 25% of all newly diagnosed breast cancers. It was anticipated that more than 51,000 new cases of DCIS would be diagnosed in 2014.

Most cases of DCIS are detected as an area of clustered calcifications on a screening mammogram without an associated palpable abnormality. Rarely, DCIS manifests as a palpable mass or as unilateral, single-duct nipple discharge.

Findings on mammography in patients with DCIS include clustered calcifications without an associated density in 75% of patients, calcifications coexisting with an associated density in 15%, and a density alone in 10%. The calcifications seen on a mammogram generally correspond to areas within the central involved duct in which there is often necrosis and debris. DCIS calcifications tend to cluster closely together, are pleomorphic, and may be linear or branching, suggesting their ductal origin.

DCIS is viewed as a precursor to invasive ductal cancer, and treatment aims to remove the DCIS to prevent progression to invasive disease. Because the prevalence of metastatic disease in patients with DCIS without demonstrable invasion is low (<1%), systemic chemotherapy is not required. Hormonal therapy may be used for prevention of new primary tumors and to improve local control after breast-conserving therapy but is generally recommended only when the DCIS is positive for ER on immunohistochemistry.

Treatment recommendations for a patient with DCIS are based on the extent of disease within the breast, histologic grade, ER status, and presence of microinvasion as well as patient age and preference. Treatment options for DCIS include mastectomy, breast-conserving surgery with irradiation, and breast-conserving surgery alone. When the patient is treated with breast conservation or unilateral mastectomy, there is also the option of adjuvant hormonal therapy with tamoxifen to reduce the risk for future breast cancers.[29]

Mastectomy

The breast cancer mortality rate after treatment of DCIS by total mastectomy is 1%. Local recurrences are rare and suggest malignant transformation of residual glandular tissue. Metastatic disease in patients with pure DCIS is suggestive of a histologically unrecognized invasive carcinoma in the mastectomy specimen or the development of a contralateral primary tumor. Reasons to select total mastectomy for treatment of DCIS include the following:

1. Diffuse suspicious mammographic calcifications suggestive of extensive disease
2. Inability to obtain clear margins with breast-conserving surgery
3. Likelihood of a poor cosmetic result after breast-conserving surgery
4. Patient not motivated to preserve her breast
5. Contraindications to radiation therapy (see Box 34-4)

Breast-Conserving Therapy

As for invasive breast cancer, breast-conserving therapy for DCIS requires resection to microscopically clear margins. The use of adjuvant whole breast radiation therapy has been demonstrated in prospective randomized trials to decrease the risk for local recurrence. The use of hormonal therapy in patients with ER-positive DCIS can decrease further the risk for local recurrence and reduces the risk for development of new contralateral and ipsilateral breast cancers.

The use of radiation therapy after lumpectomy was investigated in four prospective randomized trials (Table 34-7), the results of which are remarkably consistent. In the NSABP B-17 trial, 818 women with DCIS were randomly assigned to lumpectomy alone versus lumpectomy plus 50 Gy of postoperative whole breast irradiation. The addition of radiation to surgery decreased the ipsilateral recurrence rate from 30.8% to 14.9% ($P < .000005$) as shown by 12-year actuarial recurrence data.[30] The addition of radiation also decreased the incidence of invasive breast cancer, from 16.4% to 7.1% ($P < .00001$), and produced a smaller decrease in the incidence of in situ recurrence, from 14.1% to 7.8% ($P < .001$) (see Table 34-7). In the EORTC 10853 trial, 1010 women with DCIS were randomly assigned to lumpectomy alone versus lumpectomy plus 50 Gy of radiation therapy.[31] Radiation reduced the 10-year breast recurrence rate from 26% to 15% ($P < .0001$) and reduced the rate of invasive recurrences from 13% to 8% ($P = .0011$). The UK ANZ (United Kingdom, Australia, and New Zealand) trial, which included 1701 patients, was a large randomized trial that simultaneously evaluated the benefits of radiation therapy and tamoxifen after breast-conserving surgery for patients with DCIS.[32] This trial also demonstrated that radiation therapy reduced the risk of breast cancer recurrence (hazard ratio [HR], 0.38; $P < .0001$) and invasive breast cancer recurrence (HR, 0.45; $P = .01$). Finally, the SweDICS trial included 1067 patients with DCIS. After a median follow-up of 5 years, the cumulative incidence of breast recurrence was 22% in the group

TABLE 34-7 Randomized Trials of Lumpectomy for Ductal Carcinoma in Situ: Impact of Radiation Therapy and Tamoxifen

			LOCAL RECURRENCE RATES (%)			
TRIAL	NO. PATIENTS	FOLLOW-UP (YR)	LUMPECTOMY	LUMPECTOMY + XRT	LUMPECTOMY + XRT + TAMOXIFEN	P VALUE
NSABP B-17[a]	818	12	30.8	14.9		<.000005
EORTC 10853[b]	1010	4.25	16	9		<.005
UK ANZ	1701	5	20	8	6	<.0001
SweDCIS	1067	5	7	22		<.0001
NSABP B-24[c]	1804	7		9	6	.04

EORTC, European Organization for Research and Treatment of Cancer; *NSABP,* National Surgical Adjuvant Breast and Bowel Project; *SweDCIS,* Swedish Ductal Carcinoma In Situ trial; *UK ANZ,* United Kingdom, Australia, and New Zealand; *XRT,* radiation therapy.

[a]Fisher B, Dignam J, Wolmark N, et al: Lumpectomy and radiation therapy for the treatment of intraductal breast cancer: Findings from National Surgical Adjuvant Breast and Bowel Project B-17. *J Clin Oncol* 16:441, 1998.

[b]Julien JP, Bijker N, Fentiman IS, et al: Radiotherapy in breast-conserving treatment for ductal carcinoma in situ: First results of the EORTC randomised phase III trial 10853. EORTC Breast Cancer Cooperative Group and EORTC Radiotherapy Group. *Lancet* 355:528, 2000.

[c]Fisher B, Land S, Mamounas E, et al: Prevention of invasive breast cancer in women with ductal carcinoma in situ: An update of the National Surgical Adjuvant Breast and Bowel Project experience. *Semin Oncol* 28:400, 2001.

that underwent surgery only versus 7% in the group that underwent surgery plus radiation therapy ($P < .0001$).

Attempts have been made to identify subsets of DCIS for which wide excision without irradiation would provide sufficient local control. Silverstein[33] derived the Van Nuys criteria for classifying DCIS from a series of patients with DCIS treated by wide excision with and without radiation therapy. A system was proposed to identify patients who do not need radiation therapy because they have a low DCIS nuclear grade, a small lesion, older age, and wide surgical margins. Silverstein reported low breast recurrence rates with surgery alone for patients with favorable Van Nuys scores. However, in a prospective trial testing this approach, investigators from Harvard enrolled 158 patients from the most favorable Van Nuys subset (low-grade or intermediate-grade DCIS <2.5 cm, with a minimum 1-cm margin on excision) and were unable to reproduce the results; the Harvard investigators stopped the trial early because the rates of recurrence exceeded the predefined stopping rules. More recently, Eastern Cooperative Oncology Group investigators reported the first result of a relatively large prospective single-arm study of surgery with negative margins of at least 3 mm without radiation therapy for patients with favorable subsets of DCIS.[34] Patients with low-grade or intermediate-grade DCIS measuring 2.5 cm or smaller had a 5-year rate of ipsilateral breast recurrence of only 6.1%. In contrast, patients with high-grade disease had a much higher 5-year ipsilateral breast recurrence rate of 15.3%.

Taken together, the data from these trials of treatment for DCIS suggest that whole breast irradiation after lumpectomy should be recommended for most patients with DCIS. The one subgroup that appears to have favorable outcomes without radiation are patients with small, low-grade or intermediate-grade lesions.

Role of Tamoxifen

The use of tamoxifen has been shown to reduce the risk for development of new breast cancers in high-risk women, including women with a previous breast cancer (see "Chemoprevention for Breast Cancer" earlier). The NSABP B-24 protocol evaluated the benefit of tamoxifen for patients with DCIS. In this trial, 1804 women who had undergone lumpectomy and radiation therapy for DCIS were randomly assigned to 5 years of tamoxifen or placebo.[29] Study criteria allowed enrollment of patients with positive margins, and ER was not measured. At 7 years of follow-up, the addition of tamoxifen to lumpectomy and radiation therapy decreased the incidence of recurrent ipsilateral breast cancers from 9% to 6% and reduced the risk for a new contralateral breast cancer by 47% (an absolute reduction of 2%) (see Table 34-7).

For the NSABP B-17 and NSABP B-24 trials combined, at 7 years of follow-up, the total (ipsilateral plus contralateral) breast cancer recurrence rate was 30% for excision alone; 17% for excision with radiation therapy; and 10% for excision, irradiation, and tamoxifen. Subsequent analyses demonstrated that the benefit from tamoxifen is seen only in women with ER-positive DCIS. Patients at highest risk for local recurrence—and most likely to benefit from tamoxifen—were patients with positive margins, comedo necrosis, a mass on physical examination, and age younger than 50 years. For individual patients, the benefits of tamoxifen are weighed against its side effects, including risk for endometrial carcinoma, thromboembolic events, hot flashes, and cataracts.

Sentinel Node Surgery

DCIS, by definition, represents breast cancer contained within an intact basement membrane and without access to lymphatic or vascular channels. However, when ALND is performed during mastectomy for DCIS, positive nodes are found in 3.6% of cases, as indicated by a review of more than 10,000 patients in the National Cancer Data Base. These positive nodes probably result from microinvasive disease in the primary tumor that was not detected on routine pathologic analysis.

Sentinel node surgery is currently recommended in patients undergoing mastectomy for DCIS because 20% of patients with DCIS on a diagnostic core needle biopsy are found to have invasive cancer on detailed evaluation of the mastectomy specimen. The addition of sentinel node surgery to mastectomy adds minimal morbidity and avoids the need for ALND if invasive cancer is identified (sentinel node mapping is impossible after mastectomy). For patients undergoing breast-conserving surgery for DCIS, sentinel node surgery may be considered for patients with larger areas of DCIS, particularly patients with high-grade histology or with high suspicion of microinvasion.

RADIATION THERAPY FOR BREAST CANCER

Radiation Therapy After Breast-Conserving Surgery

For patients with invasive breast cancer treated with breast-conserving surgery, adjuvant irradiation of the breast has been conclusively demonstrated to reduce the probability of a breast recurrence and improve outcome. The EBCTCG published a meta-analysis of the data from 7300 women who participated in randomized trials of breast-conserving surgery with or without radiation therapy.[35] In this analysis, radiation was found to reduce the 10-year rate of in-breast recurrence from 29% to 10% for patients with negative lymph nodes and from 47% to 13% for patients with positive lymph nodes. This improvement in local control led to a reduction in the 15-year breast cancer mortality rate and overall death rate. On the basis of these data, radiation therapy after breast-conserving surgery should be considered as a standard. Most trials attempting to define subgroups of patients who could potentially avoid radiation after lumpectomy have been unsuccessful. The only group identified that might be able to avoid irradiation safely is patients older than 70 years who undergo lumpectomy and adjuvant hormonal therapy for a stage I ER-positive breast cancer.[36]

Historically, radiation therapy after lumpectomy has consisted of a 6- to 8-week treatment course, which can be a hardship for patients. An important Canadian trial successfully compared this historical schedule with a more abbreviated whole breast irradiation schedule. On the basis of long-term outcome results from this study, it is reasonable to treat a postmenopausal patient with a non–high-grade, ER-positive, stage I breast cancer with a 16-fraction course of treatment, which shortens the overall treatment time to approximately 3 weeks.

There has also been significant interest in shortening the treatment course to 1 week or less through an approach that focuses the radiation exclusively on the area around the tumor bed. This approach, called *partial breast irradiation,* may be performed with brachytherapy catheters, balloon catheters, or external-beam radiation. Results from large phase III clinical trials comparing partial breast irradiation with conventional whole breast treatment have yet to mature. Nonetheless, partial breast irradiation has proven to be popular with physicians and patients. The American Society for Radiation Oncology published a consensus statement highlighting appropriate selection criteria that should be considered if patients are to be treated with partial breast irradiation outside the context of a clinical trial (Table 34-8).[37]

TABLE 34-8 American Society for Radiation Oncology Guidelines for Accelerated Partial Breast Irradiation

FACTOR	"SUITABLE" GROUP	"CAUTIONARY" GROUP	"UNSUITABLE" GROUP
Patient factors			
Age (yr)	≥60	50-59	<50
Tumor factors			
Tumor size (cm)	≤2	2.1-3.0	>3
T stage	T1	T0 or T2	T3 or T4
Margins	Negative by at least 2 mm	Close (<2 mm)	Positive
Histology	Invasive ductal carcinoma or other favorable subtypes	Invasive lobular carcinoma	NA
Pure DCIS	Not allowed	≤3 cm in size	>3 cm in size
Grade	Any	NA	NA
LVI	None	Limited/focal	Extensive
ER status	Positive	Negative	NA
Multicentricity	Unicentric	NA	If present
Multifocality	Clinically unifocal with total size ≤2 cm	Clinically unifocal with total size 2.1-3 cm	Clinically multifocal or microscopically multifocal >3 cm in total size
Nodal factors			
N stage	pN0	NA	pN1-3
Treatment factors			
Neoadjuvant chemotherapy	Not allowed	NA	If used

DCIS, ductal carcinoma in situ; *ER*, estrogen receptor; *LVI*, lymphovascular invasion; *NA*, not available.
Adapted from Smith BD, Arthur DW, Buchholz TA, et al: Accelerated partial breast irradiation consensus statement from the American Society for Radiation Oncology (ASTRO). *J Am Coll Surg* 209:269, 2009.

Postmastectomy Radiation Therapy

For patients with T1N0 or T2N0 breast cancer, mastectomy and SLND provide effective local control, and radiation therapy is not required.[35] In contrast, patients with stage III breast cancer have high rates of locoregional recurrence after treatment with a modified radical mastectomy and adjuvant or neoadjuvant chemotherapy. Clinical trial data indicate that postmastectomy radiation therapy can significantly improve the outcome of patients who would be expected to have a 20% to 40% risk of locoregional recurrence without radiation therapy.

Three prospective randomized trials addressed the role of postmastectomy irradiation. In the Danish Trials, premenopausal women with stage II or III breast cancer were randomly assigned to chemotherapy alone or chemotherapy plus chest wall and nodal irradiation (protocol 82b); postmenopausal women were randomly assigned to tamoxifen alone or tamoxifen plus radiation therapy (protocol 82c).[38] In the British Columbia study, premenopausal women with node-positive breast cancer were randomly assigned to chemotherapy alone or chemotherapy plus chest wall and nodal irradiation.[39] In addition to reducing locoregional recurrences, as expected, postmastectomy irradiation significantly improved OS in all three trials (Table 34-9).

In 2005, the EBCTCG published the results of a meta-analysis of trials of postmastectomy radiation therapy, which included data from 9933 patients treated with mastectomy or axillary clearance with or without postmastectomy radiation.[35] Postmastectomy radiation therapy decreased the 15-year isolated locoregional recurrence rate for patients with lymph node–positive disease from 29% to 8% and reduced the 15-year breast cancer mortality rate from 60% to 55%. The most recent analysis from this group suggested that benefits of postmastectomy radiation therapy are similar for patients with one to three positive lymph nodes and patients with four or more positive lymph nodes.[40]

There is consensus that patients with four or more positive lymph nodes or other features characteristic of stage III disease should be counseled to undergo radiation therapy. However, the use of postmastectomy radiation therapy for patients with stage II disease is controversial because many U.S. series indicated that locoregional recurrence rates after a standard modified radical mastectomy and adjuvant chemotherapy are only 12% to 15%, much lower than rates reported in the clinical trials of postmastectomy irradiation and the EBCTCG meta-analysis. On the basis of this disparity, it is reasonable to consider postmastectomy radiation therapy only for selected patients with stage II disease, such as patients with extracapsular extension, lymphovascular invasion, age 40 years or younger, close surgical margins, or a nodal positivity ratio (ratio of positive nodes to total nodes examined) of 20% or greater and patients who have undergone less than a standard level I or II axillary dissection.

SYSTEMIC THERAPY FOR BREAST CANCER

Despite advances in locoregional therapy, a significant proportion of women with breast cancer develop metastatic disease within 5 to 10 years after diagnosis. Most patients who develop metastatic breast cancer die of their disease. Metastatic disease is the principal cause of death from breast cancer.

Systemic therapy is used to treat and prevent recurrence of microscopic metastatic breast cancer. For women with stage IV breast cancer, systemic therapy is given to palliate symptoms from cancer and potentially prolong survival. Current thinking is that metastasis occurs early in the progression of breast cancer, probably before initial clinical evaluation in most patients. This concept argues for administration of systemic therapy for breast cancer in concert with local treatment. What is missing at the present time

TABLE 34-9 Trials of Systemic Therapy With or Without Irradiation After Mastectomy

	NO. PATIENTS			LOCAL RECURRENCE RATE (%)			OS (%)		
TRIAL	SYSTEMIC THERAPY + XRT	SYSTEMIC THERAPY ALONE	TOTAL	SYSTEMIC THERAPY + XRT	SYSTEMIC THERAPY ALONE	*P* VALUE	SYSTEMIC THERAPY + XRT	SYSTEMIC THERAPY ALONE	*P* VALUE
DBCG 82b (10 yr; chemo)[a]	852	856	1708	9	32	<.001	54	45	<.001
DBCG 82c (10 yr; tamoxifen)[b]	686	689	1375	8	35	<.001	45	38	.03
DBCG 82c (combined 18 yr)[b]	1538	1545	3083	14	49	<.001	37	27	
British Columbia Trial (20 yr)[c]	164	154	318	13	25	.003*	64	54	.003*

chemo, chemotherapy; *DBCG,* Danish Breast Cancer Group; *OS,* overall survival; *XRT,* radiation therapy.
*Aggregate *P* value for comparisons at various follow-up intervals; this is the 10-year result.
[a]Overgaard M, Hansen Per S, Overgaard J, et al: Postoperative radiotherapy in high-risk premenopausal women with breast cancer who receive adjuvant chemotherapy. *N Engl J Med* 337:949, 1997.
[b]Overgaard M, Jensen M-B, Overgaard J, et al: Postoperative radiotherapy in high-risk postmenopausal breast cancer patients given adjuvant tamoxifen: Danish Breast Cancer Cooperative Group DBCG 82c randomized trial. *Lancet* 353:1641, 1999.
[c]Ragaz J, Jackson S, Le N, et al: Adjuvant radiotherapy and chemotherapy in node-positive premenopausal women with breast cancer. *N Engl J Med* 337:956, 1997.

is the ability to detect occult metastatic disease accurately and select appropriate patients to receive systemic treatment.

The first prospective trials of systemic therapy for breast cancer combined oophorectomy, to deprive patients of estrogens, with radical mastectomy. Since these early trials, hundreds of prospective studies of systemic therapy have been conducted involving thousands of women. Medications used to treat early breast cancer have their foundation as treatment for advanced disease. In general, treatments that are used effectively to improve outcome for patients with incurable breast cancer are estimated to have an increased impact on outcomes for patients with earlier stages of breast cancer, who have smaller volumes of disease and potentially less resistance to therapy. When medications are identified that improve outcomes for patients with incurable stage IV breast cancer, they are often brought forward into clinical studies for earlier stages of disease.

Goals of Therapy and Assessment of Potential Benefits and Risks from Therapy

For patients with stage I to III invasive breast cancer, the goal of treatment is cure. In selecting treatment, the potential benefits of therapy (reduction in the risk of recurrence) are considered together with the potential harms of treatment. Patient preferences, particularly preferences regarding adjuvant therapy, are carefully considered. Some patients believe that the reduction in risk of recurrence with adjuvant therapy is not worth the adverse effects of the therapy, particularly in the case of chemotherapy. Often, several long discussions with the patient are essential to determine the treatment that best suits that patient.

The risk of systemic recurrence increases with increasing stage of disease. The biologic characteristics of an individual tumor also influence the risk of systemic recurrence. The most commonly used breast cancer biomarkers—ER, PR, and HER-2—not only affect prognosis but also predict response to different systemic therapies. In general terms, tumors that have no ER or PR expression and tumors with high levels of HER-2 are associated with worse cancer outcomes than tumors that are strongly positive for ER and PR and have negative or normal levels of HER-2. For most patients, risk of recurrence is estimated on the basis of population-based statistics. Current federal and international guidelines use stage and biologic characteristics in the development of treatment recommendations to guide decisions regarding systemic therapy for breast cancer (Table 34-10).

Multigene assays, such as the 21-gene recurrence score assay (Oncotype DX Breast Cancer Assay, Genomic Health, Inc., Redwood City, CA), have been developed in an attempt to identify a specific molecular phenotype of a tumor in an individual patient and use the phenotype to predict the response to therapy or provide information regarding prognosis.[41] The Oncotype DX assay was developed from a candidate pool of 250 genes and narrowed to a specific 21-gene panel on the basis of three independent studies of the candidate genes.[18] This assay was validated first in patients with ER-positive, lymph node–negative breast cancer (NSABP B-14). The Oncotype DX assay was found to be prognostic for OS and predictive of the benefits of different systemic therapies, with higher recurrence scores predicting increased benefit from chemotherapy and lower scores predicting lesser benefit from chemotherapy and increased benefit from endocrine therapy. This assay was validated in subsequent studies. The Oncotype DX assay can help clinicians estimate the benefits of therapy for patients with lymph node–negative, ER-positive breast cancer. For patients with low recurrence scores, chemotherapy appears to have marginal benefit in terms of reducing the risk of distant recurrence, but for patients with high recurrence scores, chemotherapy offers marked benefit. For patients with intermediate recurrence scores, the magnitude of benefit from chemotherapy is uncertain. A cooperative group trial, TAILORx, was conducted to determine the benefit from chemotherapy in patients with intermediate recurrence scores. This trial has completed accrual, but results are still maturing and have not yet been reported.

Multigene assays such as Oncotype DX are used in the context of patient characteristics (e.g., general health, age) and extent of disease (e.g., tumor size) and are not the sole determinants of the type of systemic therapy prescribed. It is expected that as assays (currently available or under development) are evaluated further

TABLE 34-10 Decision Making for Systemic Therapy

STAGE	SYSTEMIC THERAPY	COMMENTS
I (<1 cm)		
Hormone receptor–positive	Endocrine therapy ± chemotherapy	Consider genomic testing
Hormone receptor—negative	Consider chemotherapy	
HER-2-positive	Strongly consider trastuzumab and chemotherapy	
I (>1 cm)		
Hormone receptor–positive	Endocrine therapy ± chemotherapy	Consider genomic testing
Hormone receptor–negative	Chemotherapy	
HER-2-positive	Trastuzumab and chemotherapy	
II (Lymph Node–Negative)		
Hormone receptor–positive	Endocrine therapy ± chemotherapy	Consider genomic testing
Hormone receptor–negative	Chemotherapy	
HER-2-positive	Trastuzumab and chemotherapy	
II (Lymph Node–Positive), III		
Hormone receptor–positive	Chemotherapy + endocrine therapy	Endocrine therapy should be recommended for all patients
Hormone receptor–negative	Chemotherapy	Decision making for chemotherapy may be influenced by results from ongoing clinical trials
HER-2-positive	Trastuzumab and chemotherapy	Consider neoadjuvant chemotherapy with dual HER-2-targeted therapy

in clinical studies, their utility for tailoring systemic therapy to an individual will improve.

Adjuvant! Online (www.adjuvantonline.com; accessed August 20, 2015) is an online tool that has been designed to help physicians determine the 10-year risk of breast cancer recurrence and breast cancer–related death for an individual patient. This validated tool also informs the clinician about how specific interventions, such as chemotherapy, hormonal therapy, or a combination of the two, are expected to affect survival.[42] These estimates of prognosis are based largely on the SEER registry estimates. The primary factors incorporated in Adjuvant! Online include age, comorbidity, ER status, grade, tumor size, and nodal status. HER-2 status is not in the model. When the clinician inputs patient-related and tumor-related information, this online tool provides graphics depicting 10-year recurrence-free survival and OS estimates for an individual patient as well as estimates adjusted for the use of chemotherapy, endocrine therapy, or both.

The Adjuvant! Online program has limitations. It is based on registry information and relapse data, and cause of death in these registries may be inaccurate. Also, Adjuvant! Online does not incorporate information about HER-2 positivity or risk-stratify for breast cancer in women younger than 35 years. For some patients, estimating the risk of recurrence and breast cancer–related death may be distressing. However, the design of Adjuvant! Online allows the physician and patient to have an interactive discussion regarding the risks and potential benefits of therapies, including how these therapies may affect the risk of recurrence and death caused by breast cancer. The website includes diagrams and patient education tools that may enhance this dialogue.

Chemotherapy

The main classes of chemotherapeutics used to treat early-stage breast cancer include anthracyclines (e.g., doxorubicin, epirubicin) and taxanes (e.g., paclitaxel, docetaxel). The anthracyclines, which act as topoisomerase II inhibitors and antimetabolites, have high levels of activity in the treatment of breast cancer. When anthracyclines are delivered as single agents for the treatment of metastatic breast cancer, responses to therapy are generally seen in 45% to 80% of patients. The 2005 EBCTCG analysis[43] noted that compared with nonanthracycline, CMF (cyclophosphamide, methotrexate, 5-fluorouracil)-type therapies, anthracyclines are associated with a 16% reduction in the risk of death and an 11% reduction in the risk of recurrence. Anthracyclines are associated with the potential long-term toxic effect of cardiomyopathy, which may lead to congestive heart failure, often many years after treatment. The risk of cardiac dysfunction resulting from anthracyclines is dose dependent, and current anthracycline-containing chemotherapy regimens are associated with a risk of cardiac dysfunction of 1.5% to 3%. An additional dangerous risk of anthracycline-based chemotherapy is the risk of development of leukemia (<1%).

Taxanes (microtubule inhibitors) have significant activity in the treatment of metastatic breast cancer and are active not only in tumors previously unexposed to chemotherapy but also in anthracycline-resistant tumors. Numerous clinical trials have evaluated the use of taxanes for treatment of early-stage breast cancer. A meta-analysis of the use of taxanes in 13 different studies found improvement in DFS (HR, 0.83; 95% CI, 0.79 to 0.87; $P < .0001$) and OS (HR, 0.85; 95% CI, 0.79 to 0.91; $P < .0001$).[44] The antitumor activity of paclitaxel depends on the timing of treatment: More frequent administration of paclitaxel improves outcomes.[45] The activity of docetaxel depends less on the timing of treatment, and docetaxel is generally administered on an every-3-week schedule. The two taxanes, when given at their optimal dose and schedule, produce equivalent outcomes. The taxanes are associated with the potential permanent toxic effect of peripheral neuropathy but do not cause long-term increased risk of cardiac dysfunction or second cancers.

Chemotherapy is generally administered with combinations of medications in an effort to take advantage of nonoverlapping toxic effects and maximize different mechanisms of action in targeting tumor cells. The largest comprehensive analysis to date of the benefits of polychemotherapy for breast cancer is the EBCTCG analysis published in 2012. This analysis summarized data from randomized trials that were initiated between 1973 and 2003. The authors presented individual patient data from trials comparing a taxane-plus-anthracycline–based regimen versus a non-taxane-containing regimen with the same or higher cumulative doses of each non-taxane component (n = 44,000), trials comparing one anthracycline-based regimen versus another (n = 7000) or versus CMF (n = 18,000), and trials comparing polychemotherapy versus no chemotherapy (n = 32,000). On the basis of the drug dosages and the anthracycline used (either doxorubicin [Adriamycin; A] or epirubicin [E]), regimens were defined as including standard CMF, standard AC, CAF, or CEF. A meta-analysis showed that compared with no chemotherapy, use of CMF or standard AC reduced the recurrence rate by one third at 8 years and produced a 20% to 25% reduction in breast cancer mortality. The addition of more chemotherapy (i.e., CAF or CEF compared with CMF or AC) resulted in an additional proportional reduction of 15% to 20% in breast cancer mortality. On average, the taxane-plus-anthracycline–based control regimens were superior to standard AC but were not superior to anthracycline regimens with extra cycles (i.e., CAF or CEF). In analyses comparing taxane-based and anthracycline-based regimens, the proportional risk reductions were not significantly affected by age, tumor size, nodal status, tumor grade, or ER status. Taken together, these data suggest that independent of age or tumor characteristics, a chemotherapy regimen that includes a taxane or anthracycline regimens with higher cumulative dosages reduced breast cancer mortality by approximately one third.

Trastuzumab-Based Targeted Therapy

Trastuzumab is a humanized monoclonal antibody developed to target the extracellular domain of the HER-2 receptor. HER-2 gene amplification or protein overexpression occurs in approximately 20% to 25% of breast cancers. Amplification leads to protein overexpression, measured clinically by immunohistochemistry and scored on a scale from 0 to 3+. Alternatively, fluorescent in situ hybridization directly detects the quantity of HER-2 gene copies; the normal copy number is two (see "Molecular Markers and Breast Cancer Subtypes" earlier).

When trastuzumab is used as a single agent for treatment of metastatic breast cancer, response is seen in approximately 30% of patients. Trastuzumab combined with chemotherapy is even more effective, with synergy seen with multiple agents. Trastuzumab-based chemotherapy regimens improve DFS and OS for patients with metastatic disease. Given the promising activity of trastuzumab against metastatic disease, numerous trials of trastuzumab for adjuvant and neoadjuvant therapy have been conducted; these trials demonstrated improved outcomes for patients with stage I to III breast cancer. The HERA (HERceptin Adjuvant) trial (N = 5090) enrolled patients with HER-2-positive breast cancer and randomly assigned them to trastuzumab treatment (for 1 or 2 years) versus observation after completion of chemotherapy.[46] In a comparison of 1 year of trastuzumab treatment versus observation, trastuzumab reduced the risk of a breast cancer–related event by 46% (HR, 0.54; 95% CI, 0.43 to 0.67; $P < .001$) and improved OS by 34% (HR, 0.66; 95% CI, 0.47 to 0.91; $P < .0115$). Treatment with trastuzumab for 2 years was not more effective than 1 year of treatment, which established 1 year of treatment as standard of care.[47]

The NSABP B-31 and NCCTG-N9831 adjuvant trials were similar in study design; the results from both studies were combined for initial analysis.[48] Patients in the control arms of these studies received AC followed by paclitaxel. Trastuzumab was added in the experimental groups, either concurrently with paclitaxel or sequentially after paclitaxel. At the time of the first analysis, after a median follow-up of 2 years, the patients who received trastuzumab had a 52% reduction in breast cancer–related events (DFS HR, 0.48; 95% CI, 0.39 to 0.61; $P < .001$) and a 33% improvement in OS (OS HR, 0.67; 95% CI, 0.48 to 0.93; P = .015). At the most recent report, after a median follow-up of approximately 4 years, there continued to be a highly statistically significant reduction in the risk of recurrence (DFS HR, 0.52; 95% CI, 0.45 to 0.60; $P < .001$) and death (HR, 0.61; 95% CI, 0.50 to 0.75; $P < .001$).[49] Patients receiving trastuzumab-based therapy in NSABP B-31 (AC followed by paclitaxel-trastuzumab) had an increased risk of cardiac dysfunction, with a 3-year event rate of 4.1% versus 0.8% in the control arm. Patients with lower ejection fraction at the initiation of therapy, older age, or hypertension were at highest risk of cardiac dysfunction.

The BCIRG 006 trial used a non-anthracycline-containing regimen as one of its treatment groups and showed equivalence in outcome between AC followed by docetaxel-trastuzumab (AC-TH) and docetaxel combined with carboplatin and trastuzumab (TCH).[50] Both trastuzumab-containing treatments were superior in terms of DFS to the control treatment of AC followed by docetaxel, with HR of 0.61 (95% CI, 0.48 to 0.76; $P < .001$) for the AC-TH group and HR of 0.67 for the TCH group (95% CI, 0.54 to 0.83). Rates of cardiac toxic effects were markedly lower in the TCH group (0.37%) than in the AC-TH group (1.87%).

Additional drugs targeting HER-2 are being evaluated, including the tyrosine kinase inhibitor lapatinib; the trastuzumab drug conjugate trastuzumab emtansine; and pertuzumab, a monoclonal antibody that inhibits dimerization of HER-2 with other HER-2 receptors. The efficacy of these agents against metastatic disease has been established, and ongoing studies are investigating their efficacy as adjuvant therapy.

Endocrine Therapy

One of the original targeted therapy approaches was the use of oophorectomy to reduce systemic estrogen production as a treatment for breast cancer. Most breast cancers (>60%) express ER or PR or both; interruption of the production of estrogen or the ability of estrogen to interact with the ER has been associated with improved DFS and OS for women with metastatic breast cancer. This therapeutic approach is associated with a generally favorable adverse effect profile compared with the adverse effects of chemotherapy.

Tamoxifen

Tamoxifen is a selective ER modulator that has antagonistic and weak agonistic effects. It is generally well tolerated; the most common side effect is hot flashes or vasomotor symptoms, which occur in less than 50% of patients. Potentially serious but rare effects include increased risk of thromboembolic disease and uterine cancer.

Clinical trials of tamoxifen as treatment for early-stage breast cancer began in the 1970s. In 2005, the EBCTCG meta-analysis reported data of more than 80,000 women treated in clinical studies.[43] Tamoxifen administered for 5 years was found to reduce the risk of recurrence of breast cancer for patients with hormone receptor–positive disease by 41% (recurrence rate ratio, 0.59; SE, 0.03). The risk of death from breast cancer was reduced by approximately one third (death rate ratio, 0.66; SE, 0.04). Tamoxifen was shown to be beneficial for premenopausal and postmenopausal women and had a similar magnitude of benefit for patients with lymph node–positive and lymph node–negative disease. The duration of therapy with tamoxifen was also evaluated; 5 years of therapy was found to be superior to only 1 to 2 years of therapy in terms of breast cancer recurrence (15.2% proportionate reduction; $P < .001$) and death from breast cancer (7.9% proportionate reduction; $P = .01$).

Tamoxifen therapy for more than 5 years has been investigated, and results from the two largest studies with the longest follow-up were reported. The ATLAS (Adjuvant Tamoxifen: Longer Against Shorter) trial showed an approximately 25% reduction in the rate of recurrence and approximately 3% reduction in mortality risk in women taking 10 years of tamoxifen versus 5 years, with the benefit being most pronounced after year 10.[51] These findings were confirmed in the aTTom (adjuvant Tamoxifen—To offer more?) trial, in which patients were also randomly assigned to 5 years versus 10 years of tamoxifen. There was a decrease in breast cancer recurrence rates and breast cancer mortality rates in patients treated for a longer duration. In light of these findings, the American Society of Clinical Oncology (ASCO) updated their guidelines regarding adjuvant endocrine therapy. For premenopausal or perimenopausal women, tamoxifen for 5 years is recommended. After 5 years, if the patient is still premenopausal, she should be offered an additional 5 years of tamoxifen therapy.[52]

Aromatase Inhibitors

AIs block the conversion of the hormone androstenedione into estrone by inhibition of the aromatase enzyme. This enzyme is present in adipose tissue, breast tissue, breast tumor cells, and other sites. Multiple generations of medications that block the aromatase enzyme have been evaluated; however, less specific agents such as aminoglutethimide also suppress production of other hormones, and this is associated with unacceptable side effects. Selective or third-generation AIs purely block the final step of conversion of hormones into estrogen and are not associated with the broad hormone suppression seen with earlier AIs. Selective AIs, which include anastrozole, exemestane, and letrozole, are unable to suppress ovarian function completely in a premenopausal or perimenopausal woman and are restricted for use in postmenopausal women. Selective AIs as a group have similar adverse effects, including hot flashes, vasomotor symptoms, joint symptoms, myalgias, bone loss, and vaginal dryness.

Several different trial designs have been used to evaluate AIs as adjuvant therapy. Direct comparisons of 5 years of a selective AI versus 5 years of tamoxifen demonstrated improvement in cancer outcomes for anastrozole and letrozole.[53] The ATAC (Arimidex, Tamoxifen, Alone or in Combination) trial demonstrated that 5 years of anastrozole significantly improved DFS by 17% compared with 5 years of tamoxifen (HR, 0.83; 95% CI, 0.73 to 94; $P = .05$). In addition to reducing the risk of distant recurrence (distant DFS HR, 0.86; 95% CI, 0.74 to 0.99; $P = .04$), anastrozole reduced the risk of development of contralateral breast cancers by 42%.[53]

Administration of selective AIs for 2 to 3 years after tamoxifen for 2 to 3 years has been compared with 5 years of tamoxifen treatment.[54] The use of all three modern AIs after 2 to 3 years of tamoxifen was associated with better cancer outcomes than the use of tamoxifen alone. In addition, extended adjuvant therapy with 5 years of the AI letrozole after 5 years of tamoxifen was shown to improve outcome compared with placebo after 5 years of tamoxifen. The use of letrozole versus placebo reduced the risk of breast cancer events by 43% ($P < .008$).

The ideal use of AIs in the treatment of postmenopausal patients with ER-positive breast cancer is unknown. The risk of recurrence of ER-positive breast cancer persists beyond 5 years after diagnosis, and there is significant interest in evaluating extended use of antiestrogen therapy to decrease the risk of recurrence. Ongoing studies are evaluating the extended use of AIs beyond 5 years as well as beyond 10 years.

It is unclear whether tamoxifen is an essential component in the adjuvant treatment of postmenopausal patients. Given the multiple studies demonstrating consistently improved outcomes with the selective AIs, the ASCO clinical practice guideline released in 2010 stated that postmenopausal women should receive a selective AI at some point during their cancer therapy.[55] The 2014 update of the ASCO guidelines recommended that postmenopausal patients with hormone receptor–positive breast cancer be offered one of the following regimens: (1) an AI for 5 years, (2) tamoxifen for 10 years, (3) tamoxifen for 5 years followed by an AI for 5 years, or (4) tamoxifen for 2 to 3 years followed by an AI for 5 years.

Ovarian Ablation

The EBCTCG meta-analysis evaluated premenopausal women who were treated with ovarian ablation or suppression and found that this treatment reduced the risk of relapse and death from breast cancer.[43] Compared with the use of CMF chemotherapy, the use of ovarian ablation with goserelin as treatment for lymph node–positive, stage II breast cancer in premenopausal women resulted in equivalent outcomes in terms of DFS (HR, 1.01; $P = .94$) and OS (HR, 0.99; $P = .94$). Even with this high level of activity, the optimal role for addition of ovarian ablation is unknown.

Results were reported from two phase III trials that evaluated use of an AI with ovarian suppression in premenopausal patients with hormone receptor–positive early breast cancer. These trials were TEXT (Tamoxifen and Exemestane Trial) and SOFT (Suppression of Ovarian Function Trial).[56] TEXT was designed to evaluate 5 years of the AI exemestane plus ovarian suppression with a gonadotropin-releasing hormone agonist versus tamoxifen plus the gonadotropin-releasing hormone agonist. SOFT was designed to evaluate 5 years of the AI exemestane plus ovarian suppression versus tamoxifen plus ovarian suppression versus tamoxifen alone. The initial combined analysis looked at AI plus ovarian suppression versus tamoxifen plus ovarian suppression; the tamoxifen-alone arm from SOFT was not included. After a median follow-up of 68 months, the combination of an AI plus ovarian suppression compared with tamoxifen plus ovarian suppression resulted in a relative reduction of 34% in the risk of breast cancer recurrence. These results compared favorably with the results of randomized trials of adjuvant AIs versus tamoxifen in postmenopausal women.

Neoadjuvant Systemic Therapy for Operable Breast Cancer

Chemotherapy is most commonly administered as adjuvant therapy after completion of surgery. Neoadjuvant chemotherapy, the administration of systemic chemotherapy or hormonal therapy before surgery, can result in a significant reduction in tumor size and convert inoperable tumors to operable ones, make tumors that would require mastectomy amenable to lumpectomy, and shrink larger tumors to allow an improved cosmetic outcome with breast-conserving surgery.

Several prospective randomized trials evaluated the efficacy of chemotherapy and hormonal therapy administered as neoadjuvant (before surgery) versus adjuvant (after surgery) therapy. These studies all demonstrated increased rates of breast conservation with the use of neoadjuvant systemic therapy. The NSABP B-18 trial included 1523 patients and found no survival advantage (or detriment) in patients who received preoperative doxorubicin and cyclophosphamide chemotherapy versus the same regimen delivered postoperatively. The breast conservation rate was higher in women completing neoadjuvant chemotherapy, and the rate of in-breast recurrence in women who underwent neoadjuvant therapy followed by lumpectomy was not significantly different from the rate of in-breast recurrence in women who underwent lumpectomy before adjuvant chemotherapy.

Delivering chemotherapy before surgery has other theoretical advantages, including the potential to lower the volume of microscopic metastatic disease, decrease drug resistance by treating tumors before resistance has developed, increase the efficacy of treatment because the vascular system has not been disrupted by surgery, and permit evaluation of the response to treatment in vivo. In theory, the ability to evaluate response to therapy in vivo may help avoid administration of ineffective therapy and allow the clinician to tailor therapy to the individual patient. In addition, it has been shown that response to neoadjuvant chemotherapy correlates with survival outcomes. In the NSABP B-18 trial, after 9 years of follow-up, the DFS rate in patients achieving a complete pathologic response in the neoadjuvant therapy arm (no evidence of tumor at surgery) was 75% compared with 58% in patients who had any residual invasive disease after chemotherapy. A meta-analysis of 12 randomized trials evaluating neoadjuvant chemotherapy found that 18% of patients had a pathologic complete response defined as no residual invasive disease in the breast or axilla, and 13% had a pathologic complete response defined as no residual invasive or in situ disease. A pathologic complete response by either definition was associated with improved event-free survival and OS.[57] The association between pathologic complete response and long-term outcomes was strongest in patients with aggressive tumor subtypes, including patients with triple-negative breast cancer and patients with HER-2-positive, hormone receptor–negative breast cancer who received trastuzumab as part of their neoadjuvant regimen.

There are several surgical considerations for patients receiving neoadjuvant chemotherapy. By the end of systemic therapy, a percentage of patients have complete resolution of their tumors by clinical examination and imaging but might have microscopic residual disease. This percentage ranges from 10% to 15% in patients with hormone receptor–positive tumors to approximately 50% in patients with HER-2-positive tumors receiving trastuzumab in combination with chemotherapy as neoadjuvant therapy. Consequently, a metallic clip is placed at the primary tumor site under image guidance before neoadjuvant chemotherapy is initiated to allow identification of the original tumor site for excision.

Management of the axilla in patients undergoing neoadjuvant therapy has evolved. The timing of SLND has been debated, with some centers performing SLND before neoadjuvant therapy in patients with clinically negative nodes to inform decisions about systemic and radiation therapy. Advocates of SLND before neoadjuvant chemotherapy cite concerns about lower successful mapping rates and higher false-negative rates after neoadjuvant therapy. Other centers favor SLND after neoadjuvant therapy for any patient whose axilla is clinically negative after therapy to obtain more information about the status of the nodes after neoadjuvant therapy. Two meta-analyses of single-institution and multicenter studies were conducted and concluded that SLND is feasible and accurate after neoadjuvant chemotherapy, resulting in sentinel node identification rates of approximately 91%.[58,59] Both of these meta-analyses included patients with clinically node-negative and node-positive disease. In one, the authors evaluated studies that included only patients with clinically node-negative disease and found a pooled sentinel node identification rate of 93%. These two meta-analyses also examined the accuracy of SLND in patients receiving neoadjuvant chemotherapy and reported false-negative rates of 10.5% to 12%. These data are consistent with the false-negative rate reported in the NSABP B-32 trial (9.8%), which established the efficacy of SLND in patients with clinically node-negative disease undergoing surgery first.

In addition, neoadjuvant chemotherapy eradicates microscopic disease in the regional nodes in 40% of patients, reducing the need for complete ALND at the time of surgical intervention. Complete ALND remains the standard for all patients receiving neoadjuvant therapy who have biopsy-proven, node-positive disease at initial presentation; however, there is significant interest in identifying patients in whom SLND might be appropriate after neoadjuvant chemotherapy. The ACOSOG reported the results of the Z1071 trial, a phase II study in which patients with clinically node-positive disease (clinical N1 disease) receiving neoadjuvant chemotherapy underwent SLND followed by planned completion ALND. This study allowed for determination of the false-negative rate for SLND, which was 12.6%—higher than the prespecified end point of 10%.[60] The false-negative rate was lower when dual tracers were used for mapping (false-negative rate, 10.8%) and when three or more sentinel nodes were identified (false-negative rate, 9.1%). These data are consistent with two other trials that evaluated SLND in patients with clinically node-positive disease, the SENTINA (SENTinel NeoAdjuvant) trial and the SN FNAC (Sentinel Node biopsy Following NeoAdjuvant Chemotherapy in biopsy-proven node-positive breast cancer) trial. The results of these studies suggest that surgical technique is critical in reducing the false-negative rate for SLND in patients with clinically node-positive disease receiving neoadjuvant chemotherapy.

Some key concepts have been gleaned from the results of neoadjuvant therapy trials. The use of neoadjuvant chemotherapy as a research platform has led to the identification of patient and tumor characteristics that can predict response to therapy. This information allows clinicians to define better the population of patients who are most likely to benefit from neoadjuvant chemotherapy. Targeted therapies, such as trastuzumab, can be safely administered in combination with chemotherapy for neoadjuvant treatment in patients with HER-2-positive breast cancer, resulting in markedly increased rates of pathologic complete response. More recently, studies showed the benefit of dual HER-2 targeting. In the NeoSphere trial, patients with operable, HER-2-positive breast cancer were randomly assigned to one of four neoadjuvant regimens: (1) trastuzumab plus docetaxel, (2) pertuzumab and trastuzumab plus docetaxel, (3) pertuzumab and trastuzumab, or (4) pertuzumab plus docetaxel.[61] The study included 417 patients, and the primary end point was pathologic complete response, which was seen in 46% of patients in the pertuzumab and trastuzumab plus docetaxel arm versus 29% of patients in the trastuzumab plus docetaxel arm. On the basis of these results, the Food and Drug Administration granted pertuzumab accelerated approval as the first drug approved for the neoadjuvant treatment of breast cancer. A pathologic complete response was shown in 17% of patients in the trastuzumab plus pertuzumab arm, suggesting that some patients with HER-2-positive breast cancer could be treated with targeted therapy alone without chemotherapy.

In the context of targeted therapy, patients with ER-positive disease can be treated with endocrine therapy as neoadjuvant therapy, and this approach produces significant response rates and increased rates of breast-conserving surgery. This approach is optimal in postmenopausal women with ER-positive tumors for whom endocrine therapy provides more protection than standard chemotherapy against risk of recurrence and death caused by breast cancer. Finally, because new and more targeted regimens have led to an increasing population of patients with a clinical complete response to neoadjuvant therapy, accurately assessing the residual tumor burden in the breast and regional nodes will become increasingly important in terms of defining prognosis and determining what further therapy is needed. Neoadjuvant chemotherapy has potential disadvantages in terms of loss of prechemotherapy prognostic information (e.g., axillary lymph node status, actual invasive tumor size), which may have an impact on decision making with respect to postmastectomy radiation therapy.

Systemic Therapy for Early-Stage Breast Cancer

Most patients with a diagnosis of early-stage (I to III) invasive breast cancer are offered systemic therapy in an effort to improve DFS and OS. In addition, the use of antiestrogen therapy as treatment of hormone receptor–positive breast cancer helps reduce the risk of new breast cancers. The use of systemic therapy is guided by tumor characteristics (e.g., stage, molecular markers), patient characteristics (e.g., age, general health, personal preferences), and a careful balance of the potential benefits versus potential risks of treatment. As molecular analysis of tumors continues to advance, it is likely that treatment recommendations and options will be refined toward a patient's tumor profile and more general guidelines, as are currently used, will not be implemented as often.

TREATMENT OF LOCALLY ADVANCED AND INFLAMMATORY BREAST CANCER

Patients with locally advanced breast cancer include patients with large primary tumors (>5 cm), tumors involving the chest wall, skin involvement, ulceration or satellite skin nodules, inflammatory carcinoma, bulky or fixed axillary nodes, and clinically apparent internal mammary or supraclavicular nodal involvement (stages IIB, IIIA, and IIIB disease). Central to treatment is the concept that the disease is advanced on the chest wall, in regional lymph nodes, or both with no evidence of metastasis to distant sites. These patients are recognized to be at significant risk for the development of subsequent metastases, and treatment must address the risk for local and systemic relapse. Experience before the 1970s demonstrated that surgery alone provided poor local control, with local relapse rates of 30% to 50% and mortality rates of 70%. Similar results were reported when radiation therapy was the sole modality of treatment. Current management includes surgery, radiation therapy, and systemic therapy, with the sequence and extent of treatment determined by specifics of the patient's circumstance.

Although inflammatory breast cancer is rare, accounting for approximately 1% to 5% of all breast tumors, it is the most aggressive subtype of breast cancer. The hallmark of inflammatory breast cancer is diffuse tumor involvement of the dermal lymphatic channels within the breast and overlying skin, often without an underlying tumor mass. Inflammatory breast cancer manifests clinically as erythema, edema, and warmth of the breast as a result of lymphatic obstruction. There may be no abnormality on mammography beyond skin thickening, and a palpable mass is not required for the diagnosis. The term *peau d'orange* is used to describe the orange-peel appearance of the skin resulting from edema and dimpling at sites of hair follicles (see Fig. 34-5*D*). The history should reveal a rapid onset of the disease, with progression over weeks to 3 months. Neglected primary breast tumors that lead to secondary inflammatory changes within the breast should not be categorized as inflammatory breast cancer. Inflammatory cancer is a clinical diagnosis and can occur with tumors of ductal or lobular histology. The pathologic hallmark of inflammatory cancer is the presence of tumor cells within dermal lymphatics, but this is often missed because of sampling error and is not a prerequisite for diagnosis. Axillary nodal metastases are common, and there is a significant risk for distant metastases.

Current treatment approaches emphasize aggressive use of combined-modality treatment, including neoadjuvant chemotherapy, mastectomy, and radiation therapy, with hormonal therapy for ER-positive tumors and trastuzumab for HER-2-positive tumors. With multimodality treatment, relapse-free survival rates are 50% or higher at 5 years; in contrast, a single-institution historical series showed a 5-year survival rate of 7% in patients receiving less aggressive treatment.[62]

TREATMENT OF SPECIAL CONDITIONS

Breast Cancer in Older Adults

Several studies have explored options that reduce the extent of surgery and radiation therapy for older women with breast cancer. In two trials, older women were randomly assigned to lumpectomy with or without irradiation. In the CALGB (Cancer and Leukemia Group B) 9343 trial, 636 women 70 years or older with ER-positive tumors 2 cm or smaller and clinically negative nodes received lumpectomy and tamoxifen and were randomly assigned to irradiation or no irradiation.[63] At 10 years, the in-breast recurrence rate was 9% in the no-radiation arm versus 2% in the radiation arm. This difference in in-breast recurrence did not translate into a survival benefit: The 10-year breast cancer–specific survival estimates were 98% in the no-radiation arm and 97% in the radiation arm.

Fyles and colleagues reported the results of a Canadian trial with more inclusive eligibility criteria in which 769 women 50 years or older with tumors up to 5 cm and positive or negative ER status were enrolled. All patients underwent wide excision and received tamoxifen and were randomly assigned to irradiation or no irradiation. Recurrence rates were significantly higher overall in patients who did not receive radiation therapy. However, in an unplanned analysis of a subset of 193 women older than 60 years, the local recurrence rate was only 1.2% without radiation therapy, and there were no recurrences with radiation therapy. These low rates of local recurrence and the significant rates of death from other comorbid conditions led to the acceptance of wide excision and hormonal therapy without irradiation for selected older patients with small ER-positive tumors and clinically negative axillary nodes. Axillary surgery was omitted in such patients in the past; however, SLND can easily be incorporated, with minimal morbidity.

Paget Disease

Paget disease accounts for 1% or less of breast malignancies. It is characterized clinically by nipple erythema and irritation with associated pruritus and may progress to crusting and ulceration. The condition may spread outward from the nipple and onto the areola and surrounding skin of the breast (see Fig. 34-5). The differential diagnosis of scaling skin and erythema of the nipple-areola complex includes eczema, contact dermatitis, post-radiation dermatitis, and Paget disease. A biopsy of the skin of the nipple should be performed; a specimen containing Paget cells confirms the diagnosis.

Pathologically, a Paget cell is a large, pale-staining cell with round or oval nuclei and large nucleoli located between the normal keratinocytes of the nipple epidermis. Paget cells spread into the lactiferous sinuses under the nipple and upward to invade the overlying epidermis of the nipple. Paget cells do not invade through the dermal basement membrane and are categorized as carcinoma in situ. More than 95% of patients with Paget disease have an underlying breast carcinoma. Paget disease may be accompanied by a palpable mass in slightly more than 50% of patients. Invasive breast cancer is identified in more than 90% of patients with a palpable mass and Paget disease.

Treatment of Paget disease includes mastectomy with axillary staging or wide local excision of the nipple and areola to achieve clear margins, axillary staging, and radiation therapy. For many patients, lumpectomy and irradiation provide an acceptable cosmetic appearance and obviate mastectomy and breast reconstruction. Nipple-areolar reconstruction can be performed 4 to 6 months after radiation therapy. For patients considering lumpectomy, thorough preoperative evaluation is required to rule out occult multicentric disease.

Breast Cancer in Men

Breast cancer occurring in the mammary gland of men is infrequent; it accounts for 0.8% of all breast cancers, less than 1% of all newly diagnosed cancers in men, and 0.2% of cancer deaths in men. In the United States, 1500 new cases of breast cancer in men and 400 deaths from this disease are reported annually. The median age at diagnosis is 68 years, 5 years older than in women. Risk factors include increasing age; radiation exposure; and factors related to abnormalities in estrogen and androgen balance, including testicular disease, infertility, obesity, and cirrhosis. Risk factors related to a genetic predisposition include Klinefelter syndrome (47,XXY karyotype); family history; and *BRCA* gene mutations, particularly *BRCA2* mutations. Gynecomastia is not a risk factor.

Histologically, 90% of breast cancers in men are invasive ductal carcinomas. Approximately 80% are ER positive, 75% are PR positive, and 35% overexpress HER-2. The remaining 10% are DCIS. Given the absence of terminal lobules in the normal breast in men, invasive and in situ lobular carcinoma is rarely seen.

Most men with breast cancer have a breast mass. The differential diagnosis includes gynecomastia, primary breast carcinoma, metastasis to the breast from carcinoma at another site, sarcoma, and breast abscess. In addition to local pain and axillary adenopathy, initial symptoms may include nipple retraction, ulceration, bleeding, and discharge. Evaluation includes breast imaging studies and diagnostic core needle biopsy. Prognostic factors for breast cancer in men are the same as prognostic factors for breast cancer in women and include nodal involvement, tumor size, histologic grade, and hormone receptor status. Survival in men with breast cancer is similar to survival in women with breast cancer matched for age and stage.

Treatment of breast carcinoma in men depends on the stage and local extent of the tumor, with treatment options similar to the options for women. Small tumors may be treated by local excision and irradiation or by mastectomy. Sentinel node biopsy has been shown to be effective for staging breast cancer in men. Breast tumors in men more commonly involve the pectoralis major muscle, probably because breast tissue in men is scant. If the underlying pectoral muscle is involved, modified radical mastectomy with excision of the involved portion of muscle is adequate treatment, but it may be combined with postoperative radiation therapy. Adjuvant systemic therapy for breast cancer in men is the same as adjuvant therapy for breast cancer in women. Most breast cancers in men are hormone receptor positive. Adjuvant hormonal therapy with tamoxifen or AIs is indicated for patients with node-positive disease and high-risk patients with node-negative disease. Adjuvant chemotherapy is used in men at substantial risk for metastatic disease.

SELECTED REFERENCES

Clarke M, Collins R, Darby S, et al: Early Breast Cancer Trialists' Collaborative Group (EBCTCG): Effects of radiotherapy and of differences in the extent of surgery for early breast cancer on local recurrence and 15-year survival: An overview of the randomized trials. *Lancet* 366:2087–2106, 2005.

This overview analysis by the Early Breast Cancer Trialists' Collaborative Group showed the benefit of radiotherapy on survival in patients with breast cancer.

Domchek S, Friebel TM, Singer CF, et al: Association of risk-reducing surgery in BRCA1 or BRCA2 mutation carriers with cancer risk and mortality. *JAMA* 304:967–975, 2010.

This was the first trial to demonstrate the survival benefit of risk-reducing surgery in BRCA1 and BRCA2 mutation carriers.

Early Breast Cancer Trialists' Collaborative Group (EBCTCG): Effects of chemotherapy and hormonal therapy for early breast cancer on recurrence and 15-year survival: An overview of the randomised trials. *Lancet* 365:1687–1717, 2005.

This overview analysis by the Early Breast Cancer Trialists' Collaborative Group showed the benefit of chemotherapy and hormonal therapy on survival based on stage of disease and hormone receptor status.

Fisher B, Anderson S, Bryant J, et al: Twenty-year follow-up of a randomized trial comparing total mastectomy, lumpectomy, and lumpectomy plus irradiation for the treatment of invasive breast cancer. *N Engl J Med* 347:1233–1241, 2002.

This randomized trial showed no difference in survival between total mastectomy and breast-conserving surgery with or without radiation.

Fisher B, Costantino JP, Wickerham DL, et al: Tamoxifen for prevention of breast cancer: Report of the National Surgical Adjuvant Breast and Bowel Project P-1 Study. *J Natl Cancer Inst* 90:1371–1388, 1998.

In this first randomized trial for breast cancer prevention in a high-risk population, patients were assessed for risk based on the Gail model and randomly assigned to receive 5 years of tamoxifen or placebo. The use of tamoxifen reduced breast cancer incidence by approximately 50%.

Fisher B, Jeong JH, Anderson S, et al: Twenty-five-year follow-up of a randomized trial comparing radical mastectomy, total mastectomy, and total mastectomy followed by irradiation. *N Engl J Med* 347:567–575, 2002.

This report showed no difference in survival between radical mastectomy and total mastectomy with or without radiation.

Giuliano AE, Hunt KK, Ballman KV, et al: Axillary dissection vs no axillary dissection in women with invasive breast cancer and sentinel node metastasis. *JAMA* 305:569–575, 2011.

This randomized trial showed no benefit to completion axillary lymph node dissection in selected patients with early-stage breast cancer and positive sentinel lymph nodes.

Hartmann LC, Sellers TA, Frost MH, et al: Benign breast disease and the risk of breast cancer. *N Engl J Med* 353:229–237, 2005.

This study identified risk factors for breast cancer development after a diagnosis of benign breast disease based on histologic classification and family history.

Krag DN, Anderson SJ, Julian TB, et al: Sentinel-lymph-node resection compared with conventional axillary-lymph-node dissection in clinically node negative patients with breast cancer: Overall survival findings from the NSABP B-32 randomised phase 3 trial. *Lancet Oncol* 11:927–933, 2010.

In this randomized trial of sentinel lymph node dissection versus axillary dissection in early-stage breast cancer, there was no difference in overall survival or locoregional recurrence among patients undergoing sentinel node surgery versus standard axillary surgery.

Perou CM, Sorlie T, Eisen MB, et al: Molecular portraits of human breast tumours. *Nature* 406:747–752, 2000.

This article provided the first description of molecular subtypes of breast cancer using microarray analysis.

Rossouw JE, Anderson GL, Prentice RL, et al: Risks and benefits of estrogen plus progestin in healthy postmenopausal women: Principal results from the Women's Health Initiative randomized controlled trial. *JAMA* 288:321–333, 2002.

In this long-term follow-up study of participants in the Women's Health Initiative, the risks and benefits of hormone replacement therapy in postmenopausal women were demonstrated.

Weaver DL, Ashikaga T, Krag DN, et al: Effect of occult metastases on survival in node-negative breast cancer. *N Engl J Med* 364:412–421, 2011.

This study demonstrated that occult metastases identified in sentinel lymph nodes of patients with early-stage breast cancer do not have clinical relevance.

REFERENCES

1. Haagensen C: *Diseases of the breast*, Philadelphia, 1986, Saunders.
2. Nelson HD, Tyne K, Naik A, et al: Screening for breast cancer: An update for the U.S. Preventive Services Task Force. *Ann Intern Med* 151:727–737, W737–742, 2009.
3. Berg WA, Blume JD, Cormack JB, et al: Combined screening with ultrasound and mammography vs mammography alone in women at elevated risk of breast cancer. *JAMA* 299:2151–2163, 2008.
4. Turnbull L, Brown S, Harvey I, et al: Comparative effectiveness of MRI in breast cancer (COMICE) trial: A randomised controlled trial. *Lancet* 375:563–571, 2010.
5. Murphy JO, Moo TA, King TA, et al: Radioactive seed localization compared to wire localization in breast-conserving surgery: Initial 6-month experience. *Ann Surg Oncol* 20:4121–4127, 2013.
6. Rosen PR: *Rosen's breast pathology*, ed 2, Philadelphia, 2001, Lippincott Williams & Wilkins.
7. Fisher B, Costantino JP, Wickerham DL, et al: Tamoxifen for prevention of breast cancer: Report of the National Surgical Adjuvant Breast and Bowel Project P-1 Study. *J Natl Cancer Inst* 90:1371–1388, 1998.
8. Hartmann LC, Sellers TA, Frost MH, et al: Benign breast disease and the risk of breast cancer. *N Engl J Med* 353:229–237, 2005.
9. Rossouw JE, Anderson GL, Prentice RL, et al: Risks and benefits of estrogen plus progestin in healthy postmenopausal women: Principal results from the Women's Health Initiative randomized controlled trial. *JAMA* 288:321–333, 2002.
10. Stefanick ML, Anderson GL, Margolis KL, et al: Effects of conjugated equine estrogens on breast cancer and mammography screening in postmenopausal women with hysterectomy. *JAMA* 295:1647–1657, 2006.
11. Vogel VG, Costantino JP, Wickerham DL, et al: Effects of tamoxifen vs raloxifene on the risk of developing invasive breast cancer and other disease outcomes: The NSABP Study of Tamoxifen and Raloxifene (STAR) P-2 trial. *JAMA* 295:2727–2741, 2006.
12. Cuzick J, Powles T, Veronesi U, et al: Overview of the main outcomes in breast-cancer prevention trials. *Lancet* 361:296–300, 2003.
13. Goss PE, Ingle JN, Ales-Martinez JE, et al: Exemestane for breast-cancer prevention in postmenopausal women. *N Engl J Med* 364:2381–2391, 2011.
14. Hartmann LC, Schaid DJ, Woods JE, et al: Efficacy of bilateral prophylactic mastectomy in women with a family history of breast cancer. *N Engl J Med* 340:77–84, 1999.
15. Domchek SM, Friebel TM, Singer CF, et al: Association of risk-reducing surgery in BRCA1 or BRCA2 mutation carriers with cancer risk and mortality. *JAMA* 304:967–975, 2010.
16. Bedrosian I, Hu CY, Chang GJ: Population-based study of contralateral prophylactic mastectomy and survival outcomes of breast cancer patients. *J Natl Cancer Inst* 102:401–409, 2010.
17. Perou CM, Sorlie T, Eisen MB, et al: Molecular portraits of human breast tumours. *Nature* 406:747–752, 2000.
18. Paik S, Shak S, Tang G, et al: A multigene assay to predict recurrence of tamoxifen-treated, node-negative breast cancer. *N Engl J Med* 351:2817–2826, 2004.

19. Fisher B, Jeong JH, Anderson S, et al: Twenty-five-year follow-up of a randomized trial comparing radical mastectomy, total mastectomy, and total mastectomy followed by irradiation. *N Engl J Med* 347:567–575, 2002.
20. Fisher B, Anderson S, Bryant J, et al: Twenty-year follow-up of a randomized trial comparing total mastectomy, lumpectomy, and lumpectomy plus irradiation for the treatment of invasive breast cancer. *N Engl J Med* 347:1233–1241, 2002.
21. Moran MS, Schnitt SJ, Giuliano AE, et al: Society of Surgical Oncology-American Society for Radiation Oncology consensus guideline on margins for breast-conserving surgery with whole-breast irradiation in stages I and II invasive breast cancer. *Ann Surg Oncol* 21:704–716, 2014.
22. Piper M, Peled AW, Foster RD, et al: Total skin-sparing mastectomy: A systematic review of oncologic outcomes and postoperative complications. *Ann Plast Surg* 70:435–437, 2013.
23. Krag DN, Anderson SJ, Julian TB, et al: Sentinel-lymph-node resection compared with conventional axillary-lymph-node dissection in clinically node-negative patients with breast cancer: Overall survival findings from the NSABP B-32 randomised phase 3 trial. *Lancet Oncol* 11:927–933, 2010.
24. Weaver DL, Ashikaga T, Krag DN, et al: Effect of occult metastases on survival in node-negative breast cancer. *N Engl J Med* 364:412–421, 2011.
25. Giuliano AE, Hawes D, Ballman KV, et al: Association of occult metastases in sentinel lymph nodes and bone marrow with survival among women with early-stage invasive breast cancer. *JAMA* 306:385–393, 2011.
26. Hunt KK, Yi M, Mittendorf EA, et al: Sentinel lymph node surgery after neoadjuvant chemotherapy is accurate and reduces the need for axillary dissection in breast cancer patients. *Ann Surg* 250:558–566, 2009.
27. Kim T, Giuliano AE, Lyman GH: Lymphatic mapping and sentinel lymph node biopsy in early-stage breast carcinoma: A metaanalysis. *Cancer* 106:4–16, 2006.
28. Giuliano AE, Hunt KK, Ballman KV, et al: Axillary dissection vs no axillary dissection in women with invasive breast cancer and sentinel node metastasis: A randomized clinical trial. *JAMA* 305:569–575, 2011.
29. Fisher B, Dignam J, Wolmark N, et al: Tamoxifen in treatment of intraductal breast cancer: National Surgical Adjuvant Breast and Bowel Project B-24 randomised controlled trial. *Lancet* 353:1993–2000, 1999.
30. Fisher B, Dignam J, Wolmark N, et al: Lumpectomy and radiation therapy for the treatment of intraductal breast cancer: Findings from National Surgical Adjuvant Breast and Bowel Project B-17. *J Clin Oncol* 16:441–452, 1998.
31. Julien JP, Bijker N, Fentiman IS, et al: Radiotherapy in breast-conserving treatment for ductal carcinoma in situ: First results of the EORTC randomised phase III trial 10853. EORTC Breast Cancer Cooperative Group and EORTC Radiotherapy Group. *Lancet* 355:528–533, 2000.
32. Houghton J, George WD, Cuzick J, et al: Radiotherapy and tamoxifen in women with completely excised ductal carcinoma in situ of the breast in the UK, Australia, and New Zealand: Randomised controlled trial. *Lancet* 362:95–102, 2003.
33. Silverstein MJ: The University of Southern California/Van Nuys prognostic index for ductal carcinoma in situ of the breast. *Am J Surg* 186:337–343, 2003.
34. Hughes LL, Wang M, Page DL, et al: Local excision alone without irradiation for ductal carcinoma in situ of the breast: A trial of the Eastern Cooperative Oncology Group. *J Clin Oncol* 27:5319–5324, 2009.
35. Clarke M, Collins R, Darby S, et al: Effects of radiotherapy and of differences in the extent of surgery for early breast cancer on local recurrence and 15-year survival: An overview of the randomised trials. *Lancet* 366:2087–2106, 2005.
36. Hughes KS, Schnaper LA, Berry D, et al: Lumpectomy plus tamoxifen with or without irradiation in women 70 years of age or older with early breast cancer. *N Engl J Med* 351:971–977, 2004.
37. Smith BD, Arthur DW, Buchholz TA, et al: Accelerated partial breast irradiation consensus statement from the American Society for Radiation Oncology (ASTRO). *Int J Radiat Oncol Biol Phys* 74:987–1001, 2009.
38. Danish Breast Cancer Cooperative Group, Nielsen HM, Overgaard M, et al: Study of failure pattern among high-risk breast cancer patients with or without postmastectomy radiotherapy in addition to adjuvant systemic therapy: Long-term results from the Danish Breast Cancer Cooperative Group DBCG 82 b and c randomized studies. *J Clin Oncol* 24:2268–2275, 2006.
39. Ragaz J, Olivotto IA, Spinelli JJ, et al: Locoregional radiation therapy in patients with high-risk breast cancer receiving adjuvant chemotherapy: 20-year results of the British Columbia randomized trial. *J Natl Cancer Inst* 97:116–126, 2005.
40. EBCTCG (Early Breast Cancer Trialists' Collaborative Group), McGale P, Taylor C, et al: Effect of radiotherapy after mastectomy and axillary surgery on 10-year recurrence and 20-year breast cancer mortality: Meta-analysis of individual patient data for 8135 women in 22 randomised trials. *Lancet* 383:2127–2135, 2014.
41. van de Vijver MJ, He YD, van't Veer LJ, et al: A gene-expression signature as a predictor of survival in breast cancer. *N Engl J Med* 347:1999–2009, 2002.
42. Ravdin PM, Siminoff LA, Davis GJ, et al: Computer program to assist in making decisions about adjuvant therapy for women with early breast cancer. *J Clin Oncol* 19:980–991, 2001.
43. Early Breast Cancer Trialists' Collaborative Group: Effects of chemotherapy and hormonal therapy for early breast cancer on recurrence and 15-year survival: An overview of the randomised trials. *Lancet* 365:1687–1717, 2005.
44. De Laurentiis M, Cancello G, D'Agostino D, et al: Taxane-based combinations as adjuvant chemotherapy of early breast cancer: A meta-analysis of randomized trials. *J Clin Oncol* 26:44–53, 2008.
45. Citron ML, Berry DA, Cirrincione C, et al: Randomized trial of dose-dense versus conventionally scheduled and sequential versus concurrent combination chemotherapy as postoperative adjuvant treatment of node-positive primary breast cancer: First report of Intergroup Trial C9741/Cancer and Leukemia Group B Trial 9741. *J Clin Oncol* 21:1431–1439, 2003.
46. Piccart-Gebhart MJ, Procter M, Leyland-Jones B, et al: Trastuzumab after adjuvant chemotherapy in HER2-positive breast cancer. *N Engl J Med* 353:1659–1672, 2005.
47. Goldhirsch A, Gelber RD, Piccart-Gebhart MJ, et al: 2 years versus 1 year of adjuvant trastuzumab for HER2-positive breast cancer (HERA): An open-label, randomised controlled trial. *Lancet* 382:1021–1028, 2013.

48. Romond EH, Perez EA, Bryant J, et al: Trastuzumab plus adjuvant chemotherapy for operable HER2-positive breast cancer. *N Engl J Med* 353:1673–1684, 2005.
49. Perez EA, Romond EH, Suman VJ, et al: Four-year follow-up of trastuzumab plus adjuvant chemotherapy for operable human epidermal growth factor receptor 2-positive breast cancer: Joint analysis of data from NCCTG N9831 and NSABP B-31. *J Clin Oncol* 29:3366–3373, 2011.
50. Slamon D, Eiermann W, Robert N, et al: Adjuvant trastuzumab in HER2-positive breast cancer. *N Engl J Med* 365:1273–1283, 2011.
51. Davies C, Pan H, Godwin J, et al: Long-term effects of continuing adjuvant tamoxifen to 10 years versus stopping at 5 years after diagnosis of oestrogen receptor-positive breast cancer: ATLAS, a randomised trial. *Lancet* 381:805–816, 2013.
52. Burstein HJ, Temin S, Anderson H, et al: Adjuvant endocrine therapy for women with hormone receptor-positive breast cancer: American Society of Clinical Oncology clinical practice guideline focused update. *J Clin Oncol* 32:2255–2269, 2014.
53. Howell A, Cuzick J, Baum M, et al: Results of the ATAC (Arimidex, Tamoxifen, Alone or in Combination) trial after completion of 5 years' adjuvant treatment for breast cancer. *Lancet* 365:60–62, 2005.
54. Boccardo F, Rubagotti A, Aldrighetti D, et al: Switching to an aromatase inhibitor provides mortality benefit in early breast carcinoma: Pooled analysis of 2 consecutive trials. *Cancer* 109:1060–1067, 2007.
55. Burstein HJ, Prestrud AA, Seidenfeld J, et al: American Society of Clinical Oncology clinical practice guideline: Update on adjuvant endocrine therapy for women with hormone receptor-positive breast cancer. *J Clin Oncol* 28:3784–3796, 2010.
56. Pagani O, Regan MM, Walley BA, et al: Adjuvant exemestane with ovarian suppression in premenopausal breast cancer. *N Engl J Med* 371:107–118, 2014.
57. Cortazar P, Zhang L, Untch M, et al: Pathological complete response and long-term clinical benefit in breast cancer: The CTNeoBC pooled analysis. *Lancet* 384:164–172, 2014.
58. Xing Y, Foy M, Cox DD, et al: Meta-analysis of sentinel lymph node biopsy after preoperative chemotherapy in patients with breast cancer. *Br J Surg* 93:539–546, 2006.
59. van Deurzen CH, Vriens BE, Tjan-Heijnen VC, et al: Accuracy of sentinel node biopsy after neoadjuvant chemotherapy in breast cancer patients: A systematic review. *Eur J Cancer* 45:3124–3130, 2009.
60. Boughey JC, Suman VJ, Mittendorf EA, et al: Sentinel lymph node surgery after neoadjuvant chemotherapy in patients with node-positive breast cancer: The ACOSOG Z1071 (Alliance) clinical trial. *JAMA* 310:1455–1461, 2013.
61. Gianni L, Pienkowski T, Im YH, et al: Efficacy and safety of neoadjuvant pertuzumab and trastuzumab in women with locally advanced, inflammatory, or early HER2-positive breast cancer (NeoSphere): A randomised multicentre, open-label, phase 2 trial. *Lancet Oncol* 13:25–32, 2012.
62. Cristofanilli M, Gonzalez-Angulo AM, Buzdar AU, et al: Paclitaxel improves the prognosis in estrogen receptor negative inflammatory breast cancer: The M. D. Anderson Cancer Center experience. *Clin Breast Cancer* 4:415–419, 2004.
63. Hughes KS, Schnaper LA, Bellon JR, et al: Lumpectomy plus tamoxifen with or without irradiation in women age 70 years or older with early breast cancer: Long-term follow-up of CALGB 9343. *J Clin Oncol* 31:2382–2387, 2013.

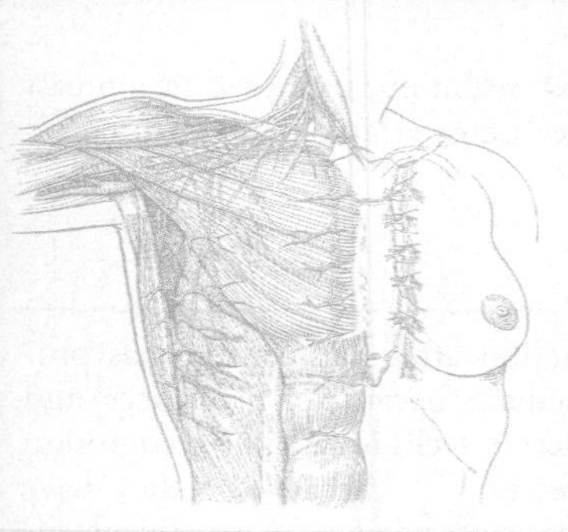

CHAPTER 35

Breast Reconstruction

Karen L. Powers, Linda G. Phillips

OUTLINE

ROLE OF THE GENERAL SURGEON IN BREAST RECONSTRUCTION

Breast cancer is an extremely emotional topic because of its anatomic location and the importance of the female breast in today's society. It is imperative for surgeons performing breast surgery to have a basic understanding of which patients are candidates for breast reconstruction and of the reconstructive options. Most patients start their inquiry about breast reconstruction with the surgeon who will be performing the mastectomy. They might ask, "What will it look like when you are done?" or "Will I have to live without a breast?" It is at this point that a general surgeon greatly influences a woman's decision to pursue breast reconstruction.

Although the reconstructive surgeon goes into detail about the surgical options, risks, and expected outcomes, ablative surgeons must be prepared for at least a basic discussion with patients. Questions that most patients want answered include whether breast implants versus autogenous tissue will be used, where the scars will be, and how long the recovery will take. The decision whether a patient undergoes breast reconstruction can be influenced by the bias of ablative surgeons. Oncologic surgeons are trained to place priority on ablation of the tumor; however, care standards now dictate that we also be sensitive to the resulting deformity. The patient's emotional, physical, and oncologic needs can be addressed only through a close alliance between the surgical oncologist and reconstructive surgeon.

HISTORY

In the late 1800s, the prognosis of patients with breast cancer was poor. Notable surgeons such as Volkmann, Czerny, and Billroth reported local recurrence rates ranging from 52% to 85%. Within 2 decades of these reports, Halsted presented his successful treatment of breast cancer, with only a 6% recurrence rate. The halstedian theory of breast cancer treatment would remain the mainstay of breast cancer surgery for the next 60 years. He believed that "the slightest inattention to detail and or attempts to hasten convalescence by such plastic operations as are feasible only when a restricted amount of skin is removed may sacrifice his patient to the disease." Concerned with the possibility of inadequate skin excision, Halsted said, "To attempt to close the breast wound more or less regularly by any plastic method is hazardous, and in my opinion, to be vigorously discounted." True attempts at breast reconstruction did not occur until almost 50 years later.

Despite Halsted's condemnation of reconstructive procedures, it was recognized that the sizable defects left after this radical surgery did need to be closed. Although primary closure was often used, skin grafting of larger wounds was acceptable. Although plastic procedures had been reported by Legueu and Graeve in France and Warren in the United States, these were merely chest wall closure techniques and not true breast mound reconstructions.

The first attempt at true breast reconstruction occurred in 1895, when Czerny transplanted a large lipoma from his patient's flank to the mastectomy site. In recounting this case, Goldwyn noted that 1 year after surgery, the patient was doing well and had good breast symmetry. In this particular case, the mastectomy was performed for fibrocystic disease and not cancer. Tansini described the first use of the latissimus dorsi myocutaneous flap in 1906. However, this remarkable operation would not gain acceptance for another 70 years.

In 1942, Gillies in England started using a tubed pedicle technique of breast reconstruction. In this operation, he "waltzed" a flap from the abdomen to the chest to reconstruct the breast. Although this technique was successful, the multiple procedures and prolonged treatment course precluded its widespread application.

Since approximately 1970, many advances in reconstructive surgery have occurred and been applied to breast reconstruction. The development of breast implants was the first of these revolutions. In 1963, the silicone breast implant was introduced for breast augmentation and was quickly adopted for breast reconstruction. In 1963, Cronin and Gerow[1] presented a series of patients who received implants for reconstruction of mastectomy defects. For the first time, the plastic surgeon had a procedure that could simulate the missing breast without the need for multiple procedures and a prolonged treatment course. In many ways, interest in breast reconstruction was ignited by the simplicity and safety of breast implants. By the later 1970s, reconstruction was being performed immediately after breast ablation.[2-4]

The development of muscle, musculocutaneous, and fasciocutaneous flaps and microsurgical transplantation has had a tremendous impact on breast reconstruction. The ideal material to reconstruct any defect is similar to tissue. Until the early 1970s, such tissue was available only in limited quantities for breast reconstruction. The landmark work by Manchot[5] on vascular territories of the body was rediscovered, and surgeons were able to exploit this basic knowledge to design flaps based on the axial patterns of named blood vessels. These technical developments allowed surgeons to rearrange tissues reliably and reconstruct more precisely all types of defects, including defects of the breast.[6]

PATIENT SELECTION

Women have many reasons for choosing to undergo breast reconstruction, including no need for an external prosthesis, fewer limitations with regard to clothing, regaining femininity, and feeling whole again. Other women choose not to undergo reconstruction because they feel too old for the procedure or are afraid of complications.[7,8] Given the myriad options in breast reconstruction, the surgery should be tailored to the patient's wishes and her underlying health. There are a few relative contraindications to breast reconstruction, including extreme age, severe cardiovascular disease or other comorbidities, extreme obesity, and advanced breast disease.

Early in the disease course, women are often faced with the choice of breast conservation therapy (BCT) versus mastectomy. Studies have shown equivalent survival outcomes when comparing the modalities of BCT with radiation and mastectomy. These decisions are often made in conjunction with the ablative surgeon. Patient satisfaction with these two modalities varies. Pusic and colleagues[9] surveyed women who underwent lumpectomy with radiation therapy, mastectomy, and mastectomy with reconstruction. Similar to the report by Reaby,[7] women who chose reconstruction were younger, white, and more educated. Comfort with nudity was much lower in the mastectomy-alone group, and quality of life varied with age. Younger women (<55 years old) were least satisfied with mastectomy alone, whereas women older than 55 years were least satisfied with lumpectomy. Ultimately, the choice is that of the patient with breast cancer and must be individualized.

Reconstruction in conjunction with BCT continues to evolve. It is now possible to minimize the effects of radiation on the breast after lumpectomy via oncoplastic techniques. These include breast reduction strategies to obliterate the dead space of lumpectomy–segmental mastectomy and to counteract the contractile forces seen after radiation therapy. These techniques are used by a breast surgeon or plastic surgeon and are discussed later in this chapter.[10,11]

TIMING

The timing of breast reconstruction after mastectomy has progressed from delayed to immediate because of advances and refinements in breast reconstructive techniques and recognition of beneficial psychological effects.[7,9,10,12] Because studies have shown a psychological benefit, cost-effectiveness, cosmetic advantage, and no increased risk for complications or oncologic risk with immediate breast reconstruction, it has become the preferred timing of reconstruction, with 75% of reconstructions being performed immediately.[13]

Because most local tumor recurrences are in the skin or subcutaneous adipose tissue or in the axilla, there are few reasons to delay reconstruction. Immediate reconstruction has become common in the United States.[14] It affords psychological benefits to women and is the opportune time to preserve the normal footprint of the breast—most importantly, the inframammary fold. This preservation can be more difficult in a delayed reconstruction setting. Skin flaps are also more pliable in the immediate setting. At the present time, most women with stage I or II cancer are candidates for immediate reconstruction. Immediate reconstruction is impossible with certain chemotherapeutic agents and the need for adjuvant radiotherapy because these can interfere with postoperative healing and outcome, respectively.

One must also consider the possibility of complications with immediate reconstruction. In patients in whom reconstructions have complications, such as delayed wound healing, infection, mastectomy flap loss, and flap necrosis, the initiation of chemotherapy and radiation therapy may require delay, and thus compromise, in cancer treatment. All these possibilities must be considered by the ablative and reconstructive surgeons as well as the patient to determine the appropriate timing of reconstruction.

PROCEDURE SELECTION AND SURGICAL PLANNING

The options for surgical breast reconstruction are varied and include partial and total reconstruction. Total breast reconstruction typically uses an expander or implant, autologous tissue, or some combination of the two. Any of these procedures must not delay adjuvant cancer therapies. The most common procedures performed are the following (Box 35-1):

- Tissue expander placement, with later exchange for an implant
- Immediate permanent implant placement
- Latissimus dorsi with implant
- Autologous tissue (pedicled)
- Autologous tissue (free)

The choice among these therapies must take into account the need for skin resection, adjuvant radiation therapy, patient size and esthetic desires, and activity level. The opposite breast and available donor tissue must be considered. Ideally, reconstructive surgeons would merely be filling the empty space left after removal of the gland, with preservation of the normal footprint of the breast; however, this is not always the case. Usually, except for advanced and inflammatory disease, some version of skin-sparing mastectomy can be performed. Breast surgeons also offer nipple-sparing and areolar-sparing mastectomies. These procedures allow

BOX 35-1 Options for Breast Reconstruction

Autogenous
- Abdominal-based flaps
- TRAM
- Single pedicle
- Double pedicle
- Free flap*
- Deep inferior epigastric perforator flap*
- Upper abdominal horizontal flap
- Vertical abdominal flap
- Tubed abdominal flap

Latissimus dorsi musculocutaneous flap
Gluteal flap*
- Superiorly based
- Inferiorly based

Rubens flap*
Thoracoepigastric flap
Lateral thigh flap*
Breast-splitting procedure†
Alloplastic
- Silicone gel implant
- Silicone implant with saline fill
- Smooth wall
- Textured wall
- Round
- Anatomic shaped
- Silicone injection†

Combination procedures
- Latissimus dorsi flap with implant
- TRAM flap with implant

*Requires microsurgical procedure.
†Historical note only.

BOX 35-2 Implant Reconstruction

Indications
Bilateral reconstruction
Patient requesting augmentation in addition to reconstruction
Patient not suited for long surgery
Lack of adequate abdominal tissue
Patient unwilling to have additional scars on back or abdomen
Small breast mound, with minimal ptosis

Relative Contraindications
Young age (may need implant replaced multiple times)
Patient unwilling to adhere to follow-up
Very large breast
Very ptotic breast
Silicon allergy
Implant fear
Previous failed implants
Need for adjuvant radiation therapy

for more esthetically pleasing reconstructions because they confine the scar to the area around the skin paddle of a flap, if used. There is no increased cancer risk or recurrence with skin-sparing mastectomy as long as the skin flaps are not too thick. Conversely, the thickness of the skin determines flap survival, and very thin flaps often become necrotic. In large-breasted women, the skin incisions for mastectomy may be modified to allow easy access for the general surgeon and the ability to have scar symmetry for the reconstructive surgeon. Breast reduction patterns can be used for the mastectomy as well as the contralateral symmetry procedure.

Breast reconstruction is more than just providing a mound on the chest wall. Of utmost importance is the ability to create symmetry. Good reconstructions can be a great disappointment if they do not match the contralateral native breast. For the most part, autologous reconstruction provides better symmetry. Symmetry is less of an issue in the case of bilateral reconstruction. In planning reconstructions, one must consider not only the size and shape of the opposite breast but also the position on the chest wall; location of the inframammary fold; height, size, and color of the nipple-areolar complex; and amount of breast ptosis.

Implant-Based Reconstructions

Implant reconstructions are performed in women who have a reasonable amount of good-quality skin after mastectomy, enough to cover an implant completely and provide a natural shape. They are advantageous in that they are relatively quick procedures, with minimal morbidity to the patient. Implant reconstruction is best used for a bilateral reconstruction because it is the best opportunity for symmetry. With implant-only reconstructions, it is difficult to mimic the natural ptosis and contour of the contralateral breast except in cases of young women with relatively small, youthful-appearing breasts (Box 35-2).

Initially, these reconstructive procedures were performed with placement of the implant in the subcutaneous pocket. This placement fell out of favor because of visible rippling of the implant beneath a thin layer of skin and a greater complication risk of capsular contracture. At the present time, these implants are placed in a submuscular pocket beneath the pectoralis major. Some surgeons provide for full muscle coverage, with the assistance of the serratus anterior and rectus abdominis fascia. Others provide coverage of the inferior pole of the implant with bioprosthetic material (e.g., human, porcine, bovine dermal allografts) to help create a natural inframammary fold and contoured reconstruction and provide an additional layer between the implant and inferior mastectomy skin flap. This material is sutured to the pectoralis major muscle superiorly and inferiorly to the previously marked or designated inframammary fold (Figs. 35-1 and 35-2).[13,15,16] Either method helps fix the pectoralis major and keeps it from migrating superiorly, exposing more of the implant.

These forms of reconstruction often are begun with placement of a tissue expander at the time of mastectomy. The tissue expander is to allow for little stress on the tenuous mastectomy flaps initially or for progressive stretching of the skin to place a larger implant than would have been safe at the time of mastectomy. Expanders are silicone shell prostheses that have an integrated or remote port for the injection of saline in the clinical setting. Most surgeons expand the skin to a slightly larger size to provide for a large pocket with some ptosis. Expanders are exchanged for implants after expansion and any adjuvant treatments are completed.

In general, implant-based reconstructions provide for a round-shaped, youthful breast mound without ptosis (Fig. 35-3). It requires multiple clinic visits to provide for expansion and then a subsequent procedure to place the permanent implants, which requires a time commitment from the patient. Over time, implant reconstructions tend to change because of the effects of gravity, the body's response to foreign objects (capsule formation), and aging of the implants themselves. This change occurs linearly with

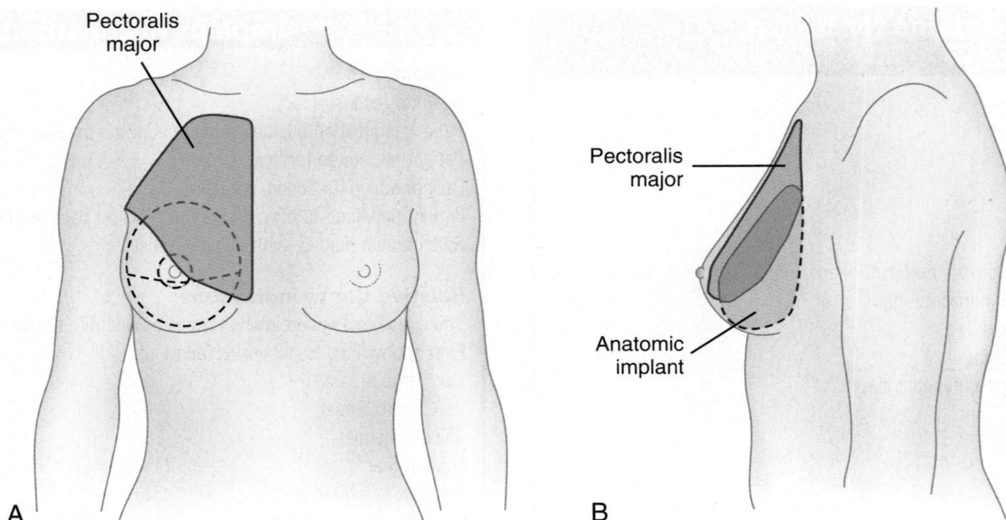

FIGURE 35-1 A, B, Schematic representation of implant position, pectoralis position, and chest wall. The pectoralis muscle cannot cover the inferior pole of the breast, and bioprosthetic material is needed in the area of greatest expansion. (From Breuing KH, Warren SM: Immediate bilateral breast reconstruction with implants and inferolateral AlloDerm slings. *Ann Plast Surg* 55:232–239, 2005.)

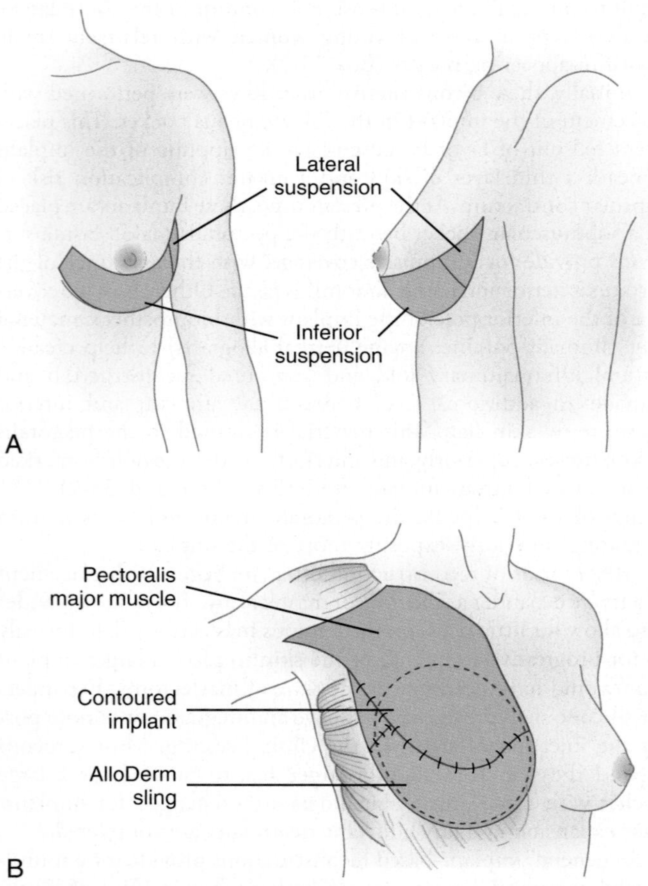

FIGURE 35-2 A, B, Schematic representation of chest wall, breast, pectoralis muscle, bioprosthetic sling, and implant. Bioprosthetic material is sutured to the inferior border of the pectoralis muscle superiorly, the inframammary fold inferiorly, and curved laterally along the chest wall to re-create the footprint of the breast for expansion. (From Breuing KH, Warren SM: Immediate bilateral breast reconstruction with implants and inferolateral AlloDerm slings. *Ann Plast Surg* 55:232–239, 2005.)

time, so that 86% of women are pleased with their results at 2 years versus 54% at 5 years.[17]

Combination Reconstruction

Use of autologous tissue in conjunction with an implant was first done in the 1970s. There is often a need for additional tissue after mastectomy to create a sizable breast and a natural breast drape to prevent the development of ptosis or to counter radiation-induced skin changes. This form of reconstruction generally uses myocutaneous latissimus dorsi muscle flap based on the thoracodorsal artery pedicle, as described by Schneider and associates.[18] It is a broad flat muscle that spans the back from the tip of the scapula superiorly to the spine medially and the iliac crest inferiorly. The muscle usually is taken with an overlying skin paddle to replace the removed nipple-areolar complex or larger deficits in the case of traditional mastectomy, as popularized by Bostwick and Scheflan.[19] The skin paddle is centered over the muscle, and attempts are made to hide the donor site scar within the bra line. In smaller breasted women, entire reconstructions can be made of the latissimus dorsi and its overlying fat plus an implant if necessary. The latissimus dorsi serves as a sling inferiorly, attached to the superior pectoralis to provide full muscle coverage of the implant (Fig. 35-4).

This flap, performed in a single-stage fashion, is ideal for relatively small-breasted women with some ptosis, but it can be used to create larger reconstructed breasts in a staged fashion. It is also used for the reconstruction of lateral partial mastectomy defects. The latissimus flap is advantageous because of its proximity to the breast and reliable circulation. It is the workhorse for reconstruction of unilateral defects in thin women with minimal donor sites and in smaller breasted women and as salvage for any failed breast reconstruction. Its disadvantages are a large scar on the back and the possibility of donor site complications (see later; Box 35-3).

Autologous Reconstruction

Pedicled Flap

At the present time, the gold standard in breast reconstruction with autogenous tissue is the transverse rectus abdominis

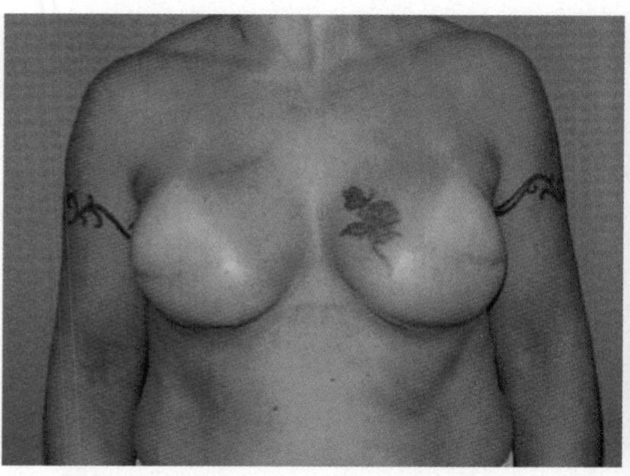
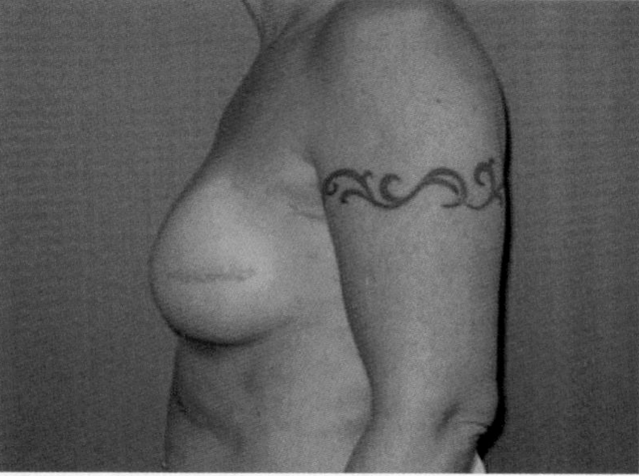

FIGURE 35-3 A 41-year-old woman with left breast cancer who underwent bilateral mastectomy with immediate placement of bilateral tissue expanders with bioprosthetic slings. Final reconstruction was carried out with the exchange of expanders for 533-mL silicone gel breast prostheses. (From Roehl KR: Breast reconstruction. *Open Breast Cancer J* 2:25–37, 2010. Photos courtesy John D. Bauer, MD.)

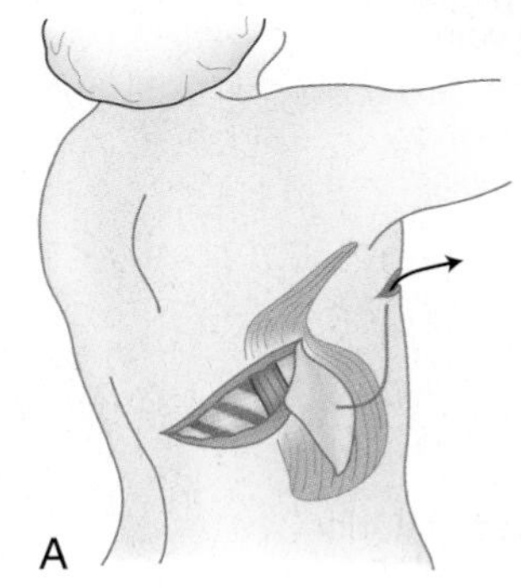

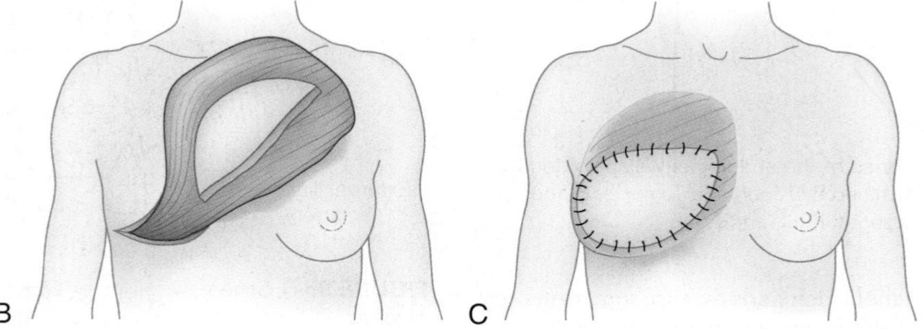

FIGURE 35-4 Schematic representation of latissimus dorsi flap. **A,** Flap elevation. **B,** Flap transposition. **C,** Flap inset.

myocutaneous (TRAM) flap because lower abdominal tissues are similar in consistency to breast tissue. The first description of the rectus abdominis myocutaneous flap used in breast reconstruction, by Robbins in 1979, was with a vertical skin island. The TRAM flap as we know it, with a horizontal lower abdominal skin paddle, was first described by Hartrampf and colleagues in 1982.[20] The TRAM flap orients the donor scar into a more acceptable abdominoplasty location. Although this location of the skin paddle provides for a better arc of rotation, the ensuing blood supply to this large volume of tissue is more distal and tenuous. This donor area of skin and adipose tissue has a dual blood supply for the superior and inferior epigastric systems. Pedicled flaps are supplied by the proximal superior epigastric vessels, and the inferior system must be divided for transfer. The small vessels connecting the superior and inferior systems, known as choke vessels, are dilated to increase perfusion when the deep system is ligated. Studies by Moon and Taylor[21] further elucidated the perfusion zones of the lower abdomen skin territory. They found rich perforating blood vessels that arise out of the rectus to supply the overlying skin and fat. Perfusion is best overlying the rectus muscle (zone I) on the side (pedicle) used, followed by the region overlying the contralateral rectus muscle (zone II). Next is the ipsilateral outer region of tissue (zone III), and the region perfused the least is the farthest from the rectus pedicle (zone IV) (Fig. 35-5).

This type of reconstruction is advantageous in that it replaces like with like tissue and provides an acceptable donor scar and improvement of abdominal contour. The limitations include the following:

BOX 35-3 Latissimus Dorsi Reconstruction

Indications
Small breast
Minor breast ptosis
Abdominal donor site unavailable (e.g., scars, lack of tissue)
Salvage of previous breast reconstruction

Relative Contraindications
Planned postoperative radiation therapy
Bilateral reconstruction
Significant breast ptosis

Contraindications
Previous lateral thoracotomy
Very large breast in patient who does not desire reduction

BOX 35-4 Transverse Rectus Abdominis Muscle Flap Reconstruction

Indications
Breasts of all sizes
Breast ptosis

Relative Contraindications
Smoking
Abdominal liposuction
Previous abdominal surgery
Pulmonary disease
Obesity

Contraindications
Previous abdominoplasty
Patient unable to tolerate 4- to 6-week recovery period
Patient unable to tolerate longer procedure

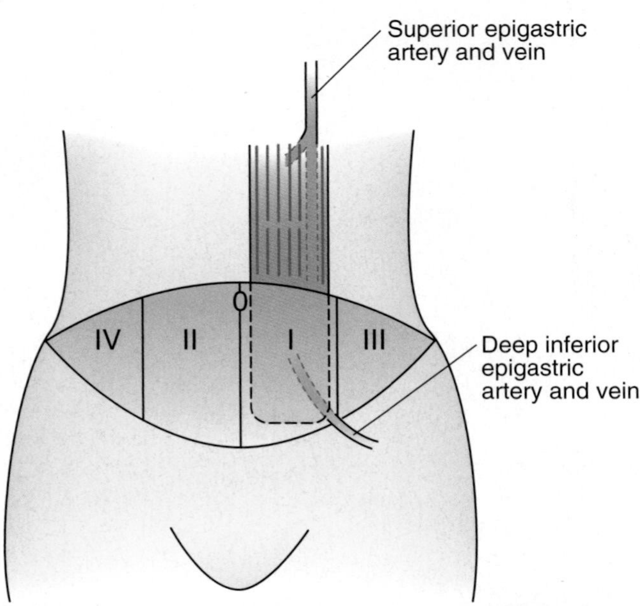

FIGURE 35-5 Vascular territories of the abdominal wall provided by a unilateral TRAM flap (as determined by Moon and Taylor[21]). Blood flow is best in zone I, followed by zones II, III, and IV.

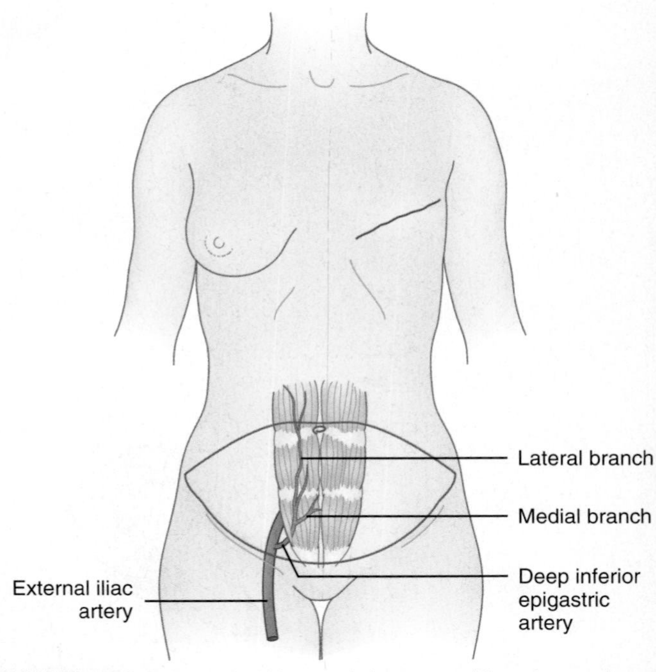

FIGURE 35-6 Schematic of lower abdomen markings for autologous reconstruction based on the medial and lateral row of perforators, which are based on the deep inferior epigastric artery system.

1. This tissue has high metabolic demands that are sometimes not met, so that portions of the flap form fat necrosis or die.
2. There is a longer recovery period after this surgery, with increased abdominal discomfort and the risk for abdominal weakness or hernia formation or both.

Use of a pedicled flap can also be limited by previous abdominal operations and scars. Women who are obese, smoke, or have medical comorbidities (especially diabetes) are at greater risk for these complications (Box 35-4).

Abdominal-Based, Gluteal-Based, and Inner Thigh–Based Flaps

Abdominal-based flaps. As noted, the dominant blood supply to the lower abdomen is the deep inferior epigastric system. Perfusion of the skin and fat based on this system is more reliable. It became evident that performing this flap as a free tissue transfer would be beneficial. Free abdominal-based flaps have less partial flap and fat necrosis than pedicled flaps and avoid the epigastric bulge of the muscle that occurs in pedicled flaps. In free TRAM flaps, the skin and fat of the lower abdomen are connected via the deep inferior epigastric artery and vein to the blood supply in the axilla (thoracodorsal vessels, originally) or, more recently, with the internal mammary artery and vein. This procedure is often done in conjunction with the mastectomy except in advanced disease, for which adjuvant radiation may be required (Figs. 35-6 to 35-8).

Holmstrom[22] was the first to perform this type of reconstruction in 1979, and further refinements have made it the gold standard for microvascular autologous breast reconstruction. Original reports from this procedure revealed a partial flap loss rate of 7.1%, total flap loss rate of 1.4%, and fat necrosis in 12% of smokers but only 3% of nonsmokers. Abdominal bulge occurred in approximately 5% initially but became less as smaller amounts of rectus muscle were harvested, transitioning to the muscle-sparing (ms) TRAM.[23] Further refinements of this operation have been made to preserve abdominal wall strength.

The quest to minimize abdominal wall morbidity led to the development of the msTRAM flap, in which only the muscle surrounding the perforating vessels is taken; the deep inferior epigastric artery perforator (DIEP) flap, in which no muscle is taken and the perforating vessels are dissected out in a chain; and the superficial inferior epigastric artery (SIEA) flap, when a suitable SIEA is available (approximately 30%) that provides a pedicle that does not penetrate the rectus muscle at all (and there is no abdominal wall morbidity and shorter recovery time) (Fig. 35-9).[24-26]

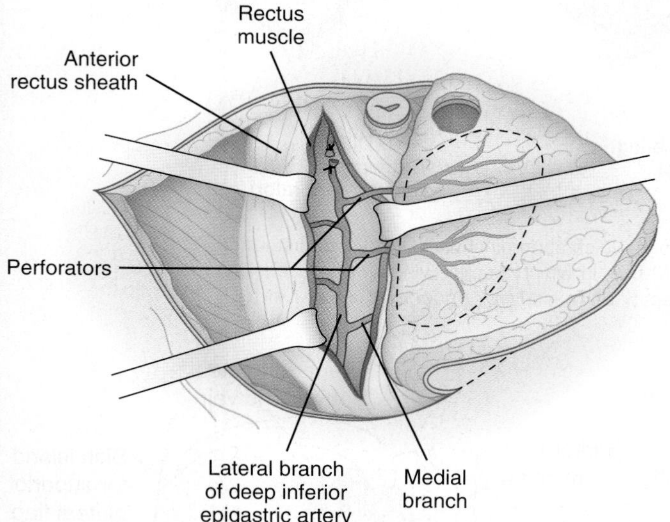

FIGURE 35-7 Anatomy of the deep inferior epigastric artery flap. Shown are perforating vessels of the lateral row, after splitting the rectus abdominis muscle, as they enter the skin and subcutaneous tissue.

The choice of flap is often determined by the patient's anatomy. When the SIEA flap is available and of reasonable caliber, often more than 1.5 mm, it is often chosen because it results in the least amount of abdominal morbidity. Difficulties with this flap can occur because the artery is small, and there may be some discrepancy between the SIEA and internal mammary artery. In addition, the SIEA supports only half of the abdominal skin and fat, so it is favorable for small breast reconstructions and for bilateral cases. The choice between DIEP and msTRAM is made by the surgeon. When the anatomy is favorable and perforators of reasonable caliber are available in a formation that allows for minimal disruption of rectus muscle, a DIEP flap is chosen. When the vessels are smaller or their orientation is unfavorable for muscular dissection, a msTRAM flap is used. Flap perfusion is often better with a msTRAM. DIEP rates of partial flap loss and fat necrosis are often higher, and abdominal wall preservation is sometimes at the expense of flap perfusion and overall breast outcome.[27] Often, preoperative imaging studies are used to evaluate the vascular system of the anterior abdominal wall. Computed tomography angiography, conventional angiography, and staging computed tomography scans performed during cancer workup have been used to visualize the perforators supplying the anterior abdominal skin and subcutaneous tissue. These can provide some guidance for perforator selection and often decrease dissection times.

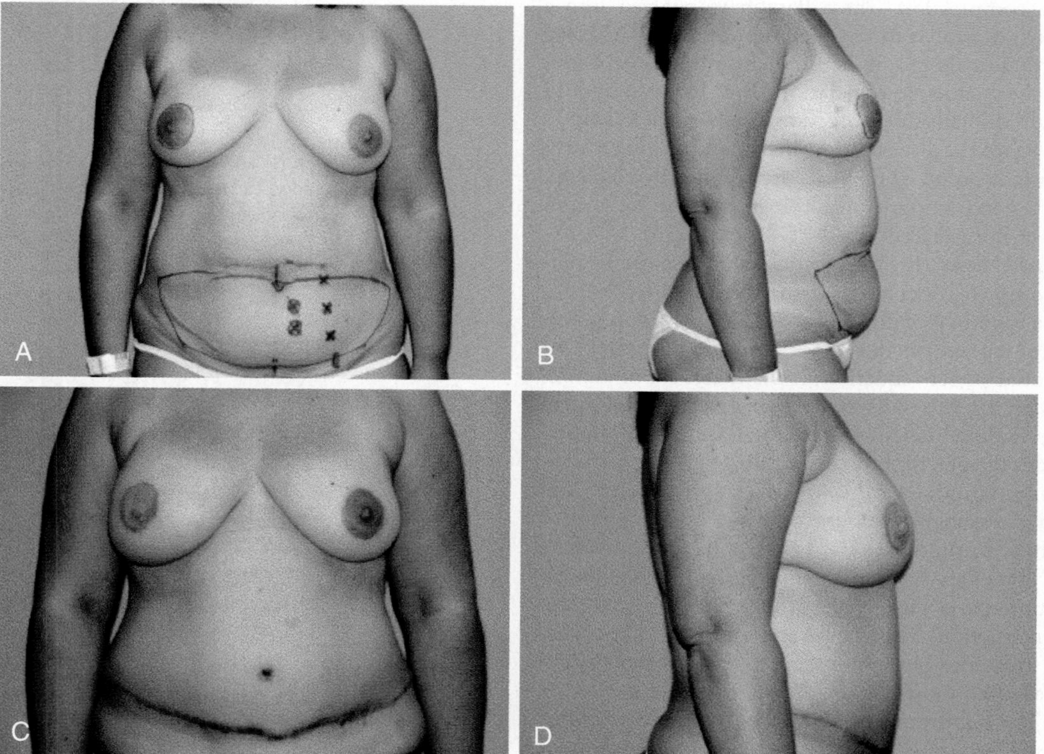

FIGURE 35-8 **A, B,** Preoperative views of a patient with right breast cancer for mastectomy and DIEP reconstruction. **C, D,** Patient approximately 3 months after breast revision, nipple creation, and tattooing. (From Granzow JW, Levine JL, Chiu ES, et al: Breast reconstruction with the deep inferior epigastric perforator flap: History and an update on current technique. *J Plast Reconstr Aesthet* Surg 59:571–579, 2006.)

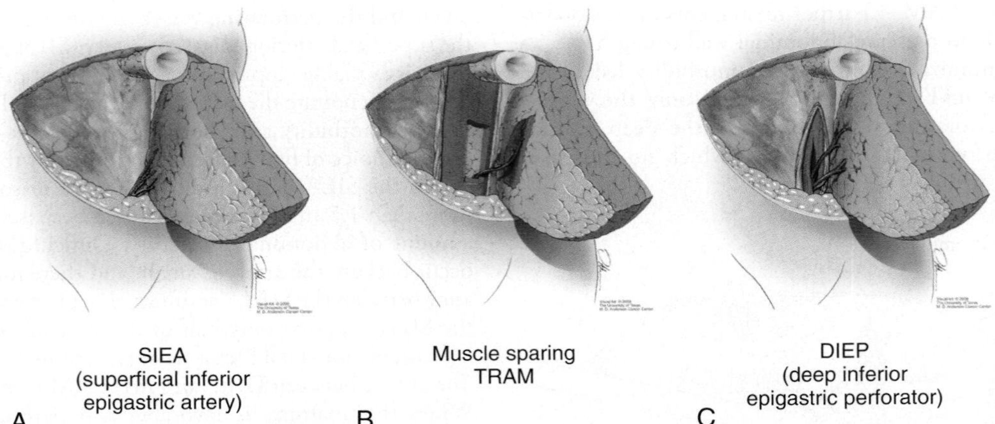

FIGURE 35-9 Schematic representation of the SIEA flap in which abdominal wall fascia is undisturbed **(A);** DIEP flap, in which all muscle is spared **(B);** and msTRAM flap, in which a small window of muscle is taken around the supplying perforators **(C).** (© 2009 The University of Texas M.D. Anderson Cancer Center.)

Gluteal-based flaps. Breast reconstruction can also be performed using tissue from the gluteal region based on the superior or the inferior gluteal arteries and their overlying skin and subcutaneous tissue. This procedure is commonly performed in women who desire autologous breast reconstruction but have little adiposity in the lower abdomen. The buttock provides a reasonable amount of fat that is firm and provides sufficient volume and projection in breast reconstruction. Originally described as a musculocutaneous flap, gluteal artery perforator (GAP) flaps (superior GAP and inferior GAP flaps) had numerous donor site complications, including significant seroma, contour deformity, and sciatica from nerve compression. These flaps have evolved into a perforator flap design, similar to the evolution of the TRAM flap to the DIEP. Perforator design limits the deformity at the donor site and lessens the incidence of sciatica. The disadvantages of these flaps include difficulty of dissection, short pedicle length, and size discrepancy of the gluteal vein when anastomosing it with the internal mammary vein. These flaps are technically challenging but provide a good amount of autologous tissue for reconstruction of one or both breasts (Figs. 35-10 to 35-13).[28-31]

Inner thigh–based flaps. Breast reconstruction also can be performed using the upper inner thigh tissue. This flap is ideal for women without abdominal or gluteal tissue to use as a donor site. Some women are opposed to the donor scar on the buttock or abdomen and would prefer reduction in the excess fat or skin in the inner thigh region. The transverse upper gracilis (TUG) flap is based on the ascending branch of the medial circumflex femoral artery and includes the gracilis muscle and the overlying horizontal paddle of skin or fat. The scar is camouflaged in the groin and gluteal fold, and a reasonable amount of tissue can be obtained to reconstruct small to moderate-sized breasts in the immediate setting. Because TUG flaps are slightly smaller than their abdominal or gluteal counterparts with regard to skin, they are less useful for delayed reconstruction. This flap is straightforward, and dissection is easier than the perforator flaps of the abdomen and buttock. Minimal to no morbidity is noticed with sacrifice of the gracilis muscle. The disadvantages of this flap include a shorter pedicle length, smaller skin island, possible contour deformity of the medial thigh, and widened donor site scar. TUG flaps are ideal for women in whom the abdominal donor site is unavailable or as a salvage procedure after reconstruction failure (Figs. 35-14 and 35-15).[32,33]

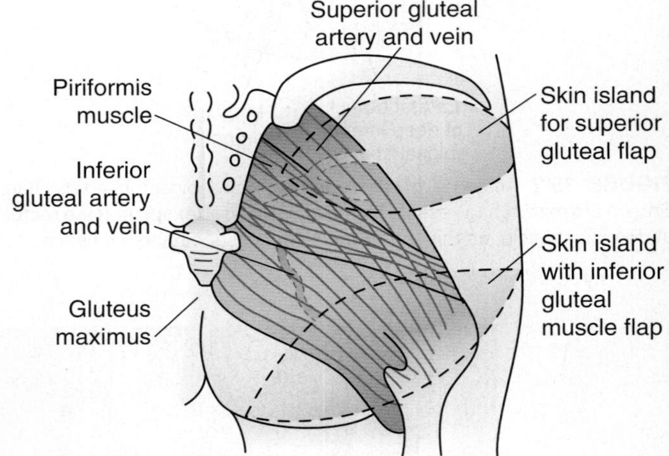

FIGURE 35-10 Skin island location of superior GAP and inferior GAP flaps. The skin paddle can be oriented over the superior or inferior gluteal artery.

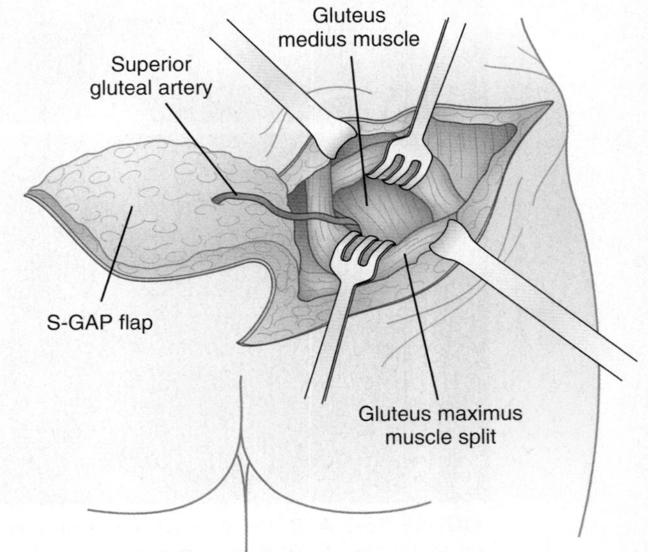

FIGURE 35-11 Superior gluteal vessel dissection through the retracted gluteus maximus muscle.

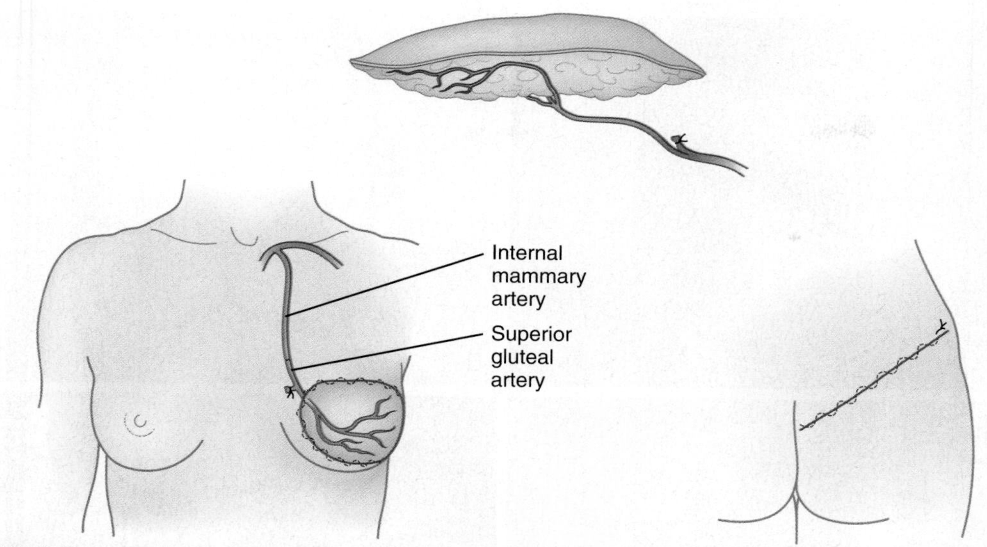

FIGURE 35-12 Schematic of the gluteal perforator flap, inset into the defect via the internal mammary vessels, and donor site closure. (From Granzow JW, Levine JL, Chiu ES, et al: Breast reconstruction with gluteal artery perforator flaps. *J Plast Reconstr Aesthet Surg* 59:614–621, 2006.)

Oncoplastic Surgery

Breast conservation has comparable outcomes in cancer treatment, and approximately half of eligible women chose it over mastectomy.[34] BCT is a reasonable choice for many women because they preserve much of their native breast and often the nipple-areolar complex. However, the adjunctive radiation that accompanies lumpectomy is not without consequence. At least 30% of women who choose BCT require some form of reconstructive surgery to achieve better symmetry.[35] Breast revision can be difficult after radiation therapy, with complication rates of 50% in the radiated breast. Women were historically offered reduction of the normal breast for symmetry in clothing and minimal to no surgery on the radiated side. In an attempt to improve cosmetic outcomes, surgeons can provide preemptive treatment at the time of lumpectomy to improve contour and esthetic deformity after the effects of radiation. This preemptive treatment takes the form of breast rearrangement after the cancerous tissue is removed. These types of procedures are ideal for large-breasted women, when resection is 20% of breast volume; when tumor location is central, medial, or inferior; when the woman desires smaller breasts; or when the woman has significant breast ptosis or asymmetry or both (Fig. 35-16).

Oncoplastic procedures are performed immediately or 1 to 2 weeks after lumpectomy, once final pathology is available. Procedures include rearrangement of the remaining breast tissue using various techniques, often adhering to breast reduction principles. In addition, more tissue can be brought into the breast to correct the volume deficit, often in the form of a latissimus dorsi flap. Indications for these procedures depend on the patient's preoperative breast size, available remaining breast tissue, and overall goals for ultimate breast size and shape. All these procedures are done before radiation to prevent the contracture of the lumpectomy defect and distortion of the nipple-areolar complex. In many cases, these women still require contralateral balancing procedures after completion of radiation.[36-38]

Complications

Complications, including partial or total flap loss, mastectomy flap loss, wound breakdown, and infection, can be encountered with any form of breast reconstruction and may cause delay in adjuvant chemotherapy. Complications are known to be higher in women who require adjuvant radiation therapy and, more commonly, with implant-based reconstructions (15% without radiation and 42% with radiation).[17,39,40] Symmetry is also affected by radiation therapy; implant-based reconstructions are not the best option for women requiring radiation therapy.

The most common complication with implant-based reconstructions is capsular contracture, which can occur regardless of implant type or placement position. Treatment may require capsulectomy, capsulotomy, change in implant position or type, or implant removal, with some other form of reconstruction. Additional complications include infection, seroma, skin slough, necrosis, deflation, and unacceptable appearance.

Satisfaction with this modality of reconstruction tends to decline over time regardless of type, volume, patient age, or type of mastectomy.[17] Implant-based reconstruction is best suited for thin patients with inadequate autologous donor sites or for women who opt not to undergo more lengthy procedures. Implants can also be used to enhance autologous reconstructions to improve symmetry and esthetic wishes of women.

Complications associated with flap reconstruction include mastectomy flap issues, partial or total flap loss, and problems related to the flap donor site. For the latissimus dorsi flap, back seroma is the most common complication. In addition, many women require the addition of an implant to achieve adequate volume and accrue all the possible implant-related complications. Abdominal-based reconstructions have possible partial flap loss, total flap loss, and fat necrosis, which can manifest later as a firm suspicious nodule. Fat necrosis occurs in approximately 50% of pedicled TRAMs versus 17% in procedures performed in a free fashion.[41] Complications associated with the abdominal donor site include flap necrosis, abdominal weakness, bulge, and hernia. Partial flap loss is more common with pedicled reconstructions, and total flap loss is more common with free transfer of the abdominal tissue. Partial flap loss rates for free tissue transfers are approximately 2% for msTRAM, 7% for DIEP, 3% for SIEA, and 4% for GAP flaps. Fat necrosis also occurs in approximately 3% of msTRAM, 7% of SIEA, and 9% of DIEP flaps. Abdominal

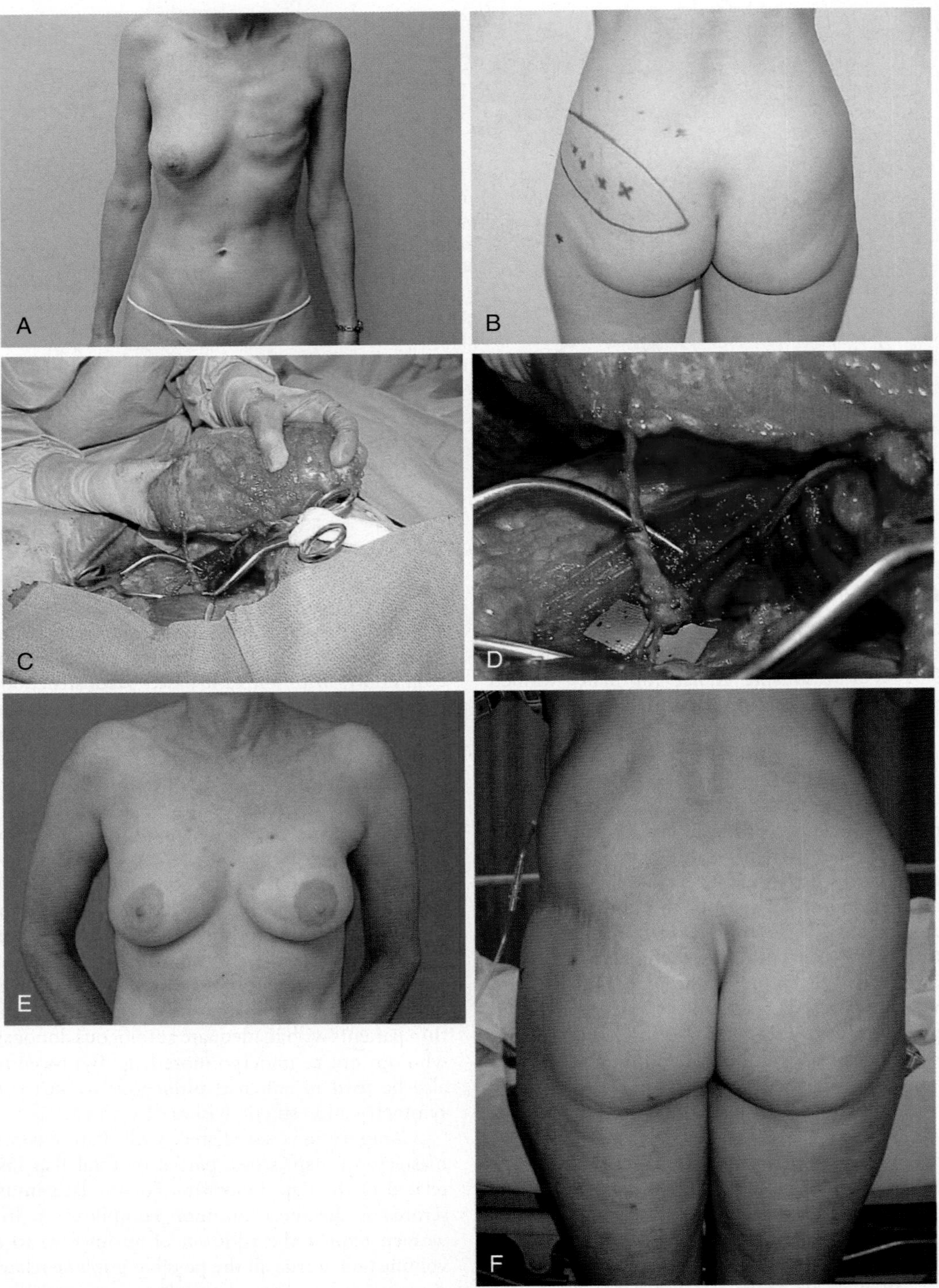

FIGURE 35-13 **A, B,** Preoperative view and markings. **C, D,** Intraoperative views of flap and superior gluteal artery perforator vessels. **E, F,** Postoperative views (anterior and posterior) 21 months after surgery. (From Granzow JW, Levine JL, Chiu ES, et al: Breast reconstruction with gluteal artery perforator flaps. *J Plast Reconstr Aesthet Surg* 59:614–621, 2006.)

weakness and bulge have been reported to occur less with DIEP flaps, especially with bilateral breast reconstruction. Studies revealed that bulge or hernia formation occurs in approximately 15% of pedicled TRAMs versus less than 5% of DIEP flaps.[41-44]

Complications of mastectomy flaps and the abdominal wall in autologous reconstructions are much higher in smokers. Smoking is believed to cut down on the microvascular distal circulation of flaps and has little impact on the anastomosis of free flaps. Similar complications are seen in obese and morbidly obese women. They also have higher mastectomy flap loss and abdominal donor site complications. Chemotherapy has little effect on the outcomes of breast reconstruction as long as surgical procedures are delayed

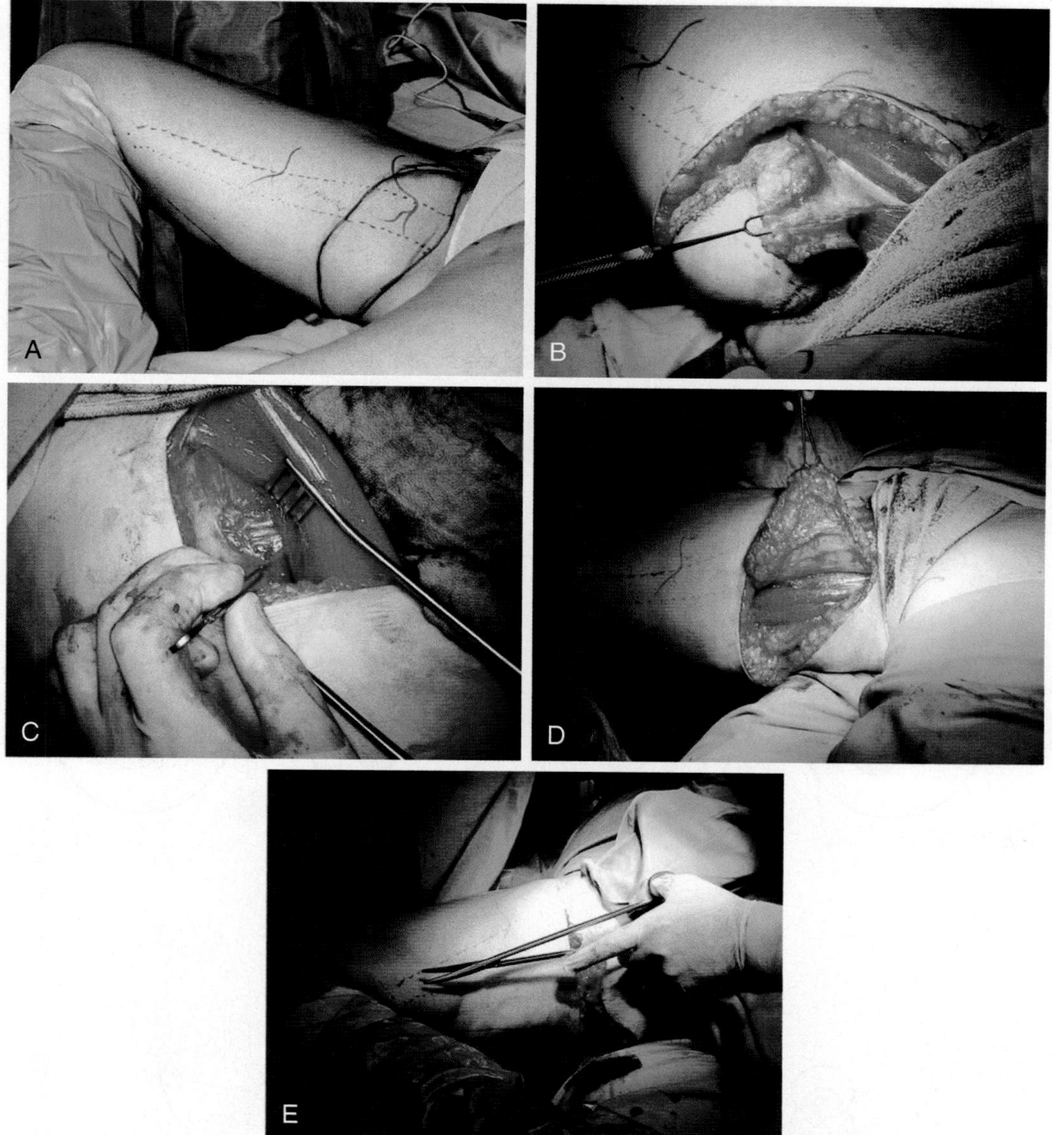

FIGURE 35-14 **A,** Typical marking of the TUG flap. **B,** The anterior portion of the flap is dissected first off the underlying adductor longus. The pedicle, medial circumflex femoral artery, is identified at the dorsal border of this muscle. **C,** Posterior portion of the skin island is lifted off the underlying muscle. The overlying skin is supplied by multiple perforators arising from within the gracilis. **D, E,** After complete skin dissection, the gracilis muscle is cut at its tendinous junction. (From Schoeller T, Huemer GM, Wechselberger G: The transverse musculocutaneous gracilis flap for breast reconstruction: Guidelines for flap and patient selection. *Plast Reconstr Surg* 122:29–38, 2008.)

after neoadjuvant chemotherapy, with return of immunologic function, and little intervention is performed during the course of adjuvant chemotherapy.

Radiation therapy can have an impact on reconstruction. It limits the options for reconstruction in that implant-based procedures have high failure rates. If implants are used, additional and larger surgeries are often required to salvage the breast reconstruction. Similarly, complications associated with irradiated autologous reconstructions are higher. Early complications are similar in delayed and immediate reconstruction with adjuvant radiation therapy. Immediate reconstruction followed by radiation has complication rates of 87% versus 8.6% in patients who have delayed reconstruction after radiation therapy. In patients who have immediate reconstruction, 28% require additional flap surgery to correct contour deformities.[45]

NIPPLE-AREOLAR RECONSTRUCTION

The focus of all the procedures described is creation of a breast mound. A breast mound provides the woman with symmetry in clothing and a bra, and for many women, this is satisfactory, and they desire no further operative intervention. Other women would like completion of their reconstruction to mirror the normal contralateral breast, which requires the creation of a nipple and areolar complex. These procedures often are done

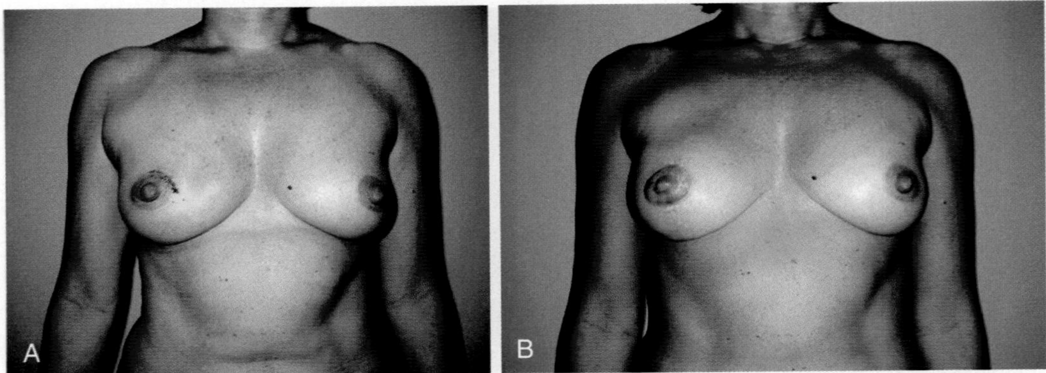

FIGURE 35-15 Patient with right breast cancer before **(A)** and after **(B)** unilateral right breast reconstruction using TUG flap. **A,** Before reconstruction. **B,** 33 months after reconstruction. (From Schoeller T, Huemer GM, Wechselberger G: The transverse musculocutaneous gracilis flap for breast reconstruction: Guidelines for flap and patient selection. *Plast Reconstr Surg* 122:29–38, 2008.)

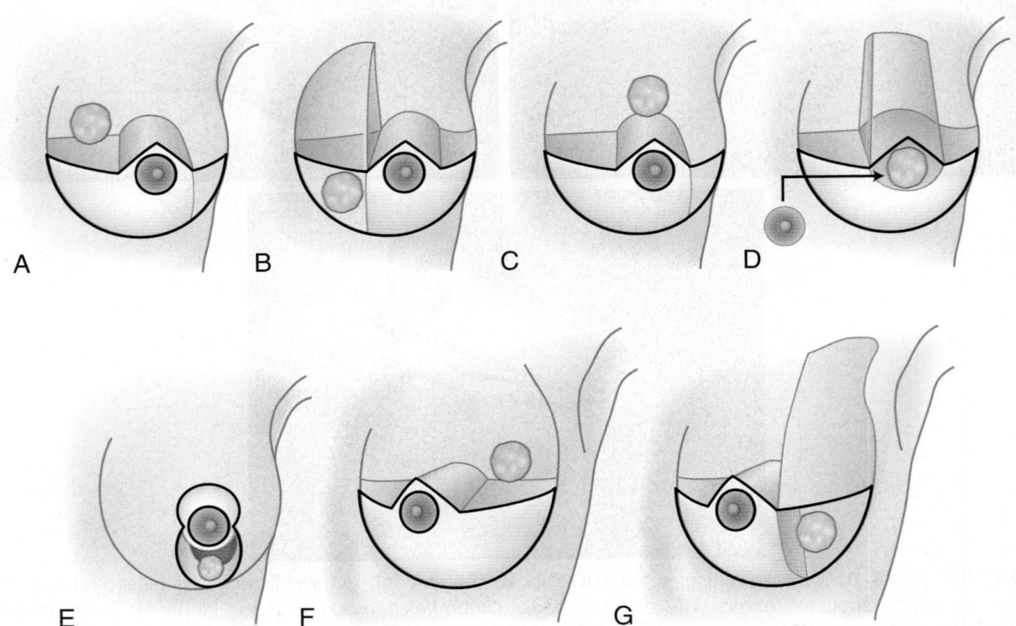

FIGURE 35-16 Guidelines for design of the nipple pedicle to repair a partial mastectomy defect using the breast reduction technique by tumor location *(pink)*. **A,** Upper inner quadrant, showing the inferomedial pedicle *(white)*. The retained medial component *(yellow)* fills the defect on closure of the Wise skin pattern and maintains the cleavage of the breast. **B,** Lower inner quadrant, showing the inferolateral pedicle. The retained lateral component provides additional blood supply to the nipple-areolar complex. A thick layer of subcutaneous tissue is maintained on the medial aspect of the Wise skin pattern flap to fill the defect on closure of the Wise skin pattern and maintain cleavage of the breast. **C,** Upper central quadrant, showing the inferomedial pedicle. The retained medial component provides a cosmetic advantage and additional blood supply to the nipple-areolar complex in patients with very large ptotic breasts. **D,** Middle central quadrant, showing the amputative design with a free nipple graft and maintenance of a thick layer of subcutaneous tissue on the central aspect of the Wise skin pattern flap *(yellow)*. **E,** Lower central quadrant, showing the vertical scar reduction mammaplasty. **F,** Upper outer quadrant, showing the inferomediolateral pedicle. The retained lateral component fills the defect on closure of the Wise skin pattern. **G,** Lower outer quadrant, showing the inferomedial pedicle. The retained medial component provides a cosmetic advantage and additional blood supply to the nipple-areolar complex. A thick layer of subcutaneous tissue is maintained on the lateral aspect of the Wise skin pattern flap to fill the defect *(yellow)*. (From Kronowitz SJ, Kuerer HM, Buchholz TA, et al: A management algorithm and practical oncoplastic surgical techniques for repairing partial mastectomy defects. *Plast Reconstr Surg* 122:1631–1647, 2008.)

months after the initial mound reconstruction to allow for settling of the reconstruction; this allows for symmetrical positioning of the created nipple. In addition, a period of time after radiation should be allotted because the breast reconstruction undergoes some amount of contraction. This time is usually 2 to 3 months after creation of the breast mound or completion of adjuvant therapy.

The nipple itself can be created via myriad local flap techniques using the skin of the reconstructed breast mound. Numerous local flap designs have been proposed, and all have had relatively similar results. Over the first year, the flaps undergo some amount of contraction, up to 50%, so all are initially made large. The areolar reconstruction can be performed in one of two ways. Some surgeons opt to use a full-thickness skin graft, usually from the groin for the native darker pigmentation. Others choose to use medical tattoo pigments that are chosen from a color wheel to match the contralateral native areola. Creation of the areola usually occurs 4 to 6 weeks after creation of the nipple. Nipple tattoo tends to fade over time and requires occasional touchup.

In general, nipple-areolar reconstruction is the least satisfying portion of the overall breast reconstruction experience. The reconstructed nipple and areola have little projection compared with normal and is insensate and less than the esthetic normal. This situation has led surgical oncologists and plastic surgeons to attempt to preserve the areola or the entire nipple-areolar complex. There is some controversy because the ducts in the nipple can harbor residual cancer, and blood supply can be tenuous after mastectomy; nipple-areolar complex survival is not guaranteed. Nonetheless, cancer is found in a few nipple specimens, especially when tumors are small, peripherally located, and have a negative nodal status. This procedure may be applicable to early-stage peripheral breast cancers and is more valuable in prophylactic mastectomies.

MANAGEMENT OF THE CONTRALATERAL BREAST

The goal in any breast reconstruction is symmetry, most importantly in clothing, but plastic surgeons strive for symmetry even out of clothing. In many cases, some revision of the breast mound reconstruction is warranted to improve shape, and surgeries on the native contralateral breast are also necessary. Mastectomy and reconstruction often meet the patient's desires with regard to breast size, whether smaller or larger. Complete reconstruction of very ptotic or a large breast is often difficult with any reconstructive technique. The techniques used are augmentation mammaplasty, mastopexy (lifting), and reduction mammaplasty.

The incidence of contralateral cancer is approximately 1%/year. Therefore, young women often choose a prophylactic mastectomy. Also, *BRCA*-positive women are encouraged to undergo bilateral mastectomies because their incidence of breast cancer is 80% or greater in their lifetime. In the case of bilateral mastectomies, reconstruction is best when the same procedure is performed on both sides.

SURVEILLANCE

Reconstructed breasts are easy to monitor for local recurrence because recurrence is most often within the skin. Biopsy should be performed of any firm or suspicious mass without delay. The result is often fat necrosis in autologous tissue reconstructions. Routine mammography of breast reconstructions is unnecessary. Ultrasound and magnetic resonance imaging are the most commonly used radiographic modalities. Recurrence is usually managed with surgical excision, adjuvant chemotherapy, or radiation therapy. The reconstruction infrequently has to be removed in its entirety—only in the case of multifocal recurrence or involvement of the flap pedicle itself.

CONCLUSIONS

Breast reconstruction is a vital component in the treatment of breast cancer for many women. It is often the optimistic portion of a devastating diagnosis. Reconstruction lessens the psychological and physical burden of the diagnosis for many women. When possible, immediate reconstruction is preferred because it has not been shown to increase oncologic risk or delay adjuvant therapy, it provides for better esthetic outcomes, and it results in less depression. Immediate reconstruction is also more cost-effective. Planning and decision making for reconstruction must be individualized to each patient to achieve her desires in the safest and most reasonable fashion. There are advantages and disadvantages of each procedure; decision making should be individualized for the patient and her reconstructive surgeon to determine the most rational radiotherapy.

SELECTED REFERENCES

Granzow JW, Levine JL, Chiu ES, et al: Breast reconstruction using perforator flaps. *J Surg Oncol* 94:441–454, 2006.

The authors describe the use of superficial inferior epigastric artery, deep inferior epigastric artery perforator, and gluteal artery perforator flaps for breast reconstruction with preservation of muscle at donor sites. The procedures and donor sites are well described and illustrated.

Khoo A, Kroll SS, Reece GP, et al: A comparison of resource costs of immediate and delayed breast reconstruction. *Plast Reconstr Surg* 101:964–968, 1998.

This report evaluated the cost of delayed versus immediate breast reconstruction in 276 patients and concluded that mastectomy with immediate breast reconstruction is significantly less expensive than mastectomy followed by delayed reconstruction.

Singletary SE: Skin-sparing mastectomy with immediate breast reconstruction: The M. D. Anderson Cancer Center experience. *Ann Surg Oncol* 3:411–416, 1996.

This report on 545 patients undergoing skin-sparing mastectomies and immediate breast reconstruction indicated a low regional recurrence rate of 2.6%. This recurrence was found to be a function of tumor biology and disease stage, not use of immediate breast reconstruction or skin-sparing mastectomy.

Warren AG, Morris DJ, Houlihan MJ, et al: Breast reconstruction in a changing breast cancer treatment paradigm. *Plast Reconstr Surg* 121:1116–1126, 2008.

This article provides an overview of the current trends in breast cancer treatment, including breast conservation, oncoplastic surgery, sentinel lymph node biopsy, and skin-sparing mastectomy. With regard to reconstruction, new silicone implants, perforator flap reconstructions, and the use of acellular dermal matrix in implant reconstructions are discussed.

Zhong T, McCarthy C, Price AN, et al: Evidence-based medicine: Breast reconstruction. *Plast Reconstr Surg* 132:1658–1669, 2013.

This article provides an overview of the most clinically important areas of breast reconstruction in the past decade, presented in a balanced and evidence-based fashion.

REFERENCES

1. Cronin TD, Gerow FJ: Augmentation mammaplasty: A new natural feel prosthesis. In Broadbent TR, editor: *Transactions of the Third International Congress of Plastic Surgery*, Amsterdam, 1963, Excerpta Medica.
2. Mandel MA: Subcutaneous mastectomy with immediate reconstruction of the large breast. *Surg Gynecol Obstet* 146:90–92, 1978.
3. Pontes R: Single-stage reconstruction of the missing breast. *Br J Plast Surg* 26:377–380, 1973.
4. Snyderman RK, Guthrie RH: Reconstruction of the female breast following radical mastectomy. *Plast Reconstr Surg* 47:565–567, 1971.
5. Manchot C: *Die Hautarterien des Menschlichen Korpers*, Leipzig, 1889, Vogel.
6. Ryan JJ: A lower thoracic advancement flap in breast reconstruction after mastectomy. *Plast Reconstr Surg* 70:153–160, 1982.
7. Reaby LL: Reasons why women who have mastectomy decide to have or not to have breast reconstruction. *Plast Reconstr Surg* 101:1810–1818, 1998.
8. Stevens LA, McGrath MH, Druss RG, et al: The psychological impact of immediate breast reconstruction for women with early breast cancer. *Plast Reconstr Surg* 73:619–628, 1984.
9. Pusic A, Thompson TA, Kerrigan CL, et al: Surgical options for the early-stage breast cancer: Factors associated with patient choice and postoperative quality of life. *Plast Reconstr Surg* 104:1325–1333, 1999.
10. McGuire KP, Santillan AA, Kaur P, et al: Are mastectomies on the rise? A 13-year trend analysis of the selection of mastectomy versus breast conservation therapy in 5865 patients. *Ann Surg Oncol* 16:2682–2690, 2009.
11. Warren AG, Morris DJ, Houlihan MJ, et al: Breast reconstruction in a changing breast cancer treatment paradigm. *Plast Reconstr Surg* 121:1116–1126, 2008.
12. Khoo A, Kroll SS, Reece GP, et al: A comparison of resource costs of immediate and delayed breast reconstruction. *Plast Reconstr Surg* 101:964–968, 1998.
13. Gamboa-Bobadilla GM: Implant breast reconstruction using acellular dermal matrix. *Ann Plast Surg* 56:22–25, 2006.
14. Singletary SE: Skin-sparing mastectomy with immediate breast reconstruction: The M. D. Anderson Cancer Center experience. *Ann Surg Oncol* 3:411–416, 1996.
15. Breuing KH, Warren SM: Immediate bilateral breast reconstruction with implants and inferolateral AlloDerm slings. *Ann Plast Surg* 55:232–239, 2005.
16. Spear SL, Parikh PM, Reisin E, et al: Acellular dermis-assisted breast reconstruction. *Aesthetic Plast Surg* 32:418–425, 2008.
17. Clough KB, O'Donoghue JM, Fitoussi AD, et al: Prospective evaluation of late cosmetic results following breast reconstruction: I. Implant reconstruction. *Plast Reconstr Surg* 107:1702–1709, 2001.
18. Schneider WJ, Hill HL, Jr, Brown RG: Latissimus dorsi myocutaneous flap for breast reconstruction. *Br J Plast Surg* 30:277–281, 1977.
19. Bostwick J, 3rd, Scheflan M: The latissimus dorsi musculocutaneous flap: A one-stage breast reconstruction. *Clin Plast Surg* 7:71–78, 1980.
20. Hartrampf CR, Scheflan M, Black PW: Breast reconstruction with a transverse abdominal island flap. *Plast Reconstr Surg* 69:216–225, 1982.
21. Moon HK, Taylor GI: The vascular anatomy of rectus abdominis musculocutaneous flaps based on the deep superior epigastric system. *Plast Reconstr Surg* 82:815–832, 1988.
22. Holmstrom H: The free abdominoplasty flap and its use in breast reconstruction. An experimental study and clinical case report. *Scand J Plast Reconstr Surg* 13:423–427, 1979.
23. Garvey PB, Buchel EW, Pockaj BA, et al: DIEP and pedicled TRAM flaps: A comparison of outcomes. *Plast Reconstr Surg* 117:1711–1719, 2006.
24. Chevray PM: Breast reconstruction with superficial inferior epigastric artery flaps: A prospective comparison with TRAM and DIEP flaps. *Plast Reconstr Surg* 114:1077–1083, 2004.
25. Man LX, Selber JC, Serletti JM: Abdominal wall following free TRAM or DIEP flap reconstruction: A meta-analysis and critical review. *Plast Reconstr Surg* 124:752–764, 2009.
26. Grotting JC, Urist MM, Maddox WA, et al: Conventional TRAM flap versus free microsurgical TRAM flap for immediate breast reconstruction. *Plast Reconstr Surg* 83:828–841, 1989.
27. Granzow JW, Levine JL, Chiu ES, et al: Breast reconstruction using perforator flaps. *J Surg Oncol* 94:441–454, 2006.
28. Guerra AB, Metzinger SE, Bidros RS, et al: Breast reconstruction with gluteal artery perforator (GAP) flaps: A critical analysis of 142 cases. *Ann Plast Surg* 52:118–125, 2004.
29. Allen RJ, Levine JL, Granzow JW: The in-the-crease inferior gluteal artery perforator flap for breast reconstruction. *Plast Reconstr Surg* 118:333–339, 2006.
30. Granzow JW, Levine JL, Chiu ES, et al: Breast reconstruction with gluteal artery perforator flaps. *J Plast Reconstr Aesthet Surg* 59:614–621, 2006.
31. Guerra AB, Soueid N, Metzinger SE, et al: Simultaneous bilateral breast reconstruction with superior gluteal artery perforator (SGAP) flaps. *Ann Plast Surg* 53:305–310, 2004.
32. Arnez ZM, Pogorelec D, Planinsek F, et al: Breast reconstruction by the free transverse gracilis (TUG) flap. *Br J Plast Surg* 57:20–26, 2004.
33. Fattah A, Figus A, Mathur B, et al: The transverse myocutaneous gracilis flap: Technical refinements. *J Plast Reconstr Aesthet Surg* 63:305–313, 2010.
34. Mahmood U, Morris C, Neuner G, et al: Similar survival with breast conservation therapy or mastectomy in the management of young women with early-stage breast cancer. *Int J Radiat Oncol Biol Phys* 83:1387–1393, 2012.

35. Bajaj AK, Kon PS, Oberg KC, et al: Aesthetic outcomes in patients undergoing breast conservation therapy for the treatment of localized breast cancer. *Plast Reconstr Surg* 114:1442–1449, 2004.
36. Losken A, Hamdi M: Partial breast reconstruction: Current perspectives. *Plast Reconstr Surg* 124:722–736, 2009.
37. Kronowitz SJ, Kuerer HM, Buchholz TA, et al: A management algorithm and practical oncoplastic surgical techniques for repairing partial mastectomy defects. *Plast Reconstr Surg* 122:1631–1647, 2008.
38. Berry M, Fitoussi AD, Curnier A, et al: Oncoplastic breast surgery: A review and systematic approach. *J Plast Reconstr Aesthet Surg* 63:1233–1243, 2010.
39. Chawla AK, Kachnic LA, Taghian AG, et al: Radiotherapy and breast reconstruction: Complications and cosmesis with TRAM versus tissue expander/implant. *Int J Radiat Oncol Biol Phys* 54:520–526, 2002.
40. Benediktsson K, Perbeck L: Capsular contracture around saline-filled and textured subcutaneously-placed implants in irradiated and non-irradiated breast cancer patients: Five years of monitoring of a prospective trial. *J Plast Reconstr Aesthet Surg* 59:27–34, 2006.
41. Schusterman MA, Kroll SS, Miller MJ, et al: The free transverse rectus abdominis musculocutaneous flap for breast reconstruction: One center's experience with 211 consecutive cases. *Ann Plast Surg* 32:234–241, 1994.
42. Blondeel N, Vanderstraeten GG, Monstrey SJ, et al: The donor site morbidity of free DIEP flaps and free TRAM flaps for breast reconstruction. *Br J Plast Surg* 50:322–330, 1997.
43. Nahabedian MY, Dooley W, Singh N, et al: Contour abnormalities of the abdomen after breast reconstruction with abdominal flaps: The role of muscle preservation. *Plast Reconstr Surg* 109:91–101, 2002.
44. Bottero L, Lefaucheur JP, Fadhul S, et al: Electromyographic assessment of rectus abdominis muscle function after deep inferior epigastric perforator flap surgery. *Plast Reconstr Surg* 113:156–161, 2004.
45. Tran NV, Chang DW, Gupta A, et al: Comparison of immediate and delayed free TRAM flap breast reconstruction in patients receiving postmastectomy radiation therapy. *Plast Reconstr Surg* 108:78–82, 2001.

SECTION VIII

Endocrine

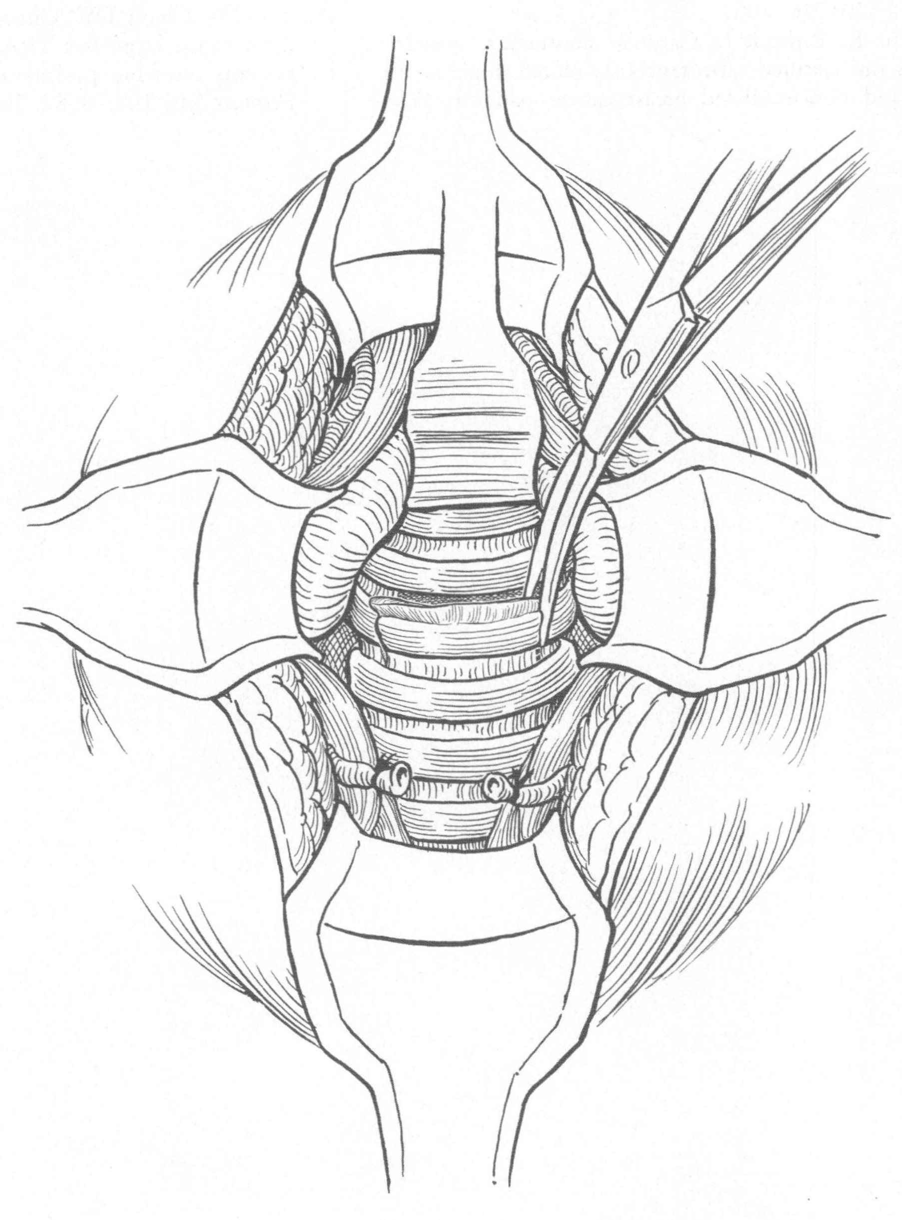

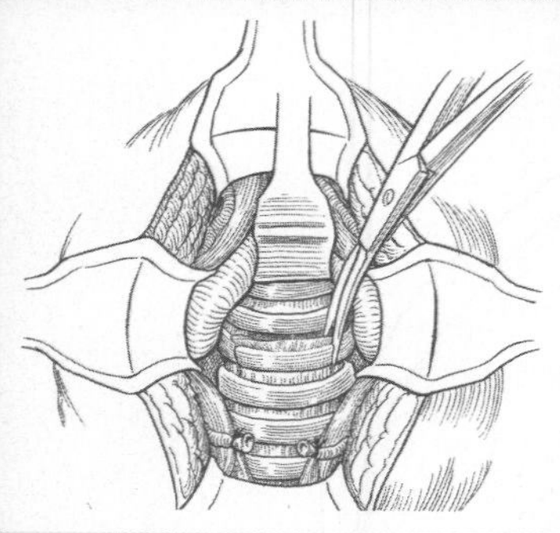

CHAPTER 36

Thyroid

Philip W. Smith, Laura R. Hanks, Leslie J. Salomone, John B. Hanks

OUTLINE

HISTORICAL PERSPECTIVE

The term *thyroid* is derived from the Greek description of a shield-shaped gland in the anterior neck ("thyreoiedes"). Classic anatomic descriptions of the thyroid were available in the 16th and 17th centuries, but the function of the gland was not understood. By the 19th century, pathologic enlargement of the thyroid, or goiter, was described, and iodine-rich seaweed was used to treat this condition. Early surgical approaches to thyroid masses had extremely high complication and mortality rates.

In the late 19th century, two surgeon-physiologists revolutionized understanding and treatment of thyroid diseases. Billroth and Kocher established large clinics in Europe and applied skilled surgical technique combined with newer anesthetic and antiseptic principles. Their surgical results proved the safety and efficacy of thyroid surgery for benign and malignant diseases. When Kocher began his series, it was expected that approximately 1 out of 6 thyroid resections would result in mortality; with his advances, this improved to a mortality rate of less than 1 out of 500 in his hands. As a result of his pioneering developments in the understanding of thyroid physiology and surgery, Kocher received the Nobel Prize in 1909.

The 20th century started with the contributions of Kocher and Billroth. Over the course of the past century, there were marked improvements in the understanding of thyroid pathophysiology, including hypothyroidism, hyperthyroidism, and thyroid cancer. There also were major advances in imaging, epidemiology, and diagnostic and surgical techniques. The 21st century has been notable so far for further refinements of the above-mentioned improvements, a focus on understanding the genetic drivers of these disease processes, and harnessing this knowledge to improve diagnosis and treatment. These advances have allowed the diagnosis and treatment of thyroid diseases to become rapid and cost-effective with low morbidity.

ANATOMY

Embryology

The tissue bud that becomes the thyroid gland initially arises as a midline diverticulum in the floor of the pharynx. This tissue originates in the primitive alimentary tract and consists of cells of endodermal origin. This point of origin corresponds to the foramen cecum of the base of the tongue in a fully developed human. The main portion of this cellular structure descends into the neck and develops into a bilobed solid organ. This structure becomes the thyroglossal duct, which is usually reabsorbed after 6 weeks of age. The distal aspect of this path of descent may be retained as a pyramidal lobe in the adult thyroid.

Calcitonin-producing C cells arise from the fourth pharyngeal pouch and migrate from the neural crest into the thyroid. These cells migrate into the lateral and posterior upper two thirds of the thyroid lobes and are distributed among the follicles. In adults, they remain limited to the upper and middle areas of the gland, usually in the posterior and medial aspects. These C cells are the only component of the adult gland not of endodermal origin.

Microscopic thyroid follicles first appear as the lateral lobes develop. When the embryo is approximately 6 cm in length, these follicles begin to develop colloid. In the third month, the follicular cells first demonstrate iodine trapping, and thyroid hormone secretion begins.

Knowledge of basic embryology is essential for understanding certain conditions, including thyroglossal duct cysts and fistulas, which result from retained tissue along the path of descent of the thyroid. A lingual thyroid is another anomaly that occurs when the median thyroid anlage does not descend in a normal fashion. Ectopic thyroid tissue also may be found occasionally in the central compartment of the neck. Small amounts of ectopic tissue may be located under the lower poles of a normal thyroid and sometimes in the anterior mediastinum. Historically, thyroid tissue found in lateral neck compartments was known as "lateral aberrant thyroid" and was explained as an embryologic variation. This concept has essentially been disproved, and it is thought that thyroid tissue found in the neck lateral to the jugular vein represents metastatic deposits from differentiated thyroid carcinoma (DTC), typically papillary cancer, and may be the initial presentation of this disease. Small thyroid follicles located at the periphery of central neck lymph nodes may occasionally occur in the absence of thyroid cancer.

Adult Surgical Anatomy

A normally developed adult thyroid weighs 10 to 20 g and is a bilobed structure that lies next to the thyroid cartilage in a position anterior and lateral to the junction of the larynx and trachea. In this position, the thyroid encircles approximately 75% of the diameter of the junction of the larynx and the upper part of the trachea. The lobes lie lateral to the trachea and esophagus; anteromedial to the carotid sheath; and posteromedial to the sternocleidomastoid, sternohyoid, and sternothyroid muscles. The two lateral lobes are joined at the midline by an isthmus, whose superior edge is situated at or just below the cricoid cartilage. A pyramidal lobe is present in approximately 30% of patients and represents the most distal portion of the thyroglossal duct. In an adult, a pyramidal lobe may be a prominent structure that can extend from the midline of the isthmus as far cephalad as the hyoid bone. When present, a pyramidal lobe typically lies on either side of midline, not directly in the midline.

A thin layer of connective tissue surrounds the thyroid. This tissue is part of the fascial layer that invests the trachea. This fascia is different from the thyroid capsule, and it can easily be separated from the capsule during surgery, whereas the true capsule of the thyroid cannot be separated. This fascia coalesces with the thyroid capsule posteriorly and laterally to form a suspensory ligament termed the *ligament of Berry*, which is the primary point of fixation of the thyroid to surrounding structures. The ligament of Berry is closely attached to the cricoid cartilage and has important surgical implications because of its relationship to the recurrent laryngeal nerve (RLN).

Innervation

The laryngeal complex is innervated by branches of the vagus nerve. The vagus nerve arises from the medulla in the brainstem and exits the skull base via the jugular foramen. It then enters the carotid sheath and lies posterior to, and between, the internal jugular vein and internal carotid artery. As the main trunk of the vagus descends from the skull base into the chest, there are two branches of relevance to the thyroid surgeon: the superior laryngeal nerve and the RLN (also known as the inferior laryngeal nerve).

Superior Laryngeal Nerve

The superior laryngeal nerve (Fig. 36-1) separates from the vagus nerve at the base of the skull and descends toward the superior pole of the thyroid medial to the carotid sheath. At the level of the cornu of the hyoid, approximately 2 to 3 cm above the superior pole of the thyroid, it divides into two branches. The larger internal branch penetrates the thyrohyoid membrane, where it provides sensory innervation to the larynx cranial to the vocal folds. The smaller external branch continues to travel along the lateral surface of the inferior pharyngeal constrictor muscle and usually descends anteriorly and medially along with the superior thyroid artery. Within 1 cm of the entrance of the superior thyroid artery into the thyroid capsule, the nerve generally takes a medial course and enters the cricothyroid muscle, which it innervates. This relationship is important because the external branch is not always visualized during thyroidectomy, as it has already entered the inferior pharyngeal muscle fascia. This nerve is at risk of being severed or entrapped if the superior pole vessels are ligated at too great a distance above the superior pole of the thyroid. Damage to the external branch can result in severe loss of voice quality or strength. The specific pattern of branching relative to the insertion of the superior thyroid vessels puts this nerve at greater or lesser risk of injury.[1] Although such loss may not be as clinically devastating as RLN damage, it is extremely bothersome to patients whose occupation or avocation demands good voice quality.[2]

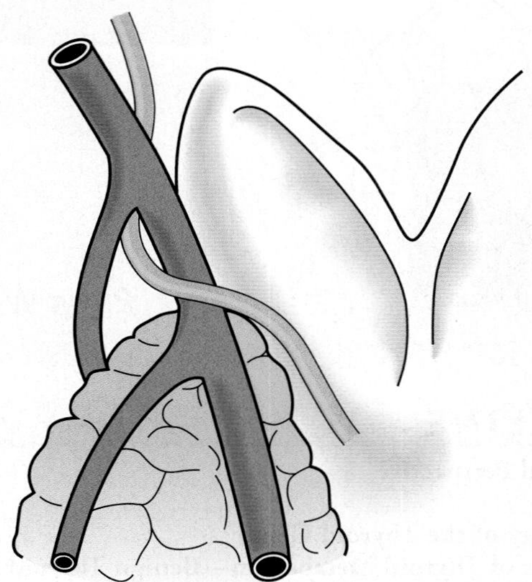

FIGURE 36-1 Relationship between the external branch of the superior laryngeal nerve *(yellow)* and the superior thyroid artery. The nerve can course inferiorly and medially and may run partly along with or around the artery or branches of the artery as they enter the superior lobe of the thyroid. (From Duh QY: Surgical anatomy and embryology of the thyroid and parathyroid glands and recurrent and external laryngeal nerves. In Clark OH, Duh QY, editors: *Textbook of endocrine surgery*, Philadelphia, 1997, Saunders, p 11.)

Recurrent Laryngeal Nerve

The RLNs (Fig. 36-2) are so named because of their course cranially into the neck after branching from the vagus nerve more caudally. The course of this recurrence and the usual course in the neck are asymmetrical. On the right side, the RLN originates from the vagus nerve as it crosses anterior to the subclavian artery. The RLN passes inferior and then posterior to the right subclavian artery and ascends in a position lateral to the trachea along the tracheoesophageal groove. During thyroidectomy, at the level of the lower border of the thyroid, the right RLN can usually be found within 1 cm lateral to or within the tracheoesophageal groove. Compared with the left side, the course of the RLN on the right is less predictable in the lower portions of the field of thyroid surgery and follows a more oblique course. However, as it ascends to the midportion of the thyroid, the right RLN assumes its position within the tracheoesophageal groove. The nerve can usually be found immediately anterior or posterior to a main arterial trunk of the inferior thyroid artery at this level.

On the left side, the RLN separates from the vagus as that nerve passes anterior to the arch of the aorta. The left RLN passes inferior and posteromedial to the aorta at the ligamentum arteriosum and begins to ascend toward the larynx. The left RLN

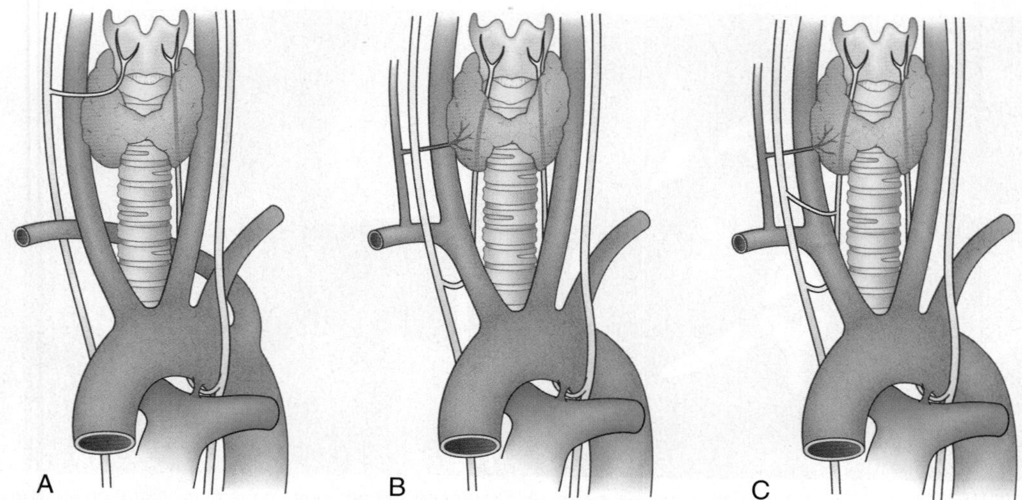

FIGURE 36-2 Anomalous variations in the course of the right recurrent laryngeal nerve. **A,** A nonrecurrent laryngeal nerve arises from the vagus and courses medially into the larynx in the setting of an aberrant origin of the right subclavian artery. **B,** The normal course of the recurrent laryngeal nerve arises from the vagus after it passes beneath the subclavian artery. **C,** The unusual coexistence of a nonrecurrent laryngeal nerve and the recurrent laryngeal nerve forms a common distal nerve.

enters the tracheoesophageal groove as it ascends to the level of the lower pole of the thyroid. Compared with the right RLN, the left RLN is more predictably directly within the tracheoesophageal groove in the lower portions of the surgical field for thyroidectomy.

Both RLNs are consistently found within the tracheoesophageal groove when they are within 2.5 cm of their entrance into the larynx. These nerves pass either anterior or posterior to a branch of the inferior thyroid artery and enter the larynx at the level of the cricothyroid articulation on the caudal border of the cricothyroid muscle. At this level, the nerve courses immediately adjacent to the superior parathyroid gland, the inferior thyroid artery, and the ligament of Berry. Great care is needed during surgical dissection in this area because the nerve is essentially tethered as it dives beneath the cricothyroid muscle and can be stretched by overly vigorous dissection. In approximately 25% of patients, the nerve is contained within the ligament of Berry, which may further exacerbate this issue, particularly with medial retraction of the thyroid. A small branch of the inferior laryngeal artery crosses the nerve at the level of the ligament of Berry. Bleeding from this small artery can be problematic, and hemostasis should be addressed with great caution in this area to avoid nerve injury.

In approximately one fourth to one third of patients, the bilateral RLNs branch before their insertion into the larynx. Although this branching more often occurs distally in the course of the nerve, there also may be branches inferior to the level of the inferior thyroid artery. When there is branching, the more anterior of the branches carries the predominance of the motor fibers, even when it is more diminutive than the posterior branch. The thyroid surgeon must carefully seek these anterior branches because they are at greater risk in the course of thyroidectomy. When branching occurs, it frequently is symmetrical.

A nonrecurrent right laryngeal nerve is an important anatomic variant. In this situation, the right inferior laryngeal nerve arises directly from the vagus and courses medially into the larynx following the course of the superior thyroid artery or of the inferior thyroid artery (see Fig. 36-2). This nonrecurrent anatomy is found in 0.5% to 1.5% of patients and occurs in the setting of arterial anomalies, most commonly an aberrant right subclavian artery, also known as arteria lusoria. An aberrant right subclavian artery arises as a separate branch from the aortic arch, distal to the left subclavian, and passes from left to right, posterior to the esophagus. This anomaly may be well demonstrated on computed tomography (CT) or magnetic resonance imaging (MRI) if those studies have been performed (Fig. 36-3). A standard cervical ultrasound scan also can detect a normal origin of the right subclavian and right common carotid from the innominate artery, which predicts a normal right RLN; the absence of this finding raises concern for a nonrecurrent nerve (Fig. 36-4). There also are reports of patients who have a right RLN and a nonrecurrent right laryngeal nerve. These two nerves normally would join in a position beneath the lower border of the thyroid.[2] A nonrecurrent left laryngeal nerve is quite rare and is associated with more extensive and less common arch and great vessel anomalies than nonrecurrent right laryngeal nerves.

The RLN has mixed motor, sensory, and autonomic functions and innervates the intrinsic laryngeal muscles. Damage to a RLN results in mixed pathology, the most important of which is paralysis of the vocal cord on the affected side. Such damage might result in a cord that remains in a midline position or paramedian position. A grossly normal voice may occur if the remaining functioning contralateral cord is able to approximate the paralyzed cord; this is particularly important to note because a completely paralyzed vocal cord may be clinically inapparent in a preoperative or postoperative patient. If the vocal cord remains paralyzed in an abducted position and closure cannot occur, a severely impaired voice and ineffective cough also may result. If the RLNs are damaged bilaterally, complete loss of voice or airway obstruction may occur and possibly require an emergency surgical airway. Occasionally, bilateral damage can result in cords taking an abducted position; although this allows airway movement, it may result in upper respiratory infection as a result of ineffective cough and aspiration.[2]

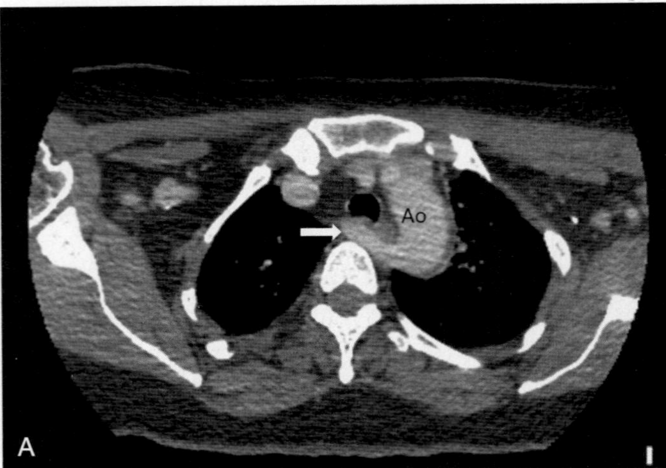

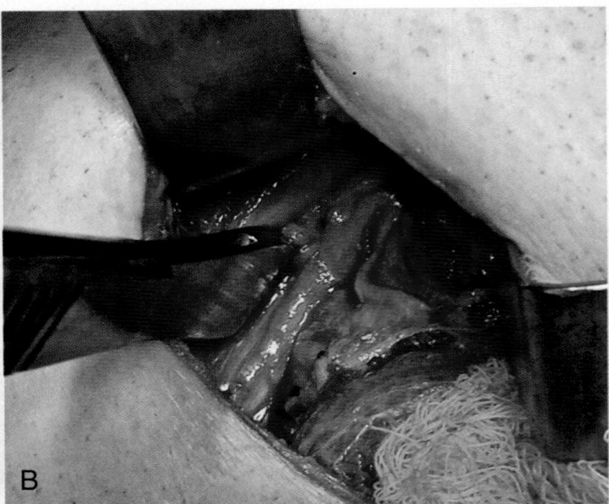

FIGURE 36-3 Nonrecurrent right laryngeal nerve. **A,** Computed tomography image demonstrating an aberrant right subclavian artery *(white arrow)* originating from the distal aortic arch and passing posterior to the trachea and esophagus. *Ao,* aorta. **B,** The nonrecurrent right laryngeal nerve passing from laterally into the central neck in the same patient.

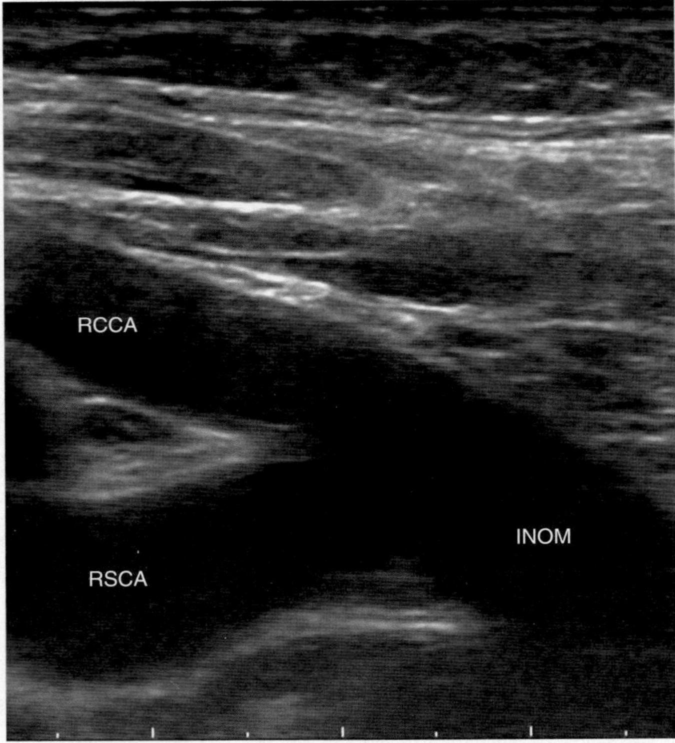

FIGURE 36-4 Ultrasound image demonstrating normal branching pattern of the innominate artery (INOM) into the right common carotid artery (RCCA) and the right subclavian artery (RSCA). This view is achievable in the course of office-based, surgeon-performed ultrasound of the thyroid by following the RCCA caudally. If the RCCA and the RSCA do not have a common trunk, an aberrant right subclavian and nonrecurrent right laryngeal nerve should be anticipated.

Blood Supply

The arterial supply to the thyroid gland consists of four main arteries, two superior and two inferior. The superior thyroid artery is the first branch of the external carotid artery after the bifurcation of the common carotid artery. The superior thyroid artery gives off the superior laryngeal artery and courses medially onto the surface of the inferior pharyngeal constrictor muscle and enters the apex of the superior pole. As the superior thyroid artery proceeds medially, it is adjacent to the external branch of the superior laryngeal nerve, and care must be taken not to damage it when controlling the artery (see Fig. 36-1). The superior thyroid artery and external branch of the superior laryngeal nerve lie immediately deep to the sternothyroid muscle as this muscle inserts on the thyroid cartilage.

The inferior thyroid artery takes its origin from the thyrocervical trunk. This artery originates from the subclavian artery and ascends into the neck on either side posterior to the carotid sheath and then arches medially and enters the thyroid gland posteriorly, usually near the ligament of Berry. Despite the name "inferior thyroid artery," no direct arterial supply generally enters the inferior aspect of the thyroid. However, an arteria thyroidea ima may be present in less than 5% of patients and usually arises directly from the innominate artery or from the aorta.

The inferior thyroid artery has important anatomic relationships. The RLN is usually directly adjacent (in either an anterior or a posterior position) to the inferior thyroid artery, within 1 cm of its entrance into the larynx. Careful dissection of the artery is mandatory and cannot be completed until the position of the RLN is absolutely defined. Additionally, the inferior thyroid artery typically supplies the superior and the inferior parathyroid glands, and care must be taken to evaluate the parathyroids after division of the inferior thyroid artery. For this reason, the inferior thyroid artery should be divided at the distal branches into the thyroid, rather than at its main trunk.

Three pairs of venous systems drain the thyroid. Superior venous drainage is immediately adjacent to the superior arteries and joins the internal jugular vein at the level of the carotid bifurcation. Middle thyroid veins may be single or multiple and course immediately laterally into the internal jugular vein. The inferior thyroid veins are usually two or three in number and descend directly from the lower pole of the gland into the innominate and brachiocephalic veins. These veins often descend in association with the cervical horn of the thymus gland.

Lymphatic System

The relationship of the thyroid gland to its lymphatic drainage is most important when considering surgical treatment of thyroid carcinoma. The thyroid gland and its neighboring structures have rich lymphatics that drain the thyroid in almost every direction. Within the gland, lymphatic channels are present immediately beneath the capsule and communicate between lobes through the isthmus. This drainage connects to structures directly adjacent to the thyroid, with numerous lymphatic channels into the regional lymph nodes. It is useful clinically to divide the lymph nodes between the central and lateral neck, with the boundary between these marked by the carotid sheath. The lateral neck zones are further subdivided as shown in Figure 36-5. Most thyroid cancers drain directly to central nodal basins (level VI) except for cancers in the superior third of the gland, which may drain directly to the lateral compartment (so-called skip metastases). Central compartment level VI lymph nodes include prelaryngeal nodes (also known as delphian nodes); pretracheal nodes inferior to the isthmus; paratracheal nodes; tracheoesophageal groove lymph nodes; retropharyngeal, retroesophageal lymph nodes; and anterior/superior mediastinal lymph nodes. The upper mediastinal nodes are variably considered as level VII or may be considered as part of level VI. The lateral neck nodes include levels II through V, which are defined as described in Figure 36-5. It is important to use these anatomically defined compartments for clear communication between physicians as well as when performing lateral neck dissections.

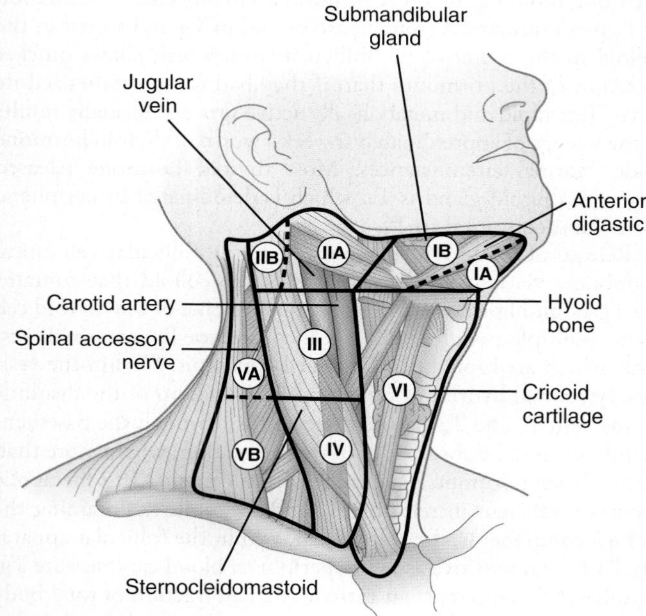

FIGURE 36-5 Lymph node compartments separated into levels and sublevels. Level VI contains the thyroid gland and the adjacent nodes bordered superiorly by the hyoid bone, inferiorly by the innominate (brachiocephalic) artery, and laterally on each side by the carotid sheaths. Level II, III, and IV nodes are arrayed along the jugular veins on each side, bordered anteromedially by level VI and laterally by the posterior border of the sternocleidomastoid muscle. Level III nodes are bounded superiorly by the level of the hyoid bone and inferiorly by the inferior aspect of the cricoid cartilage; levels II and IV are above and below level III, respectively. The level I node compartment includes the submental and submandibular nodes, above the hyoid bone and anterior to the posterior edge of the submandibular gland. Level V nodes are in the posterior triangle, lateral to the lateral edge of the sternocleidomastoid muscle. Levels I, II, and V can be further subdivided as noted in the figure. The inferior extent of level VI is defined as the suprasternal notch. Many authors also include the pretracheal and paratracheal superior mediastinal lymph nodes above the level of the innominate artery (sometimes referred to as level VII) in central neck dissection.

Parathyroid Glands

Most patients have at least four parathyroid glands; approximately one in six patients have more than four glands. It is quite rare to have fewer than four parathyroid glands; this finding most often indicates that an existing gland has yet to be located. The normal parathyroid gland is small, weighing approximately 40 mg. These glands typically have a light yellow to reddish brown appearance, and the fine vascular matrix on their surface may help the surgeon to distinguish them from surrounding fat.

The thyroid sheath encases the lateral and posterior portion of each thyroid lobe and frequently provides a covering for the superior parathyroid gland. When the superior portion of the thyroid lobe is dissected and rolled medially, an area containing fat beneath this fascia is apparent. The superior parathyroid gland typically lies within this fat beneath the thyroid sheath in a posterior position relative to the superior part of the thyroid lobe.

The inferior parathyroid gland may also be located within the thyroid sheath on the posterior aspect of the lower portion of the lobe and, similar to the superior gland, is usually associated with a small amount of fat. The position of the inferior parathyroid is more variable and can be along the branches of the inferior thyroid vein lateral or inferior to the lowermost portion of the thyroid lobe and frequently lies in the thyrothymic tract or the superior thymus. Because of the similar consistency and color of the parathyroids and the fat that surrounds them, identification of parathyroids in both positions may be aided by following the smaller branches of the inferior thyroid artery into the parathyroid substance.

The designation of a parathyroid gland as "superior" or "inferior" is not based on the relative cranial to caudal position of the gland. The embryologic superior parathyroid may actually lie caudal to the inferior gland. What is more consistent is that the inferior parathyroid glands lie anterior to the RLN, and the superior parathyroid glands lie posterior to the RLN. This holds true for low-lying glands, with descended superior glands being found posteriorly in the mediastinum and descended inferior glands being found in the anterior mediastinum.

The superior and inferior parathyroid glands most often have a single end artery that supplies them medially from the inferior thyroid artery. If the main trunk of the inferior thyroid artery is sacrificed for dissection, both parathyroids on that side become devascularized because there is no collateral blood supply in most cases to maintain viability. Careful dissection should attempt to divide only the branches of the inferior thyroid entering the thyroid capsule during excision. With careful technique, it is possible to maintain a good vascular supply to the superior and inferior parathyroid even when total thyroidectomy is performed. The inferior parathyroid blood supply is invariably from the inferior thyroid artery, whereas 15% to 20% of superior parathyroids have significant arterial supply from the superior thyroid artery.

PHYSIOLOGY OF THE THYROID GLAND

The thyroid gland weighs 10 to 20 g in normal adults and is responsible for the production of three metabolic hormones: thyroxine (T_4), triiodothyronine (T_3), and calcitonin. The spherical

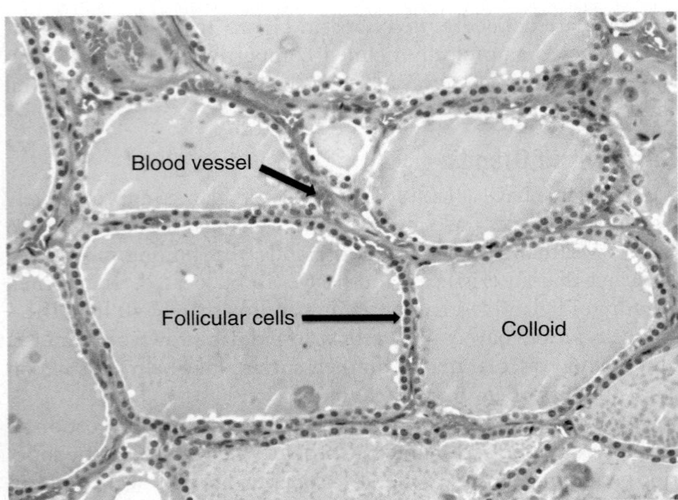

FIGURE 36-6 Photomicrograph of normal thyroid parenchyma with hematoxylin-eosin staining. The follicular unit contains colloid at the center, and each follicle is surrounded by a single layer of well-ordered, cytologically normal follicular cells. The parafollicular spaces contain blood vessels and parafollicular cells.

thyroid follicular unit is the important site of thyroid hormone production (Fig. 36-6). The follicular unit is composed of a single layer of cuboidal follicular cells that encompass a central depository of colloid filled mostly with thyroglobulin (Tg), the protein in which T_4 and T_3 are synthesized and stored. In between these units are parafollicular cells, or C cells, that generate calcitonin.

Iodine Metabolism

Iodine is essential for the production of thyroid hormones. Dietary sources of iodine include dairy products, eggs, iodized table salt, saltwater fish, shellfish, soy products, and multivitamins. Iodine is efficiently absorbed from the gastrointestinal tract in the form of inorganic iodide and rapidly enters the extracellular iodide pool. The thyroid gland is responsible for storing 90% of total body iodide at any given time, with less than 10% existing in the extracellular pool. Iodide is stored in the thyroid as preformed thyroid hormone or as an iodinated amino acid.

Iodide is transported from the extracellular space into the follicular cells against a chemical and electrical gradient via an intrinsic transmembrane protein located in the basolateral membrane of the thyroid follicular cells. Once inside the cells, iodide rapidly diffuses to the apical surface, where it is quickly moved to exocytic vesicles. Here, it is rapidly oxidized and bound to Tg. Transport of iodide into follicular cells is regulated by thyroid-stimulating hormone (TSH) from the pituitary gland as well as by the follicular content of iodide.

The relationship between iodine ingestion and thyroid disease has been known for more than 100 years. At the turn of the 20th century, iodine supplementation of food and water was implemented as a result of careful study in areas in which iodine insufficiency was linked to endemic goiter. Significant iodine deficiency still occurs in various undeveloped parts of the world. In the United States, dietary iodine was adequate in the 1970s, but then decreased in the 1980s and 1990s because of changes in diet and food production. More recent evaluations demonstrated stabilization, but a substantial number of people in the United States still have inadequate dietary iodine consumption.[3] Iodine deficiency can result in nodular goiter, hypothyroidism, cretinism, and possibly the development of follicular thyroid carcinoma (FTC). The World Health Organization has been involved in providing dietary iodine supplementation to treat entire populations in certain areas of the world. In situations in which iodine excess occurs, disorders such as Graves disease and Hashimoto thyroiditis can occur.

Thyroid Hormone Synthesis

Once organic iodide is oxidized and bound, it couples to Tg with tyrosine moieties to form iodotyrosines in a single conformation (monoiodotyrosine [MIT]) or a coupled conformation (diiodotyrosine [DIT]). The formation of DIT and MIT depends on an important intracellular catalytic agent, thyroid peroxidase, which is an integral part of the initial process of organification and storage of inorganic iodide. This enzyme, along with Tg, is remarkably specific to the thyroid follicular cells, making both important in the diagnosis and management of autoimmune thyroid disease and the follow-up of DTC.

MIT and DIT are biologically inert. Coupling of these two residues gives rise to the two biologically active thyroid hormones, T_4 and T_3. T_4 is formed by the coupling of two molecules of DIT, whereas T_3 is formed by the coupling of one molecule of MIT with one molecule of DIT. In normal circumstances, formation of T_4 predominates. T_3 and T_4 are bound to Tg and stored in the colloid in the center of the follicular unit, which allows quicker secretion of the hormones than if they had to be synthesized de novo. This rapid and metabolically active process normally results in the storage of approximately 2 weeks' worth of thyroid hormone under normal circumstances. Most thyroid hormone released from the thyroid gland is T_4, which is deiodinated in peripheral tissues and converted to T_3.

Release of T_4 and T_3 is regulated at the follicular cell apical membrane via lysosomal hydrolysis of the colloid that contains the Tg-bound hormones. The apical membrane of the thyroid cell forms multiple pseudopodia and incorporates Tg into small vesicles, which are brought into the cell apparatus. Within the vesicles, lysosomal hydrolysis results in the reduction of the disulfide bonds, and T_3 and T_4 are then free to pass through the basement membrane and be absorbed into the circulation, where more than 99% of each hormone is bound to serum protein. This metabolic process is efficient in releasing T_3 and T_4, while maintaining the storage components, Tg and colloid, within the follicular apparatus. Although sensitive assays of peripheral blood can measure Tg, peripheral Tg represents an extremely small fraction of total body stores. Residual iodotyrosines undergo peripheral breakdown, deiodination, and recycling and can be added to the recently absorbed iodide stores and become available for the synthesis of new thyroid hormone (Fig. 36-7).

Thyroglobulin

Tg is a 660-kDa glycoprotein specific to the follicular cell that is the primary component of the colloid matrix necessary for iodination and hormonogenesis. Tg facilitates the conversion of MIT and DIT into T_3 and T_4. This process is accompanied by the escape of small amounts of Tg into peripheral blood, where it can be measured. Excess peripheral levels of iodine inhibit further release by enhancing Tg resistance to proteolysis.

Peripheral Tg can be measured to evaluate benign or malignant thyroid neoplasms. Measurement of peripheral Tg has predictive value for the recurrence of DTC locally or in metastatic deposits after initial total thyroidectomy.[4] However, the usefulness of measuring serum Tg levels before the initial resection of a known or

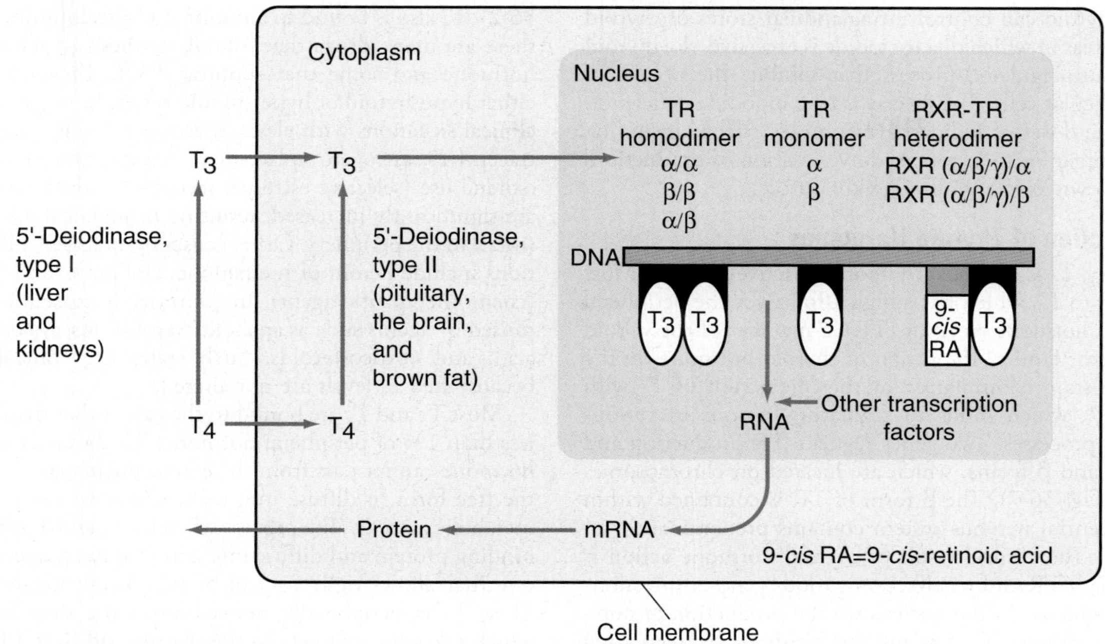

FIGURE 36-7 Cellular and molecular events involved in thyroid hormone function. Thyroxine (T_4) is converted in the periphery and in the cytoplasm of the cell into triiodothyronine (T_3). T_3 travels to the nucleus, where it binds to the thyroid hormone receptor (TR), homodimer, monomer, or heterodimer. TR binding leads to RNA transcription in association with other transcription factors; messenger RNA is subsequently expressed and then translated into protein.

suspected DTC is unknown, and its routine measurement is not recommended.[5]

Calcitonin

Calcitonin is a 32–amino acid polypeptide secreted by the parafollicular cells, or C cells, located superolaterally in each thyroid lobe. Calcitonin acts on the surface receptors of osteoclasts to inhibit calcium absorption and to lower peripheral serum calcium levels. Increased peripheral levels of serum calcium stimulate calcitonin secretion, which can be stimulated clinically by the infusion of calcium, pentagastrin, and alcohol. In normal human physiology, calcitonin does not appear to have a significant role. Patients with clinical calcitonin excess syndromes, such as medullary thyroid carcinoma (MTC), usually have little alteration in peripheral calcium metabolism. Similarly, patients who have had a thyroidectomy do not require any supplementation to replace the lost calcitonin production. Basal or stimulated calcitonin levels are sensitive markers for primary or recurrent MTC.

Regulation of Thyroid Hormone Secretion

The hypothalamic-pituitary-thyroid axis regulates thyroid hormone production and release in a classic endocrine feedback system. The major regulator of thyroid gland activity is the glycoprotein TSH, which is a major growth factor for the thyroid. TSH stimulates thyroid cell growth and differentiation as well as iodine uptake and organification and release of T_3 and T_4 from Tg. Additionally, TSH has been shown to stimulate the growth and invasive characteristics of DTC cell lines.

TSH is a 28-kDa glycoprotein secreted in a pulsatile fashion by the anterior pituitary gland. It has two components; the α subunit is common to other anterior pituitary hormones, but the β subunit is unique to TSH and determines the biologic specificity of the hormone. Once TSH activates the receptor (TSH-R) on thyroid cells, it interacts with a guanine nucleotide–binding protein (G protein), stimulating the production of cyclic adenosine monophosphate (cAMP). This cAMP pathway is an important hormone-synthesizing event. The receptors that respond to TSH have been identified and cloned. Specific mutations in the genetics of this system have been identified and are associated with follicular thyroid neoplasms.[6]

The feedback loop is an important regulator of TSH secretion. Increased thyrotropin-releasing hormone (TRH) from the paraventricular nucleus of the hypothalamus and reduced levels of T_3 stimulate release of TSH from the anterior pituitary. TRH is a three–amino acid peptide that passes through the hypothalamic portal system into the median eminence and through the pituitary stalk to the anterior pituitary. Peripheral thyroid hormone levels may, in addition to stimulating release of TSH from the anterior pituitary, enhance TRH secretion.

Many pathologic states result in increased peripheral levels of T_3 and T_4, which decrease TSH secretion by a negative feedback loop. Peripheral T_4 is locally deiodinated in the pituitary and converted to T_3, which then directly inhibits the release and synthesis of TSH. The condition that usually decreases TSH secretion is classified as primary hyperthyroidism. It has many causes, including many types of thyroiditis, Graves disease, autonomously functioning thyroid nodules, conditions that increase human chorionic gonadotropin (hCG) levels, and overuse of exogenous thyroid hormone. Decreased levels of TSH can also be caused by abnormalities at the level of the pituitary or hypothalamus, or both, which are collectively termed *central hypothyroidism*. Central hypothyroidism is much rarer than primary hypothyroidism.

Although TSH is the primary regulator of thyroid hormone synthesis, there also are intrinsic autoregulatory mechanisms whereby the thyroid can control intraglandular stores of thyroid hormones. In areas in which dietary iodide is excessive, the thyroid gland has an autoregulated process that inhibits the uptake of iodide into follicular cells. The reverse is true in iodide deficiency. Excessively large doses of iodide have complex effects, including an increase in organification followed by cessation of production, a syndrome known as the Wolff-Chaikoff effect.

Peripheral Action of Thyroid Hormones

In the periphery, T_3 is significantly more bioactive than T_4. Most T_4 is converted to T_3, which has a high affinity for the peripheral nuclear thyroid hormone receptor (TR), a member of the steroid hormone receptor family. The action of thyroid hormones in the periphery consists predominantly of the interaction of T_3 with the nuclear TR, which binds to regulatory regions in various gene-regulated processes. Two genes regulate TR production and activity, the α and β forms, which are located on chromosomes 17 and 3 (see Fig. 36-7). The β form of TR is contained within the liver; the central nervous system contains predominantly an α form of TR. The clinical result of thyroid hormone action is regulated through TR and its effect on various genes, expressions of which are regulated in the nucleus via the production of polypeptides. For example, T_3 acts on the pituitary by regulating transcription of the genes for the α and β subunits of TSH, which results in TSH secretion. T_3 affects cardiac contractility by regulating the transcription of myosin heavy chain production in cardiac muscle.

Of circulating T_3 and T_4, 80% is bound to thyroxine-binding globulin (TBG) in the periphery. Numerous medications and clinical scenarios alter serum levels of TBG or the affinity of TBG for circulating thyroid hormone as well as adversely affect extrathyroidal deiodination of thyroid hormone (Boxes 36-1 and 36-2). T_4 also is bound to albumin and prealbumin. Additionally, there are many drugs that inhibit synthesis or release of thyroid hormone and some that suppress TSH. These effects result in either hypothyroid or hyperthyroid states. In pregnancy and other clinical situations with elevated estrogen levels, such as oral contraceptives, estrogen replacement therapy, and tamoxifen or raloxifene use (selective estrogen receptor modulators), TBG levels are significantly increased, resulting in higher levels of bound T_4 (total) in the periphery. Other causes of increased TBG concentrations include heroin or methadone, clofibrate, and 5-fluorouracil (chemotherapeutic agent). In contrast, decreased TBG levels are caused by agents such as anabolic steroids (testosterone), nicotinic acid, and corticosteroids. Such states are clinically euthyroid because free T_4 levels are not altered.

Most T_3 and T_4 are bound to the extent that free T_4 constitutes less than 1% of peripheral hormone. The bound form of thyroid hormone cannot pass from the extracellular space and must be in the free form to diffuse into extracellular tissues to affect major metabolic activity. The process whereby T_3 and T_4 dissociate from binding protein and diffuse into extracellular tissues is an efficient one that allows tight control of peripheral metabolic activities. Most T_3 is peripherally derived from the deiodination of T_4, which takes place largely in the plasma and liver. Other deiodination processes are found in the central nervous system, especially the pituitary gland and brain tissues, as well as in brown adipose tissue. Peripheral conversion of T_4 to T_3 can be impaired in many clinical circumstances, such as overwhelming sepsis and malnutrition, thionamide (propylthiouracil [PTU]) use, high-dose corticosteroids, beta blockers, iodinated contrast agents, and amiodarone use resulting in thyroid imbalance (see Box 36-2).

BOX 36-1 Drugs That Affect Thyroid Hormone Serum Transport Proteins

Increased TBG Concentrations
- Estrogen
- Heroin, methadone
- Clofibrate
- 5-Fluorouracil
- Tamoxifen

Decreased TBG Concentrations
- Androgens and anabolic steroids
- Glucocorticoids
- Nicotinic acid

Interfere With Binding to TBG
- Salicylates
- Carbamazepine
- Diazepam
- Furosemide
- Sulfonylureas
- NSAIDs
- Heparin (intravenous)
- Enoxaparin

Adapted from Degroot LJ, Jameson JL: *Endocrinology*, ed 5, Philadelphia, 2005, Saunders.
NSAIDs, nonsteroidal anti-inflammatory drugs; *TBG*, thyroxine-binding globulin.

BOX 36-2 Agents That Affect Extrathyroidal Metabolism of Thyroid Hormone

Inhibit Conversion of Thyroxine to Triiodothyronine
- Propylthiouracil
- Glucocorticoids
- Propranolol
- Interleukin-6
- Iodinated contrast agents
- Amiodarone
- Clomipramine

Stimulate Thyroid Hormone Degradation
- Diphenylhydantoin
- Carbamazepine
- Phenobarbital
- Rifampin
- Ritonavir
- Sertraline

Decrease Gastrointestinal Absorption of Thyroid Hormone
- Cholestyramine
- Calcium carbonate
- Ferrous sulfate
- Sucralfate
- Aluminum hydroxide

Adapted from Degroot LJ, Jameson JL: *Endocrinology*, ed 5, Philadelphia, 2005, Saunders.

The half-life of T_3 is approximately 8 to 12 hours, and free levels disappear rapidly from the peripheral circulation. In adults, the half-life of T_4 is approximately 7 days because of the efficient and significant degree of binding to carrier proteins. Thyroid hormones generally have a slow turnover time in the peripheral circulation, and the body is ensured of at least a 7- to 10-day supply of T_4 available for peripheral metabolism.

Tests of Thyroid Function

Evaluation of the Pituitary-Thyroid Feedback Loop

Measurement of serum TSH by an ultrasensitive radioimmunoassay is an important screening test for the diagnosis of thyroid dysfunction. This assay is especially important for the delineation of hypothyroidism and hyperthyroidism from euthyroid states. Because of its sensitivity, TSH values can detect thyroid dysfunction before clinical manifestations are noted (e.g., subclinical hypothyroidism or hyperthyroidism). The sensitivity of the TSH assay is less affected by nonthyroidal disease processes and remains unaffected by changes in thyroid hormone–binding proteins.

Serum Triiodothyronine and Thyroxine Levels

Thyroid production is initially screened by measuring serum free T_4 and T_3 levels directly by radioimmunoassay. Assays for total T_4 and T_3, which measure free and protein-bound hormone, can be affected by changes in hormone production or hormone binding to serum proteins; therefore, accurate evaluation of thyroid function requires measurement of free T_4 and T_3 levels.

Calcitonin

In patients with thyroid masses and in whom multiple endocrine neoplasia type 2 (MEN2) syndrome or isolated medullary carcinoma is suspected, a baseline calcitonin level can be obtained. If there is doubt about the diagnosis, pentagastrin-stimulated or calcium-stimulated calcitonin evaluation, which is a 4- to 5-hour test, can be performed. Also, calcitonin can be used as a screening test in families with MEN2 syndrome to document clinically inapparent disease. The routine use of calcitonin determination in the workup of thyroid nodules in otherwise nonsuspicious clinical scenarios is not cost-effective and is not recommended.[5]

Radioactive Iodine Uptake

Radioactive iodine (RAI) uptake directly evaluates thyroid gland function; however, it has become less widely used because of more precise biochemical measurements of T_3, T_4, and TSH and improved thyroid ultrasonography. RAI uptake involves the oral administration of iodine-123 (^{123}I) and calculated uptake with radioscintigraphy. A normal result is 15% to 30% uptake of the radionuclide after approximately 24 hours. Many clinical situations alter the 24-hour uptake of RAI, leading to an abnormal result (Box 36-3). ^{123}I is preferable because of its shorter half-life and lesser radiation exposure with use than ^{131}I, which is used for radioablation of thyroid neoplasms. Indications for the use of radioscintigraphy include the evaluation of a solitary thyroid nodule when the initial TSH is low (Fig. 36-8), to help delineate the cause of hyperthyroidism and, detection of functioning thyroid cancer metastases after remnant iodine ablation.

Thyroid Autoantibody Levels

Thyroid antigens (thyroid-stimulating immunoglobulin, antimicrosomal and antithyroid peroxidase antibodies) are produced in autoimmune thyroid disorders, including Graves disease and Hashimoto thyroiditis. Detection of autoantibodies can be extremely important if either of these autoimmune conditions is suspected. Approximately 95% of patients with Hashimoto thyroiditis and 80% with Graves disease have detectable antimicrosomal antibodies. In Graves disease, circulating antibodies have a high affinity for TSH-R on thyroid follicular cells. Assays have greater sensitivity and may allow earlier detection of Graves disease and more accurate monitoring of the effects of thyroid medication.

BOX 36-3 Factors Affecting 24-Hour Radioactive Iodine Uptake

Increased Uptake

Hyperthyroidism—including Graves toxic nodule, thyroid hormone resistance
Nontoxic goiter—Hashimoto thyroiditis
Decreased renal clearance of iodine (renal insufficiency, severe heart failure)
Iodine deficiency (endemic or sporadic dietary, pregnancy)
TSH administration

Decreased Uptake

Hypothyroidism (primary or secondary)
TSH resistance
Thyroid hormone replacement/suppression
Iodine excess (dietary, drugs)

From Degroot LJ, Jameson JL: *Endocrinology*, ed 5, Philadelphia, 2005, Saunders.
TSH, thyroid-stimulating hormone.

DISORDERS OF THYROID METABOLISM—BENIGN THYROID DISEASE

Hypothyroidism

A delicate balance between central production and peripheral action of T_3 and T_4 is required for a euthyroid state in the periphery. Clinical hypothyroidism is usually a result of failure of the thyroid to produce sufficient hormone (i.e., primary hypothyroidism). States of limited activity or resistance to thyroid hormone in the periphery can also occur, although these are extremely rare. In many underdeveloped countries, lack of sufficient iodine intake results in a large proportion of hypothyroid conditions. In more developed countries, most cases of adult hypothyroidism are caused by Hashimoto thyroiditis, RAI therapy, or surgical removal. An increasing number of commonly used pharmacologic agents also cause primary hypothyroidism (see Boxes 36-1 and 36-2).

Metabolic Consequences of Iodine Deficiency

The chronic physiologic changes that result from a lifetime of iodine deficiency involve anatomic and metabolic alterations of varying significance. As a result of chronic deficient iodine intake, production of T_4 and T_3 is decreased, resulting in gradually increasing thyroid clearance of iodine and decreased renal excretion. Chronic preferential production of T_3 rather than T_4 and enhanced peripheral conversion of T_4 to T_3 occur. By making the production of T_3 and clearance of the metabolically active hormone as efficient as possible, clinical hypothyroidism is largely avoided by a biochemical pattern of low serum T_4 levels with elevated TSH levels and normal or above-normal levels of T_3. In the most severe cases, serum T_3 and T_4 concentrations are low, and the serum TSH level is elevated. Iodine deficiency can lead to a preventable disease termed *endemic goiter*, which in its most

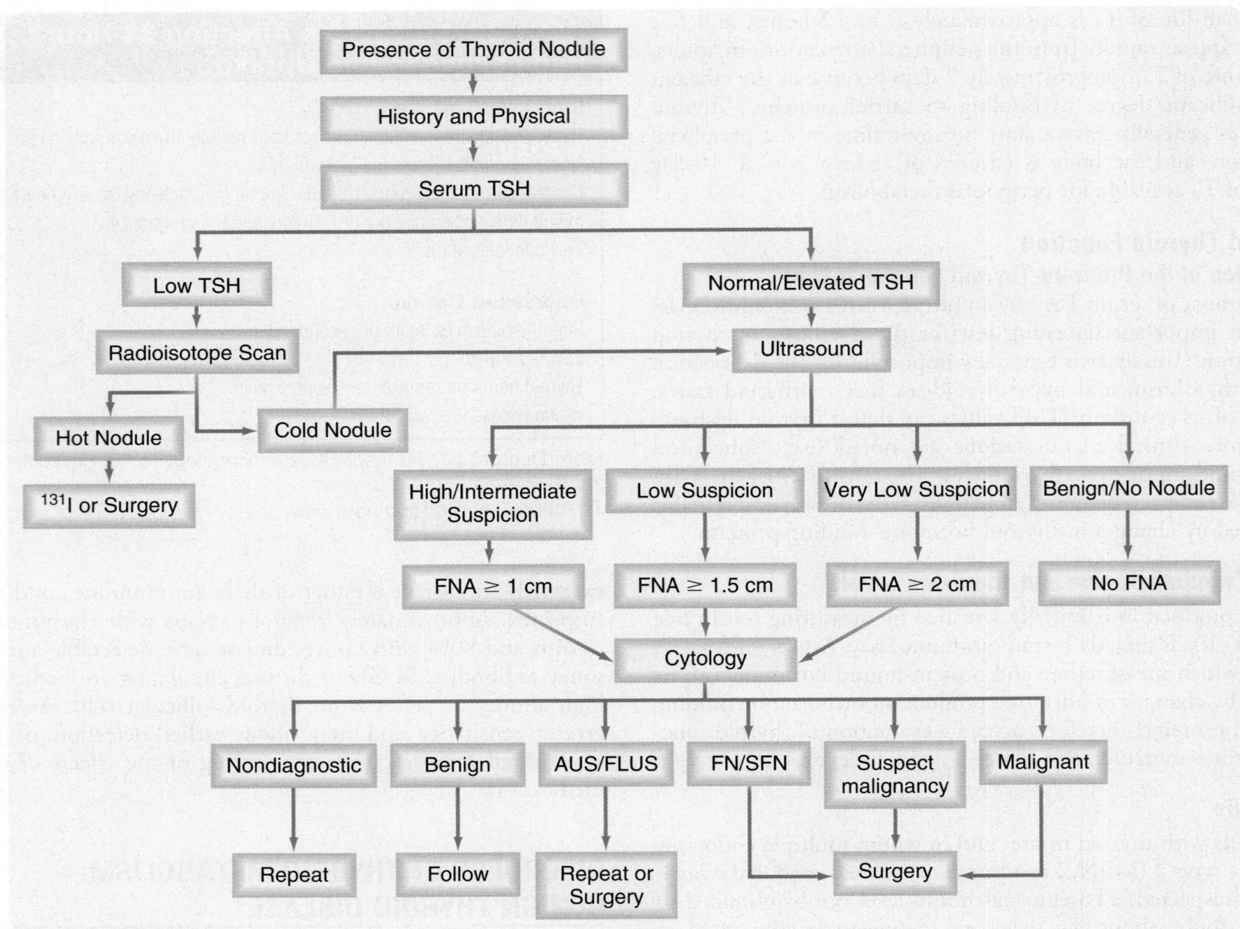

FIGURE 36-8 Workup of a thyroid nodule. *AUS*, atypia of undetermined significance; *FLUS*, follicular lesion of undetermined significance; *FN*, follicular neoplasm; *FNA*, fine-needle aspiration biopsy; *SFN*, suspicious for follicular neoplasm; *TSH*, thyroid-stimulating hormone.

severe form results in endemic cretinism. This clinical scenario includes neurologic impairment, stunted growth, mental deficiency, and overt hypothyroidism caused by profound iodine deficiency in utero.

Although countries in Southeast Asia, including India, Indonesia, and China, account for most of the total population of the world at risk for iodine deficiency (approximately 12 million), mild to moderate iodine deficiency can still be seen in many European countries, including Italy, Spain, Hungary, and Poland. In areas with the most severe iodine deficiency, clinical signs and symptoms of goiter appear at an earlier age.

The prevalence of goiter increases dramatically in the later childhood years, with a peak at puberty. The incidence decreases during adulthood but remains slightly higher in women. Diffuse enlargement of the thyroid gland often occurs, accompanying the physiologic changes in response to iodine deficiency. Thyroid follicles demonstrate a hypertrophic response, with a reduction in follicular spaces. As iodine deficiency becomes more severe, follicles can become inactive and distended with colloid. Focal areas of nodular hyperplasia may develop and form nodules, some of which may become hot nodules and have an autonomous function. Others become inactive and inert. Necrosis, scarring, and hemorrhage can occur and result in fibrous ingrowth; all these disorders are accompanied by marked enlargement of the gland, often in an asymmetrical pattern.

Postradiation Hypothyroidism

Planned clinical hypothyroidism can be the result of treatment of certain disorders by ^{131}I. This treatment has become increasingly popular for patients with hyperthyroid conditions, especially Graves disease and toxic multinodular goiter. Of patients who receive more than 10 mCi, 50% to 70% are at risk of becoming clinically hypothyroid. For patients undergoing this type of treatment, continued thyroid monitoring is necessary, at least on an annual basis. External-beam mediastinal radiation for lymphoma or for head and neck cancer is associated with subclinical hypothyroidism, particularly in patients who have previously undergone thyroid resection for a benign or malignant disease process.

Postsurgical Hypothyroidism

If ^{131}I therapy is not utilized for patients with hyperthyroidism or Graves disease, subtotal or total thyroidectomy effectively produces hypothyroidism. The incidence of permanent postoperative hypothyroidism varies with the skill of the operating surgeon and amount of thyroid that is ablated. The rate of complications, such as RLN damage and hypocalcemia, is increased with more aggressive surgical ablation. Other factors affecting postoperative development of hypothyroidism include antithyroid drug administration, dietary iodine availability, and lymphocytic infiltration of the remaining tissue.

Pharmacologic Hypothyroidism

Antithyroid drugs. If administered in excess, methimazole and PTU can cause hypothyroidism. Careful monitoring of patients taking these drugs is mandatory as well as understanding the disease process for which the drugs are given.

Amiodarone, lithium, interferon-α, interleukin-2, antineoplastic drugs. Most drugs cause hypothyroidism by interfering with thyroid hormone release from the gland or direct toxicity to the thyroid itself. The commonly used antiarrhythmic, amiodarone, is iodine-rich, containing 37% iodine by weight. Patients taking amiodarone receive a 50-fold to 100-fold excess of iodine daily. In 14% to 18% of patients treated with amiodarone, there is clinically apparent thyroid dysfunction, which can be a hyperthyroid or hypothyroid state. Amiodarone-induced thyrotoxicosis occurs more frequently in populations that are iodine-depleted at baseline, whereas in the United States, an area of higher iodine intake, hypothyroidism predominates.[7]

Although amiodarone-induced thyrotoxicosis is rare in the United States, it represents a clinical challenge when it occurs. The presentation often is not of typical hyperthyroidism, but rather patients may present with an exacerbation of the cardiac disease that is being treated with amiodarone. Depending on the specific presentation, treatment of amiodarone-induced thyrotoxicosis may include discontinuation of amiodarone, administration of methimazole or glucocorticoids, and potassium perchlorate. In cases in which amiodarone withdrawal is not feasible and medical therapy is unsuccessful, total thyroidectomy may be indicated.[7]

Lithium, used to treat bipolar disorder, inhibits the cAMP-dependent pathway of hormone formation and may inhibit the formation of thyroid hormone. Hypothyroidism in patients taking lithium is seen more frequently in patients with underlying Hashimoto thyroiditis, although it can occur in patients with normal thyroid function.

Hypothyroidism can develop in patients undergoing treatment with interferon-α or interleukin-2 for hepatitis. It can also occur in patients receiving treatment for malignancy with antineoplastic agents such as alemtuzumab, sunitinib, and sorafenib. In particular, patients with underlying Hashimoto thyroiditis are at higher risk of thyroid disruption while taking these drugs.

Diagnosis

If primary hypothyroidism is suspected based on the clinical scenario, serum TSH and free T_4 levels should be assessed. These laboratory tests demonstrate low free T_4 and elevated TSH levels.

Treatment

Levothyroxine is a safe and effective treatment for hypothyroidism after diagnosis. It is available in oral, intramuscular, and intravenous preparations. Most patients can be treated with oral medication once daily. The initial dose is calculated according to the patient's weight. Patients with severe clinical hypothyroidism are monitored closely and gradually started on increasing doses because of sensitivity to the hormone as a result of chronic depletion of catecholamines in the myocardium, especially in older patients and patients with a history of cardiac disease.

Thyroiditis

Hashimoto Thyroiditis

The major cause of hypothyroidism in adults is Hashimoto thyroiditis, autoimmune-mediated destruction of thyrocytes. The disorder predominates in women (4 to 10 : 1). A complex immunologic phenomenon results in the formation of immune complexes and complement in the basement membrane of follicular cells. Alterations in thyroid cell function result that impair T_3 and T_4 production. These cellular reactions ultimately result in the infiltration of lymphocytes and resultant fibrosis, which decreases the number and efficiency of individual follicles. As this immune phenomenon continues, the presence of TSH-blocking antibodies, such as thyroid peroxidase antibodies, can be detected. Thyroid peroxidase antibodies are probable key mediators in the initial complement fixation process. As the immune process continues, thyroid function can be altered by levels of these antibodies. Ultimately, a clinical hypothyroid state can occur in patients with persistent TSH-blocking antibodies.

Acute Suppurative Thyroiditis

Acute suppurative thyroiditis is extremely rare and is usually the result of a severe pyogenic infection of the upper airway. It may be related to a pyriform sinus fistula or other congenital anomaly. The process results in severe localized pain and is generally unilateral. The most common organisms are *Staphylococcus* species including methicillin-resistant *Staphylococcus aureus* and *Streptococcus* species. Abscess drainage followed by the administration of antibiotics is effective, and long-term deleterious effects on thyroid function are rare.

Subacute Thyroiditis

Subacute thyroiditis occurs predominantly in women (2 : 1) in the United States, England, and Japan. The mean age of patients is in the 40s in most series. The exact cause is unknown, although it is believed to have a viral or autoimmune origin. In most patients, a history of an upper respiratory infection before the onset of thyroiditis can be elicited. Patients have diffuse swelling in the cervical area and a sudden increase in pain. Approximately two thirds of patients have fever, weight loss, and severe fatigue. Fine-needle aspiration (FNA) can be diagnostic if it demonstrates giant cells of an epithelioid foreign body type, which characterize the lesion. Microscopic pathology shows large follicles infiltrated by mononuclear cells, neutrophils, and lymphocytes. Treatment with corticosteroids or nonsteroidal anti-inflammatory drugs (NSAIDs) is effective in relieving symptoms. However, the disease process generally continues, unaffected by these medications.

Riedel Struma

Riedel thyroiditis (struma) is a rare entity characterized by a firm thyroid secondary to a chronic inflammatory process involving the entire gland. Symptoms of severe discomfort can occur because of extension into the trachea, esophagus, and laryngeal nerve. As a result, patients may have impending airway obstruction or dysphagia. Unilateral involvement of symptoms may suggest a malignancy and lead to surgical intervention. The findings at surgery can also be impressive because the process can extend into the trachea and esophagus, with the obliteration of anatomic planes and landmarks. Surgical pathology reveals dense fibrous tissue and almost total obliteration of normal follicular architecture. Grossly, direct involvement of the process can result in severe tracheal and esophageal obstruction.

Treatment with thyroid hormone replacement, corticosteroids, or tamoxifen may be effective. Immediate tracheal or esophageal obstruction may require a surgical approach to relieve symptoms. Surgery should be performed by an experienced thyroid surgeon. No consensus exists on the surgical management of this rare disease, but, in general, only the constricting portion of the thyroid is removed.

Hyperthyroidism

Disease processes associated with increased thyroid secretion result in a predictable hypermetabolic state. Increased thyroid secretion can be caused by primary alterations within the gland (e.g., Graves disease, toxic nodular goiter, toxic thyroid adenoma) or central nervous system disorders and increased TSH-produced stimulation of the thyroid. Most hyperthyroid states occur because of primary malfunction. Even more unusual hyperthyroid states can result from mismanaged exogenous thyroid ingestion, molar pregnancy with increased release of hCG, and, very unusually, thyroid malignancy with overproduction of thyroid hormone. Classic symptoms of hyperthyroidism or thyrotoxicosis include sweating, unintentional weight loss despite increased appetite, heat intolerance, increased thirst, menstrual disturbance, anxiety, diarrhea, palpitations, hair loss, and sleep disturbance. More severe signs of thyrotoxicosis are high-output cardiac failure, congestive heart failure with peripheral edema, and arrhythmias such as ventricular tachycardia and atrial fibrillation.

Hyperthyroid Disorders

Graves disease. Graves disease is the most common cause of hyperthyroidism (diffuse toxic goiter). This disease entity was originally described by Graves, an Irish physician, in 1835. Women between the ages of 20 and 40 years are most commonly affected. Hyperthyroidism in Graves disease is caused by stimulatory autoantibodies to TSH-R. Although several theories about the stimulus that initiates production of these antibodies have been proposed, there is no universal agreement about the cause of the process. Genetic susceptibility to this disease is possible, as evidenced by the increased probability of Graves disease in monozygotic twins.[8] Graves disease generally manifests with the following classic triad of complaints: (1) signs and symptoms of thyrotoxicosis, (2) a visibly enlarged neck mass consistent with a goiter that may demonstrate an audible bruit secondary to increased vascular flow, and (3) exophthalmos. Tracheal compression can result in symptoms of airway obstruction, although acute compression with respiratory distress is exceedingly rare.

The ocular consequences of prolonged and untreated thyrotoxicosis, such as proptosis, supraorbital and infraorbital swelling, and conjunctival swelling and edema, can be severe. The ophthalmopathy is believed to be caused by stimulation of the overexpressed TSH-R in the retro-orbital tissues of patients with Graves disease. In its most severe form, spasm of the upper eyelid, resulting in retraction and visualization of a larger amount of sclera than normal, can lead to lid lag and exacerbation of the already swollen conjunctiva. All these pressure-related phenomena can progress to decreased oculomuscular movements, ophthalmoplegia, and diplopia. Optic nerve damage and blindness can be a long-term consequence if the underlying condition is not corrected; however, this is rarely seen with improved screening assays that detect Graves disease at early stages. Sustained hyperthyroidism is treated aggressively to remove the stimulus to the retro-orbital tissues.

Toxic nodular goiter and toxic adenoma. Toxic nodular goiter, also known as Plummer disease, refers to a nodule contained in an otherwise goitrous thyroid gland that has autonomous function. Increased thyroid hormone production occurs independently of TSH control. Patients generally have a milder course and are older than patients with Graves disease. The thyroid in these patients may be diffusely enlarged or associated with retrosternal goiters. Initial symptoms are mild, peripheral thyroid hormone levels are elevated, and TSH levels are suppressed.

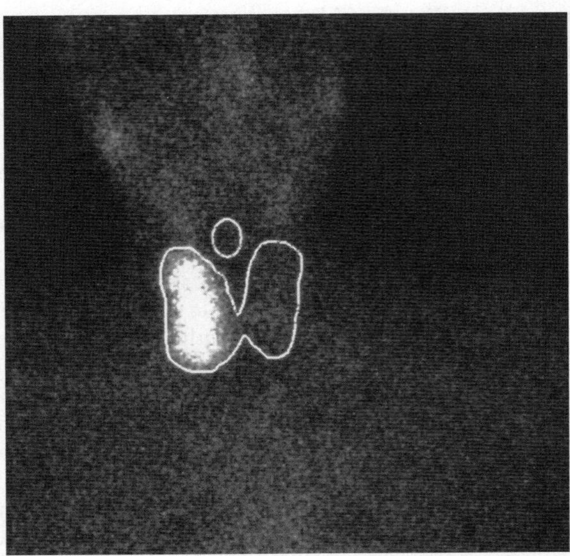

FIGURE 36-9 ^{131}I scan demonstrating an area of increased uptake in the right lobe of a 32-year-old woman with increased thyroid function test values and a palpable nodule. This scan is consistent with a toxic or hyperfunctioning nodule.

Antithyroid antibody levels are usually not detected. The diagnosis is generally confirmed after clinical suspicion, and an RAI scan is performed to localize one or two autonomous areas of function while the rest of the gland is suppressed (Fig. 36-9). Toxic nodular goiter can be treated with thionamides, RAI therapy, or surgery; the latter two are preferred because these nodules rarely resolve with prolonged thionamide therapy. RAI is widely used for patients with toxic adenomas, and most patients are euthyroid after RAI therapy because the RAI preferentially accumulates in hyperfunctioning nodules. The surrounding normal thyroid is not RAI avid because the TSH is suppressed. When resection is chosen for therapy, the surgical approach is lobectomy or near-total thyroidectomy, particularly when clinical symptoms are pronounced. In the case of a single hyperfunctioning adenoma, lobectomy is generally curative.

Diagnosis. An enlarged smooth thyroid mass and signs and symptoms of thyrotoxicosis suggest the diagnosis of hyperthyroidism. A cost-effective workup includes an extensive history, physical examination, and thyroid function tests. In addition to elevated levels of T_3 and T_4, a decreased or undetectable level of TSH is demonstrated. Depending on the cause of the hyperthyroidism, thyroid antibodies may or may not be elevated. In Graves disease, an ^{123}I radionuclide scan demonstrates elevated uptake throughout an enlarged gland versus an isolated area of increased uptake in a hyperfunctioning nodule versus low uptake in exogenous thyroid misuse or thyroiditis. Ultrasound or CT scan of the neck can be performed to evaluate clinical landmarks if needed for surgical planning, although caution is required in the administration of intravenous contrast agents if hyperthyroidism is untreated.

Treatment. When a diagnosis of hyperthyroidism has been made, therapy is initiated rapidly to ameliorate symptoms and decrease thyroid hormone synthesis. Multiple therapeutic modalities are effective, and the selection of which agents to use depends on the degree of thyrotoxicosis and other patient factors.

Patients with thyrotoxicosis have increased adrenergic stimulation. The peripheral adrenergic effects of thyrotoxicosis can be modulated by the use of beta-blocking agents such as propranolol, which should be initiated particularly in patients with tachycardia and in elderly patients. Beta blockers do not directly inhibit thyroid hormone synthesis. Although adrenergic symptoms such as an increased pulse rate, tremor, and anxiety can be improved, the hypermetabolic state can remain or progress with beta blocker treatment alone.

The thionamide class of antithyroid drugs includes PTU and methimazole (Tapazole). This class of drugs effectively blocks synthesis of thyroid hormone and acts by inhibiting the organification of intrathyroid iodine as well as the coupling of iodotyrosine molecules to form T_3 and T_4 (see Fig. 36-7). Methimazole is preferred over PTU except for during the first trimester of pregnancy and in life-threatening thyroid storm for the treatment of hyperthyroidism because it can reverse hyperthyroidism more quickly, can be dosed once daily, and has fewer concerns for hepatotoxicity. Both drugs can cause agranulocytosis, but this occurs in less than 1% of cases. Other side effects include rash, arthralgias, neuritis, and liver dysfunction (potentially worse with PTU).

Exogenous corticosteroids can effectively suppress the pituitary-thyroid axis. Also, they act in the periphery to inhibit the peripheral conversion of T_4 to T_3; this effectively lowers serum T_3 levels, allowing steroids to be used as a rapid inhibitory agent for hyperthyroid conditions. Steroids can also lower serum TSH concentration. The rapid action of steroids makes them a potentially important primary treatment of severe, previously untreated, or resistant hyperthyroidism, usually in conjunction with supportive care and the other above-mentioned agents.

Iodine, given in large doses in the form of SSKI or Lugol solution after the administration of an antithyroid medication, can inhibit thyroid hormone release by altering the organic binding process (Wolff-Chaikoff effect). This effect is transient, but iodine supplementation can be used to treat hyperactivity of the gland in preparation for surgery.

Following initial medical therapy, a decision must be made about long-term management of the hyperthyroid state. In conditions such as Graves disease, in which hyperthyroidism is expected to persist, several options exist for definitive control. Some patients may opt for medical therapy alone. In patients treated with thionamides alone, after 1 to 2 years of treatment, approximately one third of patients may be able to stop medication and have a long-term remission of their Graves disease. However, these medications are problematic, and a more definitive ablation of Graves disease via RAI or thyroidectomy is recommended for most patients.

Radioiodide ablation with ^{131}I is considered by many physicians in the United States to be the therapy of choice for Graves disease. It is also a treatment option for the treatment of toxic adenoma and toxic multinodular goiter. It ablates the thyroid within 6 to 18 weeks. Patients with mild, well-tolerated hyperthyroidism can safely proceed to RAI ablation immediately. However, patients who are older or severely thyrotoxic may require pretreatment with a thionamide. The overall cure rate with RAI is 90%. Hypothyroidism develops in cured individuals—hence the need for careful measurement of thyroid hormone and TSH levels at regular intervals after therapy. Most patients are candidates for RAI; exceptions include women who are pregnant or lactating or patients with a suspicious nodule.

Advantages of ^{131}I therapy include avoidance of surgery and the associated risks of RLN damage, hypoparathyroidism, or postsurgical recurrence. The use of ^{131}I therapy might be more cost-effective over time, but the financial advantage is not as clear if repeated ^{131}I therapy is needed. Additional disadvantages include exacerbation of cardiac arrhythmias, particularly in older patients, possible fetal damage in pregnant women, worsening ophthalmic problems, and rare but possibly life-threatening thyroid storm.

Practice patterns have varied, but thyroidectomy as a first-line treatment for Graves disease is again gaining popularity in the United States, at least in some centers.[9] Patients most typically considered candidates for thyroidectomy in the setting of Graves disease include patients with large goiters, patients who are pregnant or may become pregnant within the next 6 months, breast-feeding mothers, patients with a thyroid nodule concerning for malignancy, patients with concomitant hyperparathyroidism needing operative intervention, and patients with social factors that would expose family members to RAI. Ophthalmopathy may be transiently worsened by RAI therapy, and it may be the case that surgery more rapidly stabilizes ophthalmopathy. Patient and physician preferences also play an important role in this decision. Patients who have Graves disease refractory to RAI also should be considered for thyroidectomy. Advantages of surgical ablation of the thyroid include rapid, effective treatment of thyrotoxicosis without the necessity for long-term antithyroid medications and their potential side effects. The amount of residual tissue is a subject of some debate. Complete ablation of thyroid tissue requires total thyroidectomy, which is associated with the highest rates of hypoparathyroidism and RLN damage but also has the lowest likelihood of recurrent Graves disease. Other subtotal resections include near-total thyroidectomy or subtotal thyroidectomy. We favor total or near-total thyroidectomy.

Thyrotoxicosis must be managed medically before thyroidectomy. TSH may remain suppressed, but tachycardia and other clinical thyrotoxic symptoms must be controlled, and the circulating levels of thyroid hormone ideally should be within normal range. If the patient is not properly treated preoperatively, thyroid storm can be life-threatening. This complication is rarely encountered if appropriately anticipated. Thyroid storm is manifested by severe tachycardia, fever, confusion, vomiting to the point of dehydration, and adrenergic overstimulation to the point of mania and coma after thyroid resection in a patient with uncontrolled hyperthyroidism. Treatment of a patient with overt thyroid storm includes rapid fluid replacement and institution of antithyroid drugs, beta blockers, iodine solutions, and steroids. In life-threatening circumstances, plasmapheresis or plasma exchange may be effective in reducing T_4 and T_3 levels.

Nonfunctioning Goiter

Multinodular Goiter

The term *multinodular goiter* describes an enlarged, diffusely heterogeneous thyroid gland. Initial findings include diffuse enlargement, but asymmetric nodularity of the mass often develops. The cause of this mass is usually iodine deficiency. Initially, the mass is euthyroid, but with increasing size, elevations in T_3 and T_4 levels can occur and gradually progress to clinical hyperthyroidism. The workup and diagnosis involve evaluation of thyroid function test results. Ultrasound and radioisotopic scanning demonstrate heterogeneous thyroid substance. Nodules with poor uptake can appear as lesions suggestive of malignancy. The incidence of carcinoma in multinodular goiter has been reported to be 5% to 10%. FNA for diagnosis and resection for suspicious lesions should be strongly considered.

Substernal Goiter

A substernal goiter is an intrathoracic extension of an enlarged thyroid that generally occurs as a result of multinodular goiter.

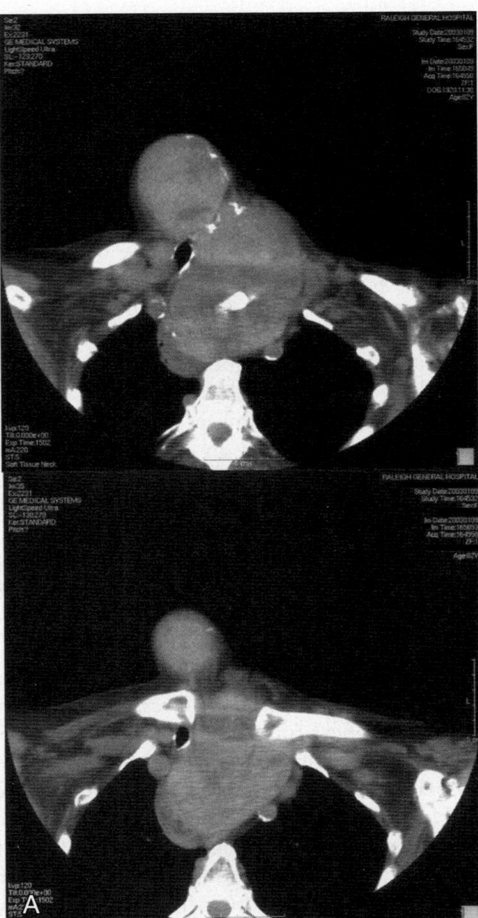

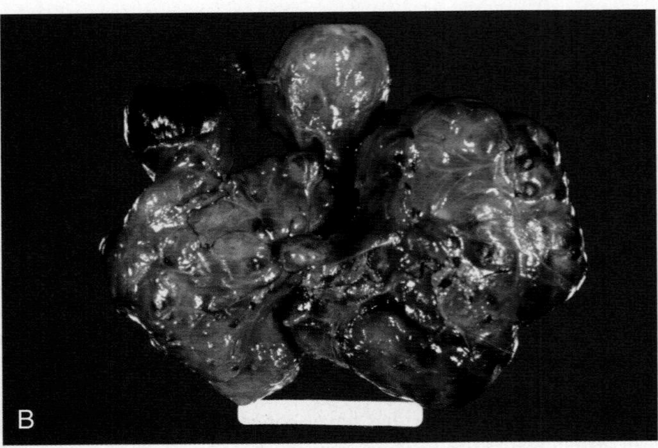

FIGURE 36-10 **A,** Computed tomography scan at the level of the thoracic inlet demonstrating a heterogeneous, large thyroid mass that involves both lobes of the thyroid and displaces the trachea. It has extended into the anterior mediastinum. This patient ultimately proved to have a large multinodular goiter. **B,** Gross picture of the resected multinodular goiter.

Most intrathoracic or substernal goiters are termed secondary because they are enlargements or extensions of multinodular goiters based on the inferior thyroid vasculature. They expand downward into the anterior mediastinum (Fig. 36-10). The rare (approximately 1%) primary substernal goiter arises as aberrant thyroid tissue within the anterior or posterior mediastinum; it is based on the intrathoracic vasculature and not supplied by the inferior thyroid artery.

EVALUATION OF A THYROID NODULE

A thyroid nodule is a discrete and radiographically definable lesion within the thyroid. Many thyroid nodules are not palpable, and not all palpable thyroid lesions correspond to a distinct radiographically definable lesion. Only findings truly definable radiographically may be classified as a thyroid nodule. Although thyroid nodules are common, most do not require any intervention, and only a few require thyroid resection. The ultimate decision to proceed to surgical intervention after detection of a thyroid nodule depends on the findings of a structured and cost-effective workup (see Fig. 36-8). The algorithm may appear complicated, but it is simplified by keeping a focus on the fact that ultimately there are three classes of indication for thyroid resection: (1) local compressive or inflammatory symptoms, (2) hyperfunction, and (3) malignancy or concern for malignancy. The structured workup systematically addresses these issues. Most patients with a solitary thyroid nodule have an asymptomatic, nonfunctioning, benign lesion; however, thyroid cancer must be considered in all patients. Deciding between conservative management and surgical therapy relies on careful analysis of the clinical findings, risk assessment, imaging, and diagnostic testing. The content of the 2015 revision of the American Thyroid Association guidelines is reflected in this chapter and serves to guide the practice of many medical thyroidologists and thyroid surgeons.[5]

Incidence

Increasing numbers of thyroid nodules are being found incidentally, possibly because of the increasing availability and sophistication of imaging techniques. Palpable thyroid nodules are present in 1% of men and 5% of women, and ultrasound-detectable thyroid nodules are present in 19% to 67% of unselected patients. The frequency of palpable and nonpalpable thyroid nodules increases with age. Most of these nodules are benign, but overall approximately 5% are thyroid cancers.[5]

Initial Evaluation

The workup of a patient with a solitary nodule begins with a careful history and physical examination. Clinical evidence of hyperthyroidism should be evaluated on the history and physical examination. The physician should enquire about local symptoms including dysphagia, subjective dyspnea, positional dyspnea, pressure or choking sensation, pain, globus sensation, or symptoms precipitated by raising the arms over the head (a subjective Pemberton sign).

An important part of the evaluation focuses on risk factors for malignancy. The highest risk for malignancy in a thyroid nodule exists in children, male patients, adults younger than 30 or older than 60 years, and patients exposed to radiation. The examiner should seek a thorough history of exposure to radiation, either through occupational sources or through therapeutic irradiation of the head or neck, especially during childhood. A personal and family history should be assessed for specific endocrine disorders, including familial medullary carcinoma, MEN2, PTC, or a history of polyposis, including Gardner syndrome or Cowden syndrome.

The physical examination of the thyroid requires an understanding of the location of the thyroid. It is not unusual for a reported thyroid nodule on physical examination to represent normal anatomy, such as laryngeal cartilage or ptotic salivary glands. This type of error is readily avoided. We start the examination by palpating the cricoid ring because the isthmus is reliably palpable immediately inferior to this. The bilateral lobes may be palpated directly lateral to this. We advocate standing on the contralateral side and slightly behind the patient to examine each lobe, placing both hands around the neck with the fingers of each hand sliding laterally off of the isthmus, displacing the sternocleidomastoid muscle laterally and lying directly over the thyroid lobe. Giving the patient a sip of water at this point causes the thyroid to move under the examining fingers with swallowing. This maneuver can reveal many lesions not appreciable by static palpation. It also allows the opportunity to appreciate if a substernal goiter may be "trapped" above the clavicular heads with swallowing. In all patients with thyroid pathology, the anterior and posterior cervical triangles should be assessed for pathologic lymphadenopathy. When a thyroid nodule is detected on physical examination, the size and consistency of the nodule should be determined. Multiple nodules and diffuse nodularity are more often associated with a benign diagnosis, whereas a firm solitary nodule, particularly in older men, is more suggestive of malignancy. It sometimes is possible to determine if a nodule is adherent to surrounding muscle, which would be concerning for malignancy. Nodules that are present on ultrasound but not palpable on physical examination have the same size-adjusted risk of malignancy as nodules that are palpable. Rapid growth and clinical indicators of potential invasion, such as pain or hoarseness, are suggestive, but not diagnostic, of malignancy.

Other important aspects of the history and physical examination focus on the suitability of the patient for operative intervention. The neck range of motion should be demonstrated, and all items related to the patient's risk of perioperative adverse events should be evaluated.

Laboratory Evaluation

Thyroid function tests can identify patients with unsuspected hyperthyroid states and dictate the appropriate workup (see Fig. 36-8). If a thyroid nodule 1 cm or larger is identified, serum TSH should be tested. Low serum TSH denotes overt or subclinical hyperthyroidism, and a radioisotope scan generally is indicated. Low serum TSH also correlates with a lower likelihood of malignancy in a thyroid nodule, and thyroid cancers are rarely thyrotoxic.[10] High serum TSH suggests hypothyroidism, most commonly the result of Hashimoto thyroiditis.

Serum Tg is important in the follow-up of patients after initial treatment of thyroid cancer but should not be checked routinely in the initial evaluation of a thyroid nodule. When there is clinical suspicion of medullary carcinoma, either by family history or by FNA, the serum calcitonin level should be measured; however, few data support the routine measurement of calcitonin in the workup of a thyroid nodule, and we do not routinely obtain this test.[5]

Thyroid Imaging

Ultrasound

Ultrasound imaging is central to the evaluation of most thyroid nodules. All nonthyrotoxic nodules should be evaluated with a diagnostic ultrasound scan (see Fig. 36-8). Ultrasound uses a high-frequency probe in the 7.5- to 16-MHz range. Ultrasound is portable and available to use in the clinic and the operating room in addition to the radiology suite and may be used successfully by radiologists, surgeons, and medical endocrinologists. Ultrasound is viewed by many physicians as an extension of the physical examination and is commonly used to assist in FNA.

Advantages of ultrasound over other imaging modalities include portability, cost-effectiveness, and lack of ionizing radiation. It is extremely useful in patients who are being managed conservatively because it can reproducibly determine whether a nodule has increased in size or has suspicious characteristics. Ultrasound findings within a nodule that are considered suspicious for malignancy include microcalcifications, hypervascularity, infiltrative margins, being hypoechoic compared with surrounding parenchyma, and having a shape that is taller than its width on transverse view (Table 36-1).[11] Patterns of sonographic features may be used to classify a given thyroid nodule as having high, intermediate, low, or very low suspicion for malignancy (Fig. 36-11 and Table 36-2). A purely cystic lesion with no solid component may be classified as benign. When combined with the size of the nodule, these characteristics can be used to guide decisions to proceed with FNA biopsy.

When a thyroid nodule is detected, it also is appropriate to evaluate the central and lateral neck sonographically for pathologic adenopathy. If pathologic nodes are detected, biopsy may be targeted to the pathologic node. If metastatic thyroid cancer is found in a node, surgical planning may proceed from there.

TABLE 36-1 Ultrasonographic Features Associated With Thyroid Carcinoma

IMAGING FEATURE	SENSITIVITY (%)	SPECIFICITY (%)	PPV (%)	NPV (%)
Microcalcifications	26-59	86-95	24-71	42-94
Hypoechogenicity	27-87	43-94	11-68	74-94
Irregular margins or no halo	17-78	39-85	9-60	39-98
Solid	69-75	53-56	16-27	88-92
Intranodular vascularity	54-74	79-81	24-42	86-97
More tall than wide	33	93	67	75

From Frates MC, Benson CB, Charboneau JW, et al: Management of thyroid nodules detected at US: Society of Radiologists in Ultrasound consensus conference statement. *Radiology* 237:794–800, 2005.
NPV, negative predictive value; *PPV*, positive predictive value.

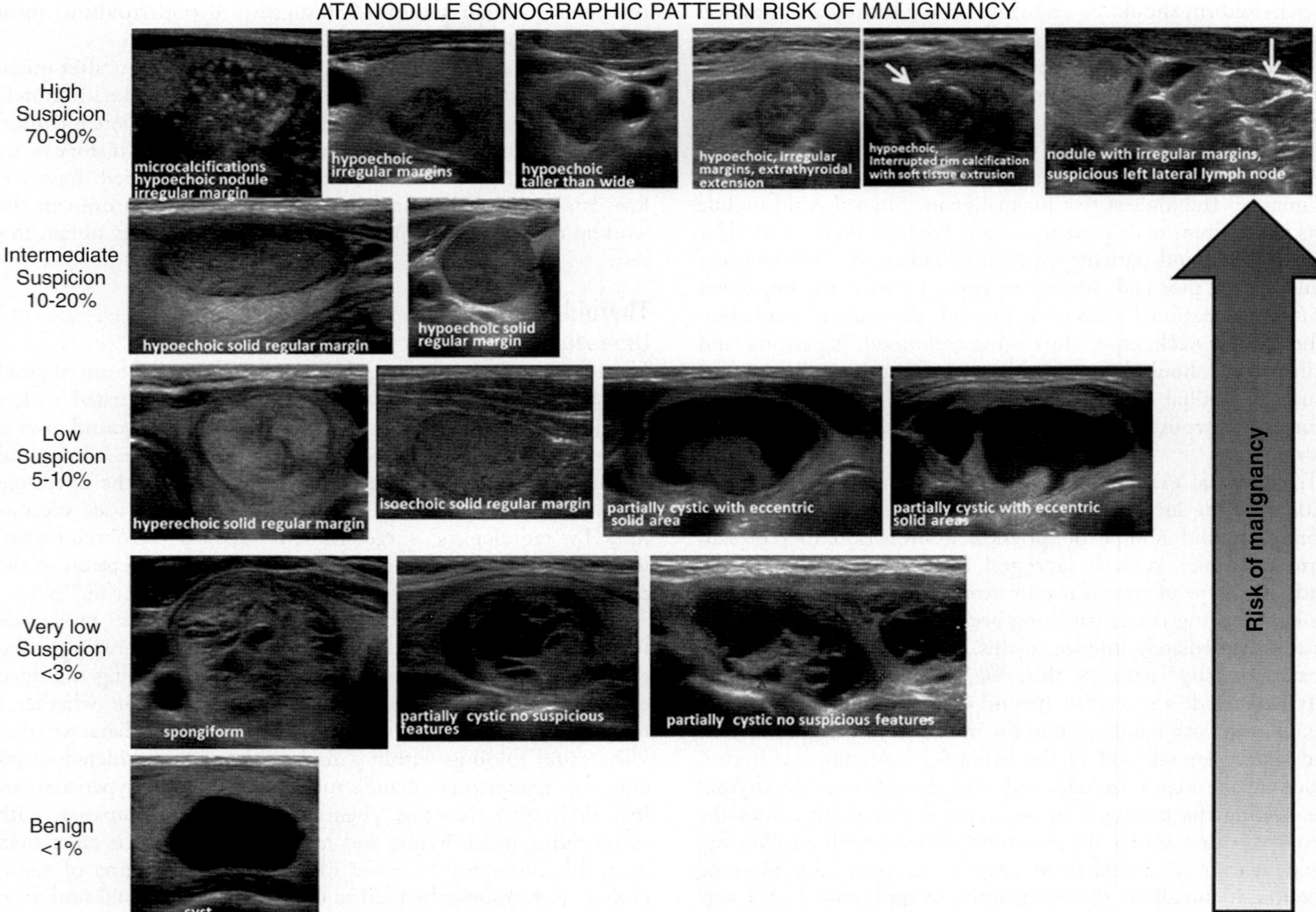

FIGURE 36-11 American Thyroid Association (ATA) nodule sonographic patterns and risk of malignancy. (From Haugen BR, Alexander EK, Bible KC, et al: 2015 American Thyroid Association management guidelines for patients with thyroid nodules and differentiated thyroid cancer. *Thyroid* [Epub ahead of print; 2015].)

TABLE 36-2 American Thyroid Association Sonographic Patterns and Estimated Risk of Malignancy for Thyroid Nodules

SONOGRAPHIC PATTERN	SONOGRAPHIC FEATURES	ESTIMATED RISK OF MALIGNANCY (%)	CONSIDER BIOPSY
High suspicion	Solid hypoechoic nodule or solid hypoechoic component of a partially cystic nodule *with* one or more of the following features: irregular margins (infiltrative, microlobulated), microcalcifications, taller than wide shape, rim calcifications with small extrusive soft tissue component, evidence of extrathyroidal extension	>70-90*	≥1 cm
Intermediate suspicion	Hypoechoic solid nodule with smooth margins *without* microcalcifications, extrathyroidal extension, or taller than wide shape	10-20	≥1 cm
Low suspicion	Isoechoic or hyperechoic solid nodule or partially cystic nodule with eccentric solid areas *without* microcalcification, irregular margin or extrathyroidal extension, or taller than wide shape	5-10	≥1.5 cm
Very low suspicion	Spongiform or partially cystic nodules *without* any of the sonographic features described in low, intermediate, or high suspicion patterns	<3	≥2 cm
Benign	Purely cystic nodules (no solid component)	<1	No biopsy†

From Haugen BR, Alexander EK, Bible KC, et al: 2015 American Thyroid Association management guidelines for patients with thyroid nodules and differentiated thyroid cancer. *Thyroid* (Epub ahead of print; 2015).

*The estimate is derived from high-volume centers; the overall risk of malignancy may be lower given interobserver variability in sonography.

†Aspiration of the cyst may be considered for symptomatic or cosmetic drainage. Ultrasound-guided fine-needle aspiration should be considered for lymph nodes that are sonographically suspicious for thyroid cancer.

Ultrasound elastography is a promising technique that may prove to have utility in risk stratification of sonographically detected thyroid nodules. Ultrasound elastography requires an appropriately configured device and is highly operator dependent, and not all nodules are anatomically appropriate for this technique. At the present time, this technique cannot be recommended for widespread application in the evaluation of all thyroid nodules.

Radioisotope Scanning

Ultrasound allows anatomic evaluation, whereas radionuclide scans allow assessment of thyroid function. If a dominant thyroid nodule larger than 1 cm is found to be associated with suppressed serum TSH, a diagnostic RAI scan should be obtained to determine whether the nodule is hyperfunctioning (see Figs. 36-8 and 36-9). In euthyroid or hypothyroid patients with thyroid nodules, radioisotope scanning is not indicated in the initial workup of a thyroid nodule.

Technetium 99m pertechnetate (^{99m}Tc) is taken up rapidly by the normal activity of follicular cells. It is trapped by follicular cells but not organified. ^{99m}Tc has a short half-life and low radiation dose. Its rapid absorption allows quick evaluation of increased uptake ("hot") or hypofunctioning ("cold") areas of the thyroid. Because screening with ^{99m}Tc shows uptake in the salivary glands and major vascular structures, interpretation of thyroid pathology requires expertise.

Iodine scintigraphy with ^{123}I and ^{131}I is also used to evaluate the functional status of the gland. ^{123}I and ^{131}I are trapped by active follicular cells and organified. Advantages of scanning with ^{123}I include a low dose of radiation (30 mrad) and short half-life (12 to 13 hours). ^{123}I is a good choice for evaluating suspected lingual thyroids or substernal goiters. ^{131}I has a longer half-life (8 days) and emits higher levels of β-radiation. ^{131}I is optimal for imaging thyroid carcinoma and is the screening modality of choice for the evaluation of distant metastasis. Malignancy is present in 15% to 20% of cold nodules and in less than 5% of hot nodules. Although suggestive, malignancy of a nodule can be neither confirmed nor excluded based on radionuclide uptake.

Positron emission tomography with ^{18}F-fluorodeoxyglucose (FDG-PET) is being used increasingly in benign and malignant diseases. FDG-PET does not have a role in the initial evaluation of thyroid nodules. However, 1% to 2% of PET scans obtained for other reasons identify discrete thyroid incidentalomas, and approximately 2% of patients have diffuse thyroid FDG-PET activity. Although most PET avid incidentalomas in the thyroid are benign, the incidence of malignancy in tumors that have progressed to resection is reported to be 33%.[12] Focal FDG-PET activity should prompt thyroid ultrasound and subsequent FNA biopsy if an ultrasound-detectable thyroid nodule is confirmed. Diffuse thyroid FDG-PET activity should prompt an ultrasound scan. Ultrasound findings typically are consistent with lymphocytic thyroiditis. If lymphocytic thyroiditis is clinically suspected, no further evaluation is needed for incidental diffuse thyroid FDG-PET activity.[5]

Computed Tomography and Magnetic Resonance Imaging

CT and MRI do not add significantly to the workup of uncomplicated thyroid nodules that are otherwise well characterized by ultrasound. However, either modality may be helpful in evaluating local extension in more advanced stages of thyroid cancer. CT or MRI is particularly appropriate for a suspicious mass (or biopsy-proven cancer) with bulky cervical lymph nodes. Additionally, either modality can be used for postoperative follow-up, particularly for suspicion of recurrent disease. CT is advisable in preoperative planning for larger thyroid masses that are believed to have a substernal component based on physical examination, ultrasound, or chest radiograph (see Fig. 36-10).

One concern with CT is the large iodine load associated with intravenous contrast agents. A typical chest or neck CT scan with iodinated contrast agent may deliver 15,000 to 30,000 mg of iodine to the patient. This iodine load is a particular concern in a patient with hyperthyroidism. If a patient with uncontrolled hyperthyroidism is given a large iodine load without appropriate medical management, there is the potential to trigger thyroid storm, which may be life-threatening. Another concern related to iodinated contrast agents is that patients must be iodine depleted before therapeutic RAI treatment of thyroid cancer. The large iodine load decreases the target cell avidity for further iodine uptake after iodinated contrast agent administration. In most cases, 4 weeks is adequate time for the clearance of iodine after a CT scan.[13] Because RAI ablation typically is performed more than 4 weeks after thyroidectomy, it is safe and appropriate to use CT with an intravenous contrast agent if needed to permit appropriate operative planning to achieve safe and complete resection of a thyroid cancer.[5]

Fine-Needle Aspiration Biopsy

FNA is a cost-effective and valuable tool and is a key diagnostic technique in the evaluation of thyroid nodules. The decision to perform FNA for a thyroid nodule is made based on a combination of patient factors, ultrasound characteristics, and size. In general, nodules that are less than 1 cm in greatest dimension are not evaluated further (see Fig. 36-8). Examples where further workup of nodules less than 1 cm may be indicated include nodules with suspicious characteristics on ultrasound; nodules associated with suspicious lymphadenopathy based on ultrasound or clinical examination; nodules in patients with family history of PTC, history of radiation exposure, or prior personal history of thyroid cancer; and lesions positive on FDG-PET. Otherwise, the size of the nodule may be coupled with the sonographic risk classification to determine the need for further evaluation with FNA biopsy. Patients with nodules with high-risk or intermediate-risk sonographic features should undergo FNA biopsy if the nodules are 1 cm or larger in size, patients with nodules with low-risk sonographic features should undergo FNA biopsy if the nodules are 1.5 cm or larger, and patients with nodules with very low suspicion sonographic features should undergo FNA biopsy if the nodules are 2 cm or larger. Purely cystic nodules do not require biopsy. This stratification is detailed in Figures 36-8 and 36-11 and Table 36-2.[5] If a decision already has been made for operative intervention based on patient preference or symptoms, FNA may be foregone if it would not change the plan to operate or the extent of the resection.

FNA is performed with a small-gauge needle (23 to 27 gauge) and may be performed with capillary or suction technique. Use of small-gauge needles has resulted in a marked decrease in the complication rate associated with the use of large-bore or core needle biopsies, while maintaining diagnostic accuracy. For palpable nodules, FNA biopsy may be performed without image guidance. However, ultrasound guidance may be used for FNA biopsy of palpable lesions, especially for heterogeneous lesions. Ultrasound guidance is recommended for nonpalpable, posteriorly located, or cystic nodules and results in a lower rate of nondiagnostic cytology and sampling error.

TABLE 36-3 Bethesda Criteria for Reporting Thyroid Cytopathology

BETHESDA CATEGORY	IMPLIED MALIGNANCY RATE ACCORDING TO BETHESDA SYSTEM (%)[55]	META-ANALYSIS REPORTED MALIGNANCY RATE IN EXCISED LESIONS (%) (MEDIAN)[56]	PERCENT OF FNA SPECIMENS IN META-ANALYSIS (% [RANGE])[56]	USUAL MANAGEMENT[55]
1—Nondiagnostic or unsatisfactory	1-4	17	13 (2-24)	Repeat FNA with image guidance
2—Benign	0-3	4	59 (39-74)	Clinical follow-up
3—AUS/FLUS	5-15	16	10 (1-27)	Repeat FNA or lobectomy
4—FN or SFN (specify if Hürthle cell type)	15-30	26	10 (1-25)	Lobectomy
5—Suspicious for malignancy (specify type)	60-75	75	3 (1-6)	Lobectomy or total thyroidectomy
6—Malignant (specify type)	97-99	99	5 (2-16)	Total thyroidectomy

AUS/FLUS, atypia of undetermined significance/follicular lesion of undetermined significance; *FN,* follicular neoplasm; *FNA,* fine-needle aspiration; *SFN,* suspicious for follicular neoplasm.

Results of FNA biopsy should be reported using the Bethesda System for Reporting Thyroid Cytology. Before the introduction of this system, descriptive cytology findings often could not be associated with a specific malignancy risk or management guideline. Analogous to the Breast Imaging Reporting and Data System in breast imaging, the Bethesda System standardized reporting to allow consistency in clinical decision making and in research. The six categories within the Bethesda System are summarized in Table 36-3, along with the predicted malignancy risk, the reported malignancy risk in a meta-analysis, the frequency of each category in a meta-analysis, and the typical management guidelines.

Although the Bethesda System must be understood and used by all physicians who manage patients with thyroid neoplasia, several considerations exist regarding thyroid cytopathology in general and the Bethesda System in particular. The first consideration is that FNA permits an analysis of cellular features and does not permit an analysis of tissue architecture. PTC is the most common thyroid cancer and has discrete cellular cytologic characteristics that make FNA extremely accurate in securing this particular diagnosis (Fig. 36-12). In contrast, the diagnosis of FTC is not made based on cellular features and instead is based on demonstration of capsular or vascular invasion by follicular cells. This architectural finding cannot be determined by FNA. Although FTCs do not have the same cytologic appearance as benign thyroid tissue, they often are categorized as suspicious for follicular neoplasm, and the diagnosis not made until final pathology is available.

Another issue that must be understood is sampling error. A fine needle by definition is sampling only a small portion of a lesion. Tissue immediately adjacent to or contained within another part of the nodule may harbor malignant cells. The false-negative rate of FNA has been reported to be 1% to 6%.[14] Benign nodules diagnosed based on FNA are monitored with ultrasound to ensure that their characteristics do not change, as further detailed subsequently.

Another issue with the Bethesda System is demonstrated in Table 36-3. The various diagnostic categories are used with varied frequencies in different centers, and different centers have reported variable rates of malignancy for a given category. The most troublesome category appears to be Bethesda 3, atypia of undetermined significance/follicular lesion of undetermined significance (AUS/FLUS). Ongoing efforts are required that likely will result in modification and further standardization of this system in the future.

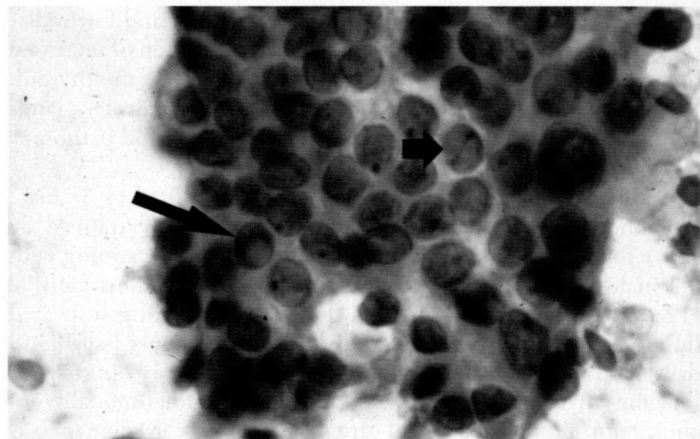

FIGURE 36-12 Fine-needle aspiration of a thyroid mass allows determination of individual cellular morphology. Cells in this aspirate demonstrate intranuclear grooving *(short arrow)* and ground-glass cytoplasmic inclusions *(long arrow)* (so-called Orphan Annie eyes). These cellular features confirm the diagnosis of papillary carcinoma of the thyroid.

Purely cystic lesions do not require FNA biopsy, but a needle may be used to aspirate the cystic fluid to relieve mass effect. Examination of most cystic fluid yields benign cytologic findings; however, an occasional papillary carcinoma can be manifested as a cyst and diagnosed by cytologic examination of cystic fluid. These lesions typically have a solid component and are not purely cystic. Cysts that have a residual mass after aspiration and cysts that are aspirated with benign cytology but then recur should be considered for resection.[5]

Patients with multiple thyroid nodules have equivalent risk of harboring malignancy as patients with a solitary nodule, but each individual nodule has lower risk than a solitary nodule. A reasonable approach for patients with multiple thyroid nodules larger than 1 cm is preferential FNA biopsy of nodules with suspicious ultrasound features. Furthermore, if radionuclide scanning demonstrates a hypofunctioning nodule in a patient with multiple nodules, FNA should be considered for the cold nodules.[5]

Decision Making and Treatment

Decision making regarding thyroid nodules depends on the structured use of the above-described modalities and consideration of the clinical setting. The three basic indications for resection of thyroid pathology must be considered in every patient. The presence of local compressive or inflammatory symptoms is largely determined by history. The presence of hyperfunction is screened by measuring serum TSH. If the patient has hyperthyroidism, a RAI uptake scan is used to guide further diagnosis and management. The evaluation for malignancy is based on clinical, ultrasound, and FNA findings as described earlier.

For a patient with a thyroid goiter and local compressive symptoms, it is appropriate to offer resection if the patient is a suitable surgical candidate. Compressive symptoms include dyspnea, wheezing, cough, dysphagia, or a pressure sensation that may be worse in the supine position. For patients with a unilateral compressive mass and a benign biopsy, thyroid lobectomy and total thyroidectomy are appropriate options. For patients with bilateral goiter or nodules, total thyroidectomy usually is recommended. Patients with Hashimoto thyroiditis may report compressive symptoms disproportionately to the size of the thyroid. Most of these patients experience relief of symptoms after thyroidectomy.[15] However, whenever operating for symptoms of compression or inflammation, the patient must be informed that some or all of his or her symptoms may not be relieved by thyroidectomy. Patients with large goiters, substernal goiters, and Hashimoto thyroiditis also should be cautioned that there is a marginally higher risk of technical complications compared with thyroidectomy performed for other indications.

The management for nodules that warrant FNA biopsy based on imaging criteria may be guided by the standard management recommendations noted in Table 36-3. In all cases, these standard guidelines also must take into account patient preference and other clinical features of the thyroid and of the patient as a whole.

A patient with a thyroid nodule with a nondiagnostic biopsy should undergo repeat FNA under image guidance and with real-time cytologic evaluation for sample adequacy. This approach results in a diagnostic specimen in 80% of such nodules. Some physicians favor waiting 3 months before repeat biopsy, but others have found waiting to be unnecessary. For patients with nodules with persistently nondiagnostic biopsy, either continued close clinical and sonographic follow-up or diagnostic lobectomy may be elected based on patient preference and concern for malignancy based on ultrasound findings.[5]

For patients with a benign FNA biopsy finding, repeat ultrasound should be performed. The interval in which to pursue repeat ultrasound may be adjusted based on ultrasound risk group (see Table 36-2). For nodules with high sonographic suspicion, repeat evaluation should be within 3 to 6 months. For nodules with low to intermediate suspicion, ultrasound should be repeated in 12 to 24 months. For nodules with very low suspicion ultrasound findings and a benign FNA specimen, it is reasonable not to repeat ultrasound; if ultrasound is repeated, it should be performed at least 2 years later. When a repeat ultrasound scan is performed for nodules with prior benign biopsy, if ultrasound shows greater than 50% change in volume or a 20% increase in two dimensions, FNA should be repeated under ultrasound guidance.[5]

For thyroid nodules with Bethesda System category 3 or 4 results, mutation testing has been explored with the hope of definitively confirming or excluding a malignancy. The two most explored approaches include testing for *BRAF* mutation and using a 167-gene messenger RNA–based gene expression classifier. These approaches are available in clinical practice and are actively used by some physicians. The goal of these tests is to avoid unnecessary surgery (e.g., diagnostic lobectomy for what proves to be benign disease) and to be able to accomplish adequate resection for malignancy in a single operation (e.g., avoided diagnostic lobectomy followed by completion thyroidectomy when final pathology demonstrates malignancy). The primary critique of these modalities is inadequate ability to rule out malignancy with an adequate negative predictive value (NPV). The current role of these tests continues to be debated at the present time. Although long-term data are unavailable, the best current use of these tests is likely to guide a patient toward a more complete resection when FNA would dictate diagnostic lobectomy, but genetic testing is indicative of a malignancy. When these tests are used, patients should be counseled carefully regarding the strengths and weaknesses, and the test results always should be interpreted with an understanding of the entire clinical picture. Although other very experienced physicians find these tests to be of great utility, we have not found them to be helpful and reliable in our practice. Based on the aforementioned considerations, the most recent American Thyroid Association guidelines do not recommend either for or against these tests.[5]

In the absence of another test to guide management, patients with indeterminate biopsy results require careful counseling because the only way at the present time for definitive diagnosis or exclusion of malignancy is a diagnostic resection. One reasonable option for a Bethesda System category 3 lesion is repeat biopsy, which frequently results in classification into a more definitive cytologic category. Other options include close observation with ultrasound surveillance versus diagnostic excision, typically in the form of a thyroid lobectomy. The decision regarding which option to pursue involves consideration of patient preference, ultrasound findings, and the whole clinical picture. If genetic testing is used to inform this discussion, the above-described considerations must be kept in mind and shared with the patient.

Bethesda System category 4 lesions typically are lesions with many follicular cells, a paucity of colloid, and absent macrophages that may demonstrate microfollicle formation and lack cytologic features of PTC. These lesions also may be considered for genetic testing, keeping in mind the above-mentioned considerations. The more time-tested approach is to pursue diagnostic excision of these lesions. For most of these lesions, an ipsilateral thyroid lobectomy is recommended. Category 4 lesions for which the standard recommendation would be total thyroidectomy rather than lobectomy include lesions that are greater than 4 cm, lesions with contralateral nodules, or lesions with other concerning clinical features such as prior significant radiation exposure. The results of genetic testing, if performed, also may sway the surgeon and the patient to pursue total thyroidectomy. As always, the extent of surgery also is affected by patient preference, and patients must be informed of the potential need for a second operation after lobectomy versus the definite need for thyroid hormone replacement and a slightly higher complication rate after total thyroidectomy. If lobectomy is performed, the patient also must accept the need for ongoing surveillance of any disease present in the contralateral lobe.

Bethesda System category 5 lesions typically are managed surgically similar to lesions with biopsy results that are diagnostic of malignancy. Category 6 lesions are diagnostic of malignancy, and the management of thyroid malignancy is further detailed subsequently.

The practice of using exogenous thyroid replacement to suppress TSH with the goal of suppressing a thyroid nodule is losing favor. It previously was believed that nodules that grew on suppressive therapy were likely malignant, whereas nodules that shrank were likely benign; this is neither sensitive nor specific because only 20% to 30% of nodules shrink on suppressive therapy, and up to 13% of proven papillary cancers in one series decreased in size on suppressive therapy. Furthermore, there are detrimental consequences to health of inducing subclinical hyperthyroidism, and the risks outweigh the potential benefit for most patients. Suppressive therapy is not considered appropriate treatment for thyroid nodules.[5]

The finding of a thyroid nodule in a child or a pregnant woman can be of particular concern to the patient, family, and referring physicians. Although the frequency of malignancy may be higher in children than in adults, the evaluation should generally proceed in the same fashion as for an adult.[5] This approach also generally holds true in pregnant patients with certain caveats, which are detailed further in "Thyroid Disease in Pregnancy."

THYROID MALIGNANCIES

Thyroid carcinoma represents 4% of all malignancies in the United States, with approximately 62,000 cases expected in 2015 and 1950 deaths predicted in 2015 resulting from thyroid cancer.[16] Greater than 75% of cases occur in women making this the fifth most common malignancy in women. Although less than 25% of thyroid carcinomas occur in men, men account for 45% of mortality from thyroid carcinoma. The incidence of PTC has been increasing rapidly in men and women, increasing 189% in the United States during the period 1973-2003 with a more recent 5.3% annual increase in men and 4.5% annual increase in women.[16,17]

Of thyroid carcinomas, 90% to 95% are categorized as DTCs that arise from follicular cells. Papillary, follicular, and Hürthle cell carcinomas are included in this category. The management of these DTCs is discussed together. MTC accounts for approximately 6% of thyroid cancers (20% to 30% of which occur on a familial basis including MEN2A and MEN2B). Anaplastic thyroid carcinoma (ATC) is an aggressive malignancy that is responsible for less than 1% of thyroid carcinomas in the United States. In the different subtypes of thyroid carcinoma, prognosis mirrors incidence in that PTC, which is the most common thyroid malignancy, also carries an excellent prognosis in most patients, whereas ATC is far less common and carries a dismal prognosis.

Thyroid Oncogenesis

Genetic Alterations

Genetic processes that lead to thyroid neoplasia include two important categories: mutated proto-oncogenes, which result in altered protein production and accelerated growth, and loss of function in growth suppression genes allowing unregulated cell growth. Most of these genetic abnormalities are acquired, but 5% to 10% of PTCs are thought to be familial. The working model for oncogenes causing papillary and follicular carcinomas is becoming better understood, and several gene categories appear to be important (Fig. 36-13 and Table 36-4).

Genetic alterations that lead to constitutive activation of mitogen-activated protein kinase (MAPK) and phosphatidylinositol-3′-kinase (PI3K)/AKT are causative in the most common forms of thyroid carcinoma. This is a downstream effect of a pathway that includes the RET and NTRK1 transmembrane proteins.

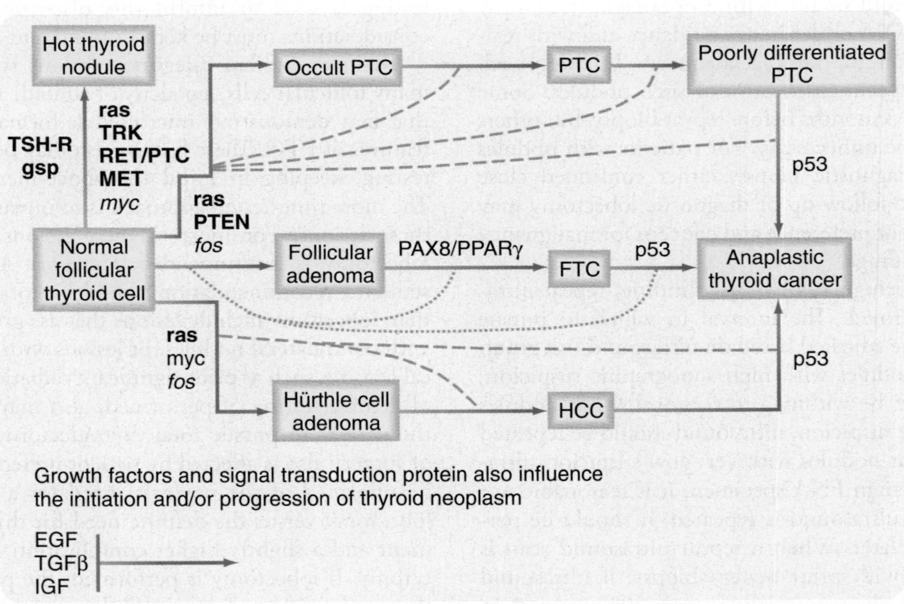

FIGURE 36-13 Genetic events that occur in thyroid oncogenesis (the main genetic events are in *bold*). The *dashed lines* for each histologic type of thyroid cancer indicate that an adenoma-to-carcinoma progression is not always the sequence of progression in carcinogenesis. *EGF,* epidermal growth factor; *FTC,* follicular thyroid carcinoma; *HCC,* Hürthle cell carcinoma; *IGF,* insulin-like growth factor; *PPARγ,* peroxisome proliferator–activated receptor γ; *PTC,* papillary thyroid carcinoma; *TGFβ,* transforming growth factor-β; *TSH-R,* thyroid-stimulating hormone receptor. (From Kebebew E: Thyroid oncogenesis. In Clark OH, editor: *Textbook of endocrine surgery,* ed 2, Philadelphia, 2005, Saunders, p 289.)

TABLE 36-4 Main Genes Involved in Thyroid Oncogenesis: Classification, Tumor Types, and Prevalence

GENES	HISTOLOGIC TYPE	PREVALENCE	COMMENTS
Receptor			
TSH	Autonomous follicular adenoma	3%-82%	TSH activation mutations are not oncogenic
TRK	PTC	6%-20%	Tyrosine kinase receptor, somatic mutation absent in benign thyroid neoplasms
RET/PTC	PTC	2.5%-85%, higher with radiation exposure	Tyrosine kinase receptor, somatic mutation Higher prevalence with radiation exposure Possibly associated with more aggressive tumors Five chimeric subtypes have been identified
Met	PTC, FTC	~75% PTC ~25% FTC	Tyrosine kinase receptor, somatic mutation Possibly associated with aggressive tumors Overexpressed mostly in PTC and poorly DTC
c-erb-2	PTC	~50% PTC	Tyrosine kinase activity, similar to epidermal growth factor receptor Overexpressed in PTC, but oncogene is not overamplified
Signal Transduction Proteins			
ras	PTC, FTC, HCC, autonomous follicular adenoma	7%-92% (~30% overall)	Early event in carcinogenesis May be associated with aggressive PTC
BRAF	PTC	40%-50% PTC	*BRAF*^{V600E} most common mutation; may confer worse prognosis
gsp	Autonomous follicular adenoma	7%-28%	Early event in carcinogenesis Similar frequency in benign and malignant thyroid neoplasms Coexisting *ras* and *gsp* mutations in same tumor may be associated with aggressive DTC
Tumor Suppressor Genes and Nuclear Oncogenes			
PAX8/PPARγ	FTC	75%	Presence of this fusion oncoprotein may be used to differentiate follicular adenoma from carcinoma
p53	Poorly DTC, ATC	~75%	p53 immunohistochemistry may be predictive of tumor aggressiveness Thought to occur as a late genetic event in thyroid carcinogenesis
PTEN	Benign follicular adenoma, infrequently in DTC	26% of benign, 6% of malignant	Higher rate in benign than malignant tumor questions the presence of strict adenoma-to-carcinoma sequence

From Kebebew E: Thyroid oncogenesis. In Clark OH, editor: *Textbook of endocrine surgery*, ed 2, Philadelphia, 2005, Saunders, p 289.
ATC, anaplastic thyroid carcinoma; *DTC*, differentiated thyroid carcinoma; *FTC*, follicular thyroid carcinoma; *HCC*, Hürthle cell carcinoma; *PTC*, papillary thyroid carcinoma; *TSH*, thyroid-stimulating hormone.

Mutations in the RET and NTRK1 tyrosine kinases result in chimeric products known as RET/PTC and TRK, respectively. These rearrangements occur in 40% of sporadic papillary carcinomas with mutations in RET being more common.[18]

The *PTC/RET* proto-oncogene perhaps has received the most attention in thyroid tumorigenesis studies and has been well characterized.[19] The *PTC/RET* proto-oncogene encodes for a membrane receptor tyrosine kinase and is the most frequent genetic alteration in PTC despite the absence of the RET protein product in normal thyroid follicular cells. This proto-oncogene may be involved in the normal differentiation of neuronal cells. Cells of neural crest origin appear to have increased expression of this gene because it has been found in neuroblastoma, pheochromocytoma, and MTC tissue. Alterations in this system have been shown to result in developmental abnormalities in many other neuronal tissues as well as in patients with Hirschsprung's disease. Expression of the *RET* oncogene is predominantly found in malignant tissue. It has not been detected to any substantial degree in nonmalignant thyroid disease processes. Thyroid malignancies expressing this oncogene may have a predilection for distant metastasis. In addition, the *RET* proto-oncogene is associated with a high frequency of missense mutations in patients with MEN2A, and genetic analysis for this mutation allows a secure diagnosis in children before the clinical appearance of MTC.

The downstream pathway of the *RET* and *NTRK1* mutations includes RAS, BRAF, MEK, and ultimately activation of MAPK. Of all the isoforms of RAF kinase, the B type (BRAF) is the most potent stimulator of MAPK signaling. BRAF is implicated in PTC and has been seen in ATC, but not FTC. The *BRAF*^{V600E} mutation is the most common in thyroid malignancy and is present in 40% to 50% of PTCs, including 60% of classic PTCs, 10% to 15% of follicular variant PTCs, greater than 90% of tall cell variant PTCs, and 25% of ATCs.[20] The role of *BRAF* mutation status to guide therapy in DTC continues to be elucidated.

The *ras* gene family encodes signal transduction G proteins that play an important role in the regulation of cell growth and differentiation. Mutational activation of this oncogene results in the production of an inactive form of an enzyme (guanosine triphosphatase) that is ineffective in inactivating protein degradation. Of thyroid tumors, 40% may have one of three *ras* gene point mutations (H-*ras*, K-*ras*, or N-*ras*), and *ras* mutations may occur in benign and malignant thyroid neoplasms, including follicular adenomas, FTCs, and follicular variant PTCs.[21] Patients who live in iodine-deficient areas may have an incidence of *ras* mutations that is slightly decreased compared with patients in iodine-sufficient areas. K-*ras* mutations appear more frequently in radiation-induced PTCs. FTCs with *ras* mutations are more aggressive than FTCs without *ras* mutations, and *ras* mutations may be found in undifferentiated thyroid carcinomas and ATCs.[22]

Tumor suppressor genes also play a role in thyroid malignancy. Loss of function of the *p53* tumor suppressor gene is one of the most common genetic alterations seen across all human cancer and is associated with radiation exposure. The *p53* gene product plays an important role in cell cycle progression. Inactivating mutations of *p53* appear to be associated with more aggressive PTC and FTC, are a late event in thyroid carcinoma progression, and have been associated with the development of ATC.[23]

Ionizing Radiation

Ionizing radiation can cause genetic mutations leading to malignant transformation. This association is much stronger for thyroid cancer than for other malignancies, and radiation is the only clearly established environmental risk factor for thyroid malignancy. The risk of developing thyroid cancer after exposure to radiation is greater in people exposed during childhood and increases with higher doses of radiation delivered to the thyroid; this is true for exposure to ionizing radiation given for medical purposes as well as environmental exposures. The association with radiation is much stronger for papillary than for follicular carcinoma.

The use of external-beam irradiation in children and young adults in the 1950s and 1960s for acne and tonsillitis was shown to result in an increased incidence of DTC (usually papillary) at any time, generally 5 years after exposure. Additionally, patients who have received external irradiation for soft tissue malignancy, such as Hodgkin lymphoma, have an increased incidence of thyroid nodules and cancer (30% to 35% of exposed patients). Acute environmental exposures, such as the Chernobyl nuclear event, also have significant impact. The incidence of thyroid cancer in children in some areas affected by Chernobyl peaked at 100 times that seen before the accident.[24,25]

Papillary Thyroid Carcinoma

PTC is the most common thyroid malignancy and usually is associated with an excellent prognosis, particularly in young female patients (Fig. 36-14). Of thyroid carcinomas diagnosed, 70% to 80% are PTC. PTC may occur much more commonly than it is diagnosed with autopsy series finding small (<1 cm) PTCs in 30% of people who died of other causes. This suggests that small PTCs may be of minimal clinical significance.

The most important risk factor for PTC is childhood radiation exposure from either medical or environmental sources. Other important risk factors for PTC include a history of thyroid carcinoma in a first-degree relative and the presence of a familial syndrome that includes thyroid carcinoma, such as Werner syndrome, Cowden syndrome, Carney complex, and familial polyposis. PTC occurs in a 2.5:1 female-to-male ratio, and the peak incidence occurs between ages 30 and 50 years.

Pathologic Classification

The pathologic diagnosis of PTC depends on the findings of well-recognized papillary cytomorphology. Individual cellular morphology may be used to make the diagnosis of PTC, and therefore the diagnosis may be made definitively based on FNA cytology. Findings of intranuclear inclusion bodies and nuclear grooving on the FNA specimen confirm the diagnosis of PTC (see Fig. 36-12). Additionally, the finding of calcified clumps of cells, known as psammoma bodies, which are most likely caused by sloughed papillary projections, is diagnostic of PTC. The neoplasm also

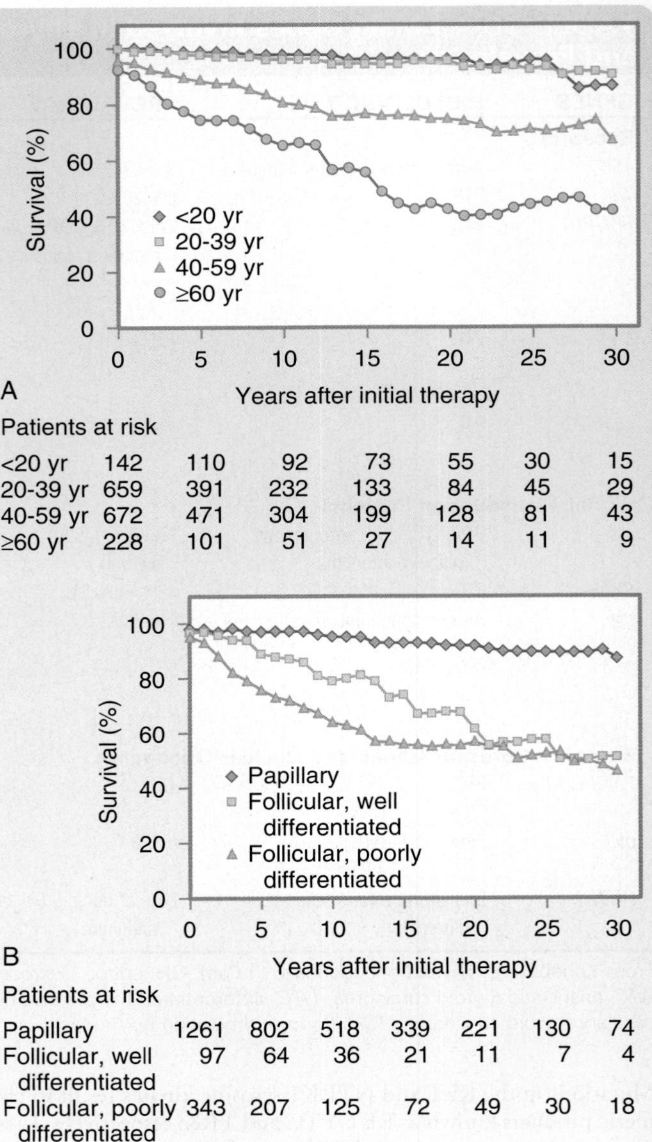

FIGURE 36-14 Survival rates of 1701 patients with papillary or follicular carcinoma (no distant metastasis at time of diagnosis). Overall survival rates were 82% at 10 years, 72% at 20 years, and 60% at 30 years. Patients were followed at the Institut Gustav-Roussy in France. **A,** Effect of age at diagnosis on mortality for combined groups. **B,** Survival rate according to histologic subtype. (From Schlumberger ML: Medical progress: Papillary and follicular thyroid carcinoma. *N Engl J Med* 338:300, 1998.)

may form well-defined follicles with only minimal papillary architecture. The latter group is classified as the follicular variant of PTC and constitutes approximately 10% of PTCs. Classic PTC and the follicular variant of PTC have similar prognostic implications. The encapsulated follicular variant of PTC is usually quite indolent with an excellent prognosis.[5]

Other subtypes of papillary carcinoma include columnar, hobnail, and tall cell carcinomas, which are more aggressive in their biologic behavior. Although these subtypes are rare, they tend to occur in older patients, and the prognosis is less favorable. These latter groups represent perhaps less than 1% of all PTCs

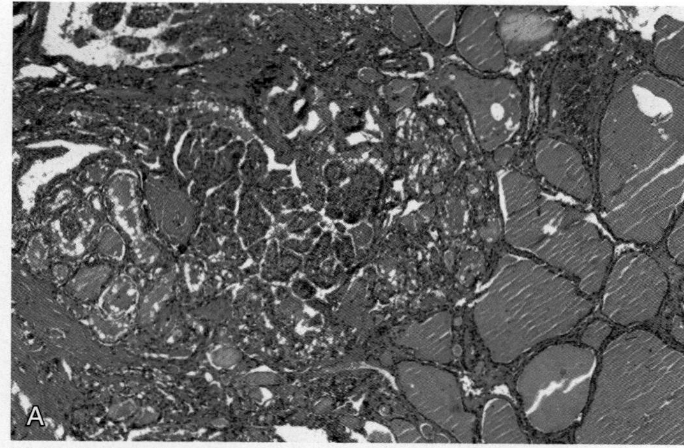

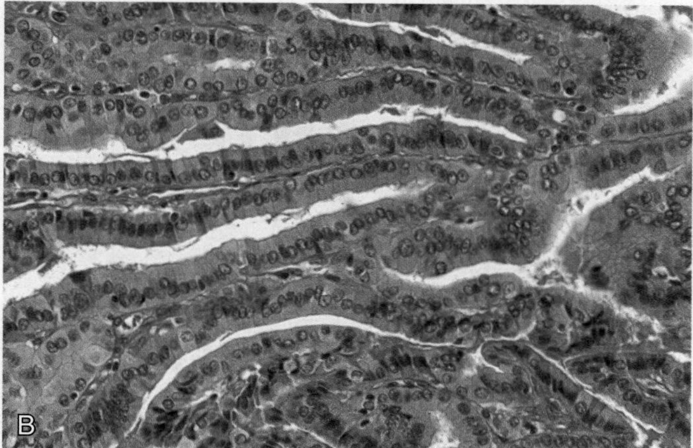

FIGURE 36-15 **A,** Hematoxylin-eosin (H&E) staining of a thyroid mass reveals papillary projections consistent with papillary carcinoma. **B,** H&E staining of a papillary carcinoma shows cells with an increased height-to-width ratio in a single row of cells. This is the so-called tall cell variant of papillary carcinoma, which is associated with a poorer prognosis than differentiated papillary cancer.

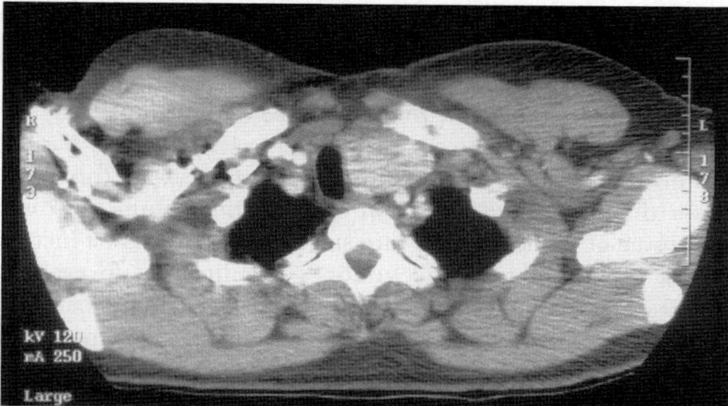

FIGURE 36-16 Computed tomography findings of a 4-cm mass in the left lobe of a 40-year-old man suggesting an infraclavicular or substernal location. The mass ultimately proved to be papillary carcinoma.

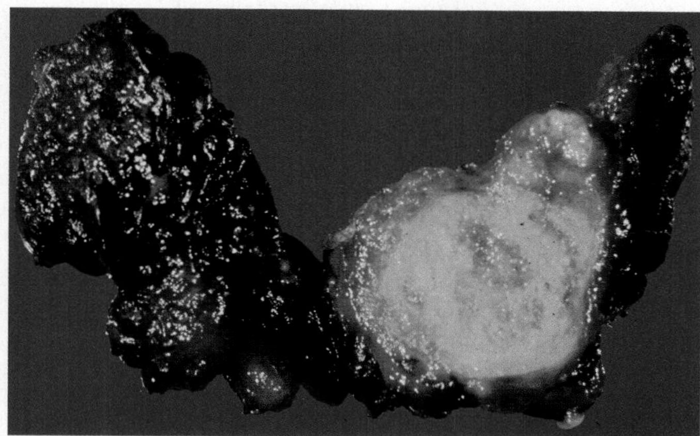

FIGURE 36-17 This 4- to 5-cm right lobe mass was removed as part of a total thyroidectomy. Permanent section pathology revealed papillary carcinoma.

(Fig. 36-15). The solid variant and the diffuse sclerosing variants of PTC have less clear prognostic implications but likely have more aggressive biologic behavior than classic PTC.

Clinical Features

PTC most typically manifests either as a palpable thyroid nodule or as an incidental imaging finding (Figs. 36-16 and 36-17). Occasionally, a metastatic PTC manifests as a painless lateral neck mass that is clinically detected before detecting the primary thyroid lesion. The evaluation of these lesions proceeds with history, physical examination, imaging, and FNA as described earlier. The FNA diagnosis of PTC has an almost 100% correlation to a diagnosis of PTC on final pathology.

Most patients with PTC can expect an excellent prognosis, with the 10-year survival rate greater than 95% for the most favorable stages (see Fig. 36-14). However, various factors in the clinical findings and pathologic staging may alter the excellent prognosis (Table 36-5). In 1979, Cady and associates[26] first evaluated a clinical scoring system and reported a 30-year study of a group of patients in which the investigators attempted to place the patients into risk stratification groups. These studies described the AMES clinical scoring system, which is based on patient age, distant metastasis, extent of primary tumor, and size of primary

TABLE 36-5 Prognostic Risk Classification for Patients With Differentiated Thyroid Carcinoma (AMES or AGES)

	LOW RISK	HIGH RISK
Age	<40 years	>40 years
Sex	Female	Male
Extent	No local extension, intrathyroidal, no capsular invasion	Capsular invasion, extrathyroidal extension
Metastasis	None	Regional or distant
Size	<2 cm	>4 cm
Grade	Well differentiated	Poorly differentiated

AGES, patient age, pathologic grade of tumor, extent of primary tumor, size of primary tumor; *AMES,* patient age, distant metastasis, extent of primary tumor, size of primary tumor.

tumor. Hay[27] reported the Mayo Clinic experience and developed his own scoring scale, the AGES clinical scoring system, which was based on patient age, pathologic grade of tumor, extent of primary tumor, and size of primary tumor. The AMES and AGES clinical scoring systems have proved beneficial in predicting the prognosis of papillary and follicular carcinomas (see Table 36-5).

Age at diagnosis is the most important prognostic factor in DTC. Diagnosis at an age younger than 40 years is associated with excellent survival. This age benefit is extended to 50 years in women. Absence of distant metastasis at the time of initial treatment and size less than 4 cm are similarly important positive predictors. Even patients with distant spread to the lungs still have significant survival of up to 50% at 10 years; however, patients with brain metastases have a median 1-year survival. Tumor size greater than 4 cm and extension of the primary tumor through the capsule of the lesion and into surrounding soft tissue increase the risk for mortality. Small tumors generally have an excellent prognosis but may still manifest with clinically evident recurrence. The impact of lymphatic metastases on prognosis depends on patient age. In a large series in younger patients (<45 years old), the presence of lymph node metastases had no effect on the excellent overall survival, but the presence of lymph node metastases increased the risk of death by 46% in patients older than 45.[28]

Multicentricity can be anticipated in 70% of patients with PTC and may represent either intraglandular metastasis or multiple primary tumors. Additionally, cervical lymph node metastases are common, particularly in children, who may have a 50% incidence of clinically detectable nodal disease at presentation. The presence of lymph node metastasis in patients with contained intrathyroidal primary papillary carcinoma also does not affect long-term survival. If there is gross or microscopic extension of a primary PTC through the thyroid capsule, a poor prognosis and possibly a higher rate of lymph node metastasis may be anticipated.[29] Although PTC typically disseminates via lymphatic spread, distant metastases can occur and are present in 3% to 5% of patients at the time of diagnosis. The two most common sites of spread are to the lungs and bones.

The TNM staging system for DTC is depicted in Table 36-6. The unique role of age in the TNM staging of thyroid carcinoma reflects the overwhelming implications of age on disease prognosis. A patient who presents at younger than 45 years old is stage 1 regardless of T stage and N stage as long as there are no distant metastases. The American Thyroid Association also has provided a risk stratification system after thyroidectomy for DTC that uses several pathologic and clinical variables to stratify patients into low, intermediate, or high risk of disease recurrence or persistence.[5] These systems may be used to guide subsequent treatment and follow-up plans for a given patient.

TABLE 36-6 TNM Components for Differentiated Thyroid Carcinoma

Primary Tumor (T)	
TX	Primary cannot be assessed
T0	No primary tumor
T1a	≤1 cm, intrathyroidal
T1b	1-2 cm, intrathyroidal
T2	2-4 cm, intrathyroidal
T3	>4 cm limited to the thyroid or any size with minimal extrathyroidal extension (muscle, soft tissue)
T4a	Invades subcutaneous tissue, larynx, trachea, esophagus, or RLN
T4b	Invades prevertebral fascia or encases carotid or mediastinal vessels
Regional Lymph Nodes (N)	
NX	Nodes cannot be assessed
N0	Negative nodes
N1a	Positive in level VI
N1b	Positive beyond level VI
Distant Metastasis (M)	
M0	No distant metastasis
M1	Distant metastasis

Stage Grouping for Differentiated Thyroid Carcinoma			
<45 Years Old			
Stage I	Any T	Any N	M0
Stage II	Any T	Any N	M1
≥45 Years Old			
Stage I	T1	N0	M0
Stage II	T2	N0	M0
Stage III	T3	N0	M0
	T1	N1a	M0
	T2	N1a	M0
	T3	N1a	M0
Stage IVA	T4a	N0	M0
	T4a	N1a	M0
	T1	N1b	M0
	T2	N1b	M0
	T3	N1b	M0
	T4a	N1b	M0
Stage IVB	T4b	Any N	M0
Stage IVC	Any T	Any N	M1

RLN, recurrent laryngeal nerve.

Follicular Thyroid Carcinoma

FTC is the second category of DTC and constitutes approximately 10% of all thyroid malignancies. FTC is a disease of an older population compared with PTC, with a peak incidence between ages 40 and 60 years. It occurs more commonly in women, with a ratio of approximately 3 : 1. Although FTC also is a follicular cell–derived DTC, there are some differences in diagnosis, behavior, and prognosis compared with PTC. There appears to be an increased incidence of FTC in geographic distributions associated with iodine deficiency. In contrast to PTC, FTC is not strongly associated with radiation exposure.

Pathologic Classification

FTC is a malignant neoplasm of the thyroid epithelium that can have a wide spectrum of microscopic changes ranging from virtually normal follicular architecture and function to severely altered cellular architecture. Histologic diagnosis of FTC depends on the demonstration of follicular cells occupying abnormal positions, including capsular or vascular invasion (Fig. 36-18). The cells may not demonstrate nuclear atypia; however, when present, marked nuclear atypia is associated with a worse prognosis. If these findings are not present, the diagnosis is benign follicular adenoma. Because this diagnosis depends on defining the lesion architecture, the diagnosis cannot be made on FNA biopsy.

Using these criteria, two types of FTC are usually described: minimally invasive and widely invasive. There is increasing evidence that microscopic angioinvasion is an important prognostic finding.[30] Lymph node involvement is unusual in FTC occurring in less than 10% of cases. In contrast, PTC is characterized by a high rate of lymph node involvement at the time of initial evaluation. In patients with widely invasive FTC, distant spread is more common, and lung, bone, and other solid organs are often involved (Fig. 36-19).[30]

A subtype of FTC, known as Hürthle cell carcinoma, consists of oxyphilic cells and tends to occur in older patients, usually 60 to 75 years old.[25] Hürthle cells have their characteristic appearance because of an increased number of mitochondria causing an appearance of an enlarged, granular, and eosinophilic cytoplasm. Hürthle cell cancers have a greater likelihood of having local recurrence and are less avid to absorb RAI, leading to more aggressive biologic behavior.

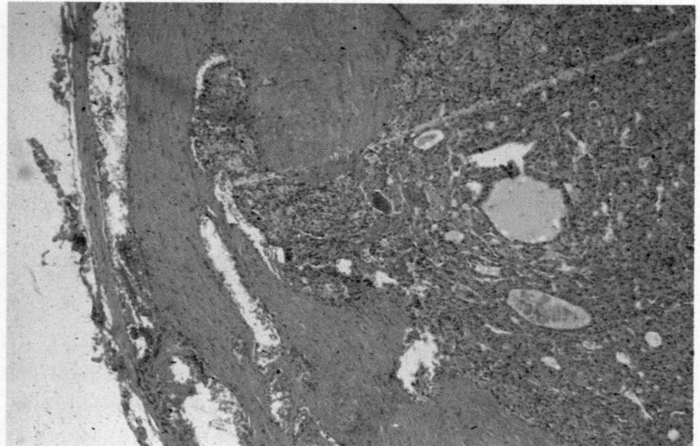

FIGURE 36-18 Hematoxylin-eosin staining of a follicular lesion. High-power examination revealing capsular invasion by follicular cells allows the diagnosis of follicular cancer.

Clinical Features

Similar to PTC, FTC typically manifests as a painless thyroid mass that is evaluated as described earlier. FTC and multinodular goiter coexist in 10% of cases. Although the findings of hoarseness and firm fixation of the mass on clinical evaluation suggest advanced disease and a poor prognosis, these circumstances are found in only a few cases. In such cases, a diligent search for aggressive extension into the trachea and for distant metastasis, particularly in older patients, is carried out with CT or MRI of the neck and chest (Fig. 36-20).[29]

Preoperative imaging may be of some assistance in assessing the extent of a palpable mass. Ultrasound can determine the size and multicentricity of the malignancy; however, FTC is usually manifested as a solitary mass. Although FNA cytology is important in the workup of thyroid nodules, it is of limited value in the preoperative diagnosis of FTC. Diagnosis of FTC requires demonstration of cellular invasion of the capsule or vascular or lymphatic channels. These structural characteristics cannot be determined with FNA. Additionally, intraoperative frozen section has been notoriously ineffective in making a definitive diagnosis of FTC.[31]

In contrast to PTC, FTC typically spreads via hematogenous routes, which occurs in 10% to 15% of cases. The most common sites for metastatic deposits are lytic bone lesions and lung (see Fig. 36-19). Prognosis is less favorable for FTC than for PTC and is best in young patients with limited capsular or vascular invasion

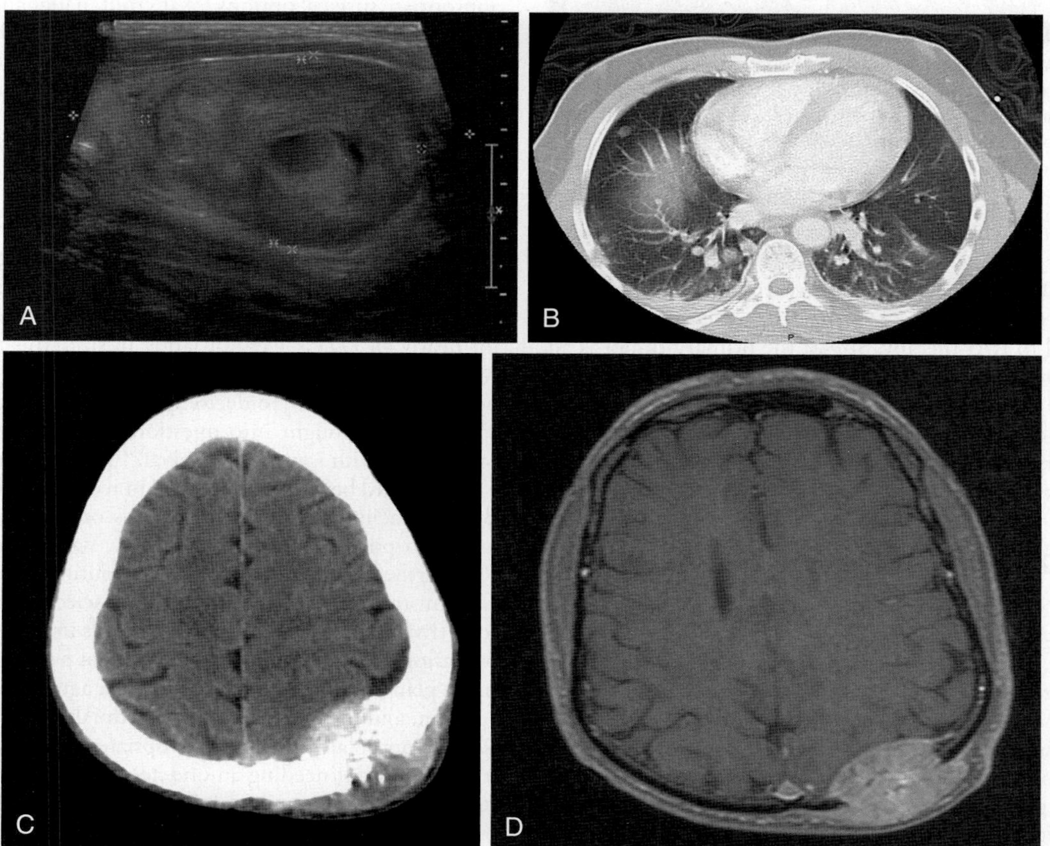

FIGURE 36-19 Metastatic follicular cancer; all images are from the same patient. **A,** Preoperative ultrasound demonstrates a 6.7-cm mass in the left lobe of the thyroid; pathology demonstrated follicular cancer. **B,** Computed tomography (CT) image of the chest demonstrates multiple pulmonary metastases. **C,** CT image of the head demonstrates left parietal bone metastasis. **D,** Magnetic resonance imaging of the head demonstrates left parietal bone metastasis with an epidural component and mass effect on the brain.

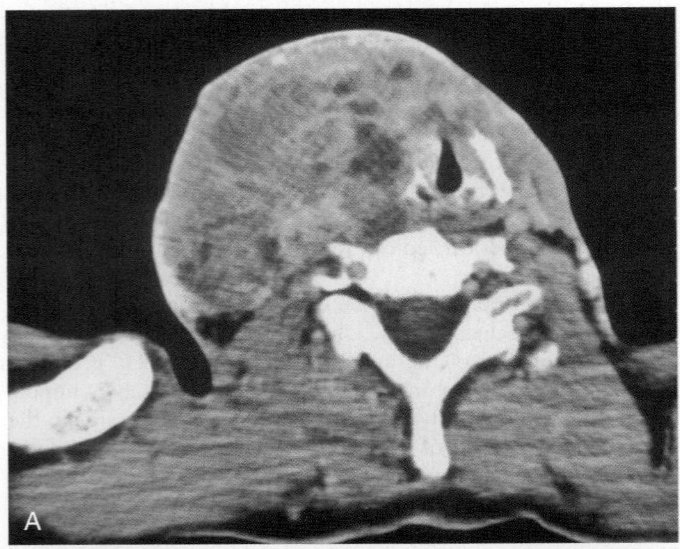

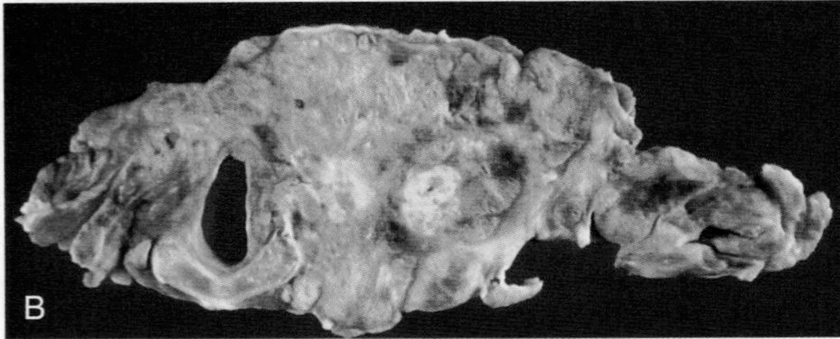

FIGURE 36-20 **A** and **B,** Rapidly enlarging thyroid mass in a 70-year-old man. Computed tomography image demonstrates displacement of the larynx and lateral involvement of both jugular veins. The patient died within 6 months of rapidly progressing follicular cancer.

(see Fig. 36-14). As with papillary cancer, age is the most important predictor of survival with a 95% 10-year survival in patients younger than 40 years and an 80% 10-year survival in patients between 40 and 60 years old. FTCs in older patients also are less likely to respond to RAI therapy. Size of the primary tumor is an important prognostic indicator, although in contrast to PTC, even small FTCs should be considered clinically significant. TNM staging for FTC is the same as for PTC; FTCs also should be risk stratified for persistence and recurrence based on the American Thyroid Association system.[5]

Treatment of Differentiated Thyroid Carcinoma (Papillary and Follicular)

The primary treatment of DTC, including PTC and FTC, is surgical ablation. The other mainstays of therapy are RAI ablation and TSH suppression. Persistent and recurrent disease also is primarily addressed using the same three modalities. External-beam radiation and systemic adjuvant chemotherapy play a role in a few cases of DTC. Targeted therapy with tyrosine kinase inhibitors may play a role in the setting of a clinical trial to manage advanced cases of metastatic DTC that are refractory to RAI, rapidly progressive, and not amenable to other means of therapy.[5,20]

Not all DTCs need all three modalities of surgery, RAI, and TSH suppression. When these therapies are recommended, not all DTCs need them to the same extent. Several factors enter into decision making, all of which must be carefully weighed. As discussed earlier, although DTCs generally have a good prognosis, there are high rates of multicentricity within the thyroid and high rates of lymph node metastases, and recurrence is frequent. Furthermore, although more aggressive resections of the thyroid and lymphatic beds expose the patient to more potential morbidity, they facilitate RAI therapy and surveillance and may limit the need for repeat operative intervention. Although RAI ablation and TSH suppression may be less morbid than radiation and traditional chemotherapies that are applied to many other malignancies, they have their own cost and morbidity. With all these considerations in mind, the objectives of initial therapy include the following: (1) remove the primary tumor and clinically significant cervical lymph nodes, (2) minimize treatment-related morbidity, (3) accurately stage the disease, (4) facilitate postoperative RAI therapy if appropriate, (5) permit accurate long-term surveillance, and (6) minimize risk of recurrence or metastasis.[5]

Extent of Thyroid Resection

Appropriate surgical options and terminology for known or suspected thyroid malignancy include the following: (1) hemithyroidectomy/thyroid lobectomy with or without isthmusectomy; (2) near-total thyroidectomy, defined by leaving less than 1 g of tissue adjacent to the RLN at the ligament of Berry on one side; and (3) total thyroidectomy, defined by removal of all visible thyroid tissue. Nodulectomy and leaving greater than 1 g of thyroid tissue in a "subtotal" thyroidectomy are not considered appropriate surgical options for thyroid malignancy (Table 36-7).[5]

For a patient with a unilateral thyroid malignancy and no evidence of metastatic disease, there are several rationales to consider total thyroidectomy, including (1) facilitation of RAI ablation, which is much less effective and requires a larger dosage if residual thyroid exists; (2) the frequent presence of occult multifocal disease; and (3) facilitating the use of Tg as a tumor marker, which is most useful if there is no remaining normal thyroid. Advantages of a procedure less than total or near-total thyroidectomy are decreased rates of bilateral RLN damage and hypoparathyroidism and preservation of functional thyroid tissue.

Previous clinical guidelines recommended total thyroidectomy for nearly all DTCs 1 cm or larger in size. This recommendation was based on the aforementioned considerations and data supporting that total thyroidectomy improved survival. More recent studies have brought into question the association of total thyroidectomy with improved survival.[32] Furthermore, there has been a shift toward being more selective in recommending RAI therapy. Because facilitating RAI therapy was one of the strongest arguments to pursue total thyroidectomy, narrowing indications for RAI further decreased the need for routine total thyroidectomy. Current trends are toward being more selective in recommending total thyroidectomy. Regardless of trends in recommendation, the operation chosen should be considered as a part of a holistic treatment plan for the patient that must be agreed by the patient, the surgeon, and the endocrinologist. If the thyroid tumor is low risk, RAI is not planned, and appropriate surveillance can be performed without needing an undetectable Tg, total thyroidectomy may not be necessary as detailed subsequently.

DTCs less than 1 cm in diameter are defined as microcarcinomas. Surgery is not clearly required for these lesions if there are no clinically involved cervical lymph nodes, no extrathyroidal extension, and no history of head and neck irradiation. Similarly, if a DTC less than 1 cm is diagnosed after thyroid lobectomy, completion thyroidectomy is not required if there are no clinically

TABLE 36-7 Indications for Interventional Procedures

PROCEDURE	ADVANTAGES	DISADVANTAGES OR COMPLICATIONS	INDICATIONS
FNA	Accurate diagnosis of malignancy	Capsular hemorrhage	Evaluation of thyroid nodule; concerning lymph node
Open biopsy	Direct visualization; large pathologic tissue volume	Requires operating room and possibly general anesthesia	Complex case in which FNA has failed to give diagnosis
Nodulectomy (less than a lobectomy)	None	Difficult second operation to complete lobectomy if diagnosis of cancer is made	None
Lobectomy (with isthmusectomy)	Preserves thyroid; protects contralateral parathyroids and nerves	May require subsequent completion thyroidectomy	Indeterminate nodules; small intrathyroidal thyroid cancer
Near-total thyroidectomy	Lower rates of hypocalcemia and nerve damage	Possible recurrence in residual thyroid tissue	Benign disease; small nodule on side of complete lobectomy; hyperthyroidism
Total thyroidectomy	Use of postoperative ^{131}I is most efficacious; use of post-thyroglobulin levels for recurrence	Higher rate of hypocalcemia and nerve damage	Extensive multinodular disease; hyperthyroidism; thyroid cancer
Modified radical lymph node dissection	Decreased rate of recurrence	Cranial nerve XI injury; loss of sensation over ear and lateral cervical area; (left) thoracic duct leak and lymphocele; Horner syndrome	Lateral neck node metastasis
Median sternotomy	Exposure of mediastinal contents	Bleeding; nonunion of sternum (if complete sternotomy); increased hospital stay	Extension of malignancy into anterior mediastinum; inability to mobilize large substernal goiter
Central neck (level VI) lymph node dissection	Decreased risk for recurrence	Increased risk for hypocalcemia and nerve damage	Medullary carcinoma, DTC with N1 disease and T3 or T4 tumors

DTC, differentiated thyroid carcinoma; *FNA*, fine-needle aspiration.

involved cervical lymph nodes, no extrathyroidal extension, and no history of head and neck irradiation.[5]

For DTCs that are 1 cm or larger, a total thyroidectomy is indicated in situations in which RAI therapy is planned. These situations include DTCs greater than 4 cm in size, DTCs with extrathyroidal extension, and DTCs with regional or distant metastases. Other factors that may make total thyroidectomy an appropriate consideration are patient and physician preference, age older than 45 years, contralateral nodules, prior irradiation, and familial DTC.[5] If none of the above-mentioned factors are concerns, thyroid lobectomy may be adequate surgical therapy for DTCs that are 1 to 4 cm after discussion with the patient and the physician who will be following the patient long-term. At the present time, many physicians still prefer to offer RAI for many of these cancers, and many of these patients receive total thyroidectomy.

Lymph Node Dissection

Because PTC is the most common thyroid carcinoma and has a high frequency of lymph node metastasis, operative planning must include consideration of cervical lymphadenectomy. When considering lymphadenectomy, distinctions should be made between the central neck (level VI) and the lateral neck and between therapeutic dissection and prophylactic dissection. A prophylactic dissection is the clearance of a clinically uninvolved nodal basin, whereas therapeutic dissection is lymph node dissection in the setting of proven nodal metastasis. The anatomically defined nodal regions of the central and lateral neck are demonstrated in Figure 36-5.

In some patients, particularly patients younger than age 45 years, lymphatic spread does not appear to have a significant impact on prognosis. However, large registry studies support that in all patients with PTC, there is a small but statistically significant decrease in long-term all-cause survival in patients with lymphatic metastases compared with patients without lymphatic metastases.[33] At the present time, it is recommended that all patients with known or suspected PTC undergo a thorough physical examination and complete ultrasound scan of the central and lateral neck before resection of the thyroid lesion.

In the evaluation of the central neck, ultrasound is not as sensitive for pathologic adenopathy as it is for lateral neck adenopathy because the central compartment nodes are in anatomically challenging locations. Therefore, if there is not already an indication for central compartment lymph dissection, the central compartment nodes should be assessed at the time of thyroidectomy by visual inspection and palpation, in addition to preoperative ultrasound. If pathologic nodes are encountered, a therapeutic central neck dissection should be performed. Many surgeons believe that prophylactic level VI dissection should be performed routinely in the setting of thyroid cancer, even in patients with clinically uninvolved nodes. Others argue against routine prophylactic dissection. In a feasibility study, it was determined that it may never be feasible to answer this question in a randomized trial, so the debate will continue.[34] Supporters of routine central neck dissection point out that there is a high frequency of pathologically positive but clinically negative nodal spread and that some studies reported lower rates of recurrent disease after routine central neck dissection. Conversely, others studies found a higher rate of transient hypocalcemia, permanent hypoparathyroidism, and nerve injury and no evidence of benefit after prophylactic central neck dissection. In the setting of clinically negative central compartment nodes, a prophylactic dissection is more clearly indicated in higher risk situations, such as tumors that are larger than 4 cm, tumors with gross extrathyroidal extension, and tumors with lateral neck nodal disease.[5]

The management of lateral neck lymph node basins must be considered separately from the central neck. In the course of thyroidectomy, the lateral compartment of the neck is not entered, and these nodes are not evaluated intraoperatively. Therefore, the lateral neck should be evaluated for malignancy before thyroidectomy. All patients with a known thyroid carcinoma or a Bethesda System category 5 FNA specimen should have careful physical examination and ultrasound evaluation of the lateral compartment for pathologic lymphadenopathy. If pathologic appearing nodes are found, FNA biopsy should be performed. In the presence of pathologically confirmed lateral neck nodal disease, an ipsilateral therapeutic lateral neck dissection is indicated. This dissection should be undertaken as a formal clearance of defined lymph node levels, rather than isolated resection of the involved node or "berry picking."[5] An operative strategy for this procedure is described later. Despite a nearly 30% rate of micrometastases in lateral lymph nodes, there is little benefit to prophylactic lateral neck dissection for clinically negative nodes, and there is significant morbidity associated with this intervention.

Completion Thyroidectomy

DTC is frequently diagnosed after completing a diagnostic thyroid lobectomy or thyroid lobectomy performed for what was thought to be benign disease such as symptomatic multinodular goiter. Similarly, more aggressive disease may be found on final pathology than was known based on preoperative evaluation. This situation presents the clinical question of whether completion thyroidectomy or lymphadenectomy should be performed. Current recommendations support that completion thyroidectomy should be performed if the original recommendation would have been total or near-total thyroidectomy if the pathology were known preoperatively. As discussed earlier, this includes the need for completion thyroidectomy if RAI is recommended as part of the treatment strategy. If RAI is not planned and if total thyroidectomy would not have been indicated even if the pathology were known preoperatively, completion thyroidectomy is not required. The potential need for completion thyroidectomy is one reason that the contralateral strap muscles should not be separated from the thyroid lobe when performing the initial thyroid lobectomy. The absence of scar formation on the thyroid and in the tracheoesophageal groove means that the complication rate for completion thyroidectomy should be low in experienced hands.

Radioactive Iodine Therapy

RAI has several particular purposes in the treatment of DTC after thyroidectomy, including (1) ablation of remnant thyroid tissue to facilitate detection of later disease recurrence by imaging and Tg assay, (2) adjuvant therapy with the intention of targeting occult metastatic disease, and (3) primary treatment of known persistent disease. There has been a general trend toward being more selective in recommending RAI and toward giving lower doses of RAI.

Most more recent guidelines state that patients with gross extrathyroidal extension or M1 disease lesions have improved disease-specific and recurrence-free survival with RAI and that RAI should routinely be recommended to these patients. For patients with tumors that are larger than 4 cm, with microscopic extrathyroidal extension, or with central or lateral compartment nodal metastasis, RAI should be considered after accounting for all clinical variables and is recommended to many of these patients. For patients with tumors that are between 1 and 4 cm, are confined to the thyroid, and do not have nodal or distant metastasis, RAI is not routinely recommended, but it should be more strongly considered in the setting of an adverse histologic subtype (e.g., tall cell) or if there is vascular invasion. RAI should not be given to patients with low-risk DTCs that are less than 1 cm without any direct extrathyroidal extension or metastases.

These recommendations are a move toward giving RAI to fewer patients with DTC than previously was the case. Actual practice patterns vary, and the ultimate decision is made after a discussion between the patient, the surgeon, and the endocrinologist or other physician who will follow the patient long-term. As discussed earlier, the decision for RAI and the extent of surgery are closely linked and should be considered together.

When RAI is recommended, several steps must be taken to ensure that the targeted cells have active uptake of the RAI. These steps include making the cells iodine avid by maintaining a low-iodine diet for 1 to 2 weeks before RAI administration. Urine iodine may be measured to ensure that the patient is iodine depleted, particularly if there was a recent large iodine exposure such as iodinated contrast agent or amiodarone.

The other consideration is that RAI uptake is stimulated by TSH, and high levels of TSH are needed before administration of RAI. The optimal TSH level is unknown, but a goal TSH greater than 30 mIU/liter has been generally adopted. This TSH elevation may be achieved either by withdrawal of thyroid hormone or by the administration of exogenous recombinant human thyroid-stimulating hormone (rhTSH). If thyroid hormone withdrawal is used, levothyroxine should be held for 3 to 4 weeks before a planned RAI therapy. Some centers prefer to use T_3 (liothyronine [Cytomel]) in the early weeks of withdrawal, which allows a shorter period off of thyroid hormone until an adequate TSH is reached. The advantage of using rhTSH is that hypothyroidism may be avoided completely. Although data are accumulating, there are significantly fewer long-term data with rhTSH compared with thyroid hormone withdrawal. However, guidelines support that rhTSH is an acceptable alternative to thyroid hormone withdrawal for patients with low-risk and intermediate-risk DTC without extensive lymph node involvement in whom RAI is planned. The available data support an improved quality of life with this approach, equivalent remnant ablation, and some data out to 10 years supporting equivalent longer term results. For patients with intermediate-risk DTCs and more extensive lymphatic metastases, rhTSH may still be considered, but the recommendation is not as strong.[5] Preparation for RAI using rhTSH rather than thyroid hormone withdrawal is likely to become a more common approach that will allow further data to accumulate to clarify the relative efficacy of these approaches.

Thyroid-Stimulating Hormone Suppression

Because DTCs continue to express the TSH receptor and TSH continues to function as a growth factor for these cancers, suppression of TSH is another element of therapy for DTCs. TSH suppression is accomplished by giving supraphysiologic doses of exogenous thyroid hormone. Given the myriad adverse effects of hyperthyroidism and subclinical hyperthyroidism, the degree of TSH suppression must be a balance between the risk posed by the malignancy compared with the adverse effects of the therapy. For patients with high-risk DTC, initial TSH suppression should be to less than 0.1 mIU/liter. For patients with intermediate-risk lesions, the initial TSH goal is 0.1 to 0.5 mIU/liter. For patients with low-risk DTC, the initial TSH goal is to be within the low half of the reference range (0.5 to 2.0 mIU/liter). As risk stratification is adjusted based on initial response to therapy, these target ranges may be adjusted. Consideration also must be given to the health of the patient, such as the increased risk of atrial fibrillation and osteoporosis in older patients with suppressed TSH.[5]

Medullary Thyroid Carcinoma

MTC accounts for 4% to 10% of thyroid carcinomas. The malignancy originates in the parafollicular cells, or C cells, which reside in the upper poles of the thyroid lobes and are of neural crest origin. MTC occurs most commonly in a sporadic form (80%); it occurs less commonly as an autosomal dominant inherited disorder such as MEN2A, MEN2B, and familial medullary thyroid carcinoma (FMTC). FMTC is a variant of MEN2A that includes MTC but not the other features of MEN2A. MTC arising in MEN2A usually has a more favorable long-term outcome than MTC arising in MEN2B or sporadic MTC.[25,35]

Clinical Features

A patient with a sporadic MTC typically has one of two manifestations: (1) a palpable mass in the thyroid that is present in most cases and for which a diagnosis can be made with FNA with immunohistochemistry or (2) the finding of an elevated calcitonin level. Excess secretion of calcitonin has been shown to be an effective marker for the presence of MTC, and the presence of a mass and an elevated calcitonin level is virtually diagnostic of MTC. The finding of an elevated basal calcitonin level in the absence of a thyroid mass might require further workup, including repeat basal calcitonin measurement and a calcium-stimulated or gastrin-stimulated test. This calcitonin excess is not clinically associated with hypocalcemia but may rarely result in symptoms of diarrhea and flushing in patients with advanced disease. Carcinoembryonic antigen may also be elevated in MTC.

The MEN2 and FMTC syndromes involve different germline activating mutations in the *RET* proto-oncogene. Additionally, 40% to 50% of sporadic MTC specimens have acquired *RET* mutations. Patients with inherited MTC syndromes initially develop C cell hyperplasia, which is a preneoplastic lesion in these patients, although C cell hyperplasia has little to no malignant potential in patients without *RET* mutations. Because of the high penetrance of MTC and the early development of C cell hyperplasia and MTC, family members of patients with MEN2 should be screened at an early age for the *RET* proto-oncogene. *RET* testing should be performed shortly after birth in MEN2B kindreds and before age 5 years in FMTC and MEN2A kindreds.[35] The workup of these patients includes a detailed and in-depth family history to inquire about the characteristics of MEN2 in the patient and family members. If MTC is suspected, the presence of other components of MEN2 syndrome must be considered; serum calcium and urinary catecholamines must be measured to evaluate for hyperparathyroidism and pheochromocytoma. Pheochromocytoma in particular must be excluded before considering interventions in patients with MTC. The consensus is that the workup of MTC should include serum calcitonin, carcinoembryonic antigen, thorough ultrasound scanning of the lateral neck including lateral compartment, genetic testing for germline *RET* mutation, and biochemical evaluation for pheochromocytoma.

Treatment

MTC can be cured only by complete resection of the primary tumor and local and regional metastases. Most patients with MTC or a syndromic predisposition to MTC should undergo at least total thyroidectomy (Fig. 36-21). Total thyroidectomy allows complete removal of the gland and a search for multicentricity. In sporadic MTC, the lesion is generally contained within one lobe, whereas in MEN2, the malignancy involves the upper halves of both lobes. Patients with the MEN2B *RET* mutation are advised to undergo prophylactic total thyroidectomy within the first year of life or at the time of diagnosis. Other patients with germline *RET* mutations should undergo prophylactic total thyroidectomy before age 5 years or at the time of diagnosis, although it may be appropriate to wait beyond 5 years with particular *RET* mutations. Level VI nodal dissection may be omitted in patients younger than 1 year with MEN2B and patients younger than 5 years with MEN2A and FMTC who are undergoing prophylactic thyroidectomy unless there are thyroid nodules larger than 5 mm, elevated calcitonin, or evidence of lymph node metastasis.[35]

Even in the absence of germline *RET* mutations, patients with known or suspected MTC without evidence of advanced disease should undergo total thyroidectomy with prophylactic level VI nodal dissection. Known nodal metastasis in the central neck mandates bilateral level VI nodal dissection and would cause some physicians to advocate the addition of a lateral neck dissection on the side ipsilateral to the level VI disease, although this is not universally recommended. The presence of clinically detectable or ultrasound-detectable disease in the lateral neck warrants total thyroidectomy and level VI and lateral compartment nodal dissection. If preoperative evaluation reveals distant metastatic disease, less aggressive surgery in the neck may be warranted to

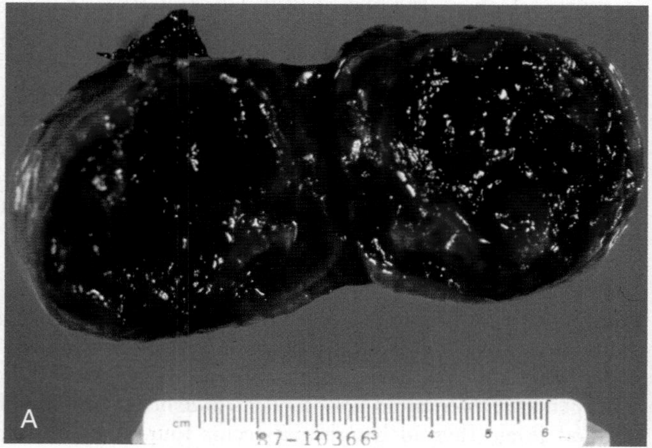

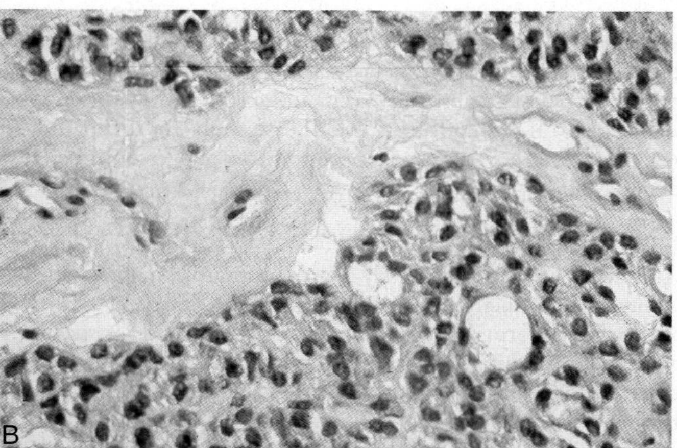

FIGURE 36-21 A, This 4-cm solitary mass in a thyroid lobe was removed by total thyroidectomy. **B,** Hematoxylin-eosin staining of the mass demonstrated cells consistent with medullary carcinoma with amyloid infiltrate.

decrease the risk of morbidity resulting from potential laryngeal nerve injury and hypoparathyroidism; however, palliative operations may be indicated in patients with neck pain or airway compromise.[35]

If MTC is diagnosed postoperatively in a patient undergoing less than total thyroidectomy, further operative intervention is indicated to complete therapy as though the diagnosis were known preoperatively, including completion thyroidectomy and nodal dissection as indicated. An exception is a patient with an incidental finding of MTC in a thyroid lobectomy where the MTC is sporadic and unifocal; there is no C cell hyperplasia; and an otherwise normal ultrasound scan of the neck, negative surgical margin, and normal serum calcitonin all are confirmed.[35]

All prophylactic thyroidectomies for patients with *RET* mutations should be performed in experienced centers, and RLN and parathyroid function should be preserved. Dissection of the central lymph node compartment allows appropriate staging of this process. A successful operation with a good prognosis is predicted for patients with smaller masses and in whom calcitonin levels are undetectable after surgery. The literature describes the use of basal and stimulated calcitonin tests to monitor for recurrence because stimulated calcitonin values may increase before basal calcitonin levels do. Documentation of recurrent MTC by biochemical means is often associated with unresectable recurrence in distant metastatic locations, including the lung and liver.[25] Because MTC is not of follicular cell origin, TSH suppression and RAI scanning and therapy have no role in MTC, unless there is a concomitant PTC or FTC.[35]

Poorly Differentiated Thyroid Carcinoma

Poorly DTC describes a lesion that previously was known as "insular" thyroid cancer. Poorly DTC may be thought of as occupying a middle ground between DTC and ATC, which is completely dedifferentiated. Poorly DTC lies between these two extremes histologically and behaviorally. Poorly DTC is defined based on a combination of cytoarchitectural and high-grade features such as mitoses and necrosis. Poorly DTCs have a significantly worse outcome than DTCs with 50% mortality at 10 years.[5,36] In a series of 91 cases of poorly DTCs that were surgically managed, 80% manifested with T3 or T4 lesions, 40% had pathologically proven nodal metastasis, and 26% had M1 disease. Although 92% of tumors were resected to grossly clear margins, only 38% had pathologically clear margins. With aggressive surgical resection, the 5-year disease-specific survival was 66%. Factors associated with mortality included locally advanced disease (T4a) and the presence of distant metastasis at presentation. Many, but not all, poorly DTCs absorb RAI, including many M1 tumors.[36] The efficacy of RAI in affecting the disease course in this pathology is unknown; however, it is appropriate to offer it until better data are available.

Anaplastic Thyroid Carcinoma

ATC accounts for approximately 1% of all thyroid malignancies. In contrast to frequently positive prognosis in DTCs, ATC is the most aggressive form of thyroid carcinoma with a disease-specific mortality approaching 100%. A typical manifestation is an older patient with dysphagia, cervical tenderness, and a painful, rapidly enlarging neck mass. Patients frequently have a history of prior or coexistent DTC, and up to 50% have history of goiter. Findings may also include superior vena cava syndrome. The clinical situation deteriorates rapidly into tracheal obstruction and rapid local invasion of surrounding structures.

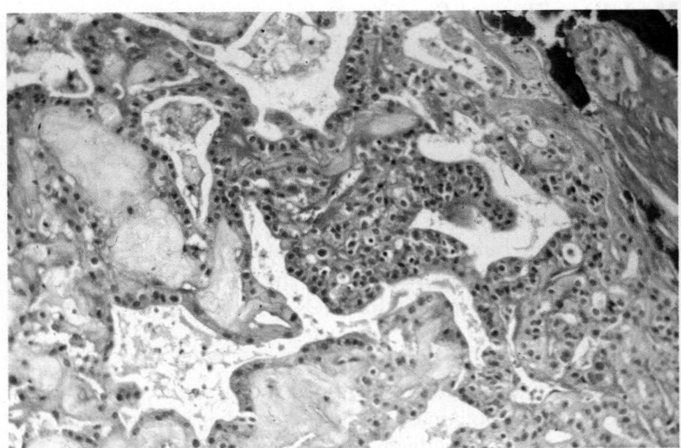

FIGURE 36-22 Hematoxylin-eosin staining of a thyroid mass reveals poorly differentiated cells, many of which are multinucleated, consistent with anaplastic carcinoma of the thyroid.

Pathology

Grossly, the tumor is locally invasive, with a firm, whitish appearance. On microscopic evaluation, giant cells with intranuclear cytoplasmic invaginations can be seen. Cell types range from moderately differentiated to extremely poorly differentiated cells (Fig. 36-22). Three types of cell populations have been classified: small spindle cell, giant cell, and squamous. All have a poor prognosis. *p53* mutations are found in 15% of tumors, a much higher rate than noted with DTCs. Occasionally, squamous cell elements or islands of more recognizable DTC, such as PTC, can be identified within the locus of the tumor. This finding led to speculation that ATC might arise from more differentiated carcinoma; however, there has been no solid proof of this theory.[25]

Treatment

The results of any surgical treatment of ATC are tempered by its rapidly progressive clinical course. Distant spread is present in 90% of patients at the time of diagnosis most commonly to the lungs, and most reports of resection are not optimistic. FNA is accurate in 90% of cases, making open biopsy an uncommon surgical indication. If ATC is initially thought to be resectable based on imaging, some small improvement in survival may be seen after resection. The finding of distant metastasis or invasion into locally unresectable structures, such as the trachea or vasculature of the anterior mediastinum, leads to a more conservative surgical approach, such as tracheostomy. Postoperative external-beam irradiation or adjunctive chemotherapy adds little to the overall prognosis but should be considered.[37] Because the prognosis is so grim in this disease, end-of-life planning and consideration of palliation must be part of very early management and counseling of these patients.

Thyroid Lymphoma

Primary thyroid lymphoma, although rare, is being recognized more frequently. The diagnosis is considered in patients with a goiter, especially one that has apparently grown significantly in a short period. Other initial symptoms include hoarseness, dysphagia, and fever. Thyroid lymphoma occurs four times more frequently in women than in men. Approximately half of primary thyroid lymphomas occur in the setting of preexisting Hashimoto thyroiditis.

Workup and Diagnosis

Patients with lymphoma undergo the standard workup for a thyroid mass or goiter. Suspicious signs are rapid enlargement and diffuse pain. Physical examination demonstrates a firm, slightly tender, fixed mass, frequently with substernal extension. There may be local symptoms including vocal cord paralysis. A few patients have "B" symptoms of lymphoma. Ultrasound may demonstrate a classic pseudocystic pattern. FNA can be diagnostic in this situation using flow cytometry for monoclonality to confirm the diagnosis. Thyroid lymphomas are almost all non-Hodgkin lymphomas, and most are B cell in origin. A subgroup of mucosa-associated lymphoid tissue (MALT) lymphomas occur in 6% to 27% of patients in some series.[38] If FNA is nondiagnostic, core needle biopsy or open biopsy can be considered. If the diagnosis is confirmed or highly suspicious, additional evaluation includes neck, chest, and abdominal CT or MRI to assess for extrathyroidal disease and may demonstrate disease completely encircling the trachea. The addition of PET imaging may be considered (Fig. 36-23). Approximately 50% of patients have disease confined to the thyroid, 5% have disease on both sides of the diaphragm or diffuse organ involvement, and the remaining patients have locoregional nodal disease.

Treatment

Patients with impending airway compromise frequently have very rapid results with the initiation of chemotherapy, particularly the glucocorticoid component, potentially avoiding the need for a surgical airway. Treatment philosophies differ with regard to chemotherapy or surgical ablation. Use of the CHOP regimen (cyclophosphamide, hydroxydaunomycin [doxorubicin], Oncovin [vincristine], and prednisolone) has been associated with excellent survival. Surgical resection, including near-total or total thyroidectomy, is thought by some authors to enhance these results, particularly for MALT lymphomas, but likely has little role in patients with extrathyroidal disease and is not pursued in most centers. There can be a significant amount of pericapsular edema and swelling with loss of normal tissue planes. There likely is no role for aggressive resections that may increase operative morbidity in the neck. In most cases, surgery is reserved for diagnostic biopsy when the diagnosis cannot be made by FNA or core biopsy.

MALT lymphomas are usually diagnosed at an earlier stage and have an indolent course. Diffuse and mixed large cell lymphomas behave more aggressively and are often initially found to have widespread involvement. For MALT lymphomas, 5-year survival rates approach 100%, whereas rates for large cell and mixed large cell lymphomas are 71% and 78%, respectively.

THYROID DISEASE IN PREGNANCY

Pregnant women and women of childbearing age constitute a subset of patients with thyroid disorders who require special

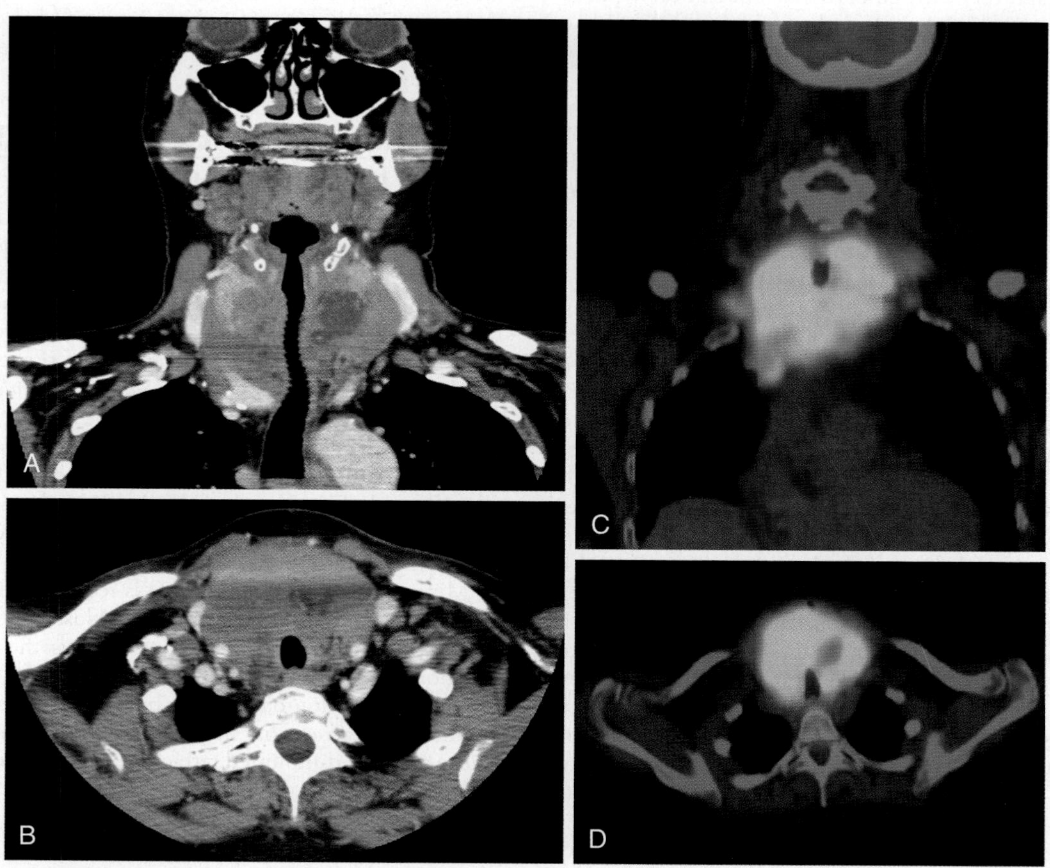

FIGURE 36-23 B cell lymphoma of the thyroid. All images are from the same patient. Computed tomography (CT) coronal **(A)** and axial **(B)** projections demonstrate a diffuse thyroid mass encasing the trachea with necrotic components. Abnormal ^{18}F-fluorodeoxyglucose positron emission tomography (PET) activity is demonstrated within this mass in PET/CT fusion imaging in coronal **(C)** and axial **(D)** projections.

attention. The prevalence of hypothyroidism in pregnant women is estimated to be 2% to 3%, and the estimated prevalence of pregnant women with hyperthyroidism is 0.4% to 1.7%.[39]

Physiologic Changes of the Thyroid Gland During Pregnancy

Pregnancy is a time of increased metabolic needs, and several factors in pregnancy also affect basic thyroid metabolism. hCG is secreted by the placenta, has significant homology with TSH, and is active at the TSH receptor. Pregnancy also results in elevated levels of serum TBG, requiring greater levels of total T_4 and T_3 to maintain adequate levels of free hormone. Overall, anticipated normal ranges of TSH concentration are lower during pregnancy with the lowest levels seen during the first trimester. Recommended ranges for TSH are 0.1 to 2.5 mIU/liter in the first trimester, 0.2 to 3.0 mIU/liter in the second trimester, and 0.3 to 3.0 mIU/liter in the third trimester.

Hypothyroidism in Pregnancy

The fetus depends entirely on maternal thyroid hormone until 10 weeks' gestation, when the fetal thyroid gland begins producing small amounts of thyroid hormone. Maternal hypothyroidism is associated with a wide range of poor pregnancy outcomes, including spontaneous abortion, fetal death, preterm delivery, pregnancy-induced hypertension, gestational diabetes, anemia, postpartum hemorrhage, placental abruption and preterm labor, preeclampsia, cesarean section, and very early embryo loss. Subclinical hypothyroidism has been associated with a threefold increased risk of placental abruption and an almost twofold increased risk of preterm labor.[40]

Pregnant women with subclinical or overt hypothyroidism should be treated with thyroid hormone to maintain serum TSH within the trimester-specific ranges. Although not universally agreed, it is recommended that thyroid function tests be measured in all women within 30 to 40 days of the first positive pregnancy test and then every 4 to 6 weeks throughout pregnancy.

Hyperthyroidism in Pregnancy

The most common cause of biochemical hyperthyroidism in pregnancy is hCG mediated. Hyperthyroidism usually is mild and resolves spontaneously, and treatment with antithyroid drugs is not recommended. Graves disease accounts for 85% to 90% of overt hyperthyroidism in pregnant women. Untreated overt maternal hyperthyroidism has been associated with the risk of low birth weight, severe preeclampsia, miscarriages, maternal congestive heart failure, stillbirth, and fetal growth restriction.

RAI at diagnostic and therapeutic doses is contraindicated in pregnancy. For medical treatment of hyperthyroidism in pregnancy, different medications are appropriate at different points in pregnancy. Methimazole should not be used in the first trimester because of associated teratogenicity. PTU is associated with hepatotoxicity. PTU is recommended in the first trimester, and methimazole is recommended in the second and third trimesters. Pregnant women being treated with antithyroid drugs should have free T_4 and TSH measured every 2 to 6 weeks during pregnancy.[41]

Thyroidectomy occasionally is required for treatment of thyrotoxicosis in pregnancy. Thyroidectomy may be performed if rapid control of hyperthyroidism is needed and antithyroid medications cannot be used because of allergies or noncompliance. If thyroidectomy is necessary during pregnancy, it is preferentially performed during the second trimester because of the risks of teratogenicity and fetal loss in the first trimester and of preterm labor in the third trimester. Preoperative treatment of pregnant women may include 10 to 14 days of iodine, antithyroid medications, and beta blockers.

Thyroid Nodules and Thyroid Carcinoma in Pregnancy

DTC occurs more frequently in women than in men and has a peak onset during female reproductive years. Therefore, thyroid carcinoma does manifest in pregnant patients. If a thyroid nodule is discovered during pregnancy, a thyroid ultrasound scan and FNA can be performed safely at any time during pregnancy. All pregnant women with a thyroid nodule should have TSH and free T_4 measured. Radionuclide scanning is contraindicated during pregnancy; however, inadvertent scanning during the first trimester does not appear to damage the fetal thyroid.[41]

If thyroid carcinoma is diagnosed during pregnancy, a sometimes emotionally difficult decision must be made in regard to performing a thyroidectomy during pregnancy or postponing thyroidectomy until after delivery. Surgery usually is not required during gestation, as deferring surgery for DTC until postpartum is not associated with a worse prognosis.[42] If surgery is deferred for FNA biopsy diagnostic of DTC, suppressive doses of thyroid hormone may be considered with a goal TSH of 0.1 to 0.5 mIU/liter. Ultrasound scans of the neck should be performed during each trimester to assess for rapid growth, which could indicate the need for surgery. Extensive local, nodal, or distant disease also may indicate the need for more urgent intervention. Thyroid nodules that are either benign or indeterminate and do not have rapid growth do not require levothyroxine suppressive therapy during pregnancy.

SURGICAL APPROACHES TO THE THYROID

Standard Cervical Thyroidectomy

Terminology for thyroid surgery is inconsistent in the literature; however, the following definitions represent consensus of appropriate terminology. *Total thyroidectomy* involves excision of all visible thyroid tissue. *Near-total thyroidectomy* is complete resection on one side while leaving a remnant of thyroid tissue on the contralateral side, leaving less than 1 g of tissue adjacent to the RLN at the ligament of Berry. *Subtotal thyroidectomy* leaves a remnant of thyroid tissue bilaterally. The typical reason to leave a remnant at the ligament of Berry is the pursuit of preservation of the RLN and blood supply to the parathyroids. *Thyroid lobectomy* typically includes removal of the thyroid isthmus and pyramidal lobe (if present). *Thyroid isthmusectomy* removes only the isthmus and is infrequently indicated.

Minimal specialized equipment is required for thyroid surgery beyond standard surgical instruments. Most surgeons prefer to use an advanced electrosurgical device such as the LigaSure or the Harmonic Scalpel, and some surgeons prefer bipolar cautery forceps. Various approaches may be used for retraction, including hand-held retractors that may be affixed in the belt of the ipsilateral surgeon, bed-mounted retractors, and self-retaining retractors such as Mahorner thyroid retractors and wound protectors. A shielded tip for the electrocautery pen may avoid inadvertent skin edge injury when working deep in the wound. Loupe magnification is standard, and at least one surgeon should wear a head-mounted light. Suction is standard, and many surgeons prefer to use the pediatric sized metal Yankauer tip. If intraoperative neuromonitoring is to be used, this complete system is required.

When general anesthesia is used, we prefer to have a large esophageal stethoscope placed because this facilitates palpation of the tracheoesophageal groove.

Before thyroidectomy, the patient must be appropriately positioned with a shoulder roll, the neck extended, and the head supported. The arms may be tucked at the sides or papoosed. Thyroid resections most commonly are performed using general anesthesia but also may be performed using cervical block regional anesthetic in experienced hands. When general anesthesia is used, some surgeons prefer paralysis; paralysis is contraindicated if intraoperative neuromonitoring is planned. Prophylactic antibiotics and chemoprophylaxis for venous thrombosis are not indicated except in unusual circumstances. After positioning and before skin preparation, an excellent opportunity to perform neck ultrasonography is available, and ultrasound can aid in ensuring that the pathology has not changed markedly from preoperative imaging as well as aiding in incision planning.

Given the sensitive cosmetic area of thyroid surgery, attention to careful incision planning and closure is appropriate. A transverse incision is placed in a way that provides a direct approach to the thyroid gland and its adjacent structures, while allowing optimal postoperative cosmetic results. Every effort should be made to place the incision in a natural skin crease to aid in optimal cosmetic healing. The cosmetic result is more enhanced by placement in a skin crease than it is by having a shorter incision. Placement of an optimal incision may be facilitated by examining and marking the candidate skin creases in the preoperative area because they will be less apparent after positioning. Ideally, the incision overlies the isthmus of the thyroid and usually lies somewhere between two finger-breadths above the clavicular heads and the level of the cricoid cartilage. A straightforward resection typically can be performed through a 3-cm incision; however, the surgeon should not hesitate to make the incision as large as required for adequate exposure to accomplish a safe and complete resection. The incision should be centered on the midline even for an asymmetrical goiter or unilateral lobectomy unless lateral neck dissection also is required. The skin incision is carried through subcutaneous fat and the platysma. Dividing the platysma beyond the edges of the skin incision allows greater access without increasing the skin incision length. A subplatysmal plane is dissected in the bloodless plane superficial to the fascia of the strap muscles. This plane is extended cephalad to the notch of the thyroid cartilage and caudally to the clavicular heads or sternal notch. The anterior jugular veins are identified, and any that are crossing or running along the midline can be divided.

The midline raphe can be identified between the sternohyoid muscles, and this raphe is opened from the thyroid cartilage superiorly to the sternal notch inferiorly. As the plane immediately deep to the sternohyoid muscles is entered, one encounters the isthmus of the thyroid in the midline and each of the lobes laterally. The cricoid ring lies at the superior aspect of the isthmus, and the cartilaginous rings of the trachea are palpable inferior to the isthmus. Any pyramidal lobe tissue should be identified and resected in its entirety regardless of whether the planned operation is a bilateral thyroidectomy, a thyroid lobectomy, or an isthmusectomy. Prelaryngeal nodal tissue frequently is included with this resection.

Some surgeons prefer to divide the isthmus at this point in the operation, whereas others do not divide the isthmus at all for a total thyroidectomy and transect the specimen from the contralateral lobe as the last step in the performance of thyroid lobectomy. Surgeons who divide the isthmus early in the operation believe that this permits greater mobility of the specimen to facilitate exposure and mobilization of large goiters. The isthmus should not be divided if there is a concerning mass or malignancy in the isthmus and division would interfere with pathologic analysis. When dividing the isthmus in the course of thyroid lobectomy, this should occur flush with the contralateral lobe such that the entire anterior trachea has no remaining thyroid tissue. If a total thyroidectomy is planned, the isthmus may be divided in the midline or on either side of a pyramidal lobe. The division is accomplished by cleanly entering the plane between the trachea and isthmus superiorly and inferiorly. Once this avascular space is well defined, an electrosurgical device may be used to divide the isthmus. The thin attachments to the anterior trachea may then be divided, but this dissection should not be carried posteriorly to avoid inadvertently entering the tracheoesophageal groove. In the relatively unusual case in which a thyroid isthmusectomy is planned, the isthmus may be divided on both sides, completing the resection.

Blunt dissection can separate the sternohyoid muscle from the thyroid capsule medially and identify the sternothyroid muscles in a deep and lateral position (Fig. 36-24). The sternothyroid muscles do not meet in the midline and must be separated off the thyroid capsule to gain lateral exposure to the thyroid. In patients who have previously undergone FNA, the planes deep to the sternothyroid muscle may be obscured by recent hemorrhage or scarring. If there is any concern for invasion of tumor into strap muscle, a portion of muscle should be left with the specimen. If the patient previously had thyroid surgery, these muscle groups

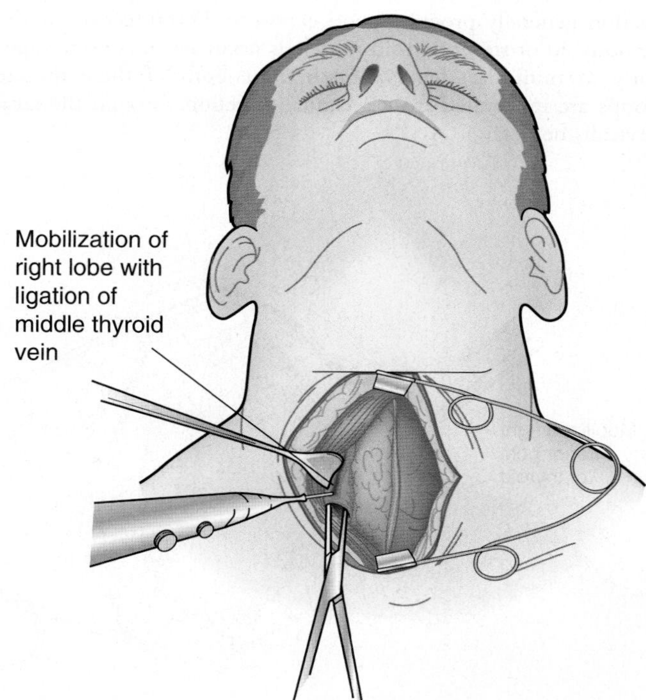

FIGURE 36-24 Image depicting a large incision to facilitate exposure. After creation of a subplatysmal plane, the strap muscles (sternohyoid and sternothyroid) are separated by dividing the tissues in the avascular midline plane from the thyroid cartilage to the suprasternal notch. The thyroid lobe is exposed by mobilizing the strap muscles away from the lobe by means of lateral retraction on the muscles. The middle vein is exposed, divided, and ligated. (From Sabiston DC, Jr, editor: *Atlas of general surgery*, Philadelphia, 1995, Saunders.)

will be densely adherent to the trachea and perhaps the tracheoesophageal groove. Great care must be used in this circumstance to identify the parathyroids and RLN.

When a thyroid lobectomy is planned, the strap muscles should not be separated from the contralateral lobe to avoid scar formation should a future completion thyroidectomy be required. When completion thyroidectomy is undertaken, it is helpful to use a different approach to the strap muscles. In completion thyroidectomy, we favor opening the strap muscles lateral to the midline, over the remaining thyroid lobe, and separating fibers of the sternohyoid muscle. This allows initial exposure of the remaining lobe in an area that has not previously been dissected, rather than attempting to dissect the scarred muscle off the midline trachea.

As the sternothyroid muscle is separated from the thyroid capsule, the thyroid should be retracted medially. The middle thyroid vein usually is encountered at this point and may be divided. This plane should be opened until the entire lobe is rolled medially leaving the carotid sheath laterally and the tracheoesophageal groove medially (Fig. 36-25). On the left side, the esophagus is more prominent because of its more lateral position at this level in the neck. Definition of this area can be enhanced by placement of an esophageal stethoscope, which allows easier palpation of the esophagus. The muscles should be well cleared off of the entire extent of the lateral upper pole to facilitate upper pole pedicle dissection.

In the case of complicated lateral thyroid masses, lymphadenopathy, or previous surgery, it may be necessary to gain exposure laterally by dividing the sternohyoid and sternothyroid muscles. It is rarely necessary to divide these two muscles because lateral traction generally provides good exposure. If transection of the sternohyoid or sternothyroid muscle is necessary, it is done superiorly to minimize denervation because both of these muscle groups are innervated from a caudal direction through the ansa cervicalis nerves.

By gaining access to the plane immediately above the thyroid sheath and placing lateral traction on the strap muscles of the neck, the operating surgeon should be able to visualize the entirety of the anterior surface of the thyroid, even in reoperative cases. To skeletonize the superior pole vessels, one needs to have good exposure laterally between the common carotid artery and the superior aspect of the ipsilateral thyroid lobe. Inferior and lateral traction on the upper pole of the thyroid facilitates identification of the avascular medial thyroid space of Reeves between the upper pole of the thyroid and the cricothyroid muscle. With this space well defined and the lateral upper pole well cleared, the adjacent sternothyroid muscle and the external branch of the superior laryngeal nerve may be swept off of the superior thyroid vascular pedicle leaving well-defined superior thyroid artery and vein. The vessels are controlled and ligated close to their insertion into the thyroid (Fig. 36-26; see Fig. 36-1). As described earlier, there is variation in location of the external branch of the superior laryngeal nerve relative to the superior thyroid artery. Some surgeons routinely identify this nerve, whereas many simply attempt to avoid this nerve by ligating the well-skeletonized vessels very close to their insertion into the thyroid parenchyma. Care must be taken to achieve secure ligation of the superior thyroid artery because this vessel may retract into the carotid sheath and be difficult to control from the existing incision. After mobilizing the upper pole vessels, in this area the superior parathyroids are usually found lying in small deposits of fat within the thyroid sheath.

For a relatively normal-sized thyroid lobe, the lobe may have been medialized and the tracheoesophageal groove exposed earlier in the procedure. For patients with large goiters and substernal goiters, it usually is impossible to mobilize the goiter into the cervical wound until after the superior pole vessels have been divided because these are an important point of fixation. After the superior thyroid vessels and middle thyroid veins have been divided, continued medial retraction of the thyroid lobe allows

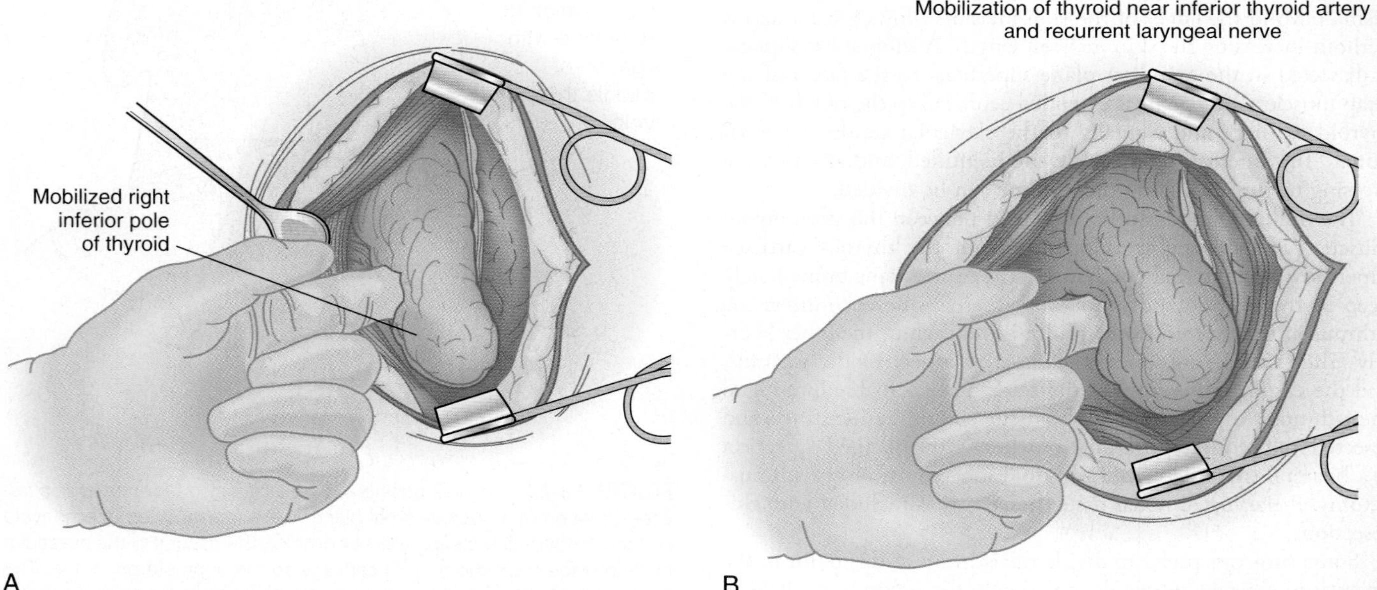

FIGURE 36-25 **A** and **B,** The thyroid lobe is retracted medially to leave the carotid sheath laterally and allow the posterolateral surface of the thyroid to be exposed. (From Sabiston DC, Jr, editor: *Atlas of general surgery*, Philadelphia, 1995, Saunders.)

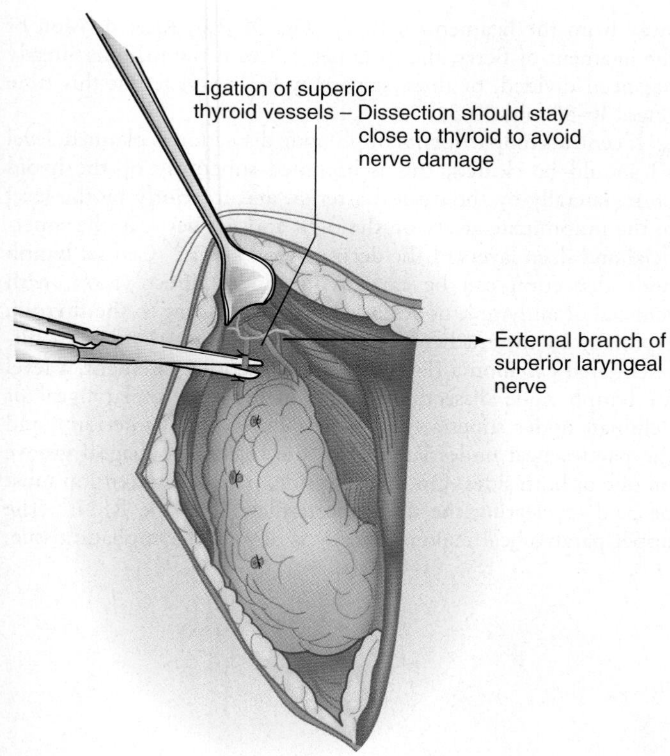

FIGURE 36-26 Downward and lateral traction exposes the superior pole vessels, including branches of the superior thyroid artery. The external branch of the superior laryngeal nerve courses along the cricothyroid muscle just medial to the superior pole vessels. To avoid injury to this nerve, the superior pole vessels are divided individually as close as possible to the point where they enter the thyroid gland. (From Sabiston DC, Jr, editor: *Atlas of general surgery*, Philadelphia, 1995, Saunders.)

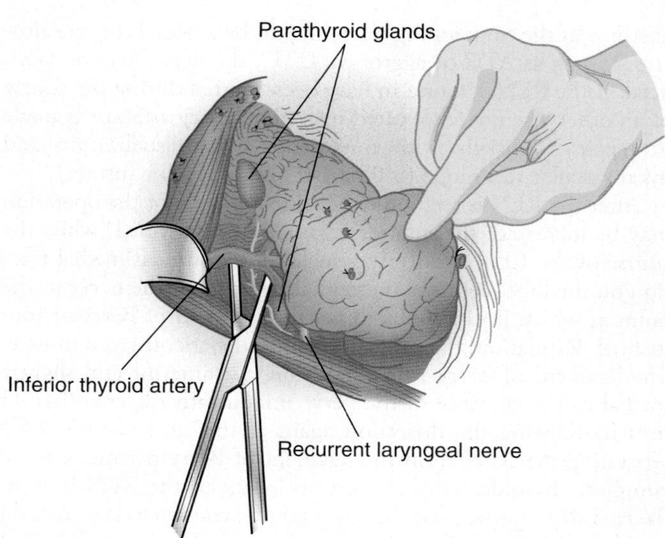

FIGURE 36-27 As the thyroid is retracted medially, gentle dissection is used to expose the parathyroid glands, inferior thyroid artery, and recurrent laryngeal nerve. The recurrent nerve usually passes deep to the inferior thyroid artery but may lie anterior to it. It is best found by careful dissection just inferior to the artery. The nerve can then be traced upward, and its position in relation to the thyroid can be determined. Parathyroid glands that lie on the thyroid surface can be mobilized with their vascular supply and preserved. (From Sabiston DC, Jr, editor: *Atlas of general surgery*, Philadelphia, 1995, Saunders.)

the posterior aspect of the thyroid lobe to be visualized, and larger goiters may be brought out through the wound.

Further mobilization of the thyroid lobe allows exposure of the tracheoesophageal groove and the RLN (Figs. 36-27 and 36-28). The upper and lower parathyroids may become evident at this point. Minimal dissection of the lower vessels entering the thyroid is undertaken, and no division is done until the RLN is seen and positively identified. On the right side, care is taken when dissecting in the posterolateral aspects of the trachea because the esophagus is not well palpated in this area. In patients undergoing thyroid reoperations, this area is extremely treacherous because of scar tissue. If the RLN is not immediately visible at the level of the thyroid lobe, it is generally advisable to proceed lower in the neck tissue in previously undissected areas to gain access to the RLN. Useful landmarks for RLN identification include the following: (1) Palpation of the tracheoesophageal groove is facilitated by having a tube such as an esophageal stethoscope in the esophagus. (2) The RLN crosses the inferior thyroid artery medial, lateral, or between branches. (3) The superior parathyroid is posterior to the RLN, and the inferior parathyroid is anterior to the RLN. (4) The RLN frequently passes immediately medial to a tubercle of Zuckerkandl. (5) The RLN enters the cricothyroid approximately 2 cm posterior to the anterior border of the trachea at approximately the level of the cricoid ring.

When the RLN has been identified on either side, it is mandatory to track it through any scar tissue or thyroid carcinoma.

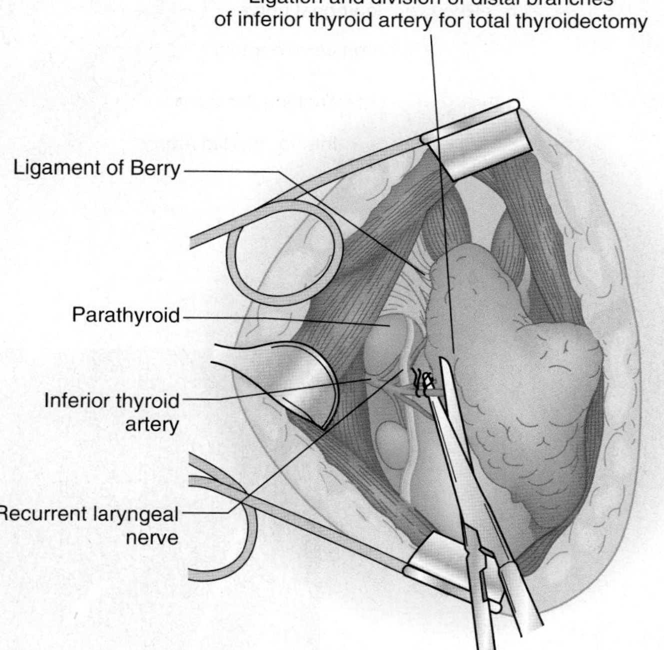

FIGURE 36-28 To perform total lobectomy, branches of the inferior thyroid artery are divided at the surface of the thyroid gland. The inferior thyroid veins can then be ligated and divided. Superiorly, the connective tissue (ligament of Berry), which binds the thyroid to the tracheal rings, is carefully divided. Several small accompanying vessels are usually present, and the recurrent nerve is closest to the thyroid and most vulnerable at this point. Division of the ligament allows the thyroid to be mobilized medially. (From Sabiston DC, Jr, editor: *Atlas of general surgery*, Philadelphia, 1995, Saunders.)

Sacrifice of the functioning nerve should be avoided. In rare situations, such as ATC or aggressive DTC, the nerve may be sacrificed. If the RLN is found to have been injured during the course of an otherwise uncomplicated operation, every attempt is made to repair it initially with microscope-aided visualization and microvascular technique (8-0 or 9-0 monofilament sutures).

After the RLN is seen on either side, the pace of the operation may be increased; the inferior vessels may be divided, while the course of the RLN is directly visualized. Continued medial traction on the lobe identifies the cephalad course of the nerve to the point at which it disappears under the ligament of Berry or into its final destination, the caudal border of the cricothyroid muscle. The ligament of Berry is in a position just anterior and slightly medial to the entrance of the nerve underneath the cricothyroid muscle. Slowing the dissection again at this area and carefully separating the RLN from the ligament of Berry permits a more complete thyroidectomy. A traction injury to the RLN is most likely at this time because the nerve may be constricted by crossing vessels and be subject to significant traction until it is dissected away from the ligament of Berry (Fig. 36-29). After division of the ligament of Berry, the specimen is free if the isthmus already has been divided, or these steps may be completed at this time (Figs. 36-30 and 36-31).

If central compartment lymph node dissection is planned, level VI should be cleared; this is bounded superiorly by the hyoid bone, laterally by the carotid arteries, and inferiorly by the level of the innominate artery on the right and lies between the superficial and deep layers of the deep cervical fascia.[43] Central lymph node dissection can be carried out under direct vision, with removal of all lymph nodes immediately adjacent to the thyroid, especially in the tracheoesophageal groove in patients with differentiated carcinoma (level VI). By consensus statement, a level VI lymph node dissection should include the prelaryngeal or delphian nodes superiorly, the pretracheal nodes inferiorly, and the paratracheal nodes laterally in the tracheoesophageal groove on one or both sides. On the right side, particular attention must be paid to clearing the nodes posterolateral to the RLN.[43] The upper paratracheal region typically is devoid of lymphatic tissue,

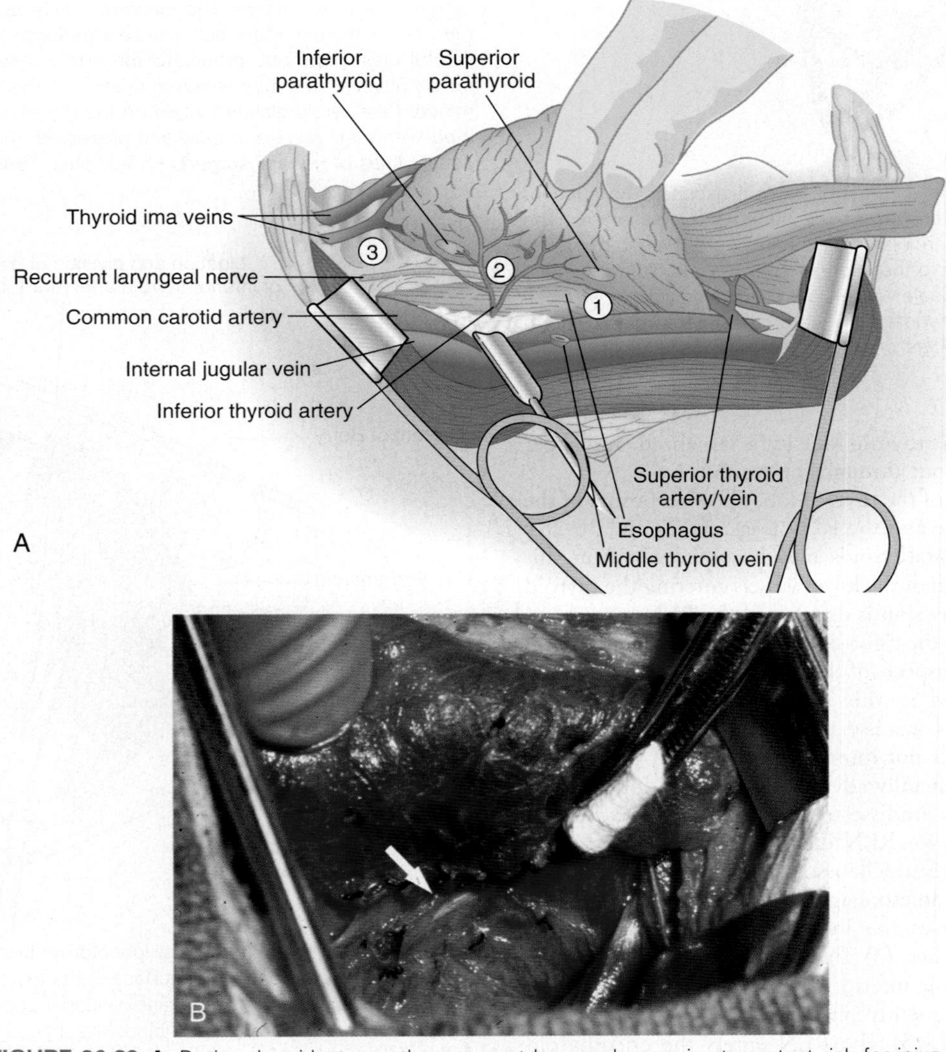

FIGURE 36-29 A, During thyroidectomy, the recurrent laryngeal nerve is at greatest risk for injury at the ligament of Berry *(1)*, during ligation of branches of the inferior thyroid artery *(2)*, and at the thoracic inlet *(3)*. **B,** Intraoperative photo of the recurrent laryngeal nerve in the tracheoesophageal groove *(arrow)*. (**A,** From Kahky MP, Weber RS: Intraoperative problems: Complications of surgery of the thyroid and parathyroid glands. *Surg Clin North Am* 73:307, 1993.)

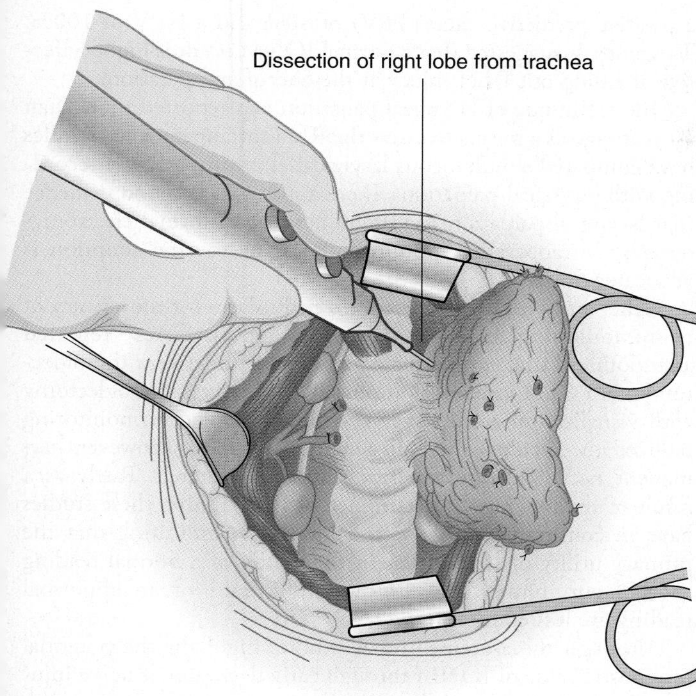

FIGURE 36-30 Dissection of the medial tracheal attachments is minimally vascular. Dissection is extended under the isthmus, and the specimen is divided so that the isthmus is included with the resected lobe. The pyramidal lobe also is included if present. (From Sabiston DC, Jr, editor: *Atlas of general surgery*, Philadelphia, 1995, Saunders.)

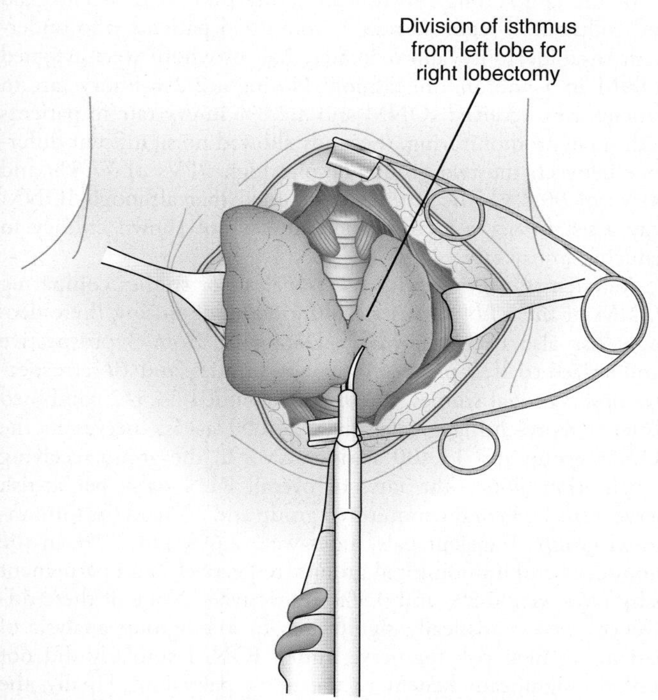

FIGURE 36-31 The thyroid can now be divided with the harmonic scalpel so that the isthmus is included in the specimen. (From Sabiston DC, Jr, editor: *Atlas of general surgery*, Philadelphia, 1995, Saunders.)

and it may be appropriate not to include this region in a central compartment dissection.[44]

Lateral Neck Dissection

In the setting of thyroid cancer, compartment-based lateral neck dissection typically is performed for known lateral neck metastatic disease. This disease may be evident by physical examination or may be detected only by lateral neck ultrasonography. Biopsy is used routinely for definitive demonstration of lateral neck metastatic spread before recommending lateral neck dissection. Prophylactic lateral neck dissection is not typically indicated, and "berry picking" of nodes from the lateral compartment should not be performed.[5]

An excellent description of lateral compartment nodal dissection for PTC is available in the literature and is reflected herein.[45] Several incisions may be used for lateral compartment dissection. Excellent exposure is provided by extending the thyroidectomy incision superiorly and laterally along the anterior border of the sternocleidomastoid muscle. We favor a lateral extension of the thyroidectomy incision in a natural skin crease to the between the lateral margin of the sternocleidomastoid and the border of the trapezius; we find that this has a better cosmetic result and provides adequate exposure in most cases. If a transverse incision is used, it occasionally is necessary to make a second, higher incision parallel to the previous surgical incision to address level II nodes. After skin incision, subplatysmal planes are raised. The anterior border of the sternocleidomastoid muscle is completely dissected, and the plane is entered between the strap muscles and the sternocleidomastoid, which is retracted laterally. The omohyoid muscle typically is divided. Nodes lying anterior to the carotid artery and vein at the level of the thyroid cartilage may be resected at this time or later in the operation. The carotid sheath contents are exposed. The carotid sheath is opened, and the lateral border of the internal jugular vein is dissected, starting several centimeters above the clavicles. With retraction of the internal jugular vein medially and dissecting down to the floor of the neck on the anterior scalene, the phrenic nerve may be found running along the anterior scalene. The transverse cervical artery passes anterior to the phrenic nerve and usually does not need to be sacrificed. The carotid artery and vagus nerve should then be well identified and cleared of nodal tissue. With these structures identified, the nodal packet should be cleared from these structures down to the base of the neck. On the left side, the thoracic duct is encountered looping up from posterior to the internal jugular vein and passing from medial to lateral to enter the subclavian vein at the junction with the internal jugular vein. The thoracic duct may be protected or may safely be ligated in an adult, particularly if injured. By dissecting laterally across the base of the neck, the nodal packet may be separated and swept superiorly off of the scalene. The brachial plexus may be identified passing between the anterior and middle scalene. The sensory branches of the cervical plexus frequently may be preserved by dissecting them out of the nodal specimen. The spinal accessory nerve is sought superiorly to this as it courses obliquely across level II. The contents inferior and medial to this nerve are included in a typical dissection for papillary cancer (level IIA), but the nodes superior and medial typically are not (level IIB). The spinal accessory nerve should be handled very carefully because even an intact motor functioning nerve may still commonly result in a constellation of troublesome symptoms known as "shoulder syndrome," which are best addressed by physical therapy. The operative bed should be inspected for residual nodal tissue and to ensure hemostasis, and then the wound may be closed in layers. We routinely leave a small-caliber, closed-suction drain such as a 10 Fr round Blake channel drain. This drain is primarily for the drainage of lymphatic fluid and remains in place until the output is low and the patient is eating a regular diet.

Substernal Goiter

Exploration of the anterior mediastinal space is within the armamentarium of an experienced thyroid surgeon. In the case of a substernal goiter, we routinely obtain preoperative cross-sectional imaging to aid in operative planning. Even impressive substernal goiters usually are amenable to resection by a cervical incision. Characteristics that might predict an inability to mobilize a thoracic goiter into a cervical incision include a reoperative field, an invasive substernal thyroid malignancy, goiters that extend below the inferior margin of the aortic arch, goiters that reach the carina, goiters that extend into the posterior mediastinum, and true ectopic mediastinal thyroid tissue.

Even in the presence of the aforementioned findings, initial exploration usually involves a cervical incision. Maneuvers that may help to mobilize the mediastinal component into the cervical incision include division of the superior thyroid vascular pedicle, division of the thyroid isthmus, and opening of the midline raphe all the way to the manubrium. The RLN is usually displaced posteriorly and inferiorly; however, it can be draped anteriorly over the mass and damaged in that position. Great care must be exercised in mobilization of the mass until the nerve is identified.

In the unusual case in which a median sternotomy is required, a midline incision is made from the middle of the cervical wound and extended inferiorly and onto the manubrium. Before dividing the sternum, access is gained on the superior border of the manubrium, and all tissues deep to the sternum are swept away bluntly. The midline sternal incision is made with a saw or splitting device and carried to the level of the second, third, or fourth intercostal space as needed. We prefer a partial sternal split of just the manubrium or of only the cephalad portion of the sternum, which usually provides excellent exposure and avoids the instability associated with full sternotomy. Substernal thyroid masses, including goiters or extension of malignancies, and ectopic parathyroid adenomatous tissue can be approached through this incision. The anteromedial fat pad and thymus can be dissected to gain visualization of the pericardium superiorly. As one proceeds laterally in this dissection, care must be taken to avoid injuring the pleura and the phrenic nerves. The innominate vein is deep to the thymus. Virtually all low-lying thyroid masses can be approached through this incision.

Intraoperative Neuromonitoring

Electronic identification and intraoperative neuromonitoring (IONM) of the RLN has gained increasing attention as an adjunct to standard visual identification of the nerve during thyroid and parathyroid surgery. As more experience with IONM has accrued, contrasting opinions about its efficacy have been reported. Proponents of the technique contend that the monitoring device aids in identification and preservation of the RLN, ultimately resulting in better outcomes such as reductions in transient and permanent voice changes. Cernea and colleagues[46] reported a prospective analysis of 447 patients who underwent thyroidectomy with IONM with endotracheal tubes that incorporated surface electrodes. Comparing IONM with vocal cord paralysis on postoperative endoscopy, the authors reported no false-negative results with a positive predictive value (PPV) of 40% and a NPV of 100%. This analysis suggested that a normal IONM result is highly effective at ruling out RLN injury at the end of an operation.

The technique of laryngeal palpation was reported more than 10 years ago as a means to assess the RLN intraoperatively. Studies have compared simultaneous laryngeal electromyography recording with laryngeal palpation. There appears to be good evidence that laryngeal palpation is a useful adjunct to formal electromyography intraoperative monitoring, and its routine adoption is advocated.

Other authors have reported less enthusiasm for the efficacy of neuromonitoring. In 2009, Barczynski and associates[47] reported a randomized trial comparing patients who underwent thyroidectomy with RLN visualization plus IONM versus thyroidectomy with visualization alone. They concluded that nerve monitoring reduced the incidence of transient nerve damage; however, permanent nerve damage was not statistically altered. Partly as a result of the low rate of occurrence of RLN injury, these studies have in common high PPV and low NPV, indicating that the primary utility of IONM lies in the ability of a normal reading to rule out injury. The clinical implications of an abnormal reading are less consistent.

Although the aforementioned studies highlight the potential prognostic value of IONM through early detection of nerve injuries, the therapeutic benefit of IONM is less commonly reported. More recent studies confirm that the use of IONM is associated with a PPV of 33% and NPV of 99%.

Large multi-institutional studies concluded that visual identification of the RLN was the gold standard of care and that IONM may have an adjunctive role in special cases as a "promising tool" for nerve identification and protection in extended thyroid resection procedures. Important risk factors of permanent RLN paralysis appear to include recurrent goiters, thyroid malignancies, and lobectomies.

In the largest single-institution study published so far, Calo and colleagues[48] reported results from 2034 patients who underwent thyroidectomy, approximately half of whom were assigned IONM in a nonrandom fashion. Noting a 2.2% injury rate in patients who received IONM and a 2.8% injury rate in patients with no neuromonitoring, the study showed no significant difference between the two groups despite high PPVs of 77.8% and NPVs of 99.8%. The authors concluded that although IONM may assist in nerve identification, it has not shown efficacy in reducing injury rate.

A systematic review with meta-analysis of studies comparing IONM of the RLN versus visualization alone during thyroidectomy has also been reported.[49] Data were from 3 prospective randomized trials, 7 prospective cohort studies, and 10 retrospective observational studies. The report included 23,512 combined patients representing greater than 24,000 at-risk nerves in the IONM group and 11,400 at-risk nerves in the group receiving visualization alone. The rates of overall RLN palsy per at-risk nerve were 3.5% in the monitored group and 3.7% in the unmonitored group. Transient palsy rates were 2.6% and 2.7% in the monitored and unmonitored groups, respectively, and permanent palsy rates were 0.8% and 0.9%, respectively. None of these differences were statistically significant. In a subgroup analysis of patients at high risk for nerve injury, IONM similarly did not confer a significant benefit to the nerve palsy rate. Finally, the authors noted a nonsignificant trend toward longer operative time from incision to closure among neuromonitored cases (97.6 minutes versus 94.6 minutes).

Taken in aggregate, we consider direct anatomic identification and protection of the RLN to be the gold standard. IONM is a technology that should be within the armamentarium of the thyroid surgeon. Some surgeons use this technology routinely; others never use it; and others (such as ourselves) use it selectively for cases with expected distorted or aberrant anatomy, cases with a preexisting deficit in vocal cord movement, and cases in which the nerve lies in a scarred surgical field. All these practices are within accepted standard of care. Further data from ongoing clinical experience may eventually prove or disprove more definitively the efficacy of IONM in preventing patient morbidity.

Postoperative Care

Evaluation and management of thyroid and parathyroid function is important. The surgeon is obligated to evaluate and inform the patient and referring physician of the details of the resection and its expected impact on postoperative function. There are several reasonable approaches to postoperative calcium supplementation. Some surgeons routinely check a calcium level the next morning and base calcium and vitamin D supplementation on that result. Other surgeons, in particular surgeons who routinely send patients home on the same day as surgery, routinely place patients on oral calcium regimens without checking an early postoperative calcium or PTH result. Other surgeons routinely use an early postoperative PTH result, even as early as in the recovery room, and base supplementation on that result.

The specific regimen of calcium supplementation also varies widely. One protocol that we have used involves routine over-the-counter calcium carbonate with vitamin D given at a dose of 1 g three times a day for 1 week and then 1 g two times a day for the subsequent 2 weeks. This is a low-cost approach, and the adverse effects are minimal, although some patients become constipated. Patients who have had a lobectomy with the contralateral side never explored should not routinely require calcium supplementation.

Previously euthyroid patients scheduled to undergo thyroid lobectomy should be informed of their risk of becoming hypothyroid despite leaving one lobe in situ; the likelihood of this occurring is related to their preoperative TSH level. Of patients with a preoperative TSH less than 1 mIU/liter, approximately 20% require postoperative thyroid supplementation; of patients with a preoperative TSH between 1 and 2 mIU/liter, approximately 40% require postoperative thyroid supplementation; of patients with a preoperative TSH between 2 and 3 mIU/liter, approximately 70% require postoperative thyroid supplementation; and of patients with a preoperative TSH between 3 and 4 mIU/liter, approximately 90% require postoperative thyroid supplementation.[50]

For patients undergoing total thyroidectomy, it is expected that the patient will be dependent on exogenous thyroid hormone. A typical physiologic replacement dose of levothyroxine is 1.6 μg/kg/day. In a 70-kg adult, this correlates to a dose of 112 μg, which is administered as a once-daily dose. Adipose tissue does not require the same degree of supplementation as lean body mass, and the weight-based dose may be adjusted in obese patients, for which several formulas are available. One method involves using the following formula:[51]

$$\mu g/kg/day = (-0.018 \times \text{body mass index}) + 2.13$$

Older patients also should be started at a lower dose. Although clinical hypothyroidism does not develop immediately, thyroid hormone supplementation typically is started on the day after total thyroidectomy. In a patient with previous hyperthyroidism, supplementation may be deferred for several days.

Calculated values for thyroid hormone replacement are imperfect, and dose monitoring and adjustment are necessary. After initiating thyroid hormone therapy or a dose adjustment, a TSH level should be checked approximately 6 weeks later. If the patient is clearly clinically hypothyroid or hyperthyroid before 6 weeks, an earlier TSH level at 2 to 3 weeks is appropriate.

In the setting of thyroid cancer, several factors must be considered regarding starting thyroid hormone. If RAI therapy is planned, one must consider whether or not to use thyroid hormone withdrawal versus exogenous rhTSH; if withdrawal is planned, one must consider whether the withdrawal will be from T_4 therapy or T_3 therapy (liothyronine) and the planned degree of TSH suppression. These plans vary depending on the pathology, the patient, and the physician, and all have implications for thyroid hormone dosing. We consider it mandatory to involve the endocrinologist, who will manage the subsequent treatment in the decision for initial thyroid hormone dosing in the setting of known or suspected thyroid carcinoma.

Alternative Approaches to Thyroid Surgery

Although the surgical techniques described in this chapter are the standard of care in the surgical management of thyroid pathology, multiple new avenues of surgical intervention are being investigated. Many surgeons, including ourselves, have found that traditional surgical technique may be accomplished through more limited skin incisions; careful positioning and appropriate use of retractors are required. Other techniques allow even more limited cervical incisions, relocation of the incision away from the neck, and potentially elimination of the skin incision. The appropriate application and safety profile of all these techniques is still being defined and must be measured against traditional thyroidectomy, which is well tolerated and has good cosmetic results in most cases.

Minimally invasive video-assisted thyroidectomy involves the use of a 1.5- to 2-cm anterior cervical incision, an endoscopic camera placed into the wound for visualization, self-retaining retractors, and dedicated surgical instruments. This technique is most commonly applied to lobectomy for benign disease, but it has been applied to total thyroidectomy including for malignancy. This approach results in longer operative times, which improve after a learning curve, and is believed to have the same rate of technical complication as traditional thyroidectomy. Prior neck surgery, a large-volume thyroid (>25 mL), a large lesion, and lymphatic metastasis are considered contraindications to this technique.

Multiple other approaches to thyroid surgery involve displacing the incision from the neck. All involve dissection planes far beyond that required for traditional thyroidectomy and introduce risks of complications not present with traditional thyroidectomy. For this reason, it is inappropriate to describe these approaches as minimally invasive; it more appropriate to describe them as "alternative access" approaches. Kang and associates[52] in South Korea championed the use of a transaxillary gasless robotically assisted approach to thyroidectomy. A 5- to 6-cm incision is made in the axilla, and a subcutaneous plane is created anterior to the pectoralis, between the heads of the sternocleidomastoid muscle, and deep to the strap muscles. Using this approach, a self-retaining retractor, and a robotic surgical system, total thyroidectomy may be performed. This approach has been applied to benign disease and small malignancies. Kang and associates included an ipsilateral level VI nodal dissection in all cases. They reported a 1% rate of permanent RLN injury and a 3-day mean hospital stay.

Other described approaches include a transaxillary approach using more traditional endoscopic instrumentation, a bilateral axillo-breast approach, a "facelift" incision approach, and a transoral approach. These approaches have variable described experience in different regions of the world and have been applied to various benign and malignant thyroid pathologies. All of them have their own associated risks, such as introducing oral flora into the central compartment of the neck with the transoral approach and introducing the potential of spinal accessory nerve injury with the facelift incision approach. Data are accumulating regarding the technical complication rates and the long-term oncologic adequacy of these approaches. They have yet to be widely adopted. We do not recommend that these approaches be introduced into a practice at this time outside of a very carefully considered and executed investigational approach.

Complications of Thyroid Surgery

The advantage of complete removal of disease-bearing tissue and efficient subsequent application of RAI ablation after total thyroidectomy must be weighed against lesser procedures such as lobectomy in terms of surgical complications. The most important complications are hypocalcemia secondary to devascularization of the parathyroid after the procedure and significant hoarseness caused by RLN injury induced by traction or division.

Hypocalcemia and Hypoparathyroidism

Rates of postprocedure hypocalcemia are approximately 5%, and it resolves in 80% of cases in approximately 12 months.[53] Every effort is made to evaluate the parathyroid tissue intraoperatively. For glands that appear to be devascularized, the use of immediate parathyroid autotransplantation of 1-mm fragments of saline-chilled tissue into pockets made in the sternocleidomastoid muscle or the brachioradialis muscle is extremely effective in avoiding permanent hypocalcemia.

Nerve Injury

All patients should undergo voice assessment before thyroid surgery including at least a description of the preoperative voice by the patient and the physician. With some experience, laryngoscopy also may readily be performed in the office setting by either mirror laryngoscopy or flexible laryngoscopy. Although some authors advocate laryngoscopy before and after every central neck procedure, we favor recommendations that support preoperative laryngoscopy in patients with preoperative onset of voice changes, patients with bulky tumor or nodal disease in the tracheoesophageal groove, and patients with a history of cervical or upper thoracic surgical intervention; this includes a prior anterior approach to the cervical spine as well as carotid procedures. A grossly normal voice does not exclude an occult nerve paralysis.

Superior Laryngeal Nerve

The superior laryngeal nerve has two branches: an internal branch that supplies sensory fibers to the larynx and an external branch that supplies motor fibers to the cricothyroid muscles and tenses the vocal cords. The external branch can run closely adherent to the superior thyroid artery, and care must be exercised during dissection in this area. Injury to the external branch causes voice changes, huskiness, poor volume and projection, voice fatigue, and inability to sing at higher ranges.[2]

Recurrent Laryngeal Nerve

As mentioned previously, the RLN arises from the vagus and is a mixed motor, sensory, and autonomous nerve that innervates the adductor and abductor muscles. Unilateral injury is classically described as a paralyzed vocal cord with loss of movement from the midline. A wide spectrum of injuries to the voice or swallowing mechanisms, or both, can occur because of the mixed fibers contained within the nerve.[2] Temporary or permanent voice change can result and is extremely distressing to the patient.

Bleeding

Wound hematoma occurs in less than 1% of patients who undergo thyroidectomy. The most important element of management of wound hematoma is early recognition; this is potentially facilitated by not closing the strap muscles completely. The typical presentation of wound hematoma is a firm swelling in the wound bed. This swelling is usually distinguishable from seroma, which is very soft and ballotable, and rarely requires intervention. Once wound hematoma is recognized, if the patient is not stridorous or in extremis, he or she should be transported immediately to the operating room. Some surgeons advocate opening the incision before intubation, whereas others favor a trial of intubation during which the surgical team is completely prepared to open the wound. If the patient has impending loss of airway, if the patient has lost the airway, or endotracheal intubation cannot be achieved, the wound should be opened immediately, even if this occurs at the bedside. When the wound is opened, this includes opening skin, platysma, and strap muscles. This may relieve the obstruction, allows endotracheal intubation, and allows placement of an emergency surgical airway if needed. Once the airway is safely secured by any of the above-described means, the patient is no longer in danger, and the reexploration may proceed in an organized fashion. The surgical team must be careful not to allow the excitement of the moment to interfere with continued protection of the parathyroids and laryngeal nerves.

Complication rates appear to be affected by a surgeon's experience. A study in Maryland comprising 5860 patients reported the lowest complication rates in patients operated on by surgeons who performed more than 100 neck explorations annually, and other studies confirmed these results.[5,54]

SELECTED REFERENCES

Adam MA, Pura J, Gu L, et al: Extent of surgery for papillary thyroid cancer is not associated with survival: An analysis of 61,775 patients. *Ann Surg* 260:601–605, discussion 605–607, 2014.

This large, well-performed analysis challenges the previously held belief that more aggressive resection alters the prognosis of papillary thyroid cancer. These and other data have informed the shift toward less aggressive resection that is reflected in the American Thyroid Association guidelines and this chapter.

Cady B, Sedgwick CE, Meissner WA, et al: Risk factor analysis in differentiated thyroid cancer. *Cancer* 43:810–820, 1979.

This classic article explores the important prognostic factors in differentiated thyroid cancer particularly highlighting the importance of age and sex.

Hartl DM, Travagli JP, Leboulleux S, et al: Clinical review: Current concepts in the management of unilateral recurrent laryngeal nerve paralysis after thyroid surgery. *J Clin Endocrinol Metab* 90:3084–3088, 2005.

This article provides an excellent discussion of the pathophysiology of surgically induced damage to the external branch of the superior laryngeal and recurrent laryngeal nerves—must reading for any thyroid surgeon.

Haugen BR, Alexander EK, Bible KC, et al: 2015 American Thyroid Association management guidelines for patients with thyroid nodules and differentiated thyroid cancer. *Thyroid* (Epub ahead of print; 2015).

This thorough update of the original 2006 and subsequent 2009 consensus statement of the American Thyroid Association on the management of thyroid nodules and differentiated thyroid cancer is a must read and an ongoing resource for anyone managing thyroid nodules or thyroid cancer.

Hay ID, Thompson GB, Grant CS, et al: Papillary thyroid carcinoma managed at the Mayo Clinic during six decades (1940-1999): Temporal trends in initial therapy and long-term outcome in 2444 consecutively treated patients. *World J Surg* 26:879–885, 2002.

This excellent contribution from the Mayo Clinic may be the longest study of thyroid cancer. The authors confirm the use of more extensive resection and postoperative radioablation and substantiate their data with 50 years of follow-up.

Porterfield JR, Factor DA, Grant CS: Operative technique for modified radical neck dissection in papillary thyroid carcinoma. *Arch Surg* 144:567–574, 2009.

This is a clear and well-written technical guide for the performance of lateral neck dissection for papillary thyroid cancer that balances oncologic principles and patient morbidity.

REFERENCES

1. Cernea CR, Ferraz AR, Furlani J, et al: Identification of the external branch of the superior laryngeal nerve during thyroidectomy. *Am J Surg* 164:634–639, 1992.
2. Hartl DM, Travagli JP, Leboulleux S, et al: Clinical review: Current concepts in the management of unilateral recurrent laryngeal nerve paralysis after thyroid surgery. *J Clin Endocrinol Metab* 90:3084–3088, 2005.
3. Caldwell KL, Miller GA, Wang RY, et al: Iodine status of the U.S. population, National Health and Nutrition Examination Survey 2003-2004. *Thyroid* 18:1207–1214, 2008.
4. Mazzaferri EL, Robbins RJ, Spencer CA, et al: A consensus report of the role of serum thyroglobulin as a monitoring method for low-risk patients with papillary thyroid carcinoma. *J Clin Endocrinol Metab* 88:1433–1441, 2003.
5. Haugen BR, Alexander EK, Bible KC, et al: 2015 American Thyroid Association management guidelines for patients with thyroid nodules and differentiated thyroid cancer. *Thyroid* (Epub ahead of print; 2015).
6. Duh QY, Grossman RF: Thyroid growth factors, signal transduction pathways, and oncogenes. *Surg Clin North Am* 75:421–437, 1995.
7. Martino E, Bartalena L, Bogazzi F, et al: The effects of amiodarone on the thyroid. *Endocr Rev* 22:240–254, 2001.
8. Tomer Y, Barbesino G, Greenberg DA, et al: Mapping the major susceptibility loci for familial Graves' and Hashimoto's diseases: Evidence for genetic heterogeneity and gene interactions. *J Clin Endocrinol Metab* 84:4656–4664, 1999.
9. Elfenbein DM, Schneider DF, Havlena J, et al: Clinical and socioeconomic factors influence treatment decisions in Graves' disease. *Ann Surg Oncol* 22:1196–1199, 2015.
10. Boelaert K, Horacek J, Holder RL, et al: Serum thyrotropin concentration as a novel predictor of malignancy in thyroid nodules investigated by fine-needle aspiration. *J Clin Endocrinol Metab* 91:4295–4301, 2006.
11. Frates MC, Benson CB, Charboneau JW, et al: Management of thyroid nodules detected at US: Society of Radiologists in Ultrasound consensus conference statement. *Radiology* 237:794–800, 2005.
12. Are C, Hsu JF, Ghossein RA, et al: Histological aggressiveness of fluorodeoxyglucose positron-emission tomogram (FDG-PET)-detected incidental thyroid carcinomas. *Ann Surg Oncol* 14:3210–3215, 2007.
13. Padovani RP, Kasamatsu TS, Nakabashi CC, et al: One month is sufficient for urinary iodine to return to its baseline value after the use of water-soluble iodinated contrast agents in post-thyroidectomy patients requiring radioiodine therapy. *Thyroid* 22:926–930, 2012.
14. Castro MR, Gharib H: Continuing controversies in the management of thyroid nodules. *Ann Intern Med* 142:926–931, 2005.
15. McManus C, Luo J, Sippel R, et al: Should patients with symptomatic Hashimoto's thyroiditis pursue surgery? *J Surg Res* 170:52–55, 2011.
16. Siegel RL, Miller KD, Jemal A: Cancer statistics, 2015. *CA Cancer J Clin* 65:5–29, 2015.
17. Albores-Saavedra J, Henson DE, Glazer E, et al: Changing patterns in the incidence and survival of thyroid cancer with follicular phenotype—papillary, follicular, and anaplastic: A morphological and epidemiological study. *Endocr Pathol* 18:1–7, 2007.
18. Bongarzone I, Vigneri P, Mariani L, et al: RET/NTRK1 rearrangements in thyroid gland tumors of the papillary carcinoma family: Correlation with clinicopathological features. *Clin Cancer Res* 4:223–228, 1998.
19. Kim DS, McCabe CJ, Buchanan MA, et al: Oncogenes in thyroid cancer. *Clin Otolaryngol Allied Sci* 28:386–395, 2003.
20. Wells SA, Jr, Santoro M: Update: The status of clinical trials with kinase inhibitors in thyroid cancer. *J Clin Endocrinol Metab* 99:1543–1555, 2014.
21. Zhu Z, Gandhi M, Nikiforova MN, et al: Molecular profile and clinical-pathologic features of the follicular variant of papillary thyroid carcinoma. An unusually high prevalence of ras mutations. *Am J Clin Pathol* 120:71–77, 2003.
22. Garcia-Rostan G, Zhao H, Camp RL, et al: ras mutations are associated with aggressive tumor phenotypes and poor prognosis in thyroid cancer. *J Clin Oncol* 21:3226–3235, 2003.
23. Parameswaran R, Brooks S, Sadler GP: Molecular pathogenesis of follicular cell derived thyroid cancers. *Int J Surg* 8:186–193, 2010.

24. Grubbs EG, Rich TA, Li G, et al: Recent advances in thyroid cancer. *Curr Probl Surg* 45:156–250, 2008.
25. Sherman SI: Thyroid carcinoma. *Lancet* 361:501–511, 2003.
26. Cady B, Sedgwick CE, Meissner WA, et al: Risk factor analysis in differentiated thyroid cancer. *Cancer* 43:810–820, 1979.
27. Hay ID, Thompson GB, Grant CS, et al: Papillary thyroid carcinoma managed at the Mayo Clinic during six decades (1940-1999): Temporal trends in initial therapy and long-term outcome in 2444 consecutively treated patients. *World J Surg* 26:879–885, 2002.
28. Zaydfudim V, Feurer ID, Griffin MR, et al: The impact of lymph node involvement on survival in patients with papillary and follicular thyroid carcinoma. *Surgery* 144:1070–1077, discussion 1077–1078, 2008.
29. Schlumberger MJ: Papillary and follicular thyroid carcinoma. *N Engl J Med* 338:297–306, 1998.
30. D'Avanzo A, Treseler P, Ituarte PH, et al: Follicular thyroid carcinoma: Histology and prognosis. *Cancer* 100:1123–1129, 2004.
31. Boyd LA, Earnhardt RC, Dunn JT, et al: Preoperative evaluation and predictive value of fine-needle aspiration and frozen section of thyroid nodules. *J Am Coll Surg* 187:494–502, 1998.
32. Adam MA, Pura J, Gu L, et al: Extent of surgery for papillary thyroid cancer is not associated with survival: An analysis of 61,775 patients. *Ann Surg* 260:601–605, discussion 605–607, 2014.
33. Podnos YD, Smith D, Wagman LD, et al: The implication of lymph node metastasis on survival in patients with well-differentiated thyroid cancer. *Am Surg* 71:731–734, 2005.
34. Carling T, Carty SE, Ciarleglio MM, et al: American Thyroid Association design and feasibility of a prospective randomized controlled trial of prophylactic central lymph node dissection for papillary thyroid carcinoma. *Thyroid* 22:237–244, 2012.
35. Kloos RT, Eng C, Evans DB, et al: Medullary thyroid cancer: Management guidelines of the American Thyroid Association. *Thyroid* 19:565–612, 2009.
36. Ibrahimpasic T, Ghossein R, Carlson DL, et al: Outcomes in patients with poorly differentiated thyroid carcinoma. *J Clin Endocrinol Metab* 99:1245–1252, 2014.
37. Pasieka JL: Anaplastic thyroid cancer. *Curr Opin Oncol* 15:78–83, 2003.
38. Bojunga J, Zeuzem S: Molecular detection of thyroid cancer: An update. *Clin Endocrinol (Oxf)* 61:523–530, 2004.
39. Nathan N, Sullivan SD: Thyroid disorders during pregnancy. *Endocrinol Metab Clin North Am* 43:573–597, 2014.
40. Casey BM, Dashe JS, Wells CE, et al: Subclinical hypothyroidism and pregnancy outcomes. *Obstet Gynecol* 105:239–245, 2005.
41. Stagnaro-Green A, Abalovich M, Alexander E, et al: Guidelines of the American Thyroid Association for the diagnosis and management of thyroid disease during pregnancy and postpartum. *Thyroid* 21:1081–1125, 2011.
42. Nam KH, Yoon JH, Chang HS, et al: Optimal timing of surgery in well-differentiated thyroid carcinoma detected during pregnancy. *J Surg Oncol* 91:199–203, 2005.
43. Carty SE, Cooper DS, Doherty GM, et al: Consensus statement on the terminology and classification of central neck dissection for thyroid cancer. *Thyroid* 19:1153–1158, 2009.
44. Holostenco V, Khafif A: The upper limits of central neck dissection. *JAMA Otolaryngol Head Neck Surg* 140:731–735, 2014.
45. Porterfield JR, Factor DA, Grant CS: Operative technique for modified radical neck dissection in papillary thyroid carcinoma. *Arch Surg* 144:567–574, discussion 574, 2009.
46. Cernea CR, Brandao LG, Hojaij FC, et al: Negative and positive predictive values of nerve monitoring in thyroidectomy. *Head Neck* 34:175–179, 2012.
47. Barczynski M, Konturek A, Cichon S: Randomized clinical trial of visualization versus neuromonitoring of recurrent laryngeal nerves during thyroidectomy. *Br J Surg* 96:240–246, 2009.
48. Calo PG, Pisano G, Medas F, et al: Identification alone versus intraoperative neuromonitoring of the recurrent laryngeal nerve during thyroid surgery: Experience of 2034 consecutive patients. *J Otolaryngol Head Neck Surg* 43:16, 2014.
49. Pisanu A, Porceddu G, Podda M, et al: Systematic review with meta-analysis of studies comparing intraoperative neuromonitoring of recurrent laryngeal nerves versus visualization alone during thyroidectomy. *J Surg Res* 188:152–161, 2014.
50. Said M, Chiu V, Haigh PI: Hypothyroidism after hemithyroidectomy. *World J Surg* 37:2839–2844, 2013.
51. Ojomo KA, Schneider DF, Reiher AE, et al: Using body mass index to predict optimal thyroid dosing after thyroidectomy. *J Am Coll Surg* 216:454–460, 2013.
52. Kang SW, Lee SC, Lee SH, et al: Robotic thyroid surgery using a gasless, transaxillary approach and the da Vinci S system: The operative outcomes of 338 consecutive patients. *Surgery* 146:1048–1055, 2009.
53. Mazzaferri EL, Kloos RT: Clinical review 128: Current approaches to primary therapy for papillary and follicular thyroid cancer. *J Clin Endocrinol Metab* 86:1447–1463, 2001.
54. Sosa JA, Bowman HM, Tielsch JM, et al: The importance of surgeon experience for clinical and economic outcomes from thyroidectomy. *Ann Surg* 228:320–330, 1998.
55. Cibas ES, Ali SZ, NCI Thyroid FNA State of the Science Conference: The Bethesda System for Reporting Thyroid Cytopathology. *Am J Clin Pathol* 132:658–665, 2009.
56. Bongiovanni M, Spitale A, Faquin WC, et al: The Bethesda System for Reporting Thyroid Cytopathology: A meta-analysis. *Acta Cytol* 56:333–339, 2012.

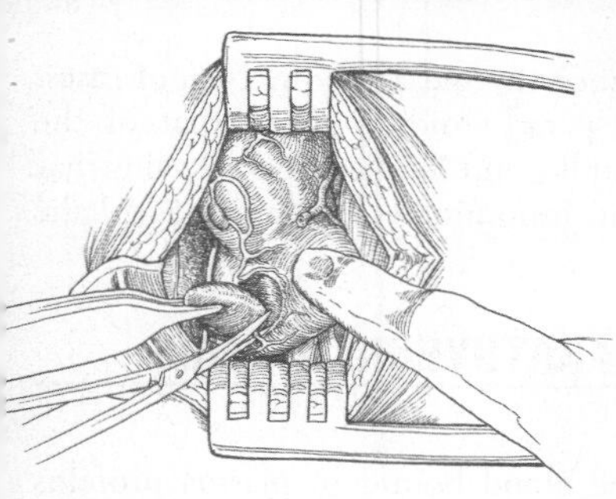

CHAPTER 37

The Parathyroid Glands

Courtney E. Quinn, Robert Udelsman

OUTLINE

HISTORY

In 1852, Owen discovered the parathyroid glands in the Indian rhinoceros. He referred to one of these glands as "a small compact yellow glandular body attached to the thyroid at the point where the veins emerged."[1] Approximately 2 decades later, Sandström, a Swedish medical student, rediscovered parathyroid glands in humans. In his monograph "On a New Gland in Man and Fellow Animals," Sandström eloquently described the glands as the "glandulae parathyroidae," noting their existence in dogs, cats, rabbits, and other animals in addition to humans.[2]

Sandström's description of the parathyroid glands received little attention until more was known about their function. Gley, a physiologist, documented the presumed function of the parathyroid glands in 1891 by observing the development of tetany after their removal. In 1908, MacCallum discerned their role in calcium metabolism. During investigation of various tumors of the parathyroid, parathyroid hormone (PTH) was first isolated by Hanson in 1923, followed by Collip in 1925, and subsequent studies by Guillemin, Schally, and Yalow led to the development of immunoassays to measure PTH levels.[3] This technologic advancement ultimately led to a Nobel Prize in 1977, a century after Sandström's discovery of the glands in humans. Further technologic advances, including the creation of a serum channel autoanalyzer, preoperative localization techniques, and rapid intraoperative PTH monitoring, facilitated earlier diagnosis and more cost-effective treatment of parathyroid disease.

ANATOMY

Embryology

The parathyroid glands arise from endodermal epithelial cells and consist of a combination of chief and oxyphil cells, adipose tissue, and fibrovascular stroma. The superior parathyroid glands are derived from the fourth branchial pouch, are closely associated with the lateral aspects of the thyroid lobes, and have a relatively abbreviated line of descent (Fig. 37-1). The inferior parathyroid glands are derived from the third branchial pouch, are closely associated with the thymus, and have a longer line of embryologic descent. This last aspect of the inferior parathyroid glands makes their anatomic position more variable; they can be found as high in the neck as the upper carotid sheath and as low in the mediastinum as the pericardium (Fig. 37-2). Despite this wide range, most inferior parathyroid glands are found near the inferior pole of the corresponding thyroid lobe.

Surgical Anatomy

Most individuals have four parathyroids: two superior and two inferior glands. However, additional (supernumerary) glands can be found, on average, in 13% of patients; fewer than four glands are found in a smaller subset (<3%). Normal parathyroid glands weigh 30 to 50 mg and are approximately the size of a grain of rice (3 to 5 mm). The color, texture, and appearance of parathyroid glands vary considerably, ranging from golden to reddish brown and becoming a more pale yellow as the fat content increases.

The superior parathyroid glands are normally located on the posteromedial surface of the middle to superior thyroid lobe, near the tracheoesophageal groove. They may reside under the superficial fascia of the thyroid, posterior to the recurrent laryngeal nerve (RLN). When a tubercle of Zuckerkandl of the thyroid lobe is present, these glands are often found posteromedial to the tubercle. The inferior parathyroid glands usually lie just below the inferior portion of the thyroid lobe and anterior to the RLN. Although there is significant variability in position, they often demonstrate bilateral symmetry; the superior and inferior glands are symmetrical compared with the contralateral side in 80% and 70% of patients, respectively.

In most cases (80%), the superior and inferior parathyroid glands receive their blood supply from the inferior thyroid artery, a branch of the thyrocervical trunk from the subclavian artery; each gland usually has its own end arterial branch. These small, fine vessels are vulnerable to injury during thyroid and parathyroid procedures. Alternatively, the blood supply to the superior

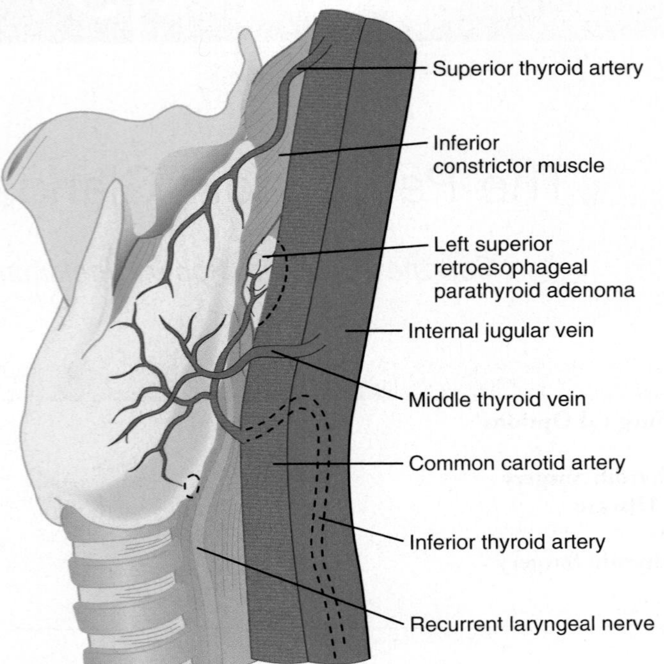

FIGURE 37-1 Anatomic relationship of a left superior parathyroid adenoma to nearby structures, including the recurrent laryngeal nerve, carotid sheath, and its blood supply from the inferior thyroid artery. Aberrantly located parathyroid glands can be found behind the esophagus and in the carotid sheath, thymus, and mediastinum.

gland can arise from the superior thyroid artery in 20% of cases. The venous drainage of the parathyroids parallels that of the thyroid, with the superior, middle, and inferior thyroid veins that drain into the internal jugular, innominate, and brachiocephalic veins.

PHYSIOLOGY OF THE PARATHYROID GLANDS

Calcium Homeostasis

Calcium is transported in the blood bound to plasma proteins (45%; largely albumin), bound to small anions such as phosphate or citrate (15%), or in the free ionized state (40%). The normal range of ionized calcium is 4.6 to 5.2 mg/dL. Total serum calcium concentrations range from 8.5 to 10.2 mg/dL. Calcium levels are maintained within the very narrow range required for optimal activity of myriad intracellular and extracellular processes, including hormone secretion, muscle contraction, synaptic function, and the coagulation cascade.

With substantial fluctuation of protein concentration, total calcium levels vary significantly, whereas ionized calcium remains relatively stable. For example, in cases of volume overload, chronic illness, or malnutrition, serum protein is often reduced. Low serum protein leads to a low total plasma calcium level; however, ionized calcium remains within normal limits—a phenomenon termed *pseudohypocalcemia*.

Additionally, changes in blood pH alter the equilibrium between calcium and albumin. Acidosis reduces calcium binding to albumin, whereas alkalosis enhances binding and can cause symptomatic hypocalcemia as a consequence of anxiety-provoked hyperventilation. Consequently, when significant shifts in pH are present, it is prudent to measure ionized calcium for accurate assessment of calcium status.

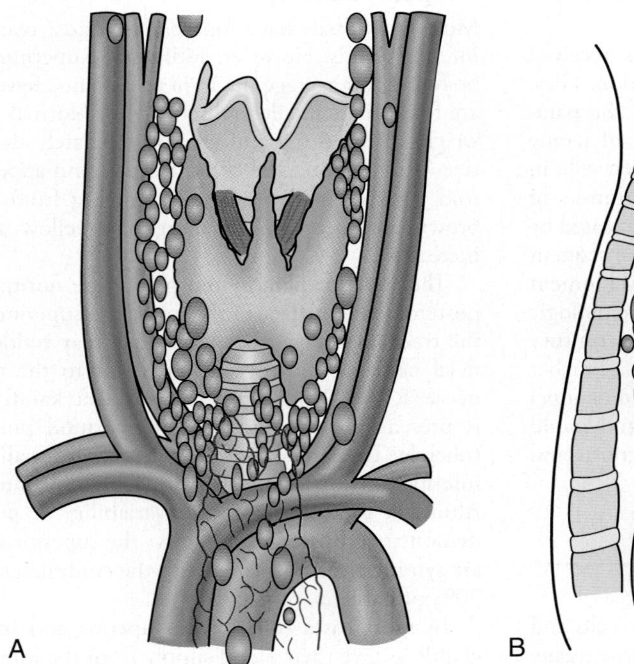

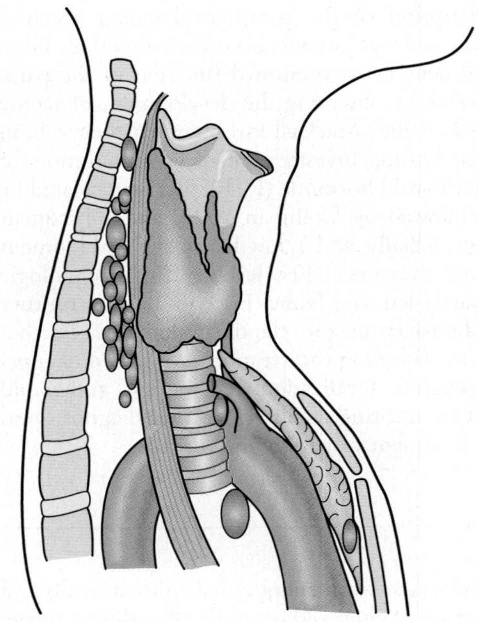

FIGURE 37-2 Locations of enlarged parathyroid glands in the neck and superior mediastinum from a series of reexplored parathyroid glands with the use of an anteroposterior projection (**A**) and a lateral projection (**B**). (From Udelsman R, Donovan PI: Remedial parathyroid surgery: Changing trends in 130 consecutive cases. *Ann Surg* 244:471–479, 2006.)

TABLE 37-1 Actions of Major Calcium-Regulating Hormones

HORMONE	BONE	KIDNEY	INTESTINE
Parathyroid hormone	Stimulates resorption of calcium and phosphate	Stimulates resorption of calcium and conversion of 25(OH)D_3; inhibits resorption of phosphate and bicarbonate	No direct effects
Vitamin D	Stimulates transport of calcium	Inhibits resorption of calcium	Stimulates calcium and phosphate absorption
Calcitonin	Inhibits resorption of calcium and phosphate	Inhibits resorption of calcium and phosphate	No direct effects

Calcium Regulation

The major regulators of serum calcium in humans are PTH and vitamin D (Table 37-1). These modulate calcium levels via their effects on target organs such as the bone, kidney, and gastrointestinal (GI) tract. Calcitonin is a 32–amino acid linear polypeptide hormone that is produced in many animals by the ultimobranchial body. In humans, calcitonin is produced by the parafollicular cells of the thyroid and opposes the effects of PTH. However, its importance in calcium homeostasis in humans is diminished compared with other animals.

PTH is synthesized as a 115–amino acid precursor (pre-pro-PTH) that is subsequently cleaved to an 84–amino acid molecule secreted by the parathyroid chief cells in response to a decrease in serum calcium. It has a plasma circulating half-life of approximately 4.5 minutes in normal individuals and exerts its action on target organs by binding to and activating one of several types of PTH receptors. The first PTH receptor, PTH1R, was cloned in 1991; it is heavily expressed in bone and kidney but is also present to some degree in breast, skin, heart, and pancreatic tissues. PTH1R recognizes intact PTH and parathyroid hormone–related peptide (PTHrP). A second, closely related receptor (PTH2R) selectively binds PTH and is heavily expressed in the GI, cardiovascular, and central nervous systems. Activation of these receptors by PTH stimulates multiple cellular signaling pathways, which stimulate the release of intracellular calcium stores.

In the kidney, PTH receptor binding leads to increased calcium resorption and increased renal production of 1,25-dihydroxyvitamin D_3 (1,25[OH]$_2D_3$). PTH acts on bone, the main reservoir of calcium, to release calcium in two phases: The immediate effect of PTH is to mobilize calcium from readily available skeletal stores in equilibrium with the extracellular fluid; later, PTH stimulates the release of calcium and phosphate through the process of bone resorption. Additionally, PTH increases calcium and phosphate absorption in the intestine (Fig. 37-3).

Vitamin D, from the diet or dermal synthesis, requires enzymatic conversion in the liver to become active. Dietary vitamin D travels to the liver, bound to vitamin D–binding protein, where it and endogenously synthesized vitamin D_3 are metabolized. The hepatic enzyme 25-hydroxylase places a hydroxyl group in the 25 position, resulting in 25-hydroxyvitamin D (25[OH]D, or calcidiol). 25-Hydroxyvitamin D_2 and 25-hydroxyvitamin D_3 produced by the liver enter the circulation and travel to the kidney. In the renal tubule, 25(OH)D is released from its binding protein and is further hydroxylated by either 1α-hydroxylase or 24α-hydroxylase, producing 1,25-dihydroxyvitamin D (calcitriol), the most active form of vitamin D.

DISORDERS OF PARATHYROID METABOLISM

Hypoparathyroidism

Hypoparathyroidism occurs when inadequate PTH secretion leads to hypocalcemia and hyperphosphatemia. It most frequently occurs as a result of damage to normal parathyroid glands (i.e., postsurgical hypoparathyroidism); it can also occur after subtotal parathyroidectomy or total parathyroidectomy with reimplantation (see "Postoperative Hypocalcemia" later).

Congenital Hypoparathyroidism

Congenital hypoparathyroidism is an extremely rare cause of hypoparathyroidism. Patients either are born without adequate parathyroid tissue (e.g., DiGeorge syndrome) or develop hypoparathyroidism secondary to in utero effects of hypercalcemia in a pregnant mother with hyperparathyroidism. DiGeorge syndrome, described by DiGeorge in 1968,[4] is caused by microdeletions occurring in chromosome region 22q11.2. The features vary widely and include congenital heart defects, defects in the palate, facial anomalies, recurrent infections, and learning disabilities. Transient neonatal hypoparathyroidism in neonates is due to primary hyperparathyroidism (PHPT) in the mother during pregnancy. Hyperparathyroidism during pregnancy can be associated with fetal complications in 80% of cases.[5] It may go unrecognized until disease is advanced because of physiologic changes that occur during pregnancy—hypoalbuminemia in the mother and calcium transport across the placenta. Ultimately, maternal hypercalcemia results in suppression of fetal parathyroid glands, leading to neonatal hypocalcemia and its sequelae (intrauterine growth retardation, preterm delivery, low birth rate, and fetal death). Most cases of neonatal hypoparathyroidism are transient and respond to medical management in the form of calcium supplementation.

Pseudohypoparathyroidism

Pseudohypoparathyroidism is a rare metabolic condition in which the body fails to respond to PTH. Patients have low serum calcium levels and hyperphosphatemia; however, the PTH level is appropriately elevated because of the hypocalcemia. The pathogenesis has been linked to a dysfunction of the G_s α subunit of G proteins,[6] and there are three types. Type 1a, also termed *Albright hereditary osteodystrophy*, has a characteristic phenotypic appearance including short fourth and fifth metacarpals and a rounded facies and is associated with thyroid-stimulating hormone resistance. Type 1b is biochemically similar but lacks the phenotypic appearance and is associated with a methylation defect. Defects in type 2 occur downstream of type 1a or 1b; a normal cyclic adenosine monophosphate response to PTH stimulation occurs despite the inherent abnormality in calcium regulation.

Hyperparathyroidism

Although hyperparathyroidism was first described and treated in the 1930s by Albright at Massachusetts General Hospital, the oldest known case was found in a cadaver from an Early Neolithic cemetery in southwest Germany.[7] Hyperparathyroidism refers to overactivity of the parathyroid glands resulting in excess production of PTH. More specifically, hyperparathyroidism is classified

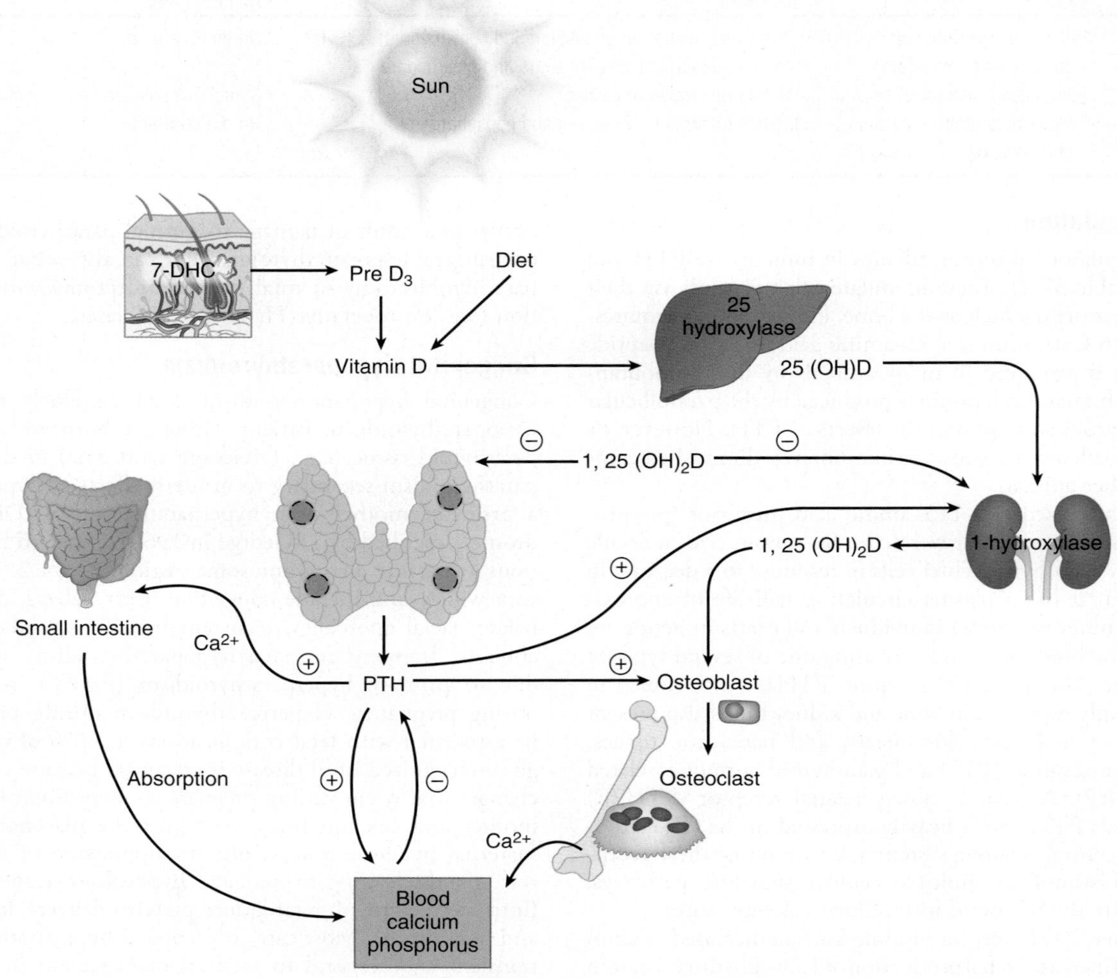

FIGURE 37-3 Calcium homeostasis.

as primary, secondary, or tertiary, depending on the cause of excess PTH synthesis.

Nonparathyroidal Hypercalcemia

Although PHPT is the most common cause of hypercalcemia in the outpatient setting, there are several other causes of elevated serum calcium levels. Nonparathyroidal hypercalcemia can be due to (1) endocrine disorders other than hyperparathyroidism, (2) granulomatous diseases, (3) medications, and (4) malignancy (Box 37-1). Hypercalcemia of malignancy represents the second most common cause of hypercalcemia after PHPT.

Hypercalcemia can occur in 30% of patients with cancer and is the most common cause of hypercalcemia in the inpatient setting.[8] It occurs in patients with either solid tumors or hematologic malignancies; the most common cancers associated with hypercalcemia are breast, lung, and multiple myeloma. There are three mechanisms by which hypercalcemia of malignancy occurs: (1) release of cytokines by osteolytic metastases, (2) tumor secretion of PTHrP, and (3) tumor production of calcitriol. Osteolytic metastases account for 20% of cases of hypercalcemia of malignancy, and breast cancer is the most frequent primary tumor. Tumor cells indirectly produce cytokines that activate osteoclasts, which mediate the bony destruction observed with osteolytic metastases. The most common cause of hypercalcemia in patients with nonmetastatic solid tumors is secretion of PTHrP by the tumor. This condition, termed *humoral hypercalcemia of malignancy*, accounts for the remaining 80% of cases of hypercalcemia caused by malignancy. Because of homology of PTHrP with PTH at the amino terminal end, PTHrP can bind to PTH1R and activate similar postreceptor pathways.[9] Endogenous PTH secretion is suppressed in patients with humoral hypercalcemia of malignancy. Patients with PTHrP-induced hypercalcemia related to cancer typically have advanced disease and a poor prognosis. Calcitriol-induced hypercalcemia typically occurs in Hodgkin lymphoma and in approximately 30% of cases of non-Hodgkin lymphoma. Under physiologic conditions, hypercalcemia suppresses the release of PTH, leading to a decrease in the production of calcitriol. This does not occur with calcitriol-induced hypercalcemia; the lack of suppression of calcitriol in lymphoma is caused by PTH-independent, extrarenal production of calcitriol from 25(OH)D by malignant lymphocytes and macrophages.

BOX 37-1 Differential Diagnosis of Nonparathyroid-Related Hypercalcemia

Endocrine Disorders and Tumors
Hyperthyroidism/thyrotoxicosis
Adrenal insufficiency
Pheochromocytoma
Vasointestinal polypeptide hormone–producing tumor (VIPoma)

Granulomatous Diseases
Sarcoidosis
Tuberculosis
Histoplasmosis
Coccidioidomycosis

Malignancy*
Solid tumors (e.g., lung, breast, bone)
Hematologic malignancies (lymphoma, leukemia)
Lytic bone metastases
Other malignancy-related factors (cytokines, growth factors, PTHrP)

Medications
Lithium
Diuretics (e.g., hydrochlorothiazide, furosemide)
Vitamin/mineral intoxication (vitamin A, D; aluminum)
Hormone therapy (estrogen, testosterone)

Other Conditions
Milk-alkali syndrome
Paget disease
Immobilization
Parenteral nutrition
Renal insufficiency (acute and chronic)
Familial hypocalciuric hypercalcemia
Dehydration
Laboratory error

PTHrP, parathyroid hormone–related peptide.
*Malignancy is the most common cause of hypercalcemia in the inpatient setting; the most common cause of hypercalcemia in the outpatient setting is primary hyperparathyroidism.

TABLE 37-2 Symptoms and Signs of Primary Hyperparathyroidism

SYMPTOMS	SIGNS
Musculoskeletal	Musculoskeletal
Bone pain	Osteoporosis
Muscle aches	Osteopenia
Renal	Renal
Polyuria	Nephrolithiasis
Gastrointestinal	Nephrocalcinosis
Nausea	Bone
Vomiting	Osteitis fibrosa cystica
Constipation	Pathologic fractures
Abdominal pain	Brown tumors/cysts
Neurocognitive dysfunction	
Fatigue	
Poor concentration	
Memory loss	
Irritability/mood swings	
Insomnia	

Primary Hyperparathyroidism

PHPT is the result of an intrinsic abnormality of one or more of the parathyroid glands. The abnormal parathyroid gland enlarges and secretes PTH inappropriately relative to the serum ionized calcium level. Excess circulating PTH results in increased serum calcium levels. Under normal conditions, the serum calcium level is tightly regulated within a narrow range as a result of the exquisite responsiveness of parathyroid cells to circulating calcium. Patients with PHPT develop a new set-point in one or more parathyroid glands, such that a higher circulating level of calcium is maintained. The higher levels of circulating PTH bind to receptors in the bone that increase osteoclast activity, and excess calcium is released into the blood. There is also increased renal absorption of calcium and increased absorption of calcium from the GI tract. The net effect is an increase in total and ionized calcium levels in the blood.

Approximately 85% of patients with PHPT have single parathyroid gland enlargement; this is termed a *parathyroid adenoma*. A subset of patients with sporadic disease has multigland disease, in which all parathyroid glands are involved. Because the intrinsic abnormality is in the parathyroid gland, this is still termed PHPT.

Most patients with PHPT develop spontaneous enlargement of a single parathyroid gland in the absence of known risk factors. A risk factor for the development of a parathyroid adenoma is a history of irradiation to the head and neck in childhood. In addition, some familial syndromes are associated with multigland PHPT, including multiple endocrine neoplasia type 1 (MEN1), which is associated with abnormalities of the parathyroid glands, endocrine pancreas, and pituitary gland. Patients with MEN type 2A (MEN2A) also have abnormalities of the parathyroid glands. Patients with MEN1 invariably have enlargement of all parathyroid glands, whereas patients with MEN2A generally have asymmetrical parathyroid gland enlargement and normal-appearing parathyroid glands. Lastly, parathyroid carcinoma (PTCA) is a malignant tumor of parathyroid parenchymal cells that is responsible for 0.7% to 2.1% of cases of PHPT. PTCA is an exceptionally rare malignancy but manifests in a similar manner to a benign atypical parathyroid adenoma (see "Parathyroid Carcinoma" later). Diagnosis is based on concurrent pathologic criteria including the presence of thick, fibrous bands; invasion into surrounding soft tissue structures; and lymphovascular and perineural invasion.[10]

Hypercalcemia is associated with an array of symptoms and signs that accompany PHPT. These include nephrolithiasis, nephrocalcinosis, and significant bone disease such as osteopenia and osteoporosis. In addition, a wide range of subtle abnormalities is associated with PHPT, including decreased cognitive function, lethargy, GI disturbances, and musculoskeletal abnormalities (Table 37-2). It is often difficult to prove that these nonspecific findings result from PHPT because they are common in the general population. An increasing number of patients is found to have PHPT with minimal (if any) overt symptoms or signs.

Secondary and Tertiary Hyperparathyroidism

Secondary hyperparathyroidism is due to physiologic secretion of PTH by the parathyroid glands in response to hypocalcemia. There are several causes of hypocalcemia that may lead to secondary hyperparathyroidism, the most common of which are vitamin

BOX 37-2 Causes of Secondary Hyperparathyroidism

Chronic renal failure
25(OH) vitamin D deficiency
Malabsorption syndromes
- Celiac disease
- Cystic fibrosis
- Short gut syndrome
- Bariatric procedures

Medications
- Lithium
- Diuretics (e.g., hydrochlorothiazide, furosemide)

Metabolic abnormalities
- Hypermagnesemia
- Hyperphosphatemia

Congenital disorders
- Transient neonatal hyperparathyroidism
- DiGeorge syndrome

D deficiency and chronic renal failure, termed *uremic hyperparathyroidism* (Box 37-2). A low serum 25(OH)D concentration is the hallmark of vitamin D deficiency and leads to a decrease in $1,25(OH)_2D$, which is necessary for adequate calcium absorption by the intestines. Consequently, PTH secretion increases in an effort to normalize $1,25(OH)_2D$. The increase in serum PTH leads to a higher rate of bone resorption, with resultant cortical bone loss; markers of bone turnover, such as urine hydroxyproline excretion, are increased in patients with low serum 25(OH)D (<30 nmol/liter).[11] Chronic renal failure leads to hyperphosphatemia and decreased renal conversion of 25-hydroxycholecalciferol to 1,25-dihydroxycholecalciferol, resulting in reduced intestinal calcium absorption, with subsequent hypocalcemia and stimulation of PTH. The mechanism by which uremic hyperparathyroidism develops is multifactorial and involves (1) mutations in calcium-sensing receptors, (2) alterations in calcium set-points, (3) decreased metabolic clearance of PTH, and (4) increased phosphate retention. Regardless of the cause of secondary hyperparathyroidism, hyperplasia of all parathyroid glands develops. However, in contrast to patients with PHPT, less than 1% of patients with uremic secondary HPT require surgical intervention. These patients are usually managed medically, until they become refractory to medical treatment, at which point subtotal parathyroidectomy is usually advised.

Tertiary hyperparathyroidism represents an advanced form of secondary HPT; it is seen in patients with long-standing chronic renal failure and in patients who have persistent autonomous secretion of PTH after renal transplantation. Loss of response to serum calcium levels leads to four-gland hyperplasia with autonomous activity. In this setting, it is not unusual to see marked asymmetry in the parathyroid gland size. Renal transplant recipients often have additional risk factors for the development of tertiary HPT, such as alterations in glomerular filtration rate or use of various transplant-associated drugs (corticosteroids, cyclosporine, and thiazide diuretics). Tertiary HPT results in elevated serum calcium and intact PTH levels. This form of HPT can be life-threatening, and all patients with tertiary HPT should be referred for surgical intervention. The surgical procedure of choice for tertiary HPT is subtotal parathyroidectomy. In addition, patients with secondary HPT who are being considered for renal transplantation should have serum calcium and PTH levels screened preoperatively.

Hypercalcemic Crisis

Hypercalcemic crisis is defined by a significantly elevated serum calcium level in association with end-organ dysfunction. Although there is no specific level of hypercalcemia, it generally occurs when serum calcium exceeds 14 mg/dL (3.5 mmol/liter) and represents a medical and surgical emergency. Such life-threatening hypercalcemia often occurs in patients with underlying malignancy, although it can also occur with long-standing, undiagnosed or untreated PHPT. The clinical presentation varies, depending on the degree of hypercalcemia as well as the underlying cause, but typically includes constitutional (fatigue), neurologic (depression, confusion, obtundation), GI (constipation, abdominal pain), and renal findings, including insufficiency caused by severe hypovolemia, oliguria/anuria, and hyperkalemia.

Treatment should be initiated immediately and concurrent with establishing the causative diagnosis. Because most patients are severely dehydrated, effective therapy begins with aggressive fluid resuscitation with normal saline, at a rate of at least 200 mL/hr to promote renal excretion of calcium as well as to restore intravascular volume. Patients with concurrent cardiac dysfunction can pose significant management challenges. Once the patient is rehydrated, a diuretic may be added to inhibit calcium resorption in the distal loop of Henle, as long as the patient's blood pressure remains stable. Dialysis is used in patients with renal failure who cannot tolerate such large-volume resuscitation.

In addition to intravenous fluids and diuresis, medications can be used in the setting of severe hypercalcemia. Glucocorticoids decrease intestinal absorption of calcium, increase renal excretion of calcium, and inhibit osteoclast-activating factor. Hydrocortisone is administered at 200 to 400 mg/day for up to 5 days. Glucocorticoids have not been shown to be effective in cases of hypercalcemia associated with malignancy. Calcitonin also reduces serum calcium levels. It lowers serum calcium levels quickly (within 24 to 48 hours) and has cumulative effects when used in combination with glucocorticoids. Bisphosphonates reduce serum calcium levels in malignancy-associated hypercalcemia. Phitayakorn and McHenry[12] noted that a rapid reduction of serum calcium could be achieved with bisphosphonate therapy. Bisphosphonates, such as pamidronate or zoledronic acid, inhibit osteoclast activity, reducing serum calcium levels. Because of the long half-life of bisphosphonates, therapy can exacerbate severe postoperative hypocalcemia and complicate surgical management.

Because these patients are usually admitted to a medical service, early surgical consultation and coordination are helpful because pharmacologic intervention may affect perioperative management. Once serum calcium level is effectively reduced, urgent parathyroidectomy should be undertaken.

Calciphylaxis

Calciphylaxis, or calcific uremic arteriolopathy, is a syndrome of vascular calcification, thrombosis, and skin necrosis. It is a rare but serious disease, seen mainly in patients with end-stage renal disease (ESRD). It results in chronic nonhealing wounds and can be fatal.

Calciphylaxis most commonly occurs in patients with ESRD who are on hemodialysis or who have recently received a kidney transplant. However, calciphylaxis does not occur exclusively in patients with ESRD. When reported in patients without ESRD,

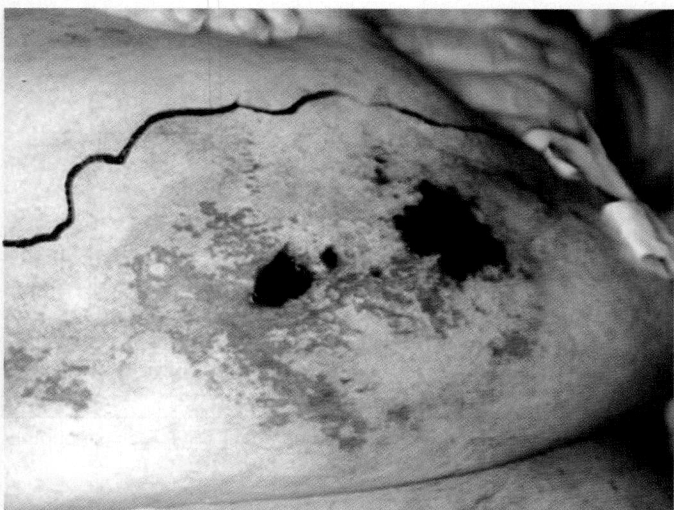

FIGURE 37-4 Calciphylaxis of the lower abdomen. Note the painful, pruritic lesion with central eschar formation and necrosis. (From Kuypers DR: Skin problems in chronic kidney desease. *Nat Clin Pract Rheumatol* 5:157–170, 2009.)

it is termed *nonuremic calciphylaxis*.[13] Nonuremic calciphylaxis has been observed in patients with PHPT, breast cancer (treated with chemotherapy), alcoholic liver cirrhosis, cholangiocarcinoma, Crohn's disease, rheumatoid arthritis, and systemic lupus erythematosus.

The diagnosis of calciphylaxis is a clinical one. Characteristic skin lesions are ischemic with areas of skin necrosis associated with severe pain. Necrotic skin appears as violaceous, leathery lesions and can be extensive (Fig. 37-4). A suspected diagnosis can be supported by a skin biopsy specimen that shows small arterial calcification and occlusion in the absence of vasculitis—although this does not ensure a definitive diagnosis. Additionally, bone scintigraphy may show increased tracer accumulation in the soft tissues. In certain patients, antinuclear antibody may play a role.[14]

Because treatment results for calciphylaxis are unpredictable, prevention is crucial. Rigorous and continuous control of phosphate and calcium balance may avoid the metabolic changes associated with calciphylaxis. However, response to treatment is variable. Also, necrotic skin areas may become infected, leading to sepsis. Overall, the clinical prognosis is poor. Urgent parathyroidectomy is usually recommended once the diagnosis is established. In this setting, an aggressive subtotal parathyroidectomy is the most commonly performed procedure.

DIAGNOSIS OF PRIMARY HYPERPARATHYROIDISM

PHPT is the third most common endocrine disorder in the United States, preceded by diabetes mellitus and thyroid disease. It most commonly affects women older than age 45; however, men and younger age groups are also at risk. PHPT is characterized by hypersecretion of PTH, which leads to hypercalcemia. The symptoms and signs of PHPT are listed in Table 37-2. The diagnosis of PHPT is biochemical—elevated intact PTH levels in the setting of elevated serum calcium confirms the diagnosis in patients with normal renal function. In equivocal cases, 24-hour urine calcium levels and calcium-creatinine ratios can aid in the diagnosis. After the diagnosis is made, all patients with symptomatic PHPT should be referred to an experienced surgeon for parathyroidectomy. In addition, a subset of patients with PHPT have hypercalcemia in the setting of a normal intact PTH level. However, in most patients, the serum PTH is "inappropriate" because it should be suppressed by hypercalcemia. A new group of patients have been characterized more recently with "normocalcemic" PHPT. Most experts agree that this subset represents the early presentation of PHPT before hypercalcemia has developed.[15]

BOX 37-3 Criteria for Surgical Referral for Asymptomatic Patients With Primary Hyperparathyroidism

Age <50 years
Serum calcium concentration >1 mg/dL (>0.25 mM/liter) above upper limit of normal
Bone density:
- T-score ≤2.5 at lumbar spine, femoral neck, total hip, or distal one third radius (perimenopausal or postmenopausal women and men ≥50 years old)
- Z-score ≤2.5 at lumbar spine, femoral neck, total hip, or distal one third radius (premenopausal women and men <50 years old)
- Vertebral fracture (including fragility fracture) present on radiologic evaluation

Renal function:
- Creatinine clearance <60 mL/min
- Radiologic evidence of renal stones or nephrocalcinosis (x-ray, ultrasound, computed tomography)

Adapted from Bilezikian JP, Brandi ML, Eastell R, et al: Guidelines for the management of asymptomatic primary hyperparathyroidism: Summary statement from the Fourth International Workshop. *J Clin Endocrinol Metab* 99:3561–3569, 2014.

Because the biochemical diagnosis of PHPT is frequently made before the onset of overt symptoms, many patients with PHPT today are "asymptomatic." Several criteria have been developed in an effort to determine which asymptomatic patients with PHPT should undergo parathyroidectomy. In 1990, a National Institutes of Health consensus conference was undertaken to solidify criteria for surgery. Despite a follow-up workshop by the National Institutes of Health in 2002 and an international workshop in 2008, there is still no consensus among endocrine surgeons and endocrinologists regarding the management of asymptomatic PHPT. The Fourth International Workshop on the Management of Asymptomatic Primary Hyperparathyroidism proposed revised guidelines regarding the advisability of parathyroid surgery in the setting of asymptomatic PHPT.[15,16] These criteria are listed in Box 37-3. All symptomatic patients should be considered surgical candidates because surgery is the only curative treatment for PHPT and has an excellent operative success and complication profile.

After the diagnosis of PHPT is made and patients meet surgical criteria, imaging studies are often undertaken to localize abnormal glands. Identification of abnormal glands preoperatively makes minimally invasive procedures possible.

PARATHYROID GLAND LOCALIZATION

Localization studies aid parathyroid surgery; they should not be used for diagnosis because the diagnostic criteria for PHPT are based on biochemical data. The purpose of imaging is to assist the

TABLE 37-3 Preoperative Imaging in Patients With Primary Hyperparathyroidism

IMAGING MODALITY	SENSITIVITY	SPECIFICITY	COST	SAFETY
Noninvasive				
^{99m}Tc sestamibi	Moderate	Moderate	Moderate	Safe
Sestamibi SPECT	High	High	Moderate	Safe
Ultrasound	Moderate	Moderate	Low	Safe
4D-CT	High	High	High	Radiation
MRI	Low	Moderate	Moderate	Safe
PET/CT	High	High	High	Radiation
Invasive				
Venous localization	High	High	Very high	Nephropathy, site-specific injury (hematoma)
Ultrasound-guided biopsy	High	High	Moderate	Site-specific injury

CT, computed tomography; *4D,* four-dimensional; *MRI,* magnetic resonance imaging; *PET,* positron emission tomography; *SPECT,* single photon emission computed tomography; *^{99m}Tc,* technetium 99m.

surgeon in planning and performing an appropriate operation. Preoperative localization studies help identify patients who are candidates for minimally invasive approaches. Such localization affords a decreased extent of surgical dissection, operative time, and length of hospital stay. Additionally, concurrent thyroid disease may be identified, allowing for combined endocrine surgical procedures. Every surgeon who performs parathyroid surgery must have experience reading the imaging studies. The list of preoperative imaging is extensive and continues to grow (Table 37-3).

Noninvasive Preoperative Localization

Technetium 99m (^{99m}Tc) sestamibi scintigraphy has long been used in the evaluation of myocardial perfusion. However, in 1989, it was noted that it had selective affinity for abnormal parathyroid glands because of their abundance of mitochondria.[17] Sestamibi is a monovalent, lipophilic cation that passively diffuses across cell membranes and accumulates in mitochondria. There are two primary techniques to differentiate sestamibi uptake by abnormal parathyroid and thyroid tissue. The first involves a dual radionuclide approach with sestamibi and either iodine-123 or ^{99m}Tc pertechnetate (subtraction imaging), and the second uses sestamibi alone with early and delayed imaging (dual phase). Sestamibi single photon emission computed tomography, owing to its improved spatial resolution, has become the most commonly used preoperative imaging study in parathyroid disease (Fig. 37-5). More recently, sestamibi combined with computed tomography (CT) offers the advantage of detecting smaller parathyroid lesions that would otherwise be undetectable with sestamibi alone. However, the overall sensitivity in detecting small lesions (<500 mg) varies considerably. Similar to neck ultrasound, the sensitivity of sestamibi is diminished by multiglandular parathyroid disease and concurrent thyroid pathology.

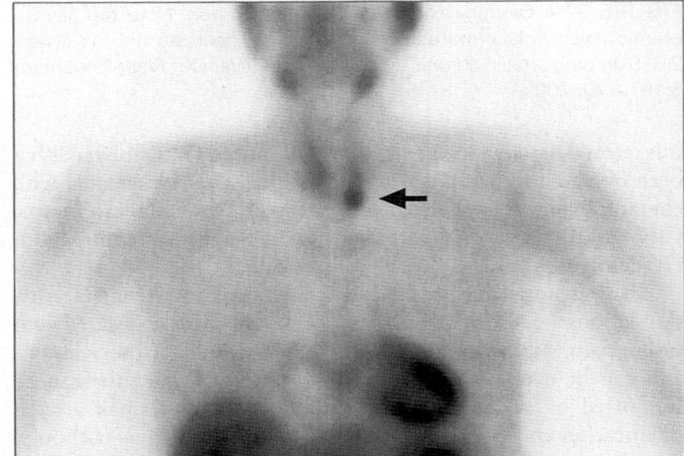

FIGURE 37-5 Technetium 99m sestamibi scan demonstrating a left inferior parathyroid adenoma *(arrow).* Physiologic areas of increased tracer uptake include the thyroid, salivary glands, heart, and liver.

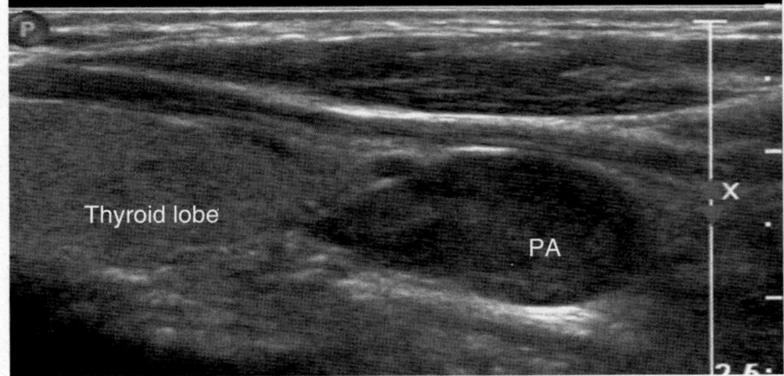

FIGURE 37-6 Ultrasound image of a hypoechoic, teardrop-shaped parathyroid adenoma *(PA)* located inferior to the inferior pole of the thyroid lobe.

Cervical ultrasound is an inexpensive, noninvasive means of evaluating parathyroid glands and has been shown to be highly sensitive in experienced hands. Sonographic characteristics of a parathyroid adenoma include a hypoechoic lesion located posterior to the thyroid gland, with an associated solitary feeding vessel (Fig. 37-6). The added advantage is that concurrent thyroid pathology, present in 30% of patients with PHPT,[18] can often be identified preoperatively. However, the major limitation of ultrasound is that its accuracy is highly operator dependent; ultrasound sensitivity for detecting abnormal parathyroid glands ranges from 70% to 96%.[19] Additionally, mediastinal parathyroid lesions cannot be identified on neck ultrasound because the ultrasound cannot penetrate the sternum or clavicles. However, when used in combination with sestamibi, the sensitivity for identifying a single parathyroid adenoma increases to 80% to 95%.[20] Many surgeons use sestamibi and neck ultrasound for preoperative localization.

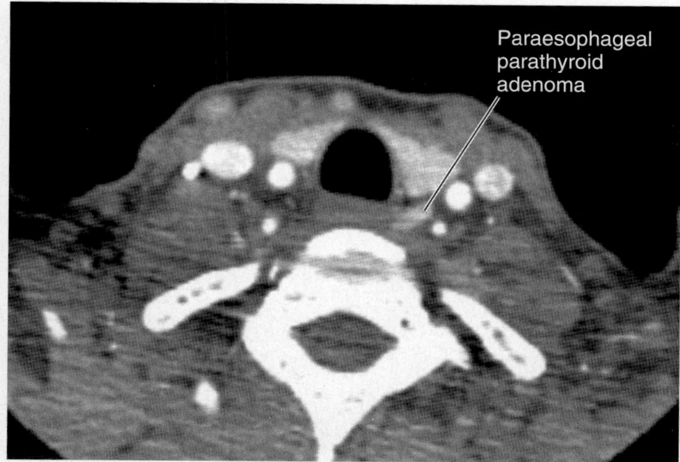

FIGURE 37-7 Four-dimensional computed tomography demonstrating a left upper ectopic (paraesophageal) parathyroid adenoma.

Standard three-dimensional CT has long been used in the preoperative localization of abnormal parathyroid glands; however, the results have been extremely variable, with a reported sensitivity ranging from 40% to 89%. In 2006, four-dimensional CT was used for parathyroid localization.[21] The fourth dimension, time, accounts for differences in perfusion characteristics between the hyperfunctioning parathyroid gland and surrounding structures, such as the thyroid gland (Fig. 37-7). An improved sensitivity of 88% for four-dimensional CT compared with the sensitivities of sestamibi and neck ultrasound (65% and 57%, respectively) was demonstrated. More recently, a combination of four-dimensional CT and ultrasound demonstrated a sensitivity of 94% and specificity of 96% for lateralizing hyperfunctioning parathyroid glands[22]; the sensitivity was 82% for localization to the correct quadrant of the neck.

Other noninvasive imaging modalities include magnetic resonance imaging (MRI) and positron emission tomography; however, these modalities are rarely indicated. Occasionally, MRI may be indicated in pregnant patients in whom ultrasound is noninformative because MRI avoids radiation exposure.

Invasive Preoperative Localization

Although noninvasive imaging studies are routinely performed before index parathyroid surgery, the results may be disappointing in the reoperative setting because they often fail to demonstrate adequate localization. Patients in this setting include patients with persistent or recurrent hyperparathyroidism and patients who have undergone prior cervical exploration, most notably total thyroidectomy. Real-time conventional selective venous sampling (SVS) is the most sensitive localization procedure in these patients.[23] The procedure involves catheterization of the common femoral vein to obtain a baseline PTH value, followed by extensive SVS of small venous branches from the neck and mediastinum. A twofold elevated PTH value compared with baseline obtained from the iliac vein defines a positive localization study (Fig. 37-8). With the institution of the rapid PTH assay in the interventional radiology suite, near real-time assay results are available, allowing for further catheterization in areas where subtle PTH gradients have been detected.[24] Although serious complications are rare, SVS is expensive, is time-consuming, and requires an experienced interventional radiologist.

Alternatively, ultrasound-guided fine-needle aspiration (FNA) of a suspicious lesion can also be used in the remedial setting. FNA is performed in the ultrasound suite, and aspirates should be tested for PTH. When FNA is positive for PTH, the patient proceeds to surgical reexploration.[25] Preoperative FNA of parathyroid glands is not recommended for most patients with PHPT because there is a theoretical risk of seeding parathyroid cells.

Negative Imaging

Negative, discordant, or equivocal noninvasive localization studies are common, even in patients who have not undergone exploration. In this setting, an experienced parathyroid surgeon can still find and cure PHPT in most patients. In patients undergoing remedial exploration, invasive imaging may be required, and it is unusual not to have a positive study.

All patients who undergo parathyroid surgery must understand that various surgical options and intraoperative adjuncts exist. It is also important that the surgeon and the patient understand that any planned procedure may be altered in the operating room, depending on the findings at surgery.

PARATHYROIDECTOMY—SURGICAL OPTIONS

Bilateral Neck Exploration

Bilateral neck exploration (BNE) has long been the gold standard operation for PHPT. It involves direct visualization of all parathyroid glands, with removal of enlarged parathyroid tissue, and has yielded cure rates of greater than 95%, with complication rates of 2% or less when performed by experienced surgeons. The principles of bilateral exploration include a thorough knowledge of parathyroid embryology and anatomy. Meticulous hemostasis and technique are required to identify normal and abnormal parathyroid glands in eutopic and ectopic locations.

BNE is usually performed under general anesthesia but can also be performed via bilateral regional cervical block. Key principles include identifying all normal and abnormal parathyroid glands; distinguishing disease involving a single gland from multiglandular disease; and resecting abnormal glands while leaving an adequate single, well-vascularized parathyroid remnant when subtotal resection is required (Box 37-4). Patients who have a single parathyroid adenoma undergo curative resection after the parathyroid adenoma is removed. In general, biopsy of normal parathyroid glands is neither recommended nor necessary because an experienced surgeon can recognize parathyroid tissue. It is reasonable to perform biopsy of normal parathyroid glands only if a surgeon is unable to locate a parathyroid adenoma, as this information would expedite subsequent exploration. Additionally, parathyroid biopsy may be undertaken in cases in which it is unclear whether resected tissue is actually parathyroid tissue. When a rapid intraoperative PTH assay is available, ex vivo parathyroid aspiration is a reliable, rapid, and inexpensive technique to prove that the tissue is of parathyroid origin. If the patient has multigland hyperplasia, either a total cervical parathyroidectomy with immediate heterotopic transplantation of parathyroid tissue to a convenient location (usually the forearm) or a subtotal parathyroidectomy is required. The goal of a subtotal parathyroidectomy is to leave a remnant of one well-vascularized parathyroid gland in situ. The remnant should ideally be the size of a normal parathyroid gland (approximately 30 mg). The choice of remnant should be a portion of the most "normal-appearing" parathyroid gland. A lower gland is ideal because of its location anterior to

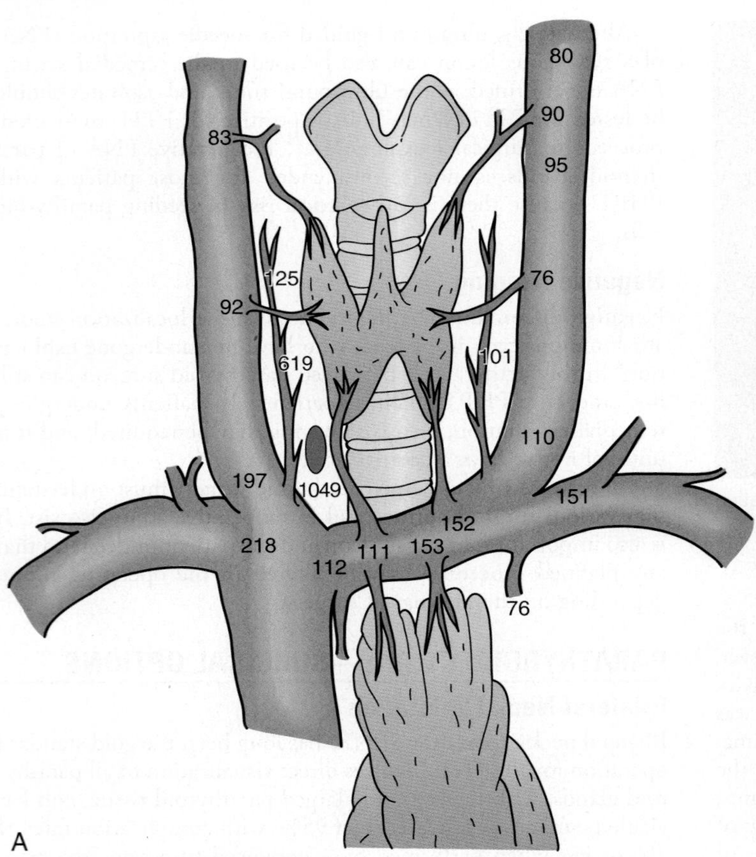

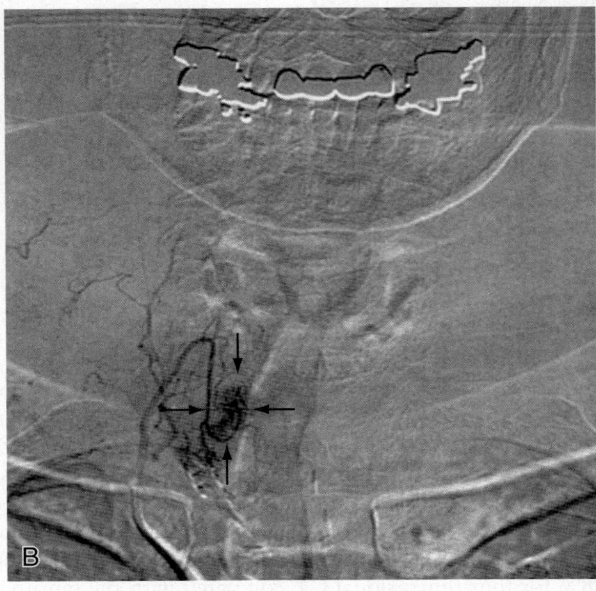

FIGURE 37-8 **A,** Venous localization mapping parathyroid hormone levels at different cervical sampling sites. The 1049 pg/mL level is consistent with a right posterior parathyroid adenoma. **B,** Corresponding angiogram showing the adenoma as a classic blush in the right posterior position *(arrows)*.

BOX 37-4 Principles of Bilateral Neck Exploration Parathyroidectomy

1. Identify all normal and abnormal parathyroid glands.
2. Distinguish between single-gland and multigland disease.
3. Resect abnormal parathyroid tissue.
   This may include cervical thymectomy to remove supernumerary parathyroid glands or parathyroid rests.
4. If a subtotal parathyroid resection is performed, leave an adequate viable remnant in one location.*
5. Avoid routine biopsy of parathyroid tissue.
   This decreases the risk of inadvertent devascularization or injury to normal parathyroid tissue.
   Biopsy occasionally is helpful to distinguish parathyroid from nonparathyroid tissue (e.g., fat or lymph nodes).
6. Most glands are found in a eutopic position.
   Exploration in ectopic locations should be carried out only after a thorough investigation of the normal locations for parathyroid glands is undertaken.

*When subtotal parathyroidectomy is performed, a remnant of "abnormal" or hypercellular parathyroid tissue must be left behind.

the RLN. This location makes subsequent surgical exploration (if necessary) easier and decreases the risk of RLN injury in remedial cases. Additionally, a titanium clip is left in place to mark the remnant. Although BNE remains a viable option, newer, less invasive techniques offer similar cure rates with less morbidity.

Minimally Invasive (Open) Parathyroidectomy

Given that approximately 85% of patients with PHPT have single-gland disease, a unilateral, minimally invasive approach has been advocated. However, the definition of minimally invasive parathyroidectomy (MIP) varies and may relate to the size of the incision, the use of local or regional anesthesia versus general anesthesia, or the institution of endoscopic or video-assisted procedures. Regardless of technique, preoperative localization is key to a successful outcome. An example of open MIP is shown in Figures 37-9 and 37-10.

Using this technique, cure rates are comparable or improved compared with standard bilateral exploration, with lower complication rates.[26,27] Additionally, MIP reduced operating time by approximately 50%, with a sevenfold reduction in length of hospital stay. These techniques require extensive experience and intraoperative adjuncts such as a rapid intraoperative PTH assay that may not be available in many hospitals. Endoscopic and video-assisted techniques have also been used as a minimally invasive approach to parathyroid surgery. Such techniques are designed to limit patient discomfort, shorten convalescence, and improve cosmesis.

Endoscopic Parathyroidectomy

Endoscopic parathyroidectomy was first described in 1996.[28] In this approach, carbon dioxide insufflation through a small (1.5 to 2 cm) cervical incision was used to provide access. However, this technique was complicated by significant hypercarbia and subcutaneous emphysema. Modifications include low-pressure

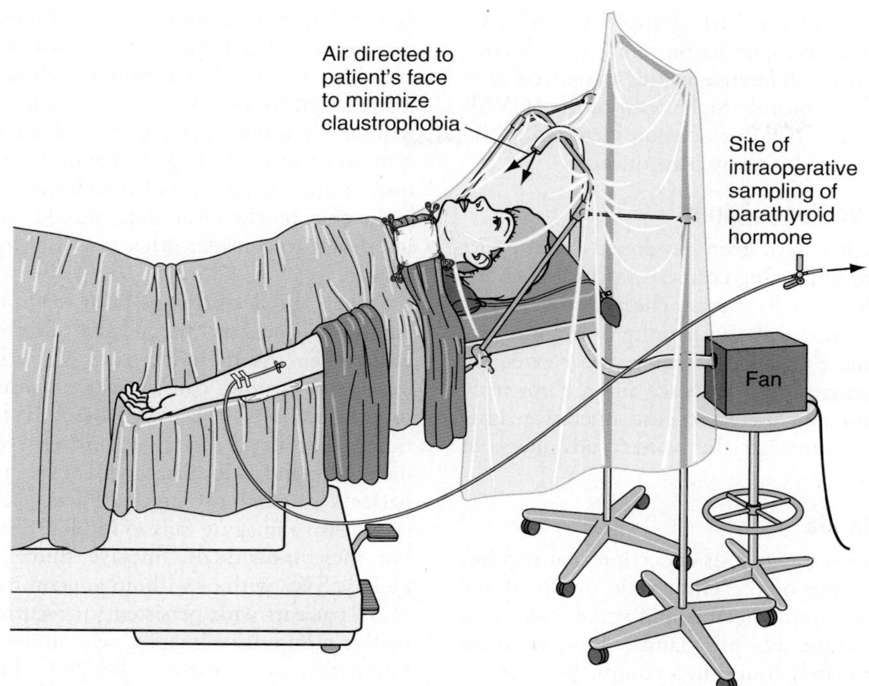

FIGURE 37-9 Organization of an ambulatory operating room used for minimally invasive parathyroidectomy. A large-bore intravenous line facilitates sedation and performance of the rapid parathyroid hormone assay. At the head of the bed, cool air blows over the patient to minimize claustrophobia.

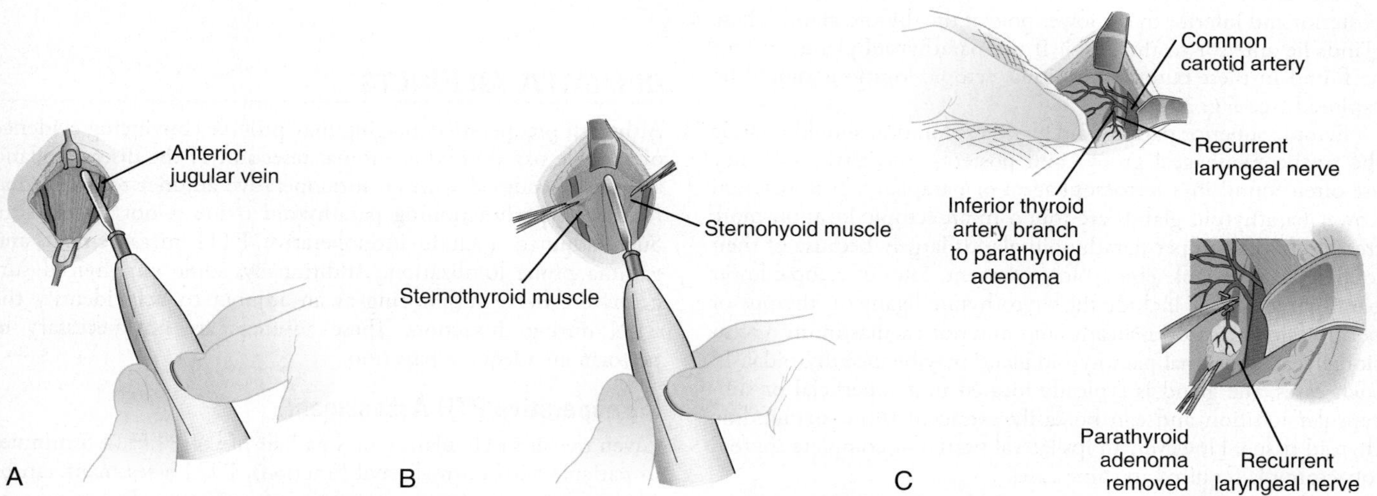

FIGURE 37-10 Technique of minimally invasive open parathyroidectomy. **A,** A small transverse cervical skin incision is made, the platysma is divided, and the anterior jugular veins are preserved. **B,** The median raphe is divided in the midline. **C,** The parathyroid adenoma is excised, with care taken to preserve the recurrent laryngeal nerve and minimize manipulation of the tumor during ligation of the end artery.

insufflation and transaxillary or postauricular approaches. Bilateral exploration can be accomplished by this technique but is time-consuming.

Video-Assisted Parathyroidectomy

Various minimally invasive, video-assisted parathyroidectomy techniques (MIVAPs) are available that differ based on location of incisions—cervical, transaxillary, transthoracic, or retroauricular. The original technique was described by Miccoli and colleagues.[29] In this procedure, a 1.5-cm transverse cervical incision is made approximately 2 cm above the sternal notch to allow for direct manual assessment of the working space. Additional 5-mm and 10-mm trocar sites are created beneath the strap muscles to allow for insertion of a 5-mm endoscope and videoscopic instruments.

A prospective, blinded trial comparing MIVAP versus open MIP randomly assigned 60 patients with PHPT and preoperative localization of a single parathyroid adenoma to either MIVAP or open MIP.[30] Both groups had similar cure and morbidity rates. The average operative time in the MIVAP group was 44 minutes (compared with 49 minutes in the MIP group). The MIVAP group reported a higher cosmetic satisfaction rate 1 month after surgery; however, there was no difference in this parameter at 6 months. Furthermore, the significantly higher cost of the MIVAP procedure resulting from use of endoscopic equipment led to the abandonment of this technique by many institutions.

Other Minimally Invasive Techniques

Various additional approaches have been developed in an effort to avoid a cervical incision, improving cosmesis, including endoscopic approaches through the axilla, breast, chest, retroauricular space, and floor of the mouth. Robotic parathyroidectomy has also been performed. All these techniques require more extensive dissection to create an adequate working space and are not truly minimally invasive. Additionally, increased cost, operative time, and potential risks largely outweigh the solitary advantage of avoiding a cervical incision.

Ectopic Parathyroid Glands

Parathyroid surgery requires a meticulous dissection that requires significant experience. Because of the embryonic origin of the parathyroid glands and their unpredictable and variable descent, it is not unusual to encounter ectopic glands; however, most parathyroid glands are ultimately found in a eutopic position.

The upper parathyroid glands are located in a more constant position than the lower glands. They are typically found at the level of cricoid cartilage, posterior to the thyroid gland, in close proximity (1 to 2 cm) to where the RLN crosses the inferior thyroid artery. The lower parathyroid glands are often located posterior and inferior to the lower pole of the thyroid gland. These glands lie anterior to the RLN. If the parathyroid glands cannot be found in these eutopic positions, ectopic locations should be explored (see Fig. 37-2).

Ectopic superior parathyroid gland exploration should include the tracheoesophageal groove and posterior mediastinum. They are often found in a retroesophageal or parapharyngeal location. Lower parathyroid glands are found in an ectopic location more frequently than upper parathyroid glands largely because of their longer, more variable embryologic descent. Sites of ectopic lower parathyroid glands include the thyrothymic ligament, thymus or perithymic fat, carotid sheath, and anterior mediastinum. Occasionally, an abnormal parathyroid gland may be intrathyroidal. In such cases, the gland is typically located in a superficial or subcapsular location and can be easily extracted from surrounding thyroid tissue. However, an ipsilateral partial or complete thyroid lobectomy is required in some cases.

Remedial Parathyroidectomy

Index parathyroid procedures for PHPT are associated with cure rates exceeding 95% and complications rates of 2% or less when performed by experienced parathyroid surgeons.[27] However, numerous patients require remedial cervical exploration for persistent or recurrent PHPT. Persistent disease is defined as failure of cure at initial exploration, as evidenced by lack of sustained normalization of serum calcium levels within 6 months postoperatively. Recurrent disease refers to initial biochemical cure, with subsequent elevation of serum calcium levels after 6 months of eucalcemia. In addition, patients who have undergone significant cervical exploration, particularly total thyroidectomy, harbor similar challenges during cervical reexploration.

Remedial parathyroid surgery can be technically challenging and is associated with increased morbidity, including operative failure. Given the complex nature of remedial parathyroid surgery, the threshold for surgical intervention should be higher and influenced by symptoms and signs as well as the ability to localize the diseased gland preoperatively. Candidates for remedial surgery require thorough evaluation and should have well-described symptoms and signs (e.g., osteoporosis, nephrolithiasis, neurocognitive impairment). Detailed review of operative notes and pathologic and biochemical data should be undertaken. It is also important to consider other causes of hypercalcemia and familial disease.

When the decision has been made to proceed with remedial parathyroid surgery, preoperative localization studies should be undertaken. As in index cases of PHPT, first-line parathyroid localization studies consist of noninvasive imaging such as ultrasound, sestamibi, CT, or MRI (see "Parathyroid Gland Localization"). For many cases of persistent or recurrent disease, the diseased gland is localized with these noninvasive measures, and patients proceed to surgery. However, in a subset of patients, noninvasive imaging fails to localize the diseased gland or glands. For these individuals, invasive studies are warranted and may include SVS, with or without concomitant angiography. A review of 31 patients with persistent or recurrent PHPT and noninformative noninvasive imaging who underwent real-time super-SVS found that the sensitivity (86.2%) and positive predictive value (92.6%) of real-time super-SVS far exceeded the results of all other noninvasive diagnostic tests.[31] The real-time super-SVS procedure extends the utility of the rapid PTH assay (see "Operative Adjuncts" next) to the interventional radiology suite to provide "real-time" PTH evaluation.

OPERATIVE ADJUNCTS

Although preoperative imaging may provide convincing evidence of a single parathyroid adenoma, resection of the diseased gland should be coupled with an intraoperative adjunct to prove that residual hyperfunctioning parathyroid tissue is not left in situ. Such adjuncts include intraoperative PTH measurement and gamma probe localization. Additionally, some parathyroid surgeons use nerve monitoring as an adjunct to help identify the RLN during dissection. These adjuncts are not necessary to perform an adequate resection.

Intraoperative PTH Assessment

Given the short circulating plasma half-life of PTH (4.5 minutes in patients with normal renal function), PTH assessment can be used intraoperatively to ensure adequate resection. The most commonly used rapid intraoperative PTH assays are immunoradiometric assays, which use chemiluminescent acridinium esters that are oxidized to an excited state in the presence of hydrogen peroxide and sodium hydroxide. Return of the oxidized acridinium to the ground state causes emission of light that can be quantified. A certified clinical laboratory technician performs the assay in close proximity to the operating room; results are typically available within 12 minutes.[32]

Various protocols exist that use intraoperative PTH measurements. The "Miami" criteria developed by Irvin and colleagues[33] describe biochemical cure as a 50% decrease in PTH levels from baseline 10 to 15 minutes after resection of the targeted parathyroid gland. Other criteria also require a decrease of PTH to within normal limits. A computerized mathematical model was developed that analyzes the slope of the curve generated by sequential

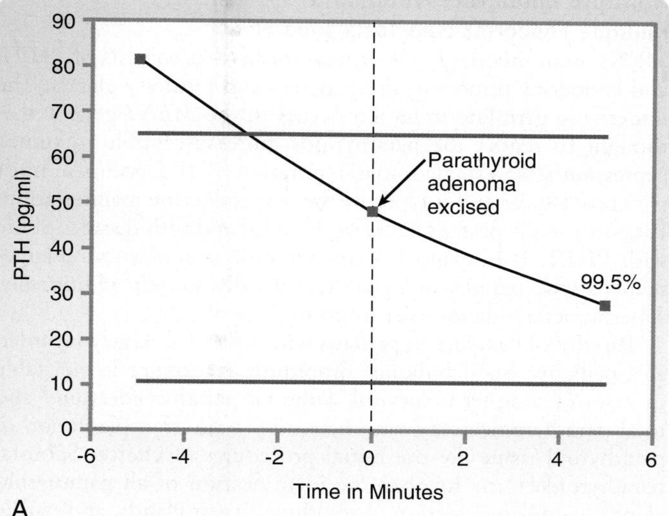

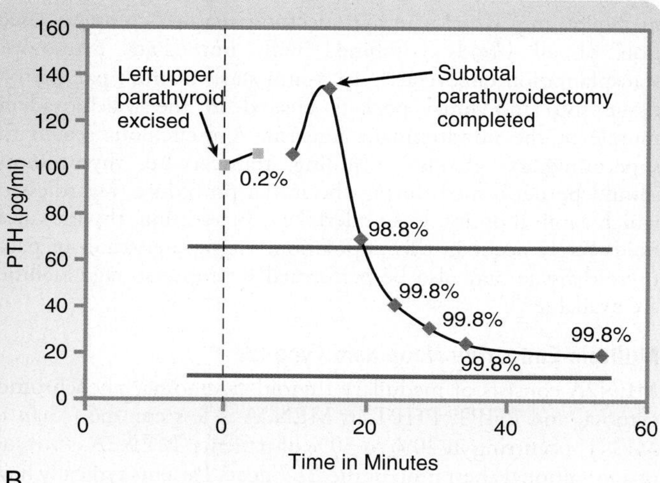

FIGURE 37-11 Intraoperative curve plotting and analysis. **A,** The parathyroid adenoma is excised at time T_0, with a curative probability of 99.5% at 5 minutes after excision. **B,** An enlarged left upper parathyroid gland was excised at time T_0; however, the plasma parathyroid hormone *(PTH)* level failed to decline, and the modeling predicted a cure rate of only 0.2%. Additional exploration was performed, confirming multigland hyperplasia. A subtotal parathyroidectomy was performed, and shortly thereafter the PTH level decreased, with a probability indicative of cure of 98.8%.

intraoperative PTH measurements after resection of the gland (Fig. 37-11).[34]

Regardless of which criteria are used, intraoperative PTH assessment has led to decreased operative failure rates in index and remedial cases. An analysis of 1650 consecutive parathyroidectomies demonstrated a 99.4% cure rate for patients who underwent MIP versus a 97.1% cure rate for patients who underwent BNE.[35] Other studies also demonstrated that increased success rates (89%) can be achieved in remedial parathyroid surgery with the aid of this intraoperative adjunctive measure.

Gamma Probe Localization

Radioguided parathyroidectomy involves a preoperative injection of 10 to 20 mCi ^{99m}Tc sestamibi followed by intraoperative localization with a hand-held quantitative gamma counter. Focused exploration proceeds in the area in which counts are highest. Intraoperative cure is suggested by radioactivity counts within the excised gland of at least 20% of background; postexcision counts in all four quadrants of the neck should subsequently equalize. Use of an intraoperative gamma probe has not been embraced by most centers that specialize in parathyroid surgery.

Recurrent Laryngeal Nerve Monitoring

One of the most dreaded complications of thyroid and parathyroid surgery is injury to the RLN. Adjunctive intraoperative RLN monitoring has been proposed as a means to reduce injury to these important nerves.

The use of electrical stimulation of the RLN during thyroid surgery was first described in 1970 by Flisberg and Lindholm.[36] Since then, several techniques have been developed; most involve electromyography and require direct contact of the laryngeal muscle by an electrode to allow for evaluation of evoked potentials with the use of a hand-held nerve stimulator. A meta-analysis comparing the effect of RLN monitoring versus RLN visual identification alone on true vocal cord palsy rates after thyroid surgery found no statistically significant difference in RLN injury rates between the two groups.[37] To date, the preponderance of data have not shown that intraoperative nerve monitoring reduces nerve injury in either thyroid or parathyroid surgery.

OUTCOMES AFTER PARATHYROID SURGERY

Parathyroidectomy is the only definitive cure for PHPT, with cure rates exceeding 95% in experienced hands. Clinical outcomes are largely related to the experience of the surgeon, with high-volume parathyroid surgeons having higher cure rates and lower complication rates.[38] The most common complications after parathyroid surgery include RLN injury, hypoparathyroidism, and neck hematoma. In addition, failure to cure must be considered as an adverse outcome.

Cure Rates

Biochemical cure is defined as normocalcemia after parathyroid surgery that lasts at least 6 months postoperatively. Cure rates after parathyroidectomy largely depend on the experience of the surgeon. The reported cure rates of 95% or greater largely come from studies reporting the experience of high-volume, experienced endocrine surgeons. A study reporting 1650 consecutive parathyroidectomies demonstrated a cure rate of 99.4% for 1037 patients who underwent MIP and 97.1% for 613 patients who underwent BNE.[27] However, most parathyroidectomies performed in the United States (and worldwide) are performed by low-volume (<30 parathyroidectomies/year) surgeons. To our knowledge, no U.S. studies directly comparing cure and complication rates between high-volume and low-volume parathyroid surgeons exist. However, it is unlikely that outcomes from low-volume surgeons are comparable to more experienced endocrine surgeons. Furthermore, data from Scandinavia demonstrate a clear association between high-volume centers and improved cure rates.[39]

Nerve Injury—Recurrent Laryngeal Nerve Injury, Bilateral Nerve Injury, Injury to External Branch of the Superior Laryngeal Nerve

Reported rates of recurrent nerve injury are variable; generally ranging from 0.5% to 1% of nerves at risk; however, rates may be 30% in less experienced hands. Manifestations of RLN injury range from variable hoarseness in cases of unilateral injury to severe airway compromise in cases of bilateral nerve injury. Bilateral RLN injury is a devastating, albeit rare, complication that often requires placement of a temporary or permanent tracheostomy. In addition to the RLN, injury to the external branch of the superior laryngeal nerve can result in subtle voice changes and voice projection compromise. These injuries can be significant for singers or professional speakers. Meticulous technique is the most important contribution to protecting the recurrent nerve and the external branch of the superior laryngeal nerve.

Postoperative Hypocalcemia

Postoperative hypocalcemia is a common event after parathyroid surgery. It often occurs because the residual parathyroid glands have undergone atrophy as a result of long-standing hypercalcemia. It also occurs from either inadvertent removal of unaffected parathyroid glands or devascularization of remaining parathyroid tissue (see "Hypoparathyroidism" earlier). Common risk factors include subtotal parathyroidectomy, BNE, concomitant thyroid surgery, and a history of prior neck dissection. Risk factors also include remedial surgery, hungry bone syndrome, and preoperative treatment with long-acting pharmacologic agents, in particular, bisphosphonates. Transient hypocalcemia is common and typically treated with calcium supplementation. However, in patients with significant, prolonged postoperative hypocalcemia, rapid administration of intravenous calcium gluconate is warranted; this is accomplished by diluting 10 ampules of calcium gluconate in 1 liter of normal saline. The initial infusion rate of 30 mL/hr is titrated, based on symptoms and serial serum calcium levels. Other electrolyte abnormalities such as hypomagnesemia and hypophosphatemia may occur and need to be addressed to facilitate reversal of hypocalcemia. Vitamin D supplementation is added for cases in which long-term management is necessary.

Bleeding or Hematoma

Significant postoperative bleeding or neck hematoma is uncommon, occurring in less than 0.5% of patients.[27] However, it is a surgical emergency. When minor oozing at the incision site is noted and there is no evidence of airway compromise, patients can be managed conservatively. Alternatively, acute airway distress requires prompt evacuation of the hematoma; this can usually be accomplished under sterile conditions in the operating room—in rare cases, bedside evacuation is warranted. It may be necessary to evacuate the hematoma before endotracheal tube placement. Signs of airway compromise may initially be subtle; skin changes such as petechial hemorrhage and ecchymosis are often mild or lacking because of patient factors (dark skin; short, obese neck) and location of the bleeding below the strap muscles. Patient anxiety is often an early symptom that may portend airway compromise. Progressive tachypnea, hypoxia, and progressive anxiety are late manifestations and signal impending airway compromise.

INHERITED PARATHYROID DISEASE

The surgical management of inherited hyperparathyroidism is complex and differs among specific syndromes. Achieving and maintaining normocalcemia, minimizing perioperative complications, and facilitating future surgery in cases of recurrent disease are basic principles in patients with inherited hyperparathyroidism.[40]

Multiple Endocrine Neoplasia

Multiple Endocrine Neoplasia Type 1

MEN1 is an inherited endocrine disorder that consists of PHPT and endocrine tumors of the pancreas and pituitary glands. The underlying germline mutation occurs in the *MEN1* gene and is thought to render the parathyroids more susceptible to tumor expression after a single somatic mutation. PHPT occurs in most patients (>90%) and is typically the first endocrine manifestation. Patients usually present between the third and fifth decades of life with PHPT. Four-gland hyperplasia with asymmetrical enlargement of the parathyroid glands is usually found; additionally, supernumerary glands exist in up to 20% of cases.

Parathyroid surgery in patients with MEN1 is largely regarded as a palliative or "debulking" procedure; recurrence is inevitable in cases of long-term survival. Subtotal parathyroidectomy and total parathyroidectomy with heterotopic autotransplantation of parathyroid tissue are the initial procedures of choice. Subtotal parathyroidectomy involves the identification of all parathyroid glands, complete resection of the three largest glands, and partial resection of the remaining gland, leaving an in situ remnant of approximately the size of a normal parathyroid gland (approximately 30 mg). Total parathyroidectomy requires complete resection of all glands combined with immediate heterotopic transplantation of several 1- to 3-mm slices of fresh parathyroid tissue into individual pockets created in the brachioradialis muscle of the nondominant forearm. A meticulous search for supernumerary glands, including transcervical thymectomy, should be performed during the initial procedure, regardless of which surgical option was undertaken. In addition, thymic carcinoids rarely occur in this population. Cryopreservation of parathyroid tissue may also be performed if proper storage facilities are available.[40]

Multiple Endocrine Neoplasia Type 2A

MEN2A consists of medullary thyroid carcinoma, pheochromocytoma, and PHPT. PHPT in MEN2A is less common than in MEN1, occurring in 20% to 30% of patients. MEN2A is a result of a mutational aberration of the *RET* gene. Patients typically have "single-gland" disease, although all parathyroid tissue is at risk, and surgical intervention is similar to intervention for sporadic PHPT and usually involves resection of a single enlarged parathyroid gland. In MEN2A, medullary thyroid carcinoma is the dominant feature (as opposed to PHPT in MEN1); PHPT is diagnosed either synchronously or after total thyroidectomy. Most experienced parathyroid surgeons resect enlarged parathyroid glands but leave normal-appearing parathyroid glands in situ during parathyroid surgery for MEN2A.

Other Familial Hyperparathyroidism Disorders

In addition to the MEN syndromes, there are other, less common forms of familial HPT, including hyperparathyroidism–jaw tumor syndrome; familial isolated hyperparathyroidism; and HPT associated with mutations in the calcium-sensing receptor such as autosomal dominant mild hyperparathyroidism, familial hypocalciuric hypercalcemia, and neonatal severe hyperparathyroidism. Recommendations regarding parathyroid surgery in the setting of these rare causes of PHPT are evolving but typically involve debulking procedures (Table 37-4).

Hyperparathyroidism–jaw tumor syndrome is an extremely rare disorder associated with a high incidence of PTCA (15%). Patients are typically young and present with PHPT during their third or fourth decade. Alternatively, they may be detected

TABLE 37-4 Familial Hyperparathyroid Disorders, Genetic Characteristics, Presentation of Hyperparathyroidism, and Associated Features

DISORDER	INHERITANCE	GENE	CHROMOSOME	HPT	ASSOCIATED TUMORS
MEN1	AD	*MEN1*	11q13	90% penetrance; multiglandular	Pituitary tumor, EPT
MEN2A	AD	*RET*	10q21	20% penetrance; multiglandular/adenoma	MTC, pheochromocytoma
HPT-JT	AD	*HRPT2*	1q21-q32	Cystic parathyroid tumors (15% risk of carcinoma)	Jaw tumor, renal tumor
FIHPT	AD	*HRPT2*	1q21-q32	Adenoma/multiglandular	—
		MEN1	11q13	Adenoma/multiglandular	
ADMH	AD	*CASR*	3q13-21	Multiglandular/adenoma	—
FHH	AD	*CASR*	3q13-21	Mildly hyperplastic	—
NSHPT	AR/AD	*CASR*	3q13-21	Markedly hyperplastic	—

From Carling T, Udelsman R: Parathyroid surgery in familial hyperparathyroid disorders. *J Intern Med* 257:27–37, 2005.
AD, autosomal dominant; *ADMH*, autosomal dominant mild hyperparathyroidism; *AR*, autosomal recessive; *EPT*, endocrine pancreatic tumor; *FHH*, familial hypocalciuric hypercalcemia; *FIHPT*, familial isolated hyperparathyroidism; *HPT*, hereditary hyperparathyroidism; *HPT-JT*, hereditary hyperparathyroidism–jaw tumor syndrome; *MEN*, multiple endocrine neoplasia; *MTC*, medullary thyroid carcinoma; *NSHPT*, neonatal severe hyperparathyroidism.

through screening of family members of an index case. Patients can be treated with single-gland resection similar to cases of sporadic PHPT, unless PTCA is suspected; in such cases, en bloc resection of the tumor and associated tissues is the mainstay of treatment (see "Parathyroid Carcinoma" next). Familial isolated hyperparathyroidism genetic mutations can involve the *MEN1* gene, *HRPT2* gene, or *CASR* gene, and surgical management varies. In general, if uniglandular disease is present, single-gland resection can be performed; subtotal parathyroidectomy is implemented to treat multiglandular disease. Similarly, surgical treatment of PHPT in syndromes associated with *CASR* mutations is variable. Patients with familial hypocalciuric hypercalcemia are largely asymptomatic and rarely benefit from surgical resection. Neonatal severe hyperparathyroidism manifests with severe hypercalcemia; this condition is typically lethal unless total parathyroidectomy is performed with the first few months of life. Patients with autosomal dominant mild hyperparathyroidism can undergo either radical subtotal parathyroidectomy or total parathyroidectomy with parathyroid autotransplantation.

PARATHYROID CARCINOMA

Parathyroid carcinoma (PTCA) was first described in 1904 by De Quervain. PTCA is an exceptionally rare malignancy, with a clinical presentation similar to benign PHPT in many cases. It is the least common endocrine malignancy, with a prevalence of 0.005% of all malignancies. Although PHPT is a common entity, affecting 1 in 500 to 1000 patients, PTCA accounts for less than 1% of cases of PHPT in the United States. These patients are at risk for recurrences throughout their lifetime and may require multiple reoperations; the disease has a significant impact on quality of life. Over time, persistent disease results in uncontrolled hypercalcemia, leading to severe morbidity, including renal failure, cardiac arrhythmias, and sometimes death.

PTCA most commonly manifests in the fourth to fifth decades of life. Preoperative findings include a palpable neck mass in the setting of a markedly elevated serum calcium. Hoarseness, suggestive of invasion of the RLN, should raise suspicion.

Distinguishing PTCA from benign PHPT intraoperatively is challenging. PTCA is often firm, is densely scarred, and obliterates normal tissue planes. Similarly, atypical adenomas may be large with significant adherence to surrounding structures, without direct invasion. Pathologic evaluation does not always distinguish benign from malignant lesions. This distinction is important because en bloc resection of PTCA at initial operation is the most effective chance of cure, and pathologic confirmation of PTCA may lead to closer postoperative surveillance and earlier detection of recurrence. Surgeons who explore patients with PHPT must be prepared to perform an initial, appropriate resection in the setting of potential PTCA.

Medical Alternatives

There are no long-term medical therapies for which data are convincing regarding their efficacy or safety in the treatment of primary HPT. Three classes of agents—bisphosphonates, selective estrogen receptor modulators, and calcimimetics—have shown preliminary efficacy on surrogate markers of severity of disease, including serum calcium and bone density, but these effects have not been verified based on clinical outcomes.

Bisphosphonates (etidronate, alendronate, pamidronate) have been used in the treatment of Paget disease, osteoporosis, and hypercalcemia of malignancy. Intravenous pamidronate appears to be the most effective for acute treatment of hypercalcemia associated with PHPT. Limitations of long-term treatment include poor GI drug absorption, increase in PTH levels with increased renal tubular resorption and GI absorption of calcium, and expense.

Bone mineral density has been a primary end point in studies of hormonal therapy in patients with PHPT. The risk-benefit equation for determining the usefulness of hormone replacement therapy is complex because estrogen replacement therapy does not reduce PTH concentrations in patients with PHPT. In addition, unopposed estrogen increases the risk for endometrial hyperplasia and carcinoma as well as the risk for venous thromboembolism and may cause vaginal bleeding or increase the risk for breast cancer. As a result, selective estrogen receptor inhibitors such as raloxifene and tamoxifen have been used only in a preliminary fashion. Lastly, cinacalcet (Sensipar) has been used to treat HPT in patients with ESRD who are on long-term hemodialysis. Sensipar has also been used to reduce serum calcium levels in patients with PTCA, particularly in cases of unresectable disease, and in rare patients who have undergone multiple operations without cure.

TABLE 37-5 Randomized Trials Comparing Minimally Invasive Parathyroidectomy With Bilateral Neck Exploration

REFERENCE	PATIENTS	RANDOMIZED GROUP (N)		RESULTS
Slepavicius et al., 2008[41]	48	MIP (24)	BNE (24)	No difference in OR time, cosmesis at ≥1 yr, or cure rate; lower cost in BNE group
Miccoli et al., 2008[42]	40	Video-assisted MIP (20)	Endoscopic BNE (20)	No difference in OR time, complication and cure rates
Aarum et al., 2007[43]	100	MIP (50)	BNE (50)	No difference in cure rate; lower cost in BNE group
Sozio et al., 2005[44]	69	Radioguided MIP (34)	BNE (35)	No difference in cure rate; shorter OR time and LOS in MIP group
Bergenfelz et al., 2005[45]	50	MIP (25)	BNE (25)	No difference in cure rate; shorter OR time, less transient hypocalcemia in MIP group
Bergenfelz et al., 2002[46]; Westerdahl and Bergenfelz, 2007[47]	91	Initial, MIP (47); 5-yr follow-up, MIP (38)	Initial, BNE (44); 5-yr follow-up, BNE (33)	No difference in cost, transient nerve injury, or short-term and long-term cure rates; shorter OR time, less transient and long-term hypocalcemia in MIP group
Miccoli et al., 1999[48]	38	Video-assisted MIP (20)	BNE (18)	No difference in cure rate; shorter OR time, less pain, improved cosmesis in MIP group

Adapted with permission from Callender GG, Udelsman R: Surgery for primary hyperparathyroidism. *Cancer* 120:3602–3616, 2014.
BNE, bilateral neck exploration; *LOS*, length of stay; *MIP*, minimally invasive parathyroidectomy; *OR*, operating room; *RLN*, recurrent laryngeal nerve.

CONTROVERSIES IN PARATHYROID SURGERY

Unilateral versus Bilateral Neck Exploration

BNE with intraoperative frozen section examination of all excised parathyroid tissue has long been considered the gold standard approach to the treatment of PHPT. Patients were admitted to the hospital and underwent general anesthesia. Although BNE is an effective operation, controversy has developed in recent years regarding the potential superiority of more focused, minimally invasive approaches.

Several randomized trials comparing MIP with BNE in the management of PHPT showed that MIP is associated with shorter operative times, decreased length of hospital stay, and decreased postoperative pain.[41-48] Cure rates were equivalent (Table 37-5). These studies provide strong evidence that MIP should be considered for patients with PHPT undergoing index parathyroidectomy.

Does Asymptomatic Primary Hyperparathyroidism Really Exist?

Although most cases of PHPT are classified as asymptomatic, defining "truly asymptomatic" PHPT can be difficult. This difficulty is largely due to the fact that many symptoms associated with PHPT (e.g., fatigue, bone pain, and GI symptoms) are nonspecific and not attributed to PHPT. Although such symptoms can have a negative impact on a person's quality of life, they are difficult to quantify. However, evidence from studies that have carefully examined preoperative and postoperative symptoms in patients with PHPT suggests that only 2% to 5% of patients are truly asymptomatic.[49,50] Most patients do not realize the severity of their symptoms until they undergo parathyroidectomy and experience symptomatic relief.

Furthermore, several studies have shown that the neurocognitive dysfunction of PHPT significantly impairs quality of life, and this is improved by surgery. Therefore, every patient with PHPT should be referred to an experienced parathyroid surgeon to discuss the risks and benefits of surgery to make informed decisions about the management of their disease. Patients should receive a strong recommendation for surgery if they have overt symptoms or if they are asymptomatic and meet guidelines.

SELECTED REFERENCES

Bilezikian JP, Brandi ML, Eastell R, et al: Guidelines for the management of asymptomatic primary hyperparathyroidism: Summary statement from the Fourth International Workshop. *J Clin Endocrinol Metab* 99:3561–3569, 2014.

This report distills an update of current information about diagnostics, clinical features, and management of primary hyperparathyroidism into a set of revised guidelines. An expert panel considered all evidence provided by the individual Workshop Panels and came to a consensus.

Carling T, Udelsman R: Parathyroid surgery in familial hyperparathyroid disorders. *J Intern Med* 257:27–37, 2005.

This thorough review of familial hyperparathyroid disorders eloquently describes the complexity of surgical management of hyperparathyroidism in these specific syndromes.

Chen H, Wang TS, Yen TW, et al: Operative failures after parathyroidectomy for hyperparathyroidism: The influence of surgical volume. *Ann Surg* 252:691–695, 2010.

This retrospective review of two prospective databases containing greater than 2000 consecutive patients who underwent parathyroidectomy demonstrated that surgical volume greatly influences the failure pattern after parathyroidectomy for primary hyperparathyroidism.

Lebastchi AH, Aruny J, Donovan PI, et al: Real-time super selective venous sampling in remedial parathyroid surgery. *J Am Coll Surg* 220:994–1000, 2015.

This retrospective review investigated the utility of real-time superselective venous sampling in the setting of negative noninvasive imaging results. The utility of the rapid parathyroid hormone assay was extended to the interventional radiology suite, generating near real-time data and facilitating on-site venous localization of diseased parathyroid glands.

Udelsman R, Akerstrom G, Biagini C, et al: The surgical management of asymptomatic primary hyperparathyroidism: Proceedings of the Fourth International Workshop. *J Clin Endocrinol Metab* 99:3595–3606, 2014.

The surgical management of primary hyperparathyroidism (PHPT) has undergone considerable advances over the past 2 decades. A subgroup was created by the Steering Committee of the Fourth International Workshop on the Management of Asymptomatic Primary Hyperparathyroidism to address key questions related to the surgical management of PHPT.

REFERENCES

1. Owen R: On the anatomy of the Indian rhinoceros. *Tran Zool Soc Lond* 4:31–58, 1862.
2. Sandstrom IV, Peters CH: On a new gland in man and several mammals. *Bull Inst Hist Med* 6:192–222, 1938.
3. Dubose J, Ragsdale T, Morvant J: "Bodies so tiny": The history of parathyroid surgery. *Curr Surg* 62:91–95, 2005.
4. Restivo A, Sarkozy A, Digilio MC, et al: 22q11 deletion syndrome: A review of some developmental biology aspects of the cardiovascular system. *J Cardiovasc Med (Hagerstown)* 7:77–85, 2006.
5. Pothiwala P, Levine SN: Parathyroid surgery in pregnancy: Review of the literature and localization by aspiration for parathyroid hormone levels. *J Perinatol* 29:779–784, 2009.
6. de Nanclares GP, Fernandez-Rebollo E, Santin I, et al: Epigenetic defects of GNAS in patients with pseudohypoparathyroidism and mild features of Albright's hereditary osteodystrophy. *J Clin Endocrinol Metab* 92:2370–2373, 2007.
7. Yip L, Seethala RR, Nikiforova MN, et al: Loss of heterozygosity of selected tumor suppressor genes in parathyroid carcinoma. *Surgery* 144:949–955, discussion 954-945, 2008.
8. Stewart AF: Clinical practice. Hypercalcemia associated with cancer. *N Engl J Med* 352:373–379, 2005.
9. Burtis WJ, Brady TG, Orloff JJ, et al: Immunochemical characterization of circulating parathyroid hormone-related protein in patients with humoral hypercalcemia of cancer. *N Engl J Med* 322:1106–1112, 1990.
10. Quinn CE, Healy JM, Lebastchi AH, et al: Modern experience with aggressive parathyroid tumors in a high-volume New England referral Center. *J Am Coll Surg* 220:1054–1062, 2015.
11. Demiaux B, Arlot ME, Chapuy MC, et al: Serum osteocalcin is increased in patients with osteomalacia: Correlations with biochemical and histomorphometric findings. *J Clin Endocrinol Metab* 74:1146–1151, 1992.
12. Phitayakorn R, McHenry CR: Hyperparathyroid crisis: Use of bisphosphonates as a bridge to parathyroidectomy. *J Am Coll Surg* 206:1106–1115, 2008.
13. Nigwekar SU, Wolf M, Sterns RH, et al: Calciphylaxis from nonuremic causes: A systematic review. *Clin J Am Soc Nephrol* 3:1139–1143, 2008.
14. Rashid RM, Hauck M, Lasley M: Anti-nuclear antibody: A potential predictor of calciphylaxis in non-dialysis patients. *J Eur Acad Dermatol Venereol* 22:1247–1248, 2008.
15. Bilezikian JP, Brandi ML, Eastell R, et al: Guidelines for the management of asymptomatic primary hyperparathyroidism: Summary Statement from the Fourth International Workshop. *J Clin Endocrinol Metab* 99:3561–3569, 2014.
16. Udelsman R, Akerstrom G, Biagini C, et al: The surgical management of asymptomatic primary hyperparathyroidism: Proceedings of the Fourth International Workshop. *J Clin Endocrinol Metab* 99:3595–3606, 2014.
17. Coakley AJ, Kettle AG, Wells CP, et al: 99Tcm sestamibi—a new agent for parathyroid imaging. *Nucl Med Commun* 10:791–794, 1989.
18. Lever EG, Refetoff S, Straus FH, 2nd, et al: Coexisting thyroid and parathyroid disease—are they related? *Surgery* 94:893–900, 1983.
19. Gilat H, Cohen M, Feinmesser R, et al: Minimally invasive procedure for resection of a parathyroid adenoma: The role of preoperative high-resolution ultrasonography. *J Clin Ultrasound* 33:283–287, 2005.
20. Patel CN, Salahudeen HM, Lansdown M, et al: Clinical utility of ultrasound and 99mTc sestamibi SPECT/CT for preoperative localization of parathyroid adenoma in patients with primary hyperparathyroidism. *Clin Radiol* 65:278–287, 2010.
21. Rodgers SE, Hunter GJ, Hamberg LM, et al: Improved preoperative planning for directed parathyroidectomy with 4-dimensional computed tomography. *Surgery* 140:932–940, discussion 940-941, 2006.
22. Mohebati A, Shaha AR: Imaging techniques in parathyroid surgery for primary hyperparathyroidism. *Am J Otolaryngol* 33:457–468, 2012.
23. Reidel MA, Schilling T, Graf S, et al: Localization of hyperfunctioning parathyroid glands by selective venous sampling in reoperation for primary or secondary hyperparathyroidism. *Surgery* 140:907–913, discussion 913, 2006.
24. Udelsman R, Aruny JE, Donovan PI, et al: Rapid parathyroid hormone analysis during venous localization. *Ann Surg* 237:714–719, 2003.
25. Maser C, Donovan P, Santos F, et al: Sonographically guided fine needle aspiration with rapid parathyroid hormone assay. *Ann Surg Oncol* 13:1690–1695, 2006.
26. Udelsman R: Six hundred fifty-six consecutive explorations for primary hyperparathyroidism. *Ann Surg* 235:665–670, discussion 670-672, 2002.
27. Udelsman R, Lin Z, Donovan P: The superiority of minimally invasive parathyroidectomy based on 1650 consecutive patients with primary hyperparathyroidism. *Ann Surg* 253:585–591, 2011.
28. Gagner M: Endoscopic subtotal parathyroidectomy in patients with primary hyperparathyroidism. *Br J Surg* 83:875, 1996.
29. Miccoli P, Berti P, Ambrosini CE: Perspectives and lessons learned after a decade of minimally invasive video-assisted thyroidectomy. *ORL J Otorhinolaryngol Relat Spec* 70:282–286, 2008.
30. Barczynski M, Cichon S, Konturek A, et al: Minimally invasive video-assisted parathyroidectomy versus open minimally invasive parathyroidectomy for a solitary parathyroid adenoma: A prospective, randomized, blinded trial. *World J Surg* 30:721–731, 2006.
31. Lebastchi AH, Aruny J, Donovan PI, et al: Real-time super selective venous sampling in remedial parathyroid surgery. *J Am Coll Surg* 220:994–1000, 2015.
32. Sokoll LJ, Drew H, Udelsman R: Intraoperative parathyroid hormone analysis: A study of 200 consecutive cases. *Clin Chem* 46:1662–1668, 2000.

33. Irvin GL, 3rd, Dembrow VD, Prudhomme DL: Operative monitoring of parathyroid gland hyperfunction. *Am J Surg* 162:299–302, 1991.
34. Udelsman R, Donovan P, Shaw C: Cure predictability during parathyroidectomy. *World J Surg* 38:525–533, 2014.
35. Richards ML, Thompson GB, Farley DR, et al: Reoperative parathyroidectomy in 228 patients during the era of minimal-access surgery and intraoperative parathyroid hormone monitoring. *Am J Surg* 196:937–942, discussion 942-943, 2008.
36. Flisberg K, Lindholm T: Electrical stimulation of the human recurrent laryngeal nerve during thyroid operation. *Acta Otolaryngol Suppl* 263:63–67, 1969.
37. Higgins TS, Gupta R, Ketcham AS, et al: Recurrent laryngeal nerve monitoring versus identification alone on post-thyroidectomy true vocal fold palsy: A meta-analysis. *Laryngoscope* 121:1009–1017, 2011.
38. Chen H, Wang TS, Yen TW, et al: Operative failures after parathyroidectomy for hyperparathyroidism: The influence of surgical volume. *Ann Surg* 252:691–695, 2010.
39. Malmaeus J, Granberg PO, Halvorsen J, et al: Parathyroid surgery in Scandinavia. *Acta Chir Scand* 154:409–413, 1988.
40. Carling T, Udelsman R: Parathyroid surgery in familial hyperparathyroid disorders. *J Intern Med* 257:27–37, 2005.
41. Slepavicius A, Beisa V, Janusonis V, et al: Focused versus conventional parathyroidectomy for primary hyperparathyroidism: A prospective, randomized, blinded trial. *Langenbecks Arch Surg* 393:659–666, 2008.
42. Miccoli P, Berti P, Materazzi G, et al: Endoscopic bilateral neck exploration versus quick intraoperative parathormone assay (qPTHa) during endoscopic parathyroidectomy: A prospective randomized trial. *Surg Endosc* 22:398–400, 2008.
43. Aarum S, Nordenstrom J, Reihner E, et al: Operation for primary hyperparathyroidism: The new versus the old order. A randomised controlled trial of preoperative localisation. *Scand J Surg* 96:26–30, 2007.
44. Sozio A, Schietroma M, Franchi L, et al: Parathyroidectomy: Bilateral exploration of the neck vs minimally invasive radio-guided treatment. *Minerva Chir* 60:83–89, 2005.
45. Bergenfelz A, Kanngiesser V, Zielke A, et al: Conventional bilateral cervical exploration versus open minimally invasive parathyroidectomy under local anaesthesia for primary hyperparathyroidism. *Br J Surg* 92:190–197, 2005.
46. Bergenfelz A, Lindblom P, Tibblin S, et al: Unilateral versus bilateral neck exploration for primary hyperparathyroidism: A prospective randomized controlled trial. *Ann Surg* 236:543–551, 2002.
47. Westerdahl J, Bergenfelz A: Unilateral versus bilateral neck exploration for primary hyperparathyroidism: Five-year follow-up of a randomized controlled trial. *Ann Surg* 246:976–980, 2007.
48. Miccoli P, Bendinelli C, Berti P, et al: Video-assisted versus conventional parathyroidectomy in primary hyperparathyroidism: A prospective randomized study. *Surgery* 126:1117–1121, 1999.
49. Okamoto T, Gerstein HC, Obara T: Psychiatric symptoms, bone density and non-specific symptoms in patients with mild hypercalcemia due to primary hyperparathyroidism: A systematic overview of the literature. *Endocr J* 44:367–374, 1997.
50. Hasse C, Sitter H, Bachmann S, et al: How asymptomatic is asymptomatic primary hyperparathyroidism? *Exp Clin Endocrinol Diabetes* 108:265–274, 2000.

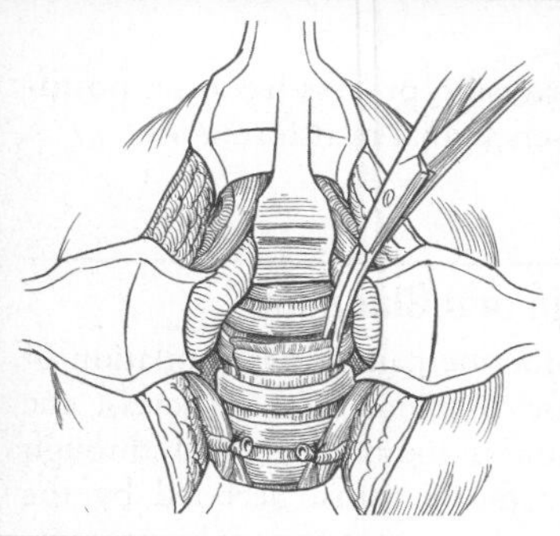

CHAPTER 38

Endocrine Pancreas

Rebekah White, Taylor S. Riall

OUTLINE

The pancreas was first identified by a Greek anatomist and surgeon, Herophilus (335-280 BC), and named 400 years later by another Greek anatomist, Rufus of Ephesus (1st century AD). The word "pancreas" is derived from a Greek word that means "sweet-bread" (pancreas as food) or literally "all flesh." Located in the retroperitoneum with the head of the pancreas lying in the C loop of the duodenum (Fig. 38-1*A* and *B*), the pancreas has distinct hormonal (endocrine) and digestive (exocrine) functions. The endocrine cells are organized in discrete clusters throughout the pancreas. These pale-staining clusters of cells (Fig. 38-1*C*) were first described by a medical student, Paul Langerhans, in 1869 and are called islets of Langerhans. The pancreatic islets secrete hormones directly into the bloodstream.

The primary physiologic function of the endocrine pancreas is regulation of glucose metabolism, through secretion of insulin and glucagon directly into the bloodstream in response to blood glucose levels and various other stimuli. In medieval Persia, in 1025, Avicenna provided the first detailed account of a patient with diabetes mellitus, who had an abnormal appetite, collapse of sexual function, and the sweet-tasting urine. In 1889, Minkowski and von Mering made the connection between diabetes and the pancreas. While studying fat absorption in dogs after pancreatectomy, they noted that surgical removal of the pancreas led to eventual coma and death, and they documented glucosuria and ketonuria. Frederick Banting and Charles Best discovered insulin in 1922. They surgically ligated the pancreas of one set of dogs, leading to atrophy of the exocrine pancreas. They then removed and homogenized the pancreas and injected the homogenized extract into a diabetic dog, temporarily reversing this condition. Banting and Best were awarded a Nobel Prize for this work. Additional pancreatic endocrine hormones play a role in the complex regulation of pancreatic exocrine secretion and digestion.

In this chapter, we describe the histomorphology, embryology, physiology, and pathophysiology of the endocrine pancreas. The focus is on the diagnosis and management of diseases relevant to surgeons, including tumors of the endocrine pancreas and diabetes, and the endocrine complications of surgical therapy.

HISTOMORPHOLOGY OF ISLETS

The adult pancreas consists of the endocrine cells, digestive enzyme–secreting acinar cells contained in clusters of acini with acinar-draining ducts, and accompanying blood vessels and lymphatics. Pancreatic endocrine cells are organized into islets of Langerhans (see Fig. 38-1*C*). The adult pancreas contains approximately 10^6 islet cells, each containing approximately 3000 cells and ranging in diameter from 40 to 900 μm. Endocrine cells comprise less than 2% of the overall pancreatic mass in the adult pancreas. The complex architecture of the pancreatic islets enables normal endocrine function. The islets are composed of four cell types: A (alpha), B (beta), D, and F cells. The four cell types are not evenly distributed within the islets or throughout the pancreas. Table 38-1 describes the cell types, their hormonal products, and their location within the islet and the pancreas.

B cells secrete insulin and constitute approximately 70% of the islet cell mass. They are located centrally within the islet. A cells, located in the periphery, secrete glucagon and constitute approximately 10% of the islet cell mass. Also located peripherally, F cells secrete pancreatic polypeptide (PP). D cells are evenly distributed throughout the islet and constitute approximately 5% of the islet cell mass. D cells secrete somatostatin, and D_2 cells secrete vasoactive intestinal peptide (VIP). B and D cells are concentrated in the body and tail of the pancreas, F cells are heavily concentrated in the uncinate process, and A cells are evenly distributed throughout the gland.

The rich portal microcirculation of the pancreatic islets allows for the endocrine-to-endocrine cell signaling necessary for hormonal regulation. Afferent arterioles enter the islet in an area of discontinuity in the peripheral, non–B cell mantle of cells. The order of islet cellular perfusion and interaction is from the B cell core outward to the mantle, which is further subordered with most D cells downstream or distal to most A cells. This order allows B cells to inhibit A cell secretion and A cells to stimulate D cell secretion.[1]

Pancreatic endocrine secretion also regulates pancreatic exocrine secretion through the islet-acinar axis of the pancreas. Insulin

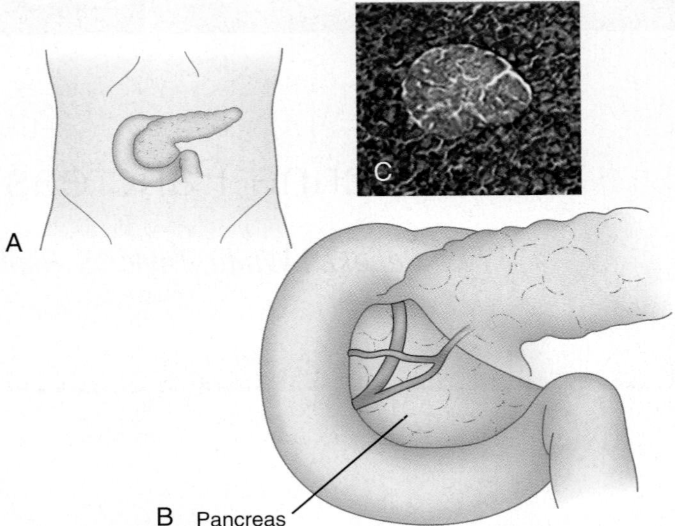

FIGURE 38-1 **A,** The pancreas in its retroperitoneal position at the level of the second lumbar vertebra. **B,** Relationship of the head of the pancreas in the C loop of the duodenum with the pancreatic duct and common bile duct emptying into the ampulla of Vater. **C,** On microscopic view, the endocrine cells are located in nests, called islets of Langerhans, which are distributed throughout the pancreas (trichrome stain, ×10).

stimulates pancreatic exocrine secretion, amino acid transport, and synthesis of protein and enzymes, whereas glucagon acts in a counterregulatory fashion, inhibiting the same processes. Based on animal studies, somatostatin, peptide YY, PP, glucagon, ghrelin, and leptin are potentially involved in inhibition of pancreatic exocrine function, although their role in humans is controversial.

EMBRYOLOGY OF THE ENDOCRINE PANCREAS

In the human fetus, pancreatic islets comprise approximately one third of the pancreatic mass. Pancreatic formation begins during week 5 of gestation as two endodermal pancreatic buds (dorsal and ventral) that form at the junction of the foregut and the midgut. The dorsal and ventral buds are composed of endoderm covered in splanchnic mesoderm. The acinar and islet cells differentiate from the endodermal cells found in the embryonic buds, whereas the splanchnic mesoderm eventually develops into the dorsal and ventral mesentery. The first glucagon-producing cells (A cells) appear in 3-week-old embryos, and the first organized islets appear at approximately 10 weeks. Subsequently, there is a major amplification of endocrine cell numbers, particularly B cells. B cell formation primarily occurs before birth with a burst of proliferation up to the first 2 years of life. Thereafter, little B cell proliferation is observed. Postnatal proliferation of A and D cells is rarely seen. The B-A cell ratio doubles neonatally, reflecting increased growth of B cells. There is a sevenfold increase in the B-D cell ratio during childhood as result of additional loss of D cells.[2]

The conversion to a nonepithelial location of endocrine cells entails a change in cell division polarity, from perpendicular to the basement membrane to parallel to the basement membrane. Endocrine cells lose their connection with the lumen and tight junctions. As endocrine progenitor cells become nonepithelial, there is downregulation of *PDX1*, found predominantly in pancreatic progenitor cells. This conversion process has been postulated to parallel epithelial-to-mesenchymal transformation.

ENDOCRINE PHYSIOLOGY

Glucose Homeostasis: Insulin and Glucagon

The primary function of the endocrine pancreas is regulation of glucose homeostasis. In response to blood glucose levels, the secretion of insulin and glucagon is tightly regulated through various feedback and regulatory mechanisms. Secreted by the endocrine pancreas, insulin functions to store energy by promoting glucose transport into cells, inhibiting glycogenolysis and fatty acid breakdown, and stimulating protein synthesis. Glucagon is the major counterregulatory hormone to insulin, increasing blood glucose levels through stimulation of glycogenolysis, lipolysis, and gluconeogenesis.

Insulin

Insulin is an anabolic hormone synthesized in the B cells of the islets. It promotes glucose transport into all cells except B cells, hepatocytes, and central nervous system cells. Insulin is a 56–amino acid polypeptide with a molecular weight of 6 kDa that is synthesized as a precursor peptide, called proinsulin. In response to pancreatic B cell stimulation by glucose, proinsulin is synthesized in the endoplasmic reticulum and transported to the Golgi complex where it is cleaved into insulin and the residual C peptide (Fig. 38-2). The resulting insulin molecule consists of two polypeptide chains (A and B) joined by two disulfide bridges. Although the amino acid sequence varies among species, the locations of the disulfide bridges are highly conserved and are critical for biologic activity of insulin. After cleavage of C peptide, insulin is moved via microtubules into secretory granules, where it is released directly into the bloodstream via exocytosis. C peptide and insulin are secreted in equimolar amounts.

The B cell is highly sensitive to changes in glucose concentration and is maximally stimulated at concentrations of 400 to 500 mg/dL. In response to glucose, the endocrine pancreas immediately reacts with a short burst of stored insulin (4 to 6 minutes), followed by a sustained secretion of insulin, which requires active synthesis of the hormone within the islet cell. Insulin has a 7- to 10-minute half-life and is primarily metabolized by the liver. Brain cells and red blood cells do not take up insulin.

Insulin binds to a specific 300-kDa glycoprotein cell surface receptor, which has been isolated and well characterized. Stimulation of the insulin receptor depends on insulin concentration. After receptor stimulation, glucose is actively transported across cell membranes throughout the body by membrane-bound glucose transporters. There are several classes of glucose transporters, with varying affinities for glucose. Insulin resistance, present in type 2 diabetes, can be the result of decreased numbers of receptors or a decreased affinity of receptors for insulin. Sulfonylurea compounds stimulate insulin secretion and are used in the treatment of type 2 diabetes, where the primary defect is peripheral insulin resistance.

Glucagon

Glucagon is a 29–amino acid, straight chain polypeptide with a molecular weight of 3.5 kDa. Secreted by the A cells, the primary function of glucagon is to elevate blood glucose levels through stimulation of glycogenolysis and gluconeogenesis in the hepatocytes. A and B cells respond primarily to serum glucose concentration, but in a reciprocal fashion. Similar to epinephrine, cortisol,

TABLE 38-1 Endocrine Cells of the Pancreas and Tumor Syndromes

CELL TYPE	% ISLET CELL MASS	LOCATION WITHIN ISLET	LOCATION WITHIN PANCREAS	MAJOR (MINOR) HORMONE SECRETED	ASSOCIATED TUMOR SYNDROME	DIAGNOSTIC HORMONE LEVELS
A (alpha)	10%	Peripheral	Evenly distributed	Glucagon (glicentin, TRH, CCK, endorphin, PP, pancreastatin)	Glucagonoma: necrolytic migratory erythema, diabetes, hypoaminoacidemia	Normal = <150 pg/mL Tumor = Fasting glucagon >1000 pg/mL
B (beta)	70%	Central	Body/tail	Insulin (TRH, CGRP, amylin, pancreastatin, prolactin)	Insulinoma: hypoglycemia and associated symptoms	>5 μU/mL in the face of hypoglycemia
D	5%*	Evenly distributed	Evenly distributed	Somatostatin (metencephalon)	Somatostatinoma: diabetes, gallstones, steatorrhea	Normal = 10-25 pg/mL Tumor = >160 pg/mL
D_2	5%*	Evenly distributed	Evenly distributed	VIP	VIPoma: high-volume secretory diarrhea, hypokalemia, metabolic acidosis, hypochlorhydria	Normal = <200 pg/mL Tumor = 225-2000 pg/mL
F	15%	Peripheral	Head and uncinate process	PP	None	NA
EC	<1%	Evenly distributed	Evenly distributed	Substance P, serotonin	None	NA
G	Not present in normal physiologic state	NA	Head, uncinate process, duodenum	Gastrin, ACTH-related peptides	Gastrinoma: acid hypersecretion, gastric/duodenal ulcers, diarrhea	Normal = <100 pg/mL Suspicious = >1000 pg/mL With secretin test, an increase of >200 pg/mL diagnostic

*Combined D and D2 islet cell mass.

Adapted from Bonner-Weir S: Anatomy of the islet of Langerhans. In Samols E, editor: *The endocrine pancreas,* New York, 1991, Raven Press, p 16; and Marx M, Newman JB, Guice KS, et al: Clinical significance of gastrointestinal hormones. In Thompson JC, Greeley GH, Jr, Rayford PL, et al, editors: *Gastrointestinal endocrinology,* New York, 1987, McGraw-Hill, p 416.

ACTH, adrenocorticotropic hormone; *CCK,* cholecystokinin; *CGRP,* calcitonin gene–related peptide; *NA,* not applicable; *PP,* pancreatic polypeptide; *TRH,* thyrotropin-releasing hormone; *VIP,* vasoactive intestinal peptide.

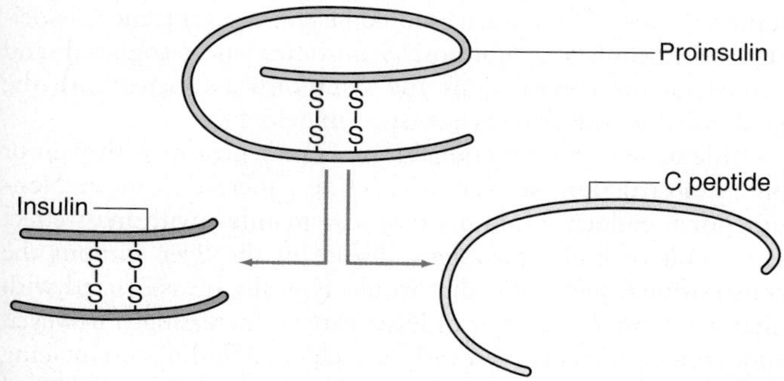

FIGURE 38-2 Diagram of insulin synthesis. Proinsulin, synthesized by the endoplasmic reticulum, is packaged within secretory granules of the beta cell, where it is cleaved to insulin and C peptide. Equimolar amounts of insulin and C peptide are secreted into the bloodstream. (From Andersen DK, Brunicardi FC: Pancreatic anatomy and physiology. In Greenfield LJ, Mulholland MW, Oldham KT, et al, editors: *Surgery: Scientific principles and practice,* ed 2, Philadelphia, 1997, Lippincott-Raven, p 869.)

and growth hormone, glucagon is considered a stress hormone because it increases metabolic fuel in the form of glucose during stress. Glucose has a strong suppressive effect on glucagon secretion.

Excess glucagon can lead to hyperglycemia, whereas insufficient glucagon can lead to profound hypoglycemia. Dysfunctional secretion of glucagon may play a role in the elevation of blood glucose levels in diabetes.

Other Influences on Glucose Homeostasis

Enteric peptide hormones released from the proximal gastrointestinal tract also influence glucose homeostasis through the enteroinsular axis. Therefore, orally administered glucose has a greater effect on insulin secretion than an equivalent amount of glucose administered intravenously, even though blood glucose levels might be similar. Insulinotropic factors, called incretins, act directly on the B cells to stimulate insulin release. They include gastric inhibitory polypeptide, glucagon, glucagon-like peptide-1, cholecystokinin (CCK), amino acids (arginine, lysine, and leucine), and free fatty acids. Humoral inhibitors of insulin secretion include somatostatin, amylin, leptin, and pancreastatin.

Ghrelin is a peptide hormone produced by ghrelin cells of the gastrointestinal tract. Evidence suggests that ghrelin primarily inhibits insulin release from the pancreas, increases hepatic glucose production, and prevents glucose disposal in muscle and adipose tissues, which collectively leads to hyperglycemia and impaired glucose tolerance. In diet-induced obesity, ghrelin exacerbates hyperglycemia; in starvation or severe calorie restriction, ghrelin increases blood glucose concentrations to maintain glucose homeostasis.[3]

Leptin is a peptide hormone produced in adipose cells. Leptin is released into the circulatory system based on energy stores and functions as a feedback mechanism that signals to regulatory centers in the brain to inhibit food intake and to regulate body weight. In response to adequate fat stores, leptin inhibits insulin secretion. In obese humans, leptin levels are increased, exacerbating hyperglycemia. Leptin resistance is thought to exist in the obese state, with lack of inhibition of food intake.

Insulin and glucagon secretion are also under neuronal control. Vagal (cholinergic) stimulation leads to the release of insulin. Alpha-sympathetic stimulation strongly inhibits insulin release, whereas beta-sympathetic fibers stimulate it. Insulin release is stimulated by the peptidergic nerve release of gastrin-releasing peptide, CCK, gastrin, enkephalin, and VIP, whereas insulin release is inhibited by neurotensin, substance P, and somatostatin. Glucagon secretion is stimulated by sympathetic neural transmitters, epinephrine, and the amino acids arginine and alanine. A loss of pancreatic innervation in the setting of pancreatic transplantation or islet cell transplantation can result in changes in the pattern and quality of insulin and glucagon secretion. Somatostatin may have a suppressive effect on glucagon secretion.

Somatostatin

Somatostatin, secreted by D cells, is a 14–amino acid polypeptide weighing 1.6 kDa. Although it is logical to think that somatostatin modulates the secretion of other islet hormones, its actual function within the pancreas is controversial. Although exogenous administration of somatostatin has been shown to inhibit the release of insulin, glucagon, and PP and to inhibit gastric, pancreatic, and biliary secretion, endogenous somatostatin has not been proven to influence the secretion of other islet hormones directly.

Long-acting and short-acting synthetic octapeptides that mimic the pharmacologic action of somatostatin have been developed. These synthetic peptides have a longer half-life in the serum than endogenous somatostatin and are more potent inhibitors of growth hormone, glucagon, and insulin secretion than the natural hormone. The potent inhibitory effect of synthetic somatostatin analogues has been used to treat exocrine and endocrine disorders of the pancreas, including secretory diarrhea, bowel fistulas, pancreatic fistulas, and endocrine hypersecretory syndromes.

Pancreatic Polypeptide

PP is a 36–amino acid, 4.2-kDa polypeptide secreted by the F cells of the pancreatic islet. PP belongs to the peptide YY/neuropeptide Y family of polypeptides. Infusion of PP in humans caused loss of appetite and reduced food intake.[4] However, its physiologic role is unclear; its clinical usefulness is limited to its role as a marker for other endocrine tumors of the pancreas. Cholinergic innervation predominantly regulates PP secretion. As a result, surgical vagotomy ablates the increased PP response normally observed after meals. In diabetes and normal aging, PP secretion is increased, resulting in increased circulating PP levels. Absence of PP may play a role in diabetes observed after total pancreatectomy or after chronic atrophic pancreatitis.

Other Peptide Hormones

Other peptide hormones secreted by the pancreatic islets include VIP, amylin, galanin, and serotonin. VIP is a 28–amino acid, 3.3-kDa polypeptide that stimulates insulin release and inhibits gastric secretion at physiologic levels. It is found not only throughout the gastrointestinal tract but also in the respiratory tract, where it causes vasodilation and bronchodilation. Amylin, a 36–amino acid polypeptide, is secreted by B cells and inhibits the secretion and uptake of insulin. Amylin deposits in the pancreas of patients with type 2 diabetes have been implicated in the pathogenesis of the disease. Pancreastatin is part of a larger ubiquitous molecule, chromogranin A, which inhibits insulin secretion. Gastrin-producing cells are present in the fetal pancreas but not in the normal adult pancreas. Many additional peptides, including thyrotropin-releasing hormone, glicentin, CCK, peptide YY, gastrin-releasing factor (GRF), calcitonin gene–related peptide, prolactin, adrenocorticotropic hormone (ACTH), parathyroid hormone–related protein, and ghrelin, have been reported in normal islets and in islet cell tumors.

PANCREATIC NEUROENDOCRINE TUMORS

Overview and History

Pancreatic neuroendocrine tumors (PNETs) are uncommon in the United States but have increased in incidence over the past few decades, with an estimated incidence of 5 to 10 cases per 1 million people annually.[5] PNETs are 1000 to 2000 times more common in autopsy series, indicating that most are indolent. Endocrine tumors of the pancreas vary greatly in presentation, severity of symptoms, location, functionality, and malignant potential.[6] Patients with PNETs may present with symptoms that result from secretion of active gastrointestinal hormones or local symptoms from tumor growth. Secretion of hormones by functional tumors leads to the characteristic syndromes and physiologic derangements associated with these rare neoplasms (see Table 38-1). Immunostaining often identifies multiple hormone products, even in the absence of clinically relevant hormone secretion. Although multiple hormones may be secreted by a single tumor, the term "functional" should be reserved for tumors associated with clinical symptoms. Syndromes are recognized and named for the clinical signs and symptoms associated with the predominant endocrine agent (see Table 38-1).

Patients with nonfunctional tumors may present with pain or biliary obstruction, similar to exocrine pancreatic cancer. Nonfunctional endocrine tumors may also manifest with mass effect as a result of bulky metastatic disease in the liver without the constitutional symptoms that would typically be associated with metastatic exocrine cancer of lesser extent. Increasingly, however, endocrine tumors manifest early as incidental findings on imaging studies performed for other reasons. Thus, the proportion of nonfunctional endocrine tumors diagnosed has increased over time.[5]

Histopathology and Staging

The staging of PNETs presents several challenges. The incidence of malignancy in these tumors ranges from approximately 10% in insulin-secreting PNETs (insulinoma) to almost 100% in glucagon-secreting or somatostatin-secreting tumors (see Table 38-1). However, in contrast to most other solid tumors, which

TABLE 38-2 World Health Organization Staging System for Neuroendocrine Tumors

	WELL-DIFFERENTIATED		POORLY DIFFERENTIATED
	LOW GRADE	INTERMEDIATE GRADE	HIGH GRADE
Appearance	Homogeneous small, round cells with abundant expression of neuroendocrine markers		Pleomorphic cells with nuclear irregularity, necrosis
Mitotic rate	<2 mitoses/10 HPF	2-20 mitoses/10 HPF	>20 mitoses/10 HPF
Ki-67 index	<3%	3-20%	>20%
Behavior	Indolent		Aggressive

HPF, high-power field.

can be classified as benign or malignant based on histopathology of the primary tumor, malignancy in PNETs can be definitely determined only by the presence of metastasis.

In an attempt to standardize staging, in 2010, the World Health Organization proposed standardized nomenclature for neuroendocrine tumors (NETs). The term *NET* replaced other terminology, including carcinoid tumor and tumor names based on functional systems (i.e., insulinoma). The WHO staging system is the most widely used staging system for NETs.[7] It includes all NETs regardless of site of origin and classifies NETs on the basis of differentiation and grade. NETs are graded as low (grade 1), intermediate (grade 2), or high (grade 3) based on appearance, mitotic rates, behavior (invasion of other organs, angioinvasion), and the Ki-67 proliferative index (Table 38-2). The distinction between well-differentiated and poorly differentiated tumors is the most important; grade 1 and grade 2 tumors are considered well differentiated and grade 3 tumors are considered poorly differentiated. High-grade/poorly differentiated PNETs are sometimes referred to as "neuroendocrine carcinoma"; these tumors account for less than 3% of PNETs. Well-differentiated tumors still have malignant potential, but the differences in behavior persist, even for patients with metastatic disease.

More recently, the American Joint Committee on Cancer (AJCC)[8,9] staging system, initially developed for pancreatic adenocarcinoma, has been applied to PNETs (Table 38-3). Similar to all AJCC staging systems, it takes into account tumor size, nodal status, and the presence or absence of metastatic disease, but it lacks information on tumor grade. However, the ability of this system to predict prognosis accurately has been documented.[8] A more recent study, proposed a tumor, grade, metastases (TGM) staging system as a more accurate prognostic tool.[10]

TABLE 38-3 American Joint Committee on Cancer Staging for Pancreatic Neuroendocrine Tumors

Primary Tumor (T)			
TX	Tumor cannot be assessed		
T0	No evidence of primary tumor		
Tis	Carcinoma in situ (includes Pan-IN 3)		
T1	Tumor limited to pancreas, ≤2 cm in size		
T2	Tumor limited to pancreas, >2 cm in size		
T3	Tumor extends beyond the pancreas but without involvement of the celiac axis or superior mesenteric artery		
Regional Lymph Nodes (N)			
NX	Regional lymph nodes cannot be assessed		
N0	No regional lymph node metastasis		
N1	Regional lymph node metastasis		
Distant Metastasis (M)			
M0	No distant metastasis		
M1	Distant metastasis		
Anatomic Stage			
Stage 0	Tis	N0	M0
Stage IA	T1	N0	M0
Stage IB	T2	N0	M0
Stage IIA	T3	N0	M0
Stage IIB	T1	N1	M0
	T2	N1	M0
	T3	N1	M0
Stage III	T4	Any N	M0
Stage IV	Any T	Any N	M1

From Edge SB, Byrd DR, Compton CC, et al, editors: *AJCC cancer staging manual,* New York, 2010, Springer. With the permission of the American Joint Committee on Cancer (AJCC), Chicago, Illinois.

Molecular Genetics of Islet Cell Tumors

Although most PNETs occur sporadically, others can be associated with genetic syndromes. The most common genetic syndrome associated with PNETs is multiple endocrine neoplasia type 1 (MEN1). The syndrome is characterized by PNETs, parathyroid adenomas or hyperplasia, and pituitary adenomas. MEN1 is caused by mutations or allelic deletions in the tumor suppressor gene, menin, on chromosome 11q13 and is inherited in an autosomal dominant fashion. Menin is a component of the histone methyltransferase complex and is involved in control of G_1-to-S phase cell cycle progression. Mutation or allelic deletion causes loss of tumor suppressor function and predisposes patients to neoplastic growth in the parathyroid, pituitary, and pancreatic endocrine tissue.

Another syndrome associated with PNETs is von Hippel-Lindau disease. Patients with inherited mutations of the *VHL* gene are at risk for the development of renal cell carcinoma; pheochromocytoma; and benign tumors of the central nervous system, retina, epididymis, and inner ear. In addition, pancreatic lesions are common, including NETs, microcystic adenomas, and simple cysts. Similar to MEN1, the management of PNETs can be challenging because they are often multifocal and associated with tumors in other locations. PNETs associated with von Hippel-Lindau disease generally behave in an indolent fashion, and it has been suggested that these tumors can be observed until they reach at least 2 to 3 cm in size. However, specific mutations may be associated with a more aggressive phenotype and warrant earlier treatment and closer surveillance.[11]

Most PNETs are not associated with a known genetic syndrome and seem to occur sporadically. Other than family history, risk factors for PNETs are not well defined. Chronic glucose elevation stimulates islet cell proliferation; a case-control study of patients with a diagnosis of predominantly sporadic PNETS and their genetically unrelated family members (spouses of patients who had cancers other than gastrointestinal, lung or head and neck cancer) demonstrated an association between insulin-requiring diabetes and the development of PNETs.[12]

Tumorigenesis of PNETs involves an accumulation of numerous genetic events, including activation of oncogenes and inactivation of tumor suppressor genes. Although several candidate genes and gene loci had previously been identified, improvements in high-throughput sequencing led to significant advancement of understanding of the molecular genetics of PNETs. The common genetic mutations and impacted signal transduction pathways in PNETs are shown in Figure 38-3. Complete exome sequencing of a discovery set of 10 sporadic PNETs revealed mutations in 149 genes, of which 6 were selected for further analysis in a validation set of 58 PNETs.[13] Inactivating mutations in *MEN1* were seen in 44% of sporadic tumors. Mutations in *DAXX* (death-domain associated protein) and *ATRX* (alpha thalassemia-mental retardation syndrome X-linked), whose protein products are involved in p53-mediated DNA damage repair, were seen in 25% and 18%, respectively. Patients with mutations in *MEN1* or *DAXX/ATRX* had prolonged survival compared with patients without mutations. Previous expression analyses had suggested dysregulation of the mammalian target of rapamycin (mTOR) pathway in a large proportion of tumors,[14,15] specifically *TSC2* (tuberous sclerosis 2) and *PTEN* (phosphatase and tensin homolog). The mutational analysis identified mutations in only 9% and 7% of these two genes, respectively. Mutational analysis has potential clinical implications because the mTOR inhibitor everolimus has been approved by the U.S. Food and Drug Administration (FDA) for advanced NETs. Potentially, mutational testing would allow selection of patients most likely to benefit from this targeted therapy. Overall, the mutational analysis was most remarkable for how distinct the genetic abnormalities were from genetic abnormalities observed in a similar study of pancreatic adenocarcinoma (Table 38-4).[16] Mutations in *KRAS* were not seen in PNETs, and mutations in *p53* were seen only rarely, at least not in these well-differentiated tumors. In a separate study comparing well-differentiated and poorly differentiated PNETs, *MEN1* and *DAXX/ATRX* expression by immunohistochemistry

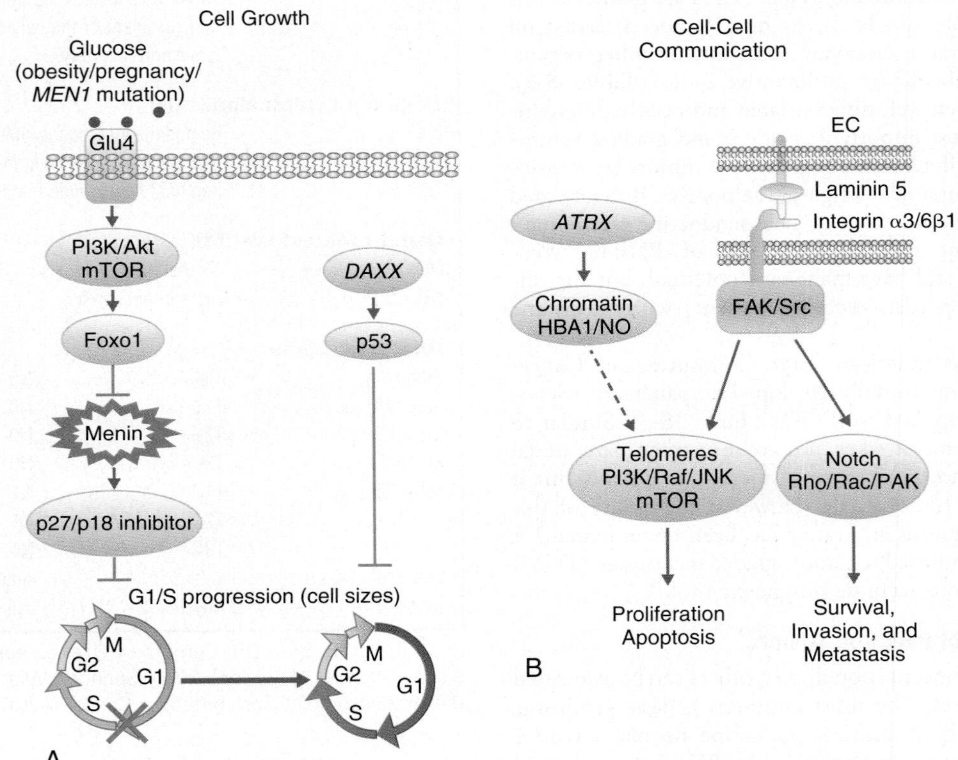

FIGURE 38-3 Common genetic mutations and impacted signal transduction pathways in pancreatic neuroendocrine tumors (PNETs). **A,** Cell growth. *MEN1* mutations decrease menin-regulated p27/p18 expression, which abrogates the glucose sensor. *DAXX* mutations decrease p53 levels, diminishing the checkpoint for cellular/DNA damages. *MEN1* and *DAXX* mutations promote cell cycle progression from the G_1 to S phase, regardless of glucose levels and damage. **B,** Cell-cell communications. Endocrine cells such as beta or alpha cells rely on the endothelium to provide extracellular matrix. This disables the attachment needed for cancer cells to invade and migrate. *ATRX* mutation–modulated chromatin modification may play a role in the abnormal activation of FAK/Src and mammalian target of rapamycin (mTOR) pathways in PNETs. *EC,* endothelial cell; *FAK,* focal adhesion kinase; *HBA1,* hemoglobin-α; *JNK,* c-Jun N-terminal kinase; *NO,* nitric oxide; *PAK,* p21-activated kinase; *PI3K/Akt,* phosphoinositide-3-kinase/protein kinase B. (From Zhang J, Francois R, Iyer R, et al: Current understanding of the molecular biology of pancreatic neuroendocrine tumors. *J Natl Cancer Inst* 105:1005–1017, 2013.)

TABLE 38-4 Comparison of Commonly Mutated Genes in Pancreatic Neuroendocrine Tumor and Pancreatic Ductal Adenocarcinoma

GENES	PNET (%)	PDAC (%)
MEN1	44	0
DAXX, ATRX	43	0
Genes in mTOR pathway	15	0.8
TP53	3	85
KRAS	0	100
CDKN2A	0	25
TGFBR1, SMAD3, SMAD4	0	38

Adapted from Jiao Y, Shi C, Edil BH, et al: DAXX/ATRX, MEN1, and mTOR pathway genes are frequently altered in pancreatic neuroendocrine tumors. *Science* 331:1199–1203, 2011.
mTOR, mammalian target of rapamycin; *PDAC,* pancreatic ductal adenocarcinoma; *PNET,* pancreatic neuroendocrine tumor.

was abnormal in approximately half of well-differentiated tumors. In contrast, staining of *DAXX/ATRX* was normal in poorly differentiated tumors, but there was a high incidence of abnormal p53 and Rb (retinoblastoma) expression as well as overexpression of the antiapoptotic protein Bcl2, implicating it as a target for therapy in these tumors.[17]

General Principles of Diagnosis and Treatment of Pancreatic Neuroendocrine Tumors

Diagnosis and Evaluation

Patients with PNETs can present with a broad range of symptoms and imaging findings. Subsequent diagnosis and evaluation depend on the history and imaging available at the time of presentation. Patients may present with classic functional hormonal syndromes associated with unregulated secretion of the tumor hormone product, where the challenge is often in identification and localization of the suspected tumor. Other patients present with abdominal symptoms, including abdominal pain, jaundice, anorexia, and weight loss. These symptoms usually prompt cross-sectional imaging, which identifies a pancreatic tumor with classic imaging findings for PNET. Until nonfunctional tumors grow large enough to cause symptoms related to mass effect, they often have no or vague symptoms, and patients present with tumors at a more advanced stage. Finally, as a result of the increase in the number of PNETs incidentally found on imaging done for other reasons, tumors may be diagnosed in patients who are completely asymptomatic. Regardless of presentation, all patients with suspected PNETs need, at minimum, (1) a careful history screening for functional tumor symptoms, with biochemical confirmation if indicated; (2) cross-sectional or more advanced imaging when necessary to localize the PNET; and (3) evaluation for metastatic disease. A general algorithm for management of patients with suspected PNETs is shown in Figure 38-4.

Screening for Functional Tumors

The diagnosis of functional PNETs can be made by elevated serum levels of the suspected peptide based on symptoms (see Table 38-1). In patients presenting with a hyperenhancing pancreatic mass suggestive of PNET on cross-sectional imaging, the history should screen for neuroglycopenic symptoms, diarrhea, ulcer diathesis, rash, and other symptoms suggestive of a classic hormonal syndrome. A family history should also be obtained to rule out the possibility of MEN1-associated PNET. In the absence of symptoms, a full hormonal screen is unnecessary.

Nonfunctional PNETs produce distinct gastrointestinal peptides including chromogranin A, neurotensin, and PP. Although these peptides are not associated with clinical symptoms or syndromes, they can aid in confirmation of the diagnosis. Chromogranin A levels have been shown to correlate with the presence of tumor in functional and nonfunctional PNETs. Similar to other biomarkers, chromogranin A is useful for confirmation of the diagnosis in a patient with suspected PNET on imaging and posttreatment surveillance for recurrence. Chromogranin A levels can also be elevated in patients taking proton pump inhibitors (PPIs), patients with atrophic gastritis, and patients with hepatic or renal insufficiency.

Localization

When a functional PNET is diagnosed, cross-sectional imaging with computed tomography (CT) or magnetic resonance imaging (MRI) is the first step in localization. Because of their rich vascular supply, PNETs are hyperattenuating compared with surrounding pancreatic tissue on contrast-enhanced multidetector CT (Figs. 38-5*A* and 38-6*A*). Most noninsulinoma or nongastrinoma pancreatic endocrine tumors are identified on cross-sectional imaging. Insulinomas and gastrinomas, which are smaller at presentation, can be more difficult to localize. CT technique, including thinner collimation (1.25-mm cuts) and multiphase imaging, is critical to improving the sensitivity of CT for these small lesions. Capturing the vascular blush in the arterial phase is critical for identification and differentiation from other types of pancreatic tumors because it is less pronounced in the venous phase. In addition, the use of water instead of an oral contrast agent may assist in identifying small duodenal gastrinomas. In general, the sensitivity of multidetector CT in the localization of PNETs is 73% to 96% and is directly related to the size and location of the tumor.[18]

MRI can also be used for localization (Fig. 38-5*B*). Pancreatic endocrine tumors demonstrate low signal intensity on T1-weighted images and high signal intensity on T2-weighted images. As with CT, size is directly related to sensitivity. In one large series of insulinomas, contrast-enhanced MRI identified all lesions larger than 3 cm, 50% of lesions 1 to 2 cm, and no lesions smaller than 1 cm.[19] The overall sensitivity of MRI for detecting PNETs is 80% to 90%.[18,20]

If a pancreatic endocrine tumor cannot be localized on CT or MRI, endoscopic ultrasound (EUS) should be performed. EUS has an overall sensitivity of approximately 90% for tumors of all sizes, and better sensitivity than CT or MRI for detecting tumors smaller than 3 cm.[20] EUS has the best diagnostic performance in detection and localization of insulinoma. However, EUS has a limited ability to detect small duodenal tumors, with a sensitivity of only 50% in this setting. EUS also allows for fine-needle aspiration of tumors for a pathologic diagnosis. Pathologic diagnosis is especially useful for nonfunctional tumors without a classic CT appearance of pancreatic endocrine tumors (Fig. 38-6*B*).

The abundance of somatostatin receptors on most PNETs makes somatostatin receptor scintigraphy (SRS) a useful adjunct in localization for tumors not evident on CT or MRI. The sensitivity for SRS is greater than 80% for all pancreatic endocrine tumors excluding insulinomas. SRS has an overall sensitivity of 80% to 100% and specificity greater than 90% for gastrinomas because somatostatin receptors are present in more than 90% of gastrin-secreting PNETs. Somatostatin receptors are also present in a significant portion of glucagon-secreting and nonfunctioning

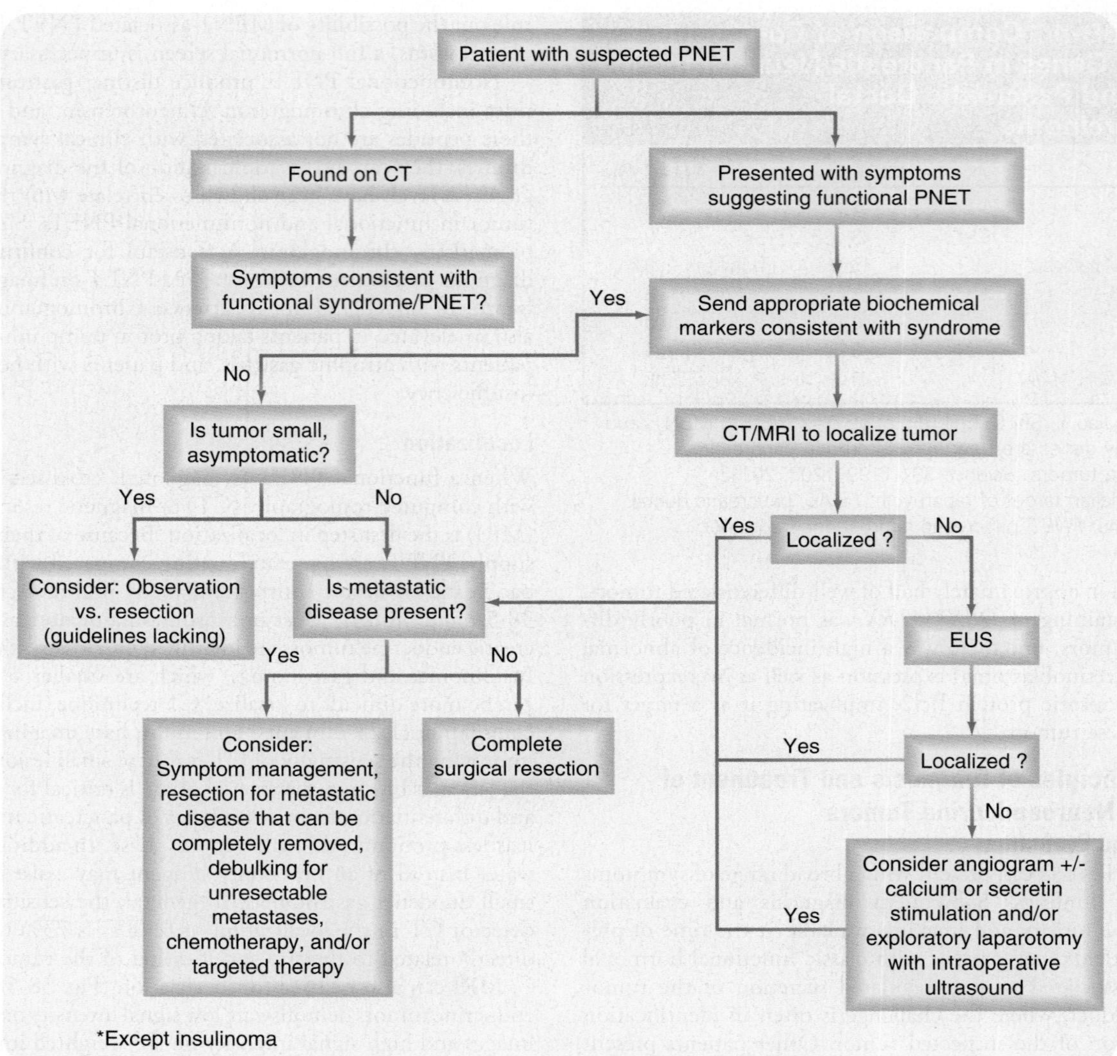

FIGURE 38-4 General algorithm for a patient with suspected pancreatic neuroendocrine tumor (PNET).

PNETs. In contrast, insulin-secreting PNETs and pancreatic adenocarcinomas do not possess somatostatin receptors. SRS is also useful for detecting hepatic metastases from noninsulinoma PNETs.

SRS is limited by physiologic sites or benign conditions that may show tracer uptake and lack anatomic precision in localization (Fig. 38-5*C*). Although sensitive, SRS may not show the exact location of a tumor but indicate only its general vicinity within a few centimeters. The shortcomings of SRS, especially those linked to the limited spatial resolution and the lack of anatomic landmarks, may be overcome by the use of hybrid single photon emission computed tomography (SPECT)/CT imaging. SPECT/CT provides better sensitivity for detection of PNETs by allowing for separation of overlying physiologic tracer accumulation from areas of interest and providing anatomic information.[21] In a study of 107 patients with suspected PNET, SPECT/CT resulted in fewer indeterminate cases than SRS (0.9% versus 13%); SPECT/CT had 88% sensitivity, 96% specificity, and 66% accuracy on a patient-based analysis, statistically better than SRS ($P < .001$). SPECT/CT provides incremental diagnostic value over SRS, mainly because of a precise anatomic localization that helps discriminate between tumor lesions and physiologic uptake (Fig. 38-5*D*).[21] SPECT/CT may detect unsuspected lesions in a small proportion of patients. SRS and SPECT/CT may potentially replace biopsy and may be useful in monitoring for recurrence and response to therapy.

For tumors not localized by other means, angiographic techniques may be useful. Angiography detects approximately 70% of insulinomas larger than 5 mm, showing a characteristic vascular blush that corresponds to the highly vascular nature of insulinomas (Fig. 38-7). If standard radiographic techniques are unsuccessful, portal venous sampling for insulin or gastrin levels may allow localization to a region of the pancreas (head, body, or tail) to aid in operative planning. Portal venous sampling does not absolutely localize the tumor, but it provides accurate information on the region of the pancreas from which the high levels of hormones are released. Calcium stimulates insulin release from insulinomas, whereas secretin stimulates gastrin release from gastrinomas. Arterial stimulation by injecting calcium or secretin into the celiac and superior mesenteric arteries can further increase the likelihood of localization with simultaneous portal venous sampling for appropriate hormone levels. Arterial stimulation venous sampling has a sensitivity greater than 90%. However, with modern localization techniques, this is rarely necessary.

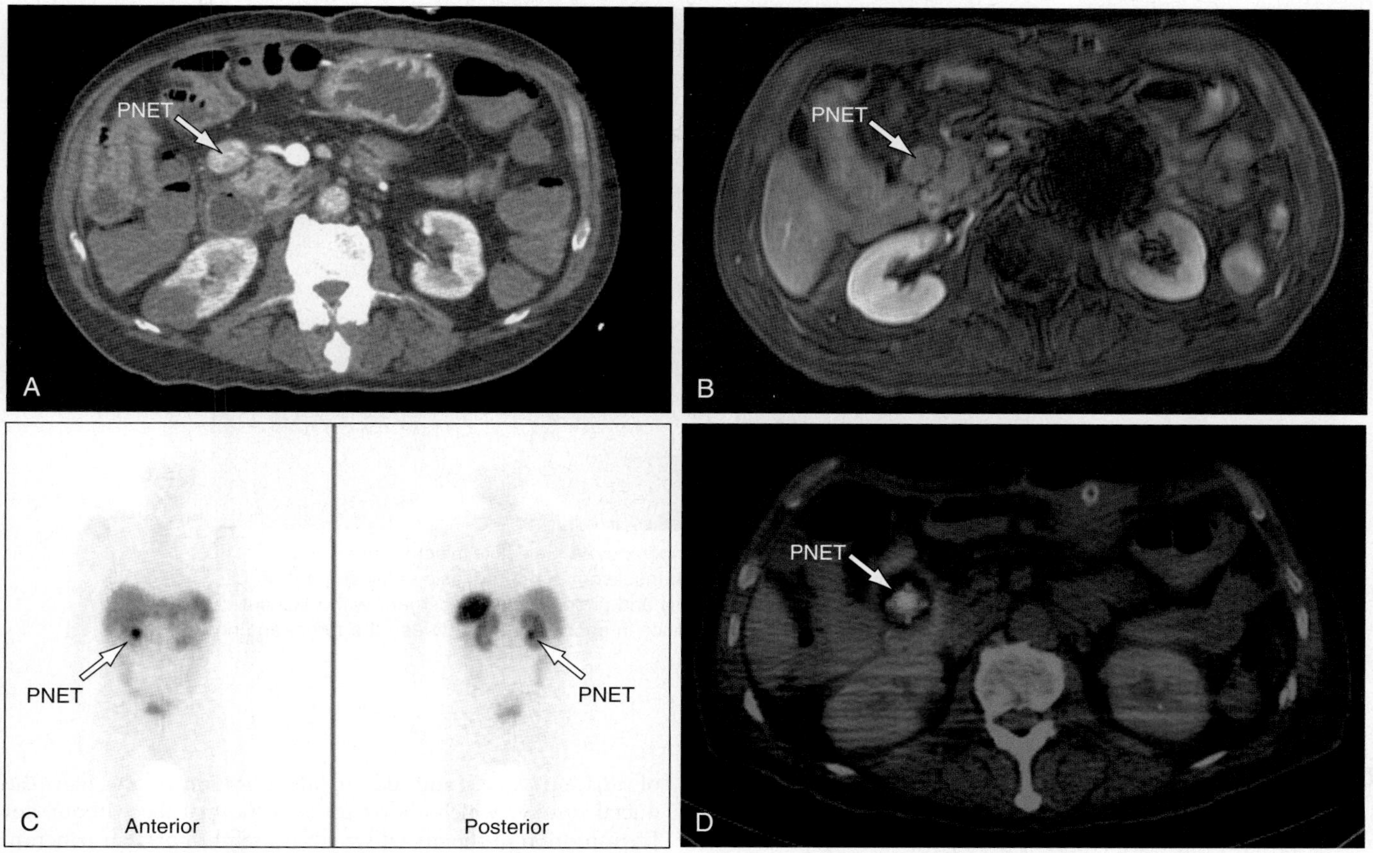

FIGURE 38-5 Patient with a pancreatic neuroendocrine tumor (PNET). **A,** CT scan demonstrating a hyperenhancing lesion adjacent to the head of the pancreas *(arrow).* **B,** Same lesion shown on MRI. **C,** Same lesion shown on SRS, anterior and posterior view; note the nonprecise anatomic localization and the physiologic uptake of tracer in the kidneys, liver, and spleen. **D,** Same lesion on SPECT/CT; note the better anatomic localization and clear identification of nonphysiologic tracer uptake.

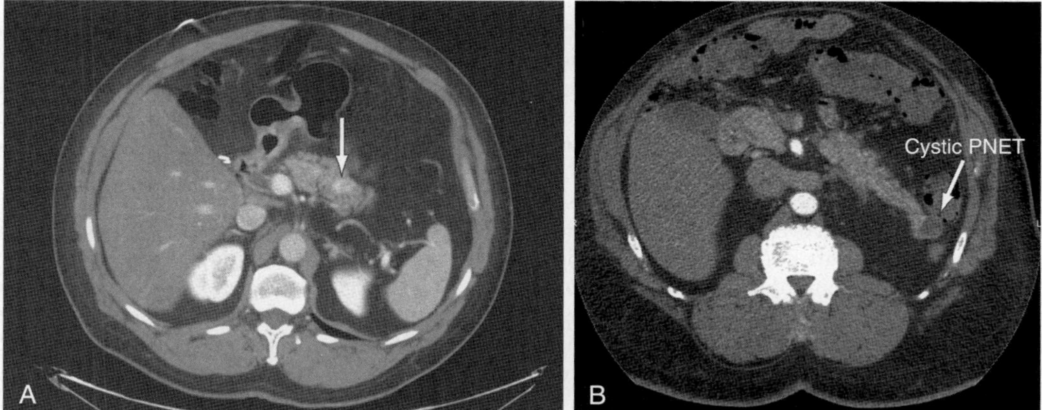

FIGURE 38-6 **A,** Three-dimensional spiral, pancreas protocol CT scan demonstrating a classic hyperattenuating 1.5-cm lesion in the tail of the pancreas *(arrow)* in a patient with a 4-year history of episodic symptomatic hypoglycemia. On a 72-hour monitored fast, the patient demonstrated symptomatic hypoglycemia and associated high insulin and C peptide levels in 22 hours. **B,** Three-dimensional spiral, pancreas protocol CT scan demonstrating a cystic 1.3-cm lesion in the tail of the pancreas *(arrow)* in a patient with a history of multiple endocrine neoplasia type 1 and bowel resection for gastrin-producing pancreatic neuroendocrine tumor (PNET). EUS biopsy was positive for PNET, leading to distal pancreatectomy, which confirmed the diagnosis of nonfunctional PNET.

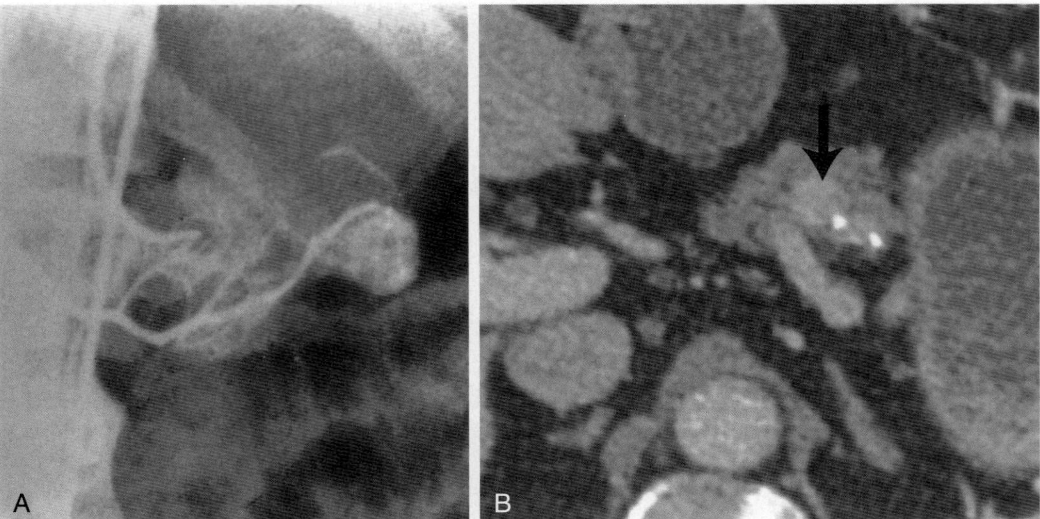

FIGURE 38-7 Demonstration of an insulinoma on arteriography. **A,** Selective injection into the specific dorsal pancreatic artery demonstrates the tumor precisely. **B,** Insulinoma with triphasic enhancement on CT. The mass in the pancreatic body *(arrow)* demonstrates early and prolonged enhancement with washout during the portal venous phase; note that the maximal difference in enhancement between the tumor and normal pancreas occurs during the pancreatic phase (shown).

Treatment

Nonmetastatic disease localized preoperatively. In the absence of metastatic disease, the primary treatment of PNETs is surgical resection. The approach and extent of resection are dictated by the type of tumor, location, and stage as well as patient factors. In most cases, a partial pancreatic resection is performed (i.e., pancreatic head resection, distal pancreatic resection, or enucleation). The goal of the procedure in most patients is to remove the primary tumor and regional lymph nodes. Several studies showed the applicability of minimally invasive approaches in pancreatic surgery, especially distal pancreatectomy and enucleation. These procedures are ideally suited to PNETs because they are often small and not locally invasive. As with open resection, the most common complication is pancreatic fistula. In most PNETs, the surrounding normal pancreas has a soft texture, increasing the risk of pancreatic fistula after partial pancreatectomy. Although generally less problematic than leaks after pancreaticoduodenectomy, leaks after distal pancreatectomy and enucleation are more common.

Although enucleation preserves pancreatic parenchyma, one theoretical disadvantage of enucleation over the more radical procedures is that regional lymph nodes are not sampled. Knowledge of lymph node status allows for a better determination of prognosis, although there is no proven therapeutic value to lymph node removal. Similarly, the importance of splenectomy with distal pancreatectomy is controversial because spleen-preserving techniques have lower lymph node yields.

Nonmetastatic disease not localized preoperatively. In cases where the PNET cannot be localized preoperatively, intraoperative ultrasonography is essential, and several reports have attested to the high degree of accuracy. Higher resolution (7.5- to 10-MHz) transducers are used for the pancreas; because of its greater depth of penetration, a 5-MHz transducer is better for the liver. Islet tumors are detected as sonolucent masses, generally of uniform consistency. The color Doppler attachment allows the detection of adjacent vessels and aids in identification of the pancreatic ductal system, which shows up as a lucent tube without flow. Identification of the ductal system is useful to prevent pancreatic fistula formation after enucleation.

If the tumor cannot be localized by other means, the entire pancreas needs to be mobilized. Mobilization is done by dividing the gastrocolic ligament from left to right, incising the posterior lining of the lesser sac along the inferior and superior margins of the pancreas, and mobilizing the C loop of the duodenum medially with an extensive Kocher maneuver. The head of the pancreas is palpated carefully and examined anteriorly and posteriorly; the body and tail of the pancreas are palpated, any ligamentous attachments to the spleen are divided, the spleen is delivered into the wound, and the tail is rotated anteriorly to allow palpation and visualization.

Metastatic disease. Although the presence of distant metastases is consistently a significant negative prognostic factor, long-term outcomes for patients with neuroendocrine liver metastases are much more favorable than for patients with liver metastases from pancreatic adenocarcinoma or other gastrointestinal tumors. The 5-year survival rates range from greater than 50% for low-grade tumors to 10% for high-grade tumors.[22]

No randomized trials have compared liver resection with other treatments for metastatic endocrine tumors, but resection is recommended if all visible tumor can be removed. Several retrospective studies demonstrated an association between liver resection and improved survival.[23] The primary criticism of these studies is that patients who are able to undergo liver resection likely have lower disease burden and higher performance status than patients who are unable to undergo resection, suggesting that these differences are possibly attributable to selection bias.

Alternatives to liver resection include other liver-directed therapies such as radiofrequency ablation and hepatic arterial therapy. Given their often multifocal and highly vascular nature, endocrine liver metastases are particularly well suited to transcatheter hepatic intra-arterial therapies, including bland arterial embolization, chemoembolization, and radioembolization.[24] There is no consensus as to which type of embolization is best, and most studies have been nonrandomized and heterogeneous. In general, intra-arterial therapies have been associated with high partial response rates and even higher rates of symptomatic improvement in patients with functional tumors. Bland arterial embolization and chemoembolization techniques have been popular for years, but drug-eluting beads and yttrium-90 microspheres are increasingly being used with the potential for more durable responses. Because intra-arterial therapies are not considered to be curative and can be associated with significant morbidity (e.g., abscess, cholecystitis, liver failure), they are generally reserved for patients with symptomatic disease that is not amenable to surgical resection. A multi-institutional retrospective study comparing resection with intra-arterial therapy for neuroendocrine liver metastases demonstrated that resection was independently associated with improved survival, even after controlling for clinicopathologic factors such as functionality, tumor burden, and resection status of the primary tumor.[25]

Because many patients with metastatic NETs die as a result of problems related to their liver disease, there is rationale for debulking procedures. However, a Cochrane review found no evidence clearly documenting a survival benefit for cytoreduction in nonresectable liver disease.[26]

In parallel with advancements in liver-directed therapy, there have been significant improvements in the systemic therapy of metastatic NETs. Traditional cytotoxic chemotherapy agents are largely ineffective in well-differentiated endocrine tumors. Poorly differentiated neuroendocrine carcinomas behave more aggressively and respond better to cytotoxic chemotherapy than well-differentiated PNETs. Similar to small cell lung cancer, the standard therapy for poorly differentiated tumors is a platinum-based agent plus etoposide.

In the PROMID study, a long-acting somatostatin analogue was demonstrated to increase time to progression in patients with metastatic well-differentiated PNETs.[27] This monthly injection is well tolerated, although cholelithiasis can develop with long-term use. For this reason, cholecystectomy should be considered at the time of resection in patients with advanced PNETs. In the RADIANT-3 trial, everolimus, an oral inhibitor of the mTOR, more than doubled progression-free survival in a similar patient population.[28] Over the same time period, the multitarget tyrosine kinase inhibitor sunitinib was also shown to be well tolerated and effective in a randomized controlled trial.[29] Both of these targeted therapies have been approved by the FDA and—together with somatostatin analogues—have largely replaced cytotoxic chemotherapy in the management of advanced well-differentiated PNETs.

Although numerous treatment options are now available for metastatic disease, resection should still be considered the first choice for patients with resectable disease. For patients with synchronous disease, the decision to perform resection of the primary and metastatic disease in one or multiple stages depends on the complexity of the respective resections. For patients with metastatic disease that is not considered resectable, resection of the primary tumor can still be justified to convert patients to "liver-only" disease so that liver-directed therapies can be employed. Additionally, in the PROMID study, patients whose primary tumor had been removed benefited more from long-acting somatostatin analogues than patients with unresected primary tumors.

PNETs tend to metastasize to the liver, and disease often does not spread beyond the liver. Even after treatment of liver metastases, most patients develop disease recurrence in the remnant liver within 2 years, demonstrating the strong predilection for PNETs to metastasize to the liver and the generally indolent nature of this disease. Total hepatectomy with allotransplantation has been proposed as a potentially curative treatment option for unresectable neuroendocrine metastases, the only metastatic indication for transplantation. The same Milan group that created the commonly used criteria for transplantation in hepatocellular carcinoma proposed criteria for transplantation in neuroendocrine metastases, which include age younger than 55, well-differentiated tumor status, Ki-67 proliferative marker index less than 5%, completely resected primary tumor with portal drainage, less than 50% liver involvement, and absence of extrahepatic disease.[30] Using these relatively strict criteria, 5-year overall survival rates of 90% were achieved. However, not all centers have adhered to these criteria, and results have been highly variable. In a multicenter study of 213 transplants for neuroendocrine metastases, the largest published to date, 5-year overall survival was 52%. Hepatomegaly, high-grade tumors, and major or minor extrahepatic tumor resection at the time of liver transplantation were associated with worse outcomes in a multivariable model.[31] Although these survival rates are comparable to rates for transplantation in hepatocellular carcinoma, they may not be significantly greater than survival rates for nonsurgical therapy of neuroendocrine metastases. Given the scarcity of organs, the role of transplantation in neuroendocrine metastases remains controversial.

Incidentally found, small pancreatic neuroendocrine tumors. Historically, all PNETs were thought to have malignant potential, and resection was recommended when these tumors were identified. However, with an increasing number of small PNETs identified incidentally, the management of small, asymptomatic lesions is controversial. PNETs are more than 1000 times more common in autopsy studies, suggesting that many of these incidentally found PNETs will behave indolently. As a result, surgeons are increasingly using more selective criteria for resection of these incidentally found lesions.

In a study of almost 4000 patients from the National Cancer Database, the strongest predictors of survival after resection of pancreatic endocrine tumors were tumor grade and the presence of distant metastases.[32] Neither tumor size nor lymph node metastasis was a significant predictor of survival in this study. In a review of 143 PNETs, of which 40% were incidentally found, the 5-year progression-free survival rate was 86% for incidentally discovered tumors versus 59% for symptomatic tumors (P = .007); the authors concluded that more selective criteria for resection may be appropriate.[33] In a review of 131 patients with small, asymptomatic nonfunctional PNETs, 77 were observed; the median tumor size (1 cm; range, 0.3 to 3.2 cm) did not change over the mean 45-month follow-up period, and there was no disease progression or disease-specific mortality. Additionally, in the operative group ($n = 56$; median tumor size 1.8 cm; range, 0.5 to 3.6 cm), 46% had a complication, most as a result of a clinically significant pancreatic leak.[34] However, in another series of 139 patients with incidentally discovered nonfunctional PNETs, 28% were found to be malignant. Even tumors less than 2 cm were associated with disease recurrence and progression. Given the limited data, the management of asymptomatic nonfunctional PNETs remains controversial. If these lesions are observed, there are no clear guidelines regarding the frequency of surveillance.

Diagnosis and Treatment of Specific Functional Pancreatic Neuroendocrine Tumors

Insulin-Secreting Pancreatic Neuroendocrine Tumor (Insulinoma)

Insulinoma is the most common functioning PNET, with an incidence of 1 to 2 per 1 million population annually in the United States. In 1935, Whipple and Frantz were the first to report an association between a clinical syndrome and an islet cell tumor. They documented (1) neuroglycopenic symptoms consistent with hypoglycemia, (2) a low plasma glucose concentration measured when symptoms were present, and (3) relief of symptoms with administration of glucose, which became known as Whipple's triad.

Symptoms may vary in patients with insulin-secreting PNETs. Some have symptoms related to sympathetic nervous system overactivity in response to hypoglycemia, including fatigue, weakness, fearfulness, hunger, tremor, diaphoresis, and tachycardia. In others, a central nervous system disturbance predominates with apathy, irritability, anxiety, confusion, excitement, loss of orientation, blurred vision, delirium, stupor, coma, or seizures. In many patients, symptoms have been present for years before diagnosis. Patients often report significant weight gain coinciding with the onset of symptoms, as they compensate by eating frequently to prevent hypoglycemia.

The average age at diagnosis is 45 years. Insulinomas are distributed equally throughout the pancreas despite predominance of beta cells in the body and tail. Rarely, they occur in the duodenum, splenic hilum, or gastrocolic ligament. Insulinomas are typically small, with an average size of 1.0 to 1.5 cm. Surgical resection of an insulinoma is usually curative because most tumors tend to be small, benign (85% to 95%), and solitary. Although insulinomas are sporadic, 5% are associated with MEN1, and these are more likely to be multiple and malignant.

Diagnosis. In any patient in whom Whipple's triad is documented, further evaluation is necessary to determine the underlying cause and guide appropriate management. The differential diagnosis of symptomatic hypoglycemia includes insulinoma, noninsulinoma pancreatogenous hypoglycemia syndrome, exogenous insulin or oral hypoglycemic agent administration (sulfonylureas, meglitinides), insulin autoimmune hypoglycemia, and insulin-like growth factor–mediated hypoglycemia (Table 38-5). In the setting of suspected hypoglycemia, blood glucose should be measured precisely and not using a home reflectance meter because reflectance meters are not sufficiently reliable in the low range.

A critical first step is to review the patient's history in detail, particularly the timing of symptoms in relationship to meals, medications taken by the patient and by family members, and family and social history. The diagnosis of insulinoma requires demonstration of inappropriately high serum insulin concentrations during a spontaneous or induced episode of hypoglycemia. During a spontaneous episode of hypoglycemia, the clinician should measure plasma glucose, insulin, C peptide, proinsulin, and beta-hydroxybutyrate levels and screen for oral hypoglycemic agents.

The gold standard for diagnosis of insulinoma is the 72-hour monitored fast. However, in cases where hypoglycemic episodes are observed and the aforementioned laboratory testing can be obtained, a monitored fast is unnecessary. Testing should be guided by the history, especially in relation to the timing of symptoms. The 72-hour fast can be initiated at home after an evening meal except for patients in whom hypoglycemia occurs after a short period of fasting. The date and time of the last meal should be noted. All nonessential medications should be stopped. Patients can drink calorie-free, caffeine-free beverages. Blood samples for measurement of plasma glucose, insulin, C peptide, proinsulin, and beta-hydroxybutyrate should be taken every 6 hours until the glucose concentration is less than 60 mg/dL. After this, blood sampling should occur every 1 to 2 hours. Insulin, C peptide, and proinsulin need to be measured only in specimens corresponding to a plasma glucose concentration of 60 mg/dL or less. Insulin antibodies should be measured, but they do not have to be measured during hypoglycemia. The fast is stopped and glucose is administered when the blood glucose level is less than 55 mg/dL or the patient becomes symptomatic. During the fast, approximately two thirds to three quarters of patients with insulinomas experience hypoglycemic symptoms in the first 24 hours, and 95% experience symptoms by 72 hours.

To interpret results, it is critical that blood samples be carefully labeled, particularly with the exact time. When hypoglycemia is documented, plasma insulin, C peptide, and proinsulin values are elevated in patients with insulinomas, noninsulinoma pancreatogenous hypoglycemia syndrome, oral hypoglycemic agent–induced hypoglycemia, and insulin autoimmune hypoglycemia. These entities can be differentiated by documented sulfonylurea or meglitinides in the plasma (oral hypoglycemia agent–induced hypoglycemia) or the presence of insulin or insulin receptor antibodies (insulin autoimmune hypoglycemia). The differentiation of insulinoma and noninsulinoma pancreatogenous hypoglycemia syndrome can be difficult in the absence of a documented pancreatic tumor consistent with an insulinoma. The latter occurs more commonly in the postprandial setting. Evaluating the insulin-glucose ratio is also useful. A ratio higher than 0.3 occurs with an insulinoma ([μU/mL of insulin/mg]/[dL of glucose]). Less commonly, a ratio of 0.3 can occur in an obese patient as a result of insulin resistance, but such patients should not be hypoglycemic. C peptide levels greater than 1.2 μg/mL with a glucose level less than 40 mg/dL are also highly suggestive of an insulinoma.

In patients who are surreptitiously administering insulin, plasma insulin values are higher than levels observed in patients with an insulinoma, but plasma C peptide and proinsulin values are low or undetectable. Because of the antiketogenic effect of insulin, all patients with an insulinoma should have serum beta-hydroxybutyrate levels of 2.7 mmol/liter or less at the end of the fast. A plasma beta-hydroxybutyrate level greater than 2.7 mmol/liter and brisk plasma glucose response to intravenous glucagon support the diagnosis of insulinoma in cases of borderline insulin/C peptide levels or suggest an insulin-like growth factor–mediated process when insulin levels are low. Hypoglycemia in the setting of low plasma concentrations of insulin, C peptide, and proinsulin suggest noninsulin or insulin-like growth factor–mediated hypoglycemia, which is rare.

Localization and treatment. The general principles for treatment of PNETs apply to insulinomas. For patients with biochemical evidence of an insulinoma, the localization and management are shown in the algorithm in Figure 38-4. The only difference in cases of insulinoma is that SRS is not indicated because these tumors rarely express somatostatin receptors. Surgical resection is the mainstay of treatment and is the only curative option for insulinoma. Preoperatively, it is important to prevent severe hypoglycemic attacks. Glucose infusions must be used in the perioperative period, especially when patients are taking nothing by mouth. Administration of diazoxide decreases beta cell release of insulin

TABLE 38-5 Interpretation of Laboratory Results and Differential Diagnosis in Patients with Whipple's Triad

DIAGNOSIS	GLUCOSE (mg/dL)	INSULIN (μU/mL)	C PEPTIDE (nmol/liter)	PROINSULIN (pmol/liter)	ANTI-INSULIN OR ANTI-INSULIN RECEPTOR ANTIBODY (+/–)	CIRCULATING ORAL HYPOGLYCEMIC AGENTS (SULFONYLUREAS, MEGLITINIDES)	BETA-HYDROXYBUTYRATE	PANCREATIC MASS (ISLET CELL TUMOR)	TIMING OF HYPOGLYCEMIA
Insulinoma	<55	≥3	≥0.2	≥5	–	No	≤2.7	Yes*	Fasting
NIPHS, post–gastric bypass hypoglycemia	<55	≥3	≥0.2	≥5	–	No	≤2.7	No	Postprandial
Surreptitious insulin administration	<55	>>>3	<0.2	<5	–	No	≤2.7	No	With administration of inappropriate insulin
Oral hypoglycemic administration	<55	≥3	≥0.2	≥5	–	Yes	≤2.7	No	With administration of oral agents
Insulin autoimmune hypoglycemia	<55	>>>3	>>>0.2	>>>5	+	No	≤2.7	No	Fasting
IGF-mediated	<55	<3	<0.2	<5	–	No	≤2.7	No	Fasting
IGF-mediated	<55	<3	<0.2	<5	–	No	>2.7	No	Fasting

*Laboratory findings consistent with insulinoma should prompt evaluation for islet cell tumor. In a few cases, the pancreatic islet cell tumor may be difficult to localize preoperatively.
IGF, insulin-like growth factor; *NIPHS*, noninsulinoma pancreatogenous hypoglycemia syndrome.

(usually 3 mg/kg/day, divided into two or three daily doses) and should be used to prevent or attenuate symptoms of hypoglycemia before surgical intervention once the diagnosis is made.

When a tumor has been identified intraoperatively, the location should correlate with preoperative localization studies. If not, multiple lesions need to be considered. Because more than 90% of insulinomas are benign, enucleation is usually preferred, when possible, to preserve functional pancreatic mass. Enucleation should not be performed if the tumor is within 2 mm of the main pancreatic duct, which can be identified on intraoperative ultrasound. Anatomic resection (i.e., distal pancreatectomy, central pancreatectomy, or pancreaticoduodenectomy) may be necessary for tumors abutting the main pancreatic duct or for large tumors.

If preoperative studies cannot localize the tumor, blind exploration with intraoperative ultrasound combined with careful palpation and exploration of the entire pancreas and duodenum will identify most tumors. Carrying out effective intraoperative pancreatic ultrasound requires complete mobilization of the pancreas. In the unlikely event in which the tumor cannot be localized with preoperative or intraoperative techniques, biopsy specimens should be taken from the pancreatic tail to evaluate for nesidioblastosis. Distal pancreatectomy should be considered in this setting, but this is controversial (see "Noninsulinoma Pancreatogenous Hypoglycemia Syndrome").

Life expectancy should be normal after complete excision of a benign insulinoma. More extensive resections are required for complete excision of malignant insulinomas. Tumor debulking in the setting of metastatic insulinoma may result in a biochemical cure because some residual disease may not be functional. Persistent hyperinsulinism after surgery for metastatic islet cell tumors may be managed with somatostatin analogues, hepatic artery tumor embolization, diazoxide, or streptozotocin plus 5-fluorouracil. Even with metastatic disease, the median survival after resection is approximately 5 years.

Gastrin-Secreting Pancreatic Neuroendocrine Tumor (Gastrinoma)

Gastrin-secreting PNET (gastrinoma) is the second most common functional pancreatic endocrine tumor, with an incidence of 1 per 2.5 million population, and was first described in 1955 by Zollinger and Ellison. The mean age of patients at diagnosis is approximately 50 years. Gastrinomas are slightly more common in men (60%), are sporadic in 75% of patients, and are associated with MEN1 in 25% of patients. The gastrin produced by islet cell tumors is not subject to the normal stimulation by amino acids and peptides in the stomach or by gastric distention. In addition, these tumors are not suppressed by a high luminal pH and can be stimulated (instead of inhibited) by secretin.

Patients with gastrinoma, also known as Zollinger-Ellison syndrome (ZES), have a fulminant peptic ulcer diathesis, acid hypersecretion, and non–beta islet cell tumors of the pancreas. Hypergastrinemia results in peptic acid hypersecretion and refractory peptic ulcer disease. Duodenal ulcers are the most common, but jejunal ulceration may also occur; the presence of jejunal ulcers should raise suspicion for a gastrin-secreting PNET. Approximately 75% of patients present with abdominal pain; almost two thirds of patients with abdominal pain have diarrhea; in 10% to 20% of patients, diarrhea is the only symptom. This acid-induced diarrhea is stopped by nasogastric aspiration of gastric secretions, differentiating it from other secretory diarrheas. More than one third of patients have signs and symptoms of gastroesophageal reflux disease, and this number appears to be increasing.

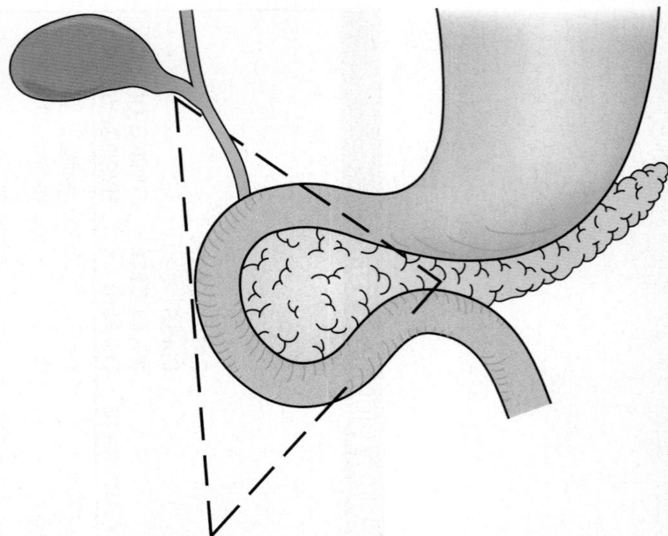

FIGURE 38-8 The anatomic triangle in which approximately 90% of gastrinomas are found. The triangle is bounded by the lines connecting the cystic duct, the junction between the second and third portions of the duodenum, and the junction between the neck and body of the pancreas.

Of gastrinomas, 90% are located within the gastrinoma triangle, bounded by the lines connecting the cystic duct, the junction between the second and third portions of the duodenum, and the junction between the neck and body of the pancreas (Fig. 38-8). More than 60% are located in the duodenum (Fig. 38-9*A*), with most arising in the first portion. Gastrinomas are occasionally localized to lymph nodes in this region, and it is unclear whether lymph nodes can be a true primary site for gastrinoma or whether they represent metastases from occult primary tumors in the duodenum or pancreas (Fig. 38-9*B*).

Diagnosis. ZES should be considered in all patients with intractable peptic ulcers (especially jejunal ulcers), severe esophagitis, or persistent secretory diarrhea. The diagnosis depends on the presence of hypergastrinemia and increased secretion of gastric acid. Most laboratories have an upper limit of normal of 100 pg/mL for fasting levels of gastrin. Levels of 100 to 1000 pg/mL are occasionally seen in patients without ZES, and levels higher than 1000 pg/mL are strongly suggestive of gastrinoma, provided that the patient demonstrated increased gastric acid secretion. Patients with pernicious anemia and patients taking PPIs have very high gastrin levels in the absence of gastric acid hypersecretion. In the workup for ZES, all PPIs should be stopped 2 weeks before testing gastrin levels. An elevated serum gastrin level coupled with a pH lower than 2 in the gastric aspirate is diagnostic of ZES. A gastric pH higher than 3 without acid-suppressing medications or prior acid-reducing operations strongly suggests that ZES is not the cause of hypergastrinemia. If the diagnosis remains in doubt despite these measures, a secretin stimulation test can be helpful. In this test, the fasting gastrin level is measured before secretin (2 IU/kg) is administered intravenously, and subsequent samples are obtained 2, 5, 10, and 20 minutes after secretin administration. Gastrin levels greater than 200 pg/mL after administration of secretin are noted in 87% of patients, with no false-positive results. False-negative results may be caused by the presence of

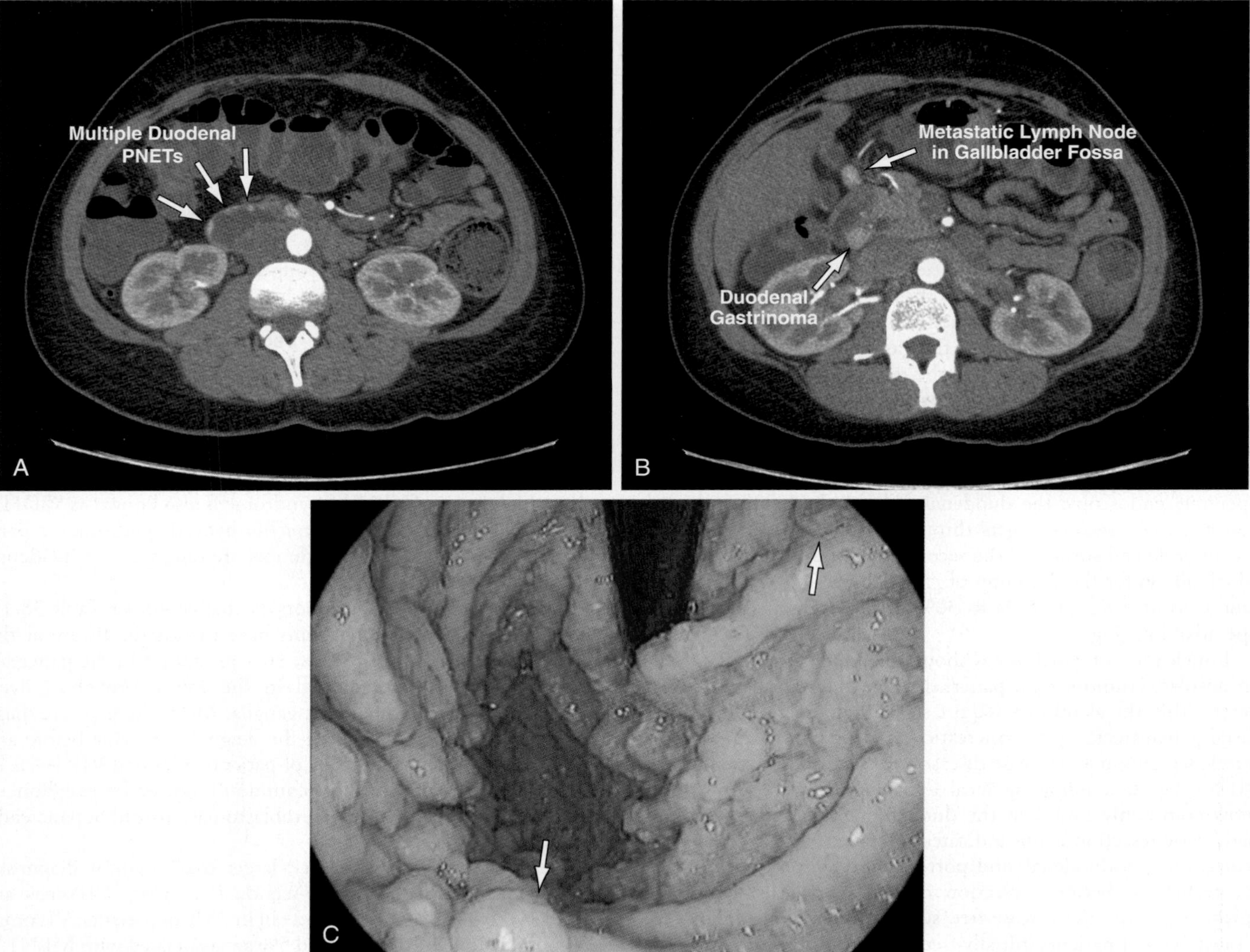

FIGURE 38-9 **A,** CT image showing multiple small duodenal pancreatic neuroendocrine tumors (PNETs) in a patient with multiple endocrine neoplasia type 1 (MEN1). **B,** CT image showing metastatic gastrinoma to a lymph node in the gallbladder fossa and a large primary duodenal gastrinoma in the same patient. **C,** Esophagogastroduodenoscopy showing multiple submucosal duodenal PNETs in a patient with MEN1; two large lesions *(arrows)* were removed endoscopically and were consistent with PNET.

Helicobacter pylori. Other causes of hypergastrinemia must be excluded; the differential diagnosis can be subdivided further into hypergastrinemia associated with high and low gastric acid output (Table 38-6).

Localization and treatment. Once the diagnosis is established, the primary goal is to prevent acid secretion and relieve symptoms. The best results are achieved with PPIs; however, higher doses than are used for simple peptic ulcer or gastroesophageal reflux disease are often required. PPIs have been shown to be safe and effective at high doses and should be given at the dosage required to decrease gastric acid output to less than 5 mEq/hr.

Similar to all PNETs, for biochemically confirmed ZES, the first step of the algorithm for localizing a gastrinoma should include CT or MRI. Water should be used as oral contrast on CT scans to allow for better visualization of hyperenhancing, small duodenal lesions. If the tumor is not localized by CT or MRI, SRS should be performed because almost all gastrinomas express somatostatin receptors. EUS may be useful to detect small pancreatic lesions. If the tumor has still not been localized, angiography with or without stimulation should be performed next. If all of these measures are unsuccessful and ZES is strongly suspected, it may be reasonable to proceed with operative exploration to localize and treat the tumor.

TABLE 38-6 Causes of Hypergastrinemia

HIGH GASTRIC ACID OUTPUT	NORMAL, LOW, OR NO GASTRIC ACID OUTPUT
ZES (gastrinoma)	H_2 receptor antagonist therapy
Gastric outlet obstruction	PPI therapy
G cell hyperplasia	Prior acid-reducing procedure
Retained gastric antrum	Atrophic gastritis, pernicious anemia, gastric cancer, vitiligo, achlorhydria, vagotomy, renal failure

PPI, proton pump inhibitor; *ZES*, Zollinger-Ellison syndrome.

Operative treatment of gastrinomas is indicated when curative resection appears to be possible based on preoperative imaging or for palliative cytoreduction for symptom control. The presence or absence of malignant disease is the most important prognostic indicator. In 5% to 8% of cases, the surgeon is unable to localize a gastrinoma intraoperatively. If the tumor is not localized preoperatively, finding it in the pancreas and duodenum may be difficult. Exploration includes the entire abdomen, from the undersurface of the diaphragm to the pelvic floor, with particular attention paid to the liver, right subhepatic and paraduodenal area, and pelvic cul-de-sac and ovaries. The entire small bowel and colon are examined carefully, with the surgeon looking for lymph nodes in the mesentery or attached to the wall of the bowel. The surgeon should carefully inspect the gastrinoma triangle (see Fig. 38-8) to confirm the location of the tumor. Intraoperative ultrasound should be routinely performed to identify small pancreatic lesions or liver metastases. Transillumination of the duodenum with intraoperative endoscopy may help identify small submucosal lesions. After transillumination of the duodenum with intraoperative endoscopy, the duodenal wall can be gently palpated between the surgeon's fingers through a 3-cm duodenotomy on the anterolateral surface of the second portion of the duodenum, which allows for the detection of gastrinomas smaller than 1 cm. Duodenotomy detects 25% to 30% of tumors not seen on preoperative imaging.

Enucleation of gastrinomas should be reserved for small, well-encapsulated tumors in the pancreas. Large unencapsulated lesions deep within the gland may require segmental resection, including distal pancreatectomy or pancreaticoduodenectomy. Pancreaticoduodenectomy may increase disease-free survival in patients with MEN1 because, following local excision, recurrent tumors are most commonly found in the duodenum.[35] In this case, blind pancreatic resection is not indicated. Detailed inspection of peripancreatic, periduodenal, and portohepatic lymph nodes should be performed because resection of grossly positive lymphatic spread may increase disease-free survival. With long follow-up, almost 50% of patients initially free of disease show symptomatic or biochemical (i.e., a positive secretin test result) recurrence by 5 years.

More than 50% of patients with gastrinomas have metastatic disease at the time of diagnosis. For patients with unresectable, symptomatic metastatic disease, treatment should focus on symptom control (i.e., reduction of acid production). Pharmacologic control of acid secretion with PPIs has rendered total gastrectomy, debulking, and other surgical acid-reducing procedures unnecessary. Symptoms are controlled in more than 90% of patients starting with dosages of 60 to 80 mg pantoprazole daily, although higher dosages may be required. The PPI dosage should be titrated to keep basal acid output less than 10 mEq/hr (or <5 mEq/hr if the patient had a prior acid-reducing procedure). One of the few remaining indications for total gastrectomy in patients with ZES is the presence of gastric carcinoid tumors, which may arise from prolonged hypergastrinemia. Gastrectomy may also be indicated for patients who are unable to tolerate PPIs and in whom control of acid secretion cannot be achieved through other means. Total gastrectomy cures all symptoms produced by excessive acid but has no effect on disease progression or survival for metastatic disease. Somatostatin analogues, used to decrease gastrin release and subsequent acid secretion, are rarely effective in suppressing acid without concurrent PPI use.

Aggressive surgical therapy is indicated because patients have been known to live more than 20 years with residual disease. Gastrinoma may take an aggressive or relatively benign clinical course. The aggressive form, seen in approximately 25% of all patients, is associated with larger pancreatic tumors, liver metastases, and worse long-term survival; 90% of aggressive tumors are located in the pancreas. The 10-year survival rate is 30% in patients with the aggressive form compared with greater than 90% in patients with the nonaggressive form. The best predictor of survival for patients with gastrinoma is the presence of liver metastases; lymph node metastases are not predictive.[6] Resection of all gross disease and metastases may provide palliation of symptoms and has been associated with long-term survival rates of greater than 50%, but cures are rare.

Vasoactive Intestinal Peptide–Secreting Pancreatic Neuroendocrine Tumor

VIP is a small peptide normally found in the brain, G cells of the antrum, adrenal medulla, gut mucosa, pancreatic neurons, and D_2 cells of the pancreas. First described by Verner and Morrison in 1958, VIPomas usually arise from pancreatic islet D_2 cells and release high levels of VIP. This syndrome is also known as WDHA (*w*atery *d*iarrhea, *h*ypokalemia, *a*chlorhydria) syndrome or pancreatic cholera. Overall, these tumors are rare, with an incidence of 1 per 10 million population.[36]

More than two thirds of tumors are malignant (see Table 38-1), and greater than 70% of patients have metastatic disease at the time of presentation. Of lesions, 90% are found in the pancreas, and 10% have been described in the colon, bronchus, liver, adrenal gland, and sympathetic ganglia. Most VIPomas are diagnosed middle-age patients, but the diagnosis is made before age 10 years in approximately 10% of patients. Elevated VIP levels in these young patients are most commonly caused by ganglioneuromas, ganglioblastomas, or neuroblastomas, instead of pancreatic tumors.

Tumors are generally solitary, larger than 3 cm at diagnosis, and easily identified on cross-sectional imaging. VIPomas are found in the pancreatic body and tail in 75% of patients. VIPomas are sporadic in 95% of cases, and 5% are associated with MEN1.[36]

Diagnosis and treatment. Normal VIP levels are less than 200 pg/mL; patients with VIPomas have levels ranging from 225 to 2000 pg/mL. Levels of VIP should be measured after an overnight fast. VIP acts directly on intestinal epithelial cells to activate adenylate cyclase, increasing cyclic adenosine monophosphate (cAMP) levels within colonocytes, which stimulates the hypersecretion of fluid into the lumen, resulting in watery diarrhea. Profuse, watery, iso-osmotic secretory diarrhea is the most common presenting symptom and may exceed a volume of 3 to 5 liters/day. The diagnosis of VIPoma is unlikely if the stool volume is less than 700 mL/day. The diarrhea is further exacerbated because cAMP inhibits sodium reabsorption and stimulates chloride secretion, causing increased fluid and electrolyte shifts into the intestinal lumen. The diarrhea persists despite fasting, which qualifies it as a secretory diarrhea, and despite nasogastric aspiration, which differentiates it from diarrhea seen with acid hypersecretion in ZES. The differential diagnosis includes laxative abuse; bacterial and parasitic diarrhea; carcinoid syndrome, which is associated with an elevated level of 5-hydroxyindoleacetic acid in the urine; and ZES, which has an elevated serum gastrin level.

Weight loss, crampy abdominal pain, dehydration, electrolyte abnormalities, and metabolic acidosis (from fluid and bicarbonate loss) are common with VIP-secreting PNETs. Hypokalemia may be profound because patients can lose more than 400 mEq of potassium per day, which may lead to disturbances of cardiac rhythm and sudden death in extreme cases. Almost 75% of patients have hypochlorhydria or achlorhydria, and decreased levels of magnesium and phosphorus are often present. The profound electrolyte abnormalities and dehydration need to be corrected before definitive surgical management.

Treatment of VIPomas begins with aggressive preoperative hydration and correction of electrolyte abnormalities and acid-base disturbances. Somatostatin analogues are commonly used preoperatively to reduce diarrhea volume and facilitate fluid and electrolyte replacement. If diarrhea persists despite somatostatin analogue therapy, addition of a glucocorticoid may be helpful.

Given the high rate of malignant disease, formal anatomic resection (not enucleation) with negative margins and including lymphadenectomy is warranted in the setting of resectable disease. There is no evidence to support debulking in the setting of metastatic disease. After resection, 5-year survival of patients with VIPomas is approximately 68%, with the presence of metastatic disease representing a poor predictive factor.[36]

Glucagon-Secreting Pancreatic Neuroendocrine Tumor (Glucagonoma)

In 1942, Becker described a patient with severe dermatitis, anemia, and diabetes who also had an islet cell tumor; McGarvan later identified the cause of the syndrome as glucagon-secreting islet cell carcinoma of the pancreas. Glucagonomas are rare, with an estimated incidence of 1 per 20 million population.[37] They are twofold to threefold more common in women. Compared with other pancreatic endocrine tumors, they tend to be larger, averaging 5 to 10 cm in size at the time of diagnosis. These tumors almost always arise in the pancreas with 65% to 75% located in the body or tail, corresponding to the normal distribution of alpha cells in the pancreas. Glucagonomas are malignant in 50% to 80% of cases; 80% of patients with malignant glucagonomas have liver metastases at the time of diagnosis. Most glucagonomas are sporadic; however, 5% to 17% are associated with MEN1.[37]

Glucagonoma syndrome is a rare syndrome, with a classic presentation of the "4 D's": diabetes, dermatitis, deep vein thrombosis, and depression. It is also characterized by a severe catabolic state with weight loss, depletion of fat and protein stores, and associated vitamin deficiencies. The characteristic skin lesion, a necrolytic migrating erythema (Fig. 38-10), is noted in approximately two thirds of patients and often appears before other symptoms of the syndrome. The cause is believed to be severe amino acid deficiency, although trace element deficiency and general malnutrition probably contribute. Parenteral administration of amino acids was found to result in the disappearance of the skin lesions. Diabetes develops in 76% to 94% of patients with glucagonoma at some point during their illness, but it is usually mild. The diagnosis of glucagonoma is established by measuring glucagon levels; normal fasting glucagon levels are less than 100 pg/mL. A fasting glucagon level higher than 1000 pg/mL is considered diagnostic.

Given their size and malignant behavior, glucagonomas are easily localized. Treatment begins with medical therapy to improve the patient's nutritional status with supplemental enteral nutrition in excess of basic caloric needs. Octreotide is often required in conjunction with enteral nutrition to reverse the catabolic state. Intravenous infusions of amino acids may be required to reverse symptoms and improve dermatitis. Prophylaxis against thromboembolism should be instituted early during hospitalization to prevent perioperative deep vein thrombosis and pulmonary embolism, which occur commonly and are significant causes of morbidity and mortality in these patients. Similar to other PNETs, complete anatomic resection is indicated for resectable disease. After resection, 5-year survival for patients with glucagonoma is almost 85% if no metastases are present. In patients with metastatic disease, the 5-year survival is approximately 60%.

Somatostatin-Secreting Pancreatic Neuroendocrine Tumor (Somatostatinoma)

Somatostatinomas are exceedingly rare, with less than 100 cases reported in the literature. Somatostatin-secreting PNET was first described in 1977, and the full syndrome of steatorrhea, diabetes mellitus, hypochlorhydria, and gallstones was characterized in 1979. Inhibition of pancreatic enzyme and hormone secretion by unregulated hypersecretion of somatostatin causes steatorrhea, diabetes, malabsorption, and cholelithiasis resulting from reduced gallbladder emptying.[38] Because the symptoms are nonspecific, the diagnosis of somatostatinoma is rarely made preoperatively. In a patient with diabetes, gallstones, and steatorrhea, with or without the finding of a pancreatic or duodenal mass on radiographic studies, a fasting plasma somatostatin level should be measured. A concentration exceeding 160 pg/mL is suggestive of the diagnosis.

Somatostatinomas are usually solitary, and 85% are larger than 2 cm. More than 60% are found in the pancreas, usually the head, with the remainder in the duodenum or elsewhere in the small intestine. Patients are typically 50 to 60 years old at the time of diagnosis. Of tumors, 90% are malignant, with metastases to the liver or lymph nodes commonly noted at the time of diagnosis. Somatostatinomas are rarely associated with MEN1 but are associated with von Recklinghausen disease and pheochromocytomas.

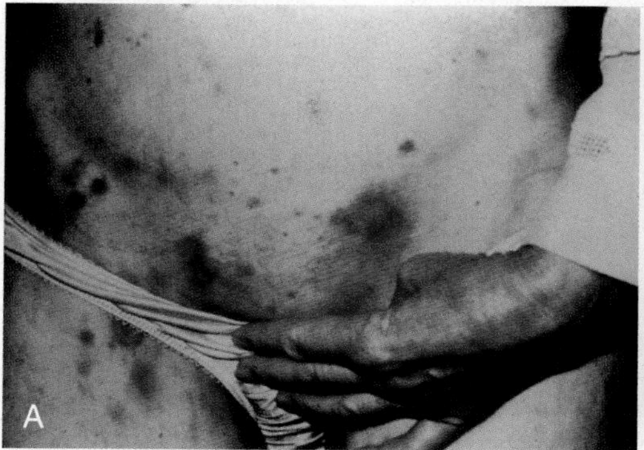

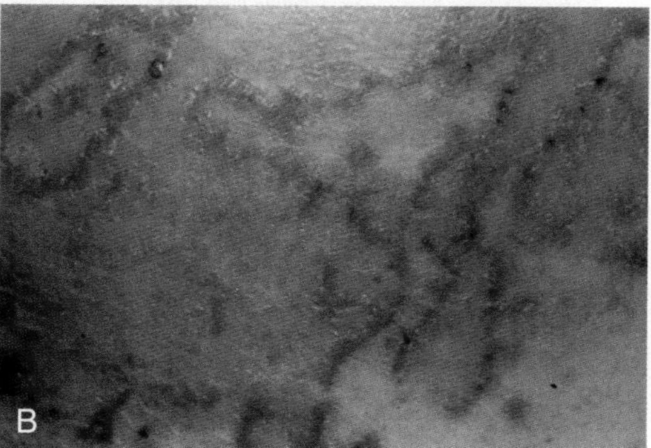

FIGURE 38-10 Characteristic necrolytic migrating erythematous dermatitis of glucagonoma syndrome. **A,** Confluent patches with superficial necrosis. **B,** Close-up showing serpiginous margins.

Given their rare nature, outcomes data are lacking, but 5-year survival is reported to be 30% to 60% after resection for patients with metastatic disease.

Other Functional Pancreatic Endocrine Tumors

Pancreatic endocrine tumors that produce other hormones have been described but are extremely rare. Case reports of pancreatic endocrine tumors that secrete GRF, parathyroid hormone–related peptide, PP, ACTH, calcitonin, enteroglucagon, CCK, gastric inhibitory peptide, luteinizing hormone, neurotensin, or ghrelin have been described. GRF-secreting pancreatic endocrine tumors are invariably associated with MEN1, and only 30% arise in the pancreas. Patients with ACTH-secreting tumors have Cushing syndrome and usually have other endocrine syndromes, most commonly ZES. Neurotensinomas are usually malignant and cause hypokalemia, weight loss, hypotension, cyanosis, flushing, and diabetes. PP-secreting pancreatic endocrine tumors are associated with high circulating levels of PP but no associated clinical syndrome. Unless associated with MEN1, these tumors are large and solitary. In addition, elevated PP levels are often seen in other endocrine tumor syndromes. PP-secreting, neurotensin-secreting, and calcitonin-secreting tumors are sometimes classified as nonfunctional because the hormone products have little biologic consequence and rarely cause symptoms.

Pancreatic Neuroendocrine Tumor Associated With Multiple Endocrine Neoplasia Type 1

The MEN1 syndrome is characterized by PNETs, parathyroid adenomas or hyperplasia, and pituitary adenomas. Pancreatic endocrine tumors occur in 30% to 80% of patients with MEN1 and are the most common cause of tumor-related death in these patients. Patients with MEN1-associated pancreatic endocrine tumors tend to be younger, more likely to have malignant disease, and more likely to have multicentric disease than patients with sporadic tumors.

Approximately 50% of patients with MEN1-associated NETs present with metastatic disease.[22] The most common pancreatic endocrine syndrome seen in patients with MEN1 is gastrinoma (54%), followed by insulinoma (21%), glucagonoma (3%), and VIPoma (1%). PP-secreting pancreatic endocrine tumors, which are not associated with a functional syndrome, occur in more than 80% of cases of MEN1.

Management of patients with MEN1 and pancreatic endocrine tumors requires recognition and staged treatment of associated tumors. Patients suspected to have MEN1 should undergo biochemical screening for gastrin, insulin and proinsulin, PP, glucagon, and chromogranin A (a tumor marker elaborated by most pancreatic endocrine tumors). All patients with suspected MEN1 should have a screening calcium level and, if calcium is elevated, a parathyroid hormone level. In the setting of hyperparathyroidism, sestamibi parathyroid scintigraphy should be performed to identify a parathyroid adenoma or hyperplasia (Fig. 38-11). Hyperparathyroidism, if present, should be treated first because correction of hyperkalemia improves the outcome of treatment for the pancreatic endocrine tumor.

It is especially important to consider the diagnosis of MEN1 in patients with ZES because 20% of patients with ZES have MEN-associated disease. The average age at onset is usually 5 to 10 years earlier with MEN-associated gastrinomas. Gastrinomas in patients with MEN1 are more likely to occur in the duodenum and are more likely to be multiple, complicating their management (see Fig. 38-9*B* and *C*). Of patients with MEN1, 60% to 80% have duodenal gastrinomas, which are metastatic to the lymph nodes in 85% at presentation (see Fig. 38-9*B*). They tend not to metastasize to the liver, whereas sporadic tumors larger than 3 cm tend to do so.

The role of routine surgical exploration for resection or cure in patients with ZES has been controversial since the original description of this disease in 1955, especially because medical therapy of acid hypersecretion is so effective. Careful surveillance

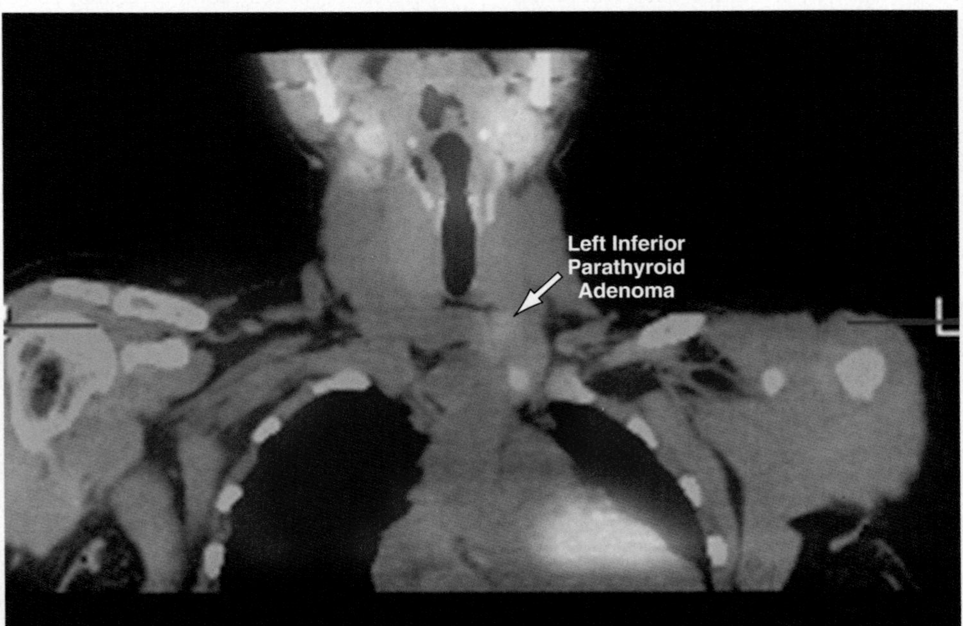

FIGURE 38-11 Sestamibi scan in the patient with multiple endocrine neoplasia type 1–associated gastrinoma in Figure 38-9. The patient had elevated calcium and parathyroid hormone levels. Sestamibi shows a left inferior parathyroid adenoma.

is indicated with annual esophagogastroduodenoscopy and removal of larger duodenal lesions; surgical resection is indicated for lesions that appear malignant, as indicated by rapid growth or new appearance.

NONINSULINOMA PANCREATOGENOUS HYPOGLYCEMIA SYNDROME

Insulinoma is the most common cause of hyperinsulinemic hypoglycemia. Noninsulinoma pancreatogenous hypoglycemia syndrome, or nesidioblastosis, is characterized by excessive pancreatic B cell function, with associated pathologic changes including pancreatic islet hyperplasia and dysplasia, with histologic identification of B cells budding from and in apposition to pancreatic ductal structures. Nesidioblastosis is usually a disease of infancy but in rare cases has been identified in adults. In an adult patient, it can be difficult to differentiate noninsulinoma pancreatogenous hypoglycemic syndrome from insulinoma. However, it is critical to do so because the surgical treatment is different.

Postprandial hypoglycemia, within 4 hours of a meal, is the hallmark of noninsulinoma pancreatogenous hypoglycemia syndrome and can help differentiate it from insulinoma, where this does not occur.[39] However, similar to patients with an insulinoma, patients with noninsulinoma pancreatogenous hypoglycemia syndrome may have a positive 72-hour fast, with episodes of hypoglycemia associated with inappropriate elevation of insulin, C peptide, and proinsulin levels. Nesidioblastosis is a clinical diagnosis of exclusion and is based on exclusion of insulinoma as described earlier. The final diagnosis can be confirmed only on pathologic examination of the pancreas and clinical response to treatment. The treatment of noninsulinoma pancreatogenous hypoglycemia syndrome includes pancreatectomy, most commonly 95% distal pancreatectomy; dietary control; and medical therapy with diazoxide and somatostatin analogues.[39]

ENDOCRINE COMPLICATIONS OF SURGICAL THERAPY

Post–Gastric Bypass Noninsulinoma Pancreatogenous Hypoglycemia Syndrome

With increasing use of Roux-en-Y gastric bypass (RYGB) to treat morbid obesity, noninsulinoma pancreatogenous hypoglycemia syndrome has been recognized more recently as a complication of this procedure. A Swedish registry study documented a 0.2% hospitalization rate for hypoglycemia after RYGB compared with only 0.04% in a reference population.[40] Although uncommon, the prevalence of hypoglycemia may be underestimated, and given the extensive use of RYGB, recognition of this complication has clinical relevance. In the setting of RYGB, the cause of nesidioblastosis is postulated to be due to obesity-induced B cell hypertrophy not reversed after RYGB, inappropriate growth factor release, or persistent altered gut hormonal signaling.

Dietary modifications and medication are the first-line treatment for post-RYGB hypoglycemia; modifications include dietary restrictions or more complex nutritional supplementation. With the addition of medical management strategies, including continuous glucose monitoring, acarbose, calcium channel blockade, diazoxide, and somatostatin analogues, hypoglycemic episodes can often be controlled. Surgery, including reversal of the gastric bypass and distal pancreatectomy, should be evaluated in the context of the perioperative risk, long-term outcome, potential weight regain, and the potential effects on obesity-related comorbidity. When surgical treatment is necessary, pancreatic resection is the most common surgical procedure used. However, the appropriate extent of resection is not defined, and symptoms often recur.

Endocrine Insufficiency After Surgical Resection

There is significant secretory reserve of insulin within the pancreas. Destruction or removal of 80% of the pancreatic islet cell mass is necessary before endocrine dysfunction becomes clinically apparent in the form of type 1 (insulin-dependent) diabetes. Approximately 20% to 50% of patients develop diabetes after pancreatic resection.[41] Pancreatectomy, most commonly performed for pancreatic/periampullary cancer or chronic pancreatitis, is often preceded by pancreatic endocrine insufficiency, although this may be subclinical. It is difficult for clinicians to predict which patients will develop pancreatic endocrine insufficiency after pancreatectomy, although studies suggest that hemoglobin A1c levels may be predictive.[42] In patients with existing chronic pancreatitis, diabetes is very common postoperatively. With pancreatic cancer, the data are less clear. Although some studies report a high incidence of diabetes after resection for cancer, others report improvements in blood glucose control attributed to relief of pancreatic ductal obstruction or other tumor-mediated factors.

In the setting of total pancreatectomy, the resulting diabetes is extremely brittle. Because of the lack of endogenous glucagon to balance exogenously administered insulin, it is very difficult to control. With the advent of longer acting insulin formulations, the management of diabetes after total pancreatectomy has significantly improved.

SURGICAL TREATMENT OF DIABETES

Autologous Islet Cell Transplantation

Autologous islet cell transplantation has a role in patients with severe chronic pancreatitis. Surgical resection of all or part of the pancreas for this disease can significantly improve quality of life by eliminating or reducing intractable pain, allowing the return of a normal appetite with subsequent weight gain, and reducing the number of hospital admissions.[43] Even without pancreatic resection, a significant number of patients with chronic pancreatitis develop diabetes or impaired glucose tolerance. Because of the loss of insulin, glucagon, and PP, the type of diabetes that develops in patients with chronic pancreatitis is similar to diabetes following pancreatic resection. Total pancreatectomy in this setting causes diabetes, but partial resections can also greatly reduce the insulin-secreting capacity of the already compromised pancreas.

Total or partial pancreatectomy with islet autotransplantation is offered in several centers. This option has the potential to treat the symptoms of chronic pancreatitis definitively, while preventing the onset of diabetes in certain patients. Other patients remain or become insulin dependent but retain significant insulin and glucagon secretion and the benefits of endogenous C peptide production, making the resulting diabetes easier to control. A diagrammatic representation of the islet isolation process is shown in Figure 38-12. Patients undergo pancreatectomy; the pancreatic tissue is immediately digested with the use of enzyme solutions containing collagenase and neutral proteases, and the islet cells are purified. The islet cells are returned to the patient via infusion into the portal vein; this can be done at the time of pancreatectomy or percutaneously after resection.[44] The islet cells engraft in the liver and produce insulin and C peptide. Glucose levels are measured to evaluate the function of the transplanted islets.

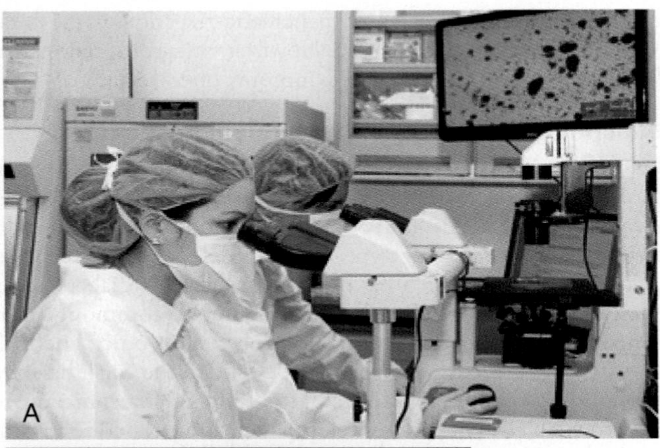

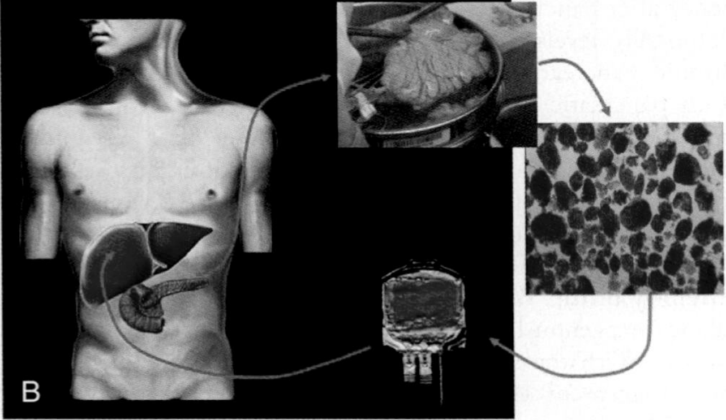

FIGURE 38-12 A, Dedicated islet isolation facility at the University of Texas Medical Branch. The screen in the upper-right-hand corner shows isolated islets stained red from a patient undergoing total pancreatectomy and islet autotransplantation. **B,** Diagram depicts pancreatic islet autotransplantation. The patient undergoes partial or total pancreatectomy. The pancreatic tissue is immediately digested with the use of enzyme solutions containing collagenase and neutral proteases, and the islet cells are purified. The islet cells are then returned to the patient via infusion into the portal vein.

Variable results after pancreatic islet autotransplantation have been reported depending on center expertise and experience. Insulin independence is 40% to 80% initially in some patients,[44-48] but there is a notable decline in islet function over time, with increased insulin requirements in the 10 years after transplantation. Only approximately 10% of patients remain insulin-independent. Although insulin independence is not always achieved, most patients are C peptide positive and have diabetes that is more manageable. In addition, most studies demonstrated improvement in pain and other symptoms of chronic pancreatitis.[43,47,48] Success rates depend on the number of isolated and transplanted islets and the cause of the pancreatic disease. Patients who are not diabetic before autotransplantation, patients who have not had prior pancreatic operations, and younger patients (especially preadolescents) achieve the best results. The most feared procedure-related complication is thrombosis of the portal vein, which occurs in less than 1% of cases.

Immune Therapy, Pancreatic Transplantation, and Islet Allotransplantation

Type 1 diabetes results from autoimmune destruction of pancreatic islets. Immune treatment for type 1 diabetes is being investigated at the present time. A growing body of evidence suggests that the autoimmunity observed in patients with type 1 diabetes is the result of an imbalance between autoaggressive and regulatory T cell subsets.[49] Vaccination with selected T cell receptor autoantigens has been shown to generate autoantibodies and the autoaggressive T cell clones, which are reacting to beta cells. The induction of a lasting, robust immune response generating autoantigen-specific regulatory T cells provides strong justification for further testing of this therapy for type 1 diabetes.

For a select group of patients with difficult-to-manage type 1 diabetes who do not respond well to conventional approaches or insulin pumps, whole pancreas transplantation is the gold standard for treatment. During the period 1966-2008, more than 40,000 pancreas transplantations were reported to the International Pancreas Transplant Registry. Recipients experience immediate normal fasting and postprandial glucose levels, and hemoglobin A1c levels return to normal. In the United States, 1-year graft survival rates have improved to 85% for simultaneous pancreas-kidney transplants, 78% for pancreas-after-kidney transplants, and 76% for pancreas-only transplants. With the observed decrease in morbidity and mortality, recipients who become insulin independent report a better quality of life, despite the need for immunosuppression. They also experience stabilization or improvements in retinopathy, nephropathy, neuropathy, and microvascular and macrovascular diseases normally associated with poor glucose control.

Allogeneic islet transplantation is a less invasive but less effective method of achieving insulin independence. At the present time, long-term insulin independence remains elusive for patients undergoing allogeneic islet transplantation. The data show that even among patients who receive multiple infusions, few remain normoglycemic over time. Data from the Collaborative Islet Transplant Registry demonstrated that 70% of patients achieve insulin independence within the first year (including patients with multiple infusions), but by the third year, the percentage of patients who remain insulin independent is closer to 35%.[50] The partial pancreatic endocrine function confers some benefit, with decreased occurrence of severe hypoglycemic events, abatement of hypoglycemic unawareness, persistent C peptide levels, improvement in glycemic control, and stabilization of diabetic complications. In addition, islet cell transplantation requires two donors per recipient to maintain graft function. Stem cell therapy offers the potential of producing an unlimited source of cells, and a growing number of studies have demonstrated successful in vitro differentiation and expansion of embryonic cells of murine and human origin from pancreatic ducts that express insulin and respond to glucose stimulation.

SELECTED REFERENCES

Bilimoria KY, Talamonti MS, Tomlinson JS, et al: Prognostic score predicting survival after resection of pancreatic neuroendocrine tumors: Analysis of 3851 patients. *Ann Surg* 247:490–500, 2008.

This large study used the National Cancer Database to define prognostic factors after resection of pancreatic neuroendocrine tumors. The article provides survival data for selected subgroups of patients and a prognostic scoring system that can be applied to individual patients.

Jiao Y, Shi C, Edil BH, et al: DAXX/ATRX, MEN1, and mTOR pathway genes are frequently altered in pancreatic neuroendocrine tumors. *Science* 331:1199–1203, 2011.

This high-impact original research study used high-throughput sequencing technology to characterize the most commonly mutated genes in sporadic pancreatic neuroendocrine tumors. The findings helped to validate several gene products and pathways as potential targets for therapy.

Klimstra DS, Modlin IR, Coppola D, et al: The pathologic classification of neuroendocrine tumors: A review of nomenclature, grading, and staging systems. *Pancreas* 39:707–712, 2010.

This review clarifies the pathologic classification of neuroendocrine tumors, including the distinction between grade and differentiation and the prognostic significance of different pathologic factors. Guidance is also included on the minimum data that should be included in neuroendocrine pathology reports.

Krampitz GW, Norton JA: Pancreatic neuroendocrine tumors. *Curr Probl Surg* 50:509–545, 2013.

This is a comprehensive review by Dr. Jeffrey Norton, a world expert on pancreatic neuroendocrine tumors (PNETs). Discussions on the diagnosis, localization, and management of functional PNETs with emphasis on differences between sporadic and multiple endocrine neoplasia type 1–associated PNETs are particularly helpful.

Mayo SC, de Jong MC, Bloomston M, et al: Surgery versus intra-arterial therapy for neuroendocrine liver metastasis: A multicenter international analysis. *Ann Surg Oncol* 18:3657–3665, 2011.

The management of neuroendocrine metastases is controversial and difficult to study because of the relative rarity of this disease and insufficient detail in national databases. This collaborative study pooled 753 patients to define prognostic factors after liver-directed therapy for neuroendocrine liver metastases.

Rinke A, Muller HH, Schade-Brittinger C, et al: Placebo-controlled, double-blind, prospective, randomized study on the effect of octreotide LAR in the control of tumor growth in patients with metastatic neuroendocrine midgut tumors: A report from the PROMID Study Group. *J Clin Oncol* 27:4656–4663, 2009.

Before this study, somatostatin analogues were known to be effective at controlling symptoms from functional tumors, but this study was the first to demonstrate a survival benefit for this approach, which has now become first-line therapy for unresectable disease.

REFERENCES

1. Samols E, Stagner JI, Ewart RB, et al: The order of islet microvascular cellular perfusion is B-A-D in the perfused rat pancreas. *J Clin Invest* 82:350–353, 1988.
2. Gregg BE, Moore PC, Demozay D, et al: Formation of a human beta-cell population within pancreatic islets is set early in life. *J Clin Endocrinol Metab* 97:3197–3206, 2012.
3. Briggs DI, Andrews ZB: A recent update on the role of ghrelin in glucose homeostasis. *Curr Diabetes Rev* 7:201–207, 2011.
4. Batterham RL, Le Roux CW, Cohen MA, et al: Pancreatic polypeptide reduces appetite and food intake in humans. *J Clin Endocrinol Metab* 88:3989–3992, 2003.
5. Halfdanarson TR, Rabe KG, Rubin J, et al: Pancreatic neuroendocrine tumors (PNETs): Incidence, prognosis and recent trend toward improved survival. *Ann Oncol* 19:1727–1733, 2008.
6. Krampitz GW, Norton JA: Pancreatic neuroendocrine tumors. *Curr Probl Surg* 50:509–545, 2013.
7. Klimstra DS, Modlin IR, Coppola D, et al: The pathologic classification of neuroendocrine tumors: A review of nomenclature, grading, and staging systems. *Pancreas* 39:707–712, 2010.
8. Bilimoria KY, Bentrem DJ, Merkow RP, et al: Application of the pancreatic adenocarcinoma staging system to pancreatic neuroendocrine tumors. *J Am Coll Surg* 205:558–563, 2007.
9. Edge S, Byrd DR, Compton CC, et al, editors: *AJCC cancer staging manual*, New York, 2010, Springer.
10. Martin RC, Kooby DA, Weber SM, et al: Analysis of 6,747 pancreatic neuroendocrine tumors for a proposed staging system. *J Gastrointest Surg* 15:175–183, 2011.
11. Libutti SK, Choyke PL, Alexander HR, et al: Clinical and genetic analysis of patients with pancreatic neuroendocrine tumors associated with von Hippel-Lindau disease. *Surgery* 128:1022–1027, discussion 1027–1028, 2000.
12. Hassan MM, Phan A, Li D, et al: Risk factors associated with neuroendocrine tumors: A U.S.-based case-control study. *Int J Cancer* 123:867–873, 2008.
13. Jiao Y, Shi C, Edil BH, et al: DAXX/ATRX, MEN1, and mTOR pathway genes are frequently altered in pancreatic neuroendocrine tumors. *Science* 331:1199–1203, 2011.
14. Missiaglia E, Dalai I, Barbi S, et al: Pancreatic endocrine tumors: Expression profiling evidences a role for AKT-mTOR pathway. *J Clin Oncol* 28:245–255, 2010.
15. Zhang J, Francois R, Iyer R, et al: Current understanding of the molecular biology of pancreatic neuroendocrine tumors. *J Natl Cancer Inst* 105:1005–1017, 2013.
16. Jones S, Zhang X, Parsons DW, et al: Core signaling pathways in human pancreatic cancers revealed by global genomic analyses. *Science* 321:1801–1806, 2008.
17. Yachida S, Vakiani E, White CM, et al: Small cell and large cell neuroendocrine carcinomas of the pancreas are genetically similar and distinct from well-differentiated pancreatic neuroendocrine tumors. *Am J Surg Pathol* 36:173–184, 2012.
18. van Essen M, Sundin A, Krenning EP, et al: Neuroendocrine tumours: The role of imaging for diagnosis and therapy. *Nat Rev Endocrinol* 10:102–114, 2014.
19. Sheth S, Hruban RK, Fishman EK: Helical CT of islet cell tumors of the pancreas: Typical and atypical manifestations. *AJR Am J Roentgenol* 179:725–730, 2002.
20. Fidler JL, Fletcher JG, Reading CC, et al: Preoperative detection of pancreatic insulinomas on multiphasic helical CT. *AJR Am J Roentgenol* 181:775–780, 2003.
21. Sainz-Esteban A, Olmos R, Gonzalez-Sagrado M, et al: Contribution of 111In-pentetreotide SPECT/CT imaging to conventional somatostatin receptor scintigraphy in the detection of neuroendocrine tumours. *Nucl Med Commun* 36:251–259, 2015.

22. Cho CS, Labow DM, Tang L, et al: Histologic grade is correlated with outcome after resection of hepatic neuroendocrine neoplasms. *Cancer* 113:126–134, 2008.
23. Gurusamy KS, Ramamoorthy R, Sharma D, et al: Liver resection versus other treatments for neuroendocrine tumours in patients with resectable liver metastases. *Cochrane Database Syst Rev* (2):CD007060, 2009.
24. Gupta S: Intra-arterial liver-directed therapies for neuroendocrine hepatic metastases. *Semin Intervent Radiol* 30:28–38, 2013.
25. Mayo SC, de Jong MC, Bloomston M, et al: Surgery versus intra-arterial therapy for neuroendocrine liver metastasis: A multicenter international analysis. *Ann Surg Oncol* 18:3657–3665, 2011.
26. Gurusamy KS, Pamecha V, Sharma D, et al: Palliative cytoreductive surgery versus other palliative treatments in patients with unresectable liver metastases from gastro-entero-pancreatic neuroendocrine tumours. *Cochrane Database Syst Rev* (1):CD007118, 2009.
27. Rinke A, Muller HH, Schade-Brittinger C, et al: Placebo-controlled, double-blind, prospective, randomized study on the effect of octreotide LAR in the control of tumor growth in patients with metastatic neuroendocrine midgut tumors: A report from the PROMID Study Group. *J Clin Oncol* 27:4656–4663, 2009.
28. Yao JC, Shah MH, Ito T, et al: Everolimus for advanced pancreatic neuroendocrine tumors. *N Engl J Med* 364:514–523, 2011.
29. Raymond E, Dahan L, Raoul JL, et al: Sunitinib malate for the treatment of pancreatic neuroendocrine tumors. *N Engl J Med* 364:501–513, 2011.
30. Mazzaferro V, Pulvirenti A, Coppa J: Neuroendocrine tumors metastatic to the liver: How to select patients for liver transplantation? *J Hepatol* 47:460–466, 2007.
31. Le Treut YP, Gregoire E, Klempnauer J, et al: Liver transplantation for neuroendocrine tumors in Europe—results and trends in patient selection: A 213-case European liver transplant registry study. *Ann Surg* 257:807–815, 2013.
32. Bilimoria KY, Talamonti MS, Tomlinson JS, et al: Prognostic score predicting survival after resection of pancreatic neuroendocrine tumors: Analysis of 3851 patients. *Ann Surg* 247:490–500, 2008.
33. Cheema A, Weber J, Strosberg JR: Incidental detection of pancreatic neuroendocrine tumors: An analysis of incidence and outcomes. *Ann Surg Oncol* 19:2932–2936, 2012.
34. Lee LC, Grant CS, Salomao DR, et al: Small, nonfunctioning, asymptomatic pancreatic neuroendocrine tumors (PNETs): Role for nonoperative management. *Surgery* 152:965–974, 2012.
35. Gibril F, Schumann M, Pace A, et al: Multiple endocrine neoplasia type 1 and Zollinger-Ellison syndrome: A prospective study of 107 cases and comparison with 1009 cases from the literature. *Medicine (Baltimore)* 83:43–83, 2004.
36. Soga J, Yakuwa Y: Vipoma/diarrheogenic syndrome: A statistical evaluation of 241 reported cases. *J Exp Clin Cancer Res* 17:389–400, 1998.
37. Kindmark H, Sundin A, Granberg D, et al: Endocrine pancreatic tumors with glucagon hypersecretion: A retrospective study of 23 cases during 20 years. *Med Oncol* 24:330–337, 2007.
38. Krejs GJ, Orci L, Conlon JM, et al: Somatostatinoma syndrome. Biochemical, morphologic and clinical features. *N Engl J Med* 301:285–292, 1979.
39. Gupta RA, Patel RP, Nagral S: Adult onset nesidioblastosis treated by subtotal pancreatectomy. *JOP* 14:286–288, 2013.
40. Marsk R, Jonas E, Rasmussen F, et al: Nationwide cohort study of post-gastric bypass hypoglycaemia including 5,040 patients undergoing surgery for obesity in 1986-2006 in Sweden. *Diabetologia* 53:2307–2311, 2010.
41. Tran TC, van Lanschot JJ, Bruno MJ, et al: Functional changes after pancreatoduodenectomy: Diagnosis and treatment. *Pancreatology* 9:729–737, 2009.
42. Hamilton L, Jeyarajah DR: Hemoglobin A1c can be helpful in predicting progression to diabetes after Whipple procedure. *HPB (Oxford)* 9:26–28, 2007.
43. Morgan K, Owczarski SM, Borckardt J, et al: Pain control and quality of life after pancreatectomy with islet autotransplantation for chronic pancreatitis. *J Gastrointest Surg* 16:129–133, discussion 133–124, 2012.
44. Morgan KA, Nishimura M, Uflacker R, et al: Percutaneous transhepatic islet cell autotransplantation after pancreatectomy for chronic pancreatitis: A novel approach. *HPB (Oxford)* 13:511–516, 2011.
45. Bellin MD, Carlson AM, Kobayashi T, et al: Outcome after pancreatectomy and islet autotransplantation in a pediatric population. *J Pediatr Gastroenterol Nutr* 47:37–44, 2008.
46. Webb MA, Illouz SC, Pollard CA, et al: Islet auto transplantation following total pancreatectomy: A long-term assessment of graft function. *Pancreas* 37:282–287, 2008.
47. Argo JL, Contreras JL, Wesley MM, et al: Pancreatic resection with islet cell autotransplant for the treatment of severe chronic pancreatitis. *Am Surg* 74:530–536, discussion 536–537, 2008.
48. Dixon J, DeLegge M, Morgan KA, et al: Impact of total pancreatectomy with islet cell transplant on chronic pancreatitis management at a disease-based center. *Am Surg* 74:735–738, 2008.
49. Orban T, Farkas K, Jalahej H, et al: Autoantigen-specific regulatory T cells induced in patients with type 1 diabetes mellitus by insulin B-chain immunotherapy. *J Autoimmun* 34:408–415, 2010.
50. Alejandro R, Barton FB, Hering BJ, et al: 2008 update from the Collaborative Islet Transplant Registry. *Transplantation* 86:1783–1788, 2008.

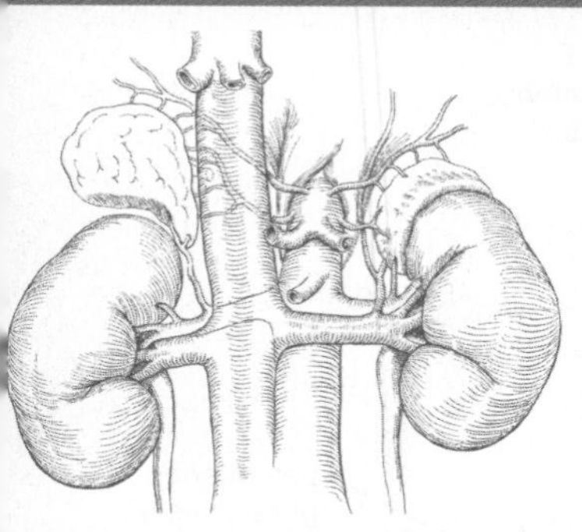

CHAPTER 39

The Adrenal Glands

Michael W. Yeh, Masha J. Livhits, Quan-Yang Duh

OUTLINE

HISTORY

The adrenal glands were first described by the Italian anatomist Bartolomeo Eustachi in 1563. The German comparative anatomist Albert von Kölliker (1817-1905), who noted the presence of the adrenals in a number of vertebrate species, is credited with first identifying two distinct portions of the adrenal gland, the cortex and the medulla. Although Thomas Addison described the clinical features of primary adrenal failure in 1855, it was not until nearly a century later that the adrenal hormones were fully isolated and characterized. Adrenaline (or epinephrine) was first isolated from adrenal extract at the turn of the century. Steroid hormones were crystallized from cortical extract ("cortin") by Swiss and American investigators in the 1930s, but their highly similar chemical structures made isolation of the individual compounds challenging. Edward Kendall, Tadeus Reichstein, and Philip Hench jointly received the 1950 Nobel Prize in Physiology or Medicine for their groundbreaking work on the adrenocortical hormones. The Austrian-born endocrinologist Hans Selye first described the stress response in mammals in 1936 and made major contributions to the understanding of the hypothalamic-pituitary-adrenal (HPA) axis. Roger Guillemin, Andrew Schally, and Rosalyn Yalow were awarded the Nobel Prize in 1977 for characterizing the peptide hormones of the brain that underlie the HPA axis as we now understand it.[1,2]

ANATOMY AND EMBRYOLOGY

General and Developmental Aspects

The adrenal glands are paired, mustard-colored structures that are positioned superior and slightly medial to the kidneys in the retroperitoneal space (Fig. 39-1). They are flattened and roughly pyramidal (right) or crescent shaped (left), weighing approximately 4 g each. The adrenals are among the most highly perfused organs in the body, receiving 2000 mL/kg/min of blood, after only the kidney and thyroid. In most respects, the cortex and medulla can be considered two completely distinct organs that happen to colocalize during development. The two portions have disparate embryologic origins. The primordial cortex arises from the coelomic mesodermal tissue near the cephalic end of the mesonephros during the fourth to fifth week of gestation. Biosynthetic activity can be detected as early as the seventh week. Cortical cell mass dominates the fetal adrenal at 4 months of development, and steroidogenesis is maximum during the third trimester. The adrenal medulla arises from the ectodermal tissues of the embryonic neural crest. It develops in parallel with the sympathetic nervous system, beginning in the fifth to sixth week of gestation. From their original position adjacent to the neural tube, neural crest cells migrate ventrally to assume a para-aortic position near the developing adrenal cortex. There, they differentiate into chromaffin cells that make up the adrenal medulla.

This course of embryologic development yields certain surgically relevant sequelae. Both cortical and medullary tissue can be found at extra-adrenal sites (Fig. 39-2). The range of potential sites is wider for chromaffin tissue than for cortical tissue. Pheochromocytomas may arise in extra-adrenal sites more commonly than previously believed (see later). When they are extra-adrenal, pheochromocytomas are also termed paragangliomas.

Relationships

The right adrenal gland abuts the posterolateral surface of the retrohepatic vena cava. The right adrenal fossa is bounded by the right kidney inferolaterally, diaphragm posteriorly, and bare area of the liver anterosuperiorly. The left adrenal gland lies between the left kidney and aorta, with its inferior limb extending farther caudad toward the renal hilum than the right adrenal. The other relationships of the left adrenal gland are the diaphragm posteriorly and the tail of the pancreas and splenic hilum anteriorly. Each adrenal gland is enveloped by its proper capsule, in addition to sharing Gerota fascia with the kidneys. The adrenal capsules are immediately associated with the perirenal fat.

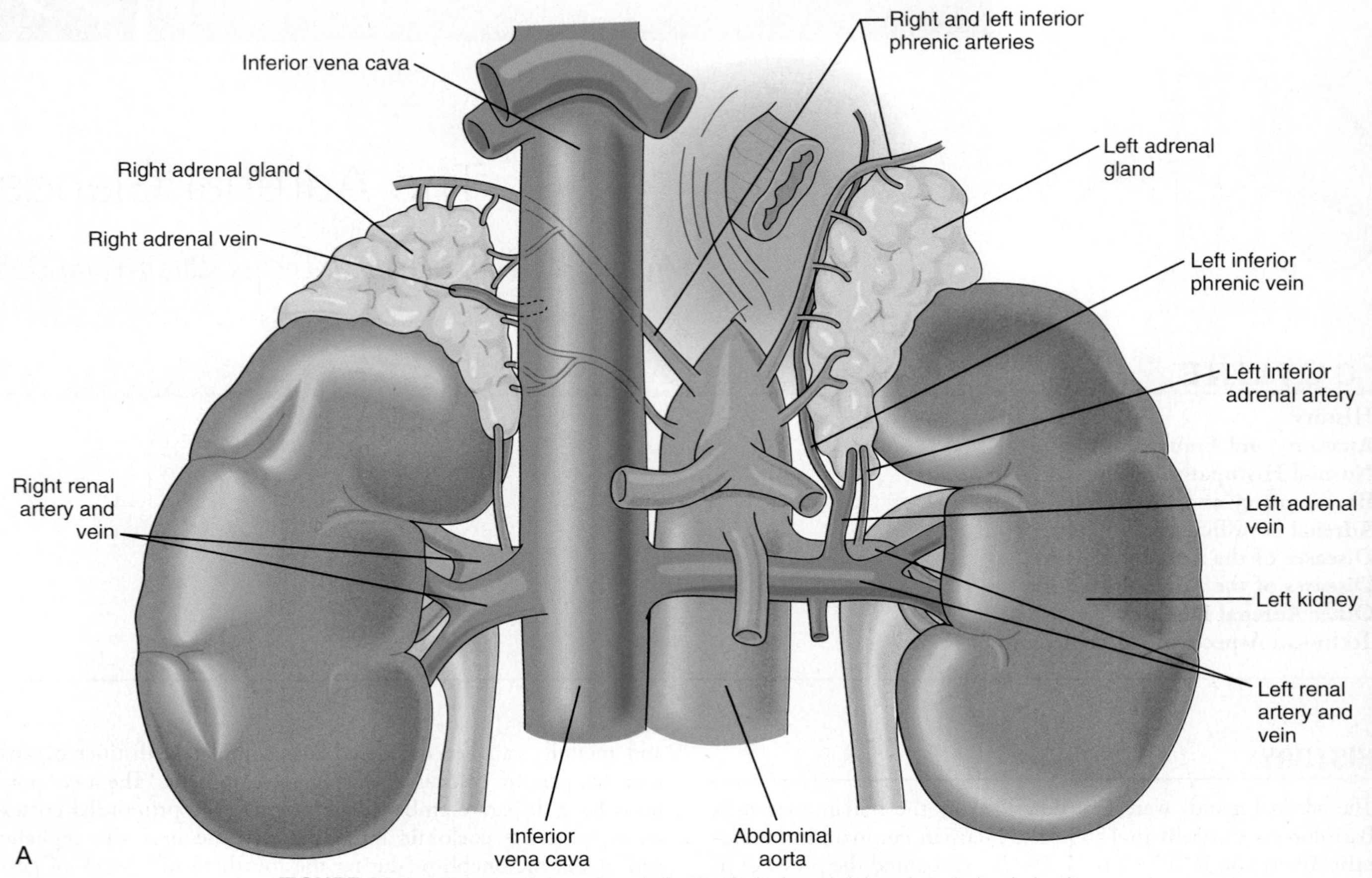

FIGURE 39-1 Anatomy of the adrenal glands. **A,** Left and right adrenal glands in situ.

Vasculature

Knowledge of the macroscopic vascular anatomy of the adrenal glands is essential to proper surgical management. It is important to conceptualize that although the arterial supply is *diffuse*, the venous drainage of each gland is usually *solitary*. The arterial supply arises from three distinct vessels—superior adrenal arteries from the inferior phrenic arteries, small middle adrenal arteries from the juxtaceliac aorta, and inferior adrenal arteries from the renal arteries. Of these, the inferior is the most prominent and is commonly a single identifiable vessel. The left adrenal vein is approximately 2 cm long and drains into the left renal vein after joining the inferior phrenic vein.[3] The right adrenal vein is typically as short as it is wide (0.5 cm) and drains directly into the vena cava. This configuration presents a surgical challenge that is discussed in more detail later in this chapter. In up to 20% of individuals, the right adrenal vein may drain into an accessory right hepatic vein or into the vena cava, at or near the confluence of such a vein. Vigilance about this variant and others (Fig. 39-3) may reduce the likelihood of intraoperative venous hemorrhage during right adrenalectomy.

NORMAL HISTOPATHOLOGY

The cortex is approximately 2 mm thick and composes more than 80% of the mass of the gland. It is made up of three layers (Fig. 39-4). The outer *zona glomerulosa* is a thin layer of relatively small cells with moderately eosinophilic, lipid-poor cytoplasm. It has an undulating inner border and normally does not form a complete circumferential layer. Most of the adrenal cortex is formed by the *zona fasciculata*, a middle layer composed of long radial columns of large, clear, lipid-laden cells. The inner *zona reticularis* is made up of small nests of compact, eosinophilic cells. The adrenal medulla consists of clusters and short cords of chromaffin cells, which are large, polyhedral, and packed with basophilic secretory granules. Catecholamines within these granules yield a brown reaction when treated with chromium salts, giving the cells their name. In contrast to the cortex, the adrenal medulla is richly endowed with autonomic nerve fibers and ganglion cells. Sympathetic fibers synapse directly with the chromaffin cells, constituting an interface between the nervous and endocrine systems.

The microvasculature of the adrenal gland functionally unifies the cortex and medulla. The adrenal arteries arborize extensively before entering the capsule to form a subcapsular plexus. Blood flows centripetally through capillaries in the zona glomerulosa and zona fasciculata before forming a deep plexus within the zona reticularis. From there, steroid-enriched postcapillary blood enters the medulla, where cortisol drives expression of phenylethanolamine *N*-methyltransferase (PNMT). PNMT is responsible for the conversion of norepinephrine to epinephrine. This microvascular arrangement is essentially a portal system between the cortex and medulla.

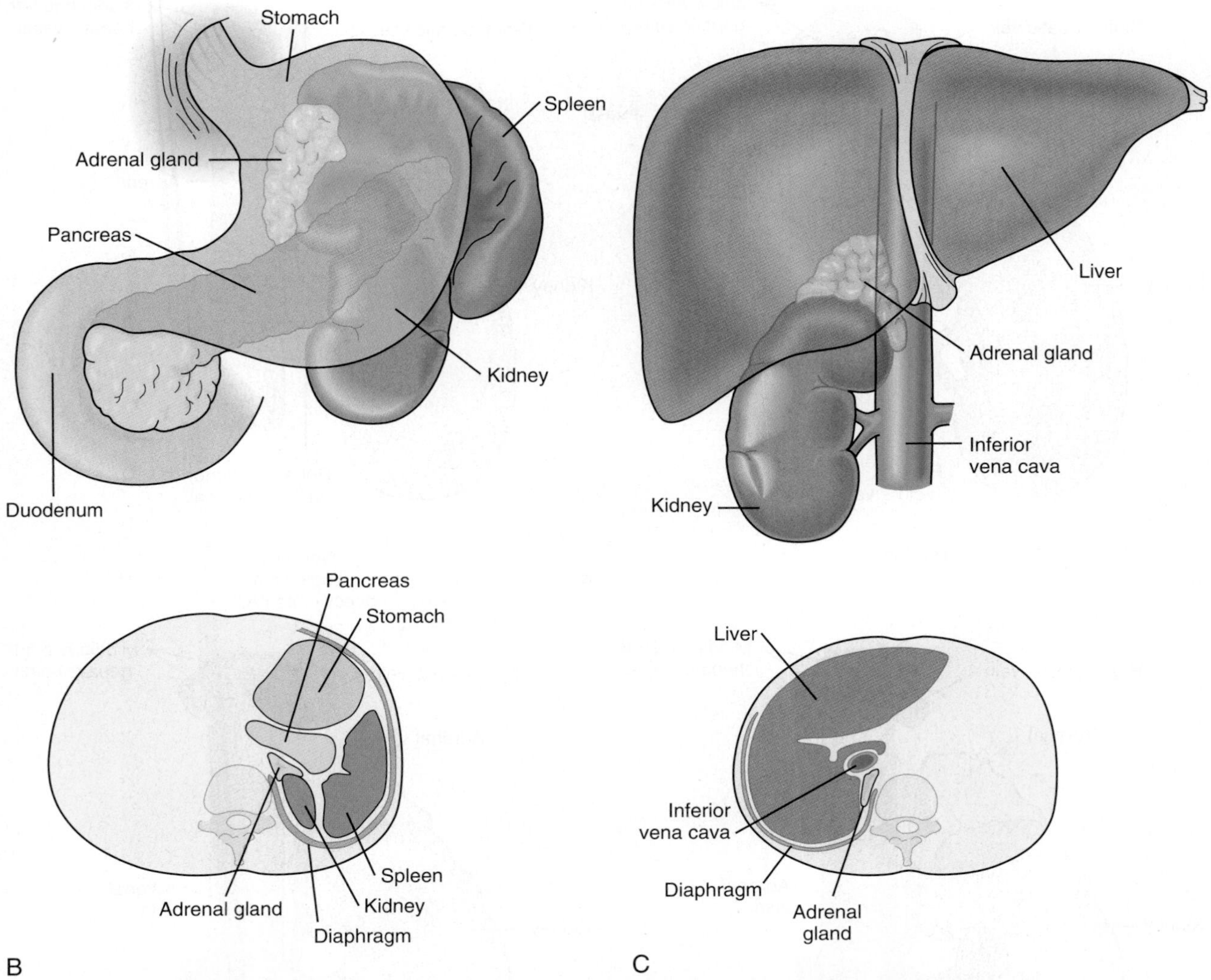

FIGURE 39-1, cont'd B, Relationships of the left adrenal gland. C, Relationships of the right adrenal gland.

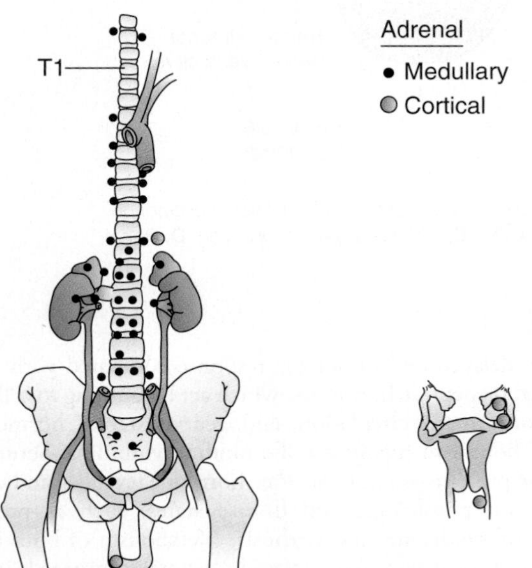

FIGURE 39-2 Sites of extra-adrenal cortical and medullary tissue.

BIOCHEMISTRY AND PHYSIOLOGY

Adrenal Steroid Biosynthesis

Adrenal steroid biosynthesis begins with the transport of cholesterol to the inner mitochondrial membrane by the steroidogenic acute regulatory protein (StAR; Fig. 39-5). Cholesterol then undergoes a series of oxidative reactions catalyzed predominantly by membrane-associated enzymes belonging to the cytochrome P450 (CYP) family. Cleavage of the cholesterol side chain yields the hormonally inactive compound pregnenolone, the immediate precursor to the adrenal steroid hormones. Serial oxidation by CYP17 converts pregnenolone and progesterone into the major adrenal sex steroids dehydroepiandrosterone (DHEA) and androstenedione. Additional enzymatic steps confined to the gonads generate testosterone, estrone, and estradiol from androstenedione. Oxidation of 17-hydroxypregnenolone by 3β-hydroxysteroid dehydrogenase followed by action of CYP21A2 and CYP11B1 yields cortisol, the active glucocorticoid hormone in humans. Aldosterone is generated by the oxidation of corticosterone by CYP11B2 within the zona glomerulosa. CYP17 expression is confined to the zona fasciculata and zona reticularis, accounting

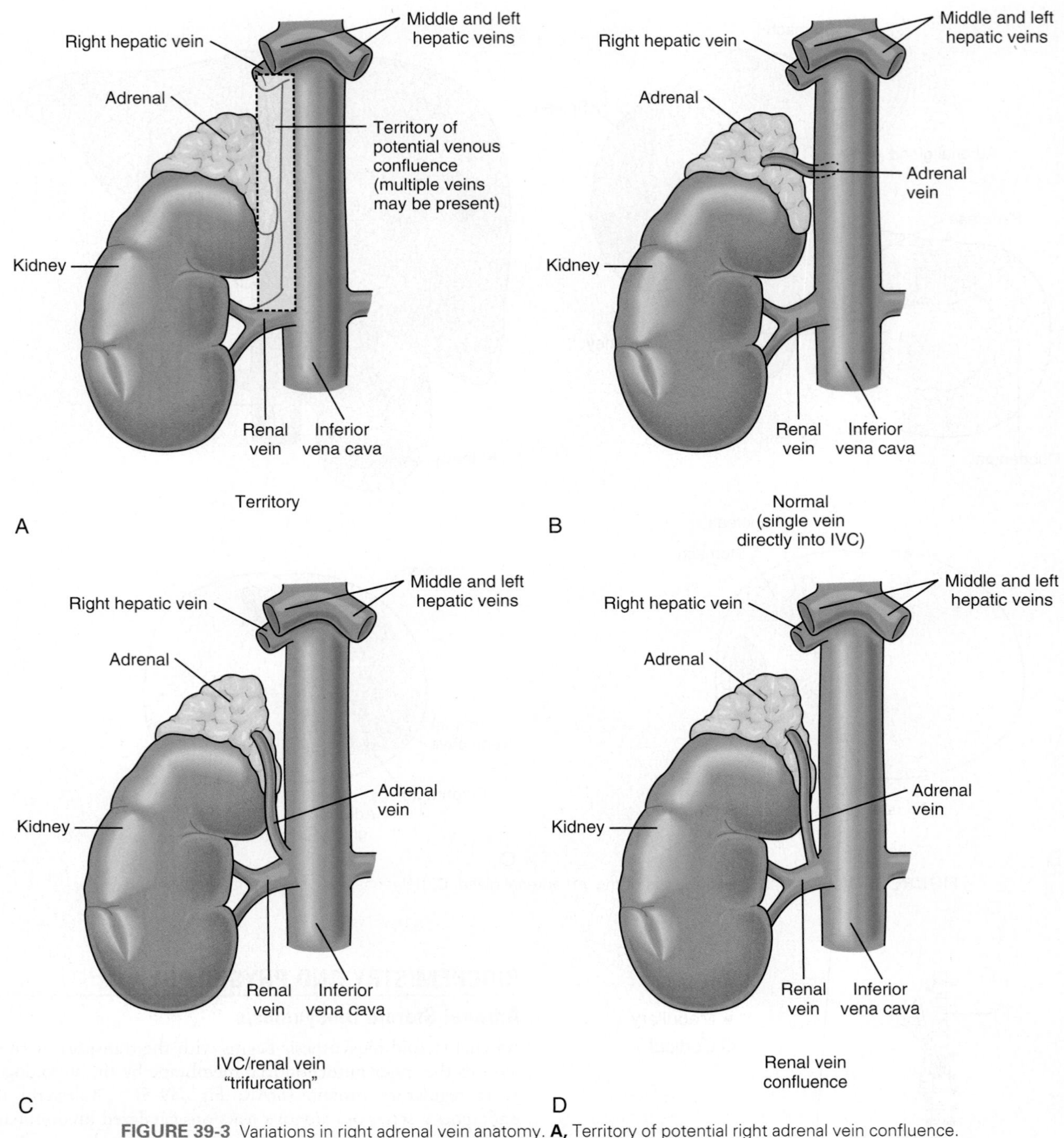

FIGURE 39-3 Variations in right adrenal vein anatomy. **A,** Territory of potential right adrenal vein confluence. **B,** Normal (>80%); single vein directly into the inferior vena cava (IVC). **C,** IVC–renal vein trifurcation. **D,** Renal vein confluence.

for the synthesis of glucocorticoids and adrenal sex steroids in these regions.

Steroid Hormone Physiology and Metabolism

Steroid hormones belong to a general class of low-molecular-weight, lipophilic signaling molecules that act by entering cells and binding to intracellular receptors. This group of hormones also includes thyroid hormone, retinoids, and vitamin D. Hormone binding results in alterations in gene expression that show a delayed and prolonged response compared with changes induced by peptide hormones, which act by binding to cell surface receptors. In the circulation, endogenous steroid hormones are largely bound to highly specific binding globulins. Serum levels of these proteins—and hence free hormone levels—can be altered by certain physiologic and disease states, such as pregnancy, nephrotic syndrome, and cirrhosis. Metabolism of both endogenous and pharmacologic steroids generally proceeds through hydroxylation, sulfonation, or conjugation to glucuronic acid in

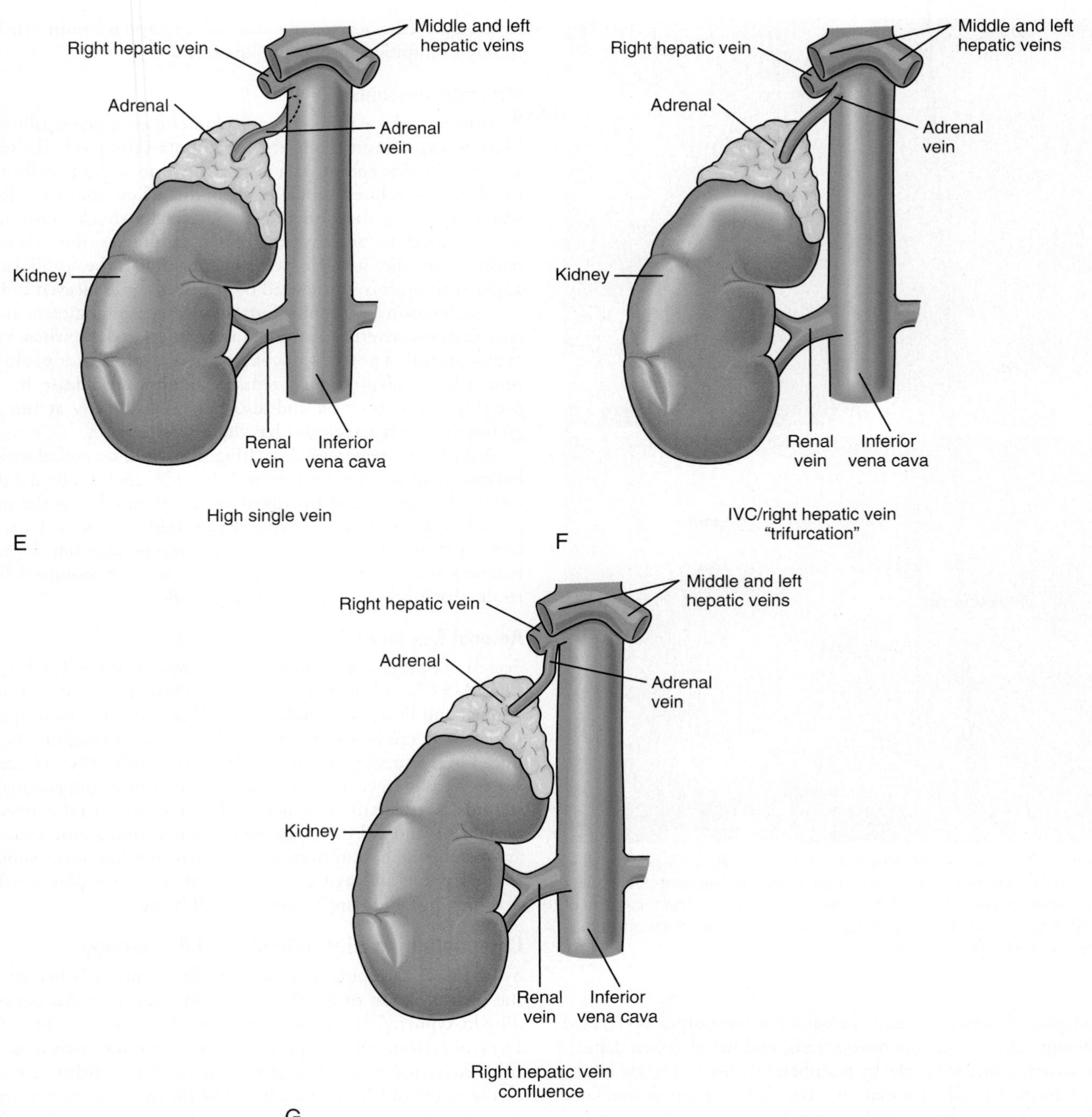

FIGURE 39-3, cont'd **E,** High single vein into the IVC. **F,** IVC–right hepatic vein trifurcation. **G,** Right hepatic vein confluence.

the liver, followed by urinary excretion. The regulation and physiologic actions of individual steroid hormones are discussed here.

Glucocorticoids

The release of corticotropin-releasing factor into the hypothalamic-pituitary portal system by hypothalamic neurons results in adrenocorticotropic hormone (ACTH) secretion by the anterior pituitary. ACTH binds to a G protein–coupled receptor on the adrenocortical cell surface and stimulates glucocorticoid secretion. Steroidogenesis is acutely upregulated by increased StAR-mediated cholesterol transport and pregnenolone synthesis by CYP11A1. ACTH is released in a pulsatile fashion that normally displays a circadian rhythm. The highest levels of ACTH and thus of cortisol are generally detected on waking, with levels gradually declining throughout the day to reach a nadir in the early evening. This pattern must be considered in evaluating patients for glucocorticoid deficiency or excess.

Glucocorticoid hormones have broad-ranging effects on almost all organ systems in the body. As a rule, they generate a catabolic state that characterizes the body's response to stress. The hormones are so named because they cause alterations in carbohydrate, protein, and lipid metabolism that have the net effect of increasing

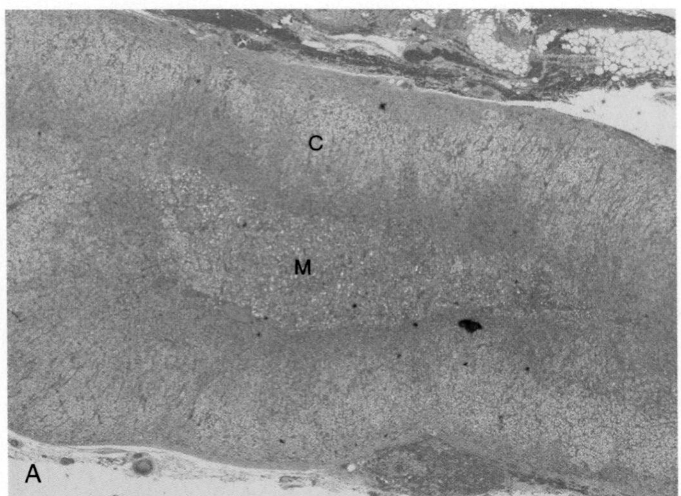

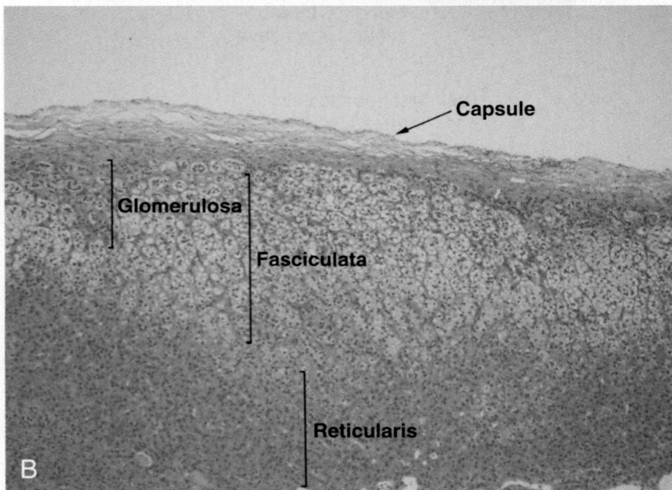

FIGURE 39-4 Normal adrenal histopathology. **A,** Low-power view showing the adrenal cortex (C) and medulla (M). **B,** Medium-power view demonstrating individual layers of the adrenal cortex. The thickness of the zona glomerulosa varies along its length (hematoxylin and eosin stain). (Courtesy Dr. Anthony Gill.)

blood glucose concentrations. Hepatic glucose output is elevated by the upregulation of gluconeogenesis, and net glycogen deposition occurs. Glucose uptake by peripheral tissues is directly inhibited. Glucocorticoids stimulate lipolysis with release of free fatty acids into the circulation, and a general state of insulin resistance is induced, resulting in protein catabolism. Fatty acids and amino acids serve as energy sources and substrates for gluconeogenesis. In the cardiovascular system, glucocorticoids exert a permissive and enhancing effect on catecholamine signaling by sensitizing arterial smooth muscle cells to β-adrenergic stimulation and increasing catecholamine concentrations in neuromuscular junctions. Cardiac contractility and peripheral vascular tone are thus maintained, explaining why the hemodynamic collapse that accompanies acute adrenal insufficiency can be remedied by glucocorticoid administration.

Glucocorticoids are potent anti-inflammatory and immunosuppressive agents. Acutely, glucocorticoids reduce circulating lymphocyte and eosinophil counts while increasing neutrophil counts. Lymphocyte apoptosis is promoted, cytokine and immunoglobulin production is decreased, and histamine release is suppressed. Glucocorticoids also reduce prostaglandin synthesis through inhibition of phospholipase A2.

Mineralocorticoids

Aldosterone release from the zona glomerulosa is principally regulated by angiotensin II and the blood potassium level. The renin-angiotensin-aldosterone axis is responsive to sodium delivery to the distal convoluted tubule of the kidney. Low sodium delivery, which occurs in states such as hypovolemia, shock, renal artery vasoconstriction, and hyponatremia, stimulates the release of renin from the juxtaglomerular apparatus. The prohormone angiotensinogen is synthesized by the liver and is cleaved to inactive angiotensin I by renin. Further cleavage of angiotensin I by angiotensin-converting enzyme in the lungs and elsewhere yields angiotensin II, a potent vasoconstrictor and stimulator of aldosterone release. Hypokalemia reduces aldosterone release by suppressing renin secretion and also by acting directly at the zona glomerulosa. Hyperkalemia has the opposite effect.

Aldosterone regulates circulating fluid volume and electrolyte balance by promoting sodium and chloride retention by the distal tubule. Potassium and hydrogen ion are secreted into the urine. Acutely, expansion of the extracellular fluid volume and a rise in blood pressure are observed after aldosterone infusion. Negative feedback occurs primarily through an increase in sodium delivery to the distal tubule, suppressing renin release.

Adrenal Sex Steroids

Secretion of the adrenal androgens androstenedione, DHEA, and DHEA-S (the sulfonated derivative of DHEA, synthesized in the adrenal and liver) is regulated by ACTH and other incompletely understood mechanisms. Of the three, androstenedione is produced in the smallest quantities. The physiologic effects of adrenal sex steroids are generally weak in comparison to the gonadal sex steroids, particularly in males. In females, peripheral conversion of DHEA and DHEA-S to more potent androgens, including androstenedione, testosterone, and dihydrotestosterone, supports normal pubic and axillary hair growth and may play a role in maintaining libido and a sense of well-being.

Catecholamine Biosynthesis and Physiology

Synthesis of catecholamines in the adrenal medulla begins with the hydroxylation of tyrosine, a rate-limiting step that generates dihydroxyphenylalanine (L-dopa) in the cytosol (Fig. 39-6). Decarboxylation of L-dopa generates dopamine, which is then β-hydroxylated to form norepinephrine. Epinephrine is created by the action of PNMT, which, unlike the other enzymes involved in catecholamine synthesis, is localized to the chromaffin cells of the adrenal medulla and organ of Zuckerkandl. Sympathetic stimulation of the adrenal medulla results in the release of stored catecholamines into the circulation. Basal levels of adrenal catecholamine secretion are normally low, although large (up to 50-fold) increases in levels may be observed in response to major physiologic or psychological stressors. Target tissue responses are mediated by α- and β-adrenergic receptors. α-Adrenergic receptors display greater affinity for norepinephrine compared with epinephrine, and the opposite is true for β-adrenergic receptors. Stimulation of β_1-adrenergic receptors in the myocardium results in increased heart rate and contractility. Stimulation of β_2-adrenergic receptors results in smooth muscle relaxation in tissues such as the uterus, bronchi, and skeletal muscle arterioles. α_1-Adrenergic receptors mediate vasoconstriction in tissues such as the skin and gastrointestinal tract. α_2-Adrenergic receptors exist

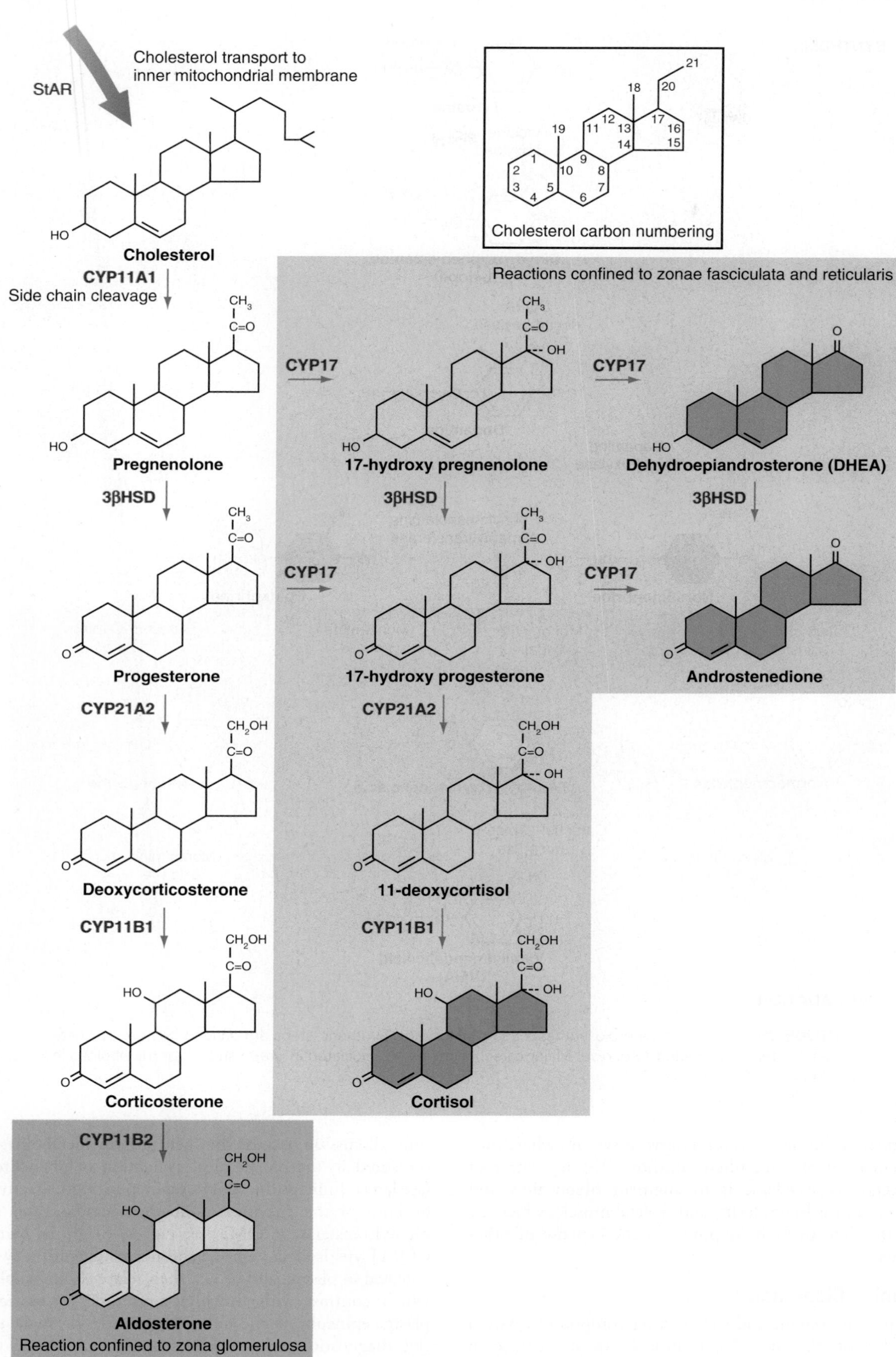

FIGURE 39-5 Adrenal steroid biosynthesis. Reactions confined to the zona glomerulosa are shaded *turquoise*, and those confined to the zonae fasciculata and reticularis are shaded *orange*. Human mineralocorticoids are indicated in *yellow*, glucocorticoids in *green*, and sex steroids in *blue*. *3β-HSD*, 3β-hydroxysteroid dehydrogenase; *StAR*, steroidogenic acute regulatory protein.

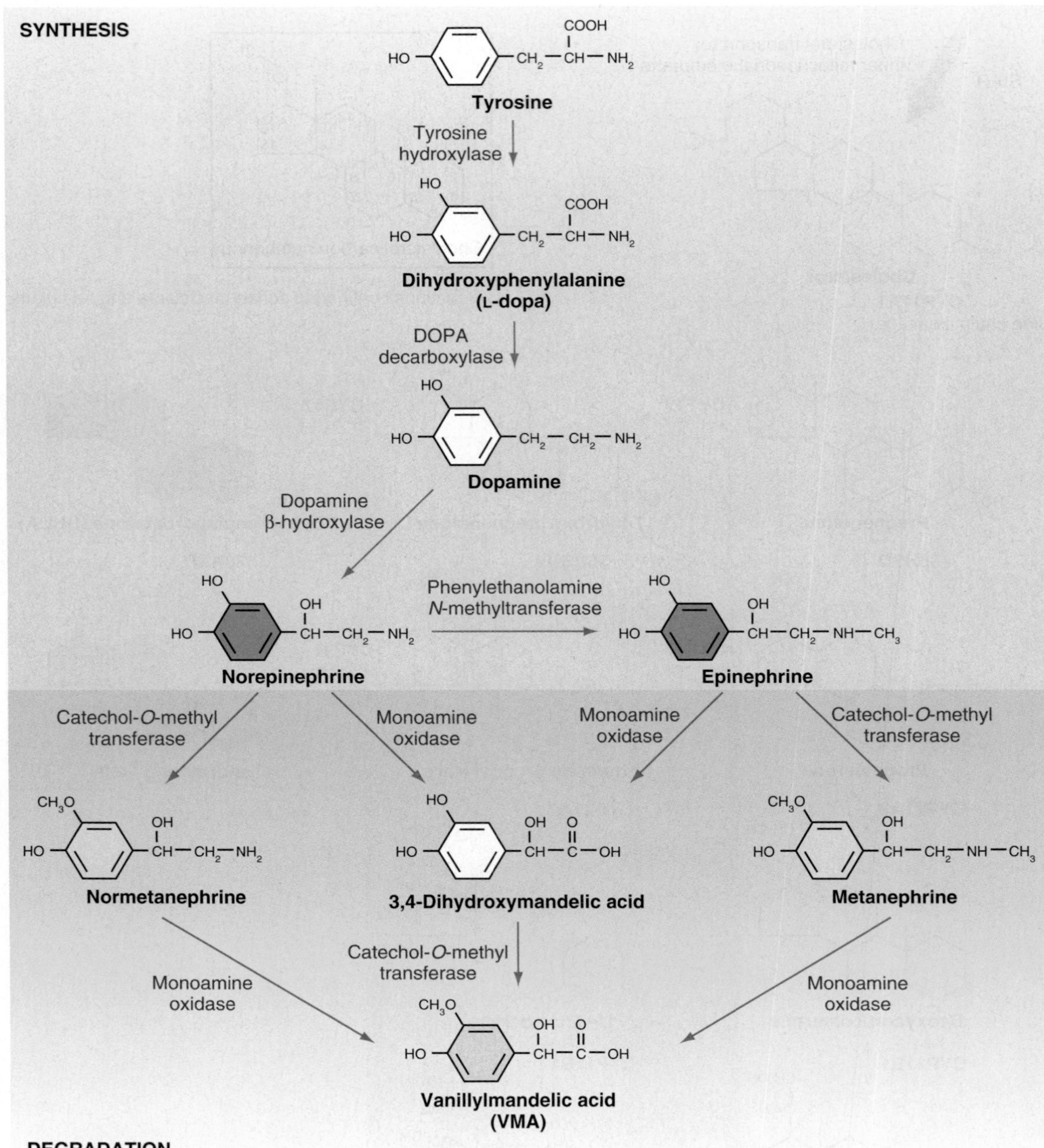

FIGURE 39-6 Catecholamine biosynthesis and metabolism. Synthetic steps are shaded *orange,* and degradative steps are shaded *turquoise.* Major catecholamines are indicated in *green* and major metabolites in *yellow.*

in presynaptic locations in the central nervous system, where they mediate attenuation of sympathetic outflow. The net effect of adrenal catecholamine release is to augment blood flow and oxygen delivery to the brain, heart, and skeletal muscle, which are essential to the fight-or-flight response, at the expense of other organ systems.

Catecholamine Clearance

Catecholamines are potent and short-acting compounds, with a plasma half-life on the order of 1 minute. Their presence in synapses and the circulation exhibits tight negative regulation by both reuptake and degradation. Degradation pathways merit some discussion because they generate the metabolites commonly measured in the biochemical evaluation of pheochromocytoma (see later). Epinephrine and norepinephrine are inactivated by one or both of the enzymes monoamine oxidase and catechol-*O*-methyltransferase (COMT; see Fig. 39-6). Initial methylation by COMT yields metanephrine and normetanephrine, which can be detected in plasma and urine. Their relatively stable plasma levels, which contrast with the high-amplitude fluctuations seen in plasma epinephrine and norepinephrine levels, make them attractive diagnostic markers.[4] The sequential action of monoamine oxidase and COMT generates the major final product, vanillylmandelic acid. Catecholamine metabolites are excreted in the urine, sometimes after sulfonation or conjugation to glucuronic acid in the liver.

ADRENAL INSUFFICIENCY

Types of Adrenal Insufficiency

Primary Adrenal Insufficiency (Addison Disease)

Originally described in patients with tuberculous destruction of the adrenal glands, this rare disease is manifested with weakness and fatigue, anorexia, nausea or vomiting, weight loss, hyperpigmentation, hypotension, and electrolyte disturbances (hyponatremia and hyperkalemia). Hyperpigmentation, previously believed to be caused by elevated levels of pro-opiomelanocortin and its cleavage product α-melanocyte-stimulating hormone, is now believed to result from ACTH-induced melanogenesis.[5] Hormonal insufficiency caused by intrinsic adrenal disease arises from three general mechanisms—congenital adrenal dysgenesis/hypoplasia, defective steroidogenesis, and adrenal destruction. Of these, adrenal destruction from autoimmune causes is the most common, followed by infectious adrenalitis (e.g., tuberculous, fungal, viral), adrenal replacement by metastatic tumor, and adrenal hemorrhage (Waterhouse-Friderichsen syndrome). The last occurs in the setting of septicemia caused by meningococcal or other organisms and is more common in pediatric and asplenic patients.

Secondary Adrenal Insufficiency

Secondary adrenal insufficiency is a relatively common disorder resulting from ACTH deficiency, often occurring in the setting of pharmacologic steroid withdrawal. Patients receiving high supraphysiologic doses of glucocorticoids (more than the equivalent of 20 mg of prednisone daily; Table 39-1) for more than 5 days and those receiving low supraphysiologic doses for more than 3 weeks are at risk for HPA axis suppression. Surgical cure of Cushing syndrome (see later) likewise results in glucocorticoid withdrawal. The rate of recovery from HPA axis suppression varies in accordance with the duration and severity of previous glucocorticoid excess, and the need for glucocorticoid supplementation may last several years.[6] Other less common causes of secondary adrenal insufficiency include panhypopituitarism caused by neoplastic or infiltrative replacement, granulomatous disease, and pituitary hemorrhage or infarction. Pituitary infarction may occur in the setting of severe postpartum hemorrhage (Sheehan syndrome).

Adrenal Insufficiency in the Critically Ill

Studies have suggested that critically ill patients with sepsis or systemic inflammatory response syndrome may be affected by acute reversible dysfunction of the HPA axis. The incidence of the disorder is approximately 30% in critically ill patients, although this figure may be higher in those with septic shock. Whether these patients incur increased mortality because of adrenal insufficiency remains to be defined. Proposed mechanisms of reversible HPA axis dysfunction include adrenal ACTH resistance and decreased responsiveness of target tissues to glucocorticoids. Glucocorticoid supplementation in septic patients has been the topic of at least 17 randomized controlled trials. Among these studies, there appears to be an inverse relationship between survival benefit and glucocorticoid dose, with physiologic (i.e., replacement) doses yielding a relative survival benefit of 1.2 and high supraphysiologic doses demonstrating significant harm. Although the data remain controversial, evidence has suggested that patients with septic shock, particularly those requiring vasopressors, may benefit from 5- to 7-day courses of glucocorticoids in the dosage range of 300 mg/day or less of hydrocortisone or equivalent.[7]

Adrenal Crisis

Acute adrenal insufficiency, or adrenal crisis, is a life-threatening condition that typically occurs in individuals with already marginal adrenocortical function who are subjected to a significant acute physiologic stressor, such as infection or trauma. Sudden and complete loss of adrenal function, as occurs with Waterhouse-Friderichsen syndrome and certain hypercoagulable states, can also be manifested with adrenal crisis. Clinical findings include shock, abdominal pain, fever, nausea and vomiting, electrolyte disturbances, and occasionally hypoglycemia. Mineralocorticoid deficiency, resulting in an inability to maintain sodium and intravascular volume, is the primary pathogenic mechanism, although diminished cardiovascular responsiveness to catecholamines caused by glucocorticoid deficiency also plays a role. The treatment of adrenal crisis centers around large-volume (>2 liters) intravenous resuscitation with isotonic saline and glucocorticoid administration in the form of hydrocortisone (100 mg intravenously every 6 to 8 hours) or dexamethasone (4 mg intravenously every 24 hours). Dexamethasone is long-acting and carries the advantage of not interfering with biochemical assays of endogenous glucocorticoid production. Ironically, mineralocorticoid replacement is not an early priority because the sodium- and fluid-retaining effects of mineralocorticoids are not manifested

TABLE 39-1 Properties of Endogenous and Commonly Used Pharmacologic Glucocorticoids

COMPOUND	IV/PO*	COMMON TRADE NAME	RELATIVE POTENCY	DAILY PHYSIOLOGIC DOSE	DOSING INTERVAL
Cortisol = hydrocortisone	Both	Cortef (PO) Solu-Cortef (IV)	1×	20 mg	q8-12h
Cortisone	PO	—	0.8×	25 mg	q8-12h
Prednisone	PO	—	4×	5 mg	q24h
Prednisolone	PO	—	4×	5 mg	q24h
Methylprednisolone	Both	Medrol (PO) Solu-Medrol (IV)	5×	4 mg	q24h
Dexamethasone†	Both	Decadron	25×	1 mg	q24h

*Oral and intravenous dosages are similar.
†Does not cross-react with the cortisol assay.

until several days after administration. Fluid and electrolyte balance can be rapidly achieved by saline infusion.

Diagnosis and Treatment

Diagnosis

As is true for most endocrine disorders, the diagnosis of adrenal insufficiency depends on maintaining sufficient clinical suspicion for the disease. The clinical manifestations have been discussed earlier. Surgeons are most likely to encounter patients with adrenal insufficiency in the intensive care unit, trauma suite, or operating room when treating patients with steroid-dependent chronic illnesses. Routine and provocative biochemical testing is necessary to confirm the diagnosis (Fig. 39-7). The first step is to document inadequate cortisol production, which can be done by measuring morning levels of cortisol in the serum or saliva. In most patients, morning serum cortisol concentration higher than 15 μg/dL or morning salivary cortisol concentration higher than 5.8 ng/mL effectively excludes adrenal insufficiency. Patients whose levels fall below these thresholds should undergo provocative testing. A high-dose cosyntropin stimulation test is performed by administering 250 μg cosyntropin and measuring serum cortisol levels 30 to 60 minutes later. A positive test result (i.e., a stimulated cortisol level lower than 18 μg/dL) is strongly suggestive of adrenal insufficiency. After the diagnosis of adrenal insufficiency has been made, a morning ACTH level is determined to differentiate between primary and secondary adrenal insufficiency.

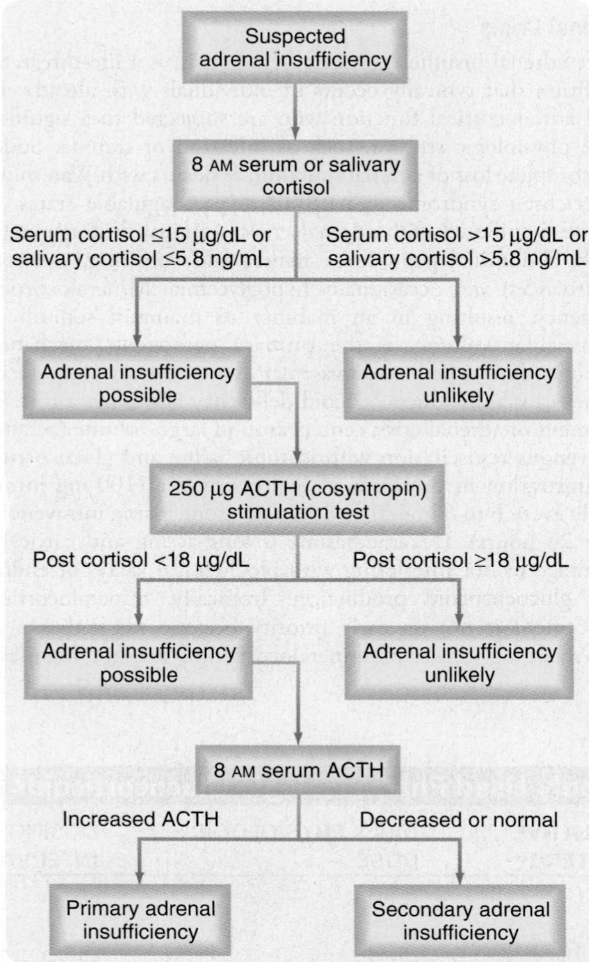

FIGURE 39-7 Algorithm for the diagnosis of adrenal insufficiency. The adequacy of cortisol production is initially assessed with morning cortisol level measurement. Patients with low or borderline values undergo provocative ACTH stimulation testing, with serum cortisol levels measured before and 30 to 60 minutes after the administration of ACTH. Failure to mount an adequate response to ACTH usually establishes the diagnosis of adrenal insufficiency. The cause of adrenal insufficiency is then investigated with a morning ACTH level measurement.

Treatment

The treatment of adrenal crisis has been discussed. The goal of maintenance therapy for chronic adrenal insufficiency is to replace physiologic glucocorticoid and mineralocorticoid levels. Daily adult cortisol production is in the range of 10 to 20 mg, which can be replaced by the long-acting, orally bioavailable agent prednisone at a dosage of 5 mg/day. Typical mineralocorticoid replacement consists of fludrocortisone, 0.1 mg/day. Commensurate increased dosages of glucocorticoids are needed during periods of minor and major physiologic stress, such as mild infections (minor) and trauma, significant infections, burns, or elective surgery (major).

Perioperative Steroid Administration

Recommendations concerning glucocorticoid administration during elective surgery have been based primarily on uncontrolled retrospective studies. The need for supraphysiologic doses of glucocorticoids in this setting has generally been overstated. Patients with primary adrenal insufficiency (Addison disease) are at increased risk for perioperative adrenal crisis because of their inability to increase endogenous cortisol production in response to stress. They generally require hydrocortisone 100 mg intravenously just before induction of anesthesia. Patients with secondary adrenal insufficiency caused by chronic glucocorticoid treatment for autoimmune or inflammatory conditions have only a 1% to 2% risk of hypotensive crisis without perioperative glucocorticoid coverage. To prevent this rare but hazardous complication, chronic glucocorticoid users should, at the least, be maintained on their usual glucocorticoid dosage throughout the perioperative period. Supplementation above this level should be given in short courses according to the guidelines listed in Table 39-2.[8] Patients undergoing unilateral adrenalectomy should be given supplemental glucocorticoids only if the underlying diagnosis is Cushing syndrome.

DISEASES OF THE ADRENAL CORTEX

Primary Hyperaldosteronism

Epidemiology and Clinical Features

Primary hyperaldosteronism, the unregulated release of excess aldosterone from one or both adrenal glands, was first described by Jerome Conn in 1954. Primary hyperaldosteronism classically is manifested with resistant hypertension and hypokalemia, although studies have revealed that most patients may be normokalemic, depending on the population screened. Hypokalemia is likely a manifestation of severe or late-stage disease. The prevalence of primary hyperaldosteronism has been the topic of considerable debate. It was generally believed to affect approximately 1% of hypertensives. Widespread application of the aldosterone-to-renin ratio (see later) as a screening test in certain centers led to reports of a 10% to 40% prevalence of primary hyperaldosteronism among hypertensive patients. There is some consensus that

TABLE 39-2 Perioperative Glucocorticoid Regimens for Patients With Secondary Adrenal Insufficiency*

DEGREE OF SURGICAL STRESS	EXAMPLES	INTRAOPERATIVE GLUCOCORTICOID DOSAGE	GLUCOCORTICOID TAPER
Minor	Procedures under local anesthetic, most outpatient procedures, inguinal hernia repair	None (take usual morning steroid dosage)	None (continue to take usual dosage)
Moderate	Routine abdominal, peripheral vascular, or orthopedic surgery	Hydrocortisone 50 mg or equivalent before procedure	Hydrocortisone 25 mg every 8 hours for 24 hours, then resume usual dosage
Major	Resection of gastrointestinal cancer, cardiopulmonary bypass	Hydrocortisone 100 mg or equivalent before procedure	Hydrocortisone 50 mg every 8 hours for 24 hours, then taper by half every day to usual dosage

*Caused by chronic pharmacologic steroid use.

these higher figures reflect strong referral bias and that the actual prevalence in unselected hypertensive patients is likely to be 7% or less.[9] Nonselective use of the aldosterone-to-renin ratio to identify patients with primary hyperaldosteronism is known to decrease the fraction of patients with surgically correctible disease (unilateral aldosteronoma) significantly, although the absolute number of surgically treatable cases has increased.

The mean age at diagnosis for primary hyperaldosteronism is approximately 50 years, and the disease has a slight male predilection. Most patients are asymptomatic, although patients with significant hypokalemia may complain of muscle cramps, weakness, or paresthesias. Patients typically have moderate to severe hypertension that is refractory to medical therapy. It is common for them to require two to four antihypertensive medications. Responsiveness to spironolactone may be seen, a feature that is predictive of a good response to surgical treatment.

Primary hyperaldosteronism is a potentially curable cause of significant cardiovascular disease. A study comparing 270 subjects with biochemically confirmed primary hyperaldosteronism with case-matched hypertensive controls has revealed that primary hyperaldosteronism is associated with a significantly increased risk of stroke, myocardial infarction, arrhythmias including atrial and ventricular fibrillation, and heart failure.[10] These results add to existing evidence indicating that the adverse cardiovascular sequelae of primary hyperaldosteronism are more pronounced than those caused by blood pressure elevation alone. Successful removal of an aldosteronoma leads to regression of many of these adverse physiologic changes.

The most common causes of primary hyperaldosteronism are unilateral aldosterone-producing adenomas (aldosteronomas; Fig. 39-8) and bilateral adrenal hyperplasia (also termed idiopathic hyperaldosteronism; Table 39-3). In the past, aldosteronoma was present in more than 60% of cases, but this number has decreased substantially as nonselective screening with the aldosterone-to-renin ratio has been applied. This phenomenon may reflect increased detection of hyperplasia, which is characterized by milder biochemical abnormalities than aldosteronoma. Recent sequencing of aldosterone-producing adrenal nodules has revealed somatic mutations in the potassium channel gene, which may provide insight into the pathogenesis of primary hyperaldosteronism.[11]

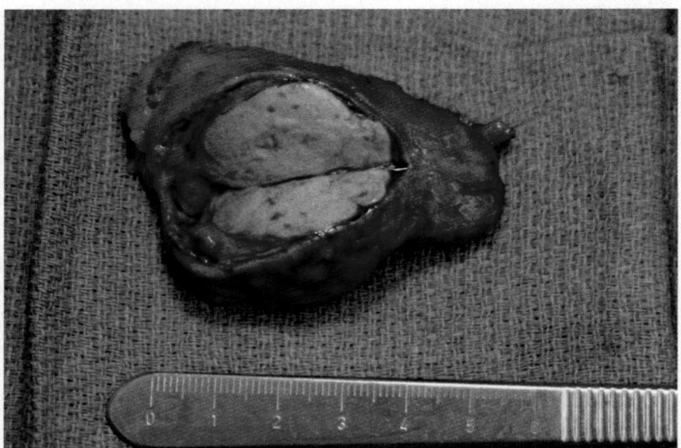

FIGURE 39-8 Classic canary-yellow aldosteronoma.

TABLE 39-3 Causes of Primary Hyperaldosteronism

	SCREENING*	
CAUSE	SELECTIVE (%)	NONSELECTIVE (%)
Aldosterone-producing adenoma	60	30
Bilateral adrenal hyperplasia (idiopathic hyperaldosteronism)	35	65
Aldosterone-producing adrenocortical carcinoma	<1	<1
Familial hyperaldosteronism		
Type I (glucocorticoid-remediable aldosteronism)	<1	<1
Type II (non–glucocorticoid-remediable aldosteronism)	<1	<1

*Rates of specific pathologic processes are highly dependent on the pattern of screening (selective versus nonselective).

Diagnosis and Localization

Biochemical diagnosis. The goal of diagnostic testing is to identify and to lateralize aldosteronomas. There is some consensus that biochemical screening should be performed in all patients with hypertension and unexplained hypokalemia as well as in those with hypertension sufficiently resistant to medical therapy to warrant investigation for secondary hypertension. Establishing the diagnosis of primary hyperaldosteronism begins with determining the ratio of plasma aldosterone concentration to plasma renin activity (expressed here as ng/dL divided by ng/[mL • hr]; Fig. 39-9). This test should be performed after discontinuation of interfering medications, such as spironolactone, angiotensin-converting enzyme inhibitors, diuretics, and β-adrenergic blockers. Variable cutoff values for the aldosterone-to-renin ratio have been used in the literature, with the most commonly cited value of 30 yielding a sensitivity of approximately 90%. Some centers have advocated a lower threshold of 20; this increases sensitivity at some cost to specificity and conceptually reflects appreciation of the clinical gravity of failing to diagnose surgically correctable hyperaldosteronism.[12] A subset of patients with essential hypertension will have suppressed renin levels, which may result in false elevations of the aldosterone-to-renin ratio. Thus, the inclusion of an absolute aldosterone concentration higher than 15 mg/dL increases the specificity of initial screening. Patients who test positive and are younger than 30 years should be genetically screened for glucocorticoid-remediable aldosteronism (familial hyperaldosteronism type I), especially if they have a family history of early-onset hypertension. This rare autosomal dominant condition results in abnormal regulation of aldosterone synthesis by ACTH and can be medically treated.

Confirmatory biochemical testing is aimed at demonstrating inappropriately high (nonsuppressible) aldosterone levels by creating a state of hypervolemia–sodium excess. This is done with intravenous saline loading (2 to 3 liters of isotonic saline given during 4 to 6 hours, followed by measurement of plasma aldosterone) or oral salt loading (200 mEq = 5000 mg sodium daily during 3 days, followed by measurement of 24-hour urine aldosterone excretion). Some centers administer high-dose fludrocortisone (0.1 mg every 6 hours) during oral salt loading to increase the specificity of suppression testing, but this method has not been widely adopted.

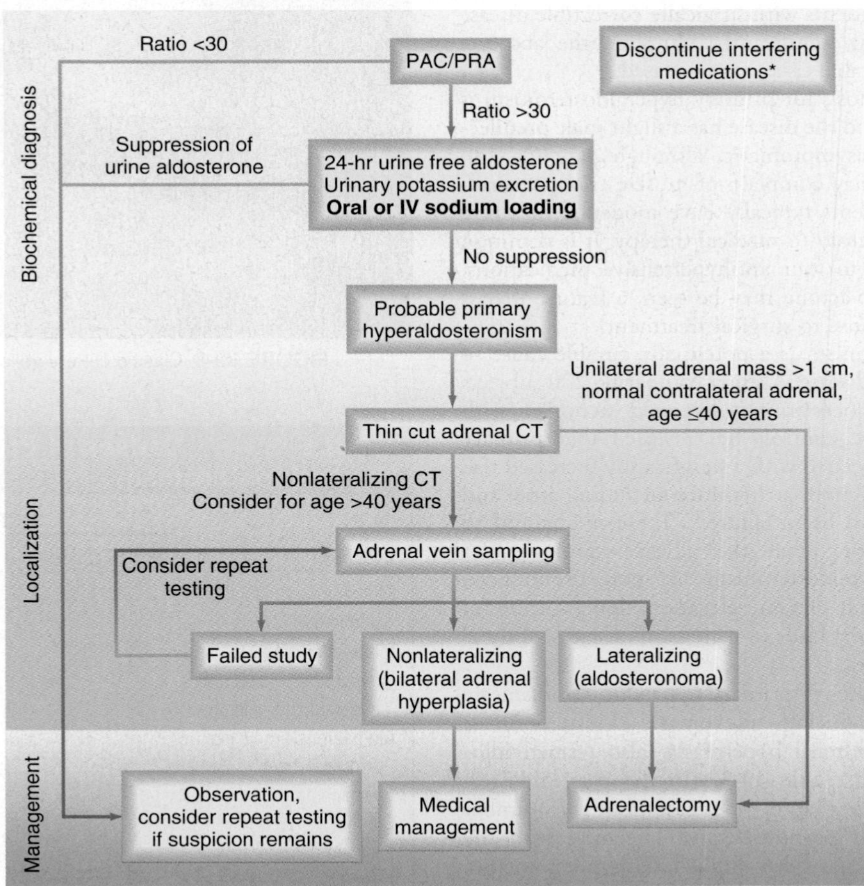

FIGURE 39-9 Algorithm for diagnosis, localization, and management of primary hyperaldosteronism. Initial screening is done with determination of the PRA/PAC ratio, followed by confirmatory testing with sodium loading. After the biochemical diagnosis has been established, noninvasive localization is attempted with computed tomography (CT). Patients with clear CT evidence of a unilateral abnormality can proceed to adrenalectomy with a more than 90% cure rate. Adrenal vein sampling is done in patients with equivocal CT findings and older patients, especially those older than 60 years, because nonfunctional cortical adenomas are found in 4% or more of this population and can cause false-positive CT localization. *ACE,* angiotensin-converting enzyme; *PAC,* plasma aldosterone concentration, in ng/dL; *PRA,* plasma renin activity, in ng/(mL • hr).

Localization. After the diagnosis has been confirmed, localization is performed with anatomic imaging, selective venous sampling, and sometimes functional scanning. The fact that most aldosteronomas are smaller than 15 mm in maximum dimension poses some challenges to localization. Thin-cut (3 mm) adrenal computed tomography (CT) scanning is the preferred initial localization test (Fig. 39-10).

The next step in the localization algorithm is selective adrenal vein sampling (AVS). This test relies on the simultaneous measurement of cortisol and aldosterone levels in the peripheral circulation and left and right adrenal veins (Fig. 39-11). More than a fivefold elevation of the cortisol concentration in a sample relative to peripheral blood indicates successful cannulation of an adrenal vein (positive control). Lateralization is indicated by an unbalanced ratio of aldosterone to cortisol in the left and right adrenal veins, with the ratio on one side being fourfold higher than the other to identify the culprit gland. Considerable controversy exists about which patients should undergo AVS, an invasive procedure with a 90% technical success rate in experienced hands. There is consensus that AVS should be applied in all cases in which the biochemical diagnosis of primary hyperaldosteronism has been confirmed and thin-cut adrenal CT reveals no abnormalities or bilateral abnormalities. Of the remaining patients who have a unilateral mass on CT scan, a small but not insignificant fraction (2% to 10%) will represent false-positive localization and have persistent hyperaldosteronism after unilateral adrenalectomy. In these patients, the adrenal mass represents a nonfunctioning cortical adenoma, and the true underlying diagnosis is a contralateral microaldosteronoma or bilateral adrenal hyperplasia, the latter of which is not surgically remediable.

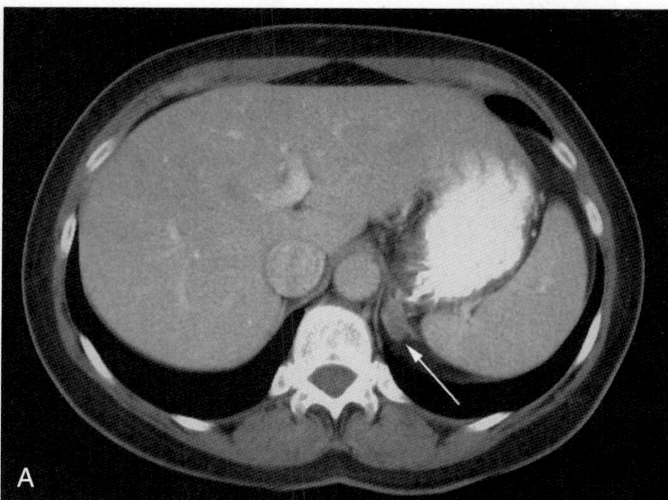

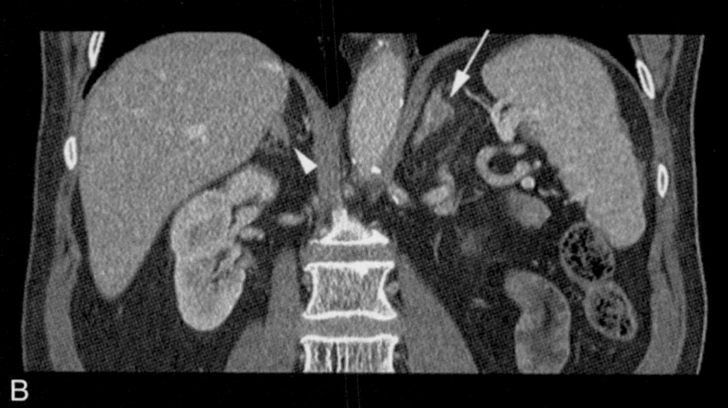

FIGURE 39-10 Appearance of aldosteronoma on anatomic imaging. **A,** Venous phase, contrast-enhanced CT scan demonstrating a 2-cm left aldosteronoma *(arrow)*. **B,** Late arterial phase, coronal CT scan demonstrating a 1.7-cm left aldosteronoma *(arrow)* and a normal right adrenal gland *(arrowhead)*.

Because patients 40 years and older are more likely to possess nonfunctioning adrenal cortical adenomas, some authors have advocated AVS in all older patients,[13] and others have recommended universal application of this test in the workup of primary hyperaldosteronism.[14] It has been our practice to perform AVS selectively. Patients found to have a unilateral cortical adrenal mass larger than 1 cm in diameter and a normal contralateral adrenal gland on CT can proceed directly to adrenalectomy, whereas those without definitive CT localization undergo AVS. This strategy has yielded cure rates in excess of 95%.[15] In consideration of the body of literature, we advocate for more liberal application of AVS for patients 40 years and older.

Practically speaking, approximately 20% to 30% of patients being evaluated for primary hyperaldosteronism undergo AVS when it is applied to select patients. The usefulness of the test is limited by its low success rate in most reports (40% to 80%), with the most common reason for incomplete AVS being failure to cannulate the right adrenal vein. Frequently, however, sufficient lateralizing information is provided during AVS to guide surgical treatment, even when the study is not bilaterally selective.[16]

Surgical Management and Outcomes

Laparoscopic adrenalectomy is the preferred procedure for the management of aldosteronoma and most other adrenal tumors.[17] Cure of primary hyperaldosteronism is defined by clinical and biochemical end points. Reductions in blood pressure, antihypertensive medication requirements, and plasma and urine aldosterone levels and resolution of hypokalemia (if previously present) are observed as soon as 24 hours after successful surgery. Overall cure rates range from 75% to 95% at subspecialty centers, depending on the specific criteria for cure that are used. In general, more than 80% of patients can expect either normalization of blood pressure or a significant reduction in antihypertensive medication requirements (typically, from three to four medications down to one). In some patients, depending on the degree of preoperative sodium overload, blood pressure may take several weeks to improve. Our practice is to stop all antihypertensive medications immediately after surgery, with the exception of beta blockers and clonidine, which must be tapered to avoid a rebound phenomenon. For those patients who continue to be hypertensive in the short term, medications may be added back temporarily, as needed, until the blood pressure gradually reaches a new equilibrium over time.

A subset of patients with the following preoperative features display reduced benefit from surgical treatment and continue to require antihypertensive medications after operation: men older than 45 years, family history of hypertension, long-standing hypertension, requirement of more than two antihypertensive medications, and nonresponse to spironolactone. These indicate a component of essential hypertension and, in some cases, irreversible cardiovascular alterations caused by chronic disease. On the basis of these features, patients should be appropriately counseled as to what they should expect to gain from surgery.

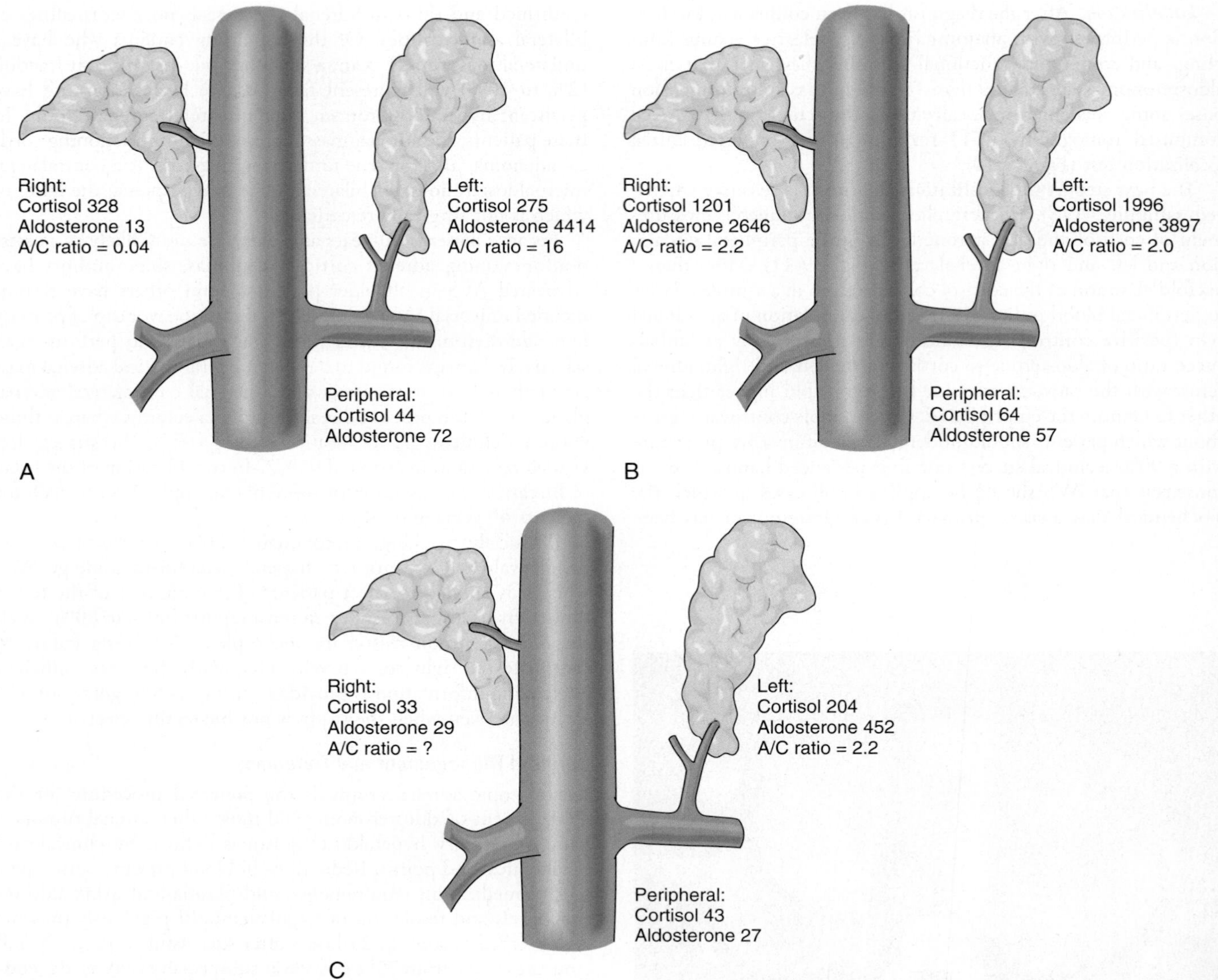

FIGURE 39-11 Possible outcomes of adrenal vein sampling for primary hyperaldosteronism. Aldosterone is expressed in ng/dL, cortisol in µg/dL. **A,** Successful study lateralizing strongly to the left adrenal. **B,** Successful study, nonlateralizing. Stimulation with ACTH yielded high adrenal vein cortisol levels. **C,** Failed study. The right adrenal vein was not cannulated.

Cushing Syndrome

Epidemiology and Clinical Features

The clinical features of glucocorticoid excess were first documented by Harvey Cushing in 1912. He described a young woman of "extraordinary appearance" who developed obesity, hirsutism, amenorrhea, easy bruising, and extreme muscle weakness. The principal differential diagnosis to be considered in evaluating patients for Cushing syndrome is obesity, an increasingly common condition. A subset of signs and symptoms, including easy bruising, muscle weakness, hypertension, plethora (a red facial appearance caused by thinning of the skin), and hirsutism, may allow discrimination between Cushing syndrome and obesity based on clinical features (Fig. 39-12). The genetic pathogenesis of cortisol-producing adrenal adenomas is not well understood. Recent next-generation sequencing on whole exome DNA has revealed a specific mutation of protein kinase A that is present in cortisol-producing adenomas, particularly in patients with overt Cushing syndrome.[18]

The most common cause of Cushing syndrome is pharmacologic glucocorticoid use for the treatment of inflammatory disorders. Endogenous Cushing syndrome is rare, affecting 5 to 10 individuals/million. Of these, most affected individuals (75%) will have Cushing *disease,* that is, glucocorticoid excess caused by an ACTH-hypersecreting pituitary adenoma. The remainder will be split between primary adrenal Cushing syndrome (15%) and ectopic ACTH syndrome (<10%), the latter of which usually is caused by neuroendocrine tumors or bronchogenic malignant neoplasms arising in the thorax.

Cushing syndrome is a lethal disease. The physiologic derangements resulting from glucocorticoid excess, including hypertension (present in >70% of cases), hyperglycemia, and truncal obesity, ultimately yield a fivefold excess mortality, primarily

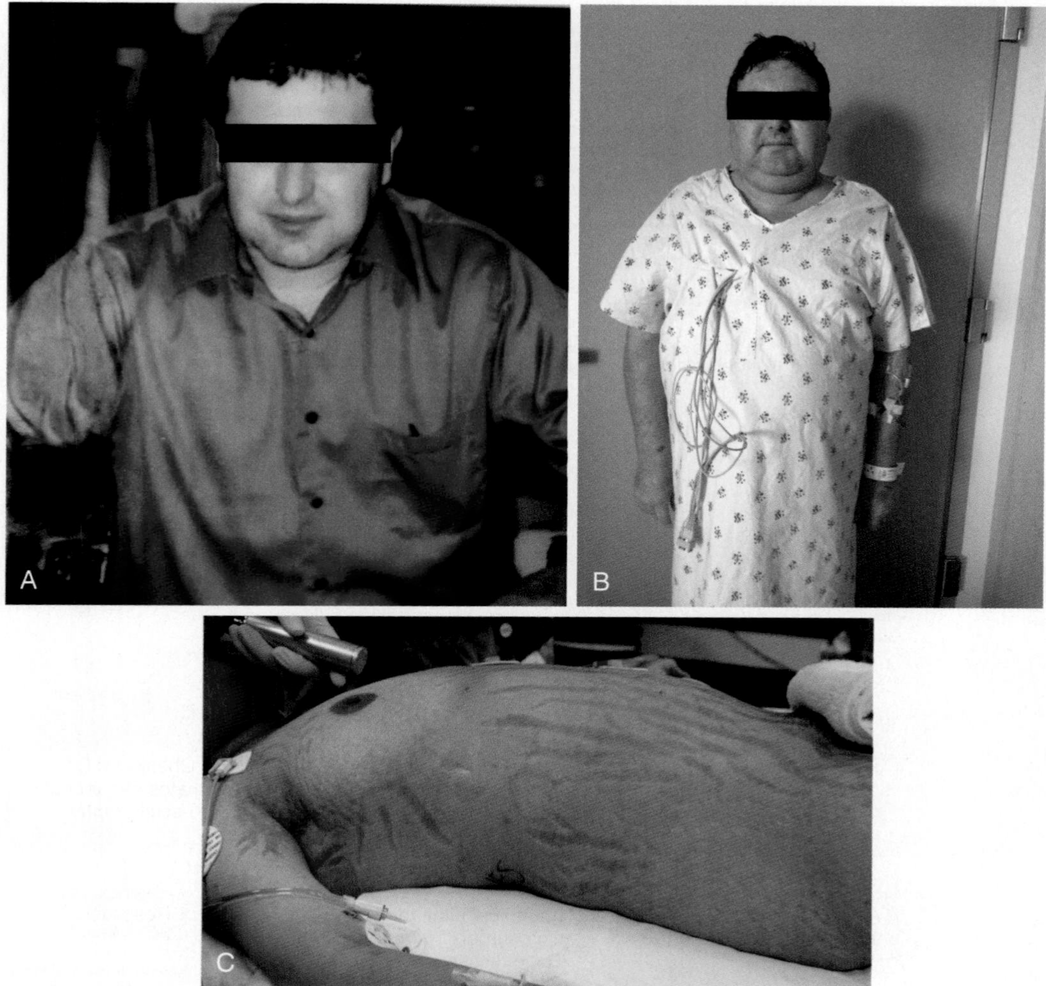

FIGURE 39-12 Clinical manifestations of Cushing syndrome. **A,** Appearance of a man before development of Cushing syndrome. **B,** Same man 1 year later, after development of Cushing syndrome. **C,** Purple abdominal and axillary striae in a man with Cushing syndrome.

because of cardiovascular complications.[19] Thus, all efforts should be made to identify and appropriately treat patients with Cushing syndrome.

Biochemical Diagnosis and Localization

The diagnosis of Cushing syndrome is reliant on demonstration of inappropriate cortisol secretion or the loss of physiologic negative feedback. Normally, cortisol release follows a predictable circadian rhythm, peaking approximately 1 hour after waking and reaching a nadir around midnight. Thus, inappropriate cortisol secretion can be detected as elevated cortisol release during a 24-hour period or as a higher than expected level in the late evening. Traditionally, lack of negative feedback has been assessed with dexamethasone suppression testing and other types of provocative tests, many of which are cumbersome and require inpatient hospitalization. The development of late evening salivary cortisol testing has provided an attractive and feasible alternative to suppression testing.

More than 90% of circulating cortisol is bound to plasma proteins. Unbound cortisol can be detected in the urine and saliva, and assessment of these body fluids forms the basis of biochemical screening for Cushing syndrome (Fig. 39-13); 24-hour urine collection for urine free cortisol should be performed at least twice for initial screening. Unequivocally elevated levels should prompt immediate further testing to determine the cause and subtype of Cushing syndrome (i.e., primary adrenal cause versus pituitary cause versus ectopic ACTH syndrome). Patients with moderately elevated 24-hour urine cortisol levels should undergo confirmatory testing with two late evening (bedtime) cortisol measurements. A high cutoff value of 550 ng/mL has a sensitivity of 93% and specificity of 100%.[20]

Primary adrenal Cushing syndrome, also termed ACTH-independent Cushing syndrome, is caused by autonomous adrenal cortisol production and therefore is generally associated with an undetectable ACTH level (<5 pg/mL) because of feedback inhibition. The underlying pathologic process is variable, with solitary adrenal adenoma found in approximately 90% of cases, adrenocortical carcinoma in less than 10%, and bilateral micronodular or macronodular hyperplasia in less than 1%. Almost all these lesions, except micronodular hyperplasia, are readily apparent on CT scans.

Hypercortisolemia associated with normal or elevated ACTH levels is indicative of ACTH-dependent Cushing syndrome, most commonly caused by a pituitary corticotroph microadenoma

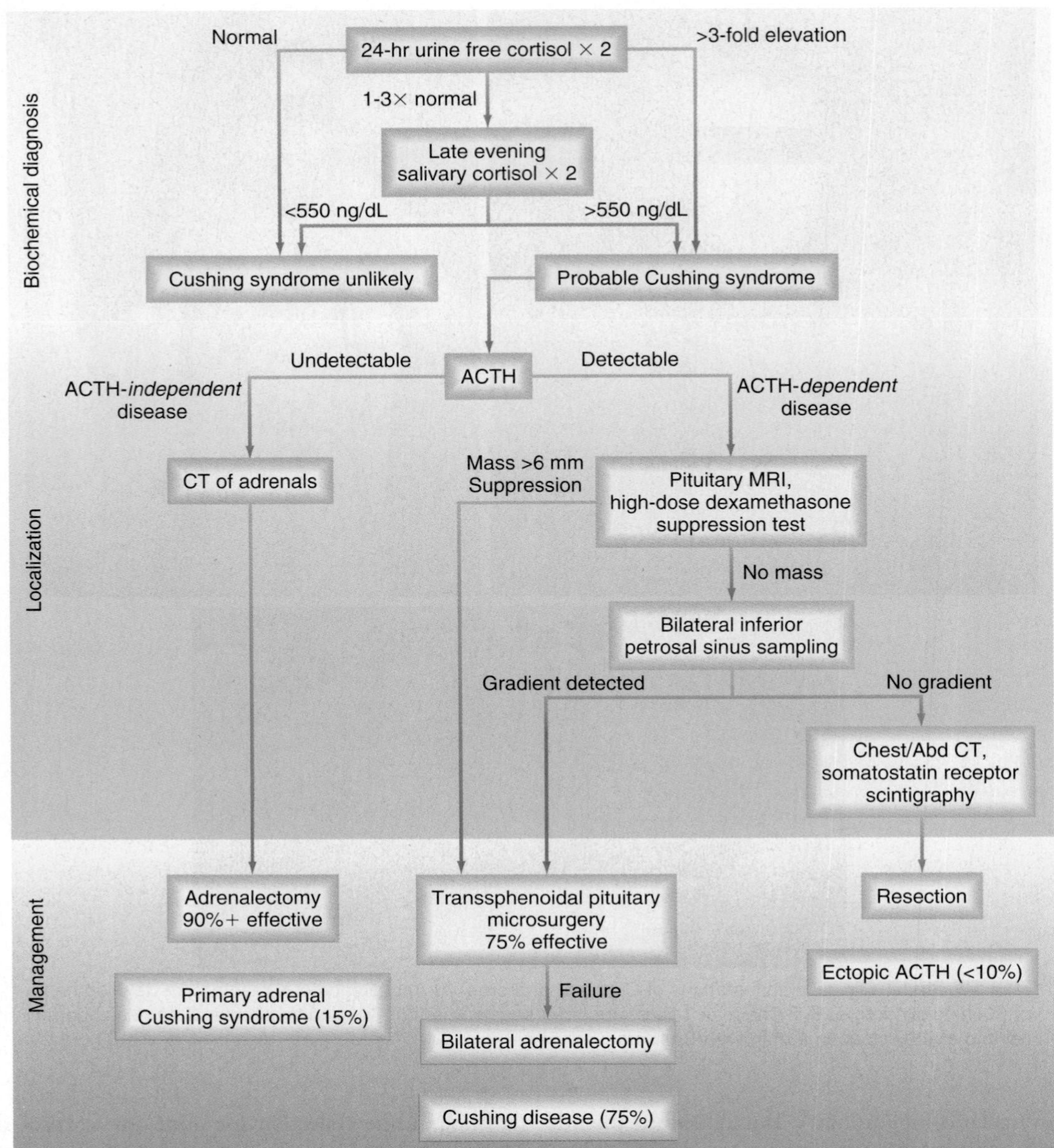

FIGURE 39-13 Algorithm for the diagnosis, localization, and management of endogenous Cushing syndrome. A biochemical diagnosis can be established with an unequivocally elevated 24-hour urine free cortisol level (greater than a threefold elevation) or an elevated late evening salivary cortisol level. Most cases of Cushing syndrome are caused by Cushing disease (pituitary corticotroph microadenoma), in which the plasma ACTH level is elevated. An undetectable ACTH level establishes the diagnosis of ACTH-independent Cushing syndrome and prompts adrenal imaging. Bilateral adrenalectomy is considered for patients with Cushing disease not cured by trans-sphenoidal surgery.

(Cushing disease). Suspicion for ACTH-dependent Cushing syndrome should prompt pituitary imaging and high-dose dexamethasone suppression testing, that is, serum or urine cortisol measurement after administration of 2 mg of dexamethasone every 6 hours during 48 hours. Dexamethasone is chosen because it does not cross-react with biochemical assays for cortisol. Corticotroph adenomas are commonly suppressed in response to high-dose dexamethasone administration, whereas ectopic ACTH sources are completely lacking in feedback inhibition. Slightly more than 50% of corticotroph microadenomas are visible on pituitary magnetic resonance imaging (MRI). Detection of a pituitary mass larger than 6 mm in diameter in a patient with ACTH-dependent Cushing syndrome that is suppressed with high-dose dexamethasone justifies proceeding to pituitary surgery.[21] In the absence of a demonstrable mass, bilateral inferior petrosal sinus ACTH sampling with corticotropin-releasing factor stimulation should be pursued. Demonstration of a central to peripheral ACTH gradient in a study performed by a skilled physician is sufficient to diagnose Cushing disease. The absence of a clear gradient should prompt CT imaging of the chest and abdomen and, occasionally, somatostatin receptor scintigraphy to identify an ectopic ACTH source.

Surgical Management and Outcomes

Perioperative and postoperative glucocorticoid administration is obviously essential in the care of patients with Cushing syndrome. For patients undergoing adrenalectomy for Cushing syndrome, perioperative stress dose steroids (e.g., hydrocortisone 100 mg intravenously every 8 hours for 24 hours) are recommended. In the most common scenario of resection of a solitary adrenal Cushing adenoma, steroids can usually be tapered to physiologic replacement levels during the course of several weeks. However, a subset of patients with Cushing syndrome of longer duration and severity will demonstrate lasting HPA axis suppression, requiring glucocorticoid supplementation for longer periods, sometimes longer than 1 year.

The management of patients who undergo pituitary surgery for Cushing disease is variable. In some centers, glucocorticoids are withheld during the immediate postoperative period to provide a window during which early remission may be assessed.[22] A subnormal morning cortisol level on postoperative day 1 or 2 is indicative of cure. Glucocorticoid supplementation is then resumed until the HPA axis recovers, usually for at least 6 months. Because of the significant risk of postoperative adrenal crisis in patients with Cushing syndrome of all subtypes, glucocorticoid management is ideally done in conjunction with an experienced endocrinologist.

Adrenalectomy is more than 90% effective in the treatment of primary adrenal Cushing syndrome. Resolution of symptoms typically takes months to years, and certain deleterious physiologic effects regarding bone density, body composition, and inflammation are extremely persistent.[23] Failures may result from local and occasionally distant tumor recurrence in the case of malignant disease. Pituitary microsurgery for Cushing disease, typically performed through a transnasal trans-sphenoidal approach, is approximately 90% successful in expert hands. Remission rates may be improved by reoperation or pituitary irradiation for patients whose basal cortisol levels do not fall appropriately after initial surgery. Laparoscopic bilateral adrenalectomy should be considered for patients in whom pituitary surgery has failed. Patients with Cushing syndrome are hypercoagulable and carry a risk of venous thromboembolism of up to 5% after pituitary or adrenal surgery. Chemical thromboprophylaxis should be considered, although there are insufficient data to determine the optimal duration and dosage.

Special Case: Subclinical Cushing Syndrome

The term *subclinical Cushing syndrome* has been used to describe patients with incidentally discovered adrenal masses (see later, "Incidentally Discovered Adrenal Mass") who display biochemical evidence of cortisol hypersecretion without overt signs or symptoms of Cushing syndrome. This disease entity has been incompletely characterized with respect to its physiologic consequences and natural history. Clear-cut definitions for the diagnosis of subclinical Cushing syndrome, such as cutoff values for biochemical tests and objective assessment guidelines for the presence or absence of clinical features, are lacking.

Hypertension, dyslipidemia, and impaired glucose tolerance appear to be more prevalent among individuals with subclinical Cushing syndrome compared with normal individuals. Retrospective studies suggest that this subset of patients experience improvement in obesity, hypertension, glycemic control, and dyslipidemia when they are treated surgically.[24] Furthermore, a randomized controlled trial comparing surgery with observation in 45 patients with subclinical Cushing syndrome noted more frequent resolution of hypertension and other metabolic conditions in the surgically treated group.[25] We observe a continuum of disease ranging from subclinical to overt Cushing syndrome, which arises as a function of both symptom severity and the perceptiveness of the treating physician. Patients along the entire spectrum appear to benefit from restoration of normal cortisol physiology. We therefore recommend surgery for patients with subclinical Cushing syndrome who are appropriate surgical candidates, especially for patients with larger (3- to 4-cm) tumors and those whose tumors enlarge on serial imaging studies.

Sex Steroid Excess

Adrenal tumors causing clinical features of sex steroid excess are rare. Most of these tumors are virilizing (as opposed to feminizing) and may be manifested at a late stage in association with an advanced adrenal malignant neoplasm. Almost all feminizing tumors are malignant, whereas approximately one third of virilizing tumors are malignant. Of adrenocortical carcinomas, 20% cause virilization, with most of these cases occurring in children. An additional 24% of adrenocortical carcinomas will display mixed features of Cushing syndrome and virilization.[26] Virilizing tumors may be biochemically detected by measurements of 24-hour urine testosterone, DHEA, and DHEA-S. Although laparoscopic adrenalectomy remains the preferred procedure for most sex steroid–secreting tumors, the high probability of malignancy merits close radiographic and intraoperative inspection for evidence of invasion or metastasis. Open adrenalectomy should be performed for malignant tumors.

Adrenocortical Carcinoma

Adrenocortical carcinoma is a rare tumor, with an annual incidence of approximately 1/million. Almost all cases occur in patients aged 40 to 50 years, although there is a minor peak in occurrence among children younger than 5 years. It demonstrates no significant gender predilection. At the time of presentation, adrenocortical carcinomas tend to be very large (mean tumor size, 9 to 13 cm) and have usually spread beyond the confines of the adrenal gland.[27] Historically, overall 5-year survival rates have been in the 15% to 20% range. Among patients who undergo surgical resection, 5-year survival is approximately 40%, a figure that has essentially remained unchanged during the past 2 decades.[28] A higher risk of death is associated with increasing age of the patient, poorly differentiated or high-grade tumors, positive surgical margins, and presence of distant metastases. More than 50% of adrenocortical carcinomas are functional. Cushing syndrome is most commonly seen, followed by virilization. Radiographic evaluation is primarily performed with CT, which typically reveals a heterogeneous mass with irregular or indistinct borders, central necrosis, and invasion of adjacent structures (Fig. 39-14). Metastases to lymph nodes, liver, and lungs may be found.

Treatment of adrenocortical carcinoma requires radical resection, which is achieved by an open approach. Complete resection can be achieved in up to 70% of patients in experienced hands. This frequently involves en bloc resection of adjacent organs or regional lymphadenectomy. Particular care must be taken in dealing with right-sided adrenocortical carcinomas larger than 9 cm because direct tumor extension into the inferior vena cava and sometimes the right side of the heart may be observed. Tumors demonstrating intravascular extension may need to be resected while the patient is on cardiopulmonary bypass to reduce the likelihood of lethal intraoperative tumor embolization.[29]

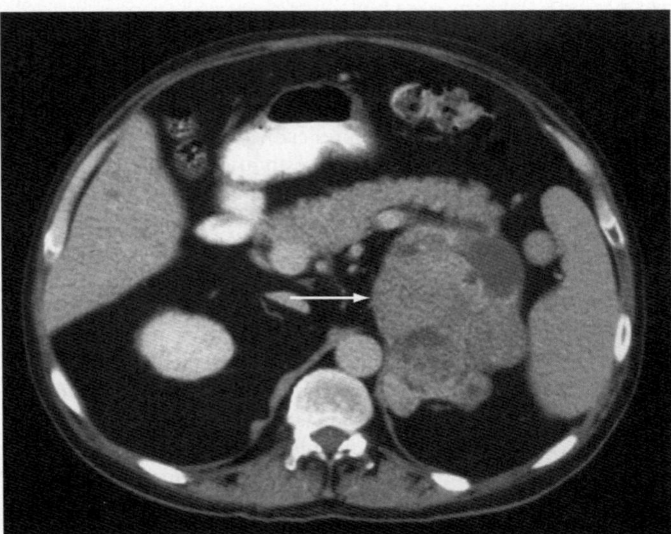

FIGURE 39-14 CT scan demonstrating a 10-cm left adrenocortical carcinoma. Note the areas of central necrosis *(arrow)*.

Patients who undergo incomplete resection of adrenocortical carcinomas have extremely limited life expectancy (median survival <1 year). Even those who undergo successful surgery are prone to development of local recurrence and metastases, which typically occur within 2 years. The principal chemotherapeutic agent for the treatment of adrenocortical carcinoma is mitotane [*o,p*-DDD, or 1,1-dichloro-2-(*o*-chlorophenyl)-2-(*p*-chlorophenyl)ethane], a derivative of the insecticide DDT that is a direct adrenocortical toxin. Mitotane has been used clinically as an adjuvant to surgery and as primary therapy in individuals with unresectable or metastatic disease. A multinational retrospective study examining the efficacy of adjuvant mitotane after radical surgery has demonstrated a significant improvement in recurrence-free survival.[30] The use of mitotane is limited by significant, dose-dependent gastrointestinal and neurologic toxicity. The multinational FIRM-ACT trial randomized 304 patients with locally advanced or metastatic adrenocortical carcinoma to receive etoposide, doxorubicin, cisplatin, and mitotane or streptozotocin and mitotane. There was a significantly improved response rate and progression-free survival in the former group, but median overall survival remained poor in both groups (14.8 versus 12.0 months).[31] A number of other trials are examining targeted agents such as epidermal growth factor inhibitors, insulin-like growth factor I inhibitors, antiangiogenic agents, and broad-spectrum tyrosine kinase inhibitors. There is also an emerging interest in individualized therapy based on genomic and expression profiling of tumors.

DISEASES OF THE ADRENAL MEDULLA

Pheochromocytoma

Epidemiology and Clinical Features

The first account of pheochromocytoma was published in 1886 by Felix Frankel, who described a young woman suffering from intermittent attacks of palpitations, anxiety, vertigo, and headache. Autopsy revealed bilateral adrenal tumors that stained brown when treated with chromium salts. Because of the characteristic positive chromaffin reaction, these adrenomedullary tumors are termed *pheochromocytoma* (dusky-colored tumor, from the Greek *phaios*, dusky). Successful surgical management of pheochromocytoma was initially described in 1926 by both César Roux and Charles Mayo.[32]

Pheochromocytoma affects approximately 0.2% of hypertensive individuals. Men and women are affected equally. The peak incidence in sporadic cases is between the ages of 40 and 50 years, whereas familial cases tend to be manifested earlier. A subset of patients present with the classic triad of headache, diaphoresis, and palpitations, although almost all patients will display at least one of these symptoms. Hypertension is present in 90% of cases and may be episodic or sustained. The principal challenge in making the diagnosis of pheochromocytoma arises from the fact that essential hypertension is common and the clinical features suggestive of pheochromocytoma are nonspecific. In fact, only 0.5% of patients with hypertension and suggestive features will ultimately prove to have the disease. The differential diagnosis of pheochromocytoma is wide, encompassing diverse processes such as hyperthyroidism, hypoglycemia, coronary artery disease, heart failure, stroke, drug-related effects, and panic disorder. Pheochromocytoma has been described as a biologic time bomb because of the potentially lethal cardiovascular effects of the bioactive compounds secreted by these tumors. Thus, despite the challenges in diagnosis, clinicians should screen for this disease aggressively and seek appropriate treatment for affected patients.

Previously, pheochromocytoma was termed the *10% tumor,* suggesting that 10% are bilateral, 10% malignant, 10% extra-adrenal, and 10% familial. Discoveries regarding the genetic underpinnings of pheochromocytoma have challenged these old axioms.

Biochemical Diagnosis and Localization

Establishing the biochemical diagnosis of pheochromocytoma is based on the detection of elevated levels of catecholamines and their metabolites in body fluids. Measurements of 24-hour urine levels of these compounds have long been the cornerstone of biochemical testing and are still the most reliable tests available today. In 2002, measurement of free (unconjugated) metanephrines in plasma was introduced as an alternative screening tool for pheochromocytoma. Plasma free metanephrine testing carries an extremely high sensitivity, approaching 99%, and being a one-time blood test, it is more convenient than 24-hour urine testing. However, the specificity of plasma free metanephrine testing is 89% at best, with specificities at most laboratories likely to be in the 85% range or below. Given that pheochromocytoma is a rare diagnosis that is sought within a large pool of hypertensive individuals, false-positive test results are a major problem. It has been estimated that false-positive test results outnumber true-positive test results by as much as 30 : 1 when plasma free metanephrine testing is used as a principal screening tool.[33]

Therefore, the primary usefulness of plasma free metanephrine testing is to exclude pheochromocytoma when the test result is negative (Fig. 39-15). When the test result is positive, confirmatory testing with 24-hour urine levels of catecholamines and their metabolites is recommended. Many drugs and conditions are capable of confounding catecholamine-based testing, contributing further to the problem of false-positive results. These include sympathomimetics (present in many cold remedies), phenoxybenzamine (frequently initiated when suspicion for pheochromocytoma is raised), acetaminophen (which interferes with the plasma free metanephrine assay), many psychotropic drugs (notably tricyclic antidepressants), and major physical or psychological stressors. Results of tests performed during episodes of acute pain,

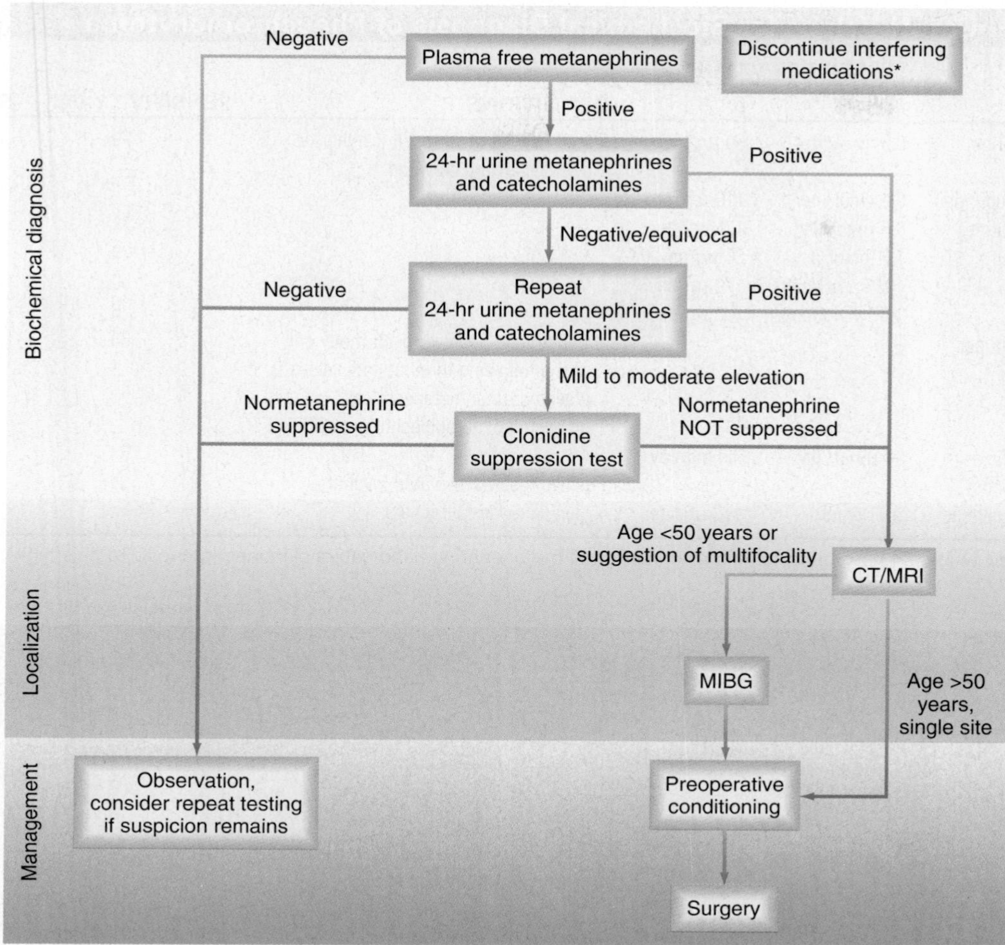

*Including sympathomimetics, phenoxybenzamine, acetaminophen, many psychotropic drugs.

FIGURE 39-15 Algorithm for the diagnosis, localization, and management of pheochromocytoma. Initial plasma free metanephrine testing can effectively exclude the diagnosis if the result is negative. A 24-hour urine collection for catecholamines and their metabolites is generally performed twice, with cutoffs approximately twice the upper limit of normal being criteria for positivity (see Table 39-4). Clonidine suppression testing can be used for the small fraction of patients in whom the diagnosis remains uncertain after urine testing. Localization with CT or MRI follows biochemical confirmation of the diagnosis, with MIBG scanning performed for younger patients and those otherwise at risk for multifocal disease. Phenoxybenzamine is given in escalating doses for at least 2 weeks before surgery.

critical illness, or urgent hospitalization may be misleading. The presence of confounding factors is extremely common in the population being screened because they represent manifestations or treatments of competing diagnoses. Clearly, biochemical testing should be ideally performed when the patient is as free as practically possible of all confounding factors.

The operating characteristics of catecholamine-based plasma and urine tests are listed, along with corresponding cutoff values, in Table 39-4. Cutoff values for 24-hour urine tests are deliberately set high to maximize specificity; these values are approximately double the upper 95% reference range in most laboratories. A urine collection may be considered positive if total metanephrines or any single catecholamine fraction (e.g., epinephrine, norepinephrine, dopamine) is elevated above its cutoff value. This approach maintains high specificity and yields an acceptable sensitivity of 88%.[34] Importantly, it takes into account the fact that pheochromocytomas synthesize and metabolize catecholamines and that tumors may possess heterogeneous secretory profiles, depending on their relative expression of synthetic and degradative enzymes (see Fig. 39-6).

Two 24-hour urine collections for catecholamines and their metabolites are sufficient to make (or to exclude) the diagnosis of pheochromocytoma in almost all cases. Clonidine suppression testing, the measurement of plasma free normetanephrine levels after the oral administration of 0.3 mg clonidine, may help clarify equivocal test results. Anatomic localization may be performed with MRI or CT. MRI is slightly more sensitive, but CT often yields better anatomic definition for operative planning (Fig. 39-16). The specificity of either modality is only 70% because of the high prevalence of incidental adrenal nodules. Scintigraphy with ^{131}I- or ^{123}I-labeled metaiodobenzylguanidine (MIBG; Fig. 39-17) should be performed in select patients in whom multifocal disease is suspected. MIBG scanning is highly specific for pheochromocytoma but carries a sensitivity of only 77% to 90%. Positron emission tomography (PET) and PET/CT using novel radionuclides such as ^{18}F-L-dihydroxyphenylalanine (^{18}F-DOPA;

TABLE 39-4 Cutoff Values for Biochemical Diagnosis of Pheochromocytoma

TEST*	CUTOFF VALUE mol	CUTOFF VALUE g	DEFINITIONS	SENSITIVITY (%)	SPECIFICITY (%)
Plasma free metanephrine	0.3 nmol/liter	59 μg/liter	Paired test, positive result if either or both values are elevated	99	85-89
Plasma free normetanephrine	0.6 nmol/liter	110 μg/liter			
Urinary total metanephrines	6.6 μmol/day	1.3 mg/day		71	99.6
Urinary epinephrine	191 nmol/day	35 μg/day		29	99.6
Urinary norepinephrine	1005 nmol/day	170 μg/day		50	99.6
Urinary dopamine	4571 nmol/day	700 μg/day		8	100
Urinary total metanephrines and catecholamines	—		Grouped test, positive result if any one of the following three urinary values is elevated: total metanephrines, epinephrine, norepinephrine, dopamine	88	99
Urinary vanillylmandelic acid	40 μmol/day	7.9 mg/day		64	95
Clonidine suppression test			Positive result = elevated level after clonidine and fall of <40	96	100
Plasma free normetanephrine	0.61 nmol/L	112 μg/liter			

*When it is performed twice, 24-hour urine testing of urinary total metanephrines and catecholamines (grouped test) is highly sensitive and highly specific.

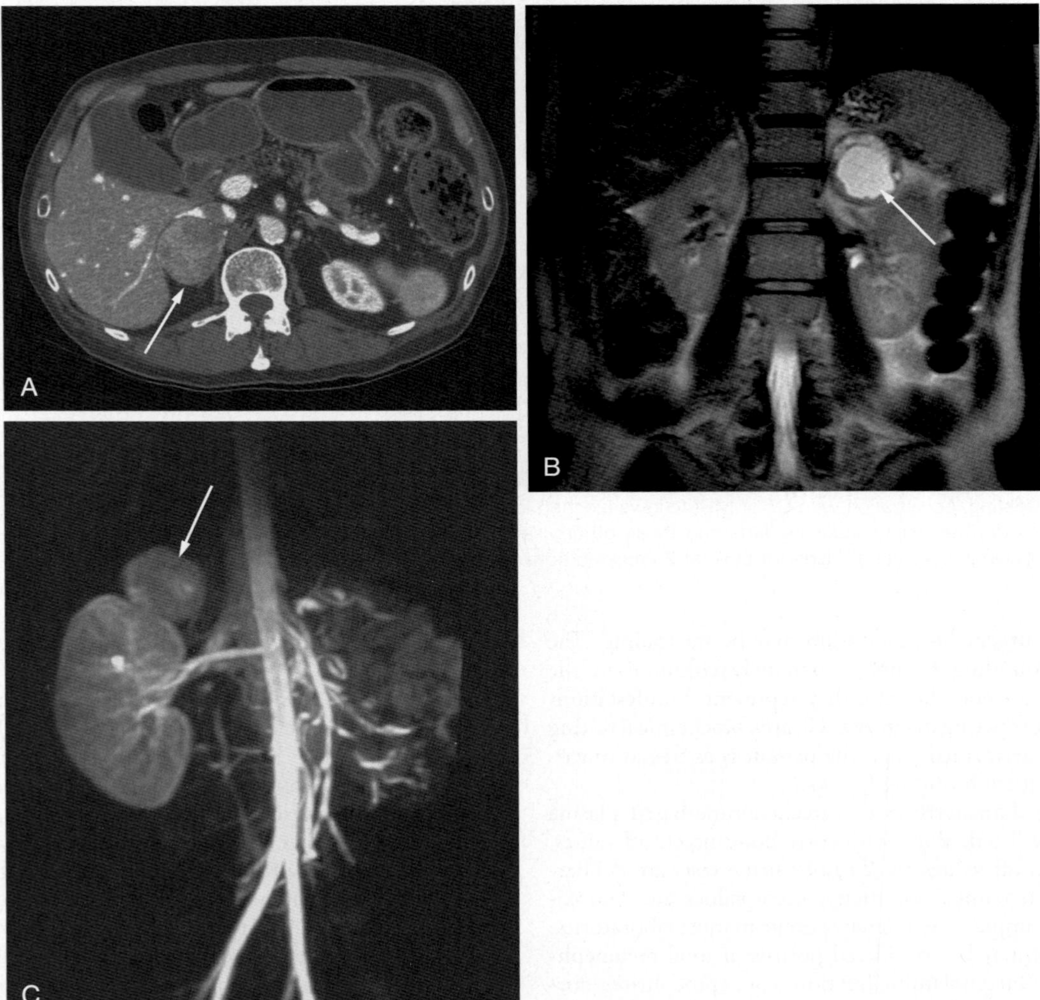

FIGURE 39-16 Appearance of pheochromocytoma on anatomic imaging. **A,** Venous phase, contrast-enhanced CT scan demonstrating a right adrenal pheochromocytoma *(arrow)*. The heterogeneity in the inferior vena cava represents swirling of contrast material, not tumor thrombus or invasion. **B,** Coronal T2-weighted MRI scan demonstrating a left adrenal pheochromocytoma with central cystic change *(arrow)*. **C,** Left anterior oblique MR angiographic reconstruction demonstrating a right adrenal pheochromocytoma *(arrow)*.

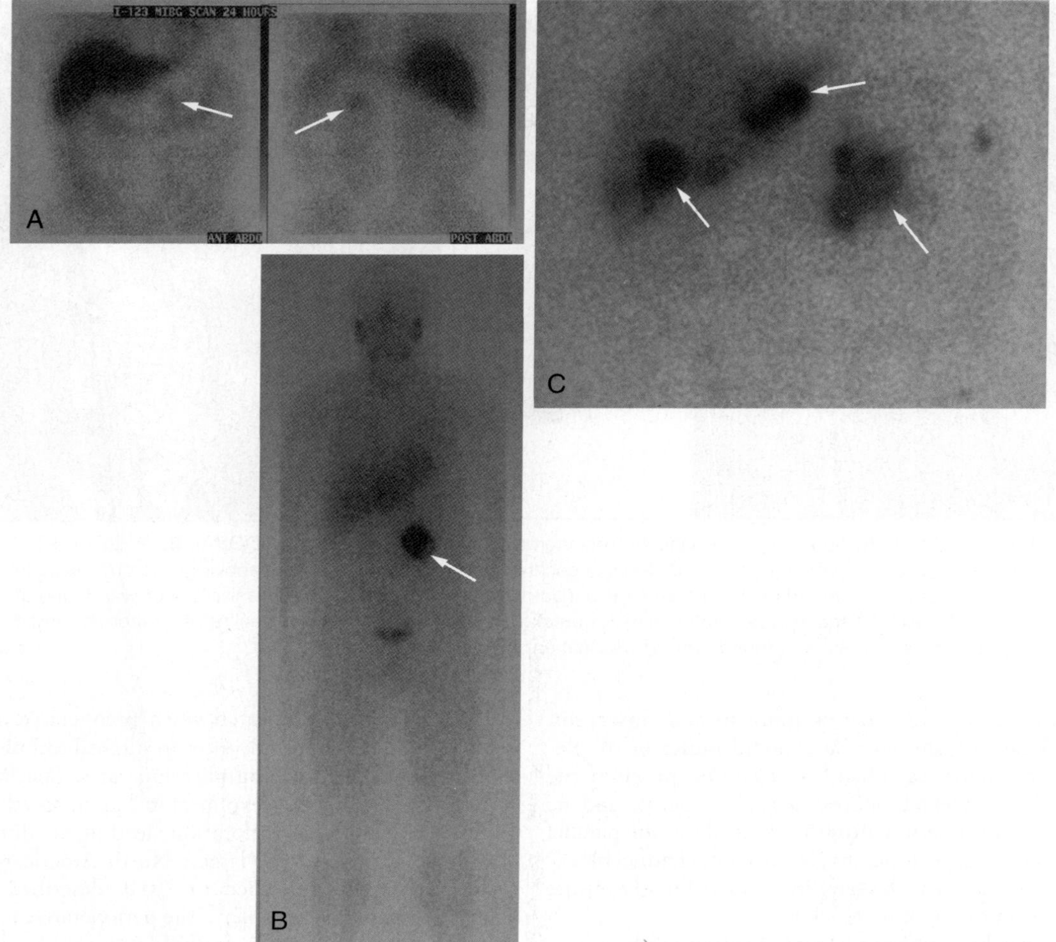

FIGURE 39-17 Appearance of pheochromocytoma on functional imaging (MIBG scanning). **A,** ^{123}I-MIBG scan of the abdomen demonstrating an isolated left adrenal pheochromocytoma *(arrows).* Physiologic radiotracer uptake is noted in the liver, right colon, and transverse colon. **B,** Whole body ^{131}I-MIBG scan demonstrating a large, left, para-aortic extra-adrenal pheochromocytoma *(arrow).* Physiologic radiotracer uptake is noted in the liver, salivary glands, and bladder. **C,** ^{131}I-MIBG scan of the abdomen demonstrating malignant pheochromocytoma, with local recurrence in the left adrenal bed and liver metastases *(arrows).*

Fig. 39-18) and ^{18}F-dopamine are highly sensitive and superior to MIBG scanning in the imaging of pheochromocytoma.[35] However, the availability of these techniques remains confined to a small number of academic centers worldwide.

Perioperative Care

Throughout the first half of the 20th century, perioperative mortality rates in the treatment of pheochromocytoma ranged from 26% to 50%. Currently, the mortality rate in most specialty centers is approximately 1%. This dramatic improvement can largely be ascribed to advances in pharmacology, physiology, anesthesia, and perioperative medical care. The adverse perioperative hemodynamic changes most commonly observed with pheochromocytoma are intraoperative hypertension and postoperative hypotension. Intraoperative hypertension may be caused by stimulation of catecholamine release by anesthetic induction agents as well as by direct manipulation of the tumor. Postoperative hypotension may be profound. It results from a state of hypovolemia created by the presence of excess circulating catecholamines. Sudden withdrawal of this stimulus after tumor removal leads to peripheral arteriolar vasodilation and a dramatic increase in venous capacitance, which together may precipitate cardiovascular collapse. In their early report of a large successful case series, investigators at the Mayo Clinic described the use of intraoperative α-adrenergic blockade followed by aggressive volume repletion and the administration of α-adrenergic agonists in the immediate postoperative period.[36]

The principles of perioperative care remain much the same. As soon as the biochemical diagnosis of pheochromocytoma has been confirmed, α-adrenergic blockade should be initiated to protect against hemodynamic lability. Our practice is to start with phenoxybenzamine 10 mg twice daily. The dosage can be titrated upward every 2 to 3 days to a maximum of 40 mg three times daily to achieve normalization of heart rate and blood pressure. The period of preoperative conditioning should last at least 2 weeks to allow adequate reversal of α-adrenergic receptor downregulation. This restores sensitivity to vasopressor agents, which can then be used to treat the patient postoperatively. Phenoxybenzamine is a nonspecific, noncompetitive (irreversible), long-acting (half-life of 24 hours) α-adrenergic antagonist. Although its use is associated with the side effects of postural hypotension and significant nasal congestion, it is generally favored over

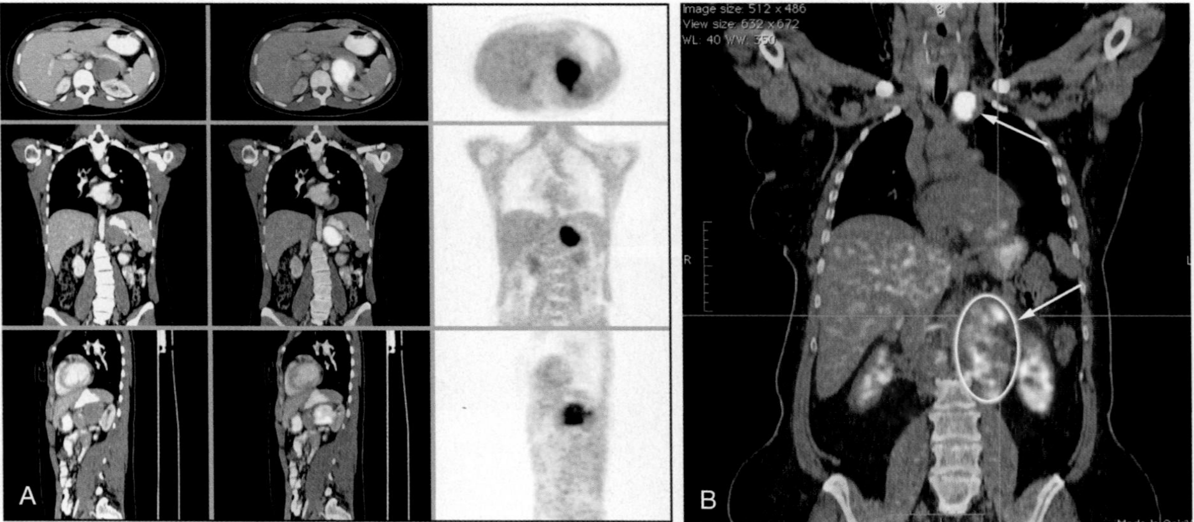

FIGURE 39-18 A, Appearance of pheochromocytoma on functional imaging (^{18}F-DOPA). **B,** ^{18}F-DOPA PET/CT scan in a patient with malignant multifocal pheochromocytoma. Diffuse uptake above background is seen in the region of the left adrenal gland and left periaortic region, where a locally invasive tumor was found at surgery *(arrow)*. A second area of intense tracer uptake is seen in the left paratracheal region, where a carotid sheath paraganglioma was found *(arrow)*. The patient is an *SDHB* mutation carrier.

α_1-adrenergic selective agents, such as prazosin and doxazosin. Nasal congestion can actually serve as a useful indicator of adequate blockade. Furthermore, phenoxybenzamine provides the most complete alpha blockade among available agents, and its pharmacokinetics permit serum drug levels to decay in parallel with catecholamine levels postoperatively. Calcium channel blockers may be added for patients who have inadequate blood pressure control after titration of an alpha blocker.

Beta blockers may be administered after adequate alpha blockade has been achieved for the subset of patients with persistent tachycardia, who often have predominantly epinephrine-secreting tumors. Beta blockers should never be the first agent administered because a decrease in peripheral vasodilatory beta receptor stimulation results in unopposed α-adrenergic tone, which may exacerbate hypertension. Preoperative volume expansion with isotonic fluids has been advocated in the past. However, in our experience, the need for this is significantly reduced when aggressive preoperative alpha blockade has been achieved because the resultant increase in venous capacitance restores euvolemia gradually by stimulating thirst. Clinical suspicion for hypovolemia should remain high in the postoperative period, and patients should be aggressively resuscitated if they become hypotensive or oliguric. Some patients may require vasopressors after tumor removal, especially if preoperative alpha blockade is incomplete.

Surgical Management and Outcomes

Successful operative treatment of pheochromocytoma is dependent on close communication between the surgeon and anesthesiologist. Invasive hemodynamic monitoring is required, and fluid management must be meticulous. Manipulation of the tumor should be minimized, and the anesthetic team should be prepared to administer supplemental intravenous alpha and beta blockers as well as vasopressors when necessary.

Surgery is curative in more than 90% of pheochromocytoma cases. Although these tumors are highly vascular and tend to adhere to adjacent structures (Fig. 39-19), most of them can be removed successfully by a laparoscopic approach. Laparoscopic resection is contraindicated when preoperative imaging demonstrates local invasion. Advances in surgical technique have resulted in reduced operative complication rates. Specifically, functional image-guided focused exploration has replaced bilateral adrenal and retroperitoneal exploration, leading to diminished rates of solid organ injury. The largest North American series on pheochromocytoma, published in 2010, described 108 operations, 90% of them laparoscopic.[37] The perioperative morbidity rate was 13%, and there were no deaths.

Molecular Genetics of Pheochromocytoma

A number of reports describing novel germline mutations have demonstrated that familial pheochromocytomas are much more common than previously believed. Before 2000, pheochromocytoma was known to be associated with multiple endocrine neoplasia type 2 syndromes (40% to 50% penetrant), von Hippel–Lindau syndrome (10% to 20% penetrant), and neurofibromatosis type 1 (1% to 5% penetrant). The discovery that neuroendocrine cells of the carotid body proliferate in response to hypoxic stimuli has led to the identification of mutations in the succinate dehydrogenase gene family in kindreds affected with pheochromocytoma or paraganglioma. Succinate dehydrogenase, which is made up of four subunits, is localized to the mitochondria and catalyzes essential steps in oxidative phosphorylation. Germline mutations in the B and D subunits, inherited in an autosomal dominant fashion, have been identified in approximately 10% of apparently sporadic pheochromocytoma cases. Thus, there is consensus that at least one third of patients with pheochromocytoma have a germline mutation.[38]

Familial cases are manifested at an earlier age and are more likely to be multifocal (Table 39-5). Succinate dehydrogenase B mutation carriers have high rates of extra-adrenal (abdominal or thoracic) pheochromocytomas and malignant disease, whereas succinate dehydrogenase D carriers tend to present with multiple tumors and hormonally inactive paragangliomas of the head and neck. The lifetime penetrance of succinate dehydrogenase mutations is estimated at more than 75%.[39] Genetic counseling should

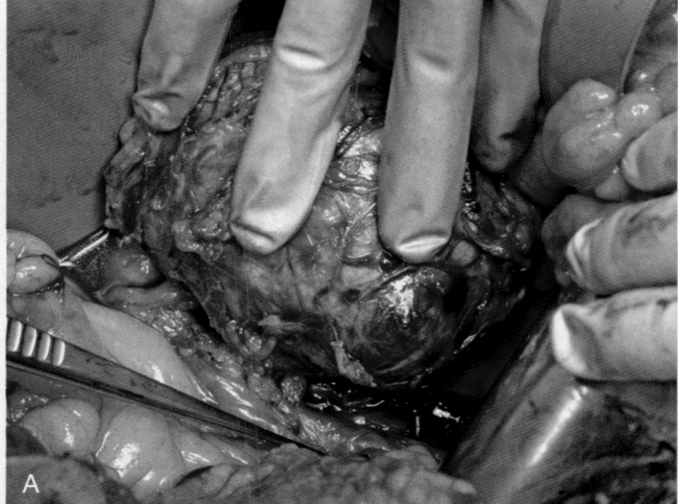

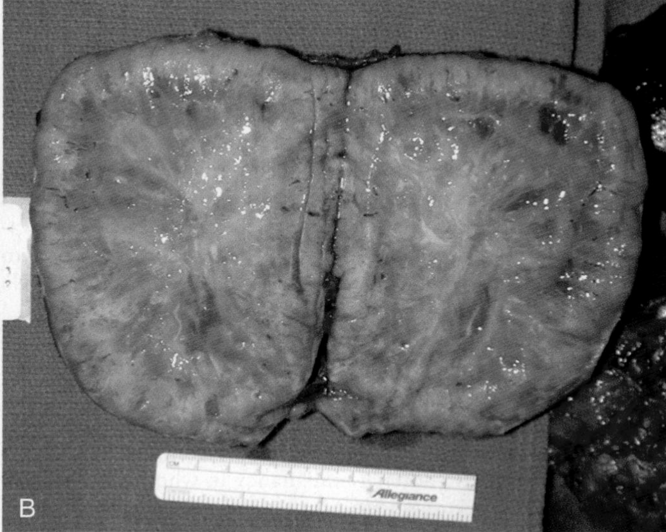

FIGURE 39-19 Gross appearance of pheochromocytoma. **A,** Open resection of a left para-aortic extra-adrenal pheochromocytoma (depicted in Fig. 39-17*B*) through an infracolic approach. The patient's head is to the right. The tumor is being rotated medially by the surgeon's hand to reveal the left ureter, indicated by forceps. **B,** Left adrenal pheochromocytoma. (**A,** Courtesy Dr. Stan Sidhu.)

be considered in all patients, particularly those younger than 45 years and those with multiple tumors, extra-adrenal location, and previous head and neck paraganglioma. The discovery of a germline mutation may influence prognosis and surveillance, prompt additional investigations, and enable early identification of affected family members.

Malignant Pheochromocytoma

Depending on the underlying genotype, 2.5% to 40% of pheochromocytomas are malignant. Survival at 5 years ranges from 20% to 45%. No histopathologic criteria for determining malignancy have demonstrated the ability to predict the clinical course accurately. Thus, malignancy is defined by the development of metastases (i.e., tumor implants distant from the primary mass in locations in which neuroectodermal tissues are not normally found). The latter criterion distinguishes metastatic disease from possible multifocal primary disease. The most common sites of metastasis are the axial skeleton, lymph nodes, liver, lung, and kidney. Treatment of primary and recurrent disease centers on surgical resection, which, even in the absence of cure, may have significant palliative benefits in terms of managing mass effect in critical anatomic locations and reducing the systemic impact of catecholamine excess.[40]

Malignant pheochromocytomas are minimally responsive to radiotherapy and chemotherapy. In a recent phase 2 study, high-dose ^{131}I-MIBG radionuclide therapy was shown to achieve a complete or partial response rate of 22% in select patients with metastatic pheochromocytoma.[41] Significant hematologic toxicities were observed, and long-term benefit remains uncommon. Chronic medical management of catecholamine excess should be performed with α_1-adrenergic selective blockers because of their favorable side-effect profile.

OTHER ADRENAL DISEASES

Incidentally Discovered Adrenal Mass (Incidentaloma)

Epidemiology and Differential Diagnosis

Incidentally discovered adrenal masses, also termed *clinically inapparent adrenal masses* or *incidentalomas,* are discovered through imaging performed for unrelated nonadrenal disease. Their existence as a clinical entity is a byproduct of advanced medical imaging. Incidentalomas were first described in the early 1980s, when CT scanners became more prevalent in developed nations, and they have become a common clinical problem as the use of CT and MRI has become widespread. Incidentalomas have been

TABLE 39-5 Hereditary Syndromes Associated With Pheochromocytoma

SYNDROME	GENE MUTATION	PHENOTYPE
Multiple endocrine neoplasia type 2A	*RET*	Medullary thyroid cancer, primary hyperparathyroidism
Multiple endocrine neoplasia type 2B	*RET*	Medullary thyroid cancer, marfanoid habitus, mucosal neuromas
Neurofibromatosis type 1 (von Recklinghausen disease)	*NF1*	Neurofibromas, café au lait spots, Lisch nodules (benign iris hamartomas)
von Hippel–Lindau	*VHL*	Retinal angioma, central nervous system hemangioblastoma, renal cell cancer, primitive neuroectodermal tumor, pancreatic and renal cysts
Familial paraganglioma syndrome	*SDHA, SDHB, SDHC, SDHD*	Gastrointestinal stromal tumor *SDHB* may be associated with renal cell cancer
Hereditary pheochromocytoma	*TMEM127*	Possibly other tumors
Hereditary pheochromocytoma	*MAX*	Possibly other tumors
Hereditary pheochromocytoma	*HIF2A*	Familial polycythemia, somatostatinomas

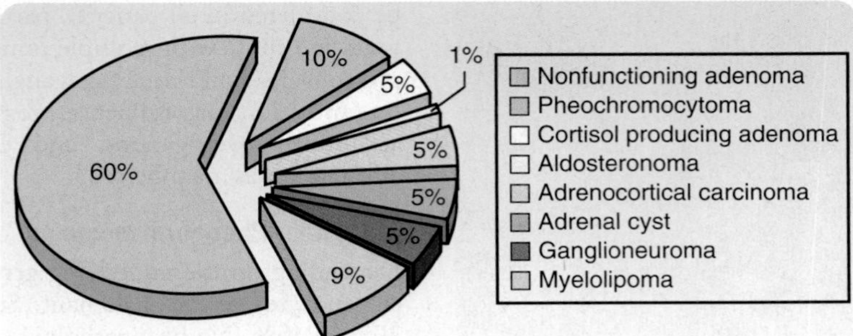

FIGURE 39-20 Differential diagnosis of adrenal incidentaloma in patients without a history of malignant disease. Approximate proportions of the various pathologic processes are shown.

found in up to 8% of autopsies and 1% to 4% of abdominal imaging studies. The prevalence increases to as high as 10% in patients older than 60 years.[42]

The differential diagnosis of adrenal incidentaloma is wide and includes secreting and nonsecreting neoplasms (Fig. 39-20). In patients with a history of malignant disease, metastatic disease is the most likely cause of adrenal masses, particularly when they are bilateral (see later, "Metastases to the Adrenal Gland"). In those without a clear history of malignant disease, at least 80% of incidentalomas will turn out to be nonfunctioning cortical adenomas or other benign lesions that do not require surgical management. Thus, in most patients, the most important aspect of management is to distinguish the subset of adrenal masses that are likely to have a clinical impact from the large proportion that are not.

Clinical Evaluation and Surgical Management

The workup of the adrenal incidentaloma integrates hormonal evaluation with size criteria. The principles and methods of hormonal evaluation have been discussed in the tumor-specific sections (see earlier) and are generally applicable to incidentalomas. However, one conceptual difference is that the biochemical thresholds that prompt operative treatment are somewhat lower in patients with an initial radiographic presentation (incidentalomas) compared with those with an initial clinical presentation. This is because tumor size, which correlates strongly with risk of malignancy, contributes an additive effect in favor of surgical management.

Evaluation begins with history taking, with a focus on prior malignant disease, hypertension, and symptoms of glucocorticoid or sex steroid excess. Biochemical investigations for hormonally active tumors are followed by consideration of size criteria (Fig. 39-21). In a general sense, surgery is recommended for hormonally active tumors and those that carry a significant risk of malignancy. Adrenocortical carcinomas represent less than 2% of adrenal tumors measuring 4 cm or smaller and roughly 6% of those measuring 4 to 6 cm. Tumors larger than 6 cm carry a more than 25% risk of malignancy. Because studies have consistently found that CT and MRI underestimate adrenal tumor size by approximately 20%, an effect that is exaggerated in smaller tumors, our practice is to remove all incidentalomas measuring 4 cm or larger in low-risk surgical patients. We strongly consider removal of those measuring 3 to 4 cm, particularly in younger patients who wish to avoid the burden of surveillance imaging.

Factors that should be considered in surgical decision making for this latter group include suspicious imaging characteristics, the patient's age and surgical risk, growth on interval imaging, and the patient's preference. Characteristics suggestive of a benign lesion on CT scan include homogeneous appearance, well-defined borders, high lipid content, rapid washout of contrast material, and low degree of vascularity. Features that are concerning for malignancy include irregular or ill-defined borders, necrosis, internal calcifications or hemorrhage, and high vascularity. ^{18}F-FDG PET is usually reserved for suspicious cases and has high sensitivity and specificity for distinguishing between benign and malignant adrenal lesions, although it cannot differentiate between a metastasis and primary adrenocortical carcinoma.[43] If observation is chosen, patients should undergo repeated imaging in 6 to 12 months and then on an annual basis, given the fact that 5% to 25% of adrenal masses may increase in size.

It must be emphasized that CT-guided fine-needle aspiration is rarely helpful in the evaluation of adrenal masses and may be hazardous. The diagnosis of primary adrenal malignancy cannot reliably be made on the basis of cytologic criteria alone. Therefore, the use of fine-needle aspiration is generally confined to patients with a history of extra-adrenal malignancy in whom the clinician seeks to establish the diagnosis of metastatic disease. In all cases, pheochromocytoma must be excluded before attempting such a procedure to avoid precipitating potentially fatal hypertensive crisis.

As with the other disease processes that have been discussed, most adrenal incidentalomas can be removed laparoscopically, except for those displaying obvious malignant features on imaging. No upper size limit to this approach has been established, and tumors measuring 15 cm have been successfully removed laparoscopically by experienced surgeons.

Metastases to the Adrenal Gland

Epidemiology and Clinical Features

The adrenal glands are common sites of metastasis because of their rich vascular supply. Autopsy studies have revealed that approximately 25% of patients with carcinomas eventually develop adrenal involvement. In 50% of these cases, metastatic disease is bilateral. The primary cancers that most often spread to the adrenals are those of the lung, gastrointestinal tract, breast, kidney, pancreas, and skin (melanoma). Patients with isolated adrenal metastases represent a very small subset of the total. However, these individuals are of particular interest to the surgeon and oncologist because evidence has indicated that resection of isolated adrenal metastases may improve survival. Depending on the underlying disease, 5-year survival rates of approximately 25% can be achieved after adrenalectomy.

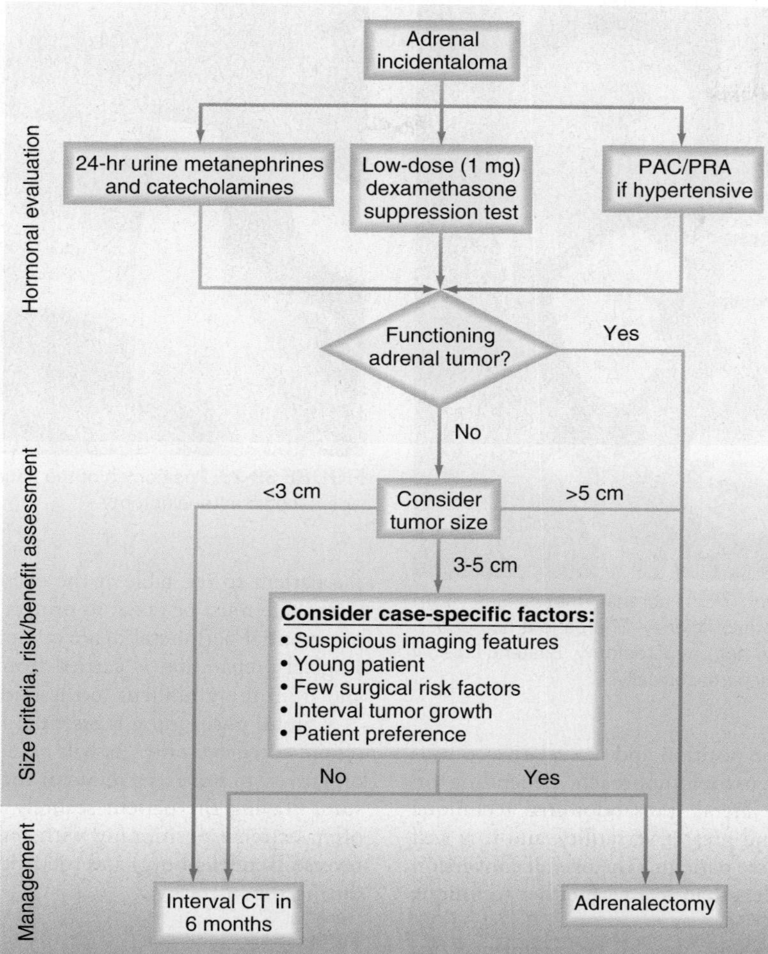

FIGURE 39-21 Algorithm for the management of an adrenal incidentaloma. Adrenalectomy is recommended for all patients with functional tumors. For nonfunctioning tumors, the risk for malignancy is assessed according to size. Tumors larger than 5 cm on CT carry a more than 25% risk for malignancy and need to be removed. Those smaller than 3 cm can be safely observed. Case-specific factors must be considered for intermediate-sized tumors. *PAC,* plasma aldosterone concentration, in ng/dL; *PRA,* plasma renin activity, in ng/(mL • hr).

Clinical Evaluation and Surgical Management

Evaluation of patients presenting with isolated adrenal metastases must involve careful exclusion of extra-adrenal disease with CT or MRI (including the head in cases of breast cancer or melanoma, and triphasic contrast-enhanced CT evaluation of the liver plus 3-mm slices through the lungs for gastrointestinal malignant neoplasms) as well as bone and PET scans, when appropriate. Patients presenting with isolated bilateral adrenal metastases (Fig. 39-22) must be evaluated for adrenal insufficiency because of replacement of all normal adrenal tissue with tumor, which may occur in up to 30% of these patients. This is best performed with measurement of morning cortisol and ACTH levels. Cortical insufficiency should be adequately treated before operation to avoid perioperative adrenal crisis.

Most adrenal metastases are well encapsulated and are thus amenable to laparoscopic resection. Complete adrenal metastasectomy has yielded mean survival rates of 20 to 30 months in most series[44] compared with 12 months for patients undergoing incomplete resection and 6 months for patients not undergoing surgical therapy.

TECHNICAL ASPECTS OF ADRENALECTOMY

Choice of Operative Approach

In our practice, approximately 90% of adrenalectomies are performed laparoscopically. Laparoscopic adrenalectomy affords many advantages, including reduced length of hospitalization, reduced pain, decreased operative blood loss, and lower rate of postoperative complications, compared with conventional open surgery.[45] Similar degrees of benefit are observed with laparoscopic transabdominal and posterior retroperitoneoscopic approaches. Randomized controlled trials have demonstrated reduced postoperative pain and faster recovery after the posterior retroperitoneoscopic approach.[46,47] We currently employ both techniques and favor the retroperitoneoscopic approach for tumors smaller than 6 cm, for bilateral tumors, and in patients with a history of extensive prior abdominal surgery. The retroperitoneoscopic approach is more challenging in older, obese male patients because of increased retroperitoneal fat, making initial entry and orientation more difficult. Severe obesity (body mass index >35) results in compression of the retroperitoneum by the abdominal viscera

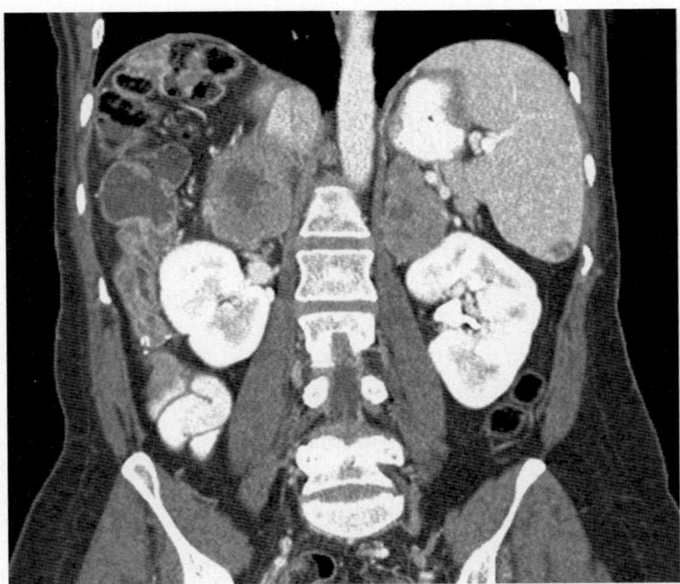

FIGURE 39-22 Isolated bilateral 7-cm adrenal metastases from colorectal cancer causing adrenal insufficiency. The patient had undergone previous right colectomy and right hepatectomy. Bilateral adrenal metastasectomy was performed laparoscopically.

when the patient is in the prone position and is a relative contraindication to the retroperitoneoscopic approach, depending on the surgeon's experience. The lateral transabdominal technique offers a wider operative field and greater versatility, and it is well suited for larger tumors and obese patients. The overall conversion rate to open adrenalectomy is less than 5% with either technique in large series.

As noted, open adrenalectomy should be performed for primary adrenal tumors demonstrating features suggestive of malignancy, such as large size (>8 cm), clinical feminization, hypersecretion of multiple steroid hormones, or any of the following imaging attributes: local or vascular invasion, regional adenopathy, and metastases. For open adrenalectomy, we prefer a transabdominal approach, which is performed through a subcostal incision (see later).

Laparoscopic Lateral Transabdominal Adrenalectomy

Patient Preparation and Positioning

Draw sheets and a full-length beanbag are placed on the operating table in advance. It is important that the table be capable of flexion and have a kidney rest that can be elevated. The patient is initially positioned supine for induction of anesthesia and placement of a urinary catheter. Intermittent pneumatic compression devices are applied to the legs. The placement of an orogastric or nasogastric tube for gastric decompression is frequently helpful, particularly in treating left-sided lesions. The patient is then turned on his or her side (80-degree lateral decubitus position), with the side of the lesion facing upward (Fig. 39-23). At this point, the patient is carefully positioned cephalocaudally so that the 10th rib is directly over the break point in the table. The table is flexed and the beanbag rigidified in a position that supports the buttocks and back while leaving the umbilicus, an important surface landmark, exposed. Flexing the table and raising the kidney rest serve to widen the space between the costal margin and iliac crest and to drop the iliac crest away from the plane of the laparoscopic instruments. Wide cloth tape is used to secure the patient to the table at the chest, hips, and lower extremities. Great care must be taken to protect bone prominences and points of potential peripheral nerve compression in the extremities. The surgical preparation is carried from the nipple line to the pubis and from the umbilicus to the midline of the back.

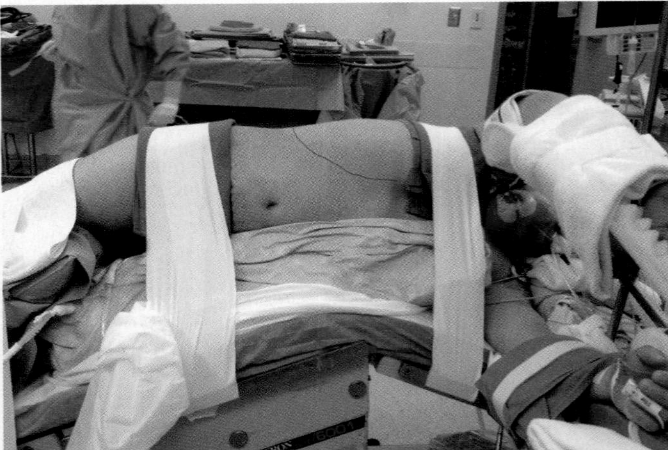

FIGURE 39-23 Positioning of the patient for left lateral transabdominal laparoscopic adrenalectomy.

Careful positioning is essential for technical success in laparoscopic adrenalectomy. As will be discussed, the surgeon is reliant on gravity to serve as a retractor for providing the necessary exposure. Having the patient securely fixed to the table permits the often extreme positioning with respect to pitch (Trendelenburg, reverse Trendelenburg) and roll (tilting left, right) that is necessary during the operation.

Technique

Left adrenal. Initial peritoneal access is achieved 2 cm inferior to the costal margin in the midclavicular line (Palmer's point). This can be performed with the Veress technique or using an optical trocar in most cases. We generally use three radially dilating trocars, and a fourth may be added in cases in which the spleen and pancreatic tail require additional retraction. The ports are equally distributed along the costal margin, with the posterior port placed as far lateral-posterior as permitted by the position of the colon (Fig. 39-24). It is advisable to leave at least 5 cm (4 fingerbreadths) between each port to minimize external interference of the laparoscopic instruments. For tissue dissection, we employ the hook monopolar cautery and an energy-based tissue sealing or dividing device.

The lateral attachments of the spleen are taken down first, with the goal of rotating the left upper quadrant viscera anteromedially. Care must be taken to avoid a capsular tear of the spleen, which may arise from undue tension on a congenital or acquired adhesive band. Splenic mobilization is continued until the greater curvature of the stomach becomes visible at its apex, at which point the spleen and tail of the pancreas are allowed to fall anteriorly with rightward tilting of the table and gentle use of the fan retractor, if necessary. It is critical to achieve the correct plane of dissection precisely during this part of the procedure because the tail of the pancreas and splenic vessels are potentially vulnerable to injury. In patients with large or inferiorly positioned tumors, the splenic flexure of the colon must be mobilized caudally by dividing the splenocolic ligament. We use an open book technique, which involves developing the cleft-like plane just medial

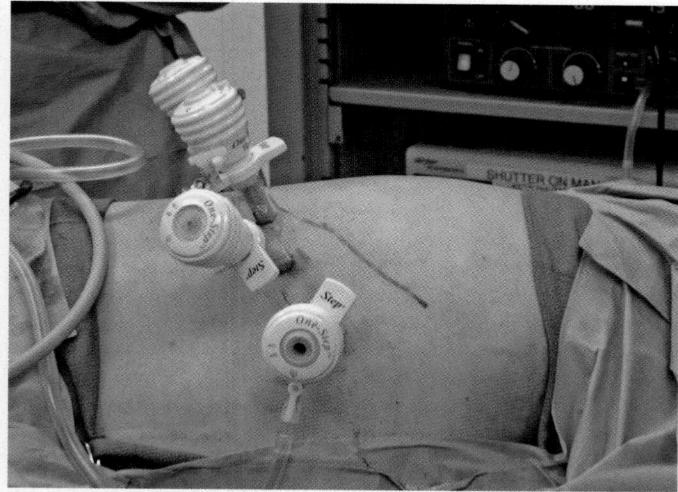

FIGURE 39-24 Port placement for right laparoscopic adrenalectomy. The patient is lying right-side up, with the head toward the right. The *marked line* denotes the costal margin. Ports are placed approximately 2 cm inferior to the costal margin, spaced about 4 fingerbreadths apart.

to the adrenal gland and lateral to the aorta (Fig. 39-25). The left-hand page of the book is composed of the spleen, tail of the pancreas, and greater curvature of the stomach. The right-hand page of the book is made up by the kidney and adrenal tumor. The left crus of the diaphragm is a useful landmark that leads the surgeon to the left inferior phrenic vein.

As mentioned in the anatomy section of this chapter, the left inferior phrenic vein courses along the medial aspect of the left adrenal gland before joining with the left adrenal vein. By developing the cleft of the open book, moving from superior to inferior, the adrenal vein is encountered at the inferomedial aspect of the adrenal gland. The small adrenal arteries that lie within this plane can be handled with energy-based coagulation. The left adrenal vein is carefully dissected out, aggressively coagulated or clipped, and divided. The inferior tip of the left adrenal gland may extend low, approaching the renal hilum within millimeters. However, because the left adrenal vein is rather long (2 cm), it is generally not necessary to expose the renal vasculature during left adrenalectomy. Many patients have a superior pole renal artery branch that approaches the inferior aspect of the left adrenal gland. Injury to this structure must be carefully avoided by keeping dissection close to the adrenal capsule while the specimen is elevated away from the medial aspect of the superior pole of the left kidney.

The adrenal gland is liberated by completing dissection circumferentially and posteriorly, taking the specimen off of the superior pole of the kidney and posterior abdominal wall. These attachments are deliberately divided last because they aid in suspending the adrenal gland on the lateral-superior wall of the operative field, providing exposure of the medial vascular plane during the critical initial portion of the procedure. The tumor is placed into a resilient catchment device, morcellated, and extracted. If noncutting trocars are used, only the skin will need to be closed.

Right adrenal. Laparoscopic right adrenalectomy is, in some respects, a mirror image of the procedure just described. During right adrenalectomy, the left-hand page of the open book is made up by the kidney and adrenal tumor and the right-hand page is composed of the bare area of the liver (Fig. 39-26). To gain access to the appropriate plane, the right triangular ligament of the liver

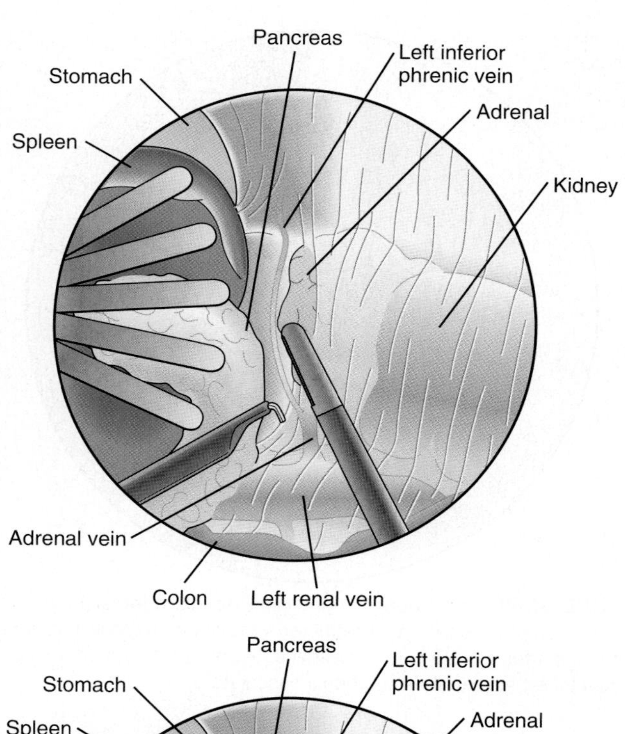

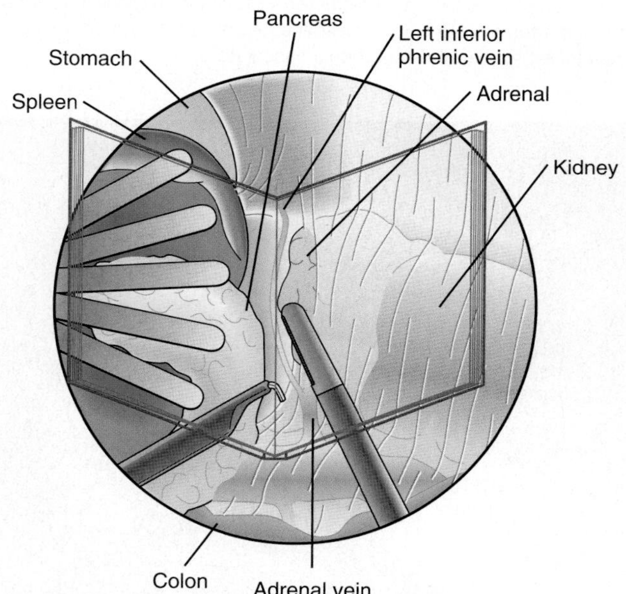

FIGURE 39-25 Technique of left laparoscopic adrenalectomy. The spleen and pancreatic tail have been mobilized and retracted anteromedially to expose the adrenal gland. The cleft of the open book is developed in a superior to inferior direction to identify the inferior phrenic vein and adrenal vein.

must first be completely mobilized and the liver allowed to rotate anteromedially. On the right side, the colon usually lies well inferior to the operative field. When developing the space between the adrenal gland and inferior vena cava from superior to inferior, the surgeon must be mindful of adrenal vein variants, as illustrated in the anatomy section of this chapter (see Fig. 39-3). The right adrenal vein is a potentially perilous structure to manage because it is short, wide, variable, and confluent with thin-walled, large-capacitance vessels (the inferior vena cava in more than 80% of cases, followed by the renal vein and, uncommonly, the right hepatic vein) that can bleed briskly if directly injured (e.g., by the cautery), lacerated from undue traction on adjacent structures, or sheared by clips. A significant second adrenal vein may be found

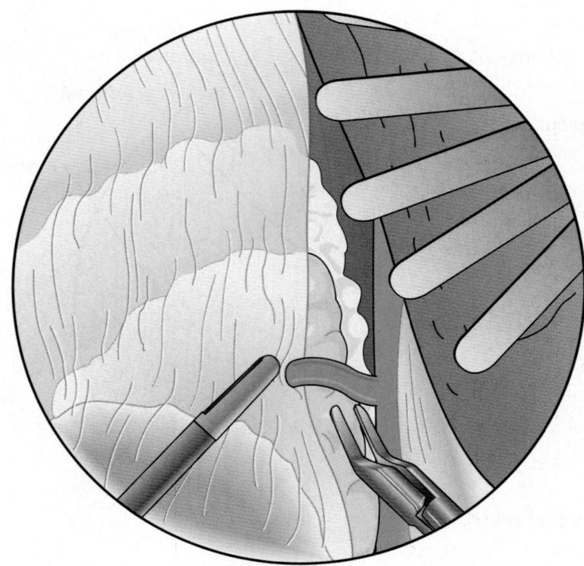

FIGURE 39-26 Technique of right laparoscopic adrenalectomy. The liver has been mobilized and retracted medially to expose the adrenal gland and inferior vena cava. The space just medial to the adrenal gland is developed to identify the adrenal vasculature.

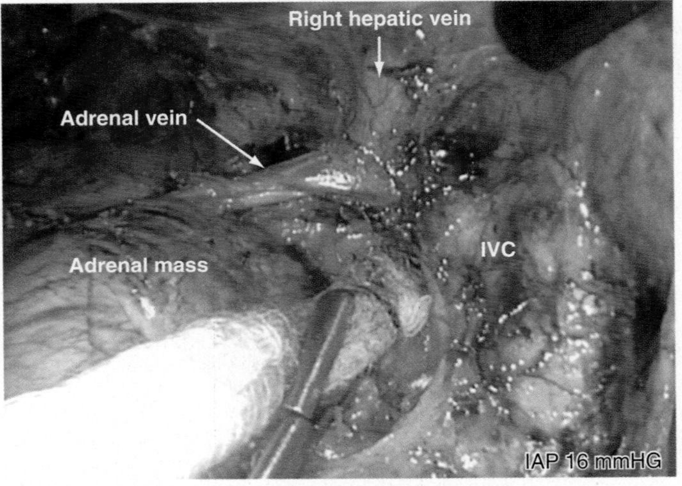

FIGURE 39-27 Right adrenal vein variant. This solitary adrenal vein arises from the superior apex of the gland and drains into the confluence of the inferior vena cava (IVC) and right hepatic vein, as shown in Figure 39-3*F*.

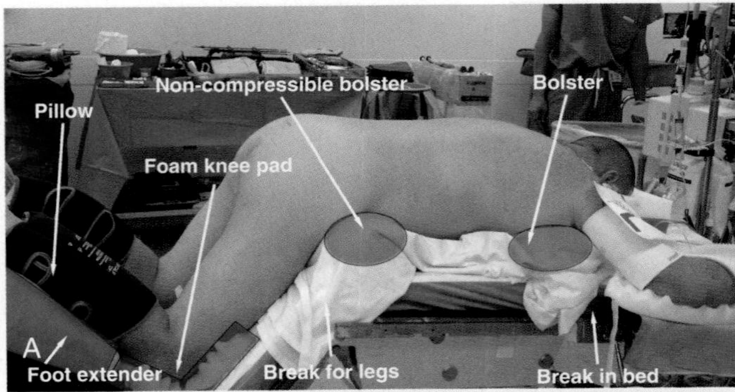

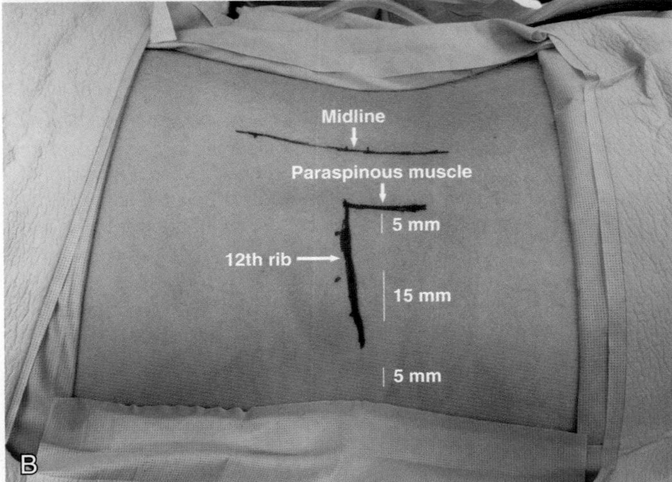

FIGURE 39-28 **A,** Positioning of the patient for posterior retroperitoneoscopic adrenalectomy. **B,** Port placement for posterior retroperitoneoscopic adrenalectomy.

in up to 10% of patients. By methodically dissecting one layer at a time and moving from superior to inferior, all potential adrenal vein variants can be encountered in a controlled fashion (Fig. 39-27). The adrenal vein must be dissected out delicately, definitively ligated (usually with two clips on the patient's side), and then divided. Loss of control of the adrenal vein stump should be avoided; should this occur, conversion to an open procedure may be necessary. A conceptual contrast between left and right adrenalectomy is that left adrenalectomy centers on identification of the correct plane of dissection and right adrenalectomy centers on the avoidance of venous bleeding.

Of note, the junction of the inferior vena cava and right renal vein is frequently difficult to identify. In vivo, the transition is a gradual curve rather than the 90-degree takeoff depicted in anatomy texts. Therefore, it cannot be used as a reliable anatomic landmark for identification of the adrenal vein. After control of the vein, the remaining mobilization of the right adrenal gland is straightforward because the inferomedial limb generally does not reach as far down toward the renal hilum as on the left side.

Posterior Retroperitoneoscopic Adrenalectomy

Posterior retroperitoneoscopic adrenalectomy was popularized in 1994 by Walz and associates.[48] The technique has undergone a series of refinements so that now a subset of lean patients with tumors smaller than 4 cm in diameter can be managed by a novel single-access technique.[49] The retroperitoneal approach has several advantages, including avoidance of mobilization of the solid organs that is necessary with transabdominal approaches, elimination of the need for repositioning during bilateral adrenalectomy, and avoidance of anterior adhesions in patients with extensive prior abdominal surgery. One disadvantage is the relatively small working space, which makes the retroperitoneal technique best suited for tumors less than 7 cm in diameter.

A prone position is used, with supports placed under the lower chest and pelvic girdle so that the abdomen is allowed to hang anteriorly (Fig. 39-28*A*). Three ports are placed inferior to the 12th rib (Fig. 39-28*B*) using a direct cut-down technique for initial access. Relatively high insufflation pressures of 20 to 28 mm Hg are used and have caused no complications in regard to air emboli, hypercapnia, or clinically significant soft tissue emphysema. The working space is initially created by bluntly dissecting

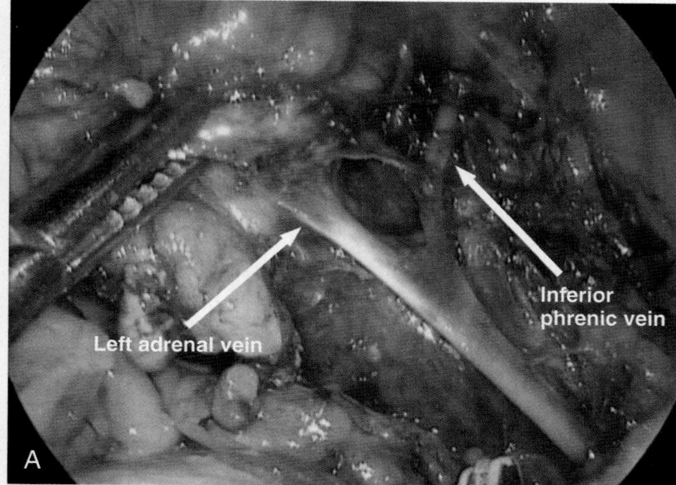

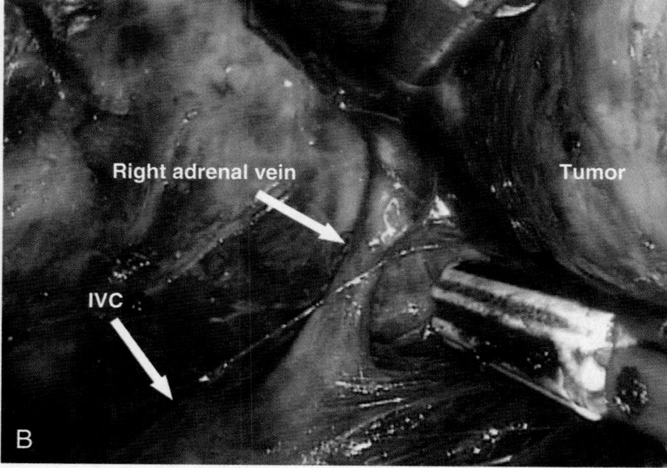

FIGURE 39-29 **A,** Posterior view of the left adrenal vein. **B,** Posterior view of the right adrenal vein. *IVC,* inferior vena cava.

the retroperitoneal contents anteriorly away from the ports. The upper pole of the kidney is mobilized and reflected inferiorly to expose the adrenal gland. Mobilization of the adrenal gland begins near the paraspinous muscles, at the inferomedial aspect of the gland. This is where the left adrenal vein is almost always encountered early in the procedure (Fig. 39-29*A*). On the right side, the vein is encountered slightly later as dissection proceeds superiorly (Fig. 39-29*B*). The small adrenal arteries that run within the medial vascular space are coagulated. After the superior apex of the adrenal gland is mobilized, dissection proceeds circumferentially to include the periadrenal fat.

Complications and Postoperative Care

Potential technical complications include venous hemorrhage and bleeding from solid organ capsular injuries. Small amounts of bleeding can often be managed with coagulation or direct pressure using a rolled Kittner gauze. Hollow viscus injuries are uncommon but may be associated with procedures performed in patients with prior major abdominal surgery. Pancreatic injuries and fistulas have been reported with left-sided procedures; these are rare complications, as are port site hernias and port site metastases in cases of malignant disease. Violation of the tumor capsule and tumor spillage can lead to tumor recurrence, especially in the case of pheochromocytoma.[50] Patients undergoing laparoscopic adrenalectomy for Cushing syndrome are at risk for surgical site infections because of their catabolic and immunosuppressed state. These include port site infections in 5% of patients and, rarely, subphrenic abscesses requiring catheter drainage. One complication specific to the retroperitoneal approach is injury of the subcostal nerve causing relaxation or hypoesthesia of the abdominal wall, which occurs in 8% of cases and is usually temporary.

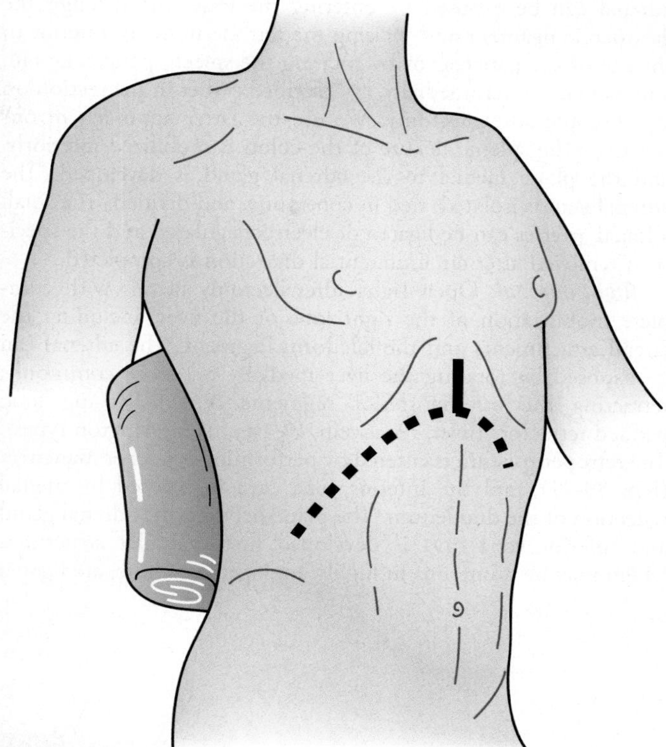

FIGURE 39-30 Positioning of the patient for open right adrenalectomy.

Patients who undergo laparoscopic adrenalectomy recover rapidly. Most patients, including approximately 50% of those treated for pheochromocytoma, can leave the hospital on the first postoperative day. In the treatment of adrenal tumors, successful outcomes hinge on excellent perioperative medical management as much as technical skill, particularly in cases of pheochromocytoma and Cushing syndrome. These considerations have been discussed earlier.

Open Anterior Transabdominal Adrenalectomy

Patient Preparation and Positioning

Neuraxial blockade (use of an epidural catheter) is routinely used for intraoperative and postoperative anesthetic or analgesic management. The patient is positioned supine, with the ipsilateral side slightly elevated on a bolster (Fig. 39-30). A urinary catheter, orogastric or nasogastric tube, and intermittent pneumatic compression devices are placed. The surgical preparation is carried from the nipple line to the pubis and down to the table on either side.

Technique

Left adrenal. We prefer to use a subcostal incision, which may be extended across the midline (chevron), with or without a vertical upper midline extension, to achieve wide exposure. The left adrenal can be exposed by entering the lesser sac through the gastrocolic ligament and incising the retroperitoneum inferior to the tail of the pancreas or by rotating the spleen, pancreatic tail, and stomach anteromedially, as described earlier in the section on laparoscopic adrenalectomy. We use the latter approach in our practice. The splenic flexure of the colon is mobilized inferiorly, and the plane medial to the adrenal gland is developed. The adrenal vein is isolated, tied in continuity, and divided. The small adrenal arteries can be ligated or electrocoagulated and the specimen removed after circumferential dissection is completed.

Right adrenal. Open right adrenalectomy begins with complete mobilization of the right lobe of the liver, including the lateral attachments and the falciform ligament. The adrenal can be exposed by rotating the liver medially or, more commonly, retracting the inferoposterior segments cephalad using long padded retractors (liver, renal vein, Deaver, or Harrington types). The retroperitoneum is entered by performing a Kocher maneuver (Fig. 39-31), and the inferior vena cava is exposed by medial reflection of the duodenum. The plane between the adrenal gland and inferior vena cava is developed first. Vascular structures, which may be numerous in highly angiogenic tumors, are ligated sequentially. The adrenal vein is isolated, securely tied, and divided. Loss of control of the adrenal vein stump may be managed with the application of a side-biting (Satinsky) vascular clamp. As noted, open adrenalectomy is generally performed in cases of suspected or known malignant disease (Fig. 39-32). Locally invasive right-sided adrenal tumors can be challenging to manage, given their frequent invasion of adjacent venous structures (Fig. 39-33*A*). It is our practice to involve an experienced vascular or liver surgeon in the management of tumors with extensive venous invasion. Locally invaded organs, most commonly the kidney, should be resected en bloc with the primary mass. Complete radical resection is a critical determinant of survival in patients with malignant adrenal tumors; in some cases, this can be achieved only if immediate venous reconstruction is performed (Fig. 39-33*B*).

Complications and Postoperative Care

Technical complications of open adrenalectomy include venous hemorrhage, tumor embolization in cases with intravascular tumor extension, and solid organ injury. Postoperative complications are similar to those associated with other major abdominal

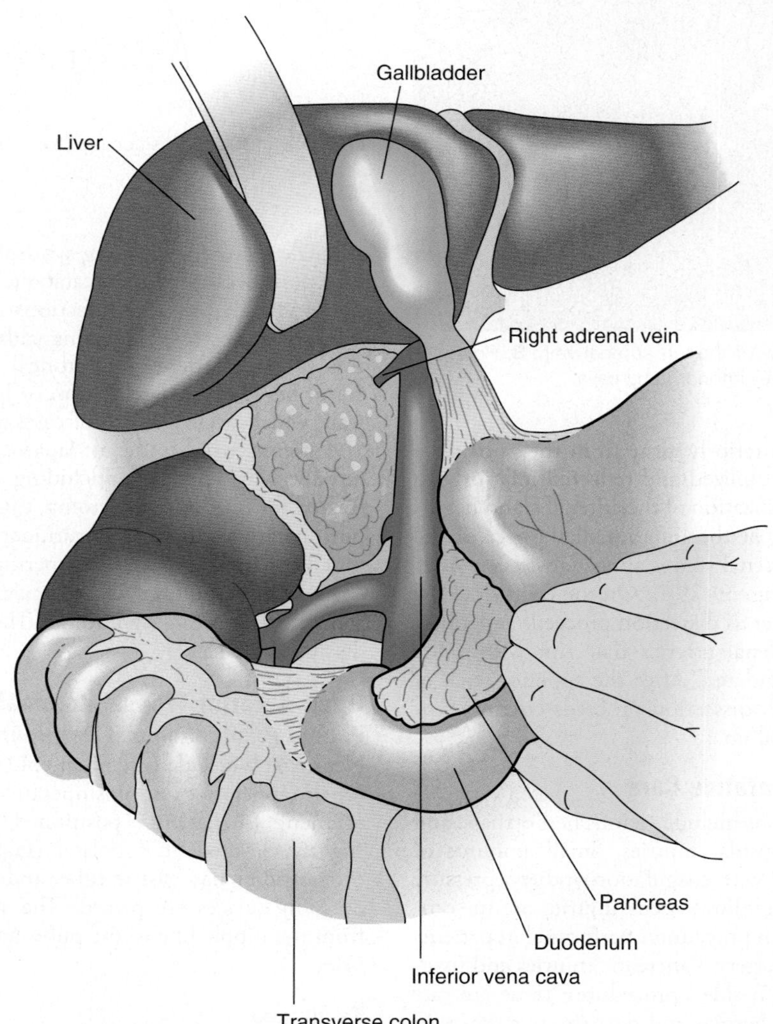

FIGURE 39-31 Open right adrenalectomy. The right lobe of the liver and the hepatic flexure of the colon have been completely mobilized. The retroperitoneum is entered, and the duodenum and head of the pancreas are reflected medially (Kocher maneuver) to expose the adrenal gland and inferior vena cava.

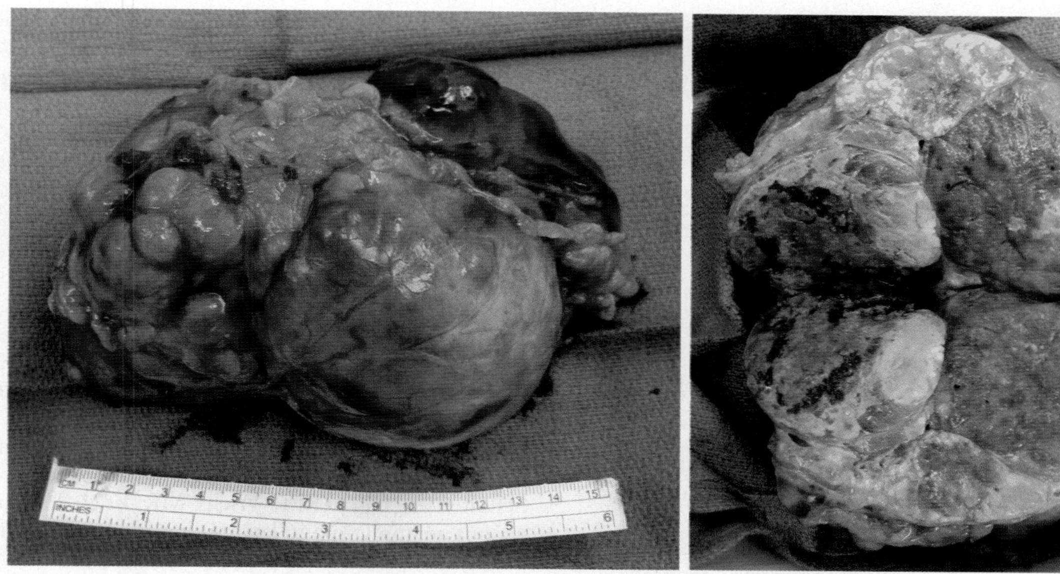

FIGURE 39-32 Gross appearance of adrenocortical carcinoma.

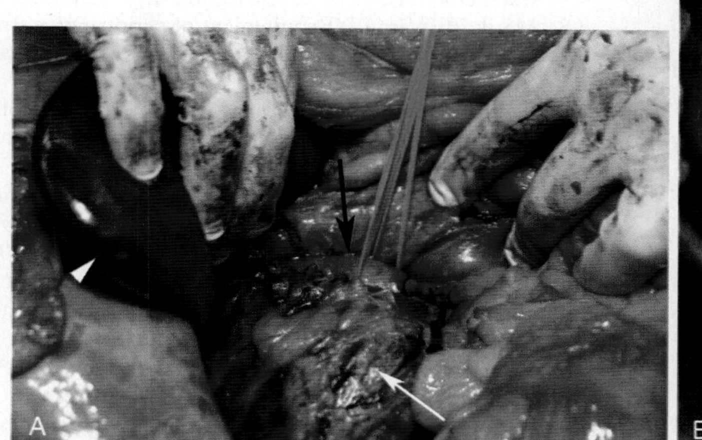

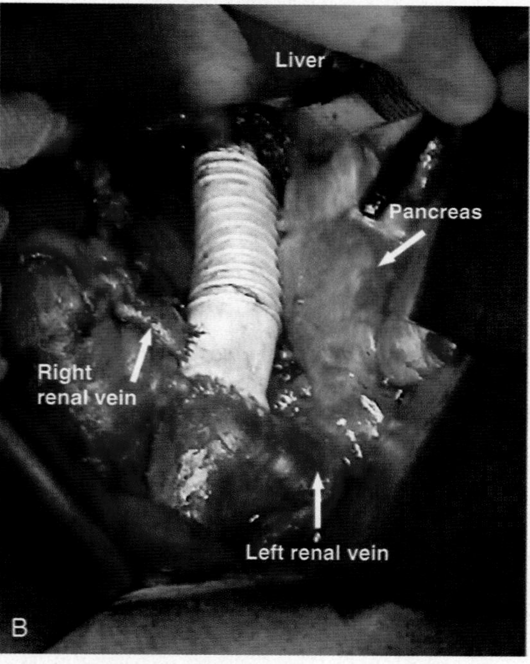

FIGURE 39-33 A, Open resection of a right adrenocortical carcinoma invading the inferior vena cava. The patient's head is to the left. The liver *(arrowhead)* is retracted cephalad. The *white arrow* indicates the tumor; the *black arrow* indicates the inferior vena cava, which is encircled with vessel loops. **B,** The infrahepatic inferior vena cava has been replaced with a polytetrafluoroethylene graft.

procedures. Most patients experience return of bowel function within 3 to 4 days and are able to leave the hospital on postoperative days 5 to 7.

SELECTED REFERENCES

Benn DE, Gimenez-Roqueplo AP, Reilly JR, et al: Clinical presentation and penetrance of pheochromocytoma/paraganglioma syndromes. *J Clin Endocrinol Metab* 91:827–836, 2006.

International SDH Consortium study elucidating genotype-phenotype associations in patients with pheochromocytoma/paraganglioma.

Fassnacht M, Terzolo M, Allolio B, et al: Combination chemotherapy in advanced adrenocortical carcinoma. *N Engl J Med* 366:2189–2197, 2012.

Until recently, mitotane has been the only accepted systemic therapy for patients with adrenocortical cancer. This randomized study of 304 patients in Europe showed improved progression-free survival in patients treated with multidrug chemotherapy in addition to mitotane.

Gifford RW, Jr, Kvale WF, Maher FT, et al: Clinical features, diagnosis and treatment of pheochromocytoma: A review of 76 cases. *Mayo Clin Proc* 39:281–302, 1964.

A landmark account of the biochemical, pharmacologic, and physiologic advances that allowed collaborators at the Mayo Clinic to treat 76 patients with pheochromocytoma while experiencing only one death.

Lenders JW, Duh QY, Eisenhofer G, et al: Pheochromocytoma and paraganglioma: An Endocrine Society clinical practice guideline. *J Clin Endocrinol Metab* 99:1915–1942, 2014.

Consensus guidelines from the Endocrine Society recommending the appropriate biochemical, imaging, and genetic evaluation as well as treatment for patients with pheochromocytoma and paraganglioma.

Nobel lectures, physiology or medicine 1942-1962, Amsterdam, 1964, Elsevier Publishing Company.

An account of the clinical discoveries and advances in organic chemistry that led to the identification, isolation, and artificial synthesis of adrenal cortical hormones. A full transcript can be found at http://nobelprize.org.

Nobel lectures, physiology or medicine 1971-1980, Amsterdam, 1992, Elsevier Publishing Company.

Documents the formidable challenges surmounted in the identification of peptide hormones, found in such minute concentrations, and the development of the radioimmunoassay necessary for their detection. A full transcript can be found at http://nobelprize.org.

Sukor N, Kogovsek C, Gordon RD, et al: Improved quality of life, blood pressure, and biochemical status following laparoscopic adrenalectomy for unilateral primary aldosteronism. *J Clin Endocrinol Metab* 95:1360–1364, 2010.

This prospective pilot study examines an array of short-term outcomes after surgical treatment of hyperaldosteronism.

Walz MK, Alesina PF, Wenger FA, et al: Posterior retroperitoneoscopic adrenalectomy—results of 560 procedures in 520 patients. *Surgery* 140:943–948, 2006.

The largest single-institution series on this procedure, written by the developers of the technique.

Welbourn RB: Early surgical history of phaeochromocytoma. *Br J Surg* 74:594–596, 1987.

Describes the initial achievements of American and European surgeons in the successful treatment of pheochromocytoma.

Zeiger MA, Thompson GB, Duh QY, et al: The American Association of Clinical Endocrinologists and American Association of Endocrine Surgeons medical guidelines for the management of adrenal incidentalomas. *Endocr Pract* 15(Suppl 1):1–20, 2009.

Consensus guidelines from the American Association of Clinical Endocrinologists and American Association of Endocrine Surgeons on workup and treatment of adrenal incidentalomas.

REFERENCES

1. *Nobel lectures, physiology or medicine 1942-1962*, Amsterdam, 1964, Elsevier Publishing Company.
2. *Nobel lectures, physiology or medicine 1971-1980*, Amsterdam, 1992, Elsevier Publishing Company.
3. Scholten A, Cisco RM, Vriens MR, et al: Variant adrenal venous anatomy in 546 laparoscopic adrenalectomies. *JAMA Surg* 148:378–383, 2013.
4. Lenders JW, Pacak K, Walther MM, et al: Biochemical diagnosis of pheochromocytoma: Which test is best? *JAMA* 287:1427–1434, 2002.
5. Nieman LK, Chanco Turner ML: Addison's disease. *Clin Dermatol* 24:276–280, 2006.
6. Shen WT, Kebebew E, Clark OH, et al: Selective use of steroid replacement after adrenalectomy: Lessons from 331 consecutive cases. *Arch Surg* 141:771–774, 2006.
7. Annane D, Bellissant E, Bollaert PE, et al: Corticosteroids in the treatment of severe sepsis and septic shock in adults: A systematic review. *JAMA* 301:2362–2375, 2009.
8. Marik PE, Varon J: Requirement of perioperative stress doses of corticosteroids: A systematic review of the literature. *Arch Surg* 143:1222–1226, 2008.
9. Douma S, Petidis K, Doumas M, et al: Prevalence of primary hyperaldosteronism in resistant hypertension: A retrospective observational study. *Lancet* 371:1921–1926, 2008.
10. Mulatero P, Monticone S, Bertello C, et al: Long-term cardio- and cerebrovascular events in patients with primary aldosteronism. *J Clin Endocrinol Metab* 98:4826–4833, 2013.
11. Choi M, Scholl UI, Yue P, et al: K^+ channel mutations in adrenal aldosterone-producing adenomas and hereditary hypertension. *Science* 331:768–772, 2011.
12. Zeiger MA, Thompson GB, Duh QY, et al: The American Association of Clinical Endocrinologists and American Association of Endocrine Surgeons medical guidelines for the management of adrenal incidentalomas. *Endocr Pract* 15(Suppl 1):1–20, 2009.
13. Young WF, Stanson AW, Thompson GB, et al: Role for adrenal venous sampling in primary aldosteronism. *Surgery* 136:1227–1235, 2004.
14. Funder JW, Carey RM, Fardella C, et al: Case detection, diagnosis, and treatment of patients with primary aldosteronism: An endocrine society clinical practice guideline. *J Clin Endocrinol Metab* 93:3266–3281, 2008.
15. Lim V, Guo Q, Grant CS, et al: Accuracy of adrenal imaging and adrenal venous sampling in predicting surgical cure of primary aldosteronism. *J Clin Endocrinol Metab* 99:2712–2719, 2014.
16. Harvey A, Kline G, Pasieka JL: Adrenal venous sampling in primary hyperaldosteronism: Comparison of radiographic with biochemical success and the clinical decision-making

with "less than ideal" testing. *Surgery* 140:847–853, discussion 853–855, 2006.
17. Sukor N, Kogovsek C, Gordon RD, et al: Improved quality of life, blood pressure, and biochemical status following laparoscopic adrenalectomy for unilateral primary aldosteronism. *J Clin Endocrinol Metab* 95:1360–1364, 2010.
18. Beuschlein F, Fassnacht M, Assié G, et al: Constitutive activation of PKA catalytic subunit in adrenal Cushing's syndrome. *N Engl J Med* 370:1019–1028, 2014.
19. Lindholm J, Juul S, Jorgensen JO, et al: Incidence and late prognosis of Cushing's syndrome: A population-based study. *J Clin Endocrinol Metab* 86:117–123, 2001.
20. Papanicolaou DA, Mullen N, Kyrou I, et al: Nighttime salivary cortisol: A useful test for the diagnosis of Cushing's syndrome. *J Clin Endocrinol Metab* 87:4515–4521, 2002.
21. Newell-Price J, Bertagna X, Grossman AB, et al: Cushing's syndrome. *Lancet* 367:1605–1617, 2006.
22. Esposito F, Dusick JR, Cohan P, et al: Clinical review: Early morning cortisol levels as a predictor of remission after transsphenoidal surgery for Cushing's disease. *J Clin Endocrinol Metab* 91:7–13, 2006.
23. Sippel RS, Elaraj DM, Kebebew E, et al: Waiting for change: Symptom resolution after adrenalectomy for Cushing's syndrome. *Surgery* 144:1054–1060, 2008.
24. Chiodini I, Morelli V, Salcuni AS, et al: Beneficial metabolic effects of prompt surgical treatment in patients with an adrenal incidentaloma causing biochemical hypercortisolism. *J Clin Endocrinol Metab* 95:2736–2745, 2010.
25. Toniato A, Merante-Boschin I, Opocher G, et al: Surgical versus conservative management for subclinical Cushing syndrome in adrenal incidentalomas: A prospective randomized study. *Ann Surg* 249:388–391, 2009.
26. Ng L, Libertino JM: Adrenocortical carcinoma: Diagnosis, evaluation and treatment. *J Urol* 169:5–11, 2003.
27. Soon PS, Sidhu SB: Adrenocortical carcinoma. *Cancer Treat Res* 153:187–210, 2010.
28. Bilimoria KY, Shen WT, Elaraj D, et al: Adrenocortical carcinoma in the United States: Treatment utilization and prognostic factors. *Cancer* 113:3130–3136, 2008.
29. Yeh MW, Lisewski D, Campbell P: Virilizing adrenocortical carcinoma with cavoatrial extension. *Am J Surg* 192:209–210, 2006.
30. Terzolo M, Angeli A, Fassnacht M, et al: Adjuvant mitotane treatment for adrenocortical carcinoma. *N Engl J Med* 356:2372–2380, 2007.
31. Fassnacht M, Terzolo M, Allolio B, et al: Combination chemotherapy in advanced adrenocortical carcinoma. *N Engl J Med* 366:2189–2197, 2012.
32. Welbourn RB: Early surgical history of phaeochromocytoma. *Br J Surg* 74:594–596, 1987.
33. Sawka AM, Prebtani AP, Thabane L, et al: A systematic review of the literature examining the diagnostic efficacy of measurement of fractionated plasma free metanephrines in the biochemical diagnosis of pheochromocytoma. *BMC Endocr Disord* 4:2, 2004.
34. Perry CG, Sawka AM, Singh R, et al: The diagnostic efficacy of urinary fractionated metanephrines measured by tandem mass spectrometry in detection of pheochromocytoma. *Clin Endocrinol (Oxf)* 66:703–708, 2007.
35. Timmers HJ, Chen CC, Carrasquillo JA, et al: Comparison of ^{18}F-fluoro-L-DOPA, ^{18}F-fluoro-deoxyglucose, and ^{18}F-fluorodopamine PET and ^{123}I-MIBG scintigraphy in the localization of pheochromocytoma and paraganglioma. *J Clin Endocrinol Metab* 94:4757–4767, 2009.
36. Gifford RW, Jr, Kvale WF, Maher FT, et al: Clinical features, diagnosis and treatment of pheochromocytoma: A review of 76 cases. *Mayo Clin Proc* 39:281–302, 1964.
37. Shen WT, Grogan R, Vriens M, et al: One hundred two patients with pheochromocytoma treated at a single institution since the introduction of laparoscopic adrenalectomy. *Arch Surg* 145:893–897, 2010.
38. Lenders JW, Duh QY, Eisenhofer G, et al: Pheochromocytoma and paraganglioma: An Endocrine Society clinical practice guideline. *J Clin Endocrinol Metab* 99:1915–1942, 2014.
39. Benn DE, Gimenez-Roqueplo AP, Reilly JR, et al: Clinical presentation and penetrance of pheochromocytoma/paraganglioma syndromes. *J Clin Endocrinol Metab* 91:827–836, 2006.
40. Ellis RJ, Patel D, Prodanov T, et al: Response after surgical resection of metastatic pheochromocytoma and paraganglioma: Can postoperative biochemical remission be predicted? *J Am Coll Surg* 217:489–496, 2013.
41. Gonias S, Goldsby R, Matthay KK, et al: Phase II study of high-dose [^{131}I]metaiodobenzylguanidine therapy for patients with metastatic pheochromocytoma and paraganglioma. *J Clin Oncol* 27:4162–4168, 2009.
42. Terzolo M, Stigliano A, Chiodini I, et al: AME position statement on adrenal incidentaloma. *Eur J Endocrinol* 164:851–870, 2011.
43. Groussin L, Bonardel G, Silvéra S, et al: ^{18}F-Fluorodeoxyglucose positron emission tomography for the diagnosis of adrenocortical tumors: A prospective study in 77 operated patients. *J Clin Endocrinol Metab* 94:1713–1722, 2009.
44. Moreno P, de la Quintana Basarrate A, Musholt TJ, et al: Adrenalectomy for solid tumor metastases: Results of a multicenter European study. *Surgery* 154:1215–1222, discussion 1222–1223, 2013.
45. Lee J, El-Tamer M, Schifftner T, et al: Open and laparoscopic adrenalectomy: Analysis of the National Surgical Quality Improvement Program. *J Am Coll Surg* 206:953–959, 2008.
46. Barczynski M, Konturek A, Nowak W: Randomized clinical trial of posterior retroperitoneoscopic adrenalectomy versus lateral transperitoneal laparoscopic adrenalectomy with a 5-year follow-up. *Ann Surg* 260:740–747, 2014.
47. Mohammadi-Fallah MR, Mehdizadeh A, Badalzadeh A, et al: Comparison of transperitoneal versus retroperitoneal laparoscopic adrenalectomy in a prospective randomized study. *J Laparoendosc Adv Surg Tech A* 23:362–366, 2013.
48. Walz MK, Alesina PF, Wenger FA, et al: Posterior retroperitoneoscopic adrenalectomy—results of 560 procedures in 520 patients. *Surgery* 140:943–948, 2006.
49. Walz MK, Groeben H, Alesina PF: Single-access retroperitoneoscopic adrenalectomy (SARA) versus conventional retroperitoneoscopic adrenalectomy (CORA): A case-control study. *World J Surg* 34:1386–1390, 2010.
50. Li ML, Fitzgerald PA, Price DC, et al: Iatrogenic pheochromocytomatosis: A previously unreported result of laparoscopic adrenalectomy. *Surgery* 130:1072–1077, 2001.

40 CHAPTER

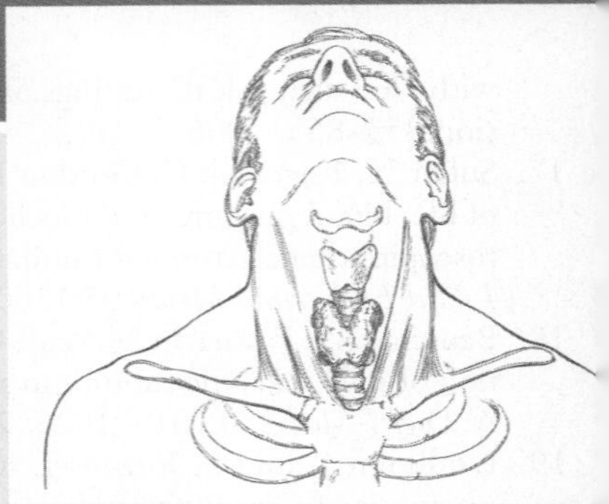

The Multiple Endocrine Neoplasia Syndromes

Terry C. Lairmore, Jeffrey F. Moley

OUTLINE

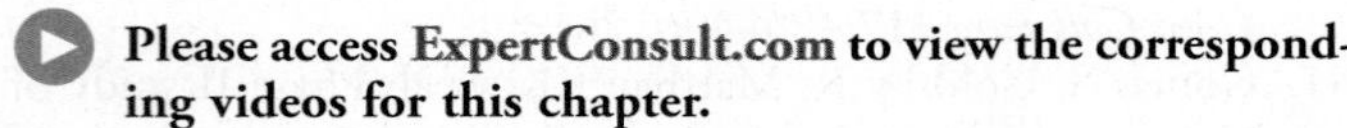

Please access ExpertConsult.com to view the corresponding videos for this chapter.

Genetic changes in a tumor suppressor gene *(MEN1)* and a proto-oncogene *(RET)* result in the multiple endocrine neoplasia (MEN) type 1 and type 2 syndromes, respectively. These hereditary cancer syndromes are characterized by neoplastic transformation in multiple target endocrine tissues as well as by pathologic involvement of some nonendocrine tissues. The associated endocrine tumors may be benign or malignant and may develop either synchronously or metachronously. Within an affected endocrine target tissue, a diffuse preneoplastic hyperplasia typically precedes the development of microscopic invasion or grossly evident multifocal carcinoma. In the MEN syndromes, the genetic predisposition to multiple endocrine neoplasms with malignant potential is conferred on otherwise healthy, young individuals. Importantly, the recent discovery of the specific genetic basis for the MEN1 and MEN2 syndromes has allowed the development of strategies for direct genetic testing, early surgical intervention, and systemic therapies. Early thyroidectomy is indicated for patients with a genetic diagnosis of MEN2, with the aim of preventing the subsequent development of regional or distant medullary thyroid carcinoma (MTC) metastases. The optimal early surgical intervention to prevent metastatic spread of the potentially malignant neuroendocrine tumors (NETs) in patients with a genetic diagnosis of MEN1 remains controversial.

The MEN syndromes are characterized by distinct patterns of endocrine organ involvement. MEN1 is characterized by the development of multiglandular parathyroid disease, NETs of the gastroenteropancreatic system, adenomas of the anterior pituitary gland, foregut and thymic carcinoids, and other associated nonendocrine neoplasms, such as facial angiofibromas, lipomas, and collagenomas. The MEN2A syndrome is characterized by thyroid C-cell hyperplasia, MTC,[1] adrenal medullary hyperplasia, pheochromocytomas, and parathyroid tumors. Features of MEN2B include C-cell hyperplasia, MTC, adrenal medullary hyperplasia, pheochromocytomas, mucosal neuromas, skeletal abnormalities, ganglioneuromatosis of the gastrointestinal tract, and a distinctive habitus (sometimes referred to as marfanoid).

MULTIPLE ENDOCRINE NEOPLASIA TYPE 1

Genetic Studies and Pathogenesis

MEN1 is an autosomal dominant hereditary cancer syndrome with a prevalence of approximately 2 or 3 per 100,000 persons. The MEN1 syndrome results from germline heterozygous loss-of-function mutations in the *MEN1* gene, leading to the development of neoplasms in multiple endocrine and nonendocrine target tissues. The *MEN1* gene encodes a protein termed menin that functions as a tumor suppressor in endocrine tissues. A tumor suppressor protein normally confers a negative influence or brake on cellular growth and proliferation, such that loss of its function results in unregulated or inappropriate cell proliferation and neoplastic transformation. Most causal mutations in the *MEN1* gene result in the production of a truncated or nonfunctional menin. According to the "two-hit" model of tumorigenesis, the first event is a mutation inherited in the germline that confers susceptibility to neoplastic change in the involved tissues. Elimination of the remaining functional copy of the gene in a single cell through a chance somatic mutational event, or *second hit* (such as a gene deletion), results in clonal expansion and cancer development. The occurrence of individual second hits in several target organ cells explains the multifocal involvement characteristically observed in affected endocrine tissues.

The *MEN1* gene[2] encodes a 610–amino acid product that is primarily a nuclear protein, but smaller amounts are present in the cytoplasm and on the cell membrane. Menin is ubiquitously expressed in both endocrine and nonendocrine tissues, but expression levels vary within different tissues. The menin protein sequence is evolutionarily conserved from *Drosophila* to humans, with the murine *MEN1* gene demonstrating 98% homology. Knockout of both *MEN1* alleles in mice results in embryonic lethality, demonstrating that menin is essential for early development and has a broader role in the regulation of cell growth that is not limited to the endocrine tissues affected in MEN1. Heterozygous *MEN1*$^{+/-}$ mice demonstrate somatic loss of the wild-type *MEN1* allele in tumors and develop a constellation of endocrine tumors remarkably similar to the human MEN1 syndrome.

Menin binds to multiple proteins with diverse functions and can act as either a repressor or activator of transcription. Although

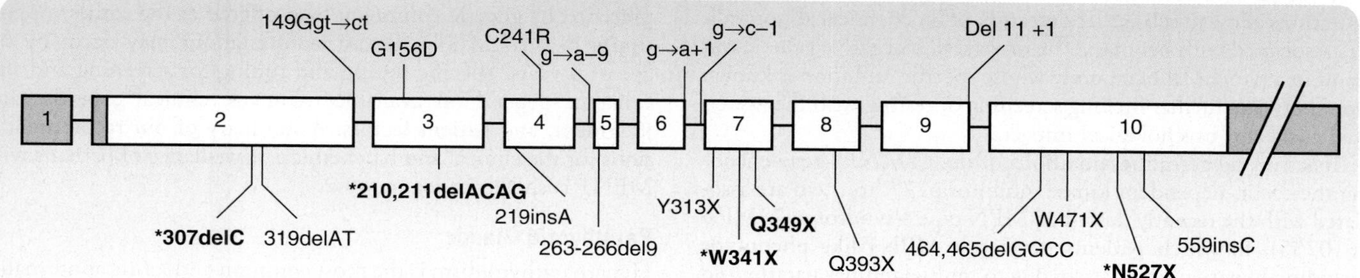

FIGURE 40-1 Germline mutations in the *MEN1* gene in a set of 25 independent kindreds. The mutations are distributed throughout the nine coding exons of the gene. The genetic alterations may include missense, nonsense, frameshift, and RNA-splicing defects that may occur anywhere throughout the coding exons and immediately flanking intron sequences. Five splicing defects and two missense mutations are depicted above the *MEN1* gene, and seven nonsense and six frameshift mutations are depicted below the *MEN1* gene. (From Mutch MG, Dilley WG, Sanjurjo F, et al: Germline mutations in the multiple endocrine neoplasia type 1 gene: Evidence for frequent splicing defects. *Hum Mutat* 13:175–185, 1999.)

menin exerts tumor suppressor actions in endocrine tissues, it is an essential cofactor of oncogenic MLL (mixed lineage leukemia) fusion proteins.[3,4] Chromosomal rearrangements of the *MLL* gene on chromosome band 11q23 result in the fusion of the *MLL* product with more than 60 different protein partners. Disruption of the *MLL* gene by these rearrangements upregulates expression of *HOXA9* and *MEIS1* homeobox genes that are critical to leukemogenesis. Menin's dichotomous role is tissue specific, as demonstrated by its tumor suppressor function in endocrine tissues and its essential role in the development of MLL-associated leukemias. Studies of the crystal structure of menin and its interacting partner proteins reveal that menin is a key scaffold protein that variously regulates gene transcription through interplay with multiple signaling pathways.[5]

Menin is involved in diverse cellular processes including the regulation of gene transcription, cell cycle progression, apoptotic pathways, DNA processing and repair, cytoskeletal integrity, and genome stability. Menin binds to JunD, a member of the AP-1 transcription factor family, and represses JunD-mediated transcription.[6] In addition, menin interacts with multiple proteins that mediate several other important cellular signaling pathways. These include SMAD proteins, which transduce transforming growth factor-β signaling; β-catenin, a member of the Wnt signaling pathway; nuclear receptors, such as estrogen receptor and peroxisome proliferator-activated receptor gamma; and Ras-activating protein SOS1. Importantly, through its interaction as a coregulator of estrogen receptor alpha, menin has been implicated in breast cancer progression. Female patients with MEN1 are at increased risk for breast cancer, and *MEN1* mutations are therefore implicated in human breast carcinogenesis.[7] Although there is now rapidly expanding knowledge about diverse menin interactions and influences on a variety of cellular functions and pathways, there is not yet a comprehensive understanding of its complex roles in these processes.

In 2008, Lemos and Thakker created a database of more than 1330 published independent *MEN1* mutations,[8] and although no additional databases have been compiled subsequently, there are nearly as many unique mutations as families. The approximate distribution of *MEN1* mutations includes 20% missense mutations, 23% nonsense mutations, 41% frameshift insertions or deletions, 6% in-frame insertions or deletions, 9% RNA splice site mutations, and 1% large deletions.[9] These diverse genetic changes occur throughout the coding sequence and intron-exon junctions of the gene[10] without mutation "hot spots," as depicted in Figure 40-1. Approximately 80% of *MEN1* mutations result in a truncated menin protein that does not reach the cell nucleus and exert is role of oncosuppressor.

Somatic mutations in the *MEN1* gene occur frequently in sporadic parathyroid adenomas, pancreatic endocrine tumors, pituitary tumors, and bronchial carcinoids, indicating that allelic loss of the *MEN1* gene is a key genetic event in the development of some nonhereditary endocrine tumors.

Direct DNA mutation testing can identify presymptomatic individuals affected with the MEN1 syndrome, allowing heightened surveillance and early intervention for the endocrine neoplasms that develop in these patients. The clinical application of genetic testing has associated limitations. DNA testing in a family with a previously defined mutation is simplified and can be accomplished by a directed test for that specific genetic change only. However, in a newly identified MEN1 family for which the specific mutation is not known in advance, a comprehensive search of the coding sequence and intron-exon junctions is necessary to search for all possible mutations, and only approximately 80% of such novel families will have the specific mutation identified by conventional testing of the entire gene. For this reason, a negative comprehensive screen for mutations in the *MEN1* gene does not exclude MEN1. Formal genetic counseling and informed consent including disclosures relevant to privacy of medical information and the potential impact of the genetic information on treatment are essential to a comprehensive program of genetic testing.

No common genotype-phenotype correlations have been established for MEN1, although phenotypic variants (isolated hyperparathyroidism, frequent prolactinomas) have been described. Because specific mutations in the *MEN1* gene have not been associated with increased disease progression in the affected patients, however, the use of genetic testing for prediction of malignant potential and prognosis is not possible currently. When an index suspected MEN1 patient is diagnosed clinically, genetic evaluation of that patient and first-degree relatives should be performed. Presymptomatic individuals who test positive for a *MEN1* mutation should then undergo more frequent and more intensive biochemical testing with special emphasis on the potentially malignant enteropancreatic and intrathoracic tumors. Close observation and frequent surveillance of patients with *MEN1* mutations allow much earlier detection of biochemical abnormalities associated with neoplasia.[11] Conversely, a negative genetic test result in a patient from a family whose specific mutation is known would obviate further lifelong screening or testing with the associated costs and psychological impact.

Inactivating germline mutations of the *CDKN1B* gene encoding the cyclin-dependent kinase inhibitor p27^{kip1} protein are associated with the recently described MEN type 4 syndrome (OMIM #610755), in which patients develop a MEN1-like phenotype including hyperparathyroidism due to multiglandular parathyroid enlargement and enteropancreatic NETs, without *MEN1* gene mutations.[12]

Clinical Features and Management

The clinical feature that develops in more than 90% of individuals with a *MEN1* mutation is hyperparathyroidism due to multiglandular parathyroid neoplasms. Patients with MEN1 also develop NETs of the pancreas and duodenum, bronchial and thymic carcinoids, and adenomas of the anterior pituitary with lesser frequency. In addition, adrenocortical nodular hyperplasia, lipomas, collagenomas, and facial angiofibromas occur with increased frequency in patients with MEN1. MEN1-associated angiofibromas, collagenomas, and lipomas have allelic loss of the *MEN1* gene, suggesting a causal relationship to the disease-associated mutations. Clinically, MEN1 is defined as the occurrence of neoplasms in at least two target endocrine tissues (parathyroid, endocrine pancreas, pituitary) in an individual, and familial MEN1 is defined as the additional occurrence of at least one tumor type in a first-degree relative.

Males and females are affected equally with MEN1, as predicted by the autosomal dominant inheritance pattern. MEN1 has been described in many geographic regions and in many ethnic groups, and no racial predilection has been demonstrated. The MEN1 trait is transmitted with essentially 100% penetrance but with variable expressivity, such that each affected person may exhibit some but not necessarily all of the components of the syndrome. Hyperparathyroidism develops in more than 90% of affected individuals. Enteropancreatic NETs (which carry a malignant potential) occur in approximately 30% to 80% of patients, whereas pituitary tumors become clinically evident in approximately 15% to 30% of affected patients. At autopsy, pathologic involvement in all three endocrine tissues has been described in essentially all patients. Compared with sporadic endocrine tumors, the endocrine tumors arising in association with the familial MEN1 syndrome are characterized by an earlier age at onset, multifocal involvement within a target endocrine tissue, and development of tumors in multiple endocrine target tissues.

The clinical manifestations of patients with MEN1 depend on the endocrine tissue involved, the specific hormone overproduced, or the local mass effect and malignant progression of the neoplasm. Previously, complications related to hormone excess, such as severe ulcer disease or hypoglycemia, were the most frequent presenting complaints. Currently, the principal cause of mortality in patients with MEN1 is malignant progression of enteropancreatic neuroendocrine cancers or intrathoracic malignant carcinoid tumors. Consensus clinical guidelines have recently been offered for the clinical evaluation, biochemical screening, and imaging surveillance of patients with MEN1.[13] *MEN1* germline mutation testing should be offered to index patients and their first-degree relatives, including patients who are asymptomatic and patients with clinically evident disease. DNA mutation testing should be preceded by genetic counseling and offered at the earliest opportunity because MEN1 disease manifestations may occur by the age of 5 years. Specific testing and timing for screening and surveillance depend on available resources, clinical expertise and judgment, and patient factors. A summary of our recommendations for the clinical and biochemical surveillance of patients with MEN1 is shown in Figure 40-2.

Parathyroid Glands

Hyperparathyroidism is the most common endocrine abnormality in patients with MEN1 (developing in more than 90% of individuals inheriting a *MEN1* mutation), with an age-dependent clinical onset beginning late in the second decade of life and peaking at approximately 21 to 30 years of age. Hyperparathyroidism in MEN1 is associated with multiglandular parathyroid disease. In contrast, less than 15% of patients with sporadic primary hyperparathyroidism have multiglandular involvement. The typical enlargement of parathyroid glands in MEN1 patients is asymmetrical (Fig. 40-3) at any one time of intervention.[14]

Hypercalcemia is usually the first biochemical abnormality detected in patients with MEN1 and may precede the clinical manifestations of a pancreatic NET by several years. The diagnosis is made by demonstrating hypercalcemia in association with an inappropriately elevated parathyroid hormone (PTH) level. The 24-hour urine calcium excretion is also elevated. Prospective, systematic genetic screening results in the diagnosis of hyperparathyroidism several years earlier than the development of clinically evident disease (Fig. 40-4).[11]

Although hyperparathyroidism is the principal endocrinopathy associated with MEN1, the parathyroid neoplasia underlying the hyperparathyroidism is benign. However, the enteropancreatic, bronchial, and thymic NET tumors that develop in these patients carry a risk of malignant progression. Operative treatment for hyperparathyroidism in MEN1 is associated with higher rates of postoperative hypoparathyroidism and recurrent hyperparathyroidism compared with the results of parathyroidectomy for sporadic hyperparathyroidism, which is most frequently due to a single adenoma. The optimal timing of surgical intervention and the extent of resection present unique features and challenges.

The surgeon should identify all four parathyroid glands and conduct a search for ectopic or supernumerary glands including a transcervical partial thymectomy in patients with MEN1. For this reason, radiographic localizing tests have limited usefulness in the preoperative evaluation. Measurement of PTH levels with quick intraoperative assays allows a biochemical test to determine the appropriate extent of parathyroid tissue resection.[15]

Two common operative procedures have been employed for the management of hyperparathyroidism in patients with MEN1. The first is total parathyroidectomy with heterotopic intramuscular autotransplantation of parathyroid tissue grafts into skeletal muscle. The rationale for this approach is to appropriately reduce the parathyroid tissue volume to achieve normocalcemia while removing all parathyroid tissue from the neck and creating vascularized autografts in a heterotopic site, such as the brachioradialis forearm muscle. If recurrent hyperparathyroidism develops, patients may then undergo reduction of the grafted parathyroid tissue under local anesthesia and without the need for repeated neck surgery. With this operative strategy, high rates of parathyroid graft function must be achieved to have an acceptably low rate of permanent hypoparathyroidism. A second operative

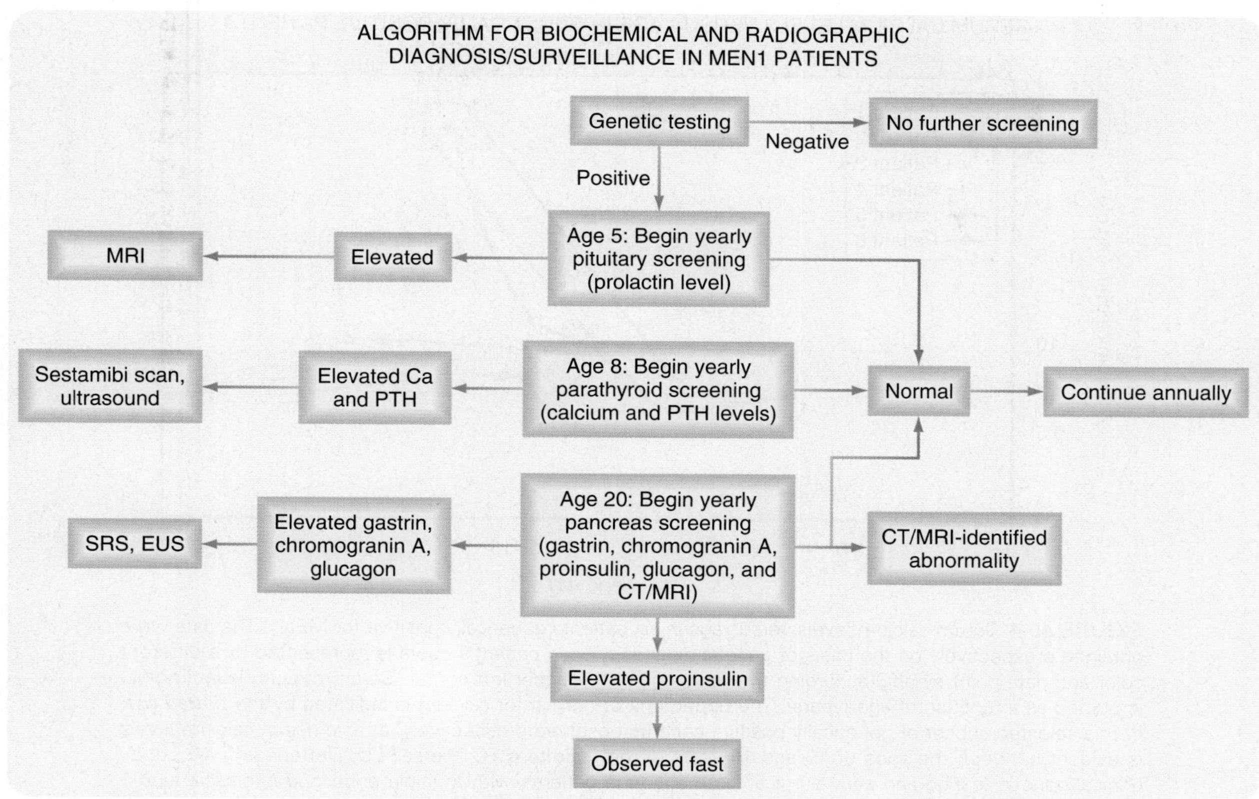

FIGURE 40-2 Clinical and biochemical surveillance in patients with MEN1. (From Whaley JG, Lairmore TC: Multiple endocrine neoplasia type 1: Current diagnosis and management. In Morita SY, Dackiw APB, Zeiger MA, editors: *McGraw-Hill's manual of endocrine surgery*, New York, 2009, McGraw-Hill, pp 334–347.)

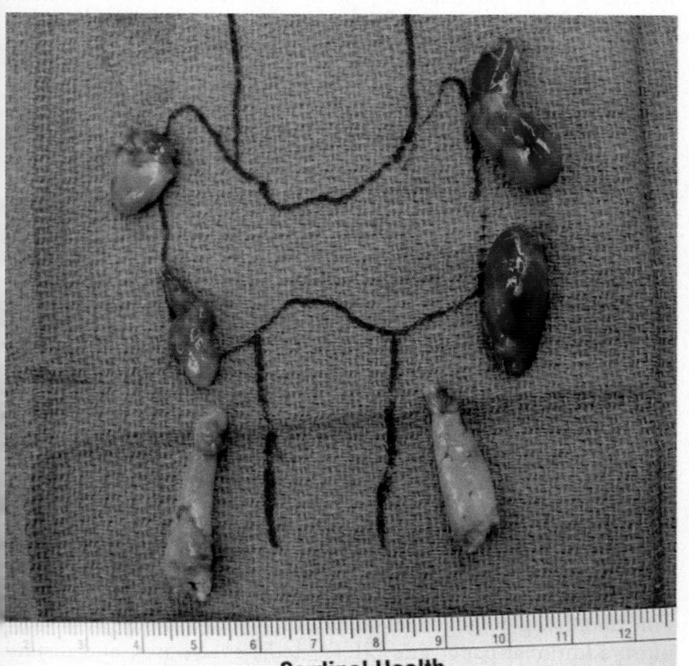

FIGURE 40-3 Photograph of four parathyroid glands and thymic horns resected from a patient with MEN1 syndrome, arranged according to location in the neck. Note the asymmetrical involvement of parathyroid tumors.

approach is a subtotal (3½-gland) parathyroidectomy, leaving a vascularized remnant of one parathyroid gland in situ in the neck. The rationale of this approach is to reduce the volume of functioning parathyroid tissue to the appropriate amount and to obviate the need for grafting of parathyroid tissue to an alternative site, thereby potentially reducing permanent hypoparathyroidism to the lowest achievable level. Despite the potential advantages and disadvantages of these two commonly practiced operations, previous retrospective studies have demonstrated similar rates of recurrent hyperparathyroidism and permanent postoperative hypoparathyroidism in patients undergoing either operation. A randomized, prospective trial[16] comparing the results of total parathyroidectomy plus autotransplantation with subtotal parathyroidectomy for the treatment of patients with hyperparathyroidism and MEN1 revealed no significant differences in outcome for the major end points of permanent hypoparathyroidism and recurrent hyperparathyroidism of the two operative strategies. Although both procedures are associated with excellent results, it was suggested that subtotal parathyroidectomy may have advantages in involving only one surgical incision and avoiding an obligate period of transient postoperative hypoparathyroidism.

Delayed transplantation of cryopreserved autologous parathyroid tissue can salvage a proportion of patients with permanent postoperative hypocalcemia after either procedure. In one study,[17] approximately 60% of delayed, cryopreserved parathyroid autografts showed evidence of graft function based on venous PTH gradients between the grafted and nongrafted arms, and 40% of autografts achieved full competency without supplements.

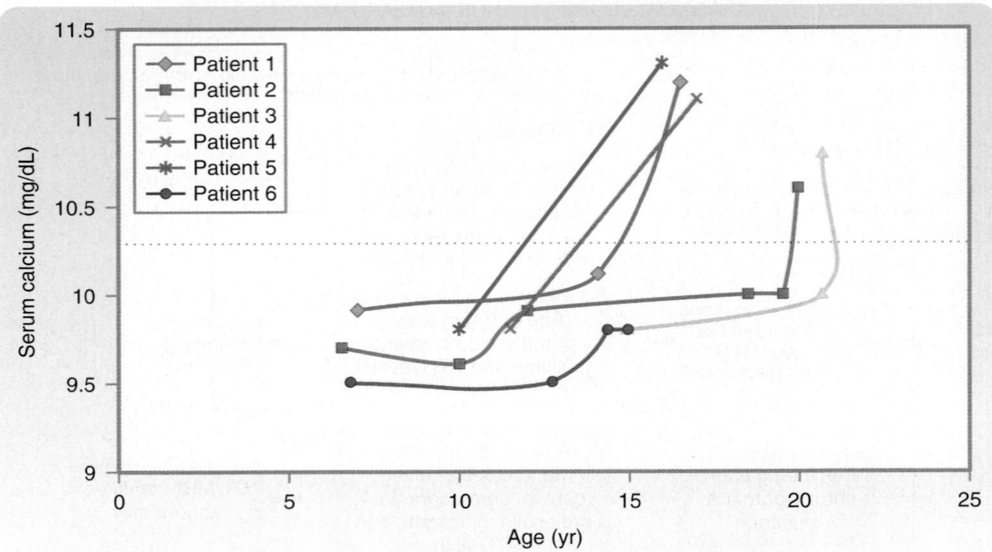

FIGURE 40-4 Serum calcium levels versus age in six patients genetically positive for MEN1. The data were obtained prospectively on the basis of genetic diagnosis. Each patient's curve is represented by a different color and data point symbol according to the legend in the upper left corner. Serum calcium level (mg/dL) is plotted as a function of age (years). The upper limit of normal for calcium is indicated by the *dotted line*. In this selected subset of genetically positive patients observed prospectively, a rapid rise in calcium levels is evident between the ages of 10 and 15 years. (From Lairmore TC, Piersall LD, DeBenedetti MK, et al: Clinical genetic testing and early surgical intervention in patients with multiple endocrine neoplasia type 1 [MEN1]. *Ann Surg* 239:637–645, 2004.)

Enteropancreatic Neuroendocrine Tumors

The second most frequent component of MEN1 is the development of NETs of the duodenum or pancreas. Depending on the method of study, 30% to 80% of patients with MEN1 develop clinically evident tumors. These tumors (along with thymic and bronchial carcinoid tumors) are associated with a risk of malignant progression and result in the majority of the MEN1 disease-related morbidity and mortality. The pathologic change is typically multifocal, and diffuse islet cell hyperplasia and microcarcinoma formation is present in areas of the pancreas distant from grossly evident tumor. Gastrinomas frequently occur within the submucosa of the duodenum and may occur rarely in extrapancreatic sites. The enteropancreatic tumors in patients with MEN1 cause symptoms due to either hormone oversecretion or the mass effects from tumor growth itself. Although a pancreatic NET results in a specific clinical syndrome based on a dominant hormone that is excessively secreted, it may stain for multiple peptides by immunohistochemistry. Some NETs are nonsecretory or secrete products such as pancreatic polypeptide that are not associated with clinical symptoms.

Several radiographic imaging methods are available for the preoperative detection of the gastroenteropancreatic NETs. A cross-sectional imaging test (computed tomography [CT] or magnetic resonance imaging [MRI]) should be performed as an initial test in essentially all patients to exclude a large primary neoplasm or metastases. Multiphasic helical CT has been reported to have a sensitivity as high as 94% for pancreatic NET. However, the sensitivity decreases with smaller tumors (<1 cm), multiple tumors (as is often the case with MEN1), tumors located in extrapancreatic locations (e.g., duodenal wall), or tumors located in the distal tail of the pancreas. MRI is advocated by some and is able to detect smaller tumors; however, no clear advantage of MRI over CT imaging has been shown.

Endoscopic ultrasonography (EUS) is a useful diagnostic test for NETs of the pancreas, with somewhat less sensitivity for small duodenal NETs, but it is dependent on availability and operator skill in selected centers. In 1992, Rosch and colleagues[18] reported a sensitivity of 82% and specificity of 95% of EUS in detecting pancreatic NETs. The sensitivity of EUS in detection of insulinomas is similar to that of helical or multislice CT, between 82% and 94%, with a combination of CT and EUS identifying 100% of the insulinomas in recent studies.[19] EUS is the preferred next diagnostic test in many centers after an initial CT scan. Small submucosal tumors in the duodenum and enlarged regional lymph nodes can be detected by EUS, and needle aspiration may be performed for a cytologic diagnosis. EUS is also useful in determining the anatomic relationship of the tumors to the main pancreatic duct. However, EUS may miss small duodenal gastrinoma tumors, and when they are detected, they may be seen on endoscopy only and not by ultrasound. Octreotide scanning, or somatostatin receptor scintigraphy (SRS), is a sensitive method for targeted localization of endocrine tumor, but its sensitivity is dependent on the number of somatostatin receptors on the tumor cell surface as well as tumor size. SRS localizes gastrinomas, which have cell surface somatostatin receptors that bind octreotide. The combination of CT or MRI and EUS provides the best information, including detection of small primary tumors in the duodenum, additional pancreatic NETs, nodal metastases, and distant metastases or unusual extrapancreatic sites within the abdomen.[20]

Finally, selective pancreatic arteriography and intra-arterial injection of a secretagogue, followed by measurement of increment hormone secretion at timed intervals through a catheter in the hepatic vein, may be performed. Selective arterial secretagogue injection (SASI) is an invasive test but may be the most accurate single localizing study. This test provides regional localization of functional tumors (insulinoma, gastrinoma) within the pancreas or duodenum and is especially useful to identify the specific functional tumor in patients with MEN1 who characteristically have multiple NETs.[21] The sensitivity and specificity of the SASI test for detection of both gastrinoma and insulinoma have been shown to be greater than 90%.[22]

Depending on the study, approximately 40% to 60% of the enteropancreatic NETs that develop in patients with MEN1 are gastrinomas. The presenting signs and symptoms in patients with hypergastrinemia, or the Zollinger-Ellison syndrome (ZES), include epigastric pain, reflux esophagitis, secretory diarrhea, and weight loss. With widespread use of proton pump inhibitors for medical therapy, active peptic ulcer disease is present in less than 20% of patients at the time of diagnosis. Patients may infrequently present with active ulcer disease or with stricture or perforation of the esophagus due to severe reflux esophagitis. The diagnosis of gastrinoma is made biochemically. Recommendations for fasting and provocative serum gastrin levels were provided from a prospective study of 309 patients at the National Institutes of Health and comparison with 2229 patients from the available literature.[23] Fasting serum gastrin (FSG) levels greater than 10 times normal indicated the presence of gastrinoma. However, two thirds of gastrinoma patients have FSG levels less than 10-fold normal that overlap with those of patients with hypergastrinemia due to other more common conditions, such as *Helicobacter pylori* infection and antral G-cell hyperplasia. In these patients, FSG levels are not diagnostic of ZES, and gastrin provocative tests are needed to establish the diagnosis.

Between 60% and 90% of MEN1-associated gastrinomas are malignant, and approximately half will have regional lymph node or distant metastases at the time of diagnosis. Gastrinomas occur 3 to 10 times more frequently in the duodenal submucosa than in an intrapancreatic location[16] (Fig. 40-5) and are almost always multiple. These tumors may be as small as 1 or 2 mm, and the primary gastrinoma may not be localized preoperatively by CT scanning or angiography. Frequently, metastatic gastrinoma in a regional lymph node is the dominant tumor mass identified on CT or SRS imaging. Possible primary gastrinomas arising in lymph nodes have been described, but these have almost all been reported in patients with sporadic ZES.[24] Although both pancreatic and duodenal gastrinomas metastasize to regional lymph nodes, liver metastases are more frequently associated with pancreatic gastrinomas, and hepatic metastases are correlated with a primary tumor larger than 3 cm as well as with decreased survival. Studies support the separation of aggressive and nonaggressive forms of gastrinoma. The aggressive form represents approximately 24% of patients and is more common in women and those without MEN1. Patients with the aggressive form of gastrinoma tend to have higher serum gastrin levels, shorter disease duration, large pancreatic primary tumors, and liver metastases.[20] The long-term survival of the aggressive form is approximately 30% compared with 96% for the nonaggressive form.

The value of surgical resection for intended cure of gastrinoma in patients with MEN1 remains controversial. Review of available series indicates that patients with ZES and MEN1 rarely demonstrate long-term biochemical cure after operation without undergoing pancreaticoduodenectomy.[20,25] Nevertheless, in selected patients, localized resection or pancreaticoduodenectomy may be indicated to control the tumoral process and to prevent subsequent malignant dissemination. With the recognition that primary gastrinomas occur frequently in the duodenal wall and are associated with a high incidence of lymph node metastases, some have suggested that pancreaticoduodenectomy combined with a complete regional lymphadenectomy may improve the cure rate of surgery for ZES in the setting of MEN1. Currently, the precise role for pancreaticoduodenectomy has not been defined, and it has not been shown to extend survival in patients with ZES with or without MEN1.[20] Total gastrectomy is not indicated for patients with gastrinoma to control acid hypersecretion because medical therapy with proton pump inhibitors effectively prevents the symptoms or complications resulting from this result of gastrin excess. Gastric carcinoids occur in hypergastrinemic conditions and in 13% to 37% of patients with ZES and MEN1. The majority of these carcinoids are small and amenable to endoscopic surveillance and resection; however, in a subset of individuals, larger, more invasive and aggressive tumors occur, and partial or total gastrectomy may be appropriate treatment for selected patients. Endoscopic surveillance is necessary because long-term administration of proton pump inhibitors to patients with MEN1 and ZES has been associated with the development of gastric carcinoid tumors.[20,26] Patients with primary hyperparathyroidism should undergo parathyroidectomy because normalization of the serum calcium level markedly ameliorates the ZES.[20]

Insulinomas account for approximately 10% to 27% of the NETs occurring in patients with MEN1 and are the second most

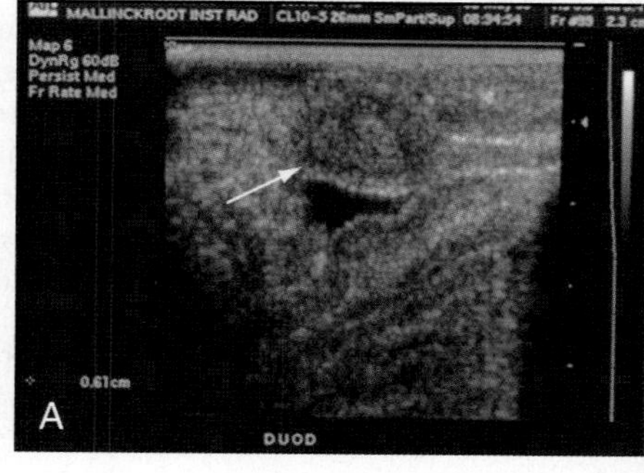

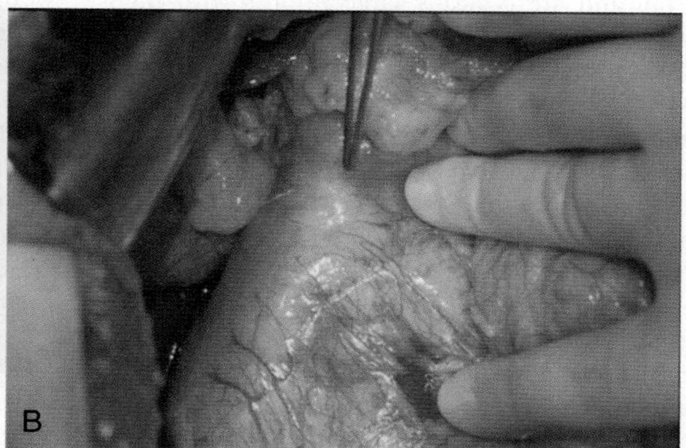

FIGURE 40-5 Gastrinoma in the duodenal wall from a patient with MEN1. **A,** Intraoperative ultrasound image of a circumscribed hypoechoic tumor in the submucosa of the duodenal wall, demonstrated just superior to the duodenal lumen. **B,** Gross appearance of the duodenal wall tumor from the serosal surface.

common functional tumor after gastrinoma. These are usually small (<2 cm) and may occur throughout the pancreas. Patients present with recurrent symptoms of neuroglycopenia: sweating, dizziness, confusion, or syncope. Documenting symptomatic hypoglycemia in association with inappropriately elevated plasma levels of insulin and C-peptide during a supervised 72-hour fast makes the diagnosis of insulinoma. Insulinomas are frequently occult and may be challenging to localize by conventional preoperative imaging studies, such as CT scanning, ultrasound, MRI, or angiography.

Medical therapies for insulinoma have limited effectiveness and are poorly tolerated; therefore, the preferred treatment is accurate localization and surgical resection of the functioning tumor to correct life-threatening hyperinsulinemia. Patients with MEN1 characteristically develop multiple NETs, a fact that may complicate identification of the specific functional tumor responsible for the hyperinsulinism. Preoperative regional localization of the functioning tumor within the pancreas may be provided by SASI using calcium gluconate as the secretagogue with measurement of insulin gradients in the hepatic veins. The operative approach includes complete mobilization of the pancreas and careful examination of the gland by inspection and palpation. Intraoperative ultrasound is essential for the identification of small tumors, especially within the pancreatic head or uncinate process. Small, benign insulinomas are amenable to enucleation. Partial pancreatectomy may be required for multiple or potentially malignant tumors.[21] In the event that the insulinoma is not identified despite an exhaustive intraoperative search, blind subtotal pancreatectomy is not recommended. Approximately 10% of insulinomas occurring in patients with MEN1 are malignant. Patients with malignant insulinoma and disseminated metastases may respond to treatment with streptozotocin, and some control of hypoglycemia may be achieved by the administration of either diazoxide or octreotide.

Other functional NETs of the pancreas, such as glucagonoma, somatostatinoma, and tumors secreting vasoactive intestinal peptide (VIP), occur rarely (less than 2% to 4%) in association with MEN1. The effects of excess hormone secretion in glucagonomas include a characteristic rash (necrolytic migratory erythema), weight loss, and anemia. Glucagon-producing NETs are usually located in the tail of the pancreas and are frequently metastatic at the time of diagnosis. VIP-producing tumors result in profuse secretory diarrhea (more than 1 liter/day during a fast), hypokalemia, achlorhydria, acidosis, and vasoactive instability (flushing and hypotension). VIPomas are also frequently located in the pancreatic tail and are typically large tumors with high malignant potential. Nonfunctional or predominantly pancreatic polypeptide–producing NETs account for approximately 20% to 55% of NETs in MEN1, depending on the series. Small, relatively indolent pancreatic polypeptide–producing tumors may be detected with increased frequency because of more sensitive imaging tests, and their natural history is not well defined. Estimated 10-year survival rates of 23% to 62% have been reported for these tumors.[27]

The involvement of NETs within the pancreas of patients with MEN1 is characteristically multifocal (Fig. 40-6). Controversy exists about the optimal timing of and most appropriate operation to perform for NETs of the pancreas and duodenum in patients with MEN1. The controversy reflects uncertainty in the natural history of small, potentially benign, or nonfunctional tumors, which must be weighed against the risks of early or repeated major pancreatic interventions carrying significant risk of morbidity.

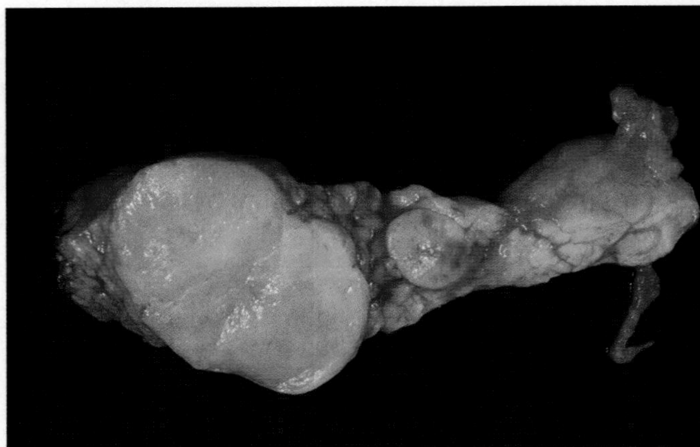

FIGURE 40-6 Multiple neuroendocrine tumors of the pancreas in a distal pancreatectomy specimen from a patient with MEN1.

Some are reluctant to advocate routine or early pancreatic exploration in young, otherwise healthy patients for small nonfunctional tumors, which are potentially clinically insignificant. On the other hand, these tumors have a malignant potential, and delay in diagnosis and effective treatment carries the risk of the development of local or distant metastasis. It is obviously desirable to intervene early to prevent malignant dissemination while minimizing morbidity and mortality (from either cancer or surgery). Complicating factors include the lack of genotype-phenotype correlation in MEN1 (that might otherwise allow genetic stratification of those at higher risk of malignant progression) and failure of studies to identify a clear relationship between size of the tumor and risk of regional lymph node or distant metastases.[28] Tumor grade and extent are the primary determinants of prognosis for malignant NETs. Ki67 is a cellular marker associated with cellular proliferation, and well and moderately differentiated neuroendocrine tumors are characterized by the presence of Ki67 antigen in less than 20%.

The spectrum of clinical strategies proposed ranges from the most aggressive approach, consisting of early surgical exploration and resection of tumors when the patient's peptide tumor markers become elevated (even without radiographically detectable tumors),[29] to the most conservative approach, advocating operation only for tumors exceeding approximately 1.0 cm in size on radiographic imaging or demonstrating hormone hyperfunction.[21,30] The malignant potential of these neoplasms is clear, with up to 50% of patients eventually developing regional lymph node or distant metastases.[21] Many groups now recommend early operation and excision of these tumors to prevent malignant progression.[21,30,31] One large retrospective study suggested improved overall survival in patients undergoing operation, especially younger patients with localized tumors and those with hormonally functional tumors. The operative strategy for NETs in patients with MEN1 must be aimed at extirpation of all grossly evident tumors with preservation of pancreatic exocrine and endocrine function and avoidance of excessive operative morbidity. These factors are complex and must be individualized to the patient.

Pituitary Gland

Adenomas of the anterior pituitary gland occur in a variable proportion (15% to 30%) of patients with MEN1. Pituitary tumors cause symptoms by either hypersecretion of hormones or compression of adjacent structures. Large adenomas may cause visual field defects by pressure on the optic chiasm or manifestations of hypopituitarism through compression of the adjacent normal gland. The most frequent pituitary tumor in patients with MEN1 is a prolactinoma. Prolactin-secreting tumors result in amenorrhea and galactorrhea in women or hypogonadism in men. MEN1 patients with pituitary tumors may exhibit acromegaly resulting from growth hormone overproduction or Cushing disease due to an adrenocorticotropic hormone–producing pituitary tumor.

Biochemical screening includes annual measurement of plasma prolactin and insulin-like growth factor I levels as well as MRI of the pituitary every 3 to 5 years, depending on clinical judgment and specific patient features. Medical treatment with a dopamine agonist such as bromocriptine or cabergoline is effective in controlling the hyperprolactinemia in most patients with prolactinomas. Medical therapy for growth hormone–producing tumors (somatotrophinomas) includes somatostatin analogues such as octreotide and lanreotide. Selective trans-sphenoidal hypophysectomy is indicated for rapidly enlarging nonfunctional macroadenomas that are unresponsive to medical therapy or result in local compressive symptoms because of their mass effect, with radiotherapy reserved for residual unresectable tumor tissue.

Other Tumors

Bronchial and thymic carcinoid tumors, type II gastric carcinoid tumors, lipomas, facial cutaneous angiofibromas and collagenomas,[32] and meningiomas and ependymomas of the central nervous system are also associated with MEN1. CT or MRI of the chest every 1 to 2 years is recommended to screen for intrathoracic carcinoid tumors. Complete surgical removal of thymic and bronchial carcinoid tumors is the preferred treatment when possible, with chemotherapy or radiotherapy used in patients with advanced tumors not amenable to curative surgery. Preventive thymectomy should be considered in male patients, especially smokers, or in families in which malignant thymic tumors have occurred.[33] Approximately 30% of patients with MEN1 develop adrenocortical nodules or bilateral nodular adrenal hyperplasia. Screening for adrenal tumors should include cross-sectional imaging (CT or MRI) every 3 years or more frequently, depending on clinical and biochemical abnormalities. Biochemical testing should be performed for adrenocortical tumors larger than 1 cm and should focus on hyperaldosteronism and hypercortisolism. The indications for surgical treatment of MEN1-associated adrenal tumors are similar to those for non-MEN1 adrenal tumors, including functioning tumors, tumors with atypical radiographic features, size greater than 4 cm, and significant interval growth on serial imaging. The optimal surveillance and treatment of gastric type II carcinoid tumors remain controversial. Current suggested guidelines include gastroscopy every 3 years in patients with hypergastrinemia and endoscopic surveillance for small lesions (<10 mm). Larger tumors should undergo endoscopic resection or local resection with partial or total gastrectomy. The role of somatostatin analogues in the treatment of type II gastric carcinoids has not been clearly defined.[13]

MULTIPLE ENDOCRINE NEOPLASIA TYPE 2 SYNDROMES

General

The MEN2 syndromes include MEN2A, MEN2B, and familial, non-MEN MTC (FMTC). The hallmark of the MEN2 syndromes is MTC,[1] in the setting of C-cell hyperplasia, which occurs with nearly complete penetrance. Additional manifestations are variably penetrant and include adrenal medullary hyperplasia and pheochromocytomas in MEN2A and MEN2B and hyperparathyroidism in MEN2A (Fig. 40-7). These features are

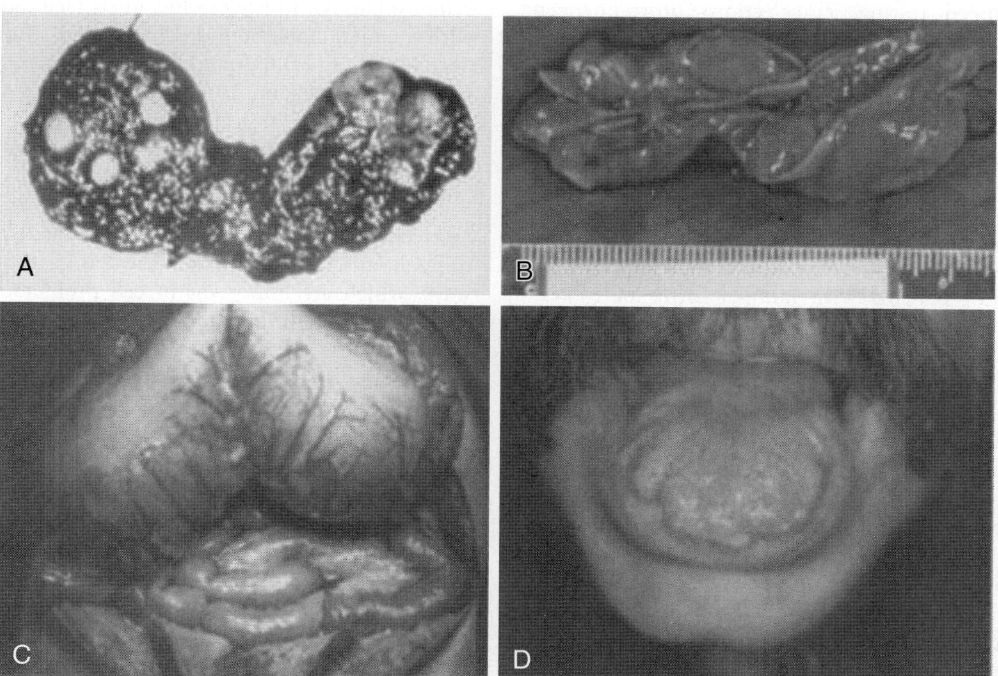

FIGURE 40-7 Features of MEN2A and 2B syndromes. **A,** Bisected thyroidectomy specimen showing multifocal, bilateral MTC tumors. **B,** Adrenalectomy specimen from patient with MEN2B showing pheochromocytoma. **C,** Megacolon in patient with MEN2B. **D,** Tongue nodules in patient with MEN2B. (**A,** Courtesy Dr. S. A. Wells. **B-D,** Courtesy Dr. R. Thompson. From Moley JF: Medullary thyroid cancer. In Clark OH, Duh QY, editors: *Textbook of endocrine surgery*, Philadelphia, 1997, WB Saunders.)

TABLE 40-1 **Clinical Features of Multiple Endocrine Neoplasia Syndromes**

CLINICAL SETTING	FEATURES OF MTC	INHERITANCE PATTERN	ASSOCIATED ABNORMALITIES	GENETIC DEFECT
Sporadic MTC	Unifocal	None	None	Somatic *RET* mutations in >20% of tumors
MEN2A	Multifocal, bilateral	Autosomal dominant	Pheochromocytomas, hyperparathyroidism	Germline missense mutations in extracellular cysteine codons of *RET*
MEN2B	Multifocal, bilateral	Autosomal dominant	Pheochromocytomas, mucosal neuromas, megacolon, skeletal abnormalities	Germline missense mutation in tyrosine kinase domain of *RET*
FMTC	Multifocal, bilateral	Autosomal dominant	None	Germline missense mutations in extracellular or intracellular cysteine codons of *RET*

Adapted from Moley JF, Lairmore TC, Phay JE: Hereditary endocrinopathies. *Curr Probl Surg* 36:653–764, 1999.

summarized in Table 40-1. The MEN2 syndromes have an autosomal dominant pattern of inheritance and are caused by activating mutations in the *RET* proto-oncogene on chromosome 10.[34] The clinical features and tumor behavior seen in the MEN2 syndromes are closely correlated with the specific germline mutation present in the *RET* gene. Management of patients and families affected by these syndromes should be informed by an understanding of the genotype-phenotype correlation associated with the specific *RET* mutation present in family members.

Understanding of the genetic basis of the MEN2 syndromes led to a paradigm shift in the screening and treatment of affected patients and their families. Treatment now focuses on early identification of *RET* mutation carriers and early thyroidectomy to prevent MTC, when possible. This section describes the genetics, clinical features, diagnosis, and management of patients with the MEN2 syndromes.

RET Proto-Oncogene

The *RET* (*RE*arranged during *T*ransfection) proto-oncogene encodes a receptor tyrosine kinase protein involved in growth, differentiation, and migration of developing tissues. The full-length protein includes an extracellular cysteine-rich ligand-binding domain, a transmembrane domain, an intracellular juxtamembrane domain, and an intracellular tyrosine kinase domain (Fig. 40-8). The mutations responsible for MTC are missense mutations that result in single amino acid changes that cause gain-of-function alterations in the protein. There are consistent associations between the specific *RET* mutation (genotype) and clinical phenotype of patients with familial forms of MTC,[35] which includes age at onset, aggressiveness of MTC, and presence or absence of other endocrine neoplasms. MEN2B patients expressing the M918T mutation have the most aggressive forms of MTC, with evidence of disease often present in early infancy. MEN2A patients have a variable course of MTC disease presentation and progression, whereas FMTC patients demonstrate an indolent form that more often is manifested in the later decades of life. *RET* mutations in MEN2 are inherited in an autosomal dominant fashion. Thus, MEN2 carriers confer a 50% risk of genetic transmission to their offspring.

RET is expressed in multiple tissues descended from the neural crest, including the thyroid parafollicular cells (C cells), parathyroid glands, adrenal chromaffin cells, enteric ganglia, and other peripheral and central neurons. Based on studies in animal models, RET signaling is necessary for the normal development of the kidney, parasympathetic nervous system, gut-associated lymphoid tissue, and enteric nervous system. RET knockout mice demonstrate features including renal agenesis and aberrant gut neurophysiology. In humans, inactivating (loss-of-function) mutations in *RET* are associated with Hirschsprung's disease (HSCR), a defect in migration and development of enteric neurons, which causes megacolon in infancy. Activating (gain-of-function) germline mutations in *RET* are associated with the MEN2 syndromes, and activating somatic mutations are associated with sporadic thyroid carcinomas. This mechanism differs from MEN1 and most other hereditary cancer syndromes (including hereditary breast cancer and colon cancer), which are caused by loss-of-function mutations in the predisposition gene (tumor suppressor genes).

The RET protein has four known ligands that induce its activation: glial cell–derived neurotrophic factor (GDNF), artemin, persephin, and neurturin, known collectively as the GDNF family ligands. RET activation by each of these GDNF family ligands is mediated through one of four ligand-specific coreceptors belonging to the GDNF family receptors alpha (GFRα). These GFRα coreceptors are anchored to the plasma membrane by a glycosylphosphatidylinositol residue, likely facilitating their interaction with the membrane-bound RET protein. Normal RET activation occurs with assembly of a dimeric complex including two RET proteins, two ligand molecules, and two GFRα coreceptors. Current evidence indicates that this entire complex is necessary for RET signaling and that ligand binding and downstream activation require the coreceptor.

The dimerized RET receptor complex activates a number of intracellular signaling pathways implicated in cell survival and differentiation. These include the Ras/ERK and PI3K/Akt pathways, which are important in cell proliferation, differentiation, and survival. Additional pathways activated by RET include p38 MAPK, phospholipase C-γ, JNK, and ERK5, suggesting additional roles for RET in cell differentiation, migration, and cytokine production. Activated RET also has a phosphorylated serine residue (S696) in the juxtamembrane domain. This site has been implicated in Rac-mediated migration of enteric neural crest cells during normal development. An inactivating mutation at this site in mice resulted in a lack of enteric neurons in the distal colon, similar to the phenotype of HSCR in humans.

MEN2A and FMTC

In the 1960s, Sipple and Steiner described the association of thyroid cancer with pheochromocytoma and hyperparathyroidism, respectively.[36] MEN2A is characterized by a hereditary predisposition to MTC. Penetrance of this feature is almost complete, that is, virtually all patients who inherit a germline MEN2A-associated mutation in the *RET* proto-oncogene develop MTC. MEN2A patients will all develop MTC during their lifetime,

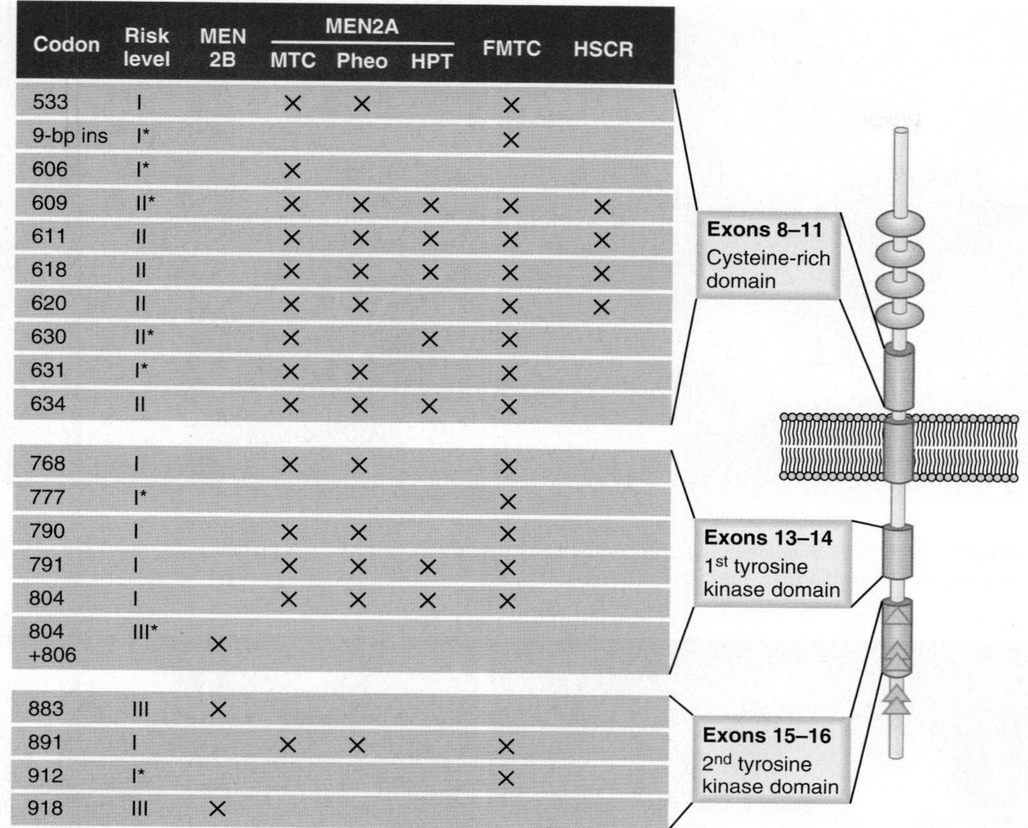

Codon	Risk level	MEN 2B	MEN2A MTC	MEN2A Pheo	MEN2A HPT	FMTC	HSCR
533	I		×	×		×	
9-bp ins	I*					×	
606	I*		×				
609	II*		×	×	×	×	×
611	II		×	×	×	×	×
618	II		×	×	×	×	×
620	II		×	×		×	×
630	II*		×		×	×	
631	I*		×	×		×	
634	II		×	×	×	×	
768	I		×	×		×	
777	I*					×	
790	I		×	×		×	
791	I		×	×	×	×	
804	I		×	×	×	×	
804 +806	III*	×					
883	III	×					
891	I		×	×		×	
912	I*					×	
918	III	×					

FIGURE 40-8 *RET* mutation sites associated with MEN2 syndromes. Codons previously reported in association with MEN2 syndromes are listed by structural domain within the RET protein. Risk level is based on consensus guidelines or more recent clinical reports. Previously reported phenotypes for each codon are shown. *FMTC,* familial medullary thyroid carcinoma; *HPT,* hyperparathyroidism; *HSCR,* Hirschsprung's disease; *MTC,* medullary thyroid carcinoma; *Pheo,* pheochromocytoma. *Risk level based on recent clinical reports (not available at publication of the consensus guidelines). (From Traugott AL, Moley JF: The RET protooncogene. *Cancer Treat Res* 153:303–319, 2010.)

although the age at onset varies from early childhood to adulthood, depending on the specific mutation and kindred (Fig. 40-9). Forty percent to 50% of MEN2A patients will develop pheochromocytoma, which may or may not be synchronous with MTC in its presentation. Pheochromocytoma occurs in 42% to 46% of MEN2A patients overall, although the prevalence varies from 5% to 100% in different kindreds. The degree of penetrance for pheochromocytoma in MEN2A correlates with specific *RET* mutations, with the highest expression in carriers of mutations at codon 634.[37] Parathyroid hyperplasia, in one or multiple glands, results in primary hyperparathyroidism in 20% to 35% of MEN2A patients overall, although this also varies by kindred (Fig. 40-10).

Cutaneous lichen amyloidosis (CLA) has been described in several kindreds and patients with MEN2A. CLA is a rare disorder characterized by amyloid deposition in the papillary dermis, resulting in pruritic cutaneous plaques, often localized to the interscapular region or extensor surfaces of the extremities. In these MEN2A kindreds, CLA phenotype cosegregates with the clinical features of MEN2A. To date, all reported *RET* mutations in kindreds with combined MEN2A and CLA features have been in codon 634.

HSCR has been associated with MEN2A and FMTC. This relatively common disease (1 in 5000 births) is characterized by the congenital absence of ganglion cells within the myenteric and submucosal plexus of the distal colon. Newborn HSCR patients present with distal bowel obstruction and megacolon. HSCR not associated with MEN2 is often associated with inactivating (loss-of-function) *RET* mutations. Kindreds with cosegregating MEN2A or FMTC and HSCR have mutations in *RET* codons 609, 618, and 624.[35,38] Within the affected kindreds, reported penetrance of HSCR in *RET* mutation carriers is 16% to 50%.

Patients who inherit FMTC also develop MTC but do not have pheochromocytoma or parathyroid hyperplasia. FMTC is caused by the same mutations as MEN2A as well as by less common mutations in the intracellular portion of the protein. MEN2A patients have a variable course of MTC disease presentation and progression, whereas FMTC patients demonstrate an indolent form that more often is manifested in the later decades of life. There is considerable overlap between the RET codons affected in FMTC and those in MEN2A, which supports the theory that FMTC is a variant of MEN2A and not a distinct clinical entity.[39] Occasional patients with FMTC will never manifest clinical evidence of MTC (symptoms or a palpable neck mass), although biochemical testing and histologic evaluation of the thyroid demonstrate MTC.

The most common mutations associated with MEN2A and FMTC occur in exons 10 and 11, within the extracellular

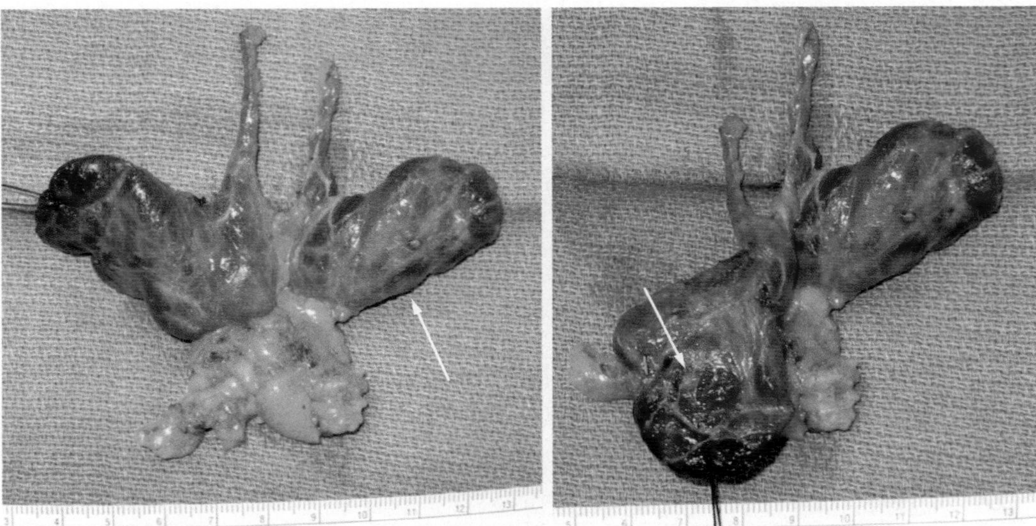

FIGURE 40-9 Total thyroidectomy and central neck dissection in a MEN2A patient with multifocal MTC. *Arrows* point to visible MTC tumors.

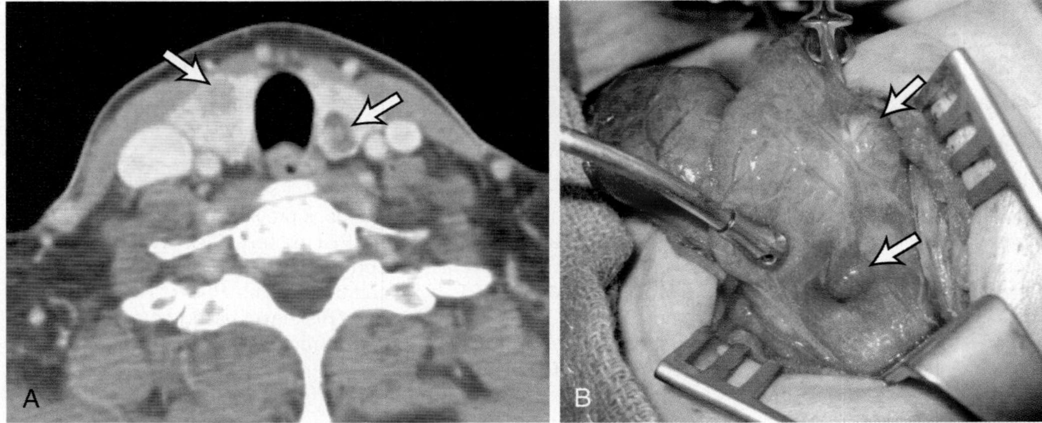

FIGURE 40-10 **A,** CT scan showing multiple bilateral foci of medullary thyroid carcinoma in an older patient with MEN2A. **B,** Operative photograph of the same patient showing focus of MTC in thyroid *(top arrow)* and enlarged parathyroid *(bottom arrow).*

cysteine-rich domain of the RET protein. Cysteine residues at codons 609, 611, 618, 620, 630, and 634 fall within this region. The amino acid changes caused by these mutations destabilize the normal tertiary structure of the RET protein, which results in ligand-independent dimerization and persistent intracellular signaling by RET.

MEN2B

In MEN2B, as in MEN2A, all patients develop MTC. All MEN2B individuals have mucosal neuromas and megacolon, and 40% to 50% of patients develop pheochromocytomas. MEN2B patients do not develop hyperparathyroidism. MTC in MEN2B is manifested at a very young age—in infancy—and appears to be the most aggressive form of hereditary MTC. These patients often have a distinct physical appearance with a prominent mid–upper lip, everted eyelids, multiple tongue nodules, and marfanoid body habitus with long, thin extremities and digits. The mucosal neuromas are unencapsulated, thickened proliferations of nerves that occur principally on the lips and tongue but can also be found on the gingiva, buccal mucosa, nasal mucosa, vocal cords, and conjunctiva. MEN2B patients also develop ganglioneuromas of the intestine in the submucosal and myenteric plexus. They have enlarged nerves (Fig. 40-11). All MEN2B patients have a megacolon and usually have chronic bowel problems. Intestinal dysfunction may be manifested early in life with poor feeding, failure to thrive, constipation, or pseudo-obstruction. Adults with this disorder may have dysphagia from esophageal dysmotility. Rarely, a patient can present with toxic megacolon. MEN2B patients, however, do not develop HSCR, as do some patients with MEN2A.

RET Mutations in Sporadic Thyroid Carcinomas

Somatic mutations or rearrangements involving *RET* have been identified in 40% to 50% of sporadic MTCs and up to 70% of sporadic papillary thyroid carcinomas (PTCs).[40] Most of the mutations identified in sporadic MTCs are point mutations involving the same codons associated with the MEN2 syndromes, including 918, 634, and 883. Of sporadic MTCs with alterations of *RET*, 60% to 80% are found to have the M918T mutation.[40,41] Patients with sporadic MTCs bearing a *RET* mutation (particularly M918T) have a more advanced stage at diagnosis, increased

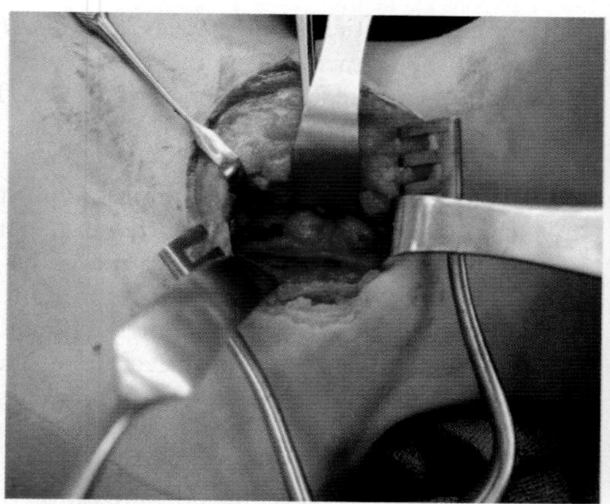
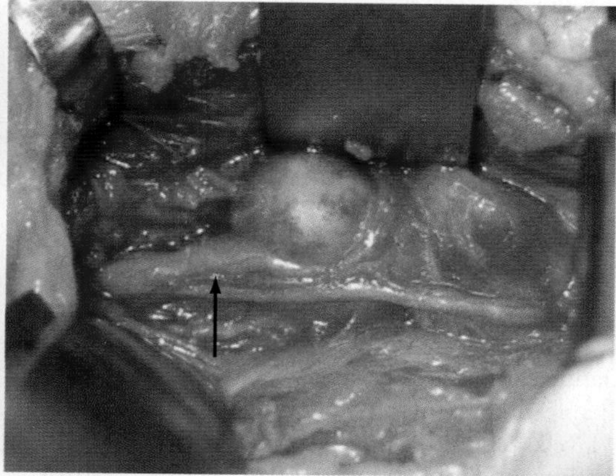

FIGURE 40-11 Reoperation, left central neck dissection in a young patient with MEN2B. Note the large size of the recurrent laryngeal nerve *(arrow)* and the nodule of recurrent medullary thyroid carcinoma adjacent to the cricoid. (From Moley JF: Medullary thyroid carcinoma: Management of lymph node metastases. *J Natl Compr Canc Netw* 8:549–556, 2010.)

rates of recurrent or persistent disease after resection, and poorer long-term survival (10 to 20 years) than those without a *RET* mutation.[40,41]

Chromosomal rearrangements of *RET*, rather than point mutations, are associated with sporadic PTCs. A number of rearrangements have been reported that result from the fusion of the *RET* tyrosine kinase domain to activating portions of other genes. Collectively, these fusion genes are referred to as RET/PTC, and to date 13 distinct variants, resulting from rearrangement events from different genes, have been described.[42]

Screening and Genetic Testing for MEN2

Before the genetic basis of MEN2 was well characterized, pentagastrin-stimulated calcitonin testing was used to screen for MEN2 and MTC in patients at risk for inheriting an MEN2 syndrome. Occasional false-positive and false-negative test results, however, resulted in either unnecessary surgery or missed opportunities to intervene early. Sequencing of the *RET* gene to detect germline mutations is now the standard screening test for MEN2 syndromes. *RET* mutation testing can identify young carriers at an earlier stage of disease, often before they develop cancer, and it has lower false-positive and false-negative rates than calcitonin testing. It is recommended that patients or their parents meet with a genetic counselor before testing. Genetic counseling is an important component of informed consent and education for these patients, who are facing a major event that will affect their own and their family's lives.

RET mutation testing should be performed routinely for at-risk members of MEN2 and FMTC families. If possible, testing should occur at birth because carrier status determines the need for clinical screening and preventive surgery. In families in which the inherited *RET* mutation is already known, *RET* sequencing can be limited to the site of the known mutation. Those family members who are negative for their kindred's known mutation have the same risk for MEN2 as the general population, and they need no other screening. When an MTC patient with no known family history of MTC or MEN2 is found to have a *RET* mutation (index case), all first-degree family members should be offered genetic counseling and testing.

RET mutation testing also is indicated for adult or pediatric patients who present with MTC or pheochromocytoma, regardless of any family history of endocrine tumors. Approximately 5% to 7% of patients thought to have sporadic MTC are found to have a germline *RET* mutation. Up to 24% of pheochromocytomas are hereditary, with 5% resulting from *RET* mutations.[43] Infants presenting with HSCR should undergo *RET* mutation testing. All reported cases of MEN2A associated with HSCR have occurred in patients with mutations in exon 10 of *RET*, at codons 609, 618, and 620.

Medullary Thyroid Carcinoma

MTC[1] represents 3% to 9% of all thyroid cancers and arises from thyroid C cells. MTC may be sporadic (75% of cases) or hereditary, occurring in all patients with the MEN2 syndromes (25% of cases). Hereditary MTCs are often multifocal and bilateral. Multicentric C-cell hyperplasia has been shown to precede development of hereditary MTC.[44] MTC is a relatively indolent malignant neoplasm, with reported 10-year survival rates of 69% to 89%.[45] Unlike differentiated thyroid cancer, MTC cells do not concentrate radioactive iodine and are not sensitive to manipulation of thyroid-stimulating hormone. These features must be considered in planning therapy for a patient with MTC.[46]

Patients with established MTC may present with a palpable thyroid mass or nodule. Symptoms of dysphagia, shortness of breath, or hoarseness are present in approximately 15% of cases. Metastases to regional cervical lymph nodes are present in up to 75% of patients who present with palpable disease.[47] The most frequent sites of lymphatic spread are to the central compartment of the neck (levels VI), followed by the ipsilateral jugular nodes (levels II to V), and then the contralateral cervical nodes. Other frequent metastatic sites are the mediastinum, lungs, liver, and bone.[48]

Calcitonin is made by thyroid C cells and MTC cells. It is a sensitive and specific tumor marker that may be measured in blood in the basal state or after the administration of the secretagogues calcium and pentagastrin (no longer available in the United States). Calcitonin levels are almost always elevated in patients with MTC. Measurement of calcitonin levels is helpful in screening patients at risk for MTC and in follow-up of patients after treatment. After primary surgery for MTC, persistent or recurrent elevation of calcitonin levels indicates persistent regional nodal metastasis or distant metastasis. Some MTCs also secrete carcinoembryonic antigen, but its long half-life and lower specificity make it a less useful marker.

On CT imaging, MTCs appear as nodules with calcifications and may demonstrate extrathyroidal disease. Fine-needle aspiration of the palpable thyroid nodule or cervical lymph node metastasis is a sensitive means for establishing the diagnosis of MTC. Ultrasound examination of the neck is a sensitive technique for identifying cervical lymph node metastases.

Surgery for Established Medullary Thyroid Carcinoma in MEN2 and FMTC

Recently published guidelines contain recommendations for management of MTC in multiple relevant clinical settings that will be useful to clinicians treating these patients.[39] Patients with established MTC (palpable or present on imaging studies, with elevated calcitonin levels) should undergo total thyroidectomy, central neck dissection, and unilateral or bilateral dissection of levels II through V nodes. The decision to resect lateral nodes depends on the extent of central neck node involvement and on the results of preoperative imaging.[39,47,49] Ultrasound examination of cervical nodes with preoperative marking of abnormal or suspicious nodes is helpful in planning the extent of surgery.[50] In patients with central lymph node metastases and normal findings on imaging of the lateral neck, however, consideration should be given to at least an ipsilateral level II to IV compartment lymph node dissection because of the high likelihood of microscopic nodal involvement.[47]

Central node dissection often compromises the blood supply of parathyroid glands. Preservation of parathyroid function may be achieved by a combination of careful preservation of glands on a vascular pedicle when possible and autotransplantation of devascularized glands. At the author's institution, the approach has been to resect and autotransplant the two parathyroids on the side of the primary tumor as well as the contralateral lower parathyroid, leaving the contralateral upper parathyroid in situ on a vascular pedicle if possible. All removed parathyroids should be carefully minced into 1 × 3-mm fragments, and fragments should be transplanted into individual muscle pockets (two or three fragments per pocket) that are then closed with a suture.[51] Transplantation of whole minced glands into a single pocket is discouraged. Parathyroid fragments may be transplanted into individual muscle pockets in the sternocleidomastoid muscle in cases of sporadic disease, FMTC, or MEN2B. They may be transplanted into the nondominant forearm in cases of MEN2A when there is a significant risk of future hyperparathyroidism (e.g., codon 634 *RET* mutation carriers). The reason for this difference is the risk of subsequent graft-dependent hyperparathyroidism in some MEN2A patients, which is more easily localized and treated if the grafts are in the forearm.

Preventive Surgery

Whereas the age at onset and rate of disease progression may differ, the lifetime penetrance of MTC is nearly 100% in carriers of *RET* mutations associated with MEN2 syndromes. For this reason, all patients diagnosed with MEN2 should undergo total thyroidectomy. A number of studies have demonstrated improved biochemical cure rates or decreased recurrence rates from early thyroidectomy, performed after positive screening by calcitonin testing or *RET* mutation testing.[52]

The American Thyroid Association risk categories for hereditary MTC have been changed. The former level D category has been changed to highest risk (HST), which includes patients with MEN2B and the *RET* codon M918T mutation. The former level C category has been changed to a new category, high risk (H), which includes patients with MEN2A and *RET* codon C634 mutations. The former level A and B categories have been combined into a new category, moderate risk (MOD), which includes patients with hereditary MTC and *RET* codon mutations other than M918T and C634.[39]

Patients with MEN2B (HST) have the most aggressive form of MTC, with invasive disease reported in patients younger than 1 year.[48] These patients should have preventive surgery early in the first year of life if possible.[53] Identification and preservation of parathyroid glands can be extremely difficult in these infants because of their small size, translucent appearance, and presence of exuberant thymic and perithyroidal nodal tissue. These procedures should be performed by surgeons experienced in parathyroid operations and pediatric thyroidectomy.

Patients with MEN2A due to mutations in codons 634 are considered at high risk (H). These patients should undergo a total thyroidectomy at 5 to 6 years of age. There is evidence that the risk of lymph node metastasis is very low in MEN2A patients younger than 8 years who have normal calcitonin levels.[54,55] Central lymph node dissection is associated with higher risk of hypoparathyroidism and recurrent laryngeal nerve injury and should be reserved for patients with elevated calcitonin levels.[39,44,56]

A larger subset of *RET* mutations, associated with MEN2A or FMTC, are considered moderate risk (MOD). These include mutations at codons other than 918 and 634.[39,48] For patients with moderate risk, total thyroidectomy is recommended, and surgery before the age of 5 to 10 years is appropriate. As with the high-risk (H) mutations, the need for central lymph node dissection should be guided by calcitonin levels and clinical features of the patient and kindred.

Our group at Washington University reported long-term follow-up of a series of 50 young patients with MEN2A after total thyroidectomy, central node dissection, and total parathyroidectomy, with autotransplantation of all of the parathyroid tissue into the muscle of the nondominant forearm during the primary surgical procedure.[51] Long-term disease control was excellent. Long-term parathyroid function was normal (no supplementation) in 47 of 50 patients. Other groups reported good results with selective removal of lymph nodes and parathyroids in young at-risk patients.[1,57] Recent follow-up studies indicate that the likelihood of nodal metastases in MEN2A and FMTC patients is extremely low in patients younger than 8 years and in patients with basal calcitonin levels less than 40 pg/mL.[51,54] Because of this, it is now our practice to perform total thyroidectomy, leaving the parathyroids in situ, if possible, in children with a low calcitonin level (<40 pg/mL). In patients with an elevated calcitonin level, we perform total thyroidectomy, central node dissection, and parathyroid autotransplantation. In either case, these operations should be performed only by surgeons experienced in thyroid and parathyroid operations in children.

Since publication of the consensus guidelines, a number of new mutations have been described in association with MEN2 syndromes, at codons 912, 630, 631, 606, and 533 and a 9–base pair duplication in exon 8. These are uncommon mutations, and because of lack of clinical experience, their penetrance and aggressiveness are not well characterized.

Follow-Up

After thyroidectomy, thyroid hormone replacement is required for life. Patients may need several weeks of oral calcium and vitamin D until parathyroid function recovers. Intermittent calcitonin testing may be done to monitor for persistent or recurrent MTC.

The term *biochemical cure* is used to refer to patients with normal calcitonin levels after surgery for MTC. Complete postoperative normalization of calcitonin has been associated with decreased long-term risk of MTC recurrence, although the evidence is less clear for a survival benefit. A persistent or recurrent elevation in calcitonin indicates residual or recurrent MTC and warrants additional investigation by imaging, at a minimum. However, as most MTC has a fairly indolent course, patients with biochemical evidence of recurrent disease may not have corollary imaging findings for some time.

Management of Recurrent and Metastatic Disease

Patients with findings indicating recurrent disease localized to the neck should undergo reoperation when possible with the goal of removing all remaining disease. These operations may result in long-term survival benefit and prevent complications of recurrence in the neck.[47] External beam radiation therapy is effective in palliation of bone metastases, but consistent benefit has not been shown for recurrent disease in the neck.[58] Previous clinical response rates for chemotherapy in patients with locally advanced or metastatic MTC have been disappointing. The understanding of MTC molecular oncogenesis, however, has resulted in identification of novel molecular targets for treatment. The majority of current targeted molecular therapies fall under the classification of tyrosine kinase inhibitors. Vandetanib (ZD6474, Zactima) is a novel anilinoquinazoline compound engineered to selectively inhibit vascular endothelial growth factor receptor, endothelial growth factor receptor, and RET tyrosine kinases. In a study of 30 patients with advanced hereditary MTC, Wells and colleagues reported a 20% partial response rate and a more than 50% reduction of calcitonin level in 24 of 30 patients.[59] At present, there are several other ongoing and completed institutional and multi-institutional phase 2 and 3 trials for MTC patients with unresectable, measurable, and locally advanced MTC.

Pheochromocytoma

Pheochromocytomas are neoplasms arising from chromaffin cells in the adrenal medulla, which synthesize and secrete catecholamines. Patients with pheochromocytoma may present with symptoms of catecholamine excess, including headache, hypertension, palpitations, tremors, and anxiety. This unregulated catecholamine secretion can have devastating consequences including stroke, myocardial infarction, and sudden death.

Approximately 40% to 50% of all patients with MEN2A or MEN2B develop pheochromocytomas, with a mean age at diagnosis between 30 and 40 years. In rare cases, the age at onset may be as young as 5 to 10 years, although this is usually in the setting of MEN2B.[48,56] Two studies indicate that the penetrance and age at diagnosis differ between kindreds and correlate somewhat with specific *RET* mutations, with the highest penetrance associated with mutations at codons 918 and 634.[37,55] Pheochromocytomas are rarely seen in patients with mutations of exon 10 (codons 609, 611, and 620). The specific amino acid change within the codon may also affect expression of features in MEN2. In MEN2A patients with amino acid substitutions at codon 618, the penetrance of pheochromocytoma is variable; C618R shows 41% penetrance, C618G 24%, and C618Y 0%.[37]

Unlike sporadic presentations of pheochromocytoma, which may be malignant or in an extra-adrenal location (paraganglioma), cases associated with MEN2 are almost always benign and confined to the adrenal medulla. These tumors are usually multifocal in MEN2 patients and are bilateral in more than half of cases.

Screening for pheochromocytomas should be done in all patients diagnosed with MEN2A or MEN2B. Numerous studies show that measurement of plasma or 24-hour urine metanephrines is more sensitive and specific than measurement of catecholamines or other metabolites for detection of pheochromocytoma.[60] Pheochromocytoma screening should begin at the age when thyroidectomy would be considered on the basis of the risk level of the patient's *RET* mutation and family history.[48] If the result is negative, testing should be done annually thereafter. Positive or borderline results mandate additional investigation by imaging, usually adrenal CT or MRI.

MEN2 patients with pheochromocytoma should undergo partial or total adrenalectomy. The surgical management of unilateral disease has been the subject of some controversy because many patients will eventually develop pheochromocytoma on the contralateral side. Some authors recommended bilateral adrenalectomies for all MEN2 patients with pheochromocytoma. Patients who have had both adrenals removed, however, have a significant risk of adrenal insufficiency and addisonian crisis. Pheochromocytomas are not malignant in MEN2 patients, and the interval in the development of a pheochromocytoma between one side and the other side is more than 10 years.[61] For these reasons, most surgeons now recommend removal of only the affected adrenal in the setting of unilateral pheochromocytoma in MEN2 patients, with annual screening thereafter.

Laparoscopic adrenalectomy has gained favor as a preferred surgical approach for many MEN2 patients. The conversion rate to an open procedure is less than 10%.[61] It is considered appropriate for lesions confined to the adrenal and less than 9 to 10 cm, depending on the capabilities of the surgeon. Laparoscopic adrenalectomy has been associated with shorter hospital stay, decreased postoperative pain, and faster recovery compared with open adrenalectomy.[62]

Primary Hyperparathyroidism

The overall reported prevalence of primary hyperparathyroidism in MEN2A patients is between 10% and 35%, although this is highly variable between kindreds. This is not a clinical feature of FMTC or MEN2B. The age at onset tends to be later than for MTC, so hyperparathyroidism is rarely the initial presenting complaint that leads to a diagnosis of MEN2A. In more than 80% of cases, parathyroid hyperplasia will be identified in multiple glands. Inappropriate secretion of PTH leads to hypercalcemia and can result in osteoporosis, kidney stones, musculoskeletal pain, depression, and a host of nonspecific symptoms. Hyperparathyroidism in MEN2A is most commonly associated with the C634R mutation.

Patients known to have MEN2A should be screened with a serum calcium measurement annually. If the calcium concentration is elevated, a PTH level should be measured. Inappropriate elevation of PTH is diagnostic in a patient with MEN2A.

The treatment for hyperparathyroidism in MEN2A is four-gland parathyroidectomy with autotransplantation to the nondominant forearm muscle. This is done even if one or more glands appear grossly normal because of the likelihood that parathyroid hyperplasia will also develop in the normal-appearing glands in the future. Patients with a new diagnosis of MEN2A should be screened before undergoing thyroidectomy as a positive finding will preclude preservation of the parathyroids in situ. Many MEN2A patients who underwent preventive thyroidectomy in childhood will have had their parathyroids removed and autotransplanted at the time of the previous surgery. If hyperparathyroidism is manifested in a patient with a forearm graft, the graft can be explored and partly excised. Patients who previously underwent thyroidectomy without removal of the parathyroids will need a reexploration of the neck.

CONCLUSIONS

The management of MEN2 syndromes has changed significantly since the syndromes were first characterized in the mid-20th century. The advent of mutation testing in the *RET* and menin proto-oncogenes and our growing understanding of the relationships between genotype and phenotype have refined our diagnostic and prognostic capabilities for the MEN syndromes. Preventive surgery based on mutation analysis may prove to be a cure for MTC in young MEN2 patients. More accurate identification of those at risk has reduced the need for screening in many members of MEN kindreds. As more is learned about the pathogenesis of this disease, treatment can be further tailored to improve outcomes for individual patients.

SELECTED REFERENCES

Brunt LM, Lairmore TC, Doherty GM, et al: Adrenalectomy for familial pheochromocytoma in the laparoscopic era. *Ann Surg* 235:713–720; discussion 720–721, 2002.

Summary of a large institutional experience with laparoscopic removal of pheochromocytomas from patients with the MEN2 syndrome.

Matkar S, Thiel A, Hua X: Menin: A scaffold protein that controls gene expression and cell signaling. *Trends Biochem Sci* 38:394–402, 2013.

Comprehensive review of menin's diverse functions. Menin is a key scaffold protein that interacts with numerous protein partners and possesses dichotomous functions to positively or negatively influence gene transcription through interplay with multiple signaling pathways.

Norton JA, Jensen RT: Resolved and unresolved controversies in the surgical management of patients with Zollinger-Ellison syndrome. *Ann Surg* 240:757–773, 2004.

Excellent summary of relevant studies addressing current controversies in the management of ZES and sporadic as well as MEN1-associated gastrinomas.

Wells SA Jr, Asa SL, Dralle H, et al: Revised American thyroid association guidelines for the management of medullary thyroid carcinoma. *Thyroid* 25:567–610, 2015.

Recently published guidelines for management of patients with MEN2 written by a panel of experts.

REFERENCES

1. Bergholm U, Adami HO, Bergstrom R, et al: Clinical characteristics in sporadic and familial medullary thyroid carcinoma: A nationwide study of 249 patients in Sweden from 1959 through 1981. *Cancer* 63:1196–1204, 1989.
2. Chandrasekharappa SC, Guru SC, Manickam P, et al: Positional cloning of the gene for multiple endocrine neoplasia-type 1. *Science* 276:404–407, 1997.
3. Stewart C, Parente F, Piehl F, et al: Characterization of the mouse *Men1* gene and its expression during development. *Oncogene* 17:2485–2493, 1998.
4. Yokoyama A, Somervaille TC, Smith KS, et al: The menin tumor suppressor protein is an essential oncogenic cofactor for MLL-associated leukemogenesis. *Cell* 123:207–218, 2005.
5. Matkar S, Thiel A, Hua X: Menin: A scaffold protein that controls gene expression and cell signaling. *Trends Biochem Sci* 38:394–402, 2013.
6. Agarwal SK, Guru SC, Heppner C, et al: Menin interacts with the AP1 transcription factor JunD and represses JunD-activated transcription. *Cell* 96:143–152, 1999.
7. Dreijerink KM, Goudet P, Burgess JR, et al: Breast-cancer predisposition in multiple endocrine neoplasia type 1. *N Engl J Med* 371:583–584, 2014.
8. Lemos MC, Thakker RV: Multiple endocrine neoplasia type 1 (MEN1): Analysis of 1336 mutations reported in the first decade following identification of the gene. *Hum Mutat* 29:22–32, 2008.
9. Marini F, Giusti F, Brandi ML: Genetic test in multiple endocrine neoplasia type 1 syndrome: An evolving story. *World J Exp Med* 5:124–129, 2015.
10. Mutch MG, Dilley WG, Sanjurjo F, et al: Germline mutations in the multiple endocrine neoplasia type 1 gene: Evidence for frequent splicing defects. *Hum Mutat* 13:175–185, 1999.
11. Lairmore TC, Piersall LD, DeBenedetti MK, et al: Clinical genetic testing and early surgical intervention in patients with multiple endocrine neoplasia type 1 (MEN 1). *Ann Surg* 239:637–645, discussion 645–647, 2004.
12. Pardi E, Mariotti S, Pellegata NS, et al: Functional characterization of a *CDKN1B* mutation in a Sardinian kindred with multiple endocrine neoplasia type 4 (MEN4). *Endocr Connect* 4:1–8, 2015.
13. Thakker RV, Newey PJ, Walls GV, et al: Clinical practice guidelines for multiple endocrine neoplasia type 1 (MEN1). *J Clin Endocrinol Metab* 97:2990–3011, 2012.
14. Doherty GM, Lairmore TC, DeBenedetti MK: Multiple endocrine neoplasia type 1 parathyroid adenoma development over time. *World J Surg* 28:1139–1142, 2004.
15. Nilubol N, Weisbrod AB, Weinstein LS, et al: Utility of intraoperative parathyroid hormone monitoring in patients with multiple endocrine neoplasia type 1—associated primary hyperparathyroidism undergoing initial parathyroidectomy. *World J Surg* 37:1966–1972, 2013.
16. Lairmore TC, Govednik CM, Quinn CE, et al: A randomized, prospective trial of operative treatments for hyperparathyroidism in patients with multiple endocrine neoplasia type 1. *Surgery* 156:1326–1334, discussion 1334–1335, 2014.
17. Cohen MS, Dilley WG, Wells SA, Jr, et al: Long-term functionality of cryopreserved parathyroid autografts: A 13-year prospective analysis. *Surgery* 138:1033–1040, discussion 1040–1041, 2005.
18. Rosch T, Lightdale CJ, Botet JF, et al: Localization of pancreatic endocrine tumors by endoscopic ultrasonography. *N Engl J Med* 326:1721–1726, 1992.
19. McLean A: Endoscopic ultrasound in the detection of pancreatic islet cell tumours. *Cancer Imaging* 4:84–91, 2004.

20. Norton JA, Jensen RT: Resolved and unresolved controversies in the surgical management of patients with Zollinger-Ellison syndrome. *Ann Surg* 240:757–773, 2004.
21. Lairmore TC, Chen VY, DeBenedetti MK, et al: Duodenopancreatic resections in patients with multiple endocrine neoplasia type 1. *Ann Surg* 231:909–918, 2000.
22. Imamura M: Recent standardization of treatment strategy for pancreatic neuroendocrine tumors. *World J Gastroenterol* 16:4519–4525, 2010.
23. Berna MJ, Hoffmann KM, Serrano J, et al: Serum gastrin in Zollinger-Ellison syndrome: I. Prospective study of fasting serum gastrin in 309 patients from the National Institutes of Health and comparison with 2229 cases from the literature. *Medicine (Baltimore)* 85:295–330, 2006.
24. Norton JA, Alexander HR, Fraker DL, et al: Possible primary lymph node gastrinoma: Occurrence, natural history, and predictive factors: A prospective study. *Ann Surg* 237:650–657, discussion 657-659, 2003.
25. Norton JA, Fraker DL, Alexander R, et al: Surgery to cure the Zollinger-Ellison syndrome. *N Engl J Med* 341:635–644, 1999.
26. Norton JA, Melcher ML, Gibril F, et al: Gastric carcinoid tumors in multiple endocrine neoplasia-1 patients with Zollinger-Ellison syndrome can be symptomatic, demonstrate aggressive growth, and require surgical treatment. *Surgery* 136:1267–1274, 2004.
27. Kouvaraki MA, Shapiro SE, Cote GJ, et al: Management of pancreatic endocrine tumors in multiple endocrine neoplasia type 1. *World J Surg* 30:643–653, 2006.
28. Lowney JK, Frisella MM, Lairmore TC, et al: Pancreatic islet cell tumor metastasis in multiple endocrine neoplasia type 1: Correlation with primary tumor size. *Surgery* 124:1043–1048, discussion 1048-1049, 1998.
29. Skogseid B, Oberg K, Eriksson B, et al: Surgery for asymptomatic pancreatic lesion in multiple endocrine neoplasia type I. *World J Surg* 20:872–876, discussion 877, 1996.
30. Bartsch DK, Fendrich V, Langer P, et al: Outcome of duodenopancreatic resections in patients with multiple endocrine neoplasia type 1. *Ann Surg* 242:757–764, discussion 764–766, 2005.
31. Tonelli F, Fratini G, Nesi G, et al: Pancreatectomy in multiple endocrine neoplasia type 1—related gastrinomas and pancreatic endocrine neoplasias. *Ann Surg* 244:61–70, 2006.
32. Darling TN, Skarulis MC, Steinberg SM, et al: Multiple facial angiofibromas and collagenomas in patients with multiple endocrine neoplasia type 1. *Arch Dermatol* 133:853–857, 1997.
33. Ferolla P, Falchetti A, Filosso P, et al: Thymic neuroendocrine carcinoma (carcinoid) in multiple endocrine neoplasia type 1 syndrome: The Italian series. *J Clin Endocrinol Metab* 90:2603–2609, 2005.
34. Mulligan LM, Kwok JB, Healey CS, et al: Germ-line mutations of the RET proto-oncogene in multiple endocrine neoplasia type 2A. *Nature* 363:458–460, 1993.
35. Eng C, Clayton D, Schuffenecker I, et al: The relationship between specific RET proto-oncogene mutations and disease phenotype in multiple endocrine neoplasia type 2. International RET mutation consortium analysis. *JAMA* 276:1575–1579, 1996.
36. Sipple J: The association of pheochromocytoma with carcinomas of the thyroid gland. *Am J Med* 31:163–166, 1961.
37. Quayle FJ, Fialkowski EA, Benveniste R, et al: Pheochromocytoma penetrance varies by RET mutation in MEN 2A. *Surgery* 142:800–805, discussion 805.e1, 2007.
38. Moore SW, Zaahl MG: Multiple endocrine neoplasia syndromes, children, Hirschsprung's disease and RET. *Pediatr Surg Int* 24:521–530, 2008.
39. Wells SA, Jr, Asa SL, Dralle H, et al: Revised American Thyroid Association guidelines for the management of medullary thyroid carcinoma. *Thyroid* 25:567–610, 2015.
40. Elisei R, Cosci B, Romei C, et al: Prognostic significance of somatic RET oncogene mutations in sporadic medullary thyroid cancer: A 10-year follow-up study. *J Clin Endocrinol Metab* 93:682–687, 2008.
41. Zedenius J, Larsson C, Bergholm U, et al: Mutations of codon 918 in the RET proto-oncogene correlate to poor prognosis in sporadic medullary thyroid carcinomas. *J Clin Endocrinol Metab* 80:3088–3090, 1995.
42. Arighi E, Borrello MG, Sariola H: RET tyrosine kinase signaling in development and cancer. *Cytokine Growth Factor Rev* 16:441–467, 2005.
43. Neumann HP, Bausch B, McWhinney SR, et al: Germ-line mutations in nonsyndromic pheochromocytoma. *N Engl J Med* 346:1459–1466, 2002.
44. Dralle H, Gimm O, Simon D, et al: Prophylactic thyroidectomy in 75 children and adolescents with hereditary medullary thyroid carcinoma: German and Austrian experience. *World J Surg* 22:744–750, discussion 750–751, 1998.
45. Hundahl SA, Fleming ID, Fremgen AM, et al: A National Cancer Data Base report on 53,856 cases of thyroid carcinoma treated in the U.S., 1985-1995 [see comments]. *Cancer* 83:2638–2648, 1998.
46. Moley JF, Fialkowski EA: Evidence-based approach to the management of sporadic medullary thyroid carcinoma. *World J Surg* 31:946–956, 2007.
47. Moley JF: Medullary thyroid carcinoma: Management of lymph node metastases. *J Natl Compr Canc Netw* 8:549–556, 2010.
48. Kloos RT, Eng C, Evans DB, et al: Medullary thyroid cancer: Management guidelines of the American Thyroid Association. *Thyroid* 19:565–612, 2009.
49. Dralle H: Lymph node dissection and medullary thyroid carcinoma. *Br J Surg* 89:1073–1075, 2002.
50. Kouvaraki MA, Shapiro SE, Fornage BD, et al: Role of preoperative ultrasonography in the surgical management of patients with thyroid cancer. *Surgery* 134:946–954, discussion 954–955, 2003.
51. Skinner MA, Moley JA, Dilley WG, et al: Prophylactic thyroidectomy in multiple endocrine neoplasia type 2A. *N Engl J Med* 353:1105–1113, 2005.
52. Gagel RF, Tashjian AH, Jr, Cummings T, et al: The clinical outcome of prospective screening for multiple endocrine neoplasia type 2a. An 18-year experience. *N Engl J Med* 318:478–484, 1988.
53. Brandi ML, Gagel RF, Angeli A, et al: Guidelines for diagnosis and therapy of MEN type 1 and type 2. *J Clin Endocrinol Metab* 86:5658–5671, 2001.
54. Machens A, Niccoli-Sire P, Hoegel J, et al: Early malignant progression of hereditary medullary thyroid cancer. *N Engl J Med* 349:1517–1525, 2003.
55. Machens A, Brauckhoff M, Holzhausen HJ, et al: Codon-specific development of pheochromocytoma in multiple

endocrine neoplasia type 2. *J Clin Endocrinol Metab* 90:3999–4003, 2005.
56. Sosa JA, Tuggle CT, Wang TS, et al: Clinical and economic outcomes of thyroid and parathyroid surgery in children. *J Clin Endocrinol Metab* 93:3058–3065, 2008.
57. Lips CJ, Landsvater RM, Hoppener JW, et al: Clinical screening as compared with DNA analysis in families with multiple endocrine neoplasia type 2A. *N Engl J Med* 331:870–871, 1994.
58. Brierley J, Tsang R, Simpson WJ, et al: Medullary thyroid cancer: Analyses of survival and prognostic factors and the role of radiation therapy in local control. *Thyroid* 6:305–310, 1996.
59. Wells SA, Gosnell JE, Gagel RF, et al: Vendetanib for the treatment of patients with locally advanced or metastatic hereditary medullary thyroid carcinoma. *J Clin Oncol* 28:767–772, 2010.
60. Eisenhofer G, Lenders JW, Linehan WM, et al: Plasma normetanephrine and metanephrine for detecting pheochromocytoma in von Hippel–Lindau disease and multiple endocrine neoplasia type 2. *N Engl J Med* 340:1872–1879, 1999.
61. Rodriguez JM, Balsalobre M, Ponce JL, et al: Pheochromocytoma in MEN 2A syndrome. Study of 54 patients. *World J Surg* 32:2520–2526, 2008.
62. Brunt LM, Lairmore TC, Doherty GM, et al: Adrenalectomy for familial pheochromocytoma in the laparoscopic era. *Ann Surg* 235:713–720, discussion 720–721, 2002.

SECTION IX

Esophagus

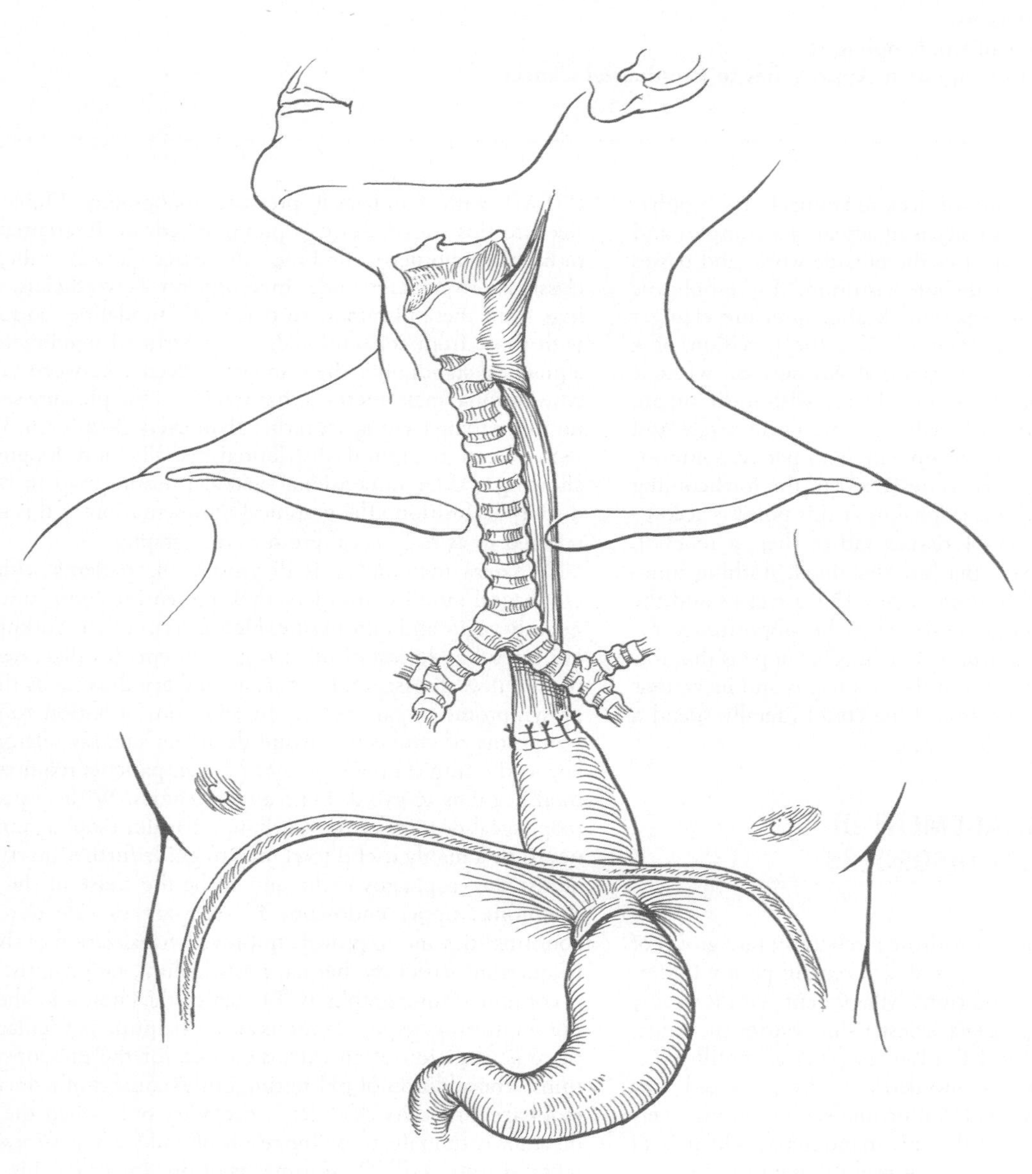

41 CHAPTER

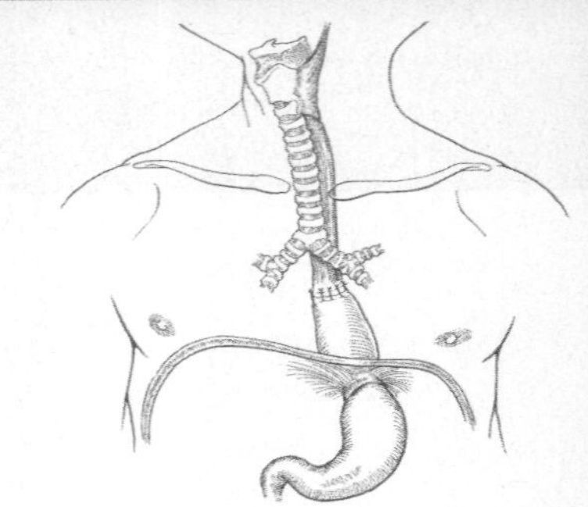

Esophagus

Jonathan D. Spicer, Rajeev Dhupar, Jae Y. Kim, Boris Sepesi, Wayne Hofstetter

OUTLINE

An organ that spans the distance of neck to stomach, the esophagus for all of its tube-like simplicity is in actuality a complex and relatively durable organ. It traverses the outside world and passes through precious territory in the mediastinum. The esophagus functions within areas that transition through pressure changes ranging from atmospheric to vacuum. Yet, the precision of a normal esophagus is virtually unrecognized. We swallow without effort, pain, or thought; but introduce disease within the organ, and we incur various degrees of malady, some quite severe and invariably chronic. We have yet to come up with perfect solutions for most of the dysfunction that is described in the forthcoming section, and replacement of the esophagus at this point is accomplished only by substitution of tissues rather than a renewal. Ultimately, among the "fixes" that are described, nothing functions as well as the original healthy organ. This leaves us and the future generation of esophagologists with the opportunity for innovation and much needed improvement. Our hope is that this chapter serves as an introduction to the esophagus and its various forms of function and dysfunction. One could literally spend a lifetime delving into each of these areas.

DIAGNOSIS AND MANAGEMENT OF ESOPHAGEAL MOTILITY DISORDERS

Diagnosis

Esophageal motility disorders constitute a relatively rare group of conditions, the underlying causes of which remain poorly understood. Patients with these conditions will present with a variety of symptoms including dysphagia, chest pain, heartburn, regurgitation, and weight loss. By definition, esophageal motility disorders are diagnosed when manometric findings exceed two standard deviations from normal. Unfortunately, symptom severity does not always correlate well with manometry, which is of critical importance in planning for surgical intervention in these generally complicated patients. Esophageal motility disorders are probably best classified by the Chicago classification, which was derived from data obtained by high-resolution manometry (HRM) with esophageal pressure topography (Table 41-1).[1] Because this classification is purely based on differentiating patterns of manometric findings, the exact clinical utility of this classification remains under investigation. Nevertheless, the findings from these ultramodern diagnostic modalities correlate well with those from conventional, water-perfused manometry. From a practical standpoint, the primary difference between HRM and conventional manometry is that in HRM, the pressure sensors are no more than 1 cm apart rather than every 3 to 5 cm. Up to 36 sensors can be found distributed radially and longitudinally, allowing a three-dimensional spatial pressure map to be drawn during deglutition. The graphical representation of this is what is referred to as esophageal pressure topography.

Whereas manometry is diagnostic for patients with named esophageal motility disorders, their presenting complaints are frequently vague and nonspecific. Hence, a complete workup including careful exclusion of other organ systems (cardiac, respiratory, peptic ulcer disease, and pancreaticobiliary disease) as the source of symptoms is paramount. In addition, attention to systemic symptoms of connective tissue disorders such as scleroderma is key as the surgical management of such patients requires specific modifications to avoid disastrous outcomes. With respect to the esophageal portion of the workup, a barium esophagram continues to be a highly useful road map to guide further investigations. When the esophagus is thought to be the cause of the patient's symptoms, upper endoscopy is necessary to rule out mucosal abnormalities and to provide improved visualization of the defects in question (stricture, hernia, diverticulum, esophagitis, masses). A computed tomography (CT) scan of the chest and abdomen is not uniformly required but may be helpful, particularly when there is suspicion of an extrinsic cause for the presenting symptoms. The addition of pH testing in the context of a documented esophageal motility disorder is necessary only when the motility disorder is thought to be the result of end-stage gastroesophageal reflux disease (GERD) as a means of documenting this.

Classically, esophageal motility disorders have been classified into primary and secondary causes. Primary disorders fall into five categories of motor disorders: achalasia, diffuse esophageal spasm

TABLE 41-1 The Chicago Classification of Esophageal Motility

	CRITERIA
Achalasia and Esophagogastric Junction Outflow Obstruction	
Type I achalasia (classic)	Median IRP >15 mm Hg; 100% failed peristalsis (DCI <100 mm Hg•s •cm); premature contractions with DCI <450 mm Hg•s •cm satisfy criteria for failed peristalsis
Type II achalasia (with esophageal compression)	Median IRP >15 mm Hg; 100% failed peristalsis, panesophageal pressurization with ≥20% of swallows
Type III achalasia (spastic achalasia)	Median IRP >15 mm Hg; no normal peristalsis, spastic contractions with DCI >450 mm Hg•s •cm with ≥20% of swallows
Esophagogastric junction outflow obstruction (achalasia in evolution)	Median IRP >15 mm Hg; sufficient evidence of peristalsis such that criteria for types I-III are not met
Major Disorders of Peristalsis	
Absent contractility	Normal median IRP, 100% failed peristalsis
Distal esophageal spasm	Normal median IRP; ≥20% premature contractions with DCI >450 mm Hg•s•cm
Hypercontractile esophagus (jackhammer)	At least 2 swallows with DCI >8000 mm Hg•cm •s
Minor Disorders of Peristalsis	
Ineffective esophageal motility	≥50% ineffective swallows
Fragmented peristalsis	≥50% fragmented contractions with DCI >450 mm Hg•cm
Normal esophageal motility	None of the above criteria are met

Integrated relaxation pressure (IRP) is the mean of the 4 seconds of maximal deglutitive relaxation in the 10-second window beginning at the upper esophageal sphincter relaxation referenced to gastric pressure; distal contractile integral (DCI) is the amplitude × duration × length (mm Hg•s •cm) of the distal esophageal contraction exceeding 20 mm Hg from the transition zone to the proximal margin of the lower esophageal sphincter.

Data from Roman S, Gyawali CP, Xiao Y, et al: The Chicago classification of motility disorders. *Gastrointest Endosc Clin N Am* 24:545–561, 2014.

(DES), nutcracker (jackhammer) esophagus, hypertensive lower esophageal sphincter (LES), and ineffective esophageal motility (IEM). Secondary conditions result from progressive damage induced by an underlying collagen vascular or neuromuscular disorder; they include scleroderma, dermatomyositis, polymyositis, lupus erythematosus, Chagas disease, and myasthenia gravis. Whereas such a classification is rooted in the basic etiology of this collection of diseases, it does not help much with interpreting manometric results, nor is it helpful as a guide to treatment strategies. For this reason, we suggest an anatomic approach to classifying esophageal motility disorders based on involvement of the esophageal body or LES as this is the basis for understanding basic esophageal manometry and often the key to guide surgical therapy.

Motility Disorders of the Esophageal Body

Diffuse Esophageal Spasm

DES is a poorly understood hypermotility disorder of the esophagus. Under the Chicago classification, this would now be called distal esophageal spasm. Although it is manifested in a similar fashion to achalasia, it is five times less common. It is seen most often in women and is often found in patients with multiple medical complaints. The cause of the neuromuscular physiology is unclear. The basic pathology is related to a motor abnormality of the esophageal body that is most notable in the lower two thirds of the esophagus. Muscular hypertrophy and degeneration of the branches of the vagus nerve in the esophagus have been observed. As a result, the esophageal contractions are repetitive, simultaneous, and of high amplitude.

The clinical presentation of DES is typically that of chest pain and dysphagia. These symptoms may be related to eating or exertion and may mimic those of angina. Patients will complain of a squeezing pressure in the chest that may radiate to the jaw, arms, and upper back. The symptoms are often pronounced during times of heightened emotional stress. Regurgitation of esophageal contents and saliva is common but acid reflux is not. However, acid reflux can aggravate the symptoms, as can cold liquids. Other functional gastrointestinal complaints, such as irritable bowel syndrome and pyloric spasm, may accompany DES, whereas other gastrointestinal problems, such as gallstones, peptic ulcer disease, and pancreatitis, all trigger DES.

The diagnosis of DES is made by radiographic and manometric studies. The classic picture of the corkscrew esophagus or pseudodiverticulosis on an esophagram is caused by the presence of tertiary contractions and indicates advanced disease. A distal bird beak narrowing of the esophagus and normal peristalsis can also be noted. The classic manometry findings in DES are simultaneous multipeaked contractions of high amplitude (>120 mm Hg) or long duration (>2.5 seconds). These erratic contractions occur after more than 10% of wet swallows. Because of the spontaneous contractions and intermittent normal peristalsis, standard manometry may not be enough to identify DES. Correlation of subjective complaints with evidence of spasm (induced by a vagomimetic drug, bethanechol) on manometric tracings is also convincing evidence of this capricious disease.

The treatment for DES is far from ideal as symptom relief is often partial. Today, the mainstay of treatment for DES is nonsurgical, and pharmacologic or endoscopic intervention is preferred. All patients are evaluated for psychiatric conditions, including depression, psychosomatic complaints, and anxiety. Control of these disorders and reassurance of the esophageal nature of the chest pain that the patient is experiencing is often therapeutic in and of itself. If dysphagia is a component of a patient's symptoms, steps must be taken to eliminate trigger foods or drinks from the diet. Similarly, if reflux is a component, acid suppression medications are helpful. Nitrates, calcium channel blockers, sedatives, and anticholinergics may be effective in some cases, but the relative efficacy of these medicines is not known. Peppermint may also provide temporary symptomatic relief. Bougie dilation of the esophagus up to 50 or 60 Fr provides relief for severe dysphagia and is 70% to 80% effective. Botulinum toxin injections have also been tried with some success, but the results are not sustainable.

Surgery is indicated for patients with incapacitating chest pain or dysphagia who have failed to respond to medical and endoscopic therapy or in the presence of a pulsion diverticulum of the thoracic esophagus. A long esophagomyotomy is performed through a left thoracotomy or a video-assisted technique through the abdomen or left side of the chest. Esophageal manometry is a useful tool to guide the extent of the myotomy. Some surgeons advocate extending the myotomy up into the thoracic inlet, but most agree that the proximal extent generally should be high enough to encompass the entire length of the abnormal motility, as determined by manometric measurements. The distal extent of the myotomy is extended down onto the LES, but the need to include the stomach is not agreed on uniformly. A Dor fundoplication is recommended to provide reflux protection as the surgery itself interrupts the phrenoesophageal ligament and encourages reflux. Results of the long esophagomyotomy for DES are variable, but it is reported to provide relief of symptoms in up to 80% of patients.

Nutcracker Esophagus

Recognized in the late 1970s as a distinct entity and known as hypercontractile esophagus in the Chicago classification, nutcracker or jackhammer esophagus is a disorder characterized by excessive contractility. It is described as an esophagus with hypertensive peristalsis or high-amplitude peristaltic contractions. It is seen in patients of all ages, with equal gender predilection, and is the most common of all esophageal hypermotility disorders. Like DES, the pathophysiologic process is not well understood. It is associated with hypertrophic musculature that results in high-amplitude contractions of the esophagus and is the most painful of all esophageal motility disorders.

Patients with nutcracker esophagus present in a similar fashion to those with DES and frequently complain of chest pain and dysphagia. Odynophagia is also noted, but regurgitation and reflux are uncommon. An esophagram may or may not reveal any abnormalities, depending on how well "behaved" the esophagus is during the examination. The Chicago classification characterizes the diagnosis of nutcracker esophagus as the subjective complaint of chest pain with at least one swallow showing a distal contractile integral greater than 8000 mm Hg•s•cm with single or multi-peaked contractions on HRM. The LES pressure is normal, and relaxation occurs with each wet swallow (Fig. 41-1). Ambulatory monitoring can help distinguish this disorder from DES. This is of critical importance because a subset of DES patients with dysphagia can be helped with esophagomyotomy, but surgery is of questionable value in patients with a nutcracker esophagus.

The treatment of nutcracker esophagus is medical. Calcium channel blockers, nitrates, and antispasmodics may offer temporary relief during acute spasms. Bougie dilation may offer some temporary relief of severe discomfort but has no long-term benefits. Patients with nutcracker esophagus may have triggers and are counseled to avoid caffeine, cold, and hot foods.

Motility Disorders of the Lower Esophageal Sphincter

Hypertensive Lower Esophageal Sphincter

Hypertensive LES was first described as a distinct entity by Code and colleagues.[2] According to the Chicago classification, this entity has been renamed esophagogastric junction (EGJ) outflow obstruction and is defined as a median integrated relaxation pressure greater than 15 mm Hg (hypertensive, poorly relaxing sphincter). Thought by some to be achalasia in evolution, the diagnosis differs by evidence of effective peristalsis that is not present in classic achalasia. Hypertensive LES may be observed in patients presenting with dysphagia, chest pain, and manometric findings of an elevated LES. Patients with hypertensive LES will infrequently present with acid reflux and regurgitation. The

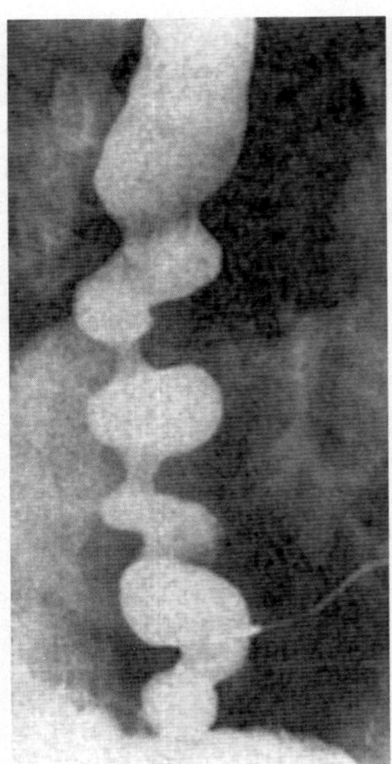

FIGURE 41-1 Barium esophagram of diffuse esophageal spasm. (Adapted from Peters JH, DeMeester TR: Esophagus and diaphragmatic hernia. In Schwartz SI, Fischer JE, Spencer FC, et al, editors: *Principles of surgery*, ed 7, New York, 1998, McGraw-Hill.)

diagnosis is made by manometry. Conventional manometry will demonstrate LES pressures above normal (>26 mm Hg), and relaxation will be incomplete but may not be consistently abnormal. Motility of the esophageal body may be hyperperistaltic or normal. An esophagram may show narrowing at the gastroesophageal junction (GEJ) with delayed flow and abnormalities of esophageal contraction; however, these are nonspecific findings. About 50% of the time, peristalsis in the esophageal body is normal. In the remainder, abnormal contractions are noted to be hypertensive peristaltic or simultaneous waveforms. The pathogenesis is not well understood.

The treatment of hypertensive LES is with endoscopic and surgical intervention. Botox injections alleviate symptoms temporarily, and hydrostatic balloon dilation may provide long-term symptomatic relief. Surgery is indicated for patients who fail to respond to interventional treatments and those with significant symptoms. A laparoscopic modified Heller esophagomyotomy is the operation of choice. In patients with normal esophageal motility, a partial antireflux procedure (e.g., Dor or Toupet fundoplication) is added. Recently, some have advocated the use of per-oral endoscopic myotomy for such patients (discussed further in the section on achalasia).[3]

Motility Disorders Affecting Both Body and Lower Esophageal Sphincter

Achalasia

The literal meaning of the term *achalasia* is "failure to relax." It is the best understood of all esophageal motility disorders. The incidence is 6/100,000 persons/year, with a predilection to affect young women. Its pathogenesis is presumed to be idiopathic or infectious neurogenic degeneration. Severe emotional stress, trauma, drastic weight reduction, and Chagas disease (parasitic infection with *Trypanosoma cruzi*) have also been implicated. Regardless of the cause, the muscles of the esophagus and LES are affected. Prevailing theories support the model that the destruction of the nerves to the LES is the primary pathologic process and that degeneration of the neuromuscular function of the body of the esophagus is secondary. This degeneration results in hypertension of the LES and failure of the LES to relax on pharyngeal swallowing as well as pressurization of the esophagus, esophageal dilation, and resultant loss of progressive peristalsis.

Vigorous (or spastic/type III) achalasia is seen in a subset of patients presenting with chest pain. In these patients, the LES is hypertensive and fails to relax, as seen in achalasia. Furthermore, the contractions of the esophageal body continue to be simultaneous and nonperistaltic. However, the amplitude of the contractions in response to swallowing is normal or high, which is inconsistent with classic achalasia (Fig. 41-2). It is postulated that patients in the early phases of achalasia may not have abnormalities in the esophageal body that are seen in later stages of the disease. Patients presenting with vigorous achalasia may be in this early phase and will go on to develop abnormal esophageal body contractions predicated on the presence of outflow obstruction of the esophagus.

Achalasia is also known to be a premalignant condition of the esophagus. During a 20-year period, a patient will have up to an 8% chance for development of carcinoma. Squamous cell carcinoma is the most common type identified and is thought to be the result of long-standing retained undigested fermenting food in the body of the esophagus, causing mucosal irritation. If the histology is adenocarcinoma, it tends to appear in the middle third of the esophagus, below the air-fluid level, where the mucosal irritation is the greatest. In contrast to these theories of carcinogenesis, it appears that even in patients with treated achalasia, there is an ongoing cancer incidence risk. Although no specific surveillance program for patients with treated achalasia has yet been endorsed by any of the gastroenterology societies, long-term surveillance is strongly recommended to monitor for recurrent achalasia and cancer.

The classic triad of presenting symptoms of achalasia consists of dysphagia, regurgitation, and weight loss. Heartburn, postprandial choking, and nocturnal coughing are commonly seen. The dysphagia that patients experience often begins with liquids and progresses to solids. Most patients describe eating as a laborious process during which they must pay special attention to the process. They eat slowly and use large volumes of water to help wash the food down into the stomach. As the water builds up pressure, retrosternal chest pain is experienced and can be severe until the LES opens, which provides quick relief. Regurgitation of undigested, foul-smelling food is common, and with progressive disease, aspiration can become life-threatening. Pneumonia, lung abscess, and bronchiectasis often result from long-standing achalasia. The dysphagia progresses slowly during years, and patients adapt their lifestyle to accommodate the inconveniences that accompany this disease. Patients often do not seek medical attention until their symptoms are advanced and will present with marked distention of the esophagus.

The diagnosis of achalasia is usually made from an esophagram and a motility study. The findings may vary, depending on the degree to which the disease has advanced. The esophagram will often show a dilated esophagus with a distal narrowing referred to as the classic bird's beak appearance of the barium-filled esophagus (Fig. 41-3). Sphincter spasm and delayed emptying through the LES as well as dilation of the esophageal body are observed. A lack of peristaltic waves in the body and failure of relaxation of the LES (the sine qua non of this disease) are noted. Lack of a gastric air bubble is a common finding on the upright portion of the esophagram and is a result of the tight LES not allowing air to pass easily into the stomach. In the more advanced stage of disease, massive esophageal dilation, tortuosity, and sigmoidal esophagus (megaesophagus) are seen (Fig. 41-4).

Manometry is the "gold standard" test for diagnosis and will help differentiate other potential esophageal motility disorders. In typical achalasia (type I), the manometry tracings show five classic

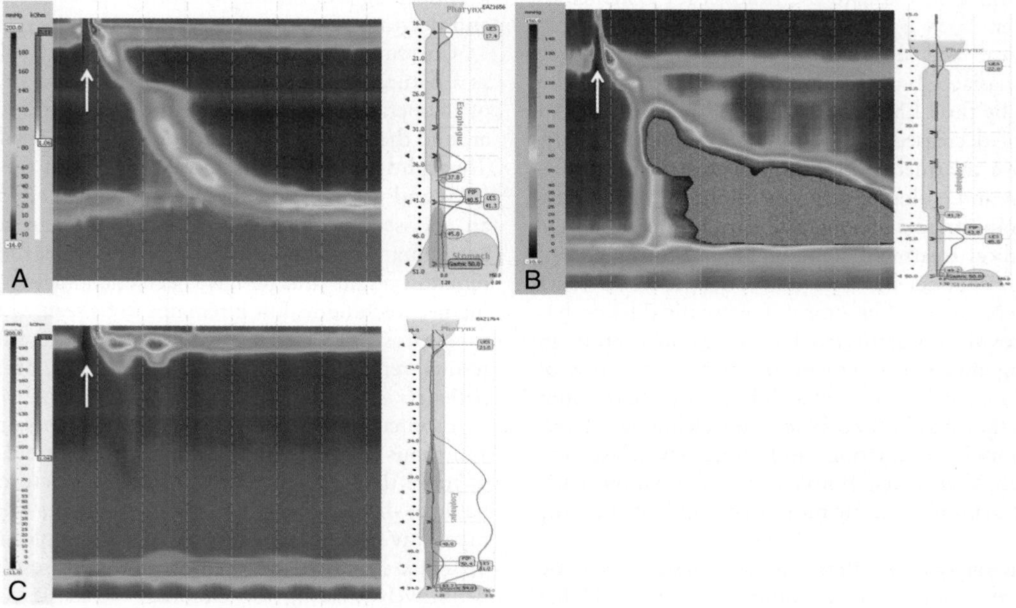

FIGURE 41-2 High-resolution esophageal manometry. **A,** A normal swallowing pattern. **B** and **C,** Classic (type I) achalasia and atypical spastic or vigorous achalasia (type III). The *arrows* denote initiation of swallowing.

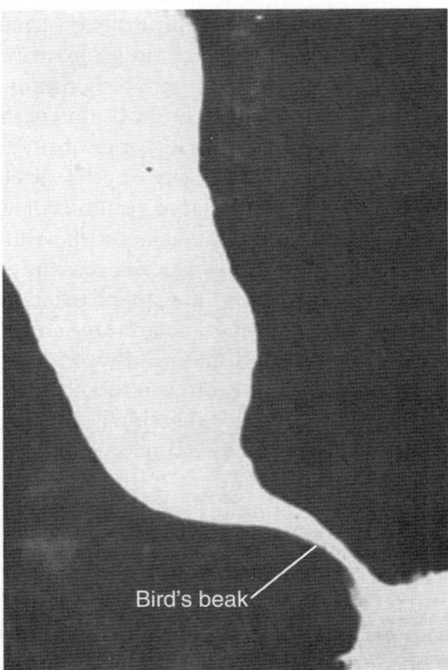

FIGURE 41-3 Barium swallow showing achalasia. (Adapted from Dalton CB: Esophageal motility disorders. In Pearson FG, Cooper JD, Deslauriers J, et al, editors: *Esophageal surgery*, ed 2, New York, 2002, Churchill Livingstone.)

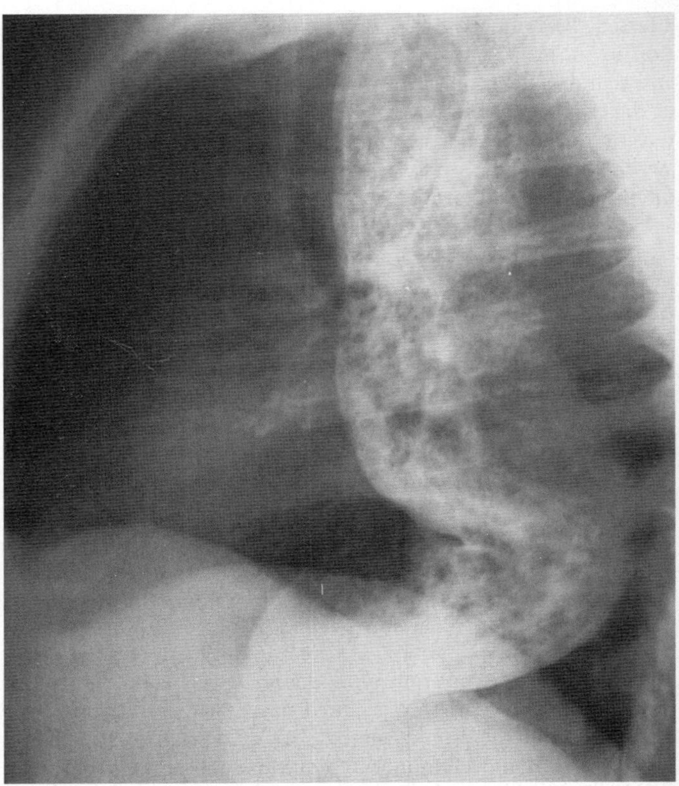

FIGURE 41-4 Barium swallow showing megaesophagus. (From Orringer MB: Disorders of esophageal motility. In Sabiston DC, editor: *Textbook of surgery*, ed 15, Philadelphia, 1997, WB Saunders.)

findings, two abnormalities of the LES and three of the esophageal body. The LES will be hypertensive, with pressures usually higher than 35 mm Hg (integrated relaxation pressure >15 mm Hg), but more important, it will fail to relax with deglutition. The body of the esophagus will have a pressure above baseline (pressurization of the esophagus) from incomplete air evacuation, simultaneous mirrored contractions with no evidence of progressive peristalsis, and low-amplitude waveforms indicating a lack of muscle tone. These five findings provide a diagnosis of achalasia. Endoscopy is performed to evaluate the mucosa for evidence of esophagitis or cancer.

There are surgical and nonsurgical treatment options for patients with achalasia; all are directed toward relieving the obstruction caused by the LES. Because none of them are able to address the issue of decreased motility in the esophageal body, they are all palliative treatments. Nonsurgical treatment options include medications and endoscopic interventions but usually are only a short-term solution to a lifelong problem. In the early stage of the disease, medical treatment with sublingual nitroglycerin, nitrates, or calcium channel blockers may offer hours of relief from chest pressure before or after a meal. Pneumatic dilation has been shown to provide excellent relief of symptoms although frequently requiring multiple interventions and with a risk of esophageal perforation of less than 4%. Injection of botulinum toxin (Botox) directly into the LES blocks acetylcholine release, prevents smooth muscle contraction, and effectively relaxes the LES. With repeated treatments, Botox may offer symptomatic relief for years, but symptoms recur more than 50% of the time within 6 months.

Surgical esophagomyotomy offers excellent results that are durable. The current technique is a modification of the Heller myotomy that was described originally through a laparotomy in 1913. Various changes have been made to the originally described procedure, but the modified laparoscopic Heller myotomy is now the operation of choice. It is done open or with video or robotic assistance. The decision to perform an antireflux procedure remains controversial. Most patients who have undergone a myotomy will experience some amount of reflux, either symptomatic or not. The addition of a partial antireflux procedure, such as a Toupet or Dor fundoplication, will restore a barrier to reflux and decrease postoperative symptoms.

Currently, per-oral endoscopic myotomy is being investigated as a natural orifice approach to perform the myotomy. With use of an operating endoscope, the mucosa of the esophagus is divided around the mid to distal third, and a submucosal tunnel is created. Through this tunnel, the muscular layer of the distal esophagus, LES, and cardia is visualized and divided, effectively performing an endoscopic myotomy. Although concern for the lack of an antireflux procedure and the possibility of debilitating reflux remains, results thus far have been encouraging.[4] This is a promising new technique, but it remains to be seen whether it is superior to laparoscopic Heller myotomy and the excellent long-term results reported in multiple large series of surgically treated patients.

Esophagectomy is considered in any symptomatic patient with a tortuous esophagus (megaesophagus), sigmoid esophagus, failure of more than one myotomy, or reflux stricture that is not amenable to dilation. Less than 60% of patients undergoing repeated myotomy benefit from surgery, and fundoplication for treatment of reflux strictures has even more dismal results. In addition to definitively treating the end-stage achalasia patient, esophageal resection also eliminates the risk for carcinoma in the resected area. A transhiatal esophagectomy with or without preservation of the vagus nerve offers a good long-term result. However, in the setting of megaesophagus, a total esophagectomy incorporating a transthoracic dissection may be safest, given the difficulty in palpating the borders of the esophagus through a transhiatal approach.

Results of medical, interventional, and surgical procedures all point to surgery as the safest and most effective treatment of achalasia. In comparing balloon dilation to Botox injections, remission of symptoms occurred in 89% versus 38% of patients at 1 year, respectively. Studies done to compare balloon dilation versus surgery have shown perforation rates of 4% and 1% and mortality rates of 0.5% and 0.2%, respectively. Results were considered excellent in 60% of patients undergoing balloon dilation and in 85% of those undergoing surgery. However, more recently in a randomized controlled trial of the European Achalasia Trial Investigators,[5] pneumatic dilation was found to be equivalent to laparoscopic Heller myotomy and Dor fundoplication with therapeutic success rates of 86% versus 90% at 2 years. Perforation occurred in 4% of the patients during pneumatic dilations and mucosal tears occurred in 12% during laparoscopic Heller myotomy, but all were repaired intraoperatively. Patients in the pneumatic dilation cohort had a 25% rate of redilation to achieve treatment success. Clinicians need to remain wary and vigilant with achalasia patients, even after "successful" intervention. Continued asymptomatic outflow obstruction will lead to dilation. Close monitoring of these patients is appropriate.

Ineffective Esophageal Motility

IEM was first recognized as a distinct motility disturbance by Castell in 2000. It is defined as a contraction abnormality of the distal esophagus and is usually associated with GERD. It may be secondary to inflammatory injury of the esophageal body because of increased exposure to gastric contents. Dampened motility of the esophageal body leads to poor acid clearance in the lower esophagus. Once altered motility is present, the condition appears to be irreversible.

The symptoms of IEM are mixed, but patients usually present with symptoms of reflux and dysphagia. Heartburn, chest pain, and regurgitation are noted. Diagnosis is made by manometry. IEM is defined by greater than 50% of swallows being deemed ineffective (distal contractile integral <450 mm Hg). A barium esophagram demonstrates nonspecific abnormalities of esophageal contraction but will not further distinguish IEM from other motor disorders.

The best treatment of IEM is prevention, which is associated with effective treatment of GERD. Once altered motility occurs, it appears to be irreversible. Similarly, scleroderma may be manifested manometrically as IEM and is best treated by addressing the underlying condition. In cases in which the motility disorder has become irreversible and intractable, the surgical approach must be tailored to the manometric findings. However, great caution must be taken in approaching surgical therapy in this cohort of patients as the likelihood of a favorable result remains low.

DIVERTICULAR DISORDERS

It is now well established that most diverticula are a result of a primary motor disturbance or an abnormality of the upper esophageal sphincter or LES. Diverticula were originally classified according to their location, and as a convention, these are classifications to which we still adhere. The three most common sites of occurrence are pharyngoesophageal (Zenker), parabronchial (midesophageal), and epiphrenic (supradiaphragmatic). True diverticula involve all layers of the esophageal wall, including mucosa, submucosa, and muscularis. A false diverticulum consists of mucosa and submucosa only. Pulsion diverticula are false diverticula that occur because of elevated intraluminal pressures generated from abnormal motility disorders. These forces cause the mucosa and submucosa to herniate through the esophageal musculature. Both a Zenker diverticulum and an epiphrenic diverticulum fall under the category of false pulsion diverticula. Traction, or true, diverticula result from external inflammatory mediastinal lymph nodes adhering to the esophagus as they heal and contract, pulling the esophagus during the process. Over time, the esophageal wall herniates, forming an outpouching, and a diverticulum ensues. These are more common in the midesophageal region around the carinal lymph nodes.

Pharyngoesophageal (Zenker) Diverticulum

Originally described by Zenker and von Ziemssen,[6] the pharyngoesophageal diverticulum (Zenker diverticulum) is the most common esophageal diverticulum found today (Fig. 41-5). It is usually manifested in older patients in the seventh decade of life and has been postulated to be a result of loss of tissue elasticity and muscle tone with age. It is specifically found herniating from Killian's triangle, between the oblique fibers of the thyropharyngeus muscle and the horizontal fibers of the cricopharyngeus muscle. As the diverticulum enlarges, the mucosal and submucosal layers dissect down the left side of the esophagus into the superior mediastinum, posteriorly along the prevertebral space. Zenker diverticulum is often referred to as cricopharyngeal achalasia and is managed accordingly.

Until the Zenker diverticulum begins to enlarge, patients are often initially asymptomatic. Commonly, patients complain of a sticking in the throat. A nagging cough, excessive salivation, and intermittent dysphagia often are signs of progressive disease. As the sac increases in size, regurgitation of foul-smelling, undigested material is common. Halitosis, voice changes, retrosternal pain, and respiratory infections are especially common in older adults. The most serious complication from an untreated Zenker diverticulum is aspiration pneumonia or lung abscess. In an older patient, this can be morbid and sometimes fatal.

Diagnosis is made by barium esophagram. At the level of the cricothyroid cartilage, the diverticulum can be seen filled with barium resting posteriorly alongside the esophagus (the "cricopharyngeal bar"). Lateral views are critical because this is usually a posterior structure. Neither esophageal manometry nor endoscopy is needed to diagnose Zenker diverticulum.

Surgical or endoscopic repair of a Zenker diverticulum is the gold standard of treatment. Traditionally, an open repair through the left side of the neck was advocated. However, endoscopic exclusion has gained popularity in many centers. Two types of open repair are performed, resection and surgical fixation of the diverticulum. The diverticulectomy and diverticulopexy are performed through an incision in the left side of the neck. In all cases, a myotomy of the proximal and distal thyropharyngeus and cricopharyngeus muscles is performed. In cases of a small diverticulum (<2 cm), a myotomy alone is often sufficient. In most patients with good tissue or a large sac (>5 cm), excision of the sac is indicated. Should a diverticulopexy be performed, it is important to suture the diverticulum to the posterior pharynx as opposed to the prevertebral fascia to allow free vertical movement of the pharynx during deglutition. The postoperative stay is approximately 2 or 3 days, during which the patient remains unable to eat or to drink.

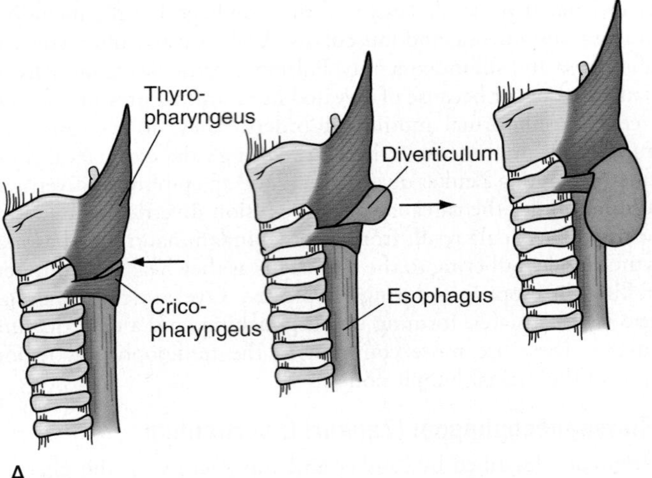

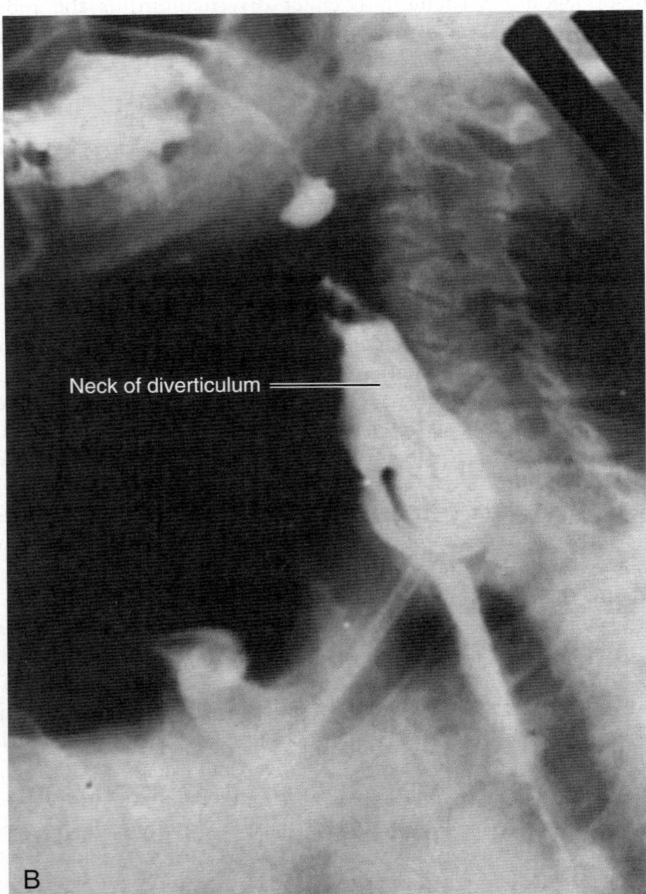

FIGURE 41-5 **A,** Zenker diverticulum. **B,** Barium swallow showing Zenker diverticulum. (Adapted from Trastek VF, Deschamps C: Esophageal diverticula. In Shields TW, Locicero J III, Ponn RB, editors: *General thoracic surgery*, ed 5, Philadelphia, 1999, Lippincott Williams & Wilkins.)

An alternative to open surgical repair is the endoscopic Dohlman procedure, which has become more popular. Endoscopic division of the common wall between the esophagus and diverticulum using a laser, electrocautery, or stapler device has been similarly successful. Because of the configuration of the inline stapling device, this approach has been advocated for larger diverticula. The risk for an incomplete myotomy increases with diverticula smaller than 3 cm. This method divides the distal cricopharyngeus muscle while obliterating the sac. The esophagus and diverticulum ultimately form a common channel. The technique requires maximal extension of the neck and can be difficult to perform in older patients with cervical stenosis. For this reason, many have advocated the use of the needle knife by flexible endoscopy to perform the myotomy. Overall, the postoperative course is slightly shorter for transoral approaches, with patients taking liquids the following day and requiring only a single overnight hospital stay. Thus, these techniques have gained favor and are advocated for patients with diverticula between 2 and 5 cm.

The results of open repair versus endoscopic repair have been well studied.[7] For diverticula 3 cm or smaller, surgical repair is superior to endoscopic repair in eliminating symptoms. For any diverticulum larger than 3 cm, the results are the same. Both the hospital stay and length of inanition are shorter with an endoscopic procedure. Regardless of the method of repair, patients do well and the results are excellent.

Midesophageal Diverticula

Midesophageal diverticula were first described in the 19th century. Historically, inflamed mediastinal lymph nodes from an infection with tuberculosis accounted for most cases. Infections with histoplasmosis and resultant fibrosing mediastinitis have now become more common. Inflammation of the lymph nodes exerts traction on the wall of the esophagus and leads to the formation of a true diverticulum in the midesophagus. This continues to be an important mechanism for these traction diverticula, but it is now believed that some may also be caused by a primary motility disorder, such as achalasia, DES, or other esophageal motility disorders.

Most patients with a midesophageal diverticulum are asymptomatic. They are often incidentally found during a workup for some other complaint (Fig. 41-6). Dysphagia, chest pain, and regurgitation can be present and are usually indicative of an underlying primary motility disorder. Patients presenting with a chronic cough are under suspicion for development of a bronchoesophageal fistula. Rarely, hemoptysis can be a presenting symptom, indicating infectious erosion of lymph nodes into major vasculature and the bronchial tree. In this case, the diverticulum is an incidental finding of lesser importance.

The diagnosis of the anatomic structure as well as of the size and location of an esophageal diverticulum is made through barium esophagram. Midesophageal diverticula typically are on the right because of the overabundance of structures in the midthoracic region of the left side of the chest. A CT scan is helpful to identify any mediastinal lymphadenopathy and may help lateralize the sac. Endoscopy is important to rule out mucosal abnormalities, including cancer that may be hidden in the sac. In addition, endoscopy may aid in identifying a fistula. Manometric studies are undertaken in all patients, symptomatic or not, to identify a primary motor disorder. Treatment is guided by the results of the manometric findings.

Determining the cause for midesophageal diverticula is critical for guiding treatment. In asymptomatic patients who have inflamed mediastinal lymph nodes, treatment of the underlying cause is the management of choice. If the diverticulum is smaller than 2 cm, it can be observed. If patients progress to become symptomatic or if the diverticulum is 2 cm or larger, surgical intervention is indicated. Usually, midesophageal diverticula have a wide mouth and rest close to the spine. Therefore, a diverticulopexy can be performed, whereby the diverticulum is suspended

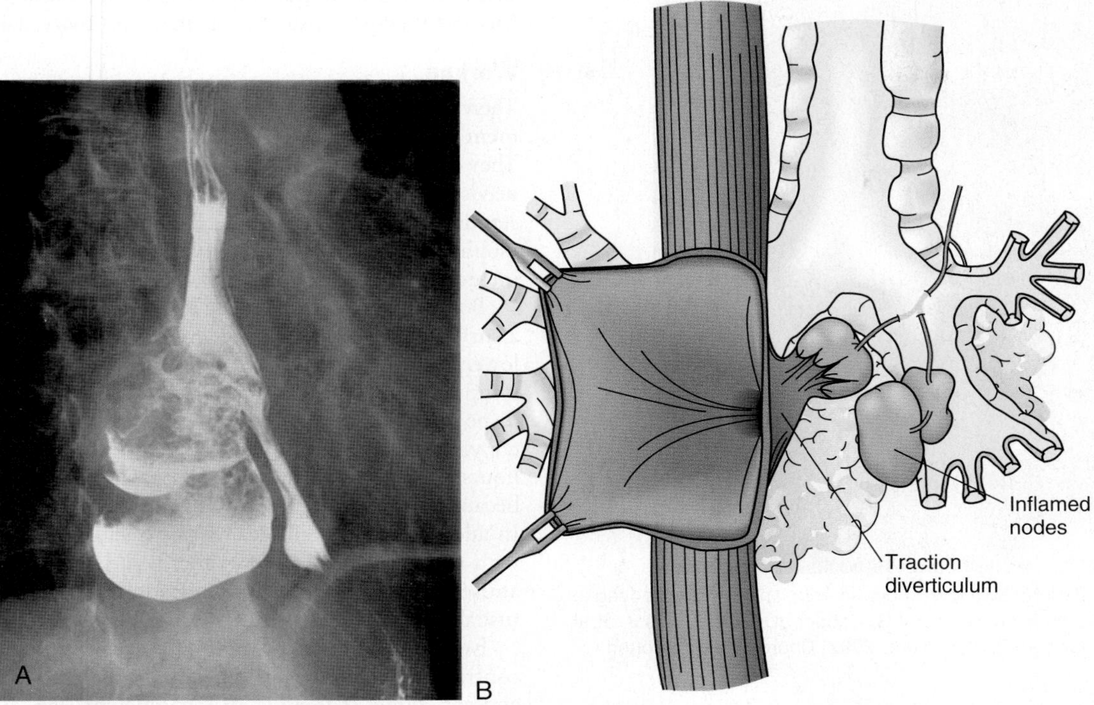

FIGURE 41-6 A, Barium esophagram demonstrating a giant midesophageal diverticulum. (Courtesy Dr. Lorenzo E. Ferri). **B,** Midesophageal diverticulum. (Adapted from Peters JH, DeMeester TR: Esophagus and diaphragmatic hernia. In Schwartz SI, Fischer JE, Spencer FC, et al, editors: *Principles of surgery*, ed 7, New York, 1998, McGraw-Hill.)

from the thoracic vertebral fascia. In patients with severe chest pain or dysphagia and a documented motor abnormality, a long esophagomyotomy is also indicated.

Epiphrenic Diverticula

Epiphrenic diverticula are found adjacent to the diaphragm in the distal third of the esophagus, within 10 cm of the GEJ. They are most often related to thickened distal esophageal musculature or increased intraluminal pressure. They are pulsion, or false, diverticula that are often associated with DES, achalasia, or IEM disorders. In patients in whom a motility abnormality cannot be identified, a congenital (Ehlers-Danlos syndrome) or traumatic cause is considered. As with midesophageal diverticula, epiphrenic diverticula are more common on the right side and tend to be wide-mouthed.

Most patients with epiphrenic diverticula present asymptomatically. They may present with dysphagia or chest pain, which is indicative of a motility disturbance. The diagnosis is often made during the workup for a motility disorder, and the diverticulum is found incidentally. Other symptoms, such as regurgitation, epigastric pain, anorexia, weight loss, chronic cough, and halitosis, are indicative of an advanced motility abnormality resulting in a sizable epiphrenic diverticulum.

A barium esophagram is the best diagnostic tool to detect an epiphrenic diverticulum (Fig. 41-7). The size, position, and proximity of the diverticulum to the diaphragm can all be clearly delineated. The underlying motility disorder is often identified as well; however, manometric studies need to be undertaken to evaluate the overall motility of the esophageal body and LES. Endoscopy is performed to evaluate for mucosal lesions, including esophagitis, Barrett esophagus, and cancer.

The treatment of an epiphrenic diverticulum is similar to that of a midesophageal diverticulum. These types of diverticula also have a wide mouth and rest close to the spine. Small (<2 cm) diverticula can also be suspended from the vertebral fascia and need not be excised. If a diverticulopexy is performed, a myotomy is begun at the neck of the diverticulum and extended onto the LES. If a diverticulectomy is pursued, a vertical stapling device is placed across the neck and the diverticulum is excised. It is essential during this process to have an esophageal bougie in place to avoid narrowing the esophageal lumen while stapling. The muscle is closed over the excision site, and a long myotomy is performed on the opposite esophageal wall, extending from the level of the diverticulum onto the LES. If a large hiatal hernia is also present, the diverticulum is excised, a myotomy performed, and the hiatal hernia repaired. Failure to repair the hernia results in a high incidence of postoperative reflux. It is essential to relieve outflow obstruction in patients with diverticula; failure to do so can result in significant complications of leak or recurrence.

GASTROESOPHAGEAL REFLUX DISEASE

GERD is the most common benign condition of the esophagus, affecting millions of people worldwide. It occurs when there is retrograde flow of gastric contents through the LES that most commonly is manifested as "heartburn." The disease is characterized by progressive worsening of heartburn symptoms until they

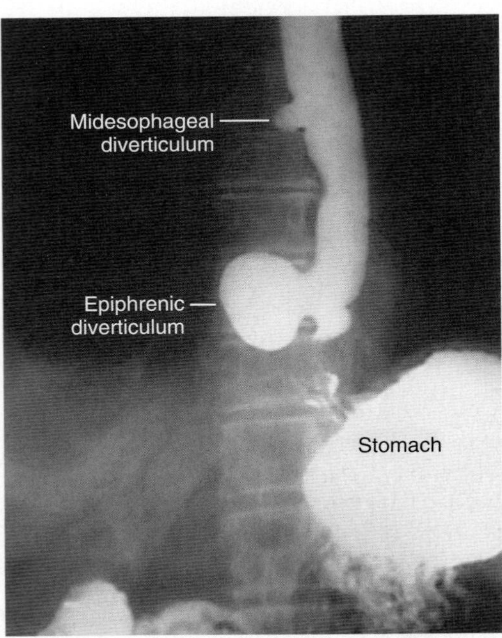

FIGURE 41-7 Barium swallow showing mid and distal esophageal diverticula. (Adapted from Pearson FG, Cooper JD, Deslauriers J, et al: *Esophageal surgery*, ed 2, New York, 2002, Churchill Livingstone.)

are frequent, persistent, and troublesome and possibly result in primary or secondary complications. Some of these complications include strictures, ulcers, metaplasia, dysplasia, carcinoma, and pulmonary disease (asthma, fibrosis).

The treatment of GERD has evolved significantly in the last several decades with the improved efficacy of antisecretory medications and refinement of surgical procedures. For many, the symptoms can be managed with medication and lifestyle modification alone. However, some people will experience symptoms that are refractory to these treatments or complications that are not medically treatable and require surgical intervention. The following sections explore the workup and surgical management of GERD in the context of failed medical management.

Medical Management

Although some patients wish to have antireflux surgery to avoid taking medication, most referrals to a surgeon are because of uncontrolled, persistent symptoms of heartburn or regurgitation despite medication. Commonly, patients will have tried proton pump inhibitors (PPIs) once daily and have progressed to twice daily. Frequently, patients will have tried several brands of PPI and have mixed multiple antacid medications. Cessation of PPIs will often result in heartburn or regurgitation that is prohibitive to normal function. However, to appropriately select patients who will have successful surgical intervention, it is critical to ensure that maximal medical therapy has been attempted and has failed with time. Patients for whom medical therapy never relieved symptoms or who demonstrate atypical symptoms should be further investigated for other causes before surgery is offered. It has been observed that the patients with the greatest likelihood of successful surgical therapy are those who have typical symptoms and good response to antisecretory therapy.[8]

Lifestyle modifications will rarely eliminate GERD symptoms, but they can decrease severity and duration and result in greater efficacy of medication. The modifications include weight loss (if overweight), smoking cessation, elimination of inciting foods, smaller and more frequent meals, and elimination of constipation. Medical therapy is usually maximal with twice-daily PPI therapy.

Workup

There are several components to the workup for surgical management of GERD that will promote successful selection of therapy. They allow tailoring of the surgical procedure to the patient's needs and avoidance of unanticipated events during surgery. The standard studies include pH test, esophageal motility test, video esophagram, and endoscopy with biopsy. Additional tests may include gastric emptying study or CT scan.

Because gastric contents are acidic, measurement of pH acts as a surrogate for reflux. Not only will it document exposure of the lower esophagus to gastric refluxate, but it will also correlate symptoms with this exposure. The test is performed by placing a disposable probe in the distal esophagus (commonly by endoscopy) and allowing a remote recorder to collect data for 24 to 48 hours. It is critical to document abnormal refluxate exposure because other disease processes can have GERD-like symptoms. In addition, several studies have correlated abnormal pH testing with successful surgical outcomes.[9] The patient should be off of antisecretory and antacid medications at the time of testing (usually cease medications 5 days to 2 weeks prior).

Esophageal motility testing allows the surgeon to evaluate if contractions are strong and effective, if there is a motility disorder, and sometimes if there is an incompetent LES. Not only is this important in distinguishing GERD from other disorders (such as achalasia or scleroderma), but it can allow tailoring of surgery for patients with coexistent GERD and motility disorder. For example, a patient with mildly impaired motility in the setting of positive pH testing might be suited to a floppy or partial fundoplication procedure rather than a full wrap. Often, patients with long-standing GERD will have esophageal dysmotility, and they must be counseled about postoperative dysphagia after fundoplication. Patients with severe dysmotility should be considered for further workup or nonsurgical therapy.

Video esophagography shows both structure and function. It will diagnose abnormalities that would modify surgical treatment, such as strictures, masses, hiatal hernia, foreshortened esophagus, or diverticula. Functionally, video esophagography confirms reflux and correlates it with symptoms and can be suggestive of motility disorders or achalasia. It is considered the "road map" before surgery, can be obtained immediately after surgery, and is useful in long-term follow-up.

Finally, endoscopy allows the surgeon to evaluate the shape and course of the esophagus, to evaluate for signs of reflux such as esophagitis and metaplasia, and to rule out masses and strictures as a cause of symptoms. A particularly dilated and tortuous esophagus can be indicative of motility disorders, and hiatal hernias not seen on esophagram can be seen on retroflexed views in the stomach. Biopsy of abnormal findings will evaluate for metaplasia, dysplasia, and carcinoma, which might alter plans for surgery and surveillance.

If there are inconsistencies between the findings on workup and the patient's symptoms, it is important to revise the diagnosis, to continue investigation, or to obtain second opinions. Surgical procedures when the diagnosis is incorrect can result in additional new symptoms without resolution of the initial complaint, leading to a dissatisfying outcome. Adjunct studies to consider include CT scan of the chest and abdomen, small bowel follow-through, gastric emptying study, and colonoscopy.

Surgical Therapy

Several operations termed "antireflux" procedures have been developed over the years as surgeons have tailored them to symptoms of patients. This section will not discuss transthoracic approaches because these are rarely indicated as primary procedures for reflux. Rather, it outlines the basic concepts of the most commonly performed transabdominal fundoplication procedure and some variations.

After it is verified that the patient's symptoms are due to reflux (see earlier) and the patient is deemed a safe surgical candidate, the surgeon has several options. Regardless of the procedure chosen, the basic tenets of antireflux surgery remain constant: (1) preserve natural tissue planes and linings, (2) identify and preserve both vagus nerves, (3) identify the true EGJ for placement of the wrap, (4) have sufficient length of intra-abdominal esophagus, and (5) reestablish the angle of His.

The Nissen fundoplication, first described in the 1950s, has become a standard in antireflux surgery (Fig. 41-8*A*). Conceptually, it is the re-creation of a sphincter around the EGJ, done by wrapping the fundus around the esophagus. Whether by laparoscopy or laparotomy, the procedure is the same. The gastrohepatic ligament is incised until the phrenoesophageal ligament is visualized, with care taken to avoid replaced hepatic arteries. The esophagus is circumferentially mobilized, with great care to preserve both vagus nerves and the peritoneal lining along the crura. Short gastric vessels are taken, and the gastrosplenic ligament is mobilized to meet the dissection along the left crus, with care taken to remain far from the splenic hilum. Any hiatal hernia will require dissection in the mediastinum to bring down sufficient esophageal length. The fat pad is then mobilized from the anterior stomach or esophagus to visualize the true EGJ and to be able to exclude both vagus nerves from the wrap.

With sufficient esophageal and gastric mobilization as well as exposure of the true EGJ, the fundic tip along the line of the short gastrics can be passed posterior to the esophagus (excluding the vagus nerves in the fat pad) to create the wrap. A "shoeshine maneuver" ensures adequate mobility and lack of tension. A 50 to 54 Fr bougie is usually in the esophagus while the stomach is then sutured to the anterior esophagus. After the bougie is removed, the diaphragmatic hiatus is assessed and is closed with suture anterior and posterior to the esophagus, ensuring not to kink or impinge too heavily on the esophagus. Usually, the passage of instruments easily through the hiatus ensures that it is not too tight. An nasogastric tube should be inserted overnight for decompression.

Some surgeons have advocated the use of mesh at the hiatus as "reinforcement" or if there is excessive tension at the crural closure. Mesh is not usually necessary if the natural linings are preserved along the crus. If there is tension on closure, this can be overcome by inducing a left-sided pneumothorax with a small amount of carbon dioxide insufflation, which will relax the left diaphragm and usually allows tension-free closure. Relaxing incisions on the diaphragm have also been described.

The wrap can be individualized to the patient's symptoms. Full 360-degree wraps are particularly important when reflux causes respiratory compromise, such as the lung transplant population. A floppy wrap, whereby there is space for the passage of an instrument between the stomach and esophagus, will result in less dysphagia but may create a less competent valve. A partial or near Nissen, with a wrap of 300 or 320 degrees, will allow some ability to belch and possibly to vomit and will lessen symptoms of dysphagia and bloat.

Variations on this classic procedure exist that allow an operation to be individualized to the patient's needs. Toupet fundoplication involves posterior partial wrap of 180 to 270 degrees, with additional tacking sutures to fix the stomach to the crura in the abdomen (Fig. 41-8*B*). Dor fundoplication is most commonly used in the setting of esophageal myotomy but consists of an anterior 180-degree wrap (Fig. 41-8*C*). A newer device named LINX can be used in patients with minimal or no hiatal hernia.[10] It is a series of magnetic beads that are placed around the EGJ that will stretch with slight pressure in the esophagus, thereby mimicking the natural LES. Long-term results of this device are not available, but short-term efficacy is promising.

A consideration for patients with bile or gastric reflux, obesity, diabetes, or esophageal dysmotility is Roux-en-Y reconstruction.[11] A near-esophagojejunostomy (with small gastric pouch) allows the passage of almost all gastric and biliary contents far downstream from the esophagus, thereby preventing symptoms related to reflux. In this population, there will be additional benefits of impact on obesity and diabetes. This is also an option in revisional surgery, in which there is a lot of scarring or the integrity of the vagus nerves is questionable.

Finally, the patient undergoing fundoplication in whom there is less than adequate intra-abdominal esophagus may require partial gastric tubularization, or Collis gastroplasty (Fig. 41-8*D-F*). This involves stapling the fundus of the stomach with a bougie in the esophagus to create a few centimeters of additional length around which the stomach can be wrapped. Both transthoracic and transabdominal approaches have been described, and although this technically difficult maneuver should be approached with caution, it is imperative to realize when it should be done.

Complicated GERD

Long-standing reflux will cause complications to the esophagus, which require management that extends beyond antireflux surgery. In the patient with esophagitis, biopsy specimens from endoscopy can reveal medically treatable problems, such as candidiasis or eosinophilic infiltrative processes. Often, these patients can have relief of symptoms without surgical intervention, and surgical intervention may not relieve their symptoms. All strictures should be biopsied to rule out malignant processes and can frequently be managed with dilation if they are benign. Metaplastic changes (Barrett esophagus) should be biopsied in four quadrants every centimeter to evaluate for dysplasia and cancer. Fundoplication procedures can still be performed in this setting, but surveillance must continue at regular intervals because regression is rare (Table 41-2).[12]

Some patients with heartburn or dysphagia will have partial or complete intrathoracic stomach. The workup and surgical therapy for these patients can be significantly different from that for standard GERD, depending on the degree of hiatal herniation. Small hernias where the GEJ is above the diaphragmatic hiatus can be manifested with classic GERD symptoms, and the workup and therapy can be the same. When there is a moderate to large hiatal hernia, consideration must be given to the degree of symptoms related to the mechanical component versus the reflux. This can be a confusing picture because patients often have symptoms from both, but if the main complaints are dysphagia, food sticking, early satiety, regurgitation, and vomiting, the mechanical component may be the dominant pathologic process. This is particularly true of nearly total intrathoracic stomach. Workup may include pulmonary function tests because of compromised lung function and thorough cardiac evaluation because of overlapping

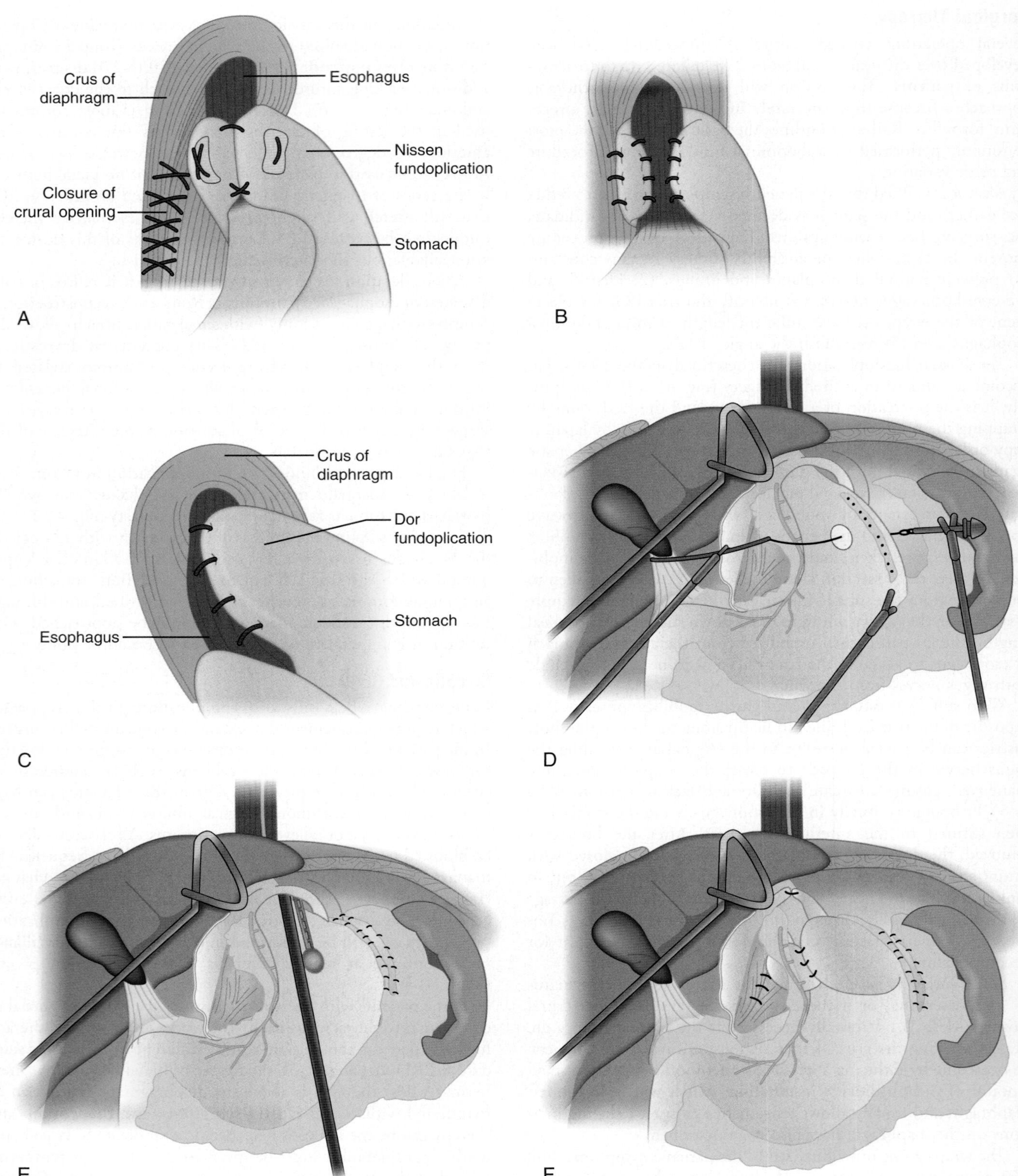

FIGURE 41-8 A, Nissen fundoplication. **B,** Toupet fundoplication. **C,** Dor fundoplication. **D-F,** Collis gastroplasty.

TABLE 41-2 American Gastroenterological Association Guidelines for Surveillance After Fundoplication for Barrett Esophagus

VARIABLE	SCORE
Age >75 years	1
Tachycardia (>100 beats/min)	1
Leukocytosis (>10,000 white blood cells/mL)	1
Pleural effusion	1
Fever (>38.5° C)	2
Noncontained leak (barium swallow or CT scan)	2
Respiratory compromise (respiratory rate >30, increasing oxygen requirement, or mechanical ventilation)	2
Time to diagnosis >24 hours	2
Presence of cancer	3
Hypotension	3

symptoms. Manometry testing is often not possible with large hernias.

During reduction of the hernia, the esophagus might be foreshortened, and the options of gastropexy versus fundoplication or Collis gastroplasty/fundoplication will have to be weighed. With dominant mechanical symptoms, patients have relief with return of the stomach to the abdominal cavity with gastropexy. However, they may subsequently suffer from reflux symptoms and require antisecretory medication thereafter. Most patients would likely benefit from a partial or floppy fundoplication procedure, keeping in mind that esophageal motility will likely be unknown.

ACQUIRED BENIGN DISORDERS OF THE ESOPHAGUS

Acquired Esophageal Disease

Perforation

Esophageal perforation is a potentially lethal condition that can have poor outcomes if there is a delay in diagnosis or improper treatment. Most series have reported overall mortality between 20% and 30%, frequently with strong correlations to etiology and interval from event to intervention.[13] The most commonly recognized cause is iatrogenic perforation during endoscopy, with others being forceful retching (Boerhaave syndrome), traumatic injury, foreign body ingestion, and tumor perforation. It is generally regarded that better outcomes are possible if the intervention is within 24 hours of the event, and poor outcomes are associated with cancer-related perforations. The key to management and patient survival is early recognition with timely diagnosis and therapy.

Suspicion of esophageal perforation begins with symptoms of epigastric or chest pain, neck or throat pain, and dysphagia. Physical examination findings might include crepitus on the chest, neck, or face; neck swelling; epigastric tenderness; nasal voice; or sometimes normal examination findings. Other early evidence might include a chest radiograph with mediastinal or cervical air, free abdominal air, or pleural effusion. A CT scan may show mediastinal air and periesophageal air or fluid. Of course, the mechanism of injury can be the greatest clue that would initiate further workup.

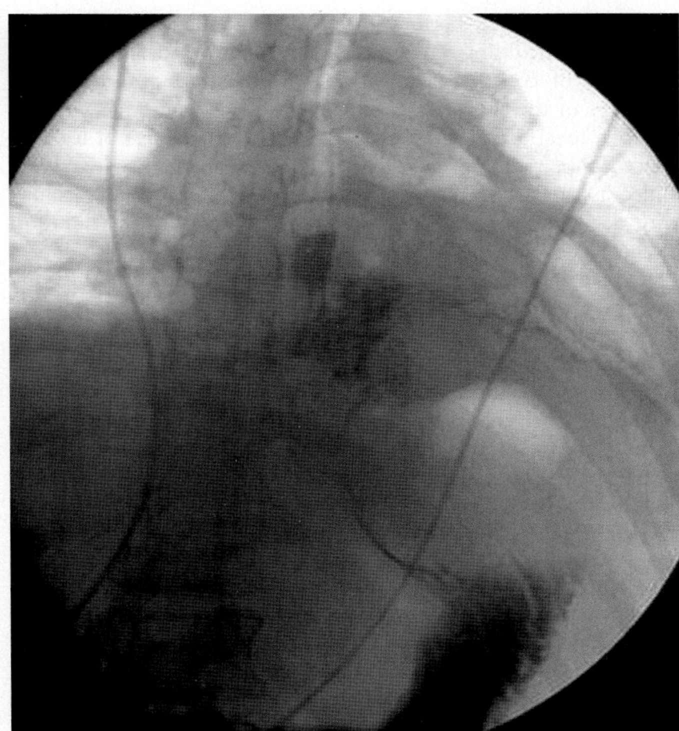

FIGURE 41-9 Barium esophagram demonstrating an esophageal perforation.

TABLE 41-3 Pittsburgh Esophageal Perforation Score

SCORE	<3	3-5	>5
Morbidity (%)	53	65	81
Mortality (%)	2	6	27
Duration of stay (days)	10	16	28

Once there is suspicion, the diagnostic workup must proceed on the basis of the index of suspicion. Barium esophagram is the standard for diagnosis (Fig. 41-9), but CT scan with oral administration of contrast material is sometimes acceptable if the diagnosis is clear. If the results of these studies are normal but the level of suspicion is high, patients may require evaluation by direct laryngoscopy or endoscopy, depending on the clinical circumstance. Of note, procedural evaluation can convert a small or partial perforation into a more clinically significant process, so caution must be used with these procedures. Once the diagnosis is made, there are several therapeutic options that must be considered on an individual basis by a team of experienced surgeons as the subtleties of management preclude algorithmic treatment. Determining severity of injury to prognosticate morbidity and mortality can be done with a clinical severity score proposed by the Pittsburgh group (Table 41-3).[14] This score has been correlated with lower morbidity, lower mortality, and shorter hospital stay and can be used to guide treatment.

The principles of management after diagnosis include (1) treatment of contamination, (2) wide local drainage, (3) source control, and (4) enteral feeding access. In the circumstance of small perforations with contained leaks and no fluid collections in the mediastinum or chest, contamination might be minimal.

In general, though, perforation is treated with broad-spectrum antibiotics, including antifungals, with duration that will vary on the basis of control of infection and the patient's condition. Drainage of the area with chest tubes is most common, with the number, location, and duration to vary by the degree of leak. In select cases, radiologically guided drains can be used as well. Video-assisted thoracoscopic surgery or open thoracic washout with decortication may be necessary, depending on the duration of the leak and amount of pleural space soiling.

Source control will also depend on the patient's condition, the severity and location of perforation, and the surgeon's experience. Endoluminal therapy with covered stents has become more widely popularized and can give good results when it is used in the appropriate patient population. Although the criteria are still debated, stents can be considered in patients with early, small perforations, with minimal contamination in a location amenable to stenting.[15] Surgical control would be considered the gold standard, with approach depending on the location of the leak.[16] In general, high perforations are approached through a left-sided neck incision, midesophageal through a right thoracotomy, and distal esophageal through a left thoracotomy or laparotomy. Radiographic studies that demonstrate a right- or left-sided leak may modify the approach. Minimally invasive approaches are reasonable, depending on the surgeon's preference.

After the area of perforation is identified, assessment continues with myotomy to expose the injury, débridement of devitalized tissues, assessment of extent of injury, and considerations for repair. Any sign of obstruction (achalasia, stricture, tumor) must be remedied at the time of the initial operation, else the perforation will not heal. Small injuries with healthy tissues can be repaired primarily in two layers with tissue flap coverage (intercostal muscle, pericardial fat, pleura, omentum), but extensive injuries with devitalized areas can be managed with controlled fistulization by T-tube. Very large or devitalized defects will require esophageal exclusion with creation of a cervical esophagostomy and gastrostomy tube, with plans for future reconstruction by esophagectomy with gastric, colon, or small bowel conduit. Gastrostomy and jejunostomy tubes at the first operation can provide decompression and drainage near the perforation as well as enteral access for nutrition.

Caustic Ingestion

The majority of caustic ingestion is accidental small-volume drinking of household products by young children. In adults, it is more commonly a suicide attempt with large volumes, and therefore more extensive injury is usually present. The injury pattern can vary from short-segment superficial injury to full-thickness necrosis of the proximal gastrointestinal tract. There are many factors that affect the extent of injury (pH, volume, duration of exposure), and the evaluation and management after the ingestion are challenging and require experience and sound judgment.

The initial evaluation should involve a surgeon immediately. Physical examination findings of upper airway compromise (dyspnea, drooling, stridor, hoarseness) will likely require endotracheal intubation. However, this should be done with bronchoscopic guidance and preparation to perform cricothyroidotomy as there is danger of inability to secure a safe airway or iatrogenic perforation. Nasogastric and orogastric tubes should not be inserted blindly. Subsequent evaluation should include radiographic studies to guide the first procedure, ideally a CT scan of chest and abdomen with intravenous and oral administration of contrast material, followed by a barium swallow study.

TABLE 41-4 Classification Scheme for Caustic Ingestion

ENDOSCOPIC FINDING	GRADE
Normal	0
Superficial edema/erythema	1
Mucosal/submucosal ulceration	2
Superficial edema/erythema	2A
Deep or circumferential	2B
Transmural ulcerations with necrosis	3
Focal necrosis	3A
Extensive necrosis	3B
Perforation	4

Evaluation continues in the operating room. With rare exception, most patients should have an endoscopic evaluation of the degree and extent of injury. It is recommended that this be done early in the hospital course as the risk of perforation increases after 48 hours. Pediatric endoscopes are useful to minimize insufflation and mechanical stresses. The traditional teaching is that endoscopy should not proceed past an area of circumferential injury; however, an experienced endoscopist can cautiously proceed to complete the evaluation if it is thought that management will change with additional information. It is important to note location and degree of injury at all locations because subsequent evaluations are frequently necessary (Table 41-4).

All patients should be treated with broad-spectrum antibiotics. Depending on the clinical course, patients may benefit from repeated endoscopy 48 to 72 hours after the event to assess for signs of worsening injury. Of paramount importance is frequent clinical reassessment as deterioration at any time should prompt resumption of workup and surgical intervention as indicated. Surgical intervention can vary from endoscopy only to placement of gastrostomy or jejunostomy tubes or esophagectomy, gastrectomy, and small bowel resection with proximal diversion and feeding tube. Reconstruction can be complicated, sometimes requiring several months of recovery and the use of colon or small bowel conduits. In the long term, patients may develop strictures that require repeated dilation or eventual resection, fistulas that require surgical interventions, or esophageal cancer (>1000 times increased risk). The use of routine corticosteroids is no longer advocated. Early dilation, esophageal stents, and other adjunctive measures must be considered on a case-by-case basis.

Foreign Body Ingestion, Benign Tracheoesophageal Fistula, and Schatzki Ring

The patient with foreign body ingestion can require technical expertise to prevent iatrogenic perforation. If the object is lodged in the esophagus, careful endoscopy under general anesthesia is preferred. Forceful pushing to move the object into the stomach can result in perforation. Full relaxation, lubrication with water, and gentle pressure can sometimes be enough. Bringing the object proximally requires special large endoscopic graspers, nets, or lassoes along with patience and full visualization as the object is removed to prevent injury in the esophagus and oropharynx. Over-tubes are frequently useful in this setting, as is rigid esophagoscopy. If the object is not retrievable, laparoscopy or laparotomy with gastrotomy may be necessary. Evaluation of the full gastrointestinal tract is recommended with radiographs and CT scan before an intervention. Inpatient psychiatric evaluation and occasionally involuntary commitment are needed for the patient's safety.

Benign tracheoesophageal fistula can be seen in patients with multiple procedures or foreign objects in the upper mediastinum. A classic example of benign tracheoesophageal fistula is in the patient with endotracheal tube (or tracheostomy) and nasogastric tube. It is manifested most commonly with recurrent or persistent respiratory infection and bilious or salivary contents emanating from the tracheostomy. CT scan and barium swallow can be helpful in determining the diagnosis. Further evaluation is done with bronchoscopy and endoscopy, ensuring that bronchoscopy is performed such that the entire airway is evaluated; the tracheostomy may have to be temporarily removed during the endoscopy. If tracheoesophageal fistula is identified, treatment principles are (1) discontinuation of the causative agent, (2) consideration of exclusion of the fistula by stent or diversion, and finally (3) repair or delayed healing. In a stable patient, definitive repair may preclude the need for temporary exclusion or diversion. If the fistula was caused by a tracheostomy balloon, a longer or cuffless tracheostomy will be required. Antibiotics are usually employed as well. Enteral access and gastric decompression can be achieved with gastrostomy and jejunostomy tubes. Repair can be undertaken when the patient is medically suitable by either thoracotomy or cervical approach with resection of the fistula, possible primary repair or resection, and vascularized tissue interposition. Attempts at definitive repair in a compromised patient are not optimal. Delayed healing can occur if the offending agents are removed and diversion is successful. Esophageal stents can occasionally be used in this setting as well, although this must be determined on a case-by-case basis.

A Schatzki ring is a concentric, nonmalignant, fibrous thickening and narrowing of the GEJ with squamous epithelium above and columnar cells below (Fig. 41-10). The cause is unknown, with correlations to reflux disease and hiatal hernia that are still debated. Presence of a ring is not pathologic, but these can be seen in patients suffering from dysphagia or obstruction. In the symptomatic patient, whether the diagnosis is by esophagram or endoscopy, treatment is usually with dilation (bougie or balloon). The area should always be biopsied to rule out malignancy. Repeated dilation is often necessary and is a reasonable way to manage symptomatic rings as there are few permanent surgical options. Persistent strictures should always raise suspicion for malignant disease.

ESOPHAGEAL NEOPLASMS AND DIAGNOSTIC APPROACHES TO ESOPHAGEAL CANCER

Epidemiology

Approximately 17,000 cases of esophageal cancer occur annually in the United States and about 480,000 cases occur worldwide.[17] Unfortunately, esophageal cancer typically is manifested at an advanced stage, and the majority of patients ultimately die of their disease. Worldwide, squamous cell carcinoma (SCC) is the most common histology, but in the United States, adenocarcinoma is more frequent. During the last 20 years, the incidence of adenocarcinoma has risen dramatically in Western countries with a concomitant decline in the incidence of SCC (Fig. 41-11).[18] This appears to be a true increase in incidence of adenocarcinoma rather than overdiagnosis as the overall stage distribution has not significantly shifted during this time. Other types of esophageal tumors, including mesenchymal tumors, neuroendocrine cancers, and benign tumors, are much more rare.

Tobacco and alcohol are strong risk factors for SCC, and they have a synergistic effect on risk. The disease is four times more prevalent in men, and race also appears to be a factor. The incidence of SCC is much higher among African Americans compared with their white counterparts, even after adjusting for socioeconomic status and tobacco and alcohol use. Worldwide, parts of the Middle East, central Asia, and China have the highest rates of SCC, after adjusting for tobacco and alcohol use,

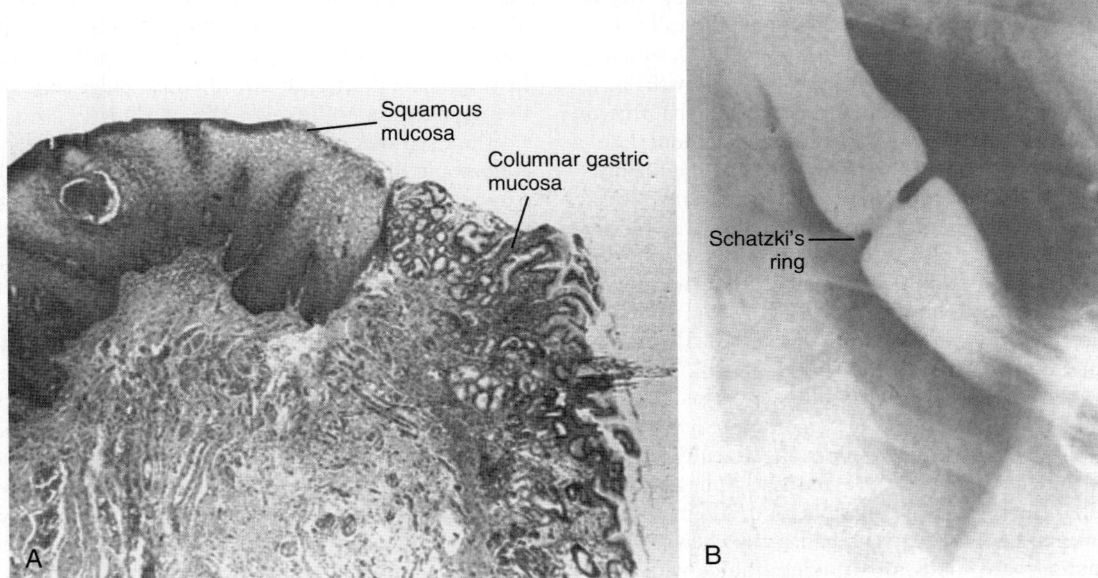

FIGURE 41-10 **A,** Histology of a Schatzki ring. **B,** Barium esophagram of a Schatzki ring. (**A** and **B,** Adapted from Wilkins EW Jr: Rings and webs. In Pearson FG, Cooper JD, Deslauriers J, et al, editors: *Esophageal surgery*, ed 2, New York, 2002, Churchill Livingstone.)

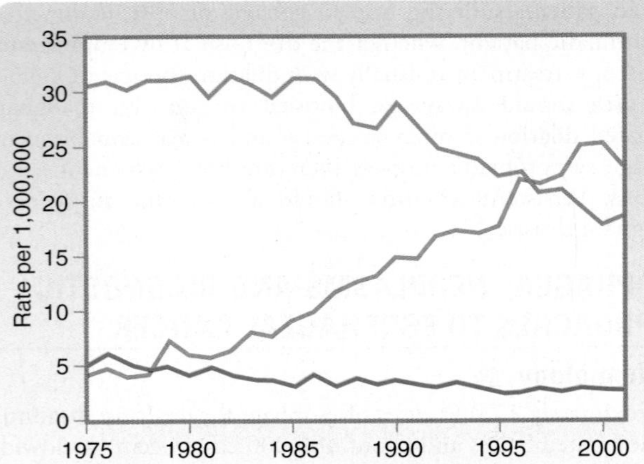

FIGURE 41-11 Trends in incidence of esophageal cancer histologic types (1975-2001). *Red line,* adenocarcinoma; *blue line,* squamous cell carcinoma; *green line,* not otherwise specified. (From Pohl H, Welch HG: The role of overdiagnosis and reclassification in the marked increase of esophageal adenocarcinoma incidence. *J Natl Cancer Inst* 97:142–146, 2005).

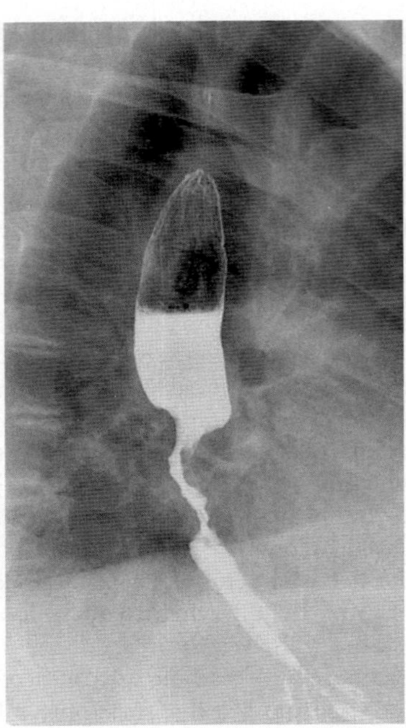

FIGURE 41-12 Barium esophagram demonstrating advanced carcinoma with abrupt, irregular narrowing in the distal esophagus, with more proximal dilation and air-fluid level.

indicating that there may be some genetic predisposition or other environmental factors. The recognition of the importance of human papillomavirus (HPV) in the pathogenesis of SCC in other organs has spurred an interest in its role in esophageal SCC. Currently, it appears that HPV-related SCC represents only a small subset of esophageal SCC. For those tumors that are HPV related, the clinical implications of HPV association are unclear. SCC is associated with certain intrinsic disorders of the esophagus, such as Plummer-Vinson syndrome and achalasia. Other hereditary cancer syndromes associated with esophageal SCC include tylosis and Fanconi anemia. Patients with a history of caustic ingestion are at significantly increased risk for SCC.

During the last 30 years, the incidence of esophageal adenocarcinoma has risen faster than any other cancer in the United States. It is now the most common histologic type of esophageal cancer in the United States. It is still relatively rare among African Americans and Asian Americans. Adenocarcinoma typically arises in the setting of Barrett esophagus. In addition to GERD, smoking and obesity are risk factors for adenocarcinoma. As with SCC, there is a male predominance. There are also familial forms of Barrett esophagus that increase the risk of adenocarcinoma.

SCC may arise in any part of the esophagus, but the majority of cases arise in the proximal and middle esophagus. In contrast, the majority of adenocarcinomas arise in the distal esophagus or GEJ. Under current American Joint Committee on Cancer (AJCC) and National Comprehensive Cancer Network staging guidelines, GEJ adenocarcinomas are staged and classified as esophageal cancers, with the exception of Siewert III tumors (tumors with an epicenter 2 to 5 cm below the GEJ).[19,20]

The majority of esophageal cancers are symptomatic at the time of diagnosis. Dysphagia is the most common symptom at presentation, with 74% of patients reporting difficulty in swallowing.[21] Often, patients will report progressive dysphagia, beginning with an initial episode after eating solid food. After the initial episode of dysphagia, many patients will adapt by chewing more thoroughly, avoiding hard foods, or drinking liquids with swallows. Thus, it is only after the dysphagia has worsened significantly that patients seek medical attention, by which point the majority have weight loss. Many patients with adenocarcinoma will endorse a long history of reflux symptoms including heartburn and regurgitation. Other associated findings may include fatigue, retrosternal pain, and anemia. Locally advanced tumors may be manifested with laryngeal nerve involvement causing hoarseness or with tracheoesophageal fistula. A careful physical examination should be performed with particular attention to cervical and supraclavicular lymph nodes. Early-stage tumors are often asymptomatic and are sometimes discovered during endoscopy done for Barrett esophagus.

Diagnosis and Staging

Barium esophagram may demonstrate irregular narrowing or ulceration (Fig. 41-12). The classic "apple-core" filling defect is seen only if there is symmetrical, circumferential narrowing. Instead, there is often an asymmetrical bulge seen with an infiltrative appearance.

The diagnosis of esophageal cancer is almost always made by endoscopic biopsy. Endoscopy should be performed in any patient with dysphagia, even if the barium esophagram is suggestive of a motility disorder. Classically, esophageal cancers appear as friable, ulcerated masses, but the endoscopic appearance can be varied. Early-stage tumors may appear as ulcerations or small nodules. More advanced tumors are more likely to be friable masses but may also appear as strictures or ulcerations. In many cases, the initial endoscopist may not recognize the presence of cancer and a single biopsy may not be diagnostic. Therefore, multiple biopsies should be performed for any suspicious lesions. During endoscopy, the location of the tumor relative to the incisors and GEJ should be noted, as well as the length of the tumor and degree of obstruction. The most proximal extent and circumferential extent of any Barrett esophagus should also be noted according to the Prague criteria. For small tumors or nodules, an experienced endoscopist should perform endoscopic mucosal resection (EMR) to provide a specimen that accurately assesses depth of invasion.

Once a diagnosis of esophageal cancer is made, accurate staging is essential to guide appropriate therapy and to predict prognosis. The most recent, seventh edition AJCC staging system acknowledged differences in the biology of adenocarcinoma and SCC by creating separate stage groupings for the two histologic types (Tables 41-5 to 41-7). The seventh edition staging classifies GEJ tumors as esophageal cancers as long as the tumor epicenter is within 5 cm of the GEJ. Tumor location also affects stage for SCC but not for adenocarcinoma (Fig. 41-13). The cervical esophagus begins at the hypopharynx and extends to the thoracic inlet, which is the level of the sternal notch. On endoscopy, this corresponds to approximately 15 to 20 cm from the incisors. The upper thoracic esophagus begins at the thoracic inlet and extends to the azygos vein. This is approximately 20 to 25 cm from the incisors. Midthoracic tumors arise from the lower border of the azygos vein to the inferior pulmonary vein. This is approximately 25 to 30 cm from the incisors. Lower tumors arise distal to the lower border of the inferior pulmonary vein to the GEJ. This is usually more than 30 cm from the incisors. Tumor grade is included in stage classification for earlier stage tumors.

Another major change in the staging system was the shift in nodal staging. The previous staging system classified celiac nodes as metastatic (M1a) for tumors of the lower esophagus, whereas cervical nodes were considered M1a for tumors of the upper thoracic esophagus. In the current system, all these nodes are considered regional regardless of the location of the primary tumor. Furthermore, nodal stage is based on the total number of involved nodes.

TABLE 41-5 Esophageal Carcinoma Stage Classifications

Primary Tumor (T)	
TX	Tumor cannot be assessed
T0	No evidence of tumor
Tis	High-grade dysplasia
T1	Tumor invades the muscularis mucosa (T1a) or submucosa (T1b)
T2	Tumor invades into but not beyond the muscularis propria
T3	Tumor invades the adventitia
T4a	Tumor invades adjacent structures that are usually resectable (diaphragm and pericardium)
T4b	Tumor invades unresectable structures
Regional Lymph Nodes (N)	
NX	Regional lymph nodes cannot be assessed
N0	No regional lymph node metastasis
N1	Metastasis in 1-2 regional lymph nodes
N2	Metastasis in 3-6 regional lymph nodes
N3	Metastasis in ≥7 regional lymph nodes
Distant Metastasis (M)	
M0	No distant metastasis
M1	Distant metastasis
Histologic Grade	
GX	Grade cannot be assessed—stage grouping as G1
G1	Well differentiated
G2	Moderately differentiated
G3	Poorly differentiated
G4	Undifferentiated—stage grouping as G3 squamous

The depth of invasion of the tumor defines the T stage (Fig. 41-14). High-grade dysplasia encompasses all noninvasive neoplastic epithelium that was formerly classified as carcinoma in situ. T1a tumors invade the muscularis mucosa, whereas T1b tumors invade into the submucosa. T2 tumors invade the muscularis propria, and T3 tumors invade the adventitia but not surrounding structures. T4a tumors invade adjacent structures that are usually resectable (diaphragm and pericardium). T4b tumors invade adjacent structures that are typically unresectable (trachea and aorta).

TABLE 41-6 Stage Groupings for Esophageal Adenocarcinoma

STAGE	T	N	M	G
0	HGD	0	0	1
IA	1	0	0	1-2
IB	1	0	0	3
	2	0	0	1-2
IIA	2	0	0	3
IIB	3	0	0	Any
	1-2	1	0	Any
IIIA	1-2	2	0	Any
	3	1	0	Any
	4a	0	0	Any
IIIB	3	2	0	Any
IIIC	4a	1-2	0	Any
	4b	Any	0	Any
	Any	3	0	Any
IV	Any	Any	1	Any

From Edge S, Byrd DR, Compton CR, et al, editors: *AJCC cancer staging manual,* ed 7, New York, 2010, Springer-Verlag.
T, tumor status; *N,* lymph node status; *M,* metastasis; *G,* grade; *HGD,* high-grade dysplasia.

TABLE 41-7 Stage Groupings for Esophageal Squamous Cell Carcinoma

STAGE	T	N	M	G	LOCATION
0	HGD	0	0	1	Any
IA	1	0	0	1	Any
IB	1	0	0	2-3	Any
	2-3	0	0	1	Lower
IIA	2-3	0	0	1	Upper, middle
	2-3	0	0	2-3	Lower
IIB	2-3	0	0		Upper, middle
	1-2	1	0	Any	Any
IIIA	1-2	2	0	Any	Any
	3	1	0	Any	Any
	4a	0	0	Any	Any
IIIB	3	2	0	Any	Any
IIIC	4a	1-2	0	Any	Any
	4b	Any	0	Any	Any
	Any	3	0	Any	Any
IV	Any	Any	1	Any	Any

From Edge S, Byrd DR, Compton CR, et al, editors: *AJCC cancer staging manual,* ed 7, New York, 2010, Springer-Verlag.
T, tumor status; *N,* lymph node status; *M,* metastasis; *G,* grade; *HGD,* high-grade dysplasia.

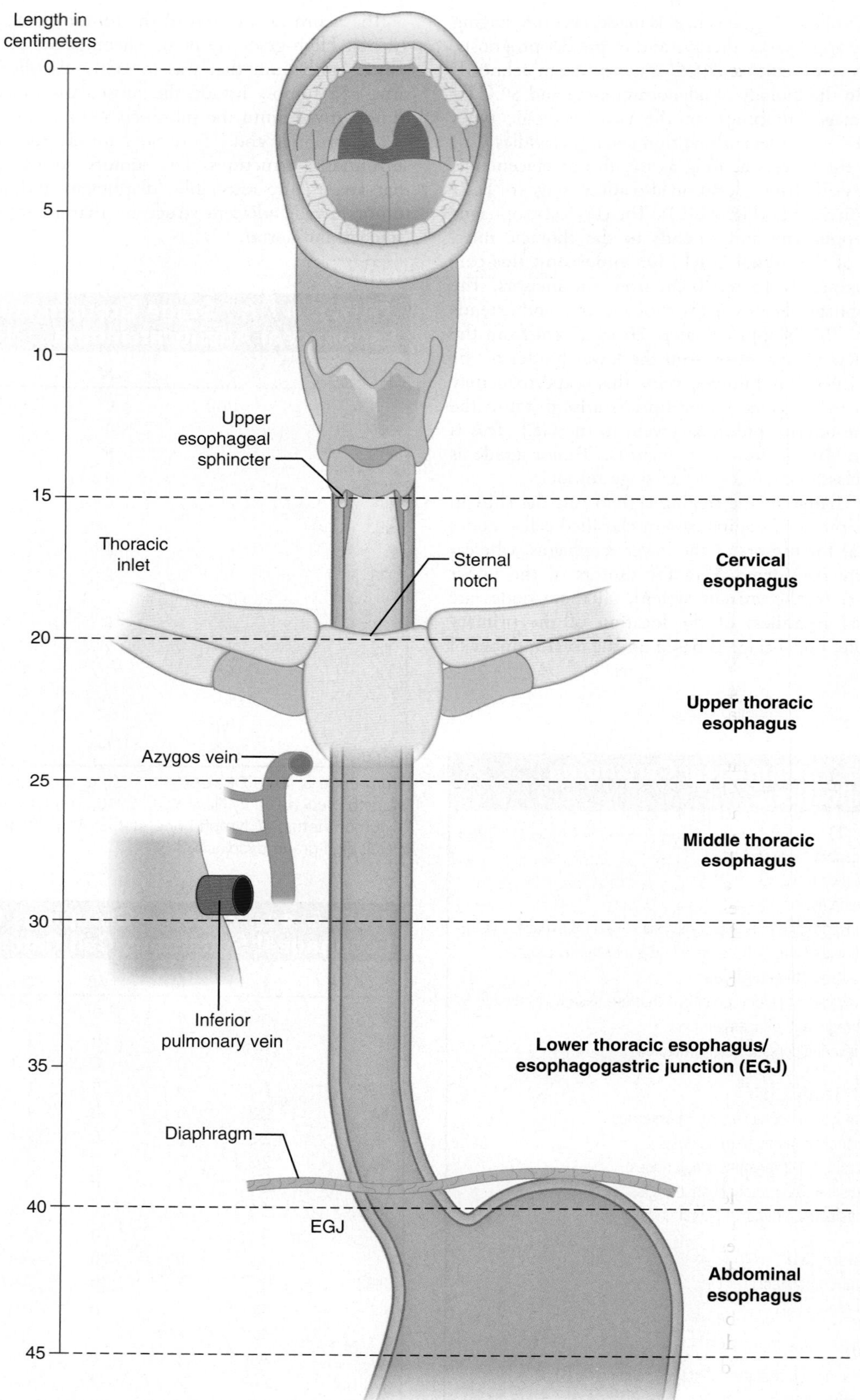

FIGURE 41-13 Regions of the esophagus. The cervical esophagus extends from the upper esophageal sphincter to the thoracic inlet. The upper thoracic esophagus extends from the thoracic inlet to the azygos vein. The midthoracic esophagus extends from the lower border of the azygos vein to the inferior pulmonary vein. The lower thoracic esophagus extends from the lower border of the inferior pulmonary vein to the gastroesophageal junction.

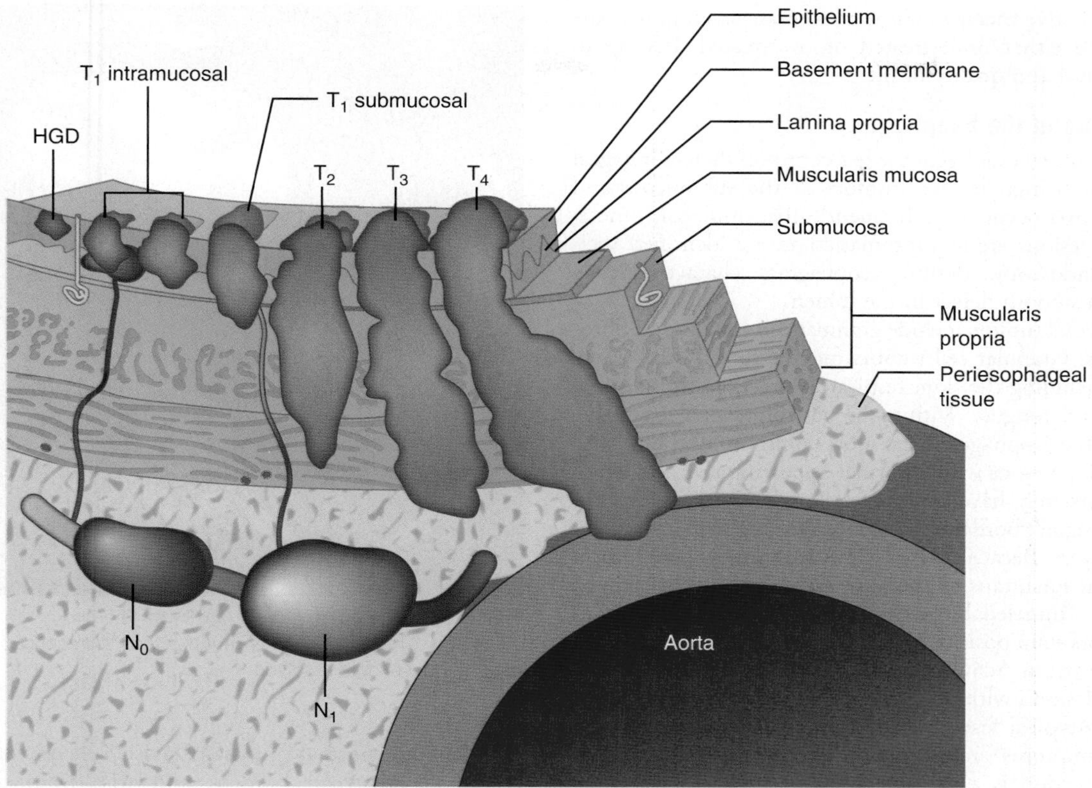

FIGURE 41-14 Tumor classification for esophageal carcinoma as defined by depth of invasion. *HGD*, high-grade dysplasia.

Small, superficial lesions that are evaluated by an experienced endoscopist may be resected by EMR without additional staging. In this setting, EMR provides adequate staging for depth of penetration (T stage) and may provide additional information about the risk of nodal metastasis. Endoscopic ultrasound (EUS) has less accuracy for superficial disease and will seldom obviate the need for EMR.[22,23] For T1a tumors resected by EMR, the risk of lymph node metastasis is very low, and additional staging studies are not required.

Most tumors, however, will be manifested as larger lesions. For these, we recommend further staging with a contrast-enhanced CT scan of the chest and abdomen and positron emission tomography (PET)/CT to evaluate for distant metastatic disease. If there is no evidence of distant metastatic disease, EUS should be performed to assess T stage and regional lymph nodes. Obtaining the PET/CT scan before EUS has several advantages. The PET/CT scan may demonstrate distant metastatic disease, eliminating the need for the patient to undergo EUS. The PET/CT scan may also identify a suspicious lymph node that can be specifically examined and sampled during the EUS procedure (Fig. 41-15). EUS is superior to CT or PET for assessment of both T and N stage. It is highly accurate for celiac nodal status with a sensitivity of 85% and specificity of 96%.[24] The accuracy rate is slightly lower for other regional lymph nodes because it is often impossible to biopsy peritumoral lymph nodes without traversing the tumor. Obstructing lesions may preclude EUS assessment. In these cases, dilation to perform EUS is associated with a risk of perforation. These risks must be weighed against the benefits of obtaining additional staging information. Most tumors with such tight stenoses are locally advanced and should likely be treated with multimodality therapy. Although EUS provides information about invasion of adjacent structures, bronchoscopy should also be performed for tumors above the carina to assess for direct tracheal invasion.

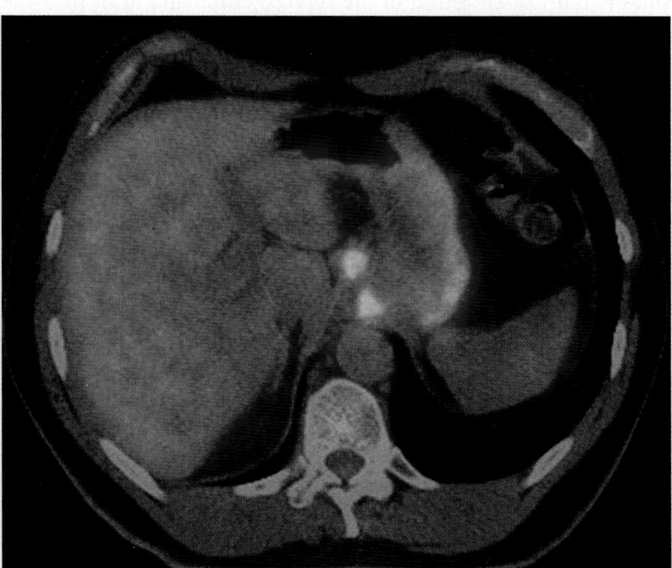

FIGURE 41-15 Fused transaxial PET/CT image demonstrating increased FDG activity in a gastroesophageal junction tumor and celiac lymphadenopathy.

Appropriate staging is critical for treatment decisions. Superficial, T1a tumors can usually be treated with EMR. Locally advanced tumors (T3 tumors or T2 tumors with nodal involvement) require multimodality therapy. Stage IV disease requires systemic or palliative therapy. Without accurate staging, patients are likely to be either undertreated or overtreated, leading to decreased survival and quality of life.

Benign Tumors of the Esophagus

Benign tumors of the esophagus are less common than esophageal cancer. Among benign lesions, tumors of the submucosa and muscularis propria occur more frequently than mucosal tumors. Most of these lesions are asymptomatic and are identified incidentally on endoscopy. Barium esophagram characteristically demonstrates a smooth defect in the lumen.

Benign mucosal tumors include granular cell tumors and fibrovascular polyps. Granular cell tumors may be found in a variety of locations, including the skin, respiratory tract, gastrointestinal tract, breast, and tongue. Within the gastrointestinal tract, the distal third of the esophagus is the most common location. They appear as bulging lesions with a normal-appearing mucosa. Up to 11% of patients may have multiple lesions.[25] On EUS, lesions typically have regular borders and arise within the first and second sonographic layers. Because these lesions are usually covered by a layer of normal squamous epithelium, standard biopsies may be nondiagnostic. Tunneled biopsies will reveal eosinophilic granules. The tumors stain positive for S100, and it has been proposed that they arise from Schwann cells. Granular cell tumors are largely benign lesions, with only 1% to 2% having been described as malignant. Atypical features on EUS, large size (>2 cm), and presence of symptoms are reasonable indications for excision. Endoscopic resection is a valuable tool for these lesions when diagnosis is in question and for lesions smaller than 3 cm.[26]

Fibrovascular polyps are a heterogeneous group of soft tissue tumors most often found in the cervical esophagus at or near the cricopharyngeus. They appear cylindrical or elongated, with a stalk. Symptoms are rare, but large tumors may cause dysphagia and some may even prolapse into the hypopharynx, causing airway obstruction. Even large tumors can usually be resected endoscopically after securing the airway.

Squamous papillomas most often occur in the distal esophagus and are usually associated with some underlying inflammation. They appear as colorless, exophytic projections. Complete excision is warranted to rule out carcinoma and can usually be performed endoscopically.[27]

Benign submucosal tumors include lipomas, hemangiomas, and neural tumors. Lipomas have a characteristic, homogeneous, hyperechoic, smooth appearance on EUS. Symptoms are rare even with large tumors. Resection is seldom warranted. Hemangiomas typically appear as a purple or reddish nodule. EUS will demonstrate a smooth, hypoechoic, submucosal mass. Most tumors are asymptomatic. Lesions causing either dysphagia or bleeding can usually be treated endoscopically. Neural tumors including neurofibromas and schwannomas are rare in the esophagus. The majority are benign, with a handful of case reports on malignant esophageal schwannoma.[28] Symptomatic tumors can usually be resected by enucleation. Large tumors may require esophagectomy.

Leiomyomas are the most common benign tumors of the esophagus. They have a 2:1 male predominance. Although they are usually asymptomatic, large tumors may cause dysphagia or discomfort (Fig. 41-16). The tumors arise in the muscularis propria and are usually found in the mid to distal esophagus. Like most other benign esophageal tumors, they will demonstrate a smooth filling defect on barium esophagram. The endoscopic appearance is a round protrusion into the lumen of the esophagus with smooth, normal mucosa. On EUS, leiomyomas are hypoechoic, have regular borders, and arise from the muscularis mucosa, submucosa, or muscularis propria. Small, asymptomatic lesions with this appearance may be safely observed without biopsy. Symptomatic lesions may be enucleated, and even large lesions can usually be removed with a minimally invasive approach.[29] One must keep in mind the differential diagnosis of a larger submucosal smooth tumor, including leiomyosarcoma, gastrointestinal stromal tumor (GIST), and leiomyoma.

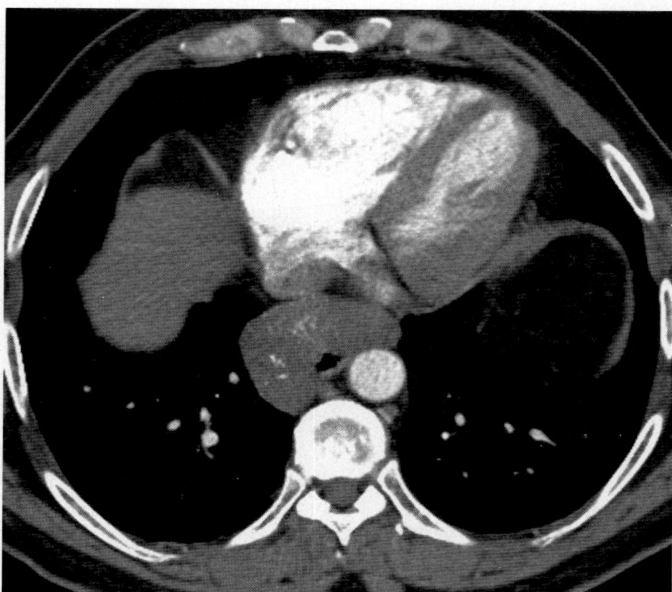

FIGURE 41-16 CT image of an 8-cm leiomyoma that was causing dysphagia. The lesion was enucleated thoracoscopically, and the patient's dysphagia resolved.

Other Malignant Tumors of the Esophagus

Although SCC and adenocarcinoma represent the overwhelming majority of esophageal cancers, a variety of other malignant histologic types may be encountered. Small cell carcinomas of the esophagus account for 0.6% of esophageal cancers.[30] These tumors have the same aggressive phenotype and histologic appearance of other poorly differentiated neuroendocrine cancers. The tumors typically are manifested at an advanced stage, but stage-specific survival may be comparable to that of non–small cell esophageal carcinomas. Long-term survival is possible in earlier stage tumors treated with surgery. Neoadjuvant therapy appears to improve survival as well.

Primary melanoma of the esophagus is even rarer than small cell carcinoma, accounting for 0.1% to 0.2% of esophageal malignant neoplasms.[31] Similar to small cell carcinoma, most tumors are manifested at a late stage, and prognosis is generally poor.

GISTs and sarcomas of the esophagus are far less common than benign leiomyomas. GISTs have similar appearance to leiomyomas but can be distinguished histologically by CD117 stain positivity. Although well-differentiated leiomyosarcomas may be difficult to distinguish from leiomyomas, higher grade sarcomas often erode through the mucosa and will appear as an ulcerated or exophytic mass on endoscopy. EUS may show more irregular borders or a heterogeneous appearance that is uncharacteristic for leiomyoma. Local resection of small GISTs may be reasonable if negative margins can be achieved, but because of the propensity of the tumors to recur locally, formal esophagectomy should be performed for larger tumors.[32] Imatinib should be considered for any GIST larger than 3 cm or with other high-risk features. Imatinib may also be considered in the neoadjuvant setting for locally advanced tumors. In general, esophagectomy is the treatment of choice for leiomyosarcomas. Other sarcomas of the esophagus have been reported but are much more rare. Lymph node metastasis is an unusual event in these mesenchymal tumors.

Approach to Early-Stage Esophageal Cancer

In the last 10 years, there has been a significant shift in the way early-stage esophageal cancers are treated.[33] Improved endoscopic technology as well as a better understanding of the biology of early-stage tumors has led to the increased use of endoscopic therapies for the diagnosis, staging, and treatment of early-stage esophageal cancers. It is likely that surgery will play a smaller role for superficial cancers as endoscopic and ablative therapies continue to evolve and biomarkers of prognosis are refined. Given the changing nature of these treatments, multidisciplinary care with surgeons, gastroenterologists, and pathologists is essential to providing patients with the best long-term outcomes.

High-Grade Dysplasia and Superficial Cancers

Dysplasia arising in Barrett esophagus is characterized by cytologic malignant changes including atypical nuclei, increased mitoses, and lack of surface maturation. High-grade dysplasia is distinguished from low-grade dysplasia by more prominent cytologic or architectural derangements. As long as the cells are confined to the epithelium without invasion of the basement membrane, the pathology should be described as dysplasia regardless of the degree of abnormality. This encompasses what was previously referred to as carcinoma in situ. Historically, esophagectomy was often recommended for patients with high-grade dysplasia for a number of reasons. In the past, endoscopic biopsies were relatively inaccurate, and up to 50% of patients who underwent esophagectomy for high-grade dysplasia were found to have invasive cancer in the surgical specimen. Also, therapies to reverse or to halt the progression of dysplasia to invasive cancer were unavailable. Although esophagectomy had very high rates of cure for high-grade dysplasia, it was associated with significant morbidity.

Overtreatment has also been a concern. Despite the data that many patients with high-grade dysplasia have invasive cancer found on esophagectomy, there is evidence from other groups reporting that only a minority of patients with flat high-grade dysplasia develop invasive cancer on follow-up endoscopy.[34] Some of the conflict may be due to interobserver variation in the diagnosis of high-grade dysplasia versus invasive adenocarcinoma on biopsy specimens and the practice of diligent search for cancer at some institutions. Any biopsy specimens with high-grade dysplasia or invasive adenocarcinoma should be reviewed by a specialty pathologist experienced with Barrett esophagus and esophageal cancer. In contrast to the high rates of cancer development in patients with high-grade dysplasia, the incidence of cancer with nondysplastic Barrett esophagus appears to be low. The largest study of endoscopic surveillance in patients with Barrett esophagus found that the annual risk for development of cancer was 0.39% in patients with no dysplasia versus 0.77% in patients with low-grade dysplasia.[35]

The Seattle biopsy protocol is still widely accepted for mapping of Barrett esophagus with high-grade dysplasia. This involves four-quadrant biopsies at 1-cm intervals along the entire length of Barrett esophagus in addition to targeted biopsies of all visible lesions. Emerging endoscopic imaging techniques increase the sensitivity for detection of dysplasia. Many specialty centers routinely use high-resolution endoscopy and some sort of chromoendoscopy or simulated chromoendoscopy, such as narrow-band imaging (Olympus), to evaluate Barrett esophagus. Narrow-band imaging uses light filters to allow more narrow wavelengths of light. The wavelengths penetrate only superficially and are absorbed well by hemoglobin, better revealing irregular mucosal vascular patterns (Fig. 41-17). Additional technologies include autofluorescence endoscopy, confocal endomicroscopy, and optical coherence tomography. These techniques hold promise for even greater resolution but require more specialized training and equipment compared with the relatively user-friendly technology of high-resolution endoscopy and narrow-band imaging.

Therapeutics

Ablation. Various endoscopic ablative and resection techniques have been developed that have largely supplanted the role of esophagectomy for high-grade dysplasia. The most commonly used technology today is radiofrequency ablation (RFA). RFA is much more effective than photodynamic therapy with a lower stricture (and overall complication) rate. RFA may be delivered

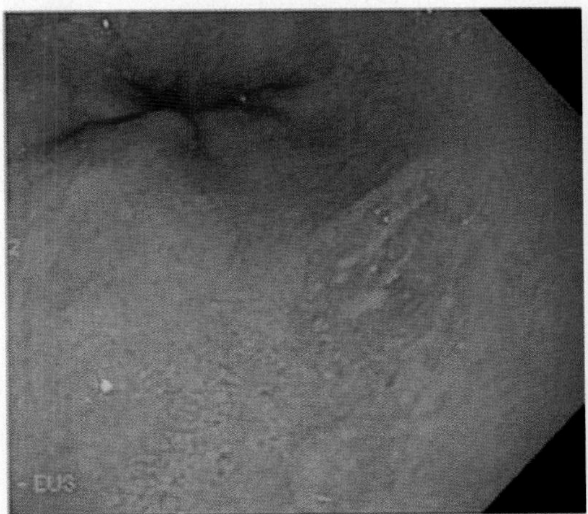

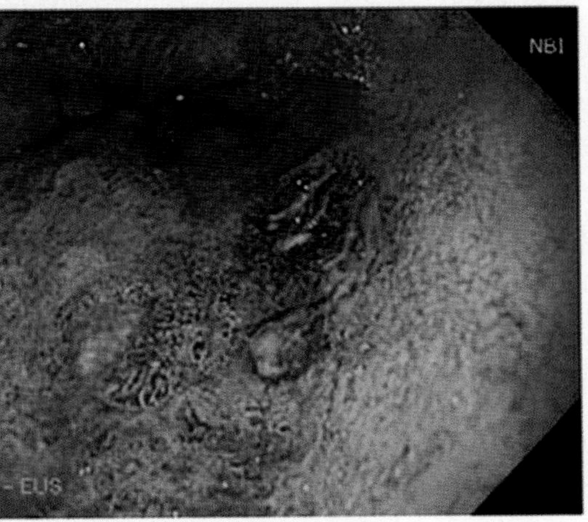

FIGURE 41-17 Traditional, white light view of Barrett esophagus with high-grade dysplasia *(left)* and narrow-band imaging of the same area *(right)*.

with a circumferential balloon or an electrical plate using a bipolar electrode that transmits radiofrequency energy, which generates heat and destroys superficial tissue. The treated mucosa is replaced by neosquamous mucosa. The standard ablation program uses two double pulses of 12 J/cm^2. The balloon is then repositioned distally, and the procedure is repeated until the entire segment of Barrett esophagus is treated. If there are areas of residual Barrett esophagus on follow-up endoscopy, those segments may be treated with more focal ablation.

Multiple studies have demonstrated the effectiveness of RFA for eradicating Barrett esophagus and dysplasia. In the Ablation of Intestinal Metaplasia (AIM-II) trial, 81% of patients with high-grade dysplasia and 90% of patients with low-grade dysplasia had eradication of dysplasia.[36] Only 4% of patients had their dysplasia progress to a higher grade of dysplasia or cancer. In a multicenter European trial of 136 patients randomly assigned to RFA versus surveillance, 1.5% of patients treated with ablation progressed to cancer versus 8.8% in the surveillance arm.[37] RFA was able to eradicate dysplasia in 93% of patients.

Cryotherapy. Cryotherapy is an alternative ablative technique that uses extreme cold rather than heat to destroy tissue. There have been no head-to-head comparisons between cryotherapy and RFA, but reports indicate similar efficacy to RFA.[38] Cryotherapy is generally well tolerated with little pain and low stricture rates. One advantage of cryotherapy compared with RFA is that cryotherapy does not require a probe to be in contact with the tissue. However, a decompression tube is required to prevent overdistention of the stomach and intestine with gas.

Regardless of what ablation technology is used, patients should have close surveillance and long-term acid suppression after ablation. A repeated endoscopy should be performed 3 months after ablative therapy, preferably with high-resolution endoscopy and some form of chromoendoscopy. Many patients will require more than one ablation session to eradicate all Barrett esophagus. There is also a small risk that areas of Barrett epithelium could be hidden beneath areas of the new squamous epithelium, known as buried glands. Malignancy can arise within these buried glands, and these cancers may be more difficult to identify during endoscopy. The clinical significance of this phenomenon is unknown, and the incidence of malignancy developing within these areas of buried glands appears to be very low.[39] Nevertheless, the potential implications of unrecognized incomplete eradication justifies future surveillance of ablated patients. After eradication of Barrett esophagus, fundoplication may also be considered for the treatment of reflux, although studies have not conclusively demonstrated effectiveness of antireflux surgery for prevention of esophageal cancer.

Endoscopic mucosal resection. One limitation of ablative therapies is the limited depth of penetration. Another disadvantage is the lack of definitive pathologic analysis. Therefore, patients with nodular or raised Barrett esophagus or other abnormalities suggestive of superficial invasive cancer should undergo EMR rather than ablation. EMR provides larger specimens to accurately determine the depth of invasion. EMR resects the full thickness of the mucosa, down into the submucosa (Fig. 41-18). Therefore, it is a good therapeutic option for superficial lesions with a low risk of nodal metastases. Depending on the size of the lesion, degree of differentiation, and lymphovascular invasion, the overall risk of nodal metastasis for lesions confined to the mucosa (T1a) ranges from less than 2% to more than 15% (Table 41-8).[40] For selected T1a lesions, EMR is highly effective (Fig. 41-19).[41] Although EMR can technically remove lesions involving the submucosa (T1b), the risk of lymph node involvement increases with depth of submucosal invasion. Therefore, EMR is generally not considered adequate for tumors involving the submucosa. Lesions involving only the most superficial third of the submucosa (SM1) have relatively low rates of nodal metastases, typically reported as less than 30%. On the other hand, lesions involving the deepest third of the submucosa (SM3) may have nodal involvement in more than 50% of cases.[42] T1b cancers with squamous cell histology also appear to have a higher risk of nodal metastasis compared with adenocarcinoma (45% versus 26%).[43] Thorough and accurate pathologic assessment is critical to formulating treatment plans. In patients who are poor surgical candidates, EMR of SM1 adenocarcinomas with low-risk features may be a reasonable treatment option. Likewise, for patients who are good surgical candidates, esophagectomy is a reasonable option for T1a lesions with high-risk features. EUS has low accuracy for assessing T stage for superficial tumors, so patients with suspected T1 lesions should have EMR performed by a qualified endoscopist to obtain accurate staging. Complications of EMR include bleeding, stricture, pain, and perforation. The stricture risk is increased for patients requiring circumferential resection. Although EMR may be performed for the entire segment of Barrett esophagus, complication

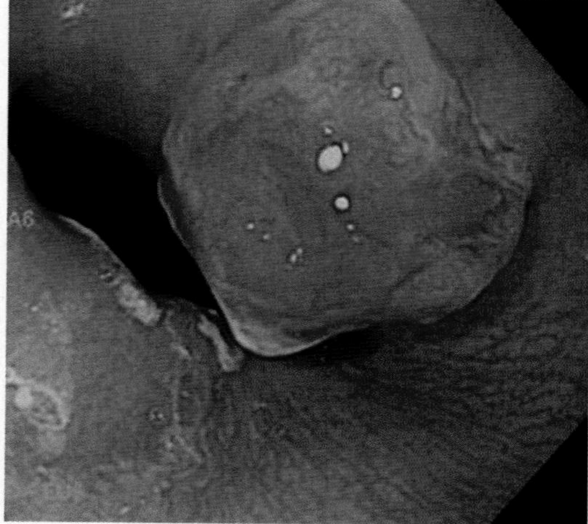

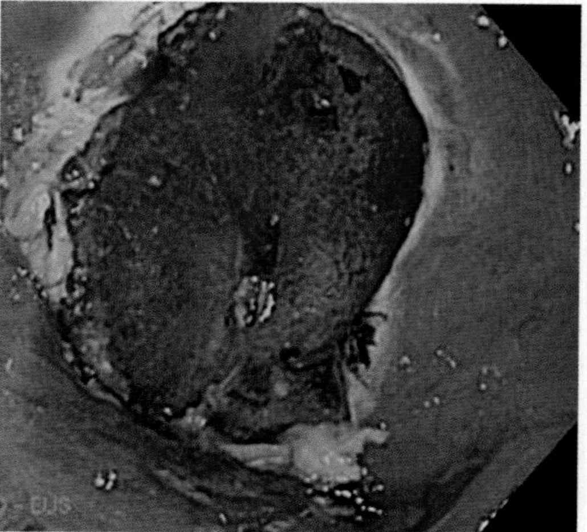

FIGURE 41-18 A superficial T1a adenocarcinoma arising in the setting of Barrett esophagus *(left)* and submucosal defect after endoscopic mucosal resection *(right)*.

TABLE 41-8 Nomogram for Prediction of Lymph Node Metastases in Early-Stage Esophageal Cancer

VARIABLE	POINTS
Size, per cm	+ 1 (per cm)
Depth	
T1a	+ 0
T1b	+ 2
Differentiation	
Well	+ 0
Moderate	+ 3
Poor	+ 3
Lymphovascular invasion	+ 6

RISK CATEGORY	POINTS	PREDICTED RISK OF LYMPH NODE METASTASES (%)
Low	0-1	≤2
Moderate	2-4	3-6
High	5+	≥7

Adapted from Lee L, Ronellenfitsch U, Hofstetter WL, et al: Predicting lymph node metastases in early esophageal adenocarcinoma using a simple scoring system. *J Am Coll Surg* 217:191–199, 2013.

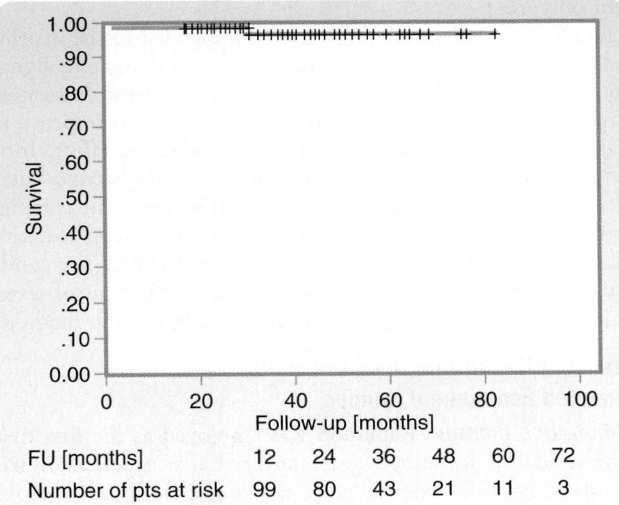

FIGURE 41-19 Survival curve of patients undergoing endoscopic mucosal resection for low-risk, superficial esophageal adenocarcinoma. (From Ell C, May A, Pech O, et al: Curative endoscopic resection of early esophageal adenocarcinomas [Barrett's cancer]. *Gastrointest Endosc* 65:3–10, 2007.)

rates are lower if EMR is focused on specific areas combined with ablation for residual Barrett esophagus.

EMR may be performed with a submucosal lifting technique, which raises the target lesion by injecting fluid into the submucosa beneath the lesion. This allows the lesion to be suctioned more easily into a cap, creating a pseudopolyp, allowing resection with a snare. Another technique uses suction to raise the lesion, allowing a band to be placed at the base of the pseudopolyp that is created and then using a snare to resect. One drawback of EMR is that larger lesions are typically removed piecemeal. Reports describe the efficacy of endoscopic submucosal dissection using an endoscopic needle knife that allows greater submucosal dissection and en bloc resection of larger lesions.[44] The safety of this technique outside a few specialized centers is unknown.

Surveillance is an important component of the treatment for superficial esophageal cancers. Patients should receive high-dose acid suppression therapy with a PPI to help EMR and ablation sites to heal. Many patients require multiple procedures to completely eradicate Barrett epithelium. Short-interval follow-up endoscopy should be performed 3 months after endoscopic treatment is completed. Any residual Barrett epithelium may be focally ablated at that time. Surveillance endoscopies should be performed frequently (i.e., every 3 months) for the first year after endoscopic treatment for high-grade dysplasia or intramucosal cancer, after which time the frequency of endoscopic surveillance may be spaced out. For superficial lesions treated endoscopically, radiologic imaging, such as fluorodeoxyglucose (FDG) PET, has no value.

Esophagectomy. The role of esophagectomy as a single-modality treatment for esophageal cancer is diminishing. Most tumors are found after symptoms develop, at which point they are usually locally advanced or metastatic. Locally advanced tumors should be treated with multimodality therapy. Asymptomatic tumors are usually found during surveillance for Barrett esophagus. These are typically superficial and can be treated with EMR with lower complication rates than with esophagectomy. This leaves a relatively narrow subset of tumors that are treated appropriately with surgery only. As discussed earlier, T1b tumors have significant risk for nodal metastasis and in general should be treated with esophagectomy. High-risk T1a lesions (larger tumors or lesions with lymphovascular invasion) could also be considered for esophagectomy. Extensive, multifocal lesions and ulcerated tumors may also be difficult to eradicate endoscopically and would be appropriate candidates for esophagectomy.

An area of controversy is the optimal treatment for clinical T2N0 tumors. Esophagectomy with an adequate lymphadenectomy would be expected to confer an overall 5-year survival of anywhere between 40% and 65% for a pathologic T2N0 cancer, depending on histology, grade, and location of tumor.[20] Unfortunately, a clinical stage of T2N0 is inaccurate in the majority of cases, and many patients are found to have node-positive disease on final pathology after esophagectomy. Clinical T2N0 patients were included in the CROSS trial, which compared neoadjuvant chemoradiation followed by surgery versus surgery alone for esophageal and GEJ cancer. Although the trial demonstrated a survival benefit for the neoadjuvant chemoradiation arm, clinical T2N0 patients represented only a small subset of the study cohort, and it is unclear how much benefit these patients in particular received.[45] It is clear that many patients with clinical T2N0 disease are understaged, but retrospective analyses indicate that there may not be a survival advantage for neoadjuvant therapy in this group.[46] One management strategy may be to selectively offer neoadjuvant therapy to patients with clinical T2N0 disease based on other high-risk factors, such as long T2N0 tumors. Similarly, an equal number of patients with cT2N0 are actually overstaged, so liberal use of diagnostic EMR is appropriate.

The advent of EMR also influences the type of esophagectomy that should be performed in early-stage esophageal cancer. Because of the potential for decreased complication and improved physiologic outcomes, vagal-sparing esophagectomy has been advocated by some for intramucosal adenocarcinoma and high-grade dysplasia. However, most low-risk lesions are now resected by EMR. Because standard lymphadenectomy is not performed as part of vagal-sparing esophagectomy, it is not appropriate for the majority of patients who are undergoing surgery for higher risk lesions. Minimally invasive esophagectomy is also a technique that is gaining favor. Long-term survival has not been directly compared with open esophagectomy in a prospective fashion, but one small, randomized trial reported reduced postoperative complications with a minimally invasive approach.[36]

Patients have increasing options for the treatment of early-stage esophageal cancers. Care needs to be individualized so patients may make informed decisions, balancing the effectiveness of therapies with their risks and impact on quality of life.

Locally Advanced Esophageal Cancer

Despite improved awareness of the increasing trend in esophageal adenocarcinoma and more frequent detection of early esophageal adenocarcinoma on surveillance endoscopies, the majority of patients with esophageal cancer still present with locally advanced or metastatic disease. Usually, it is not until patients experience dysphagia, which generally signifies transmural tumor involvement (T3), that an esophageal cancer is diagnosed. In this setting, the probability of lymph node metastases reaches 80%, so the majority of patients present with clinical stage T3N1-3 according to the seventh edition (AJCC) of esophageal cancer staging. It should be stressed that the seventh edition of esophageal cancer staging is based on the pathology specimen from patients treated with surgical therapy alone, and therefore its utility in the clinical pretreatment setting in the era of multimodality therapy is arguably limited. However, compared with the sixth edition, which grouped all patients with positive nodal disease into N1 status, current staging recognized the prognostic value in the number of metastatic lymph nodes and grouped patients into three categories: N1 (one to three positive nodes), N2 (four to six positive nodes), and N3 (seven or more positive nodes). The anatomic location of the regional nodal disease relative to the primary tumor is no longer considered an important factor; however, in clinical practice, nodal disease location continues to influence treatment decisions. This confusion is partly due to the lack of consensus and definition of which nodal stations represent regional versus distant metastatic disease. In the era of multimodality therapy and selective surgery, the rigorous definition of locally advanced esophageal cancer is necessary to guide pretreatment therapeutic decisions before committing to either aggressive locoregional therapy or initiating systemic treatment.

For esophageal adenocarcinoma, mostly located in the distal esophagus or GEJ, we consider nodal disease located in the area from the celiac axis up to the paratracheal region to represent regional disease; nodal disease located outside of these boundaries is regarded as distant disease. For esophageal SCC, which mostly arises in the mid or proximal esophagus, periesophageal cervical lymphadenopathy is still considered a regional disease. Whereas the current staging system takes the tumor differentiation into account, it is mainly the disease burden that dictates the decisions about the treatment strategy, and therapeutic decisions are best discussed in a multidisciplinary setting.

The Evolution and Principles of Multimodality Therapy for Locally Advanced Esophageal Carcinoma

Surgical resection of the esophagus was the mainstay of esophageal cancer treatment in the past. However, we have learned that even the most radical resections with extensive lymph node dissections are not adequate to cure locoregionally advanced disease in the majority of cases. Distant recurrence or metastatic disease continues to be the main cause of death in patients with esophageal cancer.

Our understanding and treatment of esophageal cancer have evolved significantly during the last 100 years. The initial recognition that a localized esophageal cancer may be cured with surgical resection dates back to the first successful esophagectomy performed by Franz Torek in 1913. Despite rather poor perioperative outcomes at that time, surgery became a supplement to radiation as the treatment of choice for localized esophageal cancer in the early 20th century. Over time, more extensive en bloc esophageal resections and lymphadenectomy became favored with the hope that radical resection of disease would result in a cure more frequently. However, similar to Halstead's radical mastectomy, we have learned that whereas extended esophagectomy may lead to better locoregional control, it fails to achieve cure in patients destined to die of metastatic disease. Today, technical aspects of esophagectomy are still passionately debated as the technologic advances enable us to perform these procedures safely even with less invasive or robotically assisted techniques. From an oncologic standpoint, however, surgical therapy has its limits in what it can contribute to the cure rate of esophageal cancer. Moreover, there continues to be a tremendous variability in the performance of surgical resection of the esophagus among surgeons, with some favoring transthoracic and some transabdominal approaches with varied extents of lymph node dissections. This lack of procedural standardization confounds the analysis of esophageal cancer treatment outcomes.

Increased understanding of cancer biology led to the development of nonsurgical treatment strategies for solid organ malignant neoplasms, including esophageal carcinoma. Chemotherapy was combined concomitantly with radiation therapy to improve the local-regional efficacy and potentially for systemic effect. Intuitively, this strategy targets both local disease and systemic micrometastases. The demonstrated efficacy of this treatment paradigm subsequently stimulated interest in combining surgery, radiation, and chemotherapy to maximize the treatment effect. The combination of these treatment modalities became the focus of several clinical trials investigating the role and timing of each method.

Treatment Modalities Used in Locally Advanced Esophageal Cancer

Radiation therapy. Radiation was employed as the first treatment modality for esophageal cancer. Early experiences with radium bougies and external beam radiation demonstrated esophageal tumor regression with occasional complete tumor responses. With the evolution of surgical care, radiation became a part of a multidisciplinary approach to esophageal cancer therapy with the goal of sterilizing areas within or around the operative field. Early randomized trials of neoadjuvant radiation administered doses of 20 to 40 Gy before resection in an attempt to decrease local recurrence and to improve survival rates. With one exception, all of these trials included patients with SCC only, and none of the trials demonstrated significant benefits of adding radiation therapy to resection.

Although the lower radiation doses (20 to 40 Gy) may have been inadequate, clinicians were wary of combining higher dose radiation before surgery, given the toxicity risks (note that radiation delivery and particles used in therapy were very different in the past compared with current therapy). Nonetheless, high rates of locoregional recurrence after surgery led to the consideration of adjuvant radiation therapy for esophageal cancer. The rationale for this approach was the ability to deliver higher doses (40 to

60 Gy) of radiation postoperatively without worsening perioperative complications. Postoperative radiation therapy for esophageal cancer appeared to be potentially beneficial in several trials, although the data are conflicting and subject to selection bias.

Chemotherapy. The cause of death from esophageal cancer is mainly due to metastatic disease. Intuitively, systemic chemotherapy has the potential to target micrometastatic deposits. Even in the setting of a seemingly localized disease, it usually downstages marginally resectable tumors, allowing improved complete (R0) resection rates, and decreases the incidence of locoregional recurrence.[47] The synergistic effect of chemotherapy with radiation strengthens the argument for its use. Importantly, when it is administered preoperatively, the biologic response can be evaluated and quantified pathologically in terms of pathologic tumor histoviability, and the degree of this response has been correlated as an indicator of outcome. Current chemotherapeutic regimens are based on platinum compounds (cisplatin and carboplatin) in combination with 5-fluorouracil or taxanes as a doublet. In several prospective randomized trials, researchers compared chemotherapy followed by surgery with surgery alone for both esophageal adenocarcinoma and SCC (Table 41-9).[48] The landmark trial by Roth and colleagues demonstrated longer median survival durations in patients with major or complete response to chemotherapy, which highlighted the biologic diversity of esophageal cancers and their varied susceptibility to chemotherapy.[49] One of the largest randomized trials using chemotherapy and surgery versus surgery alone in esophageal cancer patients was the North American Intergroup Trial (INT 0113).[50] This trial did not demonstrate better survival with chemotherapy plus surgery than with surgery alone in either histologic type. However, inaccurate staging, response evaluation, and high toxicity rates leading to a low surgical incidence confound the results of the study. Contrary to the INT 0113 trial, a phase 3 study run by the Medical Research Council (MRC) in the United Kingdom consisting of chemotherapy plus surgery versus surgery alone in locally advanced esophageal cancer demonstrated survival benefit of chemotherapy.[51] The largest trial of its kind, the MRC trial included 802 patients randomized to receive chemotherapy plus esophagectomy versus esophagectomy alone. The survival benefit of chemotherapy persisted at the updated median follow-up duration of 6 years, with 5-year survival rates of 23% with chemotherapy plus surgery and 17% with surgery alone ($P = .03$). Both adenocarcinoma and SCC patients experienced benefit. Another commonly referenced trial that demonstrated survival advantage and better R0 resection rate of neoadjuvant chemotherapy and surgery over surgery alone was the MRC Adjuvant Gastric Infusional Chemotherapy (MAGIC) trial by Cunningham and colleagues.[52] The majority of the enrolled patients had gastric carcinoma, with only a subgroup having esophageal or GEJ tumors.

In the adjuvant setting, the results of chemotherapy have not been convincing. The majority of trials were in the esophageal SCC setting, such as a phase 3 multicenter Japan Clinical Oncology Group trial (JCOG 9204), or JCOG 9907, which randomized 330 patients comparing the effects of neoadjuvant (164 patients) and adjuvant (166 patients) chemotherapy for stage II and stage III esophageal SCC.[53] Patients received the same two cycles of cisplatin and 5-fluorouracil as in JCOG 9204 before or after radical resection. The interim analysis demonstrated a significantly better ($P = .044$) median progression-free survival duration in the neoadjuvant group (3 years) than in the adjuvant group (2 years) and the difference in estimated 5-year overall survival rate of 60% versus 38% in the neoadjuvant and adjuvant arms, respectively ($P = .013$). On the basis of these findings, it was recommended to terminate the trial. The limitations of this study included disproportionate compliance with therapy between the two groups, omission of postoperative chemotherapy in patients with pN0 disease based on the JCOG 9204 results, and premature termination of the trial. In adenocarcinoma histology, the effects of adjuvant chemotherapy on survival after R0 resection was studied in a phase 2 Eastern Cooperative Oncology Group trial (E8296).[54] The median 2-year overall survival rate was 60%, which appeared to be better than that in historical controls. Similarly, Ferri and colleagues demonstrated a greater than 60% 3-year overall survival, with a preponderance of stage III patients (AJCC sixth edition), treated with perioperative docetaxel, cisplatin, and 5-fluorouracil.[55]

Chemoradiation alone. Chemoradiation may be administered in a preoperative or postoperative setting, as definitive bimodality therapy, or as part of trimodality therapy when combined with surgery. Concomitant administration of chemotherapy and radiation has a synergistic effect with increased tumor cytotoxicity at low doses. The validity of chemoradiation use for all locations

TABLE 41-9 Randomized Trials Comparing Chemotherapy and Surgery versus Surgery Alone

TRIAL	N	HISTOLOGY	CHEMOTHERAPY	R0 (%)	SURVIVAL
MRC		SCC, ADC	Cisplatin, 5-FU		Median (months)
CT	400			60	17
Sx	402			54	13
RTOG 8911		SCC, ADC	Cisplatin, 5-FU		Median (months)
CT	213			63	14.9
Sx	227			59	16.1
MAGIC		ADC	Epirubicin, cisplatin, 5-FU	NA	5 years (%)
CT	250				36*
Sx	253				23
FFCD		ADC	Cisplatin, 5-FU		5 years (%)
CT	113			84	38*
Sx	111			74	24

Adapted from Cools-Lartigue J, Spicer J, Ferri LE: Current status of management of malignant disease: Current management of esophageal cancer. *J Gastrointest Surg* 19:964–972, 2015.

ADC, adenocarcinoma; *CT,* chemotherapy; *5-FU,* 5-fluorouracil; *SCC,* squamous cell carcinoma; *Sx,* surgery.

*$P < .05$.

of esophageal cancer is based on encouraging results of definitive chemoradiation for cervical esophageal SCC. Randomized trials of chemoradiation versus radiation alone include RTOG 85-01 by Herskovic and colleagues, which established that a group of patients with esophageal SCC or adenocarcinoma could be cured with bimodality therapy alone. To improve on the favorable outcomes observed in the RTOG 85-01 trial, researchers attempted to increase locoregional disease control rates in the subsequent Intergroup 0123/RTOG 94-05 trial by modifying the intensity of radiation therapy to high-dose 64.8 Gy given concurrently with chemotherapy. Unfortunately, at a median follow-up duration of 16 months, the survival and locoregional disease control rates with the higher radiation dose did not differ significantly from those in the RTOG 85-01 trial, but the toxicity and treatment-related deaths were worse in the high-dose radiation therapy group. This study established that 50.4 Gy of radiation used concomitantly with chemotherapy is both a neoadjuvant and potentially definitive dose.[56]

Chemoradiation and surgery. When used alone, each cancer treatment modality has its limitations, ranging from inadequate therapeutic effect to excessive toxicity. The synergistic effect of chemoradiation combined with surgical resection maximizes the chances of effectively treating both locoregional disease and potential undetectable metastases (Table 41-10). Early clinical trials testing a trimodality treatment paradigm did not demonstrate a survival advantage over surgery alone. Many of these trials were underpowered and mixed SCC and esophageal adenocarcinoma histology as well as varied radiation and chemotherapy regimens. Some trials suffered from poor patient accrual or inconsistent surgical outcomes. The most notable and frequently quoted trial that compared chemoradiation followed by surgery with surgery alone for esophageal and EGJ cancer was the Chemoradiotherapy for Oesophageal Cancer Followed by Surgery Study (CROSS).[57] This trial enrolled an impressive 368 patients during a 4-year period, and 366 patients were included in the final analysis. The surgery-alone group consisted of 188 patients, whereas 178 underwent chemoradiation followed by surgery. The majority (75%) of the patients had adenocarcinoma, and 22% had SCC. The chemoradiation regimen consisted of a 5-week course of carboplatin and paclitaxel administered concurrently with radiation therapy at a dose of 41.4 Gy given in 23 fractions 5 days a week. Esophagectomy was performed within 4 to 6 weeks in the treatment group and immediately after randomization in the control group. The completeness (R0) of resection was higher in the trimodality group than in the surgery-alone group (92% versus 69%; $P < .001$). Patients with SCC experienced complete pathologic response (ypT0N0M0) significantly more than patients with adenocarcinoma (49% versus 29%; $P < .001$). Expectedly, nodal positivity was higher in patients with surgery alone compared with the trimodality group (75% versus 31%; $P < .001$). At a median follow-up duration of 45 months, patients receiving the trimodality therapy had significantly longer median overall survival

TABLE 41-10 Randomized Trials Comparing Chemoradiation and Surgery versus Surgery Alone

TRIAL	N	HISTOLOGY	CHEMOTHERAPY	RT (Gy)	pCR (%)	R0 (%)	SURVIVAL
Walsh		ADC	Cisplatin, 5-FU	40	25	NA	3 years (%)
CT-RT-Sx	58						32*
Sx	55						6
Bosset		SCC	Cisplatin	37	26	NA	Median (months)
CT-RT-Sx	143						18.6
Sx	149						18.6
Urba		SCC, ADC	Cisplatin, 5-FU, vinblastine	45	28	90	3 years (%)
CT-RT-Sx	50					90	30*
Sx	50						16
Lee		SCC	Cisplatin, 5FU	45.6	43		Median (months)
CT-RT-Sx	51					100	27.3
Sx	50					87.5	28.2
Burmeister		SCC, ADC	Cisplatin, 5-FU	35	16		Median (months)
CT-RT-Sx	128					80*	22.2
Sx	128					59	19.3
Tepper		SCC, ADC	Cisplatin, 5-FU	50.4	33	NR	5 years (%)
CT-RT-Sx	30						39*
Sx	26						16
CROSS		SCC, ADC	Carboplatin, paclitaxel	41.4	29		5 years (%)
CT-RT-Sx	178					92*	47*
Sx	188					69	34
Mariette		SCC, ADC	Cisplatin, 5-FU	45	33.3		3 years (%)
CT-RT-Sx	98					93.8	47.5
Sx	97					92.1	53

Adapted from Cools-Lartigue J, Spicer J, Ferri LE: Current status of management of malignant disease: Current management of esophageal cancer. *J Gastrointest Surg* 19:964–972, 2015.

ADC, adenocarcinoma; *CT,* chemotherapy; *5-FU,* 5-fluorouracil; *NA,* not available; *NR,* not reported; *pCR,* pathologic complete response; *RT,* radiotherapy; *SCC,* squamous cell carcinoma; *Sx,* surgery.

*$P > .05$.

duration (49.4 months) than did patients undergoing surgery alone (24 months; hazard ratio [HR], 0.65; 95% confidence interval [CI], 0.49-0.87; $P = .003$). The estimated 5-year survival rate in the trimodality therapy group was 47% compared with 34% (HR, 0.65; 95% CI, 0.49-0.87; $P = .003$) in the surgery group. Interestingly, trimodality therapy did not significantly benefit patients with adenocarcinoma histology (HR, 0.74; 95% CI, 0.53-1.02; $P = .07$), and inexplicably it benefited patients with clinically node-negative disease (HR, 0.42; 95% CI, 0.23-0.74; $P = .003$) but not those with node-positive disease (HR, 0.80; 95% CI, 0.57-1.13; $P = .21$).

The Role of Surgery in Trimodality Therapy and Salvage Surgery

Subsequent to the CROSS trial report, many Western centers adopted the trimodality therapy as the standard of care for the treatment of esophageal carcinoma. However, this trial still left many questions unanswered about the treatment strategy for locoregional esophageal carcinoma. Whereas we have observed that neoadjuvant chemoradiation improves R0 resection and locoregional recurrence rates and results in pathologic complete responses in many patients, other subgroups of patients clearly derive no benefit from neoadjuvant therapy over surgery alone. Equally, patients who are "cured" by neoadjuvant chemoradiation derive no additional survival benefit from further surgical extirpation of the esophagus. We are currently unable to identify these groups of patients and must search for simple, reproducible, and validated surrogate markers predictive of treatment outcome. So far, only histopathologic tumor response after neoadjuvant therapy has emerged as a predictor of survival in esophageal cancer patients.[58] Surgical resection and evaluation of histopathologic tumor response will therefore continue to play a role in the treatment of esophageal cancer in upcoming years.

Nevertheless, both randomized trials comparing preoperative chemotherapy versus preoperative chemoradiation failed to show a significant difference between the two treatment approaches (Table 41-11).[59,60] Indeed, the latest meta-analysis inclusive of 24 trials and 4188 patients focusing on survival after neoadjuvant chemotherapy or chemoradiotherapy for resectable esophageal carcinoma provided strong evidence for survival benefit of multimodality therapy versus surgery alone.[61] The ideal preoperative treatment regimen, however, has yet to be determined, with no clear benefit of neoadjuvant chemoradiation over chemotherapy having been demonstrated.

Some authors have debated the value of surgery after bimodality therapy. Two trials of chemoradiation versus chemoradiation and surgery suggested that there was no advantage to surgical resection. However, both these trials had unacceptably high perioperative mortality rates.[62,63] Murphy and colleagues[64] subsequently showed that surgical resection and tumor differentiation were the only independent predictors of survival in a retrospective analysis. Clearly, impeccable perioperative outcomes are necessary to demonstrate oncologic benefit of surgical therapy. Hence, one strategy is to use esophageal resection selectively, only in the setting of disease persistence or recurrence after definitive chemoradiation. This treatment paradigm was the focus of the RTOG 0246 phase 2 trial by Swisher and colleagues.[65] The study was designed to detect improvement in 1-year survival from 60% to 77.5% in patients undergoing selective or salvage esophagectomy. More than 70% of enrolled patients had T3 or N1 disease stage. Forty-one patients were included in the analysis, of whom 21 (51%) underwent salvage esophagectomy because of residual or recurrent disease; one patient requested resection. Patients with complete clinical response after definitive chemoradiation had overall survival of 53%, with clinical incomplete response of 33% and clinical incomplete response salvaged by surgery of 41%. Salvage esophagectomy after definitive chemoradiation is a feasible treatment strategy and seems to provide additional survival benefit in patients with incomplete clinical response after definitive chemoradiation.

Surveillance

Patients who have received definitive chemoradiation therapy (bimodality therapy) for esophageal cancer continue to suffer from the fear that the disease may reappear again either as locoregional or distant metastatic recurrence. The purpose behind the periodic surveillance of patients who completed definitive bimodality therapy is to potentially implement salvage therapy for locoregional failure. Evidence-based surveillance algorithms are not available; however, most providers observe patients every 3 to 6 months with clinical examination and a variety of imaging or endoscopy studies. This strategy is often costly and anxiety-provoking for patients, and it may not change the ultimate outcome for the patient. Considering the fact that more than 98% of local recurrences occur in the first 36 months, most authors suggest vigilant surveillance during this time after bimodality therapy to potentially catch recurrences early enough to render salvage surgery a feasible strategy.

Palliative Options for Esophageal Carcinoma

Patients with poor performance status or distant metastatic disease at the time of diagnosis are not candidates for aggressive

TABLE 41-11 Randomized Trials Comparing Chemoradiation and Surgery versus Chemotherapy and Surgery

TRIAL	N	HISTOLOGY	CHEMOTHERAPY	CHEMORADIOTHERAPY	pCR (%)	R0 (%)	SURVIVAL
Stahl		ADC	Cisplatin, 5-FU	Induction: cisplatin, 5-FU			3 years (%)
CT-RT	60			Concurrent: cisplatin, etoposide	15.6*	72	47.4
CT	59			(30 Gy)	2	69	27.7
Burmeister		ADC	Cisplatin, 5-FU	Cisplatin			Median (months)
CT-RT	39			5-FU (35 Gy)	31*	84.6	32
CT	36				8	80.5	29

Adapted from Cools-Lartigue J, Spicer J, Ferri LE: Current status of management of malignant disease: Current management of esophageal cancer. *J Gastrointest Surg* 19:964–972, 2015.

ADC, adenocarcinoma; *CT*, chemotherapy; *5-FU*, 5-fluorouracil; *pCR*, pathologic complete response; *RT*, radiotherapy.

*$P < .05$.

locoregional therapy. The goal of treatment in these circumstances is either to palliate existing symptoms or potentially to avoid future complications related to the disease extent. Metastatic esophageal carcinoma may be manifested with a variety of symptoms, depending on the disease spread; however, dysphagia, odynophagia, chest pain, fatigue, and weight loss are likely to be among the most common symptoms. Palliative treatment is always individualized on the basis of a patient's physiologic status, symptoms, disease extent, and wishes. Options for palliation range from best supportive care for symptom control to the use of chemotherapy or radiation, esophageal stent placement, and enteral nutrition support. With advancements in image-guided percutaneous and endoscopic procedures, surgical procedures for palliation of esophageal carcinoma have become exceedingly rare.

SUMMARY

Multimodality therapy using a combination of neoadjuvant chemotherapy with or without radiation followed by surgery is presently regarded as the standard of care for either locally advanced esophageal adenocarcinoma or SCC. Whereas some patients benefit from this aggressive locoregional treatment strategy, the majority of patients continue to develop distant metastatic disease, which is presently incurable. As the search for molecular predictors and targeted therapies for this cancer continues, we will have to rigorously test novel agents to determine their places in the therapeutic armamentarium. Standardized perioperative care in well-designed clinical trials will be imperative so the potential therapeutic benefit of surgery is not offset by unacceptably high perioperative mortality rates. The heterogeneity of esophageal adenocarcinoma will require novel treatment strategies to improve personalized treatment outcomes of this cancer.

SELECTED REFERENCES

Banki F, Mason RJ, DeMeester SR: Vagal-sparing esophagectomy: A more physiologic alternative. *Ann Surg* 236:324–335, 2002.

This was the first paper to document physiologic outcomes of vagal-sparing esophagectomy in detail (the surgery was first described by Akiyama).

Gu Y, Swisher SG, Ajani JA, et al: The number of lymph nodes with metastasis predicts survival in patients with esophageal cancer or esophagogastric junction adenocarcinoma who receive preoperative chemoradiotherapy. *Cancer* 106:1017–1025, 2006.

This paper discusses the notion that in addition to location and response to neoadjuvant therapy, the number of lymph nodes may be one of the most significant predictors of outcome.

Orringer MB, Sloan H: Esophagectomy without thoracotomy. *J Thorac Cardiovasc Surg* 76:643–654, 1978.

This landmark paper was the first to describe the transhiatal esophagectomy and to document the outcomes in detail.

Park W, Vaezi MF: Cause and pathogenesis of achalasia: The current understanding. *Am J Gastroenterol* 101:202–203, 2006.

This concise review of achalasia gives a thorough overview of the evolution of the cause and pathogenesis of this disease.

Yammamoto S, Kawahara K, Maekawa T: Minimally invasive esophagectomy for stage I and II esophageal cancer. *Ann Thorac Surg* 80:2070–2075, 2005.

This is one of the largest series of esophageal cancer patients undergoing a minimally invasive procedure to treat early-stage disease. It has become an important study, suggesting that minimally invasive surgery may be a viable option in these patients.

REFERENCES

1. Kahrilas PJ, Bredenoord AJ, Fox M, et al: The Chicago Classification of esophageal motility disorders, v3.0. *Neurogastroenterol Motil* 27:160–174, 2015.
2. Code CF, Schlegel JF, Kelley ML, Jr, et al: Hypertensive gastroesophageal sphincter. *Proc Staff Meet Mayo Clin* 35:391–399, 1960.
3. Stavropoulos SN, Desilets DJ, Fuchs KH, et al: Per-oral endoscopic myotomy white paper summary. *Surg Endosc* 28:2005–2019, 2014.
4. Inoue H, Sato H, Ikeda H, et al: Per-oral endoscopic myotomy: A series of 500 patients. *J Am Coll Surg* 221:256–264, 2015.
5. Boeckxstaens GE, Annese V, des Varannes SB, et al: Pneumatic dilation versus laparoscopic Heller's myotomy for idiopathic achalasia. *N Engl J Med* 364:1807–1816, 2011.
6. Zenker FA, von Ziemssen HW: Krankheiten des Oesophagus. *Leipzig* 1867.
7. Bonavina L, Bona D, Abraham M, et al: Long-term results of endosurgical and open surgical approach for Zenker diverticulum. *World J Gastroenterol* 13:2586–2589, 2007.
8. Campos GM, Peters JH, DeMeester TR, et al: Multivariate analysis of factors predicting outcome after laparoscopic Nissen fundoplication. *J Gastrointest Surg* 3:292–300, 1999.
9. Richter JE, Pandolfino JE, Vela MF, et al: Utilization of wireless pH monitoring technologies: A summary of the proceedings from the esophageal diagnostic working group. *Dis Esophagus* 26:755–765, 2013.
10. Ganz RA, Peters JH, Horgan S, et al: Esophageal sphincter device for gastroesophageal reflux disease. *N Engl J Med* 368:719–727, 2013.
11. Awais O, Luketich JD, Reddy N, et al: Roux-en-Y near esophagojejunostomy for failed antireflux operations: Outcomes in more than 100 patients. *Ann Thorac Surg* 98:1905–1911, discussion 1911–1913, 2014.
12. Kahrilas PJ, Shaheen NJ, Vaezi MF, et al: American Gastroenterological Association Medical Position Statement on the management of gastroesophageal reflux disease. *Gastroenterology* 135:1383–1391, 1391.e1–5, 2008.
13. Skinner DB, Little AG, DeMeester TR: Management of esophageal perforation. *Am J Surg* 139:760–764, 1980.
14. Abbas G, Schuchert MJ, Pettiford BL, et al: Contemporaneous management of esophageal perforation. *Surgery* 146:749–755, discussion 755–756, 2009.

15. Sepesi B, Raymond DP, Peters JH: Esophageal perforation: Surgical, endoscopic and medical management strategies. *Curr Opin Gastroenterol* 26:379–383, 2010.
16. Rice R, Dubose JJ, Spicer JD, et al: Perforated esophageal intervention focus (PERF) study: A multi-center study of contemporary management. *J Thorac Cardiovasc Surg* 2015. [in press].
17. Siegel RL, Miller KD, Jemal A: Cancer statistics, 2015. *CA Cancer J Clin* 65:5–29, 2015.
18. Pohl H, Welch HG: The role of overdiagnosis and reclassification in the marked increase of esophageal adenocarcinoma incidence. *J Natl Cancer Inst* 97:142–146, 2005.
19. Strong VE, D'Amico TA, Kleinberg L, et al: Impact of the 7th Edition AJCC staging classification on the NCCN clinical practice guidelines in oncology for gastric and esophageal cancers. *J Natl Compr Canc Netw* 11:60–66, 2013.
20. Rice TW, Rusch VW, Ishwaran H, et al: Cancer of the esophagus and esophagogastric junction: Data-driven staging for the seventh edition of the American Joint Committee on Cancer/International Union Against Cancer Cancer Staging Manuals. *Cancer* 116:3763–3773, 2010.
21. Daly JM, Fry WA, Little AG, et al: Esophageal cancer: Results of an American College of Surgeons Patient Care Evaluation Study. *J Am Coll Surg* 190:562–572, discussion 572–573, 2000.
22. Pouw RE, Heldoorn N, Alvarez Herrero L, et al: Do we still need EUS in the workup of patients with early esophageal neoplasia? A retrospective analysis of 131 cases. *Gastrointest Endosc* 73:662–668, 2011.
23. Dhupar R, Rice RD, Correa AM, et al: Endoscopic ultrasound estimates for tumor depth at the gastroesophageal junction are inaccurate: Implications for the liberal use of endoscopic resection. *Ann Thorac Surg* 2015. [Epub ahead of print].
24. van Vliet EP, Heijenbrok-Kal MH, Hunink MG, et al: Staging investigations for oesophageal cancer: A meta-analysis. *Br J Cancer* 98:547–557, 2008.
25. Orlowska J, Pachlewski J, Gugulski A, et al: A conservative approach to granular cell tumors of the esophagus: Four case reports and literature review. *Am J Gastroenterol* 88:311–315, 1993.
26. Chen WS, Zheng XL, Jin L, et al: Novel diagnosis and treatment of esophageal granular cell tumor: Report of 14 cases and review of the literature. *Ann Thorac Surg* 97:296–302, 2014.
27. Carr NJ, Monihan JM, Sobin LH: Squamous cell papilloma of the esophagus: A clinicopathologic and follow-up study of 25 cases. *Am J Gastroenterol* 89:245–248, 1994.
28. Murase K, Hino A, Ozeki Y, et al: Malignant schwannoma of the esophagus with lymph node metastasis: Literature review of schwannoma of the esophagus. *J Gastroenterol* 36:772–777, 2001.
29. Bonavina L, Segalin A, Rosati R, et al: Surgical therapy of esophageal leiomyoma. *J Am Coll Surg* 181:257–262, 1995.
30. Kukar M, Groman A, Malhotra U, et al: Small cell carcinoma of the esophagus: A SEER database analysis. *Ann Surg Oncol* 20:4239–4244, 2013.
31. Hu YM, Yan JD, Gao Y, et al: Primary malignant melanoma of esophagus: A case report and review of literature. *Int J Clin Exp Pathol* 7:8176–8180, 2014.
32. Lott S, Schmieder M, Mayer B, et al: Gastrointestinal stromal tumors of the esophagus: Evaluation of a pooled case series regarding clinicopathological features and clinical outcome. *Am J Cancer Res* 5:333–343, 2015.
33. Berry MF, Zeyer-Brunner J, Castleberry AW, et al: Treatment modalities for T1N0 esophageal cancers: A comparative analysis of local therapy versus surgical resection. *J Thorac Oncol* 8:796–802, 2013.
34. Schnell TG, Sontag SJ, Chejfec G, et al: Long-term nonsurgical management of Barrett's esophagus with high-grade dysplasia. *Gastroenterology* 120:1607–1619, 2001.
35. de Jonge PJ, van Blankenstein M, Looman CW, et al: Risk of malignant progression in patients with Barrett's oesophagus: A Dutch nationwide cohort study. *Gut* 59:1030–1036, 2010.
36. Shaheen NJ, Sharma P, Overholt BF, et al: Radiofrequency ablation in Barrett's esophagus with dysplasia. *N Engl J Med* 360:2277–2288, 2009.
37. Phoa KN, van Vilsteren FG, Weusten BL, et al: Radiofrequency ablation vs endoscopic surveillance for patients with Barrett esophagus and low-grade dysplasia: A randomized clinical trial. *JAMA* 311:1209–1217, 2014.
38. Shaheen NJ, Greenwald BD, Peery AF, et al: Safety and efficacy of endoscopic spray cryotherapy for Barrett's esophagus with high-grade dysplasia. *Gastrointest Endosc* 71:680–685, 2010.
39. Gray NA, Odze RD, Spechler SJ: Buried metaplasia after endoscopic ablation of Barrett's esophagus: A systematic review. *Am J Gastroenterol* 106:1899–1908, quiz 1909, 2011.
40. Lee L, Ronellenfitsch U, Hofstetter WL, et al: Predicting lymph node metastases in early esophageal adenocarcinoma using a simple scoring system. *J Am Coll Surg* 217:191–199, 2013.
41. Ell C, May A, Pech O, et al: Curative endoscopic resection of early esophageal adenocarcinomas (Barrett's cancer). *Gastrointest Endosc* 65:3–10, 2007.
42. Shimada H, Nabeya Y, Matsubara H, et al: Prediction of lymph node status in patients with superficial esophageal carcinoma: Analysis of 160 surgically resected cancers. *Am J Surg* 191:250–254, 2006.
43. Gockel I, Sgourakis G, Lyros O, et al: Risk of lymph node metastasis in submucosal esophageal cancer: A review of surgically resected patients. *Expert Rev Gastroenterol Hepatol* 5:371–384, 2011.
44. Hirasawa K, Kokawa A, Oka H, et al: Superficial adenocarcinoma of the esophagogastric junction: Long-term results of endoscopic submucosal dissection. *Gastrointest Endosc* 72:960–966, 2010.
45. van Hagen P, Hulshof MC, van Lanschot JJ, et al: Preoperative chemoradiotherapy for esophageal or junctional cancer. *N Engl J Med* 366:2074–2084, 2012.
46. Speicher PJ, Ganapathi AM, Englum BR, et al: Induction therapy does not improve survival for clinical stage T2N0 esophageal cancer. *J Thorac Oncol* 9:1195–1201, 2014.
47. Ajani JA, Roth JA, Ryan B, et al: Evaluation of pre- and postoperative chemotherapy for resectable adenocarcinoma of the esophagus or gastroesophageal junction. *J Clin Oncol* 8:1231–1238, 1990.
48. Cools-Lartigue J, Spicer J, Ferri LE: Current status of management of malignant disease: Current management of esophageal cancer. *J Gastrointest Surg* 19:964–972, 2015.
49. Roth JA, Pass HI, Flanagan MM, et al: Randomized clinical trial of preoperative and postoperative adjuvant chemotherapy with cisplatin, vindesine, and bleomycin for carcinoma

of the esophagus. *J Thorac Cardiovasc Surg* 96:242–248, 1988.

50. Kelsen DP, Winter KA, Gunderson LL, et al: Long-term results of RTOG trial 8911 (USA Intergroup 113): A random assignment trial comparison of chemotherapy followed by surgery compared with surgery alone for esophageal cancer. *J Clin Oncol* 25:3719–3725, 2007.
51. Medical Research Council Oesophageal Cancer Working Group: Surgical resection with or without preoperative chemotherapy in oesophageal cancer: A randomised controlled trial. *Lancet* 359:1727–1733, 2002.
52. Cunningham D, Allum WH, Stenning SP, et al: Perioperative chemotherapy versus surgery alone for resectable gastroesophageal cancer. *N Engl J Med* 355:11–20, 2006.
53. Ando N, Kato H, Igaki H, et al: A randomized trial comparing postoperative adjuvant chemotherapy with cisplatin and 5-fluorouracil versus preoperative chemotherapy for localized advanced squamous cell carcinoma of the thoracic esophagus (JCOG9907). *Ann Surg Oncol* 19:68–74, 2012.
54. Armanios M, Xu R, Forastiere AA, et al: Adjuvant chemotherapy for resected adenocarcinoma of the esophagus, gastro-esophageal junction, and cardia: Phase II trial (E8296) of the Eastern Cooperative Oncology Group. *J Clin Oncol* 22:4495–4499, 2004.
55. Ferri LE, Ades S, Alcindor T, et al: Perioperative docetaxel, cisplatin, and 5-fluorouracil (DCF) for locally advanced esophageal and gastric adenocarcinoma: A multicenter phase II trial. *Ann Oncol* 23:1512–1517, 2012.
56. Minsky BD, Pajak TF, Ginsberg RJ, et al: INT 0123 (Radiation Therapy Oncology Group 94-05) phase III trial of combined-modality therapy for esophageal cancer: High-dose versus standard-dose radiation therapy. *J Clin Oncol* 20:1167–1174, 2002.
57. Shapiro J, van Lanschot JJ, Hulshof MC, et al: Neoadjuvant chemoradiotherapy plus surgery versus surgery alone for oesophageal or junctional cancer (CROSS): Long-term results of a randomised controlled trial. *Lancet Oncol* 16:1090–1098, 2015.
58. Francis AM, Sepesi B, Correa AM, et al: The influence of histopathologic tumor viability on long-term survival and recurrence rates following neoadjuvant therapy for esophageal adenocarcinoma. *Ann Surg* 258:500–507, 2013.
59. Stahl M, Walz MK, Stuschke M, et al: Phase III comparison of preoperative chemotherapy compared with chemoradiotherapy in patients with locally advanced adenocarcinoma of the esophagogastric junction. *J Clin Oncol* 27:851–856, 2009.
60. Burmeister BH, Thomas JM, Burmeister EA, et al: Is concurrent radiation therapy required in patients receiving preoperative chemotherapy for adenocarcinoma of the oesophagus? A randomised phase II trial. *Eur J Cancer* 47:354–360, 2011.
61. Sjoquist KM, Burmeister BH, Smithers BM, et al: Survival after neoadjuvant chemotherapy or chemoradiotherapy for resectable oesophageal carcinoma: An updated meta-analysis. *Lancet Oncol* 12:681–692, 2011.
62. Bedenne L, Michel P, Bouche O, et al: Chemoradiation followed by surgery compared with chemoradiation alone in squamous cancer of the esophagus: FFCD 9102. *J Clin Oncol* 25:1160–1168, 2007.
63. Stahl M, Stuschke M, Lehmann N, et al: Chemoradiation with and without surgery in patients with locally advanced squamous cell carcinoma of the esophagus. *J Clin Oncol* 23:2310–2317, 2005.
64. Murphy CC, Correa AM, Ajani JA, et al: Surgery is an essential component of multimodality therapy for patients with locally advanced esophageal adenocarcinoma. *J Gastrointest Surg* 17:1359–1369, 2013.
65. Swisher SG, Winter KA, Komaki RU, et al: A phase II study of a paclitaxel-based chemoradiation regimen with selective surgical salvage for resectable locoregionally advanced esophageal cancer: Initial reporting of RTOG 0246. *Int J Radiat Oncol Biol Phys* 82:1967–1972, 2012.

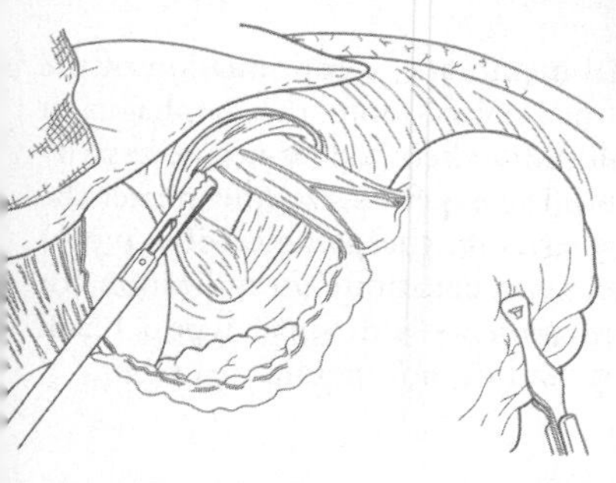

CHAPTER 42

Gastroesophageal Reflux Disease and Hiatal Hernia

Robert B. Yates, Brant K. Oelschlager, Carlos A. Pellegrini

OUTLINE

Gastroesophageal reflux disease (GERD) is the most common benign medical condition of the stomach and esophagus. In patients with GERD who experience persistent life-limiting symptoms despite maximal medical therapy, antireflux surgery should be strongly considered. The application of laparoscopy to antireflux surgery has decreased perioperative morbidity, hospital length of stay, and cost compared with open operations. Conceptually, laparoscopic antireflux surgery (LARS) is straightforward; however, the correct construction of a fundoplication requires significant operative experience and skills in complex laparoscopy. In patients who present with late complications of antireflux surgery, including recurrent GERD and dysphagia, reoperative antireflux surgery can be effectively performed. Compared with first-time operations, however, reoperative antireflux surgery is technically more challenging, is associated with higher risk of perioperative complications, and results in less durable symptom improvement. Consequently, surgeons should have a higher threshold for performing reoperative antireflux surgery, and reoperations should be performed by experienced, high-volume gastroesophageal surgeons. To decrease perioperative risk and to maximize long-term relief of GERD symptoms, surgeons must be familiar with all aspects of preoperative evaluation and operative management of patients with GERD.

Hernias at the esophageal hiatus span the spectrum from a small sliding hiatal hernia to a large paraesophageal hernia (PEH). Similarly, the symptoms of PEH can vary from mild gastroesophageal obstructive symptoms to severe, acute complications, including gastric volvulus, which requires immediate intervention. The repair of a large PEH is challenging, but when it is performed at high-volume centers by experienced surgeons, hiatal hernia and PEH can be repaired safely and provide patients with long-lasting control of gastroesophageal symptoms.

GASTROESOPHAGEAL REFLUX DISEASE

Pathophysiology

Endogenous antireflux mechanisms include the lower esophageal sphincter (LES) and spontaneous esophageal clearance. GERD results from the failure of these endogenous antireflux mechanisms.

The LES has the primary role of preventing reflux of gastric contents into the esophagus. Rather than a distinct anatomic structure, the LES is a zone of high pressure located in the lower end of the esophagus. The LES can be identified with esophageal manometry.

The LES is made up of four anatomic structures:

1. The *intrinsic musculature of the distal esophagus* is in a state of tonic contraction. Within 500 milliseconds of the initiation of a swallow, these muscle fibers relax to allow passage of liquid or food into the stomach, and then they return to a state of tonic contraction.
2. *Sling fibers of the gastric cardia* are oriented diagonally from the cardia-fundus junction to the lesser curve of the stomach. Located at the same anatomic depth as the circular muscle fibers of the esophagus, the sling fibers contribute significantly to the high-pressure zone of the LES (Fig. 42-1).
3. The *crura of the diaphragm* surround the esophagus as it passes through the esophageal hiatus. During inspiration, when intrathoracic pressure decreases relative to intra-abdominal pressure, the anteroposterior diameter of the crural opening is decreased, compressing the esophagus and increasing the measured pressure at the LES. Because of this fluctuation in LES pressure, it is important to measure the LES pressure at mid-expiration or end-expiration.
4. When the gastroesophageal junction (GEJ) is firmly anchored in the abdominal cavity, *increased intra-abdominal pressure* is transmitted to the GEJ, which increases the pressure on the distal esophagus and prevents spontaneous reflux of gastric contents.

Gastroesophageal reflux (GER) occurs when intragastric pressure is greater than the high-pressure zone of the distal esophagus. This can develop under two conditions: the LES resting pressure is too low (i.e., hypotensive LES); and the LES relaxes in the absence of peristaltic contraction of the esophagus (i.e., spontaneous LES relaxation). Hypotensive LES is frequently associated with hiatal hernia because of displacement of the GEJ into the posterior mediastinum. However, hypotensive LES can occur in its normal anatomic position, and even small changes in the high-pressure zone can compromise its effectiveness. Consequently, it is important to recognize that GER is a normal physiologic process that occurs even in the setting of a normal LES. The distinction between physiologic reflux (i.e., GER) and pathologic reflux (i.e., GERD) hinges on the total amount of esophageal acid exposure, the patient's symptoms, and the presence of mucosal damage of the esophagus.

Hiatal hernias are often associated with GERD because their abnormal anatomy compromises the efficacy of the LES. Hiatal hernias are classified into four types (I to IV). Type I hiatal hernia (Fig. 42-2*A*), also called a sliding hiatal hernia, is the most common. A type I hernia is present when the GEJ migrates cephalad into the posterior mediastinum. This occurs because of laxity of the phrenoesophageal membrane, a continuation of the endoabdominal peritoneum that reflects onto the esophagus at the hiatus (Fig. 42-3). A small sliding hernia does not necessarily imply an incompetent LES, but the larger its size, the greater the risk for abnormal GER. Furthermore, the presence of a type I sliding hiatal hernia alone does not constitute an indication for operative repair. In fact, many patients with small type I hiatal hernias do not have symptoms and do not require treatment.

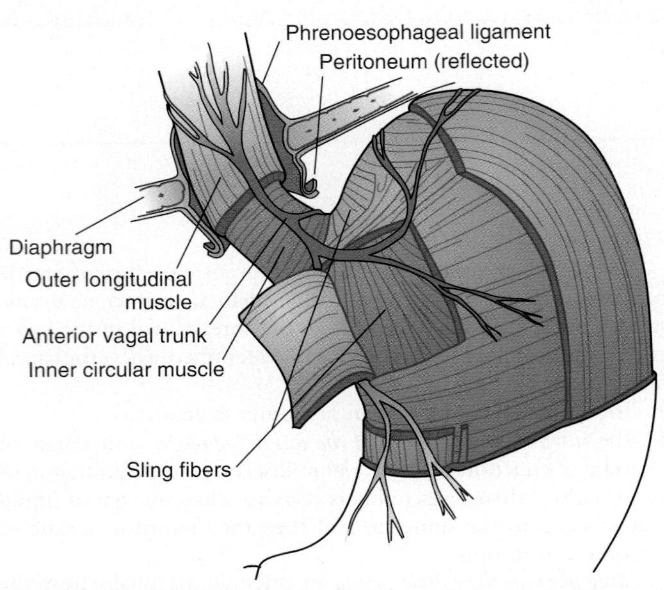

FIGURE 42-1 Schematic drawing of the muscle layers at the gastroesophageal junction. The intrinsic muscle of the esophagus, diaphragm, and sling fibers contribute to lower esophageal sphincter pressure. The circular muscle fibers of the esophagus are at the same depth as the sling fibers of the cardia.

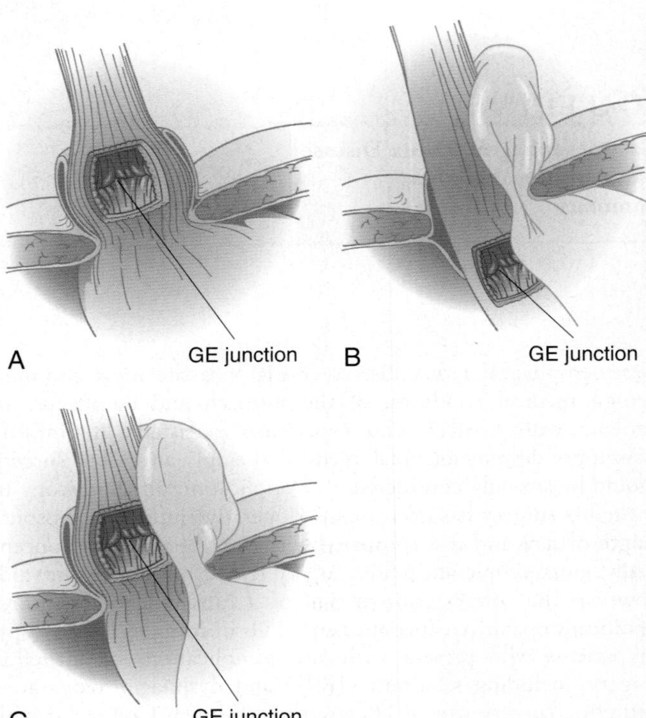

FIGURE 42-2 The three types of hiatal hernia. **A,** Type I is also called a sliding hernia. **B,** Type II is known as a rolling hernia. **C,** Type III is referred to as a mixed hernia. *GE,* gastroesophageal.

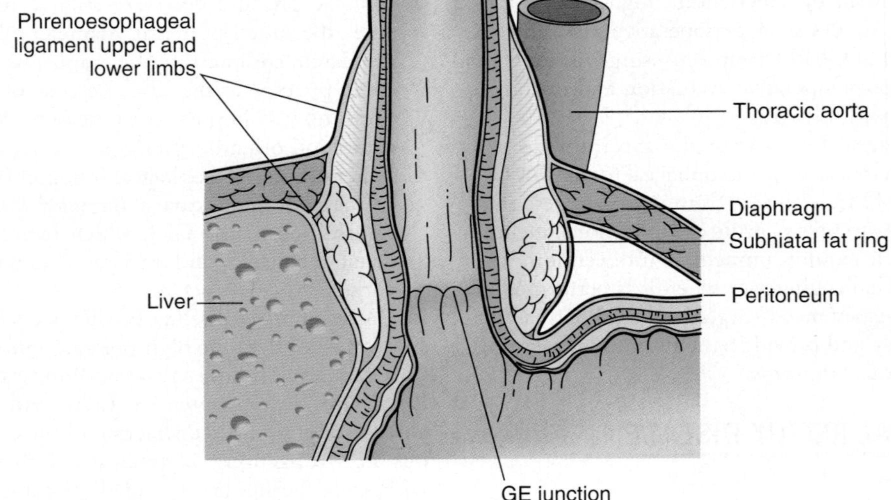

FIGURE 42-3 Section of the gastroesophageal (GE) junction demonstrates the relationship of the peritoneum to the phrenoesophageal membrane. The phrenoesophageal membrane continues as a separate structure into the posterior mediastinum. The parietal peritoneum continues as the visceral peritoneum as it reflects onto the stomach.

Hiatal hernia types II to IV, also referred to as PEH, are frequently associated with gastroesophageal obstructive symptoms (e.g., dysphagia, early satiety, and epigastric pain). However, they can also be associated with GERD. A type II hernia (Fig. 42-2*B*) occurs when the GEJ is anchored in the abdomen, and the gastric fundus migrates into the mediastinum through the hiatal defect. A type III hernia (Fig. 42-2*C*) is characterized by both the GEJ and fundus located in the mediastinum. Finally, a type IV hernia occurs when any visceral structure (e.g., colon, spleen, pancreas, or small bowel) migrates cephalad to the esophageal hiatus and is located in the mediastinum. For more information on PEH, refer to the last section of this chapter.

Clinical Presentation

Typical Symptoms of GERD

The prevalence of symptoms among 1000 patients with GERD is presented in Table 42-1. Heartburn, regurgitation, and water brash are the three typical esophageal symptoms of GERD. Heartburn and regurgitation are the most common presenting symptoms. Heartburn is specific to GERD and described as an epigastric or retrosternal caustic or stinging sensation. Typically, it does not radiate to the back and is not described as a pressure sensation, which are more characteristic of pancreatitis and acute coronary syndrome, respectively. It is important to ask the patient about his or her symptoms in detail to differentiate typical heartburn from symptoms of peptic ulcer disease, cholelithiasis, or coronary artery disease.

The presence of regurgitation often indicates progression of GERD. In severe cases, patients will be unable to bend over without experiencing an episode of regurgitation. Regurgitation of gastric contents to the oropharynx and mouth can produce a sour taste that patients will describe as either acid or bile. This phenomenon is referred to as water brash. In patients who report regurgitation as a frequent symptom, it is important to distinguish between regurgitation of undigested food and regurgitation of digested food. Regurgitation of undigested food is not common in GERD and suggests the presence of a different pathologic process, such as an esophageal diverticulum or achalasia.

Extraesophageal Symptoms of GERD

Extraesophageal symptoms of GERD arise from the respiratory tract and include both laryngeal and pulmonary symptoms (Box 42-1). Two mechanisms may lead to extraesophageal symptoms of GERD. First, proximal esophageal reflux and microaspiration of gastroduodenal contents cause direct caustic injury to the larynx and lower respiratory tract; this is the most common mechanism. Second, distal esophageal acid exposure triggers a vagal nerve reflex that results in bronchospasm and cough. The latter mechanism is due to the common vagal innervation of the trachea and esophagus.

Unlike typical GERD symptoms (i.e., heartburn and regurgitation), extraesophageal symptoms of reflux are not specific to GERD. Before LARS is performed, it is necessary to determine whether a patient's extraesophageal symptoms are due to abnormal GER or a primary laryngeal, bronchial, or pulmonary cause. This can be challenging. A lack of response of extraesophageal symptoms to proton pump inhibitor (PPI) therapy cannot reliably refute GERD as the cause of these symptoms. Although PPI therapy can improve or completely resolve *typical* GERD symptoms, patients with *extraesophageal symptoms* experience variable response to medical treatment. This may be explained by recent evidence suggesting that acid is not the only underlying caustic agent resulting in laryngeal and pulmonary injury.[1] PPI therapy will suppress gastric acid production, but microaspiration of nonacid refluxate, which contains caustic bile salts and pepsin, can cause ongoing injury and symptoms. Therefore, in patients with extraesophageal symptoms of GERD, a mechanical barrier to reflux (i.e., esophagogastric fundoplication) may be necessary to prevent ongoing laryngeal, tracheal, or bronchial injury.

In patients who present with abnormal GER and bothersome extraesophageal symptoms, a thorough evaluation must be completed to rule out a primary disorder of the upper or lower respiratory tract. This should be completed whether or not typical GERD symptoms are also present. At the University of Washington Center for Esophageal and Gastric Surgery, we frequently refer patients with GERD and extraesophageal symptoms to a laryngologist or a pulmonologist to determine if a nongastrointestinal condition is causing these symptoms. If a nonreflux cause of the extraesophageal symptoms cannot be identified, then proceeding with an antireflux operation is acceptable. We counsel these patients a 70% likelihood of improvement in extraesophageal symptoms after LARS.[2] If a patient's laryngeal or pulmonary

TABLE 42-1 Prevalence of Symptoms Occurring More Frequently Than Once per Week in 1000 Patients With GERD

SYMPTOM	PREVALENCE (%)
Heartburn	80
Regurgitation	54
Abdominal pain	29
Cough	27
Dysphagia for solids	23
Hoarseness	21
Belching	15
Bloating	15
Aspiration	14
Wheezing	7
Globus	4

BOX 42-1 Extraesophageal Symptoms of GERD

Laryngeal Symptoms of Reflux

Hoarseness or dysphonia
Throat clearing
Throat pain
Globus
Choking
Postnasal drip
Laryngeal and tracheal stenosis
Laryngospasm
Contact ulcers

Pulmonary Symptoms of Reflux

Cough
Shortness of breath
Wheezing
Pulmonary disease (asthma, idiopathic pulmonary fibrosis, chronic bronchitis, and others)

symptoms are not due to abnormal GER, an antireflux operation is not performed.

Pulmonary Disease, GERD, and Antireflux Surgery

Increasing evidence suggests that GERD is a contributing factor to the pathophysiologic mechanism of several pulmonary diseases. In their extensive review, Bowrey and colleagues[3] examined medical and surgical antireflux therapy in patients with GERD and asthma. In these patients, the use of antisecretory medications is associated with improved respiratory symptoms in only 25% to 50% of patients with GERD-induced asthma. Furthermore, less than 15% of these patients experience objective improvement in pulmonary function. One explanation for these results is that most of these studies lasted 3 months or less, which is potentially too short to see any improvement in pulmonary function. In addition, in several trials, gastric acid secretion was incompletely blocked by acid suppression therapy, and patients experienced ongoing GERD.

In patients with asthma and GERD, antireflux surgery appears to be more effective than medical therapy at managing pulmonary symptoms. Antireflux surgery is associated with improvement in respiratory symptoms in nearly 90% of children and 70% of adults with asthma and GERD. Several randomized trials have compared histamine 2 receptor antagonists and antireflux surgery in the management of GERD-associated asthma. Compared with patients treated with antisecretory medications, patients treated with antireflux surgery were more likely to experience relief of asthma symptoms, to discontinue systemic steroid therapy, and to improve peak expiratory flow rate.

Idiopathic pulmonary fibrosis (IPF) is a severe, chronic, and progressive lung disease that generally results in death within 5 years of diagnosis. Proximal esophageal reflux with microaspiration of acid and nonacid gastric contents has been implicated as one possible cause of alveolar epithelial injury that can lead to IPF. The incidence of GERD in patients with IPF has been reported to be as high as 94%.[4] Because typical symptoms of GERD are not sensitive for abnormal reflux in patients with IPF, the threshold for testing patients with IPF for GERD should be low.

Medical treatment of GERD in patients with IPF is associated with longer survival and slower pulmonary decline.[5] Whereas this is promising, PPI therapy does not prevent reflux of nonacid gastroduodenal contents, which may contribute to ongoing pulmonary injury in some patients. Therefore, in IPF patients with significant GERD, the argument could be made that a mechanical barrier to both acid and nonacid reflux (i.e., LARS) is more appropriate than PPI therapy. Although very little literature exists on LARS in patients with IPF, it appears to be safe and to provide effective control of distal esophageal acid exposure, and it may mitigate decline in pulmonary function.[6] At the time of this publication, a National Institutes of Health–funded multicenter prospectively randomized trial in patients with IPF and GERD is comparing LARS with PPI therapy. The results of this study may profoundly affect the management of these patients.

Physical Examination

Except in patients with severely advanced disease, the physical examination rarely contributes to confirmation of the diagnosis of GERD. In such patients, several observations may suggest the presence of GERD. For example, a patient who constantly drinks water during the interview may be facilitating esophageal clearance, which can suggest frequent reflux. Other patients with advanced disease will sit leaning forward and carry out the interview with their lungs inflated to almost vital capacity. This maneuver flattens the diaphragm, narrows the anteroposterior diameter of the hiatus, and increases the LES pressure to counteract GER. Patients who have severe proximal esophageal reflux and regurgitation of gastric contents into the mouth may develop erosion of their dentition (revealing yellow teeth caused by the loss of dentin), injected oropharyngeal mucosa, or signs of chronic sinusitis.

Although physical examination findings are generally not specific for GERD, the physical examination may be helpful in determining the presence of other disease processes. For example, supraclavicular lymphadenopathy in a patient with heartburn and dysphagia may suggest esophageal or gastric cancer. Similarly, if the patient's retrosternal pain is reproducible with palpation, a musculoskeletal source of the pain should be investigated. Short of these extreme presentations, the physical examination is generally not helpful in confirming or excluding GER as a pathologic entity.

Preoperative Diagnostic Testing

Frequently, the diagnosis of GERD is based on the presence of typical symptoms and improvement in those symptoms with PPI therapy. However, when a surgeon evaluates a patient for antireflux surgery, four diagnostic tests are useful to establish the diagnosis of GERD and to identify abnormalities in gastroesophageal anatomy and function that may have an impact on the performance of LARS.

Ambulatory pH and Impedance Monitoring

Ambulatory pH monitoring quantifies distal esophageal acid exposure and is the "gold standard" test to diagnose GERD. A 24-hour pH monitoring is conducted with a thin catheter that is passed into the esophagus through the patient's nares. The simplest catheter is a dual-probe pH catheter, which contains two solid-state electrodes that are spaced 10 cm apart and detect fluctuations in pH between 2 and 7. To ensure valid study results, the distal electrode must be placed 5 cm proximal to the LES; the location of the LES is identified on esophageal manometry (see next section). Alternatively, 48-hour ambulatory pH monitoring can be performed using an endoscopically placed wireless pH monitor.

Ambulatory pH monitoring generates a large amount of data concerning esophageal acid exposure, including total number of reflux episodes (pH < 4), longest episode of reflux, number of episodes lasting longer than 5 minutes, and percentage of time spent in reflux in the upright and supine positions. A formula assigns each of these data points a relative weight according to its capacity to cause esophageal injury, and the composite DeMeester score is calculated. Abnormal distal esophageal acid exposure is defined by a DeMeester score of 14.7 or higher.

In addition to these objective data, the patient can keep track of reflux-related symptoms by pressing a button on an electronic data recorder. During the interpretation of the pH study, symptom index and symptom-associated probability are calculated on the basis of the temporal relationship between the symptom event and episodes of distal esophageal acid exposure (Fig. 42-4). A symptom episode that occurs within 2 minutes of a reflux episode is defined as a close temporal relationship and suggests but does not confirm a cause and effect relationship between GER and the patient's symptoms. When interpreting these studies, it should be remembered that patients often do not maintain their normal activities and eating patterns when they have the catheter in place.

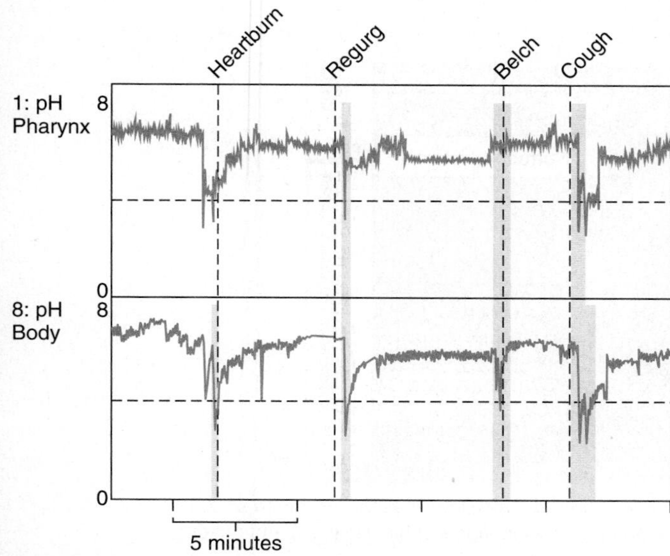

FIGURE 42-4 A 1-hour segment from a 24-hour ambulatory pH study. Time is marked on the x-axis, and pH is marked on the y-axis. Symptom events are marked along the top of the tracing. (Courtesy University of Washington Center for Esophageal and Gastric Surgery, Seattle.)

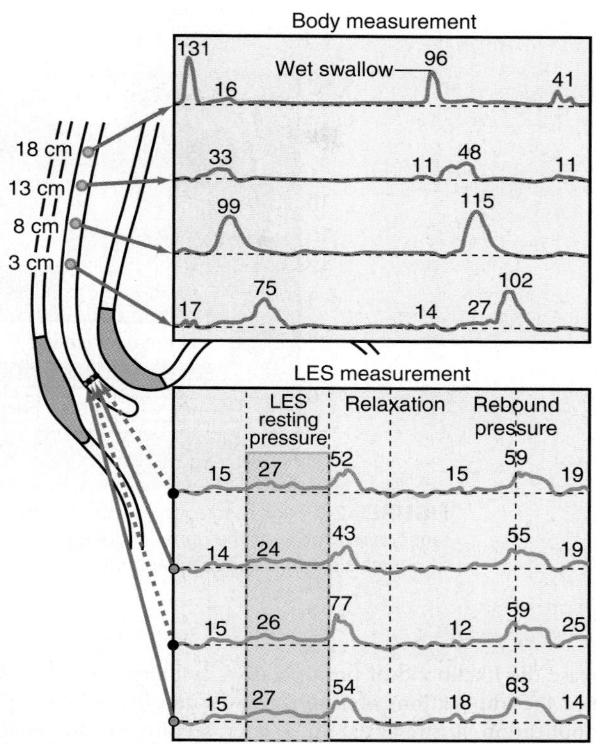

FIGURE 42-5 Representative linear tracings from standard esophageal manometry. A wet swallow initiates both esophageal peristalsis and lower esophageal sphincter (LES) relaxation.

Consequently, their symptoms may not be as prevalent during the study period. Whereas the decision to perform LARS should not hinge on symptom correlation, it can help predict symptom improvement after LARS.[7]

Esophageal impedance monitoring identifies episodes of nonacid reflux. Similar to 24-hour pH monitoring, esophageal impedance is performed with a thin, flexible catheter placed through the patient's nares into the esophagus. Impedance catheters use electrodes placed at 1-cm intervals to detect changes in the resistance to flow of an electrical current (i.e., impedance). Impedance increases in the presence of air and decreases in the presence of a liquid bolus. Therefore, this technology can detect both gas and liquid movement in the esophagus.

Some impedance catheters also have one or more pH sensors, allowing the simultaneous detection of acid and nonacid reflux. When pH-impedance catheters are used, it is possible to determine the direction of movement of esophageal acid exposures and therefore to differentiate between an antegrade event (as in a swallow) and a retrograde event (as in GER). There also exists a specialized pH-impedance catheter with a very proximal pH sensor that detects pharyngeal acid reflux. This catheter can be useful in the evaluation of patients with extraesophageal symptoms, such as cough, throat clearing, hoarseness, and wheezing. One disadvantage of impedance technology, however, is that the automated analytic software is very sensitive and tends to overestimate the number of nonacid reflux episodes, mandating that these studies be manually reviewed and edited, which can be time-consuming.

Combined impedance-pH monitoring has been shown to identify reflux episodes with greater sensitivity than pH testing alone.[8] Although there is no consensus on whether impedance-pH testing should be performed on or off acid suppression therapy, our practice is to perform all impedance-pH testing off acid suppression. Furthermore, how impedance-pH monitoring should guide the management of GERD is unknown. Patel and colleagues[9] attempted to determine the parameters on esophageal impedance-pH monitoring that predict response of GERD symptoms to both medical and surgical treatment. They showed that acid exposure time, and not the number of nonacid reflux events, best predicted symptom improvement with both medical and surgical therapy. Although the addition of impedance monitoring increased the sensitivity of the study, nonacid reflux measurements alone were unable to accurately predict symptom response to medical or surgical therapy for GERD.

Esophageal Manometry

Esophageal manometry is the most effective way to assess function of the esophageal body and the LES. Standard esophageal manometry provides linear tracings of pressure waves of the esophageal body and LES (Fig. 42-5). High-resolution esophageal manometry gathers data using a 32-channel flexible catheter with pressure-sensing devices arranged at 1-cm intervals, placed into the esophagus through the nares; the study is conducted in approximately 15 minutes, during which time the patient performs 10 swallows. A color-contour plot is generated and shows the response of the upper esophageal sphincter and LES as well as of the esophageal body; time is on the x-axis, esophageal length is on the y-axis, and pressure is represented by a color scale (Fig. 42-6). In patients undergoing evaluation for GERD, esophageal manometry can exclude achalasia and identify patients with ineffective esophageal body peristalsis. Repeated exposure of the esophagus to gastric reflux can lead to esophageal motility disorders; in one study, 25% of patients with mild esophagitis demonstrated esophageal dysmotility, whereas 48% of patients with severe esophagitis had impaired motility on manometry.[10] In patients with significant esophageal dysmotility who are undergoing LARS, the surgeon should consider a partial fundoplication to

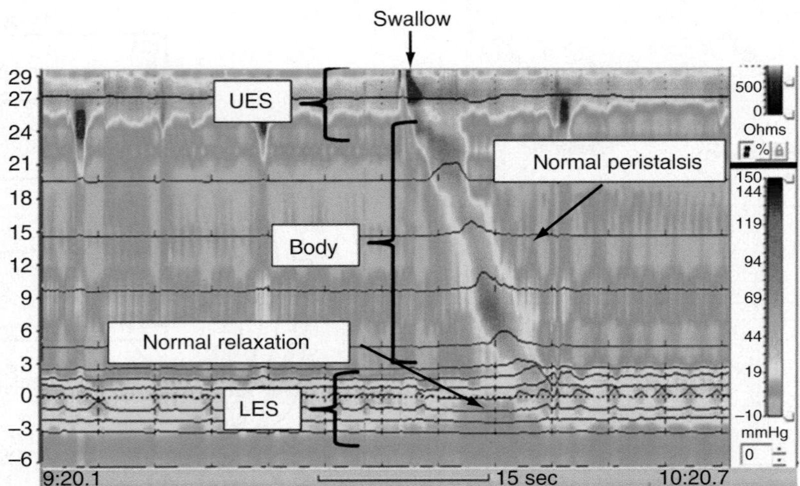

FIGURE 42-6 High-resolution esophageal manometry. The initiation of a swallow is associated with simultaneous relaxation of the upper esophageal sphincter (UES) and lower esophageal sphincter (LES) and onset of peristalsis in the esophageal body.

decrease the likelihood of postoperative dysphagia. A full discussion of the implications of esophageal dysmotility on the type of fundoplication is presented in a later section of this chapter. Esophageal manometry also measures the LES resting pressure and assesses the LES for appropriate relaxation with deglutition. Because the LES is the major barrier to GER, a defective LES is common in patients with GERD.

Esophagogastroduodenoscopy

Endoscopy is an essential step in the evaluation of patients with GERD who are being considered for LARS. The esophagus should be examined for evidence of mucosal injury due to GER, including ulcerations, peptic strictures, and Barrett esophagus. Esophagitis can be reported according to several scoring systems, including the Savary-Miller and Los Angeles (LA) classifications.[11] Both peptic strictures and LA class C and D esophagitis can be considered pathognomonic for GERD. Consequently, ambulatory pH monitoring is unnecessary in these patients. However, because of significant interobserver variability in LA class A and B esophagitis, these forms of mild esophagitis cannot be considered reliable markers of GERD.[12] As such, patients found to have LA class A and B esophagitis should undergo pH testing to confirm abnormal distal esophageal acid exposure.

Endoscopic evaluation should also include an assessment of the GEJ flap valve. To do this, the endoscope is retroflexed 180 degrees in the stomach to visualize the GEJ from below. The flap valve is graded 1 to 4, according to the length of the valve and how tightly it adheres to the endoscope. The endoscopist should make note of the presence of a hiatal hernia, and the hernia should be measured in both cranial-caudal and lateral dimensions. In patients who are being evaluated for persistent or recurrent gastroesophageal symptoms after an antireflux operation or PEH repair, it is recommended that the surgeon who is evaluating the patient perform the endoscopy. This allows the operating surgeon to correlate endoscopic findings with the patient's symptoms and data obtained on 24-hour pH monitoring, esophageal manometry, and upper gastrointestinal (UGI) series to determine if a functional or anatomic abnormality exists that can be corrected with reoperation.

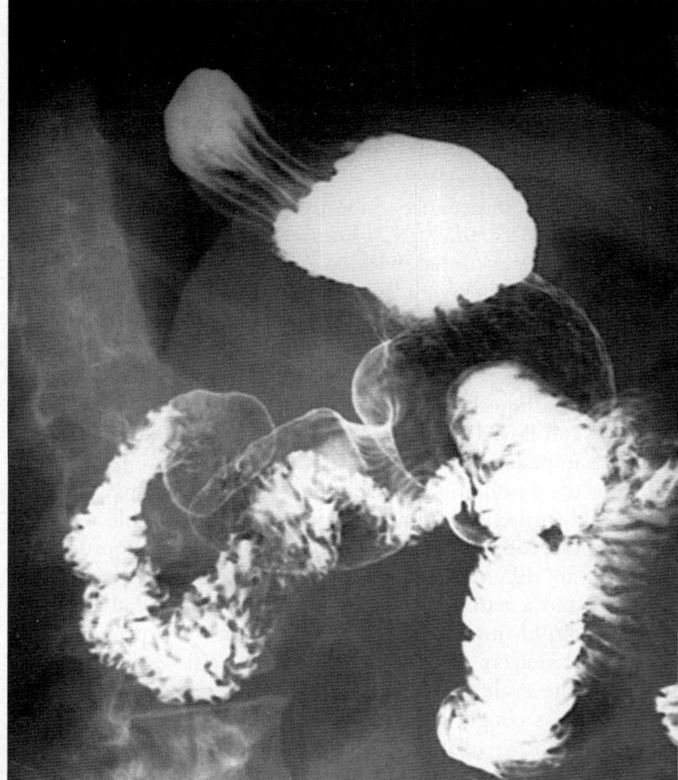

FIGURE 42-7 Upper gastrointestinal series demonstrating a large hiatal hernia. The rugal folds of the stomach clearly transgress the shadow of the left hemidiaphragm.

Barium Esophagram

Barium esophagram provides a detailed anatomic evaluation of the esophagus and stomach that is useful during preoperative evaluation of patients with GERD. Of particular importance are the presence, size, and anatomic characteristics of a hiatal hernia or PEH (Fig. 42-7). For example, a GEJ that is fixed in the posterior mediastinum on esophagography can suggest a more difficult operation that may require a more extensive intrathoracic esophageal mobilization. Despite its ability to identify episodes of GER, which can occur spontaneously or in response to positioning of the patient during the study, barium esophagram cannot confirm or refute the diagnosis of GERD. On occasion, patients presenting to the surgical clinic for evaluation of GERD may have already undergone computed tomography scan of the chest or abdomen to evaluate atypical symptoms of GERD (e.g., chest or abdominal pain). Horizontal images as well as coronal and sagittal reconstructions can provide information concerning the anatomic relationship of the stomach and esophagus to other abdominal and thoracic structures. However, we still prefer to obtain a barium esophagram as computed tomography scan frequently fails to identify important anatomic and functional gastroesophageal disease.

Additional gastroesophageal conditions that can be identified on barium esophagram are esophageal diverticula, tumors, peptic strictures, achalasia, dysmotility, and gastroparesis. If any one of these is found in a patient undergoing evaluation for GERD, LARS should be delayed until appropriate evaluation of the unexpected findings is completed.

Additional Preoperative Considerations

Dysphagia

Patients with GERD will occasionally experience dysphagia. The causes of dysphagia are listed in Box 42-2. In patients with GERD, the most common cause of dysphagia is a reflux-associated inflammatory process of the esophageal wall. This inflammation can be manifested as a Schatzki ring, a diffuse distal esophageal inflammation, or a peptic stricture. Although relatively rare since the widespread adoption of PPI therapy, peptic strictures are pathognomonic for long-standing reflux and develop from the chronic mucosal inflammation that occurs with GERD. When strictures result in significant dysphagia, patients can experience weight loss and protein-calorie malnutrition. In addition, strictures can be associated with esophageal shortening, which makes obtaining adequate intra-abdominal esophageal length at the time of operation more difficult (see "Intraoperative Management of Short Esophagus").

In patients with peptic strictures, it can be challenging to document abnormal GER on ambulatory pH monitoring because the presence of a tight stricture may prevent reflux of acid, resulting in a false-negative pH study. In patients with typical GERD symptoms and a peptic stricture, it is reasonable to forego ambulatory pH monitoring because the presence of a peptic stricture is considered pathognomonic for severe GER. If pH monitoring is performed, it is ideally completed after dilation of the stricture to increase the validity of the test. Importantly, because they are associated with long-standing GER, peptic strictures should be biopsied to rule out intestinal metaplasia, dysplasia, and malignancy.

The majority of peptic strictures are effectively treated with dilation and PPI therapy. Successful dilation can be performed with either a balloon dilator or Savary dilator, and no strong data exist to support the superiority of one dilation technique over another. Refractory peptic strictures are defined as strictures that recur despite dilation and PPI therapy. Although rare, refractory strictures can pose a significant challenge to surgeons and gastroenterologists. In these patients, LARS should strongly be considered. For patients who are unfit for or do not wish to undergo an operation, steroid injections of the stricture have been shown to result in fewer dilations.[13]

Another cause of dysphagia in patients with GERD is a Schatzki ring. Similar to peptic strictures, these are located in the distal esophagus. However, Schatzki rings are submucosal fibrotic bands (as opposed to mucosal strictures). Typically, peptic strictures and Schatzki rings can be differentiated on endoscopy. Both should be dilated to relieve obstruction, but Schatzki rings develop in the submucosal space, so in the absence of other endoscopically identified mucosal abnormalities, biopsies do not need to be performed. Furthermore, Schatzki rings are not pathognomonic for GERD, so abnormal distal esophageal acid exposure must be documented on ambulatory pH monitoring to confirm the presence of abnormal GER before LARS is performed.

Dysphagia in patients with GERD may not have a clear anatomic cause, and mild dysphagia in these patients may simply be due to the esophageal inflammation that results from persistent GER. This type of dysphagia tends to resolve after abnormal reflux is controlled. In patients who present with dysphagia and GERD, other causes of dysphagia must be excluded, including tumors, diverticula, and esophageal motor disorders. Although these conditions are much less common than peptic stricture and Schatzki ring, they require dramatically different treatments. In patients who report simultaneous onset of dysphagia to liquids and solids, one must have a high suspicion for a neuromuscular or autoimmune disorder as the etiology. Finally, some patients with severe GERD experience dysphagia without exhibiting an anatomic or physiologic abnormality of the esophagus. This is believed to be caused by inflammation associated with reflux, and we have found that such patients typically experience improvement in dysphagia after LARS.

BOX 42-2 Potential Causes of Dysphagia in Patients Undergoing Evaluation for GERD

Esophageal Obstruction
- Peptic strictures
- Schatzki ring
- Malignant neoplasm
- Benign neoplasm
- Foreign body

Esophageal Motility Disorders
- Diffuse esophageal spasm
- Hypercontractile ("Jackhammer") esophagus
- Ineffective esophageal motility
- Achalasia

Obesity

Obesity is a significant risk factor for the development of GERD. Compared with patients of normal weight, obese patients have increased intra-abdominal pressure, decreased LES pressure, and more frequent transient LES relaxations. Obese patients with GERD present a particular challenge to surgeons. Whereas it is clear that LARS can be performed safely in obese patients, the literature is mixed on the ability of LARS to provide long-term control of GERD-related symptoms. In appropriately selected patients, laparoscopic Roux-en-Y gastric bypass is the most durable method of weight loss and control of obesity-related comorbidities, including GERD. In severely obese patients with GERD, serious consideration should be given to performing a laparoscopic Roux-en-Y gastric bypass instead of a fundoplication. Ultimately, the decision to pursue gastric bypass instead of fundoplication must include a careful balance of the patient's interest in bariatric surgery, presence of other medical comorbidities, and availability of a surgeon to perform the operation.

Partial versus Complete Fundoplication

Antireflux operations include partial posterior (180- and 270-degree), partial anterior (90- and 180-degree), and 360-degree esophagogastric fundoplications. In the field of antireflux surgery, there has been a long-standing debate about which fundoplication provides superior control of GERD symptoms while mitigating postoperative side effects (e.g., dysphagia and gas-bloat). Furthermore, studies have attempted to determine whether the type of fundoplication performed should be tailored to the patient's preoperative esophageal motility and symptoms.

In patients with GERD and esophageal dysmotility, it has been suggested that partial fundoplication should be performed because of concern that a Nissen fundoplication will lead to greater postoperative dysphagia. Booth and colleagues[14] completed a randomized controlled trial to compare laparoscopic Nissen fundoplication with Toupet fundoplication in patients who were stratified on the basis of preoperative manometry. At 1 year postoperatively, there were no differences between Nissen and Toupet groups for heartburn and regurgitation. Dysphagia was more frequent in patients who underwent Nissen fundoplication. However, when a Nissen fundoplication was constructed, patients with normal and impaired esophageal motility experienced similar rates of postoperative dysphagia. Similarly, we have shown that a Nissen fundoplication can be performed in patients with ineffective esophageal motility without an increase in development of dysphagia.[15]

Fein and Seyfried[16] reviewed nine randomized trials that evaluated laparoscopic anterior, partial posterior, and total fundoplications in the management of GERD. Anterior fundoplication was associated with greater risk of recurrent GERD symptoms. In several studies, Nissen fundoplication was associated with increased postoperative dysphagia, but these patients required minimal treatment and no reoperations. In randomized trials, no difference in gas-bloat symptoms was seen between Nissen and Toupet fundoplications. However, more gas-bloat was reported in nonrandomized trials.

Shan and colleagues[17] reviewed 32 studies, including 9 randomized controlled trials, that compared laparoscopic Nissen fundoplication with laparoscopic Toupet fundoplication. No differences were noted between groups concerning patient satisfaction with the operation or perioperative morbidity and mortality. In 24 studies that assessed postoperative dysphagia, no difference was noted between fundoplication types when esophageal motility was normal. However, in patients with abnormal esophageal motility, laparoscopic Nissen fundoplication was associated with greater rates of dysphagia. An additional analysis was performed that assessed for dysphagia in patients with normal motility who underwent a Nissen fundoplication and patients with abnormal motility who underwent a Toupet fundoplication. In this comparison, the patients who underwent a Nissen fundoplication reported more dysphagia. Finally, this meta-analysis found increased rates of postoperative gas-bloat and inability to belch in patients who underwent Nissen fundoplication. This review would suggest that Toupet fundoplication is the treatment of choice, leading to effective GERD symptom control and fewer postoperative side effects.

Despite numerous randomized clinical trials and two meta-analyses, there still remains conflicting evidence about the fundoplication that provides the most durable control of reflux and the best side-effect profile. The reason for this is likely to be the heterogeneity of these studies in terms of patient characteristics, patient selection, and operative technique. For example, in the studies evaluated by Fein and Seyfried,[16] four different bougie sizes are used (34 Fr to 60 Fr), fixation of the stomach to the esophagus and hiatus is inconsistent among surgeons, and division of the short gastric vessels is not always performed. Currently, the only consistent finding in these studies is that anterior fundoplications provide less durable control of GERD than posterior partial and total fundoplications. Otherwise, surgeons should perform the fundoplication that they are most comfortable performing and not tailor fundoplication type to esophageal dysmotility.

Barrett Esophagus

In some patients, long-standing acid (and perhaps alkaline) reflux is associated with a histologic change of the distal esophageal mucosa from its normal squamous epithelium to a columnar configuration. This histologic alteration is called intestinal metaplasia or Barrett esophagus. On endoscopic evaluation, Barrett esophagus appears as velvety-red "tongues" of mucosa that extend cephalad from the GEJ. Based on endoscopic measurements, it can be classified into long segment (≥3 cm) and short segment (<3 cm). If Barrett esophagus is suspected on the basis of endoscopic appearance of the esophageal mucosa, multiple biopsy specimens should be taken to histologically establish the diagnosis and to determine the presence of dysplasia. When dysplasia is present, there is an increased risk for development of adenocarcinoma. Although the incidence of adenocarcinoma in patients with Barrett esophagus is about 40 times greater than that in the general population, the overall incidence of cancer in these patients is still very low.

Because Barrett esophagus is the result of repeated injury of the mucosa due to GER, it would be expected that an antireflux operation might cause regression of intestinal metaplasia or decrease the rate of dysplasia and cancer. However, the evidence in the literature is not conclusive. Studies have reported regression of intestinal metaplasia in up to 55% of patients after antireflux surgery.[18] At the University of Washington, we have seen regression in 55% of patients with short-segment Barrett esophagus (<3 cm). Just as important, patients with Barrett esophagus experienced excellent long-term clinical relief of GERD symptoms.

Rossi and colleagues[19] compared the efficacy of Nissen fundoplication and medical therapy in the regression of low-grade dysplasia in patients with Barrett esophagus. At 18 months after therapy with high-dose PPIs or laparoscopic Nissen fundoplication, 12 of 19 patients (63%) in the medical arm and 15 of 16 (94%) in the surgery arm had regression from low-grade dysplasia to Barrett esophagus ($P = .03$). Despite these promising results, the pathologic findings on preoperative endoscopy should still dictate postoperative endoscopic surveillance.

Treatment of Gastroesophageal Reflux Disease

Medical Management

For patients who present with typical symptoms of GERD, an 8-week course of PPI therapy is recommended.[20] However, before empirically prescribing a PPI, it is necessary to ensure that the patient does not have symptoms that may indicate the presence of a gastroesophageal malignant neoplasm or other non-GERD diagnosis, including rapidly progressive dysphagia, regurgitation of undigested food, anemia, extraesophageal symptoms of GERD, and weight loss. If the symptoms improve with PPI therapy, the trial is considered both diagnostic and therapeutic. If the symptoms persist after a trial of medical therapy, a more extensive evaluation, as described earlier, is indicated. Although lifestyle modification has been advocated before or as an adjunct to medical therapy, the efficacy of such changes in the treatment of esophagitis has not been proved.[21]

PPIs have revolutionized the pharmacologic treatment of GERD. As one of the most widely prescribed drugs worldwide, the annual expenditure on PPI therapy has reached approximately $24 billion.[22] These drugs stop gastric acid production by irreversibly binding the proton pump in the parietal cells of the stomach. The maximal pharmacologic effect occurs approximately 4 days after initiation of therapy, and the effect lasts for the life of the parietal cell. For this reason, patients must stop PPI therapy 1 week before ambulatory pH monitoring to avoid a false-negative test result.

PPIs are well tolerated medications. Immediate side effects of PPI therapy are relatively rare and generally mild, including headache, abdominal pain, flatulence, constipation, and diarrhea. This relatively safe side-effect profile and their effectiveness at controlling GERD symptoms have led to overprescription of these medications in both the outpatient and inpatient settings.[23] Although there are published evidence-based recommendations that might limit this practice of overprescription, including on-demand dosing and step-down therapy, clinicians frequently do not follow these guidelines.

Despite their short-term safety, there has been concern about the long-term effects of PPI use since their initial preclinical trials.[24] The most concerning long-term complication of PPI use is hypergastrinemia leading to enterochromaffin cell hyperplasia and ultimately carcinoid tumors. The first case of neuroendocrine tumor of the stomach in a patient with 15-year history of PPI use has just been published,[25] so it seems that the true risk of this is exceptionally low. However, additional associations have recently been made between PPI use and enteric infections, antiplatelet medication interactions, bone fractures, nutritional deficiencies, and community-acquired pneumonia.[23] Importantly, however, no cause and effect relationship has been established, and patients prescribed PPI therapy have more comorbid conditions than the general population, which may explain some of these associations. Therefore, until further studies better elucidate PPI as a contributing factor to these conditions, the results of these studies should be interpreted with caution.

Surgical Management

For patients who exhibit elevated distal esophageal acid exposure and persistent typical GERD symptoms despite maximal medical therapy, antireflux surgery should be strongly considered. The application of laparoscopy to antireflux surgery has decreased patient morbidity and hospital length of stay. Furthermore, several studies have shown that LARS is cost-effective compared with prolonged PPI therapy.[12] In patients who experience absolutely no improvement in their symptoms with the use of PPIs, the diagnosis of GERD should be questioned, and surgeons must carefully consider alternative causes before offering surgical treatment. In patients with extraesophageal symptoms of GERD that do not improve with PPI therapy, consultation with an otolaryngologist or pulmonologist should be considered to determine if a primary laryngeal, bronchial, or pulmonary cause of the symptoms is present. Endoscopic evidence of severe esophageal injury (e.g., ulcerations, peptic strictures, and Barrett esophagus) can be considered evidence of abnormal distal esophageal acid exposure and may make ambulatory pH monitoring unnecessary in patients who exhibit these findings; however, endoscopic findings should not be considered an indication for operative therapy by themselves.

Operative technique. We perform all laparoscopic antireflux operations with the patient in low lithotomy position. This provides the surgeon improved ergonomics by standing between the patient's legs; the assistant stands at the patient's left. In addition, the patient is placed in steep reverse Trendelenburg position, which allows improved visualization of the esophageal hiatus. The patient is appropriately padded to prevent pressure ulcers and neuropathies. Preoperative antibiotics are administered to reduce the risk of surgical site infection, and subcutaneous heparin and sequential compression devices are used to reduce the risk of venous thromboembolic events.

Access to the abdomen is obtained with a Veress needle at Palmer's point in the left upper quadrant of the abdomen. Three additional trocars are placed. The surgeon operates through the two most cephalad ports, and the assistant operates through the two caudad ports. A Nathanson liver retractor does not require a trocar and is placed through a small epigastric incision (Fig. 42-8).

We begin our dissection at the left crus by dividing the phrenogastric membrane and then enter the lesser sac at the level of the inferior edge of the spleen. This allows early ligation of the short gastric vessels and mobilization of the gastric fundus (Fig. 42-9). After the fundus is mobilized, the phrenoesophageal membrane is divided to expose the entire length of the left crus (Fig. 42-10).

Right crural dissection is then performed. The gastrohepatic ligament is divided, and the right phrenoesophageal membrane is opened to expose the right crus (Fig. 42-11). A retroesophageal window is created. Care is taken to preserve the anterior and posterior vagus nerves during this mobilization. A Penrose drain is placed around the esophagus to facilitate the posterior mediastinal dissection and to assist with creation of the fundoplication.

The esophagus is mobilized in the posterior mediastinum to obtain a minimum of 3 cm of intra-abdominal esophagus. Then, the crura are approximated posteriorly with permanent sutures (Fig. 42-12). The esophagus should maintain a straight orientation without angulation, and a 52 Fr bougie should easily pass

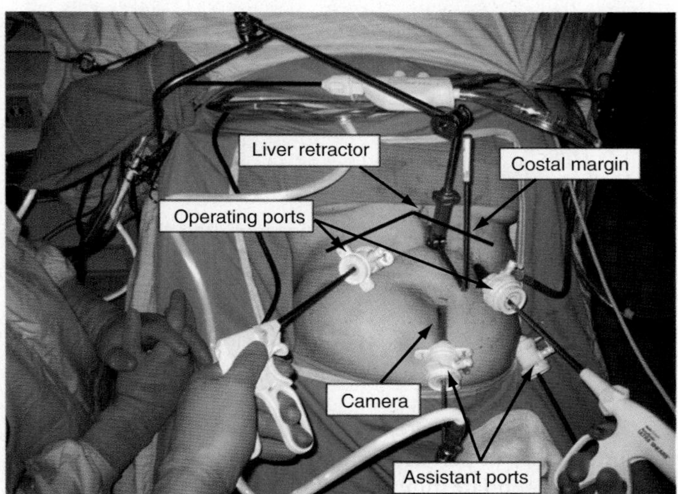

FIGURE 42-8 Port placement for laparoscopic antireflux surgery. The surgeon operates through the two cephalad ports, and the assistant operates through the two caudad ports.

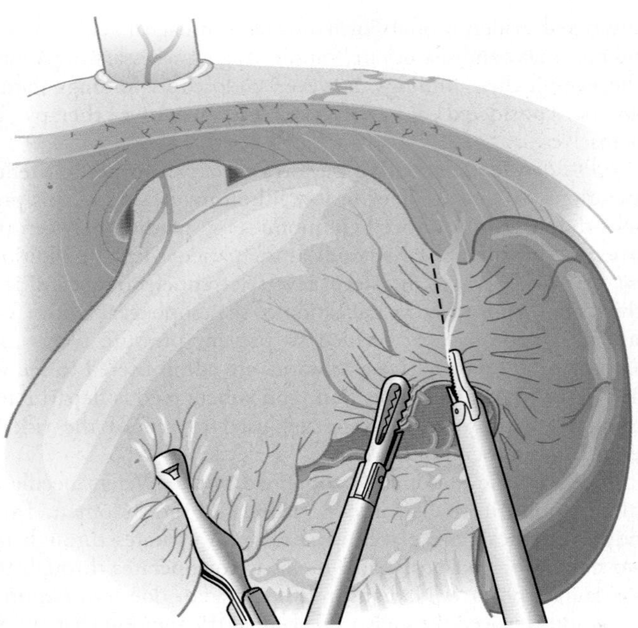

FIGURE 42-9 In the left crus approach to the esophageal hiatus, the fundus of the stomach is mobilized early during the operation to provide early visualization of the spleen, which helps prevent splenic injury.

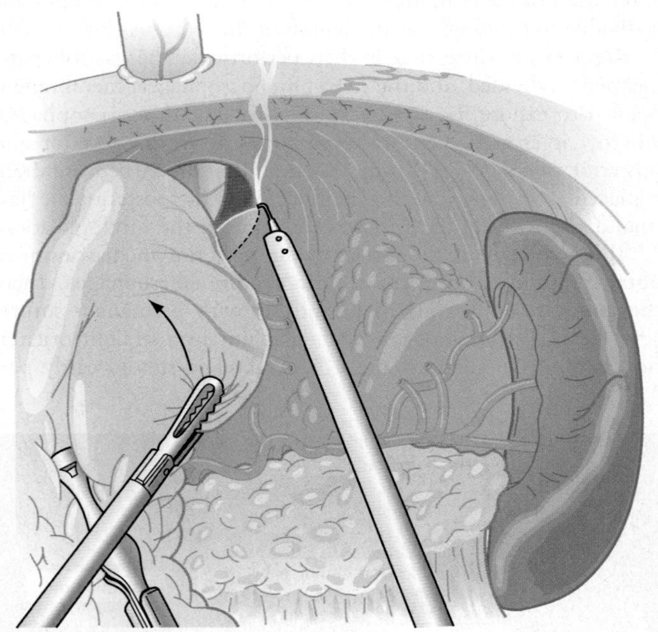

FIGURE 42-10 After the fundus has been mobilized, the phrenoesophageal membrane is incised at the left crus, with care taken to avoid injury to the esophagus, posterior vagus nerve, and aorta.

beyond the esophageal hiatus and into the stomach. At this point, the fundoplication is created.

Creation of a 360-degree fundoplication. The most common technical failure in performing a Nissen fundoplication is failure to create appropriate fundoplication anatomy. The description that follows clearly explains our method of performing a correct, effective, and reproducible Nissen fundoplication. To maintain appropriate orientation of the fundus during the creation of the

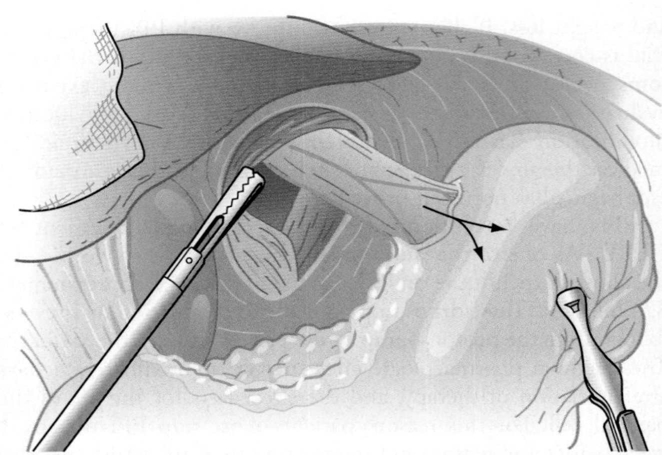

FIGURE 42-11 The phrenoesophageal membrane is incised at the right crus to complete the exposure of the hiatus. Performing the dissection immediately adjacent to the crura decreases the likelihood of injury to adjacent structures.

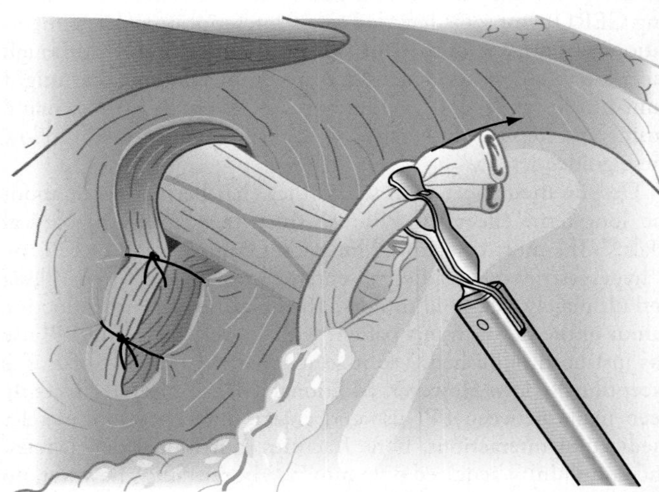

FIGURE 42-12 Posterior crural closure is performed with heavy permanent suture. Note how the peritoneum overlying the crura is incorporated into the closure. The exposure is facilitated by displacement of the esophagus anteriorly and to the left.

fundoplication, the posterior aspect of the fundus is marked with a suture 3 cm distal to the GEJ and 2 cm off the greater curvature (Fig. 42-13). The posterior fundus is then passed behind the esophagus from the patient's left to right. The anterior fundus on the left side of the esophagus is then grasped 2 cm from the greater curvature and 3 cm from the GEJ, and both portions of the fundus are positioned on the anterior aspect of the esophagus. It is of paramount importance that the two points at which the fundus is grasped are equidistant from the greater curvature (Fig. 42-14). Creation of the fundoplication in this manner decreases the chance of constructing the fundoplication with the body of the stomach, which creates a redundant posterior aspect of the wrap that can impinge on the distal esophagus and cause dysphagia. With use of three or four interrupted permanent sutures, the fundoplication is created to a length of 2.5 to 3 cm. Similar to the crural repair, the completed fundoplication should allow the easy passage of a 52 Fr bougie. After removal of the bougie, the wrap is anchored to the esophagus and crura (Fig. 42-14, *inset*)

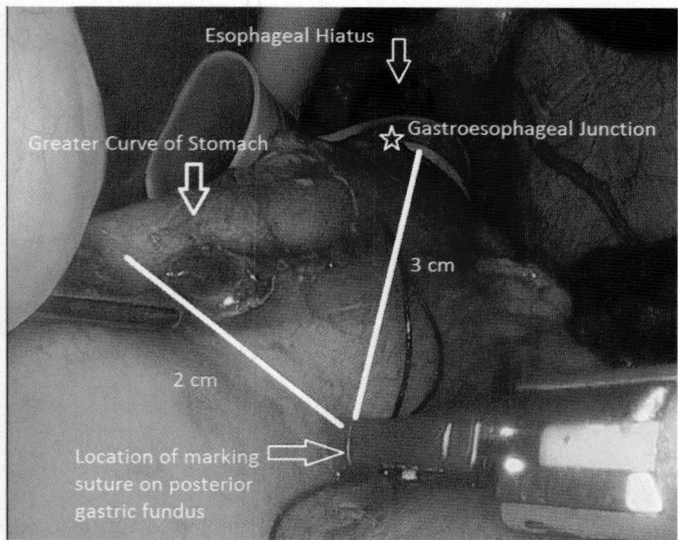

FIGURE 42-13 A posterior gastric marking suture is helpful to ensure proper geometric configuration of the fundoplication. With the greater curvature of the stomach rotated to the patient's right, the posterior stomach is exposed, and a marking stitch is placed on the posterior fundus 3 cm from the gastroesophageal junction and 2 cm from the greater curvature of the stomach.

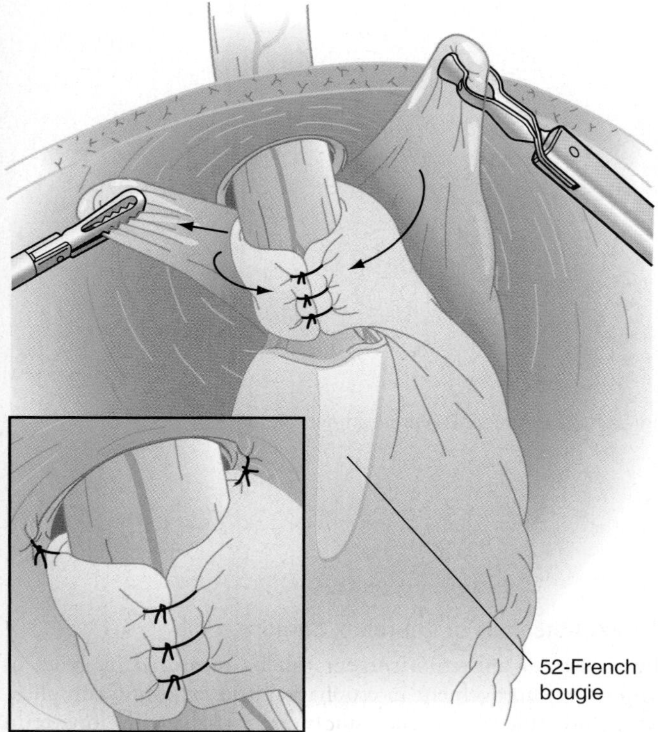

FIGURE 42-14 Creation of a 360-degree Nissen fundoplication. The anterior and posterior fundus must be grasped equidistant from the greater curvature posterior to the esophagus. After placement of the first suture of the fundoplication, a 52 Fr bougie is passed into the stomach, and the fundoplication is completed. With the bougie removed from the patient, the fundoplication is secured to the diaphragm with right and left coronal sutures *(inset)* and a single posterior suture (not shown).

to help prevent herniation into the mediastinum and slipping of the fundoplication over the body of the stomach. The suture line of the fundoplication should lie parallel to the right anterior aspect of the esophagus.

Creation of a partial fundoplication. There are several types of partial fundoplications. The most commonly performed is the Toupet fundoplication. In this operation, the gastric and esophageal dissections as well as the repair of the crura are the same as for a 360-degree fundoplication. In addition, the fundoplication must be created with the fundus, not the body, of the stomach. The key difference is that the stomach is wrapped 180 to 270 degrees (compared with 360 degrees) around the posterior aspect of the esophagus (Fig. 42-15*A* and *C*). On both sides of the esophagus, the most cephalad sutures of the fundoplication incorporate the fundus, crus, and esophagus; the remaining sutures anchor the fundus to either the crura or the esophagus.

If an anterior fundoplication is to be performed (e.g., Thal or Dor), there is no need to disrupt the posterior attachments of the esophagus, and the fundus is folded over the anterior aspect of the esophagus and anchored to the hiatus and esophagus (Fig. 42-15*B*).

Intraoperative management of short esophagus. Normal esophageal length exists when the GEJ rests at or below the esophageal hiatus. As the GEJ becomes displaced cephalad to the esophageal hiatus, the esophagus effectively shortens. At the time of LARS, a minimum of 3 cm of intra-abdominal esophagus should be obtained. When the GEJ is mildly displaced cephalad to the GEJ, adequate intra-abdominal esophageal length can be obtained with distal esophageal mobilization in the posterior mediastinum. However, if the GEJ migrates high into the posterior mediastinum, as occurs with a large hiatal hernia or PEH, the effective length of the esophagus can decrease significantly. Furthermore, this process causes adhesions to develop between the esophagus and the mediastinum that anchor the contracted esophagus in the chest. When this occurs, extensive mobilization of the esophagus must be undertaken, sometimes to the level of the inferior pulmonary veins. However, even in the case of a large hiatal hernia or PEH, mediastinal dissection alone can return the GEJ to the abdominal cavity.

In some cases, despite extensive mediastinal mobilization of the esophagus, intra-abdominal esophageal length still appears inadequate. In these rare cases, a unilateral vagotomy can result in an additional 1 to 2 cm of esophageal length, and division of both vagus nerves typically yields 3 to 4 cm of additional esophagus. Many surgeons hesitate to electively transect the vagus nerves because of concern for the development of postoperative delayed gastric emptying. However, we have shown this not to be the case. In our study of 102 patients who underwent reoperative LARS (n = 50) or PEH repair (n = 52), we performed a vagotomy in 30 patients (29%) to increase intra-abdominal esophageal length after extensive mediastinal mobilization.[26] Compared with patients who did not undergo vagotomy, patients who underwent vagotomy reported similar severity of abdominal pain, bloating, diarrhea, and early satiety.

Finally, if adequate intra-abdominal esophageal length cannot be accomplished with these techniques, a stapled wedge gastroplasty may be performed (Fig. 42-16). Since the widespread adoption of laparoscopy in the management of GERD and PEH, wedge gastroplasty has generally supplanted the traditional Collis gastroplasty that used a double-staple technique (circular and linear stapler). However, we have found this technique unnecessary in all but a very small number of patients.

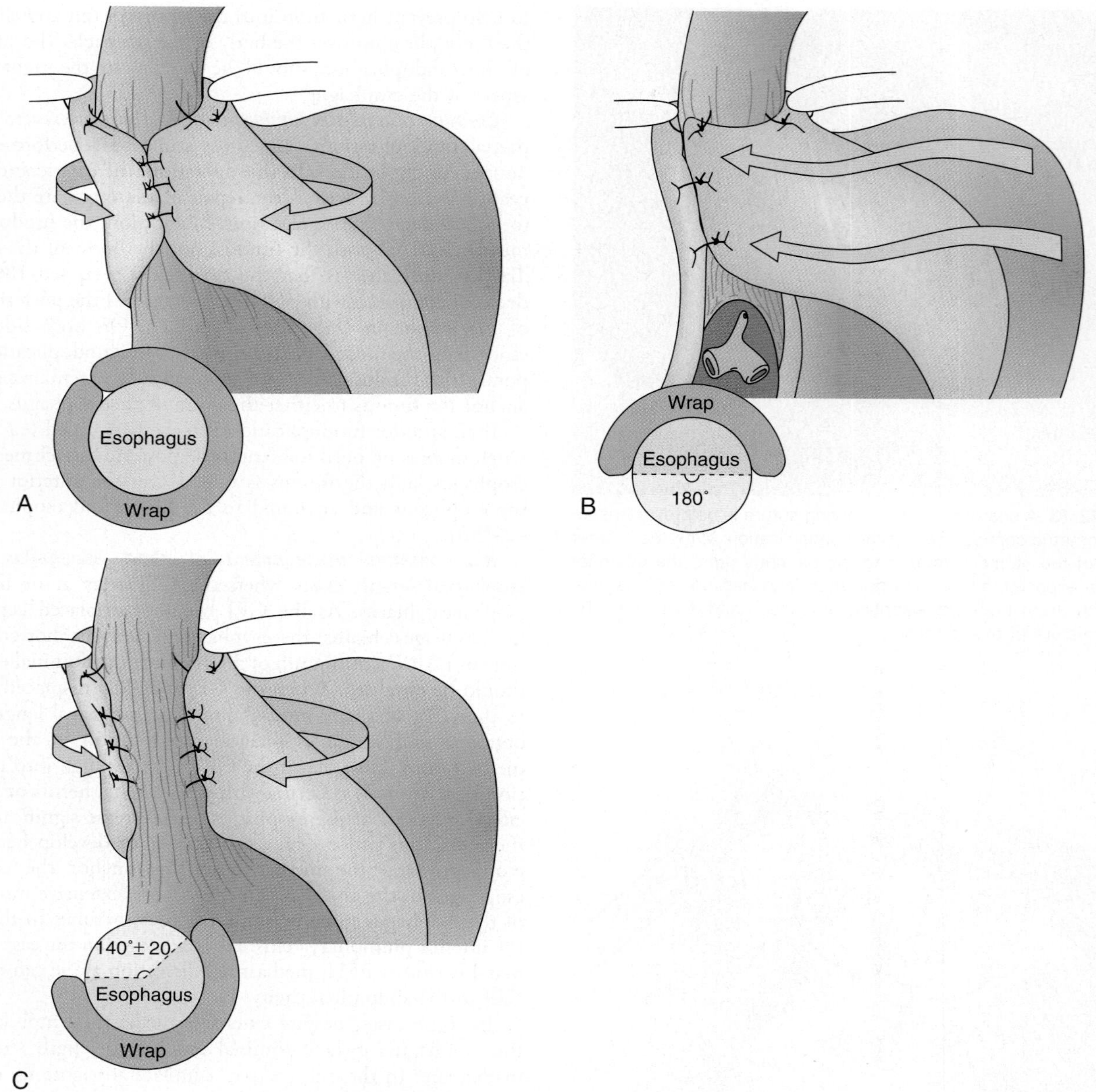

FIGURE 42-15 Three types of fundoplication. **A,** A 360-degree fundoplication. **B,** Partial anterior fundoplication. **C,** Partial posterior fundoplication.

Postoperative Care and Recovery

Except when the patient's comorbid medical conditions dictate otherwise, postoperatively patients are admitted to a general surgical ward without cardiac or pulmonary monitoring. Patients are given a clear liquid diet the evening of the operation and are advanced to a full liquid diet on postoperative day 1. Discharge requirements include tolerance of a diet to maintain hydration and nutrition, adequate pain control with oral analgesics, and ability to void without a Foley catheter. After discharge from the hospital, patients can slowly introduce soft foods into their diet, and they should expect to resume a diet without limitations in about 4 to 6 weeks.

Clinical Outcomes of Antireflux Surgery

The success of antireflux surgery can be measured by relief of symptoms, improvement in esophageal acid exposure, complications, and failures. Several randomized trials with long-term follow-up have compared medical and surgical therapy for GERD (Table 42-2). LARS is a safe operation that provides durable improvement in typical symptoms of GERD that are refractory to medical management.

Spechler and colleagues[27] found that surgical therapy results in good symptom control after 10-year follow-up. Although 62% of patients in the surgical group were taking antisecretory medications at long-term follow-up, GERD symptoms were not the

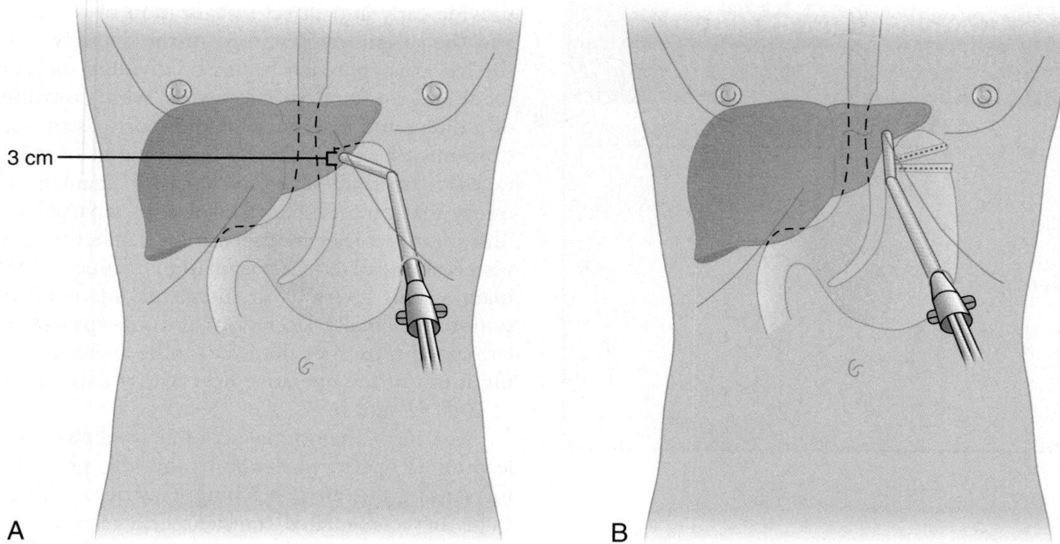

FIGURE 42-16 Laparoscopic stapled wedge gastroplasty for esophageal lengthening. **A,** With a 48 Fr bougie placed beyond the gastroesophageal junction and into the stomach, a linear stapler is used to transect the fundus perpendicular to the bougie approximately 3 to 4 cm distal to the angle of His. **B,** A second linear stapler is used to resect the portion of gastric fundus parallel to the bougie.

TABLE 42-2 Randomized Controlled Trials Comparing Surgical and Medical Therapies for GERD

STUDY	STUDY GROUPS	FOLLOW-UP	OUTCOME
Anvari et al,[46] 2011	PPI, $n = 52$ ARS, $n = 52$	3 years	ARS and PPI provided equal symptom control; ARS provided more heartburn-free days
Grant et al,[47] 2008	PPI, $n = 179$ ARS, $n = 178$	1 year	Reflux score: PPI, 73; ARS, 85; $P <$ .05
Lundell et al,[29] 2009	Omeprazole, $n = 71$ ARS, $n = 53$	12 years	Treatment failure: Omeprazole, 55%; ARS, 47%; $P = .022$
Lundell et al,[28] 2007	Omeprazole, $n = 119$ ARS, $n = 99$	7 years	Treatment failure: Omeprazole, 53%; ARS, 33%; $P = .002$

ARS, antireflux surgery; *PPI,* proton pump inhibitor.

indication for this medication use in all patients, and reflux symptoms did not change significantly when these patients stopped taking these medications.

Lundell and colleagues[28] randomized patients with erosive esophagitis into surgical or medical therapy. Treatment failure was defined as moderate or severe symptoms of heartburn, regurgitation, dysphagia, or odynophagia; recommencement of PPI therapy; reoperation; or grade 2 esophagitis. At 7-year follow-up, fewer treatment failures were seen in patients managed with fundoplication than with omeprazole (33% versus 53%; $P = .002$). In patients who did not respond to the initial dose of omeprazole, dose escalation was completed; however, surgical intervention remained superior. Patients treated with fundoplication experienced more obstructive and gas-bloat symptoms (e.g., dysphagia, flatulence, inability to belch) compared with the medically treated cohort. At 12-year follow-up, the durability of these results remained; patients who underwent fundoplication had fewer treatment failures compared with patients treated with medical therapy (47% versus 55%; $P = .022$).[29]

During the past 25 years, the experience of surgeons with LARS has increased dramatically. With increased experience, the durability of symptom improvement has increased, and perioperative complications have decreased. This is especially true in high-volume centers. In one single-institution study that observed 100 patients for 10 years after LARS, 90% of patients remained free of GERD symptoms.[30] We published our experience in a cohort of 288 patients undergoing LARS. With median follow-up of more than 5 years, symptom improvement was 90% for heartburn and 92% for regurgitation.[31] These results confirm that LARS can provide excellent durable relief of GERD when patients are appropriately selected and excellent technique is employed.

Operative Complications and Side Effects of Antireflux Surgery

LARS is a safe operation when it is performed by experienced surgeons. Using the American College of Surgeons National Surgical Quality Improvement Program, Niebisch and colleagues[32] reviewed more than 7500 patients who underwent laparoscopic fundoplication between 2005 and 2009. Overall, 30-day mortality was rare (0.19%). In patients older than 70 years, mortality was statistically significantly higher (0.8%; $P < .0001$). Complications were also more frequent in older patients (2.2% in patients <50 years and 7.8% in patients >70 years; $P < .0001$) and in patients with higher American Society of Anesthesiologists classification (2% in class 2 and 14% in class 4).

Complications of LARS are typically minor and not related specifically to antireflux surgery; they include urinary retention, wound infection, venous thrombosis, and ileus. Complications

TABLE 42-3 Complications in 400 Laparoscopic Antireflux Procedures at the University of Washington

COMPLICATION	NO. OF PATIENTS (%)
Postoperative ileus	28 (7)
Pneumothorax	13 (3)
Urinary retention	9 (2)
Dysphagia	9 (2)
Other minor complications	8 (2)
Liver trauma	2 (0.5)
Acute herniation	1 (0.25)
Perforated viscus	1 (0.25)
Death	1 (0.25)
Total	72 (17.25)

that are specific to antireflux surgery include pneumothorax, gastric or esophageal injury, and splenic or liver injury. In addition, LARS can result in postoperative side effects, including bloating and dysphagia. Complications in 400 patients who have undergone LARS at the University of Washington are listed in Table 42-3.

Operative Complications

Pneumothorax. Pneumothorax is one of the most common intraoperative complications, yet it is reported to occur in less than 2% of patients.[33] Although postoperative chest radiographs are not obtained in all patients, pneumothorax should rarely be missed as intraoperative identification of pleural violation that causes pneumothorax should be identified. The pleural violation results in intrathoracic infusion of carbon dioxide, which is absorbed rapidly. Because no underlying lung injury exists, the lung will reexpand without incident. When violation of the pleura is identified intraoperatively, the pleura should be closed with a suture, and a postoperative radiograph should be obtained. If a pneumothorax is identified on this radiograph, the patient may be maintained on oxygen therapy to facilitate its resolution. Unless the patient experiences shortness of breath or persistent oxygen therapy to maintain normal hemoglobin oxygenation saturation, no further radiographs are obtained.

Gastric and esophageal injuries. Gastric and esophageal injuries have been reported to occur in approximately 1% of patients undergoing LARS.[33] Typically, these injuries result from overaggressive manipulation of these organs or at the time the bougie is passed into the stomach. Gastric and esophageal injuries are more likely to occur in reoperative cases and should be rare during initial operations. If they are identified at the time of operation, these injuries can be repaired with suture (more commonly) or stapler (if the injury involves the stomach) without sequelae. If the injury is not identified intraoperatively, the patient will likely need a second operation to repair the viscus, unless the leak is small and contained.

Splenic and liver injuries or bleeding. The incidence of splenic parenchymal injury that results in bleeding is about 2.3% in population-based studies; major liver injury is rarely reported.[34] Whereas splenic bleeding is relatively uncommon, in rare cases, it can require splenectomy. Most commonly, splenic parenchymal injury occurs during mobilization of the fundus and greater curvature of the stomach. For this reason, we prefer beginning laparoscopic Nissen fundoplication with the "left crus approach" to provide early and direct visualization of the short gastric vessels and the spleen. As described in the operative technique section, the left crus approach begins by dividing the phrenogastric ligament and the short gastric vessels, which provides the advantage of a direct and early view of the short gastric vessels and spleen. Care must be taken during mobilization of the fundus to avoid excessive traction on the splenogastric ligament. A second type of injury that can occur to the spleen is a partial splenic infarction. This injury typically occurs during transection of the short gastric vessels and inadvertent coagulation of superior pole branch of the main splenic artery.[34] Partial splenic infarction rarely causes any symptoms. Finally, lacerations and subcapsular hematomas of the left lateral section of the liver can be avoided by carefully retracting it out of the operative field with a fixed retractor.

Side Effects

Bloating. The normal act of air swallowing is the main factor leading to gastric distention, and the physiologic mechanism for venting this air is belching. Gastric belching occurs through vagus nerve–mediated transient LES relaxation. After antireflux surgery, patients experience fewer transient LES relaxations and therefore decreased belching. Consequently, patients can experience abdominal bloating. Kessing and colleagues[35] investigated the impact of gas-related symptoms on the objective and subjective outcomes of both Nissen and Toupet fundoplications. Interestingly, they demonstrated that preoperative belching and air swallowing were not predictive of postoperative gas-related symptoms, including bloating. They concluded that gas-related symptoms are, in part, due to gastrointestinal hypersensitivity to gaseous distention. In this study, all patients experienced postoperative normalization of esophageal acid exposure. However, these authors found that patients who developed postoperative gas symptoms were less satisfied with LARS compared with patients who did not experience these symptoms.

During the early postoperative period, patients who report persistent nausea and demonstrate inadequate intake of a liquid diet should undergo abdominal radiography. If significant gastric distention is identified, a nasogastric tube can safely be placed to decompress the stomach for 24 hours. Few patients require further intervention for gastric bloating.

Dysphagia. It is expected that patients will experience mild, temporary dysphagia during the first 2 to 4 weeks postoperatively. This is thought to be a result of postoperative edema at the fundoplication and esophageal hiatus. In the majority of these patients, this dysphagia spontaneously resolves. A second but less common cause of dysphagia in the early postoperative period is the presence of a hematoma of the stomach or esophageal wall that develops during the placement of the sutures to create the fundoplication. Although this may create more severe dysphagia, it typically resolves in several days. In both these situations, surgeons should ensure that the patient can maintain nutrition and hydration on a liquid or soft diet; however, additional interventions are rarely needed. If the patient cannot tolerate liquids, a UGI series should be obtained to ensure that no anatomic abnormality, such as an early hiatal hernia, exists. Assuming that there is no early recurrent hiatal hernia and the patient can tolerate liquids, patience should be employed for 3 months. If the patient cannot maintain hydration or dysphagia persists beyond 3 months, a UGI series should be obtained to ensure no anatomic abnormality that could explain the dysphagia. If the UGI series demonstrates an appropriately positioned fundoplication below the diaphragm, esophagogastroduodenoscopy with empirical dilation of the GEJ should be performed.

Failed Antireflux Surgery

Patients who have undergone antireflux surgery may present back to the physician with recurrent, persistent, or completely new foregut symptoms. The most common symptoms of failed LARS are typical symptoms of GERD (i.e., heartburn, regurgitation, and water brash sensation) and dysphagia. During the first 2 months after the operation, most symptoms, particularly when they are mild, are of little significance, and the majority of these will abate with time. One large retrospective review of more than 1700 patients who underwent antireflux surgery found that only 5.6% of patients ultimately required a reoperation for symptoms of recurrent GERD or dysphagia.[36] Persistent symptoms should be investigated by the surgeon to evaluate for functional and anatomic problems associated with the fundoplication or the hiatal closure. Anatomic problems after a fundoplication that can cause symptoms include persistent or recurrent hiatal hernia, slipped fundoplication, and incorrectly constructed fundoplication.

All patients who present with recurrent or persistent symptoms of GERD should be evaluated with esophageal manometry and ambulatory pH study. If the pH study demonstrates elevated distal esophageal acid exposure, an esophagram and upper endoscopy should be performed. Once the diagnosis of persistent or recurrent GERD is made, PPI therapy should be instituted. Most of these patients experience resolution of their symptoms with resumption of PPI therapy. If the patient's symptoms are not effectively managed by medical therapy, reoperation should be performed to create an effective antireflux valve.

The late development of dysphagia after LARS suggests esophageal obstruction. In this setting, esophageal obstruction most frequently results from a recurrent hiatal hernia or a slipped fundoplication. A UGI series and esophagogastroduodenoscopy should be the initial studies obtained in these patients. If a clear anatomic abnormality is visualized (Fig. 42-17), reoperation can be performed without further investigation. If concurrent GERD symptoms are present, ambulatory pH testing and manometry should be performed. To achieve resolution of symptoms, reoperation is almost always necessary in these patients.

Some patients experience no improvement or even worsened symptoms after initial LARS. In these patients, one ought to examine the indication for the original procedure and the technique of the operation as these are the two most important factors associated with success or failure. An incorrectly constructed fundoplication (generally created out of the body of the stomach and not the fundus) can do nothing to prevent GER and cause new-onset gastroesophageal obstructive symptoms. Failure to completely excise the sac of a hiatal hernia or PEH frequently leads to an early recurrence of hiatal hernia. In our experience, patients who present with persistent symptoms or early recurrence of symptoms after LARS typically require operative management. After appropriate evaluation with pH testing, manometry, UGI series, and esophagogastroduodenoscopy, the patient should undergo operative correction of the anatomic problem with creation of an appropriately constructed fundoplication.

It is important to understand that reoperative antireflux surgery comes with higher stakes than first-time antireflux surgery. Tissues are less pliable, making it more challenging for surgeons to construct an effective antireflux valve. In addition, adhesions and less visible tissue planes contribute to increased rates of intraoperative injury of the stomach and esophagus. Consequently, we have a higher threshold to perform reoperative antireflux surgery. With the exceptions described before, we reserve reoperation for patients with significant symptoms despite maximal nonoperative management.

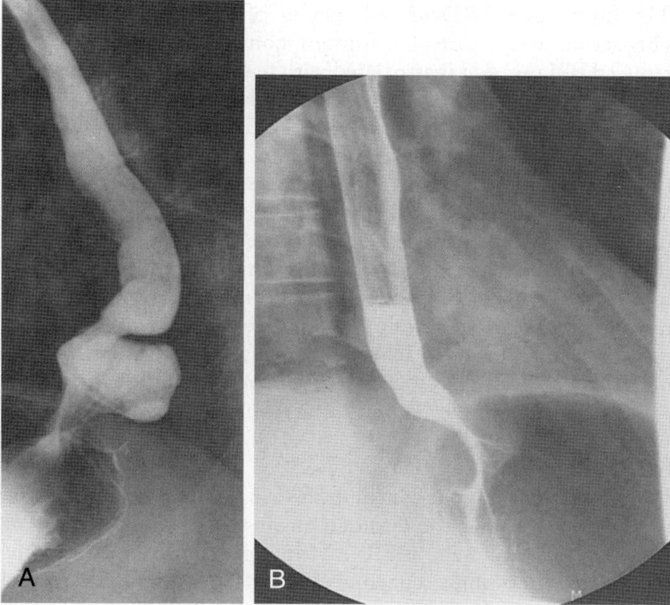

FIGURE 42-17 An upper gastrointestinal series provides invaluable anatomic information in patients with persistent or recurrent postoperative symptoms. **A,** Upper gastrointestinal series demonstrating a 360-degree fundoplication that has both slipped down around the stomach and herniated into the mediastinum. **B,** Normal anatomic appearance of 360-degree fundoplication. Note the smooth tapering of the distal esophagus.

Novel Therapies for GERD

Despite the fact that LARS provides durable symptom relief with an excellent safety profile, the last decade has seen a drive to develop new therapies for GERD. These therapies have focused on augmenting the LES by modalities such as radiofrequency energy (Mederi Therapeutics Inc, Greenwich, Conn), injection of inert biopolymers (Enteryx; Boston Scientific, Natick, Mass), creation of gastroplications (EndoCinch, Bard, Warwick, RI; EsophyX, EndoGastric Solutions, Redmond, Wash; Plicator, NDO Surgical, Mansfield, Mass), and implantation of a magnetic sphincter augmentation device (LINX, Torax Medical, Shoreview, Minn). The two most studied therapies that are currently available clinically are the endoscopic suturing device used to complete transoral incisionless fundoplication (TIF), EsophyX, and the only implantable magnetic sphincter augmentation device (MSAD), LINX.

EsophyX

EsophyX is a flexible, multichannel endoluminal device that uses fasteners to construct a full-thickness gastric plication and to create an antireflux valve at the GEJ. The endoluminal fundoplication can be created up to 4 cm in length and 270 degrees. The procedure is performed under general anesthesia; the device is inserted over a gastroscope, and because multiple fasteners are loaded on the end of the device, the entire antireflux valve can be created during a single device insertion.

Since the initial studies evaluating the safety of TIF were published in 2008, additional investigation has demonstrated that

TIF improves GERD-related quality of life, results in patient satisfaction with GERD symptom control, is associated with reduced PPI use, and is associated with few side effects.[37] However, whereas it appears that TIF is associated with significant *reduction* in acid exposure and improvement in GERD symptoms, *normalization* of esophageal acid exposure and complete cessation of PPI use have not been demonstrated in these short-term studies. In a long-term (3-year) follow-up study, Muls and colleagues[38] demonstrated similar results. Patients reported durable improvement in GERD-related quality of life and significant reduction in PPI use; however, 48% of patients had normalization of pH study results. Furthermore, 12 of 66 patients required revisional procedures (11 redo TIF and 1 Nissen) because of inadequate control of GERD symptoms associated with esophagitis (92%), PPI use (83%), and Hill grade III or IV antireflux valve (92%).

LINX

LINX is an MSAD that consists of a string of magnetic beads that is positioned around the distal esophagus to increase LES resting pressure to counteract GER. During peristaltic swallows, the propagated food bolus separates the beads, opening the GEJ and allowing the bolus to pass into the stomach, after which the beads return to their original position.

Several characteristics of the MSAD make it attractive. First, it can be sized to the esophagus of the individual patient, which creates LES augmentation to prevent pathologic GER but permits the passage of a food bolus and allows the patient to belch. Second, unlike springs and elastics, magnetic forces are inversely proportional to the distance between them, allowing easier passage of larger food boluses. In addition, magnetic forces do not decay over time, so the antireflux effects should not diminish with the age of the device. Third, the device can be placed laparoscopically, and the placement of the device is reproducible, eliminating the variability that can occur among surgeons with the creation of a fundoplication.

Two studies have evaluated the short-term outcomes comparing MSAD with Nissen fundoplication. These studies demonstrate that MSAD controls typical and extraesophageal symptoms as effectively as Nissen fundoplication but with greater rate of early postoperative dysphagia that resolves with endoscopic dilation. Louie and colleagues[39] retrospectively compared 34 patients who underwent MSAD with 32 patients who underwent Nissen fundoplication. Operative time was shorter for MSAD compared with Nissen fundoplication (73 versus 118 minutes; $P = .001$). At mean postoperative follow-up of 6 months for MSAD and 10 months for Nissen fundoplication, both groups reported significantly improved typical and extraesophageal symptoms of GERD. Objectively, both groups experienced normalization of DeMeester score and total percentage time of pH below 4. However, patients who underwent MSAD experienced significantly more total esophageal acid exposure and higher DeMeester scores than patients who underwent Nissen fundoplication. Furthermore, 44% of patients who underwent MSAD had a DeMeester score above 14.7 (threshold for normal). The total number of reflux episodes was higher for MSAD than for Nissen fundoplication (60.1 versus 21.5; $P = .002$), and the majority of these reflux episodes were postprandial. This exemplifies the trade-off that is seen with MSAD; patients experience greater ability to belch in the postprandial state but experience decreased control of reflux. It also suggests that MSAD is a more "physiologic" antireflux procedure that allows postprandial gastric venting yet is not associated with worse GERD symptoms.

At 6 weeks postoperatively, dysphagia was more severe in Nissen patients; however, by 6 months, swallowing returned to baseline in both groups. Incidence of other side effects (including gas-bloat) was similar between groups; however, patients who underwent MSAD were significantly more likely to be able to belch than patients who underwent Nissen fundoplication.

Sheu and colleagues[40] found similar results in comparing MSAD with Nissen fundoplication in a case-controlled study of 12 patients. MSAD was performed in less operative time (64 versus 90 minutes; $P < .001$), and neither group experienced any morbidity, mortality, or readmission during the first 30 days postoperatively. At mean postoperative follow-up of 7 months, both groups experienced resolution of both typical and extraesophageal symptoms of GERD, and symptom resolution was similar between the groups (MSAD 75% versus Nissen fundoplication 83%; $P = .99$). Patients undergoing Nissen fundoplication experienced significantly more gas-bloat symptoms. There was no difference in the rate of overall postoperative dysphagia (MSAD 83% versus Nissen fundoplication 58%; $P = .37$); however, endoscopic dilation for the management of dysphagia was more frequent in patients who underwent MSAD (50% versus 0%; $P = .014$). No routine objective postoperative testing for GERD was completed; two patients underwent postoperative pH testing for recurrent symptoms, but both demonstrated normal esophageal acid exposure.

Postoperative rates of dysphagia appear similar between MSAD and Nissen fundoplication; however, the need for dilation is more frequent with MSAD. The fact that dysphagia associated with MSAD improves with dilation suggests that the cause of the dysphagia is not from the placement of an undersized device. An alternative explanation is that a fibrous band develops around the MSAD. This fixed ring resists passage of food. Dilation disrupts this scar tissue and relieves dysphagia. This mechanism is supported by the time course for dysphagia between the two groups; patients undergoing Nissen fundoplication experience early dysphagia that resolves without intervention (probably because of edema at the fundoplication), whereas patients undergoing MSAD develop dysphagia relatively later postoperatively, it is progressive, and it resolves only after dilation.

Because LINX is a medical device approved by the U.S. Food and Drug Administration (FDA), all adverse events related to LINX must be reported to the FDA's safety database. Lipham and colleagues[41] reviewed the FDA database and all published surgical literature on the safety of LINX. Between 2007 and 2013, 1048 patients underwent LINX implantation. There were no intraoperative complications; however, one patient experienced an immediate postoperative respiratory arrest that was deemed unrelated to the device itself. The overall readmission rate was 1.4%, and all but one readmission occurred within 90 days postoperatively. Reasons for readmission included dysphagia, pain, nausea, and vomiting. Esophageal dilation was performed in 5.6% of patients; the majority of these were completed within 90 days postoperatively, and no further interventions were required.

Device removal has occurred in 3.6% of patients. Indications for removal were persistent dysphagia (most common), odynophagia, recurrent GERD and desire to undergo fundoplication, nausea or emesis, and need for magnetic resonance imaging. There have been no reported complications with device removal, and the operative technique appears uncomplicated.[42] One instance of device erosion into the esophageal lumen was managed with endoscopic removal of the exposed portion of the device, and the patient subsequently underwent laparoscopic removal of the remainder of the MSAD. The patient experienced no further clinical sequelae. No reported cases of device migration have been reported.

PARAESOPHAGEAL HERNIA

The anatomic definitions of PEH are discussed in a previous section and can be reviewed in Figure 42-2. PEH is frequently associated with obstructive symptoms and, less frequently, typical symptoms of GERD. On occasion, a PEH is identified incidentally on imaging performed for another purpose, and the patient's PEH is asymptomatic. Indication for operative repair of PEH is based on the size of the hernia and the presence and severity of symptoms. To prevent acute gastric volvulus and gastric strangulation, a case can be made for operative repair of a large but minimally symptomatic PEH. Otherwise, the presence of a small asymptomatic hiatal hernia or PEH does not constitute an indication for operative correction.

Pathophysiology

The two key events that facilitate the formation of a PEH are the widening of the diaphragmatic crura at the esophageal hiatus and stretching of the phrenoesophageal membrane. As the hernia enlarges, the phrenoesophageal membrane balloons into the posterior mediastinum like a parachute. After repeated episodes of the viscera entering the hernia sac, adhesions develop between the wall of the sac and the surrounding thoracic structures, thus preventing the herniated abdominal contents from returning to their normal position in the peritoneal cavity. The most common structure to herniate through the esophageal hiatus is the fundus of the stomach; however, the entire stomach as well as other abdominal organs including spleen, colon, pancreas, small bowel, and omentum can migrate into the chest.

Gastric volvulus develops because of laxity in the stomach's peritoneal attachments and subsequent rotation of the gastric fundus on the organoaxial or mesenteric axis of the stomach. The frequency with which this occurs is a matter of debate. Historically, surgeons believed that a large PEH would inevitably volvulize, become incarcerated, and result in gastric strangulation; the mere presence of a PEH was an indication for operative repair. However, more recent evidence suggests that the risk for acute strangulation is approximately 1% per year.[43] We recommend operative repair of completely asymptomatic large hernias only in young (<60 years) and otherwise healthy patients.

Clinical Presentation

The most common symptoms attributed to PEH are gastroesophageal obstructive symptoms, including dysphagia, odynophagia, and early satiety. Intermittent epigastric and chest pain can develop secondary to visceral torsion and distention, which leads to ischemia of the hernia contents. Spontaneous reduction then provides relief of these symptoms. Gastrointestinal bleeding can result from mucosal ischemia or mechanical ulceration of the gastric mucosa. Respiratory symptoms, primarily shortness of breath, can be explained by the mass effect of the hernia contents in the chest. Finally, heartburn and regurgitation are also reported by patients with PEH. These symptoms can be present individually or in combination. Because the symptoms of PEH are diverse and nonspecific, the diagnosis of PEH is often made only after performance of a barium esophagram or UGI endoscopy.

Preoperative Evaluation

The clinical investigations obtained in patients with PEH are similar to those of patients undergoing workup for GERD. A barium esophagogram provides the operating surgeon the most accurate image of the gastroesophageal anatomy (Fig. 42-18). Endoscopy evaluates the gastric and esophageal mucosa for Barrett esophagus and mechanical gastric mucosal erosions (i.e., Cameron ulcers) that can result in gastrointestinal blood loss. Manometry is necessary to determine the motor function of the esophageal body, which can affect the type of antireflux operation performed at the time of PEH repair. Even if a large PEH prevents the passage of the manometry catheter through the LES, it is generally possible to determine the degree of esophageal peristalsis. Finally, in patients with typical symptoms of GERD, ambulatory pH monitoring is indicated to document the presence of abnormal distal esophageal acid exposure. Although the results of ambulatory pH monitoring rarely change the decision for operative repair of PEH, preoperative documentation of GERD is particularly useful as a baseline for comparison in patients who have recurrent symptoms postoperatively.

Operative Repair

PEH can be repaired through the left side of the chest or the abdomen and with open or minimally invasive techniques. Laparoscopy has decreased perioperative morbidity associated with elective PEH repair, and most PEH repairs are currently performed by a laparoscopic approach. This is of particular importance because PEH occurs frequently in older patients with multiple medical comorbidities. Regardless of the operative approach, there are four key steps to PEH repair: (1) reduction of the hernia contents to the abdominal cavity; (2) complete excision of the hernia sac from the posterior mediastinum; (3) mobilization of

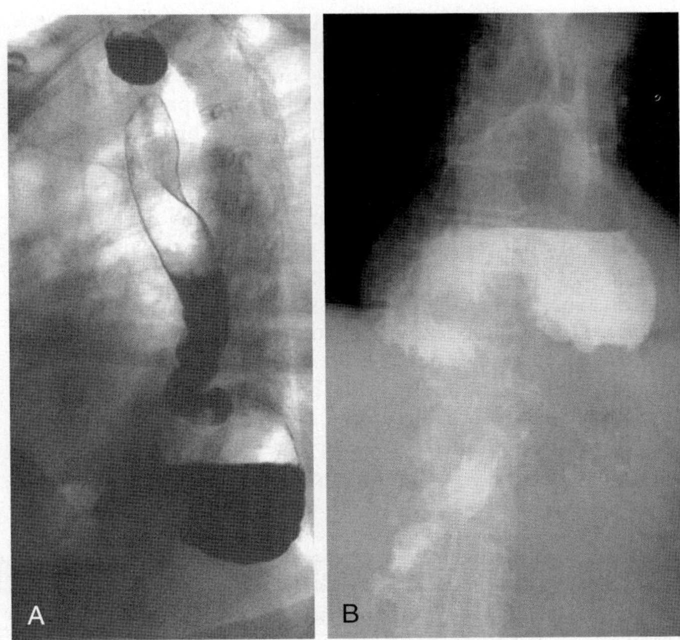

FIGURE 42-18 Upper gastrointestinal series is essential to understand the anatomy of a paraesophageal hernia. **A,** Oblique view demonstrating a distended stomach with an air-fluid level anterior to the esophagus and well into the mediastinum. **B,** Anteroposterior view demonstrating complete organoaxial volvulus with a completely intrathoracic stomach and the pylorus at the hiatus.

the distal esophagus to achieve a minimum of 3 cm of intra-abdominal esophageal length; and (4) an antireflux operation.

Our preferred approach is laparoscopic PEH repair. Only in the very rare patient have we found the need to perform either an open abdominal operation or a thoracotomy. Patient positioning and trocar placement for laparoscopic PEH repair are the same as for LARS. However, several important variations in operative technique must be made because of the unique anatomy of PEH.

The operation begins by reducing the hernia contents to the abdominal cavity using gentle traction and only to the extent that the contents can be easily reduced. Frequently, however, the hernia contents cannot be fully reduced because adhesions develop between the hernia sac and the posterior mediastinum. This prevents clear visualization of the left crus. Consequently, we divide the short gastric vessels to mobilize the fundus of the stomach and safely expose the left crus.

Once the left crus is exposed, it is necessary to enter the posterior mediastinum outside the hernia sac, which will facilitate complete excision of the hernia sac from the chest. This plane lies between the phrenoesophageal membrane and the left crus. Visualization of the muscle fibers of the left crus is confirmation that the surgeon is in the correct plane. At this point, the peritoneal sac should be divided anteriorly, parallel to the left crus. Further dissection of the sac from its mediastinal attachments will free the stomach and allow it to be delivered into the peritoneal cavity. During this mobilization, the surgeon and assistant must avoid vigorous traction on the sac, which is still attached to the esophagus and can result in esophageal tears. After the hernia contents are returned to the peritoneal cavity, the hernia sac must be transected circumferentially at the hiatus.

The most challenging aspect of the sac dissection is encountered during the mobilization of the posterior sac. The esophagus and posterior vagus nerve are intimately associated with the sac posteriorly and can be easily injured during this dissection. A lighted bougie helps identify the exact location of the esophagus. Once the esophagus is clearly identified, the bougie should be pulled back to avoid unnecessarily thinning the esophageal wall and maximizing the posterior mediastinal space to facilitate further dissection. After the sac is freed at the hiatus, a concerted effort is made to remove as much of the hernia sac from the mediastinum as possible. However, the pleura, esophagus, pericardium, aorta, and inferior pulmonary veins are intimately related to the hernia sac, and these vital structures may be injured during this dissection. The surgeon's desire to remove the entire sac must be tempered by the possibility of injuring these vital structures. Once the sac is excised from the mediastinum, the esophagus is further mobilized to obtain a minimum of 3 cm of intra-abdominal length. Then, the crura are reapproximated with interrupted nonabsorbable suture.

Tension-free closure of the esophageal hiatus is a key step in the repair of PEH. In some patients, lack of pliability of the diaphragmatic crura makes a tension-free closure of the hiatus impossible. In our experience, the size of the hernia does not accurately predict the ability to close the hiatus without tension. However, scarred and poorly pliable crura are frequently encountered during repair of recurrent hiatal hernias. If a tension-free closure is not possible, two options are available: (1) close the hiatus under tension and reinforce the closure with biologic mesh; and (2) perform a diaphragmatic relaxing incision to allow primary tension-free closure of the hiatus and reinforce the relaxing incision and hiatal closure with biologic mesh. Importantly, permanent synthetic mesh should never be used at the esophageal hiatus as it is associated with esophageal erosion and stenosis.

If the hiatus can be closed primarily but under some tension, biologic mesh should be placed to reinforce this closure. To do this, a 7 × 10-cm piece of biologic mesh is cut into the shape of a horseshoe. The mesh is then placed at the hiatus. This can be done in a U configuration, with the base overlying the posterior hiatal closure, or in a C configuration, with the base overlying the right crus and limbs of the mesh lying anterior and posterior to the esophagus. The C configuration has the advantage of reinforcing the anterior and posterior hiatus. The orientation of the mesh placement should be according to the surgeon's preference. The mesh is sutured to the diaphragm, and fibrin glue is used to reinforce the mesh placement (Fig. 42-19).

Several studies have investigated the use of mesh to reinforce hiatal closure in PEH repair (Table 42-4). A multi-institutional randomized clinical trial compared primary hiatal closure and reinforcement of primary closure with biologic mesh. At 6 months

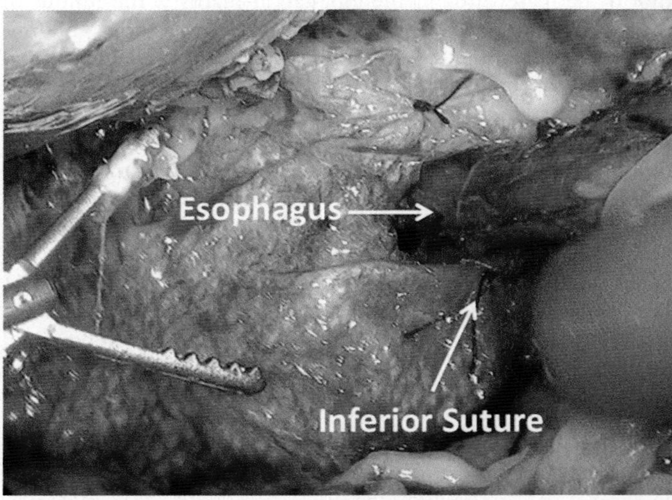

FIGURE 42-19 When the closure of the esophageal hiatus is met with mild to moderate tension, we place a 7 × 10-cm piece of biologic mesh to reinforce the hiatal closure.

TABLE 42-4 Studies of Biologic Mesh in Patients Undergoing Paraesophageal Hernia Repair

STUDY	STUDY DESIGN	ARMS	MEDIAN FOLLOW-UP	RECURRENCE
Oelschlager et al,[45] 2011	RCT	Surgisis, $n = 26$; no mesh, $n = 34$	59 months	Surgisis, 54%; no mesh, 59%; $P = .7$
Oelschlager et al,[48] 2006	RCT	Surgisis, $n = 51$; no mesh, $n = 57$	6 months	Surgisis, 9%; no mesh, 24%; $P = .04$
Ringley et al,[49] 2006	Retrospective	Alloderm, $n = 22$; no mesh, $n = 22$	7 months	Alloderm, 0%; no mesh, 9%; $P < .05$
Jacobs et al,[50] 2007	Retrospective	Surgisis, $n = 127$; no mesh, $n = 93$	38 months	Surgisis, 3%; no mesh, 20%; $P < .01$

RCT, randomized controlled trial.

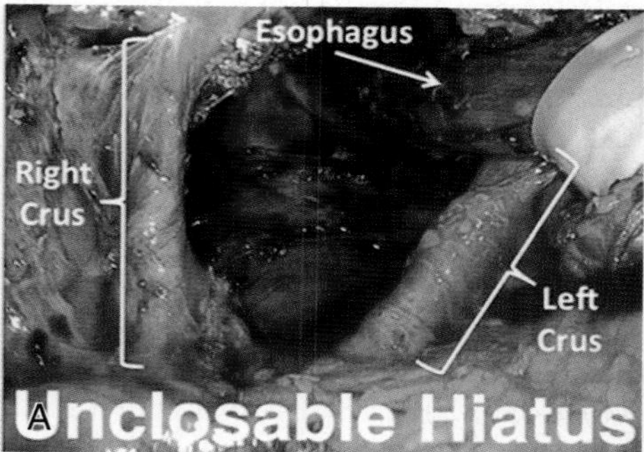

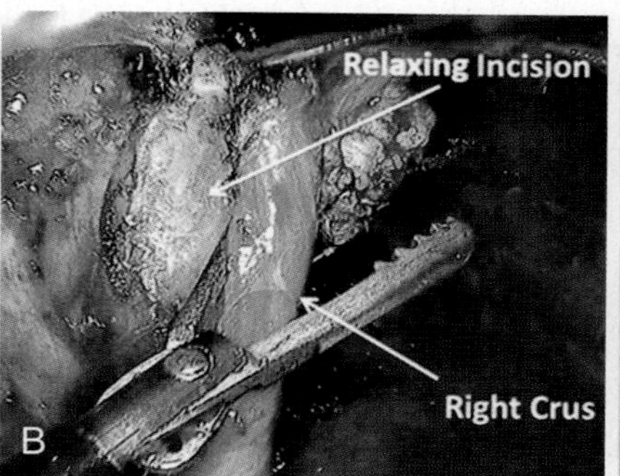

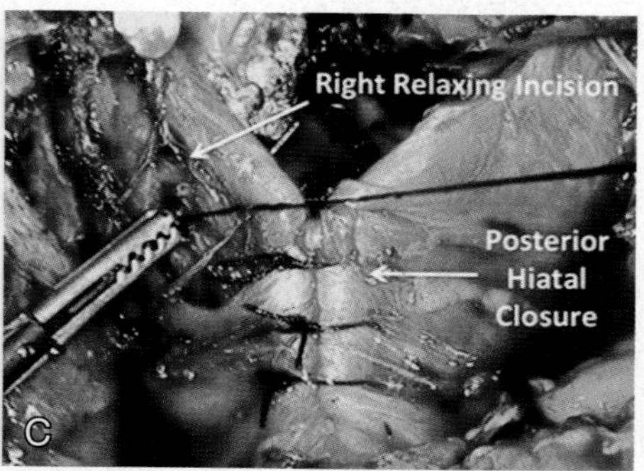

FIGURE 42-20 When poorly pliable crura prevent primary closure of the esophageal hiatus *(left)*, a relaxing incision is placed on the right crus *(middle)* to facilitate closure *(right)*.

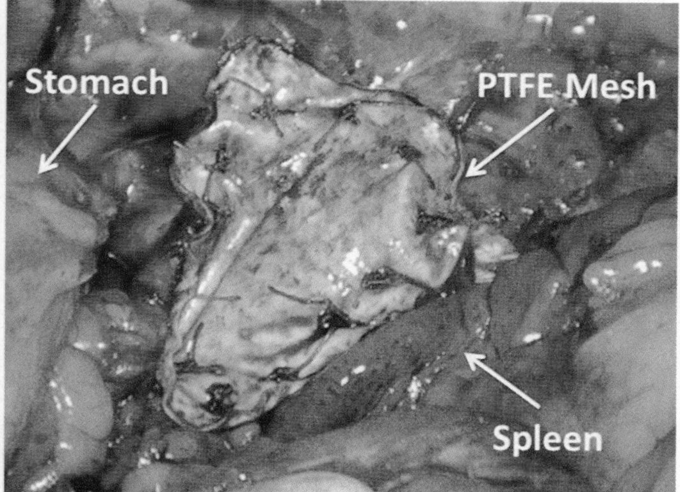

FIGURE 42-21 When bilateral relaxing incisions are necessary to facilitate hiatal closure, the left-sided relaxing incision is covered with permanent mesh to prevent the development of a diaphragmatic hernia. *PTFE*, polytetrafluoroethylene.

of follow-up, hiatal hernia recurrence rate was significantly lower when the hiatus was reinforced with biologic mesh compared with primary closure alone (9% versus 24%; $P = .04$).[44] However, at 5-year follow-up, there was no significant difference in hiatal hernia recurrence rates between patients with and without mesh.[45] This suggests that biologic mesh reinforcement of the hiatal closure in PEH repair decreases early but not late recurrent hiatal hernias. In this randomized trial using biologic mesh, there were no mesh-related complications.

On occasion, the pliability of the crura is so poor that the hiatus cannot be closed primarily. In this situation, a crural relaxing incision is performed to facilitate closure. Relaxing incisions have been described on the right and left crura. We prefer to perform a relaxing incision on the right crus (Fig. 42-20) and to patch the defect with a U-shaped biologic mesh, as described before. In very few patients, when the hiatus will not close with a right-sided relaxing incision, a left-sided relaxing incision is performed, which facilitates medialization of the left crus and primary closure. In our experience, coverage of the left-sided relaxing incision with biologic mesh is associated with the development of diaphragmatic hernias and need for reoperation. Therefore, we now patch this defect with permanent synthetic polytetrafluoroethylene mesh (Fig. 42-21). We have not encountered any complications with permanent mesh placement in this location.

After the hiatus is closed, an antireflux procedure is performed. A Nissen fundoplication is performed in all patients except those with severely ineffective motility or aperistaltic esophagus. In such patients, a Toupet fundoplication is performed. Although the need for an antireflux procedure is controversial, many patients with PEH have abnormal reflux, and the fundoplication will seal the hiatus, preventing access by other viscera. Postoperative care is the same as for patients who have undergone LARS.

Acute Gastric Volvulus and Strangulation

A relatively rare occurrence, acute gastric volvulus is a clinical emergency. Patients present with sudden onset of chest or epigastric pain associated with retching without the production of emesis. The development of fever, tachycardia, and leukocytosis suggests gastric strangulation and impending perforation. Gastric volvulus is necessary but not sufficient for gastric ischemia to develop. More often, patients present with subacute or chronic recurrent gastric volvulus, which causes gastroesophageal obstructive symptoms but never results in gastric ischemia.

Initial management of acute gastric volvulus should include placement of a nasogastric tube for gastric decompression. If bedside placement of a nasogastric tube is not possible, esophagoscopy can facilitate gastric decompression and nasogastric tube placement. On occasion, endoscopic reduction of volvulus is possible. Endoscopy also allows assessment of the gastric mucosa; if gastric ischemia is present, emergent operation is indicated.

The operative management of acute gastric volvulus should follow the same tenets as for PEH repair. In otherwise healthy patients, a formal laparoscopic PEH repair should be performed. In high operative risk patients who may not tolerate a prolonged general anesthetic necessary for PEH repair, consideration should be given to laparoscopic reduction of the gastric volvulus and anterior abdominal wall gastropexy.

SUMMARY

Operative treatment of GERD and PEH has become more common in the era of laparoscopic procedures. Careful selection of patients based on symptom assessment, response to medical therapy, and preoperative testing will optimize chances for effective and durable postoperative control of symptoms. Complications of LARS and repair of PEH are rare and generally can be managed without reoperation. When reoperation is necessary for operative failures, it should be performed by high-volume surgeons.

SELECTED REFERENCES

Jobe BA, Richter JE, Hoppo T, et al: Preoperative diagnostic workup before antireflux surgery: An evidence and experience based consensus of the Esophageal Diagnostic Advisory Panel. *J Am Coll Surg* 217:586–597, 2013.

A consensus statement from experienced surgeons and gastroenterologists in the field of GERD on the preoperative diagnostic testing of patients with GERD.

Niebisch S, Fleming FJ, Galey KM, et al: Perioperative risk of laparoscopic fundoplication: Safer than previously reported—analysis of the American College of Surgeons National Surgical Quality Improvement Program 2005-2009. *J Am Coll Surg* 215:61–68, 2012.

An observational study of more than 7500 patients who underwent laparoscopic fundoplication demonstrating a 30-day mortality and morbidity of 0.18% and 3.8%, respectively.

Oelschlager BK, Pellegrini CA, Hunter JG, et al: Biologic mesh to prevent recurrence after laparoscopic paraesophageal hernia repair: Long-term follow-up from a multicenter, prospective, randomized trial. *J Am Coll Surg* 213:461–468, 2011.

Long-term follow-up to a randomized trial evaluating the effectiveness of biologic mesh reinforcement of the esophageal hiatus at the time of paraesophageal hernia repair.

Oelschlager BK, Petersen RP, Brunt LM, et al: Laparoscopic paraesophageal hernia repair: Defining long-term clinical and anatomic outcomes. *J Gastrointest Surg* 16:453–459, 2012.

A multicenter randomized trial that evaluated the symptomatic response to laparoscopic paraesophageal hernia repair as well as the relationship between recurrent symptoms and recurrent hiatal hernia.

Richenbacher N, Kotter T, Kochen MM, et al: Fundoplication versus medical management of gastroesophageal reflux disease: A systemic review and meta-analysis. *Surg Endosc* 28:143–155, 2014.

Meta-analysis of trials comparing surgical fundoplication with medical management of GERD.

Smith CD: Antireflux surgery. *Surg Clin North Am* 88:943–958, 2008.

Comprehensive review of the diagnostic workup, patient selection criteria, surgical technique, and postoperative management for patients with GERD.

Soper NJ, Teitelbaum EN: Laparoscopic paraesophageal hernia repair: Current controversies. *Surg Laparosc Endosc Percutan Tech* 23:442–445, 2013.

Review of laparoscopic paraesophageal hernia repair operative technique and discussion of controversies in repair, including use of mesh cruroplasty and performance of esophagogastric fundoplication.

Wileman SM, McCann S, Grant AM, et al: Medical versus surgical management for gastro-oesophageal reflux disease (GORD) in adults. *Cochrane Database Syst Rev* (3):CD003243, 2010.

Comprehensive review of major studies investigating whether medical or surgical management is the most clinically and cost-effective treatment for patients with GERD.

Worrell SG, Greene CL, DeMeester TR: The state of surgical treatment of gastroesophageal reflux disease after five decades. *J Am Coll Surg* 219:819–830, 2014.

A clear, concise, and thorough description of the approach to the surgical management of patients with GERD, including selection of the appropriate operation and avoidance of operative technical pitfalls.

REFERENCES

1. Mainie I, Tutuian R, Shay S, et al: Acid and non-acid reflux in patients with persistent symptoms despite acid suppressive therapy: A multicentre study using combined ambulatory impedance-pH monitoring. *Gut* 55:1398–1402, 2006.
2. Worrell SG, DeMeester SR, Greene CL, et al: Pharyngeal pH monitoring better predicts a successful outcome for extra-esophageal reflux symptoms after antireflux surgery. *Surg Endosc* 27:4113–4118, 2013.
3. Bowrey DJ, Peters JH, DeMeester TR: Gastroesophageal reflux disease in asthma: Effects of medical and surgical antireflux therapy on asthma control. *Ann Surg* 231:161–172, 2000.
4. Raghu G, Freudenberger TD, Yang S, et al: High prevalence of abnormal acid gastro-oesophageal reflux in idiopathic pulmonary fibrosis. *Eur Respir J* 27:136–142, 2006.
5. Lee JS, Ryu JH, Elicker BM, et al: Gastroesophageal reflux therapy is associated with longer survival in patients with idiopathic pulmonary fibrosis. *Am J Respir Crit Care Med* 184:1390–1394, 2011.
6. Raghu G, Yang ST-Y, Spada C, et al: Sole treatment of acid gastroesophageal reflux in idiopathic pulmonary fibrosis: A case series. *Chest* 129:794–800, 2006.
7. Campos GMR, Peters JH, DeMeester TR, et al: Multivariate analysis of factors predicting outcome after laparoscopic Nissen fundoplication. *J Gastrointest Surg* 3:292–300, 1999.
8. Bredenoord AJ, Weusten BL, Timmer R, et al: Addition of esophageal impedance monitoring to pH monitoring increases the yield of symptom association analysis in patients off PPI therapy. *Am J Gastroenterol* 101:453–459, 2006.
9. Patel A, Sayuk GS, Gyawali CP: Parameters on esophageal pH-impedance monitoring that predict outcomes of patients with gastroesophageal reflux disease. *Clin Gastroenterol Hepatol* 13:884–891, 2015.
10. Kahrilas PJ, Dodds WJ, Hogan WJ, et al: Esophageal peristaltic dysfunction in peptic esophagitis. *Gastroenterology* 91:897–904, 1986.
11. Armstrong D: Endoscopic evaluation of gastro-esophageal reflux disease. *Yale J Biol Med* 72:93–100, 1999.
12. Epstein D, Bojke L, Sculpher MJ, et al: Laparoscopic fundoplication compared with medical management for gastro-oesophageal reflux disease: Cost effectiveness study. *BMJ* 339:b2576, 2009.

13. Wong RK, Hanson DG, Waring PJ, et al: ENT manifestations of gastroesophageal reflux. *Am J Gastroenterol* 95(Suppl):S15–S22, 2000.
14. Booth MI, Stratford J, Jones L, et al: Randomized clinical trial of laparoscopic total (Nissen) versus posterior partial (Toupet) fundoplication for gastro-oesophageal reflux disease based on preoperative oesophageal manometry. *Br J Surg* 95:57–63, 2008.
15. Oleynikov D, Eubanks TR, Oelschlager BK, et al: Total fundoplication is the operation of choice for patients with gastroesophageal reflux and defective peristalsis. *Surg Endosc* 16:909–913, 2002.
16. Fein M, Seyfried F: Is there a role for anything other than a Nissen's operation? *J Gastrointest Surg* 14(Suppl 1):S67–S74, 2010.
17. Shan CX, Zhang W, Zheng XM, et al: Evidence-based appraisal in laparoscopic Nissen and Toupet fundoplications for gastroesophageal reflux disease. *World J Gastroenterol* 16:3063–3071, 2010.
18. Kaufman JA, Houghland JE, Quiroga E, et al: Long-term outcomes of laparoscopic antireflux surgery for gastroesophageal reflux disease (GERD)–related airway disorder. *Surg Endosc* 20:1824–1830, 2006.
19. Rossi M, Barreca M, de Bortoli N, et al: Efficacy of Nissen fundoplication versus medical therapy in the regression of low-grade dysplasia in patients with Barrett esophagus: A prospective study. *Ann Surg* 243:58–63, 2006.
20. Katz PO, Gerson LB, Vela MF: Guidelines for the diagnosis and management of gastroesophageal reflux disease. *Am J Gastroenterol* 108:308–328, quiz 329, 2013.
21. Finley K, Giannamore M, Bennett M, et al: Assessing the impact of lifestyle modification education on knowledge and behavior changes in gastroesophageal reflux disease patients on proton pump inhibitors. *J Am Pharm Assoc* 49:544–548, 2009.
22. Ali T, Roberts DN, Tierney WM: Long-term safety concerns with proton pump inhibitors. *Am J Med* 122:896–903, 2009.
23. Heidelbaugh JJ, Kim AH, Chang R, et al: Overutilization of proton-pump inhibitors: What the clinician needs to know. *Ther Adv Gastroenterol* 5:219–232, 2012.
24. Havu N: Enterochromaffin-like cell carcinoids of gastric mucosa in rats after life-long inhibition of gastric secretion. *Digestion* 35(Suppl 1):42–55, 1986.
25. Jianu CS, Lange OJ, Viset T, et al: Gastric neuroendocrine carcinoma after long-term use of proton pump inhibitor. *Scand J Gastroenterol* 47:64–67, 2012.
26. Oelschlager BK, Yamamoto K, Woltman T, et al: Vagotomy during hiatal hernia repair: A benign esophageal lengthening procedure. *J Gastrointest Surg* 12:1155–1162, 2008.
27. Spechler SJ, Lee E, Ahnen D, et al: Long-term outcome of medical and surgical therapies for gastroesophageal reflux disease: Follow-up of a randomized controlled trial. *JAMA* 285:2331–2338, 2001.
28. Lundell L, Miettinen P, Myrvold HE, et al: Seven-year follow-up of a randomized clinical trial comparing proton-pump inhibition with surgical therapy for reflux oesophagitis. *Br J Surg* 94:198–203, 2007.
29. Lundell L, Miettinen P, Myrvold HE, et al: Comparison of outcomes twelve years after antireflux surgery or omeprazole maintenance therapy for reflux esophagitis. *Clin Gastroenterol Hepatol* 7:1292–1298, 2009.
30. Dallemagne B, Weerts J, Markiewicz S, et al: Clinical results of laparoscopic fundoplication at ten years after surgery. *Surg Endosc* 20:159–165, 2006.
31. Oelschlager BK, Eubanks TR, Oleynikov D, et al: Symptomatic and physiologic outcomes after operative treatment for extraesophageal reflux. *Surg Endosc* 16:1032–1036, 2002.
32. Niebisch S, Fleming FJ, Galey KM, et al: Perioperative risk of laparoscopic fundoplication: Safer than previously reported—analysis of the American College of Surgeons National Surgical Quality Improvement Program 2005 to 2009. *J Am Coll Surg* 215:61–68, discussion 68–69, 2012.
33. Bizekis C, Kent M, Luketich J: Complications after surgery for gastroesophageal reflux disease. *Thorac Surg Clin* 16:99–108, 2006.
34. Odabasi M, Abuoglu HH, Arslan C, et al: Asymptomatic partial splenic infarction in laparoscopic floppy Nissen fundoplication and brief literature review. *Int Surg* 99:291–294, 2014.
35. Kessing BF, Broeders JA, Vinke N, et al: Gas-related symptoms after antireflux surgery. *Surg Endosc* 27:3739–3747, 2013.
36. Lamb PJ, Myers JC, Jamieson GG, et al: Long-term outcomes of revisional surgery following laparoscopic fundoplication. *Br J Surg* 96:391–397, 2009.
37. Bell RCW, Mavrelis PG, Barnes WE, et al: A prospective multicenter registry of patients with chronic gastroesophageal reflux disease receiving transoral incisionless fundoplication. *J Am Coll Surg* 215:794–809, 2012.
38. Muls V, Eckardt AJ, Marchese M, et al: Three-year results of a multicenter prospective study of transoral incisionless fundoplication. *Surg Innov* 20:321–330, 2013.
39. Louie BE, Farivar AS, Shultz D, et al: Short-term outcomes using magnetic sphincter augmentation versus Nissen fundoplication for medically resistant gastroesophageal reflux disease. *Ann Thorac Surg* 98:498–504, discussion 504–505, 2014.
40. Sheu EG, Nau P, Nath B, et al: A comparative trial of laparoscopic magnetic sphincter augmentation and Nissen fundoplication. *Surg Endosc* 29:505–509, 2015.
41. Lipham JC, DeMeester TR, Ganz RA, et al: The LINX reflux management system: Confirmed safety and efficacy now at 4 years. *Surg Endosc* 26:2944–2949, 2012.
42. Harnsberger CR, Broderick RC, Fuchs HF, et al: Magnetic lower esophageal sphincter augmentation device removal. *Surg Endosc* 29:984–986, 2015.
43. Stylopoulos N, Gazelle GS, Rattner DW: Paraesophageal hernias: Operation or observation? *Ann Surg* 236:492–500, discussion 500–501, 2002.
44. Oelschlager BK, Pellegrini CA, Hunter J, et al: Biologic prosthesis reduces recurrence after laparoscopic paraesophageal hernia repair: A multicenter, prospective, randomized trial. *Ann Surg* 244:481–490, 2006.
45. Oelschlager BK, Pellegrini CA, Hunter JG, et al: Biologic prosthesis to prevent recurrence after laparoscopic paraesophageal hernia repair: Long-term follow-up from a multicenter, prospective, randomized trial. *J Am Coll Surg* 213:461–468, 2011.
46. Anvari M, Allen C, Marshall J, et al: A randomized controlled trial of laparoscopic Nissen fundoplication versus proton pump inhibitors for the treatment of patients with

chronic gastroesophageal reflux disease (GERD): 3-year outcomes. *Surg Endosc* 25:2547–2554, 2011.

47. Grant AM, Wileman SM, Ramsay CR, et al: Minimal access surgery compared with medical management for chronic gastro-oesophageal reflux disease: UK collaborative randomised trial. *BMJ* 337:a2664, 2008.
48. Oelschlager BK, Pellegrini CA, Hunter J, et al: Biologic prosthesis reduces recurrence after laparoscopic paraesophageal hernia repair: A multicenter, prospective, randomized trial. *Ann Surg* 244:481–490, 2006.
49. Ringley CD, Bochkarev V, Ahmed SI, et al: Laparoscopic hiatal hernia repair with human acellular dermal matrix patch: Our initial experience. *Am J Surg* 192:767–772, 2006.
50. Jacobs M, Gomez E, Plasencia G, et al: Use of Surgisis mesh in laparoscopic repair of hiatal hernias. *Surg Laparosc Endosc Percutan Tech* 17:365–368, 2007.

SECTION X

Abdomen

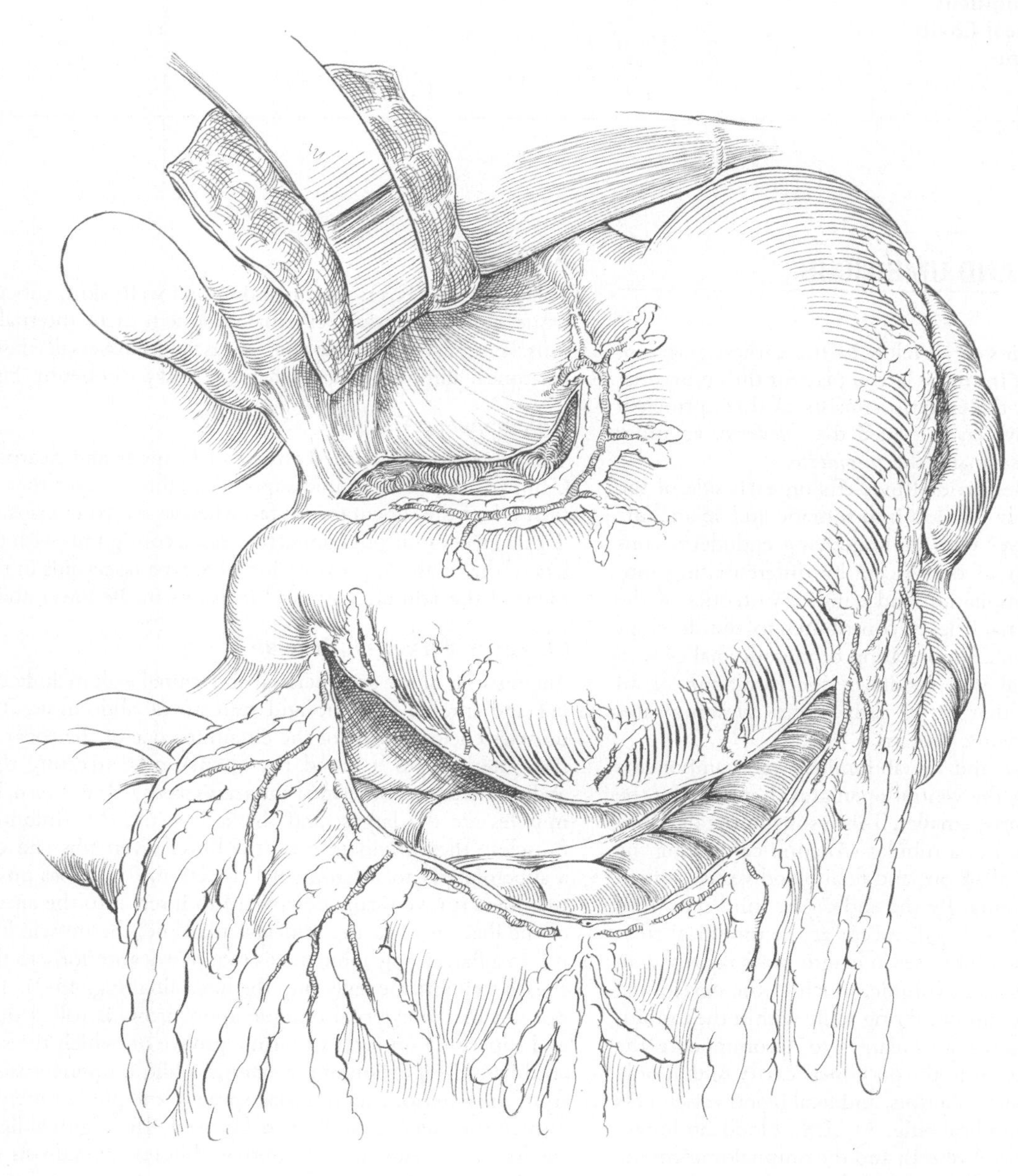

43 CHAPTER

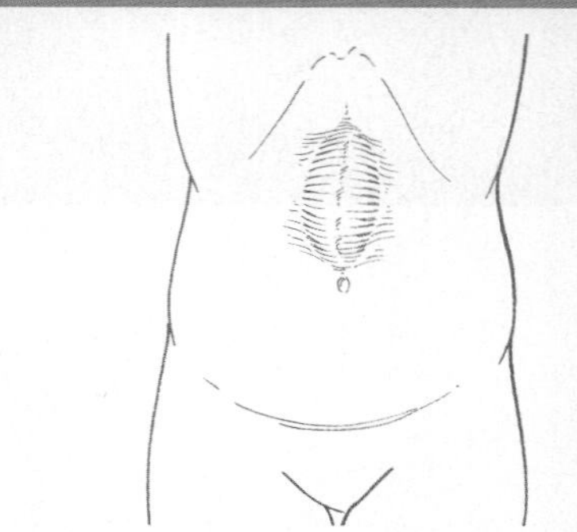

Abdominal Wall, Umbilicus, Peritoneum, Mesenteries, Omentum, and Retroperitoneum

Richard H. Turnage, Jason Mizell, Brian Badgwell

OUTLINE

ABDOMINAL WALL AND UMBILICUS

Embryology

The abdominal wall begins to develop in the earliest stages of embryonic differentiation from the lateral plate of the embryonic mesoderm. At this stage, the embryo consists of three principal layers—an outer protective layer termed the *ectoderm;* an inner nutritive layer, the *endoderm;* and the *mesoderm.*

The mesoderm becomes divided by clefts on each side of the lateral plate that ultimately develop into somatic and splanchnic layers. The splanchnic layer with its underlying endoderm contributes to the formation of the viscera by differentiating into muscle, blood vessels, lymphatics, and connective tissues of the alimentary tract. The somatic layer contributes to the development of the abdominal wall. Proliferation of mesodermal cells in the embryonic abdominal wall results in the formation of an inverted U-shaped tube that in its early stages communicates freely with the extraembryonic coelom.

As the embryo enlarges and the abdominal wall components grow toward one another, the ventral open area, bounded by the edge of the amnion, becomes smaller. This results in the development of the umbilical cord as a tubular structure containing the omphalomesenteric duct, allantois, and fetal blood vessels, which pass to and from the placenta. By the end of the third month of gestation, the body wall has closed, except at the umbilical ring. Because the alimentary tract increases in length more rapidly than the coelomic cavity increases in volume, much of the developing gut protrudes through the umbilical ring to lie within the umbilical cord. As the coelomic cavity enlarges to accommodate the intestine, the intestine returns to the peritoneal cavity so that only the omphalomesenteric duct, allantois, and fetal blood vessels pass through the shrinking umbilical ring. At birth, blood no longer courses through the umbilical vessels, and the omphalomesenteric duct has been reduced to a fibrous cord that no longer communicates with the intestine. After division of the umbilical cord, the umbilical ring heals rapidly by scarring.

Anatomy

There are nine layers to the abdominal wall: skin, subcutaneous tissue, superficial fascia, external oblique muscle, internal oblique muscle, transversus abdominis muscle, transversalis fascia, preperitoneal adipose and areolar tissue, and peritoneum (Fig. 43-1).

Subcutaneous Tissues

The subcutaneous tissue consists of Camper and Scarpa fasciae. Camper fascia is the more superficial adipose layer that contains the bulk of the subcutaneous fat, whereas Scarpa fascia is a deeper, denser layer of fibrous connective tissue contiguous with the fascia lata of the thigh. Approximation of Scarpa fascia aids in the alignment of the skin after surgical incisions in the lower abdomen.

Muscle and Investing Fasciae

The muscles of the anterolateral abdominal wall include the external and internal oblique and transversus abdominis. These flat muscles enclose much of the circumference of the torso and give rise anteriorly to a broad flat aponeurosis investing the rectus abdominis muscles, termed the *rectus sheath.* The external oblique muscles are the largest and thickest of the flat abdominal wall muscles. They originate from the lower seven ribs and course in a superolateral to inferomedial direction. The most posterior of the fibers run vertically downward to insert into the anterior half of the iliac crest. At the midclavicular line, the muscle fibers give rise to a flat, strong aponeurosis that passes anteriorly to the rectus sheath to insert medially into the linea alba (Fig. 43-2). The lower portion of the external oblique aponeurosis is rolled posteriorly and superiorly on itself to form a groove on which the spermatic cord lies. This portion of the external oblique aponeurosis extends from the anterior superior iliac spine to the pubic tubercle and is termed the *inguinal* or *Poupart ligament.* The inguinal ligament is the lower free edge of the external oblique aponeurosis posterior to which pass the femoral artery, vein, and nerve and the iliacus, psoas major, and pectineus muscles. A femoral hernia passes posterior to the inguinal ligament, whereas an inguinal hernia passes

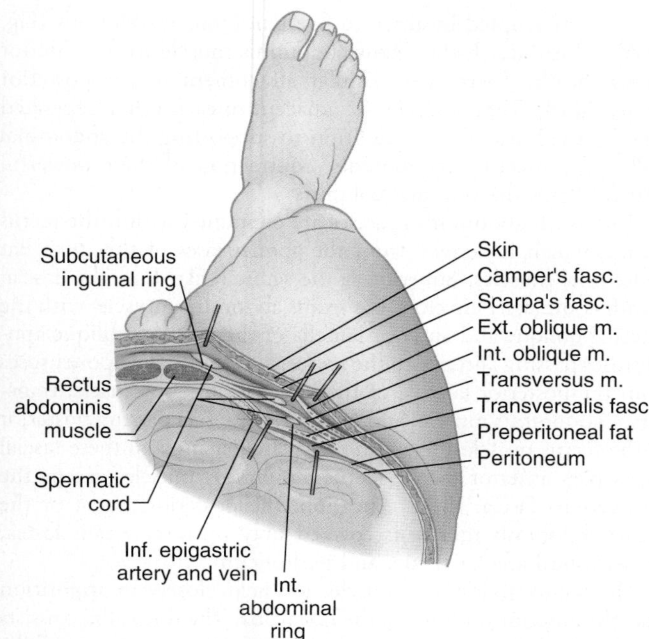

FIGURE 43-1 The nine layers of the anterolateral abdominal wall. (From Thorek P: *Anatomy in surgery,* ed 2, Philadelphia, 1962, JB Lippincott, p 358.)

anterior and superior to this ligament. The shelving edge of the inguinal ligament is used in various repairs of inguinal hernia, including the Bassini and the Lichtenstein tension-free repairs (see Chapter 44).

The internal oblique muscle originates from the iliopsoas fascia beneath the lateral half of the inguinal ligament, from the anterior two thirds of the iliac crest and lumbodorsal fascia. Its fibers course in a direction opposite to those of the external oblique, that is, inferolateral to superomedial. The uppermost fibers insert into the lower five ribs and their cartilages (Fig. 43-3; see Fig. 43-2*A*). The central fibers form an aponeurosis at the semilunar line, which, above the semicircular line (of Douglas), is divided into anterior and posterior lamellae that envelop the rectus abdominis muscle. Below the semicircular line, the aponeurosis of the internal oblique muscle courses anteriorly to the rectus abdominis muscle as part of the anterior rectus sheath. The lowermost fibers of the internal oblique muscle pursue an inferomedial course, paralleling that of the spermatic cord, to insert between the symphysis pubis and pubic tubercle. Some of the lower muscle fascicles accompany the spermatic cord into the scrotum as the cremasteric muscle.

The transversus abdominis muscle is the smallest of the muscles of the anterolateral abdominal wall. It arises from the lower six costal cartilages, spines of the lumbar vertebrae, iliac crest, and iliopsoas fascia beneath the lateral third of the inguinal ligament. The fibers course transversely to give rise to a flat aponeurotic sheet that passes posterior to the rectus abdominis muscle above the semicircular line and anterior to the muscle below it (Fig. 43-4). The inferiormost fibers of the transversus abdominis originating from the iliopsoas fascia pass inferomedially along with the lower fibers of the internal oblique muscle. These fibers form the aponeurotic arch of the transversus abdominis muscle, which lies superior to Hesselbach triangle and is an important anatomic landmark in the repair of inguinal hernias, particularly the Bassini operation and Cooper ligament repairs. Hesselbach triangle is the

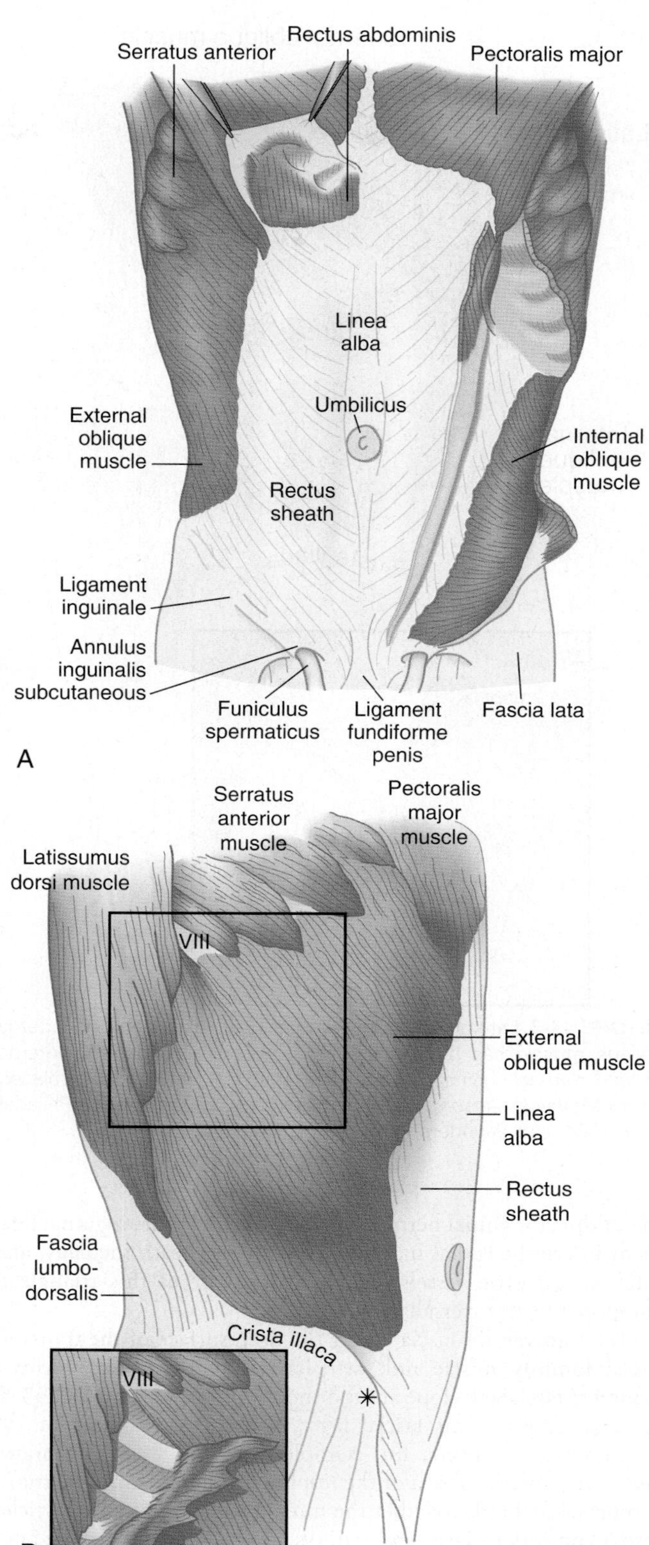

FIGURE 43-2 A, External oblique, internal oblique, and rectus abdominis muscles and anterior rectus sheath. **B,** Lateral view of the external oblique muscle and its aponeurosis as it enters the anterior rectus sheath. *Inset,* Origin of the external oblique muscle fibers from the lower ribs and their costal cartilages. (From McVay C: *Anson and McVay's surgical anatomy,* ed 6, Philadelphia, 1984, WB Saunders, pp 477–478.)

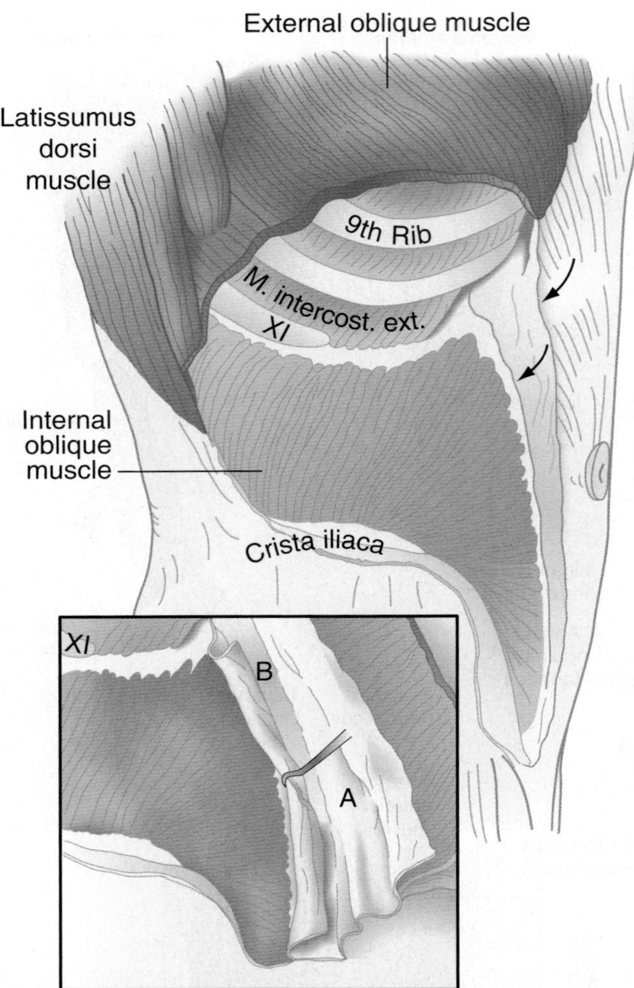

FIGURE 43-3 Lateral view of the internal oblique muscle. The external oblique muscle has been removed to show the underlying internal oblique muscle originating from the lower ribs and costal cartilages. (From McVay C: *Anson and McVay's surgical anatomy*, ed 6, Philadelphia, 1984, WB Saunders, p 479.)

site of direct inguinal hernias and is bordered by the inguinal ligament inferiorly, lateral margin of the rectus sheath medially, and inferior epigastric vessels laterally. The floor of this triangle is composed of transversalis fascia.

The transversalis fascia covers the deep surface of the transversus abdominis muscle and, with its various extensions, forms a complete fascial envelope around the abdominal cavity (Fig. 43-5; see Fig. 43-4*B*). This fascial layer is regionally named for the muscles that it covers, for example, iliopsoas fascia, obturator fascia, and inferior fascia of the respiratory diaphragm. The transversalis fascia binds together the muscle and aponeurotic fascicles into a continuous layer and reinforces weak areas where the aponeurotic fibers are sparse. This layer is responsible for the structural integrity of the abdominal wall, and by definition, a hernia results from a defect in the transversalis fascia.

The rectus abdominis muscles are paired muscles that appear as long, flat, triangular ribbons wider at their origin on the anterior surfaces of the fifth, sixth, and seventh costal cartilages and the xiphoid process than at their insertion on the pubic crest and pubic symphysis. Each muscle is composed of long parallel fascicles interrupted by three to five tendinous inscriptions (Fig. 43-5), which attach the rectus abdominis muscle to the anterior rectus sheath. There is no similar attachment to the posterior rectus sheath. These muscles lie adjacent to each other, separated only by the linea alba. In addition to supporting the abdominal wall and protecting its contents, contraction of these powerful muscles flexes the vertebral column.

The rectus abdominis muscles are contained within the rectus sheath, which is derived from the aponeuroses of the three flat abdominal muscles. Superior to the semicircular line, this fascial sheath completely envelops the rectus abdominis muscle, with the external oblique and anterior lamella of the internal oblique aponeuroses passing anterior to the rectus abdominis and aponeuroses from the posterior lamella of the internal oblique muscle, transversus abdominis muscle, and transversalis fascia passing posterior to the rectus muscle. Below the semicircular line, all these fascial layers pass anterior to the rectus abdominis muscle, except the transversalis fascia. In this location, the posterior aspect of the rectus abdominis muscle is covered only by transversalis fascia, preperitoneal areolar tissue, and peritoneum.

The rectus abdominis muscles are held closely in apposition near the anterior midline by the linea alba. The linea alba consists of a band of dense, crisscrossed fibers of the aponeuroses of the broad abdominal muscles that extends from the xiphoid to the pubic symphysis. It is much wider above the umbilicus than below, thus facilitating the placement of surgical incisions in the midline without entering the right or left rectus sheath.

Preperitoneal Space and Peritoneum

The preperitoneal space lies between the transversalis fascia and parietal peritoneum and contains adipose and areolar tissue. Coursing through the preperitoneal space are the following:

- Inferior epigastric artery and vein
- Medial umbilical ligaments, which are the vestiges of the fetal umbilical arteries
- Median umbilical ligament, which is a midline fibrous remnant of the fetal allantoic stalk or urachus
- Falciform ligament of the liver, extending from the umbilicus to the liver

The round ligament, or ligamentum teres, is contained within the free margin of the falciform ligament and represents the obliterated umbilical vein, coursing from the umbilicus to the left branch of the portal vein (Fig. 43-6). The parietal peritoneum is the innermost layer of the abdominal wall. It consists of a thin layer of dense, irregular connective tissue covered on its inner surface by a single layer of squamous mesothelium. The peritoneum is covered in more depth later in the chapter.

Vessels and Nerves of the Abdominal Wall

Vascular Supply

The anterolateral abdominal wall receives its arterial supply from the last six intercostals and four lumbar arteries, superior and inferior epigastric arteries, and deep circumflex iliac arteries (Fig. 43-7). The trunks of the intercostal and lumbar arteries together with the intercostal, iliohypogastric, and ilioinguinal nerves course between the transversus abdominis and internal oblique muscles. The distalmost extensions of these vessels pierce the lateral margins of the rectus sheath at various levels and communicate freely with branches of the superior and inferior epigastric arteries. The superior epigastric artery, one of the terminal branches of the internal mammary artery, reaches the posterior surface of the rectus abdominis muscle through the costoxiphoid space in the

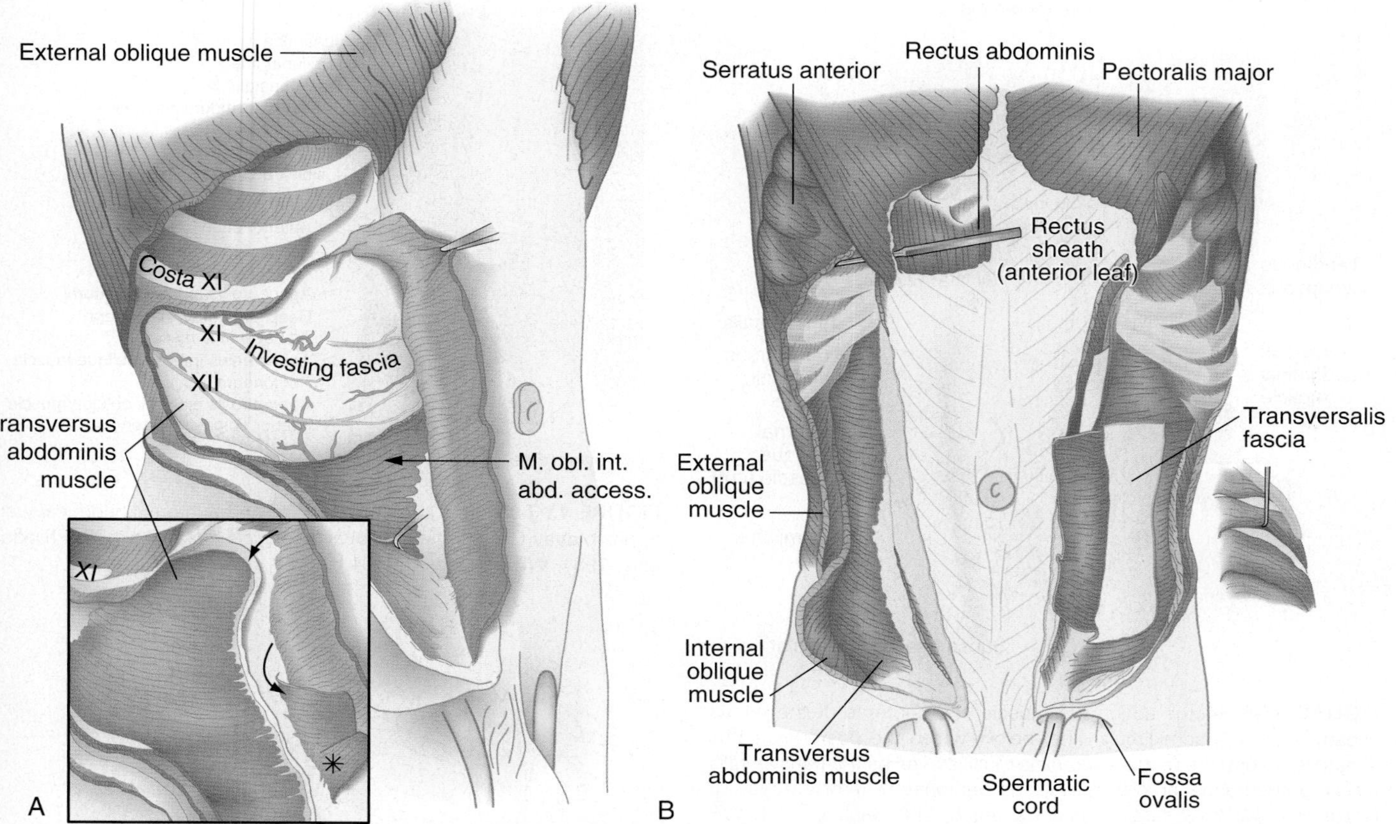

FIGURE 43-4 **A,** Anterolateral view of the investing fascia of the transversus abdominis muscle and the muscle itself with the fascia removed *(inset)*. The external and internal oblique muscles have been removed. Also note the appearance of the intercostal nerves lying between the fascia of the transversus abdominis muscle and internal oblique muscle. **B,** Anterior view of the transversus abdominis muscle *(left)* and the transversalis fascia *(right)*. Note that the transversalis fascia is shown by reflecting the overlying transversus abdominis muscle medially. (From McVay C: *Anson and McVay's surgical anatomy,* ed 6, Philadelphia, 1984, WB Saunders, pp 480–481.)

diaphragm. It descends within the rectus sheath to anastomose with branches of the inferior epigastric artery. The inferior epigastric artery, derived from the external iliac artery just proximal to the inguinal ligament, courses through the preperitoneal areolar tissue to enter the lateral rectus sheath at the semilunar line of Douglas. The deep circumflex iliac artery, arising from the lateral aspect of the external iliac artery near the origin of the inferior epigastric artery, gives rise to an ascending branch that penetrates the abdominal wall musculature just above the iliac crest, near the anterior superior iliac spine.

The venous drainage of the anterior abdominal wall follows a relatively simple pattern in which the superficial veins above the umbilicus empty into the superior vena cava by way of the internal mammary, intercostal, and long thoracic veins. The veins inferior to the umbilicus—the superficial epigastric, circumflex iliac, and pudendal veins—converge toward the saphenous opening in the groin to enter the saphenous vein and become a tributary to the inferior vena cava (Fig. 43-8). The numerous anastomoses between the infraumbilical and supraumbilical venous systems provide collateral pathways whereby venous return to the heart may bypass an obstruction of the superior or inferior vena cava. The paraumbilical vein, which passes from the left branch of the portal vein along the ligamentum teres to the umbilicus, provides important communication between the veins of the superficial abdominal wall and portal system in patients with portal venous obstruction. In this setting, portal blood flow is diverted away from the higher pressure portal system through the paraumbilical veins to the lower pressure veins of the anterior abdominal wall. The dilated superficial paraumbilical veins in this setting are termed *caput medusae.*

The lymphatic supply of the abdominal wall follows a pattern similar to the venous drainage. Those lymphatic vessels arising from the supraumbilical region drain into the axillary lymph nodes, whereas those arising from the infraumbilical region drain toward the superficial inguinal lymph nodes. The lymphatic vessels from the liver course along the ligamentum teres to the umbilicus to communicate with the lymphatics of the anterior abdominal wall. It is from this pathway that carcinoma in the liver may spread to involve the anterior abdominal wall at the umbilicus (Sister Mary Joseph node or nodule).

Innervation

The anterior rami of the thoracic nerves follow a curvilinear course forward in the intercostal spaces toward the midline of the body (see Fig. 43-7). The upper six thoracic nerves end near the sternum as anterior cutaneous sensory branches. Thoracic nerves 7 to 12 pass behind the costal cartilages and lower ribs to enter a plane between the internal oblique muscle and the transversus

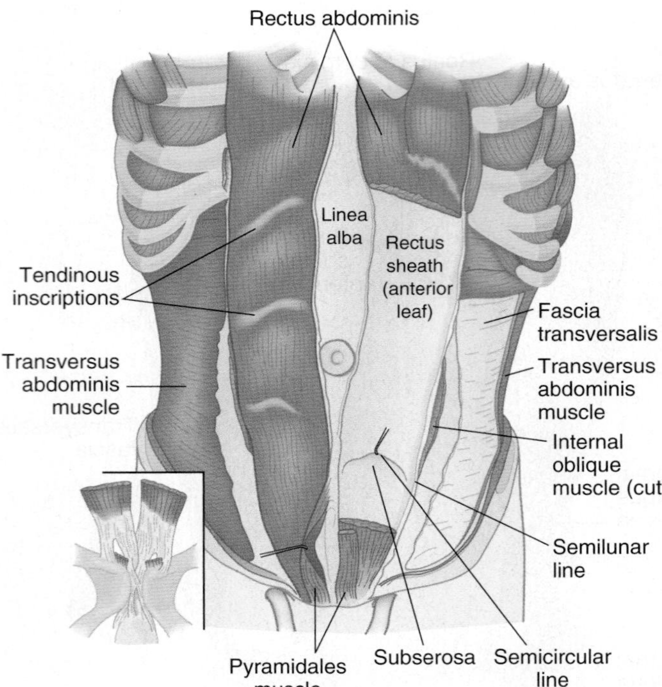

FIGURE 43-5 Rectus abdominis muscle and contents of the rectus sheath. Note the semicircular line, below which the posterior rectus sheath is absent; the rectus abdominis muscle overlies the transversalis fascia, preperitoneal areolar tissue, and peritoneum. (From McVay C: *Anson and McVay's surgical anatomy,* ed 6, Philadelphia, 1984, WB Saunders, p 482.)

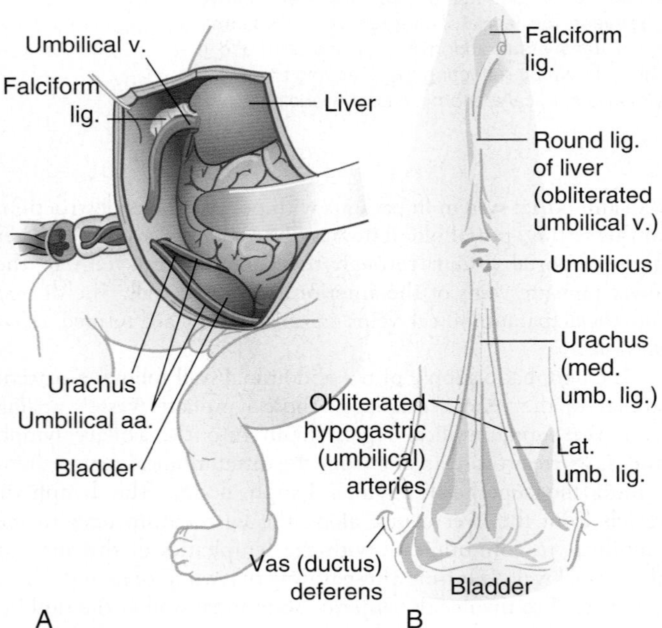

FIGURE 43-6 Umbilicus. A, In the fetus, the umbilical vein superiorly and the two umbilical arteries and urachus inferiorly radiate from the umbilicus. **B,** View of the umbilicus from within the peritoneal cavity showing the round ligament of the liver (derived from the obliterated umbilical vein) superiorly and the median umbilical ligament (derived from the obliterated urachus) and medial umbilical ligaments (also called the lateral umbilical ligaments, derived from the obliterated umbilical arteries). (From Thorek P: *Anatomy in surgery,* ed 2, Philadelphia, 1962, JB Lippincott, p 375.)

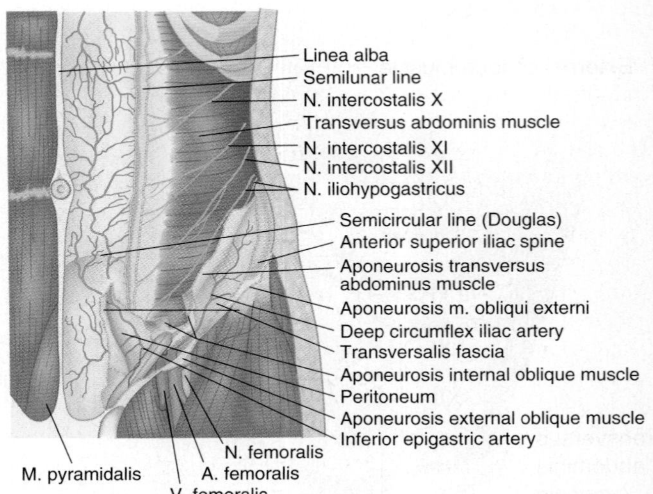

FIGURE 43-7 Arteries and nerves of the anterolateral abdominal wall. (From McVay C: *Anson and McVay's surgical anatomy,* ed 6, Philadelphia, 1984, WB Saunders, p 501.)

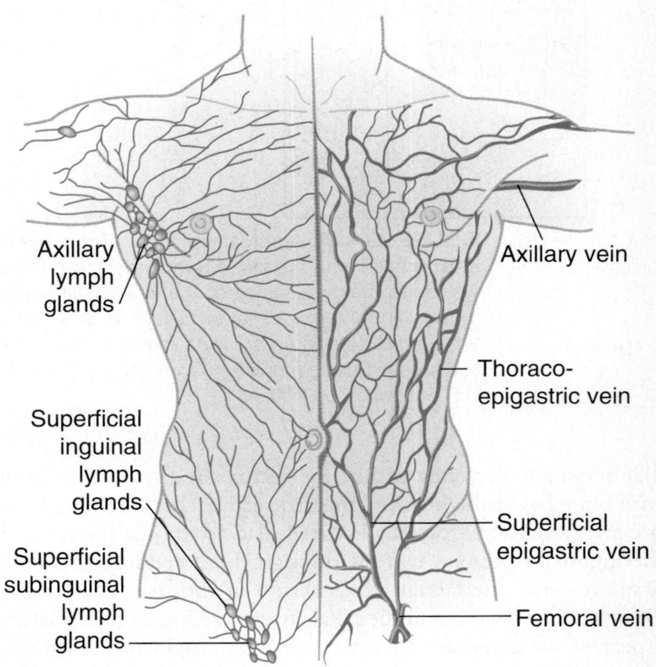

FIGURE 43-8 Venous and lymphatic drainage of the anterolateral abdominal wall. (From Thorek P: *Anatomy in surgery,* ed 2, Philadelphia, 1962, JB Lippincott, p 345.)

abdominis. The seventh and eighth nerves course slightly upward or horizontally to reach the epigastrium, whereas the lower nerves have an increasingly caudal trajectory. As these nerves course medially, they provide motor branches to the abdominal wall musculature. Medially, they perforate the rectus sheath to provide sensory innervation to the anterior abdominal wall. The anterior ramus of the 10th thoracic nerve reaches the skin at the level of the umbilicus, and the 12th thoracic nerve innervates the skin of the hypogastrium.

The ilioinguinal and iliohypogastric nerves often arise in common from the anterior rami of the 12th thoracic and first lumbar nerves to provide sensory innervation to the hypogastrium and lower abdominal wall. The iliohypogastric nerve runs parallel to the 12th thoracic nerve to pierce the transversus abdominis muscle near the iliac crest. After coursing between the transversus abdominis muscle and internal oblique for a short distance, the nerve pierces the internal oblique to travel under the external oblique fascia toward the external inguinal ring. It emerges through the superior crus of the external inguinal ring to provide sensory innervation to the anterior abdominal wall in the hypogastrium. The ilioinguinal nerve courses parallel to the iliohypogastric nerve but closer to the inguinal ligament than the iliohypogastric nerve. Unlike the iliohypogastric nerve, the ilioinguinal nerve courses with the spermatic cord to emerge from the external inguinal ring, with its terminal branches providing sensory innervation to the skin of the inguinal region and scrotum or labium. The ilioinguinal nerve, iliohypogastric nerve, and genital branch of the genitofemoral nerve are commonly encountered during the performance of inguinal herniorrhaphy.

Abnormalities of the Abdominal Wall

These can be congenital or acquired.

Congenital Abnormalities

Umbilical hernias. Umbilical hernias may be classified into three distinct forms: omphalocele and gastroschisis, infantile umbilical hernia, and acquired umbilical hernia.

Omphalocele. An omphalocele is a funnel-shaped defect in the central abdomen through which the viscera protrude into the base of the umbilical cord. It is caused by failure of the abdominal wall musculature to unite in the midline during fetal development. The umbilical vessels may be splayed over the viscera or pushed to one side. In larger defects, the liver and spleen may lie within the cord, along with a major portion of the bowel. There is no skin covering these defects, only peritoneum and, more superficially, amnion. Of infants who are born with an omphalocele, 50% to 60% will have concomitant congenital anomalies of the skeleton, gastrointestinal (GI) tract, nervous system, genitourinary system, or cardiopulmonary system.

Gastroschisis. Gastroschisis is another congenital defect of the abdominal wall in which the umbilical membrane has ruptured in utero, allowing the intestine to herniate outside the abdominal cavity. The defect is almost always to the right of the umbilical cord, and the intestine is not covered with skin or amnion. Typically, the intestine has not undergone complete mesenteric rotation and fixation; hence, the infant is at risk for mesenteric volvulus, with resultant intestinal ischemia and necrosis. Concomitant congenital anomalies occur in about 10% of these patients. Both omphalocele and gastroschisis are discussed in greater detail in Chapter 66.

Infantile umbilical hernia. The infantile umbilical hernia appears within a few days or weeks after the stump of the umbilical cord has sloughed. It is caused by a weakness in the adhesion between the scarred remnants of the umbilical cord and umbilical ring. In contrast to omphalocele, the infantile umbilical hernia is covered by skin. In general, these small hernias occur in the superior margin of the umbilical ring. They are easily reducible and become prominent when the infant cries. Most of these hernias resolve within the first 24 months of life, and complications such as strangulation are rare. Operative repair is indicated for those children in whom the hernia persists beyond the age of 3 or 4 years. This condition and its management are discussed further in Chapters 44 and 66.

Acquired umbilical hernia. In this condition, an umbilical hernia develops at a time remote from closure of the umbilical ring. This hernia occurs most commonly at the upper margin of the umbilicus and results from weakening of the cicatricial tissue that normally closes the umbilical ring. This weakening can be caused by excessive stretching of the abdominal wall, which may occur with pregnancy, vigorous labor, or ascites. In contrast to infantile umbilical hernias, acquired umbilical hernias do not spontaneously resolve but gradually increase in size. The dense fibrous ring at the neck of this hernia makes strangulation of herniated intestine or omentum an important complication.

Abnormalities resulting from persistence of the omphalomesenteric duct. During fetal development, the midgut communicates widely with the yolk sac through the vitelline or omphalomesenteric duct. As the abdominal wall components approximate one another, the omphalomesenteric duct narrows and comes to lie within the umbilical cord. Over time, communication between the yolk sac and intestine becomes obliterated, and the intestine resides free within the peritoneal cavity. Persistence of part or all of the omphalomesenteric duct results in a variety of abnormalities related to the intestine and abdominal wall (Fig. 43-9).

Persistence of the intestinal end of the omphalomesenteric duct results in Meckel's diverticulum. These true diverticula arise from the antimesenteric border of the small intestine, most often the ileum. A rule of 2s is often applied to these lesions in that they are found in approximately 2% of the population, are within 2 feet of the ileocecal valve, are often 2 inches in length, and contain 2 types of ectopic mucosa (gastric and pancreatic). Meckel's diverticula may be complicated by inflammation, perforation, hemorrhage, or obstruction. GI bleeding is caused by peptic ulceration

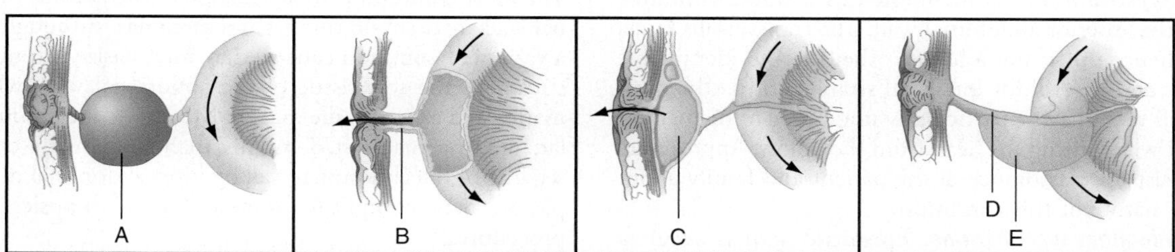

FIGURE 43-9 Abnormalities resulting from persistence of the omphalomesenteric duct. **A,** Omphalomesenteric duct cyst. **B,** Persistent omphalomesenteric duct with an enterocutaneous fistula. **C,** Omphalomesenteric duct cyst and sinus. **D,** Fibrous cord between the small intestine and the posterior surface of the umbilicus. **E,** Meckel's diverticulum. (From McVay C: *Anson and McVay's surgical anatomy,* ed 6, Philadelphia, 1984, WB Saunders, p 576.)

of adjacent intestinal mucosa from hydrochloric acid secreted by ectopic parietal cells within the diverticulum. Intestinal obstruction associated with Meckel's diverticulum is usually caused by intussusception or volvulus around an abnormal fibrous connection between the diverticulum and posterior aspect of the umbilicus. These lesions are discussed in Chapter 49.

The omphalomesenteric duct may remain patent throughout its course, thus producing an enterocutaneous fistula between the distal small intestine and umbilicus. This condition is manifested with the passage of meconium and mucus from the umbilicus in the first few days of life. Because of the risk for mesenteric volvulus around a persistent omphalomesenteric duct, these lesions are promptly treated with laparotomy and excision of the fistulous track. Persistence of the distal end of the omphalomesenteric duct results in an umbilical polyp, which is a small excrescence of omphalomesenteric ductal mucosa at the umbilicus. Such polyps resemble umbilical granulomas except that they do not disappear after silver nitrate cauterization. Their presence suggests that a persistent omphalomesenteric duct or umbilical sinus may be present, and hence they are most appropriately treated by excision of the mucosal remnant and underlying omphalomesenteric duct or umbilical sinus, if present. Umbilical sinuses result from the persistence of the distal omphalomesenteric duct. The morphology of the sinus track can be delineated by a sinogram. Treatment involves excision of the sinus. Finally, the accumulation of mucus in a portion of a persistent omphalomesenteric duct may result in the formation of a cyst, which may be associated with the intestine or umbilicus by a fibrous band. Treatment consists of excision of the cyst and associated persistent omphalomesenteric duct.

Abnormalities resulting from persistence of the allantois. The allantois is the cranialmost component of the embryologic ventral cloaca. The intra-abdominal portion is termed the *urachus* and connects the urinary bladder with the umbilicus, whereas the extra-abdominal allantois is contained within the umbilical cord. At the end of gestation, the urachus is converted into a fibrous cord that courses between the extraperitoneal urinary bladder and umbilicus as the median umbilical ligament. Persistence of part or all of the urachus may result in the formation of a vesicocutaneous fistula, with the appearance of urine at the umbilicus, an extraperitoneal urachal cyst presenting as a lower abdominal mass, or a urachal sinus with the drainage of a small amount of mucus. Because of the risk of complications including transformation into malignancy, treatment is excision of the urachal remnant with closure of the bladder, if necessary.

Acquired Abnormalities

Diastasis recti. Diastasis recti refers to a thinning of the linea alba in the epigastrium and is manifested as a smooth midline protrusion of the anterior abdominal wall. The transversalis fascia is intact, and hence this is not a hernia. There are no identifiable fascial margins and no risk for intestinal strangulation. The presence of diastasis recti may be particularly noticeable to the patient on straining or when lifting the head from the pillow. Appropriate treatment consists of reassurance of the patient and family about the innocuous nature of this condition.

Anterior abdominal wall hernias. Epigastric hernias occur at sites through which vessels and nerves perforate the linea alba to course into the subcutaneum. Through these openings, extraperitoneal areolar tissue and, at times, peritoneum may herniate into the subcutaneous tissue. Although these hernias are often small, they may produce significant localized pain and tenderness because of direct pressure of the hernia sac and its contents on the nerves emerging through the same fascial opening. Spigelian hernias occur through the fascia in the region of the semilunar line and are manifested with localized pain and tenderness. The hernia sac is only rarely palpable because it is often small and tends to remain beneath the external oblique aponeurosis. Ultrasonography of the abdominal wall or computed tomography (CT) with thin cuts through the abdomen, after careful marking of the suspected site, should be diagnostic. Treatment consists of simple operative closure of the fascial defect. These hernias are discussed in Chapter 44.

Rectus sheath hematoma. Rectus sheath hematoma is an uncommon condition characterized by acute abdominal pain and the appearance of an abdominal wall mass. It is more common in women than in men and in older than in younger individuals. A review of 126 patients with rectus sheath hematomas treated at the Mayo Clinic found that almost 70% were receiving anticoagulants at the time of diagnosis. A history of nonsurgical abdominal wall trauma or injury is common (48%), as is the presence of a cough (29%).[1] In young women, rectus sheath hematomas have been associated with pregnancy.

Patients with rectus sheath hematomas usually present with the sudden onset of abdominal pain, which may be severe and is often exacerbated by movements requiring contraction of the abdominal wall. Physical examination will demonstrate tenderness over the rectus sheath, often with voluntary guarding. An abdominal wall mass may be noted in some patients, 63% in the Mayo Clinic series. Abdominal wall ecchymosis, including periumbilical ecchymosis (Cullen sign) and blue discoloration in the flanks (Grey Turner sign), may be present if there is a delay from the onset of symptoms to presentation. The pain and tenderness associated with this process may be severe enough to suggest peritonitis. In those cases in which the hematoma expands into the perivesical and preperitoneal spaces, the hematocrit level may fall, although hemodynamic instability is uncommon.

Ultrasonography or CT will confirm the presence of the hematoma and localize it to the abdominal wall in almost all cases. Usually, these patients may be managed successfully with rest and analgesics and, if necessary, blood transfusion. In the Mayo Clinic series, almost 90% of patients were managed successfully in this manner. In general, coagulopathies are corrected, although continued anticoagulation of selected patients may be prudent, depending on the indications for anticoagulation and seriousness of the bleeding. Progression of the hematoma may necessitate angiographic embolization of the bleeding vessel or, uncommonly, operative evacuation of the hematoma and hemostasis.

Malignant Neoplasms of the Abdominal Wall

The most common primary malignant neoplasms of the abdominal wall are desmoid tumors and sarcomas. Although it is unusual, a variety of common cancers may metastasize through the bloodstream to the soft tissue of the abdominal wall, where they are manifested as soft tissue masses. Metastatic melanoma, in particular, may be manifested in this manner. Finally, transperitoneal seeding of the abdominal wall by intra-abdominal malignant neoplasms may complicate transabdominal biopsies or operative procedures.

Desmoid Tumor

Desmoid tumor, also known as *fibromatosis*, *aggressive fibromatosis*, or *desmoid-type fibromatosis*, is an uncommon neoplasm that occurs sporadically or as part of an inherited syndrome, most notably familial adenomatous polyposis (FAP) and Gardner syndrome, an autosomal dominant syndrome of GI adenomatous polyps or adenocarcinoma, osteomas, and skin and soft tissue tumors. These tumors arise from fibroaponeurotic tissue and typically are manifested as a slowly growing mass. Although they lack metastatic potential, they can be multifocal as well as locally aggressive and invasive, with a high propensity for recurrence.

Desmoid tumors are typically classified by location as extra-abdominal or extremity desmoids (i.e., those tumors occurring in the proximal extremities or limb girdle), abdominal wall tumors, and intra-abdominal desmoids (see "Mesenteric and Intra-abdominal Desmoid Tumors"), which involve the mesentery, pelvis, or bowel wall. The frequency of desmoid tumors in the general population is 2.4 to 4.3 cases/million; this risk increases 1000-fold in patients with FAP.[2,3] The majority of desmoid tumors are sporadic, typically in young women during pregnancy or within a year of childbirth. Oral contraceptive use has also been associated with the occurrence of these tumors. These associations, combined with the detection of estrogen receptors within the tumor, suggest a regulatory role for estrogen in this disease.

Patients with a desmoid tumor present with an asymptomatic mass or with symptoms related to mass effect from the tumor. There is often a temporal association between the discovery of the tumor and an antecedent history of abdominal trauma or operation.[3] Imaging (CT or magnetic resonance imaging [MRI]) is necessary to delineate the extent of tumor involvement fully, but otherwise there is no need to perform staging for metastatic disease. On CT, a desmoid tumor appears as a homogeneous mass arising from the soft tissue of the abdominal wall (Fig. 43-10). A desmoid tumor will appear as a homogeneous and isointense mass compared with muscle on T1-weighted MRI images, whereas T2-weighted images demonstrate greater heterogeneity and a signal slightly less intense than fat.

Biopsy is required to establish the diagnosis. Core needle biopsy or incisional biopsy will demonstrate a tumor composed of bundles of spindle cells and an abundant fibrous stroma. The center of the tumor is often acellular, whereas the periphery contains most of the fibroblasts. The histology can be similar to that of a low-grade fibrosarcoma, but diagnosis is usually not difficult because the fibroblasts are highly differentiated and lack the mitotic activity found in malignancy. Immunohistochemistry can help clarify difficult diagnoses; the tumors typically stain positive for β-catenin, actin, and vimentin and stain negative for cytokeratin and S-100.

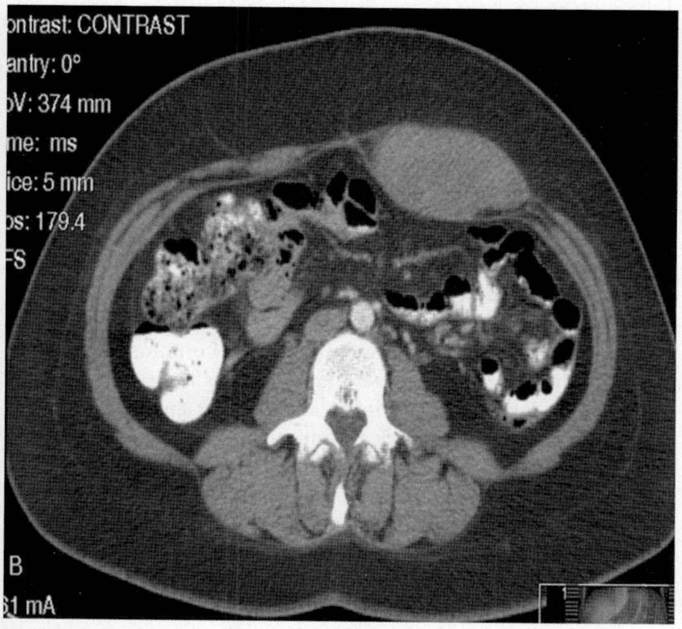

FIGURE 43-10 CT scan of the abdomen demonstrating a desmoid tumor arising within the left rectus sheath. The tumor appears as a homogeneous soft tissue mass.

Resection of the tumor with a wide margin of normal tissue was historically considered the optimal treatment. The extent of this resection will often require abdominal wall reconstruction with local tissue flaps or mesh prostheses. The completeness of resection is an important prognostic factor; Stojadinovic and colleagues[4] have reported that 68% of desmoid tumors resected with a positive margin recur within 5 years, compared with none of the tumors in which the resection margin was free of disease.

Recently, however, an approach to postpone surgery for patients with desmoid tumors, particularly for those patients who would require surgery with considerable risk of morbidity and loss of function, has gained acceptance.[5] This approach, centered on an initial observation period for all patients, was based on contemporary data that contradicted the relevance of negative surgical margins and was further supported by high recurrence rates despite optimal local treatment.[6,7] Patients undergoing observation require close follow-up to identify tumor growth early and must agree to frequent imaging. Studies suggest that approximately 50% of patients will not progress at short-term follow-up, with spontaneous regression occurring in up to 10%.[5,8,9] A conservative approach to selection of patients for surgery in desmoid-type fibromatosis is becoming the new standard of care, with further research needed in identifying select subgroups that would benefit from surgery.[10,11]

Abdominal wall desmoids are responsive to radiation therapy, although the treatment effect is slow and may be progressive for several years. Radiotherapy alone is an acceptable treatment option for patients with unresectable desmoid tumors or tumors for which resection will be associated with high morbidity risks or major functional loss. A retrospective review from the M.D. Anderson Cancer Center has reported 10-year recurrence rates of 38% for surgery alone (27% for those with negative margins), 25% for combined surgery and radiation, and 24% for radiation therapy alone.[6] It was also concluded that radiation therapy can assuage the adverse effect of positive margins on local tumor recurrence. Similar large studies have reported local control rates of approximately 80% with radiotherapy alone, rates that are consistently equivalent with or even superior to surgery alone.[12]

Adjuvant radiation therapy is controversial; most centers reserve this modality for patients with positive margins or close margins because of critical structures. The use of neoadjuvant radiation therapy is less well accepted than adjuvant radiation therapy because of the slow response times, often 1 year or more, with the potential for making subsequent abdominal wall reconstruction more difficult, and few studies demonstrated a clear benefit.

Estrogen receptor antagonists, nonsteroidal anti-inflammatory drugs, and systemic chemotherapy have been used successfully in the treatment of patients with locally advanced, recurrent, or unresectable desmoid tumors. The use of these agents in an adjuvant or neoadjuvant setting is not well studied, and they would be best used in the setting of a clinical trial.

The detection of estrogen receptors on desmoid tumors and the association with pregnancy and oral contraceptives provide some support for the use of antiestrogens, such as tamoxifen. Clinical improvement has been reported in 43% of patients receiving antiestrogens, although the response rate varies among studies. Tumor responses to antiestrogens are slow in onset but often last for several years.[13,14] Most reports of nonsteroidal anti-inflammatory drug treatment use sulindac, but indomethacin has also been used. A study using combination high-dose tamoxifen and sulindac recommended this regimen as initial treatment for FAP-associated desmoid tumors.[15]

Various cytotoxic chemotherapy regimens have been used in the treatment of patients with inoperable desmoids. Methotrexate with vinblastine, doxorubicin-based therapy, and ifosfamide-based regimens have been reported, with positive responses in 20% to 40% of patients.[13,16] For desmoids with rapid growth, medical oncologists may recommend therapies typically used for sarcomas, such as doxorubicin and dacarbazine. Reports have also suggested imatinib, a tyrosine kinase inhibitor, as another effective treatment option for patients with these tumors.[17]

Abdominal Wall Sarcoma

Abdominal wall sarcomas are classified as truncal sarcomas, including the chest and abdominal wall, and account for 10% to 20% of sarcomas overall. In general, sarcomas are rare, and abdominal wall sarcomas are exceedingly rare. Similar to desmoid tumors, these neoplasms most often are manifested as a painless mass, although as many as one third of patients with abdominal wall sarcomas will have pain at the site of the tumor. Pertinent history, such as a history of retinoblastoma, FAP, neurofibromatosis, radiation therapy, or Li-Fraumeni syndrome, should be sought. The differential diagnosis includes many common conditions, such as lipomas, hematomas, ventral hernias, endometriosis, and inflammatory processes, such as needle site granulomas in diabetics. Histologic subtypes include liposarcoma, fibrosarcoma, leiomyosarcoma, rhabdomyosarcoma, and malignant fibrous histiocytoma.

Axial imaging with MRI or CT will provide important information about the location and extent of the tumor as well as involvement of contiguous structures. Chest CT should be included to rule out metastatic disease. Definitive diagnosis requires biopsy, which may be performed with a core needle or by incision. The accuracy of core needle biopsy is consistently reported as more than 90% and can be performed under CT guidance for deep lesions. If an incisional biopsy is performed, it is optimally done by the surgeon who will perform the definitive resection; it should be oriented in the same plane as the underlying muscle to minimize unnecessary tissue loss during the definitive procedure and to facilitate reconstruction. No attempt is made to develop tissue flaps around the lesion, and hemostasis is meticulous to avoid dissemination of the tumor along the tissue planes by a postoperative hematoma.

Definitive treatment of abdominal wall sarcomas is resection with tumor-free margins; most surgeons attempt to obtain at least a 2-cm margin around the tumor. The extent of resection and associated morbidity must be balanced, however, as metastatic disease and not local recurrence represents the greatest risk of death. Lymph node metastases are rare (2% to 3%). Reconstruction of the abdominal wall defect may be accomplished primarily with myocutaneous flaps or with prosthetic meshes, depending on the site and extent of resection. Response rates with radiation and chemotherapy are generally low, although specific response rates depend on histology and grade.

Soft tissue sarcomas are discussed in greater detail in Chapter 31.

Metastatic Disease

Metastases to the abdominal wall may occur by direct seeding of the abdominal wall during biopsy or resection of an intra-abdominal malignant neoplasm or by hematogenous spread of an advanced tumor. The risk of tumor implantation at the port site after laparoscopic colon resection for adenocarcinoma is 0.9% and has been shown in randomized controlled trials to be no different from the risk of tumor recurrence in the wound after open colon resections.[18] Wound implantation with tumor can have particular relevance during cytoreductive surgery with hyperthermic intraperitoneal chemotherapy applied to the treatment of a peritoneal surface malignant neoplasm. Patients undergoing cytoreductive surgery have typically received prior surgery with abdominal wall scar or tumor formation and often require abdominal wall resection with complex reconstruction.

The most common tumors that metastasize to soft tissue are lung, colon, melanoma, and renal cell tumors. Although metastases to soft tissue are unusual, the abdominal wall is the site of such recurrence in approximately 20% of cases.[19] Similar to desmoid tumors or sarcomas, metastases to the abdominal wall are manifested as a painless mass. Immunohistochemistry staining of the tumor may allow specific identification of the type of primary tumor and facilitate differentiation from primary sarcomas of the abdominal wall. The Sister Mary Joseph nodule is often described and seldom seen; it is a palpable nodule in the region of the umbilicus representing metastatic abdominal or pelvic cancer.

Symptoms of Intra-abdominal Disease Referred to the Abdominal Wall

Abdominal pain may be categorized as visceral, somatoparietal, and referred. Visceral pain is caused by stimulation of visceral nociceptors by inflammation, distention, or ischemia. The pain is dull in nature and poorly localized to the epigastrium, periumbilical regions, or hypogastrium, depending on the embryonic origin of the organ involved. Inflammation of the stomach, duodenum, and biliary tract (derivatives of the embryonic foregut) localizes visceral pain to the epigastrium. Stimulation of nociceptors in midgut-derived organs (small intestine, appendix, right colon, proximal transverse colon) causes the sensation of pain in the periumbilical region, whereas inflammation or distention of hindgut-derived organs (distal transverse colon, left colon, rectum) causes hypogastric pain. The pain is felt in the midline because these organs transmit sympathetic sensory afferents to both sides of the spinal cord. The pain is poorly localized because the innervation of most viscera is multisegmental and contains fewer nerve receptors than highly sensitive organs such as the skin. The pain is often characterized as cramping, burning, or gnawing and may be accompanied by secondary autonomic effects, such as sweating, restlessness, nausea, vomiting, perspiration, and pallor.

Somatoparietal pain arises from inflammation of the parietal peritoneum; it is more intense and more precisely localized than visceral pain. The nerve impulses mediating parietal pain travel within the somatosensory spinal nerves and reach the spinal cord in the peripheral nerves corresponding to the cutaneous dermatomes from the T6 to the L1 region. Lateralization of parietal pain is possible because only one side of the nervous system innervates a given part of the parietal peritoneum.

The difference between visceral and somatoparietal pain is well illustrated by the pain associated with acute appendicitis, in which the early, vague, periumbilical visceral pain is followed by the localized somatoparietal pain at McBurney point. The visceral pain is produced by distention and inflammation of the appendix, whereas the localized somatoparietal pain in the right lower quadrant of the abdomen is caused by extension of the inflammation to the parietal peritoneum.

Referred pain is felt in anatomic regions remote from the diseased organ. This phenomenon is caused by convergence of visceral afferent neurons innervating an injured or inflamed organ with somatic afferent fibers arising from another anatomic region. This occurs within the spinal cord at the level of second-order neurons. Well-known examples of referred pain include shoulder pain on irritation of the diaphragm, scapular pain associated with acute biliary tract disease, and testicular or labial pain caused by retroperitoneal inflammation.

PERITONEUM AND PERITONEAL CAVITY

Anatomy

The peritoneum consists of a single sheet of simple squamous epithelium of mesodermal origin, termed *mesothelium,* lying on a thin connective tissue stroma. The surface area is 1.0 to 1.7 m^2, approximately that of the total body surface area. In males, the peritoneal cavity is sealed, whereas in females, it is open to the exterior through the ostia of the fallopian tubes. The peritoneal membrane is divided into parietal and visceral components. The parietal peritoneum covers the anterior, lateral, and posterior abdominal wall surfaces and the inferior surface of the diaphragm and the pelvis. The visceral peritoneum covers most of the surface of the intraperitoneal organs (i.e., stomach, jejunum, ileum, transverse colon, liver, spleen) and the anterior aspect of the retroperitoneal organs (i.e., duodenum, left and right colon, pancreas, kidneys, adrenal glands).

The peritoneal cavity is subdivided into interconnected compartments or spaces by 11 ligaments and mesenteries. The peritoneal ligaments or mesenteries include the coronary, gastrohepatic, hepatoduodenal, falciform, gastrocolic, duodenocolic, gastrosplenic, splenorenal, and phrenicocolic ligaments and the transverse mesocolon and small bowel mesentery (Fig. 43-11). These structures partition the abdomen into nine potential spaces: right and left subphrenic, subhepatic, supramesenteric and inframesenteric, right and left paracolic gutters, pelvis, and lesser space. These ligaments, mesenteries, and peritoneal spaces direct the circulation of fluid in the peritoneal cavity and thus may be useful in predicting the route of spread of infectious and malignant diseases. For example, perforation of the duodenum from peptic ulcer disease may result in the movement of fluid (and the development of abscesses) in the subhepatic space, right paracolic gutter, and pelvis. The blood supply to the visceral peritoneum is derived from the splanchnic blood vessels, whereas the parietal peritoneum is supplied by branches of the intercostal, subcostal, lumbar, and iliac vessels. The innervation of the visceral and parietal peritoneum is discussed earlier.

Physiology

The peritoneum is a bidirectional, semipermeable membrane that controls the amount of fluid in the peritoneal cavity, promotes the sequestration and removal of bacteria from the peritoneal cavity, and facilitates the migration of inflammatory cells from the microvasculature into the peritoneal cavity. Normally, the peritoneal cavity contains less than 100 mL of sterile serous fluid. Microvilli on the apical surface of the peritoneal mesothelium markedly increase the surface area and promote the rapid absorption of fluid from the peritoneal cavity into the lymphatics and portal and systemic circulations. The amount of fluid in the peritoneal cavity may increase to many liters in some diseases, such as cirrhosis, nephrotic syndrome, and peritoneal carcinomatosis.

The circulation of fluid in the peritoneal cavity is driven in part by the movement of the diaphragm. Intercellular pores in the peritoneum covering the inferior surface of the diaphragm (termed *stomata*) communicate with lymphatic pools in the diaphragm. Lymph flows from these diaphragmatic lymphatic channels through subpleural lymphatics to the regional lymph nodes and ultimately the thoracic duct. Relaxation of the diaphragm during

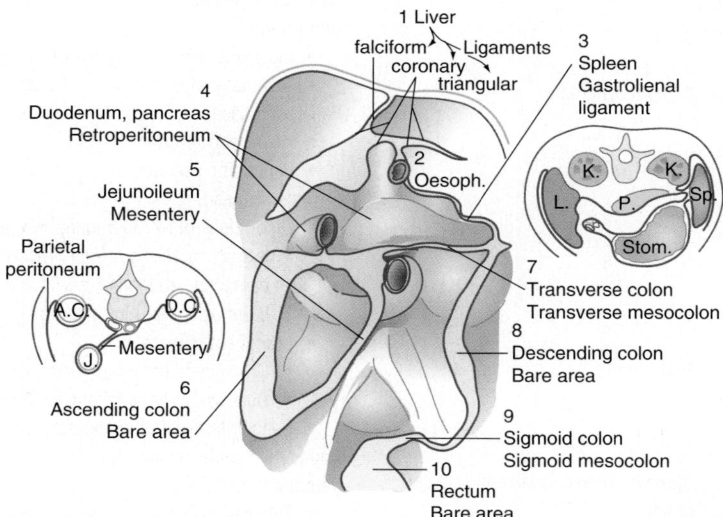

FIGURE 43-11 Peritoneal ligaments and mesenteric reflections in the adult. These attachments partition the abdomen into nine potential spaces: right and left subphrenic, subhepatic, supramesenteric, and inframesenteric spaces; and right and left paracolic gutters, pelvis, and omental bursa *(inset, right).* (From McVay C: *Anson and McVay's surgical anatomy,* ed 6, Philadelphia, 1984, WB Saunders, p 589.)

exhalation opens the stomata, and the negative intrathoracic pressure draws fluid and particles, including bacteria, into the stomata. Contraction of the diaphragm during inhalation propels the lymph through the mediastinal lymphatic channels into the thoracic duct. It is postulated that this so-called diaphragmatic pump drives the movement of peritoneal fluid in a cephalad direction toward the diaphragm and into the thoracic lymphatic vessels. This circulatory pattern of peritoneal fluid toward the diaphragm and into the central lymphatic channels is consistent with the rapid appearance of sepsis in patients with generalized intra-abdominal infections as well as the perihepatitis of Fitz-Hugh–Curtis syndrome in patients with acute salpingitis.

The peritoneum and peritoneal cavity respond to infection in five ways:

1. Bacteria are rapidly removed from the peritoneal cavity through the diaphragmatic stomata and lymphatics.
2. Peritoneal macrophages release proinflammatory mediators that promote the migration of leukocytes into the peritoneal cavity from the surrounding microvasculature.
3. Degranulation of peritoneal mast cells releases histamine and other vasoactive products, causing local vasodilation and the extravasation of protein-rich fluid containing complement and immunoglobulins into the peritoneal space.
4. Protein in the peritoneal fluid opsonizes bacteria, which, along with activation of the complement cascade, promotes neutrophil- and macrophage-mediated bacterial phagocytosis and destruction.
5. Bacteria become sequestered within fibrin matrices, thereby promoting abscess formation and limiting the generalized spread of the infection.

Peritoneal Disorders

Ascites

Pathophysiology and cause. Ascites is the pathologic accumulation of fluid in the peritoneal cavity. The principal causes of ascites formation and their pathophysiologic bases are listed in Box 43-1. Cirrhosis is the most common cause of ascites in the United States, accounting for approximately 85% of cases. Ascites is the most common complication of cirrhosis, with approximately 50% of compensated cirrhotic patients developing ascites within 10 years of diagnosis. The onset of ascites is an important prognostic factor for poor outcome in patients with cirrhosis because of its association with the occurrence of spontaneous bacterial peritonitis, renal failure, worsened quality of life, and increased likelihood of death within 2 to 5 years.

In cirrhotic patients, the two principal factors underlying the formation of ascites in cirrhotic patients are renal sodium and water retention and portal hypertension. Renal sodium retention is driven by activation of the renin-angiotensin-aldosterone and sympathetic nervous systems, which cause proximal and distal renal tubule sodium reabsorption. It is postulated that the abnormal release of nitric oxide within the splanchnic circulation causes vasodilation and a decrease in the effective circulating blood volume. Renin, aldosterone, and other hormones are generated as a counterregulatory mechanism to restore the effective circulating blood volume to normal. Portal hypertension is produced by postsinusoidal vascular obstruction from the deposition of collagen in the cirrhotic liver. Increased hydrostatic pressure within the hepatic sinusoids and splanchnic vasculature drives the extravasation of fluid from the microvasculature into the extracellular compartment. Ascites results when the capacity of the lymphatic

BOX 43-1 Principal Causes of Ascites Formation Categorized According to Underlying Pathophysiology

Portal Hypertension

Cirrhosis

Noncirrhotic

- Prehepatic portal venous obstruction
  - Chronic mesenteric venous thrombosis
  - Multiple hepatic metastases
- Posthepatic venous obstruction: Budd-Chiari syndrome

Cardiac

Congestive heart failure

Chronic pericardial tamponade

Constrictive pericarditis

Malignant Disease

Peritoneal carcinomatosis

- Primary peritoneal malignant neoplasms
  - Primary peritoneal mesothelioma
  - Serous carcinoma
- Metastatic carcinoma
  - Gastrointestinal carcinomas (e.g., gastric, colonic, pancreatic cancer)
  - Genitourinary carcinomas (e.g., ovarian cancer)

Retroperitoneal obstruction of lymphatic channels

- Lymphoma
- Lymph node metastases (e.g., testicular cancer, melanoma)

Obstruction of the lymphatic channels at the base of the mesentery

- Gastrointestinal carcinoid tumors

Miscellaneous

Bile ascites

- Iatrogenic after operations of the liver or biliary tract
- Traumatic after injuries to the liver or biliary tract

Pancreatic ascites

- Acute pancreatitis
- Pancreatic pseudocyst

Chylous ascites

- Disruptions of retroperitoneal lymphatic channels
  - Iatrogenic during retroperitoneal dissections: retroperitoneal lymphadenectomy, abdominal aortic aneurysmorrhaphy
  - Blunt or penetrating trauma
- Malignant disease
  - Obstruction of retroperitoneal lymphatic channels
  - Obstruction of lymphatic channels at the base of the mesentery
- Congenital lymphatic abnormalities

Primary lymphatic hypoplasia

Peritoneal infections

- Tuberculous peritonitis
- Myxedema
- Nephrotic syndrome
- Serositis in connective tissue disease

system to return this fluid to the systemic circulation is overwhelmed. Studies have reviewed the pathophysiologic mechanism underlying fluid retention, hyponatremia, and ascites formation that characterize patients with cirrhosis.[20,21]

Obstruction of the portal or hepatic venous blood flow in the absence of cirrhosis (e.g., portal vein thrombosis or Budd-Chiari syndrome, respectively) also causes ascites formation by increasing hydrostatic pressure within the splanchnic microvasculature. A similar pressure-based mechanism contributes to ascites formation in patients with heart failure, although the release of vasopressin and renin-angiotensin-aldosterone also promotes sodium and water retention in these patients. Patients with malignant neoplasms develop ascites by one of three mechanisms:

1. Multiple hepatic metastases cause portal hypertension by narrowing or occluding branches of the portal venous system.
2. Malignant cells scattered throughout the peritoneal cavity release protein-rich fluid into the peritoneal cavity, as in peritoneal carcinomatosis.
3. Obstruction of retroperitoneal lymphatics by a tumor, such as lymphoma, causes rupture of major lymphatic channels and the leakage of chyle into the peritoneal cavity.

Finally, ascites may result from the leakage of pancreatic fluid, bile, or lymph into the peritoneal cavity after an iatrogenic or inflammatory disruption of a major pancreatic, bile, or lymphatic duct.

Clinical presentation and diagnosis. The diagnosis of ascites is made on the basis of the medical history and appearance of the abdomen. Obviously, risk factors for hepatitis or cirrhosis are sought, as is evidence of cardiac disease, renal disease, or malignant disease. A full bulging abdomen with dullness of the flanks on percussion is suggestive of the presence of ascites. Approximately 1.5 liters of fluid must be present before dullness can be detected by percussion. Physical evidence of cirrhosis is also sought, such as palmar erythema, dilated abdominal wall collateral veins, and multiple spider angiomas. Patients with cardiac ascites have impressive jugular venous distention and other evidence of congestive heart failure.

Ascitic fluid analysis. Paracentesis with ascitic fluid analysis is the most rapid and cost-effective method of determining the cause of ascites and should be performed for patients with new-onset ascites. Another important indication for early paracentesis in a patient with ascites is the occurrence of signs and symptoms of infection, such as abdominal pain or tenderness, fever, encephalopathy, hypotension, renal failure, acidosis, or leukocytosis. Paracentesis can be performed safely in most patients, including those with cirrhosis and mild coagulopathy. It is usually performed in the lower abdomen, with the left lower quadrant preferred to the right. Ultrasound guidance may be useful in obese patients and in those with a history of laparotomy. Runyon[22] has suggested that only ongoing disseminated intravascular coagulation or clinically evident fibrinolysis is a contraindication to paracentesis in patients with ascites. In this study, no cases of hemoperitoneum, death, or infection after more than 229 paracenteses performed in 125 cirrhotic patients were reported; abdominal hematomas occurred in 2% of cases, with only 50% of these requiring blood transfusion.

Examination of the ascitic fluid begins with its gross appearance. Normal ascitic fluid is slightly yellow and transparent. The presence of more than 5000 leukocytes/mm^3 will cause the fluid to be cloudy, whereas ascitic fluid specimens with fewer than 1000 cells/mm^3 are almost clear. Blood in the ascitic fluid may be caused by a traumatic tap, in which case the fluid may be blood streaked and will often clot unless it is immediately transferred to a tube containing an anticoagulant. Nontraumatic blood-tinged ascitic fluid does not clot because the required factors have been depleted by previous clotting in the peritoneal cavity. Lipid in the ascitic fluid, such as that which accompanies chylous ascites, causes the fluid to appear opalescent, ranging from cloudy to completely opaque. If it is placed in the refrigerator for 48 to 72 hours, the lipids usually layer out.

The most valuable laboratory tests on ascitic fluid are the cell count, differential, and determination of ascitic fluid albumin and total protein concentrations. Studies vary, but most state that a normal total leukocyte count is between 100 and 300 cell/mm^3 in uncomplicated cirrhotic ascites, and approximately 50% of these cells are neutrophils. An increased polymorphonuclear neutrophil count (>250 cells/mm^3) suggests an acute inflammatory process, the most common of which is spontaneous bacterial peritonitis.

The serum-ascites albumin gradient (SAAG) is the most reliable method to differentiate causes of ascites due to portal hypertension from those not due to portal hypertension. The SAAG is calculated by measuring the albumin concentration of serum and ascitic fluid specimens and subtracting the ascitic fluid value from the serum value. If the SAAG is 1.1 g/dL or more, the patient has portal hypertension; a SAAG of less than 1.1 g/dL is consistent with the absence of portal hypertension. Examples of high- and low-gradient causes of ascites are shown in Table 43-1. The accuracy of this measurement in predicting the presence or absence of portal hypertension is approximately 97%.[23]

Treatment of ascites in cirrhotic patients. The standard treatment protocol for patients with ascites caused by portal hypertension (as opposed to patients with a SAAG of <1.1 g/dL) is a stepwise approach beginning with sodium restriction, diuretic therapy, and paracentesis.[20,21,24,25] The initial goal of medical therapy is to induce a state in which renal sodium excretion exceeds sodium intake, a situation that will reduce the extracellular volume and improve ascites. A reasonable dietary sodium restriction for most cirrhotic patients with ascites is 88 mEq (2 g) per day. The patient's compliance may be assessed by measuring the 24-hour urinary sodium excretion. Patients who are compliant with their dietary restriction and excrete more than 78 mmol/day of sodium in their urine lose weight. However, most patients will require a combination of sodium restriction and diuretics.

TABLE 43-1 Classification of Ascites by Serum-Ascites Albumin Gradient

HIGH GRADIENT (≥1.1 g/dL)	LOW GRADIENT (<1.1 g/dL)
Cirrhosis	Peritoneal carcinomatosis
Alcoholic hepatitis	Tuberculous peritonitis
Cardiac failure	Pancreatic ascites
Massive liver metastases	Biliary ascites
Fulminant hepatic failure	Nephrotic syndrome
Budd-Chiari syndrome	Postoperative lymphatic leak
Portal vein thrombosis	Serositis in connective tissue diseases
Myxedema	

From Runyon B: Ascites: spontaneous bacterial peritonitis. In Sleisenger MH, Feldman M, Friedman LS, editors: *Sleisenger and Fordtran's gastrointestinal and liver disease: Pathophysiology, diagnosis, management,* ed 7, Philadelphia, 2002, WB Saunders, p 1523.

Spironolactone and furosemide, when given in a dosing ratio of 100:40, will promote natriuresis while maintaining normokalemia. In general, spironolactone (100 mg/day) and furosemide (40 mg/day) are begun initially. If this regimen is ineffective in increasing urinary sodium excretion and decreasing body weight, the dosages of these drugs may be increased while maintaining the 100:40 ratio.

Large-volume paracentesis, in which more than 5 liters of ascites fluid is removed from the peritoneal cavity, may be useful for patients with ascites that has been unresponsive to sodium restriction and diuretic treatment; this occurs in less than 10% of patients. The intravenous infusion of albumin (6 to 8 g/liter of ascitic fluid removed) at the time of paracentesis will minimize the symptoms of intravascular volume depletion and renal insufficiency, which may accompany the removal of more than 5 liters of ascitic fluid. The continuation of diuretics and salt restriction will prevent or delay the reaccumulation of ascites after paracentesis. Others have suggested that weekly albumin administration, independent of large-volume paracentesis, may be a useful adjunct to salt restriction and diuretic therapy in patients with refractory ascites. Transjugular intrahepatic portosystemic shunt and, ultimately, hepatic transplantation have been used to manage ascites refractory to simpler, less invasive options. These modalities are discussed in Chapter 53.

Chylous ascites. Chylous ascites is the collection of chyle in the peritoneal cavity and may result from one of three principal mechanisms: (1) obstruction of major lymphatic channels at the base of the mesentery or the cisterna chyli, with exudation of chyle from dilated mesenteric lymphatics; (2) direct leakage of chyle through a lymphoperitoneal fistula caused by abnormal or injured retroperitoneal lymphatic vessels; and (3) exudation of chyle through the walls of retroperitoneal megalymphatics, without a visible fistula or thoracic duct obstruction.

In adults, the most common cause of chylous ascites is an intra-abdominal malignant neoplasm obstructing the lymphatic channels at the base of the mesentery or in the retroperitoneum. Lymphoma is the most common malignant neoplasm associated with chylous ascites, although chylous ascites has also been associated with ovarian, colon, renal, prostate, pancreatic, and gastric malignant neoplasms. Carcinoid tumors may cause chylous ascites by obstructing the lymphatics at the base of the mesentery through direct invasion and the dense fibrosis characteristic of this neoplasm. Chylous ascites may also result from injury of the retroperitoneal lymphatics during surgical procedures, such as operations on the abdominal aorta and retroperitoneal lymph node dissections. Blunt and penetrating traumatic injuries are also important causes of chylous ascites, particularly in children. Chylous ascites in children may be caused by congenital lymphatic abnormalities, such as primary lymphatic hypoplasia, resulting in lower extremity lymphedema, chylothorax, and chylous ascites.

Patients with chylous ascites most often present with painless abdominal distention. Malnutrition and dyspnea occur in approximately 50% of cases. Paracentesis yields a characteristic milky fluid with a high protein and fat content. The SAAG will be less than 1.1 mg/dL, and the triglyceride level will be higher than that of plasma, often two to eight times higher than that of plasma. CT, lymphoscintigraphy, and lymphangiography may provide information about the site of obstruction, although the last two modalities are rarely available.

Although large studies are lacking on ideal practices, management of patients with chylous ascites includes the maintenance or improvement of nutrition, reduction in the rate of chyle formation, and correction of the underlying disease process. Most patients will be successfully treated with either a high-protein, low-fat diet and diuretics or fasting with total parenteral nutrition with or without somatostatin. A low-fat, medium-chain triglyceride diet combined with diuretics has been used successfully to treat adults with chylous ascites complicating retroperitoneal lymph node dissections. It is postulated that reducing the intake of long-chain triglycerides will reduce the rate of chyle flow because their metabolites are transported through the splanchnic lymphatics as chylomicrons. In contrast, medium-chain triglycerides are directly absorbed by enterocytes and transported to the liver through the splanchnic blood vessels as free fatty acids and glycerol. Paracentesis may temporarily relieve the dyspnea and abdominal discomfort associated with chylous ascites; however, repeated paracentesis leads to hypoproteinemia and malnutrition. Experience with peritoneovenous shunts to treat chylous ascites has generally been disappointing. Surgical exploration of the abdomen and retroperitoneum is generally reserved for patients who fail to improve with nonoperative management. In rare cases, the application of fibrin glue has been a beneficial adjunct to surgical exploration of the retroperitoneum.

Peritonitis

Peritonitis is inflammation of the peritoneum and peritoneal cavity, usually caused by a localized or generalized infection. Primary peritonitis results from bacterial, chlamydial, fungal, or mycobacterial infection in the absence of perforation of the GI tract, whereas secondary peritonitis occurs in the setting of GI perforation. Frequent causes of secondary bacterial peritonitis include peptic ulcer disease, acute appendicitis, colonic diverticulitis, and pelvic inflammatory disease.

Spontaneous bacterial peritonitis. Spontaneous bacterial peritonitis (SBP) is defined as a bacterial infection of ascitic fluid in the absence of an intra-abdominal source of infection, such as visceral perforation, abscess, acute pancreatitis, or cholecystitis. Although it is usually associated with cirrhosis, SBP may also occur in patients with nephrotic syndrome and, less commonly, congestive heart failure. It is extremely rare for patients with ascitic fluid containing a high protein concentration to develop SBP, such as those with peritoneal carcinomatosis. The most common pathogens in adults with SBP are the aerobic enteric flora *Escherichia coli* and *Klebsiella pneumoniae.* In children with nephrogenic or hepatogenic ascites, group A streptococcus, *Staphylococcus aureus*, and *Streptococcus pneumoniae* are common isolates. SBP is seldom produced by anaerobic microorganisms because of their incapacity to translocate to the intestinal mucosa and because of the high volume of oxygen in the intestinal wall and in the tissues that surround it.[26-30]

Bacterial translocation from the GI tract is thought to be an important step in the pathogenesis of SBP. Impaired GI motility in cirrhotics is thought to alter normal gut microflora, and impaired local and systemic immune function prevents the effective clearance of translocated bacteria from the mesenteric lymphatics and bloodstream. A low protein concentration in ascitic fluid prevents effective opsonization of bacteria and hence clearance by macrophages and neutrophils.

The diagnosis of SBP is made initially by demonstrating more than 250 neutrophils/mm^3 of ascitic fluid in a clinical setting consistent with this diagnosis, that is, abdominal pain, fever, or leukocytosis in a patient with low-protein ascites. In addition, cultured fluid can be only monomicrobial as polymicrobial infections, particularly with gram-negative enteric organisms, raise the suspicion of secondary peritonitis. It is unusual to document bacterascites on Gram staining of ascitic fluid, and delay of appropriate antibiotic management until the ascitic fluid cultures grow bacterial isolates risks the development of overwhelming infection and death. Bedside screening of ascitic fluid for leukocyte esterase, using colorimetric leukocyte esterase reagent strips, has been used to shorten the time from paracentesis to treatment, although its widespread use remains controversial.[31,32]

Broad-spectrum antibiotics, such as a third-generation cephalosporin, are started immediately in patients suspected of having ascitic fluid infection. These agents cover approximately 95% of the flora most commonly associated with SBP and are the antibiotics of choice for patients thought to have SBP.[33,34] The spectrum of the antibiotic coverage may be narrowed once the results of antibiotic sensitivity tests are known. Repeated paracentesis with ascitic fluid analysis is not needed when there is typical rapid improvement in response to antibiotic therapy. If the setting, symptoms, ascitic fluid analysis, and response to therapy are atypical, repeated paracentesis may be helpful for detecting secondary peritonitis. The immediate mortality risk caused by SBP is low, particularly if it is recognized and treated expeditiously. However, the development of other complications of hepatic failure, including GI hemorrhage and hepatorenal syndrome, contributes to the death of many of these patients during the hospitalization in which SBP is detected. The occurrence of SBP is an important landmark in the natural history of cirrhosis, with 1- and 2-year survival rates of approximately 30% and 20%, respectively. Several studies, including a randomized controlled trial, have shown that plasma expansion with albumin improves circulatory function and reduces the risk for hepatorenal syndrome and hospital mortality in patients with SBP.[35]

Tuberculous peritonitis. Tuberculosis is common in impoverished areas of the world and is encountered with increasing frequency in the United States and other developed countries because of factors such as HIV infection and increasing use of immunosuppressive medications. Others have described an association between peritoneal tuberculosis and alcoholic cirrhosis and chronic renal failure.[36] Peritoneal tuberculosis is the sixth most common site of extrapulmonary tuberculosis, after lymphatic, genitourinary, bone and joint, miliary, and meningeal. Most cases result from reactivation of latent peritoneal disease that had been previously established hematogenously from a primary pulmonary focus. Only approximately 17% of cases are associated with active pulmonary disease.

The illness often is manifested insidiously, with patients having had symptoms for several weeks to months at the time of presentation. Its clinical presentation mimics inflammatory conditions such as Crohn's disease and malignant diseases, so obtaining a diagnosis can be problematic at times. Abdominal swelling caused by ascites formation is the most common symptom, occurring in more than 80% of cases. Similarly, most patients complain of a nonlocalized, vague abdominal pain. Constitutional symptoms such as low-grade fever and night sweats, weight loss, anorexia, and malaise are reported in approximately 60% of patients. The concomitant presence of other chronic conditions, such as uremia, cirrhosis, and AIDS, makes these symptoms difficult to interpret. Abdominal tenderness is present on palpation in approximately 50% of patients with peritoneal tuberculosis.[36] A positive tuberculin skin test response is present in most cases, whereas only approximately 50% of these patients will have an abnormal chest radiograph. The ascitic fluid SAAG is less than 1.1 g/dL, consistent with a high protein concentration in the ascitic fluid. Microscopic examination of the ascites shows erythrocytes and an increased number of leukocytes, most of which are lymphocytes. Measurement of ascitic fluid adenosine deaminase activity, even in the presence of cirrhosis, and polymerase chain reaction assays have been used as noninvasive and rapid tests for tuberculous peritonitis. Ascitic fluid adenosine deaminase activity, in particular, appears to be highly sensitive and specific for tuberculous peritonitis.

Abdominal imaging with ultrasound or CT may suggest the diagnosis but lacks the sensitivity and specificity to be diagnostic. Ultrasound may demonstrate the presence of echogenic material in the ascitic fluid, seen as fine mobile strands or particulate matter. CT will demonstrate the thickened and nodular mesentery with mesenteric lymphadenopathy and omental thickening.

The diagnosis is made by laparoscopy with directed biopsy of the peritoneum. In more than 90% of cases, laparoscopy demonstrates a number of whitish nodules (<5 mm) scattered over the visceral and parietal peritoneum; histologic examination demonstrates caseating granulomas. Multiple adhesions are commonly present between the abdominal organs and parietal peritoneum. The gross appearance of the peritoneal cavity is similar to that of peritoneal carcinomatosis, sarcoidosis, and Crohn's disease, thus reiterating the importance of biopsy. Blind percutaneous peritoneal biopsy has a much lower yield than directed biopsy, and laparotomy with peritoneal biopsy is reserved for cases in which laparoscopy has been nondiagnostic or cannot be safely performed. Microscopic examination of ascitic fluid for acid-fast bacilli identifies the organism in less than 3% of cases, and culture results are positive in less than 20% of cases. Furthermore, the diagnostic usefulness of mycobacterial cultures is further limited by the time it may take for the cultures to yield definitive information, up to 8 weeks.

Treatment of peritoneal tuberculosis consists of antituberculous drugs. Drug regimens useful in treating pulmonary tuberculosis are also effective for peritoneal disease; a commonly used and effective regimen is isoniazid and rifampin daily for 9 months. The presence of associated alcoholic cirrhosis may complicate the use of these agents because of hepatotoxicity.

Peritonitis associated with chronic ambulatory peritoneal dialysis. In the United States, approximately 6% of patients with chronic renal failure undergo peritoneal dialysis. Peritonitis is one of the most common complications of chronic ambulatory peritoneal dialysis, occurring with an incidence of approximately one episode every 1 to 3 years. A study of all patients undergoing peritoneal dialysis in Scotland between 1999 and 2002 found that one episode of peritonitis occurred in every 19.2 months of peritoneal dialysis. Importantly, refractory or recurrent peritonitis was the most common cause of technical failure, accounting for 43% of all cases of technique failure.[37]

Patients present with abdominal pain, fever, and cloudy peritoneal dialysate containing more than 100 leukocytes/mm^3, with more than 50% of the cells being neutrophils. Gram staining detects organisms only in approximately 10% to 40% of cases. Approximately 75% of infections are caused by gram-positive organisms, with *Staphylococcus epidermidis* accounting for 30% to 50% of cases. *S. aureus,* gram-negative bacilli, and fungi are also important causes of dialysis-associated peritonitis.[37]

Peritoneal dialysis–associated peritonitis is treated by the intraperitoneal administration of antibiotics, usually a first-generation cephalosporin. Overall, 75% of infections are cured by culture-directed antibiotic therapy. The cure rate for peritonitis using antibiotics without catheter removal varies according to the causative organism; one study showed rates of 90% with coagulase-negative staphylococcus compared with rates of 66%, 56%, and 0% for *S. aureus,* gram-negative bacilli, and fungi, respectively.[37] Recurrent or persistent peritonitis requires removal of the dialysis catheter and resumption of hemodialysis.

Malignant Neoplasms of the Peritoneum

Primary malignant neoplasms of the peritoneum are rare; these include malignant mesothelioma, primary peritoneal carcinoma, and sarcomas (e.g., angiosarcoma). Most malignant neoplasms that involve the peritoneum are transperitoneal metastases originating from carcinomas of the GI tract (especially the stomach, colon, and pancreas), the genitourinary tract (usually, ovarian), or, more rarely, an extra-abdominal site (e.g., breast). When metastatic cancer deposits diffusely coat the visceral and parietal peritoneum, these peritoneal metastases are referred to as *carcinomatosis.*

Pseudomyxoma peritonei. Pseudomyxoma peritonei describes mucinous ascites arising from a ruptured ovarian or appendiceal adenocarcinoma. In this disease, the peritoneum becomes coated with a mucus-secreting tumor that fills the peritoneal cavity with tenacious semisolid mucus and large, loculated cystic masses. Although the term *pseudomyxoma peritonei* is often used to describe any condition with accumulation of intraperitoneal mucin or mucinous ascites, here we focus on pseudomyxoma peritonei resulting from ruptured epithelial neoplasms of the appendix. The pathologic classification of appendiceal epithelial tumors can be confusing as there are differing classification systems. It is easier to consider these as tumors that extend along a spectrum from benign mucinous cystadenoma (also referred to as disseminated peritoneal adenomucinosis) to malignant cystadenocarcinoma, similar to the adenoma to carcinoma sequence in colorectal cancer.[38] The histology of appendiceal tumors is an important predictor of survival; adenomucinosis has the best survival rate (75% at 5 years) and peritoneal mucinous carcinomatosis the worst (14% at 5 years).[39]

Pseudomyxoma peritonei occurs most commonly in patients who are 40 to 50 years of age and occurs with equal frequency in men and women. Patients are often asymptomatic until late in the course of their disease. On presentation, they will often describe a global deterioration in their health long before the diagnosis is made. Symptoms of abdominal pain and distention and nonspecific complaints are common. Physical examination may reveal a new hernia, ascites, distended abdomen with non-shifting dullness, and, occasionally, a palpable abdominal mass.

CT of the chest, abdomen, and pelvis may provide important information about the diagnosis and the ability to resect the tumor completely or to perform an adequate cytoreduction, which is often limited by involvement of the small bowel or porta hepatis by tumor. Preoperative colonoscopy will differentiate a mucinous neoplasm of the appendix from that arising from the colon. The diagnosis is often made at laparotomy, when the surgeon is presented with a peritoneal cavity containing tenacious semisolid mucus and large, loculated cystic masses. If the surgeon is unprepared to perform a definitive procedure, the best approach is to establish the diagnosis by the least invasive procedure possible and to relieve symptoms of intestinal obstruction, if present. The patient can then be referred to a center experienced in the management of these patients.

The current treatment of patients with pseudomyxoma peritonei involves resection of as much of the tumor as possible (cytoreduction) and intraperitoneal heated chemotherapy (IPHC). Operative management includes omentectomy, stripping of involved peritoneum, resection of involved organs, and appendectomy, if not previously performed. There should be no residual tumor nodules larger than 2 mm in diameter after resection to facilitate penetration of the chemotherapy into any residual disease. In general, a right hemicolectomy is performed for these tumors, although a review of 501 patients with mucinous tumors of the appendix has suggested that this is unnecessary if the resection margin at appendectomy is negative.[40] IPHC can be performed by an open technique, in which the abdomen is left open to ensure adequate chemotherapy distribution throughout the peritoneal cavity, or a closed technique, in which the abdomen is closed after inflow and outflow cannulas are placed. The latter allows easier maintenance of hyperthermia (Fig. 43-12). There are many variations of surgical technique and chemotherapy administration, but one commonly used technique has been reported extensively by Stewart and associates.[41]

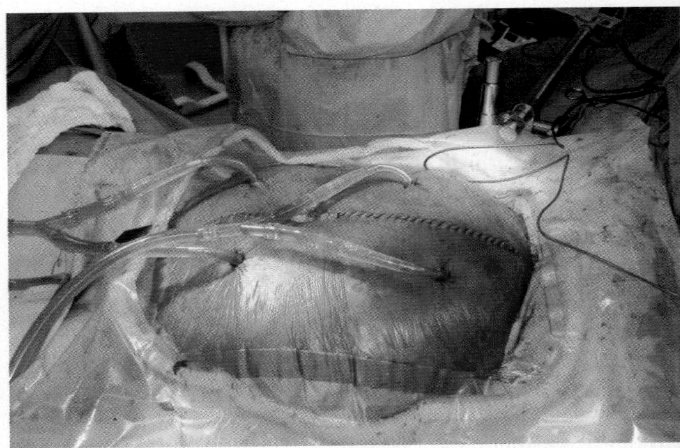

FIGURE 43-12 Placement of peritoneal catheters during the performance of intraperitoneal hyperthermic chemotherapy using the closed technique for chemotherapy administration.

Cytoreduction with IPHC is associated with improved survival for patients with pseudomyxoma peritonei compared with historical controls. Before cytoreduction and IPHC, most studies reported long-term survival rates of 20% to 30% for patients with this disease undergoing serial debulking of the tumor with systemic chemotherapy. Gonzalez-Moreno and Sugarbaker[40] have reported 10-year survival rates of 55% in 501 patients undergoing cytoreduction and IPHC. Unfortunately, there are not likely to be any randomized controlled trials for this technique, given the infrequency with which this disease is encountered and the improved survival rates reported with IPHC compared with historical treatment with surgery alone. Furthermore, reported experiences are complicated by the use of various chemotherapy regimens, surgical techniques, and preoperative and intraoperative staging protocols.[42] At centers with experience in this technique, 30-day mortality rates are 2% to 3%, with 25% to 35% of patients developing a complication. The most common postoperative complications are prolonged ileus and pulmonary complications, although bleeding, intra-abdominal infections, enterocutaneous fistula, pancreatitis, and bone marrow suppression have also been reported.

Malignant peritoneal mesothelioma. The most common primary malignant peritoneal neoplasm is malignant mesothelioma, which results from malignant transformation of the simple squamoid epithelium covering the peritoneal cavity. Peritoneal mesothelioma is rare, with approximately 400 new cases per year, with a slight male predominance and a median age at presentation of approximately 50 years.[43] As with mesothelioma of the pleura, most patients with peritoneal mesothelioma will have had exposure to asbestos.

Most patients present with abdominal pain and weight loss. Ascites is common and often intractable. The omentum may become diffusely involved with tumor and present as an epigastric mass. CT demonstrates mesenteric thickening, peritoneal studding, hemorrhage within the tumor, and ascites. At laparotomy, the ascitic fluid ranges from a serous transudate to a viscous fluid rich in mucopolysaccharides. The neoplasm tends to involve all peritoneal surfaces, producing masses and plaques of tumor that are hard and white. In contrast to pseudomyxoma peritonei, local invasion of intra-abdominal organs, such as the liver, intestine, bladder, and abdominal wall, can occur, and encasement of bowel can create a malignant bowel obstruction. In some cases, it may be difficult to differentiate malignant peritoneal mesothelioma from diffuse peritoneal carcinomatosis arising from an intra-abdominal organ such as the stomach, pancreas, colon, or ovary. Careful examination of the pattern of spread and histologic examination of the biopsy specimen will often allow this distinction to be made. Furthermore, malignant peritoneal mesothelioma will generally remain confined to the abdomen, whereas advanced-stage intra-abdominal carcinomas frequently have pulmonary and other extra-abdominal metastases. Extension of the mesothelioma into one or both pleural cavities is more likely than hematogenous dissemination. Levy and colleagues[44] have reviewed the pathologic and radiographic features of peritoneal malignant neoplasms.

Complete surgical resection is difficult because of the extent of disease. Historically, operative management consisted of debulking of the tumor and enteroenterostomies to bypass areas of actual or impending intestinal obstruction. Systemic chemotherapy and abdominal radiation have been tried, without significant improvement in survival. Radiation therapy alone, whether by open-field techniques, intraperitoneal instillation of radioactive agents, or external beam irradiation, has had limited success and substantial associated morbidity.

As with pseudomyxoma peritonei, combined-modality approaches using surgery and IPHC may offer substantial improvements compared with historical controls. There have been several retrospective series using this technique, with median survival rates of 30 to 60 months and even 5-year survival rates of up to 50%. In light of these findings and the rarity of the disease, a multi-institutional data registry from eight institutions was created, including 405 patients treated with cytoreductive surgery and perioperative intraperitoneal chemotherapy.[45] Chemotherapeutic regimens varied (cisplatin, mitomycin, and doxorubicin were most commonly used), as did the timing and administration of the chemotherapy. The morbidity rate was 46%, and the mortality rate was 2%. Median survival was impressive at 53 months. The 3- and 5-year survival rates were 60% and 47%, respectively, offering significant improvement over what was previously considered a preterminal condition.

MESENTERY AND OMENTUM

Embryology and Anatomy

The greater and lesser omenta are complex peritoneal folds that pass from the stomach to the liver, transverse colon, spleen, bile duct, pancreas, and diaphragm. They originate from the dorsal and ventral midline mesenteries of the embryonic gut. In the very early stages of development, the alimentary canal traverses the future coelomic cavity as a straight tube, suspended posteriorly by an uninterrupted dorsal mesentery and anteriorly by a ventral mesentery in the cranial portion of its extent. The embryonic stomach rotates 90 degrees on its longitudinal axis so that the lesser curvature faces to the right and the greater curvature to the left. Much of the embryonic ventral mesentery is resorbed; however, the portion extending from the fissure of the ligamentum venosum and porta hepatis to the proximal duodenum and lesser curvature of the stomach (gastrohepatic ligament) persists as the lesser omentum. The right border of the lesser omentum is a free edge that forms the anterior border of the opening into the lesser sac, termed the *foramen of Winslow.* Between the layers of the lesser omentum, and at its right border, are the common hepatic duct, portal vein, and hepatic artery.

The embryonic dorsal mesogastrium grows as a sheet of peritoneum extending from the greater curvature of the stomach over the anterior surface of the small intestine. After passing inferiorly almost to the pelvis, the peritoneal membrane turns up on itself to pass upward to a line of attachment on the transverse colon slightly above that of the transverse mesocolon. Fat is laid down in this omental apron and provides an insulating layer of protection of the abdominal viscera.

Early in its development, the small intestine elongates to form an anteriorly oriented intestinal loop, which then rotates counterclockwise so that the cecum and ascending colon move to the right side of the peritoneal cavity, and the descending colon assumes a vertical position on the left wall of the peritoneal cavity. The jejunum and ileum are supported by the peritoneum-covered dorsal mesentery carrying the mesenteric blood vessels and lymphatics. The posterior line of attachment of the mesentery extends obliquely from the duodenojejunal junction at the left side of the second lumbar vertebra toward the right iliac fossa to terminate anterior to the sacroiliac articulation.

Physiology

The omentum and intestinal mesentery are rich in lymphatics and blood vessels. The omentum contains areas with high concentrations of macrophages, which may aid in the removal of foreign material and bacteria. Furthermore, the omentum becomes densely adherent to intraperitoneal sites of inflammation, often preventing diffuse peritonitis during cases of intestinal gangrene or perforation, such as acute diverticulitis or acute appendicitis.

Diseases of the Omentum

Omental Cysts

Omental cysts are unilocular or multilocular cysts containing serous fluid that are thought to arise from congenital or acquired obstruction of omental lymphatic channels. They are lined by a lymphatic endothelium similar to that of cystic lymphangiomas. These lesions are most common in children and young adults, in whom small cysts are usually asymptomatic and discovered incidentally; larger cysts are manifested as a palpable abdominal mass. Uncomplicated cysts usually lie in the lower midabdomen and are freely movable, smooth, and nontender. Complications are more common in children and include torsion, infection, and rupture.

Plain radiographs of the abdomen may show a well-circumscribed soft tissue density in the midabdomen, and contrast studies of the intestine may show displacement of intestinal loops and extrinsic compression on adjacent bowel. Ultrasound or CT will show a fluid-filled, complex, cystic mass with internal septations. The differential diagnosis of these lesions includes cysts and solid tumors of the mesentery, peritoneum, and retroperitoneum, including desmoid tumors. Ultimately, the diagnosis is made by excision of the cyst and histologic examination of the wall. Local excision, either laparoscopically or open, is curative.

Omental Torsion and Infarction

Torsion of the greater omentum is defined as the axial twisting of the omentum along its long axis. If the twist is tight enough or the venous obstruction is of sufficient duration, arterial inflow will become compromised, leading to infarction and necrosis. Omental torsion is classified as primary when no coexisting causative condition is identified or secondary when the torsion occurs in association with a causative condition, such as a hernia, tumor, or adhesion. Primary omental torsion usually involves the right side of the omentum.

Omental torsion occurs twice as often in men as in women and is most frequent in patients in their fourth or fifth decade of life. Patients present with the acute onset of severe abdominal pain localized to the right side of the abdomen in 80% of patients. Nausea and vomiting may be present but are not predominant findings. The patient's temperature is usually normal, and palpation of the abdomen demonstrates localized abdominal tenderness with guarding, suggesting peritonitis. A mass may be palpable if the involved omentum is sufficiently large.

The differential diagnosis includes any disease associated with right-sided abdominal pain and tenderness, most notably acute appendicitis, acute cholecystitis, and torsion of an ovarian cyst. CT often demonstrates an omental mass with signs of inflammation. Usually, the patient's clinical presentation justifies laparotomy or laparoscopy, at which time a segment of the omentum appears congested and acutely inflamed. Serosanguineous fluid is often present in the peritoneal cavity. Treatment consists of resection of the involved omentum and correction of any related condition.

Omental Neoplasms

Primary malignant neoplasms of the omentum are extremely rare and are usually of soft tissue origin. The omentum is usually invaded by metastatic tumor that has spread transperitoneally from an intra-abdominal carcinoma.

Omental Grafts and Transpositions

The arterial and venous blood supplies to the greater omentum are derived from omental branches of the right and left gastroepiploic arteries, which course along the greater curvature of the stomach. Division of the right or left gastroepiploic artery and vasa recta along the greater curvature of the stomach, with mobilization of the omentum from the transverse colon, allows the development of a vascularized omental pedicle flap. This graft may be used to cover chest and mediastinal wounds after chest wall resections and to prevent the small intestine from entering the pelvis after abdominal perineal resection, thus preventing radiation enteritis during radiation therapy for rectal carcinoma. Finally, the formation of dense adhesions between the omentum and sites of perforation or inflammation facilitates its use as a patch for duodenal perforations from ulcer disease (Graham patch; Fig. 43-13).

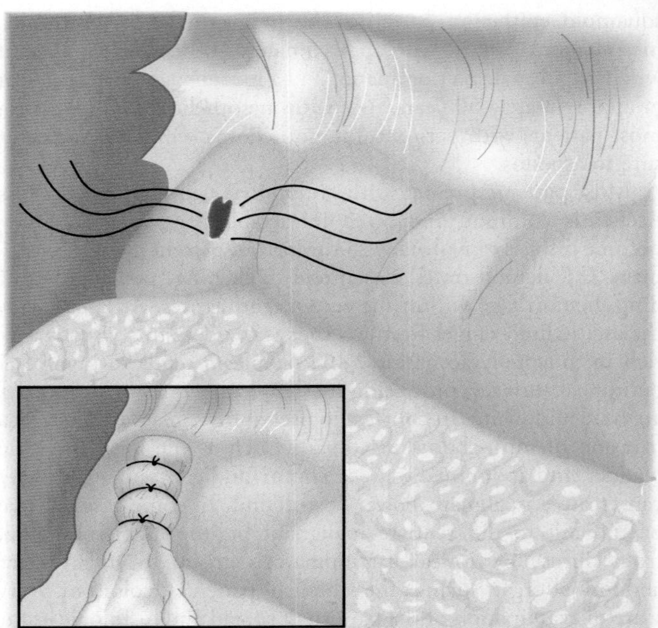

FIGURE 43-13 Closure of a perforated duodenal ulcer with an omental (Graham) patch. (From Graham RR: The treatment of perforated duodenal ulcers. *Surg Gynecol Obstet* 64:235–238, 1937.)

Diseases of the Mesentery

Mesenteric Cysts

The most common non-neoplastic mesenteric cysts are termed *mesothelial cysts* on the basis of the ultrastructure of the cells lining the cyst. The cysts contain chyle or a clear serous fluid and may occur in the mesentery of the small intestine (60%) or colon (40%). These cysts usually occur in adults, with a mean age of 45 years, and are twice as common in women as in men. Depending on the size of the cyst, patients may present with complaints of abdominal pain, fever, and emesis. A midabdominal mass may be palpable on examination of the abdomen. The diagnosis can usually be made preoperatively with ultrasonography or CT. Enucleation of the cyst at laparotomy is curative and can generally be accomplished because the mesenteric blood vessels and intestinal wall are usually not adherent to the cyst wall. Internal drainage of the cyst into the peritoneal cavity has also been successfully used in the treatment of very large cysts. Aspiration alone has a high rate of cyst recurrence. In those cases in which the cyst is not completely excised, the contents of the cyst and the internal architecture of the cyst wall must be carefully inspected and the cyst wall examined histologically to rule out a non-neoplastic cause.

Acute Mesenteric Lymphadenitis

Acute mesenteric lymphadenitis is a syndrome of acute right lower quadrant abdominal pain associated with mesenteric lymph node enlargement and a normal appendix. In general, the diagnosis is made on exploration of the abdomen of a patient suspected of having acute appendicitis, at which time a normal appendix and enlarged mesenteric lymph nodes are discovered. This syndrome occurs most commonly in children and young adults, with equal frequency in males and females.

Numerous causative agents have been implicated in the pathobiology of acute mesenteric lymphadenitis, including viral, bacterial, parasitic, and fungal infections. *Yersinia enterocolitica* in particular has been associated with this syndrome in children. Culture and histologic examination of the enlarged lymph nodes, stool culture, and antibody titers have been used to identify causative agents but are not routinely used in the treatment of these patients.

The symptom complex associated with acute mesenteric lymphadenitis is similar to that of acute appendicitis; it includes the acute onset of periumbilical pain, which shifts to the right lower quadrant over time. Physical examination demonstrates right lower quadrant tenderness, with abdominal wall muscle rigidity and rebound tenderness. Nausea, vomiting, and anorexia may also be present but are not dominant symptoms. In general, the patient's temperature and white blood cell count are normal or only slightly elevated.

The diagnosis is made at the time of operation for presumed acute appendicitis, at which time a normal-appearing appendix is found, with enlarged mesenteric lymph nodes. Excision of an enlarged lymph node with culture and nodal histology may provide information about the cause but is not routinely used.

Sclerosing Mesenteritis

Sclerosing mesenteritis is a rare inflammatory disease of the mesentery characterized histologically by sclerosing fibrosis, fat necrosis with lipid-laden macrophages, chronic inflammation with germinal centers, and focal calcification. Early in the course of the disease, sclerosing mesenteritis has a loose myxomatous appearance that progresses to chronic inflammation and dense sclerosis. This condition is characterized grossly by marked thickening of the mesentery of the small intestine, with irregular areas of discoloration suggesting fat necrosis. There may also be multiple discrete nodules on the mesentery, or the disease may appear as a single matted mass. The process most often involves the root of the small bowel mesentery and frequently encompasses the mesenteric vessels. It affects the small bowel by retraction and shortening of the mesentery without invasion. In advanced cases, mesenteric venous and lymphatic obstruction may be present. The mesocolon may also be affected but less frequently than the small bowel mesentery.[44]

Sclerosing mesenteritis is twice as common in men as in women and usually occurs in the fifth decade of life. Most patients are asymptomatic, and the diagnosis is discovered incidentally on imaging for an unrelated condition. When symptoms are present, abdominal pain or symptoms of intestinal obstruction with nausea, vomiting, and abdominal distention are most common. An abdominal mass is palpable in more than 50% of patients. Laboratory studies are usually normal, except that the erythrocyte sedimentation rate and C-reactive protein levels may be elevated.

The differential diagnosis of sclerosing mesenteritis includes a heterogeneous group of conditions that alter the density of the mesenteric fat, including inflammatory and neoplastic causes. Differentiation from peritoneal carcinomatosis, carcinoid tumor, and mesenteric and retroperitoneal sarcomas is particularly important. The CT characteristics of sclerosing mesenteritis are well described[46,47] and include the following:

- A fatty mass arising from the base of the mesentery that has well-delineated margins separating it from normal mesentery, a feature described as a *tumoral pseudocapsule*
- The presence of normal adipose tissue surrounding mesenteric vessels, termed *fat ring sign*
- The presence of normal mesenteric vessels coursing through the fatty mass, without evidence of vascular involvement or deviation
- An intra-abdominal mass that displaces adjacent bowel loops without invading them

Laparotomy or laparoscopy with biopsy of the involved mesentery remains necessary for definitive diagnosis.

Most patients with mesenteric panniculitis experience spontaneous resolution of their symptoms. If patients do not improve, corticosteroids and other anti-inflammatory and immunosuppressive agents have been reported to be successful in improving the symptoms and radiographic findings. Operative management is indicated only for patients in whom there is confusion about the diagnosis and for treatment of intestinal obstruction.

Intra-abdominal (Internal) Hernias

Internal Hernias Caused by Developmental Defects

There are three general mechanisms whereby developmental abnormalities result in the formation of internal hernias: (1) abnormal retroperitoneal fixation of the mesentery resulting in anomalous positioning of the intestine (e.g., mesocolic or paraduodenal hernia); (2) abnormally large internal foramina or fossae (e.g., foramen of Winslow, supravesical hernia); and (3) incomplete mesenteric surfaces with the presence of an abnormal opening through which the intestine herniates (e.g., mesenteric hernia).

The anatomic and radiographic features of acquired and congenital internal hernias have been reviewed by Martin and associates.[48]

Mesocolic (paraduodenal) hernias. Mesocolic hernias are unusual congenital hernias in which the small intestine herniates behind the mesocolon. They result from abnormal rotation of the midgut and have been categorized as right or left. A right mesocolic hernia occurs when the prearterial limb of the midgut loop fails to rotate around the superior mesenteric artery. This results in most of the small intestine remaining to the right of the superior mesenteric artery. Normal counterclockwise rotation of the cecum and proximal colon into the right side of the abdomen and fixation to the posterolateral peritoneum cause the small intestine to become trapped behind the mesentery of the right side of the colon. The ileocolic, right colic, and middle colic vessels lie within the anterior wall of the sac, and the superior mesenteric artery courses along the medial border of the neck of the hernia (Fig. 43-14*A*).

Left mesocolic hernias are thought to be caused by in utero herniation of the small intestine between the inferior mesenteric vein and posterior parietal attachments of the descending mesocolon to the retroperitoneum. The inferior mesenteric artery and vein are integral components of the hernia sac (Fig. 43-14*B*). Approximately 75% of mesocolic hernias occur on the left side.

Patients with paraduodenal hernias usually present with symptoms of acute or chronic small bowel obstruction. Barium radiographs will demonstrate displacement of the small intestine to the left or right side of the abdomen. CT with intravenous administration of contrast material may demonstrate displacement of the mesenteric vessels and evidence of intestinal obstruction, if present.

The operative treatment of patients with a right mesocolic hernia involves incision of the lateral peritoneal reflections along the right colon, with reflection of the right colon and cecum to the left. The entire gut then assumes a position simulating that of nonrotation of the prearterial and postarterial segments of the midgut. Opening the neck of the hernia will injure the superior mesenteric vessels and fails to free the herniated bowel (Fig. 43-14*C*).

The operative treatment of patients with a left mesocolic hernia consists of incision of the peritoneal attachments and adhesions

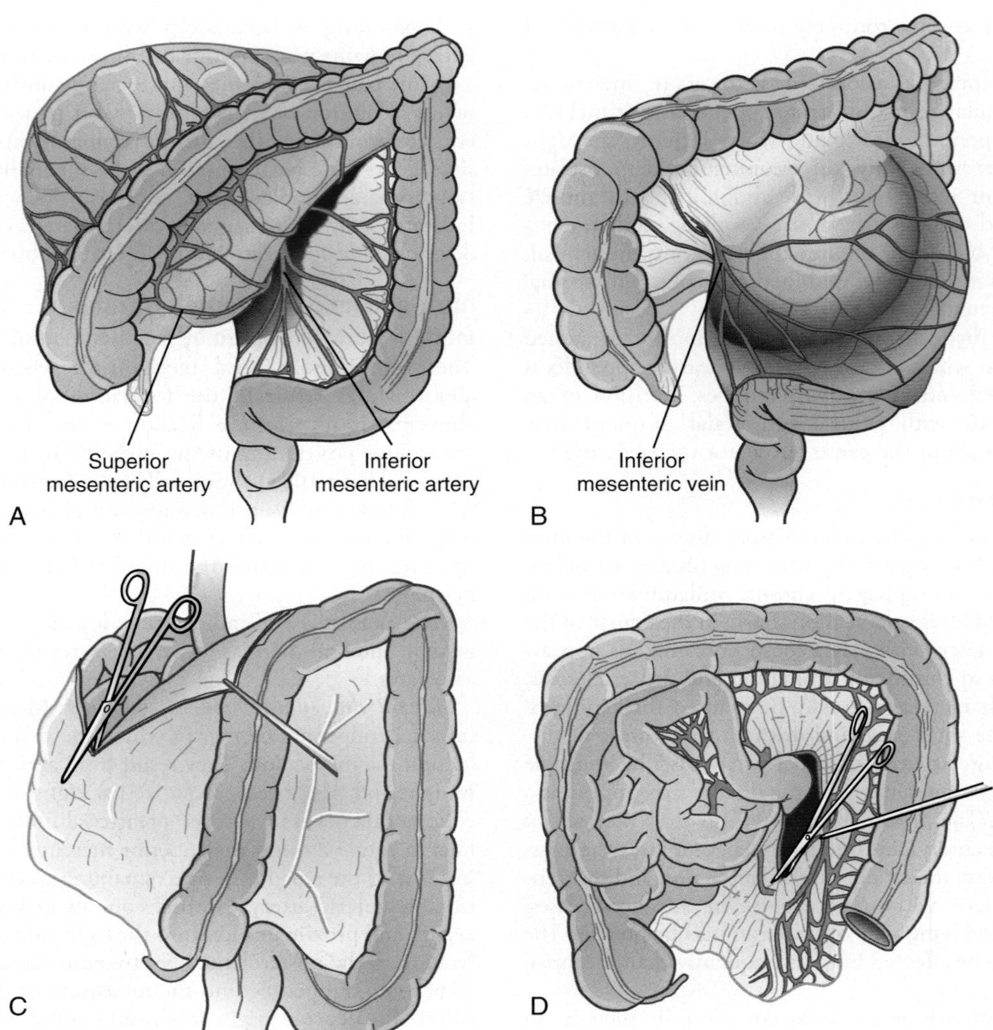

FIGURE 43-14 A, Right mesocolic (paraduodenal) hernia. Note that the anterior wall of a right mesocolic hernia is the ascending mesocolon. The hernia orifice lies to the right of the midline, and the superior mesenteric artery and ileocolic artery course along the anterior border of the hernia neck. **B,** Left mesocolic (paraduodenal) hernia. The hernia orifice is to the left of the midline, and the herniated intestine lies behind the anterior wall of the descending mesocolon. **C,** A right mesocolic hernia is repaired by division of the lateral peritoneal attachments of the ascending colon, reflecting it toward the left side of the abdomen. The small and large intestine then assume a position simulating that of nonrotation of the prearterial and postarterial segments of the midgut. Opening the neck of the hernia will injure the superior mesenteric vessels and fail to free the herniated bowel. **D,** A left mesocolic hernia is reduced by incising the hernia sac along an avascular plane immediately to the right of the inferior mesenteric vessels. (**A, B,** From Brigham RA, d'Avis JC: Paraduodenal hernia. In Nyhus LM, Condon RE, editors: *Hernia,* ed 3, Philadelphia, 1989, JB Lippincott, pp 484–485. **C, D,** From Brigham R, Fallon WF, Saunders JR, et al: Paraduodenal hernia: Diagnosis and surgical management. *Surg* 96:498–502, 1984.)

along the right side of the inferior mesenteric vein, with reduction of the herniated small intestine from beneath the inferior mesenteric vein. The vein is then allowed to return to its normal position on the left side of the base of the mesentery of the small intestine. The neck of the hernia may be closed by suturing the peritoneum adjacent to the vein to the retroperitoneum (Fig. 43-14*D*).

Mesenteric hernias. Mesenteric hernias occur when the intestine herniates through an abnormal orifice in the mesentery of the small intestine or colon. The most common location for these hernias is near the ileocolic junction, although defects in the sigmoid mesocolon have also been described. Patients present with intestinal obstruction resulting from compression of the loops of bowel at the neck of the hernia or torsion of the herniated segment. Treatment involves reduction of the hernia and closure of the mesenteric defect.

Acquired Internal Hernias

Acquired internal hernias result from the creation of abnormal mesenteric defects after operative procedures or trauma. These usually result from inadequate closure (or dehiscence) of mesenteric defects created during the performance of gastrojejunostomy, colostomy, ileostomy, or bowel resection. The creation of a small space allows the herniation of the small intestine through the mesenteric rent and development of intestinal obstruction. Depending on the type of surgery performed, variation exists in routine closure of the mesenteric defect. For instance, herniation after laparoscopic colectomy is uncommon (approximately 1%), so the defect is usually not closed. However, hernia rates after laparoscopic Roux-en-Y gastric bypass (i.e., Peterson hernia) are reported as high as 9%, so the defect is usually closed.[49] Treatment of these patients is operative reduction of the hernia and closure of the peritoneal defect.

Malignant Neoplasms of the Mesentery

Similar to the peritoneum and omentum, the most common neoplasm involving the mesentery is metastatic disease from an intra-abdominal adenocarcinoma. This may result from the direct invasion of the primary tumor (or its lymphatic metastases) into the mesentery or from the transperitoneal spread of the malignant neoplasm into the mesentery. Distortion and fixation of the mesentery by the tumor itself or by the resultant desmoplastic reaction, as in carcinoid tumors of the GI tract, may cause intestinal obstruction. The most common primary malignant neoplasm of the mesentery is a desmoid tumor.

Mesenteric and Intra-abdominal Desmoid Tumors

Mesenteric desmoids account for less than 10% of sporadic desmoid tumors, although they are reported to occur in 10% to 15% of patients with FAP. In this group of patients, 70% of the desmoid tumors are intra-abdominal, and 50% to 75% of these involve the mesentery.[2,3] The association between desmoid tumor and FAP is particularly strong in the subset of patients with Gardner syndrome. Patients with FAP and a family history of desmoid tumors have a 25% chance for development of a desmoid tumor. Several studies have shown intra-abdominal surgery to be a significant risk factor (as high as a threefold risk) for development of desmoids.[50] Levy and coworkers[46] have reviewed the pathologic and radiographic findings of these uncommon tumors.

Intra-abdominal desmoids are more lethal than those that occur at other anatomic sites because of the possibility of bowel obstruction or ischemia. Resection is less frequently possible, involves greater risk to critical structures, and may be associated with causing more aggressive growth and progression in these tumors. Intra-abdominal desmoid tumors are also more often multiple than those at other anatomic sites. Resection of mesenteric desmoids may require sacrifice of significant lengths of intestine, thus leaving the patient with an inadequate absorptive surface to maintain adequate nutrition. Finally, ureteral involvement of the tumor may require resection with reconstruction.

Although mesenteric desmoid tumors tend to be aggressive, there is considerable variability in their growth rate during the course of the disease. In fact, the biology of intra-abdominal desmoid tumors may be characterized by initial rapid growth followed by stability or even regression. Mesenteric desmoid tumors, by virtue of their relationship to vital structures and ability to infiltrate adjacent organs, may cause significant local complications, including intestinal obstruction, ischemia and perforation, hydronephrosis, and even aortic rupture, requiring operative management. Despite these complications, the overall 10-year survival rate for patients with intra-abdominal desmoid tumors is 60% to 70%.[51]

Establishing the rate of growth can be helpful in determining the optimal treatment of intra-abdominal desmoid tumors. The American Society of Clinical Oncology and Society of Surgical Oncologists have reviewed the current role of risk-reducing surgery in common hereditary cancer syndromes.[52] These recommendations, in addition to practice parameters from the Standards Task Force of the American Society of Colon and Rectal Surgeons, suggest that surgery should be reserved for small tumors with a well-defined and a clearly resectable margin.[53] Reported recurrence rates for intra-abdominal desmoids are higher than for other sites and range from 57% to 86%, although surgery can be curative in select patients.[51] Small bowel transplantation has been described for otherwise unresectable lesions.

Given the high likelihood of recurrence and prolonged survival, even in the setting of advanced disease, some have suggested that a trial of watchful waiting, along with minimally toxic agents such as sulindac and antiestrogen therapy, may be the best strategy, particularly in patients with minimal symptoms. In this nascent era of target-specific biologic therapy, clinical response to imatinib by patients with heavily treated desmoid tumor has been reported. Imatinib mesylate, specifically designed to inhibit the Bcr-Abl tyrosine kinase rendered constitutive by the Philadelphia chromosome translocation in chronic myeloid leukemia, also inhibits the tyrosine kinase receptor for platelet-derived growth factor and c-kit. The observation that patients with desmoid tumors have partial tumor response and arrest of disease progression while receiving oral imatinib offers an alternative to surgical resection of desmoid tumors arising in the mesentery.[17]

RETROPERITONEUM

Anatomy

The retroperitoneal space lies between the peritoneum and posterior parietal wall of the abdominal cavity, extending from the diaphragm to the pelvic floor. This space contains the contiguous lumbar and iliac fossae. The lumbar fossa extends from the 12th thoracic vertebra and lateral lumbocostal arch superiorly to the base of the sacrum, iliac crest, and iliolumbar ligament inferiorly. The floor of the space is formed by the fascia overlying the quadratus lumborum and psoas major muscles. This space contains varying amounts of fatty areolar tissue and the adrenal glands, kidneys, ascending and descending colon, and duodenum. It is also traversed by the ureter, renal vessels, gonadal vessels, inferior vena cava, and aorta. The iliac fossa is contiguous with the lumbar fossa superiorly, lateral and anterior preperitoneal spaces of the abdominal wall, and pelvis inferiorly. The iliacus muscle with its investing fascia is the floor of the iliac fossa, which contains the iliac vessels, ureter, genitofemoral nerve, gonadal vessels, and iliac lymph nodes.

Operative Approaches

The aorta, vena cava, iliac vessels, kidneys, and adrenal glands may be approached operatively through the retroperitoneal space. Specific operative procedures performed through the retroperitoneum include extirpative procedures, such as adrenalectomy and nephrectomy, and aortic aneurysmorrhaphy and renal transplantation. The advantages to this approach over a transabdominal approach are as follows: less postoperative ileus, facilitating a more rapid resumption of diet and earlier discharge from the hospital; no intra-abdominal adhesions, thus reducing the likelihood of subsequent small bowel obstruction; less intraoperative evaporative fluid losses, with less dramatic intravascular fluid shifts; and fewer respiratory complications, such as atelectasis and pneumonia.

Retroperitoneal Disorders

Retroperitoneal Abscesses

Retroperitoneal abscesses may be classified as primary if the infection results from hematogenous spread or secondary if it is related to an infection in an adjacent organ. The conditions associated with the development of retroperitoneal abscesses are shown in Table 43-2; the anatomic relationship of retroperitoneal abscesses to surrounding structures is shown in Figure 43-15. Most retroperitoneal abscesses originate as inflammatory processes in the kidney and GI tract. Renal causes include infections related to renal lithiasis or previous urologic operative procedures. GI causes include appendicitis, diverticulitis, pancreatitis, and Crohn's disease. In one series from an urban center, tuberculosis of the spine was a common cause of retroperitoneal abscesses, with *Mycobacterium tuberculosis* being the second most common bacterial isolate after *E. coli.*[54]

The bacteriology of retroperitoneal abscesses is related to the cause. Infections originating from the kidney are often monomicrobial, involving gram-negative rods such as *Proteus mirabilis* and *E. coli.* Abscesses associated with diseases of the GI tract involve *E. coli*, *Enterobacter* spp., enterococci, and anaerobic species such as *Bacteroides*. These infections are multimicrobial and involve gram-negative bacilli, enterococci, and anaerobic species. Infections from hematogenous spread are usually monomicrobial and related to staphylococcal species. Tuberculosis of the spine is an important cause of retroperitoneal abscesses in immunocompromised individuals and in those immigrating from underdeveloped countries.

The most common symptoms of retroperitoneal abscesses include abdominal or flank pain (60% to 75%), fever and chills (30% to 90%), malaise (10% to 22%), and weight loss (12%). Patients with psoas abscesses may have referred pain to the hip, groin, or knee. The duration of symptoms is usually longer than 1 week. Patients with retroperitoneal abscesses often have concurrent, chronic illnesses, such as renal lithiasis, diabetes mellitus, HIV infection, or malignant neoplasms. CT demonstrates a low-density mass in the retroperitoneum, with surrounding inflammation. Gas may be present in as many as one third of these lesions.[54] CT provides important information about the location of the abscess and its relationship to contiguous organs and hence likely sources of the infection.

Treatment of retroperitoneal abscesses includes appropriate antibiotics and adequate drainage. Many reports have demonstrated the efficacy of CT-guided drainage in managing this aspect of treatment. Operative drainage through a retroperitoneal approach is indicated for lesions not amenable to percutaneous drainage or those that fail percutaneous drainage. The mortality rate for patients with retroperitoneal abscesses is related, in large part, to the presence of significant medical comorbidities.

TABLE 43-2 Cause and Relative Frequency of Retroperitoneal Abscesses*

CAUSE	FREQUENCY (%)
Renal diseases	47
Gastrointestinal diseases, including diverticulitis, appendicitis, and Crohn's disease	16
Hematogenous spread from remote infections	11
Abscesses complicating operative procedures	8
Bone infections, including tuberculosis of the spine	7
Trauma	4.5
Malignant neoplasms	4
Miscellaneous causes	3

*Data are from three retrospective reviews[55-57] of 134 patients treated between 1971 and 2001.

Retroperitoneal Hematomas

Retroperitoneal hematomas usually occur after blunt or penetrating injuries, in the setting of abdominal aortic or visceral artery aneurysms, or after acute or chronic anticoagulation or fibrinolytic therapy. The diagnosis and management of retroperitoneal hematomas occurring in the setting of trauma or aneurysmal rupture are considered in detail in Chapters 16, 61, and 63.

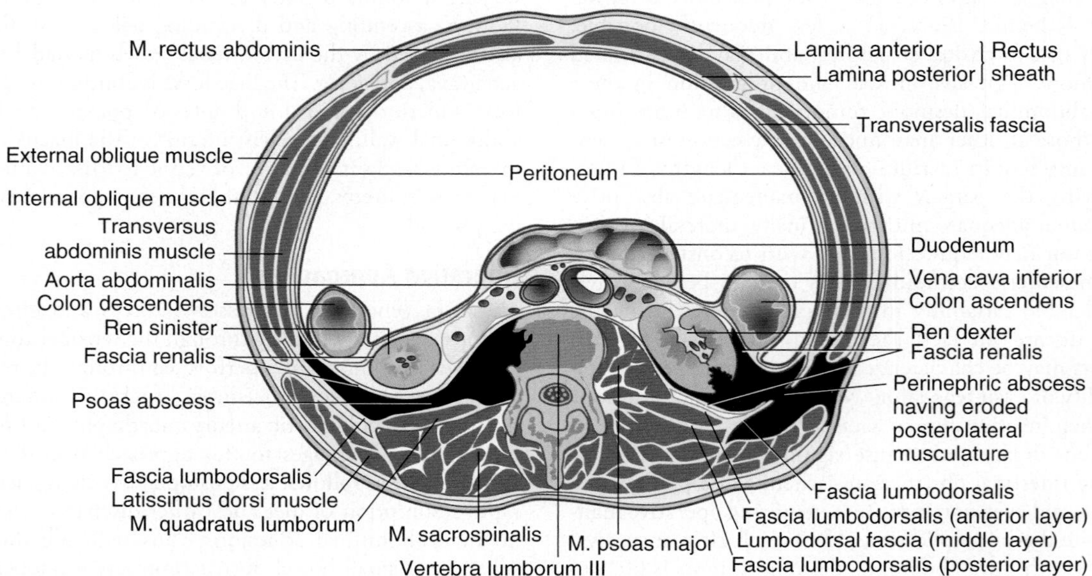

FIGURE 43-15 Anatomic relationships of retroperitoneal abscesses to surrounding structures. A psoas abscess *(left)* and perinephric abscess *(right)* are shown. (From McVay C: *Anson and McVay's surgical anatomy,* ed 6, Philadelphia, 1984, WB Saunders, p 735.)

Bleeding into the retroperitoneum may also complicate anticoagulant therapy for atrial fibrillation, deep venous thrombosis, or arterial catheterization during cardiac catheterization and endovascular procedures. Retroperitoneal hematomas have also been described in patients undergoing fibrinolytic therapy for peripheral or coronary arterial thrombosis and in patients with bleeding diatheses, such as hemophilia.

Patients present with abdominal or flank pain that may radiate into the groin, labia, or scrotum. Clinical evidence of acute blood loss may be present, depending on the volume of blood lost and the rapidity with which the patient bled. A palpable abdominal mass as well as physical evidence of ileus may be present. As many as 20% to 30% of patients will develop evidence of a femoral neuropathy.[55] The complete blood count may provide evidence of subacute or chronic blood loss or platelet deficiency. The prothrombin and partial thromboplastin times may demonstrate a coagulopathy. Microscopic hematuria is a common finding on urinalysis. CT establishes the diagnosis by demonstrating a high-density mass in the retroperitoneum, with surrounding stranding in the retroperitoneal tissue planes. These findings are readily distinguishable from the low-density mass characteristic of retroperitoneal abscesses.

Patients who develop retroperitoneal hematomas as a result of anticoagulation are best managed by the restoration of circulating blood volume and correction of the underlying coagulopathy. In rare circumstances, arteriography with embolization of a bleeding artery or operative exploration is required to stop the bleeding.

Retroperitoneal Fibrosis

Retroperitoneal fibrosis is characterized by chronic inflammation and fibrosis surrounding the abdominal aorta and iliac arteries that extend laterally to envelop surrounding structures, especially the ureters. Seventy percent of cases are idiopathic (Ormond disease), whereas 30% are associated with various drugs (most notably, ergot alkaloids or dopaminergic agonists), infections, trauma, retroperitoneal hemorrhage or retroperitoneal operations, radiation therapy, or primary or metastatic neoplasms. Many idiopathic cases are associated with inflammatory abdominal aortic aneurysms; thus, idiopathic retroperitoneal fibrosis might best be categorized with inflammatory abdominal aortic aneurysms and perianeurysmal retroperitoneal fibrosis as a form of chronic periaortitis.[56] The fibrosis is usually confined to the central and paravertebral spaces between the renal arteries and sacrum and tends to encase the aorta, inferior vena cava, and ureters. The process usually begins at the level of the aortic bifurcation and spreads cephalad. In 15% of cases, the fibrotic process extends outside the retroperitoneum to involve the peripancreatic and periduodenal spaces, pelvis, and mediastinum.

There is considerable evidence to suggest that idiopathic retroperitoneal fibrosis is a manifestation of a systemic autoimmune disease. A case-control study of 35 patients found that the disease is associated with HLA-DRB1*03, an allele linked to various autoimmune diseases, such as type 1 diabetes mellitus, myasthenia gravis, and systemic lupus erythematosus.[57] In some patients, disease will develop in the setting of a well-defined systemic autoimmune disorder (e.g., systemic lupus erythematosus) or so-called organ-specific autoimmune diseases (e.g., Hashimoto thyroiditis, sclerosing cholangitis). There are also histologic similarities between idiopathic retroperitoneal fibrosis and other systemic inflammatory conditions, such as large-vessel vasculitides.[56] Finally, systemic or constitutional symptoms are often present, such as fatigue, low-grade fever, weight loss, and myalgias.

Men are affected two to three times as often as women are. The mean age at presentation is 50 to 60 years, although the condition has also been reported in children and older adults. Patients may present with localized symptoms of side, back, or abdominal pain or lower extremity edema. Scrotal swelling is common, as is the occurrence of a varicocele or hydrocele. In most patients, localized symptoms are preceded by or coexist with systemic or constitutional symptoms (see earlier). Laboratory tests may demonstrate azotemia, and 80% to 100% of patients will have elevated concentrations of acute-phase reactants (e.g., erythrocyte sedimentation rate, C-reactive protein). The nonspecific nature of the clinical features of this disease contributes to the considerable delay between the onset of symptoms and the diagnosis. As such, ureteral involvement is present in 80% to 100% of cases.[56]

Evaluation of patients thought to have retroperitoneal fibrosis often starts with a CT scan. Without intravenous administration of contrast material, the CT scan will demonstrate a homogeneous fibrous plaque surrounding the lower abdominal aorta and the iliac arteries, which is usually isodense compared with surrounding muscle. MRI of early benign retroperitoneal fibrosis may show areas of high signal intensity on T2-weighted images as a result of the abundant fluid content and hypercellularity associated with the acute inflammation. In the mature and quiescent stages of benign retroperitoneal fibrosis, the low signal intensity on T1- and T2-weighted images is similar to that of psoas muscle.

The primary goals of treatment for patients with idiopathic retroperitoneal fibrosis are to stop the progression of retroperitoneal inflammation and fibrosis, to prevent or to relieve ureteral obstruction, to inhibit the systemic inflammatory response, and to improve the constitutional manifestations of the disease. The mainstay of treatment has been the administration of corticosteroids, which suppress the synthesis of proinflammatory cytokines and inhibit collagen synthesis and maturation. This will often result in a prompt improvement in symptoms, reduction in the size of the retroperitoneal mass, and relief of ureteral obstruction. Unfortunately, the optimal dose and duration of treatment have not been well established. Immunosuppressants such as mycophenolate mofetil, cyclophosphamide, azathioprine, methotrexate, cyclosporine, and tamoxifen have also been used to treat patients with idiopathic retroperitoneal fibrosis, particularly patients whose disease is unresponsive to steroids. Operative management of retroperitoneal fibrosis is generally performed to relieve ureteral obstruction by open ureterolysis, with intraperitoneal transposition and omental wrapping of the ureters. In most cases, when the clinical findings and imaging suggest the diagnosis of retroperitoneal fibrosis, the temporary placement of ureteral stents followed by medical therapy is the recommended course of action. Operative ureterolysis would be reserved for patients with refractory disease.

When retroperitoneal fibrosis is associated with an abdominal aortic aneurysm, repair of the aneurysm is warranted when the aortic diameter exceeds 4.5 to 5 cm. The effect of aneurysm repair of the periaortic fibrosis is unclear; some reports indicate resolution, and others report persistence or even progression of the inflammatory process.

Retroperitoneal Malignant Neoplasms

Malignant neoplasms in the retroperitoneum may result from the following:

- Extracapsular growth of a primary neoplasm of a retroperitoneal organ, such as the kidney, adrenal, colon, or pancreas

- Development of a primary germ cell neoplasm from embryonic rest cells
- Development of a primary malignant neoplasm of the retroperitoneal lymphatic system (e.g., lymphoma)
- Metastases from a remote primary malignant neoplasm into a retroperitoneal lymph node (e.g., testicular cancer)
- Development of a malignant neoplasm of the soft tissue of the retroperitoneum (e.g., sarcomas and desmoid tumors)

The most common primary malignant neoplasm of the retroperitoneum is a sarcoma.

Retroperitoneal sarcoma. Approximately 12,000 soft tissue sarcomas were diagnosed in the United States in 2014, of which 15% were retroperitoneal sarcomas.[58] The most common histologic subtypes are liposarcoma and leiomyosarcoma. Radiation is a known risk factor for the development of sarcomas, with radiation-associated sarcomas usually occurring approximately 10 years after exposure. Patients with von Recklinghausen disease (neurofibromatosis type 1) can develop malignant transformation of neurofibromas into malignant peripheral nerve sheath tumors; patients with Li-Fraumeni syndrome and hereditary retinoblastoma also have an increased incidence of sarcoma.

Most patients with a retroperitoneal sarcoma present with an asymptomatic abdominal mass, often after the primary tumor has reached a considerable size. Abdominal pain is present in 50% of patients; less common symptoms include GI hemorrhage, early satiety, nausea, vomiting, weight loss, and lower extremity swelling. Symptoms related to nerve compression by the tumor, such as lower extremity paresthesia and paresis, have also been associated with retroperitoneal sarcoma.

CT and MRI provide important information about the size and precise location of the primary tumor and its relationship to major vascular structures (Fig. 43-16). These studies will also document the presence or absence of metastatic disease in the lung or liver. These imaging modalities will also usually provide important diagnostic clues, thus obviating the need for image-guided biopsy in most cases.

Several findings can help distinguish retroperitoneal sarcomas from other retroperitoneal tumors. Lymphoma, especially with bulky retroperitoneal adenopathy, may appear as a mass arising from the retroperitoneum. The presence of constitutional symptoms, including fevers, night sweats, and weight loss, may suggest the diagnosis of lymphoma. A careful search for other evidence of lymphadenopathy is warranted in these patients. The spread of testicular cancer to the retroperitoneal lymph nodes may also be manifested as a large retroperitoneal mass. Hence, workup of male patients should include a testicular examination and serologic testing for α-fetoprotein and human chorionic gonadotropin. Finally, the local extension of tumors arising in the adrenal gland or pancreas may also be considered in the differential diagnosis of patients with large retroperitoneal tumors.

Prognostic staging is difficult for sarcomas because there are many histologic types of sarcomas, with variables grades and locations. The latest edition of the American Joint Commission cancer staging system is notable in that it includes grade and depth to the fascia in addition to standard staging criteria, such as tumor size, nodal status, and distant metastasis.[59] Most retroperitoneal sarcomas are deep to the fascia and large, so grade is the main determinant of stage in nonmetastatic disease. Nodal disease had previously been classified as stage IV but is currently reassigned to stage III.

The goal of sarcoma treatment is complete en bloc resection of the tumor and any involved adjacent organs. As retroperitoneal sarcomas are rare tumors with several different histologic subtypes that may influence surgical treatment, a consensus approach from an international group of established experts was recently constructed to assist with management strategy.[60] Recommendations found within this consensus statement address preoperative assessment and biopsy, surgical approach, adjuvant and neoadjuvant therapy, and follow-up and may serve as a resource in addition to standard National Comprehensive Cancer Network guidelines. Lymph node metastases by sarcoma are rare (<5%); therefore, lymphadenectomy is not required unless there is evidence of lymph node involvement. The main prognostic factors for patients with retroperitoneal sarcomas are the size of the tumor, histologic grade, and resection status.[61] The difficulty of obtaining resection margins free of tumor is related to the juxtaposition or invasion of the tumor and retroperitoneal structures, such as the aorta, inferior vena cava, intra-abdominal viscera (colon, duodenum, kidney, pancreas, spleen), and adjacent muscles (psoas, rectus abdominis, diaphragm). The kidney is the most commonly resected organ; series have reported multiorgan resection in approximately 50% of cases.[62] A thoracoabdominal incision may be required for upper quadrant sarcomas, but this does not appear to increase morbidity greatly. It can be difficult pathologically to determine a negative margin resulting from the large surface area and anatomic constraints of the tumor. Most experts in treating this disease consider the goal of surgery to be complete resection, defined by removal of all gross disease (macroscopically negative

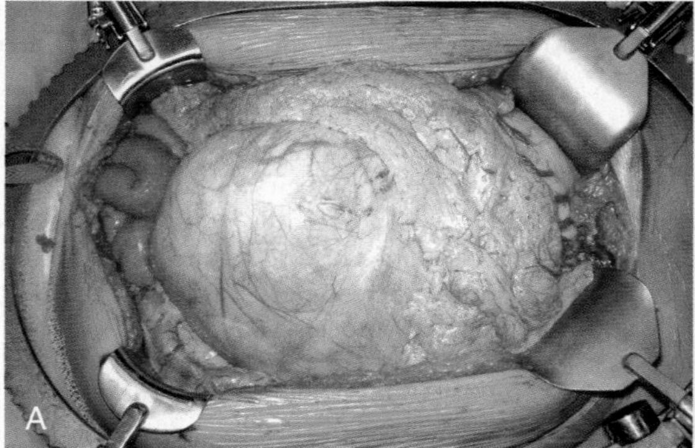

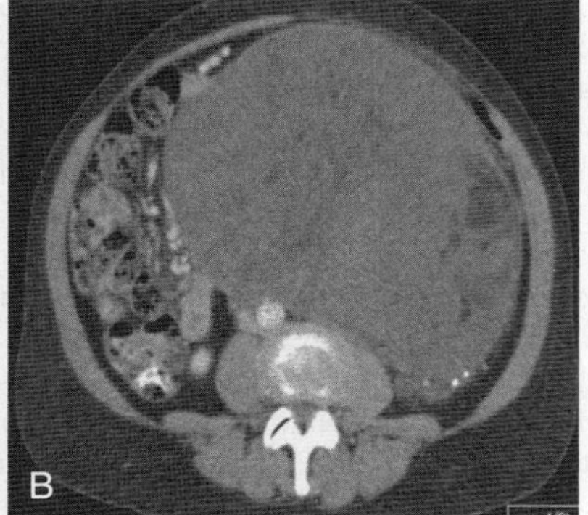

FIGURE 43-16 A, Intraoperative photograph of a large retroperitoneal sarcoma. **B,** CT scan of the same patient demonstrating the displacement of the aorta, inferior vena cava, and bowel to the right of the abdomen.

margin), with en bloc resection of adherent organs. Rates of resectability of the primary retroperitoneal sarcoma vary widely on the basis of the extent of disease at presentation, the surgeon's experience, and the institution's referral pattern. A review of several large series has reported complete resectability rates of 50% to 67%.[63]

There is no difference in survival for patients who undergo incomplete resection compared with those who are unresectable. Incomplete resection should be undertaken only for palliative purposes for all histologic types other than liposarcoma.[61] Incomplete resection of well-differentiated liposarcoma may prolong survival and has been shown to improve symptoms.[64] Local recurrence after surgery occurs in approximately 50% of patients, and distant metastases occur in 20% to 30%. The 5-year survival rate is approximately 50%.[64]

In patients with recurrent disease, complete resection of recurrent tumor is beneficial. In a report by Lewis and colleagues[61] at the Memorial Sloan Kettering Cancer Center, 35 of 61 patients with recurrent sarcoma underwent complete resection. This group of patients had a significantly higher survival rate than those undergoing incomplete resection (60% versus 18% 5-year disease-specific survival).

Unlike for extremity sarcoma, the role of external beam radiation for local control after surgical resection is limited by the low tolerance for radiation injury of the surrounding normal tissue. Postoperative radiotherapy and combined postoperative and intraoperative radiotherapy have been shown to improve recurrence rates but have not been clearly shown to have an effect on survival. Preoperative radiotherapy has some theoretical benefits, but there have been no prospective randomized trials of preoperative radiotherapy. Neoadjuvant or adjuvant chemotherapy is supported by limited and conflicting data, but unfortunately most agents used for sarcoma therapy have significant toxicity.

SELECTED REFERENCES

Chua TC, Moran BJ, Sugarbaker PH, et al: Early- and long-term outcome data of patients with pseudomyxoma peritonei from appendiceal origin treated by a strategy of cytoreductive surgery and hyperthermic intraperitoneal chemotherapy. *J Clin Oncol* 30:2449–2456, 2012.

This large multi-institutional retrospective study highlights the safety and improved outcomes using cytoreductive surgery with pseudomyxoma peritonei.

Fiore M, Rimareix F, Mariani L, et al: Desmoid-type fibromatosis: A front-line conservative approach to select patients for surgical treatment. *Ann Surg Oncol* 16:2587–2593, 2009.

This multi-institutional paper highlights the utility of a watch and wait approach for managing patients with desmoids.

Fleshman J, Sargent DJ, Green E, et al: Laparoscopic colectomy for cancer is not inferior to open surgery based on 5-year data from the COST Study Group trial. *Ann Surg* 246:655–662, 2007.

This important paper defined the incidence of port site recurrence after laparoscopic colectomy for colon cancer and established the equivalency of laparoscopic and open colectomy for the treatment of curable colon cancer.

Guillem JG, Wood WC, Moley JF, et al: ASCO/SSO review of current role of risk-reducing surgery in common hereditary cancer syndromes. *J Clin Oncol* 24:4642–4660, 2006.

This task force consensus statement outlines the current recommendations from the American Society of Clinical Oncology and Society of Surgical Oncology regarding surgery for desmoid tumors in patients with familial adenomatous polyposis.

Koulaouzidis A, Bhat S, Saeed AA: Spontaneous bacterial peritonitis. *World J Gastroenterol* 15:1042–1049, 2009.

This is a well-written and thorough review of the pathophysiology, bacteriology, and treatment of spontaneous bacterial peritonitis.

Martin LC, Merkle EM, Thompson WM: Review of internal hernias: Radiographic and clinical findings. *AJR Am J Roentgenol* 186:703–717, 2006.

This is a thorough and well-illustrated review of the types of congenital and acquired internal hernias.

Moller S, Henriksen JH, Bendtsen F: Ascites: Pathogenesis and therapeutic principles. *Scand J Gastroenterol* 44:902–911, 2009.

This is a well-written and thorough review of the pathophysiology of ascites formation in cirrhotics and the basic tenets of medical management.

Runyon BA, Montano AA, Akriviadis EA, et al: The serum-ascites albumin gradient is superior to the exudate-transudate concept in the differential diagnosis of ascites. *Ann Intern Med* 117:215–220, 1992.

This well-written paper established the use of serum-ascites albumin gradient in the elucidation of the pathophysiology of ascites formation.

Stewart JH, Shen P, Levine EA: Intraperitoneal hyperthermic chemotherapy for peritoneal surface malignancy: Current status and future directions. *Ann Surg Oncol* 12:765–777, 2005.

This review covers the rationale, technical aspects, and outcomes for intraperitoneal hyperthermic chemotherapy for several types of malignant neoplasms.

Trans-Atlantic RPS Working Group: Management of primary retroperitoneal sarcoma (RPS) in the adult: A consensus approach from the Trans-Atlantic RPS Working Group. *Ann Surg Oncol* 22:256–263, 2015.

This paper provides updated consensus statements on the management of retroperitoneal sarcoma.

Vaglio A, Salvarani C, Buzio C: Retroperitoneal fibrosis. *Lancet* 367:241–251, 2006.

This is a well-written and thorough review of the pathophysiology, immunology, and clinical features of retroperitoneal fibrosis.

REFERENCES

1. Cherry WB, Mueller PS: Rectus sheath hematoma: Review of 126 cases at a single institution. *Medicine (Baltimore)* 85:105–110, 2006.
2. Gurbuz AK, Giardiello FM, Petersen GM, et al: Desmoid tumors in familial adenomatous polyposis. *Gut* 35:377–381, 1994.
3. Kulaylat MN, Karakousis CP, Keaney CM, et al: Desmoid tumour: A pleomorphic lesion. *Eur J Surg Oncol* 25:487–497, 1999.
4. Stojadinovic A, Hoos A, Karpoff HM, et al: Soft tissue tumors of the abdominal wall: Analysis of disease patterns and treatment. *Arch Surg* 136:70–79, 2001.
5. Fiore M, Rimareix F, Mariani L, et al: Desmoid-type fibromatosis: A front-line conservative approach to select patients for surgical treatment. *Ann Surg Oncol* 16:2587–2593, 2009.
6. Lev D, Kotilingam D, Wei C, et al: Optimizing treatment of desmoid tumors. *J Clin Oncol* 25:1785–1791, 2007.
7. Gronchi A, Casali PG, Mariani L, et al: Quality of surgery and outcome in extra-abdominal aggressive fibromatosis: A series of patients surgically treated at a single institution. *J Clin Oncol* 21:1390–1397, 2003.
8. Bonvalot S, Ternes N, Fiore M, et al: Spontaneous regression of primary abdominal wall desmoid tumors: More common than previously thought. *Ann Surg Oncol* 20:4096–4102, 2013.
9. Bonvalot S, Eldweny H, Haddad V, et al: Extra-abdominal primary fibromatosis: Aggressive management could be avoided in a subgroup of patients. *Eur J Surg Oncol* 34:462–468, 2008.
10. Crago AM, Denton B, Salas S, et al: A prognostic nomogram for prediction of recurrence in desmoid fibromatosis. *Ann Surg* 258:347–353, 2013.
11. Salas S, Dufresne A, Bui B, et al: Prognostic factors influencing progression-free survival determined from a series of sporadic desmoid tumors: A wait-and-see policy according to tumor presentation. *J Clin Oncol* 29:3553–3558, 2011.
12. Nuyttens JJ, Rust PF, Thomas CR, Jr, et al: Surgery versus radiation therapy for patients with aggressive fibromatosis or desmoid tumors: A comparative review of 22 articles. *Cancer* 88:1517–1523, 2000.
13. Janinis J, Patriki M, Vini L, et al: The pharmacological treatment of aggressive fibromatosis: A systematic review. *Ann Oncol* 14:181–190, 2003.
14. Clark SK, Neale KF, Landgrebe JC, et al: Desmoid tumours complicating familial adenomatous polyposis. *Br J Surg* 86:1185–1189, 1999.
15. Hansmann A, Adolph C, Vogel T, et al: High-dose tamoxifen and sulindac as first-line treatment for desmoid tumors. *Cancer* 100:612–620, 2004.
16. Azzarelli A, Gronchi A, Bertulli R, et al: Low-dose chemotherapy with methotrexate and vinblastine for patients with advanced aggressive fibromatosis. *Cancer* 92:1259–1264, 2001.
17. Heinrich MC, McArthur GA, Demetri GD, et al: Clinical and molecular studies of the effect of imatinib on advanced aggressive fibromatosis (desmoid tumor). *J Clin Oncol* 24:1195–1203, 2006.
18. Fleshman J, Sargent DJ, Green E, et al: Laparoscopic colectomy for cancer is not inferior to open surgery based on 5-year data from the COST Study Group trial. *Ann Surg* 246:655–662, discussion 662–664, 2007.
19. Plaza JA, Perez-Montiel D, Mayerson J, et al: Metastases to soft tissue: A review of 118 cases over a 30-year period. *Cancer* 112:193–203, 2008.
20. Kashani A, Landaverde C, Medici V, et al: Fluid retention in cirrhosis: Pathophysiology and management. *QJM* 101:71–85, 2008.
21. Moller S, Henriksen JH, Bendtsen F: Ascites: Pathogenesis and therapeutic principles. *Scand J Gastroenterol* 44:902–911, 2009.
22. Runyon BA: Paracentesis of ascitic fluid. A safe procedure. *Arch Intern Med* 146:2259–2261, 1986.
23. Runyon BA, Montano AA, Akriviadis EA, et al: The serum-ascites albumin gradient is superior to the exudate-transudate concept in the differential diagnosis of ascites. *Ann Intern Med* 117:215–220, 1992.
24. Gines P, Cardenas A, Arroyo V, et al: Management of cirrhosis and ascites. *N Engl J Med* 350:1646–1654, 2004.
25. Kuiper JJ, de Man RA, van Buuren HR: Review article: Management of ascites and associated complications in patients with cirrhosis. *Aliment Pharmacol Ther* 26(Suppl 2):183–193, 2007.
26. Caruntu FA, Benea L: Spontaneous bacterial peritonitis: Pathogenesis, diagnosis, treatment. *J Gastrointestin Liver Dis* 15:51–56, 2006.
27. Berg RD: Bacterial translocation from the gastrointestinal tract. *Adv Exp Med Biol* 473:11–30, 1999.
28. Guarner C, Soriano G: Bacterial translocation and its consequences in patients with cirrhosis. *Eur J Gastroenterol Hepatol* 17:27–31, 2005.
29. Moore K: Spontaneous bacterial peritonitis (SBP). In Warrel DA, editor: *Oxford textbook of medicine* (vol 2), ed 4, New York, 2003, Oxford University Press, pp 739–741.
30. Levison ME, Bush LM: Peritonitis and intraperitoneal abscesses. In Mandell GL, Bennett JE, Dolin R, editors: *Principles and practice of infectious diseases* (vol 1), ed 6, Philadelphia, 2005, Elsevier Churchill Livingstone, pp 927–951.
31. Koulaouzidis A, Leontiadis GI, Abdullah M, et al: Leucocyte esterase reagent strips for the diagnosis of spontaneous bacterial peritonitis: A systematic review. *Eur J Gastroenterol Hepatol* 20:1055–1060, 2008.
32. Nguyen-Khac E, Cadranel JF, Thevenot T, et al: Review article: The utility of reagent strips in the diagnosis of infected ascites in cirrhotic patients. *Aliment Pharmacol Ther* 28:282–288, 2008.
33. Chavez-Tapia NC, Soares-Weiser K, Brezis M, et al: Antibiotics for spontaneous bacterial peritonitis in cirrhotic patients. *Cochrane Database Syst Rev* (1):CD002232, 2009.
34. Koulaouzidis A, Bhat S, Saeed AA: Spontaneous bacterial peritonitis. *World J Gastroenterol* 15:1042–1049, 2009.
35. Fernandez J, Navasa M, Garcia-Pagan JC, et al: Effect of intravenous albumin on systemic and hepatic hemodynamics and vasoactive neurohormonal systems in patients with cirrhosis and spontaneous bacterial peritonitis. *J Hepatol* 41:384–390, 2004.
36. Sanai FM, Bzeizi KI: Systematic review: Tuberculous peritonitis—presenting features, diagnostic strategies and treatment. *Aliment Pharmacol Ther* 22:685–700, 2005.
37. Kavanagh D, Prescott GJ, Mactier RA: Peritoneal dialysis–associated peritonitis in Scotland (1999-2002). *Nephrol Dial Transplant* 19:2584–2591, 2004.

38. Misdraji J, Yantiss RK, Graeme-Cook FM, et al: Appendiceal mucinous neoplasms: A clinicopathologic analysis of 107 cases. *Am J Surg Pathol* 27:1089–1103, 2003.
39. Ronnett BM, Yan H, Kurman RJ, et al: Patients with pseudomyxoma peritonei associated with disseminated peritoneal adenomucinosis have a significantly more favorable prognosis than patients with peritoneal mucinous carcinomatosis. *Cancer* 92:85–91, 2001.
40. Gonzalez-Moreno S, Sugarbaker PH: Right hemicolectomy does not confer a survival advantage in patients with mucinous carcinoma of the appendix and peritoneal seeding. *Br J Surg* 91:304–311, 2004.
41. Stewart JH, Shen P, Levine EA: Intraperitoneal hyperthermic chemotherapy for peritoneal surface malignancy: Current status and future directions. *Ann Surg Oncol* 12:765–777, 2005.
42. Chua TC, Moran BJ, Sugarbaker PH, et al: Early- and long-term outcome data of patients with pseudomyxoma peritonei from appendiceal origin treated by a strategy of cytoreductive surgery and hyperthermic intraperitoneal chemotherapy. *J Clin Oncol* 30:2449–2456, 2012.
43. Teta MJ, Mink PJ, Lau E, et al: US mesothelioma patterns 1973-2002: Indicators of change and insights into background rates. *Eur J Cancer Prev* 17:525–534, 2008.
44. Levy AD, Arnaiz J, Shaw JC, et al: From the archives of the AFIP: Primary peritoneal tumors: Imaging features with pathologic correlation. *Radiographics* 28:583–607, quiz 621–622, 2008.
45. Yan TD, Deraco M, Baratti D, et al: Cytoreductive surgery and hyperthermic intraperitoneal chemotherapy for malignant peritoneal mesothelioma: Multi-institutional experience. *J Clin Oncol* 27:6237–6242, 2009.
46. Levy AD, Rimola J, Mehrotra AK, et al: From the archives of the AFIP: Benign fibrous tumors and tumorlike lesions of the mesentery: Radiologic-pathologic correlation. *Radiographics* 26:245–264, 2006.
47. Horton KM, Lawler LP, Fishman EK: CT findings in sclerosing mesenteritis (panniculitis): Spectrum of disease. *Radiographics* 23:1561–1567, 2003.
48. Martin LC, Merkle EM, Thompson WM: Review of internal hernias: Radiographic and clinical findings. *AJR Am J Roentgenol* 186:703–717, 2006.
49. Cabot JC, Lee SA, Yoo J, et al: Long-term consequences of not closing the mesenteric defect after laparoscopic right colectomy. *Dis Colon Rectum* 53:289–292, 2010.
50. Nieuwenhuis MH, Mathus-Vliegen EM, Baeten CG, et al: Evaluation of management of desmoid tumours associated with familial adenomatous polyposis in Dutch patients. *Br J Cancer* 104:37–42, 2011.
51. Smith AJ, Lewis JJ, Merchant NB, et al: Surgical management of intra-abdominal desmoid tumours. *Br J Surg* 87:608–613, 2000.
52. Guillem JG, Wood WC, Moley JF, et al: ASCO/SSO review of current role of risk-reducing surgery in common hereditary cancer syndromes. *J Clin Oncol* 24:4642–4660, 2006.
53. Church J, Simmang C: Practice parameters for the treatment of patients with dominantly inherited colorectal cancer (familial adenomatous polyposis and hereditary nonpolyposis colorectal cancer). *Dis Colon Rectum* 46:1001–1012, 2003.
54. Paley M, Sidhu PS, Evans RA, et al: Retroperitoneal collections—a cause and radiological implications. *Clin Radiol* 52:290–294, 1997.
55. Loor G, Bassiouny H, Valentin C, et al: Local and systemic consequences of large retroperitoneal clot burdens. *World J Surg* 33:1618–1625, 2009.
56. Vaglio A, Salvarani C, Buzio C: Retroperitoneal fibrosis. *Lancet* 367:241–251, 2006.
57. Martorana D, Vaglio A, Greco P, et al: Chronic periaortitis and HLA-DRB1*03: Another clue to an autoimmune origin. *Arthritis Rheum* 55:126–130, 2006.
58. Siegel R, Ma J, Zou Z, et al: Cancer statistics, 2014. *CA Cancer J Clin* 64:9–29, 2014.
59. Soft tissue sarcoma. In Edge SB, Byrd DR, Compton CC, et al, editors: *AJCC cancer staging manual*, ed 7, New York, 2010, Springer, pp 291–298.
60. Trans-Atlantic RPS Working Group: Management of primary retroperitoneal sarcoma (RPS) in the adult: A consensus approach from the Trans-Atlantic RPS Working Group. *Ann Surg Oncol* 22:256–263, 2015.
61. Lewis JJ, Leung D, Woodruff JM, et al: Retroperitoneal soft-tissue sarcoma: Analysis of 500 patients treated and followed at a single institution. *Ann Surg* 228:355–365, 1998.
62. Russo P, Kim Y, Ravindran S, et al: Nephrectomy during operative management of retroperitoneal sarcoma. *Ann Surg Oncol* 4:421–424, 1997.
63. Mendenhall WM, Zlotecki RA, Hochwald SN, et al: Retroperitoneal soft tissue sarcoma. *Cancer* 104:669–675, 2005.
64. Shibata D, Lewis JJ, Leung DH, et al: Is there a role for incomplete resection in the management of retroperitoneal liposarcomas? *J Am Coll Surg* 193:373–379, 2001.

44 CHAPTER

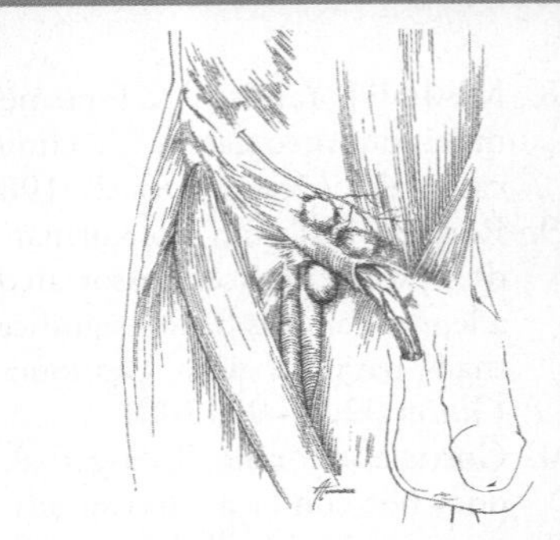

Hernias

Mark A. Malangoni, Michael J. Rosen

OUTLINE

More than 600,000 hernias are repaired annually in the United States, making hernia repair one of the most common operations performed by general surgeons. Despite the frequency of this procedure, no surgeon has ideal results, and complications such as postoperative pain, nerve injury, surgical site infection, and recurrence remain.

Hernia is derived from the Latin word for rupture. A hernia is defined as an abnormal protrusion of an organ or tissue through a defect in its surrounding walls. Although a hernia can occur at various sites of the body, these defects most commonly involve the abdominal wall, particularly the inguinal region. Abdominal wall hernias occur only at sites at which the aponeurosis and fascia are not covered by striated muscle (Box 44-1). These sites most commonly include the inguinal, femoral, and umbilical areas; linea alba; lower portion of the semilunar line; and sites of prior incisions (Fig. 44-1). The so-called neck or orifice of a hernia is located at the innermost musculoaponeurotic layer, whereas the hernia sac is lined by peritoneum and protrudes from the neck. There is no consistent relationship between the area of a hernia defect and the size of a hernia sac.

A hernia is reducible when its contents can be replaced within the surrounding musculature, and it is irreducible or incarcerated when it cannot be reduced. A strangulated hernia has compromised blood supply to its contents, which is a serious and potentially fatal complication. Strangulation occurs more often in large hernias that have small orifices. In this situation, the small neck of the hernia obstructs arterial blood flow, venous drainage, or both to the contents of the hernia sac. Adhesions between the contents of the hernia and peritoneal lining of the sac can provide a tethering point that entraps the hernia contents and predisposes to intestinal obstruction and strangulation. A more unusual type of strangulation is a Richter hernia. In Richter hernia, a small portion of the antimesenteric wall of the intestine is trapped within the hernia, and strangulation can occur without the presence of intestinal obstruction.

An external hernia protrudes through all layers of the abdominal wall, whereas an internal hernia is a protrusion of intestine through a defect in the peritoneal cavity. An interparietal hernia occurs when the hernia sac is contained within a musculoaponeurotic layer of the abdominal wall. In broad terms, most abdominal wall hernias can be separated into inguinal and ventral hernias. This chapter focuses on the specific aspects of each of these conditions individually.

INGUINAL HERNIAS

Inguinal hernias are classified as direct or indirect. The sac of an indirect inguinal hernia passes from the internal inguinal ring obliquely toward the external inguinal ring and ultimately into the scrotum. In contrast, the sac of a direct inguinal hernia protrudes outward and forward and is medial to the internal inguinal ring and inferior epigastric vessels. As indirect hernias enlarge, it sometimes can be difficult to distinguish between indirect and direct inguinal hernias. This distinction is of little importance because the operative repair of these types of hernias is similar. A pantaloon-type hernia occurs when there is both an indirect and direct hernia component.

Incidence

Hernias are a common problem; however, their true incidence is unknown. It is estimated that 5% of the population will develop an abdominal wall hernia, but the prevalence may be even higher. About 75% of all hernias occur in the inguinal region. Two thirds of these are indirect and the remainder are direct inguinal hernias. Femoral hernias represent only 3% of all groin hernias.

Men are 25 times more likely to have a groin hernia than women. An indirect inguinal hernia is the most common hernia, regardless of gender. In men, indirect hernias predominate over direct hernias at a ratio of 2 : 1. Indirect hernias are by far the most common type of hernia in women. The female-to-male ratio for femoral and umbilical hernias, however, is about 10 : 1 and 2 : 1, respectively. Although femoral hernias occur more frequently in women than in men, inguinal hernias remain the most common hernia in women. Femoral hernias are rare in men. Ten percent of women and 50% of men who have a femoral hernia have or will develop an inguinal hernia.

Indirect inguinal and femoral hernias occur more commonly on the right side. This is attributed to a delay in atrophy of the processus vaginalis after the normal slower descent of the right testis to the scrotum during fetal development. The predominance of right-sided femoral hernias is thought to be caused by the tamponading effect of the sigmoid colon on the left femoral canal.

The prevalence of hernias increases with age, particularly for inguinal, umbilical, and femoral hernias. The likelihood of strangulation and need for hospitalization also increase with aging.

BOX 44-1 Primary Abdominal Wall Hernias

Groin
- Inguinal
  - Indirect
  - Direct
  - Combined
- Femoral

Anterior
- Umbilical
- Epigastric
- Spigelian

Pelvic
- Obturator
- Sciatic
- Perineal

Posterior
- Lumbar
  - Superior triangle
  - Inferior triangle

Strangulation, the most common serious complication of a hernia, occurs in only 1% to 3% of groin hernias and is more common at the extremes of life. Most strangulated hernias are indirect inguinal hernias; however, femoral hernias have the highest rate of strangulation (15% to 20%) of all hernias, and it is therefore recommended that all femoral hernias be repaired at the time of discovery.

Anatomy of the Groin

The surgeon must have a comprehensive understanding of the anatomy of the groin to select and to use various options for hernia repair properly. In addition, the relationships of muscles, aponeuroses, fascia, nerves, blood vessels, and spermatic cord structures in the inguinal region must be completely understood to obtain the lowest incidence of recurrence and to avoid complications. These anatomic considerations must be understood from the anterior and posterior approaches because both are useful in different situations (Figs. 44-2 and 44-3).

From anterior to posterior, the groin anatomy includes the skin and subcutaneous tissues, below which are the superficial circumflex iliac, superficial epigastric, and external pudendal arteries and accompanying veins. These vessels arise from and drain to the proximal femoral artery and vein, respectively, and are directed superiorly. If encountered during operation, these vessels can be retracted or even divided when necessary.

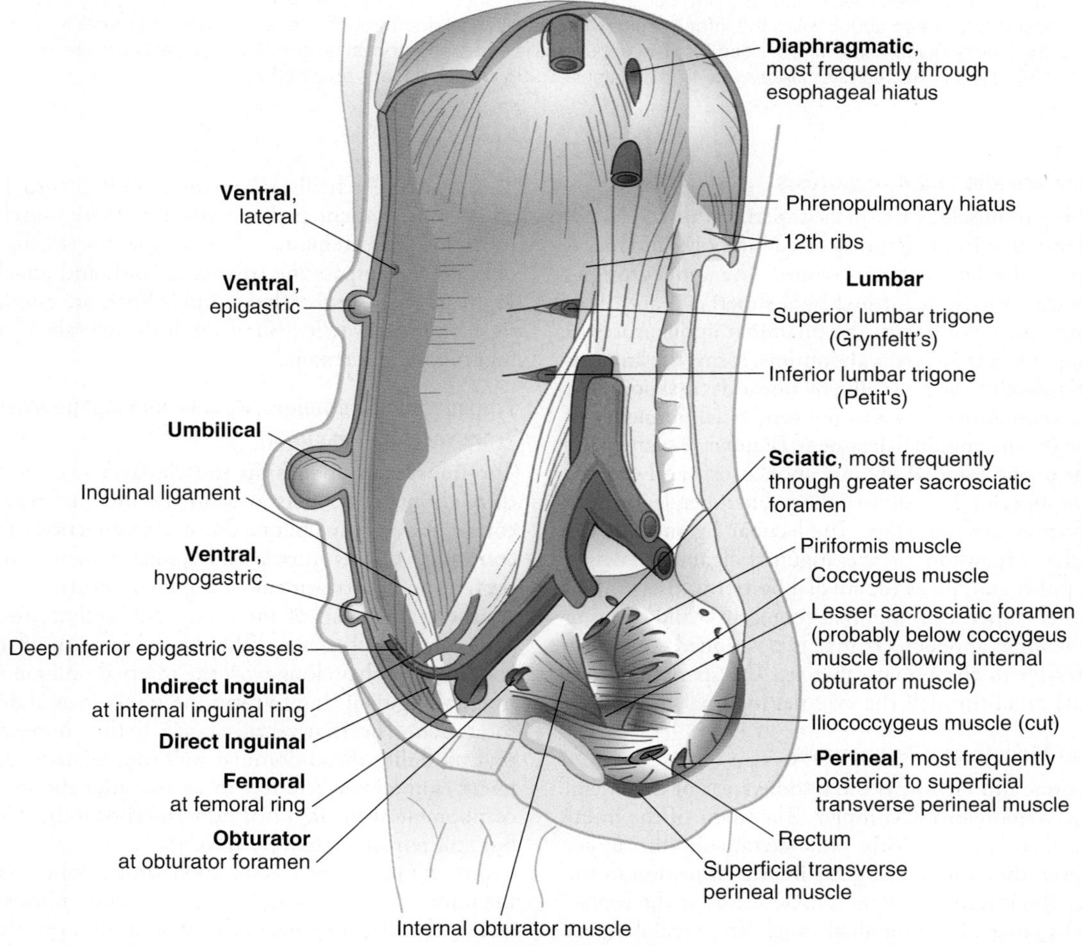

FIGURE 44-1 Types of abdominal wall hernias. (From *Dorland's illustrated medical dictionary*, ed 31, Philadelphia, 2007, WB Saunders, Plate 21.)

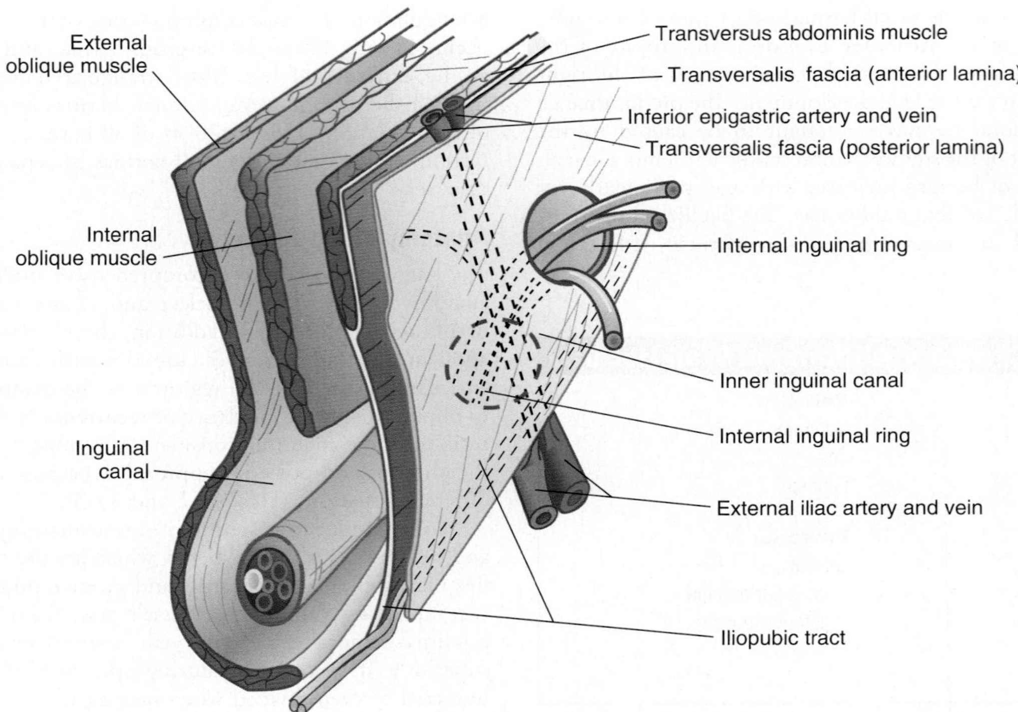

FIGURE 44-2 Nyhus's classic parasagittal diagram of the right midinguinal region illustrating the muscular aponeurotic layers separated into anterior and posterior walls. The posterior laminae of the transversalis fascia have been added, with the inferior epigastric vessels coursing through the abdominal wall medially to the inner inguinal canal. (From Read RC: The transversalis and preperitoneal fasciae: A re-evaluation. In Nyhus LM, Condon RE, editors: *Hernia*, ed 4, Philadelphia, 1995, JB Lippincott, pp 57-63.)

External Oblique Muscle and Aponeurosis

The external oblique muscle is the most superficial of the lateral abdominal wall muscles; its fibers are directed inferiorly and medially and lie deep to the subcutaneous tissues. The aponeurosis of the external oblique muscle is formed by a superficial and deep layer. This aponeurosis, along with the bilaminar aponeuroses of the internal oblique and transversus abdominis, forms the anterior rectus sheath and, finally, the linea alba by linear decussation. The external oblique aponeurosis serves as the superficial boundary of the inguinal canal. The inguinal ligament (Poupart ligament) is the inferior edge of the external oblique aponeurosis and extends from the anterior superior iliac spine to the pubic tubercle, turning posteriorly to form a shelving edge. The lacunar ligament is the fan-shaped medial expansion of the inguinal ligament, which inserts into the pubis and forms the medial border of the femoral space. The external (superficial) inguinal ring is an ovoid opening of the external oblique aponeurosis that is positioned superiorly and slightly laterally to the pubic tubercle. The spermatic cord exits the inguinal canal through the external inguinal ring.

Internal Oblique Muscle and Aponeurosis

The internal oblique muscle forms the middle layer of the lateral abdominal musculoaponeurotic complex. The fibers of the internal oblique are directed superiorly and laterally in the upper abdomen; however, they run in a slightly inferior direction in the inguinal region. The internal oblique muscle serves as the cephalad (or superior) border of the inguinal canal. The medial aspect of the internal oblique aponeurosis fuses with fibers from the transversus abdominis aponeurosis to form a conjoined tendon. This structure actually is present in only 5% to 10% of patients and is most evident at the insertion of these muscles on the pubic tubercle. The cremaster muscle fibers arise from the internal oblique, encompass the spermatic cord, and attach to the tunica vaginalis of the testis. These muscle fibers are essential to maintain the cremasteric reflex but have little relevance to the results of inguinal hernia repairs.

Transversus Abdominis Muscle and Aponeurosis and Transversalis Fascia

The transversus abdominis muscle layer is oriented horizontally throughout most of its area; in the inguinal region, these fibers course in a slightly oblique downward direction. The strength and continuity of this muscle and aponeurosis are important for the prevention and treatment of inguinal hernia.

The aponeurosis of the transversus abdominis covers anterior and posterior surfaces. The lower margin of the transversus abdominis arches along with the internal oblique muscle over the internal inguinal ring to form the transversus abdominis aponeurotic arch. The transversalis fascia is the connective tissue layer that underlies the abdominal wall musculature. The transversalis fascia, sometimes referred to as the endoabdominal fascia, is a component of the inguinal floor. It tends to be denser in this area but still remains relatively thin.

The iliopubic tract is an aponeurotic band that is formed by the transversalis fascia and transversus abdominis aponeurosis and fascia. The iliopubic tract is located posterior to the inguinal ligament and crosses over the femoral vessels and inserts on the anterior superior iliac spine and inner lip of the wing of the ilium.

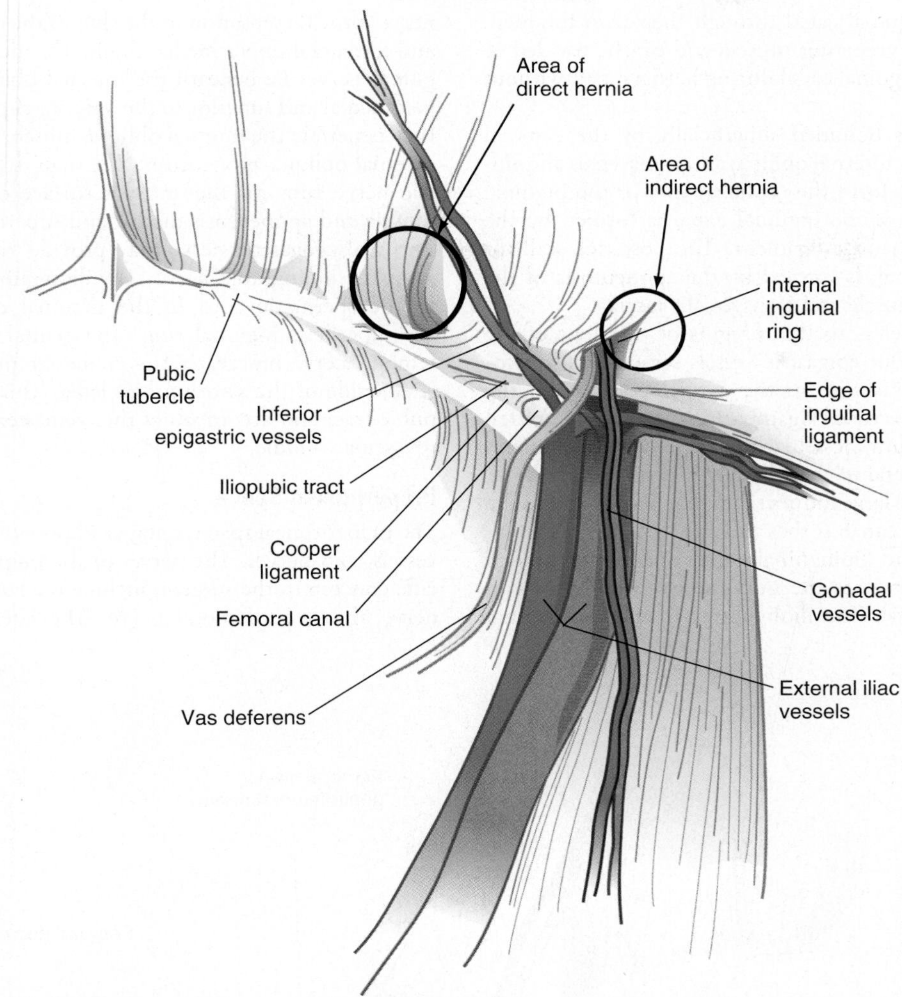

FIGURE 44-3 Anatomy of the important preperitoneal structures in the right inguinal space. (From Talamini MA, Are C: Laparoscopic hernia repair. In Zuidema GD, Yeo CJ, editors: *Shackelford's surgery of the alimentary tract*, ed 5, vol 5, Philadelphia, 2002, WB Saunders, p 140.)

The inferior crus of the deep inguinal ring is composed of the iliopubic tract; the superior crus of the deep ring is formed by the transversus abdominis aponeurotic arch. The lateral border of the internal ring is connected to the transversus abdominis muscle, which forms a shutter mechanism to limit the development of an indirect hernia.

The iliopubic tract is an extremely important structure in the repair of hernias from the anterior and posterior approaches. It composes the inferior margin of most anterior repairs. The portion of the iliopubic tract lateral to the internal inguinal ring serves as the inferior border below which staples or tacks are not placed during a laparoscopic repair because the femoral, lateral femoral cutaneous, and genitofemoral nerves are located inferior to the iliopubic tract. Although it cannot always be visualized during posterior repairs, if the tacking device cannot be palpated on the anterior abdominal wall, one must assume it is below the iliopubic tract.

Pectineal (Cooper) Ligament

The pectineal (Cooper) ligament is formed by the periosteum and aponeurotic tissues along the superior ramus of the pubis. This structure is posterior to the iliopubic tract and forms the posterior border of the femoral canal. In approximately 75% of patients, there will be a vessel that crosses the lateral border of Cooper ligament that is a branch of the obturator artery. If this vessel is injured, troublesome bleeding can result. Cooper ligament is an important landmark for open and laparoscopic repairs and is a useful anchoring structure, particularly in laparoscopic repairs.

Inguinal Canal

The inguinal canal is about 4 cm in length and is located just cephalad to the inguinal ligament. The canal extends between the internal (deep) inguinal and external (superficial) inguinal rings. The inguinal canal contains the spermatic cord in men and the round ligament of the uterus in women.

The spermatic cord is composed of the cremaster muscle fibers, testicular artery and accompanying veins, genital branch of the genitofemoral nerve, vas deferens, cremasteric vessels, lymphatics, and processus vaginalis. These structures enter the cord at the internal inguinal ring, and vessels and vas deferens exit the external inguinal ring. The cremaster muscle arises from the lowermost fibers of the internal oblique muscle and encompasses the spermatic cord in the inguinal canal. The cremasteric vessels are branches of the inferior epigastric vessels and pass through the posterior wall of the inguinal canal through their own foramen. These vessels supply the cremaster muscle and can be divided to expose the floor of the inguinal canal during hernia repair without damaging the testis.

The inguinal canal is bounded superficially by the external oblique aponeurosis. The internal oblique and transversus abdominis musculoaponeuroses form the cephalad wall of the inguinal canal. The inferior wall of the inguinal canal is formed by the inguinal ligament and lacunar ligament. The posterior wall, or floor of the inguinal canal, is formed by the aponeurosis of the transversus abdominis muscle and transversalis fascia.

Hesselbach triangle refers to the margins of the floor of the inguinal canal. The inferior epigastric vessels serve as its superolateral border, the rectus sheath as the medial border, and the inguinal ligament and pectineal ligament as the inferior border. Direct hernias occur within Hesselbach triangle, whereas indirect inguinal hernias arise lateral to the triangle. It is not uncommon, however, for medium and large indirect inguinal hernias to involve the floor of the inguinal canal as they enlarge.

The iliohypogastric and ilioinguinal nerves and genital branch of the genitofemoral nerve are the important sensory nerves in the groin area (Fig. 44-4). The iliohypogastric and ilioinguinal nerves provide sensation to the skin of the groin, base of the penis, and ipsilateral upper medial thigh. The iliohypogastric and ilioinguinal nerves lie beneath the internal oblique muscle to a point just medial and superior to the anterior superior iliac spine, where they penetrate the internal oblique muscle and course beneath the external oblique aponeurosis. The main trunk of the iliohypogastric nerve runs on the anterior surface of the internal oblique muscle and aponeurosis medial and superior to the internal ring. The iliohypogastric nerve may provide an inguinal branch that joins the ilioinguinal nerve. The ilioinguinal nerve runs anterior to the spermatic cord in the inguinal canal and branches at the superficial inguinal ring. The genital branch of the genitofemoral nerve innervates the cremaster muscle and skin on the lateral side of the scrotum and labia. This nerve lies on the iliopubic tract and accompanies the cremaster vessels to form a neurovascular bundle.

Preperitoneal Space

The preperitoneal space contains adipose tissue, lymphatics, blood vessels, and nerves. The nerves of the preperitoneal space of specific concern to the surgeon include the lateral femoral cutaneous nerve and genitofemoral nerve. The lateral femoral cutaneous

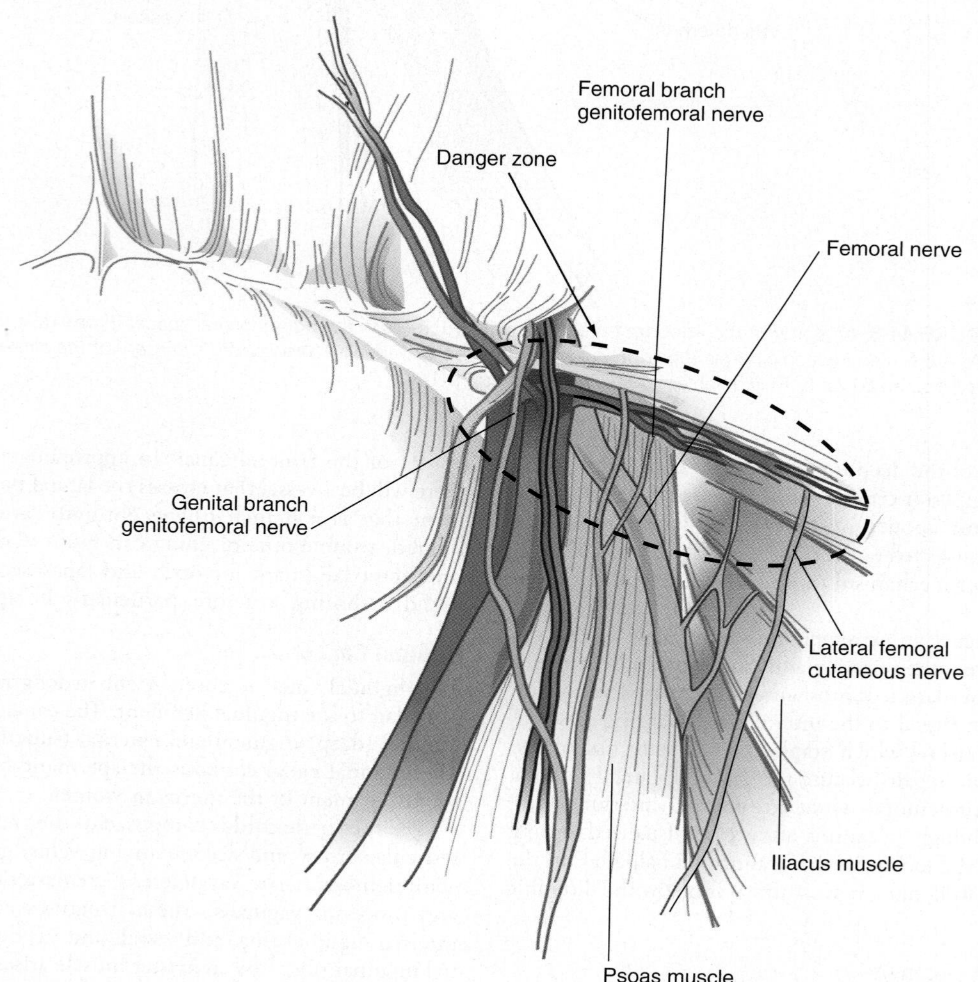

FIGURE 44-4 Important nerves and their relationship to inguinal structures (the right side is illustrated). (From Talamini MA, Are C: Laparoscopic hernia repair. In Zuidema GD, Yeo CJ, editors: *Shackelford's surgery of the alimentary tract*, ed 5, vol 5, Philadelphia, 2002, WB Saunders, p 140.)

nerve originates as a root of L2 and L3 and is occasionally a direct branch of the femoral nerve. This nerve courses along the anterior surface of the iliac muscle beneath the iliac fascia and passes under or through the lateral attachment of the inguinal ligament at the anterior superior iliac spine. This nerve runs beneath or occasionally through the iliopubic tract, lateral to the internal inguinal ring.

The genitofemoral nerve usually arises from the L2 or L1-L2 nerve roots. It divides into genital and femoral branches on the anterior surface of the psoas muscle. The genital branch enters the inguinal canal through the deep ring, whereas the femoral branch enters the femoral sheath lateral to the artery.

The inferior epigastric artery and vein are branches of the external iliac vessels and are important landmarks for laparoscopic hernia repair. These vessels course medial to the internal inguinal ring and eventually lie beneath the rectus abdominis muscle, immediately superficial to the transversalis fascia. The inferior epigastric vessels serve to define the types of inguinal hernia. Indirect inguinal hernias occur lateral to the inferior epigastric vessels, whereas direct hernias occur medial to these vessels.

The deep circumflex iliac artery and vein are located below the lateral portion of the iliopubic tract in the preperitoneal space. These vessels are branches of the inferior epigastric or external iliac artery and vein. It is important to dissect only above the iliopubic tract during a laparoscopic hernia repair to avoid injury to these vessels.

The vas deferens courses through the preperitoneal space from caudad to cephalad and medial to lateral to join the spermatic cord at the deep inguinal ring.

Femoral Canal

The boundaries of the femoral canal are the iliopubic tract anteriorly, Cooper ligament posteriorly, and femoral vein laterally. The pubic tubercle forms the apex of the femoral canal triangle. This canal usually contains connective tissue and lymphatic tissue. A femoral hernia occurs through this space and is medial to the femoral vessels.

Diagnosis

A bulge in the inguinal region is the main diagnostic finding in most groin hernias. Most patients will have associated pain or vague discomfort in the region, but one third of patients will have no symptoms. Groin hernias are usually not extremely painful unless incarceration or strangulation has occurred. In the absence of physical findings, alternative causes for pain need to be considered. On occasion, patients may experience paresthesias related to compression or irritation of the inguinal nerves by the hernia. Masses other than hernias can occur in the groin region. Physical examination alone often differentiates between a groin hernia and these masses (Box 44-2).

The inguinal region is examined with the patient in the supine and standing positions. The examiner visually inspects and palpates the inguinal region, looking for asymmetry, bulges, or a mass. Having the patient cough or perform a Valsalva maneuver can facilitate identification of a hernia. The examiner places a fingertip over the inguinal canal and repeats the examination. Finally, a fingertip is placed into the external inguinal ring by invaginating the scrotum to detect a small hernia. A bulge moving lateral to medial in the inguinal canal suggests an indirect hernia. If a bulge progresses from deep to superficial through the inguinal floor, a direct hernia is suspected. This distinction is not critical because repair is approached the same way, regardless of the type of hernia. A bulge identified below the inguinal ligament is consistent with a femoral hernia.

BOX 44-2 Differential Diagnosis of Groin and Scrotal Masses

Inguinal hernia
Hydrocele
Varicocele
Ectopic testis
Epididymitis
Testicular torsion
Lipoma
Hematoma
Sebaceous cyst
Hidradenitis of inguinal apocrine glands
Inguinal lymphadenopathy
Lymphoma
Metastatic neoplasm
Femoral hernia
Femoral lymphadenopathy
Femoral artery aneurysm or pseudoaneurysm

A bulge of the groin described by the patient that is not demonstrated on examination presents a dilemma. Having the patient stand or ambulate for a time may allow an undiagnosed hernia to become visible or palpable. If a hernia is strongly suspected but undetectable, repeated examination at another time may be helpful.

Ultrasonography also can aid in the diagnosis. There is a high degree of sensitivity and specificity for ultrasound in the detection of occult direct, indirect, and femoral hernias.[1] Other imaging modalities are less useful. Computed tomography (CT) of the abdomen and pelvis may be useful for the diagnosis of obscure and unusual hernias as well as atypical groin masses.[2] On occasion, laparoscopy can be diagnostic and therapeutic for particularly challenging cases.

Classification

There are numerous classification systems for groin hernias. One simple and widely used system is the Nyhus classification (Box 44-3). Although their purpose is to promote a common language and understanding for communication of physicians and to allow appropriate comparisons of therapeutic options, these classifications are incomplete and contentious. Most surgeons continue to describe hernias by their type, location, and volume of the hernia sac.

Treatment

Nonoperative Management

Most surgeons recommend operation on discovery of a symptomatic inguinal hernia because the natural history of a groin hernia is that of progressive enlargement and weakening, with a small potential for incarceration and strangulation. However, in patients with minimal symptoms, the clinician is often faced with balancing the risk for hernia-related complications, such as incarceration and bowel strangulation, with the potential for complications in the short and long term. Fitzgibbons and colleagues[3] reported a prospective randomized trial of a watchful waiting strategy for men with asymptomatic or minimally symptomatic inguinal hernias. These investigators randomized more than 700 men to a watchful waiting or open tension-free hernia repair. At 2 years of

BOX 44-3 Nyhus Classification of Groin Hernia

Type I
Indirect inguinal hernia: internal inguinal ring normal (e.g., pediatric hernia)

Type II
Indirect inguinal hernia: internal inguinal ring dilated but posterior inguinal wall intact; inferior deep epigastric vessels not displaced

Type III
Posterior wall defect
- A. Direct inguinal hernia
- B. Indirect inguinal hernia: internal inguinal ring dilated, medially encroaching on or destroying the transversalis fascia of Hesselbach triangle (e.g., scrotal, sliding, or pantaloon hernia)
- C. Femoral hernia

Type IV
Recurrent hernia
- A. Direct
- B. Indirect
- C. Femoral
- D. Combined

follow-up, there were no deaths attributed to the study, and the risk for hernia incarceration in the watchful waiting group was extremely low, 0.3% of study participants or 1.8 events/1000 patient-years. Almost 25% of patients assigned to watchful waiting crossed over to the surgical group, usually for pain related to the hernia that limited activity. In a later report, the crossover rate had increased to 68% at 10 years, with nearly 80% of men older than 65 years having an operation.[4] Patients who later had surgery did not have increased surgical site infections or higher recurrence rates than those who were initially assigned to early repair. A prospective randomized trial at a single institution in Great Britain had similar long-term results.[5] These studies provide conclusive evidence that a strategy of watchful waiting is safe for older patients with asymptomatic or minimally symptomatic inguinal hernias and that even though most patients eventually undergo repair, when they do, the operative risks and complication rates are no different from those of patients undergoing immediate repair. Watchful waiting can be a cost-effective management strategy for selected patients with no or minimal symptoms or who have suboptimal risk for operation. These results should not be applied to women, as women have not been included in these studies, or to patients with femoral hernias, which have a greater risk of strangulation than inguinal hernias.

Patients electing nonoperative management can occasionally have symptomatic improvement with the use of a truss. This approach is more commonly used in Europe. Spring trusses are more versatile than elastic ones, although most information on their use has been anecdotal. Correct measurement and fitting are important. Symptom control has been reported in about 30% of patients. Complications associated with the use of a truss include testicular atrophy, ilioinguinal or femoral neuritis, and hernia incarceration.

It is generally agreed that nonoperative management is not used for femoral hernias because of the high incidence of associated complications, particularly strangulation.

Operative Repair

Anterior repairs. Anterior repairs are the most common operative approach for inguinal hernias. Tension-free repairs are now standard, and there are a variety of different types. Older tissue types of repair are rarely indicated, except for patients with simultaneous contamination or concomitant bowel resection, when placement of a mesh prosthesis may be contraindicated.

There are some technical aspects of the operation common to all anterior repairs. Open hernia repair is begun by making a transversely oriented linear or slightly curvilinear incision above the inguinal ligament and a fingerbreadth below the internal inguinal ring. The internal inguinal ring is located topographically at the midpoint between the anterior superior iliac spine and ipsilateral pubic tubercle. Dissection is continued through the subcutaneous tissues and Scarpa fascia. The external oblique fascia and external inguinal ring are identified. The external oblique fascia is incised through the superficial inguinal ring to expose the inguinal canal. The genital branch of the genitofemoral nerve and the ilioinguinal and iliohypogastric nerves are identified and avoided or mobilized to prevent transection and entrapment. The spermatic cord is mobilized at the pubic tubercle by a combination of blunt and sharp dissection. Improper mobilization of the spermatic cord too lateral to the pubic tubercle can cause confusion in the identification of tissue planes and essential structures and may result in injury to the spermatic cord structures or disruption of the floor of the inguinal canal.

The cremaster muscle of the mobilized spermatic cord is separated parallel to its fibers from the underlying cord structures. The cremaster artery and vein, which join the cremaster muscle near the inguinal ring, can usually be avoided but may need to be cauterized or ligated and divided. When an indirect hernia is present, the hernia sac is located deep to the cremaster muscle and anterior and superior to the spermatic cord structures. Incising the cremaster muscle in a longitudinal direction and dividing it circumferentially near the internal inguinal ring help expose the indirect hernia sac. The hernia sac is carefully separated from adjacent cord structures and dissected to the level of the internal inguinal ring. The sac is opened and examined for visceral contents if it is large; however, this step is unnecessary in small hernias. The sac can be mobilized and placed within the preperitoneal space, or the neck of the sac can be ligated at the level of the internal ring and any excess sac excised. If a large hernia sac is present, it can be divided with use of electrocautery to facilitate ligation. It is not necessary to excise the distal portion of the sac. If the sac is broad based, it may be easier to displace it into the peritoneal cavity rather than to ligate it. Direct hernia sacs protrude through the floor of the inguinal canal and can be reduced below the transversalis fascia before repair. A "lipoma" of the cord actually represents retroperitoneal fat that has herniated through the deep inguinal ring; this should be suture ligated and removed.

A sliding hernia presents a special challenge in handling the hernia sac. With a sliding hernia, a portion of the sac is composed of visceral peritoneum covering part of a retroperitoneal organ, usually the colon or bladder. In this situation, the grossly redundant portion of the sac (if present) is excised and the peritoneum reclosed. The organ and sac then can be reduced below the transversalis fascia, similar to the procedure for a direct hernia.

Tissue repairs. Although tissue repairs have largely been abandoned because of unacceptably high recurrence rates, they remain useful in certain situations. In strangulated hernias, for which bowel resection is necessary, mesh prostheses are contraindicated and a tissue repair is necessary. Available options for tissue repair include iliopubic tract, Shouldice, Bassini, and McVay repairs.

The iliopubic tract repair approximates the transversus abdominis aponeurotic arch to the iliopubic tract with the use of interrupted sutures (Fig. 44-5). The repair begins at the pubic tubercle and extends laterally past the internal inguinal ring. This repair was initially described using a relaxing incision (see later); however, many surgeons who use this repair do not perform a relaxing incision.

The Shouldice repair emphasizes a multilayer imbricated repair of the posterior wall of the inguinal canal with a continuous running suture technique. After completion of the dissection, the posterior wall of the inguinal canal is reconstructed by superimposing running suture lines progressing from deep to more superficial layers. The initial suture line secures the transversus abdominis aponeurotic arch to the iliopubic tract. Next, the internal oblique and transversus abdominis muscles and aponeuroses are sutured to the inguinal ligament. The Shouldice repair is associated with a very low recurrence rate and a high degree of patient satisfaction in highly selected patients.

The Bassini repair is performed by suturing the transversus abdominis and internal oblique musculoaponeurotic arches or conjoined tendon (when present) to the inguinal ligament. This once popular technique is the basic approach to nonanatomic hernia repairs and was the most popular type of repair done before the advent of tension-free repairs.

Cooper ligament repair, also known as the McVay repair, has traditionally been popular for the correction of direct inguinal hernias, large indirect hernias, recurrent hernias, and femoral hernias. Interrupted nonabsorbable sutures are used to approximate the edge of the transversus abdominis aponeurosis to Cooper ligament. When the medial aspect of the femoral canal is reached, a transition suture is placed to incorporate Cooper ligament and the iliopubic tract. Lateral to this transition stitch, the transversus

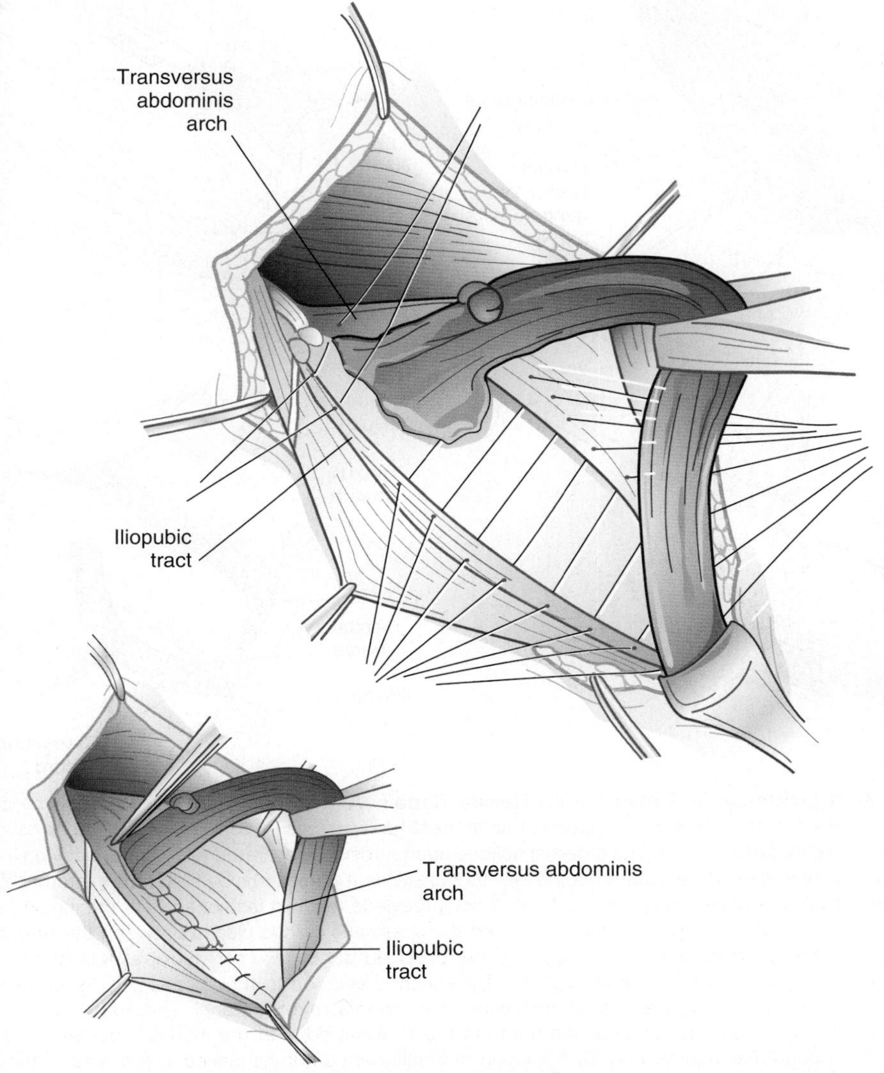

FIGURE 44-5 Iliopubic Tract Repair. *Top,* Sutures lateral to the cord complete reconstruction of the deep inguinal ring. These sutures encompass the transversus abdominis arch above and the cremaster origin and iliopubic tract below. *Bottom,* The complete repair is ready for wound closure. The reconstruction of the deep ring should be snug but also loose enough to admit the tip of a hemostat. (From Condon RE: Anterior iliopubic tract repair. In Nyhus LM, Condon RE, editors: *Hernia,* ed 2, Philadelphia, 1974, JB Lippincott, p 204.)

abdominis aponeurosis is secured to the iliopubic tract. An important principle of this repair is the need for a relaxing incision. This incision is made by reflecting the external oblique aponeurosis cephalad and medial to expose the anterior rectus sheath. An incision is then made in a curvilinear direction, beginning 1 cm above the pubic tubercle throughout the extent of the anterior sheath to near its lateral border. This relieves tension on the suture line and results in decreased postoperative pain and hernia recurrence. The fascial defect is covered by the body of the rectus muscle, which prevents herniation at the relaxing incision site. The McVay repair is particularly suited for strangulated femoral hernias because it provides obliteration of the femoral space without the use of mesh.

Tension-free anterior inguinal hernia repair. The tension-free repair has become the dominant method of inguinal hernia repair (Fig. 44-6). Recognizing that tension in a repair is the principal cause of recurrence, current practices in hernia management use a synthetic mesh prosthesis to bridge the defect, a concept popularized by Lichtenstein. There are several options for placement of mesh during anterior inguinal herniorrhaphy, including the Lichtenstein approach, plug and patch technique, and sandwich technique, with both an anterior and preperitoneal piece of mesh.

In the Lichtenstein repair,[6] a piece of prosthetic nonabsorbable mesh is fashioned to fit the canal. A slit is cut into the distal lateral edge of the mesh to accommodate the spermatic cord. There are

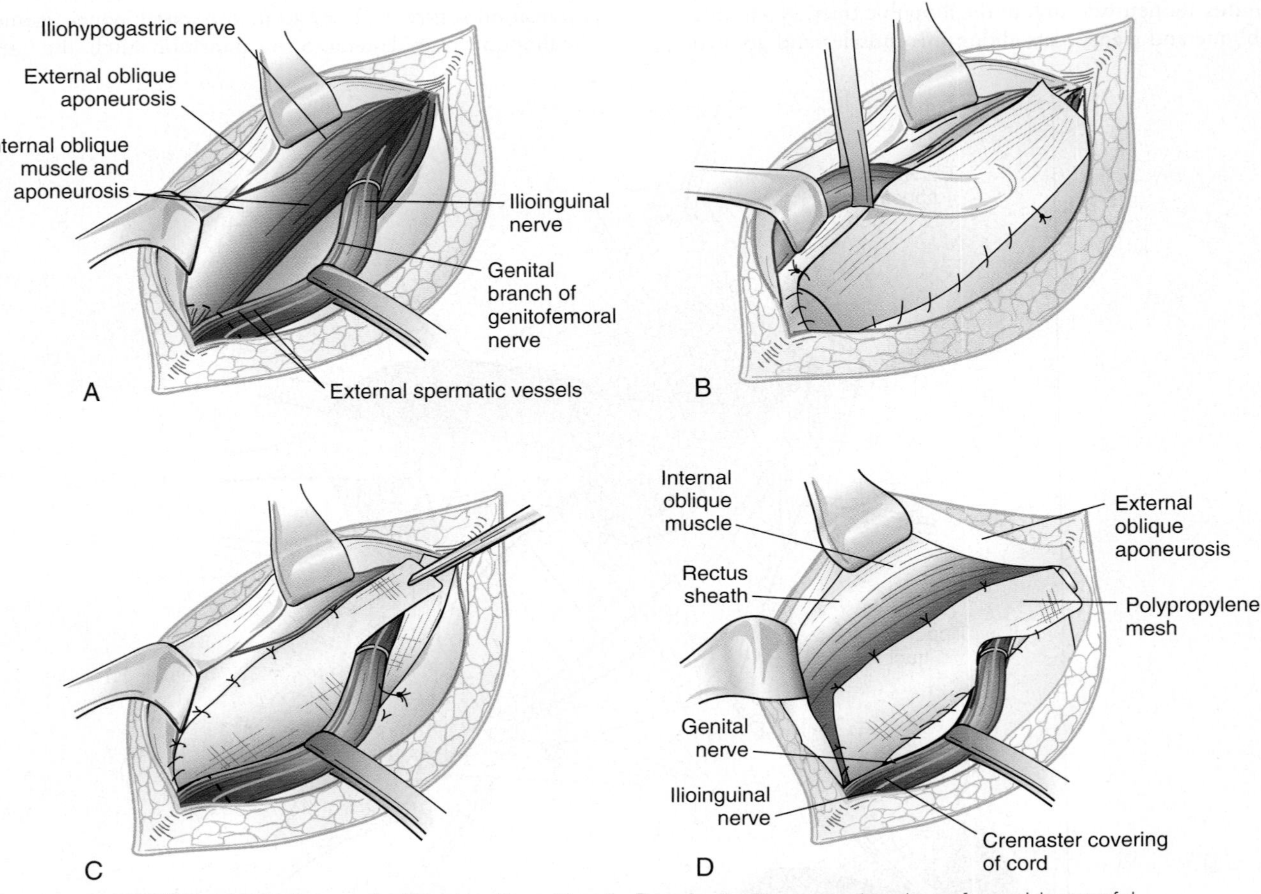

FIGURE 44-6 Lichtenstein Tension-Free Hernia Repair. A, This procedure is performed by careful dissection of the inguinal canal. High ligation of an indirect hernia sac is performed, and the spermatic cord structures are retracted inferiorly. The external oblique aponeurosis is separated from the underlying internal oblique muscle high enough to accommodate a 6- to 8-cm-wide mesh patch. Overlap of the internal oblique muscle edge by 2 to 3 cm is necessary. A sheet of polypropylene mesh is fashioned to fit the inguinal canal. A slit is made in the lateral aspect of the mesh, and the spermatic cord is placed between the two tails of the mesh. **B,** The spermatic cord is retracted in the cephalad direction. The medial aspect of the mesh overlaps the pubic bone by approximately 2 cm. The mesh is secured to the aponeurotic tissue overlying the pubic tubercle by a running suture of nonabsorbable monofilament material. The suture is continued laterally by suturing the inferior edge of the mesh to the shelving edge of the inguinal ligament to a point just lateral to the internal inguinal ring. **C,** A second monofilament suture is placed at the level of the pubic tubercle and continued laterally by suturing the mesh to the internal oblique aponeurosis or muscle approximately 2 cm from the aponeurotic edge. **D,** The lower edges of the two tails are sutured to the shelving edge of the inguinal ligament to create a new internal ring made of mesh. The spermatic cord structures are placed within the inguinal canal overlying the mesh. The external oblique aponeurosis is closed over the spermatic cord. (From Arregui ME, Nagan RD, editors: *Inguinal hernia: Advances or controversies?* Oxford, England, 1994, Radcliffe Medical.)

various preformed, commercially available prostheses available for use. Monofilament nonabsorbable suture is used to secure the mesh, beginning at the pubic tubercle and running a length of suture in both directions toward the superior aspect above the internal inguinal ring to the level of the tails of the mesh. The mesh is sutured to the aponeurotic tissue overlying the pubic tubercle medially, continuing superiorly along the transversus abdominis or conjoined tendon. The inferolateral edge of the mesh is sutured to the iliopubic tract or shelving edge of the inguinal ligament to a point lateral to the internal inguinal ring. At this point, the tails created by the slit are sutured together around the spermatic cord, snugly forming a new internal inguinal ring. It is important to protect the ilioinguinal nerve and genital branch of the genitofemoral nerve from entrapment by placing them with the cord structures as they are passed through this newly fashioned internal inguinal ring or avoiding their enclosure in the repair.

Adapting the principles of tension-free repair, Gilbert[7] has reported using a cone-shaped plug of polypropylene mesh that when inserted into the internal inguinal ring would deploy like an upside-down umbrella and occlude the hernia. This plug is sewn to the surrounding tissues and held in place by an additional overlying mesh patch. This patch may not need to be secured by sutures; however, to do so requires dissection to create a sufficient space between the external and internal oblique muscles for the patch to lie flat over the inguinal canal. This so-called plug and patch repair, an extension of Lichtenstein's original mesh repair, has now become the most commonly performed primary anterior inguinal hernia repair. Although this repair can be done without suture fixation by some experienced surgeons, most secure plug and patch with several monofilament nonabsorbable sutures, especially for very weak inguinal floors or large defects.

The sandwich technique involves a bilayered device, with three polypropylene components. An underlay patch provides a posterior repair similar to that of the laparoscopic approach, a connector functions similar to a plug, and an onlay patch covers the posterior inguinal floor. The use of interrupted fixating sutures is not mandatory, but most surgeons place three or four fixation sutures in this repair.

Another option for a tension-free mesh repair involves a preperitoneal approach using a self-expanding polypropylene patch.[8] A pocket is created in the preperitoneal space by blunt dissection, and then a preformed mesh patch is inserted into the hernia defect, which expands to cover the direct, indirect, and femoral spaces. The patch lies parallel to the inguinal ligament. It can remain without suture fixation, or a tacking suture can be placed.

The Stoppa-Rives repair uses a subumbilical midline incision to place a large mesh prosthesis into the preperitoneal space.[9] Blunt dissection is used to create an extraperitoneal space that extends into the prevesical space, beyond the obturator foramen, and posterolateral to the pelvic brim. This technique has the advantage of distributing the natural intra-abdominal pressure across a broad area to retain the mesh in a proper location. The Stoppa-Rives technique is particularly useful for large, recurrent, or bilateral hernias.

Preperitoneal repair. The open preperitoneal approach is useful for the repair of recurrent inguinal hernias, sliding hernias, femoral hernias, and some strangulated hernias.[10] A transverse skin incision is made 2 cm above the internal inguinal ring and is directed to the medial border of the rectus sheath. The muscles of the anterior abdominal wall are incised transversely, and the preperitoneal space is identified. If further exposure is needed, the anterior rectus sheath can be incised and the rectus muscle retracted medially. The preperitoneal tissues are retracted cephalad to visualize the posterior inguinal wall and the site of herniation. The inferior epigastric artery and veins are generally beneath the midportion of the posterior rectus sheath and usually do not need to be divided. This approach avoids mobilization of the spermatic cord and injury to the sensory nerves of the inguinal canal, which is particularly important for hernias previously repaired through an anterior approach. If the peritoneum is incised, it is sutured closed to avoid the evisceration of intraperitoneal contents into the operative field. The transversalis fascia and transversus abdominis aponeurosis are identified and sutured to the iliopubic tract with permanent sutures. Femoral hernias repaired by this approach require closure of the femoral canal by securing the repair to Cooper ligament. A mesh prosthesis is frequently used to obliterate the defect in the femoral canal, particularly with large hernias.

Laparoscopic repair. Laparoscopic inguinal hernia repair is another method of tension-free mesh repair based on a preperitoneal approach. The laparoscopic approach provides the mechanical advantage of placing a large piece of mesh behind the defect, covering the myopectineal orifice, and using the natural forces of the abdominal wall to disperse intra-abdominal pressure over a larger area to support the mesh in place. Proponents have touted quicker recovery, less pain, better visualization of anatomy, and usefulness for fixing all inguinal hernia defects. Critics have emphasized longer operative times, technical challenges, increased risk of recurrence, and increased cost. Laparoscopic repair is also associated with an approximately 0.3% risk of visceral or vascular injury.[11] Although controversy exists about the usefulness of laparoscopic repair for primary unilateral inguinal hernias, most agree that this approach has advantages for patients having bilateral or recurrent hernia repairs.[12] Adopting practice guidelines for the performance of laparoscopic hernia repairs could help control costs.

When considering the laparoscopic approach for repair of inguinal hernias, the surgeon has several options. The most popular techniques are totally extraperitoneal (TEP) and transabdominal preperitoneal (TAPP) approaches. The main difference between these two techniques is the sequence of gaining access to the preperitoneal space. In the TEP approach, the dissection begins in the preperitoneal space using a balloon dissector. With the TAPP repair, the preperitoneal space is accessed after initially entering the peritoneal cavity. Each approach has its merits. With the TEP approach, the preperitoneal dissection is quicker, and the potential risk for intraperitoneal visceral damage is minimized. However, the use of dissection balloons is costly, the working space is more limited, and it may not be possible to create a working space if the patient has had a prior preperitoneal operation. Also, if a large tear in the peritoneum is created during a TEP approach, the potential working space can become obliterated, necessitating conversion to a TAPP approach. For these reasons, knowledge of the transabdominal technique is essential in performing laparoscopic inguinal hernia repairs. The transabdominal approach allows identification of the groin anatomy before extensive dissection and disruption of natural tissue planes. The larger working space of the peritoneal cavity can make early experience with the laparoscopic approach easier.

There are no absolute contraindications to laparoscopic inguinal hernia repair other than the patient's inability to tolerate general anesthesia. Patients who have had extensive prior lower abdominal surgery can require significant adhesiolysis and may be best approached anteriorly. In particular, in patients who have had a radical retropubic prostatectomy with the preperitoneal space previously dissected, accurate and safe dissection can be challenging.

In the TEP approach, an infraumbilical incision is used. The anterior rectus sheath is incised, the ipsilateral rectus abdominis muscle is retracted laterally, and blunt dissection is used to create a space beneath the rectus. A dissecting balloon is inserted deep to the posterior rectus sheath, advanced to the pubic symphysis, and inflated under direct laparoscopic vision (Fig. 44-7). After it is opened, the space is insufflated, and additional trocars are placed. A 30-degree laparoscope provides the best visualization of the inguinal region (see Fig. 44-3). The inferior epigastric vessels are identified along the lower portion of the rectus muscle and serve as a useful landmark. Cooper ligament must be cleared from the pubic symphysis medially to the level of the external iliac vein. The iliopubic tract is also identified. Care must be taken to avoid injury to the femoral branch of the genitofemoral nerve and lateral femoral cutaneous nerve, which are located lateral to and below the iliopubic tract (see Fig. 44-4). Lateral dissection is carried out to the anterior superior iliac spine. Finally, the spermatic cord is skeletonized.

In the TAPP approach, an infraumbilical incision is used to gain access to the peritoneal cavity directly. Two 5-mm ports are placed lateral to the inferior epigastric vessels at the level of the umbilicus. A peritoneal flap is created high on the anterior abdominal wall, extending from the median umbilical fold to the anterior superior iliac spine. The remainder of the operation proceeds similar to a TEP procedure.

A direct hernia sac and associated preperitoneal fat are gently reduced by traction if not already reduced by balloon expansion of the peritoneal space. A small, indirect hernia sac is mobilized from the cord structures and reduced into the peritoneal cavity. A large sac may be difficult to reduce. In this case, the sac is divided with cautery near the internal inguinal ring, leaving the distal sac in situ. The proximal peritoneal sac is closed with a loop ligature to prevent pneumoperitoneum from occurring. After all hernias are reduced, a 12 × 14-cm piece of polypropylene mesh is inserted through a trocar and unfolded. It covers the direct, indirect, and femoral spaces and rests over the cord structures. It is imperative that the peritoneum be dissected at least 4 cm off

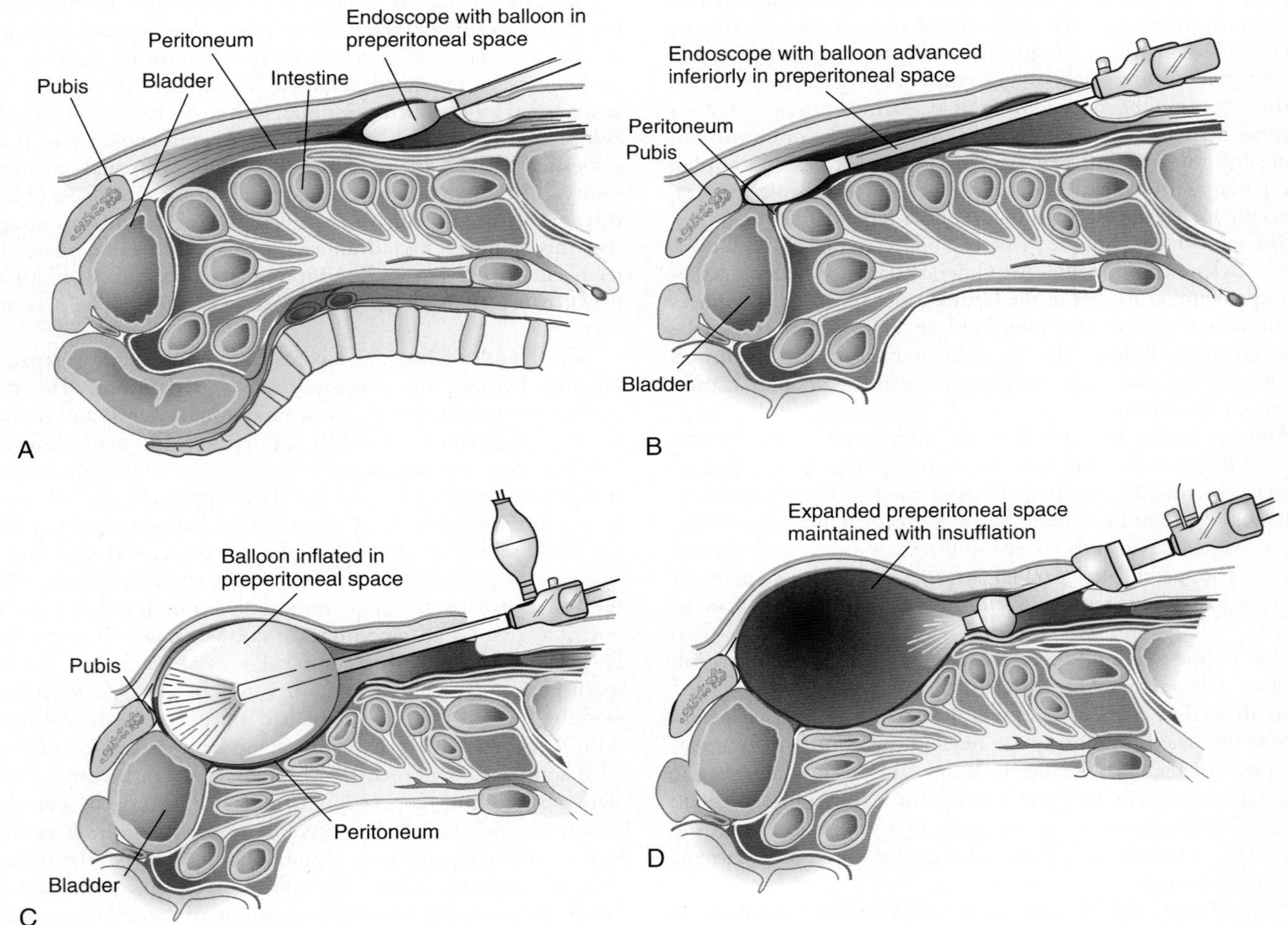

FIGURE 44-7 TEP Laparoscopic Hernia Repair. A, Access to the posterior rectus sheath is gained in the periumbilical region. A balloon dissector is placed on the anterior surface of the posterior rectus sheath. **B,** The balloon dissector is advanced to the posterior surface of the pubis in the preperitoneal space. **C,** The balloon is inflated, thereby creating an optical cavity. **D,** The optical cavity is insufflated by carbon dioxide, and the posterior surface of the inguinal floor is dissected.

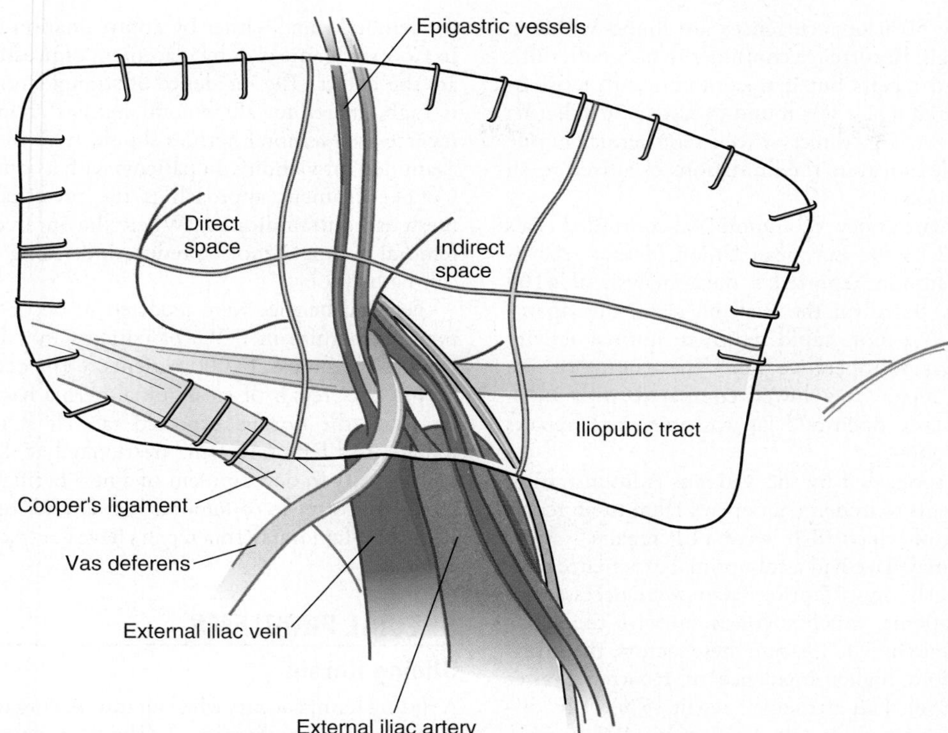

FIGURE 44-8 Prosthetic mesh placement for TEP hernia repair. (From Corbitt J: Laparoscopic transabdominal transperitoneal patch hernia repair. In Ballantyne GH, editor: *Atlas of laparoscopic surgery,* Philadelphia, 2000, WB Saunders, p 511.)

the cord structures to prevent the peritoneum from encroaching beneath the mesh, which can lead to recurrence. The mesh is carefully secured with a tacking stapler to Cooper ligament from the pubic tubercle to the external iliac vein, anteriorly to the posterior rectus musculature and transversus abdominis aponeurotic arch at least 2 cm above the hernia defect, and laterally to the iliopubic tract. The mesh extends beyond the pubic symphysis and below the spermatic cord and peritoneum (Fig. 44-8). The mesh is not fixed in this area and tacks are not placed inferior to the iliopubic tract beyond the external iliac artery. Staples placed in this area may injure the femoral branch of the genitofemoral nerve or lateral femoral cutaneous nerve. Staples are also avoided in the so-called triangle of doom, bounded by the ductus deferens medially and spermatic vessels laterally, to avoid injury to the external iliac vessels and femoral nerve. As long as one can palpate the tip of the tacking device, these structures are not likely to be injured.

Results of Hernia Repair

The true measure of success for the various types of hernia repair is based on the results. The best information on the results of hernia repair is available from large prospective randomized trials, meta-analyses of clinical trials, and two large national registries, the Danish Hernia Database and the Swedish Hernia Register. The Danish Hernia Database includes more than 98% of inguinal hernia repairs; the capture rate of the Swedish Hernia Register is approximately 80%.[13,14] In spite of the randomized nature of some trials, caution must be used in interpreting the results. Many of these patients were highly selected, and most trials excluded recurrent hernias, obese individuals, and large inguinal hernias. Also, some follow-up results were completed by telephone interviews and not by physical examination. The national registries collect information only on operations, so the incidence of recurrence is lower than if all patients had been interviewed and examined.

The mortality of all types of repair is low, and there are no significant differences reported among the various techniques. There is a greater mortality associated with the repair of strangulated hernias. Otherwise, the risk of death is related to individual comorbid conditions and should be evaluated in each patient. The type of anesthetic does not affect the recurrence rate.[14] Open repairs can be performed under local anesthesia, which can be an advantage in operating on high-risk patients.

There are important differences in the results of primary hernia repair. Hernia recurrence is the primary outcome assessed by most studies. Large series, including multiple types of repairs, have suggested that recurrence ranges from 1.7% to 10%.[13-15]

The results of tissue repairs were often based on reports consisting of personal or single institutional series that were not prospective or randomized and had erratic follow-up periods. Not surprisingly, recurrence was variable.

Tension-free repairs have a lower rate of recurrence than tissue repairs.[14,16,17] Results from the Danish Hernia Database have demonstrated that hernia recurrence resulting in reoperation after the Lichtenstein repair is only 25% that of nonmesh repairs.[13] A Cochrane review reported that prosthetic mesh repairs have a 50% to 75% lower risk of hernia recurrence, a lower risk of chronic postherniorrhaphy groin pain, and an earlier return to work than open repairs.[16] The Shouldice repair has a higher recurrence rate than mesh repairs unless mesh is used.[17] A meta-analysis comparing the Lichtenstein, mesh plug, and bilayered repairs has reported no significant differences in the rate of recurrence, chronic groin pain, other complications, or time to return to work.[18] Approximately 50% of recurrences are found within 3 years after primary repair. Recurrence continues to occur after this time in nonmesh-based repairs but is uncommon with tension-free repairs. The bilayered repair was found to have a 20% hernia recurrence when used for large direct or recurrent hernias in one study.[19] These results demonstrate the limitations of a fixed mesh size in these circumstances.

An extensive systematic review of randomized controlled trials was published in 2002 by the European Union Hernia Trialists Collaboration.[20] The authors reported a meta-analysis of 4165 patients in 25 studies. Based on the available data, the laparoscopic repair resulted in a more rapid return to normal activity and decreased persistent postoperative pain. The recurrence rate for the laparoscopic repair was lower compared with open nonmesh repairs; however, open and laparoscopic mesh repairs had similar recurrence rates.

A prospective trial sponsored by the Veterans Administration randomized 1983 patients to undergo an open Lichtenstein repair or laparoscopic repair, of which 90% were TEP repairs.[15] Most surgeons in this study may have had a suboptimal experience with the laparoscopic approach; only 25 prior repairs were necessary to be eligible to enroll patients, which is consistent with the seemingly high conversion rate of 5%. Despite these factors, the investigators found a twofold higher incidence of recurrence after laparoscopic repair (10%) than after open repair (5%). This difference in recurrence remained for primary hernias (10% laparoscopic versus 4% open); however, recurrent hernias repaired by the laparoscopic approach tended to have fewer re-recurrences (10% versus 14%). In another study by this group, surgeon inexperience with laparoscopy and surgeon age older than 45 years were both predictors of recurrence after laparoscopic repair.[18] A large cohort study and a recent meta-analysis have found a significantly higher risk of recurrence after laparoscopic repair that is nearly twice that of open repairs (4.1% versus 2.1%).[21,22] What can be concluded from these results? These results demonstrate that the laparoscopic repair of inguinal hernias has a definite learning curve to achieve an acceptably low recurrence rate.

In a Cochrane review of more than 1000 patients in eight nonrandomized trials, there was no difference in hernia recurrence between TAPP and TEP repairs.[23] TAPP procedures were associated with more port site hernias and vascular injuries, whereas the TEP approach had a greater conversion rate.

FEMORAL HERNIAS

A femoral hernia occurs through the femoral canal, which is bounded superiorly by the iliopubic tract, inferiorly by Cooper ligament, laterally by the femoral vein, and medially by the junction of the iliopubic tract and Cooper ligament (lacunar ligament). A femoral hernia produces a mass or bulge below the inguinal ligament. On occasion, some femoral hernias will present over the inguinal canal. In this case, the femoral hernia sac still exits inferior to the inguinal ligament through the femoral canal but ascends in a cephalad direction. Approximately 50% of men with a femoral hernia will have an associated direct inguinal hernia, whereas this relationship occurs in only 2% of women.

A femoral hernia can be repaired by the standard Cooper ligament repair, a preperitoneal approach, or a laparoscopic approach. The essential elements of femoral hernia repair include dissection and reduction of the hernia sac and obliteration of the defect in the femoral canal, either by approximation of the iliopubic tract to Cooper ligament or by placement of prosthetic mesh to obliterate the defect. The incidence of strangulation in femoral hernias is high; therefore, all femoral hernias should be repaired, and incarcerated femoral hernias should have the hernia sac contents examined for viability. In patients with a compromised bowel, the Cooper ligament approach is the preferred technique because mesh is contraindicated. When the incarcerated contents of a femoral hernia cannot be reduced, dividing the lacunar ligament can be helpful.

Femoral hernias were reported to occur in conjunction with inguinal hernias in 0.3% of patients in a large national hernia database of almost 35,000 patients.[24] The occurrence of a femoral hernia after repair of an inguinal hernia has been reported to be 15 times the normal expected rate. It is unclear whether this represents a femoral hernia overlooked at the prior operation or a propensity to development of a new hernia after inguinal hernia repair. Recurrence of femoral hernia after operation is only 2%. Recurrent femoral hernia repairs have a re-recurrence rate of about 10%.

SPECIAL PROBLEMS

Sliding Hernia

A sliding hernia occurs when an internal organ composes a portion of the wall of the hernia sac. The most common viscus involved is the colon or urinary bladder. Most sliding hernias are a variant of indirect inguinal hernias, although femoral and direct sliding hernias can occur. The primary danger associated with a sliding hernia is the failure to recognize the visceral component of the hernia sac before injury to the bowel or bladder. The sliding hernia contents are reduced into the peritoneal cavity, and any excess hernia sac is ligated and divided. After reduction of the hernia, one of the techniques described earlier can be used for repair of the inguinal hernia.

Recurrent Hernia

The repair of recurrent inguinal hernias is challenging, and results are associated with a higher incidence of secondary recurrence. Recurrent hernias almost always require placement of prosthetic mesh for successful repair. The exception is when infected mesh is associated with a recurrent hernia. Recurrences after anterior hernia repair using mesh are best managed by a laparoscopic or open posterior approach, with placement of a second prosthesis.

Strangulated Hernia

Repair of a suspected strangulated hernia is most easily done using a preperitoneal approach (see earlier). With this exposure, the hernia sac contents can be directly visualized and their viability assessed through a single incision. The constricting ring is identified and can be incised to reduce the entrapped viscus with minimal danger to the surrounding organs, blood vessels, and nerves. If it is necessary to resect strangulated intestine, the peritoneum can be opened and resection done without the need for a second incision.

Bilateral Hernias

The approach to repair of bilateral inguinal hernias is based on the extent of the hernia defect. Simultaneous repair of bilateral hernias has a similar recurrence rate to unilateral repair, regardless of whether the open or laparoscopic technique is used.[25] The use of a giant prosthetic reinforcement of the visceral sac (Stoppa repair)[9] or the laparoscopic repair is preferred for simultaneous repair of bilateral inguinal hernias.

Complications

There are myriad complications related to open and laparoscopic inguinal hernia repair (Table 44-1). Some are general complications that are related to underlying diseases and the effects of anesthesia. These vary by patient population and risk. In addition, there are technical complications that are directly related to the repair. Technical complications are affected by the experience of the surgeon and are more frequent during and after the repair of recurrent hernias. There is increased scarring and disturbed anatomy with hernia recurrence that can result in an inability to identify important structures at operation. This is the principal reason that we recommend using a different approach for recurrent hernias.

Although the overall complication rate from hernia repair has been estimated to be approximately 10%, many of these complications are transient and can be easily addressed. More serious complications from a large experience are listed in Table 44-1.

Surgical Site Infection

The risk for surgical site infection is estimated to be 1% to 2% after open inguinal hernia repair and slightly less with laparoscopic repairs. These are clean operations, and the risk for infection is primarily influenced by associated patient diseases. Most would agree that there is no need to use routine antimicrobial prophylaxis for hernia repair.[20] Prospective randomized clinical trials have not supported the routine use of perioperative antimicrobial prophylaxis for inguinal hernia repair for patients at low risk for infection.[26] Patients who have significant underlying disease, as reflected by an American Society of Anesthesiology score of 3 or more, receive perioperative antimicrobial prophylaxis

TABLE 44-1 Complications After Open and Laparoscopic Inguinal Hernia Repair (%)

COMPLICATION	OPEN REPAIR ($N = 994$)	LAPAROSCOPIC REPAIR ($N = 989$)
Intraoperative complications	1.9	4.8
Postoperative complications	19.4	24.6
Urinary retention	2.2	2.8
Urinary tract infection	0.4	1.0
Orchitis	1.1	1.4
Surgical site infection	1.4	1.0
Neuralgia, pain	3.6	4.2
Life-threatening complications	0.1	1.1
Long-term complications	17.4	18.0
Seroma	3.0	9.0
Orchitis	2.2	1.9
Infection	0.6	0.4
Chronic pain	14.3	9.8
Recurrence	4.9	10.1

From Neumayer L, Giobbie-Hurder A, Jonassen O, et al: Open mesh versus laparoscopic mesh repair of inguinal hernias. *N Engl J Med* 350:1819–1827, 2004.

with cefazolin, 1 to 2 g, given intravenously 30 to 60 minutes before the incision. Clindamycin, 600 mg intravenously, can be used for patients allergic to penicillin. Only a single dose of antibiotic is necessary. The placement of prosthetic mesh does not increase the risk for infection and does not affect the need for prophylaxis. Superficial surgical site infections are treated by opening the incision, local wound care, and healing by secondary intention. Some mesh infections will be manifested as a chronic draining sinus that tracks to the mesh or occur with extruded mesh. Deep surgical site infections usually involve the prosthetic mesh, which should be explanted.

The risk for infection can be decreased by using proper operative technique, preoperative antiseptic skin preparation, and appropriate hair removal. There is an increased risk for infection for patients who have had prior hernia incision infections, chronic skin infections, or infection at a distant site. These infections are treated before elective surgery.

Nerve Injuries and Chronic Pain Syndromes

Nerve injuries are an infrequent and underrecognized complication of inguinal hernia repair. Injury can occur from traction, electrocautery, transection, and entrapment. The use of prosthetic mesh can result in dysesthesias, which are usually temporary. The nerves most commonly affected during open hernia repair are the ilioinguinal, genital branch of the genitofemoral, and iliohypogastric nerves. During laparoscopic repair, the lateral femoral cutaneous and genitofemoral nerves are most often affected.[27] Rarely, the main trunk of the femoral nerve can be injured during open or laparoscopic inguinal hernia repair.

Transient neuralgias involving sensory nerves can occur and are usually self-limited and resolve within a few weeks after surgery. Persistent neuralgias usually result in pain and hyperesthesia in the area of distribution. Symptoms are often reproduced by palpation over the point of entrapment or hyperextension of the hip and may be relieved by flexion of the thigh. Transection of a sensory nerve usually results in an area of numbness corresponding to the distribution of the involved nerve.

With more attention to patient outcomes, chronic groin pain has replaced recurrence as the primary complication after open inguinal hernia repair. Approximately 10% of patients will have chronic postherniorrhaphy pain, defined as pain persisting more than 3 months after operation,[28] and pain has been reported to interfere with activities of daily living in 2% to 4%.[29] Strategies of routine nerve division in open surgery have not been associated with a reduction in chronic pain in mesh-based anterior repairs.[30] In contrast, routine ilioinguinal nerve division is associated with significantly more sensory disturbances. In laparoscopic repairs, by operating in a remote area to the commonly injured nerves and with judicious use of appropriately placed tacks, chronic groin pain intuitively is less common. Some reports comparing laparoscopic and open repairs have reported lower rates of chronic postoperative inguinal pain, but this observation remains controversial.

Various approaches to management of residual neuralgia have been described. Early symptoms are treated with anti-inflammatory agents, analgesics, and local anesthetic nerve blocks. Patients with nerve entrapment syndromes are best treated by repeated exploration with neurectomy and mesh removal through an anterior approach. Laparoscopic nerve injuries are minimized by not placing any tacks or staples below the lateral portion of the iliopubic tract. If nerve entrapment occurs, patients undergo reoperation to remove the offending tack or staple.

Ischemic Orchitis and Testicular Atrophy

Ischemic orchitis usually occurs from thrombosis of the small veins of the pampiniform plexus within the spermatic cord. This results in venous congestion of the testis, which becomes swollen and tender 2 to 5 days after surgery. The process may continue for an additional 6 to 12 weeks and usually results in testicular atrophy. Ischemic orchitis also can be caused by ligation of the testicular artery. It is treated with anti-inflammatory agents and analgesics. Orchiectomy is rarely necessary.

The incidence of ischemic orchitis can be minimized by avoiding unnecessary dissection within the spermatic cord. The incidence increases with dissection of the distal portion of a large hernia sac and in patients who have anterior operations for hernia recurrence or for spermatic cord disease. In these situations, the use of a posterior approach is preferred.

Testicular atrophy is a consequence of ischemic orchitis. It is more common after repair of recurrent hernias, particularly when an anterior approach is used. The incidence of ischemic orchitis increases by a factor of three or four with each subsequent hernia recurrence.

Injury to the Vas Deferens and Viscera

Injury to the vas deferens and intra-abdominal viscera is unusual. Most of these injuries occur in patients with sliding inguinal hernias when there is failure to recognize the presence of intra-abdominal viscera in the hernia sac. With large hernias, the vas deferens can be displaced in an enlarged inguinal ring before its entry into the spermatic cord. In this situation, the vas deferens is identified and protected.

Hernia Recurrence

Hernia recurrences are usually caused by technical factors, such as excessive tension on the repair, missed hernias, failure to include an adequate musculoaponeurotic margin in the repair, and improper mesh size and placement. Recurrence also can result from failure to close a patulous internal inguinal ring, the size of which is always assessed at the conclusion of the primary surgery. Other factors that can cause hernia recurrence are chronically elevated intra-abdominal pressure, a chronic cough, deep incisional infections, and poor collagen formation in the wound. Recurrences are more common in patients with direct hernias and usually involve the floor of the inguinal canal near the pubic tubercle, where suture line tension is greatest. The use of a relaxing incision when there is excessive tension at the time of primary hernia repair is helpful to reduce recurrence. A femoral hernia is found in approximately 5% to 10% of patients with an inguinal hernia recurrence and should always be investigated at surgery.[13]

Most recurrent hernias require the use of prosthetic mesh for successful repair.[30,31] Choosing a different approach (usually posterior) avoids dissection through scar tissue, improves visualization of the defect and reduction of the hernia, and decreases the incidence of complications, particularly ischemic orchitis and injury to the ilioinguinal nerve. Recurrences after initial prosthetic mesh repairs can be caused by displaced prostheses or the use of a prosthetic of inadequate size. Recurrences are best managed by placing a second prosthesis through a different approach.

A meta-analysis of 58 reports comparing synthetic mesh techniques with nonmesh repairs has demonstrated an almost 60% reduction in recurrence with the use of mesh.[20] This report concluded that there was no difference in the rate of hernia recurrence between laparoscopic and open approaches that used mesh. A recent meta-analysis of recurrent hernia repairs reported no difference between open and laparoscopic mesh repairs in re-recurrence or chronic groin pain.[32]

Recurrence is more common after repair of recurrent hernias and is directly related to the number of previous attempts at repair. Large population-based studies have reported a re-recurrence rate of 4% to 5% in the first 24 months, which increases to 7.5% at 5 years.[31,33] Tension-free and mesh-based repairs have the lowest rates of reoperation after recurrence and result in a reduction in recurrence of approximately 60% compared with more traditional repairs.[30]

There is a successive decrease in the time to hernia recurrence with each subsequent repair.[33] Re-recurrences are associated with increased operative times and a greater rate of complications.

Quality of Life

The major quality indicators that have been assessed for hernia repair are postoperative pain and return to work. Tension-free and laparoscopic mesh-based approaches have been demonstrated to be less painful than nonmesh repairs. Laparoscopic repairs have the least amount of postoperative pain and have been shown to provide a marginal advantage in reducing time off work.[12]

VENTRAL HERNIAS

A ventral hernia is defined by a protrusion through the anterior abdominal wall fascia. These defects can be categorized as spontaneous or acquired or by their location on the abdominal wall. Epigastric hernias occur from the xiphoid process to the umbilicus, umbilical hernias occur at the umbilicus, and hypogastric hernias are rare spontaneous hernias that occur below the umbilicus in the midline. Acquired hernias typically occur after surgical incisions and are therefore termed incisional hernias. Although not a true hernia, diastasis recti can present as a midline bulge. In this condition, the linea alba is stretched, resulting in bulging at the medial margins of the rectus muscles. Abdominal wall diastasis can occur at other sites in addition to the midline. There is no fascial ring or hernia sac, and unless it is significantly symptomatic, surgical correction is avoided.

Incidence

Based on national operative statistics, incisional hernias account for 15% to 20% of all abdominal wall hernias; umbilical and epigastric hernias constitute 10% of hernias. Incisional hernias are twice as common in women as in men. As a result of the almost 4 million laparotomies performed annually in the United States and the 2% to 30% incidence of incisional hernia, almost 150,000 ventral hernia repairs are performed each year. Several technical and patient-related factors have been linked to the occurrence of incisional hernias. There is no conclusive evidence demonstrating that the type of suture at the primary operation affects hernia formation.[34] Patient-related factors linked to ventral hernia formation include obesity, older age, male gender, sleep apnea, emphysema, and prostatism. It has been proposed that the same factors associated with destruction of the collagen in the lung result in poor wound healing, with increased hernia formation. Wound infection has been linked to hernia formation. Recent data suggest that the surgical technique used to close a midline laparotomy is highly associated with incisional hernia formation. The use of a suture to wound length ratio of 4 : 1 has been shown to significantly reduce incisional hernia formation compared with the 1-cm bites and 1-cm advancement suturing technique typically employed by most surgeons.[35]

Whether the type of initial abdominal incision influences the incisional hernia rate remains controversial. As noted, the incidence of ventral herniation after midline laparotomy ranges from 3% to 20% and doubles if the operation is associated with a surgical site infection. A meta-analysis of 11 studies examining the incidence of ventral hernia formation after various types of abdominal incisions has concluded that the risk is 10.5% for midline, 7.5% for transverse, and 2.5% for paramedian incisions.[36] A recently published prospective randomized trial has reported no difference in hernia formation in comparing midline versus transverse incisions after 1 year but noted a higher wound infection rate in the transverse incisions.[37] Given the likely similar rates of incisional hernia formation after transverse and midline incisions, the surgeon should plan the incision on the basis of the operative exposure desired to complete the procedure safely.

Few data are available about the natural history of untreated ventral hernias. As noted, asymptomatic or minimally symptomatic inguinal hernias purposely observed during 2 years have a low incidence of complications.[3] Whether this paradigm applies for asymptomatic ventral or incisional hernias is unclear. Because there is no prospective cohort available to determine the natural history of untreated ventral hernias, most surgeons recommend that these hernias be repaired when discovered.

Anatomy

The anatomy of the anterior abdominal wall is straightforward and considerably easier to grasp than the anatomy of the inguinal area. However, a clear understanding of the blood supply and innervation of the abdomen is important in performing advanced abdominal wall reconstruction. The lateral musculature is composed of three layers, with the fascicles of each directed obliquely at different angles to create a strong envelope for the abdominal contents. Each of these muscles forms an aponeurosis that inserts into the linea alba, a midline structure joining both sides of the abdominal wall. The external oblique is the most superficial muscle of the lateral abdominal wall. Deep to the external oblique lies the internal oblique muscle. The fibers of the external oblique course in an inferomedial direction (like hands in pockets), whereas those of the internal oblique muscle run deep to and opposite the external oblique. The deepest muscle layer of the abdominal wall is the transversus abdominis muscle. Its fibers course in a horizontal direction. These three lateral muscles give rise to aponeurotic layers lateral to the rectus, which contribute to the anterior and posterior layers of the rectus sheath.

The medial extension of the external oblique aponeurosis forms the anterior layer of the rectus sheath. At the midline, the two anterior rectus sheaths form the tendinous linea alba. On either side of the linea alba are the rectus abdominis muscles, whose fibers are directed longitudinally and run the length of the anterior abdominal wall. Below each rectus muscle lies the posterior layer of the rectus sheath, which also contributes to the linea alba.

Another important anatomic structure of the anterior abdominal wall is the arcuate line, which is located 3 to 6 cm below the umbilicus. The arcuate line delineates the point below which the posterior rectus sheath is absent. Above the arcuate line, the aponeurosis of the internal oblique muscle contributes to the anterior and posterior rectus sheaths, and the aponeurosis of the transversus abdominis muscle passes posterior to the rectus muscle to form the posterior rectus sheath. Below the arcuate line, the internal oblique and transversus abdominis aponeuroses pass completely anterior to the rectus muscle (Fig. 44-9). The posterior rectus sheath below the arcuate line is composed of the transversalis fascia and peritoneum only.

The abdominal wall receives most of its innervation from intercostal nerves 7 through 12 and the first and second lumbar nerves. These rami provide innervation to the lateral abdominal muscles and the rectus muscle and overlying skin. The nerves traverse through the lateral abdominal wall between the transversus abdominis and internal oblique muscles and penetrate the posterior rectus sheath just medial to the linea semilunaris.

The lateral abdominal muscles receive their blood supply from the lower three or four intercostal arteries, deep circumflex iliac artery, and lumbar arteries. The rectus abdominis has a more complex blood supply derived from the superior epigastric artery (a terminal branch of the internal mammary artery), inferior epigastric artery (a branch of the external iliac artery), and lower intercostal arteries. The superior and inferior epigastric arteries anastomose near the umbilicus. The periumbilical area provides critical perforator vessels that, if preserved, can decrease skin flap necrosis during extensive skin undermining (Fig. 44-10).

Diagnosis

The evaluation of abdominal wall hernias requires diligent physical examination. As with the inguinal region, the anterior abdominal wall is evaluated with the patient in standing and supine positions, and a Valsalva maneuver is also useful to demonstrate the site and size of a hernia. Imaging modalities may play a greater role in the diagnosis of more unusual hernias of the abdominal wall.

Classification

Umbilical Hernia

The umbilicus is formed by the umbilical ring of the linea alba. Intra-abdominally, the round ligament (ligamentum teres) and paraumbilical veins join into the umbilicus superiorly and the median umbilical ligament (obliterated urachus) enters inferiorly. Umbilical hernias in infants are congenital and are common. They close spontaneously in most cases by the age of 2 years. Those that persist after the age of 5 years are frequently repaired surgically, although complications related to these hernias in children are unusual. There is a strong predisposition toward the development of these hernias in individuals of African descent. In the United States, the incidence of umbilical hernia is eight times higher in African American than in white infants.

Umbilical hernias in adults are largely acquired. These hernias are more common in women and in patients with conditions that result in increased intra-abdominal pressure, such as pregnancy, obesity, ascites, or chronic abdominal distention. Umbilical hernia is more common in those who have only a single midline aponeurotic decussation compared with the normal decussation of fibers from all three lateral abdominal muscles. Strangulation is unusual in most patients; however, strangulation or rupture can occur in chronic ascitic conditions. Small asymptomatic umbilical hernias barely detectable on examination need not be repaired. Adults who have symptoms, a large hernia, incarceration, thinning of the overlying skin, or uncontrollable ascites should have a hernia repair. Spontaneous rupture of umbilical hernias in patients with ascites can result in peritonitis and death.

Classically, repair was done using the vest over pants repair proposed by Mayo, which uses imbrication of the superior and inferior fascial edges. Because of increased tension on the repair and recurrence rates of almost 30% with long-term follow-up,

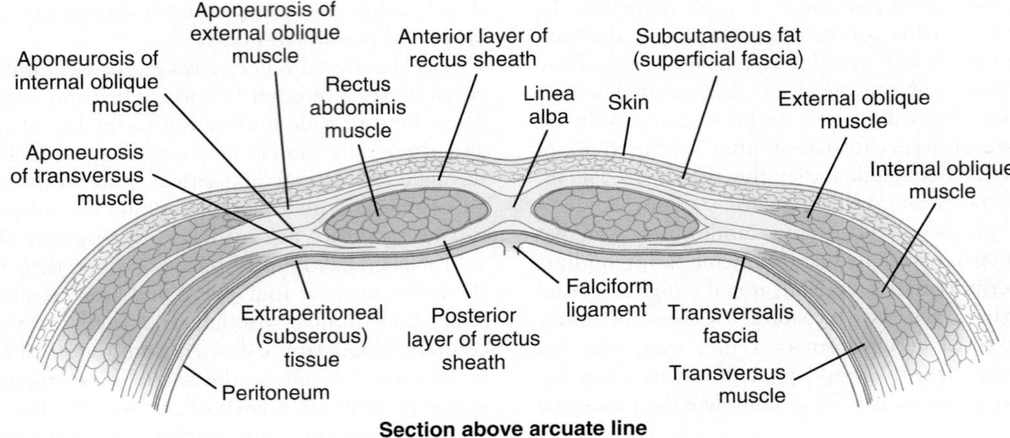

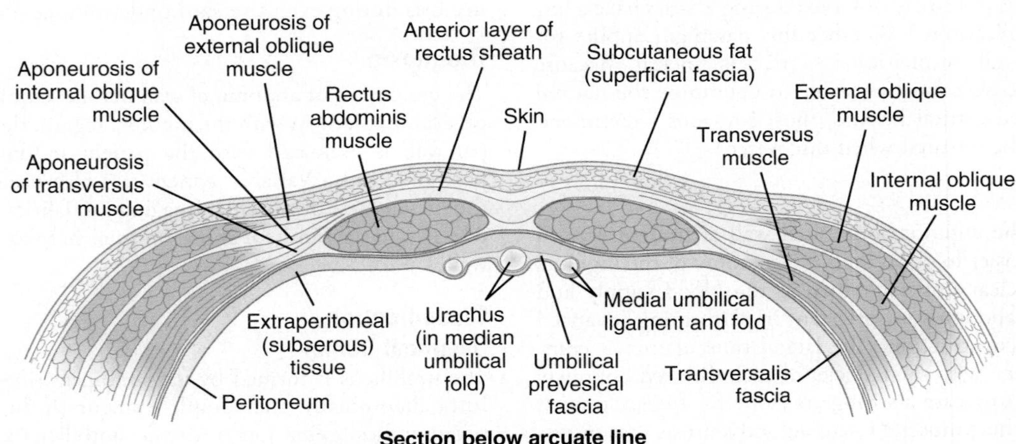

FIGURE 44-9 Cross sections of the rectus abdominis muscle and aponeurosis above and below the arcuate line. (From Netter FT: *Atlas of human anatomy*, Summit, NJ, 1989, Ciba-Geigy, Plate 235.)

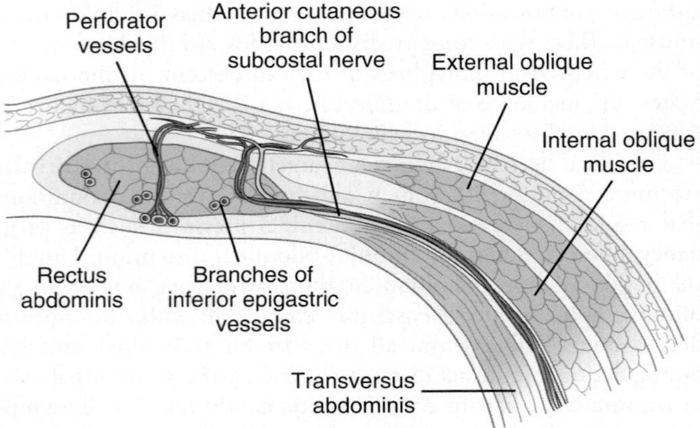

FIGURE 44-10 Cross section of the lateral abdominal wall detailing location of intercostal neurovascular bundle traveling between the transversus abdominis and internal oblique muscles.

however, the Mayo repair is rarely performed today. Instead, small defects are closed primarily after separation of the sac from the overlying umbilicus and surrounding fascia. Defects larger than 3 cm are closed using prosthetic mesh.[38] There are a number of techniques to place this mesh, and no prospective data have conclusively found clear advantages of one technique over another. Options for mesh implantation include bridging the defect, placing a preperitoneal underlay of mesh reinforced with suture repair, and placing it laparoscopically. The laparoscopic technique requires general anesthesia and is reserved for large defects or recurrent umbilical hernias.[39] There is no universal consensus on the most appropriate method of umbilical hernia repair.

Epigastric Hernia

Approximately 3% to 5% of the population has epigastric hernias. Epigastric hernias are two to three times more common in men. These hernias are located between the xiphoid process and umbilicus and are usually within 5 to 6 cm of the umbilicus. Like umbilical hernias, epigastric hernias are more common in individuals with a single aponeurotic decussation. The defects are small and often produce pain out of proportion to their size because of incarceration of preperitoneal fat. They are multiple in up to 20% of patients, and approximately 80% are in the midline. Repair usually consists of excision of the incarcerated preperitoneal tissue and simple closure of the fascial defect, similar to that for umbilical hernias. Small defects can be repaired under local anesthesia. Uncommonly, these defects can be sizable, can contain omentum or other intra-abdominal viscera, and may require mesh repairs. Epigastric hernias are better repaired anteriorly because the defect is small and fat that has herniated from within the peritoneal cavity is difficult to reduce.

Incisional Hernia

Of all hernias encountered, incisional hernias can be the most frustrating and difficult to treat. Incisional hernias occur as a result of excessive tension and inadequate healing of a previous incision, which may be associated with surgical site infection. These hernias enlarge over time, leading to pain, bowel obstruction, incarceration, and strangulation. Obesity, advanced age, malnutrition, ascites, pregnancy, and conditions that increase intra-abdominal pressure are factors that predispose to the development of an incisional hernia. Obesity can cause an incisional hernia to occur because of increased tension on the abdominal wall from the excessive bulk of a thick pannus and large omental mass. Chronic pulmonary disease and diabetes mellitus have also been recognized as risk factors for the development of incisional hernia. Medications such as corticosteroids and chemotherapeutic agents and surgical site infection can contribute to poor wound healing and increase the risk for development of an incisional hernia.

Large hernias can result in loss of abdominal domain, which occurs when the abdominal contents no longer reside in the abdominal cavity. These large abdominal wall defects also can result from the inability to close the abdomen primarily because of bowel edema, abdominal packing, peritonitis, and repeated laparotomy. With loss of domain, the natural rigidity of the abdominal wall becomes compromised and the abdominal musculature is often retracted. Respiratory dysfunction can occur because these large ventral defects cause paradoxical respiratory abdominal motion. Loss of abdominal domain can also result in bowel edema, stasis of the splanchnic venous system, urinary retention, and constipation. Return of displaced viscera to the abdominal cavity during repair may lead to increased abdominal pressure, abdominal compartment syndrome, and acute respiratory failure.

There is no simple mechanism for communicating the complexity of a ventral incisional hernia. Defect size, location on the abdominal wall, loss of domain, patient comorbidities, presence of contamination, necessity for an ostomy, acuity of the presentation, and history of prior repairs with or without a prosthetic allow an infinite number of permutations. The absence of a universal classification system has hindered comparisons within the literature and at meetings, indirectly delaying meaningful conversations about repair techniques and prosthetic choice. The TNM model for cancer staging is an enviable model to strive for in hernia repair. As such, a recent group sought to stratify ventral hernias into stages using a limited number of preoperative variables to accurately predict the two most meaningful surgical outcomes: surgical site occurrence (SSO) and long-term hernia recurrence rates.

Two of the most popular ventral hernia classification tools to date have been generated from expert opinion: the Ventral Hernia Working Group grading scale and the European Hernia Society system. The Ventral Hernia Working Group grading scale uses patient comorbidities and wound class to predict SSO risk. The European Hernia Society system assesses hernia width and location; it was initially designed to gather data on recurrence risk.[40] Using data from 333 ventral hernia repairs with no filter for technique, investigators presented a multivariate analysis that identified hernia width (<10 cm, 10 to 20 cm, ≥20 cm) and the presence of contamination as the two variables associated with wound morbidity (SSO) and hernia recurrence. Hernia location and patient comorbidities were not significant in this model for either outcome measure. Hernias could be grouped into stages (I to III) using width and wound class alone (Table 44-2), with ordinal increments in both outcome measures. Stage I hernias are smaller than 10 cm/clean and associated with low SSO and recurrence risk. Stage II hernias are 10 to 20 cm/clean or smaller than 10 cm/contaminated and carry an intermediate risk of SSO and recurrence. Stage III hernias are either 10 cm and larger/contaminated or any hernia 20 cm or larger, and these are associated with high SSO and recurrence risk. Table 44-3 demonstrates the reported rates for SSO and recurrence using this system.

The staging system is simple but comprehensive in its ability to stratify patients by risk of wound morbidity and recurrence, the two chief outcome parameters of repair. Importantly, this system does not include intraoperative details, such as approach (open versus laparoscopic), mesh choice (biologic versus synthetic), or mesh position (onlay versus sublay). It is hoped that this platform can be the basis of future inclusion and exclusion criteria for studies regarding technique.

Treatment: Operative Repair

Primary repair of incisional hernias can be done when the defect is small (≤2 to 3 cm in diameter) and there is viable surrounding tissue or in cases in which the hernia was clearly a result of a technical error at the initial operation, such as a suture fracturing. Larger defects (>2 to 3 cm in diameter) have a high recurrence rate if closed primarily and are repaired with a prosthesis.[39] Recurrence rates vary between 10% and 50% and are typically reduced

TABLE 44-2 Incisional Hernia Staging System

Stage I Risk: low recurrence, low SSO	<10 cm, clean
Stage II Risk: moderate recurrence, moderate SSO	<10 cm, contaminated 10-20 cm, clean
Stage III Risk: high recurrence, high SSO	≥10 cm, contaminated Any ≥20 cm

SSO, surgical site occurrence.

TABLE 44-3 Surgical Site Occurrence (SSO) and Recurrence Rates

	SSO RATE	RECURRENCE RATE
Stage I Risk: low recurrence, low SSO <10 cm, clean	7/77 (10%)	7/77 (10%)
Stage II Risk: moderate recurrence, moderate SSO <10 cm, contaminated 10-20 cm, clean	30/151 (20%)	22/151 (15%)
Stage III Risk: high recurrence, high SSO ≥10 cm, contaminated Any ≥20 cm	44/105 (42%)	27/105 (26%)

by more than 50% with the use of prosthetic mesh.[41] Prosthetic material may be placed as an onlay patch to buttress a tissue repair, interposed between the fascial defect, sandwiched between tissue planes, or put in a sublay position. Depending on its location, several important properties of the mesh must be considered.

Prosthetic Materials for Ventral Hernia Repair

Synthetic materials. Various synthetic mesh products are available. Desirable characteristics of a synthetic mesh include its being chemically inert, resistant to mechanical stress while maintaining compliance, sterilizable, and noncarcinogenic; it should incite minimal inflammatory reaction and be hypoallergenic. The ideal mesh has yet to be defined. When selecting the appropriate mesh, the surgeon must consider the position of the mesh, whether it will be in direct contact with the viscera, and the presence or risk of infection. Mesh constructs can be classified on the basis of weight of the material, pore size, water angle (hydrophobic or hydrophilic), and whether there is an antiadhesive barrier present. In placing a mesh in the extraperitoneal position without the risk of bowel erosion, a macroporous unprotected mesh is appropriate. Both polypropylene and polyester mesh have been successfully placed in the extraperitoneal position. Polypropylene mesh is a hydrophobic macroporous mesh that allows the ingrowth of native fibroblasts and incorporation into the surrounding fascia. It is semirigid, somewhat flexible, and porous. Placing polypropylene mesh in an intraperitoneal position directly apposed to the bowel is avoided because of unacceptable rates of enterocutaneous fistula formation.[42] Recently, lighter weight polypropylene mesh has been introduced to address some of the long-term complications of heavyweight polypropylene mesh. The definition of lightweight mesh was arbitrarily chosen at less than 50 g/m^2, with heavyweight mesh weighing more than 80 g/m^2. These lightweight mesh products often have an absorbable component of material that provides initial handling stability, typically composed of Vicryl (polyglactin 910) or Monocryl (poliglecaprone 25; Ethicon, Somerville, NJ).

Whether lightweight mesh results in improved patient outcomes is controversial. Two prospective randomized trials evaluating the incidence of postoperative pain after open inguinal hernia repair have shown mixed results.[43] In a randomized controlled trial evaluating lightweight versus heavyweight polypropylene mesh for ventral hernia repair, the recurrence rate in the lightweight group was more than twice that in the heavyweight group (17% for lightweight mesh versus 7% for heavyweight mesh), which approached statistical significance (P = .052).[44] Several investigators have reported concerning rates of central mesh failures with ultra-lightweight polypropylene mesh and lightweight polyester mesh.[45,46] Another recent finding with regard to large-pore lightweight mesh is its ability to resist bacterial contamination. Several animal studies have reported high rates of bacterial clearance with large-pore synthetic mesh when it is exposed to gastrointestinal flora and methicillin-resistant *Staphylococcus aureus*.[47,48] A large multicenter retrospective experience with 100 cases of large-pore polypropylene mesh used in clean contaminated and contaminated ventral hernia repairs was reported.[49] These authors noted excellent medium-term results with a 7% recurrence rate. Longer term data to verify the safety and durability of this approach are needed.

Polyester mesh is composed of polyethylene terephthalate and is a hydrophilic, heavyweight, macroporous mesh. This mesh has several different weaves that can yield a two-dimensional flat screen-like mesh and a three-dimensional multifilament weave. Unprotected polyester mesh should not be placed directly on the viscera because unacceptable rates of erosion and bowel obstruction have been reported.[42] When it is placed in the preperitoneal position in complex ventral hernia repairs, complication rates are low.[9,50]

When mesh is placed in an intraperitoneal position, several options are available. A single sheet of mesh with both sides constructed to reduce adhesions and a composite-type mesh with one side made to promote tissue ingrowth and the other to resist adhesion formation are available. Single-sheet mesh is composed of expanded polytetrafluoroethylene (ePTFE). This prosthetic has a visceral side that is microporous (3 μm) and an abdominal wall side that is macroporous (17 to 22 μm) and promotes tissue ingrowth. This product differs from other synthetic meshes in that it is flexible and smooth. Some fibroblast proliferation occurs through the pores, but PTFE is impermeable to fluid. Unlike polypropylene, PTFE is not incorporated into the native tissue. Encapsulation occurs slowly, and infection can occur during the encapsulation process. When it is infected, PTFE almost always must be removed.

To promote better tissue integration, composite mesh was developed. This product combines the attributes of polypropylene and PTFE by layering the two substances on top of one another. The PTFE surface serves as a permanent protective interface against the bowel and the polypropylene side faces superficially to be incorporated into the native fascial tissue. These materials have variable rates of contraction and, when placed together, can result in buckling of the mesh and visceral exposure to the polypropylene component. Other composite meshes recently have been developed that combine a macroporous mesh with a temporary, absorbable antiadhesive barrier. Basic constructs of these mesh materials include heavyweight or lightweight polypropylene or polyester. Absorbable barriers are typically composed of oxidized regenerated cellulose, omega-3 fatty acids, or collagen hydrogels. A number of small animal studies have validated the antiadhesive properties of these barriers, but currently no human trials exist evaluating the ability of these composite materials to resist adhesion formation.

Biologic materials. Biologic prostheses for ventral hernia repair are nonsynthetic, natural tissue mesh. There are numerous biologic grafts available for abdominal wall reconstruction (Table 44-4). These products can be categorized on the basis of the source material (e.g., human, porcine, bovine), postharvesting processing techniques (e.g., cross-linked, non–cross-linked), and sterilization techniques (e.g., gamma radiation, ethylene oxide gas sterilization, nonsterilized). These products are largely composed of acellular collagen and theoretically provide a matrix for neovascularization and native collagen deposition. These properties may provide advantages in infected or contaminated cases in which synthetic mesh is thought to be contraindicated. Ideal placement techniques are yet to be defined for these relatively new products; however, some general principles apply. These products function best when used as a fascial reinforcement rather than as a bridge or interposition repair.[51] The long-term durability of biologic mesh has recently been questioned in the largest series of biologic mesh use in a contaminated setting.[52] There are no prospective randomized data comparing the effectiveness of these natural tissue alternatives with that of synthetic mesh repairs in various settings of complex hernia repairs.

Operative Technique

Ventral hernias. It is generally agreed that all but the smallest incisional hernias can be repaired with mesh, and the surgeon has

TABLE 44-4 Biologic Mesh for Abdominal Wall Reconstruction and Postharvesting Processing Techniques

PRODUCT	SOURCE	CROSS-LINKED	STERILIZATION METHOD
AlloDerm (LifeCell, Branchburg, NJ)	Human dermis	No	Ionic
AlloMax (Davol, Warwick, RI)	Human dermis	No	E beam
FlexHD (Ethicon, Sommerville, NJ)	Human dermis	No	Ethanol
Strattice (LifeCell, Branchburg, NJ)	Porcine dermis	No	Gamma irradiation
Permacol (Covidien, Norwalk, CT)	Porcine dermis	Yes	Ethanol
CollaMend (Davol, Warwick, RI)	Porcine dermis	Yes	Ethanol
XenMatrix (Davol, Warwick, RI)	Porcine dermis	No	Gamma irradiation
SurgiMend (TEI Biosciences, Boston, MA)	Bovine fetal dermis	No	Ethanol
Veritas (Synovis, St. Paul, MN)	Bovine	No	
Peri-Guard (Synovis, St. Paul, MN)	Bovine	Yes	
Surgisis (Cook, Bloomfield, IN)	Porcine intestine	No	Ethanol

various options for placing the mesh. The onlay technique involves primary closure of the fascia defect and placement of a mesh over the anterior fascia. The major advantage of this approach is that the mesh is placed outside the abdominal cavity, avoiding direct interaction with the abdominal viscera. However, disadvantages include the large subcutaneous dissection, the increased likelihood of seroma formation, the superficial location of the mesh (which places it in jeopardy of contamination if the incision becomes infected), and the repair is usually under tension. Prospective analysis of this technique is not available, but a retrospective review has reported recurrence rates of 28%.[53] Interposition prosthetic repairs involve securing the mesh to the fascial edge without overlap. This results in a predictably high recurrence rate; the synthetic often pulls away from the fascial edge because of increased intra-abdominal pressure. A sublay or underlay technique involves placing the prosthetic below the fascial components. The mesh can be placed intraperitoneally, preperitoneally, or in the retrorectus (retromuscular) space. It is highly desirable to have the mesh placed beneath the fascia. With a wide overlap of mesh and fascia, the natural forces of the abdominal cavity act to hold the mesh in place and prevent migration. This can be accomplished by several techniques (Fig. 44-11).

Intraperitoneal mesh placement. After reopening of the prior incision and with the use of available dual-type mesh or composite mesh, the mesh can be placed in an intraperitoneal position at least 4 cm beyond the fascial margin and secured with interrupted mattress sutures. This technique requires raising subcutaneous flaps, and the mesh may be in direct contact with the abdominal contents.

The laparoscopic approach for ventral hernia repair relies on the same principles as the retrorectus repair; however, the mesh is placed within the peritoneal cavity. This repair is useful, particularly for large defects. Trocars are placed as far laterally as feasible based on the size and location of the hernia. The hernia contents are reduced, and adhesions are lysed. The surface area of the defect is measured, and a barrier-coated mesh is fashioned with at least 4 cm of overlap around the defect. The mesh is rolled, placed into the abdomen, and deployed. It is secured to the anterior abdominal wall with preplaced mattress sutures that are passed through separate incisions; tacking staples are placed between these sutures to secure the mesh 4 cm beyond the defect. There are fewer incisional complications with the laparoscopic approach because large incisions and subcutaneous undermining are avoided.

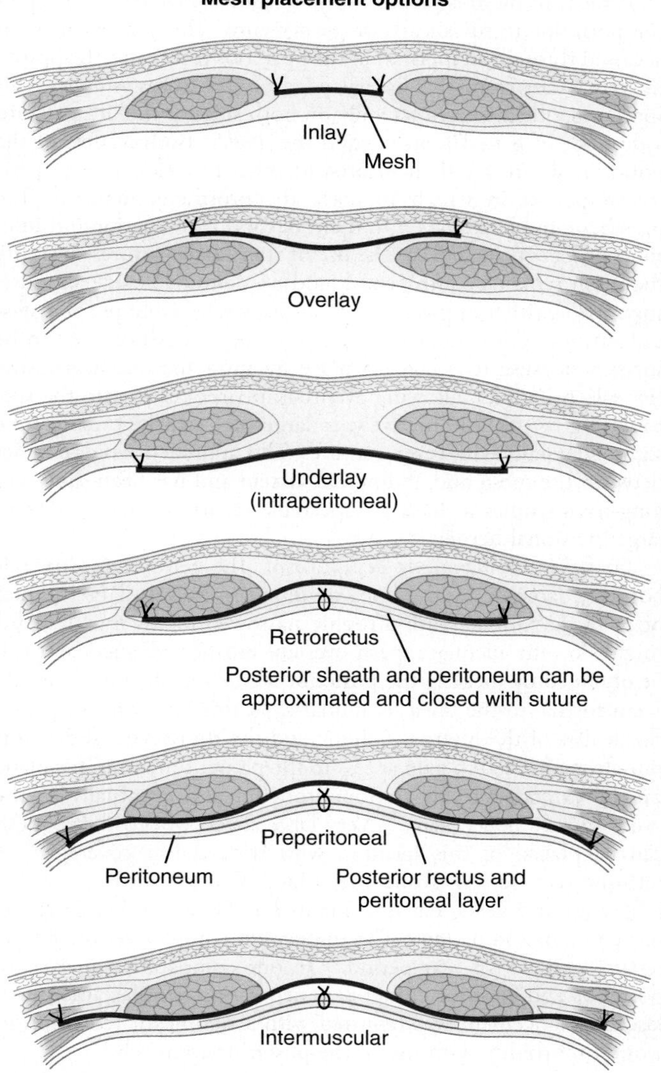

FIGURE 44-11 Mesh placement options for abdominal wall reconstruction.

Myofascial releases. One of the underlying principles of abdominal wall reconstruction is to reestablish the linea alba. Restoring the linea alba to the midline provides the advantage of a functional abdominal wall, often protects the mesh from superficial wound issues, and might result in a more durable repair. In larger hernias, there are several options to provide the myofascial advancement necessary to reconstruct the midline and to restore contour to the abdominal wall. The basic tenets of these procedures are that the abdominal wall and rectus muscle are bounded by several different myofascial compartments, and by releasing one or more fascial bundles, advancement of the rectus muscle to the midline is possible. In essence, each of these procedures creates a local advancement flap of the rectus muscle. Great care should be taken to identify and to preserve the neurovascular structures to the rectus muscle to ensure a functional well-vascularized graft.

Posterior rectus sheath incision with retromuscular mesh placement. This technique involves placing prosthetic mesh in the extraperitoneal position in the preperitoneal space or retrorectus position. This technique was initially described by Stoppa.[9] A large piece of mesh is placed in the retromuscular space on top of the posterior rectus sheath or peritoneum. The compartment is accessed through an incision in the posterior rectus sheath approximately 1 cm from the medial edge of the rectus muscle. This space must be dissected laterally on both sides of the linea alba to a distance of 8 to 10 cm beyond the defect. Both leaflets of the posterior sheath are then sutured together to create an extraperitoneal pocket in which to place the prosthetic material. The prosthetic mesh extends 5 to 6 cm beyond the superior and inferior borders of the defect. The use of transfascial sutures to secure the mesh remains controversial, and no definitive evidence exists supporting either approach. The authors selectively use transfascial sutures. With smaller defects, the mesh does not need to be sutured because it is held in place by intra-abdominal pressure (Pascal's principle), allowing eventual incorporation into the surrounding tissues. Alternatively, in larger defects, the mesh can be secured laterally with several sutures. This approach avoids contact between the mesh and abdominal viscera and has been shown in long-term studies to have a respectable recurrence rate (14%) in large incisional hernias.

Posterior component separation. The retrorectus space is bordered laterally by the linea semilunaris. In very large hernias or in those patients with atrophic narrowed rectus muscles, this might prevent adequate mesh overlap. Further advancement can be obtained by incising the posterior rectus sheath approximately 1 cm medial to the linea semilunaris. At this location, the posterior leaflet of the internal oblique and the transversus abdominis muscle are incised to gain access to the preperitoneum. This plane can be extended to the retroperitoneum and eventually to the psoas muscle if necessary.[54] Very large sheets of prosthetic mesh can be placed in this location with wide defect coverage.[55] A retrospective review from the Mayo Clinic, with a median follow-up of 5 years, has documented a 5% overall hernia recurrence rate in 254 patients who underwent complex ventral hernia repair during a 13-year period.[43] In one comparative analysis of posterior and anterior component separation, similar amount of fascial advancement was reported with a significant reduction in wound morbidity with use of the posterior approach.[55]

Anterior component separation. Another option for the repair of complex or large ventral defects is the anterior component separation technique (Fig. 44-12). This involves separating the lateral muscle layers of the abdominal wall to allow their advancement. Primary fascial closure at the midline is often possible. The procedure is performed by raising large subcutaneous flaps above the external oblique fascia. These flaps are carried laterally past the linea semilunaris. This lipocutaneous dissection itself can provide some advancement of the abdominal wall. Large perforating subcutaneous vessels can be preserved to prevent ischemic necrosis of the skin flaps. A relaxing incision is made 2 cm lateral to the linea semilunaris on the lateral external oblique aponeurosis from several centimeters above the costal margin to the pubis. The external oblique is then bluntly separated in the avascular plane, away from the internal oblique, allowing its advancement. Further relaxing incisions have been described to the aponeurotic layers of the internal oblique or transversus abdominis, but this can result in problematic lateral bulges or herniation at this site. Additional release can be safely achieved by incising the posterior rectus sheath. These techniques, when applied to both sides of the abdominal wall, can yield up to 20 cm of mobilization. Although this technique often allows tension-free closure of these large defects, recurrence rates as low as 20% have been reported with the use of prosthetic reinforcement in large hernias.[56] It is important that patients understand that a lateral bulge can occur after release of the external oblique aponeurosis. Recognizing the high recurrence rates with component separation alone, several authors have reported small series of biologic mesh reinforcement of these repairs.[51] To date, no randomized controlled trials have supported a lower recurrence rate with biologic prosthetic reinforcement. If a bioprosthetic is placed, it can be secured with an underlay or onlay technique. No comparative data exist demonstrating the superiority of either repair technique.[57]

Endoscopic component separation. One of the major limitations of open component separation is that large skin flaps are necessary to access the lateral abdominal wall musculature. Recognizing these limitations, innovative, minimally invasive approaches to component separation have been described.[58] The basic principle of a minimally invasive component separation is to gain direct access to the lateral abdominal wall without creating a lipocutaneous flap. Typically, this is performed by a direct cutdown through a 1-cm incision off the tip of the 11th rib overlying the external oblique muscle (Fig. 44-13). The external oblique is split in the line of its fibers, and a standard bilateral inguinal hernia balloon dissector is placed in between the external and internal oblique muscles, toward the pubis. Three laparoscopic trocars are placed in the space created, and the dissection is carried from the pubis to several centimeters above the costal margin. The linea semilunaris is carefully identified, and the external oblique is incised from beneath the muscle, at least 2 cm lateral to the linea semilunaris. The muscle is released from the pubis to several centimeters above the costal margin. This procedure is performed bilaterally. Synthetic or biologic mesh can be used to reinforce the repair of the midline closure. These relatively new techniques are feasible, but long-term data demonstrating equivalency to open techniques are lacking.

Results of Incisional Hernia Repairs

Several prospective randomized trials have compared laparoscopic and open ventral hernia repairs (Table 44-5).[59-63] Although most of these studies were small, with fewer than 100 patients, the results tend to favor a laparoscopic approach for small to medium-sized defects. The incidences of postoperative complications and recurrence were less in hernias repaired laparoscopically. Several retrospective reports have demonstrated similar advantages for a laparoscopic approach. Based on the comparative trials listed in

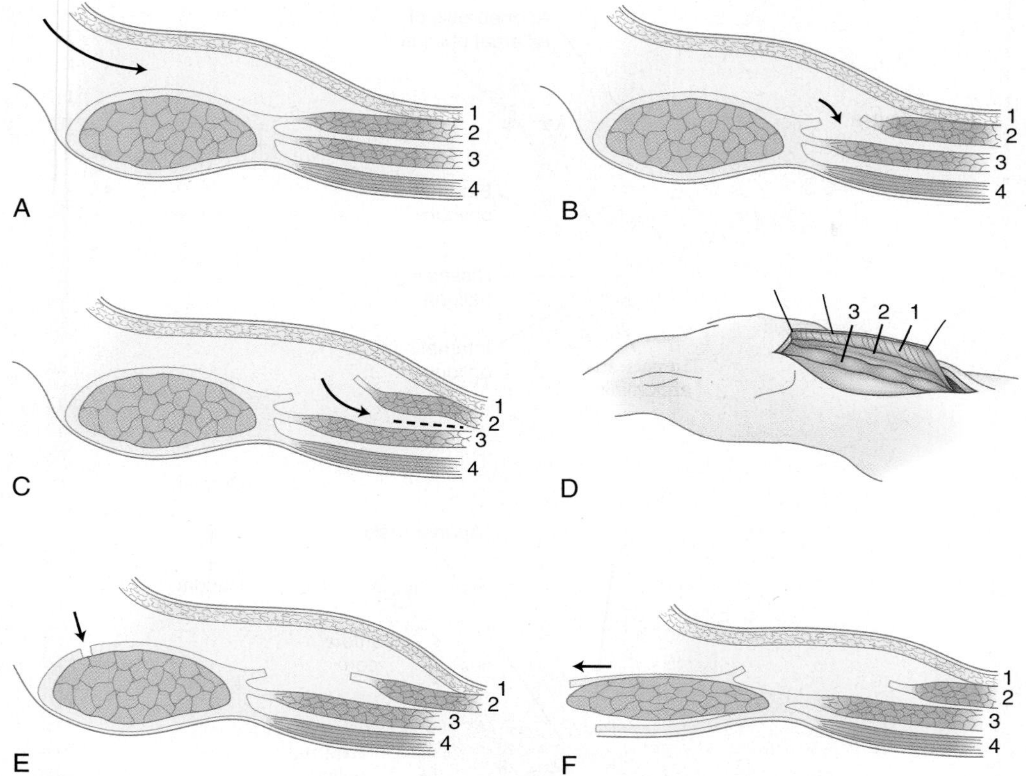

FIGURE 44-12 Component Separation Technique. A, The skin and subcutaneous fat are dissected free from the anterior sheath of the rectus abdominis muscle and the aponeurosis of the external abdominal oblique muscle. **B,** The external abdominal oblique is incised 1 to 2 cm lateral to the rectus abdominis muscle. **C,** The external abdominal oblique is separated from the internal abdominal oblique. **D,** The dissection is carried to the posterior axillary line. **E,** Additional length can be achieved by incising the posterior rectus sheath above the arcuate line. **F,** Care must be taken to avoid damaging the nerves and blood supply that enter the rectus abdominis posteriorly. (From de Vries Reilingh TS, van Goor H, Rosman C, et al: Components separation technique for the repair of large abdominal wall hernias. *J Am Coll Surg* 196:32–37, 2003.)

Table 44-5, laparoscopic incisional hernia repair results in fewer postoperative complications, lower infection rate, and decreased hernia recurrence.[54,56-60,64] Until an appropriately powered prospective randomized trial is performed, the ideal approach will largely be based on surgeon expertise and preference. In addition, these trials will need to provide guidance on the most appropriate hernia size to be repaired by either an open or a laparoscopic approach.

UNUSUAL HERNIAS

There are a number of hernias that occur infrequently, of various types.

Types

Spigelian Hernia

A spigelian hernia occurs through the spigelian fascia, which is composed of the aponeurotic layer between the rectus muscle medially and semilunar line laterally. Almost all spigelian hernias occur at or below the arcuate line. The absence of posterior rectus fascia may contribute to an inherent weakness in this area. These hernias are often interparietal, with the hernia sac dissecting posterior to the external oblique aponeurosis. Most spigelian hernias are small (1 to 2 cm in diameter) and develop during the fourth to seventh decades of life. Patients often present with localized pain in the area without a bulge because the hernia lies beneath the intact external oblique aponeurosis. Ultrasound or CT of the abdomen can be useful to establish the diagnosis.

A spigelian hernia is repaired because of the risk for incarceration associated with its relatively narrow neck. The hernia site is marked before operation. A transverse incision is made over the defect and carried through the external oblique aponeurosis. The hernia sac is opened, dissected free of the neck of the hernia, and excised or inverted. The defect is closed transversely by simple suture repair of the transversus abdominis and internal oblique muscles, followed by closure of the external oblique aponeurosis. Larger defects are repaired with a mesh prosthesis. Recurrence is uncommon.

Obturator Hernia

The obturator canal is formed by the union of the pubic bone and ischium. This canal is covered by a membrane pierced at the medial and superior border by the obturator nerve and vessels. Weakening of the obturator membrane may result in enlargement of the canal and formation of a hernia sac, which can lead to intestinal incarceration and strangulation. The patient can present with evidence of compression of the obturator nerve, which causes pain in the anteromedial aspect of the thigh (Howship-Romberg sign) that is relieved by thigh flexion. Almost 50% of patients

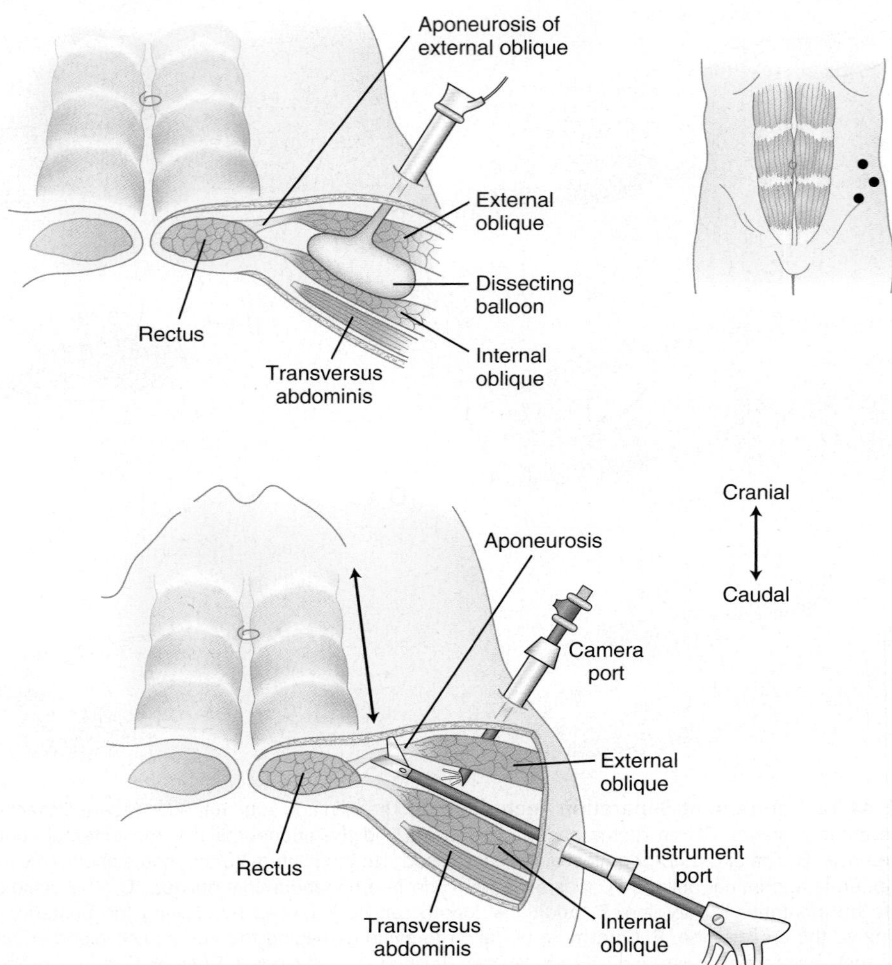

FIGURE 44-13 Endoscopic component separation: port placement and surgical technique.

TABLE 44-5 Comparative Randomized Studies Between Open and Laparoscopic Ventral Hernia Repair

STUDY	NO. OF PATIENTS LAP	NO. OF PATIENTS OPEN	MESH USED LAP	MESH USED OPEN	INTRAOPERATIVE COMPLICATIONS (%) LAP	INTRAOPERATIVE COMPLICATIONS (%) OPEN	LOS (DAYS) LAP	LOS (DAYS) OPEN	POSTOPERATIVE COMPLICATIONS (%) LAP	POSTOPERATIVE COMPLICATIONS (%) OPEN	FOLLOW-UP (MONTHS) LAP	FOLLOW-UP (MONTHS) OPEN	RECURRENCE (%) LAP	RECURRENCE (%) OPEN
McGreevy et al,[60] 2003	65	71	ePTFE or polyester + collagen	PP	N/A	N/A	1.1	1.5	7.70	21.10	N/A	N/A	N/A	N/A
Lomanto et al,[61] 2006	50	50	Polyester + collagen	ePTFE	2	2	2.74	4.7	26	40	19.6	21	2	10
Bingener et al,[62] 2007	127	233	ePTFE, PP, or ePTFE	PP	N/A	N/A	N/A	N/A	33.10	43.30	36	36	13	9
Olmi et al,[59] 2007	85	85	Polyester + collagen	PP	N/A	N/A	2.7	9.9	16.50	29.40	24	24	2	4
Pring et al,[73] 2008	31	27	PTFE	PTFE	N/A	N/A	1	1	33	49	28	28	3.30	4.20
Asencio et al,[74] 2009	45	39	PTFE or PP	PP	6.70	0	3.46	3.33	5.20	33.30	12	12	9.70	7.90

ePTFE, expanded polytetrafluoroethylene; *LAP*, laparoscopic; *LOS*, length of stay; *N/A*, not available; *PP*, polypropylene.

with obturator hernia present with complete or partial bowel obstruction. An abdominal CT scan can establish the diagnosis, if necessary.

A posterior approach, open or laparoscopic, is preferred. This approach provides direct access to the hernia. After reduction of the hernia sac and contents, any preperitoneal fat within the obturator canal is reduced. If necessary, the obturator foramen is opened posterior to the nerve and vessels. The obturator nerve can be manipulated gently with a blunt nerve hook to facilitate reduction of the fat pad. The obturator foramen is repaired with prosthetic mesh, with care taken to avoid injury to the obturator nerve and vessels. Patients with compromised bowel usually require laparotomy.

Lumbar Hernia

Lumbar hernias can be congenital or acquired after an operation on the flank and occur in the lumbar region of the posterior abdominal wall. Hernias through the superior lumbar triangle (Grynfeltt triangle) are more common. The superior lumbar triangle is bounded by the 12th rib, paraspinal muscles, and internal oblique muscle. Less common are hernias through the inferior lumbar triangle (Petit triangle), which is bounded by the iliac crest, latissimus dorsi muscle, and external oblique muscle. Weakness of the lumbodorsal fascia through either of these areas results in progressive protrusion of extraperitoneal fat and a hernia sac. Lumbar hernias are not prone to incarceration. Small lumbar hernias are frequently asymptomatic. Larger hernias may be associated with back pain. CT is useful for diagnosis.

Both open and laparoscopic repairs are useful. Satisfactory suture repair is difficult because of the immobile bone margins of these defects. Repair is best done by placement of prosthetic mesh, which is sutured beyond the margins of the hernia. There is usually sufficient fascia over the bone to anchor the mesh.

Interparietal Hernia

Interparietal hernias are rare and occur when the hernia sac lies between layers of the abdominal wall. These hernias most frequently occur in previous incisions. Spigelian hernias are almost always interparietal.

The correct preoperative diagnosis of interparietal hernia can be difficult. Many patients with complicated interparietal hernias present with intestinal obstruction. Abdominal CT can assist in the diagnosis. Large interparietal hernias usually require placement of prosthetic mesh for closure. When this cannot be done, the component separation technique may be useful to provide natural tissues to obliterate the defect.

Sciatic Hernia

The greater sciatic foramen can be a site of hernia formation. These hernias are extremely unusual and difficult to diagnose and frequently are asymptomatic until intestinal obstruction occurs. In the absence of intestinal obstruction, the most common symptom is the presence of an uncomfortable or slowly enlarging mass in the gluteal or intragluteal area. Sciatic nerve pain can occur, but sciatic hernia is a rare cause of sciatic neuralgia.

A transperitoneal approach is preferred if bowel obstruction or strangulation is suspected. Hernia contents can usually be reduced with gentle traction. Prosthetic mesh repair is usually preferred. A transgluteal approach can be used if the diagnosis is certain and the hernia is reducible, but most surgeons are not familiar with this approach. With the patient prone, an incision is made from the posterior edge of the greater trochanter across the hernia mass. The gluteus maximus muscle is opened, and the sac is visualized. The muscle edges of the defect are reapproximated with interrupted sutures, or the defect is obliterated with mesh.

Perineal Hernia

Perineal hernias are caused by congenital or acquired defects and are uncommon. These hernias may also occur after abdominoperineal resection or perineal prostatectomy. The hernia sac protrudes through the pelvic diaphragm. Primary perineal hernias are rare, occur most commonly in older multiparous women, and can be quite large. Symptoms are usually related to protrusion of a mass through the defect that is worsened by sitting or standing. A bulge is frequently detected on bimanual rectal-vaginal examination.

Perineal hernias are generally repaired through a transabdominal approach or combined transabdominal and perineal approaches. After the sac contents are reduced, small defects may be closed with nonabsorbable suture, whereas large defects are repaired with prosthetic mesh.

Loss of Domain Hernias

Loss of domain implies a massive hernia in which the herniated contents have resided for so long outside the abdominal cavity that they cannot simply be replaced into the peritoneal cavity. We typically classify loss of domain hernias into patients with and without preoperative contamination. Each group is then subcategorized into two groups. Patients with a small hernia defect and a massive hernia sac (e.g., large inguinoscrotal hernias) require restoration of peritoneal cavity domain, whereas patients with a large defect and a massive hernia sac (open abdomen with skin graft) require restoration of peritoneal domain and complex reconstruction of the abdominal wall.

Before repair of these complex defects, the patient must undergo careful preoperative evaluation. A clear understanding of the morbidity and mortality associated with these reconstructive procedures is critical. Weight reduction, smoking cessation, optimization of nutrition, and glucose control are all important aspects of complex abdominal wall reconstruction. Previously, methods to stretch the abdominal wall gradually were used to allow the restoration of abdominal domain and closure. This was accomplished by insufflation of air into the abdominal cavity to create a progressive pneumoperitoneum. Repeated administrations of increasing volumes of air during 1 to 3 weeks allowed the muscles of the abdominal wall to become lax enough for primary closure of the defect. This technique is particularly suited for small defects and massive hernia sacs.[65] For large defects, some authors have also described a staged approach using ePTFE dual mesh for patients with loss of abdominal domain and lateral retraction of the abdominal wall musculature. The initial stage involves reduction of the hernia and placement of a large sheet of ePTFE dual mesh secured to the fascial edges with a running suture. Subsequent stages involve serial elliptical excision of the mesh until the fascia can be approximated in the midline without tension. Finally, the mesh is completely excised, and the fascia is reapproximated with component separation and a biologic underlay patch, if necessary.[66] This approach is technically feasible but does require multiple operations and long hospital stays, and it is associated with a fairly high morbidity rate.

Parastomal Hernia Repair

Parastomal hernia is a common complication of stoma creation. In fact, the creation of a stoma by strict definition is an abdominal wall hernia. The incidence of parastomal hernias is highest for colostomies and occurs in up to 50% of stomas. Fortunately, most patients remain asymptomatic, and life-threatening complications, such as bowel obstruction and strangulation, are rare. Unlike midline incisional hernia repair, routine repair of parastomal hernias is not recommended. Surgical repair should be reserved for patients experiencing symptoms of bowel obstruction, problems with pouch fit, or cosmetic issues.

Three general approaches are available for parastomal hernia repair. These techniques include primary fascial repair, stoma relocation, and prosthetic repair. Primary fascial repair involves hernia reduction and primary fascial reapproximation through a peristomal incision. This technique carries a predictably high recurrence rate. The advantage of this approach is that the abdomen often is not entered, making the operation less complex. Because of the high recurrence rate with this technique, it should be reserved for patients who will not tolerate a laparotomy. Stoma relocation improves results; however, it requires a laparotomy and predisposes to another parastomal hernia in the future. To reduce the rate of recurrent herniation, some surgeons reinforce the repair with biologic or synthetic mesh in a keyhole fashion around the new stoma site. Early results are promising, but long-term outcomes have not yet been reported.[67] Prosthetic repairs of parastomal hernias can provide excellent long-term results with a lower rate of hernia recurrence, but a higher rate of prosthetic complications must be accepted.

Regardless of the technique, a permanent foreign body placed in apposition to the bowel can result in erosion, obstruction, and disastrous complications. Several approaches to prosthetic mesh placement have been described. The mesh can be placed as an onlay patch, intra-abdominally, or in the retrorectus position. When the mesh is placed intraperitoneally, a keyhole is fashioned around the stoma site or placed as a flat sheet, lateralizing the stoma as it exits the abdomen, as described by Sugarbaker.[68] Several authors have described laparoscopic approaches to parastomal hernia repair, including keyhole and Sugarbaker-type repairs[69,70] (Fig. 44-14). A retromuscular repair that takes advantage of many of the advanced reconstructive techniques described in this chapter has recently been reported. In this approach, a laparotomy is performed, and the stoma is taken down and eventually resited to the contralateral side of the abdomen. A posterior component separation is then performed; a large mesh is deployed in the retromuscular space to cover the old stoma site and the entire midline incision, and it is used to prophylactically reinforce the new stoma site. The stoma is eventually brought out through a keyhole incision in the mesh and matured.[71] All these series are fairly small with fewer than 100 patients and have reported only short-term to medium-term follow-up, limiting our ability to make clear recommendations for this difficult problem.

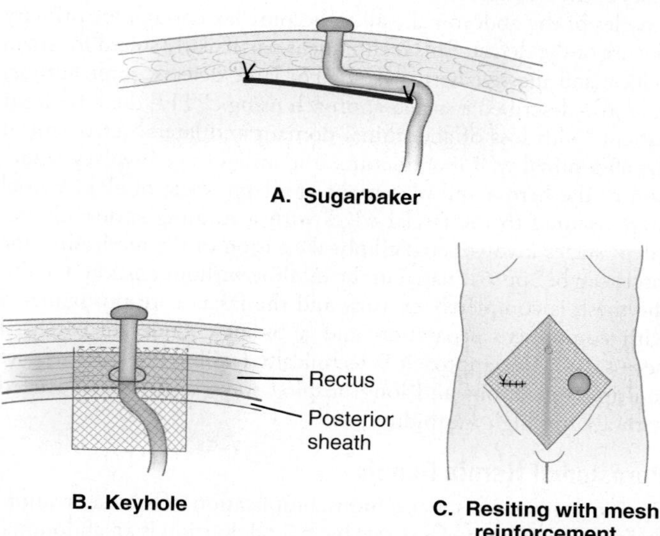

FIGURE 44-14 Surgical approaches for parastomal hernia repair.

Complications

Mesh Infection

Mesh infections are serious complications that can be difficult to treat. If ePTFE becomes infected, it requires removal with the resultant morbidity of another defect, which often must be closed under tension, leading to inevitable recurrence. In open ventral hernia repair, incisional and mesh infections are not infrequent. Use of the laparoscopic technique and placement of a large piece of mesh without undermining large subcutaneous tissue flaps avoid wound complications. In a series of almost 1000 patients who had laparoscopic ventral hernia repair, mesh infections occurred in less than 1% of cases.[72] Perhaps the greatest advantage of the laparoscopic approach for repairing ventral hernias is this reduction in infectious complications. Two randomized controlled trials have compared laparoscopic and open ventral hernia repair.[73,74]

Seromas

Seroma formation can occur after laparoscopic and open ventral hernia repair. In open ventral hernia repair, drains are often placed in an attempt to obliterate the dead space caused by the hernia and tissue dissection. These drains can cause mesh contamination, and seromas can form after drain removal. With laparoscopic repair, the hernia sac is not resected, and a seroma cavity will result. Most of these seromas will resolve over time as the mesh becomes incorporated on the hernia sac. Preoperative discussions with the patient describing the expectations of a temporary seroma are imperative before laparoscopic ventral hernia repair. We reserve aspiration for symptomatic or persistent seromas after 6 to 8 weeks.

Enterotomy

Intestinal injury during adhesiolysis can be catastrophic. Management of an enterotomy during a hernia repair is controversial and depends on the segment of intestine injured (small versus large bowel) and amount of spillage. Options include aborting the hernia repair, using a primary tissue or biologic tissue repair, and performing a delayed repair with prosthetic mesh in 3 to 4 days. When there is gross contamination, the use of synthetic mesh is contraindicated.

SELECTED REFERENCES

Anson BJ, McVay CB: Inguinal hernia: The anatomy of the region. *Surg Gynecol Obstet* 66:186–191, 1938.

Condon RE: Surgical anatomy of the transversus abdominis and transversalis fascia. *Ann Surg* 173:1–5, 1971.

Nyhus LM: An anatomic reappraisal of the posterior inguinal wall, with special consideration of the iliopubic tract and its relation to groin hernias. *Surg Clin North Am* 44:1305, 1960.

These three references are classic descriptions of the anatomy of the groin. All are well illustrated.

Bisgaard T, Bay-Nielsen M, Kehlet H: Re-recurrence after operation for recurrent inguinal hernia. A nationwide 8-year follow-up study on the role of type of repair. *Ann Surg* 247:707–711, 2008.

This long term population-based study provides useful information about the results of recurrent inguinal hernia repairs.

de Vries Reilingh TS, van Goor H, Charbon JA, et al: Repair of giant midline abdominal wall hernias: "Components separation technique" versus prosthetic repair: Interim analysis of a randomized controlled trial. *World J Surg* 31:756–763, 2007.

This is a prospective randomized trial evaluating outcomes of open ventral hernia repair with synthetic mesh versus component separation without reinforcement.

Fitzgibbons RJ, Jr, Forse RA: Clinical practice. Groin hernias in adults. *N Engl J Med* 372:756–763, 2015.

Recent review of the diagnosis and management of groin hernias in adults.

Forbes SS, Eskicioglu C, McLeod RS, et al: Meta-analysis of randomized controlled trials comparing open and laparoscopic ventral and incisional hernia repair with mesh. *Br J Surg* 96:851–858, 2009.

This is a meta-analysis evaluating eight prospective randomized trials comparing laparoscopic with open ventral hernia repair.

Itani KM, Hur K, Kim LT, et al: Veterans Affairs Ventral Incisional Hernia Investigators: Comparison of laparoscopic and open repair with mesh for the treatment of ventral incisional hernia: A randomized trial. *Arch Surg* 145:322–328, 2010.

This is a prospective randomized trial evaluating laparoscopic versus open ventral hernia repairs.

Neumayer L, Giobbie-Hurder A, Jonasson O, et al: Open mesh versus laparoscopic mesh repair of inguinal hernia. *N Engl J Med* 350:1819–1827, 2004.

Excellent prospective randomized trial comparing these two types of hernia repairs in Veterans Administration hospitals.

Zhao G, Gao P, Ma B, et al: Open mesh techniques for inguinal hernia repair: A meta-analysis of randomized controlled trials. *Ann Surg* 250:35–42, 2009.

Excellent meta-analysis of various techniques of tension-free repairs.

REFERENCES

1. Bradley M, Morgan D, Pentlow B, et al: The groin hernia—an ultrasound diagnosis? *Ann R Coll Surg Engl* 85:178–180, 2003.
2. Della Santa V, Groebli Y: [Diagnosis of non-hernia groin masses]. *Ann Chir* 125:179–183, 2000.
3. Fitzgibbons RJ, Jr, Giobbie-Hurder A, Gibbs JO, et al: Watchful waiting vs repair of inguinal hernia in minimally symptomatic men: a randomized clinical trial. *JAMA* 295:285–292, 2006.
4. Fitzgibbons RJ, Jr, Ramanan B, Arya S, et al: Long-term results of a randomized controlled trial of a nonoperative strategy (watchful waiting) for men with minimally symptomatic inguinal hernias. *Ann Surg* 258:508–515, 2013.
5. Chung L, Norrie J, O'Dwyer PJ: Long-term follow-up of patients with a painless inguinal hernia from a randomized clinical trial. *Br J Surg* 98:596–599, 2011.
6. Lichtenstein IL, Shulman AG, Amid PK, et al: The tension-free hernioplasty. *Am J Surg* 157:188–193, 1989.
7. Gilbert AI: Sutureless repair of inguinal hernia. *Am J Surg* 163:331–335, 1992.
8. Kugel RD: Minimally invasive, nonlaparoscopic, preperitoneal, and sutureless, inguinal herniorrhaphy. *Am J Surg* 178:298–302, 1999.
9. Stoppa RE: The treatment of complicated groin and incisional hernias. *World J Surg* 13:545–554, 1989.
10. Malangoni MA, Condon RE: Preperitoneal repair of acute incarcerated and strangulated hernias of the groin. *Surg Gynecol Obstet* 162:65–67, 1986.
11. Ahmad G, Duffy JM, Phillips K, et al: Laparoscopic entry techniques. *Cochrane Database Syst Rev* (2):CD006583, 2008.
12. Voyles CR, Hamilton BJ, Johnson WD, et al: Meta-analysis of laparoscopic inguinal hernia trials favors open hernia repair with preperitoneal mesh prosthesis. *Am J Surg* 184:6–10, 2002.
13. Bisgaard T, Bay-Nielsen M, Kehlet H: Re-recurrence after operation for recurrent inguinal hernia. A nationwide 8-year follow-up study on the role of type of repair. *Ann Surg* 247:707–711, 2008.
14. Nordin P, Haapaniemi S, van der Linden W, et al: Choice of anesthesia and risk of reoperation for recurrence in groin hernia repair. *Ann Surg* 240:187–192, 2004.
15. Neumayer L, Giobbie-Hurder A, Jonasson O, et al: Open mesh versus laparoscopic mesh repair of inguinal hernia. *N Engl J Med* 350:1819–1827, 2004.
16. McCormack K, Scott NW, Go PM, et al: Laparoscopic techniques versus open techniques for inguinal hernia repair. *Cochrane Database Syst Rev* (1):CD001785, 2003.
17. Amato B, Moja L, Panico S, et al: Shouldice technique versus other open techniques for inguinal hernia repair. *Cochrane Database Syst Rev* (4):CD001543, 2012.
18. Zhao G, Gao P, Ma B, et al: Open mesh techniques for inguinal hernia repair: A meta-analysis of randomized controlled trials. *Ann Surg* 250:35–42, 2009.
19. Schroder DM, Lloyd LR, Boccaccio JE, et al: Inguinal hernia recurrence following preperitoneal Kugel patch repair. *Am Surg* 70:132–136, discussion 136, 2004.
20. EU Hernia Trialists Collaboration: Repair of groin hernia with synthetic mesh: Meta-analysis of randomized controlled trials. *Ann Surg* 235:322–332, 2002.
21. El-Dhuwaib Y, Corless D, Emmett C, et al: Laparoscopic versus open repair of inguinal hernia: A longitudinal cohort study. *Surg Endosc* 27:936–945, 2013.
22. O'Reilly EA, Burke JP, O'Connell PR: A meta-analysis of surgical morbidity and recurrence after laparoscopic and open repair of primary unilateral inguinal hernia. *Ann Surg* 255:846–853, 2012.

23. Wake BL, McCormack K, Fraser C, et al: Transabdominal pre-peritoneal (TAPP) vs totally extraperitoneal (TEP) laparoscopic techniques for inguinal hernia repair. *Cochrane Database Syst Rev* (1):CD004703, 2005.
24. Mikkelsen T, Bay-Nielsen M, Kehlet H: Risk of femoral hernia after inguinal herniorrhaphy. *Br J Surg* 89:486–488, 2002.
25. Kald A, Fridsten S, Nordin P, et al: Outcome of repair of bilateral groin hernias: A prospective evaluation of 1,487 patients. *Eur J Surg* 168:150–153, 2002.
26. Aufenacker TJ, van Geldere D, van Mesdag T, et al: The role of antibiotic prophylaxis in prevention of wound infection after Lichtenstein open mesh repair of primary inguinal hernia: A multicenter double-blind randomized controlled trial. *Ann Surg* 240:955–960, discussion 960–961, 2004.
27. Grant AM, Scott NW, O'Dwyer PJ, et al: Five-year follow-up of a randomized trial to assess pain and numbness after laparoscopic or open repair of groin hernia. *Br J Surg* 91:1570–1574, 2004.
28. Fitzgibbons RJ, Jr, Forse RA: Clinical practice. Groin hernias in adults. *N Engl J Med* 372:756–763, 2015.
29. Simons MP, Aufenacker T, Bay-Nielsen M, et al: European Hernia Society guidelines on the treatment of inguinal hernia in adult patients. *Hernia* 13:343–403, 2009.
30. Shulman AG, Amid PK, Lichtenstein IL: The 'plug' repair of 1402 recurrent inguinal hernias. 20-year experience. *Arch Surg* 125:265–267, 1990.
31. Haapaniemi S, Gunnarsson U, Nordin P, et al: Reoperation after recurrent groin hernia repair. *Ann Surg* 234:122–126, 2001.
32. Karthikesalingam A, Markar SR, Holt PJ, et al: Meta-analysis of randomized controlled trials comparing laparoscopic with open mesh repair of recurrent inguinal hernia. *Br J Surg* 97:4–11, 2010.
33. Sevonius D, Gunnarsson U, Nordin P, et al: Repeated groin hernia recurrences. *Ann Surg* 249:516–518, 2009.
34. Rucinski J, Margolis M, Panagopoulos G, et al: Closure of the abdominal midline fascia: Meta-analysis delineates the optimal technique. *Am Surg* 67:421–426, 2001.
35. Muysoms FE, Antoniou SA, Bury K, et al: European Hernia Society guidelines on the closure of abdominal wall incisions. *Hernia* 19:1–24, 2015.
36. Carlson MA, Ludwig KA, Condon RE: Ventral hernia and other complications of 1,000 midline incisions. *South Med J* 88:450–453, 1995.
37. Seiler CM, Deckert A, Diener MK, et al: Midline versus transverse incision in major abdominal surgery: A randomized, double-blind equivalence trial (POVATI: ISRCTN60734227). *Ann Surg* 249:913–920, 2009.
38. Luijendijk RW, Hop WC, van den Tol MP, et al: A comparison of suture repair with mesh repair for incisional hernia. *N Engl J Med* 343:392–398, 2000.
39. Wright BE, Beckerman J, Cohen M, et al: Is laparoscopic umbilical hernia repair with mesh a reasonable alternative to conventional repair? *Am J Surg* 184:505–508, discussion 508–509, 2002.
40. Petro CC, O'Rourke CP, Posielski NM, et al: Designing a ventral hernia staging system. *Hernia* 2015. [Epub ahead of print].
41. Anthony T, Bergen PC, Kim LT, et al: Factors affecting recurrence following incisional herniorrhaphy. *World J Surg* 24:95–100, discussion 101, 2000.
42. Leber GE, Garb JL, Alexander AI, et al: Long-term complications associated with prosthetic repair of incisional hernias. *Arch Surg* 133:378–382, 1998.
43. Koch A, Bringman S, Myrelid P, et al: Randomized clinical trial of groin hernia repair with titanium-coated lightweight mesh compared with standard polypropylene mesh. *Br J Surg* 95:1226–1231, 2008.
44. Conze J, Kingsnorth AN, Flament JB, et al: Randomized clinical trial comparing lightweight composite mesh with polyester or polypropylene mesh for incisional hernia repair. *Br J Surg* 92:1488–1493, 2005.
45. Petro CC, Nahabet EH, Criss CN, et al: Central failures of lightweight monofilament polyester mesh causing hernia recurrence: A cautionary note. *Hernia* 19:155–159, 2015.
46. Cobb WS, Warren JA, Ewing JA, et al: Open retromuscular mesh repair of complex incisional hernia: Predictors of wound events and recurrence. *J Am Coll Surg* 220:606–613, 2015.
47. Diaz-Godoy A, Garcia-Urena MA, Lopez-Monclus J, et al: Searching for the best polypropylene mesh to be used in bowel contamination. *Hernia* 15:173–179, 2011.
48. Harth KC, Blatnik JA, Anderson JM, et al: Effect of surgical wound classification on biologic graft performance in complex hernia repair: An experimental study. *Surgery* 153:481–492, 2013.
49. Carbonell AM, Criss CN, Cobb WS, et al: Outcomes of synthetic mesh in contaminated ventral hernia repairs. *J Am Coll Surg* 217:991–998, 2013.
50. Rosen MJ: Polyester-based mesh for ventral hernia repair: Is it safe? *Am J Surg* 197:353–359, 2009.
51. Jin J, Rosen MJ, Blatnik J, et al: Use of acellular dermal matrix for complicated ventral hernia repair: Does technique affect outcomes? *J Am Coll Surg* 205:654–660, 2007.
52. Rosen MJ, Krpata DM, Ermlich B, et al: A 5-year clinical experience with single-staged repairs of infected and contaminated abdominal wall defects utilizing biologic mesh. *Ann Surg* 257:991–996, 2013.
53. de Vries Reilingh TS, van Geldere D, Langenhorst B, et al: Repair of large midline incisional hernias with polypropylene mesh: Comparison of three operative techniques. *Hernia* 8:56–59, 2004.
54. Novitsky YW, Porter JR, Rucho ZC, et al: Open preperitoneal retrofascial mesh repair for multiply recurrent ventral incisional hernias. *J Am Coll Surg* 203:283–289, 2006.
55. Krpata DM, Blatnik JA, Novitsky YW, et al: Posterior and open anterior components separations: A comparative analysis. *Am J Surg* 203:318–322, discussion 322, 2012.
56. de Vries Reilingh TS, van Goor H, Charbon JA, et al: Repair of giant midline abdominal wall hernias: "Components separation technique" versus prosthetic repair : Interim analysis of a randomized controlled trial. *World J Surg* 31:756–763, 2007.
57. Ewart CJ, Lankford AB, Gamboa MG: Successful closure of abdominal wall hernias using the components separation technique. *Ann Plast Surg* 50:269–273, discussion 273–274, 2003.
58. Rosen MJ, Jin J, McGee MF, et al: Laparoscopic component separation in the single-stage treatment of infected abdominal wall prosthetic removal. *Hernia* 11:435–440, 2007.
59. Olmi S, Scaini A, Cesana GC, et al: Laparoscopic versus open incisional hernia repair: An open randomized controlled study. *Surg Endosc* 21:555–559, 2007.

60. McGreevy JM, Goodney PP, Birkmeyer CM, et al: A prospective study comparing the complication rates between laparoscopic and open ventral hernia repairs. *Surg Endosc* 17:1778–1780, 2003.
61. Lomanto D, Iyer SG, Shabbir A, et al: Laparoscopic versus open ventral hernia mesh repair: A prospective study. *Surg Endosc* 20:1030–1035, 2006.
62. Bingener J, Buck L, Richards M, et al: Long-term outcomes in laparoscopic vs open ventral hernia repair. *Arch Surg* 142:562–567, 2007.
63. DeMaria EJ, Moss JM, Sugerman HJ: Laparoscopic intraperitoneal polytetrafluoroethylene (PTFE) prosthetic patch repair of ventral hernia. Prospective comparison to open prefascial polypropylene mesh repair. *Surg Endosc* 14:326–329, 2000.
64. Iqbal CW, Pham TH, Joseph A, et al: Long-term outcome of 254 complex incisional hernia repairs using the modified Rives-Stoppa technique. *World J Surg* 31:2398–2404, 2007.
65. McAdory RS, Cobb WS, Carbonell AM: Progressive preoperative pneumoperitoneum for hernias with loss of domain. *Am Surg* 75:504–508, discussion 508–509, 2009.
66. Lipman J, Medalie D, Rosen MJ: Staged repair of massive incisional hernias with loss of abdominal domain: A novel approach. *Am J Surg* 195:84–88, 2008.
67. Taner T, Cima RR, Larson DW, et al: The use of human acellular dermal matrix for parastomal hernia repair in patients with inflammatory bowel disease: A novel technique to repair fascial defects. *Dis Colon Rectum* 52:349–354, 2009.
68. Sugarbaker PH: Peritoneal approach to prosthetic mesh repair of paraostomy hernias. *Ann Surg* 201:344–346, 1985.
69. Byers JM, Steinberg JB, Postier RG: Repair of parastomal hernias using polypropylene mesh. *Arch Surg* 127:1246–1247, 1992.
70. Janes A, Cengiz Y, Israelsson LA: Randomized clinical trial of the use of a prosthetic mesh to prevent parastomal hernia. *Br J Surg* 91:280–282, 2004.
71. Raigani S, Criss CN, Petro CC, et al: Single-center experience with parastomal hernia repair using retromuscular mesh placement. *J Gastrointest Surg* 18:1673–1677, 2014.
72. Heniford BT, Park A, Ramshaw BJ, et al: Laparoscopic repair of ventral hernias: Nine years' experience with 850 consecutive hernias. *Ann Surg* 238:391–399, discussion 399–400, 2003.
73. Pring CM, Tran V, O'Rourke N, et al: Laparoscopic versus open ventral hernia repair: A randomized controlled trial. *ANZ J Surg* 78:903–906, 2008.
74. Asencio F, Aguilo J, Peiro S, et al: Open randomized clinical trial of laparoscopic versus open incisional hernia repair. *Surg Endosc* 23:1441–1448, 2009.

45 CHAPTER

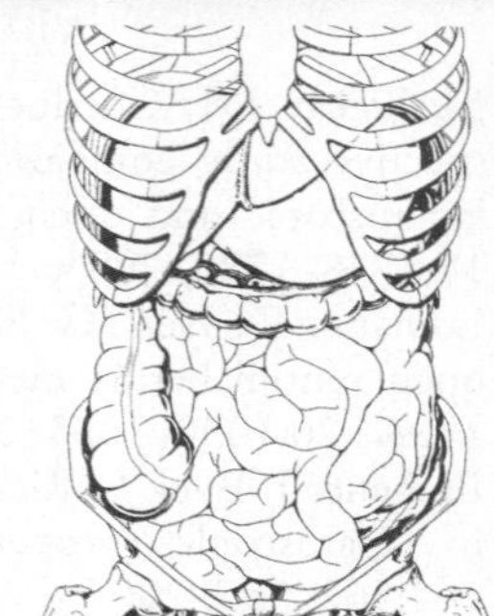

Acute Abdomen

Ronald Squires, Steven N. Carter, Russell G. Postier

OUTLINE

The term *acute abdomen* refers to signs and symptoms of abdominal pain and tenderness, a clinical presentation that often requires emergency surgical therapy. This challenging clinical scenario requires a thorough and expeditious workup to determine the need for operative intervention and to initiate appropriate therapy. Many diseases, some of which are not surgical or even intra-abdominal,[1] can produce acute abdominal pain and tenderness. Therefore, every attempt should be made to make a correct diagnosis so that the chosen therapy, often a laparoscopy or laparotomy, is appropriate. Despite improvements in laboratory and imaging studies, history and physical examination remain the mainstays of determining the correct diagnosis and initiating proper and timely therapy.

The diagnoses associated with an acute abdomen vary according to age and gender.[2] Appendicitis is more common in the young, whereas biliary disease, bowel obstruction, intestinal ischemia and infarction, and diverticulitis are more common in the elderly. Most of these diagnoses result from infection, obstruction, ischemia, or perforation.

Nonsurgical causes of an acute abdomen can be divided into three categories: endocrine and metabolic, hematologic, and toxins or drugs (Box 45-1).[3] Endocrine and metabolic causes include uremia, diabetic crisis, addisonian crisis, acute intermittent porphyria, acute hyperlipoproteinemia, and hereditary Mediterranean fever. Hematologic disorders are sickle cell crisis, acute leukemia, and other blood dyscrasias. Toxins and drugs causing an acute abdomen include lead and other heavy metal poisoning, narcotic withdrawal, and black widow spider poisoning. It is important to keep these possibilities in mind when evaluating a patient with acute abdominal pain (Box 45-1).

Because of the potential surgical nature of the acute abdomen, an expeditious workup is necessary (Box 45-2). The workup proceeds in the usual order of history, physical examination, and laboratory and imaging studies. Whereas imaging studies have increased the accuracy with which the correct diagnosis can be made, the most important part of the evaluation remains a thorough history and careful physical examination. Laboratory and imaging studies, although usually needed, are directed by the findings on history and physical examination.

ANATOMY AND PHYSIOLOGY

Abdominal pain is conveniently divided into visceral and parietal components. Visceral pain tends to be vague and poorly localized to the epigastrium, periumbilical region, or hypogastrium, depending on its origin from the primitive foregut, midgut, or hindgut (Fig. 45-1). It is usually the result of distention of a hollow viscus. Parietal pain corresponds to the segmental nerve roots innervating the peritoneum and tends to be sharper and better localized. Referred pain is pain perceived at a site distant from the source of stimulus. For example, irritation of the diaphragm may produce pain in the shoulder. Common referred pain sites and their accompanying sources are listed in Box 45-3. Determining whether the pain is visceral, parietal, or referred is important and can usually be done with a careful history.

Introduction of bacteria or irritating chemicals into the peritoneal cavity can cause an outpouring of fluid from the peritoneal membrane. The peritoneum responds to inflammation by increased blood flow, increased permeability, and the formation of a fibrinous exudate on its surface. The bowel also develops local or generalized paralysis. The fibrinous surface and decreased intestinal movement cause adherence between the bowel and omentum or abdominal wall and help to localize inflammation. As a result, an abscess may produce sharply localized pain with normal bowel sounds and gastrointestinal function, whereas a diffuse process, such as a perforated duodenal ulcer, produces generalized abdominal pain with a quiet abdomen. Peritonitis may affect the entire abdominal cavity or a portion of the visceral or parietal peritoneum.

Peritonitis is peritoneal inflammation from any cause. It is usually recognized on physical examination by severe tenderness to palpation, with or without rebound tenderness, and guarding. Peritonitis is usually secondary to an inflammatory insult, most

BOX 45-1 Nonsurgical Causes of the Acute Abdomen

Endocrine and Metabolic Causes
Uremia
Diabetic crisis
Addisonian crisis
Acute intermittent porphyria
Hereditary Mediterranean fever

Hematologic Causes
Sickle cell crisis
Acute leukemia
Other blood dyscrasias

Toxins and Drugs
Lead poisoning
Other heavy metal poisoning
Narcotic withdrawal
Black widow spider poisoning

often gram-negative infections with enteric organisms or anaerobes. It can result from noninfectious inflammation, a common example being pancreatitis. Primary peritonitis occurs more commonly in children and is most often due to pneumococcus or hemolytic streptococcus.[4] Adults with end-stage renal disease on peritoneal dialysis can develop infections of their peritoneal fluid, with the most common organisms being gram-positive cocci. Adults with ascites and cirrhosis can develop primary peritonitis, and in these cases the organisms are usually *Escherichia coli* and *Klebsiella*.

HISTORY

A detailed and organized history is essential to formulating an accurate differential diagnosis and subsequent treatment regimen. Modern advancements in imaging cannot and will never replace the need for a skilled clinician's careful history and bedside examination. The history must focus not only on the investigation of the pain complaints but also on past problems and associated symptoms as well. Questions should be open ended whenever possible and structured to disclose the onset, character, location, duration, radiation, and chronology of the pain experienced. It is tempting to ask a question such as, Is the pain sharp? or Does eating make it worse? This specific yes or no style can speed up the history taking by not allowing the patient to narrate, but it stands to miss vital details and potentially to skew the responses. A much better questioning style would be, How does the pain feel to you? or Does anything make the pain better or worse? Often, additional information can be gained by observing how the patient describes the pain that is experienced. Pain identified with one finger is often much more localized and typical of parietal innervation or peritoneal inflammation compared with an area of discomfort illustrated with the palm of the hand, which is more typical of the visceral discomfort of bowel or solid organ disease.

The intensity and severity of the pain are related to the underlying tissue damage. Sudden onset of excruciating pain suggests conditions such as intestinal perforation and arterial embolization with ischemia, although other conditions, such as biliary colic, can be manifested suddenly as well. Pain that develops and worsens during several hours is typical of conditions of progressive inflammation or infection, such as cholecystitis, colitis, and bowel obstruction. The history of progressive worsening versus intermittent episodes of pain can help differentiate infectious processes that worsen with time compared with the spasmodic colicky pain associated with bowel obstruction, biliary colic from cystic duct obstruction, or genitourinary obstruction (Figs. 45-2 to 45-4). Equally important as the character of the pain is its location and radiation. Tissue injury or inflammation can trigger both visceral and somatic pain. Solid organ visceral pain in the abdomen is generalized in the quadrant of the involved organ, such as liver pain across the right upper quadrant of the abdomen. Small bowel pain is perceived as poorly localized periumbilical pain, whereas colon pain is centered between the umbilicus and the pubic symphysis. As inflammation expands to involve the peritoneal surface,

BOX 45-2 Surgical Acute Abdominal Conditions

Hemorrhage
Solid organ trauma
Leaking or ruptured arterial aneurysm
Ruptured ectopic pregnancy
Bleeding gastrointestinal diverticulum
Arteriovenous malformation of gastrointestinal tract
Intestinal ulceration
Aortoduodenal fistula after aortic vascular graft
Hemorrhagic pancreatitis
Mallory-Weiss syndrome
Spontaneous rupture of spleen

Infection
Appendicitis
Cholecystitis
Meckel's diverticulitis
Hepatic abscess
Diverticular abscess
Psoas abscess

Perforation
Perforated gastrointestinal ulcer
Perforated gastrointestinal cancer
Boerhaave syndrome
Perforated diverticulum

Blockage
Adhesion induction small or large bowel obstruction
Sigmoid volvulus
Cecal volvulus
Incarcerated hernias
Inflammatory bowel disease
Gastrointestinal malignant neoplasm
Intussusception

Ischemia
Buerger disease
Mesenteric thrombosis or embolism
Ovarian torsion
Ischemic colitis
Testicular torsion
Strangulated hernias

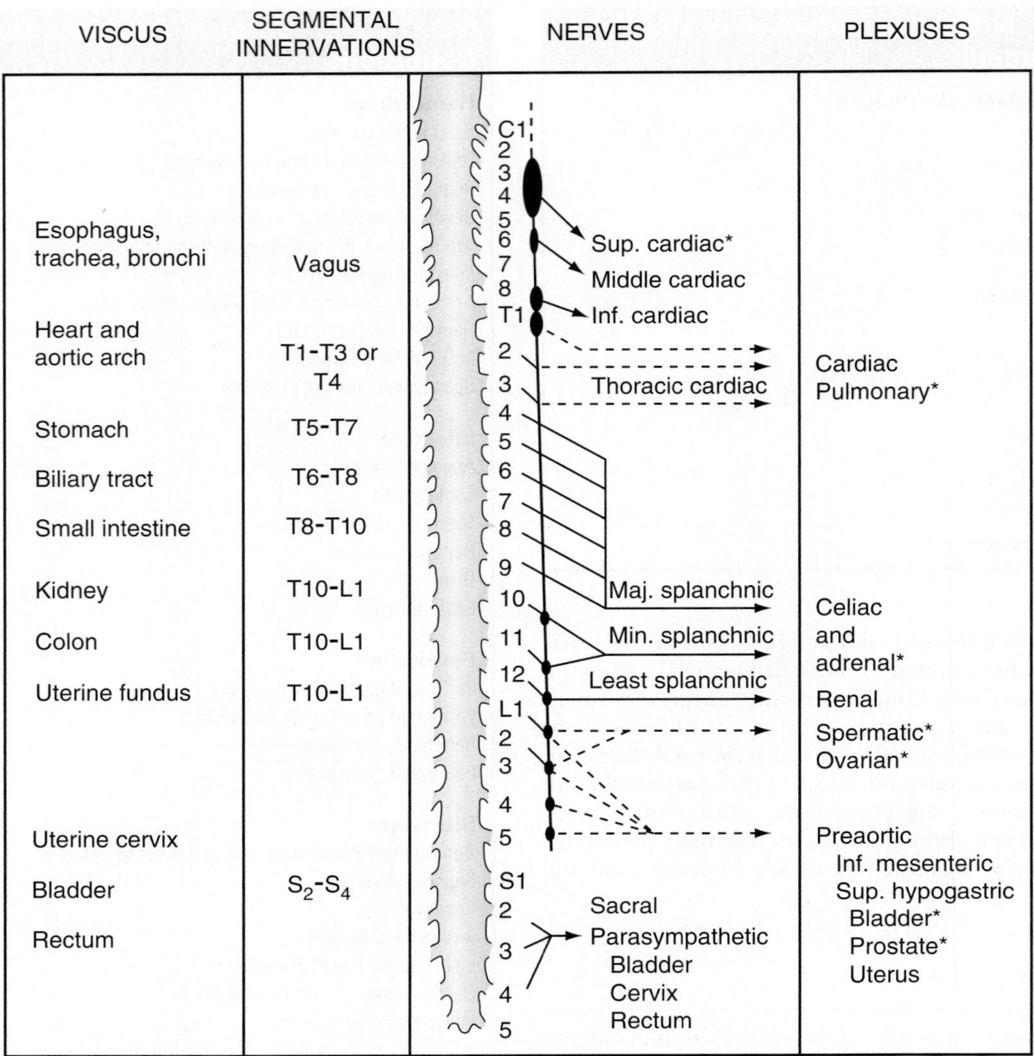

FIGURE 45-1 Sensory innervation of the viscera. (From White JC, Sweet WH: *Pain and the neurosurgeon*, Springfield, Ill, 1969, Charles C Thomas, p 526.)

parietal nerve fibers from the spine allow focal and intense sensation. This combination of innervation is responsible for the classic diffuse periumbilical pain of early appendicitis that later shifts to become an intense focal pain in the right lower abdomen at McBurney point. If clinicians focus on the character of the current pain and do not thoroughly investigate its onset and progression, they will miss these strong historical clues (Figs. 45-5 and 45-6). Pain may also extend well beyond the diseased site. The liver shares some of its innervation with the diaphragm and may create referred pain to the right shoulder from the C3-C5 nerve roots. Genitourinary pain is another source of pain that commonly has a radiating pattern. Symptoms are primarily in the flank region originating from the splanchnic nerves of T11-L1, but pain often radiates to the scrotum or labia through the hypogastric plexus of S2-S4.

Activities that exacerbate or relieve the pain are also important. Eating will often worsen the pain of bowel obstruction, biliary colic, pancreatitis, diverticulitis, or bowel perforation. Food can provide relief from the pain of nonperforated peptic ulcer disease or gastritis. Clinicians will often recognize that they are evaluating

BOX 45-3 Locations of Referred Pain and Its Causes

Right Shoulder
Liver
Gallbladder
Right hemidiaphragm

Left Shoulder
Heart
Tail of pancreas
Spleen
Left hemidiaphragm

Scrotum and Testicles
Ureter

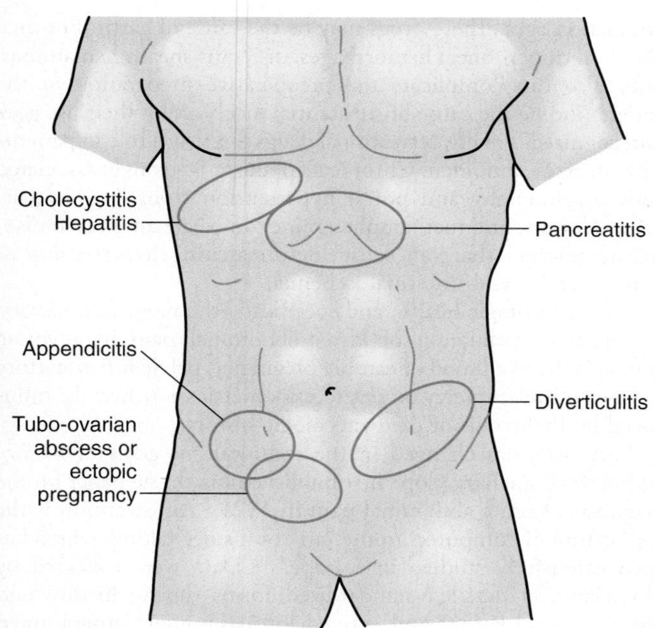

FIGURE 45-2 Character of pain: gradual, progressive pain.

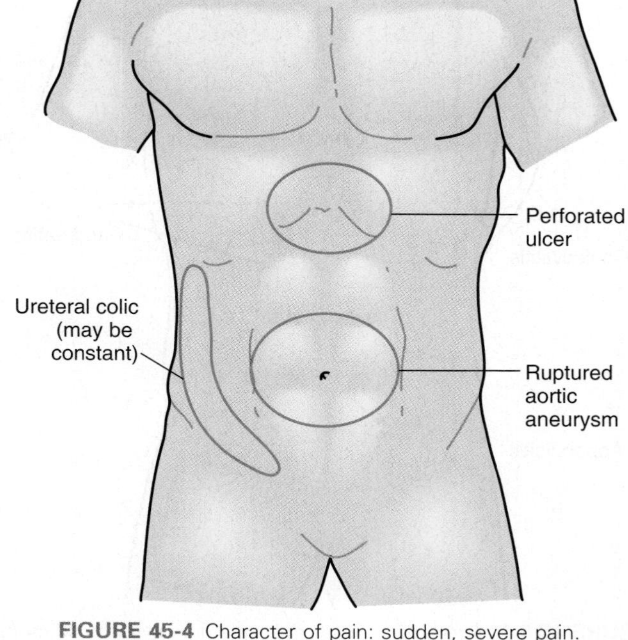

FIGURE 45-4 Character of pain: sudden, severe pain.

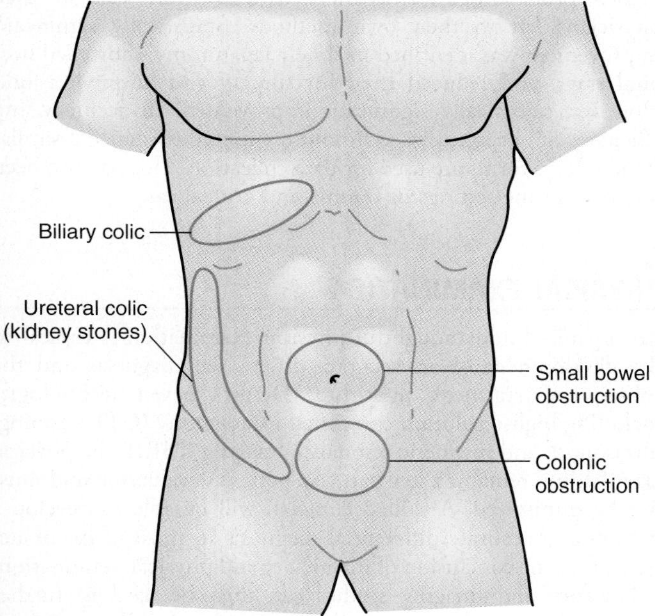

FIGURE 45-3 Character of pain: colicky, crampy, intermittent pain.

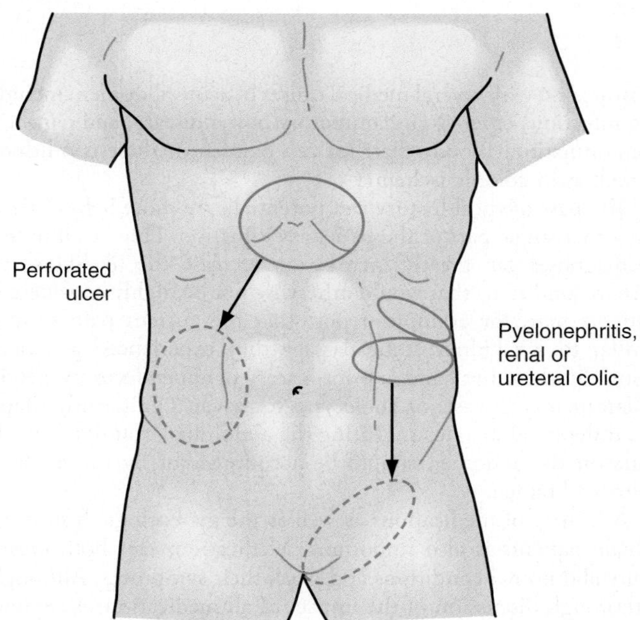

FIGURE 45-5 Referred pain. *Solid circles* are primary or most intense sites of pain.

peritonitis during the history. Patients with peritoneal inflammation will avoid any activity that stretches or jostles the abdomen. They describe worsening of the pain with any sudden body movement and will realize that there is less pain if their knees are flexed. The car ride to the hospital can be agonizing, with the patient feeling every bump along the way.

Associated symptoms can be important clues to the diagnosis. Nausea, vomiting, constipation, diarrhea, pruritus, melena, hematochezia, and hematuria can all be helpful symptoms if they are present and recognized. Vomiting may occur because of severe abdominal pain of any cause or as a result of mechanical bowel obstruction or ileus. Vomiting is more likely to precede the onset of significant abdominal pain in many medical conditions, whereas the pain of an acute surgical abdomen is manifested first and stimulates vomiting through medullary efferent fibers that are triggered by the visceral afferent pain fibers. Constipation or obstipation can be a result of either mechanical obstruction or decreased peristalsis. It may represent the primary problem and require laxatives and prokinetic agents or merely be a symptom of an underlying condition. A careful history should include whether the patient is continuing to pass any gas or stool from the rectum. A complete obstruction is more likely to be associated with subsequent bowel ischemia or perforation related to either massive distention or a closed loop of small bowel that can occur. Diarrhea

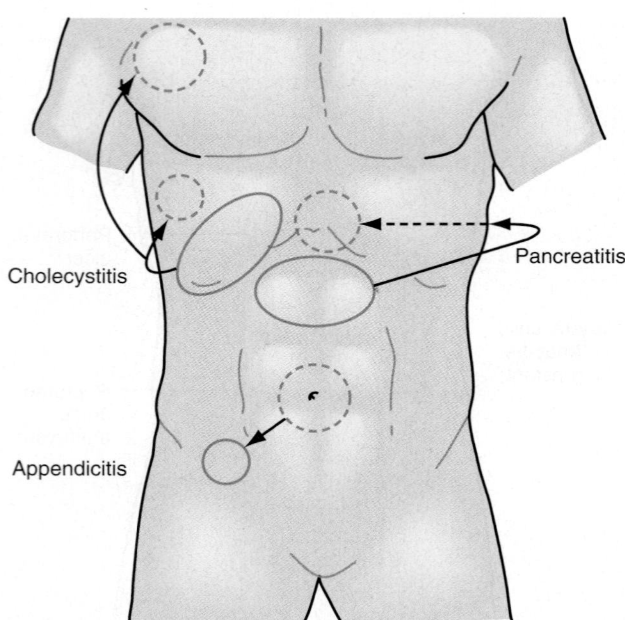

FIGURE 45-6 Referred pain. *Solid circles* are primary or most intense sites of pain.

is associated with several medical causes of acute abdomen, including infectious enteritis, inflammatory bowel disease, and parasitic contamination. Bloody diarrhea can be seen in these conditions as well as in colonic ischemia.

The past medical history can potentially be more helpful than any other single part of the patient's evaluation. Previous illnesses or diagnoses can greatly increase or decrease the likelihood of certain conditions that would otherwise not be highly considered. Patients may, for example, report that the current pain is very similar to the kidney stone passage they experienced a decade prior. On the other hand, a prior history of appendectomy, pelvic inflammatory disease, or cholecystectomy can significantly shape the differential diagnosis. During the abdominal examination, all scars on the abdomen should be accounted for by the medical history obtained.

A history of medications as well as the gynecologic history of female patients is also important. Medications can both create acute abdominal conditions and mask their symptoms. Although a thorough discussion of the impact of all medications is beyond the scope of this chapter, several common drug classes deserve mention. High-dose narcotic use can interfere with bowel activity and lead to obstipation and obstruction. Narcotics also can contribute to spasm of the sphincter of Oddi and exacerbate biliary or pancreatic pain. Clearly, they also may suppress pain sensation and alter mental status, which can impair the ability to accurately diagnose the condition. Nonsteroidal anti-inflammatory agents are associated with an increased risk of upper gastrointestinal inflammation and perforation, whereas steroid medications can block protective gastric mucus production by chief cells and reduce the inflammatory reaction to infection, including advanced peritonitis. Immunosuppressant agents as a class both increase a patient's risk of acquiring a variety of bacterial or viral illnesses and also blunt the inflammatory response, diminishing the pain that is present and the overall physiologic response. Anticoagulants are much more prevalent in our emergency patients as the population ages. These drugs may be the cause of gastrointestinal bleeds, retroperitoneal hemorrhages, or rectus sheath hematomas. They also can complicate the preoperative preparation of the patient and be the cause of substantial morbidity if their use goes unrecognized. Finally, recreational drugs can play a role in patients with an acute abdomen. Chronic alcoholism is strongly associated with coagulopathy and portal hypertension from liver impairment. Cocaine and methamphetamine can create an intense vasospastic reaction that can cause life-threatening hypertension as well as cardiac and intestinal ischemia.

The gynecologic health, and specifically the menstrual history, is crucial in evaluation of lower abdominal pain in a young woman. The likelihood of ectopic pregnancy, pelvic inflammatory disease, mittelschmerz, or severe endometriosis is heavily influenced by the details of the gynecologic history.

Very little has changed in the technique or goals of history taking since Zachary Cope first published his classic paper on the diagnosis of acute abdominal pain in 1921.[5] An exception is the application of computers to the "art" of history taking, which has been extensively studied in Europe.[6-10] Data were collected by physicians on detailed standardized forms during history and physical examinations and entered into computers programmed with a medical database of diseases and their associated signs and symptoms. The computer-generated diagnosis based on mathematical probabilities was as much as 20% more accurate than physicians left to their own methods. Statistically significant improvement was identified in timely laparotomy, shortened hospital stays, and reduced need for surgery and hospitalization.[6] However, statistically significant improvement in accuracy and efficiency has been realized without computer assistance if similar standardized forms are used for data collection. This has also been observed in the settings of trauma and critical care.

PHYSICAL EXAMINATION

An organized and thoughtful physical examination is critical to the development of an accurate differential diagnosis and the subsequent treatment algorithm. Despite newer technologies including high-resolution computed tomography (CT) scanning, ultrasound, and magnetic resonance imaging (MRI), the physical examination remains a key part of a patient's evaluation and must not be minimized. A skilled clinician will be able to develop a narrow and accurate differential diagnosis in most of his or her patients at the conclusion of the history and physical examination. Laboratory and imaging studies can then be used to further confirm the suspicions, to reorder the proposed differential diagnosis, or, less commonly, to suggest unusual possibilities not yet considered.

The physical examination should always begin with a general inspection of the patient to be followed by inspection of the abdomen itself. Patients with peritoneal irritation will experience worsened pain with any activity that moves or stretches the peritoneum. These patients will typically lie very still in the bed during the evaluation and often maintain flexion of their knees and hips to reduce tension on the anterior abdominal wall. Disease states that cause pain without peritoneal irritation, such as ischemic bowel or ureteral or biliary colic, typically cause patients to continually shift and fidget in bed while trying to find a position that lessens their discomfort (Fig. 45-7). Other important clues, such as pallor, cyanosis, and diaphoresis, may be observed during the general inspection as well.

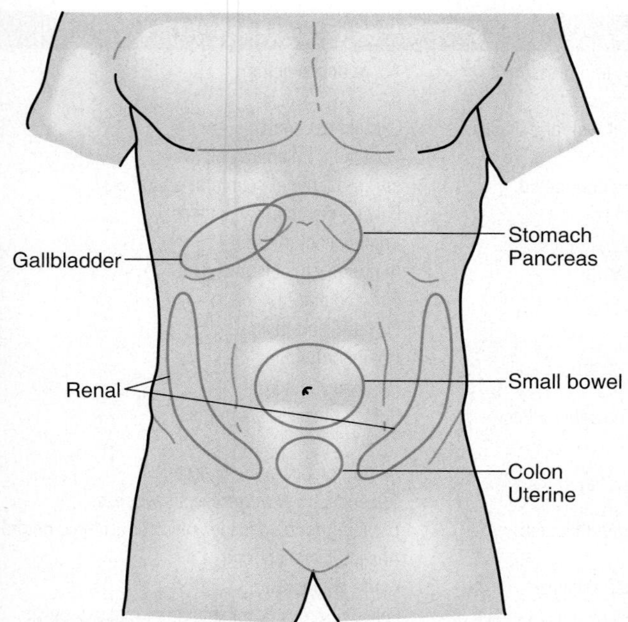

FIGURE 45-7 Common locations for visceral pain.

Abdominal inspection should address the contour of the abdomen, including whether it appears distended or scaphoid and whether a localized mass effect is observed. Special attention should be paid to all scars present; if they are surgical in nature, they should correlate with the past surgical history provided. Fascial hernias may be suspected and can be confirmed during palpation of the abdominal wall. Evidence of erythema or edema of skin may suggest cellulitis of the abdominal wall; ecchymosis is sometimes observed with deeper necrotizing infections of the fascia or abdominal structures, such as the pancreas.

Auscultation can provide useful information about the gastrointestinal tract and the vascular system. Bowel sounds are typically evaluated for their quantity and quality. A quiet abdomen suggests an ileus, whereas hyperactive bowel sounds are found in enteritis and early ischemic intestine. The pitch and pattern of the sounds are also considered. Mechanical bowel obstruction is characterized by high-pitched tinkling sounds that tend to come in rushes and are associated with pain. Far-away echoing sounds are often present when significant luminal distention exists. Bruits heard within the abdomen reflect turbulent blood flow within the vascular system. These are most frequently encountered in the setting of high-grade arterial stenoses of 70% to 95% but can also be heard if an arteriovenous fistula is present. The clinician can also subtly test for the location and degree of pain during the auscultatory examination by varying the position and amount of pressure applied with the stethoscope. These data can then be compared with the findings during palpation and evaluated for consistency. Even though few patients will intentionally try to deceive the physician, some may exaggerate their pain complaints so as not to be disregarded or taken lightly.

Percussion is used to assess for gaseous distention of the bowel, free intra-abdominal air, degree of ascites, or presence of peritoneal inflammation. Hyperresonance, commonly referred to as tympany to percussion, is characteristic of underlying gas-filled loops of bowel. In the setting of bowel obstruction or ileus, this tympany is heard throughout all but the right upper quadrant where the liver lies beneath the abdominal wall. If localized dullness to percussion is identified anywhere other than the right upper quadrant, an abdominal mass displacing the bowel should be considered. When liver dullness is lost and resonance is uniform throughout, free intra-abdominal air should be suspected. This air rises and collects beneath the anterior abdominal wall when the patient is in a supine position. Ascites is detected by looking for fluctuance of the abdominal cavity. A fluid wave or ripple can be generated by a quick firm compression of the lateral abdomen. The resulting wave should then travel across the abdominal wall. Movement of adipose tissue in the obese abdomen can be mistaken for a fluid wave. False-positive examinations can be reduced by first pressing the ulnar surface of the examiner's open palm into the midline soft tissue of the abdominal wall to minimize any movement of the fatty tissue while generating the wave with the opposite hand.

Peritonitis is also assessed by percussion. Older, traditional writings teach a technique of deep compression of the abdominal wall followed by abrupt release. This practice is excruciating in the setting of peritoneal inflammation and can create significant discomfort even in its absence. More sensitive and reliable methods can and should be used. Firmly tapping the iliac crest, the flank, or the heel of an extended leg will jar the abdominal viscera and elicit characteristic pain when peritonitis is present.

The final major step in the abdominal examination is palpation. Palpation typically provides more information than any other single component of the abdominal examination. In addition to revealing the severity and exact location of the abdominal pain, palpation can further confirm the presence of peritonitis as well as identify organomegaly or an abnormal mass lesion. Palpation should always begin gently and away from the reported area of pain. If considerable pain is induced at the outset of palpation, the patient is likely to voluntarily guard and continue to do so, limiting the information obtained. Involuntary guarding, or abdominal wall muscle spasm, is a sign of peritonitis and must be distinguished from voluntary guarding. To accomplish this, the examiner applies consistent pressure to the abdominal wall away from the point of maximal pain while asking the patient to take a slow, deep breath. In the setting of voluntary guarding, the abdominal muscles will relax during the act of inspiration; if guarding is involuntary, they remain spastic and tense.

Pain, when focal, suggests an early or well-localized disease process; diffuse pain on palpation is present with extensive inflammation or late presentations. If pain is diffuse, careful investigation should be carried out to determine where the pain is greatest. Even in the setting of extreme contamination from perforated peptic ulcers or colonic diverticula, the site of maximal tenderness often points to the underlying source.

Numerous unique physical findings have come to be associated with specific disease conditions and are well described as examination "signs" (Table 45-1). Murphy sign of acute cholecystitis results when inspiration during palpation of the right upper quadrant results in sudden worsening of pain because of descent of the liver and gallbladder toward the examiner's hand. Several signs help to localize the site of underlying peritonitis, including the obturator sign, the psoas sign, and Rovsing sign. Others, such as Fothergill sign and Carnett sign, help distinguish intra-abdominal disease from that of the abdominal wall.

Digital rectal examination needs to be performed in all patients with acute abdominal pain, checking for the presence of a mass, pelvic pain, or intraluminal blood. A pelvic examination should be included in all women in evaluating pain located below the umbilicus. Gynecologic and adnexal processes are best characterized by a thorough speculum and bimanual evaluation.

TABLE 45-1 Abdominal Examination Signs

Sign	Description	Condition
Aaron sign	Pain or pressure in epigastrium or anterior chest with persistent firm pressure applied to McBurney point	Acute appendicitis
Bassler sign	Sharp pain created by compressing appendix between abdominal wall and iliacus	Chronic appendicitis
Blumberg sign	Transient abdominal wall rebound tenderness	Peritoneal inflammation
Carnett sign	Loss of abdominal tenderness when abdominal wall muscles are contracted	Intra-abdominal source of abdominal pain
Chandelier sign	Extreme lower abdominal and pelvic pain with movement of cervix	Pelvic inflammatory disease
Charcot sign	Intermittent right upper abdominal pain, jaundice, and fever	Choledocholithiasis
Claybrook sign	Accentuation of breath and cardiac sounds through abdominal wall	Ruptured abdominal viscus
Courvoisier sign	Palpable gallbladder in presence of jaundice	Periampullary tumor
Cruveilhier sign	Varicose veins at umbilicus (caput medusae)	Portal hypertension
Cullen sign	Periumbilical bruising	Hemoperitoneum
Danforth sign	Shoulder pain on inspiration	Hemoperitoneum
Fothergill sign	Abdominal wall mass that does not cross midline and remains palpable when rectus is contracted	Rectus muscle hematomas
Grey Turner sign	Local areas of discoloration around umbilicus and flanks	Acute hemorrhagic pancreatitis
Iliopsoas sign	Elevation and extension of leg against resistance create pain	Appendicitis with retrocecal abscess
Kehr sign	Left shoulder pain when supine and pressure placed on left upper abdomen	Hemoperitoneum (especially from splenic origin)
Mannkopf sign	Increased pulse when painful abdomen is palpated	Absent if malingering
Murphy sign	Pain caused by inspiration while applying pressure to right upper abdomen	Acute cholecystitis
Obturator sign	Flexion with external rotation of right thigh while supine creates hypogastric pain	Pelvic abscess or inflammatory mass in pelvis
Ransohoff sign	Yellow discoloration of umbilical region	Ruptured common bile duct
Rovsing sign	Pain at McBurney point when compressing the left lower abdomen	Acute appendicitis
ten Horn sign	Pain caused by gentle traction of right testicle	Acute appendicitis

LABORATORY STUDIES

A number of laboratory studies are considered routine in the evaluation of a patient with an acute abdomen (Box 45-4). They help confirm that inflammation or an infection is present and also aid in the elimination of some of the most common nonsurgical conditions. A complete blood count with differential is valuable as most but not all patients with an acute abdomen will have either a leukocytosis or bandemia. Serum electrolyte, blood urea nitrogen, and creatinine measurements will assist in evaluating the effect of such factors as vomiting and third space fluid losses. In addition, they may suggest an endocrine or metabolic diagnosis as the cause of the patient's problem. Serum amylase and lipase determinations may suggest pancreatitis as the cause of the abdominal pain, but levels can also be elevated in other disorders, such as small bowel infarction and duodenal ulcer perforation. Normal serum amylase and lipase levels do not exclude pancreatitis as a possible diagnosis because of the effects of chronic inflammation on enzyme production and timing factors. Liver function tests including total and direct bilirubin, serum aminotransferase, and alkaline phosphatase are helpful in evaluating potential biliary tract causes of acute abdominal pain. Lactate levels and arterial blood gas determinations can be helpful in diagnosis of intestinal ischemia or infarction. Urine testing, such as urinalysis, is helpful in the diagnosis of bacterial cystitis, pyelonephritis, and certain endocrine abnormalities, such as diabetes and renal parenchymal disease. Urine culture, although it can confirm a suspected urinary tract infection and direct antibiotic therapy, is not available in time to be helpful in the evaluation of an acute abdomen. Urinary measurements of human chorionic gonadotropin can either suggest pregnancy as a confounding factor in the patient's presentation or aid in decision making about therapy. The fetus of a pregnant patient with an acute abdomen is best protected by providing the best care to the mother, including an operation if indicated.[11] Stool testing for occult blood can be helpful in the evaluation of these patients but is nonspecific. Stool for ova and parasite evaluation as well as culture and toxin assay for *Clostridium difficile* can be helpful if diarrhea is a component of the patient's presentation.

BOX 45-4 Helpful Laboratory Studies in the Acute Abdomen

- Hemoglobin
- White blood cell count with differential
- Electrolyte, blood urea nitrogen, and creatinine concentrations
- Urinalysis
- Urine human chorionic gonadotropin
- Amylase and lipase levels
- Total and direct bilirubin concentration
- Alkaline phosphatase
- Serum aminotransferase
- Serum lactate levels
- Stool for ova and parasites
- *C. difficile* culture and toxin assay

IMAGING STUDIES

Improvements in imaging techniques, especially multidetector CT scans, have revolutionized the diagnosis of the acute abdomen. The most difficult diagnostic dilemmas of the past, appendicitis in young women and ischemic bowel in the elderly, can now be diagnosed with much greater certainty and speed (Figs. 45-8 and 45-9).[12-14] This has resulted in more rapid operative correction of the problem with less morbidity and mortality. Despite its

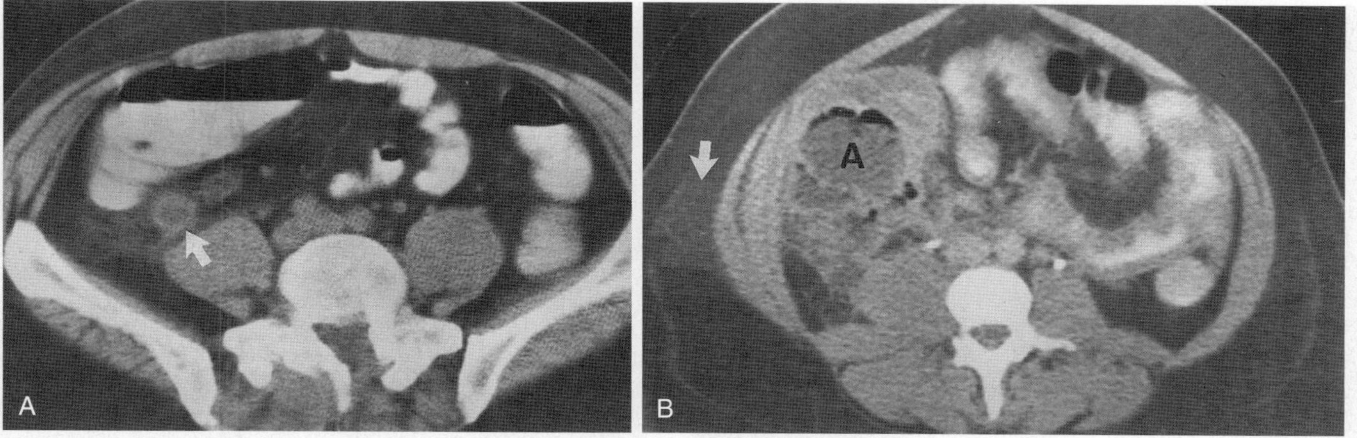

FIGURE 45-8 Appendicitis. A, CT scan of uncomplicated appendicitis. A thick-walled, distended, retrocecal appendix *(arrow)* is seen with inflammatory change in the surrounding fat. **B,** CT scan of complicated appendicitis. A retrocecal appendiceal abscess (A) with an associated phlegmon posteriorly found in a 3-week postpartum, obese woman. Inflammatory change extends through the flank musculature into the subcutaneous fat *(arrow).*

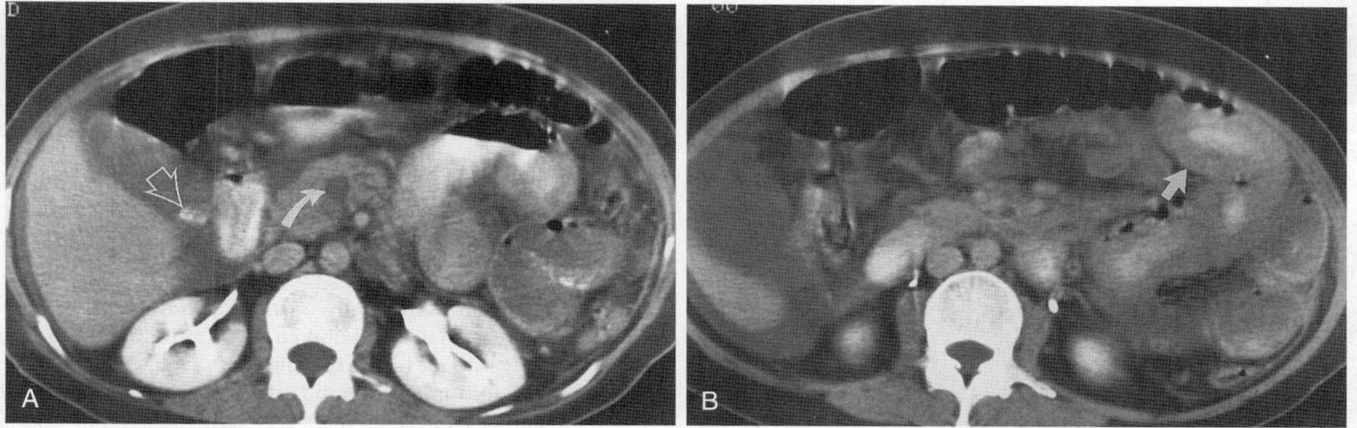

FIGURE 45-9 Small bowel infarction associated with mesenteric venous thrombosis. **A,** Note the low-density thrombosed superior mesenteric vein *(solid arrow)* and incidental gallstones *(open arrow)*. **B,** Thickening of proximal small bowel wall *(arrow)* coincided with several feet of infarcting small bowel at time of operation.

usefulness, CT is not the only imaging technique available and is also not the first step in imaging for most patients. In addition, none of the imaging techniques take the place of a careful history and physical examination.

Plain radiographs continue to play a role in imaging in patients with acute abdominal pain. Upright chest radiographs can detect as little as 1 mL of air injected into the peritoneal cavity. Lateral decubitus abdominal radiographs can also detect pneumoperitoneum effectively in patients who cannot stand. As little as 5 to 10 mL of gas may be detected with this technique.[15] These studies are particularly helpful in patients suspected of having a perforated duodenal ulcer as about 75% of these patients will have a large enough pneumoperitoneum to be visible (Fig. 45-10).[16] This obviates the need for further evaluation in most patients, allowing laparotomy with little delay.

Plain films also show abnormal calcifications. Approximately 5% of appendicoliths, 10% of gallstones, and 90% of renal stones contain sufficient amounts of calcium to be radiopaque. Pancreatic calcifications seen in many patients with chronic pancreatitis are visible on plain films, as are the calcifications in abdominal aortic aneurysms, visceral artery aneurysm, and atherosclerosis in visceral vessels.

Upright and supine abdominal radiographs are helpful in identifying gastric outlet obstruction and obstruction of the proximal, mid, or distal small bowel. They can also aid in determining whether a small bowel obstruction is complete or partial by the presence or absence of gas in the colon. Colonic gas can be differentiated from small intestinal gas by the presence of haustral markings from the taeniae coli in the colonic wall. Obstructed colon appears as distended bowel with haustral markings (Fig. 45-11). Associated distention of small bowel may also be present, especially if the ileocecal valve is incompetent. Plain films can also suggest volvulus of either the cecum or sigmoid colon. Cecal volvulus is identified by a distended loop of colon in a comma shape with the concavity facing inferiorly and to the right. Sigmoid volvulus characteristically has the appearance of a bent inner tube with its apex in the right upper quadrant (Fig. 45-12).

Abdominal ultrasonography is extremely accurate in detecting gallstones and in assessing gallbladder wall thickness and the presence of fluid around the gallbladder.[17] It is also good at

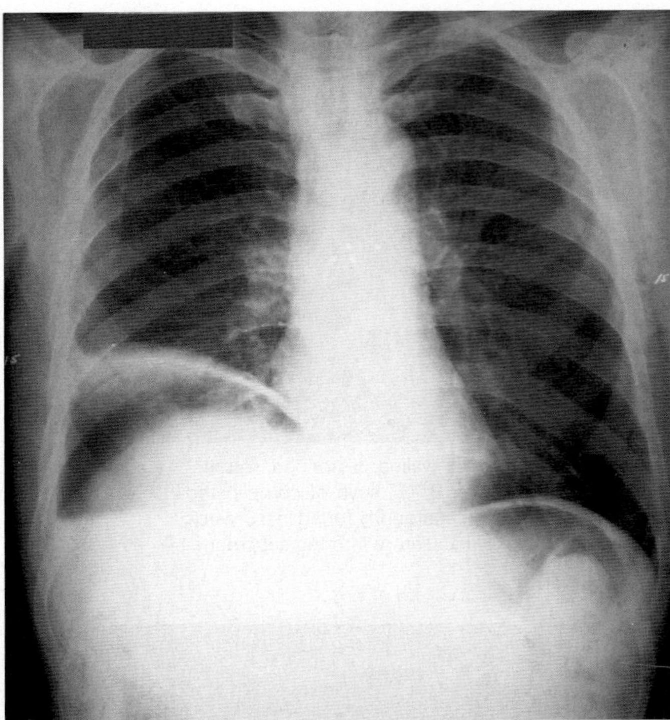

FIGURE 45-10 Upright chest radiograph depicting moderate-sized pneumoperitoneum consistent with perforation of abdominal viscus.

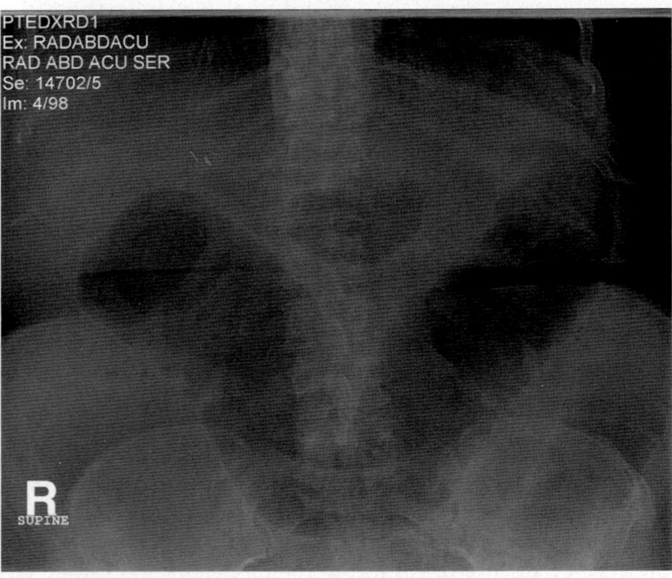

FIGURE 45-11 Upright abdominal radiograph in a patient with an obstructing sigmoid adenocarcinoma. Note the haustral markings on the dilated transverse colon that distinguished this from small intestine.

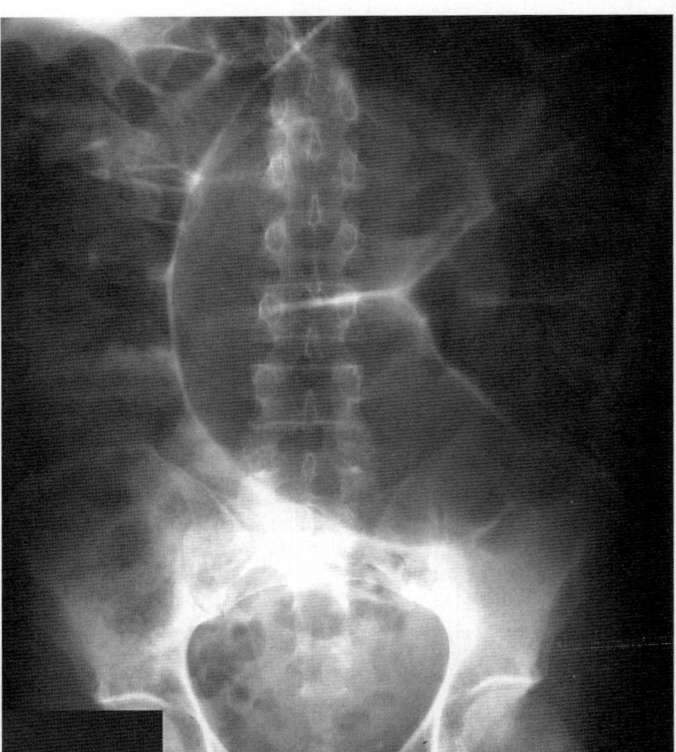

FIGURE 45-12 Upright abdominal radiograph in a patient with a sigmoid colon volvulus. Note the characteristic appearance of a bent inner tube with its apex in the right upper quadrant.

determining the diameter of the extrahepatic and intrahepatic bile ducts. Its usefulness in detecting common bile duct stones is limited. Abdominal and transvaginal ultrasonography can aid in the detection of abnormalities of the ovaries, adnexa, and uterus. Ultrasound can also detect intraperitoneal fluid. The presence of abnormal amounts of intestinal air in most patients with an acute abdomen limits the ability of ultrasonography to evaluate the pancreas or other abdominal organs. There are important limits to the value of ultrasonography in the diagnosis of diseases that are manifested as an acute abdomen. Ultrasound has been found to be clinically inferior to CT scanning for the diagnosis of appendicitis.[18] In addition, ultrasound images are more difficult for most surgeons to interpret than are plain radiographs and CT images. Many hospitals have radiologic technologists available at all times to perform CT, but this is often not the case with ultrasonography. As CT has become more widely available and less likely to be hindered by abdominal air, it is becoming the secondary imaging modality of choice in the patient with an acute abdomen, following plain abdominal radiographs.

A number of studies have demonstrated the accuracy and utility of CT of the abdomen and pelvis in the evaluation of acute abdominal pain.[12-14] Many of the most common causes of the acute abdomen are readily identified by CT scanning, as are their complications. A notable example is appendicitis. Plain films and even barium enemas add little to the diagnosis of appendicitis; however, a well-performed CT scan is highly accurate in this disease. Prior experience suggested that optimal CT imaging for appendicitis should include intravenous, oral, and rectal contrast agents. Most recently, a large retrospective review of more than 9000 patients from 56 hospitals representing both urban and rural practices found no added diagnostic accuracy with the addition of enteral contrast material. Operative findings correlated with the CT observations 90% of the time whether or not enteral contrast material was used.[19]

It is equally important that an experienced radiologist, accustomed to reading abdominal CT scans, interpret the study to maximize the sensitivity and specificity of the examination. A prospective study from The Netherlands illustrated the variability of CT interpretation in the diagnosis of appendicitis. Three blinded groups of radiologists read CT scans of patients suspected of having appendicitis. All patients then underwent exploratory laparoscopy; 83% of patients were found to have appendicitis at surgery. Radiology group A was made up of radiology residents on call and trained in CT interpretation. Group B were on-call staff radiologists. Group C was represented by expert abdominal radiologists. For group A, B, and C radiologists, the sensitivity of CT scanning for the diagnosis of acute appendicitis was 81%, 88%, and 95%, respectively; the specificity was 94%, 94%, and 100%; and the negative predictive value was 50%, 68%, and 81%. Differences between groups A and C were statistically significant.[14] CT is also excellent in differentiating mechanical small bowel obstruction from paralytic ileus and can usually identify the transition point in mechanical obstruction (Fig. 45-13). Some of the most difficult diagnostic dilemmas, including acute intestinal ischemia and bowel injury after blunt abdominal trauma, can often be identified by this method.

Traumatic small bowel injuries can be a challenging clinical diagnosis. Associated abdominal wall, pelvic, or spinous injuries can be significant distracters that compromise an otherwise careful history and physical examination. In addition, many patients suffering a blunt abdominal trauma will have altered mental states from coexisting closed head injuries or from intoxicating substances. When a bowel injury is suspected, optimal CT scanning uses both oral and intravenous contrast agents. Zissin and colleagues[17] reported an overall sensitivity of 64%, specificity of 97%, and accuracy of 82% when diagnosing small bowel injury after blunt trauma using dual contrast CT scanning. Keys to the diagnosis include bowel wall thickening, any gas outside the lumen of the intestine, or a moderate to large amount of intraperitoneal fluid without visible solid abdominal organ injury.

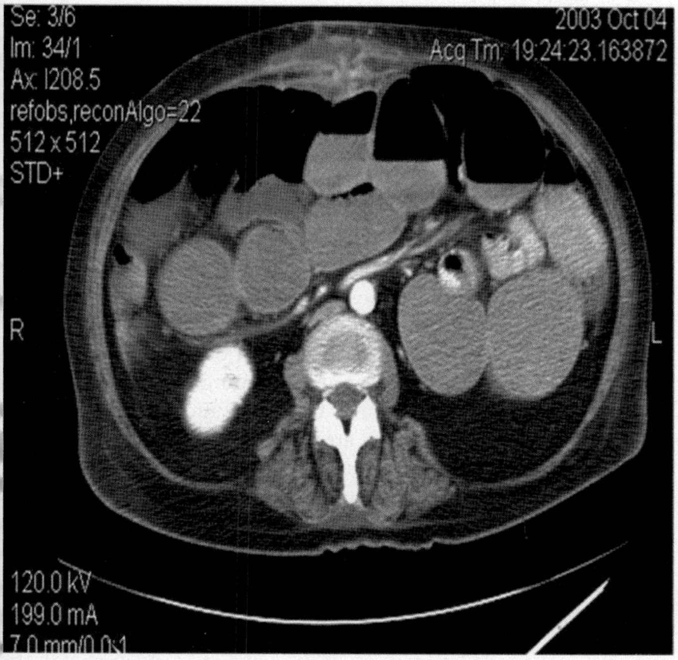

FIGURE 45-13 CT scan of a patient with a partial small bowel obstruction. Note the presence of dilated small bowel and decompressed small bowel. The decompressed bowel contains air, indicating a partial obstruction.

INTRA-ABDOMINAL PRESSURE MONITORING

An elevated intra-abdominal pressure can be a symptom of an acute abdominal process or it can be the cause of the process. Abnormally increased intra-abdominal pressures diminish the blood flow to abdominal organs and decrease venous return to the heart while increasing venous stasis. Increased pressure in the abdomen can also press upward on the diaphragm, thereby increasing peak inspiratory pressures and decreasing ventilatory efficiency. Risk of esophageal reflux and pulmonary aspiration has also been associated with abdominal hypertension. It is important to consider the possibility of abdominal hypertension in any patient who presents with a rigid or significantly distended abdomen.

Normal intra-abdominal pressure is considered to be 5 to 7 mm Hg for a relaxed individual of average body build lying in a supine position. Obesity and elevation of the head of the bed can increase the normal resting abdominal pressure. Morbid obesity has been shown to increase "normal pressures" by 4 to 8 mm Hg; elevating the head of the bed to 30 degrees raises the pressure by 5 mm Hg on average.[20] Pressures are most commonly measured through the bladder by pressure transducer attached to a Foley catheter. Pressure readings are obtained at the end-expiration after instillation of 50 mL of saline into an otherwise empty bladder. Abnormally elevated pressures are those above 11 mm Hg and are graded 1 to 4 by severity (Table 45-2). Abdominal hypertension grades 1 and 2 can most always be treated adequately with medical interventions focusing on maintaining euvolemia, gut decompression with nasogastric tubes or laxatives and enemas, withholding of enteral feedings, catheter aspiration of ascitic fluid, abdominal wall relaxation, and judicious use of hypotonic intravenous fluids. Grades 3 and 4 often require surgical decompression by laparotomy with open packing of the abdomen if the severe hypertension and organ dysfunction do not respond promptly to aggressive medical intervention.

TABLE 45-2 **Abdominal Hypertension**

	MESENTERIC PRESSURE	CO	CVP	PIP	GFR	PERFUSION	TREATMENT
Normal pressure	5-7 mm Hg	↔	↔	↔	↔	↔	None
Grade 1 hypertension	12-15 mm Hg	↔	↔/↑	↔/↑	↓	↓	Maintain euvolemia
Grade 2 hypertension	16-20 mm Hg	↓	↑*	↑	↓	↓	Nonsurgical decompression
Grade 3 hypertension	21-25 mm Hg	↓↓	↑↑*	↑↑	↓↓	↓↓	Surgical decompression
Grade 4 hypertension	>25 mm Hg	↓↓↓	↑↑*	↑↑	↓↓↓	↓↓↓	Surgical decompression; reexplore

CO, cardiac output; *CVP,* central venous pressure; *GFR,* glomerular filtration rate; *PIP,* peak inspiratory pressure.
*Misleadingly elevated and not reflective of intravascular volume.

DIAGNOSTIC LAPAROSCOPY

A number of studies have confirmed the utility of diagnostic laparoscopy in patients with acute abdominal pain.[21-23] The purported advantages include high sensitivity and specificity, ability to treat a number of the conditions causing an acute abdomen laparoscopically, decreased morbidity and mortality, decreased length of stay, and decreased overall hospital costs. It may be particularly helpful in the critically ill, intensive care patient, especially if a laparotomy can be avoided.[24] Diagnostic accuracy is high, and reports show the accuracy ranges between 90% and 100%, with the primary limitation being recognition of retroperitoneal processes. This compares favorably with other diagnostic studies showing superiority to peritoneal lavage, CT scanning, or ultrasound of the abdomen.[25] Because of advances in equipment and increased availability, this technique is being used with greater frequency in these patients.

DIFFERENTIAL DIAGNOSIS

The differential diagnosis for acute abdominal pain is extensive. Conditions range from the mild and self-limited to the rapidly progressive and fatal. All patients must therefore be seen and evaluated immediately on presentation and reassessed at frequent intervals for changes in condition. Although many "acute abdomen" diagnoses will require surgical intervention for resolution, it is important to keep in mind that many causes of acute abdominal pain are medical in etiology (see Figs. 45-2 and 45-4).[26] Development of the differential diagnosis begins during the history and is further clarified during the physical examination. Refinements are then made with the assistance of laboratory analysis and imaging studies so that typically, one or two diagnoses rise above the rest. To be successful, this process requires a comprehensive knowledge of the medical and surgical conditions that create acute abdominal pain to allow individual disease features to be matched to patient demographics, symptoms, and signs.

Certain physical examination, laboratory, and radiographic findings are highly correlated with surgical disease (Box 45-5). At times, some patients will be too unstable to undergo comprehensive evaluations that require transportation to other departments, such as radiology. In this setting, peritoneal lavage can provide information suggesting pathologic processes requiring surgical intervention. The lavage can be performed under local anesthesia at the patient's bedside. A small incision is made in the midline adjacent to the umbilicus, and dissection is carried down to the peritoneal cavity. A small catheter or intravenous tubing is inserted, and 1000 mL of saline is infused. A sample of fluid is then allowed to siphon back out into the empty saline bag and is then analyzed for cellular or biochemical anomalies. This technique can provide sensitive evidence of hemorrhage or infection as well as of some types of solid or hollow organ injury.

Patients having emergency or life-threatening surgical disease are taken for immediate laparotomy; urgent diagnoses allow time for stabilization, hydration, and preoperative preparation as needed. The remaining acute abdominal patients are grouped as those with surgical conditions that sometimes require surgery, those with medical diseases, and those who as yet remain unclear. Hospitalized patients who do not go urgently to the operating room must be reassessed frequently and preferably by the same examiner to recognize potentially serious changes in condition that alter the diagnosis or suggest development of complications.

BOX 45-5 Findings Associated With Surgical Disease in the Setting of Acute Abdominal Pain

Physical Examination and Laboratory Findings

Abdominal compartment pressures >30 mm Hg
Worsening distention after gastric decompression
Involuntary guarding or rebound tenderness
Gastrointestinal hemorrhage requiring >4 units of blood without stabilization
Unexplained systemic sepsis
Signs of hypoperfusion (acidosis, pain out of proportion to examination findings, rising liver function test results)

Radiographic Findings

Massive dilation of intestine
Progressive dilation of stationary loop of intestine (sentinel loop)
Pneumoperitoneum
Extravasation of contrast material from bowel lumen
Vascular occlusion on angiography
Fat stranding or thickened bowel wall with systemic sepsis

Diagnostic Peritoneal Lavage (1000 mL)

>250 white blood cells per milliliter of aspirate
>300,000 red blood cells per milliliter of aspirate
Bilirubin level higher than plasma level (bile leak) within aspirate
Presence of particulate matter (stool)
Creatinine level higher than plasma level in aspirate (urine leak)

Although the goal of every surgeon is to make the correct diagnosis preoperatively and to have planned the best possible surgical procedure before entering the operating suite, it must be emphasized that a clear diagnosis will not be able to be developed in every patient. Surgeons must always be willing to accept uncertainty and commit to abdominal exploration when examination findings warrant. Laboratory and imaging studies, although helpful, should never replace the bedside clinical judgment of an experienced surgeon. Patients are far more likely to be seriously or fatally harmed by delay of surgical treatment to perform confirmatory tests than by misdiagnoses discovered at operation. Laparoscopy has proved to be a valuable tool when the diagnosis is unclear. The presence of surgical disease can be confirmed in all but the most hostile abdominal environments, and as the surgeon's experience grows, more and more conditions are able to be treated laparoscopically as well. Even when conversion to open technique is required, laparoscopic evaluation facilitates more accurate positioning of the laparotomy incision, thereby reducing its length.

PREPARATION FOR EMERGENCY OPERATION

Patients with an acute abdomen vary greatly in their overall state of health at the time the decision to operate is made. Regardless of the patient's severity of illness, all patients require some degree of preoperative preparation. Intravenous access should be obtained and any fluid or electrolyte abnormalities corrected. Nearly all patients will require antibiotic infusions. The bacteria common in acute abdominal emergencies are gram-negative enteric organisms and anaerobes. Infusions of antibiotics to cover these organisms should be begun once a presumptive diagnosis is made. Patients with generalized paralytic ileus or vomiting benefit from nasogastric tube placement to decrease the likelihood of vomiting and aspiration. Foley catheter bladder drainage to assess urine output, a measure of adequacy of fluid resuscitation, is indicated in most patients. Preoperative urine output of 0.5 mL/kg/hr, systolic blood pressure of at least 100 mm Hg, and a pulse rate of 100 beats/min or less are indicative of an adequate intravascular volume. A common electrolyte abnormality requiring correction is hypokalemia. Preoperative acidosis may respond to fluid repletion and intravenous bicarbonate infusion. Acidosis due to intestinal ischemia or infarction may be refractory to preoperative therapy. Placement of a central venous catheter may facilitate resuscitation and allow accelerated correction of potassium concentration. Significant anemia is uncommon, and preoperative blood transfusions are usually unnecessary. However, most patients should have blood typed and crossmatched and available at operation. There is an inherent uncertainty in the operation that will be required in these patients, and having crossmatched blood available avoids transfusion delay if unexpected intraoperative events occur. The need for preoperative stabilization of patients must be weighed against the increased morbidity and mortality associated with a delay in the treatment of some of the surgical diseases that are manifested as an acute abdomen. The underlying nature of the disease process, such as infarcted bowel, may require surgical correction before stabilization of the patient's vital signs and restoration of acid-base balance can occur. Resuscitation should be viewed as an ongoing process and continued after the surgery is completed. Deciding when the maximum benefit of preoperative therapy in these patients has been achieved requires good surgical judgment.

ATYPICAL PATIENTS

Pregnancy

Acute abdominal pain in the pregnant patient creates several unique diagnostic and therapeutic challenges. Special emphasis must be placed on the possibility of gynecologic and surgical diseases when acute abdominal pain develops during pregnancy because of their frequency and morbidity if left unrecognized. Laparoscopy has had a major impact on the diagnosis and treatment of the gravid woman with acute abdominal pain and is now routinely employed for many clinical situations. Although case reports of fetal demise after laparoscopic surgery continue to be reported, its safety has been considered equal or superior to an open surgical approach in all trimesters of pregnancy.[27,28] A retrospective study and meta-analysis did call into question the safety of laparoscopic appendectomy compared with laparotomy, highlighting the need for more research into this area.[29,30] The greatest threat facing the pregnant patient with acute abdominal pain is the potential for delayed diagnosis. Delays in receiving surgical treatment have proved far more morbid than the operations themselves.[11,31] Delays occur for several reasons. Many times, symptoms are attributed to the underlying pregnancy, including abdominal pains, nausea, vomiting, and anorexia. Pregnancy can also alter the presentation of some disease processes and make the physical examination more challenging because of the enlarged uterus in the pelvis. The appendix rises out of the pelvis to within a few centimeters of the right anterolateral costal margin late in the third trimester (Fig. 45-14).[32] Laboratory studies such as white blood cell counts and other chemistries are also altered in pregnancy, making recognition of disease more difficult. In addition, physicians may hesitate to perform typical imaging studies, such as plain abdominal films or CT scans, because of concern over

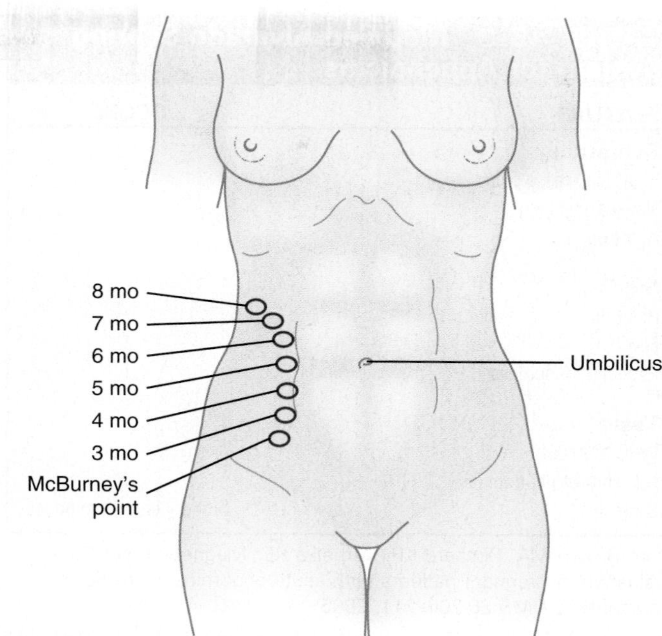

FIGURE 45-14 Location of maternal normal appendix during fetal gestation.

radiation exposure to the developing fetus. The lack of radiologic information can take a physician out of his or her diagnostic routine and cause extra emphasis to be placed on other modalities, such as vital signs and laboratory studies, which can confuse or underestimate the existing condition. Finally, physicians naturally tend to be more conservative in treating pregnant patients. First trimester miscarriage rates from nonobstetric surgeries have been reported to be as high as 38%, but most reports place the surgical miscarriage rate similar to spontaneous first trimester miscarriage rates of 8% to 16%.[27] Without controls, it is unclear if some of the increased miscarriage rates noted are secondary to the disease or the surgery itself. Surgery has not been associated with increased stillbirths and congenital abnormalities.[28] Abdominal surgery has been associated with an increased incidence of preterm labor in both the second and third trimesters of pregnancy, with the highest incidence in the third trimester. It is thought that preterm labor is less in the second trimester because of less uterine manipulation. Intraoperative care during pregnancy is focused on optimal care of the mother. If the fetus is previable, fetal heart tones should be measured before and after the surgery. If the fetus is viable, fetal heart sounds should be measured throughout the surgery with a provider capable of performing an emergent cesarean section readily available.[33]

Appendicitis is the most common nonobstetric disease requiring surgery, occurring in 1/1500 pregnancies.[29,33] Its symptoms typically consist of right lateral abdominal pain, nausea, and anorexia, yet "typical" presentations account for only 50% to 60% of cases.[34] Fever is uncommon unless the appendix is perforated with abdominal sepsis. Symptoms are sometimes attributed to the underlying pregnancy, and a high index of suspicion must be maintained. Laboratory studies can also be misleading. Leukocytosis as high as 16,000 cells/μL is common in pregnancy, and labor can increase the count to 21,000 cells/μL. Many authors have suggested that a neutrophil shift of more than 80% is suggestive of an acute inflammatory process such as appendicitis, yet others have observed that only 75% of patients with proven

TABLE 45-3 **Modified Alvarado Scoring System for Appendicitis**

FEATURE	SCORE
Symptoms	
Right iliac fossa pain	1
Nausea/vomiting	1
Anorexia	1
Signs	
Right iliac fossa tenderness	2
Fever	1
Rebound tenderness	1
Tests	
WBC ≥ 10,000	2
Left shift of neutrophils	1
Score ≥ 7	Surgery is recommended

From Brown MA, Birchard KR, Semelka RC: Magnetic resonance evaluation of pregnant patients with acute abdominal pain. *Semin Ultrasound CT MR* 26:206–211, 2005.

appendicitis had a shift, whereas as many as 50% of patients with a shift and pain were found to have a normal appendix.[11,30] Scoring systems have been advocated that assign numerical scores to certain symptoms, signs, and laboratory values to predict the likelihood of appendicitis. Although systems such as the Modified Alvarado Scoring System (Table 45-3) help predict the need for surgical intervention, they have not been validated in a model of pregnancy.[34] Ultrasound has been relied on as the first imaging tool in many centers. Graded compression ultrasound has been shown to have a sensitivity of 86% in the nonpregnant patient.[29] In a case series of 42 pregnant women with suspected appendicitis, graded compression ultrasound was found to be 100% sensitive, 96% specific, and 98% accurate.[35] Three women were excluded from the analysis because of a technically inadequate examination due to advanced gestational age (>35 weeks). Helical CT scanning has been established as a valuable tool for evaluation of the nonpregnant patient and shows promise as a second-line study in pregnancy. Compared with traditional CT scans, helical CT can provide a much faster study with radiation exposures of approximately 300 mrad to the fetus.[29] MRI now plays an important role in the diagnosis as well. MRI is not only capable of demonstrating the normal appendix, but it can also recognize an enlarged appendix, periappendiceal fluid, and inflammation.[36] The sensitivity and specificity reported in a retrospective review of 148 patients suspected of having acute appendicitis were 100% and 93%, respectively.[37]

The added difficulties in evaluating the pregnant patient with right lower quadrant abdominal pain have resulted in a significantly higher negative appendectomy rate compared with nonpregnant peers in the past. Although this diagnostic error rate would be unacceptable in a typical young healthy woman, it is widely accepted because of the fetal mortality suffered when appendicitis progresses to perforation before surgery. Perioperative fetal loss associated with appendectomy for early appendicitis is 3% to 5%, whereas it climbs to more than 20% in the setting of perforation.[31] With modern imaging, especially MRI, negative appendectomies have decreased without an associated increase in perforations.[36,37]

The second and third most common surgical diseases seen in pregnancy are biliary tract disorders and bowel obstructions. Surgery for biliary disease occurs in 1 to 6/10,000 pregnancies.[38] Symptoms of pain, nausea, and anorexia are the same as in nonpregnant patients. Even though the elevated estrogen levels should be more lithogenic, the incidence of disease is similar to that in nongravid women.[28] With few exceptions, the evaluation and treatment during pregnancy are similar to the evaluation and treatment of all patients with biliary disease. Ultrasound is the diagnostic test of choice. Alkaline phosphatase is elevated secondary to elevated estrogen, and normal values must be adjusted.

Laparoscopic cholecystectomy is the preferred technique for cholecystectomy.[28,38,39] Many studies have suggested laparoscopic cholecystectomy for all symptomatic disease secondary to high antepartum and postpartum recurrence and complications regardless of trimester.[28,38] Still, most surgeons try to treat simple biliary colic with conservative management in the first and third trimesters and plan elective laparoscopic cholecystectomy for the second trimester or the postpartum period to minimize fetal risk.[38] Gallstone pancreatitis and acute cholecystitis should be managed more carefully. Gallstone pancreatitis has been associated with fetal loss as high as 60%. If a woman does not respond quickly to conservative treatment with hydration, bowel rest, analgesia, and judicious use of antibiotics, further evaluation should be performed as surgery may be indicated.

Bowel obstructions are much less common, occurring in approximately 1 to 2/4000 pregnancies; the underlying cause is adhesions in two thirds of cases. Volvulus is the second most common cause, occurring in 25% of cases compared with only 4% of the nonpregnant population.[30] Signs and symptoms are typical but must not be attributed to "morning sickness." Colicky abdominal pain with rapid abdominal distention should key the clinician to the diagnosis. Three periods during gestation are associated with an increased risk of obstruction and correlate with rapid changes in uterine size.[30] The first is from 16 to 20 weeks when the uterus grows beyond the pelvis; the second is from 32 to 36 weeks when the fetal head descends; and the third is in the early postpartum period. The evaluation should be the same as for any patient, and there should be no hesitation to obtain abdominal radiographs if the situation warrants. As with other acute inflammatory processes in the abdomen, the maternal and fetal morbidity is most affected by delayed definitive treatment.

Pediatrics

Strategies for diagnosis of the acute abdomen in the pediatric population are the same as for adults. Appendicitis remains one of the primary causes of the acute abdomen in this age group. Although bowel obstructions and gallstone disease are seen, these entities are far less frequent than in adults. Intussusception should be maintained in the differential diagnosis, especially for those younger than 3 years. Gastroenteritis, perforations from foreign body ingestion, food poisoning, Meckel's diverticulitis, and *C. difficile* colitis are also potential causes. Presentations and examination findings are similar to those of adult patients. The primary challenge to making the correct diagnosis lies in obtaining an accurate history. Children will often be poor historians because of age, fear, or their general ability to describe their experience. A thorough history must therefore be also obtained from the child's parents as well. Diagnostic testing choices as well as treatments may be influenced by the age of the patient. Clinicians may be less inclined to perform studies that deliver ionizing radiation to young children. A retrospective study of 1228 children with suspected appendicitis evaluated the use of ultrasound as a first-line tool, with CT scanning used as an adjunct for equivocal studies.[40] This study showed that CT scanning was avoided in more than half of patients while maintaining a negative appendectomy rate of 8.1%. Finally, there is a growing experience in treating early appendicitis nonoperatively with antibiotics. A recent prospective nonrandomized study of 77 children with appendicitis found the immediate and 30-day success rates of nonoperative treatment to be 93% and 90%. Of the three patients who failed to respond to medical management, none progressed to perforated or complicated appendicitis. Children in the medically managed group were found to return to school 2 days sooner, had 14 fewer disability days, but incurred an 18-hour longer hospitalization on average.[41]

Acute Abdomen in the Critically Ill

The critically ill patient with a potential acute abdomen is a difficult challenge for intensivists and surgeons alike. Many of the underlying diseases and treatments encountered in the intensive care unit can predispose to acute abdominal disease. At the same time, unrecognized abdominal illness can be responsible for patients lingering in a critical state. Critically ill patients are often unable to appreciate symptoms to the same degree as healthy peers because of nutritional or immune compromise, narcotic analgesia, or antibiotic use. Many of these patients have an altered mental status or are intubated and cannot provide detailed information to their providers.

Cardiopulmonary bypass has been associated with several acute abdominal illnesses. Mesenteric ischemia, paralytic ileus, Ogilvie syndrome, stress peptic ulceration, acute acalculous cholecystitis, and acute pancreatitis have all been linked to the low-flow state of cardiopulmonary bypass, and incidence appears tied to the length of the cardiac procedure.[42,43] Vasoactive medications and ventilator support have also been linked to hypoperfusion and similar abdominal processes. When an acute abdominal complication occurs in an intensive care unit patient, it has a dramatic effect on outcome. Intensivists should maintain a high index of suspicion for the development of intra-abdominal disease and consult with surgeons early to maximize recovery potential. Surgeons must then work to exclude the possibility of abdominal disease using all of the methods described in this chapter as well as bedside ultrasound, paracentesis, or mini-laparoscopy so that early surgical intervention can be appropriately undertaken.[44]

Immunocompromised Patients With Acute Abdomen

Immunocompromised patients have variable presentations with acute abdominal diseases. The variability is highly correlated to the degree of immunosuppression. There is no reliable test for determining the degree of immunosuppression experienced by a given patient, so estimates are made by associations with certain disease states or medications. Mild to moderate compromise is experienced by the elderly, the malnourished, diabetics, transplant recipients on routine maintenance therapy, cancer patients, renal failure patients, and HIV patients with CD4 counts above 200/mm^3. Although patients in this group have the same types of illnesses and infections as their immunocompetent peers, they still can present in an atypical fashion. Abdominal pain and systemic signs and symptoms are often tied to the development of inflammation. These patients may not be able to mount a full inflammatory response and therefore may experience less abdominal pain, have delayed development of fever, and have a blunted leukocytosis. Severely compromised patients typically include transplant recipients having received high-dose therapy for rejection in the past 2 months, cancer patients on chemotherapy especially with neutropenia, and HIV patients with CD4 counts below 200/mm^3. These patients present very late in their course, often with little or no pain, no fever, and vague constitutional symptoms followed by an overwhelming systemic collapse.

Pseudomembranous colitis has traditionally been associated with recent broad-spectrum antibiotic use, although it is increasingly seen in immunocompromised patients with diseases such as lymphoma, leukemia, and AIDS. Clinical manifestations commonly include diarrhea, dehydration, abdominal pain, fever, and leukocytosis, yet immunocompromised patients may fail to exhibit many of these findings because of their inability to mount a normal inflammatory response. Imaging studies such as CT of the abdomen become increasingly important in making early, accurate diagnoses when presentations are atypical. CT scans are useful in patients with complicated colitis without obvious operative indications. CT scans are useful to evaluate for megacolon, ileus, ascites, perforation, and colon wall thickening (Table 45-4).[45] These findings, when present, can greatly assist the clinician with forming the diagnosis of colitis. However, up to 14% of patients with proven pseudomembranous colitis will have had normal findings on CT examination, and therefore the diagnosis should not be ruled out solely on the basis of a negative scan. Early surgical consultation has been shown to decrease mortality.[46]

In addition, these patients may suffer from atypical infections, including peritoneal tuberculosis, fungal infections including aspergillus, endemic mycoses, and a variety of viral infections including cytomegalovirus and Epstein-Barr virus (Box 45-6). When an abdominal infection does occur, it is less likely to be walled off as a localized infection because of the lack of inflammatory reaction. All severely immunocompromised patients require prompt and thorough evaluation for any persistent abdominal complaints. All patients requiring hospitalization should receive a surgical consult to aid in timely diagnosis and treatment. High-resolution CT scanning can be of great benefit in these patients, but a low threshold for laparoscopy or laparotomy should be maintained for those with equivocal diagnostic test results and persistent symptoms that remain unexplained.

Acute Abdomen in the Morbidly Obese

Morbid obesity creates numerous challenges to the accurate diagnosis of acute abdominal processes. Many authors describe alterations in the signs and symptoms of peritonitis in the morbidly

TABLE 45-4 Frequency of Common CT Scan Observations in Pseudomembranous Colitis

CT FINDINGS	FREQUENCY (%)
Bowel wall thickening (>4 mm)	86
Pancolic distribution	46
Pericolic stranding	45
Ascites	38
Nodular or polypoid wall thickening	38
Mucosal enhancement	18
Bowel dilation	14
Accordion sign	14

From Tsiotos GG, Mullany CJ, Zietlow S, et al: Abdominal complications following cardiac surgery. *Am J Surg* 167:553–557, 1994.

obese.[47-49] Findings of overt peritonitis are often late and usually ominous, leading to sepsis, organ failure, and death.[47] Abdominal sepsis is a much more subtle diagnosis in this population and may be associated only with symptoms such as malaise, shoulder pain, hiccups, or shortness of breath.[48] Physical examination findings can also be difficult to interpret. Severe abdominal pain is not common, and less specific findings, such as tachycardia, tachypnea, pleural effusion, and fever, may be the primary observation.[49] Appreciation of distention or intra-abdominal mass is also difficult because of the size and thickness of the abdominal wall.

Abdominal imaging is also adversely affected by obesity. Plain abdominal radiographs can require multiple images to view the entire abdomen, and clarity is reduced. CT and MRI scanning may be impossible to perform as a patient's girth or weight exceeds the size of the scanning aperture or the weight limit of the mechanized bed. In these settings, a high index of suspicion and low threshold for surgical exploration must be maintained. Laparoscopy is a valuable tool in these patients.

BOX 45-6 Causes of Acute Abdominal Pain in the Immunocompromised Patient

Opportunistic Infections

Endemic mycoses (coccidioidomycosis, blastomycosis, histoplasmosis)
Tuberculin peritonitis
Aspergillosis
Neutropenic colitis (typhlitis)
Pseudomembranous colitis
Cytomegalovirus colitis, gastritis, esophagitis, nephritis
Epstein-Barr virus
Hepatic abscesses (fungal or pyogenic)

Iatrogenic Conditions

Graft-versus-host disease with hepatitis or enteritis
Peptic ulcer or perforation from steroid use
Pancreatitis caused by steroids or azathioprine
Hepatic veno-occlusive disease (secondary to primary immunodeficiency or chemotherapy)
Nephrolithiasis caused by indinavir treatment of HIV

ALGORITHMS IN THE ACUTE ABDOMEN

Algorithms can aid in the diagnosis of the patient with an acute abdomen. As stated earlier, computer-assisted diagnosis has been shown to be more accurate than clinical judgment alone in a number of acute abdominal disease states. Algorithms are the basis for computer diagnosis and can be useful in making clinical decisions. The algorithms presented in Figures 45-15 to 45-20 are helpful in acute abdomen patients and can allow both a focused workup and expeditious therapy.

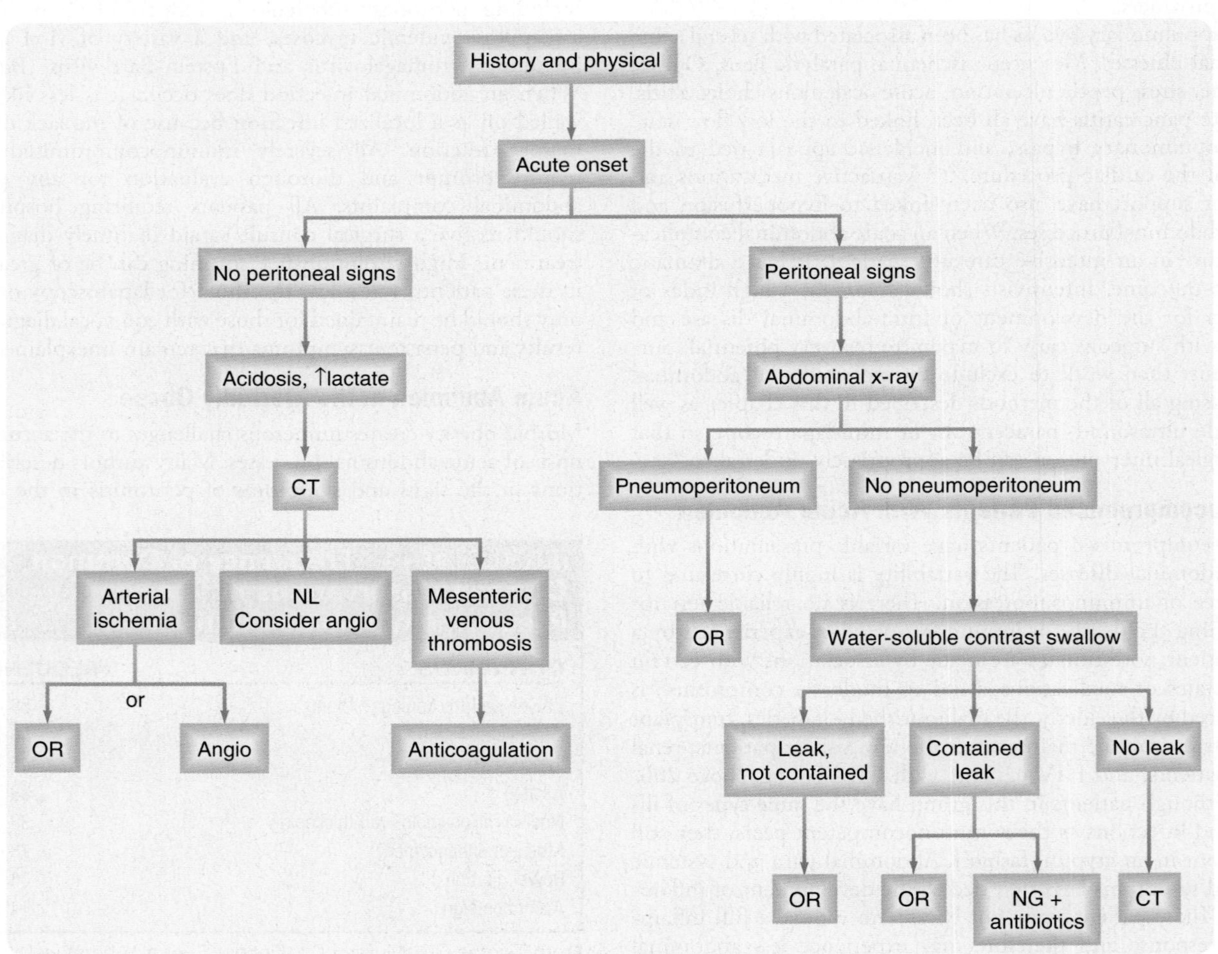

FIGURE 45-15 Algorithm for the treatment of acute-onset severe, generalized abdominal pain. *CT*, computed tomography; *NG*, nasogastric tube; *NL*, normal study; *OR*, operation.

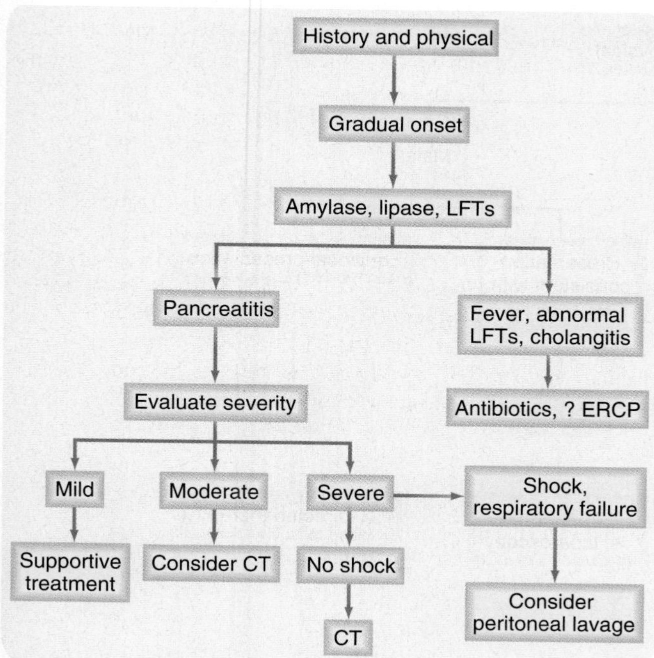

FIGURE 45-16 Algorithm for the treatment of gradual-onset severe, generalized abdominal pain. *CT,* computed tomography; *ERCP,* endoscopic retrograde cholangiopancreatography; *LFTs,* liver function tests.

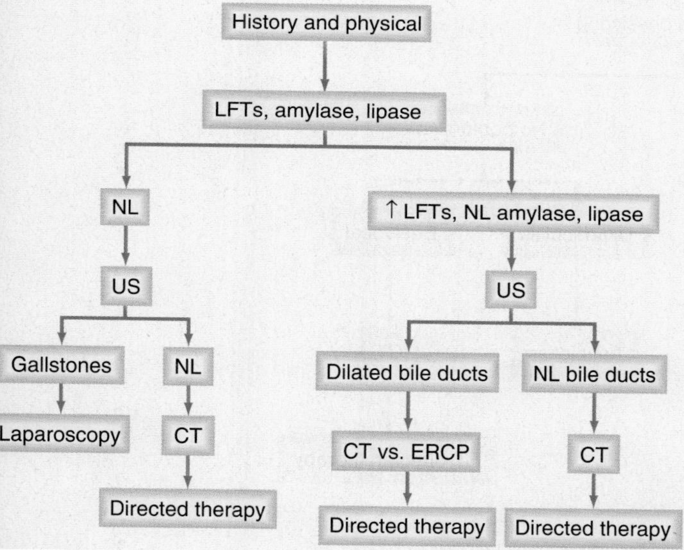

FIGURE 45-17 Algorithm for the treatment of right upper quadrant abdominal pain. *CT,* computed tomography; *ERCP,* endoscopic retrograde cholangiopancreatography; *LFTs,* liver function tests; *NL,* normal study; *US,* ultrasound.

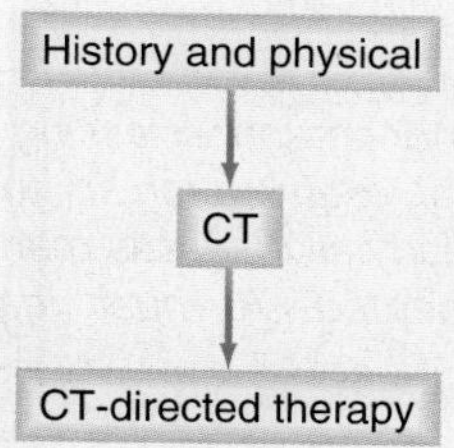

FIGURE 45-18 Algorithm for the treatment of left upper quadrant abdominal pain. *CT,* computed tomography.

SUMMARY

Evaluation and management of the patient with acute abdominal pain remain a challenging part of a surgeon's practice. Whereas advances in imaging techniques, use of algorithms, and computer assistance have improved the diagnostic accuracy for the conditions causing the acute abdomen, a careful history and physical examination remain the most important part of the evaluation. Even with these tools at hand, the surgeon must often make the decision to perform a laparoscopy or laparotomy with a good deal of uncertainty as to the expected findings. Increased morbidity and mortality associated with a delay in the treatment of many of the surgical causes of the acute abdomen argue for an aggressive and expeditious surgical approach.

Common Pitfalls

- Failure to thoroughly examine *and* document findings
- Failure to perform a rectal or vaginal examination when appropriate
- Failure to evaluate for hernias, including the scrotal region
- Failure to conduct a pregnancy test or to consider pregnancy in the diagnosis
- Failure to reassess the patient frequently while developing a differential diagnosis
- Failure to reconsider an established diagnosis when the clinical situation changes
- Failure to recognize immune compromise and to appreciate its masking effect on the historical and examination findings
- Allowing a normal laboratory value to dissuade a diagnosis when there is cause for clinical concern
- Failure to consult colleagues when appropriate
- Failure to take age- and situation-specific diagnoses into consideration
- Failure to make specific and concrete follow-up arrangements when monitoring a clinical situation on an outpatient basis
- Hesitancy to go to the operating room without a firm diagnosis when the clinical situation suggests surgical disease

SELECTED REFERENCES

Ahmad TA, Shelbaya E, Razek SA, et al: Experience of laparoscopic management in 100 patients with acute abdomen. *Hepatogastroenterology* 48:733–736, 2001.

A description of the usefulness of laparoscopy in a large series of patients with acute abdomen. A good review of this important diagnostic and therapeutic tool.

Cademartiri F, Raaijmaker RHJM, Kuiper JW, et al: Multidetector row CT angiography in patients with abdominal angina. *Radiographics* 24:969–984, 2004.

A good review of the computed tomographic characteristics of acute mesenteric ischemia. This outlines the radiographic findings that have greatly assisted in the diagnosis of this otherwise difficult condition.

Graff LG, Robinson D: Abdominal pain and emergency department evaluation. *Emerg Med Clin North Am* 19:123–136, 2001.

Good review of the spectrum of patients presenting with acute abdominal pain.

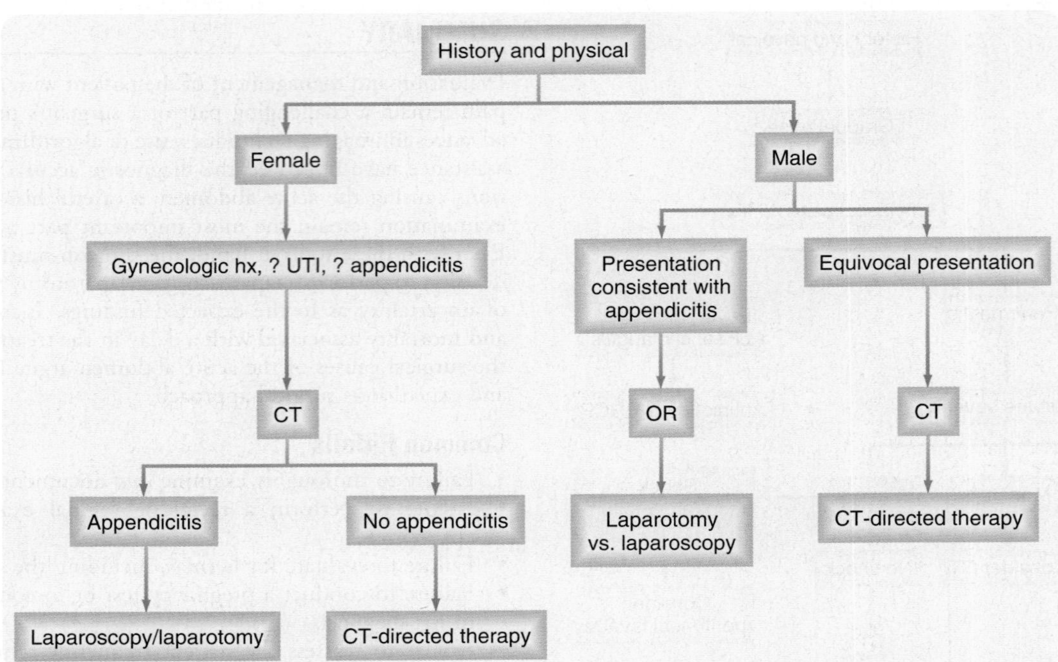

FIGURE 45-19 Algorithm for the treatment of right lower quadrant abdominal pain. *CT*, computed tomography; *hx*, history; *OR*, operation; *UTI*, urinary tract infection.

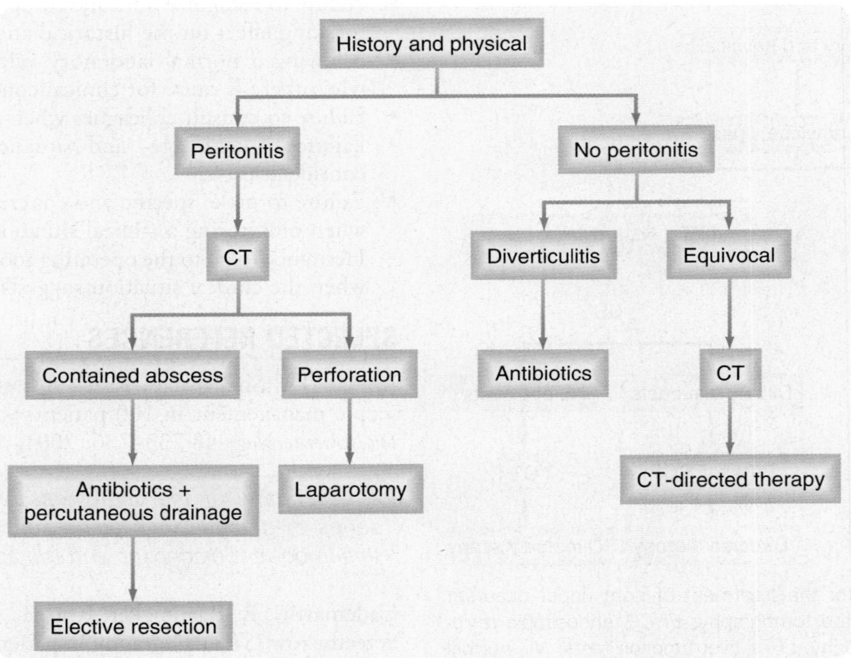

FIGURE 45-20 Algorithm for the treatment of left lower quadrant abdominal pain. *CT*, computed tomography.

Macari M, Balthazar EJ: The acute right lower quadrant: CT evaluation. *Radiol Clin North Am* 41:1117–1136, 2003.

A modern discussion of the role of computed tomography in the evaluation of patients with right lower quadrant abdominal pain.

Silen W: *Cope's early diagnosis of the acute abdomen*, ed 21, New York, 2005, Oxford University Press.

This is a classic monograph stressing the importance of history and physical examination in the diagnosis of the acute abdomen. Nearly all diseases manifesting as an acute abdomen are presented. A must read for the surgical resident.

Steinheber FU: Medical conditions mimicking the acute surgical abdomen. *Med Clin North Am* 57:1559–1567, 1973.

This classic article nicely reviews the various medical conditions that can be manifested as an acute abdomen. It is well written and remains pertinent to the evaluation of these patients.

REFERENCES

1. Sethuraman U, Siadat M, Lepak-Hitch CA, et al: Pulmonary embolism presenting as acute abdomen in a child and adult. *Am J Emerg Med* 27:514.e1–514.e5, 2009.
2. Graff LG, 4th, Robinson D: Abdominal pain and emergency department evaluation. *Emerg Med Clin North Am* 19:123–136, 2001.
3. Steinheber FU: Medical conditions mimicking the acute surgical abdomen. *Med Clin North Am* 57:1559–1567, 1973.
4. Gilbert JA, Kamath PS: Spontaneous bacterial peritonitis: An update. *Mayo Clin Proc* 70:365–370, 1995.
5. Silen W: *Cope's early diagnosis of the acute abdomen*, ed 21, New York, 2005, Oxford University Press.
6. Paterson-Brown S, Vipond MN: Modern aids to clinical decision-making in the acute abdomen. *Br J Surg* 77:13–18, 1990.
7. de Dombal FT: Computers, diagnoses and patients with acute abdominal pain. *Arch Emerg Med* 9:267–270, 1992.
8. Adams ID, Chan M, Clifford PC, et al: Computer aided diagnosis of acute abdominal pain: A multicentre study. *Br Med J (Clin Res Ed)* 293:800–804, 1986.
9. Wellwood J, Johannessen S, Spiegelhalter DJ: How does computer-aided diagnosis improve the management of acute abdominal pain? *Ann R Coll Surg Engl* 74:40–46, 1992.
10. McAdam WA, Brock BM, Armitage T, et al: Twelve years' experience of computer-aided diagnosis in a district general hospital. *Ann R Coll Surg Engl* 72:140–146, 1990.
11. Kort B, Katz VL, Watson WJ: The effect of nonobstetric operation during pregnancy. *Surg Gynecol Obstet* 177:371–376, 1993.
12. Macari M, Balthazar EJ: The acute right lower quadrant: CT evaluation. *Radiol Clin North Am* 41:1117–1136, 2003.
13. Cademartiri F, Raaijmakers RH, Kuiper JW, et al: Multidetector row CT angiography in patients with abdominal angina. *Radiographics* 24:969–984, 2004.
14. Lee R, Tung HK, Tung PH, et al: CT in acute mesenteric ischaemia. *Clin Radiol* 58:279–287, 2003.
15. Hof KH, Krestin GP, Steijerberg EW, et al: Interobserver variability in CT scan interpretation for suspected acute appendicitis. *Emerg Med J* 26:92–94, 2009.
16. Hanbidge AE, Buckler PM, O'Malley ME, et al: From the RSNA refresher courses: Imaging evaluation for acute pain in the right upper quadrant. *Radiographics* 24:1117–1135, 2004.
17. Zissin R, Osadchy A, Gayer G: Abdominal CT findings in small bowel perforation. *Br J Radiol* 82:162–171, 2009.
18. van Randen A, Bipat S, Zwinderman AH, et al: Acute appendicitis: Meta-analysis of diagnostic performance of CT and graded compression US related to prevalence of disease. *Radiology* 249:97–106, 2008.
19. Drake FT, Alfonso R, Bhargava P, et al: Enteral contrast in the computed tomography diagnosis of appendicitis: Comparative effectiveness in a prospective surgical cohort. *Ann Surg* 260:311–316, 2014.
20. De Keulenaer BL, De Waele JJ, Powell B, et al: What is normal intra-abdominal pressure and how is it affected by positioning, body mass and positive end-expiratory pressure? *Intensive Care Med* 35:969–976, 2009.
21. Ahmad TA, Shelbaya E, Razek SA, et al: Experience of laparoscopic management in 100 patients with acute abdomen. *Hepatogastroenterology* 48:733–736, 2001.
22. Perri SG, Altilia F, Pietrangeli F, et al: Laparoscopy in abdominal emergencies. Indications and limitations. *Chir Ital* 54:165–178, 2002.
23. Riemann JF: Diagnostic laparoscopy. *Endoscopy* 35:43–47, 2003.
24. Pecoraro AP, Cacchione RN, Sayad P, et al: The routine use of diagnostic laparoscopy in the intensive care unit. *Surg Endosc* 15:638–641, 2001.
25. Stefanidis D, Richardson WS, Chang L, et al: The role of diagnostic laparoscopy for acute abdominal conditions: An evidence-based review. *Surg Endosc* 23:16–23, 2009.
26. Hickey MS, Kiernan GJ, Weaver KE: Evaluation of abdominal pain. *Emerg Med Clin North Am* 7:437–452, 1989.
27. de Bakker JK, Dijksman LM, Donkervoort SC: Safety and outcome of general surgical open and laparoscopic procedures during pregnancy. *Surg Endosc* 25:1574–1578, 2011.
28. Pearl J, Price R, Richardson W, et al: Guidelines for diagnosis, treatment, and use of laparoscopy for surgical problems during pregnancy. *Surg Endosc* 25:3479–3492, 2011.
29. McGory ML, Zingmond DS, Tillou A, et al: Negative appendectomy in pregnant women is associated with a substantial risk of fetal loss. *J Am Coll Surg* 205:534–540, 2007.
30. Wilasrusmee C, Sukrat B, McEvoy M, et al: Systematic review and meta-analysis of safety of laparoscopic versus open appendicectomy for suspected appendicitis in pregnancy. *Br J Surg* 99:1470–1478, 2012.
31. Sadot E, Telem DA, Arora M, et al: Laparoscopy: A safe approach to appendicitis during pregnancy. *Surg Endosc* 24:383–389, 2009.
32. Hunt MG, Martin JN, Jr, Martin RW, et al: Perinatal aspects of abdominal surgery for nonobstetric disease. *Am J Perinatol* 6:412–417, 1989.
33. ACOG Committee on Obstetric Practice: ACOG Committee Opinion No. 474: Nonobstetric surgery during pregnancy. *Obstet Gynecol* 117:420–421, 2011.
34. Brown JJ, Wilson C, Coleman S, et al: Appendicitis in pregnancy: An ongoing diagnostic dilemma. *Colorectal Dis* 11:116–122, 2009.
35. Lim HK, Bae SH, Seo GS: Diagnosis of acute appendicitis in pregnant women: Value of sonography. *AJR Am J Roentgenol* 159:539–542, 1992.
36. Dewhurst C, Beddy P, Pedrosa I: MRI evaluation of acute appendicitis in pregnancy. *J Magn Reson Imaging* 37:566–575, 2013.
37. Pedrosa I, Lafornara M, Pandharipande PV, et al: Pregnant patients suspected of having acute appendicitis: Effect of MR imaging on negative laparotomy rate and appendiceal perforation rate. *Radiology* 250:749–757, 2009.
38. Veerappan A, Gawron AJ, Soper NJ, et al: Delaying cholecystectomy for complicated gallstone disease in pregnancy is associated with recurrent postpartum symptoms. *J Gastrointest Surg* 17:1953–1959, 2013.
39. Kuy S, Roman SA, Desai R, et al: Outcomes following cholecystectomy in pregnant and nonpregnant women. *Surgery* 146:358–366, 2009.

40. Krishnamoorthi R, Ramarajan N, Wang NE, et al: Effectiveness of a staged US and CT protocol for the diagnosis of pediatric appendicitis: Reducing radiation exposure in the age of ALARA. *Radiology* 259:231–239, 2011.
41. Minneci PC, Sulkowski JP, Nacion KM, et al: Feasibility of a nonoperative management strategy for uncomplicated acute appendicitis in children. *J Am Coll Surg* 219:272–279, 2014.
42. Guler M, Yamak B, Erdogan M, et al: Risk factors for gastrointestinal complications in patients undergoing coronary artery bypass graft surgery. *J Cardiothorac Vasc Anesth* 25:637–641, 2011.
43. Viana FF, Chen Y, Almeida AA, et al: Gastrointestinal complications after cardiac surgery: 10-year experience of a single Australian centre. *ANZ J Surg* 83:651–656, 2013.
44. Hecker A, Uhle F, Schwandner T, et al: Diagnostics, therapy and outcome prediction in abdominal sepsis: Current standards and future perspectives. *Langenbecks Arch Surg* 399:11–22, 2014.
45. Surawicz CM, Brandt LJ, Binion DG, et al: Guidelines for diagnosis, treatment, and prevention of *Clostridium difficile* infections. *Am J Gastroenterol* 108:478–498, quiz 499, 2013.
46. Sailhamer EA, Carson K, Chang Y, et al: Fulminant *Clostridium difficile* colitis: patterns of care and predictors of mortality. *Arch Surg* 144:433–439, 2009.
47. Mehran A, Liberman M, Rosenthal R, et al: Ruptured appendicitis after laparoscopic Roux-en-Y gastric bypass: Pitfalls in diagnosing a surgical abdomen in the morbidly obese. *Obes Surg* 13:938–940, 2003.
48. Byrne TK: Complications of surgery for obesity. *Surg Clin North Am* 81:1181–1193, 2001.
49. Hamilton EC, Sims TL, Hamilton TT, et al: Clinical predictors of leak after laparoscopic Roux-en-Y gastric bypass for morbid obesity. *Surg Endosc* 17:679–684, 2003.

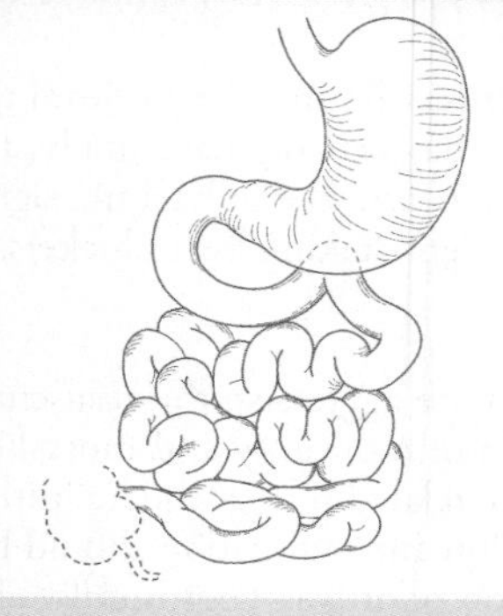

CHAPTER 46

Acute Gastrointestinal Hemorrhage

Ali Tavakkoli, Stanley W. Ashley

OUTLINE

Acute gastrointestinal (GI) hemorrhage is a common clinical problem with diverse manifestations. Such bleeding may range from trivial to massive and can originate from virtually any region of the GI tract, including the pancreas, liver, and biliary tree. The site of bleeding is typically classified by the location relative to the ligament of Treitz. Upper GI hemorrhage from proximal to the ligament of Treitz is the most common site of acute GI bleeding. Peptic ulcer disease and variceal hemorrhage are the most common causes. Most of the lower GI bleeding is from the colon, with diverticula and angiodysplasias accounting for the majority of cases. In other cases, the small intestine is responsible. Obscure bleeding is defined as hemorrhage that persists or recurs after negative evaluation with endoscopy. Occult bleeding is not apparent to the patient until symptoms related to the anemia are manifested.

During the past 20 years, multiple factors have influenced the incidence of this disease. Increased use of certain medications (e.g., nonsteroidal anti-inflammatory drugs [NSAIDs] and selective serotonin reuptake inhibitors [SSRIs]) has increased prevalence of GI bleeding, whereas the use of proton pump inhibitors (PPIs) and agents that eradicate *Helicobacter pylori* has decreased the incidence of bleeding. The overall result is that the rate of hospitalization for GI bleeding has declined modestly by 4% between 1998 and 2006.[1] A national estimate of patient discharges with a primary diagnosis of GI bleeding in 2006 was 187 discharges per 100,000 capita. The incidence of GI bleeding increased with age, occurring in approximately 1% of those 85 years or older (1187 hospital discharges with primary diagnosis of GI bleeding per 100,000 capita).[1] Although the total economic burden of GI hemorrhage has not been formally assessed, cost of a hospital admission for upper GI bleeding has been estimated to be about $20,000 per admission with a direct in-hospital economic burden of $7.6 billion in 2009.[2] Importantly, patients who experience an upper GI bleed also have significantly higher health resource utilization and costs during the subsequent 12 months than patients without bleeding.[3]

Management of these patients is frequently multidisciplinary, involving emergency medicine, gastroenterology, intensive care, surgery, and interventional radiology. The importance of early surgical consultation in the care of these patients cannot be overemphasized. In addition to aiding in the resuscitation of the unstable patient, the surgical endoscopist in some settings establishes the diagnosis and initiates therapy. Even when the gastroenterologist assumes this role, early surgical consultation is recommended, especially in high-risk patients. Approximately 5% of patients, usually those who are often older and sicker, require surgical intervention.[4] Early consultation allows the establishment of treatment goals and limits for the initial nonoperative therapy and more time for preoperative preparation and evaluation as well as patient and family education should urgent surgical intervention become necessary.

Most patients with an acute GI hemorrhage stop bleeding spontaneously. This allows time for a more elective evaluation. However, in almost 15% of cases, major bleeding persists, requiring emergent resuscitation, evaluation, and treatment. Improvements in the management of such patients, primarily by means of endoscopy and directed therapy, have significantly reduced the length of hospitalization and overall mortality in the United States to 3%, with mortality rates of 10% reported by other groups, especially in the older patients.[4]

Determination of the site of bleeding is important for directing diagnostic interventions with minimal delay. However, attempts to localize the source should never precede appropriate resuscitative measures.

MANAGEMENT OF PATIENTS WITH ACUTE GASTROINTESTINAL HEMORRHAGE

In patients with GI bleeding, several fundamental principles of initial evaluation and management must be followed. A well-defined and logical approach to the patient with GI hemorrhage is outlined in Figure 46-1. On presentation, a rapid initial assessment permits a determination of the urgency of the situation. Resuscitation is initiated with stabilization of the patient's hemodynamic status and the establishment of a means for monitoring ongoing blood loss. A careful history and physical examination should provide clues to the cause and source of the bleeding and identify any complicating conditions or medications. Specific investigation should then proceed to refine the diagnosis.

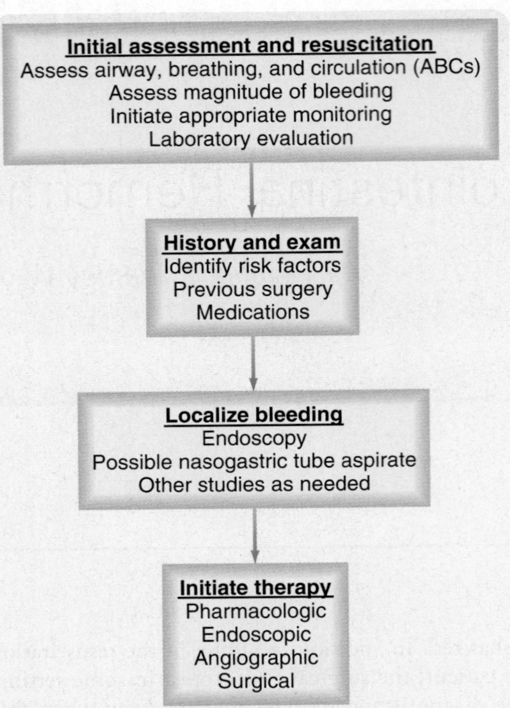

FIGURE 46-1 General approach to patients with acute GI hemorrhage.

Therapeutic measures are then initiated, and bleeding is controlled and recurrent hemorrhage prevented.

Initial Assessment

The presentation of GI bleeding is variable, ranging from hemoccult-positive stool on rectal examination to exsanguinating hemorrhage; thus, a structured approach to the assessment is important. Adequacy of the patient's airway and breathing take first priority.[5] Once these are ensured, the patient's hemodynamic status becomes the dominant concern and forms the basis for further management. Initial evaluation should focus on rapid assessment of the magnitude of both the preexisting deficits and ongoing hemorrhage. Continuous reassessment of the patient's circulatory status determines the aggressiveness of subsequent evaluation and intervention. The history of the bleeding, both its magnitude and frequency, should also provide some guidance.

The severity of the hemorrhage can be generally determined on the basis of simple clinical parameters. Obtundation, agitation, and hypotension (systolic blood pressure <90 mm Hg in the supine position) associated with cool, clammy extremities are consistent with hemorrhagic shock and suggest a loss of more than 40% of the patient's blood volume. A resting heart rate above 100 beats/min with a decreased pulse pressure implies a 20% to 40% volume loss. In patients without shock, postural changes should be elicited by allowing the patient to sit up with the legs dangling for 5 minutes. A fall in blood pressure of more than 10 mm Hg or an elevation of the pulse of more than 20 beats/min again reflects at least a 20% blood loss. Patients with lesser degrees of bleeding may have no detectable alterations.

The hematocrit is not a useful parameter for assessing the degree of hemorrhage in the acute setting because the proportion of red blood cells (RBCs) and plasma initially lost is constant. The hematocrit does not fall until plasma is redistributed into the intravascular space and resuscitation with crystalloid solution is begun. Likewise, the absence of tachycardia may be misleading; some patients with severe blood loss may actually have bradycardia secondary to vagal slowing of the heart. Hemodynamic signs are less reliable in the elderly and patients taking beta blockers.

Resuscitation

The more severe the bleeding, the more aggressive the resuscitation. In fact, the single leading cause of morbidity and mortality in these patients is multiorgan failure related to inadequate initial or subsequent resuscitation. Intubation and ventilation should be initiated early if there is any question of airway compromise. In patients with evidence of hemodynamic instability or those in whom ongoing bleeding is suspected, two large-bore intravenous lines should be placed, preferably in the antecubital fossae. Unstable patients should receive a 2-liter bolus of crystalloid solution, usually lactated Ringer solution , which most closely approximates the electrolyte composition of whole blood. The response to the fluid resuscitation should be noted. Blood should immediately be sent for type and crossmatch, hematocrit, platelet count, coagulation profile, routine chemistries, and liver function tests. A Foley catheter should also be inserted for assessment of end-organ perfusion. The oxygen-carrying capacity of the blood can be maximized by administering supplemental oxygen. Frequently, these patients benefit from early admission to and management in the intensive care unit (ICU).

The decision to transfuse blood depends on the response to the fluid challenge, the age of the patient, whether concomitant cardiopulmonary disease is present, and whether the bleeding continues. The initial effects of crystalloid infusion and the patient's ongoing hemodynamic parameters should be the primary criteria. Once again, this process requires an element of clinical judgment. For example, a young, healthy patient with an estimated blood loss of 20% who responds to the fluid challenge with a normalization of hemodynamics may not need any blood products, whereas an elderly patient with a significant cardiac history and the same blood loss probably requires a transfusion. In general, the hematocrit should be maintained above 30% in the elderly and above 20% in young, otherwise healthy patients. Likewise, the propensity of the suspected lesion to continue bleeding or to rebleed must play a role in this decision. For example, esophageal varices are very likely to continue to bleed and transfusion might be considered earlier than if a Mallory-Weiss tear, which has a low rebleeding rate, is considered the culprit. In general, packed RBCs are the preferred form of transfusion, although whole blood, preferably warmed, may be employed in circumstances of massive blood loss. Defects in coagulation and platelets should be replaced as they are detected, and patients who require high-volume transfusion should empirically receive both fresh-frozen plasma and platelets and calcium.

History and Physical Examination

Once the severity of the bleeding is assessed and resuscitation initiated, attention is directed to the history and physical examination. The history helps to make a preliminary assessment of the site and cause of bleeding and of significant medical conditions that may determine or alter the course of management.

Obviously, the characteristics of the bleeding provide important clues. The time at onset, volume, and frequency are important in estimating blood loss. Hematemesis, melena, and hematochezia are the most common manifestations of acute hemorrhage. Hematemesis is the vomiting of blood and is usually caused by bleeding from the upper GI tract, although rarely bleeding from the nose or pharynx can be responsible. It may be bright red or older and therefore take on the appearance of coffee grounds. Melena, the passage of black, tarry, and foul-smelling stool, generally suggests bleeding from the upper GI tract. Although the melanotic appearance typically results from gastric acid degradation, which converts hemoglobin to hematin, and from the actions of digestive enzymes and luminal bacteria in the small intestine, blood loss from the distal small bowel or right colon may have this appearance, particularly if transit is slow enough. Melena should not be confused with the greenish character of the stool in patients taking iron supplements. One way to distinguish these two is by performing a guaiac test, the result of which is negative in those receiving iron supplementation. Hematochezia refers to bright red blood from the rectum that may or may not be mixed with stool. Although this typically reflects a distal colonic source, if the magnitude is significant, even upper GI bleeds may produce hematochezia.

The medical history may provide a variety of clues to the diagnosis. Antecedent vomiting may suggest a Mallory-Weiss tear, whereas weight loss raises the specter of malignant disease. Even demographic data may prove useful; the elderly bleed from lesions such as angiodysplasias, diverticula, ischemic colitis, and cancer, whereas younger patients bleed from peptic ulcers, varices, and Meckel's diverticula. A past history of GI disease, bleeding, or operation should immediately begin to focus the differential diagnosis. Antecedent epigastric distress may point to a peptic ulcer, whereas previous aortic surgery suggests the possibility of an aortoenteric fistula. A history of liver disease prompts a consideration of variceal bleeding. Medication use may also be revealing. A history of ingestion of salicylates, NSAIDs, and SSRIs is common, particularly in the elderly.[6] These medications are associated with GI mucosal erosions that are typically seen in the upper GI tract but that occasionally can be seen in the small bowel and colon. GI bleeding in the setting of anticoagulation therapy, either warfarin or low-molecular-weight heparin, is still most commonly the result of GI disease and should not be ascribed to the anticoagulation alone.[7]

Physical examination may also be revealing. The oropharynx and nose can occasionally simulate symptoms of a more distal source and should always be examined. Abdominal examination is only occasionally helpful, but it is important to exclude masses, splenomegaly, and adenopathy. Epigastric tenderness is suggestive but not diagnostic of gastritis or peptic ulceration. The stigmata of liver disease, including jaundice, ascites, palmar erythema, and caput medusae, may suggest bleeding related to varices, although these patients commonly bleed from other sources as well. On occasion, the physical examination may reveal clues to more obscure diagnoses, such as the telangiectasias of Osler-Weber-Rendu syndrome or the pigmented lesions of the oral mucosa in Peutz-Jeghers syndrome. A rectal examination and anoscopy should be performed to exclude a low-lying rectal cancer or bleeding from hemorrhoids.

Localization

Subsequent management of the patient with acute GI hemorrhage depends on localization of the site of the bleeding. An algorithm for the diagnosis of acute GI hemorrhage is shown in Figure 46-2.

Although melena is usually from the upper GI tract, it can be the result of bleeding from the small bowel or colon. Likewise, hematochezia is sometimes the consequence of brisk upper GI

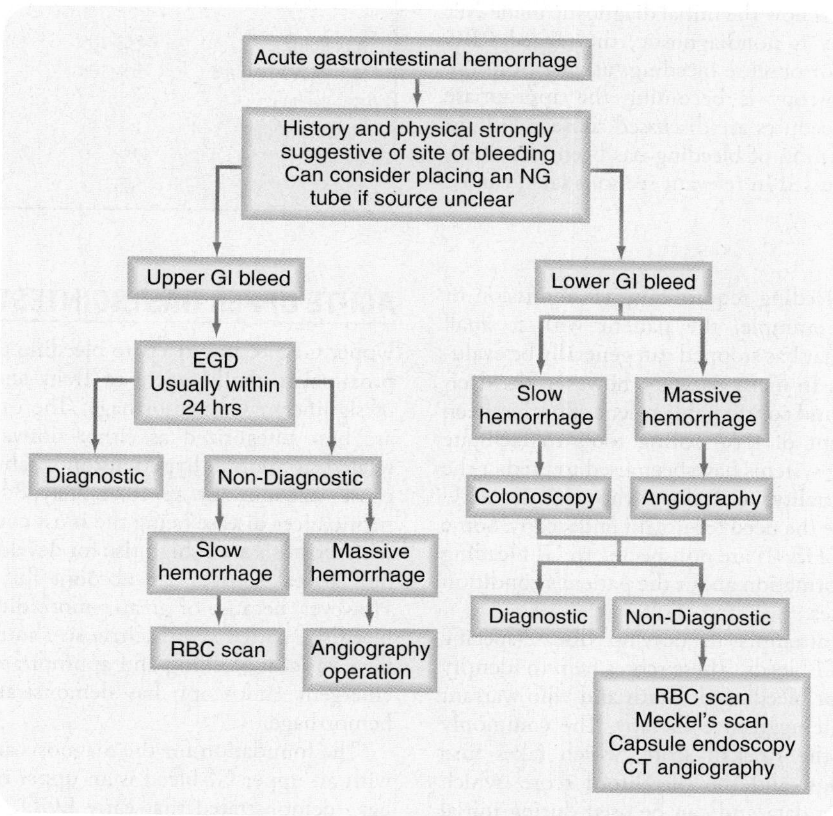

FIGURE 46-2 Algorithm for the diagnosis of acute GI hemorrhage.

bleeding. One approach to distinguishing these possibilities has been to insert a nasogastric (NG) tube and to perform a gastric lavage with examination of the aspirate. Increasing data, however, have shown that an NG tube is unreliable in localizing the bleeding site, and virtually all patients with significant bleeding should undergo upper endoscopy for direct visualization.

Upper endoscopy under these circumstances is highly accurate both in identifying an upper GI lesion and, if evaluation is negative, in directing attention to a lower GI source. Early endoscopy with directed therapy has been shown to reduce resource utilization and transfusion requirements and to shorten hospital stay. The exact definition and timeline of an "early" endoscopy have been well studied and refined. There is little argument that in an unstable patient, an urgent endoscopy is often required; however, in those patients with overt signs of bleeding but who are otherwise stable, endoscopy within 6 or 12 hours has not been shown to be of any additional benefit compared with endoscopy performed within 24 hours.[8,9]

Clinicians should be aware that esophagogastroduodenoscopy (EGD) in the urgent or emergent setting is associated with reduced accuracy, often because of poor visualization, and a significant increase in the incidence of complications, including aspiration, respiratory depression, and GI perforation, compared with elective procedures. Airway protection is critical and may require endotracheal intubation if it has not been performed previously. Volume resuscitation should not be interrupted by the examination.

As shown in Figure 46-2, subsequent evaluation depends on the results of the upper endoscopy and the magnitude of the bleeding. Angiography or even surgery may prove necessary for massive hemorrhage, precluding endoscopy, from either the upper or lower GI tract. For slow or intermittent bleeding from the lower GI tract, colonoscopy is now the initial diagnostic maneuver of choice. When endoscopy is nondiagnostic, the tagged RBC scan is usually employed. For obscure bleeding, usually from the small bowel, capsule endoscopy is becoming the appropriate study. These diagnostic procedures are discussed subsequently in greater detail. Once the location of bleeding has been identified, appropriate therapy, as discussed in relevant sections later, can be initiated.

Risk Stratification

Not all patients with GI bleeding require hospital admission or emergent evaluation. For example, the patient with a small amount of rectal bleeding that has stopped can generally be evaluated on an outpatient basis. In many patients, however, the decision is less straightforward, and considerable recent effort has been devoted to the development of risk scoring tools to facilitate patient triage. These scoring systems have been used to predict the risk of rebleeding and mortality, to evaluate the need for ICU admission, and to determine the need for urgent endoscopy. Some scoring systems (e.g., APACHE II) are nonspecific to GI bleeding but can provide general information about the patient's condition and risk of adverse outcomes.

There have also been attempts to develop disease-specific scoring systems for upper GI bleeds. These scores help to identify those at higher risk of major bleeding or death and who warrant closer observation and more aggressive therapy. The commonly used scoring systems are the Rockall score, which takes into account endoscopic findings, and the Blatchford score, which does not require endoscopic data and can be used during initial assessment. Box 46-1 summarizes these scoring systems.

BOX 46-1 Commonly Used Risk Stratification Systems for Upper Gastrointestinal Bleeds

Blatchford Score

Blood urea nitrogen
Hemoglobin
Systolic blood pressure
Pulse
Presence of melena, syncope, hepatic or cardiac dysfunction

Rockall Score

Age (<60 years, 60-79 years, >80 years)
Comorbid disease (cardiac, hepatic, renal, or disseminated cancer)
Magnitude of the hemorrhage (systolic blood pressure <100 mm Hg, heart rate >100 beats/min) on presentation
Transfusion requirement
Endoscopic findings (Mallory-Weiss tears, nonmalignant lesions, or malignant lesions)
Stigmata of recent bleed

TABLE 46-1 Common Causes of Upper Gastrointestinal Hemorrhage

NONVARICEAL BLEEDING	80%	PORTAL HYPERTENSIVE BLEEDING	20%
Gastric and duodenal ulcers	30%-40%	Gastroesophageal varices	>90%
Gastritis or duodenitis	20%	Hypertensive portal gastropathy	<5%
Esophagitis	5%-10%	Isolated gastric varices	Rare
Mallory-Weiss tears	5%-10%		
Arteriovenous malformations	5%		
Tumors	2%		
Others	5%		

ACUTE UPPER GASTROINTESTINAL HEMORRHAGE

Upper GI bleeding refers to bleeding that arises from the GI tract proximal to the ligament of Treitz and accounts for nearly 80% of significant GI hemorrhage. The causes of upper GI bleeding are best categorized as either nonvariceal sources or bleeding related to portal hypertension (Table 46-1). The nonvariceal causes account for approximately 80% of such bleeding, with peptic ulcer disease being the most common.[10] Although patients with cirrhosis are at high risk for development of variceal bleeding, nonvariceal sources can account for up to 50% of GI bleeds. However, because of greater morbidity and mortality of variceal bleeding, patients with cirrhosis should generally be assumed to have variceal bleeding and appropriate therapy initiated until an emergent endoscopy has demonstrated another cause for the hemorrhage.

The foundation for the diagnosis and management of patients with an upper GI bleed is an upper endoscopy. Multiple studies have demonstrated that early EGD, within 24 hours, results in reductions in blood transfusion requirements, a decrease in the need for surgery, and a shorter length of hospital stay. Endoscopic identification of the source of bleeding also permits an estimate of the risk of subsequent or persistent hemorrhage as well as facilitates operative planning should that prove necessary. It is somewhat surprising that studies have not shown any benefits in performing the endoscopies sooner (within 6 or 12 hours) than within 24 hours.[8,9] Although the best tool for localization of the bleeding source is EGD, this intervention is associated with increased risk and poor visualization in the acute setting, which may offset some of its benefits. In 1% to 2% of patients with upper GI hemorrhage, the source cannot be identified because of the excessive blood impairing the visualization of the mucosal surface.[11] Aggressive lavage of the stomach with room temperature normal saline solution before the procedure can be helpful. Use of promotility agents to enhance endoscopic visualization is not recommended.[12] If upper GI bleed is confirmed but identification of the actual source is still not possible, angiography may be appropriate in the reasonably stable patient, although operative intervention should be seriously considered if the blood loss is extreme or the patient is hemodynamically unstable. Tagged RBC scan is seldom necessary with a confirmed upper GI bleed, and contrast studies are usually contraindicated because they will interfere with subsequent maneuvers.

Specific Causes of Upper Gastrointestinal Hemorrhage

Nonvariceal Bleeding

Peptic ulcer disease. Peptic ulcer disease still represents the most frequent cause of upper GI hemorrhage, accounting for approximately 40% of all cases.[13] Approximately 10% to 15% of patients with peptic ulcer disease develop bleeding at some point in the course of their disease. Bleeding is the most frequent indication for operation and the principal cause for death in peptic ulcer disease.[14] Peptic ulcer disease is discussed in more detail in Chapter 48; this discussion focuses only on bleeding from ulcer disease.

The epidemiology of peptic ulcer has continued to change. The incidence of uncomplicated peptic ulcer disease has declined dramatically. This recent change has been attributed to better medical therapy, including the PPIs and regimens for eradication of *H. pylori*. Along with this decline, there has also been a decline in the number of hospitalizations for complicated peptic ulcer disease and number of surgical interventions, including suture repair of bleeding ulcers. When surgery for upper GI hemorrhage is undertaken, however, such operations are now typically performed in older patients with higher comorbidities.[14]

Bleeding develops as a consequence of acid-peptic erosion of the mucosal surface. Whereas chronic blood loss is common with any ulcer, significant bleeding typically results when there is involvement of an artery of the submucosa or, with penetration of the ulcer, of an even larger vessel. The most significant hemorrhage occurs when duodenal or gastric ulcers penetrate into branches of the gastroduodenal artery or left gastric arteries, respectively.

Management. Figure 46-3 outlines an approach to management. As stated previously, patients with clinical evidence of a GI bleed should receive an endoscopy within 24 hours, and while awaiting the EGD, they should be treated with a PPI. Although this approach has been shown to reduce the stigmata of a recent hemorrhage at index endoscopy, it had no impact on clinical outcomes such as transfusion requirements, mortality, or need for surgery; despite this, it is believed to be a cost-effective intervention for those suspected to have an upper GI bleed.[15]

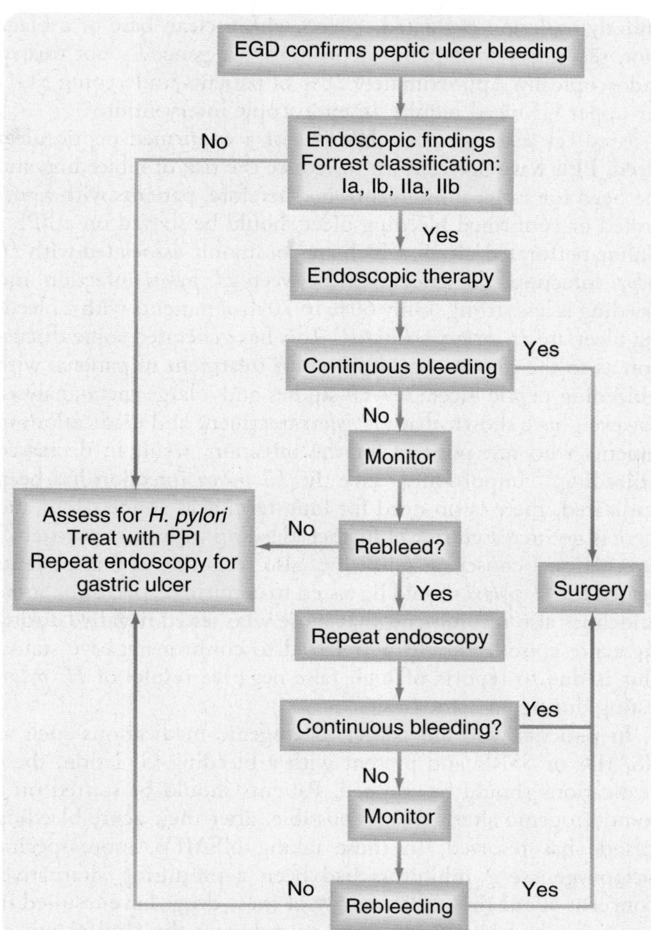

FIGURE 46-3 Algorithm for the diagnosis and management of nonvariceal upper GI bleeding.

TABLE 46-2 The Forrest Classification for Endoscopic Findings and Rebleeding Risks in Peptic Ulcer Disease

CLASSIFICATION		REBLEEDING RISK
Grade Ia	Active, pulsatile bleeding	High
Grade Ib	Active, nonpulsatile bleeding	High
Grade IIa	Nonbleeding visible vessel	High
Grade IIb	Adherent clot	Intermediate
Grade IIc	Ulcer with black spot	Low
Grade III	Clean, nonbleeding ulcer bed	Low

After the index endoscopy, treatment strategies depend on the appearance of the lesion at endoscopy. Endoscopic therapy is instituted if bleeding is active or, when bleeding has already stopped, if there is a significant risk of rebleeding. The ability to predict the risk of rebleeding permits prophylactic therapy, closer monitoring, and earlier detection of hemorrhage in high-risk patients. The Forrest classification was developed in an attempt to assess this risk on the basis of endoscopic findings and to stratify the patients into low-, intermediate-, and high-risk groups (Table 46-2). Endoscopic therapy is recommended in cases of active bleeding as well as for a visible vessel (Forrest I-IIa). In cases of an adherent clot (Forrest IIb), the clot is removed and the underlying lesion evaluated. Ulcers with a clean base or a black spot, secondary to hematin deposition, are generally not treated endoscopically. Approximately 25% of patients undergoing EGD for upper GI bleed require an endoscopic intervention.[14]

Medical management. In cases of a confirmed peptic ulcer bleed, PPIs have been shown to reduce the risk of rebleeding and the need for surgical intervention. Therefore, patients with a suspected or confirmed bleeding ulcer should be started on a PPI.[12] Unlike perforated ulcers, which are commonly associated with *H. pylori* infection, the association between *H. pylori* infection and bleeding is less strong. Only 60% to 70% of patients with a bleeding ulcer are *H. pylori* positive.[16] This has generated some discussion as to the importance of *H. pylori* treatment in patients with a bleeding peptic ulcer. Several studies and a large meta-analysis, however, have shown that *H. pylori* treatment and eradication, in patients who test positive for the infection, result in decreased rebleeding.[17] Importantly, once the *H. pylori* infection has been eradicated, there is no need for long-term acid suppression, and there is no increased risk of further bleeding with this approach.[18] International consensus guidelines also recommend that patients treated for *H. pylori* should be tested to confirm eradication. Some guidelines also recommend that those who tested negative during the acute episode should be retested to confirm negative status. This is due to reports of high false-negative results of *H. pylori* testing during an acute bleed.[12]

In patients who are taking ulcerogenic medications such as NSAIDs or SSRIs and present with a bleeding GI lesion, these medications should be stopped. Patients should be started on a nonulcerogenic alternative, if possible, after their acute bleeding episode has resolved. In those taking NSAIDs, more specific cyclooxygenase 2 inhibitors had been a promising alternative. Concerns about the cardiotoxicity of these drugs have resulted in their withdrawal from the market, reducing the clinical use of these alternative medicines. Further affecting the popularity of these medications have been population-based studies showing that not all cyclooxygenase 2 inhibitors result in a decreased incidence of upper GI complications.[19] Therefore, an alternative approach has been to identify ways to reduce the adverse GI side effects of NSAIDs. To this end, studies have shown that *H. pylori* eradication in patients who are about to start these medications can reduce the incidence of adverse GI side effects, including bleeding.[20] These studies highlight the synergistic effect of *H. pylori* eradication and NSAID use. Although this approach can have a preventive role in regard to GI bleeding, NSAIDs cannot be recommended for those who present with a bleed, even after *H. pylori* eradication.[21]

Endoscopic management. Once the bleeding ulcer has been identified, effective local therapy can be delivered endoscopically to control the hemorrhage. The available endoscopic options include epinephrine injection, heater probes, and coagulation as well as the application of clips. Epinephrine injection (1 : 10,000) to all four quadrants of the lesion is successful in controlling the hemorrhage. It has been shown that large-volume injection (>13 mL) is associated with better hemostasis, suggesting that the endoscopic injection works, in part, by compressing the bleeding vessel and inducing tamponade. Epinephrine injection alone is associated with a high rebleeding rate; therefore, the standard practice as recommended by international consensus guidelines is to provide combination therapy. This usually means the addition of thermal therapy to the injection. The sources of thermal energy can be heater probes, monopolar or bipolar electrocoagulation, and laser or argon plasma coagulation (APC). The most

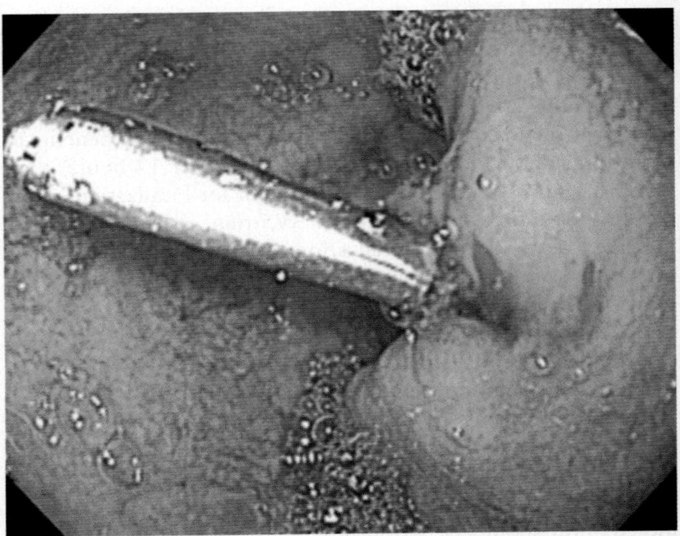

FIGURE 46-4 Hemoclip applied to a bleeding duodenal lesion. (Courtesy Linda S. Lee, MD, Brigham and Women's Hospital.)

commonly used energy sources are electrocoagulation for bleeding ulcers and APC for superficial lesions. A combination of injection with thermal therapy achieves hemostasis in 90% of bleeding peptic ulcer disease. Hemoclips (Fig. 46-4), which can be difficult to apply, may be particularly effective in dealing with a spurting vessel as they provide immediate control of hemorrhage.

Rebleeding of an ulcer is associated with a significant increase in mortality, and careful observation of patients at high risk of rebleeding using criteria previously described is important. In those who rebleed, a second attempt at endoscopic control has been validated and is recommended. A second attempt at endoscopic hemostasis is successful in 75% of patients.[22] Although this will fail in 25% of patients who will then require emergent surgery, there does not appear to be any increase in morbidity or mortality with this treatment approach. Therefore, most clinicians would encourage a second attempt at endoscopic control before subjecting the patient to surgery.

Surgical management. Despite significant advances in endoscopic therapy, approximately 10% of patients with bleeding ulcers still require surgical intervention for effective hemostasis.[14] However, identifying patients who are likely to fail to respond to endoscopic therapy is difficult, and the timing of surgery is much debated. To assist in this decision making, several clinical and endoscopic parameters have been proposed that are thought to identify patients at high risk for failed endoscopic therapy. The clinical factors to consider are shock and a low hemoglobin level at presentation. At the time of endoscopy, although the Forrest classification is the most important indicator of rebleeding risk, the location and size of the ulcer are also significant. Ulcers larger than 2 cm, posterior duodenal ulcers, and gastric ulcers have significantly higher risk of rebleeding.[23,24] Patients with these characteristics need closer monitoring and possibly earlier surgical intervention. Clearly, clinical judgment and local expertise must play a critical role in this decision.

Indications for surgery have traditionally been based on the blood transfusion requirements. Increased blood transfusions have been clearly associated with increased mortality. Although a less definitive criterion than it was in the past, most surgeons still consider an ongoing blood transfusion requirement in excess of 6 units an indication for surgical intervention, particularly in the

BOX 46-2 Indications for Surgery in Gastrointestinal Hemorrhage

- Hemodynamic instability despite vigorous resuscitation (>6-unit transfusion)
- Failure of endoscopic techniques to arrest hemorrhage
- Recurrent hemorrhage after initial stabilization (with up to two attempts at obtaining endoscopic hemostasis)
- Shock associated with recurrent hemorrhage
- Continued slow bleeding with a transfusion requirement exceeding 3 units/day

elderly, although an 8- to 10-unit loss may be more acceptable for the younger population. Current indications for surgery for peptic ulcer hemorrhage are summarized in Box 46-2. Secondary or relative indications include a rare blood type or difficult crossmatch, refusal of transfusion, shock on presentation, advanced age, severe comorbid disease, and a bleeding chronic gastric ulcer for which malignancy is a concern.

The first priority at operation should be control of the hemorrhage. Once this is accomplished, a decision must be made about the need for a definitive acid-reducing procedure. Each of these steps varies, depending on whether the lesion is a duodenal or gastric ulcer.

Duodenal ulcer. The first step in the operative management for a duodenal ulcer is exposure of the bleeding site. Because most of these lesions are in the duodenal bulb, longitudinal duodenotomy or duodenopyloromyotomy is performed. Hemorrhage can typically be controlled initially with pressure and then direct suture ligation with nonabsorbable suture. When ulcers are positioned anteriorly, four-quadrant suture ligation usually suffices. A posterior ulcer eroding into the pancreaticoduodenal or gastroduodenal artery may require suture ligature of the vessel proximal and distal to the ulcer as well as placement of a U-stitch underneath the ulcer to control the pancreatic branches.

Once the bleeding has been addressed, a definitive acid-reducing operation was traditionally considered. With the identification of the role of *H. pylori* infection in duodenal ulcer disease, the utility of such a procedure has been questioned on the basis of the argument that simple closure and subsequent treatment for *H. pylori* infection should be sufficient to prevent recurrence. This is reflected in current surgical practice, wherein rates of definitive ulcer therapy (gastrectomy or vagotomy) in patients hospitalized for peptic ulcer disease have declined significantly.

Historically, the choice between various operations has been based on the hemodynamic condition of the patient and on whether there is a long-standing history of refractory ulcer disease. The various operations for peptic ulcer disease are discussed in greater detail in Chapter 48. Because the pylorus has often been opened in a longitudinal fashion to control the bleeding, closure as a pyloroplasty combined with truncal vagotomy is the most frequently used operation for bleeding duodenal ulcer. There is some evidence to suggest that a parietal cell vagotomy may represent a better therapy for a bleeding duodenal ulcer in the stable patient, although some of this benefit may be abrogated if the pylorus has been divided. Today, inexperience of the surgeon with this procedure may be the determining factor. In a patient who has a known history of refractory duodenal ulcer disease or who has failed to respond to more conservative surgery, antrectomy with truncal vagotomy may be more appropriate. However, this procedure is more complex and should be undertaken rarely in a hemodynamically unstable patient.

Gastric ulcer. For bleeding gastric ulcers, control of bleeding is the immediate priority. Although this may initially require gastrotomy and suture ligation, this alone is associated with a high risk of rebleeding of almost 30%. In addition, because of a 10% incidence of malignancy, gastric ulcer resection is generally indicated. Simple excision alone is associated with rebleeding in as many as 20% of patients, so distal gastrectomy is generally preferred, although ulcer excision combined with vagotomy and pyloroplasty may be considered in the high-risk patient. Bleeding ulcers of the proximal stomach near the gastroesophageal junction are more difficult to manage. Proximal or near-total gastrectomies are associated with a particularly high mortality in the setting of acute hemorrhage. Options include distal gastrectomy combined with resection of a tongue of proximal stomach to include the ulcer or vagotomy and pyloroplasty combined with either wedge resection or simple oversewing of the ulcer.

Mallory-Weiss tears. Mallory-Weiss tears are mucosal and submucosal tears that occur near the gastroesophageal junction. Classically, these lesions develop in alcoholic patients after a period of intense retching and vomiting following binge drinking, but they can occur in any patient who has a history of repeated emesis. The mechanism, proposed by Mallory and Weiss in 1929, is forceful contraction of the abdominal wall against an unrelaxed cardia, resulting in mucosal laceration of the cardia as a result of the increased intragastric pressure.

Such lesions account for 5% to 10% of cases of upper GI bleeding. They are usually diagnosed on the basis of history. Endoscopy is frequently employed to confirm the diagnosis. To avoid missing the diagnosis, it is important to perform a retroflexion maneuver and to view the area just below the gastroesophageal junction. Most tears occur along the lesser curvature and less commonly on the greater curve. Supportive therapy is often all that is necessary because 90% of bleeding episodes are self-limited, and the mucosa often heals within 72 hours.

In rare cases of severe ongoing bleeding, local endoscopic therapy with injection or electrocoagulation may be effective. Angiographic embolization, usually with absorbable material such as a gelatin sponge, has been successfully employed in cases of failed endoscopic therapy. If these maneuvers fail, high gastrotomy and suturing of the mucosal tear are indicated. It is important to rule out the diagnosis of variceal bleeding in cases of failed endoscopic therapy by a thorough examination of the gastroesophageal junction. Recurrent bleeding from a Mallory-Weiss tear is uncommon.

Stress gastritis. Stress-related gastritis is characterized by the appearance of multiple superficial erosions of the entire stomach, most commonly in the body. It is thought to result from the combination of acid and pepsin injury in the context of ischemia from hypoperfusion states, although NSAIDs produce a similar appearance. In the 1960s and 1970s, it was a commonly encountered lesion in critically ill patients, with significant morbidity and mortality from bleeding. These lesions are different from the solitary ulcerations, related to acid hypersecretion, that occur in patients with severe head injury (Cushing ulcers). When stress ulceration is associated with major burns, these lesions are referred to as Curling ulcers. In contrast to NSAID-associated lesions, significant hemorrhage from stress ulceration was a common phenomenon. With improvements in the management of shock and sepsis as well as widespread use of acid suppressive therapy, significant bleeding from such lesions is rarely encountered.

In those who develop significant bleeding, acid suppressive therapy is often successful in controlling the hemorrhage. In rare cases when this fails, consideration should be given to administration of octreotide or vasopressin, endoscopic therapy, or even angiographic embolization. Historically, such cases were more commonly seen and, at times, dealt with surgically. The surgical choices included vagotomy and pyloroplasty with oversewing of the hemorrhage or near-total gastrectomy. These procedures carried mortality rates as high as 60%. Fortunately, they are seldom necessary today.

Esophagitis. The esophagus is infrequently the source for significant hemorrhage. When it does occur, it is most commonly the result of esophagitis. Esophageal inflammation secondary to repeated exposure of the esophageal mucosa to the acidic gastric secretions in gastroesophageal reflux disease leads to an inflammatory response that can result in chronic blood loss. Ulceration may accompany this, but the superficial mucosal ulcerations generally do not bleed acutely and are manifested as anemia or guaiac-positive stools. Various infectious agents may also cause esophagitis, particularly in the immunocompromised host (Fig. 46-5). With infection, hemorrhage can occasionally be massive. Other causes of esophageal bleeding include medications, Crohn's disease, and radiation.

Treatment typically includes acid suppressive therapy. Endoscopic control of the hemorrhage, usually with electrocoagulation or heater probe, is often successful. In patients with an infectious cause, targeted therapy is appropriate. Surgery is seldom necessary.

Dieulafoy lesion. Dieulafoy lesions are vascular malformations found primarily along the lesser curve of the stomach within 6 cm of the gastroesophageal junction, although they can occur elsewhere in the GI tract (Fig. 46-6). They represent rupture of unusually large vessels (1 to 3 mm) found in the gastric submucosa. Erosion of the gastric mucosa overlying these vessels leads to hemorrhage. The mucosal defect is usually small (2 to 5 mm) and may be difficult to identify.[25] Given the large size of the underlying artery, bleeding from a Dieulafoy lesion can be massive (Fig. 46-7).

Initial attempts at endoscopic control are often successful. Application of thermal or sclerosant therapy is effective in 80% to 100% of cases. In cases that fail endoscopic therapy, angiographic coil embolization can be successful. If these approaches are unsuccessful, surgical intervention may be necessary; because of difficulties in visualization and palpation of these lesions, prior endoscopic tattooing can facilitate the procedure. A gastrostomy is performed, and attempts are made at identifying the bleeding source. The lesion can then be oversewn. In cases in which the bleeding point is not identified, a partial gastrectomy may be necessary.

Gastric antral vascular ectasia. Also known as watermelon stomach, gastric antral vascular ectasia (GAVE) is characterized by a collection of dilated venules appearing as linear red streaks converging on the antrum in longitudinal fashion, giving it the appearance of a watermelon. Acute severe hemorrhage is rare in GAVE, and most patients present with persistent, iron deficiency anemia from continued occult blood loss. Endoscopic therapy is indicated for persistent, transfusion-dependent bleeding and has been reportedly successful in up to 90% of patients. The preferred endoscopic therapy is APC (Fig. 46-8). Patients failing

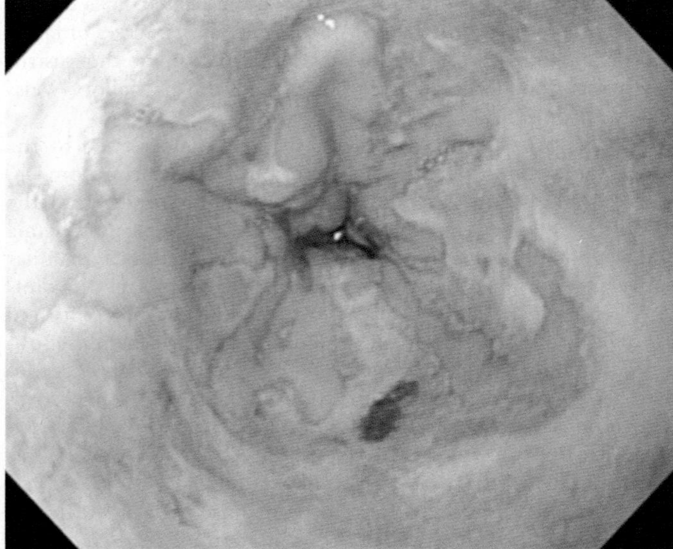

FIGURE 46-5 Bleeding esophageal ulcer secondary to herpes esophagitis. (Courtesy Scott A. Hande, MD, Brigham and Women's Hospital.)

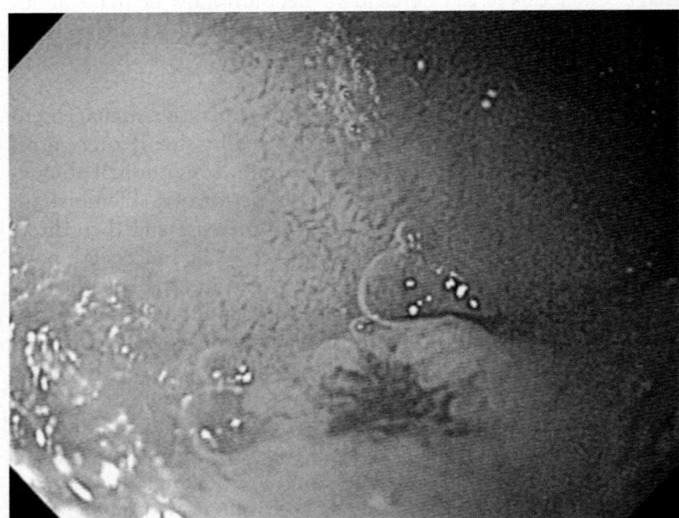

FIGURE 46-6 Dieulafoy lesion of the stomach. (Courtesy Linda S. Lee, MD, Brigham and Women's Hospital.)

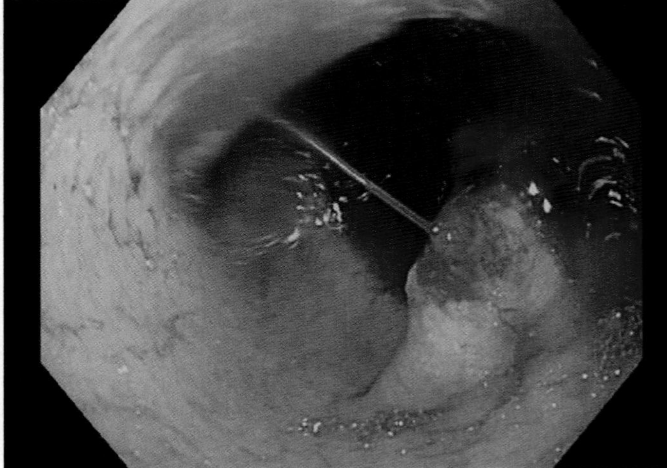

FIGURE 46-7 Bleeding Dieulafoy lesion with a spurting vessel. (Courtesy Marvin Ryou, MD, Brigham and Women's Hospital.)

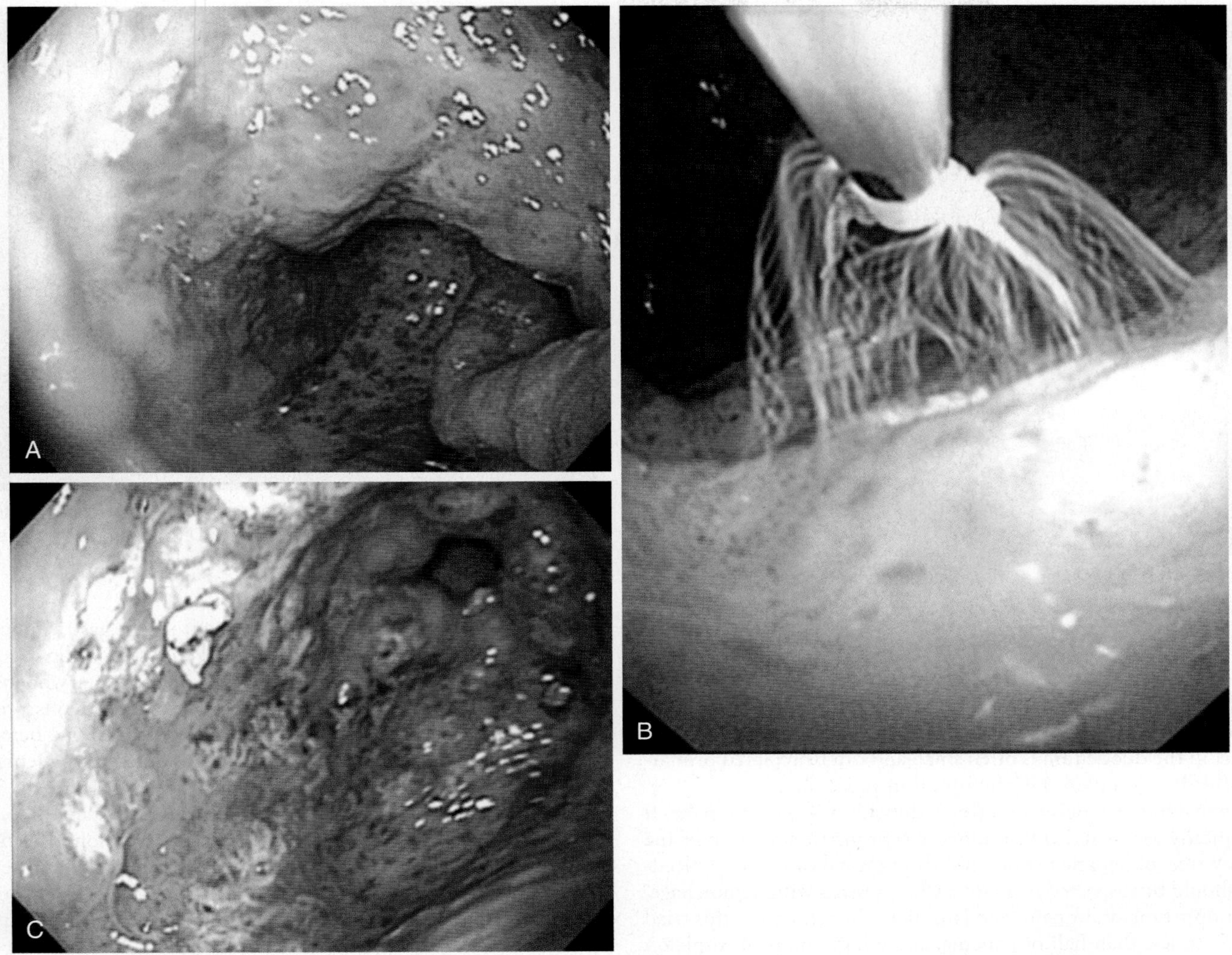

FIGURE 46-8 **A,** GAVE can be seen in the gastric antrum, giving the stomach a watermelon appearance. **B,** APC therapy of GAVE. **C,** Post-therapy appearance of GAVE. (Courtesy David L. Carr-Locke, MD, Brigham and Women's Hospital.)

to respond to endoscopic therapy should be considered for antrectomy.

Malignancy. Malignant neoplasms of the upper GI tract are usually associated with chronic anemia or hemoccult-positive stool rather than episodes of significant hemorrhage. On occasion, malignant neoplasms will be manifested as ulcerative lesions that bleed persistently. This is perhaps most characteristic of the GI stromal tumor (GIST), although it may occur with a variety of other lesions including leiomyomas and lymphomas. Although endoscopic therapy is often successful in controlling these bleeds, the rebleeding rate is high; therefore, when a malignant neoplasm is diagnosed, surgical resection is indicated. The extent of resection is dependent on the specific lesion and whether the resection is believed to be curative or palliative. Palliative resections for control of bleeding usually entail wedge resections. Standard cancer operations are indicated when possible, although this may depend on the hemodynamic stability of the patient.

Aortoenteric fistula. Primary aortoduodenal fistulas are rare lesions and likely to be fatal as they represent a rupture of the aorta to the bowel. The more common entity seen clinically is a graft-enteric erosion, which may develop in up to 1% of aortic graft cases and can be manifested as a GI bleed (Fig. 46-9). Although the interval between surgery and hemorrhage can be days to years, the median interval is about 3 years. The sequence is thought to involve development of a pseudoaneurysm at the proximal anastomotic suture line in the setting of an infection, with subsequent fistulization into the overlying duodenum.

This diagnosis should be considered in all bleeding patients with a known abdominal aortic aneurysm or a previous prosthetic aneurysm repair. Hemorrhage in this situation is often massive and fatal unless immediate surgical intervention is undertaken. Typically, patients with bleeding from an aortoenteric fistula will present first with a "sentinel bleed." This is a self-limited episode that heralds the subsequent massive and often fatal hemorrhage. This should prompt urgent upper endoscopy because diagnosis at this stage can be lifesaving. Any evidence of bleeding in the distal duodenum (third or fourth portion) on EGD should be considered diagnostic. A computed tomography (CT) scan with intravenous administration of contrast material will demonstrate air around the graft (suggestive of an infection), possible pseudoaneurysm, and rarely intravenous contrast material in the duodenal lumen.

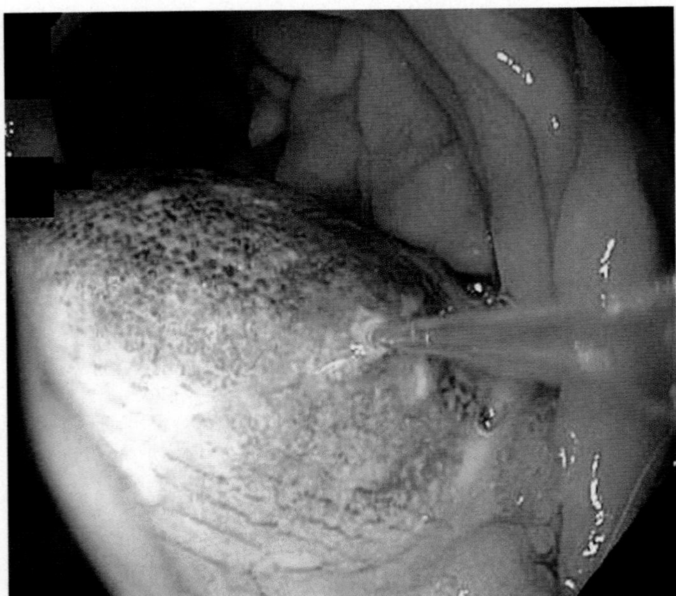

FIGURE 46-9 A vascular graft visualized during upper endoscopy for bleeding. (Courtesy Konrad Rajab, MD, Brigham and Women's Hospital.)

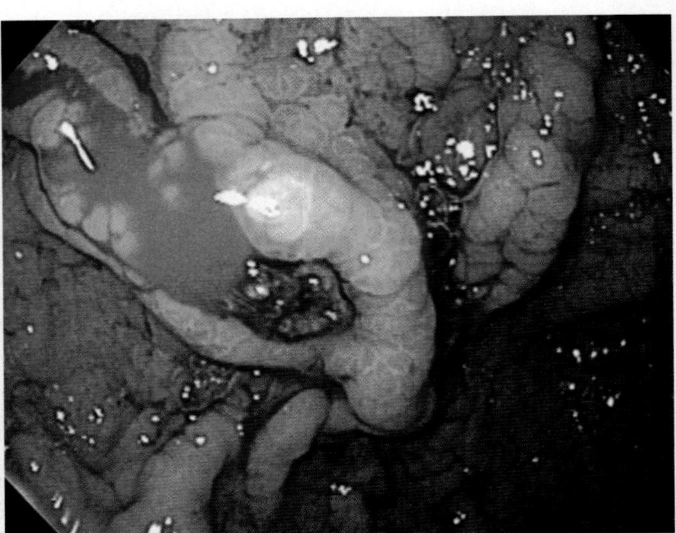

FIGURE 46-10 Bleeding from a percutaneous endoscopic gastrostomy site. (Courtesy David L. Carr-Locke, MD, Brigham and Women's Hospital.)

Therapy includes ligation of the aorta proximal to the graft, removal of the infected prosthesis, and extra-anatomic bypass. The defect in the duodenum is often small and can be repaired primarily. This is a complex and often morbid procedure.

Hemobilia. Hemobilia is often a difficult diagnosis to make. It is typically associated with trauma, recent instrumentation of the biliary tree, or hepatic neoplasms. This unusual cause of GI bleeding should be suspected in anyone who presents with hemorrhage, right upper quadrant pain, and jaundice. Unfortunately, this triad is seen in less than half of patients, and a high index of suspicion is required. Endoscopy can be helpful by demonstrating blood at the ampulla. Angiography is the diagnostic procedure of choice. If diagnosis is confirmed, angiographic embolization is the preferred treatment.

Hemosuccus pancreaticus. Another rare cause of upper GI bleeding is bleeding from the pancreatic duct. This is often caused by erosion of a pancreatic pseudocyst into the splenic artery. It is manifested with abdominal pain and hematochezia. As with hemobilia, it is a difficult diagnosis to make and requires a high index of suspicion in patients with abdominal pain, blood loss, and a past history of pancreatitis. Angiography is diagnostic and permits embolization, which is often therapeutic. In cases that are amenable to a distal pancreatectomy, the procedure often results in cure.

Iatrogenic bleeding. Upper GI bleeding may follow therapeutic or diagnostic procedures. As noted, hemobilia may be iatrogenic in nature, particularly after percutaneous transhepatic procedures. Endoscopic sphincterotomy represents another common cause for iatrogenic bleeding, which can occur in up to 2% of cases. It is often mild and self-limited. Late hemorrhage usually occurs within the first 48 hours and may require injection of the area with epinephrine. This is usually successful. Surgical intervention is rarely required.

Percutaneous endoscopic gastrostomy placement is an increasingly common procedure. Bleeding rates of up to 3% have been reported. Although the majority of these cases reflect bleeding from the incision site, some are due to bleeding from the gastric mucosa (Fig. 46-10). This can often be controlled endoscopically.

Upper GI bleeding can also be seen in patients who have recently undergone upper GI surgery. Any of the lesions previously mentioned could be responsible for postoperative hemorrhage, and these possibilities should be considered. In patients in whom a resection and anastomosis have been performed, the source of the bleeding may be the suture line or staple line. In patients in whom this is persistent and an intervention is needed, endoscopists are often concerned for the potential of suture or staple line disruption. However, it is safe to do this diagnostic or even therapeutic endoscopy, provided minimal insufflation is used and the procedure is done with care.[26]

Bleeding Related to Portal Hypertension

Upper GI bleeding is a serious complication of portal hypertension, most often in the setting of cirrhosis. Cirrhosis and portal hypertension are covered in more detail in Chapter 53; only bleeding related to portal hypertension is discussed here.

Hemorrhage related to portal hypertension is most commonly the result of bleeding from varices. These dilated submucosal veins develop in response to the portal hypertension, providing a collateral pathway for decompression of the portal system into the systemic venous circulation. They are most common in the distal esophagus and can reach sizes of 1 to 2 cm. As they enlarge, the overlying mucosa becomes increasingly tenuous, excoriating with minimal trauma (Fig. 46-11).

Although these varices are most commonly seen in the esophagus, they may also develop in the stomach and the hemorrhoidal plexus of the rectum. Portal hypertensive gastropathy, diffuse dilation of the mucosal and submucosal venous plexus of the stomach associated with overlying gastritis, is an incompletely understood entity in which the stomach acquires a snakeskin-like appearance with cherry-red spots. Unlike esophageal varices, it rarely causes major hemorrhage.

Gastroesophageal varices develop in approximately 30% of patients with cirrhosis and portal hypertension, and 30% in this group develop variceal bleeding. Compared with nonvariceal bleeding, variceal hemorrhage is associated with an increased risk of rebleeding, increased need for transfusions, longer hospital stays, and increased mortality. Hemorrhage is frequently massive, accompanied by hematemesis and hemodynamic instability. The hepatic functional reserve, estimated by Child criteria (see Chapter 53), correlates closely with outcomes in these patients. Recent advances in the field have resulted in a decrease in hospitalization rates for variceal bleeding.[27] Mortality rates have also improved but still remain high; the 6-week mortality rate after the first bleeding episode is almost 20%.[28] Treatment of variceal bleeding focuses on two aspects of care: control the acute hemorrhage and reduce the risk of rebleeding.

Management. Figure 46-12 provides an algorithm for management. As with other causes of GI bleeding, adequate resuscitation is imperative. Fluid resuscitation in patients with cirrhosis is a delicate balance. These patients frequently have hyperaldosteronism associated with fluid retention and ascites. For most of these patients, early admission to an ICU setting should be considered. A low threshold for intubation is appropriate. Defects in coagulation are common and should be aggressively corrected. A significant percentage of patients with variceal bleeding have underlying sepsis that may be associated with an aggravation in portal hypertension and lead to variceal bleeding. Studies have demonstrated that a 7-day empirical course of a broad-spectrum antibiotic (e.g., ceftriaxone) will lower the risk of rebleeding.[28]

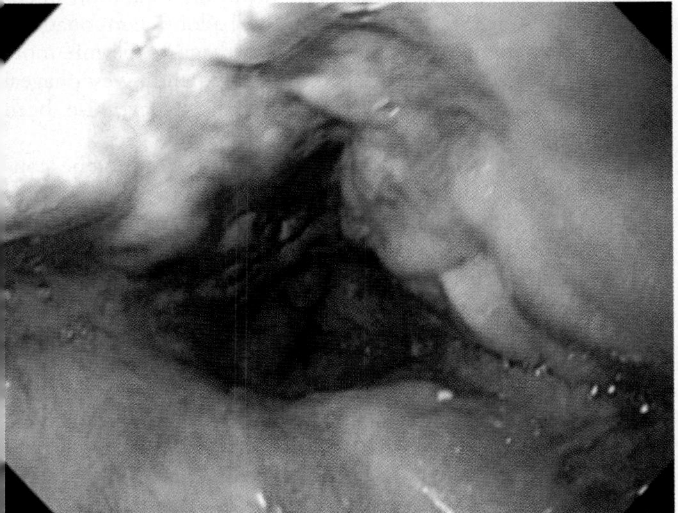

FIGURE 46-11 Nonbleeding esophageal varices secondary to cirrhosis. (Courtesy David L. Carr-Locke, MD, Brigham and Women's Hospital.)

Medical management. In patients with cirrhosis, pharmacologic therapy to reduce portal hypertension should be considered even while preparing for emergent upper endoscopy. Vasopressin produces splanchnic vasoconstriction and has been shown to significantly reduce bleeding compared with placebo. Unfortunately, this agent results in significant cardiac vasoconstriction, with resulting myocardial ischemia. Although vasopressin has been combined with nitroglycerin in clinical practice, somatostatin or its synthetic analogue, octreotide, is now the vasoactive agent of choice in the United States. Terlipressin is a newer vasopressin analogue with reduced side effects that does not need to be used as a continuous infusion. Terlipressin provides a 3% to 4% relative risk reduction in mortality in patients with acute variceal hemorrhage but is not currently available in the United States.[28]

Administration of these pharmacologic agents results in temporary control of bleeding and allows time for resuscitation and performance of the appropriate diagnostic and therapeutic maneuvers.

Endoscopic management. Early EGD is critical to evaluate the source of bleeding because more than half of bleeding is caused by nonvariceal sources, including peptic ulcer, gastritis, and Mallory-Weiss tears. In fact, studies have suggested that unlike in peptic ulcer bleeding, early endoscopy (within 15 hours of presentation) can affect survival in cases of variceal bleeding.[29]

Subsequent management is based on the endoscopic findings. If bleeding esophageal varices are identified, sclerotherapy and

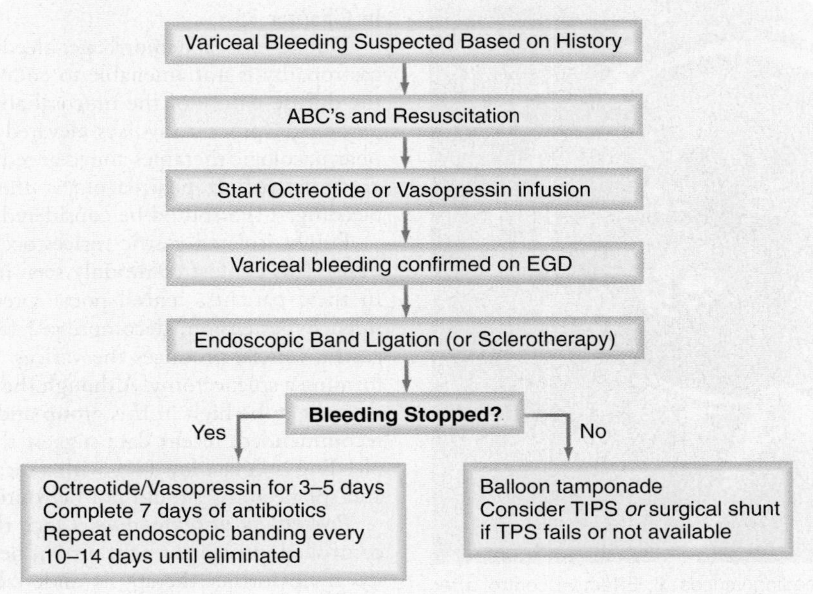

FIGURE 46-12 Algorithm for diagnosis and management of GI hemorrhage related to portal hypertension.

variceal banding have been shown to control hemorrhage effectively. Although sclerotherapy, which may use a variety of agents, is an easier procedure to perform, it is also associated with perforation, mediastinitis, and stricture. Banding seems to have a lower complication rate and, when expertise is available, should be the therapy of choice (Fig. 46-13). These endoscopic approaches, sometimes with up to three treatments during 24 hours, control the hemorrhage in up to 90% of patients with esophageal varices.

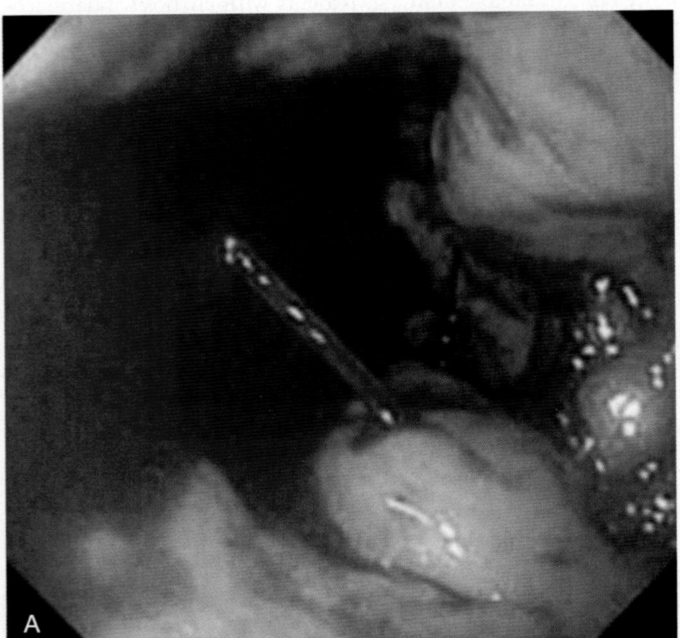

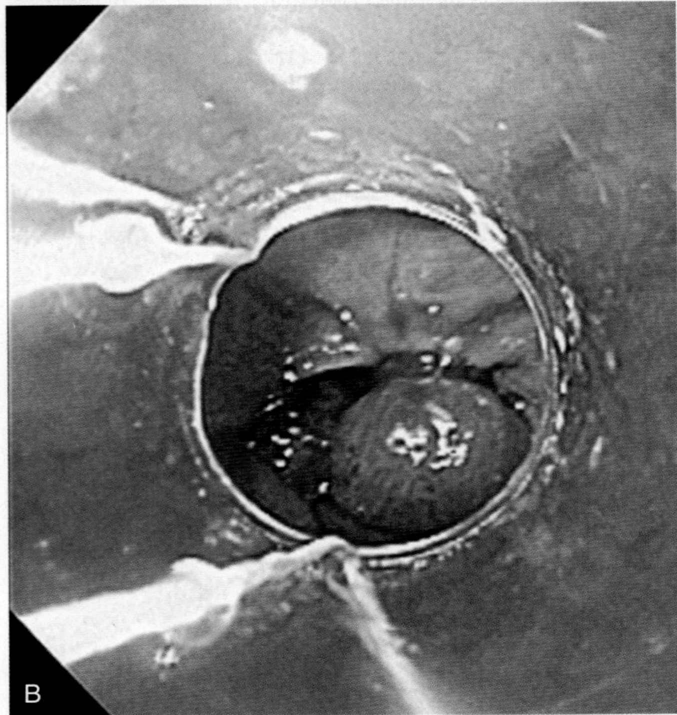

FIGURE 46-13 A, Actively bleeding varices. **B,** Effective control after variceal banding. (Courtesy David L. Carr-Locke, MD, Brigham and Women's Hospital.)

Unfortunately, gastric varices are not effectively managed by endoscopic techniques.

Other management. In cases in which pharmacologic or endoscopic therapies fail to control the hemorrhage, balloon tamponade can be successful in temporizing the hemorrhage. The Sengstaken-Blakemore tube consists of a gastric tube with esophageal and gastric balloons. The gastric balloon is inflated and tension is applied on the gastroesophageal junction. If this does not control the hemorrhage, the esophageal balloon is inflated as well, compressing the venous plexus between them. The Minnesota tube includes a proximal esophageal lumen for aspirating swallowed secretions. These tubes are associated with a high rate of complications related to both aspiration and inappropriate placement with esophageal perforation. Hemorrhage recurs on deflation in up to 50% of patients, and the balloon therapy itself has a 20% to 30% complication rate including aspiration pneumonia and esophageal tears. Currently, balloon tamponade is reserved for patients with massive hemorrhage to permit more definitive therapies. Recent trials using self-expanding esophageal stents to control massive variceal hemorrhage have also been encouraging, but their use remains experimental.[30]

In cases of refractory variceal bleeding that cannot be controlled endoscopically, emergent portal decompression is indicated. This is required in approximately 10% of patients with variceal bleeding.[31] Although randomized studies have shown equivalence between a transjugular intrahepatic portosystemic shunt (TIPS) and surgical shunting in these refractory cases,[32] this is most commonly achieved by means of a percutaneous TIPS, especially in an unstable patient. The TIPS procedure can be lifesaving in patients who are hemodynamically unstable from refractory variceal bleeding and is associated with significantly less morbidity and mortality than surgical decompression. Studies have shown that TIPS can control bleeding in 95% of cases. Rebleeding occurs in up to 20% within the first month, usually related to occlusion. Long-term patency rates are even lower, although many can be salvaged with careful surveillance and percutaneous techniques. In patients for whom TIPS is not available or fails, emergent surgical intervention is indicated, although this is seldom necessary today. Emergent surgical options are discussed in Chapter 53.

Unlike variceal hemorrhage, bleeding from portal hypertensive gastropathy is not amenable to endoscopic treatment because of the diffuse nature of the mucosal abnormalities. The underlying pathologic process involves elevated portal venous pressures, so pharmacologic therapies aimed at reducing portal venous pressure are indicated. If pharmacologic therapy fails to control acute bleeding, TIPS should be considered.[33]

Rarely, isolated gastric varices occur after splenic vein thrombosis. This is most commonly seen in the setting of pancreatitis. In these patients, central portal pressures are normal, but left-sided hypertension, decompressed from the spleen to the short gastric vessels, produces the varices. This is best treated by performing a splenectomy. Although the risk of variceal bleeding was thought to be high in this group and splenectomy was routinely recommended, recent data suggest that the incidence of variceal bleeding is in fact low (4% with a mean follow-up of 34 months), and splenectomy should not be routinely undertaken.[34]

Prevention of rebleeding. Once the initial bleeding has been controlled, prevention of recurrent hemorrhage should be a priority. If no further therapy is undertaken, approximately 70% of patients will have another bleed within 2 months. The risk of rebleeding is highest in the initial few hours to days after a first episode. Medical therapy to prevent recurrence includes a nonselective beta blocker, such as nadolol, and an antiulcer agent, such as a PPI or sucralfate. These are combined with endoscopic band ligation repeated every 10 to 14 days until all varices have been eradicated.

Although this aggressive approach results in a significant lowering of the rebleeding rate to less than 20%, it requires intensive medical follow-up and supervision.[35] In patients who are medically noncompliant or unable to tolerate such therapy, elective portal decompression should be considered if it has not already been performed. The choice between TIPS and operative decompression in the stable patient depends on the residual liver function. In general, patients with poor liver reserve who are on the liver transplant list should be considered for TIPS. This procedure provides a temporizing measure and avoids postoperative scarring of the porta hepatis, which could complicate the transplant procedure. Unfortunately, TIPS is associated with hepatic encephalopathy in up to 50% of patients within 1 year of the procedure.[36] Other shunt complications, such as thrombosis, can also occur in up to 30% of patients at 1 year. In those with good liver function who do not qualify for a transplant, surgical decompression is therefore preferred. This provides a more endurable long-term decompression, with a lower rate of hepatic encephalopathy. In those with good hepatic reserve, these advantages are thought to counterbalance the increased operative morbidity and mortality. The preferred elective shunt is a selective distal splenorenal shunt.

ACUTE LOWER GASTROINTESTINAL HEMORRHAGE

Compared with upper GI hemorrhage, lower GI bleeding is a less frequent reason for hospitalization; in fact, in looking at hospital discharge data in the United States, it is about half as common as bleeding from a location proximal to the ligament of Treitz.[1] The number of hospitalizations for this diagnosis, however, is slowly rising, increasing by 2% between 1998 and 2006. The mortality rate of lower GI bleeding is similar to that of upper GI bleeding at around 3%, but this rate increases with age to more than 5% in those 85 years or older. In more than 95% of patients with lower GI bleeding, the source of hemorrhage is the colon. The small intestine is only occasionally responsible, and because these lesions are not typically diagnosed with the combination of upper and lower endoscopy, they are considered in the section on obscure causes of GI bleeding. In general, the incidence of lower GI bleeding increases with age, and the cause is often age related (Table 46-3). Specifically, vascular lesions and diverticular disease affect all age groups but have an increasing incidence in middle-aged and elderly adults. In the pediatric population, intussusception is most commonly responsible, whereas Meckel's diverticulum must be considered in the differential in the young adult. The clinical presentation of lower GI bleeding ranges from severe hemorrhage with diverticular disease or vascular lesions to a minor inconvenience secondary to anal fissure or hemorrhoids.[37]

Diagnosis

Lower GI bleeding typically is manifested with hematochezia that can range from bright red blood to old clots. If the bleeding is slower or from a more proximal source, lower GI bleeding often is manifested as melena. Hemorrhage from the lower GI tract tends to be less severe and more intermittent and more commonly ceases spontaneously than upper GI bleeding. Compared with endoscopy in upper GI bleeding, no diagnostic modality is as

TABLE 46-3 Differential Diagnosis of Lower Gastrointestinal Hemorrhage

COLONIC BLEEDING	95%	SMALL BOWEL BLEEDING	5%
Diverticular disease	30%-40%	Angiodysplasias	
Anorectal disease	5%-15%	Erosions or ulcers (potassium, NSAIDs)	
Ischemia	5%-10%	Crohn's disease	
Neoplasia	5%-10%	Radiation	
Infectious colitis	3%-8%	Meckel's diverticulum	
Post-polypectomy	3%-7%	Neoplasia	
Inflammatory bowel disease	3%-4%	Aortoenteric fistula	
Angiodysplasia	3%		
Radiation colitis or proctitis	1%-3%		
Other	1%-5%		
Unknown	10%-25%		

sensitive or specific in making an accurate diagnosis in lower GI bleeding. Diagnostic evaluation is further complicated by the observation that in up to 40% of patients with lower GI bleeding, more than one potential source for bleeding is identified. If more than one source is identified, it is critical to confirm the responsible lesion before initiating aggressive therapy. This approach may occasionally require a period of observation with several episodes of bleeding before a definitive diagnosis can be made. In fact, in up to 25% of patients with lower GI hemorrhage, the bleeding source is never accurately identified.

An algorithm for the evaluation of lower GI hemorrhage is shown in Figure 46-14. Once resuscitation has been initiated, the first step in the workup is to rule out anorectal bleeding with a digital rectal examination and anoscopy or sigmoidoscopy. With significant bleeding, it is also important to eliminate an upper GI source. An NG aspirate that contains bile and no blood effectively rules out upper tract bleeding in most patients. However, when emergent surgery for life-threatening hemorrhage is being contemplated, preoperative or intraoperative EGD is usually appropriate.

Subsequent evaluation depends on the magnitude of the hemorrhage. With major or persistent bleeding, the workup should progress according to the patient's hemodynamic stability. The truly unstable patient who continues to bleed and requires ongoing aggressive resuscitation belongs in the operating room for expeditious diagnosis and surgical intervention. When hemorrhage is intermediate, resuscitation and hemodynamic stability permit a more directed evaluation and therapeutic intervention. Colonoscopy is the mainstay here because it allows both visualization of the pathologic process and therapeutic intervention in colonic, rectal, and distal ileal sources of bleeding. The usual adjuncts to colonoscopy include tagged RBC scan and angiography. If these modalities are not diagnostic, the source of the hemorrhage is considered obscure; such lesions and their evaluation are considered in the last section of this chapter.

Colonoscopy

Colonoscopy is most appropriate in the setting of minimal to moderate bleeding; major hemorrhage interferes significantly with visualization, and the diagnostic yield is low. In addition, in the unstable patient, sedation and manipulation may be associated with additional complications and can interfere with resuscitation. Although the blood is cathartic, gentle preparation with

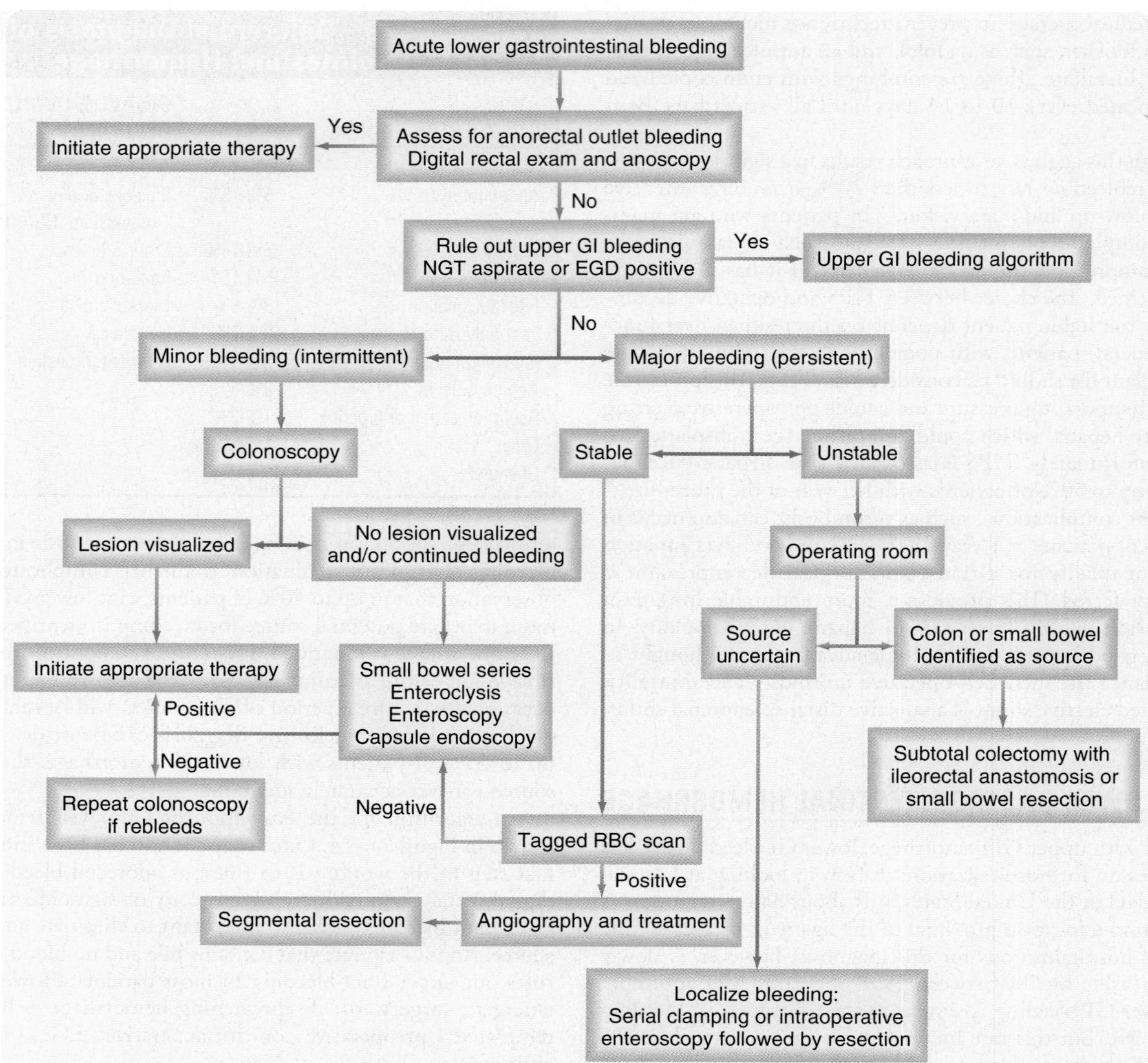

FIGURE 46-14 Algorithm for diagnosis and management of lower GI hemorrhage.

polyethylene glycol, either orally or through an NG tube, can improve visualization. Findings may include an actively bleeding site, clot adherent to a focus of mucosa or a diverticular orifice, or blood localized to a specific colonic segment, although this can be misleading because of retrograde peristalsis in the colon. Polyps, cancers, and inflammatory causes can frequently be seen. Unfortunately, angiodysplasias are often difficult to visualize, particularly in the unstable patient with mesenteric vascular constriction. Diverticula are identified in most patients, whether or not they are the source of the hemorrhage. Despite these limitations, the diagnostic yield of colonoscopy in experienced hands is reasonable. Because the majority of lower GI bleeds are self-limited, the timing of colonoscopy (within 24 hours) and experience of the colonoscopist are important in identifying the site of hemorrhage or stigmata of recent hemorrhage.[38]

Radionuclide Scanning

Radionuclide scanning with technetium Tc 99m (^{99m}Tc-labeled RBC) is the most sensitive but least accurate method for localization of GI bleeding. With this technique, the patient's own RBCs are labeled and reinjected. The labeled blood is extravasated into the GI tract lumen, creating a focus that can be detected scintigraphically. Initially, images are collected frequently and then at 4-hour intervals, for up to 24 hours. The RBC scan can detect bleeding as slow as 0.1 mL/min and is reported to be more than 90% sensitive (Fig. 46-15).[39] Unfortunately, the spatial resolution is low, and blood may move retrograde in the colon or distally in the small bowel. Reported accuracy of localization is in the range of only 40% to 60%, and it is particularly inaccurate in distinguishing right-sided from left-sided colonic bleeding. The RBC scan is not usually employed as a definitive study before surgery but instead as a guide to the utility of angiography; if the RBC scan is negative or only positive after several hours, angiography is unlikely to be revealing. Such an approach avoids the significant morbidity of angiography.

Computed Tomography Angiography

A study has shown that CT angiography may be better than scintigraphy at localizing the site of GI bleeding. Although sensitivity and specificity of the tests were similar, CT was better at localizing the site of bleeding, and the findings were more consistent to those at the time of subsequent therapeutic angiography.

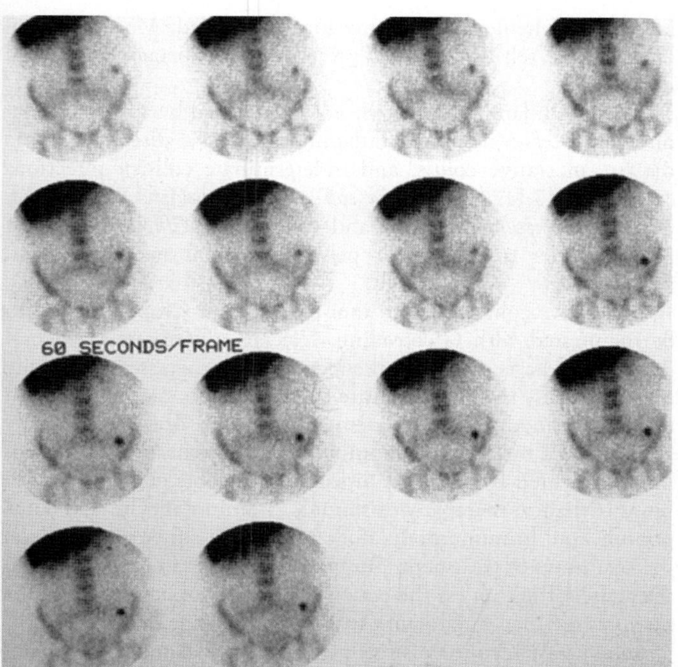

FIGURE 46-15 A positive RBC scan localizing the bleeding to the left lower quadrant. (Courtesy Richard A. Baum, MD, Brigham and Women's Hospital.)

Although patients in this group received a greater amount of contrast dye, there was no adverse outcome on renal function.[40]

Mesenteric Angiography

Selective angiography, using either the superior or inferior mesenteric arteries, can detect hemorrhage in the range of 0.5 to 1.0 mL/min and is generally employed only in the diagnosis of ongoing hemorrhage. It can be particularly useful in identifying the vascular patterns of angiodysplasias. It may also be used for localizing actively bleeding diverticula. In addition, it has therapeutic capabilities. Catheter-directed vasopressin infusion can provide temporary control of bleeding, permitting hemodynamic stabilization, although as many as 50% of patients will rebleed when the medication is discontinued. It can also be used for embolization. Although the more limited collateral circulation of the colon has made this less appealing than in the upper GI tract, it has been suggested that such techniques can be applied safely in most patients. Typically, such therapy is reserved for patients whose underlying condition precludes surgical therapy. Unfortunately, angiography is associated with significant risk of complications, including hematomas, arterial thrombosis, contrast dye reactions, and acute renal failure.

Treatment

Therapeutic approaches with lower GI bleeding are clearly dependent on the lesion identified. The criteria for operation, shown in Box 46-2, are similar to those with upper GI hemorrhage, although there is a stronger tendency to delay until the site is clearly localized.

Specific Causes of Lower Gastrointestinal Tract Bleeding

Colonic Bleeding

Diverticular disease. In the United States, diverticula are the most common cause of significant lower GI bleeding. In the past, diverticula were thought to be rare in patients younger than 40 years, but it is now an increasingly common diagnosis in this age group. Only 3% to 15% of individuals with diverticulosis experience any bleeding.[41] Bleeding generally occurs at the neck of the diverticulum and is believed to be secondary to bleeding from the vasa recti as they penetrate through the submucosa. Of those that bleed, more than 75% stop spontaneously, although approximately 10% will rebleed within a year and almost 50% within 10 years.[39] Although diverticular disease is much more common on the left side, right-sided disease is responsible for more than half the bleeding.

The best method of diagnosis and treatment is colonoscopy, although success is sometimes limited by the large amount of bleeding. If the bleeding diverticulum can be identified, epinephrine injection may control the bleeding. Electrocautery can also be used, and most recently, endoscopic clips have been successfully applied to control the hemorrhage. If bleeding ceases with these maneuvers or spontaneously, expectant management may be appropriate; however, this requires clinical judgment based on the magnitude of the hemorrhage and the patient's comorbidities, particularly cardiac disease.

If none of these maneuvers is successful or if hemorrhage recurs, angiography with embolization can be considered. Superselective embolization of the bleeding colonic vessel has gained popularity with high success rates (>90%), although the risk of ischemic complications continues to be of concern.[42] Under these circumstances, colonic resection is indicated. Certainty of the site of bleeding is critical. Blind hemicolectomy is associated with rebleeding in more than 50% of patients, and operation based on RBC scan localization alone can result in recurrent hemorrhage in up to one third of patients.[43] Subtotal colectomy does not eliminate the risk of recurrent hemorrhage and, compared with segmental resection, is accompanied by a significant increase in morbidity, particularly diarrhea in older patients, in whom the remaining rectum may never adapt.

Angiodysplasia. Angiodysplasias of the intestine, also referred to as arteriovenous malformations, are distinct from hemangiomas and true congenital arteriovenous malformations. They are thought to be acquired degenerative lesions secondary to progressive dilation of normal blood vessels within the submucosa of the intestine. Angiodysplasias have an equal gender distribution and are almost uniformly found in patients older than 50 years. These lesions are notably associated with aortic stenosis and renal failure, especially in the elderly. The hemorrhage tends to arise from the right side of the colon, with the cecum being the most common location, although they can occur in the rest of the colon and small bowel. Most patients present with chronic bleeding, but in up to 15%, hemorrhage may be massive. Bleeding stops spontaneously in most cases, but approximately 50% will rebleed within 5 years.

These lesions can be diagnosed by either colonoscopy or angiography. During colonoscopy, they appear as red stellate lesions with a surrounding rim of pale mucosa and can be treated with sclerotherapy or electrocautery. Angiography demonstrates dilated, slowly emptying veins and sometimes early venous filling. If these lesions are discovered incidentally, no further therapy is indicated. In acutely bleeding patients, they have been successfully treated with intra-arterial vasopressin, selective gel foam embolization, endoscopic electrocoagulation, or injection with sclerosing agents. If these measures fail or bleeding recurs and the lesion has been localized, segmental resection, most commonly right colectomy, is effective.

Neoplasia. Colorectal carcinoma is an uncommon cause of significant lower GI hemorrhage but is probably the most important one to rule out as more than 150,000 Americans are diagnosed each year with this cancer. The bleeding is usually painless, intermittent, and slow in nature. Frequently, it is associated with iron deficiency anemia. Polyps can also bleed, but more commonly the bleeding occurs after a polypectomy. Although bleeding in the pediatric population is discussed in Chapter 66, juvenile polyps are the second most common cause of bleeding in patients younger than 20 years. On occasion, other colonic neoplasms, most notably GISTs, can be associated with massive hemorrhage. The best diagnostic tool is colonoscopy. If the bleeding is attributable to a polyp, it can be treated with endoscopic therapy.

Anorectal disease. The major causes of anorectal outlet bleeding are internal hemorrhoids, anal fissures, and colorectal neoplasia. Although hemorrhoids are by far the most common of these entities, they account for only 5% to 10% of all acute lower GI bleeding. In general, anorectal hemorrhage is low-volume bleeding that is bright red blood per rectum seen in the toilet bowl and on the toilet paper. Most hemorrhoidal bleeding arises from internal hemorrhoids; these are painless and often accompanied by prolapsing tissue that reduces spontaneously or has to be manually reduced by the patient (Fig. 46-16). Anal fissure, on the other hand, produces painful bleeding after a bowel movement; bleeding is only occasionally the main symptom in these patients (Fig. 46-17).

Because anorectal disease is common, a careful investigation to rule out all other sources of bleeding, especially malignant neoplasia, is imperative before lower GI bleeding is attributed to such disease. Anal fissure can be treated medically with stool bulking agents (e.g., psyllium [Metamucil]), increased water intake, stool softeners, and topical nitroglycerin ointment or diltiazem to relieve sphincter spasm and to promote healing. Internal hemorrhoids should be treated with bulking agents, increased dietary fiber, and adequate hydration. A variety of office-based interventions, including rubber band ligation, injectable sclerosing agents, and infrared coagulation, have also been used. If these measures fail, surgical hemorrhoidectomy may be needed. Most anorectal bleeding is self-limited and responds to dietary and local measures.

Colitis. Inflammation of the colon is caused by a multitude of disease processes including inflammatory bowel disease (Crohn's disease, ulcerative colitis, and indeterminate colitis), infectious colitis (O157:H7 *Escherichia coli*, cytomegalovirus, *Salmonella*, *Shigella*, *Campylobacter* spp., and *Clostridium difficile*), radiation proctitis after treatment for pelvic malignant neoplasms, and ischemia.

Ulcerative colitis is much more likely than Crohn's disease to be manifested with GI bleeding. Ulcerative colitis is a mucosal disease that starts distally in the rectum and progresses proximally to occasionally involve the entire colon. Patients can present with up to 20 bloody bowel movements per day. These are usually accompanied by crampy abdominal pain and tenesmus. The diagnosis is secured by a careful history and flexible endoscopy with biopsy. Medical therapy with steroids, 5-aminosalicylic acid compounds, and immunomodulatory agents and supportive care are the mainstays of treatment. Surgical therapy is rarely indicated in the acute setting unless the patient develops a toxic megacolon or hemorrhage that is refractory to medical management.

In contrast, Crohn's disease typically is associated with guaiac-positive diarrhea and mucus-filled bowel movements but not with bright red blood. Crohn's disease can affect the entire GI tract. It is characterized by skip lesions, transmural thickening of the bowel wall, and granuloma formation. The diagnosis is made with endoscopy and contrast studies. Medical management consists of steroids, antibiotics, immunomodulators, and 5-aminosalicylic acid compounds. Because Crohn's disease is a relapsing and remitting disease, surgical therapy is used as a last resort. Massive colonic hemorrhage complicates ulcerative colitis in up to 15% of affected patients, whereas it occurs in only 1% of those with Crohn's colitis.[44]

Infectious colitis can cause bloody diarrhea. The diagnosis is usually established from the history and stool culture. *C. difficile* and cytomegalovirus colitis deserve special attention. *C. difficile* colitis usually is manifested with explosive, foul-smelling diarrhea in a patient with prior antibiotic use or hospitalization. Bloody bowel movements are not common but can be present, especially in severe cases in which there is associated mucosal sloughing. In

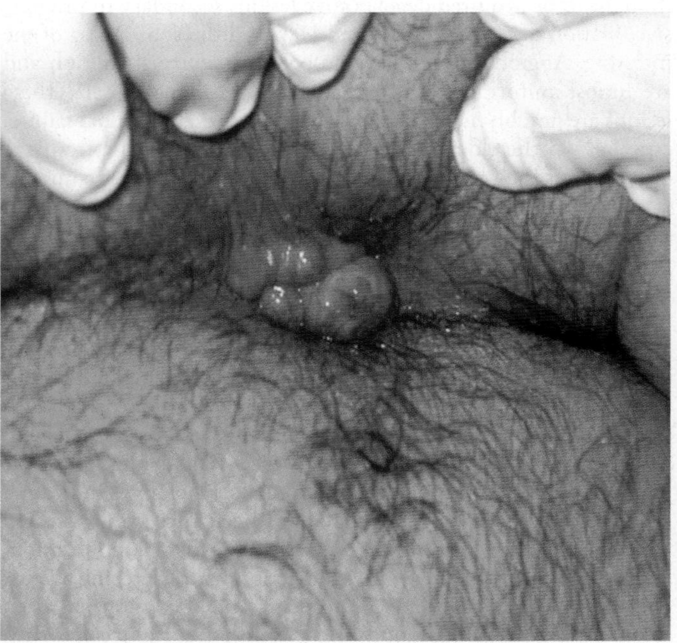

FIGURE 46-16 Bleeding and prolapsed hemorrhoids.

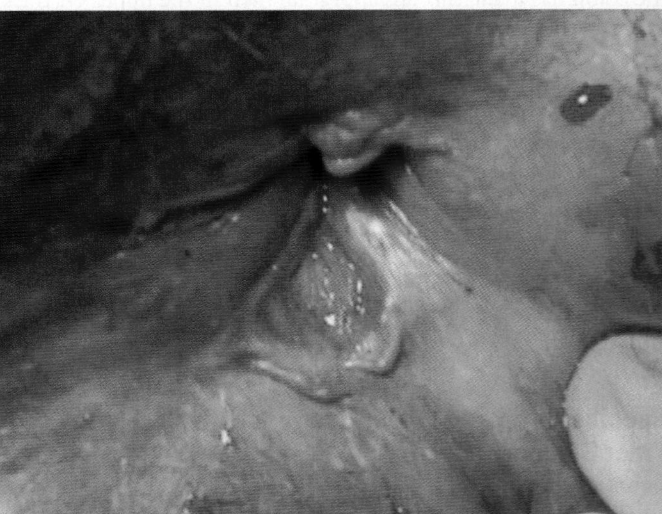

FIGURE 46-17 Anal fissures can be a source of lower GI bleeding.

North America, there has been an upsurge in the frequency and severity of *C. difficile*–associated colitis. Treatment consists of stopping antibiotics, supportive care, and oral or intravenous metronidazole or oral vancomycin. Cytomegalovirus colitis should be suspected in any immunocompromised patient who presents with bloody diarrhea. Endoscopy with biopsy confirms the diagnosis; treatment is intravenous ganciclovir.

Radiation proctitis has become much more common in the last several decades as the use of radiation to treat rectal cancer, prostate cancer, and gynecologic malignant neoplasms has increased. Patients present with bright red blood per rectum, diarrhea, tenesmus, and crampy pelvic pain. Flexible endoscopy reveals the characteristic bleeding telangiectasias (Fig. 46-18). Treatment consists of antidiarrheals, hydrocortisone enemas, and endoscopic APC. In cases of persistent bleeding, ablation with 4% formalin solution usually works well.

Mesenteric ischemia. Mesenteric ischemia can be secondary to either acute or chronic arterial or venous insufficiency. Predisposing factors include preexisting cardiovascular disease (atrial fibrillation, congestive heart failure, and acute myocardial infarction), recent abdominal vascular surgery, hypercoagulable states, medications (e.g., vasopressors and digoxin), and vasculitis. Acute colonic ischemia is the most common form of mesenteric ischemia. It tends to occur in the watershed areas of the splenic flexure and the rectosigmoid colon but can be right sided in up to 40% of patients. Patients present with abdominal pain and bloody diarrhea. CT will often show a thickened bowel wall. The diagnosis is generally confirmed with flexible endoscopy, which reveals edema, hemorrhage, and a demarcation between the normal and abnormal mucosa. Treatment focuses on supportive care consisting of bowel rest, intravenous antibiotics, cardiovascular support, and correction of the low-flow state. In 85% of cases, the ischemia is self-limited and resolves without incident, although some patients develop a colonic stricture. In the other 15% of cases, surgery is indicated because of progressive ischemia and gangrene. Marked leukocytosis, fever, a fluid requirement, tachycardia, acidosis, and peritonitis indicate a failure of the ischemia to resolve and the need for surgical intervention. During the surgery, resection of the ischemic intestine and creation of an end ostomy are indicated.[45]

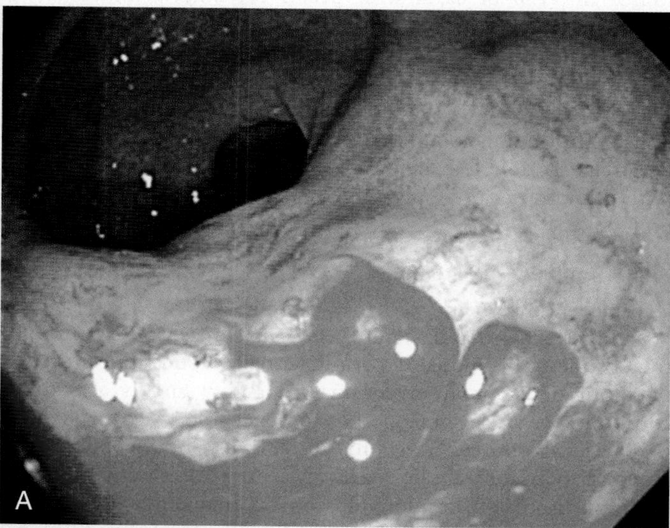

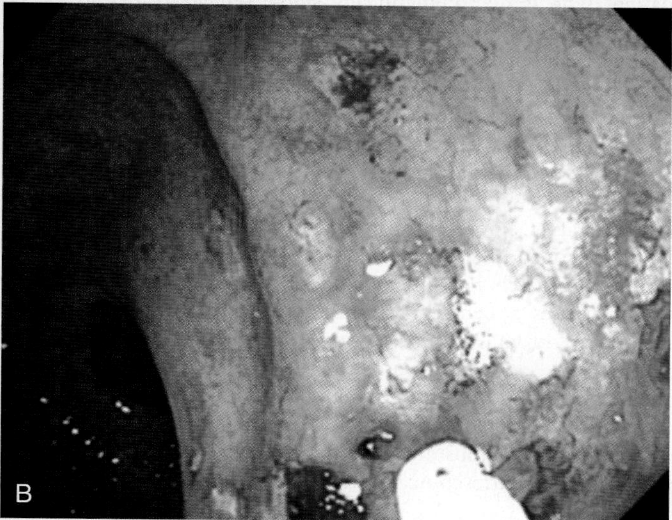

FIGURE 46-18 A, Rectal bleeding secondary to radiation damage. **B,** Effective control after application of APC treatment. (Courtesy David L. Carr-Locke, MD, Brigham and Women's Hospital.)

ACUTE GASTROINTESTINAL HEMORRHAGE FROM AN OBSCURE SOURCE

Obscure GI hemorrhage is defined as bleeding that persists or recurs after an initial negative evaluation with EGD and colonoscopy. Obscure bleeding can be further subdivided into obscure-occult or obscure-overt bleeding. Obscure-occult bleeding is characterized by iron deficiency anemia or guaiac-positive stools without visible bleeding. If initial upper and lower endoscopy fails to identify a source for obscure-occult bleeding and the patient has no systemic signs of disease, these patients are often treated with iron therapy, and more than 80% resolve their symptoms in less than 2 years. Obscure-overt bleeding is characterized by recurrent or persistent visible bleeding.[46]

Obscure bleeding can be frustrating for both the patient and the clinician, particularly for obscure-overt bleeding, which cannot be localized despite obvious signs of bleeding that can be concerning to patients and necessitate aggressive diagnostic measures. Despite improved imaging technology including video capsule endoscopy, a source of bleeding may never be found in some patients. Those patients in whom a diagnosis is reached often have had multiple tests and several hospitalizations and have received blood transfusions. Further complicating the management of these patients is that obscure GI bleeds have a high rate of rebleeding; in one study evaluating patients with a negative capsule endoscopy, the rebleeding rates were 12.9%, 25.6%, and 31.5% at 1, 3, and 5 years, respectively.[47] Fortunately, obscure-overt bleeding is responsible for only about 1% of all GI bleeding. The differential diagnosis of obscure-overt bleeding is long and varied (Box 46-3) and includes a variety of small bowel lesions not previously described. In a series of 200 patients with obscure bleeding, the small bowel was identified as the source of bleeding in more than 60% of cases. In these patients, the most common cause was small bowel ulcers and erosions secondary to Crohn's disease, Meckel's diverticulum, or NSAIDs.[48]

Diagnosis

Repeated Endoscopy

The cause of obscure-overt bleeding is often a common lesion that is missed on initial evaluation. Repeated upper endoscopy and lower endoscopy are valuable tools in identifying missed lesions

BOX 46-3 Differential Diagnosis of Obscure Gastrointestinal Bleeding

Upper Gastrointestinal Tract
- Angiodysplasia
- Peptic ulcer disease
- Aortoenteric fistula
- Neoplasia
- HIV-related causes
- Dieulafoy lesion
- Lymphoma
- Sarcoidosis
- Hemobilia
- Hemosuccus pancreaticus
- GAVE
- Metastatic cancer

Small Bowel
- Crohn's disease
- Meckel's diverticulum
- Lymphoma
- Radiation enteritis
- Ischemia
- HIV-related causes
- Bacterial infection
- Metastatic disease
- Angiodysplasia
- NSAID-induced erosions

Colon
- Colitis
  - Ulcerative colitis
  - Crohn's colitis
  - Ischemic colitis
  - Radiation colitis
  - Infective colitis
- Solitary rectal ulcer
- Amyloidosis
- Lymphoma
- Endometriosis
- Angiodysplasia
- Neoplasia
- HIV-related causes
- Hemorrhoids

as up to 35% of patients will have the bleeding source identified on second-look endoscopy. Most obscure GI hemorrhage is from a source distal to the ligament of Treitz. When repeated endoscopy fails to identify an obscure-overt bleeding source, investigation of the small bowel is warranted. This should proceed in an orderly fashion, depending on the degree of bleeding and the patient's hemodynamic status.

Conventional Imaging

The next step is probably a tagged RBC scan, although its utility in this setting has not been established, and as discussed previously, it may be misleading. Angiography may be more useful but usually requires significant ongoing hemorrhage. Provocative testing, which involves administration of anticoagulants, fibrinolytics, or vasodilators to increase hemorrhage during angiography, has been employed in small series with favorable results, but reluctance to induce uncontrolled hemorrhage has limited its use. Small bowel enteroclysis, which uses a tube to infuse barium, methylcellulose, and air directly into the small bowel, provides better imaging than simple small bowel follow-through. Because the yield has been reported to be very low and the test is poorly tolerated, it is now rarely used. An alternative to small bowel enteroclysis is CT enterography, which can identify gross lesions such as small bowel tumors and inflammatory conditions such as Crohn's disease. The limitation of small bowel radiography is that it cannot visualize angiodysplasias, the main cause of obscure small bowel hemorrhage.

In younger patients, usually younger than 30 years, part of the initial evaluation should be a Meckel's diverticulum scan. A Meckel's diverticulum with ectopic acid-secreting mucosa can ulcerate the small bowel and produce bleeding. This scan is performed by administration of ^{99m}Tc-pertechnetate that is taken up by the ectopic gastric mucosa in the diverticulum and localized with scintigraphy.

Small Bowel Endoscopy

The hemodynamically stable patient should undergo small bowel enteroscopy. Usually performed with a pediatric colonoscope, this is referred to as push endoscopy. It can reach about 50 to 70 cm past the ligament of Treitz in most cases and permits endoscopic management of some lesions. Overall, push enteroscopy is successful in 40% of patients. Sonde pull endoscopy uses an enteroscope that passes passively into the very distal small bowel. A balloon on the end of the scope permits normal small bowel peristalsis to carry the scope into the ileum; the mucosa is visualized as the scope is removed. This technique is cumbersome, does not permit intervention, and has largely been abandoned with the advent of capsule endoscopy.

Double-balloon endoscopy is another technique gaining in popularity. Although technically difficult, this approach is capable of providing a complete examination of the small bowel. In expert hands, double-balloon enteroscopy can identify a bleeding source in 77% of cases with occult bleeding, with the yield increasing to more than 85% if the endoscopy is performed within 1 month of an overt bleeding episode.[48] In cases of acute obscure-overt GI bleed, a study found that more bleeding lesions were identified by double-balloon endoscopy performed within 72 hours of admission than by video capsule endoscopy.[49] The advantage of double-balloon endoscopy is that as well as visualization, biopsies can be performed and therapeutic interventions undertaken.

Video Capsule Endoscopy

Capsule endoscopy uses a small capsule with a video camera, which is swallowed and acquires video images as it passes through the GI tract. This modality permits visualization of the entire GI tract but offers no interventional capability and is also time-consuming because someone has to watch the video to identify the bleeding source. This procedure is usually well tolerated, although it is contraindicated in patients with obstruction or a motility disorder. Capsule endoscopy is frequently used in the patient who is hemodynamically stable but continues to bleed. This technique has reported success rates as high as 90% in identifying small bowel disease. However, in a large national review of capsule endoscopy in obscure GI bleeding, the test failed to identify a source of bleeding in 30% to 40% of both obscure-occult and obscure-overt cases.[50]

Intraoperative Endoscopy

Intraoperative enteroscopy should be reserved for patients who have transfusion-dependent obscure-overt bleeding in whom an exhaustive search has failed to identify a bleeding source. This typically uses a pediatric colonoscope introduced through the mouth or through an enterotomy in the small bowel made by the surgeon. In the latter case, a sterile colonoscope is passed onto the field, introduced into the small bowel, and passed bidirectionally with the surgeon assisting to pass the bowel over the endoscope. Any suspicious areas are marked for possible resection or are dealt with endoscopically if feasible.

Treatment

Obscure GI hemorrhage requires a careful approach to diagnosis and management. Specific causes and their management are listed in the following section. Up to 25% of cases of obscure lower GI hemorrhage remain without a diagnosis, and 33% to 50% of patients will rebleed within 3 to 5 years.[46] Management strategies generally depend on the identification of a lesion. Iron replacement combined with intermittent transfusion is occasionally necessary, although this approach is not appealing. If possible, patients who are taking anticoagulants (e.g., warfarin, NSAIDs, aspirin, or clopidogrel) should be encouraged to stop these medications to lower rebleeding risks.[50]

Specific Causes of Small Bowel Bleeding

Angiodysplasias

Angiodysplasias are a common cause of small intestinal bleeding, accounting for 10% to 20%.[50] Most small intestinal vascular ectasias appear to occur in the jejunum, followed by the ileum and then the duodenum. The usual diagnostic tools are generally unsuccessful in identifying these lesions. Angiography is rarely positive. Instead, most small bowel vascular lesions require enteroscopy or capsule endoscopy for identification. In cases of severe hemorrhage requiring emergent operative intervention, intraoperative endoscopy may be helpful. These lesions have a high rebleeding rate, and segmental small bowel resection may be required. On occasion, these lesions may be diffuse; this may occur in heredity hemorrhagic telangiectasia (Osler-Weber-Rendu syndrome), acute renal failure, or von Willebrand disease. In this situation, there has been limited experience with estrogen and progesterone treatment, but it has been suggested that these agents may be of benefit.

Neoplasia

Small bowel tumors are not common but can be sources of occult or frank GI bleeding. Bleeding typically results from erosion of the mucosa overlying the tumor. GISTs have the greatest propensity for bleeding. Small bowel tumors are typically diagnosed by small bowel contrast series or spiral CT scan. Treatment involves surgical resection.

Crohn's Disease

Patients with Crohn's disease may also present with small bowel bleeding in association with terminal ileitis. Bleeding is not generally significant, nor is it usually the only presenting symptom. It is diagnosed by small bowel contrast series, and initial treatment is medical.

Meckel's Diverticulum

Meckel's diverticulum is a true diverticulum in that it contains all layers of the small bowel wall. It is a congenital remnant of the omphalomesenteric duct, occurring in approximately 2% of the general population. Often, heterotopic tissue is present at the base of the diverticulum. Bleeding from a Meckel's diverticulum is usually from an ulcerative lesion on the ileal wall opposite the diverticulum, resulting from acid production by ectopic gastric mucosa. If nuclear medicine imaging is negative and bleeding is relatively brisk, angiography may be helpful in the diagnosis. Surgical management usually requires a segmental resection to incorporate the opposing ileal mucosa, which is typically the site of bleeding.

Diverticula

Unlike a Meckel's diverticulum, small intestinal diverticula are false diverticula that do not involve all layers of the bowel. Bleeding from small bowel diverticula can present a diagnostic challenge. Capsule endoscopy or small intestinal contrast studies can confirm the diagnosis of diverticula, and in the absence of other sources of bleeding, it may be assumed that the diverticula are the source of bleeding. In cases of profuse bleeding, angiography or intraoperative endoscopy may be used to identify the bleeding source.

SELECTED REFERENCES

Barkun AN, Bardou M, Kuipers EJ, et al: International consensus recommendations on the management of patients with nonvariceal upper gastrointestinal bleeding. *Ann Intern Med* 152:101–113, 2010.

An update on international consensus on management of upper GI bleeds.

Gralnek IM: Obscure-overt gastrointestinal bleeding. *Gastroenterology* 128:1424–1430, 2005.

A concise discussion of the diagnostic approach to obscure bleeding, including the roles of small bowel fiberoptic and capsule endoscopy.

Herrera JL: Management of acute variceal bleeding. *Clin Liver Dis* 18:347–357, 2014.

A review on current management of variceal bleeding.

Rockey DC: Gastrointestinal bleeding. *Gastroenterol Clin North Am* 34:581–588, 2005.

A monograph covering all aspects of gastrointestinal hemorrhage.

Sung JJ: Marshall and Warren Lecture 2009: Peptic ulcer bleeding: An expedition of 20 years from 1989–2009. *J Gastroenterol Hepatol* 25:229–233, 2010.

A review archiving the evolution of current endoscopic, pharmacologic, and surgical management of upper GI bleeding. There is also a discussion of some of the current controversies.

REFERENCES

1. Zhao Y, Encinosa W: *Hospitalizations for gastrointestinal bleeding in 1998 and 2006: Statistical brief #65*, Rockville, Md, 2006, Healthcare Cost and Utilization Project (HCUP) Statistical Briefs.
2. Abougergi MS, Travis AC, Saltzman JR: The in-hospital mortality rate for upper GI hemorrhage has decreased over 2 decades in the United States: A nationwide analysis. *Gastrointest Endosc* 81:882–888, e1, 2015.
3. Cryer BL, Wilcox CM, Henk HJ, et al: The economics of upper gastrointestinal bleeding in a US managed-care setting: A retrospective, claims-based analysis. *J Med Econ* 13:70–77, 2010.
4. Quan S, Frolkis A, Milne K, et al: Upper-gastrointestinal bleeding secondary to peptic ulcer disease: Incidence and outcomes. *World J Gastroenterol* 20:17568–17577, 2014.

48 CHAPTER

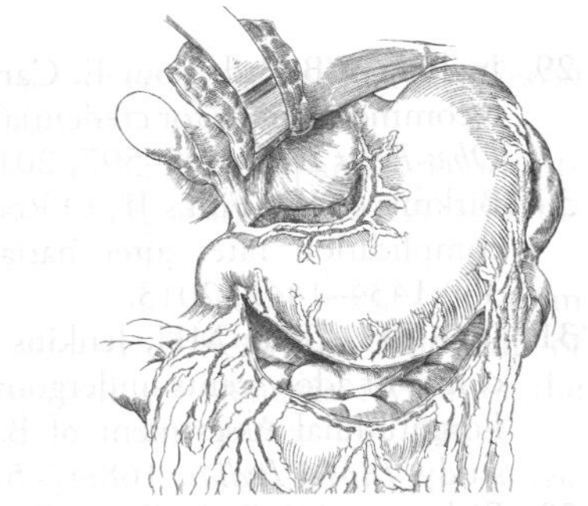

Stomach

Ezra N. Teitelbaum, Eric S. Hungness, David M. Mahvi

OUTLINE

ANATOMY

Gross Anatomy

Divisions

The stomach begins as a dilation in the tubular embryonic foregut during the fifth week of gestation. By the seventh week, it descends, rotates, and further dilates with a disproportionate elongation of the greater curvature into its normal anatomic shape and position. Following birth, it is the most proximal abdominal organ of the alimentary tract. The most proximal region of the stomach is called the *cardia* and attaches to the esophagus. Immediately proximal to the cardia is a physiologically competent lower esophageal sphincter. Distally, the pylorus connects the distal stomach (antrum) to the proximal duodenum. Although the stomach is fixed at the gastroesophageal (GE) junction and pylorus, its large midportion is mobile. The fundus represents the superiormost part of the stomach and is floppy and distensible. The stomach is bounded superiorly by the diaphragm and laterally by the spleen. The body of the stomach represents the largest portion and is also referred to as the *corpus*. The body also contains most of the parietal cells and is bounded on the right by the relatively straight lesser curvature and on the left by the longer greater curvature. At the angularis incisura, the lesser curvature abruptly angles to the right. The body of the stomach ends here and the antrum begins. Another important anatomic angle (angle of His) is the angle formed by the fundus with the left margin of the esophagus (Fig. 48-1).

Most of the stomach resides within the upper abdomen. The left lateral segment of the liver covers a large portion of the stomach anteriorly. The diaphragm, chest, and abdominal wall bound the remainder of the stomach. Inferiorly, the stomach is attached to the transverse colon, spleen, caudate lobe of the liver, diaphragmatic crura, and retroperitoneal nerves and vessels. Superiorly, the GE junction is found approximately 2 to 3 cm below the diaphragmatic esophageal hiatus in the horizontal plane of the seventh chondrosternal articulation, a plane only slightly cephalad to the plane containing the pylorus. The gastrosplenic ligament attaches the proximal greater curvature to the spleen.

Blood Supply

The celiac artery provides most of the blood supply to the stomach (Fig. 48-2). There are four main arteries—the left and right gastric arteries along the lesser curvature and the left and right gastroepiploic arteries along the greater curvature. In addition, a substantial quantity of blood may be supplied to the proximal stomach by the inferior phrenic arteries and by the short gastric arteries from the spleen. The largest artery to the stomach is the left gastric artery; it is not uncommon (15% to 20%) for an aberrant left hepatic artery to originate from it. Consequently, proximal ligation of the left gastric artery occasionally results in acute left-sided hepatic ischemia. The right gastric artery arises from the hepatic artery (or gastroduodenal artery). The left gastroepiploic artery originates from the splenic artery, and the right gastroepiploic artery originates from the gastroduodenal artery. The extensive anastomotic connection between these major vessels ensures that in most cases the stomach will survive if three out of four arteries are ligated, provided that the arcades along the greater and lesser curvatures are not disturbed. In general, the veins of the stomach parallel the arteries. The left gastric (coronary) and right gastric veins usually drain into the portal vein. The right gastroepiploic vein drains into the superior mesenteric vein, and the left gastroepiploic vein drains into the splenic vein.

Lymphatic Drainage

The lymphatic drainage of the stomach parallels the vasculature and drains into four zones of lymph nodes (Fig. 48-3). The superior gastric group drains lymph from the upper lesser curvature into the left gastric and paracardial nodes. The suprapyloric group of nodes drains the antral segment on the lesser curvature of the stomach into the right suprapancreatic nodes. The pancreaticolienal group of nodes drains lymph high on the greater curvature into the left gastroepiploic and splenic nodes. The inferior gastric and subpyloric group of nodes drains lymph along the right gastroepiploic vascular pedicle. All four zones of lymph nodes drain into the celiac group and into the thoracic duct. Although these lymph nodes drain different areas of the stomach, gastric cancers may metastasize to any of the four nodal groups, regardless of the cancer location. In addition, the extensive submucosal plexus of lymphatics accounts for the fact that there is frequently microscopic evidence of malignant cells several centimeters from gross disease.

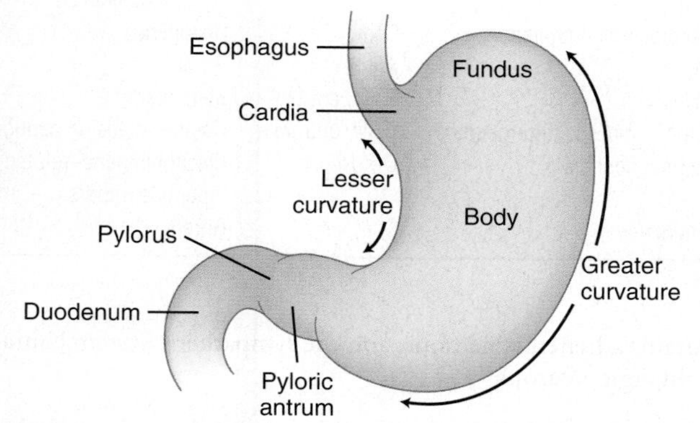

FIGURE 48-1 Divisions of the stomach. (From Yeo C, Dempsey DT, Klein AS, et al, editors: *Shackelford's surgery of the alimentary tract*, ed 6, Philadelphia, 2007, Saunders.)

Innervation

As shown in Figure 48-4, the extrinsic innervation of the stomach is parasympathetic (via the vagus) and sympathetic (via the celiac plexus). The vagus nerve originates in the vagal nucleus in the floor of the fourth ventricle and traverses the neck in the carotid sheath to enter the mediastinum, where it divides into several branches around the esophagus. These branches coalesce above the esophageal hiatus to form the left and right vagus nerves. It is not uncommon to find more than two vagal trunks at the distal esophagus. At the GE junction, the *l*eft vagus is *a*nterior, and the *r*ight vagus is *p*osterior (LARP).

The left vagus gives off the hepatic branch to the liver and continues along the lesser curvature as the anterior nerve of Latarjet. Although not shown, the so-called *criminal nerve of Grassi* is the first branch of the right or posterior vagus nerve; it is recognized as a potential cause of recurrent ulcers when left undivided. The right nerve gives a branch off to the celiac plexus and continues posteriorly along the lesser curvature. A truncal vagotomy is performed above the celiac and hepatic branches of the vagi, whereas a selective vagotomy is performed below. A highly selective vagotomy is performed by dividing the crow's feet to the proximal stomach while preserving the innervation of the antral and pyloric parts of the stomach. Most (90%) of the vagal fibers are afferent, carrying stimuli from the gut to the brain. Efferent vagal fibers originate in the dorsal nucleus of the medulla and synapse with neurons in the myenteric and submucosal plexuses.

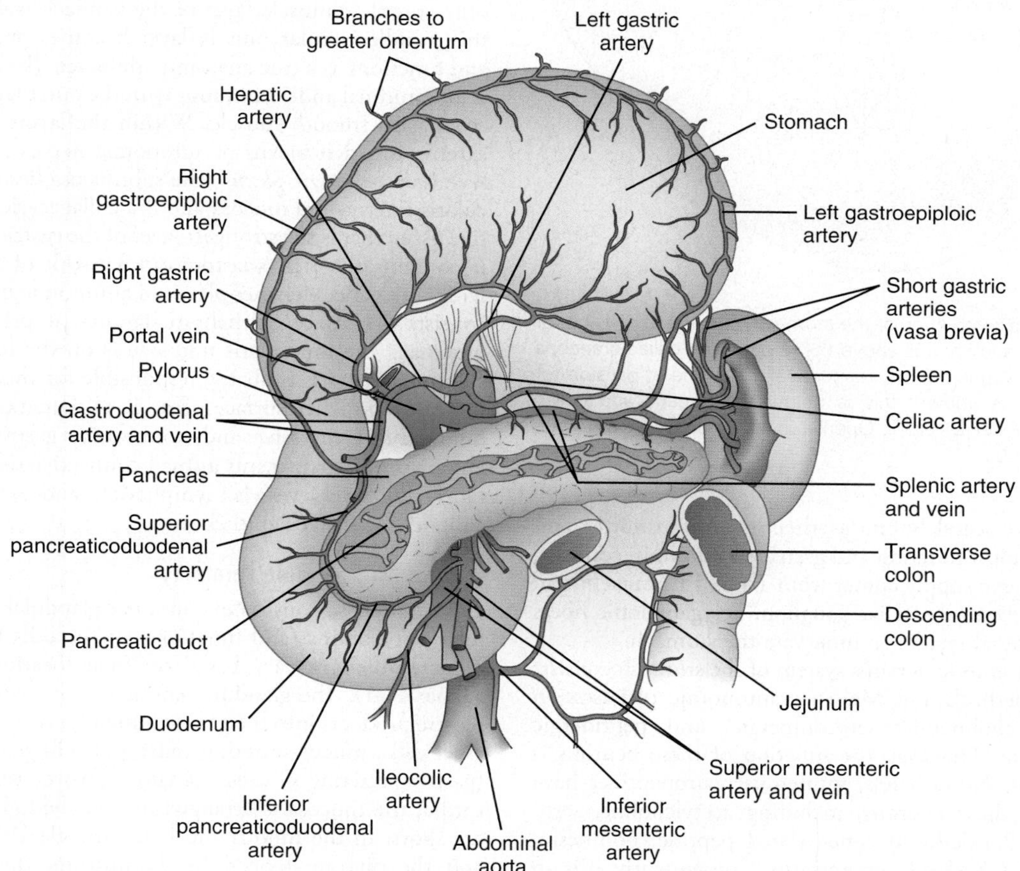

FIGURE 48-2 Blood supply to the stomach and duodenum showing anatomic relationships to the spleen and pancreas. The stomach is reflected cephalad. (From Yeo C, Dempsey DT, Klein AS, et al, editors: *Shackelford's surgery of the alimentary tract*, ed 6, Philadelphia, 2007, Saunders.)

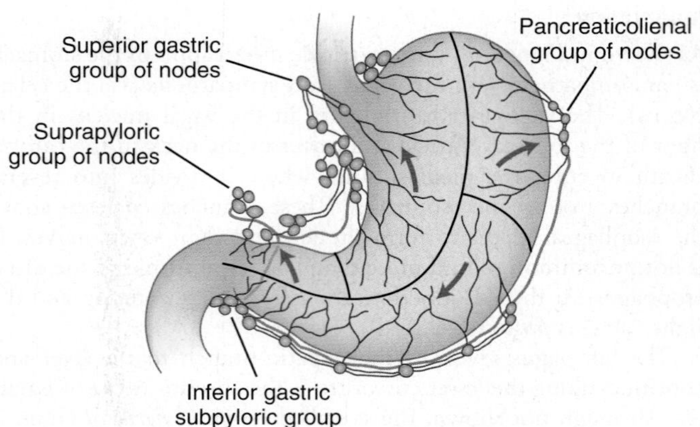

FIGURE 48-3 Lymphatic drainage of the stomach.

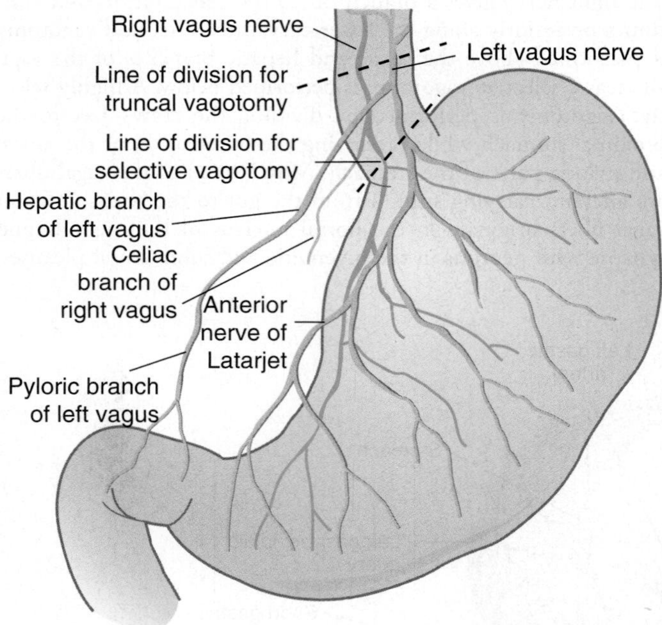

FIGURE 48-4 Vagal innervation of the stomach. The line of division for truncal vagotomy is shown; it is above the hepatic and celiac branches of the left and right vagus nerves, respectively. The line of division for selective vagotomy is shown; this is below the hepatic and celiac branches. (From Mercer D, Liu T: Open truncal vagotomy. *Oper Tech Gen Surg* 5:8–85, 2003.)

These neurons use acetylcholine as their neurotransmitter and influence gastric motor function and gastric secretion. In contrast, the sympathetic nerve supply comes from T5 to T10, traveling in the splanchnic nerve to the celiac ganglion. Postganglionic fibers travel with the arterial system to innervate the stomach.

The intrinsic or enteric nervous system of the stomach consists of neurons in Auerbach and Meissner autonomic plexuses. In these locations, cholinergic, serotoninergic, and peptidergic neurons are present. However, the function of these neurons is poorly understood. Nevertheless, numerous neuropeptides have been localized to these neurons, including acetylcholine, serotonin, substance P, calcitonin gene–related peptide, bombesin, cholecystokinin (CCK), and somatostatin. Consequently, it is an oversimplification to think of the stomach as containing only parasympathetic (cholinergic input) and sympathetic (adrenergic input) supply. Moreover, the parasympathetic nervous system contains adrenergic neurons, and the sympathetic system contains cholinergic neurons.

TABLE 48-1 Gastric Cell Types, Location, and Function

CELL TYPE	LOCATION	FUNCTION
Parietal	Body	Secretion of acid and intrinsic factor
Mucus	Body, antrum	Mucus
Chief	Body	Pepsin
Surface epithelial	Diffuse	Mucus, bicarbonate, prostaglandins (?)
Enterochromaffin-like	Body	Histamine
G	Antrum	Gastrin
D	Body, antrum	Somatostatin
Gastric mucosal interneurons	Body, antrum	Gastrin-releasing peptide
Enteric neurons	Diffuse	Calcitonin gene–related peptide, others
Endocrine	Body	Ghrelin

Gastric Morphology

The stomach is covered by peritoneum, which forms the outer serosa of the stomach. Below it is the thicker muscularis propria, or muscularis externa, which is composed of three layers of smooth muscles. The middle layer of smooth muscle is circular and is the only complete muscle layer of the stomach wall. At the pylorus, this middle circular muscle layer becomes progressively thicker and functions as a true anatomic sphincter. The outer muscle layer is longitudinal and continuous with the outer layer of longitudinal esophageal smooth muscle. Within the layers of the muscularis externa is a rich plexus of autonomic nerves and ganglia, called *Auerbach myenteric plexus*. The submucosa lies between the muscularis externa and mucosa and is a collagen-rich layer of connective tissue that is the strongest layer of the gastric wall. In addition, it contains the rich anastomotic network of blood vessels and lymphatics and Meissner plexus of autonomic nerves. The mucosa consists of surface epithelium, lamina propria, and muscularis mucosae. The muscularis mucosae is on the luminal side of the submucosa and is probably responsible for the rugae that greatly increase epithelial surface area. It also marks the microscopic boundary for invasive and noninvasive gastric carcinoma. The lamina propria represents a small connective tissue layer and contains capillaries, vessels, lymphatics, and nerves necessary to support the surface epithelium.

Gastric Microscopic Anatomy

Gastric mucosa consists of columnar glandular epithelia. The cellular populations (and functions) of the cells forming this glandular epithelium vary based on their location in the stomach (Table 48-1). The glandular epithelium is divided into cells that secrete products into the gastric lumen for digestion (parietal cells, chief cells, mucus-secreting cells) and cells that control function (gastrin-secreting G cells, somatostatin-secreting D cells). In the cardia, the mucosa is arranged in branched glands, and the pits are short. In the fundus and body, the glands are more tubular, and the pits are longer. In the antrum, the glands are more branched. The luminal ends of the gastric glands and pits are lined with mucus-secreting surface epithelial cells, which extend down into the necks of the glands for variable distances. In the cardia,

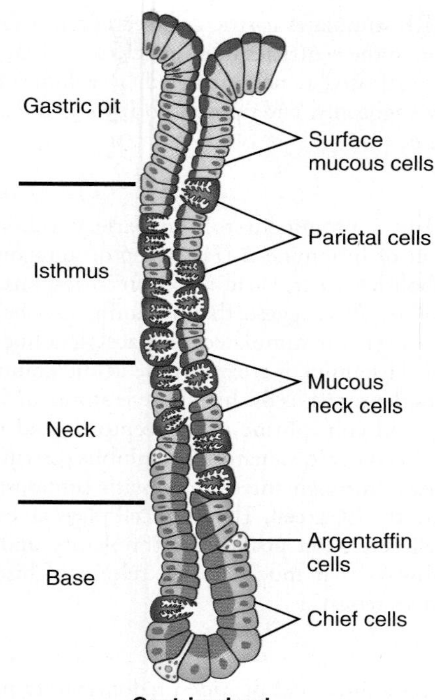

FIGURE 48-5 Cells residing within a gastric gland. (From Yeo C, Dempsey DT, Klein AS, et al, editors: *Shackelford's surgery of the alimentary tract*, ed 6, Philadelphia, 2007, Saunders.)

the glands are predominantly mucus-secreting. In the body, the glands are mostly lined from the neck to the base with parietal and chief cells (Fig. 48-5). There are a few parietal cells in the fundus and proximal antrum, but none in the cardia or prepyloric antrum. The endocrine G cells are present in greatest quantity in the antral glands.

PHYSIOLOGY

The principal function of the stomach is to prepare ingested food for digestion and absorption as it is propulsed into the small intestine. The initial period of digestion requires that solid components of a meal be stored for several hours while they undergo a reduction in size and break down into their basic metabolic constituents.

Receptive relaxation of the proximal stomach enables the stomach to function as a storage organ. Receptive relaxation refers to the process whereby the proximal portion of the stomach relaxes in anticipation of food intake. This relaxation enables liquids to pass easily from the stomach along the lesser curvature, whereas the solid food settles along the greater curvature of the fundus. In contrast to liquids, emptying of solid food is facilitated by the antrum, which pumps solid food components into and through the pylorus. The antrum and pylorus function in a coordinated fashion, allowing entry of food components into the duodenum and returning material to the proximal stomach until it is suitable for delivery into the duodenum.

In addition to storing food, the stomach begins digestion of a meal. Starches undergo enzymatic breakdown through the activity of salivary amylase. Peptic digestion metabolizes a meal into fats, proteins, and carbohydrates by breaking down cell walls. Although the duodenum and proximal small intestine are primarily responsible for digestion of a meal, the stomach facilitates this process.

Regulation of Gastric Function

Gastric function is under neural (sympathetic and parasympathetic) and hormonal control (peptides or amines that interact with target cells in the stomach). An understanding of the roles of endocrine and neural regulation of digestion is critical to understanding gastric physiology. Abnormal secretion of gastrin and pepsin was thought to be the major causative factor in peptic ulcer disease (PUD). The discovery of *Helicobacter pylori* and the effect of this organism on ulcer disease have rendered moot many of the theoretical rationales for acid hypersecretion. However, a general understanding of gastric physiology and the specific impact of peptides on acid secretion is still critical to understanding the physiologic effects of gastric surgical procedures on digestion. We initially focus here on peptide regulation of gastric function and then describe the interactions of these peptides with neural inputs in regard to acid secretion and gastric function.

Gastric Peptides

Gastrin

Gastrin is produced by G cells located in the gastric antrum (see Table 48-1). It is synthesized as a prepropeptide and undergoes post-translational processing to produce biologically reactive gastrin peptides. Several molecular forms of gastrin exist. G-34 (big gastrin), G-17 (little gastrin), and G-14 (minigastrin) have been identified; 90% of antral gastrin is released as the 17–amino acid peptide, although G-34 predominates in the circulation because its metabolic half-life is longer than that of G-17. The pentapeptide sequence contained at the carboxyl terminus of gastrin is the biologically active component and is identical to that found on another gut peptide, CCK. CCK and gastrin differ by tyrosine sulfation sites. The release of gastrin is stimulated by food components in a meal, especially protein digestion products. Luminal acid inhibits the release of gastrin. In the antral location, somatostatin and gastrin release are functionally linked, and an inverse reciprocal relationship exists between these two peptides.

Gastrin is the major hormonal regulator of the gastric phase of acid secretion after a meal. Histamine, released from enterochromaffin-like (ECL) cells, is also a potent stimulant of acid release from the parietal cell. Gastrin also has considerable trophic effects on the parietal cells and gastric ECL cells. Prolonged hypergastrinemia from any cause leads to mucosal hyperplasia and an increase in the number of ECL cells and, under some circumstances, is associated with the development of gastric carcinoid tumors.

The detection of hypergastrinemia may suggest a pathologic state of acid hypersecretion but generally is the result of treatment with agents to reduce acid secretion, such as proton pump inhibitors (PPIs). Table 48-2 lists common causes of chronic hypergastrinemia. Hypergastrinemia that results from the administration of acid-reducing drugs is an appropriate response caused by loss of feedback inhibition of gastrin release by luminal acid. Lack of acid causes a reduction in somatostatin release, which causes increased release of gastrin from antral G cells. Hypergastrinemia can also occur in the setting of pernicious anemia or uremia or after surgical procedures such as vagotomy or retained gastric antrum after gastrectomy. In contrast, gastrin levels increase inappropriately in patients with gastrinoma (Zollinger-Ellison syndrome [ZES]). These gastrin-secreting tumors are not located in the antrum and secrete gastrin autonomously.

TABLE 48-2 Causes of Hypergastrinemia

ULCEROGENIC CAUSES	NONULCEROGENIC CAUSES
Antral G cell hyperplasia or hyperfunction	Antisecretory agents (PPIs)
Retained excluded antrum	Atrophic gastritis
Zollinger-Ellison syndrome	Pernicious anemia
Gastric outlet obstruction	Acid-reducing procedure (vagotomy)
Short-gut syndrome	*Helicobacter pylori* infection
	Chronic renal failure

PPIs, Proton pump inhibitors.

Gastrin initiates its biologic actions by activation of surface membrane receptors. These receptors are members of the classic G protein–coupled seven-transmembrane–spanning receptor family and are classified as type A or B CCK receptors. The gastrin or CCK-B receptor has high affinity for gastrin and CCK, whereas type A CCK receptors have an affinity for sulfated CCK analogues and a low affinity for gastrin. Binding of gastrin with the CCK-B receptor has been associated with elevated intracellular calcium levels.

Somatostatin

Somatostatin is produced by D cells and exists endogenously as the 14–amino acid peptide or 28–amino acid peptide. The predominant molecular form in the stomach is somatostatin-14. It is produced by diffuse neuroendocrine cells located in the fundus and antrum. In these locations, D cell cytoplasmic extensions have direct contact with the parietal cells and G cells, where somatostatin presumably exerts its actions through paracrine effects on acid secretion and gastrin release.[1] Somatostatin is able to inhibit parietal cell acid secretion directly but can also indirectly inhibit acid secretion through inhibition of gastrin release and downregulation of histamine release from ECL cells. The principal stimulus for somatostatin release is antral acidification, whereas acetylcholine from vagal fibers inhibits its release.

Somatostatin receptors are also seven-transmembrane–spanning receptors. Binding of somatostatin with its receptors is coupled to one or more inhibitory guanine nucleotide–binding proteins. Parietal cell somatostatin receptors appear to be a single subunit of glycoproteins with a molecular weight of 99 kDa, with equal affinity for somatostatin-14 and somatostatin-28. Somatostatin can inhibit parietal cell secretion through G protein–dependent and G protein–independent mechanisms. However, the ability of somatostatin to exert its inhibitory actions on cellular function is primarily thought to be mediated through the inhibition of adenylate cyclase, with a resultant reduction in cyclic adenosine monophosphate (cAMP) levels.

Gastrin-Releasing Peptide

Bombesin was discovered in 1970 in an extract prepared from skin of the amphibian *Bombina bombina* (European fire-bellied toad). Its mammalian counterpart is gastrin-releasing peptide (GRP). GRP is particularly prominent in nerves ending in the acid-secreting and gastrin-secreting portions of the stomach and is found in the circular muscular layer. In the antral mucosa, GRP stimulates gastrin and somatostatin release by binding to receptors located on the G and D cells, respectively. It is rapidly cleared from the circulation by a neutral endopeptidase and has a half-life of approximately 1.4 minutes. Peripheral administration of exogenous GRP stimulates gastric acid secretion, whereas central administration in the ventricles inhibits acid secretion. The inhibitory pathway activated is not mediated by a humoral factor, is unaffected by vagotomy, and appears to involve the sympathetic nervous system.

Histamine

Histamine plays a prominent role in parietal cell stimulation. Administration of histamine 2 (H_2) receptor antagonists almost completely abolishes gastric acid secretion in response to gastrin and acetylcholine. This suggests that histamine may be a necessary intermediary of gastrin-stimulated and acetylcholine-stimulated acid secretion. Histamine is stored in the acidic granules of ECL cells and in resident mast cells. Its release is stimulated by gastrin, acetylcholine, and epinephrine after receptor-ligand interactions on ECL cells. In contrast, somatostatin inhibits gastrin-stimulated histamine release through interactions with somatostatin receptors located on the ECL cell. The ECL cell plays an essential role in parietal cell activation possessing stimulatory and inhibitory feedback pathways that modulate the release of histamine and therefore acid secretion.

Ghrelin

Ghrelin is a 28–amino acid peptide predominantly produced by endocrine cells of the oxyntic mucosa of the stomach, with substantially lower amounts from the bowel, pancreas, and other organs. Removal of the acid-producing part of the stomach decreases circulating ghrelin by 80%. Ghrelin appears to be under endocrine and metabolic control, has a diurnal rhythm, likely plays a major role in the neuroendocrine and metabolic responses to changes in nutritional status, and may be a major anabolic hormone.

In human volunteers, ghrelin administration enhances appetite and increases food intake. In patients who have undergone a gastric bypass, ghrelin levels are 77% lower than levels in matched obese control subjects, a finding not seen after other forms of antiobesity surgery. Although the mechanism responsible for suppression of ghrelin levels after gastric bypass is unknown, it is suggested that ghrelin may be responsive to the normal flow of nutrients across the stomach. Other studies have suggested that ghrelin leads to a switch toward glycolysis and away from fatty acid oxidation, which would favor fat deposition. Ghrelin appears to be upregulated in times of negative energy balance and downregulated in times of positive energy balance, although the precise role of ghrelin in energy metabolism is unclear. Ghrelin may come to have a role in the treatment and prevention of obesity.

Gastric Acid Secretion

Gastric acid secretion by the parietal cell is regulated by three local stimuli—acetylcholine, gastrin, and histamine. These three stimuli account for basal and stimulated gastric acid secretion. Acetylcholine is the principal neurotransmitter modulating acid secretion and is released from the vagus and parasympathetic ganglion cells. Vagal fibers innervate not only parietal cells but also G cells and ECL cells to modulate release of their peptides. Gastrin has hormonal effects on the parietal cell and stimulates histamine release. Histamine has paracrine-like effects on the parietal cell and, as shown in Figure 48-6, plays a central role in the regulation of acid secretion by the parietal cell after its release from ECL cells. As depicted, somatostatin exerts inhibitory actions on gastric acid secretion. Release of somatostatin from antral D cells is stimulated in the presence of intraluminal acid to a pH of 3 or lower. After

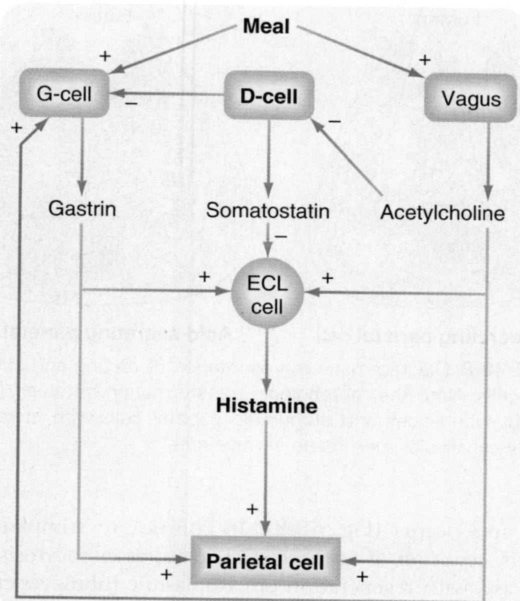

FIGURE 48-6 Central role of the enterochromaffin-like (ECL) cell in regulation of acid secretion by the parietal cell. As shown, ingestion of a meal stimulates vagal fibers to release acetylcholine (cephalic phase). Binding of acetylcholine to M_3 receptors located on the ECL cell, parietal cell, and G cell results in the release of histamine, hydrochloric acid, and gastrin. Binding of acetylcholine to M_3 receptors on D cells results in the inhibition of somatostatin release. After a meal, G cells are also stimulated to release gastrin, which interacts with receptors located on ECL cells and parietal cells to cause the release of histamine and hydrochloric acid (gastric phase). Release of somatostatin from D cells decreases histamine release and gastrin release from ECL cells and G cells. In addition, somatostatin inhibits parietal cell acid secretion (not shown). The principal stimulus for the activation of D cells is antral luminal acidification (not shown). (From Yeo C, Dempsey DT, Klein AS, et al, editors: *Shackelford's surgery of the alimentary tract*, ed 6, Philadelphia, 2007, Saunders.)

its release, somatostatin inhibits gastrin release through paracrine effects and modifies histamine release from ECL cells. In some patients with PUD, this negative feedback response is defective. Consequently, the precise state of acid secretion by the parietal cell depends on the overall influence of the positive and negative stimuli.

In the absence of food, there is always a basal level of acid secretion that is approximately 10% of maximal acid output. Under basal conditions, 1 to 5 mmol/hr of hydrochloric acid is secreted, and this is reduced after vagotomy or H_2 receptor blockade. Thus, it appears likely that basal acid secretion is caused by a combination of cholinergic and histaminergic input.

Stimulated Acid Secretion

Cephalic phase. Ingestion of food is the physiologic stimulus for acid secretion. Three phases of the acid secretory response to a meal have been described—cephalic, gastric, and intestinal. These three phases are interrelated and occur concurrently, not consecutively.

The cephalic phase originates with the sight, smell, thought, or taste of food, which stimulates neural centers in the cortex and hypothalamus. Although the exact mechanisms whereby senses stimulate acid secretion are not yet fully elucidated, it is hypothesized that several sites are stimulated in the brain. These higher centers transmit signals to the stomach by the vagus nerves, which release acetylcholine that activates muscarinic receptors located on target cells. Acetylcholine directly increases acid secretion by the parietal cells and can inhibit and stimulate gastrin release, the net effect being a slight increase in gastrin levels. Although the intensity of the acid secretory response in the cephalic phase surpasses that of the other phases, it accounts for only 20% to 30% of the total volume of gastric acid produced in response to a meal because of the short duration of the cephalic phase.

Gastric phase. The gastric phase of acid secretion begins when food enters the gastric lumen. Digestion products of ingested food interact with microvilli of antral G cells to stimulate gastrin release. Food also stimulates acid secretion by causing mechanical distention of the stomach. Gastric distention activates stretch receptors in the stomach to elicit the long vagovagal reflex arc. It is abolished by proximal gastric vagotomy and is, at least in part, independent of changes in serum gastrin levels. However, antral distention also causes gastrin release in humans, a reflex that has been called the *pyloro-oxyntic reflex*. In humans, mechanical distention of the stomach accounts for approximately 30% to 40% of the maximal acid secretory response to a peptone meal, with the remainder caused by gastrin release. The entire gastric phase accounts for most (60% to 70%) of meal-stimulated acid output because it lasts until the stomach is empty.

Intestinal phase. The intestinal phase of gastric secretion is poorly understood but appears to be initiated by entry of chyme into the small intestine. It occurs after gastric emptying and lasts as long as partially digested food components remain in the proximal small bowel. It accounts for only 10% of the acid secretory response to a meal and does not appear to be mediated by serum gastrin levels. It has been hypothesized that a distinct acid stimulatory peptide hormone (entero-oxyntin) released from small bowel mucosa may mediate the intestinal phase of acid secretion.

Activation and Secretion by the Parietal Cell

The two second messengers principally involved in stimulation of acid secretion by parietal cells are intracellular cAMP and calcium. Synthesis of these two messengers activates protein kinases and phosphorylation cascades. The intracellular events following ligand binding to receptors on the parietal cell are shown in Figure 48-7. Histamine causes an increase in intracellular cAMP, which activates protein kinases to initiate a cascade of phosphorylation events that culminate in activation of H^+, K^+-ATPase. In contrast, acetylcholine and gastrin stimulate phospholipase C, which converts membrane-bound phospholipids into inositol triphosphate to mobilize calcium from intracellular stores. Increased intracellular calcium activates other protein kinases that ultimately activate H^+, K^+-ATPase in a similar fashion to initiate the secretion of hydrochloric acid.

H^+, K^+-ATPase is the final common pathway for gastric acid secretion by the parietal cell. It is composed of two subunits, a catalytic α-subunit (100 kDa) and a glycoprotein β-subunit (60 kDa). During the resting, or nonsecreting, state, gastric parietal cells store H^+, K^+-ATPase within intracellular tubulovesicular elements. Cellular relocation of the proton pump subunits through cytoskeletal rearrangements must occur for acid secretion to increase in response to stimulatory factors. The subsequent insertion and heterodimer assembly of the H^+, K^+-ATPase subunits into the microvilli of the secretory canaliculus causes an increase in gastric acid secretion. A KCl efflux pathway must exist to supply potassium to the extracytoplasmic side of the pump. Cytosolic hydrogen is secreted by H^+, K^+-ATPase in exchange for

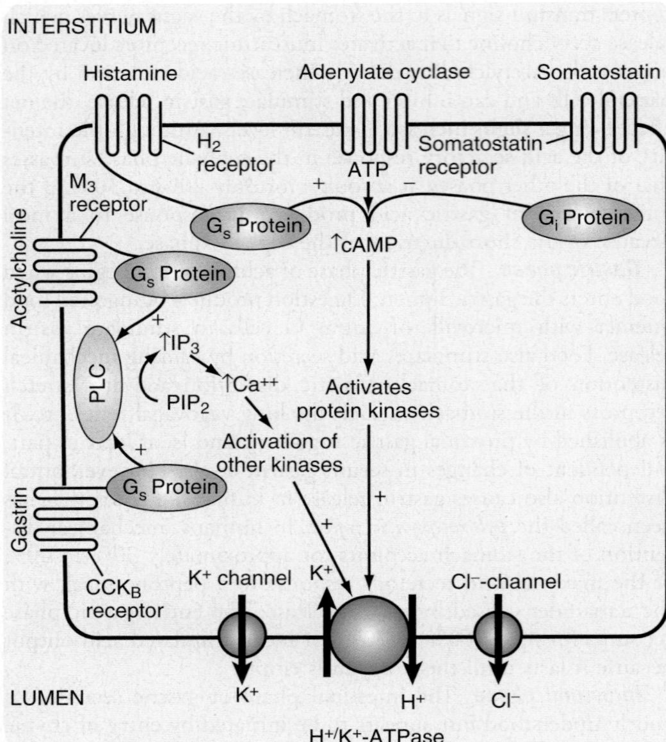

FIGURE 48-7 Intracellular signaling events in a parietal cell. As shown, histamine binds to H_2 receptors, stimulating adenylate cyclase through a G protein–linked mechanism. Adenylate cyclase activation causes an increase in intracellular cyclic adenosine monophosphate (cAMP) levels, which activates protein kinases. Activated protein kinases stimulate a phosphorylation cascade, with a resultant increase in levels of phosphoproteins that activate the proton pump. Activation of the proton pump leads to extrusion of cytosolic hydrogen in exchange for extracytoplasmic potassium. In addition, chloride is secreted through a chloride channel located on the luminal side of the membrane. Gastrin binds to type B cholecystokinin receptors, and acetylcholine binds to M_3 receptors. Following the interaction of gastrin and acetylcholine with their receptors, phospholipase C is stimulated through a G protein–linked mechanism to convert membrane-bound phospholipids into inositol triphosphate (IP_3). IP_3 stimulates the release of calcium from intracellular calcium stores, leading to an increase in intracellular calcium that activates protein kinases, which activate the H^+, K^+-ATPase. *ATP,* Adenosine triphosphate; *ATPase,* adenosine triphosphatase; *G_i,* inhibitory guanine nucleotide protein; *G_s,* stimulatory guanine nucleotide protein; *PIP_2,* phosphatidylinositol 4,5-diphosphate; *PLC,* phospholipase C. (From Yeo C, Dempsey DT, Klein AS, et al, editors: *Shackelford's surgery of the alimentary tract,* ed 6, Philadelphia, 2007, Saunders.)

extracytoplasmic potassium (see Fig. 48-7), which is an electroneutral exchange and does not contribute to the transmembrane potential difference across the parietal cell. Secretion of chloride is accomplished through a chloride channel moving chloride from the parietal cell cytoplasm to the gastric lumen. However, the secretion or exchange of hydrogen for potassium requires energy in the form of adenosine triphosphate (ATP) because hydrogen is being secreted against a gradient of more than a million-fold. Because of this large energy requirement, the parietal cell also has the largest mitochondrial content of any mammalian cell, with a mitochondrial compartment representing 34% of its cell volume. In response to a secretagogue, the parietal cell undergoes a conformational change, and a several-fold increase in the canalicular

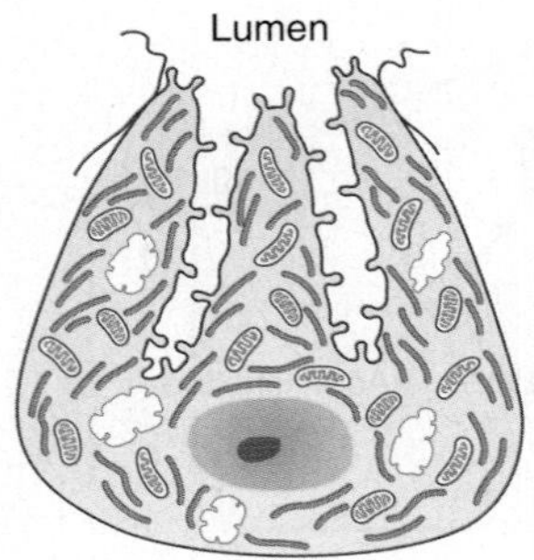

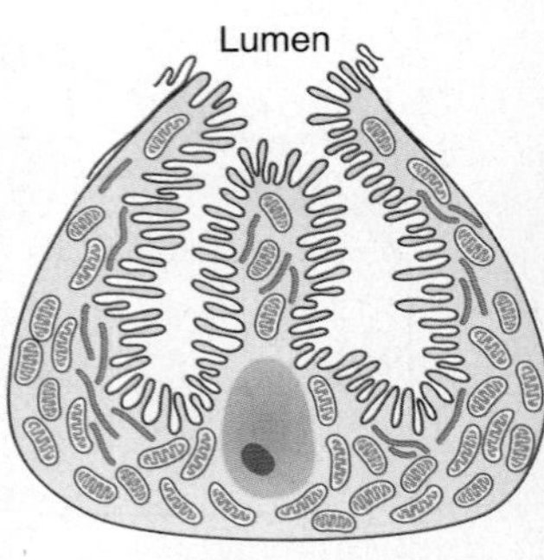

FIGURE 48-8 Diagrammatic representation of resting and stimulated parietal cells. Note the morphologic transformation between the nonsecreting parietal cell and stimulated parietal cell, with increases in secretory canalicular membrane surface area.

surface area occurs (Fig. 48-8). In contrast to stimulated acid secretion, cessation of acid secretion requires endocytosis of H^+, K^+-ATPase, with regeneration of cytoplasmic tubulovesicles containing the subunits, and this occurs through a tyrosine-based signal. The tyrosine-containing sequence is located on the cytoplasmic tail of the β-subunit and is highly homologous to the motif responsible for internalization of the transferrin receptor.

More than 1 billion parietal cells are found in the normal human stomach and are responsible for secreting approximately 20 mmol/hr of hydrochloric acid in response to a protein meal. Each individual parietal cell secretes 3.3 billion hydrogen ions/second, and there is a linear relationship between maximal acid output and parietal cell number. However, gastric acid secretory rates may be altered in patients with upper gastrointestinal (GI) disease. For example, gastric acid is often increased in patients with duodenal ulcer or gastrinoma, whereas it is decreased in patients with pernicious anemia, gastric atrophy, gastric ulcer, or gastric cancer. The lower secretory rates observed in patients with gastric ulcers are typically associated with proximal gastric ulcers, whereas distal, antral, or prepyloric ulcers are associated with acid secretory rates similar to rates in patients with duodenal ulcers.

Gastric acid plays a critical role in the digestion of a meal. It is required to convert pepsinogen into pepsin, elicits the release of secretin from the duodenum, and limits colonization of the upper GI tract with bacteria.

Pharmacologic Regulation

The diversity of mechanisms that stimulate acid secretion has resulted in the development of many site-specific drugs aimed at decreasing acid output by the parietal cell. The best-known site-specific antagonists are the group collectively known as the *H_2 receptor antagonists.* The most potent of the H_2 receptor antagonists is famotidine, followed by ranitidine, nizatidine, and cimetidine. The half-life for famotidine is 3 hours, and the half-life for the other H_2 receptor antagonists is approximately 1.5 hours. All H_2 receptor antagonists undergo hepatic metabolism, are excreted by the kidney, and do not differ much in bioavailability.

The PPIs represent the newest class of antisecretory agents. These substituted benzimidazoles, of which omeprazole is a prime example, inhibit acid secretion more completely because of their irreversible inhibition of the proton pump. PPIs are weak acids with a pK_a of 4 and become selectively localized in the secretory canaliculus of the parietal cell, which is the only structure in the body with a pH lower than 4. After oral administration, these agents are absorbed into the bloodstream as prodrugs and selectively concentrate in the secretory canaliculus. At low pH, they become ionized and activated, with the formation of an active sulfur group. Because the proton pump is located on the luminal surface, the transmembrane pump proteins are also exposed to acid or low pH. The cysteine residues on the α-subunit form a covalent disulfate bond with activated benzimidazoles, which irreversibly inhibits the proton pump. Because of the covalent nature of this bond, these PPIs have more prolonged inhibition of gastric acid secretion than H_2 blockers. For recovery of acid secretion to occur, new protein pumps need to be synthesized. As a result, these agents have a longer duration of action than their plasma half-life, with the intragastric pH being maintained higher than 3 for 18 hours or longer.

One notable side effect of all antisecretory agents is the elevation of serum gastrin levels. Serum gastrin levels are higher after treatment with PPIs than with H_2 receptor antagonists. This effect is accompanied by hyperplasia of G cells and ECL cells with long-term administration of these agents. Long-term administration of omeprazole has been found to cause ECL hyperplasia that could progress to carcinoid tumors in rats. However, this effect was not specific for omeprazole and was reproduced by other agents that caused prolonged inhibition of acid secretion and resultant hypergastrinemia.

Other Gastric Secretory Products

Gastric juice. Gastric juice is the result of secretion by the parietal cells, chief cells, and mucous cells, in addition to swallowed saliva and duodenal refluxate. The electrolyte composition of parietal and nonparietal gastric secretion varies with the rate of gastric secretion. Parietal cells secrete an electrolyte solution that is isotonic with plasma and contains 160 mmol/liter. The pH of this solution is 0.8. The lowest intraluminal pH commonly measured in the stomach is 2 because of dilution of the parietal cell secretion by other gastric secretions, which also contain sodium, potassium, and bicarbonate.

Intrinsic factor. Intrinsic factor is a 60-kDa mucoprotein secreted by the parietal cell that is essential for the absorption of vitamin B_{12} in the terminal ileum. It is secreted in amounts that far exceed the amounts necessary for vitamin B_{12} absorption. In general, secretion of intrinsic factor parallels gastric acid secretion, yet the secretory response is not linked to acid secretion. For example, PPIs do not block intrinsic factor secretion in humans, and they do not alter the absorption of labeled vitamin B_{12}. Intrinsic factor deficiency can develop in the patients with pernicious anemia or in patients undergoing total gastrectomy, and both groups of patients require vitamin B_{12} supplementation.

Pepsinogen. Pepsinogens are proteolytic proenzymes with a molecular weight of 42,500 that are secreted by the glands of the gastroduodenal mucosa. Two types of pepsinogens are secreted. Group 1 pepsinogens are secreted by chief cells and by mucous neck cells located in the glands of the acid-secreting portion of the stomach. Group 2 pepsinogens are produced by surface epithelial cells throughout the acid-secreting portion of the stomach, antrum, and proximal duodenum. Consequently, group 1 pepsinogens are secreted by the same glands that secrete acid, whereas group 2 pepsinogens are secreted by acid-secreting and gastrin-secreting mucosa. In the presence of acid, both forms of pepsinogen are converted to pepsin by removal of a short amino-terminal peptide. Pepsins become inactivated at a pH higher than 5, although group 2 pepsinogens are active over a wider range of pH values than group 1 pepsinogens. As a result, group 2 pepsinogens may be involved in peptic digestion in the presence of increased gastric pH, which commonly occurs in the setting of stress or in patients with gastric ulcer.

Mucus and bicarbonate. Mucus and bicarbonate combine to neutralize gastric acid at the gastric mucosal surface. They are secreted by the surface mucous cells and mucous neck cells located in the acid-secreting and antral portions of the stomach. Mucus is a viscoelastic gel that contains approximately 85% water and 15% glycoproteins. It provides a mechanical barrier to injury by contributing to the unstirred layer of water found at the luminal surface of the gastric mucosa. It also acts as an impediment to ion movement from the lumen to the apical cell membrane and is relatively impermeable to pepsins. Mucus is in a constant state of flux because it is secreted continuously by mucosal cells on one hand and solubilized by luminal pepsin on the other hand. Mucus production is stimulated by vagal stimulation, cholinergic agonists, prostaglandins, and some bacterial toxins. In contrast, anticholinergic drugs and nonsteroidal anti-inflammatory drugs (NSAIDs) inhibit mucus secretion. *H. pylori* secretes various proteases and lipases that break down mucin and impair the protective function of the mucous layer.

In the acid-secreting portion of the stomach, bicarbonate secretion is an active process, whereas in the antrum, active and passive secretion of bicarbonate occurs. However, the magnitude of bicarbonate secretion is considerably less than acid secretion. Although the luminal pH is 2, the pH observed at the surface epithelial cell is usually 7. The pH gradient found at the epithelial surface is a result of the unstirred layer of water in the mucous gel and of the continuous secretion of bicarbonate by the surface epithelial cells. Gastric cell surface pH remains higher than 5 until the luminal pH is less than 1.4. However, the luminal pH in patients with duodenal ulcers is frequently less than 1.4, so the cell surface is exposed to a lower pH in these patients. This reduction in pH may reflect a reduction in gastric bicarbonate secretion and decreased duodenal bicarbonate secretion and may explain why some patients with duodenal ulcers have a higher relapse rate after treatment.

Gastric Motility

Gastric motility is regulated by extrinsic and intrinsic neural mechanisms and by myogenic control. The extrinsic neural controls are mediated through parasympathetic (vagus) and sympathetic pathways, whereas the intrinsic controls involve the enteric nervous system (see "Anatomy"). In contrast, myogenic control resides in the excitatory membranes of the gastric smooth muscle cells.

Fasting Gastric Motility

The electrical basis of gastric motility begins with the depolarization of pacemaker cells located in the midbody of the stomach along the greater curvature. Once initiated, slow waves travel at 3 cycles/minute in a circumferential and antegrade fashion toward the pylorus. In addition to these slow waves, gastric smooth muscle cells are capable of producing action potentials, which are associated with larger changes in membrane potential than slow waves. Compared with slow waves, which are not associated with gastric contractions, action potentials are associated with actual muscle contractions. During fasting, the stomach goes through a cyclical pattern of electrical activity composed of slow waves and electrical spikes, which has been termed the *myoelectric migrating complex*. Each cycle of the myoelectric migrating complex lasts 90 to 120 minutes. The net effects of the myoelectric migrating complex are frequent clearance of gastric contents during periods of fasting. The exact regulatory mechanisms of myoelectric migrating complex activities are unknown, but these activities remain intact after vagal denervation.

Postprandial Gastric Motility

Ingestion of a meal results in a decrease in the resting tone of the proximal stomach and fundus, referred to as *receptive relaxation* and *gastric accommodation,* respectively. Because these reflexes are mediated by the vagus nerves, interruption of vagal innervation to the proximal stomach, such as by truncal vagotomy or proximal gastric vagotomy, can eliminate these reflexes, with resultant early satiety and rapid emptying of ingested liquids. In addition to its storage function, the stomach is responsible for the mixing and grinding of ingested solid food particles. This activity involves repetitive forceful contractions of the midportion and antral portion of the stomach, causing food particles to be propelled against a closed pylorus, with subsequent retropulsion of solids and liquids. The net effect is a thorough mixing of solids and liquids and sequential shearing of solid food particles to smaller than 1 mm.

The emptying of gastric contents is influenced by well-coordinated neural and hormonal mediators. Systemic factors, such as anxiety, fear, depression, and exercise, can affect the rate of gastric motility and emptying. Additionally, the chemical and mechanical properties and temperature of the intraluminal contents can influence the rate of gastric emptying. In general, liquids empty more rapidly than solids, and carbohydrates empty more readily than fats. An increase in the concentration or acidity of liquid meals causes a delay in gastric emptying. In addition, hot and cold liquids tend to empty at a slower rate than ambient temperature fluids. These responses to luminal stimuli are regulated by the enteric nervous system. Osmoreceptors and pH-sensitive receptors in the proximal small bowel have also been shown to be involved in the activation of feedback inhibition of gastric emptying. Inhibitory peptides proposed to be active in this setting include CCK, glucagon, vasoactive intestinal peptide, and gastric inhibitory polypeptide.

Abnormal Gastric Motility

Symptoms of abnormal gastric motility are nausea, fullness, early satiety, abdominal pain, and discomfort. Although mechanical obstruction can and should be ruled out with upper endoscopy or radiographic contrast studies, objective evaluation of a patient with a suspected motility disorder can be accomplished with gamma scintigraphy, real-time ultrasound, and magnetic resonance imaging (MRI). Gastric motility disorders usually encountered in clinical practice are gastric dysmotility after vagotomy, gastroparesis (secondary to diabetes, idiopathic, or medication related), and gastric motility dysfunction related to *H. pylori* infection. Vagotomy results in loss of receptive relaxation and gastric accommodation in response to meal ingestion, with resultant early satiety, postprandial bloating, accelerated emptying of liquids, and delay in emptying of solids. Clinical manifestations of diabetic gastropathy, which can occur in insulin-dependent or non–insulin-dependent patients, closely resemble the clinical picture of postvagotomy gastroparesis. Furthermore, structural changes have been identified in the vagus nerve of patients with diabetes, suggesting that a diabetic autonomic neuropathy may be responsible. However, the metabolic effects of diabetes have also been implicated. Specifically, hyperglycemia has been shown to cause a decrease in contractility of the gastric antrum, increase in pyloric contractility, and suppression of the migrating motor complex. Suppression of migrating motor complex activity is thought to be responsible for the accumulation of gastric bezoars seen in some diabetic patients. In contrast, hyperinsulinemia, which is often associated with non–insulin-dependent diabetes, may play a role in the gastroparesis seen in non–insulin-dependent diabetes because it also leads to suppression of migrating motor complex activity.

Patients with *H. pylori* infection and nonulcer dyspepsia have also been demonstrated to have impaired gastric emptying accompanied by a reduction in gastric compliance. In rats, lipopolysaccharide derived from *H. pylori* causes a reduction in gastric emptying of a liquid meal for up to 12 hours by an unknown mechanism.

Gastric-Emptying Studies

There are numerous ways to assess gastric emptying. The saline load test is perhaps the simplest and is accomplished by instilling a known volume of saline into the stomach and aspirating the amount remaining at a certain time. Fluoroscopic procedures can also provide information on gastric emptying and may reveal mechanical causes that could contribute to a delay, such as gastric outlet obstruction. However, computerized radionucleotide scans are more commonly used to assess gastric emptying. This scintigraphy study is performed using a meal of radiolabeled egg whites. Scans are obtained immediately after ingestion of the meal, and at 1, 2, and 4 hours after the meal. Measurement of residual gastric contents at 4 hours provides the most sensitive means for diagnosing gastroparesis, as many patients with gastroparesis have equivocal results at 2 hours. Retention of greater than 60% of the meal at 2 hours or 10% at 4 hours indicates an abnormal study. At 4 hours, retention of 10% to 15% signifies mild gastroparesis; 15% to 35%, moderate; and greater than 35%, severe.

Treatment

Regardless of the cause of gastroparesis, initial treatment consists of modification of diet and environmental factors. Patients should be encouraged to eat multiple, small meals with little fat or fiber. Medications that affect gastric motility, such as opioids, calcium channel blockers, tricyclic antidepressants, and dopamine agonists, should be avoided and stopped when possible. Glycemic control should be optimized in diabetic patients. First-line medical therapy consisting of metoclopramide (Reglan), a dopamine antagonist that stimulates antral contractions, and erythromycin, a motilin agonist that acts by stimulating fundal contraction, has been shown to have some benefit, although the evidence is more compelling in diabetic patients.

Surgery for gastroparesis is rarely required, partly because poor improvement in symptoms was observed historically after traditional open operations including gastrojejunostomy and even gastrectomy. However, several less invasive and more effective options have been introduced more recently suggesting that surgery may play a larger role in the treatment of gastroparesis in the future. Pyloromyotomy and pyloroplasty are options for the surgical management of gastroparesis that function by lowering outflow resistance at the pylorus and enhancing any remaining gastric contractility. These operations can be performed laparoscopically, and a series of laparoscopic Heineke-Mikulicz pyloroplasties showed symptom improvement in 82% of patients with a reduction in gastric-emptying half-time from 180 minutes to 60 minutes, with few perioperative complications.[2] Surgical implantation of gastric electrostimulators has also been used as a treatment for refractory idiopathic and diabetic gastroparesis. In this technique, electrical leads are placed onto the antrum laparoscopically and connected to a subcutaneously positioned simulator that delivers high-frequency, low-energy current. In an initial crossover blinded study, patients had less vomiting when their simulator was activated compared with the off period of the study.[3] Although two subsequent trials, one involving patients with diabetes and the other patients with idiopathic gastroparesis, were unable to replicate these positive results during their blinded crossover periods, both showed an improvement in symptoms during a year-long unblinded stimulation period. Based on these data, the ultimate role and benefit of gastric simulation in the treatment of gastroparesis have yet to be conclusively determined.

Gastric Barrier Function

Gastric barrier function depends on physiologic and anatomic factors. Blood flow plays a critical role in gastric mucosal defense by providing nutrients and delivering oxygen to ensure that the intracellular processes that underlie mucosal resistance to injury can proceed unabated. Decreased gastric mucosal blood flow has minimal effects on ulcer formation until it approaches 50% of normal. When blood flow is reduced by more than 75%, marked mucosal injury results, which is exacerbated in the presence of luminal acid. After damage occurs, injured surface epithelial cells are replaced rapidly by the migration of surface mucous cells located along the basement membranes. This process is referred to as *restitution* or *reconstitution*. It occurs within minutes and does not require cell division.

Exposure of the stomach to noxious agents causes a reduction in the potential difference across the gastric mucosa. In normal gastric mucosa, the potential difference across the mucosa is −30 to −50 mV and results from the active transport of chloride into the lumen and sodium into the blood by the activity of Na^+, K^+-ATPase. Damage disrupts the tight junctions between mucosal cells, causing the epithelium to become leaky to ions (i.e., Na^+ and Cl^-) and a resultant loss of the high transepithelial electrical resistance normally found in gastric mucosa. In addition, damaging agents such as NSAIDs or aspirin possess carboxyl groups that are nonionized at a low intragastric pH because they are weak acids. Consequently, they readily enter the cell membranes of gastric mucosal cells because they are now lipid-soluble, whereas they will not penetrate the cell membranes at neutral pH because they are ionized. On entry into the neutral pH environment found in the cytosol, they become reionized, do not exit the cell membrane, and are toxic to the mucosal cells.

PEPTIC ULCER DISEASE

Epidemiology

Peptic ulcers are defined as erosions in the gastric or duodenal mucosa that extend through the muscularis mucosae. The incidence and prevalence of PUD in developed countries, including the United States, have been declining in recent years, as has the progression to complicated PUD, such as perforation and gastric outlet obstruction. This change is likely due to increases in the detection and eradication of *H. pylori* infection, the primary cause of PUD. A systematic review of epidemiologic studies of PUD reported a pooled annual incidence of 0.10% to 0.19% and an overall prevalence of 0.12% to 1.50%, with most studies showing a decline in rates of PUD over the last several decades. Although the incidence and hospitalization rates for PUD have been decreasing since the 1980s, it remains one of the most prevalent and costly GI diseases. Medical costs associated with PUD are an estimated $5.65 billion annually. An estimated 15,000 operations are performed each year in patients hospitalized with PUD. Significant progress has been made over the past 2 decades, with total admissions for PUD decreasing by almost 30%. Admissions for complications of ulcer disease have also been decreasing, which has led to a significant decrease in ulcer-related mortality, from 3.9% in 1993 to 2.7% in 2006. Although overall mortality remains low, this still represents more than 4000 deaths caused by PUD each year.

The role of surgery in the treatment of ulcer disease has also decreased primarily as a result of a marked decline in elective surgical therapy for chronic disease, as the percentage of patients who require emergent surgery for complicated disease has remained constant, at 7% of hospitalized patients. This represents greater than 11,000 surgical procedures annually.

Much of this decline in ulcer incidence and the need for hospitalization has stemmed from increased knowledge of ulcer pathogenesis. Specifically, the role of *H. pylori* has been defined, and the risks of long-term NSAID use have been better elucidated. It is hoped that an increase in *H. pylori* eradication will result in not only a decrease of elective surgical procedures but also a decline in complications and mortality from emergent complications.

Pathogenesis

Peptic ulcers are caused by increased aggressive factors, decreased defensive factors, or both. Mucosal damage and subsequent ulceration result. Protective (or defensive) factors include mucosal bicarbonate secretion, mucus production, blood flow, growth factors, cell renewal, and endogenous prostaglandins. Damaging (or aggressive) factors include hydrochloric acid secretion, pepsins, ethanol ingestion, smoking, duodenal reflux of bile, ischemia, NSAIDs, hypoxia, and, most notably, *H. pylori* infection. Although it is now clear that most ulcers are caused by *H. pylori* infection or NSAID use, it is still important to understand all of the other protective and causative factors to optimize treatment and ulcer healing and prevent disease recurrence.

Helicobacter pylori Infection

It is now believed that 80% to 95% of duodenal ulcers and approximately 75% of gastric ulcers are associated with *H. pylori* infection. Infection with *H. pylori* has been shown to temporally precede ulcer formation, and when this organism is eradicated as part of ulcer treatment, ulcer recurrence is extremely rare. These observations have secured the place of *H. pylori* as the primary causative factor in the pathogenesis of PUD. *H. pylori* is a spiral or helical gram-negative rod with four to six flagella that resides in gastric-type epithelium within or beneath the mucous layer. This location protects the bacteria from acid and antibiotics. Its shape and flagella aid its movement through the mucous layer, and it produces enzymes that help it adapt to this hostile environment. Most notably, *H. pylori* is a potent producer of urease, which is capable of splitting urea into ammonia and bicarbonate, creating an alkaline microenvironment in the setting of an acidic gastric milieu. However, the secretion of this enzyme facilitates detection of the organism. *H. pylori* organisms are microaerophilic and can live only in gastric epithelium. Thus, *H. pylori* can also be found in heterotopic gastric mucosa in the proximal esophagus, in Barrett esophagus, in gastric metaplasia in the duodenum, within a Meckel's diverticulum, and in heterotopic gastric mucosa in the rectum.

The mechanisms responsible for *H. pylori*–induced GI injury are not fully elucidated, but the following four potential mechanisms have been proposed and likely interact to cause a derangement of normal gastric and duodenal physiology that leads to subsequent ulcer formation:

1. Production of toxic products that cause local tissue injury. Locally produced toxic mediators include breakdown products from urease activity (e.g., ammonia); cytotoxins; a mucinase that degrades mucus and glycoproteins; phospholipases that damage epithelial cells and mucous cells; and platelet-activating factor, which is known to cause mucosal injury and thrombosis in the microcirculation.
2. Induction of a local mucosal immune response. *H. pylori* can also cause a local inflammatory reaction in the gastric mucosa, attracting neutrophils and monocytes, which then produce numerous proinflammatory cytokines and reactive oxygen metabolites.
3. Increased gastrin levels with a resultant increase in acid secretion. In patients with *H. pylori* infection, basal and stimulated gastrin levels are significantly increased, presumably secondary to a reduction in antral D cells because of infection with *H. pylori*. However, the association of acid secretion with *H. pylori* is not as straightforward. Although *H. pylori*–positive healthy volunteers had a small increase or no increase in acid secretion compared with *H. pylori*–negative volunteers, *H. pylori*–infected patients with duodenal ulcers did have a marked increase in acid secretion. A decrease in serum levels of somatostatin as a result of *H. pylori* infection, which increases gastrin and acid secretion, could be the underlying causative mechanism behind the gastric hyperacidity.
4. Gastric metaplasia occurring in the duodenum. Metaplastic replacement of areas of duodenal mucosa with gastric epithelium likely occurs as a protective response to decreased duodenal pH, resulting from the above-described acid hypersecretion; this allows for *H. pylori* to colonize these areas of the duodenum, which causes duodenitis and likely predisposes to duodenal ulcer formation. The presence of *H. pylori* in the duodenum is more common in patients with ulcer formation compared with patients with asymptomatic infections isolated to the stomach.

Peptic ulcers are also strongly associated with antral gastritis. Studies performed before the *H. pylori* era demonstrated that almost all patients with peptic ulcers have histologic evidence of antral gastritis. It was later found that the only patients with gastric ulcers and no gastritis were those ingesting aspirin. It is now recognized that most cases of histologic gastritis are caused by *H. pylori* infection. Of patients with NSAID-associated ulcers, 25% have evidence of a histologic antral gastritis compared with 95% of patients with non–NSAID-associated ulcers. In most cases, the infection tends to be confined initially to the antrum and results in antral inflammation. The causative role of *H. pylori* infection in the pathogenesis of gastritis and PUD was first elucidated by Marshall and Warren in Australia in 1984. To prove this connection, Marshall himself ingested inocula of *H. pylori* after first confirming that he had normal gross and microscopic gastric mucosa. Within days, he developed abdominal pain, nausea, and halitosis as well as histologically confirmed presence of gastric *H. pylori* infection. Acute inflammation was observed histologically on days 5 and 10. By 2 weeks, acute inflammation had been replaced by chronic inflammation with evidence of a mononuclear cell infiltration. For their pioneering work, Marshall and Warren were jointly awarded the Nobel Prize in Medicine in 2005.

H. pylori infection usually occurs in childhood, and spontaneous remission is rare. There is an inverse relationship between infection and socioeconomic status. The reasons for this relationship are poorly understood, but it seems to be the result of factors such as sanitary conditions, familial clustering, and crowding. Such factors likely explain why developing countries have a comparatively higher rate of *H. pylori* infection, especially in children.

Numerous studies have demonstrated what appears to be a steady linear increase in the acquisition of *H. pylori* infection with age, especially in the United States and northern European nations. In the United States, *H. pylori* prevalence also varies among racial and ethnic groups.

H. pylori infection is associated with many common upper GI disorders, but most infected individuals are asymptomatic. Healthy U.S. blood donors have an overall prevalence of approximately 20% to 55%. *H. pylori* infection is almost always present in the setting of active chronic gastritis and is present in most patients with duodenal (80% to 95%) and gastric (60% to 90%) ulcers. Noninfected patients with gastric ulcers tend to be NSAID users. There is a weaker association with nonulcer dyspepsia. In addition, most patients with gastric cancer have current or past *H. pylori* infection. Although the association between *H. pylori* and cancer is strong, no causal relationship has been proven. However, *H. pylori*–induced chronic gastritis and intestinal metaplasia are thought to play a role. A meta-analysis of case-control studies comparing *H. pylori*–positive and *H. pylori*–negative individuals found that infection was associated with a twofold increased risk of developing gastric cancer. There is also a strong association between mucosa-associated lymphoid tissue (MALT) lymphoma and *H. pylori* infection. Regression of these lymphomas has been demonstrated after eradication of *H. pylori*.

Limited data are available to estimate the lifetime risk of PUD in patients with *H. pylori* infection. In a longitudinal study from Australia with a mean evaluation period of 18 years, 15% of *H. pylori*–positive subjects developed verified duodenal ulcer compared with 3% of seronegative individuals. In a 10-year study of patients with asymptomatic gastritis, 11% of patients with histologic gastritis developed PUD over a 10-year period compared with only 1% of patients without gastritis. Another factor implicating a causative role for *H. pylori* and ulcer formation is that eradication of *H. pylori* dramatically reduces ulcer recurrence. Many prospective trials showed that patients with *H. pylori* infection and non–NSAID-related ulcer disease who have documented eradication of the organism almost never (<2%) develop recurrent ulcers.

Nonsteroidal Anti-Inflammatory Drugs

Hospitalizations for bleeding upper GI lesions have increased together with the increased use of NSAIDs. The risk for bleeding and ulceration is proportional to the daily dosage of NSAIDs. The risk also increases with age older than 60 years, patients having a prior GI event, or concurrent use of steroids or anticoagulants. Consequently, the ingestion of NSAIDs is an important factor in ulcer pathogenesis, especially in regard to the development of complications and death.

NSAIDs are absorbed through the stomach and small intestine and function as systemic inhibitors of the cyclooxygenase enzymes. Cyclooxygenase enzymes form the rate-limiting step of prostaglandin synthesis in the GI tract. Prostaglandins promote gastric and duodenal mucosal protection via numerous mechanisms, including increasing mucin and bicarbonate secretion and increasing blood flow to the mucosal endothelium. The presence of NSAIDs disrupts these naturally protective mechanisms, increasing the risk of peptic ulcer formation in the stomach and the duodenum.

More than 3 million people in the United States use NSAIDs daily. Compared with the general population, NSAID users have a 2-fold to 10-fold increased risk for GI complications. The risk for mucosal injury or ulceration is roughly proportional to the anti-inflammatory effect associated with each NSAID. Compared with *H. pylori* ulcers, which are more frequently found in the duodenum, NSAID-induced ulcers are more often found in the stomach. *H. pylori* ulcers are also almost always associated with chronic active gastritis, whereas gastritis is not frequently found with NSAID-induced ulcers, occurring only approximately 25% of the time. When NSAID use is discontinued, the ulcers usually do not recur.

Acid

Acid plays an important but likely noncausative role in the formation of ulcers. In duodenal ulcers, there is a large overlap of acid levels between patients with ulcers and normal subjects. Almost 70% of patients with duodenal ulcers have an acid output within the normal range. Acid levels alone provide little information, and acid secretory testing is of little value in establishing a diagnosis of duodenal ulcer.

For types I and IV gastric ulcers, which are not associated with excessive acid secretion, acid acts as an important cofactor, exacerbating the underlying ulcer damage and attenuating the ability of the stomach to heal. For patients with type II or III gastric ulcers, gastric acid hypersecretion seems to be more common, and consequently these ulcers behave more like duodenal ulcers.

Duodenal Ulcer

Duodenal ulcer is a disease with numerous causes. The only requirements are acid and pepsin secretion in combination with infection by *H. pylori* or ingestion of NSAIDs.

Clinical Manifestations

Abdominal pain. Patients with duodenal ulcer disease can present in various ways. The most common symptom associated with duodenal ulcer disease is midepigastric abdominal pain that is usually well localized. The pain is generally tolerable and frequently relieved by food. The pain may be episodic, seasonal in the spring and fall, and worse during periods of emotional stress. Many patients do not seek medical attention until they have had the disease for many years. When the pain becomes constant, this suggests that there is deeper penetration of the ulcer. Referral of pain to the back is usually a sign of penetration into the pancreas. Diffuse peritoneal irritation is usually a sign of free perforation.

Diagnosis

History and physical examination are of limited value in distinguishing between gastric and duodenal ulceration. Routine laboratory studies include complete blood count; liver chemistries; and serum creatinine, serum amylase, and calcium levels. A serum gastrin level should also be obtained in patients with ulcers that are refractory to medical therapy or require surgery. An upright chest radiograph is usually performed when ruling out perforation. The two principal means of diagnosing duodenal ulcers are upper GI radiography and flexible upper endoscopy. Upper GI radiography is less expensive, and most (90%) ulcers can be diagnosed accurately by this means. However, approximately 5% of ulcers that appear radiographically benign are malignant. Because of the need to perform a biopsy to rule out malignancy, upper endoscopy has replaced upper GI radiography as the primary test for the diagnosis and evaluation of PUD. Also, endoscopy has the advantage of being able to evaluate for other pathologies of the esophagus, stomach, and duodenum in addition to PUD that may be causing the patient's symptoms, such as esophagitis and gastritis. *H. pylori* testing should also be done in all patients with suspected PUD.

Upper gastrointestinal radiography. Diagnosis of duodenal ulcer by upper GI radiography requires the demonstration of barium within the ulcer crater, which is usually round or oval and may or may not be surrounded by edema. This study is useful to determine the location and depth of penetration of the ulcer and the extent of deformation from chronic fibrosis. A characteristic barium radiograph of a peptic ulcer is shown in Figure 48-9. The ability to detect ulcers on radiography requires the technical skills and abilities of the radiologist but also depends on the size and location of the ulcer. With single-contrast radiographic techniques, 50% of duodenal ulcers may be missed, whereas with double-contrast studies, 80% to 90% of ulcer craters can be detected. Despite this increased accuracy with double-contrast techniques, upper GI radiography has largely been replaced by flexible upper endoscopy as the method of choice for diagnosis and evaluation of gastric and duodenal ulcers.

Flexible upper endoscopy. Endoscopy is the most reliable method for diagnosing gastric and duodenal ulcers. In addition to providing a visual diagnosis, endoscopy provides the ability to sample tissue to evaluate for malignancy and *H. pylori* infection and may be used for therapeutic purposes in the setting of GI bleeding or obstruction.

Endoscopic evaluation of the stomach and duodenum has been shown to confirm a visual diagnosis of more than 90% of peptic ulcers, and this value is likely higher today with the use of high-definition endoscopes. When an ulcer has been detected

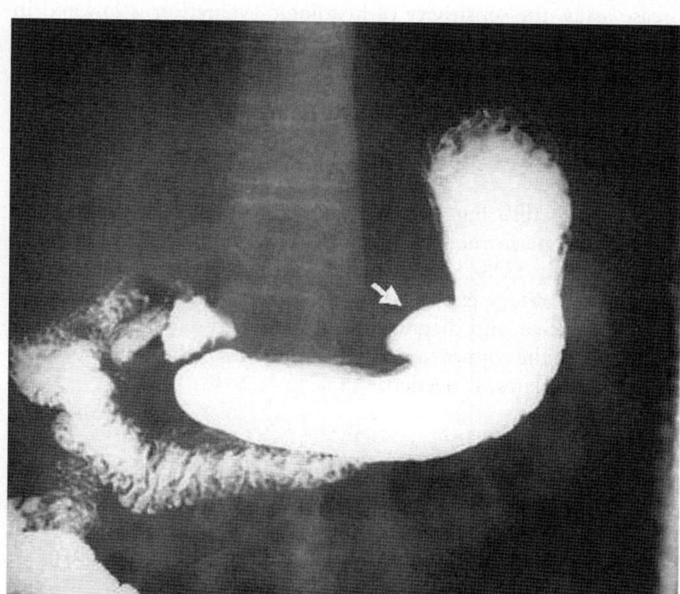

FIGURE 48-9 A large, benign-appearing gastric ulcer protrudes medially from the lesser curvature of the stomach *(arrow)*, just above the gastric incisura. (Courtesy Dr. Agnes Guthrie, Department of Radiology, University of Texas Medical School, Houston, TX.)

endoscopically, biopsy is recommended in all cases to rule out malignancy. Larger ulcers and ulcers with irregular or heaped edges are more likely to harbor cancers. Multiple biopsy specimens should be taken of the ulcer for maximum diagnostic yield. An early study of the usefulness of endoscopic biopsy showed that the first biopsy sample taken of an ulcer had only a 70% sensitivity in detecting gastric cancer, whereas taking four biopsy specimens increased this yield to 95% and taking seven specimens increased it to 98%.

Helicobacter pylori *testing*. The gold standard for diagnosis of *H. pylori* is mucosal biopsy performed during upper endoscopy, but noninvasive tests offer an effective screening tool and do not require an endoscopic procedure. If endoscopy is to be performed, evaluation of biopsy samples with either a urease assay or histologic examination offers excellent diagnostic accuracy. Evaluation of serum antibodies is the test of choice for initial diagnosis when endoscopy is not required but has the drawback of remaining positive after treatment and eradication of infection. For monitoring treatment efficacy, stool antigen and urea breath testing are better choices.

Invasive Tests

Urease assay. Endoscopic biopsy specimens should be taken from the gastric body and the antrum and are then tested for urease. Sensitivity in diagnosing infection is greater than 90%, and specificity is 95% to 100%, meaning there are almost never false-positive results. However, the sensitivity of the test is lowered in patients who are taking PPIs, H_2 antagonists, or antibiotics. Rapid urease test kits are commercially available and can detect urease in gastric biopsy specimens within 1 hour with a similar level of diagnostic accuracy.

Histology. Endoscopy can also be performed with biopsy samples of gastric mucosa, followed by histologic visualization of *H. pylori* using routine hematoxylin-eosin stains or special stains (e.g., silver, Giemsa, Genta stains) for improved visibility. Sensitivity is approximately 95% and specificity is 99%, making histology slightly more accurate than the urease assay testing. Similar to urease assay, the sensitivity of histologic evaluation is lowered in patients taking PPIs or H_2 antagonists, but it remains the most accurate test available even in this setting. Histology additionally affords the physician the ability to assess the severity of gastritis and confirm the presence or absence of the organism; however, it is a more expensive option for evaluation of biopsy samples than the urease assay.

Culture. Culturing of gastric mucosa obtained at endoscopy can also be performed to diagnose *H. pylori*. The sensitivity is approximately 80%, and specificity is 100%. However, culture requires laboratory expertise, is not widely available, and is relatively expensive, and diagnosis requires 3 to 5 days. Nevertheless, it provides the opportunity to perform antibiotic sensitivity testing on isolates, if needed.

Noninvasive Tests

Serology. There are various enzyme-linked immunosorbent assay laboratory-based tests available and some rapid office-based immunoassays that are used to test for the presence of IgG antibodies to *H. pylori*. Serology has a 90% sensitivity but a more variable specificity rate between 76% and 96%, and tests need to be locally validated based on the prevalence of specific bacterial strains. Antibody titers can remain high for 1 year or longer; consequently, this test cannot be used to assess eradication after therapy. For these reasons, stool antigen and urea breath tests are the preferred modalities for diagnosis and evaluation of treatment efficacy in patients with PUD and suspected *H. pylori* infection.

Urea breath test. The carbon-labeled urea breath test is based on the ability of *H. pylori* to hydrolyze urea as a result of its production of urease. Both sensitivity and specificity are greater than 95%. As with other testing modalities, the sensitivity of the urea breath test is reduced in patients taking antisecretory medications and antibiotics. It is recommended that patients discontinue antibiotics for 4 weeks and PPIs for 2 weeks to ensure optimal test accuracy. The urea breath test is less expensive than endoscopy and samples the entire stomach. In evaluating treatment efficacy, false-negative results can occur if the test is performed too soon after treatment, so it is usually best to perform this test 4 weeks after therapy is completed.

Stool antigen. *H. pylori* bacteria are present in the stool of infected patients, and several assays have been developed that use monoclonal antibodies to *H. pylori* antigens to test fecal specimens. These tests have demonstrated sensitivities of greater than 90% and sensitivities of 86% to 92%.[1] Several studies demonstrated that stool antigen testing has an accuracy of greater than 90% in detecting eradication of infection after treatment, on par with invasive histology and noninvasive urea breath testing. Additionally, stool antigen testing is likely the most cost-effective method for assessing treatment efficacy.

Treatment

Medical management. Antiulcer drugs fall into three broad categories—drugs targeted against *H. pylori*, drugs that reduce acid levels by decreasing secretion or chemical neutralization, and drugs that increase the mucosal protective barrier. In patients with PUD and *H. pylori* infection, the focus of therapy is on eradication of the bacteria. In addition to medications, lifestyle changes, such as smoking cessation, discontinuing NSAIDs and aspirin, and avoiding coffee and alcohol, help promote ulcer healing.

Antacids. Antacids are the oldest form of therapy for PUD that reduce gastric acidity by reacting with hydrochloric acid, forming a salt and raising the gastric pH. Antacids differ greatly in their buffering ability, absorption, taste, and side effects. Magnesium antacids tend to be the best buffers but can cause significant diarrhea, whereas acids precipitated with phosphorus can occasionally result in hypophosphatemia and sometimes constipation. Antacids are most effective when ingested 1 hour after a meal because they can be retained in the stomach and exert their buffering action for longer periods. If taken on an empty stomach, antacids are emptied rapidly and have only a transient buffering effect. Because of this transient efficacy, the use of buffering antacids has largely been replaced by antisecretory therapy (either H_2 receptor antagonists or PPIs) for the treatment of PUD.

Sucralfate. Sucralfate is structurally related to heparin but does not have any anticoagulant effects. It has been shown to be effective in the treatment of ulcer disease, although its exact mechanism of action is not entirely understood. It is an aluminum salt of sulfated sucrose that dissociates under the acidic conditions in the stomach. It is hypothesized that the sucrose polymerizes and binds to protein in the ulcer crater to produce a protective coating that can last for 6 hours. It has also been suggested that it may bind and concentrate endogenous basic fibroblast growth factor, which appears to be important for mucosal healing. Treatment with sucralfate for 4 to 6 weeks results in duodenal ulcer healing that is superior to placebo and comparable to treatment with H_2 receptor antagonists such as cimetidine. However, the efficacy and role of sucralfate in healing gastric ulcers and ulcers caused by *H.*

pylori infection has not been clearly established, and sucralfate is not included as part of initial treatment guidelines for PUD.

H_2 receptor antagonists. The H_2 receptor antagonists are structurally similar to histamine. Variations in ring structure and side chains cause differences in potency and side effects. Currently available H_2 receptor antagonists differ in their potency but only modestly in half-life and bioavailability. All undergo hepatic metabolism and are excreted by the kidney. Famotidine is the most potent, and cimetidine is the weakest. Continuous intravenous infusion of H_2 receptor antagonists has been shown to produce more uniform acid inhibition than intermittent administration. Many randomized controlled trials have indicated that all H_2 receptor antagonists result in duodenal ulcer healing rates of 70% to 80% after 4 weeks of therapy and 80% to 90% after 8 weeks.

Proton pump inhibitors. The most potent antisecretory agents are PPIs. These agents negate all types of acid secretion from all types of secretagogues. As a result, they provide a more complete and prolonged inhibition of acid secretion than H_2 receptor antagonists. H_2 receptor antagonists and PPIs are effective at night, but PPIs are more effective during the day. PPIs have a healing rate of 85% at 4 weeks and 96% at 8 weeks and produce more rapid healing of ulcers than standard H_2 receptor antagonists (14% advantage at 2 weeks and 9% advantage at 4 weeks). Because of this, PPIs have generally replaced H_2 receptor antagonists as primary therapy for PUD in the presence of and in the absence of *H. pylori* infection. PPIs require an acidic environment within the gastric lumen to become activated; thus, using antacids or H_2 receptor antagonists in combination with PPIs could have deleterious effects by promoting an alkaline environment and preventing activation of the PPIs. Consequently, antacids and H_2 receptor antagonists should not be used in combination with PPIs.

Treatment of* helicobacter pylori *infection. Before the discovery of *H. pylori* infection as the causative agent in greater than 95% of duodenal peptic ulcers, the primary form of treatment was the reduction of acid in the stomach, with or without increasing the protective barrier with drugs such as sucralfate. After it became clear that increased acid secretion was an effect of *H. pylori* infection, there was a paradigm shift that saw PUD as an infectious disease, rather than a consequence of pathologic acid secretion. Accordingly, treatment philosophy has shifted to focus on eradication of the infectious agent.

Current therapy is twofold in its approach, combining antibiotics against *H. pylori* with antacid medications. The primary goal of the antacids is to promote short-term healing by reducing pathologic acid levels and improve symptoms. *H. pylori* eradication helps with initial healing, but its primary efficacy is in preventing recurrence. There have been numerous trials comparing eradication therapy with ulcer-healing drugs alone or no treatment. Eradication of *H. pylori* has shown recurrence rates of 2%, with initial healing rates of 90%. Eradication rates after an initial course of therapy have been increasing, likely as a result of increased prevalence of antibiotic-resistant strains of *H. pylori;* at the present time, approximately 20% of patients fail initial therapy. For this reason, monitoring for infection eradication with a urea breath test, stool antigen, or repeat endoscopy with biopsy at 4 to 6 weeks after therapy is important, and many patients will require further treatment with alternative regimens.

The treatment of *H. pylori*–positive peptic duodenal ulcer disease is triple therapy aimed at the eradication of *H. pylori*, along with acid suppression (Box 48-1). This triple therapy includes a PPI and two antibiotics, usually amoxicillin (1 g BID) with clarithromycin (500 mg twice daily). In patients with penicillin allergies, metronidazole (500 mg twice daily) is substituted for amoxicillin. In areas with high rates of clarithromycin resistance (>15% to 20%), it may be beneficial to substitute tetracycline, or another antibiotic, for initial therapy. Clinical guidelines generally recommend treatment with a 14-day course of triple therapy[4]; however, this is controversial, as a meta-analysis of randomized trials comparing treatment lengths found no significant increase in eradication rates when regimens of 7 days were compared with 10-day and 14-day schedules.[5] Side effects, which are generally mild and resolve with cessation of treatment, include diarrhea, nausea and vomiting, rash, and altered taste. For the 20% of patients with refractory disease, a treatment course with new antibiotics, such as metronidazole and tetracycline, is initiated, and quadruple therapy with the addition of bismuth is recommended.

BOX 48-1 National Institutes of Health Consensus Panel Recommendations for *Helicobacter pylori* Treatment

Patients with active PUD who are *H. pylori*–positive
- Use of NSAIDs should not alter treatment
- Document eradication in patients with complications

Ulcer patients in remission who are *H. pylori*–positive, including patients on maintenance H_2 receptor antagonist therapy

H. pylori–positive patients with MALT lymphoma

Controversial issues in *H. pylori*–positive patients
- First-degree relatives of patients with gastric cancer
- Immigrants from countries with high prevalence of gastric cancer
- Individuals with gastric cancer precursor lesions (intestinal metaplasia)
- Patients with dyspepsia not resulting from ulcer who insist on eradication (benefit versus risk)
- Patients on long-term antisecretory therapy for reflux disease

BOX 48-2 Surgical Treatment Recommendations for Complications Related to Peptic Duodenal Ulcer Disease

Intractable: Parietal cell vagotomy ± antrectomy
Bleeding: Oversewing of bleeding vessel with treatment of *H. pylori*
Perforation: Patch closure with treatment of *H. pylori*
Obstruction: Rule out malignancy and gastrojejunostomy with treatment of *H. pylori*

Complicated Ulcer Disease

Ulcer disease was previously within the scope of the general surgeon, with ulcer surgery forming a major part of general surgery practice. With the shift in understanding of the disease from one primarily of aberrant acid physiology to one of infectious disease, this situation has changed significantly, with most patients with ulcers being treated and cured medically. The surgeon's role now is primarily to treat the approximately 20% of patients who have a complication from their disease, which includes hemorrhage, perforation, and obstruction (Box 48-2). Frequently included in discussions of complicated ulcer disease is an intractable ulcer. Although intractable disease no doubt exists, its definition is nebulous, and determining exactly when and what type of surgical intervention are required is primarily a matter of judgment. In the current era of excellent treatment options for *H. pylori* infection and acid suppression, few patients who are truly compliant with medical therapy develop intractable ulcer disease in the absence of malignancy.

Hemorrhage. Upper GI bleeding is a relatively common problem, with an annual incidence of approximately 1 per 1000. Most nonvariceal bleeding (70%) is attributable to peptic ulcers. Most bleeding stops spontaneously and requires no intervention. However, persistent bleeding is associated with a 6% to 8% mortality. Several clinical scores have been created to risk-stratify patients presenting with upper GI bleeding to predict risk of rebleeding and overall morbidity and mortality. The most commonly used scores are the Blatchford and Rockall prediction scores.[6,7] The Blatchford score (Table 48-3) incorporates the patient's blood urea, hemoglobin, blood pressure, and other clinical parameters to predict the need for therapeutic intervention with transfusion, endoscopy, or surgery. A score of greater than zero has a sensitivity of 99% in predicting the need for such an intervention, and the score can serve as a useful screening tool for determining which patients are at risk for serious bleeding on initial presentation. The Rockall score (see Table 48-3) uses clinical variables and the findings of initial upper endoscopy to predict the risk of rebleeding and in-hospital mortality and is more helpful in determining whether a surgical intervention may be required after the patient has been initially resuscitated and evaluated.

The initial approach to an upper GI bleed is similar to the approach to a trauma patient. Large-bore intravenous access, rapid restoration of intravascular volume with fluid and blood products as the clinical situation dictates, and close monitoring for signs of rebleeding all are essential to effective management of these patients. The role of nasogastric (NG) lavage remains debatable; however, it can be useful as a predictor of high-risk patients and as an aid for later endoscopic intervention. Patients with bright red blood on NG lavage, as opposed to clear or coffee-ground lavage, are at much higher risk for persistent bleeding or rebleeding and warrant endoscopic intervention. If the NG lavage returns bilious fluid without blood, indicating the duodenal as well as gastric contents have been sampled, a lower GI source of bleeding (i.e., one distal to the ligament of Treitz) should be considered. In addition to its diagnostic usefulness, the NG tube can be used to lavage the stomach and duodenum before endoscopy, removing the clot and old blood that could obscure visualization of the source of bleeding. Given its relatively low risk and potential benefit, NG tube placement should be part of the treatment algorithm for these patients after appropriate intravascular access has been established and resuscitation begun.

Upper flexible endoscopy is the best initial procedure for diagnosis of the source of upper GI bleeding and for therapeutic intervention, especially in the setting of bleeding ulcers. Almost all patients with a potentially substantial acute upper GI bleed should undergo endoscopy within 24 hours. Although the data are inconclusive, early endoscopy has been shown to be a cost-effective strategy by triaging patients to more rapid intervention, if warranted, and by identifying low-risk patients without the need for prolonged observation (and therefore earlier hospital discharge). Additionally, more recent data from retrospective series using multivariate regression analysis to adjust for confounding variables suggest that early endoscopic intervention (within 12 hours from presentation) results in shorter hospital length of stay and possibly lower mortality in high-risk patients.[8]

Patients who are noted on endoscopy to have active bleeding, via an arterial jet or oozing, an adherent clot, or a visible vessel within the ulcer, are at high risk, and intervention is required. Patients without active bleeding, no visible vessel, and a clean ulcer base are low risk and do not require further intervention.

TABLE 48-3 Blatchford and Rockall Prediction Scores for Upper Gastrointestinal Bleeding

BLATCHFORD CLINICAL PREDICTION SCORE FOR UPPER GI BLEEDING[6]

	SCORE					
VARIABLE	**0**	**1**	**2**	**3**	**4**	**6**
Blood urea (mmol/liter)	<6.5		6.5-8	8-10	10-25	>25
Hemoglobin (g/dL) for men	>13	12-13		10-12		<10
Hemoglobin (g/dL) for women	>12	10-12				<10
Systolic BP (mmHg)	>109	100-109	90-99	<90		
Other factors		Pulse >100, presentation with melena	Presentation with syncope, hepatic disease, cardiac failure			

ROCKALL CLINICAL PREDICTION SCORE FOR UPPER GI BLEEDING[7]

	SCORE			
VARIABLE	**0**	**1**	**2**	**3**
Age	<60	60-79	>79	
Shock	Systolic BP ≥100 mm Hg and pulse <100	Systolic BP ≥100 mm Hg and pulse ≥100	Systolic BP <100 mm Hg	
Comorbidities	No major comorbidities		Heart failure, ischemic heart disease, other major comorbidity	Renal failure, liver failure, metastatic cancer
Diagnosis	Mallory-Weiss tear, no lesion identified, and no stigmata of recent bleeding	All other diagnoses	Upper GI malignancy	
Stigmata of recent hemorrhage	None or dark spot only		Blood in upper GI tract, adherent clot, visible or spurting vessel	

BP, Blood pressure.

TABLE 48-4 **Forrest Classification of Stigmata of Recent Hemorrhage on Endoscopic Examination of Peptic Ulcers and Relative Prevalence**

STIGMATA OF RECENT HEMORRHAGE	FORREST CLASSIFICATION	PREVALENCE (%) ON INPATIENT ENDOSCOPY PERFORMED FOR UPPER GI BLEEDING*
Active bleeding		10.7 (both spurting and oozing)
Active spurting	IA	
Active oozing	IB	
Recent hemorrhage		
Nonbleeding vessel	IIA	7.2
Adherent clot	IIB	7.1
Flat pigmented spot	IIC	14.3
No signs of hemorrhage		
Clean-based ulcer	III	48.6

From Enestvedt BK, Gralnek IM, Mattek N, et al: An evaluation of endoscopic indications and findings related to nonvariceal upper-GI hemorrhage in a large multicenter consortium. *Gastrointest Endosc* 67:422–429, 2008.

*The ulcer appearance was not described in 12.1% of patients.

The most commonly used system for classifying the endoscopic appearance of bleeding ulcers is the Forrest classification (Table 48-4), which stratifies the risk of rebleeding based on observed "stigmata of recent hemorrhage." Lower risk ulcers are much more frequently encountered than actively bleeding ones, even in the setting of inpatients undergoing endoscopy for diagnosis of upper GI bleeding. All patients undergoing endoscopic examination should be tested for *H. pylori* status. For high-risk patients requiring intervention, the best initial approach is endoscopic control, which results in primary hemostasis in approximately 90% of patients. The most common method of control is injection of a vasoconstrictor at the site of bleeding. With this method alone, primary hemostasis rates are high, but up to 30% of patients have rebleeding. This situation has led to the development of new techniques, including use of a second vasoconstrictor or sclerosing agent, thermocoagulation, and placement of clips at the site of bleeding. A 2009 meta-analysis compared the use of epinephrine alone with other forms of endoscopic monotherapy, most commonly thermal therapy or clips, and found these other approaches to be more effective in preventing rebleeding.[9] A dual approach, using epinephrine injection along with either thermal therapy or clips, showed an even better reduction in rebleeding rate, with a relative risk of 0.3 compared with epinephrine injection alone.

Guidelines for endoscopic control of bleeding published in 2010 advocate either the use of epinephrine plus an additional method or monotherapy with either thermocoagulation or clipping, but discourage the use of epinephrine alone. Although routine repeat endoscopy has not been shown to be beneficial, for patients who have rebleeding, repeat endoscopy does not increase their mortality and should be attempted before surgical intervention as long as the patient remains hemodynamically stable.

All high-risk patients should be placed in a monitored setting, preferably an intensive care unit, until all bleeding has stopped for 24 hours. As part of the 2010 consensus guidelines, all high-risk patients should be placed on a PPI administered intravenously, with an initial bolus followed by continuous infusion or intermittent dosing for up to 72 hours. Compared with a histamine blocker and placebo, intravenous PPI therapy showed lower rebleeding rates, a lower rate of emergency surgery, and decreased mortality. Additionally, high-dose intravenous PPIs were shown to be more effective than PPIs at standard dosing in preventing recurrent bleeding. Patients deemed high risk based on clinical factors who are awaiting endoscopy should begin therapy before endoscopy.

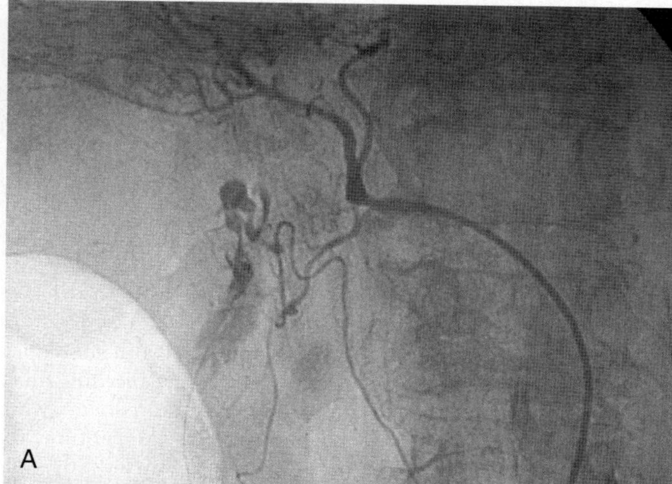

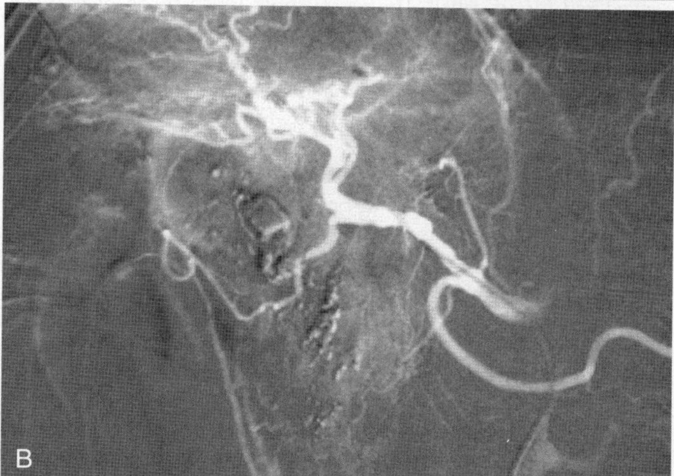

FIGURE 48-10 Endovascular control of a bleeding duodenal ulcer. **A,** An angiogram is obtained, which shows extravasation from a branch off of the gastroduodenal artery. **B,** A completion angiogram after glue embolization of the vessel shows resolution of the bleed with preservation of flow through the gastroduodenal artery. (From Loffroy R, Guiu B, Cercueil JP, et al: Refractory bleeding from gastroduodenal ulcers: Arterial embolization in high-operative-risk patients. *J Clin Gastroenterol* 42:361–367, 2008.)

Although flexible upper endoscopy remains the standard first-line therapy for upper GI bleeding, another option for nonsurgical control of bleeding duodenal ulcers is catheter-directed angiography and endovascular embolization (Fig. 48-10). A meta-analysis of studies examining the use of arterial embolization of upper GI bleeding found a pooled technical success rate of 84% in stopping hemorrhage, with prevention of rebleeding in 67% of patients.[10]

Another study retrospectively compared the effectiveness of arterial embolization and surgery for recurrent peptic ulcer bleeding after initial endoscopic therapy. Endovascular embolization was found to have higher rates of rebleeding (34% versus 13%, $P = .01$) but with fewer postintervention complications (41% versus 68%, $P = .01$). Mortality, transfusion requirements, and hospital length of stay were similar with the two approaches. Although it remains a relatively novel interventional modality, endovascular therapy for peptic ulcer bleeding offers an attractive approach in patients with recurrent bleeding after endoscopy who remain hemodynamically stable, especially patients who are poor surgical candidates based on other medical comorbidities.

Despite the use of PPIs and improved methods of endoscopic control, 5% to 10% of patients have persistent bleeding that requires surgical intervention. This group includes patients who become hemodynamically unstable and patients who continue to bleed and require ongoing blood transfusions (usually >6 U of packed red blood cells). The vessel most likely to be bleeding is the gastroduodenal artery because of erosion from a posterior ulcer. Although bleeding duodenal ulcers can be treated laparoscopically, the more typical approach is through an upper midline laparotomy, especially in patients who are hemodynamically unstable. A Kocher maneuver is performed to mobilize the duodenum. The anterior wall of the duodenal bulb is opened longitudinally, and the incision can be carried across the pylorus. The gastroduodenal artery is oversewn, with a three-point U stitch technique, which effectively ligates the main vessel (superior and inferior stitches) and prevents back-bleeding from any smaller branches (medial stitch), such as the transverse pancreatic artery, that head to the patient's left toward the body of the pancreas. One must be careful to avoid incorporating the common bile duct into the stitch. The course of the common bile duct can be identified by inserting a probe through the ampulla of Vater transduodenally or performing either a retrograde or an anterograde intraoperative cholangiogram. After the bleeding has been controlled, the duodenotomy is closed transversely to avoid narrowing (see Fig. 48-10).

Perforation. Patients with perforation typically complain of sudden-onset, frequently severe epigastric pain. For many, it is their first symptom of ulcer disease. Patients frequently have free air visible on the chest radiograph and have localized peritoneal signs on examination. Patients with more widespread spillage have diffuse peritonitis. For a small subset of patients, the perforation may seal spontaneously; however, operative intervention is required in almost all cases. Perforation has the highest mortality rate of any complication of ulcer disease, approaching 15%.

Perforation is a surgical disease, and conservative management means emergent surgical intervention. The perforation is usually in the first portion of the duodenum and can easily be accessed through an upper midline incision. Perforations smaller than 1 cm can generally be closed primarily and buttressed with a well-vascularized omentum. For larger perforations or ulcers with fibrotic edges that cannot be brought together without tension, a Graham patch repair with a tongue of healthy omentum is performed. Multiple stay sutures are placed that incorporate a bite of healthy tissue on the proximal and the distal side of the ulcer. The omentum is placed underneath these sutures, and they are tied to secure it in place and seal the perforation (Fig. 48-11). For very large perforations (>3 cm), control of the duodenal defect can be difficult. The defect should be closed by the application of healthy tissue, such as omentum or jejunal serosa from a Roux-en-Y type limb. In such cases, a pyloric exclusion is typically performed by oversewing the pylorus using absorbable suture or stapling across it using a noncutting linear stapler. A gastrojejunostomy is created to bypass the duodenum in a Billroth II or Roux-en-Y fashion. Over several weeks, the pyloric exclusion stitches or staples give way, restoring normal GI anatomy after the perforation site has been given time to heal. Alternatively, a duodenostomy tube can be placed through the perforation with wide peritoneal drainage. Leakage of GI contents into the drain is likely, but in most cases sepsis will resolve. An alternative in this difficult situation is antrectomy and a Billroth II or Roux-en-Y reconstruction.

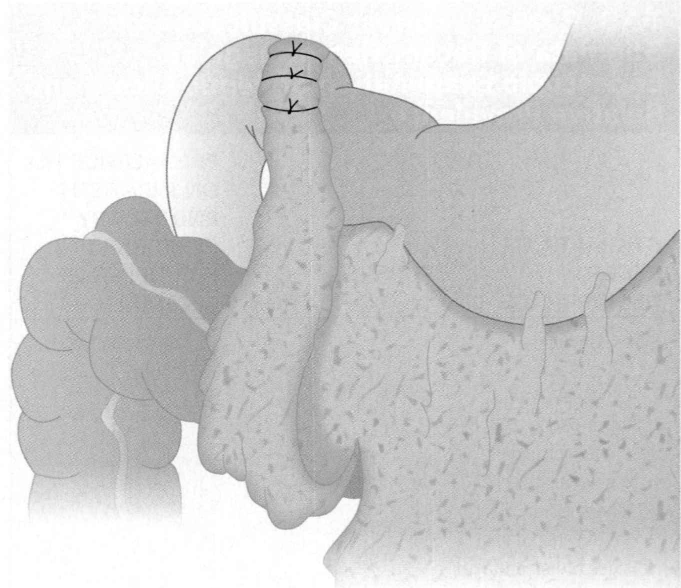

FIGURE 48-11 Graham patch repair of a perforated duodenal ulcer. A "tongue" of omentum is brought up to cover the ulcer defect and secured in position with a series of interrupted sutures. In Graham's original description, the ulcer defect is not closed, but if the tissue edges are healthy and come together without undue tension, a primary closure can be performed and reinforced with an omental patch. (From Baker RJ: Operation for acute perforated duodenal ulcer. In Nyhus LM, Baker RJ, Fischer JE, editors: *Mastery of surgery*, London, 1997, Little, Brown and Company.)

Perforations can also be treated laparoscopically. The results of two randomized controlled trials showed that patients undergoing laparoscopic repair have, as expected, less pain and parenteral narcotic use. They also have an earlier time to discharge. There was no difference in pulmonary complications or abdominal septic complications. A meta-analysis of studies comparing laparoscopic repair versus open repair, which included the randomized controlled trials along with prospective and retrospective cohort studies, showed overall similar outcomes, with longer operative times for laparoscopic repair.[11] However, these operating times have been decreasing in studies performed after 2001; in a recent randomized controlled trial, laparoscopic repair was faster than open repair. The conversion rate ranged from 10% to 15% in most reports. A case-matched analysis of the National Surgical Quality Improvement Program database comparing the two approaches found shorter hospital length of stay after laparoscopic repair with a trend toward decreased infectious complications postoperatively.[12] Based on these data, in experienced hands, laparoscopy appears to be the superior approach in patients with duodenal perforations who are hemodynamically stable.

For patients who are known to be negative for *H. pylori*, are taking long-term NSAIDs that they cannot discontinue, or have failed medical therapy in the past for their ulcer disease, an acid-reducing procedure can be added at the time of repair. These procedures are discussed later in the chapter and must be based on the clinical situation and comfort of the surgeon.

After repair, the stomach is decompressed until bowel activity returns. Drains should be kept in place until patients have eaten without a change in drain output or quality, which would suggest a leak. A routine contrast radiograph is not required before initiating eating but can be used to evaluate the security of the perforation closure should the patient exhibit symptoms or signs of enteric leak. All *H. pylori*–positive patients should undergo eradication with appropriate triple-therapy regimens.

Gastric outlet obstruction. Acute inflammation of the duodenum can lead to mechanical obstruction, with a functional gastric outlet obstruction manifested by delayed gastric emptying, anorexia, nausea, and vomiting. In cases of prolonged vomiting, patients may become dehydrated and develop a hypochloremic-hypokalemic metabolic alkalosis secondary to the loss of gastric juice rich in hydrogen and chloride. Chronic inflammation of the duodenum may lead to recurrent episodes of healing followed by repair and scarring, ultimately leading to fibrosis and stenosis of the duodenal lumen. In this situation, the obstruction is accompanied by painless vomiting of large volumes of gastric contents, with metabolic abnormalities similar to abnormalities seen in acute obstruction. The stomach can become massively dilated in this setting, and it rapidly loses its muscular tone. Marked weight loss and malnutrition are also common.

Gastric outlet obstruction from ulcer disease is now less common than obstruction from cancer. Cancer must be ruled out with endoscopy. Endoscopic dilation and *H. pylori* eradication are the mainstays of therapy. A study with an almost 5-year follow-up showed that patients who have an identifiable cause (e.g., *H. pylori* infection) that could be treated have good long-term results with endoscopic dilation, with a median of five dilations required, but no subsequent surgical therapy.[13] Patients with idiopathic duodenal ulcer disease causing gastric outlet obstruction who are treated with lifetime acid suppression also have good long-term results with endoscopic dilation. Patients with refractory obstruction are best managed with primary antrectomy and reconstruction along with vagotomy.

Intractable peptic ulcer disease. Intractability is defined as failure of an ulcer to heal after an initial trial of 8 to 12 weeks of therapy or if patients relapse after therapy has been discontinued. Intractable PUD is unusual for duodenal ulcer disease in the *H. pylori* era. Benign gastric ulcers that persist must be evaluated for malignancy. For any intractable ulcer, adequate duration of therapy, *H. pylori* eradication, and elimination of NSAID use must be confirmed. A serum gastrin level should also be determined in patients with ulcers refractory to medical therapy to rule out gastrinoma. Although rarely seen today, intractable duodenal ulcer should be treated with an acid-reducing operation. This can be a truncal vagotomy, selective vagotomy, or highly selective vagotomy, with or without an antrectomy.

Surgical procedures for peptic ulcers. Elective operative intervention has become rare as medical therapy has become more effective. The recognition of *H. pylori* and its eradication suggest that the intractability indication for surgery may apply only to patients in whom the organism cannot be eradicated or who cannot be taken off NSAIDs. Patients who are noncompliant with acid suppression therapy may also fall into this category.

The goal of operative ulcer therapy is to reduce gastric acid secretion and this can be accomplished by removing vagal stimulation via vagotomy, gastrin-driven secretion by performing an antrectomy, or both. Vagotomy decreases peak acid output by approximately 50%, whereas vagotomy plus antrectomy decreases peak acid output by approximately 85%.

Truncal vagotomy. As shown in Figure 48-4, truncal vagotomy is performed by division of the left and right vagus nerves above the hepatic and celiac branches, just above the GE junction. Truncal vagotomy is probably the most common operation performed for duodenal ulcer disease. Most surgeons use some form of drainage procedure in association with truncal vagotomy. Pyloric relaxation is mediated by vagal stimulation, and a vagotomy without a drainage procedure can cause delayed gastric emptying. Classic truncal vagotomy, in combination with a Heineke-Mikulicz pyloroplasty, is shown in Figure 48-12. When the duodenal bulb is scarred, a Finney pyloroplasty or Jaboulay gastroduodenostomy may be a useful alternative. In general, there is little difference in the side effects associated with the type of drainage procedure performed, although bile reflux may be more common after gastroenterostomy, and diarrhea is more common after pyloroplasty. The incidence of dumping is the same for both.

Selective vagotomy. Selective vagotomy divides the main right and left vagus nerves just distal to the celiac and hepatic branches, and a pyloric drainage procedure is also performed. However, selective vagotomy results in higher ulcer recurrence

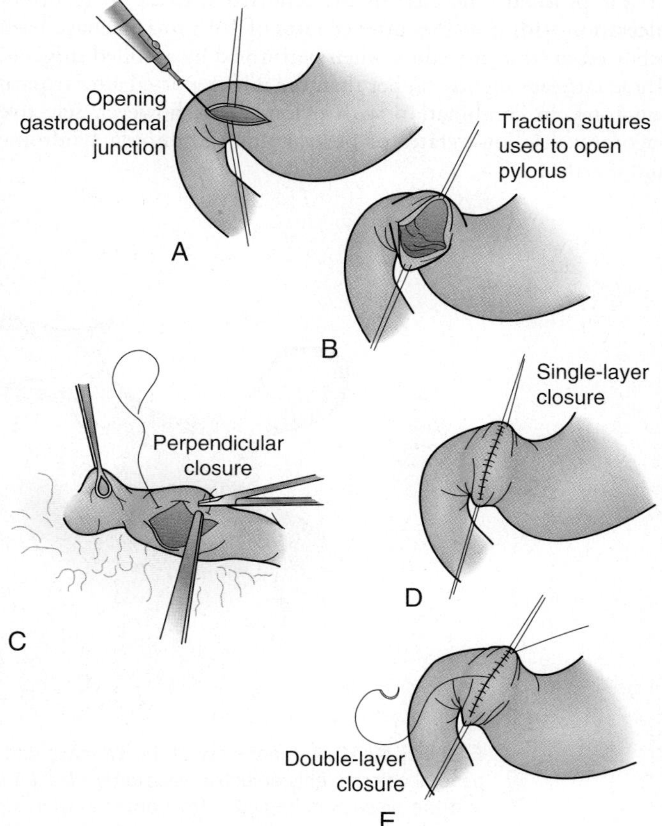

FIGURE 48-12 A-E, Heineke-Mikulicz pyloroplasty. (From Soreide JA, Soreide A: Pyloroplasty. *Oper Tech Gen Surg* 5:65–72, 2003.)

rates than truncal vagotomy, with no advantage in terms of decreased postgastrectomy symptoms. For these reasons, selective vagotomy has largely been abandoned as an option for acid-reducing surgery.

Highly selective vagotomy (parietal cell vagotomy). Highly selective vagotomy is also called *parietal cell vagotomy* or *proximal gastric vagotomy*. This procedure was developed after recognition that truncal vagotomy, in combination with a drainage procedure or gastric resection, adversely affects the pyloral antral pump function. A highly selective vagotomy divides only the vagus nerves supplying the acid-producing portion of the stomach within the corpus and fundus. This procedure preserves the vagal innervation of the gastric antrum and pylorus, so there is no need for routine drainage procedures. Consequently, the incidence of postoperative complications is lower. In general, the nerves of Latarjet are identified anteriorly and posteriorly, and the crow's feet innervating the fundus and body of the stomach are divided. These nerves are divided up until a point approximately 7 cm proximal to the pylorus or the area in the vicinity of the gastric antrum. Superiorly, division of these nerves is carried to a point at least 5 cm proximal to the GE junction on the esophagus (Fig. 48-13). Ideally, two or three branches to the antrum and pylorus should be preserved. The criminal nerve of Grassi represents a very proximal branch of the posterior trunk of the vagus, and great attention is needed to avoid missing this branch in the division process because it is frequently cited as a predisposition for ulcer recurrence if left intact.

The recurrence rates after highly selective vagotomy are variable and depend on the skill of the surgeon and duration of follow-up. Lengthy longitudinal follow-up is necessary to evaluate the results of this procedure because of the reported increase in recurrent ulceration with time. Recurrence rates of 10% to 15% have been reported for this procedure when performed by a skilled surgeon. These rates are slightly higher than the rates reported after truncal vagotomy in combination with pyloroplasty; however, selective vagotomy has lower rates of postvagotomy dumping syndrome and diarrhea.

Truncal vagotomy and antrectomy. Antrectomy is generally not performed for duodenal ulcers and is more commonly performed for gastric ulcers. Relative contraindications include cirrhosis; extensive scarring of the proximal duodenum that leaves a difficult or tenuous duodenal closure; and previous operations on the proximal duodenum, such as choledochoduodenostomy. When done in combination with truncal vagotomy, it is more effective at reducing acid secretion and recurrence than truncal vagotomy in combination with a drainage procedure or highly selective vagotomy. The recurrence rate for ulceration after truncal vagotomy and antrectomy is 0% to 2%. However, this low recurrence rate needs to be balanced against the 20% rate of postgastrectomy and postvagotomy syndromes in patients undergoing antrectomy, longer operative times, and increased postoperative morbidity.

Antrectomy requires reconstruction of GI continuity that can be accomplished by a gastroduodenostomy (Billroth I procedure [Fig. 48-14]) or gastrojejunostomy (either Billroth II procedure [Fig. 48-15] or Roux-en-Y reconstruction). For benign disease, gastroduodenostomy is generally favored because it avoids the problem of retained antrum syndrome, duodenal stump leak, and afferent loop obstruction associated with gastrojejunostomy after resection. If the duodenum is significantly scarred, gastroduodenostomy may be technically more difficult, necessitating gastrojejunostomy. If a gastrojejunostomy is performed, the loop of jejunum chosen for anastomosis is usually brought through the transverse mesocolon in a retrocolic fashion. The retrocolic anastomosis minimizes the length of the afferent limb and decreases the likelihood of twisting or kinking that could lead to afferent loop obstruction and predispose to the devastating complication of a duodenal stump leak. Although vagotomy and antrectomy are effective at managing ulcerations, they are used infrequently today in the treatment of patients with PUD. In general, operations of lesser magnitude are performed more frequently in the *H. pylori* era. The overall mortality rate for antrectomy is approximately 2% but is higher in patients with comorbid conditions, such as insulin-dependent diabetes or immunosuppression.

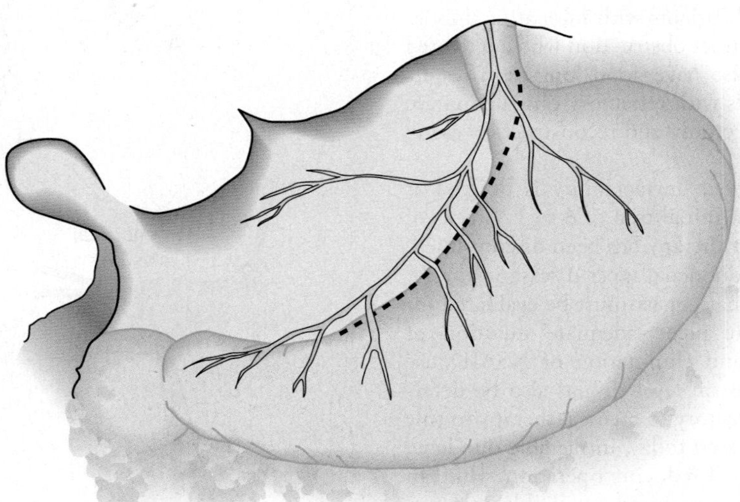

FIGURE 48-13 Anterior view of the stomach and anterior nerve of Latarjet. Note the line of dissection for parietal cell or highly selective vagotomy *(dashed line)*. The last major branches of the nerve are left intact, and the dissection begins 7 cm from the pylorus. At the gastroesophageal junction, the dissection is well away from the origin of the hepatic branches of the left vagus. (From Kelly KA, Teotia SS: Proximal gastric vagotomy. In Baker RJ, Fischer JE, editors: *Mastery of surgery*, Philadelphia, 2001, Lippincott Williams & Wilkins.)

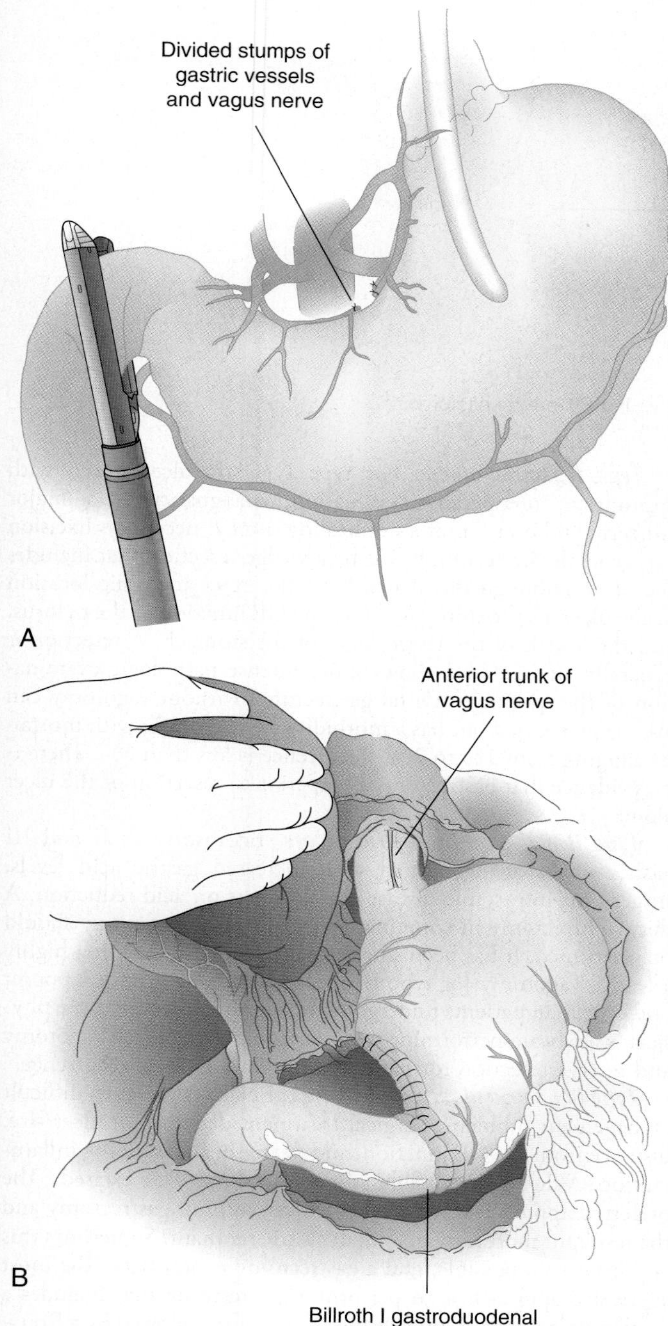

FIGURE 48-14 Hemigastrectomy with a Billroth I (gastroduodenal) anastomosis. (From Dempsey D, Pathak A: Antrectomy. *Oper Tech Gen Surg* 5:86–100, 2003.)

Approximately 20% of patients develop some form of postgastrectomy or postvagotomy complications (see later).

Gastric Ulcers

The modified Johnson anatomic classification system for gastric ulcers (i.e., types I through V, described in Table 48-5) was developed before the modern understanding that most ulcers are the consequence of *H. pylori* infection or NSAID usage. However, despite having an increased understanding of the mechanisms of how and why most ulcers develop, this historical classification system is still relevant to surgical treatment because it dictates what operation should be performed in the setting of complications of such ulcers, most commonly perforation.

Gastric ulcers can occur at any location in the stomach, although they usually manifest on the lesser curvature, near the incisura. Approximately 60% of ulcers are in this location and are classified as type I gastric ulcers. These ulcers are generally not associated with excessive acid secretion and may occur with low to normal acid output. Most occur within 1.5 cm of the histologic transition zone between the fundic and antral mucosa and are not associated with duodenal, pyloric, or prepyloric mucosal abnormalities. In contrast, type II gastric ulcers (approximately 15%) are located in the body of the stomach in combination with a duodenal ulcer. These types of ulcers are usually associated with excess acid secretion. Type III gastric ulcers are prepyloric ulcers and account for approximately 20% of the lesions. They also behave similar to duodenal ulcers and are associated with hypersecretion of gastric acid. Type IV gastric ulcers occur high on the lesser curvature, near the GE junction. The incidence of type IV gastric ulcers is less than 10%, and they are not associated with excessive acid secretion. Type V gastric ulcers can occur at any location and are associated with long-term NSAID use. Finally, some ulcers may appear on the greater curvature of the stomach, but the incidence is less than 5%.

Gastric ulcers rarely develop before the age of 40 years, and the peak incidence occurs in individuals 55 to 65 years old. Gastric ulcers are more likely to occur in individuals in a lower socioeconomic class and are slightly more common in the nonwhite than white population. The exact pathogenesis of a benign gastric ulcer is less well understood than duodenal ulcers, but most are caused by *H. pylori* or NSAID use. Some clinical conditions that may predispose to gastric ulceration include chronic alcohol intake, smoking, long-term corticosteroid therapy, infection, and intra-arterial therapy. With regard to acid and pepsin secretion, the presence of acid appears to be essential to the production of a gastric ulcer; however, the total secretory output appears to be less important. In contrast to the acidification of the duodenum leading to ulcer formation, patients with gastric ulcers caused by *H. pylori* have normal or reduced gastric acid production. Ulcer formation is more likely due to an inflammatory response to the bacterial infection itself, which is most densely concentrated at the junction between the stomach body and antrum. Nevertheless, rapid healing follows antacid therapy, antisecretory therapy, or vagotomy even when the lesion-bearing portion of the stomach is left intact because in the presence of gastric mucosal damage, acid is ulcerogenic, even when present in normal or less than normal amounts.

Clinical Manifestations

The clinical challenge of gastric ulcer management is the differentiation between gastric carcinoma and benign ulcer. This is in contrast to duodenal ulcers, in which malignancy is extremely rare. Similar to duodenal ulcers, gastric ulcers are also characterized by recurrent episodes of quiescence and relapse. They also cause pain, bleeding, and obstruction and can perforate. Occasionally, benign ulcers have also been found to result in spontaneous gastrocolic fistulas. Surgical intervention is required in 8% to 20% of patients who develop complications from gastric ulcer disease. Hemorrhage occurs in approximately 35% to 40% of patients. Patients who develop significant bleeding from gastric ulcers usually are older, are less likely to stop bleeding spontaneously, and have higher morbidity and mortality rates than patients

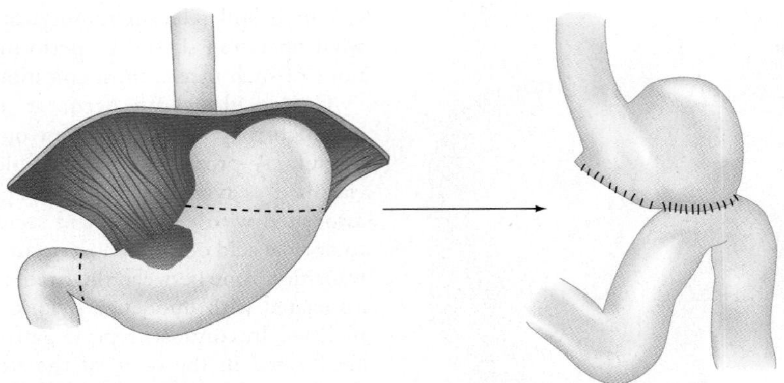

FIGURE 48-15 Subtotal gastrectomy with a Billroth II anastomosis.

TABLE 48-5 Gastric Ulcer Types

TYPE	LOCATION	ACID LEVEL
I	Lesser curve at incisura	Low to normal
II	Gastric body with duodenal ulcer	Increased
III	Prepyloric	Increased
IV	High on lesser curve	Normal
V	Anywhere	Normal, NSAID-induced

NSAID, Nonsteroidal anti-inflammatory drug.

with bleeding from a duodenal ulcer. The most frequent complication of gastric ulceration is perforation. Most perforations occur along the anterior aspect of the lesser curvature. In general, older patients have increased rates of perforations, and larger ulcers are associated with higher morbidity and mortality. Similar to duodenal ulcers, gastric outlet obstruction can also occur in patients with type II or III gastric ulcers. However, one must carefully differentiate between benign obstruction and obstruction secondary to antral carcinoma.

Diagnosis and Treatment

The diagnosis and treatment of gastric ulceration generally mirror diagnosis and treatment of duodenal ulcer disease. The significant difference is the possibility of malignancy in a gastric ulcer. This critical difference demands that cancer be ruled out in acute and chronic presentations of gastric ulcer disease. Acid suppression and *H. pylori* eradication are important aspects of any treatment.

As with duodenal ulcers, intractable nonhealing ulcers are becoming increasingly less common. It is important to ensure that adequate time has elapsed and appropriate therapy has been administered to allow healing of the ulcer to occur; this includes confirmation that *H. pylori* has been eradicated and that NSAIDs have been eliminated as a potential cause. The presentation of a nonhealing gastric ulcer in the *H. pylori* era should raise serious concerns about the presence of an underlying malignancy. These patients should undergo a thorough evaluation with multiple biopsies to exclude malignancy before any surgical intervention (Fig. 48-16). The approach for a complicated gastric ulcer varies depending on the type of ulcer and its association with pathophysiologic acid levels. Types I and IV ulcers, which are not associated with increased acid levels, do not require acid-reducing vagotomy. Figure 48-17 is an algorithm for managing complicated gastric ulcers.

Type I gastric ulcers. For type I gastric ulcers, even with appropriate preoperative evaluation, malignancy is a major concern, and excision of a nonhealing ulcer is necessary. Excision can generally be accomplished by a wedge resection that includes the ulcer, although this depends on the exact anatomic location of the ulcer, its proximity to either the GE junction or the pylorus, and the length of the lesser curve of the stomach. A resection is generally curative and allows more intense pathologic examination of the specimen. Distal gastrectomy without vagotomy can also be performed but has a morbidity of 3% to 5%, with mortality ranging from 1% to 2%. Recurrence is less than 5%. There is no evidence that gastrectomy is superior to resection of the ulcer alone.

Type II and type III gastric ulcers. Because types II and III gastric ulcers are associated with increased gastric acid levels, surgery for intractable disease should focus on acid reduction. A distal gastrectomy in combination with truncal vagotomy should be performed. It has been shown that patients undergoing highly selective vagotomy for type II or III gastric ulcers have a poorer outcome than patients undergoing resection. However, some physicians advocate performing a laparoscopic parietal cell vagotomy and reserve resection for patients who develop ulcer recurrence.

Type IV gastric ulcers. Type IV gastric ulcers present a difficult management problem. Surgical treatment depends on ulcer size, distance from the GE junction, and degree of surrounding inflammation. Whenever possible, the ulcer should be excised. The preferred approach is to resect the ulcer without gastrectomy and the resultant morbidity of a small gastric remnant. Sometimes this approach is impossible, and a gastrectomy is necessary. The most aggressive approach is to perform a gastrectomy that includes a small portion of the esophageal wall and ulcer followed by a Roux-en-Y esophagojejunostomy to restore intestinal continuity. For type IV gastric ulcers that are located 2 to 5 cm from the GE junction, a distal gastrectomy with a vertical extension of the resection to include the lesser curvature with the ulcer can be performed (the Csendes procedure). After resection, bowel continuity is restored with an end-to-end gastroduodenostomy or gastrojejunostomy.

Bleeding gastric ulcers. Treatment of bleeding gastric ulcers depends on their cause and location; however, the initial approach is similar to duodenal ulcers. Patients require resuscitation, monitoring, and endoscopic investigation. Up to 70% of gastric ulcers are *H. pylori*–positive, so an attempt should be made to control the bleeding endoscopically, with multiple biopsy specimens of the ulcer obtained to rule out malignancy and concurrently obtained biopsy specimens of the body and antrum to test for *H.*

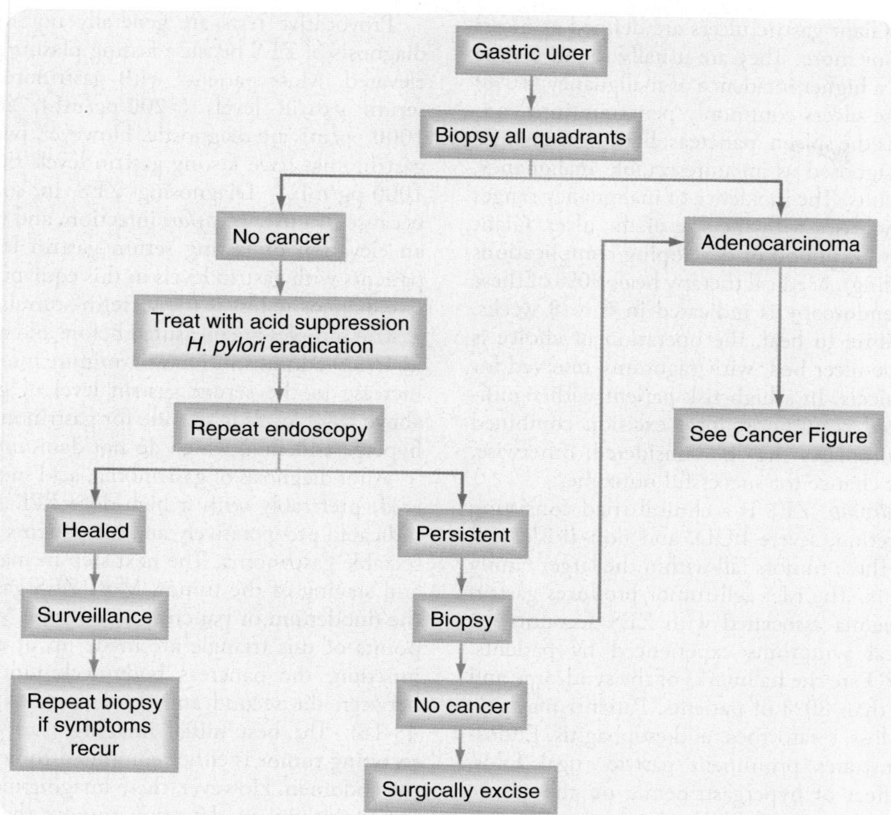

FIGURE 48-16 Algorithm for evaluation, treatment, and surveillance of a patient with a gastric ulcer.

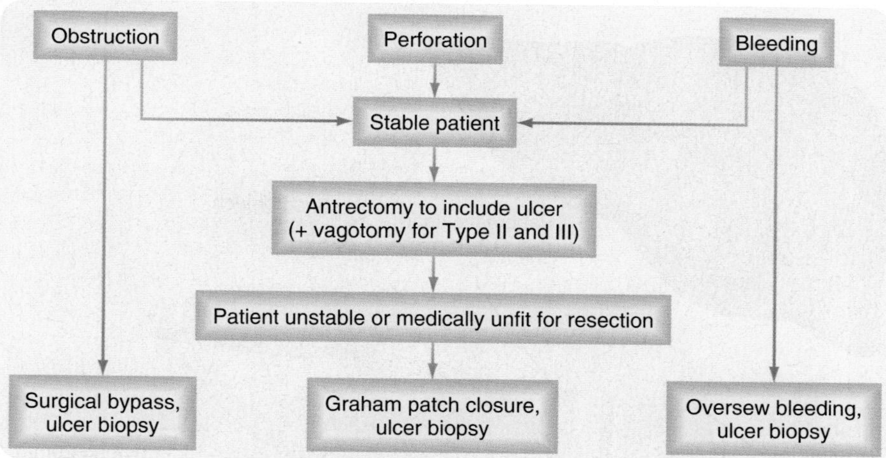

FIGURE 48-17 Algorithm for the management of complicated gastric ulcer disease.

pylori infection. Patients whose bleeding can be controlled and who are *H. pylori*–positive should undergo subsequent treatment for *H. pylori* infection. For bleeding that cannot be controlled, operative intervention again depends on the type of gastric ulcer. In all cases, the ulcer should ideally be excised with the addition of vagotomy depending on the cause of the ulcer (mostly for intractable ulcers that are not due to *H. pylori* infection or NSAID usage that can be stopped).

Perforated gastric ulcer. For perforated type I gastric ulcers that occur in patients in stable condition, distal gastrectomy with a Billroth I anastomosis is recommended. In unstable patients, simple patching of the gastric ulcer with biopsy and treatment for *H. pylori*, if positive, is recommended. However, even if the biopsy is negative, the risk for malignancy still needs to be ruled out; therefore, documentation of healing is required with repeat endoscopy and biopsy. Adding vagotomy for perforated type I gastric ulcers is unlikely to be of any value. Because they behave similar to duodenal ulcers, types II and III gastric ulcers can be simply treated with patch closure, with or without truncal vagotomy and pyloroplasty, depending on the medical condition, hemodynamic status, and extent of peritonitis, followed by treatment for *H. pylori* if positive.

Giant gastric ulcers. Giant gastric ulcers are defined as ulcers with a diameter of 2 cm or more. They are usually found on the lesser curvature and have a higher incidence of malignancy (10%) than smaller ulcers. These ulcers commonly penetrate into contiguous structures, such as the spleen, pancreas, liver, or transverse colon, and are falsely diagnosed as an unresectable malignancy, despite normal biopsy results. The incidence of malignancy ranges from 6% to 30% and increases with the size of the ulcer. Giant gastric ulcers have a high likelihood of developing complications (e.g., perforation or bleeding). Medical therapy heals 80% of these ulcers, although repeat endoscopy is indicated in 6 to 8 weeks. For complications or failure to heal, the operation of choice is gastrectomy including the ulcer bed, with vagotomy reserved for types II and III gastric ulcers. In a high-risk patient with significant underlying comorbid conditions, local excision combined with vagotomy and pyloroplasty may be considered; otherwise, resection has the highest chance for successful outcome.

Zollinger-ellison syndrome. ZES is a clinical triad consisting of gastric acid hypersecretion, severe PUD, and non–β-islet cell tumors of the pancreas. These tumors fall within the larger family of neuroendocrine tumors. The islet cell tumor produces gastrin and PUD. Hypergastrinemia associated with ZES accounts for most, if not all, clinical symptoms experienced by patients. Abdominal pain and PUD are the hallmarks of the syndrome and typically occur in more than 80% of patients. Patients may also exhibit diarrhea, weight loss, steatorrhea, and esophagitis. Endoscopy frequently demonstrates prominent gastric rugal folds, reflecting the trophic effect of hypergastrinemia on the gastric fundus in addition to evidence of PUD. Approximately one quarter of patients have ZES as part of multiple endocrine neoplasia type 1, an autosomal dominant syndrome.

Provocative tests are generally not required to establish the diagnosis of ZES because fasting plasma gastrin levels are usually elevated. Most patients with gastrinoma have elevated fasting serum gastrin levels (>200 pg/mL), and values higher than 1000 pg/mL are diagnostic. However, two thirds of patients with gastrinomas have fasting gastrin levels that are between 150 and 1000 pg/mL.[14] Diagnosing ZES in such patients is difficult because PPI use, *H. pylori* infection, and renal failure all can cause an elevation of fasting serum gastrin levels into this range. In patients with gastrin levels in this equivocal range, the most sensitive diagnostic test is the secretin-stimulated gastrin level. Serum gastrin samples are measured before and after intravenous secretin (2 U/kg) administration at 5-minute intervals for 30 minutes. An increase in the serum gastrin level of greater than 200 pg/mL above basal levels is specific for gastrinoma versus other causes of hypergastrinemia, which do not demonstrate this response.

After diagnosis of gastrinoma, acid suppression therapy is initiated, preferably with a high-dose PPI. Medical management is indicated preoperatively and for patients with metastatic or unresectable gastrinoma. The next step in management is localization and staging of the tumor. Most ZES gastrinomas are located in the duodenum or pancreas, within the "gastrinoma triangle"; the points of this triangle are made up of the cystic-common duct junction, the pancreas body-neck junction, and the junction between the second and third portions of the duodenum (Fig. 48-18). The best initial imaging study to localize the gastrin-secreting tumor is either computed tomography (CT) or MRI of the abdomen. However, these imaging modalities have a relatively low sensitivity in detecting tumors that are less than 1 cm in diameter as well as small liver metastases.[15] If initial imaging is nondiagnostic, localization can sometimes be achieved using

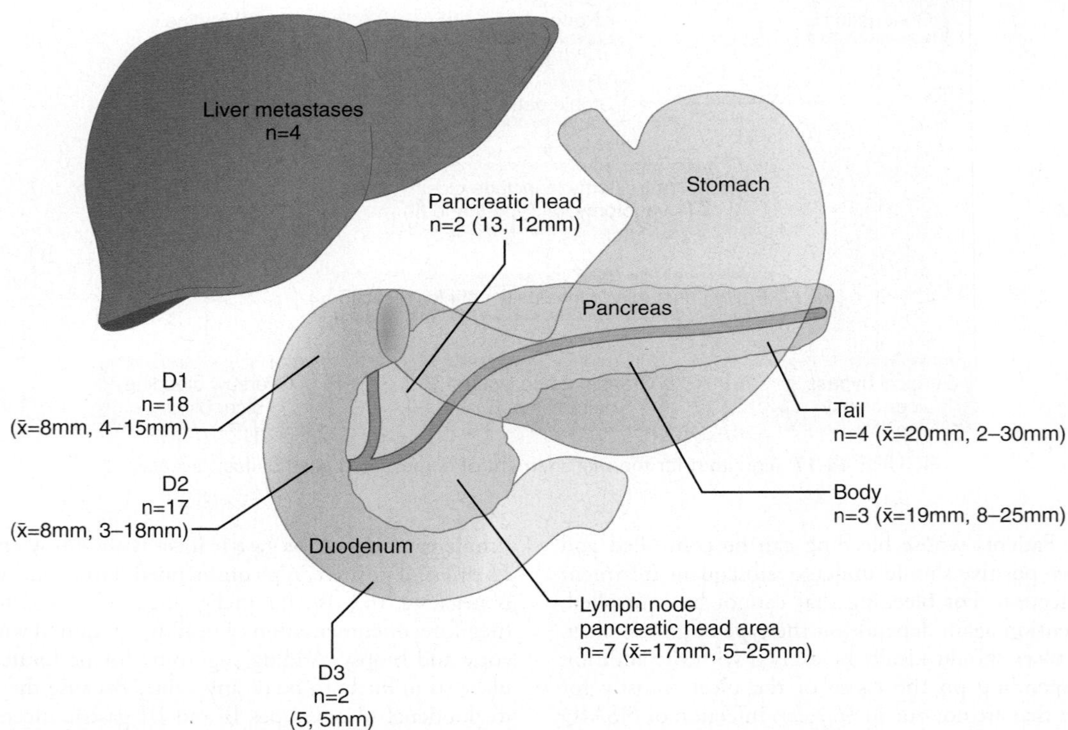

FIGURE 48-18 The location of gastrinomas at surgery that were not detected on preoperative imaging. Most tumors were located in the first and second portions of the duodenum and the head of the pancreas, within the so-called gastrinoma triangle. (From Norton JA, Fraker DL, Alexander HR, et al: Value of surgery in patients with negative imaging and sporadic Zollinger-Ellison syndrome. *Ann Surg* 256:509–517, 2012.)

somatostatin receptor scintigraphy or endoscopic ultrasound (EUS). Somatostatin receptor scintigraphy uses radionucleotide-labeled octreotide, which binds to the ZES tumor cells and can detect hepatic metastases in 85% to 95% of patients, as opposed to 70% to 80% using conventional cross-sectional imaging.

Localized gastrinoma should be resected; however, long-term cure rates are less than 40%. Although preoperative imaging is helpful in planning surgical resection, it is not necessary in all cases. In patients with ZES confirmed by gastrin levels but with negative imaging studies, the primary tumor can be localized on operative exploration in 98% of cases.[16] Once the tumor is located intraoperatively, a resection according to oncologic principles should be performed (rather than a tumor enucleation) because lymph node metastases are present in 43% to 82% of cases; however, this point is controversial. The role of surgery in patients with ZES and multiple endocrine neoplasia type 1 is also an area of debate, as these patients have higher recurrence rates and resection is rarely curative. Patients with tumor recurrence or metastatic disease are treated with chemotherapy (streptozotocin with 5-fluorouracil or doxorubicin or both), which results in clinical response rates of 20% to 45% but is never curative.

STRESS GASTRITIS

Stress gastritis, by definition, occurs after physical trauma, shock, sepsis, hemorrhage, or respiratory failure and may lead to life-threatening gastric bleeding. Stress gastritis is characterized by multiple superficial (nonulcerating) erosions that begin in the proximal or acid-secreting portion of the stomach and progress distally. They may also occur in the setting of central nervous system disease (Cushing ulcer) or as a result of thermal burn injury involving more than 30% of the body surface area (Curling ulcer).

Stress gastritis lesions typically change with time. They are considered early lesions if they appear within the first 24 hours. These early lesions are typically multiple and shallow, with discrete areas of erythema along with focal hemorrhage or an adherent clot. If the lesion erodes into the submucosa, which contains the blood supply, frank bleeding may result. On microscopy, these lesions appear as wedged-shaped mucosal hemorrhages with coagulation necrosis of the superficial mucosal cells. They are almost always seen in the fundus of the stomach and only rarely in the distal stomach. Acute stress gastritis can be classified as late if there is a tissue reaction or organization around a clot, or if an inflammatory exudate is present. This picture may be seen by microscopy 24 to 72 hours after injury. Late lesions appear identical to regenerating mucosa around a healing gastric ulcer. Both types of lesions can be seen endoscopically.

Pathophysiology

Although the precise mechanisms responsible for the development of stress gastritis remain to be fully elucidated, evidence suggests a multifactorial cause. Stress-induced gastric lesions appear to require the presence of acid. Other factors that may predispose to their development include impaired mucosal defense mechanisms against luminal acid, such as a reduction in blood flow, mucus, bicarbonate secretion by mucosal cells, or endogenous prostaglandins. All these factors render the stomach more susceptible to damage from luminal acid, with the resultant hemorrhagic gastritis. Stress is considered present when hypoxia, sepsis, or organ failure occurs. When stress is present, mucosal ischemia is thought to be the main factor responsible for the breakdown of these normal defense mechanisms. There is little evidence to suggest that increased gastric acid secretion occurs in this situation. However, the presence of luminal acid appears to be a prerequisite for this form of gastritis to evolve. Moreover, complete neutralization of luminal acid or antisecretory therapy precludes the development of experimental stress gastritis.

Presentation and Diagnosis

Stress gastritis develops within 1 to 2 days after a traumatic event in more than 50% of patients. The only clinical sign may be painless upper GI bleeding that may be delayed at onset. The bleeding is usually slow and intermittent and may be detected by only a few flecks of blood in the NG tube or an unexplained decrease in hemoglobin level. Occasionally, there may be profound upper GI hemorrhage accompanied by hypotension and hematemesis. The stool is frequently guaiac-positive, although melena and hematochezia are rare. Endoscopy is required to confirm the diagnosis and differentiate stress gastritis from other sources of GI hemorrhage.

Prophylaxis

Because of the high mortality rate in patients with acute stress gastritis who develop massive upper GI hemorrhage, high-risk patients should be treated prophylactically. Because mucosal ischemia may alter many mucosal defense mechanisms that enable the stomach to withstand luminal irritants and protect itself from injury, every effort should be made to correct any perfusion deficits secondary to shock. The two strongest risk factors for developing clinically significant bleeding from gastric stress ulcers are coagulopathy and respiratory failure requiring prolonged mechanical ventilation (>48 hours). Patients in the intensive care unit without these risk factors are unlikely to develop significant bleeding (0.1% incidence). Additionally, prophylactically increasing the gastric pH may increase rates of ventilator-associated pneumonia and *Clostridium difficile* infection. For these reasons, only critically ill patients with coagulopathy or prolonged mechanical ventilation should receive prophylaxis.[17] Enteral nutrition reduces the risk of stress ulcer formation and should be initiated as soon as possible. Some experts advocate not administering prophylaxis to patients who are being fed enterally even if they have risk factors, although this is controversial. If prophylaxis is indicated, a PPI, rather than H_2 antagonists or sucralfate, should be used, although the evidence supporting this is weak, and further head-to-head comparisons are needed.

Treatment

Any patient with upper GI bleeding requires prompt and definitive fluid resuscitation with correction of any coagulation or platelet abnormalities. Treatment of the underlying sepsis plays a major role in treating the underlying gastric erosions. More than 80% of patients who present with upper GI hemorrhage stop bleeding with only supportive care. There is little evidence to suggest that endoscopy with electrocautery or heater probe coagulation has any benefit in the treatment of bleeding from acute stress gastritis. However, some studies suggested that acute bleeding can be effectively controlled by selective infusion of vasopressin into the splanchnic circulation through the left gastric artery. Vasopressin is administered by continuous infusion through the catheter at a rate of 0.2 to 0.4 IU/min for a maximum of 48 to 72 hours. If the patient has underlying cardiac or liver disease, vasopressin should not be used. Although vasopressin may decrease blood loss, it has not been shown to result in improved survival. Another angiographic technique that can be used is embolization of the left gastric artery if bleeding is identified on angiography. However, the extensive plexus of submucosal arterial vessels within the stomach makes this approach less appealing and not as successful.

Bleeding that recurs or persists, requiring more than 6 U of blood (3000 mL), is an indication for surgery. Because most lesions are in the proximal stomach or fundus, a long anterior gastrotomy should be made in this area. The gastric lumen is cleared of blood, and the mucosal surface is inspected for bleeding points. All bleeding areas are oversewn with figure-of-eight stitches taken deep within the gastric wall. Most superficial erosions are not actively bleeding and do not require ligation unless a blood vessel is seen at its base. The operation is completed by closing the anterior gastrotomy and performing a truncal vagotomy and pyloroplasty to reduce acid secretion. The incidence of rebleeding is less than 5% if bleeding points are carefully identified and secured. Less commonly, a partial gastrectomy combined with vagotomy is performed. Total gastrectomy should be performed rarely and only in patients with life-threatening hemorrhage refractory to other forms of therapy.

POSTGASTRECTOMY SYNDROMES

Gastric surgery results in numerous physiologic derangements caused by loss of reservoir function, interruption of the pyloric sphincter mechanism, and vagal nerve transection. These physiologic changes usually cause no long-term symptoms. The GI and cardiovascular symptoms may result in disorders collectively referred to as *postgastrectomy syndromes*. Approximately 25% of patients who undergo surgery for PUD subsequently develop some degree of postgastrectomy syndrome, although this frequency is much lower in patients who undergo highly selective vagotomy. The physiologic changes are not specific to PUD and can occur after gastrectomy for resection of neoplasm or Roux-en-Y gastric bypass for treatment of severe obesity. Only approximately 1% of patients become permanently disabled from their symptoms.

Dumping Syndrome

Dumping syndrome can be early (20 to 30 minutes after eating) or late (2 or 3 hours after a meal). Early dumping is more common, with more GI and fewer cardiovascular effects. GI symptoms include nausea and vomiting, a sense of epigastric fullness, cramping abdominal pain, and often explosive diarrhea. The cardiovascular symptoms include palpitations, tachycardia, diaphoresis, fainting, dizziness, flushing, and occasionally blurred vision. This symptom complex can develop after any operation on the stomach but is more common after partial gastrectomy with the Billroth II reconstruction. It is much less commonly observed after the Billroth I gastrectomy or after vagotomy and drainage procedures.

Early dumping occurs because of the rapid passage of food of high osmolarity from the stomach into the small intestine. This occurs because gastrectomy, or any interruption of the pyloric sphincteric mechanism, prevents the stomach from preparing its contents and delivering them to the proximal bowel in the form of small particles in isotonic solution. The resultant hypertonic food bolus passes into the small intestine, which induces a rapid shift of extracellular fluid into the intestinal lumen to achieve isotonicity. After this shift of extracellular fluid, luminal distention occurs and induces the autonomic responses listed earlier.

The basic defect of late dumping is also rapid gastric emptying; however, it is related specifically to carbohydrates being delivered rapidly into the proximal intestine. When carbohydrates are delivered to the small intestine, they are quickly absorbed, resulting in hyperglycemia, which triggers the release of large amounts of insulin to control the increasing blood sugar level. An overcompensation results so that profound hypoglycemia occurs in response to the insulin. This hypoglycemia activates the adrenal gland to release catecholamines, which results in diaphoresis, tremulousness, light-headedness, tachycardia, and confusion. The symptom complex is indistinguishable from insulin shock.

The symptoms associated with early dumping syndrome appear to be secondary to the release of several humoral agents, such as serotonin, bradykinin-like substances, neurotensin, and enteroglucagon. Dietary measures are usually sufficient to treat most patients. These include avoiding foods containing large amounts of sugar, frequent feeding of small meals rich in protein and fat, and separating liquids from solids during a meal.

In some patients without a response to dietary measures, long-acting octreotide agonists have ameliorated symptoms. These peptides not only inhibit gastric emptying but also affect small bowel motility so that intestinal transit of the ingested meal is prolonged. The side effects associated with administration of these synthetic peptides are relatively benign; however, the peptides are expensive. Many operative procedures have been advocated for the surgical treatment of these patients. The paucity of patients treated for PUD with gastrectomy or vagotomy has made remedial procedures for dumping exceedingly rare.

Metabolic Disturbances

The most common metabolic defect appearing after gastrectomy is anemia. Anemia is related to iron deficiency (more common) or impairment in vitamin B_{12} metabolism. More than 30% of patients undergoing gastrectomy have iron deficiency anemia. The exact cause is not fully understood but appears to be related to a combination of decreased iron intake, impaired iron absorption, and chronic blood loss. In general, the addition of iron supplements to the patient's diet corrects this metabolic problem.

Megaloblastic anemia from vitamin B_{12} deficiency only rarely develops after partial gastrectomy but is dependent on the amount of stomach removed. Vitamin deficiency occurs secondary to poor absorption of dietary vitamin B_{12} because of the lack of intrinsic factor. Patients undergoing subtotal gastrectomy should be placed on life-long vitamin B_{12} supplementation. If a patient develops a macrocytic anemia, serum vitamin B_{12} levels should be determined and, if abnormal, treated with long-term vitamin B_{12} therapy.

Osteoporosis and osteomalacia have also been observed after gastric resection and appear to be caused by deficiencies in calcium. If fat malabsorption is also present, the calcium malabsorption is aggravated further because fatty acids bind calcium. The incidence of this problem also increases with the extent of gastric resection and is usually associated with a Billroth II gastrectomy. Bone disease generally develops approximately 4 to 5 years after surgery. Treatment of this disorder usually requires calcium supplements (1 to 2 g/day) in conjunction with vitamin D (500 to 5000 U daily). Patients with Billroth II or Roux-en-Y reconstruction that bypasses the duodenum should also receive supplementation of the fat-soluble vitamins (vitamins A, D, E, and K).

Afferent Loop Syndrome

Afferent loop syndrome occurs as a result of partial obstruction of the afferent limb, which is unable to empty its contents. After obstruction of the afferent limb, pancreatic and hepatobiliary secretions accumulate within the limb, resulting in its distention, which causes epigastric discomfort and cramping. The intraluminal pressure eventually increases enough to empty the contents of the afferent loop forcefully into the stomach, resulting in bilious vomiting that offers immediate relief of symptoms. If the obstruction has been present for a long time, it can also be aggravated by the development of the blind loop syndrome. In this situation, bacterial overgrowth occurs in the static loop, and the bacteria bind with vitamin B_{12} and deconjugated bile acids; this results in a systemic deficiency of vitamin B_{12}, with the development of megaloblastic anemia.

In contrast to the diagnosis of an acute bowel obstruction, the diagnosis of chronic afferent loop obstruction may be problematic. Failure to visualize the afferent limb on upper endoscopy is suggestive of the diagnosis. Radionuclide studies imaging the hepatobiliary tree have also been used with some success in diagnosing this syndrome. Normally, the radionuclide should pass into the stomach or distal small bowel after being excreted into the afferent limb. If it does not, the possibility of an afferent loop obstruction should be considered.

Surgical correction is indicated for this mechanical problem. A long afferent limb is usually the underlying problem, so treatment involves the elimination of this loop. Remedies include conversion of the Billroth II construction into a Billroth I anastomosis, enteroenterostomy below the stoma, and creation of a Roux-en-Y procedure. The Roux-en-Y reconstruction is a good combination of efficacy and ease, especially in a patient with a previous vagotomy. Marginal ulceration from the diversion of duodenal contents from the gastroenteric stoma is a potential complication of the Roux-en-Y conversion.

Efferent Loop Obstruction

Obstruction of the efferent limb is rare. Efferent loop obstruction may occur at any time; however, more than 50% of cases do so within the first postoperative month. Establishing a diagnosis is difficult. Initial complaints may include left upper quadrant abdominal pain that is colicky in nature, bilious vomiting, and abdominal distention. The diagnosis is usually established by a GI contrast study of the stomach, with failure of barium to enter the efferent limb. Operative intervention is almost always necessary and consists of reducing the retroanastomotic hernia if this is the cause of the obstruction and closing the retroanastomotic space to prevent recurrence of this condition.

Alkaline Reflux Gastritis

After gastrectomy, reflux of bile is common. In a small percentage of patients, this reflux is associated with severe epigastric abdominal pain accompanied by bilious vomiting and weight loss. Although the diagnosis can be made by taking a careful history, hepatoiminodiacetic acid scans usually demonstrate biliary secretion into the stomach and sometimes into the esophagus. Upper endoscopy demonstrates friable, beefy red mucosa.

Most patients with alkaline reflux gastritis have had gastric resection performed with a Billroth II anastomosis. Although bile reflux appears to be the inciting event, numerous issues remain unanswered with respect to the role of bile in its pathogenesis. For example, many patients have reflux of bile into the stomach after gastrectomy without any symptoms. Moreover, there is no clear correlation between the volume or composition of bile and the subsequent development of alkaline reflux gastritis. Although the syndrome clearly exists, caution needs to be exercised to ensure that it is not overdiagnosed. After a diagnosis is made, therapy is directed at relief of symptoms. Most medical therapies that have been tried to treat alkaline reflux gastritis have not shown any consistent benefit. For patients with intractable symptoms, the surgical procedure of choice is conversion of the Billroth II anastomosis into a Roux-en-Y gastrojejunostomy, in which the Roux limb has been lengthened to more than 40 cm. In general, a Roux-en-Y procedure should be preferred over a Billroth II for reconstruction at the time of partial or subtotal distal gastrectomy to decrease the likelihood of alkaline reflux. A meta-analysis of randomized trials found that Roux-en-Y and Billroth II reconstructions resulted in the same rates of complications in the immediate postoperative period but that patients who underwent Roux-en-Y procedures had superior long-term quality of life because of lower rates of reflux esophagitis.

Gastric Atony

Gastric emptying is delayed after truncal and selective vagotomies but not after a highly selective or parietal cell vagotomy. With selective or truncal vagotomy, patients lose their antral pump function and have a reduction in the ability to empty solids. In contrast, emptying of liquids is accelerated because of loss of receptive relaxation in the proximal stomach, which regulates liquid emptying. Although most patients undergoing vagotomy and a drainage procedure manage to empty their stomach adequately, some patients have persistent gastric stasis that results in retention of food within the stomach for several hours. This condition may be accompanied by a feeling of fullness and occasionally abdominal pain. In still rarer cases, it may be associated with a functional gastric outlet obstruction.

The diagnosis of gastroparesis is confirmed by scintigraphic assessment of gastric emptying. However, other causes of delayed gastric emptying, such as diabetes mellitus, electrolyte imbalance, drug toxicity, and neuromuscular disorders, must also be excluded. In addition, a mechanical cause of gastric outlet obstruction, such as postoperative adhesions, afferent or efferent loop obstruction, and internal herniations, must be ruled out. Endoscopic examination of the stomach also needs to be performed to rule out any anastomotic obstructions.

In patients with a functional gastric outlet obstruction and documented gastroparesis, pharmacotherapy is generally used. The agents most commonly used are prokinetic agents such as metoclopramide and erythromycin. Metoclopramide exerts its prokinetic effects by acting as a dopamine antagonist and has cholinergic-enhancing effects because of facilitation of acetylcholine release from enteric cholinergic neurons. In contrast, erythromycin markedly accelerates gastric emptying by binding to motilin receptors on GI smooth muscle cells, where it acts as a motilin agonist. One of these two agents is usually sufficient to enhance gastric tone and improve gastric emptying. In rare cases of persistent gastric atony refractory to medical management, gastrectomy may be required.

GASTRIC CANCER

Epidemiology and Risk Factors

Incidence

Gastric cancer is the 14th most common cancer and cause of cancer death in the United States, with an estimated 22,000 new

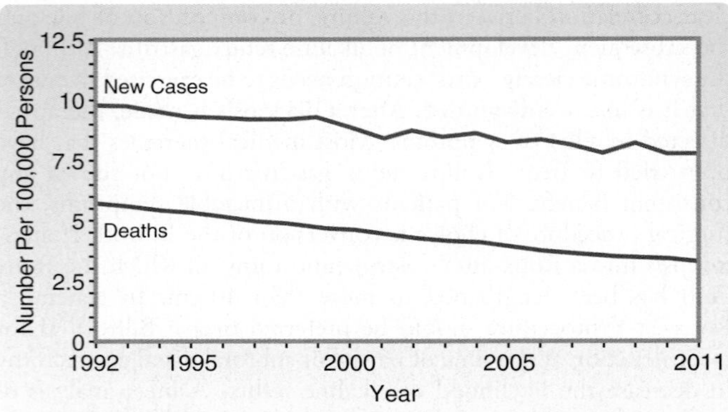

FIGURE 48-19 Age-adjusted incidence of gastric cancer, 1992-2011. (From National Cancer Institute, Surveillance Research Program: Fast Stats, 2009. <http://seer.cancer.gov/statfacts/html/stomach.html>, [Accessed October, 2014.])

cases/year and more than 10,000 deaths.[18] The disease affects men disproportionately, with more than 60% of new cases occurring in men. It is a disease of older individuals, with peak incidence in the seventh decade of life. Among racial groups, the disease is more common and has a higher mortality in African Americans, Asian Americans, and Hispanics compared with whites.

Worldwide, gastric cancer is the fourth most common cancer and the second leading cause of cancer death. It is especially prevalent in East Asia and South America and has been increasing in developing countries, which now have almost two thirds of all distal gastric cancer cases. In contrast, rates have been decreasing in the United States (Fig. 48-19). Among developed countries, Japan and Korea have the highest rates of the disease. Gastric cancer is the most common cancer in Japan. As a result, gastric cancer screening in Japan was started in the 1970s, and the mortality rate has decreased by 50% since that time. Although there has been an increase in proximal tumors in Japan, most are distal gastric cancers.

Risk Factors

The major risk factors for gastric cancer are discussed here; they include environmental and genetic factors (Box 48-3).

Helicobacter pylori Infection

In 1994, the International Agency for Research on Cancer labeled *H. pylori* a definite carcinogen. Numerous longitudinal prospective studies have demonstrated an association with the development of gastric cancer. In epidemiologic studies, *H. pylori* seropositivity has been associated with a relative risk of developing gastric cancer between 3.6 and 17. The primary mechanism is thought to be the presence of chronic inflammation. Long-term infection with the bacteria leads to gastritis, primarily within the gastric body, with ventral gastric atrophy. In some patients, gastritis progresses to intestinal metaplasia, dysplasia, and ultimately intestinal-type adenocarcinoma. A wide range of molecular alterations in intestinal metaplasia have been described and may affect the transformation into gastric cancer. These include overexpression of cyclooxygenase-2 and cyclin D2, *p53* mutations, microsatellite instability, decreased *p27* expression, and alterations in transcription factors such as CDX1 and CDX2. Intestinal metaplasia is a risk factor for the development of gastric carcinoma; however, not every patient with intestinal metaplasia develops invasive cancer. Host inflammatory responses play an important role in this process. Specifically, individuals with high levels of interleukin-1 expression are at increased risk of gastric cancer development.

BOX 48-3 Factors Associated With Increased Risk for Developing Stomach Cancer

Nutritional
Low fat or protein consumption
Salted meat or fish
High nitrate consumption
High complex carbohydrate consumption

Environmental
Poor food preparation (smoked, salted)
Lack of refrigeration
Poor drinking water (e.g., contaminated well water)
Smoking

Social
Low social class

Medical
Prior gastric surgery
H. pylori infection
Gastric atrophy and gastritis
Adenomatous polyps

Other
Male sex

Some regional variances in the development of cancer may be attributed to the prevalence and virulence of *H. pylori*. It is more common in poor areas with less sanitation, and infection rates remain high in developing countries, with a concomitant increase in gastric cancer incidence. In contrast, the prevalence in more developed countries has been decreasing. The presence of the cytoxan-associated gene A *(cagA)* is associated with increased virulence and risk of gastric cancer. Countries with high levels of gastric cancer, such as Japan, have a much higher rate of *cagA*-positive *H. pylori* infection than countries with lower rates of gastric cancer, such as the United States.

Dietary Factors

High-salt foods, particularly foods with salted or smoked meats that contain high levels of nitrate, along with low intake of fruits and vegetables are linked to an increased risk of gastric cancer. The mechanism is thought to be the conversion of nitrates in the food to N-nitroso compounds by bacteria in the stomach. N-nitroso compounds are also found in tobacco smoke, another known risk factor for gastric cancer. Fresh fruits and vegetables contain ascorbic acid, which can remove the carcinogenic N-nitroso compounds and oxygen free radicals.

There is likely synergism between diet and *H. pylori* infection, with the bacteria increasing carcinogen production and inhibiting its removal. *H. pylori* has been shown to promote the growth of the bacteria that generate the carcinogenic N-nitroso compounds. At the same time, *H. pylori* can inhibit the secretion of ascorbic acid, preventing effective scavenging of oxygen free radicals and N-nitroso compounds. The increase in refrigeration over the past 70 years has likely contributed to the decrease in gastric cancer by reducing the amount of meat preserved by salting alone and allowing the increased storage and consumption of fresh fruits and vegetables.

Hereditary Risk Factors and Cancer Genetics

Gastric cancer is associated with several rare inherited disorders. Hereditary diffuse gastric cancer is an inherited form of gastric cancer. Patients with this disorder, resulting from a gene mutation for the cell adhesion molecule E-cadherin, have an 80% lifetime incidence of developing gastric cancer. Prophylactic total gastrectomy should be considered for patients with this mutation. In familial adenomatous polyposis, approximately 85% of patients have fundic gland polyps, with 40% of these having some type of dysplasia and more than 50% containing a somatic adenomatous polyposis coli mutation, which places these patients at risk of developing gastric cancer. These polyps, combined with the much higher frequency of potentially malignant duodenal polyps, warrant upper GI surveillance. Li-Fraumeni syndrome is an autosomal dominant disorder caused by a mutation in the tumor suppressor gene *p53*. These patients are at risk for numerous malignancies, including gastric cancer. Hereditary nonpolyposis colorectal cancer, or Lynch syndrome, which accounts for 2% to 3% of all colon and rectal cancers and is associated with microsatellite instability, is also associated with an increased risk of gastric and ovarian cancers.

Several genetic alterations have been identified that are associated with gastric adenocarcinoma. These changes can be classified as the activation of oncogenes, inactivation of tumor suppressor genes, reduction of cellular adhesion, reactivation of telomerase, and presence of microsatellite instability. The c-*met* proto-oncogene is the receptor for the hepatocyte growth factor and is frequently overexpressed in gastric cancer, as are the k-*sam* and c-*erbB2* oncogenes. Inactivation of the tumor suppressor genes *p53* and *p16* has been reported in diffuse and intestinal-type cancers, whereas adenomatous polyposis coli gene mutations tend to be more frequent in intestinal-type gastric cancers. Also, a reduction or loss in the cell adhesion molecule E-cadherin can be found in approximately 50% of diffuse-type gastric cancers. Microsatellite instability can be found in approximately 20% to 30% of intestinal-type gastric cancers. Microsatellites are lengths of DNA in which a short (one to five nucleotide) motif is repeated several times. Microsatellite instability reflects a gain or loss of repeat units in a germline microsatellite allele, indicating the clonal expansion that is typical of a neoplasm.

Other Risk Factors

Patients with pernicious anemia are at increased risk for developing gastric cancer. Achlorhydria is the defining feature of this condition; it occurs when chief and parietal cells are destroyed by an autoimmune reaction. The mucosa becomes very atrophic and develops antral and intestinal metaplasia. The relative risk for a patient with pernicious anemia developing gastric cancer is 2.1 to 5.6 of the general population.

Polyps. Adenomatous polyps carry a distinct risk for the development of malignancy in the polyp. Mucosal atypia is frequent, and progression from dysplasia to carcinoma in situ has been observed. The risk for the development of carcinoma is approximately 10% to 20% and increases with increasing size of the polyp. Endoscopic removal is indicated for pedunculated lesions and is sufficient if the polyp is completely removed and there are no foci of invasive cancer on histologic examination. If the polyp is larger than 2 cm, is sessile, or has a proven focus of invasive carcinoma, operative excision is warranted.

Fundic gland polyps (Fig. 48-20) are benign lesions that are thought to result from glandular hyperplasia and decreased luminal flow. They are strongly associated with PPI use and occur in one third of patients by 1 year. Dysplasia, although common in patients whose polyps result from familial adenomatous polyposis, has been described only as individual case reports for patients whose polyps result from PPI therapy. Such cases do not require excision, regular surveillance, or cessation of therapy.

Proton pump inhibitors. The use of PPIs has increased dramatically over the past 20 years because they have been proven to be an effective treatment for patients with GI reflux disease. They are often prescribed empirically as first-line treatment for dyspepsia. The impact of PPIs on the incidence of gastric cancer has not been elucidated.

Physiologically, PPIs, as their name suggests, block the hydrogen-potassium pump within the parietal cells, effectively blocking all acid secretion in the stomach. As a result, patients taking PPIs develop hypergastrinemia, which reverses with PPI withdrawal. The potential for cancer is at the intersection between *H. pylori,* already considered a carcinogen for gastric cancer, and the physiologic changes that are a consequence of PPI use. In patients with *H. pylori* taking long-term PPIs, the low-acid environment allows the bacteria to colonize the gastric body, leading to corpus gastritis. One third of these patients develop atrophic gastritis, which is significantly more common in patients with *H. pylori* who are taking PPIs. This atrophic gastritis quickly resolves

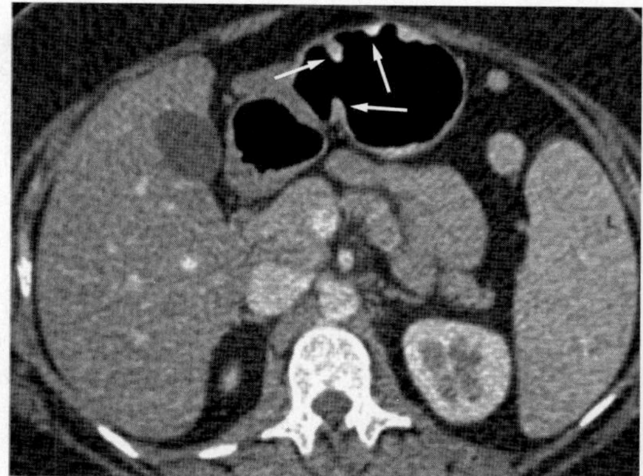
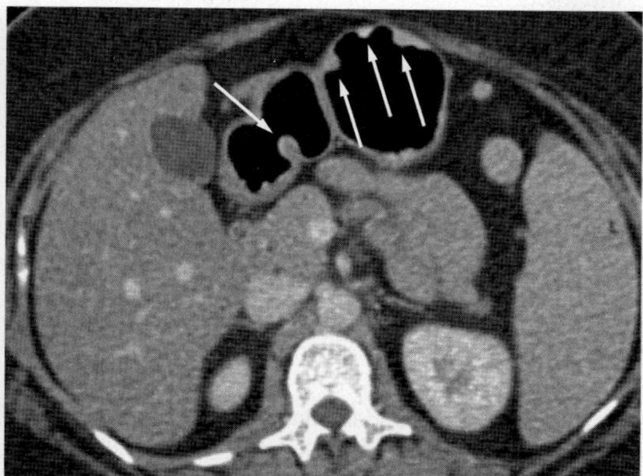

FIGURE 48-20 CT scan of fundic gland polyps. (Courtesy Dr. David Bentrem, Department of Surgery, Northwestern University Feinberg School of Medicine, Chicago, IL.)

after eradication of the *H. pylori*. At the present time, no study has shown the atrophic gastritis in this subset of patients to be associated with an increased cancer risk. However, in general, atrophic gastritis is considered a major risk factor for the development of gastric cancer. Additionally, several epidemiologic studies found an association with PPI therapy and the development of gastric cancer, although no evidence of causality has yet to be proven.[19] Therefore, PPIs are an effective first-line treatment for dyspepsia and remain an effective long-term therapy for patients with GE reflux disease. However, given the relationship between acid suppression, *H. pylori,* and the development of atrophic gastritis, a known risk factor for gastric cancer, in patients with persistent symptoms after initiation of therapy or who require long-term therapy, surveillance for and eradication of *H. pylori* is warranted.

Pathology

Numerous pathologic classification schemes of gastric cancer have been proposed. The Borrmann classification system was developed in 1926; it remains useful today for the description of endoscopic findings. This system divides gastric carcinoma into five types, depending on the lesion's macroscopic appearance (Fig. 48-21). One type, linitis plastica, describes a diffusely infiltrating lesion involving the entire stomach. Other classification systems have been proposed, but the most useful and widely used system is the one proposed by Lauren in 1965. This system separates gastric adenocarcinoma into intestinal or diffuse types based on histology, with both types having distinct pathology, epidemiology, and prognosis (Table 48-6).

The intestinal variant is more well differentiated and typically arises in the setting of a recognizable precancerous condition, such as gastric atrophy or intestinal metaplasia. Men are more commonly affected than women, and the incidence of intestinal-type gastric adenocarcinoma increases with age. These cancers are typically well differentiated, with a tendency to form glands. Metastatic spread is generally hematogenous to distant organs. The intestinal type is also the dominant histology in areas in which gastric cancer is epidemic, suggesting an environmental cause. Local rates of *H. pylori* prevalence likely play a large part in this increased environmental risk, as infection has been linked to the development of intestinal variant gastric cancer specifically.

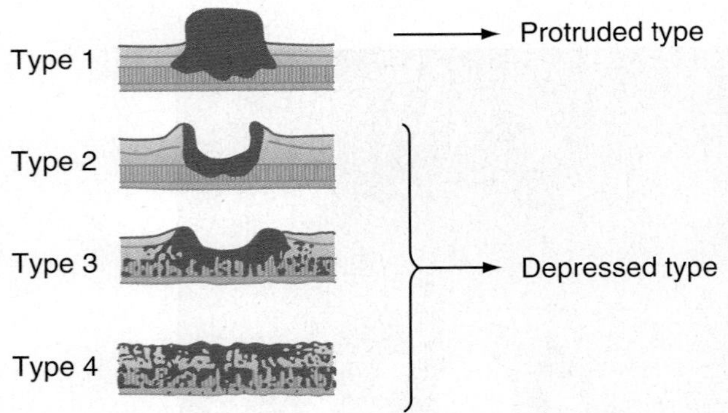

FIGURE 48-21 Borrmann's pathologic classification of gastric cancer based on gross appearance. (From Iriyama K, Asakawa T, Koike H, et al: Is extensive lymphadenectomy necessary for surgical treatment of intramucosal carcinoma of the stomach? *Arch Surg* 124:309–311, 1989.)

The diffuse form of gastric adenocarcinoma consists of tiny clusters of small, uniform signet ring cells; is poorly differentiated; and lacks glands. It tends to spread submucosally, with less inflammatory infiltration than the intestinal type, with early metastatic spread via transmural extension and lymphatic invasion. It is generally not associated with chronic gastritis, is more common in women, and affects a slightly younger age group. The diffuse form also has an association with blood type A and familial occurrence, suggesting a genetic cause. Intraperitoneal metastases are frequent, and, in general, the prognosis is less favorable than for patients with intestinal-type cancers.

In 2010, the World Health Organization (WHO) revised their alternative classification system for gastric cancers based on morphologic features. In the WHO system, gastric cancer is divided into five main categories—adenocarcinoma, adenosquamous cell carcinoma, squamous cell carcinoma, undifferentiated carcinoma, and unclassified carcinoma. Adenocarcinomas are further subdivided into five types according to their growth pattern—papillary, tubular, mucinous, poorly cohesive (including signet ring cell carcinoma), and mixed adenocarcinoma. Although widely used, the WHO classification system offers little in terms of patient management, and there are a significant number of gastric cancers that do not fit into their categories. There is little evidence that any of the above-mentioned classification systems can add to the prognostic information provided by the American Joint Cancer Commission (AJCC) tumor, node, metastasis (TNM) staging system.

Diagnosis and Workup

Signs and Symptoms

The symptoms of gastric cancer are generally nonspecific and contribute to its frequently advanced stage at the time of diagnosis. Symptoms include epigastric pain, early satiety, and weight loss. These symptoms are frequently mistaken for more common benign causes of dyspepsia including PUD and gastritis. The pain associated with gastric cancer tends to be constant and nonradiating and is generally not relieved by eating. More advanced lesions may manifest with either obstruction or dysphagia depending on the location of the tumor. Some degree of GI bleeding is common, with 40% of patients having some form of anemia and 15% having frank hematemesis.

A complete history and physical examination should be performed, with special attention to any evidence of advanced disease, including metastatic nodal disease; supraclavicular (Virchow) or periumbilical (Sister Mary Joseph node); and evidence of

TABLE 48-6 Lauren Classification System

INTESTINAL	DIFFUSE
Environmental	Familial
Gastric atrophy, intestinal metaplasia	Blood type A
Men > women	Women > men
Increasing incidence with age	Younger age group
Gland formation	Poorly differentiated, signet ring cells
Hematogenous spread	Transmural, lymphatic spread
Microsatellite instability	Decreased E-cadherin
APC gene mutations	
p53, p16 inactivation	*p53, p16* inactivation

APC, Adenomatous polyposis coli.

intra-abdominal metastases such as hepatomegaly, jaundice, or ascites. Drop metastases to the ovaries (Krukenberg tumor) may be detectable on pelvic examination, and peritoneal metastases can be felt as a firm shelf (Blumer shelf) on rectal examination. Complete blood count, chemistry panel including liver function tests, and coagulation studies should be carried out.

Staging

The most widely used staging system at the present time is the AJCC TNM staging system. This system is based on the depth of tumor invasion (T), number of involved lymph nodes (N), and presence or absence of metastatic disease (M) (Table 48-7). Before 1997, N stage was determined by the anatomic location of the nodes with respect to the primary tumor, rather than the absolute number of nodes. This staging, based on anatomy, was intimately related to the D1 versus D2 anatomic lymphadenectomy debate (see later). The revised system does not differentiate among the locations of positive nodes. In the current staging system, a minimum of 15 nodes must be evaluated for accurate staging. Some experts have suggested that other factors be included in the T and N assessment, such as the location of the primary (cardia compared with distal tumors) because this may independently predict survival and emphasis on the percentage of positive nodes (lymph node ratio) rather than the number of positive nodes. However, the current AJCC staging system does not reflect these factors.

The Siewert classification system is based on the anatomic location of adenocarcinomas (esophageal and gastric) that are in close proximity to the GE junction. This is an important distinction because such gastric cancers are more aggressive in nature and are treated in a similar manner to esophageal adenocarcinomas. There are three Siewert types: Type I tumors are tumors of the distal esophagus, within 1 to 5 cm above the GE junction; type II tumors have a tumor center located from 1 cm above the GE junction to 2 cm below it; type III tumors are termed subcardinal and are located between 2 and 5 cm caudad to the GE junction. In general, Siewert types I and II tumors are treated similar to esophageal adenocarcinoma, whereas type III tumors can be treated according to the guidelines for gastric adenocarcinoma described here, as long as the tumor does not extend into the GE junction.

Although not part of the formal AJCC staging system, the term *R status,* first described by Hermanek in 1994, is used to describe tumor status after resection and is important for determining the adequacy of surgery. R0 describes a microscopically margin-negative resection, in which no gross or microscopic tumor

TABLE 48-7 TNM Classification of Carcinoma of the Stomach

Primary Tumor (T)[†]

TX	Primary tumor cannot be assessed
T0	No evidence of primary tumor
Tis	Carcinoma in situ; intraepithelial tumor without invasion of the lamina propria
T1	Tumor invades lamina propria, muscularis mucosae, or submucosa
T1a	Tumor invades lamina propria or muscularis mucosae
T1b	Tumor invades submucosa
T2	Tumor invades muscularis propria*
T3	Tumor penetrates subserosal connective tissue without invasion of visceral peritoneum or adjacent structures[†,‡]
T4	Tumor invades serosa (visceral peritoneum) or adjacent structures[†,‡]
T4a	Tumor invades serosa (visceral peritoneum)
T4b	Tumor invades adjacent structures

Regional Lymph Nodes (N)*

NX	Regional lymph node(s) cannot be assessed
N0	No regional lymph node metastasis[§]
N1	Metastasis in 1-2 regional lymph nodes
N2	Metastasis in 3-6 regional lymph nodes
N3	Metastasis in 7 or more regional lymph nodes
N3a	Metastasis in 7-15 regional lymph nodes
N3b	Metastasis in 16 or more regional lymph nodes

Distant Metastasis (M)

M0	No distant metastasis
M1	Distant metastasis

ANATOMIC STAGE	PROGNOSTIC GROUP		
0	Tis	N0	M0
IA	T1	N0	M0
IB	T2	N0	M0
	T1	N1	M0
IIA	T3	N0	M0
	T2	N1	M0
	T1	N2	M0
IIB	T4a	N0	M0
	T3	N1	M0
	T2	N2	M0
	T1	N3	M0
IIIA	T4a	N1	M0
	T3	N2	M0
	T2	N3	M0
IIIB	T4b	N0	M0
	T4b	N1	M0
	T4a	N2	M0
	T3	N3	M0
IIIC	T4b	N2	M0
	T4b	N3	M0
	T4a	N3	M0
IV	Any T	Any N	M1

From Edge S, Byrd D, Compton C, et al, editors: *AJCC cancer staging manual*, ed 7, New York, 2010, Springer.

*A tumor may penetrate the muscularis propria with extension into the gastrocolic or gastrohepatic ligaments, or into the greater or lesser omentum, without perforation of the visceral peritoneum covering these structures. In this case, the tumor is classified T3. If there is perforation of the visceral peritoneum covering the gastric ligaments or the omentum, the tumor should be classified T4.

[†]The adjacent structures of the stomach include the spleen, transverse colon, liver, diaphragm, pancreas, abdominal wall, adrenal gland, kidney, small intestine, and retroperitoneum.

[‡]Intramural extension to the duodenum or esophagus is classified by the depth of the greatest invasion in any of these sites, including the stomach.

[§]A designation of pN0 should be used if all examined lymph nodes are negative, regardless of the total number removed and examined.

remains in the tumor bed. R1 indicates removal of all macroscopic disease, but microscopic margins are positive for tumor. R2 indicates gross residual disease. Because the extent of resection can influence survival, some include this R designation to complement the TNM system. Long-term survival can be expected only after an R0 resection.

The AJCC system is not specific for nodal location, but the debate regarding lymphadenectomies for gastric cancer has continued. In the previous version of the Union Internationale Contre le Cancer (UICC) TNM system, N categories were defined by the location of lymph node metastases relative to the primary, with pN1 defined as positive nodes 3 cm or less from the primary and pN2 as positive nodes more than 3 cm from the primary or nodal metastases along named blood vessels. The Japanese Classification for Gastric Carcinoma (JCGC) staging system was designed to describe the anatomic locations of nodes removed during gastrectomy. There are 16 distinct anatomic locations of lymph nodes described, with the recommendation for nodal basin dissection dependent on the location of the primary (Fig. 48-22). The lymph node stations, or echelons, are numbered and further classified into groups of echelons corresponding to the location of the primary and reflect the likelihood of harboring metastases. The presence of metastasis to each lymph node group determines the N classification. For example, metastasis to any of the group 1 lymph nodes in the absence of disease in more distant lymph node groups is classified as N1. This grouping of regional lymph nodes is presented in Table 48-8. This system was not adopted by the AJCC. The AJCC pathologic staging system has been widely adopted in the United States.

Staging Workup

The goal of any preoperative staging is twofold. The first is to gain information on prognosis to counsel the patient and family effectively. The second is to determine the extent of disease to determine the most appropriate course of therapy. The three main treatment paths are resection (with or without subsequent adjuvant therapy), neoadjuvant therapy followed by resection, or treatment of systemic disease without resection (Fig. 48-23).

The main modalities for staging gastric adenocarcinoma and guiding therapy are endoscopy; EUS; cross-sectional imaging such as CT, MRI, or positron emission tomography (PET); and diagnostic laparoscopy. Their roles are discussed here.

Endoscopy and endoscopic ultrasound. Flexible endoscopy is the essential tool for the diagnosis of gastric cancer. It allows visualization of the tumor, provides tissue for pathologic diagnosis, and can serve as a treatment for patients with obstruction or bleeding (Fig. 48-24). On initial diagnostic endoscopy, if a suspicious mass or ulcer is encountered in the stomach, it is essential to obtain adequate tissue to confirm the correct diagnosis histologically. Multiple biopsy specimens (six to eight) should be taken of different areas of the lesion using endoscopic biopsy forceps. A single biopsy specimen results in a diagnostic sensitivity of 70%, whereas seven biopsy specimens increases this yield to 98%.[20] Small lesions (<2 cm in diameter) can be resected at the time of initial diagnostic endoscopy using endoscopic mucosal resection (EMR) or endoscopic submucosal dissection (ESD) techniques (described in further detail later). This resection can provide a more complete specimen to aid the pathologist in obtaining an accurate diagnosis and can potentially be curative for early-stage cancers, obviating the need for any further invasive surgical intervention.

Flexible upper endoscopy combined with ultrasound is now part of the standard workup for staging and risk-stratifying patients with gastric cancer properly. EUS provides the most accurate evaluation of the depth of tumor invasion (T category of TNM staging system) and possible nodal involvement (N

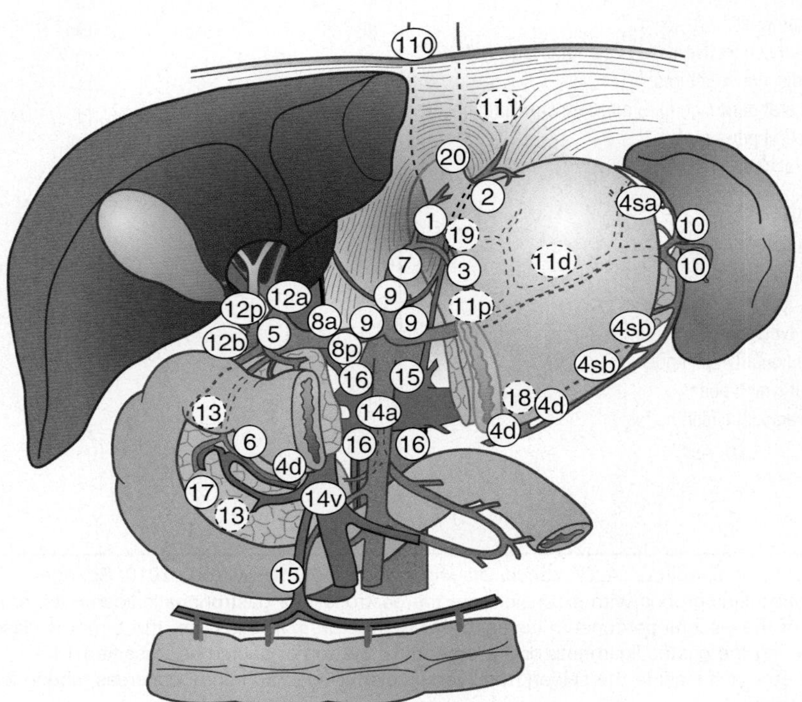

FIGURE 48-22 Lymph node station numbers as defined by the Japanese Gastric Cancer Association. (From Japanese Gastric Cancer Association: Japanese Classification of Gastric Carcinoma, 2nd English edition. *Gastric Cancer* 1:10–24, 1998.)

TABLE 48-8 Grouping of Regional Lymph Nodes (Groups 1-3) by Location of Primary Tumor*

LYMPH NODE STATION (NO.)	DESCRIPTION	LOCATION OF PRIMARY TUMOR IN STOMACH		
		UPPER THIRD	MIDDLE THIRD	LOWER THIRD
1	Right paracardial	1	1	2
2	Left paracardial	1	3	M
3	Lesser curvature	1	1	1
4sa	Short gastric	1	3	M
4sb	Left gastroepiploic	1	1	3
4d	Right gastroepiploic	2	1	1
5	Suprapyloric	3	1	1
6	Infrapyloric	3	1	1
7	Left gastric artery	2	2	2
8a	Anterior common hepatic	2	2	2
8p	Posterior common hepatic	3	3	3
9	Celiac artery	2	2	2
10	Splenic hilum	2	3	M
11p	Proximal splenic	2	2	2
11d	Distal splenic	2	3	M
12a	Left hepatoduodenal	3	2	2
12b, p	Posterior hepatoduodenal	3	3	3
13	Retropancreatic	M	3	3
14v	Superior mesenteric vein	M	3	2
14a	Superior mesenteric artery	M	M	M
15	Middle colic	M	M	M
16al	Aortic hiatus	3	M	M
16a2, b1	Para-aortic, middle	M	3	3
16b2	Para-aortic, caudal	M	M	M

M, Lymph nodes regarded as distant metastasis.
*According to the Japanese Classification of gastric carcinoma (Japanese Gastric Cancer Association: Japanese Classification of Gastric Carcinoma—2nd English edition. *Gastric Cancer* 1:10–24, 1998).

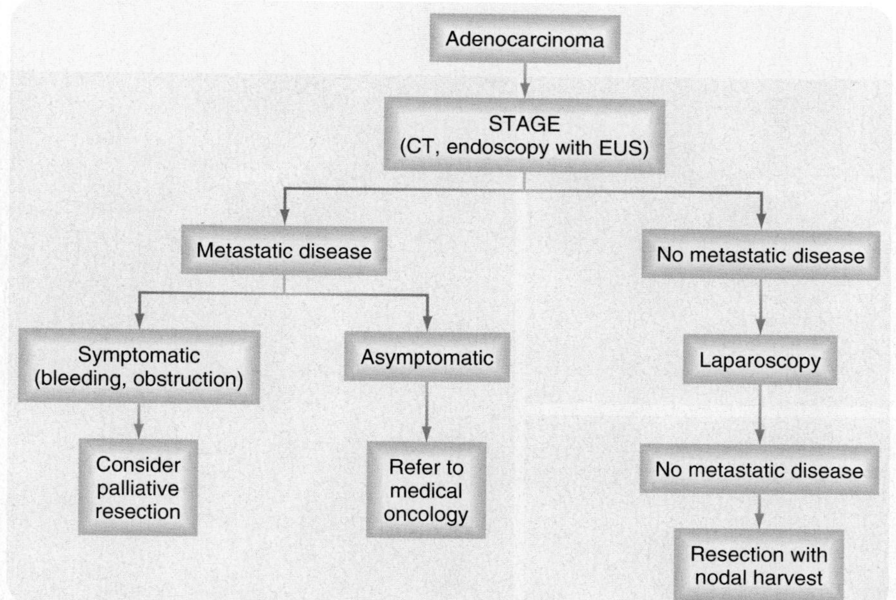

FIGURE 48-23 General staging and treatment strategy for gastric adenocarcinoma. *CT,* Computed tomography; *EUS,* endoscopic ultrasound.

category). EUS is performed using a flexible endoscope with a 7.5-MHz to 12-MHz ultrasound transducer. The stomach is filled with water to distend it and provide an acoustic window, and the stomach wall is visualized as five alternating hypoechoic and hyperechoic layers (Fig. 48-25*A*). The mucosa and submucosa represent the first three layers (T1) (Fig. 48-25*B*). The fourth layer is the muscularis propria, invasion of which is a T2 tumor. Expansion of the tumor beyond the muscularis propria causing an irregular border correlates with expansion into the subserosa, or a T3 tumor. The serosa is the fifth layer, and loss of this bright

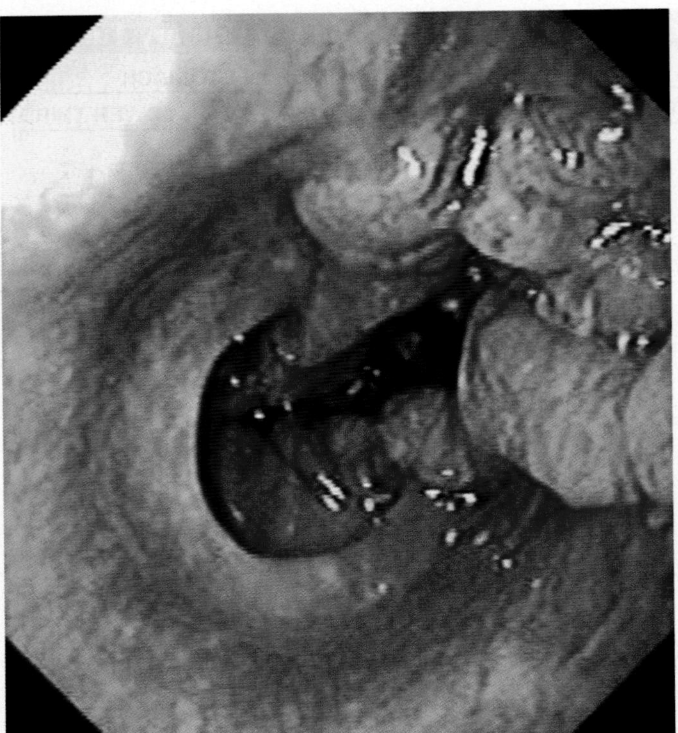

FIGURE 48-24 Endoscopic view of intestinal-type adenocarcinoma of the gastric cardia. (Courtesy Dr. David Bentrem, Department of Surgery, Northwestern University Feinberg School of Medicine, Chicago, IL.)

line correlates with penetration through it, indicating a T4a tumor. Direct invasion of surrounding structures, including named vessels, indicates a T4b tumor (Fig. 48-25*C*). Nodes are evaluated based on their size and ultrasound appearance and can additionally be sampled using fine-needle aspiration under EUS guidance.

The overall accuracy of EUS has been reported to be 85% for T stage and 80% for N stage; however, these studies considered accuracy retrospectively and not the predictive accuracy of EUS, and most were analyses of data obtained from single institutions. A larger, more recent study[21] showed lower accuracy of T and N stages. It considered the predictive accuracy of EUS for T and N stages and found them to be 57% and 50%, respectively. However, it showed improved accuracy when T and N stages were grouped together to differentiate high-risk versus low-risk disease, defined by the presence of any serosal (T3/T4) involvement or any nodal disease (>N0). When this classification system was used, the positive predictive value of EUS to identify advanced disease was 76%, and the negative predictive value to identify low-risk disease was 91% (Fig. 48-26).[21] From a prognostic and treatment standpoint, this classification may be more clinically relevant because an EUS finding indicative of advanced disease strongly correlates with decreased resectability and poorer disease-specific survival.

Another more recent study of 960 patients enrolled in a multi-institution gastric cancer database in the United States for the period 2000-2012[22] found that only 23% of patients underwent preoperative evaluation with EUS. Of patients who had preoperative EUS and then underwent resection without neoadjuvant chemotherapy or radiation therapy, the diagnostic accuracy of EUS in determining the exact T stage on pathologic examination was only 46.2% and was 66.7% for the N stage. Furthermore, the ability for EUS to differentiate between early-stage (T1/2) versus later stage (T3/4) tumors was only fair, with an area under

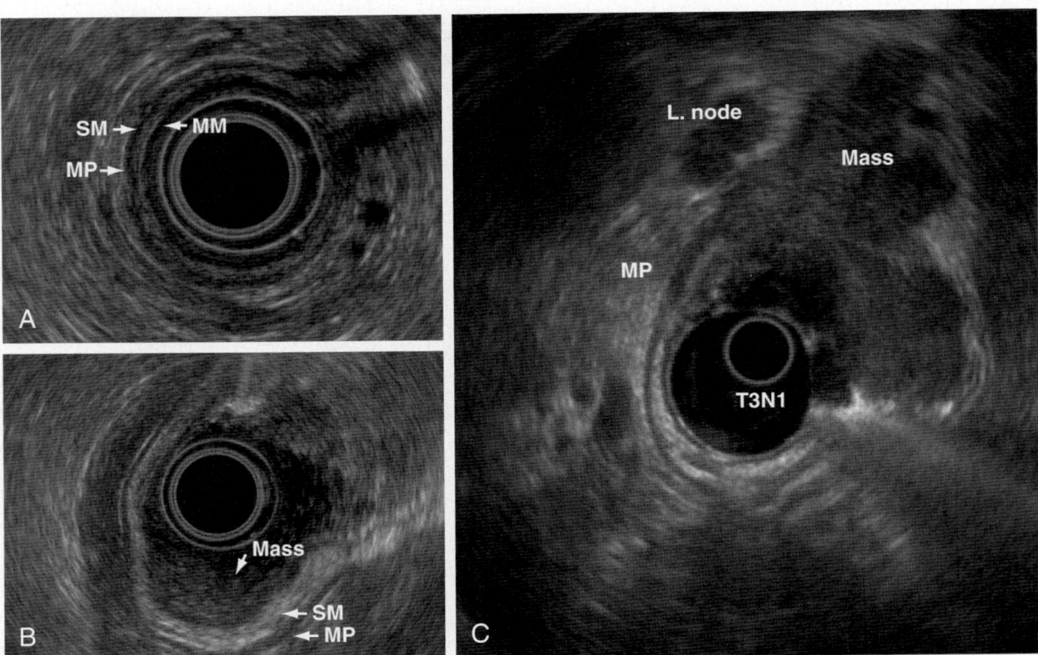

FIGURE 48-25 Endoscopic ultrasound views of normal stomach **(A)**, T1 N0 gastric cancer **(B)**, and T3 N1 gastric cancer **(C)**. *MM,* Mucosa; *MP,* muscularis propria; *SM,* submucosa. (Courtesy Dr. Rajesh Keswani, Division of Gastroenterology, Department of Medicine, Northwestern University Feinberg School of Medicine, Chicago, IL.)

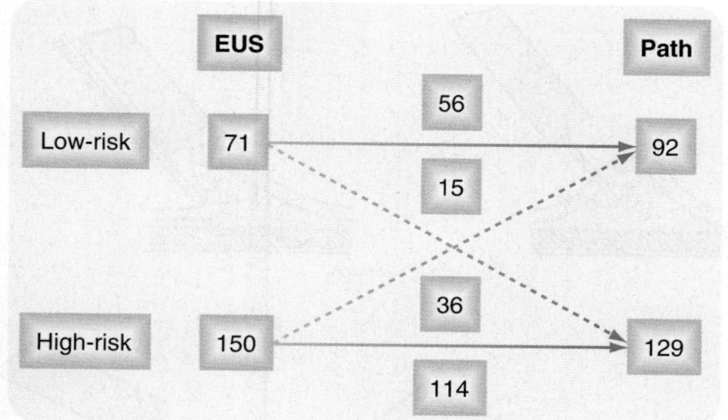

FIGURE 48-26 Predictive accuracy of endoscopic ultrasound (EUS) in gastric cancer. Of 71 patients identified as low risk (T1/2N0) on EUS, 56 were correctly staged, and 15 were understaged. Of 150 patients identified as high risk (T3/4, any N, or any T, N+) on EUS, 114 were correctly staged, and 36 were overstaged. (From Bentrem D, Gerdes H, Tang L, et al: Clinical correlation of endoscopic ultrasonography with pathologic stage and outcome in patients undergoing curative resection for gastric cancer. *Ann Surg Oncol* 14:1853–1859, 2007.)

the curve of 0.66; this is of vital importance because this distinction is often used to guide whether patients will receive neoadjuvant therapy before resection.

As the accuracy of EUS improves, it will likely play an increasing role in determining treatment algorithms in gastric cancer, much as it does in rectal cancer. At the present time, although individual T and N stage accuracy may be lacking, EUS has been shown to be a useful tool in differentiating between high-risk and low-risk patients, and this differentiation correlates with prognosis.

Computed tomography. CT of the chest, abdomen, and pelvis with oral and intravenous contrast agents is a mandatory component of the assessment of patients with gastric cancer and plays an important role in the evaluation of metastatic disease. CT is the primary method for detection of intra-abdominal metastatic disease, with an overall detection rate of approximately 85%. The sensitivity of CT for imaging peritoneal metastases is only 51%, with a high specificity of 96% if the study is positive.

CT has also been used in locoregional staging. The accuracy of T and N stages as determined by CT is less accurate than EUS. Although improved technology may increase the role for CT in locoregional evaluation and for neoadjuvant therapy, its primary role remains the evaluation of metastatic disease.

Positron emission tomography. The use of PET/CT for initial staging is limited because only 50% of gastric cancers are PET-avid. However, in patients with positive PET scans presumed to have advanced disease and patients considered for neoadjuvant therapy, there may be a role for PET. PET response to neoadjuvant therapy strongly correlates with survival, with a PET response seen within 14 days of treatment. PET may be an effective modality for monitoring response to these therapies, sparing unresponsive patients further toxic treatment. Additionally, in a study of patients with locally advanced tumors (T3/4) or N-positive on EUS, PET/CT was able to detect occult metastases that were missed on regular CT in 10% of patients.[23] Based on these data, the National Comprehensive Cancer Network guidelines now recommend PET/CT as part of routine staging for patients without evidence of metastatic disease on initial CT.

Laparoscopy. Staging laparoscopy is an integral part of the standard workup for gastric cancer. The high rate of occult metastatic disease makes laparoscopy an attractive staging modality. In the late 1990s, two large studies evaluated laparoscopy as a staging modality for patients with gastric cancer.[24,25] Both studies demonstrated high rates of occult metastatic disease (37% and 23%, respectively) in patients undergoing staging laparoscopy for gastric cancer who were previously thought to have no metastatic disease as assessed by CT. The overall sensitivity of laparoscopy for detecting metastatic disease was greater than 95%. For patients who had metastatic disease, fewer than 15% went on to require palliative gastrectomy. As a result of these studies, staging laparoscopy has been advocated as part of the workup for gastric cancer to avoid unnecessary laparotomy in patients without a clear need for laparotomy.

As CT technology has improved, the need for staging laparoscopy has been reexamined. However, a review of studies examining its usefulness showed that laparoscopy altered management in 9% to 60% of cases and specifically allowed patients to avoid an unnecessary laparotomy by detecting metastatic disease that was missed on preoperative staging in 9% to 44% of cases. Staging laparoscopy is a safe, low-risk procedure that can be planned as a single-stage procedure with resection; it can be done with minimal added risk in patients who undergo laparotomy and with no additional risk for patients who undergo an entirely laparoscopic resection. Meanwhile, there are many benefits of avoiding laparotomy, which include avoiding a delay in starting chemotherapy for patients with metastatic disease and limited life expectancy. Given the persistence of high rates of metastatic disease not detected by preoperative workup in many centers, even with improved imaging modalities, we believe that these benefits far outweigh the risk and that staging laparoscopy should be part of the workup for most patients with gastric cancer.

Treatment

Surgical Therapy

Complete resection of a gastric tumor with a wide margin of normal stomach remains the standard of care for resection with curative intent. All patients without metastatic disease or invasion of unresectable vascular structures such as the aorta, celiac trunk, proximal common hepatic, or proximal splenic arteries are candidates for curative resection. The extent of resection depends on the location of the tumor in the stomach and size of the tumor. For T4 tumors, any organ with invasion needs to be removed en bloc with the gastrectomy specimen to achieve a curative resection. The standard technique is via a laparotomy; however, minimally invasive techniques, including laparoscopy and completely endoscopic resection for very early tumors, have proven effective methods of treatment.

For cancers of the distal stomach, including the body and antrum, a distal gastrectomy is the appropriate operation. The proximal stomach is transected at the level of the incisura at a margin of at least 6 cm because studies have documented tumor spread as far as 5 cm laterally from the primary tumor, although some experts indicate that a 4-cm margin is adequate. Frozen section analysis should be performed before reconstruction. The distal margin is the proximal duodenum. The possibility of recurrence in the tumor bed (duodenal suture line and surface of the pancreas) suggests a Billroth II reconstruction rather than a Billroth I, which would result in less risk of gastric outlet obstruction secondary to tumor recurrence. If the patient is left with a small area of stomach proximal to the area of resection, a Roux-en-Y reconstruction should be performed to reduce the risk of alkaline reflux esophagitis.

For proximal lesions of the fundus or cardia, a total gastrectomy with a Roux-en-Y esophagojejunostomy or proximal gastrectomy is equivalent from an oncologic perspective. The postoperative anastomotic leak rate is higher for an esophagojejunostomy, but the margin is typically larger than for a gastrojejunostomy. When a negative margin can be achieved, a gastrojejunostomy is performed. However, to construct a tension-free anastomosis to the distal esophagus, a Roux-en-Y esophagojejunostomy is usually required. A hand-sewn or stapled technique may be used.

Minimally invasive techniques have been used for many GI tumors, and gastric cancer is no exception. Several studies have shown good short-term and long-term outcomes for the laparoscopic approach. A meta-analysis of trials comparing open and laparoscopic distal gastrectomy for treatment of gastric cancer found that a laparoscopic approach resulted in longer operative times but fewer complications and shorter hospital stays.[26] In this analysis, laparoscopy resulted in 3.9 fewer lymph nodes retrieved on average. However, a separate meta-analysis of eight trials in which D2 lymph node dissections (explained later) were specifically performed showed no difference in the number of lymph nodes resected between laparoscopic and open approaches.

Overall, laparoscopic gastrectomy has been shown to be a safe and effective treatment for gastric cancer. Although there appears to be a learning curve, when performed by an experienced surgeon, it has equivalent oncologic outcomes, with less postoperative pain, earlier initiation of oral feeding, and earlier discharge from the hospital.

Endoscopic Resection

For early gastric cancer with limited penetration of the gastric wall and no evidence of lymph node metastases, EMR can be carried out. EMR has been widely performed in Japan for decades and has been evaluated in the United States and Europe. There have been no randomized controlled trials comparing EMR with gastrectomy for early gastric cancer. Current practice is based on nonrandomized prospective studies and retrospective reviews. The most significant advantage of endoscopic resection is avoiding the need for gastrectomy, whether by laparotomy or laparoscopy. The major disadvantage is incomplete resection because of tumor size or unrecognized lymph node metastases. To avoid undertreating patients, several studies have sought to identify risk factors for harboring lymph node metastases. A Japanese study of 1196 patients with intramucosal gastric cancer without known lymph node disease who underwent resection found, in multivariate analysis, that lymphatic vessel invasion, histologic ulceration of the tumor, and larger size (≥30 mm) were independent risk factors for regional lymph node metastasis. Patients without any of these risk factors had only a 0.36% chance of having lymph node metastases.[27] Based on these data, the general guidelines for endoscopic resection of early gastric cancer are as follows: (1) tumor limited to the mucosa, (2) no lymphovascular invasion, (3) tumor smaller than 2 cm, (4) no ulceration, and (5) well or moderately well differentiated histopathology. Any of these listed findings on initial biopsy or during endoscopic resection is an indication for gastrectomy with lymph node dissection.

Endoscopic resection can be performed using one of two techniques: EMR or ESD. The basic principle for EMR involves elevating the tumor using a saline injection and then encircling the affected mucosa using a snare device to excise it with electrocautery. Perforation rates are low, and bleeding rates are approximately 15%; these can generally be controlled without the need for further intervention (Fig. 48-27).

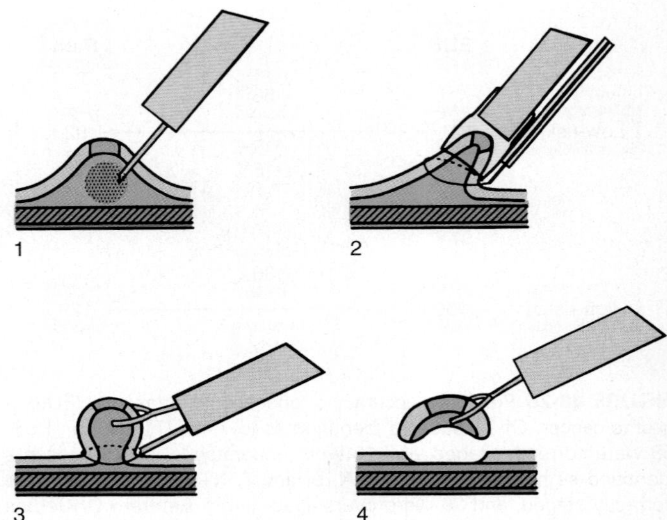

FIGURE 48-27 Endoscopic mucosal resection by strip biopsy: Saline is injected into the submucosal layer, and the area is elevated *(1)*. The top of the mound is pulled upward with forceps, and the snare is placed at the base of the lesion (*2* and *3*). Electrosurgical current is applied through the snare to resect the mucosa, and the lesion is removed *(4)*. (From Tanabe S, Koizumi W, Kokutou M, et al: Usefulness of endoscopic aspiration mucosectomy as compared with strip biopsy for the treatment of gastric mucosal cancer. *Gastrointest Endosc* 50:819–822, 1999.)

Long-term outcomes for properly selected patients are good. A 2007 multicenter retrospective review of 516 Korean patients showed complete resection in 77% of patients, 6% local recurrence rate for patients who had a complete resection, and no disease-specific mortality with 39-month median follow-up.[28] The data from the Japanese experience showed similar rates of complete resection and recurrence.

Some authors proposed expanding the eligibility criteria for endoscopic resection based on the results of several large studies of resected gastric cancer. A Japanese study of more than 5000 patients who underwent resection found that small tumors, regardless of ulcer status, and nonulcerated tumors, regardless of size, did not have associated lymph node disease.[29] It was also found that patients with submucosal invasion less than 500 μm behaved similarly to patients who had completely intramucosal tumors. Given these findings, the proposed extended criteria include all intramucosal tumors without ulceration, differentiated mucosal tumors smaller than 3 cm regardless of ulceration status, and tumors with limited (SM1) submucosal invasion that were smaller than 3 cm and without ulceration.

In treating these larger tumors or tumors with SM1 invasion, standard EMR techniques are generally ineffective. Given the size and depth, physicians treating patients under these extended criteria have used the ESD technique. This technique involves marking the borders of the lesion using electrocautery. A submucosal injection of epinephrine with indigo carmine hydrodissects the lesion, and an insulation-tipped knife is used to remove the lesion by dissecting a submucosal plane deep to the tumor and removing it en bloc. Any bleeding is controlled with electrocautery (Fig. 48-28).

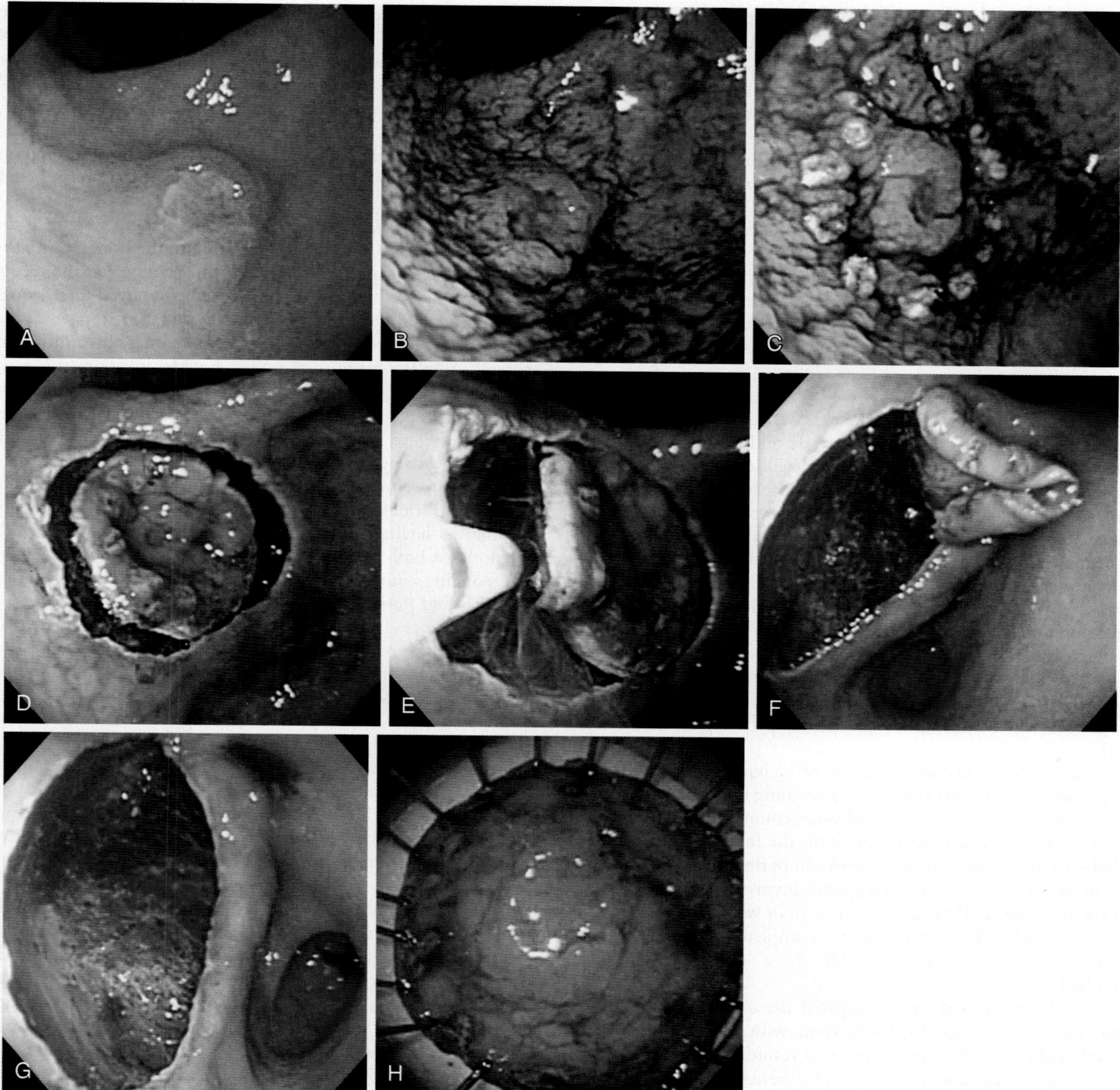

FIGURE 48-28 Procedure of endoscopic submucosal dissection. **A,** A type IIa+IIc early gastric cancer was located at the lesser curvature side of the antrum. **B,** Indigo carmine dye was sprayed around the lesion to define the margin accurately. **C,** Marking dots were made circumferentially at approximately 5 mm lateral to the margin of the lesion. **D,** After a submucosal injection of saline with epinephrine mixed with indigo carmine, a circumferential mucosal incision was performed outside the marking dots to separate the lesion from the surrounding non-neoplastic mucosa. **E** and **F,** After an additional submucosal injection, the submucosal connective tissue just beneath the lesion was directly dissected using an electrosurgical knife instead of using a snare. **G,** The lesion was completely resected, and the consequent artificial ulcer was seen. **H,** The resected specimen with a central early gastric cancer. (From Min B-H, Lee JH, Kim JJ, et al: Clinical outcomes of endoscopic submucosal dissection (ESD) for treating early gastric cancer: Comparison with endoscopic mucosal resection after circumferential precutting (EMR-P). *Dig Liver Dis* 41:201–209, 2009.)

There are limited data on the outcomes of patients undergoing EMR or endoscopic submucosal resection with extended criteria. A large series of 1627 patients who underwent resection using either EMR or ESD techniques found that patients with standard and extended criteria for endoscopic resection had similarly low local recurrence rates (0.9% and 1.1%) at median 32-month follow-up.[30] However, for patients undergoing extended criteria resection, ESD resulted in significantly higher rates of complete resection compared with EMR (83% versus 91%, $P < .01$). Based on these results, it seems reasonable to perform ESD for such extended criteria tumors. However, such procedures are technically challenging and surgeons should amass a large series of EMR resections for standard criteria tumors before attempting ESD procedures for oncologic indications, especially in the United States where fewer patients present with early-stage disease.

Clinical Decision Making

Endoscopic therapy for gastric cancer is well established in Eastern countries. Endoscopic resection is a safe and effective technique for patients who meet the criteria and will continue to play an increasing role in the treatment of this disease. Although several larger studies of patients who underwent gastrectomy with lymphadenectomy suggested that the eligibility could be safely expanded, two smaller studies of patients who underwent endoscopic resection under these criteria showed a higher rate of lymph node disease. Given that all these patients had early gastric cancer and were potentially curable with gastrectomy and lymphadenectomy, undertreatment in this group is especially concerning. As a matter of standard practice, patients with tumors larger than 2 cm, with ulceration or with any submucosal invasion, should be referred for gastrectomy with lymph node dissection if not part of a clinical trial.

Lymph node dissection. The extent of lymphadenectomy for gastric adenocarcinoma is an area of ongoing debate. Historically, lymphadenectomy for gastric adenocarcinoma was defined by, and is still often discussed in terms of, the location of the nodes relative to the primary tumor. The extent of dissection ranges from the more local D1 lymphadenectomy involving only perigastric nodes to clearance of the celiac axis, with or without splenectomy, in an extended D2 dissection to complete clearance of the celiac axis and periaortic nodes in a superextended D3 lymphadenectomy.

Several randomized trials compared the outcomes of patients undergoing D1 versus D2 dissection, with conflicting results. Whether these conflicting results are a result of different biology or of surgical technique is a matter of debate. The two large non-Japanese randomized trials (MRC and Dutch D1D2 trials) found that D2 lymphadenectomy resulted in higher rates of perioperative morbidity and increased mortality.[31,32] The MRC trial showed no difference in recurrence-free or overall survival outcomes at greater than 5-year follow-up.[33] Although the Dutch D1D2 trial showed lower recurrence rates and disease-free survival at 15-year follow-up in the D2 group, there was no difference in overall survival, possibly because of the increase in perioperative mortality for D2 patients. The results of both of these trials are confounded by the fact that patients undergoing concurrent splenectomy had much higher rates of perioperative morbidity and mortality, and the Dutch D1D2 trial group now advocates a D2 lymph node dissection with splenic preservation.

In contrast, the Japanese have shown increased survival in patients undergoing a D2 dissection, with no increased or minimal increase in morbidity. A meta-analysis of 12 randomized trials comparing lymph node dissections found that when the spleen was preserved, a D2 dissection resulted in superior recurrence-free survival, with a trend toward increased overall survival.[34] When taken together, these data illustrate that, in the absence of tumor invasion, the spleen should be spared during gastrectomy for gastric cancer and that a D2 lymph node dissection is likely oncologically superior but must be performed in a safe manner without added perioperative mortality to be of long-term benefit to the patient.

In 1997, the AJCC changed the TNM staging system so that N staging was defined not by the location of the nodes, but rather by the number of nodes. Along with this change was the recommendation that at least 15 lymph nodes be removed for adequate staging purposes. Several studies examined the impact of this change with respect to prognosis and outcomes. In multivariate analyses, only the number of nodes, not the location, was a significant predictor of mortality. When the number of nodes was used for staging, there was more consistency in survival rates, providing higher quality prognostic information for patients within a given stage (Table 48-9).

The improvement in survival rates may be caused by stage migration. Patients who were previously understaged are now classified as having node-positive disease status, improving the prognosis of both groups. Regardless, better stage homogeneity and reducing understaging are critical to clinical decisions on prognosis and potential treatments.

The number 15 nodes has become a marker for adequate lymphadenectomy. The number of nodes removed is related to hospital volume and whether the hospital is a National Comprehensive Cancer Network–National Cancer Institute institution (Table 48-10).[35] However, even at high-volume centers and National Comprehensive Cancer Network–National Cancer Institute centers, the percentage of patients who have more than 15 lymph nodes examined is less than 50%. Overall, only 23.8% of the more than 3000 patients studied had more than 15 lymph nodes examined. There is clearly room for improvement, regardless of the type of institution.

How does one achieve an adequate 15–lymph node resection? Some authors argue that the studies cited indicate evidence that a formal D2 resection should be the standard. This is also a systems issue in a given institution that depends not only on the surgeon but also on the pathology department. For the practicing surgeon, the focus should be on achieving a wide enough lymph node dissection to stage the patient adequately. Given the predominance of D1 resection in the United States and the overall failure to remove 15 lymph nodes consistently for analysis, simply clearing perigastric tissue is likely inadequate. There should be

TABLE 48-9 Median Survival According to Location of Positive Nodes Versus Number of Positive Nodes

	MEDIAN SURVIVAL (MONTHS)		
SIZE	1-6 PN	7-15 PN	>15 PN
<3 cm ($n = 402$)	38.8 ($n = 311$)	20.8 ($n = 82$)	9.5 ($n = 9$)
>3 cm ($n = 233$)	35.5 ($n = 81$)	19.7 ($n = 96$)	12.5 ($n = 56$)

Adapted from Karpeh MS, Leon L, Klimstra D, et al: Lymph node staging in gastric cancer: Is location more important than number? An analysis of 1038 patients. *Ann Surg* 232:362–371, 2000.
PN, Positive nodes.

TABLE 48-10 Lymph Node Resection Rates in Gastric Cancer*

VARIABLE	LYMPH NODES EXAMINED, MEDIAN NO. (INTERQUARTILE RANGE)	PATIENTS WITH AT LEAST 15 LYMPH NODES EXAMINED (%)
All hospitals	7 (3-14)	23.2
Hospital type		
NCCN-NCI	12 (6-20)	42.3
Other academic	8 (4-15)	25.5
Community	6 (3-12)	17.7
Hospital volume		
Highest	10 (5-18)	34.7
High	8 (4-14)	22.2
Moderate	6 (2-13)	17.8
Low	6 (3-12)	16.8

From Bilimoria KY, Talamonti MS, Wayne JD, et al: Effect of hospital type and volume on lymph node evaluation for gastric and pancreatic cancer. *Arch Surg* 143:671–678, 2008.

NCCN-NCI, National Comprehensive Cancer Network–National Cancer Institute.

*Stratified by hospital type and volume.

some attention to removing some fibrofatty tissue along named vessels. In a high-volume specialty center that can routinely perform a D2 resection without increased morbidity, wider resections are likely to be the more standard practice.

Adjuvant and Neoadjuvant Therapy

Gastric cancer remains a biologically aggressive cancer, with high recurrence and mortality rates. A review of more than 2000 patients who underwent R0 resection demonstrated recurrence rates of almost 30%, with most patients experiencing recurrence within the first 2 years (mean, 21.8 months).[36] For patients with recurrence, the prognosis was almost uniformly fatal, with a mortality rate of 94% and a mean survival time after recurrence of only 8.7 months. Other large series showed similar results.

Underlying these poor outcomes is the fact that the initial chemotherapy regimens for gastric cancer provide little benefit. Numerous primary studies and meta-analyses have shown inconclusive results. Overall, the survival for patients receiving adjuvant therapy was no better than surgery alone.

The Southwest Oncology Group (9008/INT-0116) reported a randomized controlled trial of 556 patients who had undergone curative gastrectomy alone or gastrectomy combined with adjuvant 5-fluorouracil and radiotherapy.[37] This study demonstrated a significant benefit for adjuvant therapy for overall survival (41% versus 50%) and recurrence-free survival (41% versus 64%). As a result, adjuvant chemoradiation has become the standard of care for patients undergoing curative gastrectomy in the United States. Several authors have criticized these results, noting a high rate of inadequate lymphadenectomy (54% of patients underwent a D0 resection). Given these findings, it is possible that some of the benefit from radiation was clearance of residual disease in the perigastric nodal basin. Furthermore, only 64% of patients randomly assigned to the treatment arm were able to complete therapy; 17% had to stop treatment because of toxic effects, and 5% progressed while on treatment.

Some of these study design deficiencies were addressed in the CLASSIC trial, which randomly assigned 1035 patients undergoing gastrectomy with D2 lymph node dissection to either surgery alone or surgery followed by eight 3-week cycles of capecitabine plus oxaliplatin.[38] The trial was stopped early after patients in the adjuvant therapy group were found to have significantly higher rates of disease-free survival (74% versus 59%, $P < .0001$) and overall survival (83% versus 78%, $P < .05$) at median 3-year follow-up. In the chemotherapy group, 67% of patients received all eight cycles as planned per protocol. The ARTIST trial evaluated whether the addition of adjuvant radiotherapy would be beneficial to patients undergoing gastrectomy with D2 dissection and subsequent adjuvant chemotherapy with capecitabine and cisplatin.[39] There was no difference in outcomes found between the adjuvant chemotherapy and adjuvant chemotherapy plus radiotherapy groups, but radiotherapy improved disease-free survival in patients who had lymph node metastases on resection. A follow-up study with increased power is ongoing to examine the benefit of radiotherapy in this patient subgroup alone.

Given the relatively high rate of failure to complete adjuvant treatment in these trials, there has been increased focus on combined perioperative treatment for gastric cancer, rather than postoperative adjuvant therapy. The most significant results are those of the MAGIC trial, a randomized controlled study of 503 patients with stage II or higher gastric cancer that compared perioperative chemotherapy with surgery alone.[40] The treatment group received three 3-week cycles of epirubicin, cisplatin, and a continuous infusion of 5-fluorouracil preoperatively and three additional cycles postoperatively. More than 90% of patients who started the preoperative chemotherapy were able to complete it; however, only 65% of these patients went on to receive postoperative chemotherapy, and only 50% successfully completed both.

The treatment group had significantly better pathologic results and long-term outcomes. The chemotherapy group had a higher percentage of T1 and T2 tumors in the final specimens, along with a higher proportion of limited (N0 and N1) nodal disease compared with the surgery arm alone. The rates of local recurrence, distant metastases, and 5-year overall survival were significantly improved in the chemotherapy group compared with the surgery-only group (14.4% versus 20.6%, 24.4% versus 36.8%, and 36.3% versus 23%).

Similar to the Southwest Oncology Group (9008/INT-0116; SWOG Intergroup 0116) study, MAGIC has been criticized for inadequate staging (no laparoscopy) and inadequacy of lymph node dissection. However, in contrast to the Southwest Oncology Group trial, in which greater than 50% of patients had a D0 resection, most patients in the MAGIC trial had a D2 resection, with 15% undergoing a D1 resection. Given the ongoing debate over D1 versus D2 and the shifting focus toward lymph node count rather than anatomic location, the lymphadenectomy in the MAGIC trial is generalizable to the entire population of patients with gastric cancer who undergo curative gastrectomy. Further strengthening the case for perioperative chemotherapy are the results of the French trial FFCD 9703, which also studied combined neoadjuvant and adjuvant therapy.[41] The regimen in this trial was three preoperative cycles and three postoperative cycles of 5-fluorouracil and cisplatin, with a similar survival benefit for patients who received chemotherapy (5-year survival 38% versus 24%).

One limitation of both studies is the lack of stratification. Although only patients with clinically resectable advanced gastric cancer were included (penetration through the submucosa), they were not further stratified according to stage or other prognostic factors. Other investigators have shown that factors such as serosal involvement or nodal positivity are independent negative prognostic factors. Further studies examining which groups show the most benefit from these potentially toxic regimens will be essential. However, given the results of the MAGIC trial and FFCD 9703, patients with gastric cancer should be evaluated for preoperative systemic therapy.

Palliative Therapy and Systemic Therapy

Patients with unresectable or metastatic gastric cancer represent almost 50% of patients with the disease and have only a 3- to 5-month median survival with the best supportive therapy. Palliative therapy for gastric cancer involves attempts to improve survival and palliation of the symptoms of advanced disease. Many patients with advanced disease are asymptomatic, and palliation is focused on improvement in median survival. However, a significant subset of patients with unresectable gastric cancer have debilitating symptoms and should be considered for surgical therapy even in the setting of metastatic disease.

Chemotherapy improves survival in patients with unresectable tumors. A 2006 meta-analysis showed that triple therapy with 5-fluorouracil, cisplatin, and an anthracycline-based compound, generally epirubicin, was superior to single or double therapy (hazard ratio, 0.77 and 0.83 for triple therapy versus without epirubicin and without cisplatin, respectively).[42] Adverse reactions are common, with 50% of patients having severe neutropenia or GI complaints. Because of the high rate of chemotherapy side effects, single or dual agent therapy is recommended for older patients or patients with underlying medical comorbidities or poor functional status.

Although better than supportive care alone, results of systemic treatments remain relatively poor. Investigators continue to evaluate new treatment regimens with less toxicity. Thus, there has been increased interest in directed therapies that specifically target cancer cells at the molecular level. These include the epidermal growth factor receptor inhibitor cetuximab and the human epidermal growth factor receptor 2 (HER2) antagonist trastuzumab (Herceptin), which is approved for HER2-positive breast cancer. HER2 positivity has been reported in 6% to 35% of gastric cancers. Results of a phase III trial (ToGA trial) were first presented in 2009, evaluating 594 patients with HER2-overexpressing advanced gastric cancers. These patients were randomly assigned to receive capecitabine or 5-fluorouracil with cisplatin and Herceptin or cisplatin alone. The Herceptin group had a better median survival (13.8 months versus 11.1 months), and rates of severe complications did not differ between the groups.[43]

Cetuximab has been evaluated as monotherapy and in phase II trials as part of combination therapy with FOLFIRI (5-fluorouracil, levofolinic acid, and irinotecan; FOLCETUX study) or doxatel and cisplatin (DOCETUX study). In these limited efficacy trials, there was an increased overall response rate but no increase in overall survival. Phase III trials are required to determine the role of cetuximab in gastric cancer more accurately.

Complicated Gastric Cancer

Advanced gastric cancer represents a difficult challenge for the surgeon. Advanced disease is characterized by severe symptoms such as pain, obstruction, and bleeding. Determining the optimal treatment strategy for each patient can be complex and requires input and involvement of a multidisciplinary oncology team. The general approach for these problems is discussed here.

Locally advanced gastric cancer. Patients with advanced disease that is deemed unresectable because of adjacent organ involvement, generally the pancreas or spleen, or extensive nodal disease, including the para-aortic nodes, are particularly challenging. Data from two randomized controlled trials mentioned previously, the Dutch and British trials comparing D1 and D2 lymphadenectomy, including pancreaticosplenectomy as part of D2 resection, indicated that this multiorgan resection significantly increases morbidity and perioperative mortality. As a result, multiorgan resection has generally been abandoned in patients with gastric cancer. However, in both studies, multiorgan resection was performed regardless of tumor (T) status. In the British MRC study, no patients had pathologically confirmed T4 disease, suggesting that most, if not all, patients who had a multiorgan resection would have achieved an R0 resection even without pancreaticosplenectomy. This is in contrast to the data from several retrospective studies, including a review of 1133 patients who underwent R0 resection at Memorial Sloan Kettering Cancer Center. In that study, only male sex, depth of invasion, and nodal status were predictors of poor outcome on multivariate analysis.[44] Of the 268 patients who underwent an R0 multiorgan resection, the 5-year overall survival was 32%, with a median survival of 32 months.

Underlying all these studies, and the objective of performing multiorgan resection in general, is the desire to achieve an R0 resection. Patients with proven T4 disease who achieve an R0 resection have a clinically and statistically significant survival benefit over patients undergoing palliative resection only, with the palliative resection group having survival rates similar to rates for chemotherapy alone.

In an effort to increase the number of patients for whom an R0 resection can be achieved, several investigators explored the role of neoadjuvant therapy in otherwise unresectable disease. A 2009 phase II trial by Sym and colleagues[45] treated 49 patients with clinically unresectable gastric cancer with cisplatin, docetaxel, and capecitabine and found an overall R0 resection rate of 63% compared with historical rates of 30% to 60%. These patients were prospectively stratified according to which criteria made them unresectable—adjacent organ involvement, bulky para-aortic nodal disease, or limited peritoneal disease. For patients without peritoneal disease, the R0 resection rate was greater than 70%. Of all patients who achieved R0 resection, patients with adjacent organ involvement only had significantly better outcomes. At a median follow-up of 51 months, median progression-free and overall survival have yet to be reached, with a predicted 5-year overall survival of 54%. This small phase II trial demonstrated promising results, especially for patients with T4 disease, although these outcomes need to be further validated in phase III studies.

All these data suggest that multiorgan resection is beneficial in properly selected patients. The difficulty is how to select these patients properly. The percentage of patients with clinical T4 disease who have true T4 disease on final pathology ranges from 14% to 38.5%, with CT having only a 50% positive predictive value for true T4 disease. As preoperative staging modalities improve in accuracy, so will the ability to select patients properly for various treatment modalities, including multiorgan resection. In the meantime, for patients in whom an R0 resection can be performed, aggressive surgical therapy appears warranted. However, in patients who at the time of laparoscopy or laparotomy have clearly unresectable disease and who have no symptoms that would warrant resection, palliative resection should be avoided.

Complications

Patients with unresectable disease can develop complications such as bleeding, perforation, and obstruction. Treatment should be focused on maximum palliation and minimal morbidity. For patients with bleeding, endoscopic measures (e.g., cautery, clipping, injection) should be considered first-line therapy, and, similar to any acute GI hemorrhage, multiple attempts are reasonable in hemodynamically stable patients. If endoscopy is unsuccessful, angiography with coil embolization is a reasonable but generally unsuccessful option. If the patient is unstable and other methods are unsuccessful, surgical intervention is warranted. The resection should be tailored to the clinical situation. For patients with a short expected survival, limited resection to grossly negative margins is indicated. Patients with more localized disease can be treated with more aggressive gastric resection.

For patients with a gastric outlet obstruction, several options are available. Endoscopic dilation and stent placement can provide good short-term palliation; however, tumor progression and stent migration limit the long-term efficacy. Chemoradiotherapy has shown overall response rates of 50% and may alleviate outlet obstruction. For patients predicted to have a longer survival (e.g., patients without distant metastases or high-volume peritoneal disease), bypass with a gastrojejunostomy or palliative gastrectomy is a reasonable approach.

Perforation of gastric cancer requires surgical intervention. Primary closure of perforated, frequently necrotic, tumor is not generally possible. Given the relatively poor functional status and prognosis for many of these patients, closure with healthy omentum is a reasonable approach. If it can be done without excess morbidity, such as multiorgan resection, gastrectomy can also be performed.

Linitis plastica is a particularly aggressive form of the disease. These patients frequently have increased pain, obstruction, and poor gastric function. Symptom control and palliative chemoradiotherapy should be considered as the primary treatment. For patients with intractable symptoms not responding to other measures, a total gastrectomy can be performed.

Outcomes

The overall mortality rate for gastric cancer is 3.7 deaths/100,000 people, a decline of 35% since 1992. This incidence has been declining since 1930, likely because of changes in diet such as decreased sodium intake, changes in food storage and preparation, and decreased smoking. Nonetheless, the overall 5-year survival remains less than 25%. Many of these patients present at an advanced stage. For patients who undergo a potentially curative resection, overall 5-year survival rates range from of 24% to 57%; for the subset with early gastric cancer, cure rates are greater than 80%. For patients who present with distant disease, long-term survival is only 4% (Fig. 48-29). More than 63% of patients present with locally advanced or distant disease.

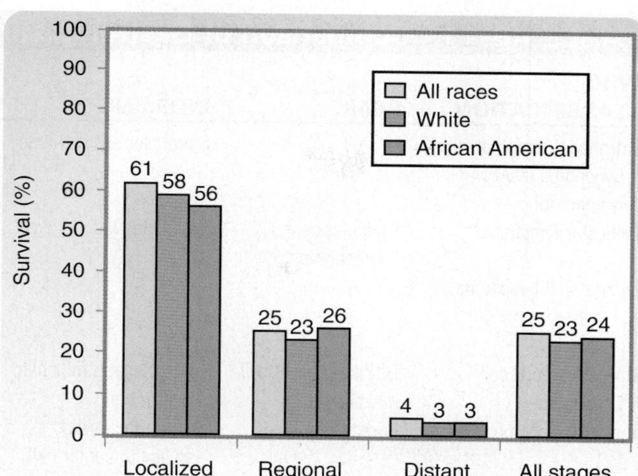

FIGURE 48-29 The 5-year relative survival rates in patients with selected cancers by race and stage at diagnosis, United States, 1996-2004. (From Jemal A, Siegel R, Ward E, et al: Cancer statistics. *CA Cancer J Clin* 59:225–249, 2009.)

Recurrence

Recurrence rates after gastrectomy are high, from 40% to 80%, depending on the series. Most recurrences occur within the first 3 years. The locoregional failure rate ranges from 38% to 45%, whereas peritoneal dissemination as a component of failure occurs in 54% of patients in several series. Isolated distant metastases are uncommon because most patients with distant failure also have locoregional recurrence. The most common sites of locoregional recurrence are the gastric remnant at the anastomosis, in the gastric bed, and in the regional nodes. Hematogenous spread occurs to the liver, lung, and bone.

Surveillance. Although all patients should be followed systematically, the evidence for how this should occur is unclear. Because most recurrences occur within the first 3 years, surveillance examinations are more frequent in the first several years. Follow-up should include a complete history and physical examination every 4 months for 1 year, every 6 months for 2 years, and annually thereafter. Laboratory tests, including complete blood counts and liver function tests, should be performed as clinically indicated. Many physicians obtain chest x-rays and CT scans of the abdomen and pelvis routinely, whereas others obtain studies only when clinically suspicious of a recurrence. Annual endoscopy should be considered for patients who have undergone a subtotal gastrectomy.

Gastric Lymphoma

Epidemiology

The stomach is the most common site of lymphomas in the GI system. However, primary gastric lymphoma is still relatively uncommon, accounting for less than 15% of gastric malignancies and 2% of lymphomas. Patients often present with vague symptoms, such as epigastric pain, early satiety, and fatigue. Constitutional B symptoms are rare. Although overt bleeding is uncommon, more than 50% of patients present with anemia. Lymphomas occur in older patients, with the peak incidence in the sixth and seventh decades, and are more common in men (male-to-female ratio of 2 : 1). Gastric lymphomas, similar to carcinomas, usually occur in the gastric antrum but can arise from any part of the stomach. Patients are considered to have gastric lymphoma if the stomach is the exclusive or predominant site of disease.

Pathology

In the management of gastric lymphomas, as in the management of nodal lymphomas, it is important to determine not only the stage of disease but also the subtype of lymphoma. There are many classification systems for lymphomas (Table 48-11). The most common gastric lymphoma is diffuse large B cell lymphoma (55%), followed by gastric MALT lymphoma (40%), Burkitt

TABLE 48-11 Comparison of Gastrointestinal Lymphoma Classifications

WHO CLASSIFICATION	REAL	WORKING	LUKES-COLLINS	KLEL	RAPPAPORT
Extranodal marginal zone lymphoma (MALT lymphoma)	—	Small cleaved cell type	Small cleaved cell type	Immunocytoma	Well-differentiated lymphocytic
Follicular lymphoma	Follicular center lymphoma	Small cleaved cell type	Small cleaved cell type	Centroblastic-centrocytic, follicular and diffuse	Nodular, poorly differentiated lymphocytic
Mantle cell lymphoma	—	—	—	Centrocytic	Intermediately or poorly differentiated lymphocytic, diffuse or nodular
Diffuse large B cell lymphoma	Diffuse large B cell lymphoma	Large cleaved follicular center cell	Large cleaved follicular center cell	Centroblastic, B-immunoblastic	Diffuse mixed lymphocytic and histiocytic
Burkitt lymphoma	Burkitt lymphoma	Small noncleaved follicular center cell	Small noncleaved follicular center cell	Burkitt lymphoma with intracytoplasmic immunoglobulin	Undifferentiated lymphoma, Burkitt type

MALT, Mucosa-associated lymphoid tissue.

TABLE 48-12 Staging Systems for Primary Gastrointestinal Non-Hodgkin Lymphoma

STAGE				
ANN ARBOR*	RAO ET AL†	MUSSHOFF‡	DESCRIPTION	RELATIVE INCIDENCE (%)
IE	IE	IE	Tumor confined to GI tract	26
IIE	IIE	IIE	Tumor with spread to regional lymph nodes	26
IIE	IIIE	IIE	Tumor with nodal involvement beyond regional lymph nodes (para-aortic, iliac)	17
IIIE-IV	IVE	IIIE-IV	Tumor with spread to other intra-abdominal organs (liver, spleen) or beyond abdomen (chest, bone marrow)	31

*Carbone PP, Kaplan HS, Musshoff K, et al: Report of the Committee on Hodgkin's Disease Staging Classification. *Cancer Res* 31:1860–1861, 1971.
†Rao AR, Kagan AR, Kagan AR, et al: Management of gastrointestinal lymphoma. *Am J Clin Oncol* 7:213–219, 1984.
‡Musshoff K: [Clinical staging classification of non-Hodgkin's lymphomas (author's trans, German)]. *Strahlentherapie* 153:218–221, 1977.

lymphoma (3%), and mantle cell and follicular lymphomas (each <1%).

Diffuse large B cell lymphomas are generally primary lesions; however, they may also occur from progression of less aggressive lymphomas, such as chronic lymphocytic leukemia–small lymphocytic lymphoma, follicular lymphoma, and MALT lymphoma. Immunodeficiencies and *H. pylori* infection are risk factors for the development of primary diffuse large B cell lymphoma.

Burkitt lymphomas of the stomach are associated with Epstein-Barr virus infections, as they are in other sites. Burkitt lymphoma is very aggressive and tends to affect younger patients than other types of gastric lymphomas. Burkitt lymphoma is usually found in the cardia or body of the stomach as opposed to the antrum.

Evaluation

Endoscopy generally reveals nonspecific gastritis or gastric ulcerations. Occasionally, a submucosal growth pattern renders endoscopic biopsies nondiagnostic. EUS is useful to determine the depth of gastric wall invasion, specifically to identify patients at risk for perforation secondary to full-thickness involvement of the gastric wall. Evidence of distant disease should be sought through upper airway examination, bone marrow biopsy, and CT of the chest and abdomen to detect lymphadenopathy. Biopsies should be performed of any enlarged lymph nodes. Histologic *H. pylori* testing should be performed and, if negative, confirmed by serology.

Staging

The best staging system is controversial. When possible, the TNM staging system should be used (using the criteria proposed for gastric carcinoma). Several other staging systems for primary gastric non-Hodgkin lymphoma are available (Table 48-12).

Treatment

Most centers use a multimodality treatment program for patients with gastric lymphoma. The role of resection in gastric lymphoma is controversial, and most patients are treated with chemotherapy alone. The risk for perforation in patients treated with chemotherapy has been overstated in the past and is now approximately 5%. The most common chemotherapeutic combination is CHOP (cyclophosphamide, hydroxydaunomycin [doxorubicin], Oncovin [vincristine], prednisone). A prospective randomized study evaluated several treatment strategies—surgical resection, resection plus radiation, resection plus chemotherapy, chemotherapy alone—in patients with early-stage (stage IE or IIE) disease.[43] The addition of chemotherapy was essential, with the surgery plus chemotherapy and chemotherapy-alone groups having significantly higher overall survival than the surgery-alone and surgery plus radiation groups. The addition of surgery to radiation therapy or chemotherapy did not improve outcomes. The primary role of surgery is for patients with limited gastric disease; patients with symptomatic recurrence of treatment failure; and patients who develop complications, such as bleeding, gastric outlet obstruction, or perforation.

The diagnosis of lymphoma discovered unexpectedly at surgery can be confirmed by frozen section. Also, fresh tissue should be sent for fluorescence-activated cell sorting, immunohistochemistry, and genetic analysis. Consideration should be given to bone marrow aspiration at the time of surgery. If isolated stage IE or IIE lymphoma is encountered, surgical removal of all gross disease is ideal. Patients with disseminated lymphoma cannot be cured surgically, and the operation should focus on obtaining enough tissue for diagnosis and the repair of perforations.

Mucosa-Associated Lymphoid Tissue Lymphomas

Numerous mucosal surfaces throughout the body have associated lymphoid tissue, including the lungs, small bowel, and stomach. In 1983, Isaacson and Wright noted that the histology of primary low-grade gastric B cell lymphoma resembled MALT. From that initial finding, it has been determined that in the setting of prolonged inflammation, these rests of lymphoid tissue can progress to low-grade lymphomas. The MALT lymphoma concept has been extended beyond the stomach to include other extranodal low-grade B cell lymphomas of the salivary gland, lung, and thyroid. These organs lack native lymphoid tissue; thus, the lymphomas at these sites arise from MALT acquired as a result of chronic inflammation.

Gastric MALT lymphoma is usually preceded by *H. pylori*–associated gastritis. Evidence of *H. pylori* infection can be found in almost every case of gastric MALT lymphoma. Epidemiologic studies have also linked *H. pylori* infection with gastric lymphomas. Genetically, MALT lymphoma is characterized by the translocations t(1;14)(p22;q32) and t(11;18)(q21;q21), both of which result in impaired responsiveness to apoptotic signaling and increased nuclear factor-κB activity. It has been suggested that t(11;18)(q21;q21) and *BCL-10* nuclear expression may predict for nonresponsiveness to treatment by *H. pylori* eradication and lymphoma regression.

Treatment

Given the strong association with *H. pylori* and the low-grade MALT lymphoma, there was interest in treating MALT lymphoma without chemotherapy. It has been suggested that early-stage MALT lymphomas and some cases of limited, diffuse large B cell lymphoma may be effectively treated by *H. pylori* eradication alone. Successful eradication resulted in remission in more than 75% of cases. However, careful follow-up is necessary, with repeat endoscopy in 2 months to document clearance of the infection and biannual endoscopy for 3 years to document regression. Some patients continued to demonstrate the lymphoma clone after *H. pylori* eradication, suggesting that the lymphoma became dormant rather than disappearing.

The presence of transmural tumor extension, nodal involvement, transformation into a large cell phenotype, t(11;18), and nuclear *BCL-10* expression all predict failure after *H. pylori* eradication alone. Additionally, a few patients with MALT lymphoma are *H. pylori*–negative. In these patients, consideration should be given to surgical resection, radiation, and chemotherapy. The 5-year disease-free survival rate with multimodality treatment is greater than 95% in stage IE disease and 75% in stage IIE disease.

Gastrointestinal Stromal Tumors

Gastrointestinal stromal tumors (GISTs) are the most common sarcomatous tumors of the GI tract. Originally thought to be a type of smooth muscle sarcoma, they are now known to be a distinct tumor derived from the interstitial cells of Cajal, an intestinal pacemaker cell. They can appear anywhere within the GI tract, although they are usually found in the stomach (40% to 60%), small intestine (30%), and colon (15%). GISTs vary considerably in their presentation and clinical course, ranging from small benign tumors to massive lesions with necrosis, hemorrhage, and wide metastases. Their pathology, presentation, and management as they relate to the stomach are discussed here.

Gastric GISTs can manifest at any age, although most typically they manifest in patients older than 50 years. They generally have an equal male-to-female ratio or a slight male predominance. They are rarely associated with familial syndromes such as GIST-paraganglioma syndrome (Carney triad), neurofibromatosis 1, and von Hippel-Lindau disease, but most develop de novo. Most GISTs manifest symptomatically, typically with bleeding or vague abdominal pain or discomfort. Bleeding is generally in the form of melena or, less frequently, frank hematemesis. Tumor rupture with intra-abdominal hemorrhage is uncommon, but when it occurs, it frequently requires emergent surgical intervention. Many patients remain asymptomatic, and their tumors are discovered incidentally at the time of other surgery or, increasingly, during imaging performed for other indications.

Patients are evaluated with upper endoscopy, on which a smooth-appearing, round, submucosal tumor can be identified, occasionally containing an area of central ulceration. Because of the submucosal nature of the tumor, obtaining tissue for histologic analysis via conventional endoscopic-forceps biopsy results in a low diagnostic yield. EUS-directed fine-needle aspiration results in superior diagnostic accuracy, with a sensitivity of 82% and specificity of 100% in diagnosing GIST.[46] Given the expense and specialized expertise involved in performing EUS-directed fine-needle aspiration, in addition to the fact that most submucosal GI tumors require surgical resection regardless of histology, some experts have argued that routine preoperative pathologic diagnosis is not needed for such tumors. CT of the abdomen and pelvis with an intravenous contrast agent is used to assess for metastatic disease. Pathologically, GISTs have smooth muscle and neuroendocrine features, consistent with their origin from the interstitial cells of Cajal. They are frequently identified by immunohistochemical staining for the c-*kit* proto-oncogene (CD117), which is overexpressed in 95% of these tumors, and for CD34, which is positive in 60% to 70% of GISTs.

The mainstay of treatment is complete surgical resection. Tumors greater than 2 cm in diameter should be resected, but the treatment for smaller tumors is controversial. Tumors that are less than 2 cm and have high-risk features on endoscopy and EUS, such as irregular borders, ulceration, and heterogeneity, should be resected, whereas tumors without such features can be observed with repeat endoscopy and EUS at 6- to 12-month intervals. Depending on tumor size, resection can include wide local excision, enucleation, sleeve gastrectomy, or total gastrectomy, with or without en bloc resection of adjacent organs. No specific surgical margin other than an R0 resection is required, and an anatomic resection according to lymph node basins is not required, as lymph node metastases are rare.

Recurrence rates are approximately 40%, and most patients who experience recurrence demonstrate metastasis to the liver, with one third having only isolated local recurrence. Recurrence can occur 20 years later, and long-term follow-up is warranted. Long-term disease-free survival is approximately 50%, with 20% to 80% of patients dying of their disease. Although there are no dichotomous criteria that are able to define benign versus malignant lesions histologically, the most important risk factors for malignancy are tumor size larger than 10 cm and more than five mitoses/50 high-power fields (HPF). Based on a long-term follow-up study of 1700 patients with gastric GISTs, guidelines for assessing malignant potential based on the combination of these two factors have been developed (Box 48-4).[47]

Adjuvant Therapy

Given the relatively high recurrence rates with increased disease-specific mortality for patients with larger lesions and increased mitotic rate, surgery alone for these patients appears inadequate.

BOX 48-4 Suggested Guidelines for Assessing Malignant Potential of Gastric Gastrointestinal Stromal Tumors of Different Sizes and Mitotic Activity

Benign (no tumor-related mortality)

- No larger than 2 cm, no more than 5 mitoses/50 HPF

Probably benign (<3% with progressive disease)

- >2 cm but ≤5 cm; no more than 5 mitoses/50 HPF

Uncertain or low malignant potential

- No larger than 2 cm; >5 mitoses/50 HPF

Low to moderate malignant potential (12%-15% tumor-related mortality)

- >10 cm; no more than 5 mitoses/HPF
- >2 cm but ≤5 cm; >5 mitoses/50 HPF

High malignant potential (49%-86% tumor-related mortality)

- >5 cm but ≤10 cm; >5 mitoses/50 HPF
- >10 cm; >5 mitoses/50 HPF

From Miettinen M, Sobin L, Lasota J: Gastrointestinal stromal tumors of the stomach: A clinicopathologic, immunohistochemical, and molecular genetic study of 1765 cases with long-term follow-up. *Am J Surg Pathol* 29:52–58, 2005.
HPF, High-power field.

However, adjuvant therapy was not effective until the discovery of the tyrosine kinase inhibitor imatinib (Gleevec). Originally designed to treat chronic myelogenous leukemia, it has proven in randomized controlled trials to be an effective treatment modality for patients with metastatic disease or disease that carries a high risk for recurrence. In patients with metastatic or unresectable disease, imatinib (400 mg daily) showed an overall 2-year survival of 70% compared with 25% for patients on traditional chemotherapy.[48] In the adjuvant setting, patients with *c-kit*–positive tumors 3 cm or larger who underwent complete resection and were treated with imatinib for 1 year had a recurrence rate of 8% compared with 20% for untreated patients.[49] This difference was even more pronounced for patients with larger tumors. The side effects were generally mild, with less than 1% of patients having any grade 3 or 4 toxicities.

The Scandinavian Sarcoma Group (SSG) XVIII trial compared an extended 36-month course of adjuvant imatinib versus a 12-month course after resection for high-risk GISTs (defined as >10 cm tumor, mitotic count >10/50 HPF, tumor >5 cm and mitotic count > per 50 HPF, or tumor rupture).[50] Patients in the extended treatment arm had higher recurrence-free survival (65.6% versus 47.9%) and overall survival (92.0% versus 81.7%) at 5 years after surgery. The results of this trial have established a 3-year course as the standard of care after surgical resection of high-risk GIST. Imatinib has also been reported to be successful in the neoadjuvant treatment of patients with nonmetastatic but unresectable disease, although this has not been evaluated in prospective randomized trials. However, as a result of current trials, for patients with metastatic disease and patients with resected primary disease at moderate risk of recurrence, indefinite treatment with imatinib has been approved by the U.S. Food and Drug Administration. Figure 48-30 is an algorithm for using imatinib in the treatment of GISTs in the neoadjuvant, adjuvant, and palliative settings.

Other Neoplasms

Gastric Carcinoid

Overall, carcinoid tumors (currently more appropriately classified as neuroendocrine tumors [NETs]) are a rare malignancy (0.49%

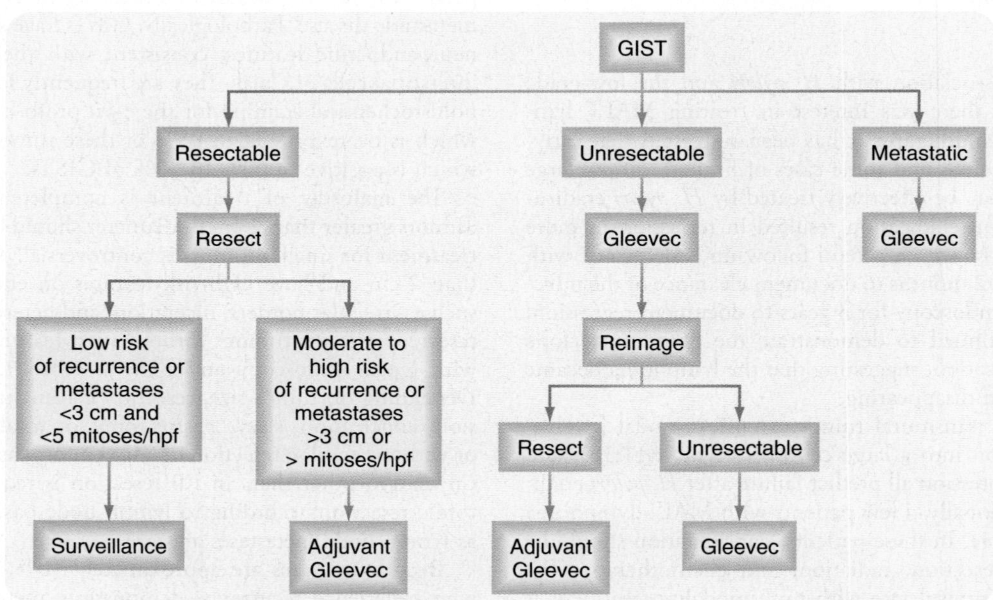

FIGURE 48-30 Algorithm for the workup and treatment of gastrointestinal stromal tumors (GISTs).

of all malignancies) that arise from neuroendocrine precursor cells and can manifest at any site in the body. The most common location is the GI tract, encompassing almost 68% of all NETs. The most common sites in the GI tract are the small intestine, rectum, and appendix.

The stomach has historically been a rare site for a GI NET; however, a marked increase has been noted over the past several decades. At the present time, the stomach is the location of almost 8% of GI NETs compared with 2% in 1950. They are also increasing as a percentage of all gastric tumors, increasing from 0.3% to 1.77% over the past 50 years. There are three types, two of which are associated with low acid and increased gastrin secretion and derive from gastric ECL cells. Type I, the most common, is associated with chronic atrophic gastritis and has a benign prognosis. These tumors are generally small and have an overall 5-year survival of greater than 95%. Type II is associated with ZES and multiple endocrine neoplasia type 1. The prognosis is still good, with long-term survival of 70% to 90% and slightly higher levels of metastases. Type III tumors are sporadic lesions with few ECL cells. They have a more than 50% rate of metastatic spread and a 5-year survival of less than 35%. The combined 5-year overall survival for all localized gastric NETs is 63%.

The treatment for localized NETs is complete removal. For small pedunculated lesions, complete removal can be accomplished endoscopically. Larger lesions may require wedge resection or partial gastrectomy. Patients with multiple gastric NETs may require total gastrectomy. For patients with recurrent or metastatic disease, somatostatin analogues can be used to decrease the burden of disease and treat carcinoid syndrome.

The incidence of gastric and small bowel NETs has increased eightfold over the past 5 to 10 years. Although more endoscopies for GI complaints account for some of the increase, there also appears to be growth in development of the disease. Given the relationship among hypergastrinemia, low-acid states, and NETs, some authors have asked whether the use of PPIs is responsible. The profound gastric acid suppression noted with PPIs has resulted in hypergastrinemia and gastric NET formation in in vivo animal studies. Although a direct causal link has not been shown in humans, database cohort studies have shown PPI use to be an independent risk factor for development of stomach and small bowel NETs. The clinical significance is unclear. With respect to small bowel NETs associated with PPI use, they tend to have a benign clinical course without any evidence of metastases, invasion of the muscle layer, or high mitotic rate. They can be treated successfully with local endoscopic excision with a low recurrence rate. Ongoing studies should define the long-term effects of PPIs and provide recommendations for surveillance of these patients.

Heterotopic Pancreas

Heterotopic pancreas (i.e., functioning pancreatic tissue is found in an abnormal anatomic location) is extremely rare, found in less than 0.2% of all autopsy specimens. Most occur in the proximal GI tract, with the stomach being the most common site. Symptomatic patients generally present with vague abdominal pain. There have been reports of pancreatitis, islet cell tumors, and pancreatic adenocarcinoma within these lesions. On endoscopy and CT, they are frequently small submucosal masses and may be confused with a GIST. The treatment is surgical excision, and the diagnosis is confirmed pathologically.

OTHER GASTRIC LESIONS

Hypertrophic Gastritis (Ménétrier Disease)

Ménétrier disease (hypoproteinemic hypertrophic gastropathy) is a rare, acquired premalignant disease characterized by massive gastric folds in the fundus and corpus of the stomach, giving the mucosa a cobblestone or cerebriform appearance. Histologic examination reveals foveolar hyperplasia (expansion of surface mucous cells), with absent parietal cells. The condition is associated with protein loss from the stomach, excessive mucus production, and hypochlorhydria or achlorhydria. The cause of Ménétrier disease is unknown, but it has been associated with cytomegalovirus infection in children and *H. pylori* infection in adults. Also, increased levels of transforming growth factor-α have been noted in the gastric mucosa of patients with the disease. Patients often present with epigastric pain, vomiting, weight loss, anorexia, and peripheral edema. Typical gastric mucosal changes can be detected by radiographic or endoscopic examination. Biopsy should be performed to rule out gastric carcinoma or lymphoma. A chromium-labeled albumin test reveals increased GI protein loss, and 24-hour pH monitoring reveals hypochlorhydria or achlorhydria. Medical treatment has yielded inconsistent results; however, some benefit has been shown with the use of anticholinergic drugs, acid suppression, octreotide, and *H. pylori* eradication. Total gastrectomy should be performed in patients who continue to have massive protein loss despite optimal medical therapy or if dysplasia or carcinoma develops.

Mallory-Weiss Tear

Mallory-Weiss tears are related to forceful vomiting, retching, coughing, or straining that results in disruption of the gastric mucosa high on the lesser curve at the GE junction. They account for 15% of acute upper GI hemorrhages and are rarely associated with massive bleeding. The overall mortality rate for the lesion is 3% to 4%, with the greatest risk for massive hemorrhage in alcoholic patients with preexisting portal hypertension. Most patients with active bleeding can be managed by endoscopic methods, such as multipolar electrocoagulation, epinephrine injection, endoscopic band ligation, or endoscopic hemoclipping. Angiographic intra-arterial infusion of vasopressin or transcatheter embolization may be useful in select high-risk cases. Operative intervention is rarely needed. If surgery is required, the lesion at the GE junction is approached through an anterior gastrotomy, and the bleeding site is oversewn with several deep 2-0 silk ligatures to reapproximate the gastric mucosa in an anatomic fashion.

Dieulafoy Gastric Lesion

Dieulafoy lesions account for 0.3% to 7% of nonvariceal upper GI hemorrhages. Bleeding from a gastric Dieulafoy lesion is caused by an abnormally large (1 to 3 mm), tortuous artery coursing through the submucosa. Erosion of the superficial mucosa overlying the artery occurs secondary to the pulsations of the large submucosal vessel. The artery is then exposed to the gastric contents, and further erosion and bleeding occur. Generally, the mucosal defect is 2 to 5 mm in size and is surrounded by normal-appearing gastric mucosa. The lesions generally occur 6 to 10 cm from the GE junction, generally in the fundus, near the cardia. In one series, 67% were located high in the body of the stomach, with 25% in the gastric fundus. Dieulafoy lesions are more common in men (2 : 1), with the peak incidence in the fifth decade. Most patients present with hematemesis. The classic presentation of a patient with a Dieulafoy lesion is sudden onset of massive, painless, recurrent hematemesis with hypotension.

Detection and identification of the Dieulafoy lesion can be difficult. The diagnostic modality of choice is esophagogastroduodenoscopy, which correctly identifies the lesion in 80% of patients. Because of the intermittent nature of the bleeding, repeated endoscopies may be needed to identify the lesion correctly. If the lesion can be identified endoscopically, attempts should be made to stop the bleeding using endoscopic modalities such as multipolar electrocoagulation, heater probe, noncontact laser photocoagulation, injection sclerotherapy, band ligation, or endoscopic hemoclipping. Angiography can be useful in cases in which endoscopy could not definitely identify the source. Angiographic findings may include a tortuous ectatic artery in the distribution of the left gastric artery, with accompanying contrast extravasation in the setting of acute bleeding. Embolization with absorbable gelatin sponge (Gelfoam) has been reported to control bleeding successfully in patients with Dieulafoy lesion, although the reported experience is limited.

Surgical therapy was once the only available treatment for Dieulafoy lesion, but it is now reserved for patients in whom other modalities have failed. Surgical management consists of gastric wedge resection to include the offending vessel. The difficulty at the time of exploration is locating the lesion, unless it is actively bleeding. The surgical procedure can be greatly facilitated by asking the endoscopist to tattoo the stomach when the lesion is identified. The traditional surgical approach has been through laparotomy with wide gastrotomy to identify the lesion with subsequent wide wedge resection. The lesion can also be approached laparoscopically, combined with intraoperative endoscopy. A wedge resection is performed with a linear stapling device using endoscopic transillumination to determine the resection margin.

Gastric Varices

Gastric varices are broadly classified into two types: GE varices and isolated gastric varices. Isolated gastric varices are subclassified into type 1 varices, located in the fundus of the stomach, and type 2, isolated ectopic varices located anywhere in the stomach.

Gastric varices can develop secondary to portal hypertension, in conjunction with esophageal varices, or secondary to sinistral hypertension from splenic vein thrombosis. In generalized portal hypertension, the increased portal pressure is transmitted by the left gastric vein to esophageal varices and by the short and posterior gastric veins to the fundic plexus and cardia veins. Isolated gastric varices tend to occur secondary to splenic vein thrombosis, which is usually the result of pancreatitis. Splenic blood flows retrograde through the short and posterior gastric veins into the varices and then hepatopetally through the coronary vein into the portal vein. Left-to-right retrograde flow through the gastroepiploic vein to the superior mesenteric vein can explain the development of ectopic varices in the stomach.

The incidence of bleeding from gastric varices has been reported to be between 3% and 30%, although it is less than 10% in most series. However, the incidence of bleeding can be as high as 78% in patients with splenic vein thrombosis and fundic varices. There are limited data on risk factors associated with hemorrhage in patients with gastric varices, although increasing size of the varices or a higher child status increases the risk for bleeding.

Gastric varices in the setting of splenic vein thrombosis are readily treated by splenectomy. Patients with bleeding gastric varices should have an imaging study to document splenic vein thrombosis before surgical intervention because gastric varices are more often associated with generalized portal hypertension.

Gastric varices in the setting of portal hypertension should be managed similarly to esophageal varices. The patient should be volume-resuscitated, with attention paid to the correction of abnormal coagulation profiles. Temporary tamponade can be attempted with a Sengstaken-Blakemore tube. Endoscopy serves as a diagnostic and therapeutic tool. Successful eradication of the esophageal varices through banding or sclerotherapy often results in obliteration of the gastric varices. Because gastric varices arise in the submucosa, a common complication associated with gastric variceal sclerotherapy is ulceration. A major problem with gastric varices is rebleeding, of which 50% is secondary to ulcers. Endoscopic variceal band ligation can achieve hemostasis in approximately 89% of patients; however, concerns about gastric perforations with this technique have tempered its use. Transjugular intrahepatic portosystemic shunting can be effective in controlling gastric variceal hemorrhage, with rebleeding rates of approximately 30%. A gastrorenal shunt between gastric varices and the left renal vein is present in 85% of patients with gastric varices. This spontaneous shunt decompresses the portal system and lessens the efficacy of transjugular intrahepatic portosystemic shunting. A balloon catheter can be inserted into the gastrorenal shunt through the left renal vein, and the shunt can be occluded by inflating the balloon. A sclerosant (e.g., ethanolamine oleate) is injected and left to remain until clots have formed in the varices. Balloon-occluded retrograde transvenous obliteration has been reported to have a high success rate (100%) with a low recurrence rate (0% to 5%). The major complication of this procedure is aggravation of esophageal varices secondary to an increase in portal pressure as a consequence of occluding the gastrorenal shunt. Also, ethanolamine oleate can cause hemolysis (treatable by haptoglobin administration), with subsequent renal damage.

Gastric Volvulus

Gastric volvulus is an uncommon condition. Torsion occurs along the stomach's longitudinal axis (organoaxial) in approximately two thirds of cases and along the vertical axis (mesenteroaxial) in one third (Fig. 48-31). Usually, organoaxial gastric volvulus occurs acutely and is associated with a diaphragmatic defect, whereas mesenteroaxial volvulus is partial (<180 degrees), recurrent, and not associated with a diaphragmatic defect. In adults, the diaphragmatic defects are usually traumatic or paraesophageal hernias, whereas in children, congenital defects such as the foramen of Bochdalek or eventration are involved. The major symptoms at presentation are abdominal pain that is acute in onset, distention, vomiting, and upper GI hemorrhage. The sudden onset of constant and severe upper abdominal pain, recurrent retching with production of little vomitus, and the inability to pass a NG tube constitute Borchardt triad. Plain films of the abdomen reveal a gas-filled viscus in the chest or upper abdomen. The diagnosis can be confirmed by barium contrast study or upper GI endoscopy. Acute volvulus is a surgical emergency. The stomach is reduced and uncoiled through a transabdominal approach. The diaphragmatic defect is repaired, with consideration given to a fundoplication in the setting of a paraesophageal hernia. In the unusual case in which strangulation has occurred (5% to 28%), the compromised segment of stomach is resected. Spontaneous volvulus, without an associated diaphragmatic defect, is treated by detorsion and fixation of the stomach by gastropexy or tube gastrostomy.

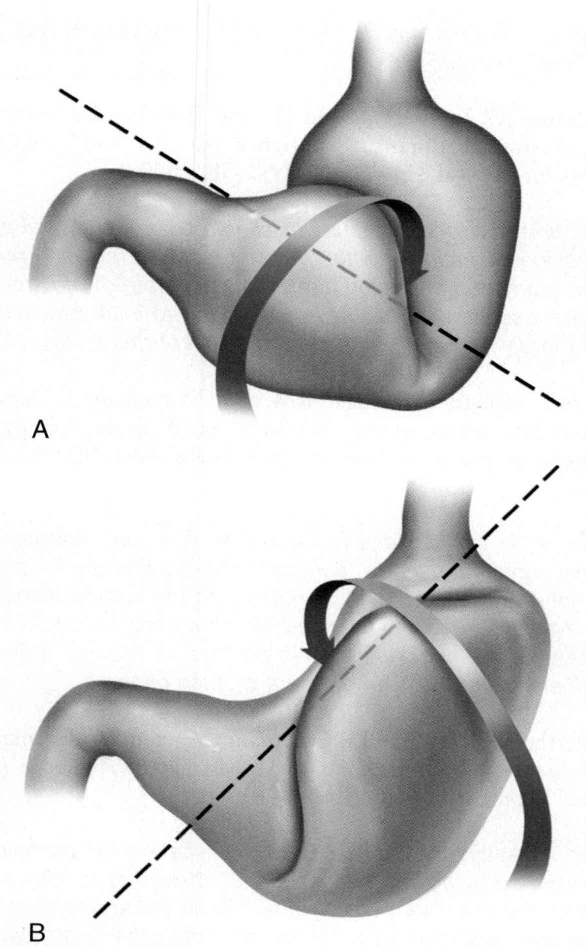

FIGURE 48-31 Torsion of the stomach along the longitudinal axis (organoaxial) **(A)** and along the vertical axis (mesoaxial) **(B)**. (From White RR, Jacobs DO: Volvulus of the stomach and small bowel. In Yeo CJ, Dempsey DT, Klein AS, et al, editors: *Shackelford's surgery of the alimentary tract*, ed 6, Philadelphia, 2007, Saunders.)

Bezoars

Bezoars are collections of nondigestible materials, usually of vegetable origin (phytobezoar) but also of hair (trichobezoar). Phytobezoars are most commonly found in patients who have undergone surgery of the stomach and have impaired gastric emptying. Diabetics with autonomic neuropathy are also at risk. The symptoms of gastric bezoars include early satiety, nausea, pain, vomiting, and weight loss. A large mass may be palpable on physical examination, and the diagnosis is confirmed by barium examination or endoscopy. In 1959, Dan and coworkers were the first to suggest enzymatic therapy to attempt dissolution of the bezoar. Papain, found in Adolph's Meat Tenderizer, is given in a dose of 1 tsp in 150 to 300 mL water several times daily. The sodium concentration in Adolph's Meat Tenderizer is high, so hypernatremia may result if large quantities are administered. Alternative enzymes such as cellulase have been used with some success. Generally, enzymatic débridement is followed by aggressive Ewald tube lavage or endoscopic fragmentation. Failure of these therapies necessitates surgical removal.

Trichobezoars are concretions of hair, generally found in long-haired girls or women who often deny eating their own hair (trichophagy). Symptoms include pain from gastric ulceration and fullness from gastric outlet obstruction, with occasional gastric perforation and small bowel obstruction. Trichobezoars tend to form a cast of the stomach, with strands of hair having been observed as far distally as the transverse colon. Small trichobezoars may respond to endoscopic fragmentation, vigorous lavage, or enzymatic therapy. However, these techniques are of limited usefulness, and larger trichobezoars require surgical removal. The small bowel should be examined to be ensure that additional bezoars are not present. Individuals with trichophagy require psychiatric care because recurrent bezoar formation is common.

SELECTED REFERENCES

Ahn JY, Jung HY, Choi KD, et al: Endoscopic and oncologic outcomes after endoscopic resection for early gastric cancer: 1370 cases of absolute and extended indications. *Gastrointest Endosc* 74:485–493, 2011.

This is a large retrospective series of patients undergoing endoscopic resection (either endoscopic mucosal resection or endoscopic submucosal dissection) for early-stage gastric cancers, generally those confined to the mucosa. This study found a very low local recurrence rate of approximately 1% at almost 3-year follow-up, suggesting these techniques are oncologically successful while obviating the need for gastrectomy in most patients. Most of the experience and data with these procedures come from East Asia, and further study is needed to determine the applicability of these procedures in Western populations, in which early-stage gastric cancer is much less frequent and endoscopic screening programs do not exist.

Bang YJ, Kim YW, Yang HK, et al: Adjuvant capecitabine and oxaliplatin for gastric cancer after D2 gastrectomy (CLASSIC): A phase 3 open-label, randomised controlled trial. *Lancet* 379:315–321, 2012.

Lee J, Lim do H, Kim S, et al: Phase III trial comparing capecitabine plus cisplatin versus capecitabine plus cisplatin with concurrent capecitabine radiotherapy in completely resected gastric cancer with D2 lymph node dissection: The ARTIST trial. *J Clin Oncol* 30:268–273, 2012.

These two large randomized controlled trials examined the role of adjuvant therapy after surgical resection for localized gastric cancer. The CLASSIC trial found that adjuvant chemotherapy (capecitabine plus oxalaplatin) improved long-term disease-free and overall survival compared with surgery alone. The ARTIST trial evaluated the addition of adjuvant radiotherapy plus chemotherapy and showed no improvement compared with adjuvant chemotherapy alone. However, radiotherapy did result in an improvement in outcomes in patients who had lymph node metastases on surgical resection.

Barkun AN, Bardou M, Kuipers EJ, et al: International consensus recommendations on the management of patients with nonvariceal upper gastrointestinal bleeding. *Ann Intern Med* 152:101–113, 2010.

This excellent overview of the prevalence of upper gastrointestinal hemorrhage includes an evidence-based assessment of various therapies. Recommendations are made regarding the role of endoscopy, methods of endoscopic control, pharmacologic interventions, proper monitoring and triaging, risk factors for rebleeding, and which patients have increased mortality.

Cunningham D, Allum WH, Stenning SP, et al: Perioperative chemotherapy versus surgery alone for resectable gastroesophageal cancer. *N Engl J Med* 355:11–20, 2006.

This major study showed a benefit to chemotherapy in gastric cancer. Patients underwent neoadjuvant treatment, and a much greater percentage were able to complete treatment compared with patients who completed the adjuvant trial. More patients had adequate lymphadenectomy than in the SWOG Intergroup 0116 trial.

Cuschieri A, Weeden S, Fielding J, et al: Patient survival after D1 and D2 resections for gastric cancer: Long-term results of the MRC randomized surgical trial. Surgical Co-operative Group. *Br J Cancer* 79:1522–1530, 1999.

Songun I, Putter H, Kranenbarg EM, et al: Surgical treatment of gastric cancer: 15-year follow-up results of the randomised nationwide Dutch D1D2 trial. *Lancet Oncol* 11:439–449, 2010.

These two randomized controlled trials were major challenges to the role of D2 lymphadenectomy in the non-Japanese population. Both studies showed increased perioperative morbidity and mortality with a D2 dissection without long-term survival benefit. They have been challenged on the grounds that patients in the D2 group were not stratified by whether they also underwent splenectomy, which later analysis showed as the major contributor to the increased operative morbidity. At 15-year follow-up in the Dutch trial, there was a benefit to D2 dissection in terms of cancer recurrence and disease-free survival, suggesting that if a spleen-sparing D2 dissection can be safely performed without adding perioperative morbidity, it will likely result in superior long-term oncologic outcomes.

DeMatteo RP, Ballman KV, Antonescu CR, et al: Adjuvant imatinib mesylate after resection of localised, primary gastrointestinal stromal tumour: A randomised, double-blind, placebo-controlled trial. *Lancet* 373:1097–1104, 2009.

Joensuu H, Eriksson M, Sundby Hall K, et al: One vs three years of adjuvant imatinib for operable gastrointestinal stromal tumor: A randomized trial. *JAMA* 307:1265–1272, 2012.

These two major randomized controlled trials established the role of adjuvant imatinib after surgical resection for the treatment of localized gastrointestinal stromal tumors (GISTs). The first study by DeMatteo and colleagues showed significantly less recurrence in patients who received imatinib compared with patients who did not; this was especially pronounced for patients at high risk of developing metastatic disease. The second trial by Joensuu and colleagues showed that a 36-month course of adjuvant imatinib was superior to a 12-month course in terms of disease-free and overall survival. These studies established long-term adjuvant treatment with imatinib as the standard of care for patients with GISTs.

DeMatteo RP, Lewis JJ, Leung D, et al: Two hundred gastrointestinal stromal tumors: Recurrence patterns and prognostic factors for survival. *Ann Surg* 231:51–58, 2000.

The first major cohort study to characterize the natural progression of patients with gastrointestinal stromal tumors. This study demonstrated a relatively high rate of recurrence and subsequent metastases, which led to increased focus on the development of improved adjuvant therapies.

Fuccio L, Minardi ME, Zagari RM, et al: Meta-analysis: Duration of first-line proton-pump inhibitor based triple therapy for *Helicobacter pylori* eradication. *Ann Intern Med* 147:553–562, 2007.

The study by Fuccio and colleagues is a meta-analysis of trials comparing shorter durations of triple therapy for eradication of H. pylori *(7 and 10 days) with the current standard of 14 days. This study found no difference in eradication rates, suggesting that shorter courses of therapy may be sufficient in the initial treatment of such patients.*

Malfertheiner P, Megraud F, O'Morain CA, et al: Management of *Helicobacter pylori* infection—the Maastricht IV/Florence Consensus Report. *Gut* 61:646–664, 2012.

The Maastricht Consensus Report is a set of guidelines developed by an international panel of experts for the diagnosis and treatment of H. pylori. *These guidelines summarize the most current evidence regarding the treatment of peptic ulcer disease caused by* H. pylori *infection.*

REFERENCES

1. Vaira D, Malfertheiner P, Megraud F, et al: Diagnosis of *Helicobacter pylori* infection with a new non-invasive antigen-based assay. HpSA European study group. *Lancet* 354:30–33, 1999.
2. Toro JP, Lytle NW, Patel AD, et al: Efficacy of laparoscopic pyloroplasty for the treatment of gastroparesis. *J Am Coll Surg* 218:652–660, 2014.
3. Abell T, McCallum R, Hocking M, et al: Gastric electrical stimulation for medically refractory gastroparesis. *Gastroenterology* 125:421–428, 2003.
4. Malfertheiner P, Megraud F, O'Morain CA, et al: Management of *Helicobacter pylori* infection—the Maastricht IV/Florence Consensus Report. *Gut* 61:646–664, 2012.
5. Fuccio L, Minardi ME, Zagari RM, et al: Meta-analysis: Duration of first-line proton-pump inhibitor based triple therapy for *Helicobacter pylori* eradication. *Ann Intern Med* 147:553–562, 2007.
6. Blatchford O, Murray WR, Blatchford M: A risk score to predict need for treatment for upper-gastrointestinal haemorrhage. *Lancet* 356:1318–1321, 2000.
7. Rockall TA, Logan RF, Devlin HB, et al: Risk assessment after acute upper gastrointestinal haemorrhage. *Gut* 38:316–321, 1996.

8. Lim LG, Ho KY, Chan YH, et al: Urgent endoscopy is associated with lower mortality in high-risk but not low-risk nonvariceal upper gastrointestinal bleeding. *Endoscopy* 43: 300–306, 2011.
9. Laine L, McQuaid KR: Endoscopic therapy for bleeding ulcers: An evidence-based approach based on meta-analyses of randomized controlled trials. *Clin Gastroenterol Hepatol* 7:33–47, quiz 31–32, 2009.
10. Mirsadraee S, Tirukonda P, Nicholson A, et al: Embolization for non-variceal upper gastrointestinal tract haemorrhage: A systematic review. *Clin Radiol* 66:500–509, 2011.
11. Lunevicius R, Morkevicius M: Systematic review comparing laparoscopic and open repair for perforated peptic ulcer. *Br J Surg* 92:1195–1207, 2005.
12. Byrge N, Barton RG, Enniss TM, et al: Laparoscopic versus open repair of perforated gastroduodenal ulcer: A National Surgical Quality Improvement Program analysis. *Am J Surg* 206:957–962, discussion 962–963, 2013.
13. Cherian PT, Cherian S, Singh P: Long-term follow-up of patients with gastric outlet obstruction related to peptic ulcer disease treated with endoscopic balloon dilatation and drug therapy. *Gastrointest Endosc* 66:491–497, 2007.
14. Berna MJ, Hoffmann KM, Serrano J, et al: Serum gastrin in Zollinger-Ellison syndrome: I. Prospective study of fasting serum gastrin in 309 patients from the National Institutes of Health and comparison with 2229 cases from the literature. *Medicine (Baltimore)* 85:295–330, 2006.
15. Ito T, Igarashi H, Jensen RT: Zollinger-Ellison syndrome: Recent advances and controversies. *Curr Opin Gastroenterol* 29:650–661, 2013.
16. Norton JA, Fraker DL, Alexander HR, et al: Value of surgery in patients with negative imaging and sporadic Zollinger-Ellison syndrome. *Ann Surg* 256:509–517, 2012.
17. Dellinger RP, Levy MM, Rhodes A, et al: Surviving sepsis campaign: International guidelines for management of severe sepsis and septic shock: 2012. *Crit Care Med* 41:580–637, 2013.
18. Jemal A, Bray F, Center MM, et al: Global cancer statistics. *CA Cancer J Clin* 61:69–90, 2011.
19. Ahn JS, Eom CS, Jeon CY, et al: Acid suppressive drugs and gastric cancer: A meta-analysis of observational studies. *World J Gastroenterol* 19:2560–2568, 2013.
20. Graham DY, Schwartz JT, Cain GD, et al: Prospective evaluation of biopsy number in the diagnosis of esophageal and gastric carcinoma. *Gastroenterology* 82:228–231, 1982.
21. Bentrem D, Gerdes H, Tang L, et al: Clinical correlation of endoscopic ultrasonography with pathologic stage and outcome in patients undergoing curative resection for gastric cancer. *Ann Surg Oncol* 14:1853–1859, 2007.
22. Spolverato G, Ejaz A, Kim Y, et al: Use of endoscopic ultrasound in the preoperative staging of gastric cancer: A multi-institutional study of the US Gastric Cancer Collaborative. *J Am Coll Surg* 220:48–56, 2015.
23. Smyth E, Schoder H, Strong VE, et al: A prospective evaluation of the utility of 2-deoxy-2-[(18)F]fluoro-D-glucose positron emission tomography and computed tomography in staging locally advanced gastric cancer. *Cancer* 118:5481–5488, 2012.
24. Burke EC, Karpeh MS, Conlon KC, et al: Laparoscopy in the management of gastric adenocarcinoma. *Ann Surg* 225:262–267, 1997.
25. Lowy AM, Mansfield PF, Leach SD, et al: Laparoscopic staging for gastric cancer. *Surgery* 119:611–614, 1996.
26. Vinuela EF, Gonen M, Brennan MF, et al: Laparoscopic versus open distal gastrectomy for gastric cancer: A meta-analysis of randomized controlled trials and high-quality nonrandomized studies. *Ann Surg* 255:446–456, 2012.
27. Yamao T, Shirao K, Ono H, et al: Risk factors for lymph node metastasis from intramucosal gastric carcinoma. *Cancer* 77:602–606, 1996.
28. Kim JJ, Lee JH, Jung HY, et al: EMR for early gastric cancer in Korea: A multicenter retrospective study. *Gastrointest Endosc* 66:693–700, 2007.
29. Gotoda T, Yanagisawa A, Sasako M, et al: Incidence of lymph node metastasis from early gastric cancer: Estimation with a large number of cases at two large centers. *Gastric Cancer* 3:219–225, 2000.
30. Ahn JY, Jung HY, Choi KD, et al: Endoscopic and oncologic outcomes after endoscopic resection for early gastric cancer: 1370 cases of absolute and extended indications. *Gastrointest Endosc* 74:485–493, 2011.
31. Cuschieri A, Fayers P, Fielding J, et al: Postoperative morbidity and mortality after D1 and D2 resections for gastric cancer: Preliminary results of the MRC randomised controlled surgical trial. The Surgical Cooperative Group. *Lancet* 347:995–999, 1996.
32. Songun I, Putter H, Kranenbarg EM, et al: Surgical treatment of gastric cancer: 15-year follow-up results of the randomised nationwide Dutch D1D2 trial. *Lancet Oncol* 11:439–449, 2010.
33. Cuschieri A, Weeden S, Fielding J, et al: Patient survival after D1 and D2 resections for gastric cancer: Long-term results of the MRC randomized surgical trial. Surgical Co-operative Group. *Br J Cancer* 79:1522–1530, 1999.
34. Jiang L, Yang KH, Guan QL, et al: Survival and recurrence free benefits with different lymphadenectomy for resectable gastric cancer: A meta-analysis. *J Surg Oncol* 107:807–814, 2013.
35. Bilimoria KY, Talamonti MS, Wayne JD, et al: Effect of hospital type and volume on lymph node evaluation for gastric and pancreatic cancer. *Arch Surg* 143:671–678, discussion 678, 2008.
36. Yoo CH, Noh SH, Shin DW, et al: Recurrence following curative resection for gastric carcinoma. *Br J Surg* 87:236–242, 2000.
37. Macdonald JS, Smalley SR, Benedetti J, et al: Chemoradiotherapy after surgery compared with surgery alone for adenocarcinoma of the stomach or gastroesophageal junction. *N Engl J Med* 345:725–730, 2001.
38. Bang YJ, Kim YW, Yang HK, et al: Adjuvant capecitabine and oxaliplatin for gastric cancer after D2 gastrectomy (CLASSIC): A phase 3 open-label, randomised controlled trial. *Lancet* 379:315–321, 2012.
39. Lee J, Lim do H, Kim S, et al: Phase III trial comparing capecitabine plus cisplatin versus capecitabine plus cisplatin with concurrent capecitabine radiotherapy in completely resected gastric cancer with D2 lymph node dissection: The ARTIST trial. *J Clin Oncol* 30:268–273, 2012.
40. Cunningham D, Allum WH, Stenning SP, et al: Perioperative chemotherapy versus surgery alone for resectable gastroesophageal cancer. *N Engl J Med* 355:11–20, 2006.
41. Ychou M, Boige V, Pignon JP, et al: Perioperative chemotherapy compared with surgery alone for resectable

gastroesophageal adenocarcinoma: An FNCLCC and FFCD multicenter phase III trial. *J Clin Oncol* 29:1715–1721, 2011.
42. Wagner AD, Grothe W, Haerting J, et al: Chemotherapy in advanced gastric cancer: A systematic review and meta-analysis based on aggregate data. *J Clin Oncol* 24:2903–2909, 2006.
43. Bang YJ, Van Cutsem E, Feyereislova A, et al: Trastuzumab in combination with chemotherapy versus chemotherapy alone for treatment of HER2-positive advanced gastric or gastro-oesophageal junction cancer (ToGA): A phase 3, open-label, randomised controlled trial. *Lancet* 376:687–697, 2010.
44. Martin RC, 2nd, Jaques DP, Brennan MF, et al: Extended local resection for advanced gastric cancer: Increased survival versus increased morbidity. *Ann Surg* 236:159–165, 2002.
45. Sym SJ, Chang HM, Ryu MH, et al: Neoadjuvant docetaxel, capecitabine and cisplatin (DXP) in patients with unresectable locally advanced or metastatic gastric cancer. *Ann Surg Oncol* 17:1024–1032, 2010.
46. Watson RR, Binmoeller KF, Hamerski CM, et al: Yield and performance characteristics of endoscopic ultrasound-guided fine needle aspiration for diagnosing upper GI tract stromal tumors. *Dig Dis Sci* 56:1757–1762, 2011.
47. Miettinen M, Sobin LH, Lasota J: Gastrointestinal stromal tumors of the stomach: A clinicopathologic, immunohistochemical, and molecular genetic study of 1765 cases with long-term follow-up. *Am J Surg Pathol* 29:52–68, 2005.
48. Blanke CD, Rankin C, Demetri GD, et al: Phase III randomized, intergroup trial assessing imatinib mesylate at two dose levels in patients with unresectable or metastatic gastrointestinal stromal tumors expressing the kit receptor tyrosine kinase: S0033. *J Clin Oncol* 26:626–632, 2008.
49. Dematteo RP, Ballman KV, Antonescu CR, et al: Adjuvant imatinib mesylate after resection of localised, primary gastrointestinal stromal tumour: A randomised, double-blind, placebo-controlled trial. *Lancet* 373:1097–1104, 2009.
50. Joensuu H, Eriksson M, Sundby Hall K, et al: One vs three years of adjuvant imatinib for operable gastrointestinal stromal tumor: A randomized trial. *JAMA* 307:1265–1272, 2012.

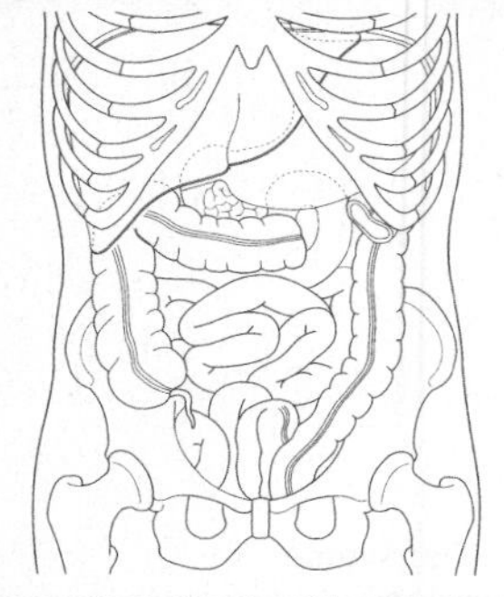

CHAPTER 49

Small Intestine

Jennifer W. Harris, B. Mark Evers

OUTLINE

The small intestine is a marvel of complexity and efficiency. The primary role of the small intestine is the digestion and absorption of dietary components after they leave the stomach. This process depends on a multitude of structural, physiologic, endocrine, and chemical factors. Exocrine secretions from the liver and pancreas enable complete digestion of the ingested dietary components. The enlarged surface area of the small intestinal mucosa then absorbs these nutrients. In addition to its role in digestion and absorption, the small bowel is the largest endocrine organ in the body and one of the most important organs of immune function. Given its essential role and complexity, it is amazing that diseases of the small bowel are not more frequent. This chapter describes the normal anatomy and physiology of the small intestine as well as disease processes involving the small bowel, which include obstruction, inflammatory and infectious diseases, neoplasms, diverticular disease, and miscellaneous disorders.

EMBRYOLOGY

The primitive gut is formed from the endodermal lining, the yolk sac, which is enveloped by the developing embryo as a result of cranial and caudal folding during the fourth week of fetal human gestation.[1] The endodermal layer gives rise to the epithelial lining of the digestive tract, and the splanchnic mesoderm surrounding the endoderm gives rise to the muscular connective tissue and all the other layers of the intestine. The splanchnic mesoderm wraps around the gut tube to form the mesenteries that suspend the gut within the body cavity; the mesoderm immediately adjacent to the endodermal tube also contributes to most of the wall of the gut tube. Nerves and neurons found in the wall are derived from the neural crest. Except for the duodenum, which is a primitive foregut structure, the small intestine is derived from the midgut. During the fifth week of fetal development, when the intestinal length is rapidly increasing, herniation of the midgut occurs through the umbilicus (Fig. 49-1). This midgut loop has a cranial and caudal limb, with the cranial limb developing into the distal duodenum, jejunum, and proximal ileum and the caudal limb becoming the distal ileum and proximal two thirds of the transverse colon. The juncture of the cranial and caudal limbs is where the vitelline duct joins to the yolk sac. This duct structure normally becomes obliterated before birth; however, it can persist as a Meckel's diverticulum in approximately 2% of the population. As the gut tube develops, the endoderm proliferates rapidly and temporarily occludes the lumen of the tube around the fifth week of gestation. Growth and expansion of mesoderm components in the wall, coupled with apoptosis of the endoderm during the seventh week, result in recanalization of the tube, and by the ninth week of gestation, the tube is again patent. This midgut herniation persists until about 10 weeks of fetal gestation, when the intestine returns to the abdominal cavity. After completing a 270-degree rotation from its initial starting point, the proximal jejunum reenters the abdomen and occupies the left side of the abdomen, with subsequent loops lying more to the right. The cecum enters last and is located temporarily in the right upper quadrant; however, with time, it descends to its normal position in the right lower quadrant.[1] Congenital anomalies of gut malrotation and fixation can occur during this process.

The primitive small bowel is lined by a sheet of cuboidal cells until about the ninth week of gestation, when villi begin to form in the proximal intestine and then proceed in a caudal fashion until the entire small bowel, and even the colon, for a time, are lined by these finger-like projections. Crypt formation begins in the tenth to twelfth weeks of gestation. The crypt layer of the small bowel is the site of continual cell renewal and proliferation. As the cells ascend the crypt-villous axis, proliferation ceases, and cells differentiate into one of the four main cell types: absorptive enterocytes, which compose about 95% of the intestinal cell population; goblet cells; Paneth cells; and enteroendocrine cells. An important distinction regarding Paneth cells is that they remain in the crypt bases, where they protect intestinal stem cells from damage by releasing signaling molecules that affect the host tissues and influence the microbial populations to maintain homeostasis in the intestine.[2] The other differentiating cells ascending the crypt-villous axis are eventually extruded into the intestinal lumen. Amazingly, with the exception of Paneth cells,

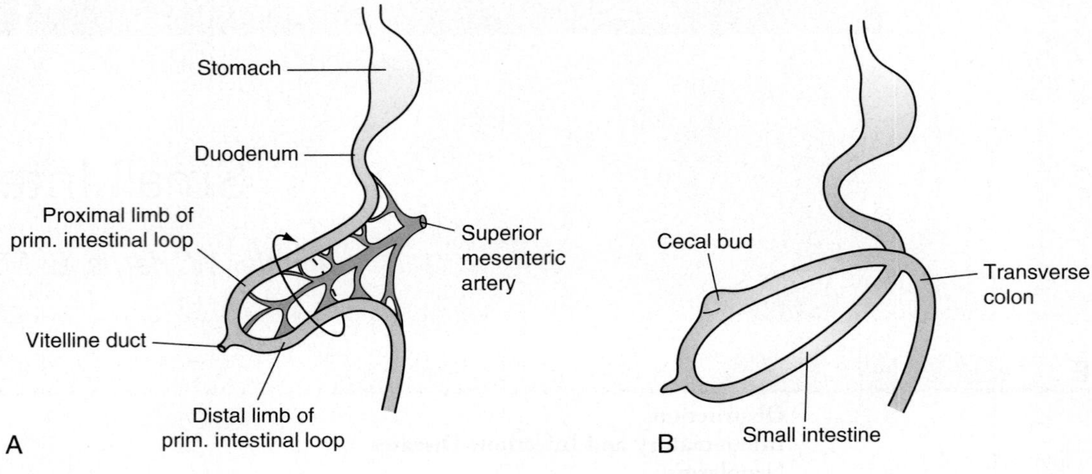

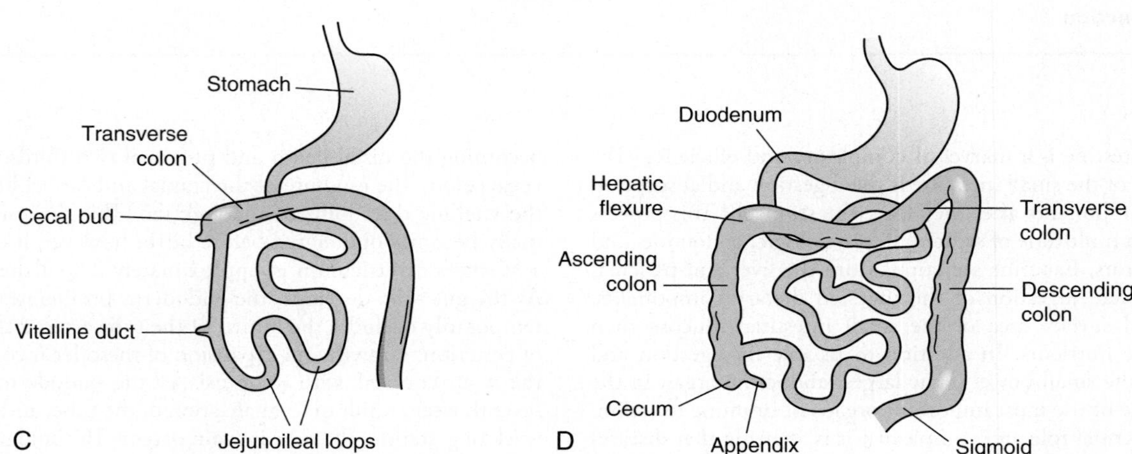

FIGURE 49-1 Rotation of the Intestine. A, The intestine after a 90-degree rotation around the axis of the superior mesenteric artery, the proximal loop on the right and the distal loop on the left. **B,** The intestinal loop after a further 180-degree rotation. The transverse colon passes in front of the duodenum. **C,** Position of the intestinal loops after reentry into the abdominal cavity. Note the elongation of the small intestine, with formation of the small intestine loops. **D,** Final position of the intestines after descent of the cecum into the right iliac fossa. (From Podolsky DK, Babyatshy MW: Growth and development of the gastrointestinal tract. In Yamada T, editor: *Textbook of gastroenterology* (vol 2). Philadelphia, 1995, JB Lippincott.)

epithelial cell turnover occurs rapidly, with a life span of 3 to 5 days in humans.

ANATOMY

Gross Anatomy

The entire small intestine, which extends from the pylorus to the cecum, measures 270 to 290 cm, with duodenal length estimated at approximately 20 cm, jejunal length at 100 to 110 cm, and ileal length at 150 to 160 cm. The jejunum begins at the duodenojejunal angle, which is supported by a peritoneal fold known as the *ligament of Treitz*. There is no obvious line of demarcation between the jejunum and the ileum; however, the jejunum is commonly considered to make up the proximal two fifths of the small intestine, and the ileum makes up the remaining three fifths. The jejunum has a somewhat larger circumference, is thicker than the ileum, and can be identified at surgery by examining mesenteric vessels (Fig. 49-2*A*). In the jejunum, only one or two arcades send out long, straight vasa recta to the mesenteric border, whereas the blood supply to the ileum may have four or five separate arcades with shorter vasa recta (Fig. 49-2*B*) The mucosa of the small bowel is characterized by transverse folds (plicae circulares), which are prominent in the distal duodenum and jejunum.

Neurovascular-Lymphatic Supply

The small intestine is served by rich vascular, neural, and lymphatic supplies, all traversing through the mesentery. The base of the mesentery attaches to the posterior abdominal wall to the left of the second lumbar vertebra and passes obliquely to the right and inferiorly to the right sacroiliac joint. The blood supply of the small bowel, except for the proximal duodenum, which is supplied by branches of the celiac axis, comes entirely from the superior mesenteric artery (Fig. 49-2*C*). The superior mesenteric artery courses anterior to the uncinate process of the pancreas and the third portion of the duodenum, where it divides to supply the pancreas, distal duodenum, entire small intestine, and ascending

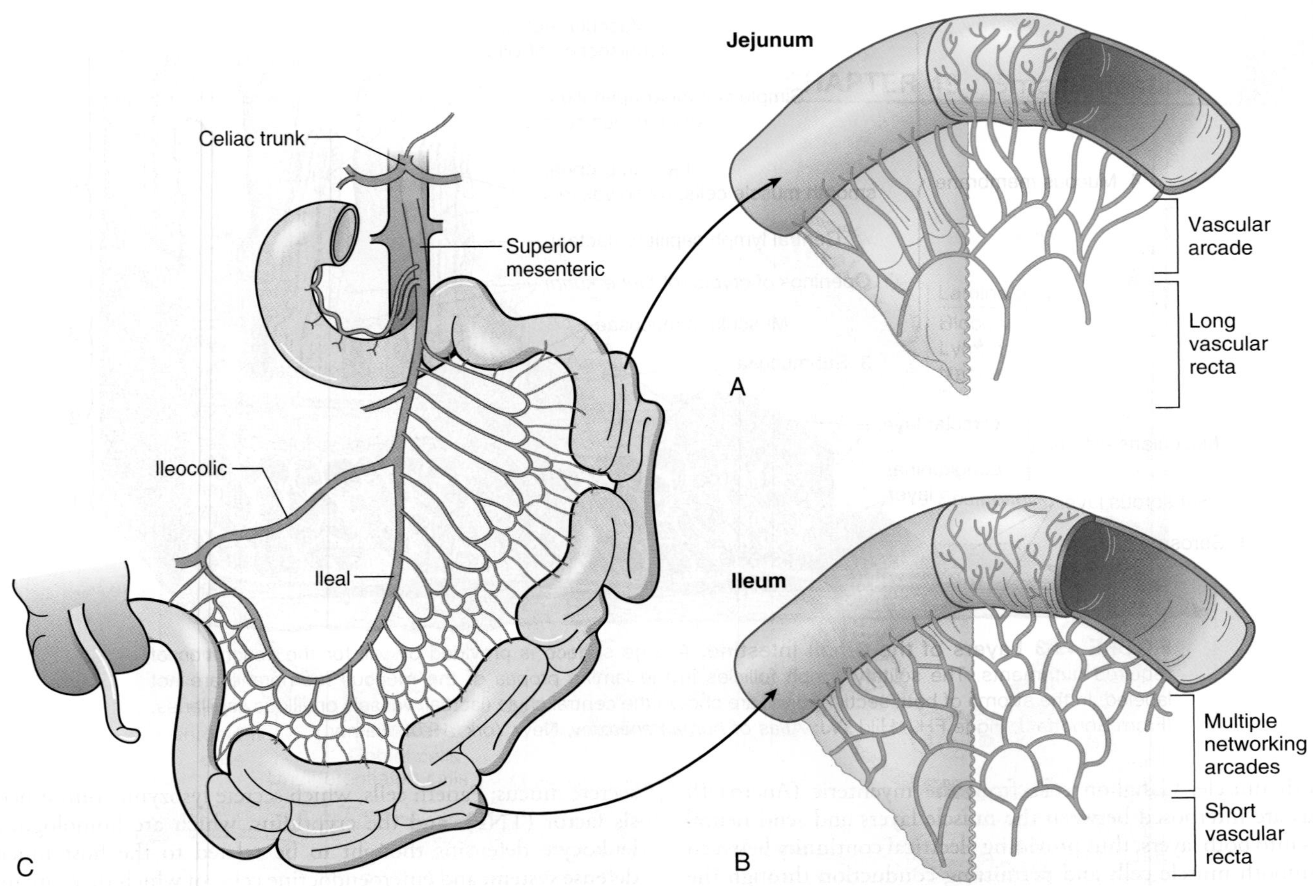

FIGURE 49-2 A, The jejunal mesenteric vessels form only one or two arcades with long vasa recta. **B,** The mesenteric vessels of the ileum form multiple vascular arcades with short vasa recta. **C,** The superior mesenteric artery, which courses anterior to the third portion of the duodenum, provides blood supply to the jejunoileum and distal duodenum. The celiac artery supplies the proximal duodenum. (Adapted from Keljo DJ, Gariepy CE: Anatomy, histology, embryology, and developmental anomalies of the small and large intestine. In Feldman M, Scharschmidt BF, Sleisenger MH, editors: *Sleisenger and Fordtran's gastrointestinal and liver disease: Pathology, diagnosis, management*, Philadelphia, 2002, WB Saunders, p 1646; illustration courtesy Matt Hazzard, University of Kentucky Medical Center, Lexington, KY.)

and transverse colons. There is an abundant collateral blood supply to the small bowel provided by vascular arcades coursing in the mesentery. Venous drainage of the small bowel parallels the arterial supply, with blood draining into the superior mesenteric vein, which joins the splenic vein behind the neck of the pancreas to form the portal vein.

The innervation of the small bowel is provided by parasympathetic and sympathetic divisions of the autonomic nervous system that, in turn, provide the efferent nerves to the small intestine. Parasympathetic fibers are derived from the vagus; they traverse the celiac ganglion and affect secretion, motility, and probably all phases of bowel activity. Vagal afferent fibers are present but apparently do not carry pain impulses. The sympathetic fibers come from three sets of splanchnic nerves and have their ganglion cells usually in a plexus around the base of the superior mesenteric artery. Motor impulses affect blood vessel motility and probably gut secretion and motility. Pain from the intestine is mediated through general visceral afferent fibers in the sympathetic system.

The lymphatics of the small intestine are noted in major deposits of lymphatic tissue, particularly in the Peyer's patches of the distal small bowel. Lymphatic drainage proceeds from the mucosa through the wall of the bowel to a set of nodes adjacent to the bowel in the mesentery. Drainage continues to a group of regional nodes adjacent to the mesenteric arterial arcades and then to a group at the base of the superior mesenteric vessels. From there, lymph flows into the cisterna chyli and then up the thoracic ducts, ultimately to empty into the venous system at the confluence of the left internal jugular and subclavian veins. The lymphatic drainage of the small intestine constitutes a major route for transport of absorbed lipid into the circulation and similarly plays a major role in immune defense and also in the spread of cells arising from cancers of the gut.

Microscopic Anatomy

The small bowel wall consists of four layers: serosa, muscularis propria, submucosa, and mucosa (Fig. 49-3).

The serosa is the outermost layer of the small intestine and consists of visceral peritoneum, a single layer of flattened meso-epithelial cells that encircles the jejunoileum, and the anterior surface of the duodenum.

The muscularis propria consists of two muscle layers, a thin outer longitudinal layer and a thicker inner circular layer of serum sodium, chloride, potassium, bicarbonate, and creatinine levels. The serial determination of serum electrolyte levels should be performed to assess the adequacy of fluid resuscitation. Dehydration may result in hemoconcentration, as noted by an elevated hematocrit value. This should be monitored because fluid resuscitation results in a decrease in the hematocrit, and some patients (e.g., those with intestinal malignant neoplasms) may require blood transfusions before surgery. In addition, the white blood cell count should be assessed. Leukocytosis may be found in patients with strangulation; however, an elevated white blood cell count does not necessarily denote strangulation. Conversely, the absence of leukocytosis does not eliminate strangulation as a possibility.

Simple Versus Strangulating Obstruction

Most patients with small bowel obstruction are classified as having simple obstructions that involve mechanical blockage of the flow of luminal contents without compromised viability of the intestinal wall. In contrast, a strangulated obstruction, which usually involves a closed loop obstruction in which the vascular supply to a segment of intestine is compromised, can lead to intestinal infarction. A strangulated obstruction is associated with an increased morbidity and mortality risk, and therefore recognition of early strangulation is important. In differentiating from simple intestinal obstruction, classic signs of strangulation have been described; these include tachycardia, fever, leukocytosis, and a constant, noncramping abdominal pain. However, a number of studies have convincingly shown that no clinical parameters or laboratory measurements can accurately detect or exclude the presence of strangulation in all cases. This reinforces the dictum that a careful history and physical examination are key for an accurate and timely diagnosis.

CT examination is useful only for detecting the late stages of irreversible ischemia (e.g., pneumatosis intestinalis, portal venous gas). Various serum determinations, including lactate dehydrogenase, amylase, alkaline phosphatase, and ammonia levels, have been assessed with no real benefit. Previous reports described limited success in discriminating strangulation by measuring serum D-lactate, creatine kinase isoenzyme (particularly the BB isoenzyme), or intestinal fatty acid–binding protein; however, these studies were ultimately abandoned as they showed no significant diagnostic benefits. Finally, noninvasive determinations of mesenteric ischemia have been described using a superconducting quantum interference device (SQUID) magnetometer to detect mesenteric ischemia noninvasively. Intestinal ischemia is associated with changes in the basic electrical rhythm of the small intestine. This technique remains investigational and is not in widespread clinical use.

Thus, it is important to remember that bowel ischemia and strangulation cannot be reliably diagnosed or excluded preoperatively in all cases by any known clinical parameter, combination of parameters, or current laboratory and radiographic examinations.

Treatment

Fluid Resuscitation and Antibiotics

Patients with intestinal obstruction are usually dehydrated and depleted of sodium, chloride, and potassium, requiring aggressive intravenous (IV) replacement with an isotonic saline solution such as lactated Ringer solution. Urine output should be monitored by the placement of a Foley catheter. After the patient has formed adequate urine, potassium chloride should be added to the infusion, if needed. Serial electrolyte level measurements as well as hematocrit and white blood cell count are performed to assess the adequacy of fluid repletion. Because of large fluid requirements, some patients, particularly older patients, may require central venous assessment and, in select cases, the placement of a Swan-Ganz catheter. Broad-spectrum antibiotics are given prophylactically by some surgeons on the basis of the reported findings of bacterial translocation occurring even in simple mechanical obstructions; however, there is no substantial evidence to support the use of antimicrobial therapy in nontoxic-appearing patients or those without suspected bacterial overgrowth of the small intestine. Antibiotics are administered preoperatively in the event that the patient requires surgery.

Tube Decompression

In addition to IV fluid resuscitation, another important adjunct to the supportive care of patients with intestinal obstruction is nasogastric suction. Suction with a nasogastric tube empties the stomach, reducing the hazard of pulmonary aspiration of vomitus and minimizing further intestinal distention from preoperatively swallowed air. Nasogastric decompression in a patient with small bowel obstruction is still considered standard of care.

The use of long intestinal tubes (e.g., Cantor or Baker tube) has been advocated by some. However, prospective randomized trials have demonstrated no significant differences with regard to the decompression achieved, success of nonoperative treatment, or morbidity rate after surgical intervention compared with the use of nasogastric tubes. Furthermore, the use of these long tubes has been associated with a significantly longer hospital stay, duration of postoperative ileus, and postoperative complications in some series. Therefore, it appears that long intestinal tubes also offer no benefit in the preoperative setting over nasogastric tubes.

Patients with a partial intestinal obstruction may be treated conservatively with resuscitation and tube decompression alone. Resolution of symptoms and discharge without the need for surgery have been reported in up to 85% of patients with a partial obstruction.[5] Enteroclysis can assist in determining the degree of obstruction, with higher grade partial obstructions requiring earlier operative intervention. Although an initial trial of nonoperative management of most patients with partial small bowel obstruction is warranted, clinical deterioration of the patient or increasing small bowel distention on abdominal radiographs during tube decompression warrants prompt operative intervention. The decision to continue to treat a patient nonoperatively with a presumed bowel obstruction is based on clinical judgment and requires constant vigilance to ensure that the clinical course has not changed.

Operative Management

In general, the patient with a complete small bowel obstruction requires operative intervention. A nonoperative approach for selected patients with complete small intestinal obstruction has been proposed by some surgeons who argue that prolonged intubation is safe in these patients, provided no fever, tachycardia, tenderness, or leukocytosis is noted. Nevertheless, one must realize that nonoperative management of these patients is undertaken at a calculated risk of overlooking an underlying strangulated obstruction. This delay of definitive treatment often necessitates an urgent surgical intervention and can result in increased morbidity and mortality compared with patients who undergo a more prompt intervention. Retrospective studies have reported that a 12- to 24-hour delay of surgery in these patients is safe but that the incidence of strangulation and other complications increases significantly after this period.

The nature of the problem dictates the approach to management of the obstructed patient. Patients with intestinal obstruction secondary to an adhesive band may be treated with lysis of adhesions. Great care should be used in the gentle handling of the bowel to reduce serosal trauma and to avoid unnecessary dissection and inadvertent enterotomies. Incarcerated hernias can be managed by manual reduction of the herniated segment of bowel and closure of the defect.

The treatment of patients with an obstruction and history of malignant tumors can be particularly challenging. In the terminal patient with widespread metastasis, nonoperative management, if successful, is usually the best course; however, only a small percentage of cases of complete obstruction can be successfully managed nonoperatively. In this case, an intestinal bypass of the obstructing lesion, by whatever means, may offer the best option rather than a long and complicated operation that might entail bowel resection.

An obstruction secondary to Crohn's disease will often resolve with conservative management if the obstruction is acute. If a chronic fibrotic stricture is the cause of the obstruction, a bowel resection or strictureplasty may be required.

Patients with an intra-abdominal abscess can present in a manner indistinguishable from those with mechanical bowel obstruction. CT is particularly useful in diagnosing the cause of the obstruction in these patients; percutaneous drainage of the abscess may be sufficient to relieve the obstruction, but laparotomy and abdominal washout may be required for large and established abscesses. Laparoscopic drainage is also an option in cases not amenable to image-guided percutaneous drainage for patients who would not otherwise tolerate a laparotomy; it has reduced wound morbidity and is also useful in multiloculated collections and allows a washout of the peritoneal cavity at the same time.

Radiation enteropathy, as a complication of radiation therapy for pelvic malignant neoplasms, may cause bowel obstruction. Most cases can be treated nonoperatively with tube decompression and possibly corticosteroids, particularly during the acute setting. In the chronic setting, nonoperative management is rarely effective; it will require laparotomy, with possible resection of the irradiated bowel or bypass of the affected area.

At the time of exploration, it can sometimes be difficult to evaluate bowel viability after the release of a strangulation. If intestinal viability is questionable, the bowel segment should be completely released and placed in a warm, saline-moistened sponge for 15 to 20 minutes and then reexamined. If normal color has returned and peristalsis is evident, it is safe to retain the bowel. A prospective controlled trial comparing clinical judgment with the use of a Doppler probe or the administration of fluorescein for the intraoperative discrimination of viability has found that the Doppler flow probe added little to the conventional clinical judgment of the surgeon. In difficult borderline cases, fluorescein fluorescence may supplement clinical judgment. Intraoperative near-infrared angiography to determine the presence of ischemic bowel has shown promising results, but this technique is currently not in wide clinical use. Another approach to the assessment of bowel viability is the so-called second-look laparotomy 18 to 24 hours after the initial procedure. This decision should be made at the time of the initial operation. A second-look laparotomy is clearly indicated for a patient whose condition deteriorates after the initial operation.

Some studies have evaluated the efficacy of laparoscopic management of acute small bowel obstruction. The laparoscopic treatment of small bowel obstruction appears to be effective and leads to a shorter hospital stay and reduced overall complications in a highly selected group of patients.[7] Patients fitting the criteria for consideration of laparoscopic management include those with the following symptoms: mild abdominal distention allowing adequate visualization; proximal obstruction; partial obstruction; and anticipated single-band obstruction.

In particular, laparoscopic treatment has been found to be of greatest benefit in patients who have undergone fewer than three previous operations, were seen early after the onset of symptoms, and were thought to have adhesive bands as the cause. Currently, patients who have advanced, complete, or distal small bowel obstructions are not candidates for laparoscopic treatment. Similarly, patients with matted adhesions or carcinomatosis or those who remain distended after nasogastric intubation should be managed with conventional laparotomy. Therefore, the future role of laparoscopic procedures in the treatment of these patients remains to be completely defined. A multicenter, prospective, randomized trial comparing laparoscopic adhesiolysis to open surgery in patients with adhesive small bowel obstruction, diagnosed by CT scan, that fails to resolve with nonoperative management is currently accruing patients for evaluation.[7]

Management of Specific Problems

Recurrent Intestinal Obstruction

All surgeons can readily remember the complicated patient with multiple previous abdominal operations and a frozen abdomen who presents with yet another bowel obstruction. An initial nonoperative trial is usually desirable and often safe. In those patients who do not respond conservatively, reoperation is required. This can often be a long and arduous procedure, with great care taken to prevent enterotomies or adjacent organ injury. In these difficult patients, various surgical procedures and pharmacologic agents have been tried in an effort to prevent recurrent adhesions and obstruction.

External plication procedures have been described, in which the small intestine or its mesentery is sutured in large, gently curving loops. Common complications have included the development of fistulas, gross leakage, peritonitis, and death. Because of frequent complications and low overall success rate, these procedures have largely been abandoned. Several series have reported moderate success with internal fixation or stenting procedures using a long intestinal tube inserted through the nose, a gastrostomy, or even a jejunostomy and left in place for 2 weeks or longer. Complications associated with these tubes include prolonged drainage of bowel contents from the tube insertion site, intussusception, and difficult removal of the tube, which may require surgical reexploration.

Pharmacologic agents, including corticosteroids and other anti-inflammatory agents, cytotoxic drugs, and antihistamines, have been used with limited success. The use of anticoagulants, such as heparin, dextran solutions, dicumarol, and sodium citrate, has modified the extent of adhesion formation, but their side effects far outweigh their efficacy. Intraperitoneal instillation of various proteinases (e.g., trypsin, papain, pepsin), which cause enzymatic digestion of the extracellular protein matrix, has been unsuccessful. Hyaluronidase has been of questionable value, and conflicting results have been obtained with fibrinolytic agents such as streptokinase, urokinase, and fibrinolytic snake venoms. In a prospective multicenter trial, the use of a hyaluronate-based, bioresorbable membrane reduced the incidence and severity of postoperative adhesion formation.[8] Another study found that placement of this membrane reduced the severity but not the incidence of postoperative adhesion in patients undergoing a Hartmann procedure. Longer term, randomized studies will be required to determine the efficacy of this material in preventing adhesions and ultimately to prevent bowel obstructions.

To date, the most effective means of limiting the number of adhesions is a good surgical technique. This includes the gentle handling of the bowel to reduce serosal trauma, avoidance of unnecessary dissection, exclusion of foreign material from the peritoneal cavity (the use of absorbable suture material when possible, the avoidance of excessive use of gauze sponges, and the removal of starch from gloves), adequate irrigation and removal of infectious and ischemic debris, and preservation and use of the omentum around the site of surgery or in the denuded pelvis.

Acute Postoperative Obstruction

Small bowel obstruction that occurs in the immediate postoperative period presents a challenge in regard to diagnosis and treatment.[5] Diagnosis is often difficult because the primary symptoms of abdominal pain and nausea or emesis may be attributed to a postoperative ileus. Electrolyte deficiencies, particularly hypokalemia, can be a cause of ileus and should be corrected. Plain abdominal films are usually not helpful in distinguishing an ileus from obstruction. CT may be useful in this regard, and in particular, enteroclysis studies may be helpful in determining whether an obstruction exists and, if so, the level of the obstruction. More than 90% of early postoperative obstructions are partial and will resolve spontaneously, given ample time. Conservative management in the form of bowel rest, fluid resuscitation, electrolyte replacement, and parenteral nutrition, if necessary, is routinely successful. However, the development of complete obstruction or signs of strangulation mandates reoperative intervention. Postoperative bowel obstruction after laparoscopic surgery is more commonly associated with a definitive obstruction point, such as a port site hernia or an internal hernia, and should prompt a high index of suspicion for the need for operative intervention.

Ileus

An ileus is defined as intestinal distention and the slowing or absence of passage of luminal contents without a demonstrable mechanical obstruction. An ileus can result from a number of causes, including drug induced, metabolic, neurogenic, and infectious factors (Box 49-2).

BOX 49-2 Causes of Ileus

- After laparotomy
- Metabolic and electrolyte derangements (e.g., hypokalemia, hyponatremia, hypomagnesemia, uremia, diabetic coma)
- Drugs (e.g., opiates, psychotropic agents, anticholinergic agents)
- Intra-abdominal inflammation
- Retroperitoneal hemorrhage or inflammation
- Intestinal ischemia
- Systemic sepsis

Adapted from Turnage RH, Bergen PC: Intestinal obstruction and ileus. In Feldman M, Scharschmidt FG, Sleisenger MH, editors: *Sleisenger and Fordtran's gastrointestinal and liver disease: Pathophysiology, diagnosis, management*, Philadelphia, 1998, WB Saunders, pp 1799–1810.

Pharmacologic agents that can produce an ileus include anticholinergic drugs, autonomic blockers, antihistamines, and various psychotropic agents, such as haloperidol and tricyclic antidepressants. One of the more common causes of drug-induced ileus in the operative patient is the use of opiates, such as morphine or meperidine. Metabolic causes of ileus are common and include hypokalemia, hyponatremia, and hypomagnesemia. Other metabolic causes include uremia, diabetic coma, and hypoparathyroidism. Neurogenic causes of an ileus include postoperative ileus, which occurs after abdominal operations. Spinal injury, retroperitoneal irritation, and orthopedic procedures on the spine or pelvis can result in an ileus. Finally, infections can result in an ileus; common infectious causes include pneumonia, peritonitis, and generalized sepsis from a nonabdominal source.

Patients often present in a manner similar to those with a mechanical small bowel obstruction. Abdominal distention, usually without the colicky abdominal pain, is the typical and most notable finding. Nausea and vomiting may occur but may also be absent. Patients with an ileus may continue to pass flatus and diarrhea, which may help distinguish these patients from those with a mechanical small bowel obstruction.

Radiologic studies may help distinguish ileus from small bowel obstruction. Plain abdominal radiographs may reveal distended small bowel as well as large bowel loops. In cases that are difficult to differentiate from obstruction, barium studies may be beneficial.

The treatment of an ileus is entirely supportive, with nasogastric decompression and IV fluids. The most effective treatment to correct the underlying condition may be aggressive treatment of the sepsis, correction of any metabolic or electrolyte abnormalities, and discontinuation of medications that may produce an ileus. Pharmacologic agents have been used but for the most part have been ineffective. Drugs that block sympathetic input (e.g., guanethidine) or stimulate parasympathetic activity (e.g., bethanechol, neostigmine) have been tried. Hormonal manipulation, using cholecystokinin or motilin, has been evaluated, but the results have been inconsistent. Erythromycin has been ineffective, and cisapride, although apparently beneficial in stimulating gastric motility, does not appear to alter intestinal ileus. Chewing gum has been suggested as an easy and inexpensive method to stimulate the cephalic phase of digestion (e.g., vagal cholinergic stimulation and the release of gastrointestinal hormones) and therefore a potential adjunct to prevent and to treat ileus. A more recent randomized trial demonstrated that chewing gum provides no benefit regarding return of bowel function or length of stay and even suggested that postoperative ileus may be further exacerbated by the use of sugared gum.

INFLAMMATORY AND INFECTIOUS DISEASES

Crohn's Disease

Crohn's disease is a chronic, transmural inflammatory disease of the gastrointestinal tract for which the definitive cause is unknown, although a combination of genetic and environmental factors has been implicated. Crohn's disease can involve any part of the alimentary tract from the mouth to the anus but most commonly affects the small intestine and colon. The most common clinical manifestations are abdominal pain, diarrhea, and weight loss. Crohn's disease can be complicated by intestinal obstruction or localized perforation with fistula formation. Medical and surgical treatments are palliative; however, operative therapy can provide effective symptomatic relief for patients with complications from Crohn's disease and produces a reasonable long-term benefit.

History

The first documented case of Crohn's disease was described by Morgagni in 1761. In 1913, the Scottish surgeon Dalziel described nine cases of intestinal inflammatory disease. However, it is the landmark paper by Crohn and colleagues in 1932 that provided, in eloquent detail, the pathologic and clinical findings of this inflammatory disease in young adults.[9] This classic paper crystallized the description of this inflammatory condition. Although many different (and sometimes misleading) terms have been used to describe this disease process, Crohn's disease has been universally accepted as its name.

Incidence and Epidemiology

Crohn's disease is the most common primary surgical disease of the small bowel. The incidence of Crohn's disease, which is rising in the United States for reasons that remain unclear, is estimated to be approximately 50 of 100,000 individuals in the general population.[10] The total direct and indirect costs for Crohn's disease in the United States have been estimated to be more than $800 million when factoring both inpatient hospital stays and outpatient visits. Crohn's disease primarily attacks young adults in the second and third decades of life. However, a bimodal distribution is apparent, with a second smaller peak occurring in the sixth decade of life. Crohn's disease is more common in urban dwellers, and although earlier reports suggested a somewhat higher female predominance, the two genders are affected equally. The risk for development of Crohn's disease is about twice as high in smokers as in nonsmokers. Several studies have indicated an increased incidence of Crohn's disease in women using oral contraceptives; however, more recent studies have shown no differences. Although Crohn's disease is uncommon in African blacks, blacks in the United States have rates similar to whites. Certain ethnic groups, particularly Jews, have a greater incidence of Crohn's disease than age- and gender-matched control subjects. Individuals born during the spring months (e.g., April to June) are more likely to develop Crohn's disease; there also appears to be a north-south gradient worldwide, and populations in higher latitudes have higher incidence rates than populations in lower latitudes. Of note, migrants moving from a low-risk region to a high-risk region have a risk for development of Crohn's disease that is similar to that in the high-risk region within one generation. There is a strong familial association, with the risk for development of Crohn's disease increased about 30-fold in siblings and 14- to 15-fold for all first-degree relatives. Other analyses supporting a genetic role for Crohn's disease have shown a concordance rate of only 3.7% in dizygotic twins but a 67% rate in monozygotic twins. More recent studies evaluating twins with and without Crohn's disease have used advanced genomic and proteomic techniques to show that intestinal microflora and epigenetic changes induced by environmental factors play an important role in disease development and progression in genetically susceptible individuals.[11]

Causes

The causes of Crohn's disease remain unknown. A number of potential causes have been proposed, with the most likely possibilities being infectious, immunologic, and genetic. Other possibilities that have met with various levels of enthusiasm include environmental and dietary factors, smoking, and psychosocial factors. Although these factors may contribute to the overall disease process, it is unlikely that they represent the primary causative mechanism for Crohn's disease.

Infectious agents. Although a number of infectious agents have been proposed as potential causes of Crohn's disease, the two that have received the most attention are mycobacterial infections, particularly *Mycobacterium paratuberculosis* and enteroadherent *E. coli*. The existence of atypical mycobacteria as a cause for Crohn's disease was proposed by Dalziel in 1913. Subsequent studies using polymerase chain reaction (PCR) techniques have confirmed the presence of mycobacteria in intestinal samples of patients with Crohn's disease. Transplantation of tissue from patients with Crohn's disease has resulted in ileitis, but antimicrobial therapy directed against mycobacteria has not been effective in ameliorating the established disease process. Strains of enteroadherent *E. coli* are in higher abundance in patients with Crohn's disease compared with the general population based on PCR analysis. More recent studies have used fluorescent in situ hybridization to demonstrate increased numbers of *E. coli* in the lamina propria of patients with active Crohn's disease compared with those with inactive disease. Furthermore, an increased number of *E. coli* has been associated with a shorter time before relapse of the disease.

Immunologic factors. Immunologic abnormalities suggested as etiologic factors in patients with Crohn's disease have included humoral and cell-mediated immune reactions directed against intestinal cells, suggesting an autoimmune phenomenon. Attention has focused on the role of cytokines, such as interleukin (IL)-1, IL-2, IL-8, and TNF-α, as contributing factors in the intestinal inflammatory response. The role of the immune response remains controversial in Crohn's disease and may represent an effect of the disease process rather than an actual cause.

Genetic factors. Genetic factors play an important role in the pathogenesis of Crohn's disease because the single strongest risk factor for development of disease is having a first-degree relative with Crohn's disease. Several genome-wide association sequencing studies have been performed and have identified more than 70 genes associated with Crohn's disease (Table 49-5). The genes with the strongest and most frequently replicated associations with Crohn's disease are *NOD2*, *IL23R*, and *ATG16L1*. Putative inflammatory bowel disease loci have been identified on chromosomes 16q, 5q, 19p, 7q, and 3p. The *CARD15/NOD2* gene, which acts as a pattern recognition receptor, has been characterized on the *IBD1* locus of 16q12-13. *CARD15* leads to impaired activation of the transcription factor NF-κB and also specifically codes for a protein expressed in monocytes, macrophages, dendritic cells, epithelial cells, and Paneth cells; *NOD2* is associated with a decreased expression of antimicrobial peptides by Paneth cells. The *NOD2* gene has been associated with increased likelihood and earlier need for surgery in Crohn's disease; *CARD15* is also helpful in distinguishing Crohn's disease from ulcerative colitis as it is more strongly associated with Crohn's disease, especially in patients of northern European descent. The *FHIT* gene located on 3p14.2 has been identified as a tumor suppressor gene and is suggested to play a role in the pathogenesis of Crohn's disease as well as in the development and progression of Crohn's disease–related cancers. A complex cellular and molecular cross-talk occurs between these genes, namely, *NOD2/CARD15* and the autophagy gene *ATG16L1*, which is associated with a synergistic increase in earlier onset and disease severity, especially in smokers.[12] Genetic profiling may be helpful in selecting patients who will benefit from intensified treatment with immunomodulators and anti-TNF therapy, thus decreasing medical nonresponse.

TABLE 49-5 Genetic Polymorphisms Related to Crohn's Disease

Genes and the Diagnosis of Crohn's Disease	
Genes related to innate pattern recognition receptors	*NOD2/CARD15, OCTN, TLR*
Genes related to epithelial barrier homeostasis	*IBD5, DLG5*
Genes related to molecular mimicry and autophagy	*ATG16L1, IRGM, LRRK2*
Genes related to lymphocyte differentiation	*IL23R, STAT3*
Genes related to secondary immune response and apoptosis	*MHC, HLA*
Genes and the Prognosis of Crohn's Disease	
Genes related to age at Crohn's disease onset	*TNFRSF6B, CXCL9, IL23R, NOD2, ATG16L1, CNR1, IL10, MDR1, DLG5, IRGM*
Genes Related to Crohn's Disease Behavior	
Stenotic/structuring behavior	*NOD2, TLR4, IL12B, CX3CR1, IL10, IL6*
Penetrating/fistulizing behavior	*NOD2, IRGM, TNF, HLADRB1, CDKAL1*
Inflammatory behavior	*HLA*
Granulomatous disease	*TLR4/CARD15*
Genes Related to Crohn's Disease Location	
Upper gastrointestinal	*NOD2, MIF*
Ileal	*IL10, CRP, NOD2, ZNF365, STAT3*
Ileocolonic	*ATG16L1, TCF4 (TCF7L2)*
Colonic	*HLA, TLR4, TLR1, TLR2, TLR6*
Other Genes Related to Crohn's Disease	
Genes related to Crohn's disease activity	*HSP702, NOD2, PAI1, CNR1*
Genes related to surgery	*NOD2, HLAG*
Genes related to dysplasia and cancer	*FHIT*
Genes related to extraintestinal manifestations	*CARD15, FcRL3, HLADRB103, HLAB27, HLA-B44, HLA-B35, TNFa-308A, TNF-1031C, STAT3*
Pharmacogenetics in Crohn's Disease	*CARD15, NAT, TPMT, MDR1, MIF, DLG5, TNF, LTA*

Adapted from Tsianos EV, Katsanos KH, Tsianos VE: Role of genetics in the diagnosis and prognosis of Crohn's disease. *World J Gastroenterol* 18:105–118, 2012.

More recent genome-wide association sequencing studies in monozygotic twins have shown no reproducible differences within twin pairs in comparing whole genome sequences and tissue-specific variants in the intestinal mucosa directly affected by the inflammation of Crohn's disease.[11] These findings suggest that it is unlikely that somatic mutations have a substantial impact on the development of the disease, and simple mendelian inheritance cannot account for the pattern of occurrence. Therefore, it is likely that multiple causes (e.g., environmental factors) contribute to the cause and pathogenesis of this disease.

Pathology

The most common sites of occurrence of Crohn's disease are the small intestine and colon. Genetic variations may determine the involvement of varying locations throughout the intestine.[13] Ileal involvement has been shown with mutations of *IL10, CRP, NOD2, ZNF365,* and *STAT3*; ileocolonic involvement has been shown with mutations of *ATG16L1, TCF4,* and *TCF7L2*; and colonic involvement has been associated with mutations of *HLA, TLR4, TLR1, TLR2,* and *TLR6*. The involvement of the large and small intestine has been noted in about 55% of patients. Thirty percent of patients present with small bowel disease alone, and in 15%, the disease appears limited to the large intestine. The disease process is discontinuous and segmental. In patients with colonic disease, rectal sparing is characteristic of Crohn's disease and helps distinguish it from ulcerative colitis. Perirectal and perianal involvement occurs in about one third of patients with Crohn's disease, particularly those with colonic involvement. Crohn's disease can also involve the mouth, esophagus, stomach, duodenum, and appendix. Involvement of these sites can accompany disease in the small or large intestine, but in only rare cases have these locations been the only apparent sites of involvement.

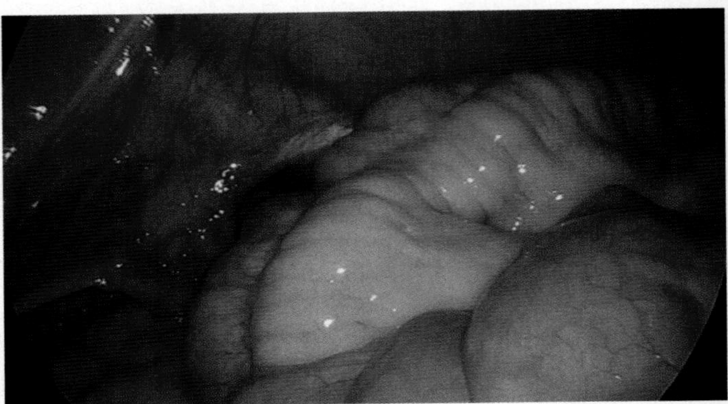

FIGURE 49-17 Laparoscopic evaluation of extensive fat wrapping caused by the circumferential growth of the mesenteric fat around the bowel wall. (Courtesy Dr. John Draus, University of Kentucky Medical Center, Lexington, KY.)

Gross pathologic features. At exploration, thickened gray-pink or dull purple-red loops of bowel are noted, with areas of thick gray-white exudate or fibrosis of the serosa. Areas of diseased bowel separated by areas of grossly appearing normal bowel, called *skip areas*, are commonly encountered. A striking finding of Crohn's disease is extensive fat wrapping caused by the circumferential growth of the mesenteric fat around the bowel wall (Fig. 49-17). As the disease progresses, the bowel wall becomes increasingly thickened, firm, rubbery, and almost incompressible (Fig. 49-18). The uninvolved proximal bowel may be dilated secondary to obstruction of the diseased segment. Involved segments often are adherent to adjacent intestinal loops or other viscera, with internal fistulas common in these areas. The mesentery of the involved segment is usually thickened, with enlarged lymph nodes often noted.

On opening of the bowel, the earliest gross pathologic lesion is a superficial aphthous ulcer noted in the mucosa. With increasing disease progression, the ulceration becomes pronounced, and complete transmural inflammation results. The ulcers are characteristically linear and may coalesce to produce transverse sinuses with islands of normal mucosa in between, thus giving the characteristic cobblestone appearance.

Microscopic features. Mucosal and submucosal edema may be noted microscopically before any gross changes. A chronic inflammatory infiltrate appears in the mucosa and submucosa and extends transmurally. This inflammatory reaction is characterized

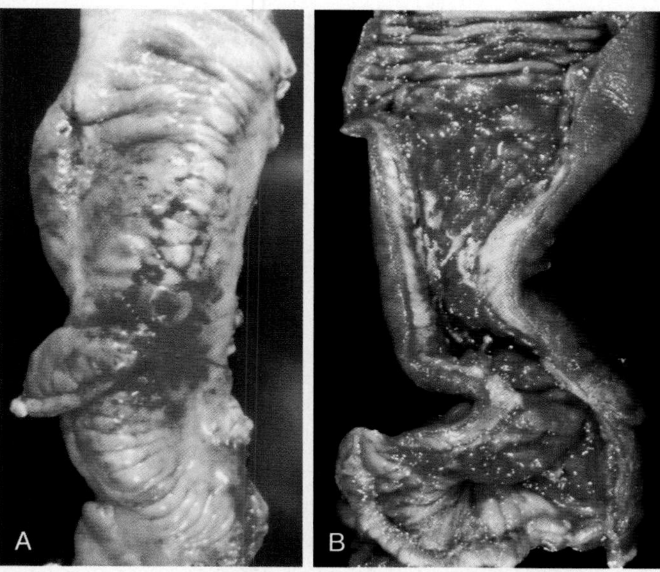

FIGURE 49-18 Gross Pathologic Features of Crohn's Disease. **A,** Serosal surface demonstrates extensive fat wrapping and inflammation. **B,** Resected specimen demonstrates marked fibrosis of the intestinal wall, stricture, and segmental mucosal inflammation. (Courtesy Dr. Mary R. Schwartz, Baylor College of Medicine, Houston, TX.)

by extensive edema, hyperemia, lymphangiectasia, intense infiltration of mononuclear cells, and lymphoid hyperplasia. Characteristic histologic lesions of Crohn's disease are noncaseating granulomas with Langerhans giant cells. Granulomas appear later in the course and are found in the wall of the bowel or in regional lymph nodes in 60% to 70% of patients (Fig. 49-19).

Clinical Manifestations

Crohn's disease can occur at any age, but the typical patient is a young adult in the second or third decade of life. The onset of disease is often insidious, with a slow and protracted course. Characteristically, there are symptomatic periods of abdominal pain and diarrhea interspersed with asymptomatic periods of varying lengths. With time, the symptomatic periods gradually become more frequent, more severe, and longer lasting. The most common symptom is intermittent and colicky abdominal pain, most commonly noted in the lower abdomen. The pain, however, may be more severe and localized and may mimic the signs and symptoms of acute appendicitis. Diarrhea is the next most frequent symptom and is present, at least intermittently, in about 85% of patients.[14] In contrast to ulcerative colitis, patients with Crohn's disease typically have fewer bowel movements, and the stools rarely contain mucus, pus, or blood. Systemic nonspecific symptoms include a low-grade fever present in about one third of the patients, weight loss, loss of strength, and malaise.

Clinically, Crohn's disease is often classified on the basis of age at onset, behavior, and site of origin. The Vienna Classification (Table 49-6) divides all patients into 24 distinct categories based on symptom onset (before or after the age of 40 years), disease behavior (nonstricturing/nonpenetrating, stricturing, or penetrating), and disease site (terminal ileum, colon, ileocolonic, upper gastrointestinal tract). This classification was developed to provide a reproducible staging of the disease, to help predict remission and relapse, and to direct therapy. The main intestinal complications of Crohn's disease include obstruction and perforation. Obstruction can occur as a manifestation of an acute exacerbation of active disease or as the result of chronic fibrosing lesions, which eventually narrow the lumen of the bowel, producing partial or near-complete obstruction. Free perforations into the peritoneal cavity leading to a generalized peritonitis can occur in patients with Crohn's disease, but this presentation is rare. More commonly, fistulas occur between the sites of perforation and adjacent organs, such as loops of small and large intestine, urinary bladder, vagina, stomach, and sometimes the skin, usually at the site of a previous laparotomy. Localized abscesses can occur near the sites of perforation. Patients with Crohn's colitis may develop toxic megacolon and present with a marked colonic dilation, abdominal tenderness, fever, and leukocytosis. Bleeding is typically indolent and chronic, but massive gastrointestinal bleeding can occasionally occur, particularly in duodenal Crohn's disease associated with chronic ulcer formation.

Long-standing Crohn's disease predisposes to cancer of the small intestine and colon. These carcinomas typically arise at sites of chronic disease and more commonly occur in the ileum. Most are not detected until the advanced stages, and prognosis is poor. Although this relative risk for small bowel cancer in Crohn's disease is approximately 100-fold, the absolute risk is still small. Of greater concern is the development of colorectal cancer in patients with colonic involvement and a long duration of disease. Dysplasia is the putative precursor lesion for Crohn's disease–associated cancer. Patients with long-standing Crohn's disease should have an equally aggressive colonoscopic surveillance regimen as patients with extensive ulcerative colitis. Small bowel adenocarcinoma associated with Crohn's disease has an aggressive behavior and a strong predominance of extracellular mucin. In surgical specimens from patients with Crohn's disease, mucinous-appearing anal fistulas and ileal areas of adhesion/retraction should always be closely examined by a pathologist to evaluate for dysplasia or malignancy.[15]

Extraintestinal cancer, such as squamous cell carcinoma of the vulva and anal canal and Hodgkin and non-Hodgkin lymphomas, may be more frequent in patients with Crohn's disease, especially those treated with immunomodulators.

Perianal disease (fissure, fistula, stricture, or abscess) is common and occurs in 25% of patients with Crohn's disease limited to the small intestine, 41% of patients with ileocolitis, and 48% of patients with colonic involvement alone. Perianal disease may be the sole presenting feature in 5% of patients and may precede the onset of intestinal disease by months or even years. Crohn's disease should be suspected in any patient with multiple, chronic perianal fistulas.

Extraintestinal manifestations of Crohn's disease may be present in 30% of patients. The most common symptoms are skin lesions (Fig. 49-20), which include erythema nodosum and pyoderma gangrenosum, arthritis and arthralgias, uveitis and iritis, hepatitis and pericholangitis, and aphthous stomatitis. In addition, amyloidosis, pancreatitis, and nephrotic syndrome may occur in these patients. These symptoms may precede, accompany, or appear independently of the underlying bowel disease.

Diagnosis

A diagnosis of Crohn's disease should be considered in patients with chronic recurring episodes of abdominal pain, diarrhea, and weight loss. Typically, the diagnostic modalities most commonly used include barium contrast studies and endoscopy. Barium radiographic studies of the small bowel reveal a number of characteristic findings, including a cobblestone appearance of the mucosa composed of linear ulcers, transverse sinuses, and clefts.

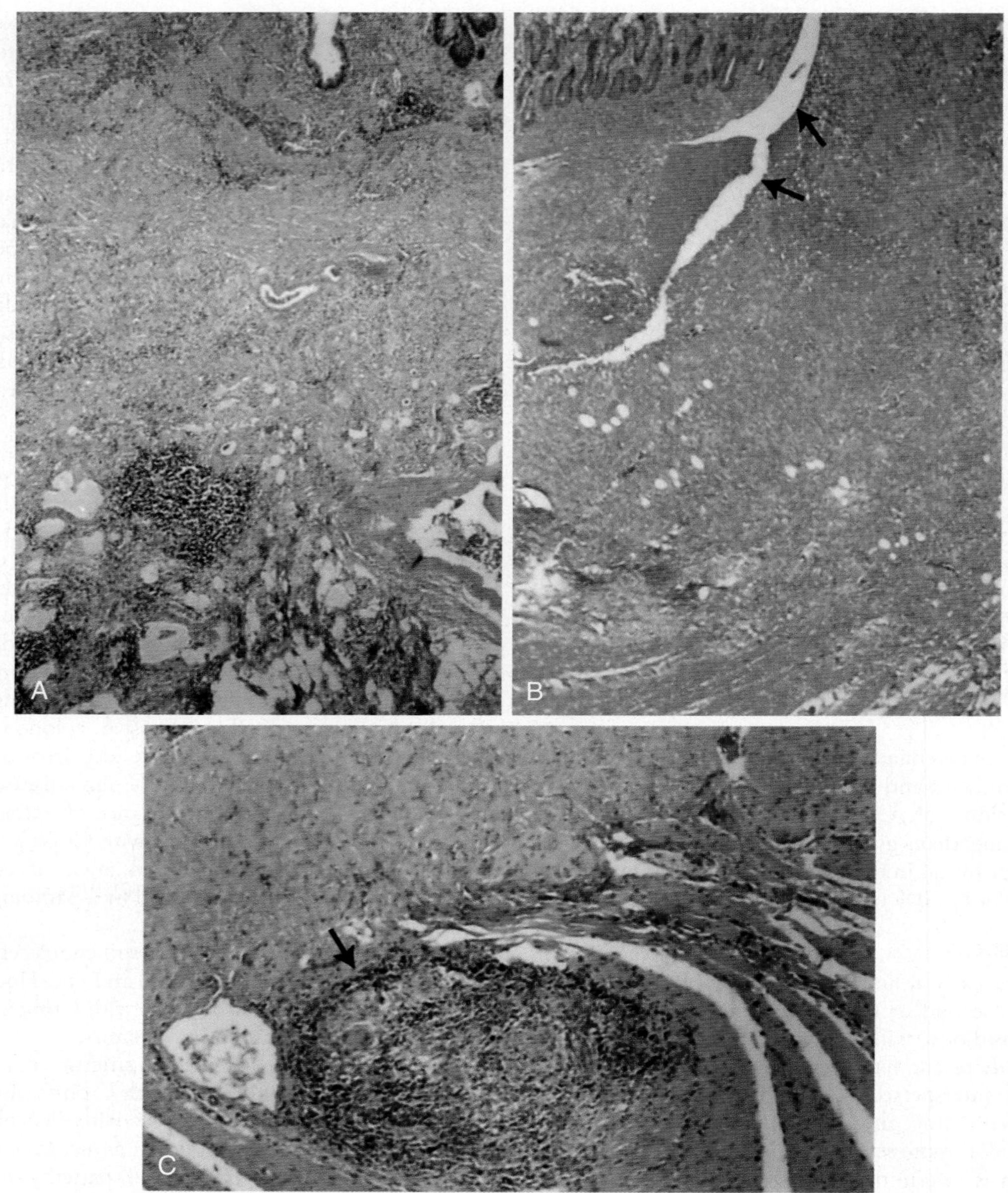

FIGURE 49-19 Microscopic Features of Crohn's Disease. A, Transmural inflammation. **B,** Fissure ulcer *(arrows)*. **C,** Noncaseating granuloma located in the muscular layer of the small bowel *(arrow)*. (Courtesy Dr. Mary R. Schwartz, Baylor College of Medicine, Houston, TX.)

TABLE 49-6 Vienna Classification of Crohn's Disease

Age at diagnosis (years)	A1: <40
	A2: ≥40
Behavior	B1: Nonstricturing/nonpenetrating
	B2: Stricturing
	B3: Penetrating
Location	L1: Terminal ileum
	L2: Colon
	L3: Ileocolon
	L4: Upper gastrointestinal tract

Adapted from Gasche C, Scholmerich J, Brynskov J, et al. A simple classification of Crohn's disease: Report of the Working Party for the World Congresses of Gastroenterology, Vienna 1998. *Inflamm Bowel Dis* 6:8–15, 2000.

Long lengths of narrowed terminal ileum (Kantor string sign) may be present in long-standing disease (Fig. 49-21). Segmental and irregular patterns of bowel involvement may be noted. Fistulas between adjacent bowel loops and organs may be apparent (Fig. 49-22).

CT may be useful in demonstrating the marked transmural thickening; it can also greatly aid in diagnosing extramural complications of Crohn's disease, especially in the acute setting (Fig. 49-23). Both MRI and CT are equally accurate in assessing disease activity and bowel damage; however, MRI may be superior to CT in detecting intestinal strictures and ileal wall enhancement. More recent studies have suggested limiting the use of CT in patients with long-standing Crohn's disease because of its significant radiation exposure and need for numerous studies during the course of the disease. Other radiation-free modalities, such as

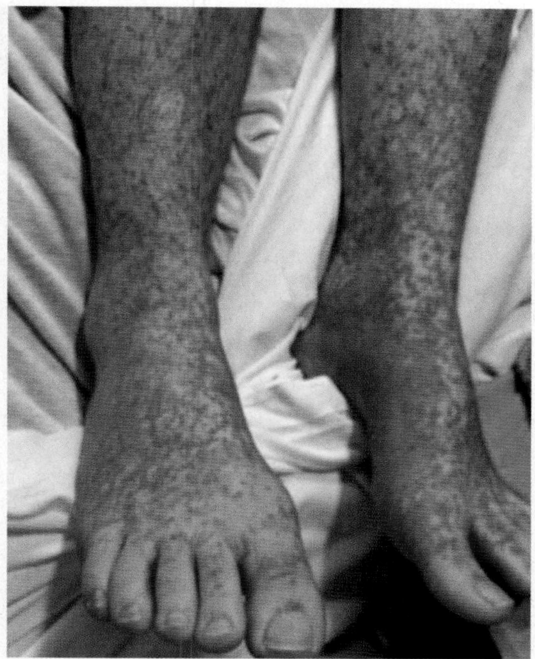

FIGURE 49-20 The most common extraintestinal presentations of Crohn's disease are skin lesions, which include erythema nodosum and pyoderma gangrenosum.

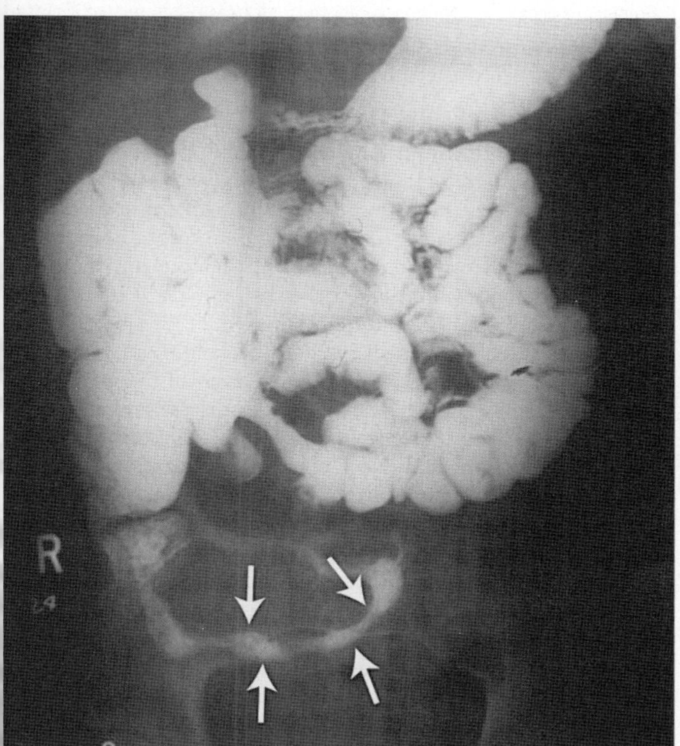

FIGURE 49-21 Small bowel series in a patient with Crohn's disease demonstrates a narrowed distal ileum *(arrows)* secondary to chronic inflammation and fibrosis. (Courtesy Dr. Melvyn H. Schreiber, The University of Texas Medical Branch, Galveston, TX.)

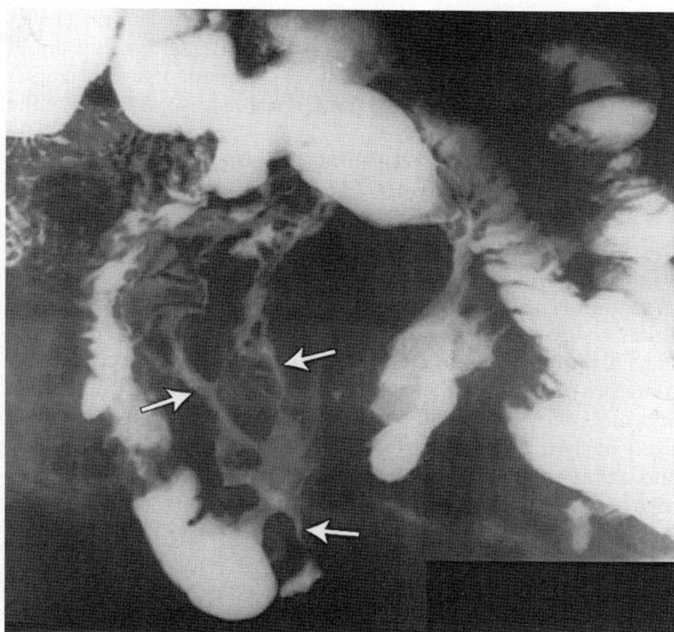

FIGURE 49-22 Crohn's disease with multiple short fistulous tracts communicating between the distal loops of ileum and the proximal colon *(arrows)*. (Courtesy Dr. Melvyn H. Schreiber, The University of Texas Medical Branch, Galveston, TX. Adapted from Evers BM, Townsend CM Jr, Thompson JC: Small intestine. In Schwartz SI, editor: *Principles of surgery*, ed 7, New York, 1999, McGraw-Hill, p 1233.)

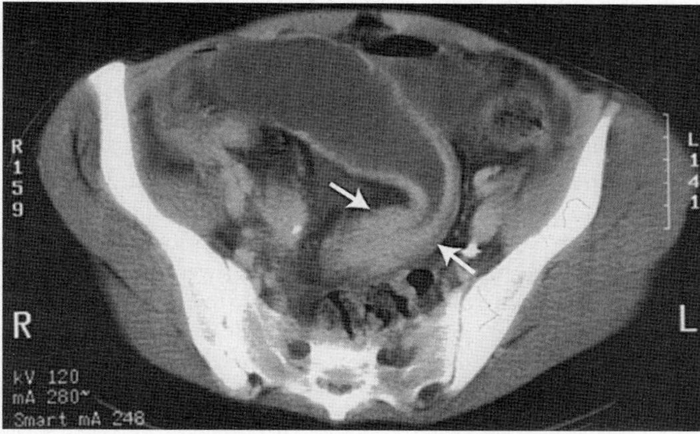

FIGURE 49-23 CT scan of a patient with Crohn's disease demonstrates marked thickening of the bowel *(arrows)* with a high-grade partial small bowel obstruction and dilated proximal intestine. (Courtesy Dr. Melvyn H. Schreiber, The University of Texas Medical Branch, Galveston, TX. Adapted from Evers BM, Townsend CM Jr, Thompson JC: Small intestine. In Schwartz SI, editor: *Principles of surgery*, ed 7, New York, 1999, McGraw-Hill, p 1233.)

MRI, ultrasound, and capsule endoscopy, should be considered in patients with long-standing Crohn's disease evaluated in an outpatient setting.[16] MRI enteroclysis is a useful adjunct to determine intestinal strictures as well as fistulas and sinus tracks; however, the relatively high cost, prolonged examination time, and limited availability may preclude many patients from receiving this procedure. Capsule endoscopy was approved by the Food and Drug Administration in 2001 and is helpful in the diagnosis of superficial mucosal abnormalities. The most commonly used criterion for an abnormal examination finding is the presence of three or more ulcers in the absence of nonsteroidal anti-inflammatory drug (NSAID) use.[17] The use of this modality is limited because of concern for capsule retention, which is defined as the presence of the capsule in the gastrointestinal tract for more than 2 weeks, which is of greater concern to patients with Crohn's disease, who have a significantly higher risk of retention (13%) compared with the general population (1% to 2.5%). Ultrasonography has limited value in the evaluation of patients with Crohn's disease and has an especially lower accuracy for detecting the disease proximal to the terminal ileum. One study determined that this modality failed to identify disease at this location in up to 67% of patients; however, ultrasound may be helpful in the assessment of undiagnosed right lower quadrant pain. When the colon is involved, sigmoidoscopy or colonoscopy may reveal characteristic aphthous ulcers with granularity and a normal-appearing surrounding mucosa. Intubation of the ileocecal valve during colonoscopy allows examination and biopsy of the terminal ileum but fails to evaluate other segments of the small intestine. With more progressive and severe disease, the ulcerations involve more and more of the bowel lumen and may be difficult to distinguish from ulcerative colitis. However, the presence of discrete ulcers and cobblestoning as well as the discontinuous segments of involved bowel favors a diagnosis of Crohn's disease. Endoscopic advances that allow better evaluation of the small intestine include single-balloon enteroscopy, double-balloon enteroscopy, and spiral enteroscopy; the most well established technique is double-balloon enteroscopy, which allows increased enteral intubation (240 to 360 cm) compared with push enteroscopy (90 to 150 cm) or ileocolonoscopy (50 to 80 cm). Limitations include specialized examiner skills and equipment, prolonged procedure times, and a 1% risk of complications (e.g., pancreatitis, perforation, or bleeding).

Serologic markers may also be useful in the diagnosis of Crohn's disease. In particular, perinuclear antineutrophil cytoplasmic antibody, anti–*Saccharomyces cerevisiae* antibody (ASCA), outer membrane porin of flagellin (anti-CBir1), and outer membrane porin of *E. coli* (OmpC-IgG) were able to predict the development of inflammatory bowel disease even in patients thought to be at low risk for development of disease.[18] ASCA has also been shown to be useful in differentiating Crohn's disease from ulcerative colitis as well as in determining patients who will require surgery in the future.

Noninvasive inflammatory markers, historically C-reactive protein and erythrocyte sedimentation rate, were used to aid in initial diagnosis, to rule out exacerbations, to monitor response to systemic therapy, and to predict relapse but were generally nonspecific and have largely been abandoned. Stool lactoferrin, an iron-binding protein in the secretory granules of neutrophils, and fecal calprotectin, a protein with antimicrobial properties released by squamous cells in response to inflammation, are inflammatory markers specific to the intestine that have shown promising results in the detection and surveillance of Crohn's disease. A prospective pilot study showed that both calprotectin and lactoferrin levels correlate well with endoscopic activity after ileocolonic resection for Crohn's disease.[19] Calprotectin had a sensitivity of 83% and a specificity of 93% to predict a risk of clinical recurrence, whereas lactoferrin had a sensitivity of 67% and a specificity of 71%. Despite being relatively inexpensive, these tests are still not widely available.

The differential diagnosis of Crohn's disease includes specific and nonspecific causes of intestinal inflammation. Bacterial inflammation (such as that caused by *Salmonella* and *Shigella*), intestinal tuberculosis, and protozoan infections (such as amebiasis) may be manifested as an ileitis. In the immunocompromised host, rare infections, particularly mycobacterial and cytomegalovirus (CMV) infections, have become more common and may cause ileitis. Acute distal ileitis may be a manifestation of early Crohn's disease, but it also may be unrelated, such as when it is caused by a bacteriologic agent (e.g., *Campylobacter*, *Yersinia*). Patients usually present in a similar fashion to those presenting with acute appendicitis, with a sudden onset of right lower quadrant pain, nausea, vomiting, and fever. These entities normally resolve spontaneously, and when they are noted during surgery, no biopsy or resection should be performed.

TABLE 49-7 Diagnosis of Crohn's Colitis versus Ulcerative Colitis

PARAMETER	CROHN'S COLITIS	ULCERATIVE COLITIS
Symptoms and Signs		
Diarrhea	Common	Common
Rectal bleeding	Less common	Almost always
Abdominal pain (cramps)	Moderate to severe	Mild to moderate
Palpable mass	At times	No (unless large cancer)
Anal complaints	Frequent (>50%)	Infrequent (<20%)
Radiologic Findings		
Ileal disease	Common	Rare (backwash ileitis)
Nodularity, fuzziness	No	Yes
Distribution	Skip areas	Rectum extending upward and continuously
Ulcers	Linear, cobblestone, fissures	Collar-button
Toxic dilation	Rare	Uncommon
Proctoscopic Findings		
Anal fissure, fistula, abscess	Common	Rare
Rectal sparing	Common (50%)	Rare (5%)
Granular mucosa	No	Yes
Ulceration	Linear, deep, scattered	Superficial, universal

In most cases, Crohn's disease of the colon can be readily distinguished from ulcerative colitis; however, in 5% to 10% of patients, the delineation between Crohn's disease and ulcerative colitis may be difficult if not impossible to make (Table 49-7). Ulcerative colitis almost always involves the rectum most severely, with lessening inflammation from the rectum to the ileocolic area. In contrast, Crohn's disease may be worse on the right side of the colon than on the left side, and sometimes the rectum is spared. Ulcerative colitis also demonstrates continuous involvement from rectum to proximal segments, whereas Crohn's disease is segmental. Although ulcerative colitis involves the mucosa of the large intestine, it does not extend deep into the wall of the bowel, as does Crohn's disease. Bleeding is a more common symptom in ulcerative colitis. Perianal involvement and rectovaginal fistulas are unusual in ulcerative colitis but are more common in Crohn's disease. Other endoscopic features of Crohn's disease are skip lesions, asymmetrical involvement of bowel, and the cobblestone appearance that results from ulcerations interspersed with islands of edematous mucosa.

Management

Medical therapy. There is no cure for Crohn's disease. Therefore, medical therapies are directed toward inducing and maintaining remission as well as preventing acute exacerbations or complications of the disease.[20] Surgery is advocated for neoplastic and preneoplastic lesions, obstructing stenoses, suppurative complications, or medically intractable disease. Narcotic analgesia should be avoided except during the perioperative period because of the potential for tolerance and abuse in the setting of chronic disease.[10] Drugs that have demonstrated efficacy in the induction or maintenance of remission in Crohn's disease include corticosteroids; TNF antagonists, such as infliximab, adalimumab, and certolizumab; aminosalicylates, such as sulfasalazine and mesalamine; immunosuppressive agents, such as azathioprine (AZT), 6-mercaptopurine (6-MP), methotrexate (MTX), and tacrolimus (FK-506); and antibiotics. Other innovative therapies, such as leukocyte trafficking inhibitors, interleukin inhibitors, and probiotics, in addition to molecular targeted therapies are currently being investigated.

Aminosalicylates. Sulfasalazine (Azulfidine) is an aminosalicylate with 5-aminosalicylic acid as the active moiety. Although a clear benefit has been noted in patients with colonic involvement, the effectiveness of sulfasalazine alone in the treatment of Crohn's disease limited to the small bowel is controversial, and its use in maintenance therapy has fallen out of favor. Mesalamine, which is also an aminosalicylate, provides a slow release of 5-aminosalicylic acid with passage through the small bowel and colon. Clinical trials have demonstrated efficacy of mesalamine at a dosage of 4 g/day without an increase in side effects. Furthermore, although mesalamine has shown some efficacy as a postoperative maintenance strategy and is an acceptable first-line therapy, most patients, especially those with relapsing disease, are treated with immunosuppressive agents with or without TNF antagonist therapy.[21] Studies are currently being conducted to evaluate the efficacy of even higher dosages of mesalamine to determine its continued utility as an appropriate first-line therapy.

Corticosteroids. Corticosteroids, particularly prednisone, are beneficial in moderate to severe Crohn's disease. Prednisone is not ideal for maintenance therapy as more than 50% of patients, particularly smokers, treated with corticosteroids become "steroid dependent," and chronic treatment is associated with osteoporosis and increased relapse rates of Crohn's disease.[10] Patients with moderate to severe disease should be treated with high-dose (40 to 60 mg daily) prednisone until resolution of symptoms and resumption of weight gain. Parenteral corticosteroids are indicated for patients with severe disease once the presence of an abscess has been excluded. IV steroids should be tapered once the patient is experiencing clinical improvement. Currently, there are no standards for corticosteroid taper, but doses are generally tapered by 5 to 10 mg per week until 20 mg, and then by 2.5 to 5 mg weekly until cessation. Dual-energy x-ray absorptiometry scan, calcium and vitamin D supplementation, and consideration of bisphosphonate therapy are warranted once corticosteroid therapy is initiated to identify baseline bone density and to prevent steroid-induced loss of bone mineral density.

Budesonide is a glucocorticoid steroid with promising implications for the symptomatic treatment of Crohn's disease. It has a high first-pass hepatic metabolism, which allows targeted delivery to the intestine while mitigating the systemic effects of steroid therapy. Controlled ileal release budesonide (9 mg/day) is effective when active disease is confined to the ileum or right colon and has been shown to be more effective than either placebo or mesalamine.[10] Given a relatively good response and its relative safety, budesonide is recommended as the preferred primary treatment to mesalamine as first-line therapy for patients with mild to moderately active Crohn's disease with localized ileal disease.

Antibiotics. Certain antibiotics have also been found to be effective in the primary therapy for Crohn's disease. Promising results were initially reported for metronidazole, but later studies determined that it was no more effective than placebo for inducing remission. Other antibiotics that have been used with varying success include ciprofloxacin, rifaximin, clofazimine, ethambutol, isoniazid, and rifabutin. Antibiotic therapy has a clear role in the septic complications associated with Crohn's disease and is beneficial in perianal disease. The mechanism of action of antibiotics in Crohn's disease is unclear, and side effects of these antibiotics preclude their long-term use. Therefore, antibiotics may play an adjunctive role in the treatment of Crohn's disease and, in selected patients, may be useful in treating perianal disease, enterocutaneous fistulas, or active colonic disease but should not be used in maintenance therapy or to induce remission.

Immunosuppressive agents. The immunosuppressive agents AZT, MTX, and 6-MP are effective in maintenance therapy for and treatment of moderate to severe Crohn's disease. AZT and 6-MP are effective for maintaining steroid-induced remission, and weekly IV MTX is effective for steroid-dependent and refractory Crohn's disease.[10] Despite their potential toxicity, these drugs have proved to be relatively safe in these patients; the most common side effects are pancreatitis, hepatitis, fever, and rash. The more disconcerting complications of immunosuppressants include chronic liver disease, bone marrow suppression, and the potential for malignant transformation. No prospective controlled trial has evaluated dose escalation or initiation of therapy using these drugs. Genetic polymorphisms for thiopurine methyltransferase (TPMT), which is the primary enzyme that metabolizes AZT and 6-MP, have been identified and can potentially be used to regulate therapy according to the measurement of their metabolites (6-thioguanine nucleotides). Patients with decreased TPMT activity have a significantly increased risk of fatal bone marrow suppression, and previous studies have reported severe myelosuppression in patients who are wild-type or heterozygous carriers for TPMT variant alleles, suggesting that TPMT genotype testing may be a safe screening tool to determine which patients may have a genetic predisposition to adverse outcomes with AZT or 6-MP treatment.

Other immunosuppressive agents that have been used with some effectiveness include cyclosporine and FK-506. FK-506 inhibits the production of IL-2 by helper T cells and was found to be effective for fistula improvement, but not fistula remission, in patients with perianal Crohn's disease. Both of these agents have been used in patients with severe disease who do not respond to IV steroids. Low-dose cyclosporine was not found to be efficacious; however, in uncontrolled studies, FK-506 demonstrated some benefit in patients with steroid-refractory disease.

Anticytokine and cytokine therapies. The introduction of anti-TNF therapy for Crohn's disease was considered to be a breakthrough in medical management. The first anti-TNF agent introduced was infliximab, a chimeric monoclonal antibody to TNF-α, which is efficacious and safe in the treatment of moderate to severe Crohn's disease and effective as a monotherapy for maintenance therapy and steroid-induced remission. Multiple studies have shown that treatment with infliximab results in perineal fistula closure in approximately two thirds of patients. Although it is highly effective in certain Crohn's disease patients with penetrating disease and extraintestinal disease, not every patient responds to infliximab. Also, there is an increased risk for tuberculosis reactivation, invasive fungal and other opportunistic infections, demyelinating central nervous system lesions, activation of latent multiple sclerosis, and exacerbation of congestive heart disease. Other promising TNF antagonists include adalimumab (humanized IgG1 monoclonal antibody), which is an effective maintenance agent and can be self-administered, and certolizumab (humanized antibody fragment [Fab]), which is ideal in pregnant and nursing women as it is linked to a polyethylene glycol moiety and does not cross the placenta and is not excreted in breast milk.

Novel therapies. Other investigational therapeutic agents include leukocyte trafficking inhibitors, interleukin inhibitors, anti–adhesion molecule antibodies, and probiotics. Natalizumab, a recombinant humanized monoclonal antibody against α_4 integrin, showed effectiveness in the induction and maintenance of remission in patients with active Crohn's disease. It was removed from the market after several patients developed progressive multifocal leukoencephalopathy but was later reinstituted for refractory Crohn's disease and is currently available only in specialized centers worldwide. Vedolizumab is a humanized monoclonal antibody that specifically binds to $\alpha_4\beta_7$ integrin and blocks its interaction with mucosal addressin cell adhesion molecule 1 (MadCAM-1), thus inhibiting the translocation of memory T lymphocytes into inflamed gastrointestinal parenchymal tissues. Results from phase 3 trials appear promising regarding the use of vedolizumab in the treatment of both Crohn's disease and ulcerative colitis. Because MadCAM-1 is preferentially expressed on blood vessels in the gastrointestinal tract, vedolizumab is more gut specific and therefore a more targeted form of immunosuppression. Also, vedolizumab prevents the gastrointestinal mucosal or transmural inflammation without the nonspecific neurologic side effects seen in less selective α_4 integrin inhibitors, such as natalizumab.[22] Ustekinumab, a humanized IgG1 monoclonal antibody that inhibits IL-12/23 through targeting of a shared p40 subunit, has been shown in two large trials to be effective in severe Crohn's disease that is refractory to anti-TNF therapies, but it has yet to be approved and is only available through compassionate use measures at some centers. Compounds are also being evaluated that block certain signaling pathways (e.g., NF-κB, mitogen-activated protein kinases, and peroxisome proliferator-activated receptor-γ); in limited studies, some of these compounds have shown clinical improvement, but results have varied, and these agents are still under development.

Nutritional therapy. Nutritional therapy in patients with Crohn's disease has been used with varying success. The use of chemically defined elemental diets has been shown in some studies to reduce disease activity, particularly in patients with disease localized to the small bowel, and they have been shown to reduce corticosteroid-induced toxicities.[10] Liquid polymeric diets may be as effective as elemental feedings and are more acceptable to patients. With few exceptions, standard elemental diets have not been effective in the maintenance of remission in Crohn's disease. Total parenteral nutrition (TPN) has also been shown to be of use in patients with active Crohn's disease; however, complication rates exceed those for enteral nutrition. Although the primary role of nutritional therapy is questionable in patients with inflammatory bowel disease, there is definitely a secondary role for nutritional supplementation to replenish depleted nutrient stores, allowing intestinal protein synthesis and healing, and to prepare patients for operation.

Smoking cessation. Although the implication of tobacco abuse as a causative factor in the development of Crohn's disease has been difficult to prove, smoking clearly affects the disease course. Smoking is associated with the late bimodal onset of disease and has been shown to increase the incidence of relapse and failure of maintenance therapy. It also appears to be associated with the severity of disease in a linear dose-response relationship. Tobacco exposure is an independent predictor of need for maintenance treatment, specifically biologic therapy. Therefore, smoking cessation therapy is an important component of medical therapy.

Surgical treatment. Although medical management is indicated during acute exacerbations of disease, most patients with chronic Crohn's disease will require surgery at some time during the course of their illness. Approximately 70% of patients will require surgical resection within 15 years after diagnosis. Indications for surgery include failure of medical treatment, bowel obstruction, and fistula or abscess formation. Most patients can be treated with elective surgery, especially with the improvement of medical management in the past decade.[22] However, patients with intestinal perforation, peritonitis, excessive bleeding, or toxic megacolon require urgent surgery. Children with Crohn's disease and resulting systemic symptoms, such as growth retardation, may benefit from resection. The extraintestinal complications of Crohn's disease, although not primary indications for operation, often subside after resection of involved bowel, with the exception of ankylosing spondylitis and hepatic complications.

The aim of surgery for Crohn's disease has shifted from radical operation to achieve inflammation-free margins of resection to minimal surgery, intended to remove just grossly inflamed tissue or to increase the luminal diameter of the bowel (i.e., strictureplasty). Even if adjacent areas of bowel are clearly diseased, they should be ignored. Early in the history of surgical therapy for Crohn's disease, surgeons tended to perform wider resections with the hope of cure or significant remission. However, repeated wide resections resulted in no greater remissions or cure and led to the short bowel syndrome, which is a devastating surgical complication. Frozen sections to determine microscopic disease are unreliable and should be performed only in the event that malignant disease is suspected. It must be emphasized that operative treatment of a complication is limited to that segment of bowel involved with the complication, and no attempt should be made to resect more bowel, even though grossly evident disease may be apparent.

Laparoscopic surgery for patients with Crohn's disease has been determined to be safe and feasible in appropriately selected patients, for example, those with localized abscesses, simple intra-abdominal fistulas, perianastomotic recurrent disease, and disease limited to the distal ileum. A large comparative study evaluating laparoscopic colectomy for Crohn's colitis determined that the laparoscopic group had a significantly shorter median operative time, earlier return of bowel function, and shorter hospital stay.[23] Other investigators caution against a laparoscopic approach in morbidly obese patients as obesity is an independent risk factor for conversion to open surgery, and obesity was also shown to increase blood loss, operative times, and incidence of incisional hernia.[24] Multiple randomized clinical trials have verified that laparoscopic surgery is associated with a more rapid recovery of bowel function and shorter hospital stay; the rate of disease recurrence is similar compared with open procedures. Randomized controlled trials with long-term follow-up have demonstrated that patients undergoing laparoscopic ileocolonic resection for Crohn's disease had improved body image and satisfaction with cosmesis of surgery and less incidence of incisional hernia compared with the open surgery group. The potential for earlier recovery after laparoscopic resection has stimulated interest in extending the role of surgical resection in inducing remission; the LIR!C trial is a randomized multicenter trial currently under way to provide evidence as to whether infliximab treatment or surgery is the best treatment for recurrent distal ileitis in Crohn's disease.[25]

The decision to perform a primary anastomosis versus initial ostomy formation with delayed reconstruction can be a difficult one for those with Crohn's disease. Patients are often malnourished, are receiving intensive immunosuppressive therapy, or present with some element of intra-abdominal sepsis. In general, standard surgical principles should direct this decision. Patients with adequate nutrition and minimal intra-abdominal sepsis can safely undergo primary anastomosis at the initial operation, whereas malnourished and septic patients are best served by diversion, if possible. Although caution should be exercised in performing an anastomosis in the setting of high-dose immunosuppression, large series have confirmed that surgery is safe for patients with Crohn's disease while they are receiving perioperative infliximab or immunosuppressive therapy. Regarding anastomotic technique, several studies suggest that creating a wider anastomosis with a stapled functional end-to-end anastomosis may decrease fecal stasis and subsequent bacterial overgrowth, which are implicated in anastomotic recurrence in Crohn's disease. However, a randomized controlled trial comparing side-to-side anastomosis versus end-to-end anastomosis determined that there was no difference in overall complication rates, anastomotic leak rates, or rates of symptomatic recurrence, with only a slight increase in endoscopic recurrence in the end-to-end anastomosis group (43% versus 38%). Kono and associates[26] introduced a new antimesenteric functional end-to-end hand-sewn anastomosis designed to minimize anastomotic restenosis in Crohn's disease. Assessment after 5 years demonstrated that the surgical recurrence rate at the anastomosis was lower than in the conventional anastomosis group, but larger randomized controlled trials are required to definitively determine its overall benefit.

Specific Problems

Acute ileitis (nonstricturing, nonpenetrating). Patients can present with acute abdominal pain localized to the right lower quadrant and signs and symptoms consistent with a diagnosis of acute appendicitis. At exploration, the appendix is found to be normal, but the terminal ileum is edematous and beefy red, with a thickened mesentery and enlarged lymph nodes. This condition, known as *acute ileitis*, is a self-limited disease. Acute ileitis may be a manifestation of early Crohn's disease but is most often unrelated. Bacteriologic agents such as *Campylobacter* and *Yersinia* may cause acute ileitis. Intestinal resection should not be performed. Although in the past the management of the appendix was controversial, it is clear now that in the absence of acute inflammatory involvement of the appendix or the cecum, appendectomy should be performed. This eliminates the appendix as a source of abdominal pain in the future.

Stricturing disease. Intestinal obstruction is the most common indication for surgical therapy in patients with Crohn's disease. Obstruction in these patients is often partial, and nonoperative management is initially indicated. The success of nonoperative management can often be predicted on the basis of the chronicity of symptoms at the affected site. In patients for whom it is difficult to determine whether the site of obstruction is caused by an acute exacerbation or a chronically strictured segment, stool lactoferrin and calprotectin levels may help identify acute inflammation, whereas certain genetic markers (e.g., *NOD2*, *TLR4*, *CX3CR1*) may predict potential success of medical therapy. In case of a chronic strictured segment, medical therapy is rarely effective.

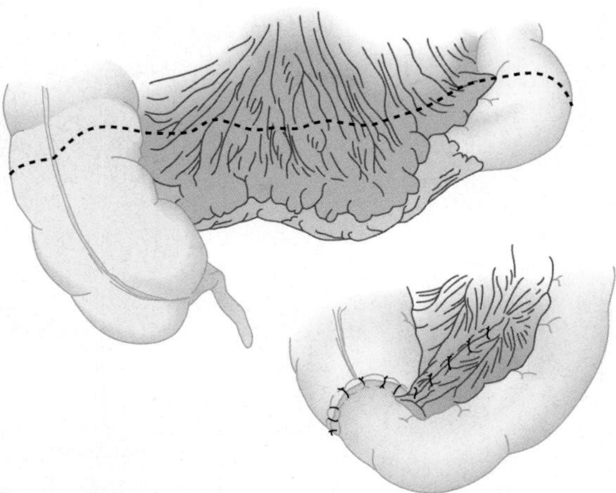

FIGURE 49-24 Resection of the ileum, ileocecal valve, cecum, and ascending colon for Crohn's disease of the ileum. Intestinal continuity is restored by end-to-end anastomosis.

Operative intervention is required for patients with complete obstruction and patients with partial obstruction whose condition does not resolve with nonoperative management. The treatment of choice for intestinal obstruction in patients with Crohn's disease is segmental resection of the involved segment with primary reanastomosis. This may involve segmental resection and primary anastomosis of a short segment of ileum if this is the site of the complication. More commonly, the cecum is involved contiguously with the terminal ileum, in which case resection of the involved terminal ileum and colon is required and the ileum is anastomosed to the ascending or transverse colon (Fig. 49-24).

In selected patients with obstruction caused by strictures (single or multiple), one option is to perform a strictureplasty that effectively widens the lumen but avoids intestinal resection. Strictureplasty is performed by making a longitudinal incision through the narrowed area of the intestine, followed by closure in a transverse fashion in a manner similar to that for a Heineke-Mikulicz pyloroplasty (Fig. 49-25*A*). For longer diseased segments (>10 cm), the strictureplasty can be performed similar to a Finney pyloroplasty (Fig. 49-25*B*) or a side-to-side isoperistaltic strictureplasty. Strictureplasty has the most application in patients in whom multiple short areas of narrowing are present over long segments of intestine, in those who have already had several previous resections of the small intestine, and when the areas of narrowing are caused by fibrous obstruction rather than by acute inflammation. This procedure preserves intestine and is associated with complication and recurrence rates comparable to those of resection and reanastomosis. Given the concerns for development of carcinoma at chronically strictured segments, full-thickness biopsy with frozen section of the stricture site has been advocated at the time of surgery to rule out malignant disease before strictureplasty is performed (Box 49-3).

In the past, bypass procedures were commonly used. There are two types of bypass operations: exclusion bypass and simple (continuity) bypass. For certain types of ileocecal disease associated with an abscess or phlegmon densely adherent to the retroperitoneum, the proximal transected end of the ileum is anastomosed to the transverse colon in an end-to-side fashion with or without construction of a mucous fistula using the distal transected end of the ileum (exclusion bypass), or an ileotransverse colonic anastomosis is made in a side-to-side fashion (continuity bypass).

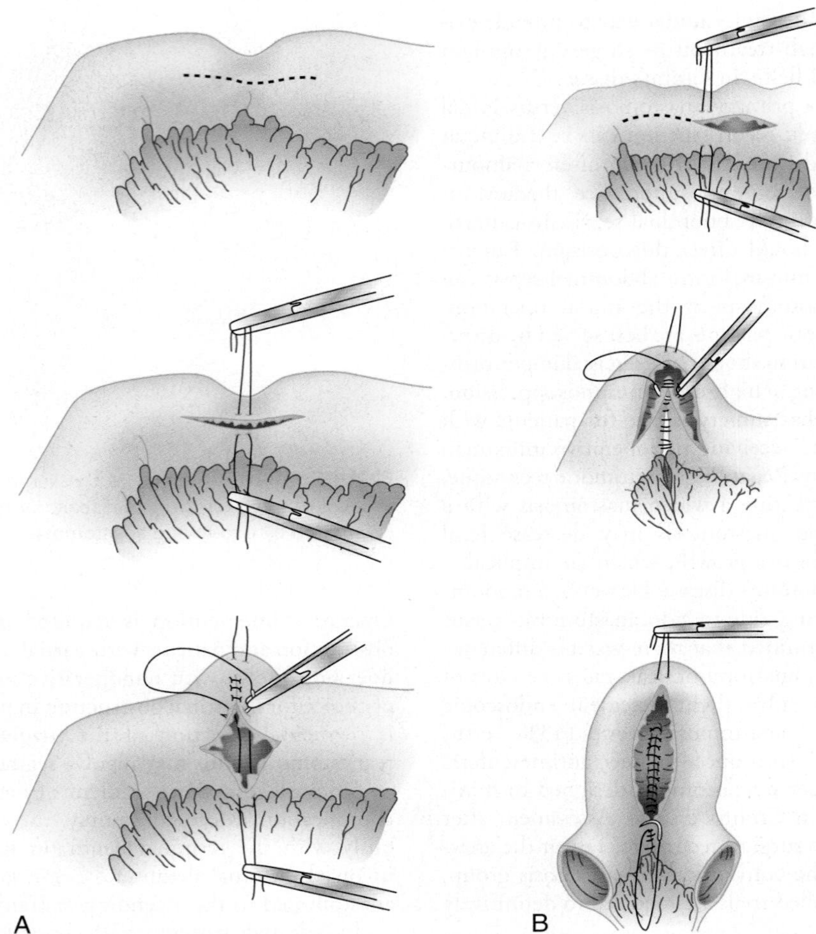

FIGURE 49-25 A, Technique of short strictureplasty in the manner of a Heineke-Mikulicz pyloroplasty. **B,** For longer diseased segments, strictureplasty may be performed in a manner similar to Finney pyloroplasty. (Adapted from Alexander-Williams J, Haynes IG: Up-to-date management of small-bowel Crohn's disease. In Mannick JA, editor: *Advances in surgery*, St. Louis, 1987, Mosby, pp 245–264.)

BOX 49-3 Contraindications to Strictureplasty

Excessive tension due to rigid and thickened bowel segments
Perforation of the intestine
Fistula or abscess formation at the intended strictureplasty site
Hemorrhagic strictures
Multiple strictures within a short segment
Malnutrition or hypoalbuminemia (<2.0 g/dL)
Suspicion of cancer at the intended strictureplasty site

Adapted from Yamamoto T, Watanabe T: Surgery for luminal Crohn's disease. *World J Gastroenterol* 20:78–90, 2014.

Currently, bypass with exclusion is used only in patients with severe gastroduodenal Crohn's disease not amenable to strictureplasty, older poor-risk patients, patients who have had several prior resections and cannot afford to lose any more bowel, and those in whom resection would necessitate entering an abscess or endangering a normal structure.

Penetrating disease. Fistula and abscess in patients with Crohn's disease are relatively common and usually involve the adjacent small bowel, colon, or other surrounding viscera (e.g., bladder). The presence of a radiographically demonstrable enteroenteral fistula without any signs of sepsis or other complications is not in itself an indication for surgery. Furthermore, penetrating disease is particularly sensitive to anticytokine therapy, and a conservative, surgical approach to Crohn's disease–related fistula is most appropriate. However, many of these patients will require eventual resection as the disease progresses and they have progressively worsening abdominal pain. Enterocutaneous fistulas may develop but are rarely spontaneous and are more likely to follow resection or drainage of intra-abdominal abscesses. Ideally, enterocutaneous fistulas should be managed by excising the fistula tract along with the diseased segment of intestine and performing a primary reanastomosis. If the fistula forms between two or more adjacent loops of diseased bowel, the involved segments should be excised. Alternatively, if the fistula involves an adjacent normal organ, such as the bladder or colon, only the segment of the diseased small bowel and fistulous tract should be resected, and the defect in the normal organ should simply be closed. Most patients with ileosigmoid fistulas do not necessarily require resection of the sigmoid because the disease is usually confined to the small bowel. However, if the segment of sigmoid is also found to have Crohn's disease, it should be resected along with the segment of diseased small bowel.

Perforation. Penetrating disease in the form of perforation into the free peritoneal cavity occurs occasionally but is not common in patients with Crohn's disease. Typically, penetration is manifested with a localized abscess densely adherent to the diseased segment of bowel. In cases of free perforation, the segment of involved bowel should be resected, and in the presence of minimal contamination, a primary anastomosis should be performed. If generalized peritonitis is present, a safer option may be to perform enterostomies until the intra-abdominal sepsis is controlled and then return for restoration of intestinal continuity. Abscesses can be treated with percutaneous drainage and antibiotics, although fistula or uncontrolled sepsis may ultimately develop, requiring resection with or without primary anastomosis.

Gastrointestinal bleeding. Although anemia from chronic blood loss is common in patients with Crohn's disease, life-threatening gastrointestinal hemorrhage is rare. The incidence of hemorrhage is more common in patients with Crohn's disease involving the colon rather than the small bowel. As with the other complications, the segment involved should be resected and intestinal continuity restored. Arteriography may be useful to localize the bleeding before surgery. In cases of bleeding associated with duodenal disease, endoscopic intervention is usually successful. However, in cases of failure, duodenotomy with oversewing of the bleeding ulcerative area is indicated.[22]

Urologic complications. Genitourinary complications occur in up to one third of patients with Crohn's disease. The most common urologic complication is ureteral obstruction, which is usually secondary to ileocolic disease with retroperitoneal abscess. Surgical treatment of the primary intestinal disease is adequate in most patients. In a few cases of long-standing inflammatory disease, periureteric fibrosis may be present and require ureterolysis with or without ureteral stenting.

Cancer. Patients with long-standing Crohn's disease of the small bowel and, in particular, the colon have an increased incidence of cancer. The management of these patients is the same as that for any patient—resection of the cancer with appropriate margins and regional lymph nodes. Patients with cancer associated with Crohn's disease commonly have a worse prognosis than those who do not have Crohn's disease, largely because the diagnosis in these patients is delayed. A strictureplasty should not be performed if malignant disease is suspected.

Colorectal disease. The same principle applies to patients with Crohn's disease limited to the colon as to those with disease to the small bowel, that is, surgical resection should be limited to the segment producing the complications. Indications for surgery include a lack of response to medical management and complications of Crohn's colitis, which include obstruction, hemorrhage, perforation, and toxic megacolon. Depending on the diseased segments, procedures commonly include segmental colectomy with colocolonic anastomosis, subtotal colectomy with ileoproctostomy, and, in patients with extensive perianal and rectal disease, total proctocolectomy with Brooke ileostomy. Laparoscopic colectomy for Crohn's colitis may be safely performed by experienced surgeons.[23] Patients with toxic megacolon should undergo colectomy, closure of the proximal rectum, and end ileostomy. Strictureplasty has limited usefulness in colonic Crohn's disease, and concerns of malignant transformation at an area of colonic obstruction should limit its application.

A particularly troubling problem after proctocolectomy in patients with Crohn's disease is delayed healing of the perineal wound. It has been found that more than half of perineal wounds are open 6 months after surgery in patients with Crohn's disease. Persistent nonhealing wounds require excision with secondary closure. Large cavities or sinuses may be filled by using well-vascularized pedicles of muscle (e.g., gracilis, semimembranosus, rectus abdominis) or omentum or by using an inferior gluteal myocutaneous graft.

Although controversial, continence-preserving operations, such as ileal pouch–anal anastomosis or continent ileostomies (Kock pouch), may be considered in very carefully selected patients with Crohn's disease isolated to the colon who undergo thorough counseling about the increased risk of anastomotic failure and wound complication. However, they should never be considered in patients with evidence of terminal ileal or perianal disease as these patients have a significantly increased rate of recurrence of Crohn's disease in the pouch, fistulas to the anastomosis, and peripouch abscesses.[22]

Perianal disease. Diseases involving the perianal region include fissures and fistulas and are common in patients with Crohn's disease, particularly those with colonic involvement. The treatment of perianal disease should be nonoperative unless an abscess or complex fistula develops, and even in these cases, surgery should be approached cautiously and limited to addressing the specific problem with minimal tissue loss. Nonsuppurative, chronic fistulization or perianal fissuring is treated with antibiotics, immunosuppressive agents (e.g., AZT or 6-MP), and infliximab, which is the most widely supported therapy as it has shown the best results in fistula closure.[10] Several uncontrolled studies have shown some benefit with cyclosporine or FK-506 treatment.

Wide excision of abscesses or fistulas is not indicated, but more conservative interventions, including the liberal placement of drainage catheters and noncutting setons, are preferable. Definitive fistulotomy is indicated for most patients with superficial, low trans-sphincteric, and low intersphincteric fistulas, although one must recognize that some degree of anal stenosis may occur as a result of chronic inflammation. High trans-sphincteric, suprasphincteric, and extrasphincteric fistulas are usually treated with noncutting setons. Fissures are usually lateral, relatively painless, large, and indolent and often respond to conservative management. Abscesses should be drained, but large excisions of tissue *should not* be performed. Advancement flap closure of perineal fistulas may be required in certain cases. Selective construction of diverting stomas has good results in combination with optimal medical therapy to induce remission of inflammation. Proctectomy may be infrequently required in a subset of patients who have persistent and unremitting disease despite conservative medical and surgical therapy.

Duodenal disease. Crohn's disease of the duodenum occurs in approximately 1% to 5% of patients with Crohn's disease and occurs most commonly in the duodenal bulb.[22] Operative intervention is uncommon. The primary indication for surgery in these patients is duodenal obstruction that does not respond to medical therapy, with endoscopic balloon dilation and surgery being the mainstays of treatment. Gastrojejunostomy to bypass the disease rather than duodenal resection is the procedure of choice. Strictureplasties have been performed with success in selected patients and may avoid the marginal ulceration and diarrhea associated with gastrojejunostomy.

Prognosis

Crohn's disease is a chronic inflammatory disorder that is not medically or surgically curable; therefore, therapeutic approaches are required to induce and to maintain symptomatic control, to improve quality of life, and to minimize long-term complications.

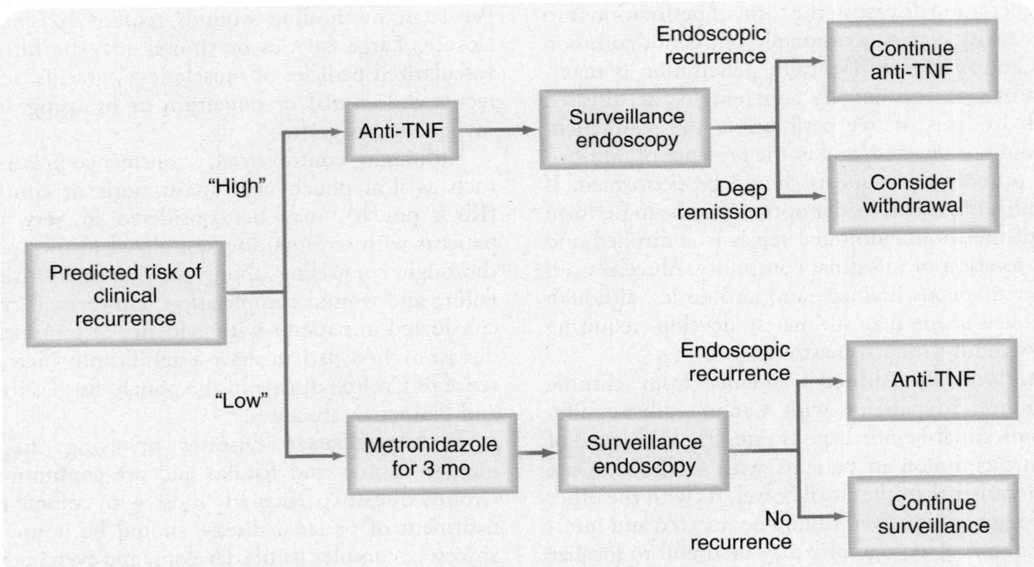

FIGURE 49-26 Suggested algorithm for deciding when to administer postoperative prophylaxis based on effectiveness of treatment. (Adapted from Vaughn BP, Moss AC: Prevention of post-operative recurrence of Crohn's disease. *World J Gastroenterol* 20:1147–1154, 2014.)

It is estimated that approximately 80% of patients will require surgery at some point in their lifetime.[27] Symptomatic recurrence varies from 40% to 80%, and endoscopic recurrence is much higher, with up to 90% of patients having visible lesions within 5 years. The only clearly modifiable risk factor is smoking cessation. Surgery is generally implicated in the event that the patient fails to respond to medical therapy or develops complications, but multiple studies have shown that patients report significant improvement in quality of life scores after surgical intervention. Although postsurgical recurrence is high, algorithms using careful endoscopic surveillance combined with biologic therapy play a role in the prevention of postoperative recurrence of Crohn's disease (Fig. 49-26). Although there is currently no cure for this disease, advances in medical and surgical therapies have clearly increased quality of life and disease-free progression.

Standardized mortality rates in patients with Crohn's disease are increased in those patients whose disease began before the age of 20 years and in those who have had disease present for longer than 13 years. Long-term survival studies have suggested that patients with Crohn's disease have a death rate approximately two to three times higher than that in the general population, which is most commonly related to chronic wound complications and sepsis. Gastrointestinal cancer remains the leading cause of disease-related death in patients with Crohn's disease; other causes of disease-related deaths include sepsis, thromboembolic complications, and electrolyte disorders.

Typhoid Enteritis

Typhoid fever remains a significant problem in developing countries, most commonly in areas with contaminated water supplies and inadequate waste disposal. It infects roughly 21.6 million people and kills an estimated 200,000 people every year worldwide. Children and young adults are most often affected. Improvements in sanitation have decreased the incidence of typhoid fever in industrialized countries. In the United States, most cases of typhoid fever arise in international travelers; however, unrecognized and untreated typhoid fever is a life-threatening illness of several weeks' duration with long-term morbidity.

Typhoid enteritis is an acute systemic infection caused primarily by *Salmonella typhi*. The pathologic events of typhoid fever are initiated in the intestinal tract after oral ingestion of the typhoid bacillus. These organisms penetrate the small bowel mucosa, making their way rapidly to the lymphatics and then systemically. Hyperplasia of the reticuloendothelial system, including lymph nodes, liver, and spleen, is characteristic of typhoid fever. Peyer's patches in the small bowel become hyperplastic and may subsequently ulcerate, with complications of hemorrhage or perforation.

The diagnosis of typhoid fever is confirmed by isolating the organism from blood (positive in 90% of the patients during the first week of the illness), bone marrow, and stool cultures. In addition, the finding of high titers of agglutinins against O and H antigens (Widal test) was used for decades but was found to be nonspecific and is no longer an acceptable clinical method. Assays for the diagnosis of *S. typhi* using PCR assay have had varying success. Combining assays of blood and urine achieved a sensitivity of 83% and reported specificity of 100%. Indirect hemagglutination, indirect fluorescent Vi antibody, and indirect enzyme-linked immunosorbent assay for IgM and IgG antibodies to *S. typhi* polysaccharide are promising, but the success rates of these assays vary greatly in the literature.

Typhoid fever and uncomplicated typhoid enteritis are treated by antibiotic administration. If a patient presents with clinical symptoms and has been in an endemic area, broad-spectrum empirical antibiotics should be started immediately. Treatment should not be delayed for confirmatory tests because prompt treatment drastically reduces the risk of complications and fatalities. Antibiotic therapy should be narrowed once more information is available. Chloramphenicol was initially the mainstay of treatment in the 1950s, but widespread antibiotic resistance occurred. Currently, the most widely used agents are fluoroquinolones and third-generation cephalosporins.

Complications requiring potential surgical intervention include hemorrhage and perforation. The incidence of hemorrhage was reported to be as high as 20% in some series, but with the availability of antibiotic treatment, this figure has decreased. When hemorrhage occurs, transfusion is indicated and usually suffices. Rarely, laparotomy must be performed for uncontrollable, life-threatening hemorrhage. Intestinal perforation through an ulcerated Peyer's patch occurs in approximately 2% of cases. Typically, it is a single perforation in the terminal ileum, and simple closure of the perforation is the treatment of choice. With multiple perforations, which occur in about 25% of patients, resection with primary anastomosis or exteriorization of the intestinal loops may be required.

Enteritis in the Immunocompromised Host

The acquired immunodeficiency syndrome (AIDS) epidemic as well as the widespread use of immunosuppressive agents after organ transplantation has resulted in a number of rare and exotic pathogens infecting the gastrointestinal tract. Almost all patients with AIDS have gastrointestinal symptoms during their illness, the most common of which is diarrhea. However, the surgeon may be asked to evaluate the immunocompromised patient with abdominal pain, an obvious acute abdomen, or gastrointestinal bleeding; a number of protozoal, bacterial, viral, and fungal organisms may be responsible.

Protozoa

Protozoa (e.g., *Cryptosporidium*, *Isospora*, and *Microsporidium*) are the most frequent class of pathogens causing diarrhea in patients with AIDS. The small bowel is the most common site of infection. Diagnosis may be established by acid-fast staining of the stool or duodenal secretions, but the introduction of specific antigen tests for stool examination has improved diagnostic capabilities. Immunochromatography cards for the rapid detection of protozoal proteins from a small sample of stool are available from several different commercial sources and are more sensitive and more specific (>90%) than the traditional microscopic examinations. Symptoms are most commonly related to diarrhea, which may be at times intractable. Current treatment regimens have not been entirely effective, but drugs such as cotrimoxazole and nitazoxanide appear to elicit a treatment response for cryptosporidiosis, and one study found no *Cryptosporidium* oocysts in the stools of patients receiving highly active antiretroviral therapy.[28]

Bacteria

Infections by enteric bacteria are more frequent and more virulent in individuals infected with human immunodeficiency virus (HIV) than in healthy hosts. *Salmonella*, *Shigella*, and *Campylobacter* are associated with higher rates of bacteremia and antibiotic resistance in the immunocompromised patient. The diagnosis of *Shigella* or *Salmonella* infection may be established by stool cultures. The diagnosis of *Campylobacter* infection is not as easily established because stool cultures are often negative, but PCR techniques evaluating stool and serum have shown promising diagnostic results in patients with negative cultures. These enteric infections are manifested clinically with high fever, abdominal pain, and diarrhea that may be bloody. Abdominal pain may mimic an acute abdomen. Bacteremia and serious infections should be treated by IV administration of imipenem antibiotics; ciprofloxacin is an attractive choice if the organisms are multiply resistant; the pregnant patient may be safely treated with erythromycin. The incidence of *Campylobacter* infection among patients with AIDS who were treated with rifabutin prophylaxis was reported to be decreased compared with untreated controls.

Diarrhea caused by *Clostridium difficile* is more common in patients with AIDS because of the increased antibiotic use in this population compared with healthy hosts. Diagnosis is by standard assays of stool for *C. difficile* enterotoxin. Treatment with metronidazole or vancomycin is usually effective.

Mycobacteria

Mycobacterial infection is a frequent cause of intestinal disease in immunocompromised hosts. This can be secondary to *Mycobacterium tuberculosis* or *Mycobacterium avium complex* (MAC), which is an atypical mycobacterium related to the type that causes cervical adenitis (scrofula). The usual route of infection is by swallowed organisms that directly penetrate the intestinal mucosa. The luminal gastrointestinal tract is affected by MAC infection, with massive thickening of the proximal small intestine often noted (Fig. 49-27). Clinically, patients with MAC present with diarrhea, fever, anorexia, and progressive wasting.

The most frequent site of intestinal involvement of *M. tuberculosis* is the distal ileum and cecum, with approximately 90% of patients demonstrating disease at this site. The gross appearance can be ulcerative, hypertrophic, or ulcerohypertrophic. The bowel wall appears thickened, and an inflammatory mass often surrounds the ileocecal region. Acute inflammation is apparent, as are strictures and even fistula formation. The serosal surface is normally covered with multiple tubercles, and mesenteric lymph nodes are frequently enlarged and thickened; on sectioning, caseous necrosis is noted. The mucosa is hyperemic, edematous, and, in some cases, ulcerated. On histologic evaluation, the distinguishing lesion is a granuloma, with caseating granulomas found most commonly in the lymph nodes. Most patients

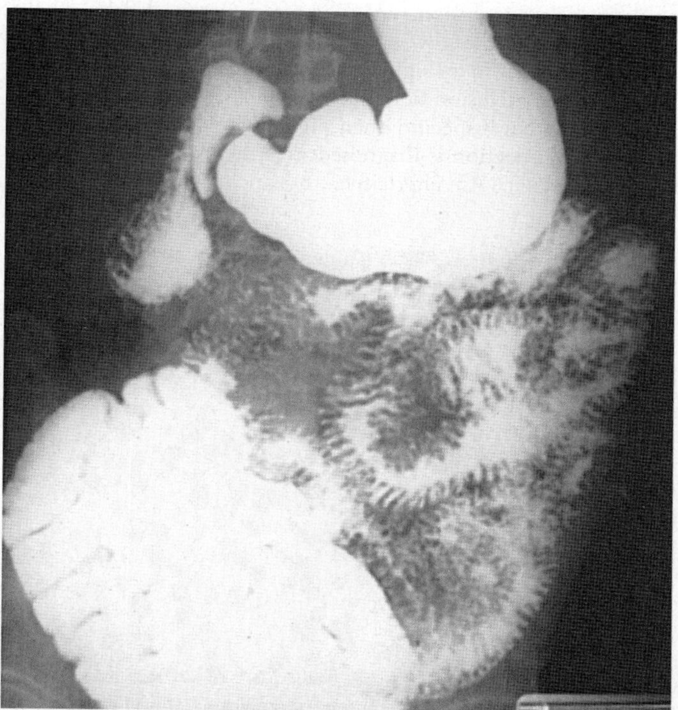

FIGURE 49-27 Barium radiograph of a patient with AIDS shows thickened intestinal folds consistent with enteritis secondary to atypical mycobacterium. (Courtesy Dr. Melvyn H. Schreiber, The University of Texas Medical Branch, Galveston, TX.)

complain of chronic abdominal pain that may be nonspecific, weight loss, fever, and diarrhea.

The diagnosis of mycobacterial infection is made by identification of the organism in tissue by direct visualization with an acid-fast stain, culture of the excised tissue, or PCR assay. Radiographic examinations usually reveal a thickened mucosa with distorted mucosal folds and ulcerations. CT may be useful and shows a thickening of the ileocecal valve and cecum.

The treatment of *M. tuberculosis* is similar in the immunocompromised or nonimmunocompromised host. The organism is usually responsive to multidrug antimicrobial therapy. The therapy for MAC infection is evolving; drugs that have been successfully used in vivo and in vitro include amikacin, ciprofloxacin, cycloserine, and ethionamide. Clarithromycin has also been successfully used in combination with other agents. Surgical intervention may be required for intestinal tuberculosis, particularly *M. tuberculosis*. Obstruction and fistula formation are the leading indications for surgery; however, with current treatment, most fistulas now respond to medical management. Surgery may be necessary for ulcerative complications when free perforation, perforation with abscess, or massive hemorrhage occurs. The treatment is usually resection with anastomosis.

Viruses

CMV is the most common viral cause of diarrhea in immunocompromised patients. Clinical manifestations include intermittent diarrhea accompanied by fever, weight loss, and abdominal pain. The manifestations of enteric CMV infection result from mucosal ischemic ulcerations, which account for the high rate of perforations noted with CMV. As a result of the diffuse ulcerating involvement of the intestine, patients may present with abdominal pain, peritonitis, or hematochezia. Diagnosis of CMV is made by demonstrating viral inclusions. The most characteristic form is an intranuclear inclusion, which is often surrounded by a halo, producing a so-called owl's eye appearance. There may also be cytoplasmic inclusions (Fig. 49-28). Cultures for CMV are usually positive when inclusion bodies are present, but these cultures are less sensitive and specific than histopathologic identification. Once CMV infection is diagnosed, treatment is usually effective with ganciclovir. An alternative to ganciclovir is foscarnet, a pyrophosphate analogue that inhibits viral replication. Infections with other less common viruses, including adenovirus, rotavirus, and novel enteric viruses such as astrovirus and picornavirus, have been reported.

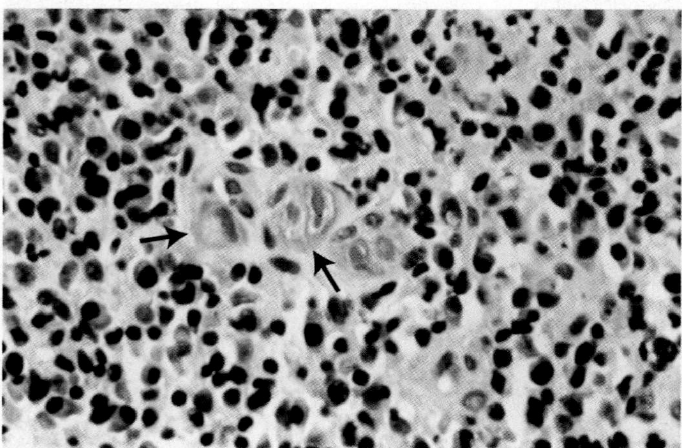

FIGURE 49-28 Microscopic section of small bowel in a patient with AIDS who has cytomegalovirus enteritis. Multiple large cells with intranuclear and intracytoplasmic inclusions typical of cytomegalovirus are demonstrated *(arrows)*. (Courtesy Dr. Mary R. Schwartz, Baylor College of Medicine, Houston, TX.)

Fungi

Fungal infections of the intestinal tract have been recognized in patients with AIDS. Gastrointestinal histoplasmosis occurs in the setting of systemic infection, often in association with pulmonary and hepatic disease. Diagnosis is made by fungal smear and culture of infected tissue or blood. The infection is most commonly treated by the administration of amphotericin B. Coccidioidomycosis of the intestinal tract is rare and, like histoplasmosis, occurs in the context of systemic infection.

NEOPLASMS

General Considerations

Despite composing 75% of the length and 90% of the surface area of the gastrointestinal tract, the small bowel harbors relatively few primary neoplasms and less than 2% of gastrointestinal malignant neoplasms. Although uncommon, rates for new small intestine cancer cases have been increasing an average of approximately 2% each year during the last 10 years. In 2015, an estimated 9160 adults (4880 men and 4280 women) in the United States will be diagnosed with small bowel cancer, and approximately 1210 individuals (640 men and 570 women) will die of this disease. The 5-year survival for localized small bowel cancer is approximately 83%. Unfortunately, only 31% of patients are diagnosed with local disease; therefore, patients with regional and distant disease have 5-year survival rates of approximately 71% and 40%, respectively. This trend may be a reflection of the spread of AIDS and the increase in neoplasms, such as lymphomas, that occur in the immunocompromised host.

The mean age at presentation is 62 years in the setting of benign tumors and approximately 57 years for malignant lesions. The mean age at onset for both is approximately 59 years. Similar to other cancers, there appears to be a geographic distribution, with the highest cancer rates found among the Maori of New Zealand and ethnic Hawaiians. The incidence of small bowel cancer is particularly low in India, Romania, and other parts of eastern Europe. The incidence of small bowel neoplasia varies considerably, with benign lesions identified more often in autopsy series. In contrast, malignant neoplasms account for 75% of symptomatic lesions that lead to surgery. This reflects the fact that most benign neoplasms are asymptomatic and are most often identified as an incidental finding. Stromal tumors and adenomas are the most frequent of the benign tumors. Benign lesions appear to be more common in the distal small bowel, but these numbers may be somewhat misleading because of the relatively short length of the duodenum. Adenocarcinoma is the most common malignant neoplasm, accounting for 30% to 50% of malignant neoplasms of the small intestine; neuroendocrine tumors (NETs) account for 25% to 30% of small intestine malignant neoplasms. Adenocarcinomas are more numerous in the proximal small bowel, whereas the other malignant lesions are more common in the distal intestine.

Numerous risk factors and associated conditions related to neoplasia of the small bowel have been described. These include patients with familial adenomatous polyposis (FAP), hereditary nonpolyposis colorectal cancer, Peutz-Jeghers syndrome, Crohn's disease, gluten-sensitive enteropathy (i.e., celiac sprue), prior peptic ulcer disease, cystic fibrosis, and biliary diversion (e.g., previous cholecystectomy). Controversial factors that may contribute to small bowel cancers include smoking, heavy alcohol consumption (>80 g/day of ethanol), and consumption of red meat or salt-cured foods.

Although the molecular genetics of small bowel neoplasms have not been entirely characterized, similar to colorectal cancers, mutations of the *KRAS* gene are commonly found. Allelic losses, particularly involving tumor suppressor genes at chromosome locations 5q (the *APC* gene), 17q (the *p53* gene), and 18q (the *DCC* [*d*eleted in *c*olon *c*ancer] and *DPC4* [*SMAD4*] genes), have been noted in some small bowel cancers. Recent findings demonstrate that approximately 15% of small intestinal adenocarcinomas have inactivation of DNA mismatch repair genes and display a high level of microsatellite instability (MSI-H). Interestingly, MSI-H is typical of small bowel carcinomas associated with celiac disease and indicates that aberrant CpG island methylation potentially links celiac disease and carcinogenesis. Furthermore, microarray analyses demonstrate a high percentage of small bowel tumors expressing both epidermal growth factor receptor and vascular endothelial growth factor (VEGF).

Clinical Manifestations

Symptoms associated with small bowel neoplasms are often vague and nonspecific and may include dyspepsia, anorexia, malaise, and dull abdominal pain, often intermittent and colicky. These symptoms may be present for months or years before surgery. Most patients with benign neoplasms remain asymptomatic, and the neoplasms are only discovered at autopsy or as incidental findings at laparotomy or upper gastrointestinal radiologic studies. Of the remainder, pain, most often related to obstruction, is the most frequent complaint. Usually, obstruction is the result of intussusception, and benign small tumors are the most common cause of this condition in adults. Hemorrhage is the next most common symptom. Bleeding is usually occult; hematochezia or hematemesis may occur, although life-threatening hemorrhage is uncommon.

Diagnosis

Because of the insidious nature of many of the small bowel neoplasms, a high index of suspicion must be present for these neoplasms to be diagnosed. In most series, a correct preoperative diagnosis is made in only 50% of symptomatic patients. An upper gastrointestinal tract series with small intestinal follow-through yields an accurate diagnosis in 53% to 83% of patients with malignant neoplasms of the small intestine (Fig. 49-29). CT enteroclysis appears to be an even more sensitive technique, with a diagnostic accuracy of approximately 95%, and MRI enteroclysis has a sensitivity and specificity of 98% and 97%, respectively.

Flexible endoscopy may be useful, particularly in diagnosing duodenal lesions, and the colonoscope can be advanced into the terminal ileum for visualization and biopsy of ileal neoplasms. Push enteroscopy has not been used routinely to evaluate lesions in the small bowel because this test may take up to 8 hours to perform and may not visualize the entire small bowel. Double-balloon enteroscopy can be a helpful adjunct; however, it should be reserved for cases in which biopsy or preoperative tattoo is required as it carries a risk of perforation, and other less invasive and highly accurate diagnostic tools are available. The sensitivity and specificity for diagnosis of a small bowel tumor by capsule endoscopy in the setting of obscure bleeding are between 89% and 95% and 75% and 95%, respectively.

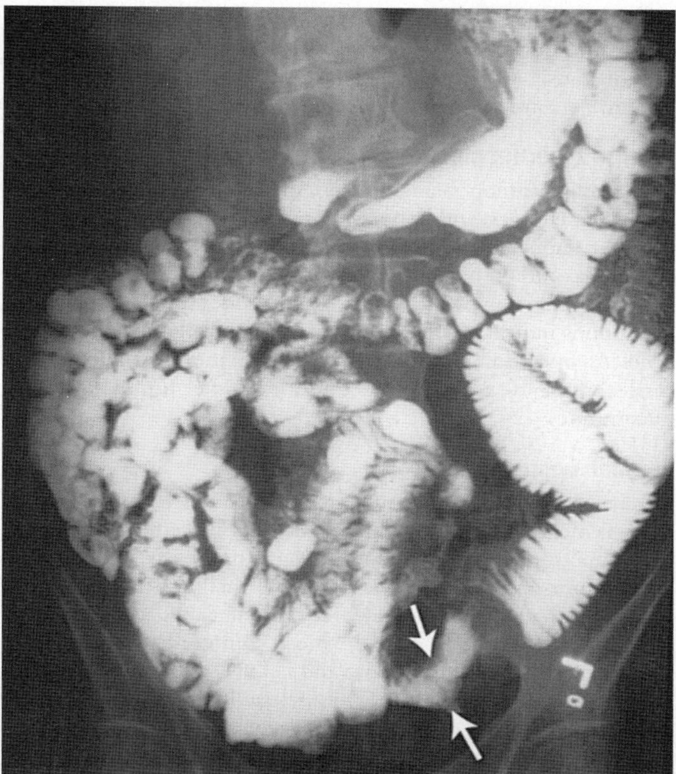

FIGURE 49-29 Barium radiograph demonstrates a typical apple core lesion *(arrows)* caused by adenocarcinoma of the small bowel, producing a partial obstruction with dilated proximal bowel. (Courtesy Dr. Melvyn H. Schreiber, The University of Texas Medical Branch, Galveston, TX.)

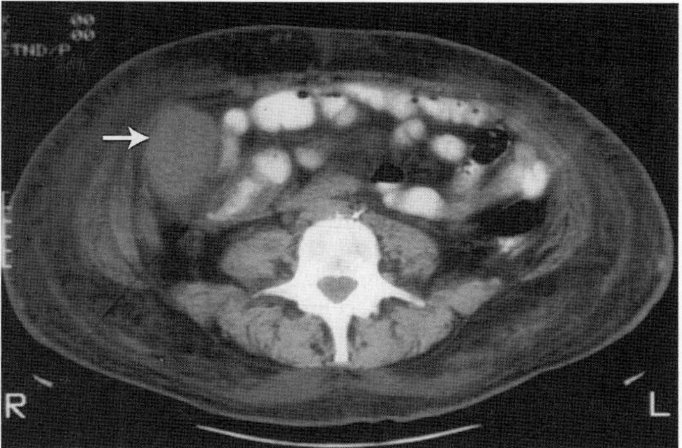

FIGURE 49-30 CT scan of abdomen demonstrates a small bowel neoplasm *(arrow)*. (Courtesy Dr. Melvyn H. Schreiber, The University of Texas Medical Branch, Galveston, TX.)

Plain films may confirm the presence of an obstruction; however, for the most part, they are useless in making a diagnosis of small bowel neoplasms. Angiography is of value in diagnosing and localizing tumors of vascular origin. CT of the abdomen can prove particularly useful in detecting extraluminal tumors, such as malignant gastrointestinal stromal tumors (GISTs), and can provide helpful information about the staging of malignant cancers (Fig. 49-30). Ultrasonography has not proved to be effective in making the preoperative diagnosis of small bowel neoplasm. Despite sophisticated imaging and diagnostic modalities, diagnosis of a small bowel tumor is often achieved only at the time of surgical exploration.

Benign Neoplasms

The most common benign neoplasms include benign stromal tumors, adenomas, and lipomas. Adenomas are the most common benign tumors reported in autopsy series, but stromal tumors are the most common benign small bowel lesions that produce symptoms. In general, when a benign tumor is identified at operation, resection is indicated because symptoms are likely to develop over time. At operation, a thorough search of the remainder of the small bowel is warranted because multiple tumors are not uncommon.

Stromal Tumors

Stromal tumors arise from the interstitial cell of Cajal, an intestinal pacemaker cell of mesodermal descent. Three histologic types of stromal tumors are noted on the basis of their cellular appearance; tumors may be fusiform (77%), epithelioid (8%), or mixed (15%).[29] Stromal tumors are three to four times more frequent than malignant GISTs and are most commonly found in the stomach (60%) and the jejunum and ileum (30%). They are rarely found in the duodenum (5%). More than 95% of stromal tumors express CD117, the c-*kit* proto-oncogene protein that is a transmembrane receptor for the stem cell growth factor, and 70% to 90% express CD34, the human progenitor cell antigen. These tumors infrequently stain positive for actin (20% to 30%), S100 (2% to 4%), and desmin (2% to 4%). The incidence is equal in men and women, and they are most frequently diagnosed in the fifth decade of life. In gross appearance, stromal tumors are firm, gray-white lesions with a whorled appearance noted on cut surface; microscopic examination demonstrates well-differentiated smooth muscle cells. These tumors may grow intramurally and cause obstruction. Alternatively, the tumors demonstrate intramural and extramural growth, sometimes achieving considerable size and eventually outgrowing their blood supply, resulting in bleeding manifestations, the most common indication for surgery in patients with benign stromal tumors. Surgical resection is necessary for appropriate treatment. The number of mitoses can vary substantially, between 0 and 150 mitoses per 50 high-power fields (hpf). Most benign tumors show a low mitotic index (<5 mitoses/50 hpf). The mitotic index is classified as low (<5 mitoses/50 hpf) or high (>5 mitoses/50 hpf); however, even mitotic counts higher than 2 mitoses/50 hpf imply an increased risk for local recurrence.

Adenomas. Adenomas account for approximately 15% of all benign small bowel tumors and are of three primary types: true adenomas, villous adenomas, and Brunner gland adenomas. Twenty percent of adenomas are found in the duodenum, 30% are found in the jejunum, and 50% are found in the ileum. Most of these lesions are asymptomatic; most occur singly and are found incidentally at autopsy. The most common presenting symptoms are bleeding and obstruction. Villous adenomas of the small bowel are rare but do occur, are most commonly found in the duodenum, and may be associated with the familial polyposis syndrome. Both true and villous adenomas are thought to proceed along a similar adenoma-carcinoma sequence as colorectal adenomas and should be considered premalignant. Villous adenomas have a particular propensity for malignant degeneration and may be of relatively large size (>5 cm) in diameter. They are usually noted secondary to abdominal pain or bleeding; obstruction may also occur. The malignant potential of these lesions is reportedly between 35% and 55%. Treatment is determined by location and adenoma type. The options for treatment are endoscopic and surgical. In the jejunum and ileum, the treatment of choice is segmental resection. Although only 5% of adenomas occur in the duodenum, they cause symptoms more frequently, and decisions about surgical management must be carefully planned because of the potential morbidity (20% to 30%) associated with duodenal resection by pancreaticoduodenectomy or pancreas-preserving duodenectomy. Endoscopic ultrasound has recently emerged as a useful modality in the preintervention evaluation and may help guide management planning. Endoscopic resection of these neoplasms is a safe alternative and may delay a more aggressive and potentially morbid surgical procedure; however, some series showed that the lifelong risk of recurrence is approximately 50% after endoscopic treatment (i.e., snare excision, thermal ablation, argon plasma coagulation, or photodynamic therapy). Endoscopic mucosal resection is gaining acceptance as a useful technique for the treatment of duodenal adenomas and Brunner gland tumors. A single-center study found that endoscopic mucosal resection, even in the setting of large (>2 cm) sessile duodenal adenomas, had a high success rate for complete removal; however, the risk of delayed bleeding is significant. Other studies have shown that endoscopic mucosal resection is associated with an approximate 17% risk of other complications, including perforation, hemorrhage, and pancreatitis. Invasive changes or a recurrence after polypectomy necessitates a more definitive approach (e.g., pancreaticoduodenectomy).

Familial adenomas typically occur in the presence of FAP syndrome and require a different algorithm. Numerous studies have shown that adenomas in the duodenum can be found in 50% to 90% of cases, and increasing age was identified as an independent risk factor for adenoma development. Although these neoplasms grow slowly, FAP patients carry a 5% lifetime risk for development of duodenal adenocarcinoma, which represents the leading cause of cancer-related mortality in these patients; therefore, routine lifelong surveillance is a priority. To direct surveillance and treatment, patients are classified by the Spigelman classification (Table 49-8). Screening endoscopy with a forward- and side-viewing endoscope is performed at regular intervals with biopsy of all suspicious, villous, or large (>3 cm) adenomas in addition to random duodenal biopsy specimens. Frequency of endoscopic screening is 1 to 5 years, depending on the Spigelman classification (Box 49-4).[30] Endoscopic or surgical polypectomy

TABLE 49-8 Spigelman Classification for Duodenal Adenomatosis

	POINTS		
PARAMETER	1	2	3
No. of polyps	1-4	5-20	>20
Polyp size (mm)	1-4	5-10	>10
Histology	Tubular	Tubulovillous	Villous
Degree of dysplasia	Mild	Moderate	Severe

Stage 0, 0 points; stage I, 1-4 points; stage II, 5-6 points; stage III, 7-8 points; stage IV, 9-12 points.

From Johnson MD, Mackey R, Brown N, et al: Outcome based on management for duodenal adenomas: Sporadic versus familial disease. *J Gastrointest Surg* 14:229, 2010.

BOX 49-4 Recommended Surveillance Interval for Upper Gastrointestinal Endoscopic Examination in Relation to Spigelman Classification

Spigelman Classification (Surveillance Interval in Years)
0/I (5)
II (3)
III (1-2)
IV (consider surgery)

Adapted from Vasen HF, Möslein G, Alonso A, et al. Guidelines for the clinical management of familial adenomatous polyposis (FAP). *Gut* 57:704–713, 2008.

can be performed for large adenomas. Ablative therapy in the form of argon beam coagulation or photodynamic therapy has been attempted for these patients but with disappointing results. The presence of high-grade dysplasia, carcinoma in situ, or a Spigelman stage IV classification necessitates pancreaticoduodenectomy or pancreas-preserving duodenectomy. Adenomas of the remaining small bowel also occur more frequently in patients with FAP but are not as prevalent as duodenal disease in this population of patients.

Brunner gland adenomas represent benign hyperplastic lesions arising from the Brunner glands of the proximal duodenum. These adenomas may produce symptoms mimicking those of peptic ulcer disease. Diagnosis can usually be accomplished by endoscopy and biopsy, and symptomatic lesions in an accessible region can be resected by simple excision, either endoscopically or surgically. There is no malignant potential for Brunner gland adenomas, and a radical resection should not be used.

Lipomas. Lipomas, which are also included in the category of stromal tumors, are most common in the ileum and are manifested as single intramural lesions located in the submucosa. They usually occur in the sixth and seventh decades of life and are more frequent in men. Less than one third of these tumors are symptomatic, and of these, the most common manifestations are obstruction and bleeding from superficial ulcerations. The treatment of choice for symptomatic lesions is excision. Lipomas do not have malignant potential and therefore, when found incidentally, should be removed only if the resection is simple.

Peutz-Jeghers syndrome. Hamartomas of the small bowel occur as part of the Peutz-Jeghers syndrome, an inherited syndrome of mucocutaneous melanotic pigmentation and gastrointestinal polyps. The pattern of inheritance is autosomal dominant, with a high degree of penetrance. The classic pigmented lesions are small, 1- to 2-mm, brown or black spots located in the circumoral region of the face, buccal mucosa, forearms, palms, soles, digits, and perianal area. The entire jejunum and ileum are the most usual portions of the gastrointestinal tract involved with these hamartomas; however, 50% of patients may also have rectal and colonic lesions, and 25% of patients have gastric lesions. The most common symptom is recurrent colicky abdominal pain, usually as a result of intermittent intussusception. Lower abdominal pain associated with a palpable mass has been reported to occur in one third of patients. Hemorrhage as a result of autoamputation of the polyps occurs less frequently and is most commonly manifested by anemia. Acute life-threatening hemorrhage is uncommon but may occur. Although once considered a purely benign disease, adenomatous changes have been reported in 3% to 6% of hamartomas. Extracolonic cancers are common, occurring in 50% to 90% of patients (small intestine, stomach, pancreas, ovary, lung, uterus, and breast). The small intestine represents the most frequent site for cancer compared with that of the general population. The treatment of complications of Peutz-Jeghers syndrome is directed mainly at the complication of obstruction or persistent bleeding. Resection should be limited to the segment of bowel that is producing complications and usually involves a limited resection. Because of the widespread nature of intestinal involvement, cure is not possible, and extensive resections are not indicated.

Hemangiomas. Hemangiomas are developmental malformations consisting of submucosal proliferation of blood vessels. They can occur at any level of the gastrointestinal tract; the jejunum is the most commonly affected small bowel segment. Hemangiomas account for 3% to 4% of all benign tumors of the small bowel and are multiple in 60% of patients. Hemangiomas of the small bowel may occur as part of an inherited disorder known as *Osler-Weber-Rendu disease*. In addition to the small bowel, hemangiomas may also be present in the lung, liver, and mucous membranes. Patients with Turner syndrome are likely also to have cavernous hemangiomas of the intestine. The most common symptom of small bowel hemangiomas is intestinal bleeding. Angiography and technetium Tc 99m red blood cell scanning are the most useful diagnostic studies. If a hemangioma is localized preoperatively, resection of the involved segment of intestine is warranted. If it is not identified, intraoperative transillumination and palpation can be helpful.

Malignant Neoplasms

Population-based analyses have shown that the incidence of malignant neoplasms of the small intestine has increased steadily during the past 3 decades. This increase has mirrored the increase in diagnosis of small bowel NETs, which have increased more than fourfold (from 2.1 to 9.3 new cases per million population) during the past 3 decades, whereas changes in the frequency of adenocarcinomas, stromal tumors, and lymphomas were less pronounced. Based on both the Surveillance, Epidemiology and End Results program and National Cancer Data Base, the distribution of typical malignant neoplasms of the small bowel from 1973 to 2004 is as follows: NETs, 37%; adenocarcinomas, 37%; lymphomas, 17%; and stromal tumors, 8%. Although the frequency of surgical intervention increased significantly for NETs (79% to 87%) and adjuvant chemotherapy increased for adenocarcinoma from 8% to 24%, the 5-year survival after resection remained unchanged over time for all histologic subtypes, even after adjustment for changes in patient demographics, tumor characteristics, and treatment approaches.[31] These findings highlight the need for more novel and effective treatment strategies.

In contrast to benign lesions, malignant neoplasms almost always produce symptoms, the most common of which are pain and weight loss. Obstruction develops in 15% to 35% of patients and, unlike the intussusception produced by benign lesions, is usually the result of tumor infiltration and adhesions. Diarrhea with tenesmus and passage of large amounts of mucus may occur. Gastrointestinal bleeding, manifested by anemia and guaiac-positive stools or occasionally by melena or hematochezia, occurs to varying degrees with malignant lesions and is more common with GISTs. A palpable mass may be felt in 10% to 20% of patients, and perforations develop in approximately 10%, usually secondary to lymphomas and sarcomas. Although presentation may be similar, each tumor type has a distinct biology that dictates management and prognosis.

Neuroendocrine Tumors

Intestinal NETs arise from enterochromaffin cells (Kulchitsky cells), which are considered neural crest cells and are situated at the base of the crypts of Lieberkühn. These cells are also known as argentaffin cells because of their staining by silver compounds. These tumors were first described by Lubarsch in 1888; in 1907, Oberndorfer coined the term *Karzinoide* to indicate the carcinoma-like appearance and the presumed lack of malignant potential. These tumors have been reported in a number of organs, including most commonly the lungs, bronchi, and gastrointestinal tract. Most patients with small bowel NETs are in their seventh decade of life. The median age for gastroenteric NET is 63 years. As noted in Chapter 38, a World Health Organization report updated the classification of NETs based on differentiation and grade of the tumor and not based on tumor site.[32] NETs are categorized as low grade (grade 1, G1), intermediate grade (grade 2, G2), or high grade (grade 3, G3) on the basis of appearance, mitotic rates, behavior (invasion of other organs, angioinvasion), and Ki-67 proliferative index. The distinction between well and poorly differentiated tumors is by far the most important; G1 and G2 tumors are considered well differentiated, and G3 tumors are poorly differentiated. The use of the word "carcinoid" to describe primary intestinal NETs is considered obsolete, although many clinicians continue to use this term. Certainly, it remains standard nomenclature to continue to refer to the syndrome as carcinoid syndrome.

NETs may be classified by the embryologic site of origin and secretory product. These tumors may be derived from the foregut (respiratory tract, thymus), midgut (jejunum, ileum and right colon, stomach, proximal duodenum), and hindgut (distal colon, rectum). Foregut NETs characteristically produce low levels of serotonin (5-hydroxytryptamine) but may secrete 5-hydroxytryptophan (5-HTP) or adrenocorticotropic hormone. Midgut NETs are characterized by having high serotonin production. Hindgut NETs rarely produce serotonin but may produce other hormones, such as somatostatin and peptide YY. The gastrointestinal tract is the most common site for NETs. After the appendix, the small intestine is the second most frequently affected site in the gastrointestinal tract. In the small intestine, NETs almost always occur within the last 2 feet of the ileum. NETs have a variable malignant potential and are composed of multipotential cells with the ability to secrete numerous humoral agents, the most prominent of which are serotonin and substance P (Table 49-9). In addition to these substances, NETs have been found to secrete corticotropin, histamine, dopamine, neurotensin, prostaglandins, kinins, gastrin, somatostatin, pancreatic polypeptide, calcitonin, and neuron-specific enolase.

TABLE 49-9 Secretory Products of Neuroendocrine Tumors*

AMINES	TACHYKININS	PEPTIDES	OTHER
5-HT	Kallikrein	Pancreatic polypeptide (40%)	Prostaglandins
5-HIAA (88%)	Substance P (32%)	Chromogranins (100%)	
5-HTP	Neuropeptide K (67%)	Neurotensin (19%)	
Histamine		HCG-α (28%)	
Dopamine		HCG-β	
		Motilin (14%)	

HCG, Human chorionic gonadotropin; *5-HIAA*, 5-hydroxyindoleacetic acid; *5-HT*, 5-hydroxytryptamine; *5-HTP*, 5-hydroxytryptophan.
*Values in parentheses represent percentage frequency.

The primary importance of NETs is the malignant potential of the tumors themselves. The carcinoid syndrome, which is characterized by episodic attacks of cutaneous flushing, bronchospasm, diarrhea, and vasomotor collapse, is present mostly in those patients with hepatic metastases. Primary sites that secrete directly into the venous system, bypassing the portal system (e.g., ovary, lung), give rise to the carcinoid syndrome without metastasis.

Pathology. Seventy percent to 80% of NETs are asymptomatic and found incidentally at the time of surgery. In the gastrointestinal tract, more than 90% of NETs are found in five typical sites: appendix (38%), small intestine (29%), colon (13%), stomach (12%), and rectum (8%). The changes in these distributions are associated with the increased incidence of NETs along with the changes of the World Health Organization classification of these tumors in 2010.[33] The malignant potential (ability to metastasize) is related to location, size, depth of invasion, and growth pattern. Only approximately 3% of appendiceal NETs metastasize, but about 35% of ileal NETs are associated with metastasis. Most (approximately 75%) gastrointestinal NETs are smaller than 1 cm in diameter, and about 2% of these are associated with metastasis. In contrast, NETs 1 to 2 cm in diameter and larger than 2 cm are associated with metastasis in 50% and 80% to 90% of cases, respectively.

In gross appearance, these tumors are small, firm submucosal nodules that are usually yellow on cut surface (Fig. 49-31*A*). They may be as subtle as a small whitish plaque seen on the antimesenteric border of the small intestine (Fig. 49-31*B*). Typically, they are associated with a larger mesenteric mass caused by nodal disease and desmoplastic invasion of the mesentery, which is often mistaken for the primary tumor. They tend to grow very slowly, but after invasion of the serosa, the intense desmoplastic reaction produces mesenteric fibrosis, intestinal kinking, and intermittent obstruction. Small bowel NETs are multicentric in 20% to 30% of patients. This tendency to multicentricity exceeds that of any other malignant neoplasm of the gastrointestinal tract. Another unusual observation is the frequent coexistence of a second primary malignant neoplasm of a different histologic type. This is usually a synchronous adenocarcinoma (most commonly in the large intestine) that can occur in 10% to 20% of patients with NETs. Multiple endocrine neoplasia type 1 is associated with NETs in approximately 10% of cases.

Clinical manifestations. In the absence of carcinoid syndrome, symptoms of patients with NETs of the small bowel are similar to those of patients with small bowel tumors of other histologic types. The most common symptom is abdominal pain, which is variably associated with partial or complete small intestinal obstruction. Obstructive symptoms can be caused by intussusception but usually occur secondary to a local desmoplastic reaction, apparently produced by humoral agents elaborated by the tumor. Diarrhea and weight loss may also occur. The diarrhea is a result of a partial bowel obstruction rather than the secretory diarrhea noted in patients with the malignant carcinoid syndrome. As mesenteric and nodal extension progresses, local venous engorgement and ultimately ischemia of the affected segment of intestine contribute to most symptoms and complications related to the tumor.

Malignant carcinoid syndrome. The malignant carcinoid syndrome is a relatively rare disease, occurring in less than 10%

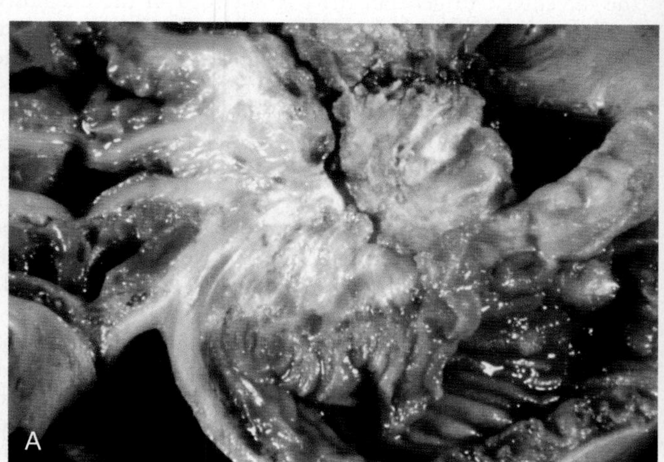

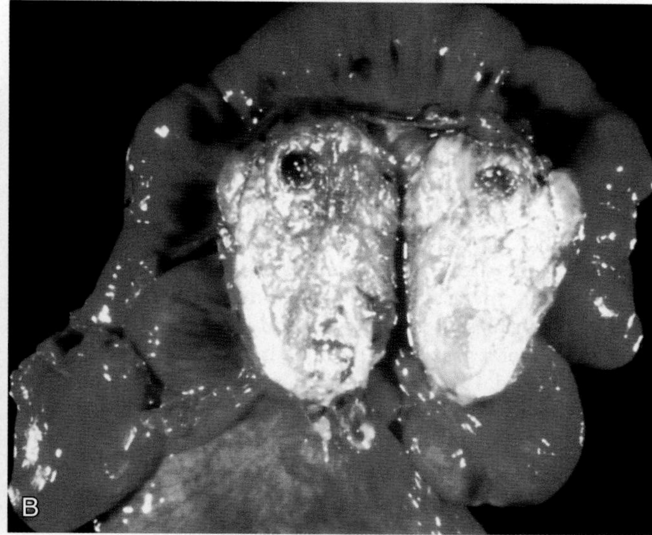

FIGURE 49-31 Gross pathologic characteristics of neuroendocrine tumor (NET). **A,** NET of the distal ileum demonstrates the intense desmoplastic reaction and fibrosis of the bowel wall. **B,** Mesenteric metastases from a NET of the small bowel. (Adapted from Evers BM, Townsend CM Jr, Thompson JC: Small intestine. In Schwartz SI, editor: *Principles of surgery*, ed 7, New York, 1999, McGraw-Hill, p 1245.)

of patients with NETs. The syndrome is usually associated with NETs of the gastrointestinal tract, particularly from the small bowel, but NETs in other locations, such as the bronchus, pancreas, ovary, and testes, have also been described in association with the syndrome. Because of the first-pass metabolism of the vasoactive peptides responsible for carcinoid syndrome, hepatic metastasis or extra-abdominal disease is necessary to elicit the syndrome. The classic description of the carcinoid syndrome typically includes vasomotor, cardiac, and gastrointestinal manifestations. A number of humoral factors are produced by NETs, but those considered to contribute to the carcinoid syndrome include serotonin, 5-HTP (a precursor of serotonin synthesis), histamine, dopamine, kallikrein, substance P, prostaglandin, and neuropeptide K. Most patients who exhibit malignant carcinoid syndrome have massive hepatic replacement by metastatic disease. However, tumors that bypass the liver, specifically ovarian and retroperitoneal NETs, may produce the syndrome in the absence of liver metastasis.

Common symptoms and signs include cutaneous flushing (80%); diarrhea (76%); hepatomegaly (71%); cardiac lesions, most commonly right-sided heart valvular disease (41% to 70%); and asthma (25%). Cutaneous flushing in the carcinoid syndrome may be of four varieties:

1. diffuse erythematous, which is short-lived and normally affects the face, neck, and upper chest;
2. violaceous, which is similar to a diffuse erythematous flush except that the attacks may be longer and patients may develop a permanent cyanotic flush, with watery eyes and injected conjunctivae;
3. prolonged flushes, which may last up to 2 or 3 days and involve the entire body and may be associated with profuse lacrimation, hypotension, and facial edema; and
4. bright-red patchy flushing, typically seen with gastric NETs.

The diarrhea associated with carcinoid syndrome is episodic (usually occurring after meals), watery, and often explosive. Increased circulating serotonin levels are thought to be the cause of the diarrhea because the serotonin antagonist methysergide effectively controls the symptom. Cardiac lesions usually involve the right side of the heart, but left-sided lesions are present in 15% of patients and can lead to congestive heart disease and symptomatic left-sided heart failure. The three most common cardiac lesions are pulmonary stenosis (90%), tricuspid insufficiency (47%), and tricuspid stenosis (42%). Asthmatic attacks are usually observed during the flushing symptom, and serotonin and bradykinin have been implicated in this symptom. Malabsorption and pellagra (dementia, dermatitis, and diarrhea) are occasionally present and are thought to be caused by excessive diversion of dietary tryptophan.

Diagnosis. The elevation of various humoral factors forms the basis for diagnostic tests in patients with NETs and the carcinoid syndrome. NETs produce serotonin, which is then metabolized in the liver and the lung to the pharmacologically inactive 5-hydroxyindoleacetic acid (5-HIAA). Elevated urinary levels of 5-HIAA measured during 24 hours with high-performance liquid chromatography are highly specific although not sensitive. For the last decade, chromogranin A (CgA) has been a well-established marker for carcinoid disease; it is elevated in more than 80% of patients with NETs. CgA alone may be used for the diagnosis of NETs, given its specificity of 95%, but some investigators suggest that other tests should be used in conjunction with CgA for diagnostic purposes because its sensitivity is only 55%. A combination of serum CgA measurement with 24-hour urine 5-HIAA is an acceptable diagnostic combination with increased sensitivity. Studies have suggested that serum CgA and N-terminal pro-brain natriuretic peptide (NT-proBNP) may also be used in combination for both diagnosis and surveillance because patients with increased NT-proBNP and CgA levels showed worse overall survival than patients with elevated CgA alone. In terms of surveillance after resection or as a prognostic marker to monitor response to therapy, CgA levels have proven efficacy over urine 5-HIAA levels.

Plasma serotonin, substance P, neurotensin, neurokinin A, and neuropeptide K levels can be measured, but these peptides may not be elevated in all patients. Provocative tests using pentagastrin, calcium, or epinephrine may be used to reproduce the symptoms of NETs. More recently, pentagastrin has been used to differentiate between NETs and chronic atrophic gastritis but is generally not used for the diagnosis of NETs, given the diagnostic reliability of 5-HIAA, CgA, and NT-proBNP.

NETs of the small intestine are rarely diagnosed preoperatively. Barium radiographic studies of the small bowel may exhibit multiple filling defects as a result of kinking and fibrosis of the bowel (Fig. 49-32). A combination of anatomic and functional imaging techniques is routinely performed to optimize sensitivity and specificity.

Traditionally, CT scanning was the imaging modality of choice for identifying the site of disease and the presence of lymphatic or hematogenous metastases. CT scan findings depend on the size, the degree of mesenteric invasion and desmoplastic reaction, and the presence of regional lymph node invasion. If these entities are not well defined, CT has limited diagnostic capabilities in this disease. However, when CT scanning reveals a solid mass with spiculated borders and radiating surrounding strands that is associated with linear strands within the mesenteric fat and kinking of the bowel, a diagnosis of gastrointestinal NET can be made fairly confidently. CT angiography may be useful in cases associated with a large mesenteric process to identify encasement and pseudoaneurysm formation, typical of a malignant process in the mesentery. In general, MRI is not used in the diagnosis of gastrointestinal NETs but can be helpful in diagnosing metastatic disease, especially in the liver. Liver metastases are well demonstrated with MRI and usually have low signal intensity on T1-weighted images and high signal intensity on T2-weighted images. After the administration of a gadolinium-based contrast agent, liver metastases enhance peripherally in the hepatic arterial phase and appear as hypointense defects in the portal venous phase. Diffusion-weighted MRI and dynamic contrast-enhanced techniques represent promising advances in radiologic imaging, although these imaging techniques have not yet been validated for monitoring therapy of NETs.

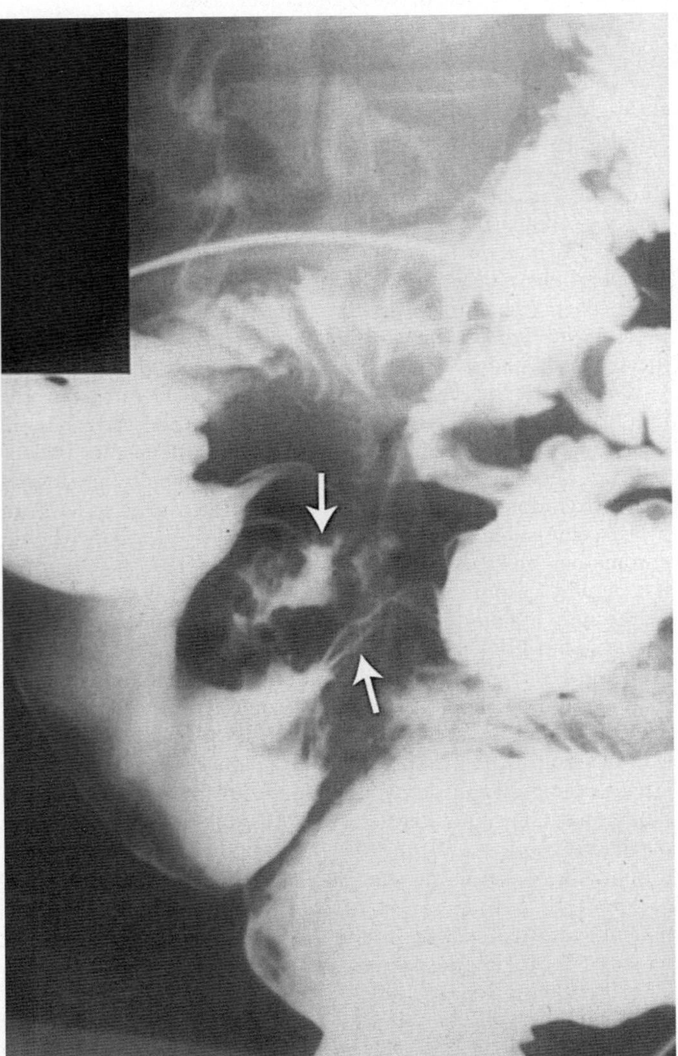

FIGURE 49-32 Barium radiograph of a NET of the terminal ileum demonstrates fibrosis with multiple filling defects and high-grade partial obstruction *(arrows)*. (Courtesy Dr. Melvyn H. Schreiber, The University of Texas Medical Branch, Galveston, TX.)

Octreotide is a synthetic analogue of somatostatin, and indium In 111–labeled pentetreotide specifically binds to somatostatin receptor subtypes 2 and 5. Functional nuclear imaging studies capitalize on the concept of somatostatin receptor positivity as these imaging techniques are used to image many NETs, including those with somatostatin-binding sites. Scintigraphic localization has a higher sensitivity than CT for delineating and localizing NETs and is particularly useful in the identification of extra-abdominal metastatic disease or in cases in which the primary tumor cannot be identified by CT scan. An area of great interest is functional imaging by ^{18}F-fluorodeoxyglucose positron emission tomography (^{18}FDG PET) scanning, although this imaging modality alone has limited capabilities because of the fact that ^{18}FDG is taken up only in high-grade NETs (e.g., high Ki-67 expression), whereas most NETs have low Ki-67 expression and are not apparent with this imaging modality. However, the addition of newer isotopes, such as ^{11}C-5-HTP and ^{18}F-L-dihydroxyphenylalanine (^{18}F-DOPA), has dramatically improved the sensitivity of PET for the diagnosis and surveillance of neuroendocrine malignant neoplasms.

Somatostatin receptor imaging with gadolinium Ga 68–DOTATATE PET/CT is increasingly used for managing patients with NETs. DOTATATE is an amide of 1,4,7,10-tetraazacyclododecane-1,4,7,10-tetraacetic acid (DOTA), which acts as a chelator for a radionuclide, and tyrosine-3-octreotate (TATE), a derivative of octreotide. The latter binds to somatostatin receptors and thus directs the radioactivity into the tumor. ^{68}Ga-DOTATATE PET/CT is a clinically useful imaging technique to localize primary tumors in patients with neuroendocrine metastases of unknown origin as well as to define the existence and extent of metastatic disease. Combining the two modalities may be even more helpful in diagnosing and managing NETs. In a study designed to investigate the relationship between PET/CT results and histopathologic findings in 27 patients with NETs, the sensitivity of ^{68}Ga-DOTATATE and ^{18}FDG PET/CT was 95% and 37%, respectively. The sensitivity in detecting liver, lymph node, and bone metastases and the primary lesion was 95%, 95%, 90%, and 93% for ^{68}Ga-DOTATATE and 40%, 28%, 28%, and 75% for ^{18}FDG, respectively. The peptide receptor radionuclide therapy agents yttrium-90 (^{90}Y) and lutetium-177 (^{177}Lu) are both diagnostic and therapeutic. The reason for developing compounds with high affinity for somatostatin receptors 2, 3, and 5 is to improve diagnostic sensitivity. These agents can also be used to adjust dosing of peptide receptor radionuclide therapy. A single-center study determined that the additional information provided by ^{68}Ga-DOTATATE PET/CT in the preoperative workup significantly influences surgical management in approximately 20% of patients treated for NET.[35] These findings are particularly important because resection is the only curative treatment in patients with NETs of the small intestine, and accurate preoperative imaging is critical for surgical planning because findings of small and distant metastases may profoundly influence surgical management.

Treatment

Surgical therapy. The treatment of patients with small bowel NETs is based on tumor size and site and presence or absence of metastatic disease. For primary tumors smaller than 1 cm in diameter without evidence of regional lymph node metastasis, a segmental intestinal resection is adequate. For patients with lesions larger than 1 cm, with multiple tumors, or with regional lymph node metastasis, regardless of the size of the primary tumor, wide excision of bowel and mesentery is required. Lesions of the terminal ileum are best treated by right hemicolectomy. Small duodenal tumors can be excised locally; however, more extensive lesions may require pancreaticoduodenectomy.[36] A single-center, prospective, longitudinal study showed that a laparoscopic approach is safe and feasible in selected patients. Laparoscopy was associated with similar R0 (i.e., without residual microscopic tumor) resection and morbidity rates but a shorter hospital stay compared with laparotomy. Median follow-up was 39 months, and progression-free survival at 1, 3, and 5 years was as follows: 95%, 83%, and 75%, respectively, for R0 patients without liver metastasis; 92%, 83%, and 57%, respectively, for R0 patients with resected liver metastasis; and 82%, 58%, and 30%, respectively, for patients with R2 resection (i.e., evidence of residual tumor on visual examination). Overall survival and progression-free survival did not show any difference in comparing the laparoscopic and open groups.[37]

In addition to treatment of the primary tumor, it is important that the abdomen be thoroughly explored for multicentric lesions. In cases in which the mesenteric disease appears to involve a large portion of the mesentery, dissection of the tumor off the mesenteric vessels, with preservation of the blood supply to unaffected bowel, is appropriate, albeit technically demanding. Not only does removal of the mesenteric disease provide a significant survival advantage, but also mesenteric debulking ensures the most durable palliation for the patient.

Caution should be exerted in the anesthetic management of patients with NETs because anesthesia may precipitate a carcinoid crisis characterized by hypotension, bronchospasm, flushing, and tachycardia predisposing to arrhythmias. The treatment of carcinoid crisis is IV octreotide given as a bolus of 50 to 100 μg, which may be continued as an infusion at 50 μg/hr.

In patients with NETs and widespread metastatic disease, surgery is still indicated. In contrast to metastases from other tumors, there is a definite role for surgical debulking, which often provides beneficial symptomatic relief. In patients with limited hepatic involvement, metastasectomy has been shown to provide the most durable survival benefit compared with other treatment modalities.[36] Unfortunately, most patients are not candidates for liver resection because of extensive disease; recurrence after metastasectomy occurs in up to 75% of patients. In these cases, transarterial chemoembolization or radioembolization has been shown to provide liver-directed control of disease. Furthermore, resection of the primary tumor, with or without mesenteric resection, has been shown to improve survival and to slow progression of hepatic metastases in patients with unresectable disease. Although there have been some small series of hepatic transplantation for extensive liver metastases from NETs, unacceptably high recurrence rates limit this approach.

Medical therapy. Medical therapy for patients with malignant carcinoid syndrome is primarily directed toward the relief of symptoms caused by the excess production of humoral factors. Table 49-10 summarizes medical therapies for NET treatment. Somatostatin analogues are the standard of care for controlling symptoms of patients with functional gastrointestinal NETs, and they control symptoms in more than 70% of patients with carcinoid syndrome.[38] Somatostatin analogues such as octreotide (Sandostatin) and lanreotide and their depot formulations (Sandostatin LAR and Somatuline, respectively) relieve symptoms of the carcinoid syndrome (e.g., diarrhea, flushing) in most patients and delay progression. The results of a randomized phase 3 trial (PROMID) of 85 patients demonstrated that the median time to progression in patients with midgut NETs treated with octreotide LAR was more than twice as long compared with that of patients treated with placebo.[39] The landmark Controlled study of Lanreotide Antiproliferative Response In NeuroEndocrine Tumors (CLARINET) trial found that lanreotide, a somatostatin analogue, was associated with significantly prolonged progression-free survival among patients with metastatic enteropancreatic NETs of grade 1 or 2 (Ki-67 proliferative marker <10%).[40] Patients were randomly assigned to receive an extended-release aqueous-gel formulation of lanreotide or placebo once every 28 days for 96 weeks. The estimated rates of progression-free survival at 24 months were 65% in the lanreotide group and 33% in the placebo group.

Second-generation somatostatin analogues have been developed to address the limitations of the current regimens. Studies are ongoing using pan-receptor agonists (e.g., pasireotide) as well as chimeric dimers, which possess features of somatostatin and

TABLE 49-10 Medical Therapies for Neuroendocrine Tumor Treatment

Approved Therapeutics	
Somatostatin analogues	Octreotide (Sandostatin; Sandostatin LAR)
	Lanreotide (Somatuline depot)
Cytotoxic therapies	Streptozotocin (pancreatic NET only)
mTOR inhibitor	Everolimus (Afinitor; pancreatic NET only)
Tyrosine kinase inhibitors	Sunitinib (Sutent; pancreatic NET only)
Used Off-Label	
Pan-receptor somatostatin agonists	Pasireotide (Signifor; approved indication for Cushing disease only)
Interferons	Interferon alfa
	Interferon alfa-2b
Cytotoxic therapies	5-Fluorouracil (5-FU)
	Cyclophosphamide (Cytoxan)
	Temozolomide (Temodar)
	Capecitabine (Xeloda)
Investigational	
Peptide receptor radionuclide therapy	^{90}Y conjugated with somatostatin analogues
	^{177}Lu isotopes conjugated with somatostatin analogues
Serotonin synthesis inhibitors	Telotristat etiprate (LX1032/LX1606)
VEGF inhibitors	Bevacizumab (Avastin)
Dopamine agonists	Dopastatins

Compiled with assistance of Lowell B. Anthony, MD, University of Kentucky.

dopamine agonists (dopastatins). These promising biologic therapies are thought to enhance symptom control by binding multiple receptors (somatostatin and dopamine receptors). Somatostatin receptor antagonists are also currently being developed for clinical use. Peptide receptor radionuclide therapy, ^{90}Y and ^{177}Lu isotopes conjugated with somatostatin analogues, appears to be efficacious in advanced NETs. These isotopes can be used for PET imaging as well as to determine the distribution of the agent and the dosimetry of the tumor. A study evaluating more than 1000 patients with metastatic NETs determined that tumor uptake is predictive for both survival after ^{90}Y-DOTA-TOC treatment and occurrence of renal toxicity as the kidney is the dose-limiting organ.[34] There is also an interest in targeting incretin receptor family members, particularly glucagon-like peptide 1 (GLP-1), which are overexpressed in NETs. The GLP-1 inhibitor Lys^{40}(Ahx-DTPA/DOTA^{111}In)NH_2-exendin-4 is highly sensitive and can be detected up to 14 days after IV injection using a probe to facilitate surgical excision.

Interferon alfa was introduced as monotherapy for NET treatment in 1983. Interferon binds to two different receptors to elicit effects that include cell cycle inhibition at G_1/S, antiangiogenesis effects through downregulation of VEGF, and upregulation of somatostatin receptors, to name a few. Although some series showed tumor regression in 10% of patients and tumor stabilization in 65%, side effects, which included chronic fatigue, pancytopenia, thyroiditis, and systemic lupus erythematosus, were not tolerable. Pegylated interferon alfa-2b showed comparable survival rates to interferon alfa, but with more tolerable side effects. Some series have shown that given the upregulation of somatostatin receptors by interferon alfa, its combination with somatostatin analogues may be efficacious. Prospective randomized controlled trials demonstrated variable findings, but one retrospective study determined that combined treatment resulted in a longer progression-free survival (58 versus 55 months). Interferon is less expensive than somatostatin analogues, but the increased incidence of side effects and variable outcomes preclude the widespread use of this drug.[34]

In the past, the only available treatment for metastatic NETs was cytotoxic chemotherapy, most frequently combinations that included streptozotocin, 5-fluorouracil (5-FU), and cyclophosphamide. These treatments resulted in a median survival of around 2 years. Currently, the role of chemotherapy is confined predominantly to patients with metastatic disease who are symptomatic, are unresponsive to other therapies, or have high tumor proliferation rates. The duration of response, however, is short-lived. Temozolomide as monotherapy has acceptable toxicity and antitumoral effects in a small series of patients with advanced NETs, and in combination with capecitabine, it was shown to prolong survival in patients with well-differentiated, metastatic NETs who experienced progression with previous therapies. The use of cisplatin and etoposide has shown some promise, but only in patients with poorly differentiated NETs. Everolimus and sunitinib are approved for pancreatic NETs; lanreotide is approved for gastroenteropancreatic NETs without carcinoid syndrome.

Serotonin receptor antagonists have been used with limited success. Methysergide is no longer used because of the increased incidence of retroperitoneal fibrosis. Ketanserin and cyproheptadine have been shown to provide some control of symptoms, and other antagonists, such as ondansetron, may be even more effective. Serotonin synthesis inhibitors, such as telotristat etiprate (LX1032/LX1606), are effective in lowering serotonin levels and are in clinical development.

The treatment of metastatic NETs requires a multidisciplinary approach; combined modalities may be the best option, including surgical debulking, hepatic artery embolization, chemoembolization, or radioembolization and medical therapy. In addition, newer and more targeted therapies are being developed that may be useful in the future. Targeted therapy has progressed down four separate pathways. Given the hypervascular nature of NETs, antiangiogenesis therapy (e.g., bevacizumab) is being investigated in combination with cytotoxic and somatostatin therapy. Sunitinib, which is a multitargeted or selective tyrosine kinase inhibitor that is active against alpha-type and beta-type platelet-derived growth factor receptor (PDGFR) and vascular endothelial growth factor receptor (VEGFR), has been noted to decrease angiogenesis and to prolong progression-free survival in pancreatic NETs in multiple clinical trials, most notably those with mutations associated with exons 9 and 11.[34]

Tyrosine kinase inhibitors have been evaluated as systemic therapy and as a liver-directed chemoembolization strategy for NETs as well. The PI3K-AKT-mTOR pathway has also recently emerged as a potential target for systemic therapy. Agents such as everolimus, a mammalian target of rapamycin (mTOR) inhibitor, although initially developed as immunosuppressant therapy, have redefined themselves as potent antitumor agents and remain under active investigation for carcinoid disease. Everolimus is approved in the United States and Europe for the treatment of patients with advanced pancreatic NETs. The activity of everolimus remains under investigation in patients with intestinal NETs. In a randomized study of patients with advanced NETs associated with carcinoid syndrome, the addition of everolimus to octreotide therapy was associated with improved yet statistically insignificant progression-free survival. Further investigation is needed to determine whether primary tumor site or other clinical and molecular factors can affect response to mTOR inhibition. Although everolimus can slow tumor progression, significant tumor reduction is rarely obtained. Targeting of multiple signaling pathways is a treatment strategy that may provide better tumor control and overcome resistance mechanisms involved with targeting of a single pathway. Results of ongoing and future studies will provide important information about the added benefit of combining mTOR inhibitors with other targeted agents, such as VEGF pathway inhibitors, and cytotoxic chemotherapy in the treatment of advanced NETs.[41]

Prognosis. NETs have the best prognosis of all small bowel tumors, whether the disease is localized or metastatic. Resection of a NET localized to its primary site approaches a 100% survival rate. Five-year survival rates are approximately 65% in patients with regional disease and 25% to 35% in those with distant metastasis. Metastatic disease at the time of diagnosis is approximately 20% to 50%, and tumors recur in 40% to 60% of patients. When widespread metastatic disease precludes cure, extensive resection for palliation is indicated. In fact, long-term palliation often can be obtained because these tumors are relatively slow growing. A number of factors have been evaluated in an attempt to identify patients with NETs who have a poor prognosis. An elevated level of CgA, which is an independent predictor of an adverse prognosis, is probably the most useful factor identified.

Adenocarcinomas

Adenocarcinomas constitute approximately 50% of the malignant tumors of the small bowel. The peak incidence is in the seventh decade of life, and most series show a slight male predominance.

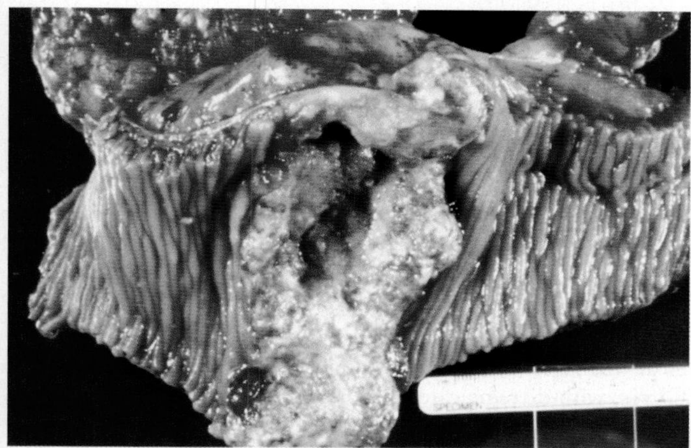

FIGURE 49-33 Large circumferential mucinous adenocarcinoma of the jejunum. (Courtesy Dr. Mary R. Schwartz, Baylor College of Medicine, Houston, TX.)

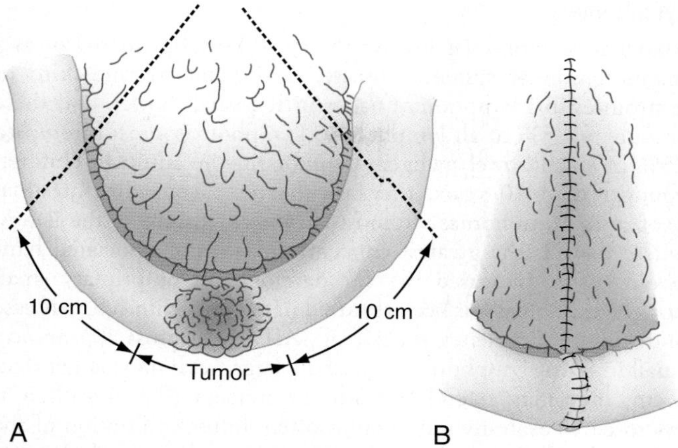

FIGURE 49-34 Surgical management of carcinoma of the small bowel. **A,** Malignant tumors should be resected with a wide margin of normal bowel and a wedge of mesentery to remove the immediate draining lymph nodes. **B,** End-to-end anastomosis of the small bowel and repair of the mesentery. (Adapted from Thompson JC: *Atlas of surgery of the stomach, duodenum, and small bowel,* St. Louis, 1992, Mosby–Year Book, p 299.)

Most of these tumors are located in the duodenum and proximal jejunum (Fig. 49-33). Those arising in association with Crohn's disease tend to occur at a somewhat younger age, and more than 70% arise in the ileum. Tumors of the duodenum tend to be manifested somewhat earlier than those in the most distal intestine because of the earlier presentation of symptoms, which are usually jaundice and chronic bleeding. Adenocarcinomas of the jejunum and ileum usually produce symptoms that may be more nonspecific and include vague abdominal pain and weight loss. Intestinal obstruction and chronic bleeding can also occur. Perforation is uncommon. As with adenocarcinomas in other organs, survival of patients with small bowel adenocarcinomas is related to the stage of disease at the time of diagnosis. Unfortunately, diagnosis is often delayed, and the disease is advanced at the time of surgery secondary to various factors (e.g., vagueness of symptoms, absence of physical findings, lack of clinical suspicion because of the rarity of these lesions).

Treatment of small bowel adenocarcinoma is determined by location and stage. Complete resection of the primary tumor with locoregional lymph node resection is mandatory. In an effort to downsize the tumor, neoadjuvant chemotherapy is appropriate to consider if there is tumor invasion into adjacent structures. Patients are then reevaluated for surgery after 2 to 3 months of treatment. Duodenal adenocarcinomas are treated with pancreaticoduodenectomy if the tumor is in the second portion of the duodenum or an infiltrating tumor in the proximal or distal duodenum. In addition, resection of the periduodenal, peripancreatic, and hepatic lymph nodes as well as resection of the involved vascular structures that originate from the celiac trunk and superior mesenteric arteries should be performed. Duodenal resection can be performed for a noninfiltrating tumor if it is located in the first, third, or fourth portion of the duodenum, but this is not recommended in the setting of residual microscopic tumor (R1 status) or grossly visible tumor after resection (R2 status) as these findings are associated with poor prognosis. An R0 resection with regional lymphadenectomy and jejunojejunal or ileoileal bypass should be performed in the setting of jejunal and ileal adenocarcinoma. If the terminal ileum is involved, an ileocecectomy with right colectomy should be performed with ligation of the ileocolic artery and subsequent regional lymphadenectomy (Fig. 49-34).

There is currently no standard adjuvant protocol for small bowel adenocarcinoma. Despite the previous lack of supporting evidence of traditional chemotherapy regimens, most guidelines suggest that patients with poorly differentiated cancers or those who had incomplete lymph node resections (<10 nodes identified) should at least be considered for adjuvant chemotherapy. Adjuvant regimens are often dictated by location, although studies have suggested that fluoropyrimidine and oxaliplatin may increase overall survival in patients with advanced disease. A prospective international phase 3 trial comparing observation versus adjuvant chemotherapy in patients with an R0 resection is currently accruing subjects. This trial proposes that in an adequately powered trial, adjuvant chemotherapy will result in an improvement in disease-free survival and overall survival compared with observation alone after potentially curative surgery for patients with stage I, II, and III small bowel adenocarcinoma. Studies have determined that FOLFOX (oxaliplatin, 5-FU, and leucovorin) and FOLFIRI (irinotecan, 5-FU, and leucovorin) significantly improve the performance status and progression-free survival in the treatment of metastatic small bowel adenocarcinoma. For metastatic small bowel adenocarcinoma, FOLFOX is considered first-line therapy, and FOLFIRI is an acceptable second-line strategy.

The prognosis of small bowel adenocarcinoma is poor, probably because of the delayed presentation and presence of advanced disease at diagnosis. Five-year survival rates are typically in the 14% to 33% range, although duodenal adenocarcinoma has a 5-year survival rate of 50%, probably because of the earlier symptom presentation and diagnosis. Lymph node invasion is the main prognostic factor for local small bowel adenocarcinoma; moreover, the number of lymph nodes assessed and the number of positive lymph nodes are of prognostic value. In stage III patients, more than three positive lymph nodes was associated with a worse 5-year disease-free survival rate than one or two positive lymph nodes (37% versus 57%, respectively). Multivariate analysis identified advanced age, advanced stage, ileal location, recovery of fewer than 10 lymph nodes, and number of positive nodes as significant predictors of poor overall survival. Thus, a curative resection at an early stage (stages I and II) should systematically include a regional lymphadenectomy.[42]

Lymphoma

Malignant lymphomas involve the small bowel primarily or as a manifestation of systemic disease. Approximately one third of gastrointestinal lymphomas occur in the small bowel, and these account for 5% of all lymphomas. Lymphomas constitute up to 25% of small bowel malignant tumors in the adult; in children younger than 10 years, they are the most common intestinal neoplasm. Lymphomas are most commonly found in the ileum, where there is the greatest concentration of gut-associated lymphoid tissue. Increased risk for development of primary small bowel lymphomas has been reported in patients with celiac disease and immunodeficiency states (e.g., AIDS). In gross appearance, small intestine lymphomas are usually large, with most larger than 5 cm; they may extend beneath the mucosa (Fig. 49-35). On microscopic examination, there is often diffuse infiltration of the intestinal wall. Symptoms of small bowel lymphoma include pain, weight loss, nausea, vomiting, and change in bowel habits. Perforation may occur in up to 25% of patients (Fig. 49-36). Fever is uncommon and suggests systemic involvement.

The treatment of small bowel lymphoma remains controversial. Traditionally, a combination of surgery, chemotherapy, and radiation therapy was used for all small bowel tumors. However, in the absence of symptoms, small bowel lymphomas are often chemoresponsive and do not require surgery. This can typically be predicted by cell type because B cell lymphomas are more chemosensitive than T cell lymphomas and have high remission rates with or without surgery. T cell lymphomas are traditionally more resistant to therapy and will progress to symptoms of obstruction or perforation if not resected. Regardless of cell type, resection is indicated at any onset of symptoms because progression to life-threatening hemorrhage or perforation portends a dismal prognosis. Five-year survival of 50% to 60% can be expected and is dictated by response to systemic therapy rather than by the success of surgical resection.

Gastrointestinal Stromal Tumors

Malignant GISTs arise from mesenchymal tissue and constitute about 20% of malignant neoplasms of the small bowel (Fig. 49-37). These tumors are more common in the jejunum and ileum, typically are diagnosed in the fifth and sixth decades of life, and occur with a slight male preponderance. Malignant GISTs are larger than 5 cm at the time of diagnosis in 80% of patients. GISTs mostly arise from the muscularis propria and generally grow extramurally. Most common indications for surgery include bleeding and obstruction, although free perforation may occur as a result of hemorrhagic necrosis in large tumor masses. Typically, GISTs tend to invade locally and to spread by direct extension into adjacent tissues and hematogenously to the liver, lungs, and bone; lymphatic metastases are unusual. The most useful indicators of survival and the risk for metastasis include the size of the tumor at presentation, mitotic index, and evidence of tumor invasion into the lamina propria.

Treatment of GISTs continues to evolve and represents one of the first breakthroughs in signal transduction manipulation. Surgical management includes complete resection for localized GISTs, with extreme care to avoid rupture of the tumor capsule, which results in relapse in 100% of these patients. If capsule rupture occurs, these patients should receive adjuvant therapy regardless of the extent of the tumor before surgery. It is advisable to perform an en bloc resection, to include adjacent organs, for prevention of tumor capsule rupture. A laparoscopic approach in patients with large tumors is strongly discouraged. Radiologic criteria for unresectability include infiltration of the celiac trunk, superior mesenteric artery, or portal vein. Lymphadenectomy is

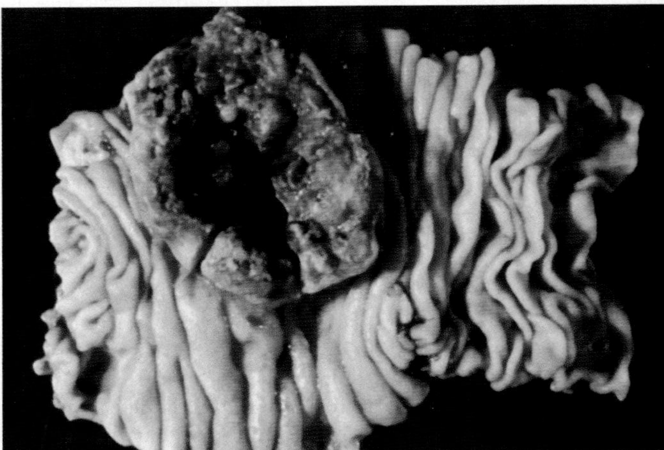

FIGURE 49-36 Small bowel lymphoma is manifested as perforation and peritonitis. (Courtesy Dr. Mary R. Schwartz, Baylor College of Medicine, Houston, TX.)

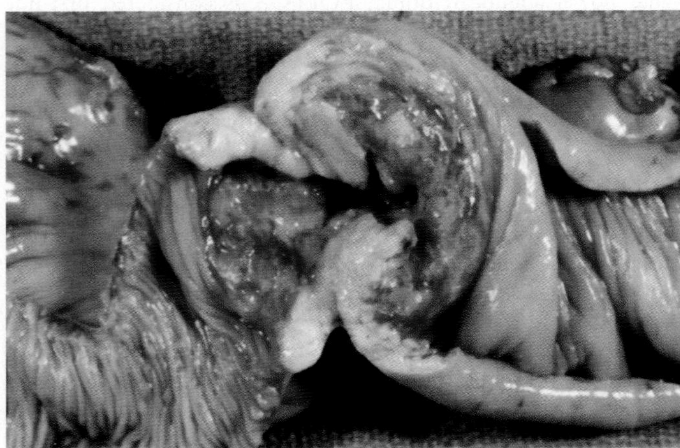

FIGURE 49-35 Gross photograph of primary lymphoma of the ileum shows replacement of all layers of the bowel wall with tumor. (Courtesy Dr. Mary R. Schwartz, Baylor College of Medicine, Houston, TX.)

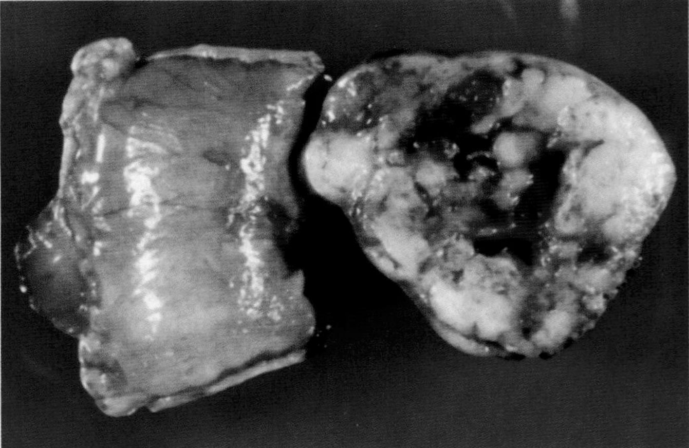

FIGURE 49-37 Small bowel GIST with hemorrhagic necrosis. (Courtesy Dr. Mary R. Schwartz, Baylor College of Medicine, Houston, TX.)

unnecessary, given the low frequency of lymph node metastasis.[29] Small GISTs (<2 cm) found incidentally in surgical specimens do not require further treatment. Before the development of tyrosine kinase inhibitors, adjuvant strategies for GISTs were lacking, and recurrence rates after resection were as high as 70%. However, the development of imatinib mesylate (Gleevec, formerly known as STI571) has significantly altered previous treatment strategies. Imatinib mesylate is a tyrosine kinase inhibitor that blocks the unregulated mutant *c-kit* tyrosine kinase and inhibits the BCR-ABL and PDGF tyrosine kinases. Multiple randomized trials have confirmed its efficacy as a first-line agent in the treatment of GIST (Fig. 49-38). Current guidelines suggest that patients with high-risk disease should receive 3 years of adjuvant treatment with imatinib, but it is not recommended for low-risk patients after an R0 resection.

Relapse-risk assessment for primary GIST is critical as it provides prognostic information as well as estimates the potential benefits of imatinib. The current American Joint Committee on Cancer staging can be found in Table 49-11. This classification does not acknowledge recent evidence indicating that the type and location of the mutation have an effect on the risk of recurrence. For example, deletions affecting exon 11, codon 557/558 of the *c-kit* gene, and D842V PDGFRα mutations have a higher risk of recurrence within the first 3 to 4 years after surgery.[29] In fact, adjuvant imatinib therapy is not recommended in patients with D842V PDGFRα mutations, given its known resistance to this agent.

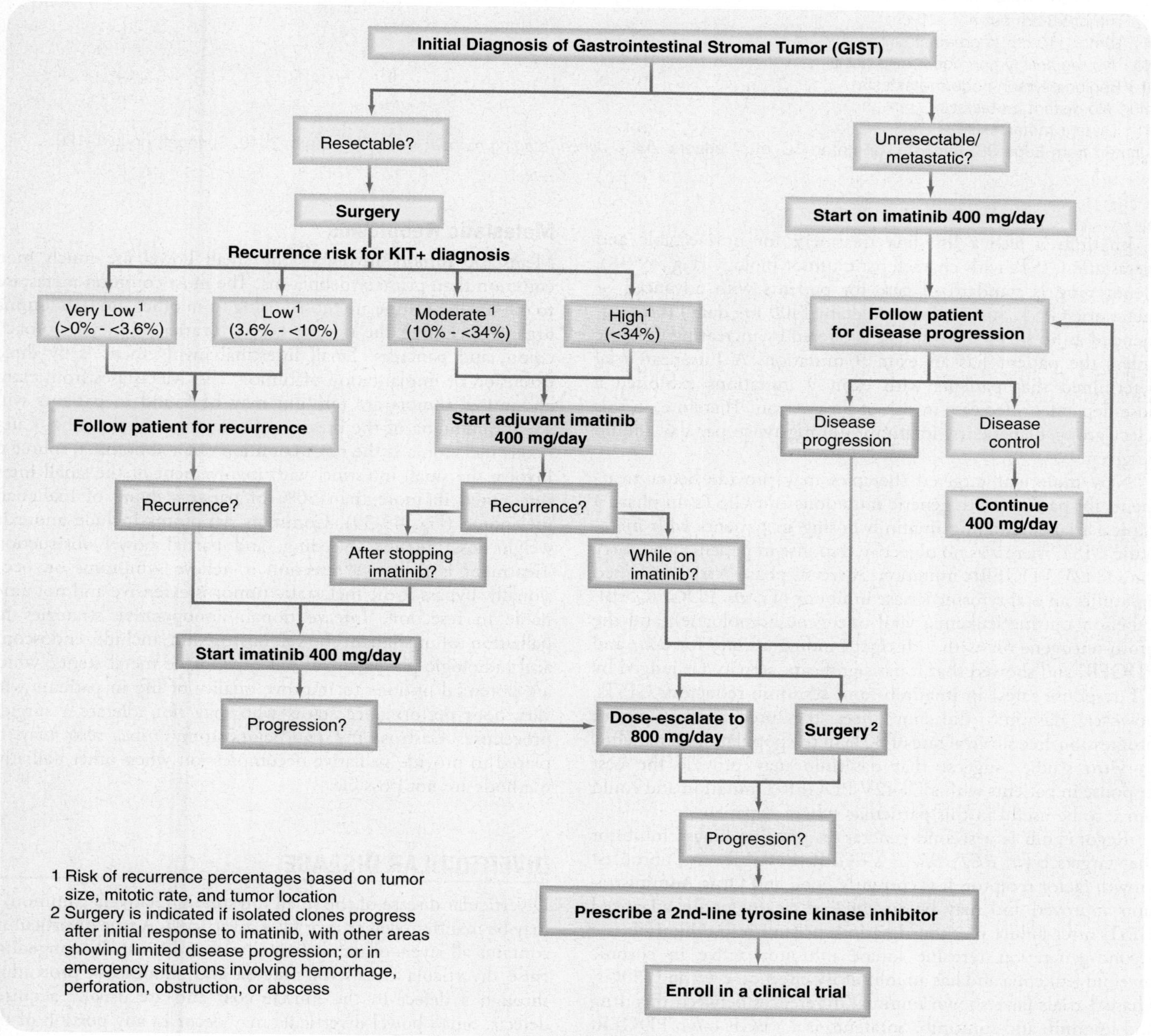

FIGURE 49-38 Current algorithm for management of GIST based on risk of recurrence. (Adapted from Pisters PW, Patel SR. Gastrointestinal stromal tumors: current management. J Surg Oncol. 2010 Jan 8. Gleevec® prescribing information. http://www.pharma.us.novartis.com/product/pi/pdf/gleevec_tabs.pdf. Accessed August 15, 2010.)

TABLE 49-11 Small Intestinal Gastrointestinal Tumor Classification

GROUP	PRIMARY TUMOR SIZE*	REGIONAL LYMPH NODE METASTASIS†	DISTANT METASTASIS‡	MITOTIC RATE
Stage I	T1 or T2	N0	M0	Low
Stage II	T3	N0	M0	Low
Stage IIIA	T1	N0	M0	High
	T4	N0	M0	Low
Stage IIIB	T2	N0	M0	High
	T3	N0	M0	High
	T4	N0	M0	High
Stage IV	Any T	N1	M0	Any rate
	Any T	Any N	M1	Any rate

*T1 Tumor ≤2 cm
T2 Tumor >2 cm but not >5 cm
T3 Tumor >5 cm but not >10 cm
T4 Tumor >10 cm in greatest dimension
†N0 No regional lymph node metastasis
N1 Regional lymph node metastasis
‡M0 No distant metastasis
M1 Distant metastasis
Adapted from Edge SB, Byrd DR, Compton CC, et al, editors: *AJCC cancer staging manual*, ed 7, New York, 2010, Springer, pp 181–189.

Imatinib is also a first-line treatment for unresectable and metastatic GISTs with characteristic tumor biology (Fig. 49-38). Genotyping is standard of care for patients with advanced or metastatic GIST. Standard-dose therapy (400 mg daily) is recommended as no survival advantage is offered by increasing the dose unless the patient has an exon 9 mutation. A European trial determined that patients with exon 9 mutations exhibited a dose-dependent decrease in risk of progression. Therefore, in this select group of patients, imatinib 400 mg twice per day should be given.

New molecular targeted therapies may provide better treatments for patients with genetic mutations and GISTs. In phase 3 clinical trials evaluating imatinib dosing in patients with metastatic GIST, there was no objective response in patients who carry the D842V PDGFRα mutation. A recent phase 2 trial evaluated dasatinib, an oral tyrosine kinase inhibitor of c-*kit*, PDGFR, ABL (Abelson murine leukemia viral oncogene homologue), and the proto-oncogene *Src* with a distinct binding affinity for c-*kit* and PDGFR, and showed that it has significant activity (as judged by CT response rates) in imatinib- and sunitinib-refractory GISTs; however, dasatinib did not meet the predefined 6-month progression-free survival rate of 30% in the population of patients. In vitro studies suggest that dasatinib may provide the best response in patients with a D842V PDGFRα mutation and could prove to be useful in this particular subset of patients.

Regorafenib is a second-generation tyrosine kinase inhibitor that targets c-*kit*, *RET*, *BRAF*, VEGFR, PDGFR, and fibroblast growth factor receptor. It is currently Food and Drug Administration approved and may be an effective treatment for advanced GISTs after failure of either imatinib or sunitinib. Nilotinib is a second-generation tyrosine kinase inhibitor active in chronic myeloid leukemia and has an inhibitory effect on c-*kit* and PDGF. Phase 3 trials have shown minimal differences between this drug and imatinib and sunitinib. Sorafenib is a VEGF, c-*kit*, PDGFR, and *BRAF* inhibitor and has been effective in imatinib- and sunitinib-resistant tumors. The combination of imatinib and doxorubicin has shown some benefit in patients with wild-type GISTs.

Metastatic Neoplasms

Metastatic tumors involving the small bowel are much more common than primary neoplasms. The most common metastases to the small intestine are those arising from other intra-abdominal organs, including the uterine cervix, ovaries, kidneys, stomach, colon, and pancreas. Small intestinal involvement is by direct extension or implantation of tumor cells. Metastases from extra-abdominal tumors are rare but may be found in patients with adenocarcinoma of the breast and carcinoma of the lung. Cutaneous melanoma is the most common extra-abdominal source to involve the small intestine, with involvement of the small intestine noted in more than 50% of patients dying of malignant melanoma (Fig. 49-39). Common symptoms include anorexia, weight loss, anemia, bleeding, and partial bowel obstruction. Treatment is palliative resection to relieve symptoms or, occasionally, bypass if the metastatic tumor is extensive and not amenable to resection. Interventional, nonoperative strategies for palliation of malignant bowel obstruction include endoscopic and radiologic placement of self-expandable metal stents, which are potential options to improve quality of life in patients with very poor performance status who may not tolerate a surgical procedure. Gastrostomy and jejunostomy tubes also may be placed to provide palliative decompression when other palliative methods are not possible.

DIVERTICULAR DISEASE

Diverticular disease of the small intestine is relatively common. It may be manifested as true or false diverticula. A true diverticulum contains all layers of the intestinal wall and is usually congenital. False diverticula consist of mucosa and submucosa protruding through a defect in the muscle coat and are usually acquired defects. Small bowel diverticula may occur in any portion of the small intestine. Duodenal diverticula are the most common acquired diverticula of the small bowel, and Meckel's diverticulum is the most common true congenital diverticulum of the small bowel.

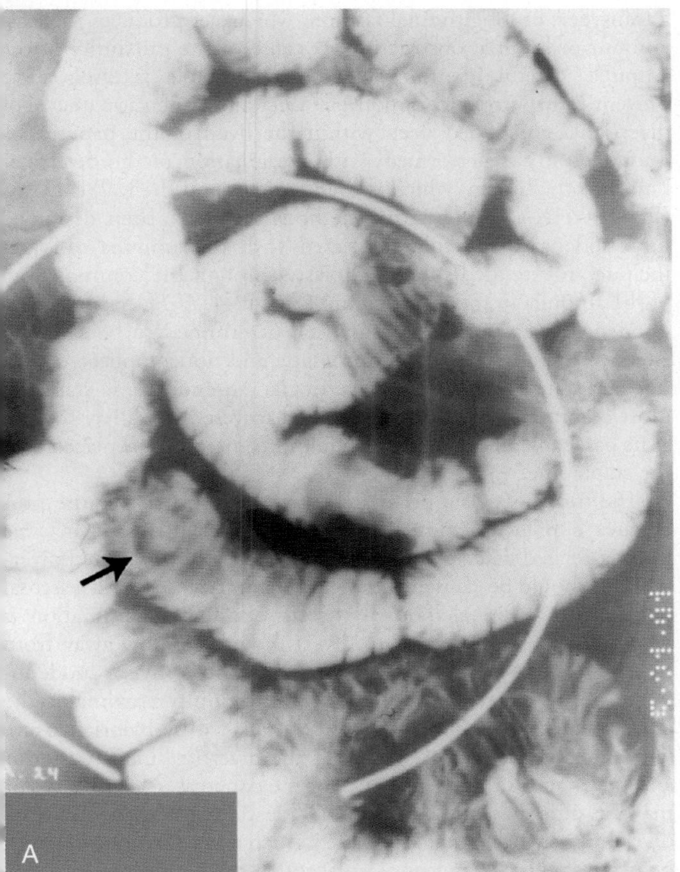

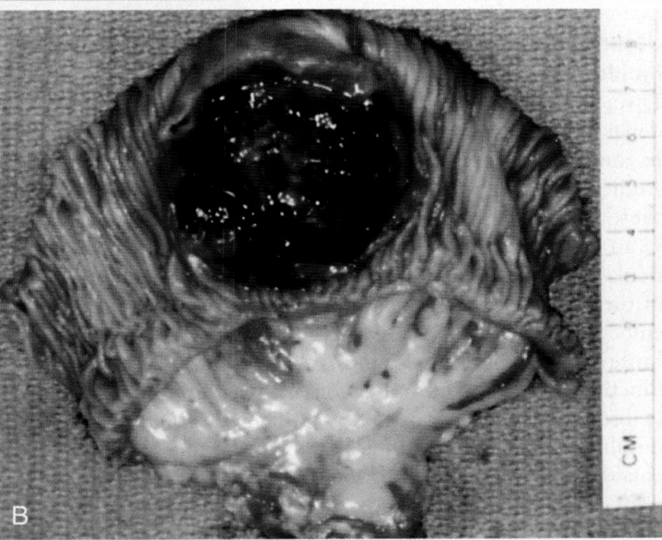

FIGURE 49-39 **A,** Barium radiograph shows target lesions consistent with metastatic melanoma of small bowel *(arrow)*. **B,** Gross specimen demonstrating metastatic melanoma to the small bowel. (**A,** Courtesy Dr. Melvyn H. Schreiber, The University of Texas Medical Branch, Galveston, TX. **B,** Courtesy Dr. Mary R. Schwartz, Baylor College of Medicine, Houston, TX.)

Duodenal Diverticula

Incidence and Cause

First described by Chomel, a French pathologist, in 1710, diverticula of the duodenum are relatively common, representing the second most common site for diverticulum formation after the colon. The incidence of duodenal diverticula varies, depending on the age of the patient and method of diagnosis. Upper gastrointestinal radiographic studies identify duodenal diverticula in 1% to 5% of all studies, whereas endoscopic retrograde cholangiopancreatography identifies 9% to 23% of cases. Previous autopsy series report the incidence as being approximately 15% to 20%. Duodenal diverticula occur twice as often in women as in men and are rare in patients younger than 40 years. They have been classified as congenital or acquired, true or false, and intraluminal or extraluminal. Extraluminal duodenal diverticula are considerably more common than intraluminal diverticula, are acquired, and consist of mucosal or submucosal outpouchings herniated through a muscle defect in the bowel wall. Intraluminal duodenal diverticula (also known as windsock diverticula) are congenital and occur as a single saccular structure that is connected to the entire circumference or part of the wall of the duodenum to create a duodenal web. Incomplete recanalization of the duodenum during fetal development leads to intraluminal diverticula, which are exceedingly rare. In general, extraluminal diverticula usually occur within the second portion of the duodenum (62%) and less commonly in the third (30%) and fourth (8%) portions. They rarely occur in the first part of the duodenum (<1%). When they occur in the second portion, most (88%) are noted on the medial wall around the ampulla (i.e., periampullary), 8% are seen posteriorly, and 4% occur on the lateral wall.

Clinical Manifestations

The important thing to remember is that the overwhelming majority of duodenal diverticula are asymptomatic and are usually noted incidentally by an upper gastrointestinal series for an unrelated problem (Fig. 49-40). Upper gastrointestinal endoscopy identifies approximately 75% of duodenal diverticula, and the use of a side-viewing scope further increases the success rate. The diagnosis may be suggested by plain abdominal films showing an atypical gas bubble; CT can identify large diverticula by the presence of a mass-like structure interposed between the duodenum and pancreatic head containing air, air-fluid levels, fluid contrast material, or debris. Magnetic resonance cholangiopancreatography is particularly helpful to demonstrate the relationship of the diverticulum to the biliary and pancreatic ducts and associated pathologic changes in the biliary system and pancreas. Hemorrhage in diverticula is best diagnosed by a combination of angiography and scanning with ^{99m}Tc-labeled red blood cells; however, surgery should not be delayed to obtain imaging in the event of hemorrhage in a hemodynamically unstable patient. Less than 5% of duodenal diverticula will require surgery because of a complication of the diverticulum itself. Major complications of duodenal diverticula include obstruction of the biliary or pancreatic ducts that may contribute to cholangitis and pancreatitis, respectively, and hemorrhage, perforation, and, rarely, blind loop syndrome. Iatrogenic injuries, most commonly acquired during endoscopic instrumentation of an asymptomatic diverticulum, can lead to perforation or hemorrhage.

Only those diverticula associated with the ampulla of Vater are significantly related to complications of cholangitis and pancreatitis. In these patients, the ampulla usually enters the duodenum at the superior margin of the diverticulum rather than through the diverticulum itself. The mechanism proposed for the increased incidence of complications of the biliary tract is the location of the perivaterian diverticulum, which may produce mechanical distortion of the common bile duct as it enters the duodenum, resulting in partial obstruction and stasis. Hemorrhage can be

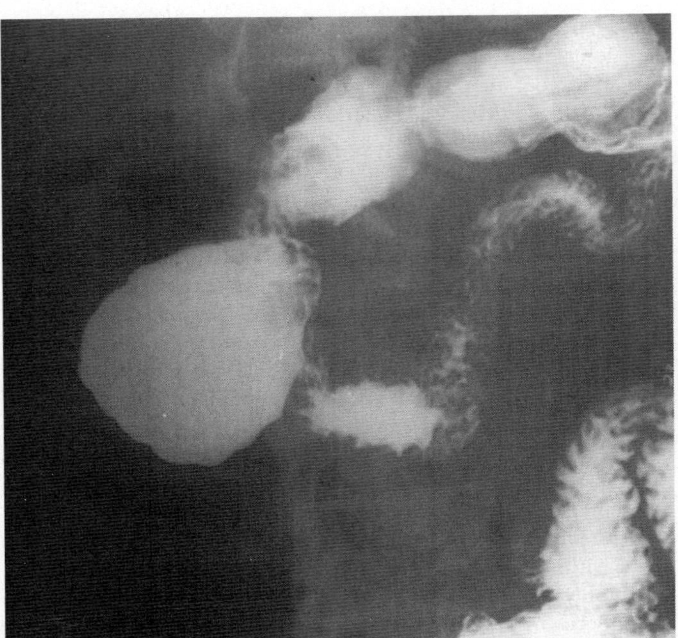

FIGURE 49-40 Large diverticulum arises from the second portion of the duodenum. (Courtesy Dr. Melvyn H. Schreiber, The University of Texas Medical Branch, Galveston, TX.)

caused by inflammation, leading to erosion of a branch of the superior mesenteric artery. Perforation of duodenal diverticula has been described but is rare. Finally, stasis of intestinal contents within a distended diverticulum can result in bacterial overgrowth, malabsorption, steatorrhea, and megaloblastic anemia (i.e., blind loop syndrome). Symptoms related to duodenal diverticula in the absence of any other demonstrable disease usually are nonspecific epigastric complaints that can be treated conservatively and may actually prove to be the result of another problem not related to the diverticulum itself.

Treatment

Most duodenal diverticula are asymptomatic and benign; when they are found incidentally, they should be left alone. For symptomatic duodenal diverticula, treatment consists of removal of the diverticulum, which can be accomplished endoscopically or surgically. Appropriate classification of these diverticula guides management. All intraluminal duodenal diverticula require treatment as recurrence of symptoms is certain. Curative treatment consists of removal of the intraluminal diverticulum by laparotomy and duodenotomy or by endoscopic resection. Large (>3 cm) or obstructing intraluminal duodenal diverticulum does not preclude endoscopic resection, but an endoscopic approach in the setting of massive hemorrhage or perforation with intra-abdominal contamination secondary to intestinal contents is discouraged. These entities are relatively rare and often require a multidisciplinary approach to determine the best treatment strategy.

Extraluminal duodenal diverticula should be resected in the setting of symptomatic disease or need for urgent surgery, such as free perforation or hemorrhage. Several operative procedures have been described for the treatment of the symptomatic extraluminal duodenal diverticula. The most common and effective treatment is diverticulectomy, which is most easily accomplished by performing a wide Kocher maneuver that exposes the duodenum. The diverticulum is then excised, and the duodenum is closed in a transverse or longitudinal fashion, whichever produces the least amount of luminal obstruction. Because of the proximity of the ampulla, careful identification of the ampulla is essential to prevent injury to the common bile duct and pancreatic duct. For diverticula embedded deep within the head of the pancreas, a duodenotomy is performed, with invagination of the diverticulum into the lumen, which is then excised, and the wall is closed (Fig. 49-41*A-C*). Alternative methods that have been described for duodenal diverticula associated with the ampulla of Vater include an extended sphincteroplasty through the common wall of the ampulla in the diverticulum (Fig. 49-41*D-F*). Laparoscopic duodenal diverticulectomy has been determined to be safe and effective in patients with symptomatic and noncomplicated (i.e., not perforated or bleeding) diverticula. An endoscopic stapler is most commonly used to traverse and to resect the diverticulum at its base, and an omental patch reinforcement can be placed over the staple line.

The treatment of a perforated diverticulum may require procedures similar to those described for patients with massive trauma-related defects of the duodenal wall. The perforated diverticulum should be excised and the duodenum closed with a serosal patch from a jejunal loop. If the surrounding inflammation is severe, it may be necessary to divert the enteric flow away from the site of the perforation with a gastrojejunostomy or duodenojejunostomy. Interruption of duodenal continuity proximal to the perforated diverticulum may be accomplished by pyloric closure with suture or a row of staples. If the diverticulum is posterior and perforates into the substance of the pancreas, operative repair may be difficult and dangerous. Wide drainage with duodenal diversion may be all that is feasible in such cases. Great care should be taken if the perforation is adjacent to the papilla of Vater.

Jejunal and Ileal Diverticula

Incidence and Cause

Diverticula of the small bowel are much less common than duodenal diverticula, with an incidence ranging from 0.1% to 1.4% in autopsy series and 0.1% to 1.5% in upper gastrointestinal studies. Jejunal diverticula are more common and are larger than those in the ileum. These are false diverticula, occurring mainly in an older age group (after the sixth decade of life). These diverticula are multiple, usually protrude from the mesenteric border of the bowel, and may be overlooked at surgery because they are embedded within the small bowel mesentery (Fig. 49-42). The cause of jejunoileal diverticulosis is thought to be a motor dysfunction of the smooth muscle or the myenteric plexus, resulting in disordered contractions of the small bowel, generating increased intraluminal pressure and herniation of the mucosa and submucosa through the weakest portion of the bowel (i.e., the mesenteric side).

Clinical Manifestations

Jejunoileal diverticula are usually found incidentally at laparotomy or during an upper gastrointestinal study (Fig. 49-43); the great majority remain asymptomatic. Acute complications, such as intestinal obstruction, hemorrhage, and perforation, can occur but are rare. Chronic symptoms include vague chronic abdominal pain, malabsorption, functional pseudo-obstruction, and chronic low-grade gastrointestinal hemorrhage. Acute complications are diverticulitis with or without abscess or perforation, gastrointestinal hemorrhage, and intestinal obstruction. Stasis of intestinal flow with bacterial overgrowth (blind loop syndrome), caused by the jejunal dyskinesia, may lead to deconjugation of bile salts and

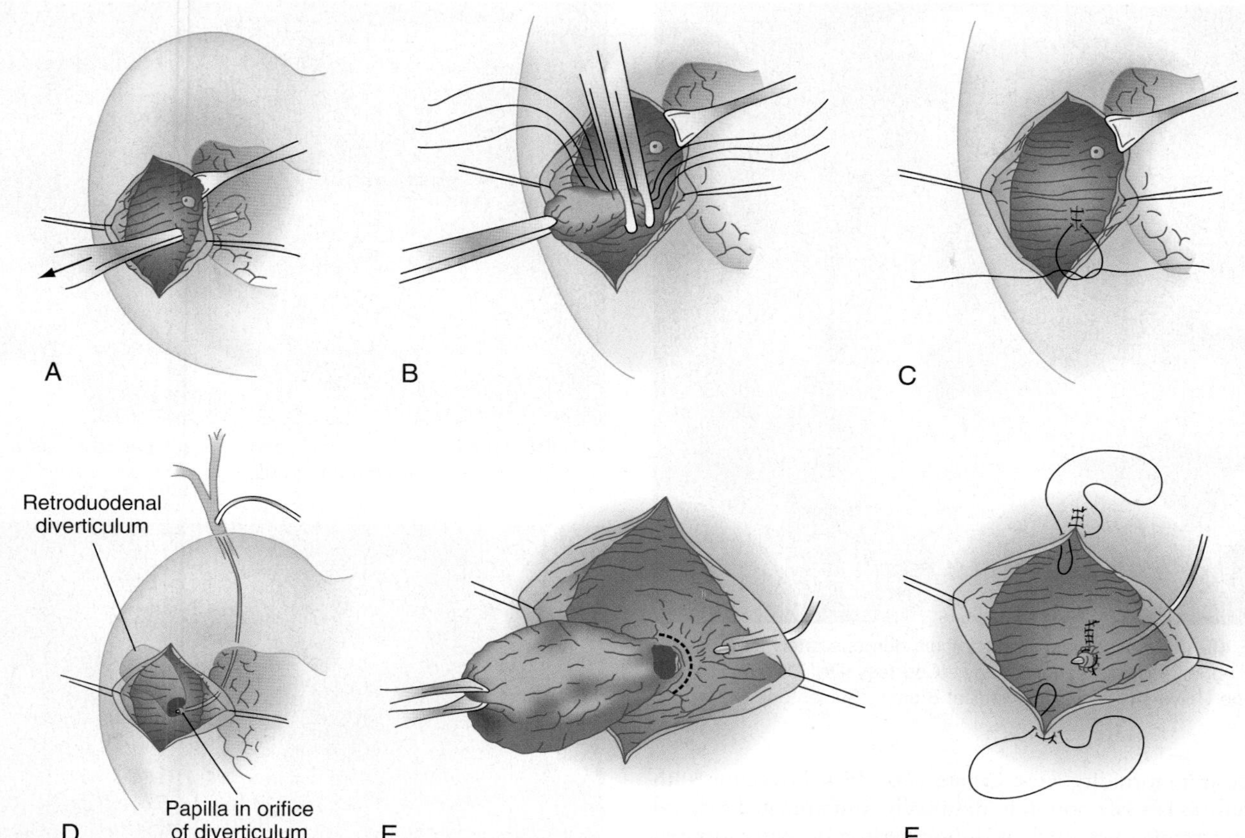

FIGURE 49-41 **A-C,** Treatment of a diverticulum protruding into the head of the pancreas. The duodenum is opened vertically. A clamp is used to invert the diverticulum into the lumen, where it is excised, and the posterior wall defect is closed. **D-F,** Management of the unusual duodenal diverticula that arise in the periampullary location. A tube stent should be placed into the common bile duct and passed distally into the duodenum to facilitate identification and later dissection of the sphincter of Oddi. The diverticulum is inverted into the lumen of the duodenum. The round opening in the wall of the base of the diverticulum is the site at which the ampullary structures were freed by a circumferential incision. **E,** Line of division of the base of the diverticulum *(heavy broken line),* which is accomplished by free-hand dissection. After the diverticulum has been removed, the stent and enveloping papilla are protruded into the defect left by the division of the base of the diverticulum. The mucosa and muscle wall of the papilla are then sewn circumferentially to the wall of the duodenum. (Adapted from Thompson JC: *Atlas of surgery of the stomach, duodenum, and small bowel,* St. Louis, 1992, Mosby–Year Book, pp 209–213.)

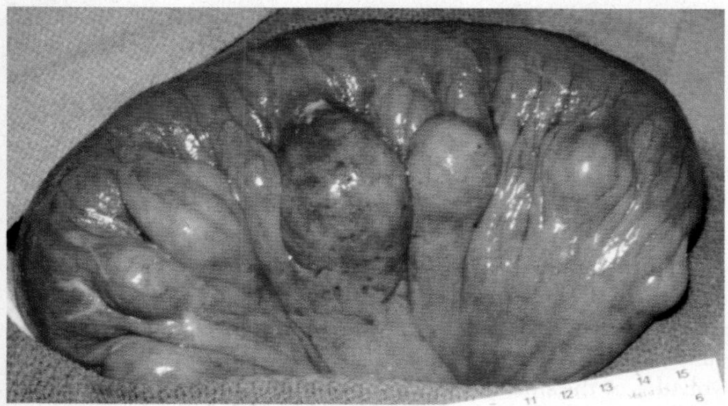

FIGURE 49-42 Multiple large jejunal diverticula located in the mesentery in an older patient presenting with obstruction secondary to an enterolith. (Adapted from Evers BM, Townsend CM Jr, Thompson JC: Small intestine. In Schwartz SI, editor: *Principles of surgery,* ed 7, New York, 1999, McGraw-Hill, p 1248.)

uptake of vitamin B_{12} by the bacterial flora, resulting in steatorrhea and megaloblastic anemia, with or without neuropathy.

Treatment

For incidentally noted, asymptomatic jejunoileal diverticula, no treatment is required. Treatment of complications of obstruction, bleeding, and perforation is usually by intestinal resection and end-to-end anastomosis. Patients presenting with malabsorption secondary to the blind loop syndrome and bacterial overgrowth in the diverticulum can usually be given antibiotics. Obstruction may be caused by enteroliths that form in a jejunal diverticulum and are subsequently dislodged and obstruct the distal intestine. This condition may be treated by enterotomy and removal of the enterolith, or sometimes the enterolith can be milked distally into the cecum. When the enterolith causes obstruction at the level of the diverticulum, bowel resection is necessary. When a perforation of a jejunoileal diverticulum is encountered, resection with reanastomosis is required because lesser procedures, such as simple closure, excision, and invagination, are associated with greater

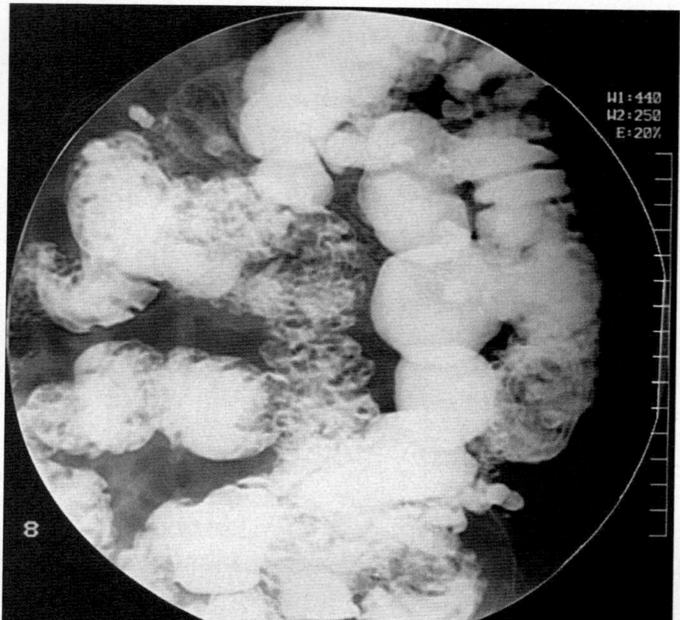

FIGURE 49-43 Multiple jejunal diverticula demonstrated by a barium contrast upper gastrointestinal study. (Courtesy Dr. Melvyn H. Schreiber, The University of Texas Medical Branch, Galveston, TX.)

mortality and morbidity rates. Laparoscopic bowel resection with reanastomosis is a safe option in minimally contaminated surgical fields. In extreme cases, such as diffuse peritonitis, enterostomies may be required if judgment dictates that reanastomosis may be risky.

Meckel's Diverticulum

Incidence and Cause

Meckel's diverticulum is the most commonly encountered congenital anomaly of the small intestine, occurring in about 2% of the population. It was reported initially in 1598 by Hildanus and then described in detail by Johann Meckel in 1809. Meckel's diverticulum is located on the antimesenteric border of the ileum 45 to 60 cm proximal to the ileocecal valve and results from incomplete closure of the omphalomesenteric, or vitelline, duct. An equal incidence is found in men and women. Meckel's diverticulum may exist in different forms, ranging from a small bump that may be easily missed to a long projection that communicates with the umbilicus by a persistent fibrous cord (Fig. 49-44) or, much less commonly, a patent fistula. The usual manifestation is a relatively wide-mouthed diverticulum measuring about 5 cm in length, with a diameter of up to 2 cm (Fig. 49-45). Cells lining the vitelline duct are pluripotent; therefore, it is not uncommon to find heterotopic tissue within the Meckel's diverticulum, the most common of which is gastric mucosa (present in 50% of all Meckel's diverticula). Pancreatic mucosa is encountered in about 5% of diverticula; less commonly, these diverticula may harbor colonic mucosa.

Clinical Manifestations

Most Meckel's diverticula are benign and are incidentally discovered during autopsy, laparotomy, or barium studies (Fig. 49-46). The most common clinical presentation of Meckel's diverticulum is gastrointestinal bleeding, which occurs in 25% to 50% of patients who present with complications; hemorrhage is the most common symptomatic presentation in children 2 years of age or younger. This complication may be manifested as acute massive hemorrhage, anemia secondary to chronic bleeding, or a self-limited recurrent episodic event. The usual source of the bleeding is a chronic acid-induced ulcer in the ileum adjacent to a Meckel's diverticulum that contains gastric mucosa.

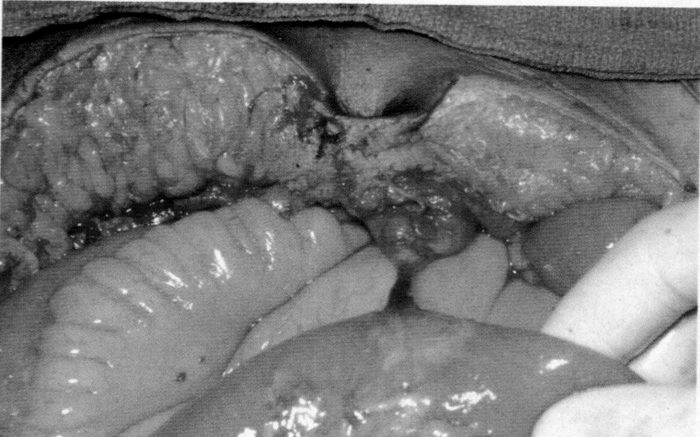

FIGURE 49-44 Omphalomesenteric remnant persisting as a fibrous cord from the ileum to the umbilicus.

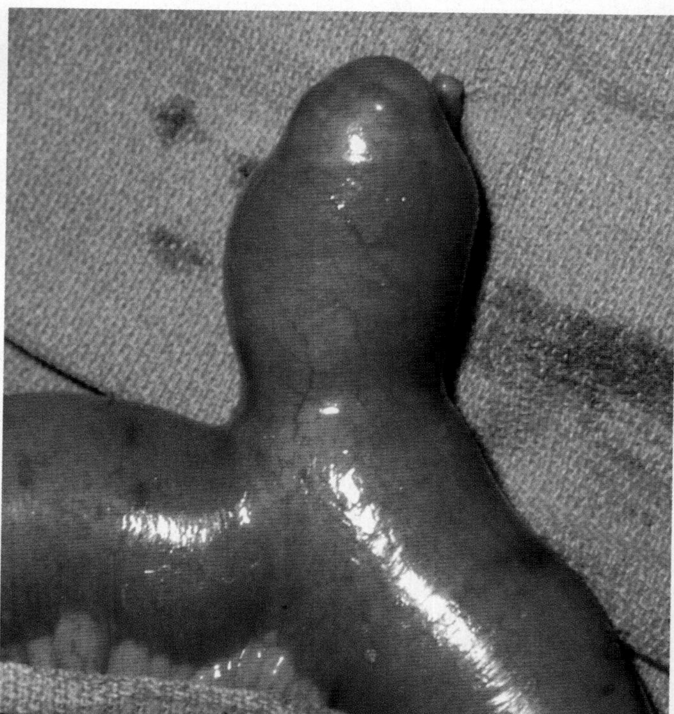

FIGURE 49-45 Common presentation of a Meckel's diverticulum projecting from the antimesenteric border of the ileum.

Another common presenting symptom of Meckel's diverticulum is intestinal obstruction, which may occur as a result of a volvulus of the small bowel around a diverticulum associated with a fibrotic band attached to the abdominal wall, intussusception, or, rarely, incarceration of the diverticulum in an inguinal hernia (Littre hernia). Volvulus is usually an acute event and, if allowed to progress, may result in strangulation of the involved bowel. In intussusception, a broad-based diverticulum invaginates and then is carried forward by peristalsis. This may be ileoileal or ileocolic

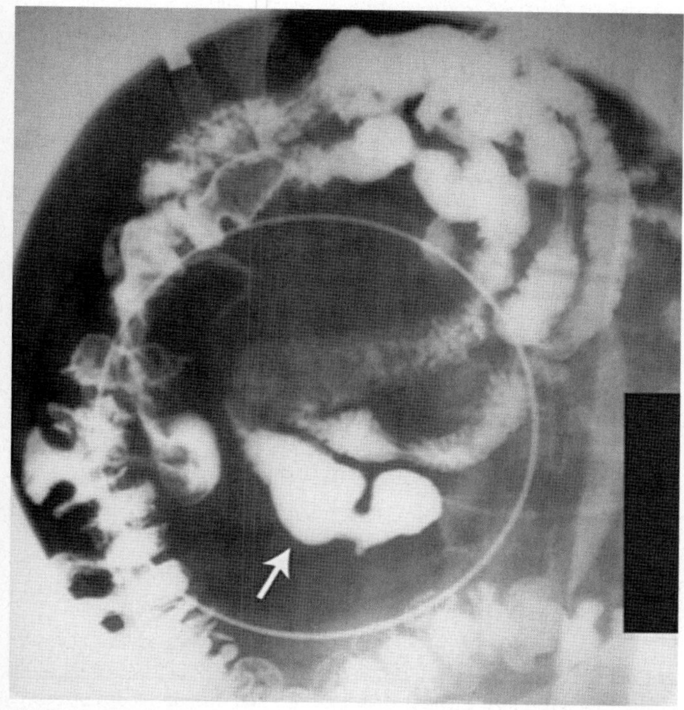

FIGURE 49-46 Barium radiograph demonstrates an asymptomatic Meckel's diverticulum *(arrow)*. (Courtesy Dr. Melvyn H. Schreiber, The University of Texas Medical Branch, Galveston, TX.)

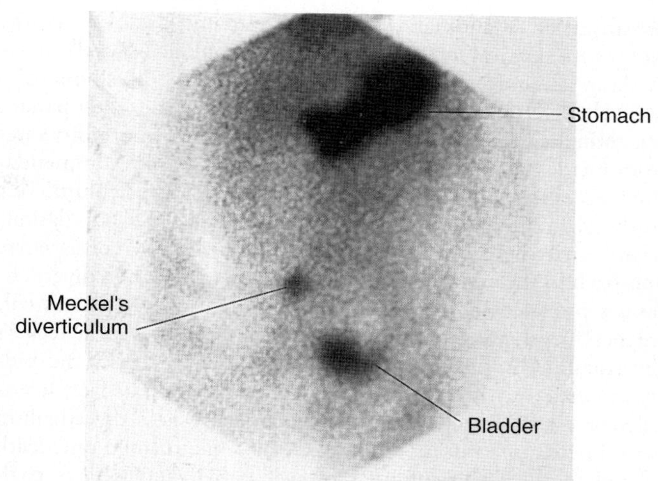

FIGURE 49-47 A ^{99m}Tc-pertechnetate scintigram from a child demonstrates a Meckel's diverticulum clearly differentiated from the stomach and bladder. (Courtesy Dr. Melvyn H. Schreiber, The University of Texas Medical Branch, Galveston, TX.)

and be manifested as acute obstruction associated with an urge to defecate, early vomiting, and occasionally the passage of the classic currant jelly stool. A palpable mass may be present. Although reduction of an intussusception secondary to Meckel's diverticulum can sometimes be performed by barium enema, the patient should still undergo resection of the diverticulum to negate subsequent recurrence of the condition.

Diverticulitis accounts for 10% to 20% of symptomatic presentations. This complication is more common in adult patients. Meckel's diverticulitis, which is clinically indistinguishable from appendicitis, should be considered in the differential diagnosis of a patient with right lower quadrant pain. Progression of the diverticulitis may lead to perforation and peritonitis. When the appendix is found to be normal during exploration for suspected appendicitis, the distal ileum should be inspected for the presence of an inflamed Meckel's diverticulum.

Neoplasms can also occur in a Meckel's diverticulum, with NET as the most common malignant neoplasm (77%). Other histologic types include adenocarcinoma (11%), which generally originates from the gastric mucosa, and GIST (10%) and lymphoma (1%).[43]

Diagnostic Studies

The diagnosis of Meckel's diverticulum may be difficult. Plain abdominal radiography, CT, and ultrasonography are rarely helpful. In children, the single most accurate diagnostic test for Meckel's diverticula is scintigraphy with sodium ^{99m}Tc-pertechnetate. The ^{99m}Tc-pertechnetate is preferentially taken up by the mucus-secreting cells of gastric mucosa and ectopic gastric tissue in the diverticulum (Fig. 49-47). The diagnostic sensitivity of this scan has been reported as high as 85%, with a specificity of 95% and an accuracy of 90% in the pediatric age group.

In adults, however, the sensitivity of ^{99m}Tc-pertechnetate scan falls to 63% because of the presence of less gastric mucosa in the diverticulum compared with that noted in the pediatric age group. The sensitivity and specificity can be improved by the use of pharmacologic agents. Cimetidine may be used to increase the sensitivity of scintigraphy by decreasing the peptic secretion, but not the radionuclide uptake, and retarding the release of pertechnetate from the diverticular lumen, thus resulting in higher radionuclide concentrations in the wall of the diverticulum. In adult patients, when nuclear medicine findings are normal, barium studies should be performed. False-negative results can occur because of inadequate gastric mucosal cells, inflammatory changes causing edema or necrosis, presence of outlet obstruction of the diverticulum, or low hemoglobin levels. In false-negative cases, mesenteric arteriography or double-balloon endoscopy can be helpful. In patients with acute hemorrhage, angiography is sometimes useful. Nevertheless, surgical intervention should not be delayed to obtain imaging for a patient with signs and symptoms of hemorrhage and hemodynamic instability.

Treatment

The treatment of a symptomatic Meckel's diverticulum should be prompt surgical intervention with resection of the diverticulum or resection of the segment of ileum bearing the diverticulum. Segmental intestinal resection is required for treatment of patients with bleeding because the bleeding site is usually in the ileum adjacent to the diverticulum. Resection of the diverticulum for nonbleeding Meckel's diverticula can be performed with a handsewn technique or stapling across the base of the diverticulum in a diagonal or transverse line to minimize the risk for subsequent stenosis. Reports have demonstrated the feasibility, effectiveness, and safety of laparoscopic diverticulectomy.

Although the treatment of complicated Meckel's diverticulum is straightforward, the optimal treatment of Meckel's diverticulum noted as an incidental finding is still debated. It is generally recommended that asymptomatic diverticula found in children during laparotomy be resected. The treatment of Meckel's diverticula encountered in the adult patient, however, remains controversial. A landmark paper by Soltero and Bill[44] formed the basis of the surgical management of asymptomatic Meckel's diverticula in adults for many years. In this study, the likelihood of a Meckel's diverticulum becoming symptomatic in the adult patient was estimated to be 2% or less, and given that the morbidity rates from incidental removal were 12% at the time, the recommendation was to not remove the incidental Meckel's diverticulum. This study was criticized, however, because it was not a population-based analysis. Further evidence supporting a conservative approach to the management of the incidental Meckel's diverticulum is provided in an analysis of 244 articles by Zani and colleagues[45] evaluating the incidence and outcomes of Meckel's diverticulum. In this study, a clear incidence of increased morbidity associated with incidental resection was noted; in fact, it was calculated that resection of an incidental Meckel's diverticulum would be required in more than 700 patients to avoid one death related to the diverticulum. However, other studies have challenged this more conservative approach to the adult patient with an incidental Meckel's diverticulum. For example, an epidemiologic population-based study by Cullen and associates[46] in 1994 initially challenged the practice of ignoring an incidentally found Meckel's diverticulum. A 6.4% rate of development of complications from the Meckel's diverticulum was calculated to occur over a lifetime. This incidence of complications did not appear to peak during childhood, as originally thought. Therefore, the recommendation from this study was that an incidentally found Meckel's diverticulum be removed at any age up to 80 years as long as no additional conditions (e.g., peritonitis) make removal hazardous. The rates of short- and long-term postoperative complications from prophylactic removal were low (~2%), and death was related to the primary operation or the general health of the patient and not to the diverticulectomy. Furthermore, in a recent population-based study evaluating patients from 1973 to 2006, the mean annual incidence of malignancy in a Meckel's diverticulum was noted to be approximately 1.44 per 10 million; therefore, the adjusted risk of cancer in the Meckel's diverticulum was at least 70 times higher than in any other ileal site, thus identifying a Meckel's diverticulum as a "hot spot" for malignant disease in the ileum.[43] Given the increased risk of malignant transformation over a lifetime, the authors advocated for removal of an incidental Meckel's diverticulum.

MISCELLANEOUS PROBLEMS

Small Bowel Ulcerations

Ulcerations of the small bowel are relatively uncommon and may be attributed to Crohn's disease, typhoid fever, tuberculosis, lymphoma, and ulcers associated with gastrinoma (Table 49-12). Drug-induced ulcerations can occur and were, in the past, attributed to enteric-coated potassium chloride tablets and corticosteroids. In addition, ulcerations of the small intestine in which no causative agent can be identified have been described. It has been suggested that small bowel complications from NSAIDs may be more common than originally considered. NSAID-induced ulcers occur more commonly in the ileum, with single or multiple ulcerations noted. Complications necessitating operative intervention include bleeding, perforation, and obstruction. In addition to ulcerations, NSAIDs are known to induce an enteropathy characterized by increased intestinal permeability leading to protein loss and hypoalbuminemia, malabsorption, and anemia. Treatment of complications from small bowel ulcerations is segmental resection and intestinal reanastomosis.

TABLE 49-12 Causes of Small Intestine Ulceration

CAUSE	EXAMPLES
Infections	Tuberculosis, syphilis, cytomegalovirus, typhoid, parasites, *Strongyloides* hyperinfection, *Campylobacter, Yersinia*
Inflammatory	Crohn's disease, systemic lupus erythematosus, celiac disease, ulcerative enteritis
Ischemia	Mesenteric insufficiency
Idiopathic	Primary ulcer, Behçet syndrome
Drug induced	Potassium, indomethacin, phenylbutazone, salicylates, antimetabolites
Radiation	Therapeutic, accidental
Vascular	Vasculitis, giant cell arteritis, amyloidosis (ischemic lesion), angiocentric lymphoma
Metabolic	Uremia
Hyperacidity	Zollinger-Ellison syndrome, Meckel's diverticulum, stomal ulceration
Neoplastic	Lymphoma, adenocarcinoma, melanoma
Toxic	Acute jejunitis (β-toxin–producing *Clostridium perfringens*), arsenic
Mucosal lesions	Lymphocytic enterocolitis

Adapted from Rai R, Bayless TM: Isolated and diffuse ulcers of the small intestine. In Feldman M, Scharschmidt BF, Sleisenger MH, editors: *Gastrointestinal and liver disease: Pathophysiology, diagnosis, management*, Philadelphia, 1998, WB Saunders, pp 1771–1778.

Ingested Foreign Bodies

Ingested foreign bodies, which can lead to subsequent perforation or obstruction of the gastrointestinal tract, are swallowed, usually accidentally, by children or adults. These include glass and metal fragments, pins, needles, toothpicks, fish bones, coins, whistles, toys, and broken razor blades (Fig. 49-48). Intentional ingestion of foreign bodies is sometimes seen in the prison population and those who are mentally unstable. For most patients, treatment is observation, which allows the safe passage of these objects through the intestinal tract. If the object is radiopaque, progress can be followed by serial abdominal films. Cathartic agents are contraindicated. Sharp pointed objects such as needles, razor blades, or fish bones may penetrate the bowel wall. If abdominal pain, tenderness, fever, or leukocytosis occurs, immediate laparotomy and surgical removal of the offending object are indicated. Laparotomy is also required for intestinal obstruction.

Small Bowel Fistulas

Despite improvements in surgical nutrition and critical care, mortality from enterocutaneous fistulas remains high, 10% in recent reports. Improvements in outcome are focused on prevention and, when fistulas occur, prompt recognition and intervention. Multidisciplinary care is critical to improve enterocutaneous fistula outcomes. Enterocutaneous fistulas are most commonly iatrogenic, as 75% to 85% occur during surgical intervention (e.g., anastomotic leakage, injury of the bowel or blood supply, erosion by suction catheters, laceration of the bowel by wire mesh or retention suture). The remaining 15% to 25% of fistula occurrences are associated with predisposing conditions such as Crohn's disease, malignant disease, radiation enteritis, diverticulitis, intra-abdominal sepsis, or trauma.

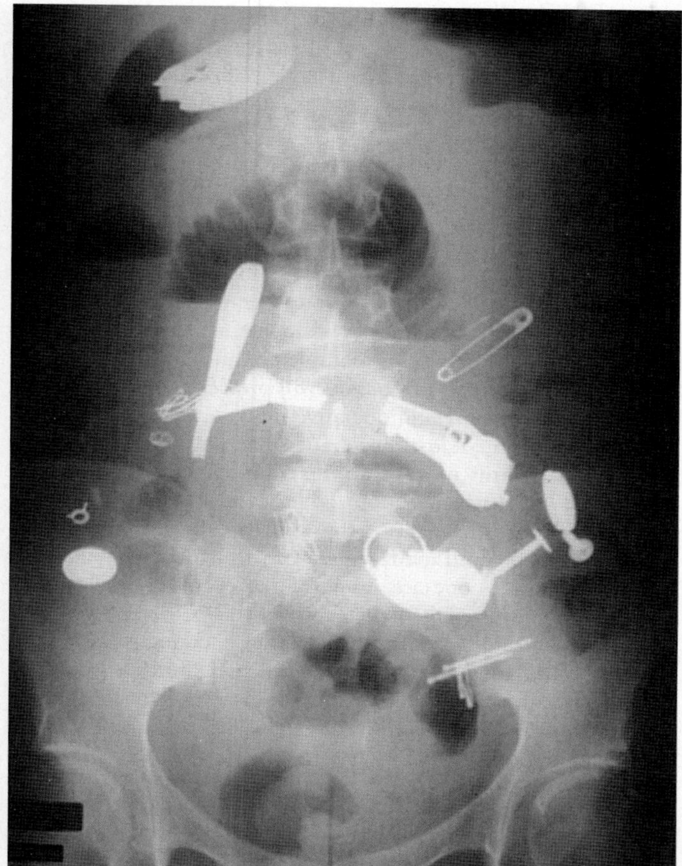

FIGURE 49-48 Plain abdominal film demonstrates a number of ingested foreign bodies in a patient presenting with a small bowel obstruction. (Courtesy Dr. Melvyn H. Schreiber, The University of Texas Medical Branch, Galveston, TX.)

Clinical Manifestations

Recognition of enterocutaneous fistulas is usually not difficult. The typical clinical presentation is that of a febrile postoperative patient with an erythematous wound. When a few skin sutures are removed, a purulent or bloody discharge is noted; leakage of enteric contents then occurs, sometimes immediately but often within 1 or 2 days. The diagnosis rarely eludes the surgeon for long. Small bowel fistulas can also be manifested with generalized peritonitis, although this is less common. Recently, the popularization of damage control laparotomy and staged management of the open abdomen has led to a more virulent form of small bowel fistula referred to as an *enteroatmospheric fistula*. These patients typically present with an open segment of intestine exposed through a large fascial defect, without a surrounding epidermal margin.

Enterocutaneous fistulas are classified according to their location and volume of daily output (Table 49-13). These factors dictate treatment and morbidity and mortality rates. Proximal fistulas are associated with higher output, greater fluid and electrolyte loss, and greater loss of digestive capacity. Distal fistulas tend to have lower output, making them easier to manage and more likely to close spontaneously. High-output fistulas are those that discharge 500 mL or more per 24 hours. Factors that prevent the spontaneous closure of fistulas are shown in Box 49-5. Once a fistula is identified, management should focus on prompt

TABLE 49-13 Fistula Classifications

CLASSIFICATION	DESCRIPTION
Category	Low: <200 mL Intermediate: 200-500 mL High: >500 mL
Anatomy	Gastric, small bowel, colon, rectum
Etiology	Radiation, inflammatory bowel diseases, foreign body (e.g., mesh), iatrogenic injury

BOX 49-5 Factors Preventing Spontaneous Fistula Closure

High output (>500 mL/24 hr)
Severe disruption of intestinal continuity (>50% of bowel circumference)
Active inflammatory bowel disease of bowel segment
Cancer
Radiation enteritis
Distal obstruction
Undrained abscess cavity
Foreign body in the fistula tract
Fistula tract <2.5 cm long
Epithelialization of fistula tract

From Visschers RGJ, van Gemert WG, Winkens B, et al: Guided treatment improves outcome of patients with enterocutaneous fistulas. *World J Surg* 36:2341–2348, 2012.

resuscitation of the patient and consideration of potential factors that could prevent spontaneous closure. Successful management of patients with intestinal fistulas requires a coordinated staged approach that can be defined in three phases—stabilization, staging and supportive care, and definitive management.

Treatment

Stabilization. Historically, malnutrition and fluid losses were the leading causes of death in patients with small bowel fistula. However, with better nutritional supplementation and critical care support, sepsis has become the most common cause of death in affected patients. Nevertheless, the fluid losses and volume depletion associated with small bowel fistula cannot be marginalized. Visschers and coworkers[47] offer a guided treatment algorithm that prolongs periods of convalescence and improves spontaneous closure rates in patients with enterocutaneous fistulas (Box 49-6). Therefore, prompt fluid resuscitation and electrolyte replacement should occur on recognition of a fistula. Sepsis control is critical, and in the early period, CT scanning may be invaluable in identifying undrained abscesses, complete distal obstructions, or generalized intra-abdominal sepsis with peritonitis. All infections should be adequately drained percutaneously or operatively, if necessary, along with appropriate antibiotic administration. Once sepsis is controlled and the patient is resuscitated, effluent control with skin protection and adequate nutrition are necessary. Fistula output is best controlled by intubation of the fistula tract with a drain. Protection of the skin around the fistulous opening is important to prevent excoriation and destruction of the skin. This is most easily accomplished by using a Stomahesive product with applications of zinc oxide, aluminum paste ointment, or karaya powder. The suction catheter can be brought out through the end of the Stomahesive bag, which is cut to just fit the fistulous opening. This will allow collection and accurate measurement of

BOX 49-6 Treatment Strategy in Patients With an Enterocutaneous Fistula

Sepsis Control
Radiologic drainage of abscess
Relaparotomy on demand, minimally invasive if possible
Consider other infectious foci: intravenous line, urinary tract infection, pulmonary

Optimization of Nutritional Status
Rehydration and electrolyte supplementation
Enteral nutrition is preferred
Parenteral nutrition to meet calorie requirements, small bowel ECF
Allow 500 mL/day clear liquids orally

Wound Care
Gauzes for low-output ECF
Collect ECF fluids with bag (wound manager, fistula bag), paste to protect the skin
Drainage of excessive ECF fluid with sump suction
Proton pump inhibitors

Anatomy of ECF
Macroscopic
Biochemical analysis of ECF fluid (bilirubin/amylase)
Methylene blue
Preoperatively: fistulography or contrast CT; length of intestine and localization of origin of ECF, stenosis, obstruction, and fluid collection

Timing of Surgery
Clinically stable (above)
Psychologically willing to undergo surgery
Albumin >25 g/liter
Period of convalescence >6 weeks

Surgical Strategy
One-stage procedure
Careful adhesiolysis
Wedge excision of intestinal resection
Limit number of anastomoses to minimum
Cover sutures with healthy, viable tissue
Keep away from compromised area

Adapted from Visschers RG, van Gemert WG, Winkens B, et al: Guided treatment improves outcome of patients with enterocutaneous fistulas. *World J Surg* 36:2341–2348, 2012.
ECF, Enterocutaneous fistula.

the output. The use of TPN has been an important advance in the management of patients with high-output enterocutaneous fistulas and significantly prevents the problems of malnutrition. TPN is particularly valuable in the stabilization period to help minimize high-output fistula losses and for immediate nutritional repletion while the fistula is being delineated. However, if the patient can meet calorie goals without the use of TPN, especially when a high-output fistula is not present, enteral feeding is preferable and recommended.

Staging and supportive care. When sepsis has been controlled and nutritional therapy has been instituted, the fistula must be adequately staged. The combined use of fluoroscopic contrast studies, fistulography if necessary, and CT, along with the patient's clinical behavior, will characterize the anatomy and underlying pathology of the fistula. Some have advocated conservative management for up to 3 months to allow spontaneous closure. However, others have shown that after sepsis is controlled, more than 90% of small intestinal fistulas that closed did so within 1 month. Less than 10% of the fistulas closed after 2 months, and none closed spontaneously after 3 months. Therefore, a reasonable management plan would be to follow a 6-week period of convalescence, at which time, if closure has not been obtained, surgical management should be considered if the preoperative albumin level is above 25 g/liter. However, knowledge that spontaneous closure is unlikely should not prompt immediate reexploration at 8 weeks. In general, a period of 3 to 6 months is beneficial to allow the profound inflammatory response associated with intra-abdominal sepsis to subside completely and for the adhesion formation to stabilize. This period will provide a better opportunity for safe and successful operative intervention. Furthermore, as is the case with enteroatmospheric small bowel fistulas, it may take several months to stabilize the complex abdominal wound associated with the fistula.

Several adjuncts have been proposed to help assist in spontaneous fistula closure and management of the associated abdominal wound, although none are supported by vigorous level I data. Studies have suggested that bowel rest with TPN therapy improves fistula closure rates and time to closure in patients with high-output fistulas. Low-output fistulas can successfully be managed with enteral therapy while avoiding the known complications of parenteral therapy. Dysmotility agents such as loperamide and codeine can also assist with attempts at enteral therapy. Furthermore, newer techniques, such as fistuloclysis, in which the distal limb of a proximal fistula is intubated and enteral therapy is delivered to the distal bowel, have proved effective. Several randomized trials have evaluated the role of octreotide in the management of fistulas. Although octreotide has been shown to decrease fistula output, which can be useful in the presence of a high-output fistula, octreotide has not convincingly provided an improvement in spontaneous closure rates. Vacuum devices are valuable in the setting of enteroatmospheric fistulas to help contract the open abdominal wound around the associated fistula. Care should be given to avoid direct contact with visceral contents as this can cause new fistulas. Skin grafting up to the fistula has also been used in cases associated with an open abdomen, with a graft success rate of up to 80% in some series.

Definitive management. Once the patient's nutritional, fluid, and wound care needs have been addressed, reoperative intervention will ultimately be necessary for some patients. Surgery is most easily accomplished by entering the previous abdominal wound, with great care taken to avoid further damage to adherent bowel. The preferred operation is fistula tract excision and segmental resection of the involved segment of intestine and reanastomosis. Simple closure of the fistula after removal of the fistula tract almost always results in a recurrence of the fistula. If an unexpected abscess is encountered or if the bowel wall is rigid and distended over a long distance, thus making primary anastomosis unsafe, exteriorization of both ends of the intestine should be accomplished. Various bypass procedures have also been described as part of a staged approach in which exclusion of the segment containing the fistula is accomplished in the first reoperation, and then another operation is required for resection of the involved segment and fistula tract. Although this may be necessary in extreme circumstances, this is certainly not the preferred surgical management. Basic surgical considerations include attempting a one-stage procedure, careful adhesiolysis, addressing compromised tissues with wedge excision or intestinal resection, covering sutures with viable tissues, and avoiding friable areas that are not directly involved with the fistula.

In summary, enterocutaneous fistulas occur most commonly as a result of a previous operative procedure. Once identified, a three-phase approach of stabilization, staging and supportive care, and, in some cases, definitive surgical intervention is necessary. Most of these fistulas heal spontaneously within 6 weeks. If closure is not accomplished after this time, surgery is indicated.

Pneumatosis Intestinalis

Pneumatosis intestinalis is an uncommon condition manifesting as multiple gas-filled cysts of the gastrointestinal tract. The cysts may be located in the subserosa, submucosa, and, rarely, muscularis layer and vary in size from microscopic to several centimeters in diameter. They can occur anywhere along the gastrointestinal tract, from the esophagus to the rectum; however, they are most common in the jejunum, followed by the ileocecal region and colon. Extraintestinal structures such as mesentery, peritoneum, and falciform ligament may also be involved. There is an equal incidence in men and women, and the condition usually occurs in the fourth to seventh decades of life. Pneumatosis in neonates is usually associated with necrotizing enterocolitis. The cause of pneumatosis intestinalis has not been completely delineated. A number of theories have been proposed, of which the mechanical, mucosal damage, bacterial, and pulmonary hypotheses seem to be most promising.

Most cases of pneumatosis intestinalis are associated with chronic obstructive pulmonary disease or the immunocompromised state (e.g., in AIDS; after transplantation; in association with leukemia, lymphoma, vasculitis, or collagen vascular disease; and in patients undergoing chemotherapy or taking corticosteroids). Other associated conditions include inflammatory, obstructive, or infectious conditions of the intestine; iatrogenic conditions, such as endoscopy and jejunostomy placement; ischemia; and extraintestinal diseases, such as diabetes. Pneumatosis not associated with other lesions is referred to as *primary pneumatosis*.

In gross appearance, the cysts resemble cystic lymphangiomas or hydatid cysts. On histologic section, the involved portion has a honeycomb appearance. The cysts are thin walled and break easily. Spontaneous rupture gives rise to pneumoperitoneum. Symptoms are nonspecific, and in pneumatosis associated with other disorders, the symptoms may be those of the associated disease. Symptoms in primary pneumatosis intestinalis, when present, usually include diarrhea, abdominal pain, abdominal distention, nausea, vomiting, weight loss, and mucus in stools. Hematochezia and constipation have also been described. Complications associated with pneumatosis intestinalis occur in about 3% of cases and include volvulus, intestinal obstruction, hemorrhage, and intestinal perforation. Usually, pneumoperitoneum occurs in these patients, generally in association with small bowel rather than large bowel pneumatosis. Peritonitis is unusual. In fact, pneumatosis intestinalis represents one of the few cases of sterile pneumoperitoneum and should be considered in the patient with free abdominal air but no evidence of peritonitis.

The diagnosis is usually made radiographically by plain abdominal or barium studies. On plain films, pneumatosis intestinalis appears as radiolucent areas within the bowel wall, which must be differentiated from luminal intestinal gas (Fig. 49-49*A*). The radiolucency may be linear or curvilinear or appear as grape-like clusters or tiny bubbles. Alternatively, barium contrast or CT studies can be used to confirm the diagnosis (Fig. 49-49*B*). Visualization of intestinal cysts has also been described by ultrasound.

No treatment is necessary unless one of the very rare complications supervenes, such as rectal bleeding, cyst-induced volvulus, or tension pneumoperitoneum. Prognosis in most patients is that of the underlying disease. The important point is to recognize that pneumatosis intestinalis is a benign cause of pneumoperitoneum. Treatment should be directed at the underlying cause of the pneumatosis, and surgical intervention should be predicated on the clinical course of the patient.

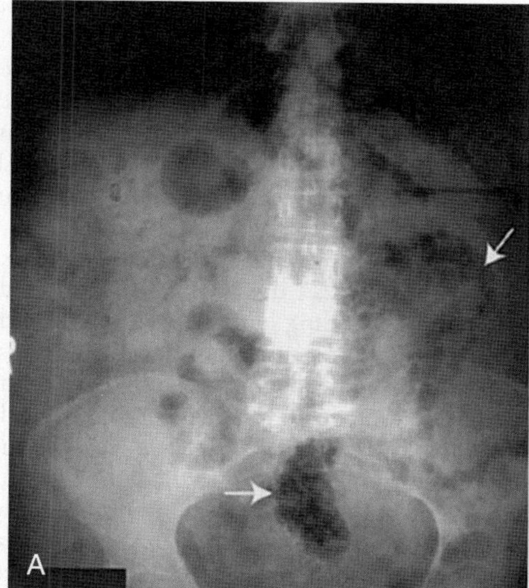

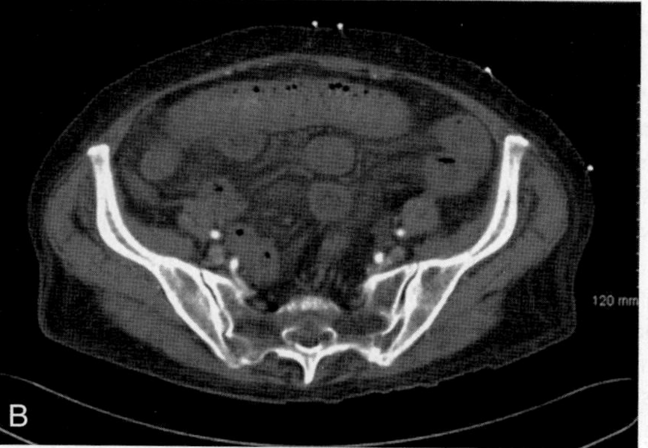

FIGURE 49-49 A, Plain abdominal film demonstrates pneumatosis intestinalis *(arrows)*. **B,** CT findings consistent with curvilinear radiolucency appearing as tiny bubbles in the antimesenteric border of the bowel consistent with pneumatosis intestinalis. (**A,** Courtesy Dr. Melvyn H. Schreiber, The University of Texas Medical Branch, Galveston, TX. **B,** Courtesy Dr. Kristin Long, University of Kentucky Medical Center, Lexington, KY.)

Blind Loop Syndrome

Blind loop syndrome is a rare condition manifested by diarrhea, steatorrhea, megaloblastic anemia, weight loss, abdominal pain, and deficiencies of the fat-soluble vitamins as well as neurologic disorders. The underlying cause of this syndrome is bacterial overgrowth in stagnant areas of the small bowel produced by stricture, stenosis, fistulas, or diverticula (e.g., jejunoileal or Meckel's diverticulum). Under normal circumstances, the upper gastrointestinal tract contains fewer than 10^5 bacteria/mL, mostly gram-positive aerobes and facultative anaerobes. However, with stasis, the number of bacteria increases, with excessive proliferation of aerobic and anaerobic bacteria; bacteroides, anaerobic lactobacilli, coliforms, and enterococci are likely to be present in varying numbers. The bacteria compete for vitamin B_{12}, producing systemic deficiency of vitamin B_{12} and megaloblastic anemia.

The syndrome can be confirmed by a series of laboratory investigations. Bacterial overgrowth can be diagnosed with cultures obtained through an intestinal tube or by indirect tests such as the ^{14}C-xylose or ^{14}C-cholylglycine breath tests. Excessive bacterial use of ^{14}C substrate leads to an increase in $^{14}C-CO_2$. After bacterial overgrowth and steatorrhea are confirmed, a Schilling test (^{57}Co-labeled vitamin B_{12} absorption) may be performed, which should reveal a pattern of urinary excretion of vitamin B_{12} resembling that of pernicious anemia (a urinary loss of 0% to 6% of vitamin B_{12} compared with the normal of 7% to 25%). In patients with blind loop syndrome, vitamin B_{12} excretion is not altered by the addition of intrinsic factor, but a course of a broad-spectrum antibiotic (e.g., tetracycline) should return vitamin B_{12} absorption to normal.

Treatment of patients with blind loop syndrome includes parenteral vitamin B_{12} therapy and broad-spectrum antibiotics. Tetracyclines have been the mainstay of treatment, but studies have shown that rifaximin and metronidazole demonstrate less resistance and are also effective. For most patients, a single course of therapy (7 to 10 days) is sufficient, and the patient may remain symptom free for months. Prokinetic agents have been used without real success. Surgical correction of the condition causing stagnation and blind loop syndrome produces a permanent cure and is indicated for patients who require multiple rounds of antibiotics or are receiving continuous therapy.

Radiation Enteritis

Radiation therapy is generally used as adjuvant therapy for various abdominal and pelvic cancers. In addition to tumor cells, however, other rapidly dividing cells in normal tissues may be affected by radiation. Surrounding normal tissue, such as the small intestinal epithelium, may sustain severe, acute, and chronic deleterious effects. Radiation injury to the small bowel can be subdivided into acute and chronic forms. Acute radiation-induced small bowel disease usually is manifested with colicky abdominal pain, bloating, loss of appetite, nausea, diarrhea, and fecal urgency during or shortly after a course of radiotherapy. Most patients notice symptoms during the second week of treatment, when tissue damage and inflammation are maximal, and symptoms peak by the fourth week when histologic changes are stable or improving.[48] Symptoms consistent with chronic radiation injury typically develop between 18 months and 6 years after a completed course of radiotherapy, but symptoms can be manifested up to 30 years after the treatment course.

The amount of radiation appears to correlate with the probability for development of radiation enteritis. Serious late complications are unusual if the total radiation dosage is less than 4000 cGy; morbidity risk increases with dosages exceeding 5000 cGy. Other factors, including previous abdominal surgeries, preexisting vascular disease, hypertension, diabetes, and adjuvant treatment with certain chemotherapeutic agents (such as 5-FU, doxorubicin, dactinomycin, and MTX), contribute to the development of enteritis after radiation treatments. A previous history of laparotomy increases the risk for enteritis, presumably because of adhesions that fix portions of the small bowel into the irradiated field. Radiation damage leads to symptoms consisting mainly of diarrhea, abdominal pain, and malabsorption. The late effects of radiation injury are the result of damage to the small submucosal blood vessels, with a progressive obliterative arteritis and submucosal fibrosis, resulting eventually in thrombosis and vascular insufficiency. This injury may produce necrosis and perforation of the involved intestine but, more commonly, leads to stricture formation with symptoms of obstruction or small bowel fistulas.

BOX 49-7 Prevention of Radiation-Induced Small Bowel Disease: Clinical Guidance

- Use of modern imaging and radiotherapy techniques to minimize radiation exposure to normal tissues
- Consideration of circadian rhythm effects and use of evening radiotherapy sessions
- Continuation of angiotensin-converting enzyme inhibitors and statins and consideration of their introduction if appropriate
- Consideration of the use of probiotics
- Consideration of surgical techniques to minimize radiation exposure to the small bowel if appropriate and surgical team is experienced and competent at the procedure involved

Adapted from Stacey R, Green JT: Radiation-induced small bowel disease: Latest developments and clinical guidance. *Ther Adv Chronic Dis* 5:15–29, 2014.

Multiple strategies are used to reduce radiation injury to the small bowel (Box 49-7). Radiation enteritis may be minimized by adjusting ports and dosages of radiation to deliver optimal treatment specifically to the tumor and not to surrounding tissues. Placement of radiopaque markers, such as titanium clips, at the time of the original operation facilitates better targeting of the radiation treatment. A reduction in field size, multiple field arrangements, conformal radiotherapy techniques, and intensity-modulated radiotherapy can reduce toxicity related to radiotherapy. Methods designed to exclude the small bowel from the irradiated field include reperitonealization, omental transposition, and placement of absorbable mesh slings.

A number of pharmacologic interventions have also been described to reduce the side effects of radiation enteritis. Angiotensin-converting enzyme inhibitors and statins significantly reduce acute gastrointestinal symptoms during radical pelvic radiotherapy. Sucralfate, a highly sulfated polyanionic disaccharide thought to stimulate epithelial healing and to form a protective barrier over damaged mucosal surfaces, may help in the treatment of bleeding from radiation proctitis, but no evidence exists supporting its use in the prevention of radiation-induced small bowel disease. Superoxide dismutase, a free radical scavenger, has been used successfully to reduce complications. Other compounds that have been evaluated include glutathione, antioxidants (e.g., vitamin A, vitamin E, beta-carotene), histamine antagonists, and the combination of pentoxifylline and tocopherols, a class of chemical compounds with vitamin E activity. In addition, early studies have supported the use of probiotics as having a radioprotective effect in the gut; however, further studies are required before a final assessment can be made. The most effective radioprotectant agent appears to be amifostine (WR-2721), a sulfhydryl compound that is converted intracellularly to an active metabolite, WR-1065, which in turn binds to free radicals and protects the cell from radiation injury. A randomized controlled trial determined that glutamine offers little benefit, even when it is used before or during radiation therapy. Agents that may prove useful in the prevention of the acute symptoms of radiation enteritis include the hormones bombesin, growth hormone, glucagon-like peptide 2 (GLP-2), and insulin-like growth factor I (IGF-I), which have demonstrated effectiveness in experimental studies in preventing or reducing symptoms associated with radiation enteritis.

The treatment of acute radiation enteritis is directed at controlling symptoms. Antispasmodics and analgesics may alleviate abdominal pain and cramping, and diarrhea usually responds to opiates or other antidiarrheal agents. The use of corticosteroids for acute radiation enteritis is of uncertain value. Dietary manipulation, including oral elemental diets, has also been advocated to ameliorate the acute effects of radiation enteritis; however, results are conflicting. Antibiotics are frequently used in the setting of bacterial overgrowth. Bile acid malabsorption, thought to be responsible for diarrheal symptoms in 35% to 72% of patients with radiation-induced small bowel disease, responds well to cholestyramine, but it is not well-tolerated and many patients voluntarily discontinue use.

Operative intervention may be required for a subgroup of patients with the chronic effects of radiation enteritis. This subgroup of patients represents only a small percentage (1% to 2%) of the total number of patients who have received abdominal or pelvic irradiation. Indications for operation include obstruction, fistula formation, perforation, and bleeding, with obstruction being the most common presentation. Operative procedures include a bypass or resection with reanastomosis. Advocates for bypass procedures contend that this procedure is safer and controls the symptoms better than resection. Advocates of resection contend that the high morbidity and mortality rates previously reported with resection and reanastomosis reflect inadequate resection and anastomosis of diseased intestine. In patients presenting with obstruction, extensive lysis of adhesions should be avoided. Obstruction caused by rigid, fixed intestinal loops in the pelvis is best bypassed. If resection and reanastomosis are planned, at least one end of the anastomosis should be from intestine outside the irradiated field. Macroscopic findings may not be accurate in evaluating the full extent of radiation damage. Frozen section and laser Doppler flowmetry techniques have been used to assist resection and anastomosis. However, reports of their clinical usefulness are conflicting. Perforation of the intestine should be treated with resection and anastomosis. When reanastomosis is thought to be unsafe, the ends should be exteriorized.

Short Bowel Syndrome

The short bowel syndrome results from a total small bowel length that is inadequate to support nutrition. Of these cases of short bowel syndrome, 75% occur from massive intestinal resection. In the adult, mesenteric occlusion, midgut volvulus, and traumatic disruption of the superior mesenteric vessels are the most frequent causes. Multiple sequential resections, usually associated with recurrent Crohn's disease, account for 25% of patients. In neonates, the most common cause of short bowel syndrome is bowel resection secondary to necrotizing enterocolitis. The clinical hallmarks of short bowel syndrome include diarrhea, fluid and electrolyte deficiency, and malnutrition. Other complications include an increased incidence of gallstones caused by disruption of the enterohepatic circulation and of nephrolithiasis from hyperoxaluria. Specific nutrient deficiencies must be prevented, and levels must be monitored closely; these nutrients include iron, magnesium, zinc, copper, and vitamins. The likelihood that a patient with short bowel syndrome will be permanently dependent on TPN is thought to be primarily influenced by the length, location, and health of the remaining intestine. In patients with short bowel syndrome, postabsorptive levels of plasma citrulline, a nonprotein amino acid produced by intestinal mucosa, may provide an indicator to differentiate transient from permanent intestinal failure.

The bowel has a remarkable capacity to adapt after small bowel resection; in many cases, this process of intestinal adaptation, termed adaptive hyperplasia, effectively prevents severe complications resulting from the markedly decreased surface area available for absorption and digestion. However, any adaptive mechanism can be overwhelmed, and adaptation can be inadequate if too much small bowel is lost. Although there is considerable individual variation, resection of up to 70% of the small bowel usually can be tolerated if the terminal ileum and ileocecal valve are preserved. Length alone, however, is not the only determining factor of complications related to small bowel resection. For example, if the distal two thirds of the ileum, including the ileocecal valve, is resected, significant abnormalities of absorption of bile salts and vitamin B_{12} may occur, resulting in diarrhea and anemia, although only 25% of the total length of the small bowel has been removed. Proximal bowel resection is tolerated better than distal resection because the ileum can adapt and increase its absorptive capacity more efficiently than the jejunum.

Treatment

The most important issue to remember about short bowel syndrome is prevention. In patients with Crohn's disease, resections limited to the particular complication should be performed. In addition, during surgery for problems related to intestinal ischemia, the smallest possible resection should be performed, and if necessary, second-look operations should be carried out to allow the ischemic bowel to demarcate, thus potentially preventing unnecessary extensive resection of the bowel.

After massive small bowel resection, the treatment course may be divided into early and late phases. In its early phase, treatment is primarily directed at the control of diarrhea, replacement of fluid and electrolytes, and prompt institution of TPN in patients who cannot safely tolerate enteral feedings. Volume losses may exceed 5 liters/day, and vigorous monitoring of intake and output with adequate replacement must be carried out. Diarrhea in this early phase can be caused by a multitude of sources. For example, hypergastrinemia and gastric hypersecretion occur after massive small bowel resection and greatly contribute to diarrhea after a massive small bowel resection. Acid hypersecretion can be managed by H_2 receptor antagonists or proton pump blockers, such as omeprazole. Diarrhea may also be caused by ileal resection, resulting in disruption of the enterohepatic circulation and excessive amounts of bile salts entering the colon. Cholestyramine may be beneficial when diarrhea is related to the cathartic effects of unabsorbed bile salts in the colon. In addition, the judicious use of agents that inhibit gut motility (e.g., codeine, diphenoxylate) may be helpful. The long-acting somatostatin analogue octreotide also appears to reduce the amount of diarrhea during the early phase of short bowel syndrome. Some studies have suggested that octreotide may inhibit gut adaptation; other studies, however, have not confirmed this deleterious effect of octreotide.

As soon as the patient has recovered from the acute phase, enteral nutrition should be started. The most common types of enteral diets are elemental (e.g., Vivonex, Flexical) and polymeric (e.g., Isocal, Ensure). Controversy exists about the optimal diet for these patients. Initially, a high-carbohydrate, high-protein diet is appropriate to maximize absorption. Milk products should be avoided, and the diet should be begun at iso-osmolar concentrations and with small amounts. As the gut adapts, the osmolality, volume, and calorie content can be increased. The provision of nutrients in their simplest forms is an important part of the treatment. Simple sugars, dipeptides, and tripeptides are rapidly absorbed from the intestinal tract. Reduction in dietary fat has long been considered to be important in the treatment of patients with short bowel syndrome. Supplementation of the diet with 100 g or more of fat, however, should be carried out, often requiring the use of medium-chain triglycerides, which are absorbed in the proximal bowel. Vitamins, especially fat-soluble vitamins, as well as calcium, magnesium, and zinc supplementation should be provided. The roles of hormones administered systemically and glutamine administered enterally have been evaluated. The hormones neurotensin, bombesin, and GLP-2 have demonstrated marked mucosal growth in various experimental studies and have been shown to prevent the gut atrophy associated with TPN in experimental studies; combination therapy appears more efficacious than single-agent administration. Randomized controlled trials have shown that teduglutide, a GLP-2 analogue that is resistant to degradation by the proteolytic enzyme dipeptidyl peptidase 4 and therefore has a longer half-life than GLP-2, is well tolerated and has led to the restoration of intestinal functional and structural integrity through significant intestinotrophic and proabsorptive effects. It is the first targeted therapeutic agent to gain approval for use in adult short bowel syndrome with intestinal failure.[49]

Two other hormones not derived from the gut that have been evaluated extensively in various experimental and limited clinical trials include growth hormone and IGF-I. A meta-analysis of randomized controlled trials using growth hormone in short bowel syndrome suggests a possible short-term benefit in terms of body weight, lean body mass, and absorptive capacity; however, long-term efficacy was not noted. Somatropin, a recombinant human growth hormone that elicits anabolic and anticatabolic influence on various cells either as a direct effect or indirectly through IGF-I, is currently indicated to treat short bowel syndrome in conjunction with nutritional support. The combination of various trophic hormones with glutamine and a modified diet may prove more efficacious in the treatment of this difficult group of patients.

A number of surgical strategies have been attempted in patients who are chronically TPN dependent, with limited success; these include procedures to delay intestinal transit time, methods to increase absorptive area, and small bowel transplantation. Methods to delay intestinal transit time include the construction of various valves and sphincters, with inconsistent results reported. Antiperistaltic segments of small intestine have been constructed to slow the transit, thus allowing additional contact time for nutrient and fluid absorption. Moderate successes have been described with this technique. Other procedures, including colonic interposition, recirculating loops of small bowel, and retrograde electrical pacing, have been tried but were found to be unsuccessful in humans and were largely abandoned. Surgical procedures to increase absorptive area include the intestinal tapering and lengthening procedure (e.g., Bianchi procedure), which improves intestinal function by correcting the dilation and ineffective peristalsis of the remaining intestine and by doubling the intestinal length while preserving the mucosal surface area.[50] Although beneficial in selected patients, potential complications can include necrosis of divided segments and anastomotic leaks.

Intestinal transplantation remains the standard of care for patients in whom intestinal rehabilitation attempts have failed and who are at risk of life-threatening complications of TPN. Patient survival after intestinal transplantation has significantly improved with the introduction of the immunosuppressive agent FK-506. The 1- and 5-year survival rates for isolated intestinal transplantation are 75% and 48%, respectively. Combined intestinal-liver transplants have comparable 1- and 5-year survival rates of approximately 66% and 54%, respectively. The challenges of small bowel transplantation continue to be the need for better immunosuppression and earlier detection of rejection.

Vascular Compression of the Duodenum

Vascular compression of the duodenum, also known as *superior mesenteric artery syndrome* or *Wilkie syndrome*, is a rare condition characterized by compression of the third portion of the duodenum by the superior mesenteric artery as it passes over this portion

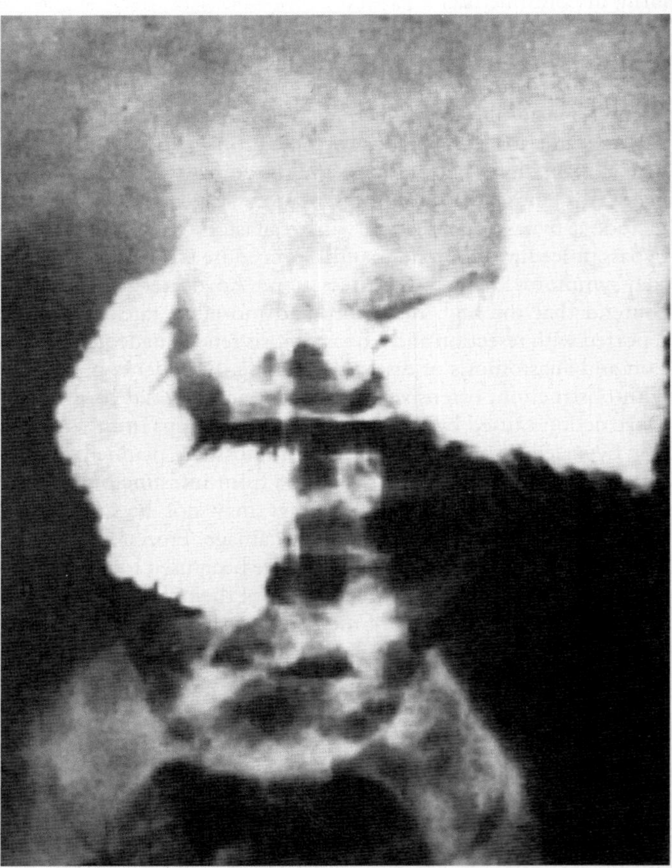

FIGURE 49-50 Barium radiograph demonstrates obstruction of the third portion of the duodenum secondary to superior mesenteric artery compression as a consequence of burn injury. (Adapted from Reckler JM, Bruck HM, Munster AM, et al: Superior mesenteric artery syndrome as a consequence of burn injury. *J Trauma* 12:979–985, 1972.)

of the duodenum. Symptoms include profound nausea and vomiting, abdominal distention, weight loss, and postprandial epigastric pain, which varies from intermittent to constant, depending on the severity of the duodenal obstruction. Weight loss usually occurs before the onset of symptoms and contributes to the syndrome.

This syndrome is most commonly seen in young asthenic individuals, with women being more commonly affected than men. Predisposing factors for vascular compression of the duodenum, aside from weight loss, include supine immobilization, scoliosis, and placement of a body cast, sometimes called the *cast syndrome*. An association between vascular compression of the duodenum and peptic ulcer has been observed. Vascular compression of the duodenum has been reported in association with anorexia nervosa and after proctocolectomy and J-pouch anal anastomosis, resection of an arteriovenous malformation of the cervical cord, abdominal aortic aneurysm repair, and orthopedic procedures, usually spinal surgery. One report in the literature described a family with a preponderance of vascular compression of the duodenum.

Diagnosis of this condition is made by a barium upper gastrointestinal series (Fig. 49-50) or hypotonic duodenography, which demonstrates abrupt or near-total cessation of flow of barium from the duodenum to the jejunum. CT has been useful in certain cases. Treatment of this syndrome varies. Conservative measures are tried initially and have been increasingly successful as definitive treatment. The operative treatment of choice for vascular compression of the duodenum is duodenojejunostomy.

SELECTED REFERENCES

Affronti A, Orlando A, Cottone M: An update on medical management on Crohn's disease. *Expert Opin Pharmacother* 16:63–78, 2015.

This represents a clear and concise review article highlighting critical issues in the management of Crohn's disease, new evidence from clinical trials, long-term prospective studies, and real-life experience, beyond the current guidelines.

Bilimoria KY, Bentrem DJ, Wayne JD, et al: Small bowel cancer in the United States: Changes in epidemiology, treatment, and survival over the last 20 years. *Ann Surg* 249:63–71, 2009.

This study represents a large, national database analysis of the overall increase of incidence of small intestine malignant neoplasms during the past two decades.

Caplin ME, Pavel M, Cwikla JB, et al: Lanreotide in metastatic enteropancreatic neuroendocrine tumors. *N Engl J Med* 371:224–233, 2014.

The landmark CLARINET trial (LanreotideAntiproliferativeResponse in patients with GEP-NET) is the largest phase 3, randomized, double-blind, placebo-controlled, multinational study that evaluated the antiproliferative effect of the somatostatin analogue lanreotide in patients with GEP-NETs. Lanreotide was associated with significantly prolonged progression-free survival among patients with grade 1 or 2 metastatic enteropancreatic neuroendocrine tumors.

Castano JP, Sundin A, Maecke HR, et al: Gastrointestinal neuroendocrine tumors (NETs): New diagnostic and therapeutic challenges. *Cancer Metastasis Rev* 33:353–359, 2014.

This paper summarizes the current understanding of the biology of somatostatin receptor, role of immunotherapy in neuroendocrine tumor (NET), new agents for peptide receptor radionuclide therapy, and methods to assess response and clinical benefit in NET.

Crohn BB, Ginzburg L, Oppenheimer GD: Regional ileitis: a pathologic and clinical entity. *JAMA* 99:1323–1329, 1932.

This landmark paper succinctly crystallizes the clinical course, differential diagnosis, and pathologic findings of regional ileitis in young adults. Although other terms have been applied to this disease process, based on the descriptions in this classic paper, Crohn's disease has been universally accepted as the name.

Thirunavukarasu P, Sathaiah M, Sukumar S, et al: Meckel's diverticulum—a high-risk region for malignancy in the ileum. Insights from a population-based epidemiological study and implications in surgical management. *Ann Surg* 253:223–230, 2011.

A national database study during 33 years that suggests Meckel's diverticulum is a high-risk area for ileal cancer and supports the resection of incidental Meckel's diverticulum.

Vasen HF, Moslein G, Alonso A, et al: Guidelines for the clinical management of familial adenomatous polyposis (FAP). *Gut* 57:704–713, 2008.

This article represents a thorough review of the literature and treatment guidelines for the clinical management of patients with FAP and their families.

REFERENCES

1. Moore KL, Persaud TVN: The digestive system. In Moore KL, Persaud TVN, editors: *The developing human: Clinically oriented embryology*, ed 9, Philadelphia, 2011, Elsevier, pp 255–286.
2. Bykov VL: Paneth cells: History of discovery, structural and functional characteristics and the role in the maintenance of homeostasis in the small intestine. *Morfologiia* 145:67–80, 2014.
3. Chung DH, Evers BM: The digestive system. In O'Leary JP, editor: *The physiologic basis of surgery*, ed 4, Philadelphia, 2007, Lippincott Williams & Wilkins, pp 475–507.
4. Field BC: Neuroendocrinology of obesity. *Br Med Bull* 109:73–82, 2014.
5. Zielinski MD, Bannon MP: Current management of small bowel obstruction. *Adv Surg* 45:1–29, 2011.
6. Maglinte DD: Fluoroscopic and CT enteroclysis: Evidence-based clinical update. *Radiol Clin North Am* 51:149–176, 2013.
7. Sallinen V, Wikstrom H, Victorzon M, et al: Laparoscopic versus open adhesiolysis for small bowel obstruction—a multicenter, prospective, randomized, controlled trial. *BMC Surg* 14:77, 2014.

8. Park CM, Lee WY, Cho YB, et al: Sodium hyaluronate–based bioresorbable membrane (Seprafilm) reduced early postoperative intestinal obstruction after lower abdominal surgery for colorectal cancer: The preliminary report. *Int J Colorectal Dis* 24:305–310, 2009.
9. Crohn BB, Ginzburg L, Oppenheimer GD: Regional ileitis: A pathologic and clinical entity. *JAMA* 99:1323–1329, 1932.
10. Lichtenstein GR: Current research in Crohn's disease and ulcerative colitis: Highlights from the 2010 ACG Meeting. *Gastroenterol Hepatol (N Y)* 6:3–14, 2010.
11. Petersen BS, Spehlmann ME, Raedler A, et al: Whole genome and exome sequencing of monozygotic twins discordant for Crohn's disease. *BMC Genomics* 15:564, 2014.
12. Vermeire S, Van Assche G, Rutgeerts P: Inflammatory bowel disease and colitis: New concepts from the bench and the clinic. *Curr Opin Gastroenterol* 27:32–37, 2011.
13. Tsianos EV, Katsanos KH, Tsianos VE: Role of genetics in the diagnosis and prognosis of Crohn's disease. *World J Gastroenterol* 18:105–118, 2012.
14. Spinelli A, Allocca M, Jovani M, et al: Review article: Optimal preparation for surgery in Crohn's disease. *Aliment Pharmacol Ther* 40:1009–1022, 2014.
15. Malvi D, Vasuri F, Mattioli B, et al: Adenocarcinoma in Crohn's disease: The pathologist's experience in a tertiary referral centre of inflammatory bowel disease. *Pathology* 46:439–443, 2014.
16. Fiorino G, Bonifacio C, Peyrin-Biroulet L, et al: Prospective comparison of computed tomography enterography and magnetic resonance enterography for assessment of disease activity and complications in ileocolonic Crohn's disease. *Inflamm Bowel Dis* 17:1073–1080, 2011.
17. Bourreille A, Ignjatovic A, Aabakken L, et al: Role of small-bowel endoscopy in the management of patients with inflammatory bowel disease: An international OMED-ECCO consensus. *Endoscopy* 41:618–637, 2009.
18. van Schaik FD, Oldenburg B, Hart AR, et al: Serological markers predict inflammatory bowel disease years before the diagnosis. *Gut* 62:683–688, 2013.
19. Yamamoto T, Shiraki M, Bamba T, et al: Faecal calprotectin and lactoferrin as markers for monitoring disease activity and predicting clinical recurrence in patients with Crohn's disease after ileocolonic resection: A prospective pilot study. *United European Gastroenterol J* 1:368–374, 2013.
20. Affronti A, Orlando A, Cottone M: An update on medical management on Crohn's disease. *Expert Opin Pharmacother* 16:63–78, 2015.
21. Terdiman JP, Gruss CB, Heidelbaugh JJ, et al: American Gastroenterological Association Institute guideline on the use of thiopurines, methotrexate, and anti-TNF-alpha biologic drugs for the induction and maintenance of remission in inflammatory Crohn's disease. *Gastroenterology* 145:1459–1463, 2013.
22. Yamamoto T, Watanabe T: Surgery for luminal Crohn's disease. *World J Gastroenterol* 20:78–90, 2014.
23. Umanskiy K, Malhotra G, Chase A, et al: Laparoscopic colectomy for Crohn's colitis. A large prospective comparative study. *J Gastrointest Surg* 14:658–663, 2010.
24. Krane MK, Allaix ME, Zoccali M, et al: Does morbid obesity change outcomes after laparoscopic surgery for inflammatory bowel disease? Review of 626 consecutive cases. *J Am Coll Surg* 216:986–996, 2013.
25. Eshuis EJ, Bemelman WA, van Bodegraven AA, et al: Laparoscopic ileocolic resection versus infliximab treatment of distal ileitis in Crohn's disease: A randomized multicenter trial (LIR!C-trial). *BMC Surg* 8:15, 2008.
26. Kono T, Ashida T, Ebisawa Y, et al: A new antimesenteric functional end-to-end handsewn anastomosis: Surgical prevention of anastomotic recurrence in Crohn's disease. *Dis Colon Rectum* 54:586–592, 2011.
27. Vaughn BP, Moss AC: Prevention of post-operative recurrence of Crohn's disease. *World J Gastroenterol* 20:1147–1154, 2014.
28. Wiwanitkit V, Srisupanant M: Cryptosporidiosis occurrence in anti-HIV-seropositive patients attending a sexually transmitted diseases clinic, Thailand. *Trop Doct* 36:64, 2006.
29. Poveda A, del Muro XG, Lopez-Guerrero JA, et al: GEIS 2013 guidelines for gastrointestinal sarcomas (GIST). *Cancer Chemother Pharmacol* 74:883–898, 2014.
30. Vasen HF, Moslein G, Alonso A, et al: Guidelines for the clinical management of familial adenomatous polyposis (FAP). *Gut* 57:704–713, 2008.
31. Bilimoria KY, Bentrem DJ, Wayne JD, et al: Small bowel cancer in the United States: Changes in epidemiology, treatment, and survival over the last 20 years. *Ann Surg* 249:63–71, 2009.
32. Reid MD, Balci S, Saka B, et al: Neuroendocrine tumors of the pancreas: Current concepts and controversies. *Endocr Pathol* 25:65–79, 2014.
33. Rindi G, Petrone G, Inzani F: The 2010 WHO classification of digestive neuroendocrine neoplasms: A critical appraisal four years after its introduction. *Endocr Pathol* 25:186–192, 2014.
34. Castano JP, Sundin A, Maecke HR, et al: Gastrointestinal neuroendocrine tumors (NETs): New diagnostic and therapeutic challenges. *Cancer Metastasis Rev* 33:353–359, 2014.
35. Ilhan H, Fendler WP, Cyran CC, et al: Impact of ^{68}Ga-DOTATATE PET/CT on the surgical management of primary neuroendocrine tumors of the pancreas or ileum. *Ann Surg Oncol* 22:164–171, 2015.
36. Coan KE, Gray RJ, Schlinkert RT, et al: Metastatic carcinoid tumors—are we making the cut? *Am J Surg* 205:642–646, 2013.
37. Figueiredo MN, Maggiori L, Gaujoux S, et al: Surgery for small-bowel neuroendocrine tumors: Is there any benefit of the laparoscopic approach? *Surg Endosc* 28:1720–1726, 2014.
38. Toumpanakis C, Caplin ME: Update on the role of somatostatin analogs for the treatment of patients with gastroenteropancreatic neuroendocrine tumors. *Semin Oncol* 40:56–68, 2013.
39. Anthony L, Freda PU: From somatostatin to octreotide LAR: Evolution of a somatostatin analogue. *Curr Med Res Opin* 25:2989–2999, 2009.
40. Caplin ME, Pavel M, Cwikla JB, et al: Lanreotide in metastatic enteropancreatic neuroendocrine tumors. *N Engl J Med* 371:224–233, 2014.
41. Chan J, Kulke M: Targeting the mTOR signaling pathway in neuroendocrine tumors. *Curr Treat Options Oncol* 15:365–379, 2014.
42. Aparicio T, Zaanan A, Svrcek M, et al: Small bowel adenocarcinoma: Epidemiology, risk factors, diagnosis and treatment. *Dig Liver Dis* 46:97–104, 2014.
43. Thirunavukarasu P, Sathaiah M, Sukumar S, et al: Meckel's diverticulum—a high-risk region for malignancy in the

ileum. Insights from a population-based epidemiological study and implications in surgical management. *Ann Surg* 253:223–230, 2011.

44. Soltero MJ, Bill AH: The natural history of Meckel's diverticulum and its relation to incidental removal. A study of 202 cases of diseased Meckel's diverticulum found in King County, Washington, over a fifteen year period. *Am J Surg* 132:168–173, 1976.
45. Zani A, Eaton S, Rees CM, et al: Incidentally detected Meckel diverticulum: To resect or not to resect? *Ann Surg* 247:276–281, 2008.
46. Cullen JJ, Kelly KA, Moir CR, et al: Surgical management of Meckel's diverticulum. An epidemiologic, population-based study. *Ann Surg* 220:564–568, discussion 568–569, 1994.
47. Visschers RG, van Gemert WG, Winkens B, et al: Guided treatment improves outcome of patients with enterocutaneous fistulas. *World J Surg* 36:2341–2348, 2012.
48. Stacey R, Green JT: Radiation-induced small bowel disease: Latest developments and clinical guidance. *Ther Adv Chronic Dis* 5:15–29, 2014.
49. Jeppesen PB: Pharmacologic options for intestinal rehabilitation in patients with short bowel syndrome. *JPEN J Parenter Enteral Nutr* 38:45S–52S, 2014.
50. Tappenden KA: Pathophysiology of short bowel syndrome: Considerations of resected and residual anatomy. *JPEN J Parenter Enteral Nutr* 38:14S–22S, 2014.

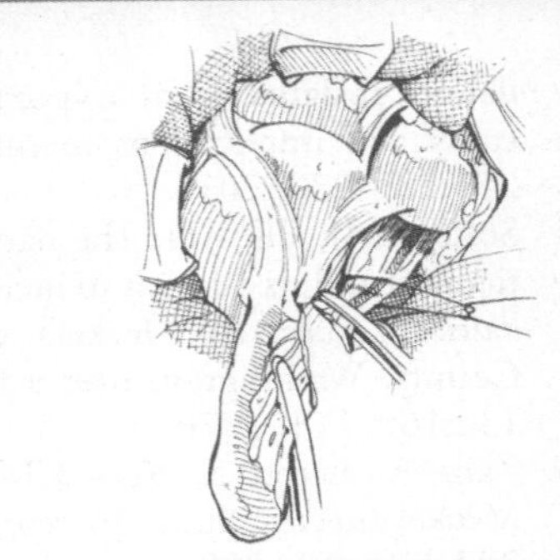

50 CHAPTER

The Appendix

Bryan Richmond

OUTLINE

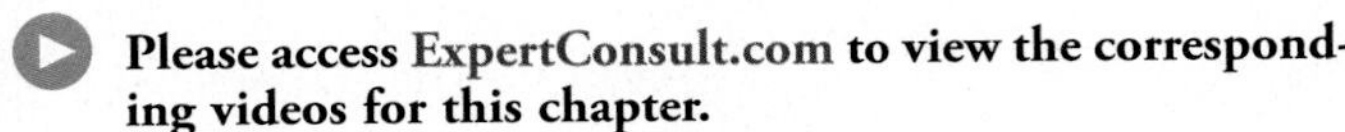

Please access ExpertConsult.com to view the corresponding videos for this chapter.

Appendicitis remains one of the most common diseases faced by the surgeon in practice. It is the most common urgent or emergent general surgical operation performed in the United States and is responsible for as many as 300,000 hospitalizations annually.[1] Although appendectomy is often the first "major" case performed by the young surgeon in training, few other operations will be learned that will have such a dramatic impact on the patient being treated.

It is estimated that as much as 6% to 7% of the general population will develop appendicitis during their lifetime, with the incidence peaking in the second decade of life.[2] Despite its high prevalence in Western countries, the diagnosis of acute appendicitis can be challenging and requires a high index of suspicion on the part of the examining surgeon to facilitate prompt treatment of this condition, thereby avoiding the substantial morbidity (and even mortality) associated with perforation. Appendicitis is much less common in underdeveloped countries, suggesting that elements of the Western diet, specifically a low-fiber, high-fat intake, may play a role in the development of the disease process.[3]

ANATOMY AND EMBRYOLOGY

The appendix is a midgut organ and is first identified at 8 weeks of gestation as a small outpouching of the cecum. As gestation progresses, the appendix becomes more elongated and tubular as the cecum rotates medially and becomes fixed in the right lower quadrant of the abdomen. The appendiceal mucosa is of the colonic type, with columnar epithelium, neuroendocrine cells, and mucin-producing goblet cells lining its tubular structure.[3] Lymphoid tissue is found in the submucosa of the appendix, leading some to hypothesize that the appendix may play a role in the immune system. In addition, evidence suggests that the appendix may serve as a reservoir of "good" intestinal bacteria and may aid in recolonization and maintenance of the normal colonic flora.[4] Consensus about this has not been achieved, however. Successful removal of the appendix has not been definitively demonstrated to have any known adverse sequelae.

As a midgut organ, the blood supply of the appendix is derived from the superior mesenteric artery. The ileocolic artery, one of the major named branches of the superior mesenteric artery, gives rise to the appendiceal artery, which courses through the *mesoappendix*. The mesoappendix also contains lymphatics of the appendix, which drain to the ileocecal nodes, along the blood supply from the superior mesenteric artery.[3,5]

The appendix is of variable size (5 to 35 cm in length) but averages 9 cm in length in adults. Its base can be reliably identified by defining the area of convergence of the taeniae at the tip of the cecum and then elevating the appendiceal base to define the course and position of the tip of the appendix, which is variable in location. The appendiceal tip may be found in a variety of locations, with the most common being retrocecal (but intraperitoneal) in approximately 60% of individuals, pelvic in 30%, and retroperitoneal in 7% to 10%. Agenesis of the appendix has been reported, as has duplication and even triplication.[3,5] Knowledge of these anatomic variations is important to the surgeon because the variable position of the appendiceal tip may account for differences in clinical presentation and in the location of the associated abdominal discomfort. For example, patients with a retroperitoneal appendix may present with back or flank pain, just as patients with the appendiceal tip in the midline pelvis may present with suprapubic pain. Both of these presentations may result in a delayed diagnosis as the symptoms are distinctly different from the classically described anterior right lower quadrant abdominal pain associated with appendiceal disease.

APPENDICITIS

History

The first appendectomy was reported in 1735 by a French Surgeon, Claudius Amyand, who identified and successfully removed the appendix of an 11-year-old boy that was found within an inguinal hernia sac and that had been perforated by a pin. Although autopsy findings consistent with perforated appendicitis appeared sporadically thereafter in the literature, the first formal description of the disease process, including the common clinical features and a recommendation for prompt surgical removal, was in 1886 by Reginald Heber Fitz of Harvard University.[3]

Notable advances in surgery for appendicitis include McBurney's description of his classic muscle-splitting incision and technique for removal of the appendix in 1894 and the description of the first laparoscopic appendectomy by Kurt Semm in 1982.[3] Laparoscopic appendectomy has become the preferred method for management of acute appendicitis among surgeons in the United States and may be accomplished using several (typically three) trocar sites or through single-incision laparoscopic surgical techniques. Finally, but of no less significance, was the development of broad-spectrum antibiotics, interventional radiologic techniques, and better surgical critical care strategies, all of which have resulted in substantial improvements in the care of patients with appendiceal perforation and its subsequent complications.

Pathophysiology and Bacteriology

Appendicitis is caused by luminal obstruction.[3] The appendix is vulnerable to this phenomenon because of its small luminal diameter in relation to its length. Obstruction of the proximal lumen of the appendix leads to elevated pressure in the distal portion because of ongoing mucus secretion and production of gas by bacteria within the lumen. With progressive distention of the appendix, the venous drainage becomes impaired, resulting in mucosal ischemia. With continued obstruction, full-thickness ischemia ensues, which ultimately leads to perforation. Bacterial overgrowth within the appendix results from bacterial stasis distal to the obstruction.[3] This is significant because this overgrowth results in the release of a larger bacterial inoculum in cases of perforated appendicitis (Table 50-1). The time from onset of obstruction to perforation is variable and may range anywhere from a few hours to a few days. The presentation after perforation is also variable. The most common sequela is the formation of an abscess in the periappendiceal region or pelvis. On occasion, however, free perforation occurs that results in diffuse peritonitis.[3]

Because the appendix is an outpouching of the cecum, the flora within the appendix is similar to that found within the colon. Infections associated with appendicitis should be considered polymicrobial, and antibiotic coverage should include agents that address the presence of both gram-negative bacteria and anaerobes. Common isolates include *Escherichia coli, Bacteroides fragilis,* enterococci, *Pseudomonas aeruginosa,* and others.[6] The choice and duration of antibiotic coverage and the controversies surrounding the need for cultures are discussed later in the chapter.

The causes of the luminal obstruction are many and varied. These most commonly include fecal stasis and fecaliths but may also include lymphoid hyperplasia, neoplasms, fruit and vegetable material, ingested barium, and parasites such as ascarids. Pain of appendicitis has both visceral and somatic components. Distention of the appendix is responsible for the initial vague abdominal pain (visceral) often experienced by the affected patient. The pain typically does not localize to the right lower quadrant until the tip becomes inflamed and irritates the adjacent parietal peritoneum (somatic) or perforation occurs, resulting in localized peritonitis.[3]

TABLE 50-1 Bacteria Commonly Isolated in Perforated Appendicitis

TYPE OF BACTERIA	PATIENTS (%)
Anaerobic	
Bacteroides fragilis	80
Bacteroides thetaiotaomicron	61
Bilophila wadsworthia	55
Peptostreptococcus spp.	46
Aerobic	
Escherichia coli	77
Viridans streptococcus	43
Group D streptococcus	27
Pseudomonas aeruginosa	18

Adapted from Bennion RS, Thompson JE: Appendicitis. In Fry DE, editor: *Surgical infections*, Boston, 1995, Little, Brown, pp 241–250.

Differential Diagnosis

Appendicitis must be considered in every patient (who has not had an appendectomy) who presents with acute abdominal pain.[7] Knowledge of disease processes that may have similar presenting symptoms and signs is essential to avoid an unnecessary or incorrect operation. Consideration of the patient's age and gender may help narrow the list of possible diagnoses. In children, other considerations include but are not limited to mesenteric adenitis (often seen after a recent viral illness), acute gastroenteritis, intussusception, Meckel's diverticulitis, inflammatory bowel disease, and (in males) testicular torsion. Nephrolithiasis and urinary tract infection may be manifested with right lower quadrant pain in either gender.[3]

In women of childbearing age, the differential diagnosis is expanded even further. Gynecologic problems may be mistaken for appendicitis and result in a higher negative appendectomy rate than in male patients of comparable age. These include ruptured ovarian cysts, *mittelschmerz* (midcycle pain occurring with ovulation), endometriosis, ovarian torsion, ectopic pregnancy, and pelvic inflammatory disease.[3,7]

Two other patient populations deserve mention. In the elderly, consideration must be given to acute diverticulitis and malignant disease as possible causes of lower abdominal pain. In the neutropenic patient, *typhlitis* (also known as neutropenic enterocolitis) should also be considered within the differential diagnosis. Appendicitis in these special populations is discussed later in the chapter.

Presentation

History

Patients presenting with acute appendicitis typically complain of vague abdominal pain that is most commonly periumbilical in origin and reflects the stimulation of visceral afferent pathways through the progressive distention of the appendix. Anorexia is often present, as is nausea with or without associated vomiting. Either diarrhea or constipation may be present as well. As the condition progresses and the appendiceal tip becomes inflamed, resulting in peritoneal irritation, the pain localizes to its classic location in the right lower quadrant. This phenomenon remains a reliable symptom of appendicitis[3,7] and should serve to further increase the clinician's index of suspicion for appendicitis (Fig. 50-1).

Whereas these symptoms represent the "classic" presentation of appendicitis, the clinician must be aware that the disease may be manifested in an atypical fashion. For example, patients with a retroperitoneal appendix may present in a more subacute manner, with flank or back pain, whereas patients with an appendiceal tip in the pelvis may have suprapubic pain suggestive of urinary tract infection.[3,7] We have on occasion encountered patients presenting with symptoms of small bowel obstruction who were found to be obstructed by multiple interloop abscesses

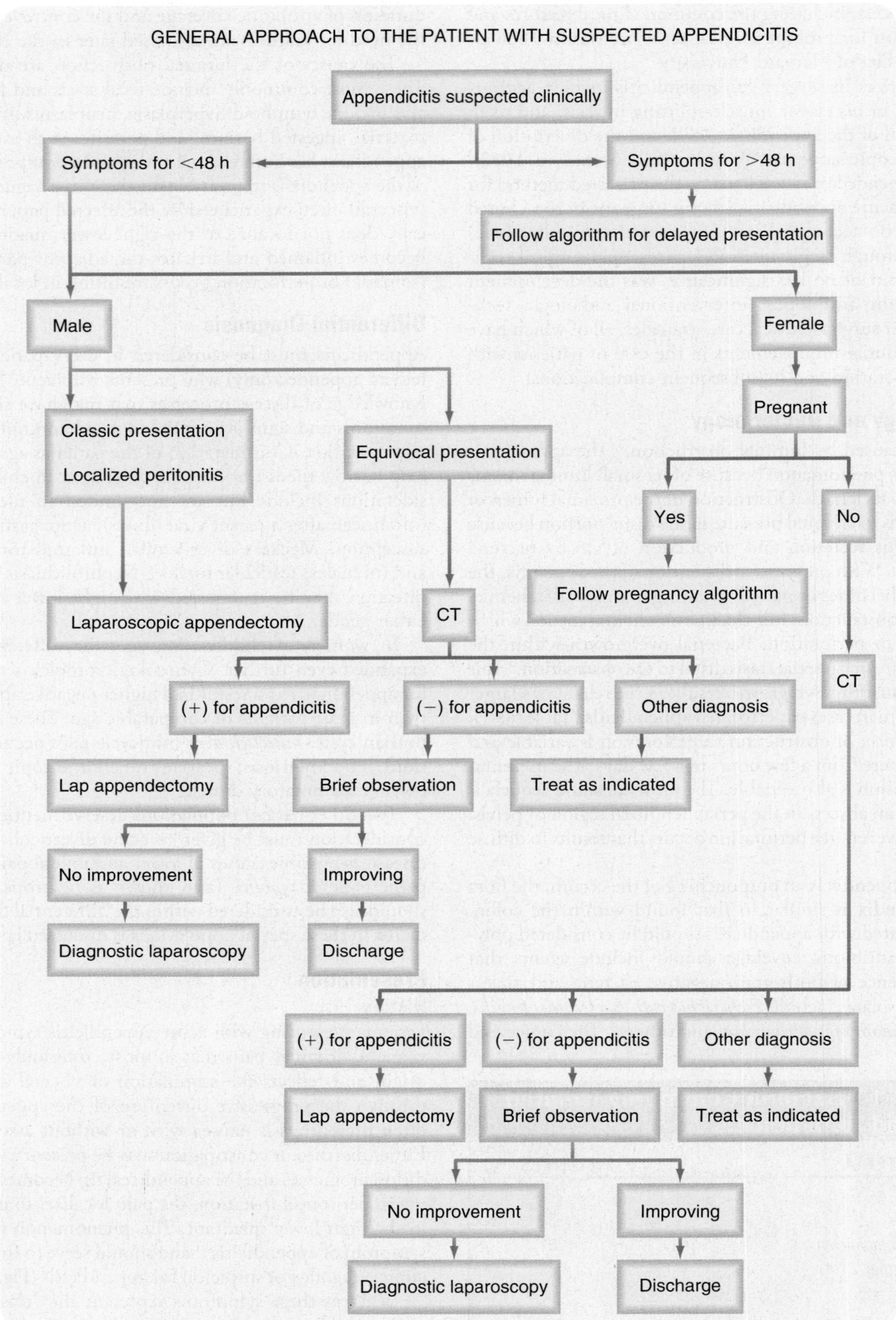

FIGURE 50-1 Suggested algorithm for the approach to the patient with possible appendicitis.

as a consequence of unrecognized appendiceal perforation. Although cases such as these are less common than the typical presentation, knowledge of these variations is essential to maintain the necessary index of suspicion to permit a prompt and accurate diagnosis.

Physical Examination

Patients with appendicitis typically appear ill. They frequently lie still because of the presence of localized peritonitis, which makes any movement painful. Tachycardia and mild dehydration are often present to varying degrees. Fever is frequently present, ranging from low-grade temperature elevations (<38.5° C) to more impressive elevations of body temperature, depending on the status of the disease process and the severity of the patient's inflammatory response. Absence of fever does not exclude a diagnosis of appendicitis.[1,3,7]

Abdominal examination typically reveals a quiet abdomen with tenderness and guarding on palpation of the right lower quadrant. The location of the tenderness is classically over McBurney point, which is located one-third the distance between the anterior superior iliac spine and the umbilicus. The pain and tenderness are typically accompanied by localized peritonitis as evidenced by the presence of rebound tenderness. Diffuse peritonitis or abdominal wall rigidity due to involuntary spasm of the overlying abdominal wall musculature is strongly suggestive of perforation.[1,3]

A number of signs have been described to aid in the diagnosis of appendicitis. These include the Rovsing sign (the presence of right lower quadrant pain on palpation of the left lower quadrant), the obturator sign (right lower quadrant pain on internal rotation of the hip), and the psoas sign (pain with extension of the ipsilateral hip), among others.[1] Although these are of historical interest, it is important to realize that they are simply indicators of localized peritonitis rather than a diagnostic of a specific disease process. Still, they are useful maneuvers to perform in examining a patient with suspected appendicitis and are supportive of the diagnosis if it is suspected clinically.

Rectal examination findings are typically normal. However, a palpable mass or tenderness may be present if the appendiceal tip is located within the pelvis or if a pelvic abscess is present. In female patients, pelvic examination is important to exclude pelvic disease. However, cervical motion tenderness, a finding typically associated with pelvic inflammatory disease, may be present in appendicitis because of irritation of the pelvic organs from the adjacent inflammatory process.[3]

Laboratory Studies

Laboratory studies should be interpreted with caution in cases of suspected appendicitis and should be used to support the clinical picture rather than definitively to prove or to exclude the diagnosis. A leukocytosis, often with a "left shift" (a predominance of neutrophils and sometimes an increase in bands), is present in 90% of cases. A normal white blood cell count is found in 10% of cases, however, and it should not be used as an isolated test to exclude the presence of appendicitis.[8] Urinalysis is typically normal as well, although the finding of trace leukocyte esterase or pyuria is not unusual and is presumably due to the proximity of the inflamed appendix to the bladder or ureter. If the presentation is strongly suggestive of appendicitis, a "positive" urinalysis should not be used as an isolated test to refute the diagnosis. Pregnancy testing is mandatory in women of childbearing age. C-reactive protein has been demonstrated to be neither sensitive nor specific in diagnosing (or excluding) appendicitis.[1,8]

No symptom or sign has been demonstrated to be discriminatory and predictive of appendicitis.[1,8] The same may be said of laboratory tests, which are also weakly predictive when considered in isolation. Rather, it is the assessment of the collective body of information that allows more precise diagnosis.[1,8]

Imaging Studies

A variety of radiographic studies may be used to diagnose appendicitis. These consist of plain radiographs, computed tomography (CT) scanning, ultrasound (US), and magnetic resonance imaging (MRI).

Plain radiographs are frequently obtained in the emergency department setting for the evaluation of acute abdominal pain but lack both sensitivity and specificity for the diagnosis of appendicitis and are rarely helpful. Findings that may support the diagnosis include the presence of a calcified fecalith in the right lower quadrant, although this finding must be placed into the appropriate clinical context and is typically present in only 5% of cases.[9] Pneumoperitoneum, if present, should alert the clinician to other causes of a perforated viscus (such as a perforated ulcer or diverticulitis), as this is not typically observed in cases of appendicitis, even with perforation.

CT scanning is the most common imaging study to diagnose appendicitis and is highly effective and accurate.[9] Modern helical CT scans have the advantage of being operator independent and easy to interpret. CT has been shown to have a sensitivity of 90% to 100%, a specificity of 91% to 99%, a positive predictive value of 92% to 98%, and a negative predictive value of 95% to 100%.[9,10] The recommended imaging protocol from the Infectious Diseases Society of America (IDSA) and the Surgical Infection Society includes the intravenous administration of contrast material only. Oral and rectal administration of contrast material is not recommended.[11]

The diagnosis of appendicitis on CT is based on the appearance of a thickened, inflamed appendix with surrounding "stranding" indicative of inflammation. The appendix is typically more than 7 mm in diameter with a thickened, inflamed wall and mural enhancement or "target sign" (Fig. 50-2). Periappendiceal fluid or air is also highly suggestive of appendicitis and suggests perforation. In cases in which the appendix is not visualized, the absence of inflammatory findings on CT suggests that appendicitis is not present.[12] Although we do not recommend CT in cases in which appendicitis is strongly suspected on clinical grounds based on supportive history and physical and laboratory findings, published data do suggest that use of CT in equivocal cases does indeed reduce the negative appendectomy rate.[13]

US has been used for diagnosis of appendicitis since the 1980s. As US technology has become more advanced, so has its ability to visualize the appendix. The US probe is applied to the area of pain in the right lower quadrant, and graded compression is used to collapse normal surrounding bowel and to diminish the interference encountered with overlying bowel gas. The inflamed appendix is typically enlarged, immobile, and noncompressible (Fig. 50-3). If the appendix cannot be visualized, the study is inconclusive and cannot be relied on to guide treatment. Although US provides the advantage of avoiding ionizing radiation, the technology is highly operator dependent. The sensitivity is reported to range from 78% to 83%, whereas the specificity ranges from 83% to 93%. Its greatest utility appears to be in the evaluation of the pediatric or pregnant patient, in whom the associated radiation exposure from CT is undesirable.[9]

MRI is typically reserved for use in the pregnant patient; the study is performed without contrast agents. If it is obtained in a pregnant woman, the study should be noncontrasted. MRI offers excellent resolution and is accurate in diagnosing appendicitis. Criteria for MRI diagnosis include appendiceal enlargement (>7 mm), thickening (>2 mm), and the presence of inflammation.[9] The sensitivity of MRI is reported to be 100%, the specificity 98%, the positive predictive value 98%, and the negative predictive value 100%. MRI is also operator independent and offers highly reproducible results. Drawbacks associated with the use of MRI include its higher cost, motion artifact, greater difficulty in interpretation by nonradiologists who may have limited

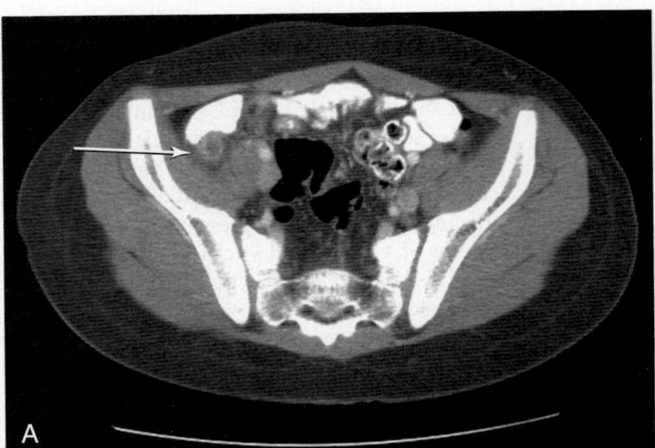

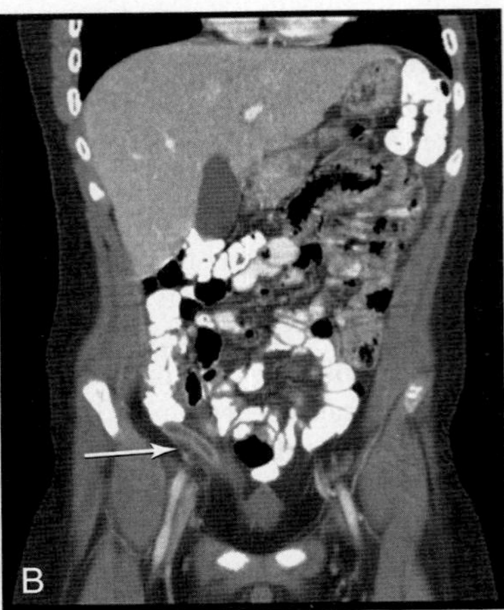

FIGURE 50-2 CT scan of the abdomen demonstrating classic findings of acute appendicitis. **A,** Sagittal view with *arrow* demonstrating a thickened, inflamed, and fluid-filled appendix (target sign). **B,** Coronal view of same patient. The *arrow* points to the thickened, elongated appendix with periappendiceal fat stranding and fluid around the appendiceal tip.

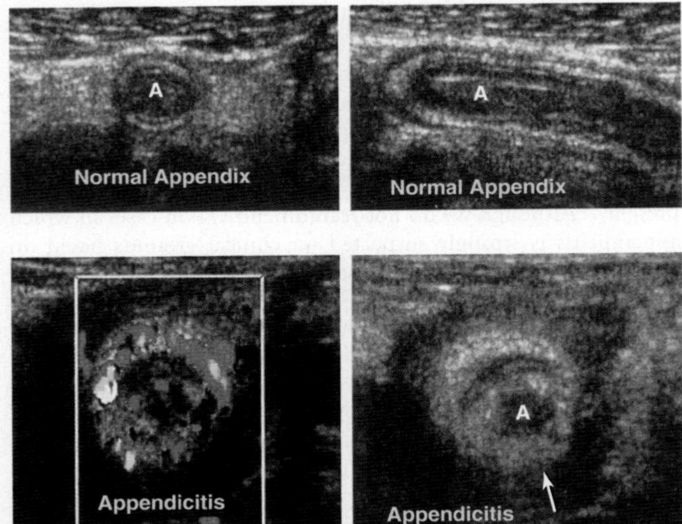

FIGURE 50-3 Ultrasound image of a normal appendix *(top)* illustrating the thin wall in coronal *(left)* and longitudinal *(right)* planes. In appendicitis, there is distention and wall thickening *(bottom, right),* and blood flow is increased, leading to the so-called ring of fire appearance. *A,* Appendix.

experience with the technology, and limited availability (especially in the after-hours emergency setting).[9]

TREATMENT OF APPENDICITIS

Acute Uncomplicated Appendicitis

The appropriate treatment of acute uncomplicated appendicitis is prompt appendectomy. The patient should undergo fluid resuscitation as indicated, and the intravenous administration of broad-spectrum antibiotics directed against gram-negative and anaerobic organisms should be initiated immediately.[11] Operation should proceed without undue delay.

For open appendectomy, the patient is placed in the supine position. The choice of incision is a matter of the surgeon's preference, whether it is an oblique muscle-splitting incision (McArthur-McBurney; Fig. 50-4), a transverse incision (Rockey-Davis), or a conservative midline incision. The cecum is grasped by the taeniae and delivered into the wound, allowing visualization of the base of the appendix and delivery of the appendiceal tip. The mesoappendix is divided, and the appendix is crushed just above the base, ligated with an absorbable ligature, and divided. The stump is then either cauterized or inverted by a purse-string or Z suture technique. Finally, the abdomen is thoroughly irrigated and the wound closed in layers.

For laparoscopic appendectomy, the patient is placed in the supine position. The bladder is emptied by a straight catheter or by having the patient void immediately before the procedure. The abdomen is entered at the umbilicus, and the diagnosis is confirmed by inserting the laparoscope (Fig. 50-5). Two additional working ports are then placed, typically in the left lower quadrant and in either the suprapubic area or supraumbilical midline, based on the surgeon's preference. We have found it to be advantageous for both the surgeon and assistant to stand to the left side of the patient with the left arm tucked. This allows optimum triangulation of the camera and working instruments. Atraumatic graspers are used to elevate the appendix, and the mesoappendix is carefully divided using the harmonic scalpel. The base is then secured with endoloops and the appendix divided. Alternatively, the appendix may be divided with an endoscopic stapler. We prefer this technique in cases in which the entire appendix is friable because it allows the staple line to be placed slightly more proximally, on the edge of the healthy cecum, thereby reducing the risk of leakage from breakdown of a tenuous appendiceal stump. Retrieval of the appendix is accomplished by the use of a plastic retrieval bag. The pelvis is irrigated, the trocars are removed, and the wounds are closed. Laparoscopic appendectomy may also be performed with single-site laparoscopic surgical techniques as well, although this technique remains less commonly performed than the traditional multitrocar approach.

Antibiotic administration is not continued beyond a single preoperative dose.[11] Oral alimentation is begun immediately and

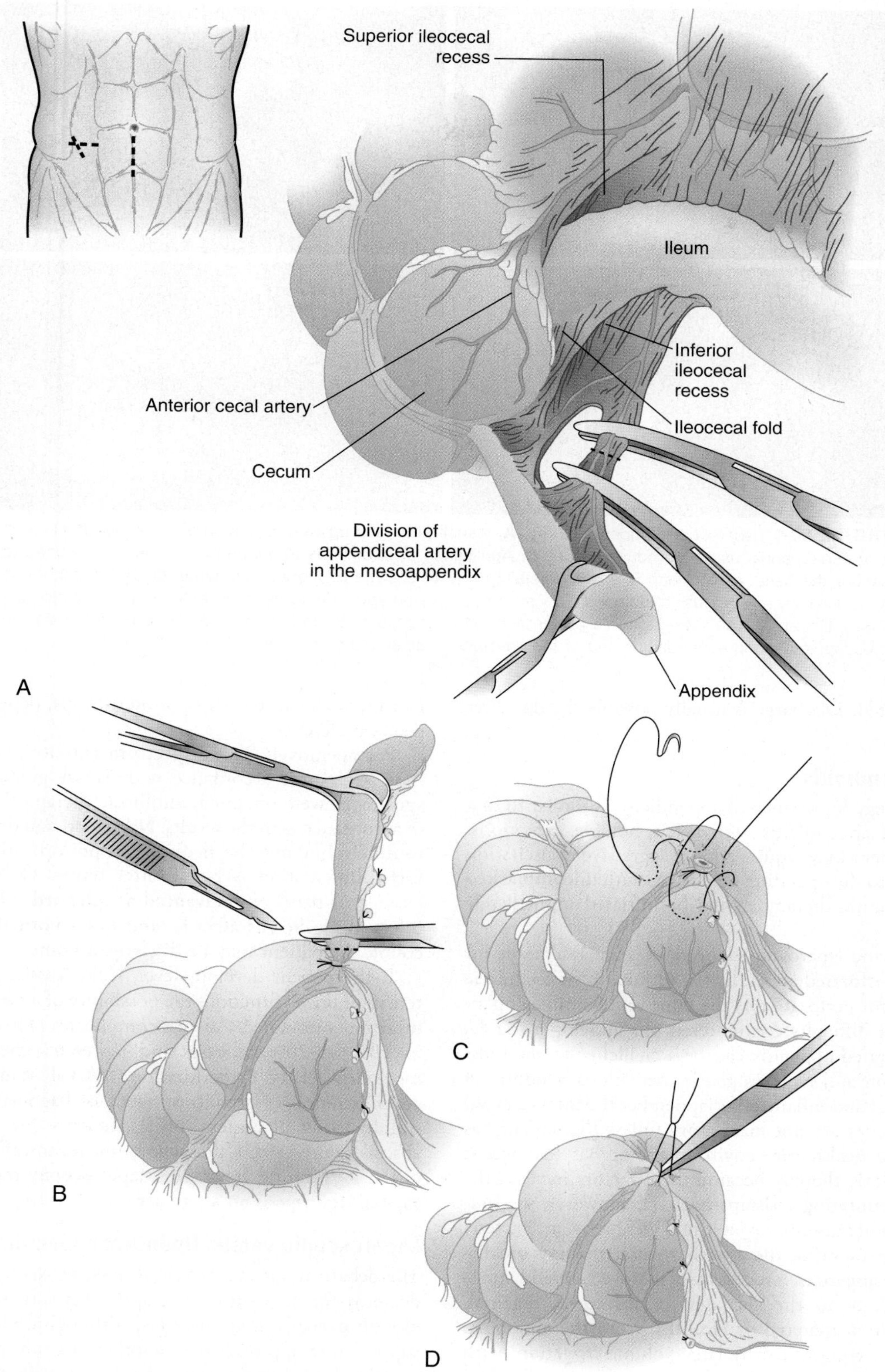

FIGURE 50-4 **A,** *Left,* Location of possible incisions for an open appendectomy. *Right,* Division of the mesoappendix. **B,** Ligation of the base and division of the appendix. **C,** Placement of purse-string suture or Z stitch. **D,** Inversion of the appendiceal stump. (From Ortega JM, Ricardo AE: Surgery of the appendix and colon. In Moody FG, editor: *Atlas of ambulatory surgery*, Philadelphia, 1999, WB Saunders.)

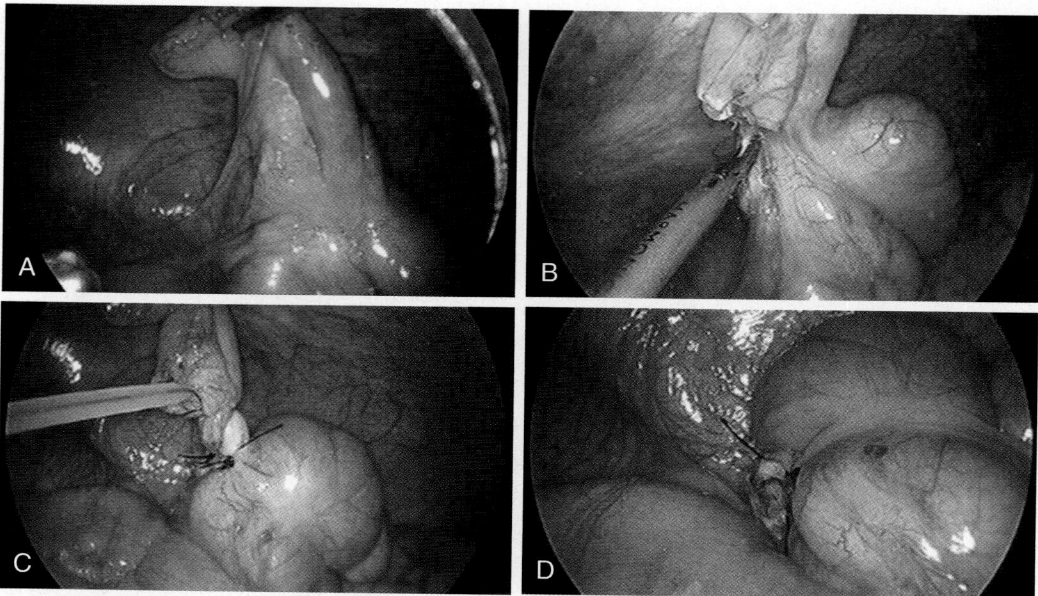

FIGURE 50-5 Laparoscopic appendectomy. **A,** Visualization and upward retraction of appendix. **B,** Division of mesoappendix using harmonic scalpel. **C,** Application of endoloops to appendix. Two loops are used to secure the base; a third loop is applied distally to avoid spillage of the luminal contents. The specimen is then divided between the endoloops. **D,** View of completed appendectomy after removal of the specimen. (*Note:* Depending on the surgeon's preference, an endoscopic stapling device may be used to divide the mesoappendix and appendix instead of the harmonic scalpel and endoloops.)

advanced as tolerated. Discharge is usually possible the day after operation.

Perforated Appendicitis

The operative strategy for perforated appendicitis is similar to that for uncomplicated appendicitis with a few notable exceptions. First of all, the patient may require a more aggressive resuscitation before proceeding to the operating theater. As with uncomplicated appendicitis, antibiotic therapy should be initiated immediately on diagnosis.[11]

Both the open and laparoscopic approaches are acceptable for the treatment of perforated appendicitis. Although the technique of appendectomy for perforation is the same as for simple appendicitis, the level of difficulty encountered in removing a friable, gangrenous, perforated appendix can be a challenge to the most experienced surgeon and requires gentle meticulous handling of the friable appendix and inflamed periappendiceal tissues to avoid tissue injury. Cultures are not mandatory unless the patient has had exposure to a health care environment or has had recent exposure to antibiotic therapy because these factors increase the likelihood of encountering resistant bacteria. However, we routinely obtain them because they sometimes yield resistant bacteria and are helpful in tailoring the switch to oral therapy on discharge.[11] Once the appendix is successfully removed, careful attention should be given to the clearance of infectious material, including spilled fecal material or fecaliths, from the abdomen. This task may be accomplished by large-volume irrigation, with special attention given to the right lower quadrant and pelvis. Drains are not routinely placed unless a discrete abscess cavity is present. If an abscess cavity is present, a single closed suction Jackson-Pratt drain is placed within its base and left for several days. If an open technique was used, the skin and subcutaneous tissues are left open for 3 or 4 days to prevent development of wound infection, at which time the wound may be closed at the bedside with sutures, clips, or Steri-Strips, depending on the surgeon's preference.

Postoperatively, broad-spectrum antibiotics are continued for 4 to 7 days in accordance with IDSA guidelines.[11] If culture specimens were obtained, antibiotic therapy should be modified in accordance with the results. Nasogastric suction is not employed routinely but may be necessary if postoperative ileus develops. Oral alimentation is begun after return of bowel sounds and passage of flatus and advanced as tolerated. Once the patient is tolerating a diet, is afebrile, and has a normal white blood cell count, the patient may be discharged home.

If the patient develops fever, leukocytosis, pain, and delayed return of bowel function, the possibility of a postoperative abscess must be entertained. Abscess complicates perforated appendicitis in 10% to 20% of cases and represents the major source of morbidity related to perforation.[1,3] A CT scan with intravenous administration of a contrast agent is diagnostic and also allows simultaneous placement of a percutaneous drain within the abscess cavity.[9] If CT drainage is not technically possible because of the location of the abscess, laparoscopic, transrectal, or transvaginal drainage is an alternative.

Laparoscopic versus Open Appendectomy

The debate about the choice of open versus laparoscopic appendectomy for the treatment of appendicitis remains a major point of controversy among surgeons. Although no level I data exist to support one approach over another, a study published in 2010 examined this issue in detail. Ingraham and colleagues[14] analyzed results from 222 hospitals comparing laparoscopic versus open appendectomy using the American College of Surgeons National Surgical Quality Improvement Program. In all, 24,969 laparoscopic and 7714 open procedures were included in the analysis. Although the data were limited by the retrospective nature, the investigators observed that laparoscopic appendectomy was associated with lower risk of wound complications and deep surgical site infection in uncomplicated appendicitis. In complicated appendicitis, laparoscopic appendectomy was associated with fewer wound complications but a slightly higher incidence of intra-abdominal abscess. The overall conclusion, however, was that the laparoscopic approach was associated with an overall lower incidence of complications than the open procedure. The conclusions evident from a number of studies indicate that both approaches are acceptable and that the advantages with laparoscopy, although small, were a lower overall morbidity, reduced wound complications, reduced postoperative pain, and perhaps a slightly shorter recovery time. The slightly higher risk of intra-abdominal abscess formation after laparoscopic appendectomy in cases of complicated appendicitis was a negative aspect of laparoscopic appendectomy, although the authors acknowledged that this has not been observed in all studies.[15]

We prefer the laparoscopic approach for several reasons. Laparoscopy allows examination of the entire peritoneal space, making it exceptionally useful to exclude other intra-abdominal disease that may be manifested in a similar fashion, such as diverticulitis or tubo-ovarian abscess, whereas visualization of these structures would not be possible through a right lower quadrant incision. We find it to be technically simpler in most patients, particularly the obese, and have been impressed with our ability to discharge patients within several hours of the operation.

The debate about the superiority of laparoscopic versus open appendectomy will likely continue as a clearly superior choice has not been conclusively demonstrated. What does appear clear, however, is that regardless of the surgeon's preferred approach, the most important aspect of appendectomy is that it be done promptly and safely.

Delayed Presentation of Appendicitis

Patients may occasionally present several days to even weeks after the onset of appendicitis. In these cases, the treatment should be individualized on the basis of the nature of the presentation (Fig. 50-6). Although rare, a patient may present with diffuse peritonitis. More commonly, however, patients present with localized right lower quadrant pain and fever, with a history that is compatible with appendicitis. A mass may be palpable in children or thin patients. Immediate exploration and attempted appendectomy in these patients may result in substantial morbidity, including failure to identify the appendix, postoperative abscess or fistula, and unnecessary extension of the operation to include ileocecectomy, all due to the extreme induration and friability of the involved tissues. For this reason, in general, treatment for these patients is initially accomplished nonoperatively.[16-20] Fluid resuscitation is initiated, and broad-spectrum antibiotic therapy is initiated. A CT scan is obtained, and perforated appendicitis with a localized abscess or phlegmon is confirmed (Fig. 50-7). If a localized abscess is identified, CT-guided percutaneous drainage is performed for source control. The drainage catheter is typically left in place for 4 to 7 days, during which the patient is treated with antibiotic therapy and after which time it is removed. If CT-guided drainage is not technically feasible, operative drainage may be accomplished through transrectal or transvaginal approaches. Laparoscopic drainage is another option that we have found to be exceptionally useful. This technique is performed by visualizing the inflammatory mass with the laparoscope and then entering the abscess with a laparoscopic suction tip, evacuating the purulent material, and placing a drain within the residual abscess cavity. Postoperative management is identical to that of patients who are successfully drained percutaneously. If a periappendiceal phlegmon is present or if the amount of fluid present is not sufficient to drain, the patient may be treated with antibiotics alone, typically for 4 to 7 days also, as recommended by IDSA guidelines for treatment of intra-abdominal infection.[11]

Traditionally, after successful nonoperative treatment of complicated appendicitis, patients were advised to undergo removal of the appendix, a procedure known as interval appendectomy, several weeks to months later. This practice has been reexamined. The rationale for interval appendectomy is based on the potential for development of recurrent appendicitis and the subsequent risks associated with emergent removal or reperforation of the appendix. However, the actual risk of recurrent appendicitis appears to be small, 8% at 8 years in one study of 6400 pediatric patients.[21] The findings in this study as well as similar results reported by others have led them to conclude that interval appendectomy should be reserved only for patients who present with symptoms of recurrent appendicitis.[21,22] In addition, the presence of an appendicolith on CT has also been shown to be predictive of a higher risk of recurrent appendicitis and has been used as a justification to proceed with interval appendectomy in that subgroup of patients. This selective approach to interval appendectomy has also been demonstrated to be more cost-effective than its routine performance in all affected patients.[22]

A systematic review published by Hall and colleagues[23] examining the role of interval appendectomy found that the overall risk of recurrent appendicitis was 20.5%. All recurrences were seen within 3 years, and 80% of these occurred within 6 months. In addition, the morbidity of interval appendectomy was significant, with complications reported in 23 of the studies, for an overall rate of 3.4%. Other authors have reported significant associated morbidity with interval appendectomy as well, with rates as high as 18%.[24]

One argument favoring interval appendectomy in adults has been the observation by some investigators of a higher incidence of appendiceal neoplasms found in interval appendectomy specimens.[8,25-27] Also, perforated tumors of the cecum may be manifested in a similar fashion as perforated appendicitis.[28] For this reason, colonoscopy is recommended in all adult patients as routine follow-up after nonoperative management of complicated appendicitis.[29] To date, no large-scale randomized controlled trials examining the outcomes of patients who do or do not undergo interval appendectomy after successful nonoperative treatment have been conducted. For this reason, this issue is likely to remain controversial for some time.

The Normal-Appearing Appendix at Operation

In cases of "negative appendectomy," in which a normal appendix is identified at operation, there is controversy as to whether the appendix should be removed.[30,31] Before that particular issue is examined, it is important to emphasize the need to thoroughly evaluate the abdomen for other causes of pain severe enough to warrant an operation. The abdominal and pelvic organs should be assessed for any abnormalities. In our experience, this is most easily done through the laparoscopic approach, which we think is a major advantage of laparoscopy over an open approach. Note should be made of any free fluid as such a finding may suggest perforation. The terminal 60 cm of ileum should be examined for a Meckel's diverticulum and the serosa of the small bowel for any stigmata of Crohn's disease, such as inflammation, stricture formation, or the characteristic "creeping fat" appearance of the mesentery. Inspection of the ileal mesentery may reveal enlarged lymph

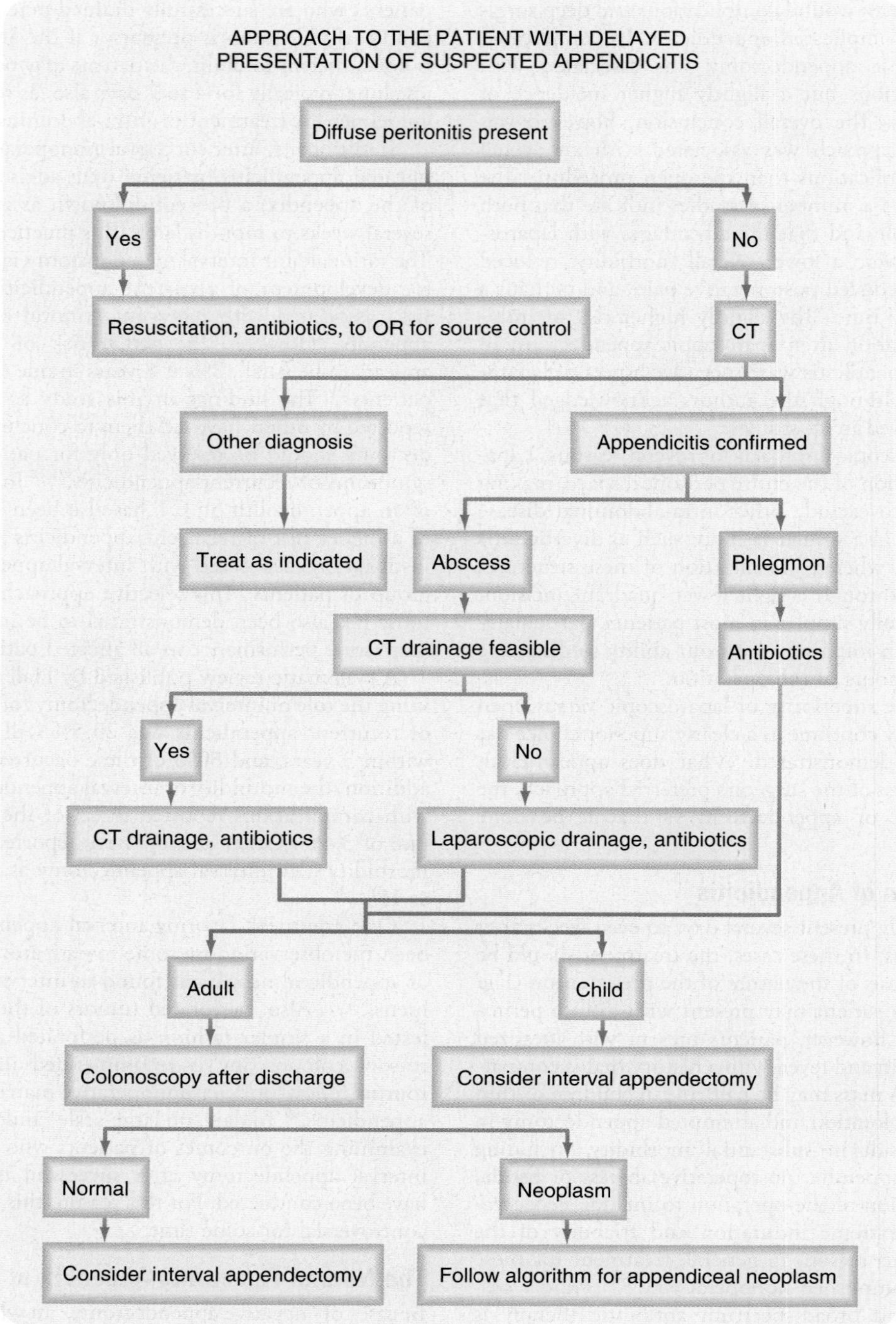

FIGURE 50-6 Suggested algorithm for managing the patient with delayed presentation of appendicitis.

nodes suggestive of mesenteric adenitis. The uterine adnexa should be examined for any evidence of tubo-ovarian or salpingeal disease, such as ovarian torsion, tubo-ovarian abscess, endometriosis, or ruptured ovarian cysts. The sigmoid colon should be examined for evidence of acute diverticulitis, especially in cases in which a redundant sigmoid colon is found in the right lower quadrant. If these are all normal, attention should be turned to the upper abdomen for examination of the gallbladder and duodenum. Inability to perform an adequate evaluation of the intra-abdominal organs or demonstration of disease of other organs requiring intervention may require conversion to a midline laparotomy if necessary.

We routinely remove the normal appendix for several reasons. First, many causes of right lower quadrant pain discussed before may be recurrent, such as pain from ruptured ovarian cysts or mesenteric adenitis. Appendectomy is also advisable in cases of Crohn's disease when suggested by findings at operation, unless the base of the appendix and cecum are involved. In this scenario, appendectomy is deferred to avoid breakdown of the inflamed stump and subsequent fistula formation. In these clinical

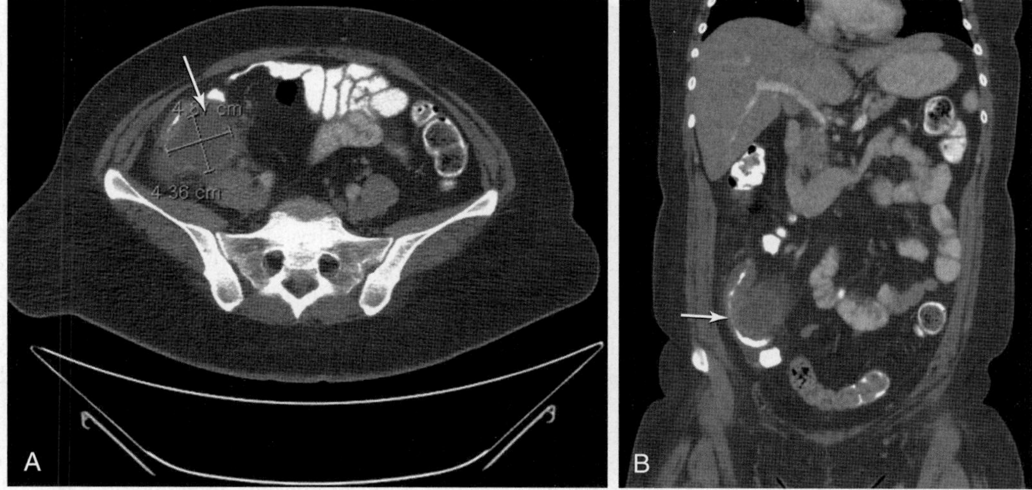

FIGURE 50-7 Sagittal **(A)** and coronal **(B)** CT images demonstrate an appendiceal abscess in a patient who presented with a 2-week history of abdominal pain and was found to have a palpable mass on examination. The *arrows* point to a periappendiceal abscess cavity. She was successfully managed with percutaneous drainage and antibiotic therapy.

circumstances, appendectomy is advisable because it removes appendicitis from the differential diagnosis when the patient presents with recurrent right lower quadrant pain. In addition, abnormalities of the appendix not apparent on gross inspection at the time of operation are sometimes identified on pathologic examination.[30,31]

Nonoperative Treatment of Uncomplicated Appendicitis

Although prompt appendectomy is the standard of care, a number of studies have challenged this concept and have supported antibiotic therapy alone as a definitive treatment for acute uncomplicated appendicitis. Two meta-analyses analyzing the results of randomized controlled trials examining this issue concluded that nonoperative treatment was associated with a lower risk of complications (12% in the nonoperative group versus 18% in the appendectomy group; $P = .001$).[32,33] Appendectomy, however, outperformed the nonoperative group in overall treatment failure rate (40% nonoperative versus 9% in the appendectomy group; $P < .001$). The authors concluded that antibiotic therapy was safe as a treatment for uncomplicated appendicitis but was associated with a significantly, perhaps prohibitively high failure rate compared with appendectomy.[32,33] For this reason, our practice is to reserve nonoperative therapy only for acute uncomplicated appendicitis for those patients in whom the operative risk is prohibitive. Failures of nonoperative therapy in these high-risk patients are then managed with adjunctive treatment measures, such as CT-guided drainage of periappendiceal abscesses.

"Chronic" Appendicitis as a Cause of Abdominal Pain

On occasion, patients will present with a history of recurrent right lower quadrant pain, and a surgical opinion will be sought as to the benefit of elective appendectomy for treatment of this condition. Modest epidemiologic data exist to suggest that appendicitis may spontaneously resolve, so it is conceivable that appendicitis may wax and wane in some patients.[1] In addition, some patients with pain are found to have a thickened appendix or an appendicolith on CT but have no evidence of a systemic illness or acute periappendiceal inflammation. In some cases, appendectomy will produce relief of symptoms, and in these cases, examination of the appendix will sometimes reveal findings consistent with chronic inflammation.[31,34] We will consider, on a case by case basis, elective appendectomy in cases in which the history is consistent with appendiceal disease and there is radiographic (CT) evidence of appendiceal disease.

More troubling, however, is the patient with pain in the absence of radiographic evidence of appendiceal disease. We typically pursue a multidisciplinary workup in these patients involving input from specialists in gastroenterology and gynecology as well as surgery. Appendectomy is typically not offered unless disease is demonstrated radiographically; however, if diagnostic laparoscopy is performed to investigate or to exclude other disease (typically by a gynecologist), we will typically perform appendectomy, an approach advocated by others.[35] We have found that as with the management of any chronic pain syndrome, management of expectations is critical in caring for this very difficult group of patients.

Incidental Appendectomy

Incidental appendectomy is the term applied when a grossly normal appendix is removed at the time of an unrelated procedure, such as a hysterectomy, cholecystectomy, or sigmoid colectomy. Once commonly performed, incidental appendectomy has become a controversial procedure. The theoretical benefit is that of eliminating the patient's risk for development of appendicitis in the future, a concept that is thought to be most beneficial in patients younger than 35 years because of their greater lifetime risk for development of the disease compared with older patients.[16] Data suggesting that incidental appendectomy may be performed with no additional morbidity have been criticized for not having been properly risk adjusted. When these data were scrutinized further, Wen and coworkers actually demonstrated that incidental appendectomy was associated with an increase in both morbidity and mortality.[36] Other investigators have demonstrated that incidental appendectomy does not appear to be cost-effective as a preventive measure.[37] Finally, the recent finding that the appendix may actually have a role in the maintenance of healthy colonic flora makes the practice of incidental appendectomy even more controversial.[4] For these reasons, we advocate careful inspection of the appendix for abnormalities during abdominal operations as part of a thorough exploration but do not advocate appendectomy unless an abnormality is detected.

APPENDICITIS IN SPECIAL POPULATIONS

Appendicitis in the Pregnant Patient

Appendicitis remains the most common nonobstetric emergency in pregnancy and is consequently the most frequent reason for general surgical intervention in this group of patients.[38] The diagnosis of appendicitis in pregnancy presents a special challenge to the surgeon. As with all conditions in pregnancy, the surgeon must consider the welfare of two patients, the mother and fetus, when considering possible diagnoses, workup, and treatment (Fig. 50-8).

In pregnancy, appendicitis has a typical clinical presentation in only 50% to 60% of cases.[38] The common symptoms of early appendicitis, such as nausea and vomiting, are nonspecific and are also often associated with normal pregnancy. The normal febrile response to illness may be blunted in pregnancy. Also, the physical examination of the pregnant patient is difficult and is altered because of the effect of the gravid uterus and its displacement of the appendix to a more cephalad location within the abdomen. Lower quadrant pain in the second trimester produced by traction on the suspensory ligaments of the uterus, a phenomenon known as round ligament pain, is a common occurrence and further complicates the clinical picture further because 50% of cases of appendicitis occur in the second trimester. Finally, biochemical and laboratory indicators used to support the diagnosis of appendicitis in the nonpregnant patient are unreliable in pregnancy. For example, a mild physiologic leukocytosis of pregnancy is a normal finding. C-reactive protein levels may also be physiologically elevated in pregnancy. In addition, the surgeon must be concerned about the possibility of obstetric emergencies as a cause of abdominal pain, such as preterm labor, placental abruption, or uterine rupture.[38-40] All of these factors have contributed to the high rate of negative appendectomy in pregnant patients, as high as 25% to 50%, when it is based on clinical presentation alone.[38]

The impact of appendicitis on the pregnant patient is severe. The risk of preterm labor has been shown to be 11% and fetal loss 6% with complicated appendicitis.[41] These data would appear to favor an aggressive, early approach to appendicitis in the pregnant patient. Complicating this approach, however, was the finding in the same series that negative appendectomy was also associated with preterm labor and fetal loss (10% and 4%, respectively). The lowest rates of preterm labor and fetal loss (6% and 2%, respectively) were seen in cases of uncomplicated

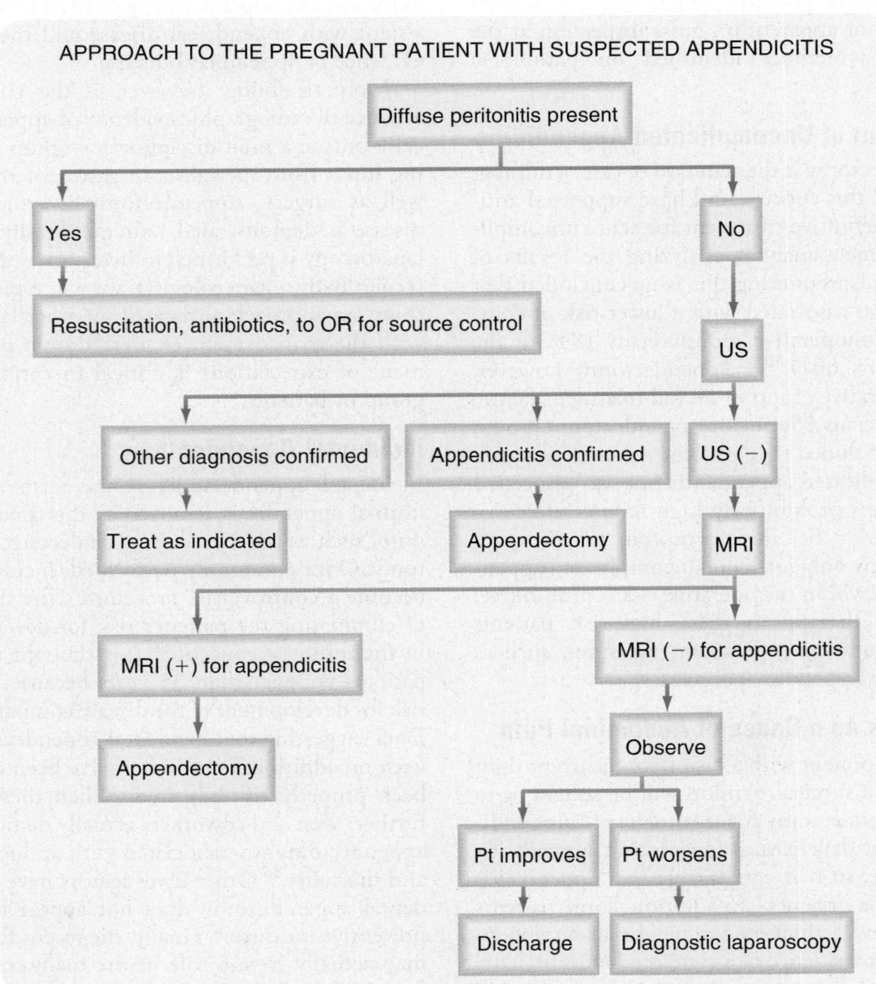

FIGURE 50-8 Suggested algorithm for managing the pregnant patient with possible appendicitis.

appendicitis.[41] For these reasons, preoperative accuracy of diagnosis is crucial in the pregnant patient with suspected appendicitis.

Routine imaging is recommended in pregnant patients. The initial study of choice is US with graded compression.[42] It has the advantage of being safe, inexpensive, and readily available. In addition, US may provide information as to fetal well-being and obstetric causes of abdominal pain, such as placental abruption. Scanning patients in a left posterior oblique or left lateral decubitus position rather than in the traditional supine position has been advocated to increase the chances of visualizing the appendix. The criteria for US diagnosis are the same as in the nonpregnant patient and have been discussed previously. Unfortunately, the sensitivity (78%) and specificity (83%) of US appear to be reduced in pregnancy because of the presence of the gravid uterus.[42]

If US examination findings are equivocal, MRI without gadolinium contrast, with its excellent soft tissue contrast resolution and lack of ionizing radiation, remains a safe alternative for confirmation or exclusion of appendicitis in the pregnant patient. In addition, the excellent sensitivity and specificity are preserved in the pregnant patient (Fig. 50-9). A patient in whom MRI findings are normal likely does not require appendectomy. Routine use of MRI in pregnant patients has been demonstrated to reduce the negative appendectomy rate by 47% without a significant increase in the perforation rate, and it has been shown to be a cost-effective study.[42] For these reasons, we encourage liberal use of MRI in pregnant patients suspected to have acute appendicitis without frank peritonitis. However, MRI may not be available in some institutions and may be available only on a limited basis or during limited times in other institutions. The decision about any delay in appendectomy to obtain an MRI study is a complex one and should be made using all available clinical and imaging data available because there are potentially severe consequences associated with both negative appendectomy and appendiceal perforation.

If US is inconclusive and MRI scanning is not immediately available, CT scanning for diagnosis of appendicitis in pregnancy has been reported. A study published in 2008 demonstrated that the use of CT was associated with an 8% negative appendectomy rate, compared with 54% by clinical assessment alone and 32% by clinical assessment combined with US. The authors concluded that CT should be used if US examination findings are equivocal and argued that the amount of radiation delivered during a limited CT examination is below the threshold required to induce fetal malformations and that most cases of appendicitis in pregnancy occur in the second or third trimester, when organogenesis in already complete.[42] Although protocols vary, if CT is used during pregnancy for equivocal cases, care should be taken to perform as limited a study as possible with avoidance of intravenous administration of contrast material. Further study is required before the routine use of CT can be accepted in this clinical scenario.

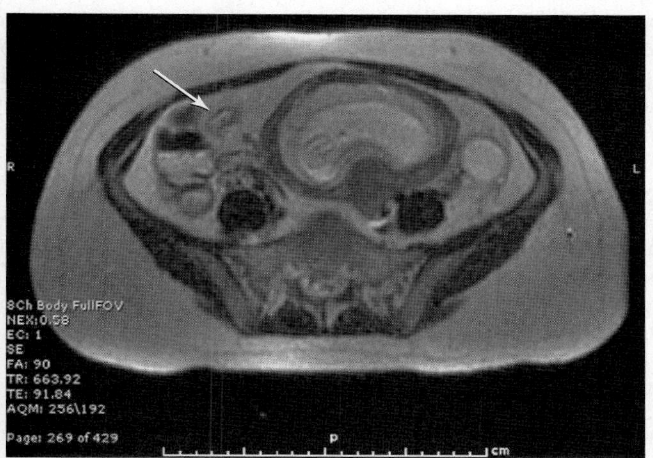

FIGURE 50-9 MRI scan with T1-weighted axial image of the abdomen in a gravid woman. The *arrow* highlights the thickened appendix. (From Parks NA, Schroeppel TJ: Update on imaging for acute appendicitis. *Surg Clin North Am* 91:141–154, 2011.)

The choice of laparoscopic versus open technique for appendectomy in pregnancy also merits discussion. Current Society of American Gastrointestinal and Endoscopic Surgeons guidelines state that laparoscopic appendectomy is safe in pregnancy and is the standard of care in pregnant patients.[43] Two studies, both small and retrospective, have shown no increased fetal loss with laparoscopic appendectomy compared with open appendectomy. Another study reported higher preterm labor and overall complication rates in the open group compared with the laparoscopic group.[40] Others have reported higher fetal loss rates with laparoscopic appendectomy (5.6% versus 3.1%) compared with open appendectomy.[44] It is apparent that this debate would be best resolved through randomized controlled trials, which to date have not been performed.

Our institutional experience with laparoscopic appendectomy in pregnancy has been positive, making it our preferred approach to the pregnant patient. In our hands, we believe it allows an easier identification of the highly variable location of the appendix, a more expeditious removal, and an opportunity for more thorough evaluation of the abdomen for any associated pathologic process. We do routinely use an open access approach (Hasson technique) for initial trocar placement to avoid any chance of injury to the gravid uterus.

Appendicitis in the Elderly

Although it is not the peak age for its occurrence, appendicitis is not infrequently seen in elderly patients and should remain in the differential diagnoses of any elderly patient presenting with acute abdominal pain who has not had an appendectomy. The most important aspect is to realize the expanded differential diagnosis that must be considered in the elderly. Other possible diagnoses include but are not limited to acute diverticulitis (uncomplicated or complicated), malignant disease, intestinal ischemia, ischemic colitis, complicated urinary tract infection, and perforated ulcer. Appendicitis may also be manifested in an atypical manner, so a high index of suspicion must be maintained. A careful history and physical examination may aid in diagnosis, but this may have little value in certain circumstances, such as in patients with dementia or an altered mental status. The higher perforation rate in the elderly population, as high as 40% to 70%, combined with the frequent coexistence of comorbidities resulting in higher morbidity makes the diagnosis and treatment of appendicitis in the elderly a challenge, to say the least.[3]

When faced with an elderly patient with diffuse peritonitis, immediate laparotomy should be performed without unnecessary delay. When the pain is localized and peritonitis is absent, CT scanning of the abdomen should be performed to confirm the diagnosis and to evaluate for other pathologic changes. Laparoscopic appendectomy is safe in the elderly and is our procedure of choice in this group of patients. Exceptions include patients with severe cardiomyopathy, in whom we prefer the open approach to avoid the deleterious effects of pneumoperitoneum in patients with marginal cardiac function.[45] We have also successfully performed open appendectomy under spinal anesthesia in patients who are "pulmonary cripples" and in whom the risk of general surgery is prohibitive and likely to result in ventilator dependence.

Appendicitis in the Immunocompromised Patient

Appendicitis in the immunocompromised patient is managed in the same manner as in the immunocompetent patient, with prompt appendectomy. The key in the evaluation of this population lies in maintenance of a high index of suspicion because the lack of the ability to mount an immune response may result in absence of fever, leukocytosis, and peritonitis. For this reason, early use of CT imaging is advisable. This allows confirmation of the diagnosis of appendicitis as well as the exclusion of diagnoses, such as neutropenic enterocolitis (typhlitis), that may be amenable to nonoperative treatment.[46]

NEOPLASMS OF THE APPENDIX

Neoplasms of the appendix, although rare, require appropriate treatment. An unanticipated appendiceal neoplasm may be encountered at any elective or emergency operation. It is estimated that 50% of appendiceal neoplasms present as appendicitis and are diagnosed on pathologic examination of the surgical specimen, but variable presentations have been reported. It is reported that appendiceal neoplasms are identified in 0.7% to 1.7% of pathology specimens. In addition, an appendiceal mass is sometimes noted as an incidental finding on abdominal CT (Fig. 50-10). The pathologic classification and biologic behavior of appendiceal neoplasms are diverse, which serves to make the classification, terminology, and treatment recommendations even more confusing.[1] Overall, appendiceal neoplasms are thought to account for 0.4% to 1% of all gastrointestinal malignant neoplasms.[1]

After appendectomy for presumed appendicitis, the incidence of unexpected findings in the surgical specimen is low. Still, if identified, appropriate counseling and treatment are essential. Carcinoid tumors are the most common tumor primary identified in the appendix.[16] These neoplasms arise from neuroendocrine cells from within the appendix and are detected in 0.3% to 0.9% of appendectomy specimens.[1] These are typically small,

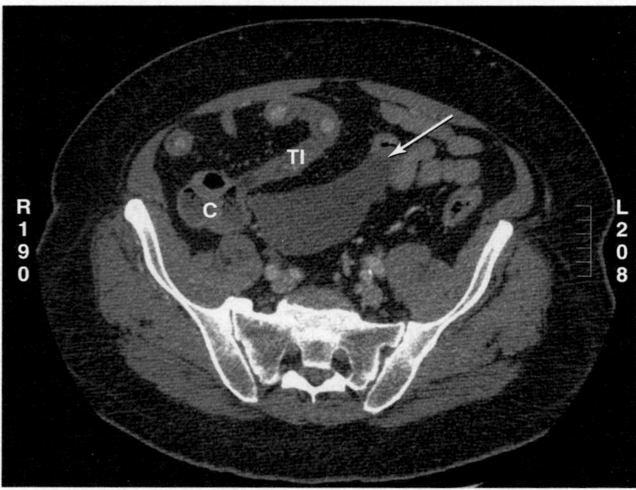

FIGURE 50-10 CT scan of the abdomen in a patient with a benign 10-cm mucocele. The axial image shows a distended fluid-filled mass medial to the appendix *(arrow)*, without associated inflammation. *C*, Cecum; *TI*, terminal ileum.

well-circumscribed lesions that are located within the more distal aspect of the appendix.

The biologic behavior of carcinoid tumors is highly variable. Size appears to be the best predictor of malignant behavior and metastatic potential, more so than histologic features, including lymphovascular invasion. Carcinoids smaller than 1 cm are typically thought to behave in a benign manner and are cured with appendectomy. Carcinoids larger than 2 cm are treated more aggressively, however. Other considerations include whether the carcinoid involves the base of the appendix or extends into the mesoappendix. Patients with carcinoids larger than 2 cm, with involvement of the base, or with extension to the mesoappendix should undergo right hemicolectomy with regional lymphadenectomy. For lesions between 1 and 2 cm in size, recommendations should be made after careful consideration of the individual tumor characteristics as metastases have been reported.[1,47]

Adenocarcinoma of the appendix is rare and occurs at a frequency of 0.08% to 0.1% of all appendectomies.[1] Treatment is identical to that of cecal adenocarcinoma and consists of right hemicolectomy with regional lymphadenectomy. Chemotherapy is also identical to that of adenocarcinoma of the colon, with adjuvant administration of 5-fluorouracil, leucovorin, and oxaliplatin (FOLFOX) to selected patients. FOLFOX has also been used in the neoadjuvant setting in patients with mucinous adenocarcinoma before cytoreductive (debulking) surgery.[48]

Mucinous tumors of the appendix are appendiceal tumors that are not frankly malignant but, if ruptured, can result in intraperitoneal spread and the development of pseudomyxoma peritonei (PMP). Classification and nomenclature of these lesions are confusing and not universally agreed on.[1] Because PMP results as a consequence of perforation and direct peritoneal seeding from the appendiceal contents, the surgeon should use great caution to avoid rupturing an intact appendix if mucocele or mucinous neoplasm is suspected on preoperative imaging or diagnosed intraoperatively. If PMP occurs, treatment by extensive cytoreductive surgery involving removal of any involved organs combined with heated intraperitoneal chemotherapy is typically employed[49] and is associated with long-term survival.

Although many appendiceal neoplasms are diagnosed on final pathologic examination, the mass will occasionally be visible at the time of appendectomy. An excellent algorithm for the management of the incidentally identified appendiceal mass was proposed by Wray and colleagues, and a modified version is provided for review (Fig. 50-11).[1] This algorithm is useful both in cases of appendicitis and in cases in which an appendiceal tumor is identified incidentally. The availability of frozen-section diagnosis may provide additional help with intraoperative decision making.

SELECTED REFERENCES

Ingraham AM, Cohen ME, Bilimoria KY, et al: Comparison of outcomes after laparoscopic versus open appendectomy for acute appendicitis at 222 ACS NSQIP hospitals. *Surgery* 148:625–635, discussion 635–637, 2010.

The authors provide one of the largest series to date, nearly 32,000 patients, comparing outcomes of laparoscopic versus open appendectomy using the ACS NSQIP database.

McGory ML, Zingmond DS, Tillou A, et al: Negative appendectomy in pregnant women is associated with a substantial risk of fetal loss. *J Am Coll Surg* 205:534–540, 2007.

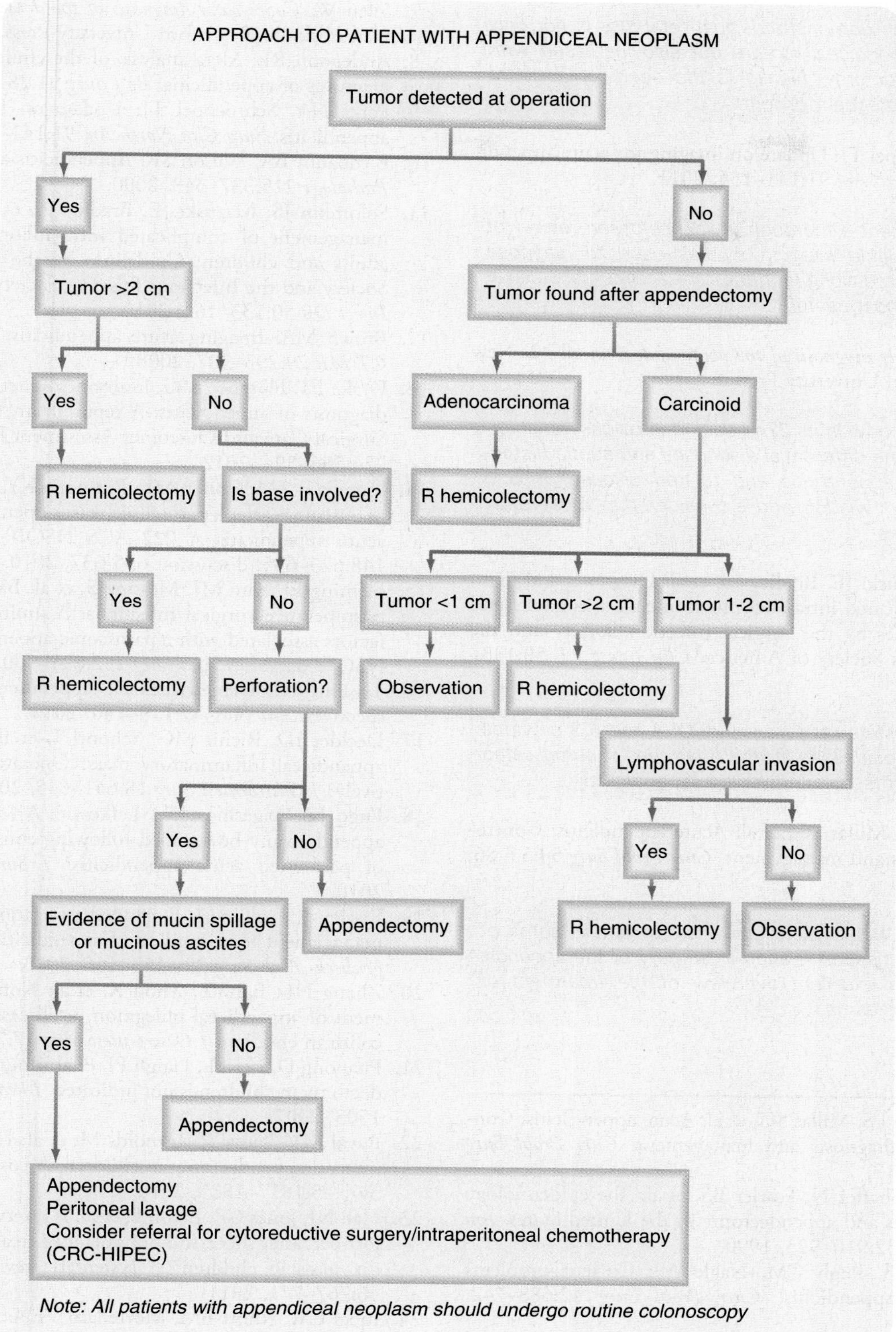

FIGURE 50-11 Suggested algorithm for managing the patient with an appendiceal neoplasm.

This article, which demonstrates that fetal loss is not only highest with appendiceal rupture but also increased with negative appendectomy, highlights the need for accurate diagnosis in the pregnant patient.

Parks NA, Schroeppel TJ: Update on imaging for acute appendicitis. *Surg Clin North Am* 91:141–154, 2011.

The authors present a thorough, evidence-based review of the current available imaging studies used to diagnose appendiceal disease along with the clinical circumstances in which they are most useful.

Silen W: *Cope's early diagnosis of the acute abdomen*, ed 22, New York, 2010, Oxford University Press.

This classic text, now in its 22nd edition, provides a masterful overview of the differential diagnoses and subtle historical findings of appendicitis and related disease. It is a timeless source of wisdom and is considered a "must read" by many surgeons.

Solomkin JS, Mazuski JE, Bradley JS, et al: Diagnosis and management of complicated intra-abdominal infection in adults and children: Guidelines by the Surgical Infection Society and the Infectious Diseases Society of America. *Clin Infect Dis* 50:133–164, 2010.

This consensus statement from the IDSA and SIS provides evidence-based guidelines for the treatment of complicated intra-abdominal infections, including appendicitis.

Wray CJ, Kao LS, Millas SG, et al: Acute appendicitis: Controversies in diagnosis and management. *Curr Probl Surg* 50:54–86, 2013.

This timely and well-written review article details some of the controversial issues relating to surgery of the appendix and includes an excellent overview of the treatment of appendiceal neoplasms.

REFERENCES

1. Wray CJ, Kao LS, Millas SG, et al: Acute appendicitis: Controversies in diagnosis and management. *Curr Probl Surg* 50:54–86, 2013.
2. Addiss DG, Shaffer N, Fowler BS, et al: The epidemiology of appendicitis and appendectomy in the United States. *Am J Epidemiol* 132:910–925, 1990.
3. Prystowsky JB, Pugh CM, Nagle AP: Current problems in surgery. Appendicitis. *Curr Probl Surg* 42:688–742, 2005.
4. Randal Bollinger R, Barbas AS, Bush EL, et al: Biofilms in the large bowel suggest an apparent function of the human vermiform appendix. *J Theor Biol* 249:826–831, 2007.
5. Deshmukh S, Verde F, Johnson PT, et al: Anatomical variants and pathologies of the vermix. *Emerg Radiol* 21:543–552, 2014.
6. Chen CY, Chen YC, Pu HN, et al: Bacteriology of acute appendicitis and its implication for the use of prophylactic antibiotics. *Surg Infect (Larchmt)* 13:383–390, 2012.
7. Silen W: *Cope's early diagnosis of the acute abdomen*, ed 22, New York, 2010, Oxford University Press.
8. Andersson RE: Meta-analysis of the clinical and laboratory diagnosis of appendicitis. *Br J Surg* 91:28–37, 2004.
9. Parks NA, Schroeppel TJ: Update on imaging for acute appendicitis. *Surg Clin North Am* 91:141–154, 2011.
10. Birnbaum BA, Wilson SR: Appendicitis at the millennium. *Radiology* 215:337–348, 2000.
11. Solomkin JS, Mazuski JE, Bradley JS, et al: Diagnosis and management of complicated intra-abdominal infection in adults and children: Guidelines by the Surgical Infection Society and the Infectious Diseases Society of America. *Clin Infect Dis* 50:133–164, 2010.
12. Brown MA: Imaging acute appendicitis. *Semin Ultrasound CT MR* 29:293–307, 2008.
13. Drake FT, Florence MG, Johnson MG, et al: Progress in the diagnosis of appendicitis: A report from Washington State's Surgical Care and Outcomes Assessment Program. *Ann Surg* 256:586–594, 2012.
14. Ingraham AM, Cohen ME, Bilimoria KY, et al: Comparison of outcomes after laparoscopic versus open appendectomy for acute appendicitis at 222 ACS NSQIP hospitals. *Surgery* 148:625–635, discussion 635-637, 2010.
15. Fleming FJ, Kim MJ, Messing S, et al: Balancing the risk of postoperative surgical infections: A multivariate analysis of factors associated with laparoscopic appendectomy from the NSQIP database. *Ann Surg* 252:895–900, 2010.
16. Teixeira PG, Demetriades D: Appendicitis: Changing perspectives. *Adv Surg* 47:119–140, 2013.
17. Deelder JD, Richir MC, Schoorl T, et al: How to treat an appendiceal inflammatory mass: Operatively or nonoperatively? *J Gastrointest Surg* 18:641–645, 2014.
18. Lugo JZ, Avgerinos DV, Lefkowitz AJ, et al: Can interval appendectomy be justified following conservative treatment of perforated acute appendicitis? *J Surg Res* 164:91–94, 2010.
19. Fawley J, Gollin G: Expanded utilization of nonoperative management for complicated appendicitis in children. *Langenbecks Arch Surg* 398:463–466, 2013.
20. Zhang HL, Bai YZ, Zhou X, et al: Nonoperative management of appendiceal phlegmon or abscess with an appendicolith in children. *J Gastrointest Surg* 17:766–770, 2013.
21. Puapong D, Lee SL, Haigh PI, et al: Routine interval appendectomy in children is not indicated. *J Pediatr Surg* 42:1500–1503, 2007.
22. Raval MV, Lautz T, Reynolds M, et al: Dollars and sense of interval appendectomy in children: A cost analysis. *J Pediatr Surg* 45:1817–1825, 2010.
23. Hall NJ, Jones CE, Eaton S, et al: Is interval appendicectomy justified after successful nonoperative treatment of an appendix mass in children? A systematic review. *J Pediatr Surg* 46:767–771, 2011.
24. Iqbal CW, Knott EM, Mortellaro VE, et al: Interval appendectomy after perforated appendicitis: What are the operative risks and luminal patency rates? *J Surg Res* 177:127–130, 2012.
25. Willemsen PJ, Hoorntje LE, Eddes EH, et al: The need for interval appendectomy after resolution of an appendiceal mass questioned. *Dig Surg* 19:216–220, discussion 221, 2002.
26. Carpenter SG, Chapital AB, Merritt MV, et al: Increased risk of neoplasm in appendicitis treated with interval

appendectomy: Single-institution experience and literature review. *Am Surg* 78:339–343, 2012.

27. Furman MJ, Cahan M, Cohen P, et al: Increased risk of mucinous neoplasm of the appendix in adults undergoing interval appendectomy. *JAMA Surg* 148:703–706, 2013.
28. Gaetke-Udager K, Maturen KE, Hammer SG: Beyond acute appendicitis: Imaging and pathologic spectrum of appendiceal pathology. *Emerg Radiol* 21:535–542, 2014.
29. Lai HW, Loong CC, Chiu JH, et al: Interval appendectomy after conservative treatment of an appendiceal mass. *World J Surg* 30:352–357, 2006.
30. Garlipp B, Arlt G: [Laparoscopy for suspected appendicitis. Should an appendix that appears normal be removed?]. *Chirurg* 80:615–621, 2009.
31. Chiarugi M, Buccianti P, Decanini L, et al: "What you see is not what you get." A plea to remove a 'normal' appendix during diagnostic laparoscopy. *Acta Chir Belg* 101:243–245, 2001.
32. Varadhan KK, Neal KR, Lobo DN: Safety and efficacy of antibiotics compared with appendicectomy for treatment of uncomplicated acute appendicitis: Meta-analysis of randomised controlled trials. *BMJ* 344:e2156, 2012.
33. Mason RJ, Moazzez A, Sohn H, et al: Meta-analysis of randomized trials comparing antibiotic therapy with appendectomy for acute uncomplicated (no abscess or phlegmon) appendicitis. *Surg Infect (Larchmt)* 13:74–84, 2012.
34. Giuliano V, Giuliano C, Pinto F, et al: Chronic appendicitis "syndrome" manifested by an appendicolith and thickened appendix presenting as chronic right lower abdominal pain in adults. *Emerg Radiol* 12:96–98, 2006.
35. Teli B, Ravishankar N, Harish S, et al: Role of elective laparoscopic appendicectomy for chronic right lower quadrant pain. *Indian J Surg* 75:352–355, 2013.
36. Wen SW, Hernandez R, Naylor CD: Pitfalls in nonrandomized outcomes studies. The case of incidental appendectomy with open cholecystectomy. *JAMA* 274:1687–1691, 1995.
37. Wang HT, Sax HC: Incidental appendectomy in the era of managed care and laparoscopy. *J Am Coll Surg* 192:182–188, 2001.
38. Brown JJ, Wilson C, Coleman S, et al: Appendicitis in pregnancy: An ongoing diagnostic dilemma. *Colorectal Dis* 11:116–122, 2009.
39. Flexer SM, Tabib N, Peter MB: Suspected appendicitis in pregnancy. *Surgeon* 12:82–86, 2014.
40. Peled Y, Hiersch L, Khalpari O, et al: Appendectomy during pregnancy—is pregnancy outcome depending by operation technique? *J Matern Fetal Neonatal Med* 27:365–367, 2014.
41. McGory ML, Zingmond DS, Tillou A, et al: Negative appendectomy in pregnant women is associated with a substantial risk of fetal loss. *J Am Coll Surg* 205:534–540, 2007.
42. Khandelwal A, Fasih N, Kielar A: Imaging of acute abdomen in pregnancy. *Radiol Clin North Am* 51:1005–1022, 2013.
43. Korndorffer JR, Jr, Fellinger E, Reed W: SAGES guideline for laparoscopic appendectomy. *Surg Endosc* 24:757–761, 2010.
44. Walsh CA, Tang T, Walsh SR: Laparoscopic versus open appendicectomy in pregnancy: A systematic review. *Int J Surg* 6:339–344, 2008.
45. Richmond BK, Thalheimer L: Laparoscopy associated mesenteric vascular complications. *Am Surg* 76:1177–1184, 2010.
46. Hernandez-Ocasio F, Palermo-Garofalo CA, Colon M, et al: Right lower quadrant abdominal pain in an immunocompromised patient: Importance for an urgent diagnosis and treatment. *Bol Asoc Med P R* 103:51–53, 2011.
47. Boudreaux JP, Klimstra DS, Hassan MM, et al: The NANETS consensus guideline for the diagnosis and management of neuroendocrine tumors: Well-differentiated neuroendocrine tumors of the jejunum, ileum, appendix, and cecum. *Pancreas* 39:753–766, 2010.
48. Sugarbaker PH, Bijelic L, Chang D, et al: Neoadjuvant FOLFOX chemotherapy in 34 consecutive patients with mucinous peritoneal carcinomatosis of appendiceal origin. *J Surg Oncol* 102:576–581, 2010.
49. Wagner PL, Austin F, Maduekwe U, et al: Extensive cytoreductive surgery for appendiceal carcinomatosis: Morbidity, mortality, and survival. *Ann Surg Oncol* 20:1056–1062, 2013.

51 CHAPTER

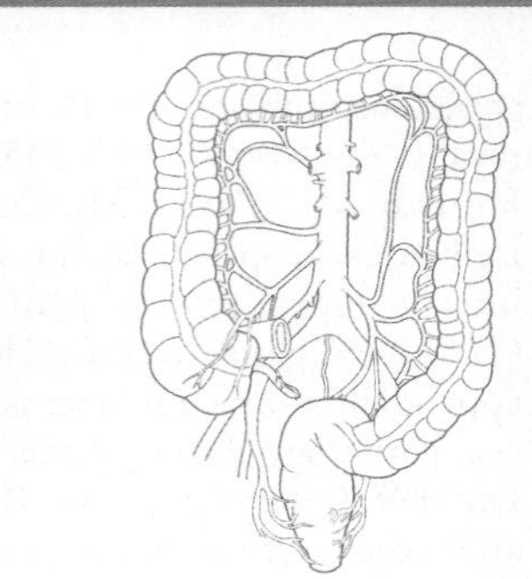

Colon and Rectum

Najjia N. Mahmoud, Joshua I.S. Bleier, Cary B. Aarons, E. Carter Paulson, Skandan Shanmugan, Robert D. Fry

OUTLINE

EMBRYOLOGY OF THE COLON AND RECTUM

No comprehensive discussion of colorectal anatomy is complete without a thorough understanding of the genesis of the gastrointestinal (GI) tract. Knowledge of the developmental anatomy of the foregut, midgut, and hindgut establishes a context in which to consider mature structural and functional anatomic relationships.

The endodermal roof of the yolk sac gives rise to the primitive gut tube. At the beginning of the third week of development, the gut tube is divided into three regions; the midgut, which opens ventrally, is positioned between the foregut in the head fold and the hindgut in the tail fold. Development progresses through the stages of physiologic herniation, return to the abdomen, and fixation. The acquisition of length and the formation of dedicated blood and lymphatic supplies take place during this time (Fig. 51-1).

Foregut-derived structures end at the second portion of the duodenum and rely on the celiac artery for blood supply. The midgut, extending from the duodenal ampulla to the distal transverse colon, is based on the superior mesenteric artery (SMA). The distal third of the transverse colon, descending colon, and rectum evolve from the hindgut fold and are supplied by the inferior mesenteric artery (IMA). Venous and lymphatic channels mirror their arterial counterparts and follow the same embryologic divisions. At the dentate line, endoderm-derived tissues fuse with the ectoderm-derived proctodeum, or ingrowth from the anal pit.

Distal rectal development is complex. The cloaca is a specialized area of the primitive distal rectum composed of endoderm- and ectoderm-derived tissues. This area is incorporated into the anal transition zone, which surrounds the dentate line in the adult. The cloaca exists in a continuum with the hindgut, but at approximately the sixth week, it begins to divide and to differentiate into anterior urogenital and posterior anal and sphincter elements. Simultaneously, the urogenital and GI tracts are separated by caudal migration of the urogenital septum. During the tenth week of development, the external anal sphincter is formed from the posterior cloaca as the descent of the urogenital septum becomes complete. The internal anal sphincter is formed by the twelfth week from enlarged circular muscle layers of the rectum.

ANATOMY OF THE COLON, RECTUM, AND PELVIC FLOOR

The colon and rectum constitute a tube of variable diameter approximately 150 cm in length. The terminal ileum empties into the cecum through a thickened, nipple-shaped invagination, the ileocecal valve. The cecum is a capacious sac-like segment of the proximal colon, with an average diameter of 7.5 cm and length of 10 cm. Although it is distensible, acute dilation of the cecum to a diameter of more than 12 cm, which can be measured by a plain abdominal radiograph, can result in ischemic necrosis and perforation of the bowel wall. Surgical intervention may be required when this degree of cecal distention is caused by obstruction or pseudo-obstruction (Fig. 51-2).

The appendix extends from the cecum approximately 3 cm below the ileocecal valve as a blind-ending elongated tube, 8 to 10 cm in length. The proximal appendix is fairly constant in location, whereas the end can be located in a wide variety of positions relative to the cecum and terminal ileum. Most commonly, it is retrocecal (65%), followed by pelvic (31%), subcecal (2.3%), preileal (1.0%), and retroileal (0.4%). Clinically, the appendix is found at the convergence of the taeniae coli. Another clinical aid useful for detecting the location of the appendix through a small abdominal incision is the identification of the fold of Treves, the only antimesenteric epiploic appendage normally found on the small intestine, marking the junction of the ileum and cecum.

The ascending colon, approximately 15 cm in length, runs upward toward the liver on the right side; like the descending colon, the posterior surface is fixed against the retroperitoneum, whereas the lateral and anterior surfaces are true intraperitoneal structures. The white line of Toldt represents the fusion of the

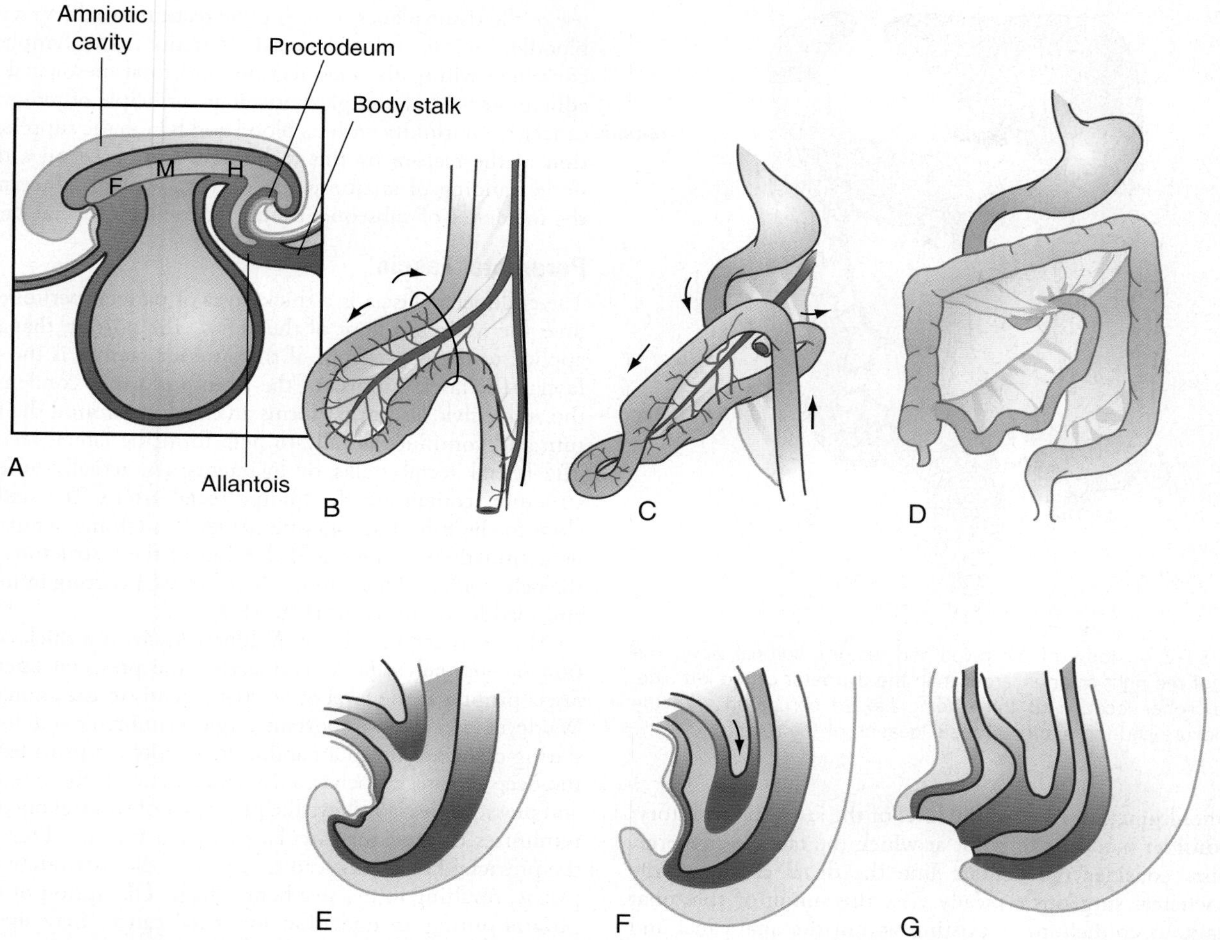

FIGURE 51-1 At the third week of development, the primitive tube can be divided into three regions **(A):** the foregut (F) in the head fold, the hindgut (H) with its ventral allantoic outgrowth in the smaller tail fold, and the midgut (M) between these two portions. Stages of development of the midgut are physiologic herniation **(B),** return to the abdomen **(C),** and fixation **(D).** At the sixth week, the urogenital septum migrates caudally **(E)** and separates the intestinal and urogenital tracts **(F, G).** (From Corman ML, editor: *Colon and rectal surgery*, ed 4, Philadelphia, 1998, Lippincott-Raven, p 2.)

mesentery with the posterior peritoneum. This subtle peritoneal landmark serves as a guide for the surgeon for mobilizing the colon and mesentery from the retroperitoneum.

The transverse colon is approximately 45 cm in length. Hanging between fixed positions at the hepatic and splenic flexures, it is completely invested in visceral peritoneum. The nephrocolic ligament secures the hepatic flexure and directly overlies the right kidney, duodenum, and porta hepatis. The phrenocolic ligament lies ventral to the spleen and fixes the splenic flexure in the left upper quadrant. The angle of the splenic flexure is higher, more acute, and more deeply situated than that of the hepatic flexure. The splenic flexure is typically approached by dissecting the descending colon along the line of Toldt from below and then entering the lesser sac by reflecting the omentum from the transverse colon. This maneuver allows mobilization of the flexure to be achieved, with minimal traction required for exposure. Attached to the superior aspect of the transverse colon is the greater omentum, a fused double layer of visceral and parietal peritoneum (four total layers) that contains variable amounts of stored fat. Clinically, it is useful in preventing adhesions between surgical abdominal wounds and underlying bowel and is often used to cover intraperitoneal contents as incisions are closed. The omentum can be mobilized and placed between the rectum and vagina after repair of a high rectovaginal fistula or used to fill the pelvic and perineal space left after excision of the rectum. The living tissue of the greater omentum makes a good patch in difficult situations, such as treatment of a perforated duodenum, when closure of inflamed and friable tissues is impossible or ill-advised.

The descending colon lies ventral to the left kidney and extends downward from the splenic flexure for approximately 25 cm. It is smaller in diameter than the ascending colon. At the level of the pelvic brim, there is a transition between the relatively thin-walled, fixed, descending colon and the thicker, mobile sigmoid colon. The sigmoid colon varies in length from 15 to 50 cm (average, 38 cm) and is very mobile. It is a small-diameter, muscular tube on a long floppy mesentery that often forms an omega loop in the pelvis. The mesosigmoid is frequently attached to the left pelvic sidewall, producing a small recess in the mesentery known as the intersigmoid fossa. This mesenteric fold is a surgical landmark for the underlying left ureter.

The rectum, along with the sigmoid colon, serves as a fecal reservoir. There is some controversy about the definition of the proximal and distal extent of the rectum. Some consider the

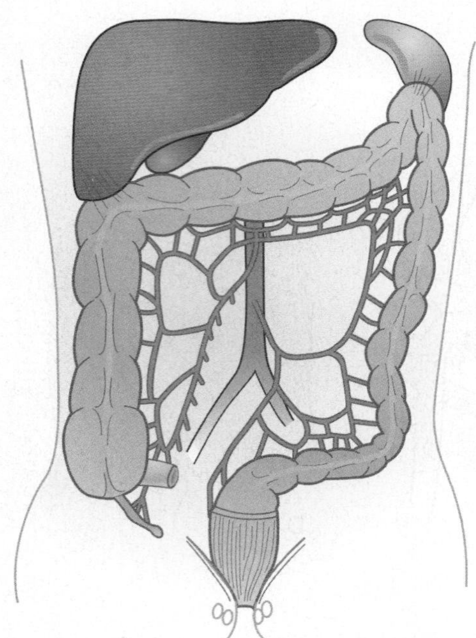

FIGURE 51-2 Anatomy of the colon and rectum, coronal view. The diameter of the right colon is larger than the diameter of the left side. Note the higher location of the splenic flexure compared with the hepatic flexure and the extraperitoneal location of the rectum.

rectosigmoid junction to be at the level of the sacral promontory; others consider it to be the point at which the taeniae converge. Anatomists consider the dentate line the distal extent of the rectum, whereas surgeons typically view this union of columnar and squamous epithelium as existing within the anal canal and consider the end of the rectum to be the proximal border of the anal sphincter complex. The rectum is 12 to 15 cm in length and lacks taeniae coli or epiploic appendices. It occupies the curve of the sacrum in the true pelvis, and the posterior surface is almost completely extraperitoneal in that it is adherent to presacral soft tissues and thus is outside the peritoneal cavity. The anterior surface of the proximal third of the rectum is covered by visceral peritoneum. The peritoneal reflection is 7 to 9 cm from the anal verge in men and 5 to 7.5 cm in women. This anterior peritonealized space is called the pouch of Douglas, pelvic cul-de-sac, or rectouterine pouch and may serve as the site of so-called drop metastases from visceral tumors. These peritoneal metastases can form a mass in the cul-de-sac (called Blumer's shelf) that can be detected by a digital rectal examination.

The rectum possesses three involutions or curves known as the valves of Houston. The middle valve folds to the left, and the proximal and distal valves fold to the right. These valves are more properly called folds because they have no specific function as impediments to flow. They are lost after full surgical mobilization of the rectum, a maneuver that may provide approximately 5 cm of additional length to the rectum, greatly facilitating the surgeon's ability to fashion an anastomosis deep in the pelvis.

The posterior aspect of the rectum is invested with a thick, closely applied mesorectum. A thin layer of investing fascia (fascia propria) coats the mesorectum and represents a distinct layer from the presacral fascia against which it lies. During proctectomy for rectal cancer, mobilization and dissection of the rectum proceed between the presacral fascia and fascia propria. Total mesorectal excision is a well-described oncologic maneuver that makes good use of the tissue planes investing the rectum to achieve a relatively bloodless rectal and mesorectal dissection. The lymphatics are contained within the mesorectum, and total mesorectal excision adheres to the basic surgical oncologic principle of removal of the cancer in continuity with its blood and lymphatic supplies. Resection of the rectum by this technique, and based on a thorough understanding of anatomy, has been shown to reduce markedly the incidence of subsequent local recurrence of rectal cancer.

Pararectal Fascia

The endopelvic fascia is a thick layer of parietal peritoneum that lines the walls and floor of the pelvis. The portion that is closely applied to the periosteum of the anterior sacrum is the presacral fascia. The fascia propria of the rectum is a thin condensation of the endopelvic fascia that forms an envelope around the mesorectum and continues distally to help form the lateral rectal stalks. The lateral rectal stalks or ligaments are actually anterolateral structures containing the middle rectal artery. The stalks reside close to the mixed autonomic nerves, containing sympathetic and parasympathetic nerves, and division of these structures close to the pelvic sidewall may injure these nerves, resulting in impotence and bladder dysfunction (Fig. 51-3).

The rectosacral fascia, or Waldeyer fascia, is a thick condensation of endopelvic fascia connecting the presacral fascia to the fascia propria at the level of S4 that extends to the anorectal ring. Waldeyer fascia is an important surgical landmark, and its division during dissection from an abdominal approach provides entry to the deep retrorectal pelvis. Dissection between the fascia propria and presacral fascia follows the principles of surgical oncology and minimizes the risk for vascular or neural injuries. Disruption of the presacral fascia may lead to injury of the basivertebral venous plexus, resulting in massive hemorrhage. Disruption of the fascia propria during an operation for rectal cancer may significantly increase the incidence of subsequent recurrence of cancer in the pelvis if mesorectum is then left behind.

Pelvic Floor

The muscles of the pelvic floor, like those of the anal sphincter mechanism, arise from the primitive cloaca. The pelvic floor, or diaphragm, consists of the pubococcygeus, iliococcygeus, and puborectalis, a group of muscles that together form the levator ani. The pelvic diaphragm resides between the sacrum, obturator fascia, ischial spines, and pubis. It forms a strong floor that supports the pelvic organs and, with the external anal sphincter, regulates defecation. The levator hiatus is an opening between the decussating fibers of the pubococcygeus that allows egress of the anal canal, urethra, and dorsal vein in men and the anal canal, urethra, and vagina in women. The puborectalis is a strong, U-shaped sling of striated muscle coursing around the rectum just above the level of the anal sphincters. Relaxation of the puborectalis straightens the anorectal angle and permits descent of feces; contraction produces the opposite effect. The puborectalis is in a state of continual contraction, a factor vital to the maintenance of continence. Puborectalis dysfunction is an important cause of defecation disorders. The pubococcygeus and iliococcygeus most likely participate in continence by applying lateral pressure to narrow the levator hiatus (Figs. 51-4 and 51-5).

Arterial Supply and Venous and Lymphatic Drainage

Knowledge of the embryologic development of the intestinal tract provides an excellent foundation for understanding the anatomic blood supply. The foregut is supplied by the celiac artery, the

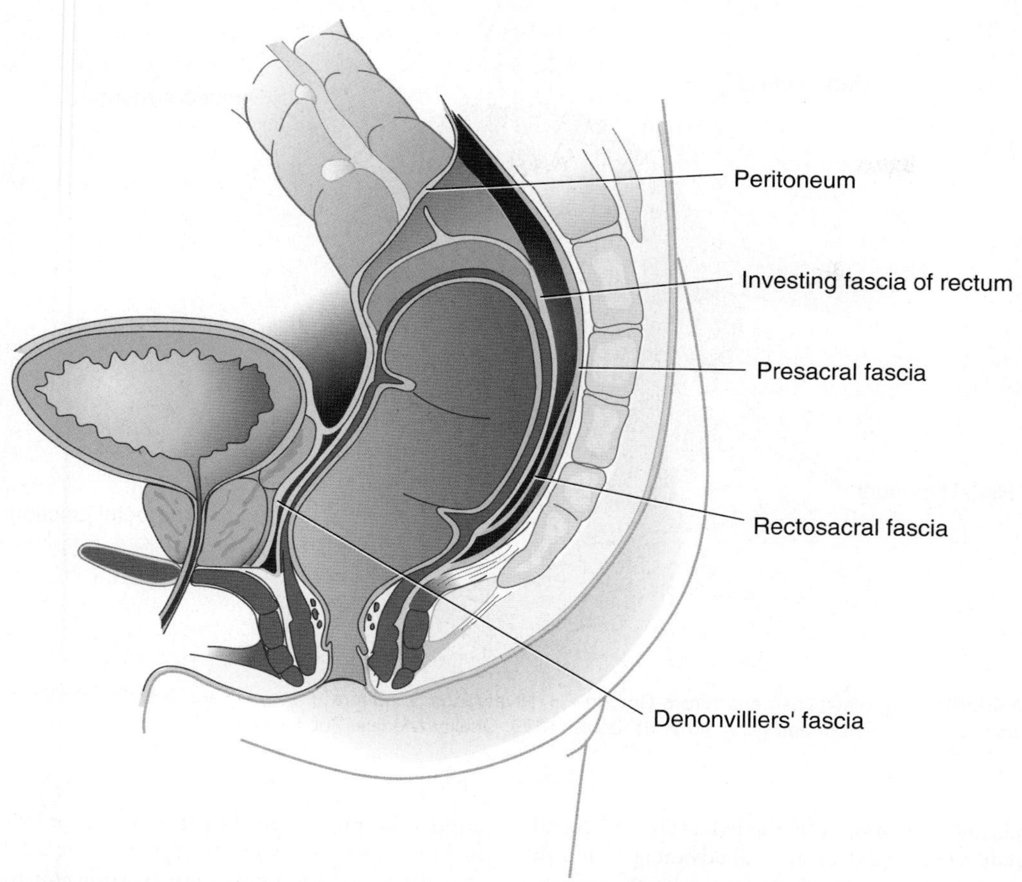

FIGURE 51-3 Endopelvic fascia. (From Gordon PH, Nivatvongs S, editors: *Principles and practice of surgery for the colon, rectum and anus*, ed 2, St. Louis, 1999, Quality Medical Publishing, p 10.)

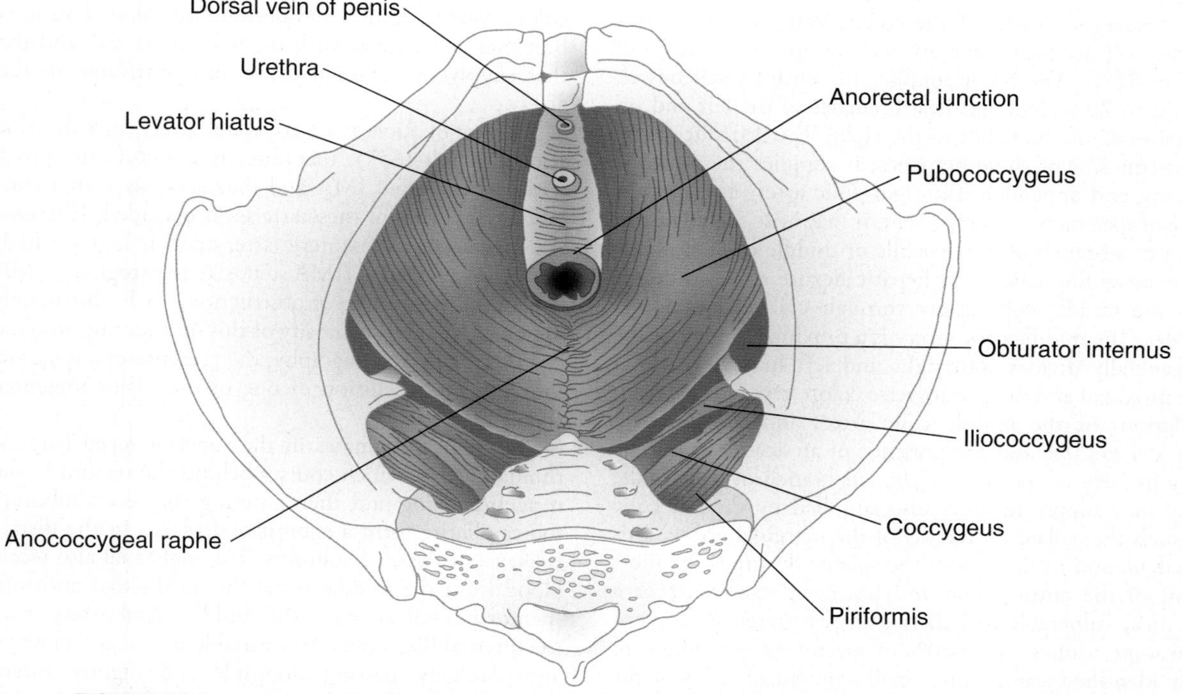

FIGURE 51-4 Levator muscles. (From Gordon PH, Nivatvongs S, editors: *Principles and practice of surgery for the colon, rectum and anus*, ed 2, St. Louis, 1999, Quality Medical Publishing, p 18.)

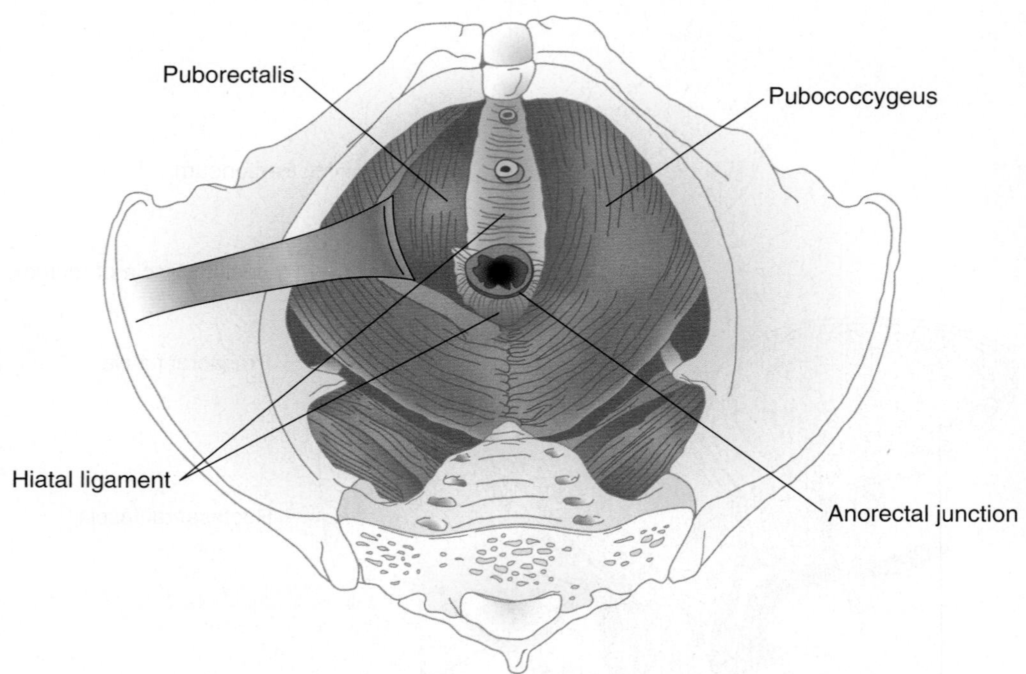

FIGURE 51-5 Hiatal ligament. (From Gordon PH, Nivatvongs S, editors: *Principles and practice of surgery for the colon, rectum and anus*, ed 2, St. Louis, 1999, Quality Medical Publishing, p 18.)

midgut by the SMA, and the hindgut by the IMA (Figs. 51-6 and 51-7). Anatomic redundancy confers survival advantages, and in the intestinal tract, this feature is provided by extensive communication between the major arteries and collateral blood supply (Fig. 51-8). The territory of the SMA ends at the distal portion of the transverse colon, and that of the IMA begins in the region of the splenic flexure. A large collateral vessel, the marginal artery, connects these two circulations and forms a continuous arcade along the mesenteric border of the colon. Vasa recta from this artery branch off at short intervals and supply the bowel wall directly (Fig. 51-9). The SMA supplies the entire small bowel, giving off 12 to 20 jejunal and ileal branches to the left and up to three main colonic branches to the right. The ileocolic artery is the most constant of these branches; it supplies the terminal ileum, cecum, and appendix. The right colic artery is absent in 2% to 18% of specimens; when present, it may arise directly from the SMA or as a branch of the ileocolic or middle colic artery. It supplies the ascending colon and hepatic flexure and communicates with the middle colic artery through collateral marginal artery arcades. The middle colic artery is a proximal branch of the SMA. It generally divides into right and left branches, which supply the proximal and distal transverse colon, respectively. Anatomic variations of the middle colic artery include complete absence in 4% to 20% and the presence of an accessory middle colic artery in 10% of specimens. The left branch of the middle colic artery may supply territory also supplied by the left colic artery through the collateral channel of the marginal artery. This collateral circulation in the area of the splenic flexure is the most inconsistent of the entire colon and has been referred to as a watershed area, vulnerable to ischemia in the presence of hypotension. In some studies, up to 50% of specimens were found to lack clearly identified arteries in a small segment of colon at the confluence of the blood supplies of the midgut and hindgut. These individuals rely on adjacent vasa recta in this area for arterial supply to the bowel wall. In practice, surgeons avoid making anastomoses in the region of the splenic flexure, fearing that the blood supply will not be sufficient to permit healing of the anastomosis, a situation that could lead to anastomotic leak and sepsis.

The IMA originates from the aorta at the level of L2 to L3, approximately 3 cm above the aortic bifurcation. The left colic artery is the most proximal branch, supplying the distal transverse colon, splenic flexure, and descending colon. Two to six sigmoid branches collateralize with the left colic artery and form arcades that supply the sigmoid colon and contribute to the marginal artery.

The arc of Riolan is a collateral artery, first described by Jean Riolan (1580-1657), that directly connects the proximal SMA with the proximal IMA and may serve as a vital conduit when one or the other of these arteries is occluded. It is also known as the meandering mesenteric artery and is highly variable in size. Flow can be forward (IMA stenosis) or retrograde (SMA stenosis), depending on the site of obstruction. Such obstruction results in increased size and tortuosity of this meandering artery, which may be detected by arteriography; the presence of a large arc of Riolan thus suggests occlusion of one of the major mesenteric arteries (Fig. 51-10).

The IMA terminates in the superior rectal (superior hemorrhoidal) artery, which courses behind the rectum in the mesorectum, branching and then entering the rectal submucosa. Here, the capillaries form a submucosal plexus in the distal rectum at the level of the anal columns. The anal canal also receives arterial blood from the middle rectal (hemorrhoidal) and inferior rectal (hemorrhoidal) arteries. The middle rectal artery is a branch of the internal iliac artery. It is variable in size and enters the rectum anterolaterally, passing alongside and slightly anterior to the lateral rectal stalks. It has been reported to be absent in 40% to 80% of specimens studied. The inferior rectal artery is a branch

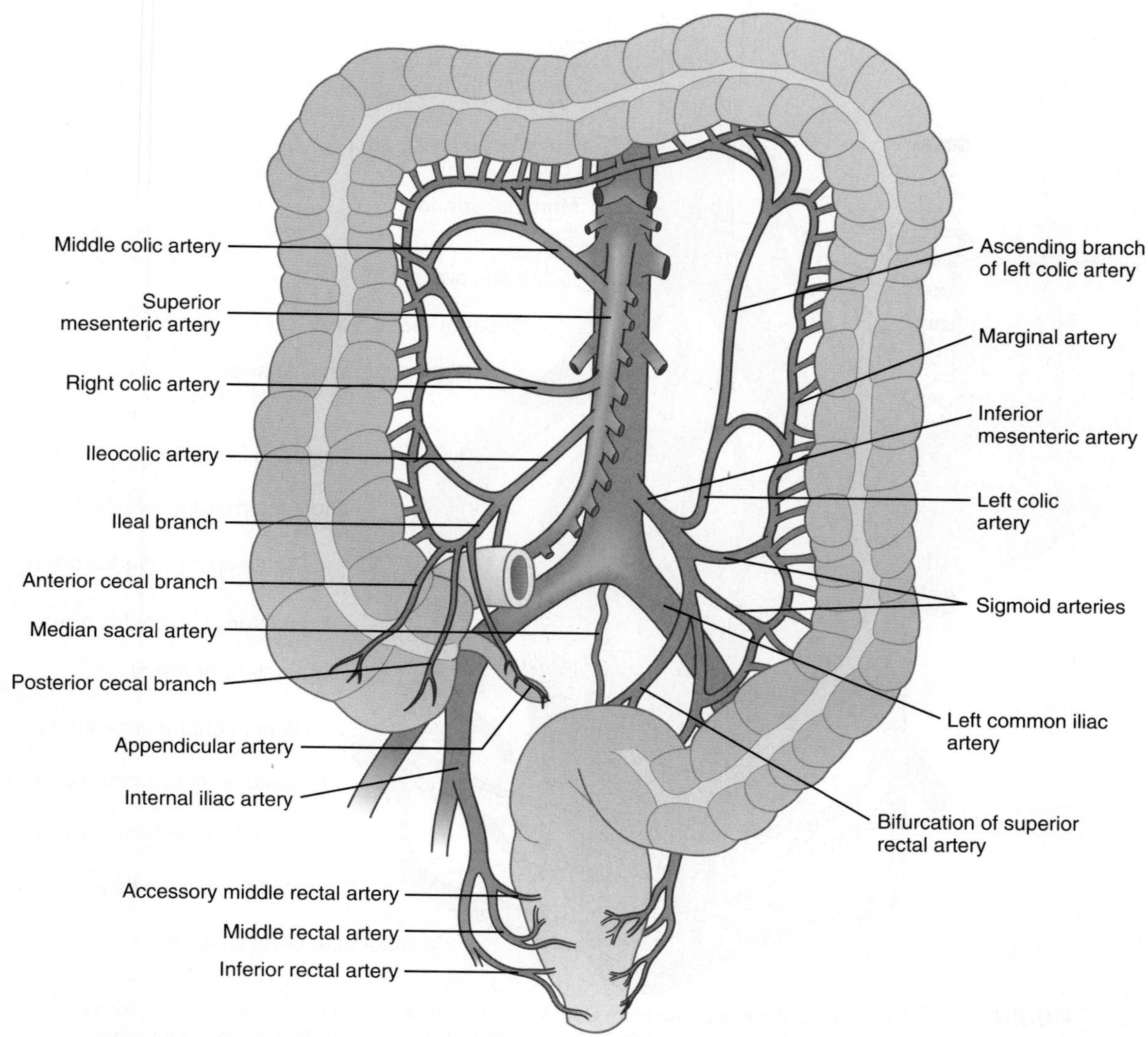

FIGURE 51-6 Arterial supply of the colon. (From Gordon PH, Nivatvongs S, editors: *Principles and practice of surgery for the colon, rectum and anus*, ed 2, St. Louis, 1999, Quality Medical Publishing, p 23.)

of the pudendal artery, which itself is a more distal branch of the internal iliac. From the obturator canal, it traverses the obturator fascia, ischiorectal fossa, and external anal sphincter to reach the anal canal. This vessel is encountered during the perineal dissection of an abdominoperineal resection.

The venous drainage of the colon and rectum mirrors the arterial blood supply. Venous drainage from the right and proximal transverse colon empties into the superior mesenteric vein, which coalesces with the splenic vein to become the portal vein. The distal transverse colon, descending colon, sigmoid, and most of the rectum drain into the inferior mesenteric vein, which empties into the splenic vein to the left of the aorta. The anal canal is drained by the middle and inferior rectal veins into the internal iliac vein and subsequently the inferior vena cava. The bidirectional venous drainage of the anal canal accounts for differences in patterns of metastasis from tumors arising in this region (Fig. 51-11).

Lymphatic drainage also follows the arterial anatomy. The wall of the large bowel is supplied with a rich network of lymphatic capillaries that drain to extramural channels paralleling the arterial supply. Lymphatics from the colon and proximal two thirds of the rectum ultimately drain into the para-aortic nodal chain, which empties into the cisterna chyli. Lymphatics draining the distal rectum and anal canal may drain to the para-aortic nodes or laterally, through the internal iliac system, to the superficial inguinal nodal basin. Although the dentate line roughly marks the level where lymphatic drainage diverges, classic studies by Block and Enquist using dye injection demonstrated that spread through lymphatic channels occurs to adjacent pelvic organs, such as the vagina and broad ligament, when injections are administered as high as 10 cm proximal to the dentate line (Figs. 51-12 and 51-13).

Lymph nodes are commonly grouped into levels according to their location. Epicolic nodes are located along the bowel wall and in the epiploic appendices. Nodes adjacent to the marginal artery are paracolic. Intermediate nodes are located along the main branches of the large blood vessels; primary nodes are located on the SMA or IMA. Lymph node invasion by metastatic cancer is an important prognostic factor for patients with colorectal cancer. Accurate pathologic assessment of lymph nodes is essential for accurate staging, which serves as a determinant for treatment of patients with colorectal cancer.

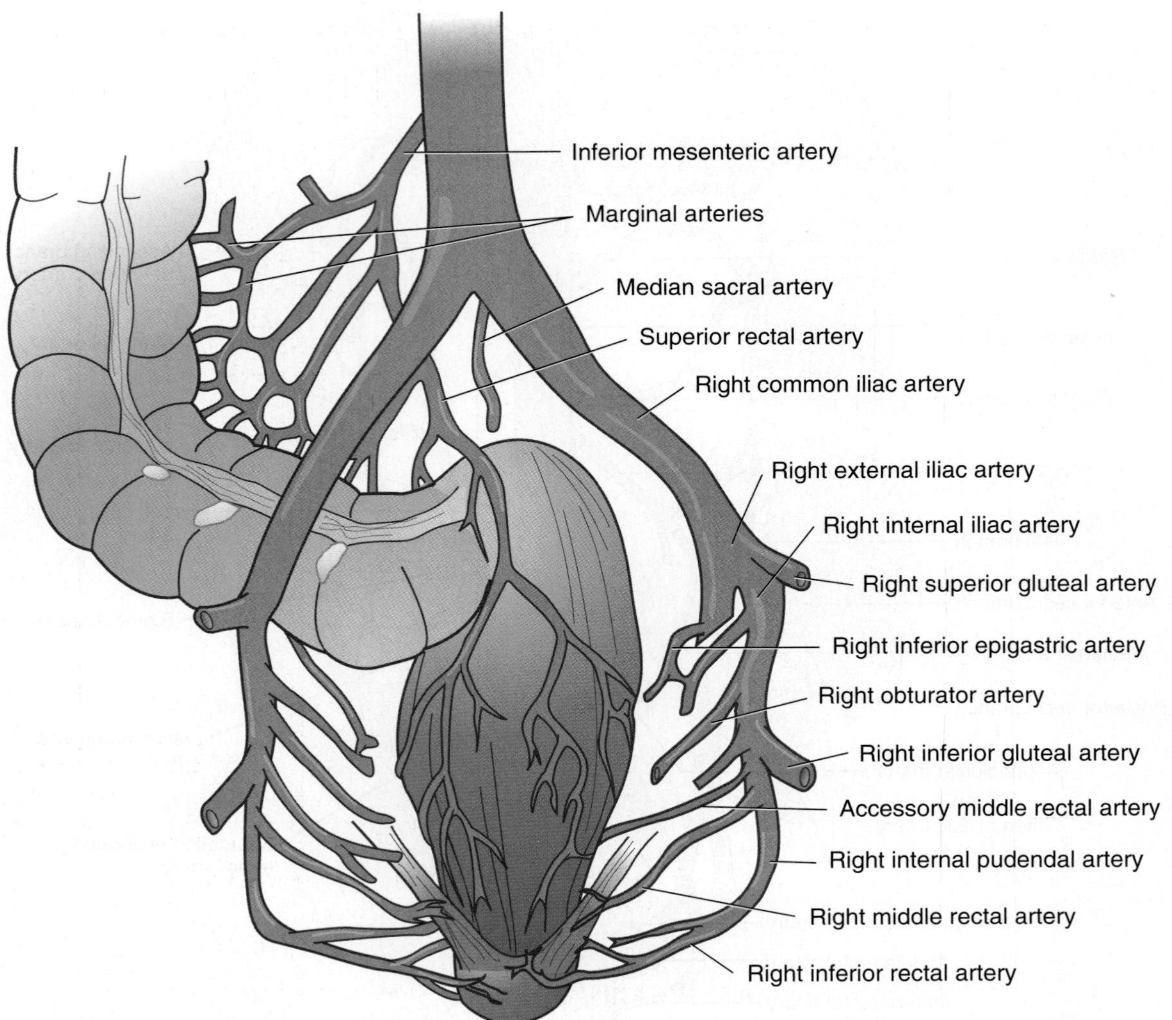

FIGURE 51-7 Arterial supply of the rectum. (From Gordon PH, Nivatvongs S, editors: *Principles and practice of surgery for the colon, rectum and anus,* ed 2, St. Louis, 1999, Quality Medical Publishing, p 24.)

Nerves

Preganglionic sympathetic nerves from T6 to T12 synapse in preaortic ganglia. Postsympathetic fibers then course along blood vessels to reach the right and transverse colon. The right and transverse colon parasympathetic supply comes from the right vagus nerve. Parasympathetic fibers follow branches of the SMA to synapse in the wall of the bowel. The left colon and rectum receive sympathetic supply from the preganglionic lumbar splanchnics of L1 to L3. These synapse in the preaortic plexus located above the aortic bifurcation, and the postganglionic elements follow the branches of the IMA and superior rectal artery to the left colon, sigmoid, and rectum. The lower rectum, pelvic floor, and anal canal receive postganglionic sympathetics from the pelvic plexus. The pelvic plexus is adherent to the pelvic sidewalls and is adjacent to the lateral stalks. It receives sympathetic branches from the presacral plexus that condense at the sacral promontory into the left and right hypogastric nerves. These sympathetic nerves, which descend into the pelvis dorsal to the superior rectal artery, are responsible for delivery of semen to the posterior prostatic urethra. Failure to preserve at least one of the hypogastric nerves during rectal dissection results in ejaculatory dysfunction in men.

The pelvic parasympathetic nerves, or nervi erigentes, arise from S2 to S4. Preganglionic parasympathetic nerves merge with postganglionic sympathetics after the latter emerge from the sacral foramina. These nerve fibers, through the pelvic plexus, surround and innervate the prostate, urethra, seminal vesicles, urinary bladder, and muscles of the pelvic floor. Rectal dissection may disrupt the pelvic plexus and its subdivisions, resulting in neurogenic bladder and sexual dysfunction. Rates of bladder and erectile dysfunction after rectal surgery are as high as 45%. The degree and type of dysfunction are affected by the level of the neurologic injury. A high IMA ligation severing the hypogastric nerves near the sacral promontory results in sympathetic dysfunction characterized by retrograde ejaculation and bladder dysfunction. Injury to the mixed parasympathetic and sympathetic periprostatic plexus results in impotence and an atonic bladder.

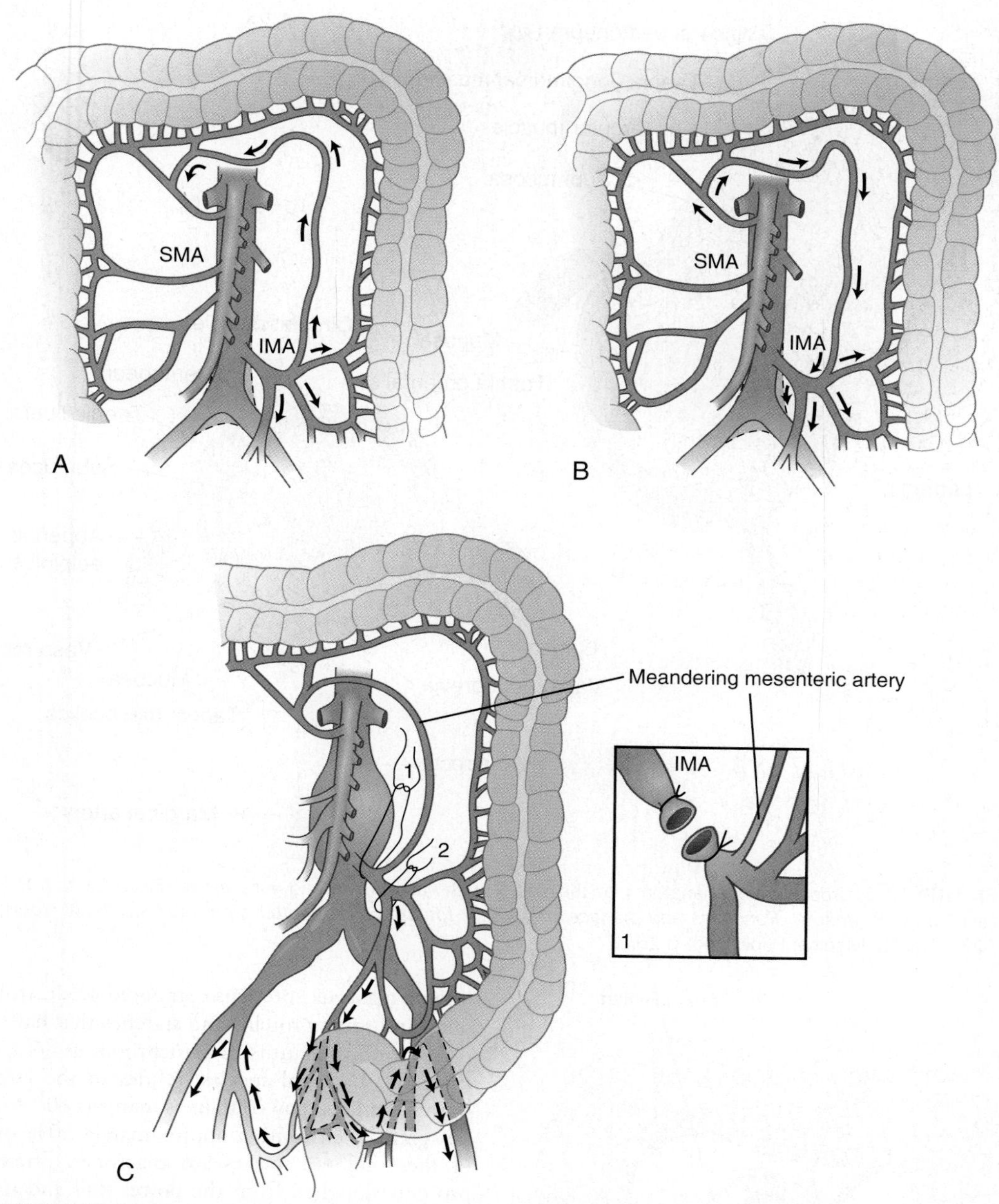

FIGURE 51-8 Pathologic anatomy and occlusion of the superior mesenteric artery (SMA) and inferior mesenteric artery (IMA). **A,** Occlusion of the SMA. **B,** Occlusion of the IMA. **C,** Ligating the IMA: *1,* correct location of ligation *(inset)*; *2,* incorrect location of ligation. (From Gordon PH, Nivatvongs S, editors: *Principles and practice of surgery for the colon, rectum and anus*, ed 2, St. Louis, 1999, Quality Medical Publishing, p 28.)

PHYSIOLOGY OF THE COLON

Generally speaking, the function of the colon is the recycling of nutrients, whereas the function of the rectum is the elimination of stool. The recycling of nutrients depends on the metabolic activity of the colonic flora, colonic motility, and mucosal absorption and secretion. Stool elimination involves dehydration of colonic contents and defecation.

Recycling of Nutrients

During the digestive process, ingested nutrients are diluted within the intestinal lumen by biliopancreatic and GI secretions. The small intestine absorbs most ingested nutrients and some of the fluid and bile salts secreted into the lumen. However, the ileal effluent is still rich in water, electrolytes, and nutrients that resist digestion. The colon has the functional ability to recover these substances to avoid unnecessary losses of fluids, electrolytes, nitrogen, and energy. To accomplish this, the colon depends highly on its bacterial flora.

Colonic Flora

Nutrients are digested within the intestinal lumen with the aid of biliopancreatic and GI secretions. By the time the chyme reaches the terminal ileum, most of the nutrients have been absorbed,

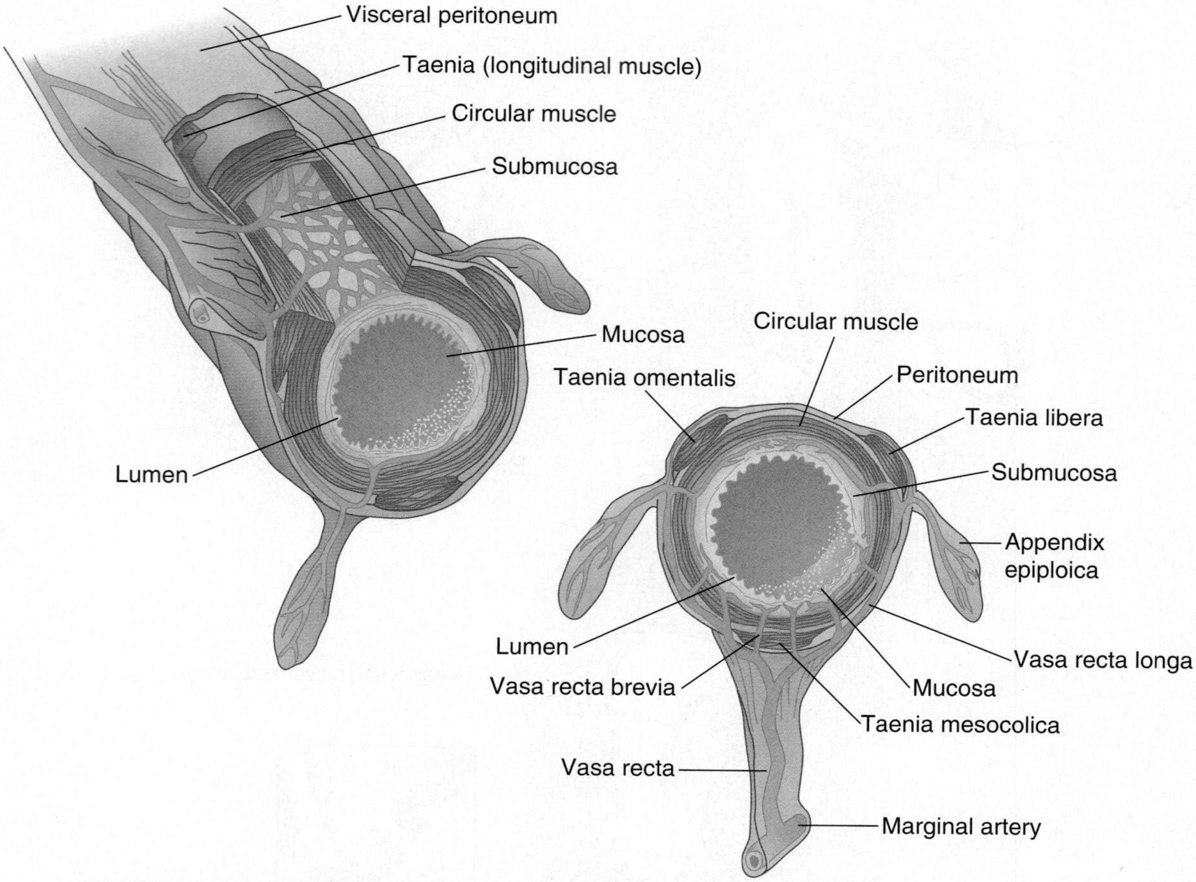

FIGURE 51-9 Cross-sectional anatomy of the colon, with vasa brevia and vasa recta. (From Gordon PH, Nivatvongs S, editors: *Principles and practice of surgery for the colon, rectum and anus*, ed 2, St. Louis, 1999, Quality Medical Publishing, p 26.)

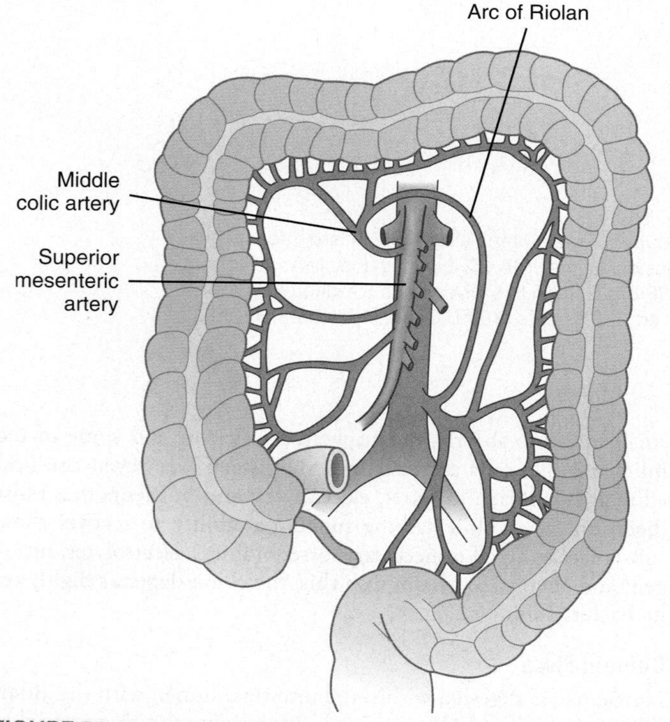

FIGURE 51-10 Arc of Riolan. (From Gordon PH, Nivatvongs S, editors: *Principles and practice of surgery for the colon, rectum and anus*, ed 2, St. Louis, 1999, Quality Medical Publishing, p 27.)

leaving a succus entericus composed of electrolyte-rich fluid, bile salts, and some proteins and starches that have resisted digestion. An enormous quantity of autochthonous flora, consisting of more than 400 bacterial species, resides in the large intestine. Large bowel contents may contain as many as 10^{11} to 10^{12} bacterial cells per gram, contributing approximately 50% of fecal mass. Most of these colonic species are anaerobes. These bacteria feed on proteins sloughed from the bowel wall and undigested complex carbohydrates.

Colonic microflora provide several important functions to the host, including barrier functions that help maintain epithelial integrity, nutritive functions that use plant polysaccharides, developmental functions that stimulate epithelial cell differentiation and angiogenesis, and, finally, immune functions through the gut. Gut-associated lymphoid tissue contributes to both innate and adaptive immunity.[1] Short-chain fatty acids (SCFAs) are produced by microbial breakdown and fermentation of dietary starches. These fatty acids are the principal source of nutrition for the colonocyte. *Bacteroides* species predominate throughout the colon, composing two thirds of the total counts of the proximal colon and almost 70% of the bacteria in the rectum. *Escherichia, Klebsiella, Proteus, Lactobacillus,* and enterococci are the predominant species of facultative anaerobes.

Prebiotics and Probiotics

Probiotics can be defined as dietary supplements that contain live cultures of bacteria and yeast that are beneficial to colonic and

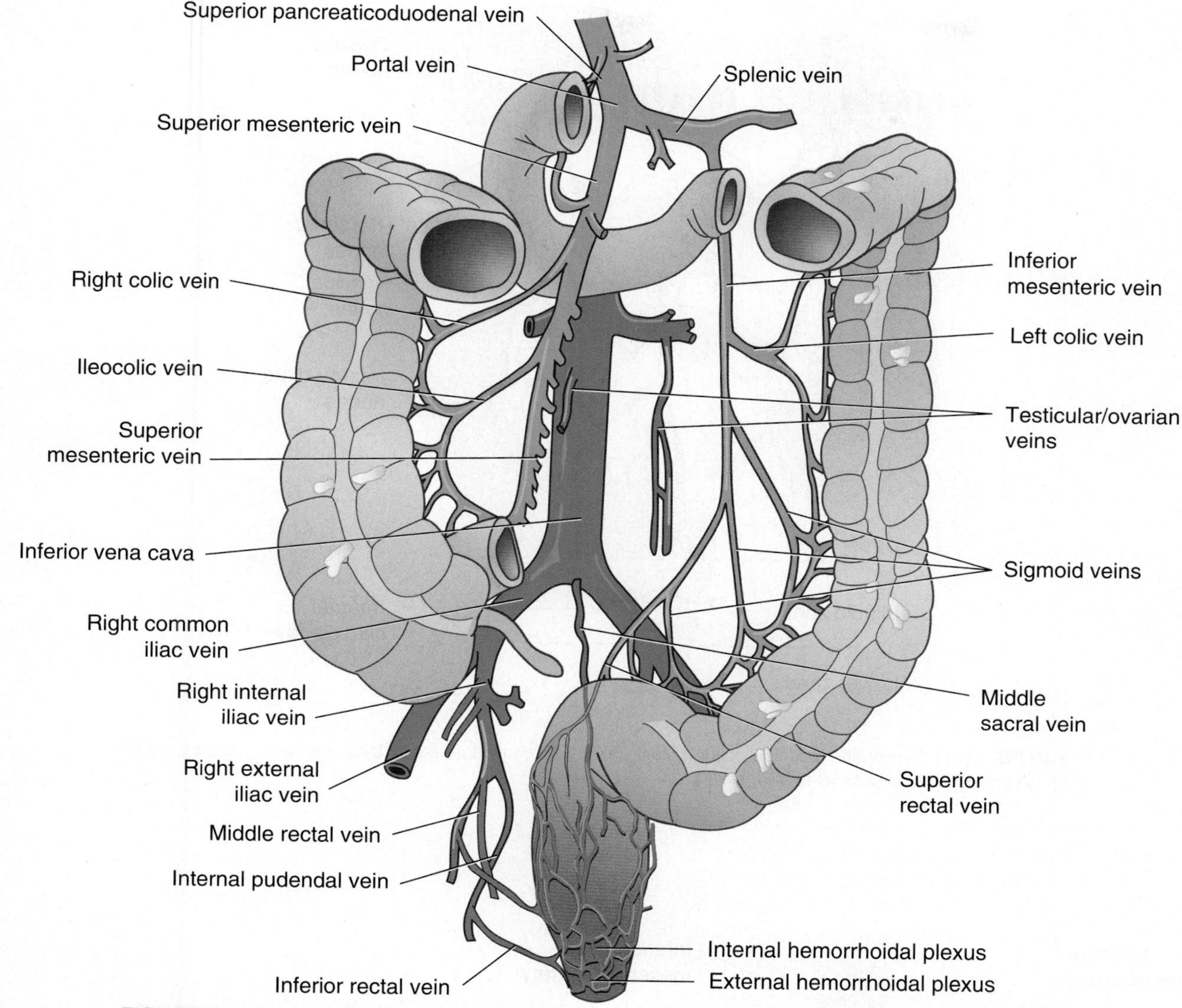

FIGURE 51-11 Venous drainage of the colon and rectum. (From Gordon PH, Nivatvongs S, editors: *Principles and practice of surgery for the colon, rectum and anus*, ed 2, St. Louis, 1999, Quality Medical Publishing, p 30.)

host function. The two most widely used agents are *Lactobacillus* and *Bifidobacterium*. Studies have indicated that probiotics may have widespread health benefits, including stimulation of immune function, anti-inflammatory effects, and suppression of enteropathogenic colonization.[2] In addition, they may increase the digestibility of dietary proteins, enhance absorption of amino acids, and play a protective or therapeutic role against *Clostridium difficile*–associated diarrhea.[3] The ultimate role of probiotics has not yet been determined. There are conflicting data in regard to whether they work more effectively as primary therapy or as prophylaxis against recurrent *C. difficile*–associated diarrhea. Indications for their use are evolving but may include necrotizing enterocolitis in neonates, patients with HIV-AIDS, and neutropenic patients undergoing chemotherapy. Further research is needed, but the evidence for probiotic use in various settings is encouraging.

Prebiotics are nondigestible oligosaccharides (e.g., inulin) that help the host by stimulating the growth of certain species of beneficial intestinal bacteria. There is a growing body of data suggesting health benefits; however, there is currently little evidence to guide recommendations for their use.

Fermentation

Unlike most of the mucosal lining of the proximal GI tract, colonic mucosa does not receive its primary nutrition from the bloodstream. Instead, nutrient requirements are fulfilled from the colonic luminal contents. The primary energy source for the colonocyte is the SCFA butyrate. The manner in which this interaction occurs illustrates the essential symbiotic interaction between the colon and its resident bacterial flora.

The main source of energy for intestinal bacteria is dietary fiber, composed of complex carbohydrates (starches and nonstarch polysaccharides [NSPs]). This fiber is metabolized by the process of fermentation. Not all complex carbohydrates are fermented in the same manner, which underlies many of the dietary recommendations for bulking agents. Lignin and psyllium are components of plants that are not fermented by human colonic flora; they are hydrophilic, thus leading to water resorption and stool

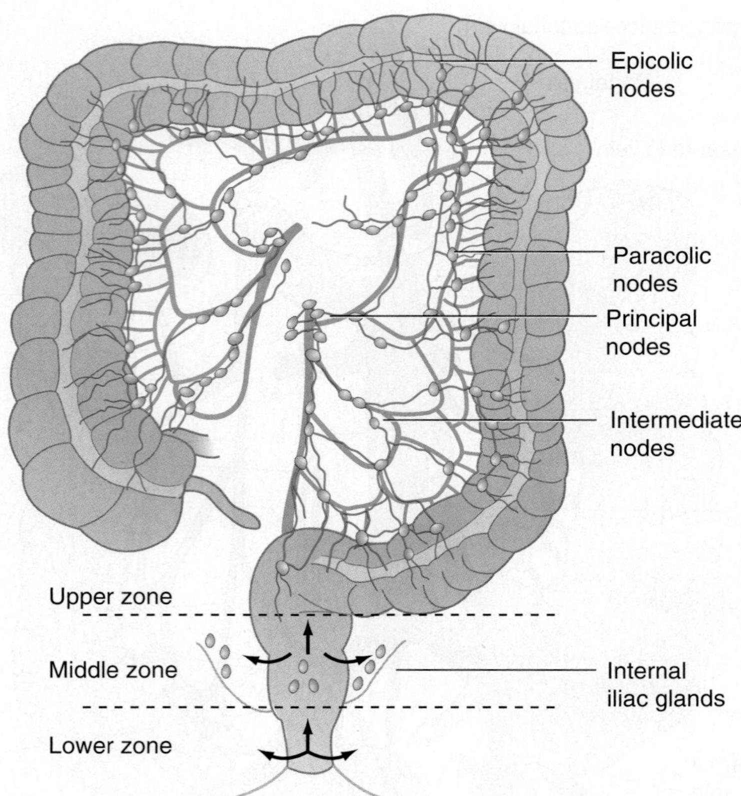

FIGURE 51-12 Lymphatic drainage of the colon. (From Corman ML, editor: *Colon and rectal surgery*, ed 4, Philadelphia,1998, Lippincott-Raven, p 21.)

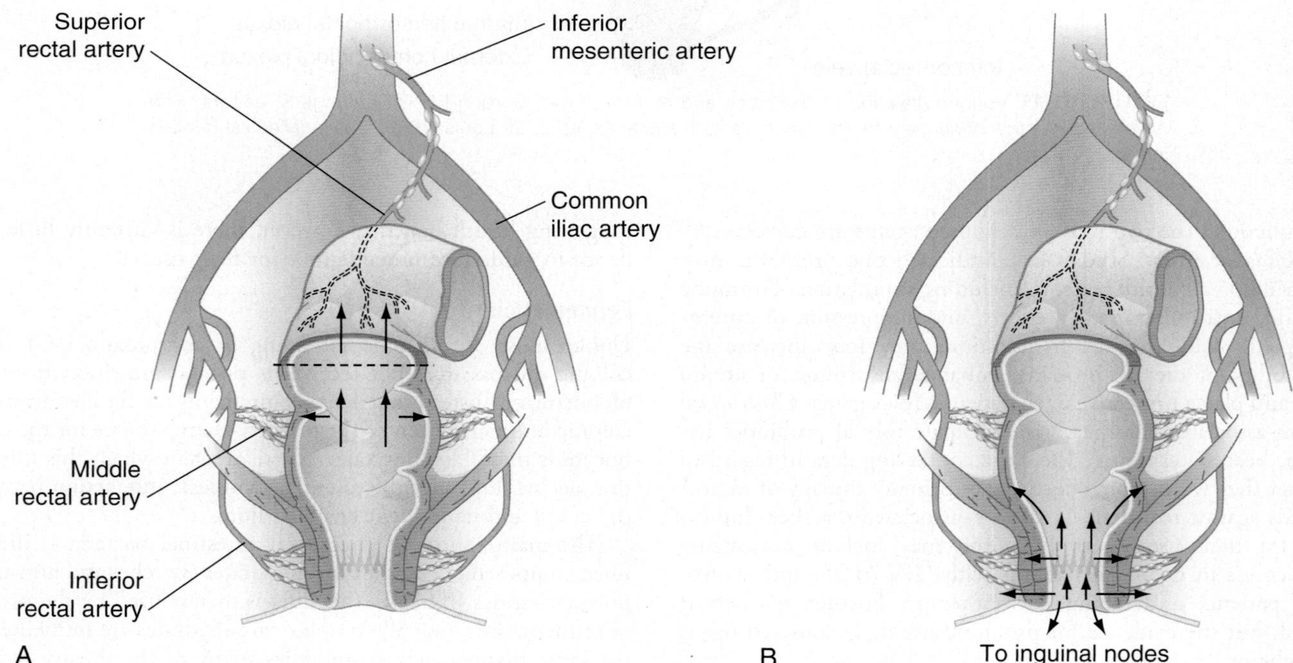

FIGURE 51-13 Lymphatic drainage of the rectum **(A)** and anal canal **(B).** (From Gordon PH, Nivatvongs S, editors: *Principles and practice of surgery for the colon, rectum and anus*, ed 2, St. Louis, 1999, Quality Medical Publishing, p 32.)

bulking. Celluloses are partially fermented, whereas fruit pectins are completely metabolized by colonic bacteria. Diets high in nonfermentable NSPs contribute to stool bulk and increased transit time; highly fermentable NSPs provide minimal bulk but enhanced colonocyte nutrition.

The end products of fermentation are SCFAs and gas—carbon dioxide, methane, and hydrogen. In addition to NSPs, colonic bacteria ferment poorly absorbed starches and proteins from the upper GI tract, known as resistant starches. Although highly variable from person to person, with daily variability dependent on diet, the gases produced by bacterial fermentation compose approximately 50% to 75% of flatus, with the remainder consisting of swallowed air.[4]

Protein fermentation, otherwise known as putrefaction, results in the formation of potentially toxic metabolites, including phenols, indoles, and amines. The production of these toxins is inhibited in many intestinal bacteria by the presence of alternative carbohydrate energy sources. This process becomes accentuated more distally in the colon as carbohydrate sources become scarcer. These deleterious end products of bacterial metabolism can lead to mucosal injury and reactive hyperproliferation, which have been hypothesized to promote carcinogenesis. Also, the presence of bulking agents decreases intracolonic pressures and may serve to prevent the formation of colonic diverticula. It can be seen, then, how providing adequate sources of various forms of dietary carbohydrates can serve positive roles in colonic health. These principles underlie the recommendations for dietary fiber, as do the evolving data on the helpful nature of probiotics and prebiotics.

Short-Chain Fatty Acids

The primary end products of bacterial fermentation are SCFAs. Absorption of SCFAs in the large intestine is efficient; only 5% to 10% is lost in the feces. The three primary fatty acids produced are acetate, propionate, and butyrate in a ratio of 3 : 1 : 1. SCFAs have key roles in colonic and also overall human metabolism. They are metabolized in three main sites: (1) colonocytes use butyrate as their primary energy source; (2) hepatocytes metabolize all three SCFAs to various degrees for use in gluconeogenesis; and (3) muscle cells oxidize acetate to generate energy. Metabolism of the SCFAs can provide up to 70% of colonocyte energy needs, reduce glucose oxidation, and spare other essential amino acids for metabolism. SCFAs also influence GI motility through the ileocolonic brake mechanism, which is defined as the inhibition of gastric emptying and nutrients reaching the ileocolonic junction.

Acetate, the principal SCFA in the colon, is primarily absorbed and transported to the liver, where it is the primary substrate for cholesterol synthesis. Nonabsorbable, nonfermentable dietary fiber, such as psyllium, may decrease the production of acetate and may have a beneficial effect on cholesterol levels. Similarly, propionate, which has a glycolytic role in the liver, may also lower serum lipid levels by inhibiting cholesterol synthesis. Butyrate is the primary energy source for colonic epithelial cells and may also play an important role in maintaining cellular health by arresting the proliferation of neoplastic colonocytes while paradoxically being trophic for normal colonocytes. In addition, butyrate serves to regulate and to stabilize cell adhesion molecules.

Urea Recycling

It was long believed that urea is the end product of nitrogen metabolism in humans. This is true in the sense that humans, and mammals in general, do not produce urease. However, colonic bacteria are rich in urease. When urea is labeled with a tracer (e.g., radioisotope, heavy isotope) and injected intravenously, 10% of the urea nitrogen is not recovered in urine but is incorporated into body protein. Bacteria firmly adherent to the colonic epithelium mediate this process of urea recycling, which produces urease. A low-protein and high-fiber diet, such as that of the Papua New Guinea highlanders, further increases urea recycling. These individuals ingest only 10 mg of protein per kilogram per day and have normal health, with normal muscle mass and serum proteins. Adaptation to this low-protein diet has made the colon efficient in recycling nitrogen to the point that it may even absorb some essential amino acids (e.g., lysine). Urea recycling has been exploited as a therapy for renal failure by excluding nonessential amino acids from the diet to promote maximal urea recycling and to diminish the need for dialysis.

However, one pathologic condition in which urea recycling is not beneficial is liver failure. When the liver cannot reuse the urea nitrogen absorbed by the colon, ammonia crosses the blood-brain barrier and produces false neurotransmitters, which results in hepatic coma.

Absorption

The total absorptive area of the colon is estimated at approximately 900 cm^2. Between 1000 and 1500 mL of fluid is poured into the cecum by the daily ileal effluent. The total volume of water in stool is only 100 to 150 mL/day. This 10-fold reduction in water across the colon represents the most efficient site of absorption in the GI tract per surface area. The net absorption of sodium is even higher. Although the ileal effluent contains 200 mEq/liter of sodium, stool contains only 25 to 50 mEq/liter. One major difference between sodium and water absorption in the colon is that although water is absorbed passively, sodium requires active transport. Sodium is transported against chemical and electrical gradients at the expense of energy consumption.

The colonic epithelium can use various fuels; however, *n*-butyrate is oxidized in preference to glutamine, glucose, or ketone bodies. Because mammalian cells do not produce *n*-butyrate, the colonic epithelium relies on luminal bacteria to produce it through the fermentation of dietary fiber. The lack of *n*-butyrate, such as that resulting from the inhibition of fermentation by broad-spectrum antibiotics, leads to less sodium and water absorption and thus diarrhea. Conversely, the perfusion of the colonic lumen with *n*-butyrate stimulates sodium and water absorption. *n*-Butyrate, acetate, and propionate are SCFAs produced through bacterial fermentation; these constitute the main anions in stool. Other physiologic effects of SCFAs on the colon include stimulation of blood flow, mucosal cell renewal, and regulation of intraluminal pH for homeostasis of the bacterial flora.

In addition to recovering sodium and water, the colonic mucosa absorbs bile acids. The colon absorbs bile acids that escape absorption by the terminal ileum, thus making the colon part of the enterohepatic circulation. Bile acids are passively transported across the colonic epithelium by nonionic diffusion. When the colonic absorptive capacity is exceeded, colonic bacteria deconjugate bile acids. Deconjugated bile acids can then interfere with sodium and water absorption, leading to secretory, or choleretic, diarrhea. Choleretic diarrhea is seen early after right hemicolectomy as a transient phenomenon and more permanently after extensive ileal resection.

Secretion

The physiologic role of colon secretion is demonstrated in patients with chronic renal failure. Uremic patients can remain normokalemic while ingesting a normal amount of potassium before requiring dialysis. This phenomenon is associated with a compensatory increase in colonic secretion and fecal excretion of potassium. This effect is blocked by spironolactone, which illustrates the effect of aldosterone on colonic potassium secretion. Potassium secretion requires both Na^+,K^+-ATPase and Na^+-K^+-$2Cl^-$ cotransport on the basolateral membrane and an apical potassium channel.

Many forms of colitis are associated with increased potassium secretion, such as inflammatory bowel disease (IBD), cholera, and shigellosis. In addition, some forms of colitis impair colonic absorption or produce secretion of chloride, such as collagenous and microscopic colitis and congenital chloridorrhea. Chloride is secreted by colonic epithelium at a basal rate, which is increased in pathologic conditions such as cystic fibrosis and secretory diarrhea. Secretion of chloride also requires the coupling of Na^+,K^+-ATPase and Na^+-K^+-$2Cl^-$ cotransport to exit passively through the apical membrane. Calcium and cyclic adenosine monophosphate both stimulate chloride secretion, whereas bicarbonate and SCFAs inhibit chloride secretion.

Colonic secretion of H^+ and bicarbonate is coupled to the absorption of Na^+ and Cl^-, respectively. It is through these exchangers that the colon is linked to systemic acid-base metabolism. The supply of H^+ and bicarbonate for these exchangers is maintained by the hydration of CO_2, catalyzed by colonic carbonic anhydrase. Changes in systemic pH induce changes in the activity of carbonic anhydrase, eliciting elimination of H^+ or bicarbonate as needed to bring the systemic pH back to normal.

Motility

Colonic motility is a highly complex process, made difficult to investigate by a lack of standardized terminology and measurements. In addition, movement through the colon is relatively slow compared with the proximal GI tract, and studies require prolonged observation.

Colonic motility patterns may be more simply divided into two primary patterns, segmental activity and propagated activity. Segmental activity consists of single contractions or rhythmic bursts of contractions. The purpose of these segmental contractions is to propel fecal matter distally through a directed pressure gradient toward the rectum in discrete distances and to allow mixing, which promotes optimal absorption. The second pattern is propagated activity, commonly classified on the basis of amplitude as low-amplitude or high-amplitude propagated contractions. High-amplitude propagated contractions have been historically referred to as mass movements, or migrating motor complexes, whose role is shifting large quantities of contents through the colon. These have an important role in defecation, with mass movements propelling larger volumes of fecal matter to the distal colon and emptying of the descending colon into the sigmoid colon and rectum. Little is known about low-amplitude propagated contractions, but they are associated with distention of the viscus and passage of flatus.[5]

There seems to be a circadian rhythm to colonic motility, with maximum peaks of activity immediately after waking and after meals. Sleep is associated with a decrease in colonic motility.

Not surprisingly, food ingestion results in an increase of overall colonic motility for approximately 2 hours. This reflex is stimulated not only by gastric distention but also by the central nervous system, initiated by visualization of food. In addition, meal composition affects colonic responses. Increased activity in response to carbohydrate meals is fairly short-lived, whereas fatty meals elicit longer term responses.

Ultimately, transit in the colon is controlled by the autonomic nervous system. Parasympathetic innervation reaches the colon through the vagus and pelvic nerves. The enteric nervous system in the colon is arranged in several plexuses—subserosal, myenteric (Auerbach), submucosal (Meissner), and mucosal plexuses. Sympathetic innervation originates in the superior and inferior mesenteric ganglia and reaches the colon through perivascular plexuses.

Formation of Stool

The frequency of defecation is just as variable among individuals as is their perception of abnormal stool frequency. An individual who passes more than three loose stools daily is considered to have diarrhea, whereas fewer than three weekly stools is considered constipation. Any frequency within that range is considered normal, although many individuals will still seek medical attention for what they perceive as diarrhea or constipation. Many factors influence colonic transit rate. Colonic transit is longer in women than in men and longer in premenopausal than in postmenopausal women. Conversely, colonic transit time is shortened in smokers. In normal subjects, supplementation with NSPs does not shorten colonic transit time, although it does increase fecal weight. In patients with idiopathic constipation, however, NSPs, in the form of psyllium seeds, shorten colonic transit time and increase stool weight.

Defecation

Normal defecation requires adequate colonic transit time, stool consistency, and fecal continence. Fecal continence implies deferment of stool elimination; discrimination among gas, liquid, and solid stool; and selective elimination of gas without stool. There is some controversy about the actual role of the rectum under resting conditions. Some have proposed that the rectum is simply a conduit, which under resting conditions should be empty. If stool arrives at the rectum, the anorectal inhibitory reflex is triggered, forcing the subject to hold defecation by voluntary contraction of the external sphincter. However, any surgeon who performs routine rigid proctosigmoidoscopies in the office is well aware that a patient can have a rectum full of stool without any awareness. This leads to the opposing view, which regards the rectum as a reservoir. Just as stool triggers the anorectal inhibitory reflex, it also triggers a rectocolic reflex. This reflex allows continuous filling of the rectum with fecal material until the colon is emptied.

The mechanisms involved in fecal continence are not fully understood. A certain reservoir capacity is needed to achieve fecal continence. A stiff nondistensible rectum, such as in radiation proctitis, may produce incontinence, even when the sphincter muscles are competent. Some of the internal and external sphincter muscle fibers are necessary for adequate continence, although many patients have part of the sphincter severed during a fistulotomy and are still continent. Probably the only factor needed for fecal continence is innervation of the sphincter. The motor nerve fibers, which produce contraction of the sphincter fibers, and also all the sensory innervation are important to empty the rectum adequately.

PREOPERATIVE WORKUP AND STOMA PLANNING

Today, routine preoperative testing guidelines exist to streamline the process to elective surgery. They are dependent on the planned procedure, the patient's comorbidities, and the American Society of Anesthesiologists class of the patient. Detailed description of preoperative management and workup for surgical patients is discussed elsewhere. However, additional preoperative evaluation specific to major colon and rectal procedures may also include the following considerations:

- Evaluation of nutritional status
- Use of a preoperative mechanical bowel preparation (MBP) or oral antibiotics
- Preoperative counseling for stoma care, education, and marking
- Colonoscopy to exclude synchronous lesions
- Postoperative fluid and pain management

Nutritional Assessment

Preoperative malnutrition is an important predictor of poor clinical outcomes in patients undergoing major colorectal operations. The additional stress of a major abdominal surgery further induces a catabolic response and insulin resistance. Therefore, nutritional parameters for chronically ill patients and especially those with IBD should be assessed before consideration for elective surgery. Serum albumin is an indicator of long-term nutrition (21 days), whereas serum prealbumin can gauge short-term nutritional status (3 to 5 days). Low preoperative albumin (<3.5 g/dL) has been further shown to be a risk factor for anastomotic leak after colorectal surgery. These two indices may also identify patients who may benefit from preoperative supplemental nutrition, such as total parenteral nutrition. The decision to initiate total parenteral nutrition should also be judicious because of its known albeit low association with infectious complications. Nonetheless, elective operations should be delayed if possible until the patient is nutritionally replete.

Preoperative Bowel Preparation

Purging the feces and reducing the concentration of colonic intraluminal bacteria before operations on the colon is a practice that has been challenged in recent years. The normal, or autochthonous, microbial organisms in the colon compose up to 90% of the dry weight of feces, reaching concentrations of up to 10^9 organisms/mL of feces. The anaerobic *Bacteroides* is the most common colonic microbe, whereas *Escherichia coli* is the most common aerobe. *Pseudomonas, Enterococcus, Proteus, Klebsiella,* and *Streptococcus* spp. are also present in large numbers.

The process of preparing the colon for an elective operation has traditionally involved two factors, purging of the fecal contents (mechanical preparation) and administration of antibiotics effective against colonic bacteria. Tradition has held that an unprepared colon (i.e., one that contains intraluminal feces) poses an unacceptably high rate of failure of the anastomosis to heal. However, experience with primary repair of traumatic colonic injuries, along with reports from Europe describing elective operations conducted safely without the use of preoperative purging, has led to reconsideration of the true value of purging the colon before colonic surgery. Because the colonocytes receive nutrition from intraluminal free fatty acids produced by fermentation from colonic bacteria, there are concerns that purging may actually be detrimental to healing of a colonic anastomosis. In the United States at present, the addition of a preoperative MBP with or without oral antibiotics is controversial and is left to the surgeon's discretion. Nonetheless, a variety of MBP regimens and antibiotic combinations are in current use. A clear superiority of one over another has not been found; however, for some patients, certain bowel preparations may have adverse physiologic consequences. Knowledge of the history of bowel preparation practices, current controversies, and data is useful.

Complete bowel obstruction and free perforation are absolute contraindications to bowel preparation. For colonoscopy, properties of preparations are judged by safety, tolerance of the patient, and efficacy or preparation quality. In the past, 4 to 5 days of clear liquids along with laxatives (such as senna, castor oil, and bisacodyl), whole bowel nasogastric irrigation, mannitol irrigation, and repeated enemas were among the regimens used. Tolerance of patients of these methods is poor; they are associated with dehydration, electrolyte abnormalities, and severe abdominal cramping and are generally not well tolerated by older or infirm patients.

In the 1980s, polyethylene glycol–electrolyte solution, a nonabsorbed, sodium sulfate–based liquid, was developed as an oral MBP. Patients are required to drink at least 2 to 4 liters of the solution, along with additional fluids. Abdominal cramping, nausea, and vomiting are common side effects of the preparation, and prophylactic antiemetics are often administered routinely. In the 1990s, oral sodium phosphate solutions and pills were developed in response to dissatisfaction of patients with the large fluid volume required for polyethylene glycol preparation, and these preparations have been found in most trials to be more tolerable, with higher rates of satisfaction and compliance of patients. Sodium phosphate, in liquid or pill form, has been linked more frequently than polyethylene glycol to rare but serious electrolyte imbalances. In patients with impaired renal function, hyperphosphatemia, hypernatremia, hypokalemia, and hypocalcemia can occur. In response to concerns about toxicity, the Food and Drug Administration removed oral sodium phosphate bowel preparations from the market in 2008; however, they are still available as over-the-counter medications in other countries. Thus, polyethylene glycol–electrolyte solution is the recommended bowel preparation in patients with renal insufficiency, cirrhosis, ascites, or congestive heart failure as well as physiologically in normal patients. Ultimately, comfort of the patient and economic factors may determine MBP practices if the efficacy is similar. Patients favor preparations that are low in volume, are palatable, have easy to complete regimens, and are either reimbursed by health insurance or are inexpensive. Physicians are advised to select a preparation that is safe to administer in light of existing comorbid conditions and those preparations that will not interact with previously prescribed medications. The ideal bowel preparation has to balance the intraoperative expectations of the surgeon with the safety profile and comfort of the patient.

For patients undergoing colonoscopy, the quality of the bowel preparation is essential for performing an accurate examination. However, for patients undergoing surgical resection, the necessity of mechanical bowel preparation has been questioned. In a 2011 update to the initial Cochrane review from 2005, Guenaga and colleagues evaluated 13 randomized controlled studies that compared MBP versus no preparation during elective colorectal surgery while looking at the primary outcome of anastomotic leakage.[6] The overall anastomotic leakage rate was 4.4% in the group with MBP (101 of 2275 participants) compared with 4.5% in the group without MBP (103 of 2258 participants) and was not statistically significant. Before conclusions are drawn, it is important to note that although the goals of many of these studies appear the same, there is significant heterogeneity in their methodology. There is significant variability among the populations of patients, and more pertinent prognostic factors for anastomotic leakage may include the indications for surgery, the patient's comorbidities and acuity, the surgeon's experience, the surgical technique, and the location of intestinal anastomosis.

Antibiotic use in colorectal surgery is a well-established practice that reduces infectious complications. Elective colorectal cases are classified as clean contaminated and, as such, benefit from routine single-dose administration of parenteral antibiotics 30 minutes before an incision to reduce rates of superficial and deep wound infection. It has been shown that when operative times are prolonged, additional doses at 4-hour intervals are required. When the operation is completed, postoperative administration of antibiotics for a clean contaminated case, such as a routine segmental resection, does not reduce infectious complications further and may promote *C. difficile* colitis, *Candida* infection, and the emergence of bacterial antibiotic resistance. Polk and Lopez-Mayer showed a reduction in postoperative infection rates from 30% to 8% with the routine use of preoperative parenteral antibiotics. Gomez-Alonzo and colleagues repeated these results, showing a decrease from 39% to 9%. Antibiotics active against both aerobes and anaerobes are ideal; a second- or third-generation cephalosporin alone or a combination of a fluoroquinolone plus metronidazole or clindamycin is typical.

The efforts to reduce surgical site infections (SSIs) have recently included the implementation of the Surgical Care Improvement Project guidelines and the push to incorporate standardized prophylactic parenteral antibiotic measures. The correct and timely administration of antibiotics has now become a performance measure for quality improvement projects nationwide. The role of appropriate parenteral antibiotics before incision is well established in reducing SSI. However, the role of oral antibiotics in conjunction with preoperative mechanical bowel preparation has been recently questioned. Despite the current trends among surgeons to omit oral nonabsorbable antibiotics, the data suggest that this omission may be premature. The use of additional oral antibiotics, theoretically to reduce the bacterial load further, is widely accepted but not as well validated. In a survey of colon and rectal surgeons, 87% indicated that both oral and parenteral antibiotic use is part of their routine preparation for elective colon operations. A typical preparation consists of erythromycin base (1 g) and neomycin (1 g) given in three preoperative doses the day before surgery. However, this regimen is associated with a high incidence of nausea and abdominal cramps, and some surgeons prefer to prescribe oral ciprofloxacin or metronidazole.

In a 2002 meta-analysis by Lewis (N = 215), the study showed a significant reduction in SSIs for patients with MBP plus oral antibiotics (from 17% to 5%); all patients received a standard preoperative parenteral antibiotic regimen.[7] Similarly, a 2012 retrospective study conducted by Cannon and colleagues showed a 57% decrease in SSIs when MBP and oral antibiotics were used in elective colon resections (N = 9940).[8] These results were echoed by Bellows and colleagues, who showed in their 2011 meta-analysis that the combination of oral antibiotics and MBP reduced the incidence of SSI after colorectal surgery by 43% compared with parenteral antibiotics alone. In 2011, the Michigan Surgical Quality Collaborative evaluated 2011 elective colectomies performed during 16 months; MBP without oral antibiotics was administered to 49.6% of patients, whereas 36.4% received MBP and oral antibiotics. In this large, well-designed study, patients receiving oral antibiotics were significantly less likely to have any SSI (4.5% versus 11.8%; $P = .0001$), to have an organ space infection (1.8% versus 4.2%; $P = .044$), or to have a superficial SSI (2.6% versus 7.6%; $P = .001$). Interestingly, they also found that patients receiving bowel preparation with oral antibiotics were also less likely to have a prolonged ileus (3.9% versus 8.6%; $P = .011$) and had similar rates of *C. difficile* colitis (1.3% versus 1.8%; $P = .58$).[5] Thus, it seems there are reliable data supporting the use of oral antibiotics as an adjunct to a preoperative MBP as a means of reducing postoperative SSI.

Planning Intestinal Stomas

The techniques of fashioning a stoma have been developed to provide diversion of waste until conditions are attained that permit the restoration of normal intestinal continuity. If it is anticipated that the creation of a stoma will be part of an operation, appropriate preparations should be made to optimize the outcome of the procedure. Preoperative consultation with an enterostomal therapist is helpful in most circumstances. This consultation provides the opportunity for education, counseling, and appropriate stoma site selection and marking. Such preparation significantly increases the patient's satisfaction and quality of life scores of patients who require permanent or temporary stomas.[9]

The preferred location of a stoma should be in an area of the anterior abdominal wall where there are no creases that could prohibit the satisfactory seal of the appliance to the peristomal skin. The stoma should be visible to the patient—not on the underside of a large pannus in an obese individual—and easily accessible. Most surgeons think that it is desirable to bring the stoma through the rectus muscle, traversing an appropriately sized aperture (2 cm) that does not constrict the blood supply to the stoma but does not result in a peristomal hernia. In a normal-sized patient, the preferred site for stoma location is through the rectus muscle, slightly inferior to the umbilicus at the apex of the naturally occurring tissue mound of the abdomen (Fig. 51-14).

Stoma Types

A colostomy is an anastomosis fashioned between the colon and skin of the abdominal wall. Colostomies may be temporary or permanent, depending on the disease and conditions for which they are created. However, appropriate planning and careful

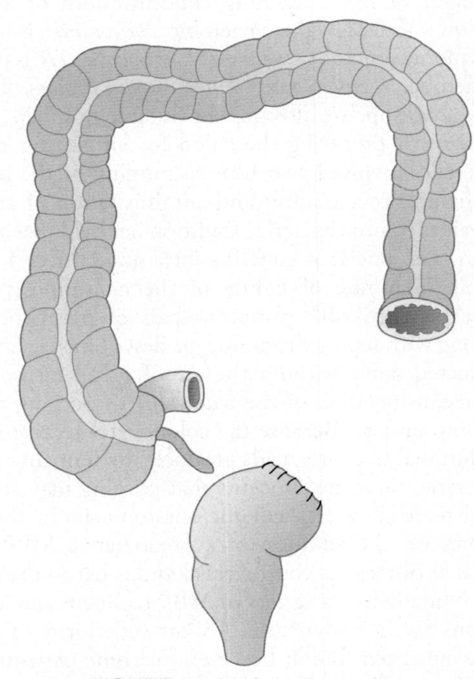

FIGURE 51-14 Selecting a site.

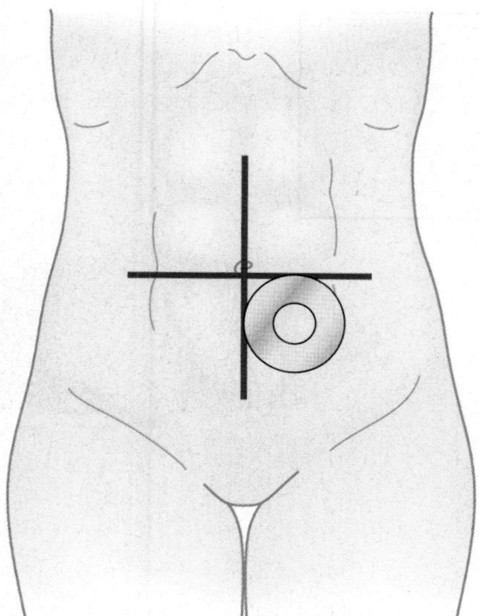

FIGURE 51-15 Hartmann operation.

technical considerations should be given to the creation of any colostomy because history has shown that even colostomies intended to be temporary may prove to be permanent in a significant number of patients.[10]

A colostomy may be indicated to divert colonic contents temporarily from a pathologic process in the distal colon or rectum, such as an obstructing rectal cancer or phlegmon of the sigmoid colon associated with diverticulitis. A loop colostomy using the sigmoid or the transverse colon can be useful for this, expedient, and able to be completed laparoscopically. Other circumstances are more appropriately treated by an end colostomy, in which the end of the sigmoid or, more commonly, descending colon is brought out the abdominal wall. An end colostomy is an essential component of an abdominal perineal proctectomy performed for rectal cancer. Resection of the sigmoid colon with closure of the rectal stump and fashioning of a descending colon is usually referred to as a Hartmann operation (Fig. 51-15). An ileostomy is the union of the terminal ileum to the skin of the abdominal wall. As described for colostomy, an ileostomy may also be fashioned as a loop or an end stoma. A temporary loop ileostomy may be fashioned to protect a distal anastomosis, such as a coloanal anastomosis in a patient who has received preoperative chemoradiation for rectal cancer, or to protect an ileal pouch–anal anastomosis (IPAA) in a patient treated with restorative proctocolectomy for ulcerative colitis. An end ileostomy is required if the colon and rectum must be removed and the anal sphincter cannot be preserved.

Physiologic Considerations and Practical Implications

Colostomy

For practical purposes, the dominant physiologic properties of the proximal colon are the completion of digestion of complex carbohydrates by fermentation, retention of electrolytes, and absorption of water. The more distal colon participates to less of an extent in these processes and serves as a reservoir for the waste products of digestion pending elimination. In some cases, the collateral communication through the marginal artery is not sufficient to sustain the sigmoid colon, so it is generally preferred to fashion a distal colostomy from the descending colon, which has a more reliable blood supply than the sigmoid colon (especially if the IMA has been divided). In addition, the sigmoid colon is often afflicted with diverticulosis and the thickening of the colonic wall associated with that disease process, so the more pliable and capacious descending colon is the preferred choice for a left-sided colostomy.

The more proximal the site of the colon that is selected to fashion a colostomy, the more likely it is that the effluent will be liquid and foul-smelling. Descending colostomies that pass formed feces are relatively easy to care for with a well-fitting enterostomal appliance, whereas transverse colostomies that expel significant amounts of feculent liquid are difficult to care for and frequently leak and prolapse. Colostomies from the right colon are particularly troublesome because there is a copious amount of liquid foul-smelling effluent that is difficult to contain with an appliance. In addition, the motility characteristics of the colon are such that the more proximal the site of the colon selected to fashion a colostomy, the higher is the likelihood of prolapse through the stoma. This is distressing to the patient and makes maintenance of the stoma exceedingly difficult. As a general rule, with modern enterostomal techniques, it is much easier to care for an ileostomy than to care for a wet colostomy or a colostomy fashioned from the proximal colon.

Transverse colostomies, although at times useful to protect a distal anastomosis or to divert colonic contents from a distal obstruction, should almost always be considered a temporary diversion to a transient problem. A transverse loop colostomy fashioned at skin level will completely divert the fecal stream for a period of at least 6 weeks, but with the passage of time and the natural maturation of the colostomy, the spur, or posterior wall of the colostomy, will retract and the stoma will no longer divert completely. In addition, the incidence of significant prolapse from a transverse loop colostomy is high and increases over time. It is usually (but not always) the distal limb of the loop colostomy that prolapses through the stoma site.

Ileostomy

The terminal ileum normally delivers up to 2 liters of succus entericus to the cecum during a 24-hour period. There is a remarkable adaptation following the construction of a stoma from the very distal ileum in that after several weeks, the absorptive capacity of the ileum increases to the extent that approximately 900 mL of effluent will be expected to be produced by the ileum during a 24-hour period. However, the intestinal adaptation cannot completely compensate for the loss of the absorptive capacity of the colon, and ileostomy patients need to recognize the need to increase their intake of fluid. Supplemental sodium chloride may often be necessary for ileostomates, although liberal addition of salt to the daily diet usually will suffice.

The ileal chyme is liquid and contains digestive substances that are normally inactivated in the colon. If the skin adjacent to the ileostomy is exposed to the effluent, significant erosion of the peristomal skin can occur. Therefore, the ileostomy is fashioned to protrude above the skin surface as a spigot that pours the ileal contents into an enterostomal appliance fitted to the abdominal skin at the base of the ileostomy to protect the skin from the corrosive properties of the ileal effluent.

Technical Considerations

End Descending Colostomy

As noted, it is generally preferable to use the descending colon, rather than the sigmoid colon, for the creation of a colostomy.

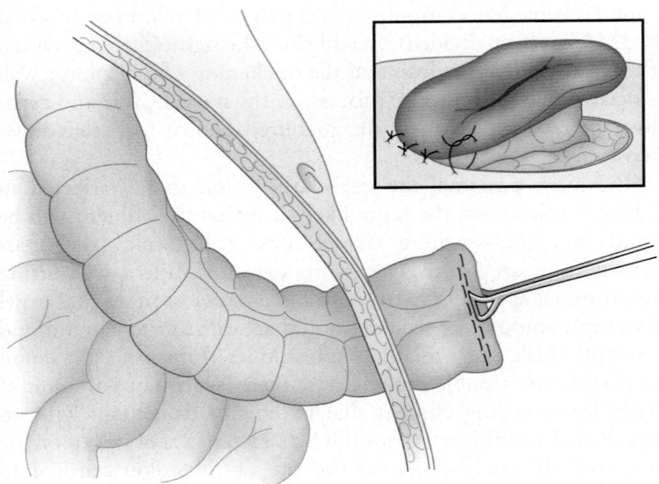

FIGURE 51-16 End colostomy.

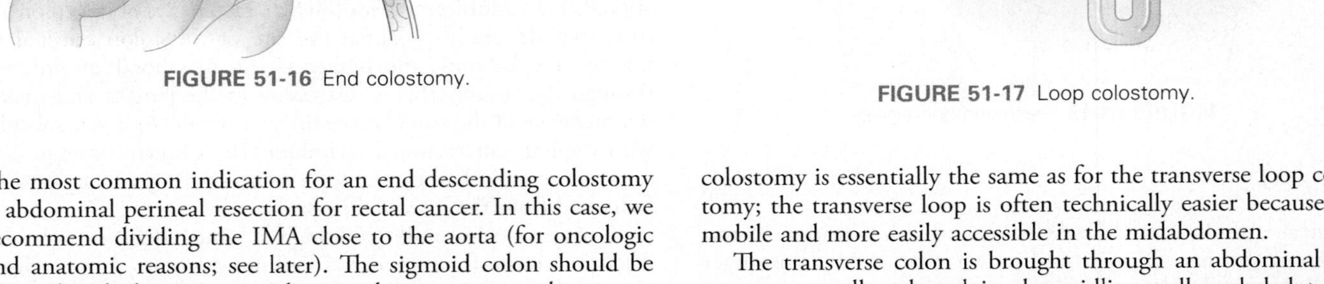

FIGURE 51-17 Loop colostomy.

The most common indication for an end descending colostomy is abdominal perineal resection for rectal cancer. In this case, we recommend dividing the IMA close to the aorta (for oncologic and anatomic reasons; see later). The sigmoid colon should be resected with the rectum, with care taken to preserve the mesentery to the descending colon. The blood supply to the descending colon will be maintained through the collateral circulation from the marginal artery, and this collateral circulation is better maintained by dividing the IMA close to its origin. The colon is then mobilized from the posterior abdominal wall and the prerenal (Gerota) fascia in such a manner that the entire descending colon and its mesentery lie anterior to the small bowel (Fig. 51-16). With use of this technique, there is no remaining lateral attachment of the colonic mesentery for the small intestine to twist around, and it is not necessary to approximate the mesentery of the descending colon to the lateral peritoneum to prevent an internal hernia.

The closed end of the descending colon is brought through an abdominal wall aperture created through the left rectus muscle at the site selected and marked before the operation. The colostomy is matured by approximating the wall of the colon to the skin with interrupted absorbable sutures. Some surgeons place the sutures in such a fashion to elevate the colostomy above skin level slightly, but this is not necessary with a descending colon because the effluent is formed and noncorrosive, and maintaining an appliance does not require eversion of the stoma.

Loop Colostomy

A loop colostomy may provide diversion from a distal obstruction (e.g., rectal cancer, diverticulitis) while simultaneously decompressing the limb of the colon leading to the obstruction. The most commonly performed type of loop colostomy is the transverse loop colostomy, but as noted, this stoma has the disadvantages of liquid effluent, eventual prolapse, and only temporary complete diversion. Although a loop transverse colostomy is certainly indicated in certain circumstances, consideration should be given to a loop ileostomy or loop descending colostomy. The loop ileostomy is easier to care for and to maintain an appliance, and the effluent of the loop descending colostomy is thicker, with less fluid loss and less chance of prolapse of the more distally placed colostomy. The technique of fashioning the descending loop colostomy is essentially the same as for the transverse loop colostomy; the transverse loop is often technically easier because it is mobile and more easily accessible in the midabdomen.

The transverse colon is brought through an abdominal wall aperture, usually selected in the midline well cephalad to the umbilicus and well above a midline incision if the operation is conducted through such an incision. The exteriorized loop of colon is supported over a plastic stoma rod (Fig. 51-17). The antimesenteric surface of the colon is incised in a longitudinal incision, and the edges of the resulting colostomy are sutured to the skin of the abdominal wall with absorbable sutures. The supporting rod is removed after the fifth postoperative day. This stoma will provide complete diversion of the feces and gas from the proximal colon while simultaneously venting the distal colon. However, after a period of approximately 6 weeks, the posterior wall of the stoma (spur) will retract, and feces from the proximal colon can spill over into the distal limb.

Ileostomy

In forming an ileostomy, the ileum is brought through the abdominal wall at a site selected before the operation to ensure that the location is ideal for maintaining the seal of an appliance (i.e., away from natural abdominal wall creases, scars, hernias). A disc of skin is excised, the dissection is carried longitudinally through the center of the rectus muscle, and the posterior fascia is divided (Fig. 51-18). The abdominal wall aperture should be approximately 2.5 cm in diameter, thus admitting two fingers (Fig. 51-19). Sufficient length of well-vascularized ileum is brought through the abdominal wall to permit creation of a spigot that will protrude well above skin level (Brooke configuration), allowing the ileal contents to pour into an appliance sealed to the adjacent skin (Fig. 51-20). The ileostomy is completed by approximating the full thickness of the divided wall of the ileum to the subcuticular tissue of the abdominal skin of the stoma site, placing sutures in so as to maintain the everted configuration of the stoma (Figs. 51-21 and 51-22).

By use of these same principles, a loop ileostomy may be fashioned (Figs. 51-23 and 51-24). The loop ileostomy can be fashioned over an ileostomy rod, but a rod is not necessary to maintain the configuration of the stoma. Some surgeons prefer not to use a supporting rod because it may interfere with maintaining the

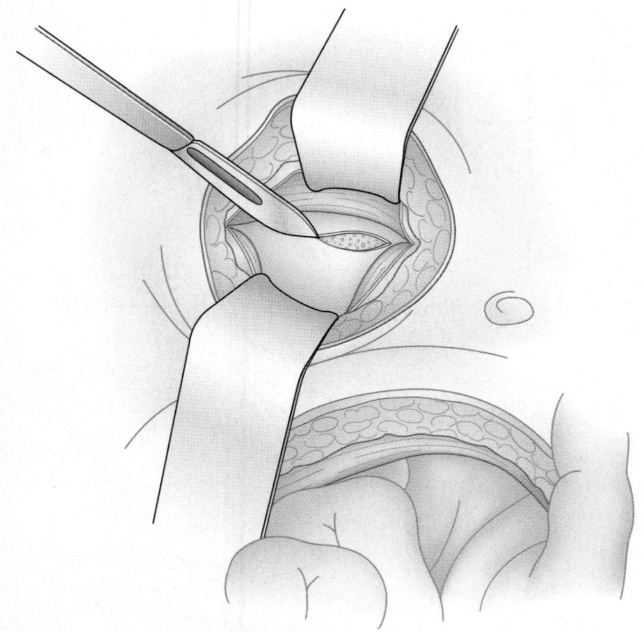

FIGURE 51-18 Dividing fascia for ileostomy.

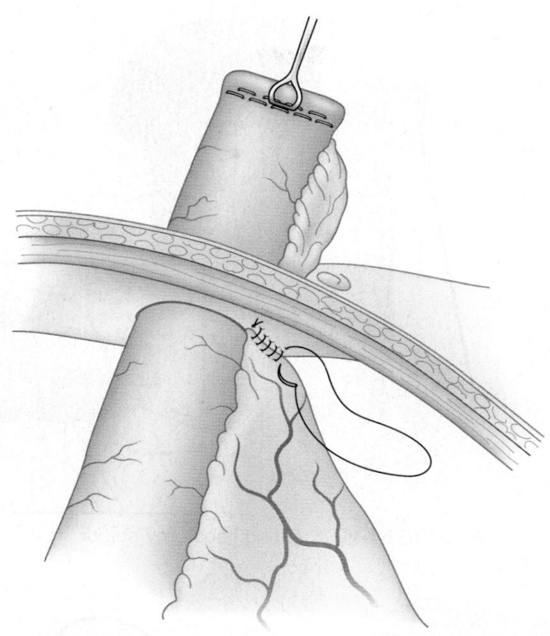

FIGURE 51-20 Ileum brought through aperture.

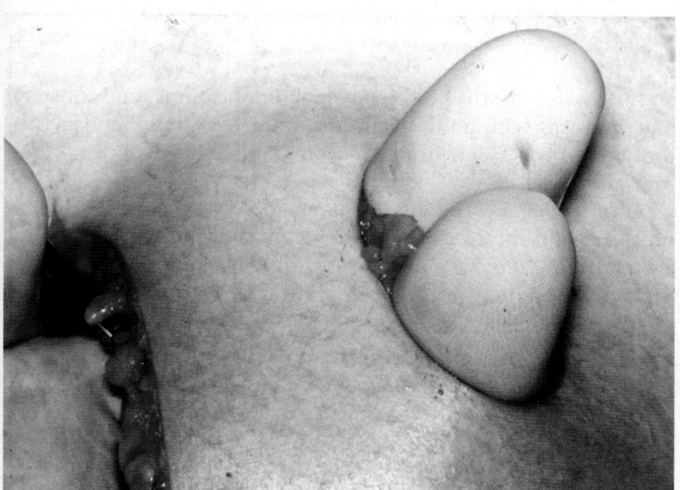

FIGURE 51-19 Aperture for ileostomy.

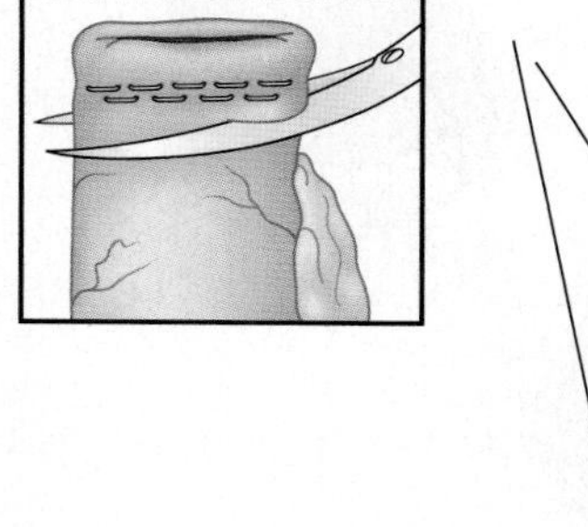

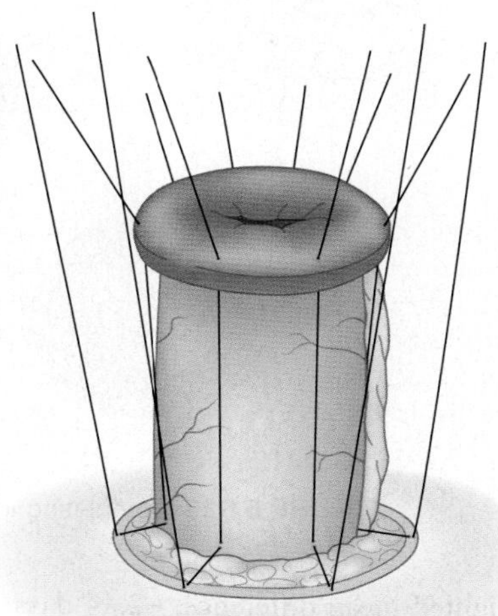

FIGURE 51-21 Maturing ileostomy.

seal of the appliance. If an ileostomy rod is used, it can be removed on the fifth postoperative day.

Postoperative Management Protocols

Major colon and rectal procedures are commonly performed in the United States, and therefore the postoperative management of these patients has come under scrutiny with the focus on decreasing morbidity, mortality, and health care cost. Evidence-based studies have now generated standardized fast-track protocols or enhanced recovery pathways to streamline the postoperative management of these patients, to limit complications, and to limit length of stay by enhancing early recovery of bowel function. These protocols include several of the following key elements:

- Appropriate selection of patients
- Minimally invasive surgery
- Perioperative fluid management
- Early enteric feeding
- Early ambulation
- Multimodality postoperative analgesia

Patients selected for inclusion in enhanced recovery pathways should understand the goals of the protocol and be able to physiologically tolerate reduced fluids and narcotics. Even so, participation in some but not all of the elements of an enhanced recovery pathway may still confer benefit. The cornerstones of the concept include intraoperative and postoperative fluid restriction as well as limitation of opiates and use of alternative pain control strategies. Acetaminophen, nonsteroidal anti-inflammatory drugs, gabapentin, and use of epidurals and cutaneous analgesic approaches have all been incorporated into various enhanced recovery protocols.

In a comprehensive meta-analysis, 13 randomized controlled studies (1910 patients) were analyzed, and in comparison with traditional care, enhanced recovery after surgery programs were associated with significantly decreased primary hospital stay

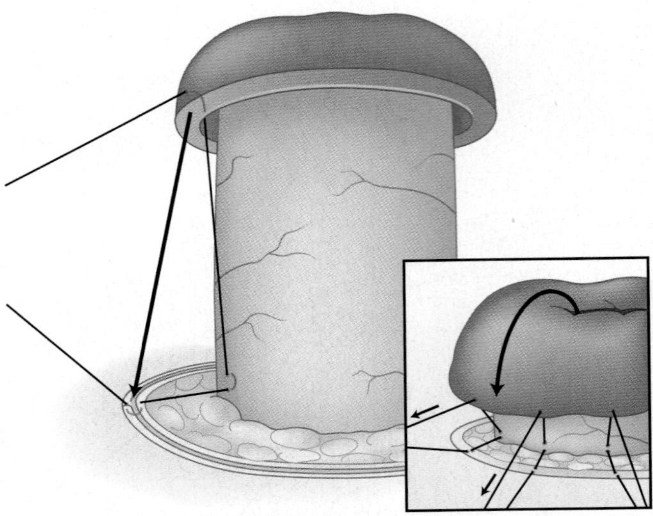

FIGURE 51-22 Creating ileostomy spigot.

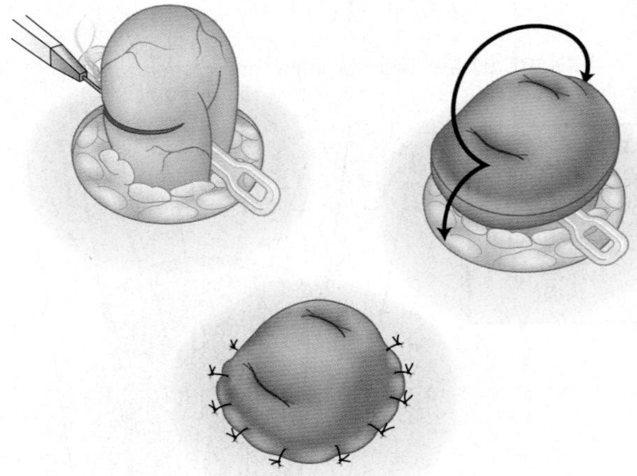

FIGURE 51-23 Completing loop ileostomy.

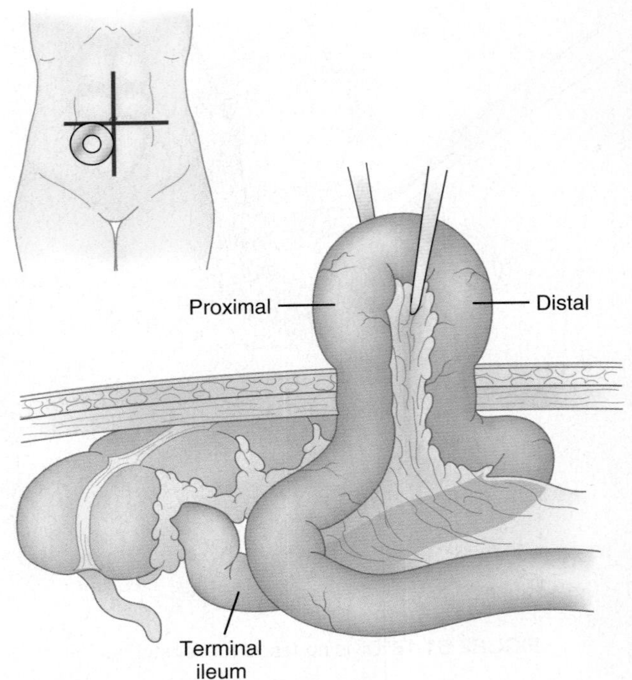

FIGURE 51-24 Loop ileostomy in continuity.

(weighted mean difference, −2.44 days; 95% confidence interval [CI], −3.06 to −1.83 days; $P < .00001$), total hospital stay (weighted mean difference, −2.39 days; 95% CI, −3.70 to −1.09 days; $P = .0003$), total complications (relative risk, 0.71; 95% CI, 0.58-0.86; $P = .0006$), and general complications (relative risk, 0.68; 95% CI, 0.56-0.82; $P < .0001$).[11] No significant differences were found for readmission rates, surgical complications, and mortality. However, despite these favorable initial results, protocols for enhanced recovery after surgery have not been widely implemented. This is not unexpected as most protocols incorporate 8 to 20 elements and require the persistence and involvement of a multidisciplinary team of surgeons, anesthesiologist, nurses, stoma therapist, and hospital administration.

More recent adjuncts to the postoperative management in major colon and rectal surgery include the abandonment of nasogastric tubes and administration of early enteral feeding. A Cochrane review in 2007 revealed that patients without a nasogastric tube after undergoing lower GI surgery experience early return of bowel function, fewer primary complications, and decreased length of stay. In addition, randomized controlled trials have shown that early postoperative enteral feeding in patients undergoing elective colorectal surgery is safe and effective and decreases both postoperative complications and hospital length of stay with no differences to the risk of anesthetic anastomotic dehiscence, pneumonia, wound infection, vomiting, and mortality.

Clearly, the implementation of enhanced recovery after surgery protocols and the contemporary evolution of postoperative management for elective colorectal surgery have significant benefits to the patient and health care costs.

DIVERTICULAR DISEASE

Background

Diverticular disease encompasses a range of signs and symptoms directly related to the presence of diverticula in the colon wall. These include infection, perforation, bleeding, fistula, and occasionally obstruction due to chronic inflammation. Diverticulosis was first described in the mid-19th century and appears to be an unfortunate product of the Industrial Revolution, which brought with it marked changes in diet. The incidence has been noted to increase with age and has been largely on the rise in the United States and other Western societies. Approximately 30% of those older than 60 years and roughly 60% to 80% of those older than 80 years may be affected. Only 10% to 20% of people with diverticula develop symptoms, which in the United States accounts for roughly 300,000 hospitalizations annually and 1.5 million outpatient visits, all of which comes at a considerable annual cost estimated to exceed $2 billion.[12]

Pathophysiology

Diverticula are abnormal outpouchings or sacs of the colon wall that occur most commonly because of interactions of high intraluminal pressures, disordered motility, alterations in colonic structure, and diets low in fiber. Diverticula are formed on the mesenteric side of the antimesenteric taeniae coli in areas of relative weakness in the bowel where small arterioles (vasa recta)

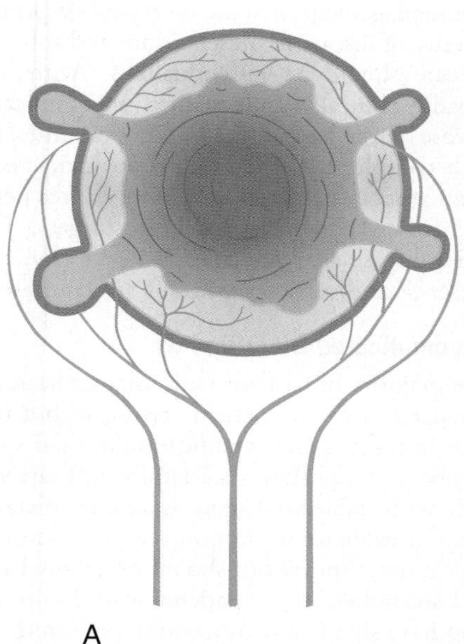

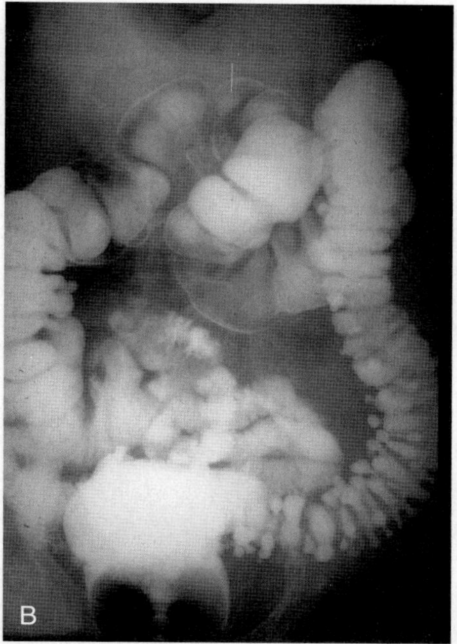

FIGURE 51-25 A, Pathogenesis of diverticular disease. Diverticula are herniations of the mucosa through the points of entry of blood vessels across the muscular wall. Because the diverticula are formed only by the mucosa rather than by the entire wall of the intestine, they are called false diverticula. Note that the diverticula form only between the mesenteric taenia and each of the two lateral taeniae. Because there are no perforating vessels, diverticula do not form on the antimesenteric side of the colon. **B,** Radiograph of barium enema with extensive sigmoid diverticulosis.

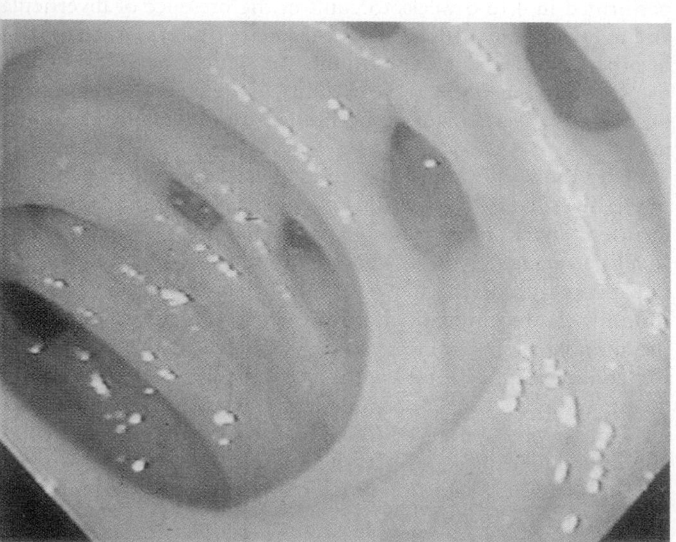

FIGURE 51-26 Colonoscopic view of diverticula.

penetrate the muscular layers as they traverse the colon wall. This results in the protrusion of the mucosa and submucosa through the layers of muscle, termed a pseudodiverticulum or false diverticulum (Fig. 51-25). A true diverticulum involves all of the layers of the intestinal wall.

The sigmoid and descending colon are the most commonly affected areas and in this disease process are characterized by hypertrophy of the muscular layers and associated decreased luminal diameter (Fig. 51-26). The resulting disordered motility in these segments and increase in luminal pressure facilitate the herniation of diverticula through the muscular coat. Deficiency in dietary fiber further aids in the overall pathogenesis of diverticulosis because there is less bulking of stool within the colon. This resulting decrease in colonic luminal content requires the generation of increased colonic pressures to propel the feces forward.

Evaluation

Diverticulitis results from the perforation of a colonic diverticulum, which leads to pericolonic inflammation as there is extravasation of feculent fluid through the ruptured diverticulum. Patients will typically present with localized abdominal pain in the left lower quadrant because the sigmoid colon is the most commonly affected site. Other symptoms may include change in bowel habits, anorexia, nausea, fever, and urinary urgency if there is associated inflammation of the bladder. Physical examination often reveals abdominal distention and localized tenderness due to focal peritonitis in the left lower quadrant if the perforation is contained. A tender mass may also be appreciated if there is a large associated phlegmon. Diffuse peritonitis with rebound and guarding is indicative of a free intra-abdominal perforation with widespread contamination. Leukocytosis is a common laboratory finding.

The diagnosis of diverticulitis can often be made by eliciting these findings on a thorough history and physical examination; however, several radiologic studies can be used to confirm the diagnosis. Barium enema studies were primarily used before the advent of computed tomography (CT) scans and have largely been abandoned as a primary tool as they provide information only about the luminal surface of the colon and cannot be performed if perforation is suspected. If a contrast enema is performed, the contrast agent should be water soluble (Fig. 51-27). CT scan of the abdomen and pelvis is now considered by most to be the standard

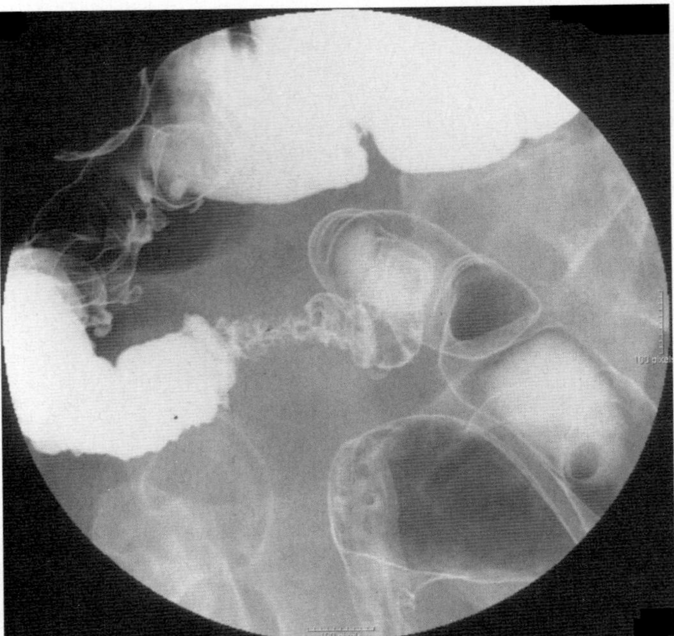

FIGURE 51-27 Radiograph of barium enema in a patient with a previous attack of diverticulitis. Note stricture in sigmoid colon. Colonoscopy was necessary to exclude cancer.

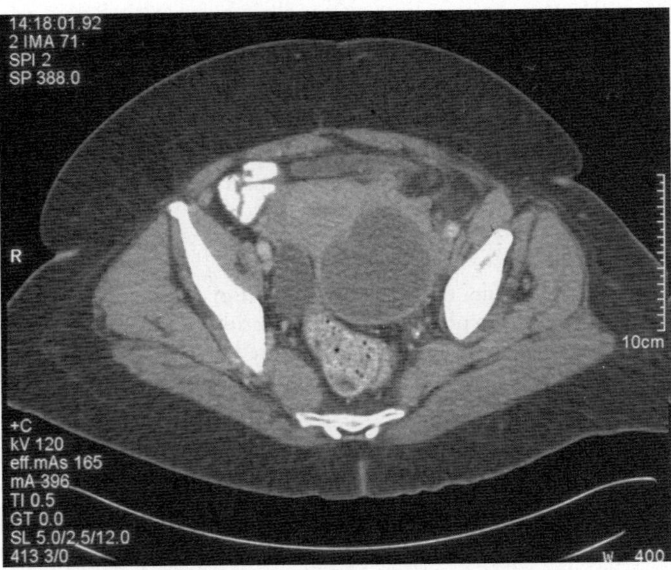

FIGURE 51-28 CT scan of pelvis showing diverticulitis with abscess.

for the evaluation of acute diverticulitis. CT scan provides useful information on the location, extent, and severity of disease as well as pathologic changes outside of the colon, such as an abscess or colovesical fistula. These findings are immensely useful in operative planning. If an abscess is detected by CT scan, it can also be a useful modality for guidance for percutaneous drainage (Fig. 51-28). Ultrasound and magnetic resonance imaging (MRI) have also been used to establish the diagnosis; however, their use varies by institution, and these procedures are not as reliable or expedient as CT scans. Sigmoidoscopy should be approached with caution in the acute setting because distention of the colon could result in worsening perforation.

Management

The management of acute diverticulitis primarily depends on the severity of disease at presentation, and subsequently the approach to care should be individualized. Acute diverticulitis is often broadly clinically divided into uncomplicated and complicated disease on the basis of the findings on initial presentation. Patients with complicated diverticulitis are characterized by the presence of an abscess, fistula, obstruction, or free perforation. The majority of these patients will require surgery. Those with uncomplicated disease are found to have pericolonic inflammation in the presence of diverticula without any of these complications.[13]

Uncomplicated Diverticulitis

The majority of patients with uncomplicated diverticulitis can be managed in the outpatient setting with a regimen of antibiotics and short-term diet modification as their symptoms resolve. This can be accomplished successfully and safely if the patient is afebrile with stable vital signs, is able to tolerate an oral diet, and is without evidence of immunosuppression or significant comorbid conditions. Antibiotics should be tailored to gram-negative rods and anaerobes. Those patients who do not meet these criteria or who have significant concerning peritonitis on physical examination should be admitted to the hospital for bowel rest, intravenous (IV) antibiotics, and judicious analgesia. Patients with uncomplicated diverticulitis usually respond promptly with marked improvement in symptoms within 48 hours; therefore, failure to improve in this interval should prompt further evaluation to ensure that there has been no progression in the severity of the disease. After the resolution of symptoms, colonoscopy should be performed in 4 to 6 weeks to confirm the presence of diverticula and to exclude any neoplasm or other colonic disease, such as IBD or other colitides, that could mimic the symptoms of diverticulitis. Contrast enema can be helpful in delineating the extent of colonic diverticula but is limited in definitely excluding neoplasms.

After the resolution of the initial episode of acute uncomplicated diverticulitis, approximately 33% of patients will have recurrent attacks or continue to have symptoms; however, only a small percentage of those who are hospitalized and roughly 1% of patients with diverticulosis will ultimately require surgery. Historically, the recommendation for elective surgery was based on the number of recurrences, as providers feared the progression to complicated disease with subsequent exacerbations of diverticulitis.[14-16] Current recommendations suggest that the decision for surgery should be individualized, taking into consideration the frequency and severity of recurrences. The patient's overall medical condition and comorbidities should also be included in the analysis.[17,18]

The goal of elective colectomy is to remove the affected segment of colon (usually the sigmoid colon) and to perform a primary anastomosis of the healthy remaining bowel. An important technical consideration after sigmoid colectomy is that the anastomosis should be made to the upper rectum to minimize the risk of recurrent disease. There is a large body of evidence to support that this can be achieved with either a laparoscopic or open approach with similar morbidity and mortality. The short-term benefits of laparoscopy, including less pain, quicker recovery of bowel function, and shorter hospital stays, can be achieved with minimally invasive sigmoid colectomy for diverticulitis. A hand-assisted laparoscopic approach has been advocated by some surgeons who believe that this technique facilitates the division of fused tissue planes while maintaining the benefits of laparoscopy.

Complicated Diverticulitis

Abscess. Diverticulitis complicated by a pelvic or pericolonic abscess is a challenging clinical entity. Patients often present with abdominal pain, fever, leukocytosis, and an ileus due to the associated inflammation of the small bowel. The management of these abscesses depends primarily on the radiographic appearance, size, and location with respect to the other intra-abdominal organs. Large (≥4 cm) pericolonic abscesses can often be managed successfully with percutaneous drainage with CT or ultrasound guidance to reduce the inflammation and to avoid a transabdominal approach by laparotomy. Smaller abscesses, which are typically not amenable to percutaneous drainage, can be managed by combining antibiotics and observation with interval imaging to ensure complete resolution. Failure of percutaneous drainage or antibiotic therapy should mandate more urgent surgical management.

The Hinchey classification is commonly used to describe the severity of diverticular disease complicated by perforation and is an additional tool that may be used to guide overall management:

Stage I: Small, confined pericolonic or mesenteric abscess
Stage II: Larger, walled-off pelvic abscess
Stage III: Generalized purulent peritonitis
Stage IV: Generalized fecal peritonitis

Hinchey stages I and II can often be managed with administration of antibiotics and percutaneous drainage, if technically feasible. If this is successful and the inflammation is allowed to subside, an urgent problem can be converted to an elective one whereby colectomy can be performed and a primary anastomosis can be achieved. Preoperative evaluation with colonoscopy is critical. Current guidelines support the recommendation of elective resection after a single episode of complicated diverticulitis.[17] Hinchey stage III and stage IV generally constitute surgical emergencies that require immediate surgical exploration as patients will present with generalized peritonitis and potentially signs of overwhelming sepsis (fever, tachycardia, hypotension). Abdominal radiographs or CT scans may reveal intraperitoneal free air in addition to inflammation associated with the perforated segment of colon. After resuscitation, operative goals should include washout of the abdominal contamination and resection of the diseased colon. In the setting of a grossly contaminated field, primary anastomosis is not a safe option; therefore, the appropriate strategy should be the Hartmann procedure: segmental resection, a proximal end colostomy, and closure of the rectal stump. Primary anastomosis with or without proximal diversion has been studied extensively in retrospective series in the setting of acute diverticulitis with peritonitis. Although it is feasible if the intra-abdominal contamination is minimal, its application should be individualized on the basis of patient and intraoperative factors.

Given the high morbidity associated with emergent colectomy for perforated diverticulitis, laparoscopic lavage has emerged as an attractive alternative therapeutic approach for patients with Hinchey stage III classification. The procedure entails a diagnostic laparoscopy followed by irrigation with warmed saline to clear the intra-abdominal contamination as well as placement of drains near the perforated segment. Neither colectomy nor colostomy is performed, and patients are treated with perioperative antibiotics. They are also monitored closely postoperatively to ensure that the peritonitis resolves. Patients who fail to improve are considered for colectomy. This has been fertile ground for study in the past decade; several studies show low morbidity and mortality rates as well as short length of hospital stay. Importantly, successful laparoscopic lavage may obviate the need for elective resection in many patients. Two large reviews showed elective resection rates of 38% and 51%, with low reported rates of recurrent diverticulitis in those who did not have elective surgery. The safety and efficacy of laparoscopic lavage have yet to be proven in a prospective, randomized fashion.

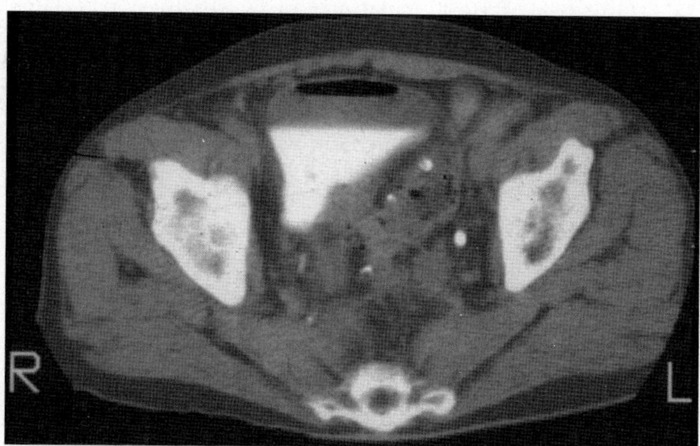

FIGURE 51-29 CT scan of pelvis. The patient has diverticulitis, and air in the bladder indicates a fistula between the sigmoid and the bladder.

Fistula. Fistulas to adjacent organs are a relatively common complication of diverticulitis as the associated inflammation of the sigmoid colon causes local attachments and ultimately communication with the bowel. The dome of the bladder is the most common site of fistulas, but the vagina and small bowel are also notable sites. On occasion, colocutaneous fistulas may be formed at the site of prior percutaneous drainage. Patients with colovesical fistulas will frequently present with recurrent urinary tract infections but may also report pneumaturia or fecaluria. Evidence on CT scan of air in the bladder that has not been instrumented is pathognomonic for a colovesical fistula (Fig. 51-29). Sigmoid-vesicular fistulas are more common in men than in women because the uterus prevents the sigmoid from adhering to the bladder. A barium enema may reveal a colovesical fistula up to 50% of the time, and cystoscopy usually reveals cystitis and bullous edema at the site of the fistula.

Initial treatment includes broad-spectrum antibiotics to ensure resolution of the inflammation. A colonoscopy to examine the affected colon and to exclude colon cancer or Crohn's disease as the cause of the fistula is important for preoperative planning. Elective resection of the involved colon and fistula tract should then be performed with subsequent primary anastomosis. If a small defect is encountered in the bladder, it may not be necessary to close this primarily, as healing will occur spontaneously if the bladder is drained with a Foley catheter for 7 days after the operation. Larger defects will require primary closure with absorbable sutures combined with Foley drainage. Fistulas to the small bowel will typically require resection and primary anastomosis.

Obstruction. Obstruction due to stricture formation is rarely associated with acute diverticulitis. However, this may occur because of chronic inflammation resulting in narrowing of the lumen. Most often, the obstruction is partial and insidious, but patients can occasionally have significant obstructive symptoms. Preoperative colonoscopy to exclude carcinoma is critical before elective resection; however, if this is not feasible because of luminal narrowing, a retrograde contrast study or CT enterography may be helpful in evaluating the remainder of the proximal colon.

Small bowel obstruction is possible in the setting of acute diverticulitis if the bowel becomes adherent to the phlegmon or abscess. In such circumstances, the appropriate treatment is to pass a nasogastric tube for decompression while addressing the obstruction by treating the infection with antibiotics or percutaneous drainage of the abscess.

Special Considerations

The Immunocompromised Patient

Diverticulitis in the immunocompromised or transplant patient represents a unique challenge for the surgeon. Whereas diverticulitis is not more prevalent in this cohort, studies indicate that they are at greater risk of presenting with recurrent and complicated disease. As a result, there should be a lower threshold for sigmoid colectomy after a single attack of diverticulitis in these patients because of their diminished ability to combat an infectious insult. Prophylactic colectomy in pretransplant patients remains controversial.

Right-Sided Diverticulitis

Diverticulitis of the right colon is relatively rare. Patients with cecal diverticulitis are typically younger by comparison to those with sigmoid diverticulitis and will present with right-sided abdominal pain. This can be a challenging clinical entity as the differential diagnosis can be broad, including acute appendicitis, Meckel's diverticulitis, cholecystitis, pelvic inflammatory disease, pyelonephritis, mesenteric adenitis, and ischemic colitis. A thorough history and evaluation with CT scan are instrumental in making the proper diagnosis. Similar to sigmoid diverticulitis, the CT scan for cecal diverticulitis will show fat stranding or associated abscess or phlegmon. Patients who have recurrent episodes or complicated disease should be considered for resection with a right colectomy.

Diverticulitis in Young Patients

Historically, diverticulitis in younger patients (<50 years) was considered more virulent and associated with worse clinical outcomes and higher recurrence rates. Therefore, elective resection was recommended after one episode even with uncomplicated disease. Further study has shown that initial reports were plagued by selection bias and missed or delayed diagnoses, making a true comparison between younger and older cohorts difficult. Current guidelines do not recommend routine elective resection on the basis of young age (<50 years).[17]

COLONIC VOLVULUS

Volvulus describes the condition in which the bowel becomes twisted on its mesenteric axis, a situation that results in partial or complete obstruction of the bowel lumen and a variable degree of impairment of its blood supply. The condition usually affects the colon. Although colonic volvulus is relatively rare in the United States, ranking behind cancer and diverticulitis, it is responsible for approximately 4% of cases of large bowel obstruction. However, in the region known as the volvulus belt, an area extending along South America, Africa, the Middle East, India, and Russia, colonic volvulus is more common and accounts for approximately 50% of all cases of colonic obstruction.

Any portion of the large bowel can twist if that segment is attached to a long and floppy mesentery that is fixed to the retroperitoneum by a narrow base of origin. However, the mesenteric anatomy is such that volvulus is most common in the sigmoid colon, with less frequent occurrences involving the right colon and terminal ileum (usually referred to as cecal volvulus), the cecum alone (the condition permitted by a highly mobile cecum, called a cecal bascule, that is mobile in a caudad to cephalad direction), and, most rarely, the transverse colon.

Sigmoid volvulus accounts for two thirds of all cases of colonic volvulus. The condition is permitted by an elongated segment of bowel accompanied by a lengthy mesentery with a narrow parietal attachment, a situation that allows the two ends of the mobile segment to come close together and to twist around the narrow mesenteric base. Associated factors include chronic constipation and aging, with the average age at presentation being in the seventh to eighth decade of life. There is an increased incidence of the condition in institutionalized patients afflicted with neuropsychiatric conditions and treated with psychotropic drugs. These medications may predispose to volvulus by affecting intestinal motility. The increased incidence of volvulus in the so-called volvulus belt countries has been attributed to a diet high in fiber and vegetables.

Patients with sigmoid volvulus may present as acute or subacute intestinal obstruction, with signs and symptoms indistinguishable from those caused by cancer of the distal colon. There is usually a sudden onset of severe abdominal pain, vomiting, and obstipation. The abdomen is generally markedly distended and tympanitic, with the distention often more dramatic than would be associated with other causes of obstruction. There is always the possibility that the condition is associated with ischemia caused by mural ischemia resulting from the increased tension of the distended bowel wall or by arterial occlusion caused by torsion of the mesenteric arterial supply. Therefore, severe abdominal pain, rebound tenderness, and tachycardia are ominous signs.

There may be a history of previous episodes of acute volvulus that spontaneously resolved. In this case, marked abdominal distention may occur with minimal tenderness.

Radiographic findings are often dramatic and enable prompt diagnosis and treatment (Fig. 51-30). Abdominal radiographs

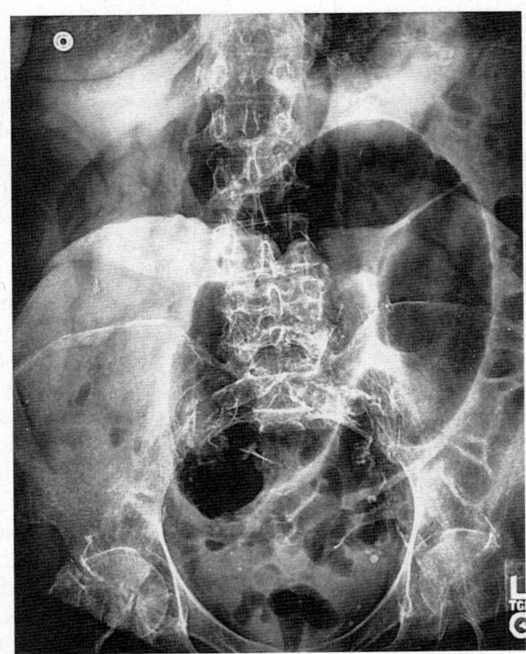

FIGURE 51-30 Plain film of sigmoid volvulus. Note bent inner tube appearance.

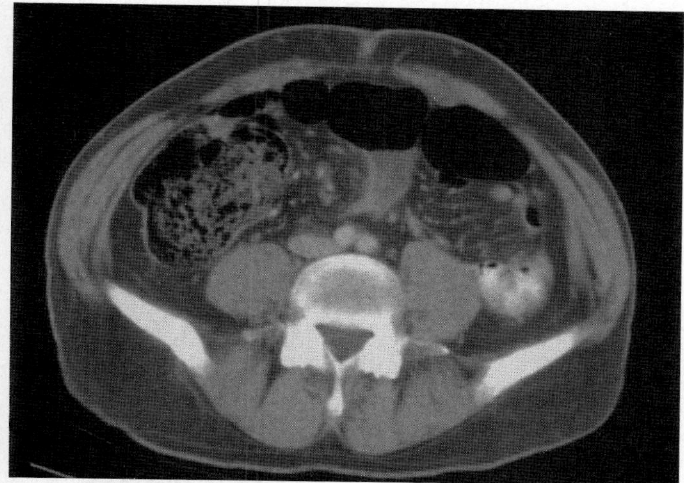

FIGURE 51-31 CT scan of abdomen in patient with sigmoid volvulus. Note characteristic whorl in mesentery.

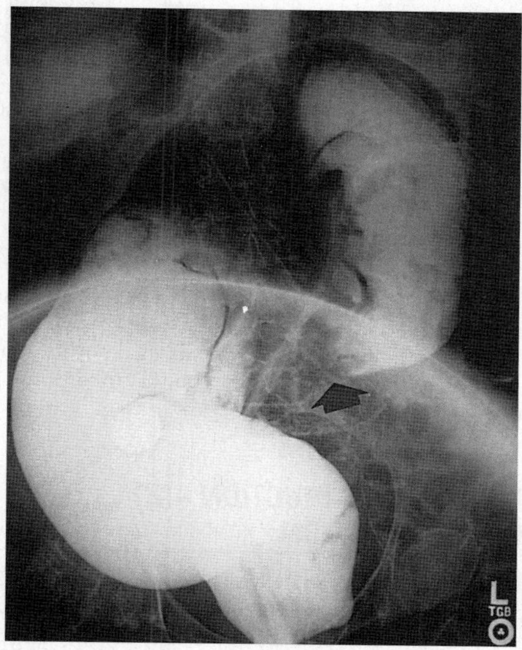

FIGURE 51-32 Radiograph of barium enema with sigmoid volvulus. Contrast material and air fill the rectum and distal sigmoid colon. The contrast material stops abruptly at the point of torsion.

reveal a markedly dilated sigmoid colon that resembles a bent inner tube, with its apex in the right upper quadrant. An air-fluid level may be seen in the dilated loop of colon, and gas is usually absent from the rectum. CT, although not necessary to establish the diagnosis, will typically reveal a characteristic mesenteric whorl (Fig. 51-31). A contrast enema typically demonstrates the point of obstruction with the pathognomonic bird's beak deformity revealing the twist that obstructs the sigmoid lumen (Fig. 51-32).

Treatment of the sigmoid volvulus begins with appropriate resuscitation and, in most cases, involves nonoperative decompression. Decompression relieves the acute problem and allows resection as an elective procedure, which can be accomplished with reduced morbidity and mortality. Patients with signs of colonic necrosis are not eligible for nonoperative decompression.

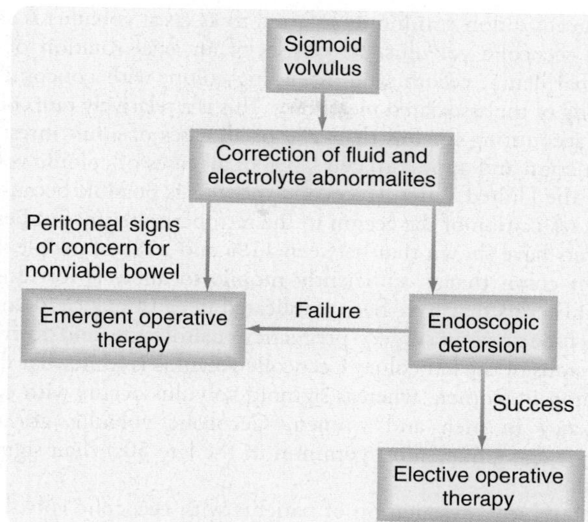

FIGURE 51-33 Algorithm for the management of volvulus.

Decompression can be achieved by placement of a rectal tube through a rigid proctoscope, but more often a flexible sigmoidoscope is used. Decompression results in a sudden gush of gas and fluid, with a decrease in the abdominal distention. The reduction should be confirmed with an abdominal radiograph. The rectal tube should be taped to the thigh and left in place for 1 or 2 days to allow continued decompression and to prevent immediate recurrence of the volvulus. The bowel can then be cleansed with cathartics and a complete colonoscopic examination performed. If detorsion of the volvulus cannot be accomplished with a rectal tube or flexible sigmoidoscope, laparotomy with resection of the sigmoid colon (Hartmann operation) is required (Fig. 51-33).

Even if detorsion of the sigmoid is successful, elective sigmoid resection is indicated in most cases because of the extremely high recurrence rate, which approaches 70%. Colonoscopy should be performed before elective resection to exclude an associated neoplasm. The operation can be conducted through a small left lower quadrant incision or by a laparoscopic approach. Because the elongated colon and mesentery require almost no mobilization, resection with primary anastomosis is easily accomplished.

For patients with signs of colonic necrosis or in whom endoscopic detorsion has failed, the traditional treatment has been a sigmoid colectomy with closure of the rectum and end colostomy (Hartmann procedure). Some surgeons have recently demonstrated, however, that resection with primary anastomosis, with or without protection from a proximal ostomy (transverse colostomy or ileostomy), may be accomplished in the acute setting. For patients who have had successful endoscopic detorsion but have significant comorbidities, endoscopic colopexy may also be an option.

Although the term *cecal volvulus* is ingrained in the literature, true volvulus of the cecum probably never occurs. There is a well-recognized condition, a cecal bascule, in which the cecum folds in a cephalad direction anteriorly over a fixed ascending colon. Although gangrene may develop, this is exceedingly rare because there is no major vessel obstruction. The cecal bascule commonly causes intermittent bouts of abdominal pain because the mobile cecum permits intermittent episodes of isolated cecal obstruction that are spontaneously relieved as the cecum falls back into its normal position.

The condition commonly referred to as cecal volvulus is actually a cecocolic volvulus. It consists of an axial rotation of the terminal ileum, cecum, and ascending colon, with concomitant twisting of the associated mesentery. This is a relatively rare condition, accounting for less than 2% of all cases of adult intestinal obstruction and approximately 25% of all cases of colonic volvulus in the United States. Cecocolic volvulus is possible because of a lack of fixation of the cecum to the retroperitoneum. Studies on cadavers have shown that between 11% and 22% of people have a right colon that is sufficiently mobile to allow a volvulus to occur. Factors that have been implicated in causing a cecal volvulus include previous surgery, pregnancy, malrotation, and obstructing lesions of the left colon. Cecocolic volvulus is somewhat more common in women, whereas sigmoid volvulus occurs with equal frequency in men and women. Cecocolic volvulus affects a younger age group (most common in the late 50s) than sigmoid volvulus.

The typical presentation of patients with cecocolic volvulus is the sudden onset of abdominal pain and distention. In the early phases of a cecocolic volvulus, the pain is mild or moderate in intensity. If the condition is not relieved and ischemia occurs, the pain increases significantly. Physical examination may reveal asymmetrical distention of the abdomen, with a tympanitic mass palpable in the left upper quadrant or midabdomen. Plain radiographs of the abdomen reveal a dilated cecum that is usually displaced to the left side of the abdomen. The distended cecum generally assumes a gas-filled comma shape, the concavity of which faces inferiorly and to the right. On occasion, the distended cecum appears as a circular shape with a narrow, triangular density pointing superiorly and to the right. Haustral markings in the distended loop indicate that the dilated bowel is colon. The torsion results in obstruction of the small bowel, and the radiographic pattern of dilated small intestine can cause diagnostic difficulty.

Although there have been reports of detorsion of cecocolic volvulus with a colonoscope, most cases require surgery to correct the volvulus and to prevent ischemia. If ischemia has already occurred, an immediate operation is obviously required. Contrast enema can sometimes be helpful to confirm the diagnosis and to exclude a carcinoma of the distal bowel as a precipitating cause of the volvulus (Fig. 51-34). Although there have been reports of endoscopic detorsion of cecal volvulus, the success rate is significantly lower than in sigmoid volvulus, and the procedure is associated with the risks of increasing distention because of insufflation of air during the procedure. Surgical intervention is therefore warranted in almost all cases of cecocolic volvulus.

Right colectomy is the procedure of choice. Primary anastomosis is usually preferred unless the volvulus has resulted in frankly gangrenous bowel, in which case resection of the gangrenous bowel with ileostomy is a safer approach. There have been many reports of correcting cecocolic volvulus with cecopexy, which should avoid the complication associated with an anastomosis. However, the procedure to provide fixation of the cecum is extensive and entails elevating and attaching a flap of peritoneum over the surface of the cecum and ascending colon. The recurrence rates are high with cecopexy, and right colectomy remains the procedure of choice for most surgeons.

Volvulus of the transverse colon is extremely rare and tends to be associated with other abnormalities, such as congenital bands and distal obstructing lesions, and pregnancy. Clinical features are indistinguishable from other causes of large bowel obstruction. Radiologic examination is not particularly useful because many cases are misdiagnosed as sigmoid volvulus. A contrast study may show a bird's beak deformity, indicating a volvulus. In such cases, colonoscopic reduction may result in detorsion and relief of obstruction. Elective resection should follow to prevent recurrence.

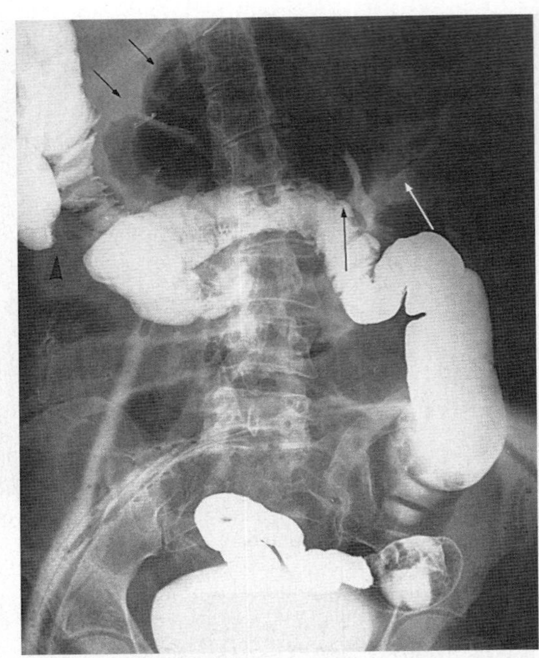

FIGURE 51-34 Radiograph of barium enema in a patient with cecal volvulus. The contrast material stops abruptly at the proximal end of the hepatic flexure *(arrowhead)*. The dilated air-filled cecum crosses the midline of the abdomen toward the left upper quadrant *(arrows)*. (Courtesy Dr. Dina F. Caroline, Temple University Hospital, Philadelphia.)

LARGE BOWEL OBSTRUCTION AND PSEUDO-OBSTRUCTION

Large bowel obstruction can be classified as dynamic (mechanical obstruction) or adynamic (pseudo-obstruction). Mechanical obstruction is characterized by blockage of the large bowel (luminal, mural, or extramural), resulting in increased intestinal contractility as a physiologic response to relieve the obstruction. Pseudo-obstruction is characterized by the absence of intestinal contractility, often associated with decreased or absent motility of the small bowel and stomach.

Colorectal cancer is the single most common cause of large intestinal obstruction in the United States, whereas colonic volvulus is the more common cause in Russia, eastern Europe, and Africa. Approximately 2% to 5% of patients with colorectal cancer in the United States present with complete obstruction. Intraluminal causes of colorectal obstruction include fecal impaction, inspissated barium, and foreign bodies. Intramural causes, in addition to carcinoma, include inflammation (e.g., diverticulitis, Crohn's disease, lymphogranuloma venereum, tuberculosis, schistosomiasis), Hirschsprung's disease (aganglionosis), ischemia, radiation, intussusception, and anastomotic stricture. Extraluminal causes include adhesions (the most common cause of small bowel obstruction but rarely a cause of colonic obstruction), hernias, tumors in adjacent organs, abscesses, and volvulus.

The signs and symptoms of large bowel obstruction depend on the cause and location of the obstruction. Cancers arising in the rectum or left colon are more likely to obstruct than those arising in the more capacious proximal colon. Regardless of the cause of the blockage, the clinical manifestations of large bowel obstruction include the failure to pass stool and flatus associated with increasing abdominal distention and cramping abdominal pain.

The colon becomes distended as gas (approximately two thirds is swallowed air, and the remainder includes the products of bacterial fermentation), stool, and liquid accumulate proximal to the site of blockage. If the obstruction is the result of a segment of colon trapped by a hernia or by a volvulus, the blood supply can become compromised, or strangulated. The venous return is blocked initially, causing localized swelling that can in turn occlude the arterial supply with resultant ischemia that, if uncorrected, can progress to necrosis or gangrene. The strangulation at first involves only the entrapped, or incarcerated, segment of bowel, but the colon proximal to that segment becomes progressively dilated because of the obstruction.

Another route to vascular compromise of the obstructed colon occurs if the bowel proximal to the point of obstruction distends to the extent that the intramural pressure within the intestinal wall exceeds the capillary pressure, depriving the bowel of adequate oxygenation. This route to ischemic necrosis can occur with mechanical obstruction and pseudo-obstruction.

A closed loop obstruction occurs when the proximal and distal parts of the bowel are occluded. A strangulated hernia or volvulus almost always leads to this condition. The more common form of closed loop obstruction, however, is seen when a cancer occludes the lumen of the colon in the presence of a competent ileocecal valve. In this situation, increasing colonic distention causes the pressure in the cecum to become so high that the vessels in the bowel wall are occluded, and necrosis and perforation can occur.

The treatment of large bowel obstruction obviously depends on the cause of the obstruction, and specific treatments are covered in the discussion of those entities (see later). However, some principles of diagnosis and treatment can be generalized. The obstruction needs to be relieved with some expediency before compromise of the blood supply results in ischemia and gangrene. The diagnosis should be established to guide appropriate treatment. History and physical examination provide important clues. The abdomen should be palpated for masses, the groins inspected for hernias, and a digital rectal examination performed to exclude rectal cancer. Plain films of the abdomen provide considerable information concerning the location of the obstruction and, in some situations, may be diagnostic of a volvulus. A CT scan is helpful in revealing an inflammatory process, such as an abscess associated with diverticulitis, and identifying the site of the obstruction. If a volvulus or distal sigmoid cancer is suspected, a water-soluble contrast enema may establish the diagnosis. Treatment options vary considerably, depending on the diagnosis, the condition of the bowel, and the status of the patient. It is helpful to establish the diagnosis before an operation to guide therapy properly. If the cause of the obstruction is a cancer of the distal or mid rectum, the preferred treatment is to relieve the obstruction with a loop sigmoid colostomy and then to treat the cancer with neoadjuvant chemoradiation, with a plan to resect the primary lesion at a later time after treatment. On the other hand, if the obstructing cancer is in the sigmoid colon, the surgical options include Hartmann operation (sigmoidectomy with descending colostomy and closure of the rectal stump or mucous fistula) and sigmoidectomy with primary colorectal anastomosis (with or without intraoperative colonic lavage if the colon is in good condition and the patient is stable).

Right-sided colonic obstruction, whether caused by cancer or the result of volvulus, is generally treated by resection and primary anastomosis of the ileum and transverse colon if the bowel is well perfused and relatively nonedematous and the patient is hemodynamically stable. If any one of those conditions is not met, temporary end ileostomy and mucous fistula or long Hartmann is indicated. In general, a stable patient with an early obstruction and well-perfused, nonedematous bowel can be considered for primary anastomosis. A safe choice and acceptable choice in emergency bowel surgery and obstruction in general is a temporary diverting stoma.

Pseudo-obstruction of the colon, also called Ogilvie syndrome, after its description by Sir William Heneage Ogilvie in 1948, describes the condition of distention of the colon, with signs and symptoms of colonic obstruction, in the absence of an actual physical cause of the obstruction. Ogilvie described two patients with clinical features of colonic obstruction despite normal findings on a barium enema study. Both patients underwent laparotomy for the condition; neither had mechanical obstruction, but both had unsuspected malignant disease involving the area of the celiac axis and semilunar ganglion. The cause of the dilation was attributed to the malignant infiltration of the sympathetic ganglia. Subsequently, there have been numerous descriptions of cases of colonic distention in the absence of mechanical obstruction and without malignant involvement of the visceral autonomic nerves. Very few cases of pseudo-obstruction have malignant infiltration of the autonomic nerves as the cause; in fact, the exact pathogenesis of the syndrome remains unknown, and it has been associated with a heterogeneous group of conditions.

Primary pseudo-obstruction is a motility disorder that is a familial visceral myopathy (hollow visceral myopathy syndrome) or a diffuse motility disorder involving the autonomic innervation of the intestinal wall. The latter may be modified by a disturbance of intestinal hormones or may be principally caused by disordered autonomic innervation.

Secondary pseudo-obstruction is more common and has been associated with neuroleptic medications, opiates, severe metabolic illness, myxedema, diabetes mellitus, uremia, hyperparathyroidism, lupus, scleroderma, Parkinson disease, and traumatic retroperitoneal hematomas. One mechanism thought to play a role in the pathogenesis is sympathetic overactivity overriding the parasympathetic system. Indirect support for this theory has been derived from the success in treating the syndrome with neostigmine, a parasympathomimetic agent. Further support comes from reports of immediate resolution of the syndrome after administration of an epidural anesthetic that provides sympathetic blockade.

Pseudo-obstruction may be manifested in an acute or chronic form. The acute variety usually affects patients with chronic renal, respiratory, cerebral, or cardiovascular disease. It generally involves only the colon, whereas the chronic form affects other parts of the GI tract, usually is manifested as bouts of subacute and partial intestinal obstruction, and tends to recur periodically.

Acute colonic pseudo-obstruction should be suspected when a medically ill patient suddenly develops abdominal distention. The abdomen is tympanitic and usually nontender, and bowel sounds are generally present. Plain abdominal radiographs reveal a distended colon, with the right and transverse segments tending to be most dramatically affected. The radiologic appearance is one of large bowel obstruction.

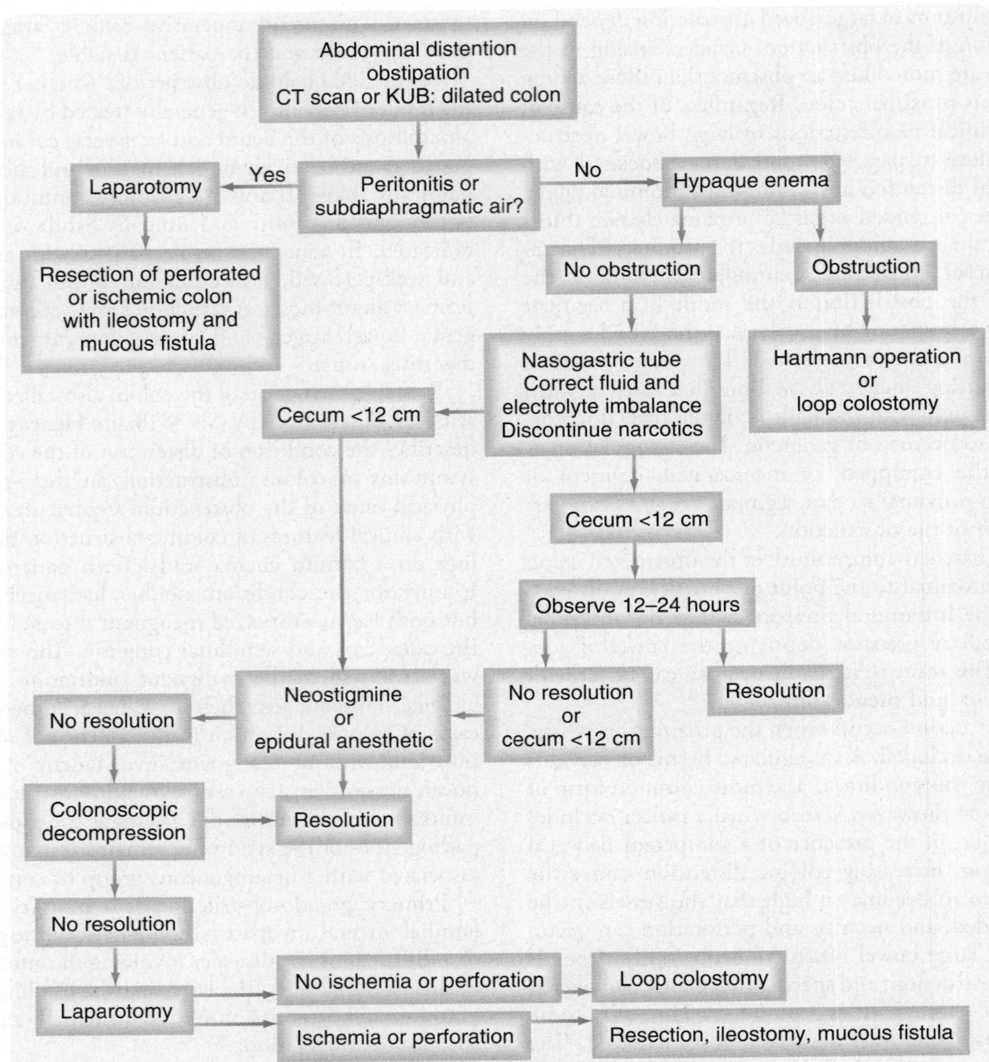

FIGURE 51-35 Algorithm for Ogilvie syndrome management.

The most useful investigation is a water-soluble contrast enema, which should be performed in all patients in whom the diagnosis is suspected, provided they are stable enough to tolerate the procedure (Fig. 51-35). The contrast enema can reliably differentiate between mechanical obstruction and pseudo-obstruction, a differentiation that is essential to guide appropriate therapy.

Colonoscopy is an alternative diagnostic investigation for pseudo-obstruction and has the attractive advantage that it can be used for treatment. However, colonoscopy runs the risk of distending the proximal colon even more, with insufflation of more air, and at present, the water-soluble contrast enema is generally the preferred initial test.

When the diagnosis of acute pseudo-obstruction is suspected, treatment should accompany the diagnostic evaluation. Initial treatment includes nasogastric decompression, replacement of extracellular fluid deficits, and correction of electrolyte abnormalities. All medications that inhibit bowel motility, such as opiates and antihistamines, should be discontinued. Ambulation, if possible, is encouraged. The patient's response is monitored by serial abdominal examinations and radiography. Most patients improve with this regimen. Until the mid-1990s, the treatment generally used when the colonic distention failed to resolve with supportive measures was colonoscopic decompression. Although this approach was usually successful, it required skilled personnel and equipment and carried the risk for colonic perforation from instrument trauma and insufflation. In addition, the procedure often had to be repeated because of recurrence of the colonic distention.

Sympathetic blockade by epidural anesthesia has been shown to relieve colonic pseudo-obstruction successfully. However, at present, the trend has been to treat this condition with neostigmine, a parasympathomimetic agent. It is obviously imperative that mechanical obstruction be excluded by water-soluble contrast enema or colonoscopy before the administration of neostigmine because the subsequent high pressures generated in the colon against a distal obstruction could cause colonic perforation.

Neostigmine enhances parasympathetic activity by competing with acetylcholine for acetylcholinesterase binding sites. In the treatment of colonic pseudo-obstruction, 2.5 mg of neostigmine is given intravenously over 3 minutes. The resolution of the condition is indicated within less than 10 minutes of administration of the drug by the passage of stool and flatus by the patient. The recurrence rates after the administration of neostigmine appear to be far lower than those associated with colonoscopic decompression, with satisfactory decompression being achieved in approximately 90% of patients after a single administration of the medication.

A significant side effect of neostigmine is bradycardia, and all patients must be monitored by telemetry during administration of the drug. Atropine must be immediately available; patients with significant cardiac disease or asthma are not candidates for this treatment.

If treatment with neostigmine, an epidural anesthetic, or colonoscopic decompression is not successful, or if signs of peritonitis or intestinal perforation occur, laparotomy is required. In the absence of perforation or ischemia, a loop colostomy is indicated to vent the proximal and distal colon. Any areas of perforation or ischemia must be resected.

INFLAMMATORY BOWEL DISEASE

The term *inflammatory bowel disease* is generally used to describe two diseases of unknown cause with similar general characteristics, ulcerative colitis and Crohn's disease. The distinction between the two entities can usually be established on the basis of clinical and pathologic criteria, including history and physical examination, radiologic and endoscopic studies, gross appearance, and histology. However, in approximately 10% to 15% of patients with inflammatory disease confined to the colon, a clear distinction cannot be made, and the disease is labeled indeterminate colitis. The medical treatment and surgical management of ulcerative colitis and Crohn's disease often differ significantly, so each entity is discussed separately here. A comparison of the characteristics of ulcerative colitis and Crohn's disease is presented in Table 51-1.

Ulcerative Colitis

Epidemiology and Cause

Ulcerative colitis occurs more commonly in developed countries and is relatively unusual in Asia, Africa, and South America. There appears to be a seasonal variation in the activity of the disease, with onset and relapse occurring statistically more often between August and January. The incidence of the disease has remained relatively stable during the past 25 years, with new cases reported as 4 to 6 cases/100,000 white adults per year, with a prevalence ranging from 40 to 100 cases/100,000. All ages are susceptible, but it more commonly affects patients younger than 30 years. A small secondary peak in the incidence occurs in the sixth decade. Both genders are equally affected, but the condition is more common in whites, Ashkenazi Jews, and persons of northern European ancestry.

Although the cause of ulcerative colitis is unknown, its prevalence in industrialized countries and the increased incidence in individuals who migrate from low-risk to high-risk areas suggest an environmental influence. Speculation on the influence of dietary factors has included inadequate fiber intake, chemical food additives, refined sugars, and cow's milk. However, none of these have been demonstrated to play a definitive role. Infectious agents, including *C. difficile* and *Campylobacter jejuni,* have been implicated as playing a causative role in the pathogenesis, but such a role has not been confirmed.

Smoking appears to confer a protective effect against the development of ulcerative colitis as well as providing a therapeutic influence; nicotine has been reported to induce remission in some

TABLE 51-1 Comparisons of Ulcerative Colitis and Crohn's Colitis

	ULCERATIVE COLITIS	CROHN'S COLITIS
Gross Appearance		
Thickened wall	0	4+
Thickened mesentery	0	3+
Serosal fat wrapping	0	4+
Segmental disease	0	4+
Microscopic Appearance		
Transmural	0	4+
Lymphoid aggregates	0	4+
Granulomas	0	3+
Clinical Features		
Bleeding per rectum	3+	1+
Diarrhea	3+	3+
Obstructive symptoms	1+	3+
Anal or perianal disease	Rare	4+
Risk for cancer	2+	3+
Small bowel disease	0	4+
Colonoscopic Features		
Distribution	Continuous	Discontinuous
Rectal disease	4+	1+
Friability	4+	1+
Aphthous ulcers	0	4+
Deep longitudinal ulcers	0	4+
Cobblestoning	0	4+
Pseudopolyps	2+	2+
Operative Treatment		
Total proctocolectomy	Curative	Combined disease: colon and rectum
Segmental resection	Rare	Absence of anorectal disease
Ileal pouch	Preferred by most patients	Contraindicated
Complications		
Postoperative recurrence	0	4+
Fistulas	Rare	4+
Sclerosing cholangitis	1+	Rare
Cholelithiasis	0	2+
Nephrolithiasis	0	2+

cases. This is in contrast to Crohn's disease, which is more common in smokers and appears to be aggravated by the habit. Both ulcerative colitis and Crohn's disease are more common in women who use oral contraceptives compared with those who do not. Patients who have had an appendectomy appear to be at decreased risk for development of ulcerative colitis.

A family history of IBD is a significant risk factor. Several studies have demonstrated the existence of family aggregates with ulcerative colitis and a high degree of concordance in monozygotic twins. The genetic predisposition for ulcerative colitis is not inherited in a classic mendelian pattern, suggesting the influence of environmental factors on an individual's susceptibility. Genetic abnormalities found to be associated with ulcerative colitis are variations in DNA repair genes and class II major histocompatibility complex genes. Patients with ulcerative colitis display specific alleles of group HLA and DR2 (HLA-DRB1), with an association between certain alleles and expression of the disease. The DR1501 allele is associated with a more benign course, whereas the DR1502 allele is associated with a more virulent form of the disease.

Another theory of the cause of IBD concerns an altered immunologic response to external and host antigens. Although anticolon antibodies have been identified in blood and tissue of patients with IBD, there is little evidence that these play a pathogenic role. Other studies have shown that defective cell-mediated immunity, leukocyte chemotactic impairment, and abnormalities of antigen-specific helper and suppressor T cells may be involved in the pathogenesis.

Pathologic Features

Gross appearance. Ulcerative colitis is a disease in which the major pathologic process involves the mucosa and submucosa of the colon, with sparing of the muscularis. Despite the name, ulceration of the mucosa is not invariably present. In fact, the typical gross appearance of ulcerative colitis is hyperemic mucosa. Friable and granular mucosa is common in more severe cases, and ulceration may not be readily evident, especially early in the course of the disease. However, ulceration may appear and vary widely, from small superficial erosions to patchy ulceration of the full thickness of the mucosa (Fig. 51-36). The rectum is invariably involved with the inflammatory process. In fact, rectal involvement (proctitis) is the hallmark of the disease, and the diagnosis should be questioned if the rectal mucosa is not affected. The mucosal inflammation extends in a continuous fashion for a variable distance into the more proximal colon. Pseudopolyps, or inflammatory polyps, represent regeneration of inflamed mucosa and are composed of a variable mixture of non-neoplastic colonic mucosa and inflamed lamina propria (Fig. 51-37).

As implied earlier, a diagnostic characteristic of ulcerative colitis is continuous uninterrupted inflammation of the colonic mucosa, beginning in the distal rectum and extending proximally to a variable distance. This is in contrast to Crohn's disease, in which normal segments of colon (skipped areas) may be interspersed between distinct segments of colonic inflammation. The entire colon, including the cecum and appendix, may be involved in ulcerative colitis. In contrast to Crohn's disease, ulcerative colitis does not involve the terminal ileum, except in cases of backwash ileitis, when the ileal mucosa may appear inflamed in the presence of extensive proximal colonic involvement. However, in such cases, contrast studies usually reveal the inflamed ileum to be dilated, in contrast to the frequently narrowed and contracted ileum characteristic of Crohn's disease.

Colonic strictures can occur in 5% to 12% of patients with chronic ulcerative colitis. Although these strictures are most often benign, caused by hypertrophy of the muscularis, cancer must be excluded as the cause of any colonic stricture occurring in the setting of ulcerative colitis. Three important features are suggestive of malignant strictures: appearance later in the course of ulcerative colitis (60% after 20 years versus 0% before 10 years); location proximal to the splenic flexure (86% malignant); and large bowel obstruction caused by the stricture (Fig. 51-38).

Histologic appearance. The typical microscopic finding in ulcerative colitis is inflammation of the mucosa and submucosa. The most characteristic lesion is the crypt abscess, in which collections of neutrophils fill and expand the lumina of individual crypts of Lieberkühn (Fig. 51-39). Crypt abscesses, however, are not specific for ulcerative colitis and can be seen in Crohn's disease and infectious colitis. Hematochezia often results from the marked vascular congestion. Crypt branching may be seen in chronic ulcerative colitis and is an important characteristic. The number of goblet cells in the crypts is diminished, as is mucus production.

It has been stressed that the inflammatory process in ulcerative colitis spares the muscular layer of the colon, a characteristic that differentiates it from Crohn's disease, which is characterized by transmural inflammation or involvement of all layers of the

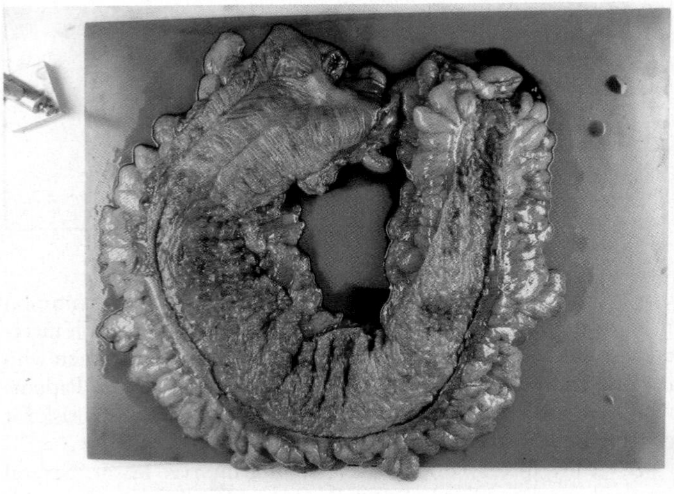

FIGURE 51-36 Ulcerative colitis: macroscopic appearance of colitis extending continuously from the rectum *(upper right)* to the mid–ascending colon *(upper left)*. The proximal colon appears spared, with normal colonic folds. Most of the colon exhibits erythema and granularity of the mucosal surface. (Courtesy Dr. Jeffrey P. Baliff, Thomas Jefferson University, Philadelphia.)

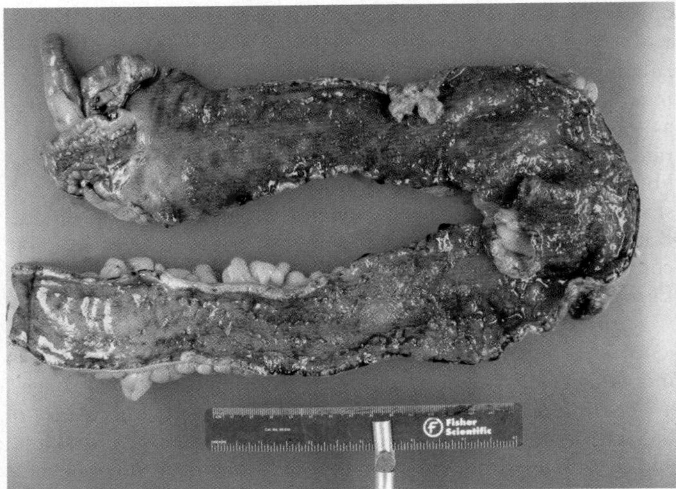

FIGURE 51-37 Ulcerative colitis: macroscopic appearance of pancolitis. The entire length of the colonic mucosa exhibits prominent flattening, erythema, and friability, with focal areas of green-yellow exudate. There is a suggestion of linear ulcerations along the bowel axis. Overall, the colon is narrowed and shortened. The terminal ileum *(upper left)* is spared. (Courtesy Dr. Jeffrey P. Baliff, Thomas Jefferson University, Philadelphia.)

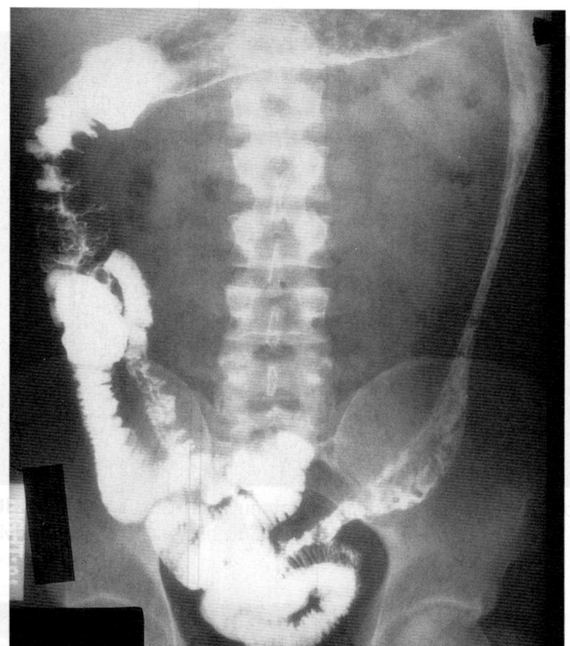

FIGURE 51-38 Radiograph of stricture in chronic ulcerative colitis. Colonoscopy revealed chronic inflammation but no dysplasia or cancer.

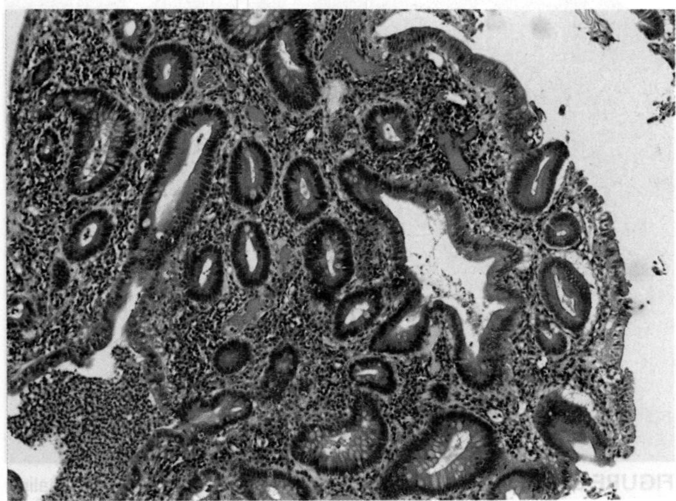

FIGURE 51-39 Histologic section of active ulcerative colitis. There is glandular architectural distortion manifested by irregular branching and orientation of glands relative to the surface. The lamina propria is expanded with inflammatory cells, and intraepithelial neutrophils are present. A crypt abscess is noted *(lower left)*. (Courtesy Dr. Jeffrey P. Baliff, Thomas Jefferson University, Philadelphia.)

intestinal wall. However, in rare cases of severe inflammation, all layers of the colon may be involved, and perforation may occur if treatment is delayed. However, the inflammatory process in such cases (toxic megacolon) is atypical and may be related to factors such as prolonged colonic distention with vascular compromise.

Numerous studies have demonstrated that antineutrophil cytoplasmic antibodies with a perinuclear staining pattern are seen in up to 86% of patients with mucosal ulcerative colitis. The presence of perinuclear antineutrophil cytoplasmic antibodies has been used as a diagnostic test to help differentiate ulcerative colitis from Crohn's disease.

Clinical Presentation

Ulcerative colitis and colonic Crohn's disease often have similar clinical presentations. Both may be manifested with diarrhea and the passage of mucus. Patients with ulcerative colitis tend to have more urgency than those with Crohn's disease, likely because ulcerative colitis is invariably associated with distal proctitis. Rectal bleeding is also common in ulcerative colitis; although it may be present in patients with Crohn's disease, it is typically not as severe. Patients with acute-onset ulcerative colitis often complain of abdominal discomfort, but the pain is seldom as severe as that found in patients with Crohn's disease. A tender abdominal mass suggestive of a phlegmon or abscess is more commonly associated with Crohn's disease.

Perianal disease is an uncommon finding in patients with ulcerative disease, whereas it may be the only presenting symptom of Crohn's disease. It is interesting and seemingly paradoxical that rectal involvement is present in almost 100% of patients with ulcerative colitis, whereas anal involvement is rare. In contrast, patients with Crohn's disease may have normal rectal mucosa (so-called rectal sparing), although anal disease (e.g., fissures, fistulas, abscesses) is common.

Extraintestinal Manifestations

Extraintestinal manifestations of ulcerative colitis include arthritis, ankylosing spondylitis, erythema nodosum, pyoderma gangrenosum, and primary sclerosing cholangitis (PSC). Arthritis, particularly of the knees, ankles, hips, and shoulders, occurs in approximately 20% of patients, typically in association with increased activity of intestinal disease. Ankylosing spondylitis occurs in 3% to 5% of patients and is most prevalent in patients who are HLA-B27 positive or have a family history of ankylosing spondylitis. Erythema nodosum arises in 10% to 15% of patients with ulcerative colitis and often occurs in conjunction with peripheral arthropathy. Pyoderma gangrenosum typically is manifested on the pretibial region as an erythematous plaque that progresses into an ulcerated painful wound. Most patients who develop this condition have underlying active IBD. Arthritis, ankylosing spondylitis, erythema nodosum, and pyoderma gangrenosum typically improve or completely resolve after colectomy.

PSC occurs in 5% to 8% of patients with ulcerative colitis. Most patients with IBD who develop PSC are younger than 40 years, and most are men. Genetics likely play a role because patients with ulcerative colitis who have the HLA-B8 or HLA-DR3 haplotype are 10 times more likely to develop PSC. Patients with PSC and ulcerative colitis typically have a more quiescent disease course; however, the risk for colon cancer in these patients is up to five times greater than in patients with ulcerative colitis alone. These tumors are more likely to arise proximal to the splenic flexure. PSC may be asymptomatic and diagnosed only by abnormal laboratory test results, or it may be manifested with symptoms of obstructive jaundice and abdominal pain. The disease is progressive and ultimately fatal unless liver transplantation is undertaken. Colectomy has no effect on the course of PSC.

Diagnosis

Endoscopic examination of the colon and rectum is essential in the diagnosis of IBD. In the acute phase of the disease, proctosigmoidoscopy is often sufficient because the rectum is invariably inflamed in patients with ulcerative colitis. Complete colonoscopy

survival rates (50% to 75%), a decrease in local recurrence rates (30% to 5%), and a decrease in the incidence of impotence and bladder dysfunction (85% to <15%).[42]

Intestinal continuity is reestablished by fashioning an anastomosis between the descending colon and rectum, which has been greatly facilitated by the introduction of the circular stapling device. After the colorectal anastomosis has been completed, it should be inspected with a proctoscope inserted through the anus. If there is concern about the integrity of the anastomosis or if the patient has received high-dose preoperative chemoradiation, a temporary proximal ileostomy should be made to permit complete healing of the anastomosis.[43] The stoma can be closed in approximately 10 weeks if proctoscopy and contrast studies verify the integrity of the anastomosis.

An end-to-end anastomosis between the descending colon and distal rectum or anus may result in significant alteration of bowel habits attributed to the loss of the normal rectal capacity (Fig. 51-78). Patients treated with this operation often experience frequent small bowel movements (low anterior resection syndrome or clustering). This problem can be partially addressed by fashioning a colonic J pouch as the proximal component of the anastomosis (Fig. 51-79). As experience has accumulated with this approach, it appears that improvement in bowel function is significant for cancers located in the distal rectum, but if the anastomosis is created above 9 cm from the anal verge, there is little benefit of a J pouch compared with an end-to-end anastomosis. The limbs of the J pouch should be relatively short (6 cm) because patients with larger pouches have a significant incidence of difficulty with evacuation. It is generally thought to be preferable to avoid using the sigmoid colon as the proximal component of a colorectal anastomosis because the blood supply to the sigmoid from the IMA may be tenuous, and the presence of diverticular disease, common in the sigmoid colon, is often considered to be a risk factor for anastomotic leak. In obese patients and in patients with a narrow pelvis, it may not be technically feasible to fashion a J pouch as the proximal component of the low pelvic anastomosis because the bulk of the pouch simply will not fit into the narrow pelvis. In such cases, a reservoir can be devised with a coloplasty.[44,45] This technique provides a rectal reservoir by making an 8- to 10-cm colotomy 4 to 6 cm from the divided end of the colon. The colotomy is closed transversely to provide increased rectal space and capacitance (Figs. 51-80 and 51-81).

Sphincter-Sparing Abdominal Perineal Resection With Coloanal Anastomosis

Abdominal perineal resection is required when a cancer in the distal rectum cannot be resected with adequate margins while preserving the anal sphincter. However, the use of preoperative radiation and chemotherapy has been shown, in some cases, to shrink the tumor to an extent that acceptable margins can be achieved.[46] If the anal sphincters do not need to be sacrificed to achieve adequate margins based on oncologic principles, a permanent stoma may be avoided with a sphincter-sparing abdominal perineal resection, with an anastomosis between the colon and anal canal. This procedure has particular application for young patients with rectal tumors who have a favorable body habitus and good preoperative sphincter function. The operation can be conducted in a variety of ways, but all methods involve mobilizing the sigmoid colon and pelvic rectum through an abdominal approach, dissecting the rectal mucosa from the anal sphincters

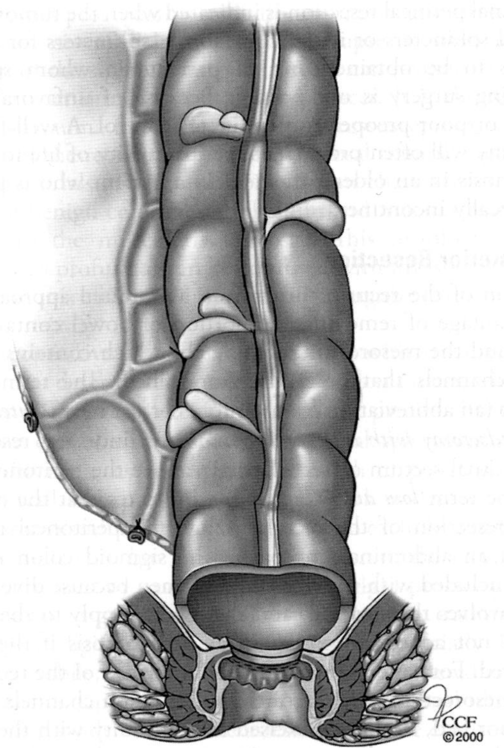

FIGURE 51-78 Anastomosis between descending colon and anus, following complete resection of the rectum. The absence of the rectum often results in frequent small bowel movements, a phenomenon known as clustering or low anterior resection syndrome. (Courtesy Cleveland Clinic Foundation, Cleveland, 2000.)

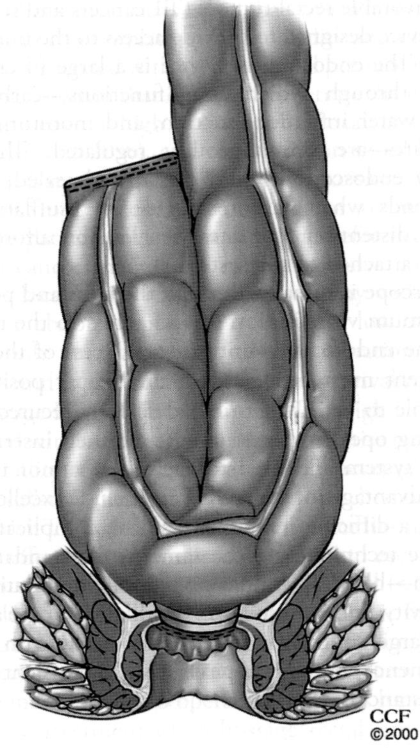

FIGURE 51-79 J pouch fashioned from descending colon to form proximal portion of coloanal anastomosis. This increases its capacitance to decrease the frequency of bowel movements. (Courtesy Cleveland Clinic Foundation, Cleveland, 2000.)

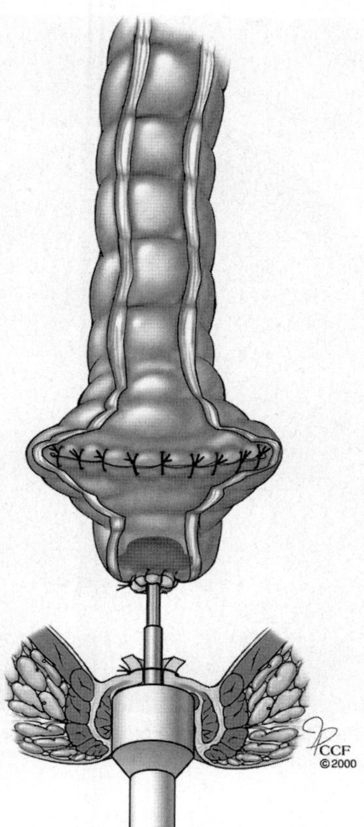

FIGURE 51-80 A coloplasty is performed by making an 8- to 10-cm colotomy 4 to 6 cm from the cut end of the colon. The longitudinal colotomy is made between the taeniae on the antimesenteric side. It is closed transversely with absorbable sutures. An end-to-end stapled anastomosis then joins the colon to the distal rectum or anus. (Courtesy Cleveland Clinic Foundation, Cleveland, 2000.)

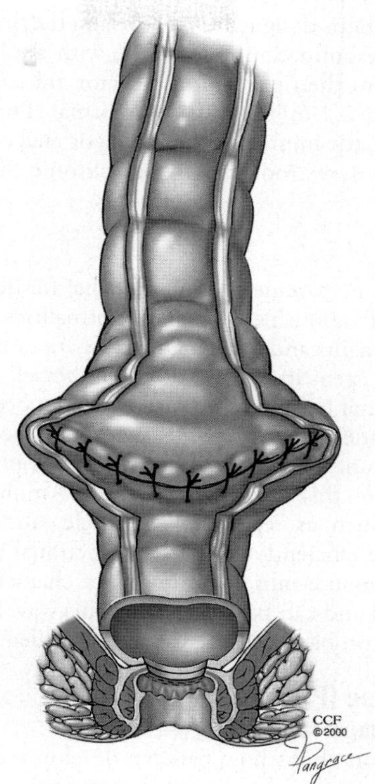

FIGURE 51-81 The completed stapled coloplasty with anastomosis. (Courtesy Cleveland Clinic Foundation, Cleveland, 2000.)

at the level of the dentate line, and completing the resection of the most distal rectum through the anal approach. An anastomosis is then fashioned between the descending colon and anus, often using a J pouch or coloplasty procedure described earlier for the low colorectal anastomosis. The anastomosis is made with sutures placed through a transanal approach by the surgeon in the perineal field. Low anterior resection syndrome describes a functional disorder created by removal of the rectum and fashioning of a coloanal anastomosis. It can occur no matter how the anastomosis is constructed, and a patient facing rectal cancer surgery with a consideration for sphincter preservation must be made aware of this as it can seriously and adversely affect quality of life.[42,47]

PELVIC FLOOR DISORDERS AND CONSTIPATION

Disorders of the pelvic floor can be classified as primarily colorectal, urologic, or gynecologic. Often, problems requiring the attention of multiple specialists present in a synchronous fashion, a condition known as complex prolapse. Rectal prolapse (procidentia), enterocele, rectocele, and functional disorders of the muscles of the pelvic floor (anismus, levator spasm) are among the pelvic floor disorders treated by surgeons. A functional disorder is defined by the concurrent presence of normal anatomy and abnormal function. Surgeons are often consulted concerning functional disorders of the large bowel or pelvic floor. These problems do not usually require operative intervention; in fact, the surgical literature is replete with examples of failed operations to correct these problems. However, the signs and symptoms of these disorders mimic surgical diseases and require proper recognition and treatment. Although chronic constipation is often considered an example of a functional problem, surgery is a consideration for some patients who fail to respond to medical management. The surgical evaluation and management of these disorders is discussed in this section.

Diagnosis: Testing and Evaluation

Anorectal Physiology Laboratory Testing

Anorectal physiology testing refers to the systematic evaluation of anal canal resting and squeeze pressures, anal reflexes, pudendal nerve conduction velocities, and electromyographic muscle fiber recruitment. Measurement of anal canal pressures (manometry) involves the use of water-filled balloons attached to catheters and transducers placed in the anal canal. The measurement of resting and squeeze pressures at various points in the anal canal reflects the strength, tone, and function of the internal and external sphincter. Normal resting and squeeze values are 40 to 80 mm Hg. Resting pressure reflects the function of the internal sphincter, whereas squeeze pressure measures external sphincter (voluntary muscle) contributions. Measurement of anal canal pressures is useful in the evaluation of conditions ranging from incontinence to obstructive defecation. Electromyographic recruitment refers to the motor unit potential of the puborectalis muscle and is compared for rest, squeeze, and push (simulated defecation). An increase in the recruitment of fibers during straining is pathognomonic for the syndrome of paradoxical puborectalis, or inappropriate puborectalis contraction. Pudendal nerve terminal motor latency times are measured with a special transducer attached to a glove-like apparatus designed to be worn on the finger and hand. A digital rectal examination is required, with application of the finger electrode to the right and left levator ani complex. Values between 1.8 and 2.2 milliseconds are normal. Prolonged values are seen in traumatic injuries of the vagina or anal canal (obstetric in cause), sacral nerve root damage, or chronic diseases such as diabetes.

Defecography

Defecography is an extremely useful modality for determining the precise nature of various pelvic floor abnormalities. Barium paste is placed in the vagina and rectum after the patient ingests a water-soluble contrast agent to opacify the small bowel. As the patient evacuates the rectal barium paste, abnormalities occurring during the act of defecation can be recorded with fluoroscopic videotaping. A vast amount of functional and anatomic information can be gathered from this test. The presence of multiple anatomic abnormalities, such as rectocele, enterocele, and vaginal vault prolapse, can be efficiently evaluated. Functional problems such as paradoxical puborectalis syndrome have characteristic defecographic patterns and can be evaluated in this way. Many contributing anatomic problems can be readily identified.

Rectal Prolapse (Procidentia)

Causes and Symptoms

Most information about how patients develop rectal prolapse is based on observation of the clinical characteristics of those suffering from this problem. The condition was documented in the Hippocratic Corpus, and since then, descriptions of causes and rectifying procedures have been numerous. However, two competing theories of rectal prolapse did evolve. In 1912, Alexis Moschcowitz proposed that a rectal prolapse was caused by a sliding herniation of the pouch of Douglas through the pelvic floor fascia into the anterior aspect of the rectum. His theory was based on the fact that the pelvic floor of prolapse patients is mobile and unsupported and on the observation that other adjacent structures can occasionally be seen alongside the rectal component of the prolapse. With the advent of defecography in 1968, however, Broden and Snellman were able to show convincingly that procidentia is basically a full-thickness rectal intussusception starting approximately 3 inches above the dentate line and extending beyond the anal verge. Both explanations take into consideration the weakness of the pelvic floor in rectal prolapse cases, the concept of herniation, and the observation that there are abnormal anatomic features that characterize this condition.

Women aged 50 years and older are six times as likely as men to present with rectal prolapse. The peak age of incidence is the seventh decade in women, whereas the relatively few men afflicted with the syndrome may develop prolapse at the age of 40 years or younger. One striking characteristic of young male patients is their tendency to have psychiatric disorders, and many are institutionalized. Young male patients with procidentia also tend to take constipating medications and report significant symptoms related to bowel function.

Anatomy and Pathophysiology

Patients with prolapse are frequently found to have specific anatomic characteristics. Diastasis of the levator ani, abnormally deep cul-de-sac, redundant sigmoid colon, patulous anal sphincter, and loss of the rectal sacral attachments are commonly described.

Large case reviews aimed at elucidating other predisposing factors have supported several observations. Chronic or lifelong

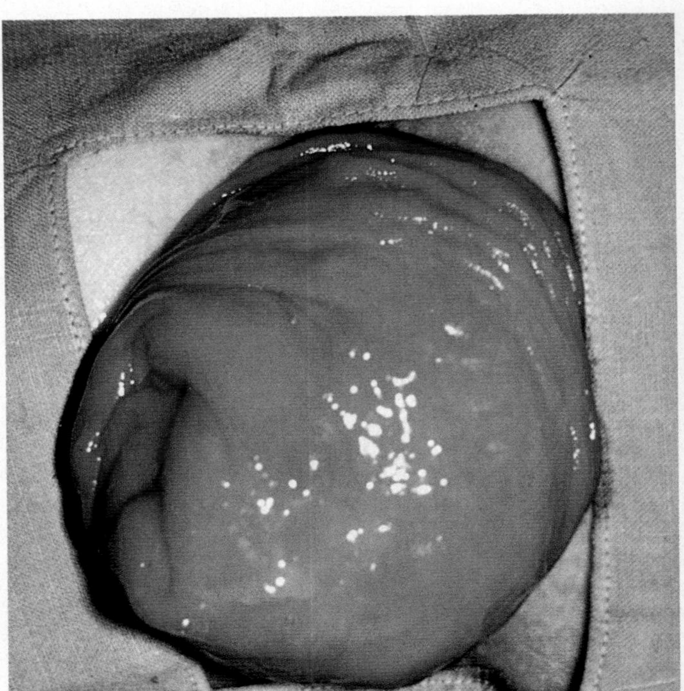

FIGURE 51-82 Procidentia, or rectal prolapse. The entire rectum has protruded through the anal canal.

constipation with a component of straining is present in more than 50% of patients, and 15% experience diarrhea. Contrary to the common assumption that rectal prolapse is a consequence of multiparity, 35% of patients with rectal prolapse are nulliparous. Once a prolapse is apparent, fecal incontinence becomes a predominant symptomatic feature, occurring in 50% to 75% of cases. Proximal bilateral pudendal neuropathy is present in incontinent prolapse patients and is responsible for denervation atrophy of the external sphincter musculature. This finding is absent in normal controls. It is speculated that pudendal nerve damage is responsible for pelvic floor and anal sphincter weakening and may be the underlying cause of a spectrum of pelvic floor disorders. Pudendal nerve damage can result from direct trauma (e.g., obstetric injury), chronic diseases (e.g., diabetes), and neoplastic processes causing sacral nerve root damage.

Symptoms of prolapse progress as the prolapse develops. Often, the prolapse initially comes down with defecation or straining, only to reduce spontaneously afterward. Patients describe a mass or large lump that they may have to push back in after defecation (Fig. 51-82). The presenting complaint may be the concurrent fecal incontinence that results from the prolapse or a sensation of chronic moisture and mucous drainage in the perineal area. Minimal or spontaneously reducible prolapses may progress to a chronically prolapsed rectum, requiring digital reduction. Chronically prolapsed rectal mucosa may become thickened or ulcerated and cause significant bleeding. On occasion, the presentation of rectal prolapse can be dramatic when the prolapsed segment becomes incarcerated below the level of the anal sphincter. Emergent operative therapy is indicated in this situation.

Differential Diagnosis and Investigation

A common pitfall in the diagnosis of rectal prolapse is the potential for confusion with prolapsed incarcerated internal hemorrhoids. These conditions may be distinguished by close inspection of the direction of the prolapsed tissue folds. In the case of rectal prolapse, the folds are always concentric, whereas hemorrhoidal tissue develops radial invaginations defining the hemorrhoidal cushions. Prolapsed incarcerated hemorrhoids produce extreme pain and can be accompanied by fever and urinary retention. Unless it is incarcerated, rectal prolapse is easily reducible and painless.

Before operative intervention, a careful history, physical examination, and colonoscopy should be performed. Of patients with rectal prolapse, 35% complain of urinary incontinence and another 15% have a significant vaginal vault prolapse. These symptoms will require evaluation and potential multidisciplinary surgical intervention.

If the diagnosis is suspected from the history but not detected on physical examination, confirmation can be obtained by asking the patient to produce the prolapse by straining while on a toilet. Inspection of the perineum with the patient in the sitting or squatting position is helpful for this purpose. In the event that the prolapse is still elusive, defecography (see earlier) may reveal the problem.

Although uncommon, a neoplasm may form the lead point for a rectal intussusception. For this reason, and because this age group has the highest incidence of colorectal neoplasia, colonoscopy or barium enema should precede an operation. A significant finding on colonoscopic inspection may change the operative approach.

Anal manometry and pudendal nerve terminal motor latency tests can be ordered preoperatively to evaluate symptoms of incontinence further. However, these test results rarely change the operative strategy. A finding of increased nerve conduction periods (nerve damage) may have postoperative prognostic significance for continence, although more studies are required to confirm this. Patients with evidence of nerve damage may have a higher rate of incontinence after surgical correction of the prolapse. Decreased anal squeeze or resting pressures are expected with this condition and may predate the actual development of the prolapse. Routine manometric studies for obvious prolapse are usually not done.

Operative Repair

The number of procedures described in the literature, historically and in recent times, is breathtaking. More than 50 types of repair have been documented, most of historical interest only. Approaches have generally included anal encirclement, mucosal resection, perineal proctosigmoidectomy, anterior resection with or without rectopexy, rectopexy alone, and a host of procedures involving the use of synthetic mesh affixed to the presacral fascia. The apparent enthusiasm and ingenuity of surgeons in their quest to define the ideal prolapse operation serve only to highlight its elusiveness. Two predominant approaches, abdominal and perineal, are considered in the operative repair of rectal prolapse. The surgical approach is dictated by the comorbidities of the patient, the surgeon's preference and experience, and the patient's age. It is generally believed that the perineal approach results in less perioperative morbidity and pain and a reduced length of hospital stay. These advantages have, until relatively recently, been considered to be offset by a higher recurrence rate, but data are unclear on this point, however, and a properly executed perineal operation may yield the same good long-term results as an abdominal procedure. This point will be clarified by ongoing long-term studies. All of the abdominal operations for prolapse can be performed laparoscopically. Data suggest that the surgical approach (laparoscopic versus open) does not influence the recurrence rates in experienced hands.

Abdominal approaches

Ripstein repair and anterior mesh repairs. The Ripstein repair involves placement of a prosthetic mesh around the mobilized rectum, with attachment of the mesh to the presacral fascia below the sacral promontory. Recurrence rates for this procedure range from 2.3% to 5%. The bowel is mechanically prepared for this procedure with a polyethylene glycol or sodium phosphate solution. The procedure involves mobilizing the rectum on both sides and posteriorly down to the levator ani muscle plate. Recent data suggest that mobilizing anteriorly down to the levators as well helps reduce rates of anterior prolapse even further. Division of the upper portion of the lateral rectal ligaments has been described, but some advocate leaving them wholly intact because the rates of postoperative constipation are 50% higher in patients with divided lateral stalks. After mobilization of the rectum, a 5-cm band of rectangular mesh is placed around its anterior aspect at the level of the peritoneal reflection, and both sides of the mesh are sutured with nonabsorbable suture to the presacral fascia, approximately 1 cm from the midline. Sutures are used to secure the mesh to the rectum anteriorly, and the rectum is pulled upward and posteriorly. Various materials have been recommended to secure the rectum, including autologous fascia lata, synthetic nonabsorbable products such as Marlex (Chevron Phillips Chemical, The Woodlands, Tex), Teflon (DuPont, Wilmington, Del), and absorbable prosthetics such as polyglycolic acid. The recurrence rates for all these materials are less than 10%, although follow-up times and evaluation criteria among studies have varied and strict comparisons cannot be made. Complications include large bowel obstruction, erosion of the mesh through the bowel, ureteric injury or fibrosis, small bowel obstruction, rectovaginal fistula, and fecal impaction. Postoperative morbidity rates are 20%, but most of these complications are minor. Although mesh rectopexy results in significant improvement in fecal incontinence (50%), no rectal prolapse operation should be advocated as a procedure to restore continence, and patients, especially those with prolapse for longer than 2 years, should be warned of the possibility that incontinence could persist.

A significant complication of this operation is the incidence of new-onset or worsened constipation. Fifteen percent of patients experience constipation for the first time after Ripstein rectopexy, and at least 50% of those who are constipated preoperatively are made worse. Although some of these difficulties are attributed to complications of the procedure, such as mesh stricture, obstruction at the level of the repair, or rectal dysfunction after lateral stalk division, a subset of patients will be found to have slow-transit constipation characterizing a global motility disorder. Some advocate routine preoperative transit studies to select these patients out, but a good bowel habit history will usually suffice. The cause of any severe, unremitting postoperative defecation or obstruction problem should be investigated with a barium enema and perhaps with a small bowel study. Strictures, obstructions, adhesions, and fistulas may be identified by radiography.

Fiber, fluids, and stool softeners are useful in the management of functional constipation after rectal prolapse repairs of any type. On occasion, mild laxatives such as milk of magnesia, magnesium citrate, or polyethylene glycol–based therapies may be necessary for short periods. Newer treatments for constipation involve oral administration of 5-HT_4 receptor agonists (e.g., tegaserod maleate) and may prove invaluable in the short-term treatment of this problem.

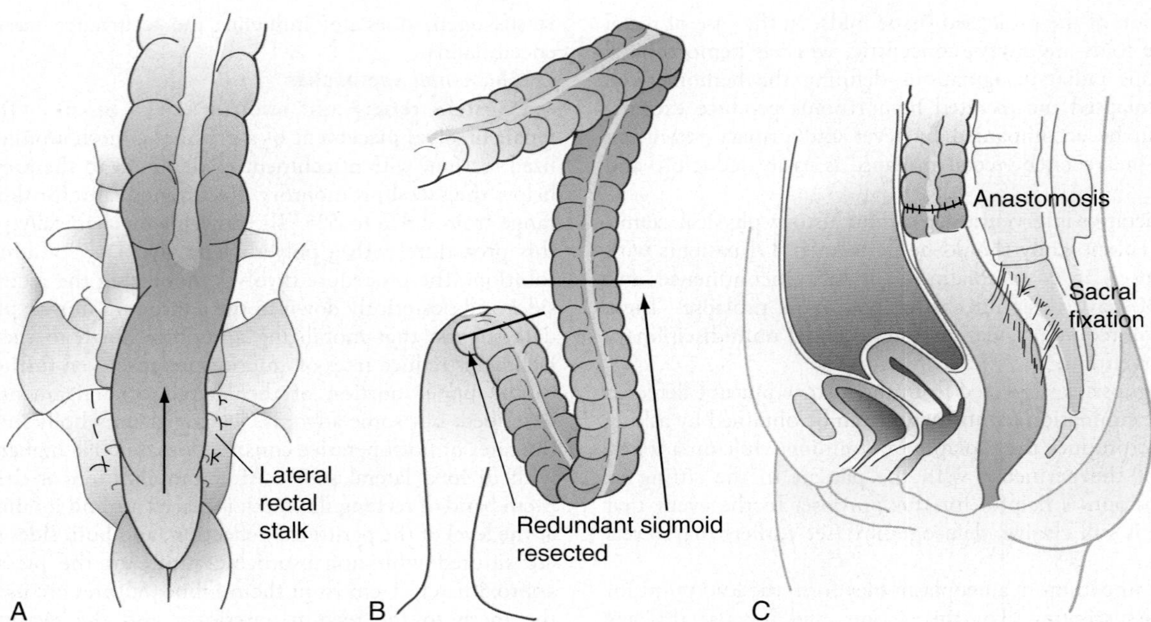

FIGURE 51-83 Anterior resection with rectopexy, or the Frykman-Goldberg procedure, for rectal prolapse. **A,** After full mobilization by sharp dissection, the tissues lateral to the rectal wall are swept away laterally. **B,** Resection of the redundant sigmoid colon. **C,** Anastomosis is completed, and rectopexy sutures are placed. (From Gordon PH, Nivatvongs S, editors: *Principles and practice of surgery for the colon, rectum and anus*, ed 2, St Louis, 1999, Quality Medical Publishing.)

Resection rectopexy. Resection rectopexy is a technique first described by Frykman and Goldberg in 1969 and popularized in the United States in the past 35 years (Fig. 51-83). Lack of artificial mesh, ease of operation, and reduction of redundant sigmoid colon are the principle advantages of the procedure. Recurrence rates are low, ranging from 2% to 5%, and major complication rates range from 0% to 20% and relate to obstruction or anastomotic leak. Basically, the sigmoid colon and rectum are mobilized to the level of the levators. The lateral ligaments are divided, elevated from the deep pelvis, and sutured to the presacral fascia. Again, as in anterior mesh repairs, anterior mobilization has gotten renewed interest because of the observed lower incidence of recurrence with this technique. The mesentery of the sigmoid colon is then divided, with preservation of the IMA, and a tension-free anastomosis is created. A revised version of this procedure involves preservation of the lateral stalks and unilateral fastening of the rectal mesentery to the sacrum at the level of the sacral promontory. Sigmoid resection is a unique feature of this procedure. It appears to reduce constipation by 50% in those who complain preoperatively of this symptom in some studies. Interestingly, in patients who complain of incontinence before surgery, this symptom consistently improves in approximately 35%, even with the sigmoid resection. A variant of this procedure involves forgoing the sigmoid resection in those who report no history of constipation and whose predominant complaint is fecal incontinence and doing the mobilization and rectopexy alone.

Perineal approaches

Perineal proctosigmoidectomy and the Altemeier procedure. Perineal proctosigmoidectomy was first introduced by Mikulicz in 1899 and remained the favored treatment for prolapse in Europe for many years. Miles advocated this procedure in the United Kingdom, and it was promoted in the United States by Altemeier at the University of Cincinnati. As the abdominal approaches gained favor, principally because of the reduced recurrence rates, the perineal approach was increasingly reserved only for those with the highest operative risk. However, renewed interest in the technique has accompanied studies showing reduced recurrence rates, and a number of surgeons believe that strong consideration should be given to this technique in repairing prolapse in young men who have an increased risk for autonomic nerve injury resulting in impotence.

The Altemeier procedure combines a perineal proctosigmoidectomy with an anterior levatorplasty (Fig. 51-84). The latter procedure is performed to correct the levator diastasis commonly associated with this condition. Theoretically, restoration of fecal continence is enhanced by this additional maneuver. As always, the large bowel is mechanically cleansed. The patient is placed in the prone jackknife position, and a Foley catheter is placed. The rectal mucosa is serially grasped with Babcock or Allis clamps until a full-thickness prolapse is demonstrated. A full-thickness circumferential incision is made 1.5 cm proximal to the dentate line. The low peritoneal reflection can usually be incised anteriorly and the peritoneal cavity entered. The mesentery of the rectum and sigmoid colon is sequentially clamped and tied until no redundant bowel remains. The colon is transected at this point, and an anastomosis is fashioned between the colon and anal canal with sutures or staples.

Patients undergoing perineal proctosigmoidectomy are generally older and have significantly more comorbidities than those who are considered for abdominal repair. Complication rates are less than 10%, and recurrence rates have been reported as high as 16%, although, as mentioned, some series have demonstrated significantly lower recurrence rates. Complications include bleeding from the staple or suture line, pelvic abscess, and, rarely, dehiscence of the suture line, with perineal evisceration. Lack of an abdominal incision, reduced pain, and reduced length of hospitalization make this procedure an attractive option.

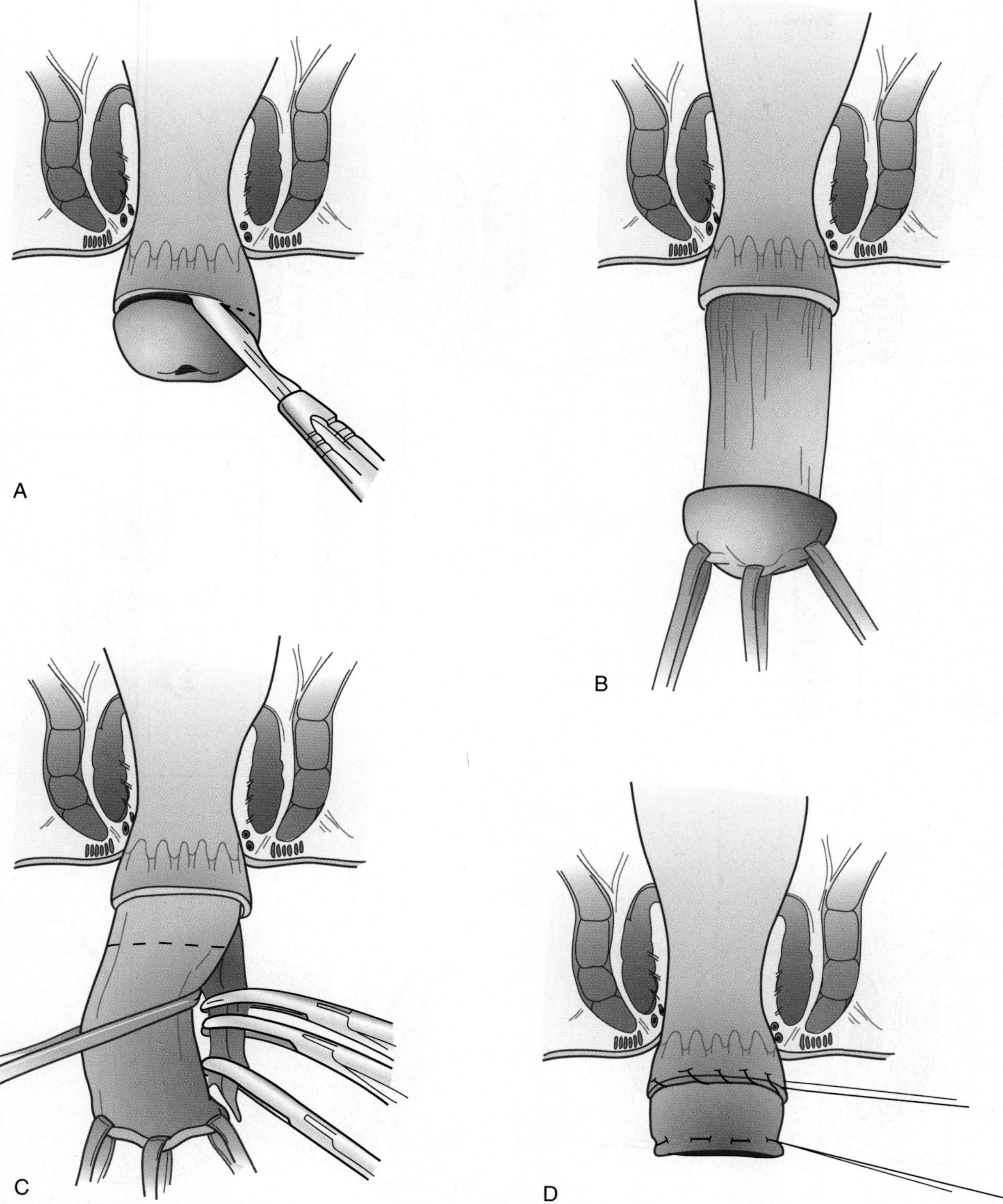

FIGURE 51-84 Altemeier perineal rectosigmoidectomy. **A,** Circumferential incision of rectum proximal to dentate line. **B,** Delivery of redundant rectum and sigmoid colon. **C,** Ligation of blood supply to rectum. **D,** Placement of purse-string suture on proximal bowels and excision of redundant colon and rectum; whip stitch placed on rectal stump.

Continued

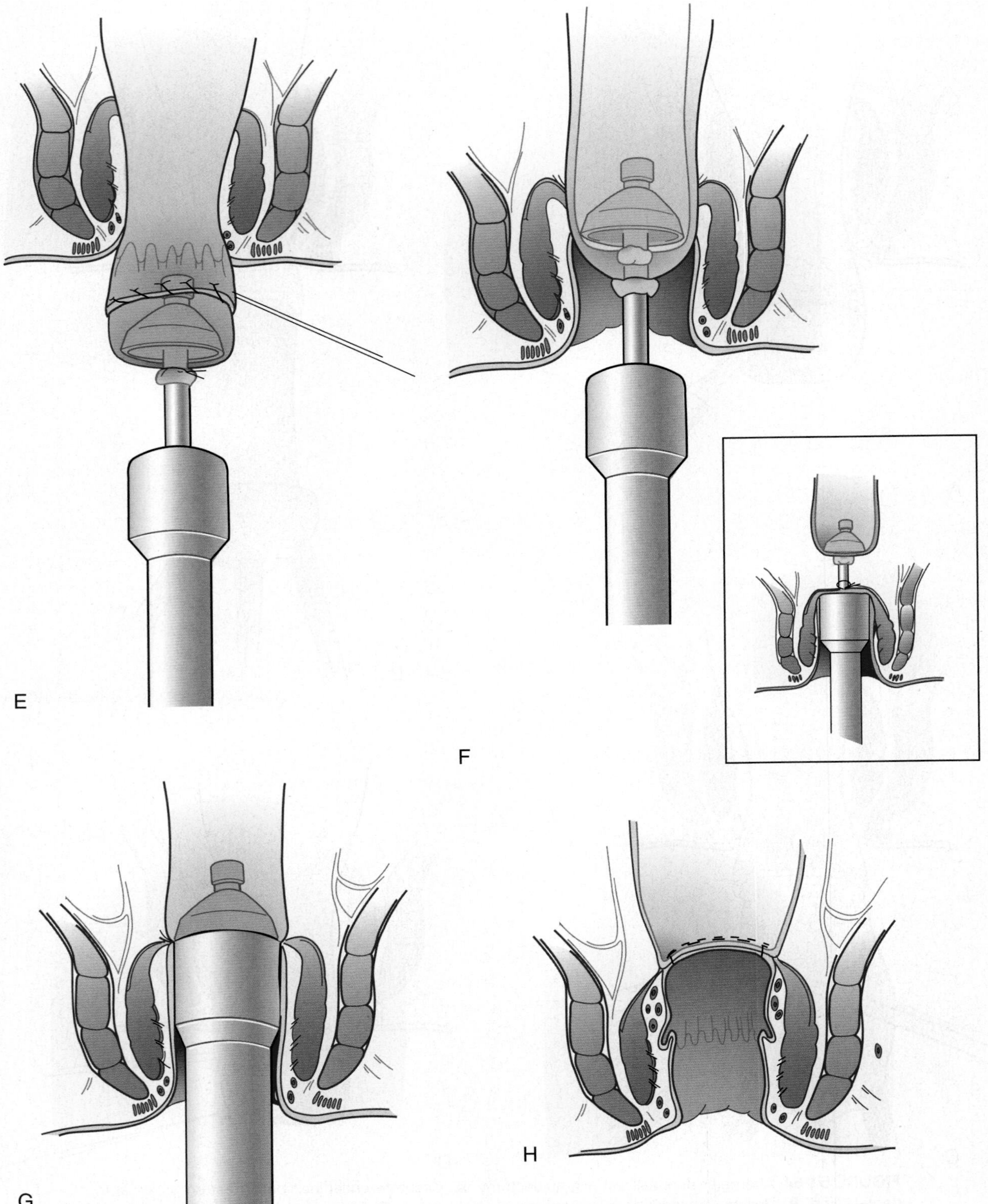

FIGURE 51-84, cont'd **E,** Proximal purse-string suture secured around central shaft. **F,** Proximal bowel advanced through anus and distal purse-string tied. **G,** Approximation of anvil to cartridge and activation of stapler. **H,** Completed anastomosis. (From Gordon PH, Nivatvongs S, editors: *Principles and practice of surgery for the colon, rectum and anus*, ed 2, St Louis, 1999, Quality Medical Publishing.)

Anal encirclement. Anal encirclement is one of the oldest surgical techniques for rectal prolapse described. Thiersch described silver wire anal encirclement in 1891. Since then, it has been tried with a wide variety of materials, including stainless steel wire, nonabsorbable mesh, small Silastic bands, nylon suture, and polypropylene. Anal encirclement does not correct the fecal incontinence associated with prolapse, and the recurrence rate is high (>30%), as is the morbidity. Erosion of the wire into the sphincter, anovaginal fistula formation, rectal prolapse incarceration, fecal impaction, and infection can occur. Reoperative rates of 7% to 59% have been reported. The safety of current anesthetic techniques and the low morbidity and relative functional success of perineal proctectomy have made anal encirclement, for the most part, a procedure of the past.

Internal Prolapse and Solitary Rectal Ulcer Syndrome

Two areas of controversy related to rectal prolapse involve the treatment of solitary rectal ulcer syndrome (SRUS) and internal intussusception of the rectal mucosa. Although identified as an ulcer, the gross pathologic features of SRUS can range from a typical crater-like ulcer with a fibrinous central depression to a polypoid lesion. It is always located on the anterior aspect of the rectum, 4 to 12 cm from the anal verge, and is thought to correspond to the location of the puborectalis sling. It is frequently although not exclusively associated with internal intussusception or full-thickness rectal prolapse. Patients are typically young and female, however, with an average age of 25 years and a history of straining and difficult evacuation.

The rectal ulcer is usually found on proctoscopy or flexible sigmoidoscopy and commonly is manifested with rectal bleeding in the setting of straining or constipation. The cause of SRUS remains somewhat unclear, but speculation centers on chronic ischemia. The fold with the ulcer is thought to form the lead point of an intussusception into the anal canal. Chronic, repeated straining or prolapse of this lead point produces ischemia, tissue breakdown, and ulceration. Possible digital self-disimpaction may also be a contributing factor. Histology reveals a thick layer of fibrosis obliterating the lamina propria and a central fibrinous exudate. Other common pathologic findings include the presence of mucus-filled glands misplaced in the submucosa and lined with normal colonic epithelium (colitis cystica profunda). Differentiating SRUS from malignant disease, infection, or Crohn's disease is important but not difficult. The anterior location in the context of classic symptoms and pathologic findings is conclusive.

Defecography is the radiologic procedure of choice for diagnostic evaluation and usually reveals the underlying disorder. Full-thickness rectal prolapse, internal prolapse, paradoxical puborectalis syndrome (failure of relaxation of the pelvic floor musculature on straining), and thickened rectal folds are common findings.

Data regarding the treatment of this unusual disorder are retrospective, and studies have been small, but several common observations have been made. In general, one third of patients with SRUS also suffer from full-thickness rectal prolapse. Abdominal prolapse repairs have resulted in a cure rate of 80% in patients with SRUS and full-thickness rectal prolapse. In the same study, patients treated with the same procedure for mucosal prolapse and SRUS fared far worse; only 25% of patients responded to operative intervention. In most studies, dietary management, pelvic floor retraining (biofeedback), and short-term use of topical anti-inflammatory medications containing mesalamine result in remission for those with internal prolapse or pelvic muscle dysfunction. Prompt diagnosis of the underlying problem and appropriate treatment can be difficult but are the keys to cure. Local excision usually results in a larger nonhealing wound and has no role in management. Rarely, symptoms of severe bleeding, pain, and spasm may require a temporary diverting sigmoid colostomy.

Internal intussusception was first described in the late 1960s, when defecography was first developed and came into widespread use. The condition is also called internal or hidden prolapse and is confined to the rectal mucosa and submucosa, which separates

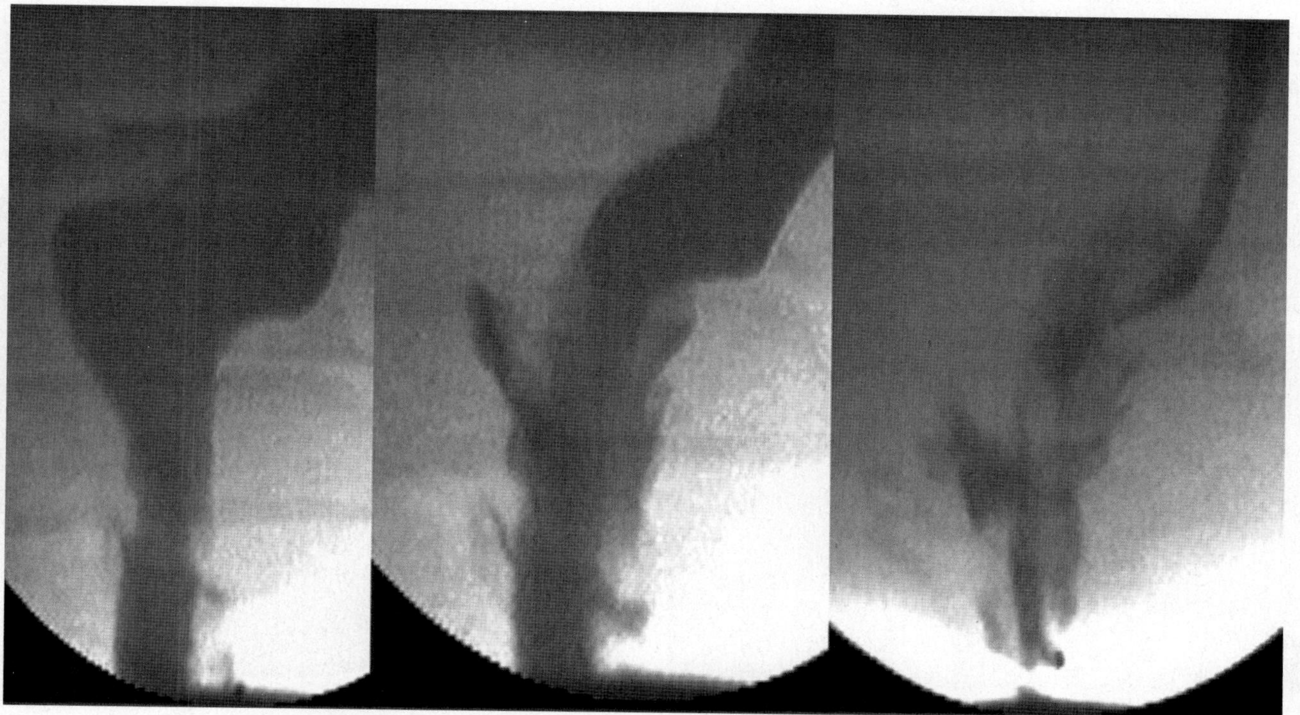

FIGURE 51-85 Defecogram showing progression of internal intussusception.

from the muscularis mucosae layer and slides down the anal canal (Fig. 51-85). Internal intussusception can be identified in a significant proportion of the asymptomatic population and appears to represent a normal variant. However, there are advocates of internal prolapse repair when it is found in patients who complain of dysfunctional defecation. The transanal Delorme mucosal resection procedure involves circumferential removal of redundant anal canal and distal rectal mucosa and imbrication of the muscularis layer with serial vertical sutures. Although satisfactory results were reported for this procedure in the 1990s, experience has been discouraging, and enthusiasm for the procedure has waned.

Abdominal repairs such as the Ripstein procedure have also been advocated as an alternative for symptomatic patients. Unfortunately, the results of these studies are not conclusive. Of patients who underwent repair by an abdominal approach, only 24% to 38% reported improvement, whereas a significant number experienced worsening. As for patients with SRUS, the treatment of patients with incomplete or obstructed defecation should be initially evaluated with defecography. Studies have not supported operative intervention for these disorders when internal intussusception alone is present.

Rectocele

A rectocele is an abnormal sac-like projection of the anterior rectum that extends from the distal rectum to the distal anal canal. It usually begins just above the sphincter complex (Figs. 51-86 and 51-87). The cause of rectoceles is multifactorial. Stretching of the endopelvic fascia from antecedent pelvic floor injury, followed by chronic increased intra-abdominal pressure, causes an anterior full-thickness herniation of the rectum into the vagina. Rectal pressures are higher than those in the vagina; therefore, pressure tends to push the rectum anteriorly and stretch and shift the rectovaginal septum as well. The major symptom of rectocele is stool trapping, a form of obstructed defecation. Women commonly describe requiring vaginal pressure to reduce the bulge, effectively stenting the anterior rectum and enabling defecation.

Criteria for operative intervention include symptomatic stool trapping requiring digital evacuation or vaginal support and the presence of large protruding rectoceles that push vaginal mucosa beyond the introitus, producing dryness, ulceration, and discomfort. Although small rectoceles are common, it is rare that a rectocele smaller than 2 cm is symptomatic.

There are two major operative approaches to rectoceles, transanal and transvaginal. Although the transvaginal approach has been criticized by surgeons because the repair is done on the low-pressure side of the rectovaginal septum, it does have certain distinct advantages. The bowel is fully prepared and the patient is placed in the lithotomy position. After the submucosal injection of lidocaine with 1% epinephrine, a swath of vagina is excised, starting at the vaginal introitus and carried to the apex of the vagina. The size of this segment is determined by the depth of the rectocele. The goal is to excise a full-thickness segment of vagina, to dissect out and to reduce an enterocele if one is found in the rectovaginal septum, and then to obliterate the deep cul-de-sac by suturing the cut edges of the vagina closed, allowing the space to contract by fibrosis.

Alternatively, several approaches for the transanal correction of rectocele have been described. This technique was probably best described by Sullivan, who expected 80% of patients to have good to excellent results. An incision is made longitudinally in the rectum over the bulge above the sphincters. The incision's length varies with the size of the rectocele. The underlying vagina is exposed and imbricated to obliterate the sac, and the rectum is separately imbricated and closed over that with absorbable sutures. Unfortunately, direct comparisons in the literature between these techniques are absent. However, the largely unsubstantiated argument has been made by surgeons that a repair based in the high-pressure or rectal side of the bulge may reduce recurrence. No matter the technique, patient selection and follow-up are crucial. In one study, only 54% of patients who underwent rectocele repair obtained relief from their symptoms of obstructive defecation. Paradoxical puborectalis syndrome was not ruled out and

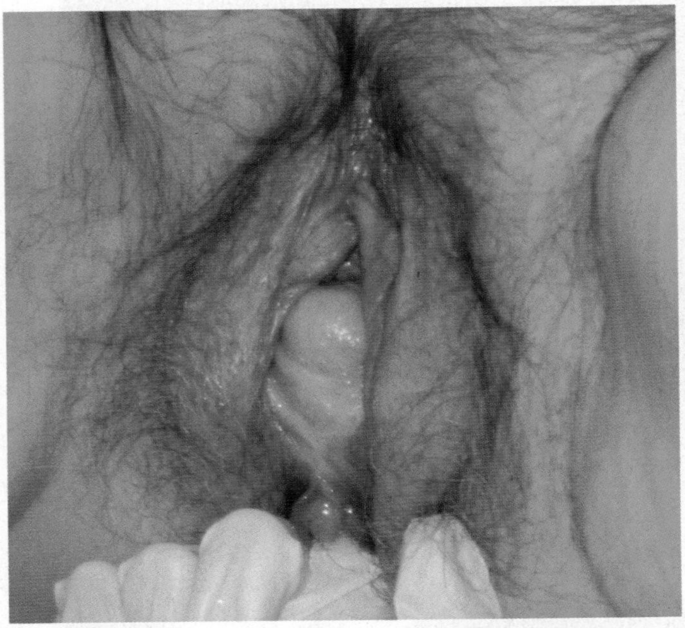

FIGURE 51-86 Digital anorectal examination demonstrating anterior rectocele protruding from the vaginal introitus.

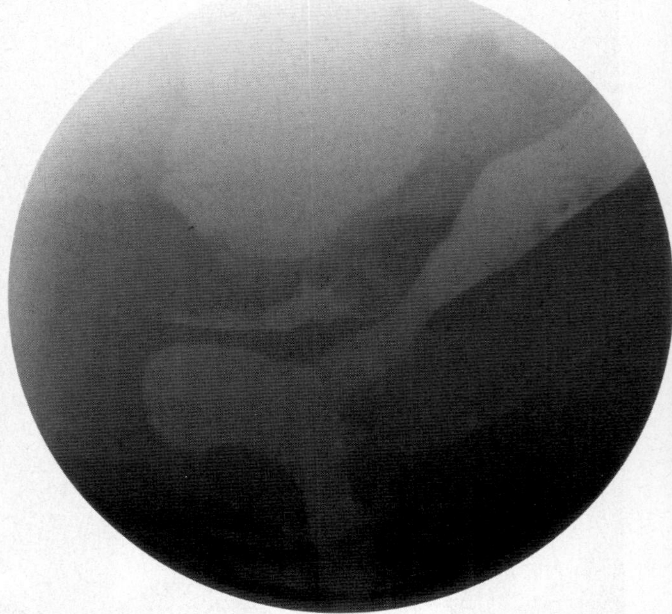

FIGURE 51-87 Triple-contrast radiograph demonstrates large anterior rectocele. Contrast material is also in the vagina and small intestine.

was responsible for continued problems. Postoperative biofeedback therapy is appropriate in these cases. Defecography evaluation is helpful to distinguish these problems before surgery.

Constipation

Constipation is a symptom, and it is often used by patients to describe different problems. It occurs frequently in older populations; in one survey, 50% of women and 30% of men older than 65 years were affected. Although functional constipation appears to occur most often in older patients, a small subset of patients present at a young age with severe unremitting symptoms. These patients are evaluated differently (see later). Although most individuals describe constipation in terms of reduced stool frequency, up to 25% use the term to indicate straining, excessive pushing, or a feeling of incomplete defecation. Normal stool frequencies range from three times weekly to three times daily. The causes of constipation are numerous, but the evaluation of constipation is relatively straightforward and the indications for surgery are few (Fig. 51-88). The initial evaluation of constipation should elicit information about acuteness of symptoms, stool frequency, changes in stool form, presence or absence of blood in the stool, new medications, and any newly diagnosed illnesses. The physical examination should always include a rectal examination and proctoscopy. New-onset constipation can be divided into categories for further diagnostic consideration. These categories are depression or debilitation, new medications, endocrine conditions such as hypothyroidism, and obstructed defecation. For our purposes, we focus on surgically correctable causes while recognizing that most constipation is chronic and functional and is rectified simply by the addition of fluid and fiber to the diet.

A patient whose symptoms include straining and incomplete defecation with a normal stool frequency should be evaluated for obstructive defecation. The best way to obtain the most information is through the physical examination and defecography. Symptomatic rectoceles are those that fail to empty completely on defecography. Associated anatomic abnormalities (e.g., vaginal

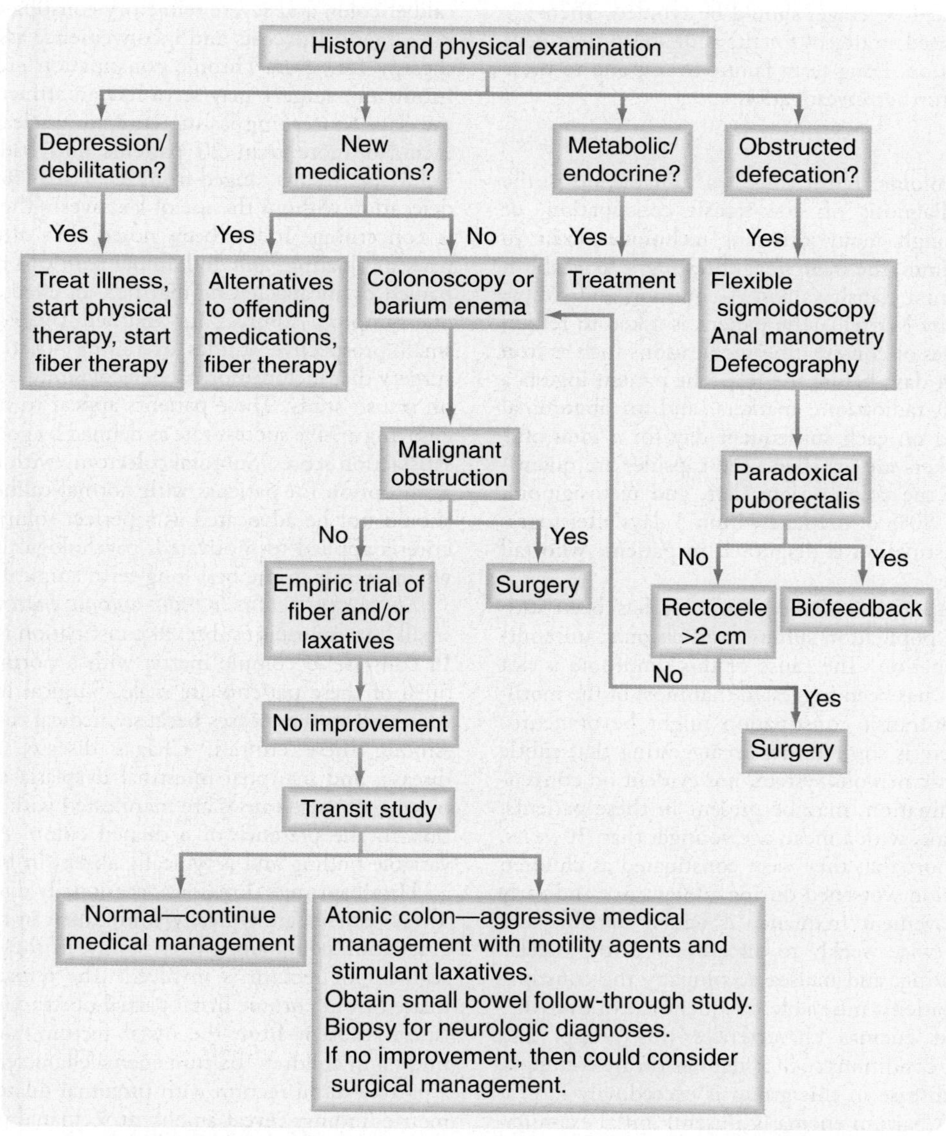

FIGURE 51-88 Algorithm for management of patients with constipation.

vault prolapse, enterocele) can be concurrently corrected. Anal manometry with electromyographic recruitment is an invaluable investigatory tool for the patient with normal anatomy and suspected paradoxical puborectalis syndrome. Biofeedback therapy is indicated in these cases. On occasion, surgically correctable rectocele and functional defecatory disorders coexist. In this situation, biofeedback is usually initiated and rectocele repair is done subsequently.

The primary concern for the physician evaluating new-onset constipation is to rule out large bowel malignant disease. A patient who presents with complaints of an acute change in bowel habits should be evaluated by colonoscopy in the absence of obvious causes, such as narcotic use. Suspect medications should be immediately stopped, and reevaluation should take place shortly thereafter. No improvement or a guaiac-positive stool should lead to a colonoscopic examination. Barium enema is acceptable as well, but flexible sigmoidoscopy, even combined with stool guaiac testing, fails to detect 25% of right-sided malignant neoplasms. A normal finding on colonoscopic examination is reassuring and should lead to trials of dietary therapy. Fluid intake should be increased to 2 liters/day at a minimum, and fiber therapy should be instituted. Caffeinated beverages should be avoided. There are many other laxative-based strategies for the short-term treatment of functional constipation. Long-term failure to respond to these strategies necessitates further investigation.

Transit Studies

Measurement of the colonic transit time is a valuable aid in the establishment of a diagnosis of slow-transit constipation, or colonic inertia. Although many different techniques exist to assess colonic transit times, the main goal of testing is to establish whole gut and segmental transit values. A common and simple test has been devised by Martelli. The patient is asked to refrain from the use of laxatives or constipating medications such as iron supplements for 3 to 4 days before the test. The patient ingests a capsule containing 20 radiopaque markers, and an abdominal radiograph is obtained on each subsequent day for a total of 7 days or until the markers are expelled. The capsules are quantified in three areas of the colon—right, left, and rectosigmoid. Normal subjects expel 80% of markers within 5 days after ingestion. Slow-transit constipation is diagnosed in patients who fail to meet these criteria.

Slow-transit constipation: colonic inertia. It has been estimated that 2% of the population suffers from chronic, unremitting functional constipation. The cause of this syndrome is not well understood, but it has been suggested that most of the motility alterations in slow-transit constipation might be of neuropathic origin, and there is some evidence suggesting that subtle alterations of the enteric nervous system, not evident on conventional histologic examination, may be present in these patients. Most patients are female, with a mean age younger than 30 years. Most of them will report that they were constipated as children and that the constipation worsened during adolescence and early adulthood. Bowel movement frequency is widely variable and ranges from once or twice weekly to once every 2 to 3 weeks. Abdominal pain, bloating, and nausea accompany the constipation and make these patients miserable. Frequent use of over-the-counter laxatives and enemas characterizes this group, and concurrent psychiatric conditions such as depression are common. Although malignant disease in this group is exceedingly rare, it should be ruled out. A barium enema is a useful initial examination; not only does it screen for large obvious lesions, but the morphology of the colon and presence of dilation can also be evaluated. A transit study is the next diagnostic step. Biopsies are usually not indicated unless a strong suspicion of neuropathic constipation is harbored. A loss of the argyrophil plexus, with a marked increase in Schwann cells indicating extrinsic damage to the myenteric plexus, may be found. This damage is thought to result from chronic laxative abuse. A delay in gastric emptying and small bowel follow-through has been noted in some patients, implying a global motility problem. This motility problem may be responsible for the mixed surgical outcomes reported.

An aggressive bowel regimen is always the first course of action after the diagnosis of slow-transit constipation. A combination of laxatives, fiber, and polyethylene glycol–based solutions can be helpful. A new class of laxative approved for short-term use is 5-HT_4 receptor agonists. These may prove beneficial and merit investigation.

Surgery for idiopathic colonic inertia is controversial. The most commonly described procedure is subtotal colectomy with ileorectal anastomosis. Traditionally, only patients with symptoms in the setting of megacolon or megarectum were considered for operative intervention, but now more patients with a normal-caliber colon and severe refractory constipation are being referred for surgery. The costs and inconvenience associated with medical therapy for severe chronic constipation are not inconsiderable. Intuitively, surgery may seem like an attractive option. However, the data concerning lasting cure are unclear. In most series that included more than 20 patients and had longer than 2-year follow-up, results ranged from 33% to 94% success rates (regular defecation without the use of laxatives). The wide range of results is concerning. It has been noted that often the symptoms of nausea, bloating, and abdominal pain can persist and be accompanied by incapacitating diarrhea. In effect, many patients trade one symptom complex for another. There have been only a few small prospective studies exercising strict selection criteria for surgery that include normal defecography results and diffuse delay on transit study. These patients appear to fare best in follow-up, enjoying a 94% success rate as defined by good or excellent patient satisfaction scores. Subtotal colectomy with ileorectal anastomosis is an option for patients with normal-caliber colonic inertia but should not be advocated as a perfect solution. Careful selection criteria applied to motivated, psychologically well-adjusted individuals result in the best long-term surgical results.

Slow-transit constipation: colonic inertia with megacolon. A small but important subset of constipation is neurologic in origin. In contrast to colonic inertia with a normal colon, as a group, 50% of these patients are male. Surgical intervention is usually indicated in these cases because medical therapy eventually fails. Among these entities, Chagas disease, adult Hirschsprung's disease, and neuronal intestinal dysplasia are considered. Commonly, all these causes are manifested with slow-transit constipation in the presence of a dilated colon. A dilated rectum is a variable finding and is typically absent in Hirschsprung's disease.

Hirschsprung's disease is occasionally diagnosed in adulthood. These patients are typically young men in their 20s with lifelong evacuation complaints. Commonly, in these cases, a short, distal segment of rectum is involved. The remainder of the colon is dilated from chronic distal partial obstruction. Stool is characteristically absent from the distal rectum, similar to the physical finding in children. Barium enema characteristically demonstrates a narrow distal rectum with proximal dilated colon. Anal manometric findings reveal an absent rectoanal inhibitory reflex, indicating that the rectum has lost its neurologically mediated ability to relax in response to the presence of a fecal load. Histologic diagnosis is made on biopsy of the distal rectal mucosa at least 3 cm above the dentate line to avoid the normal aganglionic segment in this area. Suction mucosal and superficial punch biopsies are both diagnostic and can be done in the office setting. Acetylcholinesterase staining of the submucosa and lamina propria reveals an increased number of large brown-stained nerve fibers and is considered 99% accurate in establishing the diagnosis. A discussion of surgical interventions for this problem is found elsewhere in this text (see Chapter 66).

Megacolon is the most common complication of intestinal trypanosomiasis. The organism involved is *Trypanosoma cruzi,* a parasite endemic to South America. Nerve damage resulting from trypanosomiasis causes megacolon and megarectum. Fecal impaction and sigmoid volvulus are the most common complications. Subtotal colectomy for this problem results in a residual dyskinetic rectum; therefore, pull-through procedures with excision of the colon and rectum and creation of an ileal reservoir (ileal J pouch or Park pouch) are preferable.

Neuronal intestinal dysplasia describes two distinct congenital defects of the intestinal mural ganglia. Type A is seen predominantly in children and consists of hypoplasia of the sympathetic innervation. Type B is present in children and adults and is characterized by dysplasia of the submucosal plexus, resulting in weak forward propulsion of stool. On histologic evaluation, hyperplasia and giant ganglia with 7 to 10 nerve cells are present. Acetylcholinesterase staining shows a dense plexus of parasympathetic fibers with increased activity. Laxative therapy in these individuals is usually a short-term strategy, and most patients fail to respond to treatment. Surgical resection with ileorectal anastomosis is the treatment of choice.

SELECTED REFERENCES

Clinical Outcomes of Surgical Therapy Study Group: A comparison of laparoscopically assisted and open colectomy for colon cancer. *N Engl J Med* 350:2050–2059, 2004.

A multi-institutional study demonstrating similar results for laparoscopically assisted colectomy and open colectomy performed for colon cancer.

Corman ML, editor: *Colon and rectal surgery*, ed 5, Philadelphia, 2005, Lippincott Williams & Wilkins.

A surgeon's view of the entire spectrum of colon and rectal surgery. Scattered throughout the text are 139 thumbnail biographical sketches of historical surgeons filled with fun factoids.

Feingold D, Steele SR, Lee S, et al: Practice parameters for the treatment of sigmoid diverticulitis. *Dis Colon Rectum* 57:284–294, 2014.

A comprehensive overview of evidence-based practices related to the surgical management of diverticulitis sponsored by the American Society of Colon and Rectal Surgeons.

Gordon PL, Nivatvongs S, editors: *Principles and practice of surgery for the colon, rectum, and anus*, ed 3, London, 2007, Informa Healthcare.

This text provides excellent anatomic illustrations and detailed descriptions of all aspects of diseases of the colon, rectum, and anus. The discussion of anorectal abscesses and fistula-in-ano is particularly helpful.

Haggitt RC, Glotzbach RE, Soffer EE, et al: Prognostic factors in colorectal carcinomas arising in adenomas: Implications for lesions removed by endoscopic polypectomy. *Gastroenterology* 89:328–336, 1985.

Description of Haggitt's criteria, a classification for polyps with adenocarcinoma that assesses malignant potential according to the depth of invasion.

Miles WE: Pathology of spread of cancer of rectum and its bearing on surgery of cancerous rectum. *Surg Gynecol Obstet* 52:350–359, 1931.

Classic article describing the lymphatic pathways whereby rectal cancer spreads, providing the rationale for abdominal perineal resection as a superior operation to perineal proctectomy.

Sauer R, Becker H, Hohenberger W, et al: Preoperative versus postoperative chemoradiotherapy for rectal cancer. *N Engl J Med* 351:1731–1740, 2004.

The only randomized controlled trial of preoperative versus postoperative chemoradiation that has been done, which demonstrated superiority of the neoadjuvant technique.

Vogelstein B, Fearon ER, Hamilton SR, et al: Genetic alterations during colorectal-tumor development. *N Engl J Med* 319:525–532, 1988.

An excellent description of the most common molecular pathways in the development of colorectal adenocarcinoma.

Wolff BG, Fleshman JW, Beck DE, editors: *The ASCRS textbook of colon and rectal surgery*, New York, 2016, Springer.

This text is sponsored by the American Society of Colon and Rectal Surgeons, with chapters written by recognized authorities in their field.

REFERENCES

1. Pai R, Kang G: Microbes in the gut: A digestable account of host-symbiont interactions. *Indian J Med Res* 128:587–594, 2008.
2. Parkes GC, Sanderson JD, Whelan K: The mechanisms and efficacy of probiotics in the prevention of *Clostridium difficile*–associated diarrhoea. *Lancet Infect Dis* 9:237–244, 2009.
3. McFarland LV: Evidence-based review of probiotics for antibiotic-associated diarrhea and *Clostridium difficile* infections. *Anaerobe* 15:274–280, 2009.
4. Wong JM, de Souza R, Kendall CW, et al: Colonic health: Fermentation and short chain fatty acids. *J Clin Gastroenterol* 40:235–243, 2006.
5. Englesbe MJ, Brooks L, Kubus J, et al: A statewide assessment of surgical site infection following colectomy: The role

of oral antibiotics. *Ann Surg* 252:514–519, discussion 519–520, 2010.
6. Guenaga KF, Matos D, Wille-Jorgensen P: Mechanical bowel preparation for elective colorectal surgery. *Cochrane Database Syst Rev* (9):CD001544, 2011.
7. Lewis RT: Oral versus systemic antibiotic prophylaxis in elective colon surgery: A randomized study and meta-analysis send a message from the 1990s. *Can J Surg* 45:173–180, 2002.
8. Cannon JA, Altom LK, Deierhoi RJ, et al: Preoperative oral antibiotics reduce surgical site infection following elective colorectal resections. *Dis Colon Rectum* 55:1160–1166, 2012.
9. American Society of Colon and Rectal Surgeons Committee Members, Wound Ostomy Continence Nurses Society Committee Members: ASCRS and WOCN joint position statement on the value of preoperative stoma marking for patients undergoing fecal ostomy surgery. *J Wound Ostomy Continence Nurs* 34:627–628, 2007.
10. Francone TD, Saleem A, Read TA, et al: Ultimate fate of the leaking intestinal anastomosis: Does leak mean permanent stoma? *J Gastrointest Surg* 14:987–992, 2010.
11. Zhuang CL, Ye XZ, Zhang XD, et al: Enhanced recovery after surgery programs versus traditional care for colorectal surgery: A meta-analysis of randomized controlled trials. *Dis Colon Rectum* 56:667–678, 2013.
12. Sheth AA, Longo W, Floch MH: Diverticular disease and diverticulitis. *Am J Gastroenterol* 103:1550–1556, 2008.
13. Janes SE, Meagher A, Frizelle FA: Management of diverticulitis. *BMJ* 332:271–275, 2006.
14. Anaya DA, Flum DR: Risk of emergency colectomy and colostomy in patients with diverticular disease. *Arch Surg* 140:681–685, 2005.
15. Strate LL, Liu YL, Syngal S, et al: Nut, corn, and popcorn consumption and the incidence of diverticular disease. *JAMA* 300:907–914, 2008.
16. Chapman JR, Dozois EJ, Wolff BG, et al: Diverticulitis: A progressive disease? Do multiple recurrences predict less favorable outcomes? *Ann Surg* 243:876–883, discussion 880–883, 2006.
17. Rafferty J, Shellito P, Hyman NH, et al: Practice parameters for sigmoid diverticulitis. *Dis Colon Rectum* 49:939–944, 2006.
18. Rocco A, Compare D, Caruso F, et al: Treatment options for uncomplicated diverticular disease of the colon. *J Clin Gastroenterol* 43:803–808, 2009.
19. Dignass A, Lindsay JO, Sturm A, et al: Second European evidence-based consensus on the diagnosis and management of ulcerative colitis part 2: Current management. *J Crohns Colitis* 6:991–1030, 2012.
20. Blonski W, Buchner AM, Lichtenstein GR: Treatment of ulcerative colitis. *Curr Opin Gastroenterol* 30:84–96, 2014.
21. Kiran RP, Khoury W, Church JM, et al: Colorectal cancer complicating inflammatory bowel disease: Similarities and differences between Crohn's and ulcerative colitis based on three decades of experience. *Ann Surg* 252:330–335, 2010.
22. Edge SB, Byrd DR, Compton CC, et al: *AJCC cancer staging manual*, ed 7, New York, 2010, Springer-Verlag.
23. Khan KJ, Dubinsky MC, Ford AC, et al: Efficacy of immunosuppressive therapy for inflammatory bowel disease: A systematic review and meta-analysis. *Am J Gastroenterol* 106:630–642, 2011.
24. Metcalf DR, Nivatvongs S, Sullivan TM, et al: A technique of extending small-bowel mesentery for ileal pouch–anal anastomosis: Report of a case. *Dis Colon Rectum* 51:363–364, 2008.
25. Remzi FH, Fazio VW, Gorgun E, et al: The outcome after restorative proctocolectomy with or without defunctioning ileostomy. *Dis Colon Rectum* 49:470–477, 2006.
26. Shen B, Fazio VW, Remzi FH, et al: Clinical approach to diseases of ileal pouch–anal anastomosis. *Am J Gastroenterol* 100:2796–2807, 2005.
27. Cohen SH, Gerding DN, Johnson S, et al: Clinical practice guidelines for *Clostridium difficile* infection in adults: 2010 update by the Society for Healthcare Epidemiology of America (SHEA) and the Infectious Diseases Society of America (IDSA). *Infect Control Hosp Epidemiol* 31:431–455, 2010.
28. Eaton SR, Mazuski JE: Overview of severe *Clostridium difficile* infection. *Crit Care Clin* 29:827–839, 2013.
29. Neal MD, Alverdy JC, Hall DE, et al: Diverting loop ileostomy and colonic lavage: An alternative to total abdominal colectomy for the treatment of severe, complicated *Clostridium difficile* associated disease. *Ann Surg* 254:423–427, discussion 427–429, 2011.
30. Jemal A, Siegel R, Xu J, et al: Cancer statistics, 2010. *CA Cancer J Clin* 60:277–300, 2010.
31. Sampson JR, Jones S, Dolwani S, et al: MutYH (MYH) and colorectal cancer. *Biochem Soc Trans* 33:679–683, 2005.
32. Karapetis CS, Khambata-Ford S, Jonker DJ, et al: K-ras mutations and benefit from cetuximab in advanced colorectal cancer. *N Engl J Med* 359:1757–1765, 2008.
33. Habr-Gama A, Perez RO, Nadalin W, et al: Long-term results of preoperative chemoradiation for distal rectal cancer correlation between final stage and survival. *J Gastrointest Surg* 9:90–99, discussion 99-101, 2005.
34. O'Neill BD, Brown G, Heald RJ, et al: Non-operative treatment after neoadjuvant chemoradiotherapy for rectal cancer. *Lancet Oncol* 8:625–633, 2007.
35. Guillem JG, Diaz-Gonzalez JA, Minsky BD, et al: cT3N0 rectal cancer: Potential overtreatment with preoperative chemoradiotherapy is warranted. *J Clin Oncol* 26:368–373, 2008.
36. Nyasavajjala SM, Shaw AG, Khan AQ, et al: Neoadjuvant chemo-radiotherapy and rectal cancer: Can the UK watch and wait with Brazil? *Colorectal Dis* 12:33–36, 2010.
37. Stephens RJ, Thompson LC, Quirke P, et al: Impact of short-course preoperative radiotherapy for rectal cancer on patients' quality of life: Data from the Medical Research Council CR07/National Cancer Institute of Canada Clinical Trials Group C016 randomized clinical trial. *J Clin Oncol* 28:4233–4239, 2010.
38. Okabe S, Shia J, Nash G, et al: Lymph node metastasis in T1 adenocarcinoma of the colon and rectum. *J Gastrointest Surg* 8:1032–1039, discussion 1039–1040, 2004.
39. Bentrem DJ, Okabe S, Wong WD, et al: T1 adenocarcinoma of the rectum: Transanal excision or radical surgery? *Ann Surg* 242:472–477, discussion 477-479, 2005.
40. Kesisoglou I, Sapalidis K: Treatment of early rectal cancer. *Tech Coloproctol* 14(Suppl 1):S33–S34, 2010.
41. West NP, Finan PJ, Anderin C, et al: Evidence of the oncologic superiority of cylindrical abdominoperineal excision for low rectal cancer. *J Clin Oncol* 26:3517–3522, 2008.

42. Schmidt CE, Bestmann B, Kuchler T, et al: Ten-year historic cohort of quality of life and sexuality in patients with rectal cancer. *Dis Colon Rectum* 48:483–492, 2005.
43. Matthiessen P, Hallbook O, Rutegard J, et al: Defunctioning stoma reduces symptomatic anastomotic leakage after low anterior resection of the rectum for cancer: A randomized multicenter trial. *Ann Surg* 246:207–214, 2007.
44. Ho YH: Techniques for restoring bowel continuity and function after rectal cancer surgery. *World J Gastroenterol* 12:6252–6260, 2006.
45. Remzi FH, Fazio VW, Gorgun E, et al: Quality of life, functional outcome, and complications of coloplasty pouch after low anterior resection. *Dis Colon Rectum* 48:735–743, 2005.
46. Rullier E, Laurent C, Bretagnol F, et al: Sphincter-saving resection for all rectal carcinomas: The end of the 2-cm distal rule. *Ann Surg* 241:465–469, 2005.
47. Cornish JA, Tilney HS, Heriot AG, et al: A meta-analysis of quality of life for abdominoperineal excision of rectum versus anterior resection for rectal cancer. *Ann Surg Oncol* 14:2056–2068, 2007.

52 CHAPTER

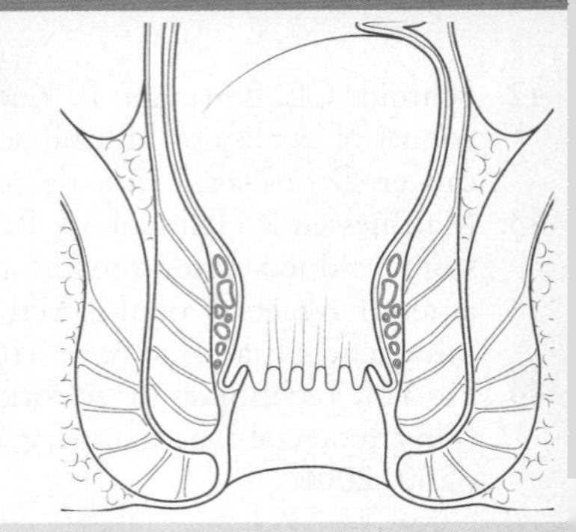

Anus

Amit Merchea, David W. Larson

OUTLINE

DISORDERS OF THE ANAL CANAL

The anal canal remains an area of medicine and surgery plagued by obscurity and limited provider knowledge. Many conditions are in fact common and benign, but some lead to incapacitating interference with the patient's daily life. Provider limitations in both experience and traditional knowledge often lead to misdiagnosis or maltreatment. Therefore, attempts to improve our fund of knowledge of the anatomy and function of the anal canal and the basic physiology of the pelvic floor should facilitate accurate diagnosis and management of both common and rare conditions.

Anatomy

The anal canal extends from the anorectal ring at the most distal aspect of the rectum to the skin of the anal verge and is approximately 4 cm in length. The internal and external sphincter muscles along with the pelvic floor structures contribute significantly to the regulation of defecation and continence. The anus is bounded by the coccyx posteriorly, the ischiorectal fossa bilaterally, and the perineal body and either vagina or urethra anteriorly.

The sphincter apparatus of the anal canal consists of the internal and external sphincters and can be considered as two tubular structures overlying each other. The circular muscle layer of the rectum continues distally to form the thickened and rounded internal sphincter, which terminates approximately 1.5 cm below the dentate line, just cephalad to the external sphincter (intersphincteric groove). The external sphincter is elliptical and surrounds the internal sphincter superiorly and is continuous with the puborectalis and levator ani muscles (Fig. 52-1). The perineal body is formed by the constitution of the external sphincter, bulbospongiosus, and transverse perineal muscles anteriorly. The paired levator ani muscles form the bulk of the pelvic floor, and their fibers decussate medially with the contralateral side to fuse with the perineal body around the prostate or vagina.

The internal sphincter is tonically contracted independent of voluntary control. It receives innervation by the autonomic nervous system. The external sphincter, under voluntary control, is innervated by the inferior rectal branch of the internal pudendal nerve and perineal branch of the fourth sacral nerve. Thus, the loss of bilateral S3 nerve roots (either surgically or otherwise) will result in incontinence. If all sacral nerve roots on either side are sacrificed, normal function is preserved. Similarly, if S1-S3 remains intact on only one side, the patient would maintain anorectal control.

Distal to the anal verge, the perianal skin becomes anoderm, which is a modified squamous lining without hair. At the dentate line, the squamous epithelium transitions to columnar epithelium; this region is referred to as the anal transition zone. Proximal to this area, the lining becomes exclusively gastrointestinal columnar epithelium.

Physiology

The process of defecation and maintenance of continence constitute the principal function of the anus. Various factors affect our ability to effectively achieve these functions—the coordinated sensory and muscular activities of the anus and pelvic floor, the compliance of the rectum, and the consistency, volume, and timing of the fecal movements are all critical to avoidance of fecal incontinence or defecatory disorders.

As the external sphincter contracts, the anal canal lengthens. With straining, it shortens. The internal anal sphincter imparts the resting pressure (~90 cm H_2O). Squeeze pressure, generated by external sphincter contraction, more than doubles resting pressure. The pressure differential between the rectum and anal canal (low to high) is the principal mechanism that provides continence. The anorectal angle is the angle between the anal canal and the rectum. This angle is approximately 75 to 90 degrees at rest and becomes more obtuse, straightening with straining and evacuation. The ability of the puborectalis to relax and to allow this straightening of the angle facilitates defecation.

Diagnostic Evaluation of the Anus

Anorectal disorders are common. Therefore, basic principles including careful history and physical examination should occur before elaborate testing.

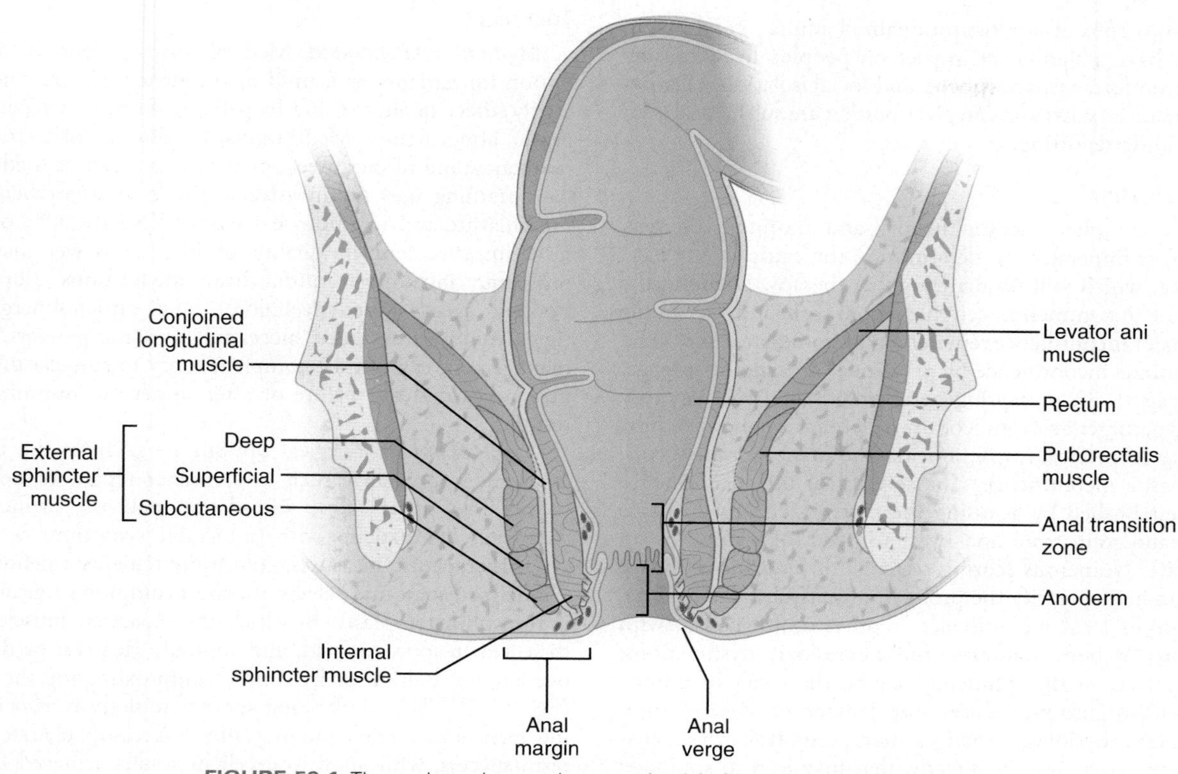

FIGURE 52-1 The anal canal musculature and pelvic floor muscles are depicted.

History

It is important to elicit symptoms of pain, bleeding, discharge (purulent or fecal), and any alteration of bowel habits (frequency, consistency). Other past medical, social (including sexual), and family history may be relevant in diagnosing anorectal disease.

Bleeding is among the most common presenting symptoms of diseases of the anus and large bowel. Specific details about the nature of the bleeding can help localize the source in the alimentary tract. Blood that drips, is separate from stools, and is bright red is usually seen with rectal outlet bleeding, as from internal hemorrhoids. Blood on toilet tissue may be associated with minor hemorrhoidal disease but also with anal fissure, although anal fissure is typically accompanied by severe pain at defecation. Passage of clots or melena may indicate a more proximal source of bleeding. One must always give consideration to evaluation of the more proximal bowel to exclude serious conditions, such as cancer. This should be of prime importance when initial anorectal examination cannot confirm a bleeding source, when the patient has greater than average risk of cancer, or when bleeding does not resolve promptly after initiation of appropriate treatment.

Anal or rectal pain occurring during or immediately after stooling is another common presenting complaint. Severe pain during defecation, often described by patients as passing glass, is usually associated with anal fissure. Pain, either with or without defecation, that is throbbing in nature is most often seen with an abscess or poorly draining fistula. Patients may also complain of purulent, mucoid, or feculent discharge. A deep-seated rectal pain unrelated to defecation often characterizes proctalgia fugax or levator ani syndrome. This is characterized by painful episodes of short duration (<20 to 30 minutes) that are often relieved by walking, warm baths, or other maneuvers.

Physical Examination

Adequate visualization of the external anal anatomy and the anal canal by anoscopy requires appropriate positioning of the patient (either left lateral or, more commonly, prone jackknife) and good lighting. Skin tags, excoriations, scars, and any changes in color or appearance of perianal skin should be easily recognized. A patulous anus may indicate incontinence and possibly prolapse. Inspection while straining (even with the patient on the commode) may help differentiate the presence of hemorrhoids from rectal prolapse. A careful and systematic digital examination allows the identification of any palpable abnormalities of the anal canal. Finally, the resting tone and strength of the squeeze pressure of the anal sphincter can be assessed.

Anoscopy or proctosigmoidoscopy (flexible or rigid) after enema preparation enables visualization of the anus, rectum, and left colon. Mucosal inflammation is identified by loss of the normal vascular pattern with erythema, granularity, friability, and even ulcerations. Gross lesions (polyps or carcinoma) should be readily identifiable. Biopsy specimens of any suspicious findings should be obtained for histologic diagnosis.

Other investigations, such as stool culture, specialized imaging (ultrasound, magnetic resonance imaging [MRI], defecography), and specialized physiologic testing, may be helpful adjuncts and should be obtained as clinically appropriate.

PELVIC FLOOR DISORDERS

Incontinence

Fecal incontinence is defined as the recurrent uncontrolled passage of fecal material for at least 1 month in an individual with a developmental age older than 4 years. The reported prevalence of fecal incontinence varies considerably. It has been estimated to occur in 2% to 15% of noninstitutionalized adults.[1] Fecal incontinence can have a significant impact on people's lives, causing physical discomfort, embarrassment, and social isolation. Furthermore, the financial costs and caregiver burden are substantial with real risk of underreporting.

Clinical Evaluation

Obtaining a complete medical history and thorough physical examination is imperative in determining the cause of the fecal incontinence, which will ultimately guide therapy. Defining the extent of the incontinence can be accomplished by a simple history—major incontinence represented by complete loss of solid stool, and minor incontinence by occasional staining or seepage. Mucus seepage from prolapsing hemorrhoids or large secretory villous polyp, urgency from colitis or proctitis, and overflow incontinence from fecal impaction may be inappropriately confused with true incontinence. The severity of the incontinence should be established by assessing the patient's control of flatus and liquid and solid stool and by the impact of symptoms on quality of life. Numerous scoring systems for fecal incontinence exist and can help quantify the problem objectively (Table 52-1).

The cause of fecal incontinence is often multifactorial with combinations of both anatomic and physiologic dysfunctions. Anatomic defects in the sphincter may be the result of trauma from previous surgical procedures, impalement, or obstetric injuries. Moreover, physiologic changes may occur from these anatomic changes, over time or directly, that may lead to sphincter dysfunction, decreased rectal compliance, or decreased sensation. All of these issues may contribute to or have an impact on the degree of incontinence even years after the inciting events.

The most common nonanatomic causes of fecal incontinence should include associated gastrointestinal disorders, such as diarrhea, which can aggravate continence.[2] A physical examination may reveal anatomic abnormalities that account for the incontinence, such as the presence of prolapse, hemorrhoids, or abscess/fistula. A proper digital rectal examination can highlight a weak resting tone and squeeze pressure or a patulous anus and the presence of scars, defects, deformities, or keyhole abnormalities. Endoscopy remains critical to exclude proctitis, impaction, neoplasia, or other rectal mucosal abnormalities that may be contributing factors.

To confirm physical examination findings, the use of focused diagnostic tests may be required. Anorectal manometry confirms the extent of impairment of the internal and external sphincters. Manometry may identify asymmetry, suggesting anatomic defects amenable to repair. Balloon expulsion testing during manometry may demonstrate impairments in rectal sensation. Endoanal ultrasound or MRI may also be employed to detect structural defects of the anal sphincters, rectal wall, and puborectalis muscle.

Treatment

Medical management. Medical management is the initial option for patients with mild incontinence that may not significantly affect quality of life in patients without a reparable anatomic abnormality. Medications to slow transit, to decrease frequency, and to increase stool consistency can be used. Biofeedback training uses noninvasive methods to strengthen the anal musculature and to improve sensation. Nearly 90% of patients note improvement in quality of life.[3] A bowel management program, including antidiarrheal medications (loperamide), bulking agents (methylcellulose), and anticholinergic agents (hyoscyamine), has been successful for some patients.[4] Medical management can also be complementary to surgical therapy and may be carried out before or after surgery to optimize surgical results.

Surgical repair. Surgical options range from the traditional anatomic approaches, such as sphincter repair, to newer techniques like sacral nerve stimulation and the artificial bowel sphincter. For patients with intractable symptoms or failure of other therapeutic measures, colostomy remains a definitive cure. For defined anatomic defects, the most common surgical approach is the sphincteroplasty, in which the separated muscle ends are dissected, reapproximated, and sutured. This can be done in an overlapping fashion or by simply reapproximating the sphincter (Fig. 52-2).[5] The overlapping sphincteroplasty is associated with low rates of morbidity and mortality and reasonable rates of short-term success, with good to excellent results achieved in 55% to 68% of patients.[6] Long-term results of sphincteroplasty have demonstrated a deterioration of continence over time, with only 40% having good to excellent control at a median follow-up of 10 years.[7]

The use of injectable materials for the treatment of fecal incontinence has recently gained attention. In this procedure, a bulking agent (silicone, collagen, carbon microbeads, or dextranomer–hyaluronic acid) is injected into the intersphincteric space to augment the internal anal sphincter. There are limited data for these approaches; however, a single randomized controlled trial did demonstrate short-term improvement in 50% of patients undergoing injection with dextranomer–hyaluronic acid (Solesta; Salix Pharmaceuticals, Raleigh, NC).[8]

More complex approaches to treatment of fecal incontinence include the dynamic graciloplasty, sacral nerve stimulator, and artificial bowel sphincter. The use of the gracilis muscle as a flap encircling the anal canal is reserved for patients in whom the bulk of the anal sphincter is missing and requires complete reconstruction. Results of graciloplasty have been favorable, with the majority of patients maintaining continence and the ability to defer defecation at 5 years.[9] Sacral nerve stimulation has been traditionally used in patients in whom the anal sphincter is intact but there

TABLE 52-1 Cleveland Clinic Fecal Incontinence Score

TYPE	NEVER	RARELY	SOMETIMES	USUALLY	ALWAYS
Solid	0	1	2	3	4
Liquid	0	1	2	3	4
Gas	0	1	2	3	4
Pad use	0	1	2	3	4
Quality of life impact	0	1	2	3	4

From Jorge JM, Wexner SD: Etiology and management of fecal incontinence. *Dis Colon Rectum* 36:77–97, 1993.
Responses are scored and summed. A score of 0 indicates perfect continence, 20 is complete incontinence; rarely, <1/month; sometimes, >1/month; usually, >1/week; always, >1/day.

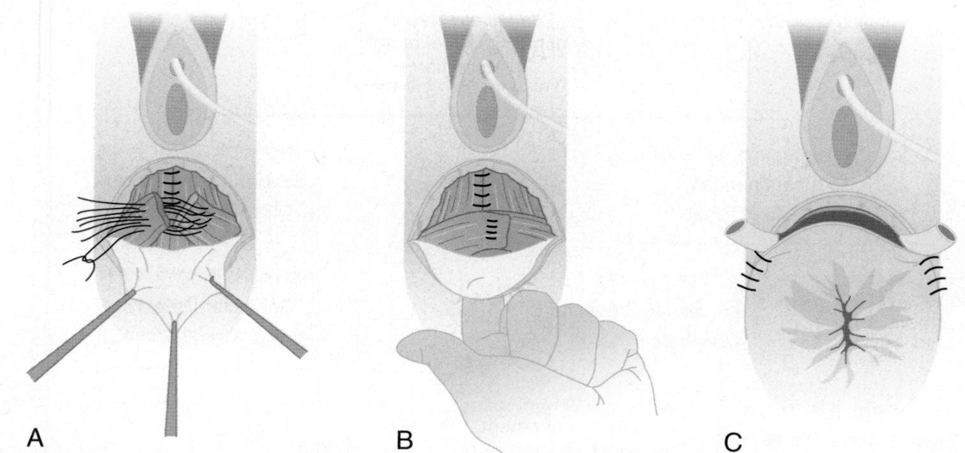

FIGURE 52-2 Overlapping Sphincteroplasty. A, An anterior curvilinear incision is made on the perineum between the anus and vagina. The disrupted ends of the external sphincter are dissected free, and the muscle ends are overlapped and reapproximated with suture. A levatorplasty is also concurrently performed. **B,** Digital rectal examination can judge for appropriate tightness of the repair. **C,** The incision is then reapproximated. Some surgeons may leave drains or a small gap in the closure to allow drainage.

is an associated neurologic injury or poor innervation. A prospective multicenter trial demonstrated success rates of up to 85% at 2 years with a decrease in the number of incontinent episodes per week by approximately 70%.[10] More recent investigation has been conducted to determine its effectiveness in the setting of a defined anal sphincter defect (<180 degrees); many patients have noted significant improvement in these settings.[11] With increasing use of sacral nerve stimulation, the use of an artificial bowel sphincter has been limited. Complications associated with its use are erosion, infection, and obstruction. A review had demonstrated little change in the rate of device explantation or infection in spite of novel surgical techniques and approaches to placement.[12] An algorithm for the treatment of fecal incontinence is presented (Fig. 52-3).

Prolapse of the Rectum

Pathogenesis and Clinical Presentation

Prolapse of the rectum, or procidentia, is an uncommon problem (incidence of 0.25% to 0.4%) characterized by eversion of the rectum through the anus.[13] The prolapse may be complete, characterized by protrusion of all layers of the rectal wall, or partial, characterized by a mucosal prolapse only. Risk factors that increase the risk of prolapse include female sex, age older than 40 years, multiparity, vaginal delivery, prior pelvic surgery, chronic straining, dementia, and pelvic floor anatomic defects.

The symptoms of early prolapse may be vague, including discomfort or a sensation of incomplete evacuation during defecation, bleeding, and seepage. Many patients have a long history of constipation and straining. When prolapse is complete, protrusion of the rectum is generally obvious. In patients with occult prolapse, a feeling of pressure and sensation of incomplete evacuation may be the only symptoms.

Preoperative Evaluation

The preoperative assessment should focus on defining the extent of the prolapse; the presence of associated conditions, such as constipation and pelvic floor dysfunction; and other potentially related complications, such as incontinence. Any of these factors may influence management. Nearly 50% of patients have constipation, and the majority have fecal incontinence.[14] If the presence and extent of the prolapse are not readily apparent, examination while straining on the commode may make it more evident. Complete prolapse demonstrates full-thickness rectal protrusion with concentric rings (Fig. 52-4); this should be differentiated from prolapsed hemorrhoids, which demonstrate radial folds. Associated complex pelvic floor abnormalities (cystocele, enterocele, rectocele, vaginal vault prolapse) can be assessed by dynamic pelvic floor MRI; identification of these additional pathologic processes may alter the surgical approach.

Complete lower gastrointestinal tract evaluations should be performed as indicated. On endoscopy, a solitary rectal ulcer 6 to 8 cm anteriorly may be evidenced by redness or ulceration of the anterior rectal wall. Additional tests can be ordered but have limited value and are not typically required. Manometry identifies the presence of sphincter damage but does not predict recovery. Despite the ability of pudendal nerve terminal motor latency to predict a high risk for postoperative anal incontinence, it rarely influences the management. In patients with severe constipation, colonic transit studies may be valuable; although it is exceedingly rare, these patients may respond better to a more extensive colonic resection.

Surgical Correction

Surgical repair of rectal prolapse may be conducted through a perineal approach (Delorme or Altemeier procedure) or an abdominal approach (rectopexy with or without resection and mesh fixation). Insufficient data exist to definitely demonstrate which surgical approach is superior.[15,16] The perineal approach is less morbid for the patient but has a higher recurrence rate; thus, it is best suited for patients with high operative risk and limited life expectancy. Abdominal approaches (laparoscopic, robotic, or open) are preferred for younger patients, particularly those with constipation or associated pelvic floor disorders.

Perineal procedures. For patients with a short (3 to 4 cm) prolapse, a mucosal sleeve resection with muscularis plication (Delorme procedure) is ideal (Fig. 52-5). Recurrence rates associated with this procedure range from 10% to 15%. Mortality and major morbidity are low, approximately 1% and 14%,

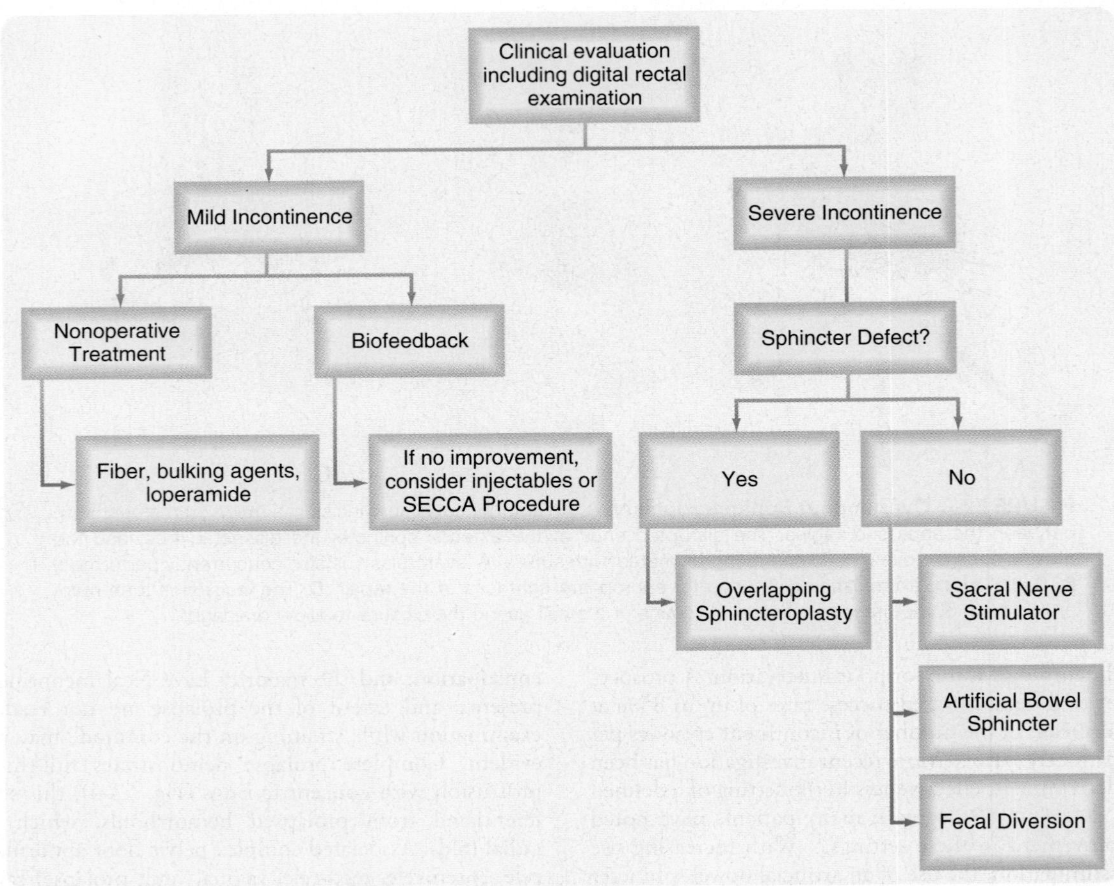

FIGURE 52-3 Algorithm for treatment of fecal incontinence.

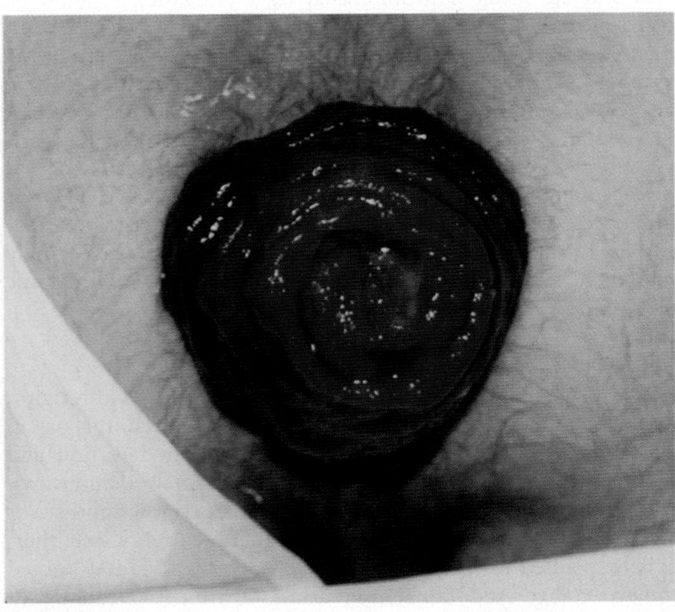

FIGURE 52-4 Full-thickness rectal prolapse. The prolapsed rectal wall appears as concentric folds circumferentially. With prolapsed hemorrhoids, these concentric rings are not seen. (Courtesy Mayo Foundation for Medical Education and Research, Rochester, Minn.)

respectively.[17] Improvement in incontinence is observed in as many as 69% of patients. Prolapse recurrence is common and is likely underestimated because this procedure is performed in patients with limited life expectancies and therefore short follow-up.

The Altemeier procedure (perineal rectosigmoidectomy) involves a full-thickness rectal resection, starting just above the dentate line. The bowel and associated mesentery are resected. Because the pelvic cavity is entered, care must be taken to avoid injury to the small bowel. A full-thickness anastomosis is completed once the prolapsed bowel is resected. For patients with incontinence, a levatorplasty may be added to the resection. Long-term results are similar to those described for the Delorme procedure.[18]

Abdominal procedures. The abdominal approaches include rectal mobilization to the pelvic floor, with or without anterior resection (dependent on the presence of constipation), followed by rectopexy of the rectum to the sacral promontory, with or without mesh. Preservation of the lateral stalks is believed to improve function but results in a greater risk for recurrence. If resection and anastomosis are being performed, they should be performed high rather than low in the rectum; this decreases the risk of anastomotic leak. Once it is completely mobilized, the rectum is retracted cephalad out of the pelvis and secured with sutures at the level of the sacral promontory. Resection with rectopexy is generally completed in those patients with symptoms of constipation and is associated with low recurrence rates (0% to 9%). Constipation has been shown to improve in up to 50% of

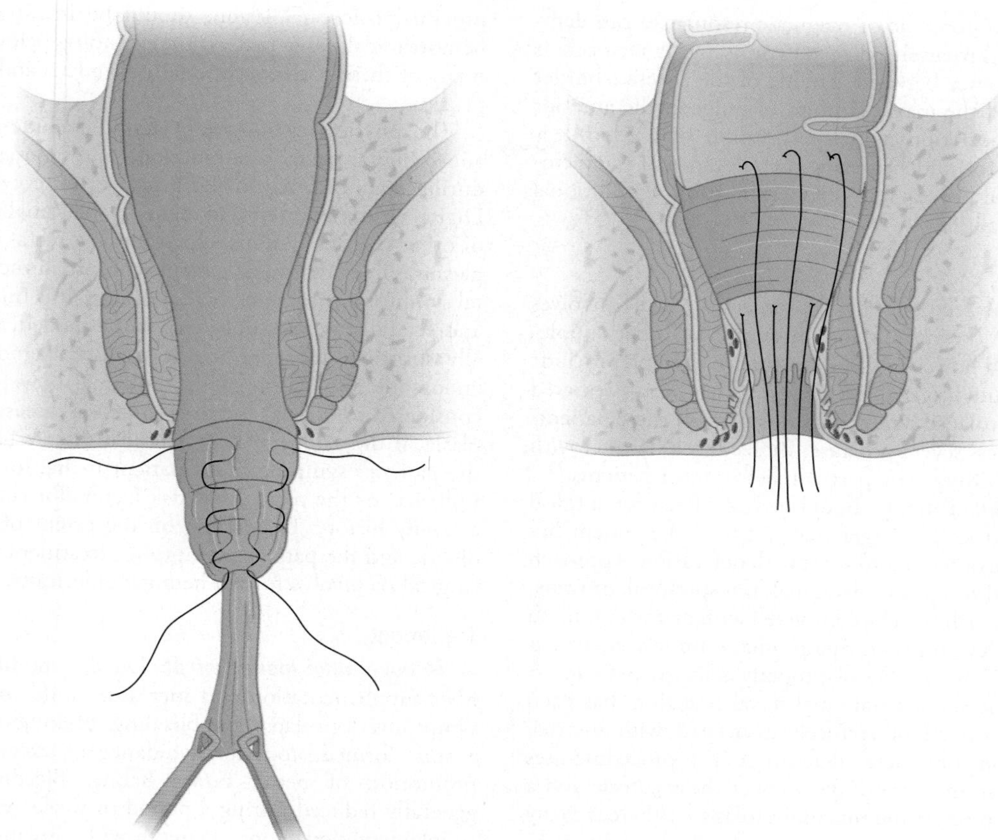

FIGURE 52-5 Delorme Repair. Mucosal sleeve resection is performed and followed by muscle plication, anastomosing the proximal mucosal resection site to the distal mucosa, proximal to the dentate. (Courtesy Mayo Foundation for Medical Education and Research, Rochester, Minn.)

patients. Minimally invasive (laparoscopic or robotic assisted) techniques have been described; however, meta-analyses have yet to identify a significant improvement in function or recurrence rates with this approach compared with more traditional open techniques.[16,19] The universal benefits of minimally invasive approaches (reduced pain, shorter return of bowel function, decreased length of stay) are still evident.

Rectopexy with mesh fixation, and no resection, avoids the risks for resection and anastomosis with low recurrence rates. The mesh can be placed anteriorly or posteriorly. Complications can result, however, from the presence of a foreign body, and symptoms of constipation are often aggravated. In one described technique of anterior mesh fixation, the rectum is minimally mobilized in an effort to avoid autonomic nerve injury and to decrease the risk of increased constipation and poor function postoperatively.[20] In this technique, the right lateral peritoneum is incised overlying the sacral promontory and extended along the rectum toward the pouch of Douglas. Denonvilliers fascia is incised, opening the rectovaginal septum. No rectal mobilization or lateral dissection is performed. A piece of permanent mesh is fixed to the ventral distal rectum and to the sacral promontory using nonabsorbable sutures. Care is taken to not place the rectum on traction. The incised peritoneum can be closed over the mesh, protecting it from the abdominal viscera. Reviews of this technique have demonstrated a low morbidity with less than 5% risk of recurrence.[21]

Incontinence and Biofeedback

Incontinence secondary to pudendal nerve damage from chronic stretching may improve after prolapse repair, except in those patients in whom the lateral stalks are divided. Although the majority of patients report excellent satisfaction with results, the most common reasons for dissatisfaction include persistent constipation or incontinence. The role of biofeedback for treating persistent postoperative incontinence or for preventing recurrent prolapse in patients with pelvic floor dysfunction has not been well established. However, it can be beneficial to some patients, and it is noninvasive.

Rectocele

Clinical Evaluation

Rectocele, like sigmoidocele and enterocele, is associated with a posterior vaginal defect. Symptoms include a vaginal bulge or prolapse of the anterior rectal wall into the vagina, obstructed defecation, and, in many cases, the need to digitally compress the vagina or to digitize the rectum or perineum to evacuate. The cause of rectocele is likely to be multifactorial as it is often associated with a number of other pelvic floor disorders, including constipation, paradoxical muscle contraction, and neuropathies or anatomic disorders from vaginal childbirth.[22] A careful rectovaginal examination will reveal the size of the defect where the rectum prolapse extends to the vagina.

Defecography (fluoroscopic or magnetic resonance) can demonstrate dynamic information on rectal emptying. A rectocele is diagnosed if the distance between the line of the anterior border of the anal canal and the maximal point of bulge of the anterior rectal wall into the posterior vaginal wall is more than 2 cm. It is the most useful test for understanding the relevance of the rectocele in the defecation process and for identification of additional pelvic floor abnormalities.

Treatment

Treatment, when the rectocele is symptomatic, initially involves the optimization of bowel function through diet, fiber supplementation, and good bowel habits. Nonsurgical therapies include the use of pessaries and biofeedback. A pessary has been associated with resolution of prolapse symptoms, but many of these patients are older and have less severe prolapse. Biofeedback has met with limited success, providing only partial relief in most patients.[23]

Surgical treatment. Patients should be considered for surgical correction if the rectocele is larger than 2 cm or the patient has to digitize the vagina or rectum to assist with defecation. Approach to surgical repair is through a transvaginal, transperineal, or transanal technique. All repairs can be completed with or without mesh and may include a levatorplasty. Symptomatic improvement has been observed in 73% to 79% of properly selected patients. A newer technique, the stapled transanal rectal resection, has been investigated for treatment of rectocele associated with internal rectal prolapse causing obstructed defecation. This procedure uses two circular staplers, one anteriorly to resect the rectocele and a second posteriorly to resect the mucosal prolapse. Whereas many patients note improvement in their symptoms, this has been associated with a high rate of fecal urgency and potential for anal stenosis.[24]

COMMON BENIGN ANAL DISORDERS

Hemorrhoids

Presentation and Evaluation

Hemorrhoids are normal, vascular tissue within the submucosa located in the anal canal. They are thought to aid in anal continence by providing bulk to the anal canal. They are typically located in the left lateral, right anterior, and right posterior quadrants of the canal. Hemorrhoids can be external or internal; the differentiation is based on physical examination. External hemorrhoids are distal to the dentate line and are covered with anoderm; these may periodically engorge, causing pain and difficulty with hygiene. Thrombosis of these external hemorrhoids results in severe pain. Internal hemorrhoids are characterized by bright red, painless bleeding or prolapse. Internal hemorrhoids are stratified into four grades that summarize their severity and influence treatment options (Table 52-2). The patient may report dripping or squirting of blood in the toilet. Occult blood loss resulting in anemia is rare, and other causes of anemia, such as a more proximal colorectal lesion, should be investigated. Prolapse of hemorrhoidal tissue may occur, extending below the dentate line; many of these patients complain of mucus and fecal leakage and pruritus.

TABLE 52-2 Internal Hemorrhoids Grading

GRADE	SYMPTOMS AND SIGNS
First degree	Bleeding; no prolapse
Second degree	Prolapse with spontaneous reduction
Third degree	Prolapse requiring manual reduction
Fourth degree	Prolapsed, cannot be reduced

The physical examination should include inspection of the anus, digital rectal examination, and anoscopy. Examination during straining may make prolapse more evident (Fig. 52-6). Digital examination should focus on anal canal tone and exclusion of other palpable lesions, especially low rectal or anal canal neoplasms. Given that most patients confuse numerous other anorectal symptoms for hemorrhoidal disease, it is imperative that other anorectal diseases be considered and excluded. Anoscopy is generally sufficient to arrive at the correct diagnosis, but complete endoscopic evaluation of the proximal bowel should always be considered to exclude proximal mucosal disease, particularly neoplasia, if the extent of hemorrhoidal disease is incongruent with the patient's symptoms, the patient is due for colonoscopic surveillance, or the patient has risk factors for colon cancer, such as a family history. Depending on the extent of the hemorrhoidal disease and the patient's symptoms, treatment can either be nonsurgical or involve formal hemorrhoidectomy.

Treatment

Nonoperative management. Dietary modifications including fiber supplementation and increasing fluid intake may improve symptoms of prolapse and bleeding. Bulking of the stool permits a soft, formed stool for avoidance of excessive straining and promotion of better bowel habits. Bleeding symptoms are generally reduced during a period of weeks with the use of fiber supplementation alone. Patients with prolapse of internal plus external hemorrhoids will generally benefit from additional interventions.

First-, second-, and some third-degree internal hemorrhoids can usually be treated with office procedures. Results are typically more favorable for lower degree hemorrhoids. Rubber band ligation remains one of the simplest and widely used office-based procedures for treatment of hemorrhoids. Sedation is not required, and ligation is carried out through an anoscope, using a ligator (Fig. 52-7). Although rare, severe perineal sepsis has been reported after rubber band ligation; thus, patients should be instructed to be aware of delayed or increasing pain, inability to void, or fever. Patients with larger hemorrhoids are likely to be better served by a surgical approach, which is more durable and effective. In patients undergoing one or more bandings, relief of symptoms was noted in 80%, with failure predicted in patients who required four or more bandings.[25] Relative contraindications to banding include immunocompromised patients (chemotherapy, HIV/AIDS), presence of coagulopathy, and patients taking anticoagulation or antiplatelet medications (excluding aspirin products).

Sclerotherapy involves the injection of a low volume (3 to 5 mL) of a sclerosant (e.g., 3% normal saline) into the internal hemorrhoid. This technique has good short-term success, but the hemorrhoidal disease tends to recur in longer follow-up. The benefit to this technique is its application in patients with bleeding tendency or who are taking anticoagulants that cannot be stopped. Infrared and laser coagulation involves the use of light energy to cause coagulation and necrosis, causing fibrosis of the submucosa in the region of the hemorrhoid.

Surgical treatment. Hemorrhoidectomy is a durable option and has the best long-term results. It should be considered whenever patients fail to respond to more conservative repeated attempts to treat the disease. Hemorrhoidectomy should

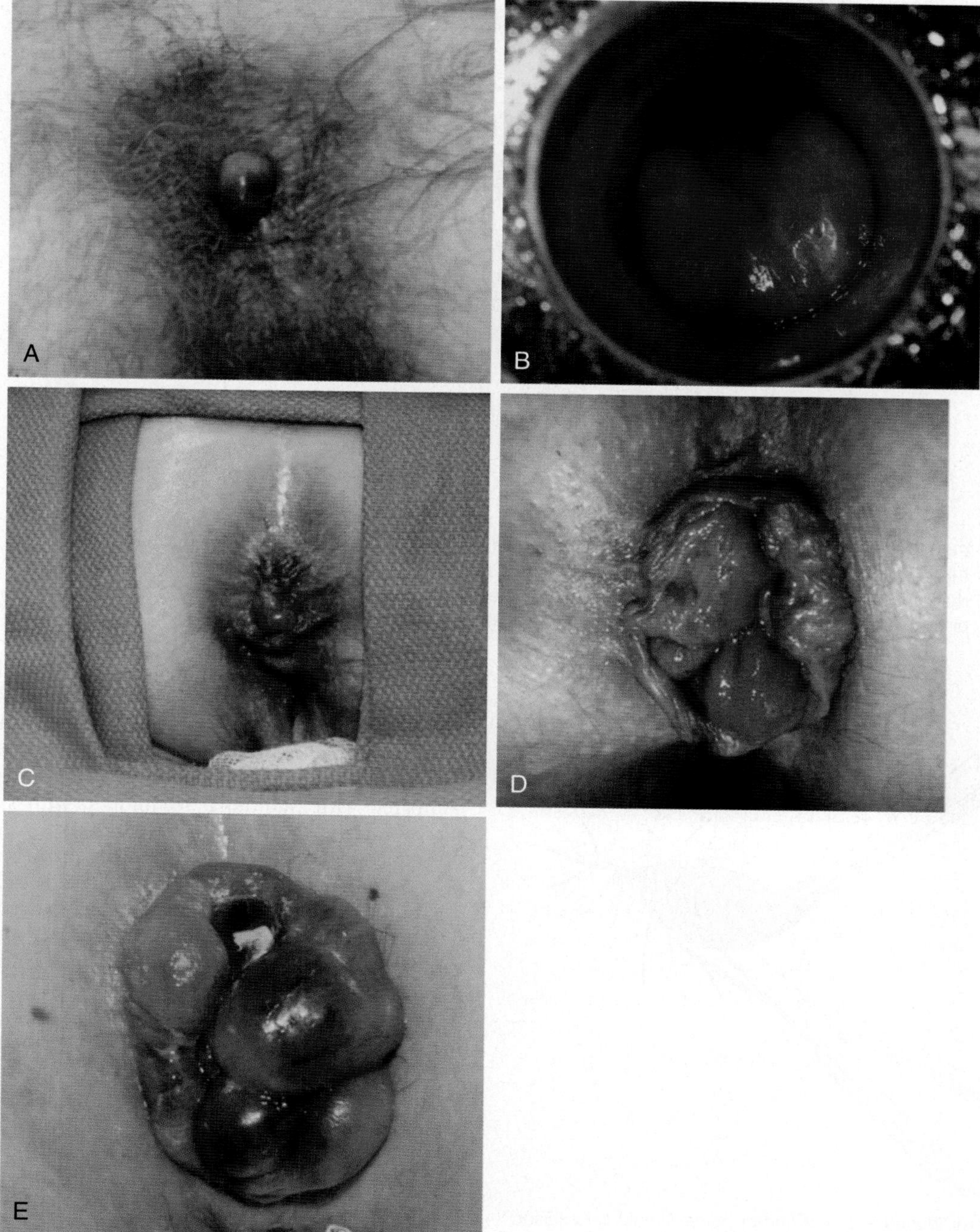

FIGURE 52-6 Hemorrhoids. **A,** Thrombosed external. **B,** Internal, first-degree internal as seen through anoscope. **C,** Internal prolapsed and reduced spontaneously, second degree. **D,** Internal prolapsed, requiring manual reduction, third degree. **E,** Inability to be reduced, strangulated, fourth degree. (Courtesy Mayo Foundation for Medical Education and Research, Rochester, Minn.)

be considered in patients who continue to present with severe prolapse and require manual reduction (grade III) or cannot be reduced (grade IV); for those hemorrhoids complicated by strangulation, ulceration, fissure, or fistula; and for those patients who have symptomatic external hemorrhoids. Patients with thrombosed external hemorrhoids may ideally undergo excision in the office, during the period of maximum pain (generally the first 72 hours). In this case, the thrombosed external hemorrhoid should be excised, not incised, as this may increase the risk of rethrombosis (Fig. 52-8). Those patients presenting after the period of maximum pain are best served by supportive measures. In patients presenting with complex internal or external hemorrhoids, operative hemorrhoidectomy can be performed as an outpatient procedure.

Closed (Ferguson) hemorrhoidectomy consists of simultaneous excision of internal and external hemorrhoids (Fig. 52-9). With use of a large anoscopic retractor, such as the Fansler, an elliptical incision is made encompassing the complete hemorrhoidal column. Care must be taken to not excise excessive amounts of tissue and to ensure that sufficient anoderm is

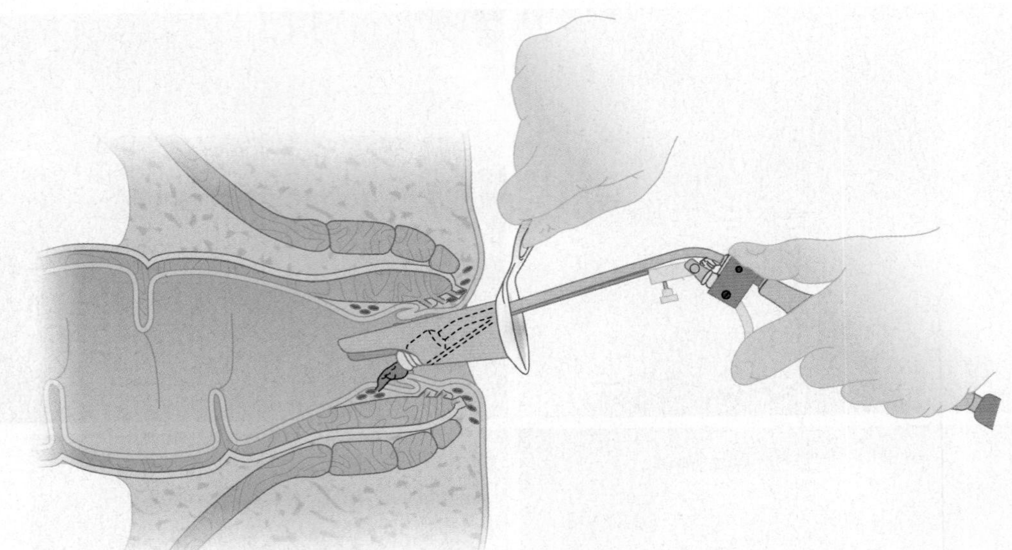

FIGURE 52-7 Rubber Band Ligation. The internal hemorrhoid is identified proximal to the dentate line; the area of proposed banding should be pinched to test for sensation before banding. The hemorrhoid is drawn into the ligator by use of either forceps or the suction device of a suction ligator. The band is then placed. (Courtesy Mayo Foundation for Medical Education and Research, Rochester, Minn.)

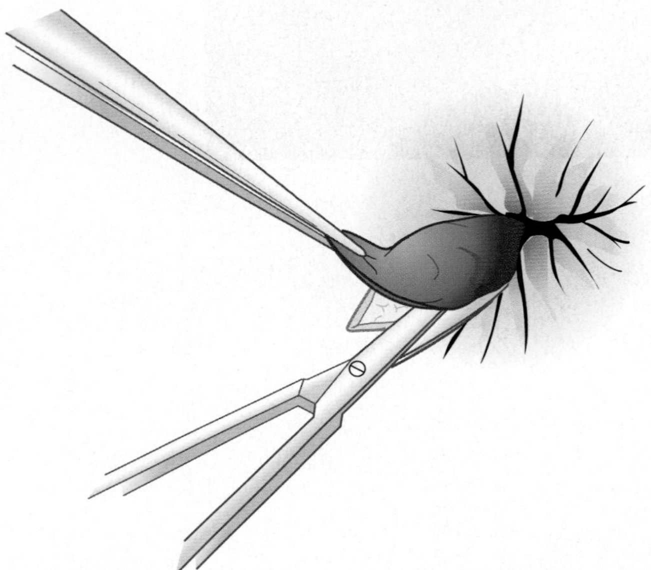

FIGURE 52-8 Thrombosed external hemorrhoids should be excised, not incised, after the area has been infiltrated with local anesthetic. There is no need to close the excision site. (Courtesy Mayo Foundation for Medical Education and Research, Rochester, Minn.)

preserved to avoid the complication of anal stenosis. The excision site is then closed with a continuous absorbable suture. The open (Milligan-Morgan) hemorrhoidectomy differs in that the excision site is not closed and left open. Postoperative complications include urinary retention (in up to 30% of patients), fecal incontinence (2%), infection (1%), delayed hemorrhage (1%), and stricture (1%). Patients typically recover quickly and are able to return to work within 1 to 2 weeks.

Other techniques involving the application of ultrasonic (Harmonic Scalpel; Soma, Bloomfield, CT) or electrical energy (LigaSure; Covidien, Boulder, CO) devices have been applied to the operative treatment of hemorrhoids. Both methods remove the excess hemorrhoidal tissue, with minimal lateral thermal injury in the hope of decreasing postoperative pain and edema. Various studies have investigated their efficacy and have demonstrated decreased postoperative pain and analgesic use in these groups compared with traditional techniques, with similar short-term success rates.[26,27]

Stapled hemorrhoidopexy is a technique that results in excision of a circumferential portion of the lower rectal and upper anal canal mucosa and submucosa with a circular stapling device (Fig. 52-10). The procedure is completed by first reducing the hemorrhoidal tissue into the anal canal. A purse-string suture is placed 3 to 4 cm above the dentate line, ensuring that all the redundant tissue is incorporated circumferentially. Overly aggressive placement of the sutures may inadvertently incorporate the vaginal wall anteriorly, resulting in a rectovaginal fistula. In addition, if the suture is placed too close to the dentate line, it could result in severe and intractable pain.

Results of stapled hemorrhoidopexy are varied. A meta-analysis of randomized controlled trials comparing this with conventional hemorrhoidectomy found that the stapled procedure was safe but on long-term follow-up was associated with a higher rate of recurrence and reoperation (Fig. 52-11).[28]

Anal Fissures

Presentation and Evaluation

An anal fissure is a linear ulcer usually found in the midline, distal to the dentate line (Fig. 52-12). These lesions are typically easily seen by visual inspection of the anal verge with gentle spreading of the buttocks. Location may vary; most fissures are identified in the posterior midline, and anterior midline fissures are still more common that lateral fissures. Other associated findings include a sentinel tag at the distal portion of the fissure and a hypertrophied anal papilla proximal to the fissure. Fissures occurring in the lateral positions should raise the possibility of other associated diseases, such as Crohn's disease, tuberculosis, syphilis, HIV/AIDS, or carcinoma. Anal fissure most often is manifested with

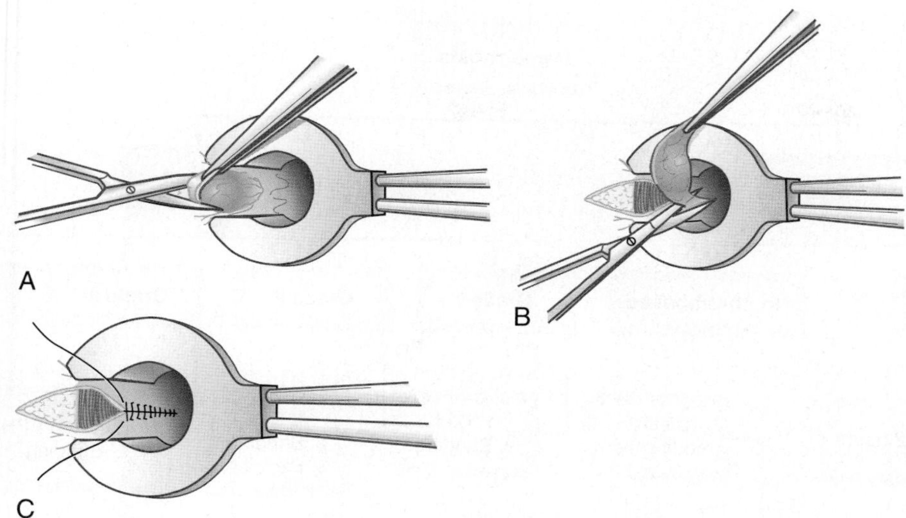

FIGURE 52-9 Closed Hemorrhoidectomy. A, An elliptical incision is made surrounding the hemorrhoidal tissues, and these are excised from distal to proximal. **B,** Care is taken to preserve the sphincter muscle. **C,** The feeding vascular pedicle at the proximal point is sutured and the defect closed with a running absorbable suture. In the open technique, this excision site is not closed with suture. (Courtesy Mayo Foundation for Medical Education and Research, Rochester, Minn.)

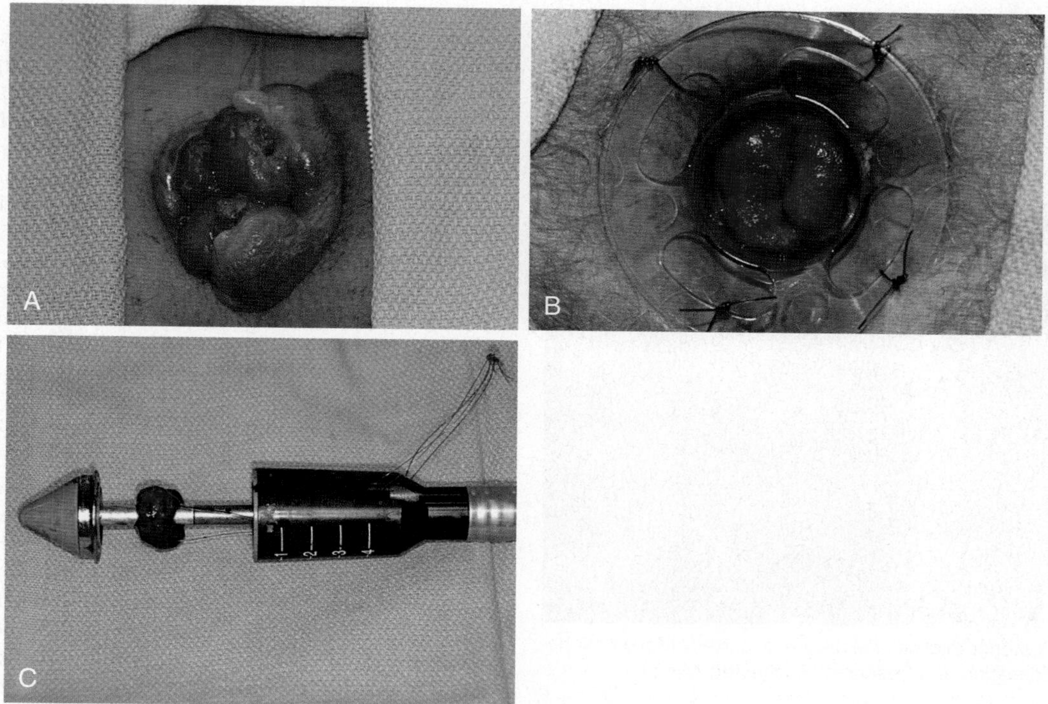

FIGURE 52-10 Procedure for Prolapsed Hemorrhoids. A, Circumferential grade IV hemorrhoids. **B,** The stapling device has an obturator that is placed in the internal canal to aid in reduction of tissue and placement of purse-string suture in the mucosa above the dentate line. **C,** Stapling device demonstrating circumferential excision of anal canal and hemorrhoid mucosa.

excruciating anal pain (because of its location extending onto the very sensitive anoderm) with defecation and bleeding.

Patients typically describe a preceding episode of constipation. Digital and anoscopic examination may result in severe pain and is not necessary if the fissure can be visualized. Examination under anesthesia, with or without biopsy of the fissure, or endoscopic examination should be performed if it is refractory to medical management.

Pathogenesis

The cause of anal fissure is likely to be multifactorial. The passage of large and hard stools, low-fiber diet, previous anal surgery,

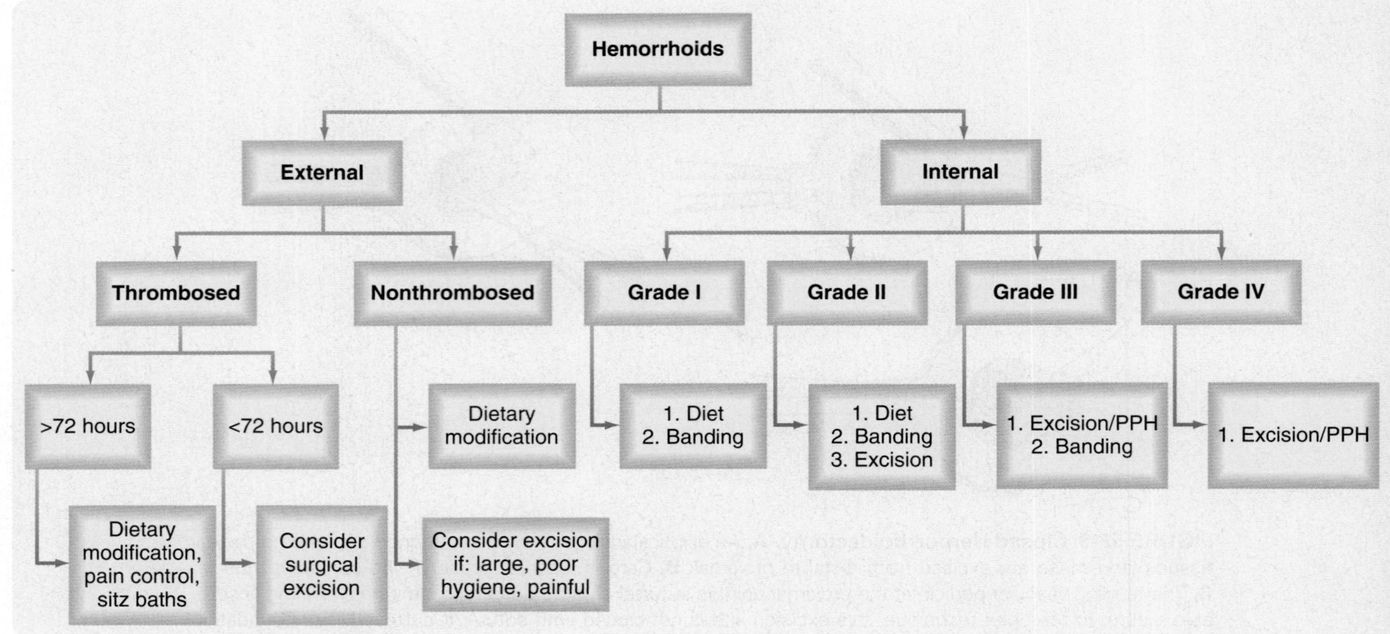

FIGURE 52-11 Algorithm for the treatment of hemorrhoids. *PPH,* procedure for prolapse and hemorrhoids.

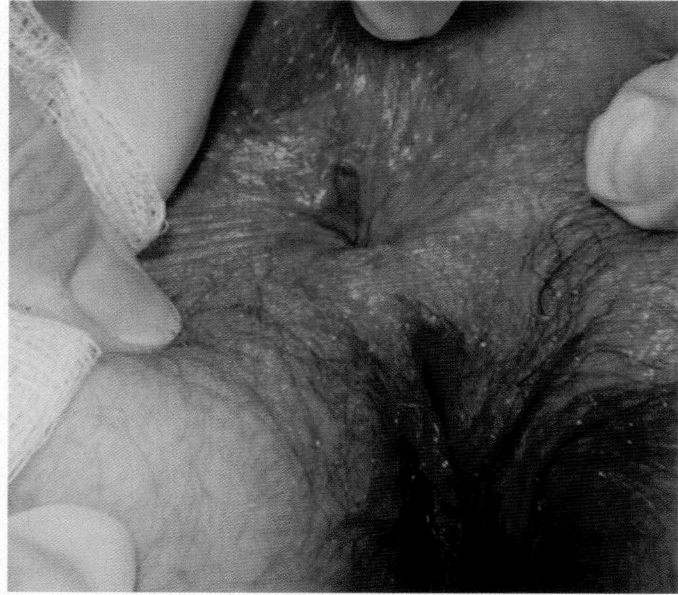

FIGURE 52-12 Posterior midline anal fissure. (Courtesy Mayo Foundation for Medical Education and Research, Rochester, Minn.)

trauma, and infection may be contributing factors. Increased resting anal canal pressures and reduced anal blood flow in the posterior midline have also been postulated as causes. These possibilities have led to the introduction of several medical approaches.

Treatment

Given that a hypertonic sphincter and large, hard stools may contribute to anal fissures, most medical therapies are directed to achieve the goals of relaxation of the anal sphincter without causing fecal incontinence, passage of soft and formed stools, and relief of pain. Many pharmacologic agents have been considered, including topical nitric oxide (e.g., nitroglycerin), calcium channel blockers (e.g., diltiazem, nifedipine), and botulinum toxin injections.

Nonsurgical therapy is safe and often effective, with limited side effects, and should be the first-line therapy for anal fissure. However, a subset of patients may benefit from upfront surgical intervention, and the treatment should generally be individualized (Fig. 52-13).

Medical management. Medical therapies for acute anal fissures (those presenting within 6 weeks of symptom onset) are effective. Medical management includes topical and oral pharmacotherapy in addition to diet modification and bulking agents.[29] Topical therapy is popular, given its fewer side effects compared with oral therapies.

Topical nitrates (0.2% to 0.4% nitroglycerin) or calcium channel blockers (0.2% nifedipine or 2% diltiazem) are commonly prescribed. A meta-analysis compared nonsurgical treatments and found that nitroglycerin was significantly better than placebo (49% versus 36%; $P < .0009$) in healing anal fissures, but there was a 50% late recurrence rate. Calcium channel blockers were equally effective but exhibited fewer side effects.[29]

Temporary chemodenervation of the internal anal sphincter can be achieved by injection of botulinum toxin (Botox). This results in relaxation of the internal anal sphincter and is believed to promote increased blood flow to the affected anoderm, allowing the fissure to heal. Success is variable, with reported rates of 60% to 80% being achieved. Up to 10% of patients may develop temporary incontinence to flatus, with rare temporary fecal incontinence. Presently, there is no agreed on standard dose, site of injection, or number or timing of injections in the administration of botulinum toxin. Our practice is to inject 20 units of botulinum toxin into the internal anal sphincter on each side of the fissure. In patients who are nonresponders to diet modification and topical pharmacotherapy, such as topical nitroglycerin or calcium channel blockers, and who wish to avoid surgery, botulinum injection may be a reasonable alternative treatment.

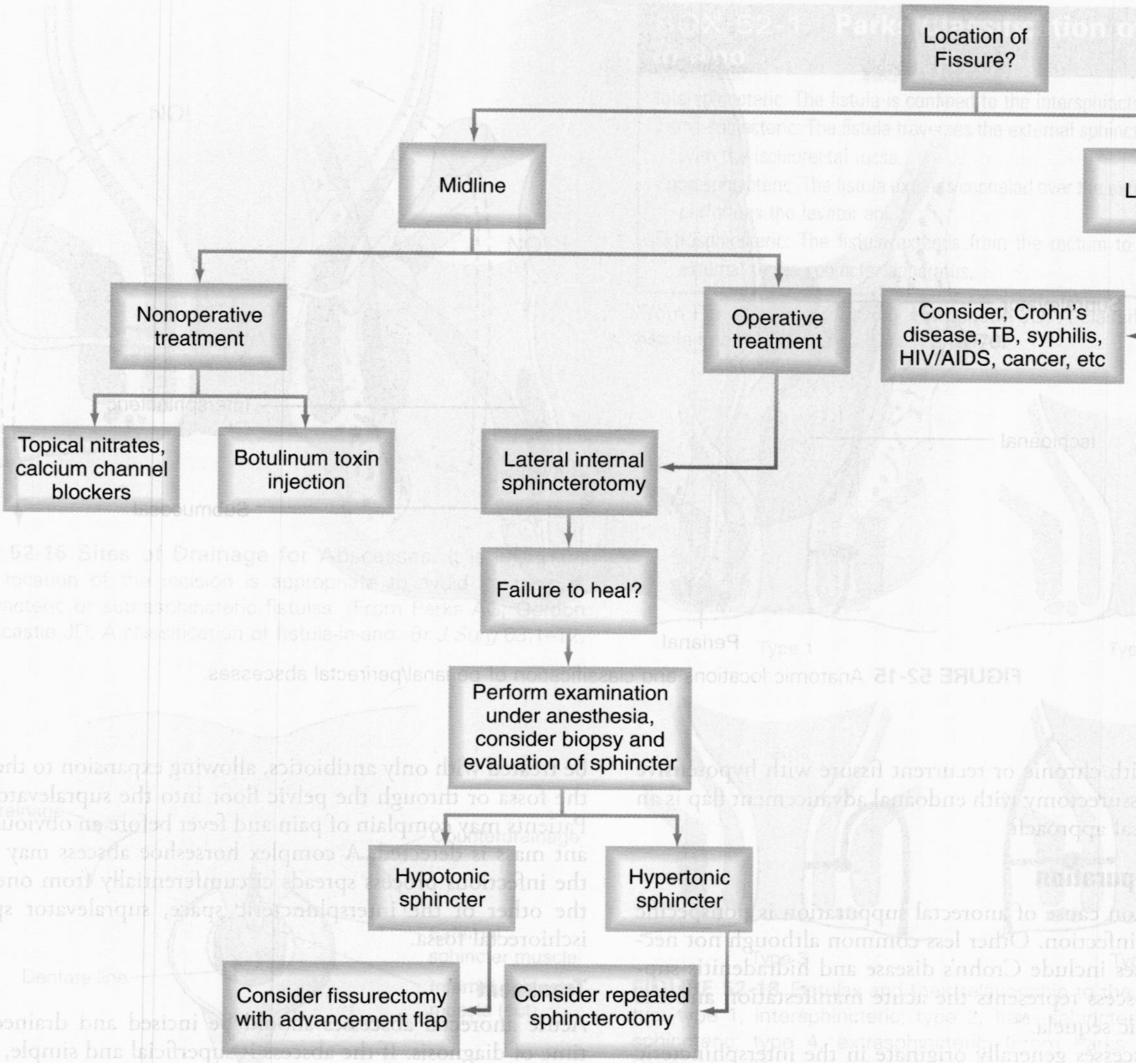

Location of Fissure?

- Midline
  - Nonoperative treatment
    - Topical nitrates, calcium channel blockers
    - Botulinum toxin injection
  - Operative treatment
    - Lateral internal sphincterotomy
      - Failure to heal?
        - Perform examination under anesthesia, consider biopsy and evaluation of sphincter
          - Hypotonic sphincter
            - Consider fissurectomy with advancement flap
          - Hypertonic sphincter
            - Consider repeated sphincterotomy
- Lateral
  - Consider, Crohn's disease, TB, syphilis, HIV/AIDS, cancer, etc

FIGURE 52-13 Algorithm for the treatment of anal fissure.

Surgical management. Patients with severe or chronic fissures and those who have failed to respond to medical therapy may benefit from surgery. Lateral internal sphincterotomy remains the operation of choice and has been shown to be superior to all other medical therapies, anal dilation, or fissurectomy.[30] Lateral internal sphincterotomy can be carried out by the closed or open (Fig. 52-14) technique, depending on the surgeon's preference. There is no significant difference between these techniques for rate of healing or rate of incontinence. In terms of the extent of sphincterotomy, studies have investigated whether sphincterotomy to the level of the dentate line is superior to sphincterotomy to the fissure apex. Those with sphincterotomy to the level of the dentate had a higher rate of fissure healing, with no statistical difference in rate of incontinence.[30] The risk of incontinence with sphincterotomy is not negligible. A meta-analysis demonstrated an overall rate of incontinence of 14%. Incontinence of flatus occurred in 9% of patients. Incontinence of liquid or solid stool occurred in 2% of all patients.[31] It is important to evaluate for any preexisting incontinence before undertaking surgical intervention so as not to further compromise sphincter function.

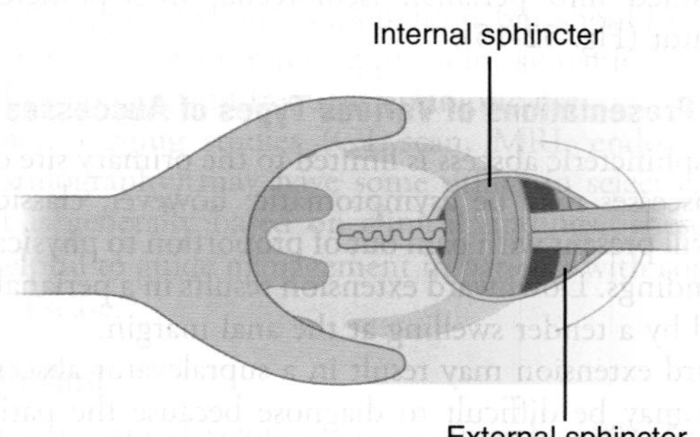

FIGURE 52-14 Lateral Internal Sphincterotomy. A large operating anoscope is placed into the anal canal. A small incision is made along the intersphincteric groove. The mucosa is elevated from the sphincter, and the underlying internal sphincter is elevated off the external sphincter. This is divided either to the level of the dentate line or to the proximal extent of the fissure. (Courtesy Mayo Foundation for Medical Education and Research, Rochester, Minn.)

Algorithm for Management of Variceal Hemorrhage

An algorithm for definitive management of variceal hemorrhage is shown in Figure 53-26. Patients are first grouped according to their transplantation candidacy. This decision is based on a number of factors, including cause of portal hypertension, abstinence for alcoholic cirrhotic patients, presence or absence of other diseases, and physiologic rather than chronologic age. Transplantation candidates with decompensated hepatic function or a poor quality of life secondary to their liver disease should undergo transplantation as soon as possible.

Most future transplantation and nontransplantation candidates should undergo initial endoscopic treatment or pharmacotherapy unless they bleed from gastric varices or portal hypertensive gastropathy or live in a remote geographic location and have

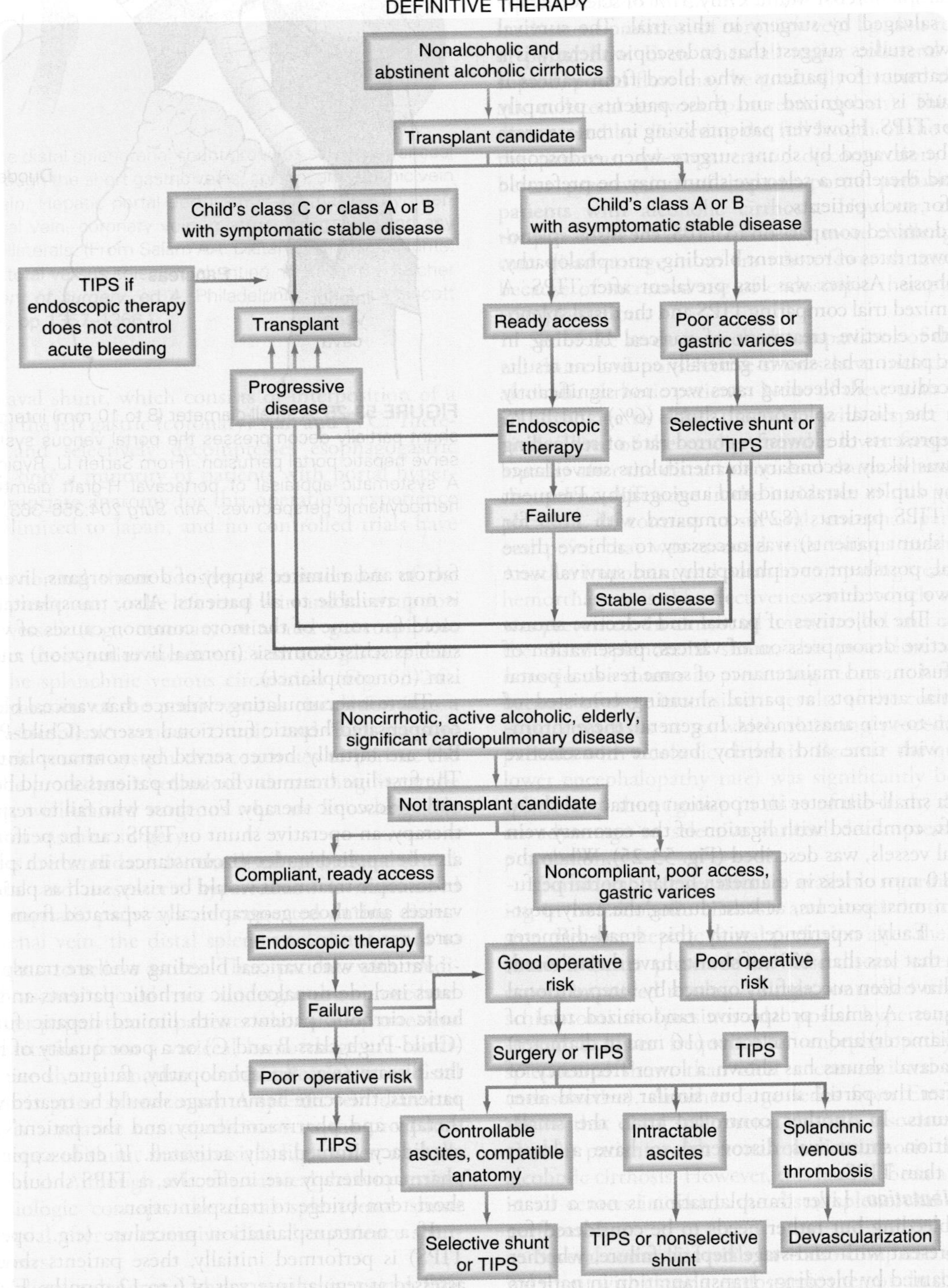

FIGURE 53-26 Algorithm for definitive therapy of variceal hemorrhage (see text for details). (Adapted from Rikkers LF: Portal hypertension. In Levine BA, Copeland E, Howard R, et al, editors: *Current practice of surgery* (vol 3), New York, 1995, Churchill Livingstone.)

limited access to emergency tertiary care. Patients who live in remote locations and those who fail to respond to endoscopic and drug therapy should receive a selective shunt or TIPS. A controlled trial has shown that if careful surveillance of TIPS patency and frequent TIPS reinterventions are done, these procedures are equally efficacious.

Until improvements in TIPS technology are fully realized, the distal splenorenal shunt is likely to remain a more durable long-term solution and a reasonable alternative for TIPS failure. However, a TIPS is more commonly done, and few surgeons who are experienced in shunt surgery remain. Therefore, it is likely that operative shunts will play an even smaller role in the management of variceal bleeding in the future than they do now. Patients with medically intractable ascites in addition to variceal bleeding are best treated with TIPS when less invasive measures fail to control bleeding. If the TIPS eventually fails, an open side-to-side shunt can then be constructed if the patient has reasonable hepatic function and is not a transplantation candidate. On the other hand, TIPS is clearly indicated for patients with endoscopic treatment failure who may require transplantation in the near future and for nontransplantation candidates with advanced hepatic functional deterioration. Future transplantation candidates should be carefully monitored so that they undergo transplantation at the appropriate time before they become poor operative risks.

The treatment algorithm for variceal bleeding has changed considerably since the 1970s, during which time endoscopic therapy, liver transplantation, and TIPS have become available to these patients. Nontransplantation operations are now less frequently necessary, the survival results are better because patients at high operative risk are managed by other means, and emergency surgery has almost been eliminated.

INFECTIOUS DISEASES

Pyogenic Abscess

Epidemiology

Ochsner and DeBakey, in their classic paper on pyogenic liver abscess in 1938, described 47 cases and reviewed the world literature. This was the largest experience at that time and the first serious attempt to study this disease. In that era, pyogenic liver abscess was largely a disease of people in their 20s and 30s, mostly the result of acute appendicitis. With the marked changes in medical care since then, notably effective antibiotics and prompt effective treatments for acute inflammatory disorders, and an aging population, the spectrum of this disease has changed. Pyogenic liver abscess is now mostly seen in patients in their 50s to 60s and is more often related to biliary tract disease or is cryptogenic in nature.

However, the incidence of pyogenic liver abscess has remained similar. In 1938, Ochsner and DeBakey reported an incidence of 8/100,000 hospital admissions, whereas in 1975, Pitt and Zuidema reported 13/100,000 hospital admissions. Two large autopsy studies, one from 1901 and another from 1960, have reported similar incidences of pyogenic liver abscess, 0.45% and 0.59%, respectively. More recent studies from the 1980s through the 2000s have suggested small but significant increases in the incidence of pyogenic liver abscess as high as 22/100,000 hospital admissions.[11] These figures may be declining on the basis of more recent data. This may reflect better, more available, and more frequently used high-quality imaging techniques. Hospital admission practices also affect these numbers. A recent population-based study from North America calculated an annual incidence of 3.6 cases/100,000 population.[12] There is no significant gender, ethnic, or geographic differences in disease frequency; the male-to-female ratio is approximately 1.5:1. Comorbid conditions associated with pyogenic abscess are cirrhosis, diabetes, chronic renal failure, and a history of malignant disease.

Pathogenesis

The liver is probably exposed to portal venous bacterial loads on a regular basis and usually clears this bacterial load without problems. The development of a hepatic abscess occurs when an inoculum of bacteria, regardless of the route of exposure, exceeds the liver's ability to clear it. This results in tissue invasion, neutrophil infiltration, and formation of an organized abscess. The potential routes of hepatic exposure to bacteria are the biliary tree, portal vein, hepatic artery, direct extension of a nearby nidus of infection, and trauma. The relative contribution of these routes to the formation of hepatic abscess is summarized in Table 53-3.

Along with cryptogenic infections, infections from the biliary tree are the most common identifiable cause of hepatic abscess. Biliary obstruction results in bile stasis with the potential for subsequent bacterial colonization, infection, and ascension into the liver. This process is known as ascending suppurative cholangitis. The nature of biliary obstruction is mostly related to stone disease or malignant disease. In Asia, intrahepatic stones and cholangitis (recurrent pyogenic cholangitis; see later) are common causes, whereas in the West, malignant obstruction has become a more predominant cause. Other factors associated with increased risk include Caroli disease, biliary ascariasis, and biliary tract surgery. The common link between all causes of hepatic abscesses from the biliary tree is obstruction and bacteria in the biliary tract. Prior biliary-enteric anastomosis has also been associated with hepatic abscess formation, likely because of unimpeded exposure of the biliary tree to enteric organisms.

The portal venous system drains the gastrointestinal tract; therefore, any infectious disorder of the gastrointestinal tract can

TABLE 53-3 Pyogenic Abscesses Attributable to Specific Cause

		CAUSE (%)					
YEAR OF REPORT	NO. OF PATIENTS	PORTAL VEIN	HEPATIC ARTERY	BILIARY TREE	DIRECT EXTENSION	TRAUMA	CRYPTOGENIC
1927-1938 (one study*)	622	42	—	—	17	4	20
1945-1982 (eight studies)	521	17	9	38	10	4	16
1970-1999 (eight studies)	1264	5	3	38	1	2	43

*Ochsner A, DeBakey M, Murray S: Pyogenic abscess of the liver. *Am J Surg* 40:292–319, 1938. This is the classic study of Ochsner and DeBakey that reviewed 286 previously reported cases and 47 new cases.

result in an ascending portal vein infection (pyelophlebitis), with exposure of the liver to large amounts of bacteria. Historically, untreated appendicitis was considered the most common cause of hepatic abscess, but with the advent of antibiotics and the development of prompt and effective treatment of acute intra-abdominal infections, portal venous infections of the liver have become less frequent. The most common causes of pyelophlebitis are diverticulitis, appendicitis, pancreatitis, inflammatory bowel disease, pelvic inflammatory disease, perforated viscus, and omphalitis in the newborn. Hepatic abscess has also been associated with colorectal malignant disease. In a case-control study from Taiwan, the incidence of gastrointestinal cancers was increased fourfold among patients with pyogenic liver abscess compared with controls.[13]

Any systemic infection (e.g., endocarditis, pneumonia, osteomyelitis) can result in bacteremia and infection of the liver through the hepatic artery. Microabscess formation is a relatively common finding at autopsy in patients dying of sepsis, but these patients are generally not included in analyses of pyogenic liver abscess. Hepatic abscess from systemic infections may also reflect an altered immune response, such as in patients with malignant disease, AIDS, or disorders of granulocyte function. Children with chronic granulomatous disease are particularly susceptible.

Hepatic abscess can be the result of direct extension of an infectious process. Common examples include suppurative cholecystitis, subphrenic abscess, perinephric abscess, and even perforation of the bowel directly into the liver.

Penetrating and blunt trauma can also result in an intrahepatic hematoma or an area of necrotic liver, which can subsequently develop into an abscess. Bacteria may have been introduced from the trauma, or the affected area may be seeded from systemic bacteremia. Hepatic abscesses associated with trauma can be manifested in a delayed fashion up to several weeks after injury. Other mechanisms of iatrogenic hepatic necrosis, such as hepatic artery embolization or, more recently, thermal ablative procedures, can be complicated by abscess. This is an uncommon complication of these procedures but is seen more often when there has been a previous biliary-enteric anastomosis.

Usually, no cause for a hepatic abscess is found. Cryptogenic abscesses predominate in many series and are more common in some case reports. Possible explanations for cryptogenic hepatic abscess are undiagnosed abdominal disease, resolved infectious process at the time of presentation, and host factors such as diabetes or malignant disease rendering the liver more susceptible to transient hepatic artery or portal vein bacteremia. In patients with cryptogenic hepatic abscess who have undergone computed tomography (CT) and ultrasonography, it has been argued whether a diligent search for a cause should ensue. In series evaluating colonoscopy and endoscopic retrograde cholangiopancreatography (ERCP) in patients with cryptogenic abscess, the yield has been low and often is only fruitful in patients with some objective finding that might have suggested a subclinical abnormality (e.g., mildly elevated bilirubin level). In general, these patients should undergo a thorough history, physical examination, and laboratory workup in search of abnormalities in the intestinal tract or biliary tree. Further invasive procedures or imaging studies should be based on clinical suspicions raised by this workup.

Pathology and Microbiology

Most hepatic abscesses involve the right hemiliver, accounting for about 75% of cases. The explanation for this is not known, but preferential laminar blood flow to the right side has been postulated. The left liver is involved in approximately 20% of the cases; the caudate lobe is rarely involved (5%). Bilobar involvement with multiple abscesses is uncommon. Approximately 50% of hepatic abscesses are solitary. Hepatic abscesses can vary in size from less than 1 mm to 3 or 4 cm in diameter and can be multiloculated or a single cavity. At abdominal exploration, hepatic abscesses appear tan and are fluctuant to palpation, although deeper abscesses may not be visible and can be difficult to palpate. Surrounding inflammation can cause adhesions to local structures.

Studies of the microbiology of hepatic abscesses have had variable results, for a number of reasons. In early series, sterile abscesses were commonly reported but probably reflected inadequate culture techniques, whereas in modern series, few abscesses are sampled before the administration of antibiotics. Also, the heterogeneity of the routes of infection makes the microbiology variable. Abscesses from pyelophlebitis or cholangitis tend to be polymicrobial, with a high preponderance of gram-negative bacilli. Systemic infections, on the other hand, usually cause infection with a single organism.

Although the rate of sterility reported by Ochsner's review in 1938 was approximately 50%, series in the 1990s reported sterile abscess rates in approximately 10% to 20% of cases. Many hepatic abscesses are polymicrobial in nature and account for approximately 40% of cases. Some have suggested that solitary abscesses are more likely to be polymicrobial. Anaerobic organisms are involved approximately 40% to 60% of the time. The most common organisms cultured are *Escherichia coli* and *Klebsiella pneumoniae*. Other commonly encountered organisms are *Staphylococcus aureus, Enterococcus* sp., viridans streptococci, and *Bacteroides* spp. *Klebsiella* is frequently associated with gas-forming abscesses. Enterococci and viridans streptococci are generally found in polymicrobial abscesses, whereas staphylococcal infections are typically caused by a single organism. Uncommonly encountered organisms (<10% of cultures) include species of *Pseudomonas, Proteus, Enterobacter, Citrobacter, Serratia,* beta-hemolytic streptococci, microaerophilic streptococci, *Fusobacterium, Clostridium,* and other rare anaerobes. Blood cultures are positive in approximately 50% to 60% of cases. Of note, highly resistant organisms in patients with indwelling biliary catheters, multiple episodes of cholangitis, and repeated use of antibiotics are being encountered as the use of these catheters becomes more common. Fungal and mycobacterial hepatic abscesses are rare and are almost always associated with immunosuppression, usually from chemotherapy.

Clinical Features

The classic description of the presenting symptoms of hepatic abscess is fever, jaundice, and right upper quadrant pain, with tenderness to palpation. Unfortunately, this presentation is present in only 10% of cases. Fever, chills, and abdominal pain are the most common presenting symptoms, but a broad array of nonspecific symptoms can be present (Table 53-4). A study from Taiwan of 133 patients found fever in 96% of patients, chills in 80%, abdominal pain in 53%, and jaundice in 20%. Many of the symptoms, such as malaise and vomiting, were constitutional in nature. Involvement of the diaphragm may result in symptoms of cough or dyspnea. Rarely, patients can present with peritonitis secondary to rupture. Cases of rupture into the pleural space or pericardium have been reported but are distinctly uncommon. The duration of presenting symptoms is variable, ranging from an acute illness to a chronic presentation lasting months. It has been

TABLE 53-4 Pyogenic Abscesses With Noted Symptoms

		SYMPTOM (%)								
YEAR OF REPORT	NO. OF PATIENTS	FEVER, CHILLS	NIGHT SWEATS	MALAISE	ANOREXIA, WEIGHT LOSS	NAUSEA, VOMITING	DIARRHEA	ABDOMINAL PAIN	CHEST PAIN	COUGH
1927-1938 (one study*)	333	94	—	—	—	33	—	92	—	—
1945-1982 (eight studies)	494	88	8	58	62	40	17	66	14	13
1970-1995 (ten studies)	1314	72	9	25	33	30	14	59	16	6

*Ochsner A, DeBakey M, Murray S: Pyogenic abscess of the liver. *Am J Surg* 40:292–319, 1938. This is the classic study of Ochsner and DeBakey that reviewed 286 previously reported cases and 47 new cases.

suggested that acute presentation is associated with identifiable abdominal disease, whereas a chronic presentation is often associated with a cryptogenic abscess. A rare complication specific to *Klebsiella* hepatic abscesses is endogenous endophthalmitis, occurring in approximately 3% of cases. This serious complication is more common in diabetics. The best chance to preserve visual function is with early diagnosis and treatment.

On physical examination, fever and right upper quadrant tenderness are the most common findings. Tenderness is present in 40% to 70% of patients. Jaundice is also found in approximately 25% of cases and is often secondary to underlying biliary disease. Chest findings are often found in approximately 25% of patients, and hepatomegaly is also commonly noted in approximately 50%. Ascites, splenomegaly, and severe sepsis are uncommon signs of hepatic abscesses.

Nonspecific abnormalities of blood tests are common in pyogenic abscesses. Leukocytosis is present in 70% to 90% of patients, and anemia is commonly encountered. Abnormalities of LFT results are generally present. The ALP level is mildly elevated in 80% of patients, whereas total bilirubin concentration is elevated 20% to 50% of the time. Transaminases are mildly elevated in approximately 60% of patients. Severe abnormalities of liver function are almost always associated with underlying biliary disease. Hypoalbuminemia or mild elevations of the PT and INR can be present and reflect a degree of chronicity. None of these blood tests specifically help diagnose a hepatic abscess. However, together they may suggest a liver abnormality that often leads to imaging studies.

The most essential element to establishing the diagnosis of hepatic abscess is radiographic imaging. Chest radiographs are abnormal approximately 50% of the time, and findings generally reflect subdiaphragmatic disease, such as an elevated right hemidiaphragm, right pleural effusion, or atelectasis. On occasion, these can be left-sided findings in the case of an abscess involving the left liver. Plain abdominal radiographs, in rare cases, can be helpful. They can show air-fluid levels or portal venous gas (Fig. 53-27).

Ultrasound and CT are the mainstays of diagnostic modalities for hepatic abscess. Ultrasound usually demonstrates a round or oval area that is less echogenic than the surrounding liver. Ultrasound can reliably distinguish solid from cystic lesions. The limitations of ultrasound are in its ability to visualize lesions high up in the dome of the liver and that it is a user-dependent modality.

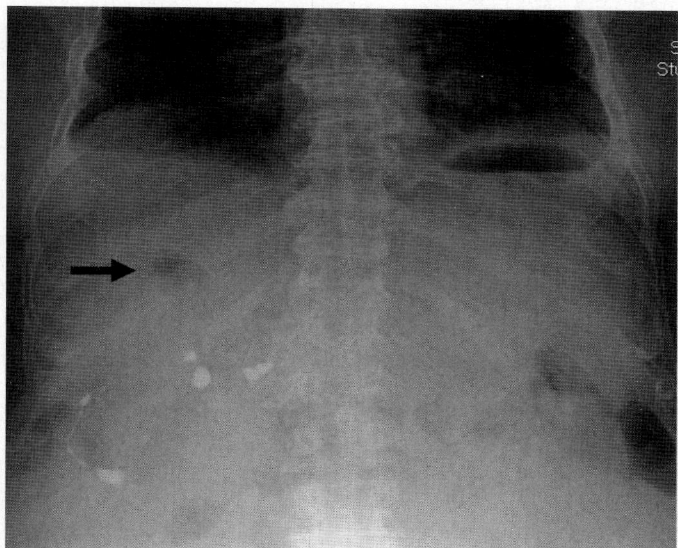

FIGURE 53-27 Plain abdominal radiograph demonstrating an abnormal collection of air in the right upper quadrant consistent with a pyogenic hepatic abscess *(arrow)*.

The sensitivity of ultrasound in diagnosing hepatic abscess is 80% to 95%. CT demonstrates similar findings to ultrasound, and lesions are of lower attenuation than surrounding hepatic parenchyma. High-quality CT scans can demonstrate very small abscesses and can more easily identify multiple small abscesses. The abscess wall usually has an intense enhancement on contrast-enhanced CT. The sensitivity of CT in diagnosing hepatic abscess is 95% to 100%. Both CT and ultrasound are useful in diagnosing other intra-abdominal pathologic processes, such as biliary disease (ultrasound) and inflammatory disorders such as appendicitis and diverticulitis (CT). Magnetic resonance imaging (MRI) can be helpful in distinguishing the cause of many hepatic masses and evaluating the biliary tree for pathologic changes, but it does not appear to have any distinct advantage over CT in diagnosing hepatic abscess.

Differential Diagnosis

Differentiating pyogenic abscess from other cystic infective diseases of the liver, such as amebic abscess or echinococcal cyst, is

TABLE 53-5 **Features of Amebic versus Pyogenic Liver Abscess**

CLINICAL FEATURES	AMEBIC ABSCESS	PYOGENIC ABSCESS
Age	20-40 years	>50 years
Male-to-female ratio	≥10:1	1.5:1
Solitary versus multiple	Solitary 80%*	Solitary 50%
Location	Usually right liver	Usually right liver
Travel in endemic area	Yes	No
Diabetes	Uncommon (≈2%)	More common (≈27%)
Alcohol use	Common	Common
Jaundice	Uncommon	Common
Elevated bilirubin	Uncommon	Common
Elevated alkaline phosphatase	Common	Common
Positive blood culture	No	Common
Positive amebic serology	Yes	No

*In acute amebic abscess, 50% are solitary.

important because of differences in treatment. Pyogenic abscess (see later) is largely treated by antibiotics and drainage. Amebic abscess is mainly treated by antibiotics, whereas echinococcal cysts often require surgical management. Fortunately, echinococcal cysts can usually be diagnosed by history and characteristic radiologic findings (see later). The presentations of amebic and pyogenic abscess, however, are more similar, with some notable exceptions that are critical in distinguishing the two (Table 53-5). Amebic abscesses generally occur in young Hispanic men, whereas pyogenic abscess tends to occur in patients 50 to 60 years of age, with no predominant gender or race. Fever is common in both, but chills and symptoms of a severe acute bacteremia are more common in pyogenic abscess. On serologic testing, *Entamoeba histolytica* antibodies are almost always present in amebic abscesses but are uncommon in patients with pyogenic abscess. A study comparing 471 patients with amebic abscess to 106 patients with pyogenic abscess found age older than 50 years, pulmonary findings on physical examination, multiple abscesses, and low amebic serology titers to be independently predictive of pyogenic abscess. On occasion, differentiating the two is not possible, and diagnostic aspiration or a trial of antiamebic antibiotics may be necessary. Unfortunately, aspiration is diagnostic in amebic abscess only approximately 10% to 20% of the time.[14]

Treatment

Before the availability of antibiotics and the routine use of drainage procedures, untreated hepatic pyogenic abscess was almost uniformly fatal. It was not until the classic review by Ochsner and DeBakey in 1938 (see earlier) that routine surgical drainage was used and dramatic reductions in mortality were noted. Open surgical drainage of pyogenic abscesses was the sole treatment (with the addition of antibiotics eventually) for hepatic abscess until the 1980s. Since then, less invasive percutaneous drainage techniques and intravenous (IV) antibiotics have been used. Laparotomy is generally reserved for failures of percutaneous drainage.

Once the diagnosis of pyogenic hepatic abscess is suspected, broad-spectrum IV antibiotics should be started immediately to control ongoing bacteremia and its associated complications. Blood samples and specimens of the abscess from aspiration should be sent for aerobic and anaerobic cultures. In immunosuppressed patients, mycobacterial and fungal cultures of the aspirate should be considered. Patients who are at risk for amebic infections should have blood samples drawn for amebic serology. Until cultures have specifically identified the offending organisms, broad-spectrum antibiotics covering gram-negative, gram-positive, and anaerobic organisms should be used. Combinations such as ampicillin, an aminoglycoside, and metronidazole or a third-generation cephalosporin with metronidazole are appropriate. The optimal duration of antibiotic treatment is not well defined and must be individualized, depending on the success of the drainage procedure. Antibiotics should certainly be continued while there is evidence of ongoing infection, such as fever, chills, or leukocytosis. Beyond this, it is unclear how long to continue antibiotics, but recommendations are usually for 2 weeks or more.

Percutaneous drainage for pyogenic hepatic abscesses was first reported in 1953 but did not gain widespread acceptance until the 1980s with the development of high-quality imaging and expertise in interventional radiologic techniques. During the last 25 years, percutaneous catheter drainage has become the treatment of choice for most patients (Fig. 53-28). Success rates range from 66% to 90%.[11,13] The obvious advantages are the simplicity of treatment (usually at the time of radiologic diagnosis) and avoidance of general anesthesia and a laparotomy. Relative contraindications to percutaneous catheter drainage include the presence of ascites, coagulopathy, and proximity to vital structures. Percutaneous drainage of multiple abscesses is usually met with a higher failure rate, but reports have demonstrated a high enough success rate that percutaneous approaches should be made first, reserving surgery for failures. A retrospective study comparing surgical with percutaneous drainage for large abscesses (>5 cm) has shown a better success rate with surgical drainage. Despite this, two thirds of percutaneous treatments were successful, and the overall morbidity and mortality rates were similar. There has never been a randomized prospective comparison between percutaneous and surgical therapy for hepatic abscess. However, case series have suggested that for most cases, there are similar success and mortality rates. Modern series attempting to compare these two techniques retrospectively must be read with caution because most patients treated surgically have failed to respond to other less invasive techniques. In general, surgery should be reserved for patients who require surgical treatment of the primary pathologic process (e.g., appendicitis) or for those who have failed to respond to percutaneous techniques. Laparoscopic drainage procedures have been reported with some success, and this can be considered a reasonable option to pursue in select cases.[11]

Percutaneous aspiration without the placement of an indwelling drain has been investigated by a number of groups. Success rates are generally 60% to 90% and are somewhat similar to those for percutaneous catheter drainage.[15] Most patients, however, require more than one aspiration, and 25% of patients require three or more aspirations. One randomized trial has evaluated percutaneous aspiration versus percutaneous catheter drainage. Success rates were 60% in the aspiration group and 100% in the catheter group. All but one patient in the aspiration group had a single aspiration. Another randomized trial of 64 patients has compared aspiration alone with catheter drainage. There were similar outcomes in terms of treatment success rate, hospital stay, antibiotic duration, and mortality. In the aspiration-only group, 40% required two aspirations and 20% required three aspirations. In general, catheter drainage remains the treatment of choice, although a trial of a single aspiration is reasonable to consider.

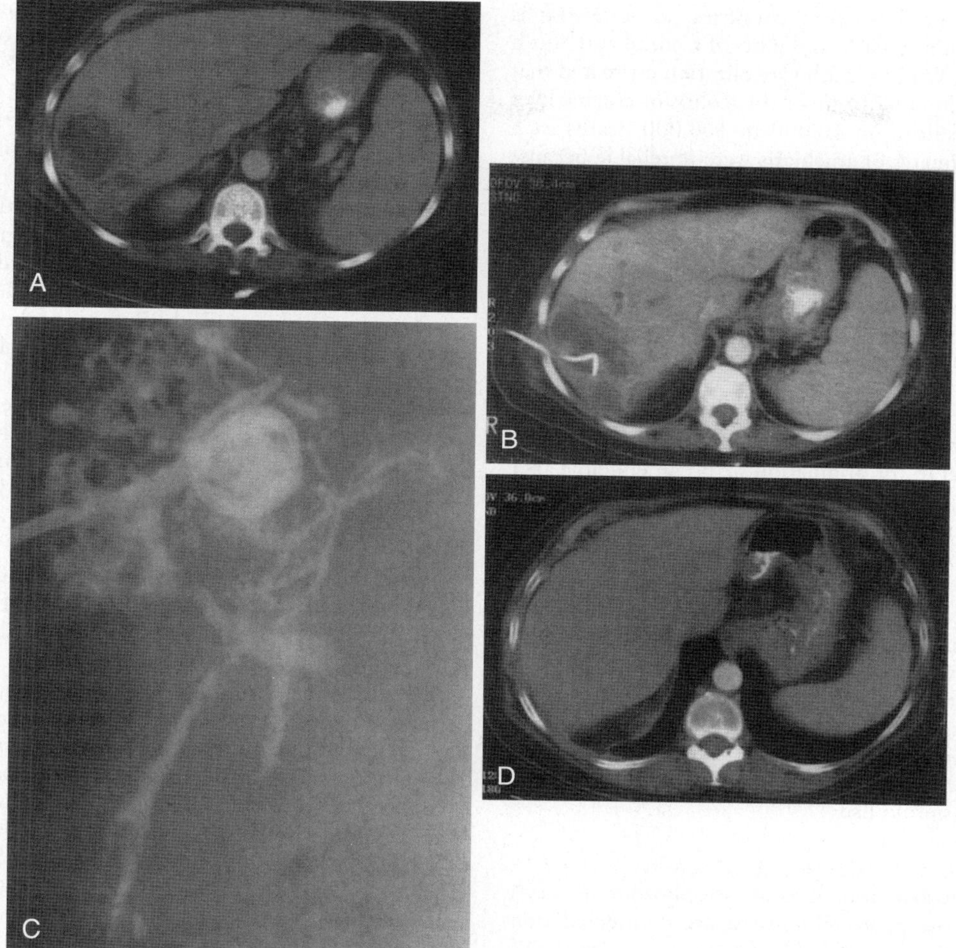

FIGURE 53-28 **A,** CT scan demonstrating multiloculated hepatic abscess in the right liver. **B,** CT scan at the time of percutaneous drainage. **C,** Contrast study through the drainage catheter demonstrating typical irregular loculated appearance as well as communication with biliary tree. **D,** Follow-up CT scan 3 months after treatment demonstrating complete resolution of abscess. (From Brown KT, Getrajdman GI: Interventional radiologic techniques in the liver and biliary tract. In Blumgart LH, Fong Y, editors: *Surgery of the liver and biliary tract,* London, 2000, WB Saunders, pp 575–594.)

Some investigators have reported success with antibiotics alone. Most of these patients, however, have had a diagnostic aspiration and thus at least a partial drainage. Also, other series have reported that antibiotic treatment without drainage carries a prohibitively high mortality (59% to 100%). In patients who are not surgical candidates or who refuse any invasive procedure, an attempt at antibiotic treatment is reasonable. However, this is not recommended in other situations.

Liver resection is occasionally required for hepatic abscess. This may be required for an infected hepatic malignant neoplasm, hepatolithiasis, or intrahepatic biliary stricture. If hepatic destruction from infection is severe, some patients may benefit from resection.

Outcomes

Mortality from pyogenic hepatic abscess has dramatically improved during the last 70 years. Before the routine use of surgical drainage, pyogenic abscess was uniformly fatal. With the routine use of surgical drainage and the use of IV antibiotics, mortality was reduced to approximately 50%, a figure that stayed relatively constant from 1945 until the early 1980s. Since then, the mortality has been reported from 10% to 20%, and series from the 1990s have demonstrated a mortality rate below 10%.[15] The most recent series from Memorial Sloan Kettering Cancer Center (MSKCC) has reported a 3% mortality. A number of studies have analyzed factors predictive of a poor outcome in patients with hepatic pyogenic abscess. The presence of malignant disease, factors associated with malignant disease (e.g., jaundice, markedly elevated LFT results), and signs of sepsis appear to be consistent markers of poor prognosis. Signs of chronic disease, such as hypoalbuminemia, are also often associated with a poor outcome. Finally, signs of severe infection, such as marked leukocytosis, APACHE II (Acute Physiology and Chronic Health Evaluation II) scores, abscess rupture, bacteremia, and shock, are also associated with mortality.

Amebic Abscess

Epidemiology

Amebiasis is largely a disease of tropical and developing countries but is also a significant problem in developed countries because of immigration and travel between countries. *E. histolytica* is endemic in Mexico, India, Africa, and parts of Central and South America. In 1995, the World Health Organization estimated that 40 to 50 million people suffer from amebic colitis or amebic liver abscess worldwide, resulting in 40,000 to 100,000 deaths each year.[14] Before this, estimates of amebiasis were unreliable because *E. histolytica* (the pathogenic form) was not differentiated from *Entamoeba dispar* (the nonpathogenic form). Male homosexuals with diarrhea, previously thought to harbor *E. histolytica,* were actually found to be infected with *E. dispar,* which requires no treatment. Epidemiologic studies specifically addressing *E. histolytica* infections have estimated that as many as 55% of those in endemic regions are infected, although less than 50% are symptomatic.

In contrast to pyogenic hepatic abscesses, patients with amebic liver abscesses tend to be Hispanic men, 20 to 40 years of age, with a history of travel to (or origination from) an endemic area. Poverty and cramped living conditions are associated with higher rates of infection. A male preponderance of more than 10 : 1 has been reported in almost all studies. For unclear reasons, menstruating women have a low incidence of invasive amebiasis, and pregnancy appears to abrogate this resistance. Heavy alcohol consumption is commonly reported and may render the liver more susceptible to amebic infection. Patients with impaired host immunity also appear to be at higher risk of infection and have higher mortality rates. Patients with amebic liver abscess without a history of travel to an endemic area often have associated immunosuppression, such as HIV infection, malnutrition, chronic infection, or chronic steroid use.[16]

Pathogenesis

E. histolytica is a protozoan and exists as a trophozoite or a cyst. All other species in the genus *Entamoeba* are considered nonpathogenic, and not all strains of *E. histolytica* are considered virulent. Ingestion of *E. histolytica* cysts through a fecal-oral route is the cause of amebiasis. Humans are the principal host, and the main source of infection is human contact with a cyst-passing carrier. Contaminated water and vegetables are also routes of human infection. Once ingested, the cysts are not degraded in the stomach and pass to the intestines, where the trophozoite is released and passed on to the colon. In the colon, the trophozoite can invade mucosa, resulting in disease.

It is thought that the trophozoites reach the liver through the portal venous system. There is no evidence for trophozoites passing through lymphatics. As implied by its name, *E. histolytica* trophozoites can lyse tissues through a complex set of events, including cell adherence, cell activation, and subsequent release of enzymes, resulting in necrosis. The principal mechanism is probably enzymatic cellular hydrolysis. Amebic liver abscesses are formed by progressing, localized hepatic necrosis producing a cavity containing acellular proteinaceous debris surrounded by a rim of invasive amebic trophozoites. Early development of an amebic liver abscess is associated with an accumulation of polymorphonuclear leukocytes, which are then lysed by the trophozoites.

Antiamebic antibodies develop rapidly in patients with invasive disease or an amebic hepatic abscess. Secretory immunoglobulin A (IgA) antibodies have been shown to inhibit adherence to colonic epithelium in vitro. However, the development of these antibodies does not halt the progression of disease. Interestingly, children who lack antiamebic IgG have innate resistance to invasive infection, suggesting an alternative immune-mediated response. There is now evidence that a cell-mediated helper T cell response is probably the major mechanism of resistance.

Pathology

Hepatic amebic abscess is essentially the result of liquefaction necrosis of the liver producing a cavity full of blood and liquefied liver tissue. The appearance of this fluid is typically described as resembling anchovy sauce; the fluid is odorless unless secondary bacterial infection has taken place. The progressive hepatic necrosis continues until Glisson capsule is reached because the capsule is resistant to hydrolysis by the amebae. Thus, amebic abscesses tend to abut the liver capsule. Because of the resistance of Glisson capsule, the cavity is typically crisscrossed by portal triads protected by this peritoneal sheath. Early on, the formed cavity is ill-defined, with no real fibrous response around the edges. However, a chronic abscess can ultimately develop a fibrous capsule and may even calcify. Like pyogenic abscesses, amebic abscesses tend to occur mainly in the right liver.

Clinical Features

Approximately 80% of patients with amebic liver abscess present with symptoms lasting from a few days to 4 weeks. The duration of symptoms has been found to be typically less than 10 days. The presenting clinical signs and symptoms are summarized in Table 53-6. The typical clinical picture is a patient 20 to 40 years of age who has recently traveled to an endemic area, with fever, chills, anorexia, right upper quadrant pain and tenderness, and hepatomegaly. The abdominal pain is typically constant, dull, and localized to the right upper quadrant. Although some studies report higher numbers, approximately 25% of patients have diarrhea despite an obligatory colonic infection. Synchronous hepatic abscess is found in one third of patients with active amebic colitis.

TABLE 53-6 Signs, Symptoms, and Laboratory Findings in Amebic Liver Abscess*

PARAMETER	AVERAGE	RANGE	NO. OF CASES REVIEWED
Symptoms and Signs			
Abdominal pain (%)	92	73-100	1701
Fever (%)	90	72-100	2192
Abdominal tenderness (%)	78	40-100	1424
Hepatomegaly (%)	62	20-100	1539
Anorexia (%)	47	28-89	499
Weight loss (%)	39	11-83	871
Diarrhea (%)	23	12-40	1426
Jaundice (%)	22	5-50	1630
Laboratory Tests			
Stool cysts, trophozoites (%)	12	4-30	4908
Amebae in cyst aspirate (%)	42	30-76	1402
Hemoglobin (g/dL)	12.1	10.2-12.8	229
Alkaline phosphatase (% >120 U/liter)	76	65-91	589
Total bilirubin (g/dL)	1.4	0.8-2.4	509
Albumin (g/dL)	2.8	2.3-3.4	404
AST (× upper limit normal)	1.7	1.0-2.5	459

*In an extensive literature review.

Jaundice, as a result of a large abscess compressing the biliary tree, is not as rare as was once thought, with an average 22% of patients presenting with this feature worldwide. Weight loss and myalgias may occur when symptoms have been present for weeks. Pleuritic or right shoulder pain can occur if there is irritation of the right hemidiaphragm. Symptoms and tenderness may be epigastric or left sided if the abscess is located in the left liver. Rupture into the peritoneum with peritonitis occurs infrequently; when it does occur, it is more often with left-sided abscesses. Rare cases of rupture into the pleural space, pericardium, and other intra-abdominal organs have also been reported.

Patients presenting acutely (symptoms <10 days) versus those with a chronic presentation (>2 weeks) differ clinically. Acute presentations are typically more dramatic, with high fevers, chills, and significant abdominal tenderness. In the acute presentation, 50% of patients have multiple lesions, whereas with the chronic presentation, more than 80% of patients have a single right-sided lesion. A more complicated course tends to ensue in the acute presentation, but response to therapy is similar in both groups.

Laboratory abnormalities are common in amebic abscess (Table 53-6). Patients typically have a mild to moderate leukocytosis, without eosinophilia. Anemia is common. Mild abnormalities of LFT results, including albumin, PT-INR, ALP, AST, and bilirubin levels, are typical. The most common LFT abnormality is an elevated PT-INR. Because more than 70% of patients with amebic liver abscess do not have detectable amebae in their stool, the most useful laboratory evaluation is the measurement of circulating antiamebic antibodies, which are present in 90% to 95% of patients. A number of serologic tests have been devised over the years. An indirect hemagglutinin test was used extensively in the past and has a sensitivity of 90%. This test has largely been replaced by enzyme immunoassays, which detect presence of antibodies against the parasite and are simple, rapidly performed, and inexpensive. An enzyme immunoassay has a reported sensitivity of 99% and specificity higher than 90% in patients with hepatic abscess. Unfortunately, the presence of antibodies may reflect prior infection, and interpretation can be difficult in endemic areas. Ongoing studies are focusing on identifying specific *E. histolytica* antigens in an attempt to identify acute infection. The antigen detection kits have been evaluated in endemic areas. These kits can detect the *E. histolytica* lectin antigen in the serum and liver abscess pus and in small studies have been shown to have high sensitivity. However, the sensitivity may decrease if the test is performed after treatment with metronidazole.[17]

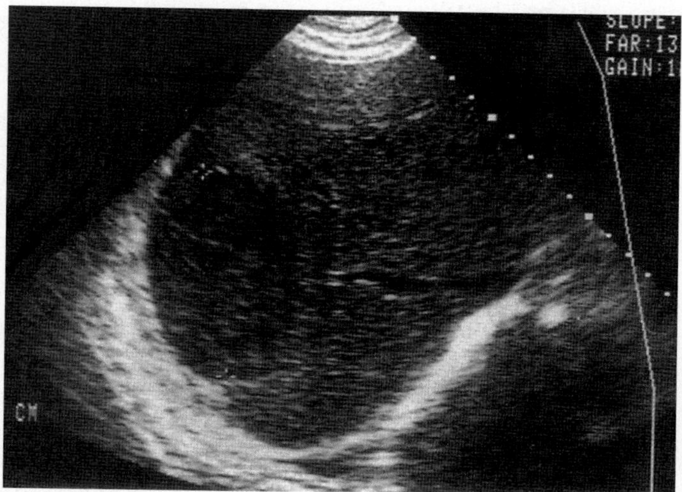

FIGURE 53-29 Typical ultrasound image of an amebic hepatic abscess. Note the peripheral location, rounded shape with poor rim, and internal echoes. (From Thomas PG, Ravindra KV: Amebiasis and biliary infection. In Blumgart LH, Fong Y, editors: *Surgery of the liver and biliary tract*, London, 2000, WB Saunders, pp 1147–1166.)

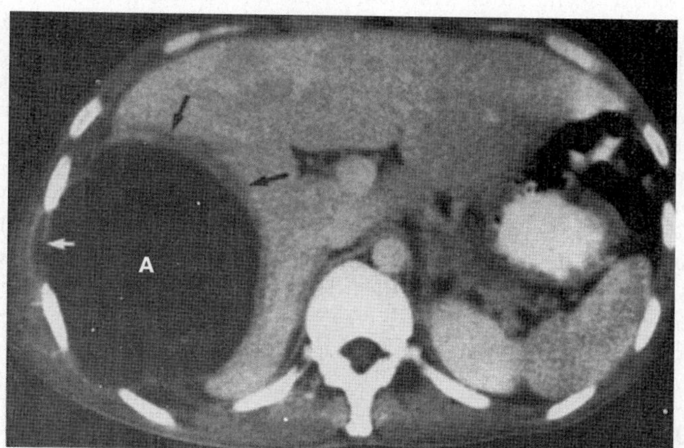

FIGURE 53-30 CT scan of amebic abscess. The lesion is peripherally located and round. The rim is nonenhancing but shows peripheral edema *(black arrows)*. Note the extension into the intercostal space *(white arrow)*.

Radiologic studies are a critical element in the diagnosis of amebic liver abscess. Plain chest radiographs are abnormal in approximately 50% of cases, usually demonstrating an elevated right diaphragm, pleural effusion, or atelectasis. Abdominal ultrasound has a reported accuracy of approximately 90% when it is combined with a typical history and clinical presentation. Typical findings on abdominal ultrasound are a rounded lesion abutting the liver capsule (see earlier) without significant rim echoes, interpreted as an abscess wall. The contents of the cavity are usually hypoechoic and nonhomogeneous (Fig. 53-29). These findings on ultrasound are found in 40% to 70% of cases. Abdominal CT scanning is probably more sensitive than ultrasound and is helpful in differentiating amebic from pyogenic abscess, with rim enhancement noted in the pyogenic abscess (Fig. 53-30). CT can also be helpful in identifying simple cysts and necrotic tumors. MRI of the liver has no distinct advantages over CT or ultrasound in typical cases but may be helpful in differentiating atypical lesions. Nuclear medicine studies, such as gallium scanning or technetium Tc 99m liver scans, can be helpful in differentiating pyogenic from amebic abscesses because the amebic abscesses typically do not contain leukocytes and therefore do not light up on these scans.[18]

When this workup is still not definitive and diagnostic uncertainty persists, two options should be considered. First, a therapeutic trial of antiamebic drugs can be used. If a rapid improvement occurs, this supports the diagnosis. In situations in which amebic serology is inconclusive and a therapeutic trial of antibiotics is deemed inappropriate or has failed to improve symptoms, the second option, a diagnostic aspiration, should be considered. A pyogenic abscess would have bacteria and leukocytes, whereas an amebic abscess would contain the typical so-called anchovy sauce. Cultures of amebic abscess are usually negative and do not contain leukocytes. In patients for whom neoplasm or hydatid disease is in the differential diagnosis, aspiration should not be performed.

Differential Diagnosis

The differential diagnosis of an amebic liver abscess can be broad and include diseases such as viral hepatitis, echinococcal disease, cholangitis, cholecystitis, and even other inflammatory abdominal disorders, such as appendicitis. Malignant lesions of the liver can also have similar presentations in atypical situations. On occasion, primary pulmonary disorders must be considered. Usually, the most important distinction to be made is between pyogenic and amebic abscess. The essential elements of this distinction are summarized in Table 53-5 and in the earlier section on pyogenic abscess.

Treatment

The mainstay of treatment for amebic abscesses is metronidazole (750 mg orally, three times daily for 10 days), which is curative in more than 90% of patients. Clinical improvement is usually seen within 3 days. Other nitroimidazoles (e.g., secnidazole, tinidazole) are also as effective and are commonly used outside the United States. If response to metronidazole is poor or the drug is not tolerated, other agents can be used. Emetine hydrochloride is effective against invasive amebiasis, particularly in the liver, but requires intramuscular injections and has serious cardiac side effects. A more attractive option is chloroquine, but this is a less effective agent. After treatment of the liver abscess, it is recommended that luminal agents such as iodoquinol, paromomycin, and diloxanide furoate be administered to treat the carrier state.

Therapeutic needle aspiration of amebic abscesses has been proposed. However, a Cochrane systematic review did not support any benefit of therapeutic aspiration in addition to metronidazole treatment over metronidazole treatment alone to hasten clinical or radiologic resolution of amebic liver abscesses.[19] In general, aspiration is recommended for diagnostic uncertainty (see earlier), with failure to respond to metronidazole therapy in 3 to 5 days, or in abscesses thought to be at high risk for rupture. Abscesses larger than 5 cm in diameter and in the left liver are thought to carry a higher risk of rupture, and aspiration should be considered.

Outcomes

Although amebic liver abscesses usually respond rapidly to treatment, there are uncommon complications of which one must be aware. The most frequent complication of amebic abscess is rupture into the peritoneum, pleural cavity, or pericardium. The size of the abscess appears to be the most important risk factor for rupture, and the overall incidence of rupture ranges from 3% to 17%. Most peritoneal ruptures tend to be contained by the diaphragm, abdominal wall, or omentum, but rupture can fistulize into a hollow viscus. A peritoneal rupture usually is manifested as abdominal pain, peritonitis, and a mass or generalized distention. Laparotomy was advocated in the past for this complication, but now many patients are treated successfully with percutaneous drainage. Laparotomy is indicated in cases of doubtful diagnosis, hollow viscus perforation, fistulization resulting in hemorrhage or sepsis, and failure of conservative therapy. Rupture into the pleural space usually results in a large and rapidly accumulated effusion that collapses the involved lung. Treatment consists of thoracentesis, but if secondary bacterial infection ensues, more aggressive surgical approaches may be necessary. Rupture can occur into the bronchi and is usually self-limited with postural drainage and bronchodilators. Rarely, a left-sided abscess may rupture into the pericardium and can be manifested as an asymptomatic pericardial effusion or even tamponade. This must be treated with aspiration or drainage through a pericardial window. Other complications include compression of the biliary tree or IVC from a very large abscess and the development of a brain abscess.

The mortality for all patients with amebic liver abscess is approximately 5% and does not appear to be affected by the addition of aspiration to metronidazole therapy or by chronicity of symptoms. When an abscess ruptures, mortality ranges from 6% to as high as 50%. Factors independently associated with poor outcome are elevated serum bilirubin level (>3.5 mg/dL), encephalopathy, hypoalbuminemia (<2.0 g/dL), multiple abscess cavities, abscess volume larger than 500 mL, anemia, and diabetes. Although clinical improvement after adequate treatment with antiamebic agents is the rule, radiologic resolution of the abscess cavity is usually delayed. The average time to radiologic resolution is 3 to 9 months, and in some patients, it can take years. Studies have shown that more than 90% of the visible lesions disappear radiologically, but a small percentage of patients are left with a clinically irrelevant residual lesion.

Hydatid Cyst

Hydatid disease or echinococcosis is a zoonosis that occurs primarily in sheep-grazing areas of the world but is common worldwide because the dog is a definitive host. Echinococcosis is endemic in Mediterranean countries, the Middle East, Far East, South America, Australia, New Zealand, and east Africa.[20] Humans contract the disease from dogs, but there is no human-to-human transmission.[21,22]

There are three species that cause hydatid disease. *Echinococcus granulosus* is the most common, and *Echinococcus multilocularis* and *Echinococcus ligartus* account for a small number of cases.[20] Dogs are the definitive host of *E. granulosus;* the adult tapeworm is attached to the villi of the ileum. Up to thousands of ova are passed daily and deposited in the dog's feces. Sheep are the usual intermediate host, but humans are an accidental intermediate host. Humans are an end stage to the parasite. In the human duodenum, the parasitic embryo releases an oncosphere containing hooklets that penetrate the mucosa, allowing access to the bloodstream. In the blood, the oncosphere reaches the liver (most commonly) or lungs, where the parasite develops its larval stage—the hydatid cyst.

Three weeks after infection, a visible hydatid cyst develops, which then slowly grows in a spherical manner. A pericyst or fibrous capsule derived from host tissues develops around the hydatid cyst. The cyst wall itself has two layers, an outer gelatinous membrane (ectocyst) and an inner germinal membrane (endocyst). Brood capsules are small, intracystic cellular masses in which future worm heads develop into scoleces. In a definitive host, the scoleces develop into an adult tapeworm; but in the intermediate host, they can differentiate only into a new hydatid cyst. Freed brood capsules and scoleces are found in the hydatid fluid and form the so-called hydatid sand. Daughter cysts are true replicas of the mother cyst. Hydatid cysts can die with degeneration of the membranes, development of cystic vacuoles, and calcification of the wall. Calcification of a hydatid cyst, however, does not always imply that the cyst is dead.

Hydatid cysts are diagnosed in equal numbers of men and women at an average age of about 45 years. Approximately 75% of hydatid cysts are located in the right liver and are solitary. The clinical presentation of a hydatid cyst is largely asymptomatic until complications occur. The most common presenting symptoms are abdominal pain, dyspepsia, and vomiting. The most frequent sign is hepatomegaly. Jaundice and fever are each present in approximately 8% of patients. Bacterial superinfection of a hydatid cyst can occur and be manifested like a pyogenic abscess. Rupture of the cyst into the biliary tree or bronchial tree or free rupture into the peritoneal, pleural, or pericardial cavities can occur. Free ruptures can result in disseminated echinococcosis or a potentially fatal anaphylactic reaction. In cases of diagnostic uncertainty, a battery of serologic tests are available to evaluate antibody response, but all are plagued by low sensitivity and specificity.

Ultrasound is most commonly used worldwide for the diagnosis of echinococcosis because of its availability, affordability, and accuracy. A number of findings on ultrasound can be diagnostic but depend on the stage of the cyst at the time of the examination. A simple hydatid cyst is well circumscribed with budding signs on the cyst membrane and may contain free-floating hyperechogenic hydatid sand. A rosette appearance is seen when daughter cysts are present. The cyst can be filled with an amorphous mass, which can be diagnostically misleading. Calcifications in the wall of the cyst are highly suggestive of hydatid disease and can be helpful in the diagnosis (Fig. 53-31). Similar findings are seen on CT or MRI scans. These cross-sectional imaging studies can also evaluate extrahepatic disease and demonstrate detailed hepatic anatomic relationships to the cyst. In patients with suspected biliary involvement, ERCP or percutaneous transhepatic cholangiography may be necessary.

Although the treatment of hepatic hydatid cysts is primarily surgical, alternative options are in evolution.[23] In general, most cysts should be treated; but in older patients with small, asymptomatic, densely calcified cysts, conservative management is appropriate. In preparation for an operation, preoperative steroids have been recommended but are not universally used. The anesthesiologist should have epinephrine and steroids available in case of an anaphylactic reaction. A number of operations have been used, but in general, the abdomen is completely explored, the liver mobilized, and the cyst exposed. Packing off the abdomen is important because rupture can result in anaphylaxis and diffuse seeding. The cyst is usually then aspirated through a closed suction system and flushed with a scolicidal agent, such as hypertonic saline. The cyst is then unroofed, which can then be followed by a number of possibilities, including excision (or pericystectomy), marsupialization procedures, leaving the cyst open, drainage of the cyst, omentoplasty, and partial hepatectomy to encompass the cyst. Total pericystectomy or formal partial hepatectomy can also be performed without entering the cyst (Fig. 53-32). Both radical (resection) and conservative (drainage and evacuation) surgical approaches appear to be equally effective at controlling disease, although a prospective comparison has never been performed. When bile duct communication is diagnosed preoperatively or at operation, it must be meticulously sought after. Simple suture repair is often sufficient, but major biliary repairs, approaches through the common bile duct, or postoperative ERCP may be necessary. Laparoscopic techniques for drainage and unroofing of cysts have been reported in a number of series, with encouraging results. Recurrence rates after surgical treatment range from 1% to 20% but are generally 5% or less in experienced centers.

In the past, percutaneous aspiration of hydatid cysts was contraindicated because of the risk of rupture and uncontrolled spillage. However, percutaneous aspiration with injection of scolicidal agents has been reported with high success rates in highly selected

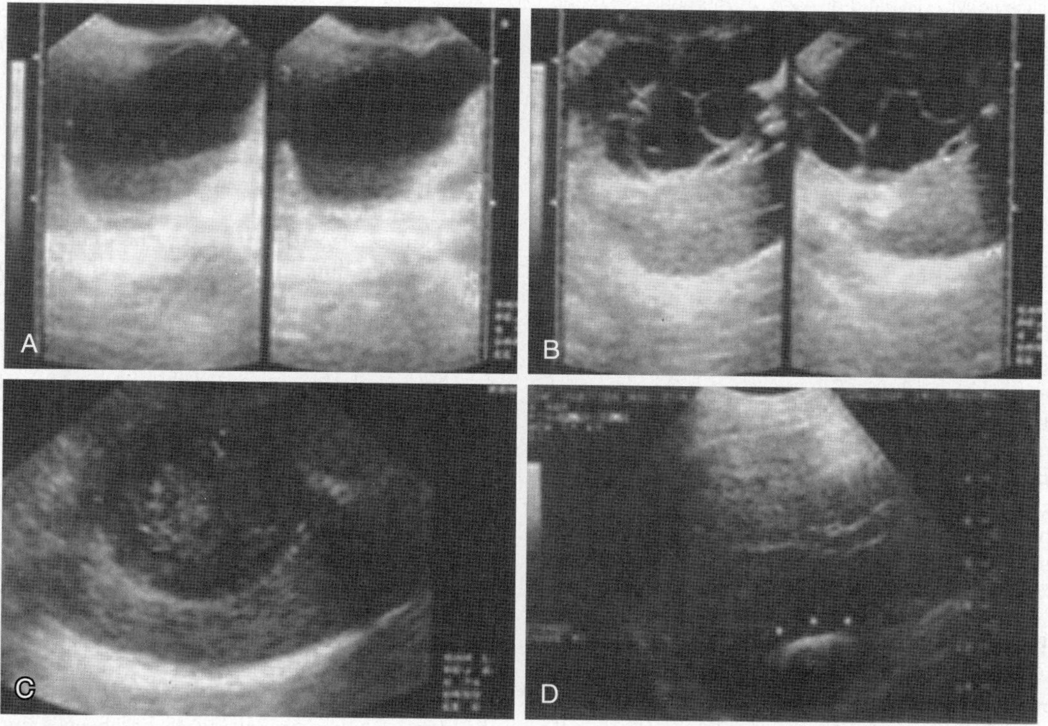

FIGURE 53-31 Ultrasound image demonstrating typical characteristics of a hydatid cyst at varying stages. **A,** Simple hydatid cyst with hydatid sand. **B,** Daughter and granddaughter cysts and typical rosette appearance. **C,** Hydatid cyst filled with amorphous mass, giving a solid or semisolid appearance. **D,** Calcified cyst with eggshell appearance. (From Thomas PG, Ravindra KV: Amebiasis and biliary infection. In Blumgart LH, Fong Y, editors: *Surgery of the liver and biliary tract,* London, 2000, WB Saunders, pp 1147–1166.)

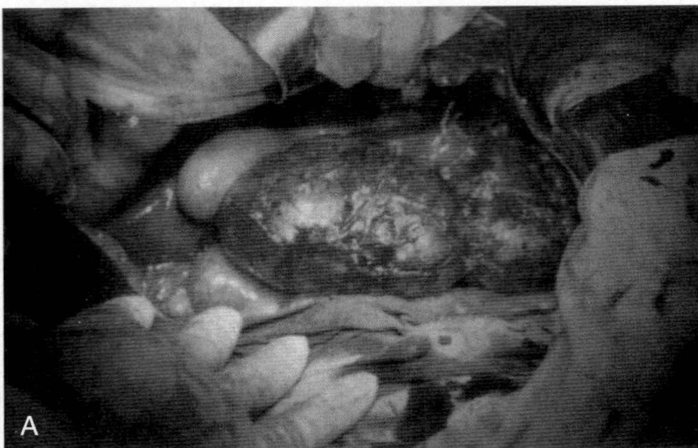

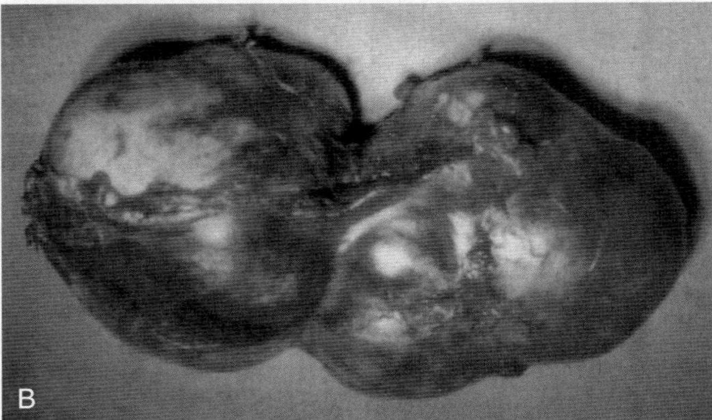

FIGURE 53-32 A, Peripheral hydatid cyst of the left liver. **B,** Intact specimen after pericystectomy. Note that the entire pericyst has been removed. (From Milicevic MN: Hydatid disease. In Blumgart LH, Fong Y, editors: *Surgery of the liver and biliary tract*, London, 2000, WB Saunders, pp 1167–1204.)

patients.[24] This technique is known as PAIR (puncture, aspiration, injection, and reaspiration) and has become more accepted in some centers. Two randomized trials, one comparing PAIR with surgery ($N = 50$) and one comparing PAIR with medical therapy, have shown similar success rates. These trials were small and had significant methodologic problems, limiting the ability to draw firm conclusions.[25] Although surgery remains the treatment of choice, further prospective trials are clearly indicated to address this interesting and potentially useful technique. Treatment of echinococcosis with albendazole or mebendazole is effective at shrinking cysts in many patients with *E. granulosus* infection, but cyst disappearance occurs in well below 50% of patients. Preoperative treatment may decrease the risk of spillage and is a reasonable and safe practice.[15] Medical therapy without definitive resection or drainage should be considered only for widely disseminated disease or poor surgical candidates.

Recurrent Pyogenic Cholangitis

Recurrent pyogenic cholangitis (RPC) is a syndrome of repeated attacks of cholangitis secondary to biliary stones and strictures that involve the extrahepatic and intrahepatic ducts. The condition has many names but is often referred to as Oriental cholangiohepatitis or hepatolithiasis. The disease is almost exclusively found in Asians and Asian medical centers. However, it is also seen in Asian immigrants throughout the world. Men and women are equally affected, and historically, the disease strikes at an early age (20 to 40 years) in patients from lower socioeconomic classes.[26]

The cause of RPC is unknown but is related to recurrent infection of biliary radicals with gut bacteria. Ultimately, stones and strictures develop in the biliary tree, but it is not known which occurs first. The stones are bilirubinate stones; in some patients, no stones are found and only biliary sludge is demonstrated. An association between RPC and *Clonorchis sinensis* and *Ascaris lumbricoides* infection has been noted, but a true causal relationship has never been proven.[27]

Strictures can be found anywhere in the biliary tree but usually involve the intrahepatic main hepatic ducts, most often the left hepatic duct. The gallbladder is involved only in approximately 20% of cases. Cirrhosis and liver failure are seen only in longstanding disease, usually after multiple operations. Other complications include choledochoduodenal fistulas and acute pancreatitis from common bile duct stones. An increased incidence of cholangiocarcinoma has been noted, but a causal relationship is difficult to prove.

The typical patient with RPC is a young Asian of a lower socioeconomic background who presents with repeated bouts of cholangitis. The symptoms and presentation are those of cholangitis. These include fever, right upper quadrant abdominal pain, and jaundice. Biliary obstruction is usually incomplete, and therefore marked jaundice and pruritus are not common. There is usually leukocytosis and abnormal LFT results consistent with biliary obstruction. Evaluation of the anatomic distribution of disease is critical to formulation of a sound therapeutic plan. A combination of ultrasound, CT, and direct cholangiography is often necessary to evaluate these patients. Direct cholangiography is performed endoscopically or transhepatically and is considered an important study complementing the cross-sectional imaging. Magnetic resonance cholangiopancreatography can combine cross-sectional imaging and cholangiography in one noninvasive test and may ultimately replace direct cholangiography.

In an acute presentation, most patients improve with conservative management, allowing time for radiologic studies and planning of a definitive operation, which is the treatment of choice. If intervention is necessary during the acute phase, it must focus on adequate decompression of the biliary tree through open common bile duct exploration or endoscopic papillotomy with stenting. Although nonoperative approaches, such as percutaneous transhepatic cholangioscopic lithotomy, have been developed, surgical treatment remains the treatment of choice. Percutaneous transhepatic cholangioscopic lithotomy is generally used for poor-risk surgical patients and those who have failed to respond to surgical treatment. Stone clearance rates are high (>80%) and necessary for a successful long-term outcome. Unfortunately, stone recurrence is common and is mostly related to the presence of biliary strictures.[28]

The goal of operative approaches is to clear the biliary tree of stones and to bypass, resect, or enlarge strictures.[29] Many cases require only exploration of the common bile duct, with or without hepaticojejunostomy. In complicated cases, providing permanent access to the biliary tree for interventional radiologic procedures by extending the end of the Roux-en-Y hepaticojejunostomy to the skin or subcutaneous space has been a successful approach (Fig. 53-33). Other potentially necessary procedures include stricturoplasty and partial hepatectomy. Partial hepatectomy is advocated for patients with intrahepatic strictures, hepatic atrophy, liver abscess, or suspicion of cholangiocarcinoma.[30]

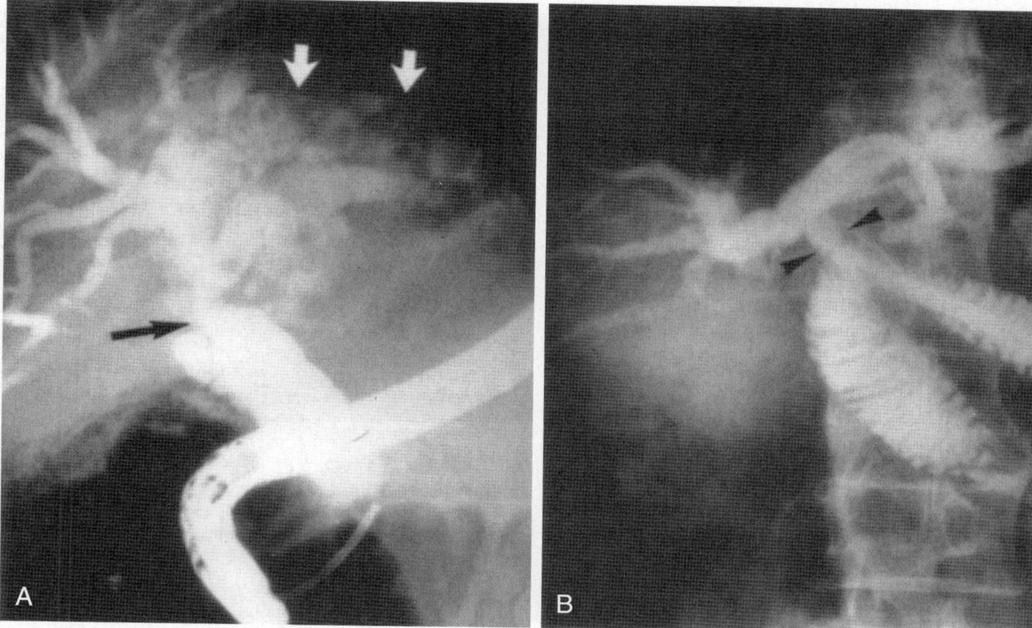

FIGURE 53-33 **A,** Cholangiogram of a patient with recurrent pyogenic cholangitis and a common hepatic duct stricture *(black arrow)*. There are numerous stones inside dilated left ducts *(white arrows)*. **B,** A hepaticojejunostomy to the segment III duct *(arrowheads)* has been performed, and a flexible choledochoscope is shown passing through the anastomosis into the peripheral left ducts. All stones have been cleared. (From Fan ST, Wong J: Recurrent pyogenic cholangitis. In Blumgart LH, Fong Y, editors: *Surgery of the liver and biliary tract*, London, 2000, WB Saunders, pp 1205–1225.)

In a large series from Asia, where surgery and hepatectomy are liberally applied, surgical mortality rates are 1%. Moreover, with aggressive treatment, there is almost a 100% stone clearance rate. Long-term outcome is excellent, with a less than 5% stone recurrence rate. Long-term survival is mostly related to the presence of cholangiocarcinoma, which is found in approximately 10% of patients. Particularly complicated cases can have a higher rate of recurrent symptoms.

NEOPLASMS

Solid Benign Neoplasms

It is estimated that benign focal liver masses are present in approximately 10% to 20% of the population in developed countries. With the increasing use of rapidly improving radiologic examinations, these entities have been encountered more frequently. Familiarity with the clinical characteristics, natural history, imaging characteristics, and indications for surgery in these tumors is essential. Many benign lesions can be adequately characterized by modern imaging studies, such as CT, ultrasound, and MRI. In unclear cases, serum tumor markers (e.g., AFP, CEA) and a search for a primary tumor in the case of suspected metastases should be carried out. A resection might be necessary to make a definitive diagnosis. Laparoscopy for assessment, biopsy, or resection has become an important diagnostic technique as well.[31,32]

Liver Cell Adenoma

Liver cell adenoma (LCA) is a relatively rare benign proliferation of hepatocytes in the context of a normal liver. It is predominantly found in young women (aged 20 to 40 years) and is often associated with steroid hormone use, such as long-term oral contraceptive pill (OCP) use. Male anabolic hormone use can also predispose to development of LCA. The female-to-male ratio is approximately 11:1. LCAs are usually singular, but multiple lesions have been reported in 12% to 30% of cases. Interestingly, cases with multiple adenomas are not associated with OCP use and do not have as dramatic a female preponderance. On histologic evaluation, LCAs are composed of cords of benign hepatocytes containing increased glycogen and fat. Bile ductules are not observed histologically, and the normal architecture of the liver is absent in these lesions. Hemorrhage and necrosis are commonly seen.[33] On the basis of detailed molecular pathology correlation studies, a French collaborative group has recently proposed a molecular-pathologic classification whereby the adenomas are classified as β-catenin mutated adenoma, *HNF1A* mutated adenoma, inflammatory adenoma, and not otherwise specified adenoma.[34,35] Molecular studies have also identified genetic signatures associated with a higher risk of malignant transformation. Specifically, highest risk of malignant transformation is observed in LCA with β-catenin activation.[35,36] Patients with LCA present with symptoms approximately 50% to 75% of the time. Upper abdominal pain is common and may be related to hemorrhage into the tumor or local compressive symptoms. The physical examination is usually unrevealing, and tumor markers are normal. Dramatic presentations with free intraperitoneal rupture and bleeding can occur. Imaging tends to be characteristic and obviates the need for tissue diagnosis most of the time.[37-39] Because of intratumoral hemorrhage, the necrosis and fat component of LCA tends to be heterogeneous on CT. On contrast-enhanced CT, LCA tends to have peripheral enhancement with centripetal progression. MRI scans of LCA also have specific imaging characteristics, including a well-demarcated heterogeneous mass containing fat or hemorrhage. Despite high-quality imaging, resection may sometimes be necessary to secure a diagnosis in difficult cases. Intriguingly, studies are elucidating a correlation between the molecular subtypes described and imaging characteristics.[40]

The two major risks of LCA are rupture, with potentially life-threatening intraperitoneal hemorrhage, and malignant transformation. Quantifying the risk of rupture is difficult, but it has been estimated to be as high as 30% to 50%, with all instances of spontaneous rupture occurring in lesions 5 cm and larger.[39] Although there are numerous reports of transformation of LCA into hepatocellular carcinoma (HCC), the true risk of transformation is probably low. Hepatic adenomas with β-catenin activation should be considered for early surgical intervention as malignant transformation most commonly occurs in this subtype.[36,41]

Patients who present with acute hemorrhage need emergent attention. If possible, hepatic artery embolization is a helpful and usually effective temporizing maneuver. Once the patient is stabilized and appropriately resuscitated, a laparotomy and resection of the mass are required. Symptomatic masses should be similarly resected. Patients with asymptomatic LCAs taking OCPs can be watched for regression after stopping of the OCPs, although progression and rupture have been observed in this setting. Behavior of LCAs during pregnancy has been unpredictable, and resection before a planned pregnancy is usually recommended. Overall, the surgeon must compare the risks of expectant management with serial imaging studies and AFP measurements against those of resection. Resection is usually recommended because of low mortality in experienced hands and the risks of observation. Margin status is not important in these resections, and limited resections can be performed. The management of adenomatosis is controversial, but large lesions should probably be resected because of the risk of rupture, whereas the risk of malignancy is low in lesions smaller than 5 cm.[42] On occasion, liver transplantation is necessary for aggressive forms of adenomatosis.[43,44]

Focal Nodular Hyperplasia

Focal nodular hyperplasia (FNH) is the second most common benign tumor of the liver after hemangioma and is predominantly discovered in young women.[39] FNH is characterized by a central fibrous scar with radiating septa, although no central scar is seen in approximately 15% of cases (Fig. 53-34). On microscopic examination, FNH contains cords of benign-appearing hepatocytes divided by multiple fibrous septa originating from a central scar. Typical hepatic vascularity is not seen, but atypical biliary epithelium is found scattered throughout the lesion. The central scar often contains a large artery that branches out into multiple smaller arteries in a spoke wheel pattern. The cause of FNH is not known, but the most common theory is that FNH is related to a developmental vascular malformation. Female hormones and OCPs have been implicated in the development and growth of FNH, but the association is weak and difficult to prove.

In most patients, FNH is an incidental finding at laparotomy or, more commonly, on imaging studies. If symptoms are noted, vague abdominal pain is most often present, but a variety of nonspecific symptoms have been described. It is often difficult to ascribe these reported symptoms to the presence of FNH, and therefore other possible causes must be sought. Physical examination is usually unrevealing, and mild abnormalities of liver function may be found. Serum AFP levels are normal.

With advances in hepatobiliary imaging, most cases of FNH can be diagnosed radiologically with reasonable certainty. Contrast-enhanced CT and MRI have become accurate methods of diagnosing FNH.[45] FNH typically shows strong hypervascularity in the arterial phase of CT or MRI with central nonenhancing scar. The enhancement fades over time, and the lesion becomes isointense to the liver parenchyma in the portal and delayed phases. When no central scar is seen, however, radiologic diagnosis is difficult, and differentiation from LCA or a malignant mass, especially fibrolamellar HCC, can sometimes be impossible. On occasion, histologic confirmation is necessary, and resection is recommended for definitive diagnosis. Fine-needle aspiration for the diagnosis of FNH has been recommended but is often unrevealing.

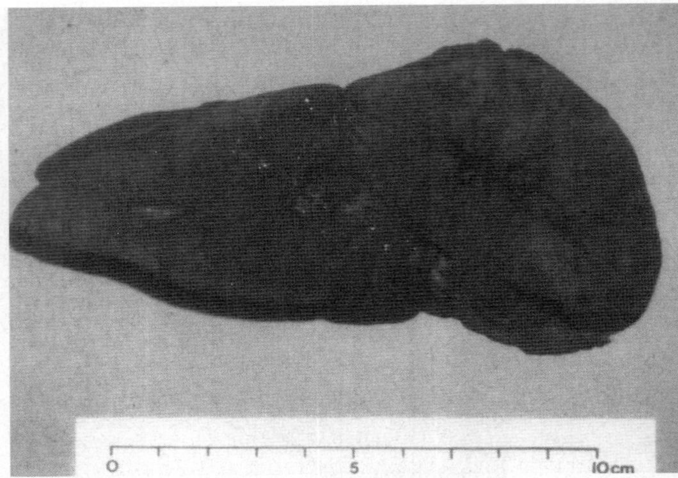

FIGURE 53-34 Cross section of resected focal nodular hyperplasia. Note the well-defined central scar. (From Hugh TJ, Poston GJ: Benign liver tumors and masses. In Blumgart LH, Fong Y, editors: *Surgery of the liver and biliary tract*, London, 2000, WB Saunders, pp 1397–1422.)

Most FNH tumors are benign and indolent. Rupture, bleeding, and infarction are exceedingly rare, and malignant degeneration of FNH has never been reported. The treatment of FNH therefore depends on diagnostic certainty and symptoms. Asymptomatic patients with typical radiologic features do not require treatment.[39] If diagnostic uncertainty exists, resection may be necessary for histologic confirmation. Symptomatic patients should be thoroughly investigated to look for other pathologic processes to explain the symptoms. Careful observation of symptomatic FNH with serial imaging is reasonable because symptoms may resolve in a significant number of cases. Patients with persistent symptomatic FNH or an enlarging mass should be considered for resection. Because FNH is a benign diagnosis, resection must be performed, with minimal morbidity and mortality.[46]

Hemangioma

Hemangioma is the most common benign tumor of the liver.[39] It occurs in women more than in men (3:1 ratio) and at a mean age of approximately 45 years. Small capillary hemangiomas are of no clinical significance, whereas larger cavernous hemangiomas more often come to the attention of the liver surgeon (Fig. 53-35). Cavernous hemangiomas have been associated with FNH and are also theorized to be congenital vascular malformations. The enlargement of hemangiomas is by ectasia rather than by neoplasia. They are usually solitary and less than 5 cm in diameter, and they occur with equal incidence in the right and left hemilivers. Lesions larger than 5 cm are arbitrarily called giant hemangiomas. Involution or thrombosis of hemangiomas can result in dense fibrotic masses that may be difficult to differentiate from malignant tumors. On microscopic examination, they are

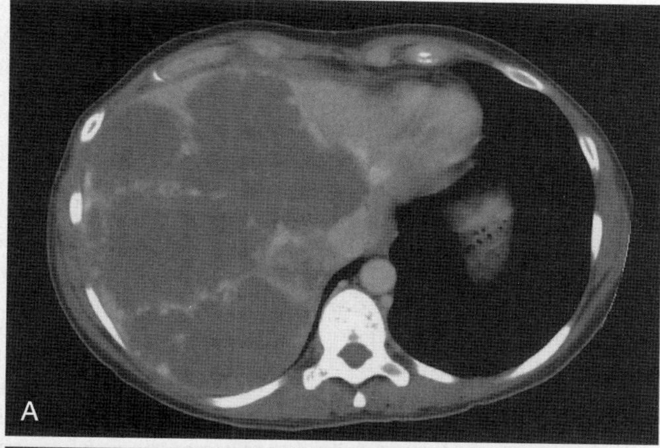

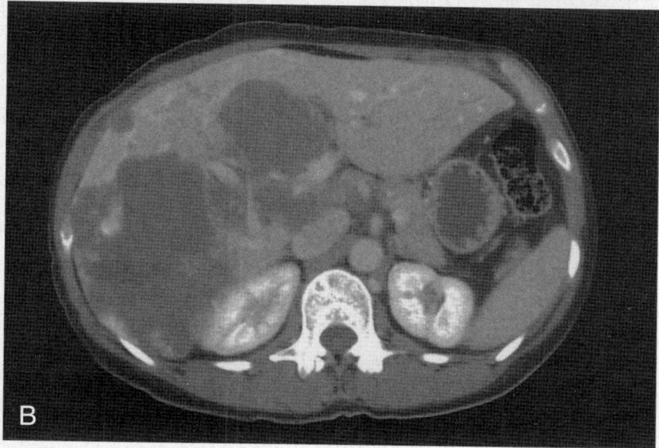

FIGURE 53-35 **A** and **B,** CT scans of a large cavernous hemangioma showing displacement of left and middle hepatic veins and abutment of the left portal vein. The mass was symptomatic and required an extended right hepatectomy for removal.

endothelium-lined, blood-filled spaces separated by thin fibrous septa.[47,48]

Hemangiomas are usually asymptomatic and found incidentally on imaging studies. Large compressive masses may cause vague upper abdominal symptoms. Symptoms ascribed to a liver hemangioma, however, mandate a search for other disease because an alternative cause of symptoms will be found in approximately 50% of cases. Rapid expansion or acute thrombosis can occasionally cause symptoms. Spontaneous rupture of liver hemangiomas is exceedingly rare. An associated syndrome of thrombocytopenia and consumptive coagulopathy known as Kasabach-Merritt syndrome is rare but well described.

LFT results and tumor markers are usually normal in liver hemangiomas. Radiologic investigation can make the diagnosis reliably in most cases. CT and MRI are usually sufficient if a typical peripheral nodular enhancement pattern is seen.[45,47] Isotope-labeled red blood cell scans are an accurate test but are rarely necessary if high-quality CT and MRI are available. Percutaneous biopsy of a suspected hemangioma is potentially dangerous and inaccurate. Therefore, biopsy is not recommended.

The natural history of liver hemangioma is generally benign; it appears that most remain stable for a long time, with a low risk of rupture or hemorrhage.[39] Growth and development of symptoms do occur, however, occasionally requiring resection. There has never been a report of malignant degeneration of a liver hemangioma. An asymptomatic patient with a secure diagnosis can therefore be simply observed.[39] Symptomatic patients should undergo a thorough evaluation looking for alternative explanations for the symptoms but are candidates for resection if no other cause is found. Rupture, significant change in size, and development of the Kasabach-Merritt syndrome are indications for resection. In rare cases of diagnostic uncertainty, resection may be necessary for a definitive diagnosis to be made. Resection of liver hemangiomas should be performed, with minimal morbidity and mortality. The preferred approach to resection is enucleation with arterial inflow control, but anatomic resections may be necessary in some cases. Surgery on large central hemangiomas can be associated with significant morbidity.

Liver hemangiomas in children are common, accounting for approximately 12% of all childhood hepatic tumors.[49] They are usually multifocal and can involve other organs. Large hemangiomas in children can result in congestive heart failure secondary to arteriovenous shunting. Untreated symptomatic childhood hemangiomas are associated with high mortality. On the other hand, almost all small capillary hemangiomas resolve. Symptomatic childhood hemangiomas may be treated with therapeutic embolization; medical therapy should be initiated for congestive heart failure. Radiation and chemotherapeutic agents have been used, but experience has been limited. Resection may be necessary for symptomatic lesions or rupture.

Other Benign Tumors

Most benign solid liver tumors are LCAs, FNHs, or hemangiomas, but there are other benign hepatic tumors. However, these are rare and can be difficult to differentiate from malignant neoplasms. Macroregenerative nodules, previously known as adenomatous hyperplasia, are single or multiple, well-circumscribed, bile-stained, bulging surface nodules that occur primarily in cirrhotics and result from the hyperplastic response to chronic liver injury. These lesions have malignant potential and can be difficult to distinguish from HCC. Nodular regenerative hyperplasia is a benign diffuse micronodular (usually <2 cm) process associated with lymphoproliferative disorders, collagen vascular diseases, and the use of steroids or chemotherapy. Nodular regenerative hyperplasia has no malignant potential and is not associated with cirrhosis. Biopsy may be necessary to distinguish these focal nodules from malignant neoplasms.

Mesenchymal hamartomas are rare solitary tumors of childhood that account for 5% of pediatric liver tumors. They are usually large cystic masses found in the right liver that present as progressive, painless, abdominal distention. Resection of mesenchymal hamartomas may be necessary in the case of large lesions causing a mass effect.

Fatty tumors of the liver are rarely encountered but can usually be distinguished by typical characteristics on CT or MRI scans. Fatty tumors of the liver include primary lipomas, myelolipomas (which contain hematopoietic tissue), angiolipomas (which contain blood vessels), and angiomyolipomas (which contain smooth muscle). Focal fatty change in the liver can be confused with a neoplastic process and is becoming more common with improved imaging and the increasing incidence of hepatic steatosis.

Benign fibrous tumors of the liver can become large and symptomatic, requiring resection. Inflammatory pseudotumors of the liver are localized masses of inflammatory cells that can mimic a neoplasm. The cause of these inflammatory lesions is unknown but may be related to thrombosed vessels or old abscesses. Other extremely rare benign hepatic tumors include leiomyomas, myxomas, schwannomas, lymphangiomas, and teratomas.

Intrahepatic biliary cystadenomas or bile duct adenomas are rare but can cause biliary symptoms. Biliary hamartomas and biliary hyperplasia are common and are often seen as small white surface lesions that can mimic small metastatic tumors at abdominal exploration. Adrenal and pancreatic rests have also been found in the liver.

Primary Solid Malignant Neoplasms

Hepatocellular Carcinoma

Epidemiology. HCC is the most common primary malignant neoplasm of the liver and one of the most common malignant neoplasms worldwide, accounting for more than 1 million deaths annually. The geographic distribution of HCC is clearly related to the incidence of hepatitis B virus (HBV) infection. The highest incidence of disease (>10 to 20 cases/100,000) is found in Southeast Asia and tropical Africa. The lowest incidence (1 to 3 cases/100,000) is found in Australia, North America, and Europe. In high-incidence areas, rates are variable. For example, Taiwan has an incidence of 150 cases/100,000, and Singapore has an incidence of 28 cases/100,000. Epidemiologic evidence strongly suggests that HCC is largely related to environmental factors; the incidence of HCC in immigrants eventually approaches that of the local population after several generations. An exception to this is that whites living in high-prevalence areas tend to have a low incidence of HCC. This is likely related to the continuation of the lifestyle and environment of their home country. It is probable that the variation in incidence rates among immigrants is related to HBV carrier rates. A significant rise in the incidence of HCC in the United States and other Western countries has been noted during the last 35 years. However, recent data suggest that at least in the United States, the epidemic may have peaked as the incidence rates have stabilized in the last few years.[50,51] The explanation for the observed increase during the last few decades is not understood, but the emergence of hepatitis C virus (HCV) infection and immigration patterns have been suggested.[52-54] Risk of HCC is further increased in obese patients and in those with nonalcoholic fatty liver disease and nonalcoholic steatohepatitis.[55] Given that obesity and its ensuing complications are increasing at epidemic proportion in the Western world, obesity as the cause of HCC is becoming more important. Recent data also suggest that addressing the environmental factors can lead to reduction in incidence of HCC. In Taiwan, treatment of chronic hepatitis B and C under the auspices of a national viral hepatitis therapy program has met with a reduction in incidence and mortality due to HCC.[56]

HCC is two to eight times more common in men than in women in low- and high-incidence areas. Although sex hormones may play a minor role in the development of HCC, the higher incidence in men is probably related to higher rates of associated risk factors, such as HBV infection, cirrhosis, smoking, alcohol abuse, and higher hepatic DNA synthesis in cirrhosis. In general, the incidence of HCC increases with age, but a tendency to development of HCC earlier in high-incidence areas has been noted. For example, in Mozambique, 50% of patients with HCC were found to be younger than 30 years. This may be related to differing ages at infection and the natural histories of hepatitis B and C.

Causative factors. A large number of associations between hepatic viral infections, environmental exposure, alcohol use, smoking, genetic metabolic diseases, cirrhosis, and OCP use and the development of HCC have been recognized. Overall, 75% to 80% of HCC cases are related to HBV (50% to 55%) or HCV (25% to 30%) infections. It is also clear from research that the development of HCC is a complex and multistep process that involves any number of these risk factors.[54,57]

Many years of research have documented a clear association between persistent HBV infection and the development of HCC.[58] Studies have estimated relative risks of 5 to 100 for the development of HCC in HBV-infected individuals compared with noninfected individuals. Other evidence includes the following observations: geographic areas high in HBV infection have high rates of HCC; HBV infection precedes the development of HCC; the sequence of HBV infection to cirrhosis to HCC is well documented; and the HBV genome is found in the HCC genome. The HBV has no known oncogenes, but insertional mutagenesis into hepatocytes may be a contributing factor to the development of HCC. Another proposed mechanism is related to cirrhosis and chronic hepatic inflammation, which is present in 60% to 90% of patients with HBV infection and HCC. Cirrhosis, however, is not a prerequisite for the development of HBV-related HCC. The risk of HCC is not simply related to HBV exposure but requires chronic infection (i.e., chronically positive HBV surface antigen). There is a higher risk of persistent infection (carrier state) when the infection is acquired at birth or during early childhood. Familial clustering of HCC is probably related to early vertical transmission of the virus and establishment of the chronic carrier state.

Hepatitis C has been discovered to be a major cause of chronic liver disease in Japan, Europe, and the United States, where there is a relatively low rate of HBV infection. Antibodies to the HCV are found in 76% of patients with HCC in Japan and Europe and in 36% of patients in the United States. HBV and HCV infections are both independent risk factors for the development of HCC but probably act synergistically when an individual is infected with both viruses. Although the natural history of HCV infection is not completely understood, it appears to be one of chronic infection, with a benign early course. However, the ultimate development of cirrhosis and HCC may ensue. Studies on the rates of progression to cirrhosis estimate a median time of 30 years, but differing progression rates yield a range of less than 20 years to more than 50 years. Factors associated with a more rapid progression include male gender, chronic alcohol use, and older age at the time of infection. HCV is an RNA virus that does not integrate into the host genome, and therefore the pathogenesis of HCV-related HCC may be related more to chronic inflammation and cirrhosis than to direct carcinogenesis.[59,60]

The true relationship of cirrhosis and HCC is difficult to ascertain, and suggestions of causation remain speculative. Cirrhosis is not required for the development of HCC, and hepatocarcinogenesis is not an inevitable result of cirrhosis. The relationship of cirrhosis and HCC is further complicated by the fact that they share common associations. Furthermore, some associations (e.g., HBV infection, hemochromatosis) are associated with higher risk of HCC, whereas others (e.g., alcohol, primary biliary cirrhosis) are associated with a lower risk of HCC. Research has demonstrated that cirrhotic livers with higher DNA replication rates are associated with the development of HCC.

Chronic alcohol abuse has been associated with an increased risk of HCC, and there may be a synergistic effect with HBV and HCV infection. Alcohol causes cirrhosis but has never been shown to be directly carcinogenic in hepatocytes. Thus, alcohol likely acts as a cocarcinogen. Cigarette smoking has been linked to the development of HCC, but the evidence is not consistent, and the contributing risk independent of viral hepatitis is likely to be small. Aflatoxin, produced by *Aspergillus* spp., is a powerful hepatotoxin. With chronic exposure, aflatoxin acts as a carcinogen and increases the risk of HCC. The offending fungi grow on grains, peanuts, and food products in tropical and subtropical regions. Ingestion of contaminated foods results in aflatoxin exposure. Levels of aflatoxin in these implicated foods are regulated in the United States.

Other chemicals have also been implicated as carcinogens related to HCC. These include nitrites, hydrocarbons, solvents, pesticide, and vinyl chloride. Thorotrast (colloidal thorium dioxide) is an angiographic medium that was used in the 1930s. It emits high levels of long-lasting radiation and has been associated with hepatic fibrosis, angiosarcoma, cholangiosarcoma, and HCC. Associations with inherited metabolic liver diseases, such as hereditary hemochromatosis, α_1-antitrypsin deficiency, and Wilson disease, have also been implicated as risk factors for HCC. Associations with hormonal manipulations, such as the use of OCPs and anabolic steroids, have been suggested but are weak and are probably better linked specifically to adenoma and well-differentiated HCC. Research has been focusing on relationships of HCC with diabetes, obesity, and metabolic syndrome.[55,61-63]

Clinical presentation. Most commonly, patients presenting with HCC are men 50 to 60 years of age who complain of right upper quadrant abdominal pain and weight loss and have a palpable mass. In countries endemic for HBV, presentation at a younger age is common and probably related to childhood infection. Unfortunately, in unscreened populations, HCC tends to be manifested at a later stage because of the lack of symptoms in early stages. Presentation at an advanced stage is often with vague right upper quadrant abdominal pain that sometimes radiates to the right shoulder. Nonspecific symptoms of advanced malignant disease, such as anorexia, nausea, lethargy, and weight loss, are also common. Another common presentation of HCC is hepatic decompensation in a patient with known mild cirrhosis or even in patients with unrecognized cirrhosis.

HCC can rarely be manifested as a rupture, with the sudden onset of abdominal pain followed by hypovolemic shock secondary to intraperitoneal bleeding. Other rare presentations include hepatic vein occlusion (Budd-Chiari syndrome), obstructive jaundice, hemobilia, and fever of unknown origin. Less than 1% of cases of HCC are manifested with a paraneoplastic syndrome, usually hypercalcemia, hypoglycemia, and erythrocytosis. Small, incidentally noted tumors have become a more common presentation because of the knowledge of specific risk factors, screening programs for diagnosed HBV or HCV infection, and increasing use of high-quality abdominal imaging.

Diagnosis. Radiologic investigation is a critical part of the diagnosis of HCC. In the past, liver radioisotope scans and angiography were common methods of diagnosis, but ultrasound, CT, and MRI have replaced these studies. Ultrasound plays a significant role in screening and early detection of HCC, but definitive diagnosis and treatment planning rely on CT or MRI. Contrast-enhanced CT and MRI protocols aimed at diagnosing HCC take advantage of the hypervascularity of these tumors, and arterial-phase images are critical to assess the extent of disease adequately.[64,65] CT and MRI also evaluate the extent of disease in terms of peritoneal metastases, nodal metastases, and extent of vascular and biliary involvement. Detection of bland or tumor thrombus in the portal or hepatic venous system is also important and can be diagnosed with any of these modalities (Fig. 53-36).

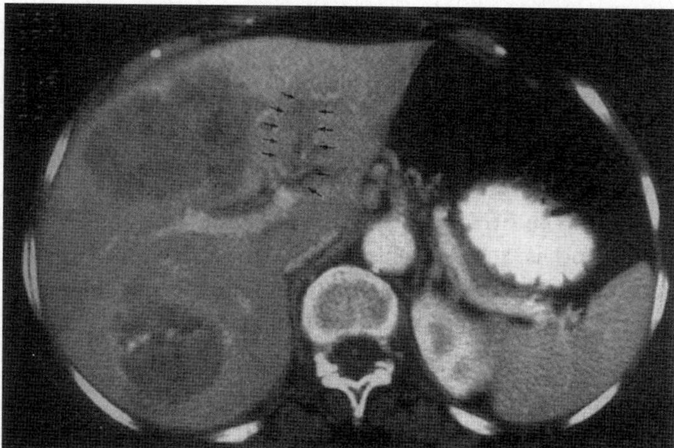

FIGURE 53-36 Contrast-enhanced CT scan demonstrating multifocal hepatocellular carcinoma. The left portal vein is invaded and expanded by tumor. (From Roddie ME, Adam A: Computed tomography of the liver and biliary tree. In Blumgart LH, Fong Y, editors: *Surgery of the liver and biliary tract*, London, 2000, WB Saunders, pp 309–340.)

AFP measurements can be helpful in the diagnosis of HCC. However, AFP measurement is associated with multiple problems. First, AFP measurements have low sensitivity and specificity. The specificity and positive predictive values of AFP improve with higher cutoff levels (e.g., 400 ng/mL) but at the cost of sensitivity. False-positive elevations of serum AFP levels can be seen in inflammatory disorders of the liver, such as chronic active viral hepatitis. Furthermore, AFP is not specific to HCC and can be elevated with intrahepatic cholangiocarcinoma and colorectal metastases. With improvements in imaging technology and the ability to detect smaller tumors, AFP is largely used as an adjunctive test in patients with liver masses. AFP levels are particularly useful in monitoring treated patients for recurrence after normalization of levels.

Since the proposal of guidelines for the diagnosis of HCC by the Barcelona-2000 European Association for the Study of the Liver conference[66] and the American Association for the Study of Liver Disease,[67] new data have accumulated and the recommendations have evolved.[68,69] AFP used to play a major role in the diagnosis of HCC larger than 2 cm.[67] However, given the excellent performance of contrast-enhanced imaging modalities, AFP does not play a critical role in the diagnosis of HCC anymore.[68,69] For hepatic nodules 1 to 2 cm in size on a background of cirrhosis, a contrast-enhanced triple-phase CT and MRI scan is now recommended.[68,69] If typical features of HCC on imaging (arterially enhancing mass with washout of contrast material in delayed phases) are observed, diagnosis of HCC is presumed. For lesions larger than 2 cm, a single study may suffice. However, for lesions 1 to 2 cm in size, contrast-enhanced CT and MRI have a sensitivity of 53% to 62%, specificity of approximately 100%, positive predictive value of 95% to 100%, and negative predictive value of 80% to 84%.[70] Performance of both MRI and CT in a sequential fashion can increase the sensitivity and may be required for difficult cases.[70]

Patients with appropriate risk factors and suggestive radiologic features, with or without an elevated AFP level, who are candidates for potentially curative surgical therapy do not require preoperative biopsy unless the diagnosis is in question. Percutaneous fine-needle aspiration of HCC does run a small risk of tumor cell spillage (estimated to be ≈1%) and rupture or bleeding, especially in cirrhotic livers and subcapsular tumors. Once the diagnosis of HCC has been made, the disease must be staged to develop an appropriate treatment plan. Most patients with HCC have two diseases, and survival is as much related to the tumor as it is to cirrhosis. Staging includes an extent of disease and extent of cirrhosis workup.

In assessing the extent of disease, the common sites of metastases must be considered. HCC largely metastasizes to the lung, bone, and peritoneum. Preoperative history should focus on symptoms referable to these areas. Extent of disease in the liver, including macrovascular invasion and the presence of multiple liver masses, must also be considered. Cross-sectional abdominal imaging, including arterial-phase images (see earlier), yields information on the extent of disease in the liver as well as peritoneal disease. Preoperative chest CT is mandatory because lung metastases are usually asymptomatic. Routine bone scans are not performed unless there are suggestive symptoms or signs.

Assessment of liver function is absolutely critical in considering treatment options for a patient with HCC. Liver resection is considered the treatment of choice for HCC, and the risk of postoperative liver failure and death must be considered. This risk is related to the degree of cirrhosis, portal hypertension, amount of liver resected (functional liver reserve), and regenerative potential response. Other successful treatments are available for HCC, such as ablative techniques, embolization techniques, and liver transplantation. Therefore, a complete assessment of tumor and liver function must be carried out. A number of tests of liver function are available, generally divided into clinical assessment and functional tests, and there are many clinical assessment schemes (see earlier). However, Child-Pugh status is used most often. Child-Pugh class C patients are not candidates for resectional therapy, whereas Child-Pugh class A patients can usually tolerate some extent of liver resection. Many consider Child-Pugh class B patients to be candidates for operation, but they are generally borderline, and therapy must be individualized.

Outside of scoring systems, it has been demonstrated that significant portal hypertension, regardless of biochemical assessments, is highly predictive of postoperative liver failure and death. Portal hypertension can be assessed directly through hepatic vein wedge pressures, but it is usually obvious on high-quality imaging in the form of splenomegaly, a cirrhotic-appearing liver, and intra-abdominal varices. Blood work usually demonstrates marked cytopenias. Most typically, patients have thrombocytopenia. Functional tests of liver function have been well described but are not routinely used in most Western centers because the results of studies evaluating their predictive value have been mixed.

Staging laparoscopy has been used as a staging tool in HCC and spares about one in five patients a nontherapeutic laparotomy. Laparoscopy yields additional information about the extent of disease in the liver, extrahepatic disease, and cirrhosis. The yield of laparoscopy is dictated by the extent of disease and is only selectively used. The presence of clinically apparent cirrhosis, radiologic evidence of vascular invasion, or bilobar tumors increases the yield to 30%, whereas without these factors, the yield is 5%.[71]

There are a number of staging systems for HCC, but none have been shown to be particularly superior; they probably depend on the specific population in which the disease is being staged as well as the cause of HCC in that particular population of patients. The TNM staging system is not routinely used for HCC because it does not accurately predict survival; it does not take liver function into account. Moreover, the TNM staging system relies on pathology that is frequently unavailable preoperatively. The Okuda staging system is an older but simple and effective system that takes liver function and tumor-related factors into account. It adds up a single point for the presence of tumor involving more than 50% of the liver, presence of ascites, albumin level less than 3 g/dL, and bilirubin level higher than 3 mg/dL. The Okuda staging system reliably distinguishes patients with a prohibitively poor prognosis from those with potential for long-term survival. The most well validated staging system is the Cancer of the Liver Italian Program (CLIP), which was rigorously developed and has been prospectively validated (Table 53-7). An example of a scoring system that is probably population specific is the Chinese University Prognostic Index (CUPI), which takes into account TNM stage, symptoms, and ascites and the levels of AFP, bilirubin, and ALP; it appears to apply mainly to HBV-related HCC in China.

Pathology. On histologic evaluation, HCC is graded as well, moderately, or poorly differentiated. The grade of HCC, however, has never been shown to predict outcome accurately. In gross appearance, the growth patterns of HCC have been classified in a number of ways. The most useful scheme divides HCC into three distinct growth patterns that have distinct relationships to outcome. The hanging type of HCC is connected to the liver by a small vascular stalk and is easily resected without sacrifice of a significant amount of adjacent non-neoplastic liver tissue. This type can grow to substantial size without involving much normal liver tissue. The pushing type of HCC is well demarcated and often contains a fibrous capsule. It is characterized by growth that displaces vascular structures rather than invading them. This type is usually resectable. The last type is called the infiltrative type of HCC, which tends to invade vascular structures, even at a small size. Resection of the infiltrative type is often possible, but positive histologic margins are common. Small tumors (<5 cm) usually do not fall into any of these groups and are often discussed as a separate entity.

Finally, HCC can be manifested in a multifocal manner. Most HCC probably starts as a single tumor, but ultimately multiple satellite lesions can develop secondary to portal vein invasion and metastases. Multifocal tumors throughout the liver probably represent the end stage of HCC, with multiple metastases and multiple primary tumors.

TABLE 53-7 Cancer of the Liver Italian Program Score*

CLINICAL PARAMETERS	CUTOFF VALUES	POINTS
Child-Pugh class	A	0
	B	1
	C	2
Tumor morphology	Uninodular, <50% extension	0
	Multinodular, <50% extension	1
	Massive or extension >50%	2
AFP level	<400 ng/dL	0
	>400 ng/dL	1
Portal vein thrombosis	No	0
	Yes	1

*Score ranges from 0 to 6; a score of 4 to 6 is generally considered advanced disease, whereas a score of 0 to 3 has the potential for long-term survival.

BOX 53-1 Treatment Options for Hepatocellular Carcinoma

Surgical
Resection
Orthotopic liver transplantation

Ablative
Ethanol injection
Acetic acid injection
Thermal ablation (cryotherapy, radiofrequency ablation, microwave)

Transarterial
Embolization
Chemoembolization

Radiotherapy
Combination transarterial and ablative: external beam radiation

Systemic
Chemotherapy
Hormonal
Immunotherapy

Treatment. There are a large number of treatment options for patients with HCC, reflecting the heterogeneity of this disease and the lack of a proven superior treatment, except complete resection (Box 53-1). Deciding on a treatment regimen for any one patient must take into consideration the stage of malignancy, condition of the patient and of the liver, and experience of the treating physician.

Complete excision of HCC by partial hepatectomy or by total hepatectomy and liver transplantation is the treatment of choice, when possible, because it has the highest chance of long-term survival. In general, however, only 10% to 20% of patients are considered to have resectable disease. Historically, mortality rates for partial hepatectomy have ranged from 1% to 20%, but if it is performed in healthy patients without advanced cirrhosis, most series have a mortality rate of less than 5%. Advances in surgical technique have also allowed the development of limited segmental resections when appropriate, which preserves liver function and improves early postoperative recovery. Selection of the appropriate patient for resection is critical and must take into account the condition of the liver and extent of disease. Patients with Child-Pugh class B or C cirrhosis or portal hypertension do not tolerate resection. The volume of the FLR is also an important consideration and is associated with postoperative complications and mortality. Preoperative portal vein embolization is an effective strategy to increase the volume and function of the FLR and should be used liberally in patients with Child-Pugh class A cirrhosis with a small FLR (i.e., <30% to 40% of the total liver volume) who are being considered for a major resection. The overall postresection survival rates for HCC are 58% to 100% at 1 year, 28% to 88% at 3 years, 11% to 75% at 5 years, and 19% to 26% at 10 years. These results obviously depend on the stage of the tumor and degree of cirrhosis in each particular series. Together, they give a sense of the possibilities.

A variety of prognostic factors predictive of survival after resection have been identified, but none are universally agreed on. The most commonly cited negative prognostic factors are tumor size, cirrhosis, infiltrative growth pattern, vascular invasion, intrahepatic metastases, multifocal tumors, lymph node metastases, margin less than 1 cm, and lack of a capsule. The best outcomes are found in patients with single small tumors, but size alone should not contraindicate resection. Especially for patients with large tumors that are outside the criteria for transplantation, not many therapeutic options are available. In such patients with adequate liver function, adequate functional liver remnant, and resectable tumors, surgical resection may offer the best possible outcomes. Multifocal tumors and major vascular invasion are generally associated with a poor outcome, but some groups advocate resection in highly select patients.[72,73] A randomized controlled trial corroborated these findings. In this study, patients with multifocal HCC outside Milan criteria were randomized to resection or transarterial chemoembolization.[74] In this study, resection provided better overall survival for patients with multifocal HCC compared with transarterial chemoembolization, suggesting that resection may be an option for these patients.

Theoretically, orthotopic liver transplantation is the ideal treatment for HCC because it addresses the liver dysfunction and cirrhosis and the HCC. The limitations of transplantation are the need for chronic immunosuppression and the lack of organ donors. There has been growing interest in the use of partial hepatectomy from live donors, which addresses the lack of organ donors but remains a somewhat controversial approach. Early series of transplantation for HCC had high recurrence rates and relatively poor long-term survival, largely attributed to the fact that most of these patients were undergoing transplantation for advanced disease. Refinements in patient selection—namely, patients with single tumors smaller than 5 cm or no more than three tumors 3 cm in size—have resulted in improved outcomes.[75,76] Long-term survival rates with more stringent selection criteria have ranged from 50% to 85%. Studies have begun to expand the indications for orthotopic liver transplantation without a major effect on long-term survival but likely an increase in overall recurrence rates. Comparison of results of resection with transplantation is difficult, and the two should be viewed as complementary rather than competitive.[77] Patients with advanced cirrhosis (Child class B and C) and early-stage HCC should be considered for transplantation, whereas those with Child class A cirrhosis have similar results with transplantation and resection and should probably be resected.[78-80]

A number of other nonsurgical local ablative therapies are available for the treatment of small tumors. Percutaneous ethanol injection (PEI) is a useful technique for ablating small tumors. The tumor is killed by a combination of cellular dehydration, coagulative necrosis, and vascular thrombosis. Most tumors smaller than 2 cm can be ablated with a single application of PEI, but larger tumors may require multiple injections. Long-term survival after PEI for tumors smaller than 5 cm has been reported to range from 24% to 40%, but no randomized trials have compared PEI with resection. Percutaneous injection of acetic acid is a technique similar to PEI but has stronger necrotizing abilities, making it more useful in septated tumors.

Thermal ablative techniques that freeze or heat tumors to destroy them have become popular. Cryotherapy uses a specialized cryoprobe to freeze and thaw tumor and surrounding liver tissue, with resulting necrosis. Cryotherapy is usually performed at laparotomy or laparoscopically, but it has been performed with percutaneous techniques. One advantage is that the ice ball formed is easily monitored with ultrasound. Disadvantages include a heat sink effect limiting the usefulness of freezing near major blood vessels and a relatively high complication rate of 8% to 41%. Reported 2-year survival rates for cryoablation of HCC range from 30% to 60%, but no comparative studies to resection have been carried out. Radiofrequency ablation (RFA) uses high-frequency alternating current to create heat around an inserted probe, resulting in temperatures higher than 60° C (140° F) and immediate cell death. Although initially limited to smaller tumors, improvements in technology have created RFA probes reportedly able to ablate tumors as large as 7 cm. Nonetheless, the efficacy of RFA for HCCs larger than 3 cm is limited because of increased local recurrence rates. RFA is also limited by the protective effect of blood vessels and does not ablate well in these areas. The procedure can easily be performed percutaneously, with low complication rates, and optimal guidance systems are being developed. Recent data suggest that resection may be superior to RFA for small HCCs in terms of both disease-free and overall survival.[81]

Transarterial therapy for HCC is based on the fact that most of the tumor's blood supply is from the hepatic artery. Today, the transarterial therapy is applied in a percutaneous fashion, thus avoiding morbidity and mortality of laparotomy. Percutaneous transarterial embolization can induce ischemic necrosis in HCC, resulting in response rates as high as 50% (Fig. 53-37). Attempts to improve the efficacy of arterial embolization have included adding chemotherapeutic agents (chemoembolization) to the bland embolization particles and oils, such as ethiodized oil (Ethiodol), that are selectively taken up by HCCs.[82] Although chemoembolization has not been shown to be superior to bland embolization with regard to survival, a trial suggested an improvement in local control with chemoembolization.[83] Seven randomized trials have compared embolization or chemoembolization with conservative management. Two of these trials and a meta-analysis have confirmed an overall survival advantage from the embolization strategies.[84-86] The selection of appropriate candidates for embolization is important, and treatment should generally be limited to patients with preserved liver function and asymptomatic multinodular tumors without vascular invasion. Poor selection will result in a higher incidence of treatment-induced liver failure, offsetting the potential benefits.

External beam radiation therapy (EBRT) has a limited role in the treatment of HCC, although occasional dramatic responses are seen. EBRT is limited by damage to normal liver parenchyma and to surrounding organs, but newer methods of conformal radiotherapy and breath-gated techniques are improving the usefulness of this treatment modality. Intra-arterial injections of iodine-131 with Ethiodol or yttrium-90 in glass microspheres have also been used to deliver localized radiation to HCCs, with reports of dramatic response rates. Transarterial radiotherapy is a potentially promising therapy for HCC as a primary or adjuvant therapy.[82]

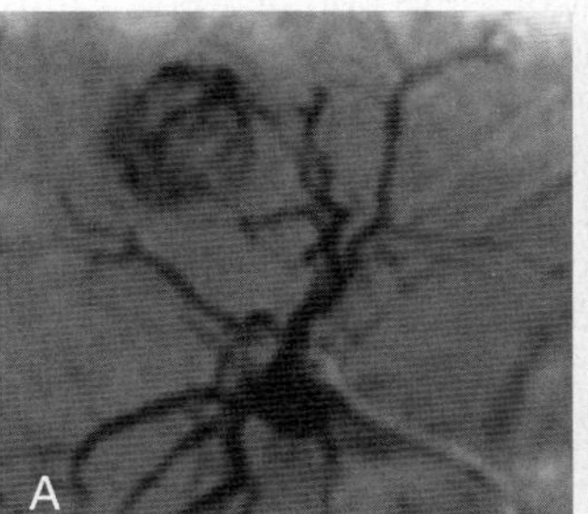

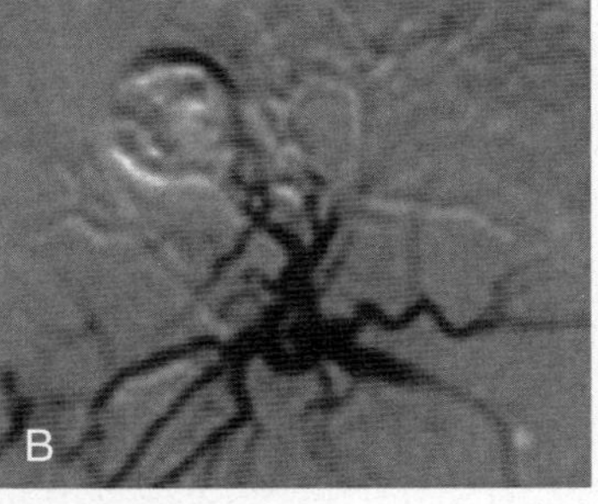

FIGURE 53-37 Angiograms demonstrating hypervascular hepatocellular carcinoma before **(A)** and after **(B)** embolization.

Systemic chemotherapy with a variety of agents (e.g., cisplatin, doxorubicin, etoposide, 5-fluorouracil [5-FU], mitomycin C, amsacrine, mitoxantrone, picibanil, tamoxifen, uracil, VM-26) has been ineffective and has had a minimal role in the treatment of HCC. Response rates are generally below 20% and of short duration. Systemic immunotherapy and hormonal therapy have been used in small numbers of patients with HCC, with some early promising results, but have not yet demonstrated superiority to standard regimens.

Most recently, sorafenib, a molecular targeted therapy that inhibits the serine-threonine kinases Raf-1 and B-Raf and the receptor tyrosine kinase activity of vascular endothelial growth factor receptors 1, 2, and 3 and platelet-derived growth factor β, was evaluated. Llovet and colleagues[87] randomized 599 patients with advanced-stage HCC and Child-Pugh level A cirrhosis to oral sorafenib or placebo. The median overall survival was 10.7 months in the sorafenib group and 7.9 months in the placebo group ($P < .001$), a difference of 2.8 months. The median time to radiologic progression was 5.5 months in the sorafenib group and 2.8 months in the placebo group ($P < .001$), a difference of 2.7 months. Neither group demonstrated any complete responses by radiologic criteria. Although the adverse event profile of sorafenib was similar to the placebo group, this and earlier studies have shown that sorafenib is best tolerated in patients with Child-Pugh class A cirrhosis. With better understanding of the molecular pathogenesis, there is hope that novel therapeutics will be increasingly evaluated in this disease.[87]

In summary, a plethora of treatment options are available for treatment of HCC. Selection of the appropriate treatment modality is based on disease extent, presence or absence of portal hypertension, and liver reserve. Patients with resectable disease with maintained liver reserve and absence of portal hypertension are best treated with resection. Patients with advanced underlying liver disease and with portal hypertension are best treated with liver transplantation. Liver transplantation is applicable only if the tumor is 5 cm or smaller or there are two or three tumors, the largest of which is 3 cm or smaller. Expanded criteria for transplantation are being increasingly used. In patients with very small tumors and with multiple comorbidities, percutaneous ablative techniques may be applied. The efficacy of ablation decreases with increasing size of the tumor. For multifocal disease in the absence of macrovascular invasion and extrahepatic disease, neither resection nor transplantation is applicable, and trans-arterial therapies offer the best results. For symptomatic patients with advanced disease, with macrovascular involvement, and in the presence of extrahepatic disease, sorafenib is an option. For patients with extensive disease who are symptomatic with deterioration of their performance status and who have severe deterioration of their liver function, any treatment modality is unlikely to provide significant benefit, and these patients should be offered supportive treatment only.

Distinct variants of HCC. Fibrolamellar HCC[88] is a variant of HCC with remarkably different clinical features, summarized in Table 53-8. This tumor generally occurs in younger patients without a history of cirrhosis. The tumor is usually well demarcated and encapsulated and may have a central fibrotic area. The central scar can make distinguishing this tumor from FNH difficult. On histologic evaluation, fibrolamellar HCC is composed of large polygonal tumor cells embedded in a fibrous stroma, forming lamellar structures (Fig. 53-38). Fibrolamellar HCC does not produce AFP but is associated with elevated neurotensin levels. In general, fibrolamellar HCC has a better prognosis than

TABLE 53-8 Comparison of Standard Hepatocellular Carcinoma and Fibrolamellar Hepatocellular Carcinoma

PARAMETER	HCC	FIBROLAMELLAR HCC
Male-to-female ratio	2:1-8:1	1:1
Median age	55 years	25 years
Tumor	Invasive	Well circumscribed
Resectability	<25%	50%-75%
Cirrhosis	90%	5%
AFP positive	80%	5%
Hepatitis B positive	65%	5%

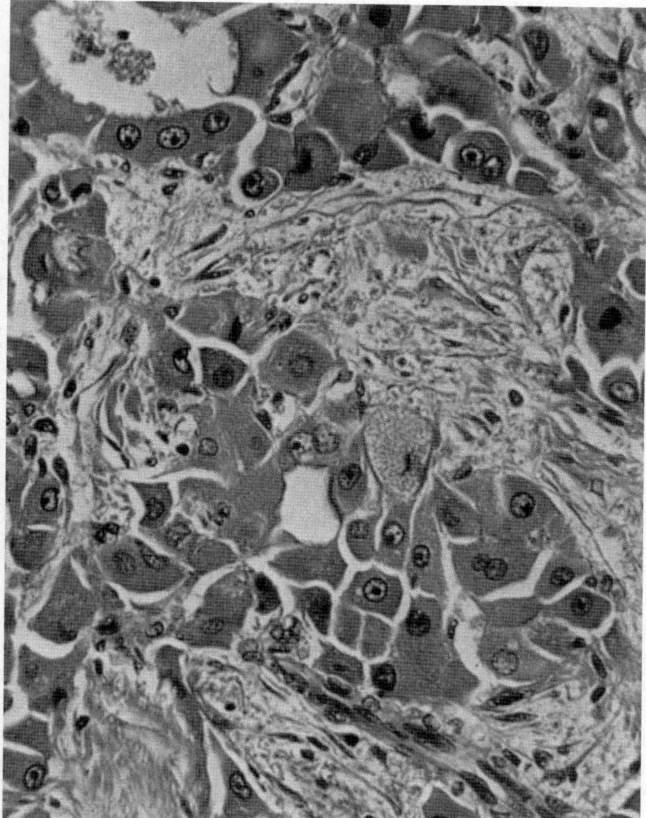

FIGURE 53-38 Fibrolamellar HCC. Abundant collagen is evident interconnecting clusters of cells. The cells are often in single-layer sheets. An acinus is present in the left upper field.

HCC, probably related to high resectability rates, lack of chronic liver disease, and a more indolent course. Long-term survival can be expected in approximately 50% to 75% of patients after complete resection, but recurrence is common and occurs in at least 80% of patients. The presence of lymph node metastases predicts a worse outcome. Resection of lymph node metastases and recurrent disease has been advocated because of a lack of alternative therapy and the possibility of long-term survival. A study identified a chimeric transcript that is expressed in fibrolamellar HCC but not in the adjacent normal liver.[89] The study also suggested that this transcript codes for a chimeric protein containing the catalytic domain of protein kinase A, thus suggesting that this gain of kinase activity may have a role in the pathogenesis of fibrolamellar HCC. Elucidation of such novel processes can lead to development of novel targeted therapies against this disease, which typically strikes young, healthy people.

Rarely, HCC can be manifested as a mixed hepatocellular-cholangiocellular tumor, with cellular differentiation of both types present. Whether this is two separate tumors growing into each other or mixed differentiation of the same tumor is not known. These mixed tumors tend to have a prognosis that is worse than for standard HCC but better than expected for intrahepatic cholangiocarcinoma.

A clear cell variant of HCC also exists, in which the cells contain a clear cytoplasm. These tumors can resemble renal cell neoplasms. The clear cell variant may have a better prognosis than standard HCC, but this is a subject of debate. A pleomorphic or giant cell variant of HCC has also been reported. Cells in this type are multinucleated, pleomorphic, and large and likely to originate from primary hepatic cells. Some HCCs show evidence of sarcomatoid differentiation and are referred to as a sarcomatoid variant or carcinosarcoma. These tumors tend not to produce AFP and have a higher incidence of metastases at presentation.

Childhood HCC is a distinct entity that represents almost 25% of pediatric liver tumors but rarely occurs in infancy. Viral hepatitis is associated with childhood HCC in Asia but less so in the United States. Other inherited metabolic liver diseases (see earlier) are often associated with childhood HCC. As in adult HCC, complete resection is the only potentially curative treatment. There is a high incidence of multifocality, vascular invasion, and extrahepatic metastases, resulting in relatively poor long-term survival rates of 10% to 20%.

Intrahepatic Cholangiocarcinoma

Cholangiocarcinoma is an uncommon neoplasm, with an incidence of 1 to 2/100,000 in the United States, and can develop anywhere along the biliary tree, from the ampulla of Vater to the peripheral intrahepatic bile ducts. Most of these tumors (40% to 60%) involve the biliary confluence (Klatskin tumor), but approximately 10% emanate from intrahepatic ducts and are known as intrahepatic cholangiocarcinoma (IHC). IHC is the second most common primary hepatic neoplasm. Studies on the incidence and natural history of IHC have been confused by the fact that in the past, many of these tumors were mistaken for metastatic adenocarcinoma because biopsy is unable to differentiate the two.

Historically, the most common risk factors for the development of cholangiocarcinoma (all types) were primary sclerosing cholangitis, choledochal cyst disease, hepatolithiasis,[90] and RPC. Recent epidemiologic evidence has now linked IHC to HBV infection,[91] HCV infection,[53] cirrhosis, nonalcoholic steatohepatitis,[92] and diabetes.[93] Increases in the diagnosis of IHC in the United States are likely related to better recognition of the disease, changed classification, and perhaps the rise in HCV infections in the 1960s and 1970s.[94,95]

The clinical presentation of IHC is similar to that of HCC. These tumors are asymptomatic in early stages. When present, the most common symptoms are right upper abdominal pain and weight loss. Jaundice occurs less commonly as these tumors tend to arise in the periphery of the liver. More commonly, patients present with incidentally found liver masses on cross-sectional imaging. Unlike in HCC, the AFP levels are normal, although CEA or CA 19-9 levels can be elevated in some cases. Because metastatic adenocarcinoma to liver is more common, IHC is a diagnosis of exclusion, and a search for a primary tumor with upper and lower gastrointestinal endoscopy and cross-sectional imaging of the chest, abdomen, and pelvis should be carried out. If a biopsy has been performed, it is often read as adenocarcinoma. Although special stains may suggest diagnosis of IHC, they are not conclusive. On CT and MRI, IHC is seen as a focal hepatic mass that may be associated with peripheral biliary dilation. The mass typically has peripheral or central enhancement on contrast-enhanced scans. Intrahepatic metastases, lymph node metastases, and growth along the biliary tree are often encountered.

Complete resection is the treatment of choice for IHC. Resectability rates generally range up to 60%, and long-term survival in unresected patients is rare. If it is completely resected, 3-year survival rates range from 16% to 61%, and 5-year survival rates range from 24% to 44%. Factors associated with a poor outcome include multifocality, lymph node metastases, vascular invasion, and positive margins. Because of the rarity of IHC, little is known about the effectiveness of radiation therapy and chemotherapy for IHC in the adjuvant setting. Thus, their application is not routine. Chemotherapy is largely considered ineffective for IHC, but it is hoped that improvements in chemotherapy for other gastrointestinal tumors will translate into improved outcomes. Regional hepatic artery chemotherapy has been under study and may be a promising approach.

Other Primary Malignant Neoplasms

Hepatoblastoma is the most common primary hepatic tumor of childhood. There are approximately 50 to 70 new cases per year in the United States. Rare cases of adult hepatoblastoma have been reported, but overall, the median age at presentation is 18 months, and almost all cases occur before the age of 3 years. Hepatoblastoma has been associated with the familial polyposis syndrome. There are a number of histologic subtypes, but in general, the tumor is derived from fetal or embryonic hepatocytic progenitors, and mesenchymal elements are often present. This tumor generally is manifested as an asymptomatic mass. Mild anemia and thrombocytosis are commonly found at presentation. Serum AFP levels are elevated in 85% to 90% of patients and can serve as a useful marker for therapeutic response. Most studies have supported the use of chemotherapy followed by resection, and survival appears to be dependent on complete resection. Chemotherapy can serve to downstage tumors, which facilitates resection. In patients without metastatic disease or the anaplastic variant, long-term survival rates of 60% to 70% can be expected with complete resection. Interestingly, 50% of patients with pulmonary metastases can be cured with resection of the hepatic tumor and chemotherapy or resection of the pulmonary metastases.

A variety of sarcomas can rarely be manifested as primary liver tumors, but they must always be considered metastatic lesions until proven otherwise. Angiosarcoma is probably the best-described primary hepatic sarcoma because of its well-known association with vinyl chloride or Thorotrast exposure. Angiosarcoma typically is manifested as multiple hepatic masses and can appear in childhood. Long-term survival is uncommon with primary hepatic angiosarcoma. Other sarcomas, including leiomyosarcoma, malignant fibrous histiocytoma, embryonic sarcoma, and primary hepatic rhabdoid tumors, have been described but are rare. The last two lesions are typically seen in the pediatric population.

Non-Hodgkin lymphoma can be manifested primarily in the liver, with or without extrahepatic disease. Primary hepatic lymphoma should be treated in the same manner as lymphoma elsewhere in the body if the diagnosis can be made before a liver resection.

Primary hepatic neuroendocrine tumors or carcinoid tumors have been described but are probably extremely rare. Distinguishing the rare primary hepatic neuroendocrine tumor from a metastatic lesion can be difficult because the extrahepatic primary tumor can be radiologically occult for many years, and the liver is the most common site of metastases.

Malignant germ cell tumors of the liver including teratomas, choriocarcinomas, and yolk sac tumors are very rare and are principally described in the pediatric population.

Epithelioid hemangioendothelioma of the liver is a rare malignant vascular tumor that is manifested with multiple bilateral hepatic masses. Extrahepatic metastases occur in approximately 25% of patients and clinical behavior is unpredictable, with some patients having a prolonged indolent course. Most patients ultimately die of liver failure, but cases of successful transplantation have been reported.

Metastatic Tumors

The most common malignant tumors of the liver are metastatic lesions. The liver is a common site of metastases from gastrointestinal tumors, presumably because of dissemination through the portal venous system. The most relevant metastatic tumor of the liver to the surgeon is colorectal cancer because of the well-documented potential for long-term survival after complete resection. However, a large number of other tumors commonly metastasize to the liver, including cancers of the upper gastrointestinal system (stomach, pancreas, biliary), genitourinary system (renal, prostate), neuroendocrine system, breast, eye (melanoma), skin (melanoma), soft tissue (retroperitoneal sarcoma), and gynecologic system (ovarian, endometrial, cervical). The large majority of metastatic liver tumors that present with concomitant extrahepatic disease will have unresectable liver disease or are not curable with resection, limiting the role of the surgeon to highly select cases. Metastatic adenocarcinoma to the liver of unknown primary is often a primary IHC, and this diagnosis must always be kept in mind.

Traditionally, cancer spread to a distant site was considered a systemic disease in which locoregional therapies (i.e., surgery) were not effective. Some metastatic tumors to the liver and, in particular, metastatic colorectal cancer have been shown to be an exception to this rule. More than 35 years of clinical research has documented that metastatic colorectal cancer isolated in the liver can be resected, with the potential for long-term survival and cure.[96-98] Advances in systemic and regional chemotherapy have also broadened the number of patients eligible for surgical therapy and probably have improved long-term survival after resection.[99] Selection of patients is the most important aspect of surgical therapy for metastatic disease in the liver, and clinical follow-up of resected patients has identified those most and least likely to benefit. Although long-term survival is common and occurs in up to 50% to 60% of patients in current series, recurrence and chronic multimodal therapy are common, occurring in approximately 75% of patients. Therefore, an important aspect of treatment is realistic expectations and honest patient education. Tumors other than colorectal cancer manifested as isolated or limited hepatic metastases can also be resected for potential long-term survival, but data on these other tumors are sparse and less compelling than for colorectal cancer.

Colorectal Metastases

There are more than 50,000 cases of colorectal liver metastases a year in the United States. Most of these cases are associated with widespread disease or unresectable hepatic disease. It is estimated that approximately 5% to 10% of these patients are candidates for a potentially curative liver resection. With improved response rates to modern chemotherapy and advances in hepatic surgery, however, more patients are now candidates for hepatectomy than in the past; at present, up to 20% of patients may be candidates. In the distant past, patients with hepatic colorectal metastases generally presented with symptoms and signs of advanced malignant disease, such as pain, ascites, jaundice, weight loss, and a palpable mass. Presentation with these symptoms is a poor prognostic sign; few of these patients are candidates for therapy aside from chemotherapy or supportive care. This has led most physicians to observe patients with resected primary colorectal cancer carefully who are potential candidates for aggressive therapy with serial physical examinations, cross-sectional imaging studies, LFTs, and determination of CEA levels. Although not supported by randomized trials, clinical observations have indicated that patients who are carefully observed with serial physical examinations, cross-sectional imaging studies, LFTs, and determination of CEA levels are those often found to have resectable metachronous disease and the greatest potential for long-term survival. In addition to these patients, some are found to have synchronous metastatic disease at the time of diagnosis of the primary colorectal cancer on preoperative imaging or at laparotomy.[100]

Although an elevated CEA level is not specific for recurrent colorectal cancer, a rising CEA level on serial examinations and a new solid mass on imaging studies are diagnostic of metastatic disease. Mild elevations in LFT results are common in metastatic colorectal cancer to the liver but are not effective as a screening tool. The levels most commonly elevated are those of ALP, GGT, and lactate dehydrogenase. Imaging of hepatic metastases with high-quality CT or MRI is important for determining resectability and operative planning. Most physicians use thin-cut (5 mm), high-resolution, dynamic, contrast-enhanced helical scanning techniques. Timing with IV administration of a contrast agent should correspond to the portal venous phase to maximize hepatic parenchymal enhancement, which improves the disparity between parenchyma and tumor.

Once a patient with colorectal liver metastases is considered a candidate for surgical therapy, a complete extent of disease workup must be performed. Colonoscopy should be performed if it has been longer than 1 year since the last examination to rule out local recurrence or metachronous colorectal lesions. Complete abdominal and pelvic cross-sectional imaging must also be performed. Chest CT is often performed but is of low yield. Many studies have evaluated the added benefit of positron emission tomography (PET) scans to detect occult extrahepatic disease. Approximately 25% of patients have a change in management based on PET scan findings, but this is highly variable, depending on the quality of cross-sectional imaging, radiologic interpretation, and patient selection (Fig. 53-39). A randomized trial of PET/CT versus CT in patients with potentially resectable colorectal liver metastases has been published.[101] In this trial, the use of PET/CT did not result in significant changes in surgical management, and there was no difference in resectability or long-term outcomes between the two groups. This trial provides definitive evidence that routine use of PET does not significantly affect outcomes among patients with potentially resectable colorectal cancer liver metastasis. With use of staging laparoscopy, 10% of patients are spared a nontherapeutic laparotomy, and the yield of laparoscopy correlates with the number of poor prognostic factors present, allowing it to be used on a selective basis.

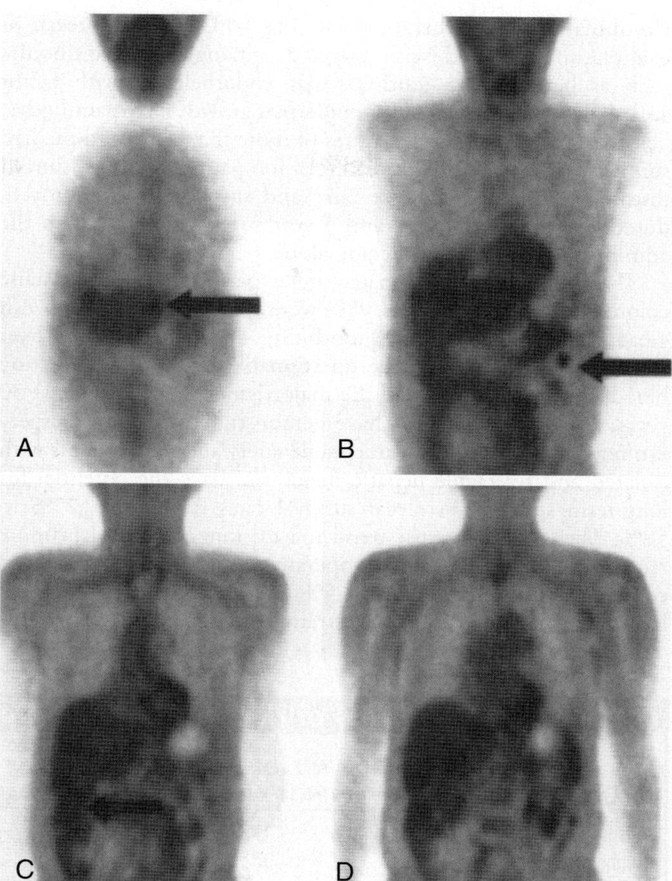

FIGURE 53-39 PET scan in a patient diagnosed with colorectal cancer synchronously metastatic to the liver after resection of the colonic tumor. The scan demonstrates hypermetabolic activity throughout the liver but also shows two areas in the left upper quadrant consistent with an omental lesion as well as an anastomotic recurrence. A recent CT scan demonstrated liver disease only. (From Akhurst T, Larson SM: The role of nuclear medicine in the diagnosis and management of hepatobiliary diseases. In Blumgart LH, Fong Y, editors: *Surgery of the liver and biliary tract*, London, 2000, WB Saunders, pp 271–308.)

To date, a prospective trial comparing surgery with no treatment or chemotherapy alone has not been performed, nor is this likely ever to be done. Therefore, the rationale for liver resection comes from retrospective comparisons of these treatment strategies. The surgeon must understand the natural history of colorectal liver metastases left untreated or treated with systemic chemotherapy to interpret survival data associated with hepatectomy appropriately. Before the 1980s, most hepatic metastases were left untreated. Two key studies retrospectively identified patients with isolated single hepatic metastases or multiple but resectable tumors who received no therapy. One study documented a 10% 3-year survival and the other a 2% 5-year survival for patients with limited and potentially resectable disease. It was clear from these studies that long-term survival is extremely rare without treatment and that survival is closely related to the extent of disease. In the past, 5-FU–based systemic chemotherapy was ineffective as sole therapy for hepatic colorectal metastases, with median survivals of approximately 12 months and response rates of 20% to 30%. Tremendous advances in systemic chemotherapy for metastatic colorectal cancer have now been achieved.

Combination chemotherapy, including 5-FU with irinotecan or oxaliplatin combined with targeted antiangiogenic antibodies such as bevacizumab (anti–vascular endothelial growth factor antibody) or cetuximab (anti–epidermal growth factor antibody), has now resulted in response rates of more than 50% and median survivals of 20 months and longer for patients with advanced disease.[97] Although response rates and survival have improved, durable complete response and 5-year survival are rare with the administration of chemotherapy alone.

The sporadic partial hepatectomies performed for metastatic colorectal cancer before the 1980s were appropriately viewed with great skepticism. The high morbidity and mortality for liver surgery at that time and the questionable rationale of resecting bloodborne metastases were the major issues. During the last 30 years, however, large series have demonstrated that liver surgery can now be practiced with acceptable safety and that patients with isolated and resectable hepatic metastases have the potential for long-term survival. Five-year survival rates range from 25% to 58%. There is also a clear trend toward longer survival in more recent series (Table 53-9). Perioperative mortality in experienced centers is consistently less than 5% and in many series has been less than 2%. Almost all demonstrate that almost 50% of patients undergoing a liver resection for metastatic colorectal cancer will survive 3 years and 20% will survive 10 years. Despite the low operative mortality, liver surgery is still associated with significant morbidity rates of 30% to 50%.[102] Complications are most commonly bleeding, bile leak, abscess, and other generalized cardiorespiratory complications. With improvements in chemotherapy, a higher proportion of patients undergoing hepatectomy have been treated preoperatively. However, some studies have shown that preoperative chemotherapy is associated with hepatic toxicity (steatohepatitis and sinusoidal obstructive syndrome) and higher rates of postoperative liver failure.

From these large series, we have learned much about prognostic factors as well as which patients are most likely to benefit from a liver resection for hepatic colorectal metastases. Although not all studies agree, it has been found that poor prognostic factors include extrahepatic metastases, involved lymph nodes with the primary colorectal tumor, synchronous presentation (or shorter disease-free interval), larger number of tumors, bilobar involvement, CEA level elevation more than 200 ng/mL, size of largest hepatic tumor more than 5 cm, and involved histologic margins. In a series of 1001 liver resections from MSKCC, a multivariate analysis[103] identified five preoperative factors as the

TABLE 53-9 Results of Hepatic Resection for Hepatic Colorectal Metastases*

STUDY	NO. OF PATIENTS	OPERATIVE MORTALITY RATE (%)	SURVIVAL RATE (%) 1-YEAR	5-YEAR	10-YEAR	MEDIAN SURVIVAL (MONTHS)
Adson, 1984	141	2	82	25	—	24
Hughes, 1986	607	—	—	33	—	—
Schlag, 1990	122	4	85	30	—	32
Doci, 1991	100	5	—	30	—	28
Gayowski, 1994	204	0	91	32	—	33
Scheele, 1995	469	4	83	33	20	40
Fong, 1995	577	4	85	35	—	40
Jenkins, 1997	131	4	81	25	—	33
Rees, 1997	150	1	94	37	—	
Jamison, 1997	280	4	84	27	20	33
Fong, 1999	1001	3	89	37	22	42
Minagawa, 2000	235	0	—	35	26	37
Scheele, 2000	597	—	—	36	—	35
Choti, 2002	226	1	—	40†	26	46
Abdalla, 2004	190	—	—	58	—	Not reached
Nicoli, 2004	228	0.9		16	9	
Andres, 2008	210	0.5	95	40	—	—
de Jong, 2009	243	—	—	47	—	36
House, 2010	1600					
1985-1998	1037	2.5	—	35	16	43
1999-2004	563	0.5	—	43	—	64
Faitot, 2014‡	272					
One stage	155	3	85	35		37.2
Two stage	117	4	82	49		34.5
Saxena, 2014	701	2	86	33	20	35
Marques, 2012§	676					
Preoperative chemotherapy‖	334	3.9	91	43		
No preoperative chemotherapy	342	3.4	93	55		

*In selected series with more than 100 patients.
†The 5-year survival rate in the patients operated on in the most current time period in this study was 58%.
‡Long-term results of two-stage hepatectomy versus one-stage hepatectomy used in combination with ablation approaches.
§Combined data from two hepatobiliary centers, data analyzed with respect to receipt of preoperative chemotherapy or not.
‖Number of tumors higher in the preoperative chemotherapy group (2.8 ± 2.2) compared with those with no preoperative therapy (1.8 ± 1.6).

TABLE 53-10 Clinical Risk Score and Survival in 1001 Patients Undergoing Liver Resection for Metastatic Colorectal Cancer*

SCORE	SURVIVAL RATE (%) 1-YEAR	3-YEAR	5-YEAR	MEDIAN SURVIVAL (MONTHS)
0	93	72	60	74
1	91	66	44	51
2	89	60	40	47
3	86	42	20	33
4	70	38	25	20
5	71	27	14	22

Adapted from Fong Y, Fortner J, Sun RL, et al: Clinical score for predicting recurrence after hepatic resection for metastatic colorectal cancer: Analysis of 1001 consecutive cases. *Ann Surg* 230:309–318, 1999.

*Each of the following five risk factors equals 1 point: node-positive primary, disease-free interval <12 months, >1 tumor, size >5 cm, carcinoembryonic antigen level >200 ng/mL. Score is total number of points in an individual patient.

most influential on outcome: size larger than 5 cm, disease-free interval less than 1 year, more than one tumor, lymph node–positive primary, and CEA level higher than 200 ng/mL. Using these five factors, we have developed a risk score predictive of recurrence after liver resection (Table 53-10).

Traditionally, the presence of extrahepatic disease, four or more hepatic metastases, close margins, and inability to resect all disease in the liver have been considered contraindications to hepatectomy. The only one of these historic contraindications that holds true today is the inability to resect all disease. Recent reports have shown that hepatectomy for four or more metastases is associated with an approximate 5-year survival of 33%, despite a high recurrence rate. Although the width of the closest margin has been shown to be associated with outcome, it is often confounded by its relationship to an overall poor prognostic tumor (i.e., multiple synchronous tumors).[104] However, close or involved margins do not appear to preclude the possibility of long-term survival, but patients with positive margins tend to fair poorly. Nonetheless, attempts at wide margins more than 1 cm are appropriate, when possible.[105] Resection of extrahepatic metastases that present simultaneously with liver metastases has been shown to be associated with long-term survival in highly select cases.[106] The sites that appear to be associated with the best outcomes in this situation are limited lung metastases, locoregional recurrences of the primary tumor, and portal lymph nodes. These results have been further confirmed in a meta-analysis of 50 studies including 3481 patients with colorectal liver metastases with extrahepatic disease.[107] Selection of patients is critical for this aggressive approach and generally requires preoperative chemotherapy to exclude progression and consideration of the overall bulk of metastatic disease.

Although long-term survival after liver resection for hepatic colorectal metastases is clearly possible, recurrence of disease is common. Overall, approximately 75% of patients have recurrence, but in high-risk situations (e.g., four or more tumors, extrahepatic disease), recurrence rates approach 100%. Approximately 50% of recurrences are isolated to the liver, and a small number of these patients (≈5% of all patients undergoing liver resection) are candidates for a second liver resection. These highly select patients who undergo a second liver resection with complete removal of all disease can expect further 5-year survival rates of 30% to 40%. Limited and isolated lung recurrences can also be resected, with the potential for further long-term survival. Furthermore, multiple lines of effective chemotherapy are now available, associated with prolongation of survival. Because of the potential for further effective therapeutic interventions after liver resection, patients eligible for such treatment should be observed with serial CEA level determinations and imaging studies to detect recurrences at an early, potentially treatable phase.

Adjuvant chemotherapy has been used in an attempt to reduce recurrence and to improve long-term survival. Prospective randomized clinical trials have shown a benefit to adjuvant hepatic intra-arterial chemotherapy. However, results of randomized controlled trials on the benefit of adjuvant systemic chemotherapy after resection of hepatic metastases have been mixed. In a multicenter randomized trial, Portier and associates[108] randomized 173 patients to hepatic resection alone (87 patients) or to hepatic resection plus adjuvant chemotherapy (5-FU–folinic acid) for 6 months (86 patients). Even though this chemotherapy regimen is no longer standard, the 5-year disease-free survival rate was 26.7% for patients who had surgery alone and 33.5% for patients who had surgery plus chemotherapy ($P = .028$). A nonsignificant trend toward improved overall survival was also observed in the chemotherapy arm. The results of this trial were pooled with another phase 3 trial that failed to accrue. This pooled analysis failed to show a statistically significant improvement in progression-free survival or overall survival.[109] In this analysis, there were 278 patients (138 in the surgery with chemotherapy arm and 140 in the surgery-alone arm). Median progression-free survival was 27.9 months in the chemotherapy arm compared with 18.8 months in the surgery arm (hazard ratio, 1.32; 95% confidence interval, 1.00-1.76; $P = .058$). Median overall survival was 62.2 months in the chemotherapy arm compared with 47.3 months in the surgery arm (hazard ratio, 1.32; 95% confidence interval, 0.95-1.82; $P = .095$).[109] Adjuvant chemotherapy was independently associated with both progression-free survival and overall survival in multivariable analysis.

In another multi-institutional randomized controlled trial (European Organization for Research and Treatment and Cancer, EORTC 40983 trial), Nordlinger and colleagues randomized 364 patients into two groups; 182 patients were treated with surgery alone, and 182 patients had surgery plus systemic chemotherapy.[110] Three cycles of systemic 5-FU–folinic acid plus oxaliplatin (FOLFOX4) were administered preoperatively and postoperatively in the chemotherapy group. Among eligible patients after randomization, the progression-free survival of patients at 3 years was 28.1% in the group with surgery alone and 36.2% in the group with surgery plus chemotherapy ($P = .041$). When analyzed by all patients, there was no significant difference in outcome. Long-term results of this trial have been released, and no difference in overall survival was observed with addition of chemotherapy.[111] Although this trial provides evidence that perioperative systemic chemotherapy can delay recurrence of disease, there is little difference in the recurrences at later time points. Also, the benefit of adjuvant chemotherapy may be related to better selection of patients. In summary, there is level 1 clinical evidence that adjuvant systemic chemotherapy, when combined with liver resection, modestly improves progression-free survival in patients with colorectal liver metastases.

Neoadjuvant chemotherapy for resectable metastases is also a common strategy to treat occult systemic disease and can be helpful in selecting the small group of patients (<10%) who progress while receiving chemotherapy and have a poor outcome after hepatectomy. A prospective randomized study by the National Surgical Adjuvant Breast and Bowel Project has begun accruing patients to study the role of adjuvant chemotherapy in these patients.

A convincing argument for adjuvant therapy with the use of hepatic arterial infusion (HAI) chemotherapy can be made.[112,113] The rationale for adjuvant hepatic artery chemotherapy is based on the fact that liver metastases derive most of their blood supply from the hepatic artery. Regional infusion of chemotherapeutic agents such as fluorodeoxyuridine has hepatic extraction rates of 90%, providing high local concentrations with minimal systemic toxicity. Furthermore, approximately 50% of all recurrences after hepatectomy involve the liver, so controlling the liver is likely to affect long-term outcome. There is clearly a higher response rate for liver tumors with HAI therapy compared with systemic therapy. A trial from MSKCC comparing HAI therapy with systemic chemotherapy to systemic chemotherapy alone has demonstrated significantly lower recurrence rates (9% and 36%) and a survival advantage at 2 years (86% versus 72%).[114] Other trials have shown HAI therapy with fluorodeoxyuridine to be more effective than hepatectomy alone, with significantly improved disease-free survival.

For patients with unresectable disease, preoperative systemic and HAI chemotherapy has been shown to convert some patients to resection candidates. A critical observation in these patients is that outcome after complete resection appears to be as good as in those who were resectable at initial presentation. Strategies to extend the limits of liver resection have used parenchyma-preserving segmental resections, two-stage operations, and thermal ablative techniques, such as cryoablation or RFA. Most recently, microwave ablation is being studied as a treatment for these patients, and long-term results suggest that recurrence rates increase with the size of the tumor and when ablation is performed for the tumor close to the vessels.[115] Recent results suggest that microwave ablation either alone or in combination with liver resection can provide good long-term results. Thus, multiple bilobar tumors can be extirpated by a combination of resection and ablation with preservation of sufficient hepatic parenchyma.

In summary, the treatment of hepatic colorectal metastases is evolving at a rapid pace, and improvements in hepatic surgery and chemotherapy have greatly improved prospects for patients. Chemotherapy has improved, but long-term survival with this modality alone is rare. Combinations of chemotherapy and complete resection of hepatic metastases are associated with long-term survival in up to 50% to 60% of patients. Long-term survival also appears to be possible in patients undergoing resection of extensive hepatic metastases and limited extrahepatic disease.[106] Complete resection of hepatic metastases appears to be a critically important treatment modality that is necessary for long-term survival.

Neuroendocrine Metastases

Liver metastases from neuroendocrine tumors are common but vary according to the primary tumor type. Examples of primary tumors that commonly metastasize to the liver are gastrinomas, glucagonomas, somatostatinomas, and nonfunctional neuroendocrine tumors. Insulinomas and carcinoid tumors metastasize to the liver less commonly.

There are two issues to consider in determining the appropriate therapy for metastatic neuroendocrine tumors. First, these are slow-growing, indolent tumors in which long-term survival is possible even in the absence of treatment. Thus, assessing the effects of any treatment is difficult. Second, these tumors often secrete functional neuropeptides that can create debilitating syndromes of hormonal excess, so the goal of treatment is focused more often on quality of life rather than on prolongation of life.

A number of effective nonsurgical therapies exist for neuroendocrine liver metastases. Long-acting somatostatin analogues are useful for alleviating hormonal symptoms and may have a cytostatic role as well. Liver tumors can also be treated by hepatic arterial embolization or thermoablative approaches. Combinations of these therapies can be effective in cytoreducing tumor loads and alleviating symptoms of hormonal excess.

Liver resection can play a role in patients whose tumor can be completely encompassed. Because these tumors are indolent, any therapy must be delivered with minimal morbidity. This has been the case in experienced hepatobiliary units.[116] Five-year survival rates in excess of 50% to 75% can be expected if a complete resection is accomplished. Retrospective comparisons have suggested that this survival is better than that in untreated patients, but selection bias accounts for at least some of this difference. Because of the rarity of this diagnosis, no prospective data exist. The other role of surgery is for those patients who have failed to respond to medical therapy and have recalcitrant symptoms of hormonal excess. If preoperative staging suggests that at least 90% of tumor can be removed without prohibitive operative risk, surgical cytoreduction is reasonable. Symptom improvement can be expected in most patients if adequate cytoreduction is achieved. Formal resections with wide margins are not necessary for neuroendocrine tumors, and techniques such as enucleation and wedge resection are reasonable options. Thermoablative approaches, such as cryoablation and RFA, are also attractive alternatives in this type of cytoreductive surgery. Laparoscopic RFA has recently been used, although long-term follow-up is not available.[117]

Noncolorectal, Non-Neuroendocrine Metastases

Other tumors can be manifested as isolated liver metastases, but these are uncommon situations and therefore data for these situations are sparse.[118,119] There are many tumors that can be manifested in this way, including breast, lung, melanoma, soft tissue sarcoma, Wilms tumor, ocular melanoma, upper gastrointestinal (gastric, pancreas, esophagus, gallbladder), adrenocortical, urologic (bladder, renal cell, prostate, testicular), and gynecologic (uterine, cervical, ovarian) tumors. General principles that should be considered in dealing with these tumors as isolated liver metastases are similar to those for metastatic colorectal cancer. Prognosis tends to be dismal if there is extrahepatic disease, multiple tumors, large tumors, or a short disease-free interval, and patients should be carefully selected for surgery on the basis of these factors.

Although there have been rare reports of long-term survival after resection of isolated liver metastases from upper gastrointestinal tumor, in general, these patients have a dismal prognosis and liver resection is not recommended. In most series, liver resection for genitourinary tumors has the best prognosis, and in well-selected patients, liver resection should be considered. Breast tumor, melanoma, and sarcoma patients rarely present with isolated liver metastases, and with a long disease-free interval or long-term stability on chemotherapy, liver resection should be considered. In general, liver resection for metastatic noncolorectal, non-neuroendocrine tumors has to be considered cytoreductive and should be used only in the most favorable situations (see earlier). Liver resection can also be an effective therapy for symptomatic tumors in patients who have a reasonable life expectancy and no other effective therapy.

Cystic Neoplasms

Simple Cyst

Simple cysts of the liver contain serous fluid, do not communicate with the biliary tree, and do not have septations. They are generally spherical or ovoid and can be as large as 20 cm. Large cysts can compress normal liver, inducing regional atrophy and sometimes compensatory contralateral hypertrophy. In 50% of cases, the cysts are singular. On histologic evaluation, a single layer of cuboidal or columnar cells without atypia lines these cysts. Simple cysts are generally regarded as congenital malformations.

Simple cysts are a relatively common finding in adults and are mostly asymptomatic incidental radiologic findings. On occasion, a large cyst will cause symptoms. Although CT demonstrates anatomic relationships, ultrasound is a helpful test of choice to confirm a single, thin-walled simple cyst. Hydatid disease, cystadenoma, and metastatic neuroendocrine tumor are the most important differential diagnoses to consider. A thick or nodular wall raises the suspicion of a cystadenoma but can also represent hemorrhage within the cyst. The most common complication is intracystic bleeding, but overall, complications are rare. The treatment of simple hepatic cysts is indicated only if they are symptomatic or there is diagnostic uncertainty. Because most cysts are asymptomatic, a thorough evaluation of the cause of the symptoms must be carried out before attributing them to the cyst. Nonsurgical treatment consists of aspiration and injection of a sclerosing agent. Few studies have documented long-term follow-up of sclerotherapy for hepatic cysts. Surgical therapy is achieved by fenestration or unroofing of the portion of the cyst that is extrahepatic. This can be performed at laparotomy with good long-term results or through laparoscopic approaches. The laparoscopic approach is favored, but long-term efficacy has not been well documented.[120] A meta-analysis including nine retrospective case-control studies involving 657 patients comparing laparoscopic fenestration with the open approach demonstrated that the laparoscopic approach was associated with shorter operative time, shorter hospital stay, and less operative blood loss with no difference in cyst recurrence rates.[121]

Cystadenoma and Cystadenocarcinoma

Cystadenoma of the liver is a rare neoplasm that generally is manifested as a large cystic mass, usually 10 to 20 cm. The cyst has a globular external surface with multiple protruding cysts and locules of various sizes. The fluid contained in these cysts is usually mucinous. On microscopic examination, atypical cuboidal or columnar cells resting on a basement membrane, with ovarian-like stroma, line the cysts. The epithelium often forms polypoid or papillary projections.

Cystadenoma of the liver mainly affects woman older than 40 years. Although many cystadenomas are asymptomatic, symptoms can include abdominal pain, anorexia, nausea, and abdominal distention. The diagnosis is usually suspected by a combination of cross-sectional imaging (CT or MRI) and ultrasound. Ultrasound usually demonstrates a cystic structure with varying wall thickness, nodularity, septations, and fluid-filled locules. Importantly, contrast-enhanced CT demonstrates enhancement of the cyst wall and septa. Hydatid disease must always be considered in the differential diagnosis. Cystadenomas tend to grow slowly but can eventually progress to their malignant counterpart, cystadenocarcinomas.

Cystadenocarcinoma is an extremely rare malignant neoplasm with little documentation of its natural history and outcome after resection. Malignant degeneration is typically suggested on imaging, with large projections and a markedly thickened wall. The treatment of cystadenoma or cystadenocarcinoma is complete excision, which can be done with an enucleation if there is no evidence of invasive malignant disease. Incomplete resection risks recurrence or the development of cystadenocarcinoma.

Polycystic Liver Disease

Liver cysts are commonly seen in patients with the autosomal dominant inherited adult polycystic kidney disease.[122] The cysts are histologically similar to simple cysts (see earlier). The main difference between the two entities is the number of cysts. When liver cysts are present in patients with adult polycystic kidney disease, they are always multiple in number. Also, there are usually numerous microscopic hepatic cysts as well as the grossly visible macrocysts. Despite the large number of liver cysts, hepatic parenchyma and function are usually preserved. Liver cysts are always preceded by kidney cysts, and their prevalence in adult polycystic kidney disease increases with age. In those younger than 20 years, the prevalence of liver cysts is 0%, whereas in those older than 60 years, it is 80%.

Liver cysts in patients with adult polycystic kidney disease are generally asymptomatic, but in a few patients, numerous large cysts may cause abdominal pain and distention. LFT results are almost always normal. Rare complications can occur; these include infection and intracystic bleeding. Ultrasound and CT reveal multiple simple cysts throughout the liver and kidneys. Treatment of polycystic liver disease is reserved for severe symptoms related to large cysts and complications. Treatment includes percutaneous aspiration with or without sclerotherapy, cyst fenestration (by laparotomy or laparoscopy), hepatic resection, and orthotopic liver transplantation. Liver transplantation is used only with progressive disease after fenestration or resection with liver or renal dysfunction. In the context of renal failure, a combined kidney and liver transplantation may be appropriate.

Bile Duct Cysts

Bile duct cysts or choledochal cysts are congenital dilations of the biliary tree that are usually diagnosed in childhood but can present in adulthood. Because of the risk of malignancy and recurrent cholangitis, treatment is excision with reestablishment of biliary-enteric continuity. Most bile duct cysts involve the extrahepatic biliary tree, but in type IV cysts, there is involvement of the extrahepatic bile duct and intrahepatic ducts. In contrast, Caroli disease (type V) is characterized by multiple intrahepatic cysts. Thus, bile duct cysts must be considered in the differential diagnosis of a patient with multiple hepatic cystic lesions. The intrahepatic lesions of type IV bile duct cysts and Caroli disease are multifocal dilations of the segmental bile ducts separated by portions of normal-caliber bile ducts. Approximately 50% of cases of Caroli disease are associated with congenital hepatic fibrosis; the cysts are diffusely located throughout the liver. In the other 50% of cases, the dilations may be confined to a portion of the liver, usually the left hemiliver. Recurrent bacterial cholangitis usually dominates the clinical course of these diseases, and death generally ensues within 5 to 10 years without adequate treatment. When intrahepatic bile duct cysts are localized, hepatic resection, with or without biliary reconstruction, is the treatment of choice. Treatment of diffuse hepatic involvement is poor; in complicated cases, the only probably effective treatment is transplantation.

Principles of Hepatic Resection

Although liver resections were performed in the late 1800s, it was not until 1952 that Lortat-Jacob was given credit for the first true anatomic right hepatectomy. This event ushered in the modern era of hepatic surgery. However, early series were plagued by high morbidity and mortality, which were largely related to massive intraoperative blood loss. Series from the 1970s and 1980s often reported mortality rates in excess of 10%, often as high as 20%, especially for major resections. This high mortality limited the use of liver resection, and there was reluctance to refer patients for such operations. During the last 3 decades, a number of advances have improved perioperative outcomes dramatically for patients undergoing major hepatic surgery. The understanding that most blood loss during a liver resection comes from the hepatic veins has prompted surgeons to perform these operations with a low central venous pressure. We perform partial hepatectomy with a central line in place, the patient in a mild Trendelenburg position, and fluid restriction and venodilators if necessary to maintain a central venous pressure lower than 5 mm Hg. The other major advance has been an improved understanding of the segmental anatomy of the liver, making intrahepatic dissection safer and more precise. There are numerous techniques to transect liver tissue and many methods to coagulate and to control vessels. The most important concept, however, is that dividing liver tissue is a dissection done by a surgeon with complete understanding of the liver's vascular anatomy.

In experienced centers, perioperative mortality is routinely 5% or less and depends on a number of factors. The three most critical factors related to perioperative morbidity are blood loss, the amount of normal liver resected, and the condition of the liver itself (e.g., cirrhosis). A partial hepatectomy must be performed with these factors in mind to minimize morbidity. In a review of more than 1800 liver resections during a 10-year period from MSKCC, the operative mortality was 3.1%.[123] The median blood loss was 600 mL, and two thirds of patients did not require a red blood cell transfusion. Overall, postoperative morbidity was 45%, but the median hospital stay was 8 days. Morbidity was mostly related to blood loss and the extent of resection. Minor resections were associated with a mortality of 1%. Most complications and deaths were seen in complex biliary tumors, cirrhotics with HCC, and extensive resections. Improving outcomes after partial hepatectomy continue, and experienced hepatobiliary centers have reported mortality rates that approach 1% to 2%, with fewer patients now requiring perioperative blood transfusions. As a result of the increasing safety of hepatic surgery, liver resection has become the treatment of choice for many malignant and benign hepatic conditions.

Bile leaks are a problem in cases requiring complex biliary reconstruction but can also occur in approximately 10% to 20% of hepatectomies without biliary reconstruction. Careful ligation of biliary radicals is of obvious importance in minimizing this complication. Because of the regenerative capacity of the liver, resections of up to 80% of normal noncirrhotic livers can be performed, with functional compensation within a few weeks. Because many resections encompass tumors and normal liver, the concepts of functional liver parenchyma and FLR volume are important because there is often compensatory hypertrophy of normal liver when tumors occupy a significant amount of the liver volume. The risk of hepatic dysfunction is minimal if the reduction of functional liver parenchyma is less than 50% but begins to rise when this figure approaches 20% to 25%. Patients with cirrhosis have much higher rates of postoperative liver dysfunction because of impaired regenerative capacity and impaired primary liver function. Liver failure, extrahepatic multiorgan failure, and death are serious hazards to performance of major liver resections in cirrhotics. In general, patients with Child class B or C cirrhosis or portal hypertension do not tolerate liver resections, and selection of patients is therefore critical. Ascites and infectious complications are also common problems after major liver resection. One strategy to minimize postoperative liver dysfunction and morbidity after major hepatectomy is to embolize the portal vein percutaneously on the side of the liver to be resected. In approximately 4 weeks, this induces atrophy of the liver parenchyma to be resected and hypertrophy of the FLR. In turn, this increases the relative volume of the FLR.

Techniques of liver resection differ according to the disease being treated. In benign hepatic diseases requiring resection, the indications for operation are usually symptoms or infection. Removal of normal liver should be kept to a minimum in these cases, and techniques such as enucleation are appropriate, although a major resection is occasionally necessary. For malignant disease, a margin of normal tissue is important, and formal anatomic resections yield the best results. Techniques such as wedge resection often result in higher rates of margin involvement and disease recurrence and should therefore be used carefully and sparingly.

Detailed knowledge of liver anatomy is essential to the practice of safe hepatic surgery (see earlier). Unfortunately, detailed and complicated descriptions of liver anatomy and common liver resections can be confusing to the student. A 2000 consensus conference conducted in Brisbane, Australia, with the assistance of the Americas Hepato-Pancreato-Biliary Association has published guidelines for this terminology (Table 53-11 and Fig. 53-40). In general, the term *lobectomy* is not preferred because there are no external markings on the liver denoting a lobe. When

TABLE 53-11 Nomenclature for Most Common Major Anatomic Hepatic Resections*

SEGMENTS†	COUINAUD, 1957	GOLDSMITH AND WOODBURNE, 1957	BRISBANE, 2000
V-VIII	Right hepatectomy	Right hepatic lobectomy	Right hemihepatectomy
IV-VIII‡	Right lobectomy	Extended right hepatic lobectomy	Right trisectionectomy
II-IV	Left hepatectomy	Left hepatic lobectomy	Left hemihepatectomy
II, III	Left lobectomy	Left lateral segmentectomy	Left lateral sectionectomy
II, III, IV, V, VIII‡	Extended left hepatectomy	Extended left lobectomy	Left trisectionectomy

Adapted from the Terminology Committee of the International Hepato-Pancreatico-Biliary Association: The Brisbane 2000 terminology of liver anatomy and resections, 2000 <http://www.ahpba.org/assets/documents/Brisbane_Article.pdf>.

*The original terminology is based on the anatomic descriptions of Couinaud and of Goldsmith and Woodburne.

†See Figure 53-40*A-E*.

‡Another common name for these operations is right or left trisegmentectomy.

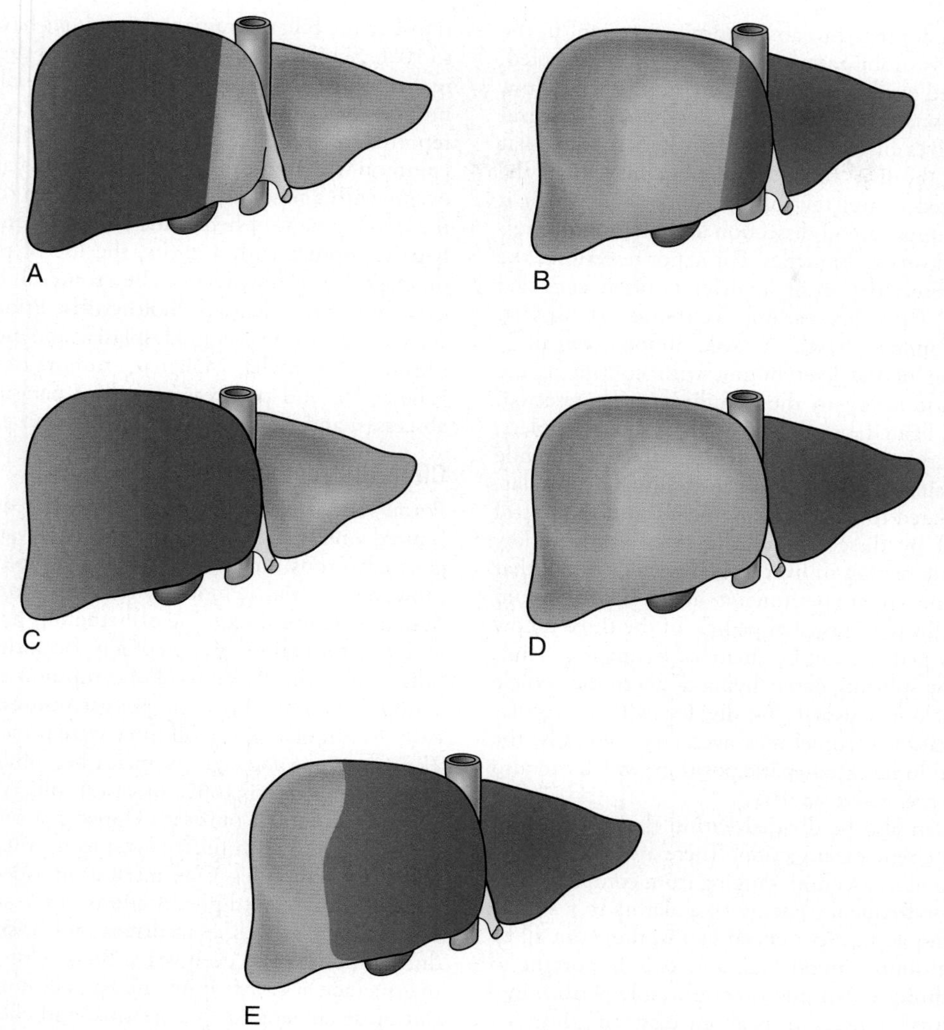

FIGURE 53-40 Commonly performed major hepatic resections are indicated by the *shaded areas.* **A,** Right hepatectomy, right hepatic lobectomy, or right hemihepatectomy (segments V to VIII). **B,** Left hepatectomy, left hepatic lobectomy, or left hemihepatectomy (segments II to IV). **C,** Right lobectomy, extended right hepatic lobectomy, or right trisectionectomy (trisegmentectomy; segments IV to VIII). **D,** Left lobectomy, left lateral segmentectomy, or left lateral sectionectomy (segments II to III). **E,** Extended left hepatectomy, extended left lobectomy, or left trisectionectomy (trisegmentectomy; segments II to V, VIII). See Table 53-11. (From Blumgart LH, Jarnagin W, Fong Y: Liver resection for benign disease and for liver and biliary tumors. In Blumgart LH, Fong Y, editors: *Surgery of the liver and biliary tract*, London, 2000, WB Saunders, pp 1639–1714.)

in doubt, one should always revert to the numeric segments of the liver if there is any confusion about the description of a liver resection. Recall that the right liver is composed of segments V through VIII, and *right hepatectomy* and *right hemihepatectomy* are appropriate terms for resection of these segments. Segments II through IV compose the left liver, and *left hepatectomy* and *left hemihepatectomy* are appropriate terms for resection of these segments. A right hepatectomy can be extended farther to the left to include segment IV, and a left hepatectomy can be extended farther to the right to include segments V and VIII. Terms such as *extended right-left hepatectomy, right-left trisectionectomy,* and *trisegmentectomy* are appropriate to describe these resections. Resection of segments II and III is a commonly performed sublobar resection and is often referred to as a left lateral segmentectomy or left lateral sectionectomy. Other common sublobar resections, such as that of the right posterior sector (segments VI and VII) or the right anterior sector (segments V and VIII), are referred to as a right posterior sectorectomy-sectionectomy and right anterior sectorectomy-sectionectomy, respectively. Single or bisegmental resections can always be simply referred to by a numeric description of the segments to be resected.

A detailed discussion of the techniques of liver resection is beyond the scope of this chapter; in general, it requires specialty training, but general principles can be discussed. A liver resection must consider the disease to be treated and the goal of the operation, whether that is a margin-negative resection of a malignant neoplasm or the removal of benign tissue to alleviate symptoms. The most basic steps can be distilled down to inflow control (portal vein, hepatic artery, bile duct), outflow control (hepatic veins), and parenchymal transection, with preservation of a liver remnant of adequate size with intact inflow, biliary drainage, and venous outflow.

The most common approach to an anatomic resection, in the most common order, is mobilization of the liver to be resected, dissection of inflow and outflow structures, division of the inflow, division of the outflow, and parenchymal transection. Mobilization of the liver involves division of the right or left triangular ligaments, freeing up the liver from the diaphragm. Often, the liver must be mobilized completely off the vena cava, which it straddles, and this requires careful dissection and division of multiple retrohepatic caval venous branches. For major resections, the hepatic vein of the resected portion of liver is often encircled before the resection. There are various techniques to dissect, control, and divide inflow vessels. Classic inflow control is obtained by dissection of the liver hilum, with control of the portal vein and hepatic artery to the hemiliver to be resected. These can be suture ligated or divided with vascular staplers. Unless tumor proximity mandates, we advocate dividing the bile duct within the liver substance to minimize absolutely contralateral biliary injuries related to anatomic anomalies. Inflow control can also be obtained by dissection of the intrahepatic inflow pedicle to the anatomic section of liver to be resected. Recall that the inflow structures invaginate peritoneum at the hepatic hilum and run intrahepatically as an invested pedicle of the three inflow structures. The inflow pedicles can be encircled by making flanking hepatotomies or by splitting parenchyma down to the pedicle of interest. The pedicle can usually be divided with a vascular stapler, but suture ligation is sometimes necessary. Typically, the hepatic vein is divided in its extrahepatic position, which can also usually be done with a vascular stapler.

The hepatic vein can also be divided within the substance of the liver during parenchymal transection. There are a number of methods of parenchymal transection, ranging from complex ultrasonic irrigators to radiofrequency energy coagulators to a simple clamp-crushing technique. In experienced hands, these can all be used effectively to minimize blood loss, and it is important to develop a specific technique that one is comfortable performing. Ultimately, parenchymal transection is about dissecting intrahepatic anatomy, controlling vascular and biliary structures, minimizing blood loss, and avoiding injury to the FLR.

HEMOBILIA

A case of lethal hemobilia secondary to penetrating abdominal trauma was first described by Glisson in 1654. It was not until 1948 that Sandblom coined the term *hemobilia* in his seminal paper on the subject. Hemobilia is defined as bleeding into the biliary tree from an abnormal communication between a blood vessel and bile duct. It is a rare condition that is often difficult to distinguish from common causes of gastrointestinal bleeding. The most common causes of hemobilia are iatrogenic trauma, accidental trauma, gallstones, tumors, inflammatory disorders, and vascular disorders. Major hemobilia is relatively uncommon, whereas minor inconsequential hemobilia is a common consequence of gallstone disease or interventional radiologic hepatic procedures.

Causes

The most common cause of hemobilia is iatrogenic trauma to the liver and biliary tree. Before the 1980s, the ratio of hemobilia attributed to accidental trauma compared with iatrogenic trauma was 2 : 1, but iatrogenic trauma is now regarded as the cause of hemobilia in 40% to 60% of cases. Percutaneous liver biopsy results in hemobilia in less than 1% of cases, but percutaneous transhepatic biliary drainage procedures have an incidence of 2% to 10%. Similarly, surgical exploration of the biliary tree can result in hemobilia from direct injury or arterial pseudoaneurysm. A number of cases of hemobilia after cholecystectomy have been reported. Hemobilia secondary to accidental trauma is more common with blunt than with penetrating abdominal trauma and occurs with a reported incidence of 0.2% to 3%. Risk factors for the development of hemobilia after accidental trauma are central hepatic rupture with a cavity, the use of packs, and inadequate drainage. The gallbladder can be a source of bleeding from trauma, gallstones, or acalculous cholecystitis. Primary vascular diseases, such as aneurysms, angiodysplasia, and hemangiomas, are rare causes of hemobilia. Malignant tumors of the liver, biliary tree, gallbladder, and pancreas as well as parasitic infections, hepatic abscesses, and cholangitis are uncommon causes of hemobilia.

Clinical Presentation

Portal venous bleeding into the biliary tree is rare and often self-limited unless the portal pressure is elevated. Minor hemobilia generally runs an uneventful asymptomatic clinical course. However, arterial hemobilia, the most common source, can be dramatic. Clinical sequelae of hemobilia are related to blood loss and the formation of potentially occlusive blood clots in the biliary tree. The classic triad of symptoms and signs of hemobilia is upper abdominal pain, upper gastrointestinal hemorrhage, and jaundice. In one report, all three were present in 22% of patients. The symptoms and signs of major hemobilia are melena (90% of cases), hematemesis (60% of cases), biliary colic (70% of cases), and jaundice (60% of cases). Upper gastrointestinal bleeding seen in conjunction with biliary symptoms must always raise the suspicion of hemobilia. One interesting aspect of hemobilia is the tendency for delayed presentations, up to weeks after the inciting causal event, as well as recurrent and brisk but limited bleeding during months and even years. Blood clots in the biliary tree can masquerade as stones if hemobilia goes unrecognized. These clots can cause cholangitis, pancreatitis, and cholecystitis.

Diagnostic Workup

Once hemobilia is suspected, the first evaluation should be upper gastrointestinal endoscopy, which rules out other sources of hemorrhage and may visualize bleeding from the ampulla of Vater. However, upper endoscopy is diagnostic of hemobilia in only approximately 10% of cases. If upper endoscopy is diagnostic and conservative management is planned, no further studies are necessary. Ultrasound or CT may be helpful in demonstrating intrahepatic tumor or hematoma. Evidence of active bleeding into the biliary tree may be seen on contrast-enhanced CT in the form of pooling contrast material, intraluminal clots, or biliary dilation. CT may also show risk factors associated with hemobilia, such as cavitating central lesions and aneurysms. Arterial angiography is now recognized as the test of choice when significant hemobilia is suspected and will reveal the source of bleeding in approximately 90% of cases. Cholangiography demonstrates blood clots in the biliary tree that may appear as stringy defects or smaller spherical defects that may be difficult to distinguish from stones.

Treatment and Outcomes

The treatment of hemobilia must be focused on stopping the bleeding and relieving biliary obstruction. Most cases of minor hemobilia can be managed conservatively with correction of coagulopathy, adequate biliary drainage (only if necessary), and close observation. In a review of 171 reported cases from 1996 to 1999,

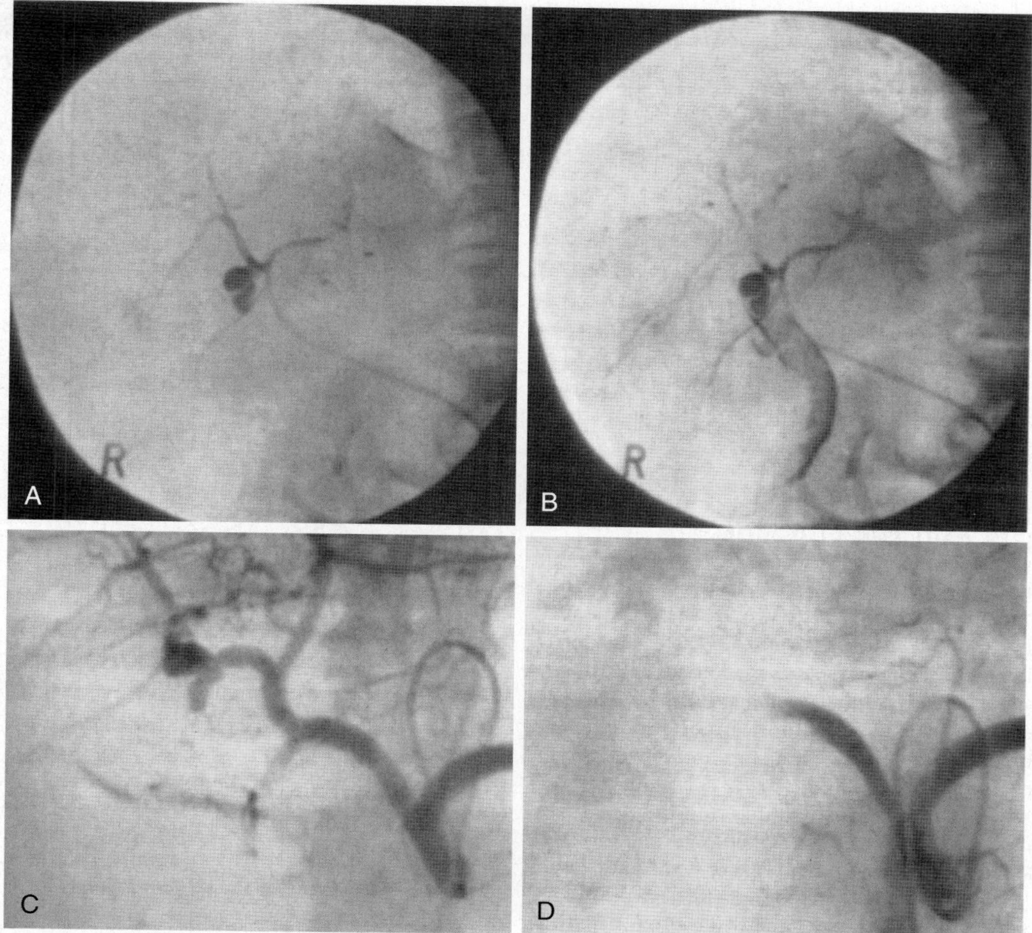

FIGURE 53-41 Classic Findings of Hemobilia. After a complicated cholecystectomy, an iatrogenic pseudoaneurysm developed and ruptured into the biliary tree. Exsanguinating hemobilia ensued; the diagnosis was made by endoscopy and then treated by arterial embolization. **A,** Arteriogram demonstrating a pseudoaneurysm of the hepatic artery at the hilum. **B,** A few seconds later, the contrast material is seen flowing down the hepatic duct, with evidence of clot in the biliary tree. **C** and **D,** The same aneurysm before **(C)** and after **(D)** successful embolization. (From Sandblom JP: Hemobilia and bilhemia. In Blumgart LH, Fong Y, editors: *Surgery of the liver and biliary tract*, London, 2000, WB Saunders, pp 1319–1342.)

43% of cases were successfully managed conservatively. The first line of therapy for major hemobilia was transarterial embolization, and success rates of 80% to 100% were reported. Angiography with transarterial embolization is indicated for major hemobilia requiring blood transfusion (Fig. 53-41).

Surgery is indicated when conservative therapy and transarterial embolization have failed. Surgical treatment of hemobilia is rarely necessary, and even in cases in which a laparotomy may be mandated for other reasons, transarterial embolization is still the therapy of choice for hemobilia because of its lower morbidity. Surgical approaches generally involve ligation of bleeding vessels, excision of aneurysms, or nonselective ligation of a main hepatic artery. Hepatic resection may be necessary for failed arterial ligation or for cases of severe trauma or tumor. Hemorrhage from the gallbladder or hemorrhagic cholecystitis mandates cholecystectomy. There have been isolated reports of successful management of hemobilia with endoscopic coagulation, somatostatin, and vasopressin. The management of hemobilia after percutaneous transhepatic biliary drainage usually consists of removal of the catheter or replacement with larger catheters but may require transarterial embolization.

At the time of Sandblom's report from the early 1970s, the mortality for hemobilia was at least 25%. A report from 1987 noted a mortality of 12%. In a review of cases from 1996 through 1999, only four deaths were reported. There has clearly been a reduction in mortality from hemobilia, which is probably related to two factors. First, the incidence of minor self-limited hemobilia has increased secondary to the rising number of percutaneous hepatic procedures. Second, improvements in selective angiography and transarterial embolization have greatly improved the treatment of major hemobilia.

Bilhemia

Bilhemia is an extremely rare condition in which bile flows into the bloodstream through the hepatic veins or portal vein branches. This flow occurs in the context of a high intrabiliary pressure exceeding that of the venous system. The cause can be gallstones eroding into the portal vein or accidental or iatrogenic trauma. The condition can be fatal secondary to embolization of large amounts of bile into the lungs. Usually, however, bile flow is low, and the fistulas close spontaneously. The clinical presentation is that of rapidly increasing jaundice, marked direct hyperbilirubinemia

TABLE 53-12 Serologic Evaluation of the Most Common Viral Hepatitides

VIRUS	ANTIGEN NAME	INTERPRETATION	ANTIBODY NAME	INTERPRETATION
HAV	HAV antigen	Acute infection	Anti-HAV IgM	Acute infection
			Anti-HAV IgG	Immunity
HBV	HBsAg	Acute or chronic infection	Anti-HBs	Immunity
	HBeAg	HBV replication, infectivity	Anti-HBc	All phases of infection
			Anti-HBe	Late convalescence
HCV	None	—	Anti-HCV	Late convalescence or chronic infection

without elevation of hepatocellular enzyme levels (e.g., AST, ALT), and septicemia. This diagnosis is best determined by ERCP. Treatment is directed at lowering intrabiliary pressures through stents or sphincterotomy.

VIRAL HEPATITIS AND THE SURGEON

Epidemics of jaundice were noted in ancient civilizations and recorded by Hippocrates. During World War II, these epidemics were called catarrhal jaundice. More than 28,000 cases were documented at that time. Epidemiologic studies in the 1940s documented the difference between bloodborne hepatitis (hepatitis B) and enteric hepatitis (hepatitis A). The most important discovery was that of the Australia antigen by Blumberg and coworkers in 1965. This antigen proved to be the hepatitis B surface antigen (HBsAg) and provided a means for differentiating the two types of hepatitis and characterizing the epidemiology of this disease. This discovery also led to the development of HBV vaccines based on this antigen, with obvious and profound effects worldwide. Further research led to the discovery of the delta virus (hepatitis D) and hepatitis C, explaining cases of non-A, non-B hepatitis. Hepatitis E has been found to be a unique enteral form of infectious hepatitis; the hepatitis G virus, discovered in 1995, is still being defined.

Viral hepatitis is a major health problem and is the most common cause of liver disease worldwide. Although fulminant acute hepatitis is uncommon, there are more than 5 million people who suffer from chronic hepatitis. It is estimated that more than 15,000 patients die each year of viral hepatitis in the United States alone. Viral hepatitis is not a surgical disease, but it has important consequences for surgeons and surgical patients. For any surgeon performing hepatic surgery, the functional state of the liver is extremely important, and patients with chronic viral hepatitis require special attention before any surgical intervention. Also, chronic viral hepatitis is a common cause of HCC. Finally, the risk of transmission from patient to surgeon and vice versa is an issue with which all surgeons should be familiar.

Definition

Viral hepatitis is an infection of the liver by one of six known viruses that have diverse genetic compositions and structures. HAV, HCV, HDV, HEV, and HGV have RNA genomes, whereas HBV has a DNA genome that replicates through RNA intermediates. HAV and HEV are both responsible for forms of epidemic hepatitis and are transmitted through the fecal-oral route. HBV is the only one with the potential to integrate into host genomes, although this is not required for replication. HCV replicates in the cytoplasm of hepatocytes and has complex mechanisms of evading host immunity through hypervariable areas in its genome.

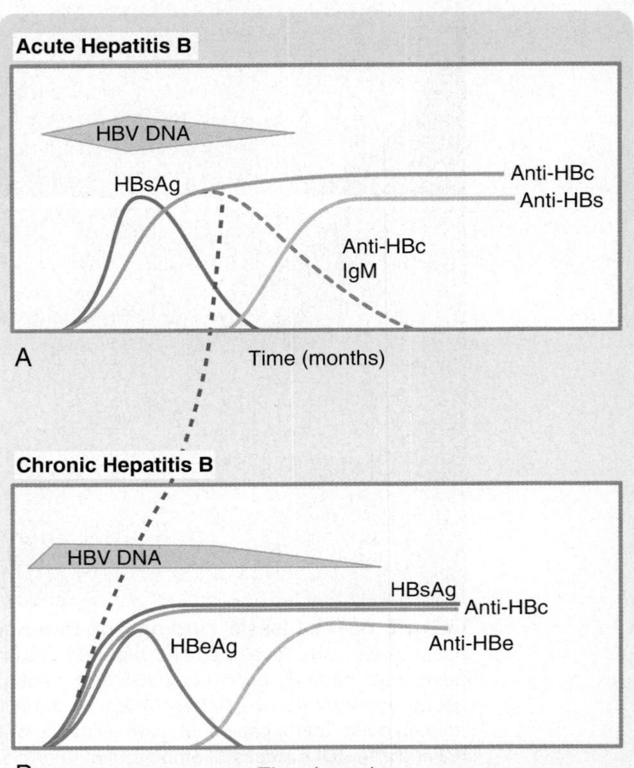

FIGURE 53-42 Serologic makers in acute **(A)** and chronic **(B)** HBV infection. (From Doo EC, Lian TJ: The hepatitis viruses. In Schiff ER, Sorrell MF, Maddrey WC, editors: *Schiff's diseases of the liver*, Philadelphia, 1999, Lippincott-Raven, pp 725–744.)

HDV requires the presence of HBV coinfection for replication and infectivity and can alter the clinical course of HBV infection. HGV was discovered more recently and has similarities to HCV but has no definitive association with clinical hepatitis.

Diagnosis

Table 53-12 summarizes the serologic tests and their implications for HAV, HBV, and HCV. The diagnosis of HAV infection relies on the determination of antibodies to HAV. Both IgM and IgG antibodies are present early in the infection, but only IgG persists long term. HAV antigens and tests for HAV RNA have been developed but are generally restricted to research laboratories.

HBV infection has been characterized by a number of antigens and antibodies (Fig. 53-42). HBsAg is the hallmark of the diagnosis of HBV infection and appears in the serum 1 to 10 weeks after infection; it usually disappears in 4 to 6 months, but persistence in the serum implies chronic infection. Anti-HBs antibodies usually appear during a window period after the disappearance of HBsAg and indicate recovery after HBV infection. Anti-HBs antibodies are also induced by the HBV vaccine. The hepatitis core antigen (HBcAg) is an intracellular antigen that is not detectable in serum. On the other hand, anti-HBc antibodies are detectable early after infection and persist after recovery and in chronic infections. Hepatitis B e antigen (HBeAg) is a secretory protein that is a marker of HBV replication and infectivity. It is usually present early and may persist for years in chronic infection but generally disappears within months in the absence of chronic infection. Seroconversion to anti-HBe antibodies is usually associated with resolution of infection. It has also been shown that many patients who have seroconverted often have measurable HBV DNA, albeit at low levels. Quantification of HBV DNA in the serum has become the most accurate way of assessing HBV activity. Evidence has shown that many patients thought to have resolved acute HBV infection may have persistent viral infection and may be at risk for ongoing hepatitis or reactivation.

The diagnosis of HCV infection relies on the detection of antibodies to a number of HCV antigens. Current immunoassays are highly specific and sensitive. No specific HCV antigen tests exist, but there are a variety of quantitative and qualitative tests for HCV RNA, which have become important in confirming the diagnosis in unclear cases and assessing responses to therapy.

HDV coinfection of HBV-infected patients is best diagnosed by detection of HDV RNA, which can be measured in serum. The HDV antigen can be detected in liver specimens. HEV infection can be diagnosed by measurement of antibodies in serum or by detection of the virus or its components in feces, serum, or the liver itself.

Epidemiology and Transmission

The incidence of hepatitis A has fallen dramatically since the introduction of effective vaccines, but vaccination is not routine in all countries. Hepatitis A is common in third-world countries, with seropositivity rates approaching 100% in some populations. Infection occurs in childhood and is facilitated by poor hygiene and sanitation. Infection rates are much lower in developed countries. In the United States, approximately 10% of children and 35% of adults have been infected with HAV. Despite vaccination availability, 6000 cases were reported in the United States in 2004, likely representing an estimated 60,000 cases nationwide. The primary route of HAV infection is the fecal-oral route. Most cases of HAV occur because of ingestion of contaminated water or food and person-to-person contact. Parenteral transmission is possible but uncommon. Sexual transmission has been documented in homosexual men.

Hepatitis B is a major worldwide health problem. There are more than 300 million carriers and 250,000 associated deaths annually. The prevalence of HBV infection has considerable geographic variation. Low prevalence areas such as the United States and western Europe have carrier rates of 0.1% to 2%. In these regions, transmission is generally through sexual intercourse or IV drug abuse. Carrier rates in intermediate-prevalence areas such as Japan and Singapore range from 3% to 5%. In high-prevalence areas such as Southeast Asia and sub-Saharan Africa, carrier rates range from 10% to 20%. Transmission in high-prevalence areas is largely perinatal and horizontal during childhood.

Transfusion-associated HBV infection was common in the 1960s, and the risk has been estimated to be as high as 50% at that time. Currently, screening programs and limitation of blood donation to voluntary donors have decreased the risk of acquiring HBV from a blood transfusion to 1 in 63,000. Percutaneous transmission through the use of any contaminated needle is a major route of HBV infection and is common in IV drug abusers. Sexual transmission is common in low-prevalence countries and is estimated to account for approximately 30% of cases in the United States. There is a particularly high incidence in male homosexuals and heterosexuals with multiple sexual partners. Perinatal HBV infection accounts for less than 10% of cases in the United States but is common in endemic regions, with rates of transmission of 90% in some areas. Horizontal transmission among children is common and is probably related to minor breaks in the skin and mucous membranes. HBV is the most commonly transmitted virus among health care personnel, and transmission is usually patient to patient or patient to worker. Needle-stick risk has been related to HBeAg positivity. Rare cases of physician to patient transmission have been reported.

Hepatitis C is the most common cause of chronic liver disease in the United States, with an estimated prevalence of 1.8% accounting for 3.9 million infected people. New infections typically occur at a younger age (20 to 39 years), and the most common risk factor is IV drug abuse. Health care workers have higher carrier rates than the general public. Transmission among health care workers is usually related to needle-stick incidents, and the risk of transmission is higher than that of HBV and HIV. In the past, blood transfusion was the major cause of HCV infection, accounting for at least 85% of cases. Currently, less than 2% of acute infections are caused by transfusions, and the risk of transfusion-associated transmission is estimated to be about 1 in 10,000. Although HCV has never been documented in semen, it is estimated that approximately 20% of HCV infections are caused by sexual transmission. Risk of sexual transmission appears to be related to the number of partners and presence of other sexually transmitted diseases. Monogamous sexual partners of HCV-infected people occasionally test positive for HCV in the absence of other risk factors, but this appears to be rare. Perinatal transmission has been documented but is also rare. No identifiable risk factors are found in 30% to 40% of HCV cases.

HDV infection occurs worldwide, with a variable distribution that parallels that of HBV infection. Approximately 5% of HBsAg-positive patients also harbor HDV infection. Transmission of HDV is parenteral and can occur only in patients previously infected with HBV.

HEV is endemic in Southeast Asia and central Asia and occurs with low frequency in other areas of the world. HEV infection outbreaks are usually large, affecting hundreds to thousands of people at once, and often follow large rains and flooding. There is a particularly high incidence and mortality in pregnant women. Transmission is fecal-oral and usually related to contaminated drinking water or food. Person-to-person transmission and vertical transmission are rare.

Pathogenesis and Clinical Presentation

The pathogenesis of hepatic injury from these viral infections is not completely understood. For all the viruses discussed in this section, hepatic inflammation appears to be caused by direct cytotoxicity or immune-related phenomena. A combination of these two mechanisms probably underlies the cause of hepatic damage.

Humans are the only host for HAV, and no reservoir of infection has been identified. After oral intake, HAV can survive the acidic gastric pH, but the mechanism of hepatic uptake is not known. HAV infection results in acute inflammation of the liver and has no associated chronic sequelae. The most recent data suggest that hepatocyte damage is most likely an immunopathologic response rather than direct hepatotoxicity. Most children with HAV infection younger than 2 years are asymptomatic, whereas in pediatric patients older than 5 years, 80% will develop symptoms. Fulminant hepatitis develops in 1% to 5% of cases, and mortality is generally below 1%.

Approximately 70% of patients with acute HBV infection have subclinical or anicteric hepatitis; the other 30% have icteric hepatitis. The incubation period for HBV infection ranges from 1 to 4 months. A prodromal serum sickness–like syndrome may develop, followed by a multitude of constitutional symptoms, such as malaise, anorexia, and nausea. The constitutional symptoms last about 10 days and are followed by jaundice in 30% of patients. Clinical symptoms usually disappear within 3 months. Fulminant hepatic failure develops in 0.1% to 0.5% of patients. Almost 80% of patients with fulminant HBV-related hepatitis will die unless liver transplantation is performed.

Risk of chronic HBV infection is related to immunocompetence and age. Immunocompetent adults have a risk of less than 5%, whereas 30% of children and 90% of infants will develop chronic disease. Most patients with chronic HBV infection are asymptomatic, but some may experience exacerbations of symptoms. Laboratory test results may be entirely normal in HBV carriers, or mild elevations of ALT and AST may be the only findings. Progression to cirrhosis is marked by hepatic synthetic dysfunction and often cytopenias, related to hypersplenism. Extrahepatic manifestations of HBV infection, caused by circulating immune complexes, occur in approximately 10% to 20% of patients; these include polyarteritis nodosa, glomerulonephritis, essential mixed cryoglobulinemia, and papular acrodermatitis. The sequelae of chronic HBV infection range from none to cirrhosis, HCC, hepatic failure, and death. It has been noted that patients thought to have previously cleared the infection can have a reactivation, especially during a period of immunosuppression. In nonendemic areas, the long-term risk appears to be low, but in endemic areas, chronic HBV infection is a significant cause of morbidity and mortality.

Acute HCV infection generally is manifested with mild elevation of hepatocellular enzyme levels. In general, 80% of cases occur 5 to 12 weeks after infection. Symptoms occur in less than 30% of patients and are usually so mild and nonspecific that they do not affect daily life. Jaundice occurs in less than 20% of patients, and fulminant hepatic failure caused by HCV is extremely uncommon. Chronic HCV infection develops in approximately two thirds of patients; the other third appear to clear the infection. Most patients with chronic HCV infection are asymptomatic without evidence of overt liver disease and present with only mildly elevated hepatocellular enzyme levels. Despite this quiet clinical course, patients with chronic HCV infection are at risk for development of cirrhosis and HCC. Estimates place the risk of cirrhosis at 2% to 20% at a 20- to 30-year interval. The risk for development of HCC from that point has been estimated at 1% to 4%/year. Progression of liver damage can be variable, and several factors appear to affect its rate. Factors associated with a more rapid progression include male gender, older age at infection, immunosuppression (e.g., HIV infection), coinfection with HBV, moderate alcohol intake, and obesity. Extrahepatic manifestations, such as autoimmune disorders and lymphoma, can occur with HCV infection and are likely related to circulating immune complexes.

The clinical presentation of HDV infection is related to a complex relationship between the degree of HBV and HDV infection. Simultaneous coinfection with high expression of HBV and HDV results in higher rates of acute fulminant hepatitis. Superinfection in a previous HBV carrier generally results in more rapidly progressive chronic liver damage. Some milder forms of acute HDV infection are associated with decreased expression of HDV and repression of HBV infection.

Hepatitis E has a histologic picture different from that of the other viral hepatitides in that a cholestatic type of hepatitis is seen in more than 50% of patients. HEV is introduced orally, and it is not known how the virus travels to the liver. The incubation period of HEV infection ranges from 2 to 9 weeks. The most common form of illness is acute icteric hepatitis; most series report jaundice in more than 90% of patients. Asymptomatic forms of the disease occur and are probably more common than the icteric form, but the actual frequency is unknown. The disease is usually self-limited, but fulminant hepatic failure can occur in a small percentage of patients. Overall, the mortality rate is probably significantly less than 1%. Pregnant women tend to have a more severe clinical course; mortality rates range from 5% to 25%.

Prevention

HAV infection prophylaxis relies on sanitary measures and administration of serum immunoglobulin. The development of safe and effective HAV vaccines, however, has made the use of preexposure immunoglobulin unnecessary. Serum immunoglobulin is still the therapy of choice for postexposure prophylaxis and may be safely given, along with active immunization. In the United States, the Centers for Disease Control and Prevention has recommended universal vaccination of children on the basis of the safety and efficacy of the vaccine in high-risk populations. Public health researchers are investigating vaccination schemes to eradicate HAV infection in high-risk populations throughout the world. However, cost-benefit analyses have not supported universal vaccination worldwide. Similarly, HEV infection prophylaxis has focused on sanitary measures, particularly strategies aimed at drinking water. Unfortunately, HEV immunoglobulin has not been successful in preexposure or postexposure prevention of HEV infection, whereas anti-HEV antibodies appear to be effective at attenuating the clinical syndrome. Vaccines for HEV infection have been developed and evaluated in clinical trials.

Remarkable advances have been made in the prevention of HBV infection. In the past, prevention of HBV infection was limited to passive immunization with immunoglobulin containing high titers of antibody to HBsAg. Currently, immunoglobulin immunization is used only in postexposure prophylaxis. HBsAg-containing vaccines have been developed, with good safety and efficacy profiles. These vaccines are used primarily for preexposure prophylaxis but can also be used in a postexposure setting along with immunoglobulin. HBV vaccination is recommended for high-risk groups such as health care workers. There are also programs for HBV vaccination to prevent perinatal transmission; currently, all children 11 or 12 years old should be vaccinated if this has not been done previously. HBV DNA–based vaccines have been developed, and a combined HBV and HAV vaccine was approved by the U.S. Food and Drug Administration in 2001. Although no vaccine is available for HDV infection, effective prevention of HBV infection prevents HDV infection.

The only effective preventive strategy for HCV infection relies on public health principles aimed at the major risk factors for transmission. Conventionally prepared anti-HCV immunoglobulin has been evaluated in a number of trials and has not been demonstrated to prevent transfusion-related non-A, non-B hepatitis. Screening of blood donors has rendered this issue irrelevant today. Unfortunately, because of various obstacles, a successful HCV vaccine has not been developed.

Treatment

Treatment of HAV or HEV infection is supportive in nature and is generally aimed at correcting dehydration and providing adequate calorie intake. Although fatigue may mandate significant periods of rest, hospitalization is usually not necessary, except in cases of fulminant liver failure.

The treatment of HBV infection is largely aimed at patients with chronic active disease. The two approved therapies are interferon alfa and the nucleoside analogue lamivudine. Interferon alfa is an immunomodulatory agent with some antiviral properties that can induce a virologic response in 35% to 40% of patients. However, long-term benefit with interferon therapy has not been proven. Many nucleoside analogues for the treatment of HBV infection have been developed and probably work through inhibition of DNA synthesis. They have similar viral response rates to interferon alfa, are inexpensive, are given orally, and have few side effects. On the other hand, nucleoside analogues often require long-term therapy (>1 year), and the development of resistant HBV mutants has been documented. Randomized trials have shown oral lamivudine to be effective at decreasing the risk of cirrhosis progression and HCC. Newer antiviral agents are in development and are likely to improve outcomes.

During the last 20 years, tremendous advances in the treatment of HCV infection have occurred. A benefit for interferon alfa in the treatment of non-A, non-B hepatitis was originally demonstrated in 1986, before the discovery of HCV. With current interferon alfa treatment regimens, complete viral response, defined as sustained loss of serum viral RNA, occurs in 12% to 20% of patients. The addition of ribavirin to interferon alfa has resulted in response rates of 35% to 45%. In the most recent trials, treatment with pegylated interferon alfa and ribavirin for 48 weeks resulted in viral clearance in 55% of patients. The specific genotype appears to be predictive of response, with some types resulting in response rates of 80% and others of 45%. Relapse can occur, but it usually occurs with monotherapy and shortened courses of therapy. Because therapy with interferon alfa has significant side effects, controversies such as indications for treatment, optimal doses, and duration of treatment are still being resolved.

SELECTED REFERENCES

Blumgart LH: *Video atlas: Liver, biliary and pancreatic surgery*, Philadelphia, 2011, Elsevier.

This video atlas includes an extensive library of narrated and captioned videos that present history, radiologic evidence, and operative procedures for hepatic and biliary surgery. It also includes laparoscopic approaches to liver resections.

Blumgart LH: *Surgery of the liver, biliary tract, and pancreas*, ed 5, Philadelphia, 2012, Elsevier.

A comprehensive and clinical review of hepatobiliary anatomy. The text is specifically oriented toward surgery of the liver and biliary tree. It covers anatomy, pathophysiology, immunology, molecular biology, genetics, diagnosis, and treatment. In addition, it is accompanied by a DVD with detailed video clips of laparoscopic procedures, effectively allowing one to use it as an operative atlas.

Bruix J, Sherman M, American Association for the Study of Liver Disease: Management of hepatocellular carcinoma: An update. *Hepatology* 53:1020–1022, 2011.

This is an update on the original AASLD guidelines on the management of hepatocellular carcinoma.

Fong Y, Fortner J, Sun RL, et al: Clinical score for predicting recurrence after hepatic resection for metastatic colorectal cancer: Analysis of 1001 consecutive cases. *Ann Surg* 230:309–318, 1999.

At the time of publication, this was the largest single-institution series of liver resection for metastatic colorectal cancer. A very useful prognostic scoring system is presented and remains critically important in evaluating patients today.

Foster JH, Berman MM: *Solid liver tumors*, Philadelphia, 1977, WB Saunders.

A classic and comprehensive monograph that contains a complete history of liver surgery.

Herrera JL: Management of acute variceal bleeding. *Clin Liver Dis* 18:347–357, 2014.

This review article discusses the management of acute variceal bleeding with special emphasis on the appropriate role of various treatment modalities in the current era and when to escalate the therapy and move to the next stage.

House MG, Ito H, Gonen M, et al: Survival after hepatic resection for metastatic colorectal cancer: Trends in outcomes for 1,600 patients during two decades at a single institution. *J Am Coll Surg* 210:744–752, 2010.

This study analyzes factors associated with differences in long-term outcomes after hepatic resection for metastatic colorectal cancer. Despite worse clinical and pathologic features, survival rates after hepatic resection for colorectal metastases have improved, which might be attributable to improvements in patient selection, operative management, and chemotherapy.

Jang HJ, Yu H, Kim TK: Imaging of focal liver lesions. *Semin Roentgenol* 44:266–282, 2009.

Imaging modalities are key in diagnosing and differentiating various focal liver lesions. This monograph covers the critical elements of ultrasonography, computed tomography, and magnetic resonance imaging of focal liver lesions.

Jarnagin WR, Gonen M, Fong Y, et al: Improvement in perioperative outcome after hepatic resection: Analysis of 1,803 consecutive cases over the past decade. *Ann Surg* 236:397–406, 2002.

One of the largest series of hepatic resections that documents the remarkable improvement in perioperative outcomes.

Kelly K, Weber SM: Cystic diseases of the liver and bile ducts. *J Gastrointest Surg* 18:627–634, quiz 634, 2014.

This review article covers the diagnosis and management of cystic disease of the liver including hydatid disease.

Leung U, Fong Y: Robotic liver surgery. *Hepatobiliary Surg Nutr* 3:288–294, 2014.

This manuscript reviews the place and evolution of robotics in the current era of minimally invasive liver surgery.

Llovet JM, Ricci S, Mazzaferro V, et al: Sorafenib in advanced hepatocellular carcinoma. *N Engl J Med* 359:378–390, 2008.

The first randomized phase 3 clinical trial in patients with advanced hepatocellular carcinoma that showed a benefit of improved median survival and time to radiologic progression for patients treated with a chemotherapeutic agent compared with patients who were given a placebo.

Mittal S, El-Serag HB: Epidemiology of hepatocellular carcinoma: Consider the population. *J Clin Gastroenterol* 47(Suppl):S2–S6, 2013.

A recent comprehensive and concise review of the subject.

Ochsner A, DeBakey M, Murray S: Pyogenic abscess of the liver. *Am J Surg* 40:292–319, 1938.

A classic landmark study on pyogenic abscesses of the liver. This was the first serious attempt to study hepatic abscesses and ushered in the modern era of treatment.

Sandhu BS, Sanyal AJ: Management of ascites in cirrhosis. *Clin Liver Dis* 9:715–732, 2005.

This is an excellent, comprehensive, and practical review of the treatment of ascites in patients with cirrhosis.

REFERENCES

1. Tsung A, Geller DA, Sukato DC, et al: Robotic versus laparoscopic hepatectomy: A matched comparison. *Ann Surg* 259:549–555, 2014.
2. Biernat J, Pawlik WW, Sendur R, et al: Role of afferent nerves and sensory peptides in the mediation of hepatic artery buffer response. *J Physiol Pharmacol* 56:133–145, 2005.
3. de Franchis R: Revising consensus in portal hypertension: Report of the Baveno V consensus workshop on methodology of diagnosis and therapy in portal hypertension. *J Hepatol* 53:762–768, 2010.
4. Garcia-Tsao G, Bosch J: Management of varices and variceal hemorrhage in cirrhosis. *N Engl J Med* 362:823–832, 2010.
5. Bureau C, Garcia-Pagan JC, Otal P, et al: Improved clinical outcome using polytetrafluoroethylene-coated stents for TIPS: Results of a randomized study. *Gastroenterology* 126:469–475, 2004.
6. Orloff MJ, Orloff MS, Orloff SL, et al: Three decades of experience with emergency portacaval shunt for acutely bleeding esophageal varices in 400 unselected patients with cirrhosis of the liver. *J Am Coll Surg* 180:257–272, 1995.
7. Bernard B, Lebrec D, Mathurin P, et al: Beta-adrenergic antagonists in the prevention of gastrointestinal rebleeding in patients with cirrhosis: A meta-analysis. *Hepatology* 25:63–70, 1997.
8. Villanueva C, Minana J, Ortiz J, et al: Endoscopic ligation compared with combined treatment with nadolol and isosorbide mononitrate to prevent recurrent variceal bleeding. *N Engl J Med* 345:647–655, 2001.
9. de la Pena J, Brullet E, Sanchez-Hernandez E, et al: Variceal ligation plus nadolol compared with ligation for prophylaxis of variceal rebleeding: A multicenter trial. *Hepatology* 41:572–578, 2005.
10. Funakoshi N, Segalas-Largey F, Duny Y, et al: Benefit of combination beta-blocker and endoscopic treatment to prevent variceal rebleeding: A meta-analysis. *World J Gastroenterol* 16:5982–5992, 2010.
11. Fong Y, Wong J: Evolution in surgery: Influence of minimally invasive approaches on the hepatobiliary surgeon. *Surg Infect (Larchmt)* 10:399–406, 2009.
12. Meddings L, Myers RP, Hubbard J, et al: A population-based study of pyogenic liver abscesses in the United States: Incidence, mortality, and temporal trends. *Am J Gastroenterol* 105:117–124, 2010.
13. Lai HC, Lin CC, Cheng KS, et al: Increased incidence of gastrointestinal cancers among patients with pyogenic liver abscess: A population-based cohort study. *Gastroenterology* 146:129–137, e1, 2014.
14. Salles JM, Salles MJ, Moraes LA, et al: Invasive amebiasis: An update on diagnosis and management. *Expert Rev Anti Infect Ther* 5:893–901, 2007.
15. Mezhir J, Fong Y, Jacks L, et al: Current management of pyogenic liver abscess: Surgery is now second-line treatment. *J Am Coll Surg* 975–983, 2010.
16. Wuerz T, Kane JB, Boggild AK, et al: A review of amoebic liver abscess for clinicians in a nonendemic setting. *Can J Gastroenterol* 26:729–733, 2012.
17. Haque R, Mollah NU, Ali IK, et al: Diagnosis of amebic liver abscess and intestinal infection with the TechLab *Entamoeba histolytica* II antigen detection and antibody tests. *J Clin Microbiol* 38:3235–3239, 2000.
18. Benedetti NJ, Desser TS, Jeffrey RB: Imaging of hepatic infections. *Ultrasound Q* 24:267–278, 2008.
19. Chavez-Tapia NC, Hernandez-Calleros J, Tellez-Avila FI, et al: Image-guided percutaneous procedure plus metronidazole versus metronidazole alone for uncomplicated amoebic liver abscess. *Cochrane Database Syst Rev* (1): CD004886, 2009.
20. Nunnari G, Pinzone MR, Gruttadauria S, et al: Hepatic echinococcosis: Clinical and therapeutic aspects. *World J Gastroenterol* 18:1448–1458, 2012.
21. Agayev RM, Agayev BA: Hepatic hydatid disease: Surgical experience over 15 years. *Hepatogastroenterology* 55:1373–1379, 2008.

22. Dziri C, Haouet K, Fingerhut A, et al: Management of cystic echinococcosis complications and dissemination: Where is the evidence? *World J Surg* 33:1266–1273, 2009.
23. Brunetti E, Kern P, Vuitton DA: Expert consensus for the diagnosis and treatment of cystic and alveolar echinococcosis in humans. *Acta Trop* 114:1–16, 2010.
24. Tamarozzi F, Vuitton L, Brunetti E, et al: Non-surgical and non-chemical attempts to treat echinococcosis: Do they work? *Parasite* 21:75, 2014.
25. Nasseri Moghaddam S, Abrishami A, Malekzadeh R: Percutaneous needle aspiration, injection, and reaspiration with or without benzimidazole coverage for uncomplicated hepatic hydatid cysts. *Cochrane Database Syst Rev* (2): CD003623, 2006.
26. Nguyen T, Powell A, Daugherty T: Recurrent pyogenic cholangitis. *Dig Dis Sci* 55:8–10, 2010.
27. Das AK: Hepatic and biliary ascariasis. *J Glob Infect Dis* 6:65–72, 2014.
28. Chen C, Huang M, Yang J, et al: Reappraisal of percutaneous transhepatic cholangioscopic lithotomy for primary hepatolithiasis. *Surg Endosc* 19:505–509, 2005.
29. Parray FQ, Wani MA, Wani NA: Oriental cholangiohepatitis—is our surgery appropriate? *Int J Surg* 12:789–793, 2014.
30. Mori T, Sugiyama M, Atomi Y: Gallstone disease: Management of intrahepatic stones. *Best Pract Res Clin Gastroenterol* 20:1117–1137, 2006.
31. Buell JF, Cherqui D, Geller DA, et al: The international position on laparoscopic liver surgery: The Louisville Statement, 2008. *Ann Surg* 250:825–830, 2009.
32. Sasaki A, Nitta H, Otsuka K, et al: Ten-year experience of totally laparoscopic liver resection in a single institution. *Br J Surg* 96:274–279, 2009.
33. Huurman VA, Schaapherder AF: Management of ruptured hepatocellular adenoma. *Dig Surg* 27:56–60, 2010.
34. Dhingra S, Fiel MI: Update on the new classification of hepatic adenomas: Clinical, molecular, and pathologic characteristics. *Arch Pathol Lab Med* 138:1090–1097, 2014.
35. Zucman-Rossi J, Jeannot E, Nhieu JT, et al: Genotype-phenotype correlation in hepatocellular adenoma: New classification and relationship with HCC. *Hepatology* 43:515–524, 2006.
36. Rebouissou S, Bioulac-Sage P, Zucman-Rossi J: Molecular pathogenesis of focal nodular hyperplasia and hepatocellular adenoma. *J Hepatol* 48:163–170, 2008.
37. Assy N, Nasser G, Djibre A, et al: Characteristics of common solid liver lesions and recommendations for diagnostic workup. *World J Gastroenterol* 15:3217–3227, 2009.
38. Curvo-Semedo L, Brito JB, Seco MF, et al: The hypointense liver lesion on T2-weighted MR images and what it means. *Radiographics* 30:e38, 2010.
39. Marrero JA, Ahn J, Rajender Reddy K: ACG clinical guideline: The diagnosis and management of focal liver lesions. *Am J Gastroenterol* 109:1328–1347, quiz 1348, 2014.
40. Katabathina VS, Menias CO, Shanbhogue AK, et al: Genetics and imaging of hepatocellular adenomas: 2011 update. *Radiographics* 31:1529–1543, 2011.
41. Bioulac-Sage P, Laumonier H, Couchy G, et al: Hepatocellular adenoma management and phenotypic classification: The Bordeaux experience. *Hepatology* 50:481–489, 2009.
42. Deneve JL, Pawlik TM, Cunningham S, et al: Liver cell adenoma: A multicenter analysis of risk factors for rupture and malignancy. *Ann Surg Oncol* 16:640–648, 2009.
43. Vetelainen R, Erdogan D, de Graaf W, et al: Liver adenomatosis: Re-evaluation of aetiology and management. *Liver Int* 28:499–508, 2008.
44. Wellen JR, Anderson CD, Doyle M, et al: The role of liver transplantation for hepatic adenomatosis in the pediatric population: Case report and review of the literature. *Pediatr Transplant* 14:E16–E19, 2010.
45. Cogley JR, Miller FH: MR imaging of benign focal liver lesions. *Radiol Clin North Am* 52:657–682, 2014.
46. Koffron A, Geller D, Gamblin TC, et al: Laparoscopic liver surgery: Shifting the management of liver tumors. *Hepatology* 44:1694–1700, 2006.
47. Harman M, Nart D, Acar T, et al: Primary mesenchymal liver tumors: Radiological spectrum, differential diagnosis, and pathologic correlation. *Abdom Imaging* 40:1316–1330, 2015.
48. Kamaya A, Maturen KE, Tye GA, et al: Hypervascular liver lesions. *Semin Ultrasound CT MR* 30:387–407, 2009.
49. Hsi Dickie B, Fishman SJ, Azizkhan RG: Hepatic vascular tumors. *Semin Pediatr Surg* 23:168–172, 2014.
50. Altekruse SF, Henley SJ, Cucinelli JE, et al: Changing hepatocellular carcinoma incidence and liver cancer mortality rates in the United States. *Am J Gastroenterol* 109:542–553, 2014.
51. Njei B, Rotman Y, Ditah I, et al: Emerging trends in hepatocellular carcinoma incidence and mortality. *Hepatology* 61:191–199, 2015.
52. El-Serag HB: Epidemiology of hepatocellular carcinoma in USA. *Hepatol Res* 37(Suppl 2):S88–S94, 2007.
53. El-Serag HB, Engels EA, Landgren O, et al: Risk of hepatobiliary and pancreatic cancers after hepatitis C virus infection: A population-based study of U.S. veterans. *Hepatology* 49:116–123, 2009.
54. Mittal S, El-Serag HB: Epidemiology of hepatocellular carcinoma: Consider the population. *J Clin Gastroenterol* 47(Suppl):S2–S6, 2013.
55. Corey KE, Kaplan LM: Obesity and liver disease: The epidemic of the twenty-first century. *Clin Liver Dis* 18:1–18, 2014.
56. Chiang CJ, Yang YW, Chen JD, et al: Significant reduction in end-stage liver diseases burden through national viral hepatitis therapy program in Taiwan. *Hepatology* 61:1154–1162, 2015.
57. Kim do Y, Han KH: Epidemiology and surveillance of hepatocellular carcinoma. *Liver Cancer* 1:2–14, 2012.
58. Riviere L, Ducroux A, Buendia MA: The oncogenic role of hepatitis B virus. *Recent Results Cancer Res* 193:59–74, 2014.
59. Hoshida Y, Fuchs BC, Bardeesy N, et al: Pathogenesis and prevention of hepatitis C virus–induced hepatocellular carcinoma. *J Hepatol* 61:S79–S90, 2014.
60. Tsai WL, Chung RT: Viral hepatocarcinogenesis. *Oncogene* 29:2309–2324, 2010.
61. Davila JA, Morgan RO, Shaib Y, et al: Diabetes increases the risk of hepatocellular carcinoma in the United States: A population based case control study. *Gut* 54:533–539, 2005.
62. Setiawan VW, Hernandez BY, Lu SC, et al: Diabetes and racial/ethnic differences in hepatocellular carcinoma risk: The Multiethnic Cohort. *J Natl Cancer Inst* 106:2014.

63. Turati F, Talamini R, Pelucchi C, et al: Metabolic syndrome and hepatocellular carcinoma risk. *Br J Cancer* 108:222–228, 2013.
64. Fowler KJ, Saad NE, Linehan D: Imaging approach to hepatocellular carcinoma, cholangiocarcinoma, and metastatic colorectal cancer. *Surg Oncol Clin N Am* 24:19–40, 2015.
65. Wald C, Russo MW, Heimbach JK, et al: New OPTN/UNOS policy for liver transplant allocation: Standardization of liver imaging, diagnosis, classification, and reporting of hepatocellular carcinoma. *Radiology* 266:376–382, 2013.
66. Bruix J, Sherman M, Llovet JM, et al: Clinical management of hepatocellular carcinoma. Conclusions of the Barcelona-2000 EASL conference. European Association for the Study of the Liver. *J Hepatol* 35:421–430, 2001.
67. Bruix J, Sherman M: Management of hepatocellular carcinoma. *Hepatology* 42:1208–1236, 2005.
68. EASL-EORTC clinical practice guidelines: Management of hepatocellular carcinoma. *J Hepatol* 56:908–943, 2012.
69. Bruix J, Sherman M: Management of hepatocellular carcinoma: An update. *Hepatology* 53:1020–1022, 2011.
70. Khalili K, Kim TK, Jang HJ, et al: Optimization of imaging diagnosis of 1-2 cm hepatocellular carcinoma: An analysis of diagnostic performance and resource utilization. *J Hepatol* 54:723–728, 2011.
71. Weitz J, D'Angelica M, Jarnagin W, et al: Selective use of diagnostic laparoscopy prior to planned hepatectomy for patients with hepatocellular carcinoma. *Surgery* 135:273–281, 2004.
72. Pawlik TM, Poon RT, Abdalla EK, et al: Critical appraisal of the clinical and pathologic predictors of survival after resection of large hepatocellular carcinoma. *Arch Surg* 140:450–457, discussion 457–458, 2005.
73. Schiffman SC, Woodall CE, Kooby DA, et al: Factors associated with recurrence and survival following hepatectomy for large hepatocellular carcinoma: A multicenter analysis. *J Surg Oncol* 101:105–110, 2010.
74. Yin L, Li H, Li AJ, et al: Partial hepatectomy vs. transcatheter arterial chemoembolization for resectable multiple hepatocellular carcinoma beyond Milan Criteria: A RCT. *J Hepatol* 61:82–88, 2014.
75. Mazzaferro V, Bhoori S, Sposito C, et al: Milan criteria in liver transplantation for hepatocellular carcinoma: An evidence-based analysis of 15 years of experience. *Liver Transpl* 17(Suppl 2):S44–S57, 2014.
76. Mazzaferro V, Regalia E, Doci R, et al: Liver transplantation for the treatment of small hepatocellular carcinomas in patients with cirrhosis. *N Engl J Med* 334:693–699, 1996.
77. Llovet JM, Fuster J, Bruix J: Intention-to-treat analysis of surgical treatment for early hepatocellular carcinoma: Resection versus transplantation. *Hepatology* 30:1434–1440, 1999.
78. Capussotti L, Ferrero A, Vigano L, et al: Liver resection for HCC with cirrhosis: Surgical perspectives out of EASL/AASLD guidelines. *Eur J Surg Oncol* 35:11–15, 2009.
79. Facciuto ME, Rochon C, Pandey M, et al: Surgical dilemma: Liver resection or liver transplantation for hepatocellular carcinoma and cirrhosis. Intention-to-treat analysis in patients within and outwith Milan criteria. *HPB (Oxford)* 11:398–404, 2009.
80. Llovet JM, Schwartz M, Mazzaferro V: Resection and liver transplantation for hepatocellular carcinoma. *Semin Liver Dis* 25:181–200, 2005.
81. Huang J, Yan L, Cheng Z, et al: A randomized trial comparing radiofrequency ablation and surgical resection for HCC conforming to the Milan criteria. *Ann Surg* 252:903–912, 2010.
82. Sangro B: Chemoembolization and radioembolization. *Best Pract Res Clin Gastroenterol* 28:909–919, 2014.
83. Malagari K, Pomoni M, Kelekis A, et al: Prospective randomized comparison of chemoembolization with doxorubicin-eluting beads and bland embolization with BeadBlock for hepatocellular carcinoma. *Cardiovasc Intervent Radiol* 33:541–551, 2010.
84. Llovet JM, Bruix J: Systematic review of randomized trials for unresectable hepatocellular carcinoma: Chemoembolization improves survival. *Hepatology* 37:429–442, 2003.
85. Llovet JM, Real MI, Montana X, et al: Arterial embolisation or chemoembolisation versus symptomatic treatment in patients with unresectable hepatocellular carcinoma: A randomised controlled trial. *Lancet* 359:1734–1739, 2002.
86. Lo CM, Ngan H, Tso WK, et al: Randomized controlled trial of transarterial lipiodol chemoembolization for unresectable hepatocellular carcinoma. *Hepatology* 35:1164–1171, 2002.
87. Llovet JM, Ricci S, Mazzaferro V, et al: Sorafenib in advanced hepatocellular carcinoma. *N Engl J Med* 359:378–390, 2008.
88. Lim II, Farber BA, LaQuaglia MP: Advances in fibrolamellar hepatocellular carcinoma: A review. *Eur J Pediatr Surg* 24:461–466, 2014.
89. Honeyman JN, Simon EP, Robine N, et al: Detection of a recurrent DNAJB1-PRKACA chimeric transcript in fibrolamellar hepatocellular carcinoma. *Science* 343:1010–1014, 2014.
90. Guglielmi A, Ruzzenente A, Valdegamberi A, et al: Hepatolithiasis-associated cholangiocarcinoma: Results from a multi-institutional national database on a case series of 23 patients. *Eur J Surg Oncol* 40:567–575, 2014.
91. Matsumoto K, Onoyama T, Kawata S, et al: Hepatitis B and C virus infection is a risk factor for the development of cholangiocarcinoma. *Intern Med* 53:651–654, 2014.
92. Reddy SK, Hyder O, Marsh JW, et al: Prevalence of nonalcoholic steatohepatitis among patients with resectable intrahepatic cholangiocarcinoma. *J Gastrointest Surg* 17:748–755, 2013.
93. Jamal MM, Yoon EJ, Vega KJ, et al: Diabetes mellitus as a risk factor for gastrointestinal cancer among American veterans. *World J Gastroenterol* 15:5274–5278, 2009.
94. Khan SA, Emadossadaty S, Ladep NG, et al: Rising trends in cholangiocarcinoma: Is the ICD classification system misleading us? *J Hepatol* 56:848–854, 2012.
95. Shaib YH, Davila JA, McGlynn K, et al: Rising incidence of intrahepatic cholangiocarcinoma in the United States: A true increase? *J Hepatol* 40:472–477, 2004.
96. Carpizo DR, D'Angelica M: Liver resection for metastatic colorectal cancer in the presence of extrahepatic disease. *Lancet Oncol* 10:801–809, 2009.
97. Maithel SK, D'Angelica MI: An update on randomized clinical trials in advanced and metastatic colorectal carcinoma. *Surg Oncol Clin N Am* 19:163–181, 2010.
98. Tomlinson JS, Jarnagin WR, DeMatteo RP, et al: Actual 10-year survival after resection of colorectal liver metastases defines cure. *J Clin Oncol* 25:4575–4580, 2007.

99. Beppu T, Miyamoto Y, Sakamoto Y, et al: Chemotherapy and targeted therapy for patients with initially unresectable colorectal liver metastases, focusing on conversion hepatectomy and long-term survival. *Ann Surg Oncol* 21(Suppl 3):S405–S413, 2014.
100. Smith DD, Schwarz RR, Schwarz RE: Impact of total lymph node count on staging and survival after gastrectomy for gastric cancer: Data from a large US-population database. *J Clin Oncol* 23:7114–7124, 2005.
101. Moulton CA, Gu CS, Law CH, et al: Effect of PET before liver resection on surgical management for colorectal adenocarcinoma metastases: A randomized clinical trial. *JAMA* 311:1863–1869, 2014.
102. Shubert CR, Habermann EB, Truty MJ, et al: Defining perioperative risk after hepatectomy based on diagnosis and extent of resection. *J Gastrointest Surg* 18:1917–1928, 2014.
103. Fong Y, Fortner J, Sun RL, et al: Clinical score for predicting recurrence after hepatic resection for metastatic colorectal cancer: Analysis of 1001 consecutive cases. *Ann Surg* 230:309–318, discussion 318–321, 1999.
104. Muratore A, Ribero D, Zimmitti G, et al: Resection margin and recurrence-free survival after liver resection of colorectal metastases. *Ann Surg Oncol* 17:1324–1329, 2010.
105. Are C, Gonen M, Zazzali K, et al: The impact of margins on outcome after hepatic resection for colorectal metastasis. *Ann Surg* 246:295–300, 2007.
106. Carpizo DR, Are C, Jarnagin W, et al: Liver resection for metastatic colorectal cancer in patients with concurrent extrahepatic disease: Results in 127 patients treated at a single center. *Ann Surg Oncol* 16:2138–2146, 2009.
107. Hwang M, Jayakrishnan TT, Green DE, et al: Systematic review of outcomes of patients undergoing resection for colorectal liver metastases in the setting of extra hepatic disease. *Eur J Cancer* 50:1747–1757, 2014.
108. Portier G, Elias D, Bouche O, et al: Multicenter randomized trial of adjuvant fluorouracil and folinic acid compared with surgery alone after resection of colorectal liver metastases: FFCD ACHBTH AURC 9002 trial. *J Clin Oncol* 24:4976–4982, 2006.
109. Mitry E, Fields AL, Bleiberg H, et al: Adjuvant chemotherapy after potentially curative resection of metastases from colorectal cancer: A pooled analysis of two randomized trials. *J Clin Oncol* 26:4906–4911, 2008.
110. Nordlinger B, Sorbye H, Glimelius B, et al: Perioperative chemotherapy with FOLFOX4 and surgery versus surgery alone for resectable liver metastases from colorectal cancer (EORTC Intergroup trial 40983): A randomised controlled trial. *Lancet* 371:1007–1016, 2008.
111. Nordlinger B, Sorbye H, Glimelius B, et al: Perioperative FOLFOX4 chemotherapy and surgery versus surgery alone for resectable liver metastases from colorectal cancer (EORTC 40983): Long-term results of a randomised, controlled, phase 3 trial. *Lancet Oncol* 14:1208–1215, 2013.
112. Kemeny N, Capanu M, D'Angelica M, et al: Phase I trial of adjuvant hepatic arterial infusion (HAI) with floxuridine (FUDR) and dexamethasone plus systemic oxaliplatin, 5-fluorouracil and leucovorin in patients with resected liver metastases from colorectal cancer. *Ann Oncol* 20:1236–1241, 2009.
113. Kemeny N, Jarnagin W, Gonen M, et al: Phase I/II study of hepatic arterial therapy with floxuridine and dexamethasone in combination with intravenous irinotecan as adjuvant treatment after resection of hepatic metastases from colorectal cancer. *J Clin Oncol* 21:3303–3309, 2003.
114. Kemeny N, Huang Y, Cohen AM, et al: Hepatic arterial infusion of chemotherapy after resection of hepatic metastases from colorectal cancer. *N Engl J Med* 341:2039–2048, 1999.
115. Leung U, Kuk D, D'Angelica MI, et al: Long-term outcomes following microwave ablation for liver malignancies. *Br J Surg* 102:85–91, 2015.
116. Que FG, Sarmiento JM, Nagorney DM: Hepatic surgery for metastatic gastrointestinal neuroendocrine tumors. *Adv Exp Med Biol* 574:43–56, 2006.
117. Mazzaglia PJ, Berber E, Milas M, et al: Laparoscopic radiofrequency ablation of neuroendocrine liver metastases: A 10-year experience evaluating predictors of survival. *Surgery* 142:10–19, 2007.
118. D'Angelica M, Jarnagin W, Dematteo R, et al: Staging laparoscopy for potentially resectable noncolorectal, nonneuroendocrine liver metastases. *Ann Surg Oncol* 9:204–209, 2002.
119. Groeschl RT, Nachmany I, Steel JL, et al: Hepatectomy for noncolorectal non-neuroendocrine metastatic cancer: A multi-institutional analysis. *J Am Coll Surg* 214:769–777, 2012.
120. Mimatsu K, Oida T, Kawasaki A, et al: Long-term outcome of laparoscopic deroofing for symptomatic nonparasitic liver cysts. *Hepatogastroenterology* 56:850–853, 2009.
121. Qiu JG, Wu H, Jiang H, et al: Laparoscopic fenestration vs open fenestration in patients with congenital hepatic cysts: A meta-analysis. *World J Gastroenterol* 17:3359–3365, 2003.
122. Gevers TJ, Drenth JP: Diagnosis and management of polycystic liver disease. *Nat Rev Gastroenterol Hepatol* 10:101–108, 2013.
123. Jarnagin WR, Gonen M, Fong Y, et al: Improvement in perioperative outcome after hepatic resection: Analysis of 1,803 consecutive cases over the past decade. *Ann Surg* 236:397–406, discussion 406–407, 2002.

54 CHAPTER

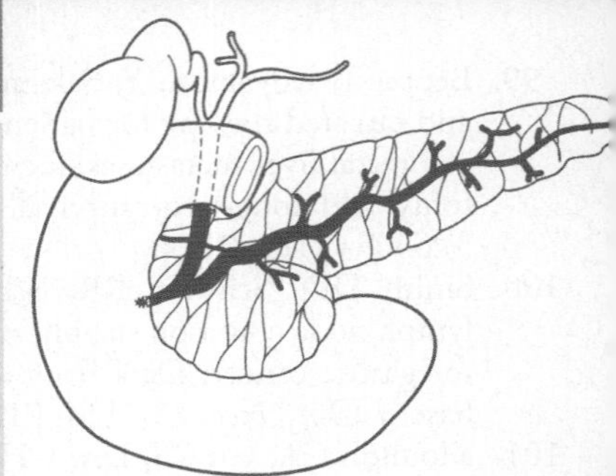

Biliary System

Patrick G. Jackson, Stephen R.T. Evans

OUTLINE

ANATOMY AND PHYSIOLOGY

As anatomic variations in biliary anatomy are common, occurring in up to 30% of patients, understanding of both normal anatomy and the variations is important for the management of patients with biliary disease. The ampulla of Vater contains the distalmost portion of the common bile duct and inserts into the wall of the duodenum. The pancreatic duct also joins the ampulla and may fuse with the bile duct before passing through the wall of the duodenum or within the wall of the duodenum, or it may have a separate orifice within the ampulla (Fig. 54-1). The most inferior portion of the common bile duct is encompassed by the head of the pancreas. Superior to the intrapancreatic portion, the common bile duct is divided into retroduodenal and supraduodenal segments. The insertion of the cystic duct marks the differentiation of the common hepatic duct above and the common bile duct below.

The cystic duct drains the gallbladder, which is divided into the neck, infundibulum with Hartmann pouch, body, and fundus. Roughly the size and shape of a common light bulb, the gallbladder holds 30 to 60 mL of bile as an extrahepatic reservoir. The gallbladder is attached to the inferior surface of the liver and is enveloped by liver for a variable portion of its circumference. Although some gallbladders are almost enveloped by liver parenchyma, others hang on a mesentery, predisposing to volvulus. The attachment of the gallbladder to the liver, known as the gallbladder fossa, identifies the separation of the left and right lobes of the liver (Fig. 54-2). Where the gallbladder attaches to the liver, Glisson capsule does not form, and this common surface provides most of the venous drainage of the gallbladder. The cystic duct drains at an acute angle into the common bile duct and can range from 1 to 5 cm in length. There are a number of anatomic variations in insertion of the cystic duct, including into the right hepatic duct (Fig. 54-3). Within the neck of the gallbladder and cystic ducts lie folds of mucosa oriented in a spiral pattern, known as the spiral valves of Heister, which act to keep gallstones from entering the common bile duct in spite of distention and intraluminal pressure. The dependent portion of Hartmann pouch may overlie the common hepatic or right hepatic ducts, thus placing these structures at risk during the performance of a cholecystectomy.

Above the cystic duct lies the common hepatic duct, draining the left and right hepatic duct systems. The confluence of these structures lies at the hilar plate, which is an extension of Glisson capsule. The absence of any vascular structures overlying the bile ducts at this location allows exposure of the bifurcation by incision of this layer at the base of segment IV, lifting the liver off these structures, known as lowering the hilar plate; this is generally used to expose the proximal extrahepatic biliary tree for resection or reconstruction.

Vascular Anatomy

The segmental anatomy of the liver parenchyma is based on the vascular supply and drainage, and the biliary drainage is described by the corresponding vascular segment. The hepatic parenchyma is divided into lobes, each of which is divided into lobar segments (Fig. 54-4) to define the basic hepatic anatomic resections. The left lobe is composed of medial and lateral segments. The right lobe is divided into posterior and anterior segments. Alternatively, the hepatic parenchyma can be divided into segments based on the specific hepatic venous drainage and portal inflow, allowing a more precise description of anatomic pathology as described by Couinaud.[1] The three hepatic veins divide the liver into four separate sectors. Each sector is then subdivided by the insertion of the portal vein, resulting in eight segments. In this classification system, the liver is composed of eight segments. Segment I refers to the caudate lobe. The left lobe of the liver, supplied by the left portal vein, constitutes segments II through IV. The left lobe is further subdivided by the falciform ligament, which separates segments II and III, also known as the left lateral segment, from segment IV. Within the left lateral segment, segment II lies superior to the insertion of the portal vein and segment III lies inferior to it. Segment IV is similarly divided into segment IVA above and segment IVB below the portal vein insertion. The right portal vein supplies the right lobe of the liver and divides it into the posterior and anterior sectors. Each sector is then subdivided on the basis of its relative location compared with the portal vein. Segment V is supplied by the inferior branch of the anterior sector, and

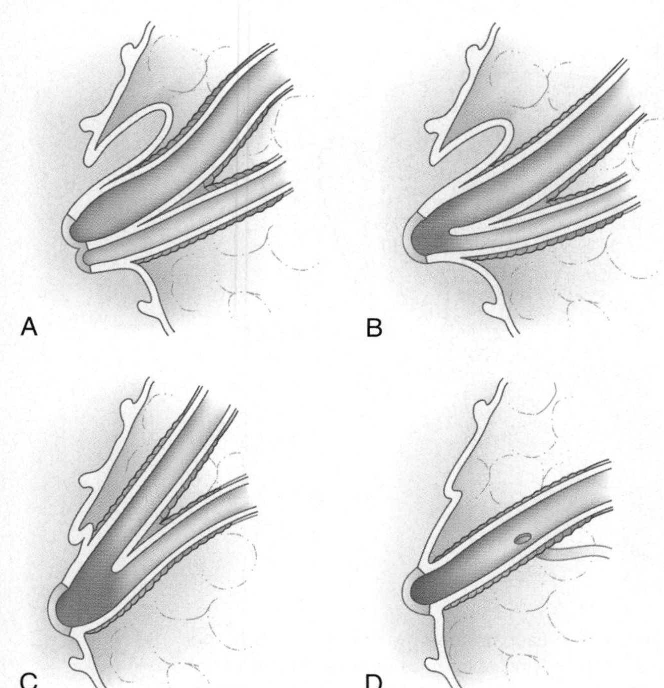

FIGURE 54-1 Patterns of biliary duct–pancreatic duct junction and insertion into the duodenal wall.

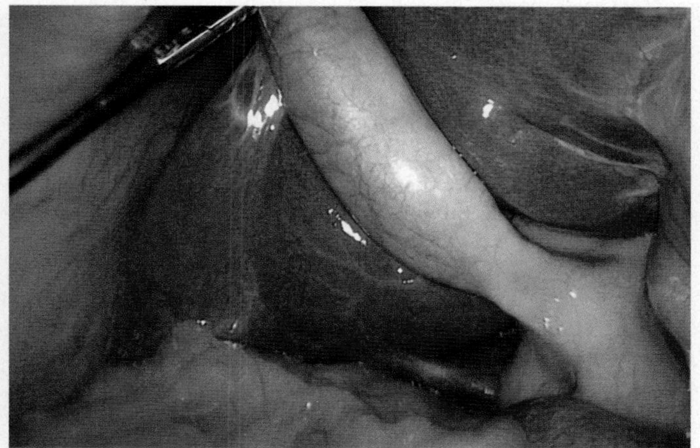

FIGURE 54-2 Laparoscopic photograph of the gallbladder in situ. The gallbladder is being suspended by the fundus to expose the infundibulum and porta hepatis.

segment VIII is supplied by the superior branch. In the posterior sector, segment VI is supplied by the inferior branch and segment VII is supplied by the superior branch. There are three major hepatic veins that drain into the inferior vena cava, in addition to a number of small veins that drain directly from the right lobe. The right hepatic vein constitutes most of the venous drainage from the right lobe and generally lies in the intersegmental fissure between the anterior and posterior sectors of the right lobe. The middle hepatic vein drains the medial segment of the left lobe and a small amount of the medial portions of segments V and VIII. In most cases, the middle hepatic vein fuses with the left hepatic vein that drains the left lateral segment.

As opposed to the hepatic parenchyma, where most perfusion comes from portal venous flow, the entire biliary tree is supplied solely by the arterial anatomy. This anatomic arrangement makes

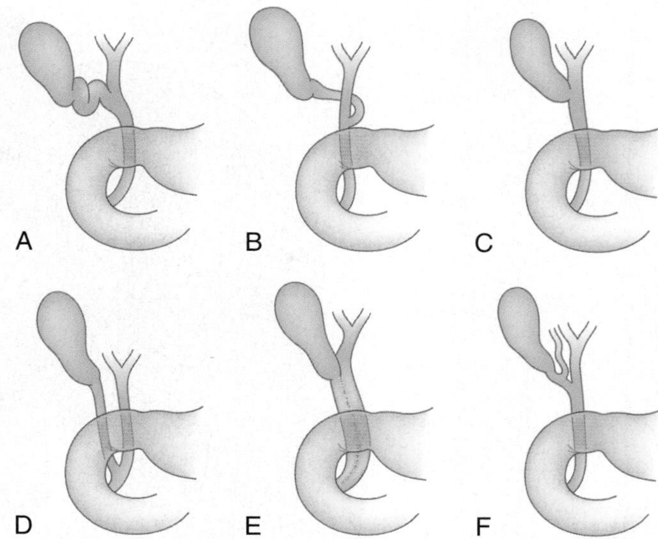

FIGURE 54-3 Variability in cystic duct anatomy. Knowledge of these variations is important to try to avoid inadvertent injury to the biliary tree during cholecystectomy.

it particularly susceptible to ischemic injury at the intrahepatic and extrahepatic levels. The inferior bile duct, below the level of the duodenal bulb, receives its perfusion from tributaries of the posterosuperior pancreaticoduodenal and gastroduodenal arteries. The small branches coalesce to form the two vessels that run along the common bile duct at the 3- and 9-o'clock positions. With close dissection of the areolar tissue surrounding the bile duct, these vessels can be damaged, leaving the bile duct at risk for ischemic injury. The supraduodenal common bile duct, from the duodenal bulb to the cystic duct, and common hepatic ducts receive their blood supply from the right hepatic and cystic arteries. As the proper hepatic artery ascends on the anterior medial side of the porta, it divides into right and left hepatic arteries. In most cases, the right hepatic artery passes posterior to the common hepatic duct to supply the right lobe of the liver. After crossing the duct, the right hepatic artery passes through the triangle of Calot, bordered by the cystic duct, common hepatic duct, and edge of liver. In this triangle, the right hepatic artery gives off the cystic artery to the gallbladder and is at risk for injury during a cholecystectomy. An accessory or replaced right hepatic artery, when present, passes through the portacaval space and ascends to the right lobe along the lateral aspect of the common bile duct. A pulsatile structure on the most lateral aspect of the porta during a Pringle maneuver identifies this anomaly. In addition, it can be noted on computed tomography (CT) as a vessel passing transversely between the portal vein and inferior vena cava behind the head of the pancreas.

The cystic artery normally arises from the right hepatic artery, which can pass posterior or anterior to the common bile duct to supply the gallbladder. Similar to the variability of the cystic duct, the cystic artery may arise from the right hepatic, left hepatic, proper hepatic, common hepatic, gastroduodenal, or superior mesenteric artery. Although variable, the cystic artery generally lies superior to the cystic duct and is usually associated with a lymph node, known as Calot node (Fig. 54-5). Because this node provides some of the lymphatic drainage of the gallbladder, it can be enlarged in the setting of gallbladder disease, whether it is inflammatory or neoplastic.

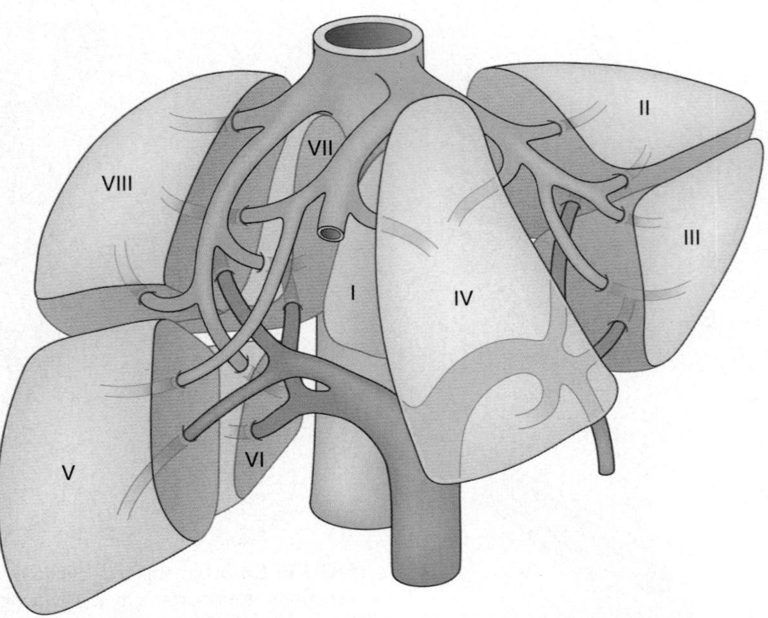

FIGURE 54-4 Couinaud Segmental Anatomy. Segment I is the caudate lobe. Segments II and III are supplied by the lateral branch of the left portal vein, with segment II lying above the passage of the portal vein and segment III below it. Segment IV is supplied by the medial branch of the left portal vein and is further subdivided into IVA above and IVB below the segmental portal vein. Segment V is supplied by the inferior distribution of the anterior branch of the right portal vein, and segment VIII receives flow from the superior distribution of this branch. Similarly, with respect to the posterior branch of the right portal vein, segment VI lies inferior to the portal vein, whereas segment VII lies superior.

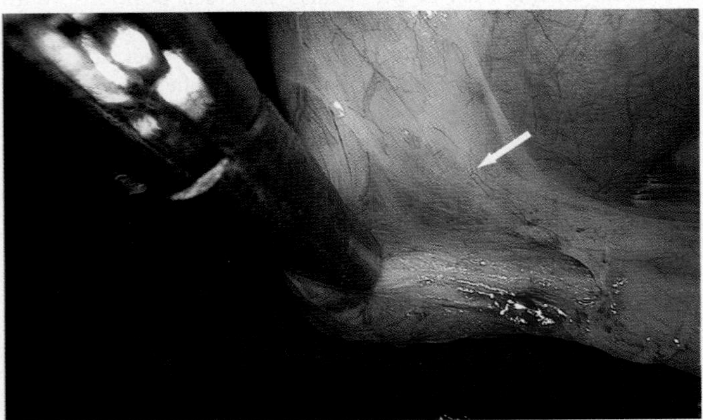

FIGURE 54-5 Operative photograph of Calot node. This node *(arrow)* is useful for identification of the common location of the cystic artery.

Both within the liver and immediately outside the parenchyma, the bile ducts generally lie superior to the corresponding portal veins, which in turn are superior to the arterial supply (Fig. 54-6). Retaining a longer extrahepatic segment before inserting into the liver, the left hepatic duct travels under the edge of segment IV before slipping superior and posterior to the left portal vein. During this transverse portion, it can receive a few subsegmental branches from segment IV. The left duct drains segments II, III, and IV, with the most distal branch draining segment IVA. Further superolateral, the ducts draining segment IVB arise, and further up the left duct are the ducts for segments II and III. These fused ducts can generally be found just posterior and lateral to the umbilical recess. The caudate lobe drains through smaller ducts that enter the right and left hepatic duct systems. The drainage of the right duct system includes segments V, VI, VII, and VIII and is substantially shorter than the left duct, bifurcating almost immediately. The fusion of two sectoral ducts, posterior and anterior, creates this short right hepatic duct. The anterior sectoral duct runs in a vertical direction to drain segments V and VIII, whereas the posterior sectoral duct follows a horizontal course to drain segments VI and VII.

Physiology

Bile secretion from the liver serves two opposing functions, namely, excretion of toxins and metabolites from the liver and absorption of nutrients from the intestinal tract. Bile is secreted into bile canaliculi, which encircle each hepatocyte. Within the hepatic lobule, these canaliculi coalesce to form small bile ducts, eventually entering a portal triad. Four to six portal triads combine to create a hepatic lobule, the smallest functional unit of the liver, identified by its central terminal hepatic venule. On the opposite aspect from the canalicular surface of the hepatocyte lies the sinusoidal surface, which contacts the space of Disse. In this contact area, the hepatocyte is responsible for the absorption of circulating components of bile, an important step in the enterohepatic circulation of bile. Once the bile components are absorbed and secreted into the bile canaliculi, the tight junctions in the biliary tree keep these components within the bile secretory pathway. The secretion of bile components into the biliary tree is a major stimulus to bile flow, and the volume of bile flow is an osmotic process. Because bile salts combine to form spherical pockets, known as micelles, the salts themselves provide no osmotic activity. Instead, the cations that are secreted into the biliary tree along with the bile salt anion provide the osmotic load to draw water into the duct and to increase flow to keep bile electrochemically neutral. For this reason, bile maintains an osmolality approximately comparable to that of plasma.

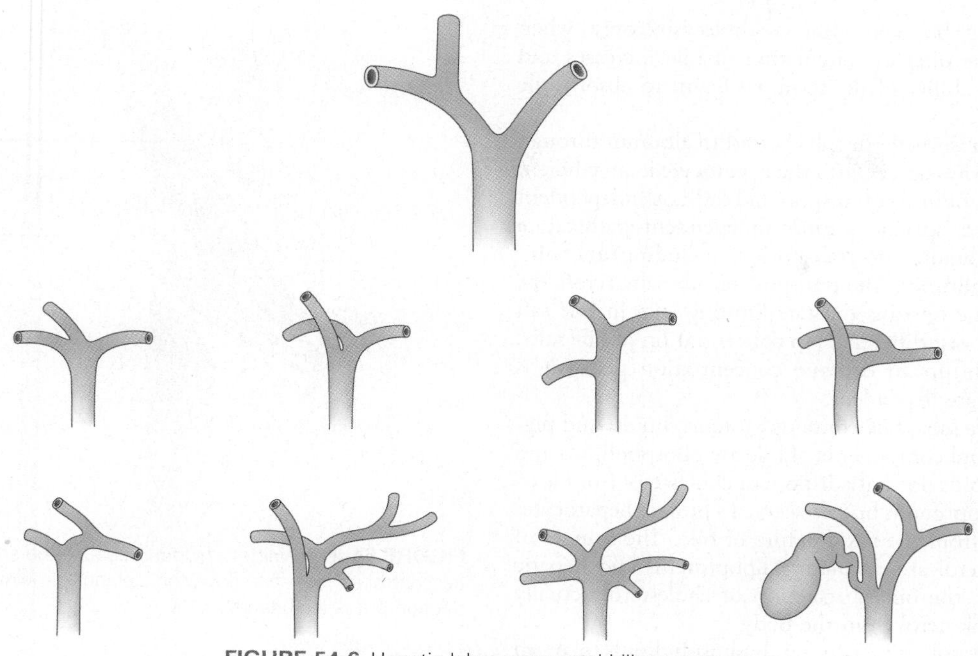

FIGURE 54-6 Hepatic lobar segmental biliary anatomy.

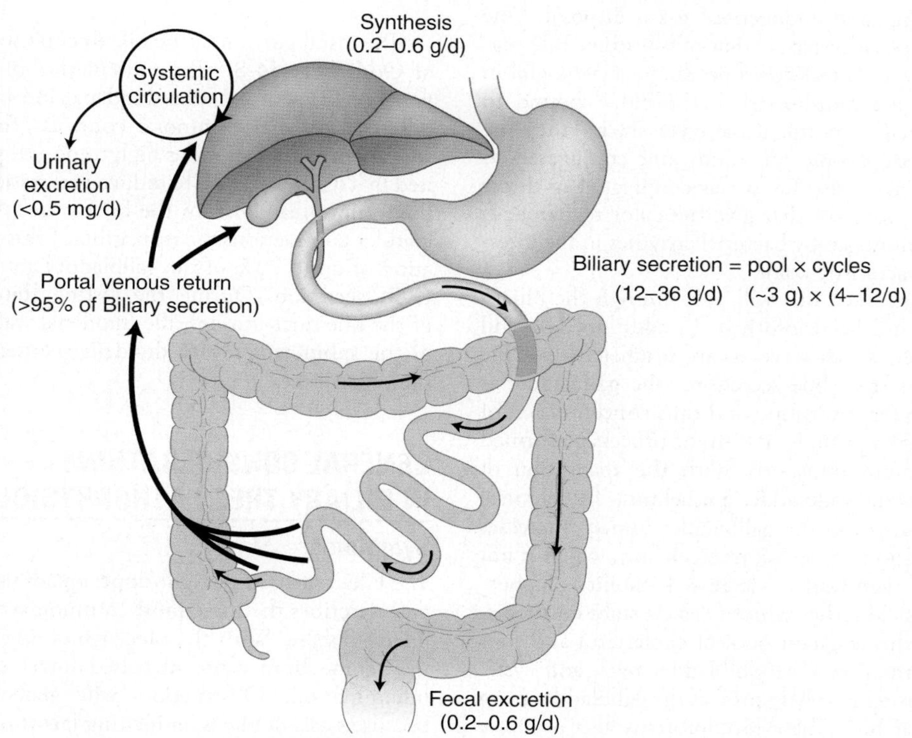

FIGURE 54-7 Enterohepatic circulation.

Although a small amount of bile flow is bile salt independent, serving to expel toxins and metabolites from the body, much of the flow is dependent on neural, humoral, and chemical stimuli. Vagal activity induces bile secretion, as does the gastrointestinal hormone secretin. Cholecystokinin (CCK), secreted by the intestinal mucosa, serves to induce biliary tree secretion and gallbladder wall contraction, thereby augmenting excretion of bile into the intestines.

Bile salts, such as cholic acid and deoxycholic acid, are originally created from cholesterol and secreted into bile canaliculi as cholic acid and its metabolite, deoxycholic acid. The liver actually makes only a small amount of the total bile salt pool used on a daily basis because most bile salts are recycled after use in the intestinal lumen, known as the enterohepatic circulation (Fig. 54-7). After passage into the intestinal tract and reabsorption by the terminal ileum, bile acids are transported back to the liver for recycling bound to albumin. Less than 5% of bile salts are lost each day in the stool. When sufficient quantities of bile salts reach the colonic lumen, the powerful detergent activity of the bile salts can cause inflammation and diarrhea.

This can sometimes be seen after a cholecystectomy when the speed of the enterohepatic circulation of bile increases and may overwhelm the ability of the terminal ileum to absorb bile salts.

The passage of reabsorbed bile salts bound to albumin through the space of Disse allows uptake into the hepatocyte in an efficient process that involves sodium cotransport and sodium-independent pathways. In the less specific sodium-independent pathway, a number of organic anions are transported, including unconjugated and indirect bilirubin. The transport of bile salts across the canalicular membrane remains the rate-limiting step in bile salt excretion. Given the vast differences in concentration of bile salts, the transport of bile up an extreme concentration gradient is adenosine triphosphate dependent.

In addition to bile salts, bile contains proteins, lipids, and pigments. The major lipid components of bile are phospholipids and cholesterol. These lipids not only dispose of cholesterol from low- and high-density lipoproteins but also serve to protect hepatocytes and cholangiocytes from the toxic nature of bile. The sources of most biliary cholesterol are circulating lipoproteins and hepatic synthesis. Therefore, the biliary secretion of cholesterol actually serves to excrete cholesterol from the body.

Although cholesterol, bile salts, and phospholipids play an important role in nutritional homeostasis, bile also serves as a major route of exogenous and endogenous toxin disposal. One such example of the disposal system is that of bilirubin. Bile pigments, such as bilirubin, are breakdown products of hemoglobin and myoglobin. These are transported in the blood bound to albumin and transported into the hepatocyte. Here, they are transferred into the endoplasmic reticulum and conjugated to form bilirubin glucuronides, also known as conjugated or direct bilirubin. It is the bile pigments that give the color to bile and, when converted to urobilinogen by bacterial enzymes in the intestines, give stool its characteristic color.

In the fasting state, secreted bile will pass through the biliary tree into the intestine and be reabsorbed. In addition, bile will collect in the gallbladder, which serves as an extrahepatic storage site of secreted bile. To store bile secretions, the gallbladder is extremely efficient in water absorption and thus concentration of bile components. This absorption is an osmotic process performed through the active sodium transport. With the absorption of sodium and water across the gallbladder epithelium, the chemical composition of bile changes in the gallbladder lumen. Increases in cholesterol concentration, in addition to calcium, which is not as efficiently absorbed, then lead to decreased stability of phospholipid cholesterol vesicles. The reduced vesicle stability predisposes to nucleation of this stagnant pool of cholesterol and thus to cholesterol stone formation. The gallbladder neck and cystic duct also secrete glycoproteins to help protect the gallbladder from the detergent activity of bile. These glycoproteins also promote cholesterol crystallization.

The gallbladder fills through a retrograde mechanism. With an increase in the tonic activity of the sphincter of Oddi in the fasting state, pressure increases in the common bile duct. This increased pressure allows filling of the lower intraluminal pressure gallbladder, which is capable of storing up to 600 mL of the daily production of bile. The passage of fat, protein, and acid into the duodenum induces CCK secretion from duodenal epithelial cells. CCK, as its name suggests, then causes gallbladder contraction, with intraluminal pressures up to 300 mm Hg. Vagal activity also induces gallbladder emptying but is a less powerful stimulus to gallbladder contraction than CCK.

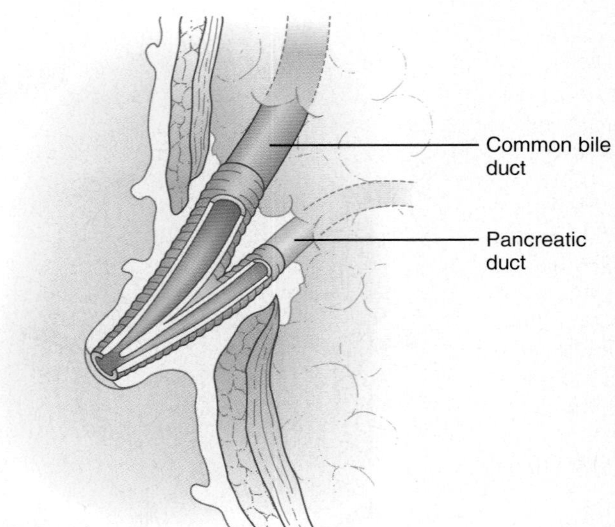

FIGURE 54-8 Sphincter of Oddi. Because the sphincter is responsible for control of most bile flow, this sphincter maintains a high tonic contraction but is inhibited by CCK.

The distal portion of the bile duct passes through the sphincter of Oddi (Fig. 54-8). The musculature of this sphincter is independent from that of the duodenal intestinal wall and responds differently to neurohumoral controls. This muscular sphincter, which normally maintains high tonic and phasic activity, is inhibited by CCK. With CCK-induced relaxation of the sphincter, bile flows more readily from the biliary tree. Coordinated with gallbladder contraction, the relaxation of this sphincter allows evacuation of up to 70% of the gallbladder contents within 2 hours of CCK secretion. During the fasting state, the oblique passage of the bile duct through the duodenal wall and the tonic activity of the sphincter prevent duodenal contents from refluxing into the biliary tree.

GENERAL CONSIDERATIONS IN BILIARY TREE PATHOPHYSIOLOGY

Symptoms

The Charcot triad of right upper quadrant pain, fever, and jaundice describes the three most common symptoms associated with biliary disease. With the blockage of any tubular structure, pain may come from acute increased intraluminal pressure or from inflammation. Obstruction will generally precede infection because stasis of bile is an inciting factor of biliary infection along with sufficient quantity of infectious inoculum in a susceptible host.

Pain

Postprandial abdominal pain is generally termed biliary colic, actually a misnomer because the pattern of pain is not colicky in nature. Because the nerve fibers to the gallbladder originate in the celiac axis, this pain can be epigastric in origin or may locate in the right upper quadrant as the inflammatory process affects the parietal peritoneum. As a meal containing fat or protein enters the duodenum, CCK is released, causing contraction of the gallbladder and increases in bile secretion. When the gallbladder lumen cannot fully empty because of a stone in the gallbladder neck, visceral pain fibers are activated, causing pain in the epigastrium or right upper quadrant. The same luminal obstruction of biliary colic but associated with sufficient stasis, pressure, and bacterial inoculum creates infection and thereby inflammation, therefore progressing to acute cholecystitis. With this infection and inflammation, the right upper quadrant pain of biliary colic will be accompanied by tenderness noted on palpation of the right upper quadrant. Specifically, the voluntary cessation of respiration when the examiner exerts constant pressure under the right costal margin, known as a Murphy sign, suggests inflammation of the visceral and parietal peritoneal surfaces and can be seen in diseases such as acute cholecystitis and hepatitis. Alternatively, biliary colic in the absence of infection and inflammation is not associated with any reproducible physical examination finding or systemic symptom.

Fever

Whereas biliary colic does not produce systemic manifestations, infection or inflammation in the gallbladder or biliary tree will usually cause fever. It can be seen in a number of inflammatory diseases, but fever associated with right upper quadrant pain is a hallmark of an infectious process in the biliary tree. With immediate and direct access to the metabolically active hepatic parenchyma, infection of the gallbladder and biliary tree induces cytokine secretion and thereby direct systemic manifestations.

Jaundice

Jaundice, caused by elevation of the serum bilirubin level, can be demonstrated in the sclera, the frenulum of the tongue, or the skin. Serum bilirubin levels above 2.5 mg/dL are necessary to detect scleral icterus routinely, and levels above 5 mg/dL will be manifested as cutaneous jaundice. Failure to excrete bile from the liver into the intestines is a prerequisite of jaundice. Therefore, although both are associated with fever and pain, acute cholecystitis does not cause the jaundice seen in infection of the biliary tree, known as ascending cholangitis. The constellation of fever, right upper quadrant pain, and jaundice, known as Charcot triad, suggests blockage of the biliary secretion from the liver, not just the gallbladder. With the addition of hypotension and altered mental status, known as Reynolds pentad, patients will demonstrate the systemic manifestations of shock from biliary origin. Jaundice is generally divided into surgical, from obstruction, and medical, from a hepatocellular process.

Laboratory Tests

Although termed liver function tests, the routine hepatic panel for most laboratories tests a number of aspects of metabolic and hepatic activity. The tests most useful for evaluation of biliary physiology include determination of levels of bilirubin and alkaline phosphatase, seen in any cholestatic process, and serum transaminases, suggesting evidence of hepatocellular injury. Bilirubin can be subdivided into the conjugated and unconjugated forms, thereby allowing delineation of cause based on cellular location of derangement. In other words, hyperbilirubinemia may be caused by increased synthesis of bilirubin, impaired hepatocyte uptake of unconjugated bilirubin, decreased intracellular conjugation, reduced intracellular transport and excretion of conjugated bilirubin, or obstruction of the biliary tree. Although this is an oversimplification of a complex process, derangements up to and including conjugation will be manifested as elevated unconjugated bilirubin levels.

Imaging Studies

Plain Films

Plain radiographs are of limited use in the overall evaluation of biliary tree disease. Gallstones are not regularly seen by plain films, and even when they are seen, it rarely changes therapy. Therefore, the role of plain radiographs in the evaluation of possible biliary disease is limited to exclusion of other diagnoses, such as a duodenal ulcer with free air, small bowel obstruction, or right lower lobe pneumonia causing right upper quadrant pain.

Ultrasound

Transabdominal ultrasound is a sensitive, inexpensive, reliable, and reproducible test to evaluate most of the biliary tree, being able to separate patients with medical jaundice, in which the source of hyperbilirubinemia is from hemoglobin breakdown through the process of conjugation, from those with surgical jaundice, in which the hyperbilirubinemia occurs from a blockage of excretion. Therefore, this modality is seen as the study of choice for the initial evaluation of jaundice or symptoms of biliary disease. The finding of a dilated common bile duct in the setting of jaundice suggests an obstruction of the duct from stones, usually associated with pain, or from a tumor, which is commonly painless (Fig. 54-9). Gallbladder diseases are regularly diagnosed by ultrasound because the superficial location of the gallbladder with no overlying bowel gas enables its evaluation by sound waves. Ultrasound has a high specificity and sensitivity for cholelithiasis, or gallstones. The density of gallstones allows crisp reverberation of the sound wave, showing an echogenic focus with a characteristic shadowing behind the stone (Fig. 54-10). Most gallstones, unless impacted, will move with positional changes in the patient. This feature allows their differentiation from gallbladder polyps, which are fixed, and from sludge, which will move more slowly and does not have the sharp echogenic pattern of gallstones. Pathologic changes seen in many gallbladder diseases can be identified by ultrasound. For example, the gallbladder wall thickening and pericholecystic fluid seen in cholecystitis are visible by ultrasound (Fig. 54-11). Porcelain gallbladder, with its calcified wall, will appear as a curvilinear echogenic focus along the entire gallbladder wall, with posterior shadowing (Fig. 54-12). In addition

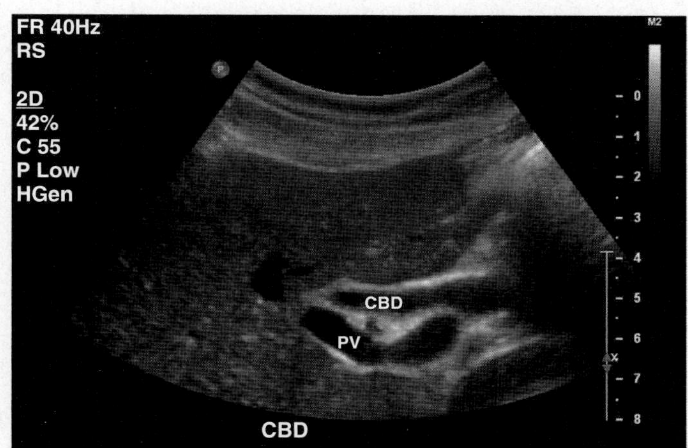

FIGURE 54-9 Ultrasound image of dilated biliary tree. The common bile duct (CBD) is dilated. As it travels parallel to the portal vein (PV), it is easy to identify. The depiction of the parallel stripes of duct and vein helps ensure that the common duct diameter is not overestimated by a tangential view, which would artificially increase the anteroposterior diameter.

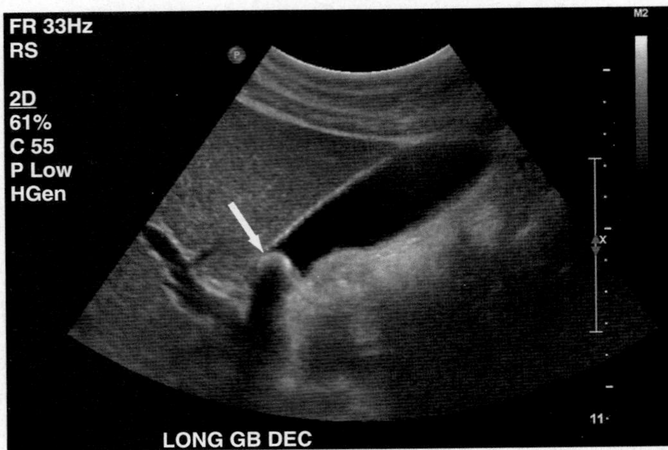

FIGURE 54-10 Ultrasound image of a gallstone in the gallbladder neck. The sharp echogenic wall of the gallstone *(arrow)*, with the characteristic posterior shadowing stripe under the stone, helps differentiate it from other intraluminal findings.

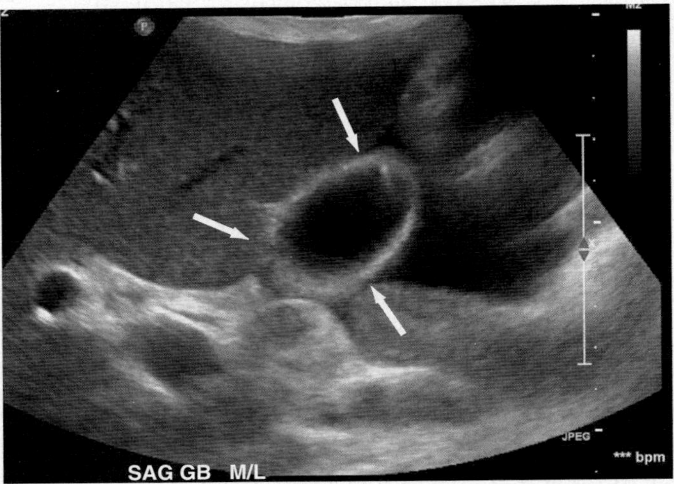

FIGURE 54-11 Ultrasound image with acute cholecystitis and thickened gallbladder wall *(arrows)*.

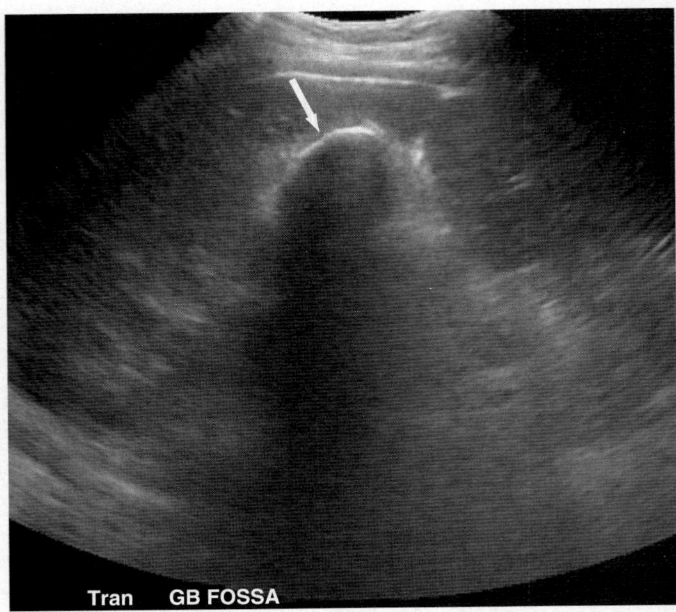

FIGURE 54-12 Ultrasound image of porcelain gallbladder. The curvilinear sharp echogenic focus *(arrow)* combined with substantial posterior shadowing helps confirm this diagnosis.

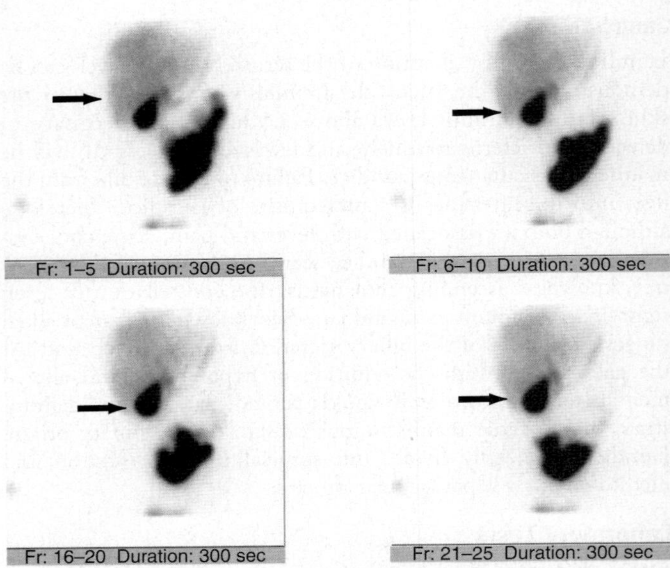

FIGURE 54-13 HIDA scan showing filling of the gallbladder. With gallbladder filling *(arrows)*, the diagnosis of acute cholecystitis is effectively eliminated.

to division of medical versus surgical jaundice, ultrasound can sometimes identify the cause of obstructive jaundice, showing common bile duct stones or even cholangiocarcinoma.

Hepatic Iminodiacetic Acid Scan

Although incapable of providing any precise anatomic delineation, biliary scintigraphy, also known as a hepatic iminodiacetic acid (HIDA) scan, can be used to evaluate the physiologic secretion of bile. The injection of an iminodiacetic acid, which is processed in the liver and secreted with bile, allows identification of bile flow. Therefore, the failure to fill the gallbladder 2 hours after injection demonstrates obstruction of the cystic duct, as seen in acute cholecystitis (Figs. 54-13 and 54-14). In addition, the scan will identify obstruction of the biliary tree and bile leaks, which may be useful in the postoperative setting. HIDA scans can also be used to determine gallbladder function because the injection of CCK during a scan will document physiologic ejection of the gallbladder. This may be useful in patients with biliary tract pain but without stones because some patients have pain from impaired emptying, known as biliary dyskinesia. As a nuclear medicine test, the test demonstrates physiologic flow but does not provide fine anatomic detail, nor can it identify gallstones.

Computed Tomography

Although ultrasound is clearly the first test of choice for delineation of biliary disease, CT provides superior anatomic information and therefore is indicated when more anatomic delineation is required. Because most gallstones are radiographically isodense to bile, many will be indistinguishable from bile. However, because ultrasound is operator dependent and provides no anatomic reconstruction of the biliary tree, CT can be used to

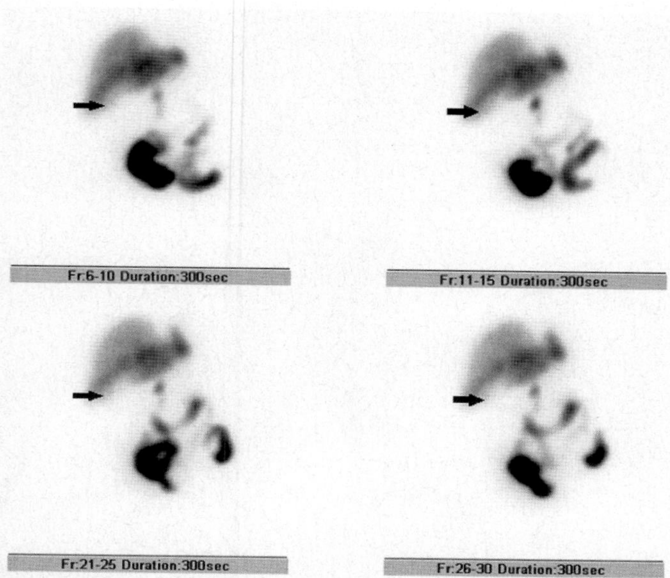

FIGURE 54-14 HIDA scan showing nonfilling of the gallbladder. With no filling of the gallbladder *(arrows)* even on delayed images, HIDA confirms occlusion of the cystic duct, the characteristic feature of acute cholecystitis.

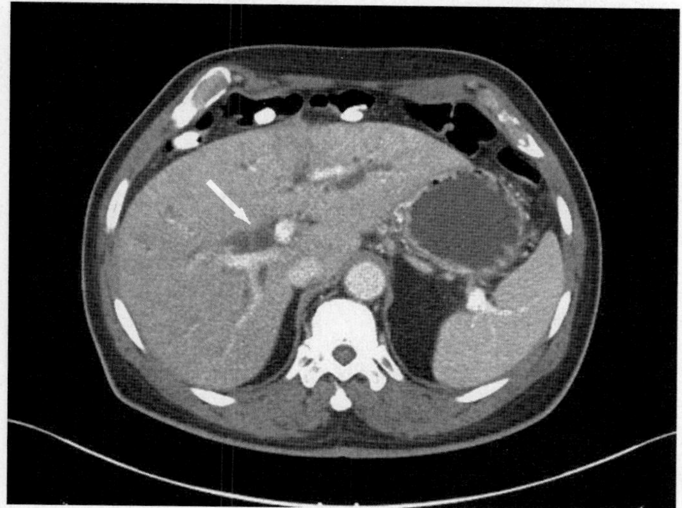

FIGURE 54-15 CT scan showing dilated biliary tree *(arrow)* at the portal confluence. This dilation continued down to the head of the pancreas.

identify the cause and site of biliary obstruction (Fig. 54-15). When it is performed for the evaluation of hepatic or pancreatic parenchyma or possible neoplastic processes, CT is invaluable in preoperative planning, and the use of arterial phase, portal venous phase, and delayed phase imaging, known as a triple-phase CT, has essentially replaced diagnostic angiography of the liver.

Magnetic Resonance Imaging and Magnetic Resonance Cholangiopancreatography

Magnetic resonance imaging uses the water in bile to delineate the biliary tree and thus provides superior anatomic definition of the intrahepatic and extrahepatic biliary tree and pancreas. Although management of most patients with biliary disease

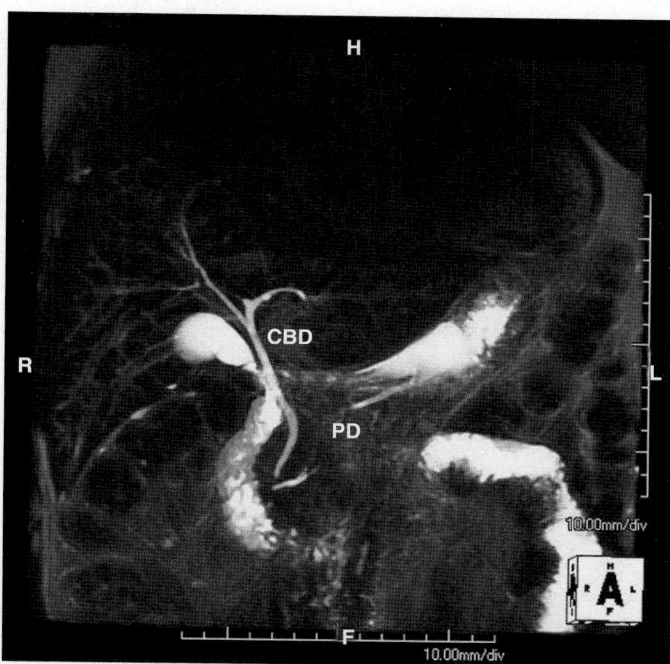

FIGURE 54-16 Normal MRCP image. Note the normal common bile duct (CBD) and pancreatic duct (PD).

does not require the fine detail of anatomic evaluation shown by cross-sectional imaging, magnetic resonance imaging is noninvasive, requires no radiation exposure, and can prove extremely useful in planning resection of biliary or pancreatic neoplasms or management of complex biliary disease. By use of the water content of bile, a cholangiopancreatogram can be created (Fig. 54-16), which makes it an excellent modality for cross-sectional imaging of the biliary tree.

Endoscopic Retrograde Cholangiopancreatography

Endoscopic retrograde cholangiopancreatography (ERCP) is an invasive test using endoscopy and fluoroscopy to inject contrast material through the ampulla to image the biliary tree (Fig. 54-17). Although it does carry a complication rate of up to 10%, its usefulness lies in its ability to diagnose and to treat many diseases of the biliary tree. For patients with malignant obstruction, ERCP can be used to provide tissue samples for diagnosis while also decompressing an obstruction, but it does not stage disease accurately. Many benign diseases, such as choledocholithiasis, can be easily treated by endoscopic means. ERCP has also proven extremely useful in the diagnosis and treatment of complications of biliary surgery.

Percutaneous Transhepatic Cholangiography

Interventional radiologic techniques can be used in the evaluation of biliary anatomy. Similar to ERCP, percutaneous transhepatic cholangiography (PTC) is an invasive procedure used to evaluate the biliary tree. A needle is passed directly into the liver to access one of the biliary radicals, and the tract is then used for insertion of transhepatic catheters. Useful for patients with intrahepatic biliary disease or in whom ERCP is not technically feasible, PTC can decompress biliary obstruction, stent obstructions nonoperatively, and provide anatomic information for biliary reconstruction (Fig. 54-18).

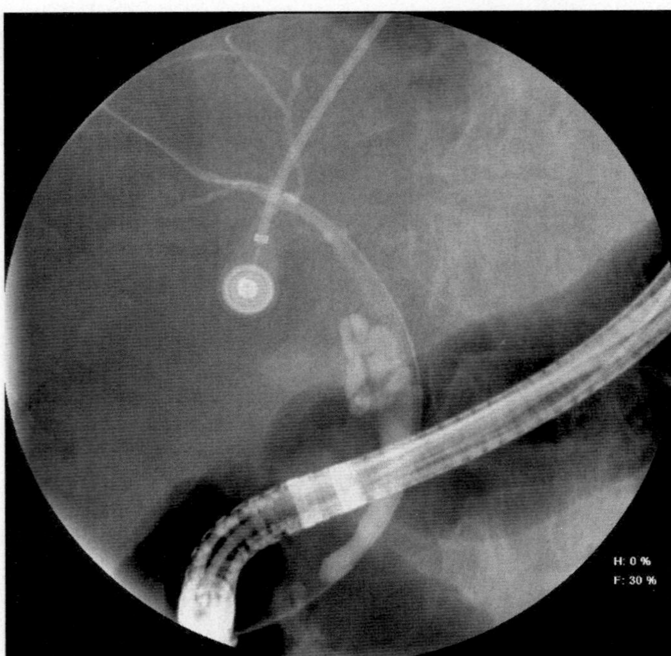

FIGURE 54-17 Normal ERCP image.

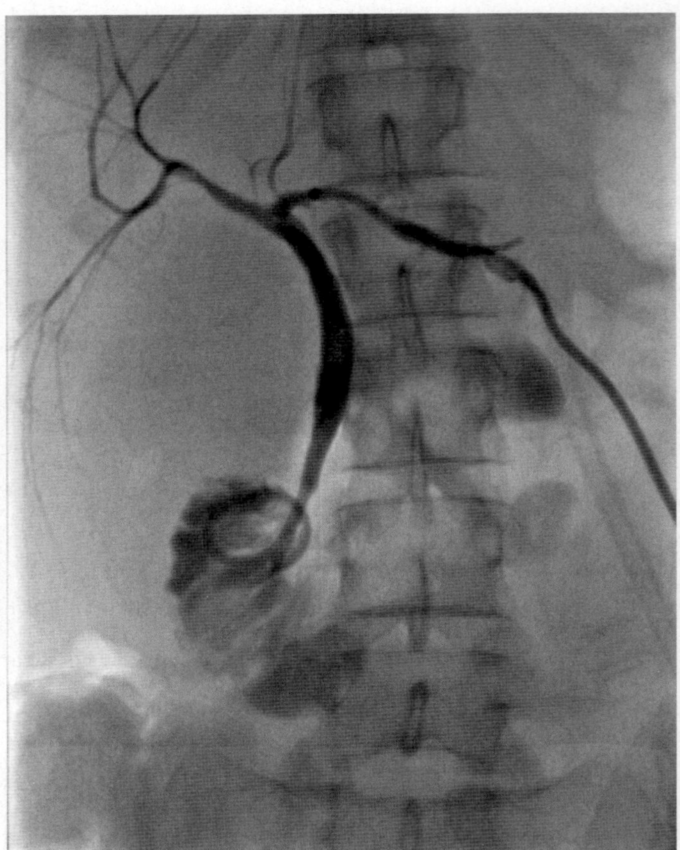

FIGURE 54-18 PTC image of hepatic biliary anatomy.

Intraoperative Cholangiography

Another imaging tool for the diagnosis of biliary tract abnormalities is intraoperative cholangiography. With the injection catheter inserted through the cystic duct during a cholecystectomy or through another point in the biliary tree, intraoperative cholangiography can help delineate anomalous biliary anatomy, identify choledocholithiasis, or guide biliary reconstruction. Some surgeons advocate routine cholangiography during cholecystectomy. Advocates for routine cholangiography note that common duct injuries can be identified and managed immediately when cholangiography is used routinely. However, because it adds operative time and fluoroscopic exposure to the operation, many surgeons use intraoperative cholangiography selectively during the performance of a cholecystectomy. Although debated, the routine use of intraoperative cholangiography does not reduce significantly the incidence of injury to the biliary tree during laparoscopic cholecystectomy. Indications for the selective use of cholangiography include pain on the day of operation, abnormal hepatic function panel, anomalous or confusing biliary anatomy, and alteration in anatomy that precludes the ability to perform ERCP after cholecystectomy, such as Roux-en-Y gastric bypass, dilated biliary tree, or any preoperative suspicion of choledocholithiasis (Box 54-1).

BOX 54-1 Indications for Selective Cholangiography

Pain at time of operation
Abnormal hepatic function panel
Anomalous or confusing biliary anatomy
Inability to perform postoperative ERCP
Dilated biliary tree
Any suspicion of choledocholithiasis

Endoscopic Ultrasound

Although of limited use in the evaluation of gallbladder disease or intrahepatic disease of the biliary tree, endoscopic ultrasound is valuable in the assessment of distal common bile duct and ampulla. With the close apposition of the distal common bile duct and pancreas to the duodenum, sound waves generated by endoscopic ultrasound provide detailed evaluation of the bile duct and ampulla; this has proved most useful in assessing tumors for invasion into vascular structures. Echoendoscopes are subdivided into those that scan perpendicular to the long axis of the endoscope, known as radial echoendoscopes, and those that scan parallel, known as linear echoendoscopes. Radial echoendoscopes are most useful for providing a tomographic evaluation, whereas linear echoendoscopes can guide interventions such as needle biopsies under real-time ultrasound guidance (Fig. 54-19).

Fluorodeoxyglucose Positron Emission Tomography

Fluorodeoxyglucose positron emission tomography (FDG PET) exploits the metabolic difference between a highly metabolically active tissue, such as a neoplasm, and normal tissue. With the injection of a radiolabeled glucose molecule, FDG PET scans can differentiate benign and malignant lesions, detect recurrence, and identify metastatic disease. Unfortunately, FDG PET is incapable of demonstrating carcinomatosis and, given the high metabolism of the immune system, is of limited value in the setting of infection or inflammation.

Bacteriology

The biliary tree inserts into the duodenum and therefore cannot be considered truly sterile. Through a low bacterial load, and with

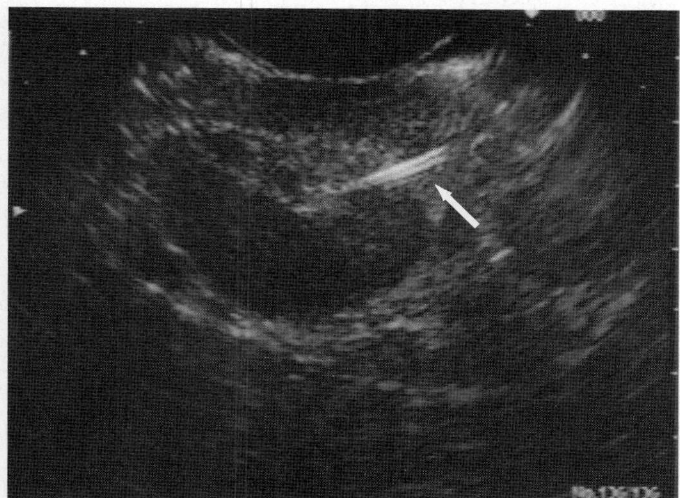

FIGURE 54-19 Linear endoscopic ultrasound with needle *(arrow)* biopsy of a lymph node.

the flow of bile, infection in the absence of obstruction is rare. However, with the presence of stones or obstruction, the likelihood of bacterial infection increases. The most common types of bacteria found in biliary infections are Enterobacteriaceae, such as *Escherichia coli, Klebsiella,* and *Enterobacter,* followed by *Enterococcus* spp.

Prophylactic antibiotics should be used in most patients undergoing interventions in the biliary tree, such as ERCP or PTC. To cover the most common bacterial species, a first- or second-generation cephalosporin or fluoroquinolone should suffice. For those undergoing elective laparoscopic cholecystectomy for biliary colic, no antibiotic prophylaxis is necessary. However, antibiotics should be used for any patient with suspected or documented infection of the biliary tree, such as acute cholecystitis or ascending cholangitis, and should be chosen to cover gram-negative bacteria and anaerobes.

BENIGN BILIARY DISEASE

Calculous Biliary Disease

By far, the most common disease state involving the gallbladder and biliary tree is that of cholelithiasis. Because the gallbladder concentrates bile, the concentration of solutes in the gallbladder differs from that in the rest of the biliary tree. This increase in solute concentration combined with stasis in the gallbladder between meals predisposes to stone formation in the gallbladder. Gallstones can be subclassified into two major subtypes, depending on the principal solute that precipitates into a stone. More than 70% of gallstones in America are formed by precipitation of cholesterol and calcium, with pure cholesterol stones accounting for only a small (<10%) portion. Pigment stones, further subclassified as black or brown stones, are caused by precipitation of concentrated bile pigments, the breakdown products of hemoglobin. Four major factors explain most gallstone formation: supersaturation of secreted bile, concentration of bile in the gallbladder, crystal nucleation, and gallbladder dysmotility. High concentrations of cholesterol and lipid in bile secretion from the liver constitute one predisposing condition to cholesterol stone formation, whereas increased hemoglobin processing is seen in most patients with pigment stones. Once in the gallbladder, bile is concentrated further through the absorption of water and sodium,

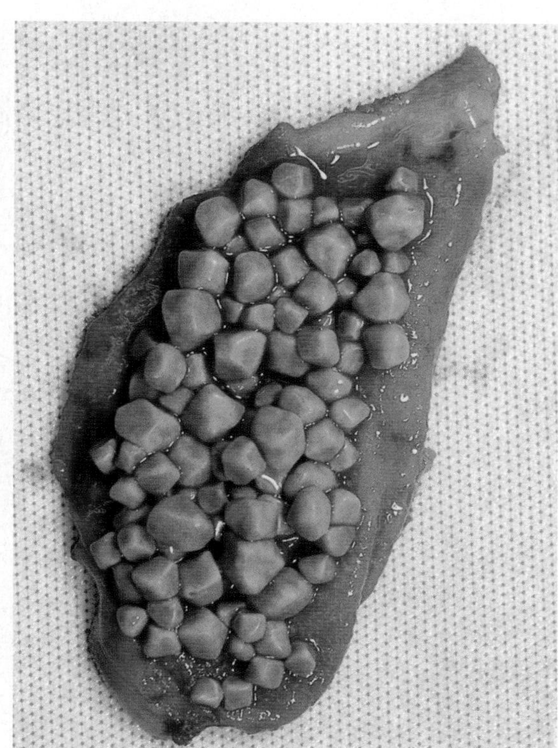

FIGURE 54-20 Gallbladder with characteristic yellow cholesterol stones.

increasing the concentrations of the bile solutes and calcium. Bile salts act to solubilize cholesterol. With respect to cholesterol stones (Fig. 54-20), cholesterol precipitates out into crystals when the concentration in the gallbladder vesicles exceeds the solubility of cholesterol (Fig. 54-21).[2] Crystal formation is further accelerated by pronucleating agents, including glycoproteins and immunoglobulins. Finally, abnormal gallbladder motility can increase stasis in the gallbladder, allowing more time for solutes to precipitate in the gallbladder. Therefore, increased stone formation can be seen in conditions associated with impaired gallbladder emptying, such as in prolonged fasting states, with use of total parenteral nutrition, after vagotomy, and with use of somatostatin analogues.

Pigment stones can be divided into black stones, as seen in hemolytic conditions and cirrhosis, and brown stones, which tend to be found in the bile ducts and are thought to be secondary to infection. The difference in color comes from incorporation of cholesterol into the brown stones. Because black pigment stones occur in hemolytic states from concentration of bilirubin, they are found almost exclusively in the gallbladder. Alternatively, brown stones occur within the biliary tree and suggest a disorder of biliary motility and associated bacterial infection.

Natural History

Most gallstones are asymptomatic, often being identified at the time of abdominal imaging for other reasons or during laparotomy. To become symptomatic, the gallstone must obstruct a visceral structure, such as the cystic duct. Biliary colic, caused by temporary blockage of the cystic duct, tends to occur after a meal, in which the secretion of CCK leads to gallbladder contraction. Stones that do not obstruct the cystic duct or pass through the entire biliary tree into the intestines without impaction do not

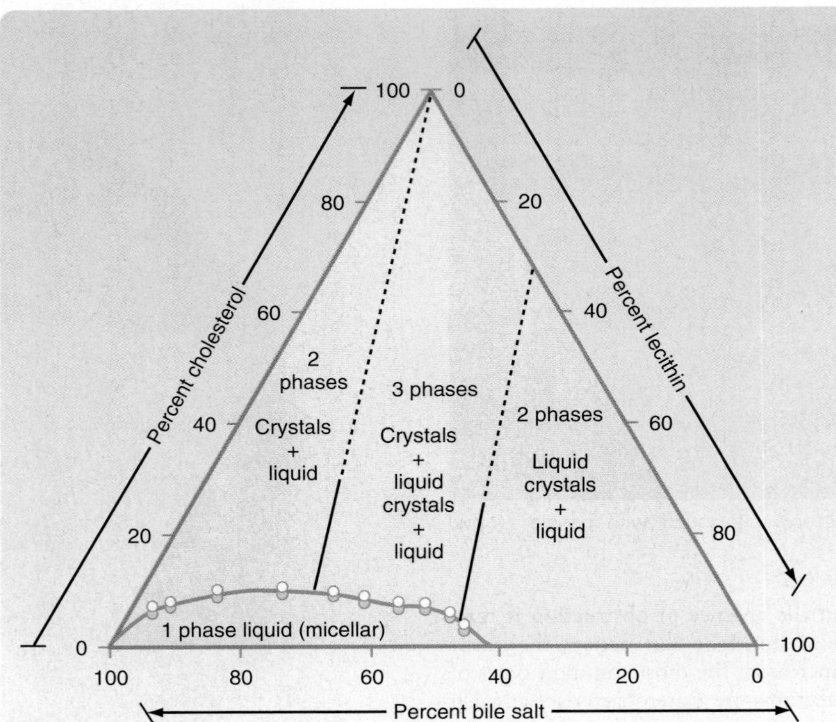

FIGURE 54-21 **Triangle of Solubility.** With the three major components of bile that determine cholesterol solubility and stability, each can be quantified by molar percentage to show a relative ratio to the other two. Cholesterol is completely soluble in only the small area in the left lower corner, where a clear micellar solution exists, below the *closed circles*. Just above this, in the area between the *open* and *closed circles*, cholesterol is supersaturated but stable and thus crystallized only with stasis. In the remainder of the triangle, cholesterol is significantly supersaturated and unstable. In this region, crystals form immediately. (From Admirand WH, Small DM: The physicochemical basis of cholesterol gallstone formation in man. *J Clin Invest* 47:1043–1052, 1968.)

cause symptoms. Only 20% to 30% of patients with asymptomatic stones will develop symptoms within 20 years, and because approximately 1% of patients with asymptomatic stones develop complications of their stones before onset of symptoms, prophylactic cholecystectomy is not warranted in asymptomatic patients.

Certain subsets of patients, however, constitute a higher risk pool, so prophylactic cholecystectomy should be considered. Among these are patients with hemolytic anemias, such as sickle cell anemia. These patients have an extremely high rate of pigment stone formation, and cholecystitis can precipitate a crisis. Patients with a calcified gallbladder wall (known as porcelain gallbladder), those with large (>2.5 cm) gallstones, and those with a long common channel of bile and pancreatic ducts all have a higher risk of gallbladder cancer and should consider cholecystectomy. In addition, patients with asymptomatic gallstones undergoing bariatric surgery may also benefit from cholecystectomy. Not only does rapid weight loss favor stone formation, but also, after gastric bypass, ERCP to remove common bile duct stones in ascending cholangitis is extremely challenging and usually unsuccessful. Finally, because severe infection can be life-threatening in the immunocompromised patient, some transplantation surgeons recommend prophylactic cholecystectomy before receipt of an organ transplant.

Nonoperative Treatment of Cholelithiasis

Medical treatment of gallstones is generally unsuccessful and is used rarely. Options include dissolution with oral bile salt therapy; contact dissolution, which requires cannulation of the gallbladder and infusion of organic solvent; and extracorporeal shock wave lithotripsy. With the dissolution strategies, unacceptable recurrence rates of up to 50% limit their application to the most select group of patients. Extracorporeal shock wave lithotripsy has a lower recurrence rate, approximately 20%, and can be used in patients with single stones 0.5 to 2 cm in size. The widespread use, safety, and efficacy of laparoscopic cholecystectomy have relegated nonoperative therapy to patients for whom general anesthesia presents a prohibitively high risk.

Chronic Cholecystitis

Recurrent attacks of biliary colic, with only temporary occlusion of the cystic duct, can cause inflammation and scarring of the neck of the gallbladder and cystic duct. This process, called chronic cholecystitis, causes fibrosis as histologic evidence of repeated self-limited episodes of inflammation. The diagnosis of chronic cholecystitis lies along a continuum with biliary colic because it results from recurrent attacks. Therefore, the presentation is that of symptomatic cholelithiasis, or biliary colic. Pain occurring after ingestion of a fatty meal, with the attendant increase in CCK secretion in response to duodenal intraluminal fat, is classic for biliary colic, although only 50% of patients will report an association with food. Pain from stones tends to locate in the epigastrium or right upper quadrant and may radiate around to the scapula. These attacks of pain generally last a few hours. Pain lasting longer than 24 hours or associated with fever

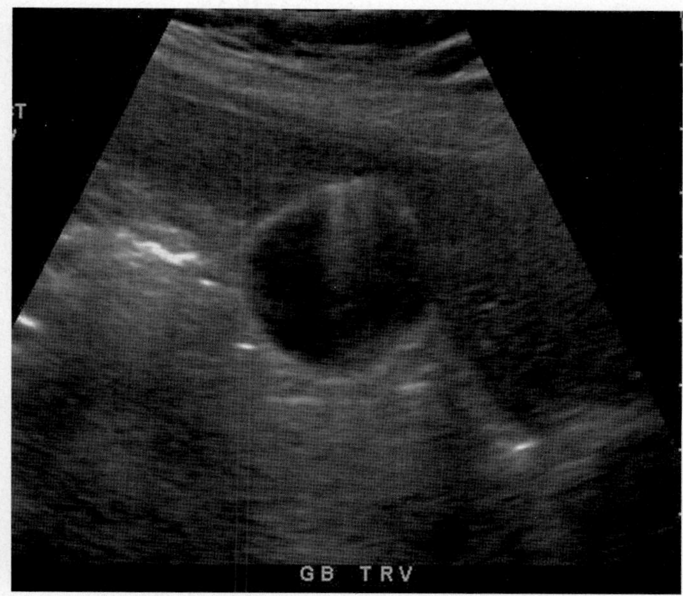

FIGURE 54-22 Ultrasound image of cholesterolosis.

suggests acute cholecystitis. The pain of biliary colic, even in the absence of cholecystitis, may also cause other gastrointestinal symptoms, such as bloating, nausea, or even vomiting.

Symptomatic stones constitute a risk profile different from that of asymptomatic stones, with a higher likelihood of complications. Therefore, symptomatic cholelithiasis is an indication for cholecystectomy. To perform a cholecystectomy for symptomatic stones, one needs presence of symptoms and documentation of stones.

Diagnosis

The diagnosis of symptomatic cholelithiasis, the clinical manifestation of chronic cholecystitis, relies on a history consistent with biliary tract disease. Transabdominal ultrasonography reliably documents the presence of cholelithiasis. Ultrasound can provide other important information, such as common bile duct dilation, gallbladder polyps, porcelain gallbladder, or evidence of hepatic parenchymal processes. Cholesterolosis, or the accumulation of cholesterol found in gallbladder mucosal macrophages, can also be seen (Fig. 54-22). Even in the absence of frank stones, so-called sludge found in the gallbladder on ultrasonography, with appropriate symptoms, is consistent with biliary colic.

Treatment

Patients with sufficient symptoms from gallstones should undergo elective cholecystectomy. Cholecystectomy carries a low-risk profile but is not without complications, so an analysis of risks and benefits is important. Because patients with mild symptoms have a low rate of complications from gallstones (1% to 3%/year), observation and dietary and lifestyle changes are appropriate in this population. Patients with more severe or recurrent symptoms have a higher rate of complications of the disease (7%/year), so elective laparoscopic cholecystectomy is warranted. In more than 90% of patients, cholecystectomy is curative, leaving them symptom free.

Acute Calculous Cholecystitis

The pathophysiologic mechanism of acute cholecystitis is blockage of the cystic duct. When the blockage occurs from an obstructing

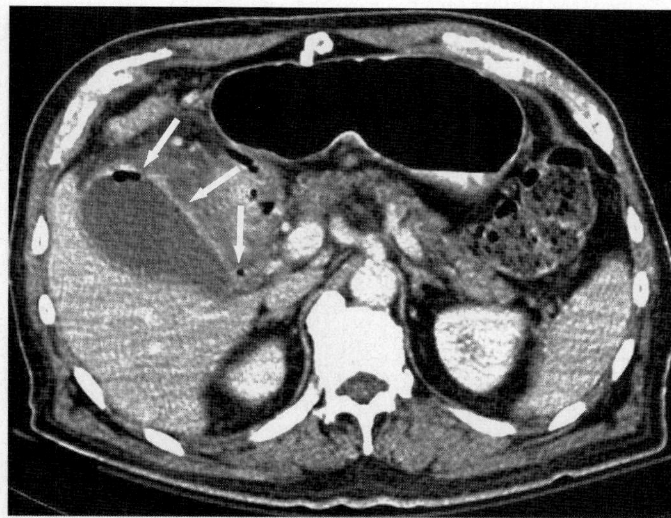

FIGURE 54-23 CT scan of emphysematous cholecystitis. Significant pericholecystic inflammatory changes and air in the gallbladder wall *(arrows)* are signs of emphysematous cholecystitis.

stone, the diagnosis is acute calculous cholecystitis. The differentiation of biliary colic from acute cholecystitis is unresolved blockage of the cystic duct. In biliary colic, the obstruction is temporary and self-limited. In acute cholecystitis, the obstruction does not resolve, and inflammation ensues, with edema and subserosal hemorrhage. Infection of the stagnant pool of bile is a secondary phenomenon; the primary pathophysiologic mechanism is unresolved cystic duct obstruction. Without resolution of the obstruction, the gallbladder will progress to ischemia and necrosis. Eventually, acute cholecystitis becomes acute gangrenous cholecystitis and, when complicated by infection with a gas-forming organism, acute emphysematous cholecystitis (Fig. 54-23).

Presentation

The inflammatory changes in the gallbladder wall are manifested as fever, right upper quadrant pain, tenderness to palpation, and guarding in the right upper quadrant. This process will cause an arrest of inspiration with gentle pressure under the right costal margin, a finding known as Murphy sign. Tenderness and the presence of Murphy sign help distinguish acute cholecystitis from biliary colic, in which there is no inflammatory process. Given that the common bile duct is not obstructed, profound jaundice in the setting of a picture of acute cholecystitis is rare and should raise the suspicion of cholangitis, with obstruction of the common bile duct, or Mirizzi syndrome, in which inflammation or a stone in the gallbladder neck leads to inflammation of the adjoining biliary system, with obstruction of the common hepatic duct. Mild elevations of alkaline phosphatase, bilirubin, and transaminase levels and a leukocytosis support the diagnosis of acute cholecystitis.

Diagnosis

Transabdominal ultrasonography is a sensitive, inexpensive, and reliable tool for the diagnosis of acute cholecystitis, with a sensitivity of 85% and specificity of 95%. In addition to identifying gallstones, ultrasound can demonstrate pericholecystic fluid (Fig. 54-24), gallbladder wall thickening, and even a sonographic Murphy sign, documenting tenderness specifically over the gallbladder. In most cases, an accurate history and physical

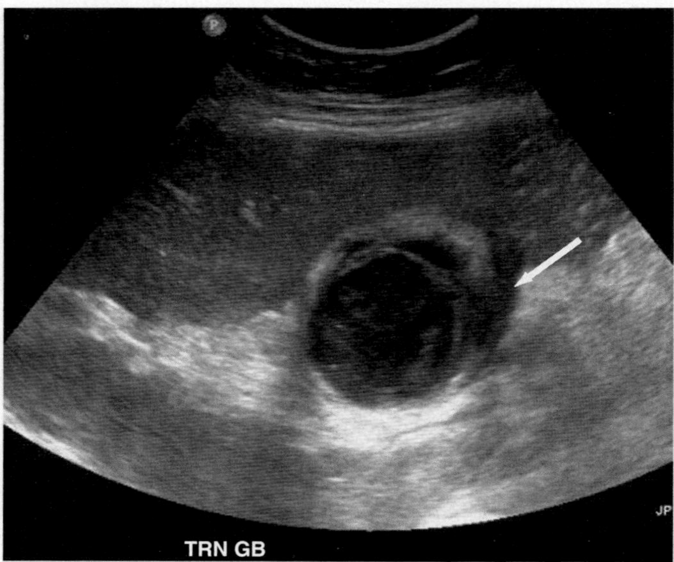

FIGURE 54-24 Ultrasound image of pericholecystic fluid. The thickened gallbladder wall with pericholecystic fluid *(arrow)* indicates acute cholecystitis.

examination, along with supporting laboratory studies and an ultrasound examination, make the diagnosis of acute cholecystitis. In atypical cases, an HIDA scan may be used to demonstrate obstruction of the cystic duct, which definitively diagnoses acute cholecystitis. Filling of the gallbladder during an HIDA scan essentially eliminates the diagnosis of cholecystitis. CT may show similar findings to ultrasound with pericholecystic fluid, gallbladder wall thickening, and emphysematous changes, but CT is less sensitive than ultrasound for the diagnosis of acute cholecystitis.

Treatment

Although the primary pathophysiologic event in acute cholecystitis is the obstruction of the cystic duct and infection is a secondary event that follows stasis and inflammation, most cases of acute cholecystitis are complicated by superinfection of the inflamed gallbladder. Therefore, patients are given nothing by mouth, and intravenous (IV) fluids and parenteral antibiotics are started. Given that gram-negative aerobes are the most common organisms found in acute cholecystitis, followed by anaerobes and gram-positive aerobes, broad-spectrum antibiotics are warranted. Parenteral narcotics are usually required to control the pain.

Cholecystectomy, whether open or laparoscopic, is the treatment of choice for acute cholecystitis. The timing of operative intervention in acute cholecystitis has long been a source of debate. In the past, many surgeons advocated for delayed cholecystectomy, with patients managed nonoperatively during their initial hospitalization and discharged home with resolution of symptoms. An interval cholecystectomy was then performed at approximately 6 weeks after the initial episode. More recent studies have shown that early in the disease process (within the first week), the operation can be performed laparoscopically with equivalent or improved morbidity, mortality, and length of stay as well as a similar conversion rate to open cholecystectomy.[3] In addition, approximately 20% of patients initially admitted for nonoperative management failed to respond to medical treatment before the planned interval cholecystectomy and required surgical intervention. Initial nonoperative therapy remains a viable option for patients who present in a delayed fashion and should be decided on an individual basis.

Given the inflammatory process occurring in the porta hepatis, early conversion to open cholecystectomy should be considered when delineation of anatomy is not clear or when progress cannot be made laparoscopically. With substantial inflammation, a partial cholecystectomy, transecting the gallbladder at the infundibulum with cauterization of the remaining mucosa, is acceptable to avoid injury to the common bile duct. Some patients present with acute cholecystitis but have a prohibitively high operative risk. For these patients, a percutaneously placed cholecystostomy tube should be considered. Frequently performed with ultrasound guidance under local anesthesia with some sedation, cholecystostomy can act as a temporizing measure by draining the infected bile. Percutaneous drainage results in improvement in symptoms and physiology, allowing a delayed cholecystectomy 3 to 6 months after medical optimization. In patients with cholecystostomy tubes, when fluoroscopy shows a patent cystic duct, the cholecystostomy tube can be removed and the decision for cholecystectomy determined by the patient's ability to tolerate surgical intervention.

Choledocholithiasis

Choledocholithiasis, or common bile duct stones, is classified by the point of origin. Primary common duct stones arise de novo in the bile duct, and secondary common duct stones pass from the gallbladder into the bile duct. Primary choledocholithiasis is generally from brown pigment stones, which are a combination of precipitated bile pigments and cholesterol. Brown stones are more common in Asian populations and are associated with a bacterial infection of the bile duct. The bacteria secrete an enzyme that hydrolyzes bilirubin glucuronides to form free bilirubin, which then precipitates. Most common duct stones found in the United States are secondary, having originated in the gallbladder, and are termed retained common duct stones when they are found within 2 years after cholecystectomy.

Many common duct stones are clinically silent and may be identified only during cholangiography if it is performed routinely during cholecystectomy (Fig. 54-25). Without pain or an abnormal liver function panel, a setting in which selective cholangiography is not performed, 1% to 2% of patients after cholecystectomy will present with a retained stone. When it is performed routinely, intraoperative cholangiography identifies choledocholithiasis in approximately 10% of asymptomatic patients, suggesting that most choledocholithiasis remains clinically silent.[4,5]

When not clinically silent, common duct stones may be manifested with symptoms ranging from biliary colic to the clinical manifestations of obstructive jaundice, such as darkening of the urine, scleral icterus, and lightening of the stools. Jaundice with choledocholithiasis is more likely to be painful because the onset of obstruction is acute, causing rapid distention of the bile duct and activation of pain fibers. Fever, a common symptom, can be associated with right upper quadrant pain and jaundice, a constellation known as Charcot triad. This triad suggests ascending cholangitis that, if untreated, may progress to septic shock. The addition of hypotension and mental status changes, both evidence of shock from a biliary source, to Charcot triad is known as Reynolds pentad.

Diagnosis

In the setting of choledocholithiasis, abnormalities of the hepatic function panel are common but neither sensitive nor specific, and with superinfection, leukocytosis may also be present. Ultrasound

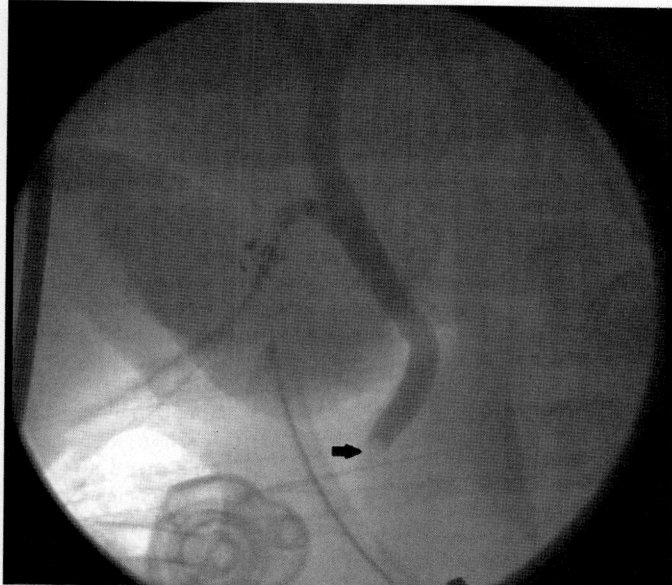

FIGURE 54-25 Intraoperative cholangiogram showing choledocholithiasis in an asymptomatic patient, with no filling of duodenum and outline of stone *(arrow)*.

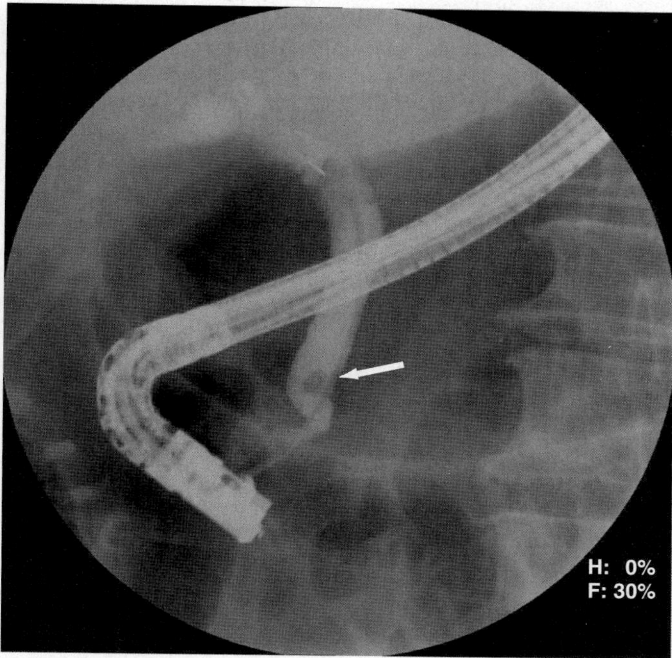

FIGURE 54-26 ERCP with choledocholithiasis. With retrograde injection of contrast material, a filling defect noted within the lumen of the common bile duct *(arrow)* identifies choledocholithiasis. ERCP can also be used to remove the stone through sphincterotomy and balloons or baskets.

may show choledocholithiasis or only biliary ductal dilation. In patients with biliary pain, gallstones, and jaundice, a dilated bile duct (>8 mm) is highly suggestive of choledocholithiasis, even if common duct stones are not documented ultrasonographically. Even without symptoms of biliary colic, a dilated bile duct in the presence of gallstones suggests choledocholithiasis.

ERCP is highly sensitive and specific for choledocholithiasis (Fig. 54-26) and can usually be therapeutic by clearing the duct of all stones in approximately 75% of patients during the first procedure and in approximately 90% with repeated ERCP. During the endoscopic procedure, a sphincterotomy is performed with a balloon sweep and extraction of the stone, all of which have a complication rate of 5% to 8%. Indications for preoperative ERCP before cholecystectomy include cholangitis, biliary pancreatitis, limited experience of the surgeon with common duct exploration, and patients with multiple comorbidities.

Alternatively, magnetic resonance cholangiopancreatography (MRCP) is highly sensitive (>90%) with an almost 100% specificity for the diagnosis of common duct stones (Fig. 54-27). As a noninvasive test, MRCP provides accurate imaging of the biliary tree, but in the setting of choledocholithiasis, it does not provide a therapeutic solution. A clear cholangiogram by MRCP eliminates the need for ERCP. However, choledocholithiasis identified by MRCP requires intervention by some other method. As many surgeons are not facile at laparoscopic common duct exploration, many have resorted to preoperative MRCP to determine the need for preoperative ERCP for duct clearance.[6] With inexperience in common duct exploration, choledocholithiasis found on cholangiography during laparoscopic cholecystectomy would necessitate postoperative ERCP and the small chance that endoscopic means could not clear the duct, necessitating reoperation.

PTC can also be used to diagnose and to treat choledocholithiasis. PTC is an invasive test with a complication rate similar to that of ERCP. Although requiring less skill, and at a lower cost, PTC is as effective in patients with a dilated biliary ductal system but less effective in the setting of a nondilated biliary tree.

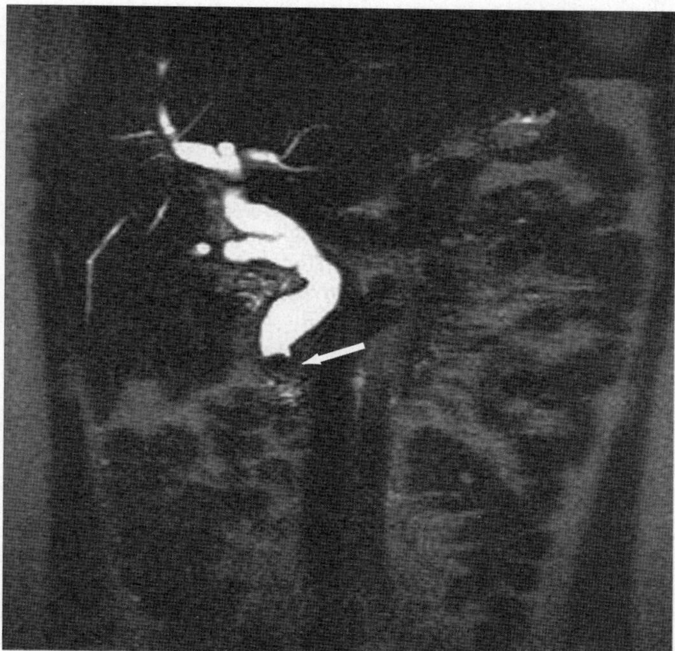

FIGURE 54-27 MRCP with choledocholithiasis. The dilated common bile duct ends abruptly, with a convex intraluminal filling defect *(arrow)* consistent with choledocholithiasis.

Ultrasound should be used routinely for evaluation of the gallbladder and biliary tree, but the remaining studies should be chosen selectively on the basis of the likelihood of finding common duct stones. Patients with highest risk, such as those with cholangitis or jaundice, should undergo ERCP. Those with lower risk can undergo laparoscopic cholecystectomy with cholangiography and possible laparoscopic common duct exploration or MRCP, depending on the surgeon's expertise. In general, choledocholithiasis identified but not removed during cholecystectomy mandates ERCP for stone extraction.

Treatment

Endoscopic retrograde cholangiopancreatography. Endoscopic sphincterotomy with stone extraction is effective for the treatment of choledocholithiasis. In the preoperative setting, it can clear the duct of stones, and when it is unsuccessful at removal of all stones, it will alter intraoperative decision making. Common reasons for endoscopic failure include large stones, intrahepatic stones, multiple stones, altered gastric or duodenal anatomy, impacted stones, and duodenal diverticula. Sphincterotomy with stone extraction does not eliminate the risk of recurrent biliary stone disease. When managed by ERCP and sphincterotomy, almost 50% of all patients have recurrent symptoms of biliary tract disease if they are not also treated by cholecystectomy.[7] More than one third of these patients eventually require cholecystectomy, suggesting that cholecystectomy should be offered to patients who present with choledocholithiasis. Interestingly, older patients (>70 years) have only a 15% rate of symptom recurrence, so cholecystectomy can be offered selectively to this population of patients.

Laparoscopic common bile duct exploration. At the time of cholecystectomy, intraoperative cholangiography will help identify choledocholithiasis. A laparoscopic common duct exploration can then be performed in an attempt to manage all calculous biliary tract disease in one setting, without the need for an additional anesthetic or procedure. Access to the common duct with a small-caliber cholangioscope is provided through the cystic duct or through a separate incision in the common duct itself. In the transcystic approach, the cystic duct is dilated, and a flexible cholangioscope is passed down into the common bile duct. For the transcystic approach in the setting of a narrow cystic duct, the duct can be dilated with a flexible dilator passed over a wire, using a Seldinger technique. Given the angle of insertion of the cystic duct into the common bile duct, stones in the common hepatic duct above the cystic duct insertion are not accessible through the transcystic route. Other contraindications for the transcystic approach include a small, friable cystic duct; numerous (more than eight) stones in the common bile duct; and large stones (>1 cm), which would be difficult or impossible to extract through the cystic duct orifice. In any of these settings, a separate incision can be made in the common bile duct, with the only contraindication being that of a small common duct that may become strictured on closure. Many studies show the high success rate of laparoscopic transcystic duct common bile duct exploration for choledocholithiasis.

Open common bile duct exploration. With greater use of endoscopic and laparoscopic methods, the frequency of open common duct exploration has decreased. Open exploration should be used when endoscopic and laparoscopic means are not feasible for documented common duct stones or when concomitant biliary drainage is required. Open exploration carries a low morbidity (8% to 15%) and mortality (1% to 2%), with a low rate of retained stones (<5%). Impacted stones at the ampulla present a difficult problem for ERCP and common duct exploration. With unsuccessful attempts to remove an impacted stone in the setting of a nondilated biliary tree, a transduodenal sphincteroplasty can provide drainage. In a similar setting but with a dilated biliary tree, drainage of the biliary tree through a separate choledochoenterostomy can be successful. The two options for drainage are a choledochoduodenostomy and Roux-en-Y choledochojejunostomy. Anastomosis to the duodenum can be performed rapidly with a single anastomosis (Fig. 54-28). This anatomic arrangement continues to allow endoscopic access to the entire biliary tree. The downside of this approach is that the bile duct distal to the anastomosis does not drain well and may collect debris that obstructs the anastomosis or the pancreatic duct, a process known as sump syndrome. Anastomosis to the jejunum in a Roux-en-Y arrangement provides excellent drainage of the biliary tree without a risk of sump syndrome but does not allow future endoscopic evaluation of the biliary tree (Fig. 54-29).

Intrahepatic stones, which are almost uniformly brown pigment stones, represent a different management challenge than secondary bile duct stones. Relatively uncommon in Western compared with Asian populations, these stones tend to occur specifically in patients with stasis of the biliary tree, such as those with strictures, parasites, choledochal cysts, or sclerosing cholangitis. Because these stones collect at sites above obstructions, the transhepatic approach to cholangiography is generally more successful. Percutaneous drainage catheters are left in place and upsized to perform percutaneous stone extraction. Long-term management of intrahepatic stones must be carefully tailored to the disease but frequently requires hepaticojejunostomy for better biliary drainage. Liberal use of choledochoscopy at the time of a drainage procedure ensures removal of all current stones. This approach allows a stone clearance rate of more than 90%.

Gallstone Pancreatitis

As a stone may pass through the common bile duct and into the duodenum, it traverses the ampulla. In the process, it may cause secondary injury to the pancreas. A generally accepted pathophysiologic mechanism involves temporary elevation of pancreatic ductal pressures, causing a secondary inflammation of the pancreatic parenchyma. Even a temporary elevation of intraluminal pressure can cause significant injury to the pancreas. As opposed to the gallbladder, in which relief of the obstruction is accompanied by pain resolution, the symptoms in pancreatitis continue in spite of passage of the stone. With the diagnosis of pancreatitis in which the cause is unclear, ultrasound will help identify gallstones and may show choledocholithiasis or a dilated bile duct. The offending stone usually passes spontaneously but may still cause severe pancreatitis. In most cases of gallstone pancreatitis, the pancreatitis is self-limited. If, by clinical assessment, the pancreatitis is severe, early ERCP to remove a stone that may not have passed is indicated and has been shown to reduce the morbidity of the episode of pancreatitis.[8] To prevent a future episode of gallstone pancreatitis, a laparoscopic cholecystectomy is warranted; this is generally recommended during the same hospitalization, just before discharge. Given the suspicion of choledocholithiasis, intraoperative cholangiography should be performed if no other imaging has been performed to confirm the passage of the gallstone.

Biliary Dyskinesia

Patients may present with classic symptoms of calculous biliary disease but have no ultrasonographic evidence of stones or sludge. In some of these cases, the dysfunction of the gallbladder creates pain, even in the absence of stones. These patients will have other diagnoses excluded by CT and upper endoscopy and should undergo a CCK-stimulated HIDA scan, in which the radiolabeled iminodiacetic acid will collect in the gallbladder. The

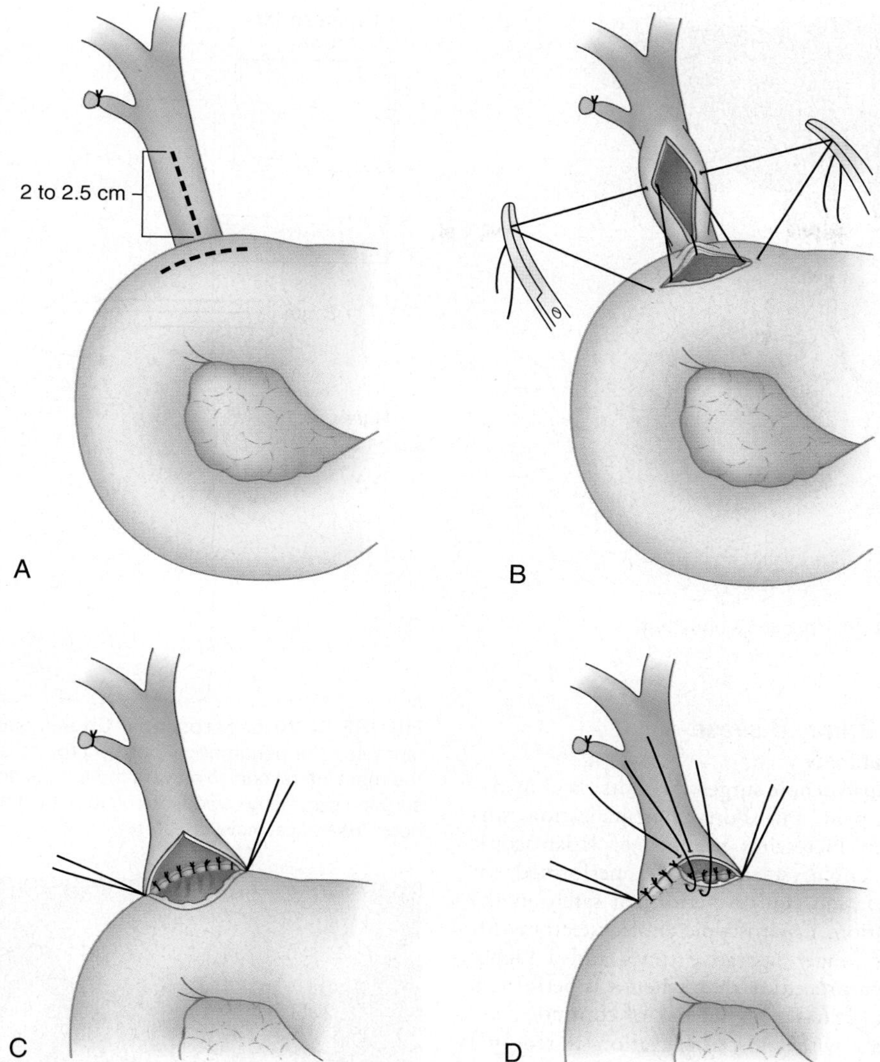

FIGURE 54-28 Choledochoduodenostomy. In the setting of a dilated common bile duct with inability to clear all the stones from the distal duct, an anastomosis can be performed between the common bile duct and adjacent duodenum. Although maintaining the possibility of future endoscopic therapy, this arrangement risks sump syndrome in the undrained distal duct.

patient is given an IV dose of CCK, and the percentage ejection of the gallbladder in response to CCK is calculated. An ejection fraction less than one third at 20 minutes after CCK administration in patients without stones is considered diagnostic of dyskinesia, which should be managed with cholecystectomy. The symptoms of dyskinesia are fairly responsive to cholecystectomy, with more than 85% of patients showing improvement or resolution. In nonresponders, ERCP with sphincterotomy may prove useful.

Sphincter of Oddi Dysfunction

Although there is considerable debate among surgeons and gastroenterologists as to the validity of this diagnosis, sphincter of Oddi dysfunction, which is manifested as biliary tract pain, with normal liver function test results and recurrent pancreatitis, may be caused by a structurally abnormal sphincter or a histologically normal but functionally abnormal one. The theoretical pathophysiologic event occurs with injury to the sphincter from trauma due to pancreatitis, gallstone passage, or congenital anomalies, which induces inflammation and subsequent fibrosis leading to elevated sphincter pressure. Alternatively, patients may have elevated sphincter pressure in the absence of fibrosis, suggesting a spasm of the muscular component. This subset of patients may have evidence of altered motility elsewhere in the gastrointestinal tract. The diagnosis of sphincter of Oddi dysfunction should be suspected in patients with biliary pain and a common duct diameter of more than 12 mm. The bile duct in these patients tends to increase in diameter in response to CCK, as does the pancreatic duct after secretin administration. Manometry has also been used to make the diagnosis, with sphincter pressure higher than 40 mm Hg predicting good response to therapy. Therapy consists of endoscopic sphincterotomy or transduodenal sphincteroplasty, with approximately equivalent results from the two approaches. In patients with objective evidence of sphincter of Oddi dysfunction, division of the sphincter will improve or resolve the pain in 60% to 80% of patients.

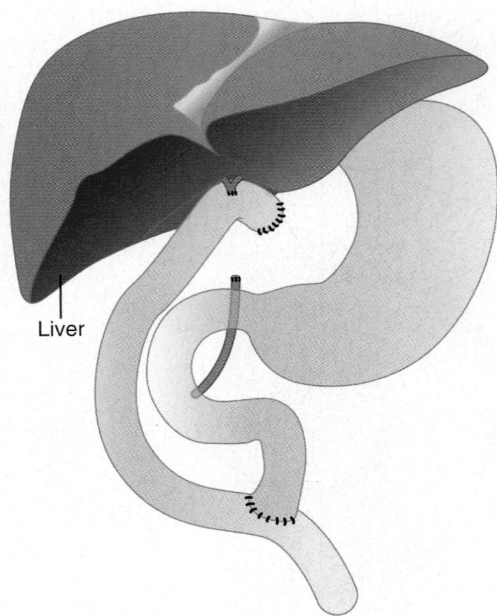

FIGURE 54-29 Hepaticojejunostomy.

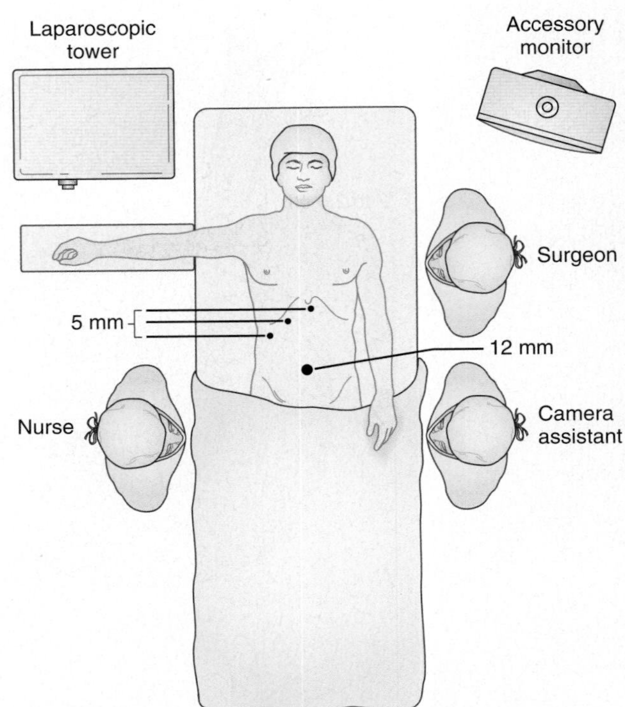

FIGURE 54-30 Laparoscopic Cholecystectomy Ports. The assistant uses the periumbilical port to provide access for the camera and the most lateral port to elevate the fundus and to expose the neck. The surgeon can then provide inferolateral traction on the infundibulum and open the critical view of safety.

Surgery for Calculous Biliary Disease

Laparoscopic Cholecystectomy

Following the advent of laparoscopic surgery, with its accompanying smaller incisions, less pain, and shorter hospitalization, surgeons have performed an increasing number of laparoscopic cholecystectomies. Most cholecystectomies are performed for biliary colic, but the operation can be performed safely in the setting of acute inflammation. Laparoscopic cholecystectomy for acute cholecystitis carries longer operative times and a higher conversion rate to the open procedure than when it is performed in the elective setting, and it has a higher risk of common duct injury.[9] General anesthesia with muscle relaxation is required when a laparoscopic cholecystectomy is performed. Therefore, one contraindication to the procedure is the inability to tolerate general anesthesia. Others include end-stage liver disease with portal hypertension, precluding safe portal dissection, and coagulopathy. Because most pneumoperitoneum laparoscopy is performed using CO_2 and has a number of adverse physiologic effects, severe chronic obstructive pulmonary disease, with poor ability for gas exchange, and congestive heart failure are considered relative contraindications.

Preparation of the patient, induction of anesthesia, and sterile draping are performed as for an open cholecystectomy. Although use of a urinary catheter depends on the clinical setting, an orogastric tube is standard to decompress the stomach and help with exposure of the upper abdomen. After the establishment of a CO_2 pneumoperitoneum, a brief exploration is performed, and additional 5-mm ports are placed in the right anterior axillary line, right midclavicular line, and subxiphoid location (Fig. 54-30). The lateral port at the anterior axillary line is used to elevate the fundus of the gallbladder toward the right shoulder. This retraction provides exposure to the infundibulum and porta hepatis. The midclavicular trocar is used to grasp the gallbladder infundibulum, retracting it inferolaterally to open the triangle of Calot (Figs. 54-31 to 54-33). By distraction of Hartmann pouch laterally, the cystic duct no longer lies almost parallel to the common hepatic duct.

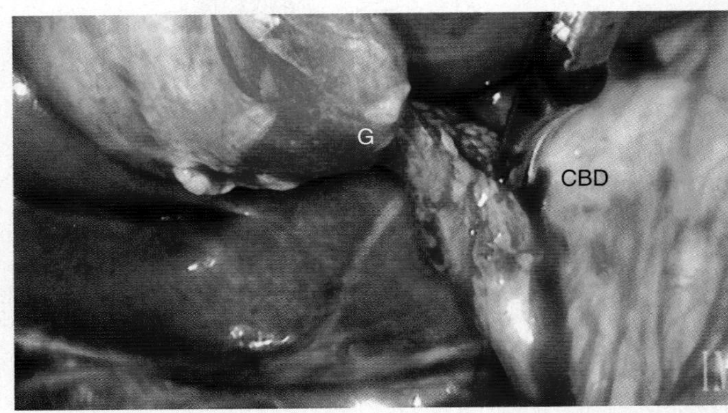

FIGURE 54-31 Laparoscopic view of the porta and gallbladder infundibulum, without inferolateral traction on the infundibulum. Note that the gallbladder infundibulum (G) lies immediately adjacent to the common bile duct (CBD).

The dissection is then carried along the infundibulum on the anterior and posterior surfaces to expose the base of the gallbladder. This dissection will eventually clear all fibrofatty tissue from the triangle of Calot. Inferolateral traction of the infundibulum then allows documentation of two structures entering the gallbladder, the cystic duct and cystic artery. A useful landmark for the cystic artery is the overlying lymph node, known as Calot node. To minimize bile duct injury, a strategy known as the critical view of safety can be employed. This process involves dissection of the infundibulum of the gallbladder and continuation of the dissection by taking down the cystic plate and separating the lower third of the gallbladder from its attachments to the liver. Once completed, the tubular structures attached to the gallbladder

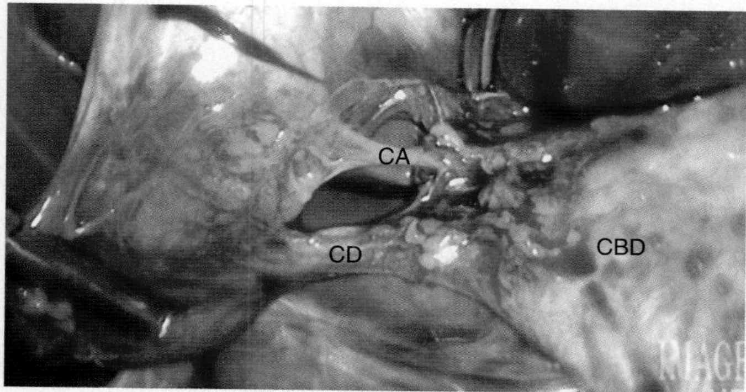

FIGURE 54-32 Laparoscopic view of the same patient as in Figure 54-31 but with inferolateral traction on the infundibulum. Note the angular change to the cystic duct (CD) compared with the common bile duct (CBD). The dissecting tool indicates the location of the right hepatic artery. The key element to this view in minimizing CBD injury is the identification of the cystic artery (CA) and duct entering the gallbladder, with the inferior aspect of segment V of the liver identified in the space on either side of the artery and duct.

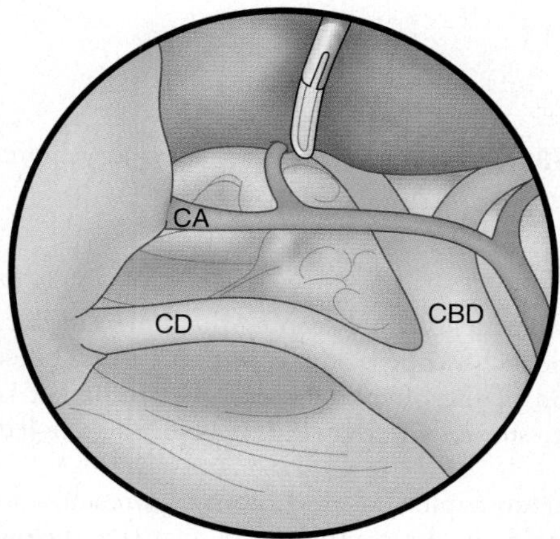

FIGURE 54-33 An artist's representation of Figure 54-32, showing hidden anatomy.

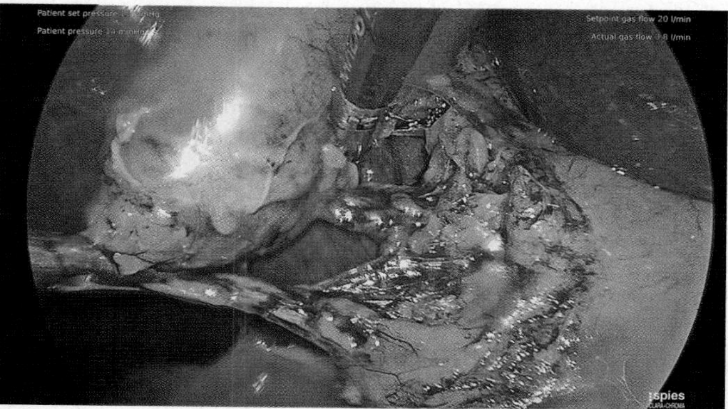

FIGURE 54-34 Wide critical view.

should be cleaned of all extraneous material. Rotating the gallbladder infundibulum laterally and then medially, there should be only two structures entering the gallbladder, and liver on the opposite side of the gallbladder should be visible through the open spaces around each structure (Fig. 54-34).[9] With sufficient dissection, clips are placed on the cystic artery and cystic duct. If

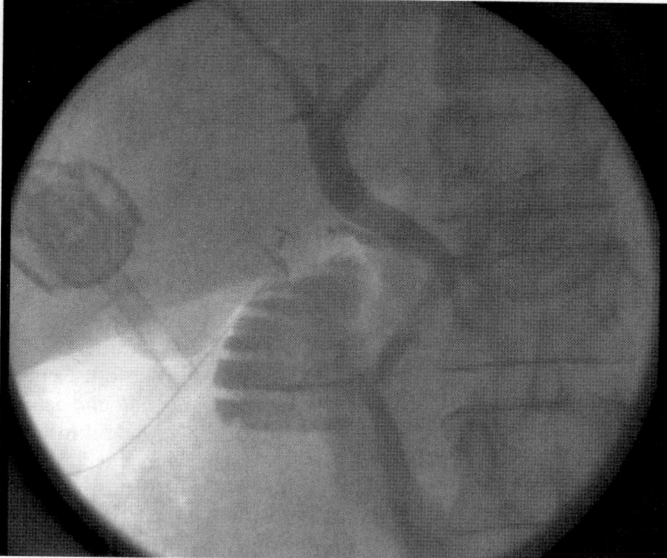

FIGURE 54-35 Normal cholangiogram.

cholangiography is performed, the cystic duct is clipped only adjacent to the gallbladder, and the cystic duct is incised but not transected. A cholangiographic catheter is then fed through the incised duct, and fluoroscopic images are obtained with injection of contrast material into the cystic duct and biliary tree (Fig. 54-35). On obtaining a normal cholangiogram or when cholangiography is not performed, the cystic duct is doubly clipped on the common duct side and transected. The previously clipped artery is also transected, and the gallbladder is dissected off the liver bed using electrocautery. Because the venous drainage of the gallbladder is directly into the liver bed through venules, excellent hemostasis must be achieved during this dissection. The cystic duct and cystic artery clips are inspected just before completion of the dissection of the fundic attachments because the superior traction of the fundus has provided exposure to the porta and triangle of Calot. The gallbladder is then brought out of the abdominal cavity through the umbilical port. In the setting of acute cholecystitis or if the gallbladder was entered during dissection, a plastic bag should be used for retrieval. Any stones that are spilled during a cholecystectomy should also be retrieved.

Opinion is sharply divided about the performance of selective versus routine cholangiography, with supportive data for each approach. Routine cholangiography will identify unsuspected stones in less than 10% of patients, and the natural history of these asymptomatic stones suggests that they will remain asymptomatic. Although vigorously debated, the incidence of biliary injury is not significantly reduced with cholangiography. Even when it is performed routinely, cholangiograms are frequently misinterpreted.[10] In many cases of laparoscopic cholecystectomy performed for biliary colic, cholangiography will not alter management. Also, it increases the operative time and adds fluoroscopic exposure. Indications for cholangiography in the selective setting include unexplained pain at the time of cholecystectomy, any suspicion of current or previous choledocholithiasis without preoperative duct clearance, any question of anatomic delineation during cholecystectomy, elevated preoperative liver enzyme levels, dilated common bile duct in preoperative imaging, and suspicion of intraoperative biliary injury. Although the routine use of cholangiography has been decreasing, many authors advocate its use in the academic setting to ensure that trainees are facile in its performance.[6] Although it is just as accurate as cholangiography for the identification of choledocholithiasis, laparoscopic ultrasonography is highly operator dependent, requires additional instrumentation, and is not widely available.

Open Cholecystectomy

As laparoscopic cholecystectomy has become the procedure of choice for the treatment of most gallbladder disease, experience with open cholecystectomy has drastically declined. Open cholecystectomy is generally performed after conversion from the laparoscopic approach or as a step during another operation, such as a pancreaticoduodenectomy. The open cholecystectomy can be performed through a midline or right subcostal incision. Retraction of segment IV provides exposure of the cystic duct and artery. With similar inferolateral traction to the gallbladder infundibulum, the cystic duct is taken out of alignment from the common duct for its identification and division. Early identification and ligation of the cystic artery limit the blood loss during the procedure but may prove difficult because of inflammation. Another approach to the gallbladder infundibulum involves dissecting the fundus off the liver in a dome-down approach. Here, the attachments of the gallbladder are divided, allowing inferolateral traction of the entire gallbladder to open the triangle of Calot and to identify the appropriate duct and artery. This approach, although intermittently useful, must be used with caution as the extension of the dissection continues inferiorly, putting portal vein and other portal structures at risk.[11] When it is performed for severe cholecystitis, the dissection of the gallbladder of the liver bed may be associated with substantial blood loss, but with removal of the infected gallbladder and packing of the area, the bleeding is usually well controlled.

Laparoscopic Common Bile Duct Exploration

Given the risk of ascending cholangitis, gallstone pancreatitis, or cystic duct stump leak, all attempts must be made to remove known bile duct stones. Many factors are relevant to the decision as to which approach to duct clearance should be used. The experience of the surgeon or endoscopist is important in determining if operative clearance or postoperative ERCP will be most effective, with lowest morbidity. Anatomic aspects such as duct size and stone size and number should be considered. As experience with laparoscopic surgery has grown, laparoscopic approaches to bile duct clearance have become more prevalent. With a common bile duct stone identified fluoroscopically, the common duct can be irrigated, and glucagon is given to relax the sphincter of Oddi. If this technique fails to flush the stone, a balloon catheter or wire basket can be passed under fluoroscopic guidance to attempt stone extraction. If this is still unsuccessful, flexible choledochoscopy is indicated. The two common laparoscopic approaches to explore the common bile duct for stone removal are the transcystic approach and choledochotomy. In the transcystic approach, at the completion of cholangiography, a wire is fed down the cystic duct into the common bile duct. Through a Seldinger technique or use of a balloon catheter, the cystic duct is gently dilated to allow passage of a flexible choledochoscope. Alternatively, a flexible ureteroscope can be used. To pass the fiberoptic scope through the duct system, a water irrigation system is attached and allowed to constantly infuse out the end of the scope. If a laparoscopic screen is available, the choledochoscopic image is projected onto a corner it. With the surgeon feeding the choledochoscope into the cystic duct and the assistant adjusting the

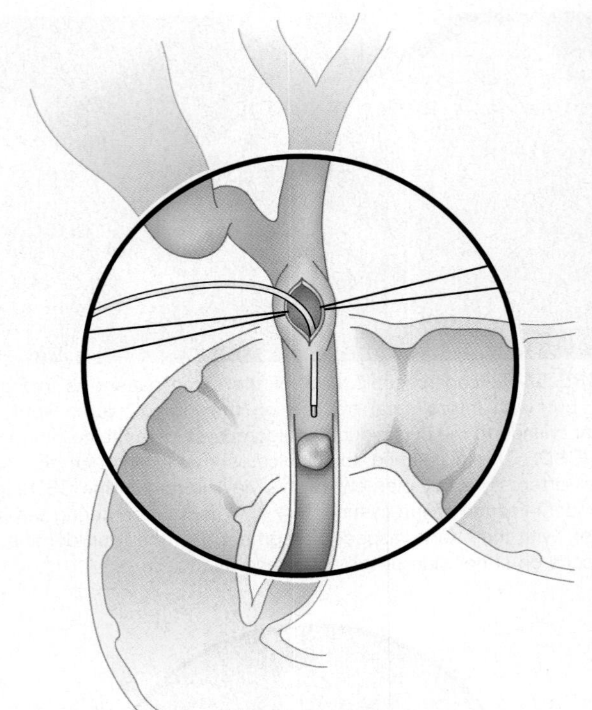

FIGURE 54-36 Laparoscopic choledochotomy for common bile duct exploration.

tip of the choledochoscope, keeping the lumen in the screen, the flexible choledochoscope is advanced to the distal bile duct. With identification of the offending stone, a wire basket is passed to ensnare the stone, withdrawing it and the choledochoscope together.

In the laparoscopic choledochotomy approach, a longitudinal incision is made in the common bile duct (i.e., below the cystic duct). To expose the common bile duct, two stay sutures are placed on either side of the planned choledochotomy (Fig. 54-36). The size of the incision should be at least as large as the diameter of the largest stone. The choledochoscope can then be fed down into the distal bile duct and stone extraction performed as described earlier. At the completion of the exploration, a T tube should be placed through the choledochotomy and the bile duct closed with 4-0 absorbable sutures. Completion cholangiography through the T tube documents stone removal.

In addition to being technically easier, because it does not require fine laparoscopic suturing, the transcystic approach avoids a T tube. Contraindications to the transcystic approach include numerous (more than eight) stones, a stone larger than 1 cm, intrahepatic stones, and a cystic duct that does not allow dilation and choledochoscope passage. Given the need for suture closure of the incision in the bile duct, the only contraindication to the choledochotomy approach is a small-caliber bile duct (<6 mm), which could be strictured by closure. Both approaches are successful at stone removal, with most studies showing a 75% to 95% rate of stone clearance. This is comparable to that of laparoscopic cholecystectomy, followed by postoperative ERCP, with the only difference being a shorter hospitalization and lower physician fees for patients undergoing common duct exploration as the cholecystectomy and clearance of stones are performed in one setting by a single physician.[12]

Open Common Bile Duct Exploration

With advanced laparoscopic, endoscopic, and percutaneous techniques, open exploration of the bile duct has become less common. When open surgery is otherwise required or previous surgery, such as gastric bypass, makes other techniques unsuccessful, clearance of choledocholithiasis must be performed by the open approach. The exposure to the bile duct is through a midline or right upper quadrant incision. A Kocher maneuver must be performed to expose the distal bile duct. Gentle palpation of the distal bile duct will frequently find the offending stone, which may be milked backward. As in the laparoscopic approach, stay sutures are placed and a choledochotomy is performed in the supraduodenal bile duct. Flushing of the duct with a soft rubber catheter will frequently remove the offending stones. Balloon catheters and, with fluoroscopic guidance, wire baskets may be useful to withdraw the stone. Flexible choledochoscopes are used to visualize the distal bile duct. With complete removal of stones, a T tube is placed and a cholangiogram obtained before closure to document clearance.

In the setting of common bile duct stones, some patients should be considered for a drainage procedure. With dilated bile ducts, multiple distal impacted stones, a distal duct stricture with stones, intrahepatic stones, or primary bile duct stones, drainage procedures provide more successful long-term outcomes. Options in this setting include choledochoduodenostomy and Roux-en-Y hepaticojejunostomy, with Roux-en-Y considered a superior drainage procedure. A side-to-side or end-to side choledochoduodenostomy is a fast and safe approach that allows future endoscopic intervention of the upper biliary tree, if necessary. In the side-to-side approach, however, by leaving of the distal bile duct in continuity, patients are at risk for sump syndrome, in which the distal bile duct that does not drain well may collect debris and even food stuffs. Occlusions of the ampulla, with subsequent pancreatitis, and anastomotic stricture with cholangitis have been reported. An alternative to duodenostomy is a Roux-en-Y choledochojejunostomy. By use of a 60-cm limb of jejunum for drainage, occlusion of the anastomosis by food debris is rare, but endoscopic treatment of the hepatic duct is impossible.

Impacted stones at the ampulla that cannot be removed through choledochotomy or several stones in a nondilated tree can be addressed by a transduodenal sphincteroplasty (Figs. 54-37 and 54-38). After completion of the Kocher maneuver, a longitudinal duodenotomy is made on the lateral wall. Compression of the lateral wall against the medial wall will allow palpation of the ampulla to plan placement of the duodenotomy appropriately. With identification of the ampulla, an incision is made at 11 o'clock, and each wall is elevated with stay sutures. The pancreatic duct usually enters at 5 o'clock on the ampulla and must be avoided. Sequential straight clamps are placed along the planned incision of the ampulla to guide visualization through hemostasis. With each step, the duodenal mucosa is sewn to the bile duct mucosa with absorbable 4-0 sutures. A 1.5-cm sphincterotomy is usually sufficient to allow stone removal and subsequent drainage. Closure of the longitudinal duodenotomy in transverse fashion avoids a future duodenal stricture.

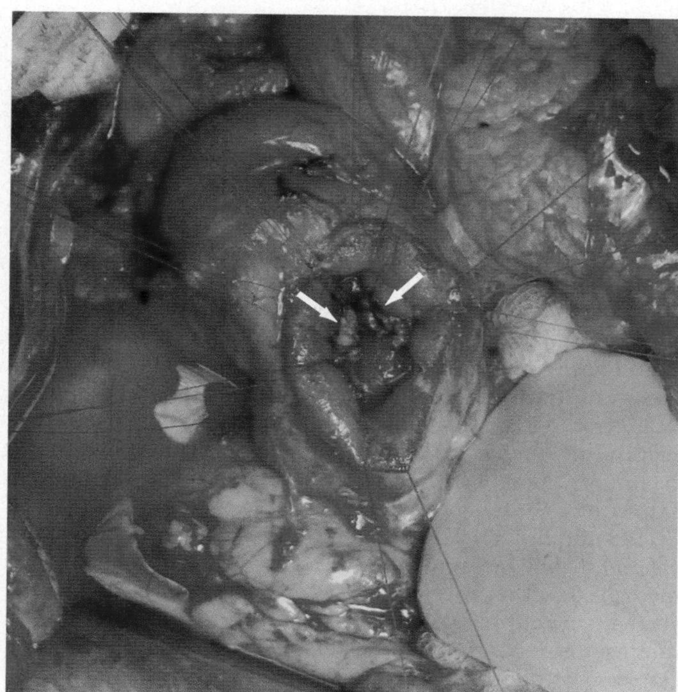

FIGURE 54-37 Transduodenal sphincteroplasty. Note the generous opening of the distal common duct with sequential duct to mucosa approximation *(arrows)*.

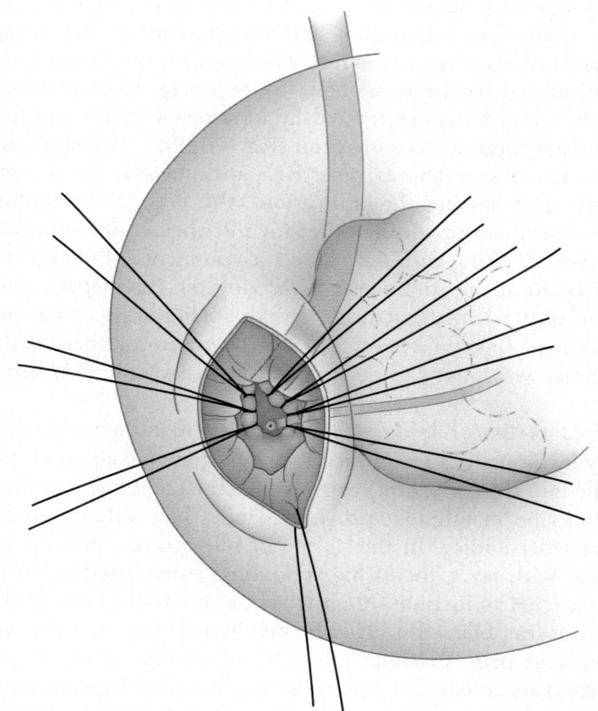

FIGURE 54-38 Transduodenal sphincteroplasty.

Postcholecystectomy Syndromes

Bile Duct Injury

The most devastating complication of any right upper quadrant operation occurring with any significant frequency is iatrogenic bile duct injury. More than 80% of all iatrogenic bile duct injuries occur during cholecystectomy, and they can occur in the open or laparoscopic setting. Inflammation in the porta, variable biliary anatomy, inappropriate exposure, aggressive attempts at hemostasis, and inexperience of the surgeon are commonly cited risk factors. Although early reports suggested that surgical inexperience (performing fewer than 20 laparoscopic cholecystectomies) was highly correlated with bile duct injury, evidence has suggested that visual misperception accounts for 97% of iatrogenic biliary injuries and technical skill or knowledge accounts for only 3%.[6] With sufficient cephalad retraction of the gallbladder fundus, the cystic duct overlies the common hepatic duct, running in a parallel path. Without inferolateral traction of the gallbladder infundibulum to dissociate these structures, dissection of the apparent cystic duct may actually include the common hepatic duct, placing it in jeopardy. By retraction of Hartmann pouch inferolaterally and opening of the triangle of Calot, the cystic duct is displaced from the porta, no longer collinear with the hepatic duct. The use of a 30-degree laparoscope provides adequate visualization of the critical view of safety during laparoscopic cholecystectomy. Also, in many of these cases, a confirmation bias occurs, in which surgeons tend to rely on evidence that supports their perception while simultaneously discounting visual cues that suggest an alternative explanation. Confirmation bias helps explain why most bile duct injuries are identified in the postoperative setting, not intraoperatively.

The multifactorial nature of biliary injury highlights the concept that injury avoidance consists of many levels of protective mechanisms. The surgeon's knowledge of biliary anatomy and aberrant anatomy, use of an angled laparoscope, appropriate and directed traction and countertraction on the gallbladder, sufficient suspicion of findings that discount the current perspective, and low threshold for conversion to an open operation can help minimize the likelihood of biliary injury. Although the use of routine versus selective cholangiography is controversial, evidence has suggested that cholangiography does not completely avoid bile duct injury but may reduce the incidence and extent of injury and allow immediate recognition and management.[13] The original analysis of biliary reconstruction was based on the Bismuth classification and has been modified by Strasberg. Classification of bile duct injuries is determined by location of injury and helps guide later surgical reconstruction (Fig. 54-39).[14] Among postoperative bile duct strictures, types E1 and E2 involve the common hepatic duct but not the bifurcation, with type E1 maintaining more than 2 cm of common hepatic duct below the bifurcation and type E2 being within 2 cm of the confluence. Type E3 strictures occur at the confluence, preserving the extrahepatic ducts, and in type E4, the stricturing process includes the extrahepatic biliary tree. Type E5 strictures involve aberrant right hepatic duct anatomy, with injury to the aberrant duct and common hepatic duct.

Presentation. Bile duct injury may be identified intraoperatively but usually is manifested in the postoperative period. Leak of bile into the peritoneal cavity, with subsequent bile peritonitis, tends to be manifested earlier than bile duct stricture and its associated jaundice. In the setting of bile leakage, patients may present with fever, increasing abdominal pain, jaundice, or bile leakage from an incision. Alternatively, injury to the bile duct that does not leak bile will usually be manifested with jaundice, with or without pain. Overall, only 10% of postoperative bile duct strictures are recognized within the first week, and approximately 70% are diagnosed within 6 months of the original operation. Regardless of timing or presentation, adequate repair and subsequent outcome depend on diagnosis, sufficient delineation of anatomy, creation of a tension-free anastomosis, and liberal use of transanastomotic stents.[15]

Treatment

Recognized at the time of cholecystectomy. When bile duct injury is suspected intraoperatively, conversion to an open operation and use of cholangiography help delineate management.

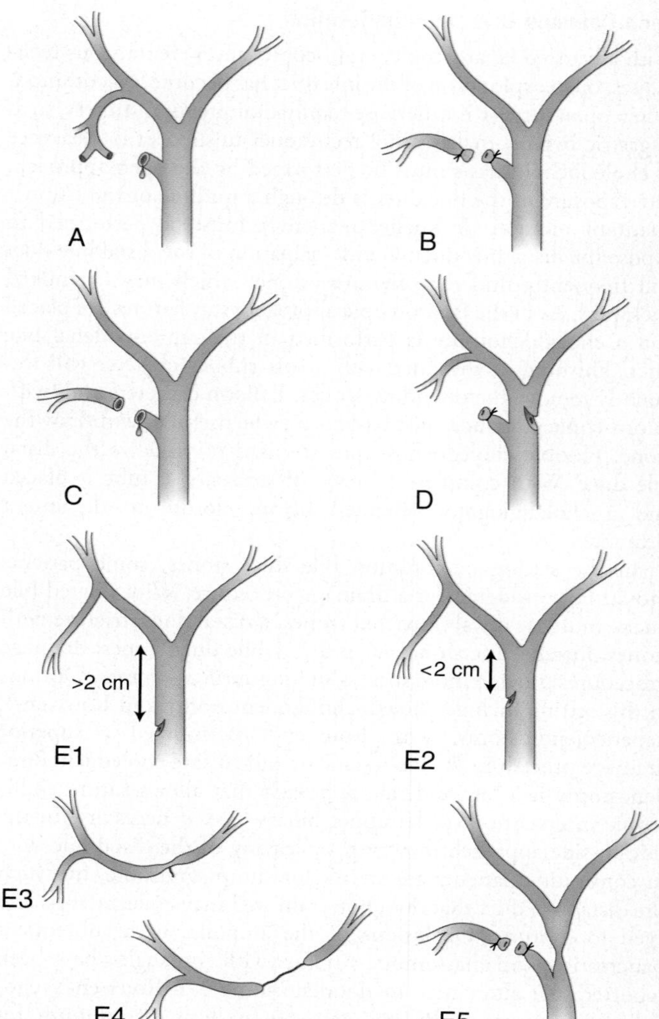

FIGURE 54-39 Strasberg classification of postoperative bile duct strictures.

Goals for the immediate treatment of bile duct injury include maintenance of ductal length, elimination of any bile leakage that would affect subsequent management, and creation of a tension-free repair.

In the adult, for ducts smaller than 3 mm that by cholangiography drain only a single segment or subsegment of liver, simple ligation should suffice for management. Ducts larger than 3 mm usually drain more than a single segment of liver and thus, if transected, should be reimplanted into the biliary tree. If the injury occurs to a larger duct but is not caused by electrocautery and involves less than 50% of the circumference of the wall, a T tube placed through the injury, which is effectively a choledochotomy, usually will allow healing without the need for subsequent biliary-enteric anastomosis. Any cautery-based injury, in which the extent of thermal damage may not be manifested immediately, or an injury involving more than 50% of the duct circumference requires resection of the injured segment with anastomosis to reestablish biliary-enteric continuity. Although it is unusual, when the defect is smaller than 1 cm and not near the hepatic duct bifurcation, mobilization with end-to-end anastomosis of the bile duct can provide acceptable reconstruction. This approach should be accompanied with transanastomotic T tube placement. The tube should be inserted through a separate choledochotomy and not exit the bile duct though the anastomosis. To ensure a tension-free anastomosis, a generous Kocher maneuver, mobilizing the duodenum and the head of the pancreas out of the retroperitoneum, is necessary.

More commonly, injuries occur adjacent to the bifurcation or involve more than a 1-cm defect between the ends of the bile duct. These injuries require reanastomosis to the gastrointestinal tract. In this setting, the distal end is oversewn and the proximal end débrided to normal tissue. The choice of reconstruction depends on location and extent of injury, history of previous attempts at repair, and preference of the surgeon. Low injuries to the bile duct can be reimplanted into the duodenum, although the new choledochoduodenostomy anastomosis risks a duodenal fistula, especially considering that these anastomoses may require significant mobilization to avoid anastomotic tension. Choledochoduodenostomy allows endoscopic intervention if necessary, but the Roux-en-Y approach to reconstruction is substantially more versatile and can be applied to injuries throughout the biliary tree. In addition, most injuries to the bile duct occur higher in the biliary tree, close to the hilum, thus not allowing tension-free anastomosis to the duodenum. Therefore, in almost all cases of bile duct injury, a resection of the injured segment with mucosa-to-mucosa anastomosis using a Roux-en-Y jejunal limb is preferred. Transanastomotic stenting has been shown to improve anastomotic patency, with longer duration of stenting providing a more favorable outcome. As concomitant vascular injuries are common, Doppler ultrasonography can confirm adequate hepatic arterial and portal venous flow to the hepatic parenchyma.

Recent data suggest that there is no significant difference in frequency of biliary injuries sustained at teaching hospitals compared with hospitals without residents.[16] Because most bile duct injuries and therefore most immediate repairs occur at centers where biliary reconstruction is performed infrequently, most immediate repairs go unreported in the literature. However, the importance of surgical judgment and experience in biliary reconstruction cannot be overemphasized. Although reports of previous failed attempts at reconstruction have not documented injuries successfully managed immediately, they do highlight the value of experience in the treatment of bile duct injuries.[17] Therefore, when one is confronted with a bile duct injury and no surgeon with experience in biliary reconstruction is available, the most appropriate management strategy is placement of a drain and immediate referral to an experienced center.

Identified after cholecystectomy

Diagnosis and management. Patients suffering a bile duct injury who present in the postoperative setting are generally found to have jaundice, with an elevated alkaline phosphatase level, or leakage from the injured duct. Leakage may be manifested as bilious drainage into a subhepatic drain placed at the time of operation or bilious drainage from a surgical incision. Without a site for external drainage, bile leakage can be manifested as a biloma, whether sterile or infected, or with biliary ascites.

The diagnosis of iatrogenic bile duct injury should be suspected in any patient who presents with new or increasing symptoms after a laparoscopic cholecystectomy. Changes in serum bilirubin and alkaline phosphatase levels can be seen, even in the first few days after injury. Symptoms of shoulder pain, postprandial pain, fever, and malaise tend to improve after the first few days because a laparoscopic cholecystectomy is generally well tolerated. Complaints that persist or increase over time should raise the suspicion of a bile duct injury.

BOX 54-2 Goals of Therapy in Iatrogenic Bile Duct Injury

1. Control of infection, limiting inflammation
   - Parenteral antibiotics
   - Percutaneous drainage of periportal fluid collections
2. Clear and thorough delineation of entire biliary anatomy
   - MRCP or PTC
   - ERCP (especially if cystic duct stump leak is suspected)
3. Reestablishment of biliary-enteric continuity
   - Tension-free, mucosa-to-mucosa anastomosis
   - Roux-en-Y hepaticojejunostomy
   - Long-term transanastomotic stents if bifurcation or higher is involved

Patients suspected of having an iatrogenic bile duct injury should undergo imaging to assess for a fluid collection and to evaluate the biliary tree. Ultrasonography can achieve both these goals, but because percutaneous drainage may be required and anatomic delineation is valuable, cross-sectional imaging by CT will generally provide more useful data. Some surgeons advocate the use of radionuclide scanning to confirm bile leakage, but with any documentation of a leak, CT will be necessary to plan management. Also, ischemia is a common cause of bile duct stricture. In the setting of a bile duct injury, 20% or more of patients will have concomitant unrecognized vascular injuries.

In the delayed presentation of a bile duct injury, three major goals guide therapy (Box 54-2). First, control of infection with drainage of any fluid collections will minimize the inflammatory process. Inflammation in the porta hepatis leads to fibrosis, which acts only to increase stricture formation. Broad-spectrum antibiotics, decompression of the biliary tree, and drainage, whether percutaneous or operative, of any fluid collections will achieve this goal. With control of sepsis, there is no urgency for biliary reconstruction. In fact, with time, resolution of the periportal inflammation helps with the execution of a durable reconstruction. In addition, the retraction of an injured bile duct into the hilum of the liver as well as inflammation in this region makes successful repair in the immediate postoperative setting unlikely. Therefore, although immediate reexploration to manage the injury as expeditiously as possible is tempting, successful long-term management of bile duct injuries identified postoperatively depends on clear and deliberate preoperative planning of the reconstruction.

A second goal of management is clear and thorough delineation of the biliary anatomy with cholangiography. Without preoperative cholangiography, any attempts at repair are unlikely to be successful. The cholangiogram must indicate the intrahepatic anatomy and bile duct bifurcation. For patients with bile duct continuity, ERCP may be possible, but PTC is generally more useful. PTC will demonstrate the intrahepatic biliary tree, identify the location of the injury, provide drainage of bile, and possibly even allow the leak to close (Fig. 54-40). Percutaneous biliary catheters can also be left in place during reconstruction to assist in dissection and to provide drainage perioperatively. PTC can be combined with ERCP as necessary, depending on the site and extent of injury. Small bile leaks with bile duct continuity and cystic duct stump leaks can be successfully managed by endoscopic stenting and sphincterotomy.

The third goal of management is to reestablish durable biliary-enteric drainage. Although a combination of percutaneous and endoscopic biliary dilations and stenting may establish continuity, surgical reconstruction has the highest patency rates. To achieve

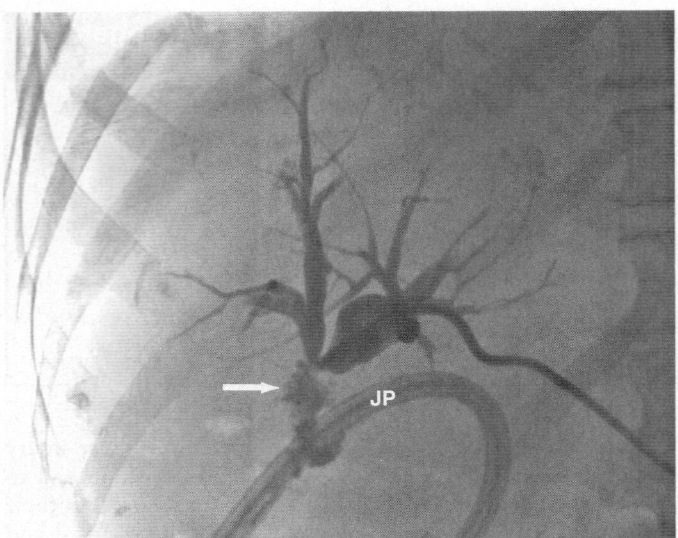

FIGURE 54-40 Percutaneous transhepatic cholangiogram of bile duct injury. Note the extravasation of contrast material *(arrow)* and the Jackson-Pratt drain (JP) placed at the time of initial operation.

a successful and durable repair, the anastomosis must be performed between a minimally inflamed bile duct to intestines in a tension-free, mucosa-to-mucosa fashion. When the anastomosis is within 2 cm of the hepatic duct bifurcation or involves intrahepatic ducts, long-term stenting appears to improve patency. If the bifurcation is involved, stenting of both right and left ducts should be performed. When the reconstruction involves the common bile duct or common hepatic duct more than 2 cm from the bifurcation, stenting is not necessary; therefore, a preoperatively placed transhepatic drain or intraoperatively placed T tube will provide adequate decompression in the immediate postoperative period.

At the time of operation, the adhesions of the duodenum and colon to the liver should be separated. The porta hepatis can be encircled with a Penrose drain. Although the bile duct should lie on the lateral border of the porta hepatis, the marked fibrosis and inflammatory process may make its identification difficult. Preoperatively placed percutaneous biliary drainage catheters can assist in the dissection. Also, clips placed at the previous operation may be identified. If necessary, a small-caliber needle attached to a syringe can be used to aspirate and to identify the bile duct while avoiding inadvertent injury to a vascular structure (Fig. 54-41). Once identified, above the stricture only a limited segment of bile duct (<5 mm) is dissected free. Any further dissection of normal duct risks vascular compromise of the segment to be used in the anastomosis. Preservation of as much normal biliary tree as possible remains a goal of the reconstruction. Next, the bile duct can be opened and the percutaneously placed catheters advanced through the incision. At this point, a wire can be used to exchange the catheters for long-term Silastic stents, if appropriate, or the catheters can be left in place for transanastomotic decompression. The mucosa-to-mucosa anastomosis can be created in an end-to-side fashion to the Roux-en-Y jejunal limb. In the setting of substantial inflammation at the bifurcation, another reconstruction option involves anastomosis of the Roux limb to the left hepatic duct. As noted, the left hepatic duct retains a substantial extraparenchymal length, allowing an anastomosis in this portion of normal duct. Before this section is used for drainage of the

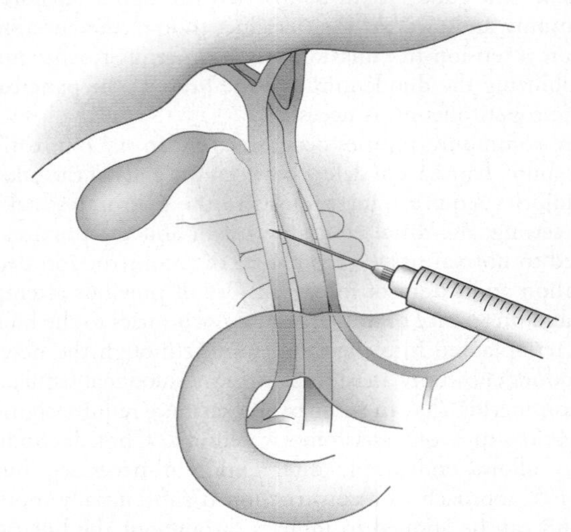

FIGURE 54-41 Needle aspiration of porta used to identify the common bile duct in the setting of substantial inflammation.

entire liver, cholangiography must confirm that the biliary bifurcation is widely patent, thus ensuring drainage of the right lobe across the bifurcation to the left duct system.

Interventional radiologic and endoscopic techniques. Although long-term patency rates are lower than those seen with surgical reconstruction, nonoperative techniques can be used when the injury has created a stricture in the biliary tree. When the duct remains in continuity, transhepatic management of bile duct strictures can be performed using fluoroscopy, with sedation and local anesthesia. With percutaneous access to the biliary tree, a wire is used to traverse the stricture. By use of balloon dilation techniques, the stricture is dilated, and a catheter is left in place to decompress the system, to allow healing, to document resolution, and, if necessary, to guide repeated dilations (Fig. 54-42). This approach is successful in up to 70% of patients.[18] Complications, although frequent, are generally limited and include cholangitis, hemobilia, and bile leaks requiring repeated intervention. Endoscopic balloon dilation of bile duct strictures is generally reserved for those with primary bile duct strictures or patients who have undergone choledochoduodenostomy for reconstruction because the Roux limb does not usually allow endoscopic strategies. Therefore, series are limited, but results are encouraging, with 88% of patients responding to therapy and a complication rate of 8% from pancreatitis and cholangitis.

Outcomes. Successful outcomes can be achieved in patients undergoing biliary-enteric reconstruction after bile duct injury, with many series showing more than 90% of patients free of jaundice and cholangitis. High success rates are generally achieved when injuries are identified early and patients are referred immediately to experienced centers. In several studies, referral to centers performing complex biliary surgery routinely was associated with better long-term success.[19] Surgical reconstruction provides a durable long-term management strategy.[20] Management of these injuries requires a multidisciplinary management and may need percutaneous techniques as well as surgical reconstruction. Sepsis at the time of reconstruction and biliary cirrhosis are predictors of stricture. In some studies, results were generally better if transanastomotic stents were used during reconstruction.[20] Chronic liver disease and hepatic fibrosis are associated with higher operative mortality and lower success rates. Although a devastating

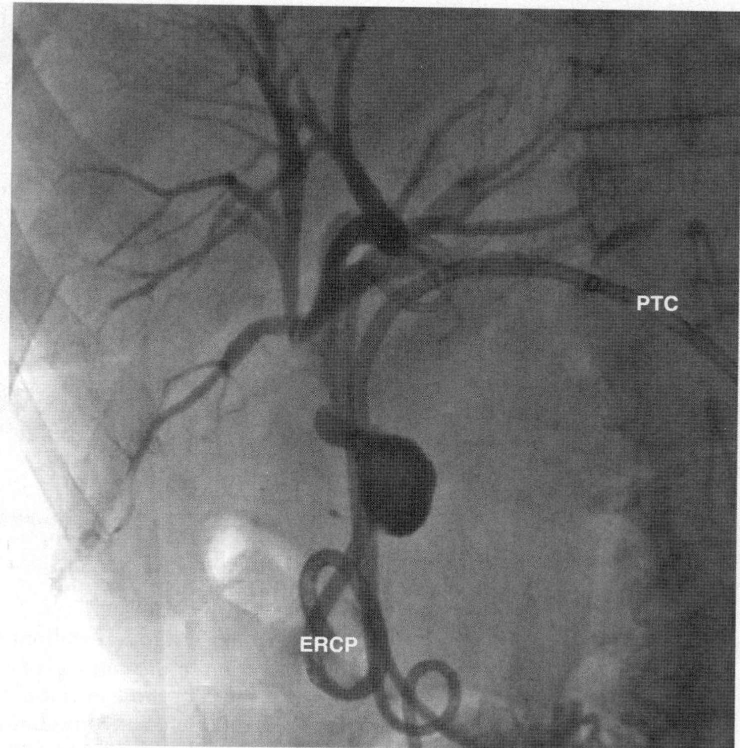

FIGURE 54-42 PTC catheter (PTC) traversing common bile duct iatrogenic injury. This catheter was used to guide ERCP stenting (ERCP) in a poor operative candidate with iatrogenic injury but common bile duct continuity.

complication, management is highly successful and restores health-related quality of life scores to preinjury levels.[21]

Lost Stones

In the era of laparoscopic cholecystectomy, inadvertent opening of the gallbladder with spillage of stones is not infrequent, occurring in 20% to 40% of cholecystectomies. Risk factors for intraoperative perforation of the gallbladder include cholecystitis, presence of pigmented stones, number of stones (>15), and performance of the operation by surgical resident. Unfortunately, stones lost during a cholecystectomy can have significant and even substantially delayed consequences, such as chronic abscess, fistula, wound infection, and bowel obstruction. Most dropped stones settle into Morison pouch or the retrohepatic space along the abdominal wall, which may develop into a chronic abscess in this location. The likelihood for development of complications from lost stones is difficult to quantify because surgeon documentation of gallbladder perforation is variable and a substantial delay frequently exists between cholecystectomy and complication from lost stones. On the basis of available studies, lost stones do not necessitate conversion to an open operation; treatment should include extensive irrigation, significant attempt to retrieve lost stones, course of antibiotics, documentation of the perforation in the operative notes, and clear communication with the patient of the small possibility of delayed presentation from erosion or abscess.[22]

Postcholecystectomy Pain

Although unusual, pain similar to biliary colic may persist or recur after cholecystectomy. A thorough evaluation of the biliary tree should be undertaken after cholecystectomy if the pain recurs. Recurrence of pain, if it is associated with other system findings of jaundice, fever, or chills within days to weeks after cholecystectomy, suggests a secondary choledocholithiasis or a bile leak. Other biliary tree phenomena may cause a similar picture, such as sphincter of Oddi dysfunction. Postoperative bile duct strictures, which usually are manifested with jaundice, are generally identified within the first year after cholecystectomy and may be manifested with pain or fever if only one lobar duct is obstructed. In the setting of a normal liver panel, other causes of right upper quadrant pain should be investigated.

Retained Biliary Stones

Retained common bile duct stones, or secondary common duct stones, can be identified for up to 2 years after cholecystectomy. Secondary common duct stones, which, by definition, originate in the gallbladder and pass into the common duct, are usually cholesterol stones and frequently become symptomatic within weeks of a cholecystectomy. Patients will complain of sharp right upper quadrant pain, with jaundice. Fever, completing Charcot triad, is also common. Hyperbilirubinemia and an elevated alkaline phosphatase level should raise the suspicion of a retained stone. Ultrasound may not show intrahepatic biliary ductal dilation if the stone does not fully occlude the duct or the obstruction is early. Endoscopic removal of these stones through a generous sphincterotomy is almost universally successful (Fig. 54-43).

Biliary Leak

After a cholecystectomy, patients may suffer a leak from the cystic duct or an unrecognized duct of Luschka. Fever, chills, right upper quadrant pain, jaundice, leakage of bile from an incision or into a drain, or persistent anorexia or bloating should raise the

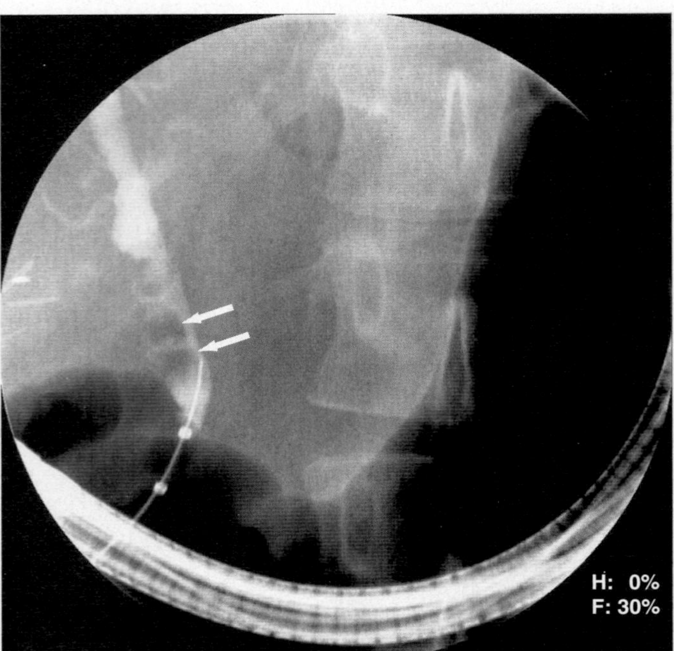

FIGURE 54-43 ERCP showing multiple retained common bile duct stones *(arrows).*

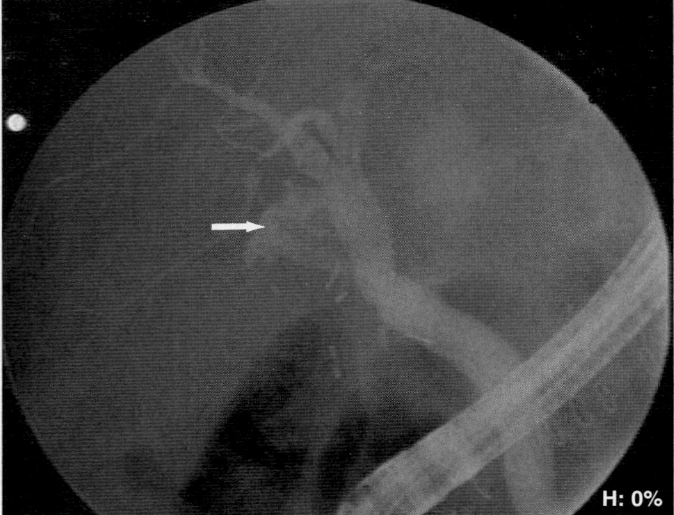

FIGURE 54-44 ERCP showing cystic duct stump leak *(arrow).*

suspicion of a bile leak. Although it can be seen after any cholecystectomy, those performed for acute cholecystitis carry the greatest risk. With inflammation and fibrosis around an obstructed cystic duct, clips placed on the duct may not fully occlude it or may be dislodged as the inflammatory process resolves. Patients will generally present within 1 week of cholecystectomy as the bile collects and becomes clinically manifested. On presentation, CT should be performed and will show ascites or a right upper quadrant fluid collection consistent with a biloma. Not only is reexploration in this setting unsuccessful, but it further complicates later reconstruction attempts that may be necessary. Endoscopic cholangiography should be performed, with percutaneous drainage of any fluid collections (Fig. 54-44). If the leak is from a cystic duct stump, sphincterotomy with stenting of the common duct

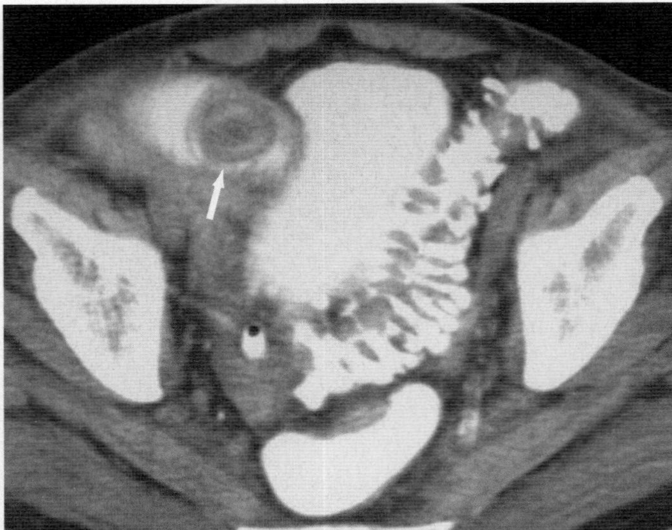

FIGURE 54-45 CT scan of stone *(arrow)* obstructing distal ileum.

will allow the leak to seal without need for surgical management.[20] Reexploration in this setting is reserved for patients with evidence of septic shock or those in whom the leakage is not percutaneously accessible. If percutaneous drainage is not feasible because of overlying bowel or the fluid is not localized and thus not amenable to percutaneous drainage, a laparoscopic washout of the abdomen and placement of subhepatic drains should be considered. No attempt should be made to fix the leak because any such intervention is almost always unsuccessful and carries a risk of further injury to the biliary tree. Persistence of a bile leak after longer than 6 weeks should raise the suspicion of an unrecognized bile duct injury, thus mandating complete cholangiography by MRCP and repeated ERCP. Similar to common bile duct injuries, surgical treatment of a duct leak is most successful once the inflammatory process has resolved.

Gallstone Ileus

Obstruction of the intestinal lumen from a gallstone carries the misnomer gallstone ileus, which is, in fact, a mechanical blockage. In order for a stone of sufficient size to obstruct the intestine, a large stone in the dependent portion of the gallbladder that has fistulized into the adjacent duodenum passes directly into the intestine. Most of these fistulas occur in older patients and may be caused by inflammation in the gallbladder or simply pressure necrosis. The blockage can be anywhere in the small intestine but occurs most commonly in the distal ileum as the ileum tapers before entering the cecum.

Presentation and diagnosis. Patients will present with clinical evidence of a mechanical small bowel obstruction in the absence of surgical history or hernias. A history of symptoms referable to the biliary tree is variable. Although most patients will have constant pain from the obstruction, others can present with only episodic discomfort because the gallstone only intermittently obstructs the intestinal tract. The most common site of stone impaction is in the distal ileum, a few centimeters proximal to the ileocecal valve, where the caliber of the ileum decreases (Fig. 54-45). Plain radiographs demonstrate air-fluid levels consistent with a small bowel obstruction, although the offending stone may or may not be identified. Pneumobilia, which may be identified only by CT scan, is a ubiquitous finding because the fistula that

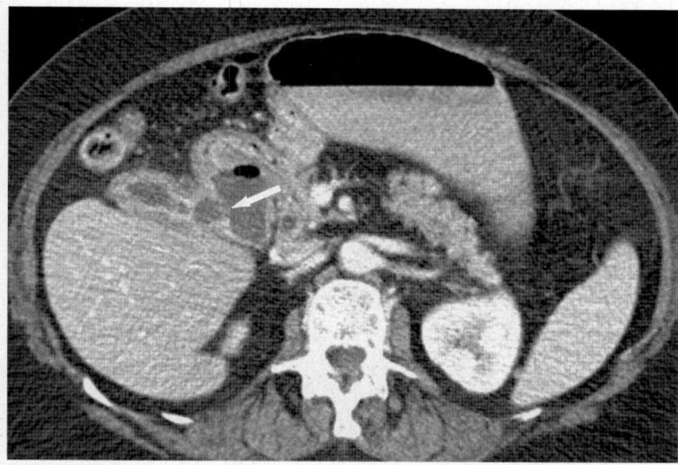

FIGURE 54-46 CT scan of cholecystoduodenal fistula *(arrow)*.

permitted a stone to pass into the duodenum allows air into the gallbladder and biliary tree (Fig. 54-46).

Treatment. Exploration and enterotomy are required to relieve the obstruction. A longitudinal incision is made on the antimesenteric border of the ileum, a few centimeters proximal to the impacted stone. The stone can then be milked back through the enterotomy. The site of impaction is at risk for ischemia and pressure necrosis, with eventual perforation. Therefore, any suggestion of nonviability of this region mandates resection. The remainder of the small intestine should be inspected because approximately 10% of patients will have multiple large stones that have passed through the fistula. Although some surgeons advocate surgical treatment of the biliary-enteric fistula at the same setting, the intense inflammatory process in the right upper quadrant may complicate the cholecystectomy and duodenal repair. In addition, because most of these patients are older, their overall physiologic status may not permit fistula repair in the emergent setting. One-stage repair should generally be performed in healthy patients without severe inflammatory changes in the right upper quadrant. Enterotomy with removal of the offending stone should suffice for patients with multiple comorbidities. Palpation of the remaining small intestine should be performed to exclude a second stone that could reobstruct the ileum. A second operation for the cholecystectomy can be considered to avoid the possibility of future biliary complications.

Acute Cholangitis

Acute cholangitis is due to an acute, ascending bacterial infection of the biliary tree caused by an obstruction. Although stones are a common cause, ascending cholangitis can be seen with any obstructing phenomenon, including a malignant neoplasm. The two absolute requirements for the development of acute cholangitis are bacteria in the biliary tree and obstruction of flow, with increased intraluminal pressure. The source of bactibilia in patients with acute cholangitis is unclear because culture of most bile is sterile. With obstruction from a stone, bactibilia can be identified in up to 90% of patients. The most common pathogens include *Klebsiella, E. coli, Enterobacter, Pseudomonas,* and *Citrobacter* spp.

The classic presentation of cholangitis is that of Charcot triad, with fever, jaundice, and right upper quadrant pain. All three findings are seen in less than 50% of patients, with jaundice being the most variable. When the infection begins to be manifested with shock, the two additional findings of mental status changes and hypotension join Charcot triad to become Reynolds pentad. With the acute obstruction of a visceral tubular structure, the pain can be severe but is not usually associated with abdominal tenderness.

Diagnosis. As with any severe intra-abdominal infection, tachycardia and manifestations of shock are not uncommon. Leukocytosis with an abnormal liver panel is common. Hepatocellular injury from the infection and inflammation elevate serum transaminase and alkaline phosphatase levels. Ultrasound should be the first screening test and will commonly show dilation of the biliary tree. HIDA scans should be interpreted with caution because infection of the biliary tree reduces the secretion of these agents into the biliary tree. CT can be helpful in identifying the site of obstruction although not always the cause. Cholangiography through ERCP or PTC is critical not only to diagnosis but also to therapy. These two modalities can usually identify the location and cause of obstruction, drain the biliary tree, and obtain culture and biopsy specimens of a lesion if necessary.

Treatment. Acute cholangitis is a severe medical condition that can progress quickly to septic shock and death. Adequate hydration and IV antibiotics should be started immediately. Many patients will respond to medical therapy, so prompt diagnostic measures should be taken to identify the location and cause of obstruction. Others, however, will not respond to medical therapy and will progress to shock. These patients require emergent decompression of the biliary tree. Historically, this could be achieved only through a surgical route, with high morbidity and mortality. Endoscopic or percutaneous drainage achieves the same goal with less morbidity. Removal of the stone can be accomplished by endoscopic means, thus providing an advantage over percutaneous methods, which simply decompress the obstructed biliary tree. If endoscopic and percutaneous means are unavailable or unsuccessful, surgical drainage consists of common duct exploration with placement of a T tube. Given the unstable nature of the patient, definitive surgical treatment of the cause is deferred until the patient is stabilized, the cholangitis is treated, and the diagnosis is confirmed.

Recurrent Pyogenic Cholangitis

Recurrent pyogenic cholangitis is caused by cholangiohepatitis or intrahepatic stones and is usually found in East Asian populations. Biliary pathogens such as *Clonorchis sinensis* and *Ascaris lumbricoides* populate the biliary tree. These and other pathogens secrete an enzyme that hydrolyzes water-soluble bilirubin glucuronides to form free bilirubin, which then precipitates to form brown pigment stones. These stones may partially or fully obstruct the biliary tree, causing recurrent episodes of cholangitis and eventually abscesses or even cirrhosis. The chronicity of the infection and inflammation places these patients at risk for the development of cholangiocarcinoma. It is unclear whether the primary inciting event is infection causing inflammatory stricture or inflammatory stricture with subsequent infection of stagnant bile.

Presentation. Recurrent pyogenic cholangitis tends to occur in the third to fourth decade of life, affecting men and women equally. The clinical presentation is that of cholangitis with fever, right upper quadrant pain, and jaundice. Because the infection, inflammation, and stones commonly present in a segmental or lobar pattern, the jaundice tends to be mild. Serum studies are similar to other causes of cholangitis, with a leukocytosis and elevated bilirubin and high alkaline phosphatase levels. Diagnosis is usually made by a combination of CT or MRCP with ERCP

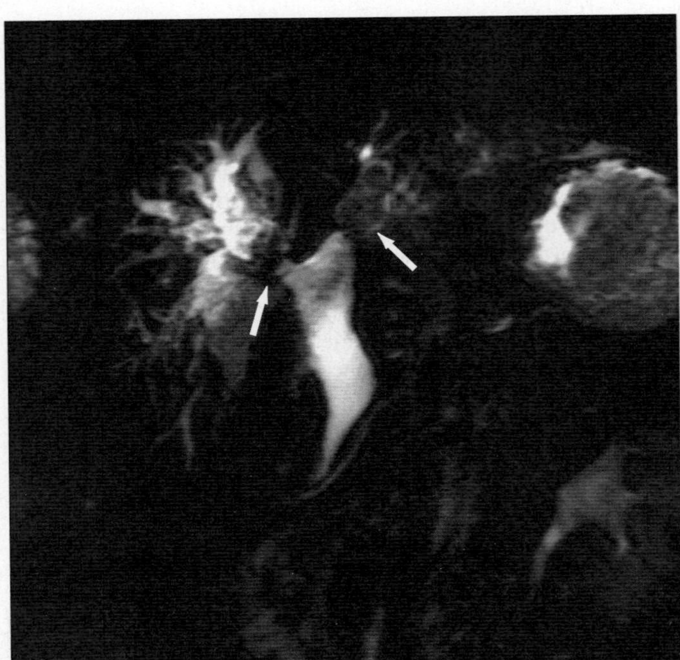

FIGURE 54-47 MRCP of recurrent pyogenic cholangitis. Intraluminal filling defects from stones are noted in both lobes *(arrows)*.

(Fig. 54-47). Lobar or segmental atrophy or hypertrophy may be seen in chronic cases.

Treatment. In the setting of an acute attack, conservative treatment with parenteral antibiotics, IV fluids, and analgesics will usually suffice. Failure of this approach, with clinical deterioration, mandates biliary drainage by ERCP or percutaneous methods. Once the attack has subsided, a thorough investigation of biliary tree anatomy will help direct treatment. Definitive operative treatment is almost always required. The goals of surgical therapy are threefold: (1) remove all stones; (2) bypass, enlarge, or resect the strictures; and (3) provide adequate biliary drainage. The variability of presentation and location of disease has spurred the development of a number of operations to achieve these goals. The presence of intrahepatic strictures connotes a complicated case and may warrant resection, stricturoplasty, or hepaticocutaneous jejunostomy. When clearance of all stones is not possible or future need for endoscopic therapy is anticipated, the terminal end of the Roux limb for a hepaticojejunostomy can be brought out as a stoma to provide easy access for choledochoscopy. Given the risk of cholangiocarcinoma, disease affecting predominantly one lobe should be resected in patients with adequate hepatic reserve. In the absence of the development of cholangiocarcinoma, surgical management is highly successful.[23]

Noncalculous Biliary Disease

Acute Acalculous Cholecystitis

Any blockage of the cystic duct is known as acute cholecystitis. When this occurs in the absence of stones, the diagnosis is acute acalculous cholecystitis. Although the exact pathophysiologic mechanism is poorly understood, concentration of biliary solutes and stasis in the gallbladder clearly play important roles. Risk factors for the development of acalculous cholecystitis include older age, critical illness, burns, trauma, prolonged use of total parenteral nutrition, diabetes, and immunosuppression. The disease process is generally more fulminant than that of calculous cholecystitis and may progress to gangrene and perforation of the gallbladder.

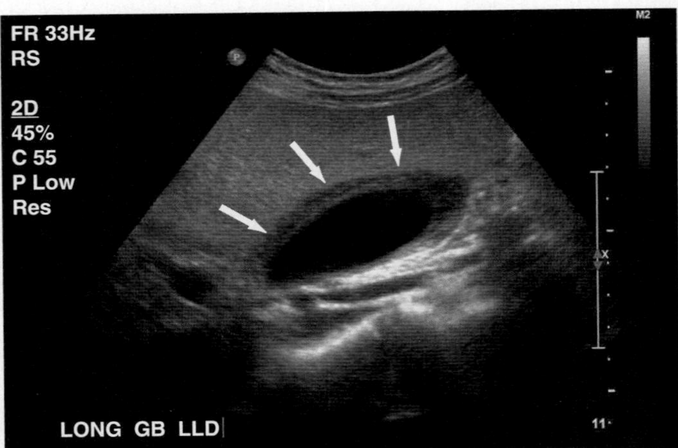

FIGURE 54-48 Ultrasound image of gallbladder with acute acalculous cholecystitis. The diffusely thickened gallbladder wall *(arrows)* is highly suggestive of cholecystitis.

The presentation of acalculous cholecystitis can be similar to that of calculous disease, with fever, anorexia, and right upper quadrant pain. Because many of these patients are critically ill, history may be impossible to obtain and the physical examination may be unreliable. The workup of fever in the intensive care patient may reveal a thickened gallbladder wall, with pericholecystic fluid (Fig. 54-48). HIDA scans may make the diagnosis but can have a false-positive rate of up to 40%.

Treatment of acalculous cholecystitis is similar to that of calculous cholecystitis, with cholecystectomy being therapeutic. Given the substantial inflammation and high risk of gallbladder gangrene, an open procedure is generally preferred. However, many of these patients are critically ill and would not tolerate the physiologic insult of a laparotomy, explaining why the mortality rate of cholecystectomy for acalculous cholecystitis is up to 40%. Accordingly, percutaneous drainage of the distended and inflamed gallbladder is carried out in patients unable to tolerate a laparotomy. The cholecystostomy tube used to drain the gallbladder can be placed by ultrasound or CT guidance. Approximately 90% of patients will improve with percutaneous drainage, and the tube can eventually be removed. If follow-up imaging continues to demonstrate no stones, interval cholecystectomy is generally unnecessary.

Primary Sclerosing Cholangitis

Primary sclerosing cholangitis (PSC) is an idiopathic, likely autoimmune process affecting the intrahepatic and extrahepatic biliary trees. Although the cause is unknown, it is associated with other autoimmune diseases, such as ulcerative colitis and Riedel thyroiditis. As its name suggests, the disease causes inflammation and scarring in the biliary tree and must be distinguished from secondary sclerosing cholangitis, which involves a similar clinical picture but has an identifiable cause, such as malignant neoplasm, infection, or ischemia. The disease of PSC is characterized by progressive chronic cholestasis and advances at an unpredictable rate to biliary cirrhosis and eventually death from liver failure. Although historically the diagnosis was made only in the late stages of disease, understanding of the disease as well as increased frequency of liver function analyses and increased use of ERCP has contributed to earlier diagnosis, frequently in the asymptomatic phase.

The microscopic picture is one of inflammation, fibrosis, and cholestasis. In the absence of previous biliary manipulation, acute ascending cholangitis is uncommon in patients presenting with PSC.

Clinical presentation. The presentation of PSC is variable, but most patients present with fatigue, pruritus, and jaundice. This symptom complex spurs the physician to perform ERCP, although many patients have symptoms for 12 to 24 months before the diagnosis is made. The abnormalities seen on cholangiography confirm the diagnosis. Asymptomatic elevations of alkaline phosphatase levels can also occur and may be associated with evidence of hepatocellular injury and hyperbilirubinemia before clinical manifestations of symptoms. Abnormal liver function tests in a patient observed for inflammatory bowel disease should suggest PSC. Elevation of perinuclear antineutrophil cytoplasmic antibodies can be seen in 80% of patients. Disease severity does not correlate with perinuclear antineutrophil cytoplasmic antibody titer.

ERCP is the preferred route for cholangiography and can demonstrate the characteristic multifocal, diffusely distributed dilations and strictures of the intrahepatic and extrahepatic biliary trees. The sequential stricturing, proximal dilation, and more proximal stricturing create a pattern described as beading or chain of lakes. PTC is frequently unsuccessful because the proximal ducts are both fibrosed and generally not dilated. Other cholangiographic findings include multiple diverticulum-like outpouchings of the bile ducts and multiple short-segment strictures. MRCP can also be useful for diagnosis and monitoring of disease but does not allow interventions that may be necessary, such as brushing, balloon dilation, or stenting (Fig. 54-49). Liver biopsy tends to show an onionskin concentric periductal fibrosis. With disease progression, periportal fibrosis occurs, progressing to bridging necrosis and eventually biliary cirrhosis. Unfortunately, PSC is associated with cholangiocarcinoma, and distinguishing the strictures of PSC fibrosis from those of cholangiocarcinoma can be challenging.

Treatment. No specific effective medical therapy exists for PSC. Although some experimental trials of ursodeoxycholic acid have shown improvement in liver function test results and histologic appearance compared with controls, this did not result in any significant clinical improvement in the long term. Early in the disease, with mild symptoms, observation is a reasonable approach. Intervention must be specifically tailored to the pattern of disease and its clinical manifestations. Medical therapies are generally targeted to the underlying hepatobiliary disease process; these include choleretic agents such as ursodeoxycholic acid, immunosuppressive agents, and antifibrogenic agents such as colchicine. However, none of these agents has shown a consistent benefit. In the symptomatic patient, endoscopic therapy, consisting of balloon dilation of the dominant strictures, has been shown to alleviate pruritus, to reduce likelihood of cholangitis, and even to prolong survival.

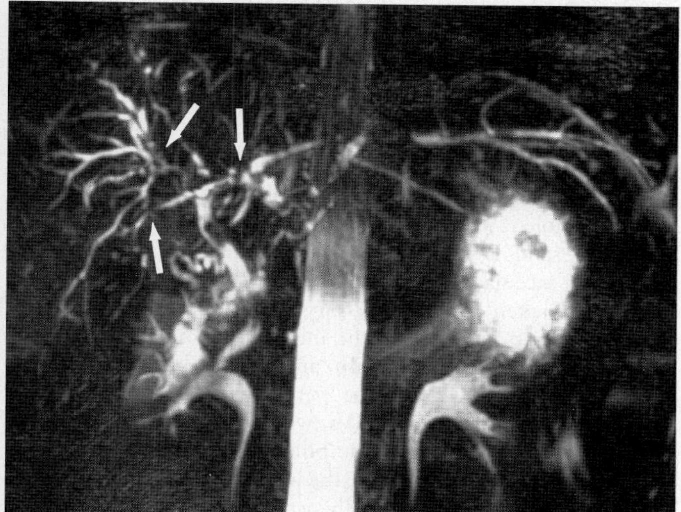

FIGURE 54-49 MRCP showing primary sclerosing cholangitis. Note the multilevel strictures *(arrows)*.

With the lack of effective, durable medical therapy in this progressive and ultimately fatal disease, an aggressive surgical approach is advocated. Options include biliary reconstructive procedures and liver transplantation. Although it is associated with ulcerative colitis, proctocolectomy does not appear to affect biliary disease progression or survival in patients with both ulcerative colitis and PSC. Biliary reconstruction is an option for patients with a dominant stricture at the hepatic bifurcation, for which resection of this region with long-term Silastic stenting can be performed. With increased success of orthotopic liver transplantation, the use of biliary reconstructive procedures has decreased.

Orthotopic liver transplantation appears to be the only lifesaving option for patients with progressive hepatic dysfunction from PSC. The survival rate for patients undergoing liver transplantation for PSC is approximately equivalent to that of those undergoing transplantation for other noninfectious end-stage liver disease causes, with 5-year survival rates ranging from 75% to 85%.[24] Although the development of cholangiocarcinoma in a PSC liver is generally considered a contraindication to transplantation, some centers have shown excellent survival rates, up to 70% at 5 years, for patients with limited disease localized within the liver who undergo an extensive neoadjuvant protocol of chemotherapy and radiation followed by transplantation.[25] Because these results have not been reproduced universally, the use of liver transplantation for the treatment of cholangiocarcinoma occurring in the setting of PSC is limited to experimental protocols. After liver transplantation, many PSC patients develop strictures, raising the possibility of recurrence of disease in the donor liver. Biopsy may show identical findings to the original disease, but this is obviously complicated by the possibility of development of secondary sclerosing cholangitis from ischemia, infection, or rejection. Even with the development of strictures, disease progression does not usually follow the aggressive course for which PSC is known.

Biliary Strictures

Benign strictures of the bile duct have a number of causes and generally affect the extrahepatic biliary tree, although cholangiohepatitis can create intrahepatic biliary strictures as well. Any inflammatory process occurring along the length of the common bile duct can cause a stricture. For example, the fibrotic inflammatory process of chronic pancreatitis can create a stricture of the intrapancreatic portion of the bile duct. The cholangiographic pattern of this stricture is that of a long (2 to 4 cm), smooth, gradually tapered narrowing affecting the distal common bile duct.

Strictures may occur in the middle portion of the common duct and are frequently associated with a process in the gallbladder. Any inflammatory process involving the gallbladder and cystic duct can secondarily inflame the common bile duct, causing an obstruction. Alternatively, a large stone in Hartmann pouch

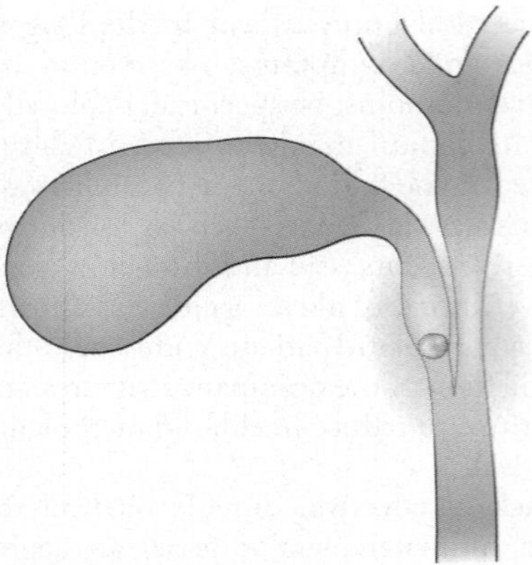

FIGURE 54-50 **Mirizzi Syndrome.** Obstruction of the bile duct from an inflammatory process is the hallmark of this syndrome; the cholecystocholedochal fistula may or may not be apparent.

can compress the adjacent bile duct and cause an apparent stricture. Both of these fall under the diagnosis of Mirizzi syndrome (Fig. 54-50). The prerequisites for this syndrome, characterized by gallbladder disease causing obstructive jaundice, include a cystic duct that courses parallel to the common hepatic duct, an impacted stone in the gallbladder neck or cystic duct, and an obstruction of the common hepatic duct caused by the stone or inflammatory response. The resultant inflammation can cause a cholecystocholedochal fistula. The treatment of Mirizzi syndrome is cholecystectomy, which may require repair of the common duct; when a large fistula exists, a choledochojejunostomy may be necessary.

Other strictures of the biliary tree include inflammatory strictures from long-standing choledocholithiasis, which tends to occur in the intrapancreatic portion of the bile duct, and stenosis of the sphincter of Oddi. ERCP with sphincterotomy, balloon dilation, and stent placement is generally regarded as primary treatment for benign bile duct strictures to make the diagnosis and potentially to treat the process. Endoscopic and percutaneous therapy can provide long-term success in more than 50% of patients. When this is unsuccessful, surgical management with anastomosis of the biliary tree to a Roux-en-Y jejunal limb has success rates of up to 90%.

Biliary Cysts

Cysts of the biliary tree are rare, occurring in fewer than 1/100,000 patients, but are more common in those of Asian descent and are three to eight times more common in women than in men. Biliary cysts, known as choledochal cysts, are considered a premalignant condition requiring surgical intervention. They are commonly diagnosed in infancy, but many present in adulthood. Although not proven, the commonly accepted theory of their pathogenesis relies on the presence of an anomalous pancreaticobiliary junction (APBJ; Figs. 54-51 and 54-52).

With APBJ, the pancreatic duct and biliary tree fuse to form a common channel before passage through the duodenal wall; APBJ is seen in up to 90% of patients with choledochal cysts. The fused duct forms a long common channel, which allows pancreatic secretions to reflux into the biliary tree. Because the pancreatic duct has higher secretory pressures than the biliary tree, exocrine pancreatic secretions reflux up into the bile duct and can inflame and damage the biliary tree, resulting in cystic degeneration.

The original classification for choledochal cysts by Alonso-Lej and colleagues has been modified by Todani and associates to

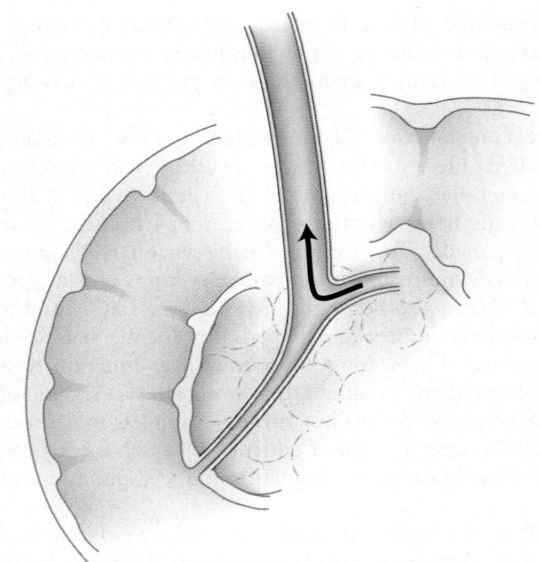

FIGURE 54-51 **Anomalous Pancreaticobiliary Junction.** With fusion of the common bile duct and pancreatic duct long before they pass through the duodenal wall, the pancreatic secretions can reflux into the common bile duct and may cause damage to the common duct through pressure or chemical injury.

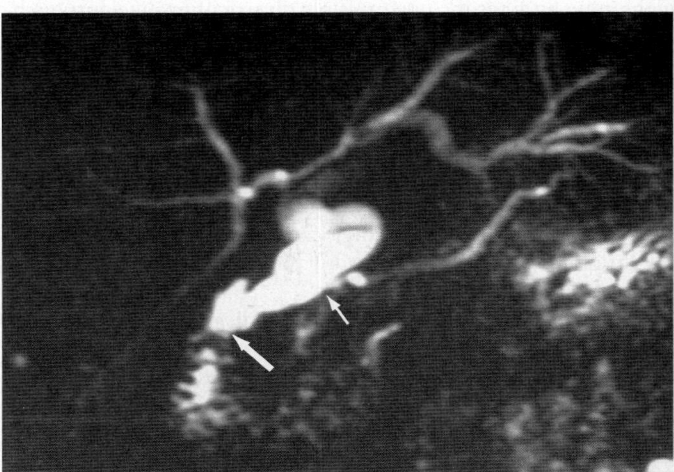

FIGURE 54-52 MRCP showing anomalous pancreaticobiliary junction with long common channel. The pancreatic duct fuses with the common bile duct *(slender arrow)*, and the common channel enters the duodenum *(bold arrow)*. Also noted in this illustration is the fusiform dilation of only the extrahepatic bile duct, as seen in a type I choledochal cyst.

include intrahepatic cystic disease (Fig. 54-53).[26] The most common choledochal cyst, type I, involves only the extrahepatic biliary tree and is generally a fusiform dilation. Type II cysts appear as a saccular diverticulum off the common bile duct and may be mistaken for an accessory gallbladder. Type III cysts appear as a cystic dilation of the intramural common bile duct, within the wall of the duodenum, and are also known as choledochoceles. Cysts involving the intrahepatic and extrahepatic biliary tree are known as type IVa, with type IVb being multiple cysts limited to the extrahepatic biliary tree. Type V cysts, also known as Caroli disease, involve the intrahepatic ducts only. Type V cysts may be solitary but usually occur diffusely in all segments. Although classified as a single disease, debate continues as to whether these constitute more than one pathologic entity.

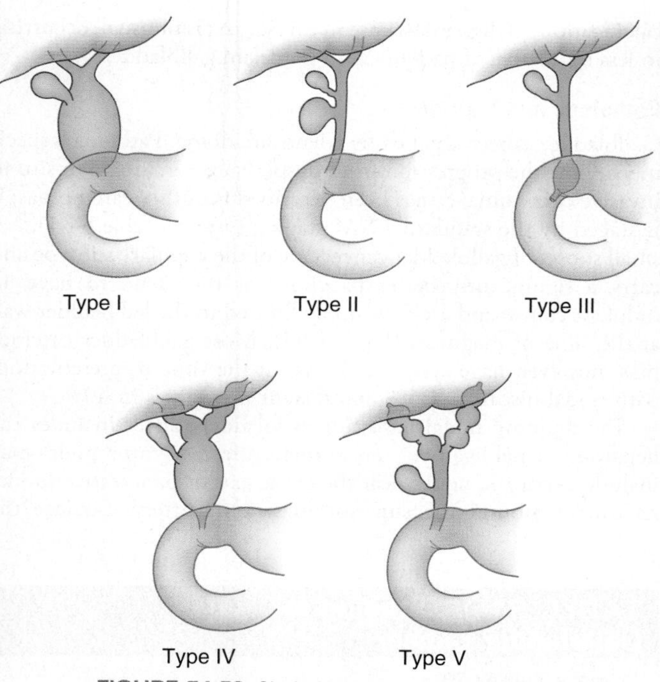

FIGURE 54-53 Choledochal cyst classification.

Presentation. The classic presentation of jaundice, right upper quadrant pain, and a palpable mass occurs rarely. Most patients have two of the three symptoms, with jaundice being the most consistent symptom, before undergoing any diagnostic imaging. Other symptoms include nausea, pruritus, and weight loss. Long-standing disease can induce a chronic injury to the liver with cirrhosis. Cholangitis, pancreatitis, hepatic fibrosis, and malignant disease have all been reported at the time of presentation. An unusual presentation is that of acute rupture of the cyst, with subsequent bile peritonitis.

Most cystic biliary lesions are originally identified and subsequently diagnosed by imaging because the common presenting symptoms are nonspecific. With the current liberal use of CT, the diagnosis of a choledochal cyst is suspected, but it is further classified by MRCP. With a choledochal cyst, the upper biliary tree is difficult to fill and therefore to evaluate by a retrograde route. Accordingly, MRCP helps create a complete cholangiogram. The distal bile duct is difficult to analyze by MRCP, so ERCP is more useful for defining the distal biliary tree and pancreatic duct–bile duct junction. Laboratory studies may identify cholestasis and jaundice. In late stages of disease, secondary hepatic injury and evidence of cirrhosis may be seen.

Because choledochal cysts are a premalignant condition, the original presentation of a choledochal cyst may be that of cholangiocarcinoma. The incidence of malignant disease in patients with biliary cysts ranges from 10% to 30%. The pathogenesis appears to be one of a field defect because the entire biliary tree is at risk, even in nondilated portions of the biliary tract, and complete excision of a benign choledochal cyst does not eliminate the risk of subsequent cholangiocarcinoma development. Malignant cyst degeneration is common and is thought to relate to chronic mucosal irritation from the refluxed pancreatic enzymes.

Treatment. Surgical management of choledochal cysts consists of resection of the entire cyst and appropriate surgical reconstruction. Historically, enteric drainage of the cyst was performed without resection, but this approach is complicated by recurrent

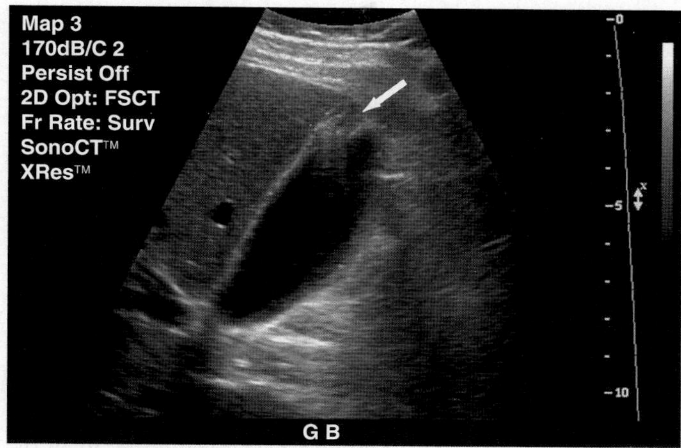

FIGURE 54-54 Ultrasound image of adenomyomatosis. Seen in the fundus of the gallbladder is a sessile thickening *(arrow)* with smaller microcysts within it, consistent with adenomyomatosis.

biliary stasis, infection, and development of malignancy. Type I cysts are treated by complete surgical excision, cholecystectomy, and Roux-en-Y hepaticojejunostomy. The proximal extent of resection should continue to the nondilated biliary tree and may require anastomosis to the left and right hepatic ducts. If there is substantial pericyst fibrosis, an intramural plane can be developed to excise the entire epithelium while leaving the fibrotic outer cyst wall in place. The distal duct is oversewn, with care taken not to injure the pancreatic duct. Type II cysts should be excised entirely, and in the presence of an APBJ, biliary-enteric diversion by Roux-en-Y hepaticojejunostomy is appropriate. Type III cysts are uncommon and may be approached transduodenally. Because the pathogenesis of type III cysts is not clear and may not involve APBJ, endoscopic drainage may suffice. In the setting of duodenal or biliary obstruction, transduodenal excision or sphincteroplasty can be performed. Surgical treatment of type IV cysts must be carefully individualized to the affected anatomy. Type IV cysts affecting only the extrahepatic bile ducts are managed similarly to type I cysts, with excision and hepaticojejunostomy. Those with intrahepatic extension involving only one lobe can be treated with partial hepatectomy and reconstruction. Surgical treatment of Caroli disease ranges from resection if the disease is unilobar to liver transplantation when diffuse disease is detected.

Polypoid Lesions of the Gallbladder

Benign masses of the gallbladder are common and consist of pseudotumors and adenomas. Pseudotumors are further divided into cholesterol polyps and adenomyomatosis. Cholesterol polyps appear as pedunculated echogenic lesions of the gallbladder, are usually smaller than 1 cm, and are frequently multiple. Alternatively, adenomyomatosis is seen as a sessile lesion, commonly in the fundus, with characteristic microcysts within the lesion, and is frequently larger than 1 cm (Fig. 54-54). Adenomas are benign growths in the wall of the gallbladder that may be difficult to differentiate from adenocarcinoma preoperatively because the only difference is that of transmural invasion, which can be challenging to detect by ultrasonography. Size larger than 10 mm is a risk factor for adenocarcinoma, along with growth, presence of gallstones, and age of the patient older than 60 years. The management of all symptomatic polypoid lesions of the gallbladder is laparoscopic cholecystectomy. Patients with a polypoid lesion and risk factors for adenocarcinoma or those suspected of having in situ or invasive cancer should undergo open cholecystectomy because perforation during laparoscopy may spread tumor cells throughout the peritoneal cavity. Asymptomatic lesions smaller than 10 mm with no other risk factors and no ultrasonographic features suggesting malignant disease can be observed with serial ultrasonography.

Benign Biliary Masses

Benign intraluminal growths of the biliary tree are unusual but mostly consist of adenomas. These lesions are soft fleshy growths occurring mostly in the periampullary bile duct arising from the glandular epithelium. The presentation is that of biliary obstruction, with jaundice and sometimes right upper quadrant pain. Treatment consists of complete resection with a small rim of normal epithelium because incomplete excision of affected epithelium carries a high risk of recurrence. These lesions occur in the periampullary duct, so a transduodenal approach can be used.

Inflammatory lesions of the biliary tree, known as pseudotumors or benign fibrosing disease, may be mistaken for cholangiocarcinoma. When this process follows surgical intervention on the biliary tree, the mass-like stricture may be the result of ischemia to the duct, with subsequent inflammation and fibrosis. Alternatively, pseudotumors may occur de novo; these commonly affect the extrahepatic biliary tree above the bifurcation.

MALIGNANT BILIARY DISEASE

Gallbladder Cancer

Gallbladder cancer is an aggressive malignant disease and carries an extremely poor prognosis. Patients have no specific presenting symptoms, and therefore presentation with late-stage disease is common. The poor prognosis corresponds to the high proportion of patients presenting with advanced disease. For patients with earlier stage disease, a more aggressive surgical approach is warranted.

Incidence

Gallbladder cancer generally is manifested in the sixth and seventh decades of life and is two to three times more common in women than in men. Ethnicity plays an important role in the development of gallbladder cancer, with the highest incidence in women from India and Pakistan. Among North American populations, Native Americans and immigrants from Latin America have the highest rates.

Cause

Although not proven scientifically, the prevailing theory of gallbladder cancer focuses on chronic inflammation with subsequent cellular proliferation. Therefore, the presence of gallstones is considered to be the primary risk factor, and larger stones (>3 cm) carry an increased risk of cancer development. More than 80% of patients with gallbladder cancer have cholelithiasis, and gallbladder cancer is approximately seven times more common in patients with gallstones than in those without stones. The type of stone does not correlate with incidence of gallbladder cancer. Other risk factors include entities that may also cause inflammation in the gallbladder wall, such as APBJ, choledochal cysts, and PSC.

Extensive calcification of the wall of the gallbladder can cause a brittle gallbladder wall, leading to what is termed porcelain gallbladder, and carries a risk of cancer development, as does the presence of a gallbladder polyp larger than 10 mm. Whereas the risk of gallbladder cancer is higher in patients with gallbladder wall calcification, malignant disease in this setting is unusual, occurring in less than 10% of patients with porcelain gallbladder.[27]

Pathology and Staging

Gallbladder cancer is generally adenocarcinoma. Pathologic specimens show the progression from dysplasia to carcinoma in situ to invasive carcinoma, as has been described for other carcinomas; it is staged by the standard TNM staging system (Table 54-1).[28] A small subset of gallbladder cancers are of the papillary subtype and carry a significantly better prognosis as they tend to have an indolent course and are commonly limited to the gallbladder wall at the time of diagnosis (Fig. 54-55). Most gallbladder carcinomas, however, have systemic disease at the time of presentation, with nodal disease in 35% and distant metastases in 40%.

The draining nodal basin for gallbladder cancer includes the hepatoduodenal ligament. From there, affected lymph nodes may include periaortic nodes near the celiac axis or pancreaticoduodenal nodes around the superior mesenteric artery. Because the

TABLE 54-1 Staging for Gallbladder Cancer

Primary Tumor (T)			
TX	Primary tumor cannot be assessed		
T0	No evidence of primary tumor		
Tis	Carcinoma in situ		
T1	Tumor invades lamina propria or muscle layer		
T1a	Tumor invades lamina propria		
T1b	Tumor invades muscle layer		
T2	Tumor invades perimuscular connective tissue; no extension beyond serosa or into liver		
T3	Tumor perforates the serosa (visceral peritoneum) and/or directly invades the liver and/or one other adjacent organ or structure, such as the stomach, duodenum, colon, pancreas, omentum, or extrahepatic bile ducts		
T4	Tumor invades main portal vein or hepatic artery or invades two or more extrahepatic organs or structures		
Regional Lymph Nodes (N)			
NX	Regional lymph nodes cannot be assessed		
N0	No regional lymph node metastasis		
N1	Metastases to nodes along the cystic duct, common bile duct, hepatic artery, and/or portal vein		
N2	Metastases to periaortic, pericaval, superior mesenteric artery and/or celiac artery lymph nodes		
Distant Metastasis (M)			
M0	No distant metastasis		
M1	Distant metastasis		
Anatomic Stage and Prognostic Groups			
Stage 0	Tis	N0	M0
Stage I	T1	N0	M0
Stage II	T2	N0	M0
Stage IIIA	T3	N0	M0
Stage IIIB	T1-3	N1	M0
Stage IVA	T4	N0-1	M0
Stage IVB	Any T	N2	M0
	Any T	Any N	M1

From Edge SB, Byrd DR, Compton CC, et al, editors: *AJCC cancer staging manual*, ed 7, New York, 2010, Springer, pp 213–214.

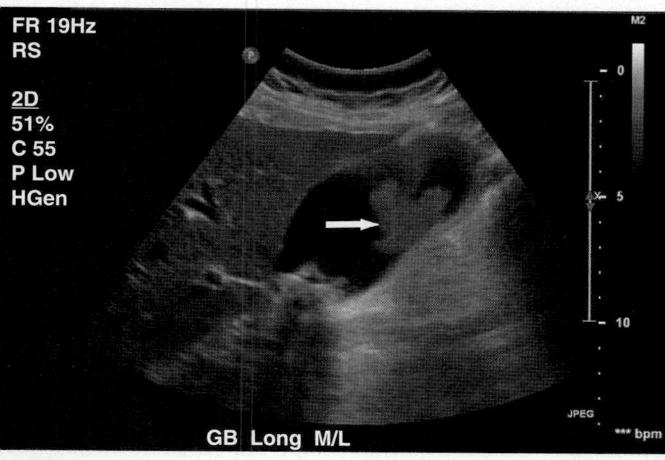

FIGURE 54-55 Ultrasound image showing intraluminal polypoid gallbladder wall mass *(arrow)* but without extraluminal extension.

venous drainage of the gallbladder includes direct venous tributaries into the liver parenchyma, these tumors may spread directly into segment IV of the liver. Transperitoneal spread is also common and can progress to carcinomatosis.

Clinical Presentation

Because 90% of gallbladder cancers originate in the fundus or body of the gallbladder, most do not produce symptoms until the disease is advanced (Fig. 54-56). Symptoms of acute cholecystitis, with obstruction of the neck of the gallbladder, may portend a better prognosis because patients with these symptoms may present with earlier stages of disease. Weight loss, jaundice, or an abdominal mass is associated with later stages of disease. Some patients describe symptoms of chronic cholecystitis in which the pain has recently changed in quality or frequency. Other common symptoms include chronic epigastric pain, early satiety, and a sense of fullness.

Diagnosis

Ultrasonography is generally the first examination used in the evaluation of right upper quadrant pain. Ultrasonographic findings of gallbladder cancer include an irregularly shaped lesion in the subhepatic space, heterogeneous mass in the gallbladder lumen, and asymmetrically thickened gallbladder wall (Fig. 54-57). The finding of a polyp larger than 10 mm should raise the suspicion of gallbladder cancer.

CT can be useful in the staging and therefore treatment of gallbladder cancer. Although the sensitivity of CT for detection of direct extension into the liver is poor, CT can demonstrate peritoneal metastases, hepatic parenchymal metastases, lymphadenopathy, and adjacent vascular involvement (Fig. 54-58). Cholangiography can help delineate the location of obstruction in patients with gallbladder cancer, but most of these patients are incurable. Triphasic CT can be used to identify hepatic arterial or portal venous involvement. In the setting of unresectability (portal vein encasement or extensive hepatic involvement) or incurability (hepatic or peritoneal metastases), percutaneous methods for confirmatory tissue diagnosis should be used.

Treatment

Resection of gallbladder cancer remains the only potential for cure. Patients with gallbladder cancer can be divided into four specific subgroups of presentation: patients with an incidental

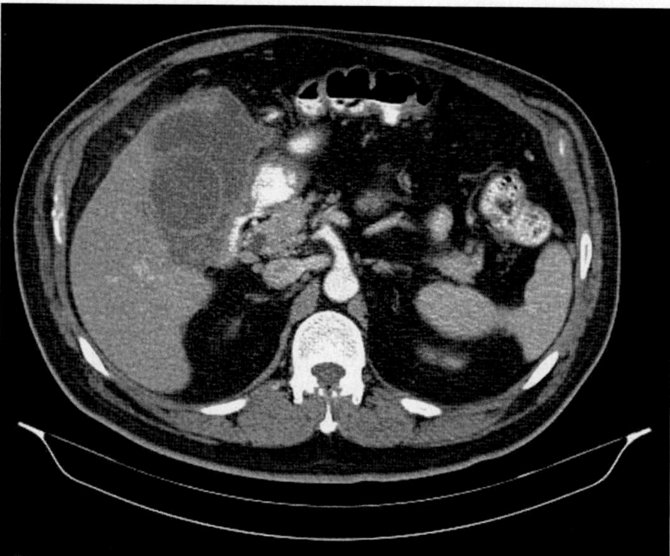

FIGURE 54-56 CT scan showing gallbladder cancer with invasion into the duodenum and liver parenchyma.

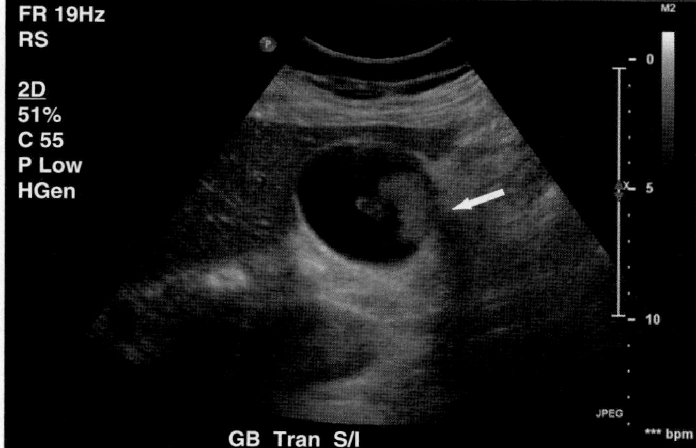

FIGURE 54-57 Ultrasound image of gallbladder mass with loss of continuity of gallbladder wall *(arrow)*, suggesting extraluminal growth.

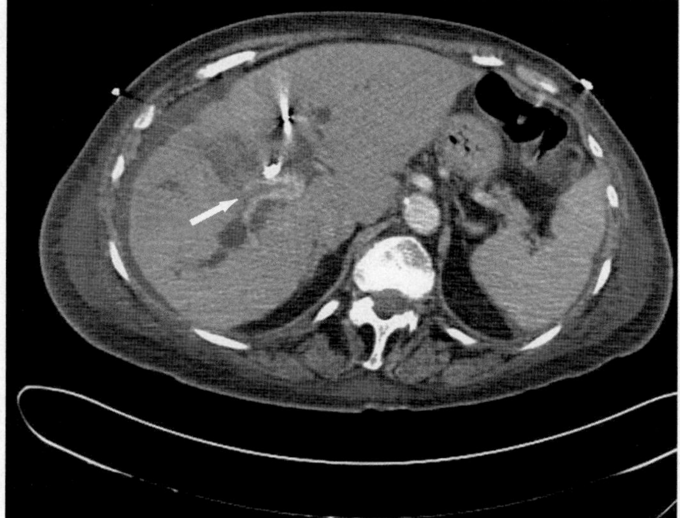

FIGURE 54-58 CT scan showing gallbladder mass with local invasion into portal vein *(arrow)*.

polyp on imaging, patients with an incidental finding of gallbladder cancer at the time of or after cholecystectomy, patients suspected of having gallbladder cancer preoperatively, and patients with advanced disease at presentation.

Patients with incidental findings

Gallbladder polyp. Because gallbladder polyps larger than 10 mm carry an increased risk of malignancy, cholecystectomy is the treatment of choice. It should be performed through an open approach because laparoscopic perforation in the setting of cancer may convert a potentially curable disease into an incurable one.

Gallbladder cancer after cholecystectomy. With the finding of carcinoma after cholecystectomy, subsequent treatment depends on depth of penetration of the gallbladder wall and surgical margins. With T1a lesions, in which the carcinoma penetrates the lamina propria but does not invade the muscle layer, cholecystectomy should suffice for therapy. The likelihood of nodal disease in this setting is less than 3%. For those penetrating the muscularis but not the deeper connective tissue or serosa, classified as T1b lesions, cholecystectomy is sufficient as long as the margins are negative. With T1b lesions and perineural, lymphatic, or vascular invasion, the likelihood of nodal disease increases significantly, and therefore an extended cholecystectomy is indicated. The extended cholecystectomy is directed at obtaining an R0 resection of the disease, including the draining lymph node basins. Therefore, removal of the pericholedochal, periportal, hepatoduodenal, right celiac, and posterior pancreaticoduodenal lymph nodes should be included. Resection of the cystic duct margin to uninvolved mucosa may require resection of the common bile duct with Roux-en-Y reconstruction. Because local extension into the hepatic parenchyma is common, 2 cm of apparently normal hepatic parenchyma from the gallbladder fossa is resected. As port site recurrences have been reported for patients with even in situ disease, all port sites should also be excised. In patients with T2 lesions, in which the cancer extends past the muscularis but not beyond the serosa, a similar approach with radical cholecystectomy is indicated because more than 40% of these patients have lymph node metastases and up to 25% have positive margins when treated with standard cholecystectomy alone. Because gallbladder cancer is generally unresponsive to other therapies, the presence of any residual disease after operative intervention predicts poor outcome.[29]

Patients suspected of having gallbladder cancer preoperatively. Patients in whom preoperative evaluation suggests possibly resectable gallbladder cancer without metastatic disease should be offered an attempt at resection, even though survival is poor compared with those found incidentally. These patients tend to present with advanced locoregional disease and may require an extended liver resection. Because surgical intervention provides the only potential for cure or prolongation of life, radical resection should be considered for adequate operative candidates. The operation begins with a diagnostic laparoscopy to identify small-volume peritoneal or hepatic metastases that would preclude a resection, thereby avoiding an unnecessary operation. In the setting of metastatic disease, nonoperative strategies should be used to palliate symptoms. Radical resection in the setting of T3 and T4 lesions includes at least segments IVB and V but more often requires a central hepatectomy, including all of segments IV, V, and VIII. If necessary to achieve R0 margin status, a right trisegmentectomy may be used. Direct extension of tumor into adjacent structures such as the hepatic flexure is not a contraindication to resection as long as negative margins can be obtained and all disease resected. Debulking without the possibility of complete resection has no role in the management of gallbladder cancer.

Patients with advanced disease at presentation. Many patients with gallbladder cancer will present with advanced disease, and therefore the goal of therapy is palliation of symptoms. Common symptoms requiring palliation include jaundice, pain, and intestinal obstruction. Jaundice can be managed by endoscopic biliary stenting, and self-expanding endobiliary metal stents can provide a durable solution, with less need for repeated interventions than with plastic stents. Pain is generally treated with oral narcotics but may progress to require parenteral opioids in the hospice setting. Percutaneous neurolysis of the celiac ganglion can help with the palliation of pain. Intestinal obstruction is usually gastric outlet obstruction from local extension of tumor and is generally managed by an endoscopic duodenal wall stent. Unfortunately, neither chemotherapy nor radiation therapy has shown a survival benefit in the management of gallbladder cancer.

Survival

Survival of patients diagnosed with gallbladder cancer is dependent on the stage of disease at presentation and whether surgical resection is performed. Independent factors affecting survival include T status, N status, histologic differentiation, and common bile duct involvement. Advances in surgical management and extent of resection have led to improvements in survival in surgical patients, although most patients present with late-stage disease and are not candidates for resection. Patients with T1a lesions, limited to the mucosa and lamina propria, have an excellent prognosis. Complete resection of T1b lesions to negative margins also affords an excellent prognosis. Survival of patients with T2 lesions depends on nodal status, and radical resection in this setting improves 5-year survival from approximately 20% to more than 60%. The 5-year survival of patients with T3 tumors is less than 20%, and patients with T4 lesions have a survival measured in months. Patients with metastatic disease at presentation have a median survival of 13 months. Because most patients with gallbladder cancer present with advanced disease, the overall survival of gallbladder cancer is less than 15%.

Bile Duct Cancer

Cholangiocarcinoma is a rare disease entity that carries a dismal prognosis. Historically, evaluation and management of cholangiocarcinoma required arbitrary division of the bile duct into thirds based on the location of obstruction. Lesions of the middle third, however, are decidedly rare, so investigations have recently focused on perihilar and intrahepatic lesions, known as proximal lesions, versus those involving the periampullary region, known as distal disease. More than two thirds of all cholangiocarcinomas involve the proximal biliary tree near the bifurcation, known as Klatskin tumor.

Risk Factors

Although most patients with cholangiocarcinoma have no identifiable cause, the risk of development of cholangiocarcinoma appears to correlate with chronic inflammation in the biliary tree and compensatory cellular proliferation. Therefore, many predisposing disease states carry an increased risk for development of cholangiocarcinoma. Congenital lesions, such as choledochal cysts, predispose to the development of cholangiocarcinoma from exposure of the biliary epithelium to toxic pancreatic secretions. Cholangiocarcinoma is more prevalent in Southeast Asia, where infection with the liver flukes *Clonorchis sinensis* and *Opisthorchis viverrini* creates chronic biliary inflammation, with obstructions and strictures. Recurrent pyogenic cholangitis is characterized by primary bile duct stone formation with infections and carries a risk of cholangiocarcinoma development. Finally, PSC, with its autoimmune multifocal strictures of the intrahepatic and extrahepatic biliary trees, carries an increased risk of cholangiocarcinoma. Although sporadic cases of cholangiocarcinoma tend to occur at the bifurcation, patients with PSC may have multifocal disease not amenable to resection. Medications and chemical carcinogens have been associated with the development of cholangiocarcinoma, including Thorotrast, oral contraceptives, asbestos, and cigarette smoke.

Staging and Classification

The three distinct pathologic subtypes include sclerosing, nodular, and papillary cholangiocarcinoma. Sclerosing cholangiocarcinoma tends to occur in the proximal bile ducts, causing periductal fibrosis in a concentric pattern and a circumferential duct occlusion. The papillary and nodular subtypes tend to occur in distal cholangiocarcinomas and are manifested with intraluminal growths. In the nodular subtype, a firm mass based in the duct wall can be seen growing into the duct lumen, whereas the more common papillary subtype appears as a polypoid lesion that is soft, with less periductal fibrosis and a better prognosis.

The staging of cholangiocarcinoma relies on the TNM staging system but is slightly different on the basis of anatomic location. The three staging subdivisions include intrahepatic (Table 54-2), extrahepatic (Table 54-3), and distal bile duct (Table 54-4).[28] Similar to many adenocarcinomas, direct local invasion and local lymph node spread are common and portend a worse prognosis. Tumors confined to the bile duct (T1) and those extending outside the bile duct but not invading adjacent structures such as the hepatic artery or portal vein (T2) carry a significantly better prognosis than those invading any nearby structure. The two pathologic factors most influencing prognosis after resection are complete (R0) resection to negative margins and absence of lymph node metastases.

Clinical Presentation

The presentation of cholangiocarcinoma depends on the site of origin and manifestations of biliary obstruction at that site. Painless jaundice is a common symptom, but patients with unilobar obstruction of a bile duct may present with unilateral lobar

TABLE 54-2 Staging for Intrahepatic Bile Duct Cancer

Primary Tumor (T)			
TX	Primary tumor cannot be assessed		
T0	No evidence of primary tumor		
Tis	Carcinoma in situ (intraductal tumor)		
T1	Solitary tumor without vascular invasion		
T2a	Solitary tumor with vascular invasion		
T2b	Multiple tumors, with or without vascular invasion		
T3	Tumor perforating the visceral peritoneum or involving local extrahepatic structures by direct extension		
T4	Tumor with periductal invasion		
Regional Lymph Nodes (N)			
NX	Regional lymph nodes cannot be assessed		
N0	No regional lymph node metastasis		
N1	Regional lymph node metastasis present		
Distant Metastasis (M)			
M0	No distant metastasis		
M1	Distant metastasis present		
Anatomic Stage and Prognostic Groups			
Stage 0	Tis	N0	M0
Stage I	T1	N0	M0
Stage II	T2	N0	M0
Stage III	T3	N0	M0
Stage IVA	T4	N0	M0
	Any T	N1	M0
Stage IVB	Any T	Any N	M1

From Edge SB, Byrd DR, Compton CC, et al, editors: *AJCC cancer staging manual*, ed 7, New York, 2010, Springer, pp 203–204.

TABLE 54-3 Staging for Perihilar Bile Duct Cancer

Primary Tumor (T)			
TX	Primary tumor cannot be assessed		
T0	No evidence of primary tumor		
Tis	Carcinoma in situ		
T1	Tumor confined to the bile duct, with extension up to the muscle layer or fibrous tissue		
T2a	Tumor invading beyond the wall of the bile duct to surrounding adipose tissue		
T2b	Tumor invades the adjacent hepatic parenchyma		
T3	Tumor invades unilateral branches of the portal vein or hepatic artery		
T4	Tumor invading main portal vein or its branches bilaterally; or the common hepatic artery; or the second-order biliary radicals bilaterally; or unilateral second-order biliary radicals with contralateral portal vein or hepatic artery involvement		
Regional Lymph Nodes (N)			
NX	Regional lymph nodes cannot be assessed		
N0	No regional lymph node metastasis		
N1	Regional lymph node metastasis (including nodes along the cystic duct, common bile duct, hepatic artery, and portal vein)		
N2	Metastasis to periaortic, pericaval, superior mesenteric artery and/or celiac artery lymph nodes		
Distant Metastasis (M)			
M0	No distant metastasis		
M1	Distant metastasis		
Anatomic Stage and Prognostic Groups			
Stage 0	Tis	N0	M0
Stage I	T1	N0	M0
Stage II	T2a-b	N0	M0
Stage IIIA	T3	N0	M0
Stage IIIB	T1-3	N1	M0
Stage IVA	T4	N0-1	M0
Stage IVB	Any T	N2	M0
	Any T	Any N	M1

From Edge SB, Byrd DR, Compton CC, et al, editors: *AJCC cancer staging manual*, ed 7, New York, 2010, Springer, p 221.

TABLE 54-4 Staging for Distal Bile Duct Cancer

Primary Tumor (T)			
TX	Primary tumor cannot be assessed		
T0	No evidence of primary tumor		
Tis	Carcinoma in situ		
T1	Tumor confined to the bile duct histologically		
T2	Tumor invades beyond the wall of the bile duct		
T3	Tumor invades the gallbladder, pancreas, duodenum, or other adjacent organs without involvement of the celiac axis or superior mesenteric artery		
T4	Tumor involves the celiac axis or superior mesenteric artery		
Regional Lymph Nodes (N)			
N0	No regional lymph node metastasis		
N1	Regional lymph node metastasis		
Distant Metastasis (M)			
M0	No distant metastasis		
M1	Distant metastasis		
Anatomic Stage and Prognostic Groups			
Stage 0	Tis	N0	M0
Stage IA	T1	N0	M0
Stage IB	T2	N0	M0
Stage IIA	T3	N0	M0
Stage IIB	T1	N1	M0
	T2	N1	M0
	T3	N1	M0
Stage III	T4	Any N	M0
Stage IV	Any T	Any N	M1

From Edge SB, Byrd DR, Compton CC, et al, editors: *AJCC cancer staging manual*, ed 7, New York, 2010, Springer, p 229.

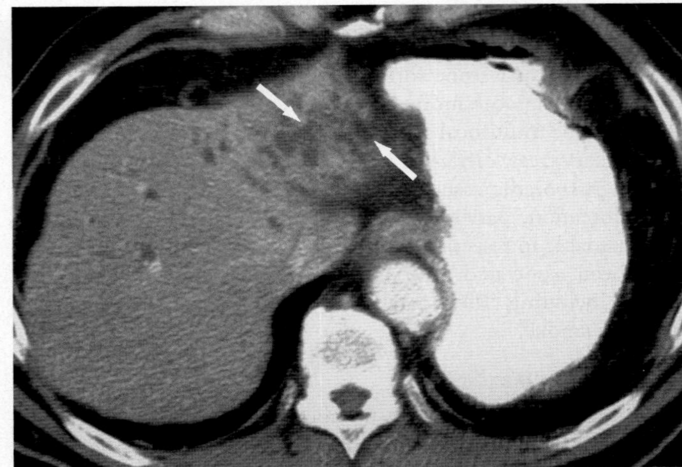

FIGURE 54-59 CT scan of cholangiocarcinoma with left lobar atrophy caused by obstruction of the left duct. Noted in the atrophied left lobe are dilated biliary radicals *(arrows)*.

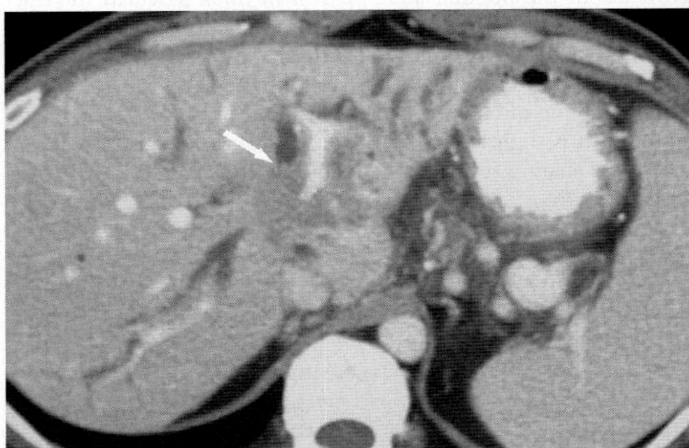

FIGURE 54-60 CT scan of Klatskin tumor *(arrow)* encasing the main portal vein, consistent with unresectable disease.

atrophy and subsequent contralateral lobar hypertrophy (Fig. 54-59). The resultant hepatic compensation can delay presentation until the later stages of disease. Therefore, cholangiocarcinoma causing obstruction at or below the hepatic bifurcation tends to be manifested at earlier stages than intrahepatic cholangiocarcinoma. With obstruction of the biliary tree, the common manifestations of direct hyperbilirubinemia, such as pruritus, dark urine, and steatorrhea, can be seen. Cholangiocarcinomas tend to extend in a submucosal route, with associated perineural invasion, but constant pain on presentation suggests more advanced disease.

Diagnosis and Assessment of Resectability

At the time of presentation, most patients will have manifestations of obstructive jaundice with hyperbilirubinemia and an elevated alkaline phosphatase level. Other markers of hepatic function, such as prothrombin time and albumin level, are generally unaffected until later in the disease or when the biliary obstruction is long-standing. Tumor markers, including carcinoembryonic antigen and carbohydrate antigen 19-9, are unreliable for diagnosis of cholangiocarcinoma but may be followed postoperatively in the surveillance of recurrence.

The radiologic evaluation of jaundice includes a right upper quadrant ultrasound examination, which may show intrahepatic biliary ductal dilation but does not usually identify the actual site of obstruction. With hilar cholangiocarcinomas, the gallbladder and visualized extrahepatic biliary tree are usually decompressed, whereas distal lesions will have extrahepatic biliary ductal dilation and gallbladder distention. Cross-sectional imaging by triphasic CT allows not only assessment of metastatic disease but also evaluation of resectability. The location of the tumor can be identified, and its relationship to vascular structures can also be assessed. Identification of aberrant anatomy and determination of segmental or lobar involvement by CT are helpful for preoperative planning.

Typically, CT alone is insufficient for the assessment of feasibility and appropriateness of resection. Cholangiography by MRCP, PTC, or ERCP helps determine the proximal extent of resection. Endoscopic cholangiography carries the additional risk of cholangitis by the introduction of enteric bacteria into an undrained portion of the biliary tree. Bilobar intrahepatic metastases and any extrahepatic disease are contraindications to resection, as is the involvement of bilateral secondary biliary radicals. Because complete (R0) resection is the only strategy that affords the possibility of cure, other contraindications to resection include encasement of the main portal vein (Fig. 54-60), bilateral hepatic lobar artery involvement, and lobar atrophy with involvement of the contralateral portal vein or biliary radicals. Involvement of unilobar vascular structures is managed with resection of the primary and affected lobe in continuity, and therefore it is not a contraindication.

Tissue diagnosis before resection in operative patients is unnecessary. With obstructive jaundice, bile cytology and brushings are unreliable, and thus a negative cytology report does not exclude malignant disease. Therefore, invasive attempts to establish a diagnosis before resection carry risk but do not alter subsequent management. Establishment of a tissue diagnosis is important only when the patient is not a surgical candidate. However, preoperative biliary drainage may be useful in select cases. In patients with distal cholangiocarcinoma, preoperative biliary drainage increases the rate of infectious complications of resection but is generally useful for those with preoperative hyperbilirubinemia (bilirubin level >10 mg/dL) and those with a prolonged time interval between presentation and resection. For patients with hilar cholangiocarcinoma, hepatic resection remains an important feature of the operative strategy. In the setting of complete biliary obstruction, hepatic resection carries an additional risk of bleeding, sepsis, and hepatic failure. Drainage of the obstructed but unaffected segments can enhance the postresection hypertrophy of the remaining liver but may increase perioperative infectious complications.

Treatment

Operative management. With the clinical suspicion of cholangiocarcinoma in adequate operative candidates without contraindications to resection, exploration should proceed, even in the absence of a confirmed tissue diagnosis. Between 7% and 15% of patients undergoing resection for suspected biliary malignant disease will prove to have benign disease. Alternatively, more than 50% of patients undergoing exploration will have findings precluding resection, such as peritoneal metastases, hepatic metastases, or locally advanced lesions.

Distal cholangiocarcinoma. Distal cholangiocarcinoma is managed by pancreaticoduodenectomy. Because these lesions tend to grow in a submucosal plane, a frozen section of the proximal bile duct margin helps ensure an R0 resection. An R0 resection remains one of the most important prognostic factors for this disease, with 5-year survival rates of up to 50% in node-negative patients with an R0 resection.

Proximal cholangiocarcinoma. Surgical management of proximal cholangiocarcinoma involves resection of regional nodal tissue and en bloc resection of the common bile duct with hepatic parenchyma as necessary to achieve negative margins. The Bismuth-Corlette classification of the tumor by assessment of the involvement of biliary radicals helps with operative planning (Fig. 54-61).[30] Types I and II lesions are treated with common duct resection, cholecystectomy, and a 5- to 10-mm margin of resection. Type II lesions may also require partial hepatic resection, which commonly includes resection of the caudate lobe. Resection of the bile duct and nodal tissue requires skeletonization of the hepatic artery and portal vein. Reconstruction is performed using a Roux limb of jejunum. Types III and IV lesions may involve complex resection and reconstruction of the portal vein, hepatic artery, or both. With resection to secondary biliary radicals, transanastomotic stenting is used liberally to allow healing and even confirmation of anastomotic integrity.

A substantial improvement in long-term survival has correlated with the increasing use of hepatic resection to achieve negative margins. Negative margin status is the most important variable associated with outcome.[31] Five-year survival rates as high as 59% have been reported in selected series, and with vascular resection and reconstruction techniques, resectability rates have also increased. Increases in the magnitude of the operation have also correlated with an expected increase in surgical mortality, from 2% to 4% to 3% to 11%.

As noted previously, an extensive neoadjuvant therapy protocol followed by transplantation has shown promising results in tightly controlled trials. In spite of these findings, the role of transplantation in the management of cholangiocarcinoma remains experimental, and substantial debate remains about the routine use of an extremely limited resource in this disease process.

Palliation. In patients found to have unresectable or incurable disease preoperatively, all attempts to palliate their symptoms nonoperatively should be used. The goals of palliation should include relief of jaundice, alleviation of pain, and relief of duodenal obstruction, if necessary. Surgical palliation has not been shown to prolong survival or to reduce complication rates and thus should be reserved for candidates found to be unresectable or metastatic at time of operation. Depending on the location of the biliary obstruction, endoscopic or percutaneous routes of drainage can be used, and placement of a self-expandable metallic stent provides a durable solution. When plastic stents are used, additional manipulation or placement of subsequent stents may be required. For distal cholangiocarcinomas, ERCP is the preferred route of nonoperative biliary drainage, whereas PTC is more useful for proximal lesions. Drainage of atrophic lobes with stents does not improve palliation of disease. Pain can be treated with oral narcotics. IV narcotics and even percutaneous destruction of the celiac plexus have shown some benefit. For distal cholangiocarcinomas, in which duodenal obstruction may occur, endoscopic duodenal stenting can relieve the obstruction in this preterminal condition.

Medical treatment. Chemotherapy has not been shown to improve survival in patients with cholangiocarcinoma. In addition, radiation therapy has not been proven in a prospective fashion to affect survival. Therefore, neither chemotherapy nor radiation therapy is used routinely in the adjuvant or neoadjuvant setting. Although some retrospective studies have shown a small

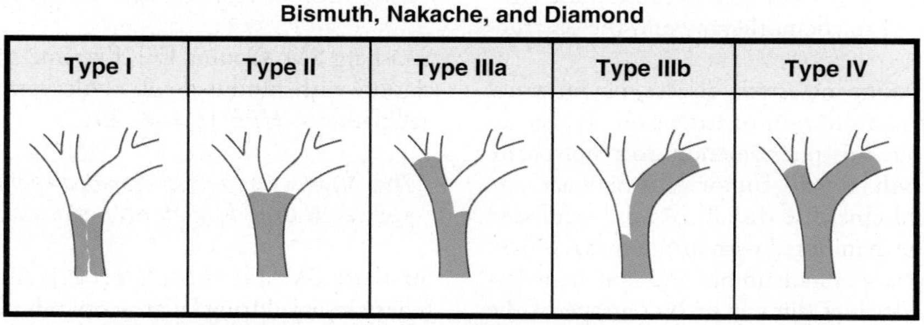

FIGURE 54-61 Bismuth-Corlette classification of tumor involvement.

survival advantage with adjuvant radiation, prospective studies of adjuvant radiotherapy have shown no benefit in completely resected patients. Radiation therapy may provide a small survival advantage as an adjunct to resection when microscopic residual disease remains. Most studies have reported a clinical response rate of less than 10%. Even in the absence of supportive data, adjuvant chemoradiation is used routinely at many centers but should be limited to patients with nodal disease, those with R1 resections, and those undergoing a clinical trial.

Outcomes

Long-term survival is highly dependent on stage at presentation and whether surgical resection to negative margins is achieved. With the use of common duct resection with partial hepatectomy, negative margin rates have increased to more than 75%. This has resulted in 5-year survival rates of 20% to 45% in most series. Although morbidity rates of 35% to 50% are common, mortality rates are generally low (<10%). In the setting of distal bile duct cancers, resection rates are generally higher, with approximately similar 5-year survival among patients undergoing R0 resections. Alternatively, because there is no reliable therapeutic alternative, the median survival of unresected patients ranges from 5 to 8 months.

Because negative margin status is easier to obtain by explanting the liver, some have advocated total hepatectomy with liver transplantation for treatment. Unfortunately, initial experience with therapeutic transplantation was plagued by early mortality and high recurrence rates. Even the most aggressive and radical resections with multivisceral transplantation have not shown a survival advantage. Therefore, without a specific clinical trial, cholangiocarcinoma is considered a contraindication to transplantation. However, some centers have attempted neoadjuvant chemoradiation followed by exploration for the evaluation of resectability and metastases, and finally transplantation, with improved survival over resection alone.[25] At present, the role of transplantation in the management of cholangiocarcinoma is at best controversial, and it should be limited to research protocols.

METASTATIC AND OTHER TUMORS

Any primary or secondary tumor affecting the liver can cause biliary obstruction. The most common examples include portal nodal disease from adenocarcinomas, such as hepatocellular carcinoma, pancreatic adenocarcinoma, and colorectal carcinoma. The metastatic nodes can compress the common bile duct at any point along its length. Lymphoma may affect the portal lymph node chain and, when isolated to periportal nodes, is notoriously difficult to differentiate from cholangiocarcinoma. Placement of temporary plastic stents to relieve the obstruction is usually the only therapeutic biliary intervention required because these lymphomas will generally respond to chemotherapy and the obstruction will usually resolve.

Primary lesions of the liver or metastatic disease may obstruct the biliary tree from direct compression or extension, as seen in hepatocellular carcinoma, but this phenomenon does not create an intraluminal biliary growth. Rarely, tumor cells may actually pass into the biliary tree and embolize distally. As the exfoliated cellular mass grows, it may be manifested with intraluminal biliary obstruction. Intrahepatic biliary cystadenomas and cystadenocarcinoma may obstruct the bile duct directly or by passage of the mucin that they produce.

SELECTED REFERENCES

Butte JM, Kingham TP, Gonen M, et al: Residual disease predicts outcomes after definitive resection for incidental gallbladder cancer. *J Am Coll Surg* 219:416–429, 2014.

This article evaluated the survival of gallbladder cancer after attempted surgical resection, noting the import of R0 resection status on survival.

Darwish Murad S, Kim WR, Harnois DM, et al: Efficacy of neoadjuvant chemoradiation, followed by liver transplantation, for perihilar cholangiocarcinoma at 12 US centers. *Gastroenterology* 143:88–98.e3, 2012.

This article evaluated the results of transplantation for cholangiocarcinoma after a rigorous neoadjuvant therapy protocol.

Fogel EL, Sherman S: ERCP for gallstone pancreatitis. *N Engl J Med* 370:150–157, 2014.

This article reviews the current status of the role of ERCP in the diagnosis and management of biliary pancreatitis, depending on severity.

Horwood J, Akbar F, Davis K, et al: Prospective evaluation of a selective approach to cholangiography for suspected common bile duct stones. *Ann R Coll Surg Engl* 92:206–210, 2010.

This article evaluates the criteria for selective cholangiography during routine cholecystectomy.

Pitt HA, Sherman S, Johnson MS, et al: Improved outcomes of bile duct injuries in the 21st century. *Ann Surg* 258:490–499, 2013.

This article reviewed a large series of iatrogenic bile duct injuries, highlighting the success of surgical intervention and the multidisciplinary approach to management.

Sirinek KR, Schwesinger WH: Has intraoperative cholangiography during laparoscopic cholecystectomy become obsolete in the era of preoperative endoscopic retrograde and magnetic resonance cholangiopancreatography? *J Am Coll Surg* 220:522–528, 2015.

This article highlights current practice patterns of imaging in the management of suspected choledocholithiasis, noting the application of MRCP as a screening tool for referral for ERCP before laparoscopic cholecystectomy.

Strasberg SM, Gouma DJ: 'Extreme' vasculobiliary injuries: Association with fundus-down cholecystectomy in severely inflamed gallbladders. *HPB* 14:1–8, 2012.

This article discusses the surgical pitfalls of a "dome down" approach to the inflamed gallbladder.

Strasberg SM, Hertl M, Soper NJ: An analysis of the problem of biliary injury during laparoscopic cholecystectomy. *J Am Coll Surg* 180:101–125, 1995.

This is the most cited article for classification of iatrogenic bile duct injuries and is considered the seminal comprehensive article on the topic.

REFERENCES

1. Couinaud C: Les envelopes vasculobiliares de foie ou capsule de Glisson: Leur interet dans la chirurgie vesiculaire, les resections hepatique et l'abord du hile du foie. *Lyon Chir* 49:589–615, 1954.
2. Admirand WH, Small DM: The physicochemical basis of cholesterol gallstone formation in man. *J Clin Invest* 47:1043–1052, 1968.
3. de Mestral C, Rotstein OD, Laupacis A, et al: Comparative operative outcomes of early and delayed cholecystectomy for acute cholecystitis: A population-based propensity score analysis. *Ann Surg* 259:10–15, 2014.
4. Verbesey JE, Birkett DH: Common bile duct exploration for choledocholithiasis. *Surg Clin North Am* 88:1315–1328, 2008.
5. Horwood J, Akbar F, Davis K, et al: Prospective evaluation of a selective approach to cholangiography for suspected common bile duct stones. *Ann R Coll Surg Engl* 92:206–210, 2010.
6. Sirinek KR, Schwesinger WH: Has intraoperative cholangiography during laparoscopic cholecystectomy become obsolete in the era of preoperative endoscopic retrograde and magnetic resonance cholangiopancreatography? *J Am Coll Surg* 220:522–528, 2015.
7. Lee JK, Ryu JK, Park JK, et al: Roles of endoscopic sphincterotomy and cholecystectomy in acute biliary pancreatitis. *Hepatogastroenterology* 55:1981–1985, 2008.
8. Fogel EL, Sherman S: ERCP for gallstone pancreatitis. *N Engl J Med* 370:150–157, 2014.
9. Strasberg SM, Hertl M, Soper NJ: An analysis of the problem of biliary injury during laparoscopic cholecystectomy. *J Am Coll Surg* 180:101–125, 1995.
10. Way LW, Stewart L, Gantert W, et al: Causes and prevention of laparoscopic bile duct injuries: Analysis of 252 cases from a human factors and cognitive psychology perspective. *Ann Surg* 237:460–469, 2003.
11. Strasberg SM, Gouma DJ: 'Extreme' vasculobiliary injuries: Association with fundus-down cholecystectomy in severely inflamed gallbladders. *HPB* 14:1–8, 2012.
12. Rogers SJ, Cello JP, Horn JK, et al: Prospective randomized trial of LC+LCBDE vs ERCP/S+LC for common bile duct stone disease. *Arch Surg* 145:28–33, 2010.
13. Nieuwenhuijs VB: Impact of routine intraoperative cholangiography during laparoscopic cholecystectomy on bile duct injury. *Br J Surg* 101:685, 2014.
14. Bismuth H, Majno PE: Biliary strictures: Classification based on the principles of surgical treatment. *World J Surg* 25:1241–1244, 2001.
15. Lillemoe KD: Current management of bile duct injury. *Br J Surg* 95:403–405, 2008.
16. Harrison VL, Dolan JP, Pham TH, et al: Bile duct injury after laparoscopic cholecystectomy in hospitals with and without surgical residency programs: Is there a difference? *Surg Endosc* 25:1969–1974, 2011.
17. Sicklick JK, Camp MS, Lillemoe KD, et al: Surgical management of bile duct injuries sustained during laparoscopic cholecystectomy: Perioperative results in 200 patients. *Ann Surg* 241:786–792, discussion 793–795, 2005.
18. Eum YO, Park JK, Chun J, et al: Non-surgical treatment of post-surgical bile duct injury: Clinical implications and outcomes. *World J Gastroenterol* 20:6924–6931, 2014.
19. Pottakkat B, Vijayahari R, Prakash A, et al: Factors predicting failure following high bilio-enteric anastomosis for post-cholecystectomy benign biliary strictures. *J Gastrointest Surg* 14:1389–1394, 2010.
20. Pitt HA, Sherman S, Johnson MS, et al: Improved outcomes of bile duct injuries in the 21st century. *Ann Surg* 258:490–499, 2013.
21. Ejaz A, Spolverato G, Kim Y, et al: Long-term health-related quality of life after iatrogenic bile duct injury repair. *J Am Coll Surg* 219:923–932.e10, 2014.
22. Pazouki A, Abdollahi A, Mehrabi Bahar M, et al: Evaluation of the incidence of complications of lost gallstones during laparoscopic cholecystectomy. *Surg Laparosc Endosc Percutan Tech* 24:213–215, 2014.
23. Co M, Pang SY, Wong KY, et al: Surgical management of recurrent pyogenic cholangitis: 10 years of experience in a tertiary referral centre in Hong Kong. *HPB* 16:776–780, 2014.
24. Carbone M, Neuberger JM: Autoimmune liver disease, autoimmunity and liver transplantation. *J Hepatol* 60:210–223, 2014.
25. Darwish Murad S, Kim WR, Harnois DM, et al: Efficacy of neoadjuvant chemoradiation, followed by liver transplantation, for perihilar cholangiocarcinoma at 12 US centers. *Gastroenterology* 143:88–98.e3, 2012.
26. Todani T, Watanabe Y, Narusue M, et al: Congenital bile duct cysts: Classification, operative procedures, and review of thirty-seven cases including cancer arising from choledochal cyst. *Am J Surg* 134:263–269, 1977.
27. Schnelldorfer T: Porcelain gallbladder: A benign process or concern for malignancy? *J Gastrointest Surg* 17:1161–1168, 2013.
28. Edge SB, Byrd DR, Compton CC, et al, editors: *AJCC cancer staging manual*, ed 7, New York, 2010, Springer.
29. Butte JM, Kingham TP, Gonen M, et al: Residual disease predicts outcomes after definitive resection for incidental gallbladder cancer. *J Am Coll Surg* 219:416–429, 2014.
30. Bismuth H, Nakache R, Diamond T: Management strategies in resection for hilar cholangiocarcinoma. *Ann Surg* 215:31–38, 1992.
31. Maithel SK, Gamblin TC, Kamel I, et al: Multidisciplinary approaches to intrahepatic cholangiocarcinoma. *Cancer* 119:3929–3942, 2013.

55 CHAPTER

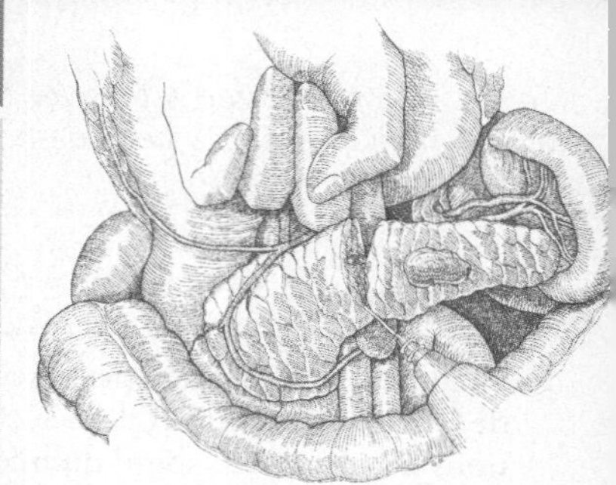

Exocrine Pancreas

Vikas Dudeja, John D. Christein, Eric H. Jensen, Selwyn M. Vickers

OUTLINE

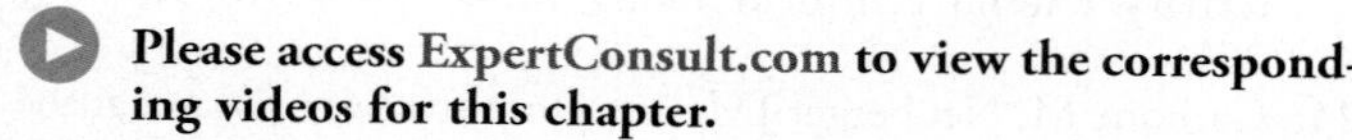

Please access ExpertConsult.com to view the corresponding videos for this chapter.

ANATOMY

The average pancreas weighs between 75 and 125 g and measures 10 to 20 cm. It lies in the retroperitoneum just anterior to the first lumbar vertebra and is anatomically divided into four portions, the head, neck, body, and tail. The head lies to the right of midline within the C loop of the duodenum, immediately anterior to the vena cava at the confluence of the renal veins. The uncinate process extends from the head of the pancreas behind the superior mesenteric vein (SMV) and terminates adjacent to the superior mesenteric artery (SMA). The neck is the short segment of pancreas that immediately overlies the SMV. The body and tail of the pancreas then extend across the midline, anterior to Gerota fascia and slightly cephalad, terminating within the splenic hilum (Fig. 55-1).

Arterial Blood Supply

The pancreas is supplied by a complex arterial network arising from the celiac trunk and SMA. The head and uncinate process are supplied by the pancreaticoduodenal arteries (anterior and posterior), which arise from the hepatic artery through the gastroduodenal artery (GDA) superiorly and the SMA inferiorly. The neck, body, and tail receive arterial supply from the splenic arterial system. Several small branches originate from the length of the splenic artery, supplying arterial blood flow to the superior portion of the organ. The dorsal pancreatic artery arises from the splenic artery and courses posterior to the body of the gland to become the inferior pancreatic artery. The inferior pancreatic artery then runs along the inferior border of the pancreas, terminating at its tail.

Venous Drainage

The venous drainage mimics the arterial supply, with blood flow from the head of the pancreas draining into the anterior and posterior pancreaticoduodenal veins. The posterior superior pancreaticoduodenal vein enters the SMV laterally at the superior border of the neck of the pancreas. The anterior superior pancreaticoduodenal vein enters the right gastroepiploic vein just before its confluence with the SMV at the inferior border of the pancreas. The anterior and posterior inferior pancreaticoduodenal veins enter the SMV along the inferior border of the uncinate process. The remaining body and tail are drained through the splenic venous system.

EMBRYOLOGY

The exocrine pancreas begins development during the fourth week of gestation. Pluripotent pancreatic epithelial stem cells give rise to exocrine and endocrine cell lines as well as the intricate pancreatic ductal network. Initially, dorsal and ventral buds appear from the primitive duodenal endoderm (Fig. 55-2*A*). The dorsal bud typically appears first and ultimately develops into the superior head, neck, body, and tail of the mature pancreas. The ventral bud develops as part of the hepatic diverticulum and maintains communication with the biliary tree throughout development. The ventral bud will become the inferior part of the head and uncinate process of the gland. Between the fourth and eighth weeks, the ventral bud rotates posteriorly in a clockwise fashion to fuse with the dorsal bud (Fig. 55-2*B*). At approximately 8 weeks of gestation, the dorsal and ventral buds are fused (Fig. 55-2*C*).

The initiation of pancreas bud formation and differentiation of the ventral bud from the hepatic-biliary fates is dependent on the expression of pancreatic duodenal homeobox 1 (PDX1)

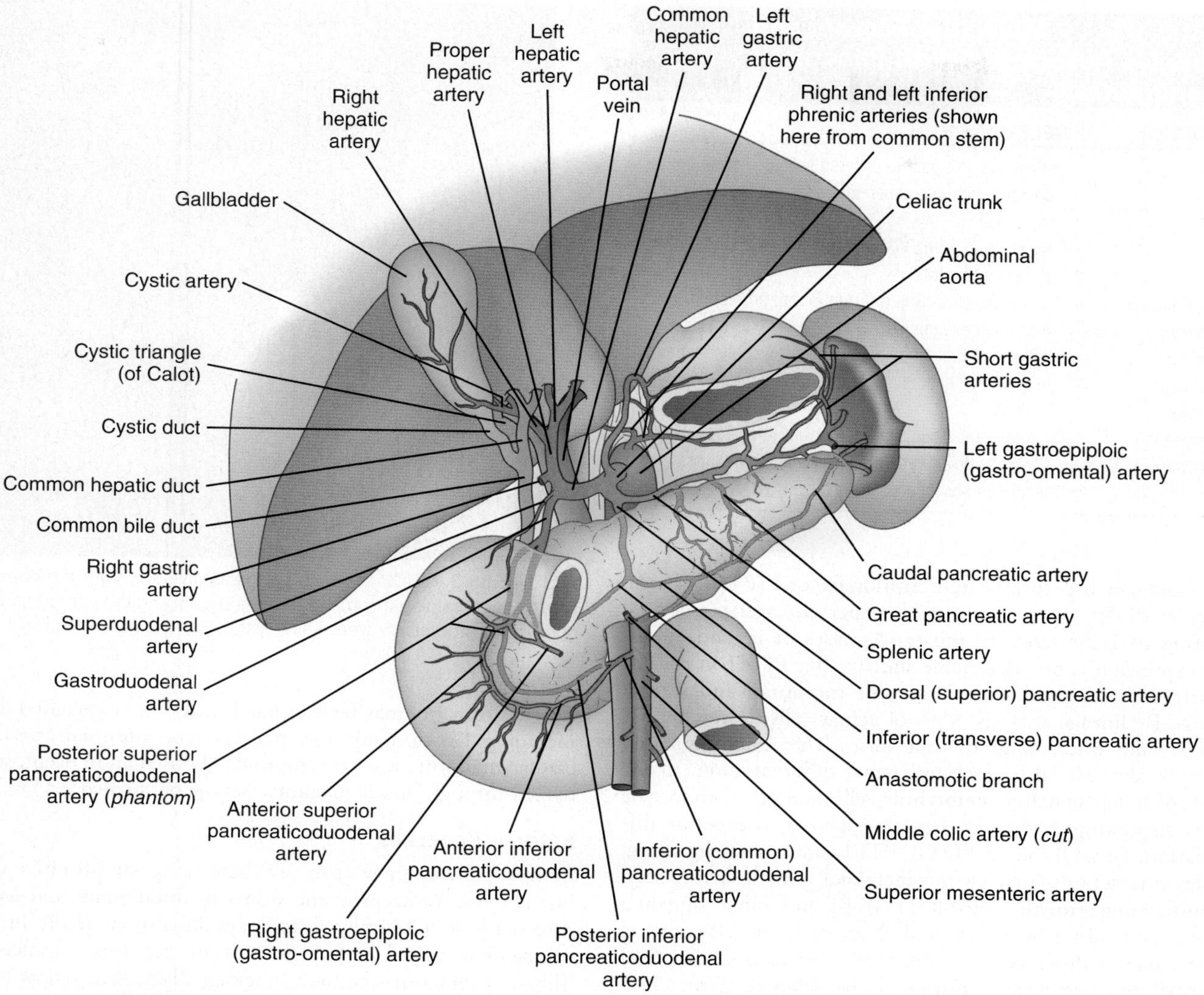

Common hepatic artery
Left gastric artery
Left hepatic artery
Proper hepatic artery
Portal vein
Right hepatic artery
Right and left inferior phrenic arteries (shown here from common stem)
Gallbladder
Celiac trunk
Abdominal aorta
Cystic artery
Cystic triangle (of Calot)
Short gastric arteries
Cystic duct
Left gastroepiploic (gastro-omental) artery
Common hepatic duct
Common bile duct
Right gastric artery
Caudal pancreatic artery
Superduodenal artery
Great pancreatic artery
Splenic artery
Gastroduodenal artery
Dorsal (superior) pancreatic artery
Inferior (transverse) pancreatic artery
Posterior superior pancreaticoduodenal artery (phantom)
Anastomotic branch
Anterior superior pancreaticoduodenal artery
Middle colic artery (cut)
Anterior inferior pancreaticoduodenal artery
Inferior (common) pancreaticoduodenal artery
Superior mesenteric artery
Right gastroepiploic (gastro-omental) artery
Posterior inferior pancreaticoduodenal artery

FIGURE 55-1 Anatomy. (Netter illustration from *www.netterimages.com*. © Elsevier Inc. All rights reserved.)

Common bile duct
Dorsal pancreatic duct
Dorsal pancreas
Ventral pancreas
Common bile duct
Ventral pancreatic duct
B
Stomach
Liver
Accessory pancreatic duct (Santorini)
Main pancreatic duct (Wirsung)
Gallbladder
Dorsal pancreas
C
Ventral pancreas
A

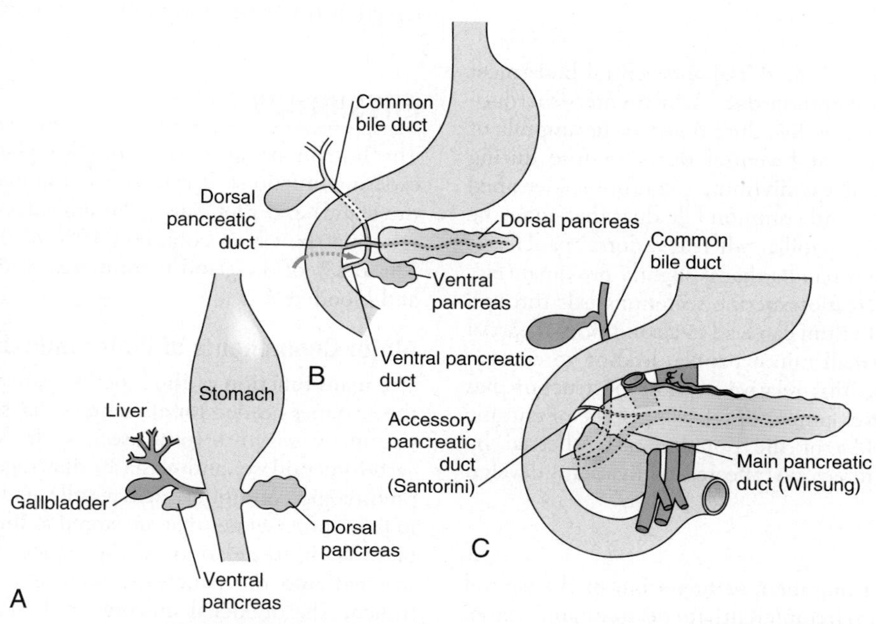

FIGURE 55-2 Embryologic development of the pancreas.

TABLE 55-1 Molecular Factors and Pathways Associated With Pancreatic Organogenesis

MUTATION	RELEVANCE
PDX1	Critical role in exocrine differentiation; knockout mice develop primitive pancreatic buds but agenesis of the organ
PTF1	Coexpression with *PDX1* determines progenitor cells to pancreatic fate
Notch signaling pathway	Suppresses endocrine differentiation, promoting exocrine development
Hedgehog signaling pathway	Inhibition of hedgehog in *PDX1*-positive cells leads to initiation of endoderm differentiation into pancreas lineage
Wnt signaling pathway	Complex Wnt signaling is important in all aspects of pancreas development; lack of Wnt signaling results in absence of acinar tissue

protein and pancreas-specific transcription factor 1 (PTF1). In the absence of PDX1 expression in mice, pancreatic agenesis occurs, indicating its importance in the early phases of organogenesis. PTF1 expression is first detectable shortly after PDX1 in cells of the early endoderm, which will become the dorsal and ventral pancreas. By lineage analysis, 95% of acinar cells express PTF1. In PTF1 null mice, acini do not form. The notch signaling pathway is also critical to duct and acinar differentiation. In the absence of notch signaling, embryonic cells commit to endocrine lineage, suggesting that notch signaling is vital to exocrine differentiation. In addition to PDX1, PTF1, and notch signaling, complex interactions between mesenchymal growth factors such as transforming growth factor-β (TGF-β) and other signaling pathways, including hedgehog and Wnt, seem to play critical roles in pancreas development.[1] The precise interactions that lead to normal organogenesis continue to be defined. Table 55-1 summarizes the factors and pathways that affect pancreas development.

Pancreas Divisum

During normal organogenesis, the dorsal and ventral buds most commonly fuse to form a common duct, which enters the duodenum along with the common bile duct through the ampulla of Vater. Failure of the dorsal and ventral ducts to fuse during embryogenesis leads to pancreas divisum, a condition identified by a ventral pancreatic duct and common bile duct that enter the duodenum through a major papilla, whereas a dorsal pancreatic duct enters through a minor papilla that is slightly proximal (Fig. 55-3). Because most pancreatic exocrine secretions exit through the dorsal duct, pancreas divisum can lead to a condition of partial obstruction caused by a small minor papilla, leading to chronic backpressure in the duct. This relative outflow obstruction has been implicated in the development of relapsing acute or chronic pancreatitis. Although 10% of the population is affected by pancreas divisum, only rarely do affected individuals develop pancreatitis.

Annular Pancreas

Annular pancreas results from aberrant migration of the ventral pancreas bud, which leads to circumferential or near-circumferential pancreas tissue surrounding the second portion of the duodenum.

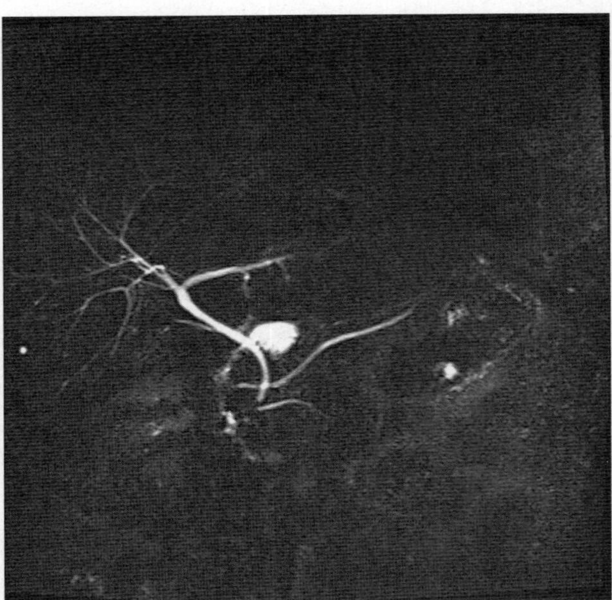

FIGURE 55-3 MRCP showing pancreas divisum, with the dorsal pancreatic duct draining through the minor papilla and the ventral pancreatic duct joining the biliary tree draining through the major papilla.

This abnormality may be associated with other congenital defects, including Down syndrome, malrotation, intestinal atresia, and cardiac malformations. If symptoms of obstruction occur, surgical bypass through duodenojejunostomy is performed.

Ectopic Pancreas

Ectopic pancreas may arise anywhere along the primitive foregut but is most common in the stomach, duodenum, and Meckel's diverticulum. Clinically, ectopic nodules may result in bowel obstruction caused by intussusception, bleeding, or ulceration. They can sometimes be found incidentally as firm yellow nodules that arise from the submucosa. Although there have been rare case reports of adenocarcinoma arising in ectopic pancreas tissue, resection is not necessary unless symptoms occur.

PHYSIOLOGY

The human pancreas is a complex gland, with endocrine and exocrine functions. It is mainly composed of acinar cells (85% of the gland) and islet cells (2%) embedded in a complex extracellular matrix, which composes 10% of the gland. The remaining 3% to 4% of the gland is composed of the epithelial duct system and blood vessels.

Major Components of Pancreatic Juice

The main function of the exocrine pancreas is to provide most of the enzymes needed for alimentary digestion. Acinar cells synthesize many enzymes (proteases), such as trypsin, chymotrypsin, carboxypeptidase, and elastase, that digest food proteins. Under physiologic conditions, acinar cells synthesize these proteases as inactive proenzymes that are stored as intracellular zymogen granules. With stimulation of the pancreas, these proenzymes are secreted into the pancreatic duct and eventually the duodenal lumen. The duodenal mucosa synthesizes and secretes enterokinase, which is the critical enzyme in the enzymatic activation of

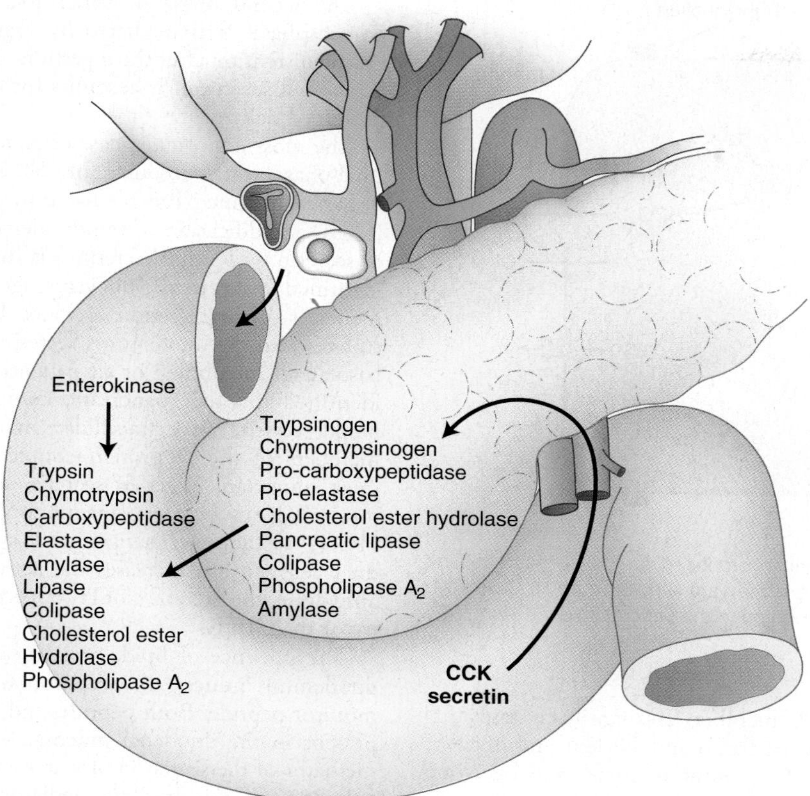

FIGURE 55-4 Physiology of the secretion of pancreatic enzymes. The presence of peptides and fatty acids from food triggers the release of cholecystokinin (CCK). CCK induces the release of pancreatic enzymes into the duodenal lumen. Conversely, S cells located in the duodenum release secretin in response to the acidification of the duodenum. Secretin induces the secretion of HCO_3^- from pancreatic cells into the duodenum.

trypsin from trypsinogen.[2] Trypsin also plays an important role in protein digestion by propagating pancreatic enzyme activation through autoactivation of trypsinogen and other proenzymes, such as chymotrypsinogen, procarboxypeptidase, and proelastase. Figure 55-4 summarizes the mechanisms of pancreatic exocrine secretion.

In addition to protease production, acinar cells also produce pancreatic amylase and lipase, also known as glycerol ester hydrolase, as active enzymes. With the exception of cellulose, pancreatic amylase hydrolyzes major polysaccharides into small oligosaccharides, which can be further digested by the oligosaccharidases present in the duodenal and jejunal epithelium. Pancreatic lipase hydrolyzes ingested fats into free fatty acids and 2-monoglycerides. In addition to pancreatic lipase, acinar cells produce other enzymes that digest fat, but they are secreted as proenzymes, like the proteases previously mentioned. These include colipase, cholesterol ester hydrolase, and phospholipase A2. The main function of colipase is to increase the activity of pancreatic lipase; cholesterol esters are cleaved by cholesterol ester hydrolase into free cholesterol and one fatty acid; and phospholipase A2 hydrolyzes phospholipids. Pancreatic acinar cells also secrete deoxyribonuclease and ribonuclease, enzymes required for the hydrolysis of DNA and RNA, respectively.

Pancreatic enzymes are inactive inside acinar cells because they are synthesized and stored as inactive enzymes. In addition to this autoprotective mechanism, acinar cells synthesize pancreatic secretory trypsin inhibitor, which also protects acinar cells from autodigestion because it counteracts premature activation of trypsinogen inside acinar cells. Pancreatic secretory trypsin inhibitor is encoded by serine protease inhibitor Kazal type 1 *(SPINK1)* gene. *SPINK1* gene mutations are associated with the development of chronic pancreatitis, especially in childhood.

The primary function of pancreatic duct cells is to provide the water and electrolytes required to dilute and to deliver the enzymes synthesized by acinar cells. Although the concentrations of sodium and potassium are similar to their respective concentrations in plasma, the concentrations of bicarbonate and chloride vary significantly according to the secretion phase.

The mechanism responsible for the secretion of bicarbonate was first described in 1988 on the basis of in vitro studies. According to this model, extracellular CO_2 diffuses across the basolateral membrane of ductal cells. Once CO_2 is inside pancreatic duct cells, it is hydrated by intracellular carbonic anhydrase; as a result of this reaction, HCO_3^- and H^+ are generated. The apical membrane of pancreatic duct cells contains an anion exchanger that secretes intracellular HCO_3^- into the lumen of the cell and favors the exchange of luminal Cl^- inside the ductal epithelium. Studies have shown that this exchanger interacts with the cystic fibrosis transmembrane conductance regulator (CFTR). This may correlate with the inability of patients with cystic fibrosis to secrete water and bicarbonate. Although the nature of this exchanger has not been completely elucidated, it is possible that this anion

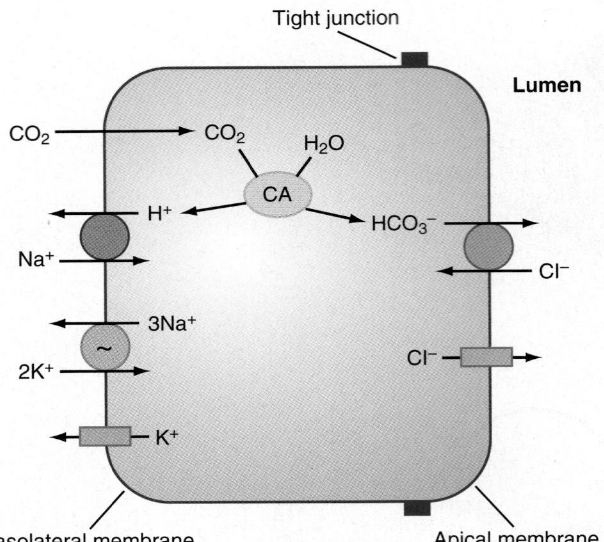

FIGURE 55-5 Cellular mechanism proposed for HCO_3^- secretion by pancreatic duct epithelium. (From Steward MC, Ishiguro H, Case RM: Mechanisms of bicarbonate secretion in the pancreatic duct. *Annu Rev Physiol* 67:377–409, 2005.)

exchanger is an SLC26 family member. This family contains different anion exchangers that transport monovalent and divalent anions, such as Cl^- and HCO_3^-. Some of these exchangers are known to interact with CFTR.

In addition to HCO_3^-, CO_2 hydration also generates H^+ ions, which are secreted by Na^+ and H^+ exchangers present in the basolateral membrane of ductal cells. These exchangers belong to the *SLC9* gene family. The main function of these exchangers is to maintain the intracellular pH within a physiologic range. In addition, the basolateral membrane of duct cells contains multiple Na^+,K^+-ATPases that provide the primary force that drives HCO_3^- secretion; the Na^+,K^+-ATPase maintains the Na^+ gradient used to extrude H^+ as well. Finally, K^+ channels present in the basolateral membrane of acinar cells maintain the membrane potential to allow recirculation of K^+ ions brought by the Na^+,K^+ pump inside the cell. Figure 55-5 illustrates HCO_3^- secretion inside pancreatic duct cells.

Once the HCO_3^- secreted by pancreatic duct cells reaches the duodenal lumen, it neutralizes the hydrochloric acid secreted by parietal cells. Pancreatic enzymes are inactivated at a low pH; therefore, pancreatic bicarbonate provides an optimal pH for acinar cell enzyme function. The optimal pH for the function of chymotrypsin and trypsin is 8.0 to 9.0; for amylase, the optimal pH is 7.0; and for lipase, it is 7.0 to 9.0.

Phases and Regulation of Pancreatic Secretion

Pancreatic exocrine secretion occurs during the interdigestive state and after the ingestion of food, which is also known as the digestive state. The same phases of secretion that have been identified in the stomach during the digestive state have also been described in pancreatic secretion. The first phase is the cephalic phase, in which the pancreas is stimulated by the vagus nerve in response to the sight, smell, or taste of food. This phase is generally mediated by the release of acetylcholine at the terminal endings of postganglionic fibers. The main effect of acetylcholine is to induce acinar cell secretion of enzymes. This phase accounts for 20% to 25% of the daily secretion of pancreatic juice.

The second phase of pancreatic secretion is known as the gastric phase. It is mediated by vagovagal reflexes triggered by gastric distention after the ingestion of food. These reflexes induce acinar cell secretion. It accounts for 10% of the pancreatic juice produced daily.

The most important phase of pancreatic secretion is the intestinal phase, which accounts for 65% to 70% of the total secretion of pancreatic juice. It is mediated by secretin and cholecystokinin (CCK). Acidification of the duodenal lumen induces the release of secretin by S cells. Secretin was the first polypeptide hormone identified more than 100 years ago. It is the most important mediator of the secretion of water, bicarbonate, and other electrolytes into the duodenum. Secretin receptors are located in the basolateral membrane of all pancreatic duct cells but cannot be identified in other pancreatic components, such as islet cells, blood vessels, or extracellular matrix. Secretin receptors are members of the G protein–coupled receptor superfamily. The most important effect of secretin stimulation is an increase of intracellular cyclic adenosine monophosphate, which activates the HCO_3^--Cl^- anion exchanger in the apical membrane of pancreatic duct cells. It also increases the activity of the enzyme carbonic anhydrase, the excretion of H^+ outside the duct cell, and the activity of the CFTR.

The presence of lipid, protein, and carbohydrates inside the duodenum induces the secretion of CCK-releasing factor and monitor peptide. Both peptides induce release of CCK by I cells present in the duodenal mucosa. Whereas secretin is the main mediator of the secretion of water and bicarbonate in the intestinal phase, CCK is the main mediator of the secretion of pancreatic enzymes. CCK exerts a number of effects:

1. CCK travels through the bloodstream and induces the release of pancreatic enzymes by acinar cells.
2. CCK induces local duodenal vagovagal reflexes that cause the release of acetylcholine, vasoactive intestinal peptide, and gastrin-releasing peptide, which promotes the release of pancreatic enzymes.
3. CCK induces the relaxation of the sphincter of Oddi. Also, CCK potentiates the effects of secretin, and vice versa.

ACUTE PANCREATITIS

The incidence of acute pancreatitis (AP) has increased during the past 20 years. AP is responsible for more than 300,000 hospital admissions annually in the United States. Most patients develop a mild and self-limited course; however, 10% to 20% of patients have a rapidly progressive inflammatory response associated with prolonged length of hospital stay and significant morbidity and mortality. Patients with mild pancreatitis have a mortality rate of less than 1%, but in severe pancreatitis, this increases up to 10% to 30%. The most common cause of death in this group of patients is multiorgan dysfunction syndrome. Mortality in pancreatitis has a bimodal distribution; in the first 2 weeks, also known as the early phase, the multiorgan dysfunction syndrome is the final result of an intense inflammatory cascade triggered initially by pancreatic inflammation. Mortality after 2 weeks, also known as the late period, is often caused by septic complications.[3]

Pathophysiology

The exact mechanism whereby predisposing factors such as ethanol and gallstones produce pancreatitis is not completely known. Most researchers believe that AP is the final result of abnormal pancreatic enzyme activation inside acinar cells.

Immunolocalization studies have shown that after 15 minutes of pancreatic injury, both zymogen granules and lysosomes colocalize inside the acinar cells. The fact that zymogen and lysosome colocalization occurs before amylase level elevation, pancreatic edema, and other markers of pancreatitis are evident suggests that colocalization is an early step in the pathophysiologic process and not a consequence of pancreatitis. Studies also suggest that lysosomal enzyme cathepsin B activates trypsin in these colocalization organelles. In vitro and in vivo studies have elucidated an intricate model of acinar cell death induced by premature activation of trypsin. In this model, once cathepsin B in lysosomes and trypsinogen in zymogen granules are brought in contact by colocalization induced by pancreatitis-inciting stimuli, activated trypsin then induces leak of colocalized organelles, releasing cathepsin B into the cytosol. It is the cytosolic cathepsin B that then induces apoptosis or necrosis, leading to acinar cell death. Thus, acinar cell death and to a degree the inflammatory response seen in AP can be prevented if acinar cells are pretreated with cathepsin B inhibitors. In vivo studies have also shown that cathepsin B knockout mice have a significant decrease in the severity of pancreatitis.[2]

Intra-acinar pancreatic enzyme activation induces autodigestion of normal pancreatic parenchyma. In response to this initial insult, acinar cells release proinflammatory cytokines, such as tumor necrosis factor-α (TNF-α) and interleukin (IL)-1, IL-2, and IL-6, and anti-inflammatory mediators, such as IL-10 and IL-1 receptor antagonist. These mediators do not initiate pancreatic injury but propagate the response locally and systemically. As a result, TNF-α, IL-1 and IL-7, neutrophils, and macrophages are recruited into the pancreatic parenchyma and cause the release of more TNF-α, IL-1 and IL-6, reactive oxygen metabolites, prostaglandins, platelet-activating factor, and leukotrienes. The local inflammatory response further aggravates the pancreatitis because it increases the permeability and damages the microcirculation of the pancreas. In severe cases, the inflammatory response causes local hemorrhage and pancreatic necrosis. In addition, some of the inflammatory mediators released by neutrophils aggravate the pancreatic injury because they cause pancreatic enzyme activation.[4]

The inflammatory cascade is self-limited in approximately 80% to 90% of patients. However, in the remaining patients, a vicious circle of recurring pancreatic injury and local and systemic inflammatory reaction persists. In a small number of patients, there is a massive release of inflammatory mediators to the systemic circulation. Active neutrophils mediate acute lung injury and induce the adult respiratory distress syndrome frequently seen in patients with severe pancreatitis. The mortality seen in the early phase of pancreatitis is the result of this persistent inflammatory response. A summary of the inflammatory cascade seen in AP is shown in Figure 55-6.

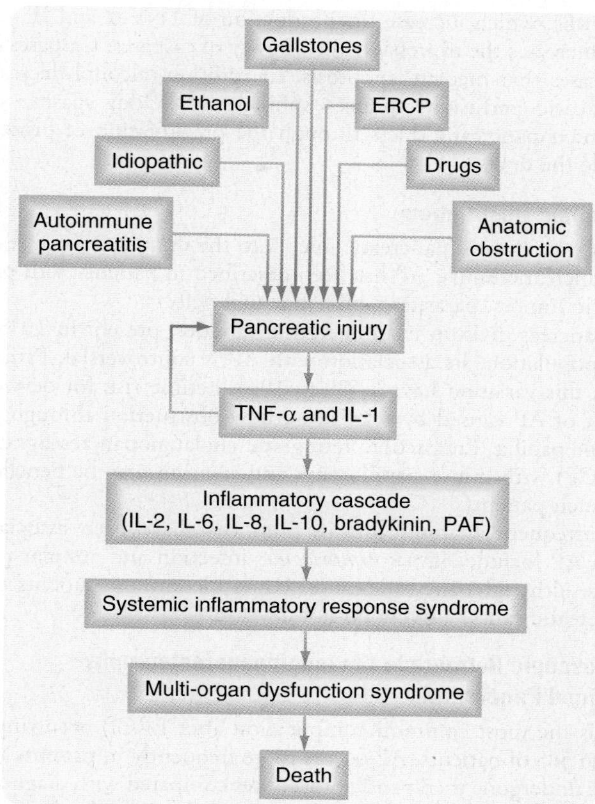

FIGURE 55-6 Pathophysiology of Severe Acute Pancreatitis. The local injury induces the release of TNF-α and IL-1. Both cytokines produce further pancreatic injury and amplify the inflammatory response by inducing the release of other inflammatory mediators, which cause distant organ injury. This abnormal inflammatory response is responsible for the mortality seen during the early phase of acute pancreatitis.

Risk Factors

Gallstones and ethanol abuse account for 70% to 80% of AP cases. In pediatric patients, abdominal blunt trauma and systemic diseases are the two most common conditions that lead to pancreatitis. Autoimmune and drug-induced pancreatitis should be a differential diagnosis in patients with rheumatologic conditions such as systemic lupus erythematosus and Sjögren syndrome.

Biliary or Gallstone Pancreatitis

Gallstone pancreatitis is the most common cause of AP in the West. It accounts for 40% of U.S. cases. The overall incidence of AP in patients with symptomatic gallstone disease is 3% to 8%. It is seen more frequently in women between 50 and 70 years of age. The exact mechanism that triggers pancreatic injury has not been completely understood, but two theories have been proposed.[5] In the obstructive theory, pancreatic injury is the result of excessive pressure inside the pancreatic duct. This increased intraductal pressure is the result of continuous secretion of pancreatic juice in the presence of pancreatic duct obstruction. The second, or reflux, theory proposes that stones become impacted in the ampulla of Vater and form a common channel that allows bile salt reflux into the pancreas. Animal models have shown that bile salts cause direct acinar cell necrosis because they increase the concentration of calcium in the cytoplasm; however, this has never been proven in humans.[2]

Alcohol-Induced Injury

Excessive ethanol consumption is the second most common cause of AP worldwide. It accounts for 35% of cases and is more prevalent in young men (30 to 45 years of age) than in women. However, only 5% to 10% of patients who drink alcohol develop AP. Factors that contribute to ethanol-induced pancreatitis include heavy ethanol abuse (>100 g/day for at least 5 years), smoking, and genetic predisposition. Compared with nonsmokers, the relative risk of alcohol-induced pancreatitis in smokers is 4.9.[6]

Alcohol has a number of deleterious effects in the pancreas. It triggers proinflammatory pathways such as nuclear factor κB

(NF-κB), which increase the production of TNF-α and IL-1. It also increases the expression and activity of caspases. Caspases are proteases that mediate apoptosis. In addition, alcohol decreases pancreatic perfusion, induces sphincter of Oddi spasm, and obstructs pancreatic ducts through the precipitation of proteins inside the ducts.

Anatomic Obstruction

Abnormal flow of pancreatic juice into the duodenum can result in pancreatic injury. AP has been described in patients with pancreatic tumors, parasites, and congenital defects.

Pancreas divisum is an anatomic variation present in 10% of the population. Its association with AP is controversial. Patients with this variation have a 5% to 10% lifetime risk for development of AP caused by relative outflow obstruction through the minor papilla. Endoscopic retrograde cholangiopancreatography (ERCP) with minor papillotomy and stenting may be beneficial for such patients.

Infrequent anatomic obstructions that have been associated with AP include *Ascaris lumbricoides* infection and annular pancreas. Although pancreatic cancer is not uncommon, patients with pancreatic cancer usually do not develop AP.

Endoscopic Retrograde Cholangiopancreatography–Induced Pancreatitis

AP is the most common complication after ERCP, occurring in up to 5% of patients. AP occurs more frequently in patients who have undergone therapeutic procedures compared with diagnostic procedures. It is also more common in patients who have had multiple attempts of cannulation, sphincter of Oddi dysfunction, and abnormal visualization of the secondary pancreatic ducts after injection of contrast material. The clinical course is mild in 90% to 95% of patients.

Drug-Induced Pancreatitis

Up to 2% of AP cases are caused by medications. The most common agents include sulfonamides, metronidazole, erythromycin, tetracyclines, didanosine, thiazides, furosemide, 3-hydroxy-3-methylglutaryl-coenzyme A (HMG-CoA) reductase inhibitors (statins), azathioprine, 6-mercaptopurine, 5-aminosalicylic acid, sulfasalazine, valproic acid, and acetaminophen. More recently, antiretroviral agents used for the treatment of AIDS have been implicated in AP.

Metabolic Factors

Hypertriglyceridemia and hypercalcemia can also lead to pancreatic damage. Direct pancreatic injury can be induced by triglyceride metabolites. It is more common in patients with type I, II, or V hyperlipidemia. It should be suspected in patients with a triglyceride level higher than 1000 mg/dL. A triglyceride level higher than 2000 mg/dL confirms the diagnosis. Hypertriglyceridemia secondary to hypothyroidism, diabetes mellitus, and alcohol does not typically induce AP.

Hypercalcemia is postulated to induce pancreatic injury through the activation of trypsinogen to trypsin and intraductal precipitation of calcium, leading to ductal obstruction and subsequent attacks of pancreatitis. Approximately 1.5% to 13% of patients with primary hyperparathyroidism develop AP.

Miscellaneous Conditions

Blunt and penetrating abdominal trauma can be associated with AP in 0.2% and 1% of cases, respectively. Prolonged intraoperative hypotension and excessive pancreatic manipulation during abdominal surgery can also result in AP. Pancreatic ischemia in association with acute pancreatic inflammation can develop after splenic artery embolization. Other rare causes include scorpion venom stings and perforated duodenal ulcers.

Clinical Manifestations

The cardinal symptom of AP is epigastric or periumbilical pain that radiates to the back. Up to 90% of patients have nausea or vomiting that typically does not relieve the pain. The nature of the pain is constant; therefore, if the pain disappears or decreases, another diagnosis should be considered.

Dehydration, poor skin turgor, tachycardia, hypotension, and dry mucous membranes are commonly seen in patients with AP. Severely dehydrated and older patients may also develop mental status changes.

The physical examination findings of the abdomen vary according to the severity of the disease. With mild pancreatitis, the physical examination findings of the abdomen may be normal or reveal only mild epigastric tenderness. Significant abdominal distention, associated with generalized rebound and abdominal rigidity, is present in severe pancreatitis. The nature of the pain described by the patient may not correlate with the physical examination findings or the degree of pancreatic inflammation.

Rare findings include flank and periumbilical ecchymosis (Grey Turner and Cullen signs, respectively). Both are indicative of retroperitoneal bleeding associated with severe pancreatitis. Patients with concomitant choledocholithiasis or significant edema in the head of the pancreas that compresses the intrapancreatic portion of the common bile duct can present with jaundice. Dullness to percussion and decreased breathing sounds in the left or, less commonly, in the right hemithorax suggest pleural effusion secondary to AP.

Diagnosis

The cornerstone of the diagnosis of AP is the clinical findings plus an elevation of pancreatic enzyme levels in the plasma. A threefold or higher elevation of amylase and lipase levels confirms the diagnosis. The serum half-life of amylase is shorter than that of lipase. In patients who do not present to the emergency department within the first 24 to 48 hours after the onset of symptoms, determination of lipase levels is a more sensitive indicator to establish the diagnosis. Lipase is also a more specific marker of AP because serum amylase levels can be elevated in a number of conditions, such as peptic ulcer disease, mesenteric ischemia, salpingitis, and macroamylasemia.

Patients with AP are typically hyperglycemic; they can also have leukocytosis and abnormal elevation of liver enzyme levels. The elevation of alanine aminotransferase levels in the serum in the context of AP confirmed by high pancreatic enzyme levels has a positive predictive value of 95% in the diagnosis of acute biliary pancreatitis.[5]

Imaging Studies

Although simple abdominal radiographs are not useful for diagnosis of pancreatitis, they can help rule out other conditions, such as perforated ulcer disease. Nonspecific findings in patients with AP include air-fluid levels suggestive of ileus, cutoff colon sign as a result of colonic spasm at the splenic flexure, and widening of the duodenal C loop caused by severe pancreatic head edema.

The usefulness of ultrasound for diagnosis of pancreatitis is limited by intra-abdominal fat and increased intestinal gas as a result of the ileus. Nevertheless, this test should always be ordered in patients with AP because of its high sensitivity (95%) in diagnosing gallstones. Combined elevations of liver transaminase and pancreatic enzyme levels and the presence of gallstones on ultrasound have an even higher sensitivity (97%) and specificity (100%) for diagnosing acute biliary pancreatitis.

Contrast-enhanced computed tomography (CT) is currently the best modality for evaluation of the pancreas, especially if the study is performed with a multidetector CT scanner. The most valuable contrast phase in which to evaluate the pancreatic parenchyma is the portal venous phase (65 to 70 seconds after injection of contrast material), which allows evaluation of the viability of the pancreatic parenchyma, amount of peripancreatic inflammation, and presence of intra-abdominal free air or fluid collections. Noncontrast CT scanning may also be of value in the setting of renal failure by identifying fluid collections or extraluminal air.

Abdominal magnetic resonance imaging (MRI) is also useful to evaluate the extent of necrosis, inflammation, and presence of free fluid. However, its cost and availability and the fact that patients requiring imaging are critically ill and need to be in intensive care units limit its applicability in the acute phase. Although magnetic resonance cholangiopancreatography (MRCP) is not indicated in the acute setting of AP, it has an important role in the evaluation of patients with unexplained or recurrent pancreatitis because it allows complete visualization of the biliary and pancreatic duct anatomy. In addition, intravenous (IV) administration of secretin increases pancreatic duct secretion, which causes a transient distention of the pancreatic duct. For example, secretin MRCP is useful in patients with AP and no evidence of a predisposing condition to rule out pancreas divisum, intraductal papillary mucinous neoplasm (IPMN), or a small tumor in the pancreatic duct.

In the setting of gallstone pancreatitis, endoscopic ultrasound (EUS) may play an important role in the evaluation of persistent choledocholithiasis. Several studies have shown that routine ERCP for suspected gallstone pancreatitis reveals no evidence of persistent obstruction in most cases and may actually worsen symptoms because of manipulation of the gland. EUS has been proven to be sensitive for identifying choledocholithiasis; it allows examination of the biliary tree and pancreas with no risk of worsening of the pancreatitis. In patients in whom persistent choledocholithiasis is confirmed by EUS, ERCP can be used selectively as a therapeutic measure.

Assessment of Severity of Disease

The earliest scoring system designed to evaluate the severity of AP was introduced by Ranson and colleagues in 1974.[7] It predicts the severity of the disease on the basis of 11 parameters obtained at the time of admission or 48 hours later. The mortality rate of AP directly correlates with the number of parameters that are positive. Severe pancreatitis is diagnosed if three or more of the Ranson criteria are fulfilled. The main disadvantage is that it does not predict the severity of disease at the time of the admission because six parameters are assessed only after 48 hours of admission. The Ranson score has a low positive predictive value (50%) and high negative predictive value (90%). Therefore, it is mainly used to rule out severe pancreatitis or to predict the risk of mortality.[8] The original scoring symptom designed to predict the severity of the disease and its modification for acute biliary pancreatitis are shown in Boxes 55-1 and 55-2.

AP severity can also be addressed by the Acute Physiology and Chronic Health Evaluation (APACHE II) score. Based on the patient's age, previous health status, and 12 routine physiologic measurements, APACHE II provides a general measure of the severity of disease. An APACHE II score of 8 or higher defines severe pancreatitis. The main advantage is that it can be used on admission and repeated at any time. However, it is complex, not specific for AP, and based on the patient's age, which easily upgrades the AP severity score. APACHE II has a positive predictive value of 43% and a negative predictive value of 89%.[8]

Using imaging characteristics, Balthazar and associates[9] have established the CT severity index. This index correlates CT findings with the patient's outcome. The CT severity index is shown in Table 55-2.

In 1992, the International Symposium on Acute Pancreatitis defined severe pancreatitis as the presence of local pancreatic complications (necrosis, abscess, or pseudocyst) or any evidence of organ failure. Severe pancreatitis is diagnosed if there is any evidence of organ failure or a local pancreatic complication (Box 55-3).

C-reactive protein (CRP) is an inflammatory marker that peaks 48 to 72 hours after the onset of pancreatitis and correlates with the severity of the disease. A CRP level of 150 mg/mL or

BOX 55-1 Ranson Prognostic Criteria for Non-Gallstone Pancreatitis

At presentation
- Age >55 years
- Blood glucose level >200 mg/dL
- White blood cell count >16,000 cells/mm^3
- Lactate dehydrogenase level >350 IU/liter
- Aspartate aminotransferase level >250 IU/liter

After 48 hours of admission
- Hematocrit*: decrease >10%
- Serum calcium level <8 mg/dL
- Base deficit >4 mEq/L
- Blood urea nitrogen level: increase >5 mg/dL
- Fluid requirement >6 liters
- PaO_2 <60 mm Hg

Ranson score ≥3 defines severe pancreatitis.

*Compared with admission value.

BOX 55-2 Ranson Prognostic Criteria for Gallstone Pancreatitis

At presentation
- Age >70 years
- Blood glucose level >220 mg/dL
- White blood cell count >18,000 cells/mm^3
- Lactate dehydrogenase level >400 IU/liter
- Aspartate aminotransferase level >250 IU/liter

After 48 hours of admission
- Hematocrit*: decrease >10%
- Serum calcium level <8 mg/dL
- Base deficit >5 mEq/L
- Blood urea nitrogen level: increase >2 mg/dL
- Fluid requirement >4 liters
- PaO_2: Not available

Ranson score ≥3 defines severe pancreatitis.

*Compared with admission value.

TABLE 55-2 Computed Tomography Severity Index (CTSI) for Acute Pancreatitis

FEATURE	POINTS
Pancreatic Inflammation	
Normal pancreas	0
Focal or diffuse pancreatic enlargement	1
Intrinsic pancreatic alterations with peripancreatic fat inflammatory changes	2
Single fluid collection or phlegmon	3
Two or more fluid collections or gas, in or adjacent to the pancreas	4
Pancreatic Necrosis	
None	0
≤30%	2
30%-50%	4
>50%	6

CTSI 0-3, mortality 3%, morbidity 8%; CTSI 4-6, mortality 6%, morbidity 35%; CTSI 7-10, mortality 17%, morbidity 92%.

BOX 55-3 Atlanta Criteria for Acute Pancreatitis

Organ Failure, as Defined by

Shock (systolic blood pressure <90 mm Hg)
Pulmonary insufficiency (Pao_2 <60 mm Hg)
Renal failure (creatinine level >2 mg/dL after fluid resuscitation)
Gastrointestinal bleeding (>500 mL/24 hr)

Systemic Complications

Disseminated intravascular coagulation (platelet count ≤100,000)
Fibrinogen <1 g/liter
Fibrin split products >80 μg/dL
Metabolic disturbance (calcium level ≤7.5 mg/dL)

Local Complications

Necrosis
Abscess
Pseudocyst

Severe pancreatitis is defined by the presence of any evidence of organ failure or a local complication.

higher defines severe pancreatitis. The major limitation is that it cannot be used on admission; the sensitivity of the assay decreases if CRP levels are measured within 48 hours after the onset of symptoms. In addition to CRP, a number of studies have shown other biochemical markers (e.g., serum levels of procalcitonin, IL-6, IL-1, elastase) that correlate with the severity of the disease. However, their main limitation is their cost, and they are not widely available.

Treatment

Regardless of the cause or the severity of the disease, the cornerstone of the treatment of AP is aggressive fluid resuscitation with isotonic crystalloid solution. The rate of administration should be individualized and adjusted on the basis of age, comorbidities, vital signs, mental status, skin turgor, and urine output. Patients who do not respond to initial fluid resuscitation or have significant renal, cardiac, or respiratory comorbidities often require invasive monitoring with central venous access and a Foley catheter.

In addition to fluid resuscitation, patients with AP require continuous pulse oximetry because one of the most common systemic complications of AP is hypoxemia caused by the acute lung injury associated with this disease. Patients should receive supplementary oxygen to maintain arterial saturation above 95%.

It is also essential to provide effective analgesia. Narcotics are usually preferred, especially morphine. One of the physiologic effects described after systemic administration of morphine is an increase in tone in the sphincter of Oddi; however, there is no evidence that narcotics exert a negative impact on the outcome of patients with AP.

There is no proven benefit in treating AP with antiproteases (e.g., gabexate mesilate, aprotinin), platelet-activating factor inhibitors (e.g., lexipafant), or pancreatic secretion inhibitors.

Nutritional support is vital in the treatment of AP. Oral feeding may be impossible because of persistent ileus, pain, or intubation. In addition, 20% of patients with severe AP develop recurrent pain shortly after the oral route has been restarted. The main options to provide this nutritional support are enteral feeding and total parenteral nutrition (TPN). Although there is no difference in the mortality rate between both types of nutrition, enteral nutrition is associated with fewer infectious complications and reduces the need for pancreatic surgery. Although TPN provides most nutritional requirements, it is associated with mucosal atrophy, decreased intestinal blood flow, increased risk of bacterial overgrowth in the small bowel, antegrade colonization with colonic bacteria, and increased bacterial translocation. In addition, patients with TPN have more central line infections and metabolic complications (e.g., hyperglycemia, electrolyte imbalance). Whenever possible, enteral nutrition should be used rather than TPN.

Given the significant increase in mortality associated with septic complications in severe pancreatitis, a number of physicians advocated the use of prophylactic antibiotics in the 1970s. Recent meta-analyses and systematic reviews that have evaluated multiple randomized controlled trials have proved that prophylactic antibiotics do not decrease the frequency of surgical intervention, infected necrosis, or mortality in patients with severe pancreatitis. In addition, they are associated with gram-positive cocci infection, such as by *Staphylococcus aureus*, and *Candida* infection, which is seen in 5% to 15% of patients.[10]

Special Considerations

Endoscopic retrograde cholangiopancreatography. Early ERCP, with or without sphincterotomy, was initially advocated to reduce the severity of pancreatitis because the obstructive theory of AP states that pancreatic injury is the result of pancreatic duct obstruction. However, three randomized trials have demonstrated that ERCP is beneficial only for patients with severe acute biliary pancreatitis. Routine use of ERCP is not indicated for patients with mild pancreatitis because the bile duct obstruction is usually transient and resolves within 48 hours after the onset of symptoms. In addition to severe acute biliary pancreatitis, ERCP is indicated for patients who develop cholangitis and those with persistent bile duct obstruction demonstrated by other imaging modalities, such as EUS. Finally, in older patients with poor performance status or severe comorbidities that preclude surgery, ERCP with sphincterotomy is a safe alternative to prevent recurrent biliary pancreatitis.

Laparoscopic cholecystectomy. In the absence of definitive treatment, 30% of patients with acute biliary pancreatitis will have recurrent disease. With the exception of older patients and those with poor performance status, laparoscopic cholecystectomy is indicated for all patients with mild acute biliary pancreatitis. Studies have shown that early laparoscopic cholecystectomy, defined as laparoscopic cholecystectomy during the initial admission to the hospital, is a safe procedure that decreases recurrence of the disease.[5] Choledocholithiasis can be excluded by intraoperative cholangiography, ERCP, or laparoscopic common bile duct exploration.

For patients with severe pancreatitis, early surgery may increase the morbidity and length of stay.[11] Current recommendations suggest conservative treatment for at least 6 weeks before laparoscopic cholecystectomy is attempted in this setting. This approach has significantly decreased morbidity.[5]

Complications

Sterile and Infected Peripancreatic Fluid Collections

The presence of acute abdominal fluid during an episode of AP has been described in 30% to 57% of patients. In contrast to pseudocysts and cystic neoplasias of the pancreas, fluid collections are not surrounded or encased by epithelium or fibrotic capsule. Treatment is supportive because most fluid collections will be spontaneously reabsorbed by the peritoneum. Fever, elevated white blood cell count, and abdominal pain suggest infection of this fluid, and percutaneous aspiration is confirmatory. Percutaneous drainage and IV administration of antibiotics should be instituted if infection is present.

Pancreatic Necrosis and Infected Necrosis

Pancreatic necrosis is the presence of nonviable pancreatic parenchyma or peripancreatic fat; it can be manifested as a focal area or diffuse involvement of the gland. Contrast-enhanced CT is the most reliable technique to diagnose pancreatic necrosis. It is typically seen as areas of low attenuation (<40 to 50 HU) after the IV injection of contrast material. Normal parenchyma usually has a density of 100 to 150 HU. Up to 20% of patients with AP develop pancreatic necrosis. It is important to identify and to provide proper treatment of this complication because most patients who develop multiorgan failure have necrotizing pancreatitis; pancreatic necrosis has been documented in up to 80% of the autopsies of patients who died after an episode of AP.[3]

The main complication of pancreatic necrosis is infection. The risk is directly related to the amount of necrosis; in patients with pancreatic necrosis involving less than 30% of the gland, the risk of infection is 22%. The risk is 37% for patients with pancreatic necrosis that involves 30% to 50% of the gland and up to 46% if more than 70% of the gland is affected.[3] This complication is associated with bacterial translocation usually involving enteric flora, such as gram-negative rods (e.g., *Escherichia coli, Klebsiella,* and *Pseudomonas* spp.) and *Enterococcus* spp.

Infected pancreatic necrosis should be suspected in patients with prolonged fever, elevated white blood cell count, or progressive clinical deterioration. Evidence of air within the pancreatic necrosis seen on a CT scan confirms the diagnosis but is a rare finding. If infected necrosis is suspected, fine-needle aspiration (FNA) may be performed if the diagnosis is equivocal; from the aspirate, a positive Gram stain or culture establishes the diagnosis. Although positive cultures are confirmatory, a review has demonstrated that despite negative preoperative cultures, 42% of patients with so-called persistent unwellness will have infected necrosis.[12] Figure 55-7 illustrates the pathophysiologic process of pancreatic necrosis infection.

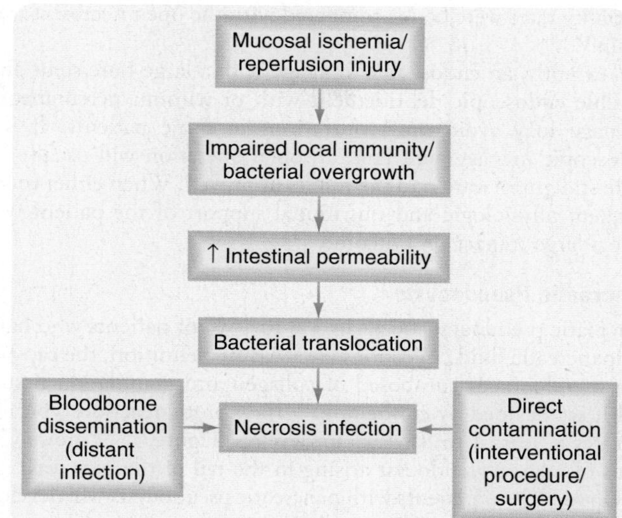

FIGURE 55-7 Pathophysiology of Pancreatic Necrosis Infection. The acute inflammatory injury that occurs during the first 48 to 72 hours causes mucosal ischemia and reperfusion injury. Both effects favor bacterial overgrowth because they alter local immunity. Mucosal ischemia also produces an increase in the permeability of intestinal cells, which is initiated 72 hours after the acute episode but typically peaks 1 week later. These transient episodes of bacteremia are associated with pancreatic necrosis infection. Less frequently, distant sources of infection, such as pneumonia and vascular or urinary tract infection associated with central lines and catheters, are associated with bacteremia and pancreatic necrosis. Finally, local contamination after surgery or interventional procedures such as ERCP is responsible for necrosis infection.

Once infection has been demonstrated, IV antibiotics should be given. Because of their penetration into the pancreas and spectrum coverage, carbapenems are the first option of treatment. Alternative therapy includes quinolones, metronidazole, third-generation cephalosporins, and piperacillin.

Historically, the definitive treatment of infected pancreatic necrosis is surgical débridement with necrosectomy, closed continuous irrigation, or open packaging (Fig. 55-8). The overall mortality rate after open necrosectomy has been as high as 25% to 30%[12] because of the severe nature of the disease as well as the high complication rate of an open débridement. Outcomes are time dependent; patients who undergo surgery in the first 14 days have a mortality rate of 75%, and those who undergo surgery between 15 and 29 days and after 30 days have mortality rates of 45% and 8%, respectively.[13] As a result of the elevated morbidity and mortality rates with open débridement, endoscopic and laparoscopic techniques are being used more often. Both may ultimately provide similar outcomes, with hopes of reducing perioperative morbidity and mortality, although level I data are lacking. In general, the longer a patient can be medically optimized and managed with enteral nutrition and antibiotics (if indicated), the more mature a fluid collection (with or without necrosis), and therefore the extent of an endoscopic or operative débridement (if needed) will be better delineated and tolerated.

In 2010, the Dutch Pancreatitis Study Group performed a randomized trial evaluating open necrosectomy versus percutaneous drainage followed by minimally invasive retroperitoneal débridement for necrotizing and infected necrotizing pancreatitis. The results showed that long-term end-point complications and mortality rates were better compared with the open necrosectomy group.[14]

Currently, an endoscopic drainage with a large-bore stent and possible endoscopic débridement with or without percutaneous drainage may avoid open operations in some patients. If the endoscopic management fails, an open operation will usually be more straightforward and the results improved. When either route is taken, physiologic and nutritional support of the patient will have a large impact on outcome.

Pancreatic Pseudocysts

Pancreatic pseudocysts occur in 5% to 15% of patients who have peripancreatic fluid collections after AP. By definition, the capsule of a pseudocyst is composed of collagen and granulation tissue, and it is not lined by epithelium.[15] The fibrotic reaction typically requires at least 4 to 8 weeks to develop. Figure 55-9 shows CT scans of a large pseudocyst arising in the tail of the pancreas.

Up to 50% of patients with pancreatic pseudocysts will develop symptoms. Persistent pain, early satiety, nausea, weight loss, and elevated pancreatic enzyme levels in plasma suggest this diagnosis. The diagnosis is corroborated by CT or MRI. EUS with FNA is indicated for patients in whom the diagnosis of pancreatic pseudocyst is not clear. Characteristic features of pancreatic pseudocysts include high amylase levels associated with the absence of mucin and low carcinoembryonic antigen (CEA) levels.

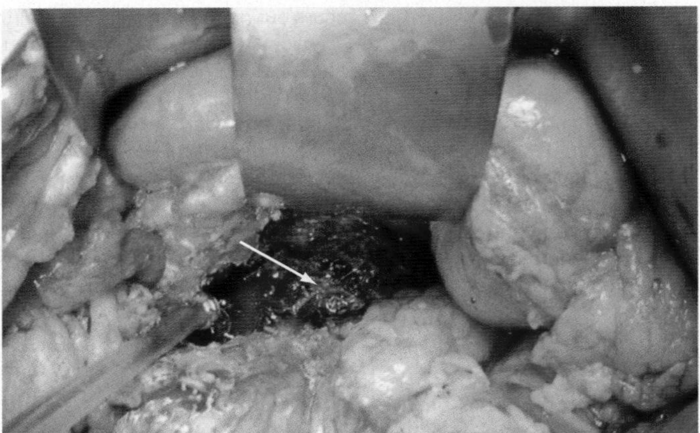

FIGURE 55-8 Infected Pancreatic Necrosis. This 45-year-old man had severe ethanol-induced pancreatitis. Four weeks after the initial episode, the patient developed fever (39.5° C [103° F]), hypotension, and leukocytosis (19,000 cells/mm^3). The CT scan documented pancreatic necrosis involving 35% of the gland. After FNA, Gram staining documented the presence of gram-negative rods. The exploratory laparotomy indicated pancreatic necrosis involving mainly the body of the gland *(arrow)*. The patient was treated with necrosectomy, closed drainage, and IV meropenem. Final culture documented the presence of *Escherichia coli*. The patient was discharged home 56 days after the initial episode.

Observation is indicated for asymptomatic patients because spontaneous regression has been documented in up to 70% of cases; this is particularly true for patients with pseudocysts smaller than 4 cm in diameter, located in the tail, and no evidence of pancreatic duct obstruction or communication with the main pancreatic duct.[15] Invasive therapies are indicated for symptomatic patients or when the differentiation between a cystic neoplasm and pseudocyst is not possible. Because most patients are treated with decompressive procedures and not with resection, it is imperative to have a pathologic diagnosis. Surgical drainage has been the traditional approach for pancreatic pseudocysts. However, there is increasing evidence that transgastric and transduodenal endoscopic drainage are safe and effective approaches for patients with pancreatic pseudocysts in close contact (defined as <1 cm) with the stomach and duodenum, respectively. In addition, transpapillary drainage can be attempted in pancreatic pseudocysts communicating with the main pancreatic duct. For patients in whom a pancreatic duct stricture is associated with a pancreatic pseudocyst, endoscopic dilation and stent placement are indicated.

Surgical drainage is indicated for patients with pancreatic pseudocysts that cannot be treated with endoscopic techniques and for patients who fail to respond to endoscopic treatment. Definitive treatment depends on the location of the cyst. Pancreatic pseudocysts closely attached to the stomach should be treated with a cystogastrostomy. In this procedure, an anterior gastrostomy is performed. Once the pseudocyst is located, it is drained through the posterior wall of the stomach using a linear stapler. The defect in the anterior wall of the stomach is closed in two layers. Pancreatic pseudocysts located in the head of the pancreas that are in close contact with the duodenum are treated with a cystoduodenostomy. Finally, some pseudocysts are not in contact with the stomach or duodenum. The surgical treatment for these patients is a Roux-en-Y cystojejunostomy. Surgical cyst enterostomy is successful in achieving immediate cyst drainage in more than 90% of cases. After initial resolution, pseudocyst formation may recur in up to 12% of cases during long-term follow-up, depending on the location of the cyst and underlying cause of the disease.[15]

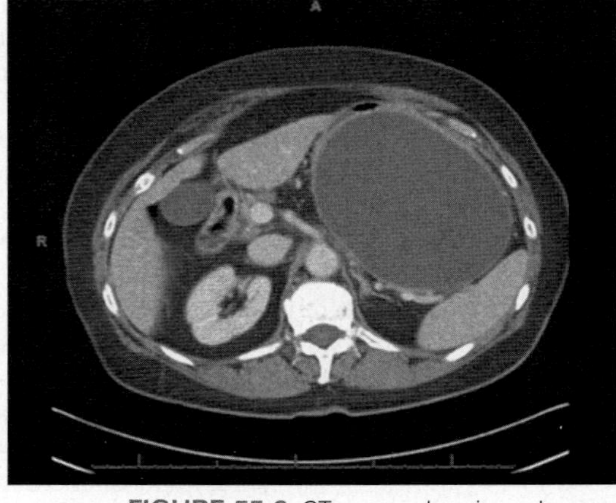

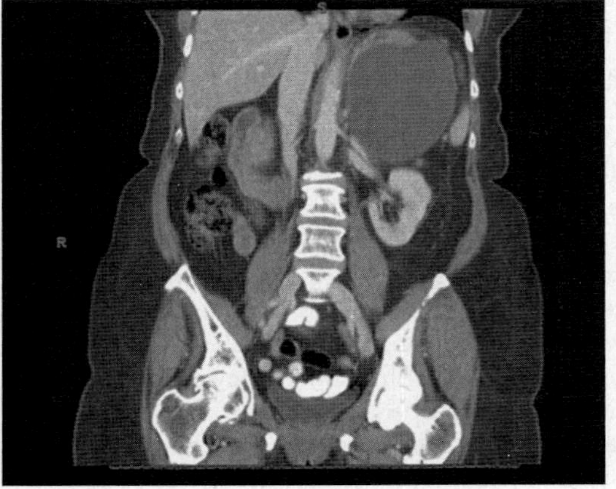

FIGURE 55-9 CT scans showing a large pseudocyst arising in the tail of the pancreas.

Complications of pancreatic pseudocysts include bleeding and pancreaticopleural fistula secondary to vascular and pleural erosion, respectively; bile duct and duodenal obstruction; rupture into the abdominal cavity; and infection. Percutaneous drainage is indicated only for septic patients secondary to pseudocyst infection because it has a high incidence of external fistula.

Pancreatic Ascites and Pancreaticopleural Fistulas

Although very rare, complete disruption of the pancreatic duct can lead to significant accumulation of fluid. This condition should be suspected in patients who have an episode of AP, develop significant abdominal distention, and have free intra-abdominal fluid. Diagnostic paracentesis typically demonstrates elevated amylase and lipase levels. Treatment consists of abdominal drainage combined with endoscopic placement of a pancreatic stent across the disruption. Failure of this therapy requires surgical treatment; it consists of distal resection and closure of the proximal stump.

Posterior pancreatic duct disruption into the pleural space has been described rarely. Symptoms that suggest this condition include dyspnea, abdominal pain, cough, and chest pain. The diagnosis is confirmed with chest radiography, thoracentesis, and CT scan. Figure 55-10 demonstrates a large, left-sided pleural effusion caused by a pancreatic-pleural fistula. Amylase levels above 50,000 IU in the pleural fluid confirm the diagnosis. It is more common after alcoholic pancreatitis and in 70% of patients is associated with pancreatic pseudocysts. Initial treatment requires chest drainage, parenteral nutritional support, and administration of octreotide. Up to 60% of patients respond to this therapy. Persistent drainage should also be treated with endoscopic sphincterotomy and stent placement. Patients who do not respond to these measures require surgical treatment, similar to that described for pancreatic ascites.

Vascular Complications

AP is rarely associated with arterial vascular complications. The most common vessel affected is the splenic artery, but the SMA, cystic artery, and GDA have also been found to be affected. It has

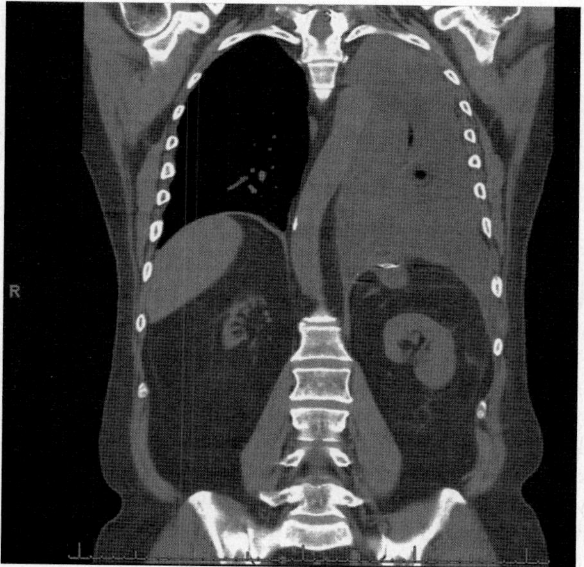

FIGURE 55-10 Massive left-sided pleural effusion secondary to a pancreaticopleural fistula.

been proposed that pancreatic elastase damages the vessels, leading to pseudoaneurysm formation. Spontaneous rupture results in massive bleeding. Clinical manifestations include sudden onset of abdominal pain, tachycardia, and hypotension. If possible, arterial embolization should be attempted to control the bleeding. Refractory cases require ligation of the vessel affected. The mortality ranges from 28% to 56%.

Pancreatic inflammation can also produce vascular thrombosis; the vessel usually affected is the splenic vein, but in severe cases, it can extend into the portal venous system. Imaging demonstrates splenomegaly, gastric varices, and splenic vein occlusion. Thrombolytics have been described in the acute early phase; however, most patients can be managed with conservative treatment. Recurrent episodes of upper gastrointestinal bleeding caused by venous hypertension should be treated with splenectomy.

Pancreatocutaneous Fistula

The frequency of pancreatic fistulas is low. Only 0.4% of patients have this complication after an acute episode. However, the incidence of this complication increases in patients with other complications after AP: 4.5% in patients with pancreatic pseudocysts (4.5%) and 40% in patients with infected necrosis after surgical débridement.[12] Treatment is conservative for most patients.

CHRONIC PANCREATITIS

In contrast to AP, the histologic hallmark of chronic pancreatitis is the persistent inflammation and irreversible fibrosis associated with atrophy of the pancreatic parenchyma. These histologic features are associated with chronic pain and endocrine and exocrine insufficiency that significantly decrease the quality of life of these patients. Chronic pancreatitis affects between 3 and 10/100,000 persons.

Risk Factors

The specific cause and frequency of each condition vary among countries, hospital populations, and referral practices. In general, heavy alcohol consumption is the most common cause of chronic pancreatitis (70% to 80% of cases), especially in urban hospitals. Conditions such as chronic duct obstruction, trauma, pancreas divisum, cystic dystrophy of the duodenal wall, hyperparathyroidism, hypertriglyceridemia, autoimmune pancreatitis, tropical pancreatitis, and hereditary pancreatitis are rare and account for less than 10% of all cases. However, hereditary, chronic, and autoimmune pancreatitis are more common in referral centers. In up to 20% of patients, a clear cause cannot be documented and cases are considered to be idiopathic.

Alcohol Abuse

Prolonged alcohol abuse is the most important risk factor associated with chronic pancreatitis. The fact that only 3% to 7% of heavy drinkers develop chronic pancreatitis suggests that alcohol is only a cofactor and that other factors are required for development of this complication. Alcohol exerts multiple noxious effects in the pancreas: it increases the total protein concentration in the pancreatic juice, it promotes the synthesis and secretion of lithostathine by acinar cells, and it increases glycoprotein 2 secretion in pancreatic juice. These factors lead to protein precipitation and subsequent formation of protein plugs and eventually stones inside the pancreatic duct. As a result of the obstruction, acinar cells are no longer able to secrete pancreatic enzymes and are predisposed to autodigestion. In addition, several products of alcohol metabolism, such as fatty acid ethyl esters and reactive oxygen species, cause fragility of intra-acinar organelles, such as zymogen granules and lysosomes, which leads to abnormal pancreatic enzyme activation inside acinar cells. Acetaldehyde, another alcohol metabolite, causes direct acinar injury. Chronic alcohol consumption is associated with enhanced NF-κB activity, decreased perfusion in the microcirculation of the pancreas, and increased intracellular calcium levels.

The identification of pancreatic stellate cells (PSCs) in the late 1990s is one of the most important discoveries in the pathophysiology of chronic pancreatitis.[16] PSCs are specialized quiescent fibroblasts found at the base of acinar cells. Once stimulated, PSCs differentiate into activated myofibroblasts, which synthesize proteins that form the extracellular matrix. Examples of these proteins include collagen I and III, fibronectin, laminin, and matrix metalloproteinases. PSCs have responses similar to hepatic stellate cells; chronic necrosis and inflammation (necroinflammation) induce the release of inflammatory mediators, such as platelet-derived growth factor, TGF-β, TNF-α, IL-1, and IL-6, which are known to activate PSCs. Consequently, the synthesis of collagen and other components of pancreatic fibrosis is increased. It has been postulated that the chronic necroinflammation induced by ethanol activates PSCs and induces pancreatic fibrosis. Interestingly, it has also been shown that alcohol and some of its metabolites (e.g., acetaldehyde) cause activation of PSCs.

Although they have been evaluated only in preclinical studies, novel therapies that target the activation of PSCs are being investigated. It has been reported that antioxidants, angiotensin-converting enzyme inhibitors, peroxisome proliferator-activated receptor gamma ligands, and vitamin A inhibit the activity of PSCs.

Smoking

Epidemiologic studies have shown that smoking increases the risk of alcohol-induced chronic pancreatitis. Active smokers develop chronic pancreatitis at a younger age compared with nonsmokers. In addition, the risk of pancreatic calcifications and diabetes mellitus is increased in patients who smoke compared with nonsmokers.

Gene Mutations

Under physiologic conditions, pancreatic enzyme activation is strictly controlled. Mutations in proteins that regulate this activation increase the risk of chronic pancreatitis. Mutations in the cationic trypsinogen gene, also known as protease serine 1 *(PRSS1)* gene, are common in hereditary chronic pancreatitis. *PRSS1* is located on chromosome 7 and regulates trypsinogen production; mutations in this gene are associated with intra-acinar trypsinogen activation. *PRSS1* mutations have been documented in hereditary pancreatitis but are uncommon in other forms of chronic pancreatitis.

SPINK-1 is a peptide secreted by acinar cells that regulates the premature activation of trypsinogen. Because *SPINK1* mutations are present in 1% to 2% of healthy patients but the prevalence of chronic pancreatitis is much lower, it has been hypothesized that *SPINK1* mutations are not enough to trigger pancreatic inflammation. However, they lower the threshold for its development and influence the severity of the disease. *SPINK1* mutations are more prevalent in alcoholic, hereditary, and idiopathic pancreatitis.

The secretion of bicarbonate and chloride in respiratory and pancreatic secretions is regulated by the *CFTR* gene. *CFTR* mutations affect the normal secretion of bicarbonate, decrease pancreatic juice volume, and augment the concentration of pancreatic enzymes inside the pancreatic duct. Homozygous *CFTR* mutations result in cystic fibrosis; heterozygous mild mutations predispose to pancreatic exocrine insufficiency and chronic pancreatitis. The prevalence of *CFTR* gene mutations is higher in patients with alcoholic, idiopathic, and hereditary pancreatitis compared with the general population.

Animal studies in trypsin knockout mice suggest that even in the absence of trypsin, chronic noxious stimuli can induce chronic pancreatitis.[17] These results suggest that alternative pathways independent of trypsin may exist that can lead to chronic injury in pancreatitis, and elucidation of these pathways may lead to development of novel therapeutics.

Types of Chronic Pancreatitis

Autoimmune Pancreatitis

Autoimmune pancreatitis is a chronic inflammatory disorder that involves the pancreas. At least two different histologic variants have been defined. Type 1 is the most common; it is characterized by dense, periductal lymphoplasmacytic infiltrates, storiform fibrosis, and obliterative venulitis. Plasmatic cells typically stain positive for immunoglobulin G4. In type 2, the pancreas is infiltrated by neutrophils, lymphocytes, and plasma cells that destroy and obliterate the epithelium in the pancreatic duct. Autoimmune pancreatitis is more common in men than in women. Up to 80% of patients are older than 50 years. Patients with autoimmune pancreatitis can develop acute symptoms such as jaundice or AP, closely mimicking patients with pancreatic adenocarcinoma. However, most patients with chronic pancreatitis develop chronic abdominal discomfort associated with abnormal elevation of amylase and lipase levels.

Tropical Pancreatitis

Tropical pancreatitis is not common in the United States; it is more common in tropical areas within 30 degrees of the equator, particularly in India. Its pathophysiology has not been completely delineated, but it has been associated with cassava ingestion and *SPINK1* mutations. Up to 45% to 50% of patients with tropical pancreatitis have *SPINK1* mutations.

Idiopathic Pancreatitis

In up to 10% to 20% of patients with chronic pancreatitis, a clear cause that predisposed to the disease is not evident. Future identification of genetic defects associated with chronic pancreatitis may allow the identification of individuals at highest risk for development of this disease.

Clinical Manifestations

Pain is the primary manifestation of chronic pancreatitis. Initially precipitated by oral intake, the intensity, frequency, and duration of pain gradually increase with worsening disease. Quality of life of these patients is significantly affected because of decreased oral intake, interference with daily activities, and dependence on narcotic pain medications. Nausea and vomiting are not common early on; however, they may appear as the disease progresses.

Pancreatic inflammation and fibrosis not only affect the pancreatic ducts but also decrease the number and function of acinar cells. At least 90% of the gland needs to be dysfunctional before steatorrhea, diarrhea, and other symptoms of malabsorption develop. In severe cases, diseases associated with fat-soluble vitamin deficiency, such as bleeding, osteopenia, and osteoporosis, develop. Exocrine insufficiency occurs in 80% to 90% of patients with long-standing chronic pancreatitis.

Chronic pancreatitis also affects islet cell populations. As a result, 40% to 80% of patients will have clinical manifestations of diabetes mellitus. The prevalence depends on the predisposing condition and onset of symptoms. Diabetes mellitus typically occurs many years after the onset of abdominal pain and pancreatic exocrine insufficiency.

Jaundice or cholangitis occurs in 5% to 10% of patients because of fibrosis of the distal common bile duct. Extensive scarring in the head of the pancreas can also obstruct the duodenum, leading to severe nausea, vomiting, and abdominal pain. Upper gastrointestinal bleeding secondary to portal or splenic vein thrombosis is a rare manifestation of chronic pancreatitis.

Diagnosis

Imaging Studies

The diagnosis of chronic pancreatitis may be challenging early in the course of the disease because the correlation between symptoms and the structural changes seen on imaging studies is poor. The most common CT findings in chronic pancreatitis include dilated pancreatic duct (68%), parenchymal atrophy (54%), and pancreatic calcifications (50%; Fig. 55-11). Other findings include peripancreatic fluid, focal pancreatic enlargement, biliary duct dilation, and irregular pancreatic parenchyma contour. CT has a sensitivity of 56% to 95% and a specificity of 85% to 100% for the diagnosis of chronic pancreatitis. In addition to establishing the diagnosis, CT is particularly useful to assess complications, such as pancreatic duct disruption, pseudocysts, portal and splenic vein thrombosis, and splenic and pancreaticoduodenal artery pseudoaneurysms.

MRI is a reliable alternative to evaluate patients with chronic pancreatitis. The sensitivity for the diagnosis of pancreatic calcifications is lower, but MRI is useful to detect changes in the pancreatic parenchyma suggestive of chronic inflammation, such as changes in intensity, pancreatic atrophy, and irregularities in the contour. In addition, MRCP with secretin injection is particularly useful to evaluate intraductal strictures and pancreatic duct disruption.

Although ERCP was historically considered the "gold standard" for the diagnosis of chronic pancreatitis, the advent of secretin MRCP and EUS has significantly decreased its role as a diagnostic test. Current indications include patients for whom other diagnostic tests, including CT and MRCP, are contraindicated or have failed to corroborate the diagnosis. ERCP should be considered a therapeutic modality in patients who develop pancreatic duct complications amenable to endoscopic therapy, such as stricture, stone, pseudocysts, and biliary stenosis.

EUS has emerged during the past 25 years as the most accurate technique to diagnose chronic pancreatitis in patients with minimal change disease or in the early stages. A panel of endosonographers has defined the criteria required for diagnosis of chronic pancreatitis, known as the Rosemont criteria (Box 55-4). Histologic evidence of inflammation, atrophy, and fibrosis is the gold standard for the diagnosis of chronic pancreatitis; however, current evidence does not support the use of EUS-guided FNA or Tru-Cut biopsies to diagnose this disease.[18]

Functional Tests

Measurement of the fecal elastase 1 level is the preferred noninvasive study to diagnose pancreatic exocrine insufficiency. It quantifies the amount of fecal elastase 1 using monoclonal or polyclonal anti–human elastase 1 antibodies. A fecal elastase 1 concentration above 200 μg/g feces is normal; a fecal elastase 1 concentration between 100 and 200 μg/g defines mild to moderate pancreatic insufficiency; and a fecal elastase 1 concentration below 100 μg/g establishes the diagnosis of severe pancreatic exocrine insufficiency.

The fecal fat and weight estimation test measures the stool content of fat after a nutritional intake of 100 g of fat per day during 3 days. If the stool fat content exceeds 7 g/day, the diagnosis of steatorrhea is established.

Treatment

Medical Treatment

The main goal in the treatment of these patients is palliation of symptoms. Optimal treatment requires that a multidisciplinary team follow a systematized and well-structured therapeutic plan. Patient counseling is an important component because current

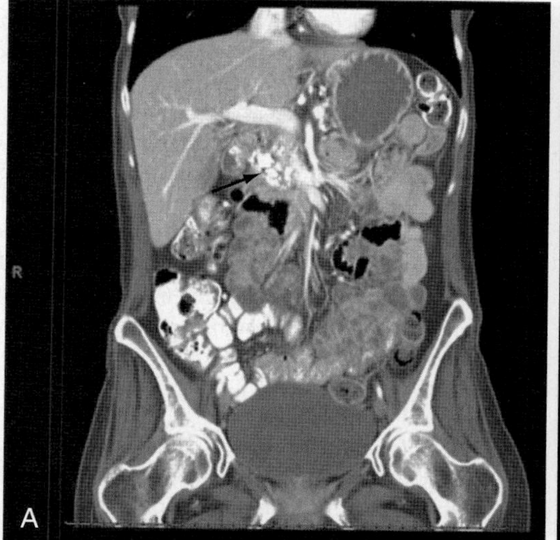

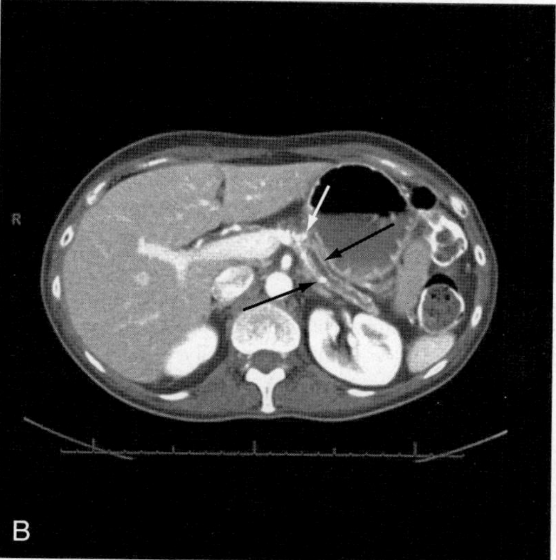

FIGURE 55-11 Typical CT findings associated with chronic pancreatitis. Shown are pancreatic duct dilation *(long arrow)* and intrapancreatic calcifications, which are also typical of chronic pancreatitis *(small arrow)*.

BOX 55-4 Rosemont Consensus-Based Endoscopic Ultrasound Features for Diagnosis of Chronic Pancreatitis

Parenchymal Features

Major A Criteria

- Hyperechoic foci with postacoustic shadowing

Major B Criteria

- Honeycombing lobularity*

Minor Criteria

- Hyperechoic, nonshadowing foci ≥3 mm in length and width
- Lobularity including three or more noncontiguous lobules in the body or tail
- Pancreatic cysts ≥2 mm in short axis
- At least three strands†

Ductal Features

Major A Criteria

- Main pancreatic duct calculi‡

Minor Criteria

- Irregular main pancreatic duct contour
- Dilated side branches§
- Main pancreatic duct dilation (≥3.5 mm in the body or ≥1.5 mm in the tail)
- Hyperechoic main pancreatic duct margin >50% of the main pancreatic duct in the body and tail*

Diagnosis of Chronic Pancreatitis

Consistent with chronic pancreatitis

- 1 major A criterion + ≥3 or more minor criteria
- 1 major A criterion + major B criterion
- 2 major A criteria

Suggestive of chronic pancreatitis¶

- 1 major A criterion + <3 minor criteria
- 1 major B criterion + ≥3 minor criteria
- ≥5 minor criteria

Indeterminate for chronic pancreatitis¶

- 3-4 minor criteria in the absence of major criteria
- Major B criterion + <3 minor criteria

Normal

- <3 minor criteria

Adapted from Catalano MF, Sahai A, Levy M, et al: EUS-based criteria for the diagnosis of chronic pancreatitis: The Rosemont classification. *Gastrointest Endosc* 69:1251–1261, 2009.
*Defined as lobularity that includes at least three contiguous lobules in the body or tail. It should be assessed in the body and tail.
†Strands are defined as hyperechoic lines ≥3 mm in length seen in at least two different directions in the body or tail of the pancreas.
‡The presence of calculi in the main pancreatic duct, regardless of location, is the most predictive finding of chronic pancreatitis.
§Defined as at least three tubular anechoic structures, each one ≥1 mm in width, budding from the main pancreatic duct.
¶With suggestive and indeterminate chronic pancreatitis, the diagnosis needs to be confirmed with another imaging modality.

evidence suggests that this disease is irreversible, but disease progression can be delayed if the predisposing condition is eradicated. Patients should be strongly encouraged to stop drinking and smoking. Furthermore, other risk factors, such as hypertriglyceridemia, should be treated, and diet modification (i.e., low-fat diet) may benefit some patients.

Because most patients develop pain during the natural history of the disease, analgesic selection is a cornerstone of treatment. Nonsteroidal anti-inflammatory drugs are the first line of treatment. Moderate to severe pain that does not respond to nonsteroidal anti-inflammatory drugs should be treated with tramadol or propoxyphene. Patients with severe pain that does not respond to these recommendations should be treated with potent long-acting narcotics. It cannot be overemphasized that adjuvant measures to prevent addiction, depression, and poor quality of life should be considered for patients with severe pain who require narcotics. Alternative drugs useful in the treatment of other conditions associated with chronic pain, such as tricyclic antidepressants, selective serotonin reuptake inhibitors, combined serotonin and norepinephrine reuptake inhibitors, and $\alpha 2\delta$ inhibitors, may also be considered.

There is no question about the digestive benefits of pancreatic enzyme replacement in patients with pancreatic exocrine insufficiency. However, it is controversial whether pancreatic enzyme replacement helps control the chronic pain seen in this condition. Therapeutic trials with pancreatic enzymes should last at least 6 weeks and should be given along with proton pump inhibitors because acid suppression improves the effects of uncoated pancreatic enzymes. For patients with unrelenting pain, celiac neurolysis has been attempted without sustained success in those with chronic pancreatitis. However, it is well established that during open operation, percutaneously, or through EUS, celiac block may diminish pain in those with unresectable or locally advanced pancreatic cancer.

Interventional Therapy: Endoscopic Treatment

ERCP is the primary modality for treating symptomatic pancreatic duct obstruction with dilation and polyethylene stent placement. A number of sessions are usually required because of symptom recurrence. Note that the differential diagnosis of pancreatic duct strictures includes pancreatic cancer. Only after a thorough evaluation, which includes CT, MRCP, or EUS, has completely ruled out the possibility of malignant disease should endoscopic treatment be considered. Surgical resection is indicated if any concern of malignant disease exists.

Endoscopic stone extraction should be considered for patients with pain and pancreatic duct dilation secondary to stones. Extracorporeal shock wave lithotripsy followed by therapeutic ERCP may be required for the treatment of large impacted stones. The success rate varies from 44% to 77% for this technique. In conjunction with stone extraction, pancreatic duct stenting may benefit patients by relieving obstruction. Although this relief may be temporary, during this interim a patient may be able to improve nutritional and functional status before further, perhaps more invasive therapy.

Biliary obstruction caused by chronic pancreatitis occurs in 10% of patients and is best treated with surgical bypass. Temporary relief of the obstruction with plastic stents is indicated for patients with cholangitis or for those who are severely malnourished.

Surgical Treatment

Several factors, including intractable pain, biliary or pancreatic duct obstruction, duodenal obstruction, pseudocyst or pseudoaneurysm formation, and the inability to rule out malignant disease, may prompt surgical intervention. The choice of surgical procedure depends on the symptoms requiring palliation and the presence or absence of pancreatic ductal dilation. In general, patients with a dilated pancreatic duct (defined as diameter >7 mm), or large duct disease, require a decompressing procedure; patients with a nondilated pancreatic duct, or small duct disease, require a resectional procedure. Several clinical scenarios that require surgical intervention are described here.

Pancreatic duct dilation secondary to duct stones or strictures. Pancreatic duct dilation is defined as a main pancreatic duct measuring at least 7 mm in diameter. Pancreatic duct dilation can be secondary to a single stone or stricture; however, it is often caused by multiple strictures and stones in the pancreatic duct. The pancreatic duct dilation observed on pancreatography for chronic pancreatitis is classically described as a chain of lakes, which reflects the presence of multiple dilations and stenoses. When it is accompanied by intractable pain, this condition is best treated with side-to-side Roux-en-Y pancreaticojejunostomy, also known as the modified Puestow procedure or lateral pancreaticojejunostomy.

The anterior surface of the pancreatic duct is opened, and the anterior surface of the duct is completely unroofed. This tissue may be sent for frozen section analysis to rule out underlying malignant disease. The proximal extent of tissue resection is within 1 cm of the duodenum, and the distal limit is within 1 to 2 cm of the end of the pancreas. Failure to cross the GDA into the neck and head of the pancreas may leave undrained pancreatic head or uncinate process ducts obstructed by stones or strictures, which may give incomplete relief or early recurrence of symptoms. After all stones are extracted, a standard Roux-en-Y is used to create a lateral pancreaticojejunostomy. The main advantage offered by this procedure is parenchymal conservation, which preserves endocrine and exocrine function. The modified Puestow procedure provides palliation of pain in 80% of cases; however, 30% of cases will recur, usually 3 to 5 years after surgery. Decompressive procedures temporarily relieve the ductal obstruction, but in most cases, they do not modify the natural history of the disease, and chronic pancreatitis progresses. Other factors associated with recurrence include smoking and alcohol ingestion after surgery, failure to decompress the head and uncinate process properly, and length of the pancreaticojejunostomy.[19]

In 1987, Andersen and Frey[20] described the local resection of the pancreatic head with longitudinal pancreaticojejunostomy as an alternative procedure. The surgical approach is similar to the Puestow procedure; however, once the anterior surface of the pancreatic duct has been completely exposed, the anterior portion of the head of the pancreas is also resected, leaving a 1-cm rim of pancreatic tissue along the duodenal margin. Figure 55-12 shows intraoperative images of a Frey procedure. This procedure is also an alternative for patients with a dilated pancreatic duct secondary to a benign stricture in the head of the pancreas associated with severe inflammation, scarring, or portal hypertension surrounding the head of the pancreas that precludes a safe pancreaticoduodenectomy. The main disadvantage is the removal of pancreatic parenchyma. A study has demonstrated that 62% of patients are completely free of pain and 95% of patients have satisfactory pain control after this procedure. In the same series, 34% of patients developed endocrine or exocrine pancreatic insufficiency.[21]

Pancreatic duct dilation secondary to a single stricture or stone. On occasion, a single stricture that is proximal to the papilla produces pancreatic duct dilation. As an alternative to a Puestow or Frey procedure, a pancreaticoduodenectomy can be performed to relieve the obstruction. This procedure is described later in the surgical treatment of pancreatic adenocarcinoma. It must be emphasized that this procedure is absolutely contraindicated if more than one obstruction is present in the duct. Single distal obstructions can occasionally be treated with a distal pancreatectomy. The main disadvantage of both procedures is that they can be associated with pancreatic insufficiency because normal parenchyma is removed.

Focal inflammatory mass without significant dilation of the pancreatic duct. In a small percentage of patients with chronic pancreatitis, a predominant mass in the head or, less commonly, in the tail of the pancreas without any evidence of pancreatic duct dilation is seen. Long-standing chronic pancreatitis is also a risk factor for development of pancreatic cancer; therefore, even in patients with a known history of chronic pancreatitis, finding a focal mass is concerning because it may represent an area of pancreatic adenocarcinoma that has developed in the setting of chronic pancreatitis. Resection is recommended for surgical candidates to avoid any error in diagnosis.

Once malignant disease is ruled out with percutaneous or EUS biopsy, resection of the pancreatic head may be done with either of two operations: pancreaticoduodenectomy or duodenum-preserving pancreatic head resection, otherwise known as the Beger procedure. The Beger procedure was designed to remove the pancreatic head while preserving the remainder of the foregut anatomy and therefore function. Once the pancreatic head is removed, a Roux-en-Y is created and anastomosed to the rim of pancreas or duodenum, pancreatic duct, and body and perhaps the bile duct if it was entered. Randomized controlled trials have

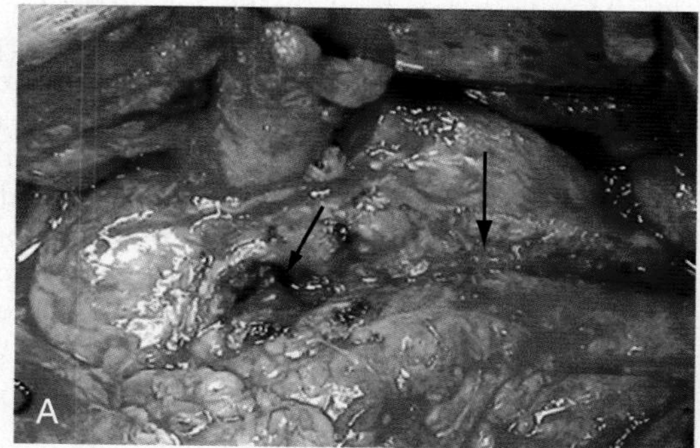

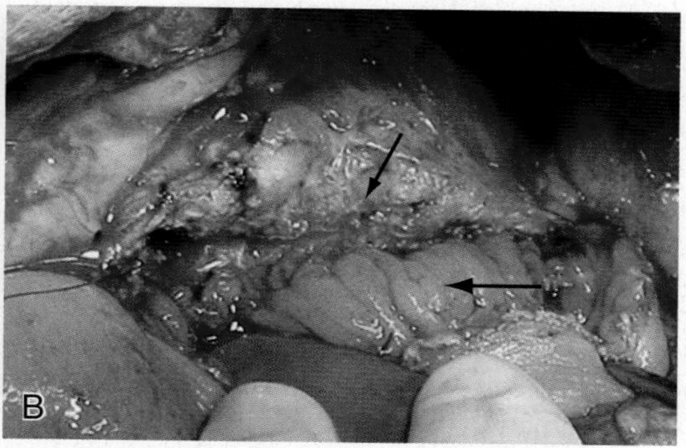

FIGURE 55-12 Frey procedure, intraoperative photographs. **A,** Significant dilation of the main pancreatic duct at the level of the head *(short arrow)* and body of the pancreas *(large arrow)* after the anterior surface of the pancreas has been opened. **B,** Side-to-side anastomosis between the pancreatic duct *(short arrow)* and jejunum *(large arrow)*.

demonstrated that the Beger procedure offers symptomatic relief that is equivalent to the pancreaticoduodenectomy and Frey procedure in appropriately selected patients.

Diffuse glandular involvement without dilation of the pancreatic duct. Decompressive procedures and local pancreatic resections are associated with an elevated failure rate in this group of patients. Patients who do not respond to medical and endoscopic therapies require surgical treatment. The most effective treatment to eliminate pain is total pancreatectomy. However, this procedure is invariably associated with diabetes mellitus. In contrast to type 1 diabetes mellitus, the severity and risk of hypoglycemia are increased in these patients.[22] In 1977, researchers at the University of Minnesota described islet autotransplantation after total pancreatectomy to prevent the effects of surgically induced diabetes. In the largest experience there, one third of patients who underwent this procedure were insulin independent, an additional one third required insulin intermittently, and the other third was fully dependent. According to this study, 90% had pain relief or reduction and 50% were able to discontinue narcotics. Similar results were demonstrated at the University of Cincinnati; up to two thirds of patients had complete or partial islet function, and 40% were insulin independent. Narcotics were discontinued in 66% of patients.[23] Although preliminary results have been encouraging, routine implementation of this operative intervention has been controversial. Major limitations associated with this procedure include the cost and lack of islet processing facilities.

As several other centers have established islet autotransplantation programs and laboratories, it has become clear that the treatment of patients with severe diffuse chronic pancreatitis should be coordinated by a multidisciplinary team. It is imperative to involve a pancreatic surgeon, pancreatologist, interventional endoscopist, radiologist, anesthesia pain specialist, and perhaps a neuropsychologist or psychiatrist. The multifaceted approach to the decision and the type of treatment is crucial to long-term success. The groups at the Medical University of South Carolina and at the University of Alabama at Birmingham[24] have shown that patients with depression or substance abuse, such as alcoholism, have a poor outcome compared with those patients without depression or alcoholism.

At the University of Minnesota,[25] a high rate of success for improvements in quality of life has been shown in pediatric patients after total pancreatectomy with islet autotransplantation. Similarly, the University of Cincinnati has described the benefit of genetic testing and the improvement in outcomes with early intervention once a genetic defect has been diagnosed.

Biliary strictures. Chronic scarring and fibrosis of the head of the pancreas result in external compression of the intrapancreatic portion of the common bile duct. Up to one third of patients with chronic pancreatitis develop radiologic evidence of bile duct dilation; however, significant biliary obstruction occurs in 6% of patients. Biliary strictures typically appear as a long symmetrical narrowing that involves the intrapancreatic portion of the common bile duct in MRCP or ERCP (Fig. 55-13). IV fluid and antibiotic therapy and temporary bile duct decompression with plastic stents is indicated for patients who present with cholangitis. Pancreaticoduodenectomy is indicated for patients in whom malignant disease cannot be excluded before surgery. A Roux-en-Y hepaticojejunostomy is an alternative treatment for patients without evidence of malignant disease or significant scarring that precludes resection of the head of the pancreas.

Duodenal stenosis. Up to 1.2% of patients with chronic pancreatitis develop duodenal strictures. Clinical manifestations include abdominal pain, nausea, vomiting, and significant weight loss. Differential diagnoses include other causes of gastric outlet obstruction secondary to upper gastrointestinal malignant neoplasms and gastroparesis. Severely malnourished patients require IV hydration, nutritional support, and gastric decompression with a nasogastric tube. Permanent treatment requires a gastrojejunostomy.

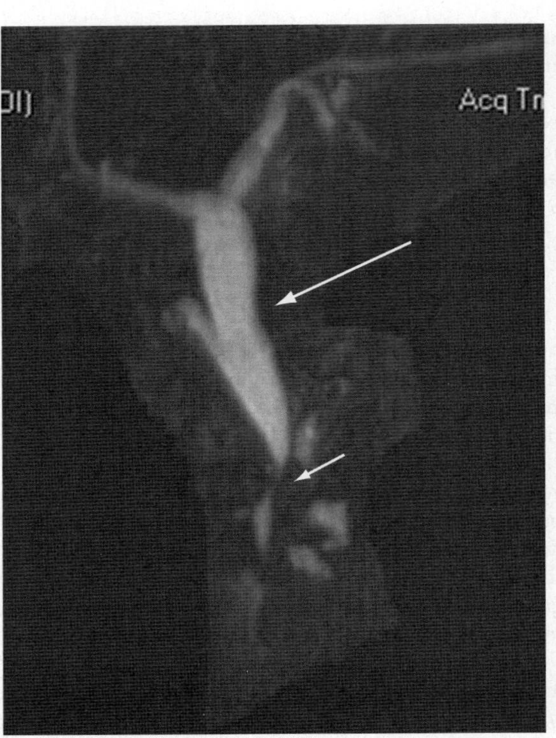

FIGURE 55-13 Bile duct stricture secondary to chronic pancreatitis. MRCP indicates common bile duct dilation *(large arrow)* secondary to a stricture at the level of the intrapancreatic portion of the common bile duct *(small arrow)*.

Pancreatic pseudocyst. Pancreatic pseudocysts develop more frequently in patients with chronic pancreatitis compared with AP. Up to 30% to 40% of patients develop pseudocysts during the course of their disease. Only 10% of patients have spontaneous pancreatic pseudocyst regression. Spontaneous regression is less likely to occur in these patients because pancreatic pseudocysts arise more frequently in the setting of pancreatic duct obstruction. Indications for treatment include symptoms secondary to gastric, duodenal, or biliary compression or associated complications, such as bleeding, pancreaticopleural fistulas, rupture, or spontaneous bleeding. Alternative modalities in the treatment include endoscopic and surgical drainage (see earlier).

Traditionally, management of a symptomatic or persistent pseudocyst has been open operation and, depending on location, drainage through either cystogastrostomy or Roux-en-Y cystojejunostomy. With advancements in interventional endoscopy, drainage has proven successful with ERCP. More recently, drainage with EUS has been shown to be more successful because of improved visualization of vasculature as well as fluid collections and necrosis. Small-caliber plastic stents may be used for simple pancreatic fluid collections or larger metal stents for complex collections or those with infection or necrosis. At the University of Alabama at Birmingham, a prospective randomized trial of endoscopic versus operative cystogastrostomy showed equal efficacy but quicker improvement in quality of life and less hospital expenditure from the endoscopic approach for simple pancreatic pseudocysts.[26]

CYSTIC NEOPLASMS OF THE PANCREAS

Cystic tumors are the second most common exocrine pancreatic neoplasm, following only adenocarcinomas of the pancreas in incidence. Given the advances in modern cross-sectional imaging, the identification of cystic lesions of the pancreas is becoming common. Surgeons must be familiar with the characteristics and treatment of these lesions to determine individual management appropriately.

Types of Cystic Neoplasms

Mucinous Cystic Neoplasm

In the 1970s, the clinicopathologic spectrums of mucinous and serous cystic tumors were described. Mucinous cystic neoplasms (MCNs) are the most common cystic neoplasms of the pancreas. These tumors span the histologic spectrum from benign to invasive carcinomas. MCNs contain mucin-producing epithelium and are identified histologically by the presence of mucin-rich cells and ovarian-like stroma (Fig. 55-14). Staining for estrogen and progesterone is positive in most cases. Frequently seen in young women, the mean age at presentation is in the fifth decade. Men are rarely affected. MCNs are typically found in the body and tail of the pancreas but infrequently can occur elsewhere. Although incidental MCN is becoming increasingly common, up to 50% of patients present with vague abdominal pain. A history of pancreatitis may be found in up to 20% of patients, which explains the common misdiagnosis of pseudocyst.

The radiologic characteristic of an MCN on a CT scan is the presence of a solitary cyst, which may have fine septations and be surrounded by a rim of calcification (Fig. 55-15). Cross-sectional imaging may not be able to distinguish between benign and malignant MCNs; however, the presence of eggshell calcification, larger tumor size, or a mural nodule on cross-sectional imaging is suggestive of malignancy.

EUS and cyst fluid analyses play an important role in the diagnosis of MCN and other cystic neoplasms. FNA with cyst fluid analysis of MCNs demonstrates mucin-rich aspirate and high CEA levels (>192 ng/mL; log scale). Figure 55-16 illustrates the sensitivity and specificity of CEA in identifying mucinous neoplasms on the basis of fine-needle fluid aspiration. Unlike pseudocysts, MCNs typically have low levels of cyst fluid amylase. These fluid analyses provide accurate diagnosis in up to 80% of cases.[27] Table 55-3 summarizes the distinguishing features of cystic neoplasms of the pancreas.[28]

Pancreatic resection is the standard treatment for MCNs, given the potential for malignant transformation. In the absence of invasive malignant disease, resection is curative and no further surveillance is required. The prognosis of patients who undergo pancreatectomy for invasive MCNs is poor although more favorable than that of patients with ductal adenocarcinoma of the pancreas. Invasive MCNs exhibit slower growth, less frequent nodal involvement, and less aggressive clinical behavior compared with ductal adenocarcinoma; a 5-year survival of 50% to 60% can

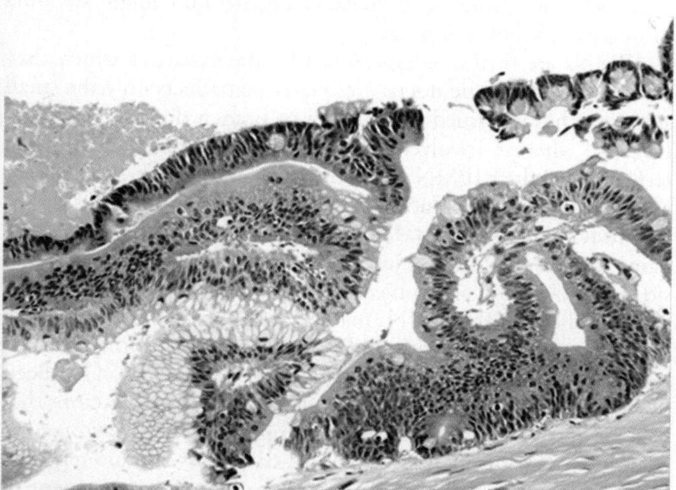

FIGURE 55-14 Ovarian-like stroma is a histologic feature often seen in MCN.

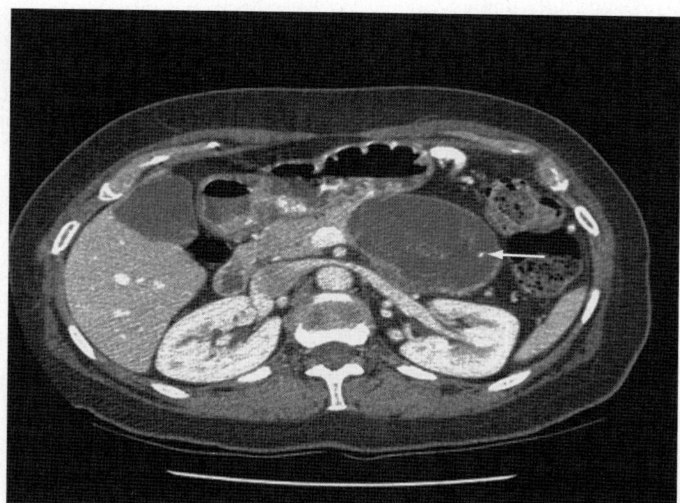

FIGURE 55-15 CT scan of the tail of the pancreas MCN showing a large multiloculated cyst in the absence of pancreatic ductal communication.

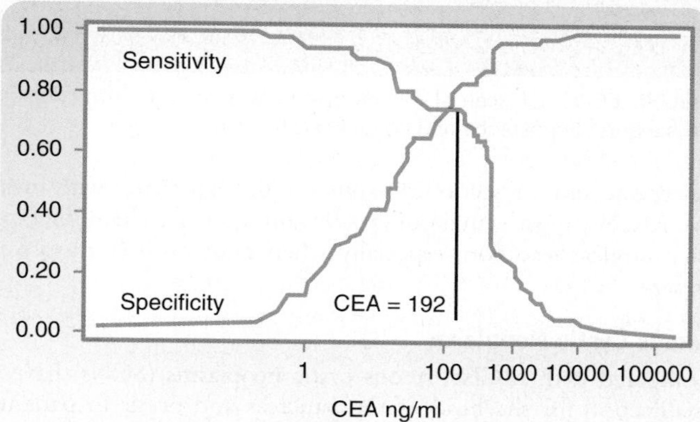

FIGURE 55-16 Sensitivity and specificity curves of cyst fluid CEA concentrations (ng/mL; log scale) for differentiating between mucinous and nonmucinous cystic lesions. An optimal cutoff value of 192 ng/mL correlated with the crossover of the sensitivity and specificity curves. (From Brugge WR, Lewandrowski K, Lee-Lewandrowski E, et al: Diagnosis of pancreatic cystic neoplasms: A report of the cooperative pancreatic cyst study. *Gastroenterology* 126:1330–1336, 2004.)

TABLE 55-3 Defining Characteristics of Pseudocysts and Pancreatic Cystic Neoplasms

CHARACTERISTICS	PSEUDOCYST	SCN	MCN	IPMN
Epidemiology				
Gender	F = M	F ≫ M (4:1)	F ⋙ M (10:1)	F = M
Age (years)	40-60	60-70	50-60	60-70
Imaging Findings				
Location	Evenly distributed	Evenly distributed	Head ≪ body/tail	Head > diffuse > body/tail
Appearance	Round, thick-walled large cyst; gland atrophy ± calcification	Multiple small cysts separated by internal septations with central starburst calcifications	Thick-walled, septated macrocyst with smooth contour; ± solid component, eggshell calcifications	Poorly demarcated, lobulated, polycystic mass with dilation of main or branch ducts
Communication with ducts	Yes	No	Very rare	Yes
Cyst Fluid Analysis				
Cytology	Inflammatory cells	Scant glycogen-rich cells, with positive periodic acid–Schiff stain	Sheets and clusters of columnar, mucin-containing cells	Tall, columnar, mucin-containing cells
Mucin stain	Negative	Negative	Positive	Positive
Amylase	Very high	Low	Low	High
CEA	Low	Low	High	High

From Tran Cao HS, Kellogg B, Lowy AM, et al: Cystic neoplasms of the pancreas. *Surg Oncol Clin N Am* 19:267–295, 2010.
IPMN, intraductal papillary mucinous neoplasm; *MCN,* mucinous cystic neoplasm; *SCN,* serous cystic neoplasm.

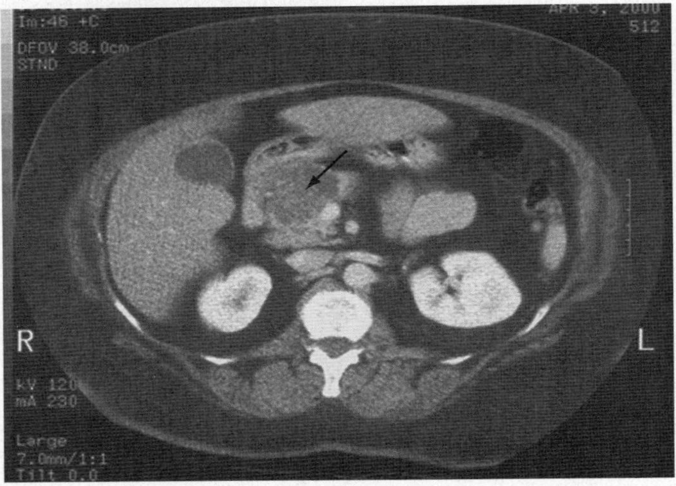

FIGURE 55-17 CT scan of serous cyst neoplasm. The *arrow* depicts the sunburst appearance and central calcification.

be expected after resection. Despite limited experience with invasive MCNs, most centers offer adjuvant systemic chemotherapy after surgical resection, especially when node-positive disease is present.

Serous Cystic Neoplasm

Compared with MCNs, serous cystic neoplasms (SCNs) have a predilection for the head of the pancreas and occur in patients with a higher median age. Patients commonly present with vague abdominal pain and less frequently with weight loss and obstructive jaundice. On gross inspection, SCNs are large, well-circumscribed masses. Microscopic examination reveals multiloculated, glycogen-rich small cysts. Central calcification, with radiating septa giving the sunburst appearance, is a radiographic sign on CT in 10% to 20% of patients (Fig. 55-17). With the advent of EUS, these features can now be better delineated. Recently, differential cyst fluid protein expression was observed between SCNs and IPMNs, with accurate discrimination in 92% of patients.[29] Although serous cystic tumors are generally considered benign, pancreatectomy is suggested when the diagnosis of malignant disease is uncertain or in symptomatic serous cystadenomas. Patients with a tumor larger than 4 cm are more likely to be symptomatic and to display a more rapid median growth rate than patients with tumors smaller than 4 cm. Thus, in select patients with large (>4 cm) or rapidly growing lesions, resection of an SCN is appropriate.

Intraductal Papillary Mucinous Neoplasm

IPMNs of the pancreas, first described by Ohashi, typically are manifested in the sixth to seventh decade of life. IPMNs encompass a wide spectrum of epithelial changes from benign adenoma to invasive adenocarcinoma.

IPMNs are further characterized by the extent to which they involve the pancreatic ducts. Neoplasia that affects only the small side branches is termed side branch or branch duct IPMN (BD-IPMN), whereas involvement of the main pancreatic duct is termed main duct IPMN (MD-IPMN). Side branch IPMNs that extend into the main duct are termed mixed-type IPMNs.

Branch duct intraductal papillary mucinous neoplasm. As the name implies, BD-IPMN involves dilation of the pancreatic duct side branches that communicate with but do not involve the main pancreatic duct. BD-IPMNs may be focal, involving a single side branch, or multifocal, with multiple cystic lesions throughout the length of the pancreas. Risk of malignant transformation has been described in BD-IPMNs and is related to multiple factors that have been stratified as worrisome and high risk. These factors have been identified through international consensus and are reported in the international consensus guidelines for the management of IPMN and MCN of the pancreas, most recently updated in 2012.[30]

Worrisome features of BD-IMPN based on imaging include cyst size larger than 3 cm, thickened enhancing cyst wall, main pancreatic duct size of 5 to 9 mm, nonenhancing mural nodule, abrupt change in caliber of main pancreatic duct with distal pancreatic atrophy, and lymphadenopathy. In addition, patients who present with clinical signs of pancreatitis due to a cystic lesion should be considered to have worrisome features. These features are summarized in Table 55-4.

High-risk imaging features of BD-IPMN include the presence of an enhancing solid component within the cyst and main pancreatic duct dilation of more than 1 cm. Patients who present with clinical signs of jaundice should also be considered at high risk.

All cysts with worrisome features on CT or MRI and any cyst larger than 3 cm with or without worrisome features should undergo EUS; all cysts with high-risk features should be resected. Recommendations for management of suspected BD-IPMN are summarized in Figure 55-18.[30]

TABLE 55-4 A Summary of Worrisome and High-Risk Features of Intraductal Papillary Mucinous Neoplasm

WORRISOME FEATURES	HIGH-RISK FEATURES
Main duct 5-9 mm	Main duct >1 cm
Nonenhancing mural nodule	Enhancing solid component
Thickened, enhancing cyst wall	Jaundice
BD-IPMN size >3 cm	
Abrupt caliber change in main duct with upstream atrophy	
Lymphadenopathy	
Pancreatitis	

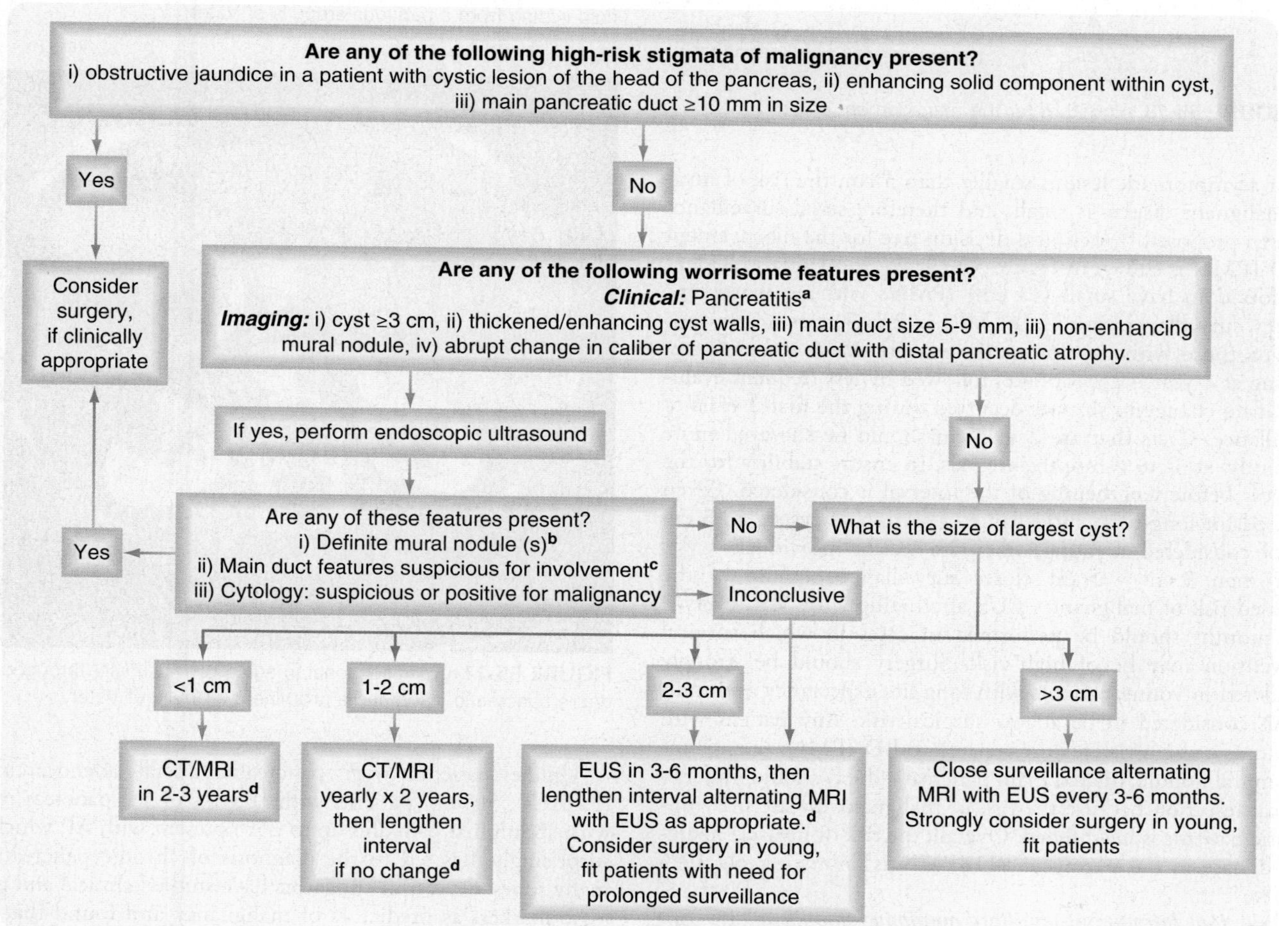

a. Pancreatitis may be an indication for surgery for relief of symptoms.
b. Differential diagnosis includes mucin. Mucin can move with change in patient position, may be dislodged on cyst lavage and does not have Doppler flow. Features of true tumor nodule include lack of mobility, presence of Doppler flow and FNA of nodule showing tumor tissue.
c. Presence of any one of thickened walls, intraductal mucin or mural nodules is suggestive of main duct involvement. In their absence main duct involvement is inconclusive.
d. Studies from Japan suggest that on follow-up of subjects with suspected BD-IPMN there is increased incidence of pancreatic ductal adenocarcinoma unrelated to malignant transformation of the BD-IPMN(s) being followed. However, it is unclear if imaging surveillance can detect early ductal adenocarcinoma, and, if so, at what interval surveillance imaging should be performed.

FIGURE 55-18 Recommendations for management of suspected BD-IPMN. (From Tanaka M, Fernandez-del Castillo C, Adsay V, et al: International consensus guidelines 2012 for the management of IPMN and MCN of the pancreas. *Pancreatology* 12:183–197, 2012.)

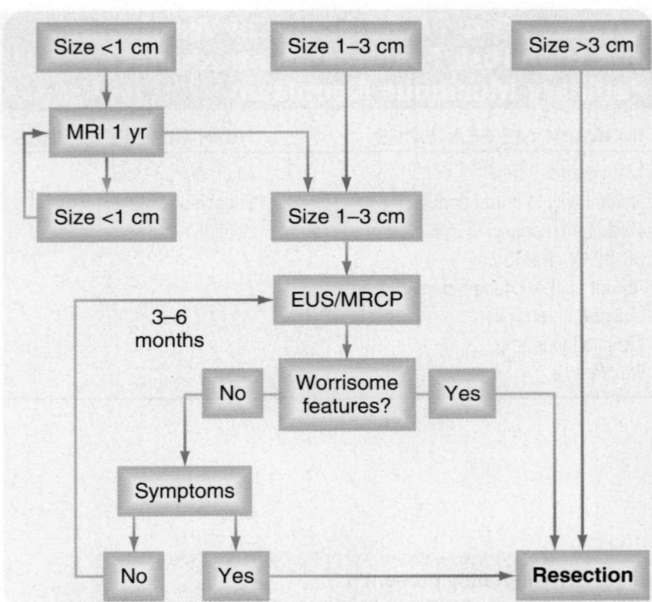

FIGURE 55-19 Algorithm for the management of BD-IPMN.

For asymptomatic lesions smaller than 3 cm, the risk of invasive malignant disease is small, and therefore serial surveillance has been proposed.[30] A clinical decision tree for the management of BD-IPMN is shown in Figure 55-19. For individuals incidentally found to have small (<1 cm) IPMNs with no worrisome features, surveillance with CT or MRI in 2 to 3 years is appropriate. For those with asymptomatic cysts between 1 and 2 cm, imaging at 1 year is appropriate, followed by less frequent evaluation if no change in size has occurred during the first 2 years of surveillance. Cysts that are 2 to 3 cm should be surveyed more frequently, at 3- to 6-month intervals, to ensure stability for the first year before lengthening of the interval is considered. Given the need for long-term surveillance, resection of cysts 2 to 3 cm may be considered in young, otherwise healthy individuals. Cysts larger than 3 cm warrant closer surveillance because of the increased risk of malignancy. EUS alternating with MRI every 3 to 6 months should be performed in cases in which surgical intervention may be of high risk. Surgery should be strongly considered in young patients with long life expectancy and individuals considered to be at low surgical risk. Any patient with symptoms or high-risk features related to BD-IPMNs (e.g., jaundice, mural nodule, dilated main pancreatic duct) should undergo surgical resection because the risk of malignant disease in symptomatic patients is heightened. Overall, the risk of invasive malignant disease in the setting of BD-IPMN is approximately 10% to 15%.

Main duct intraductal papillary mucinous neoplasm. In contrast to BD-IPMN, MD-IPMN indicates abnormal cystic dilation of the main pancreatic duct with columnar metaplasia and thick mucinous secretions, which can be seen oozing from a patulous papilla on endoscopic evaluation (Fig. 55-20). Involvement of the main pancreatic duct may be focal or diffuse; it is most relevant because of the significantly increased risk of malignant degeneration. Individuals with MD-IPMN have a 30% to 50% risk of harboring invasive pancreatic cancer at the time of presentation. Thus, surgical resection is the cornerstone of treatment. Figure 55-21 demonstrates MD-IPMN with dilation of the entire pancreatic duct.

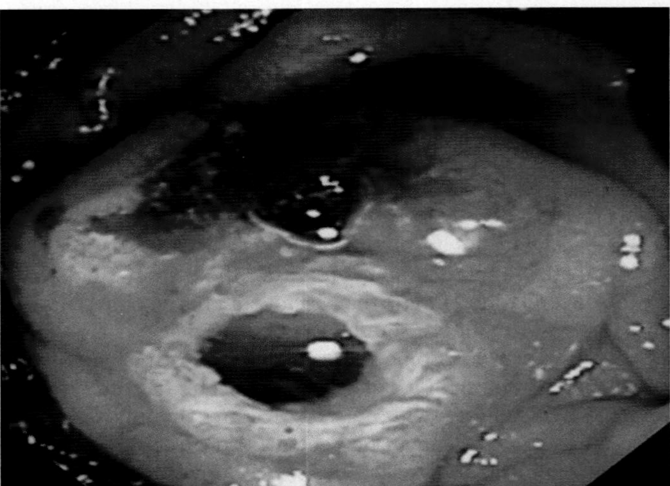

FIGURE 55-20 Classic endoscopic view of IPMN showing viscous fluid oozing from a patulous ampulla of Vater.

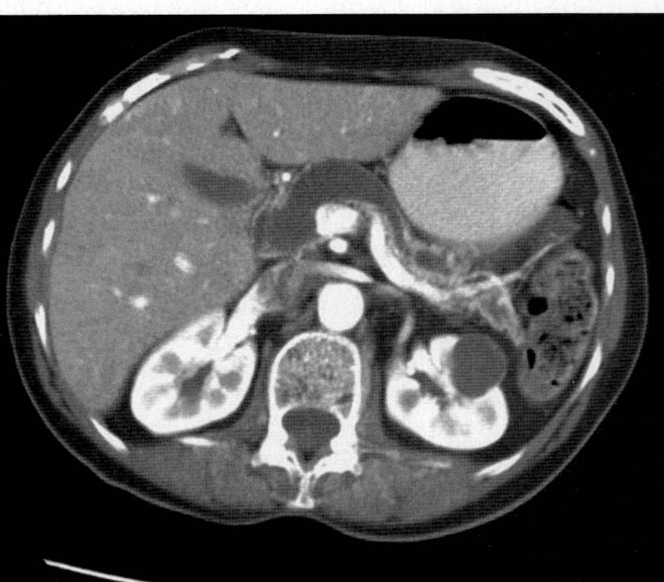

FIGURE 55-21 Cross-sectional imaging of MD-IPMN throughout the entire pancreatic gland and a prominent ampulla of Vater.

Unlike patients with pancreatic ductal adenocarcinomas (PDACs), 50% of patients with IPMNs of the pancreas present with abdominal pain and up to 25% present with AP, which, not surprisingly, has led to the diagnosis of chronic pancreatitis in many series. Several investigators have studied clinical and pathologic markers as predictors of malignancy and found that jaundice, elevated serum alkaline phosphatase level, mural nodules, diabetes, and main pancreatic duct diameter of 7 mm or larger are strongly associated with invasive IPMNs.[31] Current guidelines suggest that main duct dilation of more than 5 mm is consistent with a diagnosis of MD-IPMN, whereas 5 to 9 mm is considered worrisome and more than 1 cm is considered high risk.[30] Given the overall high risk of malignant transformation, all patients with evidence of MD-IPMN should be considered for surgical resection if they are surgically fit.

On a molecular level, investigations using genomic array analysis of pancreatic cystic neoplasms have shown that IPMN has several distinct cytogenetic alterations that separate it as an entity from ductal adenocarcinoma of the pancreas.

The radiographic features of IPMNs on pancreatic CT scans may include a dilated main pancreatic duct, cysts of varying sizes, and possibly mural nodules (Fig. 55-21). MRCP and EUS are important secondary diagnostic studies for the evaluation of patients with suspected IPMN. MRCP may allow localization of mural nodules and pretreatment classification of suspected side branch or main duct types of IPMN. EUS can evaluate the pancreatic duct and assess the fluid and solid components of the neoplasm. Aspirated fluid is typically viscous and clear and contains mucin. Cytology studies demonstrate mucin-rich fluid with variable cellularity; columnar mucinous cells with variable atypia may also be seen. As in MCNs and BD-IPMNs, fluid aspirates characteristically reveal an elevated CEA level (>192 ng/mL; log scale). This elevation of the CEA level is not predictive of invasive malignant disease, only the presence of mucinous metaplasia.

Mixed-type intraductal papillary mucinous neoplasm. Mixed-type IPMN denotes a side branch IPMN that has extended to involve the main pancreatic duct to a varying degree. Concern for mixed-type IPMNs should be raised in individuals with side branch cysts who exhibit upstream dilation of the pancreatic duct because this is an indication of main duct involvement. The biologic behavior of mixed-type IPMNs most closely resembles that of MD-IPMNs, with a significant risk of invasive malignant disease at the time of presentation (30% to 50%). As for MD-IPMN, surgical resection is indicated for the treatment of mixed-type IPMN.

Treatment: Surgical Resection for Intraductal Papillary Mucinous Neoplasm

Partial pancreatectomy is the primary treatment for high-risk lesions; however, the optimal extent of pancreatic resection for some patients remains unknown. For BD-IPMN, resection should target the lesion of concern, and therefore surgical decision making is usually straightforward. For MD-IPMN, however, it is not always possible to determine the extent of microscopic abnormality within the duct. Many pancreatic surgeons recommend right-sided partial pancreatectomy with the knowledge that the disease is most often located in the head of the gland, even though ductal changes may extend to involve other parts of the pancreas.[32] Partial pancreatectomy also eliminates the risk of brittle diabetes, which accompanies total pancreatectomy. Although some investigators continue to advocate total pancreatectomy for the treatment of any IPMN, the evidence supporting this approach is decreasing with longer follow-up of patients treated by R0 and R1 partial pancreatectomy. It is appropriate to recommend partial pancreatectomy and to discuss management of the pancreatic margin preoperatively, advising the patient that approximately 15% of patients will require conversion to total pancreatectomy to achieve negative parenchymal resection margins. The surgical margins are assessed intraoperatively, and additional margins are obtained for high-grade dysplasia or invasive cancer.

Survival outcomes are significantly better in patients with IPMNs than in patients with PDACs. Sohn and associates[33] have analyzed a series of 136 patients with IPMNs; survival rates for patients with noninvasive IPMNs are 97% at 1 year, 94% at 2 years, and 77% at 5 years. When the group of patients with noninvasive IPMNs was analyzed further, no survival differences were found between patients with IPMNs and those with borderline IPMNs. On the contrary, there was a significant difference in survival rate between patients with noninvasive IPMNs and those with invasive IPMNs. The 1-, 3-, and 5-year survival rates for patients with invasive IPMNs were 72%, 58%, and 43%, respectively. Therefore, survival is clearly dependent on the invasive component of the lesion.

It is increasingly clear that not all patients with IPMNs require surgery. Overall, for BD-IPMN, the risk of invasive malignant disease is approximately 2% to 3% per year.[34] A plan for watchful surveillance with delayed intervention in these patients is reasonable because the risk for malignant transformation with small, asymptomatic branch duct tumors is low, most patients are older, and the time required for development of invasive malignant disease may be longer than the patient's life expectancy.

ADENOCARCINOMA OF THE EXOCRINE PANCREAS

Epidemiology

In 2015, it is estimated that PDAC will affect approximately 48,960 individuals in the United States and 40,560 will die of the disease. In comparison, 2 decades ago in 1995, there were 24,000 new cases of pancreatic cancer. Whereas the increasing and aging population is the most likely cause of this increase, whether factors other than population size and age have contributed to this increase is not known. Although it is the ninth most common cancer diagnosis, pancreatic cancer ranks fourth in cancer deaths each year. Despite significant advances in the treatment of other cancers, the prognosis of pancreatic cancer remains dismal. Overall, less than 5% of individuals will survive 5 years beyond their diagnosis. One of the reasons for these dismal outcomes is that most patients with pancreatic cancer have locally advanced or distant metastatic disease at presentation. Efforts at early detection of pancreatic cancer may change these outcomes by detecting pancreatic cancer at an early and curable stage. In a recent study, the authors performed a quantitative analysis of the timing of evolution of metastatic clones in pancreatic cancer. This elegant study suggested that on average, 5 years are required for the acquisition of metastatic ability in pancreatic cancer, thus suggesting that a window of opportunity does exist when the cancer is a locoregional disease and potentially curable.[35] Men are affected slightly more commonly than women, with a 1.3:1 incidence ratio. African Americans have a slightly higher risk for development of pancreatic cancer and dying of their disease compared with whites. The risk of pancreatic cancer increases with age beyond the sixth decade; the mean age at diagnosis is 72 years.

Risk Factors

Environmental Risk Factors and Causes

Although the cause of pancreatic cancer remains unclear, several environmental risks have been associated with its increased incidence. The most notable risk factor is related to smoking. Several epidemiologic studies have shown an association of the amount and duration of smoking history with an elevated risk of pancreatic cancer. On average, smokers face a onefold to threefold increase in risk for development of pancreatic cancer compared with nonsmokers. This risk seems to be a linear association, with pancreatic cancer incidence directly related to the number of pack-years smoked (packs/day × number of years smoking). As with other cancers, the risk of pancreatic cancer persists many years beyond smoking cessation. Over the years, there have been several other factors, including chronic pancreatitis and occupational exposure, that were thought to contribute to an elevated risk of pancreatic cancer; however, population data have been somewhat controversial. It is likely that these factors are associated with an elevated risk, but the magnitude of the risk is uncertain. Obesity has recently become the focus of investigation; several authors have found that obese patients may be up to three times more likely to develop pancreatic cancer than nonobese individuals. It remains unclear whether obesity itself or one of the comorbidities related to obesity is associated with the higher incidence of pancreatic cancer seen in this population.

The relationship between diabetes and pancreatic cancer is a complicated one. Studies suggest that patients with new-onset diabetes have higher incidence of pancreatic cancer.[36] The association with pancreatic cancer is especially strong if the new diagnosis of diabetes is made in those who are elderly, have a lower body mass index, or have weight loss and in those who do not have family history of diabetes. In these patients with new-onset diabetes, diabetes may be caused by pancreatic cancer. However, the mechanism of pancreatic cancer–induced diabetes is unclear at this time. Other studies have suggested that long-term diabetes may increase the risk of pancreatic cancer. However, these observations may be confounded by the fact that factors like obesity are associated with both diabetes and pancreatic cancer. It is clear, though, that in elderly patients with new-onset diabetes in the presence of unusual symptoms like weight loss and abdominal symptoms, diagnosis of pancreatic cancer should be considered and may lead to early diagnosis of pancreatic cancer.

Hereditary Risk Factors

An inherited predisposition to pancreatic cancer is seen in a range of clinical settings. Several hereditary cancer syndromes (e.g., Peutz-Jeghers syndrome, familial atypical mole and multiple melanoma syndrome, hereditary breast and ovarian cancer syndrome) are known to be associated with increased risk of pancreatic cancer. Increased risk of pancreatic cancer is present in patients with inheritable inflammatory disease of the pancreas, namely, hereditary pancreatitis and cystic fibrosis. These patients with known genetic syndromes are responsible for about 20% of hereditary cases of pancreatic cancer. The term *familial pancreatic cancer* (FPC) applies to the remaining 80% of patients with an inherited predisposition but who do not have an identifiable genetic syndrome. Table 55-5 summarizes several known gene mutations and their clinical significance.

TABLE 55-5 Hereditary Risk Factors Associated With Development of Pancreatic Cancer

GENE	ASSOCIATED SYNDROME	CLINICAL SIGNIFICANCE
PRSS1	Familial pancreatitis	Mutation results in chronic pancreatitis and 40% lifetime risk of PDAC
STK11	Peutz-Jeghers syndrome	Mutation results in >100-fold increase in risk of PDAC
CDKN2A	Familial atypical mole and multiple melanoma syndrome	Mutation leads to increased risk of melanoma and >40-fold increase in risk of PDAC
CFTR	Cystic fibrosis	Thick secretions result in chronic pancreatitis and 30-fold increase in risk of PDAC
BRCA2	Hereditary breast and ovarian cancer	Mutation results in elevated risk of breast and ovarian cancer and 10-fold increase in risk of PDAC
MLH1	Lynch syndrome	Mismatch repair gene mutation leads to increased risk of colon cancer and eightfold increase in risk of PDAC
APC	Familial adenomatous polyposis	Mutation results in polyposis coli and colon cancer with fourfold increase in risk of PDAC

Hereditary pancreatitis (PRSS1 and SPINK1 gene mutation). It has long been noted that individuals with familial pancreatitis have an elevated risk of pancreatic cancer. Mutations in the cationic trypsinogen gene *(PRSS1)* are responsible for 80% of the cases of hereditary pancreatitis and lead to increased trypsin activity and chronic inflammation in the pancreas. The *SPINK1* gene codes for a serine protease inhibitor that inhibits active protein, and mutations in this gene have been associated with hereditary pancreatitis. Individuals with hereditary pancreatitis have a greater than 50-fold increase in their risk for development of pancreatic cancer compared with unaffected individuals.[37]

Peutz-Jeghers syndrome (STK11 gene mutation). Individuals with Peutz-Jeghers syndrome are distinguished by the development of gastrointestinal hamartomatous polyps and pigmented mucocutaneous lesions. The specific role of *STK11* is not defined, although it is thought to act as a tumor suppressor gene, with loss of heterozygosity leading to the development of gastrointestinal tumors. In addition to gastrointestinal cancers, individuals with Peutz-Jeghers syndrome are at a higher risk of lung, ovarian, breast, uterine, and testicular cancers. The risk of pancreatic cancer in the setting of Peutz-Jeghers syndrome is more than 100 times greater than that in unaffected individuals.[37]

Cystic fibrosis (CFTR gene mutation). Although the cause remains unclear, those with cystic fibrosis (*CFTR* gene mutation) are up to 30 times more likely to develop pancreatic cancer than the general population. It is postulated that this elevated risk is caused by the chronic inflammatory condition of the pancreas resulting from a lifetime of thickened secretions and partial ductal obstruction.[37]

Familial atypical mole and multiple melanoma syndrome (CDKN2A gene mutation). *CDKN2A* encodes protein p16, which normally inhibits cell proliferation by binding to cyclin-dependent kinases (CDKs). Mutations of *CDKN2A* lead to uninhibited cell cycle activation and proliferation. Although *CDKN2A* is most noted for its associated increased risk of melanoma, individuals with *CDKN2A* mutations have up to a 20-fold increase in risk for the development of pancreas cancer.[37]

Hereditary breast and ovarian cancer (BRCA2 gene mutation). Although germline *BRCA* mutations are most recognized because of their association with breast cancer, 10% of individuals from high-risk pancreatic cancer families (at least two first-degree relatives with pancreas cancer) have been found to have *BRCA2* mutations. Germline mutations of the *BRCA2* gene lead to an elevated risk for pancreatic cancer, which is up to 10 times that of the general population.[37]

Lynch syndrome (mismatch repair gene mutations). Although most strongly associated with colon cancers caused by mutations in mismatch repair genes *(MLH1, MSH2, MSH6),* Lynch syndrome also leads to an increased risk of pancreatic cancer. The microsatellite instability noted in colon cancer cells has also been seen in pancreatic cancer cells from individuals with Lynch syndrome, indicative of a common genetic cause. It is estimated that the risk of pancreatic cancer is increased eightfold in individuals with Lynch syndrome.[37]

Familial adenomatous polyposis (APC gene mutation). Familial adenomatous polyposis results from mutation of the adenomatous polyposis coli gene *(APC),* leading to the development of thousands of colonic polyps. It has been found that individuals affected by familial adenomatous polyposis are also significantly more likely to develop pancreas cancer, with a fourfold increase above that in the general population. These data remain observational because the cause of pancreatic cancer in this setting has not been defined.[37]

Familial pancreatic cancer (unknown gene). FPC is defined by families with two or more first-degree relatives with pancreatic adenocarcinoma that do not fulfill the criteria of other inherited tumor syndromes with an increased risk for the development of pancreatic adenocarcinoma. Compared with relatives of patients with sporadic pancreatic cancer, the risk for development of pancreatic cancer is markedly elevated in FPC kindreds. Family members of FPC kindreds are at an 18-fold increased risk for development of pancreatic cancer compared with the general population. Furthermore, this risk increases with increasing numbers of first-degree relatives with pancreatic cancer in FPC kindreds and if one of the affected individuals is diagnosed before 50 years of age. Segregation analysis suggests that the aggregation of pancreatic cancer in these families is due to unidentified, autosomal dominantly inherited genes with reduced penetrance. This entity is being increasingly appreciated, and guidelines for pancreatic cancer screening and management of identified suspicious lesions in this population are under evolution.

Pathogenesis of Sporadic Pancreatic Cancer

Although there are several inherited forms of PDAC, most cases are sporadic. As for many other cancers, a sequential pathway has been observed in the development of PDAC from pancreatic intraepithelial neoplasia (PanIN) to invasive cancer. A number of tumor suppressor genes and oncogenes have been identified that play a significant role in the pathogenesis of PDAC, including *PDX1, KRAS2, CDKN2A/p16, P53,* and *DPC4 (SMAD4).*

Genetic Progression of Pancreatic Intraepithelial Neoplasia to Invasive Pancreatic Ductal Adenocarcinoma

PanIN is defined histologically by progressive abnormality of the ductal epithelium from columnar metaplasia (PanIN-1A) through carcinoma in situ (PanIN-3). PanIN-1A is histologically characterized by the presence of columnar, mucin-producing ductal epithelium that maintains basally located homogeneous nuclei without atypia. The development of papillary architecture defines PanIN-1B, but it is otherwise identical to PanIN-1A. PanIN-2 denotes the progression from simple papillary growth to evidence of nuclear atypia not seen in PanIN-1B. Enlarged nuclei with nuclear crowding and loss of polarity are present. Prominent nuclear abnormalities with complete loss of polarity and marked cytologic atypia are characteristic of PanIN-3 (carcinoma in situ). Clusters of abnormal cells can usually be seen within the duct lumen.

The *KRAS2* oncogene is activated in more than 95% of pancreatic cancers and is thought to be the initiating event in tumorigenesis. *KRAS2* is activated by point mutation (codon 12, 13, or 61), which causes constitutive activation and loss of regulation of mitogen-activated protein kinase cell signal transduction. Mutation of the *KRAS2* oncogene is one of the earliest genetic abnormalities identified in the progression of PanIN to PDAC and has been noted in 36% of PanIN-1 cases, 44% of PanIN-2 cases, and 87% of PanIN-3 cases.

CDKN2A/p16, P53, and *DPC4* are tumor suppressor genes that also appear to play critical roles in the development of PDAC. *CDKN2A* encodes a protein, p16, that binds to cyclin-dependent kinases (CDK4, CDK6), resulting in cell cycle arrest. Mutation of *CDKN2A* and loss of p16 lead to a loss of cell cycle regulation. Like mutation of *KRAS,* mutation of *CDKN2A* (loss of p16 expression) has been identified in 30% of PanIN-1 cases, 55% of PanIN-2 cases, and 71% of PanIN-3 cases. Approximately 90% of PDACs demonstrate loss of p16 function. Also, *P53* encodes the protein p53, which regulates cell proliferation through cell cycle arrest and proapoptotic mechanisms. Although it is rare in PanIN, 79% of invasive PDACs demonstrate *P53* mutations, indicating its potential importance in the transition from noninvasive to invasive tumors. Similarly, *DPC4* mutations occur late in the pathway from PanIN to PDAC. Loss of *DPC4,* which normally functions as a downstream mediator related to TGF-β, leads to decreased inhibition of cell growth and proliferation. Loss of *DPC4* function has been observed in 20% to 30% of PanIN-3 and localized cancers, whereas 78% of widely metastatic tumors show loss of *DPC4.* Figure 55-22 demonstrates the molecular genetic alterations involved in the PanIN-PDAC pathway.

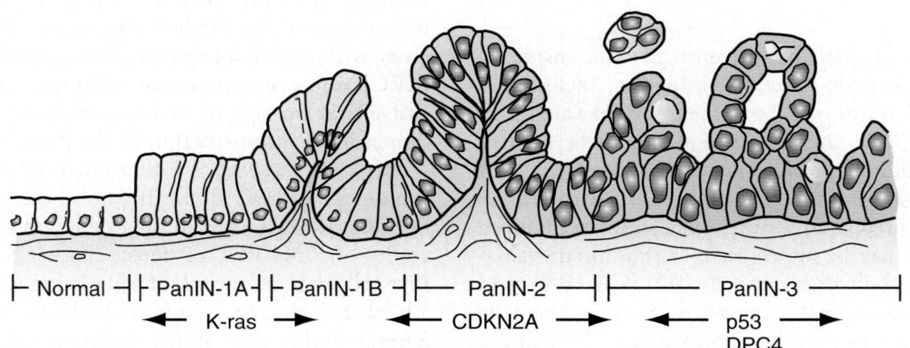

FIGURE 55-22 Molecular genetic progression from PanIN to invasive ductal adenocarcinoma. (Adapted from Wilentz RE, Iacobuzio-Donahoe CA, Argani P, et al: Loss of expression of DPC4 in pancreatic intraepithelial neoplasia: Evidence that DPC4 inactivation occurs late in neoplastic progression. *Cancer Res* 60:2002–2006, 2000.)

TABLE 55-6 Presenting Symptoms for Periampullary Tumors of the Pancreas

PRESENTING SYMPTOM	FREQUENCY (%)
Jaundice	75
Weight loss	51
Abdominal pain	39
Nausea/vomiting	13
Pruritus	11
Fever	3
Gastrointestinal bleeding	1

Clinical Presentation

The defining presenting symptom of patients with PDACs in the periampullary region is jaundice. Although painless jaundice has frequently been described, a significant number of patients present with pain in addition to jaundice, typically arising in the epigastrium and radiating to the back. Weight loss is also common at the time of presentation, affecting more than 50% of individuals. For tumors of the body and tail of the pancreas, pain and weight loss become more common at presentation. In the largest single-institution experience reported to date, Winter and coworkers[38] have described 1423 pancreaticoduodenectomies for PDAC. Table 55-6 lists the most common presenting symptoms and their frequency. As mentioned before, new-onset diabetes in an elderly patient with weight loss may be an early presenting symptom of pancreatic cancer. Except for jaundice, the physical examination findings are otherwise unremarkable for most patients with PDAC. A palpable distended gallbladder can be identified in approximately one third of patients with periampullary PDAC, an association first described by Courvoisier, a Swiss surgeon, in 1890. He noted that choledocholithiasis was commonly associated with a shrunken fibrotic gallbladder, whereas the slow progressive occlusion by other causes, including tumors, was more likely to result in ectasia of the organ. Although not diagnostic in itself, Courvoisier sign is familiar to medical students as a defining characteristic of PDACs. With widespread disease, a left supraclavicular node (Virchow node) may be palpable. Similarly, periumbilical lymphadenopathy may be palpable (Sister Mary Joseph node). In cases of peritoneal dissemination, perirectal tumor involvement may be palpable through digital rectal examination, referred to as Blumer shelf.

Diagnosis

Laboratory Evaluation

Laboratory evaluation of patients presenting with suspected PDAC should include hepatic function evaluation, including a coagulation profile and nutritional assessment. An elevated bilirubin level is expected, but careful attention should be paid to nutritional values, including prealbumin and albumin levels if surgical intervention is to be considered. Individuals with malnutrition should be given preoperative nutritional supplementation. Several tumor markers may be appropriate at the initial evaluation, including CEA, carbohydrate antigen 19-9 (CA 19-9), and α-fetoprotein. Of these, CA 19-9 is most sensitive for pancreatic adenocarcinoma, with a sensitivity of approximately 79% and a specificity of 82%. A notable limitation of CA 19-9 testing in the setting of periampullary tumors is the false elevation caused by biliary obstruction, which can be misleading. In addition, 10% to 15% of individuals do not have elevation of the CA 19-9 level, a finding that has been associated with blood Lewis antigen–negative status. Accepting these limitations, CA 19-9 continues to be the most reliable tumor marker for pretreatment evaluation and post-treatment surveillance for pancreatic adenocarcinoma.

Imaging Studies

Multidetector CT is the imaging study of choice for the evaluation of lesions arising in the pancreas. CT allows an accurate determination of the level of biliary obstruction, the relationship of the tumor to critical vascular anatomy, and the presence of regional or metastatic disease. For suspected periampullary disease, a three-phase (noncontrast, arterial, and portal venous) CT scan with 3-mm slices and coronal and three-dimensional reconstruction should be routine. Because of its widespread availability and excellent sensitivity (85%), CT has become the imaging modality of choice for the evaluation of suspected pancreatic cancer. Pancreatic adenocarcinoma is typically seen as a hypoattenuating lesion during the portal venous phase of the imaging.

ERCP is frequently used in the assessment of the jaundiced patient because of its ability to perform a biopsy and to palliate jaundice, if necessary. Although palliative biliary stenting remains routine for PDAC tumors resulting in jaundice, its usefulness is questionable for patients who are candidates for surgical resection. Preoperative biliary decompression may increase the rate of wound infection caused by bactibilia, although overall morbidity and mortality are unchanged. In modern medical practice, ERCP should be reserved for cases requiring therapeutic or palliative intervention because other imaging modalities provide superior diagnostic abilities without the invasiveness of ERCP.

EUS is becoming widely used for the evaluation of suspected pancreatic disease. Perhaps its most important ability is to provide tissue diagnosis of suspected tumors through the use of FNA before initiation of systemic therapy. FNA has a sensitivity and specificity that are far superior to those of brush cytology, with a diagnostic accuracy of 92% to 95%. It may also play a crucial role in the molecular evaluation of tumor samples from patients undergoing neoadjuvant therapy. Although the use of EUS is increasing for the evaluation of peritumoral vasculature and regional lymph nodes, it has not been shown to provide any significant benefit over CT alone in the absence of a need for tissue diagnosis. EUS may be beneficial for the identification of small tumors that do not appear on CT scans and for the delineation of more clearly suspicious lesions smaller than 2 cm; it therefore plays an important complementary role.

For cases that require detailed assessment of luminal pancreatobiliary anatomy, MRCP should be considered. MRCP has become useful for the investigation of cystic lesions of the pancreas, with sensitivity and specificity slightly superior to CT alone. MRCP also provides several advantages over ERCP; it is noninvasive, has no risk of inciting pancreatitis, and provides three-dimensional reconstruction of the ductal system.

Biologic imaging. ^{18}F-fluorodeoxyglucose positron emission tomography (FDG PET) in combination with CT scanning has been increasingly used in the evaluation of pancreatic cancer. The ability of FDG PET to detect cancers is based on the principle that cells that are actively metabolizing will preferentially take up ^{18}F-labeled glucose compared with surrounding normal tissues. Several studies have noted the potential benefits of FDG PET with CT, including the ability to differentiate between benign and malignant pancreas tumors (autoimmune pancreatitis versus adenocarcinoma) and also to identify unsuspected disease, which alters clinical planning in more than 10% of cases. False-positive findings are also possible, most notably because of inflammatory conditions, and the risk-benefit ratio of FDG PET with CT has not yet been determined. Further studies will be necessary to clarify the role of FDG PET with CT in the evaluation of pancreatic cancer before its routine use should be advocated.

Staging

Pancreatic cancer staging is based on the American Joint Committee on Cancer tumor, node, metastasis (TNM) system (Table 55-7). After biopsy confirmation, typically by EUS-FNA, accurate staging is accomplished by multidetector CT scanning of the abdomen and pelvis with three-phase administration of contrast material and three-dimensional reconstruction. Chest radiography is sufficient for the evaluation of potential pulmonary metastasis and should be followed by CT of the chest if any suspicious lesions are noted. Individuals with stages IA to IIB tumors—tumor confined to the pancreas or peripancreatic tissue without evidence of celiac artery or SMA involvement and no evidence of metastasis—are considered potential candidates for surgical resection. Individuals with stage III (T4) disease involving the celiac artery or SMA or stage IV (metastatic disease) are not candidates for immediate surgery.

After CT imaging, tumors are classified into resectable, borderline resectable, or unresectable. Resectable tumors are defined as localized to the pancreas, with no evidence of SMV or portal vein involvement (i.e., no abutment, distortion, thrombus, or encasement) and a preserved fat plane surrounding the SMA and celiac artery branches, including the hepatic artery. Patients with imaging consistent with resectable disease should proceed with operative resection.

The appropriate definition of borderline resectable tumors continues to evolve. The National Comprehensive Cancer Network defines borderline resectable as tumors that exhibit one of the following characteristics: severe unilateral or bilateral SMV-portal impingement; less than 180-degree tumor abutment on the SMA; abutment or encasement of hepatic artery, if reconstructible; and SMV occlusion, if of a short segment and reconstructible. Historically, many of these patients would be considered to have locally advanced, unresectable (T4) disease, and the benefit of arterial resection in the setting of significant vascular involvement remains to be determined. Complex procedures required for the extirpation of borderline tumors should be performed only by experienced surgeons, ideally in the setting of a clinical trial.

Unresectable tumors are those that exhibit metastasis (including lymph node metastasis outside the field of resection), ascites, or vascular involvement beyond what has been detailed here.

TABLE 55-7 Current American Joint Committee on Cancer Staging Guidelines for Pancreatic Cancer

Primary Tumor (T)			
TX	Primary tumor cannot be assessed		
T0	No evidence of primary tumor		
Tis	Carcinoma in situ*		
T1	Tumor limited to the pancreas, 2 cm or smaller in greatest dimension		
T2	Tumor limited to the pancreas, more than 2 cm in greatest dimension		
T3	Tumor extends beyond the pancreas but without involvement of the celiac axis or superior mesenteric artery		
T4	Tumor involves the celiac axis or superior mesenteric artery (unresectable primary tumor)		
Regional Lymph Nodes (N)			
NX	Regional lymph nodes cannot be assessed		
N0	No regional lymph node metastasis		
N1	Regional lymph node metastasis		
Distant Metastasis (M)			
M0	No distant metastasis		
M1	Distant metastasis		
Anatomic Stage–Prognostic Groups			
Stage 0	Tis	N0	M0
Stage IA	T1	N0	M0
Stage IB	T2	N0	M0
Stage IIA	T3	N0	M0
Stage IIB	T1	N1	M0
	T2	N1	M0
	T3	N1	M0
Stage III	T4	Any N	M0
Stage IV	Any T	Any N	M1

From Edge S, Byrd D, Compton C, et al, editors: *AJCC cancer staging manual*, ed 7, New York, 2010, Springer.

*This also includes the PanIN-3 classification.

Laparoscopy

Staging laparoscopy has been advocated by several authors as a means to reduce the frequency of nontherapeutic laparotomy for patients with unsuspected metastatic or locally advanced unresectable disease identified at the time of surgery. For patients who appear to have resectable disease on imaging studies alone, laparoscopy identifies additional unresectable disease in up to 30% of cases. Others have argued that with current imaging used properly, the benefit of additional laparoscopy only rarely alters surgical planning. Recently, there has been some consensus on a more selective use of laparoscopy for those at particularly high risk for occult disease, including those with large tumors (>3 cm), significantly elevated CA 19-9 level (>100 U/mL), uncertain findings on CT, or body or tail tumors. It may be clinically prudent also to consider laparoscopy for patients with clinical indicators of widespread disease, including significant weight loss, malnutrition, and pain.[39] There are no level I data available to define the role of staging laparoscopy, and therefore its use remains at the discretion of the surgeon. Furthermore, the role and place of peritoneal cytology are unclear at this time. However, patients with positive findings on peritoneal cytology have very poor prognosis and behave like patients with metastatic disease.[40]

Treatment

Surgical resection remains the only potentially curative treatment of pancreas cancer.

Surgery for Tumors of the Head of the Pancreas

For tumors involving the head of the pancreas, pancreaticoduodenectomy is the procedure of choice. Although first described in 1909 by Kausch, the technique became widely known after the first successful surgical resection was performed by Whipple and Parsons and presented to the American Surgical Association by Parsons in 1935. The first two attempts, in 1934, resulted in operative mortality; but in 1935, a two-stage procedure, which included biliary decompression followed by pancreaticoduodenectomy, was successful. The initial operative description included ligation of the pancreas remnant without reanastomosis.

The first one-stage Whipple procedure was reported by Trimble and colleagues at Johns Hopkins University in 1941.[41] The modern Whipple procedure maintained a perioperative mortality of 25% and morbidity of well above 50% up until the late 1970s. The advent of improved outcomes for this complex procedure can be attributed to many surgeons and institutions. Most notable on this list of early and seminal leaders in regard to improved mortality and outcome are Cameron (Johns Hopkins Hospital, Baltimore), Tredi (Mannheim Clinic, Mannheim, Germany), Warshaw (Massachusetts General Hospital, Boston), and Brennan (Memorial Sloan Kettering Cancer Center, New York). Each surgeon and center performed more than 100 procedures without any deaths in the 1980s and 1990s.

Surgical technique. The modern pancreaticoduodenectomy begins with exploration of the peritoneal surfaces for evidence of metastatic disease, which would deem the patient inoperable. The right colon is then fully mobilized and reflected medially (Cattell-Braasch maneuver), exposing the infrapancreatic SMV. A Kocher maneuver is performed to the level of the left lateral border of the aorta, with attention to clearance of the lymphatic tissue overlying the great vessels. The transverse mesocolon is separated off the head of the pancreas. Figure 55-23 shows complete mobilization of the head of the pancreas and gallbladder. The lesser sac is entered through the gastrocolic ligament, sparing the gastroepiploic vessels. The right gastroepiploic vein is ligated at its confluence with the SMV, allowing the SMV to be dissected from the inferior border and posterior neck of the pancreas. The middle colic vein may also be sacrificed, if necessary, to allow adequate dissection at this level.

Once the infrapancreatic SMV is dissected and the head of the pancreas is fully mobilized, the gallbladder is removed and the common hepatic duct is circumferentially dissected. Division of the common hepatic duct allows visualization of the suprapancreatic SMV. The duodenum is divided at least 2 cm distal to the pylorus using electrocautery or a blue load stapler. The hepatic artery is exposed proximally and distally and assessed for replacement or aberrant anatomy. The GDA and right gastric artery are visualized. Before division of the GDA, the vessel is temporarily occluded, and blood flow through the distal common hepatic artery is ensured using a Doppler device. This maneuver is vital in patients with atherosclerosis of celiac origin to ensure that the hepatic blood supply is not dependent on collateral retrograde arterial flow from the SMA through the GDA. Once hepatic arterial flow is confirmed, the right gastric artery and GDA are ligated and divided. If flow in the hepatic artery is interrupted by occlusion of the GDA, resection may proceed only with preservation of the GDA or arterial resection and bypass, typically as an aortohepatic conduit.

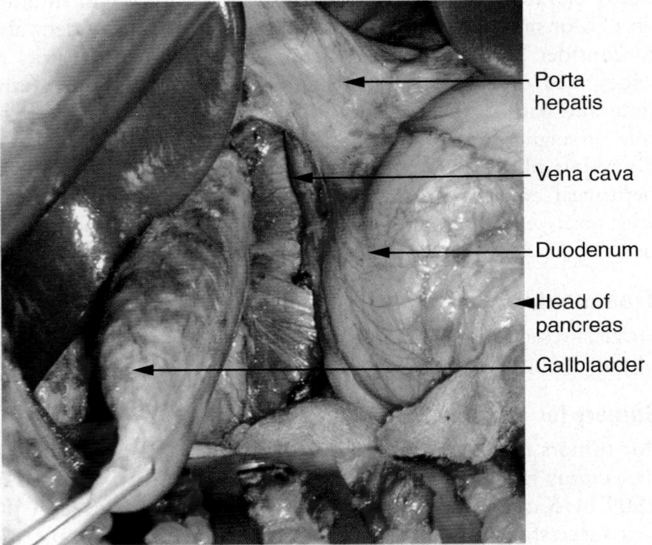

FIGURE 55-23 Complete mobilization of the head of the pancreas is shown. The vena cava is visible posteriorly. The gallbladder has been freed from the gallbladder fossa.

The pancreas is then divided after four-point ligation of the inferior and superior pancreaticoduodenal arteries. Blunt dissection is used to separate the portal vein from the uncinate process. This dissection often includes ligation of a superior and inferior branch from the portal vein and SMV to the uncinate process. The jejunum is divided approximately 10 cm distal to the ligament of Treitz, and the short mesenteric vessels are divided to allow retromesenteric rotation of the jejunum and third and fourth portions of the duodenum. The head of the pancreas and attached small bowel are then retracted to the patient's right, and the remaining portal vein and uncinate dissection is completed.

With the portal vein completely free, the gland is retracted farther to the right to allow complete visualization of the uncinate process and SMA. The retroperitoneal tissue is dissected from the SMA, allowing complete removal of the caudate and periarterial lymphatic tissue. Figure 55-24*A* shows the anatomy after removal of the head of the pancreas, and Figure 55-24*B* highlights complete clearance of periarterial tissue from the SMA. If portal venous or SMV tumor involvement is encountered, as shown in Figure 55-25*A* and *B,* venous resection should be performed. Resections that compromise less than 50% of the venous diameter can be closed primarily (Fig. 55-25*C*); otherwise, segmental resection with primary anastomosis or interposition graft using internal jugular or femoral vein should be performed.

Reconstruction. Before reconstruction, frozen section evaluation of the surgical margins is performed. Once negative margins are ensured, the proximal jejunum is brought through the transverse mesocolon or the retromesenteric defect in preparation for pancreaticojejunostomy and hepaticojejunostomy. The pancreaticojejunostomy is created in two layers, anterior and posterior, with a duct-to-mucosa anastomosis (Fig. 55-26). An internal pancreatic stent can be left in place for ducts smaller than 5 mm. The hepaticojejunostomy anastomosis is then created 6 to 8 cm downstream from the pancreaticojejunostomy in an end-to-side fashion. If the duct is smaller than 5 mm, it is spatulated to improve patency. After this, an antecolic duodenojejunostomy is completed. External drains are selectively placed adjacent to the pancreaticojejunostomy and hepaticojejunostomy. Similarly, a feeding jejunostomy is placed in selected patients with significant preoperative malnutrition (albumin level <3.5 g/dL).

Surgery for Tumors of the Body and Tail of the Pancreas

Tumors arising in the body and tail of the pancreas are rarely resectable at the time of presentation, given the lack of symptoms with small tumors. Only 5% to 7% of individuals with body or tail PDACs will ultimately undergo surgery, and median survival is significantly shorter than with PDACs of the pancreatic head because of the more advanced nature of resected tumors. Although tumor involvement of the splenic artery or vein does not preclude

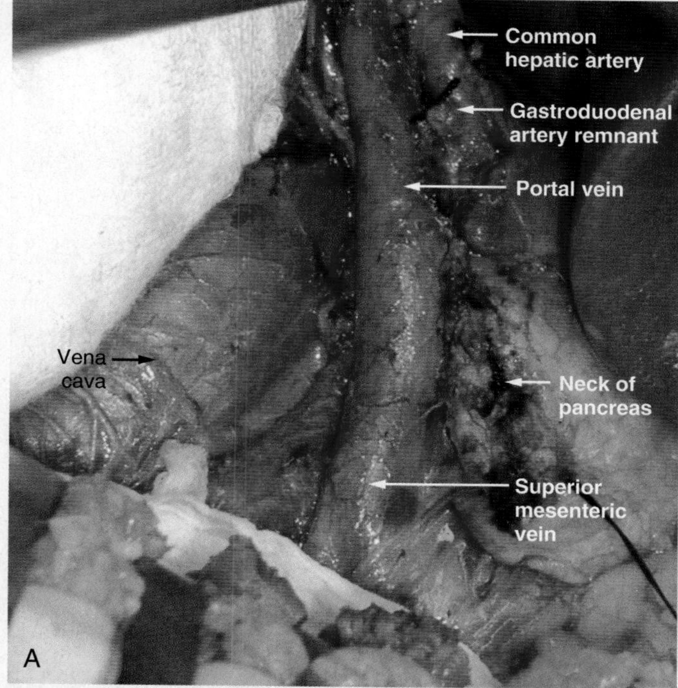

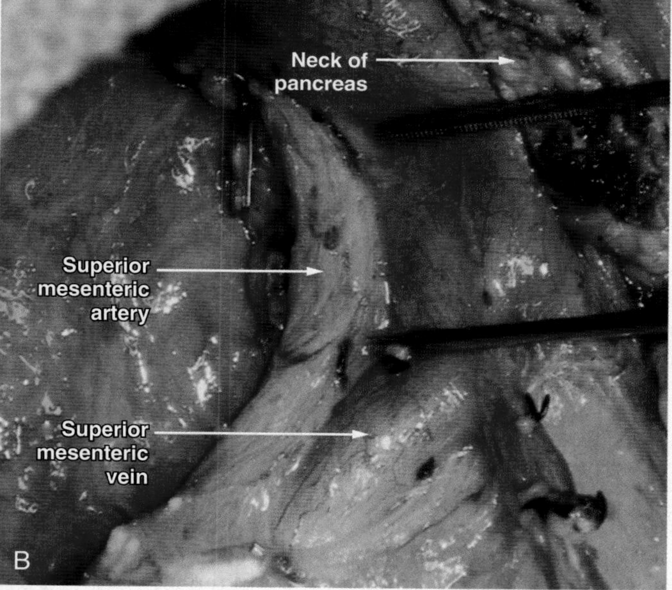

FIGURE 55-24 **A,** Surgical anatomy after pancreaticoduodenectomy. The SMV, portal vein, hepatic artery, and vena cava are visualized. Complete lymphatic clearance is noted. **B,** SMA dissection illustrating complete clearance of periarterial lymphatic tissue.

surgery, involvement of the celiac axis is a contraindication to resection. For resectable tumors, distal pancreatectomy and en bloc splenectomy should be performed. Distal pancreatectomy and splenectomy can be performed in a retrograde fashion whereby the spleen and pancreas are mobilized lateral to medial en bloc, thus providing access to splenic vasculature located superior and behind the pancreas. Alternatively, the dissection can proceed antegrade in a medial to lateral fashion. In this approach, the pancreatic neck is encircled and divided away from the tumor early in the procedure. This medial to lateral approach in combination with extensive lymph node dissection has been termed radical antegrade modular pancreatosplenectomy.[42] The medial to lateral or antegrade approach is described here, but depending on the situation, a combination of these two approaches can be used.

After inspection of the peritoneal surfaces, the gastrocolic and splenocolic ligaments and short gastric vessels are divided to expose the pancreas and spleen. The inferior border of the pancreas is dissected, exposing the retroperitoneal plane behind the gland. This anatomic plane can be used to mobilize the body and tail of the pancreas anterior to Gerota fascia completely. At the superior border of the pancreas, the splenic artery is circumferentially dissected and divided at its origin from the celiac trunk. The splenic vein is carefully dissected from the posterior wall of the pancreas at its confluence with the SMV and divided. At this point, the distal pancreas and spleen are devascularized and the neck of the pancreas is divided. A medial to lateral dissection is completed, and the spleen is detached from its posterior peritoneal attachments to allow en bloc removal of the specimen and surrounding lymph node basin. Several techniques may be used to close the pancreatic duct remnant, with the most common being direct suture ligation or use of a linear stapling device. Either technique is appropriate, with similar risk for the development of pancreatic fistula.

Laparoscopic Distal Pancreatectomy

There has been growing interest in the use of minimally invasive surgery for the resection of tumors of the distal pancreas. Laparoscopic distal pancreatectomy (LDP) may offer advantages over open resection for select patients, with smaller incisions and shorter hospital stay. In a review of more than 800 LDPs, Borja-Cacho and colleagues[43] described an overall morbidity rate of 38% and hospital length of stay of 5 days, which compare favorably with large series after open pancreatectomy. Although LDP is increasingly used for benign conditions, its usefulness for the treatment of PDAC remains to be validated. There have been no randomized trials to evaluate LDP versus open resection, and few studies have reported outcomes of LDP for PDACs. Currently, LDP in the setting of PDACs should be considered experimental.

Outcomes

Perioperative Mortality: Long-Term Survival

Perioperative mortality has become a rare event after the Whipple procedure, occurring in less than 2% of cases at high-volume centers. Despite significant reduction in mortality, however, morbidity remains common, occurring after 30% to 50% of procedures.[38] Table 55-8 lists several of the most common postoperative morbidities and their frequencies.

After surgical resection and adjuvant therapy for pancreatic cancer, the median survival is approximately 22 months, with 5-year survival of 15% to 20%. Most patients experience relapse of disease in the form of metastatic disease (85%) and, less commonly, local recurrence (40%). In the absence of surgical resection, those with locally advanced disease who receive palliative chemotherapy may survive 10 to 12 months, whereas those with metastases rarely survive beyond 6 months. The role of adjuvant chemotherapy and radiation is described later in this chapter.

Morbidity

Delayed gastric emptying characterized by the need for prolonged nasogastric decompression or inability to tolerate oral intake is a

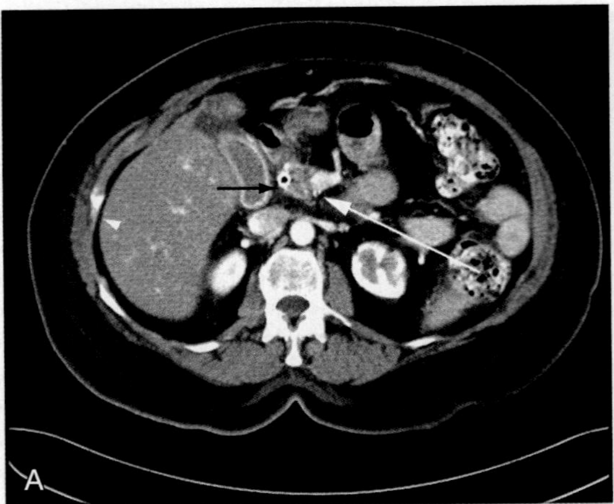

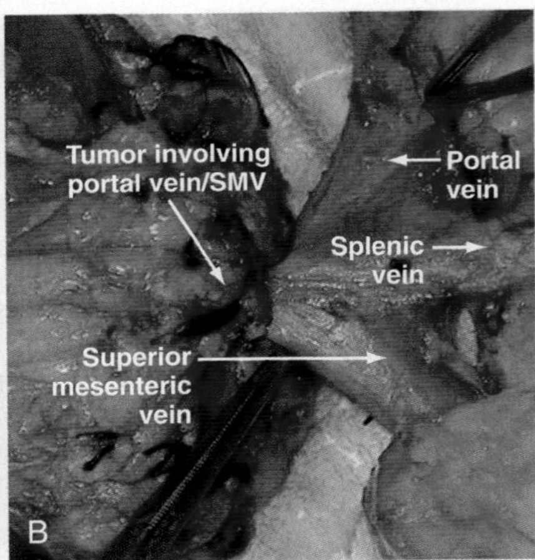

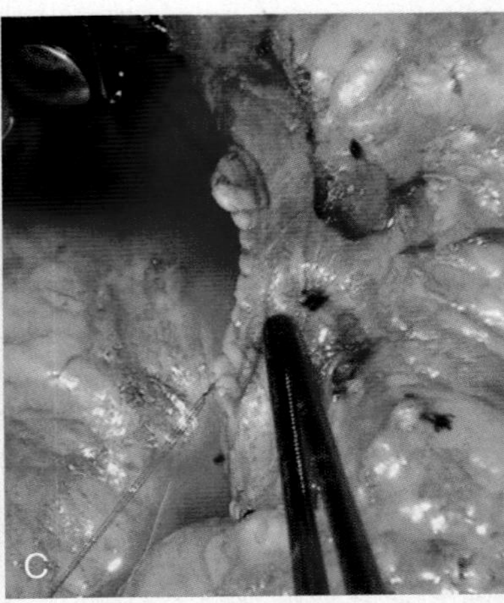

FIGURE 55-25 **A,** CT scan showing PDAC of the pancreatic head with involvement of portal vein–SMV confluence *(large arrow)*. A metal biliary stent is in place *(small arrow)*. **B,** Operative image demonstrating tumor involvement of the lateral aspect of the portal vein–SMV confluence. **C,** Primary closure of portal vein–SMV confluence after tumor removal with lateral vein resection.

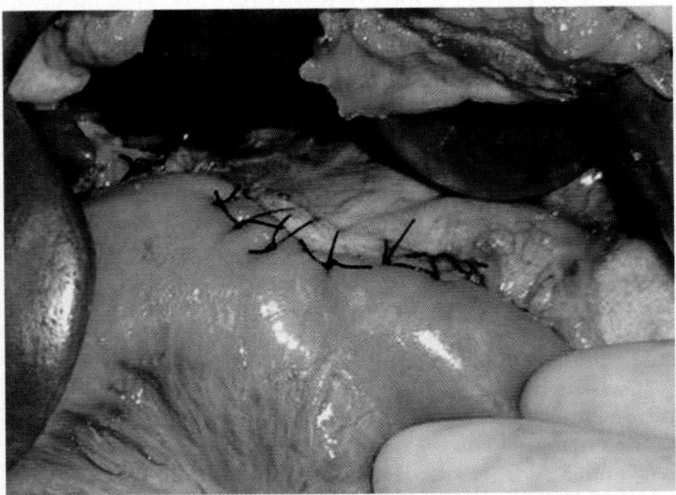

FIGURE 55-26 Completed pancreaticojejunostomy.

TABLE 55-8 Morbidity After Pancreaticoduodenectomy

COMPLICATION	FREQUENCY (%)
Delayed gastric emptying	18
Pancreas fistula	12
Wound infection	7
Intra-abdominal abscess	6
Cardiac events	3
Bile leak	2
Overall reoperation	3

frequent complication after pancreaticoduodenectomy, occurring 5% to 15% of the time. Few studies have demonstrated an association of delayed gastric emptying with pylorus preservation, but this finding has not been confirmed by all. When patients have the inability to tolerate solid foods or a prolonged nasogastric tube requirement, it is critical to perform cross-sectional imaging to rule out a secondary cause, such as pancreatic leak or intra-abdominal abscess. An underlying structural abnormality, like stricture or other anastomotic complications, is ruled out with imaging and endoscopy. Enteral feeding with a feeding tube placed during surgery or percutaneously through endoscopy is used to maintain nutrition while waiting for stomach function to return.

TABLE 55-9 International Study Group on Pancreatic Fistula Classification of Pancreatic Fistulas

	GRADE		
PARAMETER	A	B	C
Clinical conditions	Well	Often well	Ill-appearing, bad
Specific treatment	No	Yes/no	Yes
US/CT (if obtained)	Negative	Negative/positive	Positive
Persistent drainage (after 3 weeks)	No	Usually yes	Yes
Reoperation	No	No	Yes
Death related to POPF	No	No	Possibly yes
Signs of infections	No	Yes	Yes
Sepsis	No	No	Yes
Readmission	No	Yes/no	Yes/no

From Bassi C, Dervenis C, Butturini G, et al: Postoperative pancreatic fistula: An international study group (ISGPF) definition. *Surgery* 138:8–13, 2005.
POPF, postoperative pancreatic fistula.

Pancreatic leak or pancreatic fistula, which has been defined by the International Study Group on Pancreatic Fistula[44] as "output via an intraoperatively placed drain (or percutaneous drain) of any measurable volume on or after postoperative day 3, with amylase >3 times normal serum value," is a frequent complication after pancreaticoduodenectomy, occurring after 5% to 22% of surgeries. Perhaps the most predictive factor is the texture of the gland, with soft fatty glands at significantly higher risk of leak. Most fistulas are controlled by drainage catheters placed at the time of surgery and require no additional intervention. Rarely, uncontrolled fistulas require additional drain placement or operative exploration, sometimes mandating completion pancreatectomy to eliminate further abdominal contamination. The classification of pancreatic fistulas is given in Table 55-9.

Anastomotic leaks from the hepaticojejunostomy and duodenojejunostomy are rare and occur after less than 5% of procedures. Infectious complications (e.g., intra-abdominal abscess, wound infection) are slightly more common and may require intervention with percutaneous drainage or open wound dressing changes.

Pancreatic endocrine and exocrine insufficiency can occur after pancreaticoduodenectomy, but the risk of these events is unpredictable. For individuals with a normal gland, pancreatic insufficiency is rare. However, for those with preexisting chronic pancreatitis, fibrosis of the gland, or insulin resistance, exogenous enzyme and insulin replacement is usually needed.

Controversies

Pylorus-Preserving versus Non–Pylorus-Preserving Whipple Procedure

We have described the pylorus-preserving Whipple procedure, which is the operation of choice for a growing number of pancreatobiliary surgeons. It was initially proposed as a means to reduce postpancreatectomy dumping and bile reflux, which is common after a non–pylorus-preserving Whipple procedure. Although initial results were encouraging, none of the randomized controlled trials have suggested superiority of a pylorus-preserving over a non–pylorus-preserving Whipple procedure. We prefer pylorus preservation when possible but do not hesitate to proceed with a non–pylorus-preserving Whipple procedure in case of tumor involvement of the duodenum or concern for duodenal blood supply.

Pancreaticojejunostomy versus Pancreatogastrostomy

The pancreaticojejunostomy remains the Achilles heel of the Whipple procedure because of the frequency of pancreatic fistula. Several studies have reported successful outcomes with pancreatogastrostomy and reduced leak rates compared with pancreaticojejunostomy, but this finding has not been reproducible in several randomized trials, and most surgeons continue to prefer pancreaticojejunostomy.[45] In cases in which the pancreatic duct is not identified, invagination of the gland into the jejunal stump may also be performed.

Use of Somatostatin Analogues to Reduce Pancreatic Fistula

Although the mortality of pancreaticoduodenectomy has gone down, postoperative morbidity continues to be a significant problem. Pancreatic fistula is the major source of morbidity after the Whipple operation. Because pancreatic exocrine secretion is the proposed mechanism by which postoperative fistula occurs, inhibition of this secretion by means of somatostatin and its analogues has been evaluated in multiple trials with mixed results. Whereas European studies have shown that use of octreotide perioperatively leads to a decreased incidence of postoperative pancreatic fistula, North American trials have not confirmed these results. A trial evaluated the efficacy of pasireotide, a somatostatin analogue with a longer half-life (11 hours for pasireotide versus 2 hours for octreotide) and a broader binding profile (pasireotide binds to somatostatin-receptor subtypes 1, 2, 3, and 5, whereas octreotide binds only to receptor subtypes 2 and 5), in reducing pancreatic fistula, leak, or abscess of grade 3 or higher after pancreatic surgery (both pancreaticoduodenectomy and distal pancreatectomy). In this trial, pasireotide treatment significantly lowered the rate of grade 3 or higher postoperative pancreatic fistula, leak, or abscess (9% versus 21%; relative risk, 0.44; 95% confidence interval, 0.24-0.78; $P = .006$). This finding was seen consistently in patients who underwent pancreaticoduodenectomy or distal pancreatectomy as well as in patients with dilated duct versus nondilated pancreatic duct.[46]

Extent of Lymphadenectomy

Given the fact that 75% to 80% of patients are found to have lymph node involvement at the time of the Whipple procedure and, overall, 80% to 85% of patients will experience tumor recurrence and cancer-related death, some have proposed that radical lymphadenectomy may improve outcomes. Regional pancreatectomy was first proposed by Fortner in 1973 and has been used widely in Japan, where significant improvements in survival of patients undergoing extended lymphadenectomy have been reported. In addition to peripancreatic, portal, and pyloric lymph nodes, extended lymphadenectomy includes retrieval of hilar and retroperitoneal lymph nodes, extending from the celiac origin to the level of the inferior mesenteric artery and including all tissue between the renal hilum laterally. Several randomized controlled trials have since been completed, with no evidence to suggest improved survival after extended lymphadenectomy. In fact, more than one trial has shown increased morbidity associated with extended lymphadenectomy, including delayed gastric emptying, pancreatic fistula, and dumping.[47] In view of the current evidence, standard pancreaticoduodenectomy is the operation of choice for localized pancreatic adenocarcinoma.

Laparoscopic and Robotic Pancreaticoduodenectomy

The first laparoscopic pancreaticoduodenectomy was performed in 1994 by Gagner and Pomp. Since then, several case reports and small series have demonstrated the feasibility of the minimally invasive approach. In the largest U.S. series to date, Kendrick and Cusati[48] have reported outcomes of 65 laparoscopic pancreaticoduodenectomies, with an overall morbidity rate of 42%: pancreatic fistula, 18%; delayed gastric emptying, 15%; bleeding, 8%; wound infection, 6%; reoperation, 5%; and mortality, 1.5%. These results indicate that laparoscopic pancreaticoduodenectomy has similar short-term outcomes to the open approach. Recently, the authors have presented the updated experience with 108 laparoscopic pancreaticoduodenectomies. Their data suggested that the median length of hospital stay was shorter with the laparoscopic approach. Furthermore, the authors observed that compared with the laparoscopic approach, a significantly higher proportion of patients had delay in delivery of adjuvant therapy with the open approach.[49] Pancreaticoduodenectomy is one of the most complex intra-abdominal operations, and to perform it laparoscopically, the operator needs advanced training in both hepatopancreatobiliary and laparoscopic approaches, not to mention years of high-volume experience. Given the complexity of the procedure and the fact that the major morbidities that follow pancreaticoduodenectomy are not related to the size of the incision, the laparoscopic Whipple procedure has not become widely adopted.

Robotics has emerged as both an alternative and an adjunct to laparoscopy. Given the limitations of current laparoscopic technology and the need for meticulous vascular control and complex reconstruction in pancreatic surgery, robotic pancreaticoduodenectomy has been proposed as an alternative to laparoscopic pancreaticoduodenectomy. There are only a few centers in the United States that are pursuing robotics as an approach to pancreaticoduodenectomy. The largest series on robotic pancreaticoduodenectomy is from the University of Pittsburgh. Zureikat and colleagues published their experience with 132 robotic pancreaticoduodenectomies.[50] However, as mentioned before, the major morbidity of pancreaticoduodenectomy does not emanate from the incision, and it is too early to predict whether robotic pancreaticoduodenectomy will ever be widely adopted. At this time, open pancreaticoduodenectomy remains the standard of care.

Antecolic versus Retrocolic Duodenojejunostomy

Delayed gastric emptying is a common occurrence after pancreaticoduodenectomy with an elusive cause. Emerging data suggest that creation of an antecolic duodenojejunostomy may improve gastric emptying compared with the retrocolic technique.

Drain versus No Drain

Given the high frequency of pancreatic fistula after pancreatic resection and morbidity associated with uncontrolled pancreatic leak, drains are routinely used after pancreatic resections. However, surgical drains are not without untoward effects, and their use has been associated with increased rates of intra-abdominal and wound infection, increased pain, and prolonged hospital stay. Use of surgical drains after pancreatic resection has been evaluated in randomized controlled trials. In a randomized controlled trial from Memorial Sloan Kettering Cancer Center comparing outcomes in patients undergoing pancreatic resection with and without placement of surgical drains, no difference in complication rate was observed between the two groups. Furthermore, presence of a drain failed to reduce the need for radiologic intervention or surgical exploration. However, a multi-institution randomized controlled trial comparing drain versus no drain in patients undergoing pancreaticoduodenectomy had to be terminated early as a result of increased morbidity as well as a fourfold increase in mortality in the no-drain group. In this trial, the use of a drain decreased the adverse clinical impact of pancreatic fistula. Good results without use of surgical drains have been achieved only at high-volume specialized centers that have vast experience in dealing with intra-abdominal complications after pancreaticoduodenectomy. These centers have access to advanced interventional radiology techniques as well as experienced endoscopists who can drain many of the intra-abdominal collections internally through the stomach. At this time, use of a surgical drain should be considered standard of care.

Adjuvant Therapy for Pancreatic Cancer

Chemotherapy and Radiation Therapy

During the last 30 years, there have been conflicting reports about the survival benefit of adjuvant therapy after surgical resection of localized pancreatic cancer, particularly with regard to radiation therapy. Although the use of chemotherapy is widely accepted, the usefulness of radiation therapy has been increasingly questioned. In the United States, chemotherapy and radiation therapy are still widely used, whereas European centers have stopped using radiation therapy as part of standard adjuvant therapy because of lack of evidence to support a survival benefit.

Several randomized trials have attempted to clarify the roles of chemotherapy and radiation therapy for adjuvant treatment of pancreatic cancer after surgical resection. Table 55-10 summarizes the findings of several important trials. In 1974, the Gastrointestinal Tumor Study Group (GITSG) began a prospective randomized trial comparing adjuvant 5-fluorouracil (5-FU) and 40-Gy radiation with observation after curative resection.[51] The trial was terminated prematurely because of low accrual and the observation that the chemoradiation arm had a significant survival advantage. During an 8-year period, only 49 patients were accrued and randomized (43 patients were included in the final analysis because of withdrawal of 5 individuals and misdiagnosis of 1). Median survival was 20 months for the chemoradiation group compared with 11 months for the observation group. Despite its limitations, this was the first randomized controlled trial that demonstrated an overall survival benefit after chemoradiation.

TABLE 55-10 Summary of Clinical Trials Defining Role of Adjuvant Therapy After Resection of Pancreatic Cancer

TRIAL	CONCLUSIONS
GITSG	Adjuvant chemoradiation with 5-FU and 40-Gy radiation therapy improves survival compared with observation alone.
ESPAC-1	Adjuvant chemotherapy improves survival; chemoradiation is deleterious.
CONKO-001	Adjuvant gemcitabine improves disease-free survival compared with observation.
RTOG 97-04	Gemcitabine before and after 5-FU–based chemoradiation provides similar overall survival compared with 5-FU but with significantly less toxicity.
ESPAC-3	Adjuvant chemotherapy alone with gemcitabine provides similar overall survival compared with 5-FU but with significantly less toxicity.

The European Study Group for Pancreatic Cancer-1 (ESPAC-1) trial was a 2 × 2 factorial design that compared chemoradiotherapy alone (5-FU, 20 Gy during 2 weeks) versus chemotherapy alone (5-FU) versus chemoradiotherapy and chemotherapy versus observation.[52] At a median follow-up of 47 months, it was noted that the estimated 5-year survival for those who underwent chemoradiotherapy was significantly less than that for those who did not (10% versus 20%; $P = .05$). At the same time, those who received chemotherapy had a 5-year survival of 21% versus 8% for those who did not ($P < .009$). These findings led to the conclusion that although chemotherapy provided significant improvement in overall survival, the routine use of chemoradiation may be detrimental.

In 2007, the Charité Onkologie (CONKO-001) trial of 368 individuals enrolled during a 6-year period evaluated whether chemotherapy with gemcitabine (without radiation) could extend disease-free survival compared with observation.[53] Trial patients received six cycles of gemcitabine (days 1, 8, and 15 every 4 weeks for 6 months), and outcomes were compared with observation alone. Median disease-free survival was significantly improved in the gemcitabine group compared with the observation group (13.4 versus 6.9 months). There was a trend toward improved overall survival, but this did not meet statistical significance (median, 22.1 versus 20.2 months). This trial established the use of adjuvant gemcitabine for the treatment of pancreatic cancer.

The Radiation Therapy Oncology Group (RTOG 97-04) trial compared 5-FU versus gemcitabine chemotherapy before and after 5-FU–based chemoradiation.[54] The purpose of the study was to determine whether gemcitabine provided a survival benefit over 5-FU in combination with 5-FU–based chemoradiation. It was noted that although overall survival was similar (20.5 months for gemcitabine versus 16.9 months for 5-FU; $P =$ NS), the treatment-related toxicity was significantly higher in the 5-FU group. These data have led to the use of gemcitabine as the first-line agent for adjuvant chemotherapy, with or without radiation therapy.

The most recent international randomized controlled trial to be completed (ESPAC-3) was designed to evaluate overall survival comparing 5-FU (425 mg/m^2 IV bolus injection, given on days 1 to 5 every 28 days) versus gemcitabine (1000 mg/m^2 IV infusion, days 1, 8, and 15 every 4 weeks) after curative surgery. No observation arm was included because it was thought to be unethical, given the existing data suggesting a survival benefit of chemotherapy over observation alone. More than 1000 participants from 16 countries were randomized. Overall survival was similar between the groups (23.0 months for 5-FU, 23.6 months for gemcitabine), but gemcitabine was found to have less treatment-related toxicity, with fewer severe adverse events and better compliance. The current National Comprehensive Cancer Network guidelines recommend gemcitabine or 5-FU alone or in combination with 5-FU–based chemoradiation as adjuvant treatment after resection for PDAC. Given the overall poor prognosis, enrollment into clinical trials is encouraged.

Role of Neoadjuvant Therapy

It is clear that for the optimal outcome, patients with pancreatic cancer require multimodal treatment that includes a combination of surgery and chemotherapy with or without radiation treatment. The administration of chemotherapy, with or without radiation therapy, before planned surgical resection for pancreatic cancer is becoming increasingly common. The rationale for the neoadjuvant approach is multifaceted. After surgical resection, approximately 25% of patients do not receive adjuvant therapy because of refusal, surgical complications, or an inability to recover physiologically. Giving therapy before surgery ensures that all patients will receive multimodality therapy, and by delivery of therapy to an intact gland with an established blood supply, the efficacy of therapy may be maximized. In addition, by treatment of patients with measurable disease, response to therapy can be assessed more readily. Progression of disease during neoadjuvant treatment is indicative of aggressive tumor biology and may prevent these patients from undergoing extensive surgery, which is unlikely to provide any survival benefit. Finally, the administration of chemotherapy and radiation therapy before surgery has been viewed as a physiologic stress test and helps select patients who would be unlikely to tolerate the major stress of surgical resection. Neoadjuvant therapy may provide improved selection of patients, avoiding surgery for those who progress, but also improved negative margin rates and reduced lymph node metastasis.

Despite all these theoretical benefits, currently there is no level I evidence demonstrating advantage of the neoadjuvant strategy over the surgery first approach. Most of the data supporting the neoadjuvant approach are in the form of single- or multi-institutional retrospective studies. In a study from MD Anderson Cancer Center, the authors retrospectively reviewed and compared the outcomes of patients with resectable pancreatic adenocarcinoma who underwent neoadjuvant therapy followed by surgery with the outcomes of patients who were treated with the surgery first approach. In this study, 83% of patients with neoadjuvant therapy completed all components of therapy, including surgery with chemotherapy or radiotherapy, compared with 58% of patients treated with the surgery first approach. In this study, patients who completed all components of multimodal therapy had better outcomes compared with those who received only one component, whether surgery or chemotherapy. Although the rate of complications in both groups was similar, patients who received neoadjuvant therapy and suffered postoperative major complication had longer survival compared with patients with the surgery first approach who had a major postoperative complication. This may suggest that neoadjuvant therapy protects patients with pancreatic cancer who undergo pancreatectomy for pancreatic cancer from early recurrence and death. Alternatively, these results may just be a reflection of the fact that the patients who underwent surgery first and developed a complication were unable to receive adjuvant therapy, which is an equally critical component of treatment. Although these results are intriguing, this study is retrospective, and overall survival was used instead of recurrence-free survival. The neoadjuvant approach has multiple advantages, but the issue of superiority over a surgery first approach can be settled only by a randomized controlled trial.

In select patients, the role of neoadjuvant therapy is clearer, particularly for those with significant venous or limited arterial involvement whose disease is classified as borderline resectable. In these patients, for whom upfront surgical exploration has a significant risk of exposing them to nontherapeutic laparotomy, the argument for neoadjuvant therapy is strengthened. For individuals with significant SMV–portal vein involvement (>180 degrees or short-segment encasement) or hepatic arterial or SMA abutment (<180 degrees) who have been traditionally considered to have unresectable disease, neoadjuvant therapy may play an important role in identifying the subset of patients most likely to derive benefit from aggressive multimodality therapy, including surgical resection with vascular reconstruction.[55] This type of aggressive treatment should be undertaken only by an experienced multidisciplinary team in the setting of a clinical trial.

Chemotherapy for Metastatic Pancreatic Adenocarcinoma

More than 80% of patients with pancreatic cancer present with locally advanced or metastatic disease and are primarily managed with chemotherapy. There has been some progress in the chemotherapy treatment of locally advanced or metastatic pancreatic adenocarcinoma. It is vital for the surgeons taking care of patients with pancreatic cancer to know these studies as regimens used to treat locally advanced and metastatic pancreatic adenocarcinoma slowly find their way into the treatment of patients with resectable pancreatic cancer in both adjuvant and neoadjuvant settings. Gemcitabine has been the standard of care for the treatment of metastatic pancreatic cancer since the late 1990s. Few chemotherapy regimens have shown greater efficacy than gemcitabine. Compared with gemcitabine alone, FOLFIRINOX (combination of 5-FU, oxaliplatin, irinotecan, and leucovorin) improves the median overall survival (gemcitabine, 6.8 months; FOLFIRINOX, 11.1 months) and progression-free survival (gemcitabine, 3.3 months; FOLFIRINOX, 6.4 months).[56] FOLFIRINOX is being used as the neoadjuvant regimen of choice in patients with borderline resectable pancreatic cancer and good performance status who can tolerate this aggressive regimen.

In a similar vein, the combination of gemcitabine with nab-paclitaxel improves overall and progression-free survival of patients with metastatic pancreatic cancer compared with gemcitabine alone.[57] The results with targeted therapies in pancreatic cancer have not been very promising as yet. The addition of erlotinib, which targets epidermal growth factor receptor–dependent growth pathways to gemcitabine, leads to statistically significant but marginal improvement in overall survival and progression-free survival in patients with metastatic pancreatic cancer.[58] Evaluation of gemcitabine-erlotinib combination as adjuvant therapy is currently ongoing. Randomized controlled trials evaluating addition of the vascular endothelial growth factor inhibitor bevacizumab or epidermal growth factor receptor inhibitor cetuximab to gemcitabine have not demonstrated improvement in outcomes of patients with metastatic pancreatic cancer compared with gemcitabine alone.

Palliative Therapy for Pancreatic Cancer

Given that 80% to 85% of those with pancreatic cancer have locally advanced or metastatic disease at the time of presentation and are therefore not candidates for surgical resection, it is imperative that all surgeons be familiar with nonoperative and operative palliative options. In general, nonoperative management should be pursued whenever possible to expedite systemic therapy and to optimize quality of life for these patients.

Biliary Obstruction

Palliation of biliary obstruction is commonly required for patients who are not candidates for surgical resection. ERCP with metal stent placement provides excellent palliation of jaundice, and at high-volume university centers, successful biliary drainage is possible in more than 90% of cases. In patients for whom endoscopic palliation is impossible, percutaneous biliary drainage with subsequent internalization may be required. For patients who are found at laparotomy to have unresectable disease or those for whom nonsurgical measures have failed, a surgical biliary-enteric bypass may be performed by Roux-en-Y hepaticojejunostomy, with excellent long-term patency.

Gastric Outlet Obstruction

Approximately 20% of patients with locally advanced pancreatic cancer will develop gastric outlet obstruction. For those with metastatic disease or disease found to be unresectable on the basis of imaging findings who have symptoms of gastric outlet obstruction, endoscopic luminal stenting should be carried out. Palliative endoscopic stenting has excellent short-term results, with almost immediate improvement in oral intake, but is limited in its ability to provide long-term patency. For this reason, patients who are found to have unresectable cancer at the time of laparotomy may benefit from preventive gastrojejunostomy, with no increase in perioperative morbidity. For patients who require surgical intervention, a double bypass consisting of a Roux-en-Y hepaticojejunostomy and gastrojejunostomy may be performed.

Pain Relief

Pain is a common component in the natural history of pancreatic cancer, affecting most patients with advanced disease. Palliation of pain is paramount for optimizing the quality of life for patients and should be a primary goal for physicians. The initial management of pain may include anti-inflammatories or long-acting opioids, taken orally or through a cutaneous patch. For patients with pain that is not well controlled or who suffer side effects of narcotic use, celiac nerve block should be considered. The procedure involves injecting a combination of 3 mL of 0.25% bupivacaine and 10 mL of absolute alcohol into each celiac plexus. For cases that are found at exploration to be unresectable, this can be performed intraoperatively, as described by Lillemoe and coworkers.[59] For those with unresectable disease based on staging evaluation who do not undergo surgical exploration, neurolysis can be achieved through EUS guidance, with pain relief expected in 80% of patients.[60] CT-guided percutaneous neurolysis may also be performed.

PANCREATIC TRAUMA

Pancreatic injuries are uncommon. The mechanism of injury varies according to the age of the patient. The most common mechanism in pediatric patients is abdominal blunt trauma. Direct compression of the epigastrium against the vertebral column and a blunt object (handlebar) is typically seen after bicycle injuries. The most common segment of the pancreas affected is the body. Penetrating injuries into the abdomen are the most common injuries seen in adults.[61]

Isolated pancreatic injuries are not common. Up to 90% of patients present with associated hepatic, gastric, splenic, renal, colonic, or vascular lesions.[61] The diagnosis and therapy in unstable patients with severe retroperitoneal injuries, gunshot wounds, or penetrating injury into the abdomen are usually straightforward, and they do not require further evaluation. Hemodynamically stable patients represent a challenge because isolated pancreatic injuries are normally associated with subtle or absent physical symptoms and signs. Undiagnosed pancreatic injuries are associated with significant complications, such as intra-abdominal abscess, fistula, and fluid collections, in 60% of patients.[62] Pancreatic injuries should always be considered after epigastric compression during a car or bicycle accident.

The modality of choice to evaluate patients with abdominal trauma is CT scanning of the abdomen. Findings such as peripancreatic hematomas, free fluid in the lesser sac, and abnormal thickening of Gerota fascia suggest pancreatic injury. Studies have shown that MRCP provides excellent visualization of the pancreatic duct, peripancreatic fluid contiguous to fractured segments of the pancreas, and hemorrhage after nonpenetrating trauma. Its main limitations include high cost, availability, and amount of time required to perform the study. Isolated pancreatic amylase measurement is not recommended because up to 40% of patients with transected pancreatic duct have normal serum amylase levels. Serial quantification levels increase the sensitivity of the assay. Abnormal amylase level elevations require further imaging.

The most reliable test to demonstrate pancreatic duct integrity is ERCP. However, its applicability is frequently limited by the risk of inducing pancreatitis, availability, and severity of the trauma.

Pancreatic injuries are classified according to the system described by the American Association for the Surgery of Trauma (Table 55-11). Definitive treatment is based on surgical findings.

TABLE 55-11 American Association for the Surgery of Trauma Pancreatic Injury Grading

GRADE		INJURY DESCRIPTION
I	Hematoma	Minor contusion without ductal injury
	Laceration	Superficial laceration without ductal injury
II	Hematoma	Major contusion without ductal injury or tissue loss
	Laceration	Major laceration without ductal injury or tissue loss
III	Laceration	Distal transection or pancreatic parenchymal injury with ductal injury
IV	Laceration	Proximal transection or pancreatic parenchymal injury involving the ampulla
V	Laceration	Massive disruption of the pancreatic head

From Subramanian A, Dente CJ, Feliciano DV: The management of pancreatic trauma in the modern era. *Surg Clin North Am* 87:1515–1532, 2007.

Major pancreatic resections have been described in stable patients with isolated pancreatic injury. However, pancreatic resections in unstable patients are associated with significant morbidity and mortality. Therefore, damage control surgery is indicated for complex injuries or unstable patients. Most pancreatic lesions can be temporarily controlled with drains. Once the physiologic insult has been controlled, definitive treatment should be considered, if indicated. Up to 75% of deaths occur within the 48 to 72 hours after trauma, and most are related to hypovolemic shock.[61]

SELECTED REFERENCES

Abrams RA, Lowy AM, O'Reilly EM, et al: Combined modality treatment of resectable and borderline resectable pancreas cancer: Expert consensus statement. *Ann Surg Oncol* 16:1751–1756, 2009.

A consensus statement about recommending multimodality therapy to optimize outcomes for patients with resectable and borderline resectable pancreatic cancer.

Andersen DK, Frey CF: The evolution of the surgical treatment of chronic pancreatitis. *Ann Surg* 251:18–32, 2010.

A historical review of surgical techniques for the management of chronic pancreatitis.

Beger HG, Rau BM: Severe acute pancreatitis: Clinical course and management. *World J Gastroenterol* 13:5043–5051, 2007.

A review of the pathophysiology of acute pancreatitis and clinical management strategies.

Gittes GK: Developmental biology of the pancreas: A comprehensive review. *Dev Biol* 326:4–35, 2009.

A comprehensive review of pancreatic embryology and development.

IAP/APA evidence-based guidelines for the management of acute pancreatitis. *Pancreatology* 4:e1–e16, 2013.

This manuscript provides evidence-based guidelines addressing multiple issues in the management of acute pancreatitis, including role and timing of ERCP and use of antibiotics.

Tanaka M, Chari S, Adsay V, et al: International consensus guidelines for management of intraductal papillary mucinous neoplasms and mucinous cystic neoplasms of the pancreas. *Pancreatology* 6:17–32, 2006.

Tanaka M, Fernandez-del Castillo C, Adsay V, et al: International consensus guidelines 2012 for the management of IPMN and MCN of the pancreas. *Pancreatology* 12:183–197, 2012.

The first version of the consensus guidelines (2006) for diagnosis and management of cystic neoplasms of the pancreas points out the issues, provides guidelines, and provides the evidence behind the guidelines. Even though these guidelines have been updated (2012), a review of the older version provides perspective on how the diagnosis and management of this common pancreatic problem have evolved.

Winter JM, Cameron JL, Campbell KA, et al: 1423 pancreaticoduodenectomies for pancreatic cancer: A single-institution experience. *J Gastrointest Surg* 10:1199–1210, 2006.

A historic review of the largest single-institution pancreaticoduodenectomy experience.

REFERENCES

1. Gittes GK: Developmental biology of the pancreas: A comprehensive review. *Dev Biol* 326:4–35, 2009.
2. Saluja AK, Lerch MM, Phillips PA, et al: Why does pancreatic overstimulation cause pancreatitis? *Annu Rev Physiol* 69:249–269, 2007.
3. Beger HG, Rau BM: Severe acute pancreatitis: Clinical course and management. *World J Gastroenterol* 13:5043–5051, 2007.
4. Elfar M, Gaber LW, Sabek O, et al: The inflammatory cascade in acute pancreatitis: Relevance to clinical disease. *Surg Clin North Am* 87:1325–1340, vii, 2007.
5. Larson SD, Nealon WH, Evers BM: Management of gallstone pancreatitis. *Adv Surg* 40:265–284, 2006.
6. Frossard JL, Steer ML, Pastor CM: Acute pancreatitis. *Lancet* 371:143–152, 2008.
7. Ranson JH, Rifkind KM, Roses DF, et al: Prognostic signs and the role of operative management in acute pancreatitis. *Surg Gynecol Obstet* 139:69–81, 1974.
8. Gravante G, Garcea G, Ong SL, et al: Prediction of mortality in acute pancreatitis: A systematic review of the published evidence. *Pancreatology* 9:601–614, 2009.
9. Balthazar EJ, Robinson DL, Megibow AJ, et al: Acute pancreatitis: Value of CT in establishing prognosis. *Radiology* 174:331–336, 1990.
10. Charbonney E, Nathens AB: Severe acute pancreatitis: A review. *Surg Infect (Larchmt)* 9:573–578, 2008.
11. Nealon WH, Bawduniak J, Walser EM: Appropriate timing of cholecystectomy in patients who present with moderate to severe gallstone-associated acute pancreatitis with peripancreatic fluid collections. *Ann Surg* 239:741–749, discussion 749–751, 2004.
12. Rodriguez JR, Razo AO, Targarona J, et al: Debridement and closed packing for sterile or infected necrotizing pancreatitis: Insights into indications and outcomes in 167 patients. *Ann Surg* 247:294–299, 2008.
13. Besselink MG, Verwer TJ, Schoenmaeckers EJ, et al: Timing of surgical intervention in necrotizing pancreatitis. *Arch Surg* 142:1194–1201, 2007.
14. van Santvoort HC, Besselink MG, Bakker OJ, et al: A step-up approach or open necrosectomy for necrotizing pancreatitis. *N Engl J Med* 362:1491–1502, 2010.
15. Lerch MM, Stier A, Wahnschaffe U, et al: Pancreatic pseudocysts: Observation, endoscopic drainage, or resection? *Dtsch Arztebl Int* 106:614–621, 2009.
16. Apte MV, Haber PS, Applegate TL, et al: Periacinar stellate shaped cells in rat pancreas: Identification, isolation, and culture. *Gut* 43:128–133, 1998.
17. Sah RP, Dudeja V, Dawra RK, et al: Cerulein-induced chronic pancreatitis does not require intra-acinar activation of trypsinogen in mice. *Gastroenterology* 144:1076–1085.e2, 2013.

18. Catalano MF, Sahai A, Levy M, et al: EUS-based criteria for the diagnosis of chronic pancreatitis: The Rosemont classification. *Gastrointest Endosc* 69:1251–1261, 2009.
19. O'Neil SJ, Aranha GV: Lateral pancreaticojejunostomy for chronic pancreatitis. *World J Surg* 27:1196–1202, 2003.
20. Andersen DK, Frey CF: The evolution of the surgical treatment of chronic pancreatitis. *Ann Surg* 251:18–32, 2010.
21. Keck T, Wellner UF, Riediger H, et al: Long-term outcome after 92 duodenum-preserving pancreatic head resections for chronic pancreatitis: Comparison of Beger and Frey procedures. *J Gastrointest Surg* 14:549–556, 2010.
22. Heidt DG, Burant C, Simeone DM: Total pancreatectomy: Indications, operative technique, and postoperative sequelae. *J Gastrointest Surg* 11:209–216, 2007.
23. Blondet JJ, Carlson AM, Kobayashi T, et al: The role of total pancreatectomy and islet autotransplantation for chronic pancreatitis. *Surg Clin North Am* 87:1477–1501, x, 2007.
24. Dunderdale J, McAuliffe JC, McNeal SF, et al: Should pancreatectomy with islet cell autotransplantation in patients with chronic alcoholic pancreatitis be abandoned? *J Am Coll Surg* 216:591–596, discussion 596–598, 2013.
25. Bellin MD, Freeman ML, Schwarzenberg SJ, et al: Quality of life improves for pediatric patients after total pancreatectomy and islet autotransplant for chronic pancreatitis. *Clin Gastroenterol Hepatol* 9:793–799, 2011.
26. Varadarajulu S, Bang JY, Sutton BS, et al: Equal efficacy of endoscopic and surgical cystogastrostomy for pancreatic pseudocyst drainage in a randomized trial. *Gastroenterology* 145:583–590.e1, 2013.
27. Brugge WR, Lewandrowski K, Lee-Lewandrowski E, et al: Diagnosis of pancreatic cystic neoplasms: A report of the cooperative pancreatic cyst study. *Gastroenterology* 126:1330–1336, 2004.
28. Tran Cao HS, Kellogg B, Lowy AM, et al: Cystic neoplasms of the pancreas. *Surg Oncol Clin N Am* 19:267–295, 2010.
29. Allen PJ, Qin LX, Tang L, et al: Pancreatic cyst fluid protein expression profiling for discriminating between serous cystadenoma and intraductal papillary mucinous neoplasm. *Ann Surg* 250:754–760, 2009.
30. Tanaka M, Fernandez-del Castillo C, Adsay V, et al: International consensus guidelines 2012 for the management of IPMN and MCN of the pancreas. *Pancreatology* 12:183–197, 2012.
31. Salvia R, Fernandez-del Castillo C, Bassi C, et al: Main-duct intraductal papillary mucinous neoplasms of the pancreas: Clinical predictors of malignancy and long-term survival following resection. *Ann Surg* 239:678–685, discussion 685–687, 2004.
32. Katz MH, Mortenson MM, Wang H, et al: Diagnosis and management of cystic neoplasms of the pancreas: An evidence-based approach. *J Am Coll Surg* 207:106–120, 2008.
33. Sohn TA, Yeo CJ, Cameron JL, et al: Intraductal papillary mucinous neoplasms of the pancreas: An updated experience. *Ann Surg* 239:788–797, discussion 797–799, 2004.
34. Levy P, Jouannaud V, O'Toole D, et al: Natural history of intraductal papillary mucinous tumors of the pancreas: Actuarial risk of malignancy. *Clin Gastroenterol Hepatol* 4:460–468, 2006.
35. Yachida S, Jones S, Bozic I, et al: Distant metastasis occurs late during the genetic evolution of pancreatic cancer. *Nature* 467:1114–1117, 2010.
36. Chari ST, Leibson CL, Rabe KG, et al: Probability of pancreatic cancer following diabetes: A population-based study. *Gastroenterology* 129:504–511, 2005.
37. Klein AP, Hruban RH, Brune KA, et al: Familial pancreatic cancer. *Cancer J* 7:266–273, 2001.
38. Winter JM, Cameron JL, Campbell KA, et al: 1423 pancreaticoduodenectomies for pancreatic cancer: A single-institution experience. *J Gastrointest Surg* 10:1199–1210, discussion 1210–1211, 2006.
39. Callery MP, Chang KJ, Fishman EK, et al: Pretreatment assessment of resectable and borderline resectable pancreatic cancer: Expert consensus statement. *Ann Surg Oncol* 16:1727–1733, 2009.
40. Ferrone CR, Haas B, Tang L, et al: The influence of positive peritoneal cytology on survival in patients with pancreatic adenocarcinoma. *J Gastrointest Surg* 10:1347–1353, 2006.
41. Trimble IR, Parsons JW, Sherman CP: One-stage operation for the cure of carcinoma of the ampulla of Vater and the head of the pancreas. *Surg Gynecol Obstet* 73:711–722, 1941.
42. Strasberg SM, Drebin JA, Linehan D: Radical antegrade modular pancreatosplenectomy. *Surgery* 133:521–527, 2003.
43. Borja-Cacho D, Al-Refaie WB, Vickers SM, et al: Laparoscopic distal pancreatectomy. *J Am Coll Surg* 209:758–765, quiz 800, 2009.
44. Bassi C, Dervenis C, Butturini G, et al: Postoperative pancreatic fistula: An international study group (ISGPF) definition. *Surgery* 138:8–13, 2005.
45. Wente MN, Shrikhande SV, Muller MW, et al: Pancreaticojejunostomy versus pancreaticogastrostomy: Systematic review and meta-analysis. *Am J Surg* 193:171–183, 2007.
46. Allen PJ, Gonen M, Brennan MF, et al: Pasireotide for postoperative pancreatic fistula. *N Engl J Med* 370:2014–2022, 2014.
47. Farnell MB, Aranha GV, Nimura Y, et al: The role of extended lymphadenectomy for adenocarcinoma of the head of the pancreas: Strength of the evidence. *J Gastrointest Surg* 12:651–656, 2008.
48. Kendrick ML, Cusati D: Total laparoscopic pancreaticoduodenectomy: Feasibility and outcome in an early experience. *Arch Surg* 145:19–23, 2010.
49. Croome KP, Farnell MB, Que FG, et al: Total laparoscopic pancreaticoduodenectomy for pancreatic ductal adenocarcinoma: Oncologic advantages over open approaches? *Ann Surg* 260:633–638, discussion 638–640, 2014.
50. Zureikat AH, Moser AJ, Boone BA, et al: 250 robotic pancreatic resections: Safety and feasibility. *Ann Surg* 258:554–559, discussion 559–562, 2013.
51. Kalser MH, Ellenberg SS: Pancreatic cancer. Adjuvant combined radiation and chemotherapy following curative resection. *Arch Surg* 120:899–903, 1985.
52. Neoptolemos JP, Stocken DD, Friess H, et al: A randomized trial of chemoradiotherapy and chemotherapy after resection of pancreatic cancer. *N Engl J Med* 350:1200–1210, 2004.
53. Oettle H, Post S, Neuhaus P, et al: Adjuvant chemotherapy with gemcitabine vs observation in patients undergoing curative-intent resection of pancreatic cancer: A randomized controlled trial. *JAMA* 297:267–277, 2007.
54. Regine WF, Winter KA, Abrams RA, et al: Fluorouracil vs gemcitabine chemotherapy before and after fluorouracil-based chemoradiation following resection of pancreatic adenocarcinoma: A randomized controlled trial. *JAMA* 299:1019–1026, 2008.

55. Abrams RA, Lowy AM, O'Reilly EM, et al: Combined modality treatment of resectable and borderline resectable pancreas cancer: Expert consensus statement. *Ann Surg Oncol* 16:1751–1756, 2009.
56. Conroy T, Desseigne F, Ychou M, et al: FOLFIRINOX versus gemcitabine for metastatic pancreatic cancer. *N Engl J Med* 364:1817–1825, 2011.
57. Von Hoff DD, Ervin T, Arena FP, et al: Increased survival in pancreatic cancer with nab-paclitaxel plus gemcitabine. *N Engl J Med* 369:1691–1703, 2013.
58. Moore MJ, Goldstein D, Hamm J, et al: Erlotinib plus gemcitabine compared with gemcitabine alone in patients with advanced pancreatic cancer: A phase III trial of the National Cancer Institute of Canada Clinical Trials Group. *J Clin Oncol* 25:1960–1966, 2007.
59. Lillemoe KD, Cameron JL, Kaufman HS, et al: Chemical splanchnicectomy in patients with unresectable pancreatic cancer. A prospective randomized trial. *Ann Surg* 217:447–455, discussion 456–457, 1993.
60. Puli SR, Reddy JB, Bechtold ML, et al: EUS-guided celiac plexus neurolysis for pain due to chronic pancreatitis or pancreatic cancer pain: A meta-analysis and systematic review. *Dig Dis Sci* 54:2330–2337, 2009.
61. Stawicki SP, Schwab CW: Pancreatic trauma: Demographics, diagnosis, and management. *Am Surg* 74:1133–1145, 2008.
62. Subramanian A, Dente CJ, Feliciano DV: The management of pancreatic trauma in the modern era. *Surg Clin North Am* 87:1515–1532, x, 2007.

56 CHAPTER

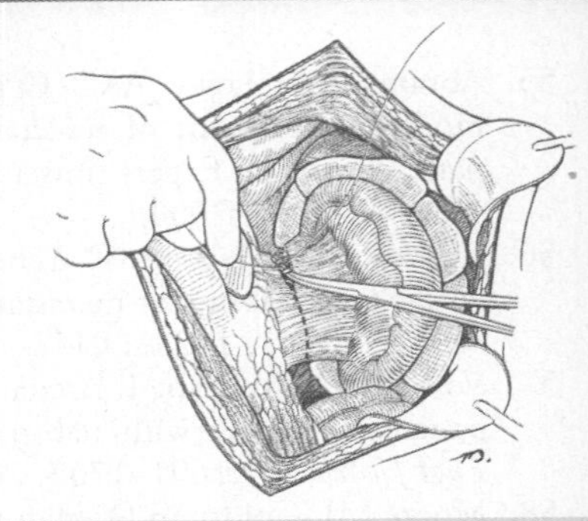

The Spleen

Benjamin K. Poulose, Michael D. Holzman

OUTLINE

SPLENIC ANATOMY

The spleen is an 80- to 300-g organ that initially develops from mesenchymal cells in the dorsal mesogastrium during week 5 of embryogenesis and settles into the left uppermost aspect of the abdomen. Its superior surface is roofed by the diaphragm, separating it from the pleura. However, the costodiaphragmatic recess extends to the inferiormost aspect of a normal-sized spleen. The spleen's visceral relationships include the greater curvature of the stomach, splenic flexure of the colon, apex of the left kidney, and tail of the pancreas (Fig. 56-1). It is protected by ribs 9, 10, and 11 and is suspended in its location by multiple peritoneal reflections, the splenophrenic, gastrosplenic, splenorenal, and splenocolic ligaments. In patients without portal hypertension, the splenophrenic and splenocolic ligaments are relatively avascular. The gastrosplenic ligament carries the short gastric vessels in its superior aspect and the left gastroepiploic in its inferior aspect. The splenorenal ligament houses the splenic artery and vein as well as the tail of the pancreas. The tail of the pancreas abuts the splenic hilum in 30% of individuals and is within 1 cm of the hilum in 70%.

The splenic artery, a branch of the celiac trunk, is a tortuous vessel that gives off multiple branches to the pancreas as it travels along its posterior aspect (Fig. 56-2). There are two common variations of the splenic artery as originally described by Michels: the magistral type, which branches into terminal and polar arteries near the hilum of the spleen; and the distributed type, which, as the name implies, gives off its branches early and distant from the hilum.[1] The magistral type of splenic arterial anatomy occurs in 30% of individuals compared with the distributed type (70%). There is typically a superior polar artery, which sometimes communicates with the short gastric arteries and the superior, middle, and inferior terminal arteries, and an inferior polar artery. Knowing these variable distributions is necessary in performing resections, especially a spleen-preserving procedure. Because of the variable nature of the splenic artery, one must be cautious when operating near this vessel and its tributaries.

The spleen is encased within a fibroelastic capsule. Trabeculae that compartmentalize the spleen pass from the splenic capsule. The spleen is also segmented by the divisions of the splenic vessels as they branch within the organ and merge with these trabeculae. The arterioles branch into even smaller vessels and leave these trabeculae to merge with the splenic pulp, where their adventitia is replaced by a covering of lymphatic tissue that continues until the vessels thin to capillaries. These lymphatic sheaths make up the white pulp of the spleen and are interspersed among the arteriolar branches as lymphatic follicles. The white pulp then interfaces with the red pulp at the marginal zone. It is in this marginal zone that the arterioles lose their lymphatic tissue and the vessels evolve into thin-walled splenic sinuses and sinusoids. The sinusoids then merge into venules, draining into veins that travel along the trabeculae to form splenic veins that mirror their arterial counterparts. The splenic vein leaves the splenic hilum and travels posteriorly to the pancreas, joining with pancreatic branches and often the inferior mesenteric vein to finally receive the superior mesenteric vein, forming the portal vein.

SPLENIC FUNCTION

During fetal development, the spleen has important hematopoietic functions, which include white and red blood cell production. This production is usurped by the bone marrow during the fifth month of gestation, and under normal conditions, the spleen has no significant hematopoietic function beyond this point. In certain pathologic conditions, such as myelodysplasia, the spleen may reacquire this function. Beyond hematopoiesis, the specialized vasculature in the spleen is directly related to its remaining functions, defense and cleansing. It is likely that the spleen's mechanical filtration contributes to control of infection by removing pathogens within cells (e.g., malaria) or circulating in the plasma. This filtration may be particularly important for removal of microorganisms for which the host does not have a specific antibody (Box 56-1).

The immune functions of the spleen become obvious after splenectomy, when patients are noted to be significantly at risk for infection. The most serious sequela is overwhelming postsplenectomy infection (OPSI), with meningitis, pneumonia, or bacteremia.[2] Older studies have demonstrated that the risk of OPSI

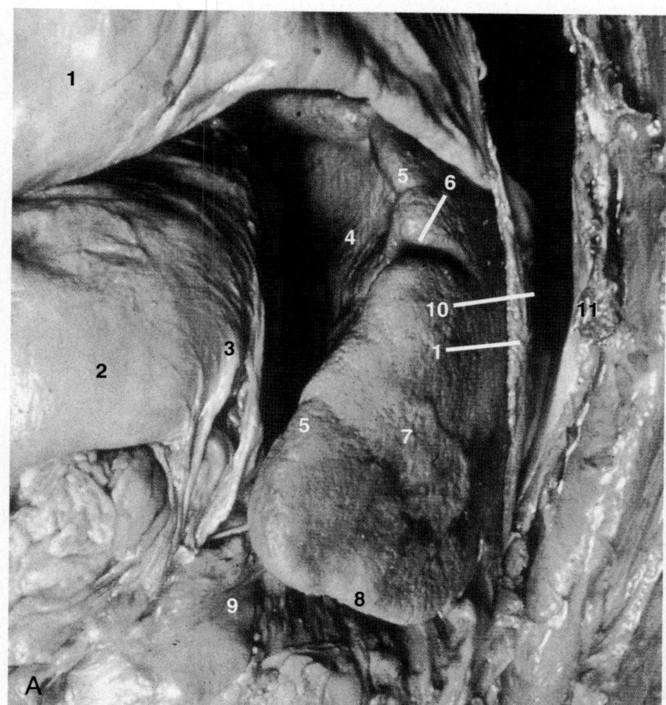

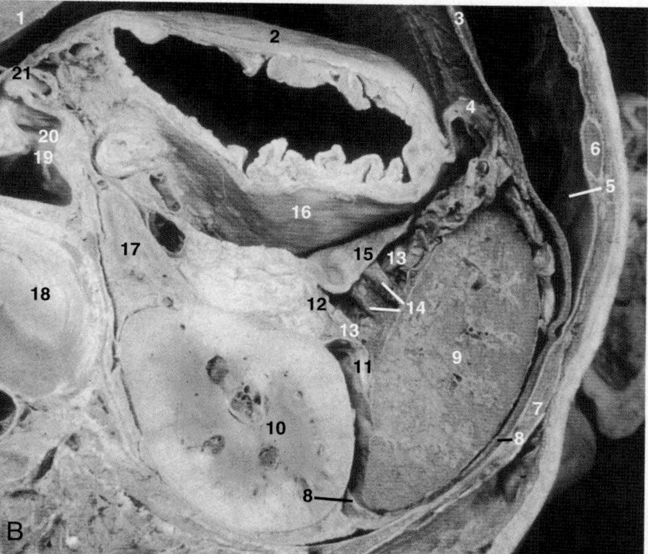

FIGURE 56-1 A, Spleen, from the front: (1) diaphragm, (2) stomach, (3) gastrosplenic ligament, (4) gastric impression, (5) superior border, (6) notch, (7) diaphragmatic surface, (8) inferior border, (9) left colic flexure, (10) costodiaphragmatic recess, and (11) thoracic wall. The left upper abdominal and lower anterior thoracic walls have been removed, and part of the diaphragm (1) has been turned upward to show the spleen in its normal position, lying adjacent to the stomach (2) and colon (9), with the lower part against the kidney (**B,** 9 and 10). **B,** Spleen, in a transverse section of the left upper abdomen: (1) left lobe of liver, (2) stomach, (3) diaphragm, (4) gastrosplenic ligament, (5) costodiaphragmatic recess of pleura, (6) ninth rib, (7) tenth rib, (8) peritoneum of greater sac, (9) spleen, (10) left kidney, (11) posterior layer of lienorenal ligament, (12) tail of pancreas, (13) splenic artery, (14) splenic vein, (15) anterior layer of lienorenal ligament, (16) lesser sac, (17) left suprarenal gland, (18) intervertebral disc, (19) abdominal aorta, (20) celiac trunk, and (21) left gastric artery. The section is at the level of the disc (18) between the twelfth thoracic and first lumbar vertebrae and is viewed from below looking toward the thorax. The spleen (9) lies against the diaphragm (3) and left kidney (10) but is separated from them by peritoneum of the greater sac (8). The peritoneum behind the stomach (2), forming part of the gastrosplenic (4) and ileorenal (15) ligaments, belongs to the lesser sac (16). (From McMinn RMH, Hutchings RT, Pegington J, Abrahams PH: *Color atlas of human anatomy*, ed 3, St Louis, 1993, Mosby–Year Book, pp 230–231.)

is greatest within the first 2 years after splenectomy, but recent studies have confirmed that a lifelong risk remains. One third of cases occur more than 5 years after surgery, with the overall incidence reported to be 3.2% to 3.5%. For those who acquire OPSI, mortality is between 40% and 50%.[3] The risk is greatest in patients with thalassemia major and sickle cell disease. OPSI is typically caused by polysaccharide-encapsulated organisms, such as *Streptococcus pneumoniae, Neisseria meningitidis,* and *Haemophilus influenzae.* These and other organisms are identified and bound by antibodies and complement components in preparation for phagocytosis by macrophages in the spleen. After splenectomy, the antibodies continue to bind, but digestion by splenic macrophages is no longer possible.

In comparing the timing of pneumococcal vaccinations in postsplenectomy trauma patients and control subjects, asplenic patients have been noted to express similar postvaccination immunoglobulin G antibody levels; functional antibody levels, however, were lower.[4] Also, asplenic patients have been found to express subnormal immunoglobulin M levels, and their peripheral blood mononuclear cells exhibit a suppressed immunoglobulin response. The risk for development of OPSI or asplenic or hyposplenic overwhelming sepsis for reasons other than surgical removal of the spleen is linked to the patient's understanding of the risks of infection.[5] Registries that allow long-term follow-up and periodic teaching of current recommendations should be considered for this high-risk population.[6,7]

Other factors involved in the immune response, such as properdin and tuftsin, opsonins produced in the spleen, exhibit reduced serum levels after splenectomy. Properdin, a globulin protein also known as factor P, initiates the alternate pathway of complement activation; this increases the destruction of bacteria and foreign or otherwise abnormal cells. Tuftsin, a tetrapeptide, enhances the phagocytic activity of mononuclear phagocytes and polymorphonuclear leukocytes. Absence of a circulating mediator appears to result in suppressed neutrophil function. The spleen also plays a key role in cleaving tuftsin from the heavy chain of immunoglobulin G; thus, circulating levels of tuftsin are subnormal in asplenic patients.

The filtration consists of two methods of blood flow within the spleen, the closed and open systems. In the closed system, blood flows directly from arteries to veins. In the open system, most of the spleen's blood flow occurs when blood flows through the

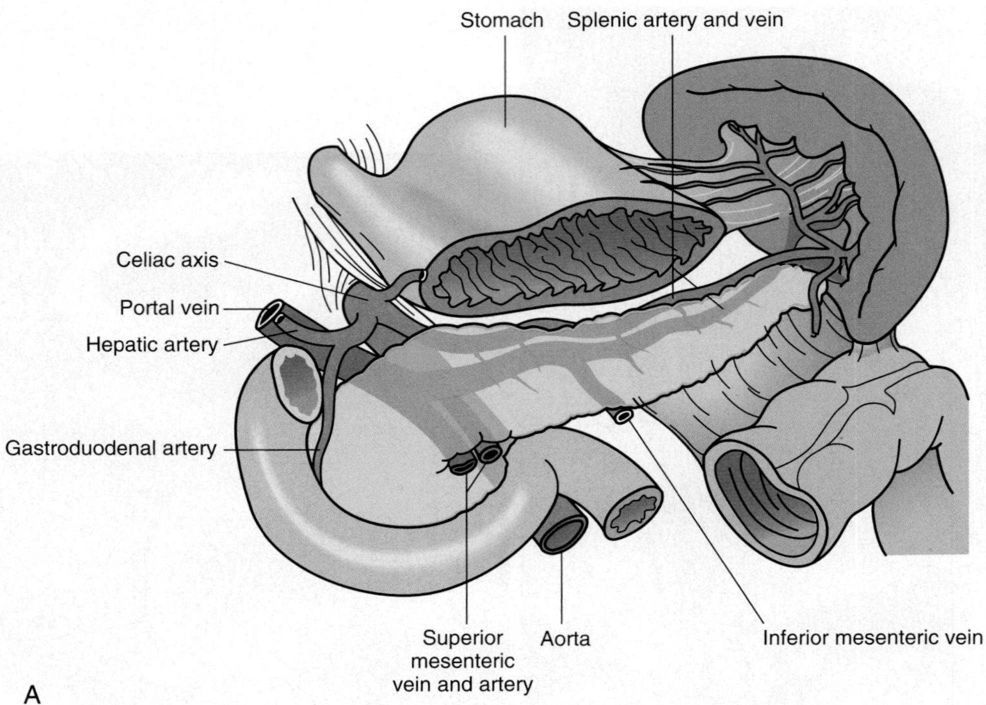

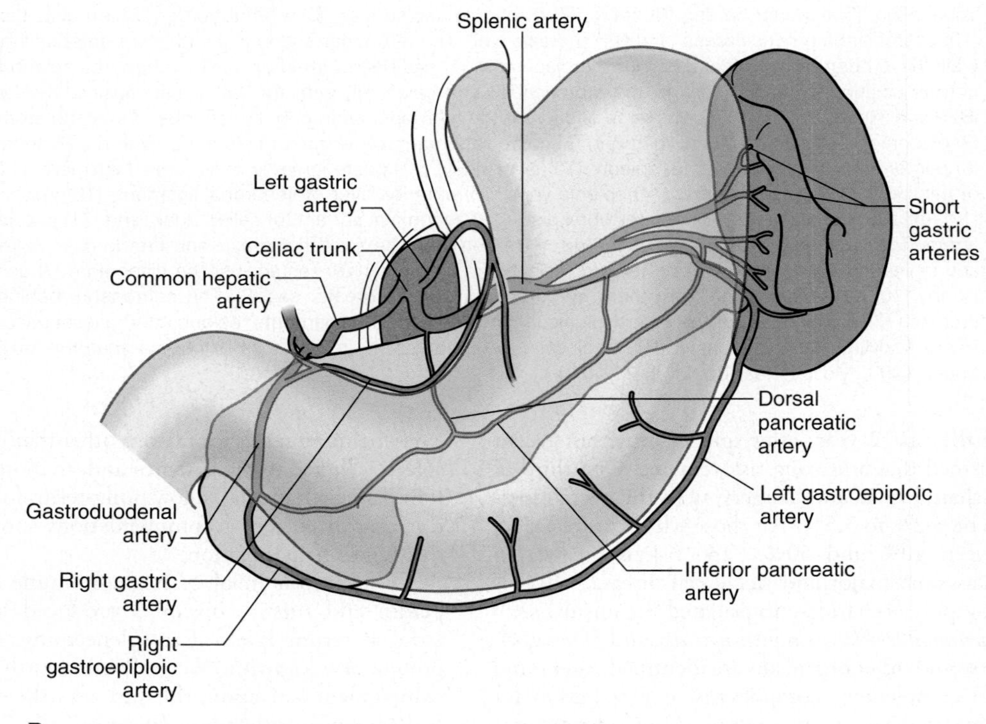

FIGURE 56-2 Anatomic relationships of the splenic vasculature. The magistral type of splenic artery anatomy **(A)** occurs in 30% of individuals. The more common distributed type of anatomy **(B)** occurs in 70% of individuals. (From Economou SG, Economou TS: *Atlas of surgical techniques*, Philadelphia, 1966, WB Saunders, p 562.)

arterioles and then trickles through a sieve-like parenchyma made up of reticuloendothelial cells into the splenic sinuses before draining into the venous system (Fig. 56-3). The cellular elements are directed toward these reticuloendothelial cells, in which cellular cleansing processes take place. These include removal of senescent cells, cellular inclusions (e.g., red blood cell nucleoli), and parasites and the sequestration of red blood cells (for maturation) and platelets (reservoir). The plasma is directed to the lymphoid tissue, where soluble antigens stimulate the production of antibodies.

Red blood cell morphology, and thus red blood cell function, is maintained by splenic filtration. Normal red blood cells are biconcave and deform easily. This plasticity allows passage through the microvasculature and optimizes the exchange of oxygen and carbon dioxide. Imperfect red blood cells with inclusions such as nucleoli, Howell-Jolly bodies (nuclear remnant), Heinz bodies (denatured hemoglobin), Pappenheimer bodies (iron granules), acanthocytes (spur cells), codocytes (target cells), and stippling cause these red blood cells to undergo cleansing in the spleen. Aged red blood cells with decreased plasticity (>120 days) become trapped and destroyed in the spleen.

Abnormal erythrocytes that result from sickle cell anemia, hereditary spherocytosis, thalassemia, or pyruvate kinase deficiency are also trapped and destroyed by the spleen. The overall effect is worsening anemia, splenomegaly, and sometimes autoinfarction of the spleen. Similarly, the spleen is involved in platelet destruction in immune thrombocytopenic purpura (ITP).

BOX 56-1 Biologic Substances Removed by the Spleen

Normal Subjects

Red blood cell membrane
Red blood cell surface pits and craters
Howell-Jolly bodies
Heinz bodies
Pappenheimer bodies
Acanthocytes
Senescent red blood cells
Particulate antigen

Patients With Disease

Spherocytes (hereditary spherocytosis)
Sickle cells, hemoglobin C cells
Antibody-coated red blood cells
Antibody-coated platelets
Antibody-coated white blood cells

Adapted from Eichner ER: Splenic function: Normal, too much and too little. *Am J Med* 66:311–320, 1979.

SPLENECTOMY

Splenectomy may be performed for a number of reasons and conditions.

Benign Hematologic Conditions

Immune Thrombocytopenic Purpura

ITP, classically known as idiopathic thrombocytopenic purpura, is characterized by a low platelet count despite normal bone marrow and the absence of other causes of thrombocytopenia that could be responsible for the finding. Autoantibodies are responsible for the disordered platelet destruction mediated by the overactivated platelet phagocytosis within the reticuloendothelial system. Within the bone marrow, normal (or sometimes increased)

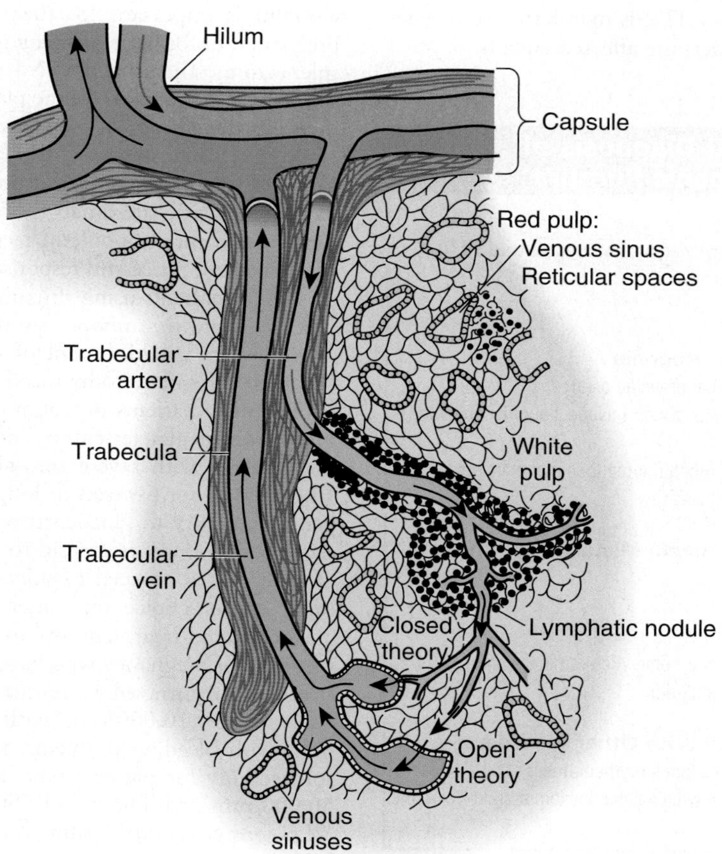

FIGURE 56-3 Structure of the sinusoidal spleen showing the open and closed blood flow routes. (From Bellanti JA: *Immunology: Basic processes.* Philadelphia, 1979, WB Saunders.)

amounts of megakaryocytes are present. There persists, however, a relative bone marrow failure in that production cannot match destruction to compensate sufficiently.

The typical presentation of ITP is characterized by purpura, epistaxis, and gingival bleeding. Less commonly, gastrointestinal bleeding and hematuria are noted. Intracerebral hemorrhage is a rare but sometimes fatal presentation. The diagnosis of ITP involves the exclusion of other relatively common causes of thrombocytopenia—pregnancy, drug-induced thrombocytopenia (e.g., heparin, quinidine, quinine, sulfonamides), viral infections, and hypersplenism (Box 56-2). Mild thrombocytopenia may be seen in approximately 6% to 8% of otherwise normal pregnancies and in up to 25% of women with preeclampsia. Drug-induced thrombocytopenia is thought to occur rarely, in approximately 20 to 40 cases/million users of common medications, such as trimethoprim-sulfonamide and quinine. Other medications, such as gold salts, have a higher incidence, almost 1% of users.[8] Viral infection (e.g., hepatitis C, HIV infection, rarely Epstein-Barr virus infection) can be responsible for thrombocytopenia independent of splenic sequestration. Once again, other processes must be ruled out, but health care providers can be confident of these causative factors if platelet counts improve with successful treatment of the responsible infection. Bacterial infection, specifically *Helicobacter pylori,* has also been linked to infection-related thrombocytopenia that improves with eradication. Other causes are listed in Box 56-2; spurious laboratory values caused by platelet clumping or the presence of giant platelets should not be ignored.

ITP is predominantly a disease of young women; 72% of patients older than 10 years are women, and 70% of affected women are younger than 40 years. ITP is manifested somewhat differently in children; both genders are affected equally, onset is sudden, thrombocytopenia is severe, and complete spontaneous remissions are seen in approximately 80% of affected children. Girls older than 10 years with more chronic purpura are those in whom the disease seems to persist.

BOX 56-2 Differential Diagnosis of Immune Thrombocytopenic Purpura

Falsely Low Platelet Count

In vitro platelet clumping caused by ethylenediaminetetraacetic acid (EDTA)–dependent or cold-dependent agglutinins
Giant platelets

Common Causes of Thrombocytopenia

Pregnancy (gestational thrombocytopenia, preeclampsia)
Drug-induced thrombocytopenia (common drugs include heparin, quinidine, quinine, sulfonamides)
Viral infections, such as HIV infection, rubella, infectious mononucleosis
Hypersplenism caused by chronic liver disease

Other Causes of Thrombocytopenia Mistaken for Immune Thrombocytopenic Purpura

Myelodysplasia
Congenital thrombocytopenias
Thrombotic thrombocytopenic purpura and hemolytic-uremic syndrome
Chronic disseminated intravascular coagulation

Thrombocytopenia Associated With Other Disorders

Autoimmune diseases, such as systemic lupus erythematosus
Lymphoproliferative disorders (chronic lymphocytic leukemia, non-Hodgkin lymphoma)

Adapted from George JN, El-Harake MA, Raskob GE: Chronic idiopathic thrombocytopenic purpura. *N Engl J Med* 331:1207–1211, 1994.

Management of ITP depends primarily on the severity of the thrombocytopenia.[9] Asymptomatic patients with platelet counts higher than 50,000/mm^3 may be observed without further intervention. Platelet counts of 50,000/mm^3 and higher are rarely associated with clinical sequelae, even with invasive procedures. Patients with slightly lower platelet counts, between 30,000 and 50,000/mm^3, may be observed but with more routine follow-up because they are at increased risk for progressing to severe thrombocytopenia. Initial medical treatment of patients with platelet counts below 50,000/mm^3 and symptoms such as mucous membrane bleeding, high-risk conditions (e.g., active lifestyle, hypertension, peptic ulcer disease), or platelet counts below 20,000 to 30,000/mm^3, even without symptoms, is glucocorticoid administration (typically, prednisone, 1 mg/kg body weight/day). Clinical response with increases in platelet levels to higher than 50,000/mm^3 is seen in up to two thirds of patients within 1 to 3 weeks of initiating treatment. Of patients treated with steroids, 25% will experience a complete response. Patients with platelet counts higher than 20,000/mm^3 who remain symptom free or who experience minor purpura as their only symptom do not require hospitalization. Hospitalization may be required for patients whose platelets counts remain below 20,000/mm^3 with significant mucous membrane bleeding and is required for those who have life-threatening hemorrhage. Platelet transfusion is indicated only for those who experience severe hemorrhage. Intravenous immune globulin is important for the treatment of acute bleeding, in pregnancy, or for patients being prepared for operation, including splenectomy. The usual dose is 1 g/kg body weight/day for 2 days. This dose usually increases the platelet count within 3 days; it also increases the efficacy of platelet transfusions.

Should initial therapy for ITP fail, medical options for refractory ITP include oral prednisone, oral dexamethasone (40 mg/day for 4 days), rituximab (375 mg/m^2/wk intravenously for 4 weeks), and thrombopoietin receptor antagonists (eltrombopag, romiplostim). Successful response for months is observed in 28% to 44% of patients using rituximab; more transient responses are observed from thrombopoietin receptor antagonists.[10]

Before the establishment of glucocorticoids for treatment of ITP in 1950, splenectomy was the treatment of choice.[9] For those two thirds of patients in whom glucocorticoids result in the normalization of platelet counts, no further treatment is necessary. For patients with severe thrombocytopenia with counts below 10,000/mm^3 for 6 weeks or longer, for those with thrombocytopenia refractory to glucocorticoid treatment, and for those who require toxic doses of steroid to achieve remission, the treatment of choice is to proceed to splenectomy. Splenectomy is also the treatment of choice for patients with incomplete response to glucocorticoid treatment and for pregnant women in the second trimester of pregnancy who have also failed to respond to steroid treatment or intravenous immune globulin therapy with platelet counts below 10,000/mm^3 without symptoms or below 30,000/mm^3 with bleeding problems. It is not necessary to proceed to splenectomy for patients who have platelet counts higher than 50,000/mm^3, who have had ITP for longer than 6 months, who are not experiencing bleeding symptoms, and who are not engaged in high-risk activities. A review of short-term and long-term failure of laparoscopic splenectomy has reported an overall approximate failure rate of 28% at 5 years after splenectomy.[11]

A systematic review of 436 published articles from 1966 to 2004 has reported that 72% of patients with ITP had a complete response to splenectomy. Relapse occurred in a median of 15% of patients (range, 1% to 51%), with a median follow-up of 33 months.[12]

In addition to relapse rates, predictors of successful splenectomy were examined. Of the variables in the multivariate model, age at the time of splenectomy was an independent variable that was most correlated with response.[12] Younger patients had improved responses. On preoperative indium In 111–labeled platelet scintigraphy, patients with platelets sequestered predominantly within the spleen had a significantly higher response rate than those noted to have hepatic sequestration.[13]

Most patients will exhibit improved platelet counts within 10 days postoperatively, and durable platelet responses are associated with patients who have platelet counts of 150,000/mm^3 by postoperative day 3 or more than 500,000/mm^3 by postoperative day 10. Even with splenectomy, however, some patients may relapse (≈12%; range, 4% to 25%).[14] A review of 1223 ITP patients has estimated the long-term failure rate of laparoscopic splenectomy at approximately 8% and approximately 44/1000 patient-years of follow-up.[11] Another study has estimated the complete response of ITP patients after splenectomy to be 66%.[12]

Although a thorough search for accessory spleens is completed during the initial surgery, evaluation for a missed accessory spleen must be undertaken in patients who experience a relapse. In their evaluation of 394 patients treated with laparoscopic splenectomy, Katkhouda and colleagues[14] noted 15% of patients with accessory spleens. In those with accessory spleens, examination of a peripheral blood smear will lack the characteristic red blood cell morphology resulting from excision of the spleen. Radionuclide imaging may also be helpful in locating the presence and location of any accessory splenic tissue. Patients with chronic ITP in whom an accessory spleen is identified should have this removed, as long as the patient can withstand the surgical risk.

Other treatment options for these patients include observation of stable nonbleeding patients with platelet counts higher than 30,000/mm^3, long-term glucocorticoid therapy, and treatment with azathioprine or cyclophosphamide. Recent evidence regarding thrombopoietin receptor agonists may offer a novel medical therapy for patients with no response to steroids, intravenous immune globulin therapy, or splenectomy.[15]

Other conditions linked to thrombocytopenia include thrombotic thrombocytopenic purpura, chronic disseminated intravascular coagulation, congenital thrombocytopenia, myelodysplasia, autoimmune disorders (e.g., systemic lupus erythematosus), and lymphoproliferative disorders (e.g., chronic lymphocytic leukemia, non-Hodgkin lymphoma).

Approximately 10% to 20% of otherwise asymptomatic patients with HIV infection will develop ITP. Splenectomy is a safe treatment option for this cohort of patients and may actually delay HIV disease progression.[16,17]

Hereditary Spherocytosis

Hereditary spherocytosis is an autosomal dominant disease affecting the production of spectrin, a red blood cell cytoskeletal protein. Loss of this protein causes red blood cells to lack their characteristic biconcave shape. This affects the deformability of red blood cells because lack of this protein results in rigid erythrocytes that are small and sphere shaped. Also, these cells have increased osmotic fragility and are more susceptible to trapping and destruction by the spleen. The resulting clinical features are anemia, occasionally with jaundice, and splenomegaly. Diagnosis is made by examination of a peripheral blood smear, increased reticulocyte count, increased osmotic fragility, and negative Coombs test result.

The resultant anemia can be successfully treated with splenectomy, but normalization of the erythrocyte morphology does not occur. Splenectomy should be delayed until the age of 5 years to preserve immunologic function of the spleen and to reduce the risk of OPSI. Just as with other hemolytic anemias, the presence of pigmented gallstones is common. The preoperative workup should include ultrasound evaluation; if gallstones are present, cholecystectomy may be performed at the same time as splenectomy.

Hereditary elliptocytosis, hereditary pyropoikilocytosis, hereditary xerocytosis, and hereditary hydrocytosis also result in anemia secondary to red blood cell membrane abnormalities. Splenectomy is indicated in cases of severe anemia with these conditions, except hereditary xerocytosis, which results in only mild anemia of limited clinical significance.

Hemolytic Anemia Caused by Erythrocyte Enzyme Deficiency

Pyruvate kinase deficiency and glucose-6-phosphate dehydrogenase (G6PD) deficiency are the predominant hereditary conditions associated with hemolytic anemia. Pyruvate kinase deficiency is an autosomal recessive disease that results in decreased red blood cell deformability and the formation of echinocytes, a type of spiculated red blood cell. This morphologic variant increases the likelihood that the cell will be trapped and destroyed by the spleen, which results in splenomegaly, hemolytic anemia, and associated transfusion requirements, which can be mitigated with splenectomy. Again, for reasons discussed earlier, splenectomy is delayed until 5 years of age.

In G6PD deficiency, however, splenectomy is rarely indicated. This X-linked condition is typically seen in people of African, Middle Eastern, or Mediterranean ancestry. Hemolytic anemia in these patients most often occurs after infection or exposure to certain foods, medications, or chemicals. Primary treatment, therefore, is avoidance of exacerbation of the condition.

Hemoglobinopathies

In addition to defects of cellular membranes or enzymes, hereditary anemias may also result from defects in hemoglobin molecules. Sickle cell disease and thalassemia are two disorders in which the hemoglobin molecules exhibit qualitative or quantitative defects. These lead to abnormally shaped erythrocytes, which may lead to splenic sequestration and subsequent destruction.

Sickle cell anemia results from a single amino acid substitution (valine for glutamic acid) in the sixth position of the β chain of hemoglobin A, which causes those hemoglobin chains, under reduced oxygen conditions, to become rigid and unable to deform within the microvasculature. This rigidity causes the red blood cells to assume the elongated crescent or sickle shape. Sickle cell disease results from homozygous inheritance of the defective hemoglobin (hemoglobin S), although sickling can also be seen when hemoglobin S is inherited along with other hemoglobin variants, such as hemoglobin C or sickle cell β-thalassemia. In African Americans, 8% are heterozygous for hemoglobin S (sickle cell trait), and approximately 0.5% are homozygous for hemoglobin S. During conditions of low oxygen tension, these hemoglobin S molecules crystallize, distorting the cell into a crescent shape. These misshapen cells are unable to pass through the microvasculature, which results in capillary occlusion, thrombosis, and ultimately microinfarction. This cascade of events frequently occurs in the spleen. These episodes of vaso-occlusion and progressive infarction result in autosplenectomy. The spleen, which is usually hypertrophied early in life, typically atrophies by adulthood, although splenomegaly may occasionally persist.

Other causes of hemolytic anemia are the thalassemias. These are inherited as autosomal dominant traits and result from a defect in hemoglobin synthesis that causes variable degrees of hemolytic anemia. Splenomegaly, hypersplenism, and splenic infarction, common in sickle cell disease, are also seen commonly in the thalassemias.

Hypersplenism and acute splenic sequestration are life-threatening disorders in children with thalassemia and sickle cell disease. In these conditions, there may be rapid splenic enlargement, which results in severe pain and may require multiple blood transfusions. Patients with acute splenic sequestration crisis present with severe anemia, splenomegaly, and an acute bone marrow response, with erythrocytosis. There may be a concurrent decrease in hemoglobin levels, abdominal pain, and circulatory collapse. Resuscitation with hydration and transfusion may be followed by splenectomy in these patients. Hypersplenism related to sickle cell disease is characterized by anemia, leukopenia, and thrombocytopenia requiring transfusions; transfusions may be reduced by performing splenectomy. Symptomatic massive splenomegaly that interferes with daily activities may also be improved by splenectomy. Finally, in children with sickle cell disease who exhibit growth delay or even weight loss because of increased metabolic rate and whole body total protein turnover, splenectomy may relieve these symptoms.

Splenic abscesses may also be seen in patients with sickle cell anemia. These patients present with fever, abdominal pain, and a tender enlarged spleen. Most patients with splenic abscesses will have a leukocytosis as well as thrombocytosis and Howell-Jolly bodies, indicating a functional asplenia. *Salmonella* and *Enterobacter* spp. and other enteric organisms are commonly seen in those with a splenic abscess. These patients require resuscitation with hydration and transfusion and may require urgent splenectomy after stabilization.

Malignant Disease

Lymphomas

Hodgkin disease. Hodgkin disease is a malignant lymphoma that usually affects young adults in their 20s and 30s. Rarely, patients present with constitutional symptoms such as night sweats, weight loss, and pruritus; but more typically, asymptomatic lymphadenopathy usually involves the cervical nodes. Hodgkin disease is characterized histologically as lymphocyte predominant, nodular sclerosing, mixed cellularity, or lymphocyte depleted. The disease is pathologically staged according to the Ann Arbor classification. Stage I is disease in a single lymphatic site. Stage II is disease in two or more lymphatic sites on the same side of the diaphragm. Stage III indicates disease on both sides of the diaphragm and includes splenic involvement. Stage IV disease is disease in which there is dissemination into extralymphatic sites, such as liver, lung, or bone marrow. The addition of a subscript E to stage I, II, or III indicates single or contiguous extralymphatic spread; subscript S indicates splenic involvement. Patients who exhibit constitutional symptoms are denoted with a B (presence), and those without symptoms are denoted with an A (absence).

Historically, patients with Hodgkin disease underwent a staging laparotomy that included splenectomy to provide pathologic staging information required to determine appropriate therapy. This was particularly common in stage I and stage II disease to rule out splenic or subdiaphragmatic involvement. In addition to splenectomy, the procedure involves splenic hilar lymphadenectomy, liver biopsy, retroperitoneal node biopsy, and biopsy of a hepatoduodenal node and oophoropexy in premenopausal women. Staging methods have evolved to include imaging techniques—computed tomography (CT), ^{18}F-fluorodeoxyglucose positron emission tomography, and lymphangiography—thus making invasive staging methods almost obsolete. Staging laparotomy remains appropriate for select patients, such as those with early clinical disease stages (IA or IIA) in whom abdominal staging will significantly alter therapeutic management. Early-stage Hodgkin disease is often cured with radiation therapy alone. Laparotomy is no longer indicated for patients likely to relapse, those with evidence of intra-abdominal involvement on imaging, and those with B symptoms. These patients should receive systemic chemotherapy.

Non-Hodgkin lymphomas. Splenomegaly or hypersplenism is a common occurrence during the course of non-Hodgkin lymphoma (NHL). Splenectomy is indicated for NHL patients with massive splenomegaly leading to abdominal pain, early satiety, and fullness. It may also be indicated for patients who develop anemia, neutropenia, and thrombocytopenia associated with hypersplenism.

Splenectomy may also be instrumental in the diagnosis and staging of patients with isolated splenic disease. The most common primary splenic neoplasm is NHL. Less than 1% of patients present with splenomegaly without lymphadenopathy; however, 50% to 80% of patients with NHL have involvement of the spleen.[18] Patients with clinically isolated splenic disease are said to have malignant lymphoma with splenic involvement. Most patients have low-grade NHL, with frequent involvement of the splenic hilar lymph nodes, extrahilar nodes, bone marrow, or liver. Approximately 75% of these patients have clinically apparent hypersplenism. In patients with spleen-predominant features, survival is significantly improved after splenectomy compared with similar patients who did not undergo splenectomy.

Leukemia

Hairy cell leukemia. Hairy cell leukemia, a rare disease that accounts for approximately 2% of adult leukemias, is characterized by splenomegaly, pancytopenia, and neoplastic mononuclear cells in the peripheral blood and bone marrow. The cells that give the disease its name are B lymphocytes that have a ruffling of the cell membrane. This ruffling causes the cells to appear to have cytoplasmic projections under the light microscope. This disease affects older men, who present with palpable splenomegaly. Approximately 10% of patients require no treatment because of the indolent course of the disease. Treatment for cytopenias or splenomegaly typically begins with purine analogue chemotherapy.[19,20] For more refractory cancers, a second-line immunotherapy may be instituted. In others, however, the extent of splenomegaly or symptoms from hypersplenism, symptomatic anemia, infections from neutropenia, or hemorrhage from thrombocytopenia can lead to splenectomy. Most patients show improvement after the procedure, with a response lasting approximately 10 years after splenectomy, and some patients (≈40% to 60%) show normalization of blood counts after splenectomy.[21] Patients with diffusely involved bone marrow without massive splenomegaly are less responsive to splenectomy. Patients with hairy cell leukemia are also at a twofold to threefold risk for development of other malignant neoplasms after their diagnosis of hairy cell leukemia. Most of these second malignant neoplasms are solid tumors, such as skin cancers, lung cancer, prostate cancer, and gastrointestinal adenocarcinomas. Hairy cell leukemia behaves like a chronic leukemia; many patients can achieve a clinical remission, with a normal or near-normal life span.

Chronic lymphocytic leukemia. Chronic lymphocytic leukemia (CLL) is a clinically heterogeneous disease of B lymphocytes characterized by the progressive accumulation of relatively mature but functionally incompetent lymphocytes. CLL is seen with a slight predominance in men, mainly after the age of 50 years. CLL is staged according to the Rai system and correlates fairly well with survival. Low-risk CLL (formerly stage 0) involves bone marrow and blood lymphocytosis only; intermediate-risk CLL (formerly stages I and II) involves lymphocytosis and lymphadenopathy in any site or splenomegaly, hepatomegaly, or hepatosplenomegaly; and high-risk CLL (formerly stages III and IV) involves lymphocytosis and anemia or thrombocytopenia. The Rai system helps clinicians determine when therapy should be started. New molecular tests, such as that for ZAP-70, zeta chain–associated protein 70 (an intracellular protein rarely found in normal B cells), are increasingly helpful for determining prognosis.[22] Medical treatment, consisting of nucleoside analogues or combination therapy, is indicated for symptomatic patients or those exhibiting evidence of rapid disease progression. Monoclonal antibodies are also used in the treatment of CLL.

Bone marrow transplantation currently offers the only known cure for CLL. Splenectomy is indicated for patients with refractory splenomegaly and pancytopenia, which results in improvements in blood counts in 60% to 70% of patients.[23]

Chronic myelogenous leukemia. Chronic myelogenous leukemia (CML) is a myeloproliferative disorder that develops as a result of a neoplastic transformation of myeloid elements. CML is characterized by the progressive replacement of normal diploid elements of the bone marrow with mature-appearing neoplastic myeloid cells. Although CML can be asymptomatic at presentation, patients commonly present with fever, fatigue, malaise, effects of pancytopenia (infections, anemia, easy bruising), and occasionally splenomegaly. A chromosomal marker, the Philadelphia chromosome, is highly associated with CML and is caused by the fusion of fragments of chromosomes 9 and 22. This fusion results in expression of the BCR-ABL gene product, a tyrosine kinase, which then accelerates cell division and inhibits DNA repair.

CML may occur in patients from childhood to old age. It usually is manifested with an asymptomatic chronic phase but may progress to an accelerated phase associated with fever, night sweats, and progressive splenomegaly. The accelerated phase may be asymptomatic and may be detectable only by changes in peripheral blood or bone marrow. The accelerated phase may then progress to the blastic phase. This phase is also characterized by fever, night sweats, and splenomegaly but is also associated with anemia, infections, and bleeding.

The BCR-ABL gene product is the target for therapy with tyrosine kinase inhibitors and other chemotherapeutic modalities. Bone marrow transplantation is an option, but prognosis has improved dramatically with the advent of recent therapies, making transplantation less common. Studies evaluating the efficacy of newer therapies and combination therapies are ongoing. Symptomatic splenomegaly and hypersplenism in CML can be effectively treated with splenectomy, but there does not appear to be a survival benefit when it is performed during the early chronic phase.[24] Surgery is therefore reserved for patients with significant symptoms.

Nonhematologic Tumors of the Spleen

The spleen can also be the site of metastatic disease, seen in up to 7% of autopsies of cancer patients. The solid tumors that most frequently spread to the spleen are carcinomas of the breast and lung and melanoma. Any primary malignant neoplasm, however, can metastasize to the spleen.[25] Metastases are often asymptomatic but may be associated with splenomegaly and even splenic rupture; thus, splenectomy may provide palliation for carefully chosen patients with symptomatic splenic metastases.

Primary tumors of the spleen are commonly vascular neoplasms and include benign and malignant variants. Hemangiomas are frequent findings in spleens removed for other reasons. Angiosarcomas (or hemangiosarcomas) of the spleen usually occur spontaneously but have been linked to environmental exposures, such as to thorium dioxide and monomeric vinyl chloride. Patients with angiosarcomas may present with splenomegaly, hemolytic anemia, ascites, pleural effusions, or even spontaneous splenic rupture. These tumors are aggressive and have a poor prognosis. Lymphangiomas, by contrast, are endothelium-lined cysts that come to attention because of splenomegaly secondary to cyst enlargement. These are usually benign tumors; however, lymphangiosarcoma has been found within lymphangiomas. Splenectomy is appropriate for the diagnosis, treatment, and palliation of these conditions.

Miscellaneous Benign Conditions

Splenic Cysts

Splenic cysts have been seen with increasing frequency since the advent of CT and ultrasound scanning. They are classified as true cysts, which can be parasitic or nonparasitic, or as pseudocysts. Tumors of the spleen may also appear to be cystic; these include lymphangiomas and cavernous hemangiomas (see earlier).[26] Primary true cysts of the spleen account for approximately 10% of all nonparasitic splenic cysts, whereas most nonparasitic cysts are pseudocysts secondary to trauma. True cysts are lined with a squamous epithelium, and many are considered congenital. These epithelial cells are often positive for carbohydrate antigen 19-9 and carcinoembryonic antigen by immunohistochemistry. Patients with splenic epidermoid cysts may have elevated serum levels of one or both of these tumor markers. These cysts, however, are benign and apparently do not have malignant potential beyond that of the surrounding native tissue.

True splenic cysts are often asymptomatic and discovered incidentally. Patients may complain of abdominal fullness, early satiety, pleuritic chest pain, shortness of breath, and left shoulder or back pain. They may also experience renal symptoms from compression of the left kidney. On physical examination, an abdominal mass may be palpable. Rarely, splenic cysts are manifested with acute symptoms related to rupture, hemorrhage, or infection. Diagnosis is best made by CT, and operative intervention is indicated for those with symptomatic or large cysts. Total or partial splenectomy may provide appropriate treatment. Partial splenectomy has the advantage of preserving splenic function; 25% of the spleen appears to be sufficient to protect against pneumococcal pneumonia. Open and laparoscopic procedures allow total or partial splenectomy, cyst wall resection, or partial decapsulation.[26,27]

Most true splenic cysts are parasitic cysts and occur in areas of endemic hydatid disease (*Echinococcus* spp.). Radiographic imaging reveals cyst wall calcifications or daughter cysts, and although hydatid disease is uncommon in North America, this diagnosis must be excluded before invasive procedures are undertaken that might result in spillage of the cyst contents. Rupture of the cyst and expulsion of contents into the abdomen may precipitate anaphylactic shock and can also lead to intraperitoneal dissemination of the infection. Serologic testing is helpful for verifying the presence of these parasites. Splenectomy is the treatment of choice. As with hydatid cysts of the liver, the cysts may be sterilized by injection of a 3% sodium chloride solution, alcohol, or 0.5% silver nitrate. Even so, great care should be taken to avoid intraoperative rupture of the cyst.

Pseudocysts represent the remaining 70% to 80% of nonparasitic splenic cysts. A history of prior trauma can typically be elicited. Pseudocysts of the spleen are not lined with epithelium. Radiologic imaging usually reveals a smooth, unilocular, thick-walled lesion, sometimes with focal calcifications. Asymptomatic, small (<4 cm) pseudocysts do not require treatment and may involute with time. Symptomatic pseudocysts are manifested in a fashion similar to true splenic cysts; these are treated surgically with total or partial splenectomy, again remembering that partial splenectomy preserves splenic function. Percutaneous drainage has also been reported for splenic pseudocysts,[28] although, in a case series, recurrence was common and subsequent complications were deemed too high.[29]

Splenic Abscess

Splenic abscess is an unusual but potentially life-threatening illness, with a 0.7% incidence in autopsy series.[30] The mortality rate for splenic abscess ranges from 15% to 20% in previously healthy patients with single unilocular lesions to 80% for multiple abscesses in immunocompromised patients. Illnesses and other factors that predispose to splenic abscess include malignant neoplasms, polycythemia vera, endocarditis, prior trauma, hemoglobinopathies, urinary tract infections, intravenous drug use, and AIDS.

Approximately 70% of splenic abscesses result from hematogenous spread of the infective organism from another location, as in endocarditis, osteomyelitis, and intravenous drug use. Spread may also occur in a contiguous fashion from local infections of the colon, kidney, or pancreas. Gram-positive cocci (commonly *Staphylococcus, Streptococcus,* or *Enterococcus* spp.) and gram-negative enteric organisms are typically involved. *Mycobacterium tuberculosis, Mycobacterium avium,* and *Actinomyces* spp. have also been found. Fungal abscesses (e.g., *Candida* spp.) also occur, typically in immunosuppressed patients.

Splenic abscesses are manifested with nonspecific symptoms—vague abdominal pain, fever, peritonitis, and pleuritic chest pain. Splenomegaly is not typical. CT is the preferred method for diagnosis; however, the diagnosis can also be made with ultrasound.

Treatment of splenic abscesses depends on whether the abscess is unilocular or multilocular. In one third of adult patients, the abscess is multilocular. In one third of children, the abscess is unilocular. Unilocular abscesses are often amenable to percutaneous drainage, along with antibiotics,[31] with success rates reported at 75% to 90% for unilocular lesions. Multilocular lesions, however, are usually treated with splenectomy, drainage of the left upper quadrant, and antibiotics.[32] Laparoscopic splenectomy for abscess has been reported.[33]

Wandering Spleen

Wandering spleen is a rare finding seen in children and in women between the ages of 20 and 40 years. One of two causes is suspected. The first is theorized to result from a failure to form normal splenic peritoneal attachments that suspend the organ securely within its usual anatomic position. Failure to form these attachments is thought to arise from lack of fusion of the dorsal mesogastrium to the posterior abdominal wall during embryogenesis. The second theory surmises that in multiparous women, hormonal changes and abdominal laxity lead to an acquired defect in splenic attachments. In either case, without these attachments, the splenic pedicle is unusually long and prone to torsion.

Intermittent abdominal pain, splenomegaly resulting from venous congestion, and severe persistent pain are suggestive of wandering spleen and tension or intermittent torsion of the splenic pedicle. A mobile mass may be palpable on physical examination. CT of the abdomen with intravenous administration of contrast material provides confirmation of the diagnosis, with the spleen located outside its usual position. A noncontrasted spleen or whorled appearance of the vascular pedicle provides additional evidence for the condition and may be helpful in choosing splenopexy or splenectomy.[34]

Other Considerations

Splenic Trauma

See Chapter 16.

Elective Laparoscopic Splenectomy

Laparoscopic splenectomy is now the preferred method for resecting the spleen. This technique was first described in 1991,[35] and many studies have supported its use in terms of outcomes and patient safety.[14] Disadvantages of the laparoscopic technique are longer operating times and difficulty in removing large organs; however, reduced hospital stay and more rapid postoperative recovery alleviate these limitations. Complications are typically linked to the patient's comorbidities.

Laparoscopic splenectomy has been reported for most splenic diseases and is the preferred method for most situations, barring trauma or cases of massive splenomegaly. In deciding whether to pursue laparoscopic methods for splenectomy, certain considerations should be taken into account, such as operative indication (e.g., benign or malignant disease), splenic size, and any potential contraindications to laparoscopy. Preoperative planning is aided by CT imaging especially regarding splenomegaly. Melman and Matthews[36] have noted that spleens measuring more than 22 cm in craniocaudal dimension or more than 19 cm in width and with an estimated weight of more than 1600 g will require hand-assisted laparoscopic procedures, if not open splenectomy. Laparoscopic splenectomy can be completed in approximately 90% of patients. The reported conversion to open splenectomy is between 0% and 20%. Most conversions are caused by intraoperative bleeding, lack of surgical experience, prohibitive adhesions,[37] massive splenomegaly,[28] and obesity.[2,17] As with other laparoscopic procedures, there is a learning curve, and with increasing experience, conversion to open splenectomy declines.[4,38] Recently published guidelines regarding laparoscopic splenectomy reiterate the importance of indications for the procedure, preoperative imaging for determining size and volume and presence of accessory splenic tissue, choices regarding hand-assisted techniques (early in cases of splenomegaly), contraindications (e.g., portal hypertension, major medical comorbidities), and splenic vaccinations.[39] Vaccinations for *N. meningitidis, S. pneumoniae,* and *H. influenzae* should be given 15 days before elective splenectomy or within 30 days of an emergent splenectomy to reduce the risk of OPSI (see earlier).

Postoperative recovery from laparoscopic splenectomy is rapid, as seen with laparoscopic cholecystectomy. The length of stay ranges from 1.8 to 6 days; shorter hospital stays are a major advantage of laparoscopic procedures.[18,20] A prospective randomized controlled trial comparing open and laparoscopic approaches was performed in patients with β-thalassemia major. This study reported a shorter median hospital stay in the laparoscopic patients but longer operative times and an increase in blood transfusions.[40] It is not known whether these results can be generalized to all patients with splenic disease. Several case series have also compared the laparoscopic with the open approach and consistently favored the laparoscopic approach, particularly in regard to earlier resumption of diet, decreased postoperative pain, and shorter hospital stay.[13]

Treatment outcomes are the primary concern in comparing these approaches. In published results to date, laparoscopic outcomes are equivalent to those of open splenectomy. In a review of laparoscopic splenectomy for malignant disease, Burch and associates[41] have reported that this population of patients benefits from laparoscopic splenectomy, similar to those with benign disease. Katkhouda and coworkers[14] have reported that in the treatment of ITP, laparoscopic and open splenectomy results appear to be similar.

As noted, laparoscopic surgery needs careful consideration for special populations. Portal hypertension and its risk of operative hemorrhage prohibit laparoscopic splenectomy. Laparoscopic splenectomy during pregnancy for refractory thrombocytopenia carries an associated fetal mortality rate of 31%. There is scant literature regarding this rare patient population, although laparoscopic splenectomy can be performed during pregnancy.[39,42]

The laparoscopic technique may be performed with the patient in the supine or lateral position or a combination. After induction of general anesthesia and endotracheal intubation, a nasogastric tube and urinary catheter are inserted. Standard antithrombotic precautions are taken. Positioning of the patient is crucial for the completion of a laparoscopic splenectomy. For all three positions, the patient is placed so that the kidney rest can be raised to maximize the space between the iliac crest and costal margin. The patient is positioned so that the table may be flexed to widen the working space. Finally, the patient is tilted in a reverse Trendelenburg position to facilitate retraction of the viscera caudally away from the left upper quadrant.

In the supine position, the surgeon stands to the patient's left, and the first assistant and camera assistant stand to the patient's right.[37] It may be easier for a right-handed surgeon to work from a position between the patient's legs, with the patient in a modified lithotomy position. The scrub nurse stands to the patient's left side, near the foot of the table. Alternatively, the patient may be placed in a 60-degree right lateral decubitus position using a beanbag and axillary roll. In this case, the patient's left arm is placed on an arm board or supported by a splint. With this approach, the surgeon and scrub nurse stand to the patient's right and the assistants stand to the patient's left. The spleen will thus be suspended from its diaphragmatic attachments; gravity retracts the stomach, omentum, and colon; and the splenic hilum will be under some degree of tension. For either approach, the video monitors are placed on either side of the table, at or above the level of the patient's shoulders.

Trocar access to the abdomen is gained, and pneumoperitoneum is established to a pressure of 12 to 15 mm Hg. Three to five 2- to 12-mm-diameter ports are used, with the camera port at the umbilicus or offset between the umbilicus and costal margin. The other port sites are positioned as depicted in Figure 56-4.

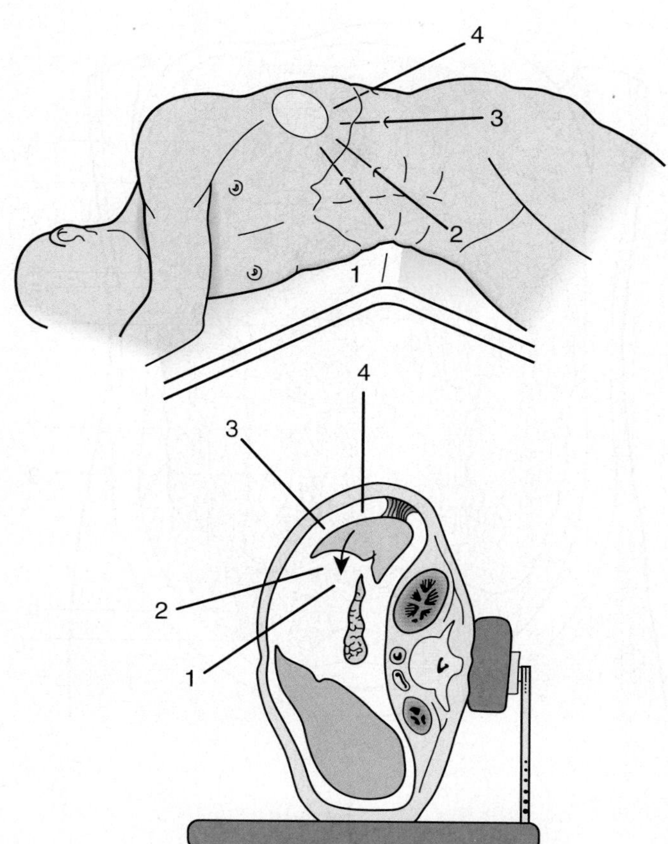

FIGURE 56-4 Right lateral decubitus position of the patient for laparoscopic splenectomy. The table is angulated, giving forced lateral flexion of the patient to open the costophrenic space. Trocars are inserted along the left costal margin more posteriorly. The spleen is suspended by its peritoneal attachments. The *numbered lines* show the position of laparoscopic ports. (From Gigot JF, Lengele B, Gianello P, et al: Present status of laparoscopic splenectomy for hematologic diseases: Certitudes and unresolved issues. *Semin Laparosc Surg* 5:147–167, 1998.)

The operation is begun with a thorough search of the abdominal cavity for the presence of accessory splenic tissue (Fig. 56-5); the stomach is retracted to the right side to facilitate examination of the gastrosplenic ligament. The splenocolic ligament, greater omentum, and phrenosplenic ligament are inspected next. The small and large bowel mesenteries, pelvis, and adnexal tissues are examined. Finally, the gastrosplenic ligament is opened, and the tail of the pancreas is confirmed to be free of splenic tissue.

Our preference has been to use the right lateral decubitus approach, with the operating room table bent 45 degrees from horizontal and the kidney rest elevated. The initial dissection is begun by mobilizing the splenic flexure of the colon. By use of sharp dissection, the splenocolic ligament is divided. The spleen can then be retracted cephalad; care should be taken not to rupture the splenic capsule during retraction. The lateral peritoneal attachments of the spleen are incised next, with use of scissors or ultrasonic shears. A 1-cm cuff of peritoneum is left along the lateral aspect of the spleen, which can then be grasped to facilitate medial retraction. The lesser sac is entered along the medial border

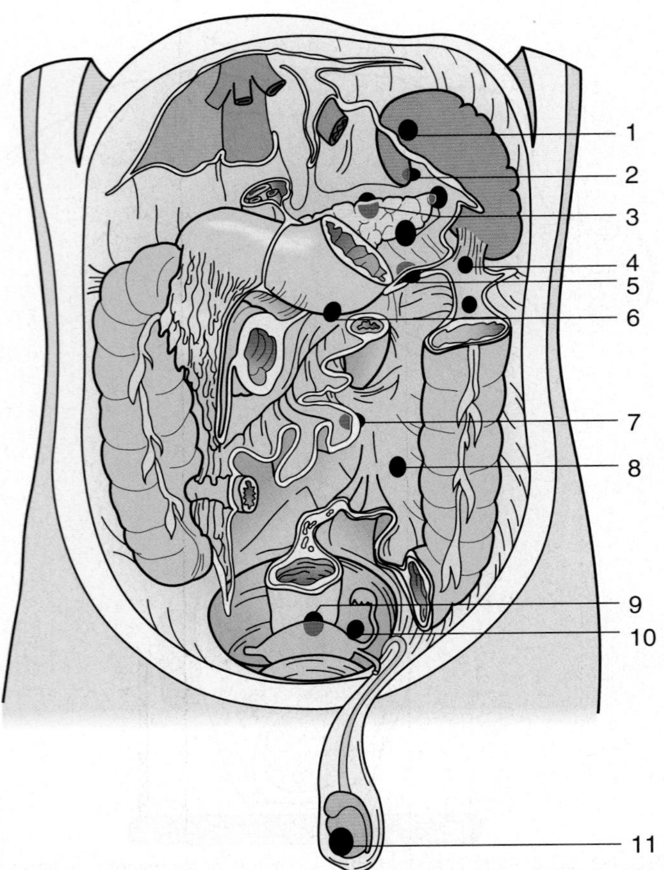

FIGURE 56-5 Usual location of accessory spleens: (1) gastrosplenic ligament, (2) splenic hilum, (3) tail of the pancreas, (4) splenocolic ligament, (5) left transverse mesocolon, (6) greater omentum along the greater curvature of the stomach, (7) mesentery, (8) left mesocolon, (9) left ovary, (10) Douglas pouch, and (11) left testis. (From Gigot JF, Lengele B, Gianello P, et al: Present status of laparoscopic splenectomy for hematologic diseases: Certitudes and unresolved issues. *Semin Laparosc Surg* 5:147–167, 1998.)

of the spleen. Continuing the cephalad retraction, the short gastric vessels and main vascular pedicle can be identified. The tail of the pancreas is also visualized, and care is taken to avoid it as it nears the splenic hilum. The short gastric vessels are divided. A number of options are currently available for this, including ultrasonic dissectors, hemoclips, bipolar devices, LigaSure (Covidien, Boulder, Colo), and endovascular stapling devices. Hemoclips are used minimally around the area of the splenic hilum to prevent interference with future use of a stapling device, which could lead to significant bleeding from improperly ligated hilar vessels.

After the short gastric vessels are divided, the splenic pedicle is carefully dissected from the medial and lateral aspects. After the artery and vein are dissected, the vessels are divided by application of endovascular staplers or suture ligatures. In the more prevalent distributed mode, there are multiple vascular branches entering the spleen close to the hilum, so the dissection is carried out approximately 2 cm from the splenic capsule. Several branches may still be encountered, but these may be individually controlled more easily. A pedicle formed by the artery and vein that enters the hilum is known as the magistral type of arterial anatomy. If this is seen, the pedicle is transected en bloc using a linear vascular stapler. The tail of the pancreas, which is within 1 cm of the splenic hilum in 75% of patients and touches the hilum in 30%, should be well visualized as the stapler is applied to avoid injury.

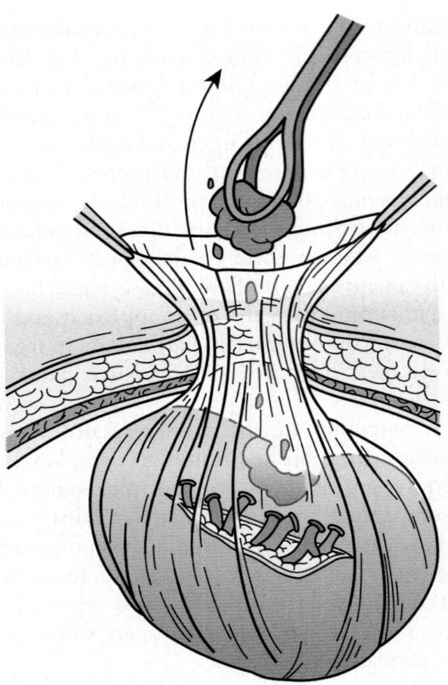

FIGURE 56-6 Extraction of the spleen within a heavy plastic bag, with instrumental morcellation of the organ with forceps. (From Gigot JF, Lengele B, Gianello P, et al: Present status of laparoscopic splenectomy for hematologic diseases: Certitudes and unresolved issues. *Semin Laparosc Surg* 5:147–167, 1998.)

The now-devascularized spleen is suspended only from a small cuff of avascular splenophrenic tissue at the superior pole. This tissue facilitates transfer of the spleen into a retrieval bag. To remove the detached spleen, the puncture-resistant nylon bag is grasped by its drawstring, which can be drawn through a port, usually the epigastric or supraumbilical site. The bag is opened slightly, providing access to the still intra-abdominal spleen. The spleen is then morcellated with ring forceps or finger fracture and removed piecemeal (Fig. 56-6). In the rare cases requiring pathologic examination of an intact spleen, an incision large enough to allow extraction of the spleen must be made. Care must be taken to avoid spillage of any splenic fragments into the abdominal cavity or wound. The laparoscope is then reinserted and the splenic bed assessed for hemostasis. Drains may be placed, if necessary. Pneumoperitoneum is then released, and the fasciae of all trocar ports larger than 5 mm are closed.

Robotic Splenectomy

There have been few reports of splenic disease treated robotically and only one report specifically comparing laparoscopic with robotic splenectomy. In their retrospective report, Bodner and colleagues[43] compared operative times, hospital stay, and cost. They concluded that although the robotic procedure is feasible and safe for the patient, cost and operative times are both higher in the robotic group. In another study, Corcione and associates[44] evaluated the use of a robotic system in common general surgical procedures. Although they noted some benefits (e.g., availability of three-dimensional vision, greater dexterity with instruments), they reported concerns about the ability to control bleeding with only two instruments available; in these cases, they were required to convert to a traditional laparoscopic procedure. Overall, the addition of the robot to a straightforward procedure such as laparoscopic splenectomy is currently deemed unnecessary.

LATE MORBIDITY AFTER SPLENECTOMY

Postsplenectomy thrombocytosis occurs particularly in patients with myeloproliferative disorders (e.g., CML, polycythemia vera, essential thrombocytosis), which can result in thrombosis of the mesenteric, portal, and renal veins and can be life-threatening because it can lead to hemorrhage and thromboembolism. The lifelong risk for deep venous thrombosis and pulmonary embolism has not been established but may be significant. Also, there have been case reports of acute myocardial infarction in postsplenectomy patients with thrombocytosis.

OPSI is the most common fatal late complication of splenectomy. Infection may occur at any time after splenectomy.[2] In one series, most infections occurred more than 2 years after splenectomy and 42% occurred more than 5 years after splenectomy, although the true incidence of OPSI has been difficult to determine because infection in postsplenectomy patients is likely to be underreported.

OPSI typically begins with a prodromal phase characterized by fever, rigors, and chills and other nonspecific symptoms, including sore throat, malaise, myalgias, diarrhea, and vomiting. Pneumonia and meningitis may be present. Many patients have no identifiable focal site of infection and present only with high-grade primary bacteremia. Progression of the illness is rapid, with the development of hypotension, disseminated intravascular coagulation, respiratory distress, coma, and death within hours of presentation. Despite antibiotics and intensive care, the mortality rate is between 50% and 70% for florid OPSI. Survivors also often have a long and complicated hospital course with multiple sequelae, such as peripheral gangrene requiring amputation, deafness from meningitis, mastoid osteomyelitis, bacterial endocarditis, and cardiac valvular destruction.

The most frequently involved organism in OPSI is *S. pneumoniae,* which is estimated to be responsible for between 50% and 90% of cases. Other organisms involved in OPSI include *H. influenzae, N. meningitidis, Streptococcus* and *Salmonella* spp., other pneumococcal organisms, and *Capnocytophaga canimorsus,* implicated in OPSI as a result of dog bites.

In an autopsy series by Pimpl and coworkers,[45] lethal pneumonia was identified twice as often in the postsplenectomy patients as in controls. Lethal sepsis with multiorgan failure was also identified in 6.9% of postsplenectomy patients compared with 1.5% of autopsies on the controls. One intriguing observation is that the risk for OPSI is greater for patients who have received splenectomy for malignant disease or hematologic conditions than for those who underwent splenectomy for trauma. The risk is also greater for young children (<4 years of age). The risk for fatal OPSI is estimated to be 1/300 to 350 patient-years of follow-up for children and 1/800 to 1000 patient-years of follow-up for adults. A review of selected reported splenectomy series of 7872 total cases, including children and adults, has revealed 270 episodes of sepsis (3.5%), with 169 septic fatalities (2.1%).[17] The incidence of nonfatal infection and sepsis is therefore likely to be significantly greater.

PROPHYLACTIC TREATMENT OF SPLENECTOMIZED PATIENTS

Immunization

Currently, the standard of care for postsplenectomy patients includes immunization with polyvalent pneumococcal vaccine (PPV23), *H. influenzae* type b conjugate, and meningococcal polysaccharide vaccine within 2 weeks of splenectomy if the patient did not receive these before surgery.[4] Despite this established standard, the literature reflects a diverse 11% to 75% postsplenectomy immunization rate. This may represent lack of understanding by patient and caregiver regarding the risk for postsplenectomy infection and sepsis.[46]

As noted, most cases of infection are caused by *S. pneumoniae, H. influenzae,* and *N. meningitidis* and thus are potentially preventable if appropriate prophylactic vaccinations are given. There are reports of other, less common organisms as the cause of postsplenectomy infection.[3] Continued education of patients, families, and caregivers must stress the need for prompt medical attention if these patients show signs of infection.

Many cases of delayed OPSI have been in nonimmunized immunocompetent patients, before the current PPV23 that was introduced in 1983, which replaced the 14-valent vaccine licensed in 1977. PPV23 is composed of purified preparations of pneumococcal capsular polysaccharide antigens of 23 types of *S. pneumoniae* (25 mg each) that cause 88% of the bacteremic pneumococcal disease in the United States.

The relationship between antibody titer and protection from invasive disease has not been established. Most healthy adults show a twofold or greater rise in type-specific antibody within 2 to 3 weeks of vaccination. However, it has been clearly documented that after vaccination with PPV23, antibody levels decline after 5 to 10 years and may fall to prevaccination levels. Even with vaccination, the development of a protective level of antibody against pneumococci is only about 50%. Currently available vaccines elicit a T cell–independent response and do not produce a sustained increase in antibody titers. Thus, the ability to define the need for revaccination based on serology continues to represent a clinical challenge.

Routine revaccination of immunocompetent persons is not recommended by the U.S. Centers for Disease Control and Prevention (CDC). Revaccination is, however, recommended for high-risk individuals. Candidates for revaccination with PPV23 include the following:

- Persons who received the 14-valent vaccine who are at highest risk for fatal pneumococcal infection (e.g., asplenic patients)
- Adults at highest risk who received the 23-valent vaccine 6 years prior
- Adults at highest risk who have shown a rapid decline in pneumococcal antibody levels (e.g., patients with nephrotic syndrome, those with renal failure, transplant recipients)
- Children at highest risk (e.g., those with asplenia, nephritic syndrome, sickle cell anemia) who would be 10 years old at revaccination

Only one PPV23 revaccination dose is recommended for these high-risk individuals, and it is administered 5 years after the initial dose. Rutherford and colleagues[47] have examined the efficacy and safety of pneumococcal revaccination after splenectomy for trauma. Of 45 patients offered revaccination 2 years or more after primary vaccination, 24 patients demonstrated a lack of understanding of the postsplenectomy state, confirming the poor understanding of patients of the postsplenectomy risk. After revaccination, 48% of patients demonstrated at least a twofold increase in at least one titer (serotypes 6 and 23 pneumococcus).

The CDC has concluded that despite physician and patient education, pamphlets, and MedicAlert bracelets, the patient's retention regarding the risks of the postsplenectomy state is poor. The CDC recommended that all splenectomy patients, including those with hereditary spherocytosis, be revaccinated and reeducated between 2 and 6 years after splenectomy. Recommendations include determination of pneumococcal antibody titers after immunization of every splenectomized patient because nonresponders to vaccination may be at high risk for OPSI. Subsequent follow-up of antibody titers is recommended at 3 to 5 years to evaluate for possible need for revaccination.

In an effort to improve host immunocompetence, partial splenic salvage or splenic autotransplantation has been considered because this may improve the humoral immune response to PPV23.[48] The difficulty with splenic salvage techniques is the lack of objective functional immune testing in humans. This is also true for patients who have undergone angiographic embolization for cessation of splenic hemorrhage in trauma. No studies are available regarding the risk of these patients for OPSI. Preclinical studies have examined the optimal site and amount of splenic tissue for autotransplantation. The most effective site of splenic autotransplantation was found to be the omental pouch, and approximately 50% of the spleen would be necessary for the prevention of pneumococcal sepsis. Although all efforts need to be made to preserve the spleen in trauma victims, the strategy of splenic autotransplantation seems to have limited applicability in humans.

Currently, it is suggested that educational intervention for patients who have undergone splenectomy is necessary; patients may require a number of instructional sessions. Communication with and educational efforts for primary care providers who assume medical care for asplenic patients are also extremely important because OPSI is preventable if appropriate precautions are taken. CDC immunization guidelines for 2010 have recommended the following vaccines for asplenic patients: tetanus (Td/Tdap); human papillomavirus; measles, mumps, rubella; varicella; zoster; influenza; pneumococcal polysaccharide; hepatitis A; hepatitis B; and meningococcal (Table 56-1).

The 2006 recommendations of the Surgical Infection Society for patients 2 to 64 years of age are *H. influenzae* type b conjugate vaccine, meningococcal vaccine, and 23-valent pneumococcal vaccine. Several sources have reported that the conjugate pneumococcal vaccine is more effective in asplenic patients than the polysaccharide vaccine and should be given immediately postoperatively as well as every 5 years to maintain efficacy. Shatz and associates[4] have evaluated antibody titers to pneumococcal vaccination in traumatic splenectomy patients randomized to receive the vaccine at 14 or 28 days postoperatively. Prior work by this group suggested that a delay in therapy might increase titer production; in the follow-up study, they determined that there was no statistically significant difference in antibody response between the two groups.

Despite lack of high-level evidence and because of the lifelong risk of OPSI, most recommend vaccines (*H. influenzae* type b conjugate vaccine, meningococcal vaccine, 23-valent pneumococcal vaccine) immediately for pneumococcal vaccination and at 14 days postoperatively or at least 2 weeks before elective splenectomy. Depending on the patient's reliability, these vaccinations may be given before hospital discharge for emergent splenectomy. The current recommendations are summarized in Figure 56-7.

TABLE 56-1 Centers for Disease Control and Prevention Vaccine Recommendations for Asplenic Patients

VACCINE	RECOMMENDATION
Tetanus (Td/Tdap)	One dose every 10 years
Human papillomavirus	Three doses for women through age 26 years (0, 2, 6 months)
Measles, mumps, rubella	One or two doses
Varicella	Two doses (0, 4-8 weeks)
Zoster	One dose
Influenza	One dose annually
Pneumococcal polysaccharide	One or two doses
Hepatitis A	Two doses (0, 6-12 months or 0, 6-18 months)
Hepatitis B	Three doses (0, 1-2 months, 4-6 months)
Meningococcal	One dose

Antibiotics

Significant controversy still exists about antibiotic prophylaxis in postsplenectomy patients. The primary goal of this prophylaxis is to prevent OPSI, particularly that secondary to pneumococcal infection, which is reported to be the cause of OPSI in 50% to 90% of patients. However, OPSI secondary to penicillin-sensitive pneumococcal infection has been reported in children and adults receiving penicillin prophylaxis.

Regardless, prophylaxis with penicillin is routinely practiced in children, at least during the first 2 years after splenectomy, and some authors advocate this practice in adults, although evidence for this is scarce. Others recommend lifelong prophylaxis in adults and children. This length of treatment may be unacceptable to patients, and there is evidence that there is no difference in the incidence of sepsis in postsplenectomy sickle cell patients when the antibiotic prophylaxis is ceased after 5 years.[49] Other studies have reported significant differences in the incidence of sepsis, with and without antibiotic prophylaxis. Again, OPSI has been reported in patients taking prophylactic medications, and patients should be made aware that even with daily antibiotics, not all infections may be preventable.

A rational approach may be to provide a supply of oral antibiotics (standby antibiotics) to postsplenectomy adults, with instructions to begin taking the medication at the onset of a febrile illness or rigors if there is no access to immediate medical evaluation. There is evidence that the risk of OPSI is lowest in patients who exhibit the greatest understanding of the infectious risks of asplenia.[5] This highlights the importance of education of the patient, particularly at follow-up visits, to ensure compliance with antibiotic and vaccine prophylaxis.

Whether the patient elects to take antibiotic prophylaxis, and because of the risk of OPSI and the extreme level of associated mortality, any asplenic patient who presents with rigors or fever must be started immediately on aggressive empirical antibiotic coverage, even without culture data.

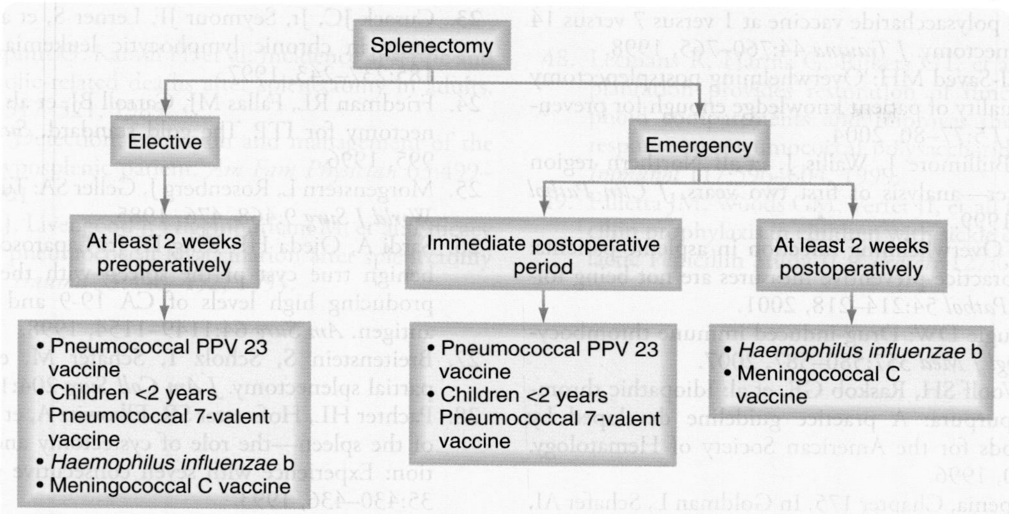

FIGURE 56-7 Splenectomy immunoprophylaxis flow chart. (From Harji DP, Jaunoo SS, Mistry P, Nesargikar PN: Immunoprophylaxis in asplenic patients. *Int J Surg* 7:421–423, 2009.)

SELECTED REFERENCES

Feldman LS: Laparoscopic splenectomy: Standardized approach. *World J Surg* 35:1487–1495, 2011.

This article provides a useful overview of indications and technique for laparoscopic splenectomy. It also provides useful tips on minimally invasive approaches to specific scenarios in splenic disease (e.g., splenomegaly, accessory spleens).

George JN, Woolf SH, Raskob GE, et al: Idiopathic thrombocytopenic purpura: A practice guideline developed by explicit methods for the American Society of Hematology. *Blood* 88:3–40, 1996.

Comprehensive summary and practice guidelines for the treatment of ITP established by the American Society of Hematology; provides a comprehensive review of the current treatment recommendations and outcomes for pediatric and adult patients with ITP.

Gigot JF, Jamar F, Ferrant A, et al: Inadequate detection of accessory spleens and splenosis with laparoscopic splenectomy. A shortcoming of the laparoscopic approach in hematologic diseases. *Surg Endosc* 12:101–106, 1998.

Despite being more than 10 years old, this article provides good technical tips for the surgeon. The article discusses numerous hematologic indications for splenectomy and their surgical outcome.

Habermalz B, Sauerland S, Decker G, et al: Laparoscopic splenectomy: The clinical practice guidelines of the European Association for Endoscopic Surgery (EAES). *Surg Endosc* 22:821–848, 2008.

Publication of an expert panel using a Delphi process to develop practice guidelines for laparoscopic splenectomy; covers indications, preoperative evaluation, management, and operative and postoperative issues.

Katkhouda N, Hurwitz MB, Rivera RT, et al: Laparoscopic splenectomy: Outcome and efficacy in 103 consecutive patients. *Ann Surg* 228:568–578, 1998.

Large series of patients with long-term follow-up demonstrating the safety and efficacy of laparoscopic splenectomy. The discussion section provides an extensive review of previously published series and compares open splenectomy with laparoscopic splenectomy.

Musallam KM, Khalife M, Sfeir PM, et al: Postoperative outcomes after laparoscopic splenectomy compared with open splenectomy. *Ann Surg* 257:1116–1123, 2013.

This study provides one of the few reliable comparative evaluations assessing the differences between open and laparoscopic splenectomy."

Spelman D, Buttery J, Daley A, et al: Guidelines for the prevention of sepsis in asplenic and hyposplenic patients. *Intern Med J* 38:349–356, 2008.

Reviews spectrum of causative organisms and recommended preventive strategies; consensus guidelines developed and discussed.

REFERENCES

1. Michels N: The variational anatomy of the spleen and splenic artery. *Am J Anat* 70:21–72, 1942.
2. Horowitz J, Smith JL, Weber TK, et al: Postoperative complications after splenectomy for hematologic malignancies. *Ann Surg* 223:290–296, 1996.
3. Spelman D, Buttery J, Daley A, et al: Guidelines for the prevention of sepsis in asplenic and hyposplenic patients. *Intern Med J* 38:349–356, 2008.
4. Shatz DV, Schinsky MF, Pais LB, et al: Immune responses of splenectomized trauma patients to the 23-valent

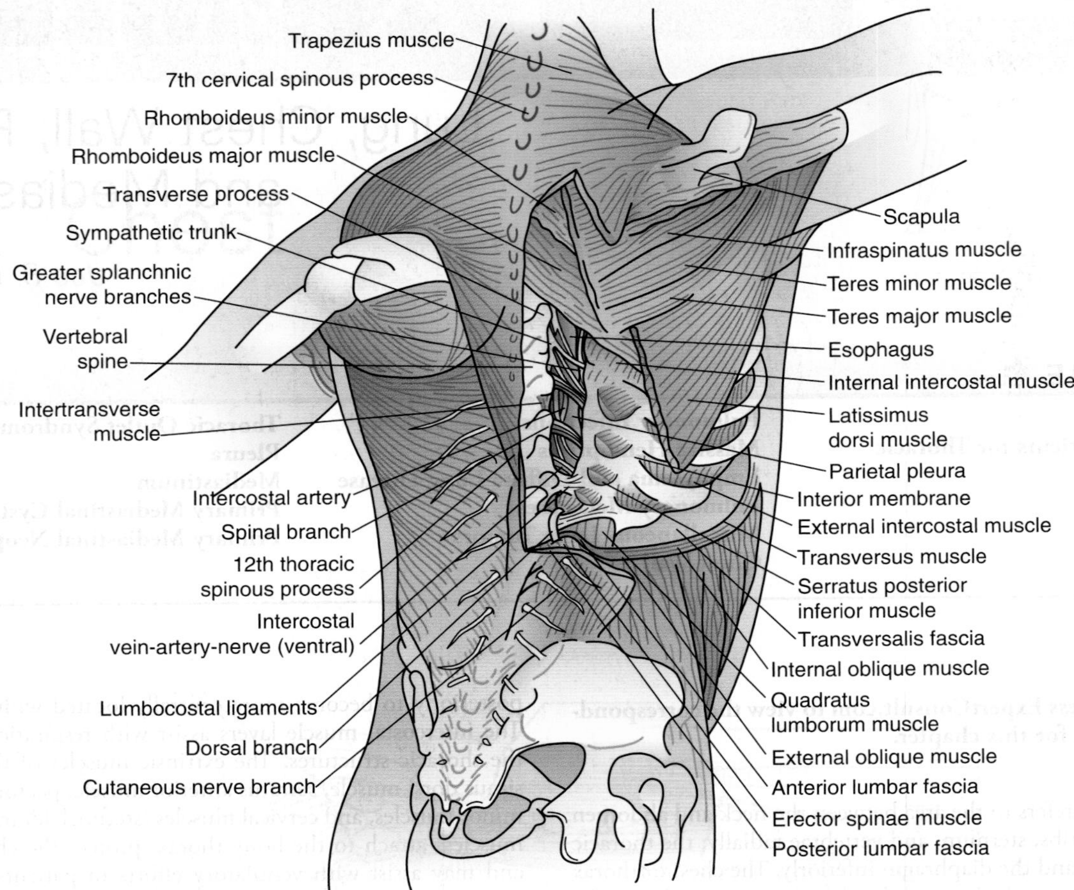

FIGURE 57-1 Musculature of the chest wall. (From Ravitch MM, Steichen FM: *Atlas of general thoracic surgery*, Philadelphia, 1988, Saunders.)

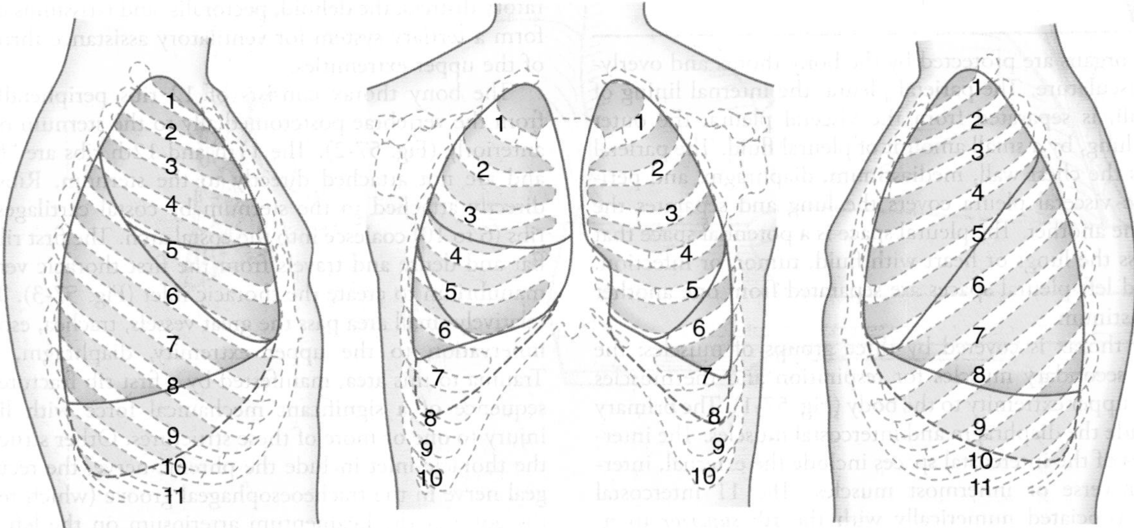

FIGURE 57-2 The relationships of the lobes of the lung to the ribs and the pleural reflections with respiration. The topographic anatomy and the relationship of the fissures of the lobes to specific ribs in inspiration and expiration are important in evaluation of routine posteroanterior and lateral chest films.

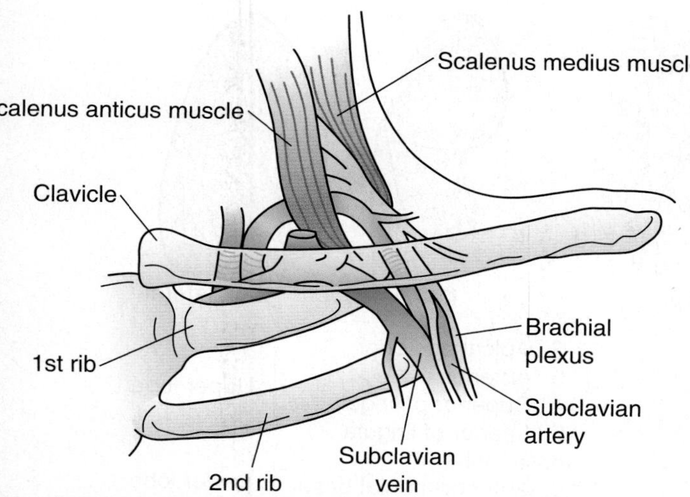

FIGURE 57-3 Relationship of the neurovascular bundle to the scalenus muscles, clavicle, and first rib. (From Urschel HC: Thoracic outlet syndromes. In Baue AE, Geha AS, Hammond GL, et al, editors: *Glenn's thoracic and cardiovascular surgery*, ed 6, Stamford, CT, 1996, Appleton & Lange, p 567.)

downward. Each rib is composed of a head, neck, and shaft. Each head has an upper facet, which articulates with the vertebral body above it, and a lower facet, which articulates with the corresponding thoracic vertebra to that rib, establishing the costovertebral joint. The neck of the rib has a tubercle with an articular facet; this articulates with the transverse process, creating the costotransverse joint and imparting strength to the posterior rib cage.

The sternum is flat, 15 to 20 cm long, and approximately 1.0 to 1.5 cm thick and comprises the manubrium, body, and xiphoid. The manubrium articulates with each clavicle and the first rib. The manubrium joins the body of the sternum at the angle of Louis, which corresponds to the anterior aspect of the junction of the second rib. The angle of Louis is a superficial anatomic landmark for the level of the carina. The anterior cartilaginous attachments of the true ribs to the sternum, along with intercostal muscles and the hemidiaphragms, allow for movement of the ribs with respiration.

The trachea in adults is approximately 12 cm long with 18 to 22 cartilaginous rings. The internal diameter is 2.3 cm laterally and 1.8 cm anteroposteriorly. The larynx ends with the inferior edge of cricoid cartilage. The cricoid is the only complete cartilaginous ring in the trachea. The trachea begins approximately 1.5 cm below the vocal cords and is not rigidly fixed to surrounding tissues. Vertical movement is easily possible. The most rigid point of fixation is where the aortic arch forms a sling over the left mainstem bronchus. The innominate artery crosses over the anterior trachea in a left inferolateral to high right anterolateral direction. The azygos vein arches over the proximal right mainstem bronchus as it travels from posterior to anterior to empty into the superior vena cava. The esophagus is closely applied to the membranous trachea and lies to the left of the midline of the trachea. The recurrent laryngeal nerves run in the tracheoesophageal groove on both the right and the left. The blood supply to the trachea is lateral and segmental from the inferior thyroid, the internal thoracic, the supreme intercostal, and the bronchial arteries. During trachea reconstruction, circumferential dissection greater than 1 to 2 cm may lead to vascular insufficiency with necrosis or anastomotic dehiscence.

Lung development begins at approximately 21 to 28 days' gestation. The true alveolar stage, with air sacs surrounded on all sides by capillaries, occurs from approximately 7 months to term. Alveolar proliferation continues after birth. There are approximately 20 million alveoli at birth, which increase to approximately 300 million by age 10 years, with no more increase after that time. There are 23 generations of bronchi between the trachea and terminal alveoli. Air accounts for 80% of the lung volume, blood accounts for 10%, and solid tissue accounts for approximately 10%. Alveoli make up approximately half of the entire lung volume.

The lungs are broadly divided into five lobes and multiple segments within each lobe (Fig. 57-4). The right lung is composed of three lobes: upper, middle, and lower. Two fissures separate these lobes. The major, or oblique, fissure separates the lower lobe from the upper and middle lobes. The minor or horizontal fissure separates the upper lobe from the middle lobe. The left lung has two lobes—the upper lobe and the lower lobe; the lingula corresponds embryologically to the right middle lobe. A single oblique fissure separates the lobes.

The bronchopulmonary segments are divisions of each lobe that contain anatomically separate arterial, venous, and bronchial supply. There are 10 bronchopulmonary segments on the right and 8 bronchopulmonary segments on the left.

The blood supply of the lung is twofold. Unoxygenated blood circulates from the right ventricle through the pulmonary artery to each lung. After oxygenation in the lung, the blood is returned to the left atrium through the pulmonary veins. Blood supply to the bronchi is from the systemic circulation by bronchial arteries arising from the superior thoracic aorta or the aortic arch, either as discrete branches or in combination with the intercostal arteries.

Lymphatic vessels are present throughout the lung parenchyma and pleura and gradually coalesce toward the hilar areas of the lungs. Generally, lymphatic drainage from the lung affects the ipsilateral lymph nodes; however, flow of lymph from the left lower lobe may drain to the right mediastinal (paratracheal) lymph nodes. Lymphatic drainage within the mediastinum moves cephalad. The pulmonary parenchyma does not contain a nerve supply.

The visceral pleura is separated from the parietal pleura by a small amount of pleural fluid, which allows nearly frictionless movement during respiration. The blood supply of the parietal pleura comes from the systemic arteries and veins, including the posterior intercostal, internal mammary, anterior mediastinal, and superior phrenic arteries and corresponding systemic veins. The blood supply of the visceral pleura is both systemic and pulmonary. The lymphatic drainage of the parietal pleura is into regional lymph nodes, including intercostal, mediastinal, and phrenic nodes. Visceral pleural lymphatics follow the superficial lung lymphatics and drain into the mediastinal lymph nodes. The parietal pleura underlying the ribs has rich nerve endings from the intercostal nerves. Generous local anesthesia is necessary for chest tube insertion. The visceral pleura is innervated by vagal branches and the sympathetic system.

The anatomic boundaries of the mediastinum include the thoracic inlet superiorly, the diaphragm inferiorly, the sternum anteriorly, the vertebral column posteriorly, and medially to the parietal pleura. Thoracic tumors that penetrate through the pleura (by definition) invade the mediastinum. Traditionally, the mediastinum can be divided into anterosuperior, middle, and posterior compartments. No specific anatomic planes define these areas. Fat and lymph nodes are found throughout the mediastinum.

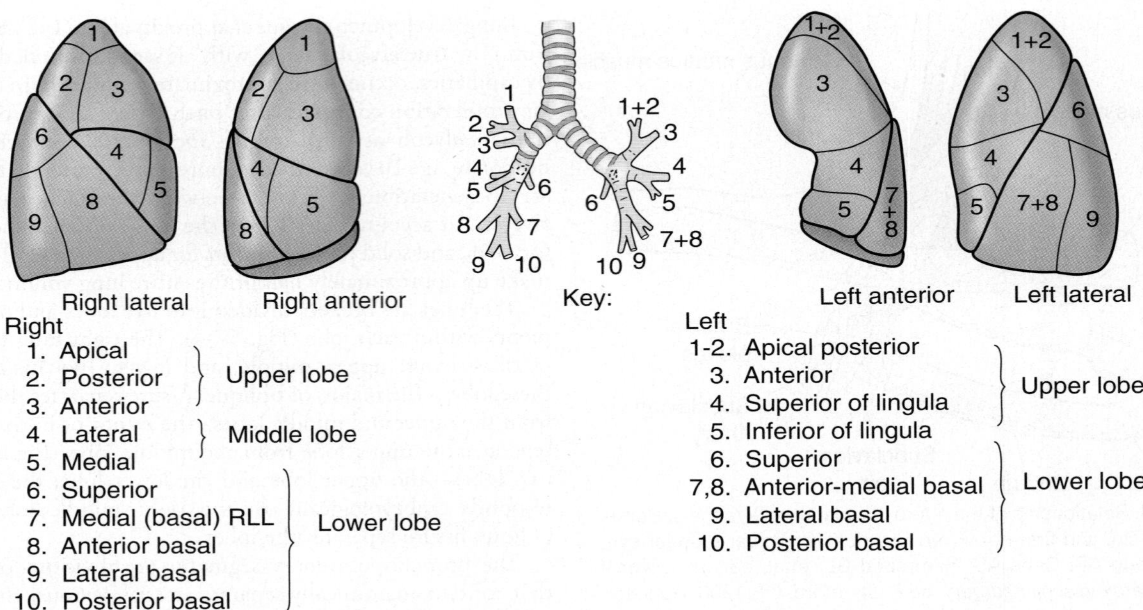

FIGURE 57-4 Segments of the pulmonary lobes. *RLL,* Right lower lobe. (Adapted from Jackson CL, Huber JF: Correlated applied anatomy of the bronchial tree and lungs with a system of nomenclature. *Dis Chest* 9:319, 1943.)

The anterosuperior compartment includes the thymus gland. The right and left lobes of the thymus extend into the cervical areas, and these portions of the thymus must be resected to provide for complete extirpation of the gland.

The middle mediastinum contains the heart; pericardium; great vessels including the descending, transverse, and descending aorta; superior and inferior vena cava; pulmonary artery and veins; trachea and bronchi; and phrenic, vagus, and recurrent laryngeal nerves. The phrenic nerve enters the thorax through the thoracic inlet on the anterior aspect of the anterior scalene muscle.

The vagus nerve enters the thoracic inlet through the carotid sheath. It lies anterior to the subclavian and posterior to the innominate artery on the right. The right recurrent laryngeal nerve loops or "recurs" around the innominate artery to innervate the right vocal cord. The vagus nerve then continues posteriorly in the tracheoesophageal groove to innervate the trachea and continues down to innervate the esophagus. On the left side, the vagus nerve enters the thorax through the thoracic inlet, and as it exits the carotid sheath, it moves along the anterior aspect of the aortic arch. The recurrent laryngeal nerve arises from the vagus nerve and loops around under the ligamentum arteriosum and continues superiorly under the aorta and lies in the tracheoesophageal groove as it innervates the left recurrent laryngeal nerve. The left vagus continues posteriorly within the mediastinum along the esophagus to innervate both the trachea and the esophagus.

The posterior mediastinum contains structures between the heart/pericardium and trachea anteriorly and the vertebral column and paravertebral spaces posteriorly. The posterior mediastinum contains the esophagus, descending aorta, azygos and hemiazygos veins, thoracic duct, sympathetic chain, and lymph nodes. The thoracic duct originates from the cisterna chyli in the abdomen. It enters into the chest through the aortic hiatus in an anterolateral position and travels superiorly just to the right of midline in the chest along the anterolateral surface of the vertebral column. At approximately the level of T5, it crosses over to the left and continues superiorly to empty, posteriorly, into the junction of the left jugular and subclavian veins.

The inferior border of the mediastinum is the diaphragm, which separates the abdominal contents from the thorax. Hernias through the esophageal hiatus (paraesophageal hernias), through the foramen of Bochdalek (posteriorly), or through the foramen of Morgagni (anteriorly) may be initially identified as a mediastinal mass.

Each spinal root exits the neural foramina of the vertebral body and bifurcates to form a branch to the intercostal nerve to innervate the skin and intercostal musculature and a branch to the sympathetic ganglion. Intercostal nerves innervate the skin and musculature of the intercostal muscles. The spinal root divides as it exits the neural foramina. One branch goes to the intercostal nerve, and one lies in the posterior vertebral gutter to form the sympathetic ganglion. The thoracic sympathetic trunk comprises several ganglia that lie along the ribs. The most superior ganglion is the stellate ganglion.

SELECTION OF PATIENTS FOR THORACIC OPERATIONS

The physiologic evaluation of the thoracic surgical patient must be individualized for each patient but generally emphasizes the pulmonary and cardiac function. The assessment of a patient's ability to tolerate lung resection from a cardiopulmonary standpoint is fundamental to patient selection for surgery. Patients with advanced pulmonary disease and severe pulmonary dysfunction may have prohibitive risk, which may exist in greater than one third of patients with otherwise resectable lung disease.[1]

Cigarette smoking is associated with increased postoperative pulmonary complications. If the patient is a smoker, he or she must stop smoking immediately. The physician must clearly communicate this message. Although there are few studies specific to pulmonary resection, there is evidence that smoking abstinence

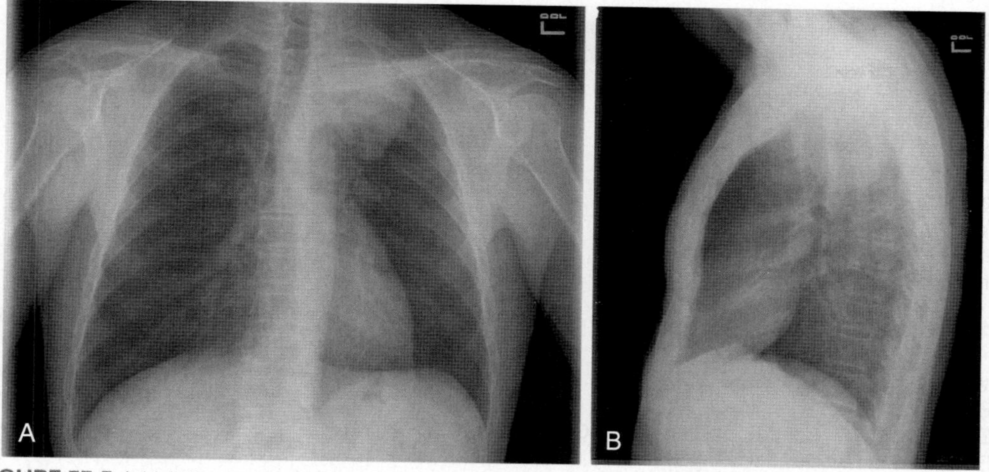

FIGURE 57-5 Initial chest x-ray. This patient is a 67-year-old man with weight loss of 10 pounds in 4 weeks and a 35 pack-year history of cigarette smoking. He quit smoking 10 year ago. He had left shoulder pain for 4 months with no dyspnea, cough, hemoptysis, or other symptoms. Massage and other musculoskeletal manipulation did not improve his symptoms. A chest x-ray with posteroanterior **(A)** and lateral views **(B)** demonstrates an 8.4-cm left upper lung mass. Some deviation of the distal trachea is noted.

of 4 to 8 weeks' duration preoperatively is necessary to reduce the incidence of complications. Ideally, patients are smoke-free for a minimum of 2 weeks and preferably for 4 to 8 weeks before surgery,[2] although smoking cessation at any time is valuable.[3,4] Smoking cessation programs may be helpful for these patients, and patients may need pharmacologic assistance. This combination may have increased efficacy in smoking cessation efforts over counseling alone.[5]

Before the operation and in the perioperative period, deep venous thrombosis prophylaxis is provided by subcutaneous heparin, sequential compression stockings, or both.[6] Perioperative antibiotics are used to minimize complications from infections. Postoperative morbidity may also be minimized by adequate pain control to facilitate early ambulation. Routine use of a thoracic epidural catheter, or intercostal rib blocks with long-acting local anesthetics, or patient-controlled analgesia provide excellent pain control. Incentive spirometry assists in expanding the lung and reducing the incidence of pulmonary morbidity. Nasal bilevel positive airway pressure for patients with obstructive sleep apnea may delay or eliminate the need for intubation or reintubation after pulmonary resection. Early mobilization is essential to avoid most perioperative complications.

Physiologic Evaluation

Before thoracic operations, patients may be evaluated by a combination of radiographic and physiologic studies.[1] A plain chest x-ray (CXR) is commonly obtained (Fig. 57-5). Spirometry measures the lung volumes (Fig. 57-6) and mechanical properties of lung elasticity, recoil, and compliance. Pulmonary function testing (Fig. 57-7) also evaluates gas exchange functions, such as carbon monoxide diffusing capacity (DLCO).

The predicted postoperative forced expiratory volume in 1 second (FEV_1) is the most commonly used as an indicator of postoperative pulmonary reserve. Depending on other evaluable factors, most patients with FEV_1 greater than 60% predicted can tolerate an anatomic lobectomy. If FEV_1 is less than 60% of predicted, further testing in an attempt to estimate postoperative FEV_1 (predicted postoperative FEV_1 [ppo-FEV_1]) could be considered. The quantitative ventilation-perfusion lung scan is used

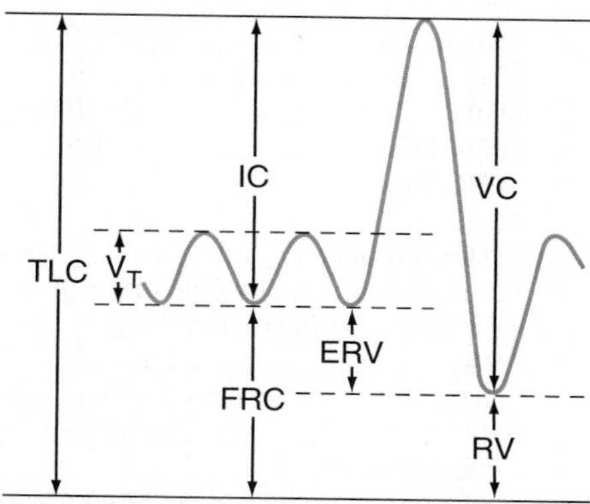

FIGURE 57-6 Spirometry with subdivisions of lung volumes. *ERV,* Expiratory reserve volume; *FRC,* functional residual capacity (i.e., lung volume at end expiration); *IC,* inspiratory capacity; *RV,* residual volume (i.e., lung volume after forced expiration from FRC); *TLC,* total lung capacity; *VC,* vital capacity (i.e., maximal volume of gas inspired from RV); V_T, tidal volume.

to assist in the calculation of postoperative residual pulmonary function after resection. Patients with a ppo-FEV_1 of 35% to 40% should functionally tolerate the operation.

Quantitative radionucleotide lung perfusion (Fig. 57-8) provides a measurement of the relative function of each lobe and lung and allows an estimation of pulmonary function after lung resection:

$$\text{ppo-FEV}_1 = \text{preop FEV}_1 \times (1 - \text{fraction of perfusion to region of planned resection})$$

A ppo-FEV_1 of 30% or less carries a greater risk for supplemental oxygen and ventilator dependence, but a decision to deny surgical resection to this group of patients must be considered on an individual basis because some will do better than expected with careful selection at experienced centers. Finally, in the immediate postoperative period, the ppo-FEV_1 is not likely to be realized secondary to limited ambulation, pain, or other emotional or physical factors.

Section of Pulmonary Medicine
Pulmonary Function Report

Last Name:		First Name:	
Identification:			
Age:	56 years	Room:	Out-patient
Sex:	Male	Race:	Caucasian
Height:	65 inches	Physician:	
Weight:	177 lbs	Operator:	
Date			
Time			

Spirometry	Pred	Pre BD	%Pred	Post BD	%Pred	%Chg
FVC....[l]	3.48	3.07	88	3.07	88	0
FEV_1....[l]	2.83	2.23	79	2.26	80	1
FEV_1/VC....[%]	80.81	72.26	89	69.78	86	–3
FEF 25–75....[l/s]	3.01	1.37	45	1.46	49	7
PEF....[l/s]	7.57	6.43	85	7.10	94	10
FIVC....[l]	3.48	3.09	89	3.24	93	5
FIV_1....[l]		3.09		3.24		5
FIV_1/FVC.... [%]		100.00		100.00		0

Lung Volumes	Pred	Measured	%Pred
SVC....[l]	3.48	3.04	87
TLC....[l]	5.51	5.54	101
RV....[l]	1.96	2.49	127
RV/TLC....[%]	35.9	45.0	125
FRC-Box....[l]	2.24	3.01	134

Diffusion SB	Pred	Measured	%Pred
DLCO SB....[ml/min/mm Hg]	22.59	23.81	105
DLCO Hb Corr[ml/min/mm Hg]	22.6	24.2	107
VA....[l]		5.27	
DLCO/VA....[ml/min/mm Hg/l]	3.93	4.52	115
Hb....[g/100ml]		14.1	

Interpretation

Spirometry reveals an isolated reduction in mid-expiratory flows consistent with an obstructive small airways defect. Increased residual volume (RV) is consistent with air trapping. Following the inhalation of a bronchodilator, there is no improvement of the obstructive airway defect. The diffusing capacity is normal.

FIGURE 57-7 The pulmonary function report provides complete spirometry data based on predicted values for height and weight. In this patient, the forced expiratory volume in 1 second (FEV_1) is 2.26 liters after bronchodilators, which is 80% of predicted. The carbon monoxide diffusing capacity (DLCO) is measured as 23.81 ml/min/mm Hg, which is 105% of predicted. *FEF,* Forced expiratory flow; *FIV_1,* forced inspiratory volume in 1 second; *FIVC,* forced inspiratory vital capacity; *FRC,* functional reserve capacity; *FVC,* forced vital capacity; *Hb,* hemoglobin; *PEF,* peak expiratory flow; *SB,* single breath; *SVC,* slow vital capacity; *TLC,* total lung capacity; *VA,* alveolar volume; *VC,* vital capacity.

DLCO can be measured by several methods, although the single-breath test is most commonly performed. DLCO measures the rate at which test molecules such as carbon monoxide move from the alveolar space to combine with hemoglobin in the red blood cells. DLCO is determined by calculating the difference between inspired and expired samples of gas. DLCO levels less than 40% to 50% are associated with increased perioperative risk.[7]

The ratio of FEV_1 to forced vital capacity (FEV_1/FVC) describes the relationship between the FEV_1 and the functional lung volume. In obstructive disease, the ratio is low (FEV_1 is low, and FVC is high); in restrictive disease, the ratio is about normal because both FEV_1 and FVC are reduced.

Flow-volume loops derived from spirometry describe the relationship between lung volume and air flow as the lung volume changes during a forced expiration and inspiration. The typical test consists of tidal breathing at rest, followed by maximal inspiratory effort to total lung capacity, then maximal expiratory effort to residual volume, concluding with maximal inspiratory effort to total lung capacity.

Cardiopulmonary Exercise Testing

Cardiopulmonary exercise testing (CPET) can be extremely useful in the evaluation of marginal candidates (ppo-FEV_1 or predicted postoperative DLCO <50% predicted) or patients who appear more disabled than expected from simple spirometry measurements. CPET includes exercise electrocardiography, heart rate response to exercise, and measurements of minute ventilation and oxygen uptake per minute. CPET allows a calculation of maximal

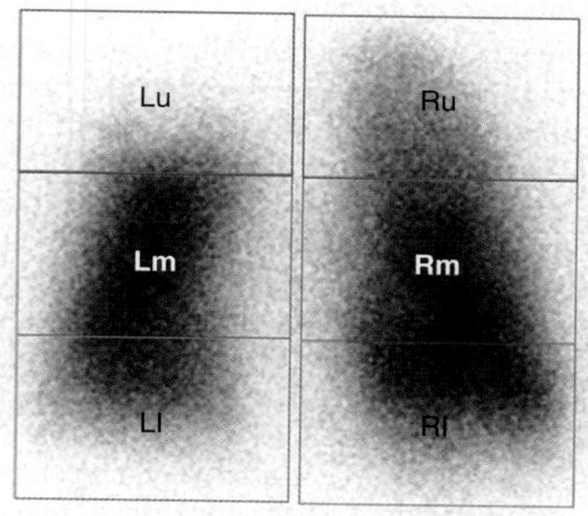

	Left lung		Right lung	
	%	Kct	%	Kct
Upper zone:	4.7	22.66	9.5	46.27
Middle zone:	24.0	116.91	28.3	138.05
Lower zone:	13.2	64.20	20.3	99.02
Total lung:	41.8	203.77	58.2	283.34

FIGURE 57-8 The quantitative perfusion lung scan report provides the lung volume and the perfusion to each lung. In a patient with a large left hilar tumor, perfusion may be reduced in the involved left lung compared with the uninvolved right lung. The predicted post–left pneumonectomy right lung function can be obtained by multiplying the right lung percent perfusion (58.2%) by the observed best FEV_1 (2.26 liters). The resulting value, 1.31 liter, 46.5% predicted, is the predicted postoperative FEV_1 (after left pneumonectomy). This value suggests that a left pneumonectomy would be functionally tolerated. *Ll,* Left lower zone; *Lm,* left middle zone; *Lu,* left upper zone; *Rl,* right lower zone; *Rm,* right middle zone; *Ru,* right upper.

oxygen consumption ($\dot{V}O_2max$) and provides insight into overall cardiopulmonary function (the "cardiopulmonary axis") that cannot be ascertained from other objective studies. CPET may identify clinically occult cardiac disease and provide a more accurate assessment of pulmonary function than spirometry and DLCO, which tend to overestimate functional loss after resection.

A patient's risk of perioperative morbidity and mortality may be stratified by $\dot{V}O_2max$. A level less than 11 to 15 mL/kg/min is associated with an increased risk, and $\dot{V}O_2max$ less than 10 mL/kg/min indicates high risk.[8] In patients undergoing evaluation for lung volume reduction surgery or for lung transplantation, a 6-minute walk test is used for a measure of the cardiac and pulmonary reserve. Patients are told to walk as far and as fast as they can during this time period. Distances of more than 1000 feet suggest an uncomplicated course.

Measurement of diaphragm function by fluoroscopy, the "sniff test," is needed to determine symmetry of effort and to exclude paradoxical movement of the diaphragm. Paradoxical movement (elevation of one hemidiaphragm with active contraction/retraction of the other diaphragm) suggests paresis or paralysis. This finding may suggest a specific reason for breathlessness. Diaphragm plication may be therapeutic.

No single test result should be viewed as an absolute contraindication to surgical resection. Although the physiologic assessment for patients undergoing normal spirometry and minimal comorbidity is straightforward, patients with marginal preoperative indices must be considered on an individual basis.

Thoracic Incisions

The choice of incision depends on the operation, the patient's underlying physiologic condition, and the anticipated benefits and limitations of the planned approach. Video-assisted thoracic surgery (VATS), robotic surgery, and other minimally invasive surgical techniques have been developed to treat most thoracic problems, including lung cancer, mediastinal tumors, pleural diseases, and parenchymal diseases, and to diagnose and stage thoracic malignancies. Various small incisions are made for the camera and other instruments depending on the location of the tumor. The ribs are not spread. Improved lighting and optics create excellent exposure and visualization. Advantages of minimally invasive surgical techniques include minimizing pain and surgical trauma from the incisions, decreasing hospitalization, and improving convalescence.

A thoracotomy requires spreading the ribs with a retractor and is used for operations on a single thorax. The patient is placed in a lateral decubitus position. The location of the incision may be posterior, axillary, or anterior. Posteriorly, an oblique incision is used with or without sparing the latissimus dorsi muscle. The chest is typically entered through the fifth interspace for pulmonary resection. A vertical axillary incision is made anterior to the latissimus dorsi muscle, and the chest is entered through the fourth interspace. This approach provides excellent hilar visualization. The anterior or anterolateral thoracotomy is created by a curvilinear incision underneath the inferior border of the pectoralis major muscle at the inframammary fold. A median sternotomy is performed using a vertical incision from the sternal notch to the xiphoid. A sternal saw is then used to divide the sternum in the midline. With gentle retraction, the sternum can be spread approximately 8 to 10 cm to allow access to the mediastinum, heart, great vessels, and right and left thorax. The pleura can be opened on either side to explore the hemithorax. The sternum is usually closed with stainless steel wire.

The transverse sternotomy or "clamshell" incision is larger than a median sternotomy and more uncomfortable for the patient. This incision combines two anterior thoracotomy incisions in the inframammary fold with transverse division of the sternum at the fourth intercostal space. Both internal mammary arteries are ligated. This approach is ideal for accessing both the right and the left hilum and providing additional exposure for large mediastinal tumors, bilateral hilar dissections, bilateral lung transplantation, or posterior-based metastases in both lungs.

LUNG

Congenital Lesions of the Lung

Various congenital lung abnormalities can occur as a consequence of disturbed embryogenesis.[9] Bilateral agenesis of the lungs is fatal. Unilateral agenesis may occur more frequently on the left (~70%) than on the right (~30%), with more than a 2:1 male-to-female ratio.

Hypoplasia of the lungs may occur as a result of interference with the development of the alveolar system during the last 2 months of gestation. Bochdalek hernia is the most frequent cause of hypoplasia. Conditions associated with hypoplasia of the lungs include oligohydramnios, prune-belly syndrome (deficiency in the abdominal musculature, genitourinary abnormalities), scimitar syndrome (abnormal pulmonary vein draining into the inferior vena cava, demonstrated as a crescent along the right heart border on cardiac angiography), and dextrocardia. Isolated pulmonary hypoplasia is rare.

Hyaline membrane disease (or infant respiratory distress syndrome) is frequent in premature infants (24 to 28 weeks' gestation) and infants of diabetic mothers. At a gestational age of 24 to 28 weeks, infants have an immature surfactant system. Hyaline membrane disease develops in the alveoli, causing congestion and a lung with a deep purple gross appearance. Respiratory distress frequently ensues, requiring high concentrations of oxygen. CXRs demonstrate a ground-glass appearance from the interstitial edema. As needs for oxygen and ventilator pressure increase to counteract this interstitial edema, pneumothorax frequently occurs. Of these infants, 10% to 30% do not survive.

Congenital Cystic Lesions

Congenital cystic lesions generally occur as a result of separation of the pulmonary remnants from airway branchings. Clinically, approximately one third of patients do not have symptoms; one third have cough; and one third have infection or, rarely, hemoptysis. Treatment may be with antibiotics or, for more severe localized cases, with resection. Any cystic lesion that enlarges on serial radiographs needs to be considered for resection.[10]

A bronchogenic cyst arises from a tracheal or bronchial diverticulum (see also "Primary Mediastinal Cysts"). This diverticulum becomes completely separated from the trachea and is frequently found as an asymptomatic mass on routine CXRs. Computed tomography (CT) scan of the chest demonstrates this abnormality as a homogeneous, well-circumscribed mass adjacent to the trachea (Fig. 57-9). The bronchogenic cyst accounts for 10% of

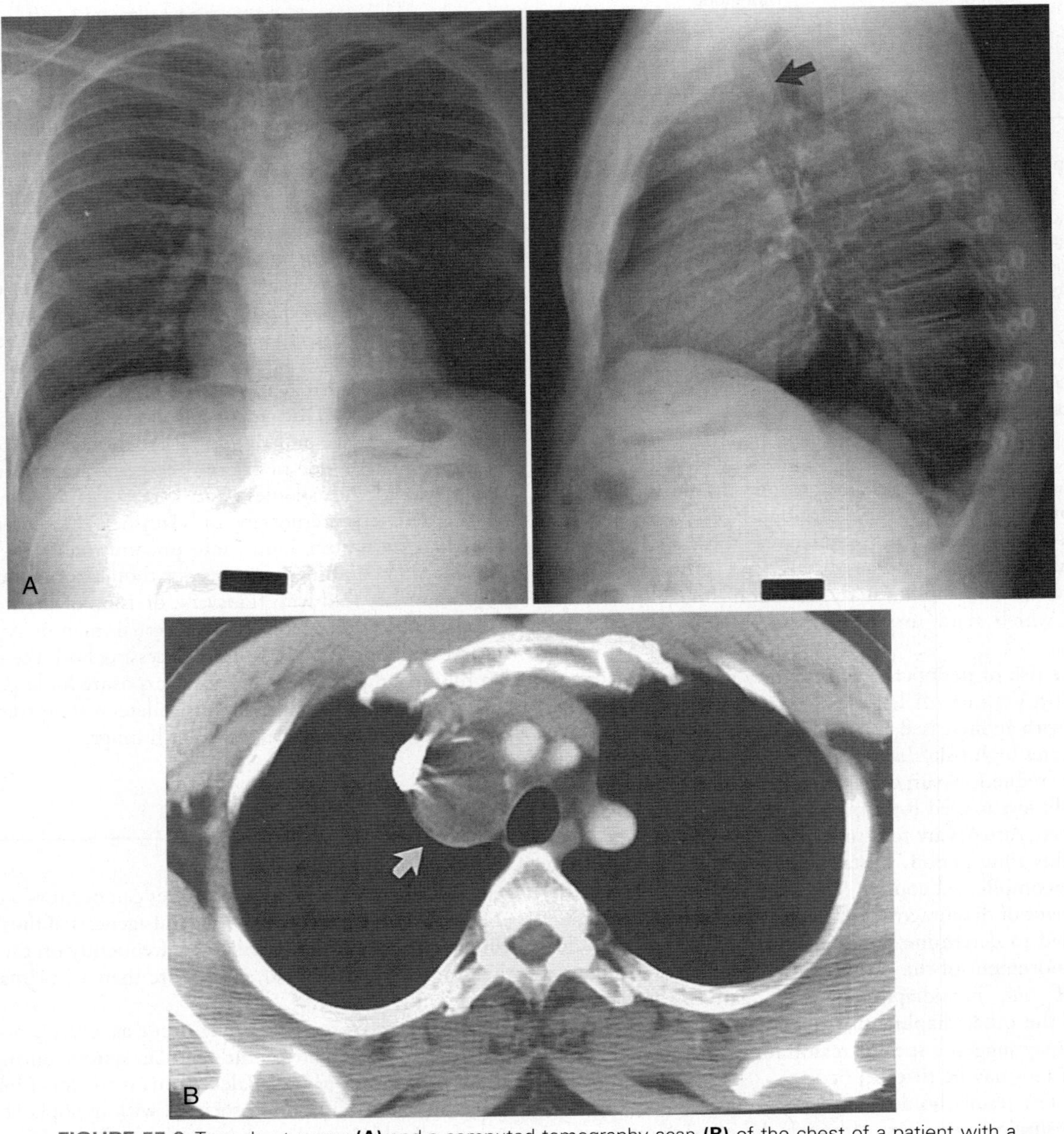

FIGURE 57-9 Two chest x-rays **(A)** and a computed tomography scan **(B)** of the chest of a patient with a bronchogenic cyst *(arrow)*.

mediastinal masses in children and is located in the midmediastinum. Treatment consists of excision, even if the patient is asymptomatic, to confirm the diagnosis.

Cystic fibrosis is an autosomal recessive disorder that is found more commonly in whites. Approximately 20% of patients with cystic fibrosis survive to the age of 30 years. Lung failure is the most frequent cause of death. Excessively thick mucus leads to inspissation, recurrent infections, bronchitis, and bronchiectasis. Pneumothorax secondary to air trapping is also found. Fibrosis and cystic changes on pathologic examinations are identified. A tension cyst may be a complication of cystic disease. A rapid increase in the size of the cyst may cause mechanical ventilation problems and mediastinal shift. Resection, usually lobectomy, corrects this problem. Pneumatoceles may develop as a result of childhood *Staphylococcus aureus* infection. They can be very large and may cause mechanical complications. These problems may resolve completely as the pneumonia resolves. Resection may be needed.

Congenital Bronchopulmonary Malformations

Lobar emphysema[9] is the most commonly resected congenital cystic lesion (50%). The onset of rapidly progressive respiratory distress usually occurs 4 to 5 days to several weeks after birth. It rarely occurs after 6 months of age. It affects the upper lobe predominately. Bronchiolitis is probably the most common cause overall. Treatment is lobectomy.

Congenital cystic adenomatoid malformations are the second most commonly resected congenital cystic lesion.[11] They are closely related to a hamartoma without cartilage. Terminal bronchioles proliferate, yielding the "adenomatoid" malformation. The lung has the appearance of Swiss cheese and feels like a large rubbery mass. With air trapping and overdistention, respiratory distress may occur, which is optimally relieved by lobectomy.

Pulmonary sequestration is an area of embryonic lung tissue, separate from the lung, which receives blood supply from an anomalous systemic artery from the aorta, not the pulmonary artery. This condition occurs secondary to an accessory lung bud caudal to the normal lung, but with a lack of absorption of primitive surrounding splanchnic vessels. During lung development, interlobar sequestration (75%) occurs early. Later, after the pleura forms, extralobar sequestration occurs (25%), primarily on the left side (66%), and is completely enclosed by its own pleura. The extralobar sequestration blood supply is usually from the thoracic or upper abdominal aorta to systemic (azygos or hemiazygos veins). Extralobar sequestration is more common in male patients. Resection is recommended. Intralobar sequestration occurs within the lower lobes predominately (>95%) and is equally distributed between the right and left lower lobes. Intralobar sequestration blood supply is from the descending thoracic aorta that usually traverses the pulmonary ligament. Venous drainage is via the pulmonary veins. The thoracic aorta provides 95% of the systemic blood supply to the pulmonary sequestration.

Congenital Abnormalities of the Trachea and Bronchi

Esophageal atresia with tracheoesophageal fistula is the most frequent abnormality of the trachea in infants (see "Pediatric Surgery"). Bronchial atresia is the second most frequent congenital pulmonary lesion after tracheoesophageal fistula.[12] The lung tissue distal to the atresia expands and becomes emphysematous as a result of air entry through the pores of Kohn. With no exit for air or mucus because of this blind bronchial stump, emphysema from air trapping or development of a mucocele may occur. CXRs may demonstrate hyperinflation of a lobe or a segment. The oval density may be identified between the hyperinflated lung and the hilum. The left upper lobe is the most frequently involved of all lobes within the lung. Diagnosis may be confirmed with bronchography or CT. The surgeon must rule out a mucous plug, adenoma, vascular compression, or sequestration.

Tracheal agenesis is a rare phenomenon and is fatal. The trachea is absent from the larynx to the carina, and bronchi communicate with the esophagus.

Tracheal stenosis is also rare and consists of generalized hypoplasia, a funnel-like trachea, and bronchial and segmental malformations. The right upper lobe bronchus may come from the trachea directly and may be associated with an aberrant left pulmonary artery (so-called pulmonary artery sling). Completely circular vascular rings are common. Repair is by incision of the trachea vertically and widening of the tracheal lumen.

Tracheomalacia can be identified by diagnostic imaging (dynamic expiratory CT) or bronchoscopy. The surgeon should notice marked variation of the tracheal lumen with inspiration and expiration. Collapse of greater than half of the lumen during expiration is consistent with this condition. Respiratory difficulty ensues from the intermittently collapsing trachea. Relief of the extrinsic compression is needed. Stent placement in adults or posterior splinting or primary tracheobronchoplasty may be required.[13] This condition may have a congenital predisposition but is most often seen in adults with COPD.

Congenital Vascular Disorders

Congenital vascular disorders of the lungs may occur.[14] In Swyer-James and Macleod syndrome, there is idiopathic hyperlucent lung. This problem develops from chronic pulmonary infections such as bronchiectasis. As the consolidation persists, decreased pulmonary artery blood supply may cause an "autopneumonectomy" and a hyperlucent lung.

Scimitar syndrome is associated with hypoplastic right lung with drainage of the pulmonary vein to the inferior vena cava. The anomaly is usually corrected using extracorporeal cardiopulmonary support. A patch from the pulmonary vein to the left atrium via an atrial septal defect corrects this problem.

Pulmonary arteriovenous malformations may exist as one or more pulmonary artery–to–pulmonary vein connections, bypassing the pulmonary capillary bed. This connection results in a right-to-left shunt. Approximately one third of these patients have hereditary hemorrhagic telangiectasia (Osler-Weber-Rendu syndrome). Approximately half of the malformations are small (<1 cm) and tend to be multiple. Half are greater than 1 cm and usually less than 5 cm and tend to be subpleural. These lesions need to be considered in the differential diagnosis of any patient with hemoptysis that is unexplained on the basis of bronchoscopy or routine imaging. Either local resection or catheter embolization of these lesions can be curative.

A pulmonary vascular sling consists of an anomalous or aberrant left pulmonary artery, which causes airway obstruction, and is associated with other anomalies. The aberrant left pulmonary artery arises from the right (main) pulmonary artery and courses between the trachea and the esophagus to supply the left lung. More than 90% of patients have wheezing and stridor. Esophagoscopy shows the anomalous vessel anterior to the esophagus; bronchoscopy or bronchography demonstrates the vessel posterior to the trachea. Surgical correction requires exploration of the left chest, division of the artery, and oversewing of the vessel as far as possible distal within the mediastinum. Reanastomosis to the main pulmonary artery is then performed.

Vascular rings[15] constitute 7% of all congenital heart problems. The most common vascular ring is a double aortic arch, which occurs in 60% of these patients. The right, or posterior, arch is the larger arch and gives rise to the right carotid and right subclavian arteries. The ring wraps around both the trachea and the esophagus. A posterior indentation is noted in the esophagus on barium swallow. Simple division corrects the anomaly. A right aortic arch with a retroesophageal left subclavian artery and left ligamentum arteriosum occurs in approximately 25% to 30% of patients with vascular rings. Intracardiac defects occur with a double aortic arch. Most of these infants require operation within the first weeks or months of life. Most patients with vascular rings require only a careful history and barium swallow for diagnosis. Typically, bronchoscopy or esophagoscopy is not ordered because it may be harmful; aortography adds little additional information. Repair is performed through the left chest. Division of the smaller arch, usually the left one, is undertaken. The ligamentum is divided, and the trachea and the esophagus are freed from the surrounding tissues. When a retroesophageal right subclavian artery with left ligament occurs, the patient may complain of dysphagia, which is referred to as *dysphagia lusoria.* The differential diagnosis includes neuromotor diseases of the esophagus or stricture.

LUNG CANCER

Lung cancer is a significant global health problem. In the United States in 2015, there were estimated to be 221,200 new cases of lung cancer.[16] Lung cancer is the most frequent cause of death from cancer in men and women and accounts for 13.0% of all cancer diagnoses and 27.0% of all cancer deaths in the United States. Lung cancer deaths exceed the combined total deaths from breast, prostate, and colorectal cancer. Since 1987, more women have died of lung cancer than breast cancer. Lung cancer deaths in men have decreased by approximately 3% per year in men and by approximately 2% per year in women. Smoking cessation in women has lagged behind smoking cessation in men, and thus the incidence of lung cancer in women has not declined as much as the incidence in men (Fig. 57-10). The decline in lung cancer

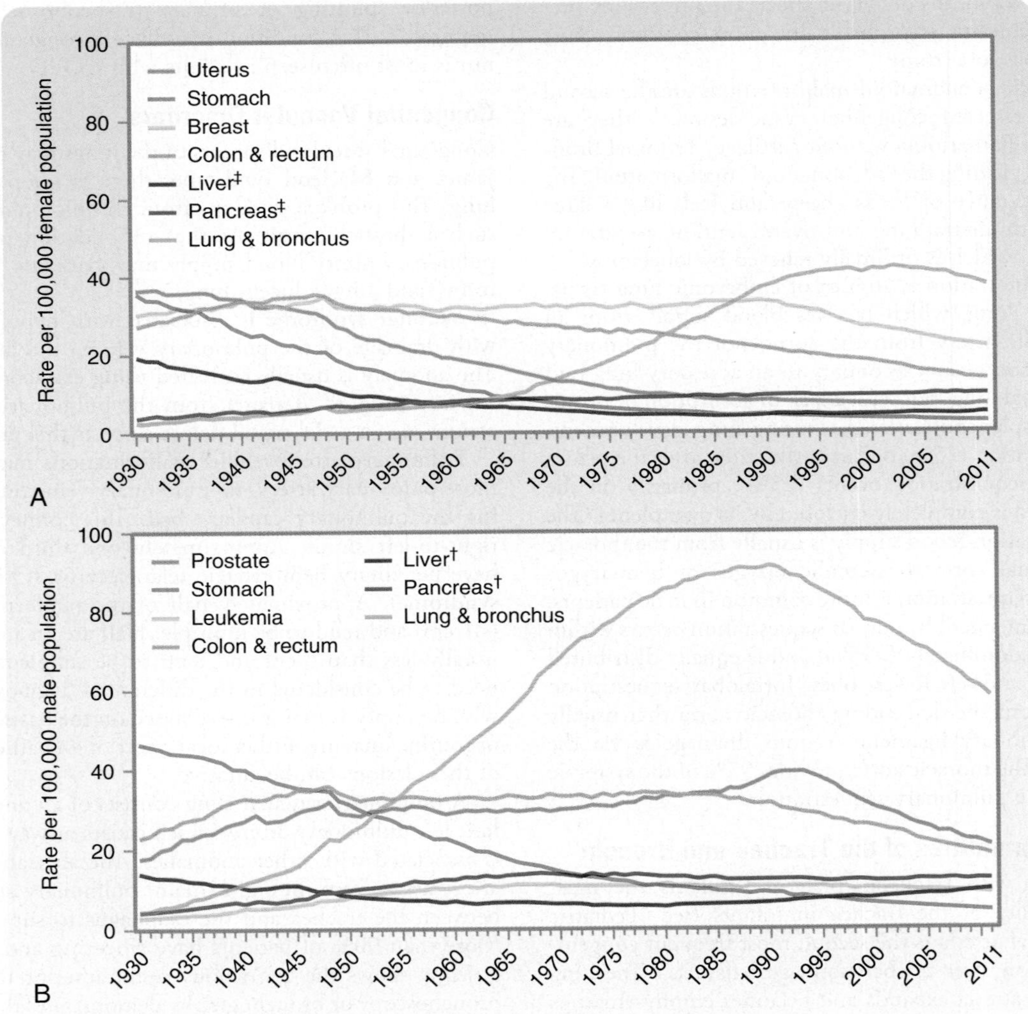

FIGURE 57-10 A, Age-adjusted cancer death rates for women, by site, in the United States (1930-2011) per 100,000, age-adjusted to the 2000 U.S. standard population. **B,** Age-adjusted cancer death rates for men, by site, in the United States (1930-2011) per 100,000, age-adjusted to the 2000 U.S. standard population. (From Siegel RL, Miller KD, Jemal A: Cancer statistics, 2015. *CA Cancer J Clin* 65:5–29, 2015.)

incidence and mortality rate likely reflects decreasing cigarette smoking and potentially earlier detection of smaller, asymptomatic lung cancers. African American men have both the highest incidence and the highest death rate from cancer of the lung and bronchus.

Lung cancer survival is stage specific. Overall, the 1-year 44%, and the 5-year relative survival rate is 17%. Localized (early-stage) lung cancer has a 5-year survival rate of 54%, although greater than 50% of all patients have advanced or distant disease at diagnosis, with 1-year and 5-year survivals of 26% and 4%, respectively.

Cigarette smoking is unequivocally the most important risk factor in the development of lung cancer. Other environmental factors may predispose to lung cancer. Environmental radon gas exposure is estimated to be the second most important risk factor. Other factors include asbestos, arsenic, chromium, nickel, organic chemicals, iatrogenic radiation exposure, air pollution, and secondary smoke from nonsmokers.

Radon is associated with approximately 18,000 lung cancer deaths a year.[17] Radon is a natural radioactive gas released from the normal decay of uranium in the soil. Inhalation is associated with health risk. Inexpensive test kits are available to determine the amount of radon present in homes.

Optimal treatment of lung cancer requires accurate diagnosis and clinical staging before treatment begins. The anatomic basis for staging (tumor, lymph nodes, and metastases) includes the physical properties of the tumor and the presence of regional or systemic metastases. The biologic basis for staging (molecular markers prognostic for survival as well as predictive for response to therapy) is expected to be incorporated into staging systems of the future. Clinical trials are available for patient enrollment to understand and evaluate various treatments better.[18] The National Cancer Institute National Clinical Trials Network conducts clinical trials for patients with lung cancer and other malignancies throughout the United States.[19]

Pathology

The pathology of lung cancer has been reviewed elsewhere.[20] Development of lung cancer follows a progression of histologic changes that results from smoking and includes (1) proliferation of basal cells, (2) development of atypical nuclei with prominent nucleoli, (3) stratification, (4) development of squamous metaplasia, (5) carcinoma in situ, and (6) invasive carcinoma.

Adenocarcinoma of the lung is the most frequent histologic type and accounts for approximately 45% of all lung cancers. Adenocarcinoma of the lung is derived from the mucus-producing cells of the bronchial epithelium. Microscopic features consist of cuboidal to columnar cells with adequate to abundant pink or vacuolated cytoplasm and some evidence of gland formation. Most of these tumors (75%) are peripherally located. Adenocarcinoma of the lung tends to metastasize earlier than squamous cell carcinoma (SCC) of the lung and more frequently to the central nervous system.

The pathology of adenocarcinoma has been revised.[21] Bronchoalveolar or bronchioloalveolar carcinoma and mixed type adenocarcinoma have been eliminated, and adenocarcinoma in situ (pure lepidic growth) and minimally invasive adenocarcinoma (predominantly lepidic growth with <5 mm invasion) have been created. A solitary focus is treated in a manner similar to adenocarcinoma. Multifocal disease generally is not amenable to surgical resection. For invasive adenocarcinomas, the predominant pattern includes lepidic, acinar, papillary, and solid growth.

SCC of the lung occurs in approximately 30% of patients with lung cancer. Approximately two thirds of these tumors are centrally located and tend to expand against the bronchus, causing extrinsic compression. These tumors are prone to undergo central necrosis and cavitation. SCC tends to metastasize later than adenocarcinoma. Microscopically, keratinization, stratification, and intercellular bridge formation are exhibited. SCC may be more readily detected on sputum cytology than adenocarcinoma.

A diagnosis of large cell undifferentiated carcinoma may be made in approximately 10% of all lung tumors. Specific cytologic features of SCC or adenocarcinoma are lacking. These tumors tend to occur peripherally and may metastasize relatively early. Microscopically, these tumors show anaplastic, pleomorphic cells with vesicular or hyperchromatic nuclei and abundant cytoplasm. Neuroendocrine histopathology in adenocarcinoma can also portend a poorer prognosis and is more common in the large cell variant.

Small cell lung cancer represents approximately 20% of all lung cancers; approximately 80% are centrally located. The disease is characterized by an aggressive tendency to metastasize. It often spreads early to mediastinal lymph nodes and distant sites, especially bone marrow and brain. Small cell lung cancer appears to arise in cells derived from the embryologic neural crest. Microscopically, these cells appear as sheets or clusters of cells with dark nuclei and little cytoplasm. The term *oat cell carcinoma* for this disease is due to the oatlike appearance under the microscope. Neurosecretory granules are evident on electron microscopy. This tumor is staged as *limited stage* (disease restricted to an ipsilateral hemithorax within a single radiation port) and *extensive stage* (obvious metastatic disease). These tumors are often advanced at presentation with an aggressive tendency to metastasize. Chemoradiotherapy is generally used for treatment. Prophylactic cranial irradiation needs to be considered in a patient with limited or extensive stage disease that responds well to first-line therapy. Complete responses may occur in approximately 30% of patients; however, the 5-year survival rate is only 5%. Patients with clinical early-stage disease (e.g., <3 cm in size, no nodal metastases, and no extrathoracic metastases) may be considered for surgical resection, followed by adjuvant systemic therapy. Staging before resection includes ^{18}F-fluorodeoxyglucose positron emission tomography (FDG-PET), brain CT or magnetic resonance imaging (MRI), and mediastinoscopy. Mediastinal metastases on clinical staging suggest advanced disease, which is best treated with chemoradiotherapy.

Lung cancers commonly metastasize to the pulmonary and mediastinal lymph nodes (lymphatic spread). Hematogenous spread of lung cancer commonly may result in metastases to the adrenal glands, brain, lung, and bone. Adenocarcinoma is more likely to metastasize to the central nervous system. Bone metastases are osteolytic. Extrathoracic metastases may occur without hilar nodes or mediastinal metastases.

Screening

Patients with lung cancer often present with advanced stage disease and symptoms. The pulmonary parenchyma does not contain nerve endings, and tumors may grow undetected until symptoms of pain, hemoptysis, or obstructive pneumonia arise. With the increased use of CT in the United States, smaller asymptomatic lung cancers are being identified.

Screening for lung cancer has been evaluated by the National Lung Screening Trial (NLST).[22,23] The NLST is a prospective randomized multicenter study evaluating annual low-dose helical

CT with annual chest radiography. The 53,454 enrolled patients were randomly assigned between the two arms. The men and women screened were asymptomatic, and were older (age range, 55 to 74 years) with 30 pack-years or more of cigarette smoking at the beginning of the trial, and either were current smokers or had recently quit (within 15 years). The NLST found that patients randomly assigned to low-dose helical CT screening for 3 years (compared with CXR) had a reduced lung cancer–specific mortality and all-cause mortality. The death rate from lung cancer in this high-risk population was reduced by 20%, and all-cause mortality was reduced by 7%. The study showed the benefit is statistically significant, as 354 lung cancer deaths occurred in the CT group compared with 442 lung cancer deaths in the CXR group (P = .0041), leading to early study closure. Screening for early lung cancer detection using low-dose helical CT in average-risk asymptomatic individuals is recommended by the U.S. Preventive Services Task Force for selected current or former smokers 55 to 74 years old in good health with at least a 30-pack-year history of cigarette smoking.[24] Various professional organizations have incorporated the U.S. Preventive Services Task Force recommendations into their guidelines.[25]

These patients may discuss testing for early-stage lung cancer on an individual basis based on consultation and evaluation by their personal physicians—the informed shared decision-making model. This discussion with the patient should include the risks, benefits, and limitations associated with lung cancer screening with low-dose helical CT and should occur before a decision is made to start any lung cancer screening. Screening is not an alternative to smoking cessation. A clear and unambiguous statement is needed from the physician that smoking cessation is essential. Pharmacologic or other strategies need to be tailored to the individual patient. Screening of asymptomatic patients may identify nonspecific findings, such as overdiagnosis of benign nodules, which could result in patient anxiety as well as additional radiation exposure.

Diagnosis

The diagnosis of lung cancer can be challenging.[26] Many benign conditions mimic lung cancer. Physical examination should focus on the cardiorespiratory system. In addition, the presence of cancer in supraclavicular lymph nodes, identified by a careful examination of the cervical and supraclavicular lymph nodes, suggests advanced disease (N3 status for non–small cell lung cancer [NSCLC]), and therapy other than resection is recommended. Paraneoplastic syndromes are distant manifestations of lung cancer (not metastases) as revealed in extrathoracic nonmetastatic symptoms. The lung cancer causes an effect on these extrathoracic sites by producing one or more biologic or biochemical substances.

NSCLC typically occurs in patients who are 50 to 70 years old with a history of cigarette smoking. Patients develop symptoms based on the physical impact of tumor growth within the lung parenchyma. Symptoms such as cough, dyspnea, chest wall pain, and hemoptysis are related to the physical presence of the tumor and its interactions with the structures of the lung and chest wall.[27]

Pathologic confirmation of NSCLC can assist the patient and physician in discussions of risk and benefit for specific treatment options. Guidelines for management of the indeterminate pulmonary nodule, or "solitary" pulmonary nodule (SPN), are available.[28,29] Under certain circumstances, a SPN may be deemed benign with adequate confidence in the absence of a pathologic diagnosis. SPNs that are entirely calcified, or radiologically stable on CT of the chest over a minimum of 2 years, are very likely to be benign. Review of old radiographs or other prior imaging studies can assist in evaluation of changes in the mass.

In patients with a clinically suspicious SPN, histologic information may be needed to assess risk and benefit of various treatment options for the patient. Various options are available, and the least invasive strategy compatible with obtaining a diagnosis would be recommended. Diagnostic bronchoscopy, transthoracic needle aspiration, or navigational bronchoscopy[30] can be selected based on the size, location, and condition of the patient. In a physiologically fit patient with a suspicious yet undiagnosed SPN, nonanatomic wedge or sublobar resection provides a diagnosis. Confirmation of NSCLC by the pathologist should be followed by definitive resection in the same setting. For a SPN in the absence of a cancer diagnosis (that cannot be removed by wedge resection), a lobectomy can be considered for diagnosis (and treatment). A pneumonectomy is not performed without a cancer diagnosis.

One third of patients with NSCLC may have a pleural effusion at the time of presentation. Pleural fluid sampling with thoracentesis is required for cytologic examination. Malignant pleural effusion (MPE) is a contraindication to resection, but many pleural effusions in this setting may be sympathetic or reactive in origin.

Bronchoscopy is recommended before any planned pulmonary resection. The surgeon independently assesses (via bronchoscopy) the endobronchial anatomy to exclude secondary endobronchial primary tumors and to ensure that all known cancer will be encompassed by the planned pulmonary resection. Secretions can be cleared with suctioning and gentle irrigation. When pneumonectomy or bronchoplastic resection is contemplated for a central tumor, the surgeon's assessment at bronchoscopy is critical to the determination of whether complete (R0) resection can be achieved.

If the patient has hard palpable lymph nodes in the cervical or supraclavicular area, fine-needle aspiration or biopsy may provide an accurate diagnosis of N3 disease. Otherwise, a superficial lymph node biopsy or a scalene node biopsy could be performed to obtain tissue for further evaluation.

Staging

Staging is a description of the extent of the cancer based on similarities in survival for the group of patients with those characteristics. The staging system creates a shorthand description of the tumor, lymph nodes, and metastatic characteristics of the patient to facilitate the choice of optimal therapy and to evaluate outcomes based on the clinical and pathologic stage. The American Joint Committee on Cancer (AJCC) and the Union for International Cancer Control work to establish and promulgate staging system guidelines. The current international staging system for NSCLC[31] provides the basis for specific patient stage groupings and is used for initial treatment recommendations based on the clinical stage and on the pathologic stage after pulmonary resection.

The clinician's responsibility is to ensure the highest possible degree of certainty of the extent of the disease and to recommend the therapy or therapeutic combination of greatest efficacy based on this clinic stage. Optimal staging assists the clinician in providing the best recommendations for therapeutic interventions for the patient. The clinical stage is the physician's best and final estimate of the extent of disease based on all available information from invasive and noninvasive studies before the initiation of definitive therapy. The pathologic stage is the determination of the physical extent of the disease based on histologic examination

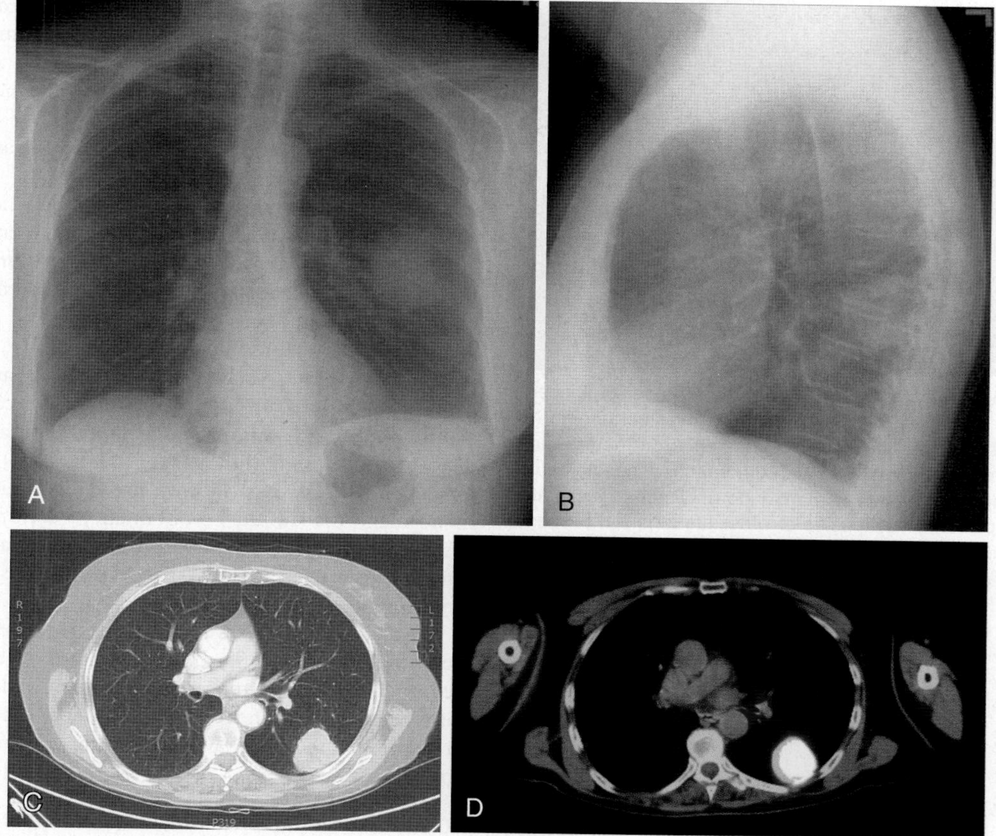

FIGURE 57-11 Radiographic evaluation for any patient with known or suspected lung cancer includes a plain chest x-ray, posteroanterior **(A)** and lateral **(B)** views. Evaluation of the plain films and computed tomography (CT) **(C)** guides subsequent evaluations. ^{18}F-Fluorodeoxyglucose positron emission tomography (FDG-PET) with fused CT **(D)** provides the ability to correlate metabolic activity with physical findings. Although FDG-PET uses the increased metabolism in most neoplasms to create the FDG-PET image, other processes, such as infection, inflammation, or sequelae of trauma or fractures, can be identified as well. Sites of increased metabolism should be carefully evaluated for metastases.

of the resected tissues, including the hilar and mediastinal lymph nodes.

Evaluation of Tumor (T) Stage

As the tumor size increases, survival decreases. Diagnostic imaging commonly includes a CXR and CT scan of the chest and upper abdomen, including the liver and adrenals (Fig. 57-11). The CXR provides information on the size, shape, density, and location of the primary tumor and its relationship to the mediastinal structures. CT scan of the chest provides more detail on tumor characteristics and provides information on the relationship of the tumor to the mediastinum, chest wall, and diaphragm as well as invasion into the vertebrae or mediastinal structures (clinical T4). MRI may complement CT in these patients (T4). MRI of the brain may be reserved for patients with stage I or II cancer with new neurologic symptoms only (vertigo, headache), all patients with stage III and IV cancer, and patients with small cell carcinoma or superior sulcus tumors (Pancoast tumor) because these patients have a higher incidence of occult brain metastases.

Evaluation of Nodal (N) Stage

Determination of metastases to mediastinal lymph nodes constitutes a critical point in staging and treatment recommendations.[32,33] Mediastinal lymph node metastases are present in 26% to 32% of patients at the time of diagnosis and initially assessed with chest CT. Lymph nodes may be enlarged normally from infection (e.g., histoplasmosis, previous bronchitis, or pneumonia) or other inflammatory processes, such as granulomatous disease. Mediastinal adenopathy is most often defined as lymph nodes with a maximal transverse diameter greater than 1 cm on axial tomographic images. In the absence of mediastinal nodes greater than 1 cm in diameter, the likelihood of N2 or N3 disease is low. If mediastinal nodes greater than 1 cm are identified, nodal tissue must be examined (e.g., with endoscopic bronchial ultrasound, cervical mediastinoscopy, endoscopic ultrasound, VATS) for histologic evidence of metastases before definitive resection.

CT has a reported sensitivity of 57% to 79% for mediastinal lymph node assessment in NSCLC, with a positive predictive value of 56%.[32] No CT size criteria are entirely reliable for the determination of mediastinal lymph node involvement. Larger mediastinal lymph nodes are more likely to be associated with metastasis (>70%); however, normal-sized lymph nodes (<1 cm) have a 7% to 15% chance of containing metastases.

PET may assist in evaluating the local extent and presence of known or occult metastases based on the differential increased metabolism of glucose by cancer cells compared with normal tissues (Fig. 57-12). A PET scan is not a cancer-specific study or a "cancer scan," as high cellular glucose metabolism is seen in

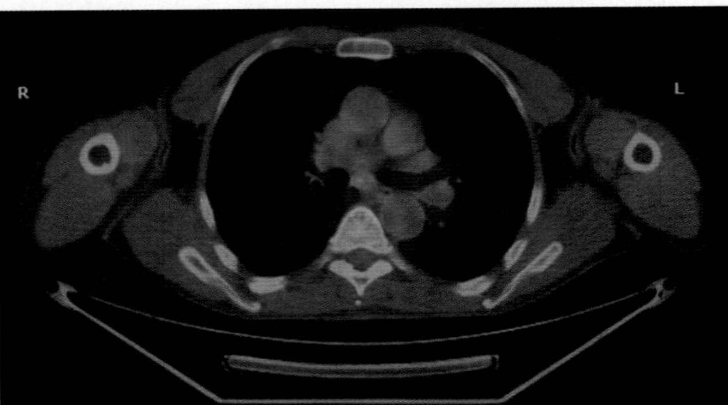

FIGURE 57-12 A subcarinal lymph node has mild ^{18}F-fluorodeoxyglucose (FDG) uptake. Based on these findings, additional invasive staging is warranted, including bronchoscopy and invasive staging of mediastinal lymph nodes. Endobronchial ultrasound with transtracheal needle aspiration can be performed with real-time ultrasound guidance to facilitate transtracheal needle placement. Biopsies of other stations can be performed as well. If needed, cervical mediastinoscopy is performed with biopsy of high paratracheal (2R and 2L), low paratracheal (4R and 4L), pretracheal (3A), and subcarinal (7) lymph nodes. If left-sided aortopulmonary lymph nodes were FDG avid, a Chamberlain procedure (anterior mediastinotomy) or video-assisted thoracic surgery with biopsy of aortopulmonary window lymph nodes or hilar lymph nodes could also be performed. Additional evaluation of the patient would be warranted if the patient would be considered a surgical candidate.

inflammatory processes in addition to malignancy. FDG-PET scan is not a consistent diagnostic test for lung cancer.[34] Histologic confirmation of FDG avid mediastinal lymph node involvement is indicated to complete clinical staging before final treatment decisions. FDG-PET scan may identify areas of occult activity that must be evaluated for histologic evidence of NSCLC. FDG-PET coupled with CT may yield increased sensitivity and specificity in determining the stage of patients with lung cancer before treatment interventions.[35] Reed and colleagues[36] identified that PET and CT together were better than either one alone in determining a patient's suitability for resection. The negative predictive value of PET for mediastinal lymph node metastases from NSCLC was 87%.

Invasive staging includes cervical mediastinoscopy or mediastinotomy (Chamberlain procedure), endoscopic bronchial ultrasound, or endoscopic ultrasound.[32] Cervical mediastinoscopy is traditionally indicated in patients with otherwise operable NSCLC with enlarged paratracheal or subcarinal lymph nodes, particularly if the cancer is proximal, if pneumonectomy is planned, or if the patient is at increased risk for the planned resection. Cervical mediastinoscopy is commonly performed for biopsy of bilateral paratracheal (level 2 and 4) and subcarinal (level 7) lymph nodes. A left anterior mediastinotomy is used to gain access to the mediastinum after resection of the second costosternal cartilage to evaluate the aortopulmonary window (level 5) or anterior mediastinum (level 6) lymph nodes. Cervical mediastinoscopy has a negative predictive value greater than 90%, may be performed as an outpatient procedure, and is associated with a low rate of significant complications. When pathologic "frozen section" evaluation fails to demonstrate malignant nodal involvement, mediastinoscopy may be followed by resection under the same anesthetic. The use of cervical mediastinoscopy regardless of radiographic evidence of nodal involvement ("routine mediastinoscopy") is not a cost-effective approach and adds little to the accuracy of staging in patients with an adequate noninvasive preoperative evaluation.[37]

Additional sampling techniques may be helpful. Endoscopic bronchial ultrasound may be more sensitive than mediastinoscopy.[38] Combining endoscopic bronchial ultrasound and surgical staging may provide greater sensitivity for mediastinal nodal metastases than surgical staging alone and avoid unnecessary thoracotomies.[39] VATS techniques can evaluate enlarged level 5 or 6 lymph nodes as well as enlarged level 8 or 9 or low level 7 lymph nodes. Endoscopic ultrasound–guided aspiration can be easily used for transesophageal needle aspiration of subcarinal and left aortopulmonary window lymph nodes.

Extrathoracic or distant metastases (M1b) are common in lung cancer. Beyond a thorough history and physical examination and standard staging techniques, additional evaluation for metastatic disease is indicated only for selected cases. In cases in which metastatic disease is suspected based on imaging techniques, a tissue diagnosis should be obtained to confirm the presence or absence of metastases. Nodules in the contralateral lung are characterized as metastatic disease (M1a) as are MPE and pleural carcinomatosis.

Up to 7% of patients have metastatic adrenal involvement at presentation. The standard CT evaluation of the chest should also include evaluation of the upper abdomen including the liver and the adrenal glands. Indeterminate adrenal lesions on CT may be further evaluated with MRI or with CT-guided percutaneous biopsy.

Current American Joint Committee on Cancer Seventh Edition Staging System

The International Association for the Study of Lung Cancer (IASLC) embarked on its lung cancer staging project to include all treatment and diagnostic groups, to collect data for analysis, and to reform future revisions.[40] The current AJCC seventh edition lung cancer staging reflects the impact of the IASLC lung cancer staging project.[41] The IASLC collected more than 100,000 NSCLC cases treated between 1990 and 2000. Each patient had a minimum of 5 years of follow-up, and all treatment modalities were included. Greater than 81,000 cases were submitted and eligible for analysis. These included 67,725 patients with NSCLC and 13,290 patients with small cell carcinoma. Survival was calculated by the Kaplan-Meier method. Prognostic groups were created using Cox regression analysis, and results were internally and externally validated.[42] Stage groupings were revised to reflect these analyses and internally and externally validated.[31] External validation was assessed against the Surveillance, Epidemiology, and End Results program database. The data collected were retrospective, and an audit of the data was not performed; however, information was provided by credible centers, which facilitated data collection, and analysis of a large patient population. Future directions will likely include prospective data collection[43] and proteomic and genomic characteristics.

The TNM definitions, nodal characteristics, and stage groupings of the TNM subsets with survival are shown in Table 57-1, Box 57-1, and Table 57-2. Other schematics have been created for the lymph node map[44] and T characteristics.[45]

The mediastinal and regional lymph node classification schema is presented in Figure 57-13. This map presents a graphic representation of mediastinal and pulmonary lymph nodes in relation to other thoracic structures for optimal dissection and anatomic labeling by the surgeon.

TABLE 57-1 T, N, and M Descriptors for Lung Cancer Staging

T (Primary Tumor)	
TX	Primary tumor cannot be assessed, or tumor proven by the presence of malignant cells in sputum or bronchial washings but not visualized by imaging or bronchoscopy
T0	No evidence of primary tumor
Tis	Carcinoma in situ
T1	Tumor ≤3 cm in greatest dimension, surrounded by lung or visceral pleura, without bronchoscopic evidence of invasion more proximal than the lobar bronchus (i.e., not in the main bronchus)*
• T1a—Tumor ≤2 cm in greatest dimension	
• T1b—Tumor >2 cm but ≤3 cm in greatest dimension	
T2	Tumor >3 cm but ≤7 cm or tumor with any of the following features (T2 tumors with these features are classified T2a if ≤5 cm)
• Involves main bronchus, ≥2 cm distal to the carina	
• Invades visceral pleura	
• Associated with atelectasis or obstructive pneumonitis that extends to the hilar region but does not involve the entire lung	
• T2a—Tumor >3 cm but ≤5 cm in greatest dimension	
• T2b—Tumor >5 cm but ≤7 cm in greatest dimension	
T3	Tumor >7 cm or one that directly invades any of the following: chest wall (including superior sulcus tumors), diaphragm, phrenic nerve, mediastinal pleura, parietal pericardium; or
• Tumor in the main bronchus <2 cm distal to the carina* but without involvement of the carina or	
• Associated atelectasis or obstructive pneumonitis of the entire lung or	
• Separate tumor nodule(s) in the same lobe	
T4	Tumor of any size that invades any of the following: mediastinum, heart, great vessels, trachea, recurrent laryngeal nerve, esophagus, vertebral body, carina; or
• Separate tumor nodule(s) in a different ipsilateral lobe	
N (Regional Lymph Nodes)	
NX	Regional lymph nodes cannot be assessed
N0	No regional lymph node metastases
N1	Metastasis in ipsilateral peribronchial and/or ipsilateral hilar lymph nodes and intrapulmonary nodes, including involvement by direct extension
N2	Metastasis in ipsilateral mediastinal and/or subcarinal lymph node(s)
N3	Metastasis in contralateral mediastinal, contralateral hilar, ipsilateral or contralateral scalene, or supraclavicular lymph node(s)
M (Distant Metastasis)	
MX	Distant metastasis cannot be assessed
M0	No distant metastasis
M1	Distant metastasis
• M1a—Separate tumor nodule(s) in a contralateral lobe; tumor with pleural nodules or malignant pleural (or pericardial) effusion†	
• M1b—Distant metastasis in extrathoracic organs	

Adapted from Goldstraw P, Crowley J, Chansky K, et al: The IASLC Lung Cancer Staging Project: Proposals for the revision of the TNM stage groupings in the forthcoming (seventh) edition of the TNM Classification of malignant tumours. *J Thorac Oncol* 2:706–714, 2007; and Edge SB, Byrd DR, Compton CC, et al: *AJCC cancer staging manual*, ed 7, New York, 2010, Springer.

*The uncommon superficial spreading tumor of any size with its invasive component limited to the bronchial wall, which may extend proximally to the main bronchus, is also classified as T1.

†Most pleural (and pericardial) effusions with lung cancer are due to tumor. In a few patients, multiple cytopathologic examinations of pleural (pericardial) fluid are negative for tumor, and the fluid is nonbloody and is not an exudate. Where these elements and clinical judgment dictate that the effusion is not related to the tumor, the effusion should be excluded as a staging element, and the patient should be classified as T1, T2, T3, or T4.

Tumor (T)

In the IASLC lung cancer staging project, more than 18,000 patients had a T1 to T4 tumor with N0 lymph node dissection and R0 resection.[46] T1 was divided into T1a (≤2 cm) and T1b (>2 to 3 cm). T2 was divided into T2a (>3 to 5 cm) and T2b (>5 to 7 cm). "T2c" would have been tumors greater than 7 cm; however, these patients had a survival that was statistically similar to survival of T3 patients, and so tumors greater than 7 cm were categorized as T3.

Other T2 descriptors, such as visceral pleural invasion and partial atelectasis (less than the entire lung), could not be evaluated because of the small number of patients and inconsistent data. In the AJCC seventh edition, nodules in the same lobe were categorized as T3; nodules in a different lobe were categorized as T4; a nodule in a contralateral lobe would be designated as M1a, *unless* there was compelling evidence to suggest synchronous primary tumors.

T3 tumors may be characterized as a tumor with invasion into the pleura, pericardium, or diaphragm; an endobronchial tumor less than 2 cm from the carina; an obstructing tumor causing atelectasis of the entire lung; or, as mentioned before, two nodules in the same lobe. T4 tumors involve the mediastinal structures, such as the heart, great vessels, esophagus, and trachea, as well as the vertebral body or the carina. Two nodules, one each in two separate ipsilateral lobes, would also be characterized as T4.

BOX 57-1 Lymph Node Map Definitions

N2 Nodes*

1. Highest mediastinal nodes: Nodes lying above a horizontal line at the upper rim of the brachiocephalic (left innominate) vein where it ascends to the left, crossing in front of the trachea at its midline.
2. Upper paratracheal nodes: Nodes lying above a horizontal line drawn tangential to the upper margin of the aortic arch and below the inferior boundary of number 1 nodes.
3. Prevascular and retrotracheal nodes: Pretracheal and retrotracheal nodes may be designated 3A and 3P. Midline nodes are considered to be ipsilateral.
4. Lower paratracheal nodes: The lower paratracheal nodes on the right lie to the right of the midline of the trachea between a horizontal line drawn tangential to the upper margin of the aortic arch and a line extending across the right main bronchus at the upper margin of the upper lobe bronchus and contained within the mediastinal pleural envelope; the lower paratracheal nodes on the left lie to the left of the midline of the trachea between a horizontal line drawn tangential to the upper margin of the aortic arch and a line extending across the left main bronchus at the level of the upper margin of the left upper lobe bronchus, medial to the ligamentum arteriosum and contained within the mediastinal pleural envelope.

Regional (N2) Lymph Node Classification

5. Subaortic (aortopulmonary window): Subaortic nodes are lateral to the ligamentum arteriosum or the aorta or left pulmonary artery and proximal to the first branch of the left pulmonary artery and lie within the mediastinal pleural envelope.
6. Para-aortic nodes (ascending aorta or phrenic): Nodes lying anterior and lateral to the ascending aorta and the aortic arch or the innominate artery, beneath a line tangential to the upper margin of the aortic arch.
7. Subcarinal nodes: Nodes lying caudad to the carina of the trachea but not associated with the lower lobe bronchi or arteries within the lung.
8. Paraesophageal nodes (below carina): Nodes lying adjacent to the wall of the esophagus and to the right or left of the midline, excluding subcarinal nodes.
9. Pulmonary ligament nodes: Nodes lying within the pulmonary ligament, including nodes in the posterior wall and lower part of the inferior pulmonary vein.

N1 Nodes†

10. Hilar nodes: The proximal lobar nodes, distal to the mediastinal pleural reflection and the nodes adjacent to the bronchus intermedius on the right; radiographically, the hilar shadow may be created by enlargement of both hilar and interlobar nodes.
11. Interlobar nodes: Nodes lying between the lobar bronchi.
12. Lobar nodes: Nodes adjacent to the distal lobar bronchi.
13. Segmental nodes: Nodes adjacent to segmental bronchi.
14. Subsegmental nodes: Nodes around the subsegmental bronchi.

From Mountain CF, Dresler CM: Regional lymph node classification for lung cancer staging. *Chest* 111:1718–1723, 1997.
*All N2 nodes (single-digit designator) lie within the mediastinal pleural envelope.
†All N1 nodes lie distal to the mediastinal pleural reflection and within the visceral pleura.

Pleural metastases or MPE was changed from T4 (in the AJCC sixth edition) to M1 in the AJCC seventh edition. Patients previously categorized as a clinical T4 based on MPE, malignant pericardial effusions, or pleural nodules, are now categorized as clinical M1 based on poor survival more closely resembling patients with metastatic disease.

TABLE 57-2 American Joint Committee on Cancer Seventh Edition TNM Stage Groupings

				PERCENT (%) 5-YEAR SURVIVAL	
STAGE	T	N	M	CLINICAL STAGE	PATH STAGE
Occult cancer	TX	N0	M0	Not calculated	
Stage 0	Tis	N0	M0	Not calculated	
Stage IA	T1a/b	N0	M0	50	73
Stage IB	T2a	N0	M0	43	58
Stage IIA	T2b	N0	M0	36	46
	T1a/b; T2a	N1	M0		
Stage IIB	T2b	N1	M0	25	36
	T3	N0	M0		
Stage IIIA	Any T1; T2	N2	M0	19	24
	T3	N1/N2	M0		
	T4	N0/N1	M0		
Stage IIIB	T4	N2	M0	7	9
	Any T	N3	M0		
Stage IV	Any T	Any N	M1a/b	2	13

From Goldstraw P, Crowley J, Chansky K, et al: The IASLC Lung Cancer Staging Project: Proposals for the revision of the TNM stage groupings in the forthcoming (seventh) edition of the TNM Classification of malignant tumours. *J Thorac Oncol* 2:706–714, 2007; and Edge SB, Byrd DR, Compton CC, et al: *AJCC cancer staging manual*, ed 7, New York, 2010, Springer.

Lymph Nodes (N)

The nodal characteristics and designations did not change in the AJCC seventh edition.[47] T, N, and M characteristics as well as histologic type and survival were available for more than 67,000 patients. Clinical nodal staging information was available for 38,265 patients, and pathologic nodal staging information was available for 28,371 patients. Clinical staging studies included tests such as diagnostic imaging, CT, and mediastinoscopy. Thoracotomy for staging was excluded. PET was not widely used internationally in this cohort during this time. A new international lymph node map was proposed combining the integral aspects of the Japanese/Naruke and the North American/Mountain lymph node maps.[48] The authors proposed radiographic regions for the location of specific mediastinal lymph nodes, particularly for integration with CT, to guide the radiologic staging of patients with NSCLC.

Metastases (M)

Metastases were divided into M1a and M1b.[49] Patients with metastasis to the contralateral lung *only* were designated as M1a; metastases to regions outside the lung/pleura were designated as M1b. A second nodule in the nonprimary ipsilateral lobe, previously designated as M1, was changed to T4M0. In this situation, the patient received the "benefit of the doubt" approach, as this might represent a second primary.

Results of Treatment of Lung Cancer

The choice of initial therapy (whether single-modality or multimodality therapy) depends on the patient's clinical stage at presentation and the availability of prospective protocols. However,

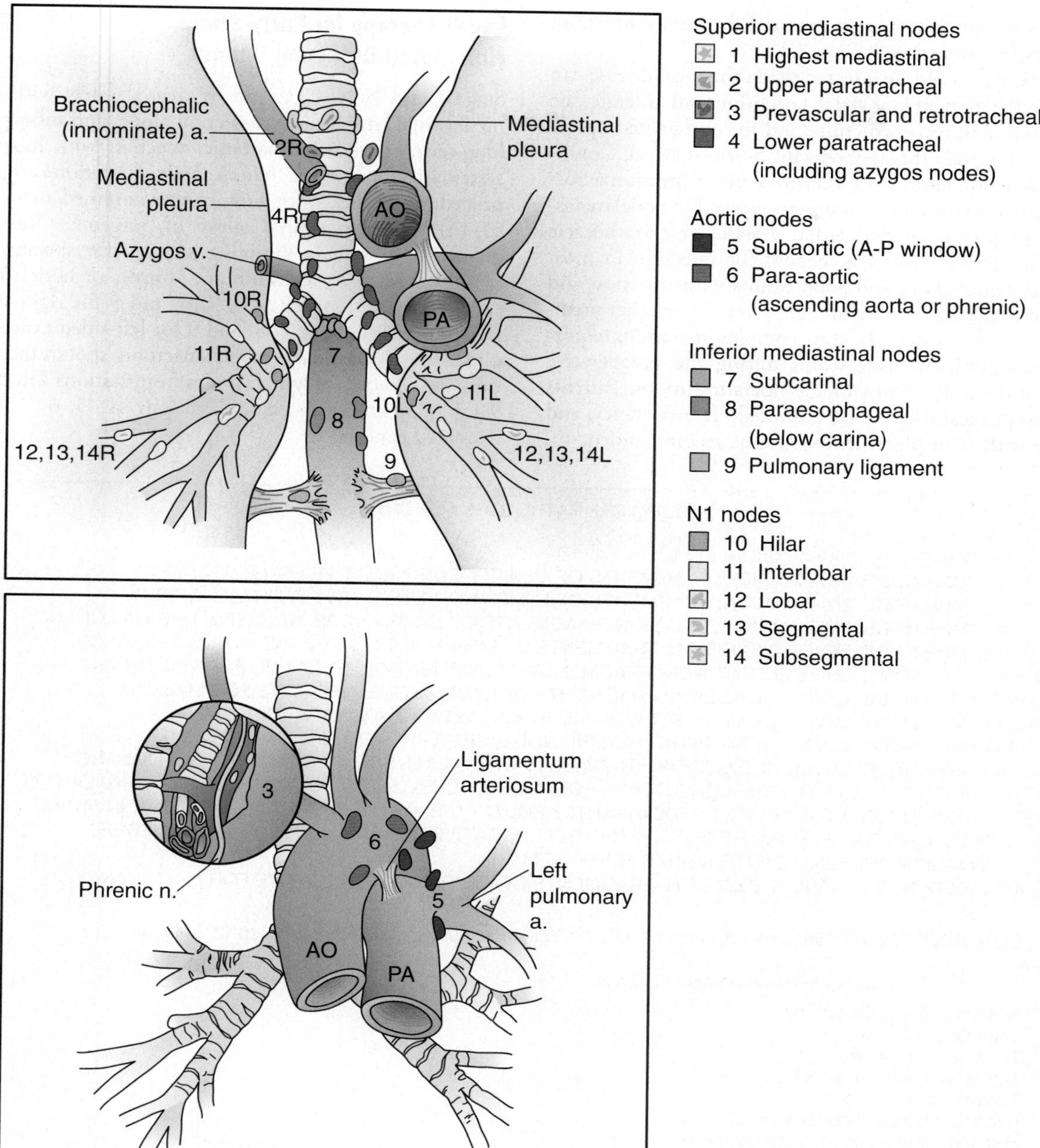

FIGURE 57-13 Regional lymph node station location. *AO*, Aorta; *A-P*, aortopulmonary; *PA*, pulmonary artery. (From Mountain CF, Libshitz HI, Hermes KE: *Lung cancer: a handbook for staging, imaging, and lymph node classification*, Houston, TX, 1999, Mountain, pp 1–71.)

treatment options may vary, even among different subsets of patients within the same clinical stage. Pretreatment staging is the critical step before initiating therapy. With current efforts, 5-year survival rates by pathologic stage are 73% for stage IA, 58% for stage IB, 46% for stage IIA, 36% for stage IIB, 24% for stage IIIA, 9% for stage IIIB, and 13% for stage IV.[31] Treatment for lung cancer can be roughly grouped into three major categories, as follows:

1. *Stage I* and *II* tumors are contained within the lung and may be completely resected with surgery. Stereotactic body radiation therapy has had good early results in selected patients not amenable to resection.[50]
2. *Stage IV* disease includes metastatic disease and is not typically treated by surgery except in patients requiring surgical palliation. Systemic therapies for metastatic disease are common. Targeted therapies have provided carefully screened patients with excellent results.
3. *Resectable stage IIIA* and *IIIB* tumors are locally advanced tumors with metastasis to the ipsilateral mediastinal (N2) lymph nodes (stage IIIA) or involving mediastinal structures (T4N0M0). These tumors, by their advanced nature, may be mechanically removed with surgery; however, surgery does not consistently control the micrometastases that exist within the general area of the operation or systemically. Combinations of

chemotherapy and radiotherapy are used for locally advanced disease or before resection.

Lung carcinoma should be resected when the local disease can be controlled, the patient's physical condition can tolerate the planned resection and reconstruction, and the anticipated operative mortality is less than the stage-specific 5-year survival. Conditions such as superior vena cava syndrome, tumor invasion across the mediastinum into the main pulmonary artery, N3 nodal metastases, malignant pleural or pericardial disease, or extrathoracic metastases carry greater risk than benefit for resection in most patients. Some centers have had good results with resection and reconstruction of the trachea, atrium, great vessels, or other mediastinal or vertebral structures. These are complex operations requiring dedicated multidisciplinary teams during the preoperative phase and multispecialty teams in the operating room. Patients with tracheoesophageal fistula have a limited life expectancy, and palliative care with stent placement would be recommended.

Local Therapy for Early-Stage Non–Small Cell Lung Cancer

Stage I and II NSCLC can be treated safely with surgery and mediastinal lymph node dissection alone, and most patients have long-term survival.[51] Anatomic resection with lobectomy, with systematic mediastinal lymph node dissection/sampling, is the procedure of choice for lung cancer confined to one lobe (Fig. 57-14). The American College of Surgeons Oncology Group defined a systematic sampling strategy for specific mediastinal lymph nodes.[52] At a minimum, samples of nodal (not adipose) tissue from stations 2R, 4R, 7, 8, and 9 for right-sided cancers and stations 4L, 5, 6, 7, 8, and 9 for left-sided cancers should be obtained. Mediastinal lymphadenectomy should include exploration and removal of lymph nodes from stations 2R, 4R, 7, 8, and 9 for right-sided cancers and stations 4L, 5, 6, 7, 8, and 9 for left-sided cancers.

SURGICAL PATHOLOGY REPORT

DIAGNOSIS:

1) LYMPH NODE, 4R, EXCISION: FRAGMENTS OF LYMPH NODE, NEGATIVE FOR MALIGNANCY.
2) LYMPH NODE, 2R, EXCISION: FRAGMENTS OF LYMPH NODE, NEGATIVE FOR MALIGNANCY.
3) LYMPH NODE, PRE-CARINAL, EXCISION: FRAGMENTS OF LYMPH NODE, NEGATIVE FOR MALIGNANCY.
4) LYMPH NODE, LEVEL 4, EXCISION: FRAGMENTS OF LYMPH NODE, NEGATIVE FOR MALIGNANCY.
5) LYMPHNODE, LEVEL 2L, EXCISION: FRAGMENTS OF LYMPH NODE, NEGATIVE FOR MALIGNANCY.
6) LYMPH NODE, LEVEL 7, EXCISION: FRAGMENTS OF LYMPH NODE, NEGATIVE FOR MALIGNANCY.
7) LYMPH NODE, LEVEL 8, EXCISION: INVOLVED BY METASTATIC ADENOCARCINOMA.
8) LYMPH NODE, LEVEL 11, EXCISION: 1 LYMPH NODE, NEGATIVE FOR MALIGNANCY (0/1).
9) LYMPH NODE, LEVEL 10, EXCISION: FRAGMENTS OF LYMPH NODE, NEGATIVE FOR MALIGNANCY.
10) LUNG, LEFT LOWER LOBE, LOBECTOMY: POORLY-DIFFERENTIATED ADENOCARCINOMA, SIMILAR TO PREVIOUS (SEE S10-37167), PREDOMINANTLY SOLID TYPE, 4.9 CM IN GREATEST EXTENT, INVADING INTO VISCERAL PLEURA; RESECTION MARGINS NEGATIVE FOR MALIGNANCY; LARGE VESSEL INVASION PRESENT; CENTRIACINAR EMPHYSEMA.
11) LYMPH NODE, LEVEL 5, EXCISION: FRAGMENTS OF LYMPH NODE, NEGATIVE FOR MALIGNANCY.

COMMENT: These findings correspond to AJCC 7th Edition pathologic Stage IIIA (pT2a, pN2, pM n/a).

Lung Carcinoma Summary Findings

Specimen Type: lobectomy
Laterality: left
Tumor site: lower lobe
Tumor size: 4.9 x 4.1 x 3.8 cm
Tumor focality: unifocal
Histologic type: adenocarcinoma
Histologic Grade: poorly-differentiated
Visceral Pleura Invasion: present (confirmed with elastin stain)
Direct extension of tumor: limited to lung and visceral pleura
Venous (large vessel invasion): present
Arterial (large vessel invasion): negative
Lymphatic (small vessel invasion): negative
Treatment effect: n/a

Margins: 1.1 cm from parenchymal margin

Ancillary testing:
EGFR mutational analysis: yes
KRAS mutational analysis: yes
Other (specify): ALK
Pathologic staging (pTNM): IIIA
Primary tumor: pT2a
Regional lymph nodes: pN2
Distant metastasis: pM n/a

FIGURE 57-14 Structured pathology report after left lower lobectomy. Lung carcinoma summary findings are helpful in identifying factors critical for pathologic staging and factors that may influence subsequent survival. Ancillary testing for mutational analysis of epidermal growth factor receptor (EGFR), KRAS, and ALK is done routinely.

Lesser operations such as wedge resection or segmentectomy may be considered for patients at greater risk for lobectomy. A prospective trial found no local control advantage for patients with wedge resection with brachytherapy radioactive iodine-131 threads placed at the suture line compared with wedge resection alone.[53] Patients with NSCLC that invades into the chest wall may undergo resection with lobectomy with en bloc chest wall resection.

Stereotactic body radiation therapy is another local control modality.[50] Treatment with 54 Gy in three fractions appears to be well tolerated with good early results. Prospective clinical trials, such as ACOSOG Z4099/RTOG 1021, were initiated to evaluate high-risk patients (unable to tolerate a lobectomy) with early-stage NSCLC randomly assigned to wedge resection or stereotactic body radiation therapy. This and other similar trials closed early without sufficient accrual to answer this important question.

Neoadjuvant and Adjuvant Therapy

Advanced stage lung cancer, particularly with nodal spread, cannot typically be considered a disease effectively treated with a single modality. Survival after resection may be improved in selected patients with adjuvant chemotherapy. The International Adjuvant Lung Trial[54] enrolled 1867 patients with completely resected stage I to III NSCLC. These patients were randomly assigned to observation or chemotherapy. Radiation therapy was at the discretion of the institution. The treatment group received one of four cisplatin-based doublet adjuvant regimens.[55] Survival was increased 5% in the adjuvant chemotherapy group. All patients staged IB and IIB should be considered for adjuvant chemotherapy after resection, and this should be discussed with a medical oncologist.

Surgery alone for stage IIIA (N2), IIIB, or IV lung cancer is infrequently performed; however, selected patients may benefit from a multidisciplinary approach to treatment.[56] Resection for isolated brain metastasis is warranted for improvement in symptoms, quality of life, and survival rate. The primary lung tumor can be treated according to T and N stage. Additional treatment beyond resection is needed.

Even with complete resection, patients with resectable NSCLC have poor survival. Preoperative therapy (induction or neoadjuvant) has been evaluated: Preoperative paclitaxel and carboplatin followed by surgery was compared with surgery alone in patients with early-stage NSCLC. Median overall survival was 41 months in the surgery-only arm and 62 months in the preoperative chemotherapy arm (hazard ratio, 0.79; 95% confidence interval, 0.60 to 1.06; $P = .11$). Median progression-free survival was 20 months for surgery alone and 33 months for preoperative chemotherapy (hazard ratio, 0.80; 95% confidence interval, 0.61 to 1.04; $P = .10$). Overall survival and progression-free survival were higher with preoperative chemotherapy, although the differences did not reach statistical significance.[57]

Induction chemoradiotherapy has been evaluated for treatment of clinical stage IIIA (N2) NSCLC.[58] In one phase III trial, concurrent chemotherapy and radiotherapy followed by resection was compared with standard concurrent chemotherapy and definitive radiotherapy without resection. The median overall survival was similar in both groups (~23 months). Progression-free survival was better in the surgery group (12.8 months median versus 10.5 months; $P = .017$). The authors reported pneumonectomy was associated with poor outcomes. In an exploratory analysis, overall survival was improved for patients who were found to have undergone induction chemoradiotherapy and lobectomy. In selected patients with resectable stage IIIA NSCLC, induction chemoradiotherapy followed by resection is an alternative treatment to chemoradiotherapy alone.[56]

Patients with local extension of lung cancer at the apex of the lung into the thoracic inlet may have characteristics of shoulder and arm pain, Horner syndrome, and occasionally paresthesia in the ulnar nerve distribution of the hand (fourth and fifth fingers) (Fig. 57-15). Patients with all these characteristics may be classified as having Pancoast syndrome. Pain comes from the C8 and T1 nerve roots. Sympathetic nerve involvement may result in Horner syndrome (miosis, ptosis, anhidrosis, and enophthalmos). Typically, the first, second, and third ribs are involved and require resection, but the bony spine and intraforaminal spaces can also be involved. MRI is necessary, in addition to CT, to plan the surgical procedure. Preoperative therapy includes chemoradiotherapy.[59,60]

Treatment of Metastatic Disease

Metastatic disease (stage IV NSCLC) is usually incurable.[61] Performance and quality of life decline. Patients and families should be informed of the diagnosis and potential outcomes of treatment. Treatment decisions should take into consideration the wishes of the patient and family, and realistic expectations should be set and monitored during therapy.

Combination chemotherapy with platinum doublets has been well tolerated and associated with a modest improvement in survival rates.[55] The addition of bevacizumab (a monoclonal antibody to the vascular endothelial growth factor receptor) to paclitaxel and carboplatin improved survival compared with treatment with paclitaxel and carboplatin alone.[62] Induction chemotherapy followed by radiation appears to improve survival rate in patients with locally advanced unresectable lung cancer. In these studies, cisplatin-based combination chemotherapy was shown to improve expected survival over and above survival achieved with radiation alone.

Additional strategies to identify the molecular characteristics of the tumor as part of the initial staging could also improve survival by creating better models for treatments of NSCLC. As a result of advances in tumor biology, predictive markers of response to epidermal growth factor receptor (EGFR) inhibitors[63] and ALK (a chimeric protein originally identified in anaplastic large cell lymphoma) receptors have become available.[64] These studies focused efforts to target specific genetic mutations in a patient's specific lung cancer. Mutations in EGFR strongly predict the response to EGFR tyrosine kinase inhibitors. In addition, there is improved outcome for patients with adenocarcinoma treated with pemetrexed. Clinical trials have shown significant progression-free survival in patients with metastatic NSCLC treated with gefitinib and platinum-based doublet chemotherapy compared with chemotherapy alone.[65,66] Targeted therapies in addition to current chemotherapeutic regimens, or alone, may limit toxicity and improve outcomes compared with the current chemotherapeutic regimens. In 2015, the U.S. Food and Drug Administration approved gefitinib for first-line treatment of patients with metastatic NSCLC with the most common types of EGFR mutations (exon 19 deletions or exon 21 L858R substitution gene mutations).[67] In addition, several clinical trials are evaluating various antibodies that target the PD-1 pathway (programmed cell death protein 1) and the PDL1 (programmed death ligand-1) and provide a "checkpoint blockade" inhibiting further cancer progression.[68]

Quality-of-life issues arise in patients with metastatic NSCLC. Dyspnea from MPE, superior vena cava syndrome, tracheoesophageal fistula, bone metastases, and pain occur. Nutrition and

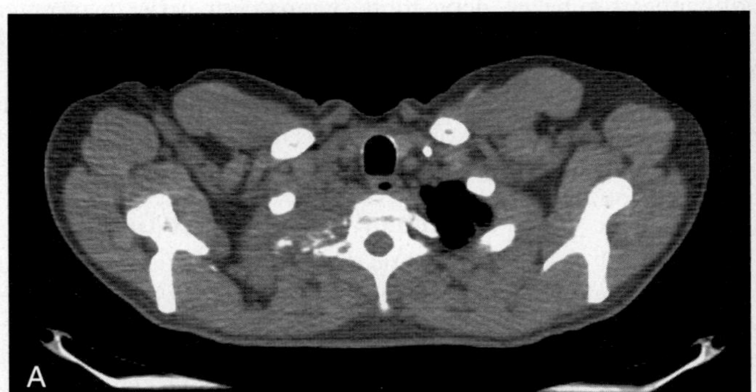

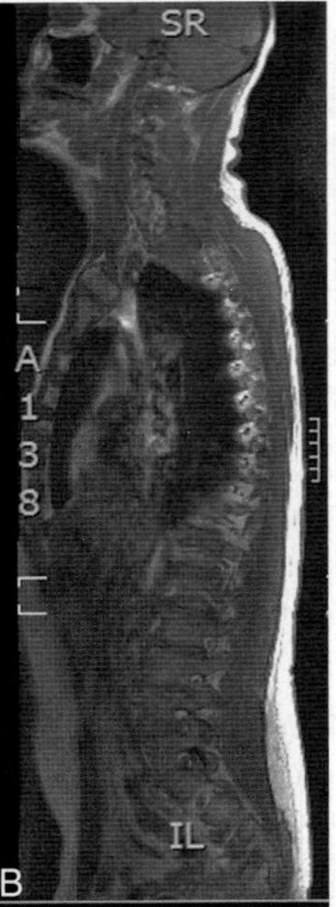

FIGURE 57-15 The patient is a 50-year-old man with a right superior sulcus tumor. Diagnostic imaging revealed a right apical mass and destruction of the posterior aspect of the second rib. Transthoracic biopsy was positive for poorly differentiated adenocarcinoma (non–small cell lung carcinoma). Endobronchial ultrasound for mediastinal staging was negative; cervical mediastinoscopy was also negative. Induction chemoradiotherapy was given with 48 Gy in 24 fractions over 1 month with chemotherapy (carboplatin AUC of 5 + pemetrexed 500 mg/m^2). **A,** Computed tomography (CT) scan of the chest demonstrates the mass is present in the apex of the chest with complete destruction of the posterior aspect of the right second rib and cortical erosion of the right T2 vertebral body secondary to the mass. The patient is left hand–dominant. **B,** Magnetic resonance imaging of the thoracic spine demonstrates a medial right apical lung mass, consistent with a Pancoast tumor involving the right lateral aspect of the T2 vertebral body, articular facet, and transverse process. There was also extension into the neural foramen and involvement of the nerve roots on the right at T1-2 and T2-3. There was no extension into the central canal or involvement of the spinal cord. CT scan of the head demonstrated no acute findings involving the brain. Complete resection was performed with a two-surgeon team, a thoracic surgeon and neurosurgeon. The patient required a right upper lobectomy with en bloc chest wall and vertebral body resection and mediastinal lymph node dissection. Spine stabilization was required.

hydration are significant issues. Palliation from symptoms may be accomplished with good results.[27,69]

TRACHEA

The position of the trachea can be up to 50% cervical with hyperextension in a young patient. The location of the carina is at the level of the angle of Louis anteriorly and the T4 vertebra posteriorly. Stenosis of the trachea implies significant functional impairment. A normal 2-cm trachea has a 100% peak expiratory flow rate. A 10-mm opening provides an 80% peak expiratory flow rate. At 5 to 6 mm, only a 30% expiratory flow rate is obtained. Tracheostomy is one of the most commonly performed operations. Percutaneous tracheostomy is frequently performed,[70] although open procedures may be selected. Infection and inflammation are uncommon causes of tracheal obstruction.

Primary neoplasms of the trachea[71] include SCC in approximately two thirds of patients and adenoid cystic carcinoma in other patients. SCC may be focal, diffuse, or multiple. The physical appearance may be exophytic or ulcerative. One third of these primary tracheal tumors have extensive local spread or metastases at initial presentation. Resection can be performed with excellent results.[72] Adenoid cystic carcinoma (previously called *cylindroma*) has a propensity for intramural and perineural spread. In adenoid cystic carcinoma, negative margins are important. Margin evaluation with frozen-section control is performed for stricture resection. Clinical features include dyspnea on exertion, wheezing, cough with or without hemoptysis, and recurrent pulmonary infections.

Involvement of the trachea because of local extension from bronchogenic carcinoma may contraindicate resection. Involvement of the trachea because of local extension of esophageal carcinoma may require palliative therapy or stent placement.

Tracheal Trauma

Penetrating injuries to the trachea are usually cervical and may involve the esophagus. Concurrent esophageal injury needs to be excluded by barium esophagography or esophagoscopy. Neck exploration may be required. Blunt trauma to the neck or trachea can produce lacerations, transections, or shattering injuries of both the cervical and the mediastinal trachea. Clinical features of a tracheal injury are suggested by subcutaneous air in the neck, respiratory distress, and hemoptysis. Diagnosis is made by bronchoscopy. Anesthetic management with laryngeal mask airway may be helpful for initial examination for full visualization of the airway before endotracheal intubation. Primary repair of tracheal injury may be accomplished with cervical exploration. Bronchial disruption may require thoracotomy for repair. Right thoracotomy provides excellent visualization of the carina and proximal left mainstem bronchus.

Postintubation tracheal stenosis may occur because of laryngeal or tracheal irritation from an indwelling endotracheal tube. Low-pressure cuffs on the endotracheal tube have reduced pressure necrosis. Tracheal stenosis may manifest with dyspnea on exertion, stridor or wheezing (which is easily noted), and sometimes episodes of obstruction by small amounts of mucus. Emergency management of obstruction may include sedation, humidified air, or racemic epinephrine by nebulizer. Dilation under general anesthesia may be helpful.

Acquired tracheoesophageal fistula can occur from cancer or from prolonged intubation with erosion posteriorly. Repair is with separation of the trachea and esophagus, repair of the fistulous tract, and interposition of normal tissue such as muscle between the two structures.

Tracheoinnominate fistula may result from prolonged cuff erosion inferiorly and anteriorly in the trachea. Inappropriate low stoma may further increase the likelihood of a direct erosion of the trachea by the innominate artery. The tip of the endotracheal tube may predispose to erosions or granulomas within the trachea. Tracheoinnominate fistula may manifest with a sentinel hemorrhage before sudden exsanguinating hemorrhage. Investigation of these sentinel hemorrhage episodes is critical. Evaluation in the operating room may provide for optimal situational control should additional interventions be required.

The surgical management of tracheal problems may be complex. General inhalational anesthesia is used, and induction may take a long time if the stenosis is tight. The patient should be maintained spontaneously breathing if possible. If the stenosis is less than 5 to 6 mm, dilation may be required before passing the endotracheal tube; the dilation may be performed with rigid bronchoscopy. If the stenosis is greater than 5 to 6 mm, the endotracheal tube may be positioned to a point above the stricture for induction. Stenoses that are subglottic must be dilated for intubation. The endotracheal tube often goes alongside tumors.

The cervical approach for tracheal resection is usually used for tumors of the upper half of the trachea plus all benign tracheal stenoses (because these usually occur as a result of endotracheal tube placement). Occasionally, an upper sternal split may be needed (Fig. 57-16). The posterolateral thoracotomy (fourth interspace) is used for tumors of the lower half of the trachea plus

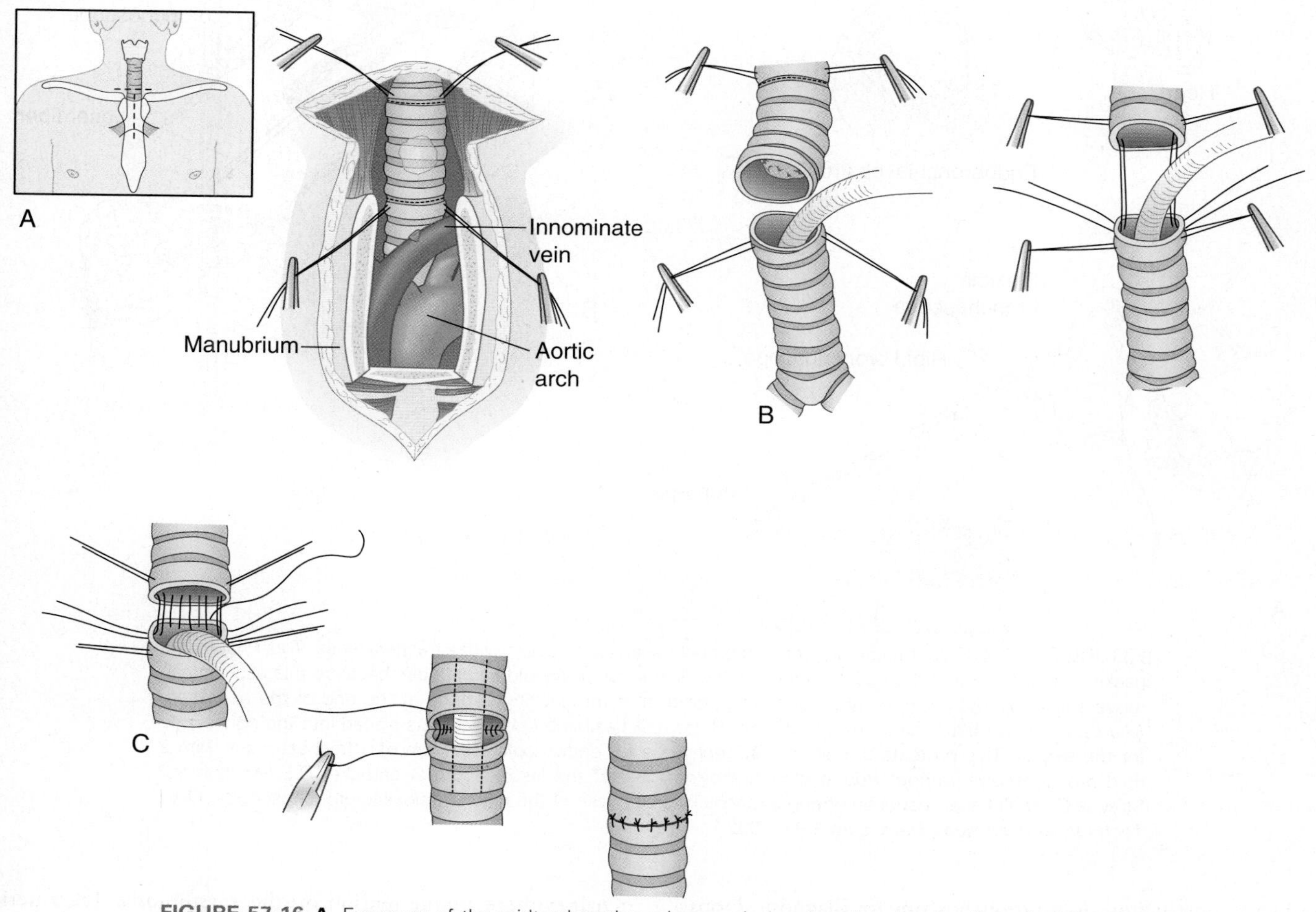

FIGURE 57-16 **A,** Exposure of the midtrachea through a cervical and partial sternal-splitting incision. The extent of the resection has been marked by sutures. **B,** After distal division, a sterile, armored endotracheal tube is placed. After proximal resection, two mattress sutures are placed in the edges of the cartilaginous rings. A simple running suture completes the membranous anastomosis. **C,** At this point, the original endotracheal tube is positioned in the distal trachea so that the anastomosis can be completed with interrupted simple sutures between cartilaginous rings.

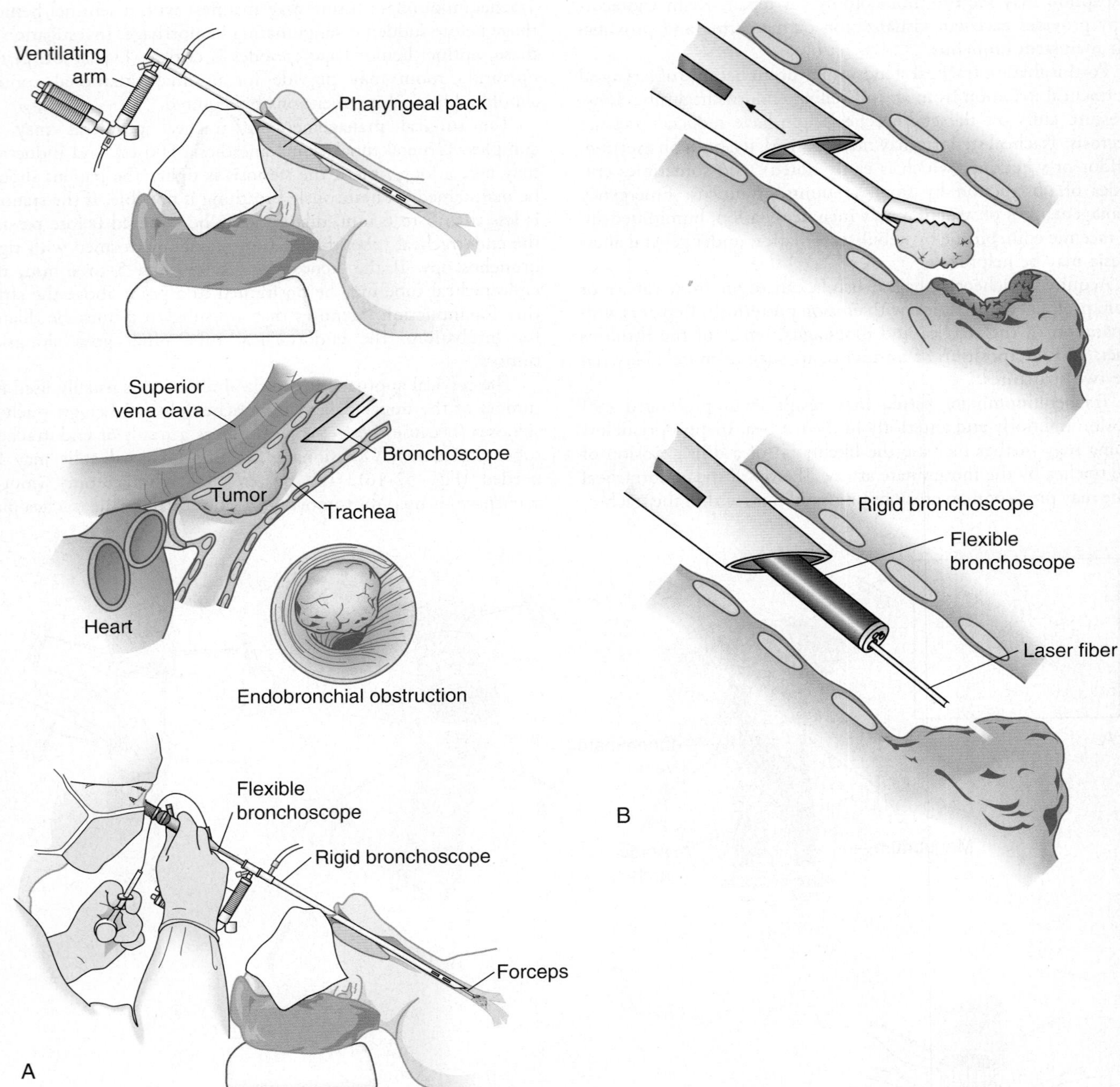

FIGURE 57-17 A, Proper technique for rigid bronchoscopy in a patient with a tracheal mass. *Top,* Pharyngeal packing used to protect the esophagus is shown. The surgeon should be cautious because this packing can move and may obstruct the larynx. Complete removal of the packing is done at the end of the operation. *Middle,* A nearly obstructing tumor is shown. *Bottom,* A flexible bronchoscope is placed into the rigid scope for the biopsy. This protects the airway. **B,** Technique for endoscopic resection of a tracheal mass with a rigid bronchoscope without *(top)* and with *(bottom)* use of the laser. (From Sugarbaker DJ, Mentzer SJ, Strauss G, et al: Laser resection of endobronchial lesions: Use of the rigid and flexible bronchoscopes. *Oper Tech Otolaryngol Head Neck Surg* 3:93, 1992.)

carinal reconstruction. Rigid bronchoscopy for diagnosis, biopsy, dilation, or morcellation of tumor or other treatment may be required if the tumor cannot be immediately resected (Fig. 57-17).

In general, the maximal amount of trachea that can be resected is approximately 5 cm, but this varies from person to person. Various techniques are used to mobilize the trachea to create a repair without undue tension on the anastomosis. The anterior cervical approach plus mobilization of the trachea and neck flexion can allow for 4 to 5 cm of trachea resection. A suprahyoid release may achieve 1 cm of additional length. Mobilization of the right hilum, together with division of the pericardium around the right hilum, may achieve an additional 1.4 cm.

Stenosis of the subglottic larynx or cricoid stenosis is a challenging technical procedure. The recurrent nerves innervate the larynx just superior to the posterolateral cricoid on each side. If the tracheal lesions involve only the anterior surface, the anterior cricoid can be removed and the distal trachea beveled to match the defect. This maneuver spares the recurrent laryngeal nerves. With circumferential involvement, it may be necessary to perform a laryngectomy.

Reconstruction of the lower trachea is performed in the right fourth intercostal space. Intubation of the distal trachea or the left mainstem is performed. Carinal reconstruction is usually performed for tumor and is the most feasible of alternative reconstructions chosen.

Contraindications to trachea repair include (1) inadequately treated laryngeal problem (which does not include single vocal cord paralysis); (2) need for ventilatory support or permanent tracheostomy for patients with amyotrophic lateral sclerosis, myasthenia gravis, or quadriplegia; (3) use of high-dose steroids; and (4) inflamed or recent tracheostomy. Poor pulmonary reserve is not a contraindication for repair in patients who have been weaned from the ventilator.

PULMONARY INFECTIONS

Pulmonary infections requiring surgical interventions are infrequent compared with pleural space infections. Clinical features are similar to pneumonia, including fever, cough, leukocytosis, pleuritic pain, and sputum production. The patient is specifically questioned about aspiration of a foreign body. Evaluation includes CXR and CT scan of the chest and upper abdomen. Bronchoscopy can be performed to clear secretions and, when the diagnosis is suspected, to rule out cancer, foreign body, bronchial stenosis, or stricture. Cultures may be obtained to facilitate antibiotic treatment. Medical treatment is optimized; this includes discontinuation of smoking and institution of postural drainage, bronchodilator medications, and oral antibiotics.

Bronchiectasis

Bronchiectasis is an infection of the bronchial wall and surrounding lung with sufficient severity to cause destruction and dilation of the air passages. As a result of the use of antibiotics, this condition is decreasing in frequency and severity. There are numerous predisposing factors, including cystic fibrosis; α_1-antitrypsin deficiency; various immunodeficiency states; Kartagener syndrome (sinusitis, bronchiectasis, situs inversus, and hypomotile cilia); and bronchial obstruction from foreign body, extrinsic lymph nodes that compress the bronchus, neoplasm, or mucous plug. The distribution is primarily in the basal segments of the lower lobes. Destructive changes and dilation of the bronchi accompany the infection. Massive hemoptysis is rare. Symptoms frequently can be controlled with medical management, such as long-term antibiotic therapy and postural drainage. Disease limited to one lobe is best treated surgically. If bilateral bronchiectasis exists, medical management is continued.

Lung Abscess

The incidence of lung abscess is decreasing in frequency as a result of use of antibiotics. A lung abscess may occur from an infection behind a blocked bronchus. *Staphylococcus* bacteremia is frequently associated with lung abscess. Necrotizing pneumonia from *Klebsiella* spp. may rapidly destroy the involved lung with minimal surrounding reaction. Rupture of a lung abscess may yield empyema and pneumothorax. Lung abscess may also be superimposed on structural abnormalities, such as a bronchogenic cyst, sequestration, bleb, or tuberculous or fungal cavities. CXR and CT scan of the chest may demonstrate an air-fluid level within the abscess cavity.

The differential diagnosis of a mediastinal or thoracic air-fluid level includes loculated empyema, epiphrenic diverticulum, tuberculous or fungal cavity, or a cavitary lung cancer (usually SCC). Tubercular and fungus cavities do not retain fluid, so no air-fluid level is present; however, they may contain debris or a fungus ball. *Aspergillus* spp. infection may manifest in this manner. Medical management is with antibiotics and pulmonary care (e.g., reexpansion). Bronchoscopy may be used for treatment to assist in drainage of the cavity either directly or via transbronchial catheterization of the cavity. Most patients (85% to 95%) respond to medical management with rapid decrease in fluid, collapse of the walls, and complete healing in 3 to 4 months. Patients with symptoms for longer than 3 months before treatment or cavities larger than 4 to 6 cm are less likely to respond.

Surgical therapy is indicated for persistent cavity (≥2 cm and thick-walled), failure to clear sepsis after 8 weeks of medical therapy, hemoptysis, and exclusion of cancer. If a lung abscess ruptures into the pleural cavity, simple drainage may suffice, and the patient is managed for empyema or bronchopleural fistula. Lobectomy is typically required; the mortality rate is 1% to 5%. Occasionally, external drainage may be required in critically ill patients if pleural symphysis has occurred.

Other Bronchopulmonary Disorders

Bronchopulmonary disorders caused by inflammatory lymph node disease are usually caused by tuberculosis or histoplasmosis. Lobar atelectasis, hemoptysis, or broncholithiasis can occur. Bronchial compressive disease typically occurs most commonly in the middle lobe. More than 20% of disorders are caused by cancer. This condition results in repeated infection in the same area of the lung, which usually responds to antibiotics. Bronchoscopy is essential to rule out cancer and foreign body and to evaluate for stricture. Medical management is required to treat infection. Surgery is indicated to treat bronchostenosis, irreversible bronchiectasis, or severe recurrent infection.

Broncholithiasis is a calcified node tightly adherent to a bronchus. An innocent hemoptysis may occur even with a negative CXR. Sudden bleeding caused by erosion of a small bronchial artery and mucosa by a spicule in the calcified node causes this hemoptysis. Bright red blood occurs and usually stops with sedation and antitussive therapy. This type of hemoptysis is almost never massive (≥600 mL in 24 hours). Bronchoscopy is possible during a bleeding episode to localize the site of the bleeding. Nasal or pharyngeal lesions or hematemesis from a gastrointestinal source should be excluded.

Organizing pneumonia may replace lung parenchyma with scar tissue or persistent atelectasis or consolidation. If the shadow or mass persists over 6 to 8 weeks, resection is performed to exclude carcinoma. The differential diagnosis includes pneumonia, congenital abnormality, and aneurysm of the aorta.

Mycobacterial Infections

Mycobacterium tuberculosis infects approximately 7% of patients exposed, and tuberculosis develops in 5% to 10% of patients who are infected. A primary infection develops. The exudative response progresses to caseous necrosis. Postprimary tuberculosis tends to occur in apical and posterior segments of the upper lobes and superior segments of the lower lobes. Healing occurs with fibrosis and contracture. Extensive caseation with cavitation may occur early. Coalescing areas of caseous necrosis may form cavities. There are frequently incomplete septations and lobulations. Erosions of septations supplied by bronchial arteries cause hemoptysis and may be secondarily infected.

Medical management is with isoniazid, rifampin, ethambutol, streptomycin, and pyrazinamide.[73] Bronchoscopy may be required for patients who do not respond to medical management. Cancer should be excluded for a newly identified mass on CXR even with a positive tuberculosis skin test and acid-fast bacillus–positive sputum.

Surgical therapy may be considered when medical therapy fails and persistent tuberculosis-positive sputum remains and when surgically correctable residua of tuberculosis may be of potential danger to the patient.[74,75] This is not the same management as for atypical mycobacteria; many of these patients remain clinically well even with positive sputum. Indications for surgery include the following:

1. Open positive cavity after 3 to 6 months of chemotherapy, especially if resistant mycobacteria.
2. Destroyed lung, atelectasis, bronchiectasis, or bronchostenosis that is amenable to resection.
3. Open negative cavities if thick-walled, slow response, or unreliable patient.
4. Exclusion of cancer.
5. Recurrent or persistent hemoptysis if greater than 600 mL of blood is lost in 24 hours or less.

Surgical options include resection with preservation of good lung tissue. Surgical complications are doubled if the sputum is positive for *M. tuberculosis* and decreased if remaining lung tissue is fully expanded within the chest. Infectious complications include empyema, bronchopleural fistula, and endobronchial spread of the disease and are associated with a higher mortality rate. Tuberculosis infection of the pleural space without lung destruction is primarily treated medically.

Thoracoplasty or muscle flap interposition may be used to control postresection empyema space. Collapse therapy, with thoracoplasty or plombage, is rarely used to manage parenchymal disease alone.

Fungal and Parasitic Infections

The surgical management of fungal infections includes diagnosis and management of complications of fungal disease. Frequently, cancer has to be excluded or other infectious or benign conditions have to be confirmed. Medical management may be considered as initial treatment of fungal diseases in the lung and as part of the patient's overall management.

Immunocompromised patients experience *Aspergillus* spp. infection as the most frequent opportunistic infection followed by *Candida* and *Nocardia* spp. and mucormycosis. Normal, or immunocompetent, patients may be affected by histoplasmosis, coccidioidomycosis, or blastomycosis. Immunocompromised and immunocompetent patients may be affected by actinomycosis and cryptococcosis. Although *Nocardia* and *Actinomyces* spp. are bacteria, they are usually discussed with fungal infections. Diagnosis is most often made by sputum examination using potassium hydroxide preparations (Fig. 57-18). Cultures may take some time for results to be obtained; Papanicolaou test cytology may be best. Silver methenamine stain is used for microscopic evaluation. Most infections are self-limited and do not require treatment. Intravenous or oral antifungal agents may be used for treatment of the diseases.

Aspergillosis is an opportunistic infection, characterized by coarse fragmented septa and hyphae (see Fig. 57-18*A*). There are three types of aspergillosis: aspergilloma, invasive pulmonary aspergillosis, and allergic bronchopulmonary aspergillosis. Aspergilloma is the most common form of aspergillosis. The fungus colonizes an existing lung cavity, commonly a tuberculosis cavity. CXR may demonstrate a crescent radiolucency next to a rounded mass. Cavities may form because of destruction of the underlying pulmonary parenchyma, and debris and hyphae may coalesce and form a fungus ball, which lies free in the cavity and can move with the patient's change in position. Invasion and destruction of parenchymal blood vessels occur within this cavity. Patients with aspergilloma fungus balls are at high risk for fatal hemorrhage; they are treated aggressively and undergo resection when possible.[76] Involvement and destruction of parenchymal blood vessels occur. Prophylactic resection is controversial, although some physicians recommend resection if isolated disease is present in low-risk patients. Surgery is indicated for treatment, for massive or recurrent hemoptysis, or to rule out neoplasm. The procedure of choice is lobectomy. The operation can be complex with a significant inflammatory response within the hilum. Invasive aspergillosis occurs in immunocompromised patients and manifests with chest pain, cough, and hemoptysis. The treatment is primarily medical, although lung biopsy may be necessary for diagnosis. Allergic aspergillosis is diagnosed by bronchoscopy and represents the allergic reaction to chronic colonization with the fungus. It is usually treated medically. Rarely, resection is performed for localized bronchiectasis.

Histoplasmosis is the most common of all fungal infections in the United States and is most frequently a serious systemic fungal disease. *Histoplasma capsulatum* is endemic to the Mississippi and Ohio River valleys as well as portions of the southwestern United States. A high percentage of patients are affected usually with a subclinical form of this disease. An inoculum (from the mycelial form found in soil, decaying materials, and bat or bird guano) can produce an acute pneumonic illness in immunocompetent hosts, which usually resolves without specific treatment. The yeast form exists in macrophages or within the cytoplasm of the alveoli. Pathologic examination demonstrates granulomas (e.g., tuberculosis) or caseating epithelioid granulomas. The lymphogenous reaction to *Histoplasma* causes mediastinal lymph node enlargement, middle lobe syndrome, bronchiectasis, esophageal traction diverticulum, broncholithiasis with hemoptysis, tracheoesophageal fistula, constrictive pericarditis, or fibrosing mediastinitis with superior vena cava syndrome or other problems relating to compression of mediastinal structures. In addition to the compressive symptoms, the lymphadenopathy caused by histoplasmosis may confound radiographic evaluation of the mediastinal lymph nodes in patients with lung cancer and may complicate lung resection.

Coccidioidomycosis is endemic to the Southwest and is localized in the soil. It is second only to histoplasmosis in frequency. Inhaling the organism results in a primary lung disease that is usually self-limited (see Fig. 57-18*B*). In endemic areas, coccidioidomycosis is a frequent cause of lung nodules, and resection may be required to rule out malignancy. Medical management is preferred. Surgery may be considered for treatment of cavitary disease or complications of cavitary disease.

Cryptococcosis is the second most common lethal fungus after histoplasmosis. Lungs are frequently involved. Central nervous

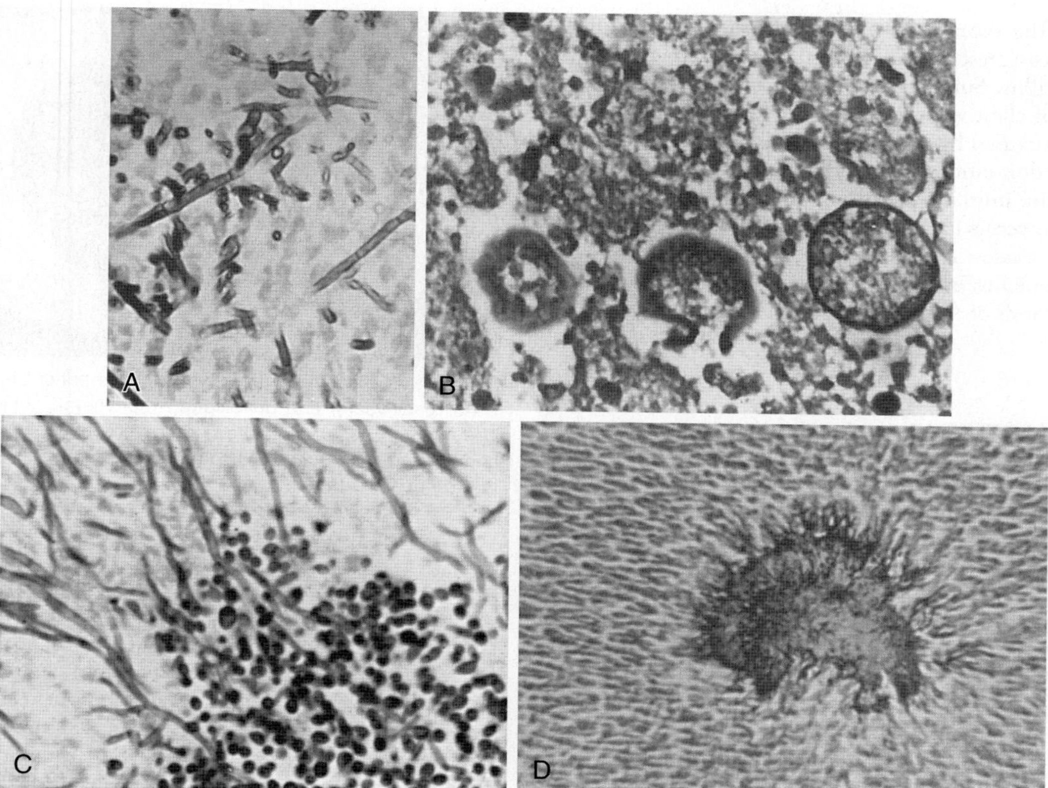

FIGURE 57-18 A, The coarse, fragmented, septate mycelia of *Aspergillus fumigatus*. **B,** Microscopic section of a coccidioidal granuloma (×400) shows spherules packed with endospores. **C,** *Candida albicans* with both the mycelial and the yeast forms. **D,** Actinomycotic granule shows branching filaments of a microscopic colony of *Actinomyces israelii*. (Gomori stain, ×250.) (**A** and **C,** From Takaro T: Thoracic mycotic infections. In *Lewis' practice of surgery*, New York, 1968, Hoeber Medical Division, Harper & Row; **B,** from Scott S, Takaro T: Thoracic mycotic and actinomycotic infections. In Shields TW, editor: *General thoracic surgery*, ed 4, Baltimore, 1994, Williams & Wilkins.)

system involvement with meningitis is the most frequent cause of death. Any patient diagnosed with pulmonary cryptococcosis undergoes lumbar puncture to rule out central nervous system involvement. Surgery may be required for open lung biopsy for diagnosis or to exclude lung cancer.

Mucormycosis is a rare, opportunistic, rapidly progressive infection; it occurs in immunocompromised patients, including patients with diabetes. The appearance is that of a black mold; it has wide nonseptate branching hyphae. The infection causes blood vessels to thrombose and lung tissue to infarct. Clinically, the rhinocerebral form occurs much more frequently than the pulmonary form of consolidation and cavities. Medical management involves cessation of steroids and antineoplastic drugs and initiation of amphotericin and control of diabetes. The disease is often too advanced for effective treatment. Aggressive surgical and medical treatment may improve what is usually a grave prognosis.

Candida is a small, thin-walled budding yeast that occurs in immunocompromised patients (see Fig. 57-18*C*). Lung involvement alone is rare. Surgery may be needed to confirm the diagnosis.

Pneumocystis carinii is an opportunistic infection that is positive on silver methenamine stain. Bronchoalveolar lavage is diagnostic in more than 90% of patients. However, lung biopsy may be required to confirm the diagnosis.

Surgery may also be used to manage the sequelae and complications of parasitic infections. Infections with *Entamoeba histolytica* are usually confined to the right lower thorax and are related to extension from a liver abscess below the diaphragm via direct extension or lymphatics to the right thorax. Metronidazole (Flagyl) is usually effective, although Flagyl and tube drainage may be required for treatment of empyema. Open resection is infrequently required. Similarly, infection with *Echinococcus* spp. may occur. The hydatid cyst may rupture, flooding the lung or producing a severe hypersensitivity reaction. A lung abscess could occur with compression of the airway, great vessels, or esophagus. Surgery, if feasible, may include simple enucleation via cleavage of planes between the cyst and the normal tissue. Aspiration and hypertonic saline 10% may be performed before enucleation. Positive pressure on the lung needs to be maintained until the cyst is out to prevent contamination, soilage, or hypersensitivity reaction. Nonoperative therapy for small asymptomatic calcified cysts may be considered. Paragonimiasis is another common infection and cause of hemoptysis in Asia. In endemic areas, prevalence may be 5%, and hemoptysis from paragonimiasis must be differentiated from tuberculosis or lung cancer.[77]

Actinomycosis is a bacterium that is not found free in nature. It produces a chronic anaerobic endogenous infection deep within a wound. "Sulfur granules" draining from infected sinuses are microcolonies (see Fig. 57-18*D*). The cervicofacial form is the most common. The thoracic form usually occurs as pulmonary parenchymal disease resembling cancer. The treatment is most commonly penicillin. Surgery may occasionally be required for radical excision of chest wall disease and empyema.

Nocardiosis is caused by an aerobic bacterium widely disseminated in soil and domestic animals; it was formerly rare, although it is increasing in immunocompromised patients. Nocardiosis resembles actinomycosis in invading the chest wall and produces subcutaneous abscesses and sinuses draining sulfur granules. Surgery is performed to exclude cancer, to obtain a diagnosis, or to treat complications of the disease. Medical therapy may include sulfonamides.

MASSIVE HEMOPTYSIS

Massive hemoptysis may be defined as greater than 500 to 600 mL of blood loss from the lungs in 24 hours.[78] However, the proximal airways may be occluded with only 150 mL of clotted blood, and even lower volume hemoptysis may be life-threatening.[79] The current mortality rate is approximately 13% and is related to drowning or suffocation rather than exsanguination. Diagnosis and treatment of massive hemoptysis typically include a CXR and emergency rigid bronchoscopy.[80] The major causes of massive hemoptysis are tuberculosis, bronchiectasis, and cancer. Flexible bronchoscopy is usually inadequate for treatment of hemoptysis, but it may be considered for diagnosis, localization of the source of the bleeding, or observation if active bleeding has stopped. Rigid bronchoscopy is recommended.[80,81] Mortality is high with urgent or emergency resection. Conservative management may consist of maintaining a functional and patent airway, bronchoscopy, clearing the airway of blood, cough suppression (with codeine), and monitoring until stabilized.

Angiographic catheterization for massive hemoptysis may be considered in patients with hemoptysis.[82,83] Risks include spinal cord ischemia and paralysis. Small particles of polyvinyl alcohol or other synthetic materials used for embolization occlude vessels at a peripheral level. Embolization may be repeated.

EMPHYSEMA AND DIFFUSE LUNG DISEASE

Emphysema

Emphysema is defined as dilation and destruction of the terminal air spaces. These air cavities are blebs (subpleural air space separated from the lung by a thin pleural covering with only minor alveolar communications) or bullae (larger than a bleb with some destruction of the underlying lung parenchyma). Bullous emphysema (Fig. 57-19) is either congenital without general lung disease or a complication of COPD with more or less generalized lung disease. The challenge is to separate the disability related to the bullae from that caused by the chronic emphysema or chronic bronchitis. DLCO is a good index of the state of severity of the generalized lung disease. On pulmonary angiography, bullae are vacant and do not contain vessels. The bullae may compress normal lung with crowding of the relatively normal pulmonary vasculature. COPD may show abrupt narrowing and tapering of vessels. Surgical therapy includes resection of the bullae to leave functioning lung tissue. Simple removal of the bullae alone is required. Lobectomy is seldom indicated because good lung tissue is removed, which is frequently needed for independent function by these patients, who have significant lung impairment.

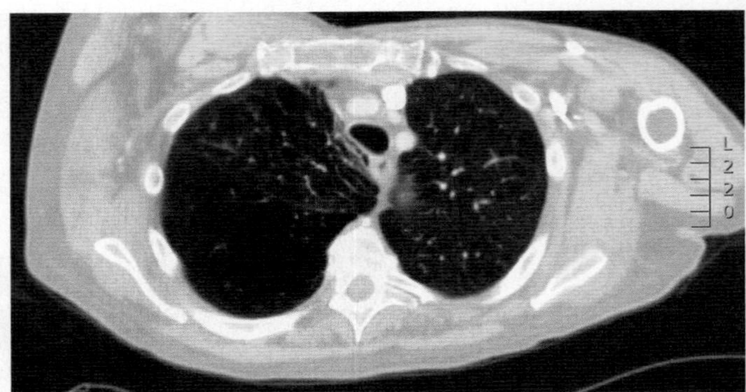

FIGURE 57-19 Bullous emphysema. The patient is a chronic smoker (>100 pack/years) and developed emphysema, which is progressing. The superior segment of the right lower lobe is completely destroyed, and the resultant bullae are compressing functioning lung parenchyma in the right and the left lung.

Treatment of emphysema is primarily medical, but there are surgical therapies. Although emphysema usually diffusely involves the lung, it may have a heterogeneous distribution within the lung. These areas may be identified by CT and perfusion scan. Often the disease predominates in the upper lobes and the superior segment of the lower lobes. Lung volume reduction surgery removes areas of greatest emphysematous involvement. The remaining lung tissue expands with improved elastic recoil, improved aeration and perfusion of the remaining lung, and improved chest wall mechanics. The National Emphysema Treatment Trial compared lung volume reduction surgery with the best medical therapy. Patients with predominantly upper lobe emphysema and low exercise capacity had lower mortality with lung volume reduction surgery than medical therapy.[84] In patients with non–upper lobe emphysema and high exercise capacity, mortality was higher in the operative group. Long-term results have been favorable.[85] Endoscopic therapies have been developed, including airway bypass and one-way valves. These devices are still in the investigational stage.

Lung transplantation is performed for COPD (including α_1-antitrypsin deficiency), pulmonary fibrosis, primary pulmonary hypertension, cystic fibrosis, and bronchiectasis. The survival rates after lung transplantation (all lungs) are approximately 78% at 1 year, 56% at 5 years, and 30% at 10 years.[86] Long-term immunosuppression is required. Unilateral lung transplantation is more readily tolerated than bilateral lung transplantation; however, bilateral lung transplantation is more frequently performed and has a survival advantage after 1 year.

Diffuse Lung Disease

The surgeon's role in diffuse lung disease is to obtain a diagnosis, typically by open lung biopsy after other methods (e.g., transthoracic needle aspiration; bronchoscopy with transbronchial biopsy) have failed. The CXR may demonstrate an alveolar pattern (fluffy with air bronchograms) or an interstitial pattern (ground-glass or granular appearance, indicating a diffuse increase in interstitial tissue) (Box 57-2). Patients may be mildly symptomatic, and biopsy may be needed to confirm or exclude a specific diagnosis before embarking on aggressive medical therapy, such as cyclophosphamide for Wegener granulomatosis, or patients may be critically ill and in the intensive care unit, requiring mechanical ventilation.

BOX 57-2 Classification of Diffuse Lung Diseases

Infections (more commonly cause focal disease, granuloma formation)
- Viruses—especially influenza, cytomegalovirus
- Bacteria—tuberculosis, all types of regular bacteria, Rocky Mountain spotted fever
- Fungi—all types can cause diffuse disease
- Parasites—*Pneumocystis* species infection, toxoplasmosis, paragonimiasis, among others

Occupational causes
- Mineral dusts
- Chemical fumes—NO_2 (silo filler's disease), Cl, NH_3, SO_2, CCl_4, Br, HF, HCl, HNO_3, kerosene, acetylene

Neoplastic disease
- Lymphangitic spread
- Hematogenous metastases
- Leukemia, lymphoma, bronchioloalveolar cell cancer

Congenital—familial
- Niemann-Pick disease, Gaucher disease, neurofibromatosis, and tuberous fibrosis

Metabolic and unknown
- Liver disease, uremia, inflammatory bowel disease

Physical agents
- Radiation, O_2 toxicity, thermal injury, blast injury

Heart failure and multiple pulmonary emboli

Immunologic causes

Hypersensitivity pneumonia
- Inhaled antigens
- Farmer's lung (actinomycosis)
- Bagassosis (sugar cane)
- Malt workers (*Aspergillus* spp.)
- Byssinosis (cotton)

Drug reactions
- Hydralazine, busulfan, nitrofurantoin (Macrodantin), hexamethonium, methysergide, bleomycin

Collagen diseases
- Scleroderma, rheumatoid disease, systemic lupus erythematosus, dermatomyositis, Wegener granulomatosis, Goodpasture syndrome

Other
- Sarcoidosis
- Histiocytosis
- Idiopathic hemosiderosis
- Pulmonary alveolar proteinosis
- Diffuse interstitial fibrosis, idiopathic pulmonary fibrosis
- Desquamative interstitial pneumonia
- Eosinophilic pneumonia (*Note:* some are caused by drugs, actinomycosis, and parasites)
- Lymphangioleiomyomatosis

Sarcoidosis affects the lungs in 90% of patients with this diagnosis, causing symptoms of dyspnea and dry cough. Foci of noncaseating epithelioid granulomas may be found in any part of the body. In 40% to 50% of cases, patients have insidious respiratory complaints without constitutional symptoms. Severe progressive pulmonary fibrosis may develop in 10% to 20% of patients. Bilateral hilar mediastinal lymph nodes are involved in 60% to 80% of patients. Bronchoscopic lung biopsy is the initial diagnostic procedure. If required, biopsy of mediastinal lymph nodes may be performed. Steroids may be used for treatment.

Lung biopsy may be required for progressive interstitial parenchymal changes for which no diagnosis can be obtained. Lung biopsies can be performed using minimally invasive techniques. Biopsy specimens are sent for routine, fungal, and acid-fast bacillus culture. In immunocompromised patients, *Nocardia* cultures are considered. If possible, the surgeon should sample more than one area of the lung. One method is to resect the worst-appearing region on radiography and the most normal-appearing area. The normal-appearing lung may exhibit early-stage disease and may aid the pathologist in making the diagnosis. Frozen section is used only to confirm that adequate samples of the pathologic process were obtained. In the acute setting of a critically ill patient, an open lung biopsy is performed only when the results would significantly modify subsequent treatment, such as the initiation of protocol-based treatment for experimental antibiotics, or to withdraw futile care.

Adult Respiratory Distress Syndrome

Adult respiratory distress syndrome is a complex biologic and clinical process. Acute deterioration of pulmonary function occurs exclusive of pulmonary edema, pneumonia, or exacerbation of COPD. Approximately 50,000 cases occur each year in the United States, with a mortality rate of 30% to 40%.

The initial clinical presentation of dyspnea, tachypnea, hypoxemia, and mild hypocapnia is nonspecific. CXR may show diffuse bilateral infiltrates secondary to increased interstitial fluid. Pathologically, vascular congestion occurs with alveolar collapse, edema, and inflammatory cell infiltration. The underlying mechanism is increased pulmonary capillary permeability with extravasation of intravascular fluid and protein into the interstitium and alveoli. The leukocyte is the most prominent mediator of this injury. Stimuli such as sepsis activate the complement pathway, causing recruitment of leukocytes to the site of the infection. The lung releases potent mediators, such as oxygen free radicals, arachidonic acid metabolites, and proteases. If the underlying disease is not controlled, these changes progress to vascular thrombosis and interstitial fibrosis and hyaline membrane deposition in the alveoli. This process causes hypoxemia; pulmonary hypertension; carbon dioxide retention; secondary infections; and eventually right heart failure, hypoxia, and death. Other criteria include impaired oxygenation with a PaO_2/FIO_2 ratio of less than 200 mm Hg. Pulmonary edema is present without cardiac failure, and pulmonary capillary wedge pressure is less than 18 mm Hg (noncardiac pulmonary edema).

Treatment is supportive and directed toward improving oxygenation. Maintaining an inspired oxygen concentration as low as possible and positive end-expiratory pressure (PEEP) as low as possible to maintain adequate oxygenation and carbon dioxide exchange is helpful.[87] Tidal volumes and PEEP are kept low; however, increased PEEP may be needed in selected patients to facilitate oxygenation.[88] Based on a more recent meta-analysis, prone or rotational therapy may improve outcomes of these patients.[89]

PULMONARY METASTASES

Isolated pulmonary metastases represent a unique manifestation of systemic spread of a primary neoplasm. Patients with metastases located only within the lungs may be more amenable to local or local and systemic treatment options than other patients with multiorgan metastases. Although primary tumors can be locally controlled with surgery or radiation, extraregional metastases are usually treated with systemic chemotherapy. Radiation therapy may be used to treat or palliate the local manifestations of metastatic disease, particularly when metastases occur within the bony skeleton and cause pain. Resection of solitary and multiple pulmonary metastases from sarcomas and various other primary neoplasms has been performed, with improved long-term survival rates in 40% of patients. Therefore, isolated pulmonary metastases are treatable.

Certain clinical characteristics (prognostic indicators) may be used to select patients with more favorable disease-free and overall survival expectations. Patients who have complete resection of all metastases have associated longer survival than patients whose metastases are unresectable. Long-term survival (>5 years) may be expected in approximately 20% to 30% of all patients with resectable pulmonary metastases. Optimal (and more consistent) survival statistics await improvements in local control, systemic therapy, or regional drug delivery to the lungs.

Surgical Treatment

Predictors for improved survival rate have been studied retrospectively for various tumor types. These predictors may allow the clinician to identify selected patients who would optimally benefit from pulmonary metastasectomy. Patients should have pulmonary parenchymal nodules consistent with metastasis, absence of uncontrolled or untreated extrathoracic metastases, control of the primary tumor, sufficient physiologic and pulmonary reserve to tolerate the operation, and the probability of complete resection. Regardless of histology, patients with pulmonary metastases isolated to the lungs that are completely resected have improved survival rates compared with patients with unresectable metastases. Resectability consistently correlates with improved post-thoracotomy survival rates for patients with pulmonary metastases. In one series of more than 5000 patients with metastases treated with resection, overall actuarial 5-year survival rate was 36%. Favorable clinical indicators included a disease-free interval of greater than 3 years, a SPN, and germ cell histology.[90] Soft tissue sarcomas of all types predominantly metastasize to the lungs. CT usually underestimates the number of metastases by 50% to 100%.

Resection can be accomplished safely. Open or minimally invasive procedures may be used. These procedures have minimal mortality and morbidity. Patients with pulmonary metastases may also undergo multiple procedures for reresection of metastases with prolonged survival expectations after complete resection. VATS procedures limit the ability of the surgeon to palpate the lung to identify occult metastases. Follow-up with radiographic screening at regular intervals is recommended to exclude recurrence.

MISCELLANEOUS LUNG TUMORS

Slow-growing lung tumors may arise from the epithelium, ducts, and glands of the bronchial tree and account for 1% to 2% of all lung neoplasms. Most are of low-grade malignant potential.

Carcinoid tumors (1% of lung neoplasms) arise from Kulchitsky (APUD [amine precursor uptake and decarboxylation]) cells in bronchial epithelium. They have positive histologic reactions to silver staining and to chromogranin. Special stains and examination can identify neurosecretory granules by electron microscopy. These typical carcinoid tumors (least malignant) are the most indolent of the spectrum of pulmonary neuroendocrine tumors that include atypical carcinoid, large cell undifferentiated carcinoma, and small cell carcinoma (most malignant).[91] Histologic findings include less than 2 to 10 mitoses per 10 high-power fields. Peripheral tumors are usually symptom-free, although central tumors may cause endobronchial obstruction with cough, hemoptysis, recurrent infection or pneumonia, bronchiectasis, lung abscess, pain, or wheezing. Symptoms may persist for many years without diagnosis, particularly if only an endobronchial component partially obstructs the airway. Carcinoid syndrome (flushing, tachycardia, wheezing, and diarrhea) is uncommon and occurs with large tumors or extensive metastatic disease. Bronchoscopy is usually positive, unless the nodule or mass is peripheral. Most carcinoids can be identified in this matter; although they tend to bleed, biopsy can usually be performed safely.

Atypical carcinoid may have lymph node or vascular invasion with metastasis. The location is in the mainstem bronchi (20%), lobar bronchi (70% to 75%), or peripheral bronchi (5% to 10%). They rarely occur in the trachea. Local invasion with involvement of peribronchial tissue occurs. At bronchoscopy, most carcinoids are sessile, although a few are polypoid. The histology is that of small uniform cells with oval nuclei and interlacing cords of vascular connective tissue stroma. Mitoses are infrequent, but occasionally bizarre cells are noted. Atypical carcinoids are more pleomorphic and have more mitoses (>2 to 10 mitoses per 10 high-power fields) than typical carcinoid. They have more prominent nucleoli but are more monotonous and have more cytoplasm than oat cell carcinoma. These tumors are more aggressive, with a 5-year survival rate of approximately 60%. Tumors tend to metastasize to the liver, bone, or adrenal. Electron microscopy can be used to identify neurosecretory granules.

Surgical resection is standard, with complete removal of the tumor and as much preservation of lung as possible.[92] Lobectomy is the most common procedure; endoscopic removal is performed only for rare polypoid tumors if thoracotomy is contraindicated. Survival rate is typically 85% at 5 to 10 years. Large cell neuroendocrine tumors and small cell cancer are not typically treated with surgery and may be best treated with combinations of chemotherapy and radiation; survival of these patients is poor.

Adenoid cystic carcinoma is a slow-growing malignancy involving the trachea and mainstem bronchi that is similar to salivary gland tumors.[93] Adenoid cystic carcinoma is more malignant than carcinoid tumors and has a slight female preponderance. The tumor typically involves the lower trachea, carina, and take-off of the mainstem bronchi. Stridor is often the presenting symptom of adenoid cystic tumors because these tumors are most often found in the trachea and mainstem bronchi. One third of patients have tumors that have metastasized at the time of treatment. These patients typically have involvement of the perineural lymphatics; regional nodes; or liver, bone, or kidneys. The tumor arises from ducts in the submucosa and extends proximally and distally in that plane. Microscopic examination demonstrates cells with large nuclei and a small cytoplasm and surrounding cystic spaces (pseudoacinar type); the medullary type has a Swiss cheese appearance. Treatment is wide en bloc resection with conservation of as much lung tissue as possible.[94] Radiation treatment alone may be effective in patients not amenable to surgical resection.

Benign tumors of the lung account for less than 1% of all lung neoplasms and arise from mesodermal origins (Box 57-3). Hamartomas are the most frequent benign lung tumor; they consist of normal tissue elements found in an abnormal location. Hamartomas are manifested by overgrowth of cartilage. Hamartomas are

BOX 57-3 Miscellaneous Lung Tumors

Hamartoma
Epithelial origin tumors
- Papilloma—single or multiple, squamous epithelium, occurs in childhood, probably viral, may require bronchial resection but frequently recur
- Polyp—inflammatory-squamous metaplasia on a stalk; bronchial resection may be needed; these do not usually recur

Mesodermal origin tumors
- Fibroma—most frequent mesodermal tumor
- Chondroma
- Lipoma
- Leiomyoma—intrabronchial or peripheral; conservative resection

Granular cell tumors
- Rhabdomyoma
- Neuroma
- Hemangioma—subglottic larynx or upper trachea of infants; radiation therapy
- Lymphangioma—similar to cystic hygroma; upper airway obstruction in neonates
- Hemangioendothelioma—newborn lungs, often progressive and lethal
- Lymphangiomyomatosis—rare, slowly progressive; death from pulmonary insufficiency; fine, multinodular lesions, loss of parenchyma and honeycombing; usually women in their reproductive years
- Arteriovenous fistula—congenital, right-to-left shunt; cyanosis, dyspnea on exertion, clubbing, brain abscess; associated with hereditary hemorrhagic telangiectasia of lower lobes

Inflammatory tumors and pseudotumors
- Plasma cell granuloma
- Pseudolymphoma
- Xanthoma

Teratoma

typically identified in patients 40 to 60 years old and have a 2:1 male-to-female predominance. They are usually peripheral and slow-growing. CXR demonstrates a 2- to 3-cm mass that is sharply demarcated and frequently lobulated. It is usually not calcified, but the "popcorn" appearance on CXR may provide the diagnosis of hamartoma. Cystic adenomatoid malformation may represent adenomatous hamartomas, which occur in infants as cysts or immature elements in the lung.

Very low-grade malignancies include hemangiopericytoma and pulmonary blastoma that arises from embryonic lung tissue. Treatment is resection. Tumorlets are epithelial proliferative lesions that may resemble oat cell carcinoma or carcinoid. These are typically incidental findings noted on examination of resected lung specimens. They rarely metastasize.

Primary sarcomas of the lung occur rarely. Resection, similar to lung carcinoma, is feasible in 50% to 60% of patients.[95] Prognosis of patients with leiomyosarcoma is excellent, with approximately a 50% survival rate at 5 years; all other sarcomas have poor survival expectations.

Lymphoma of the lung most commonly occurs as disseminated lymphoma involving the lung. Disseminated lymphoma occurs in 40% of patients with Hodgkin disease and 7% of patients with non-Hodgkin disease. Primary lymphoma of the lung is rare. The diagnosis is usually made at surgery. A thorough evaluation for other primary sites of lymphoma is done if primary pulmonary lymphoma is suspected preoperatively.

CHEST WALL

Pectus Excavatum

Pectus excavatum is the most common chest wall deformity, occurring in 1 of 400 children with a male predominance (4:1).[96] More than 30% of cases have a family history of chest wall anomalies. Pectus excavatum refers to the sternal depression (depressed dorsally) caused by unequal growth rates or development of the lower ribs and costal cartilages (usually after the third rib). The sternum is not depressed equally or symmetrically and is also rotated. This syndrome may be associated with other musculoskeletal abnormalities. Most patients are asymptomatic, but some have decreased exercise capacity or pulmonary reserve. Patients are evaluated with plain CXRs, CT scans, pulmonary function studies, ventilation-perfusion lung scans, and other physiologic studies.

Surgical repair of pectus excavatum can be accomplished by various techniques, including sternal osteotomy, osteotomy with posterior strut or other stabilization (e.g., a metal plate), removing the sternum and turning it over with stabilization, placement of a prosthesis to fill the defect, and placement of an internal (posterior) sternal support (which is more effective in younger patients than older patients). Open techniques typically reflect the overlying pectoralis major and the rectus muscles. Involved costal cartilages are removed, leaving the perichondrium. The sternum is mobilized and stabilized. The muscles are reapproximated in the midline over the repair.

Pectus carinatum (also called *pigeon breast*) refers to the anterior protrusion of the sternum and costal cartilages and occurs with a male predominance (4:1). This condition is approximately five times less likely to occur than pectus excavatum.

Poland syndrome is a rare, nonfamilial disease of unknown cause that occurs in 1 in 30,000 births. Characteristics of this syndrome include absence of the pectoralis major muscle, absence or hypoplasia of the pectoralis minor muscle, absence of costal cartilages, hypoplasia of breast and subcutaneous tissue (including the nipple complex), and various hand anomalies.

Chest Wall Tumors

Chest wall tumors[97,98] are rare. The most frequent chest wall tumors are metastatic tumors related to metastasis to the chest wall from another primary tumor. Primary chest wall tumors are typically sarcomas of the chest wall (rib). Primary bone tumors can occur in the ribs, scapula, and sternum as well (Table 57-3).

Clinical presentation of chest wall tumors can range from an enlarging painless mass to a painful and fungating mass. Pain can occur with periosteal invasion. Local tumor extension onto the lung or mediastinum can create associated symptoms. Evaluation requires diagnostic imaging such as CXR, CT, and FDG-PET. MRI is effective for tumors involving the thoracic inlet or upper chest that may involve the brachial plexus or tumors that involve or abut the vertebral bodies. Histologic confirmation is required. A core needle biopsy is frequently effective. Excisional biopsy with minimal contamination of the surgical site may be required for a larger tumor. Consideration for future resection may dictate size and location of the incisional biopsy. Resection and reconstruction with prosthesis or muscle flaps can be accomplished with excellent results. A multidisciplinary approach to treatment is complemented by a multispecialty team in the operating room.

Bone Tumors

Benign bone tumors include fibrous dysplasia of the bone, which accounts for approximately 30% of these tumors. Chondromas account for 15% to 20% of benign chest wall lesions and arise from the anterior costochondral junction. Osteochondroma occurs commonly in young men as an asymptomatic tumor originating from the cortex of the rib. Eosinophilic granuloma is a benign component of malignant fibrous histiocytosis and primarily affects men. Skull and rib involvement are common and appear as expansile lesions on radiographic evaluation. Excisional biopsy is indicated for solitary lesions, and radiotherapy is indicated for multiple lesions. Aneurysmal bone cysts occur in the ribs and may be associated with previous trauma. Radiographic characteristics include a blow-out lytic lesion (Fig. 57-20). Resection is recommended for diagnosis and for relief of pain.

Malignant bone tumors include chondrosarcoma, which is the most common malignant tumor of the chest wall, accounting for 20% of all bone tumors. Chondrosarcomas arise in the third and fourth decades of life. Radiographic characteristics include a poorly defined tumor mass that is destroying cortical bone. Resection with wide margins (3 to 5 cm) is the treatment of choice. The 5-year survival after complete resection is approximately 70%. Osteosarcoma (osteogenic sarcoma) most frequently arises in the long bones of adolescents and young adults. Primary osteosarcomas in the chest account for 10% to 15% of malignant tumors. The tumor grows rapidly, and radiographic characteristics include a sunburst pattern on CXR. Ewing sarcoma commonly arises in bones of the pelvis, humerus, or femur of young men. It is the third most common malignant chest wall tumor (5% to 10%). The radiographic characteristics include an onion-peel appearance with periosteal elevation and bony remodeling. With multimodality therapy, 5-year survival is 50%. Solitary plasmacytoma is a rare tumor that occurs in older men as a painful solitary tumor arising from plasma cells. Multiple myeloma is the same tumor arising in more than one location. Radiographic characteristics include a diffuse, moth-eaten or punched-out appearance of the bone. Systemic disease can be confirmed using serum protein electrophoresis, urinalysis (Bence-Jones protein), and bone marrow aspiration. Local radiotherapy for solitary plasmacytoma is recommended.

TABLE 57-3 Classification of Tumors of the Chest Wall

	BENIGN	MALIGNANT
Bony Tissue		
Bone	Osteoid osteoma	Osteosarcoma
	Aneurysmal bone cyst	Ewing sarcoma
Cartilage	Enchondroma	Chondrosarcoma
	Osteochondroma	
Fibrous	Fibrous dysplasia	Malignant fibrous histiocytoma
Marrow	Eosinophilic granuloma	Plasmacytoma
Vascular	Hemangioma	Hemangiosarcoma
Soft Tissue		
Adipose	Lipoma and variations	Liposarcoma
Muscle	Leiomyoma	Leiomyosarcoma
	Rhabdomyoma	Rhabdomyosarcoma
Neural	Neurofibroma	Neurofibrosarcoma
	Neurilemoma	Malignant schwannoma
		Askin tumor (primitive neuroectodermal tumor)
Fibrous	Desmoid	Fibrosarcoma

Adapted from Faber LP, Somers J, Templeton AC: Chest wall tumors. *Curr Probl Surg* 32:661–747, 1995.

Soft Tissue Tumors

Soft tissue sarcomas are the most common malignant primary chest wall tumors.[98,99] Core needle or incisional biopsy is performed to establish the diagnosis (Fig. 57-21). Resection with wide local excision (3 to 5 cm) is required. These tumors should not be shelled out despite the presence of a pseudocapsule. Complete resection is associated with excellent local control and

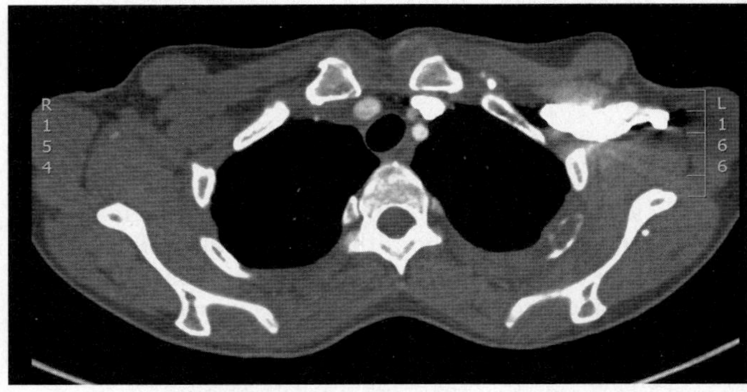

FIGURE 57-20 Aneurysmal bone cyst.

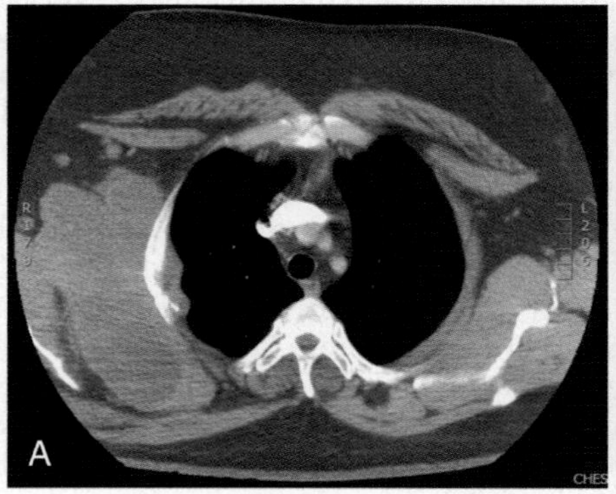

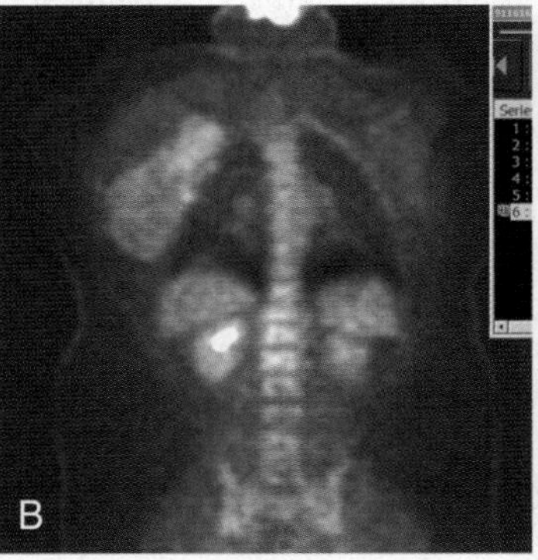

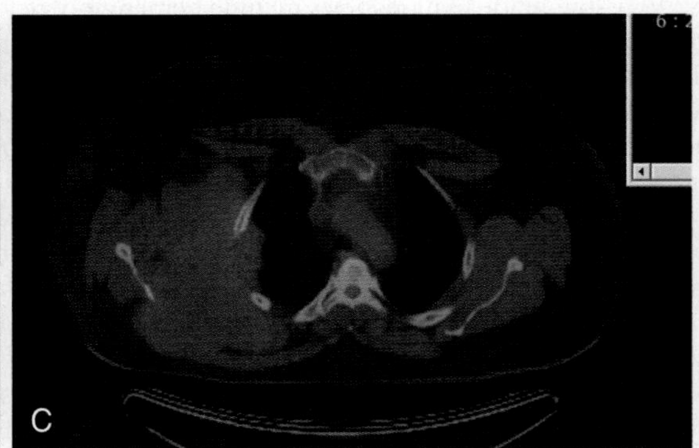

FIGURE 57-21 A, Primary chest wall tumor, desmoid tumor of the right lateral and posterior chest wall, is shown on computed tomography (CT) image. **B,** ^{18}F-Fluorodeoxyglucose positron emission tomography (FDG-PET) demonstrates mild FDG avidity. No sites of metastases were identified. **C,** A fused image of CT and FDG-PET is shown. Resection of the tumor included chest wall musculature and chest wall. Reconstruction was performed with prosthetic material, and a muscle flap was required.

prolonged survival. Combinations of chemotherapy and radiation therapy may be used as components of the multidisciplinary treatment plan.

Metastatic Tumors

Metastatic neoplasms may involve the chest wall by direct extension, by lymphatic metastasis, or by hematogenous metastasis. Lung cancer and breast cancer can involve the chest wall by direct extension, and if identified, chest wall resection should be performed concurrently with resection of the primary neoplasm.

Reconstruction

Reconstruction of the chest wall depends on the size, location, and cosmetic and functional impairment that results from resection. Prevention of flail chest and maintenance of physiologic stability requires careful judgment regarding the choice of prosthetic reconstruction, autologous tissue coverage available including myocutaneous flaps, and free tissue flap transfer.

Chest Wall Infections

Chest wall infections may occur after thoracic surgery, thoracic trauma, or other interventions. Inflammatory breast carcinoma is not an infection but may mimic a chest wall infection. Biopsy may be needed to confirm the diagnosis. Mondor disease, thrombophlebitis of the superficial veins of the breast and anterior chest wall, is also not an infection. Ultrasound or biopsy may be necessary to confirm the diagnosis. Tietze syndrome or costochondritis is usually self-limited and can be treated with nonsteroidal anti-inflammatory drugs and rest. Because of the limited blood supply to the cartilage, infection in this area may be difficult to diagnose. Débridement and reconstruction may be necessary. Sternal wound infections are complications following median sternotomy or cardiac surgery. Spontaneous primary chest wall infections can arise from various sources as a consequence of immunosuppression, drug-resistant organisms including tuberculosis, or HIV infection.

Chest Wall Trauma

Trauma to the chest wall is common. CXR and chest CT scan are obtained often as part of the secondary survey in chest wall trauma. CT can identify rib, parenchymal, or other abnormalities. Blunt chest wall trauma commonly results in contusion of the chest wall tissues and the underlying lung parenchyma. Supportive care is warranted.

Rib fractures are perhaps the most common traumatic injury sustained after blunt chest wall trauma. Symptoms include pain on inspiration and localized point tenderness. Plain films can confirm the diagnosis. Fractures of the first or second ribs may occur after significant trauma or high-velocity injury. Because of the size and thickness of the first rib, tremendous force is needed to fracture this rib. This traumatic event is associated with aortic disruption. Contusion or injury to underlying structures should be suspected with any rib fracture. Contusion of the lung parenchyma and injury to the spleen, liver, diaphragm, or kidney can occur. Treatment with analgesia and nerve blocks can be helpful. Flail chest may occur with multiple rib fractures. Flail chest results in an unstable chest wall that develops paradoxical motion during respiration (e.g., depression during the negative inspiratory phase and extrusion during the positive expiratory phase). Flail chest is often associated with an underlying pulmonary contusion and should be supported with pain relief, stabilization of the chest wall, or even mechanical ventilation.

Sternal injuries are uncommon and may result from blunt trauma to the anterior chest, typically from a steering wheel injury during a motor vehicle accident. An underlying cardiac injury, such as aortic disruption, cardiac contusion, pericardial effusion, or arrhythmia, must be considered. Heart rhythm monitoring, serial cardiac observations with electrocardiography and cardiac enzymes, and echocardiography are used to exclude these injuries. Clavicular fractures may be associated with injury to the great vessels or the brachial plexus. Supportive care and stabilization are recommended.

THORACIC OUTLET SYNDROME

Thoracic outlet syndrome (TOS) refers to compression of the subclavian vessels and nerves of the brachial plexus in the region of the thoracic inlet. Symptoms most commonly develop secondary to neural compromise; however, vascular and neurovascular symptoms are reported.[100] Middle-aged women are most commonly affected by TOS. The subclavian vessels and the brachial plexus can be compressed at various locations as they pass between the thoracic inlet and the upper extremity (Fig. 57-22). From medial to lateral, these anatomic regions are as follows:

1. Interscalene triangle (artery and nerves)
2. Costoclavicular space (vein)
3. Subcoracoid area (artery, vein, nerves)

Diagnosis

The symptoms associated with TOS vary depending on the anatomic structure that is compressed. Neurogenic manifestations are reported in more than 90% of cases. Symptoms of subclavian artery compression include fatigue, weakness, coldness, upper extremity claudication, thrombosis, and paresthesia. Thrombosis with distal embolization rarely can occur, producing vasomotor symptoms (Raynaud phenomenon) in the hand or ischemic changes. Venous compression results in edema, venous distention,

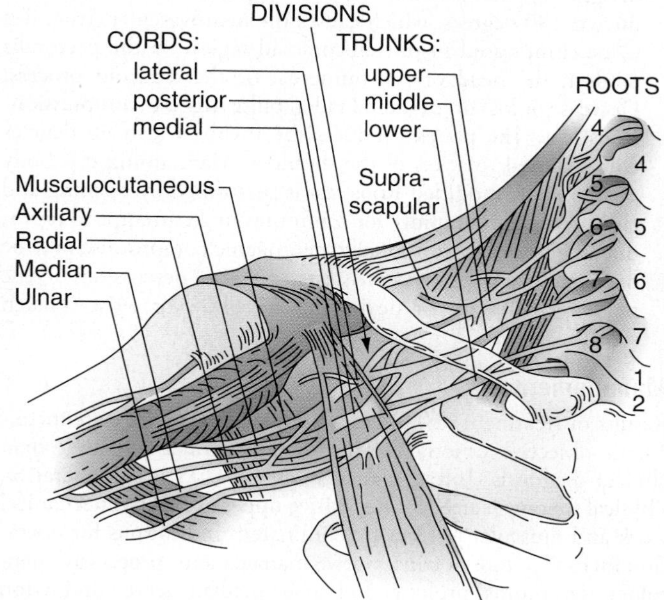

FIGURE 57-22 Detailed view of brachial plexus. (From Urschel HC, Razzuk M: Upper plexus thoracic outlet syndrome: Optimal therapy. *Ann Thorac Surg* 63:935–939, 1997.)

collateral formation, and cyanosis of the affected limb. Venous TOS may be characterized by upper extremity edema, venous distention, or effort thrombosis, also known as *Paget-Schroetter syndrome*.

The diagnosis of neurogenic TOS is initially made clinically. Objective evaluation for TOS includes chest and cervical spine films. A cervical rib or bony degenerative cervical spine changes may be present.[101] CT, MRI, and cervical myelography are sometimes helpful to rule out narrowing of the intervertebral foramina or cervical disc pathology. Doppler studies or vascular imaging (angiography/venography) may be indicated if the extent of vascular impairment cannot be determined clinically or if an aneurysm or venous thrombosis is suspected. Neurogenic TOS needs to be confirmed with nerve conduction studies to localize the area of slowing of nerve conduction and to rule out other compression syndromes, such as carpal tunnel syndrome. Electromyelography and nerve conduction studies are helpful to rule out carpal tunnel syndrome. Patients with moderate to severe slowing of nerve conduction usually respond to nonoperative therapy. Vascular TOS must be confirmed with objective studies.[102]

Clinical maneuvers to evaluate a patient suspected to have TOS are performed to identify the loss or decrease of radial pulse or to reproduce neurologic symptoms. A clear objective validated definition for TOS is needed. Evocative tests to illicit symptoms include the following:

- Adson (scalene) test. The patient inspires maximally and holds his or her breath while the neck is fully extended and the head is turned toward the affected side. This maneuver narrows the space between the scalenus anticus and medius, resulting in compression of the subclavian artery and the brachial plexus. Decrease or loss of ipsilateral radial pulse suggests compression.
- Halsted (costoclavicular) test. The patient is instructed to place his or her shoulders in a military position (drawn backward and downward) to narrow the costoclavicular space between the first rib and the clavicle, causing neurovascular compression. Reproduction of neurologic symptoms or decrease or loss of ipsilateral radial pulse suggests compression.
- Wright (hyperabduction) test. The patient's arm is hyperabducted 180 degrees, which causes the neurovascular structures to be compressed in the subcoracoid region by the pectoralis tendon, the head of the humerus, or the coracoid process. Decrease or loss of ipsilateral radial pulse suggests compression.
- Roos test. The patient abducts the involved arm 90 degrees with external rotation of the shoulder. Maintaining this body position, the modified Roos test is performed by opening and closing the hand rapidly for 3 minutes in an attempt to reproduce symptoms. Additionally, neurogenic compromise may be detected using provocative tests, such as percussion of the nerve (Tinel sign) or flexion of the elbow or wrist (Phalen sign).

Management

Results of treatment of TOS are variable because there are inconsistent objective criteria for the diagnosis of TOS other than clinical diagnosis. Initial management of TOS is nonoperative. Physical therapy is needed. Repetitive upper extremity mechanical work and muscular trauma are eliminated. Indications for operation include failure of conservative management, progressive neurologic symptoms, prolonged ulnar or median nerve conduction velocities, narrowing or occlusion of the subclavian artery, and thrombosis of the axillary or subclavian vein. Operative management can provide excellent results.[103] Objective agreed-on outcome measures and clinical trials are needed to compare outcomes of surgery for TOS compared with no surgery.[104] Success rates with surgery only approach 70% at 5 years. Recurrent symptoms may prompt operation in up to one third of patients.

PLEURA

Pleural Effusions

The pleural space is a potential space defined normally by the small amount of pleural fluid separating the visceral and parietal pleura. Many benign and malignant pleural space problems can disrupt the balance of fluid production and absorption leading to various pleural space problems, including increased mass effect from air, fluid, or tumor on the ipsilateral lung parenchyma and heart, infection, or dyspnea and pulmonary dysfunction. The cause of pleural effusions is quite varied (Box 57-4).

The movement of fluid across the pleural membranes is governed by Starling's law of capillary exchange. The amount of

BOX 57-4 Pleural Effusions

Cause of Transudative Effusions

Congestive heart failure
Cirrhosis
Nephrotic syndrome
Hypoalbuminemia
Fluid retention/overload
Pulmonary embolism
Lobar collapse
Meigs syndrome

Cause of Exudative Effusions

Malignant
- Primary lung or metastatic carcinoma
- Lymphoma
- Mesothelioma

Infectious
- Bacterial (parapneumonic)/empyema
- Tuberculosis
- Fungal
- Viral
- Parasitic

Collagen vascular disease related
- Rheumatoid arthritis
- Wegener granulomatosis
- Systemic lupus erythematosus
- Churg-Strauss syndrome

Abdominal/gastrointestinal disease related
- Esophageal perforation
- Subphrenic abscess
- Pancreatitis/pancreatic pseudocyst
- Meigs syndrome

Others
- Chylothorax
- Uremia
- Sarcoidosis
- After coronary artery bypass grafting
- Radiation/trauma
- Dressler syndrome
- Pulmonary embolism with infarction
- Asbestosis related

pleural fluid is controlled by a balance of oncotic and hydrostatic pressure within the pleural space and the pleural capillaries. Under normal circumstances, the net pressure moves fluid from the parietal pleura into the pleural space. It is estimated that 5 to 10 liters of fluid are produced and transgress the pleural space over a 24-hour period. However, the normal volume of pleural fluid is quite small. The balance of forces favors fluid reabsorption from the pleural cavity across the visceral pleura. Under physiologic conditions, most pleural fluid is reabsorbed through lymphatics of the parietal pleura because protein that enters the pleural space cannot enter the relatively impermeable visceral pleura. The parietal pleura and its lymphatics have significant capacity for protein and fluid removal. A small imbalance of accumulation and absorption can lead to the development of a pleural effusion. The causative factors include increased hydrostatic pressure, increased negative intrapleural pressure, increased capillary permeability, decreased plasma oncotic pressure, and decreased or interrupted lymphatic drainage.

Pleural fluid is characterized as a transudate or an exudate. Transudative effusions are protein-poor and result in change in fluid balance in the pleural space. Exudative effusions are protein-rich and may be related to disruption of pleural or lymphatic reabsorption. After drainage, the fluid is evaluated by Light's criteria.[105] An exudate is defined as (1) pleural fluid protein–to–serum protein ratio greater than 0.5, (2) pleural fluid lactate dehydrogenase (LDH)–to–serum LDH ratio greater than 0.6, or (3) pleural fluid LDH 1.67 times the normal serum level or higher. In addition, pleural fluid should be assessed for its visual characteristics (serous, bloody, milky, turbid, or frankly purulent). Pleural fluid should be analyzed for cytology; cell counts; Gram stain; culture for aerobic, anaerobic, and fungal organisms; tuberculosis testing; and chemistry with simultaneous pleural and serum protein, glucose, LDH, and pH. The treatment goals for patients with pleural effusion include obtaining a diagnosis, relieving or eliminating symptoms such as dyspnea, optimizing patient function, minimizing or eliminating hospitalization, and minimizing costs of care.

Benign Pleural Effusions

Most benign pleural effusions are transudates, free-flowing, without loculation, and treatment should be directed toward the underlying cause, such as congestive heart failure, ascites, or malnutrition. Symptoms are typically dyspnea or cough. Pleural fluid can be identified on CXR; the presence of 300 mL of fluid causes blunting of the costophrenic angle on upright CXR. Clinical examination can detect 500 mL of fluid or greater. Initial thoracentesis should achieve complete drainage for diagnosis and treatment. In addition, radiographic evidence of complete re-expansion of the lung should be sought. Failure of the lung to expand completely suggests a "trapped" lung, which may require decortication, particularly if symptoms, such as dyspnea, persist. Relief of symptoms with thoracentesis usually indicates the pleural effusion as the cause. Occasionally, symptoms are not relieved by thoracentesis, and an alternative diagnosis is required.

Recurrent effusions can occur, and repeat thoracenteses may be required. Alternative therapies, such as chest tube insertion (tube thoracostomy) or thoracoscopic drainage with or without mechanical and chemical pleurodesis, can be considered. Visceral and parietal pleural apposition is required to achieve pleurodesis. Drainage of the effusion can be diagnostic and therapeutic. Sclerosing agents can be placed to facilitate pleural symphysis. This pleurodesis is most effectively accomplished with slurry of 5 g of talc in 100 mL of saline placed through the chest tube. Video-assisted thoracoscopic drainage of effusions can also be diagnostic and therapeutic. Pleural biopsy or wedge resection of the lung can be easily performed to facilitate diagnosis. Mechanical pleural abrasion or chemical pleurodesis with talc is typically used. The talc is insufflated within the hemithorax to cover all visceral pleural surfaces (e.g., talc poudrage). Pleurectomy is not commonly needed; however, persistent pleural effusions and trapped lung may not be amenable to more conservative measures. Decortication may be required.

Malignant Pleural Effusion

Patients with known or previous malignancy can develop MPE. In 25% of MPEs, a histologic diagnosis of cancer is not made within the fluid after two thoracenteses. Drainage is required for relief of dyspnea (Fig. 57-23).

MPE is an effusion with positive cytopathology. Not all pleural effusions associated with malignancy are caused by direct or metastatic pleural involvement. Other mechanisms for their development (bronchial or lymphatic obstruction, hypoproteinemia, and sympathetic accumulation from infradiaphragmatic involvement) exist. Although repeated cytologic evaluation of a pleural effusion achieves high positive and negative predictive values, this diagnostic procedure has important limitations. A cancer diagnosis is obtained after three thoracenteses in 70% to 80% of patients. Thoracoscopy is diagnostic in 92% of patients.

A patient with MPE has a median survival of 90 days.[106] Patients with breast cancer and MPE have a median survival of approximately 5 months; patients with lymphoma typically have a longer median survival.[107] Local treatment of MPE does not affect the systemic disease process but may provide significant symptomatic relief. Complications of treatments include hemothorax, loculation of fluid, empyema, failure of pleurodesis with recurrence of effusion, and lung entrapment caused by inexpansile lung. Open surgical pleurectomy and pleurodesis are reserved for patients who fail other therapies and who have a reasonably long life expectancy. A phase 3 study demonstrated that a long-term indwelling pleural catheter was as effective as chest tube drainage with doxycycline pleurodesis.[108] Talc slurry following chest tube insertion and drainage of the effusion is as effective as VATS with talc pleurodesis.[109]

Empyema

Empyema is an infection of the pleural space and commonly an exudate.[110] Empyemas progress from an acute phase with fluid that is thin and can be drained completely with a chest tube or small bore catheter. This process typically worsens as the fluid becomes more turbid and thick and begins to loculate. Mucopurulent debris occurs within the pleural space and compresses the underlying lung parenchyma. The organizing or chronic phase is reflected in more lung entrapment with capillary ingrowth and creation of a pleural rind, which traps the lung.

An empyema typically occurs after a reactive pleural effusion as a consequence of a lung infection.[111] These infections historically were due to streptococcal or pneumococcal pneumonia; at the present time, gram-negative and anaerobic organisms are common causes of empyema. Tuberculous empyema can also be identified. Empyema can follow trauma or thoracic surgery (from residual pleural space or bronchopleural fistula), hematologic spread, rupture of a pulmonary or mediastinal abscess, or esophageal perforation.

Symptoms typically include constitutional symptoms of general malaise, fever, loss of appetite, and weight loss. Cough and

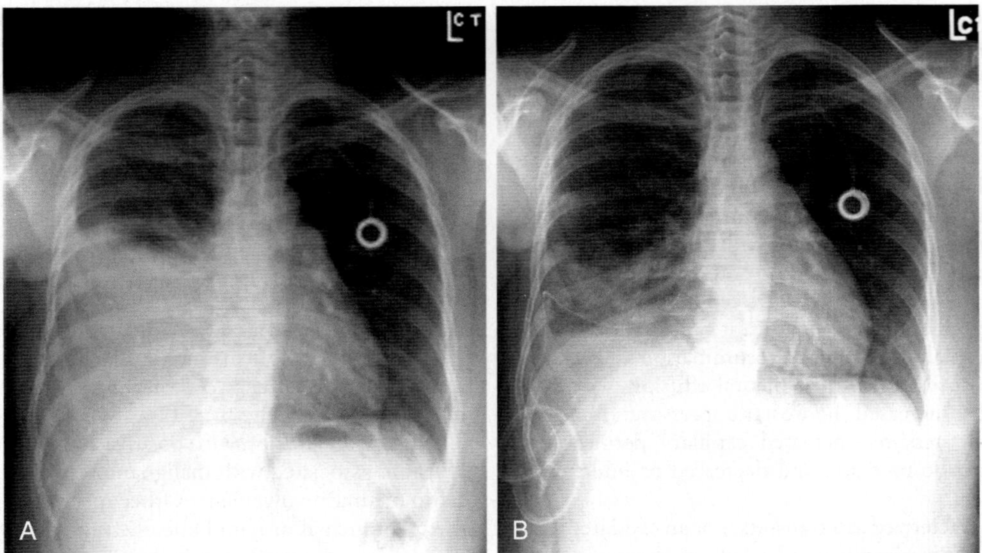

FIGURE 57-23 A, Malignant pleural effusion causing dyspnea. A long-term indwelling pleural catheter was placed as an outpatient procedure to facilitate drainage at home to prevent dyspnea. Hospitalization was not required. **B,** Following drainage. A long-term indwelling pleural catheter is effective in patients with trapped lung. Every-other-day drainage reduces impairment of the contralateral lung and prevents mediastinal shift.

dyspnea are common if lung infection is present. Evaluation includes CXR, posterior row anterior and lateral, and CT scan of the chest and upper abdomen.

Treatment of empyema depends on the extent of the disease and its location.[112] Complete and dependent drainage are required. Antibiotics and supportive care (e.g., fluids, nutrition, skin care) are commonly initiated. Use of fibrinolytic agents can be effective. Intrapleural tissue plasminogen activator and DNase when used together improve drainage of pleural fluid in patients with pleural infection or loculations and reduce the need for surgical drainage.[113]

Simple dependent and complete drainage is required for successful outcomes. This dependent drainage can be achieved easily with posterior rib resection and insertion of an empyema tube. This technique can be effective and can minimize operative time for patients who are critically ill or septic. Complete expansion of the lung may not be achieved at the time of the operation; however, with time and drainage, the lung typically reexpands, and the space closes. VATS decortication and thoracotomy with débridement or formal decortication in later stage empyema is reserved for treatment failures with persistent symptoms of dyspnea, loculations, or continued sepsis.

Bronchopleural fistula after lobectomy or pneumonectomy predisposes to empyema. Management of bronchopleural fistula requires evaluation of the underlying cause of the fistula, drainage of the infection, and obliteration of the residual pleural space along with general supportive care. Chronic empyema with a residual pleural space can be treated with drainage, gauze packing, or skin flap (Eloesser flap) with eventual muscle transposition and skin closure. Lung resection or pleuropneumonectomy is rarely required.

Chylothorax

Chylothorax occurs when chyle from the thoracic duct empties into the pleural space.[114] Chyle is a milky white fluid with a high concentration of triglycerides and chylomicrons and white blood cells. It is nutritionally rich and depends on the nutritional and dietary status of the patient. It may be clear. Chylothorax has multiple causes (Box 57-5).

BOX 57-5 Chylothorax

- Traumatic (chest and neck)
  - Blunt
  - Penetrating
- Iatrogenic
  - Catheterization, particularly subclavian vein
  - Postsurgical
  - Excision of cervical/supraclavicular lymph nodes
  - Radical lymph node dissections of the neck or chest
  - Lung, esophageal, or mediastinal resection
  - Thoracic aneurysm repair
  - Sympathectomy
  - Congenital cardiovascular surgery
- Neoplasms
  - Lymphoma, lung, esophageal, or mediastinal neoplasms
  - Metastatic carcinoma
- Infectious
  - Tuberculous lymphadenosis
  - Mediastinitis
  - Ascending lymphangitis
- Other
  - Lymphangioleiomyomatosis
  - Venous thrombosis
- Congenital

Symptoms from chylothorax include dyspnea or cough. In addition, because of the nutritional consequences of chronic chyle leak (e.g., loss of fat, protein) and the volume of the leak (0.5 to 3.0 liters per day), fluid and nutritional replacement and correction of the underlying problem are necessary. The diagnosis may be made with thoracentesis or drainage of the fluid with a chest tube. Analysis of pleural fluid with chylomicrons confirms the diagnosis. Conservative measures, such as medium-chain triglyceride diet or total parenteral nutrition, are used initially. If conservative measures fail, operative intervention may be considered between days 7 and 14. Commonly ligation of thoracic duct where it enters the chest through the diaphragmatic hiatus is achieved via a right thoracotomy or thoracoscopy. Placement of olive oil or ice cream by nasogastric tube at the time of the operation may increase chyle drainage into the operative field and help to identify the area of thoracic duct disruption. Percutaneous techniques with needle cannulation and duct occlusion have been proposed.[115]

Pneumothorax

Pneumothorax is the accumulation of air within the pleural space and may occur as a result of trauma, surgery, needle aspiration, central line insertion, increased pressure from mechanical ventilation, or lung diseases (e.g., COPD, cystic or pulmonary fibrosis) or other conditions (e.g., catamenial pneumothorax) (Box 57-6). A primary spontaneous pneumothorax occurs as a consequence of subpleural blebs or other pulmonary disease. Tension pneumothorax occurs when air continues to enter the pleural space without decompression. This problem results in positive intrathoracic pressure causing compression of the lung and mediastinum, shift of the mediastinum into the contralateral chest, and decrease in ventilation and venous return. Cardiopulmonary collapse and death ensue. Immediate decompression with needle or chest tube insertion is lifesaving.

Symptoms of pneumothorax include pain and dyspnea. Patients with spontaneous pneumothorax are usually tall and thin young men. Diagnostic imaging includes CXR and occasionally CT. Apical blebs and bullae are common. CT scan can be performed to assess for the cause of spontaneous pneumothorax or the presence of other occult lung disease. Subcutaneous emphysema may or may not be present.

Treatment depends on size and symptoms. Smaller pneumothorax may be followed and may resolve spontaneously, particularly pneumothorax that occurs after needle aspiration for lung biopsy. Progression in the size of pneumothorax requires intervention with drainage. Initial spontaneous pneumothorax may be treated with small bore catheter drainage or chest tube and drainage with resolution of the air space and cessation of air leak. Persistent air leak (>72 hours) or failure of the lung to expand fully suggests additional intervention may be needed.

Operative intervention is recommended for patients who have a persistence or recurrence of spontaneous pneumothorax or who develop a contralateral pneumothorax. High-risk professions (e.g., scuba diver, airplane pilot) should be avoided. Operative repair typically includes thoracoscopy to identify apical blebs, which are resected with endoscopic staplers. Mechanical abrasion of the parietal pleura is performed. Pleurodesis with talc in patients with malignancy or in older patients may be considered.

BOX 57-6 Pneumothorax

Spontaneous
- Primary
- Secondary
  - COPD
  - Bullous disease
  - Cystic fibrosis
  - *Pneumocystis* related
  - Congenital cysts
  - IPF
  - Pulmonary embolism
- Catamenial
- Neonatal

Traumatic
- Penetrating
- Blunt

Iatrogenic
- Mechanical ventilation
- Needle puncture: thoracentesis, FNA lung nodule, central line insertion
- Postsurgical

COPD, Chronic obstructive pulmonary disease; *FNA,* fine-needle aspiration; *IPF,* Idiopathic pulmonary fibrosis.

Mesothelioma

Mesothelioma is a rare neoplasm that arises from mesothelial cells lining the parietal and visceral pleura and can manifest in a localized or diffuse manner. Pathology of pleural tumors has been reviewed elsewhere.[20] Mesothelioma develops from the mesothelial cells that line the pleural cavity. Histologic subtypes include epithelial, sarcomatoid, or mixed histology.[116] Epithelial histology alone has a more favorable prognosis.

The localized variant, the solitary fibrous tumor of the pleura, is a rare benign neoplasm that usually manifests as a well-defined, encapsulated tumor that is not associated with asbestos exposure. Historically, this variant was classified as a benign mesothelioma. Typically, the lesions are diagnosed as an asymptomatic mass on a chest radiograph. Complete surgical resection is the treatment of choice.

Diffuse malignant pleural mesothelioma manifests as a locally aggressive tumor commonly associated with asbestos exposure (75%). A long latency period between asbestos exposure and the development of the disease has been reported. Diagnostic imaging includes CXR, CT, and FDG-PET scan to determine the extent of tumor invasion and to evaluate occult metastases, including mediastinal metastases. Echocardiography is also performed to determine cardiac involvement. The diagnosis is made with pleural biopsy, which may include thoracentesis or pleural biopsy alone or incisional biopsies via thoracoscopy or open techniques.

Survival for this disease is poor, ranging from 4 to 12 months. Treatment has included chemotherapy,[117] standard and conformal radiation therapy, and extrapleural pneumonectomy. Combinations of therapies are commonly used. Extrapleural pneumonectomy and total pleurectomy are two commonly used surgical procedures.[118,119] In patients with epithelioid histology, negative margins, and negative mediastinal lymph nodes, 5-year survival is 46% after extrapleural pneumonectomy with adjuvant chemoradiotherapy.[120] Other techniques include preoperative chemotherapy followed by extrapleural pneumonectomy and conformal radiotherapy for the pleural surface. Survival is poor even with treatment. Improved therapies are needed.

MEDIASTINUM

Mediastinal abnormalities may manifest as an asymptomatic mass identified on screening CXR or with significant symptoms, including hypoxia, facial swelling, and acute respiratory distress. Symptoms are related to the involvement of the specific mediastinal structures. A definitive diagnosis is needed to optimize treatment planning.[121] Cytology from fine-needle aspiration or core biopsy or surgical biopsy may be needed to make the diagnosis and to determine optimal therapy. Generally, a mediastinal mass should be removed prophylactically to obtain a definitive diagnosis, achieve local control, and avoid future symptoms. If cancer is identified, adjuvant therapy given after complete resection may treat microscopic disease better than bulky disease.

Mediastinal masses differ between adults and children.[122] The most common mediastinal masses (Box 57-7) in adults are

BOX 57-7 Mediastinum: Classification of Primary Mediastinal Tumors and Cysts

Thymoma
- Benign
- Malignant

Lymphoma
- Hodgkin disease
- Lymphoblastic lymphoma
- Large cell lymphoma

Germ cell tumors
- Teratodermoid (benign/malignant)
- Seminoma
- Nonseminoma
  - Embryonal
  - Choriocarcinoma
  - Endodermal

Primary carcinomas

Mesenchymal tumors
- Fibroma/fibrosarcoma
- Lipoma/liposarcoma
- Leiomyoma/leiomyosarcoma
- Rhabdosarcoma
- Xanthogranuloma
- Myxoma
- Mesothelioma
- Hemangioma
- Hemangioendothelioma
- Hemangiopericytoma
- Lymphangioma
- Lymphangiomyoma
- Lymphangiopericytoma

Endocrine tumors
- Intrathoracic thyroid
- Parathyroid adenoma/carcinoma
- Carcinoid

Cysts
- Bronchogenic
- Pericardial
- Enteric
- Thymic
- Thoracic duct
- Nonspecific

Giant lymph node hyperplasia
- Castleman disease

Chondroma

Extramedullary hematopoiesis

Neurogenic tumors
- Neurofibroma
- Neurilemoma
- Paraganglioma
- Ganglioneuroma
- Neuroblastoma
- Chemodectoma
- Neurosarcoma

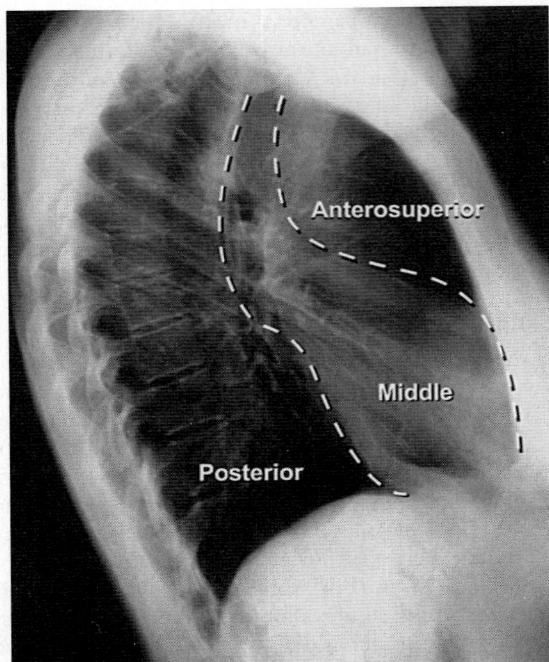

FIGURE 57-24 Lateral chest radiograph demonstrating the mediastinum divided into three anatomic subdivisions.

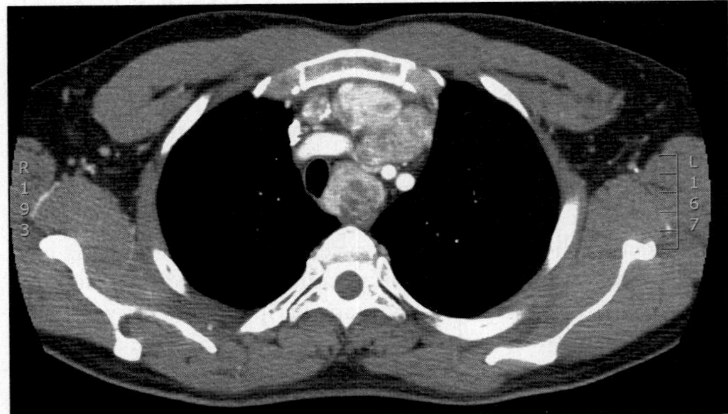
FIGURE 57-25 Thyroid carcinoma within the mediastinum. The tumor was resected via median sternotomy. No invasion was identified. A complete resection was accomplished.

thymomas and thymic cysts (26.5%), neurogenic tumors (20.0%), other cysts (16.1%), germ cell tumors (13.8%), and lymphomas (12.7%). In a combined series of 718 children with mediastinal masses, neurogenic tumors (41.6%), germ cell tumors (13.5%), primary cysts (13.4%), and lymphomas (13.4%) were diagnosed most frequently. Pericardial cysts and thymomas are uncommon in children.

Malignant mediastinal neoplasms account for 25% to 50% of mediastinal masses in adults. Lymphomas, thymomas, germ cell tumors, primary carcinomas, and neurogenic tumors are the most common. Primary carcinomas of the mediastinum constitute up to 10% of primary mediastinal masses and need to be differentiated from malignant thymomas, germ cell tumors, carcinoid tumors, lymphomas, mediastinal extension of bronchogenic carcinomas, and metastatic tumors, which may have a similar appearance by light microscopy.

Many mediastinal lesions occur in characteristic sites within the mediastinum (Fig. 57-24). Approximately half of all mediastinal masses are located in the anterosuperior mediastinum with the remainder divided between the posterior and middle mediastinum. In addition, the location of the mass explains some of the typical symptoms related to a mediastinal mass because of compression or invasion of adjacent mediastinal structures.

Anterosuperior Compartment

The anterosuperior compartment of the mediastinum borders the undersurface of the sternum ventrally, the pericardium dorsally, and the visceral pleura laterally (at the apposition of the pleura and pericardium). Tumors of the anterior mediastinum include thymomas, teratoma or germ cell tumors, a spectrum of lymphomas including Hodgkin disease, and thyroid goiter. In most cases, tissue (core biopsy) is required for diagnosis; fine-needle aspirate is usually inadequate.

Thymomas are usually the most frequently occurring neoplasm of the anterior mediastinum, and lymphomas are second. Germ cell neoplasms include benign and malignant teratomas, choriocarcinoma, seminoma, and embryonal cell neoplasm. Teratomas frequently occur in young adults. The gonads are the most common primary site, followed by the mediastinum. Most germ cell neoplasms are benign, but 20% are malignant. Malignant teratomas may produce high serum levels of α-fetoprotein (AFP) and carcinoembryonic antigen. Endocrine disease of the thyroid and parathyroid may occur in the anterior mediastinum as a result of their anatomic position in adults (substernal goiter) or embryologic development (Fig. 57-25). Carcinoid tumors may be found within the thymus. Primary carcinomas of the mediastinum are often unresectable and respond poorly to treatment.

Middle Compartment

The middle (or visceral) compartment extends from (and contains) the structures of the thoracic inlet (superiorly), the pericardium anteriorly, to the anterior surface of the vertebrae posteriorly. Lymphomas can occur in the middle mediastinum. Tumors of the heart and great vessels as well as tumors of the trachea, mainstem bronchi, and esophagus may be considered tumors of the middle compartment. Benign diseases, such as pericardial cysts and bronchogenic cysts, also occur here.

Posterior or Paravertebral Sulci Compartment

The posterior compartment is bounded by the middle compartment anteriorly and the costophrenic angle laterally. Neurogenic tumors are usually the most common primary tumors of the mediastinum, and approximately 25% of these tumors are malignant. These tumors are located within the paravertebral sulcus and may erode the adjacent vertebra or rib. Schwannomas and neurilemomas are the most common neurogenic tumors. Neurofibromas arise from the nerve sheath and fibers and occur in middle-aged patients. In children, ganglioneuroma is the most common neurogenic tumor. The tumor frequently attains a large size before presentation of symptoms. Increased levels of catecholamines may produce symptoms. Surgical resection of these neurogenic tumors is usually the procedure of choice.

Embryologic development of the neural crest cells forms the basis of neuroendocrine tumors in the mediastinum. Of pheochromocytomas, 1% occur within the mediastinum. Chemodectomas or paragangliomas may arise from chemoreceptor tissues around the aorta and great vessels, including the carotid. Symptoms may result from catecholamine production and are alleviated by surgical resection.

Clinical Manifestations and Diagnosis

Approximately one third of adult patients may develop symptoms from a mediastinal mass. Symptoms include chest pain, dyspnea, and cough. The symptoms may vary widely and relate to size (fatigue, weight loss); location; extent of compression or invasion of mediastinal structures (superior vena cava syndrome); and production of hormones, markers, or other biochemical materials (e.g., myasthenia gravis, fatigue, night sweats). Larger mediastinal tumors are more likely to produce symptoms. Benign lesions are more often asymptomatic. Superior vena cava syndrome (obstruction of the superior vena cava with head and neck and upper extremity swelling), cough, hoarseness (from involvement of the recurrent laryngeal nerve), dyspnea from tumor volume or phrenic nerve paralysis, and dysphagia occur with compression or invasion of mediastinal structures. Other manifestations include Horner syndrome and Pancoast syndrome.

Infections within the mediastinum are devastating. Because of the extensive thin areolar planes between major structures, infections within a limited portion of the mediastinum may spread vertically or horizontally to create an extensive infection. Synergistic aerobic and anaerobic infections from the perforated esophagus are particularly life-threatening. Treatment consists of surgical drainage and antibiotics.

Specific clinical syndromes may occur as a result of mediastinal tumors. Physical examination may reveal swelling of the head, neck, or upper extremities. Dyspnea may result from compression of the trachea, bronchus, or a portion of the lung parenchyma. Recurrent respiratory symptoms may occur for some time until a CXR is obtained and the abnormality is identified. Postobstructive pneumonitis or infection of benign pericardial or enteric duplication cysts may produce fever or sepsis. Myasthenia gravis may result from thymomas. In addition, thymomas may result in autoimmune problems, such as hypogammaglobulinemia, red cell aplasia, and smooth muscle degeneration. Mediastinal Hodgkin disease may produce an intermittent fever (Pel-Ebstein fever). Patients with hypertension from pheochromocytoma, thyrotoxicosis from goiter, hypercalcemia from ectopic mediastinal parathyroid adenoma or carcinoma, or hypogammaglobulinemia should be evaluated carefully; mediastinal findings may affect subsequent therapeutic recommendations.

Evaluation and Diagnostic Imaging

Diagnostic imaging typically includes a plain CXR taken in two planes (posteroanterior and left lateral), which provides basic information about the location of the mass within the mediastinum. Given the known propensity of specific lesions to occur in the anterior, visceral (middle), or paravertebral (posterior) sulcus based on the anatomy and embryologic development of cervicothoracic organs, a differential diagnosis may be obtained.

Diaphragm fluoroscopy, or "sniff test," is used to evaluate paradoxical motion of the diaphragm on rapid inspiration indicative of phrenic nerve paralysis. CT scan of the chest has replaced plain CXRs as the diagnostic procedure of choice for mediastinal masses. MRI may enhance the diagnostic abilities of chest CT. Anterior mediastinal masses, such as thymoma, can be evaluated for the extent of compression or possible invasion into the pulmonary artery, innominate vein, or superior vena cava. Evaluation of the extent of invasion into the brachial plexus, great vessels, vertebral body, neural foramina, and spinal column may be easily accomplished with MRI. Echocardiography and FDG-PET have been commonly used. High FDG uptake is more likely to correlate with invasion in both thymic carcinomas and invasive thymomas.

Mediastinal tumors may secrete specific hormones or biological markers. Parathyroid adenomas or functioning parathyroid carcinomas may secrete parathormone. Pheochromocytomas may secrete various catecholamines (in serum and urine), which may cause hypertension. Carcinomas may secrete carcinoembryonic antigen. Nonseminomatous germ cell neoplasms may secrete AFP or β-human chorionic gonadotropin (β-HCG). Skin tests for tuberculosis, histoplasmosis, and coccidioidomycosis may also yield positive results. Other diagnostic tests for mediastinal tuberculosis include sputum cytology, CXR, and urine cytology.

Histologic Diagnosis

A mediastinal mass cannot be treated until a diagnosis is made. Although radiographic diagnosis may suffice for mediastinal cysts, tissue for definitive diagnosis is needed for solid masses. Fine-needle aspiration or needle biopsy with CT guidance of a mediastinal mass may provide sufficient tissue for diagnosis for thymic carcinoma or other defined neoplasms. For lymphomas in particular as well as thymomas and neural tumors, larger amounts of tissue may be required for cellular analysis. In these patients, core needle biopsy, mediastinoscopy, or intrathoracic biopsy (via thoracoscopy or open thoracotomy) may be considered. Electron microscopy may be required for confirmation of specific histologies. For recurrent lymphomas, after chemotherapy, open techniques for incisional biopsy are often required.

Median sternotomy provides a direct visual approach to the mediastinum and may be used for management of a wide range of mediastinal disease. VATS techniques and robotic techniques of resection are increasingly used for treatment of these noninvasive tumors. More extensive approaches include the transverse sternotomy or "clam-shell" incision. Anesthetic considerations should include avoidance of airway obstruction, awake intubation, and avoidance of muscle paralytics or drugs such as fluoroquinolones with potential paralytic effects.

PRIMARY MEDIASTINAL CYSTS

Primary cysts of the mediastinum account for approximately 20% of mediastinal masses in most collected series.[122] Cysts are characterized from the organ of origin and may be bronchogenic, pericardial, enteric, or thymic or may be of an unspecified nature. More than 75% of cases are asymptomatic, and these tumors rarely cause morbidity; however, with proximity to vital structures within the mediastinum and increasing size, the cyst may cause significant problems. Benign cysts may be resected with minimally invasive techniques.

Bronchogenic cysts account for most primary cysts of the mediastinum (see Fig. 57-9). They originate as sequestrations from the ventral foregut, the antecedent of the tracheobronchial tree, and can be situated within the lung parenchyma or the mediastinum. Bronchogenic cysts are usually located proximal to the trachea or bronchi and may be just posterior to the carina. A connection to the bronchus rarely exists; however, when it occurs, these cysts may become infected. Diagnostic imaging may reveal an air-fluid level within the mediastinum. Two thirds of bronchogenic cysts are asymptomatic. In infants, cysts cause severe respiratory compromise by compressing the trachea or the bronchus. Resection is recommended.

Pericardial cysts are second in frequency to bronchogenic cysts and occur in the cardiophrenic angle mostly on the right side (70%). These cysts may or may not communicate with the pericardium. Typically, clear fluid is encountered. The characteristics of pericardial cysts include location in the cardiophrenic angle, characteristic appearance, smooth borders, and attenuation approximating water for the cyst fluid. Needle aspiration and routine surveillance may be all that is needed. Resection may be used for diagnosis and to exclude malignant tumors.

Enteric cysts or duplication cysts arise from the primitive foregut, which develops into the upper division of the gastrointestinal tract. These cysts are usually attached to the esophagus. Symptoms occur as size increases with compression of the esophagus and dysphagia. Neuroenteric cysts are associated with anomalies of the vertebral column. Excision is recommended.

PRIMARY MEDIASTINAL NEOPLASMS

Thymoma

The pathology of thymoma has been reviewed elsewhere.[20] Thymoma is the most common neoplasm of the anterosuperior compartment. The peak incidence is in the third through fifth decades, but thymomas may occur throughout adulthood. Thymoma is rare in the first 2 decades of life. A thymoma may appear on a radiograph as a small, well-circumscribed mass or as a bulky lobulated mass confluent with adjacent mediastinal structures (Fig. 57-26). Symptoms at presentation are related to local mass effects causing chest pain, dyspnea, hemoptysis, cough, and superior vena cava syndrome or systemic syndromes caused by immunologic mechanisms. The most common syndrome is myasthenia gravis, although other syndromes include pure red blood cell aplasia, pure white blood cell aplasia, aplastic anemia, Cushing syndrome, hypogammaglobulinemia and hypergammaglobulinemia, dermatomyositis, systemic lupus erythematosus, progressive systemic sclerosis, hypercoagulopathy with thrombosis, rheumatoid arthritis, megaesophagus, and granulomatous myocarditis. Early surgical treatment of myasthenia gravis and small thymomas is common. When thymectomy is performed early in the course of myasthenia gravis, a greater percentage of thymomas are benign.

Benign and malignant disease is differentiated by the presence of gross invasion of adjacent structures, metastasis, or microscopic evidence of capsular invasion. Tumors less than 3 cm in size are frequently benign; however, determination of malignancy (invasion) can be challenging for patients with tumors between 3 and 5 cm. A malignant process may be present in tumors greater than 5 cm.

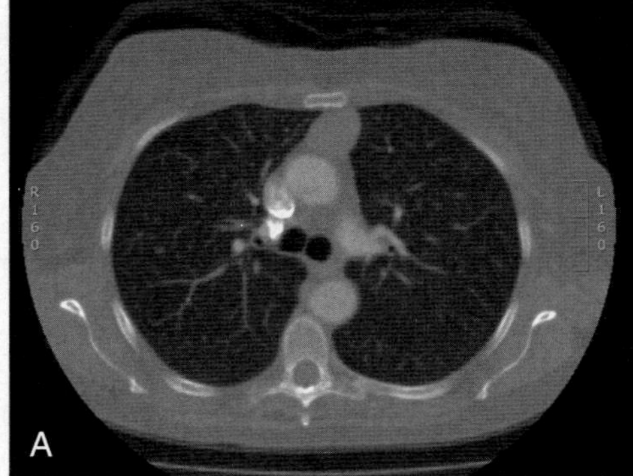

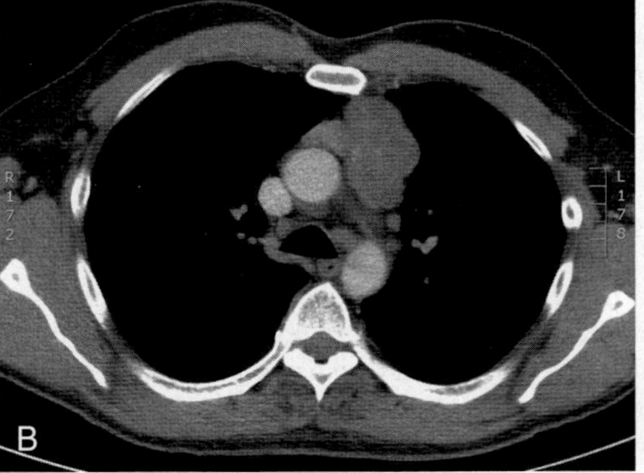

FIGURE 57-26 A, Computed tomography (CT) scan of the chest in a patient with myasthenia gravis and thymoma. The thymoma is small with a plane of separation between the tumor and the pericardium. **B,** Chest CT scan in a patient with a larger mediastinal mass. The location, character, and size are noted. Transthoracic core needle biopsy was performed. Germ cell tumor markers were normal. Pathology demonstrated thymoma. A 6.5-cm thymoma was subsequently resected. There was no invasion of the pericardium. A complete resection (R0) was accomplished.

Whenever possible, the therapy for thymoma is excision without removing or injuring vital structures.[123] Even with well-encapsulated thymomas, extended thymectomy with eradication of all accessible mediastinal fatty areolar tissue is performed to ensure removal of all ectopic thymic tissue and to reduce the number of tumor recurrences. Protection and preservation of the phrenic nerves are integral components of thymectomy.

The perioperative management in patients with myasthenia gravis is crucial to prevent complications. Anticholinesterase inhibitors are discontinued to decrease the amount of pulmonary secretions and prevent inadvertent cholinergic weakness. Plasmapheresis is used routinely within 72 hours of thymectomy. In most patients, plasmapheresis is effective in controlling generalized weakness. Survival is based on stage. Stage I is characterized by a well-encapsulated tumor without evidence of gross or microscopic capsular invasion; in stage II, tumor exhibits pericapsular growth into adjacent fat or mediastinal pleura or microscopic invasion of the thymic capsule; in stage III, tumor invades adjacent organs; stage IVa is characterized by intrathoracic metastases; and stage IVb is characterized by extrathoracic metastases (uncommon). Complete resection (R0) is required. For patients with stage I thymoma, resection alone is sufficient without the need for adjuvant therapy. For stage II and III disease, adjuvant radiation therapy is commonly used. Tumors greater than 5 cm, locally invasive tumors, unresectable tumors, and metastatic tumors are treated using protocols that include chemotherapy followed by surgical exploration with the goal of complete resection and postoperative (adjuvant) radiation therapy. Cisplatin-based regimens have excellent response rates.[124]

Invasive thymomas require radical resection of involved structures, which may include vascular reconstruction of the superior vena cava, innominate vein, or its branches.[125] Using this aggressive approach to obtain complete resection, a significant difference in 5-year survival rates is seen in patients with stage III thymomas (94%) compared with patients with incomplete resections (35%). Thymomas frequently show recurrence, and reoperation for recurrent disease has been recommended.

Germ Cell Tumors

Germ cell tumors arise from primordial germ cells that fail to complete the migration from the urogenital ridge and rest in the mediastinum. Treatment depends on histology.[126] The anterosuperior mediastinum is the most common extragonadal primary site of these tumors. Although these lesions are identical histologically to germ cell tumors originating in the gonads, they are not considered metastatic from primary gonadal tumors. The current recommendations for evaluating the testes of a patient with mediastinal germ cell tumor are careful physical examination and ultrasonography of the testes. Biopsy is reserved for positive findings. Blind biopsy or orchiectomy is contraindicated.

Teratomas

Teratomas are the most common mediastinal germ cell neoplasms and are located most commonly in the anterosuperior mediastinum. They are composed of multiple tissue elements that are derived from the three primitive embryonic layers foreign to the area in which they occur. The peak incidence is in the second and third decades of life. There is no gender predisposition. Radiographic evidence of normal tissue (e.g., well-formed teeth or globular calcifications, a fatty mass) in an abnormal location can be considered specific. The teratodermoid (dermoid) cyst is the simplest form of a teratoma and is composed of derivatives of the epidermal layer, including dermal and epidermal glands, hair, and sebaceous material. Teratomas are histologically more complex. The solid component of the tumor often contains well-differentiated elements of bone, cartilage, teeth, muscle, connective tissue, fibrous and lymphoid tissue, nerve, thymus, mucous and salivary glands, lung, liver, or pancreas. Malignant tumors are differentiated from benign tumors by the presence of primitive (embryonic) tissue or by the presence of malignant components. Immature teratomas contain combinations of mature epithelial and connective tissues with immature areas of mesenchymal and neuroectodermal tissues. Teratomas with malignant components are divided into categories based on the elements present.

Diagnosis and therapy rely on surgical excision. For benign tumors of large size or with involvement of adjacent mediastinal structures such that complete resection is impossible, partial resection has led to resolution of symptoms, frequently without relapse. For malignant teratomas, chemotherapy and radiation therapy, combined with surgical excision, are individualized for the type of malignant components contained in the tumors. The overall prognosis is poor for malignant teratomas.

Malignant Nonteratomatous Germ Cell Tumors

Malignant germ cell tumors occur predominantly in the anterosuperior mediastinum with a marked male predominance most commonly in the third and fourth decades of life.[127] Most patients have symptoms of chest pain, cough, dyspnea, and hemoptysis; the superior vena cava syndrome occurs commonly. A large anterior mediastinal mass is identified on diagnostic imaging. There is evidence of intrathoracic spread of disease. CT and MRI are helpful to define the extent of the disease and involvement of mediastinal structures. Serologic measurements of AFP and β-HCG are useful for differentiating seminomas from nonseminomatous tumors, assessing response to therapy, and diagnosing relapse or failure of therapy. Seminomas rarely produce β-HCG and never produce AFP; in contrast, more than 90% of nonseminomatous tumors secrete one or both of these hormones. This differentiation is important, as seminomas are radiosensitive, and nonseminomatous tumors are relatively radioinsensitive.

Seminomas

Seminomas constitute 50% of malignant germ cell tumors. Seminomas usually remain intrathoracic. Symptoms are related to the mechanical effects of the tumor on adjacent mediastinal and pulmonary structures. The superior vena cava syndrome occurs in 10% to 20% of patients. These tumors are sensitive to irradiation and chemotherapy. Therapy is determined by the stage of the disease. Cytoreductive resection before chemotherapy or radiation therapy is unnecessary. Treatment consists of systemic and local therapy—chemotherapy with salvage surgery or combined chemoradiotherapy. Radiation therapy may be considered for early-stage disease but is not recommended for regional disease. Platinum-based chemotherapy is common. Occasionally, excision is possible without injury to vital structures and can be recommended. When complete resection is possible, the use of adjuvant therapy is unnecessary. When excision is impossible, a biopsy sample of sufficient size to establish the diagnosis is obtained.

Nonseminomatous Tumors

Malignant nonseminomatous germ cell tumors include choriocarcinomas, embryonal cell carcinomas, immature teratomas, teratomas with malignant components, and endodermal cell (yolk sac) tumors and occur mostly in men in their third or fourth decades.

Diagnostic imaging reveals a large anterior mediastinal mass with frequent extension to the lung, chest wall, and mediastinal structures. Nonseminomatous germ cell neoplasms are more aggressive tumors and more frequently disseminated at the time of diagnosis, they are rarely radiosensitive, and more than 90% produce either β-HCG or AFP. All patients with choriocarcinoma and some patients with embryonal cell tumors have elevated levels of β-HCG. AFP is most commonly elevated in patients with embryonal cell carcinomas and yolk sac tumors. Mediastinal nonseminomatous germ cell tumors, but not testicular germ cell tumors, are associated with the development of rare hematologic malignancies, such as acute megakaryocytic leukemia, systemic mast cell disease, and malignant histiocytosis, as well as other hematologic abnormalities, including myelodysplastic syndrome and idiopathic thrombocytopenia refractory to treatment.

Treatment of these nonseminomatous tumors currently is with cisplatin and etoposide-based regimens. Advanced disease, invasion into thoracic structures, and metastasis preclude surgical resection. Serum markers, AFP or β-HCG, are followed to assess response to systemic treatment. If a complete serologic and radiologic response is achieved, patients are closely observed. If the disease progresses during therapy, salvage chemotherapy is initiated. Operative intervention may be required to establish a histologic diagnosis in patients without elevations in serum AFP or β-HCG or for salvage resection after tissue or serologic response to therapy.[126] The pathology of the resected postchemotherapy specimen appears to be the most significant predictor of survival. The presence of residual disease after chemotherapy portends a poor prognosis and the need for additional chemotherapy. When tumor necrosis or a benign teratoma is found during surgical exploration after chemotherapy, an excellent or intermediate prognosis is conferred, respectively.

Neurogenic Tumors

Neurogenic tumors are usually located in the posterior mediastinum and originate from the sympathetic ganglia (ganglioma, ganglioneuroblastoma, and neuroblastoma), the intercostal nerves (neurofibroma, neurilemoma, and neurosarcoma), and the paraganglia cells (paraganglioma). Although the peak incidence occurs in adults, neurogenic tumors make up a proportionally greater percentage of mediastinal masses in children. Although most neurogenic tumors in adults are benign, a greater percentage of neurogenic tumors are malignant in children.

The most common neurogenic tumor is neurilemoma or schwannoma, which originates from perineural Schwann cells. They are benign, slow-growing neoplasms that frequently arise from a spinal nerve root but can involve any thoracic nerve. These tumors are well circumscribed and have a defined capsule. They arise from the nerve sheath and extrinsically compress the nerve fibers. The peak incidence of these tumors is in the third through fifth decades of life; men and women are equally affected.

Many of these tumors are asymptomatic. Symptoms such as pain occur from compression or invasion of intercostal nerve, bone, and chest wall; cough and dyspnea resulting from compression of the tracheobronchial tree; Pancoast syndrome; and Horner syndrome resulting from involvement of the brachial and the cervical sympathetic chain. Approximately 10% of neurogenic tumors have extensions into the spinal column and are termed *dumbbell tumors* because of their characteristic shape with relatively large paraspinal and intraspinal portions connected by a narrow isthmus of tissue traversing the intervertebral foramen. Patients with paraspinal tumors should undergo MRI to evaluate the presence and extent of the tumor and its relationship to the neural foramen and the intraspinal space. During resection, the intraspinal component should be removed first via a posterior laminectomy. This approach minimizes the potential for spinal column hematoma, cord ischemia, and paralysis. A separate transthoracic approach is needed for resection of the intrathoracic component.

Neuroblastoma

Neuroblastomas originate from the sympathetic nervous system. The most common location for a neuroblastoma is in the retroperitoneum; however, 10% to 20% occur primarily in the mediastinum. These are highly invasive neoplasms that have frequently metastasized before diagnosis. Most of these tumors occur in children 4 years old or younger. A 24-hour urine collection to measure catecholamines is obtained in children with a posterior mediastinal mass. Therapy is determined by the stage of the disease: stage I, surgical excision; stage II, excision and radiation therapy; stages III and IV, multimodality therapy using surgical debulking, radiation therapy, and multiagent chemotherapy and a second-look exploration to resect residual disease when necessary. The usual chemotherapeutic agents are cisplatin, vincristine, doxorubicin, cyclophosphamide, and etoposide.

Ganglion Tumors

Ganglioneuroblastomas are composed of mature and immature ganglion cells. Treatment of ganglioneuroblastoma ranges from surgical excision alone to various chemotherapeutic strategies depending on histologic characteristics, age at diagnosis, and stage of disease. Ganglioneuromas are benign tumors that originate from the sympathetic chain and are composed of ganglion cells and nerve fibers. These tumors typically manifest at an early age and are the most common neurogenic tumors occurring during childhood. The usual location is the paravertebral region. These tumors are well encapsulated and, when cross-sectioned, frequently exhibit areas of cystic degeneration. Surgical excision provides cure.

Paraganglioma (Pheochromocytoma)

Mediastinal paragangliomas are rare tumors, representing less than 1% of all mediastinal tumors and less than 2% of all pheochromocytomas. Although most are found in the paravertebral sulcus, an increasing number occur in the branchial arch structures, coronary and aortopulmonary paraganglia, atria, and islands of tissue in the pericardium. Although adrenal pheochromocytomas often produce both epinephrine and norepinephrine, extra-adrenal paragangliomas rarely secrete epinephrine. Multiple paragangliomas occur in 10% of patients. These tumors are more common in patients with multiple endocrine neoplasia syndromes, a family history of disease, and Carney syndrome (pulmonary chondroma, gastric leiomyosarcoma, and functioning extra-adrenal paraganglioma). In patients who have had excision of an adrenal pheochromocytoma and continue to have symptoms, a search for an extra-adrenal lesion is undertaken, with careful attention to the mediastinum. Tumor localization has improved through the use of CT and iodine-131 metaiodobenzylguanidine scintigraphy, particularly when the tumors are hormonally active. When appropriate, surgical resection is the optimal therapy. In patients with tumors involving the middle mediastinum, cardiopulmonary bypass may be necessary to enable resection. Preoperative embolization to reduce perioperative bleeding may be considered. Although half of tumors appear malignant morphologically, metastatic disease rarely develops.

Lymphomas

Although the mediastinum is frequently involved in patients with lymphoma at some time during the course of their disease, it is infrequently the sole site of disease at the time of presentation. Hodgkin and non-Hodgkin lymphoma are distinct clinical entities with overlapping features. Patients usually have symptoms; chest pain, cough, dyspnea, hoarseness, and superior vena cava syndrome are the most common clinical manifestations. Nonspecific systemic symptoms of fever and chills, weight loss, and anorexia are frequently noted and are important in the staging of patients with Hodgkin lymphoma. Symptoms characteristic of Hodgkin lymphoma include chest pain after consumption of alcohol and Pel-Ebstein fever.

Surgical excision of all disease is rarely possible; the surgeon's primary role is to provide sufficient tissue for diagnosis and to assist in pathologic staging. A needle biopsy is often unsuccessful because larger tissue samples are needed to make a histologic diagnosis, particularly with nodular sclerosing lesions. Thoracoscopy, mediastinoscopy, or mediastinotomy and, rarely, thoracotomy or median sternotomy may be necessary to obtain sufficient tissue. The role of staging laparotomy has been minimized, and its only current indication is for patients with clinically limited disease who opt for limited treatment.

Patients with non-Hodgkin lymphoma usually have symptoms because of involvement of adjacent mediastinal structures. Superior vena cava syndrome is relatively common. Lymphoblastic lymphoma occurs predominantly in children, adolescents, and young adults and represents 60% of cases of mediastinal non-Hodgkin lymphoma.

After treatment of lymphomas, residual radiographic abnormalities within the mediastinum are commonly noted (64% to 88%). CT cannot differentiate fibrosis or necrosis from residual tumor. FDG-PET has shown promise as a noninvasive way to detect active mediastinal disease and predict relapse in patients with lymphoma, but tissue confirmation is required. Needle biopsy does not provide significant diagnostic material. Transthoracic incisional biopsy under general anesthesia is often needed given the significant fibrosis that remains after therapy.

Endocrine Tumors

Thyroid Tumors

Although substernal extension of a cervical goiter is common, totally intrathoracic thyroid tumors are rare and make up only 1% of all mediastinal masses in collected series. These tumors arise from heterotopic thyroid tissue, which occurs most commonly in the anterosuperior mediastinum but may also occur in the middle mediastinum between the trachea and the esophagus as well as in the posterior mediastinum. Although there may be a demonstrable connection with the cervical gland (usually a fibrous connective tissue band), a true intrathoracic thyroid gland derives its blood supply from thoracic vessels. Substernal extensions of a cervical goiter can usually be excised using a cervical approach.

Parathyroid Tumors

Although parathyroid glands may occur in the mediastinum in 10% of patients, they are usually accessible through the cervical incision. Most often, these adenomas are found in the anterosuperior mediastinum (80%) embedded in or near the superior pole of the thymus. This anatomic relationship is the result of the common embryogenesis of the inferior parathyroid glands from the third branchial cleft. The superior parathyroid glands and the lateral lobes of the thyroid gland are derived from the fourth branchial pouch. Because they migrate with the lateral lobes of the thyroid gland to a paraesophageal position, parathyroid adenomas can also be found in the posterior mediastinum.

Most frequently, the mediastinal parathyroid adenoma may be excised after a negative exploration of the cervical region through the existing cervical incision. Usually the vascular supply extends from cervical blood vessels. In patients with persistent hyperparathyroidism after cervical exploration, if localization studies show residual parathyroid in the mediastinum, mediastinal exploration using a median sternotomy or thoracoscopy is indicated.

Parathyroid carcinomas have been reported and are usually hormonally active. Patients differ in clinical presentation in that they often have higher serum calcium levels and manifest more severe symptoms of hyperparathyroidism. When possible, resection is the optimal therapy.

Neuroendocrine Tumors

Mediastinal neuroendocrine tumors, carcinoid tumors, arise from cells of Kulchitsky located in the thymus and commonly occur in men in their 40s and 50s; they are usually located in the anterosuperior mediastinum. These tumors are aggressive, and 20% have metastatic spread to mediastinal and cervical lymph nodes, liver, bone, skin, and lungs. More than 50% of thymic neuroendocrine tumors are hormonally active, often associated with Cushing syndrome because of production of adrenocorticotropic hormone, less frequently associated with multiple endocrine neoplasia syndromes, and only rarely associated with carcinoid syndrome (0.6%). If possible, resection is recommended; however, local invasion and metastasis often preclude complete excision. Adjuvant therapy is controversial, but irradiation should probably be added, particularly in patients with capsular invasion.

SELECTED REFERENCES

Arriagada R, Bergman B, Dunant A, et al: Cisplatin-based adjuvant chemotherapy in patients with completely resected non-small-cell lung cancer. *N Engl J Med* 350:351–360, 2004.

Adjuvant therapy after complete resection of non–small cell lung carcinoma has been shown to improve survival in selected patients. The International Lung Adjuvant Trial proved that adjuvant platinum-based chemotherapy improved survival compared with no treatment.

Diagnosis and Management of Lung Cancer: ACCP Guidelines (2nd Edition). *Chest* 132(Suppl 3):2007.

National Comprehensive Cancer Network: NCCN Clinical Practice Guidelines in Oncology. Non-small cell lung cancer, 2011 (<http://www.nccn.org/professionals/physician_gls/f_guidelines.asp>; Accessed August 20, 2015).

Guidelines for diagnosis, treatment, and surveillance are published by various organizations based on evidence and consensus of experts. Two sets of guidelines for the management of non–small cell lung cancer were published by the American College of Chest Physicians and the National Comprehensive Cancer Network.

Dresler CM, Olak J, Herndon JE, 2nd, et al: Phase III intergroup study of talc poudrage vs talc slurry sclerosis for malignant pleural effusion. *Chest* 127:909–915, 2005.

This prospective randomized study evaluated chest tube with talc slurry versus video-assisted thoracic surgery (VATS) with talc poudrage. Both groups benefited from the intervention, and neither intervention was superior. VATS has the advantage of complete drainage, pleural biopsy, and direct placement of talc.

Edge SB, Byrd DR, Compton CC, et al: *AJCC cancer staging manual*, ed 7, New York, 2010, Springer.

Goldstraw P, Crowley J, Chansky K, et al: The IASLC Lung Cancer Staging Project: Proposals for the revision of the TNM stage groupings in the forthcoming (seventh) edition of the TNM Classification of malignant tumours. *J Thorac Oncol* 2:706–714, 2007.

Pao W: Defining clinically relevant molecular subsets of lung cancer. *Cancer Chemother Pharmacol* 58(Suppl 1):s11–s15, 2006.

Staging for non–small cell lung carcinoma has changed significantly with the results of the International Association for the Study of Lung Cancer Staging Project. This data set was predominately surgery based but international in extent and both internally and externally validated. These results have formed the basis for the American Joint Committee on Cancer and Union for International Cancer Control staging systems. Future staging systems may evaluate the molecular characteristics of the tumor as both prognostic (of survival) and predictive (of response) characteristics.

Fernando HC, Schuchert M, Landreneau R, et al: Approaching the high-risk patient: Sublobar resection, stereotactic body radiation therapy, or radiofrequency ablation. *Ann Thorac Surg* 89:S2123–S2127, 2010.

Timmerman R, Paulus R, Galvin J, et al: Stereotactic body radiation therapy for inoperable early stage lung cancer. *JAMA* 303:1070–1076, 2010.

New methods of local control of non–small cell lung carcinoma are being studied. A review of local treatment options evaluated sublobar resection, stereotactic body radiation therapy, and radiofrequency. Clinical trials are underway to evaluate these treatment options prospectively.

National Lung Screening Trial Research Team, Aberle DR, Berg CD, et al: The National Lung Screening Trial: overview and study design. *Radiology* 258:243–253, 2011.

The National Lung Screening Trial tested screening for lung cancer and found that fewer lung cancer–related deaths occurred in the population screened with computed tomography compared with chest x-ray.

Walsh GL, Davis BM, Swisher SG, et al: A single-institutional, multidisciplinary approach to primary sarcomas involving the chest wall requiring full-thickness resections. *J Thorac Cardiovasc Surg* 121:48–60, 2001.

This article presents one of the largest series on primary chest wall tumors.

REFERENCES

1. Brunelli A, Kim AW, Berger KI, et al: Physiologic evaluation of the patient with lung cancer being considered for resectional surgery: Diagnosis and management of lung cancer, 3rd ed: American College of Chest Physicians evidence-based clinical practice guidelines. *Chest* 143:e166S–190S, 2013.
2. Thomsen T, Villebro N, Moller AM: Interventions for preoperative smoking cessation. *Cochrane Database Syst Rev* CD002294, 2010.
3. Mason DP, Subramanian S, Nowicki ER, et al: Impact of smoking cessation before resection of lung cancer: A Society of Thoracic Surgeons General Thoracic Surgery Database study. *Ann Thorac Surg* 88:362–370, discussion 370-371, 2009.
4. Zaman M, Bilal H, Mahmood S, et al: Does getting smokers to stop smoking before lung resections reduce their risk? *Interact Cardiovasc Thorac Surg* 14:320–323, 2012.
5. Cataldo JK, Dubey S, Prochaska JJ: Smoking cessation: An integral part of lung cancer treatment. *Oncology* 78:289–301, 2010.
6. Gould MK, Garcia DA, Wren SM, et al: Prevention of VTE in nonorthopedic surgical patients: Antithrombotic Therapy and Prevention of Thrombosis, 9th ed: American College of Chest Physicians Evidence-Based Clinical Practice Guidelines. *Chest* 141:e227S–277S, 2012.
7. Poonyagariyagorn H, Mazzone PJ: Lung cancer: Preoperative pulmonary evaluation of the lung resection candidate. *Semin Respir Crit Care Med* 29:271–284, 2008.
8. Beckles MA, Spiro SG, Colice GL, et al: The physiologic evaluation of patients with lung cancer being considered for resectional surgery. *Chest* 123:105S–114S, 2003.
9. Mendeloff EN: Sequestrations, congenital cystic adenomatoid malformations, and congenital lobar emphysema. *Semin Thorac Cardiovasc Surg* 16:209–214, 2004.
10. Fievet L, D'Journo XB, Guys JM, et al: Bronchogenic cyst: Best time for surgery? *Ann Thorac Surg* 94:1695–1699, 2012.
11. Sfakianaki AK, Copel JA: Congenital cystic lesions of the lung: Congenital cystic adenomatoid malformation and bronchopulmonary sequestration. *Rev Obstet Gynecol* 5:85–93, 2012.
12. Jaquiss RD: Management of pediatric tracheal stenosis and tracheomalacia. *Semin Thorac Cardiovasc Surg* 16:220–224, 2004.
13. Damle SS, Mitchell JD: Surgery for tracheobronchomalacia. *Semin Cardiothorac Vasc Anesth* 16:203–208, 2012.
14. Pegoli W, Mattei P, Colombani PM: Congenital intrathoracic vascular abnormalities in childhood. *Chest Surg Clin North Am* 3:529, 1993.
15. Maldonado JA, Henry T, Gutierrez FR: Congenital thoracic vascular anomalies. *Radiol Clin North Am* 48:85–115, 2010.
16. Siegel RL, Miller KD, Jemal A: Cancer statistics, 2015. *CA Cancer J Clin* 65:5–29, 2015.
17. Field RW: Environmental factors in cancer: Radon. *Rev Environ Health* 25:23–31, 2010.
18. U.S. National Institutes of Health: Information on clinical trials and human research studies, 2011 (<http://www.clinicaltrials.gov>; Accessed August 20, 2015).
19. An Overview of NCI's National Clinical Trials Network (<http://www.cancer.gov/research/areas/clinical-trials/nctn>; Accessed August 20, 2015).

20. Travis WD, Brambilla E, Muller-Hermelink HK, et al: *World Health Organization classification of tumours. Pathology and genetics of tumours of the lung, pleura, thymus, and heart*, Lyon, France, 2004, IARC Press.
21. Travis WD, Brambilla E, Noguchi M, et al: International Association for the Study of Lung Cancer/American Thoracic Society/European Respiratory Society: International multidisciplinary classification of lung adenocarcinoma: executive summary. *Proc Am Thorac Soc* 8:381–385, 2011.
22. National Lung Screening Trial Research T, Aberle DR, Berg CD, et al: The National Lung Screening Trial: Overview and study design. *Radiology* 258:243–253, 2011.
23. National Lung Screening Trial Research T, Aberle DR, Adams AM, et al: Baseline characteristics of participants in the randomized national lung screening trial. *J Natl Cancer Inst* 102:1771–1779, 2010.
24. Preventive Services Task Force: Lung cancer: Screening, 2013 (<http://www.uspreventiveservicestaskforce.org/Page/Document/UpdateSummaryFinal/lung-cancer-screening>; Accessed August 20, 2015).
25. Gould MK: Clinical practice. Lung-cancer screening with low-dose computed tomography. *N Engl J Med* 371:1813–1820, 2014.
26. Spiro SG, Gould MK, Colice GL, et al: Initial evaluation of the patient with lung cancer: Symptoms, signs, laboratory tests, and paraneoplastic syndromes: ACCP evidenced-based clinical practice guidelines (2nd edition). *Chest* 132:149S–160S, 2007.
27. Simoff MJ, Lally B, Slade MG, et al: Symptom management in patients with lung cancer: Diagnosis and management of lung cancer, 3rd ed: American College of Chest Physicians evidence-based clinical practice guidelines. *Chest* 143:e455S–497S, 2013.
28. Gould MK, Donington J, Lynch WR, et al: Evaluation of individuals with pulmonary nodules: When is it lung cancer? Diagnosis and management of lung cancer, 3rd ed: American College of Chest Physicians evidence-based clinical practice guidelines. *Chest* 143:e93S–120S, 2013.
29. Ost DE, Gould MK: Decision making in patients with pulmonary nodules. *Am J Respir Crit Care Med* 185:363–372, 2012.
30. Rivera MP, Mehta AC, Wahidi MM: Establishing the diagnosis of lung cancer: Diagnosis and management of lung cancer, 3rd ed: American College of Chest Physicians evidence-based clinical practice guidelines. *Chest* 143:e142S–165S, 2013.
31. Goldstraw P, Crowley J, Chansky K, et al: The IASLC Lung Cancer Staging Project: Proposals for the revision of the TNM stage groupings in the forthcoming (seventh) edition of the TNM Classification of malignant tumours. *J Thorac Oncol* 2:706–714, 2007.
32. Silvestri GA, Gonzalez AV, Jantz MA, et al: Methods for staging non-small cell lung cancer: Diagnosis and management of lung cancer, 3rd ed: American College of Chest Physicians evidence-based clinical practice guidelines. *Chest* 143:e211S–250S, 2013.
33. Detterbeck FC, Mazzone PJ, Naidich DP, et al: Screening for lung cancer: Diagnosis and management of lung cancer, 3rd ed: American College of Chest Physicians evidence-based clinical practice guidelines. *Chest* 143:e78S–92S, 2013.
34. Deppen SA, Blume JD, Kensinger CD, et al: Accuracy of FDG-PET to diagnose lung cancer in areas with infectious lung disease: A meta-analysis. *JAMA* 312:1227–1236, 2014.
35. Fischer B, Lassen U, Mortensen J, et al: Preoperative staging of lung cancer with combined PET-CT. *N Engl J Med* 361:32–39, 2009.
36. Reed CE, Harpole DH, Posther KE, et al: Results of the American College of Surgeons Oncology Group Z0050 trial: The utility of positron emission tomography in staging potentially operable non-small cell lung cancer. *J Thorac Cardiovasc Surg* 126:1943–1951, 2003.
37. Fernandez FG, Kozower BD, Crabtree TD, et al: Utility of mediastinoscopy in clinical stage I lung cancers at risk for occult mediastinal nodal metastases. *J Thorac Cardiovasc Surg* 149:35–41, 42.e1, 2015.
38. Harris CL, Toloza EM, Klapman JB, et al: Minimally invasive mediastinal staging of non-small-cell lung cancer: Emphasis on ultrasonography-guided fine-needle aspiration. *Cancer Control* 21:15–20, 2014.
39. Annema JT, van Meerbeeck JP, Rintoul RC, et al: Mediastinoscopy vs endosonography for mediastinal nodal staging of lung cancer: A randomized trial. *JAMA* 304:2245–2252, 2010.
40. Goldstraw P, Crowley JJ: The International Association for the Study of Lung Cancer International Staging Project on Lung Cancer. *J Thorac Oncol* 1:281–286, 2006.
41. Edge SB, Byrd DR, Compton CC, et al: *AJCC cancer staging manual*, ed 7, New York, 2010, Springer.
42. Groome PA, Bolejack V, Crowley JJ, et al: The IASLC Lung Cancer Staging Project: Validation of the proposals for revision of the T, N, and M descriptors and consequent stage groupings in the forthcoming (seventh) edition of the TNM classification of malignant tumours. *J Thorac Oncol* 2:694–705, 2007.
43. Giroux DJ, Rami-Porta R, Chansky K, et al: The IASLC Lung Cancer Staging Project: Data elements for the prospective project. *J Thorac Oncol* 4:679–683, 2009.
44. American Joint Committee on Cancer: AJCC 7th Edition Staging Posters, 2012. http://cancerstaging.org/references-tools/quickreferences/Documents/Lung%20Cancer%20Staging%20Poster%20Updated.pdf
45. Rice TW, Murthy SC, Mason DP, et al: A cancer staging primer: Lung. *J Thorac Cardiovasc Surg* 139:826–829, 2010.
46. Rami-Porta R, Ball D, Crowley J, et al: The IASLC Lung Cancer Staging Project: Proposals for the revision of the T descriptors in the forthcoming (seventh) edition of the TNM classification for lung cancer. *J Thorac Oncol* 2:593–602, 2007.
47. Rusch VW, Crowley J, Giroux DJ, et al: The IASLC Lung Cancer Staging Project: Proposals for the revision of the N descriptors in the forthcoming seventh edition of the TNM classification for lung cancer. *J Thorac Oncol* 2:603–612, 2007.
48. Rusch VW, Asamura H, Watanabe H, et al: The IASLC lung cancer staging project: A proposal for a new international lymph node map in the forthcoming seventh edition of the TNM classification for lung cancer. *J Thorac Oncol* 4:568–577, 2009.
49. Postmus PE, Brambilla E, Chansky K, et al: The IASLC Lung Cancer Staging Project: Proposals for revision of the M descriptors in the forthcoming (seventh) edition of the

TNM classification of lung cancer. *J Thorac Oncol* 2:686–693, 2007.
50. Timmerman R, Paulus R, Galvin J, et al: Stereotactic body radiation therapy for inoperable early stage lung cancer. *JAMA* 303:1070–1076, 2010.
51. Kozower BD, Sheng S, O'Brien SM, et al: STS database risk models: Predictors of mortality and major morbidity for lung cancer resection. *Ann Thorac Surg* 90:875–881, discussion 881-883, 2010.
52. Darling GE, Allen MS, Decker PA, et al: Randomized trial of mediastinal lymph node sampling versus complete lymphadenectomy during pulmonary resection in the patient with N0 or N1 (less than hilar) non-small cell carcinoma: Results of the American College of Surgery Oncology Group Z0030 Trial. *J Thorac Cardiovasc Surg* 141:662–670, 2011.
53. Fernando HC, Landreneau RJ, Mandrekar SJ, et al: Impact of brachytherapy on local recurrence rates after sublobar resection: Results from ACOSOG Z4032 (Alliance), a phase III randomized trial for high-risk operable non-small-cell lung cancer. *J Clin Oncol* 32:2456–2462, 2014.
54. Arriagada R, Bergman B, Dunant A, et al: Cisplatin-based adjuvant chemotherapy in patients with completely resected non-small-cell lung cancer. *N Engl J Med* 350:351–360, 2004.
55. Schiller JH, Harrington D, Belani CP, et al: Comparison of four chemotherapy regimens for advanced non-small-cell lung cancer. *N Engl J Med* 346:92–98, 2002.
56. Ramnath N, Dilling TJ, Harris LJ, et al: Treatment of stage III non-small cell lung cancer: Diagnosis and management of lung cancer, 3rd ed: American College of Chest Physicians evidence-based clinical practice guidelines. *Chest* 143:e314S–340S, 2013.
57. Pisters KM, Vallieres E, Crowley JJ, et al: Surgery with or without preoperative paclitaxel and carboplatin in early-stage non-small-cell lung cancer: Southwest Oncology Group Trial S9900, an intergroup, randomized, phase III trial. *J Clin Oncol* 28:1843–1849, 2010.
58. Albain KS, Swann RS, Rusch VW, et al: Radiotherapy plus chemotherapy with or without surgical resection for stage III non-small-cell lung cancer: A phase III randomised controlled trial. *Lancet* 374:379–386, 2009.
59. Deslauriers J, Tronc F, Fortin D: Management of tumors involving the chest wall including pancoast tumors and tumors invading the spine. *Thorac Surg Clin* 23:313–325, 2013.
60. Kappers I, van Sandick JW, Burgers JA, et al: Results of combined modality treatment in patients with non-small-cell lung cancer of the superior sulcus and the rationale for surgical resection. *Eur J Cardiothorac Surg* 36:741–746, 2009.
61. Socinski MA, Evans T, Gettinger S, et al: Treatment of stage IV non-small cell lung cancer: Diagnosis and management of lung cancer, 3rd ed: American College of Chest Physicians evidence-based clinical practice guidelines. *Chest* 143:e341S–368S, 2013.
62. Sandler A, Gray R, Perry MC, et al: Paclitaxel-carboplatin alone or with bevacizumab for non-small-cell lung cancer. *N Engl J Med* 355:2542–2550, 2006.
63. Pao W: Defining clinically relevant molecular subsets of lung cancer. *Cancer Chemother Pharmacol* 58(Suppl 1):s11–s15, 2006.
64. Pao W, Girard N: New driver mutations in non-small-cell lung cancer. *Lancet Oncol* 12:175–180, 2011.
65. Takeda K, Hida T, Sato T, et al: Randomized phase III trial of platinum-doublet chemotherapy followed by gefitinib compared with continued platinum-doublet chemotherapy in Japanese patients with advanced non-small-cell lung cancer: Results of a West Japan Thoracic Oncology Group trial (WJTOG0203). *J Clin Oncol* 28:753–760, 2010.
66. Mitsudomi T, Morita S, Yatabe Y, et al: Gefitinib versus cisplatin plus docetaxel in patients with non-small-cell lung cancer harbouring mutations of the epidermal growth factor receptor (WJTOG3405): An open label, randomised phase 3 trial. *Lancet Oncol* 11:121–128, 2010.
67. U.S. Food and Drug Administration: FDA approves targeted therapy for first-line treatment of patients with a type of metastatic lung cancer, July 13, 2015. (<http://www.fda.gov/NewsEvents/Newsroom/PressAnnouncements/ucm454678.htm>; Accessed August 20, 2015).
68. Harvey RD: Immunologic and clinical effects of targeting PD-1 in lung cancer. *Clin Pharmacol Ther* 96:214–223, 2014.
69. Ford DW, Koch KA, Ray DE, et al: Palliative and end-of-life care in lung cancer: Diagnosis and management of lung cancer, 3rd ed: American College of Chest Physicians evidence-based clinical practice guidelines. *Chest* 143:e498S–512S, 2013.
70. Dennis BM, Eckert MJ, Gunter OL, et al: Safety of bedside percutaneous tracheostomy in the critically ill: Evaluation of more than 3,000 procedures. *J Am Coll Surg* 216:858–865, discussion 865-857, 2013.
71. Honings J, Gaissert HA, Ruangchira-Urai R, et al: Pathologic characteristics of resected squamous cell carcinoma of the trachea: Prognostic factors based on an analysis of 59 cases. *Virchows Arch* 455:423–429, 2009.
72. Gaissert HA, Honings J, Gokhale M: Treatment of tracheal tumors. *Semin Thorac Cardiovasc Surg* 21:290–295, 2009.
73. Drugs for tuberculosis. *Treat Guidel Med Lett* 10:29–36, quiz 37-38, 2012.
74. Pezzella AT, Fang W: Surgical aspects of thoracic tuberculosis: A contemporary review—part 1. *Curr Probl Surg* 45:675–758, 2008.
75. Cummings I, O'Grady J, Pai V, et al: Surgery and tuberculosis. *Curr Opin Pulm Med* 18:241–245, 2012.
76. Passera E, Rizzi A, Robustellini M, et al: Pulmonary aspergilloma: Clinical aspects and surgical treatment outcome. *Thorac Surg Clin* 22:345–361, 2012.
77. Jeon K, Koh WJ, Kim H, et al: Clinical features of recently diagnosed pulmonary paragonimiasis in Korea. *Chest* 128:1423–1430, 2005.
78. Worrell SG, Demeester SR: Thoracic emergencies. *Surg Clin North Am* 94:183–191, 2014.
79. Dudha M, Lehrman S, Aronow WS, et al: Hemoptysis: Diagnosis and treatment. *Compr Ther* 35:139–149, 2009.
80. Sakr L, Dutau H: Massive hemoptysis: An update on the role of bronchoscopy in diagnosis and management. *Respiration* 80:38–58, 2010.
81. Shigemura N, Wan IY, Yu SC, et al: Multidisciplinary management of life-threatening massive hemoptysis: A 10-year experience. *Ann Thorac Surg* 87:849–853, 2009.
82. Chen J, Chen LA, Liang ZX, et al: Immediate and long-term results of bronchial artery embolization for hemoptysis

due to benign versus malignant pulmonary diseases. *Am J Med Sci* 348:204–209, 2014.
83. Chun JY, Morgan R, Belli AM: Radiological management of hemoptysis: A comprehensive review of diagnostic imaging and bronchial arterial embolization. *Cardiovasc Intervent Radiol* 33:240–250, 2010.
84. Fishman A, Martinez F, Naunheim K, et al: A randomized trial comparing lung-volume-reduction surgery with medical therapy for severe emphysema. *N Engl J Med* 348:2059–2073, 2003.
85. Sanchez PG, Kucharczuk JC, Su S, et al: National Emphysema Treatment Trial redux: Accentuating the positive. *J Thorac Cardiovasc Surg* 140:564–572, 2010.
86. Hertz MI, Aurora P, Christie JD, et al: Scientific Registry of the International Society for Heart and Lung Transplantation: Introduction to the 2010 annual reports. *J Heart Lung Transplant* 29:1083–1088, 2010.
87. Malhotra A: Low-tidal-volume ventilation in the acute respiratory distress syndrome. *N Engl J Med* 357:1113–1120, 2007.
88. Briel M, Meade M, Mercat A, et al: Higher vs lower positive end-expiratory pressure in patients with acute lung injury and acute respiratory distress syndrome: Systematic review and meta-analysis. *JAMA* 303:865–873, 2010.
89. Tonelli AR, Zein J, Adams J, et al: Effects of interventions on survival in acute respiratory distress syndrome: An umbrella review of 159 published randomized trials and 29 meta-analyses. *Intensive Care Med* 40:769–787, 2014.
90. Pastorino U, Buyse M, Friedel G, et al: Long-term results of lung metastasectomy: Prognostic analyses based on 5206 cases. *J Thorac Cardiovasc Surg* 113:37–49, 1997.
91. Detterbeck FC: Clinical presentation and evaluation of neuroendocrine tumors of the lung. *Thorac Surg Clin* 24:267–276, 2014.
92. Horsch D, Schmid KW, Anlauf M, et al: Neuroendocrine tumors of the bronchopulmonary system (typical and atypical carcinoid tumors): Current strategies in diagnosis and treatment. Conclusions of an expert meeting February 2011 in Weimar, Germany. *Oncol Res Treat* 37:266–276, 2014.
93. Maziak DE, Todd TR, Keshavjee SH, et al: Adenoid cystic carcinoma of the airway: Thirty-two-year experience. *J Thorac Cardiovasc Surg* 112:1522–1531, discussion 1531-1532, 1996.
94. Gaissert HA, Grillo HC, Shadmehr MB, et al: Long-term survival after resection of primary adenoid cystic and squamous cell carcinoma of the trachea and carina. *Ann Thorac Surg* 78:1889–1896, discussion 1896-1897, 2004.
95. Blackmon SH, Rice DC, Correa AM, et al: Management of primary pulmonary artery sarcomas. *Ann Thorac Surg* 87:977–984, 2009.
96. Huddleston CB: Pectus excavatum. *Semin Thorac Cardiovasc Surg* 16:225–232, 2004.
97. Shah AA, D'Amico TA: Primary chest wall tumors. *J Am Coll Surg* 210:360–366, 2010.
98. Walsh GL, Davis BM, Swisher SG, et al: A single-institutional, multidisciplinary approach to primary sarcomas involving the chest wall requiring full-thickness resections. *J Thorac Cardiovasc Surg* 121:48–60, 2001.
99. Gross JL, Younes RN, Haddad FJ, et al: Soft-tissue sarcomas of the chest wall: Prognostic factors. *Chest* 127:902–908, 2005.
100. Sanders RJ, Hammond SL, Rao NM: Diagnosis of thoracic outlet syndrome. *J Vasc Surg* 46:601–604, 2007.
101. Chang KZ, Likes K, Davis K, et al: The significance of cervical ribs in thoracic outlet syndrome. *J Vasc Surg* 57:771–775, 2013.
102. Klaassen Z, Sorenson E, Tubbs RS, et al: Thoracic outlet syndrome: A neurological and vascular disorder. *Clin Anat* 27:724–732, 2014.
103. Orlando MS, Likes KC, Mirza S, et al: A decade of excellent outcomes after surgical intervention in 538 patients with thoracic outlet syndrome. *J Am Coll Surg* 220:934–939, 2015.
104. Povlsen B, Belzberg A, Hansson T, et al: Treatment for thoracic outlet syndrome. *Cochrane Database Syst Rev* CD007218, 2010.
105. Light RW, Macgregor MI, Luchsinger PC, et al: Pleural effusions: The diagnostic separation of transudates and exudates. *Ann Intern Med* 77:507–513, 1972.
106. Putnam JB, Jr, Light RW, Rodriguez RM, et al: A randomized comparison of indwelling pleural catheter and doxycycline pleurodesis in the management of malignant pleural effusions. *Cancer* 86:1992–1999, 1999.
107. Heffner JE, Nietert PJ, Barbieri C: Pleural fluid pH as a predictor of survival for patients with malignant pleural effusions. *Chest* 117:79–86, 2000.
108. Warren WH, Kalimi R, Khodadadian LM, et al: Management of malignant pleural effusions using the pleurx catheter. *Ann Thor Surg* 85:1049–1055, 2007.
109. Dresler CM, Olak J, Herndon JE, 2nd, et al: Phase III intergroup study of talc poudrage vs talc slurry sclerosis for malignant pleural effusion. *Chest* 127:909–915, 2005.
110. Brims FJ, Lansley SM, Waterer GW, et al: Empyema thoracis: new insights into an old disease. *Eur Respir Rev* 19:220–228, 2010.
111. Light RW: Parapneumonic effusions and empyema. *Proc Am Thorac Soc* 3:75–80, 2006.
112. Molnar TF: Current surgical treatment of thoracic empyema in adults. *Eur J Cardiothorac Surg* 32:422–430, 2007.
113. Rahman NM, Maskell NA, West A, et al: Intrapleural use of tissue plasminogen activator and DNase in pleural infection. *N Engl J Med* 365:518–526, 2011.
114. Nair SK, Petko M, Hayward MP: Aetiology and management of chylothorax in adults. *Eur J Cardiothorac Surg* 32:362–369, 2007.
115. Lyon S, Mott N, Koukounaras J, et al: Role of interventional radiology in the management of chylothorax: A review of the current management of high output chylothorax. *Cardiovasc Intervent Radiol* 36:599–607, 2013.
116. Travis WD: Sarcomatoid neoplasms of the lung and pleura. *Arch Pathol Lab Med* 134:1645–1658, 2010.
117. Ellis P, Davies AM, Evans WK, et al: The use of chemotherapy in patients with advanced malignant pleural mesothelioma: A systematic review and practice guideline. *J Thorac Oncol* 1:591–601, 2006.
118. Yanagawa J, Rusch V: Surgical management of malignant pleural mesothelioma. *Thorac Surg Clin* 23:73–87, 2013.
119. Friedberg JS: The state of the art in the technical performance of lung-sparing operations for malignant pleural mesothelioma. *Semin Thorac Cardiovasc Surg* 25:125–143, 2013.
120. Sugarbaker DJ, Wolf AS: Surgery for malignant pleural mesothelioma. *Expert Rev Respir Med* 4:363–372, 2010.

121. Whitten CR, Khan S, Munneke GJ, et al: A diagnostic approach to mediastinal abnormalities. *Radiographics* 27:657–671, 2007.
122. Donahue JM, Nichols FC: Primary mediastinal tumors and cysts and diagnostic investigation of mediastinal masses. In Shields TW, LoCicero J, III, Reed CE, et al, editors: *General thoracic surgery*, ed 7, Philadelphia, 2009, Lippincott Williams & Wilkins, pp 2195–2199.
123. Falkson CB, Bezjak A, Darling G, et al: The management of thymoma: A systematic review and practice guideline. *J Thorac Oncol* 4:911–919, 2009.
124. Kim ES, Putnam JB, Komaki R, et al: Phase II study of a multidisciplinary approach with induction chemotherapy, followed by surgical resection, radiation therapy, and consolidation chemotherapy for unresectable malignant thymomas: Final report. *Lung Cancer* 44:369–379, 2004.
125. Wright CD: Extended resections for thymic malignancies. *J Thorac Oncol* 5:S344–S347, 2010.
126. Walsh GL, Taylor GD, Nesbitt JC, et al: Intensive chemotherapy and radical resections for primary nonseminomatous mediastinal germ cell tumors. *Ann Thorac Surg* 69:337–343, discussion 343-344, 2000.
127. Kesler KA, Einhorn LH: Multimodality treatment of germ cell tumors of the mediastinum. *Thorac Surg Clin* 19:63–69, 2009.

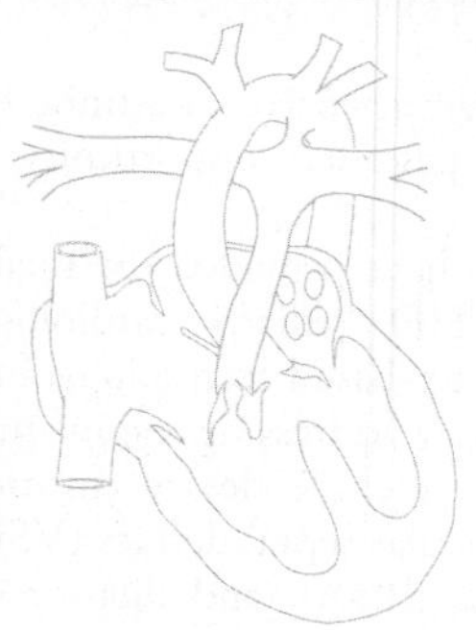

CHAPTER 58

Congenital Heart Disease

Charles D. Fraser, Jr., Lauren C. Kane

OUTLINE

This chapter is designed to provide medical students, general surgery residents, and practicing general surgeons with a working tool to aid in their understanding of the features of anatomy and physiology in patients presenting for general surgical procedures in the setting of repaired or unrepaired congenital cardiac lesions. The large scope and breadth of the evolving field of congenital heart surgery precludes an exhaustive treatise on all aspects of this specialty. Several excellent and thorough textbooks of congenital heart surgery are referenced in this chapter, and the reader is encouraged to use them for additional in-depth understanding of the lesions to be reviewed. A general surgeon practicing today needs to be well versed in the basics of cardiac anatomy, physiology, and specific derangements associated with the various known congenital cardiac lesions. Furthermore, few patients with complex congenital cardiac lesions may be considered cured of their cardiac problem, even after successful reconstructive surgery. Thus, it is imperative that a general surgeon who needs to perform a noncardiac operation on such a patient be familiar with the specific issues of ongoing concern in patients with congenital cardiac disease.

HISTORY AND OTHER CONSIDERATIONS

The era of surgical treatment for congenital cardiac anomalies was initiated in November 1944, when Alfred Blalock and associates Vivien Thomas and Helen Taussig combined their unique talents and vision to treat a young child dying of cyanotic congenital heart disease (CHD).[1] This palliative operation involved the surgical creation of a systemic–pulmonary artery connection in the patient, who had inadequate pulmonary blood flow. The procedure has since been recalled as miraculous and now more than 60 years later is known by the eponym Blalock-Taussig (BT) shunt. The striking success of this simple concept and the reproducible nature of the operation in children with otherwise fatal cardiac conditions have emboldened subsequent surgical innovators to venture inside the congenitally malformed heart. At first, the parent was asked to serve as a biologic oxygenator using the technique of controlled cross-circulation; soon thereafter, the mechanical, extracorporeal, heart-lung bypass pump was developed.[2,3] With the aid of this ability to support the patient's circulation during intracardiac exploration, surgeons have sequentially attacked almost every described congenital cardiac anomaly. The prospect of meaningful survival for patients born with otherwise devastating congenital cardiac lesions is now expected in most, if not all, cases.

As a result of this success story, there is now a large and growing population of adults with repaired or unrepaired CHD; estimates in the United States for 2010 placed the number of adult patients surviving with repaired or palliated congenital cardiac lesions at more than 1 million.[4] There has been an increase of greater than 50% in CHD prevalence since 2000, and by 2010, adults accounted for two thirds of patients with CHD in the general population.[5] This reality has been associated with new challenges in the ongoing medical maintenance of such patients, with particular focus on the care of patients with congenital cardiac lesions presenting for surgery for noncardiac illnesses. The evolving subspecialty of adult CHD points to the unique needs of this population of patients.

PATHWAYS FOR PRACTICING CONGENITAL HEART SURGERY

Before embarking on a review of the field, it is worthwhile to describe the setting in which patients with CHD seek and receive care in today's medical environment. With the development of sophisticated methods of fetal ultrasound, a large percentage of children requiring surgery for CHD are diagnosed during gestation (Fig. 58-1). A fetal diagnosis of complex CHD is extremely helpful to parents and the medical management team. Fetal diagnosis is particularly important in the setting of lesions dependent

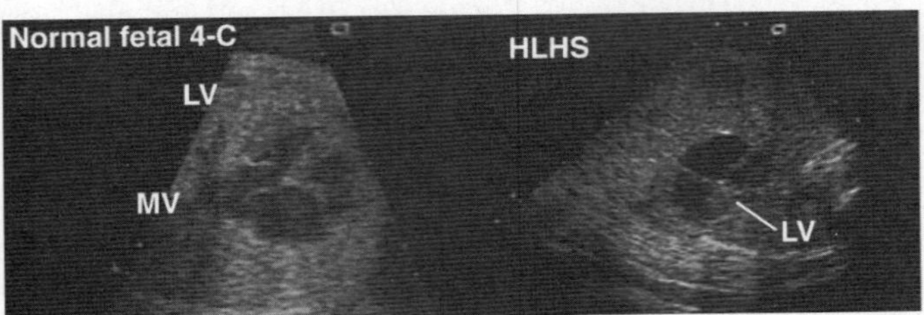

FIGURE 58-1 Normal fetal ultrasound (four chamber; *left*) and fetal ultrasound of a child with hypoplastic left heart syndrome *(right)*. *LV*, Left ventricle; *MV*, mitral valve.

on persistent patency of the ductus arteriosus for postnatal survival. In these individuals, survival after delivery is predicated on the maintenance of ductal patency through the intravenous infusion of prostaglandin E1 (PGE1) initiated in the delivery suite, often through an umbilical vein catheter. Several studies have shown a decrease in morbidity, but there is inconclusive evidence that mortality rates are decreased.[6,7]

A growing number of congenital cardiac lesions are known to be associated with specific genetic mutations, many clearly inherited and some presumed to be sporadic. A chromosomal analysis is frequently performed in individuals found to have major structural cardiac abnormalities; this analysis may be performed during gestation through amniocentesis or after delivery. The chromosomal evaluation is beneficial to the family when planning the risk of such an occurrence in future offspring. For the clinician, knowledge of chromosomal abnormalities in their patients, such as DiGeorge sequence, velocardiofacial syndrome, and Marfan syndrome, aids in the delivery of acute medical management.

In general terms, the timing of surgery for various congenital cardiac conditions depends on the presenting symptoms and expectations for further associated complications. Neonates presenting with limited pulmonary blood flow or atretic pulmonary connections typically require surgery during the first few days of life and occasionally within hours of delivery. Lesions associated with excessive pulmonary blood flow result in early heart failure, which may manifest as poor feeding, tachypnea, or respiratory failure. These patients are operated on during early infancy to ameliorate their symptoms and prevent the development of pulmonary vascular disease.

Preterm and low-birth-weight infants with CHD have been presenting for surgical consideration with more frequency. This treatment strategy requires thoughtful planning and coordination among the surgery, anesthesia, cardiology, intensive care, and neonatology teams. At our institution, the Texas Children's Hospital, we successfully operated on an 800-g infant with transposition of the great arteries (TGA).

The specialty of congenital heart surgery is now recognized as a subspecialty of cardiothoracic surgery. Congenital heart surgeons were previously certified in cardiothoracic surgery by the American Board of Thoracic Surgery and received additional fellowship training in the United States or abroad in congenital heart surgery. As of 2009, the American Board of Thoracic Surgery offers a formal certification process for subspecialty training in congenital heart surgery. At the present time, there are 12 congenital cardiac surgery residency programs approved by the Accreditation Council for Graduate Medical Education.[8] Most pediatric cardiac surgery is performed in large, multispecialty children's hospitals in association with formal programs focused on the care of these complex patients. The management team includes pediatric cardiac anesthesiologists, perfusionists, and nursing staff. Focused pediatric cardiac intensive care units have been developed to optimize the patients' opportunity for recovery.

Historically, pediatric cardiologists have provided the medical management of patients born with CHD. Pediatric cardiology is also evolving. With advances in catheter-based technology, interventional pediatric cardiologists are now addressing lesions previously treated with surgery. Examples include device closure of atrial septal defects (ASDs) and ventricular septal defects (VSDs), occlusion of patent ductus arteriosus (PDA), and dilation and stenting of stenotic vessels in the systemic and pulmonary circulation. For a more in-depth review of this specialty, see the excellent technical text by Mullins.[9]

The care for adults with CHD is in evolution. This issue is of particular relevance to the general surgeon faced with operating on an adult patient with significant CHD. One overriding message needs to be clear to the general surgeon in this setting: It must be assumed that in patients with previously repaired congenital cardiac lesions, even without overt cardiac symptoms, the potential for significant perioperative cardiorespiratory derangement exists. More simply stated, the presence of a surgical scar on the chest of a patient with known CHD does not suggest that the lesion has been cured. With this message firmly in mind, the general surgeon may find it challenging to determine the best source for a qualified consultation for such a patient. At the present time, many adult cardiologists are not adequately trained in CHD to provide competent consultation on adult patients with CHD.

Pediatric cardiologists are not educated in adult medicine and cardiology, and many feel uncomfortable providing consultation on adult patients with CHD. The subspecialty of adult CHD is currently becoming more formalized, but the number of physicians who have been educated specifically to care for these patients is still few. In 2015, the American Board of Internal Medicine offered the first certification examination in Adult Congenital Heart Disease. The Accreditation Council for Graduate Medical Education–accredited fellowship is expected to be available in 2019.[10] The practicing general surgeon needs to become familiar with the specific issues of concern for patients with CHD to ascertain that the patient's unique anatomic and physiologic issues have been evaluated properly. A pediatric cardiologist, in coordination with an adult cardiologist, must evaluate adult patients with CHD who present for care in a center without a designated qualified specialist. Of equal importance, the anesthesiologists and intensivists caring for an adult patient with CHD must have a working understanding of the complexities and nuances of the patient's cardiac condition. The anesthetic management of patients with CHD undergoing general surgical procedures is complicated and can become disastrous if managed improperly.

ANATOMY, TERMINOLOGY, AND DIAGNOSIS

Anatomy and Terminology

One of the most intimidating aspects for the student of CHD is developing a level of comfort with the terminology used for describing specific lesions. A thorough and sound understanding of normal cardiac anatomy is mandatory. There are several excellent texts on this subject; in particular, the text edited by Wilcox and coworkers[11] is especially concise and clear. One difficulty that challenges proper understanding of anatomy is the frequent use of abbreviations and eponyms for various congenital lesions—for example, congenitally corrected transposition of the great arteries (ccTGA), ventricular inversion, and L-transposition all describe the same heart, but none provides a complete anatomic description. Unless otherwise clear to all clinicians involved in the care of these complicated patients, the anatomic description needs to be segmental and complete to avoid mistakes and misinterpretations of structure.

In describing congenital cardiac lesions, a segmental approach is used to determine the relationship of the various structural elements. The situs describes the relationship of sidedness—situs solitus (normal), situs inversus (reversed), or situs ambiguus (indeterminate). The cardiac elements described include (in sequence) the atria, ventricles, and great vessels. The relationship of the connections must be understood; connections are concordant (e.g., the right atrium connecting to the right ventricle) or discordant (e.g., the right ventricle connecting to the aorta). The chamber sidedness must be clarified (e.g., a morphologic right atrium may be on the left side of the patient). The relationship and connections of the cardiac valves must then be assessed; connections may be normal, stenotic, atretic, or straddling. Of note to the general surgeon, abnormal sidedness of the cardiac structures is frequently associated with abnormal relationships of the thoracic and abdominal organs. A thorough assessment of the patient's anatomy is recommended before surgery. Commonly used tools in evaluation of anatomy include echocardiogram, computed tomography (CT), magnetic resonance imaging (MRI), and cardiac catheterization.

There are two widely accepted and applied schools of cardiac morphologic description. The Van Praagh nomenclature uses abbreviations to describe the relationship of the atria, ventricular looping, and position of the aorta sequentially. The first letter describes the situs of the atrial chambers (and usually the abdominal organs): "S" for situs solitus (normal), "I" for situs inversus (reversed), or "A" for situs ambiguus (indeterminate). The second letter describes the relationship of the embryologic looping of the ventricles: "D" for dextro looping or right-handed topology (normal) or "L" (levo) for left-handed topology. The third and last letter describes the relationship of the aortic valve to the pulmonary valve: "D" for right-sided and "L" for left-sided (Fig. 58-2).

The Anderson nomenclature is more wordy and longer but is perhaps simpler to understand. The descriptions are again of the sequential relationship of the structures. Starting with the atria, the connections and relationships are sequentially described. Thus, the atrial sidedness is described, followed by the sequence of connections to the ventricles and then great vessels. For example, "atrial situs solitus (normal) with atrioventricular discordance (reversed) and ventriculoarterial discordance (reversed)" describes the heart mentioned earlier as corrected transposition, or S,L,L by the Van Praagh classification (Fig. 58-3).

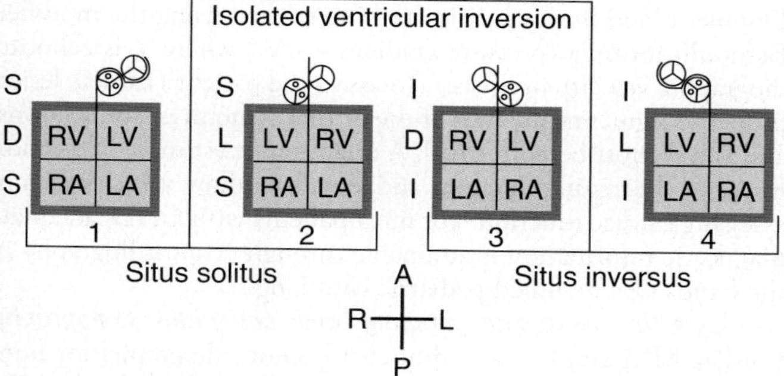

FIGURE 58-2 Model depicting cardiac morphology for normal hearts—that is, hearts with atrioventricular concordance and ventriculoarterial concordance—using Van Praagh nomenclature. The *vertical line* above the box denotes the position of the ventricular septum. (From Kirklin JW, Barratt-Boyes BG: General considerations: Anatomy, dimensions, and terminology. In *Cardiac surgery*, ed 2, New York, 1993, Churchill Livingstone.)

Diagnosis

As with all aspects of surgery, a wide variety of highly sophisticated diagnostic tools are available to examine cardiac structure and function. Despite the widespread availability and application of these tools, none has replaced or eliminated the necessity of a thorough history and physical examination. Most patients who have a history of CHD become very well informed about the specifics of their cardiac conditions, as do their parents. A detailed review of the patient's past medical history is mandatory. This review includes, when possible, securing records from all previous diagnostic and procedural reports. An incorrect assumption often is made about a patient's previous surgical history and anatomy, frequently in a setting in which a patient's old operative report or clinical summary could easily clarify the misunderstanding.

In adults with CHD, in particular, there are specific points of medical history that must be elucidated. A history of palpitations, syncope, and neurologic deficit must be investigated further. The incidence of significant dysrhythmias in certain categories of adults with CHD is high and, in many cases, warrants further investigation, including continuous monitoring (Holter), electrophysiologic study, or provocative testing.

Physical Examination

A complete physical examination in a patient with previously repaired CHD often yields critical information for the proper planning of a general surgical procedure. Patients need to be completely undressed and thoroughly examined. In many cyanotic patients, color changes may be prominent, particularly in the nail beds, lips, and mucous membranes. In other patients, cyanosis may be more subtle, giving the patient a gray or even pale appearance. Previous surgical incisions need to be noted and reconciled with the known medical history. Thoracotomy incisions on either side may indicate a previous BT shunt using the turned-down, divided subclavian artery or with a prosthetic interposition graft—the so-called modified BT shunt. In patients with a left aortic arch, a left thoracotomy incision is present if a

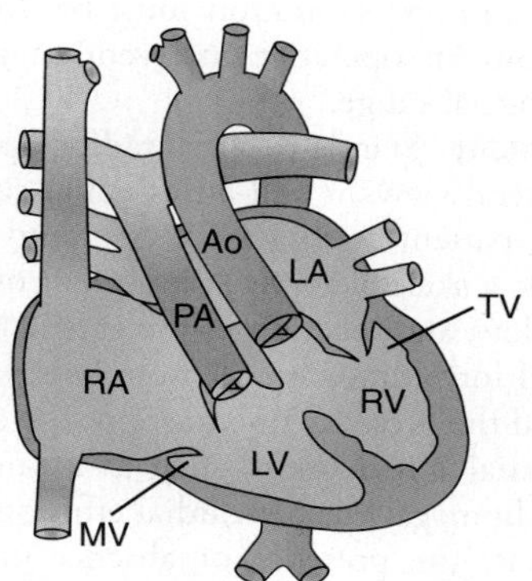

FIGURE 58-3 Congenitally corrected transposition of the great arteries. Atrial situs solitus (normal) with atrioventricular discordance and ventriculoarterial discordance using Anderson nomenclature, S,L,L by Van Praagh classification. *Ao,* Aorta; *LA,* left atrium; *LV,* left ventricle; *MV,* mitral valve; *RA,* right atrium; *RV,* right ventricle; *TV,* tricuspid valve.

previous coarctation repair has been carried out. Median sternotomy incisions or anterior thoracotomy incisions may indicate previous intracardiac or extracardiac surgery.

A complete vascular examination is often overlooked in patients with CHD. It is important to assess pulses and obtain blood pressure measurements in all four extremities. Patients who have an existing or have previously had a BT shunt often have diminished or absent pulses in the upper extremity corresponding to the previous shunt. Also, patients with previous coarctation repairs may have diminished or absent pulses in the left upper extremity, especially if a subclavian flap angioplasty was performed (Waldhausen procedure). Furthermore, a history of previous coarctation repair does not guarantee that the lower extremity pulses and blood pressures will be normal. Moreover, patients who have undergone previous cardiac catheterization may have chronically stenosed or occluded femoral vessels. All these issues may be of significance for monitoring and vascular access in a patient undergoing a general surgical procedure.

Later in this chapter, the Fontan procedure for single-ventricle palliation is reviewed. Briefly, this operation results in significant systemic venous hypertension, often in 12 to 15 mm Hg. In patients with a Fontan circulation, physical examination may reveal hepatic congestion, ascites, pedal edema, venous varicosities, and jugular venous distention. In some patients, macronodular hepatic cirrhosis may be suspected on the basis of a firm fibrotic liver edge.

Entire textbooks have been dedicated to the physical examination of patients with cardiac disease, and a thorough discussion of this issue, particularly the specifics of cardiac auscultation, is beyond the scope of this chapter. In general, the cardiac examination includes an assessment of the patient's rhythm, point of maximal impulse, and character of any auscultated murmurs. Also, the absence of a significant cardiac murmur does not rule out significant cardiac pathology.

Diagnostic Tests

Pulse oximetry. Four-extremity pulse oximetry is an essential part of the clinical assessment of a patient with suspected CHD. Patients with ductal-dependent circulation to the lower body (severe aortic coarctation or aortic arch interruption) may present with differential cyanosis. This presentation indicates the ejection of desaturated systemic venous blood through the patent ductus to the descending aorta contrasted with fully saturated pulmonary venous blood ejected to the ascending aorta and the upper extremities. Baseline (room air) saturation must be documented in all patients for whom an operative intervention is anticipated to establish their normal range.

Plain radiography. Standard chest radiography with anteroposterior and lateral views is still an essential component of the assessment of a patient with CHD. Standard elements to be examined include a skeletal survey, assessment of the diaphragms and hepatic shadow, and location of the gastric bubble. The lung fields are assessed for pulmonary plethora (arterial or venous), air space disease, and the presence of effusions. The cardiac silhouette may reveal essential information, such as a cardiothoracic ratio indicative of cardiomegaly or pericardial effusion, the presence of atrial enlargement, the presence or absence of the pulmonary artery shadow, and arch sidedness (Fig. 58-4).

Electrocardiography. The electrocardiogram (ECG) is important in assessing patients with CHD. The rate and rhythm must be noted, including the presence or absence of P wave activity and axis. Many patients with CHD, especially patients with complex

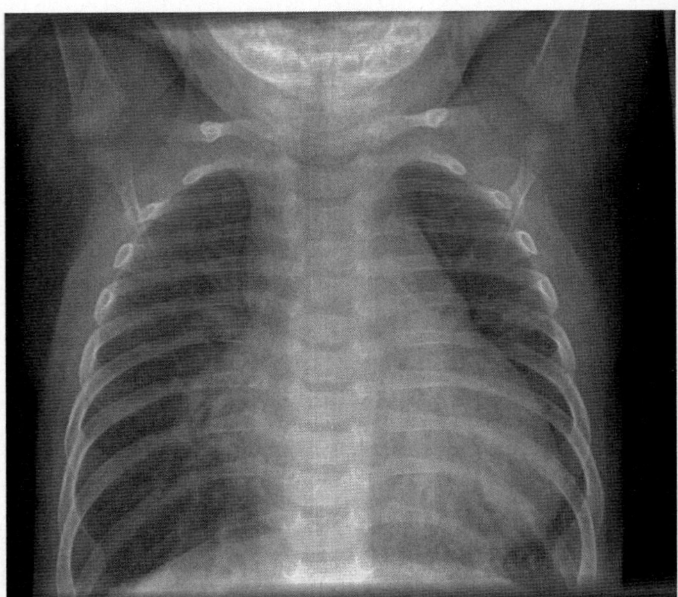

FIGURE 58-4 Cardiomegaly and increased pulmonary vascular markings in a patient with complete atrioventricular canal defect.

conditions such as heterotaxy syndrome, may exhibit deranged or absent sinus node activity, giving rise to a predominant junctional rhythm, which may significantly compromise cardiac output. The QRS duration and axis reveal information concerning conduction delay and abnormal ventricular forces. For example, patients with atrioventricular (A-V) canal defects are known to have left axis deviation. Furthermore, in patients undergoing repair of certain forms of CHD, there may be an early or late predisposition to malignant dysrhythmias. It is particularly important to elucidate a history of palpitations from a patient with repaired or unrepaired CHD; such a history may warrant further investigation with 24-hour continuous ECG monitoring (Holter).

Echocardiography. Noninvasive imaging is well established as the primary diagnostic modality for structural cardiac disease. For most patients, excellent anatomic detail may be obtained using two-dimensional transthoracic imaging. Standard images include subcostal, suprasternal, parasternal, and subxiphoid views and are oriented in long and short axis directions. Furthermore, significant hemodynamic information may be inferred using echo Doppler blood flow velocities and interpreted using the modified Bernoulli formula (pressure gradient = $4V^2$, where V is echocardiographic velocity in m/sec). To assess the patient's cardiac lesion properly, segmental analysis of the cardiac structures, connections, and valves must be performed. A quantitative estimate of ejection fraction, shortening fraction, and valvular inflow velocity aids in assessing cardiac function. For most patients with CHD, adequate diagnostic information is attainable through echocardiography in the hands of a qualified pediatric cardiologist.

Magnetic resonance imaging and computed tomography. Cardiac MRI and CT are adjuncts to echocardiography for noninvasive structural and functional assessment of the heart. MRI has been used with increasing frequency to provide anatomic detail in congenitally malformed hearts in which echocardiographic detail is lacking or unattainable. This modality has proved particularly useful for imaging the extracardiac great vessels and systemic and pulmonary venous connections and for providing accurate estimates of cardiac function, especially right ventricular ejection fraction. MRI has the added benefit of using nonionizing electromagnetic fields. CT may also be used for such imaging detail but has the potential detrimental association with significant radiation exposure. A CT scan of the chest averages 5 to 7 mSv, and CT coronary angiography averages 9 to 11 mSv.[12]

Cardiac catheterization. Cardiac catheterization was long considered the gold standard for diagnostic imaging of congenitally malformed hearts. With the current sophistication of echocardiography, this is no longer the case for most patients. Nonetheless, there are still circumstances in which diagnostic cardiac catheterization is necessary to obtain accurate anatomic detail. One such circumstance may be patients who have poor echocardiographic windows, although even this issue may be overcome using transesophageal echocardiography. More often, there are specifics of anatomic detail that neither echocardiography nor MRI can delineate, such as branch pulmonary artery (or segmental) stenosis, origin and course of aortopulmonary collateral vessels, and fistulous connections and intracardiac communications (septal defects) not clarified by other imaging modalities.

Usually, diagnostic cardiac catheterization is performed to obtain precise hemodynamic information needed to make an informed assessment of the consequences of the patient's cardiac lesions. Using oximetric measurements, pressure data, and thermodilution cardiac output determination, accurate assessment of the patient's hemodynamic profile is obtained. Measured or derived data include central venous pressure, atrial pressure, ventricular pressures (including end-diastolic pressure), shunt fraction (in the case of ASDs or VSDs), pulmonary artery pressures, pulmonary capillary wedge pressure, systemic arterial pressure, and segmental oximetry of cardiac structures, including systemic and pulmonary venous return (Fig. 58-5). Thus, critical information is obtained about the presence and degree of shunting, systemic and pulmonary vascular resistance (PVR), and cardiopulmonary function. In certain clinical settings, these data are mandatory to a successful clinical management strategy. This may be particularly true for an adult patient with CHD requiring noncardiac surgery.

A thorough understanding of normal cardiorespiratory physiology is critical in interpreting data obtained by cardiac catheterization in a patient with CHD. Specifically, the normal pressure range, pulse waveforms, and oxygen saturations for the various cardiac chambers must be compared against data obtained in a deranged circulation. The various cardiac chambers have normal pulse waveforms. In the atria, there are characteristic waveforms—a wave corresponding to atrial contraction, c wave corresponding to A-V valve closure, and v wave corresponding to atrial filling from venous return against the closed A-V valve. Typical normal right atrial mean pressures range from 1 to 5 mm Hg, and left atrial pressures range from 2 to 10 mm Hg. Right ventricular pressure tracings in normal hearts demonstrate a more gradual upstroke when compared with the left ventricle. Filling or end-diastolic pressures are between 2 and 10 mm Hg in normal hearts. The normal right ventricular systolic pressure (and thus pulmonary artery systolic pressure) is 15 to 30 mm Hg, and the left ventricular systolic pressure is 90 to 110 mm Hg.

In normal hearts, there is a small, physiologically insignificant right-to-left shunt, which results from ventilation-perfusion mismatch in the lungs and coronary venous return directly to the left ventricle (thebesian venous return). This physiologic shunt represents less than 5% of the cardiac output and, in normal circumstances, does not produce detectable systemic arterial desaturation. Thus, significant systemic arterial desaturation represents a pathologic finding, consistent with pulmonary disease, intracardiac shunting, or both. As noted, the origin and degree of intracardiac shunting may be assessed by echocardiography. However, in certain circumstances, cardiac catheterization is necessary to measure cardiac oximetry, calculate shunt fraction, and derive systemic and PVR. Using a derivation of the Fick principle, the ratio of pulmonary blood flow (Qp) to systemic blood flow (Qs) can be determined as follows:

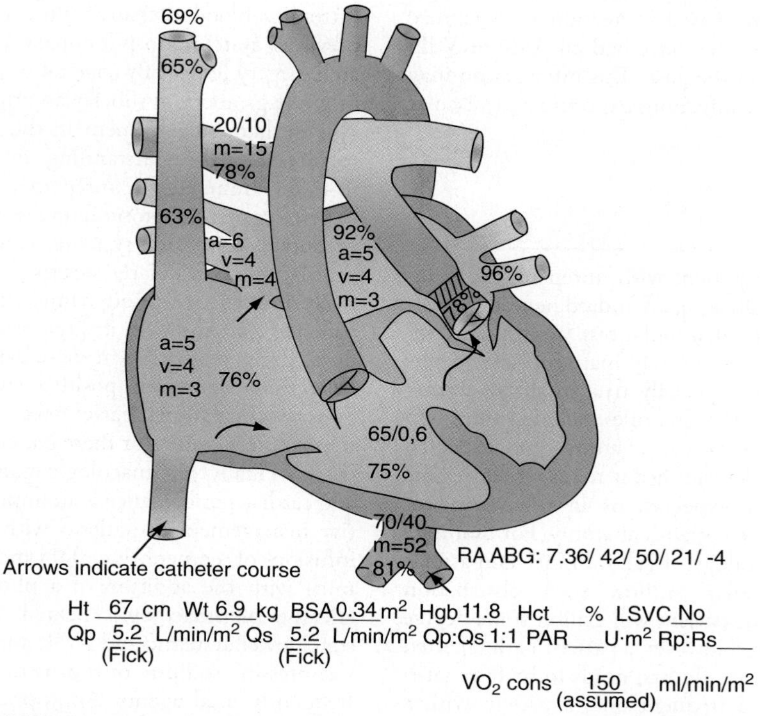

FIGURE 58-5 Hemodynamic information obtained after cardiac catheterization.

$$Qp/Qs = (SaO_2\ sat - (\bar{M}O_2\ sat)/(\bar{P}O_2\ sat) - PaO_2\ sat)$$

where SaO_2 sat is systemic arterial oxygen saturation, $\bar{M}O_2$ sat is mixed venous oxygen saturation, $\bar{P}O_2$ sat is pulmonary venous oxygen saturation, and PaO_2 sat is pulmonary arterial oxygen saturation.

Thus, in a patient with $\bar{M}O_2$ sat of 60%, $\bar{P}O_2$ sat of 100%, SaO_2 sat of 100%, and PaO_2 sat of 80%, the equation is as follows:

$$Qp/Qs = (100 - 60)/(100 - 80) = 40/20 = 2:1$$

Calculating vascular resistances may also be crucial in determining operability in a patient with CHD. In many settings, a precise measure of vascular resistance is unnecessary based on the clinical evidence. For example, in a small child with a large VSD seen on echocardiogram, the clinical findings of tachypnea, cardiomegaly, and failure to thrive confirm a large left-to-right shunt and infer acceptable PVR. However, in less clear circumstances, a precise calculation may be important in clinical decision making. The PVR may be calculated from cardiac catheterization data as follows:

Pulmonary vascular resistance (Rp)
= (mean pulmonary artery pressure [in mm Hg]
− mean left atrial pressure [in 2 mm Hg])/
(pulmonary blood flow [Qp, in liters/min/m])

In general, patients with an elevated PVR are further evaluated with pulmonary vasodilation—hyperventilation, hyperoxygenation, and inhaled nitric oxide—to determine whether the resistance is responsive. This information may be critical for patients who are otherwise marginal candidates.

Finally, cardiac catheterization has been evolving as the primary therapeutic method for many important structural cardiac defects. In many children's hospitals, including Texas Children's Hospital, most catheterizations now performed are for interventional procedures rather than diagnostic procedures. This fact may be particularly pertinent to a general surgeon faced with treating a patient with a previous catheter-based correction of a cardiac defect. For example, the patient may have had an ASD or VSD closed with an occluder device in the past. This information may have important ramifications for infectious exposure and vascular access.

PERIOPERATIVE CARE

Perioperative management of a patient with unrepaired or palliated CHD can be extremely challenging. Standard hemodynamic, respiratory, and pharmacologic manipulations appropriate for structurally normal hearts may be entirely inappropriate in settings of complex CHD; this is especially true in the operating room and intensive care settings. General rules include a thorough knowledge of the patient's intracardiac anatomy and expected physiology. It is possible to make significant management errors based on incorrect physiologic expectations in the setting of incomplete understanding of the patient's anatomy. For example, in a patient with unrepaired tetralogy of Fallot (TOF) and associated significant right ventricular outflow tract obstruction (RVOTO), it is expected that the patient will exhibit some degree of systemic arterial desaturation. However, a patient with repaired TOF, with no residual intracardiac shunts, needs to be fully saturated. This clinical scenario is a frequent one; a patient with a specific cardiac diagnosis, despite having undergone a successful correction, continues to be incorrectly presumed to have ongoing physiologic perturbation.

Anesthesia Pitfalls

Providing physiologic anesthetic management can be challenging in patients with CHD, especially in situations such as chronic single-ventricle palliation, unrepaired CHD, chronic cyanosis, and residual intracardiac pathology. Standard anesthetic management paradigms may be completely inappropriate and potentially disastrous in the setting of complex CHD. A thorough understanding of the patient's anatomy is mandatory, along with knowledge of the potential for unexpected response to anesthetic agents and ventilator settings. The field of pediatric and congenital cardiac anesthesia has evolved relative to this specific clinical need; the text by Andropoulos and colleagues[13] is an excellent resource.

Several points concerning anesthesia management warrant discussion. The first is vascular access for intraoperative and postoperative management. In patients with complex CHD, especially patients who have undergone previous complex surgical and catheterization procedures, obtaining appropriate vascular access may be challenging. Typically, a large-bore, multilumen central venous line is necessary for appropriate resuscitation and monitoring of right-sided filling pressures. In some patients, the placement of a thermodilution pulmonary artery catheter (oximetric) must be considered because one cannot presume that right-sided filling pressures correlate well with left heart volume or functional status (e.g., after a Fontan operation). Options for central access include percutaneous internal jugular or subclavian routes, with a secondary option of common femoral access to the inferior vena cava (IVC). Access may be difficult in the setting of previous catheterization or venous reconstruction; this situation may be addressed with the aid of ultrasound-guided catheter placement, which has become a standard in many cardiac operating room. Arterial access for continuous blood pressure monitoring and sampling is important for many patients. Percutaneous radial arterial cannulation can be readily achieved in most patients; however, upper extremity blood pressure values may be factitiously altered by previous systemic-to-pulmonary artery shunts, previous aortic arch surgery (especially coarctation), and abnormalities of vascular origin (e.g., aberrant subclavian origin from the descending aorta).

Ventilator management in the perioperative setting of CHD requires special understanding. In settings of large potential left-to-right shunts (e.g., unrepaired VSDs), hyperventilation and hyperoxygenation promote excessive pulmonary blood flow and potentially diminish systemic cardiac output. Positive pressure ventilation, particularly positive end-expiratory pressure, negatively influences hemodynamics in many patients, especially in palliated patients with a single ventricle after the Fontan procedure. Early extubation in these patients can be done to limit the deleterious effects of positive end-expiratory pressure on the Fontan circulation. Early data showed that early extubation improves outcomes for these patients and reduces overall hospital costs.[14] Finally, pharmacologic manipulation of systemic and PVR and cardiac performance is an important adjunct in the perioperative management of patients with CHD. In general, a low-dose infusion of epinephrine 0.05 mcg/kg/min (0.02-0.05 mcg/kg/min) with the addition of a phosphodiesterase inhibitor is an effective pharmacologic cocktail to promote a cardiac inotropic state, lower systemic and PVR, and limit tachycardia. Dopamine, vasopressin, sodium nitroprusside, and nitroglycerin are other frequently used agents. Appropriate perioperative analgesia and sedation are also important aspects of the patient's management.

Neurologic Outcomes

With expectations of almost 100% survival after surgery for CHD, emphasis has been placed on the long-term neurologic outcomes and quality of life of these patients. The potential for neurologic insult in children after CHD arises from the nature of their disease (e.g., cyanotic defects, low cardiac output state, genetic syndromes, effects of cardiopulmonary bypass, circulatory arrest). Evidence also suggests that patients with CHD may be genetically predisposed to neurologic insult. Gestational age has been found to be an important factor to consider in the optimization of neurologic outcomes.[15]

LESION OVERVIEW

Defects Associated With Increased Pulmonary Blood Flow

Persistent Arterial Duct (Patent Ductus Arteriosus)

A persistent arterial duct, or PDA, is a frequently encountered congenital cardiac condition. The arterial duct is necessary during gestation to shunt right ventricular blood away from the unventilated pulmonary vasculature; ductal flow is from the pulmonary artery to the aorta during gestation. At delivery, after the first breath of the neonate, ductal flow reverses and becomes left to right in most individuals. Over the first several hours or days of postnatal life, the PDA closes spontaneously and is completely closed in most infants by 2 to 3 weeks of age.

In the absence of other congenital cardiac lesions, a PDA becomes pathologic related to its presence and the degree of left-to-right shunting. A PDA may be present in association with other structural cardiac conditions and may sometimes be necessary for systemic or pulmonary blood flow. The amount of shunting produced relates to the size and geometry of the duct and the PVR. A PDA may be responsible for a large Qp/Qs and result in pulmonary overcirculation, left heart volume overload, and congestive heart failure (CHF). A large unrestricted PDA is associated with pulmonary hypertension; if left untreated, this proceeds to irreversible pulmonary vascular disease (Eisenmenger syndrome), ultimately proceeding to pulmonary and right heart failure, treatable only by pulmonary transplantation. Even with a small, pressure-restrictive PDA, there is an ongoing risk for pulmonary congestion and left heart volume overloading; endocarditis is always of concern even for small PDAs. Closure is recommended for all PDAs.

The gold standard of therapy for closure of PDA is surgery, usually accomplished through a left thoracotomy using ductal division, ligation, or clipping (Fig. 58-6). Surgery needs to be a low-risk procedure associated with minimal potential for persistence. Nonetheless, the invasive nature of this proven method has led to the development of alternative strategies for ductal occlusion. From a surgical perspective, many PDAs are amenable to thoracoscopic clipping through very small port incisions; robot-assisted PDA occlusion has been performed in many patients, with good results.[11] Medical treatment with indomethacin 0.1 mg/kg (0.1 mg/kg for <1 kg, 0.2 mg/kg ≥1 kg on day 1, then 0.1 mg/kg daily for days 2-7 oral or IV over 1 hr) can be attempted in a neonate but carries risk of necrotizing enterocolitis, intracranial hemorrhage, and renal toxicity. However, at the present time, most PDAs are occluded in the cardiac catheterization laboratory using occlusive devices. Even the repair of large defects in small infants has been successfully addressed. The long-term effects of the devices remaining in the vascular tree are not fully understood yet; however, successful device closure appears to be an extremely effective and durable therapy.

A PDA in an adult patient can be challenging. As noted, a long-standing large PDA may be associated with pulmonary vascular disease. A right-to-left shunt in a PDA is cause for significant

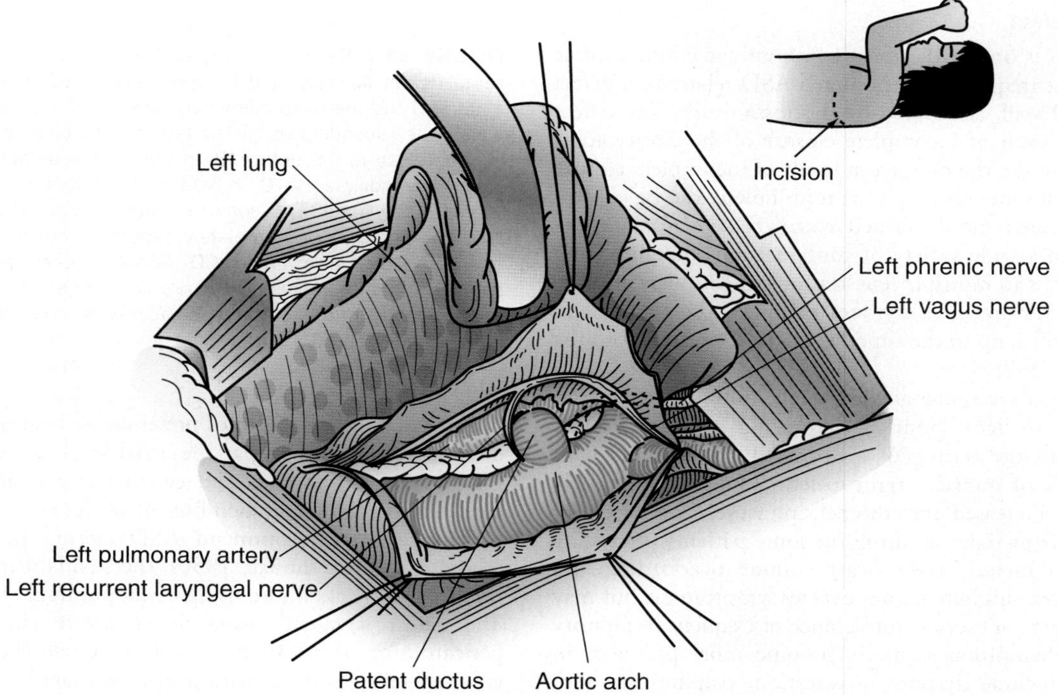

FIGURE 58-6 Anatomic relationships of a patent ductus arteriosus, exposed from a left thoracotomy. (From Castaneda AR, Jones RA, Mayer JE, Jr, et al: Patent ductus arteriosus. In *Cardiac surgery of the neonate and infant*, Philadelphia, 1994, Saunders.)

concern and warrants further investigation. In adults with PDAs, the arterial wall may calcify, making an attempt at ligation or division hazardous. In these patients, ductal occlusion may require resection of the adjacent descending aorta with patch grafting or short-segment graft replacement (Dacron).

Aortopulmonary Septal Defect (Aortopulmonary Window)

An aortopulmonary septal defect is a communication between the ascending aorta and, usually, the main pulmonary artery. This is a rare defect; it relates to the common embryologic origin of the arterial trunk and failure of complete separation into the aorta and pulmonary artery. Defects are classified by their location: Type I is proximal, just above the aortic sinuses; type II is more distal on the ascending aorta and often involves the origin of the right pulmonary artery; and type III is more distal and associated with a separate origin of the right pulmonary artery from the aorta (Fig. 58-7). An aortopulmonary septal defect may occur in isolation or in association with other conditions, including interrupted aortic arch (IAA) and anomalous origin of a coronary artery. Defects are typically large and responsible for a large left-to-right shunt with systemic pulmonary artery pressures. Children with this problem typically present with CHF, failure to thrive, and frequent respiratory infections. Echocardiography, MRI, or cardiac catheterization may be used to make the diagnosis.

All aortopulmonary septal defects are surgically closed; this lesion is not amenable to catheter-based closure, and such an attempt is hazardous. A small defect may be ligated through a thoracotomy or median sternotomy approach, but this method is not recommended because of significant risk for rupture or incomplete closure. Surgical closure is accomplished with cardiopulmonary bypass support. Options for closure include complete division and separate patch repairs of the great vessel defects or a sandwich type of closure, using a patch to construct a common intervening wall; both methods are effective (Fig. 58-8).

Atrial Septal Defect

An isolated ASD is one of the most common congenital cardiac lesions. The most frequently encountered ASD relates to a defect in the interatrial wall, as defined by the fossa ovalis. The defect develops as the result of incomplete closure of the embryologic patent foramen ovale; the defect is a result of incomplete closure of the septum primum. Although the terminology can be confusing, these defects are typically termed *secundum atrial septal defects*. They manifest in a wide variety of configurations, ranging from single small defects to multiple fenestrations to complete absence of the septum primum. The confines of the defect may extend from the IVC orifice up to the superior atrial wall adjacent to the aortic root (Fig. 58-9).

The primary pathophysiologic derangement in ASDs relates to a significant left-to-right shunt in the setting of normal PVR. However, even in the setting of a normal PVR, patients with ASDs are capable of transient right-to-left shunting, particularly during times of increased intrathoracic pressure. The effects of chronic, large left-to-right shunting (in some patients producing a Qp/Qs >3:1) include right heart volume overloading and enlargement. Most children are not overtly symptomatic but may exhibit some degree of exercise intolerance or frequent respiratory tract infection. Symptoms typically become more prevalent in adulthood and include dyspnea on exertion, palpitations, and, ultimately, evidence of right heart failure. Pulmonary vascular disease is not a typical finding in secundum ASDs, but one may demonstrate an ASD in a patient with primary pulmonary hypertension. A rare form of presentation relates to the potential of right-to-left shunting at the atrial level; the ever-present risk for paradoxical embolus and cerebrovascular accident must be considered when recommending ASD closure.

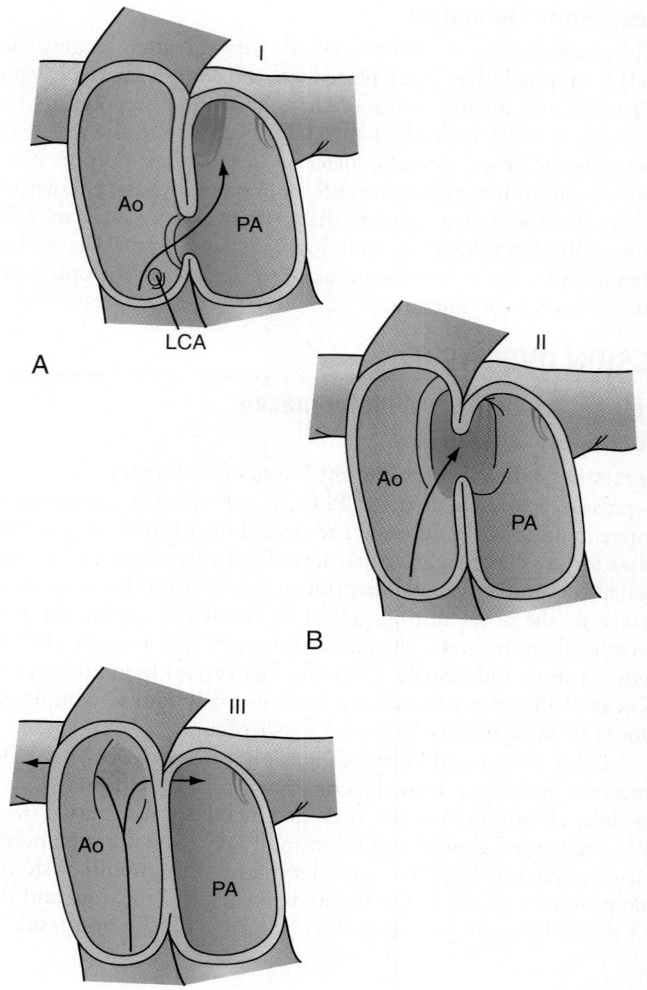

FIGURE 58-7 Native anatomy and classification of aortopulmonary septal defect. **A,** In type I, the communication is between the ascending aorta *(Ao)* and the main pulmonary artery *(PA)* on the posterior medial wall of the ascending aorta. The left main coronary artery *(LCA)* orifice may be close to the defect. **B,** In type II, the defect is more cephalic on the ascending aorta. **C,** In type III, the defect is more posterior and lateral in the aorta. The communication is with the right pulmonary artery, which may be completely separate from the main pulmonary artery. (Adapted from Fraser CD: Aortopulmonary septal defects and patent ductus arteriosus. In Nichols DG, Ungerleider RM, Spevak PJ, et al, editors: *Critical heart disease in infants and children*, Philadelphia, 2006, Mosby, pp 664–666.)

Most centers recommend ASD closure in patients before school age. Since the late 1950s, the standard therapy for ASDs has been surgical closure using cardiopulmonary bypass support. The defect is closed using direct suture closure, autologous pericardium, or prosthetic patch material (Fig. 58-10). This is an effective method, with a low associated perioperative risk, including the virtual absence of residual or recurrent defects.[16] Minimally invasive techniques for ASD closure have also gained popularity.

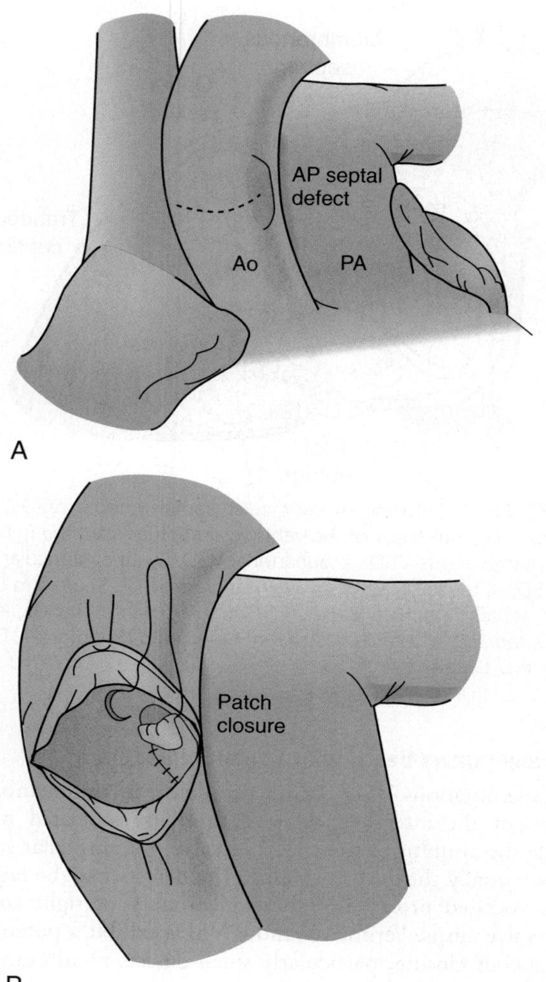

FIGURE 58-8 **A,** Surgical exposure of aortopulmonary *(AP)* septal defect includes a transverse incision in the ascending aorta *(Ao)*. **B,** The aortopulmonary septal defect is closed by suturing a patch over the aortic side of the defect. *PA,* Pulmonary artery. (Adapted from Fraser CD: Aortopulmonary septal defects and patent ductus arteriosus. In Nichols DG, Ungerleider RM, Spevak PJ, et al, editors: *Critical heart disease in infants and children,* Philadelphia, 2006, Mosby, pp 664–666.)

The potential for closing defects using nonsurgical methods has led to the development of catheter-based therapies, which are now being widely applied to large numbers of patients worldwide for the treatment of ASD. The most commonly used device is the Amplatzer septal occluder device (St. Jude Medical, St. Paul, MN), made of nitinol metal mesh, which is placed percutaneously and delivered with echocardiographic and fluoroscopic guidance. Early reports indicated an acceptable procedure-related complication rate and successful closure rate.[17] However, the long-term effects of having such a device in mobile cardiac structures are not fully understood. More recent reports have documented an alarming incidence of device erosion through the atrial wall and into the adjacent ascending aorta as well as disruption of the conduction system.[18,19] A case report showing severe endocarditis involving a previously placed Amplatzer ASD device has highlighted the need for ongoing observation of the long-term consequences of placing large prosthetic devices into the circulation.[20]

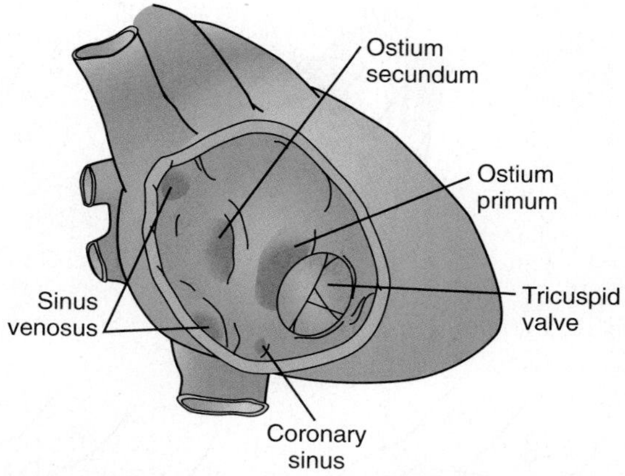

FIGURE 58-9 Types of atrial septal defects as viewed through the right atrium, ostium secundum, ostium primum, and sinus venosus. (Adapted from Redmond JM, Lodge AJ: Atrial septal defects and ventricular septal defects. In Nichols DG, Ungerleider RM, Spevak PJ, et al, editors: *Critical heart disease in infants and children*, Philadelphia, 2006, Mosby, p 580.)

Sinus venosus ASDs occur as the result of embryologic malalignment between the superior vena cava (SVC) or IVC. These defects are not associated with the ovale fossa and are frequently associated with partial anomalous pulmonary venous return. A superior sinus venosus ASD occurs high in the atrium, near the orifice of the SVC. This lesion is frequently associated with anomalous drainage of a portion of the right lung to the SVC. An inferior sinus venosus ASD is located low in the atrium, often extending into the IVC orifice. This lesion is typically associated with anomalous pulmonary venous drainage of the entire right lung to the IVC (potentially intrahepatic); pulmonary sequestration and an abnormal systemic artery perfusing the right lower lobe, with origin from the abdominal aorta, may also be present. In patients with total anomalous pulmonary venous return (TAPVR) to the IVC, the anomalous pulmonary vein may be obvious on a plain chest radiograph and has been described as appearing like a saber (scimitar syndrome), first described by Neill and colleagues.[21]

Surgery for sinus venosus ASDs is recommended for the same pathophysiologic reasons surgery is recommended for secundum ASDs. The repair is not amenable to catheter techniques, and surgery is more complicated than for an isolated secundum ASD. Superior sinus venosus defects with partial anomalous pulmonary venous return to the SVC may be treated with an intracardiac patch baffle; however, in the setting of high drainage of the anomalous pulmonary veins, an SVC translocation operation (Warden procedure) may be necessary. Surgery for an inferior sinus venosus ASD with a scimitar vein can be more complicated, potentially involving the need for a patch baffle within the intrahepatic IVC, which may require periods of hypothermic circulatory arrest.

Ventricular Septal Defect

A VSD is a pathologic communication involving a defect in the interventricular septum. Defects are classified in terms of their location and surrounding structures. Patients may be entirely asymptomatic, depending on the size and location of the VSD, along with associated lesions and PVR. In the setting of otherwise normal cardiac morphology and appropriate PVR, the net shunt in patients with VSD is left to right; the Qp/Qs depends on the size of the defect and pulmonary resistance. Large defects result

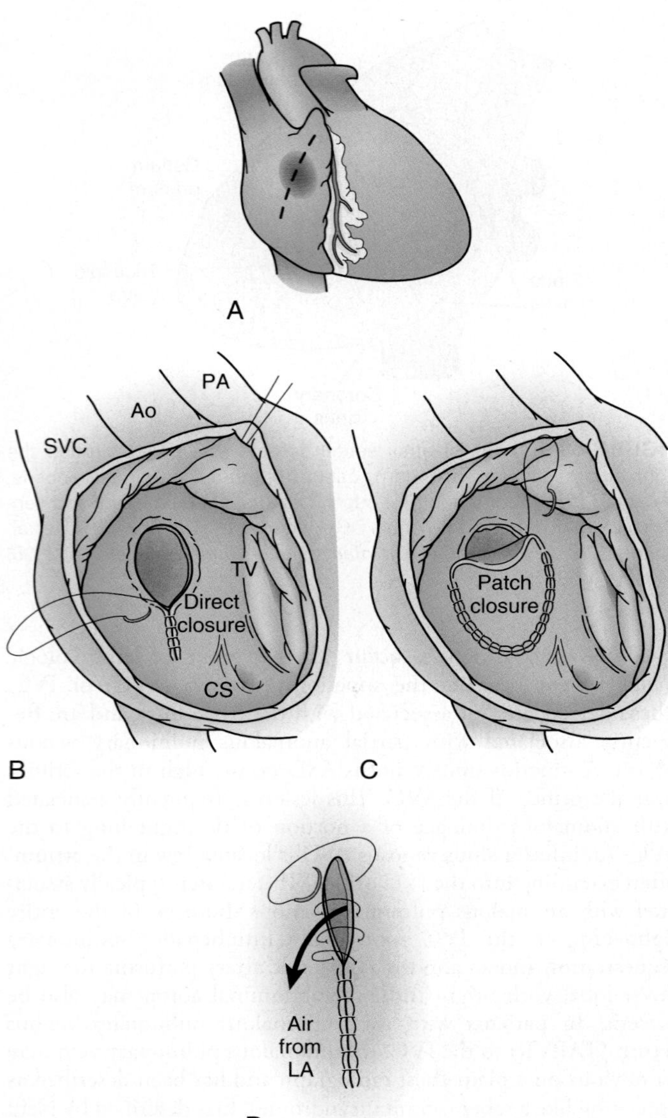

FIGURE 58-10 Surgical closure for atrial septal defect. **A,** Right atriotomy. **B,** Direct suture closure. **C,** Patch closure. **D,** Deairing the left atrium *(LA). Ao,* Aorta; *CS,* coronary sinus; *PA,* pulmonary artery; *TV,* tricuspid valve. (Adapted from Redmond JM, Lodge AJ: Atrial septal defects and ventricular septal defects. In Nichols DG, Ungerleider RM, Spevak PJ, et al, editors: *Critical heart disease in infants and children,* Philadelphia, 2006, Mosby, p 583.)

in large shunts; high right ventricular and pulmonary artery pressures; and significant pulmonary overcirculation, CHF, and left heart volume overload. In these settings, unrestrictive pulmonary blood flow exposes the patient to the risk for pulmonary vascular disease and Eisenmenger syndrome.

The ventricular septum can be best thought of in terms of the pathway of blood and associated cardiac anatomy. Thus, the right ventricular aspect of the septum has an inlet portion; midmuscular portion; apical, posterior, anterior, and outlet portions; and subaortic portion. This knowledge aids in the classification of VSDs. Furthermore, defects are understood relative to their embryologic origins and have varying propensities for spontaneous decreases in size or closure.

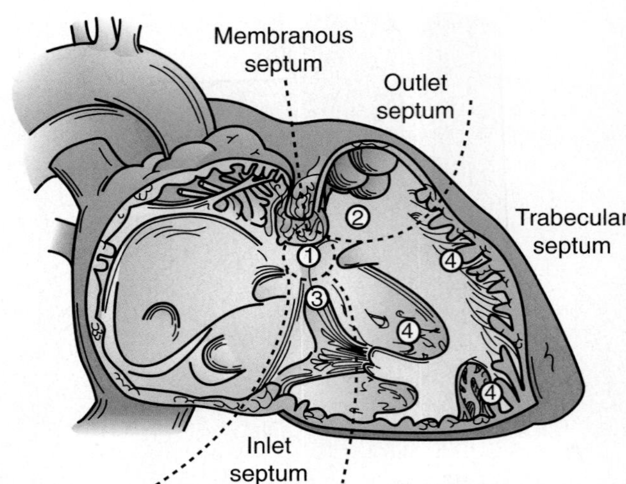

FIGURE 58-11 Location of ventricular septal defects (VSDs) in the ventricular septum (view of the ventricular septum from the right side). *1,* Perimembranous VSD; *2,* subarterial VSD; *3,* atrioventricular canal–type VSD; *4,* muscular VSD. (From Tchervenkov CI, Shum-Tim D: Ventricular septal defect. In Baue AE, Geha AS, Hammond GL, editors: *Glenn's thoracic and cardiovascular surgery,* ed 6, Stamford, CT, 1996, Appleton & Lange.)

Perimembranous Ventricular Septal Defect

A perimembranous VSD occurs as a defect in the membranous portion of the interventricular septum; its associated margins include the annulus of the tricuspid valve, the muscular septum, and potentially the aortic annulus. The defects may be large and have associated prolapse of the noncoronary or right coronary aortic valve cusps. Perimembranous VSDs exhibit a potential for spontaneous closure, particularly small defects manifesting early in childhood.

Muscular Ventricular Septal Defect

Muscular VSDs occur in all aspects of the muscular interventricular septum. Margins of these defects are entirely muscle. The lesions may be isolated or involve multiple openings in the septum (so-called Swiss cheese septum). Small defects have great potential for regression or spontaneous closure.

Subarterial (Supracristal or Outlet) Ventricular Septal Defect

Subarterial VSDs occur in association with the annulus of the aortic valve, pulmonary valve, or both. The defects are almost always associated with significant prolapse of the adjacent aortic valve cusp, usually the right coronary cusp, which may lead to significant cusp distortion, aortic valve insufficiency, and cusp perforation. The only mechanism for spontaneous closure of these defects relates to the cusp prolapse and valve distortion and is generally not complete or a favorable arrangement. All these defects are surgically closed because of the ongoing risk for aortic valve injury (Fig. 58-11).

The indications for surgery to close VSDs relate to the size of the VSD, degree of shunting, and associated lesions. Small infants presenting with large VSDs, refractory heart failure, and large shunts undergo surgical closure of the defects in the newborn period, regardless of age or size. Other defects are addressed based on the ongoing concerns of left-to-right shunting, aortic valve cusp distortion, and risk for endocarditis. Asymptomatic patients with evidence of significant shunts and cardiomegaly are proposed for surgical therapy. Prophylactic closure of small defects in asymptomatic patients with normal cardiac size and function is advocated by some surgeons because of the lifelong risk for endocarditis and comparatively low risk for surgery.

Percutaneous VSD closure is an acceptable alternative to surgical closure of VSDs with very high procedural success.[22] The complex relationship of many defects, including close association with the aortic valve and cardiac conduction tissue, makes the existing technology less than ideal. At the present time, surgery remains the primary mode of therapy for VSD closure. Defects are approached with the aid of cardiopulmonary bypass support and may be closed with various materials, including autologous pericardium (our preference), Dacron, polytetrafluoroethylene, and homograft material. Surgical closure of VSDs is a low-risk procedure with a high expectation of complete closure. Challenging anatomic situations, such as Swiss cheese septum or multiple apical muscular VSDs, may be initially palliated by limiting pulmonary blood flow with a pulmonary artery band and deferring corrective surgery to later in life.

Atrioventricular Septal Defect (Atrioventricular Canal Defect)

Atrioventricular septal defects (AVSDs) are a complex constellation of cardiac lesions involving deficiency of the atrial septum, ventricular septum, and A-V valves. This lesion results from an embryologic maldevelopment involving the endocardial cushions; thus, the term *endocardial cushion defect* is often applied. AVSDs may be partial, involving no ventricular level component; intermediate or transitional, involving a small restrictive VSD; or complete, involving a large nonrestrictive VSD. The A-V valve tissue is always abnormal in AVSD, although there is great individual variability in terms of the severity of the valvular malformation and valve function. Complete AVSDs are frequently seen in patients with trisomy 21 but also occur in patients with normal chromosomes. The morphology of the septal defects in this condition is different from that previously discussed. The ASD in this defect is termed a *primum ASD* and is distinctly separate from the ovale fossa. There is displacement of the A-V node and bundle of His to the inferior aspect of the primum defect and A-V junction, a feature of critical importance during surgical repair. Patients with AVSD have an *inlet VSD*, which may extend into the subaortic region and have a component of septal malalignment. The chordal support of the A-V valves has a variable relationship to the interventricular septum. The relationship of the chordal support and superior bridging component of the left A-V valve has been used to classify complete AVSD, as described by Rastelli and associates[23]: type A, with superior leaflet and chordal support committed to the left side of the ventricular septum; type B, with straddling and shared chordal support; and type C, with a floating left superior leaflet component and chordal support on the right side of the ventricular septum (Fig. 58-12).

Patients with complete AVSD typically present in infancy with large left-to-right shunts, cardiomegaly, and CHF. Without surgical treatment, patients exhibit severe failure to thrive, a susceptibility to severe respiratory infections, and potential for early development of pulmonary vascular disease. Surgical repair is recommended in infancy (usually before 6 months of age) but may be necessary in the newborn period for neonates with refractory heart failure, especially in association with aortic arch anomalies. Patients with partial or intermediate defects may have the surgery deferred until later in childhood, depending on the degree

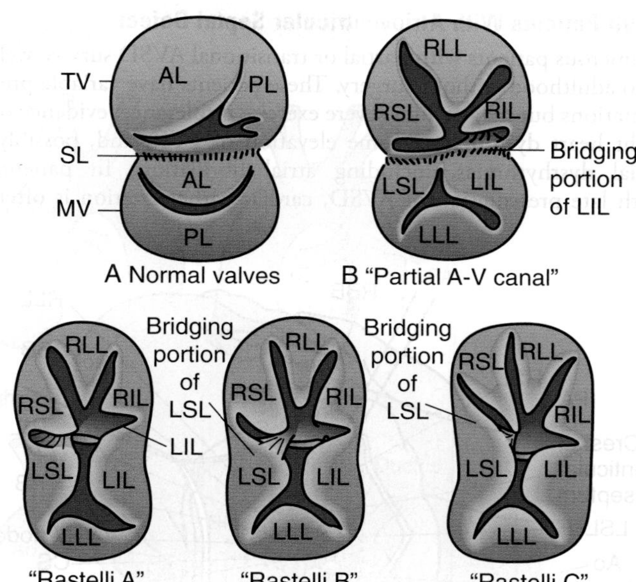

FIGURE 58-12 Rastelli classification type A, B, or C. The difference in valve morphology in a normal **(A)**, partial **(B)**, and complete **(C)** canal defect is illustrated. *AL,* Anterior leaflet; *A-V,* atrioventricular; *MV,* mitral valve; *PL,* posterior leaflet; *RIL,* right inferior leaflet; *RLL,* right lateral leaflet; *RSL,* right superior leaflet; *TV,* tricuspid valve. (From Kirklin JW, Pacifico AD, Kirklin JK: The surgical treatment of atrioventricular canal defects. In Arciniegas E, editor: *Pediatric cardiac surgery,* Chicago, 1985, Year Book Medical Publishers.)

of atrial level shunting and the presence of A-V valve regurgitation. AVSD may also manifest in unbalanced forms, with dominance of right-sided or left-sided components. In severely affected individuals, biventricular repair is not feasible, and patients are managed along a single-ventricle pathway. AVSD may also be found in association with TOF; this combination is associated with cyanosis, and repair is more challenging than for either condition considered in isolation.

Surgery is the primary mode of therapy for patients with AVSD. Operative goals include complete closure of ASDs and VSDs and effective use of available A-V valve tissue to achieve valve competence. As noted, the inferiorly displaced conduction tissue must be protected to avoid the complication of surgically induced A-V block (Fig. 58-13). Surgical intervention is performed with the use of the cardiopulmonary bypass machine. The atrial and ventricular septal components are closed with a common patch (single-patch method) or separate patches (two-patch technique). We believe the two-patch method to be superior in preserving A-V valve tissue (Fig. 58-14).[24] The critical component of the repair lies in the valve repair; typically, after suspending the valve tissue to the reconstructed septum, the line of coaptation between the superior and inferior leaflet components (cleft) is closed; however, care must be exercised to avoid valvular stenosis.

Perioperative care is predicated on an accurate and hemodynamically favorable repair. Patients with long-standing pulmonary overcirculation may have a potential for early perioperative pulmonary hypertensive crisis. This condition may require therapy, including oxygen, optimization of fluid balance, continuous sedation, hyperventilation, and, possibly, inhaled nitric oxide.

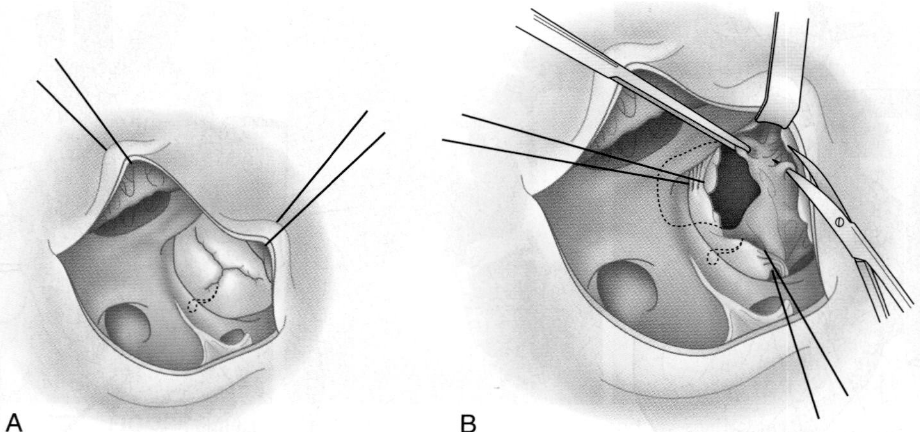

FIGURE 58-23 **A,** Surgeon's view through a transatrial incision in the transatrial/transpulmonary approach. **B,** Right ventricular outflow tract muscle resection through the right atriotomy. (From Morales DL, Zafar F, Heinle JS: Right ventricular infundibulum sparing [RVIs] tetralogy of Fallot repair: A review of over 300 patients. *Ann Surg* 250:611–617, 2009.)

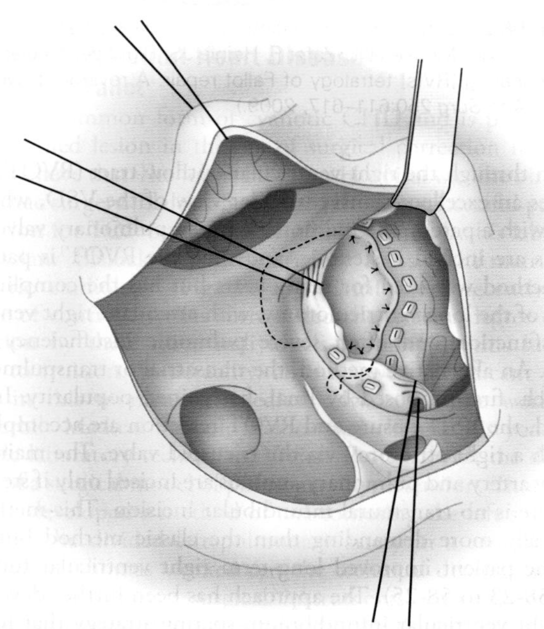

FIGURE 58-24 Ventricular septal defect patch closure with pledgets around the defect and onto the tricuspid valve annulus to avoid the conduction system. (From Morales DL, Zafar F, Heinle JS: Right ventricular infundibulum sparing [RVIs] tetralogy of Fallot repair: A review of over 300 patients. *Ann Surg* 250:611–617, 2009.)

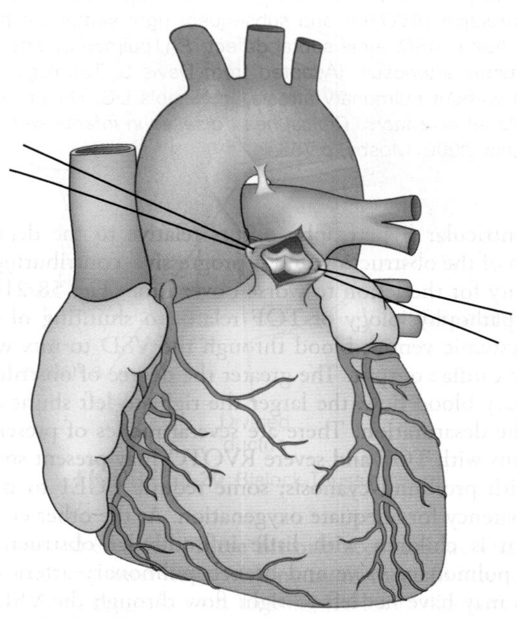

FIGURE 58-25 Mini–transannular incision in the transatrial-transpulmonary approach. (From Morales DL, Zafar F, Heinle JS: Right ventricular infundibulum sparing [RVIs] tetralogy of Fallot repair: A review of over 300 patients. *Ann Surg* 250:611–617, 2009.)

right atrial dilation may ultimately lead to atrial dysrhythmias, including atrial tachycardia and fibrillation. Relative to these and other potential issues after TOF repair, patients require careful and lifelong medical follow-up. Many need reintervention; this is frequently the case in patients with chronic, severe pulmonary insufficiency, which is indicated when right ventricular dilation and dysfunction become significant. In these patients, placing a competent pulmonary valve is necessary to relieve chronic right ventricular overload. These issues are of particular importance to a patient with repaired TOF presenting for noncardiac surgery. A careful assessment of the patient's cardiac anatomy and function is performed, including echocardiography, Holter monitoring, and occasionally cardiac catheterization.

Pulmonary Atresia and Intact Ventricular Septum

Pulmonary atresia with an intact ventricular septum manifests with profound desaturation and ductal-dependent pulmonary blood flow in newborns. The cardiac morphology in this condition varies widely. On the most severe end of the spectrum, patients have very small right ventricles, tiny tricuspid inlets, and often a right ventricle–dependent coronary circulation. In these cases, the right ventricle must remain hypertensive to provide flow to these segments of the coronary circulation. At the other end of the anatomic spectrum, patients have a relatively normal tricuspid valve and right ventricle. Most patients fall in between these extremes, with some degree of tricuspid valve and right ventricle underdevelopment.

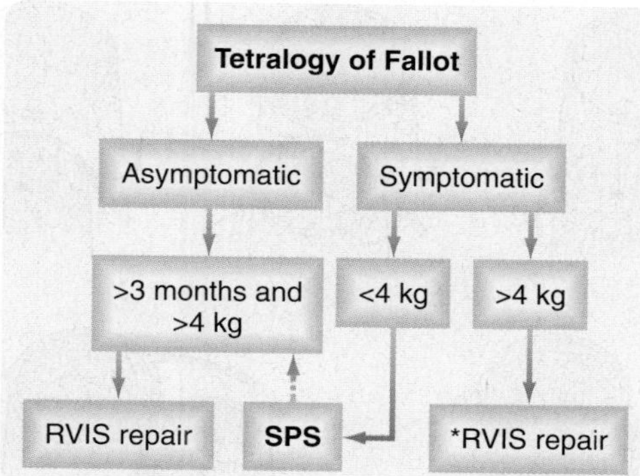

FIGURE 58-26 Algorithm for the right ventricular infundibulum-sparing (RVIS) strategy. The goal of this strategy is to minimize the right ventricular incision and preserve the pulmonary valve. It is an individualized approach that considers the patient's weight, age, and overall clinical picture. *SPS,* systemic-to-pulmonary artery shunt. (From Morales DL, Zafar F, Heinle JS: Right ventricular infundibulum sparing [RVIs] tetralogy of Fallot repair: A review of over 300 patients. *Ann Surg* 250:611–617, 2009.)

Because patients are ductal-dependent at birth, an assessment must be made as to whether the right heart will be capable of ultimately supporting a biventricular circulation. If the coronary circulation is truly right ventricle–dependent, decompressing the right ventricle would result in coronary insufficiency. In these situations, a palliative BT shunt is created in anticipation of promoting the patient down a single-ventricle pathway. In other patients, the atretic pulmonary valve must be opened with percutaneous balloon dilation or open surgical valvotomy. Over time, the hypertensive, often apparently underdeveloped right ventricle will improve in size and function and become capable of supporting all or a significant proportion of the cardiac output. At initial presentation, many patients have a large patent foramen ovale or ASD; in patients with a restrictive ASD and marginal right heart, an atrial septostomy (balloon) allows for atrial-level right-to-left shunting until the right ventricle improves. Ultimately, if the right ventricle is adequate, the ASD can be closed.

Pulmonary Atresia With Ventricular Septal Defect

Pulmonary atresia with VSD is morphologically similar to TOF, with the exception of an atretic pulmonary valve. Patients may have confluent, normal-sized pulmonary arteries perfused by a PDA. In severe cases, the pulmonary arteries are discontinuous, and the lungs are variably perfused by diminutive native branch pulmonary arteries and muscularized, collateral vessels originating from the descending aorta and brachiocephalic vessels. These major aortopulmonary collateral arteries (MAPCAs) have a propensity to develop severe stenoses as they are exposed to systemic arterial pressure. Many of these MAPCAs eventually occlude at an unpredictable rate during childhood. Because they may provide the only blood supply to some lung segments, patients become progressively desaturated.

The goal of surgical therapy for pulmonary atresia with VSD is biventricular repair to achieve normal cardiac workload and systemic arterial saturations. In patients with confluent native pulmonary arteries of adequate caliber, the VSD is surgically closed, and a valved conduit (homograft or heterograft) is interposed between the right ventricle and pulmonary bifurcation. In patients with pulmonary atresia with VSD and MAPCAs, the pulmonary arteries must be repaired by connecting the various lung segments into a common trunk through a process termed *pulmonary artery unifocalization.* Depending on the source and size of the MAPCAs and native pulmonary arteries, this may be a challenging surgical procedure, but the goal is constructing a pulmonary tree as close to normal as possible so that biventricular repair is feasible (see earlier).

The long-term issues of repair of pulmonary atresia with VSD are similar to concerns described earlier for TOF. The addition of a right ventricle–pulmonary artery conduit guarantees the need for reoperation because no currently available conduit choice offers the potential for somatic growth or an indefinitely durable valve.

Valvular Pulmonic Stenosis

Patients with isolated valvular pulmonary stenosis are almost always treated in infancy with a percutaneous balloon pulmonary valvotomy. The intermediate-term results of this treatment are good; however, all patients are left with significant pulmonary valve insufficiency and eventually require pulmonary valve replacement.

Conotruncal Anomalies

Transposition of the Great Arteries

TGA is a common cyanotic congenital cardiac lesion. In this section, our discussion relates only to TGA in which there are two good ventricles identified as being capable of independent function as the right and left ventricle. TGA is commonly referred to as D-TGA, in relationship to the typically normal D (dextro) ventricular looping that occurs in association with the discordant ventriculoarterial connection and normal A-V connection. TGA occurs in the setting of an intact ventricular septum (TGA-IVS) or with associated VSD (TGA-VSD). In TGA-VSD, there may be associated aortic arch hypoplasia and coarctation. On the other extreme, there may be severe pulmonic and subpulmonic stenosis (left ventricular outflow tract obstruction [LVOTO]) or even pulmonary atresia (TGA-VSD with pulmonary atresia).

Patients with TGA-IVS typically present in the early newborn period with profound cyanosis associated with normal perinatal PDA closure. In the absence of a significant ASD, the cyanosis is severe and progresses to death if left untreated. Administration of intravenous PGE1 is almost uniformly successful in reestablishing ductal patency to improve the patient's arterial saturation by providing left-to-right shunting and improved pulmonary blood flow.

In most patients, a balloon atrial septostomy is performed (percutaneous through the umbilical vein or femoral vein) to allow atrial-level mixing (Fig. 58-27). This procedure is usually effective in allowing sufficient atrial-level mixing so that the patient is adequately saturated (70% to 80%).

After the procedure, the prostaglandin infusion can be discontinued. In TGA-VSD, there is often sufficient shunting at the level of the VSD to promote adequate systemic saturation; in patients with large VSDs, the predominant presenting symptom may be pulmonary overcirculation and CHF. Patients with TGA with pulmonary atresia have ductal-dependent pulmonary blood flow. In patients with TGA-VSD and aortic arch hypoplasia or coarctation, PGE1 may be necessary to maintain ductal patency and systemic perfusion. Echocardiography is the primary diagnostic modality for TGA.

The treatment of TGA has evolved significantly during the past 60 years of surgical therapy for CHD. Initial success was achieved by surgical reconstruction to create a physiologic repair. The atrial switch operation involves a series of intra-atrial baffles using a

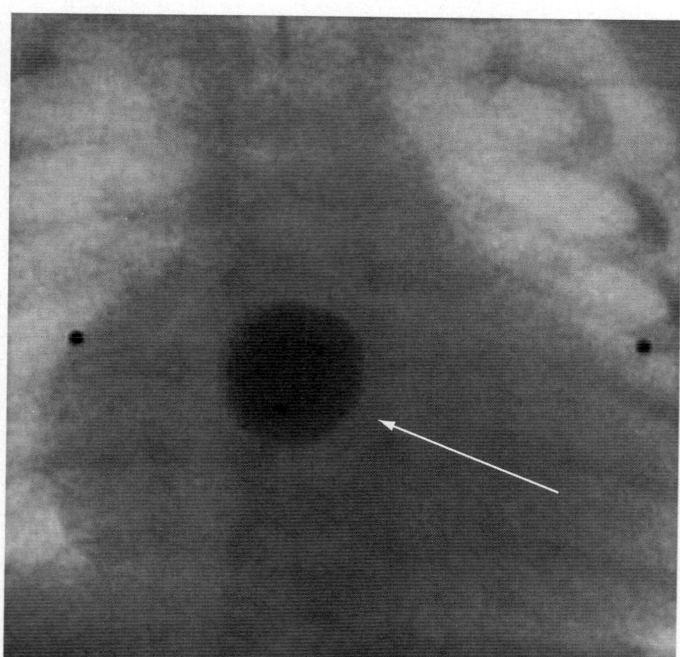

FIGURE 58-27 Angiogram during balloon atrial septostomy. The *arrow* points to the inflated balloon catheter at the atrial septum. The interventional cardiologist forcefully pulls the balloon across the patent foramen ovale to create an open, unobstructed secundum atrial septal defect.

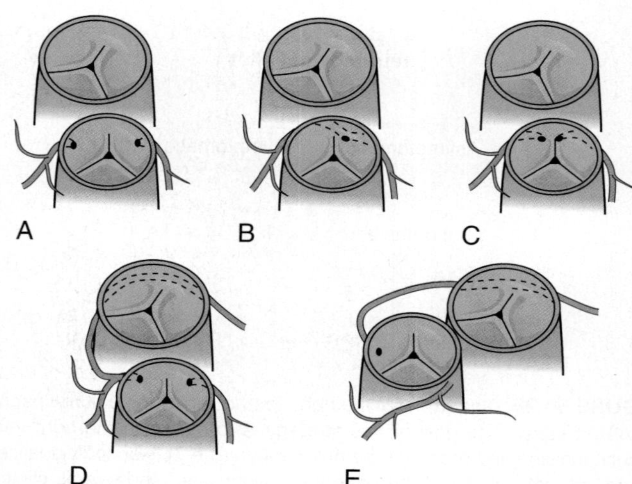

FIGURE 58-28 **(A-E)** Five basic coronary artery configurations, as described by Yacoub and Radley-Smith. (Adapted from Mee R: The arterial switch operation. In Stark J, de Leval M, editors: *Surgery for congenital heart defects*, ed 2, Philadelphia, 1994, Saunders, p 484.)

patch channel (Mustard procedure)[30] or infolding of the native atrial wall and interatrial septum (Senning procedure).[31] Both procedures achieve the same physiologic result: The systemic venous blood is redirected to the left ventricle (and the pulmonary circulation), and the pulmonary venous blood is redirected to the right ventricle. After a successful atrial switch, patients are fully saturated but are left with their morphologic right ventricle supporting the entire systemic cardiac output. In many (perhaps ultimately all) patients undergoing the atrial switch procedure, the right ventricle becomes dysfunctional over time, which is manifested by dilation, decreased ejection fraction, tricuspid insufficiency, and dysrhythmias. The observation of problems with the systemic right ventricle in patients after the atrial switch operation was the primary impetus behind the development and application of the arterial switch operation (ASO), which is now established as the surgical treatment of choice for patients with TGA. At the present time, operative survival rates for the ASO approach 100%.[32,33]

The ASO provides physiologic and anatomic correction of TGA by establishing ventriculoarterial concordance. The procedure involves transection and translocation of the malposed great vessels. The technically challenging requirement of the ASO relates to the translocation of the coronary arteries to the pulmonary root (the neoaorta). As noted, there are numerous possible branching patterns for the coronary arteries in TGA—some are easily transferred in the ASO, whereas others are more challenging (including single coronary ostium and intramural course) (Fig. 58-28).[34] Nonetheless, precise surgical techniques have been described and successfully applied to all coronary branching patterns. Given this as well as the known benefit of aligning the morphologic left ventricle with the systemic circulation, the ASO is offered to all patients with TGA regardless of the coronary branching pattern. There is no need for precise anatomic definition before surgery; all patients undergo the ASO. In most patients undergoing this procedure, the pulmonary artery bifurcation is moved anterior to the reconstructed neoaorta to minimize the potential for pulmonary artery distortion and compression of the translocated coronary arteries—the Lecompte maneuver (Fig. 58-29). Although there are interinstitutional biases in terms of nuances of treatment for TGA, the following surgical strategies are generally agreed on for this group of patients.

Transposition of the great arteries–intact ventricular septum. After balloon atrial septostomy and weaning from PGE1, if possible, newborns with TGA-IVS undergo semielective ASO in the first few days to weeks of life. Rarely, patients present with profound desaturation refractory to balloon atrial septostomy and PGE1; in this setting, an emergent ASO is indicated. We have found this to be necessary in one patient during the past decade in an experience involving more than 200 ASOs performed in newborns. For other patients, the ASO needs to be performed in a timely but nonemergent setting. Even in the presence of adequate systemic saturation, the patient's morphologic left ventricle is functioning in a low-pressure work environment—supporting the pulmonary circulation. Thus, left ventricle mass and function involute rapidly in the first few weeks of life. By 6 weeks of life, the left ventricle may be incapable of supporting the normal systemic workload after the ASO. As such, the preferred timing for the operation is in the first 1 to 2 weeks of life.

Transposition of the great arteries–ventricular septal defect with or without arch hypoplasia. There are several modes of presentation for patients with TGA-VSD. In patients with small, pressure-restrictive VSD, the presenting symptoms are similar to those of TGA-IVS. These patients require the ASO early in life, along with VSD closure before left ventricle involution. In patients with TGA and nonrestrictive VSD, there may be adequate mixing to allow reasonable systemic arterial saturation. In this setting, the left ventricle remains pressure-loaded and does not involute; thus, the necessity of early promotion to the ASO is less time-compressed. Many newborns with TGA and a large VSD are relatively asymptomatic soon after birth; they go on to develop CHF in the first 1 to 2 months of life as the normal decrease in newborn pulmonary resistance occurs. Our preference for these patients is

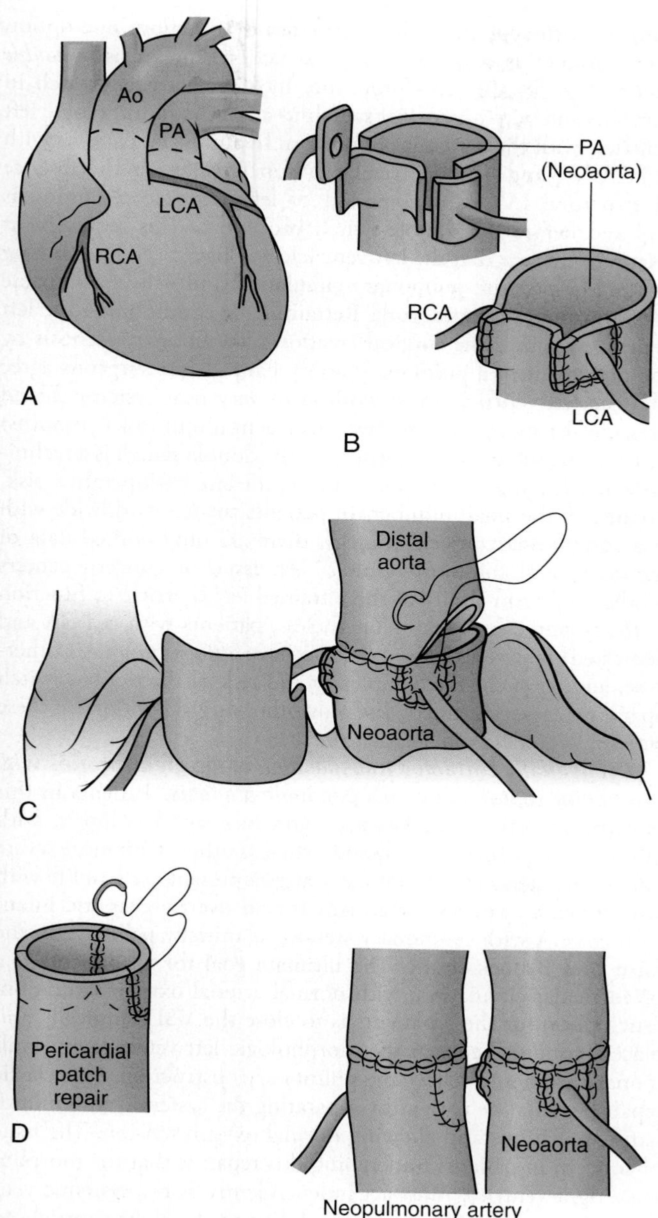

FIGURE 58-29 Arterial switch operation. **A,** The aorta *(Ao)* and pulmonary artery *(PA)* are transected above the sinuses of Valsalva. **B,** The coronaries are excised from the aorta and anastomosed to the pulmonary artery using a trapdoor technique. **C,** The distal aorta is brought behind the pulmonary artery (Lecompte maneuver) and anastomosed to the neoaorta. **D,** Separate pericardial patches are sutured to replace the excised coronary artery tissue from the aorta. **E,** Completed repair. *LCA,* Left coronary artery; *RCA,* right coronary artery. (Adapted from Karl TR, Kirshbom PM: Transposition of the great arteries and the arterial switch operation. In Nichols DG, Ungerleider RM, Spevak PJ, et al, editors: *Critical heart disease in infants and children*, Philadelphia, 2006, Mosby, p 721.)

to follow them closely for evidence of CHF and perform semielective ASO and VSD closure in the first 4 to 6 weeks of life. Some centers prefer to proceed with this surgery sooner; this appears to be a matter of surgeon preference and has not been shown to affect long-term outcome. In patients with TGA-VSD with arch hypoplasia or coarctation, early surgery is required. In this setting, the preferred treatment involves one-stage, complete correction, including ASO, VSD closure, and aortic arch repair.

Transposition of the great arteries–ventricular septal defect with pulmonary stenosis–left ventricular outflow tract obstruction or pulmonary atresia. The issue of concern in this group of patients is the degree of LVOTO. In patients with TGA-VSD and organic LVOTO, with a relatively normal pulmonary valve, the treatment strategy is as described earlier, with ASO, VSD closure, and left ventricular outflow tract (LVOT) resection. The situation becomes more complex in the setting of severe pulmonary stenosis or pulmonary atresia. These patients may be ductal-dependent as newborns (pulmonary atresia) and require newborn complete correction or a palliative Blalock shunt in the newborn period, followed by biventricular repair later in infancy (our preference). The goal in these patients is to achieve biventricular repair to create an unobstructed connection between the morphologic left ventricle and systemic circulation. Several operations have been described and successfully used in this setting.

The Rastelli procedure involves an interventricular patch baffle, which commits the left ventricle to the aorta through the VSD. Typically, a right ventricle–pulmonary artery conduit is then placed to achieve pulmonary blood flow. Issues of concern include the potential for LVOTO (at or below the level of the VSD) and the certain need for future right ventricle–pulmonary artery conduit revision. The REV procedure is designed to minimize the potential of LVOT obstruction and to use all possible native tissue-tissue connections to limit the potential need for future surgery. This procedure involves resection of the muscular conus between the aorta and pulmonary roots, interventricular baffle of the left ventricle to the aorta, and translocation of the native main pulmonary artery to the right ventricle (by a Lecompte maneuver) without the use of an intervening conduit. The final option involves aortic root translocation, which includes resection of the entire native aortic root and coronary origins, resection of the intervening muscular conus, and posterior translocation of the aortic root to the surgically enlarged pulmonary root to achieve a direct connection between the left ventricle and aorta. The VSD is then closed, and a conduit is placed or a direct connection is created between the right ventricle and pulmonary arteries.

Transposition of the great arteries in adults. The long-term prognosis of adult patients who have undergone childhood repair of TGA is still incompletely understood; however, all these patients require lifelong surveillance and have the potential of developing significant anatomic and functional cardiac problems. Patients who were treated with the atrial switch operation have a morphologic right ventricle supporting their systemic circulation, which will predictably fail in many patients. Although fully saturated, these patients may present later in life with signs and symptoms of CHF and dysrhythmia. For severely affected individuals, the only realistic treatment option may ultimately be cardiac transplantation.

The long-term issues related to the ASO are less well understood. Despite technical advances in reconstructive methods, there is still a troubling incidence of postoperative supravalvular and branch pulmonic stenosis. The neoaortic root may dilate in some patients undergoing the ASO, leading to neoaortic insufficiency and coronary artery distortion. The fate of the surgically translocated coronary ostia is unclear; there is clearly a risk for late sudden cardiac death related to unsuspected coronary insufficiency noted elsewhere in this chapter. For an adult patient undergoing noncardiac surgery after previous surgery for complex congenital cardiac disease, including TGA, a high index of suspicion is warranted.

Double-Outlet Right Ventricle

Double-outlet right ventricle occurs when both great vessels are anatomically committed to the right ventricle. This condition may occur in association with a subaortic VSD, a noncommitted (remote) VSD, or a subpulmonary VSD (Taussig-Bing anomaly). As with other complex cardiac conditions, the goal of treatment relates to the presenting hemodynamic conditions and patient symptoms. The ultimate goal is to achieve a biventricular circulation when possible. Patients may present with severe cyanosis and require corrective or palliative therapy in the newborn period. Conversely, they may present with unrestricted pulmonary blood flow and develop CHF. The challenging issue of constructing a biventricular repair relates to achieving unobstructed outlets from the right and left ventricles. In patients with double-outlet right ventricle with subaortic VSD and RVOTO, reconstruction is similar to that for TOF. More remote VSDs may require enlargement with interventricular tunnel repair. For the Taussig-Bing anomaly, the relationship of the VSD to the pulmonary artery makes the ASO the procedure of choice. These patients often have RVOTO and aortic arch hypoplasia, which require attention at the time of complete correction. For rare individuals, the relationship of the great vessels and complexity of the VSD preclude a biventricular repair, and the patient must be treated as if he or she has a functional single ventricle.

Congenitally Corrected Transposition of the Great Arteries (L-Transposition)

ccTGA, or L-TGA, describes a constellation of conditions with the common feature of A-V and ventriculoarterial discordance. ccTGA may occur in association with VSD, pulmonic and subpulmonic stenosis, and displaced left A-V valve (Ebsteinoid left A-V valve). In ccTGA, the morphologic mitral valve is right-sided and associated with the morphologic left ventricle; the morphologic tricuspid valve is associated with the morphologic right ventricle. Patients with this condition are physiologically corrected in that in the absence of ventricular-level shunting, they are fully saturated—hence, the term *corrected transposition.* The age and mode of patient presentation in this condition depend on the contribution of associated defects and the function of the morphologic right ventricle, which acts as the systemic ventricle. Controversy exists regarding the timing and mode of surgical treatment for patients presenting with various manifestations of ccTGA.

Congenitally corrected transposition of the great arteries with intact ventricular septum. Patients with ccTGA-IVS may be entirely asymptomatic throughout childhood and early adulthood. Frequently, the diagnosis is made incidentally. In other patients, the disease manifests with symptoms of CHF in association with right ventricular dysfunction or left A-V valve insufficiency. There is also a high incidence of complete heart block in patients with ccTGA, and the first manifestation may be this dysrhythmia, with associated symptoms.

Treatment for patients presenting with CHF is a challenging management scenario. For patients with ccTGA and preserved right ventricular function, left A-V valve repair or replacement may be considered. In many of these patients, the valvular insufficiency may be more a manifestation of declining systemic RV function, with septal shift and annular dilation, rather than intrinsic valve pathology. In this setting, valve replacement would not correct the progression of right ventricular dysfunction. For patients with systemic right ventricular dysfunction, one option for treatment is a complex reconstruction known as a *double switch* (Fig. 58-30). This procedure includes an atrial switch in combination with an arterial switch to align the morphologic left ventricle with the systemic circulation. In almost all patients with ccTGA-IVS and right ventricular dysfunction (and in the absence of structural LVOTO), a period of left ventricle retraining is required before the double-switch procedure. This requirement relates to the fact that the left ventricle will have been functioning in the low-pressure pulmonary circulation and will be incapable of performing systemic work. Retraining or conditioning the left ventricle requires the surgical creation of pulmonary stenosis by the placement of a pulmonary artery band. Most surgeons agree that the left ventricle must work at or very near systemic blood pressure for many months (we favor a minimum of 6 months) before the double-switch operation. The double switch is a technically challenging operation, with significant perioperative risk. Because of the small numbers of patients treated worldwide with this complicated surgical strategy, there are only limited data of the acute and midterm results.[35] An issue of concern centers on the long-term ability of the retrained left ventricle to function as the systemic ventricle. Nonetheless, patients with ccTGA and depressed right ventricular function have a poor prognosis otherwise, and, as such, the complexity and risk of the double-switch operation appear justified. The only other surgical option for these patients is cardiac transplantation.

Congenitally corrected transposition of the great arteries with ventricular septal defect and pulmonic stenosis. Patients in this category are often well balanced and have mild cyanosis, with minimal symptoms in childhood, whereas others with more severe pulmonary stenosis or pulmonary atresia present early in life with symptomatic cyanosis. Treatment for an overtly cyanotic infant with ccTGA with pulmonary stenosis is initially palliative in the form of a Blalock shunt. The ultimate goal for all patients is a biventricular circulation, with normal arterial oxygen saturation. One option for these patients is to close the VSD surgically and place a conduit between the morphologic left ventricle and pulmonary arteries to relieve the pulmonary obstruction. This classic repair benefits the patient by separating the systemic and pulmonary circulations and allowing normal oxygen tension. The issue of concern in patients undergoing this repair is that the morphologic right ventricle must act independently as the systemic ventricle after repair. As noted, the ability of the right ventricle to support the systemic circulation may be questionable over the long-term in some patients. As such, an alternative strategy in these patients is to baffle the left ventricular outflow to the aorta through the VSD, then to perform an atrial switch to reroute the systemic and pulmonary venous return, and finally to place a conduit from the morphologic right ventricle to the pulmonary arteries. This option is a modification of the double-switch arrangement, affording the patient the benefit of a systemic left ventricle. Because the left ventricle has been working at systemic pressure before correction, a period of retraining is unnecessary.

Adult patients with ccTGA, with or without previous surgery, warrant careful attention before any noncardiac operation. These patients may have various complex ongoing cardiac issues, including rhythm disturbance, ventricular dysfunction, and valvular insufficiency.

Left Ventricular Outflow Tract Obstruction

LVOTO may manifest in isolation or in combination with other complex cardiac lesions. The physiologic consequences of severe

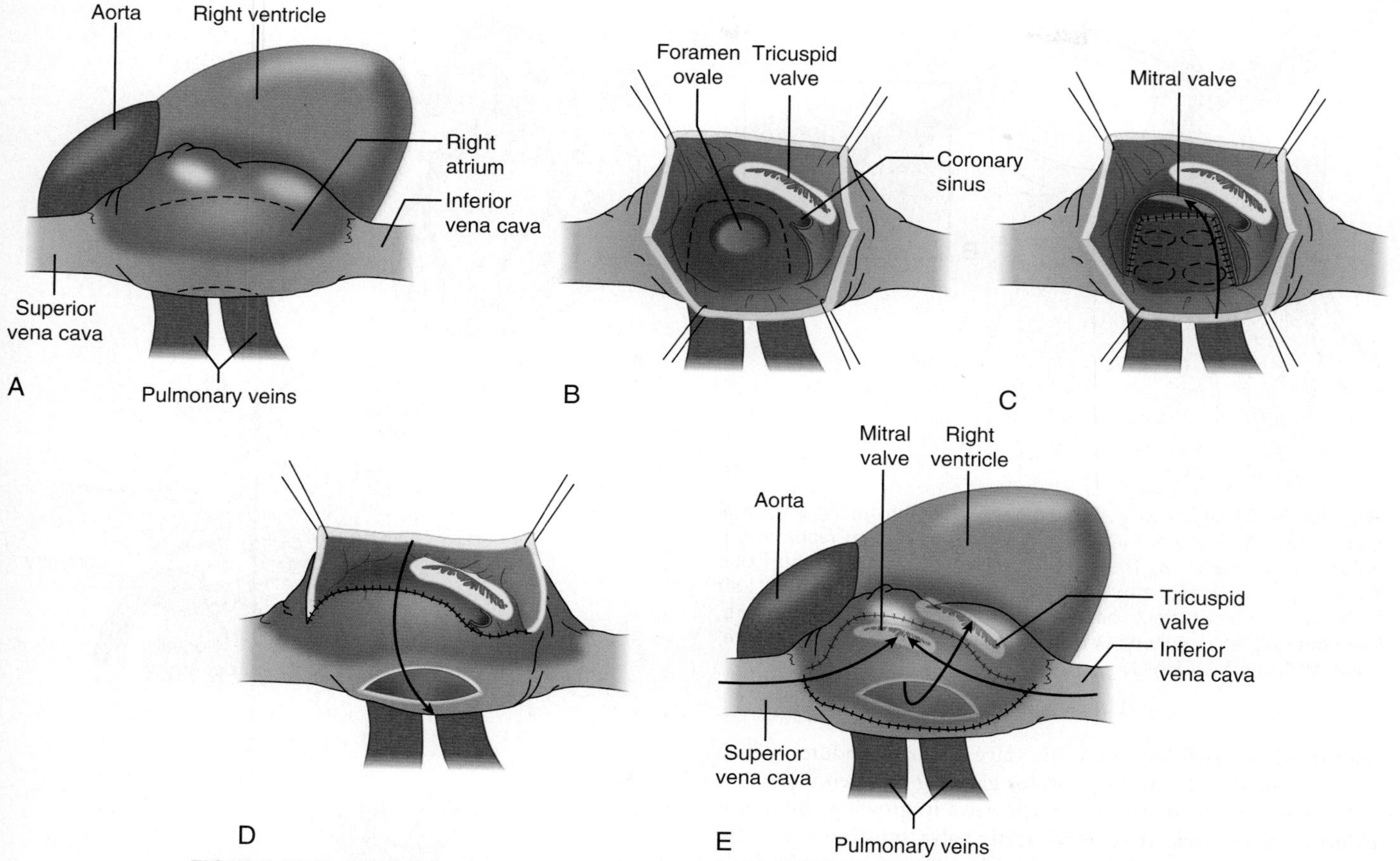

FIGURE 58-30 Schematic representation of the Senning procedure for transposition of the great arteries. **A,** Two separate incisions, one in the right atrium and the other in the left atrium near the insertion of the pulmonary veins. **B,** Location of the incision in the atrial septum. **C,** The atrial septum sewn down to the pulmonary veins preparing for oxygenated blood to be directed to the tricuspid valve. The inferior free wall of the right atrium is sewn along the cut edge of the atrial septum redirecting the deoxygenated blood to the mitral valve. **D,** The superior free wall of the right atrium is now sewn to the cut edge of the left atrium, redirecting the oxygenated blood from the pulmonary veins to the tricuspid valve. **E,** Schematic representation of the oxygenated blood and deoxygenated blood pathways. (Reprinted with permission from Texas Children's Hospital, 2016.)

LVOTO may be catastrophic, including diminished systemic cardiac output and tremendous left ventricular pressure overload. Newborns with severe LVOTO may present in shock with diminished peripheral perfusion, cardiomegaly, and pulmonary congestion. There is a significant risk for necrotizing enterocolitis in these infants. In older patients, gradual onset of LVOTO may be initially asymptomatic, only to manifest over time as decreasing exercise tolerance and declining left ventricular function. Patients with severe LVOTO and cardiomegaly are at high risk for myocardial ischemia and sudden cardiac death. The resting ECG often demonstrates left ventricular hypertrophy, with a strain pattern. If an exercise stress test is performed, it may demonstrate worrisome ST segment depression and ventricular dysrhythmias. Echocardiography is the primary diagnostic tool for patients with LVOTO. In rare cases, diagnostic cardiac catheterization may be considered to delineate the level of obstruction.

Valvular Aortic Stenosis

Congenital valvular aortic stenosis (AS) is a common cause of LVOTO. The degree of obstruction may range from mild in patients with a congenitally bicuspid aortic valve to severe in patients with critical AS with unidentifiable valve commissures and annular hypoplasia. Infants presenting with critical AS are often symptomatic early in the newborn period, presenting with shock and profoundly depressed ventricular function. At the present time, almost all patients are taken to the cardiac catheterization laboratory for balloon aortic valvotomy. This procedure may be lifesaving in relieving AS and allowing for recovery of ventricular function. However, for most patients, the procedure is palliative, with a significant incidence of recurrence of AS or development of significant aortic insufficiency after the procedure. In patients with AS refractory to balloon dilation, an open aortic valvotomy may be necessary (Fig. 58-31). A surgical valvotomy, especially in small infants with adequate annular dimension, can be accomplished by an accurate incision down a rudimentary commissure or raphe to improve cusp mobility.

Recurrent AS after previous ballooning may be amenable to repeat dilation; however, when associated with significant aortic insufficiency, the patient requires surgery. Severe aortic insufficiency after previous balloon dilation is usually related to an avulsed cusp. In these cases, valve repair may be possible, but replacement may become necessary. Published series have

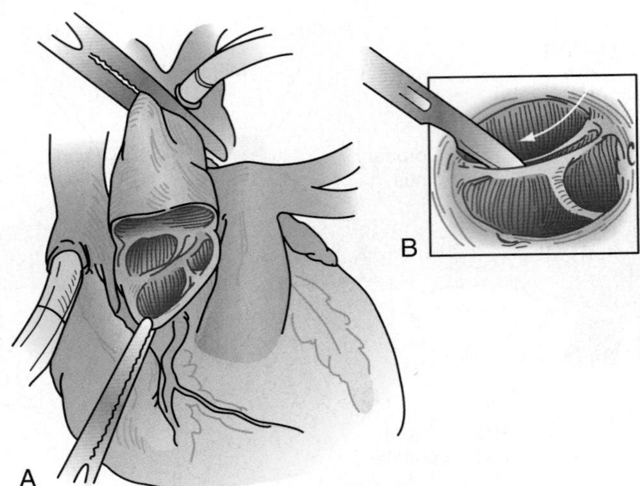

FIGURE 58-31 Close-up of the aortic valve demonstrating a surgical valvectomy. **A,** The valve is bicuspid, with a prominent raphe in the anterior valve leaflet. **B,** The orifice is enlarged by incising the fused commissure between the two leaflets. (From Chang AC, Burke RP: Left ventricular outflow tract obstruction. In Chang AC, Hanley FL, Wernovsky G, et al, editors: *Pediatric cardiac intensive care.* Baltimore, 1998, Williams & Wilkins.)

confirmed the usefulness of aortic valve repair procedures, which is a particularly attractive option for growing children.[36-38]

The decision to replace the aortic valve in growing children is clouded by the lack of an ideal aortic valve substitute—a valve capable of lifelong durability, appropriate somatic growth, easily implantable, and not requiring anticoagulation. Criteria for aortic valve replacement are beyond the scope of this chapter; however, severe valvular AS not amenable to catheter or open valvotomy is an appropriate indication. Options for aortic valve replacement in children include a mechanical prosthesis, heterograft, homograft, and pulmonary autograft. A mechanical prosthesis may be considered in childhood; however, the valve size must be sufficient to provide adequate function as the patient grows. Most surgeons and cardiologists recommend therapeutic anticoagulation in children with a mechanical valve prosthesis, but this can be challenging and potentially dangerous in growing children and adolescents. Many surgeons believe the risk for such medical treatment outweighs the potential benefit of a theoretically durable valve.

Heterograft aortic valve prostheses historically have been associated with limited durability in children and are not capable of somatic growth. Currently available heterograft prostheses have not undergone sufficient use in children to provide useful data concerning improved durability. Human cadaver aortic valves (aortic homograft) have been used extensively in children and young adults. These valves are usually implanted as a complete aortic root replacement, which requires coronary ostial implantation. Thus, surgery to place an aortic homograft is considerably more complex and with potentially higher risk. The positive features of an aortic homograft include improved durability compared with heterograft and avoidance of anticoagulation. Nonetheless, these valves eventually fail, necessitating a complicated reoperative aortic root replacement.

Pulmonary autograft aortic root replacement (Ross operation) involves translocation of the pulmonary valve to the aortic position with subsequent replacement of the pulmonary valve with a homograft or heterograft valved conduit (Fig. 58-32). The

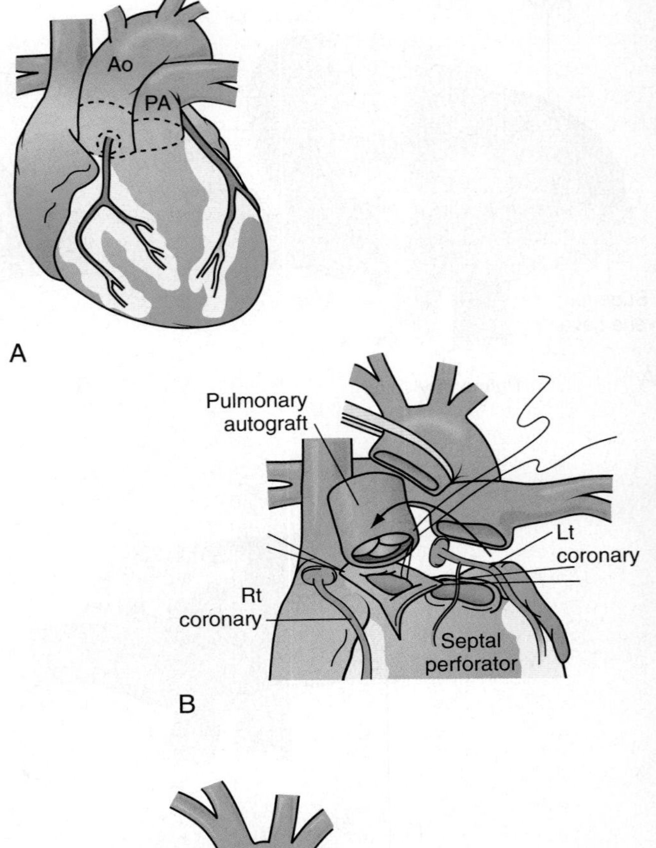

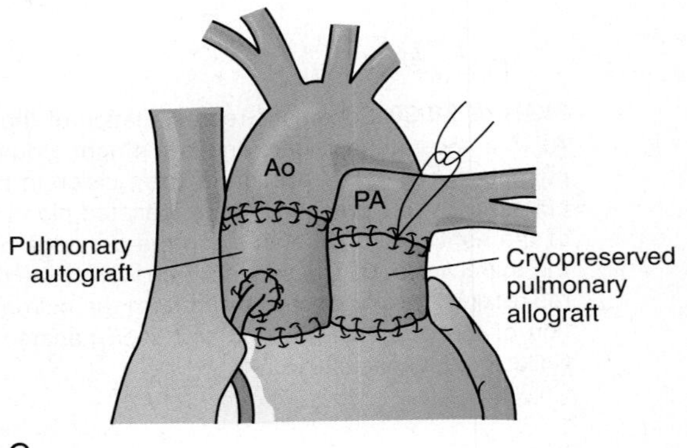

FIGURE 58-32 Ross procedure. **A,** The great arteries are transected above the sinotubular ridge. The coronary arteries are excised using coronary artery buttons. **B,** The pulmonary autograft is excised from the right ventricular outflow tract, and the proximal end of the autograft is anastomosed to the annulus. **C,** The coronary artery buttons are anastomosed to the pulmonary autograft. *Ao,* Aorta; *PA,* pulmonary artery. (Adapted from St Louis JD, Jaggers J: Left ventricular outflow tract obstruction. In Nichols DG, Ungerleider RM, Spevak PJ, et al, editors: *Critical heart disease in infants and children,* Philadelphia, 2006, Mosby, p 615.)

theoretical advantages of the Ross procedure include the potential for somatic growth, avoidance of anticoagulation, and possibility of extended durability. Enthusiasm for this procedure has been tempered by the recognition that the need for extension cardiac dissection to harvest the autograft, along with a more complex implantation, is associated with increased operative risk. Furthermore, the unsupported pulmonary root may dilate in the presence of systemic arterial pressure, leading to progressive autograft aortic insufficiency. This observation has led to various modifications of the implantation technique to support the aortic annulus and the sinus segment. Given these considerations and the certain need for reoperation to replace the right ventricular–pulmonary artery conduit, great caution must be exercised in the application of the Ross operation.[39]

Fibromuscular Subaortic Stenosis

This condition is a progressive narrowing of the LVOT related to a dense fibrous membrane usually found in association with asymmetrical protrusion of the interventricular septum into the outflow tract. The membrane is often concentric and becomes densely adherent to the septum and mitral valve. The membrane progresses toward and eventually onto the undersurface of the aortic valve cusps, which leads to progressive LVOTO, aortic valve cusp retraction, and aortic insufficiency.

Echocardiography is the primary diagnostic tool when assessing the degree of obstruction and progression of subaortic stenosis. However, it is not accurate for assessing subtle degrees of cusp extension.[40] Cardiac catheterization is rarely needed to diagnose this condition; balloon dilation is of no use in treating LVOTO.

Surgery is the mainstay of treatment for subaortic stenosis, but there is disagreement about surgical indications. Most surgeons believe that new onset of any degree of aortic insufficiency in association with a subaortic membrane, regardless of the pressure gradient, is an indication for surgery. In other patients, an escalating LVOT gradient, associated left ventricular hypertrophy, and appropriate anatomic substrate are acceptable indications for operation.

The surgical procedure for subaortic stenosis involves a transaortic resection of the subaortic membrane, including all attachments to the mitral valve, septum, and aortic valve cusps. A septal myectomy is performed, along with membrane resection, in most patients (Fig. 58-33). Complications include membrane recurrence, injury to the bundle of His, and iatrogenic VSD creation. Nonetheless, with careful technique, the risk for these complications is minimized.

Tunnel Subaortic Stenosis

Tunnel subaortic stenosis is a more severe form of LVOTO that is often associated with aortic annular hypoplasia and valvular AS. In severe cases, the LVOTO is not amenable to subaortic resection alone. In this situation, an aortic root–enlarging procedure may be necessary to relieve the obstruction (aortoventriculoplasty, or Konno procedure). This complex reconstruction generally is associated with the necessity of aortic valve replacement using one of the aforementioned options. Moreover, all degrees of LVOTO may be seen in association with numerous left heart obstructive lesions (Shone syndrome[41]) that may require extensive reconstruction.

Aortic Arch Anomalies

Aortic Coarctation

Coarctation of the aorta is one of the most frequently encountered congenital cardiac lesions. This condition has a wide range of presentations, from a severely symptomatic newborn with CHF and depressed ventricular function to an adult with proximal hypertension and minimal symptoms. Coarctation is classified relative to its association with the ligamentum arteriosus and aortic arch. An infantile or preductal aortic coarctation is seen in combination with a large PDA, which may have predominantly right-to-left flow to the lower descending aorta. In this setting, the patient is ductal-dependent for systemic blood flow until the coarctation is repaired, and a PGE1 infusion must be maintained to prevent ductal closure. A periductal or juxtaductal coarctation occurs in the region of the ductal insertion and is distal to the aortic isthmus, which may be normal or hypoplastic (Fig. 58-34).

Aortic coarctation with or without aortic arch hypoplasia is frequently associated with intracardiac anomalies, including

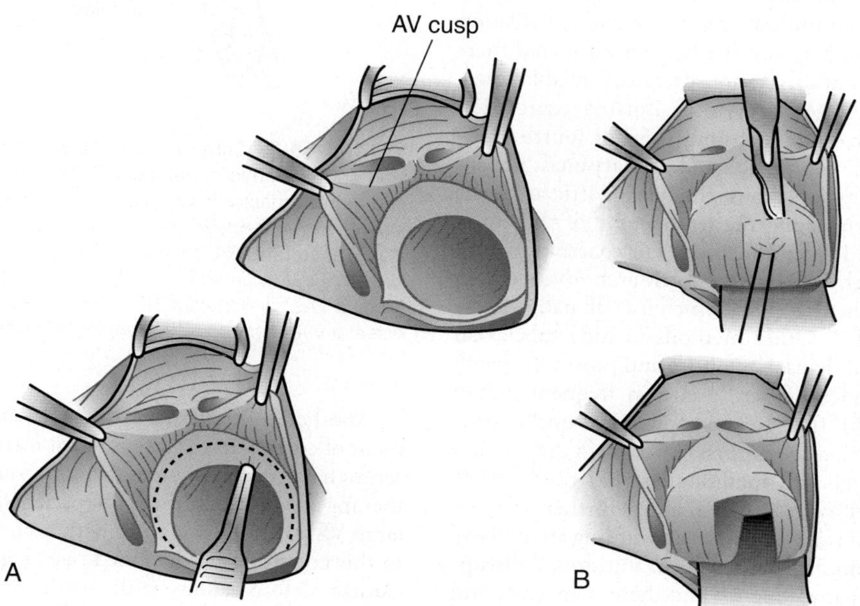

FIGURE 58-33 **A,** Excision of discrete subaortic stenosis. The aorta is opened obliquely, and the aortic valve leaflets are retracted to expose the subaortic membrane. The membrane is excised circumferentially *(dotted line)*. **B,** This is usually combined with a muscle resection. (From de Leval M: Surgery of the left ventricular outflow tract. In Stark J, de Leval M, editors: *Surgery for congenital heart defects,* ed 2, Philadelphia, 1994, Saunders.)

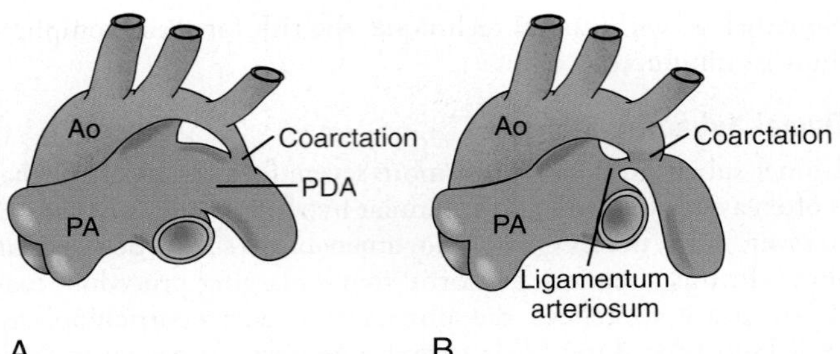

FIGURE 58-34 Coarctation of the aorta *(Ao)*. **A,** Infantile or preductal coarctation. **B,** Adult coarctation. *PA,* Pulmonary artery; *PDA,* patent ductus arteriosus. (From Backer CL, Mavroudis C: Coarctation of the aorta. In Mavroudis C, Backer CL, editors: *Pediatric heart surgery*. Philadelphia, 2003, Mosby, p 252.)

multiple left heart obstructive lesions (e.g., mitral stenosis, left ventricular hypoplasia or endocardial fibroelastosis, subaortic stenosis or AS) known as Shone syndrome.[41] Patients with large VSDs may present in infancy with severe aortic coarctation, with or without subaortic stenosis.

Aortic coarctation may be suspected on clinical examination by a significant upper extremity–lower extremity blood pressure gradient and diminished or absent femoral and pedal pulses. In older patients with well-developed intercostal collateral arteries, a continuous murmur may be auscultated over the posterior thorax. Echocardiography is now the primary diagnostic modality for aortic coarctation. MRI and CT angiography may also be useful in some patients. In rare cases, cardiac catheterization is required to define the anatomy, but this modality is now used more frequently for treatment, including balloon dilation with or without stenting.

Treatment strategies for aortic coarctation have evolved significantly since the first successful surgical treatment almost 70 years ago. Newborns presenting with severe aortic coarctation with or without associated ductal-dependent systemic blood flow are best treated by surgery. Initial enthusiasm regarding balloon dilation in these patients has diminished as it has become clear that there is a high incidence of recurrent coarctation after neonatal dilation.[42] Most congenital cardiac surgeons perform isolated coarctation repair through a left thoracotomy incision (third or fourth interspace) using resection of the coarctation and primary anastomosis. For patients with relative hypoplasia of the distal aortic arch, the anastomosis can be brought along the lesser curve of the aortic arch using an extended end-to-end method. For coarctation with a hypoplastic transverse arch, we favor the aortic arch advancement procedure at Texas Children's Hospital, which uses all native tissue repair to allow for growth.[43] Other methods include subclavian artery flap aortoplasty (Waldhausen method) and prosthetic patch aortoplasty. These latter methods are used less frequently than primary repair (Fig. 58-35). Catheter therapy as a primary treatment for aortic coarctation is a controversial therapy in the opinion of most surgeons. Although this methodology has been widely applied, its true comparability to surgery requires further prospective study. There are several issues of concern regarding angioplasty for coarctation. The balloon dilation results in transmural disruption of the aortic wall in many patients, and there is an acute and ongoing risk for aneurysm formation. To limit this risk and minimize the potential of recurrence, off-label use of stents has been done for treatment of coarctation. Obvious issues of concern include somatic growth and lifetime risk potential of a metal device in the descending aorta.

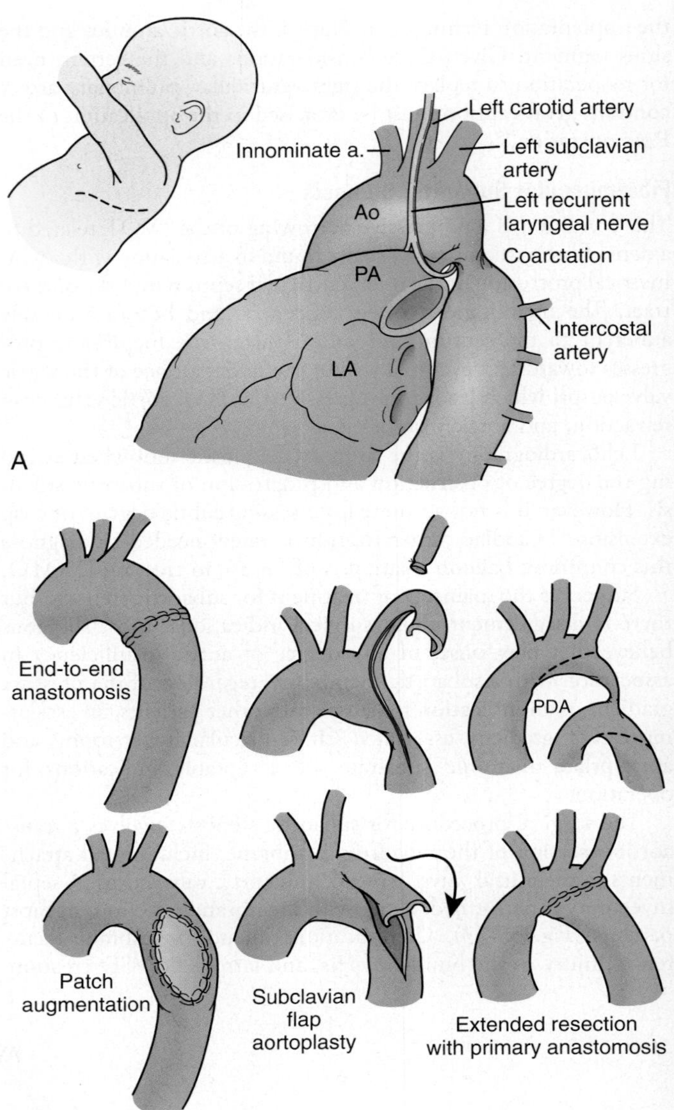

FIGURE 58-35 Surgical repair for aortic coarctation. **A,** Surgical incision and anatomic orientation. **B,** Four different methods are shown: end-to-end anastomosis, patch augmentation, subclavian flap aortoplasty, and extended resection with primary anastomosis. *Ao,* Aorta; *LA,* left atrium; *PA,* pulmonary artery. (Adapted from Hastings LA, Nichols DG: Coarctation of the aorta and interrupted aortic arch. In Nichols DG, Ungerleider RM, Spevak PJ, et al, editors: *Critical heart disease in infants and children*, Philadelphia, 2006, Mosby, p 635.)

Another controversial issue surrounds the concomitant treatment of coarctation and significant intracardiac pathology. Several series have demonstrated superior outcomes for simultaneous therapy in selected groups of patients, including neonates with large VSDs and coarctation with arch hypoplasia. Our approach to this condition has included one-stage complete repair of intracardiac defects along with aortic arch advancement through median sternotomy on cardiopulmonary bypass.

Interrupted Aortic Arch

IAA results from lack of proper fusion and involution of the fetal aortic arches. This is a fatal condition without treatment, and IAA

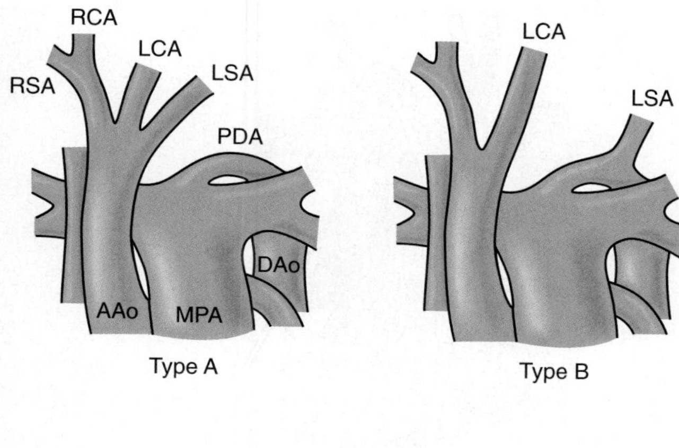

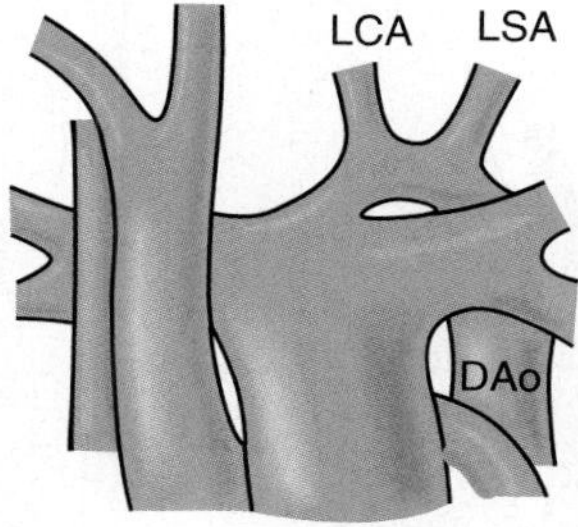

FIGURE 58-36 Classification of interrupted aortic arch. *AAo,* Ascending aorta; *DAo,* descending aorta; *LCA,* left common carotid artery; *LSA,* left subclavian artery; *MPA,* main pulmonary artery; *RCA,* right common carotid artery; *RSA,* right subclavian artery. (Adapted from Monro JL: Interruption of aortic arch. In Stark J, de Leval M, editors: *Surgery for congenital heart defects,* ed 2, Philadelphia, 1994, Saunders, p 299.)

is frequently associated with serious intracardiac pathology. IAA is classified based on the level of the interruption. Type A is distal to the left subclavian artery, type B occurs between left subclavian and common carotid arteries, and type C occurs proximal to the left subclavian artery (Fig. 58-36). There is a frequent finding of an aberrant right subclavian artery (retroesophageal) from the descending aorta. Survival for patients with IAA is initially predicated on ductal patency; thus, a PGE1 infusion is required to stabilize the patient. Diagnosis is confirmed by echocardiography; other methods, including cardiac catheterization, are needed infrequently.

IAA requires surgical treatment in the newborn period, which typically involves simultaneous repair of intracardiac lesions (Fig. 58-37). Repair may be accomplished with the aid of an aortic arch augmentation patch, although researchers at Texas Children's Hospital reported a series confirming that a primary tissue-tissue repair can be performed in most patients and minimizes the potential for recurrent aortic arch obstruction.[44]

SINGLE VENTRICLE

Single-ventricle physiology is a frequently encountered form of CHD. Patients may present as newborns with inadequate pulmonary blood flow, excessive pulmonary blood flow, or balanced circulations. The single ventricle may be of right, left, or indeterminate morphology. Surgical treatment is required to provide adequate systemic oxygen delivery, while protecting the pulmonary vasculature. The function of the single ventricle must be preserved to afford the patient the best possible long-term outcome.

The rapid evolution of successful palliation for patients with various forms of single-ventricle physiology since the late 1970s has led to a large and growing population of adults with a single ventricle. For most of these patients, lifelong cardiac attention is needed, and the potential for subsequent cardiac reoperation is high. Patients in this category who present for noncardiac surgery may be especially difficult to manage because of their challenging physiology.

An exhaustive discussion of the various forms of single ventricle is well beyond the scope of this chapter. This discussion is limited to common forms of single right and left ventricles to provide examples of the surgical management strategies for a single ventricle.

Tricuspid Atresia

Tricuspid atresia is the template of a single-ventricle lesion for which most current palliative strategies were developed. Patients with tricuspid atresia have a single morphologic left ventricle and may have normally related or transposed great vessels (Fig. 58-38). They may present with excessive pulmonary blood flow and require pulmonary artery banding early in infancy to relieve pulmonary overcirculation and CHF. Conversely, patients may have pulmonary stenosis or pulmonary atresia and require creation of a Blalock shunt to provide adequate pulmonary blood flow and systemic oxygenation.

As noted, the initial palliative goals in patients with tricuspid atresia include adequate systemic oxygenation, protection of ventricular function, and adequate pulmonary arterial growth. Patients with ductal-dependent pulmonary blood flow require a Blalock shunt in the newborn period. We prefer to construct the shunt to the morphologic right pulmonary artery through a right thoracotomy. This construction allows shunt flow to be governed by the size of the subclavian artery. Furthermore, the right pulmonary artery is typically longer and runs in a more horizontal plane compared with the left pulmonary artery; this facilitates avoiding distortion of a lobar branch. The goal of the shunt is to protect the pulmonary arteries, promote adequate pulmonary artery development, and support systemic arterial oxygenation for the first 4 to 6 months of life until the next planned stage of palliation (see later discussion of Glenn and Fontan operations). The shunt is not designed for long-term use; thus, in most patients, a small interposition graft (expanded polytetrafluoroethylene, 3.0 to 4.0 mm) is selected. In the early era of single-ventricle palliation, less well-controlled shunts were constructed, including classic Blalock (divided native subclavian artery-to-branch pulmonary artery), Pott's (side-to-side left pulmonary artery to descending aorta), and Waterston (side-to-side right pulmonary artery to ascending aorta) shunts (Fig. 58-39). These native tissue-tissue connections are capable of somatic growth but have the confounding risks for pulmonary overcirculation, pulmonary artery hypertension (potentially irreversible), and branch pulmonary artery distortion with hypoplasia. During the early stages of development of single-ventricle palliation, many patients were treated with these poorly controlled shunts. Thus, significant numbers of adult patients present with complications of these palliations, including chronic cardiac volume overload and decreased ventricular function, severe pulmonary artery distortion or isolation, pulmonary vascular disease, and profound cyanosis. These patients may present for surgery for noncardiac illness and are extremely difficult to manage.

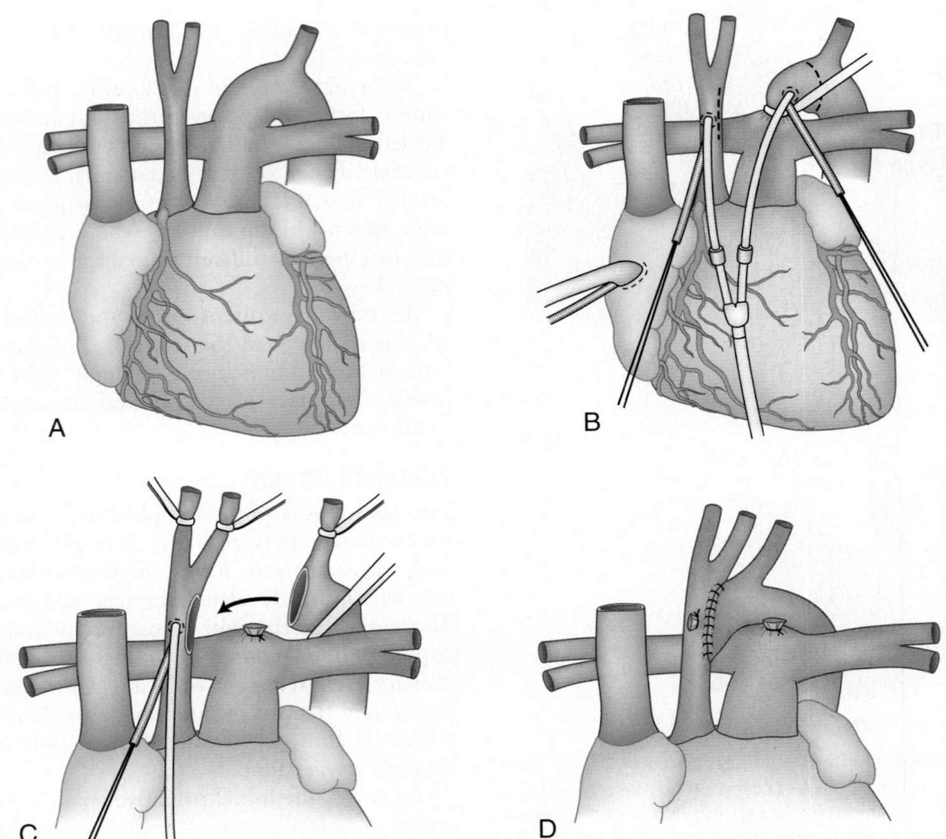

FIGURE 58-37 **A,** Type B interrupted aortic arch. **B,** Cannulation and site of incision for repair. The descending thoracic aorta is brought upward into the mediastinum **(C)** and then anastomosed to the ascending aorta in an end-to-side fashion **(D)**. (From Hirooka K, Fraser CD: One-stage neonatal repair of complex aortic arch obstruction or interruption. *Tex Heart Inst J* 24:317–321, 1997.)

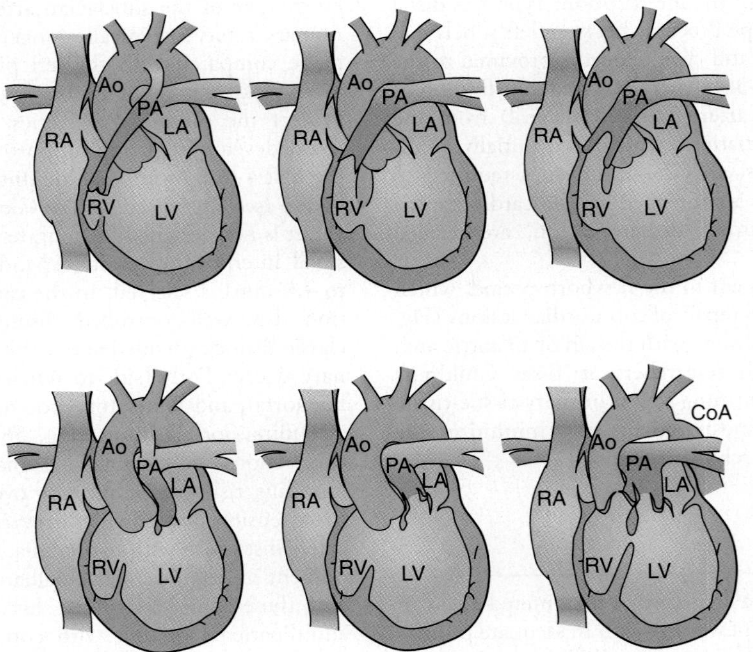

FIGURE 58-38 Anatomy of the various types of tricuspid atresia. *Top,* Normally related great vessels. *Bottom,* D-Transposition of the great vessels. *Ao,* Aorta; *CoA,* coarctation of the aorta; *LA,* left atrium; *LV,* left ventricle; *PA,* pulmonary artery; *RA,* right atrium; *RV,* right ventricle. (Adapted from Lok JM, Spevak PJ, Nichols DG: Tricuspid atresia. In Nichols DG, Ungerleider RM, Spevak PJ, et al, editors: *Critical heart disease in infants and children*, Philadelphia, 2006, Mosby, pp 800–801.)

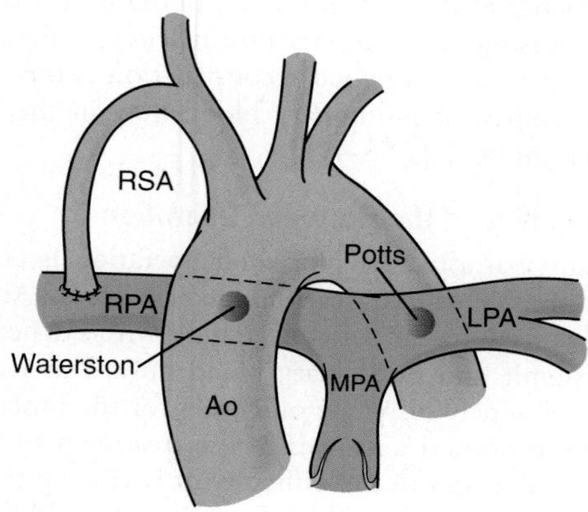

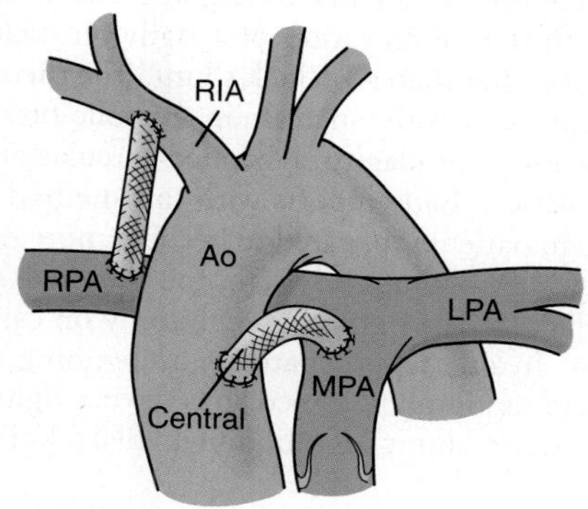

FIGURE 58-39 Systemic-to-pulmonary artery shunts. *Ao,* Aorta; *LPA,* left pulmonary artery; *MPA,* main pulmonary artery; *RIA,* right innominate artery; *RPA,* right pulmonary artery; *RSA,* right subclavian artery. (Adapted from Marino BS, Wernovsky G, Greeley WJ: Single-ventricle lesions. In Nichols DG, Ungerleider RM, Spevak PJ, et al, editors: *Critical heart disease in infants and children*, Philadelphia, 2006, Mosby, p 793.)

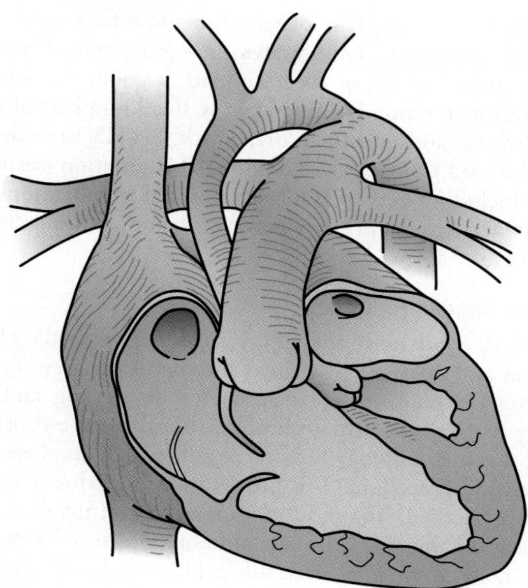

FIGURE 58-40 Anatomy of hypoplastic left heart syndrome. The tiny ascending aorta is seen arising from a markedly hypoplastic left ventricle. The ductus arteriosus is large, providing forward flow to the systemic circuit. The right ventricle is hypertrophied, and the pulmonary artery is enlarged. (From Wernovsky G, Bove EL: Single ventricle lesions. In Chang AC, Hanley FL, Wernovsky G, et al, editors: *Pediatric cardiac intensive care*, Baltimore, 1998, Williams & Wilkins.)

Hypoplastic Left Heart Syndrome

Hypoplastic left heart syndrome (HLHS) is the prototypical single right ventricle. Patients with this condition present with inadequate left heart structures ranging from mitral stenosis and AS with left ventricular hypoplasia to almost complete absence of the left heart structures with aortic and mitral atresia. In the case of aortic and mitral atresia, the ascending aorta is typically small (1 to 2 mm) and is perfused through retrograde aortic arch flow provided by the PDA. In HLHS, ductal closure results in rapid cardiovascular collapse, with profound systemic hypoperfusion and hypoxia, followed quickly by death. Therefore, in cases of prenatal diagnosis, patients must be born in a facility qualified to institute appropriate medical management immediately, including the establishment of suitable vascular access (umbilical artery catheter) and institution of intravenous PGE1 to maintain ductal patency. Patients with HLHS undiagnosed at birth typically have an early grace period of a few hours, but with the initiation of ductal closure, these children become critically ill and require aggressive resuscitation for survival. Although most children with HLHS are otherwise normal, without treatment, HLHS is a uniformly fatal condition (Fig. 58-40).

After delivery, medical treatment is directed at maintaining ductal patency and balancing systemic and pulmonary blood flow. Balancing the circulations becomes increasingly challenging with the normal decline in neonatal PVR, resulting in massive pulmonary overcirculation. As the overcirculation progresses, infants become tachypneic and may exhibit decreased systemic perfusion. Necrotizing enterocolitis is a significant risk in these children, and if there is any question of visceral malperfusion, many centers avoid enteral nutrition in an effort to minimize this potential. Other medical maneuvers include deliberate hypoventilation, low inspired oxygen concentration, and additional carbon dioxide in an attempt to increase PVR and limit pulmonary flow. These options are of limited use in newborns with HLHS; over days to weeks, the infants become progressively ill, with pulmonary congestion and marginal systemic cardiac output. Patients who are maintained have the potential of developing increased PVR as they age, and there is a known association with advanced age (>30 days) and increased operative mortality.

Surgery in the newborn period is the only realistic option for long-term survival in infants born with HLHS. Outcomes for surgical palliation of HLHS have come to be synonymous with the reputation of the treating center and surgeons. As with tricuspid atresia, patients with HLHS require a staged palliative approach. In the experiences of all centers, the first stage is the most challenging and risk-laden. The various first-stage options are described in the following sections.

Neonatal Cardiac Transplantation

Transplantation is a theoretically attractive option in infants with HLHS that replaces the malformed heart with a structurally normal one. Leonard Bailey has been an influential champion of this approach and was the first to report exciting results with transplantation in newborns with HLHS.[45] Furthermore, although there is an ever-present risk for rejection and infection in children with heart transplants, long-term meaningful survival is possible, and the quality of life of the recipients is good. The option of cardiac transplantation is limited by the small numbers of suitable donor hearts, and most children with HLHS are unable to survive the wait time for a donor graft. This situation has led most centers, including Texas Children's Hospital, to abandon cardiac transplantation as the primary mode of therapy for most neonates with HLHS.

Norwood Reconstruction

After initial work and success at Boston Children's Hospital, Norwood and colleagues[46] gained international attention at the Children's Hospital of Philadelphia for developing and implementing a reconstructive technique to palliate newborns with HLHS; this methodology now carries the widely used eponym of the Norwood procedure. This procedure was gradually refined as experience accrued. The most common method involves surgical connection of the divided main pulmonary artery to the reconstructed aortic arch. In almost all children with HLHS, there is associated aortic arch hypoplasia with coarctation. A critical feature of the operation is to reconstruct the aortic arch to provide unrestricted systemic blood flow. Most surgeons use some form of prosthetic material, usually pulmonary artery homograft patching. Some surgeons have reported accomplishing the arch reconstruction without the necessity of additional material. After reconstructing the aortic arch, the divided main pulmonary artery is anastomosed to the arch and small ascending aorta to create a neoaortic confluence providing systemic output from the right ventricle. The challenging feature of the reconstruction involves the accurate connection of this often-miniscule ascending aorta to the confluence of the arch and main pulmonary artery stump. The risk for torsion and coronary insufficiency is high. The final element of the classic Norwood reconstruction is the creation of a controlled source of pulmonary blood flow in the form of a modified BT shunt (Fig. 58-41).

Sano Modification of the Norwood Operation

Achieving survival after the Norwood operation is challenging, involving innumerable technical and medical details. At best, after a Norwood procedure, the patient is fragile, with a delicate balance between systemic and pulmonary blood flow. This fact and the observation of widely disparate outcomes for the procedure have led to many important advances in the treatment of these children. One issue relates to the difficulty of balancing the systemic to pulmonary artery shunt, which lowers diastolic blood pressure (and coronary perfusion pressure) and volume loads the heart. Sano and associates[47] from Okayama University in Japan were the first to report a series of infants undergoing a successful Norwood procedure with the modification of a right ventricle–pulmonary artery conduit rather than a Blalock shunt. The theoretical advantage of this approach is the increase in diastolic pressure, creating a physiology more similar to a banded circulation rather than shunted circulation. Early reports with this method were encouraging, although patients appeared to become more rapidly desaturated as they aged compared with the shunted patients. The long-term effects of the right ventriculotomy on cardiac function are unknown. In one report, patients undergoing the Norwood operation were randomly assigned to receive a right ventricle-to-pulmonary artery shunt or modified Blalock-Taussig shunt.

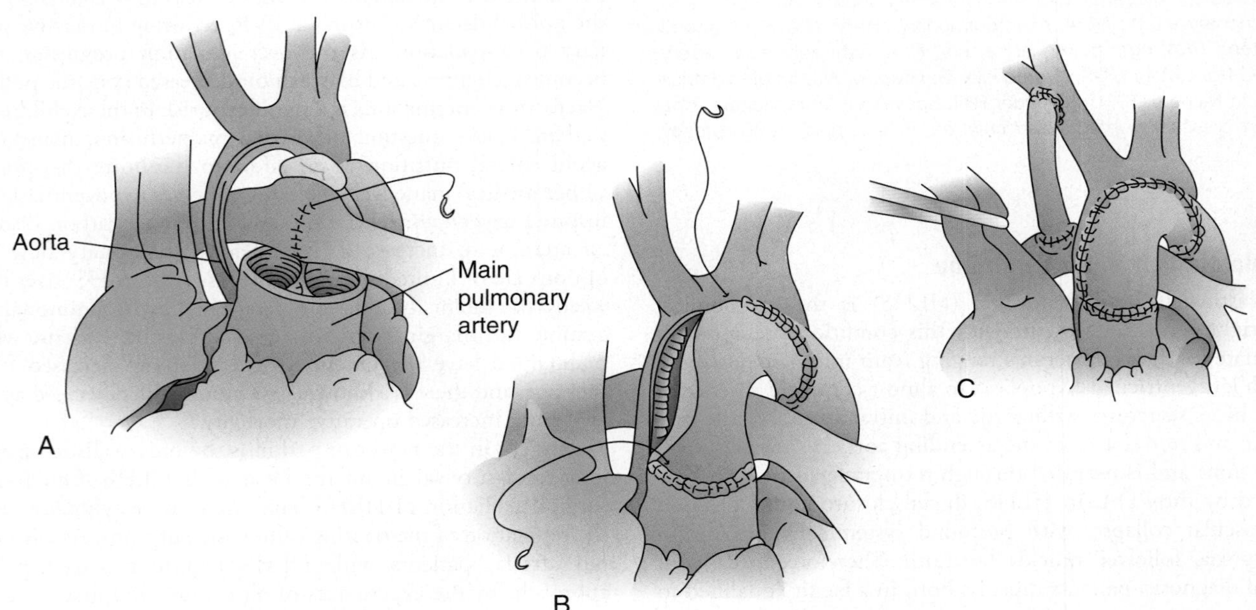

FIGURE 58-41 Norwood procedure for first-stage palliation of hypoplastic left heart syndrome. **A,** The main pulmonary artery is divided proximal to the bifurcation, the ductus arteriosus is ligated and divided, and the aortic arch is opened from the level of the transected main pulmonary artery to a point distal to the ductal insertion in the descending aorta. **B,** A segment of homograft is cut to an appropriate size and shape. This is sutured into place, creating an unobstructed outflow from the right ventricle to the pulmonary artery and aorta. **C,** Polytetrafluoroethylene tube graft is placed from the innominate artery to the right pulmonary artery. The atrial septectomy is done while the patient is under circulatory arrest. (From Castaneda AR, Jonas RA, Mayer JE, et al: Hypoplastic left heart syndrome. In *Cardiac surgery of the neonate and infant*, Philadelphia, 1994, Saunders.)

Transplantation-free survival was higher 12 months after randomization in the right ventricle-to-pulmonary artery shunt group, as was the rate of unplanned reinterventions and complications.[48] Midterm results are being analyzed and preliminarily show possible midterm survival benefit.

Hybrid Procedure

The notion of a combined therapy between interventional cardiology and surgery for the first-stage palliation of HLHS has achieved significant attention. The idea is to minimize the risk of the first operation by banding the branch pulmonary arteries and delivering a stent into the ductus to maintain patency. This hybrid arrangement is designed to allow newborn survival so that a more complete reconstruction may be performed later in infancy in a larger child. There appears to be a significant learning curve with this approach, as with any new procedure, and the incidence of complications warrants further study. Data have shown that the prevalence of necrotizing enterocolitis after the hybrid procedure is significant and comparable to reports after the Norwood procedure.[49] In addition, concerning features include the effect of the banding on long-term pulmonary artery growth, the fact that cardiac perfusion is still retrograde through the aortic arch, and the risk profile of the more extensive reconstruction later in life. The true place for this mode of therapy is unclear at the present time, but it represents an important direction of advancement to optimize the opportunity of survival for these children.

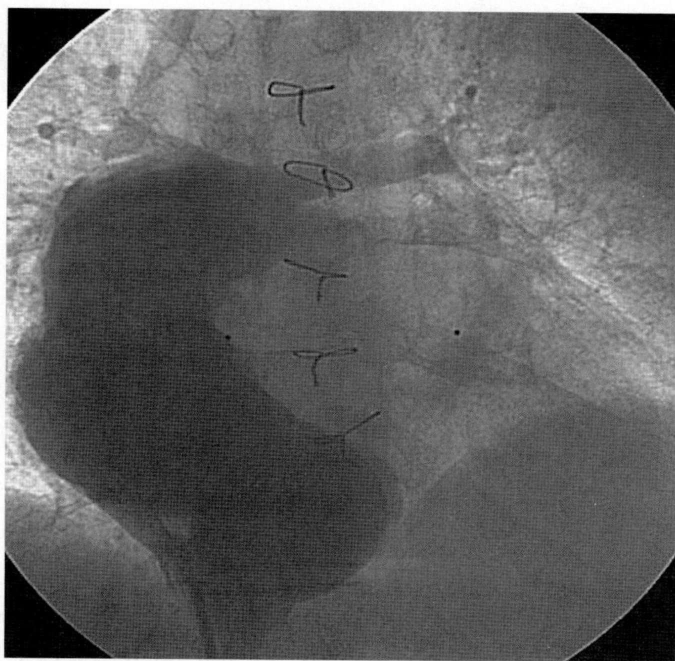

FIGURE 58-42 Angiogram of a dilated right atrium in a patient with an atriopulmonary Fontan connection.

Fontan Operation

The long-term goal of single-ventricle palliation is to optimize ventricular function and promote systemic oxygen delivery. As noted earlier, patients with a single ventricle who are shunted or banded have ongoing concerns, including systemic desaturation, continued intracardiac mixing, and chronic cardiac volume overload. The current strategy for addressing these concerns uses a direct connection between the branch pulmonary arteries and systemic venous return, as initially proposed by Fontan in the early 1970s.[50] The Fontan operation is now the treatment of choice for children born with all varieties of single ventricle and provides acceptable long-term palliation in suitable patients. However, the Fontan circulation is not normal and even in the best of circumstances results in significant alteration in normal cardiorespiratory physiology.

The Fontan circulation is established by connecting the systemic venous return directly into isolated branch pulmonary arteries without an intervening power source. Thus, blood flow in the Fontan circuit is passive, being promoted only by the pressure differential between the systemic venous system and pulmonary venous atrium. An impediment to flow in the systemic-to-pulmonary pathway results in a poor Fontan outcome. Established criteria for creating an effective Fontan circulation include the ability to connect the systemic venous return surgically to the pulmonary arteries in an unobstructed manner, normal pulmonary artery architecture and resistance, normal pulmonary venous drainage and low left atrial pressure, absence of significant A-V valve regurgitation, good ventricular function (and low ventricular end-diastolic pressure), an unobstructed systemic arterial outlet, and good aortic valve function. Compromise of any of these elements may compromise the quality of the Fontan circulation.

The Fontan operation has undergone several technical modifications in the almost 40 years of successful application to patients with single-ventricle physiology. Many patients underwent an atriopulmonary connection in which the open right atrial appendage was directly anastomosed to the pulmonary artery bifurcation with surgical closure of the ASD. Many of these patients present as adults with extreme dilation of the right atrium, with resulting sluggish flow, hepatic congestion, and atrial dysrhythmias (Fig. 58-42). Today, the most widely practiced modification of the Fontan operation is the total cavopulmonary connection. First described by DeLeval, this operation involves connection of the divided SVC to the superior and inferior aspects of the right pulmonary artery (typically offset), along with the creation of a channel to direct the IVC flow into the pulmonary arteries. The channel may be created using a surgically created lateral tunnel in the right atrium (Fig. 58-43) or interposing a conduit between the IVC and pulmonary arteries (extracardiac Fontan) (Fig. 58-44).

The change from a volume-loaded circulation in patients with a single ventricle who are shunted or banded to a Fontan circulation results in acute volume unloading of the systemic ventricle. In the chronic overloaded heart, this acute change may be poorly tolerated, with resultant diastolic dysfunction and decreased ventricular compliance. To deal with this problem, patients with a single ventricle typically undergo an intervening stage of palliation in the form of a bidirectional, superior cavopulmonary anastomosis (Glenn shunt). The bidirectional Glenn shunt is constructed by anastomosing the cephalad end of the divided SVC to the superior aspect of the right pulmonary artery (Fig. 58-45). Other sources of pulmonary blood flow are typically eliminated, and the heart is volume-unloaded; however, systemic cardiac output is maintained because the IVC return is preserved. After the Glenn shunt, the patients are not fully saturated; typically, patients have saturations of approximately 80%. Over time, the unloaded ventricle remodels, and the patient is promoted to reoperation and completion of the Fontan circulation.

Perioperative care of a patient after a Fontan procedure can be challenging. The acute changes in cardiac volume loading may negatively affect cardiac output. Even in patients with supposedly

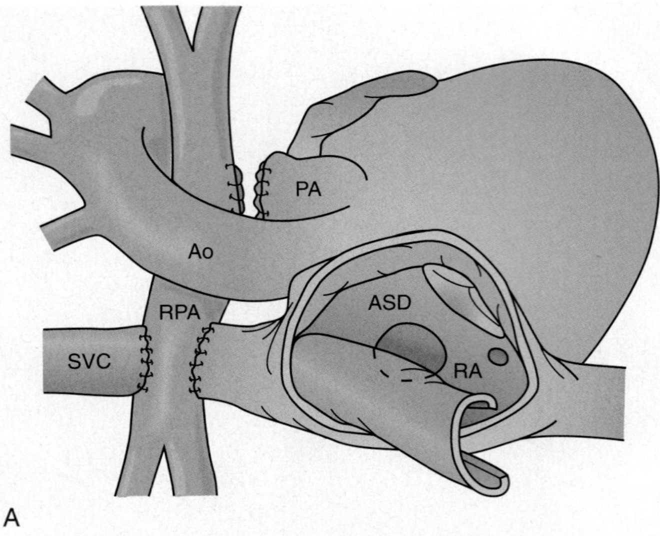

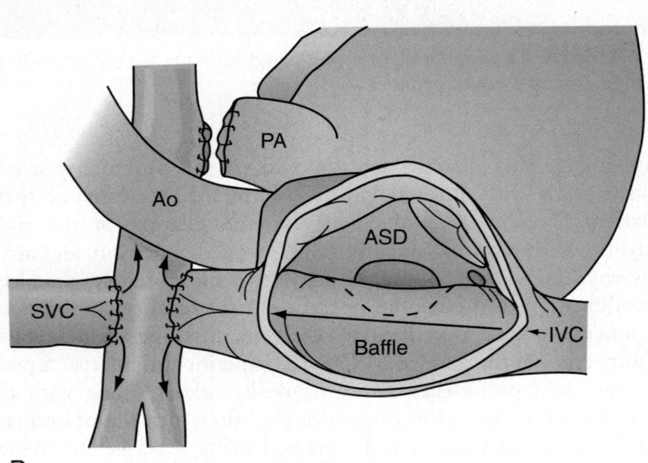

FIGURE 58-43 A and **B,** Lateral tunnel Fontan procedure. *Ao,* Aorta; *ASD,* atrial septal defect; *IVC,* inferior vena cava; *PA,* pulmonary artery; *RA,* right atrium; *RPA,* right pulmonary artery; *SVC,* superior vena cava. (Adapted from Lok JM, Spevak PJ, Nichols DG: Tricuspid atresia. In Nichols DG, Ungerleider RM, Spevak PJ, et al, editors: *Critical heart disease in infants and children,* Philadelphia, 2006, Mosby, p 813.)

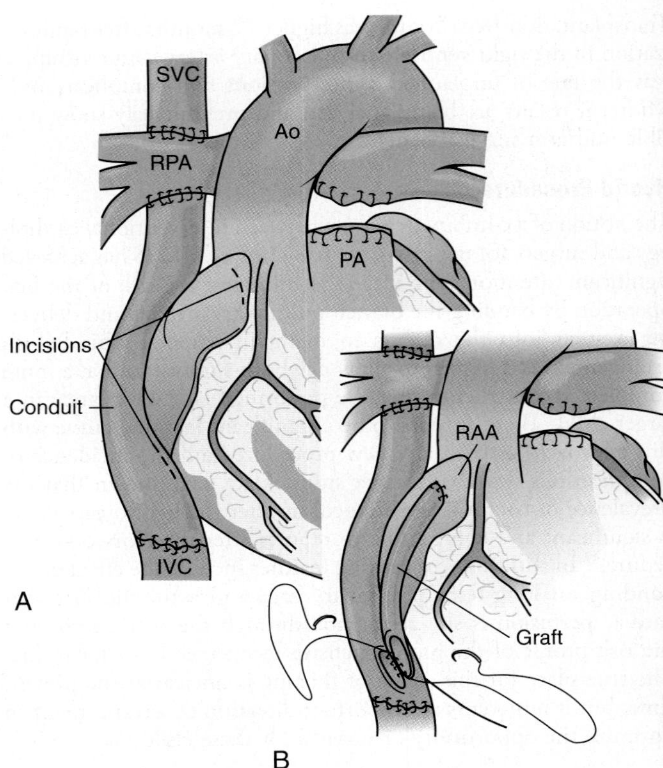

FIGURE 58-44 A, Extracardiac Fontan procedure. **B,** Creation of a fenestration in an extracardiac Fontan procedure using a graft between the extracardiac conduit and right atrial appendage *(RAA). Ao,* Aorta; *IVC,* inferior vena cava; *PA,* pulmonary artery; *RPA,* right pulmonary artery; *SVC,* superior vena cava. (Adapted from Lok JM, Spevak PJ, Nichols DG: Tricuspid atresia. In Nichols DG, Ungerleider RM, Spevak PJ, et al, editors: *Critical heart disease in infants and children,* Philadelphia, 2006, Mosby, p 814.)

ideal Fontan connections, the central venous pressure acutely increases to 12 to 15 mm Hg. Consequences of this increased venous pressure include pleural effusions, hepatic congestion, and ascites. In marginal Fontan candidates, some surgeons routinely place an intentional leak, or fenestration; the goal here is to preserve systemic ventricular volume loading and decrease systemic venous congestion at the expense of some degree of desaturation caused by the right-to-left shunting. The practice of routine fenestration after the Fontan operation has been examined, and some early data have shown that excellent outcomes can be achieved with highly selective application of a fenestration, which mitigates the risks associated with such a procedure, including hypoxia and systemic embolism.[51] Any impediment to passive pulmonary blood flow will inhibit Fontan flow and result in right heart failure. Positive pressure ventilation, especially elevated levels of positive end-expiratory pressure, impedes pulmonary blood flow in the Fontan patient. Conversely, early extubation and effective spontaneous ventilation will improve pulmonary blood flow in the Fontan patient. Data have suggested that early extubation in the operating room for patients after the Fontan procedure improves hemodynamics, decreases the length of stay for patients, and decreases hospital costs.[14]

The chronic complications of living with a Fontan circulation are still unfolding and include chronic hepatic congestion and cirrhosis, protein-losing enteropathy, atrial dysrhythmias, and venous stasis disease. Management of patients with failing Fontan circulations is especially challenging. These patients are at high risk for severe cardiac compromise while undergoing general anesthesia with positive pressure ventilation or any procedure involving large fluid shifts, including abdominal surgery. Patients with chronic hepatic congestion may develop a coagulopathy related to a decrease in factor production.

MISCELLANEOUS ANOMALIES

Vascular Rings and Pulmonary Artery Slings

Vascular Rings

Vascular rings are abnormalities of the aortic arch and its branches, compressing the trachea, esophagus, or both. The ring may be

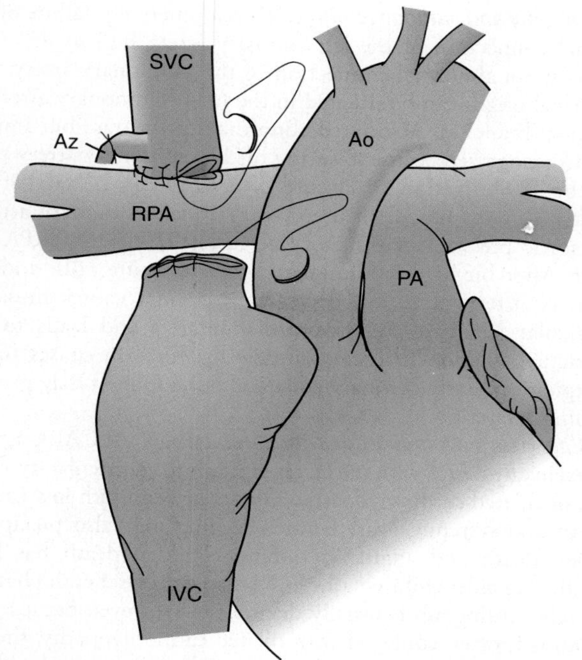

FIGURE 58-45 Bidirectional Glenn shunt. *Ao,* Aorta; *Az,* azygos vein; *IVC,* inferior vena cava; *PA,* pulmonary artery; *RPA,* right pulmonary artery; *SVC,* superior vena cava. (Adapted from Lok JM, Spevak PJ, Nichols DG: Tricuspid atresia. In Nichols DG, Ungerleider RM, Spevak PJ, et al, editors: *Critical heart disease in infants and children,* Philadelphia, 2006, Mosby, p 809.)

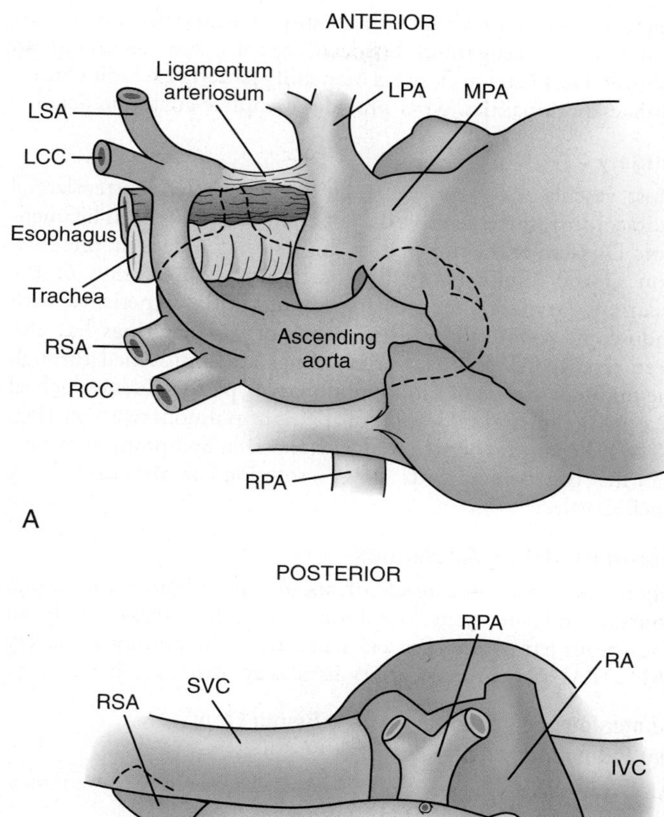

FIGURE 58-46 Double aortic arch, posterior **(A)** and superior **(B)** views. *IVC,* inferior vena cava; *LCC,* Left common carotid artery; *LPA,* left pulmonary artery; *LSA,* left subclavian artery; *MPA,* main pulmonary artery; *RA,* right atrium; *RCC,* right common carotid artery; *RSA,* right subclavian artery; *SVC,* superior vena cava. (Adapted from Jonas RA: *Comprehensive surgical management of congenital heart disease.* New York, 2004, Oxford University Press, p 499.)

complete or partial. Categorization of the defects is useful for description:

- Complete vascular rings
  - Double arch: Equal arches or left or right arch dominant (Fig. 58-46)
  - Right arch: Left ligamentum arteriosus from anomalous left subclavian artery
  - Right arch: Mirror image branching, with left ligamentum from descending aorta
- Partial vascular rings
  - Left arch: Aberrant right subclavian artery
  - Left arch: Innominate artery compression

The double aortic arch is the most common form of complete ring. Two arches arise from the ascending aorta, forming a true ring. The left arch is usually smaller. The right arch–left ligamentum complex is formed from persistence of the right fourth arch and regression of the left fourth arch. The anomalously arising left subclavian artery is often associated with a diverticulum at its base (Kommerell diverticulum). In partial rings, the most common form is an aberrant right subclavian artery arising distal to the left subclavian artery with a left arch. The right subclavian artery passes behind the esophagus from left to right. Innominate artery compression arises from a more posterior and leftward origin of the innominate artery from a left arch, leading to anterior compression of the trachea.

Pulmonary Artery Slings

A pulmonary artery sling occurs when the left pulmonary artery arises from the right pulmonary artery, passing leftward between the trachea and the esophagus. The ligamentum arteriosum attachment from the main pulmonary artery to the undersurface of the aorta forms a vascular ring around the trachea but not the esophagus. The trachea may be compressed, the cartilage may be soft, or there may be intrinsic stenosis of the trachea in the form of complete cartilage rings.

Diagnosis and Indications for Intervention

Symptoms reflect the degree of tracheal and esophageal compression from complete rings as well as the presence of coexistent tracheomalacia or stenosis. Upper respiratory symptoms predominate, with a characteristic brassy cough, recurrent respiratory infections, failure to thrive, and sometimes esophageal motility problems. In children, documentation of a ring is an indication for surgery. Older patients are often asymptomatic. Initially, the diagnosis is based on a high index of suspicion, and barium swallow is the first investigation. Echocardiography can document an abnormal head and neck vessel branching pattern, excluding intracardiac abnormalities. MRI provides complete anatomic detail.

Surgery

Most vascular rings are accessible through a left posterolateral thoracotomy; the exception is a left arch with right-sided ligamentum. Division of the ring and, in the case of double arch, preservation of the dominant arch is performed. Preservation of the recurrent laryngeal nerve is important. Initial experience with endoscopic robotically assisted repair of vascular rings has also been reported. Pulmonary artery slings are approached through the midline; the use of cardiopulmonary bypass facilitates tracheal reconstruction and relocation of the right pulmonary artery (Fig. 58-47). Repair can be achieved with low risk. Symptoms may take months to resolve, with slow resolution of the underlying tracheomalacia.

Coronary Artery Anomalies

Anomalies occur as a result of anomalous origin, termination, courses, and aneurysm formation. Of these variables, only an anomalous left coronary artery rising from the pulmonary artery (ALCAPA) and coronary artery fistulas are discussed here.

Anomalous Left Coronary Artery Rising From the Pulmonary Artery

An ALCAPA is a rare, often lethal lesion in early infancy. Untreated, the mortality rate approaches 90%.

Anatomy and pathophysiology. Developmentally, failure of the normal connection of the left coronary artery bud to the aorta results in an abnormal connection to the pulmonary artery. The abnormal origin can be situated in the main pulmonary artery or proximal branches. Associated abnormalities are rare but important to recognize because lowering of the pulmonary artery pressure by PDA ligation or closure of a VSD can be fatal if the ALCAPA is not noted. In utero, with equal pulmonary arterial and aortic pressures, satisfactory perfusion of the ALCAPA can occur. After birth, the pulmonary artery pressure falls, and left coronary artery perfusion decreases. Ischemia causes impaired ventricular function and myocardial infarcts and leads to left ventricular dilation. Papillary muscle dysfunction causes mitral regurgitation. Early coronary collateral development may prevent ongoing infarction.

Diagnosis and indications for intervention. ALCAPA is suspected in any infant with mitral regurgitation, ventricular dysfunction, or dilated cardiomyopathy. Infants present with low cardiac output and systemic heart failure. Feeding may also precipitate sudden death and angina in infants. Sudden death has been described in older children. The ECG may reflect ischemic changes. The echocardiogram is usually diagnostic. However, because this diagnosis is often confused with dilated cardiomyopathy, there is an argument in favor of catheterizing all patients with dilated cardiomyopathy in whom the coronary artery anatomy cannot be clearly defined on echocardiography. Secondary findings of dilated cardiac chambers and segmental wall motion abnormalities together with mitral regurgitation prompt a search for an ALCAPA. Diagnosis of an ALCAPA is an indication for intervention.

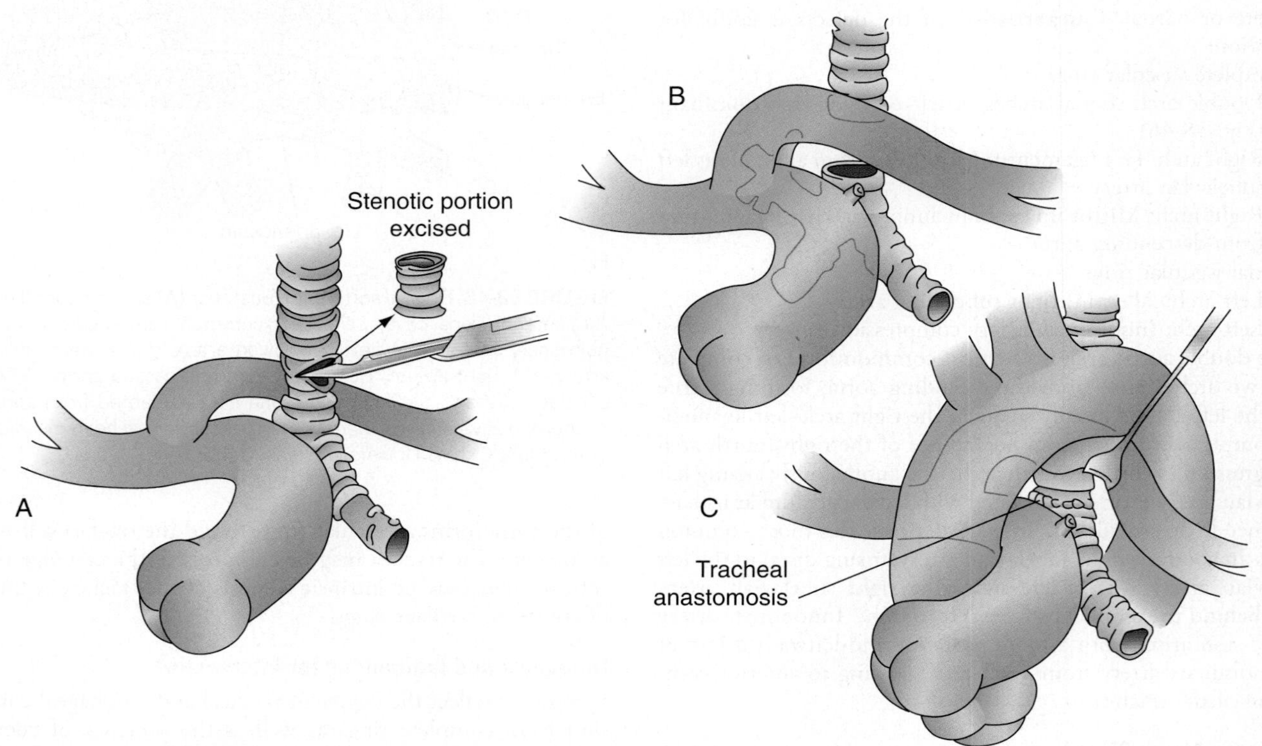

FIGURE 58-47 Method for the management of a pulmonary artery sling with associated tracheal stenosis, using cardiopulmonary bypass. **A,** Tracheal resection of the involved segment. **B,** Anterior translocation of the left pulmonary artery after transection of the trachea. **C,** Direct anastomosis of the trachea. (From Castaneda AR, Jonas RA, Mayer JE, et al: Vascular rings, slings, and tracheal anomalies. In *Cardiac surgery of the neonate and infant*, Philadelphia, 1994, Saunders.)

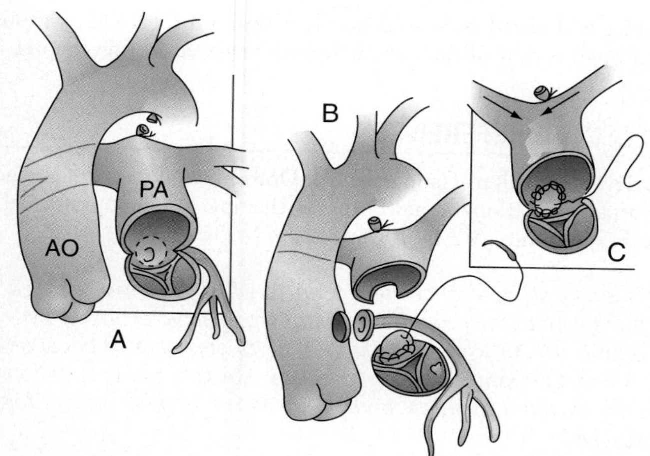

FIGURE 58-48 Direct reimplantation of anomalous left coronary artery rising from the pulmonary artery (ALCAPA). **A,** Excision of ALCAPA from the pulmonary artery *(PA)*. **B,** Aortic reimplantation of the coronary ostium into the aorta. **C,** Reconstruction of the PA with autologous pericardium. *AO,* Aorta. (From Vouhe PR, Tamisier D, Sidi D, et al: Anomalous left coronary artery from the pulmonary artery: Results of isolated aortic reimplantation. *Ann Thorac Surg* 54:621–626, 1992.)

Surgery. A degree of ventricular dysfunction is usually present. Preoperative inotropic support and optimization of hemodynamics may be required before surgical intervention. Severe cardiomyopathy rarely may necessitate cardiac transplantation. Current experience indicates that creation of a dual coronary system is safe and reproducible and offers the best opportunity for recovery of function.[52] Operative considerations include optimal myocardial protection and prevention of left heart distention. Direct reimplantation of the ALCAPA into the ascending aorta is the procedure of choice (Fig. 58-48). Sometimes, limited mobility of the coronary artery precludes reimplantation, and a surgically created aorta–pulmonary artery–coronary artery tunnel is created; this is known as the *Takeuchi procedure*. Ligation of the ALCAPA is not recommended.

Postoperative management is directed toward maintaining adequate coronary perfusion and cardiac output. Mechanical support of the heart may be temporarily required. Mitral regurgitation usually improves, and valve replacement is rarely necessary. Current intervention has a low operative mortality. Risks for nonsurvival relate to preoperative ventricular dysfunction and cardiogenic shock. The Takeuchi repair is associated with tunnel complications such as obstruction, leak, aortic valve damage, and RVOTO in the long-term.

Coronary Arteriovenous Fistula and Aneurysms

Isolated coronary artery fistula is more rare than ALCAPA. Drainage of coronary artery fistula is reported to terminate more commonly in the right side of the heart or pulmonary artery than in the left side of the heart. A shunt from the high-pressure coronary artery system into a low-pressure cardiac chamber may result in coronary steal and some degree of cardiac volume overload. Coronary artery aneurysms are associated with Kawasaki disease.

Diagnosis and indications for intervention. Presentation depends on the amount of functional compromise produced by the ischemia and volume overload. Echocardiography may be able to delineate the anomaly, but coronary angiography is diagnostic. Details of coronary anatomy are essential for determining intervention. Interventional catheterization is useful for the obliteration of fistulas and terminal aneurysms.

Surgery. If the lesion is not amenable to transcatheter intervention, surgery is indicated. Options include suture ligation without bypass, cardiopulmonary bypass, and aneurysmectomy with closure of the fistula. Early and late mortality rates are low. Risk factors for death and ventricular dysfunction relate to coronary artery insufficiency and infarction after fistula ligation or aneurysmectomy.[53]

Ebstein Anomaly of the Tricuspid Valve

Ebstein anomaly of the tricuspid valve is a rare defect in which the tricuspid valve attachments are displaced into the right ventricle to varying degrees. Ebstein anomaly includes a spectrum of abnormalities involving a degree of displacement of the tricuspid valve, variable right ventricular size, and variable pulmonary outflow obstruction. Associated abnormalities are ASD, pulmonary atresia, and ccTGA. The posterior and septal leaflets of the tricuspid valve are variably displaced to the apex of the right ventricle, which results in an atrialized portion of the right ventricle. The anterior leaflet remains large and sail-like. The major hemodynamic issue is tricuspid incompetence with decreased pulmonary blood flow and, if an ASD is present, right-to-left shunting causing cyanosis. Long-standing tricuspid incompetence leads to volume overload of an abnormal right ventricle. Variable pulmonary outflow tract obstruction limits effective pulmonary blood flow. If adequate pulmonary blood flow requires continued ductal patency, the need for neonatal intervention is almost certain.

Diagnosis and Intervention

The more severe forms of Ebstein anomaly manifest with cyanosis in infancy. Critically ill neonates tend to have a severe form of the disease, with a grossly inefficient right ventricle compounded by the high pulmonary resistance of the neonate or by pulmonary valve atresia. The mortality rate in this group is high. Older patients present in heart failure and may have cyanosis. Supraventricular dysrhythmias and the pre-excitation syndrome (Wolff-Parkinson-White syndrome) are associated with Ebstein anomaly. Echocardiography is diagnostic. Critically ill neonates have poor survival rates, and surgery is indicated only after stabilization with PGE1 and controlled ventilation. In older patients, cyanosis and heart failure are indications to intervene, although earlier intervention in asymptomatic patients, before excessive right ventricular dilation, is being more actively pursued.

Surgery

In critically ill neonates, after stabilization, palliation with a systemic-to-pulmonary artery shunt may be required. The Starnes operation has allowed salvage in previously hopeless cases. This operation consists of patch closure of the tricuspid orifice, atrial septectomy, and a systemic-to-pulmonary artery shunt.[54] In patients with less severe forms of this disease, tricuspid valve repair or replacement is also an option. Surgical techniques for the treatment of Ebstein anomaly have been evolving, and outcomes are improving for this challenging group of patients (Fig. 58-49).[55]

Mitral Valve Anomalies

Most abnormalities of the mitral valve are associated with other complex lesions (e.g., Shone complex). More commonly, mitral disease in children is inflammatory in nature—that is, rheumatic disease or infective endocarditis. It may also be associated with collagen vascular disease and Marfan syndrome.

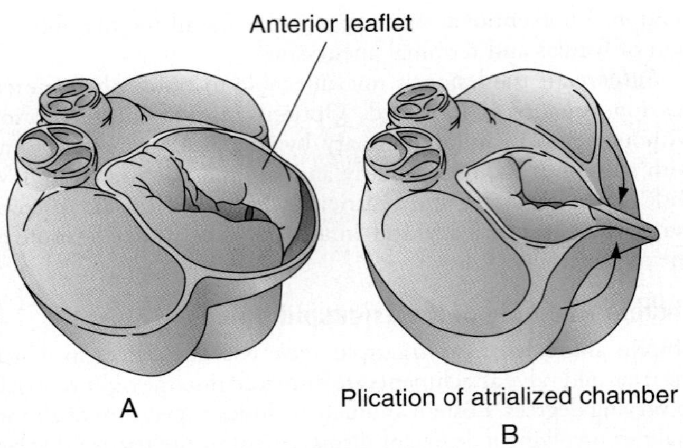

FIGURE 58-49 Repair of Ebstein malformation using the Carpentier method. **A,** The anterior and posterior leaflets of the tricuspid valve are detached from the annulus. **B,** The atrium is plicated, reducing the annular diameter. The detached leaflets are reattached to the annulus. (From Castaneda AR, Jonas RA, Mayer JE, et al: Ebstein's anomaly. In *Cardiac surgery of the neonate and infant*, Philadelphia, 1994, Saunders.)

Mitral Stenosis

Mitral stenosis is caused by obstruction at a supravalvular, valvular, or subvalvular level, singly or in combination. Supravalvular stenosis is caused by a ring of fibrous tissue above the annulus of the mitral valve or attached to the proximal leaflets. Valvular stenosis involves the leaflets, with commissural fusion occurring with or without hypoplasia of the valve ring. Hypoplasia of the mitral valve is often associated with left ventricular hypoplasia. Frequently, the leaflets and subvalvular apparatus are also dysplastic. Fusion of the leaflets can lead to an accessory orifice and produce mitral stenosis at a purely valvular level (so-called double-orifice mitral valve). Three types of subvalvular stenosis have been recognized—parachute mitral valve, hammock valve, and absence of one or both papillary muscles. Mitral regurgitation is a result of secondary annular dilation, congenital isolated clefts of the valve, and prolapse of the leaflets from abnormal chordae or papillary muscle insertion.

Echocardiography is diagnostic. Intervention includes balloon valvuloplasty, particularly for selected forms of rheumatic mitral stenosis, and surgical intervention. Intervention is timed to avoid irreversible sequelae related to chronic volume overload or pulmonary hypertension. Surgical intervention is aimed at preserving the mitral valve, and valvuloplasty techniques have a valuable place in children. Prosthetic valves are the least desirable option. Bioprosthetic or tissue valves need to be avoided in children. Supra-annular placement of the prosthesis may be necessary. Repeat placement is ensured.

SUMMARY

This chapter provides a basic overview of the major congenital cardiac lesions and a framework for the diagnosis and treatment of these conditions. For most patients, the diagnosis of CHD, whether surgically treated or not, carries lifelong implications. For patients with CHD presenting for noncardiac surgery, a thorough understanding of the patient's unique anatomy and physiology is mandatory when planning a rational management strategy. The reader is directed to several excellent texts on CHD for a more thorough review of each of the lesions reviewed in this chapter.

SELECTED REFERENCES

Bailey LL, Nehlsen-Cannarella SL, Doroshow RW, et al: Cardiac allotransplantation in newborns as therapy for hypoplastic left heart syndrome. *N Engl J Med* 315:949–951, 1986.

This classic reference describes the first report of cardiac transplantation in newborns with hypoplastic left heart syndrome (HLHS). Although limited in its applicability because of limited donor organs, neonatal cardiac transplantation has provided children born with HLHS a new option for survival.

Blalock A, Taussig HB: The surgical treatment of malformations of the heart in which there is pulmonary stenosis or pulmonary atresia. *JAMA* 128:189–202, 1945.

This landmark article describes the surgical procedure that initiated the era of elective cardiac surgery. The study reported the initial experience with palliative surgical treatment of patients with pulmonary stenosis or pulmonary atresia using the Blalock-Taussig shunt.

Fontan F, Baudet E: Surgical repair of tricuspid atresia. *Thorax* 26:240–248, 1971.

This article represents a milestone in the evolution of surgical management of patients with single-ventricle physiology. It described the first corrective operation for patients with tricuspid atresia. Although previous palliative procedures, provided by various systemic-to-pulmonary artery shunts, improved the clinical condition of patients, systemic blood was still a mixture of oxygenated and deoxygenated blood. The Fontan operation redirected superior and inferior vena cava blood flow to the lungs so that only oxygenated blood returned to the heart and subsequently to the systemic circulation.

Kirklin JW, Dushane JW, Patrick RT, et al: Intracardiac surgery with the aid of a mechanical pump-oxygenator system (gibbon type): Report of eight cases. *Mayo Clin Proc* 30:201–206, 1955.

This landmark article demonstrated that open repairs of congenital cardiac defects using mechanical pump oxygenator systems could be performed with minimal risk to patients.

Mustard W: Successful two-stage correction of transposition of the great vessels. *Surgery* 55:469–472, 1964.

This classic reference describes one of the initial surgical approaches to the treatment of transposition of the great arteries (D-TGA). Although the arterial switch operation is now the surgical treatment of choice for D-TGA, there are many adult patients with congenital heart disease who have been palliated with the Mustard operation. Understanding the operation and resulting physiology is critical to general surgery management strategies for noncardiac operations.

Nichols DG, Ungerleider RM, Spevak PJ, et al, editors: *Critical heart disease in infants and children*, ed 2, Philadelphia, 2006, Mosby.

This text provides a comprehensive and current review of heart disease in infants and children. It contains numerous surgical drawings and diagnostic images to supplement the didactic material.

Norwood WI, Lang P, Casteneda AR, et al: Experience with operations for hypoplastic left heart syndrome. *J Thorac Cardiovasc Surg* 82:511–519, 1981.

In this landmark article, Norwood and colleagues reported the outcomes of what was then a new reconstructive surgical technique to palliate newborns with hypoplastic left heart syndrome (HLHS). Until the Norwood operation, the only option for survival of patients with HLHS was cardiac transplantation. At most centers today, the Norwood operation is the primary mode of therapy for most neonates with HLHS.

Sano S, Ishino K, Kawada M, et al: Right ventricle-pulmonary artery shunt in first-stage palliation of hypoplastic left heart syndrome. *J Thorac Cardiovasc Surg* 126:504–509, 2003.

This classic reference describes the right ventricle–to–pulmonary artery conduit used in the Norwood procedure. This novel procedure, named after the author, Sano, allowed for more hemodynamic stability postoperatively from the Norwood procedure and improved intrastage survival.

Senning A: Surgical correction of transposition of the great vessels. *Surgery* 45:966–980, 1959.

This classic reference describes the initial surgical approach to management of transposition of the great arteries (D-TGA). Although the arterial switch operation is currently the surgical treatment of choice for D-TGA, there are many adult patients with congenital heart disease in the community who have had the Senning operation. Understanding the operation and resulting physiology is critical to general surgery management strategies for noncardiac operations.

Starnes VA, Pitlick PT, Bernstein D, et al: Ebstein's anomaly appearing in the neonate. A new surgical approach. *J Thorac Cardiovasc Surg* 101:1082–1087, 1991.

This classic reference describes the first report of a new surgical approach to Ebstein anomaly in neonates. The procedure was named after the surgeon, Starnes. This approach has provided children born with severe Ebstein anomaly a new option for survival.

Warden HE, Cohen M, Read RC, et al: Controlled cross circulation for open intracardiac surgery: Physiologic studies and results of creation and closure of ventricular septal defects. *J Thorac Surg* 28:331–341, 1954.

This landmark article described the technique of cross-circulation to facilitate cardiopulmonary bypass and intracardiac repair of congenital heart lesions. Warden and colleagues documented the successful use of cross-circulation to correct defects such as ventricular septal defect.

Wilcox B, Cook A, Anderson R: *Surgical anatomy of the heart*, ed 3, Cambridge, England, 2004, Cambridge University Press.

This text provides an excellent reference manual for understanding the complex anatomy of the heart. It contains color photographs and diagrams and is an invaluable resource for any student of cardiac surgery.

REFERENCES

1. Blalock A, Taussig HB: The surgical treatment of malformations of the heart in which there is pulmonary stenosis or pulmonary atresia. *JAMA* 128:189–202, 1945.
2. Warden HE, Cohen M, Read RC, et al: Controlled cross circulation for open intracardiac surgery: Physiologic studies and results of creation and closure of ventricular septal defects. *J Thorac Surg* 28:331–341, discussion 341–343, 1954.
3. Kirklin JW, Dushane JW, Patrick RT, et al: Intracardiac surgery with the aid of a mechanical pump-oxygenator system (gibbon type): Report of eight cases. *Proc Staff Meet Mayo Clin* 30:201–206, 1955.
4. Marelli A, Gilboa S, Devine O, et al: Estimating the congenital heart disease population in the United States in 2010—what are the numbers? *J Am Coll Cardiol* 59:E787–E787, 2012.
5. Marelli AJ, Ionescu-Ittu R, Mackie AS, et al: Lifetime prevalence of congenital heart disease in the general population from 2000 to 2010. *Circulation* 130:749–756, 2014.
6. Levey A, Glickstein JS, Kleinman CS, et al: The impact of prenatal diagnosis of complex congenital heart disease on neonatal outcomes. *Pediatr Cardiol* 31:587–597, 2010.
7. Morris SA, Ethen MK, Penny DJ, et al: Prenatal diagnosis, birth location, surgical center, and neonatal mortality in infants with hypoplastic left heart syndrome. *Circulation* 129:285–292, 2014.
8. American Board of Thoracic Surgery. <https://www.abts.org/root/home.aspx>; (Accessed August 6, 2015).
9. Mullins CE: *Cardiac catheterization in congenital heart disease: Pediatric and adult*, Malden, MA, 2006, Blackwell Futura.
10. American Board of Internal Medicine. <www.abim.org>; (Accessed August 6, 2015).
11. Wilcox BR, Cook AC, Anderson RH: *Surgical anatomy of the heart*, ed 3, Cambridge, 2004, Cambridge University Press.
12. Morin RL, Gerber TC, McCollough CH: Radiation dose in computed tomography of the heart. *Circulation* 107:917–922, 2003.
13. Andropoulos DB, Stayer SA, Russell IA: *Anesthesia for congenital heart disease*, ed 2, Hoboken, NJ, 2010, Wiley-Blackwell.
14. Morales DL, Carberry KE, Heinle JS, et al: Extubation in the operating room after Fontan's procedure: Effect on practice and outcomes. *Ann Thorac Surg* 86:576–581, discussion 581–582, 2008.
15. Licht DJ, Shera DM, Clancy RR, et al: Brain maturation is delayed in infants with complex congenital heart defects.

J Thorac Cardiovasc Surg 137:529–536, discussion 536–527, 2009.
16. Hopkins RA, Bert AA, Buchholz B, et al: Surgical patch closure of atrial septal defects. *Ann Thorac Surg* 77:2144–2149, author reply 2149–2150, 2004.
17. Knepp MD, Rocchini AP, Lloyd TR, et al: Long-term follow up of secundum atrial septal defect closure with the Amplatzer septal occluder. *Congenit Heart Dis* 5:32–37, 2010.
18. Clark JB, Chowdhury D, Pauliks LB, et al: Resolution of heart block after surgical removal of an Amplatzer device. *Ann Thorac Surg* 89:1631–1633, 2010.
19. Piatkowski R, Kochanowski J, Scislo P, et al: Dislocation of Amplatzer septal occluder device after closure of secundum atrial septal defect. *J Am Soc Echocardiogr* 23:1007.e1–1007.e2, 2010.
20. Slesnick TC, Nugent AW, Fraser CD, Jr, et al: Images in cardiovascular medicine. Incomplete endothelialization and late development of acute bacterial endocarditis after implantation of an Amplatzer septal occluder device. *Circulation* 117:e326–e327, 2008.
21. Neill CA, Ferencz C, Sabiston DC, et al: The familial occurrence of hypoplastic right lung with systemic arterial supply and venous drainage "scimitar syndrome". *Bull Johns Hopkins Hosp* 107:1–21, 1960.
22. Balzer D: Current status of percutaneous closure of ventricular septal defects. *Pediatr Therapeut* 2:112–114, 2012.
23. Rastelli GC, Weidman WH, Kirklin JW: Surgical repair of the partial form of persistent common atrioventricular canal, with special reference to the problem of mitral valve incompetence. *Circulation* 31(Suppl 1):31–35, 1965.
24. Bakhtiary F, Takacs J, Cho MY, et al: Long-term results after repair of complete atrioventricular septal defect with two-patch technique. *Ann Thorac Surg* 89:1239–1243, 2010.
25. Morales DL, Braud BE, Gunter KS, et al: Encouraging results for the Contegra conduit in the problematic right ventricle-to-pulmonary artery connection. *J Thorac Cardiovasc Surg* 132:665–671, 2006.
26. Chen JM, Glickstein JS, Davies RR, et al: The effect of repair technique on postoperative right-sided obstruction in patients with truncus arteriosus. *J Thorac Cardiovasc Surg* 129:559–568, 2005.
27. Vezmar M, Chaturvedi R, Lee KJ, et al: Percutaneous pulmonary valve implantation in the young 2-year follow-up. *JACC Cardiovasc Interv* 3:439–448, 2010.
28. Balasubramanian S, Marshall AC, Gauvreau K, et al: Outcomes after stent implantation for the treatment of congenital and postoperative pulmonary vein stenosis in children. *Circ Cardiovasc Interv* 5:109–117, 2012.
29. Morales DL, Zafar F, Heinle JS, et al: Right ventricular infundibulum sparing (RVIS) tetralogy of Fallot repair: A review of over 300 patients. *Ann Surg* 250:611–617, 2009.
30. Mustard WT: Successful two-stage correction of transposition of the great vessels. *Surgery* 55:469–472, 1964.
31. Senning A: Surgical correction of transposition of the great vessels. *Surgery* 45:966–980, 1959.
32. Dibardino DJ, Allison AE, Vaughn WK, et al: Current expectations for newborns undergoing the arterial switch operation. *Ann Surg* 239:588–596, discussion 596–598, 2004.
33. Angeli E, Formigari R, Pace Napoleone C, et al: Long-term coronary artery outcome after arterial switch operation for transposition of the great arteries. *Eur J Cardiothorac Surg* 38:714–720, 2010.
34. Yacoub MH, Radley-Smith R: Anatomy of the coronary arteries in transposition of the great arteries and methods for their transfer in anatomical correction. *Thorax* 33:418–424, 1978.
35. Ly M, Belli E, Leobon B, et al: Results of the double switch operation for congenitally corrected transposition of the great arteries. *Eur J Cardiothorac Surg* 35:879–883, discussion 883–884, 2009.
36. Bacha EA, McElhinney DB, Guleserian KJ, et al: Surgical aortic valvuloplasty in children and adolescents with aortic regurgitation: Acute and intermediate effects on aortic valve function and left ventricular dimensions. *J Thorac Cardiovasc Surg* 135:552–559, 559.e551–553, 2008.
37. d'Udekem Y: Aortic valve repair in children. *Ann Cardiothorac Surg* 2:100–104, 2013.
38. Brown JW, Rodefeld MD, Ruzmetov M, et al: Surgical valvuloplasty versus balloon aortic dilation for congenital aortic stenosis: Are evidence-based outcomes relevant? *Ann Thorac Surg* 94:146–153, discussion 153–155, 2012.
39. Shinkawa T, Bove EL, Hirsch JC, et al: Intermediate-term results of the Ross procedure in neonates and infants. *Ann Thorac Surg* 89:1827–1832, discussion 1832, 2010.
40. Booth JH, Bryant R, Powers SC, et al: Transthoracic echocardiography does not reliably predict involvement of the aortic valve in patients with a discrete subaortic shelf. *Cardiol Young* 20:284–289, 2010.
41. Shone JD, Sellers RD, Anderson RC, et al: The developmental complex of "parachute mitral valve," supravalvular ring of left atrium, subaortic stenosis, and coarctation of aorta. *Am J Cardiol* 11:714–725, 1963.
42. Cowley CG, Orsmond GS, Feola P, et al: Long-term, randomized comparison of balloon angioplasty and surgery for native coarctation of the aorta in childhood. *Circulation* 111:3453–3456, 2005.
43. Mery CM, Guzman-Pruneda FA, Carberry KE, et al: Aortic arch advancement for aortic coarctation and hypoplastic aortic arch in neonates and infants. *Ann Thorac Surg* 98:625–633, discussion 633, 2014.
44. Morales DL, Scully PT, Braud BE, et al: Interrupted aortic arch repair: Aortic arch advancement without a patch minimizes arch reinterventions. *Ann Thorac Surg* 82:1577–1583, discussion 1583–1584, 2006.
45. Bailey LL, Nehlsen-Cannarella SL, Doroshow RW, et al: Cardiac allotransplantation in newborns as therapy for hypoplastic left heart syndrome. *N Engl J Med* 315:949–951, 1986.
46. Norwood WI, Lang P, Casteneda AR, et al: Experience with operations for hypoplastic left heart syndrome. *J Thorac Cardiovasc Surg* 82:511–519, 1981.
47. Sano S, Ishino K, Kado H, et al: Outcome of right ventricle-to-pulmonary artery shunt in first-stage palliation of hypoplastic left heart syndrome: A multi-institutional study. *Ann Thorac Surg* 78:1951–1957, discussion 1957–1958, 2004.
48. Ohye RG, Sleeper LA, Mahony L, et al: Comparison of shunt types in the Norwood procedure for single-ventricle lesions. *N Engl J Med* 362:1980–1992, 2010.
49. Luce WA, Schwartz RM, Beauseau W, et al: Necrotizing enterocolitis in neonates undergoing the hybrid approach to complex congenital heart disease. *Pediatr Crit Care Med* 12:46–51, 2011.

50. Fontan F, Baudet E: Surgical repair of tricuspid atresia. *Thorax* 26:240–248, 1971.
51. Salazar JD, Zafar F, Siddiqui K, et al: Fenestration during Fontan palliation: Now the exception instead of the rule. *J Thorac Cardiovasc Surg* 140:129–136, 2010.
52. Alsoufi B, Sallehuddin A, Bulbul Z, et al: Surgical strategy to establish a dual-coronary system for the management of anomalous left coronary artery origin from the pulmonary artery. *Ann Thorac Surg* 86:170–176, 2008.
53. Valente AM, Lock JE, Gauvreau K, et al: Predictors of long-term adverse outcomes in patients with congenital coronary artery fistulae. *Circ Cardiovasc Interv* 3:134–139, 2010.
54. Starnes VA, Pitlick PT, Bernstein D, et al: Ebstein's anomaly appearing in the neonate. A new surgical approach. *J Thorac Cardiovasc Surg* 101:1082–1087, 1991.
55. Brown ML, Dearani JA, Danielson GK, et al: The outcomes of operations for 539 patients with Ebstein anomaly. *J Thorac Cardiovasc Surg* 135:1120–1136, 1136.e1121–1127, 2008.

59 CHAPTER

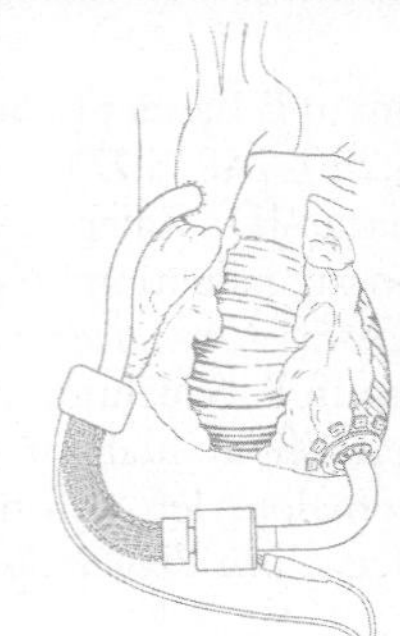

Acquired Heart Disease: Coronary Insufficiency

Shuab Omer, Lorraine D. Cornwell, Faisal G. Bakaeen

OUTLINE

Ischemic heart disease (IHD) is the predominant public health problem worldwide. In the United States, 1 in 3 adults (about 83.6 million) has cardiovascular disease; 15.4 million of these persons have coronary artery disease (CAD).[1] Despite improved survival among CAD patients,[2] CAD is responsible for approximately 380,000 deaths in the United States every year, with an age-adjusted mortality rate of 113 per 100,000 population.[3] CAD is the leading cause of death in both men and women, and IHD accounts for most of the mortality and morbidity associated with CAD.[1] The costs of caring for patients with IHD are enormous, with hundreds of billions of dollars spent every year in the United States in taking care of these patients. Although recent advances in percutaneous intervention have reduced the number of referrals for surgical intervention, coronary artery bypass grafting (CABG) still remains the most effective treatment for CAD and is the most commonly performed open cardiac procedure in the United States.

CORONARY ARTERY ANATOMY AND PHYSIOLOGY

Anatomic Considerations

The coronary arteries, the predominant blood supply to the heart, arise from the sinuses of Valsalva. They are the first arterial branches of the aorta, and two are usually present. The coronary arteries are designated right and left according to the embryologic chamber that they predominantly supply. The left coronary artery (LCA) arises from the left coronary sinus, which is located posteromedially; the right coronary artery (RCA) arises from the right coronary sinus, which is located anteromedially. The LCA, also called the left main coronary artery, averages approximately 2 to 3 cm in length and courses in a left posterolateral direction, winding behind the main pulmonary artery trunk and then splitting into the left anterior descending (LAD) and left circumflex arteries. The LAD courses in an anterolateral direction to the left of the pulmonary trunk and runs anteriorly over the interventricular septum. The diagonal branches of the LAD supply the anterolateral wall of the left ventricle (LV). The LAD is considered the most important surgical vessel because it supplies more than 50% of the LV mass and most of the interventricular septum. The LAD has several septal perforating branches that supply the interventricular septum from its anterior aspect. The LAD extends over the interventricular septum up to the apex of the heart, where it may form an anastomosis with the posterior descending artery (PDA), which is typically a branch of the right coronary system (Fig. 59-1).

The circumflex artery passes through the atrioventricular (AV) groove and follows a clockwise course. Where the circumflex artery courses through the AV groove, it gives off branches that extend toward but do not quite reach the apex of the heart. These branches, the obtuse marginal branches, are designated numerically from proximal to distal. The circumflex coronary artery usually terminates as the left posterolateral branch after taking a perpendicular turn toward the apex.

The term *ramus intermedius* is used to designate a dominant coronary vessel that arises from the occasional trifurcation of the LCA. This branch can be intramyocardial and difficult to locate at times.

The RCA supplies most of the right ventricle as well as the posterior part of the LV. The RCA emerges from its ostium in the right coronary sinus and passes deep in the right AV groove. At the superior end of the acute margin of the heart, the RCA turns posteriorly toward the crux and usually bifurcates into the PDA over the posterior interventricular sulcus and right posterolateral artery. The RCA also supplies multiple right ventricular branches (i.e., the acute marginal branches). On occasion, the PDA arises from both the RCA and LCA, and the circulation is considered to be codominant. The AV node artery arises from the RCA in approximately 90% of patients. The sinoatrial node artery arises from the proximal RCA in 50% of patients. Although the source of the PDA is often used clinically to define dominance of circulation in the heart, anatomists define it according to where the sinoatrial node artery arises. Table 59-1 summarizes the hierarchy of the coronary artery anatomy.

All the epicardial conductance vessels and septal perforators from the LAD give rise to a multitude of branches, termed

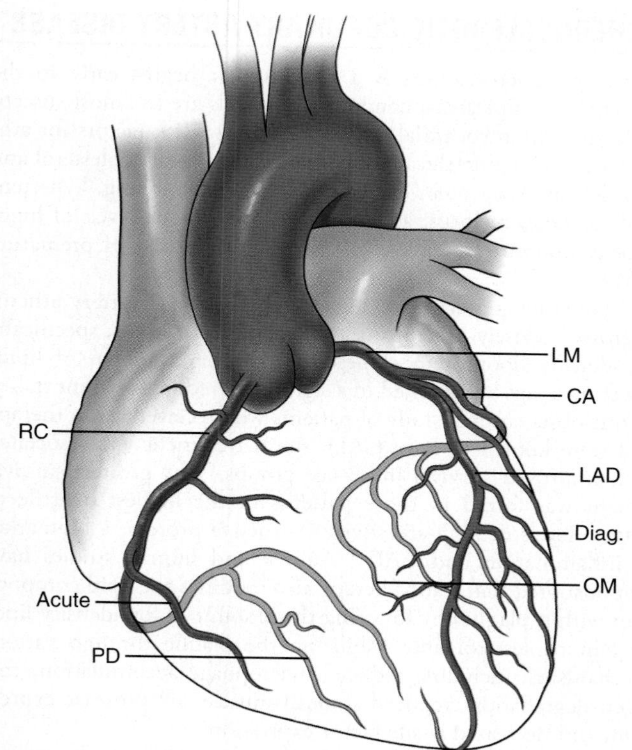

FIGURE 59-1 Anatomy of normal coronary artery vasculature. *CA*, circumflex artery; *LAD*, left anterior descending; *LM*, left main; *OM*, obtuse marginal; *PD*, posterior descending; *RC*, right coronary.

TABLE 59-1 Anatomic Architecture of Coronary Arteries

NAMED VESSELS	BRANCHES
Left main coronary artery	Left anterior descending Circumflex coronary Ramus intermedius
Left anterior descending	Diagonal arteries Septal perforators
Circumflex coronary artery	Obtuse marginal branches Left posterolateral artery
Right coronary artery	Acute marginal artery Posterior descending artery Right posterolateral artery

resistance vessels, that penetrate into the ventricular wall. These vessels play a crucial role in oxygen and nutrient exchange with the myocardium by forming a rich capillary plexus. This plexus offers a low-resistance sink that allows arterial blood flow to increase unimpeded when oxygen demand rises. This is important because the myocardial vascular bed extracts oxygen at its full capacity, even in low-demand circumstances, thereby allowing no margin for further oxygen extraction when demand is high.

An intricate network of veins drains the coronary circulation, and the venous circulation can be divided into three systems: the coronary sinus and its tributaries, the anterior right ventricular veins, and the thebesian veins. The coronary sinus predominantly drains the LV and receives 85% of coronary venous blood. It lies within the posterior AV groove and empties into the right atrium.

BOX 59-1 Unique Features of Coronary Blood Flow

- Autoregulated over wide pressure ranges
- Blood flow: 0.7-0.9 mL per gram of myocardium per minute
- 75% oxygen extraction
- Coronary sinus blood is the most deoxygenated blood in the body
- 4- to 7-fold increase in flow with increased demand
- 60% blood flow occurs during diastole
- Flow-limited oxygen supply

The anterior right ventricular veins travel across the right ventricular surface to the right AV groove, where they enter directly into the right atrium or form the small cardiac vein, which enters into the right atrium directly or joins the coronary sinus just proximal to its orifice. The thebesian veins are small venous tributaries that drain directly into the cardiac chambers and exit primarily into the right atrium and right ventricle. Understanding of the anatomy of the coronary sinus is essential for placement of the retrograde cardioplegia cannula during cardiopulmonary bypass (CPB).

Physiology and Regulation of Coronary Blood Flow

Aortic pressure is a driving force in the maintenance of myocardial perfusion. During resting conditions, coronary blood flow is maintained at a fairly constant level over a wide range of aortic perfusion pressures (70 to 180 mm Hg) through the process of autoregulation.

Because the myocardium has a high rate of energy use, normal coronary blood flow averages 225 mL/min (0.7 to 0.9 mL per gram of myocardium per minute) and delivers 0.1 mL/g/min of oxygen to the myocardium. Under normal conditions, more than 75% of the delivered oxygen is extracted in the coronary capillary bed, so any additional oxygen demand can be met only by increasing the flow rate. This highlights the importance of unobstructed coronary blood flow for proper myocardial function. Box 59-1 summarizes the unique features of coronary blood flow.

In response to increased load, such as that caused by strenuous exercise, the healthy heart can increase myocardial blood flow fourfold to sevenfold. Blood flow is increased through several mechanisms. Local metabolic neurohumoral factors cause coronary vasodilation when stress and metabolic demand increase, thereby lowering the coronary vascular resistance. This results in increased delivery of oxygen-rich blood, mimicking the phenomenon of reactive hyperemia. When a transient occlusion to the coronary artery is released (e.g., during the performance of a beating-heart operation), blood flow immediately rises to exceed the normal baseline flow and then gradually returns to its baseline level. The autoregulatory mechanism responsible is guided by several metabolic factors, including carbon dioxide, oxygen tension, hydrogen ions, lactate, potassium ions, and adenosine. Adenosine, a potent vasodilator and a degradation product of adenosine triphosphate, accumulates in the interstitial space and relaxes vascular smooth muscle. This results in vasomotor relaxation, coronary vasodilation, and increased blood flow. Another substance that plays an important role is nitric oxide, which is produced by the endothelium. Without the endothelium, coronary arteries do not autoregulate, suggesting that the mechanism for vasodilation and reactive hyperemia is endothelium dependent.

Extravascular compression of the coronaries during systole also plays an important role in the regulation of blood flow. During systole, the intracavitary pressures generated in the LV wall exceed intracoronary pressure, and blood flow is impeded. Hence, approximately 60% of coronary blood flow occurs during diastole. During exercise, increased heart rate and reduced diastolic time can compromise flow time, but this can be offset by vasodilatory mechanisms of the coronary vessels. Buildup of atherosclerotic plaques and fixed coronary occlusion significantly impair coronary arterial compensatory mechanisms while heart rate is elevated. This forms the basis for exercise-induced stress tests, in which abnormal physiologic responses to increased physical activity unmask underlying CAD.

HISTORY OF CORONARY ARTERY BYPASS SURGERY

One of the first attempts at myocardial revascularization was made by Arthur Vineberg from Canada. He operated on a series of patients who presented with symptoms of myocardial ischemia and implanted the left internal mammary artery (LIMA) into the myocardium by creating a pocket. The operation did not entail a direct anastomosis to any coronary vessel and was performed on a beating heart through a left anterolateral thoracotomy. Michael DeBakey performed a successful aortocoronary saphenous vein graft in 1964. Mason Sones, who is credited with inventing cardiac catheterization, helped establish CABG surgery as a planned and consistent therapy in patients with angiographically documented CAD.

The development of the heart-lung machine and its successful clinical use by John Heysham Gibbon in the 1950s, along with the advancement of cardioplegia techniques in later years by Gerald Buckberg, allowed surgeons to perform coronary anastomosis on an arrested (nonbeating) heart with a relatively bloodless field, thus increasing the safety and accuracy of the coronary bypass. In the 1990s, the advent of devices that could atraumatically stabilize the heart provided another pathway for the development of off-pump techniques of myocardial revascularization. Today, an armamentarium of techniques ranging from conventional on-pump CABG to minimally invasive robotic and percutaneous approaches is available to manage CAD. Table 59-2 summarizes the timeline of major historical events in the development of surgery for myocardial revascularization.

TABLE 59-2 Evolution of Surgical Coronary Artery Interventions: Timeline

1950	A. Vineberg	Direct implantation of mammary artery into myocardium
1953	J. H. Gibbon	First successful use of cardiopulmonary bypass machine
1962	F. M. Sones	Successful cineangiography
1964	M. E. DeBakey	First successful coronary artery bypass grafting
1964	T. Sondergaard	Introduced routine use of cardioplegia for myocardial protection
1964	D. A. Cooley	Routine use of normothermic arrest for all cardiac cases
1968	R. Favoloro	First large series showing success of coronary artery bypass grafting
1973	V. Subramanian	Beating-heart coronary artery bypass grafting
1979	G. Buckberg	First use of blood cardioplegia as preferred method for arrested myocardial protection

ATHEROSCLEROTIC CORONARY ARTERY DISEASE

Coronary atherosclerosis is a process that begins early in the patient's life. Epicardial conductance vessels are the most susceptible and intramyocardial arteries, the least. Risk factors for atherosclerosis include elevated plasma levels of total cholesterol and low-density lipoprotein cholesterol, cigarette smoking, hypertension, diabetes mellitus, advanced age, low plasma levels of high-density lipoprotein cholesterol, and family history of premature CAD.

Epidemiologic evidence suggests that coronary artery atherosclerosis is closely linked to the metabolism of lipids, specifically low-density lipoprotein cholesterol. The development of lipid-lowering drugs has resulted in a significant reduction in mortality. In one observational study of patients who received statin therapy and were known to have CAD, statin treatment was associated with improved survival in all age groups.[4] The greatest survival benefit was found in those patients in the highest quartile of plasma levels of high-sensitivity C-reactive protein, a biomarker of inflammation and CAD.[5] Animal and human studies have demonstrated that statin therapy also modifies the lipid composition within plaques by lowering the amount of low-density lipoprotein cholesterol and stabilizing the plaque through various mechanisms, including reduced macrophage accumulation, collagen degradation, reduced smooth muscle cell protease expression, and decreased tissue factor expression.

Pathogenesis

The primary cause of CAD is endothelial injury induced by an inflammatory wall response and lipid deposition. There is evidence that an inflammatory response is involved in all stages of the disease, from early lipid deposition to plaque formation, plaque rupture, and coronary artery thrombosis. Vulnerable or high-risk plaques that are prone to rupture have the following characteristics: a large, eccentric, soft lipid core; a thin fibrous cap; inflammation within the cap and adventitia; increased plaque neovascularity; and evidence of outward or positive vessel remodeling.

Thinner fibrous caps are at a higher risk for rupture, probably because of an imbalance between the synthesis and the degradation of the extracellular matrix in the fibrous cap that results in an overall decrease in the collagen and matrix components (Fig. 59-2). Increased matrix breakdown caused by matrix degradation by an inflammatory cell-mediated metalloproteinase or reduced production of extracellular matrix results in thinner fibrous caps. Not all plaque ruptures are symptomatic; whether they are depends on the thrombogenicity of the plaque's components. Tissue factor within the lipid core of the plaque, secreted by activated macrophages, is one of the most potent thrombogenic stimuli. Rupture of a vulnerable plaque may be spontaneous or caused by extreme physical activity, severe emotional distress, exposure to drugs, cold exposure, or acute infection.

Fixed Coronary Obstructions

More than 90% of patients with stable IHD (SIHD) have advanced coronary atherosclerosis caused by a fixed obstruction. Atherosclerotic plaques of the coronary arteries are concentric (25%) or eccentric (75%). Eccentric lesions compromise only a portion of the lumen; through vascular remodeling, the arterial lumen may remain patent until late in the disease process. The impact of an arterial stenosis on coronary blood flow can be appreciated in the context of Poiseuille's law. Reductions in

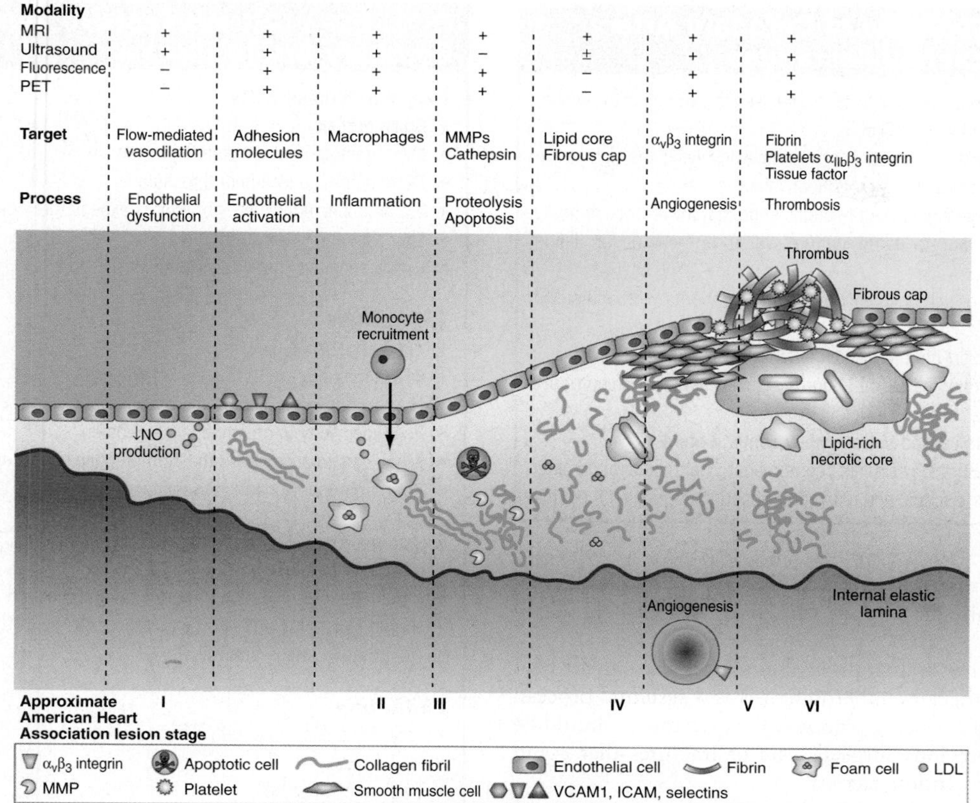

FIGURE 59-2 Components of Atherosclerotic Plaque. Thinning of the fibrous cap eventually results in plaque rupture and extrusion of highly thrombogenic lipid-laden material into the coronary artery. This causes an acute occlusion of the coronary artery, resulting in myocardial infarction. (Adapted from Choudhury RP, Fuster V, Fayad ZA: Molecular, cellular and functional imaging of atherothrombosis. *Nat Rev Drug Discov* 3:913–925, 2004.)

luminal diameter up to 60% have minimal impact on flow, but when the cross-sectional area of the vessel has decreased by 75% or more, coronary blood flow is significantly compromised. Clinically, this loss of flow often coincides with the onset of exertional angina. A 90% reduction in luminal diameter results in resting angina.

CLINICAL MANIFESTATIONS AND DIAGNOSIS OF CORONARY ARTERY DISEASE

Clinical Presentation

Clinically, IHD has two predominant modes of presentation:

- Stable angina
- Acute coronary syndrome: ST-segment elevation myocardial infarction (STEMI) and its complications, non–ST-segment myocardial infarction (NSTEMI), and unstable angina (UA)

Anginal pain is the main presenting symptom of IHD. It typically lasts minutes. The location is usually substernal, and pain can radiate to the neck, jaw, epigastrium, or arms. Anginal pain is precipitated by exertion or emotional stress and relieved by rest. Sublingual nitroglycerin also usually relieves angina within 30 seconds to several minutes.

On presentation, angina must be classified as stable or unstable.[6] Patients are said to be having UA if the pain is increasing (in frequency, intensity, or duration) or occurring at rest. Such patients should be transferred promptly to an emergency department.

Patients, especially female and elderly patients, sometimes present with atypical symptoms, such as nausea, vomiting, mid-epigastric discomfort, or sharp (atypical) chest pain. In the WISE (Women's Ischemic Syndrome Evaluation) study, 65% of women with ischemia presented with atypical symptoms.[7]

The term *acute coronary syndrome* has evolved to refer to a constellation of clinical symptoms that represent myocardial ischemia. It encompasses both STEMI and NSTEMI. Myocardial infarction (MI) often is manifested as crushing chest pain that may be associated with nausea, diaphoresis, anxiety, and dyspnea. Symptoms of the hypoperfusion that follows MI may include dizziness, fatigue, and vomiting. Heart rate and blood pressure may be initially normal, but both increase in response to the duration and severity of pain. Loss of blood pressure is indicative of cardiogenic shock and indicates a poorer prognosis. At least 40% of the ventricular mass must be involved for cardiogenic shock to occur.

Mechanical complications of MI include acute ventricular septal defect (VSD), papillary muscle rupture, and free ventricular rupture. They usually occur approximately 7 to 10 days after the initial MI.

Physical Examination

Some clinical findings are generic and are related to the systemic manifestations of atherosclerosis. Eye examination may reveal a copper wire sign, retinal hematoma or thrombosis secondary to vascular occlusive disease, and hypertension. Corneal arcus and

BOX 59-2 Sequelae of Coronary Artery Disease: Clinical Manifestations

- Abnormal neck vein pulsations, which may be seen in patients with second- or third-degree heart block or CHF
- Bradycardia—a subtle presentation of ischemia involving the right coronary territories and a possible sign of heart block
- Weak or thready pulse suggestive of ectopic or premature ventricular beats
- Third heart sound that is noted with elevated left ventricular filling pressures/CHF
- Fourth heart sound, which is commonly heard in patients with acute and chronic CAD
- Mitral regurgitant heart murmurs caused by ischemic papillary muscles
- Ejection systolic murmur indicative of aortic stenosis, which can contribute to coronary ischemia
- Holosystolic murmurs caused by ventricular septal rupture
- Manifestations of CHF, such as rales, hepatomegaly, right upper abdominal quadrant tenderness, ascites, and marked peripheral and presacral edema

xanthelasma are features noticed in cases of hypercholesterolemia. Other clinical manifestations are caused by sequelae of CAD (Box 59-2).

A thorough vascular evaluation is essential for any patient who presents with CAD because atherosclerosis is a systemic process. In addition, if surgery is being planned, the extremities should be evaluated for any previous surgical scars or fractures that could potentially preclude conduit harvest.

Diagnostic Testing

Biochemical Studies

Patients suspected of having an acute coronary syndrome should undergo appropriate blood testing. Levels of creatine kinase muscle and brain subunits (CK-MB) and troponin T or I should be assessed at least 6 to 12 hours apart. Additional laboratory tests include a complete blood count, comprehensive metabolic panel, and lipid profile (total cholesterol, triglycerides, low-density lipoprotein cholesterol, high-density lipoprotein cholesterol). Elevated brain natriuretic peptide and C-reactive protein levels suggest a worse outcome.

Chest Radiography

The chest radiograph is helpful in identifying causes of chest discomfort or pain other than CAD. Chest radiography does not detect CAD directly; it only identifies sequelae, such as cardiomegaly, pulmonary edema, and pleural effusions, that are indicative of heart failure. From a surgical standpoint, preoperative chest radiography is important because it can identify obvious abnormalities, such as porcelain aorta, lung masses, effusion, and pneumonias, that may affect further workup or prompt a change in operative strategy.

Resting Electrocardiography

A 12-lead resting electrocardiogram (ECG) should be obtained in all patients with suspected IHD or sequelae thereof. The ECG is evaluated for evidence of LV hypertrophy, ST-segment depression or elevation, ectopic beats, or Q waves. In addition, arrhythmias (atrial fibrillation or ventricular tachycardia) and conduction defects (left anterior fascicular block, right bundle branch block, left bundle branch block) are suggestive of CAD and MI. Persistent ST-segment elevation or an evolving Q wave is consistent with myocardial injury and ongoing ischemia. Fifty percent of patients with significant CAD nonetheless have normal electrocardiographic results, and 50% of ECG recordings obtained during chest pain at rest will be normal, indicating the inaccuracy of the test. Patients with SIHD tend to have a worse prognosis if they have the following abnormalities on a resting ECG: evidence of prior MI, especially Q waves in multiple leads or an R wave in V_1 indicating a posterior infarction; persistent ST-T wave inversions, particularly in leads V_1 to V_3; left bundle branch block, bifascicular block, second- or third-degree AV block, or ventricular tachyarrhythmia; or LV hypertrophy.[8-10]

BOX 59-3 Stress Tests to Identify Coronary Artery Disease

Exercise Stress ECG

- Bruce protocol
- Five 3-minute bouts of treadmill exercise
- Determines the ischemia threshold
- 12 metabolic equivalents of energy expenditure needed for complete test
- Low cost and short duration
- Highly sensitive in multivessel disease

Limitations

- Suboptimal sensitivity
- Low detection rate of one-vessel disease
- Nondiagnostic with abnormal baseline ECG
- Poor specificity in premenopausal women
- Many cannot accomplish the 12 metabolic equivalents for a complete test or an appropriate heart rate response

Exercise and Pharmacologic Stress SPECT Perfusion Imaging

- Simultaneous evaluation of perfusion and function
- Higher sensitivity and specificity than exercise ECG
- Quantitative image analysis

Limitations

- Long procedure time with ^{99m}Tc
- Higher cost
- Radiation exposure
- Poor-quality images in obese patients

Exercise and Pharmacologic Stress Echocardiography

- Higher sensitivity and specificity than exercise ECG
- Comparable value with dobutamine stress
- Short examination time
- Identification of structural cardiac abnormalities
- Simultaneous evaluation of perfusion with contrast agents
- No radiation

Limitations

- Decreased sensitivity for detection of one-vessel disease or mild stenosis
- Highly operator dependent
- No quantitative image analysis
- Poor imaging in some patients
- Infarct zone poorly defined

Functional (Stress) Tests

In patients with suspected stable ischemic CAD, functional or stress testing is used to detect inducible ischemia. These are the most common noninvasive tests used to diagnose SIHD (Box 59-3). All functional tests rely on the principle of inducing cardiac ischemia by using exercise or pharmacologic stress agents, which increase myocardial work and oxygen demand, or by causing vasodilation-elicited heterogeneity in induced coronary flow. Whether ischemia is induced, however, depends on the severity of both the stress imposed (e.g., submaximal exercise can fail to produce ischemia) and the flow disturbance. Approximately 70% of coronary stenoses are not detected by functional testing. Because abnormalities of regional or global ventricular function occur later in the ischemic cascade, they are more likely to indicate severe stenosis; thus, such abnormalities have a higher diagnostic specificity for SIHD than do perfusion defects, such as those seen on nuclear myocardial perfusion imaging (MPI).

Exercise versus pharmacologic testing. In patients capable of performing routine activities of daily living without difficulty, exercise testing is preferred to pharmacologic testing because it induces greater physiologic stress than drugs can. This may make exercise testing the better means of detecting ischemia as well as providing a correlation to a patient's daily symptom burden and physical work capacity not offered by pharmacologic stress testing.

The treadmill protocols initiate exercise at 3.2 to 4.7 metabolic equivalents (METs) of work and increase by several METs every 2 to 3 minutes of exercise (e.g., modified or standard Bruce protocol). Performance of most activities of daily living requires approximately 4 to 5 METs of physical work. Patients unable to perform moderate physical activity and those with disabling comorbidities should undergo pharmacologic stress imaging instead.

Diagnostic accuracy of stress testing for SIHD

Exercise electrocardiography (Bruce protocol). The criterion for diagnosis of ischemia is an ECG showing 1-mm horizontal or downsloping (at 80 ms after the J point) ST-segment depression at peak exercise. The diagnostic sensitivity and specificity of this sign is 61% (range, 70% to 77%). It is lower in women than in men[11,12] and lower than that of stress imaging modalities.

Exercise and pharmacologic stress echocardiography. These tests rely on detecting new or worsening wall motion abnormalities and changes in global LV function during or immediately after stress. In addition to the detection of inducible wall motion abnormalities, most stress echocardiography includes screening images to evaluate resting ventricular function and valvular abnormalities.

Pharmacologic stress echocardiography is usually performed using dobutamine with an end point of producing wall motion abnormalities. Vasodilator agents such as adenosine can be used to the same effect.

The diagnostic sensitivity is 70% to 85% for exercise and 85% to 90% for pharmacologic stress echocardiography.[13,14] The use of intravenous ultrasound contrast agents, by improving endocardial border delineation, can result in improved diagnostic accuracy.

Exercise and pharmacologic stress nuclear myocardial perfusion imaging. Myocardial perfusion single-photon emission computed tomography (SPECT) generally is performed with rest and with stress. Technetium Tc 99m agents are generally used; one of these, thallium Tl 201, has limited applications (e.g., viability) because of its higher radiation exposure. Pharmacologic stress is generally induced with vasodilator agents administered by continuous infusion (adenosine, dipyridamole) or bolus injection (regadenoson).

The diagnostic end point of nuclear MPI is a reduction in myocardial perfusion after stress. The diagnostic accuracy for detection of obstructive CAD of exercise and pharmacologic stress nuclear MPI has been studied in detail.[15-17] Studies suggest that nuclear MPI's sensitivity ranges from 82% to 88% for exercise and 88% to 91% for pharmacologic stress, and its diagnostic specificity ranges from 70% to 88% and 75% to 90% for exercise and pharmacologic stress nuclear MPI, respectively.

For myocardial perfusion SPECT, global reductions in myocardial perfusion, such as in the patients with left main or three-vessel CAD, can result in balanced reduction and an underestimation of ischemic burden.

Echocardiography

From a surgical standpoint, most patients with SIHD should undergo preoperative echocardiography. Echocardiography provides information not only for surgical planning but also regarding prognosis. A resting LV ejection fraction (LVEF) of 35% is associated with an annual mortality rate of 3% per year. Resting two-dimensional Doppler echocardiography provides information on cardiac structure and function, including identifying the mechanism of heart failure and differentiating systolic from diastolic LV dysfunction. Echocardiography can identify LV or left atrial dilation, identify aortic stenosis (a potential non-CAD cause of angina-like chest pain), measure pulmonary artery pressure, quantify mitral regurgitation, identify LV aneurysm, identify LV thrombus (which increases the risk of death), and measure LV mass and the ratio of wall thickness to chamber radius—all of which predict cardiac events and mortality.[18-20]

Multidetector Computed Tomography

From a surgical standpoint, multidetector computed tomography (CT) has two pertinent applications in the management of CAD: to detect CAD and to inform the planning of grafting sites for CABG by providing additional information about coronary lesions, especially calcification and the course of coronary arteries. It also gives additional pertinent information about aortic disease and calcification, which might profoundly influence surgical decision making. However, the timing of cardiac CT should be carefully weighed against the risk of renal failure as a result of contrast nephropathy. Although revascularization decisions are currently made on the basis of coronary angiography, there have been tremendous improvements in temporal and spatial resolution of cardiac CT that make it useful for this purpose as well. Coronary computed tomography angiography (CCTA) can now provide high-quality images of the coronary arteries.[21] When it is performed with 64-slice CT, CCTA has a sensitivity of 93% to 97% and a specificity of 80% to 90% for detecting obstructive CAD.[22-28] Factors such as image quality, extent of coronary calcification, and body mass index adversely affect accuracy; in addition, coronary stenosis measurements are not well correlated between CT angiography and traditional angiography. This is an important fact to consider because current recommendations state that only vessels with stenosis greater than 50% to 70% should be bypassed.

The potential advantages of CCTA over standard functional testing for CAD screening include the high negative predictive value of CCTA for obstructive CAD. This can reassure caregivers that it is a sensible strategy to provide guideline-directed medical therapy (GDMT) and to defer consideration of revascularization. Among the greatest potential advantages of CCTA over conventional angiography, in addition to documentation of stenotic lesions, is that CCTA can assess remodeling and identify nonobstructive plaque, including calcified, noncalcified, and mixed plaque.[29,30]

Magnetic Resonance Imaging

Myocardial first-pass perfusion magnetic resonance imaging has been considered a good alternative to nuclear cardiac ischemia and viability testing. However, the procedure has not gained widespread popularity because special training and expertise are required to perform this type of imaging and to interpret the results.

Cardiac Catheterization and Intervention

Coronary catheterization is the "gold standard" for diagnosis of CAD. Coronary angiography defines coronary anatomy, including the location, length, diameter, and contour of the epicardial coronary arteries; the presence and severity of coronary luminal obstructions; the nature of the obstruction; the presence and extent of angiographically visible collateral flow; and coronary blood flow.

The classification for defining coronary anatomy that is still used today was developed for the Coronary Artery Surgery Study (CASS)[31] and further modified by the Balloon Angioplasty Revascularization Investigation (BARI) study group.[32] This scheme assumes that there are three major coronary arteries: the LAD, the circumflex, and the RCA, with a right-dominant, left-dominant, or codominant circulation. The extent of disease is defined as one-vessel, two-vessel, three-vessel, or left main disease; a luminal diameter reduction of at least 70% is considered to be significant stenosis (Figs. 59-3 and 59-4). Left main disease, however, is defined as stenosis of at least 50% (Fig. 59-5). Despite being recognized as the traditional gold standard for clinical assessment of coronary atherosclerosis, this test is not without limitations. There is marked variation in interobserver reliability, and investigators have found only 70% overall agreement among readers with regard to the severity of stenosis; this was reduced to 51% when restricted to coronary vessels rated as having some stenosis by any reader. Also, angiography provides only anatomic data and is not a reliable indicator of the functional significance of a given coronary stenosis unless a technique such as fractional flow reserve (FFR) is used to provide information about the physiologic effects of the stenosis. FFR is measured by passing a sensor guidewire into the LAD or circumflex vessels for LCA lesions. Thereafter, the flow reserve in the artery is checked by using adenosine to induce hyperemia in the coronary system, which is discussed in the next section on FFR. In addition, angiography cannot distinguish between vulnerable and stable plaques. In angiographic studies performed before and after acute events and early after MI, plaques causing UA and MI commonly were found to be 50% obstructive before the acute event and were therefore

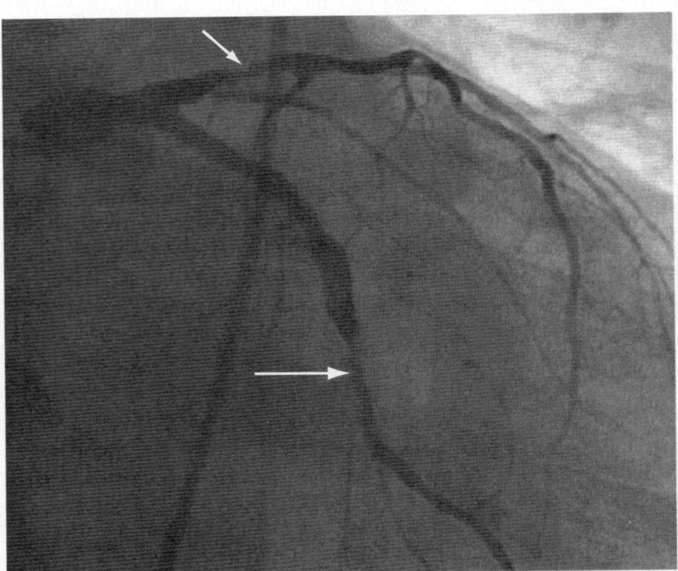

FIGURE 59-3 Left coronary angiogram showing hemodynamically severe lesions in the left anterior descending artery *(small arrow)* and the circumflex artery *(large arrow)*.

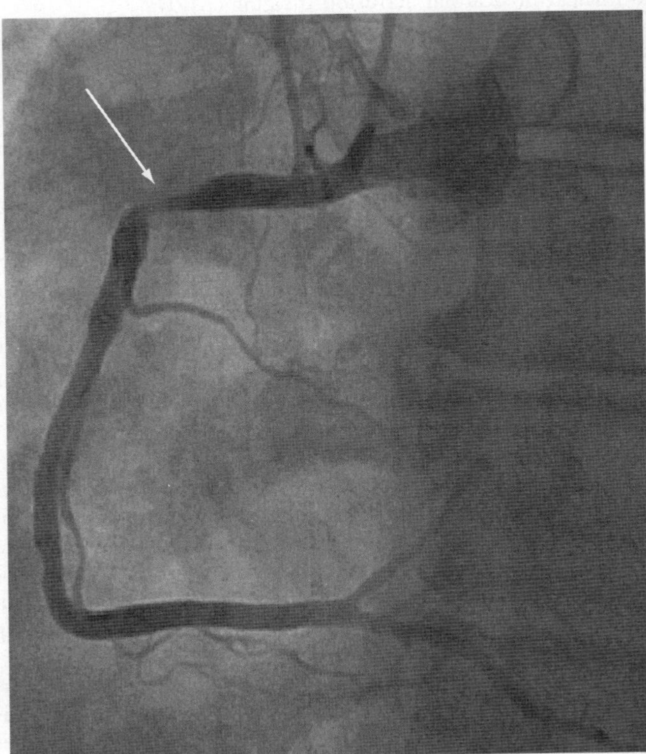

FIGURE 59-4 Right coronary angiogram showing hemodynamically significant lesion *(arrow)*. The right coronary artery terminates as a posterior descending artery in the right dominant system.

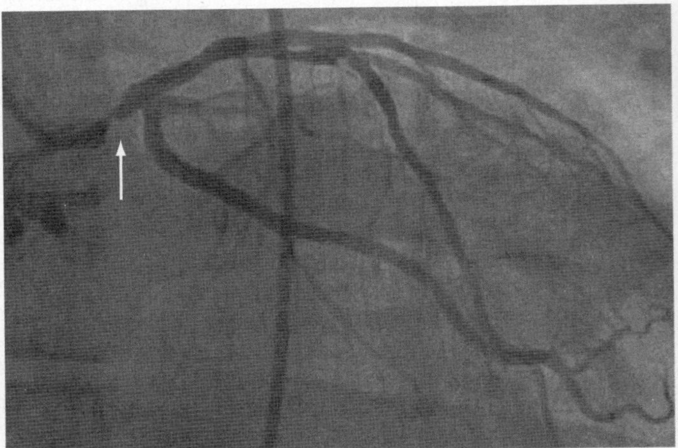

FIGURE 59-5 Coronary angiogram showing critical left main coronary artery stenosis *(arrow)*.

angiographically "silent."[31,32] Diagnostic testing methods to identify vulnerable plaque and therefore the patient's risk of MI are being intensely studied, but no gold standard has yet emerged. Despite these limitations of coronary angiography, the extent and severity of CAD as revealed angiographically remain important predictors of long-term patient outcomes.[33,34]

In the CASS registry[35] of medically treated patients, the 12-year survival rate of patients with normal coronary arteries was 91% compared with 74% for those with one-vessel disease, 59% for those with two-vessel disease, and 40% for those with three-vessel disease.

Importantly, besides informing the decision whether to intervene surgically or with percutaneous coronary intervention (PCI), the salient characteristics of coronary lesions (e.g., stenosis severity, length, and complexity and presence of thrombus), the number of lesions threatening regions of contracting myocardium, the effect of collaterals, and the volume of jeopardized viable myocardium also can afford some insight into the potential consequences of subsequent vessel occlusion and therefore the haste with which surgery should be scheduled. For example, a patient with a noncontracting inferior or lateral wall and severe proximal stenosis of a large LAD artery is presumably at substantial risk for development of cardiogenic shock if the LAD artery were to become occluded. Thus, such a patient should be scheduled relatively quickly for surgery.

Right-sided heart catheterization is used to measure central venous, right atrial, right ventricular, pulmonary artery, and pulmonary wedge pressures as well as cardiac output. It can also be used to identify intracardiac shunts, to assess arrhythmias, and to initiate temporary cardiac pacing. Preoperative right-sided heart catheterization is used selectively and is generally not necessary unless right ventricular dysfunction or pulmonary vascular disease is suspected.

PCI techniques in current use include balloon dilation, stent-supported dilation, atherectomy and plaque ablation with a variety of devices, thrombectomy with aspiration devices, specialized imaging, and physiologic assessment with intracoronary devices.

Coronary artery stents were the first substantial breakthrough in the prevention of restenosis after angioplasty. Although stent recoil and compression are not completely insignificant problems, the greatest cause of lumen loss in stented coronary arteries is neointimal hyperplasia. This is the principal mechanism of in-stent stenosis and results from inappropriate cell proliferation—hence, the advent of cytotoxic drug-eluting stents (DES).

Fractional Flow Reserve

Angiography can underestimate the severity of CAD, especially LCA disease. This underestimation may be due to the lack of a reference segment or to very ostial or distal disease. Therefore, in cases with intermediate lesions, FFR has emerged as a helpful modality.[36,37]

FFR is measured by passing a sensor guidewire into the LAD or circumflex vessels for LCA lesions. Thereafter, the flow reserve in the artery is checked by using adenosine to induce hyperemia in the coronary system. An FFR below 0.75 is considered to signify ischemia-producing lesions. Some studies have used a threshold of 0.8.

Intravascular Ultrasonography

Intravascular ultrasonography (IVUS) provides high-quality cross-sectional images of the coronary system.[38] It is done by inserting an IVUS wire into the LAD or circumflex artery and gradually pulling it out while obtaining real-time images of the coronary system. In indeterminate lesions of the LCA, an IVUS minimum luminal diameter of 2.8 or a minimum luminal area of 6 mm^2 suggests a physiologically significant lesion.

Hybrid Imaging

Hybrid imaging has the potential of taking coronary artery assessment one step further by combining the advantages of two different modalities to give both anatomic and physiologic information in one snapshot. Hybrid imaging can combine positron emission tomography (PET) and CT or SPECT and CT, thus allowing combined anatomic and functional testing. In addition, novel scanning techniques make it possible to use CCTA alone to assess perfusion and FFR, in addition to coronary anatomy.[39-41] Interestingly, these combined assessments can produce a fused image in which physiologic information about flow is combined with information about the anatomic extent and severity of CAD, plaque composition, and arterial remodeling. Robust evidence to support the use of hybrid imaging is lacking at this point, despite its reported accuracy in predicting cardiac events with both ischemic and anatomic markers.[42] The strength of combined imaging is that it provides anatomic information to guide the interpretation of ischemic and scarred myocardium as well as information to guide therapeutic decision making. Hybrid imaging also can overcome technical limitations of myocardial perfusion SPECT or myocardial perfusion PET by providing anatomic correlates to guide interpretative accuracy,[43] and it can provide the functional information that an anatomic technique like CCTA or magnetic resonance angiography lacks; however, use of hybrid techniques requires increasing the radiation dose.

INDICATIONS FOR CORONARY ARTERY REVASCULARIZATION

Per the most current American College of Cardiology/American Heart Association guidelines, the only class Ia indication for PCI is acute STEMI. In all other indications, CABG has superior class based on current evidence (Table 59-3). These guidelines are based on the existing literature, which spans 4 decades. Many of the studies on which current recommendations are based were conducted in the 1970s and 1980s.

Coronary Artery Bypass Grafting versus Contemporaneous Medical Therapy

In the 1970s and 1980s, three landmark randomized controlled trials (RCTs) established the survival benefit of CABG compared with medical therapy without revascularization in certain patients with SIHD: the Veterans Affairs Cooperative Study,[44] European Coronary Surgery Study,[45] and CASS.[35] Subsequently, a 1994 meta-analysis of seven studies in which 2649 patients were randomly assigned to medical therapy or CABG[36] showed that CABG offered a survival advantage over medical therapy for patients with LCA or three-vessel CAD. The studies also established that CABG is more effective than medical therapy for relieving anginal symptoms. These studies have been replicated only once during the past decade. In MASS II (Medicine, Angioplasty, or Surgery Study II), patients with multivessel CAD who were treated with CABG were less likely than those treated with

TABLE 59-3 Guidelines for Coronary Revascularization

CORONARY ARTERY LESIONS	RECOMMENDATIONS
Unprotected left main	
CABG	I
PCI	IIa—For SIHD when both of the following are present: • Cardiac catheterization reveals a low risk of PCI procedural complications with a high likelihood of good long-term outcome (low SYNTAX score 22, ostial or trunk left main). • Significantly increased risk of adverse surgical outcomes (STS-predicted risk of operative mortality 5%) IIa—For UA/NSTEMI if not a CABG candidate IIa—For STEMI when distal coronary flow is TIMI flow grade 3 and PCI can be performed more rapidly and safely than CABG IIb—For SIHD when both of the following are present: • Cardiac catheterization reveals a low to intermediate risk of PCI procedural complications and an intermediate to high likelihood of good long-term outcome (low-intermediate SYNTAX score of 33, bifurcation left main) • Increased risk of adverse surgical outcomes (moderate—severe COPD, disability from prior stroke, or prior cardiac surgery; STS-predicted operative mortality 2%) III: Harm—For SIHD in patients (versus performing CABG) with unfavorable anatomy for PCI and who are good candidates for CABG
3-vessel disease with or without proximal LAD artery disease	
CABG	I IIa—It is reasonable to choose CABG over PCI in patients with complex 3-vessel CAD (SYNTAX score 22) who are good candidates for surgery
PCI	IIb—Of uncertain benefit
2-vessel disease with proximal LAD artery disease	
CABG	I
PCI	IIb—Of uncertain benefit
2-vessel disease without proximal LAD artery disease	
CABG	IIa—With extensive ischemia IIb—Of uncertain benefit without extensive ischemia
PCI	IIb—Of uncertain benefit
1-vessel proximal LAD artery disease	
CABG	IIa—With LIMA for long-term benefit
PCI	IIb—Of uncertain benefit
1-vessel disease without proximal LAD artery involvement	
CABG	III: Harm
PCI	III: Harm
LV dysfunction	
CABG	IIa—LVEF 35% to 50% IIb—LVEF 35% without significant left main CAD
PCI	Insufficient data
Survivors of sudden cardiac death with presumed ischemia-mediated VT	
CABG	I
PCI	I
No anatomic or physiologic criteria for revascularization	
CABG	III: Harm
PCI	III: Harm

Class I Benefit >>> Risk. Procedure should be performed.
Class IIa Benefit >> Risk. Additional studies with focused objectives needed. It is reasonable to perform procedure.
Class IIb Benefit ≥ Risk. Additional studies with broader objectives and additional registry data may be needed. Procedure treatment may be considered.
Class III No Benefit
or
Class III Harm

From reference 45a.

CABG, coronary artery bypass graft (major adverse events occurred less frequently with CABG); *CAD,* coronary artery disease; *COPD,* chronic obstructive pulmonary disease; *LAD,* left anterior descending; *LIMA,* left internal mammary artery; *LV,* left ventricle; *LVEF,* left ventricular ejection fraction; *PCI,* percutaneous coronary intervention; *SIHD,* stable ischemic heart disease; *STEMI,* ST-elevation myocardial infarction; *STS,* Society of Thoracic Surgeons; *SYNTAX,* Synergy between Percutaneous Coronary Intervention with Taxus and Cardiac Surgery; *TIMI,* Thrombolysis In Myocardial Infarction; *UA/NSTEMI,* unstable angina/non–ST-elevation myocardial infarction; *VT,* ventricular tachycardia.

medical therapy to have a subsequent MI, to need additional revascularization, or to experience cardiac death in the 10 years after randomization.[37] Surgical techniques and medical therapy have improved substantially during the intervening years. Some critics state that if CABG were compared with GDMT in RCTs today, the relative benefits in terms of survival and angina relief observed several decades ago might no longer be observed. However, it should also be understood that the concurrent administration of GDMT, which most post–cardiac surgery patients now receive, may also substantially improve long-term outcomes in patients treated with CABG in comparison with those receiving medical therapy alone. Thus, the survival difference might still favor CABG over GDMT.

Percutaneous Coronary Intervention versus Medical Therapy

Although contemporary interventional treatments have lowered the risk of restenosis compared with earlier techniques, meta-analyses have not shown that the use of bare-metal stents (BMS) confers a survival advantage over balloon angioplasty[38,39] or that the use of DES confers a survival advantage over BMS.[40] Evaluation of trials of PCI conducted during the last 30 years shows that despite improvements in PCI technology and pharmacotherapy, PCI has not reduced the risk of death or MI in patients without recent acute coronary syndrome. The findings from individual studies and systematic reviews of PCI versus medical therapy can be summarized as follows:

- PCI reduces the incidence of angina.
- PCI has not been demonstrated to improve survival in stable patients.
- PCI may increase the short-term risk of MI.
- PCI does not lower the long-term risk of MI.

Coronary Artery Bypass Grafting versus Balloon Angioplasty or Bare-Metal Stents

From a review of multiple RCTs comparing CABG with balloon angioplasty or BMS, the following conclusions can be drawn[41]:

- Survival was similar for CABG and PCI (with balloon angioplasty or BMS) at 1 year and 5 years. Survival was similar for CABG and PCI in patients with one-vessel CAD (including those with disease of the proximal portion of the LAD artery) or multivessel CAD.
- Incidence of MI was similar at 5 years.
- Procedural stroke occurred more commonly with CABG than with PCI (1.2% versus 0.6%).
- Relief of angina was more effective with CABG than with PCI at 1 year and 5 years.
- At 1 year after the index procedure, repeated coronary revascularization was performed less often after CABG than after PCI (3.8% versus 26.5%). This was also found after 5 years of follow-up (9.8% versus 46.1%). This difference was more pronounced with balloon angioplasty than with BMS.

Coronary Artery Bypass Grafting versus Drug-Eluting Stents

Multiple observational studies comparing CABG and DES implantation have been published, but most of them had short (12 to 24 months) follow-up periods. Only one large RCT comparing CABG and DES implantation has been published, called the Synergy between Percutaneous Coronary Intervention with Taxus and Cardiac Surgery (SYNTAX) trial,[42] in which 1800 patients (of a total of 4337 who were screened) were randomly assigned to undergo DES implantation or CABG. Major adverse cardiac events (a composite of death, stroke, MI, or repeated revascularization during the 3 years after randomization) occurred less frequently in CABG patients (20.2%) than in DES patients (28.0%; $P = .001$). The rates of death and stroke were similar; however, MI (3.6% for CABG, 7.1% for DES) and repeated revascularization (10.7% for CABG, 19.7% for DES) were more likely to occur with DES implantation. In SYNTAX, the extent of CAD was assessed by using the SYNTAX score, which is based on the location, severity, and extent of coronary stenoses, with a low score indicating less complicated anatomic CAD. In post hoc analyses, a low score was defined as 22 or lower; intermediate, 23 to 32; and high, 33 or higher. The occurrence of major adverse cardiac events correlated with the SYNTAX score for DES patients but not for those undergoing CABG. At 12-month follow-up, the primary end point was similar for CABG and DES in those with a low SYNTAX score. In contrast, major adverse cardiac events occurred more often after DES implantation than after CABG in those with an intermediate or high SYNTAX score. At 3 years of follow-up, the mortality rate was greater in patients with three-vessel CAD treated with PCI than in those treated with CABG (6.2% versus 2.9%). The differences in major adverse cardiac events of those treated with PCI or CABG increased with an increasing SYNTAX score. Although the utility of using a SYNTAX score in everyday clinical practice remains uncertain, it seems reasonable to conclude from SYNTAX and other data that outcomes of patients undergoing PCI or CABG in those with relatively uncomplicated and lesser degrees of CAD are comparable, whereas in those with complex and diffuse CAD, CABG appears to be preferable.

Left Main Coronary Artery Disease

CABG or PCI versus Medical Therapy for Left Main CAD

CABG confers a survival benefit over medical therapy in patients with LCA CAD. Subgroup analyses from RCTs performed 3 decades ago demonstrated a 66% reduction in relative risk of death with CABG, with the benefit extending to 10 years.[36,46]

Studies Comparing PCI versus CABG for Left Main CAD

Of all patients undergoing coronary angiography, approximately 4% are found to have LCA CAD, 80% of whom have significant (70% diameter) stenoses in other epicardial coronary arteries. Published cohort studies have found that major clinical outcomes for ostial LCA are similar with PCI or CABG 1 year after revascularization and that mortality rates are similar at 1 year, 2 years, and 5 years of follow-up; however, the risk of needing target vessel revascularization is significantly higher with stenting than with CABG.

Three RCTs have looked at this topic: the SYNTAX trial, the Study of Unprotected Left Main Stenting versus Bypass Surgery (LE MANS) trial,[43] and the Premier of Randomized Comparison of Bypass Surgery versus Angioplasty Using Sirolimus-Eluting Stent in Patients with Left Main Coronary Artery Disease (PRECOMBAT) trial. The results from these three RCTs suggest (but do not definitively prove) that major clinical outcomes in *selected* patients with LCA CAD are similar with CABG and PCI at 1- to 2-year follow-up, but repeated revascularization rates are higher after PCI than after CABG. RCTs with extended follow-up of 5 years are required to provide definitive conclusions about the optimal treatment of LCA CAD.

Revascularization Options for LCA CAD

Although CABG has been considered the gold standard for unprotected LCA CAD revascularization, PCI has more recently emerged as a possible alternative mode of revascularization in carefully selected patients. Lesion location is an important determinant when PCI is considered for unprotected LCA CAD. Stenting of the LCA ostium or trunk is more straightforward than treatment of distal bifurcation or trifurcation stenoses, which generally requires a greater degree of operator experience and expertise.[47] In addition, PCI of bifurcation disease is associated with higher restenosis rates than PCI of disease confined to the ostium or trunk. Although lesion location influences technical success and long-term outcomes after PCI, location exerts a negligible influence on the success of CABG. In subgroup analyses, patients with LCA CAD and a SYNTAX score of 33 with more complex or extensive CAD had a higher mortality rate with PCI than with CABG. Physicians can estimate operative risk for all CABG candidates by using a standard instrument, such as the risk calculator from the Society of Thoracic Surgeons (STS) database. These considerations are important factors when one is choosing among revascularization strategies for unprotected LCA CAD and have been factored into revascularization recommendations. Use of a Heart Team approach has been recommended in cases in which the choice of revascularization is not straightforward. The patient's ability to tolerate and to comply with dual antiplatelet therapy is also an important consideration in revascularization decisions.

Experts have recommended immediate PCI for unprotected LCA CAD in the setting of STEMI.[48] The impetus for such a strategy is greatest when LCA CAD is the site of the culprit lesion, antegrade coronary flow is diminished (e.g., Thrombolysis In Myocardial Infarction [TIMI] flow grade 0, 1, or 2), the patient is hemodynamically unstable, and it is believed that PCI can be performed more quickly than CABG. When possible, the interventional cardiologist and cardiac surgeon should decide together on the optimal form of revascularization for these patients, although it is recognized that they are usually critically ill and therefore not amenable to a prolonged deliberation or discussion of treatment options.

Proximal Left Anterior Descending Artery Disease

Multiple studies have suggested that CABG confers a survival advantage over contemporaneous medical therapy for patients with disease in the proximal segment of the LAD artery. Cohort studies and RCTs as well as collaborative analyses and meta-analyses have shown that PCI and CABG result in similar survival rates in these patients.

Completeness of Revascularization

Most patients undergoing CABG receive complete or nearly complete revascularization, which seems to influence long-term prognosis positively.[49,50] In contrast, complete revascularization is accomplished less often in patients receiving PCI (e.g., in 70% of patients), and the extent to which the incomplete initial revascularization influences outcome is less clear. Rates of late survival and survival free of MI appear to be similar in patients with and without complete revascularization after PCI. Nevertheless, the need for subsequent CABG is usually higher in those whose initial revascularization procedure was incomplete (compared with those with complete revascularization) after PCI.

Left Ventricular Systolic Dysfunction

Several older studies and a meta-analysis of the data from these studies reported that patients with LV systolic dysfunction (predominantly mild to moderate in severity) had better survival with CABG than with medical therapy alone. For patients with more severe LV systolic dysfunction, however, the evidence that CABG results in better survival compared with medical therapy is lacking. In the Surgical Treatment for Ischemic Heart Failure (STICH) trial of CABG and GDMT in patients with an LVEF of 35% with or without viability testing, both treatments resulted in similar rates of survival (i.e., freedom from death from any cause, the study's primary outcome) after 5 years of follow-up. The data suggest the possibility that outcomes would differ if the follow-up were longer; as a result, the study is being continued to provide follow-up for up to 10 years.[51,52]

Only limited data are available comparing PCI with medical therapy in patients with LV systolic dysfunction. The data that exist at present on revascularization in patients with CAD and LV systolic dysfunction are more robust for CABG than for PCI, although data from contemporary RCTs in this population of patients are lacking. Therefore, the choice of revascularization method in patients with CAD and LV systolic dysfunction is best based on clinical variables (e.g., coronary anatomy, presence of diabetes mellitus, presence of chronic kidney disease), magnitude of LV systolic dysfunction, preferences of the patient, clinical judgment, and consultation between the interventional cardiologist and the cardiac surgeon.

Revascularization Options for Previous CABG

In patients with recurrent angina after CABG, repeated revascularization is most likely to improve survival in patients at highest risk, such as those with obstruction of the proximal LAD artery and extensive anterior ischemia. Patients with ischemia in other locations and those with a patent LIMA to the LAD artery are unlikely to experience a survival benefit from repeated revascularization.[53] Cohort studies comparing PCI and CABG among post-CABG patients report similar rates of midterm and long-term survival after the two procedures. In patients with previous CABG who are referred for revascularization for medically refractory ischemia, factors that may support the choice of repeated CABG include vessels unsuitable for PCI, multiple diseased bypass grafts, availability of the internal mammary artery (IMA) for grafting of chronically occluded coronary arteries, and good distal targets for bypass graft placement. Factors favoring PCI over CABG include limited areas of ischemia causing symptoms, suitable PCI targets, patent graft to the LAD artery, poor CABG targets, and comorbid conditions.

Unstable Angina/Non–ST-Segment Elevation Myocardial Infarction

The main difference between treating a patient with SIHD and a patient with UA/NSTEMI is that the impetus for revascularization is stronger in the treatment of UA/NSTEMI because myocardial ischemia occurring as part of an acute coronary syndrome is potentially life-threatening, and associated angina symptoms are more likely to be reduced with a revascularization procedure than with GDMT.[54] Thus, the indications for revascularization are strengthened by the acuity of presentation, the extent of ischemia, and the likelihood of achieving full revascularization. The choice of revascularization method is generally dictated by the same considerations used to decide between PCI or CABG for patients with SIHD.

ST-Segment Elevation Myocardial Infarction–Acute Myocardial Infarction

Percutaneous Coronary Intervention versus Medical Management for Acute Myocardial Infarction

In general, PCI confers a greater survival advantage than thrombolytics as an initial treatment for STEMI–acute myocardial infarction (AMI), and the use of delayed PCI as an adjunct to therapy, including therapy with thrombolytics, does not affect survival. In the Global Use of Strategies to Open Occluded Coronary Arteries in Acute Coronary Syndromes (GUSTO) IIb trial,[55] the 30-day rate of the composite end point of death, nonfatal MI, and nonfatal disabling stroke was 9.6% for PCI patients and 13.7% for recipients of thrombolytics.

Prospective observational data collected from the Second National Registry of Myocardial Infarction between June 1994 and March 1998 included data from a cohort of 27,080 consecutive patients with AMI associated with ST-segment elevation or left bundle branch block. These patients were all treated with primary angioplasty. The study revealed that the adjusted odds of mortality were significantly higher (62% versus 41%) for patients with door-to-balloon times longer than 2 hours. The longer the door-to-balloon time, the higher the mortality risk, emphasizing that door-to-balloon time has a significant impact on outcomes for patients with AMI.[56]

On the basis of this evidence, PCI facilities have been required to establish a target door-to-balloon time of no longer than 90 minutes. Depending on the available facilities in a particular region, it is the responsibility of emergency medical services personnel to determine whether that goal can be achieved by transferring the patient to a PCI-capable facility. If this cannot be accomplished, a medical management strategy should be considered, with the goal being a door-to-needle time of 30 minutes or less.[46]

Role of Coronary Artery Bypass Grafting

Although an increasing number of patients undergo catheterization early after AMI, the initial treatment is directed by the interventionalist, which has significantly diminished the role of emergency CABG. In general, patients who undergo CABG early after AMI are sicker, and efforts to improve myocardial function are typically refractory to medical therapy. These patients typically have a higher incidence of comorbidities and are more likely to require intra-aortic balloon pump (IABP) insertion. The optimal timing of CABG after AMI is not well established. A review of California discharge data identified 9476 patients who were hospitalized for AMI and subsequently underwent CABG. Of these, 4676 (49%) were in the early CABG group and 4800 (51%) were in the late CABG group. The mortality rate was highest (8.2%) among patients who underwent CABG on day 0 and declined to a nadir of 3.0% among patients who underwent CABG on day 3. The mean time to CABG was 3.2 days. Early CABG was an independent predictor of mortality, suggesting that CABG may best be deferred for 3 days or more after admission for AMI in nonurgent cases.[57]

The SHOCK (Should We Emergently Revascularize Occluded Coronaries for Cardiogenic Shock) trial has shown the survival advantage of emergency revascularization versus initial medical stabilization in patients in whom cardiogenic shock developed after AMI. A subanalysis that compared the effects of PCI and CABG on 30-day and 1-year survival showed that survival rates were similar at both time points. Among SHOCK trial patients randomly assigned to undergo emergency revascularization, those treated with CABG had a greater prevalence of diabetes and worse CAD than those treated with PCI. However, survival rates were similar.[58]

In patients with AMI, CABG is usually performed in conjunction with an operation to treat a specific complication, such as refractory postinfarction angina, papillary muscle rupture with mitral regurgitation, and infarction VSD. The rationale for urgent or emergent surgery is often based on high early mortality risk from mechanical complications.

Preoperative Evaluation

The success of coronary artery revascularization depends on proper workup and patient selection. Currently, a multidisciplinary approach with cardiologists and cardiac surgeons is needed to give the patient the most appropriate form of revascularization based on guidelines (Fig. 59-6). Comorbidities that affect CABG outcomes and that are typically incorporated into risk models include age, gender, urgency of the procedure, ejection fraction, need for mechanical circulatory support, MI, smoking status, use of immunosuppressive drugs, prior coronary interventions, hypertension, diabetes, peripheral vascular disease (PVD), and cerebrovascular disease. In addition, the severity of angina, as designated by the Canadian Cardiovascular Society classification of angina, and the New York Heart Association classification of congestive heart failure (CHF) are important risk variables.

The following are essential components of a preoperative workup for CABG patients:

- Detailed history and physical examination, including conduit evaluation
- Review of medications, including angiotensin-converting enzyme inhibitors, beta blockers, antiplatelet agents, and anticoagulants
- Carotid duplex ultrasonography in patients who have clinical bruit or are at high risk for cerebrovascular disease
- Cardiac echocardiography to evaluate ventricular function and the structural integrity of valves and chambers
- Cardiac viability study in patients with depressed LVEF, chronic total occlusions, frailty, and high-risk operations to decide between PCI and CABG
- Cardiac catheterization to delineate the coronary anatomy
- Chest radiography
- Coagulation and platelet profile, comprehensive metabolic panel, and complete blood count

Depending on the findings of these tests, patients may need additional workup. In emergency circumstances, several of these tests may be skipped so that immediate revascularization can be performed.

Technique of Myocardial Revascularization: Conventional On-Pump Cardiopulmonary Bypass

Box 59-4 outlines all the major steps of an on-pump CABG operation.

Positioning and Draping

General anesthesia with a single-lumen endotracheal tube is the anesthetic technique of choice. After anesthetic induction and placement of necessary access and monitoring lines, the patient is positioned supine, with or without a roll underneath the shoulder blades according to the surgeon's preference. The arms are tucked beside the patient with appropriate padding to minimize the

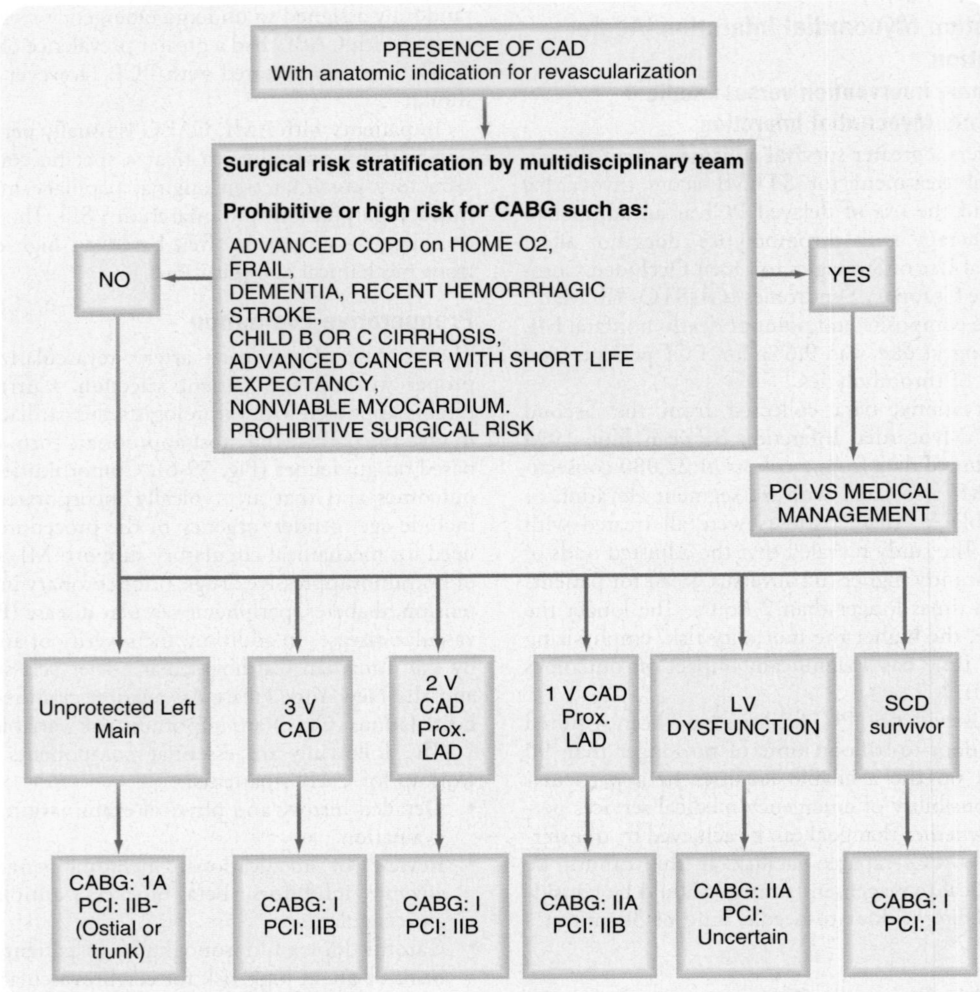

FIGURE 59-6 Surgical decision-making tree for coronary revascularization.

BOX 59-4 Major Steps in On-Pump Coronary Artery Bypass Grafting

- Induction of anesthesia and establishment of intraoperative monitoring adjuncts
- Positioning and draping
- Median sternotomy or appropriate approach
- Harvest and evaluation of blood conduits
- Heparinization and cannulation for cardiopulmonary bypass
- Establishment of cardiopulmonary bypass
- Myocardial arrest and protection
- Identification of target vessels and construction of distal anastomoses
- Restoration of myocardial electromechanical activity
- Creation of proximal anastomoses
- Weaning from cardiopulmonary bypass
- Evaluation for and establishment of necessary adjuncts—inotropes, IABP, pacing wires
- Reversal of anticoagulation and establishment of hemostasis
- Evaluation of surgical sites and establishment of surgical drainage
- Closure of sternotomy

chance of any nerve injury. A warming blanket is typically placed underneath the patient to assist in rewarming after controlled hypothermia during CPB. The entire chest, abdomen, and lower extremities are prepared. Circumferential preparation of the lower extremities is important because the leg may have to be maneuvered during harvesting of the saphenous vein conduit. If radial artery harvesting is being contemplated, the arm also has to be circumferentially prepared and positioned 90 degrees from the bedside on an arm board. Because most patients have a multilumen central line in the internal jugular vein or a Swan-Ganz catheter, the anesthesiologist must have continuous access to these lines, but without compromising the domain of the surgeon. Anchor points on the drapes are designated appropriately to allow CPB circuit lines to be secured without compromising sterility.

Cardiopulmonary Bypass

CPB is the establishment of extracorporeal oxygenation and perfusion of the human body by diverting all returning venous blood from the body to the heart-lung machine and returning the oxygenated blood in a controlled, pressurized manner. In essence, most blood flow to the heart and lungs is bypassed. Establishment

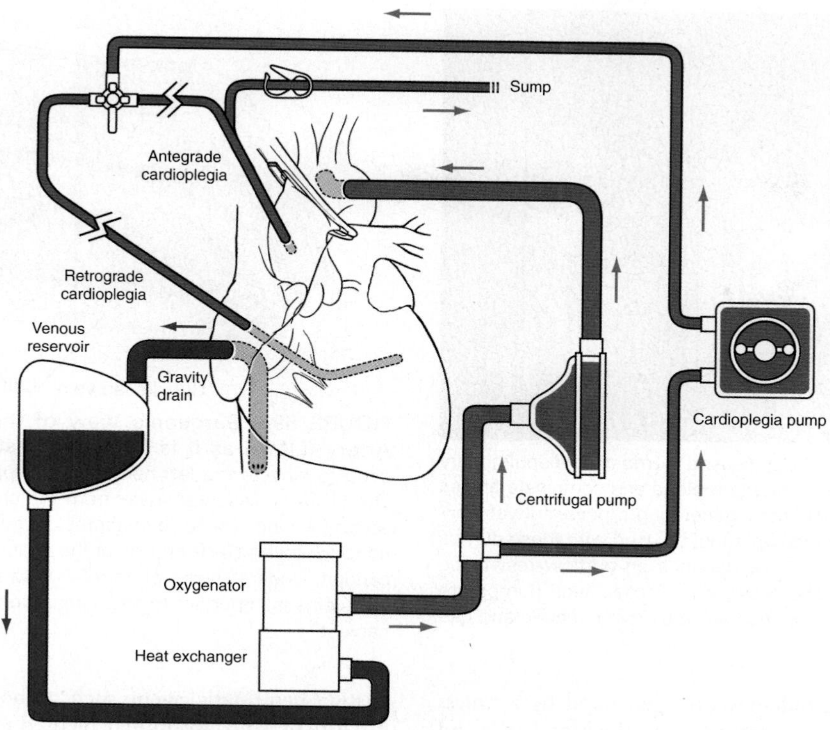

FIGURE 59-7 Schematic of Total Cardiopulmonary Bypass Circuit. All returning venous blood is siphoned into a venous reservoir and is oxygenated and temperature regulated before being pumped back through a centrifugal pump into the arterial circulation. The most common site for inflow cannulation is the ascending aorta; alternative sites include the femoral arteries and the right axillary artery in special circumstances. A parallel circuit derives oxygenated blood that is mixed with cold (4° C) cardioplegia solution in a 4 : 1 ratio and administered in antegrade or retrograde fashion to induce cardiac arrest. Cardioplegia solution is administered antegrade into the aortic root and retrograde through the coronary sinus. During the retrograde administration of cardioplegia solution, the efflux of blood from the coronary ostium is siphoned off through the sump drain, a return parallel circuit connected to the venous reservoir (not shown) that also helps to keep the heart decompressed during the arrest phase.

of CPB is a critical step for any major cardiac procedure and allows complete control of the operation.

The basic components of an extracorporeal heart pump circuit are venous cannulas to drain the returning venous blood, venous reservoir that collects blood by gravity, oxygenator and heat exchanger, perfusion pump, blood filter in the arterial line, and arterial cannula (Fig. 59-7). The blood conduits are designed to minimize turbulence, cavitation, and changes in blood flow velocity, which are detrimental to the integrity of component blood cells. Because the circuit contains a dead space created by the tubing and pump, a certain volume of nonblood solution is necessary to prime the pump and tubing. The priming solution consists of a balanced salt solution and, often, a starch solution. Homologous blood or fresh-frozen plasma may be added if the patient is anemic or if a bleeding problem is anticipated. The circuit has multiple access ports or sites from which to obtain blood samples for laboratory studies and into which to infuse blood, blood products, crystalloids, or drugs.

Supplemental components include a cardiotomy suction system to collect undiluted or clean blood from open cardiac chambers and the surgical field. This blood is filtered, de-aired, and returned to the bypass pump. Diluted field blood and blood that has mixed with inflammatory cytokines or fat is collected through a separate device that concentrates washed red cells before returning them directly to the patient.

A cardioplegia infusion device consists of a separate pump, reservoir, and heat exchanger. It is used to deliver cold, potassium-enriched blood or crystalloid solutions into the coronary circulation to arrest and to protect the heart.

Use of CPB requires suppression of the clotting cascade with heparin because the surgical wound and components of the bypass pump are powerful stimuli for thrombus formation. A strict anticoagulation protocol should be enforced before CPB is initiated. The pump prime is premixed with 4 U/mL heparin, and the patient is systemically heparinized with 300 U/kg before cannulation. An activated clotting time obtained approximately 3 minutes after heparin administration should be more than 400 seconds before cannulation is begun and should be maintained for more than 450 seconds throughout CPB, with intermittent doses given as needed during the operation.

The usual pumps are roller head pumps, which consist of circumferential tubing that is compressed by a roller on the outside, thereby forcing blood in one direction. This pump mechanism is associated with higher rates of hemolysis compared with centrifugal pumps, so roller head pumps are used only in cardiotomy suction and cardioplegia pumps. The main systemic pump is a centrifugal pump that consists of a vortex polyurethane-embedded magnetic cone housed in a conical chamber. The vortex spins at approximately 2000 to 5000 rpm, thereby generating enough centrifugal force to pump blood. Because the flow is

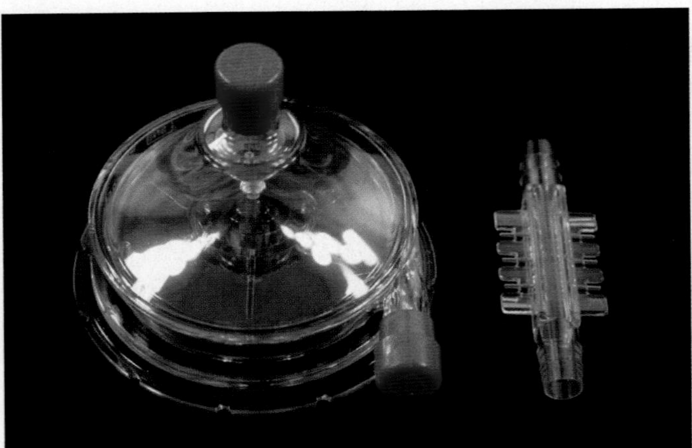

FIGURE 59-8 Main centrifugal pump used in most cardiopulmonary bypass circuits. The entire unit is sterile molded and contains a finless cone that spins at 2000 to 5000 rpm, generating a powerful yet nonturbulent vortex. A flow meter (shown) must be used with these pumps because the ultimate volume of flow depends on outflow resistance rather than on pump speed. The conventional roller head pumps are still used for the auxiliary circuits, such as cardiotomy suction and cardioplegia circuits.

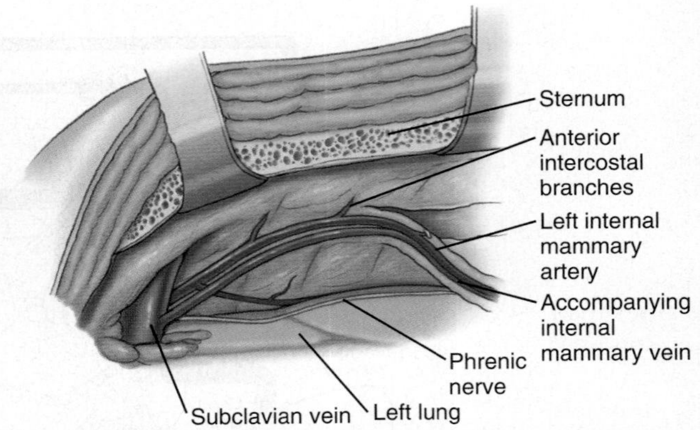

FIGURE 59-9 Surgeon's View of the Left Internal Mammary Artery (LIMA) as It Is Being Harvested. A mammary retractor is used to elevate the left hemithorax to provide adequate visualization. The LIMA is dissected away from the chest wall as a pedicle with its accompanying venae comitantes. Low-voltage electrocautery with no-touch technique is crucial for the atraumatic harvest of this important conduit. Understanding of its relation to the phrenic nerve and subclavian veins is important to avoid injury to these structures during LIMA harvest.

entirely caused by a nonturbulent vortex generated by a finless cone, this mechanism is almost atraumatic to the blood cells and is therefore associated with less hemolysis than the roller head pump mechanism (Fig. 59-8).

Neurologic Protection During Cardiopulmonary Bypass

The incidence of stroke after CPB is approximately 2.5%, but neurocognitive deficits are more frequent. Thus, several steps should be taken during CPB to minimize the risk of neurologic insult, including maintaining adequate cerebral perfusion, minimizing fat microemboli by eliminating the unnecessary use of cardiotomy suction, minimizing aortic manipulation by using single-clamp techniques when feasible, and instituting moderate hypothermia.

The oxygen consumption of a patient on CPB at normal temperatures averages 80 to 125 mL/min/m^2, similar to that of an anesthetized adult not on bypass. However, with the use of hypothermia, the oxygen consumption is markedly lower, and the flow rate can be reduced to less than 2.2 L/min/m^2. This is because the mean oxygen consumption of the body decreases by 50% for every 10° C decrease in body temperature. Below 28° C, a flow rate of 1.6 L/min/m^2 may be safe for as long as 2 hours. Significant disadvantages of using systemic hypothermia to accommodate lower flow rates include the extra time required to rewarm the patient and associated changes in the reactivity of blood elements, particularly platelets. These changes may increase the rewarmed patient's propensity for bleeding.

Median Sternotomy

The most common approach for performing CABG is a median sternotomy, although anterolateral thoracotomy is used in certain circumstances. A traditional sternotomy incision commences at the midpoint of the manubrium and is carried down to the xiphoid. The sternum is split through the middle with a sternal saw. It is essential that gentle upward force and a backward tilt be applied to the saw to prevent it from engaging the lung or soft tissues in the anterior mediastinum. Once the sternotomy is completed, the periosteum of the posterior table is cauterized, and a passive hemostatic agent such as bone wax or a reconstituted mixture of vancomycin may be used to prevent bleeding from the marrow. The most important consideration during the sternotomy is staying in the midline because the most common cause of sternal dehiscence is an off-midline sternotomy and the consequent technically suboptimal closure. Other potential problems associated with the sternotomy include indirect injury to the liver and direct injury to the heart, innominate vein, and lungs.

Conduit Choice and Harvesting

Left internal mammary artery. In a seminal study from the Cleveland Clinic, Loop and colleagues[59] have shown improved 10-year survival in patients who received a LIMA graft; patients who received a saphenous vein graft (SVG) had 1.6 times the risk of death that LIMA graft recipients had. The long-term patency rate of the LIMA graft has been shown to be approximately 95% and 90% at 10 and 20 years, respectively. The best patency rates are achieved when the LIMA is used as an in situ pedicled graft and is anastomosed to the LAD.

Bilateral internal mammary artery. Observational studies from major CABG centers suggested that the use of bilateral IMA (BIMA) grafts improves survival and significantly reduces the need for reoperation without increasing mortality. However, early results from a randomized trial demonstrated that compared with SVGs, BIMA grafts are associated with a higher (twofold) incidence of deep sternal wound infection. BIMA grafts are best used by experienced surgeons in younger, nondiabetic, nonobese patients. Four major studies that tilted the balance in favor of BIMA grafts were the two Cleveland Clinic studies (1999 and 2004), in which propensity scores were used to match single and bilateral IMA graft recipients; the Oxford meta-analysis (2001); and a retrospective study from Japan (2001). Skeletonization of the IMA grafts may reduce the wound complication rate.

The IMA is harvested after the sternotomy is completed. A specially designed mammary retractor is used to elevate the appropriate hemithorax, typically the left for harvesting the LIMA. Adequately exposing the undersurface of the sternum is essential for successful harvest of the IMA (Fig. 59-9). The artery may be harvested as a pedicle that includes the two venae comitantes and surrounding soft tissue from the level of the subclavian vein to the level of the bifurcation of the artery into the superior epigastric and musculophrenic branches. The alternative method of harvesting is the skeletonized harvest, in which only the IMA is dissected away from the chest wall.

The basic principle of harvesting the IMA relies exclusively on the no-touch technique, use of low-voltage electrocautery, and clipping of the anterior intercostal branches. Care must be taken during the harvest to identify the course of the phrenic nerves and to avoid injury to them. This is particularly important while harvesting the right IMA because the phrenic nerve is more closely related to it at the level of the second or third intercostal space. The IMA is a fragile vessel, and direct handling or undue traction should be avoided because it may cause traumatic dissection of the vessel. The distal end of the IMA should be divided only after the patient is fully heparinized to avoid thrombosis of the conduit. Once the IMA is divided, the distal end is spatulated appropriately to fashion the anastomosis.

Greater saphenous vein. Grafts made from this vein have a patency rate of 90% at 1 year.[60] Beyond 5 years after surgery, graft atherosclerosis develops in a substantial number of SVGs. By 10 years, only 60% to 70% of SVGs are patent, and 50% of those have angiographic evidence of atherosclerosis.

While the sternotomy is being done, a separate team begins harvesting saphenous or radial artery conduits. Saphenous vein harvesting can be performed by open or endoscopic techniques. The conventional method of open vein harvesting involves making a long incision along the entire length of the harvested vein. Alternatively, a bridging technique can be used in which multiple 1- to 2-inch incisions are made, with intact bridges of skin between them. The most common complications associated with long open incisions are pain, slow wound healing, and dehiscence, which is compounded by the fact that a significant number of CABG patients have diabetes or PVD. The use of endoscopic or bridging techniques significantly alleviates but does not entirely eliminate these problems. There are some centers that avoid endoscopic vein harvesting entirely on the assumption that the technique is too traumatic to the vein itself, may be associated with intimal trauma, and may impair the long-term patency of the conduit. However, studies have shown reduced graft patency in endoscopically harvested veins. These reports were based on post hoc analyses of data from trials designed to address other aspects of coronary revascularization. Once the vein is extracted and the branches are ligated, the graft is soaked in a heparin solution while awaiting implantation. The veins are typically used in a reversed fashion and hence may not require valvotomy. A typical configuration of a three-vessel coronary artery bypass graft is shown in Figure 59-10.

Alternative conduits may be needed in patients who have had previous coronary bypass, peripheral vascular surgery with the use of vein conduits, or lower extremity amputations and in those who have unusable saphenous vein conduits because of severe varicosities of the saphenous vein. Other manifestations of venous insufficiency or disease may also pose problems. In addition, patients who have severely calcified ascending aortas may not be amenable to a vein-based aortocoronary bypass because anastomosis to the ascending aorta is complicated. In these cases, alternative bypass strategies include total arterial revascularization with BIMA pedicles (Fig. 59-11). In addition, the IMA may be used as the main conduit from which further arterial conduits may be Christmas-treed in an off-pump setup so that any aortic manipulation is avoided.

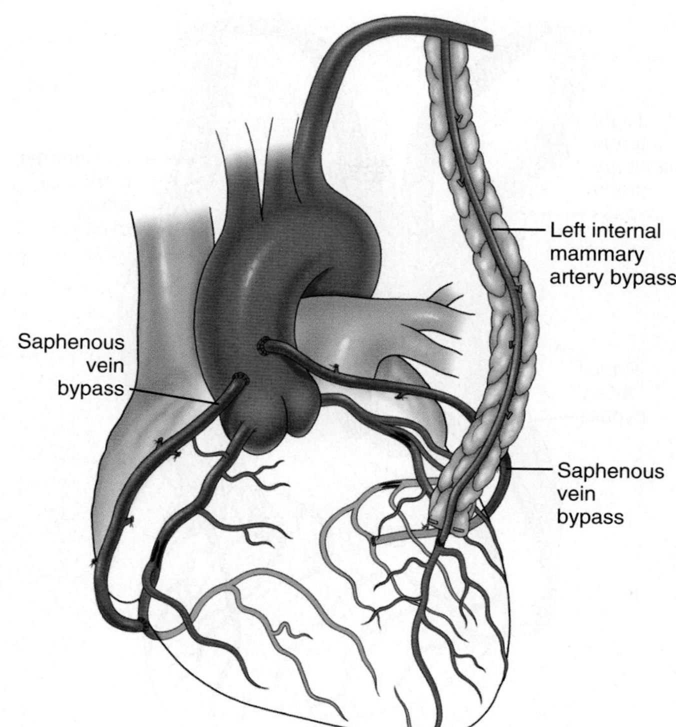

FIGURE 59-10 Typical Configuration for a Three-Vessel Coronary Artery Bypass. The left internal mammary artery is anastomosed to the left anterior descending artery. Aortocoronary bypasses are created with reversed saphenous vein to the distal right coronary artery and an obtuse marginal branch of the circumflex coronary artery. The circumflex coronary artery is usually avoided as a target for bypass because its location well inside the atrioventricular groove makes it difficult to visualize.

Other conduits

Radial artery. The radial artery graft is easily harvested and can reach all coronary territories, making it an attractive option for an arterial conduit. Both the Radial Artery Patency Study and the Radial Artery versus Saphenous Vein Patency study showed radial artery grafts to have better patency than SVGs on 5-year angiographic follow-up. However, the radial artery is associated with a significantly higher incidence of string sign. In addition, to date, no study has shown a survival advantage of radial artery over SVG grafting. Also, patency is much worse if the radial grafts are not placed on critically stenotic vessels.

Gastroepiploic artery. The gastroepiploic artery is rarely used today, although some centers in Asia still use gastroepiploic grafts and continue to report acceptable outcomes associated with them. Evidence from RCTs and a recent meta-analysis suggests that the saphenous vein has better early (6-month) and midterm (3-year) graft patency than the right gastroepiploic artery when it is used for RCA revascularization.

Total Arterial Revascularization

More than 95% of all CABG operations performed in the United States and more than 90% of those performed in the United Kingdom and Australia involve only one arterial graft.[61,62] The LIMA and SVG remain the standard CABG grafts; SVGs account for most of the conduits used. Of these SVGs, 40% to 50% become occluded at 10 years, and more than 75% are occluded

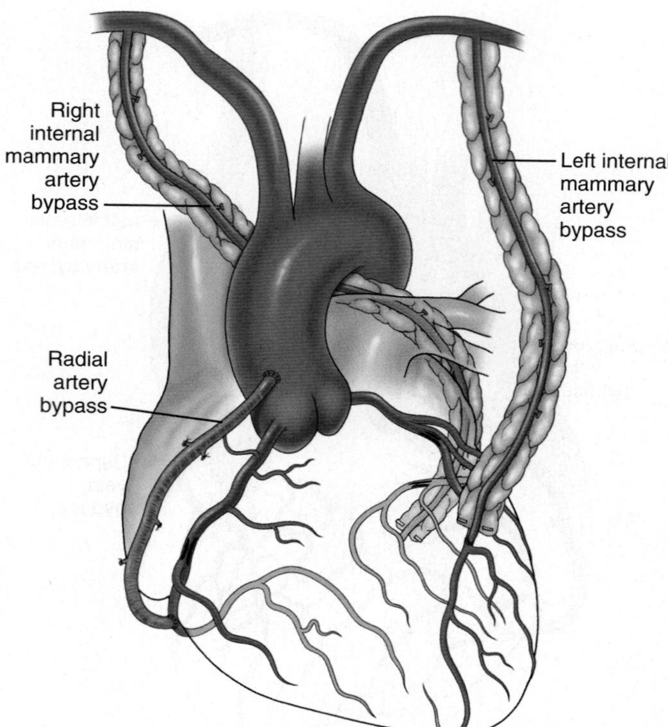

FIGURE 59-11 Total arterial revascularization by use of bilateral mammary artery and radial artery conduits. The right internal mammary artery, bypassed to an obtuse marginal branch, is routed behind the aorta, and the pulmonary artery is routed through the transverse sinus.

at 15 years. In an effort to ameliorate these shortcomings of SVGs, some centers have been heavily emphasizing total arterial revascularization in which the LIMA, right IMA, and radial arteries are used.

Results from retrospective series have shown some survival benefit with total arterial revascularization, as would be expected. However, there are certain pragmatic reasons that total arterial revascularization has not totally replaced the use of SVGs:

- Concern about arterial spasm: Most arterial grafts are prone to spasm, and their use necessitates vasodilator administration, both locally and systemically, for a prolonged period. This can interfere with achieving stable hemodynamics in the immediate postoperative period.
- Use of arterial grafts appropriate only for severely stenotic arteries: Most experts would not use an arterial graft other than the LAD unless the stenosis was at least 80% and probably 90% or more because of the risk of competitive flow. It is well known that venous grafts work with less critical lesions.
- Inadequate length: As an in situ graft, the right IMA is not long enough to reach the PDA, distal RCA, mid or distal circumflex, or distal LAD and cannot be used easily as a sequential graft. It can, however, be used as a free graft.
- Concern about sternal nonunion and mediastinitis: There is a higher risk of sternal nonunion and mediastinitis with the use of BIMA grafts versus SVGs. Most experts will not use BIMA grafts in patients with diabetes, severe PVD, use of steroids, severe chronic obstructive pulmonary disease, or morbid obesity. Also, in the event that BIMA is used, most would recommend the skeletonized technique of BIMA harvest with preservation of the intercostal blood supply.
- Longer operative times: Using BIMA grafts obviously prolongs operative times.

Because of all these practical considerations, total arterial revascularization has not become as popular as would be expected, and most surgeons would offer total arterial revascularization only to younger patients because of their longer life expectancy.

Cannulation for Cardiopulmonary Bypass

Cannulation for establishment of CPB commences after conduit harvest and preparation are completed, the pericardium is opened, and the thymus is divided along the embryologic fusion plane. The patient is fully heparinized at a dose of 3 mg/kg. A purse-string is created on the anterior surface of the distal ascending aorta at the cannulation site. The aortic purse-string should involve only a partial thickness of the aorta, incorporating the adventitia and media but entirely avoiding the intimal layer. It is essential that the cannulation site be free of calcified plaques or atheroma to minimize the chance of embolization and cannulation site bleeding. Manual palpation, the commonly practiced method of assessment, is unreliable. Doppler transesophageal or epiaortic ultrasonographic guidance should be used whenever aortic disease is suspected. Also, the presence of calcium elsewhere in the ascending aorta may preclude safe clamp application. Although cannulation of the aorta may be a simple task, loss of control of the aortic cannulation site or inadvertent dissection could lead to a disastrous situation.

With a sharp scalpel, the adventitia is teased, and a full-thickness stab incision is made. The aortic cannula is inserted with the outflow bevel aimed toward the aortic arch. Tourniquet snares are used to secure the cannula in position and are tied. After the cannula is de-aired, it is connected to the arterial line of the CPB circuit. Alternative sites of arterial cannulation include the femoral artery and right axillary artery, which are used in reoperations or cases in which concomitant complex aortic and arch reconstruction may be required. Axillary artery cannulation is usually achieved with an 8-mm graft anastomosed end to side to the axillary artery.

For venous cannulation, a purse-string is then placed around the right atrial appendage. The tip of this appendage is amputated, and a dual-stage venous cannula is inserted and positioned with the tip at the level of the diaphragm. The basket of the dual-stage cannula should rest in the main chamber of the right atrium to capture drainage from the superior vena cava into the right atrium (Figs. 59-12 and 59-13).

Cardiac Arrest and Myocardial Protection

The initiation of CPB allows the heart to be stopped. To achieve cardiac arrest, a large dose of potassium solution (cardioplegia) is injected into the coronary vessels. This requires the coronary blood flow to be completely isolated from the systemic circulation, which is done by applying a cross-clamp to the ascending aorta proximal to the aortic cannula.

There are several different delivery options for cardioplegia solutions. One involves taking a balanced approach; the cardioplegia solution is administered antegrade through the ascending aorta proximal to the cross-clamp and then retrograde through a coronary sinus catheter inserted through a purse-string suture placed in the right atrium by use of special cannulas (Fig. 59-14). The extensive collateralization among the coronary veins and arteries and the paucity of valves in the coronary vein system ensure a relatively homogeneous distribution of cardioplegia solution when the retrograde approach is used. Patients with high-grade

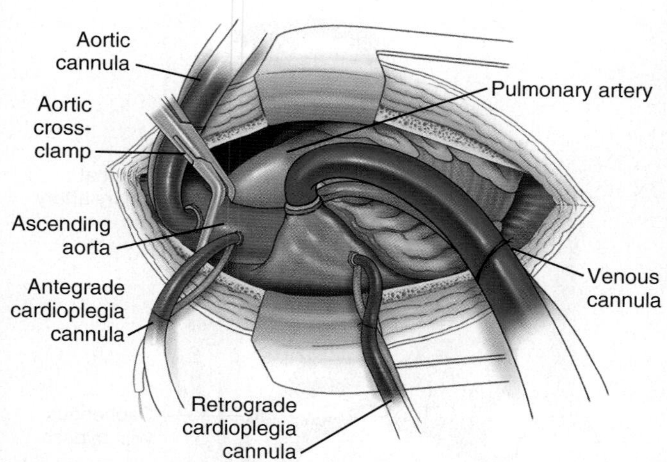

FIGURE 59-12 Surgeon's View of the Heart After Cannulation. The cross-clamp isolates the aortic root and coronary vessels from the rest of the systemic circulation. This allows administration of cardioplegia solution in a closed circuit and prevents the systemic blood from washing the cardioplegia solution out of the coronary system during the arrest phase. Applying the cross-clamp prevents active blood flow through the coronary arteries and thus allows the surgeon to perform the distal anastomoses in a bloodless field.

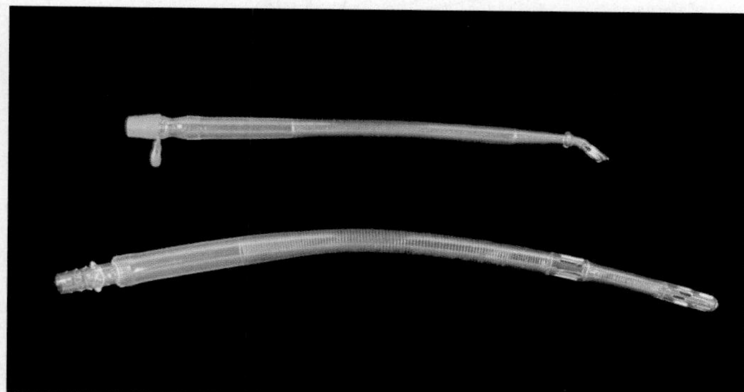

FIGURE 59-13 Aortic cannula *(top):* The specially designed tip is angulated to allow laminar flow of blood into the aortic arch. Dual-stage venous cannula *(bottom):* The first stage is the fenestrated basket that usually rests at the level of the hepatic veins and captures all venous return from the inferior vena cava. The second-stage basket is located such that it remains within the right atrium and captures venous return from the superior vena cava, azygos vein, coronary sinus, and direct collateral drainage into the right atrium. The venous drainage is a passive siphon aided by gravity.

proximal lesions, especially those with suboptimal collateral vessels, may benefit from the application of both techniques. After the initial administration of cardioplegia solution, additional doses are usually administered every 15 to 20 minutes.

An antegrade cardioplegia line with a Y-connector to the circuit is inserted into the ascending aorta. This allows antegrade administration of cardioplegia solution and also sumping and decompression of the ascending aorta while cardioplegia solution is administered retrogradely into the coronary sinus. The sump drain also functions to keep the coronary arteries free of any blood, thus providing the surgeon with a bloodless field in which to fashion the distal anastomoses. In addition, the sump drain performs the important function of decompressing the LV while the heart is arrested (see Figs. 59-7 and 59-12).

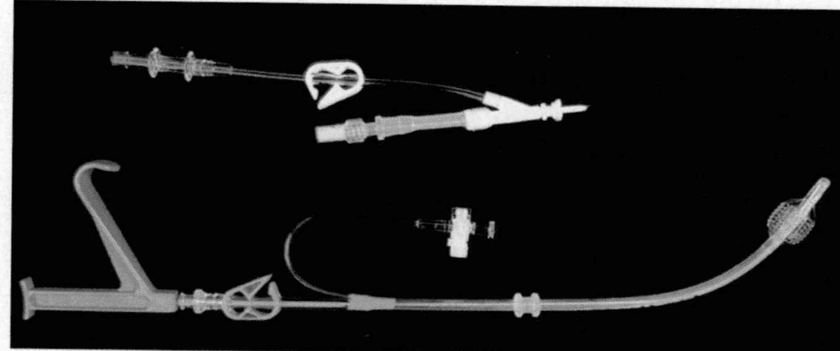

FIGURE 59-14 Retrograde cardioplegia cannula *(bottom)* used to administer cardioplegia solution into the coronary sinus. The self-inflating balloon distends, forming a seal only when cardioplegia solution is administered. Antegrade cardioplegia cannula *(top)* used to administer cardioplegia solution into the aortic root. The side port functions as a sump.

The most important task for ensuring myocardial protection is establishing complete diastolic arrest with an unloaded heart. In this state, the myocardial consumption of adenosine triphosphate is extremely low and allows maximal preservation of myocytes. In conventional CABG with total CPB, the decompression of the ventricle by off-loading, systemic cooling, topical cooling, and diastolic arrest of the heart with potassium cardioplegia solution serves to decrease myocardial oxygen consumption. Approximately 40% of the myocardial metabolic demand is eliminated when total CPB is established before diastolic arrest and cooling are instituted.

Target Identification and Distal Anastomosis

Once successful diastolic arrest of the heart is accomplished, the target coronary arteries to be bypassed are identified. Some of the epicardial conductance vessels are intramyocardial and therefore may not be directly visible. Once a target vessel is identified, it is opened with a sharp blade. Typically, the arteriotomy is approximately 5 mm long. The conduit, which is prepared and spatulated, is then grafted in an end-to-side fashion with running 7-0 Prolene suture. This component of the operation is technically the most challenging and requires precision. The flow and integrity of each vein conduit are tested by flushing it with cold blood or cardioplegia solution mix. The LIMA to left descending artery anastomosis is usually the last one to be performed (Fig. 59-15) because it is best to avoid manipulating the heart once this anastomosis is completed in case avulsion of the LIMA conduit occurs. Bypassing the PDA and obtuse marginal targets requires lifting the apex of the heart out of the pericardium.

Typically, a single segment of conduit is anastomosed to each planned distal target. On occasion, a single conduit can be used to supply blood to two targets, which is known as a sequential anastomosis. This is a good technique to use when there is a shortage of available vein conduits or when the target vessels are small; in these cases, use of this technique ensures a higher rate of blood flow through the vein conduit, reducing the risk of graft thrombosis (Fig. 59-16).

As the last distal anastomosis is being completed, the patient is warmed back to physiologic temperature. The cross-clamp is released after the final dose of warm cardioplegia solution is administered, which helps in scavenging the accumulated free radicals in the myocardium. A partial clamp is then applied to the ascending aorta, and the proximal anastomoses are constructed in an end-to-side fashion with running 5-0 Prolene suture. If there

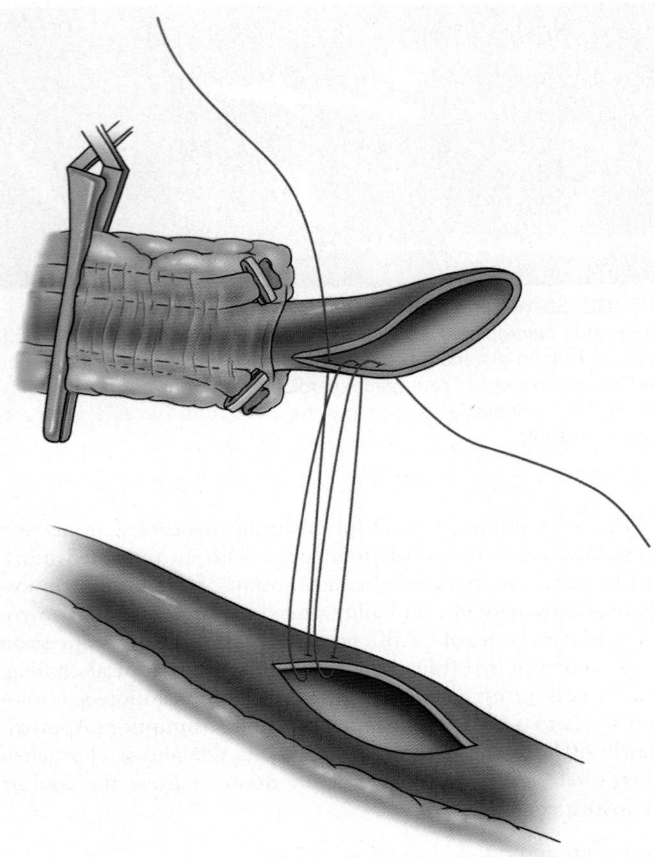

FIGURE 59-15 Technique of constructing the distal anastomoses: left internal mammary artery to left anterior descending artery, magnified surgeon's view. A 5-mm longitudinal arteriotomy is made on the coronary artery to be bypassed. The distal end of the left internal mammary artery is spatulated to an appropriate size match. A 7-0 Prolene suture is used to create the anastomosis with a parachuting technique.

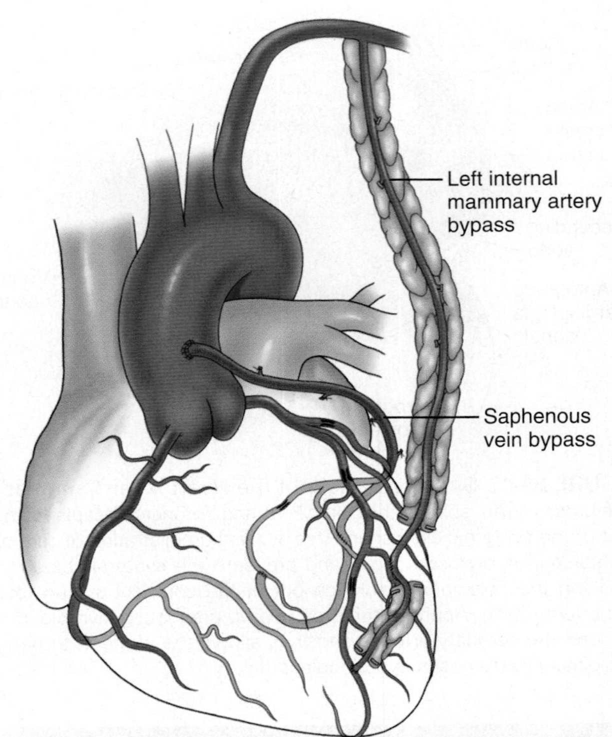

FIGURE 59-16 Alternative Configuration for a Three-Vessel Coronary Artery Bypass. The left internal mammary artery is anastomosed sequentially to a diagonal branch and to the distal left anterior descending artery. Aortocoronary bypasses are constructed with reversed saphenous vein in sequential configuration to the left posterolateral artery and an obtuse marginal branch of the circumflex coronary artery. The ideal configuration depends on the extent and distribution of the coronary blockages.

are concerns about the quality of the aorta, use of a partial clamp is typically avoided in favor of a single-clamp technique, which involves constructing the proximal anastomoses on an arrested heart, as for the distal anastomoses.

In patients in whom the ascending aorta is calcified or a free IMA pedicle needs to be used, a branching pattern of proximal anastomoses is made. This conserves vein length to a certain extent but also minimizes the number of aortotomies, especially if the ascending aorta is short or a concomitant aortic procedure has been performed. The ascending aorta is allowed to de-air as the aortic clamp is released, after which the vein grafts are de-aired.

Separation from Cardiopulmonary Bypass

Separation from CPB commences once the following physiologic criteria have been met:

- Resumption of rhythmic electromechanical activity
- Attainment of physiologic temperature above 36.5° C
- Availability of adequate reserve blood volume
- Restoration of normal systemic potassium levels
- Resumption of ventilation with an acceptable arterial blood gas level

A few other actions that may be considered at this point are placement of temporary pacing wires and insertion of an IABP, if needed. Typically, the CPB flows are progressively decreased as the following parameters are closely observed:

- Data from the Swan-Ganz catheter
- Direct visual observations of cardiac function and chamber volume
- The transesophageal echocardiogram

Most patients have a transient systemic inflammatory response, causing vasodilation that becomes more pronounced as they are warmed. Thus, restoration of volume with intravascular fluids or administration of vasopressors may be necessary to maintain systemic blood pressure. Inotropic agents may be used if ventricular function is not adequate. Separating patients from CPB is primarily the surgeon's responsibility but requires dynamic communication with the perfusionist and anesthesiologist.

After CPB is discontinued, the venous cannula is removed and the purse-string is tied down. Once it is confirmed that the heart is providing satisfactory perfusion, protamine is administered. Close monitoring is needed because adverse reactions to protamine range from transient hypotension to fatal anaphylaxis. Such reactions necessitate the resumption of CPB.

Hemostasis

As protamine is being administered, hemostasis is expeditiously accomplished. As the patient rewarms, blood vessels that had been hemostatic may dilate and rebleed. Persistent bleeding should alert the surgeon to the following possible causes: aspects of the surgical technique; platelet dysfunction; inadequate protamine reversal; and hypothermia. The administration of blood and blood products may be necessary.

Sternal Closure and Completion of Surgery

The chest tube and temporary pacing wires should be checked for appropriate positioning. The sternum is approximated with stainless steel wires. The soft tissues and skin are closed in layers with absorbable sutures.

ADJUNCTS TO CORONARY ARTERY BYPASS GRAFTING

Transesophageal Echocardiography

Use of transesophageal echocardiography (TEE) enables the assessment of ventricular wall motion abnormalities and the detection of any chamber or valve anomalies that may change the strategy of the operation. Examples of TEE findings that may affect the conduct of the operation include an incidentally discovered large patent foramen ovale or fibroelastoma of the valves. New-onset or worsening mitral regurgitation after CABG suggests inferior wall ischemia and may indicate reevaluation of the bypass grafts or valve repair or replacement. Also, TEE helps in assessing ejection fraction and the volume status of the heart after surgery.

Inotropes and Pharmacotherapy

Cardioplegic arrest causes transient myocardial ischemia and lactic acid accumulation. After perfusion is reestablished, the ventricles are stiffer and require higher filling pressures to maintain adequate stroke volume. Also, CPB may cause significant third spacing and vasodilation. Thus, epinephrine as an inotropic agent is ideal to maintain adequate contractility in the initial recovery phase and during separation from CPB. Alpha agonists such as norepinephrine, phenylephrine, and vasopressin may be used to counteract the effects of inflammatory vasodilation. In patients with depressed myocardial function, such as left- or right-sided heart failure, dobutamine or a phosphodiesterase inhibitor such as milrinone may be required to enhance myocardial contractility and to decrease afterload or pulmonary vascular resistance. Because hypotension is a common side effect of these drugs, the systemic volume must be adequate, and an alpha agonist may be required. Calcium channel blockers or nitroglycerin may be needed in patients with preexisting hypertension.

It is essential to maintain a mean arterial pressure higher than 60 mm Hg in the initial postoperative period, but hypertension should be avoided because it puts stress on a myocardium that is trying to recover and increases the risk of bleeding from anastomotic suture lines. Blood pressure management requires a thorough understanding of physiologic and pharmacologic principles. It is a balancing act geared toward maintaining adequate systemic pressure, cardiac output, and peripheral perfusion while minimizing myocardial stress. Urine output is the most reliable indicator of peripheral organ perfusion.

Intra-Aortic Balloon Pump

For patients whose profound myocardial dysfunction is unresponsive to volume resuscitation and significant pharmacologic therapy, IABP support may be indicated. The IABP is a special Silastic balloon with a capacity of 40 to 60 mL that is positioned in the descending aorta just beyond the origin of the left subclavian artery. The balloon is designed to be actively inflated and deflated during each cardiac cycle; its timing is controlled by a specially designed computer with input from an arterial line tracing or ECG. Intra-aortic balloon counterpulsation has the benefit of decreasing myocardial work and oxygen consumption while increasing coronary perfusion.

The balloon is actively deflated just before systolic contraction begins, thereby decreasing LV impedance and assisting in the ejection of blood. The balloon then actively inflates at the time of aortic valve closure, that is, it is timed to occur at the dicrotic notch of the arterial line tracing. This increases the diastolic perfusion pressure and improves coronary blood flow, both of which decrease the time-tension index and increase the diastolic pressure-time index, thereby increasing the myocardial oxygen supply-to-demand ratio. The use of IABP is absolutely contraindicated in patients with aortic regurgitation and aortic dissection. It is relatively contraindicated in patients with PVD or aortic aneurysm.

POSTOPERATIVE CARE

Postoperative care in the intensive care unit (ICU) begins with a thorough physical and hemodynamic assessment. Mediastinal chest tube drainage should be recorded and assessed hourly. Initial ventilator settings should be set to match those in the operating room. Further adjustments in ventilator settings are made according to the postoperative blood gases. High positive end-expiratory pressure should be avoided in patients with hemodynamic instability. The ideal mode of ventilation is that with which the surgical or intensive care team is comfortable. A portable chest radiograph is obtained to confirm the position of the endotracheal tube, central lines, Swan-Ganz catheter, and IABP and to identify any pneumothorax, atelectasis, pulmonary edema, or pleural effusions. Initial laboratory studies should include hemoglobin, hematocrit, electrolyte, blood urea nitrogen, creatinine, and arterial blood gas levels and platelet count, prothrombin time, and partial thromboplastin time.

The patient should have an ECG monitor that can assess ST-T wave abnormalities; an arterial line to measure arterial blood pressure; and a line to measure central venous pressure, pulse oximetry, and core temperature. In select patients, pulmonary artery pressures and cardiac output are monitored continuously with a Swan-Ganz catheter. Neurologic assessment should be completed as soon as the patient wakes up to ensure that no cerebrovascular accident has occurred.

The primary considerations during the first 12 hours after the operation should be maintaining adequate blood pressure and cardiac output, correcting coagulation defects and electrolyte levels, stabilizing intravascular volume, and normalizing the peripheral vascular resistance. This often involves administration of crystalloid solutions, blood or blood products, inotropic agents, calcium, and vasodilators or vasoconstrictors.

Some of the goals in the postoperative period are as follows:

- Avoiding marked elevations in blood pressure
- Maintaining adequate perfusion pressure (60-80 mm Hg)
- Maintaining core body temperature higher than 36.5°C by warming the patient with forced hot air blankets
- Maintaining adequate cardiac output and a cardiac index of 2.2 L/min/m^2
- Keeping mixed venous oxygenation at 60%
- Reducing afterload, as appropriate, to minimize myocardial work

- Volume resuscitation with crystalloid or blood products, as necessary
- Maintaining hemoglobin level higher than 8 g/dL, or higher than 10 g/dL in older patients or those with severe cerebrovascular disease
- Maintaining homeostatic pH. Metabolic acidosis may be caused by hypoperfusion from low cardiac output, poor resuscitation, hypovolemia, or end-organ ischemia from embolism.
- Monitoring neurologic and peripheral vascular status
- Maintaining a sinus or perfusing rhythm at a rate of 70 to 100 beats/min
- Monitoring for and treating postoperative cardiac arrhythmias
- Ensuring adequate pain control to minimize fluctuations in blood pressure and myocardial stress
- Keeping blood glucose levels below 180 mg/dL. Standardized insulin-infusion regimens should be initiated, if needed.

Pulmonary Care

It is desirable to separate patients from the ventilator as soon as they awaken, are hemodynamically stable with minimal chest tube drainage, and can maintain a satisfactory spontaneous tidal volume and respiratory rate. Coughing and deep breathing exercises with appropriate sternal precautions are essential for postoperative recovery. Suboptimal postoperative pulmonary function may indicate additional therapy, including the use of bronchodilators, mucolytics, and chest physical therapy. Although β-adrenergic bronchodilators and *N*-acetylcysteine are useful adjuncts, they also can induce atrial fibrillation.

After extubation, it is important to provide the patient with sufficient pain relief to minimize emotional distress, poor coughing, and reluctance to begin ambulation. Unrelieved pain can also be a source of tachycardia, hypertension, myocardial ischemia, atelectasis, hypoxia, and pneumonia.

Discharge from the Intensive Care Unit

Before the patient leaves the ICU, unnecessary lines and catheters should be removed. Chest tubes are removed approximately 48 hours postoperatively, when the combined drainage is less than 200 mL per shift and chest radiography reveals no effusion. Removal of temporary atrial and ventricular pacing wires is often deferred to the third postoperative day.

Outcomes

Hospital Mortality

Seven core variables—emergency of operation, age, prior heart surgery, gender, LVEF, percentage stenosis of LCA, and number of major coronary arteries with more than 70% stenosis—have the greatest impact on CABG mortality. Other variables are important but have minimal impact when added to these core variables; these include recent MI (<1 week), angina severity, ventricular arrhythmia, CHF, mitral regurgitation, diabetes, PVD, renal insufficiency, and creatinine level.

In cardiac surgery, operative mortality has traditionally included 30-day and in-hospital mortality. The mortality figure for CABG is 1% to 3% in most modern series. Risk-adjusted outcomes have become the gold standard for reporting and comparing cardiac surgery outcomes. The STS database is the largest and most authoritative voluntary national database to date. The STS has developed a risk calculator that estimates morbidity and mortality for a given patient's risk profile. The observed-to-expected mortality ratio for a given surgeon or institution can then be determined.

Long-Term Survival

Survival after CABG is related to cardiac and noncardiac comorbidities. Risk factors for atherosclerosis, particularly cigarette smoking, hypercholesterolemia, hypertension, and diabetes, are associated with decreased survival.

In no longitudinal study has CABG obliterated the negative impact of abnormal LV function on late survival. Incomplete revascularization is associated with decreased survival, whereas complete revascularization, the use of the LIMA, and, in some studies, the use of BIMA are associated with improved survival.

The CASS documented overall survival of 96%, 90%, 74%, 56%, and 45% at 1, 5, 10, 15, and 18 postoperative years, respectively. These figures are inferior to those for the age-matched U.S. population and for modern series of patients who receive single or bilateral mammary grafts.

Morbidity

Tamponade. Pericardial tamponade is caused by the formation of pericardial clot and compression of the heart. The condition should be suspected if there is evidence of low cardiac output, hypotension coincident with tachycardia, and elevated central venous pressure. The quantity of mediastinal drainage is an unreliable predictor of tamponade, although an abrupt decline in mediastinal chest tube drainage should raise suspicion of tamponade caused by absence of an exit path for the blood. Widening of the mediastinum on chest radiography and echocardiographic evidence of a pericardial effusion should confirm the diagnosis.

If a Swan-Ganz catheter is in place and right- and left-sided heart pressures are monitored, the central venous pressure and pulmonary capillary wedge pressure are usually elevated and equal. The earliest manifestation of tamponade is an acute drop in mixed venous oxygen saturation. After the diagnosis is made, the patient should be returned to the operating room for evacuation of the clot and relief of the compression. If the patient's condition is rapidly deteriorating, the sternotomy incision may have to be reopened at the bedside.

Postoperative bleeding. The combination of heparinization, hypothermia, CPB, and protamine reversal is associated with increased risk for bleeding after CABG. Post-CABG bleeding that requires transfusion or reoperation is associated with a significant increase in morbidity and mortality risk. A minority of patients having cardiac procedures (15% to 20%) consume more than 80% of all blood products transfused at operation. Blood must be viewed as a scarce resource that carries significant risks and unproven benefits. There is a high-risk subset of patients who require multiple preventive measures to reduce the chance of postoperative bleeding. Nine variables stand out as important indicators of risk (Box 59-5).

Available evidence-based blood conservation techniques include the following:

- Administration of drugs that increase preoperative blood volume (e.g., erythropoietin) or decrease postoperative bleeding (e.g., ε-aminocaproic acid). Aprotinin is currently banned in the United States because some studies have associated it with increased mortality, stroke, and renal failure when it is administered to cardiac surgery patients.
- Intraoperative blood salvage and blood-sparing interventions
- Interventions that protect the patient's own blood from the stress of operation (e.g., autologous predonation, normovolemic hemodilution)
- Institution-specific blood transfusion algorithms supplemented with point-of-care testing

BOX 59-5 Risk Factors for Postoperative Bleeding

- Advanced age
- Low preoperative red blood cell volume (preoperative anemia or small body size)
- Preoperative antiplatelet or antithrombotic drugs
- Reoperative or complex procedures
- Emergency operations
- Noncardiac patient comorbidities
- Renal failure
- Chronic obstructive pulmonary disease
- Congestive heart failure

BOX 59-6 Causes of Immediate Postoperative Bleeding

Surgical
- Conduit
- Anastomoses
- Cannulation sites
- Mammary bed
- Thymic veins
- Pericardial edge
- Sternal wire sites

Platelet dysfunction
Inadequate protamine reversal
Hypothermia

Despite efforts at blood conservation to limit perioperative bleeding and blood transfusions, 2% to 3% of patients will require reexploration for bleeding, and as many as 20% will have excessive bleeding and blood transfusion postoperatively. Bleeding of more than 500 mL in the first hour or persistent bleeding of more than 200 mL/hr for 4 hours is an indication for mediastinal exploration. Exploration is also indicated if a large hemothorax is identified on chest radiography or pericardial tamponade occurs. Usually, a specific bleeding site is not identified. Box 59-6 summarizes the common causes of immediate postoperative bleeding.

Neurologic complications. There are two types of neurologic deficits after CABG: type I deficit, which is a focal neurologic deficit; and type II deficit, which is manifested as nonspecific encephalopathy. In a 1996 multi-institutional prospective study, 6% of patients had these adverse outcomes, which were evenly distributed between the two types of deficit. Associated mortality was 20% for type I, which was twice the mortality for type II deficit. Age (especially >70 years) and hypertension are consistent risk factors for both types. History of previous neurologic abnormality, diabetes, and atherosclerosis of the aorta are risk factors for type I. Significant atherosclerosis of the ascending aorta mandates a surgical approach that will minimize the possibility of atherosclerotic emboli. Patients with concomitant carotid stenosis are at an elevated risk for neurologic complications. One approach used in such patients involves a staged procedure in which the more symptomatic and more critical vascular bed is addressed first. Otherwise, a combined approach may be used, but this poses a greater overall risk.

Mediastinitis. The incidence of deep sternal wound infection is 1% to 4% in CABG patients. Risk factors include obesity, reoperation, diabetes, and duration and complexity of operation. Using a BIMA graft can increase the risk of sternal wound complications in high-risk patients. The use of perioperative antibiotics and a strict protocol aimed at controlling the blood glucose level to less than 180 mg/dL by continuous intravenous infusion of insulin has been shown to reduce the incidence of mediastinitis significantly. Early débridement and muscle flap closure improve outcome. More recently, good outcomes have also been reported with the use of wound vacuum-assisted closures after adequate débridement.

Renal dysfunction. Mangano and coworkers have reported a 7.7% incidence of postoperative renal dysfunction (PRD) in CABG patients and mortality rates of 0.9%, 19%, and 63% in patients without PRD, patients with PRD but without need for dialysis, and patients who required dialysis, respectively. The 63% figure was confirmed in a large Veterans Administration study.

Medical Adjuncts for Postoperative Management

The following drugs are considered essential components of the postoperative management of CABG patients:

- Aspirin administration, 81 to 325 mg orally or rectally, is begun on the same day after CABG, unless the patient is bleeding because of platelet dysfunction. This is a quality-of-care index and has been shown to improve long-term graft patency.
- Beta blocker administration should begin after all inotropes have been discontinued. The goal is to maintain a heart rate of 60 to 80 beats/min and adequate mean perfusion pressures.
- Afterload reduction is important in all patients with a low LVEF. Afterload reduction is commenced after all inotropes are discontinued and adequate beta blockade is achieved. The angiotensin-converting enzyme inhibitors are first-line drugs for afterload reduction. Creatinine levels should be monitored.
- For antiarrhythmic treatment, amiodarone is used in many cardiac centers as prophylaxis against or treatment of atrial fibrillation. This drug should be used with caution in patients with preexisting interstitial lung disease and those taking warfarin. A prolonged Q-T interval is a contraindication.
- Administration of furosemide, a diuretic, is begun on the first postoperative day; the goal is to maintain a negative fluid balance. Chest radiography, creatinine levels, physical examination, and input-output charts help guide the dose of furosemide.

ALTERNATIVE METHODS FOR MYOCARDIAL REVASCULARIZATION

Cardiopulmonary Bypass With Hypothermic Fibrillatory Arrest

Hypothermic fibrillatory arrest is a good on-pump alternative to conventional cardioplegic arrest and avoids the use of the aortic cross-clamp. Although cardioplegic arrest offers maximal myocardial protection while providing a stable, immobile target for the distal anastomoses, not all patients are amenable to cardioplegia-based arrest. In patients with an extensively calcified aorta, cross-clamp application may be precarious and associated with an elevated incidence of stroke.

In these cases, a hypothermic fibrillatory arrest strategy may be used in which aortic manipulation is minimized. Once CPB is initiated, the patient is cooled to 28° C. The heart typically begins fibrillating at approximately 32° C. An LV sump is usually introduced through the right superior pulmonary vein to ensure LV decompression. Handling of the distal and proximal targets is similar to off-pump CABG (OPCAB) techniques because the coronary arteries are still fully perfused while the anastomoses are being performed. Vessel loops or occluders may be needed. In patients with extensive aortic calcification, there may not be any room to place an aortic cannula in or a proximal vein graft on the ascending aorta. In these cases, the right axillary artery may be used for arterial perfusion, and the saphenous vein can be anastomosed to the innominate artery if it is free of disease, or a total arterial vascularization approach should be considered with the use of one or both mammary arteries.

Once the anastomoses are completed, the patient is rewarmed to physiologic temperature and the heart is defibrillated into sinus rhythm. The use of hypothermic fibrillatory arrest is contraindicated in patients with significant aortic valve incompetence because the ventricle would distend with the regurgitant blood once fibrillation sets in, and no stroke volume is generated. Increased ventricular wall tension and energy consumption could lead to myocardial ischemia.

On-Pump Beating-Heart Bypass

On-pump beating-heart bypass is a selective strategy used for patients who have a very low LVEF and have suffered a recent MI. The logic behind this approach is that the myocardium is severely compromised and would poorly tolerate further ischemic compromise. Despite currently available techniques for myocardial protection, cardioplegic arrest is always associated with a certain degree of ischemia. This is especially true in patients with severe CAD and a stunned myocardium, in whom uniform protection of the ventricle with cardioplegia may be difficult to achieve, and an on-pump beating-heart strategy can be considered. The coronary arteries continue to be perfused, and exposure and handling of the anastomoses are similar to those for OPCAB. The use of CPB offloads the ventricle and offers a safety margin to manipulate the heart and to visualize all the targets that need to be bypassed. Use of IABP should be considered for most of these patients because their hemodynamic state is precarious to begin with.

Off-Pump Coronary Artery Bypass Grafting

The main rationale for using OPCAB was to avoid the adverse effects of CPB related to the systemic inflammatory response caused by contact of blood components with the surface of the bypass circuit. This hypothesis, although not supported by much sound scientific clinical data, spawned the belief that CPB contributed to various adverse outcomes, including postoperative bleeding, neurocognitive dysfunction, thromboembolism, fluid retention, and reversible organ dysfunction. Because OPCAB eliminated the use of a CPB circuit and could potentially reduce some of these pump-associated complications, there was a great enthusiasm for OPCAB. In fact, throughout Asia and particularly in India, 95% of CABG operations are still performed off-pump.

In a recent nationwide review of the STS database by Bakaeen et al, the use of off-pump procedures peaked in 2002 (23%) and again in 2008 (21%), followed by a progressive decline in off-pump frequency to 17% by 2012. Interestingly, after 2008, off-pump rates declined among both high-volume and intermediate-volume centers and surgeons, and currently in the United States, this technique is used in fewer than one in five patients who undergo surgical coronary revascularization. A minority of surgeons and centers, however, continue to perform OPCAB in most of their patients.

This decline in OPCAB is presumably due not only to the procedure's technical complexity and steep learning curve but also, and more important, to the decreased long-term patency, higher rate of incomplete revascularization, and inferior long-term survival associated with OPCAB.

Data from multiple studies have not supported the belief that OPCAB decreases inflammatory mediator release. Some investigators have shown that even though complement activation may be reduced, there is no difference in production of cytokines and chemokines that modulate neutrophils and platelets.[63,64] In addition, myocardial ischemia by itself activates complement such as C5b-9. Thus, great caution should be used in interpreting studies regarding activation of the inflammatory cascade.

Three recent RCTs—the ROOBY trial, the SMART trial, and the CORONARY trial—have also shown worse outcomes with OPCAB than with CABG. In addition, the GOPCADE trial showed no benefit of OPCAB in elderly patients.

The Randomized On/Off Bypass (ROOBY) trial was a prospective RCT of CABG and OPCAB that involved 2203 patients at 18 Veterans Affairs medical centers. There was no difference in 30-day mortality or short-term major adverse cardiovascular events. The OPCAB patients received significantly fewer grafts per patient. One-year rates of cardiac-related death (8.8% versus 5.9%; $P = .01$) and major adverse events (9.9% versus 7.4%; $P = .04$) were significantly higher in the OPCAB group. Furthermore, graft patency was significantly lower in the OPCAB group (82.6% versus 87.8%; $P < .001$). The results did not differ when the operation was performed by a resident or attending physician or by a high- or low-volume surgeon. Critics noted that women were excluded from the study, and there were no data regarding low-density lipoprotein levels, the use of statins and aspirin, or whether glycemic control was practiced in these patients.

The Surgical Management of Arterial Revascularization Therapy (SMART) trial examined long-term survival and graft patency in a prospective RCT involving 297 patients who underwent isolated elective CABG or OPCAB. After 7.5 years of follow-up, there was no difference in mortality or late graft patency between OPCAB and on-pump CABG. Although recurrent angina was more common in the OPCAB group, this difference did not reach statistical significance. Hence, this study, performed by one of the world's experts in OPCAB surgery, could not demonstrate any superiority of OPCAB over on-pump CABG.

Another prospective study, the Coronary Artery Bypass Surgery Off or On Pump Revascularization Study (CORONARY) trial, involved 4752 patients randomly assigned to either CABG or OPCAB at 79 centers in 19 countries. There were no significant differences in the incidence of recurrent angina between the OPCAB (0.9%) and CABG (1.0%) groups, but the need for repeated revascularization was higher in the OPCAB group, and the difference approached statistical significance (1.4% OPCAB versus 0.8% CABG; $P = .07$).

The CORONARY trial included twice as many participants as the ROOBY trial. Each off-pump procedure was performed by an experienced surgeon who had more than 2 years of experience and had performed more than 100 OPCAB cases. Trainees were not allowed to be the primary surgeon. The rate of crossover from the off-pump to the on-pump group was lower in the CORONARY trial (7.9% versus 12.4%), suggesting a higher level of surgical expertise. Despite the improved technical experience of highly qualified off-pump surgeons, the need for revascularization remained higher in the off-pump group.

In the German Off-Pump Coronary Artery Bypass Grafts in Elderly Patients (GOPCADE) trial, patients aged 75 years and older scheduled for isolated bypass surgery were randomly assigned to on-pump or off-pump surgery. The trial was undertaken to attempt to define the potential benefits of OPCAB in an elderly group of high-risk patients with multiple comorbidities. The study involved 2539 patients from 12 centers. The primary end point was the composite of death or major adverse events (MI, cerebrovascular accident, acute renal failure requiring renal replacement therapy, or need for repeated revascularization) within 30 days and within 12 months after surgery. The secondary end points included operating room time, duration of mechanical ventilation, transfusion requirements, and ICU and hospital length of stay.

There was no difference in the primary composite end point (7.0% off-pump versus 8.0% on-pump; $P = .40$). However, additional revascularization procedures within 30 days were more frequent in the off-pump group (1.3% versus 0.3%; $P = .03$). Patients in the off-pump group were less likely to receive blood products; however, the study had no protocols to determine when transfusions should be given. There was no difference in any of the other secondary end points. The mean number of grafts was significantly lower in the off-pump group (2.7 versus 2.8; $P < .001$). The investigators concluded that OPCAB did not improve outcomes in these elderly high-risk patients. Furthermore, concerns were raised that the increased need for early repeated revascularization and the decreased number of grafts in the off-pump group would lead to an increased incidence of future cardiovascular events, thus exposing these elderly patients to increased morbidity and mortality.

These findings have dampened the enthusiasm for OPCAB at most centers. However, it is our practice to offer OPCAB to patients with single-vessel CAD in the LAD system.

The technique and operative strategy of OPCAB differ significantly from those of on-pump CABG. Certain adjuncts are needed to provide adequate exposure of the coronary vessels. Because the heart is fully contractile and maintaining systemic perfusion, the manipulation should proceed in a planned and systematic manner. Both the pleural spaces are opened to allow the heart to rotate into either side to allow the surgeon to visualize the targets, especially the lateral and inferior wall. The more critical areas of the myocardium are revascularized first, which minimizes ischemia time, improves myocardial reserve, and permits more complex manipulation of the heart for the other targets. Mammary artery–based pedicles are typically approached first because these do not require a proximal anastomosis, thus providing immediate coronary blood flow to the bypassed vessel.

Once the target vessel is selected, a small area of the coronary artery is exposed proximal and distal to the planned area of anastomosis to allow placement of vessel loops or bulldog clamps for proximal and distal control. A coronary occluder may also be used. Two stabilizers are used to stabilize the myocardium (Fig. 59-17). The fork-octopus has a suction padded tip and is attached to a multifunctional arm. The fork is positioned so that the limbs straddle the coronary target, and suction is applied, which attaches the device to the myocardium while the arm is secured in position. The other device consists of a suction cup that is applied to the apex of the heart and is used to lift it out of the chest to expose its posterior aspect. A sling attached to the posterior pericardium allows the heart to be elevated out and enhances visualization of the posterior targets.

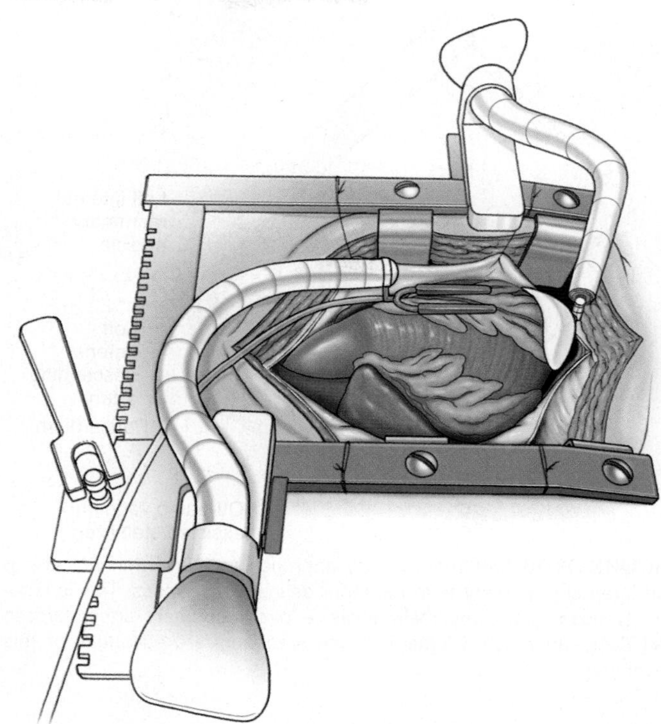

FIGURE 59-17 Off-pump coronary artery bypass with vacuum-assisted multiarticulating arms to position and to stabilize the myocardium. This minimizes the movement of the heart, allowing the surgeon to feasibly perform the distal anastomoses. Here, the stabilizer is positioned in preparation for creating a bypass to the left anterior descending artery.

Full heparinization is not needed; in general, 50% of the usual dose is used. Success of the operation requires coordinated efforts between the surgeon and anesthesiologist so that adequate systemic perfusion is maintained throughout the operation while allowing a comfortable milieu in which the surgeon can operate. Short-acting beta blockers to slow the heart rate and alpha constrictors to maintain systemic perfusion pressures are important adjuncts for this procedure.

The postoperative management of OPCAB patients is significantly different from that of patients who undergo conventional CABG, primarily because of the reduced inflammatory effects, which are more prominent in patients who have undergone CPB. The OPCAB patients do not manifest the vasodilatory response or massive fluid shifts seen with CPB. Rather, these patients are more like those who have undergone major general surgery and require early deep venous thrombosis and balanced postoperative fluid management. In our practice, all patients who undergo OPCAB are given aspirin and clopidogrel (Plavix) on the day of surgery.

Minimally Invasive Direct Coronary Artery Bypass

Minimally invasive direct coronary artery bypass (MIDCAB) describes any technique of coronary artery bypass that uses a minimally invasive approach, such as an anterolateral thoracotomy (Fig. 59-18), ministernotomy, or subxiphoid approach, without the use of a robot. Most MIDCABs are performed on the beating heart and involve vascularization of the anterior wall.

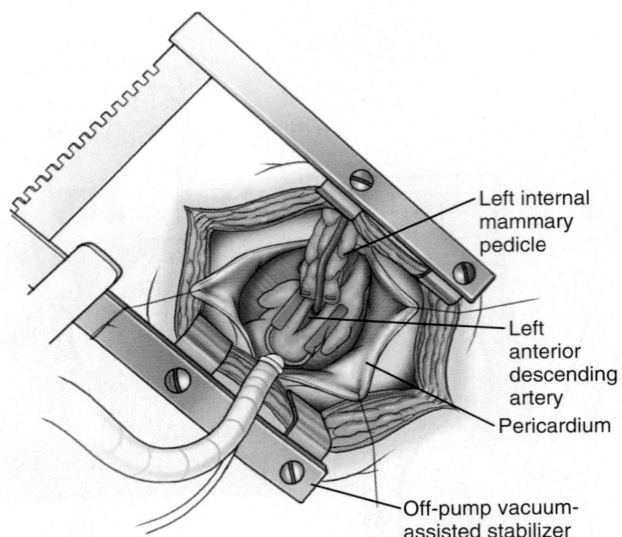

FIGURE 59-18 Left thoracotomy approach for performing off-pump left internal mammary to left anterior descending bypass. This is commonly used in the minimally invasive direct coronary artery bypass (MIDCAB) approach. Multiarticulating stabilizers are essential for this technique.

A meta-analysis of all published outcome studies of MIDCAB grafting performed from January 1995 through October 2007 has revealed early and late (>30 days) death rates of 1.3% and 3.2%, respectively. Of the grafts that were studied angiographically immediately after surgery, 4.2% were occluded and 6.6% had a significant stenosis (50% to 99%). At 6-month follow-up, 3.6% were occluded and 7.2% had significant stenosis. Long-term follow-up results and further prospective RCTs comparing MIDCABs with standard revascularization procedures in large patient cohorts are needed. Although MIDCAB offers several advantages, such as the avoidance of sternotomy and CPB, it is subject to the same limitations as OPCAB in addition to its own technical challenges and limited revascularization territory.

Robotics: Totally Endoscopic Coronary Artery Bypass

With the popularity of robotic technology in other surgical specialties, robotic totally endoscopic coronary artery bypass (TECAB) has been in vogue for several years. Robotically assisted microsurgical systems have the theoretical advantage of enhancing surgical dexterity and minimizing the invasiveness of otherwise conventional coronary artery surgery. The da Vinci system (Intuitive Surgical, Mountain View, Calif) is the most commonly used system. It consists of three major components: surgeon-device interface module, computer controller, and specific patient interface instrumentation. It allows real-time surgical manipulation of tissue, advanced dexterity in multiple degrees of freedom, and optical magnification of the operative field, all through minimal access ports. The technology has seen significant use in valve repair operations and other surgical specialties as well.

With regard to coronary artery bypass, TECAB can be performed on-pump or totally off-pump, and multivessel TECAB is currently a reality. However, operating times and conversion rates are much higher with this technology. More important, it is technically more difficult and expensive, and it has a steep learning curve. Long-term data regarding its durability and safety are unavailable at this point.

In the largest TECAB series to date (about 500 cases), success and safety rates were 80% ($n = 400$) and 95% ($n = 474$), respectively. Intraoperative conversion to larger thoracic incisions was required in 49 (10%) patients. The median operative time was 305 minutes (range, 112-1050 minutes), and the mean lengths of stay in the ICU and in the hospital were 23 hours (range, 11-1048 hours) and 6 days (range, 2-4 days), respectively. Independent predictors of success were single-vessel TECAB ($P = .004$), arrested-heart TECAB ($P = .027$), non–learning curve case ($P = .049$), and transthoracic assistance ($P = .035$). The only independent predictor of safety was EuroSCORE ($P = .002$). Interestingly, the mean time per anastomosis was 27 minutes (range, 10-100 minutes), which is significantly longer than an average surgeon would take to accomplish an open anastomosis (i.e., well below 10 minutes per anastomosis). Also, the LIMA injury rate was high ($n = 24$; 5%).[65] All these data point to less than perfect procedures and technology that require further development before they can replace open CABG, which has an excellent track record and is an elegant, fast, and reproducible procedure.

The current limitations of robotic TECAB include its lack of applicability to all patients, prolonged operating room time, limited access to all vessels, cost, and limited training opportunities. However, over time, robotic surgery is likely to become a niche specialty for a subset of surgeons who treat a specific population of patients.

Transmyocardial Laser Revascularization

Patients with chronic, severe angina refractory to medical therapy who cannot be completely revascularized with percutaneous catheter intervention or CABG present clinical challenges. Transmyocardial laser revascularization (TMLR), either as sole therapy or as an adjunct to CABG surgery, may be appropriate for some of these patients. The STS Evidence-Based Workforce has reviewed available evidence and recommends the use of TMLR for patients with an LVEF greater than 0.30 and Canadian Cardiovascular Society class III or class IV angina that is refractory to maximal medical therapy. These patients should have reversible ischemia of the LV free wall and CAD corresponding to the regions of myocardial ischemia. In all regions of the myocardium, the CAD must not be amenable to CABG or PCI.

The TMLR procedure uses a high-energy laser beam to create myocardial transmural channels that were originally thought to provide direct access to oxygenated blood in the LV cavity. This is no longer considered to be the mechanism whereby TMLR reduces the symptoms of IHD. Although some local neovascularization has been documented, the magnitude of changes does not account for any substantive increases in myocardial perfusion. One mechanism that has been proposed relates to a local effect on cardiac neuronal signaling. It has been hypothesized that local tissue injury by TMLR damages ventricular sensory neurons and autonomic efferent axons, which leads to local cardiac denervation and anginal relief. Regardless of the mechanism, TMLR therapy is associated with a reproducible improvement in symptoms. Patients who undergo TMLR show a persistent improvement in Canadian Cardiovascular Society angina class. This improvement is observed in 60% to 80% of patients within 6 months after the operation.

Hybrid Procedures

It is generally accepted that the LIMA to LAD anastomosis is the single most important component of CABG and confers long-term benefits unmatched by those of any other intervention. State-of-the-art PCIs with DES have produced outcomes competitive with those of vein grafts to non-LAD targets. This has led to an integrated approach to coronary revascularization, termed the hybrid procedure. The hybrid procedure consists of a minimally invasive LIMA to LAD anastomosis in conjunction with PCI of non–LAD-obstructed coronary arteries.

This approach has met with initial success, but many potential pitfalls exist. The procedural costs may be greater than those of either CABG or DES implantation alone. The timing and staging of the procedures are uncertain, and limited data are available on long-term outcomes.

Technical Aspects of Reoperative Coronary Artery Bypass Grafting

Within 5 years, 15% of CABG patients experience a recurrence of symptoms, typically angina. This increases to approximately 40% within 10 years. Recurrent symptoms almost always indicate either progression of disease in the native coronary circulation or graft disease. In most cases, the indications for coronary angiography, PCI with or without stenting, or repeated CABG are the same as for the first operation. Patients who are considered candidates for reoperative CABG are usually older, have more diffuse CAD, and have diminished ventricular function. Factors that increase the risk for reoperation include the absence of an IMA graft, younger age at the time of the index operation, prior incomplete revascularization, CHF, and New York Heart Association class III or class IV angina.

The technical aspects of reoperative CABG differ significantly from those of the index procedure. Reentry into the chest and dissection of the old grafts are sometimes challenging. Preparation for femoral cannulation for femorofemoral bypass or axillary cannulation should be considered with preemptive availability of blood products. Redo sternotomy is typically completed with an oscillating saw or after the heart is dissected away from the sternum through a subxiphoid approach. Injury to the right ventricle or to the aorta or vein grafts is of potential concern. A poorly placed LIMA graft from the prior operation is also at risk during the sternotomy. If a cardiac or vascular injury is identified, an assistant holds the sternum together to prevent further bleeding, and expeditious cannulation of alternative sites is begun with the institution of CPB. Preoperative CT scans are helpful in planning the operation.

Once the sternotomy is completed, the rest of the adherent cardiac structures are dissected away from the underside of the sternum to allow placement of a sternal retractor. No retractor should be placed unless the heart is adequately dissected away; this will result in disruption of the aorta or right ventricle, which may be difficult to control.

The next steps are geared toward establishing sites for cannulation. The right atrium and aorta are dissected first; then, the rest of the heart is dissected away from the pericardium, which may be performed on CPB. The areas of previous cannulation and vein grafts are the most adherent regions, whereas the diaphragmatic aspect is least adherent and provides a good starting point to gain entry into the correct plane.

Manipulation of the old grafts should be kept to a minimum to avoid distal coronary bed microembolization. Isolation of the LIMA pedicle is often necessary and should be carefully performed, with the ability to start bypass rapidly if an inadvertent injury occurs (Fig. 59-19). The rest of the operation proceeds in a similar fashion to primary CABG and can be performed on-pump or off-pump. In some cases, the procedure can be performed through a left anterolateral thoracotomy approach. Typically, this approach is used in patients with previous mediastinitis or multiple sternotomies or when an extensive area of the heart is adherent to the sternum, precluding a safe entry. The vein conduit is anastomosed to the descending aorta in these cases (Fig. 59-20).

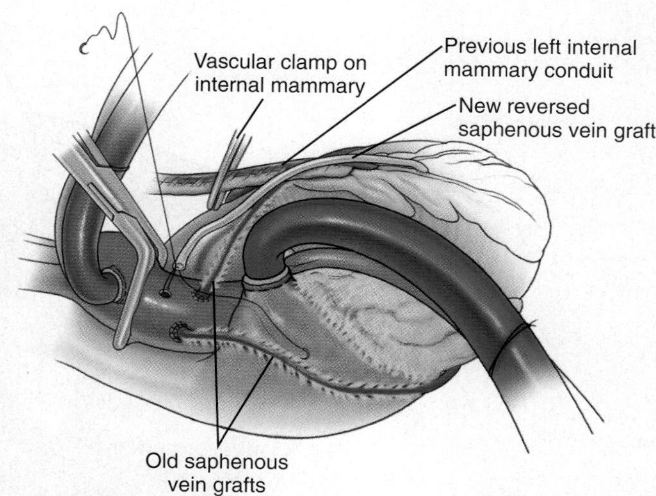

FIGURE 59-19 Redo Coronary Artery Bypass Grafting. The cannulation is similar to that used in a first-time coronary artery bypass operation in most cases. However, identification of coronary targets is much more difficult because of scarring. The course of the prior grafts is useful in identifying the targets. In addition to clamping of the aorta above the previous vein grafts, the left internal mammary pedicle should be dissected and clamped separately, if feasible. A single-clamp technique is preferred because it avoids the tedious and potentially dangerous dissection around the proximal aorta that may be needed to place a partial side-biting clamp.

To summarize, some of the unique difficulties that can be encountered in redo CABG are as follows:

- Injury to heart during sternotomy
- Injury to mammary pedicle
- Limited space on ascending aorta for placement of new grafts
- Inability to identify distal targets because of scars and adhesions
- Limited availability of conduits
- Increased risk of perioperative MI because atheroembolic embolization from diseased vein grafts and diffuse CAD preclude optimal cardioplegia
- Increased bleeding because of higher inflammatory response and more raw surface
- Injury to pulmonary artery during cross-clamping of the aorta

In most published series, the mortality rate of reoperative CABG patients exceeds that of primary CABG patients.

MECHANICAL COMPLICATIONS OF CORONARY ARTERY DISEASE

Left Ventricular Aneurysm

The incidence of ventricular aneurysm after AMI has been declining because of early interventional therapies. Of LV aneurysms, 90% are the result of a transmural MI secondary to an acute

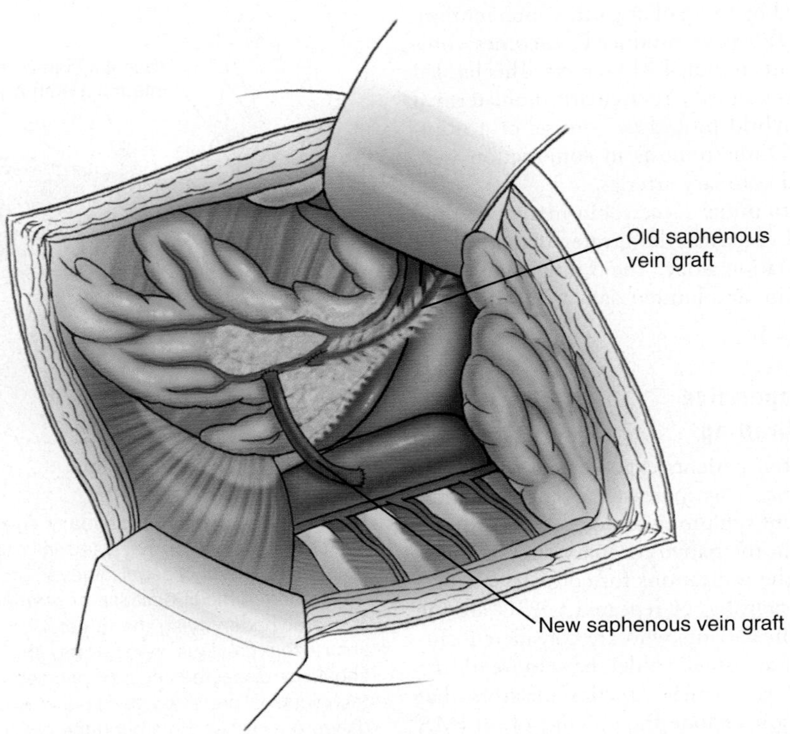

FIGURE 59-20 Left Thoracotomy Approach for Recurrent Coronary Artery Disease. This approach avoids the hazards of a difficult redo sternotomy and is used as an alternative in some cases. New saphenous vein graft: descending thoracic aorta to obtuse marginal bypass.

occlusion of the LAD. Patients may develop an aneurysm (pseudoaneurysm) as early as 48 hours after infarction, but most patients develop one within weeks. Approximately two thirds of patients who develop ventricular aneurysms remain asymptomatic.

The 10-year survival rate is 90% for asymptomatic patients and 50% for symptomatic patients. The most common causes of death are arrhythmias (>40%), CHF (>30%), and recurrent MI (>10%). The risk of thromboembolism is low, so long-term anticoagulation is not recommended unless there is a mural thrombus. The diagnosis is usually made by echocardiography. Thallium imaging or PET is useful for determining the extent of the aneurysm and viability of adjacent regions.

Surgery for LV aneurysm is indicated if the patient is scheduled to undergo CABG for symptomatic CAD, there is contained rupture or evidence of a false aneurysm, or the patient has a thromboembolic event despite anticoagulation. The 5-year postoperative survival rate has been reported to range between 60% and 80%. In general, surgical repair or resection in conjunction with CABG results in angina relief and resolution of heart failure symptoms for most patients.

Surgical ventricular restoration is a technical term that describes the surgical resection of the aneurysm and reconstruction of the native ventricular geometric shape. This is ideally performed with CPB and without cardioplegic arrest, as long as the aortic valve is competent. The aneurysm is usually recognized by the paradoxical movement of the walls compared with the rest of the viable LV myocardium. The aneurysm is opened, and a purse-string Fontan stitch is placed at the junction of the viable and nonviable myocardium, which can be manually palpated on the beating heart. A Dacron or bovine pericardial patch is used to exclude the aneurysm, and the aneurysm is closed over the patch. Two potentially acute complications that require surgical intervention are postinfarction VSD and postinfarction mitral regurgitation caused by papillary muscle rupture.

Ventricular Septal Defect

This occurs in less than 1% of patients and is associated with acute LAD occlusion. The defect is more common in men than in women (3 : 2) and typically is manifested within 2 to 4 days of the infarction. However, a VSD that occurs in the first 6 weeks after an infarct is still considered acute. The VSD is usually located in the anterior or apical aspect of the ventricular septum. Approximately 25% of affected patients have a posterior VSD caused by an inferior wall MI due to occlusion of the RCA system or a distal branch LCA. A full-thickness infarct is a prerequisite for VSD formation. A new, loud, systolic cardiac murmur after an MI suggests the diagnosis; echocardiography is effective for determining the size and character of the VSD as well as the degree of left-to-right shunting. Right-sided heart catheterization typically shows an increase in oxygen saturation levels in the right ventricle and pulmonary artery. The defect is usually approximately 1 to 2 cm in size.

After the diagnosis is established, patients should undergo immediate left-sided heart catheterization to characterize the degree of CAD and the magnitude of LV dysfunction and to detect any mitral valve insufficiency. Approximately 60% of patients with an infarction VSD have significant CAD in an unrelated vessel. The mortality rate in untreated patients is high; 25% of patients die within 24 hours of refractory heart failure. Survival rates of patients at 1 week, 1 month, and longer than 1 year are 50%, 20%, and less than 3%, respectively.

Patients who are considered candidates for surgery should be treated early with closure of the defect and concomitant CABG.

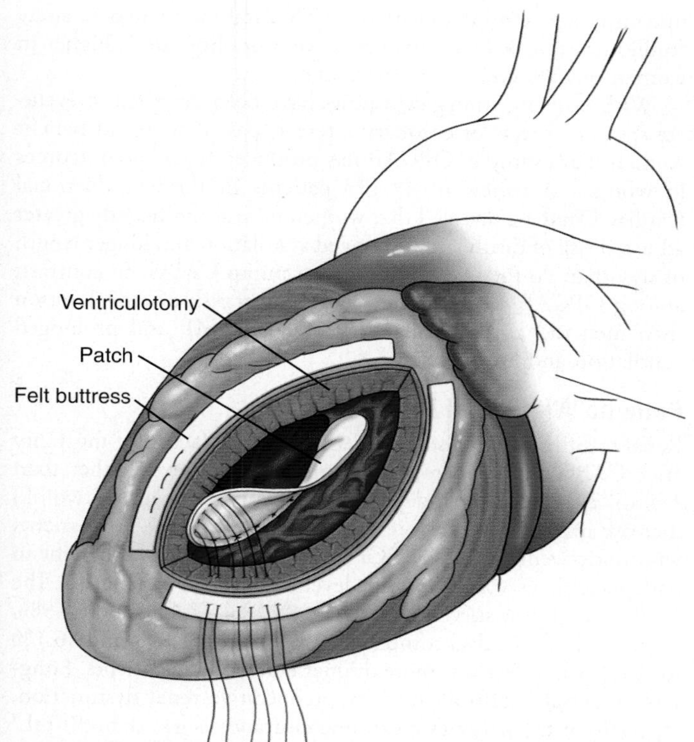

FIGURE 59-21 Infarct exclusion technique for repair of acute ventricular septal defect secondary to acute myocardial infarction. A ventriculotomy is made through the zone of infarct, and all necrotic muscle is débrided. The repair is accomplished with a patch placed on the left ventricular aspect of the septum. Felt buttresses are used to reinforce the closure of the ventriculotomy, and it is essential that all sutures be incorporated into healthy myocardium to ensure durability of the repair.

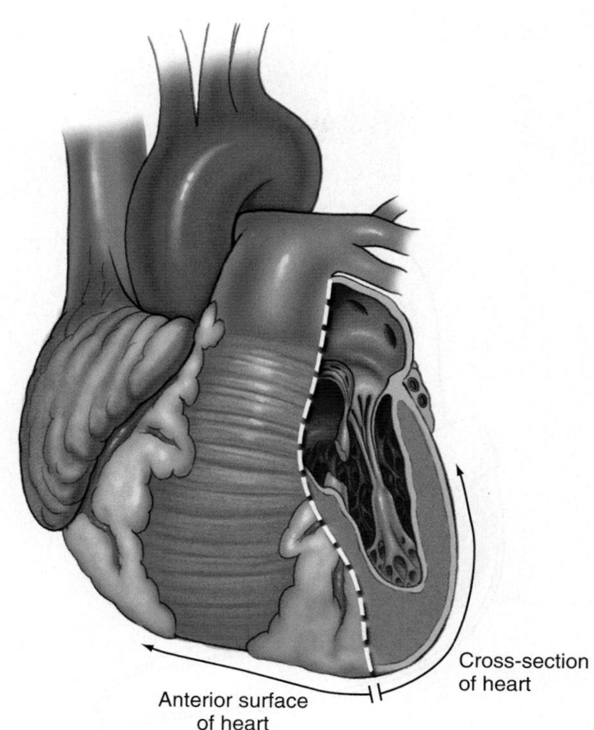

FIGURE 59-22 Mechanical Complication of Acute Myocardial Infarction. Acute papillary muscle rupture (shown here) and acute ventricular septal defect are two sequelae in a patient with extensive zones of infarct. Acute papillary muscle rupture results in acute mitral regurgitation that is manifested as cardiogenic shock and immediate pulmonary decompensation. If the patient is a surgical candidate, mitral valve replacement is the only option.

In the absence of refractory heart failure and hemodynamic instability, the survival rate may be as high as 75%. The infarct exclusion technique is used to repair the VSD and is one of the most technically challenging procedures. The LV is opened longitudinally on the infarct, and the defect is evaluated. Multiple VSDs may be present, and necrotic myocardium is débrided to viable tissue. A prosthetic Dacron patch or bovine pericardium is then sutured to the LV side of the septal defect and brought out through the ventriculotomy, where it is incorporated into the closure (Fig. 59-21). In this method, the posterior aspect of the patch is thus anchored to the remnant viable septum, and the anterior aspect is incorporated with the free ventricular wall, forming the neo–interventricular septum. Felt strips are used to buttress the closure.

In addition to the traditional repair of postinfarction VSD, there has been recent enthusiasm about transcatheter closure of postinfarction VSD. This obviates a pump run in an otherwise tenuous patient. In both the patients treated surgically and with transcatheter closure, temporary circulatory support in the form of extracorporeal membrane oxygenation or ventricular assist device can be lifesaving.

Mitral Regurgitation

Approximately 40% of patients who sustain an AMI develop chronic ischemic mitral regurgitation (IMR) detectable by color flow Doppler echocardiography. In 3% to 4% of cases, the degree of mitral regurgitation is moderate or severe.

The cause of chronic IMR is ischemic papillary muscle dysfunction and LV dilation associated with mitral annular dilation and restriction of the posterior leaflet. The operation for chronic IMR is usually performed on an elective basis. It consists of complete myocardial revascularization and mitral valve repair with the use of an annuloplasty ring.

Acute IMR may result from papillary muscle necrosis and rupture caused by occlusion of the overlying epicardial arteries that give rise to the penetrating vessels that supply the papillary muscles. The posterior papillary muscle is involved three to six times more often than the anterior muscle (Fig. 59-22), and either the entire trunk of the muscle or one of the heads to which chordae attach may rupture partially or totally.

In most cases, prompt surgical intervention provides the best chance for survival. Predictors of in-hospital death include CHF, renal insufficiency, and multivessel CAD. Emergent surgical treatment usually involves mitral valve replacement and concomitant CABG. The hospital mortality rate may be as high as 50% in acute cases. Mitral repair should not be attempted in such cases because it may not be feasible in papillary muscle rupture; it requires prolonging the cross-clamp time (compared with replacement), which is not ideal in acute cases. Operations on patients with acute mechanical complications from MI are challenging; the surgeon has to anticipate and be prepared for placement of an LV assist device if the patient cannot be separated from CPB (Fig. 59-23).

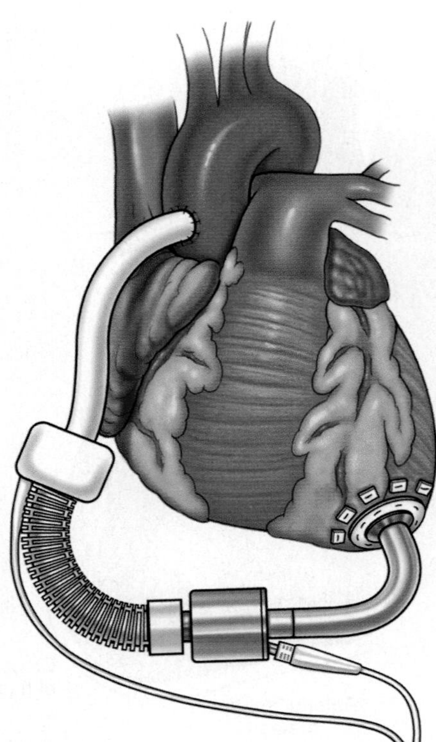

FIGURE 59-23 An axial flow left ventricular assist device, which can be used as temporary mechanical support or a bridge to transplantation for a patient in end-stage cardiomyopathy due to coronary artery disease not amenable to bypass surgery. The inflow of blood into the pump is from the apex of the left ventricle. The blood is then pumped into the ascending aorta through specially designed grafts that are incorporated into the pump. The axial flow pumps are less bulky and relatively easy to implant. They have only a single moving part, which is the axial impeller.

CORONARY ARTERY BYPASS GRAFTING AND SPECIAL POPULATIONS OF PATIENTS

Patients With Diabetes

Mortality and morbidity rates after CABG are higher in diabetic patients than in the general population. The BARI trial showed that diabetic patients with multivessel disease benefit more from CABG than from any other treatment. Similarly, the FREEDOM trial also demonstrated superiority of CABG over PCI.

Older Patients

Approximately 10% of patients who undergo CABG are older than 80 years. Older age is an independent predictor of surgical morbidity and mortality and a nonroutine discharge status. Although CABG should not be denied to patients on the basis of age alone, it should be considered during risk assessment. Appropriate arrangements should be made beforehand with the expectation that only one in five postoperative patients will be able to go home without additional support.

Women

Although women in every age group have a lower incidence of CAD than men, CAD is still the leading cause of death in women in the United States. Historically, serious manifestations and associated complications of CAD in women were considered uncommon. Examination of the STS database in two separate studies has revealed that the operative mortality rate is higher in women, 3.15% versus 2.61% in men.

With evolving strategies, studies have been designed to evaluate specific aspects of coronary artery bypass that would benefit women. For example, OPCAB has produced favorable outcomes in women. A review of 42,477 patients in the STS National Cardiac Database revealed that women have a significantly greater adjusted risk of death and prolonged ventilation and longer length of stay than do men who undergo on-pump CABG. In contrast, among OPCAB cases, women had a lower risk of reexploration than men did and a similar risk of death, MI, and prolonged ventilation and hospital stay.

Patients With Renal Disease

Renal insufficiency is also an independent risk factor for mortality after CABG. A preoperative serum creatinine level higher than 1.4 to 2.5 mg/dL is independently associated with a twofold increase in mortality. In a retrospective study of 59,576 patients who underwent CABG or PCI, CABG had a survival benefit in patients with a serum creatinine level higher than 2.5 mg/dL. The 1-, 2-, and 3-year survival rates were 84.1%, 77.4%, and 65.9%, respectively, for CABG compared with 70.8%, 51.9%, and 46.1% for PCI. This effect was more dramatic in diabetic patients. Long-term survival is also affected by preoperative renal dysfunction, especially if the patient's creatinine clearance is less than 30 mL/min. Although CABG in patients with renal insufficiency or failure is associated with increased morbidity and mortality, CABG is nonetheless associated with better survival than PCI in such patients.

Obese Patients

The incidence of postoperative renal failure, prolonged ventilation, and sternal wound infection is significantly higher in obese patients than in normal-weight patients. Both extremes of weight are risk factors for CABG-related mortality.

ACKNOWLEDGMENTS

We would like to acknowledge Scott Weldon and Michael DeLaflor for graphic services, Johnny Airheart for photographic support, Dr. Chinnapapu Muthusamy for assistance with review questions, and Dr. Stephen N. Palmer for editorial assistance.

SELECTED REFERENCES

Chu D, Bakaeen FG, Dao TK, et al: On-pump versus off-pump coronary artery bypass grafting in a cohort of 63,000 patients. *Ann Thorac Surg* 87:1820–1826, 2009.

This study was a nationwide comparison of on-pump versus off-pump coronary artery bypass surgery in the United States. The study highlighted the fact that off-pump coronary artery bypass does not produce lower postoperative mortality or stroke rates than conventional on-pump coronary artery bypass. Furthermore, off-pump coronary artery bypass was associated with longer hospital stays and higher hospital costs.

Edwards FH, Carey JS, Grover FL, et al: Impact of gender on coronary bypass operative mortality. *Ann Thorac Surg* 66:125–131, 1998.

This study analyzed the outcomes of more than 300,000 patients from the Society of Thoracic Surgeons database and used multivariate analysis and risk model stratification to examine the outcomes of female patients. Female gender was shown to be an independent predictor of higher mortality in low- to moderate-risk patients but not in high-risk patients.

Influence of diabetes on 5-year mortality and morbidity in a randomized trial comparing CABG and PTCA in patients with multivessel disease: The Bypass Angioplasty Revascularization Investigation (BARI). *Circulation* 96:1761–1769, 1997.

Follow-up results from the initial randomized controlled trial established that patients with treated diabetes mellitus who were assigned to undergo CABG had a striking reduction in mortality compared with patients who underwent percutaneous transluminal coronary angioplasty. This benefit was attributed predominantly to the use of the left internal mammary artery conduit in CABG.

Loop FD, Lytle BW, Cosgrove DM, et al: Influence of the internal-mammary-artery graft on 10-year survival and other cardiac events. *N Engl J Med* 314:1–6, 1986.

This retrospective study of 5931 CABG patients operated on at a single institution compared the outcomes of patients who had an internal mammary artery graft with those of patients who had only vein grafts. The findings of this landmark study established the superiority of the internal mammary artery over any other conduit. During a 10-year period, patients who had only vein grafts had a 1.6 times higher risk of mortality than those who had mammary grafts.

Lopes RD, Hafley GE, Allen KB, et al: Endoscopic versus open vein-graft harvesting in coronary-artery bypass surgery. *N Engl J Med* 361:235–244, 2009.

This retrospective study evaluated the effects of endoscopic vein harvesting on the rate of vein graft failure and on clinical outcomes. Endoscopic vein harvesting was shown to be independently associated with vein graft failure and adverse clinical outcomes compared with open vein harvesting.

Parisi AF, Khuri S, Deupree RH, et al: Medical compared with surgical management of unstable angina: 5-year mortality and morbidity in the Veterans Administration Study. *Circulation* 80:1176–1189, 1989.

This prospective, multicenter Veterans Administration randomized controlled trial compared surgical and medical management and established that for patients with triple-vessel coronary disease, surgical intervention better promotes survival than medical management.

Peduzzi P, Kamina A, Detre K: Twenty-two-year follow-up in the VA Cooperative Study of Coronary Artery Bypass Surgery for Stable Angina. *Am J Cardiol* 81:1393–1399, 1998.

This study compared the 22-year results of initial CABG surgery with saphenous vein grafts with those of initial medical therapy with regard to survival, the incidences of myocardial infarction and reoperation, and symptomatic status in 686 patients with stable angina who participated in the Veterans Affairs Cooperative Study of Coronary Artery Bypass Surgery. This trial provided strong evidence that initial bypass surgery did not improve survival for low-risk patients and did not reduce the overall risk of myocardial infarction. The early survival benefit with surgery in high-risk patients did not translate to comparable long-term survival rates for both treatment groups.

Serruys PW, Morice MC, Kappetein AP, et al: Percutaneous coronary intervention versus coronary-artery bypass grafting for severe coronary artery disease. *N Engl J Med* 360:961–972, 2009.

This was a landmark contemporary study of PCI with drug-eluting stents versus CABG. The primary end point was a major adverse cardiac or cerebrovascular event (i.e., death from any cause, stroke, myocardial infarction, or repeated revascularization) during the 12-month period after randomization. Rates of major adverse cardiac or cerebrovascular events at 12 months were significantly higher in the PCI group (17.8% versus 12.4% for CABG; P = .002), in large part because of an increased rate of repeated revascularization (13.5% versus 5.9%; P < .001); as a result, the criterion for noninferiority was not met. At 12 months, the rates of death and myocardial infarction were similar between the two groups; stroke was significantly more likely to occur with CABG (2.2% versus 0.6% with PCI; P = .003). The investigators concluded that CABG remains the standard of care for patients with three-vessel or left coronary artery disease because the use of CABG, compared with PCI, resulted in lower rates of the combined end point of major adverse cardiac or cerebrovascular events at 1 year.

Serruys PW, Ong AT, van Herwerden LA, et al: Five-year outcomes after coronary stenting versus bypass surgery for the treatment of multivessel disease: The final analysis of the Arterial Revascularization Therapies Study (ARTS) randomized trial. *J Am Coll Cardiol* 46:575–581, 2005.

The final results of the ARTS were summarized and showed that the overall rate of major adverse cardiac and cerebrovascular events was higher in patients who underwent coronary artery stenting than in CABG patients. This difference was driven by the increased need for repeated revascularization in the stent group.

Shroyer AL, Grover FL, Hattler B, et al: On-pump versus off-pump coronary-artery bypass surgery. *N Engl J Med* 361:1827–1837, 2009.

This study was a randomized, multicenter Veterans Affairs trial that compared conventional CABG with off-pump coronary artery bypass (OPCAB) in 2203 patients. The primary end point was a composite of death from any cause, repeated revascularization, or nonfatal myocardial infarction within 1 year after surgery. At 1-year follow-up, the OPCAB patients had worse composite outcomes and poorer graft patency. The presumed benefit of fewer neuropsychological adverse outcomes was not found in OPCAB patients.

White HD, Assmann SF, Sanborn TA, et al: Comparison of percutaneous coronary intervention and coronary artery bypass grafting after acute myocardial infarction complicated by cardiogenic shock: Results from the Should We Emergently Revascularize Occluded Coronaries for Cardiogenic Shock (SHOCK) trial. *Circulation* 112:1992–2001, 2005.

This randomized controlled trial was designed to compare CABG surgery with PCI in patients who presented with cardiogenic shock. The trial evaluated 30-day and 1-year mortality and found comparable results between the two groups, even though the CABG patients had a higher prevalence of diabetes and worse coronary artery disease preoperatively.

REFERENCES

1. Lloyd-Jones D, Adams RJ, Brown TM, et al: Executive summary: Heart disease and stroke statistics—2010 update: A report from the American Heart Association. *Circulation* 121:948–954, 2010.
2. Ford ES, Capewell S: Coronary heart disease mortality among young adults in the U.S. from 1980 through 2002: Concealed leveling of mortality rates. *J Am Coll Cardiol* 50:2128–2132, 2007.
3. Murphy SL, Xu J, Kochanek K: Deaths: Preliminary data for 2010. *Natl Vital Stat Rep* 60:1–52, 2012.
4. Maycock A, Muhlestein JB, Horne BD, et al: Statin therapy is associated with reduced mortality across all age groups of individuals with significant coronary disease, including very elderly patients. *J Am Coll Cardiol* 40:1777–1785, 2002.
5. de Winter RJ, Windhausen F, Cornel JH, et al: Early invasive versus selectively invasive management for acute coronary syndromes. *N Engl J Medicine* 353:1095–1104, 2005.
6. Jneid H, Anderson JL, Wright RS, et al: 2012 ACCF/AHA focused update of the guideline for the management of patients with unstable angina/non-ST-elevation myocardial infarction (updating the 2007 guideline and replacing the 2011 focused update): A report of the American College of Cardiology Foundation/American Heart Association Task Force on Practice Guidelines. *J Am Coll Cardiol* 60:645–681, 2012.
7. Pepine CJ, Balaban RS, Bonow RO, et al: Women's Ischemic Syndrome Evaluation: Current status and future research directions: Report of the National Heart, Lung and Blood Institute workshop: October 2-4, 2002: Section 1: Diagnosis of stable ischemia and ischemic heart disease. *Circulation* 109:e44–e46, 2004.
8. Daly C, Norrie J, Murdoch DL, et al: The value of routine non-invasive tests to predict clinical outcome in stable angina. *Eur Heart J* 24:532–540, 2003.
9. Daly CA, De Stavola B, Sendon JL, et al: Predicting prognosis in stable angina—results from the Euro heart survey of stable angina: Prospective observational study. *BMJ* 332:262–267, 2006.
10. Hammermeister KE, DeRouen TA, Dodge HT: Variables predictive of survival in patients with coronary disease. Selection by univariate and multivariate analyses from the clinical, electrocardiographic, exercise, arteriographic, and quantitative angiographic evaluations. *Circulation* 59:421–430, 1979.
11. Kwok Y, Kim C, Grady D, et al: Meta-analysis of exercise testing to detect coronary artery disease in women. *Am J Cardiol* 83:660–666, 1999.
12. Shaw LJ, Mieres JH, Hendel RH, et al: Comparative effectiveness of exercise electrocardiography with or without myocardial perfusion single photon emission computed tomography in women with suspected coronary artery disease: Results from the What Is the Optimal Method for Ischemia Evaluation in Women (WOMEN) trial. *Circulation* 124:1239–1249, 2011.
13. Imran MB, Palinkas A, Picano E: Head-to-head comparison of dipyridamole echocardiography and stress perfusion scintigraphy for the detection of coronary artery disease: A meta-analysis. Comparison between stress echo and scintigraphy. *Int J Cardiovasc Imaging* 19:23–28, 2003.
14. Marcassa C, Bax JJ, Bengel F, et al: Clinical value, cost-effectiveness, and safety of myocardial perfusion scintigraphy: A position statement. *Eur Heart J* 29:557–563, 2008.
15. Fleischmann KE, Hunink MG, Kuntz KM, et al: Exercise echocardiography or exercise SPECT imaging? A meta-analysis of diagnostic test performance. *JAMA* 280:913–920, 1998.
16. Sabharwal NK, Stoykova B, Taneja AK, et al: A randomized trial of exercise treadmill ECG versus stress SPECT myocardial perfusion imaging as an initial diagnostic strategy in stable patients with chest pain and suspected CAD: Cost analysis. *J Nucl Cardiol* 14:174–186, 2007.
17. Underwood SR, Anagnostopoulos C, Cerqueira M, et al: Myocardial perfusion scintigraphy: The evidence. *Eur J Nucl Med Mol Imaging* 31:261–291, 2004.
18. Badran HM, Elnoamany MF, Seteha M: Tissue velocity imaging with dobutamine stress echocardiography—a quantitative technique for identification of coronary artery disease in patients with left bundle branch block. *J Am Soc Echocardiogr* 20:820–831, 2007.
19. Leischik R, Dworrak B, Littwitz H, et al: Prognostic significance of exercise stress echocardiography in 3329 outpatients (5-year longitudinal study). *Int J Cardiol* 119:297–305, 2007.
20. Levy D, Garrison RJ, Savage DD, et al: Prognostic implications of echocardiographically determined left ventricular mass in the Framingham Heart Study. *N Engl J Med* 322:1561–1566, 1990.
21. Mark DB, Berman DS, Budoff MJ, et al: ACCF/ACR/AHA/NASCI/SAIP/SCAI/SCCT 2010 expert consensus document on coronary computed tomographic angiography: A report of the American College of Cardiology Foundation Task Force on Expert Consensus Documents. *Catheter Cardiovasc Interv* 76:E1–E42, 2010.
22. Budoff MJ, Dowe D, Jollis JG, et al: Diagnostic performance of 64-multidetector row coronary computed tomographic angiography for evaluation of coronary artery stenosis in individuals without known coronary artery disease: Results from the prospective multicenter ACCURACY (Assessment by Coronary Computed Tomographic Angiography of Individuals Undergoing Invasive Coronary Angiography) trial. *J Am Coll Cardiol* 52:1724–1732, 2008.
23. Hamon M, Biondi-Zoccai GG, Malagutti P, et al: Diagnostic performance of multislice spiral computed tomography of coronary arteries as compared with conventional invasive coronary angiography: A meta-analysis. *J Am Coll Cardiol* 48:1896–1910, 2006.

24. Janne d'Othee B, Siebert U, Cury R, et al: A systematic review on diagnostic accuracy of CT-based detection of significant coronary artery disease. *Eur J Radiol* 65:449–461, 2008.
25. Meijboom WB, Meijs MF, Schuijf JD, et al: Diagnostic accuracy of 64-slice computed tomography coronary angiography: A prospective, multicenter, multivendor study. *J Am Coll Cardiol* 52:2135–2144, 2008.
26. Miller JM, Rochitte CE, Dewey M, et al: Diagnostic performance of coronary angiography by 64-row CT. *N Engl J Med* 359:2324–2336, 2008.
27. Schuijf JD, Bax JJ, Shaw LJ, et al: Meta-analysis of comparative diagnostic performance of magnetic resonance imaging and multislice computed tomography for noninvasive coronary angiography. *Am Heart J* 151:404–411, 2006.
28. Stein PD, Beemath A, Kayali F, et al: Multidetector computed tomography for the diagnosis of coronary artery disease: A systematic review. *Am J Med* 119:203–216, 2006.
29. Motoyama S, Sarai M, Harigaya H, et al: Computed tomographic angiography characteristics of atherosclerotic plaques subsequently resulting in acute coronary syndrome. *J Am Coll Cardiol* 54:49–57, 2009.
30. Shmilovich H, Cheng VY, Tamarappoo BK, et al: Vulnerable plaque features on coronary CT angiography as markers of inducible regional myocardial hypoperfusion from severe coronary artery stenoses. *Atherosclerosis* 219:588–595, 2011.
31. Ambrose JA, Tannenbaum MA, Alexopoulos D, et al: Angiographic progression of coronary artery disease and the development of myocardial infarction. *J Am Coll Cardiol* 12:56–62, 1988.
32. Little WC, Constantinescu M, Applegate RJ, et al: Can coronary angiography predict the site of a subsequent myocardial infarction in patients with mild-to-moderate coronary artery disease? *Circulation* 78:1157–1166, 1988.
33. Eleven-year survival in the Veterans Administration randomized trial of coronary bypass surgery for stable angina. The Veterans Administration Coronary Artery Bypass Surgery Cooperative Study Group. *N Engl J Med* 311:1333–1339, 1984.
34. Ringqvist I, Fisher LD, Mock M, et al: Prognostic value of angiographic indices of coronary artery disease from the Coronary Artery Surgery Study (CASS). *J Clin Invest* 71: 1854–1866, 1983.
35. Passamani E, Davis KB, Gillespie MJ, et al: A randomized trial of coronary artery bypass surgery. Survival of patients with a low ejection fraction. *N Engl J Med* 312:1665–1671, 1985.
36. Yusuf S, Zucker D, Peduzzi P, et al: Effect of coronary artery bypass graft surgery on survival: Overview of 10-year results from randomised trials by the Coronary Artery Bypass Graft Surgery Trialists Collaboration. *Lancet* 344:563–570, 1994.
37. Hueb W, Lopes N, Gersh BJ, et al: Ten-year follow-up survival of the Medicine, Angioplasty, or Surgery Study (MASS II): A randomized controlled clinical trial of 3 therapeutic strategies for multivessel coronary artery disease. *Circulation* 122:949–957, 2010.
38. Brophy JM, Belisle P, Joseph L: Evidence for use of coronary stents. A hierarchical bayesian meta-analysis. *Ann Intern Med* 138:777–786, 2003.
39. Trikalinos TA, Alsheikh-Ali AA, Tatsioni A, et al: Percutaneous coronary interventions for non-acute coronary artery disease: A quantitative 20-year synopsis and a network meta-analysis. *Lancet* 373:911–918, 2009.
40. Kastrati A, Mehilli J, Pache J, et al: Analysis of 14 trials comparing sirolimus-eluting stents with bare-metal stents. *N Engl J Med* 356:1030–1039, 2007.
41. Bravata DM, Gienger AL, McDonald KM, et al: Systematic review: The comparative effectiveness of percutaneous coronary interventions and coronary artery bypass graft surgery. *Ann Intern Med* 147:703–716, 2007.
42. Serruys PW, Morice MC, Kappetein AP, et al: Percutaneous coronary intervention versus coronary-artery bypass grafting for severe coronary artery disease. *N Engl J Med* 360:961–972, 2009.
43. Buszman PE, Kiesz SR, Bochenek A, et al: Acute and late outcomes of unprotected left main stenting in comparison with surgical revascularization. *J Am Coll Cardiol* 51:538–545, 2008.
44. VA Coronary Artery Bypass Surgery Cooperative Study Group: Eighteen-year follow-up in the Veterans Affairs Cooperative Study of Coronary Artery Bypass Surgery for stable angina. *Circulation* 86:121–130, 1992.
45. Varnauskas E: Twelve-year follow-up of survival in the randomized European Coronary Surgery Study. *N Engl J Med* 319:332–337, 1988.
45a. Fihn SD, Gardin JM, Abrams J, et al: 2012 ACCF/AHA/ACP/AATS/PCNA/SCAI/STS guideline for the diagnosis and management of patients with stable ischemic heart disease: a report of the American College of Cardiology Foundation/American Heart Association Task Force on practice guidelines, and the American College of Physicians, American Association for Thoracic Surgery, Preventive Cardiovascular Nurses Association, Society for Cardiovascular Angiography and Interventions, and Society of Thoracic Surgeons. *Circulation* 126:e354–e471, 2012.
46. Antman EM, Hand M, Armstrong PW, et al: 2007 Focused update of the ACC/AHA 2004 guidelines for the management of patients with ST-elevation myocardial infarction: A report of the American College of Cardiology/American Heart Association Task Force on Practice Guidelines: Developed in collaboration with the Canadian Cardiovascular Society endorsed by the American Academy of Family Physicians: 2007 Writing Group to review new evidence and update the ACC/AHA 2004 guidelines for the management of patients with ST-elevation myocardial infarction, writing on behalf of the 2004 Writing Committee. *Circulation* 117:296–329, 2008.
47. Chieffo A, Park SJ, Valgimigli M, et al: Favorable long-term outcome after drug-eluting stent implantation in nonbifurcation lesions that involve unprotected left main coronary artery: A multicenter registry. *Circulation* 116:158–162, 2007.
48. Lee MS, Bokhoor P, Park SJ, et al: Unprotected left main coronary disease and ST-segment elevation myocardial infarction: A contemporary review and argument for percutaneous coronary intervention. *JACC Cardiovasc Interv* 3:791–795, 2010.
49. Jones EL, Craver JM, Guyton RA, et al: Importance of complete revascularization in performance of the coronary bypass operation. *Am J Cardiol* 51:7–12, 1983.
50. Omer S, Cornwell LD, Rosengart TK, et al: Completeness of coronary revascularization and survival: Impact of age and off-pump surgery. *J Thorac Cardiovasc Surg* 148:1307–1315.e1, 2014.

51. Bonow RO, Maurer G, Lee KL, et al: Myocardial viability and survival in ischemic left ventricular dysfunction. *N Engl J Med* 364:1617–1625, 2011.
52. Velazquez EJ, Lee KL, Deja MA, et al: Coronary-artery bypass surgery in patients with left ventricular dysfunction. *N Engl J Med* 364:1607–1616, 2011.
53. Subramanian S, Sabik JF, 3rd, Houghtaling PL, et al: Decision-making for patients with patent left internal thoracic artery grafts to left anterior descending. *Ann Thorac Surg* 87:1392–1398, discussion 1400, 2009.
54. Choudhry NK, Singh JM, Barolet A, et al: How should patients with unstable angina and non-ST-segment elevation myocardial infarction be managed? A meta-analysis of randomized trials. *Am J Med* 118:465–474, 2005.
55. Berger PB, Ellis SG, Holmes DR, Jr, et al: Relationship between delay in performing direct coronary angioplasty and early clinical outcome in patients with acute myocardial infarction: Results from the global use of strategies to open occluded arteries in Acute Coronary Syndromes (GUSTO-IIb) trial. *Circulation* 100:14–20, 1999.
56. Cannon CP, Gibson CM, Lambrew CT, et al: Relationship of symptom-onset-to-balloon time and door-to-balloon time with mortality in patients undergoing angioplasty for acute myocardial infarction. *JAMA* 283:2941–2947, 2000.
57. Weiss ES, Chang DD, Joyce DL, et al: Optimal timing of coronary artery bypass after acute myocardial infarction: A review of California discharge data. *J Thorac Cardiovasc Surg* 135:503–511, 511.e1–511.e3, 2008.
58. White HD, Assmann SF, Sanborn TA, et al: Comparison of percutaneous coronary intervention and coronary artery bypass grafting after acute myocardial infarction complicated by cardiogenic shock: Results from the Should We Emergently Revascularize Occluded Coronaries for Cardiogenic Shock (SHOCK) trial. *Circulation* 112:1992–2001, 2005.
59. Loop FD, Lytle BW, Cosgrove DM, et al: Influence of the internal-mammary-artery graft on 10-year survival and other cardiac events. *N Engl J Med* 314:1–6, 1986.
60. Comparison of coronary bypass surgery with angioplasty in patients with multivessel disease. The Bypass Angioplasty Revascularization Investigation (BARI) Investigators. *N Engl J Med* 335:217–225, 1996.
61. Tabata M, Grab JD, Khalpey Z, et al: Prevalence and variability of internal mammary artery graft use in contemporary multivessel coronary artery bypass graft surgery: Analysis of the Society of Thoracic Surgeons National Cardiac Database. *Circulation* 120:935–940, 2009.
62. Tatoulis J, Buxton BF, Fuller JA: The right internal thoracic artery: Is it underutilized? *Curr Opin Cardiol* 26:528–535, 2011.
63. Castellheim A, Hoel TN, Videm V, et al: Biomarker profile in off-pump and on-pump coronary artery bypass grafting surgery in low-risk patients. *Ann Thorac Surg* 85:1994–2002, 2008.
64. Hoel TN, Videm V, Mollnes TE, et al: Off-pump cardiac surgery abolishes complement activation. *Perfusion* 22:251–256, 2007.
65. Bonaros N, Schachner T, Lehr E, et al: Five hundred cases of robotic totally endoscopic coronary artery bypass grafting: Predictors of success and safety. *Ann Thorac Surg* 95:803–812, 2013.

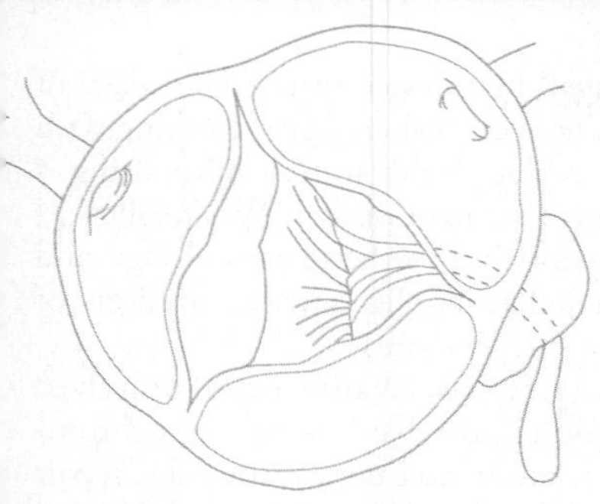

CHAPTER 60

Acquired Heart Disease: Valvular

Todd K. Rosengart, Jatin Anand

OUTLINE

The heart contains four one-way valves that regulate the flow of blood into and out of its chambers. Normal cardiac pumping activity is dependent on the proper functioning of these valves. The atrioventricular (AV) valves (mitral and tricuspid valves), when closed, allow stepwise pressure gradients to be maintained between the atria and ventricles; the semilunar valves (aortic and pulmonic valves) likewise allow pressure gradients between the ventricles and great arteries.

The heart beats 100,000 times per day on average and more than 2.5 billion times throughout an average life span. Given the great number of open-close cycles to which the heart valves are subjected and the relative infrequency of cardiac valvular heart disease (reported at a prevalence of <2% of the population[1]), it must be concluded that the cardiac valvular structures are exceedingly well designed to meet the hemodynamic demands to which they are exposed.

The cardiac valves may nevertheless succumb to injury or degeneration from a number of pathophysiologic processes. The advent in the past century of open surgical valve repair and replacement procedures and more recently of percutaneous interventions to repair or to replace damaged valves has meant life and health to countless millions of individuals with cardiac valve disease. Today, for example, approximately 90,000 patients in the United States and 280,000 worldwide undergo valve replacement each year.

HISTORY OF HEART VALVE SURGERY

The possibility of human intervention to abort the fulminant sequelae of cardiac valve disease was well recognized at least a century ago. The ravages of heart failure secondary to mitral stenosis caused by rheumatic disease became an obvious initial target for such interventions, which were first considered in detail as early as the late 19th century. Conceptualization of such interventions was at first limited to blind procedures incorporating remote manipulation of the valve through surgically created apertures in the heart wall. Later, beginning in the middle of the 20th century, the development of the heart-lung machine provided open access to the interior of the heart and the possibility of precise manipulations of the heart valves under direct vision in a still, bloodless field.

Sir Thomas Lauder Brunton, a Scottish physician, was in 1902 one of the first to describe a technique for closed mitral repair, proposing access to the mitral valve by passing a dilator through the left ventricular (LV) wall. This idea was shunned by his colleagues and never attempted.

After significant experimentation in the research laboratories of the Peter Bent Brigham Hospital in Boston, Elliot Cutler and Peter Levine followed up on Brunton's early surgical theory and performed the first surgical correction of the mitral valve in 1923. Their technique involved the blind insertion of a neurosurgical tenotomy knife through a transventricular approach to divide the stenotic valve commissures. Although their first clinical attempt at valve repair was successful, subsequent procedures had less promising results, and this specific technique was also abandoned.

A new era of cardiac intervention was ushered in soon after Cutler and Levine's false start by the innovation of closed digital commissurotomy. In this procedure, the operator's index finger was inserted into the left atrial (LA) appendage through a purse-string suture and across the mitral valve as a means for mechanical dilation. The first successful clinical report was by Henry Souttar of England in 1925. Although the procedure was technically successful, it was still not until 1948, when Charles Bailey of Philadelphia and Dwight Harken of Boston both reported successful closed digital mitral commissurotomies, that the procedure became a widespread technique for treatment of mitral stenosis (Fig. 60-1).

Techniques for blinded aortic valvular surgery were also attempted as early valve interventions, with varying degrees of success. In 1912, Theodore Tuffier of Paris reported the first clinical attempt to dilate a stenotic aortic valve, reportedly by pushing his finger against the aorta and invaginating the aortic wall through the valve. This report met with considerable skepticism, but then mechanical dilation using an instrument passed retrograde through the innominate artery was reported by Russell

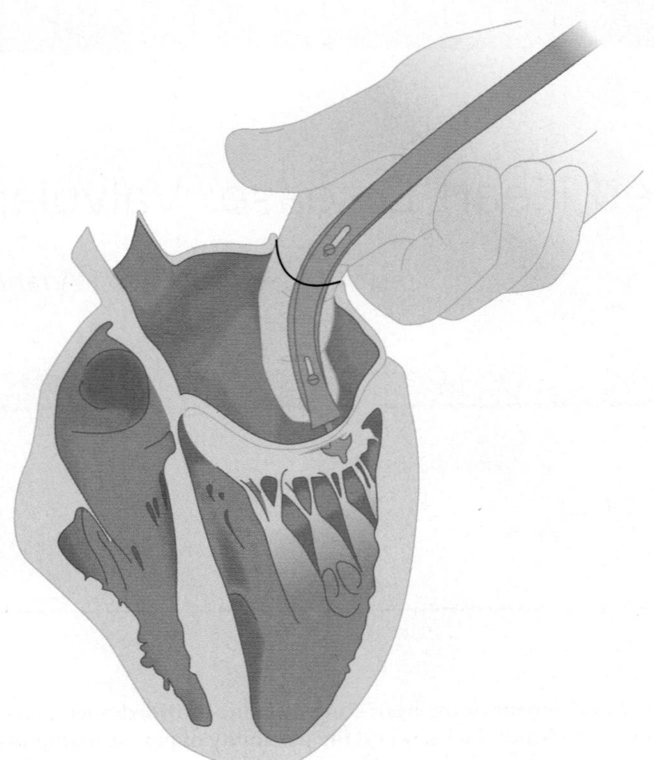

FIGURE 60-1 Closed Mitral Commissurotomy. Dwight Harken developed a closed mitral commissurotomy procedure to correct rheumatic mitral stenosis that became the first widespread approach to treatment of valvular heart disease. (From Muller WH, Jr: The surgical treatment of mitral stenosis. *Calif Med* 75:285–289, 1951.)

Brock of London in 1940. Although this technique led to poor results and was abandoned, it opened the door to new, more compelling possibilities.

In 1948, Horace Smithy of Charleston, South Carolina, performed the first successful aortic valvotomy using a valvulotome inserted through a purse-string suture in the LV apex. Three years later, Charles Bailey of Philadelphia reported the first successful aortic valvotomy using a transventricular expanding dilator, and "closed" approaches to treatment of cardiac valve disease continued to proliferate until further advances overtook these early endeavors.

Two major milestones occurring in the middle of the 20th century marked the beginning of the modern era of successful heart valve surgery: the development of a prosthetic valve and the advent of cardiopulmonary bypass. The first successful implantation of a prosthetic valve was reported by Charles Hufnagel of Georgetown University in 1952. Given the then absence of a means to access the aortic valve in situ, Hufnagel innovated the implantation of a caged-ball valve into the *descending aorta* in a series of patients with aortic insufficiency. In this ingenious design, the forward flow of blood pushed the ball out of the orifice to open the valve during systole, while regurgitant flow was prevented when the ball fell back into the orifice to seal the valve during diastole. Although this extra-anatomic device served to prevent aortic regurgitation, the replacement of cardiac valves in situ would still need to await the advent of cardiopulmonary bypass.

Following the first successful clinical use of the heart-lung machine by Gibbon in 1953 to repair an atrial septal defect, Harken in 1960 finally reported the first successful in situ aortic valve replacement, using a caged-ball device inserted in place of an excised aortic valve. That same year, Albert Starr, working with Lowell Edwards in Oregon, replaced the mitral valve using a similar caged-ball prosthesis of their own design. What followed was an explosion of improvements in prosthetic valve design and implantation techniques that led to applications in millions of patients worldwide during the next 50 years.

Advances in heart valve surgery have spanned ever-improved tissue valve preservation techniques, mechanical valve antithrombotic and durability properties, mitral and now aortic valve repair techniques, and the modern era of percutaneous interventions. These improvements have made survival from cardiac valve disease possible for an ever-expanding spectrum of patients previously considered inoperable, with ever-improving results.

VALVE ANATOMY

The four human heart valves follow similar early embryologic development, beginning as early as 4 weeks of gestation with the formation of the valve primordia in the primitive heart tube. This development is closely linked to the division of the heart tube into its chambers, including septation of the outflow tract (truncus arteriosus) and fusion of the AV canal cushions (Fig. 60-2).

The majority of the cells that migrate into the valve primordia originate from the endocardial cushion, although epicardial and neural crest cells also appear to contribute. Between 20 and 39 weeks of gestation, the valve primordia grow and elongate, thinning to form leaflets and cusps. In late gestation and early after birth, the valve leaflets become stratified into highly organized collagen-, proteoglycan-, and elastin-rich compartments (Fig. 60-3). Valve maturation and remodeling continue into the juvenile stages of life.

In the fully formed heart, the bileaflet mitral and the trileaflet (tricuspid) AV valves are positioned at the inflow to the left and right ventricles, and the three-leaflet aortic and pulmonic semilunar valves are seated atop the outflow tracts of these ventricles, respectively. The AV valves are tethered at their origin to fibrous annular rings (the annuli fibrosi). In comparison, the aortic and pulmonic semilunar valves do not have discrete, ring-like annuli, instead attaching in a curvilinear fashion to the wall of the aorta or pulmonary artery at their junction with the left or right ventricular (RV) outflow tracts, respectively.

The three *cusps* of the semilunar valves (aortic and pulmonic) have a semilunar shape from which they derive their name (Fig. 60-4). Each cusp is in turn made up of four components: the hinge region, where the cusp connects to the annulus; the belly, which makes up the majority of the cusp; the coapting surface at the cusp periphery; and the lunulae, which are thin, crescent-shaped segments of the cusp surrounding a central fibrous nodule at the midpoint of its free edge (termed the nodes of Arantius in the aortic valve).

The mitral valve proper has two *leaflets* possessing approximately equal surface area (Fig. 60-5). The square-shaped anterior leaflet originates from approximately the anterior third of the valve annulus. The posterior mitral leaflet is less wide ("tall") but is longer than the anterior leaflet, attaching to approximately two thirds of the annulus. The anterior and posterior leaflets have three scallops each (e.g., A1, P1), based on indentations found in the posterior leaflet (Fig. 60-5). In comparison, the tricuspid valve is composed of anterior, posterior, and septal leaflets, of which the anterior leaflet is the largest and the septal leaflet the smallest.

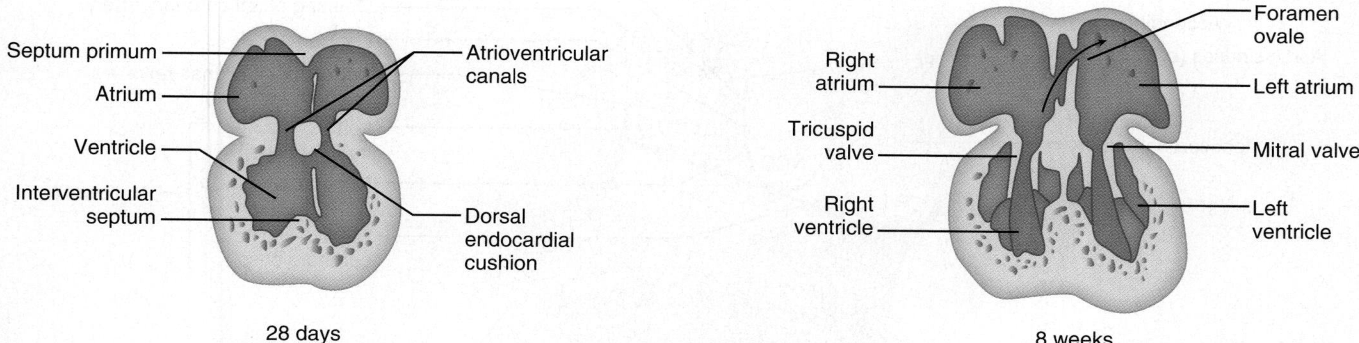

FIGURE 60-2 Embryology of the Cardiac Valves. The development of the valve primordia is closely linked to the division of the heart tube into its chambers, including septation of the outflow tract (truncus arteriosus) and fusion of the atrioventricular canal cushion.

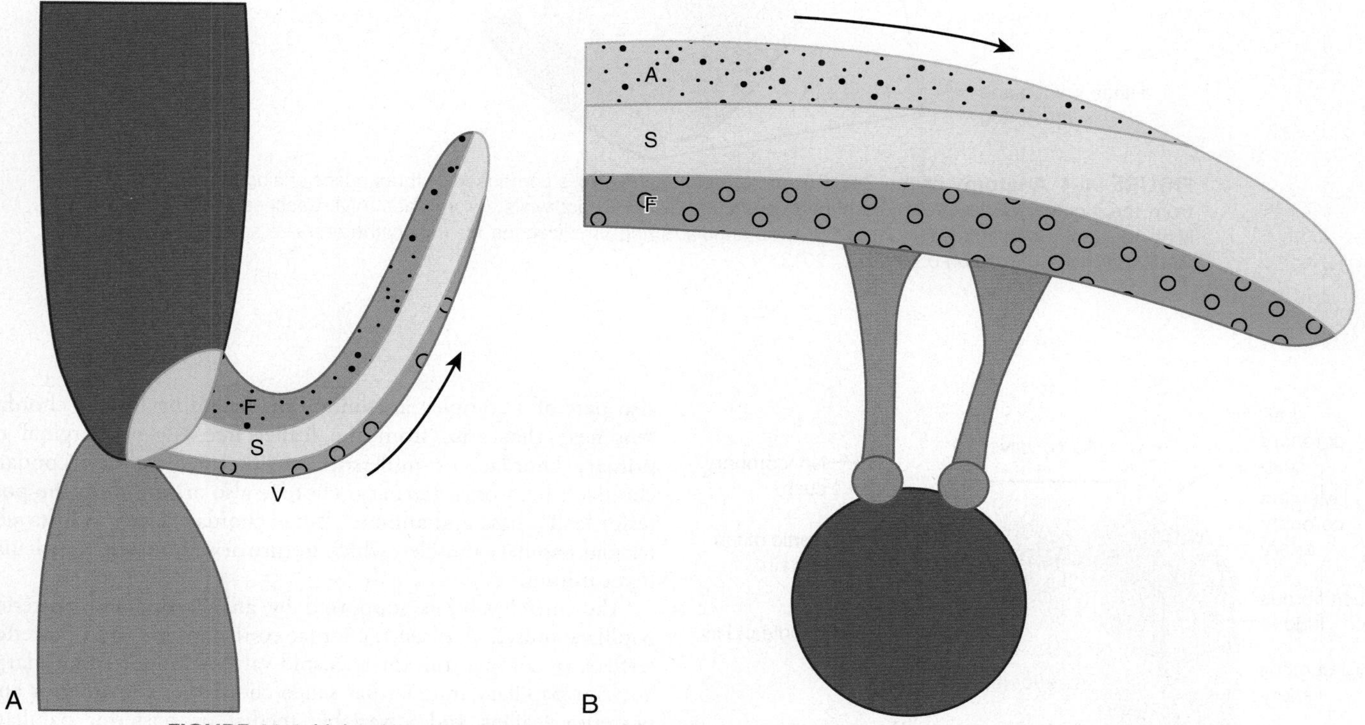

FIGURE 60-3 Valve Histology. The mature valve is composed of a highly organized extracellular matrix, which is compartmentalized into three layers: the fibrosa (F), made of fibrillar collagen; the spongiosa (S), made of proteoglycans; and either the ventricularis (V) of the semilunar valves or the atrialis (A) of the atrioventricular valves, made of elastin fiber. (From Combs MD, Yutzey KE: Heart valve development: Regulatory networks in development and disease. *Circ Res* 105:408–421, 2009.)

All four cardiac valves are supported by internal plates of dense collagen and elastin-rich connective tissue that are continuous with the fibrous cardiac skeleton at the base of the heart. This highly organized extracellular matrix is compartmentalized into three layers: the fibrosa, made of fibrillar collagen; the spongiosa, made of proteoglycans; and either the ventricularis of the semilunar valves or the atrialis of the AV valves, made of elastin fibers (see Fig. 60-3).

In contrast to the free-standing semilunar valves, the mitral and tricuspid valve leaflets and their adjoining fibrous annuli are

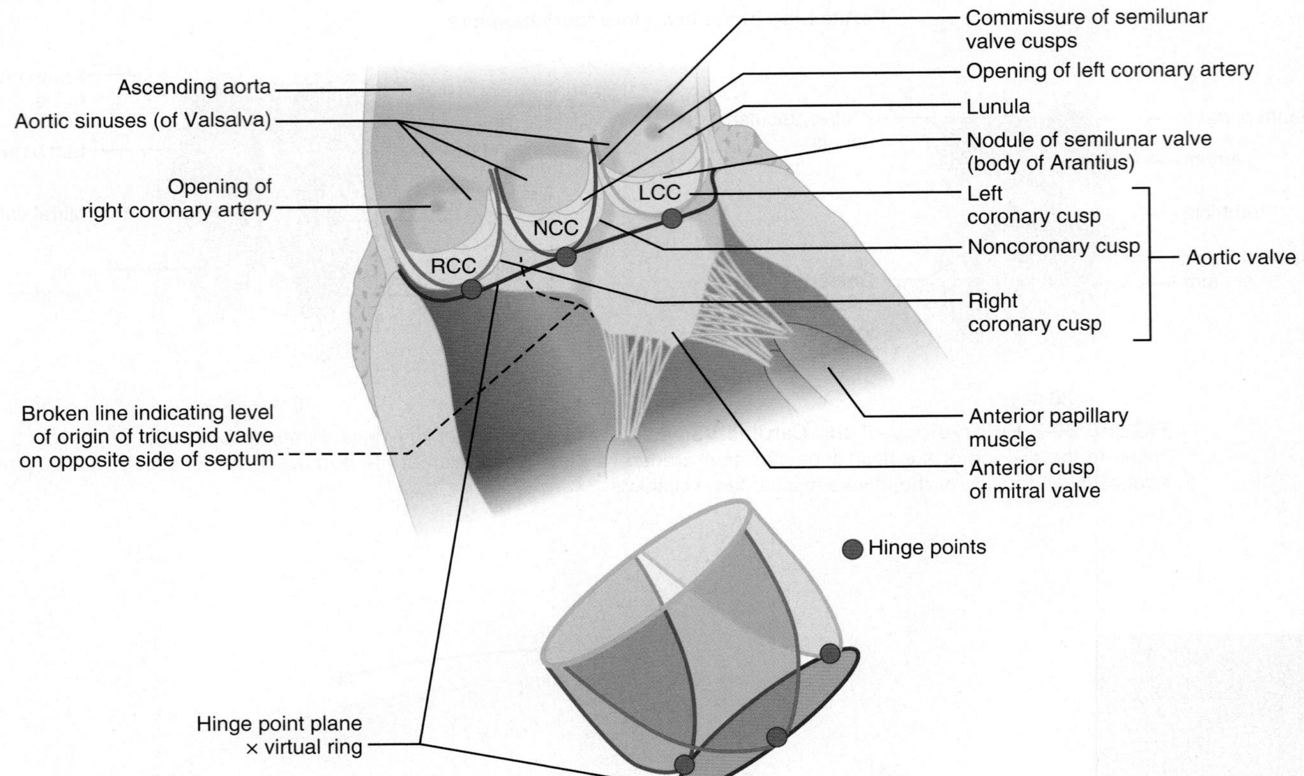

FIGURE 60-4 Anatomy of the Semilunar Valves. Each valve is composed of three cusps arising directly from the juncture of the great vessel and ventricular outflow tract walls. (From Kasel AM, Cassese S, Bleiziffer S, et al: Standardized imaging for aortic annular sizing: Implications for transcatheter valve selection. *JACC Cardiovasc Imaging* 6:249–262, 2013.)

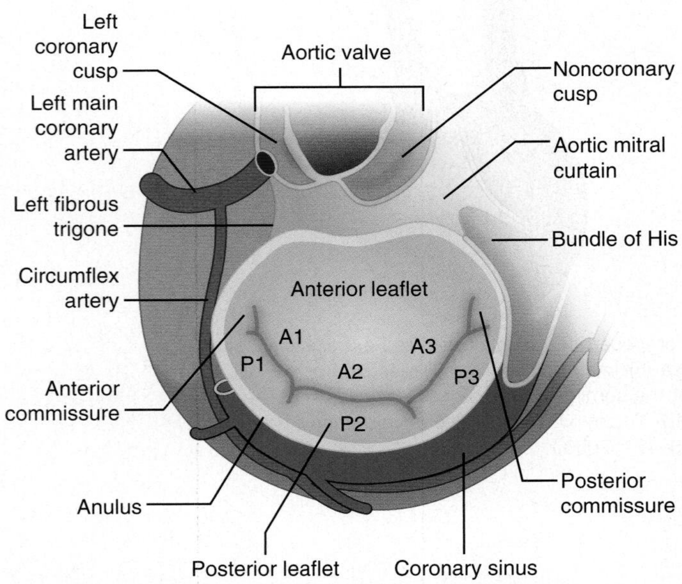

FIGURE 60-5 Anatomy of the AV Valves. The AV valves are composed of leaflets arising from a distinct fibrous annulus. The depicted mitral valve is composed of an anterior and posterior leaflet, each subdivided into three scallops. (From http://www.sciamsurgery.com/sciamsurgery/institutional/figTabPopup.action?bookId=ACS&linkId=part11_ch01_fig20&type=fig.)

also part of a complex anatomic unit including fibrous chordae tendineae that arise from the leaflet free edges (marginal or primary chordae) or undersurface (intermediate or secondary chordae), with basal (tertiary) chordae also arising from the posterior leaflet base and annulus. These chordae attach to intraventricular papillary muscles, which in turn arise from the ventricular myocardium.

The mitral valve is supported by an anterior and posterior papillary muscle that sends chordae to the anterior and posterior leaflets. In comparison, the tricuspid valve is supported by a large anterior papillary muscle that sends chordae to the anterior and posterior leaflets and a variable medial or posterior papillary muscle that provides chordae to the posterior and septal leaflets. The RV septal wall also provides chordae to the anterior and septal tricuspid leaflets, but there is no formal septal papillary muscle.

As suggested by their contrasted anatomy, the semilunar and AV valves differ in their mechanisms of maintaining coaptation. The semilunar valve cusps are dependent largely on coaptation mechanisms intrinsic to the cusps themselves, falling passively to the central arterial lumen in diastole and there sealing the orifice by coapting with the corresponding midpoint nodules on adjoining cusps. The AV valves are tethered in their closed position by their chordal attachments to the papillary muscles, which contract during systole to maintain leaflet coaptation and to prevent leaflet prolapse into the atria (Fig. 60-6).

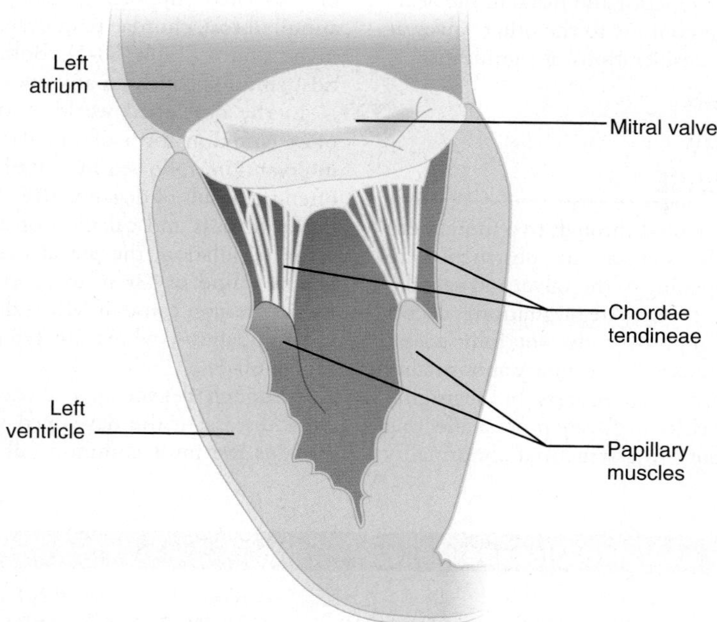

FIGURE 60-6 Subvalvular Apparatus of the AV Valves. The mitral and tricuspid valves are supported by a robust subvalvular apparatus featuring the chordae tendineae that tether the leaflets and annuli to the papillary muscles, which contract during systole to maintain leaflet coaptation and to prevent leaflet prolapse into the atria. (From Filsoufi F, Carpentier A. TheMitralValve.org.)

Surgical Anatomic Relationships

The central location of the aortic valve at the base of the heart imparts to it important anatomic as well as clinical surgical relationships to the other cardiac chambers and valves. The coronary arterial circulation originates at the sinuses of Valsalva, gentle dilations of the aorta just distal to the valve proper that impart important facilitation to valve closure and coronary and blood flow. The right and left coronary arteries arise from the right and left sinuses, respectively. The aortic valve cusps are named with respect to these sinusoidal and coronary relationships, that is, the right coronary, left coronary, and noncoronary (posterior) cusps. (The pulmonic valve cusps are analogously termed the right, left, and anterior cusps.)

In direct continuity with the left and noncoronary cusps of the aortic valve, from about 5 to 8 o'clock in the traditional surgical perspective, is the anterior leaflet of the mitral valve. The noncoronary cusp of the aortic valve and the anterior leaflet of the mitral valve are therefore at risk of injury during mitral and aortic valve surgery, respectively. Likewise, the AV node lies embedded in the top of the ventricular membranous septum, just beneath the commissure between the noncoronary and right coronary aortic leaflets, from 3 to 5 o'clock in the surgical perspective. Only the remaining circumference of the aortic annulus is relatively free anatomically from surgical injury during aortic valve surgery.

The mitral valve bears two additional anatomic relationships of important surgical consideration. The posterior (mural or lateral) leaflet is in continuity with the posterior LV wall. Deep (posterior) to the posterior leaflet lies the AV groove, within which lies the circumflex coronary artery, which is thereby at risk of surgical injury. The AV node likewise lies deep to the posteromedial commissure of the mitral valve.

Tricuspid valve surgery entails risks to two additional structures, found superior to the valve in the right atrium. The coronary sinus ostium lies adjacent to the commissure of the septal and posterior leaflets of the valve and can be inadvertently oversewn if it is not carefully identified. The AV node lies in the apex of a triangular area first described by Koch, which is bounded by the septal annulus of the tricuspid valve anteriorly, the tendon of Todaro posteriorly, and the central fibrous body containing the bundle of His superiorly, leading to the coronary sinus inferiorly (Fig. 60-7). A suture placed within the triangle may lead to complete heart block.

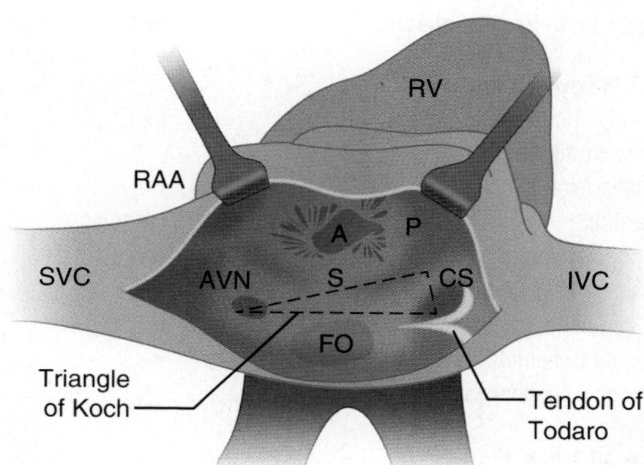

FIGURE 60-7 Surgical Anatomy of the Tricuspid Valve. The AV node lies in the apex of a triangular area first described by Koch, which is bounded by the septal annulus of the tricuspid valve anteriorly, the tendon of Todaro posteriorly, and the central fibrous body containing the bundle of His superiorly, leading to the coronary sinus inferiorly. *A*, anterior tricuspid valve leaflet; *AVN*, atrioventricular node; *CS*, coronary sinus ostium; *FO*, foramen ovale; *IVC*, inferior vena cava; *P*, posterior tricuspid valve leaflet; *RAA*, right atrial appendage; *RV*, right ventricle; *S*, septal tricuspid valve leaflet; *SVC*, superior vena cava. (From Rogers JH, Bolling SF: The tricuspid valve: Current perspective and evolving management of tricuspid regurgitation. *Circulation* 119:2718–2725, 2009.)

Because the pulmonic valve lies superior and distal to the heart proper in the embryonic conus, in contrast to the other valves, it shares limited surgical anatomic considerations of significance.

PATHOLOGY AND ETIOLOGY OF VALVULAR HEART DISEASE

The cardiac valves may become impaired through two fundamental forms of dysfunction: valvular stenosis, an obstruction to forward flow due to incomplete opening of the valve; and valvular insufficiency, in which backward flow (regurgitation) occurs through a valve when its cusps or leaflets do not fully coapt. Valvular stenosis is almost always caused by a primary abnormality of the cusp or leaflet from a chronic disease process, but regurgitation may be caused by an acute or chronic disease process affecting the valve itself or may be secondary to a structural abnormality of associated supporting structures, such as the great arteries, annuli fibrosi, chordae tendineae, papillary muscles, or ventricular myocardium (Table 60-1). Both stenosis and insufficiency may exist simultaneously in any one valve.

In the developed world, aortic valvular stenosis (AS) is the most common form of valvular heart disease requiring surgical intervention, followed by mitral regurgitation (MR). AS is most often the result of degenerative changes to the aortic valve, resulting in fibrosis and calcification in older patients. Because of the aging population, the prevalence of AS continues to rise, and it is now found in 4% of the population older than 85 years. The most common cause of MR is degenerative changes to the mitral valve apparatus, which are typically found in younger patients (Table 60-1).

Although degenerative disease is a more prevalent cause of valve disease in the developed world, rheumatic fever probably remains the most common (albeit decreasing) cause of valvular

TABLE 60-1 Etiology of Valve Disease

	LEAFLETS	ANNULUS	CHORDAE TENDINEAE	VENTRICULAR WALL/ PAPILLARY MUSCLE	AORTIC ROOT
Mitral Stenosis					
Rheumatic valve disease	++	++	++	± (PM fusion/shortening)	NA
Endocarditis (vegetation)	±	–	–	–	NA
Congenital*	++	–	–	±	NA
Supravalvular (thrombus, myxoma)	++	–	–	–	NA
Mitral Regurgitation					
Mitral valve prolapse (myxomatous/ connective tissue disorder)	++	++	++	–	NA
Rheumatic fever	++	–	±	–	NA
Endocarditis	++	±	++	+	NA
Congenital anomaly†	++	–	±	–	NA
Systemic lupus erythematosus‡	++	±	±	± (PM)	NA
Mitral annular calcification	±	++	–	–	NA
Myocardial ischemia/infarction	–	±	–	++	NA
Hypertrophic cardiomyopathy				++	NA
Aortic Stenosis					
Degenerative disease (trileaflet)	++	+	NA	–	–
Bicuspid valve disease	++	+	NA	–	–
Rheumatic valve disease	++	+	NA	–	–
Endocarditis (vegetation)	++	+	NA	–	–
Other congenital anomaly§	++	+	NA	++	+
Hypertrophic cardiomyopathy	–	–	–	++	–
Aortic Insufficiency					
Degenerative/connective tissue disease‖	++	++	NA	–	++
Rheumatic disease	++	–	NA	–	–
Inflammatory disease¶	+	–	NA	–	++
Endocarditis	++	+	NA	–	+
Congenital (bicuspid, unicuspid)	++	–	NA	–	+
Aortic dissection/aortic aneurysm	–	++	NA	–	++

++ common; + fairly common; ± possibly involved; – rarely involved. *NA,* not applicable; *PM,* papillary muscle.
*Parachute mitral valve, supramitral ring.
†Cleft leaflet, endocardial cushion defect, parachute mitral valve.
‡Libman-Sacks lesion.
§Unicuspid/unicommissural valve, hypoplastic annulus/root, subaortic membrane/stenosis.
‖Marfan syndrome, myxomatous degeneration, osteogenesis imperfecta, Ehlers-Danlos syndrome.
¶Ankylosing spondylitis, Reiter syndrome, Takayasu disease, giant cell aortitis.

dysfunction worldwide. Despite the increasing application of antibiotics to treat rheumatic fever, rheumatic heart disease (RHD) will still occur in 30% of those with the acute illness. RHD is still prevalent in part because of the decades-long lag time between the occurrence of rheumatic fever in the first decade of life (mean age, 8 to 12 years) and the subsequent manifestation of rheumatic valvular disease as a sequel in the third or fourth decade of life.[2] The basis of RHD is a chronic inflammatory insult against laminin, a valvular basement membrane protein typically exposed by an initial group A beta-hemolytic streptococcal infection and subsequently targeted through a cross-reactive antibody formation process known as molecular mimicry.

RHD is the most common cause of regurgitant valve lesions, primary multivalvular disease, and mixed (stenotic and regurgitant) lesions. Although RHD may be manifested as MR acutely, chronic disease most commonly is manifested as mitral valve stenosis (MS) or mixed valve lesions and affects women in two thirds of cases. RHD next most frequently directly leads to AS, although indirect upstream hemodynamic stresses caused by MS (see later) make tricuspid regurgitation (TR) a common secondary valvular abnormality.

RHD is the most common cause of MS, and it is uncommon to have rheumatic valvular disease without mitral valve involvement. In 50% of cases, rheumatic mitral valve disease presents as a pathognomonic, mixed stenotic and regurgitant "fish mouth" funnel valve lesion, often associated with fusion and shortening of the leaflets and chordae tendineae (Fig. 60-8). Congenital anomalies, such as parachute deformities and supramitral rings, are far more unusual causes of MS in the adult.

Stenotic disease of the aortic valve is relatively equally divided between that affecting initially normal trileaflet valves and that arising in congenitally bicuspid valves. It occurs as a degenerative process at increasing frequency with age, with more than 90% of AS seen in patients older than 60 years and more than 80% of patients with trileaflet AS presenting for surgery after the age of 60 years.[3] The progression of degenerative (calcific) AS (previously termed senile or wear-and-tear disease) is now thought to be an actively regulated phenomenon related to atherosclerotic disease, wherein turbulent blood flow at leaflet attachment points induces endothelial injury, which leads to accumulation of lipids,

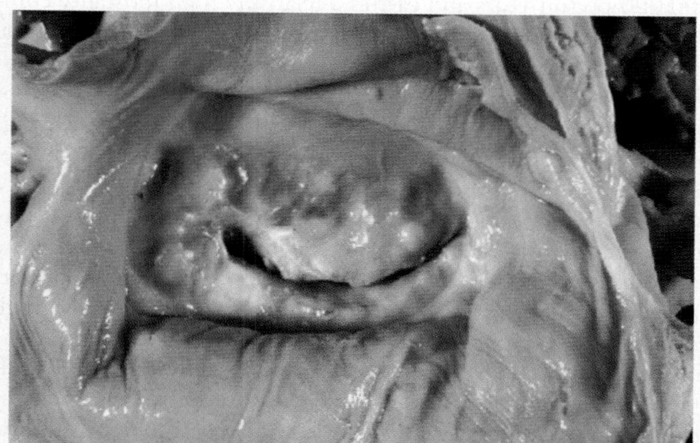

FIGURE 60-8 Mitral Valve in Rheumatic Heart Disease. Typical rheumatic mitral valve disease presenting as a pathognomonic, mixed stenotic and regurgitant "fish mouth" funnel valve lesion, often associated with fusion and shortening of the leaflets and chordae tendineae. (From http://library.med.utah.edu/WebPath/CVHTML/CV061.html.)

infiltration of macrophages and T cells, and transformation of cells to an osteoblastic phenotype.[4] It is believed that this process leads to aortic leaflet calcification, which may involve the aortic and mitral annuli as well as the mitral leaflets.

AS occurs in 20% to 30% of patients born with bicuspid aortic valves, which are more commonly found in males than in females and are present in 1% to 2% of the population, making this anomaly the most prevalent of the congenital valve lesions. Less commonly, unicuspid aortic valves or other congenital anomalies of the LV outflow tract may also be manifested as AS early in life.

Degenerative disease of bicuspid aortic valves is manifested as AS about 2 decades earlier than it is with tricuspid valves, peaking in the fifth and sixth decades of life. Increased hemodynamic stresses associated with the abnormally configured bicuspid valve leaflets are thought to accelerate degenerative valve changes in this anomaly.

Although AS is the most common pathologic presentation of a congenitally bicuspid valve, regurgitant lesions may also occur, typically at a much younger age and with a lower rate of progression requiring surgical intervention. Importantly, mendelian inheritance of a bicuspid aortic valve anomaly is also associated with dilation of the proximal ascending aorta because of pathologic alterations of the aortic media in up to 50% of patients with bicuspid aortic valves.

MR leads to surgical intervention far less often than does AS, but MR is actually the most frequently occurring form of valve dysfunction, with at least trivial MR present in most healthy adults. MR necessitating surgical intervention is related to degenerative disease in 60% to 70% of cases, to ischemic disease in 20% of cases, and to endocarditis or rheumatic disease in 2% to 5%.[5] Congenital anomalies, such as cleft leaflets and AV canal or endocardial cushion defects, may lead to MR as well. Carpentier described a functional classification of MR based on abnormal patterns of leaflet motion (Table 60-2), which together with MR etiology and the specific valve lesion can be used to plan treatment and to predict prognosis.

A wide variety of connective tissue diseases may lead to degenerative disease of the mitral valve, most prominently including Marfan syndrome. Myxomatous disease describes a common pathologic end point of connective tissue disruption that typically is manifested as MR in the third and fourth decades of life. This process is characterized by glycosaminoglycan infiltration of the valve leaflets, thickening of the spongiosa, and separation of collagen bundles in the fibrosa.

Myxomatous disease of the mitral valve typically leads to excessive, "billowing" valve leaflets, annular dilation, and chordae enlargement or elongation and consequent abnormal systolic leaflet "prolapse" into the atrium. This syndrome typically occurs in young women and is termed Barlow disease after the clear identification in 1963 of the cause of this "click-murmur syndrome."[6] Mitral disease is the most common manifestation of myxomatous disease, but it may also present as aortic and tricuspid valve disease. It is often differentiated from fibroelastic deficiency syndrome, which is typically characterized by thinned leaflets and chordal rupture presenting in older patients. Prolapse or flail of the middle posterior leaflet cusp (P2) due to chordae rupture is a common manifestation of this syndrome.[7]

MR may also be caused by secondary, "functional" disorders, in which the morphology of the valve itself is normal. Typically, functional MR is a result of myocardial ischemic events or infarction or ventricular enlargement, which leads to outward (lateral) and apical displacement of the posteromedial papillary muscle

TABLE 60-2 Carpentier Classification of Mitral Valve Regurgitation

CARPENTIER CLASSIFICATION	DYSFUNCTION	LESIONS	ETIOLOGY
Type I	Normal leaflet motion	Annular dilation Leaflet perforation/tear	Dilated cardiomyopathy Endocarditis
Type II	Excessive leaflet motion (prolapse)	Elongation/rupture of chordae Elongation/rupture of papillary muscle	Degenerative valve disease Fibroelastic deficiency Barlow disease Marfan disease Rheumatic (acute) Endocarditis Trauma Ischemic cardiomyopathy
Type IIIa	Restricted leaflet motion (diastole and systole)	Leaflet thickening/retraction Leaflet calcification Chordal thickening/retraction/fusion Commissural fusion	Rheumatic (chronic) Carcinoid heart disease
Type IIIb	Restricted leaflet motion (systole)	Left ventricular dilation/aneurysm Papillary muscle displacement Chordae tethering	Ischemic/dilated cardiomyopathy

Carpentier AF: Cardiac valve surgery—the "French correction." *J Thorac Cardiovasc Surg* 86:323–337, 1983.
Carpentier AF, Lessana A, Relland JY, et al: The "physio-ring": An advanced concept in mitral valve annuloplasty. *Ann Thorac Surg* 60:1177–1186, 1995.

and malapposition of the leaflets because of "tethering" of the leaflets by the chordae (Carpentier type IIIb lesion).

Ischemia or rupture of a papillary muscle secondary to coronary ischemia or acute myocardial infarction, particularly in the inferior distribution, can also lead to functional MR (Carpentier type II). This typically involves the posterior muscle, leading to prolapse or flail of the posterior leaflet because the blood supply to the posterior papillary muscle is from only a single (terminal) branch of the posterior descending coronary artery, compared with dual blood supply to the anterolateral papillary muscle from the left anterior descending and circumflex arteries.

Aortic valve insufficiency (AI) may be caused by myxomatous disease leading to thinning, enlargement, perforation, or prolapse of the aortic valve cusps themselves. AI may also be caused by dilation of the aortic root, which prevents proper aortic valve coaptation by increasing intravalvular closing distances. Root enlargement is typically caused by hypertension or connective tissue disorders, such as cystic medial necrosis, Marfan syndrome, Ehlers-Danlos syndrome, or Loeys-Dietz syndrome, either directly or as a result of aortic dissection.

Bicuspid valve disease is also frequently associated with aortic root enlargement, potentially either through a currently unidentified common genetic defect causing abnormalities in aortic wall elasticity or through hemodynamic "blast" effects of abnormal flow through the bicuspid valve orifice. Less common causes of aortic root enlargement and aortic dissection include trauma, syphilitic aortitis, rheumatoid arthritis, lupus erythematosus, and other systemic vasculopathies, such as Takayasu and giant cell aortitis and osteogenesis imperfecta.

Mitral annular calcification (MAC) is an extremely common degenerative change found in older patients that is typically without functional sequelae. It may be associated with similar changes involving the aortic or mitral valves. However, on occasion, MAC can produce MR by reducing annulus pliability and systolic contraction, which prevents appropriate leaflet coaptation. Less frequently, MAC may be associated with mitral or aortic valve disorders through a more widespread degenerative process.

Endocarditis can also lead to valve destruction and insufficiency or, less frequently, to valve orifice obstruction by endocarditic vegetations—masses of platelets, fibrin, microcolonies of microorganisms, and inflammatory cells. Platelets and fibrin initially become deposited on normal or deformed valves as part of a normal healing process after normal disruptions of the valvular endothelium, typically caused by hemodynamic or metabolic injury. Endocarditis results from subsequent seeding onto the valve of a microbiologic organism, most commonly staphylococci, streptococci, and enterococci, after bacteremia or fungemia.

The incidence of endocarditis varies from 3 to 10 episodes per 100,000 person-years and carries a relatively high mortality compared with other valve lesions.[8] It may affect previously normal valves, but it typically affects valves deformed by congenital or rheumatic disease, degenerative processes such as calcification, or previously replaced prosthetic valves. Infectious endocarditis is usually left sided, reflecting the normal distribution of such preexisting valvular disease.

Acute endocarditis, increasingly affecting normal valves, may follow an aggressive course with valvular perforation or more extensive destruction of the leaflet or surrounding support structures, resulting in acute valvular regurgitation. Although endocarditis is typically relatively indolent, endocarditis is the most common cause of death secondary to acute AI in the adult population. With subacute presentations, valve insufficiency may result from residual leaflet deformities caused by fibrotic healing of endocarditic lesions. The growth of large vegetations may also uncommonly lead to improper leaflet coaptation and insufficiency.

Nearly all of the pathophysiologic mechanisms causing left-sided valve disease may analogously lead to primary right-sided valve disease, but the most common presentation of right-sided valve disease is functional TR caused by RV failure arising from left-sided dysfunction and pulmonary hypertension. Less commonly, functional TR may also be caused by RV infarction or ischemia. Less frequently, transvalvular pacemaker or cardioverter-defibrillator leads can also cause mild or even higher grade TR.

Tricuspid stenosis (TS) occurs infrequently in developed countries because rheumatic disease accounts for more than 90% of such lesions. Carcinoid syndrome is the most common of a group of unusual disorders that lead to the deposition of pathologic materials in the tricuspid and pulmonic leaflets as a far less frequent cause of primary TR, TS, or pulmonic valve disease. Congenital anomalies causing pulmonic valve stenosis are often associated with tetralogy of Fallot, TS, and TR, typically occurring as part of Ebstein anomaly, three of the most common of the congenital disorders leading to right-sided valve disease.

PATHOPHYSIOLOGY OF VALVULAR HEART DISEASE

Two fundamental pathophysiologic derangements may affect the heart valves: stenosis and insufficiency. The hemodynamic hallmark of cardiac valve stenosis is the occurrence of a pressure gradient between an upstream pumping chamber and a downstream receiving chamber or artery caused by the resistance to normal laminar blood flow introduced by the stenotic valve during the time that the valve is normally open. The hemodynamic hallmark of regurgitant valvular disease is the retrograde flow of blood from downstream structures (ventricle or great vessel) into an upstream chamber during the diastolic interval during which the malfunctioning valve should normally be closed. Uncompensated, both stenotic and regurgitant lesions cause an increase in upstream chamber afterload and consequent wall stress—predominating either during ventricular systolic ejection against the resistance of stenotic valves or with increased chamber filling by regurgitant volumes peaking at the end of diastole, respectively.

Two compensatory mechanisms provide robust reserves in cardiac function before the volume and pressure overload stresses of valve disease translate into significant cardiac physiologic derangements. The first, described by the Frank-Starling law (Fig. 60-9), produces increases in ventricular contractile force as a function of end-diastolic volume (EDV), or preload, which enhances stroke volume and ventricular emptying. The second involves stress-induced ventricular hypertrophy, which leads to increased wall thickness. By decreasing chamber radius (volume) or increasing wall thickness, respectively, each of these processes can improve wall stress, as described by Laplace's law: wall stress α = (pressure $\times$ radius)/(2 $\times$ wall thickness). Decreased wall stress, in turn, translates into decreased myocardial work and oxygen demand and improved cardiac function.

The microanatomic basis of the Frank-Starling relationship relates to the orientation between cardiomyocyte sarcomeric actin and myosin fibers, which become ideally aligned to generate contractile force as cardiac muscle is stretched from a "zero-load" status. At a sarcomere length of 2.2 μm, contractile proteins become optimally sensitized to calcium fluxes, resulting in maximized sarcomere contractility as well as rates of contraction and relaxation. As valve-induced cardiomyopathies progress, however, contractile function diminishes at a given level of stretch on the macroanatomic and microanatomic level, and eventually heart failure ensues.

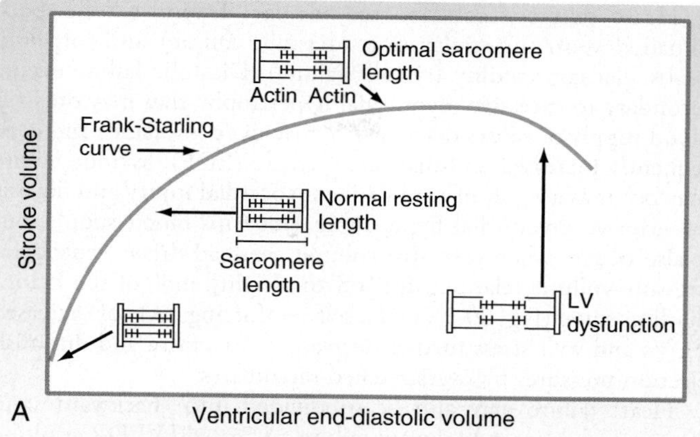

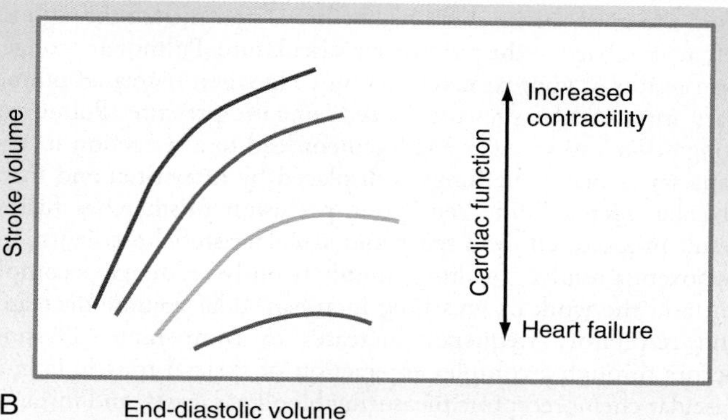

FIGURE 60-9 Frank-Starling Curve. The Frank-Starling law describes a generally linear relationship between increasing end-diastolic volume, or preload, and generated ventricular pressure. **A,** Shifts in volume change generated pressure or stroke volume along a given pressure-volume curve. **B,** Cardiomyopathy shifts the curve downward. (From http://cardiovascres.oxfordjournals.org/content/cardiovascres/77/4/627/F1.large.jpg.)

Heart Failure

Heart failure is defined as the inability of the heart to adequately fill or to pump blood in quantities sufficient to support the metabolic demands of the body under tolerable preload (volume filling) conditions. In the setting of cardiac valvular disease, congestive heart failure ultimately occurs when increases in ventricular volume loading (EDV) or decreases in myocardial contractile function (i.e., change in pressure over time [dp/dt]) exceed the adaptive range of Frank-Starling pressure responses or when excessive ventricular hypertrophy exceeds available nutritive blood supply, causing myocardial ischemia.

Precipitous, fulminant or even fatal heart failure may occur despite relatively normal intrinsic ventricular function in the setting of acute valvular dysfunction when there is insufficient time for compensatory mechanisms to adapt to excessive hemodynamic stresses. More typically, with the chronic progression of valvular dysfunction, heart failure develops after a prolonged, asymptomatic period during which hemodynamic stresses are initially well compensated. In this scenario, profound changes in cardiac functional anatomy (i.e., hypertrophy, enlargement) occur before the onset of symptoms. In modern treatment models, interventions are therefore increasingly indicated before the onset of symptoms.

Heart failure secondary to valvular disease reflects both impaired ventricular relaxation (diastolic failure) and impaired ventricular contractility (systolic failure). Diastolic failure occurs secondary to excessive myocardial hypertrophy that may outstrip blood supply or causes decreased ventricular compliance and consequently increased end-diastolic pressure (EDP). Systolic failure may occur as a result of cumulative myocardial injury and fibrosis as excessive myocardial hypertrophy outstrips blood supply, but it also occurs when excessive volume overload drives ventricular pressure-volume relationships "off the [right] end" of the Frank-Starling curve (Fig. 60-9), and a self-reinforcing cycle of increased EDVs and wall stress further decrease contractility and diminish ejection pressures by overstretched sarcomeres.

Heart failure may also be subdivided into "backward" and "forward" failure. In backward failure, increased LVEDP resulting from the mechanisms described before is transmitted through the left atrium back to the pulmonary vasculature. Pulmonary congestion results at approximately 25 mm Hg when increased pulmonary intravascular pressure exceeds oncotic pressure. Pulmonary congestion and vascular engorgement lead to a reduction in vital capacity as air in the lungs is displaced by interstitial and intra-alveolar edema fluid. Ventilation-perfusion mismatches further result in increased dead space and alveolar-arterial gradients, and hypoxemia results. The lungs simultaneously become less compliant and the work of breathing increases, tidal volume decreases, and respiratory frequency increases to compensate. Dyspnea occurs through a complex interaction of skeletal muscle fatigue, vascular chemoreceptors measuring blood gas levels, and intrapulmonary, chest wall, and skeletal muscle stretch receptors.

Long-standing increases in LVEDP can eventually lead to pulmonary hypertension. Pulmonary hypertension, representing an increase in RV afterload, can eventually precipitate right-sided failure. Right-sided heart failure leads to increased central venous pressure, peripheral venous congestion, and ultimately peripheral organ (e.g., hepatic and renal) failure as a result of decreased capillary–central venous pressure gradients and impaired peripheral emptying.

Typical backward/right-sided heart failure symptoms of orthopnea (dyspnea on recumbency) and paroxysmal nocturnal dyspnea (intermittent nighttime dyspnea associated with recumbency) occur when increases in venous return associated with gravity-neutral recumbency exacerbate pulmonary congestion as otherwise peripherally pooled blood returns to the central circulation.

Forward heart failure—inadequate cardiac output resulting as ventricular systolic dysfunction progresses—leads to further increases in end-systolic volume as ejection fraction (EF) decreases, which in turn leads to further exacerbation of the decompensatory processes described before. Right-sided forward failure impairs left-sided heart filling, furthering inadequate LV ejection and forward output. Left-sided forward failure can be manifested by end-organ hypoperfusion symptoms, such as fatigue, and can trigger a number of systemic components of heart failure that are initially adaptive but typically lead to a number of the maladaptive sequelae of heart failure.

With left-sided forward failure, decreased inhibitory inputs from the carotid and aortic arch baroreceptors and cardiopulmonary mechanoreceptors as well as increased excitatory inputs from peripheral chemoreceptors and mechanoreceptors lead to an increase in sympathetic tone. Together with increased circulating plasma norepinephrine, adrenergic activation causes an increase in heart rate (chronotropy), conduction velocity (dromotropy), contractility (inotropy), and rate of relaxation (lusitropy) as compensatory responses to decreased cardiac output.

Decreased effective arterial blood volume resulting from left-sided forward failure causes renal hypoperfusion, decreased filtered sodium at the macula densa, and increased renal sympathetic tone, all contributing to increased release of renin from the juxtaglomerular apparatus. Renin-angiotensin system activation leads to sodium retention, activation of thirst centers in the brain, and secretion of aldosterone, increasing cardiac preload from salt and water retention.

Both adrenergic and renin-angiotensin system activation leads to vasoconstriction, hypertension, and increased afterload. With elevated preload and afterload, ventricular wall stress increases, leading to further myocyte hypertrophy. Eventually, myocyte hypertrophy, necrosis, apoptosis, and fibrosis combine with desensitization of β-adrenergic receptors and other maladaptive changes in gene expression and biomolecular mechanisms, such as those affecting intracellular calcium handling, to further propagate decreasing cardiac function.

VALVE DISEASE SYNDROMES

Mitral Stenosis

The nondiseased mitral valve orifice has a cross-sectional area of 4 to 6 cm^2. Under normal conditions, there is no gradient across the mitral valve, and LA pressure is typically less than 10 to 15 mm Hg. MS, typically occurring as a result of rheumatic disease, causes a pressure gradient to develop across the diseased mitral valve. More specifically, as the mitral valve orifice narrows to a cross-sectional area of 2 to 2.5 cm^2 (mild MS), resistance to flow leads to increased LA blood volume "pooling." Increased LA pressure generated by Frank-Starling mechanics maintains adequate diastolic flow across the resistive valve orifice.

When progressive MS leads to a transvalvular gradient of more than 5 to 10 mm Hg, typically corresponding to a valve orifice of less than 1.5 cm^2, MS is classified as severe. The resultant increase in LA pressure is transmitted upstream to the pulmonary veins, capillaries, and arteries. At an LA pressure of 25 mm Hg, pulmonary edema typically develops.

With chronically increased pulmonary pressure, arterial vasoconstriction and vascular remodeling lead to fixed pulmonary hypertension. Elevated pulmonary arterial systolic pressure higher than 60 mm Hg imparts significant RV afterload and may ultimately lead to RV dilation, TR, and RV failure as well. MS, on the other hand, is the most sparing of left-sided valvular lesions in regard to sparing intrinsic left ventricle function. LVEDP is normal or below normal in 85% of cases, and LV chamber size is normal or smaller than normal in most cases. Cardiac output is impaired in one third of cases, but primarily because of restricted LV inflow.

Several changes in cardiac hemodynamics can acutely exacerbate this pathophysiologic process. Any increase in cardiac output, as with exercise, will lead to an increase in transvalvular pressure gradients according to the law of Poiseuille: flow $\alpha = \Delta p$/resistance, where Δp signifies pressure gradient. At a given cardiac output, decreased diastolic filling time caused by increased heart rates, such as with exercise or the onset of atrial fibrillation, will cause a similar increase in transvalvular gradient as more flow must occur per unit time.

Chronically increased transmitral pressure gradients caused by MS typically lead to atrial hypertrophy and dilation. Associated LA fibrosis and disorganization of the atrial muscle fibers cause abnormal atrial conduction velocities and refractory times. Increased automaticity, ectopic foci, and reentry circuits eventually lead to supraventricular tachycardias and atrial fibrillation in nearly 40% of patients with MS. Loss of the "kick" generated by normal atrial contraction, responsible for 30% of ventricular diastolic filling, results in a 20% decrease in cardiac output and necessitates increased atrial pressure to allow adequate ventricular loading. Atrial fibrillation consequently causes increased diastolic pressures and volume overload, potentially leading to worsening congestion.

Diagnosis of Mitral Stenosis

Symptoms and signs. MS patients may remain asymptomatic for many years. As valvular stenosis gradually worsens, however, symptoms characteristic of low cardiac output and pulmonary venous congestion eventually develop, including fatigue, dyspnea, orthopnea, and paroxysmal nocturnal dyspnea. Ultimately, peripheral edema and other congestive symptoms caused by volume overload and right-sided heart failure ensue. Increased heart rate caused by atrial fibrillation or supraventricular tachycardia, exercise, or other factors may exacerbate or precipitate earlier symptoms.

Patients with MS who develop atrial fibrillation may complain of palpitations and symptomatic tachycardia. More ominously, thromboembolization will occur in 20% of patients with MS and may be its first symptom in 10% of cases, presenting as stroke, myocardial ischemia or infarction, renal infarction, and gut or limb ischemia. Half of all thromboembolic events will involve the cerebral circulation. Rarely, a large, pedunculated atrial thrombus may form and obstruct the valve inlet, resulting in hemodynamic collapse and sudden death.

With advanced disease, LA enlargement may cause hoarseness from left recurrent laryngeal nerve compression onto the pulmonary artery, dysphagia from esophageal compression, or persistent cough from bronchial compression. Pulmonary venous congestion may induce hemoptysis from sudden rupture of a dilated bronchial vein. RV failure and TR can cause abdominal pain and swelling from hepatomegaly and ascites or even florid peripheral edema.

Physical examination. The characteristic physical finding of MS is a low-pitched, rumbling diastolic murmur that is best heard at the apex with the patient in the left lateral decubitus position. In patients who are in sinus rhythm, the murmur increases in intensity during late diastole (known as presystolic accentuation) because of the increased flow across the stenotic valve with atrial contraction. As severity of MS progresses, the diastolic rumble may be of longer duration or even holodiastolic. The Graham Steell diastolic murmur of MS can result from pulmonary regurgitation caused by pulmonary hypertension and right-sided overload.

A high-pitched "opening snap" or an accentuated first heart sound caused by forceful opening or closing, respectively, of an inflexible but still mobile mitral leaflet may be heard with early MS. As MS progresses, LA pressure rises and the mitral valve opens earlier in diastole. As pulmonary arterial pressure increases, a loud pulmonic component of second heart sound (P2) may be appreciated.

Advanced MS is typically associated with rales developing with the onset of pulmonary edema. As RV failure develops, an RV heave, jugular venous distention, hepatomegaly, ascites, and lower extremity edema may be found.

Diagnostic testing. The earliest appreciable changes of MS discernible by routine chest radiography include evidence of an enlarged left atrium seen as a straightening of the left cardiac border, a double shadow in the cardiac silhouette, and an elevated left mainstem bronchus. Prominent pulmonary vessels may also be appreciated. If stenosis is severe, congested pulmonary lymphatics in the lower lung fields may be present as horizontal linear opacities, known as Kerley B lines. Mitral valve calcification may also be visible. Stigmata of heart failure, such as opacification of the lung fields and pleural effusions, may follow.

The electrocardiographic recording of MS patients is often grossly normal, although 90% of patients will demonstrate evidence of LA enlargement as a widened, notched P wave (P mitrale). Atrial arrhythmias may also be appreciated if present. With advanced MS, RV hypertrophy may be associated with right axis deviation.

Echocardiography, as with other valve lesions, is the primary diagnostic method to determine the presence and severity of MS and associated abnormalities. Commissural fusion, leaflet immobility, and leaflet as well as annular and subvalvular thickening and calcification can be well assessed by transthoracic and especially by transesophageal echocardiography. Newer, three-dimensional echocardiography provides further definition of valve morphology and function, although the role for this technology has not as yet been fully defined.

Doppler echocardiography has largely replaced cardiac catheterization in accurately assessing the hemodynamic parameters of MS as well as other valve lesions. Doppler blood velocity measurement allows mean and peak transvalvular mitral pressure gradient determination as a function of the simplified Bernoulli equation: $p = 4v^2$. Orifice area can be measured by planimetry (tracing the valve opening orifice on a still echocardiographic image) or as a derivative of velocity measurements, based on continuity equations. Mitral valve area can also be calculated on the basis of the pressure half-time, the time in which the transvalvular velocity decreases by half. Pressure half-time will become prolonged with increasing severity of stenosis.

Natural History

Ten-year patient survival is greater than 80% in the asymptomatic patient with MS, and interventional treatment is consequently not recommended in this setting. In comparison, 10-year survival for symptomatic patients with severe MS who forgo intervention is less than 15%, and mean survival is less than 3 years in patients with MS and severe pulmonary hypertension. All MS patients are therefore recommended to receive careful clinical surveillance, including serial echocardiography.

Treatment

Medical management. Medical management of patients with symptomatic MS includes the use of diuretics to reduce LA pressure and vascular congestion. Beta blockers and calcium-blocking agents are recommended to provide heart rate control and to help maintain sinus rhythm. Anticoagulation therapy is guided by $CHADS_2$ scoring in patients developing atrial fibrillation (Table 60-3) and in patients without atrial fibrillation but who have suffered a prior embolic event or have a documented LA thrombus.[9]

Interventional management. Early operation is associated with improved long-term survival compared with patients in whom intervention is delayed until the development of class III symptoms, in whom 5-year survival is 62%, and compared with class IV patients, in whom 5-year survival is 15%.[10] Mechanical relief of MS is accordingly indicated for symptomatic patients with severe MS (mitral valve area 1.5 cm^2) or even in asymptomatic patients with critical MS (orifice area < 1 cm^2) or those who have significant elevation of mean transvalvular gradient (>15 mm Hg) or pulmonary capillary wedge pressure (>25 mm Hg) during provocative testing.[9,11] The onset of atrial fibrillation and systemic embolization, especially if recurrent, are other considerations for intervention.

Options for mechanical intervention include percutaneous balloon mitral commissurotomy (PBMC), open mitral commissurotomy (OMC) and surgical repair, and replacement of the mitral valve.

Percutaneous balloon mitral commissurotomy. The first clinical application of mitral commissurotomy by a balloon catheter was reported by Inoue and colleagues in 1984.[12] This endovascular procedure introduces a balloon catheter into the left atrium through transseptal puncture or retrograde transaortic delivery with subsequent dilation of the mitral valve. Randomized clinical trials have clearly established the safety and efficacy of PBMC compared with surgical commissurotomy, and PBMC has largely replaced surgical interventions in patients with appropriate (Wilkins) echocardiographic criteria (Table 60-4), which include the presence of mobile, noncalcified, thin valves with minimal fusion, scarring, or calcification of the subvalvular apparatus and the absence of moderate to severe MR or LA thrombus.[9]

Successful PBMC, defined as a valve area of more than 1.5 cm^2 with no MR higher than grade 2/4, is achieved in more than 80% of appropriately selected patients undergoing this procedure. Mortality risk is 0.5%, and there is a less than 10% risk of cardiac or peripheral vascular complications, embolization, or creation of severe MR.[11] Although reintervention is often ultimately required, more than half of patients can expect to remain free from surgery at 20 years.[13]

TABLE 60-3 $CHADS_2$ Score for Atrial Fibrillation Stroke Risk and Recommended Anticoagulation

$CHADS_2$ SCORE	POINTS
Congestive heart failure	1
Hypertension	1
Age ≥ 75 years	1
Diabetes mellitus	1
Stroke or TIA history	2

Points are additive for each risk factor. Score of 0, low risk; 1, moderate risk; 2-6, high risk. Recommended therapy for low risk is aspirin, 75 to 325 mg daily; for moderate risk, warfarin or aspirin; for high risk, warfarin (international normalized ratio, 2-3).
TIA, transient ischemic attack.

Open mitral commissurotomy. Although it is seldom performed in lieu of PBMC or valve replacement, OMC is the primary form of surgical repair for patients with MS in whom intervention is needed but PBMC is contraindicated or for patients in whom previous percutaneous intervention has failed. OMC under cardiopulmonary bypass provides for careful inspection of the mitral valve apparatus, débridement of calcium deposits, sharp division of fused commissures and leaflets, mobilization of scarred chordae, removal of LA thrombus, and ligation of the LA appendage as indicated. It can be performed through a median sternotomy or minimally invasive access. The mortality rate for open commissurotomy is less than 2%, and the 10-year freedom from reoperation rate after OMC is approximately 90%.[14,15]

Mitral valve replacement. For patients in whom PBMC or OMC is contraindicated, mitral valve replacement with a bioprosthetic or mechanical valve is today a safe procedure providing excellent long-term results (Table 60-5). Regardless of whether a mechanical or tissue valve is employed, there is well-documented evidence that preservation of the subvalvular apparatus is critical for the maintenance of optimal LV geometry and function and improving 30-day and long-term survival.[9,16]

Mitral Regurgitation

Pathologic changes to any portion of the mitral valve apparatus or its function may cause improper systolic coaptation between the anterior and posterior mitral leaflets with subsequent valvular regurgitation. Importantly, disease of the mitral annulus or leaflets proper, termed primary MR and classified as type I or type II disease in the Carpentier system (see Table 60-2), is distinct in terms of pathophysiology, natural history, and treatment approach from functional MR, which is typically caused by abnormal LV function and classified as a Carpentier type IIIb lesion.

The severity of MR depends on the size of the mitral orifice, the pressure gradient between the left ventricle and left atrium, and the systemic afterload. Because LV pressure exceeds LA pressure well before it exceeds systemic pressure, mitral valve incompetency may allow a significant amount of regurgitant volume (up

TABLE 60-4 Wilkins Score for Assessing Appropriateness of Percutaneous Balloon Mitral Commissurotomy

WILKINS SCORE GRADE	MOBILITY	THICKENING	CALCIFICATION	SUBVALVULAR THICKENING
1	Highly mobile valve with only leaflet tips restricted	Leaflets nearly normal in thickness (4-5 mm)	A single area of increased echocardiographic brightness	Minimal thickening just below the mitral leaflets
2	Leaflet mid and base portions have normal mobility	Midleaflets normal, considerable thickening of margins (5-8 mm)	Scattered areas of brightness confined to leaflet margins	Thickening of chordal structures extending to one-third the chordal length
3	Valve continues to move forward in diastole, mainly from the base	Thickening extending through the entire leaflet (5-8 mm)	Brightness extending into the midportions of the leaflets	Thickening extended to distal third of the chords
4	No or minimal forward movement of the leaflets in diastole	Considerable thickening of all leaflet tissue (>8-10 mm)	Extensive brightness throughout much of the leaflet tissue	Extensive thickening and shortening of all chordal structures extending down to the papillary muscles

Sum of the four items ranges between 4 and 16. With a score of 8 or less, percutaneous balloon mitral valvuloplasty is likely to be successful. If the score is higher than 8, surgery is recommended.

TABLE 60-5 Outcomes of Surgery for Valvular Heart Disease

VALVE SURGERY	VALVE LESION	OPERATIVE MORTALITY	SURVIVAL AFTER SURGERY	FREEDOM FROM REOPERATION
Aortic valve replacement	Aortic stenosis	1%-3%[a]	85% at 10 years[b]	75% (lifetime; biologic) 97% (lifetime; mechanical)[c]
	Aortic insufficiency	1%-4%[a]	63% at 10 years[d]	75% (lifetime; biologic) 97% (lifetime; mechanical)[c]
Aortic valve repair	Aortic insufficiency	1%-4%[a]	95% at 13 years[d]	83% to 93% at 8 years[e]
Mitral valve replacement	Mitral stenosis	3%-10%[a]	15%-62% at 5 years[f]	92% at 10 years[g]
	Primary mitral regurgitation	4%[h]	60% at 10 years[g]	92% at 10 years[g]
	Functional mitral regurgitation	3%-5%[i,j]	66% at 5 years[k]	70%-85% at 4 years[i]
Mitral valve repair	Primary mitral regurgitation	0%-1%[l]	87% at 10 years[g]	94% at 10 years[g]
	Functional mitral regurgitation	~5%[m]	50%-75% at 5 years[k,n]	63% at 10 years[j]
Percutaneous balloon mitral commissurotomy	Mitral stenosis	0.5%-2%[a]	80% at 9 years[o]	50% at 20 years[p]
Open mitral commissurotomy	Mitral stenosis	<2%[o]	96% at 10 years[q]	98% at 9 years[j]

[a]Vahanian A, Alfieri O, Andreotti, et al: Guidelines on the management of valvular heart disease (version 2012): The Joint Task Force on the Management of Valvular Heart Disease of the European Society of Cardiology (ESC) and the European Association for Cardio-Thoracic Surgery (EACTS). *Eur J Cardiothorac Surg* 42:S1–S44, 2012. Patients younger than 70 years.
[b]Kvidal P, Bergström R, Hörte LG, et al: Observed and relative survival after aortic valve replacement. *J Am Coll Cardiol* 35:747–756, 2000.
[c]van Geldorp MW, Eric Jamieson WR, Ye J, et al: Patient outcome after aortic valve replacement with a mechanical or biological prosthesis: Weighing lifetime anticoagulant-related event risk against reoperation risk. *J Thorac Cardiovasc Surg* 137:881–886, 2009.
[d]Chaliki HP, Mohty D, Avierinos JF, et al: Outcomes after aortic valve replacement in patients with severe aortic regurgitation and markedly reduced left ventricular function. *Circulation* 106:2687–2693, 2002.
[e]Talwar S, Saikrishna C, Saxena A, et al: Aortic valve repair for rheumatic aortic valve disease. *Ann Thorac Surg* 79:1921–1925, 2005.
[f]Olesen KH: The natural history of 271 patients with mitral stenosis under medical treatment. *Br Heart J* 24:349–357, 1962.
[g]Gillinov AM, Blackstone EH, Nowicki ER, et al: Valve repair versus valve replacement for degenerative mitral valve disease. *J Thorac Cardiovasc Surg* 135:885–893, 2008.
[h]Gammie JS, Sheng S, Griffith BP, et al: Trends in mitral valve surgery in the United States: Results from the Society of Thoracic Surgeons Adult Cardiac Surgery Database. *Ann Thorac Surg* 87:1431–1439, 2009.
[i]Lorusso R, Gelsomino S, Vizzardi E, et al: Mitral valve repair or replacement for ischemic mitral regurgitation? The Italian Study on the Treatment of Ischemic Mitral Regurgitation (ISTIMIR). *J Thorac Cardiovasc Surg* 145:128–139, 2013.
[j]DiBardino DJ, ElBardissi AW, McClure RS, et al: Four decades of experience with mitral valve repair: Analysis of differential indications, technical evolution, and long-term outcome. *J Thorac Cardiovasc Surg* 139:76–84, 2010.
[k]Calafiore AM, Di Mauro M, Gallina S, et al: Mitral valve surgery for chronic ischemic mitral regurgitation. *Ann Thorac Surg* 77:1989–1997, 2004.
[l]Tourmousoglou C, Lalos S, Dougenis D: Is aortic valve repair or replacement with a bioprosthetic valve the best option for a patient with severe aortic regurgitation? *Interact Cardiovasc Thorac Surg* 18:211–218, 2014.
[m]Braunberger E, Deloche A, Berrebi A, et al: Very long-term results (more than 20 years) of valve repair with Carpentier's techniques in nonrheumatic mitral valve insufficiency. *Circulation* 104:I8–I11, 2001.
[n]Oliveira JM, Antunes MJ: Mitral valve repair: Better than replacement. *Heart* 92:275–281, 2006.
[o]Song JK, Kim MJ, Yun SC, et al: Long-term outcomes of percutaneous mitral balloon valvuloplasty versus open cardiac surgery. *J Thorac Cardiovasc Surg* 139:103–110, 2010.
[p]Bouleti C, Iung B, Himbert D, et al: Reinterventions after percutaneous mitral commissurotomy during long-term follow-up, up to 20 years: The role of repeat percutaneous mitral commissurotomy. *Eur Heart J* 34:1923–1930, 2013.
[q]Antunes MJ, Vieira H, Ferrão de Oliveira J: Open mitral commissurotomy: The 'golden standard.' *J Heart Valve Dis* 9:472–477, 2000.

to half of the ventricular preload) into the left atrium well before the opening of the aortic valve and forward flow into the aorta.

In the acute phase of MR, retrograde flow into the small, low-compliance left atrium receiving chamber may be poorly tolerated, and high atrial pressures may be transmitted into the pulmonary vasculature. Pulmonary hypertension with fulminant heart failure can ensue and even prove to be fatal. When the onset of MR is more insidious, the left atrium has time to dilate and hypertrophy, and a chronic compensated state without pulmonary hypertension may be sustained for many years. On the other hand, LA dilation may be accompanied by atrial fibrillation with the potential for thrombosis and episodic embolization.

Critical compensatory changes in LV hemodynamics are characteristic of chronic MR. Regurgitant volumes returning to the left ventricle during diastole result in increased LVEDV and supranormal EFs, based on standard Frank-Starling mechanics as well as the presence of LV ejection into the relatively low-resistance/low-afterload left atrium. Although net forward blood flow is reduced, this supranormal ejection serves to marginally unload the left ventricle and normalize LVEDV. Wall stress resulting from increased LVEDV also leads to compensatory myocardial hypertrophy and restoration of normal wall tension per Laplace's law.

Whereas a hypertrophied or hyperdynamic left ventricle is typical of acute or compensated chronic MR, the finding of diminished EF despite the afterload reduction associated with MR is suggestive of a decompensated state with rightward or downward shifts in Frank-Starling curve pressure-volume relationships (Fig. 60-9). In this setting, net forward flows continue to decrease and LVEDV increases. Consequent LA and LV dilation leads to an increase in mitral orifice size. A self-perpetuating cycle of worsening heart failure with worsened MR eventually takes hold. LV failure may then lead to pulmonary hypertension and right-sided heart failure.

Diagnosis of Mitral Regurgitation

Symptoms and signs. Acute decompensated MR may cause the sudden onset of dyspnea secondary to pulmonary venous hypertension and congestion. An associated decrease in forward cardiac output may cause hypotension or even hemodynamic collapse. More typically, patients with chronic, mild MR may be asymptomatic for most of their lives. When MR more gradually becomes moderate to severe, typical symptoms of left-sided heart failure, atrial fibrillation, or even right-sided heart failure may become manifested.

Physical examination. Palpation of patients with MR may reveal a hyperdynamic, laterally displaced cardiac impulse. Auscultation typically reveals a holosystolic, high-pitched, blowing apical murmur that radiates to the axilla. Isolated posterior leaflet dysfunction may cause the murmur to radiate to the sternum or aortic area, whereas isolated anterior leaflet dysfunction may cause the murmur to radiate to the back or head. Other findings may include a diminished first heart sound, wide splitting of the second heart sound due to early aortic valve closure, and a third heart sound due to increased blood flow across the mitral valve.

Diagnostic testing. Echocardiography is the primary method for diagnosis and monitoring of MR, although cardiac magnetic resonance imaging can also provide useful regurgitant volume and cardiac function data. Routine chest radiography may demonstrate an enlarged cardiac silhouette and LA enlargement or signs of pulmonary congestion associated with heart failure. Electrocardiography may reveal atrial fibrillation or signs of LA enlargement (P mitrale) and QRS or ST-T interval changes reflective of ventricular hypertrophy or bundle branch conduction abnormalities.

Transthoracic and in particular transesophageal echocardiography studies allow precise visualization of the mechanisms responsible for inducing MR and classification according to the Carpentier system (see Table 60-2), including single-leaflet or bileaflet prolapse or flail, enlarged or billowing leaflets, annular dilation, chordal rupture, papillary muscle rupture, and restricted leaflet motion and tethering caused by an enlarged or infarcted ventricle. Leaflet disruption or perforation, valvular vegetations, or annular abscesses secondary to infective endocarditis may also be visualized.

Doppler analysis provides important prognostic data on regurgitant jet localization and quantification, typically measured by the proximal isovolumetric surface area (PISA) metric. The PISA measurement is based on the principle that flow through an orifice (mitral valve) will produce a hemispheric area of flow convergence proximal to the orifice (on the ventricular side of the leaking mitral valve). Measuring the radius of this zone allows estimated calculation of the regurgitant flow, effective regurgitant orifice area, and regurgitant volume on the basis of the equation flow = velocity × area.

Natural History

Acute MR is poorly tolerated and typically requires urgent intervention. In the absence of intervention, severe pulmonary edema, cardiac decompensation, and development of pulmonary hypertension often lead to rapid deterioration and poor outcomes.

It was long thought that the asymptomatic MR patient was not at decreased survival risk, but a rich body of new data now clearly demonstrates that even in the asymptomatic patient, the presence of severe MR with ventricular dysfunction, pulmonary hypertension, or atrial fibrillation carries a diminished prognosis. For example, it has been shown prospectively that asymptomatic patients with severe MR have significantly reduced 5-year survival with medical management compared with the general population.[17] Even moderate primary MR has now been shown to be associated with an annual mortality risk of 3%, representing excessive risk in the context of outstanding results now achievable with mitral repair.[5]

Patients with functional MR, typically occurring on the basis of ischemic disease, carry a far worse prognosis than patients with primary MR.[5] Retrospective data from the STICH trial examining patients undergoing coronary artery bypass grafting (CABG) with diminished EF demonstrated that mortality during approximately 4.5 years was about twofold greater in patients with moderate to severe MR compared with those with mild or no MR.[18]

Treatment

Medical treatment. The medical management of acute MR involves intravenous vasodilator therapy, typically with nitroprusside. The resultant decrease in aortic pressure and afterload enhances forward cardiac output and decreases regurgitant flow into the LA. When vasodilator use is limited by systemic hypotension, intra-aortic balloon counterpulsation effectively lowers systolic afterload and increases forward flow. Prompt mitral valve surgery is typically needed in acute MR, particularly in the symptomatic or hemodynamically compromised patient.

In symptomatic patients with chronic MR, standard vasodilator and diuretic medical therapy can be useful in improving ventricular hemodynamics and reducing pulmonary congestion. Diuretics may be particularly effective in reducing volume overload and ventricular distention and thus annular orifice size and regurgitant MR fractions. Contrary to popular practice, however, there is no evidence to support the use of vasodilator or other afterload-reducing medications in an attempt to delay the need for surgery in asymptomatic patients with chronic MR and normal LV systolic function.[9] In fact, vasodilators may decrease LV size and therefore reduce the mitral valve closing force, potentially increasing mitral valve prolapse and worsening rather than decreasing the severity of regurgitation.

For patients with functional MR, medical therapy should specifically address underlying ventricular dysfunction. Treatment should include carefully titrated use of nitrates, diuretics, angiotensin-converting enzyme inhibitors or angiotensin receptor antagonists, beta blockers (carvedilol is preferred), and aldosterone antagonists in the presence of heart failure.[11]

Surgical treatment. The onset of symptoms is a class I indication for surgical intervention in the setting of severe MR, but even patients with asymptomatic severe MR have a class II indication if mitral repair can be performed, given the risk for the insidious development of LV dysfunction in these individuals and a deteriorated prognosis (Table 60-6). Some evidence suggests that these considerations hold for moderate MR as well.[9]

Because a supranormal EF is typically associated with severe MR before the onset of ventricular dysfunction, an EF less than 60% or an LV end-systolic volume greater than 40 to 45 mm should also prompt consideration of surgery, even in the asymptomatic patient with severe MR (class I indication). The presence of pulmonary hypertension and the new onset of atrial fibrillation represent other indications for repair of MR lesions (Table 60-6).

Importantly, it has been traditional to defer surgical treatment of functional MR, especially in the setting of CABG, under the

TABLE 60-6 Indications for Intervention for the Treatment of Valvular Heart Disease (excerpted)

VALVE LESION	PROCEDURE	INDICATION	INDICATION CLASS	LEVEL OF EVIDENCE
Mitral stenosis	Percutaneous balloon mitral commissurotomy (PBMC)[a]	Symptomatic patients with severe MS (MVA 1.5 cm^2)	I	A[c]
		Asymptomatic patients with very severe MS (MVA 1.0 cm^2) or	IIa	C
		Severe MS (MVA 1.5 cm^2) and new onset of AF	IIb[c]	C
		Severely symptomatic patients (NYHA class III/IV) with severe MS (MVA 1.5 cm^2) who have suboptimal valve anatomy and are at high risk for surgery	IIb[c]	C
		Symptomatic patients with MVA >1.5 cm^2 if there is evidence of hemodynamically significant MS during exercise	IIb	C
	Mitral valve surgery[b]	Severely symptomatic patients (NYHA class III/IV) with severe MS (MVA 1.5 cm^2)	I	B
		Severe MS (MVA 1.5 cm^2) in patients who have had recurrent embolic events while receiving adequate anticoagulation[d]	IIb	C
Mitral regurgitation, chronic primary	Mitral valve surgery	Symptomatic patients with severe primary MR:	I	B
		With severe primary MR and LVEF >30%	I	B
		Undergoing cardiac surgery for other indications; may be considered with LVEF ≤30%	IIb	C
		Asymptomatic patients with severe primary MR and LV dysfunction (LVEF 30%-60% and/or LVESD ≥40 mm[e])	I	Be
	Mitral valve repair	Severe primary MR	I	B
		Limited to the posterior leaflet		
		Involving the anterior leaflet or both leaflets when a successful and durable repair can be accomplished		
		Reasonable in asymptomatic patients with severe primary MR with preserved LV function (LVEF >60% and LVESD <40 mm) in whom the likelihood of a successful and durable repair without residual MR is >95%	IIa	B
		With an expected mortality rate of <1% when performed at a Heart Valve Center of Excellence		
		With nonrheumatic disease and (1) new onset of AF or (2) resting pulmonary hypertension (systolic pulmonary arterial pressure >50 mm Hg)		
		Moderate primary MR in patients undergoing cardiac surgery for other indications	IIa	C
Mitral regurgitation, chronic severe secondary	Mitral valve surgery	Reasonable as concomitant procedure when undergoing CABG or AVR[f]	IIa[f]	C
	Mitral valve repair	Severely symptomatic patients (NYHA class III/IV)	IIb[f]	B[f]
		May be considered for patients with chronic moderate secondary MR who are undergoing other cardiac surgery	IIb[f]	C
Aortic stenosis	AVR	Severe high-gradient AS in patients who have symptoms by history or on exercise testing	I	B
		Severe AS and LVEF <50% in asymptomatic patients	I	B[g]
		Severe AS (stage C or D) when undergoing other cardiac surgery	I	B[g]
		Reasonable for asymptomatic patients with very severe AS (aortic velocity ≥5.0 m/s) and low surgical risk	IIa	B
		Reasonable in asymptomatic patients with severe AS and decreased exercise tolerance or an exercise fall in blood pressure	IIa	B[g]
		Reasonable in symptomatic patients with low-gradient severe AS with reduced LVEF with aortic velocity ≥4.0 m/s (or mean pressure gradient ≥40 mm Hg) with a valve area ≤1.0 cm^2 on dobutamine study	IIa[g]	B[g]
		Reasonable with moderate AS (aortic velocity 3.0-3.9 m/s) who are undergoing other cardiac surgery	IIa	C
		May be considered for asymptomatic patients with severe AS and rapid disease progression and low surgical risk	IIb[g]	C

Continued

TABLE 60-6 Indications for Intervention for the Treatment of Valvular Heart Disease (excerpted)—cont'd

VALVE LESION	PROCEDURE	INDICATION	INDICATION CLASS	LEVEL OF EVIDENCE
	TAVR	Recommended in patients who meet an indication for AVR who have a prohibitive surgical risk and a predicted post-TAVR survival >12 months	I	B
		Reasonable alternative to surgical AVR in patients who meet an indication for AVR and who have high surgical risk	IIa	B
Aortic insufficiency	AVR	Symptomatic patients with severe AI regardless of LV systolic function	I	B
		Asymptomatic patients with chronic severe AI and LV systolic dysfunction (LVEF <50%)	I	B
		Severe AR while undergoing cardiac surgery for other indications	I	C
		Reasonable for asymptomatic patients with severe AI with LVEF ≥50% but with severe LV dilation (LVESD >50 mm)	IIa	B[h]
		Reasonable for moderate AI for patients undergoing other cardiac surgery	IIa	C
		Consider for asymptomatic patients with severe AI and LVEF ≥50% with progressive severe LV dilation (LVEDD >65 mm) if surgical risk is low	IIb	C

Adapted from References 9 and 11.

AF, atrial fibrillation; *AI,* aortic insufficiency; *AR,* aortic regurgitation; *AS,* aortic stenosis; *AVR,* aortic valve replacement; *CABG,* coronary artery bypass grafting; *LV,* left ventricular; *LVEDD,* left ventricular end-diastolic diameter; *LVEF,* left ventricular ejection fraction; *LVESD,* left ventricular end-systolic diameter; *MR,* mitral regurgitation; *MS,* mitral stenosis; *MVA,* mitral valve area; *NYHA,* New York Heart Association; *TAVR,* transcatheter aortic valve replacement.

[a]PBMC is indicated if valve morphology is favorable based on Wilkins score (Table 60-4) in the absence of contraindications.

[b]If appropriate risk and not candidates for PBMC.

[c]In the ESC/EACTS guidelines, PBMC for symptomatic patients with favorable characteristics is Class I, Level of Evidence B. In the ESC/EACTS guidelines, PBMC is indicated in symptomatic patients with contraindication or high risk for surgery—Class I, Level C. In the ESC/EACTS guidelines, PBMC should be considered in asymptomatic patients without unfavorable characteristics and high thromboembolic risk (previous history of embolism, dense spontaneous contrast in the left atrium, recent or paroxysmal atrial fibrillation)—Class IIa, Level C.

[d]With excision of the left atrial appendage.

[e]In the ESC/EACTS guidelines, indicated in asymptomatic patients with LV dysfunction (LVESD ≥45 mm and/or LVEF ≤60%)—Class I, Level C.

[f]In the ESC/EACTS guidelines, indicated in patients with severe MR undergoing CABG and LVEF >30%—Class I, Level C. In the ESC/EACTS guidelines, surgery should be considered in symptomatic patients with severe MR, LVEF <30%, option for revascularization, and evidence of viability— Class IIa, Level C. In the ESC/EACTS guidelines, surgery should be considered in patients with moderate MR undergoing CABG—Class IIa, Level C.

[g]In the ESC/EACTS guidelines, indicated for asymptomatic patients with severe AS and systolic LV dysfunction (LVEF <50%) not due to another cause—Class I, Level C; indicated for severe AS if undergoing CABG, surgery of the ascending aorta or another valve—Class I, Level C; considered in asymptomatic patients with severe AS and abnormal exercise test showing fall in blood pressure below baseline—Class IIa, Level C; considered in symptomatic patients with severe AS and LV dysfunction without flow reserve—Class IIb, Level C.

[h]In the ESC/EACTS guidelines, considered for asymptomatic patients with resting EF >50% with severe LV dilation—Class IIa, Level C.

presumption that improvements in the ischemic milieu after CABG would lead to the resolution of functional MR. Although the literature remains contradictory, data from studies such as the STICH trial suggest, however, that deferring intervention for moderate to severe MR leads to worse outcomes in the setting of concomitant CABG.[18] Isolated intervention for correction of functional MR likewise remains controversial, with no clear evidence of survival benefit as yet identified.

Mitral valve repair is the procedure of choice in the 90% of individuals with primary MR amenable to this approach when they are treated at high-volume, experienced centers. A wide variety of well-validated, relatively easy to perform procedures are available to repair regurgitant mitral valves. Valve repair minimizes the risks of prosthetic valve complications, such as endocarditis, as well as a potential need for long-term anticoagulation.[9] Importantly, operative mortality should be close to 0%, and 10-year freedom from reoperation or recurrent moderate to severe MR should exceed 90% with successful repair documented by (mandatory) intraoperative transesophageal echocardiography and when the repair also includes the mandatory use of a reinforcing annuloplasty ring (see Table 60-5).

When valve replacement is required for MR, it is generally associated with an operative mortality rate about double that of patients undergoing repair, although these data are solely from retrospective studies (see Table 60-5).[19] However, valve replacement may be preferable to repair for functional MR in light of discouraging recent survival and freedom from reoperation with repair.[20] Recurrent moderate to severe MR has been reported in at least 20% to 30% of mitral repairs for functional MR, even with the use of annuloplasty rings designed specifically to correct the apicolateral posterior leaflet displacement associated with this syndrome.[21] Alternative procedures to restore ventricular-annular dimensions using papillary muscle anchoring and other similar techniques remain largely investigational.[22]

Aortic Stenosis

The normal aortic valve orifice measures 3 to 5 cm^2. Aortic valve stenosis to less than half this size causes hemodynamic obstruction and a transvalvular pressure gradient. Increased ventricular pressure, generated through Frank-Starling mechanisms (see earlier), leads to an increase in myocardial wall tension, and the left ventricle undergoes compensatory concentric hypertrophy through parallel replication of sarcomeres. Wall tension thereby normalizes according to the law of Laplace, and a compensated state preserving the systolic function of a hypertrophied but nondilated left ventricle may persist for many years.

Progressive AS is associated with several pathophysiologic sequelae. Two thirds of patients with severe AS develop myocardial ischemia as a result of the elevated myocardial oxygen demand and the increased work of a hypertrophied ventricle generating increased ejection pressures over prolonged systolic intervals against the increased afterload of the narrowed aortic valve. Myocardial ischemia, particularly in the subendocardial region, is accentuated by the reduction of perfusion gradients during diastolic coronary flow intervals. AS patients likewise demonstrate severely impaired coronary arterial flow reserve—decreased from normal values of up to 800% to often less than double the resting coronary flow. Consequent cell death and myocardial fibrosis can lead to a cardiomyopathy and exacerbate AS-induced heart failure.

Myocardial hypertrophy can also precipitate ventricular diastolic dysfunction, which typically occurs before the onset of systolic dysfunction. Decreased ventricular compliance leads to increased LVEDP, prolonged LV relaxation time, and shortened diastolic filling time. These increased pressures are transmitted back through the left atrium and pulmonary circulation, leading to pulmonary congestion. Pulmonary hypertension and right-sided heart failure may develop in severe cases. Eventually, maximal ventricular hypertrophy is reached and an adequate pressure gradient can no longer be achieved, resulting in inadequate cardiac outputs and overt, self-reinforcing systolic LV failure.

Increased LA pressure and consequent LA dilation also increase the risk for atrial arrhythmias. The loss of normal atrial contraction severely compromises filling of the noncompliant ventricle, leading to a sometimes precipitous decrease in cardiac output. Reduced forward flow can further increase LVEDP and aggravate the symptoms of heart failure.

Presyncope and syncope are unusual sequelae of AS related to inadequate (cerebral) organ perfusion, typically caused by inadequate forward flow through the restrictive aortic valve. Symptoms are typically associated with periods of peripheral vasodilation, such as during exercise or in changing from a recumbent to standing positioning when increased cardiac output is required to maintain peripheral vascular filling.

Diagnosis of Aortic Stenosis

Symptoms and signs. Patients with AS will typically remain asymptomatic for an extended time. The onset of symptoms occurs when the valve orifice area decreases to approximately 1 cm^2, which marks a critical point in the natural history of the disease. The classic symptoms of AS typically progress from the appearance of *angina* and (pre-)*syncope* to the occurrence of *dyspnea* associated with heart failure (mnemonic: ASD). Whereas angina is the presenting symptom of AS in 35% of patients, syncope is a relatively sporadic event that is the presenting symptom in 15% of patients. Although heart failure typically appears late in the course of AS, dyspnea or other heart failure symptoms are presenting signs in 50% of patients.

Physical examination. The diagnosis of AS is frequently made before the onset of symptoms. The typical finding is a crescendo-decrescendo ejection murmur best heard along the left sternal border and that radiates to the upper right sternal border and carotid arteries. The apical impulse in AS is forceful and slightly enlarged. If heart failure develops, the apical impulse may become laterally displaced. The characteristic carotid upstroke of AS has a slow rate of rise and a reduced peak (pulsus parvus et tardus) and may have an associated thrill.

As AS progresses, its murmur peaks progressively later in systole and may actually decrease in intensity because of diminished stroke volume. The second heart sound may become singular because the aortic and pulmonic components are superimposed, or the aortic valve component may be absent because of the immobility of the calcified valve. A third or fourth heart sound may become audible in patients in sinus rhythm.

Diagnostic testing. Nonspecific findings of AS on chest radiography include a boot-shaped heart typical of concentric hypertrophy of the left ventricle, calcification of the valvular cusps, and poststenotic dilation of the aorta. As heart failure ensues, cardiomegaly and pulmonary vascular congestion may be seen. The right-sided heart border may become more prominent in severe failure. Electrocardiographic changes are similar to those seen for MR.

Echocardiography allows the precise assessment of aortic valve anatomy, calcification, and effective orifice size, measured by planimetry. Ventricular hypertrophy and function can also be assessed. As with MS, Doppler echocardiography allows measurement of transvalvular pressure gradients and valve area as a derived function (e.g., Doppler velocity >4 m/sec = valve area <1 cm^2). Pressure gradients may be decreased in AS patients with low cardiac output, leading to miscalculated (falsely increased) aortic valve areas. Low-dose dobutamine may be used during echocardiography to increase cardiac output and to assess the true severity of the AS lesion in these patients.

Cardiac catheterization may occasionally be needed to measure pressure gradients in ambiguous cases. Simultaneous pressure readings can be obtained in such instances with one pressure measuring port in the body of the left ventricle and a second device in the proximal aorta. Valvular area may then be determined by the Gorlin formula. Catheterization may be needed to assess the presence of coronary artery disease, coexistent in up to 50% of AS patients.

Natural History

Calcific AS is a progressive disease marked by a long, asymptomatic latent period. The duration of the asymptomatic period varies greatly between individuals. Ross and Braunwald's classic 1968 report first described the onset of symptoms of heart failure, syncope, or angina in patients with AS as a marker of impending death (Fig. 60-10).[23] Although mean survival after the appearance of angina is about 5 years, it is less than 3 years after the onset of syncope and only 1 to 2 years once heart failure symptoms develop. Since Ross and Braunwald's report, other studies have confirmed that nearly 50% of patients will die within 3 to 5 years after the onset of symptoms from AS.[24,25] Sudden death may occur in symptomatic patients at a rate of 2%/month but appears to be rare (<1% per year) in asymptomatic patients.[24] Significantly, echocardiography-based population studies have demonstrated that aortic jet velocity can effectively predict progression to symptoms and surgery.[24]

Treatment

Medical management. Medical therapy is important in the treatment of early signs and symptoms of heart failure and other common comorbidities, such as hypertension. Treatment of hypertension may also serve to unload the AS ventricle, helping to relieve adverse ventricular remodeling. Although there are no medical therapies currently proven to alter the natural history of

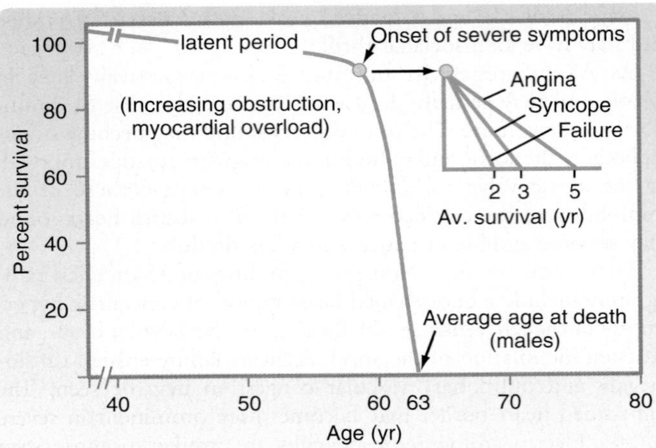

FIGURE 60-10 Symptoms and Survival in AS. Ross and Braunwald's classic 1968 report first described the onset of symptoms of heart failure, syncope, and angina in patients with AS as a marker of impending death. (From Ross J, Jr, Braunwald E: Aortic stenosis. *Circulation* 38:61–67, 1968.)

calcific AS, multiple ongoing investigations are seeking to slow disease progression through an apparent endothelial injury/atherosclerosis AS pathway.

Surgical treatment. Because the natural history of untreated symptomatic AS is grave, mechanical relief of AS is recommended as a class I indication in all symptomatic patients, and a careful history noting the onset of symptoms in AS patients is essential (see Table 60-6). Aortic valve surgery improves symptoms, increases life expectancy, and often improves or normalizes systolic function and has transformed the outlook for this disease.

Surgical intervention now also carries a class I indication in the asymptomatic patient with severe AS and evidence of LV dysfunction (LVEF <50%). Other class IIb indications have also been proposed for patients with severe asymptomatic disease who demonstrate rapid disease progression and are at low surgical risk, given evidence that these patients will likely go on to develop symptoms and that the risk of death without surgery remains significant even before the onset of symptoms.[9,11] Ongoing investigations are attempting to identify other subgroups of patients who are at high risk for disease progression and who may benefit from valve replacement rather than watchful waiting. For example, exercise or dobutamine stress echocardiography has been shown to elicit abnormal physiology or symptoms in as many as 30% of patients tested.[26]

Surgery for AS almost always requires valve replacement, with either a mechanical or tissue valve (see later), and is associated with excellent immediate and long-term outcomes (see Table 60-5), especially when it is conducted before the onset of ventricular dysfunction. Earlier efforts at valve débridement met with disastrous intermediate-term outcomes with delayed onset of regurgitation and led to the general abandonment of this technique. Patients in whom surgical valve replacement is considered too risky may alternatively be candidates for percutaneous, catheter-based valve replacement (see later section on transcatheter aortic valve replacement).

Aortic Insufficiency

Competency of the aortic valve, like that of the mitral valve, is dependent on the coordinated function of a complex and dynamic anatomy. It includes the valve cusps, annulus, sinuses of Valsalva, and sinotubular junction above the sinuses. Aortic regurgitation, or aortic insufficiency (AI), may be induced by pathologic processes that may alter any one or more of these components or their anatomic relationships with each other.

Acute AI, usually the consequence of endocarditis or aortic dissection, produces sudden increases in LVEDV caused by acute regurgitant flow into a relatively small, nonadapted, noncompliant ventricle. Even greater increases in LVEDP result, and equalization of systemic and ventricular pressure may occur. Transmission of increased LVEDP into the pulmonary circuit may produce fulminant pulmonary edema, particularly in the setting of coexisting MR. Increased wall tension typically leads to myocardial ischemia, especially if aortic dissection extends to the coronary ostia, and hemodynamic collapse or early death may ensue.

Chronic AI, like chronic MR, is an insidious process that triggers a number of compensatory mechanisms to maintain net forward stroke volume, and patients with chronic AI often remain well compensated for many years. Ventricles can ultimately weigh as much as three times normal and have a capacitance of more than 200 mL to accommodate massive regurgitant volumes. Marked decreases in systemic diastolic pressure, with reciprocal increases in pulse pressure, are typically found with massive regurgitant flow back into the ventricle. The sum effect of myocardial hypertrophy and LV enlargement in AI patients is a dramatically enlarged heart known as cor bovinum, characterized by the largest EDV and mass of any form of heart disease.

These changes associated with chronic AI begin with increases in afterload and wall stress caused by mild or moderate regurgitant flow and increases in LVEDV less severe than those associated with acute AI. Compensation occurs through Frank-Starling shifts in contractility (see earlier) and stress-induced eccentric ventricular hypertrophy characterized by sarcomere replication in series and elongation of myofibers. This hypertrophy tends to preserve ventricular compliance and to minimize increases in LVEDP while still decreasing wall tension. Increases in heart rate and decreases in peripheral vascular resistance that reduce diastolic filling time and decrease afterload also act to decrease regurgitant flow.

Over time, however, progressive increases in LVEDV eventually exhaust preload reserve and overwhelm compensation mechanisms. Progressive increases in LVEDV and LVEDP lead to ventricular dilation, increased wall tension, and increased myocardial oxygen demand. Decreased systemic diastolic pressure and increased intramyocardial wall tension decrease coronary perfusion gradients and further exacerbate myocardial ischemia. Ultimately, ischemia may lead to myocardial fibrosis and cardiomyopathy. When the ventricle can no longer maintain adequate forward flow, overt heart failure ensues.

Diagnosis and Treatment of Aortic Insufficiency

Symptoms and signs. Severe acute AI may be difficult to recognize clinically, although acute AI patients may present with dyspnea, hemodynamic instability, or shock. Frequently, symptoms reflecting the underlying cause of the AI, such as fever from endocarditis or chest pain from aortic dissection, may mask AI symptoms and obscure a correct diagnosis.

Although chronically compensated AI patients remain asymptomatic for long periods, symptoms of heart failure often eventually develop. Those with severe AI may also experience angina pectoris, nocturnal angina, and palpitations during stress or exertion.

Physical examination. Acute AI may yield few if any diagnostic signs other than those of fulminant heart failure or hemodynamic collapse. In comparison, chronic AI typically offers many physical findings, primarily related to the increases in stroke volume, systolic blood pressure, and pulse pressure associated with this condition. These include peripheral pulses that rise abruptly and rapidly collapse (water-hammer pulse), a bounding carotid pulse (Corrigan pulse), head bobbing with each heartbeat (de Musset sign), pulsation of the uvula (Müller sign), a "pistol shot" auscultated with compression of the femoral artery (Traube sign), and capillary pulsations seen with fingernail compression using a glass slide (Quincke sign).

Cardiac examination typically reveals an apical impulse that is diffuse, hyperdynamic, and displaced inferiorly and laterally. It may be associated with a systolic thrill at the base of the heart, suprasternal notch, and carotid arteries due to high stroke volume. Auscultation reveals a high-frequency blowing, decrescendo diastolic murmur best heard with the diaphragm at the left sternal border with the patient sitting up, leaning forward, and at end-exhalation. The murmur is increased by maneuvers such as squatting or hand-grip, which increase diastolic pressure. The examiner may appreciate a mid and late diastolic apical rumble (Austin Flint murmur), which is thought to be secondary to vibration of the anterior mitral leaflet caused by a posteriorly directed AI jet. The second heart sound may be soft or absent, and a third heart sound may be present.

Diagnostic testing. Chest radiography in patients with acute AI may reveal only pulmonary edema, and electrocardiography may reveal evidence of LV strain, but echocardiography may be the only test useful in diagnosis of this condition. With chronic AI, chest radiography typically shows a significantly enlarged cardiac silhouette. The ascending aorta may be enlarged if AI is due to an aortic aneurysm. Electrocardiography will typically show signs of increased LV mass, with left axis deviation and increased QRS amplitude with strain patterns and conduction abnormalities.

Echocardiography allows the comprehensive evaluation of aortic apparatus abnormalities as well as the character and magnitude of the regurgitant jet. Severe AI, for example, may be diagnosed by a jet width of 65% or more of the LV outflow tract, vena contracta (the narrowest central flow region of a jet that occurs at or just downstream to the orifice of a regurgitant valve) of more than 0.6 cm, regurgitant fraction of 50% or more, or an effective regurgitant orifice area (derived from the PISA radius) of 0.3 cm^2 or more. Echocardiography also allows assessments of LV size and compliance important to prognostic calculations.

Natural History

Whereas acute AI may lead to the sudden onset of heart failure or hemodynamic collapse, patients with chronic AI typically enjoy years of asymptomatic, compensated LV function. The combined likelihood of onset of adverse events for such patients (LV dysfunction, onset of symptoms, or death) is less than 5% per year. Overall, the freedom from ventricular dysfunction or death incidence rate in asymptomatic patients is about 75% at 5 years, but this incidence decreases to 60% at 10 years.[27] Furthermore, once the end-systolic diameter of the left ventricle is greater than 50 mm, adverse event rates increase to about 20% per year.[9,11,27] Once symptoms develop in AI patients, mortality rates rise to more than 10% per year.[27]

Treatment

Medical management. Medical therapy should be considered only a temporizing measure for patients with acute severe AI and acute volume overload, hypotension, or pulmonary edema who will require emergent surgery. In this scenario, vasodilators and inotropes may be valuable in augmenting forward flow and reducing LVEDP. Beta blockers used for aortic dissection should be employed with great caution in other causes of acute AI because they block compensatory tachycardia and could cause a significant drop in blood pressure. Importantly, intra-aortic balloon counterpulsation is contraindicated in patients with AI because it will worsen regurgitation and compromise forward output.

Patients with chronic severe AI may benefit from medical management with the primary goal of reducing systolic hypertension, therefore reducing wall stress and improving ventricular function. Vasodilator therapy is also indicated in patients with severe AI who have symptoms or LV dysfunction, although surgical intervention should not be delayed if it is indicated.[9,11] Furthermore, although vasodilating drugs may improve hemodynamic abnormalities and forward flow, their effect in favorably prolonging the asymptomatic period in patients with chronic severe AI and normal ventricular function is uncertain.[9,11] Medical treatment of symptomatic patients with AI is appropriate only until surgical intervention can be undertaken.

Surgical treatment. Urgent or emergent surgical intervention to repair or to replace the aortic valve and to address underlying pathologic mechanisms (e.g., endocarditis, aortic dissection) is nearly always indicated in patients with acute severe AI. Surgery is also indicated (class I) for symptomatic patients with severe chronic AI (see Table 60-6). Importantly, on the basis of improved current understandings of the natural history of chronic AI, aortic valve surgery now also carries a class I indication for asymptomatic chronic severe AI patients with LV systolic dysfunction (LVEF <50%) and a class IIa and class IIb indication, respectively, for asymptomatic severe AI with normal LV systolic function (LVEF ≥50%) but with severe LV dilation (LV end-systolic diameter >50 mm) or progressive severe LV dilation (LV end-diastolic diameter >65 mm).

Valve replacement with mechanical or biologic prostheses has yielded excellent results in correcting isolated AI (see Table 60-5); however, during the past 2 decades, increasing numbers of centers are employing repair strategies in selected patients, as described later.[28] For patients with aortic root disease, these procedures are typically combined with root repair or replacement and coronary reimplantation, as discussed elsewhere in this text.

In selected patients, the aortic valve may alternatively be replaced with a pulmonary autograft, with heterograft substitution of the native pulmonic valve (Ross procedure). Excellent results with this procedure have been demonstrated in highly experienced centers, especially for younger (<30 years) patients in whom traditional valve replacement procedures carry high risks of valve-related complications over time. However, given the lack of reproducibility of these results more generally because of technical challenges, this procedure is likely best performed for selected patients undergoing surgery at experienced centers.[9]

Tricuspid Regurgitation and Other Right-Sided Valve Disease

Functional TR is by far the most prevalent right-sided valve disease. It typically occurs as the result of left-sided valve disease or heart failure, and like primary right-sided valve disease, it is due to pathophysiologic mechanisms very similar to left-sided equivalents. Unlike in left-sided disease, altered RV mechanics and geometry associated with RV failure may cause irreversible dilation of the saddle-shaped ellipsoid of a healthy tricuspid annulus into a more planar circular shape, leading to persistence of TR despite the correction of inciting hemodynamics. Increased central venous pressure resulting from tricuspid valve disease can lead to venous congestion, hepatic enlargement, ascites, and peripheral edema as well as right atrial enlargement and arrhythmias. Decreased RV output can lead to LV underfilling and inadequate left-sided output.

Diagnosis of Tricuspid Valve Disease

Symptoms and signs. Because patients with tricuspid disease almost invariably have coexisting left-sided valve disease, it is difficult to separate symptoms of tricuspid disease from those of multivalvular disease, and tricuspid valve disease itself may frequently be asymptomatic. Dyspnea, fatigue, and exercise intolerance may, however, result as heart failure develops.

Physical examination. A classic holosystolic murmur that increases with inspiration (Carvallo sign) and that may be heard along the sternal border is typical of TR. With TS, an opening snap followed by a diastolic rumble may be heard at the right sternal border. The physical examination of patients with tricuspid valve disease may otherwise reveal only jugular venous distention with a prominent systolic *v* wave. With progressive central venous congestion, physical findings that may be out of proportion to symptoms may include pleural effusions, hepatic enlargement (with a pulsatile liver typical of TR), abdominal tenderness, ascites, and peripheral edema.

Diagnostic testing. Because of the overlay of concomitant left-sided disease, echocardiography is the sole reliable testing modality useful in assessing tricuspid disease, similar in application to that for assessing mitral disease. Estimation of pulmonary arterial systolic pressure based on the velocity of the TR jet measured by continuous-wave Doppler is a useful prognostic criterion. An annular diameter of more than 40 mm defines significant tricuspid annular dilation, an important consideration in selecting appropriate treatment of TR.[29]

Natural History

Decreased survival is associated with increasing TR severity, regardless of other indices of cardiac function.[30] Although patients who undergo surgical treatment of left-sided valve disease may experience improved or resolved functional TR, such improvement is highly unpredictable, and survival for patients with uncorrected moderate to severe TR is less than 50% at 4 years.[30] The natural history of other right-sided valve lesions is poorly documented because such lesions typically require surgical correction as congenital anomalies or with rheumatic disease of the mitral and aortic valves.

Treatment

Medical management. The medical treatment of tricuspid valve disease involves optimization of RV preload and afterload, using diuretics and angiotensin-converting enzyme inhibitors, respectively. If atrial fibrillation is present, rate control may optimize diastolic filling. With functional TR, medical treatment to reduce pulmonary hypertension may also improve cardiac output.

Surgical treatment. The timing and method for surgical treatment of functional TR are controversial. Until recent years, the notion that functional TR would improve or disappear after the primary left-sided heart disease was treated led to recommendations of avoiding tricuspid surgery. However, the improvement of functional or primary forms of severe TR has not been predictable after left-sided heart surgery. Left uncorrected, secondary TR may worsen in about 25% of patients, which has functional and survival implications because of irreversible progression of RV damage and organ failure.[30]

Adding tricuspid repair during left-sided heart surgery does not significantly increase operative risk. However, reoperation due to persistent TR after left-sided heart surgery carries a perioperative mortality of 10% to 25%. Therefore, severe TR has emerged as a class I indication for concomitant tricuspid valve surgery in patients who are undergoing left-sided heart surgery.[9,11] Concomitant repair is also probably indicated in those with mild or greater TR and either tricuspid annular dilation or evidence of right-sided heart failure.[30]

Tricuspid valve repair is generally preferred to replacement whenever possible. For severe TR due to isolated annular dilation, annuloplasty using a prosthetic ring has been shown in a number of studies to have better long-term results than traditional suture annuloplasty.[31] Valve replacement should be considered for functional TR due to leaflet tethering and RV remodeling.

Symptomatic patients with isolated TS do not benefit from medical management and are best treated with valve replacement. Those with TS and left-sided valve disease should likewise undergo concomitant correction during the same operation.[9,11] Percutaneous tricuspid valvulotomy may be considered, but outcomes are less optimistic than those seen with MS and may induce significant TR.[32]

Mixed Valve Disease

Patients with mixed valve disease typically present with a predominant lesion that dictates symptoms and pathophysiologic changes. There are limited data on the natural history of mixed valve disease, and therefore the optimal timing of serial evaluation is not clear. Therapy should be targeted to the predominant lesion while considering the severity of concomitant valve disease.

Patients with multivalvular disease present even more complex diagnostic and therapeutic challenges. The coexistence of aortic valve disease and MR, for example, will mitigate LV changes induced by aortic valve disease but worsen pulmonary and right-sided complications. Limited data are available to guide treatment in these cases, and indications for interventions should be based on symptoms and objective analysis of surgical outcome rather than on severity indices for the individual lesions.[11]

OPERATIVE APPROACHES

Surgery for valvular heart disease is today associated with excellent short- and long-term outcomes, with some evidence suggesting even better outcomes for surgery performed at high-volume centers.[33] The risk of operative mortality, which in the modern era is generally less than 5% for all types of valve disease, can now be accurately predicted by several widely available multivariable risk calculation scoring systems, such as those provided by the Society of Thoracic Surgeons and the European Association for Cardiothoracic Surgery.

In general, operative mortality is predicted by risk factors such as age, female gender, emergency surgery, symptoms, concomitant procedures, decreased EF, and comorbidities, such as diabetes mellitus, renal dysfunction or pulmonary disease, peripheral vascular disease, or prior operation (Table 60-7). Typically, MR is associated with the poorest operative mortality risk, followed by AI, with surgery for AS and MS offering the best operative mortality outcomes. Complications most frequently associated with

TABLE 60-7 European System for Valvular Surgery Operative Risk Evaluation (EuroSCORE)

	DEFINITION	SCORE
Patient-Related Factors		
Age	Per 5 years or part thereof over 60 years	1
Sex	Female	1
Chronic pulmonary disease	Long-term bronchodilators or steroids	1
Extracardiac arteriopathy	Claudication; carotid occlusion or >50% stenosis; intervention on abdominal aorta, limb arteries, carotids	2
Neurologic dysfunction	Severely affecting ambulation or day-to-day functioning	2
Previous cardiac surgery	Requiring opening of the pericardium	3
Serum creatinine concentration	>200 mmol/liter preoperatively	2
Active endocarditis	Antibiotic treatment for endocarditis at the time of surgery	3
Critical preoperative state	Ventricular tachycardia, fibrillation, aborted sudden death; preoperative cardiac massage, ventilation, inotropic support, IABP, or acute renal failure (anuria or oliguria <10 mL/hr)	3
Cardiac-Related Factors		
Unstable angina	Rest angina requiring intravenous nitrates preoperatively	2
LV dysfunction	Moderate or LVEF 30-50%	1
	Poor or LVEF <30%	3
Recent myocardial infarct	Within 90 days	2
Pulmonary hypertension	Systolic pulmonary artery pressure >60 mm Hg	2
Operation-Related Factors		
Emergency	Carried out on referral before next working day	2
Other than isolated CABG	Major cardiac procedure other than or in addition to CABG	2
Surgery on thoracic aorta	For disorder of ascending, arch, or descending aorta	3
Postinfarct septal rupture		4

Adapted from Roques F, Nashef SA, Michel P, et al: Risk factors and outcome in European cardiac surgery: Analysis of the EuroSCORE multinational database of 19030 patients. *Eur J Cardiothorac Surg* 15:816–822, 1999.
Interpretation: low risk, 0-2; medium risk, 3-5; high risk, 6 or more.
CABG, coronary artery bypass graft surgery; *IABP*, intra-aortic balloon counterpulsation; *LV*, left ventricular; *LVEF*, left ventricular ejection fraction.

TABLE 60-8 Complications Associated With Valvular Heart Surgery

OUTCOME	AVR	MVR
Prolonged ventilation	7%	10.8%
Renal failure	3.7%	5.2%
Reoperation for bleeding	4.1%	4.7%
Permanent stroke	1.6%	2.2%
Deep sternal infection	0.5%	0.3%
Postoperative hospital stay*	8.5 ± 8.4	9.9 ± 10.3
Overall hospital stay*	10.6 ± 9.6	12.8 ± 12.6

Adapted from data from the Society of Thoracic Surgeons national database (N = 49,073 patients). Edwards FH, Peterson ED, Coombs LP, et al: Prediction of operative mortality after valve replacement surgery. *J Am Coll Cardiol* 37:885–892, 2001.
AVR, aortic valve replacement; *MVR*, mitral valve replacement.
*Mean days ± standard deviation.

surgery for valvular heart disease include infection, bleeding, stroke, conduction block (potentially requiring permanent pacemaker placement), and heart failure (Table 60-8).

Long-term outcomes and resolution of ventricular hemodynamic pathophysiology can likewise generally be predicted by the duration or severity of symptoms as well as by the extent of ventricular dysfunction or the presence and severity of pulmonary hypertension.[9,11] Complete hemodynamic recovery from valvular disease, including resolution of ventricular hypertrophy and enlargement, may be seen as early as the first several weeks postoperatively but may progress for up to a year after surgery. The long-term complications frequently associated with valve surgery are thromboembolic events including stroke, reoperation for valve deterioration or perivalvular leaks, bleeding associated with anticoagulant medications, and endocarditis (Table 60-8).

Conduct of Surgery

A full midline median sternotomy has traditionally been the predominant means to obtain wide exposure for heart valve surgery. More recently, partial upper or lower sternotomies or small third or fourth interspace thoracotomies have been popularized as minimally invasive access approaches, using either direct visualization with specialized instruments or indirect, robotic surgical techniques (Fig. 60-11). In all cases, intraoperative transesophageal echocardiography is essential in the assessment of valve anatomy and function.

Cardiopulmonary bypass and hypothermic cardioplegic arrest of the heart are standard to performance of open heart procedures on the cardiac valves. Bicaval cannulation is typically used for mitral or tricuspid valve surgery. Minimally invasive approaches generally use peripheral cannulation of the femoral or axillary arteries for cardiopulmonary bypass, although direct aortic cannulation may also be possible.

Mitral Valve Replacement and Repair

The mitral valve is typically exposed through a left lateral atriotomy made just anterior to the pulmonary veins (Fig. 60-12). Alternatively, a right atriotomy and a second incision through the atrial septum also provide excellent exposure to the mitral valve.

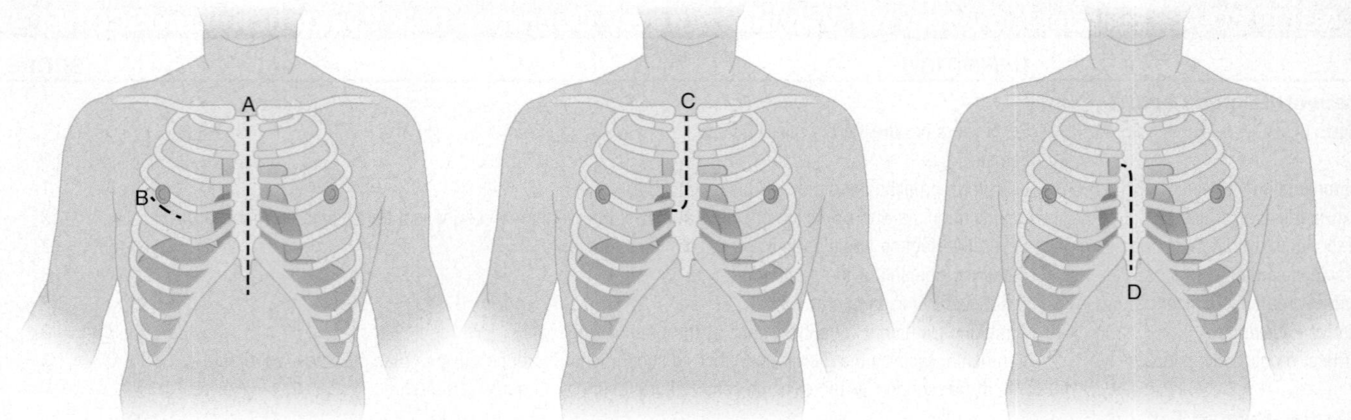

FIGURE 60-11 Surgical Access for Valvular Heart Surgery. Median sternotomy (A) versus minimally invasive access through minithoracotomy (B) or partial upper (C) or lower (D) sternotomy. (From Byrne JG, Leacche M, Vaughan DE, et al: Hybrid cardiovascular procedures. *JACC Cardiovasc Interv* 1:459–468, 2008.)

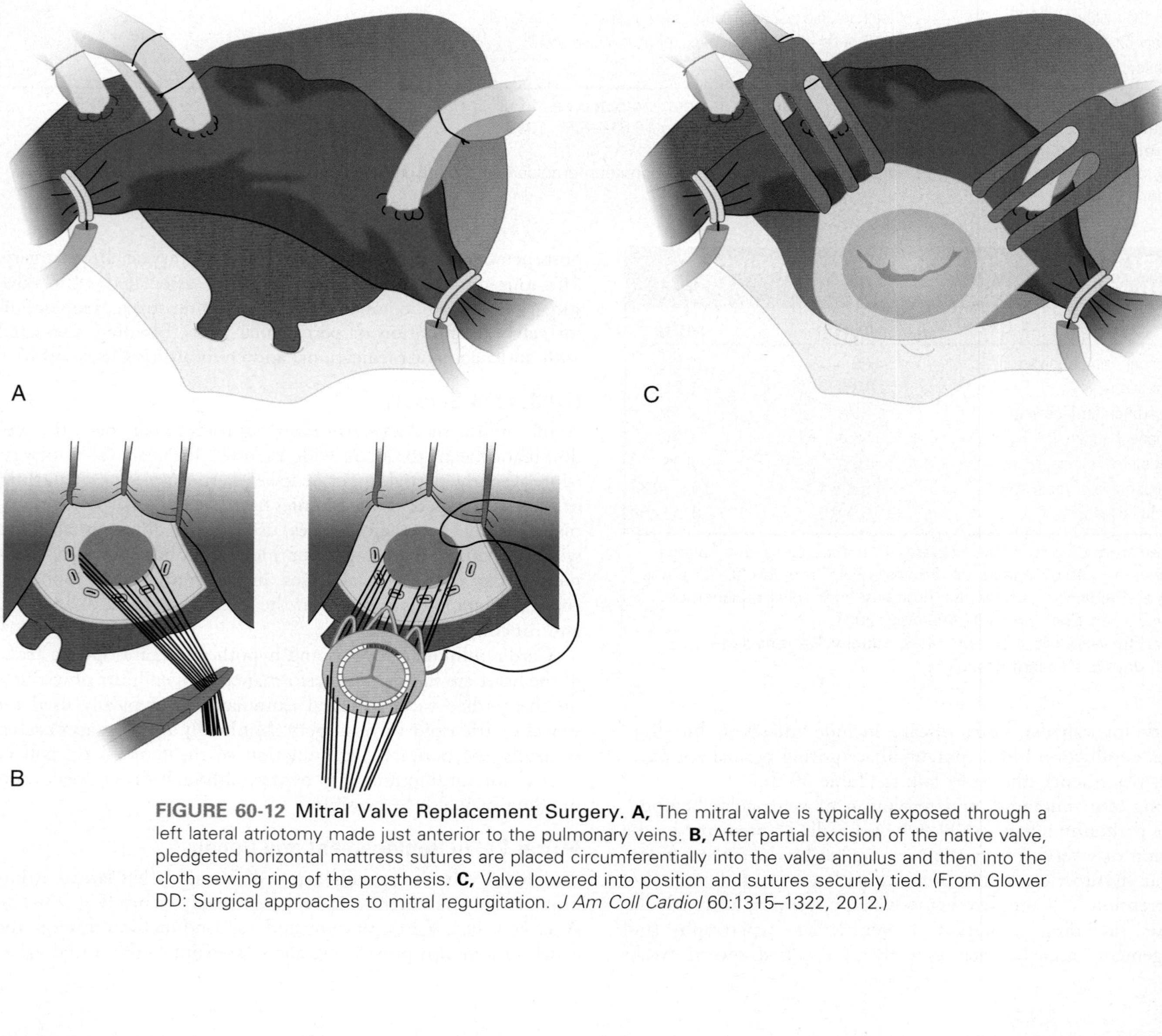

FIGURE 60-12 Mitral Valve Replacement Surgery. A, The mitral valve is typically exposed through a left lateral atriotomy made just anterior to the pulmonary veins. **B,** After partial excision of the native valve, pledgeted horizontal mattress sutures are placed circumferentially into the valve annulus and then into the cloth sewing ring of the prosthesis. **C,** Valve lowered into position and sutures securely tied. (From Glower DD: Surgical approaches to mitral regurgitation. *J Am Coll Cardiol* 60:1315–1322, 2012.)

Even greater exposure can be provided by a "superior septal" approach joining the right atrial and septostomy incisions onto the dome of the left atrium, but this approach requires more extensive closure. Once the mitral valve has been exposed and appropriate retraction applied, typically including rotation of the heart toward the left side of the chest, the surgeon carefully inspects all components of the mitral valve apparatus to select valve repair versus replacement.

Mitral Valve Replacement

If valve replacement is necessary, minimal resection (typically of a portion of the anterior leaflet) should be performed, making best efforts to preserve the subvalvular apparatus in continuity with the valve leaflets and annulus. Calcified or fused fibrotic leaflet or annular tissue is excised as needed to allow implantation of an adequately sized valve prosthesis without perivalvular leak.

Typically, after sizing of the annulus with a plastic avatar and selection of an appropriate prosthesis, nonabsorbable braided pledgeted horizontal mattress sutures are placed circumferentially into the valve annulus and then into the cloth sewing ring of the prosthesis (Fig. 60-12*B*). The sutures are tied securely to make sure there is no perivalvular defect that would allow a regurgitant leak, and the atriotomy is closed after de-airing of the heart (Fig. 60-12*C*).

Mitral Valve Repair

A wide variety of surgical techniques may be employed to repair primary MR lesions. Most commonly, flail or prolapsing (typically posterior [P2]) segments of the valve can be excised through a limited (triangular) or more extensive (quadrangular) resection, and leaflet continuity is restored simply by suturing the resected leaflet edges back together (Fig. 60-13*A*). Often, relaxing incisions along the posterior leaflet base (sliding annuloplasty) may be used to take tension off this repair or to decrease the "height" of the posterior leaflet. This helps prevent postresection MR resulting from systolic anterior motion of the anterior mitral leaflet, which may become displaced toward the aortic outflow tract after inadequate resections.

More recently, a number of authors have validated the use of artificial chordae, instead of or in addition to valve resection, to help support normal leaflet function. Typically made of polytetrafluoroethylene and now available as presized lengths selected on the basis of pre-repair measurements, these are sutured between the papillary muscles and leaflet edges to correct flail or prolapsing leaflet segments.

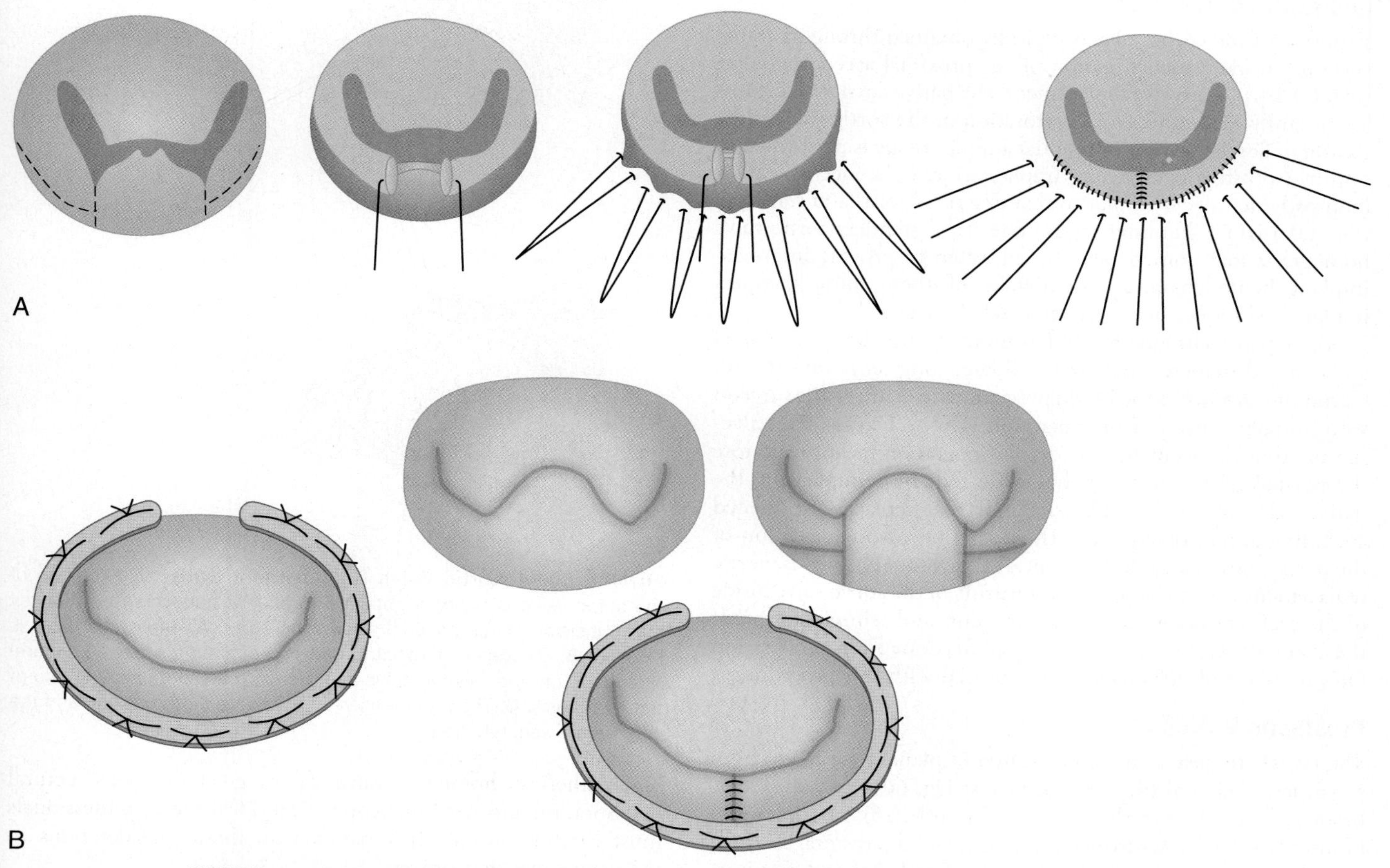

FIGURE 60-13 Mitral Valve Replacement Surgery. A, Exposure of the left atrium is obtained from the right side of the heart by developing Sondergaard's plane at the interatrial groove. **B,** The mitral valve is exposed through a left lateral atriotomy made just anterior to the pulmonary veins. **C,** After partial excision of the native valve, pledgeted horizontal mattress sutures are placed circumferentially into the valve annulus and then into the cloth sewing ring of the prosthesis. The valve is then lowered into position and the sutures securely tied.

An annuloplasty ring is almost always implanted, in a manner analogous to valve implantation, to supplement resectional repairs, or it may be used alone to address MR arising from a dilated annulus (Fig. 60-13*B*). Insertion of an annuloplasty ring dramatically helps re-form normal annular geometry to "compress" the anterior and posterior leaflets together, providing a minimum coaptation length of 6 to 8 mm between anterior and posterior leaflets.

Annuloplasty rings are generally sized to approximate the surface area of the anterior mitral leaflet but may be "undersized" to maximize leaflet coaptation while care is taken to avoid an inadequately sized ring, which can create systolic anterior motion from redundancy in the anterior leaflet. The author typically uses complete, semirigid rings to maximally stabilize the annulus, but more flexible or partial rings are preferred by many surgeons and may provide comparable results.

A number of specially configured rings have also been developed to correct the apical and lateral displacement of the posterior valve leaflet associated with functional MR. In general, intermediate- and long-term results with these repair strategies have been discouraging. More complex techniques to correct papillary muscle–annular relationships have been proposed.[22]

Surgical Aortic Valve Replacement and Aortic Valve Repair

Exposure of the aortic valve is typically obtained through a transverse or "hockey stick" incision of the proximal ascending aorta (Fig. 60-14*A*). For valve replacement, the native aortic valve cusps are carefully excised to avoid perforation of the aortic wall, and a thorough decalcification of residual annular tissue is performed to improve prosthetic valve fit. Implantation of a mechanical or bioprosthetic valve is similar to that described for the mitral valve (Fig. 60-14*B,C*). Homografts or "free-style" stentless aortic valve homografts may sometimes be used, often to provide improved implant hemodynamics. The details of these more complex implant techniques may be referenced elsewhere.[34]

The repair technique for AI has more recently been developed and attained an increasingly well-validated long-term track record. Commonly known as the David procedure (in credit to the surgeon who initially conceived the operation, Tirone David), the valve-sparing root replacement is a complex operation meant to restore the normal relationships of the aortic root by reimplanting the native valve inside of a Dacron graft that replaces the dilated ascending aorta causing AI.[35] The operation involves excision of the aortic sinuses and detachment of the coronary arteries, aortic replacement with a Dacron graft, securing of the aortic valve inside of the graft above and below the annulus, and reimplantation of the coronary vessels. Overall 20-year freedom from reoperation rates in excess of 90% have been reported with this procedure.[36]

Prosthetic Valves

The prosthetic heart valves most often implanted are made from a synthetic material (mechanical valves; Fig. 60-15*A*), allogeneic biologic tissue (bioprosthetic valves; Fig. 60-15*B*), or (cadaveric) homografts. Each has distinct advantages and disadvantages. Anticoagulation with a vitamin K antagonist (warfarin) and monitoring of the international normalized ratio are recommended in nearly all patients with mechanical prosthetic valves and typically for the first 3 months after bioprosthetic mitral implants (Table 60-9). Aspirin may be added to warfarin therapy to reduce rates of major embolism, stroke, and overall mortality. In comparison, bioprosthetic or homograft valves carry a greater risk of structural deterioration and need for reoperation. Health care professionals must carefully advise their patients on these considerations in their valve selection process.

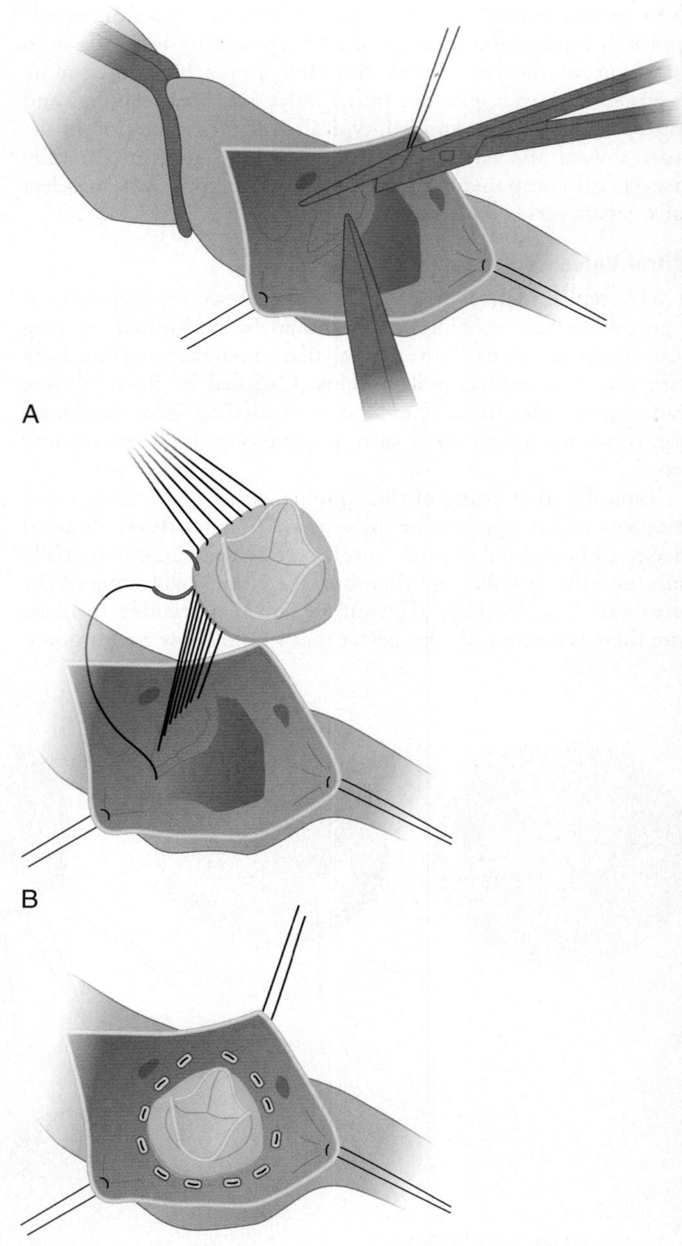

FIGURE 60-14 Aortic Valve Replacement Surgery. Exposure of the aortic valve is typically obtained through a transverse or "hockey stick" incision of the proximal ascending aorta. **A,** The aortic valve is excised. **B,** Pledgeted horizontal mattress sutures are placed circumferentially into the valve annulus and then into the cloth sewing ring of the prosthesis. **C,** The prosthetic valve is lowered into position and the sutures are securely tied.

The current generation of mechanical valves, nearly all bileaflet pyrolytic carbon in design, can be expected to provide an extremely low incidence of structural deterioration but a 0.6% to 2.3% per patient-year incidence of thromboembolic complications, even with warfarin anticoagulation.[37] The need for anticoagulation

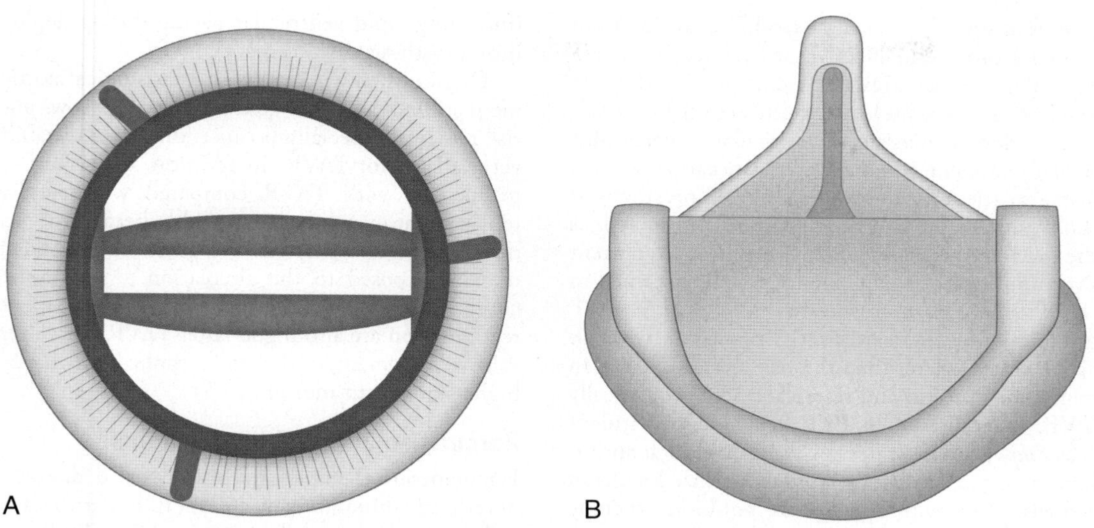

FIGURE 60-15 Prosthetic Valves. Prosthetic heart valves most often implanted are made from synthetic material (**A**), such as pyrolytic carbon (mechanical valve), or allogeneic biologic tissue (**B**), such as bovine pericardium (bioprosthetic valve). (From http://circ.ahajournals.org/content/119/7/1034/F1.expansion.html.)

TABLE 60-9 Anticoagulation Recommendation With Prosthetic Valves

	ANTICOAGULATION RECOMMENDATION			
VALVE TYPE	ASPIRIN*	WARFARIN (INR GOAL)	DURATION	INDICATION CLASS
Mechanical				
MVR	+	(3.0)	Long-term	I
AVR (+ risk factors)†	+	(3.0)	Long-term	I
AVR (– risk factors)†	+	(2.5)	Long-term	I
Bioprosthetic				
MVR		(2.5)	3 months	IIa
AVR		(2.5)	3 months	IIb
MVR	+	–	Long-term	IIa
AVR	+	–	Long-term	IIa
TAVR	+‡		6 months	IIb

Adapted from Nishimura RA, Otto CM, Bonow RO, et al: 2014 AHA/ACC guideline for the management of patients with valvular heart disease: A report of the American College of Cardiology/American Heart Association Task Force on Practice Guidelines. *J Thorac Cardiovasc Surg* 148:e1–e132, 2014.

AVR, aortic valve replacement; *INR,* international normalized ratio; *MVR,* mitral valve replacement; *TAVR,* transcatheter aortic valve replacement.

*Recommended aspirin dose, 75-100 mg daily.

†Risk factors: atrial fibrillation, previous thromboembolism, left ventricular dysfunction, hypercoagulable condition, older-generation valve.

‡For TAVR, lifelong aspirin plus clopidogrel 75 mg daily for 6 months.

with warfarin in turn is associated with approximately a 1% annual risk of bleeding complications. Both bleeding and thromboembolic complications may be reduced through more frequent (e.g., weekly) surveillance of international normalized ratio or home testing.[38]

Bioprosthetic valves are almost universally fabricated from preserved (bovine) pericardium or from porcine valves specially harvested for this use. Anticoagulation is typically not needed with the implantation of bioprosthetic valves beyond an initial 3-month period to allow sewing ring endothelialization to occur, unless other indications such as atrial fibrillation exist.[37]

Modern antimineralization and tissue preservation techniques involving treatment of valves with alpha-oleic acid reduce cusp calcification and typically provide approximately 90% freedom from structural valve deterioration and reoperation at 10 years in patients older than 65 years.[39] Failure rates may be higher in younger patients as a result of greater hemodynamic stresses or metabolic (calcium turnover) rates, but many surgeons now recommend implantation of bioprosthetic valves in patients younger than the recommended cutoff of 60 to 70 years of age (class IIa), accepting the risk of reintervention by open or percutaneous technique as being less than the lifelong risk of anticoagulation/mechanical valve thromboembolism. Relative contraindications to anticoagulation, including pregnancy, may influence choice of prosthesis.

Regardless of implant type, similar excellent early and long-term survival outcomes have been achieved after valve implantation (see Tables 60-5 and 60-8), and the technical considerations in implantation are generally considered similar between valve types, except for xenograft stentless aortic bioprosthetic roots and homografts. In particular, improved valve designs have largely eliminated differences in the hemodynamic profile of bioprostheses versus historically better-performing mechanical valves.

Patient-prosthesis mismatch describes a syndrome arising from an undersized (aortic) prosthetic effective orifice area compared with the patient's body surface area (0.65 cm^2/m^2). Inadequate prosthetic valve effective orifice area can lead to residual transvalvular gradients, resulting in persistent ventricular hypertrophy, impaired ventricular remodeling, and excessive late cardiac events. Charts are available to select the appropriately sized prosthesis as a function of body surface area. Patient-prosthesis mismatch is unusual with the excellent hemodynamic performance of current valves, but native annulus/root enlargement can be performed to accommodate a sufficiently large prosthesis.

Finally, prosthetic valve endocarditis (PVE) occurs with an incidence that is 50 times greater than the risk of endocarditis in the general population. Excision and re-replacement are typically indicated for PVE, especially when PVE is caused by virulent organisms such as *Staphylococcus aureus* or fungi, although antibiotic therapy alone may occasionally be used to sterilize lesions in high-risk individuals. Even with appropriate antibiotic therapy and surgical intervention, PVE carries a mortality rate approaching 40% at 1 year. Accordingly, practitioners and patients with prosthetic valves as well as individuals at increased risk for native valve endocarditis should be well versed in and strictly adhere to recommendations for antibiotic prophylaxis against endocarditis.

Transcatheter Aortic Valve Replacement and Other Emerging Technologies

Transcatheter aortic valve replacement (TAVR) describes a new procedure coupling balloon aortic valvuloplasty, which of itself does not provide long-term relief of AS, with implantation of an expandable bioprosthesis delivered and expanded into the aortic annulus using catheter technology. This technology has rapidly evolved since early reports of the clinical applicability of catheter-based pulmonic and aortic valve replacements in 2000 and 2002.[40,41] Compelling evidence of the efficacy of TAVR was provided by the PARTNER (Placement of Aortic Transcatheter Valves) trial, the world's first randomized, controlled study of this new procedure.[42,43] On the basis of data from PARTNER, the Food and Drug Administration (FDA) granted approval for TAVR in 2011 for inoperable (>50% predicted mortality or irreversible morbidity) patients and in 2012 for high-risk (>10% predicted mortality) patients with a predicted postprocedural survival longer than 12 months. Involvement of a Heart Team, consisting of both cardiologists and cardiac surgeons, in evaluation and treatment of TAVR patients is a critical, FDA-mandated component of TAVR protocols.

More specifically, PARTNER A demonstrated that TAVR mortality rates were noninferior to surgery (24% versus 27% at 1 year and 34% versus 35% at 2 years). PARTNER B demonstrated a 40% mortality reduction at 1 year after TAVR compared with standard therapy (31% versus 51%; $P < .001$). This mortality benefit persisted at 2 years (43% versus 68%), although the risk of stroke was significantly higher (14% versus 6% at 2 years) in the TAVR group.[44]

TAVR is being applied today with improving results to increasing numbers of high-risk and even moderate-risk AS patients. These outcomes have been aided by the introduction of new, smaller caliber valves and catheters and ventricular transapical deployment techniques that have decreased vascular complications and improved patient selection and deployment strategies (including rapid ventricular pacing during deployment to minimize prosthesis displacement).

Despite these encouraging data, surgical aortic valve replacement still remains the "gold standard" for low- and intermediate-risk patients, especially because long-term durability data are not yet available for TAVR. In addition, the risk of stroke continues to increase with TAVR compared with surgical aortic valve replacement over time, presumably because of vascular injury or thromboembolic material from the native calcified valve that remains exposed to the circulation.[43,44] Complications such as complete heart block, left bundle branch block, and paravalvular regurgitation are also higher after TAVR than after surgical aortic valve replacement, and these complications have been linked to higher long-term mortality.[42-46]

Percutaneous Mitral Interventions

Percutaneous therapies for mitral valve disease are also being developed, although they lag TAVR, in part because of the greater difficulty in successfully accessing the mitral as opposed to the aortic annulus. Most therapies are adaptations of current surgical techniques, including the Alfieri stitch (edge-to-edge leaflet repair) and annuloplasty.

The MitraClip System, clinically introduced in 2003, has seen the greatest advancement of all percutaneous mitral valve therapies, receiving FDA approval for high-risk patients in 2013. With use of a catheter-based clip delivery system, an intra-atrial septal puncture is performed to gain access to the left atrium and to cross the mitral valve. The catheter then grasps the mitral valve leaflet edges and places a clip that emulates the edge-to-edge leaflet repair (Fig. 60-16). Although the reduction of severe MR is less effective than with surgical therapy, this technology has brought therapeutic options with demonstrable hemodynamic improvement to many who are not surgical candidates.[47]

Other experimental mitral valve therapies include "indirect annuloplasty" strategies using compression devices placed inside the coronary sinus (because of its anatomic proximity to the mitral annulus) designed to apply radial forces onto the annulus to decrease the size of an enlarged mitral orifice in functional regurgitation. Results with this approach have been inconsistent.

Sutureless valves are another emerging technology that has already seen significant advancement in clinical trials. These valves are placed surgically, under direct vision, but with an implantation technique similar to current catheter-based technology. Because sutureless valves do not require meticulous sewing to the native annulus, their major benefits include decreased cardiopulmonary bypass and aortic cross-clamp times, reduced risk of iatrogenic injury to structures surrounding the diseased valve, and preserved options to perform concomitant open procedures such as CABG.[48,49] Reports of shorter intubation times, fewer days in the intensive care unit, and decreased incidence of postoperative atrial fibrillation, pleural effusion, and respiratory insufficiency have recently emerged.[50] Much like for transcatheter valve replacements, long-term outcomes data will be important in guiding the appropriate use of this new technology.

ACKNOWLEDGMENT

The authors would like to acknowledge Ana María Rodríguez, PhD, for her outstanding assistance in providing editorial support.

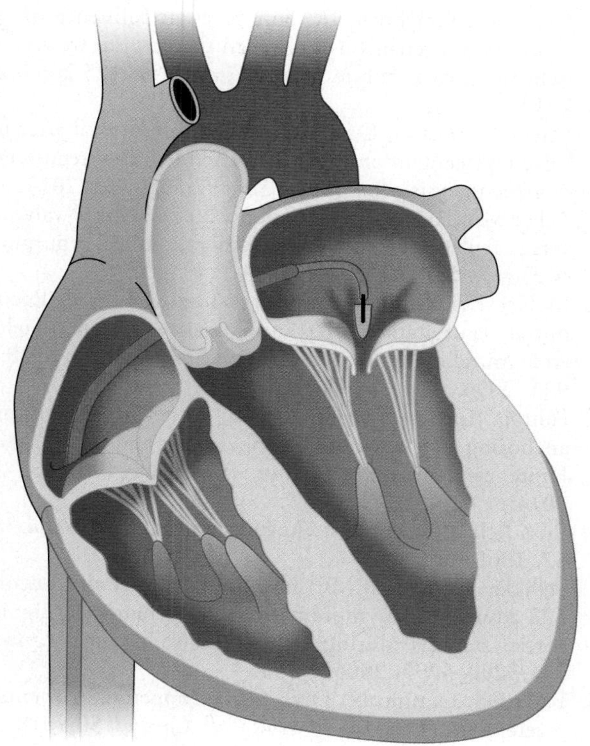
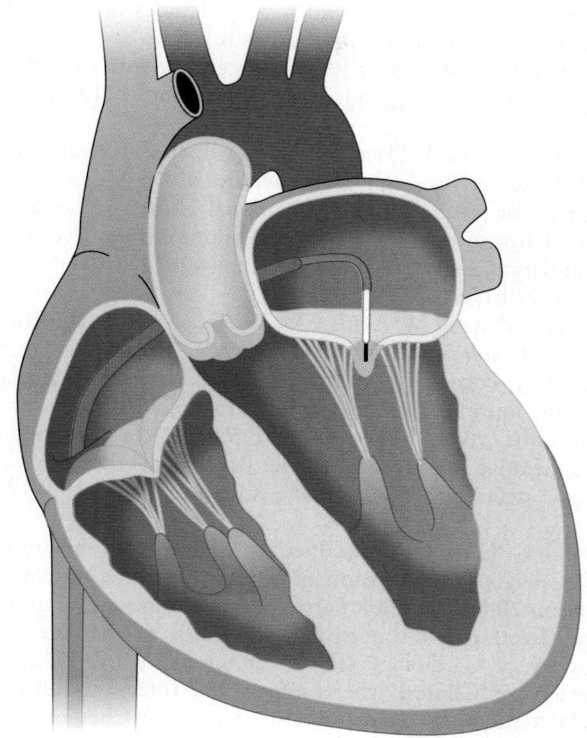

FIGURE 60-16 Percutaneous Mitral Valve Repair. Using a catheter-based clip delivery system, the operator grasps the mitral valve leaflet edges and places a clip that emulates the edge-to-edge leaflet repair. (From http://www.cathlabdigest.com/files/mitra1.png.)

SELECTED REFERENCES

Carpentier A: Cardiac valve surgery—the "French correction". *J Thorac Cardiovasc Surg* 86:323–337, 1983.

This seminal work by Alain Carpentier for the first time described a comprehensive strategy for repairing regurgitant lesions of the mitral valve. It remains a relevant classic today.

David TE, Feindel CM: An aortic valve-sparing operation for patients with aortic incompetence and aneurysm of the ascending aorta. *J Thorac Cardiovasc Surg* 103:617–622, 1992.

In this seminal article, David and Feindel reported their initial cohort of patients treated with a novel technique for aortic valve-sparing root replacement. David has shown excellent results 20 years later in several hundred patients. This technique is used around the world as retaining the native valve avoids prosthetic structural valve degeneration or the need for anticoagulation.

Leon MB, Smith CR, Mack M, et al: Transcatheter aortic-valve implantation for aortic stenosis in patients who cannot undergo surgery. *N Engl J Med* 363:1597–1607, 2010.

This is the original prospective randomized study report from the PARTNER investigators demonstrating the feasibility of percutaneous aortic valve replacement.

Nishimura RA, Otto CM, Bonow RO, et al: 2014 AHA/ACC guideline for the management of patients with valvular heart disease: A report of the American College of Cardiology/American Heart Association Task Force on Practice Guidelines. *J Thorac Cardiovasc Surg* 148:e1–e132, 2014.

These are the most recent American College of Cardiology/American Heart Association Task Force guidelines on current knowledge and treatment of valvular heart disease.

Ross J, Braunwald E: Aortic stenosis. *Circulation* 38:61–67, 1968.

This classic article first described the onset of symptoms of heart failure, syncope, or angina in patients with aortic stenosis as a marker of impending death and indicated a mean survival of 5 years after onset of angina, 3 years after onset of syncope, and 1 to 2 years after onset of heart failure symptoms.

REFERENCES

1. Nkomo VT, Gardin JM, Skelton TN, et al: Burden of valvular heart diseases: A population-based study. *Lancet* 368:1005–1011, 2006.
2. Seckeler MD, Hoke TR: The worldwide epidemiology of acute rheumatic fever and rheumatic heart disease. *Clin Epidemiol* 3:67–84, 2011.

3. Roberts WC, Ko JM: Frequency by decades of unicuspid, bicuspid, and tricuspid aortic valves in adults having isolated aortic valve replacement for aortic stenosis, with or without associated aortic regurgitation. *Circulation* 111:920–925, 2005.
4. Rajamannan NM, Evans FJ, Aikawa E, et al: Calcific aortic valve disease: Not simply a degenerative process: A review and agenda for research from the National Heart and Lung and Blood Institute Aortic Stenosis Working Group. Executive summary: Calcific aortic valve disease—2011 update. *Circulation* 124:1783–1791, 2011.
5. Enriquez-Sarano M, Akins CW, Vahanian A: Mitral regurgitation. *Lancet* 373:1382–1394, 2009.
6. Barlow J, Pocock W, Marchand P, et al: The significant late systolic murmurs. *Am Heart J* 66:443–452, 1963.
7. Anyanwu AC, Adams DH: Etiologic classification of degenerative mitral valve disease: Barlow's disease and fibroelastic deficiency. *Semin Thorac Cardiovasc Surg* 19:90–96, 2007.
8. Habib G, Hoen B, Tornos P, et al: Guidelines on the prevention, diagnosis, and treatment of infective endocarditis (new version 2009): The Task Force on the Prevention, Diagnosis, and Treatment of Infective Endocarditis of the European Society of Cardiology (ESC). Endorsed by the European Society of Clinical Microbiology and Infectious Diseases (ESCMID) and the International Society of Chemotherapy (ISC) for Infection and Cancer. *Eur Heart J* 30:2369–2413, 2009.
9. Nishimura RA, Otto CM, Bonow RO, et al: 2014 AHA/ACC guideline for the management of patients with valvular heart disease: A report of the American College of Cardiology/American Heart Association Task Force on Practice Guidelines. *J Thorac Cardiovasc Surg* 148:e1–e132, 2014.
10. Olesen KH: The natural history of 271 patients with mitral stenosis under medical treatment. *Br Heart J* 24:349–357, 1962.
11. Vahanian A, Alfieri O, Andreotti F, et al: Guidelines on the management of valvular heart disease (version 2012): The Joint Task Force on the Management of Valvular Heart Disease of the European Society of Cardiology (ESC) and the European Association for Cardio-Thoracic Surgery (EACTS). *Eur J Cardiothorac Surg* 42:S S1–S44, 2012.
12. Inoue K, Owaki T, Nakamura T, et al: Clinical application of transvenous mitral commissurotomy by a new balloon catheter. *J Thorac Cardiovasc Surg* 87:394–402, 1984.
13. Bouleti C, Iung B, Himbert D, et al: Reinterventions after percutaneous mitral commissurotomy during long-term follow-up, up to 20 years: The role of repeat percutaneous mitral commissurotomy. *Eur Heart J* 34:1923–1930, 2013.
14. Song JK, Kim MJ, Yun CS, et al: Long-term outcomes of percutaneous mitral balloon valvuloplasty versus open cardiac surgery. *J Thorac Cardiovasc Surg* 139:103–110, 2010.
15. Antunes MJ, Vieira H, Ferrão de Oliveira J: Open mitral commissurotomy: The 'golden standard.' *J Heart Valve Dis* 9:472–477, 2000.
16. Sá MP, Ferraz PE, Escobar RR, et al: Preservation versus non-preservation of mitral valve apparatus during mitral valve replacement: A meta-analysis of 3835 patients. *Interact Cardiovasc Thorac Surg* 15:1033–1039, 2012.
17. Enriquez-Sarano M, Avierinos JF, Messika-Zeitoun D, et al: Quantitative determinants of the outcome of asymptomatic mitral regurgitation. *N Engl J Med* 352:875–883, 2005.
18. Deja MA, Grayburn PA, Sun B, et al: Influence of mitral regurgitation repair on survival in the surgical treatment for ischemic heart failure trial. *Circulation* 125:2639–2648, 2012.
19. Dayan V, Soca G, Cura L, et al: Similar survival after mitral valve replacement or repair for ischemic mitral regurgitation: A meta-analysis. *Ann Thorac Surg* 97:758–765, 2014.
20. Acker MA, Parides MK, Perrault LP, et al: Mitral-valve repair versus replacement for severe ischemic mitral regurgitation. *N Engl J Med* 370:23–32, 2014.
21. McGee EC, Gillinov AM, Blackstone EH, et al: Recurrent mitral regurgitation after annuloplasty for functional ischemic mitral regurgitation. *J Thorac Cardiovasc Surg* 128:916–924, 2004.
22. Pantoja JL, Ge L, Zhang Z, et al: Posterior papillary muscle anchoring affects remote myofiber stress and pump function: Finite element analysis. *Ann Thorac Surg* 98:1355–1362, 2014.
23. Ross J, Jr, Braunwald E: Aortic stenosis. *Circulation* 38:61–67, 1968.
24. Pellikka PA, Sarano ME, Nishimura RA, et al: Outcome of 622 adults with asymptomatic, hemodynamically significant aortic stenosis during prolonged follow-up. *Circulation* 111:3290–3295, 2005.
25. Bach DS, Cimino N, Deeb GM: Unoperated patients with severe aortic stenosis. *J Am Coll Cardiol* 50:2018–2019, 2007.
26. Gillam LD, Marcoff L, Shames S: Timing of surgery in valvular heart disease: Prophylactic surgery vs watchful waiting in the asymptomatic patient. *Can J Cardiol* 30:1035–1045, 2014.
27. Bekeredjian R, Grayburn PA: Valvular heart disease: Aortic regurgitation. *Circulation* 112:125–134, 2005.
28. David TE: Surgical treatment of aortic valve disease. *Nat Rev Cardiol* 10:375–386, 2013.
29. Van de Veire NR, Braun J, Delgado V, et al: Tricuspid annuloplasty prevents right ventricular dilatation and progression of tricuspid regurgitation in patients with tricuspid annular dilatation undergoing mitral valve repair. *J Thorac Cardiovasc Surg* 141:1431–1439, 2011.
30. Nath J, Foster E, Heidenreich PA: Impact of tricuspid regurgitation on long-term survival. *J Am Coll Cardiol* 43:405–409, 2004.
31. De Bonis M, Taramasso M, Lapenna E, et al: Management of tricuspid regurgitation. *F1000Prime Rep* 6:58, 2014.
32. Yeter E, Ozlem K, Kiliç H, et al: Tricuspid balloon valvuloplasty to treat tricuspid stenosis. *J Heart Valve Dis* 19:159–160, 2010.
33. Goodney PP, O'Connor GT, Wennberg DE, et al: Do hospitals with low mortality rates in coronary artery bypass also perform well in valve replacement? *Ann Thorac Surg* 76:1131–1137, 2003.
34. El-Hamamsy I, Clark J, Stevens LM, et al: Late outcomes following freestyle versus homograft aortic root replacement: Results from a prospective randomized trial. *J Am Coll Cardiol* 55:368–376, 2010.
35. David TE, Feindel CM: An aortic valve-sparing operation for patients with aortic incompetence and aneurysm of the ascending aorta. *J Thorac Cardiovasc Surg* 103:617–622, 1992.
36. David TE: Aortic valve sparing operations: Outcomes at 20 years. *Ann Cardiothorac Surg* 2:24–29, 2013.

37. Pibarot P, Dumesnil JG: Prosthetic heart valves: Selection of the optimal prosthesis and long-term management. *Circulation* 119:1034–1048, 2009.
38. Garcia-Alamino JM, Ward AM, Alonso-Coello P, et al: Self-monitoring and self-management of oral anticoagulation. *Cochrane Database Syst Rev* (4):CD003839, 2010.
39. Flameng W, Rega F, Vercalsteren M, et al: Antimineralization treatment and patient-prosthesis mismatch are major determinants of the onset and incidence of structural valve degeneration in bioprosthetic heart valves. *J Thorac Cardiovasc Surg* 147:1219–1224, 2014.
40. Cribier A, Eltchaninoff H, Bash A, et al: Percutaneous transcatheter implantation of an aortic valve prosthesis for calcific aortic stenosis: First human case description. *Circulation* 106:3006–3008, 2002.
41. Bonhoeffer P, Boudjemline Y, Saliba Z, et al: Percutaneous replacement of pulmonary valve in a right-ventricle to pulmonary-artery prosthetic conduit with valve dysfunction. *Lancet* 356:1403–1405, 2000.
42. Leon MB, Smith CR, Mack M, et al: Transcatheter aortic-valve implantation for aortic stenosis in patients who cannot undergo surgery. *N Engl J Med* 363:1597–1607, 2010.
43. Smith CR, Leon MB, Mack MJ, et al: Transcatheter versus surgical aortic-valve replacement in high-risk patients. *N Engl J Med* 364:2187–2198, 2011.
44. Kodali SK, Williams MR, Smith CR, et al: Two-year outcomes after transcatheter or surgical aortic-valve replacement. *N Engl J Med* 366:1686–1695, 2012.
45. Généreux P, Webb JG, Svensson LG, et al: Vascular complications after transcatheter aortic valve replacement: Insights from the PARTNER (Placement of AoRTic TraNscathetER Valve) trial. *J Am Coll Cardiol* 60:1043–1052, 2012.
46. Houthuizen P, Van Garsse LA, Poels TT, et al: Left bundle-branch block induced by transcatheter aortic valve implantation increases risk of death. *Circulation* 126:720–728, 2012.
47. Munkholm-Larsen S, Wan B, Tian DH, et al: A systematic review on the safety and efficacy of percutaneous edge-to-edge mitral valve repair with the MitraClip system for high surgical risk candidates. *Heart* 100:473–478, 2014.
48. Shrestha M, Folliquet TA, Pfeiffer S, et al: Aortic valve replacement and concomitant procedures with the Perceval valve: Results of European trials. *Ann Thorac Surg* 98:1294–1300, 2014.
49. Englberger L, Carrel TP, Doss M, et al: Clinical performance of a sutureless aortic bioprosthesis: Five-year results of the 3f Enable long-term follow-up study. *J Thorac Cardiovasc Surg* 148:1681–1687, 2014.
50. Pollari F, Santarpino G, Dell'Aquila AM, et al: Better short-term outcome by using sutureless valves: A propensity-matched score analysis. *Ann Thorac Surg* 98:611–617, 2014.

SECTION XII

Vascular

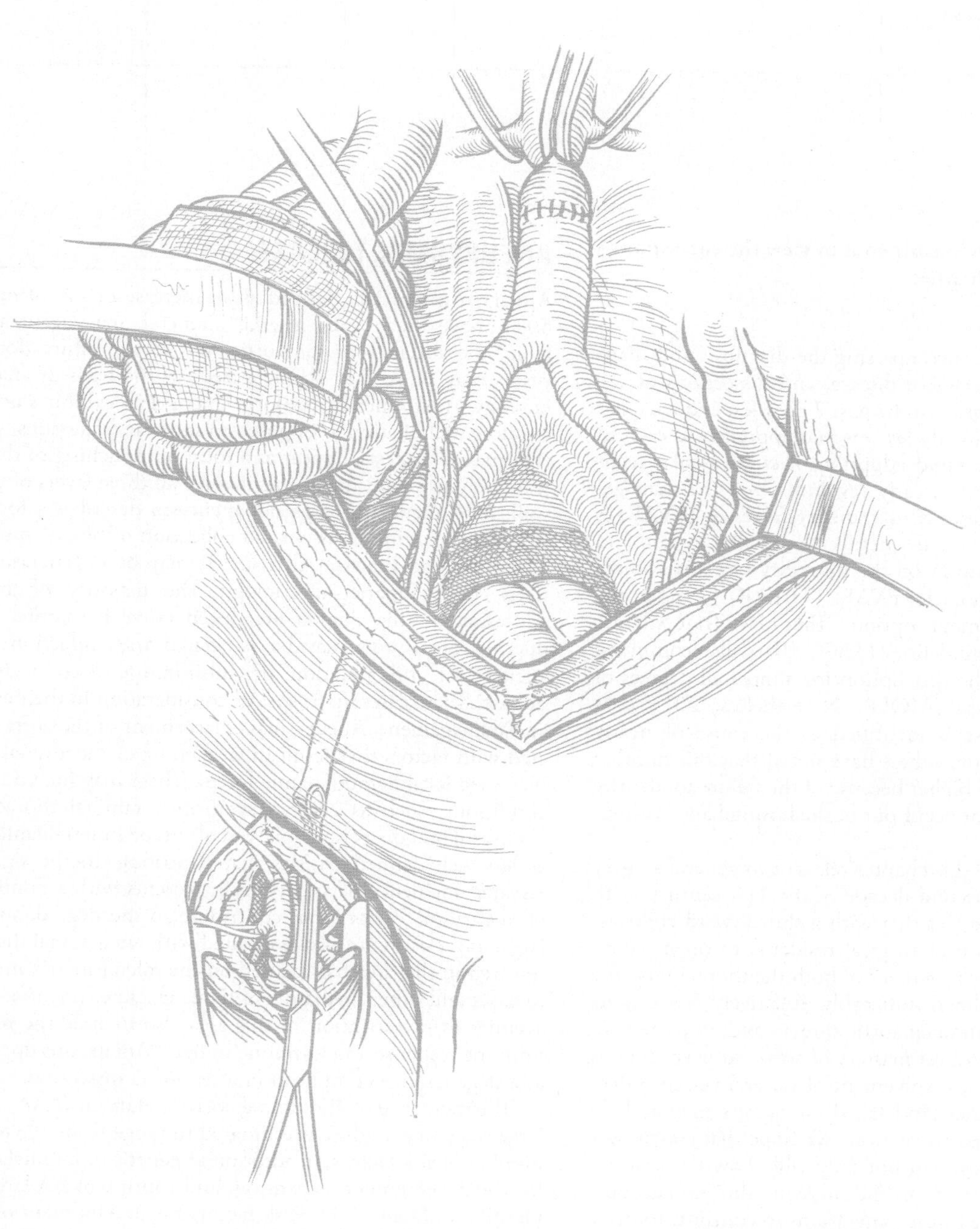

61 CHAPTER

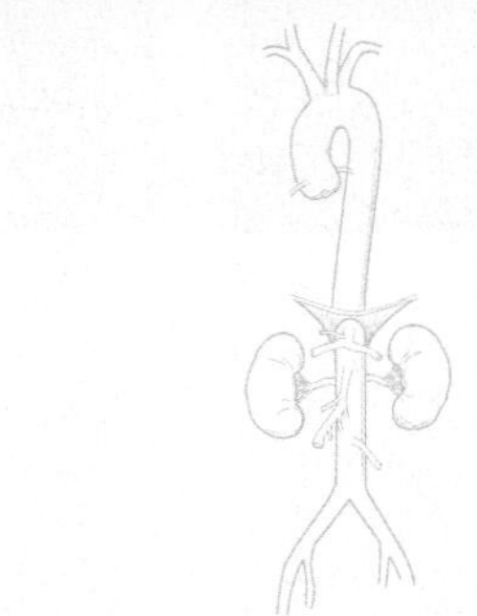

The Aorta

Margaret C. Tracci, Kenneth J. Cherry

OUTLINE

 **Please access ExpertConsult.com to view the corresponding video for this chapter.**

The aorta is a broad topic encompassing the diagnosis and management of aneurysms, occlusive disease, and dissections of the abdominal and thoracic aorta. In the past 2 decades, endovascular therapy has offered a frequently less morbid approach to each of these disease entities. The rapid adoption of endovascular techniques and technologies has clearly revolutionized the management of aortic disease. Endovascular aneurysm repair (EVAR) is now performed much more frequently than open repair and appears to have had an impact on the mortality rate attributable to aortic aneurysm.[1] Thoracic EVAR (TEVAR) is now the recommended first treatment option. The new TransAtlantic Inter-Society Consensus guidelines (TASC III) will recommend endovascular therapy as the first option for almost all degrees of aortoiliac occlusive disease (AIOD). Nevertheless, 2013 data suggest that aortic disease is identified as the cause of nearly 10,000 deaths per year,[2] and others have noted that this number is likely to be significantly higher because of the failure to identify aortic disease in deaths that occur out of the hospital and without autopsy.

We have tried to make this chapter relevant to general surgery residents training in the second decade of the 21st century, with particular attention to the fact that with a shift toward endovascular therapy, the exposure of surgical residents to open reconstructive techniques for management of both the thoracic and the abdominal aorta has declined noticeably. Relatively few centers still offer rich experience in open aortic surgery and, in particular, the most complex cases, and yet mastery of aortic surgery remains a necessity. Dense calcium, involvement of visceral vessels, infections, trauma, small arteries, and failed endografts may and do necessitate formal open reconstruction. We hope that concurrent changes in the training regimen not only will allow the maintenance of standards with regard to the surgeon's skill set and outcomes but also will enable future generations to continue to drive advances in the state of the art of vascular surgery.

ANEURYSMAL DISEASE

Aneurysms, typically defined as an increase in size of more than 50% above the normal arterial diameter, may occur anywhere along the aorta, from the aortic root to the bifurcation. Aneurysms may be further characterized on the basis of anatomy or etiology. Anatomically, fusiform aneurysms exhibit smooth, circumferential dilation as opposed to saccular aneurysms, which, as their name suggests, appear as a focal outpouching of the arterial wall. Whereas true aneurysms involve all three layers of the vessel wall, false aneurysm or pseudoaneurysm describes a focal defect in the artery with an associated collection of blood contained by adventitia and periarterial tissue; it may be degenerative, infectious, or traumatic in etiology. The majority of aneurysms addressed in this chapter are degenerative in nature. Less frequently, aneurysms may be associated with infection (mycotic aneurysms), inflammation, or autoimmune or connective tissue disease. These cases merit special consideration in their evaluation and management. Aneurysmal enlargement of the aorta is associated with factors that result in weakening of the arterial wall and increased local hemodynamic forces. These may include heritable conditions, such as Marfan syndrome, familial thoracic aortic aneurysm and dissection, and vascular-type Ehlers-Danlos, as well as less well defined entities that contribute to the significantly elevated incidence of aneurysm in patients with a family history of aneurysm. Factors that contribute to the degradation of collagen and elastin are also associated with aneurysmal disease, and research in this area has focused on the role of matrix metalloproteinases and other mediators of tissue enzyme function. Ongoing avenues of investigation in this area also include the role of the immune response and hormone milieu.[3] Aneurysms do also occur as a degenerative complication after aortic dissection.

The incidence of abdominal aortic aneurysm (AAA), based on large screening studies, is estimated to range from 3% to 10%. A number of risk factors, in addition to genetic or familial disorders, for the development, expansion, and rupture of AAAs have been identified (Table 61-1). Risk factors for development of an AAA include age, male gender, concurrent aneurysms, family history,

TABLE 61-1 Risk Factors for Aneurysm Development, Expansion, and Rupture

SYMPTOM	RISK FACTORS
AAA development	Tobacco use
	Hypercholesterolemia
	Hypertension
	Male gender
	Family history (male predominance)
AAA expansion	Advanced age
	Severe cardiac disease
	Previous stroke
	Tobacco use
	Cardiac or renal transplantation
AAA rupture	Female gender
	↓ FEV_1
	Larger initial AA diameter
	Higher mean blood pressure
	Current tobacco use (length of time smoking ≫ amount)
	Cardiac or renal transplantation
	Critical wall stress–wall strength relationship

Adapted from Chaikof EL, Brewster DC, Dalman RL, et al: The care of patients with an abdominal aortic aneurysm: The Society for Vascular Surgery practice guidelines. *J Vasc Surg* 50:S2–S49, 2009.

TABLE 61-2 Estimated Annual Rupture Risk

AAA DIAMETER (cm)	RUPTURE RISK (%/yr)
<4	0
4-5	0.5-5
5-6	3-15
6-7	10-20
7-8	20-40
>8	30-50

Adapted from Brewster DC, Cronenwett JL, Hallett JW Jr, et al: Guidelines for the treatment of abdominal aortic aneurysms. Report of a subcommittee of the Joint Council of the American Association for Vascular Surgery and Society for Vascular Surgery. *J Vasc Surg* 37:1106–1117, 2003.

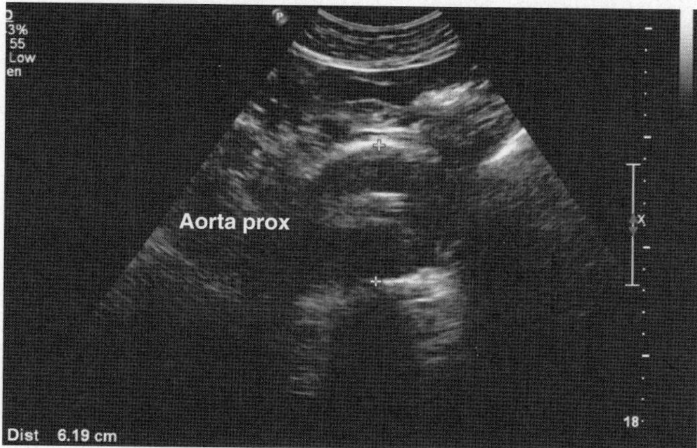

FIGURE 61-1 Gray-scale cross-sectional ultrasound image of an infrarenal aortic aneurysm measuring 6.19 cm in maximal anteroposterior diameter.

tobacco use, hypertension, hyperlipidemia, and height. Female gender, black race, and diabetes appear to be protective.[4-14]

Gender differences extend to the presentation, associations, and natural history of aneurysms. Men with AAA, for instance, are more likely to present with concurrent iliac or femoropopliteal aneurysms.[15] Women are more likely to experience rupture and consistently demonstrate poorer outcomes after repair, perhaps because of a significantly higher incidence of challenging anatomy.[16,17]

Risk of Rupture

Predicting the behavior of an aneurysm over time is difficult. Published risk factors for rupture include chronic obstructive pulmonary disease (COPD), current tobacco use, larger initial AAA diameter, female gender, cardiac or renal transplantation, and certain patterns of wall stress.[4,18-26]

The most widely adopted surrogate for rupture risk is maximal cross-sectional aneurysm diameter (Table 61-2), although the implications for rupture risk of a particular aortic diameter remain debated. Some data suggest that surgeons tend to overestimate rupture risk.[27] In addition, an observational study suggested that even broadly accepted estimates of risk may overstate the rupture rates of untreated AAA and noted, in patients deemed medically unfit for elective repair, that the risk of death from non–aneurysm-related causes exceeded the risk of death from rupture.[28]

In addition, despite a relative paucity of natural history data regarding growth rate and rupture, most clinicians do consider the rate of enlargement a risk factor for rupture. A rate of growth of more than 5 mm in 6 months or more than 1 cm per year has been widely adopted as an indication for repair, independent of aneurysm size. Size is an imperfect predictor of rupture risk; autopsy studies have discovered evidence of rupture in up to 12% of aneurysms less than 5 cm in diameter.[29] A number of investigational models attempt to quantify rupture risk by calculations of wall stress, observation of particular wall or thrombus characteristics, or the combination of multiple factors thought to contribute to increased wall stress or decreased strength.

Diagnosis

Abdominal aneurysm may be detected on physical examination as a palpable pulsatile mass, most commonly supraumbilical and in the midline. The location may be variable, however, as aortic tortuosity can result in a lateral or infraumbilical location. The sensitivity of physical examination is, as one might expect, dependent on the aneurysm's size and the patient's habitus.

The detection and characterization of aneurysms are greatly aided by modern imaging techniques. Ultrasound examination has been demonstrated to afford excellent sensitivity and specificity (Fig. 61-1). Ultrasound may be limited by the patient's habitus or bowel gas, but as it avoids the complications associated with invasive testing, radiation, and contrast media, it is an excellent choice for screening. Ultrasound is not an ideal method for detecting rupture; it is unable to image all portions of the aortic wall, and the nonfasting status of emergently examined patients may further preclude ideal image acquisition. It has been estimated that ultrasound may fail to detect up to 50% of aneurysm ruptures.

Computed tomography (CT) provides excellent imaging of AAA, with greater reproducibility of diameter measurements than by ultrasound. CT, particularly with the adjunctive use of iodinated contrast agents to perform CT angiography (CTA), provides a wealth of anatomic information; it detects vessel calcification, thrombus, and concurrent arterial occlusive disease and permits multiplanar and three-dimensional reconstruction and analysis for operative planning (Fig. 61-2). Drawbacks include substantial radiation exposure, particularly in the setting of serial examinations, and the use of iodinated contrast media in a population with a high incidence of comorbid kidney disease.[4]

Magnetic resonance imaging (MRI) and magnetic resonance angiography (MRA) are, like CT, sensitive in the detection of AAA (Fig. 61-3). Unlike CT, MRI does not demonstrate aortic wall calcification, which may be important in operative planning. Although the study does not require the use of iodinated contrast material, MRA uses gadolinium, which has been associated with the development of nephrogenic systemic fibrosis in patients with low glomerular filtration rate. The availability of MRI may also be limited by the presence of incompatible metallic implants or foreign bodies. The ability to acquire dynamic images throughout the cardiac cycle may ultimately prove clinically useful.[30]

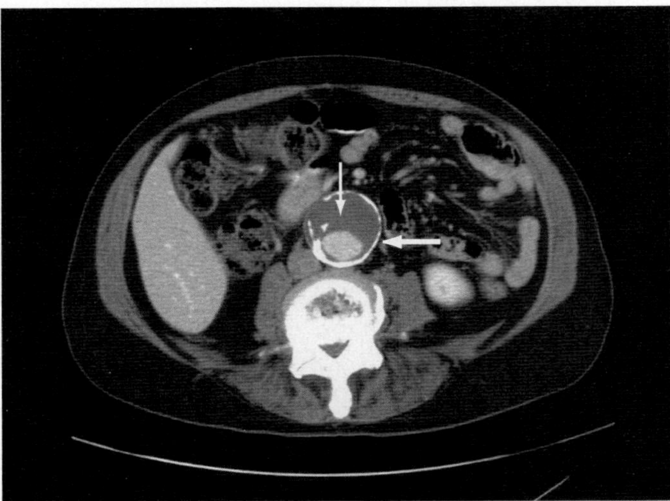

FIGURE 61-2 CTA axial plane image of an infrarenal abdominal aortic aneurysm demonstrating aortic wall calcification *(thick arrow)* and intraluminal thrombus *(thin arrow)*.

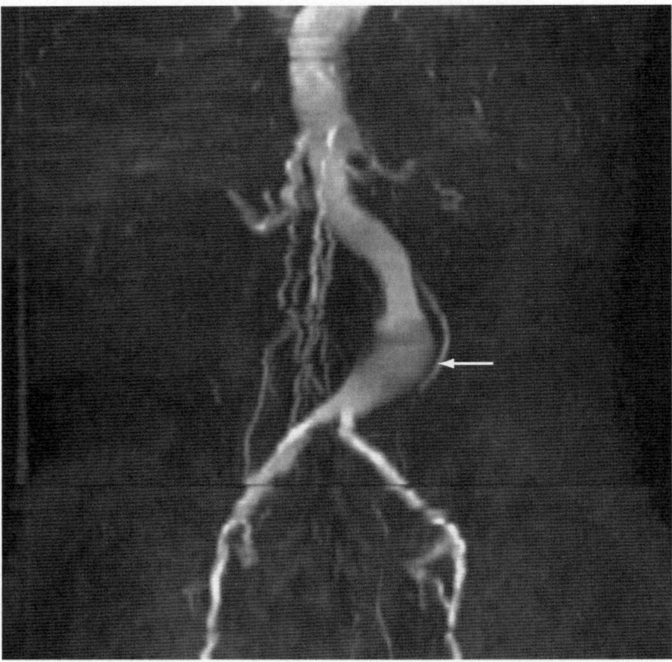

FIGURE 61-3 MRA coronal view of an infrarenal aneurysm *(arrow)*.

Screening and Surveillance Recommendations

Screening recommendations for AAA are informed by the sensitivity and specificity of ultrasound screening, the detection yield of screening based on various risk factor selection criteria, and cost. A major recent compilation of evidence-based recommendations for screening and surveillance of AAA is provided by the 2009 Practice Guidelines developed by the Clinical Practice Council of the Society for Vascular Surgery. The Society for Vascular Surgery committee charged with reviewing available data regarding screening made a strong recommendation for one-time screening of all men aged 65 years and older or men 55 years and older with a family history of AAA. Screening of women is also strongly recommended for those aged 65 years and older with a family history of AAA or a personal smoking history. The evidence basis of these recommendations was deemed to be strong in the former case and moderate in the latter.[4]

The U.S. Preventive Services Task Force issued a more limited recommendation for one-time screening of men between 65 and 75 years of age who have a personal smoking history.[31]

Screening of women remains controversial. Although there is evidence that women may exhibit a stronger association between smoking and aneurysm, it is known that the incidence of aneurysm in women who have smoked exceeds that of men who have never smoked, and mortality data reflect that gender differences in aneurysm-related mortality narrow with advanced age.[4] Payer policies regarding reimbursement may not track either of these recommendations. Medicare, for instance, as a result of the Screening Abdominal Aortic Aneurysms Very Efficiently (SAAAVE) Act, reflects an intermediate approach in offering a screening benefit for men with a personal smoking history and men or women with a family history of AAA, although only as a part of the initial Welcome to Medicare physical examination.

Once an aneurysm has been detected, the Society for Vascular Surgery Clinical Practice Council recommends further screening intervals as follows, based on aneurysm size (maximum external aortic diameter) and associated risk of rupture[4]:

<2.6 cm: no further screening recommended
2.6-2.9 cm: reexamination at 5 years
3-3.4 cm: reexamination at 3 years
3.5-4.4 cm: reexamination at 12 months
4.5-5.4 cm: reexamination at 6 months

The recommendation for follow-up of aortic diameters less than 3 cm is controversial and has been criticized on the basis of cost-effectiveness analyses. It is based on findings that a significant proportion of 65-year-old men (13.8%) with an initial aortic diameter of 2.6 to 2.9 cm developed aneurysms exceeding 5.5 cm at 10 years. Given current life expectancy projections, it is evident that a subset of patients deemed "normal" at screening will go on to develop large aneurysms.[32]

Medical Therapy

Once an aneurysm has been diagnosed, the optimization of medical therapy serves a dual purpose: to potentially minimize the rate of aneurysm expansion or rupture and to medically prepare for potential repair. Many avenues have been investigated in the search for effective medical treatment to prevent the progression of aortic aneurysm, leading to a recent editorial statement that "the bottom line is that no drug can currently be recommended for the indication of reducing AAA enlargement."[33] A highly anticipated, randomized trial of doxycycline, an antibiotic and inhibitor of matrix metalloproteinase activity, not only failed to demonstrate benefit but found increased AAA enlargement primarily in the first 6 months of follow-up.[34] Investigation is ongoing, particularly with regard to the role of anti-inflammatory agents.

Currently, many continue to incorporate beta blockade in an effort to control blood pressure and dP/dT that may contribute to harmful wall stress. Studies using propranolol demonstrated mixed results and low patient compliance. Angiotensin-converting enzyme inhibitors and angiotensin receptor blockers have yielded mixed results in clinical studies, but their use is based on the goal of blood pressure management as well as on evidence for their utility in the management of patients with aortic disease associated with Marfan syndrome.[35] HMG–coenzyme A reductase inhibitor (statin) therapy has been associated with reduced rates of AAA enlargement and is otherwise appropriate in a population with a high prevalence of concurrent atherosclerotic disease. Antiplatelet therapy using aspirin does, like beta blockers and statins, offer secondary preventive benefit in this population and should be considered. Perhaps the most important intervention, in both regards, is smoking cessation. Current tobacco use has been associated with an increased rate of aneurysm expansion. Smoking cessation may also yield benefits with regard to perioperative morbidity and mortality in the event that the aneurysm ultimately requires repair.

Surgical Treatment

Surgical treatment is generally recommended for aneurysms more than 5.5 cm in maximal diameter, those demonstrating more than 5 mm of growth in 6 months or more than 1 cm in a year, and aneurysms with a saccular rather than the typical fusiform anatomy. Gender differences in a variety of factors have led some to advocate for consideration of aneurysm repair at a smaller size in women. It has been observed that the average size of "normal" aorta tends to be slightly smaller in women. Evaluation of several indices relating aortic diameter to body build, such as body surface area or wrist circumference, also suggests that measures other than aortic diameter alone may be more accurate in predicting AAA.[36] These observations are consistent with evidence suggesting more rapid aneurysm growth and rupture at smaller sizes in women (average diameter of 5 cm rather than one of 6 cm in male patients).[37,38] The presence of significant aneurysm-related anxiety associated with awareness of the presence of an unrepaired aneurysm has also been cited as affecting quality of life and presenting a potential consideration in managing aneurysms below 5.5 cm in diameter.[38]

Preoperative Evaluation

The preoperative evaluation of patients with AAA comprises operative planning as well as identification and management of important medical comorbidities, such as coronary artery disease, renal insufficiency, peripheral arterial occlusive disease, diabetes, and obstructive lung disease. As coronary artery disease is the primary cause of mortality after either open or endovascular repair of AAA, a great deal of attention has been focused on the preoperative evaluation and management of comorbid coronary artery disease. The guiding principles in this evaluation have traditionally been the identification of information that will alter management and the institution of therapy that will improve cardiac-related mortality. In 2007, the American College of Cardiology/American Heart Association (ACC/AHA) published guidelines regarding the preoperative cardiac evaluation of patients undergoing noncardiac vascular surgery.[39] These guidelines stratify patients according to the presence or absence of symptomatic cardiac disease, the presence of significant clinical risk factors (mild angina, prior myocardial infarction, compensated congestive heart failure, diabetes mellitus, or renal insufficiency), and the level (quantified in metabolic equivalents) of the patient's functional capacity. Resting electrocardiography is typically performed before high-risk surgery, such as open aneurysm repair, but it is no longer recommended by the ACC/AHA or European Society of Cardiology for patients without clinical risk factors who are undergoing low-risk surgery. Echocardiography may be used to evaluate the cardiac function of those with a history of heart failure or current dyspnea. Heart failure is a significant consideration; left ventricular ejection fraction less than 35% has been found to have 50% sensitivity and 91% specificity for predicting perioperative cardiac events.[40]

The decision to proceed with noninvasive testing in patients without symptoms of active cardiac disease should be based on the patient's functional capacity and the presence of three or more significant additional risk factors. Coronary angiography should be considered in patients with evidence of active cardiac disease based on screening questions or evidence of ischemia on noninvasive stress testing. Adjunctive medical therapy may also serve to reduce the risk of perioperative cardiac events. Perioperative beta blockade, statin use, and aspirin use are widely accepted, and there is also evidence to support the use of other antihypertensives during this period (Fig. 61-4). An important caveat has been added to the perioperative use of beta blockade, with the 2009 American College of Cardiology Foundation/American Heart Association Focused Update on Perioperative Beta Blockade advising continuation of previously prescribed beta blockers in the perioperative period and titration of beta blockers to desired heart rate and blood pressure, noting that routine perioperative high-dose beta blockers without titration may be harmful.[41] The withdrawal of statins in the perioperative period may be associated with an increased risk of coronary events.[42]

Renal insufficiency related to renovascular or medical renal disease is a well-established risk factor for morbidity and mortality after AAA repair. Coexisting renal artery occlusive disease may be present in 20% to 38% of patients with AAA.[43] In addition, both open and endovascular repair of AAA may result in further deterioration in the renal function of patients with preexisting renal disease. Concurrent repair of clinically significant renal occlusive disease is appropriate at the time of either open repair or EVAR. A number of strategies for intraoperative renal protection have been proposed. Current recommendations include adequate hydration, perioperative discontinuation of angiotensin-converting enzyme inhibitors and angiotensin receptor blockers, and avoidance of hypotension. There is also evidence of increased perioperative mortality associated with postoperative nonresumption of angiotensin-converting enzyme inhibitors.[44] There is mixed evidence regarding the benefits of antioxidants (mannitol, ascorbic acid, vitamin E, *N*-acetylcysteine, and allopurinol) and some data supporting the beneficial effects of infused fenoldopam.[45,46] When suprarenal clamp placement is necessary, the

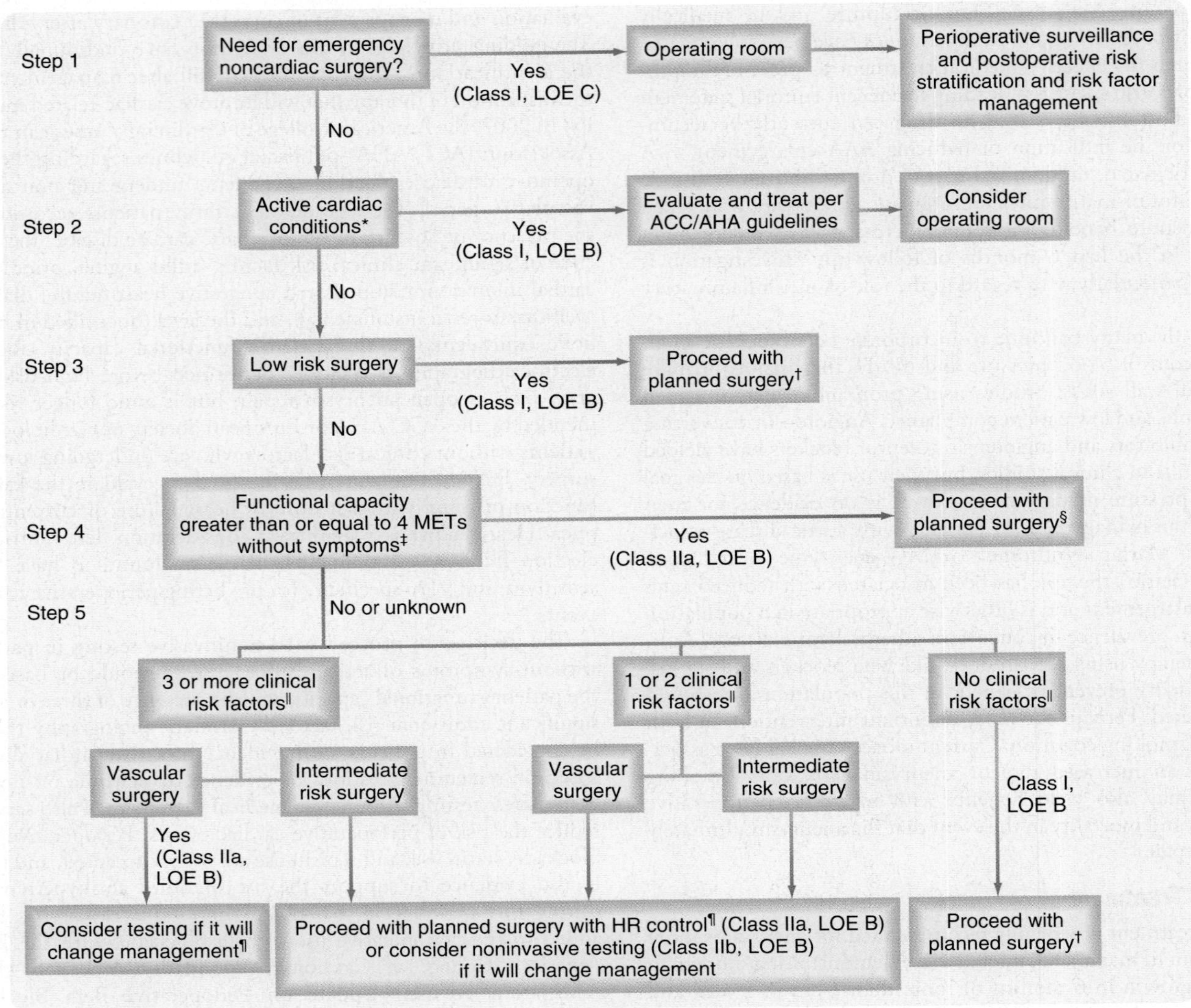

*See Table 2 for active clinical conditions.
†See Class III recommendations in Section 5.2.3, Noninvasive Stress Testing.
‡See Table 3 for estimated MET level equivalent.
§Noninvasive testing may be considered before surgery in specific patients with risk factors if it will change management.
‖Clinical risk factors include ischemic heart disease, compensated or prior heart failure, diabetes mellitus, renal insufficiency, and cerebrovascular disease.
¶Consider perioperative beta blockade (see Table 12) for populations in which this has been shown to reduce cardiac morbidity/mortality.
ACC/AHA indicates American College of Cardiology/American Heart Association; HR, heart rate, LOE, level of evidence; and MET, metabolic equivalent.

FIGURE 61-4 Cardiac evaluation and care algorithm for noncardiac surgery based on active clinical conditions, known cardiovascular disease, or cardiac risk factors for patients 50 years of age or older. (From Fleisher LA, Beckman JA, Brown KA, et al: ACC/AHA 2007 guidelines on perioperative cardiovascular evaluation and care for noncardiac surgery: A report of the American College of Cardiology/American Heart Association Task Force on Practice Guidelines [Writing Committee to Revise the 2002 Guidelines on Perioperative Cardiovascular Evaluation for Noncardiac Surgery]: Developed in collaboration with the American Society of Echocardiography, American Society of Nuclear Cardiology, Heart Rhythm Society, Society of Cardiovascular Anesthesiologists, Society for Cardiovascular Angiography and Interventions, Society for Vascular Medicine and Biology, and Society for Vascular Surgery. *Circulation* 116:e418–e499, 2007.)

authors endorse the use of cold saline perfusion of the kidneys, preclamp administration of furosemide and mannitol, and selective use of fenoldopam. An additional consideration, particularly in patients with preexisting renal dysfunction, is contrast-induced nephropathy associated with administration of iodinated contrast agents for CT imaging or angiography. Current data support intravenous hydration with sodium bicarbonate or normal saline and possibly the use of antioxidants, such as ascorbic acid or *N*-acetylcysteine. When EVAR is contemplated, carbon dioxide may be used as an imaging agent to alleviate or to minimize the need for iodinated agents as the rate of contrast-induced nephropathy is related to the amount of agent administered as well as age and prior renal function.

Data are mixed with regard to the impact of pulmonary disease, particularly COPD, on mortality after AAA repair. However, there is evidence that optimal management of comorbid COPD may improve morbidity and mortality.[47] The authors support obtaining a preoperative pulmonary function assessment, including arterial blood gases, to assess risk and to guide management in the perioperative period. Patients with poor pulmonary function must be made aware of the increased risk that they will require prolonged ventilatory support postoperatively and the attendant possibility that tracheostomy will be required during this period. Smoking cessation before surgery may be beneficial and can be aided by counseling and a variety of pharmacologic therapies. Although several studies have suggested that initiating smoking cessation less than 2 weeks before surgery may actually be associated with worse outcomes, a meta-analysis suggests that smoking cessation at any time within 8 weeks of surgery is not associated with a higher rate of either overall complications or pulmonary complications postoperatively.[48]

The preoperative evaluation should also include a chest radiograph, complete blood count, blood chemistries, and coagulation studies as well as urinalysis. The chest radiograph may demonstrate evidence of infection, thoracic aortic disease, or malignant disease, all of which should be thoroughly investigated before AAA repair. The use of various anticoagulant agents is common in patients with AAA, and management is tailored to the indication for use. Vitamin K antagonists should be stopped 5 to 7 days before surgery and bridging anticoagulation provided, if indicated, with low-molecular-weight or unfractionated heparin. Thienopyridines are typically stopped 7 to 10 days before surgery, although patients receiving thienopyridine therapy for drug-eluting coronary stents necessitate careful consideration of the merits of delaying surgery until therapy is discontinued in light of the additional bleeding risk associated with these drugs. Aspirin is typically continued perioperatively as it may confer some degree of benefit with regard to cardiac complications in the perioperative period.

Careful evaluation of preoperative imaging is crucial in planning repair. Anatomic variations, such as a retroaortic renal vein, variant inferior vena cava, or horseshoe kidney, may significantly affect the selection of surgical approach and, if not appreciated preoperatively, can lead to disastrous complications. CT imaging affords the additional advantage of demonstrating vascular calcification, thus permitting the surgeon to assess the feasibility of clamping the aorta and iliac arteries at various levels (Fig. 61-5). Occlusion balloons may be substituted for arterial clamp placement, most frequently at the iliac arteries, should severe calcification render clamp placement untenable. Finally, the size and patency of branch vessels, such as the inferior mesenteric, accessory renal, iliac, and lumbar arteries, can be assessed and may further contribute to preoperative planning.

Technique of Open Surgical Repair of Abdominal Aortic Aneurysms

Open surgical repair of AAA may be accomplished by either a transperitoneal or a retroperitoneal approach. The choice of technique is guided by technical advantages and disadvantages afforded by each as well as by the surgeon's experience and preference. Transperitoneal repair through a midline laparotomy incision is the most widely used approach to the usual infrarenal aneurysm

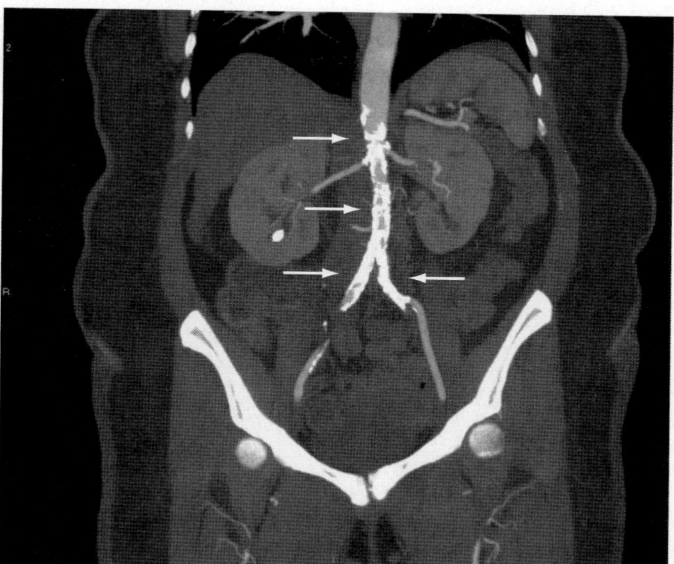

FIGURE 61-5 Reconstruction of coronal CTA image demonstrating heavy calcification *(arrows)* extending from above the renal arteries distally through both common iliac arteries.

and offers a rapid exposure, excellent access to renal and iliac vessels, and the ability to fully examine the abdominal contents. Adjunctive measures to improve exposure at or above the level of the renal arteries may include ligation and division of the tributaries (gonadal, lumbar, and adrenal) of the left renal vein, if the vein is to be preserved, or division of the proximal left renal vein itself. Although data are mixed regarding the effect of left renal vein ligation on postoperative renal function, it is essential that these tributaries be preserved to provide collateral outflow should renal vein ligation be planned. Alternatively, repair of the left renal vein after ligation has been reported.

The infrarenal transperitoneal repair begins with the perioperative administration of an antibiotic, typically a first-generation cephalosporin, and scrupulous skin preparation from the nipples to the thighs. If a ruptured aneurysm is being treated, skin preparation and draping are accomplished before the induction of general anesthesia to permit rapid exposure and control should induction incite hemodynamic collapse. The patient is draped, and a generous midline laparotomy incision is made from the xiphoid to just above the pubis. Extension of this incision along the xiphoid may facilitate supraceliac exposure, if necessary. If repair is elective and preoperative imaging has demonstrated iliac disease necessitating extension of a bifurcated graft to the femoral artery on one or both sides, the femoral artery dissection should be accomplished before laparotomy (Fig. 61-6).

If supraceliac clamp placement is anticipated, the left lobe of the liver is mobilized by division of the triangular ligament, and the esophagus is identified and reflected to the patient's left. Placement of a nasogastric tube facilitates identification and protection of the esophagus. The crural fibers of the diaphragm are divided proximal to the celiac artery to provide adequate exposure and mobilization of the aorta for supraceliac clamp placement. Once these steps have been accomplished, the neck of the aneurysm may be approached. In some cases, the proximal clamp may be moved down to a suprarenal or infrarenal position at this stage, permitting perfusion of visceral and, ideally, renal vessels.

The surgeon may then proceed with iliac dissection and clamp placement.

The surgeon's preference guides the decision with regard to intravenous administration of heparin in rupture. Typical systemic administration of heparin in the elective setting consists of 100 units/kg, administered intravenously and permitted to circulate before clamp placement.

Elective repair permits controlled exposure of the iliac arteries and aneurysm neck before heparinization and clamp placement. Exposure of the infrarenal neck of the aneurysm requires careful

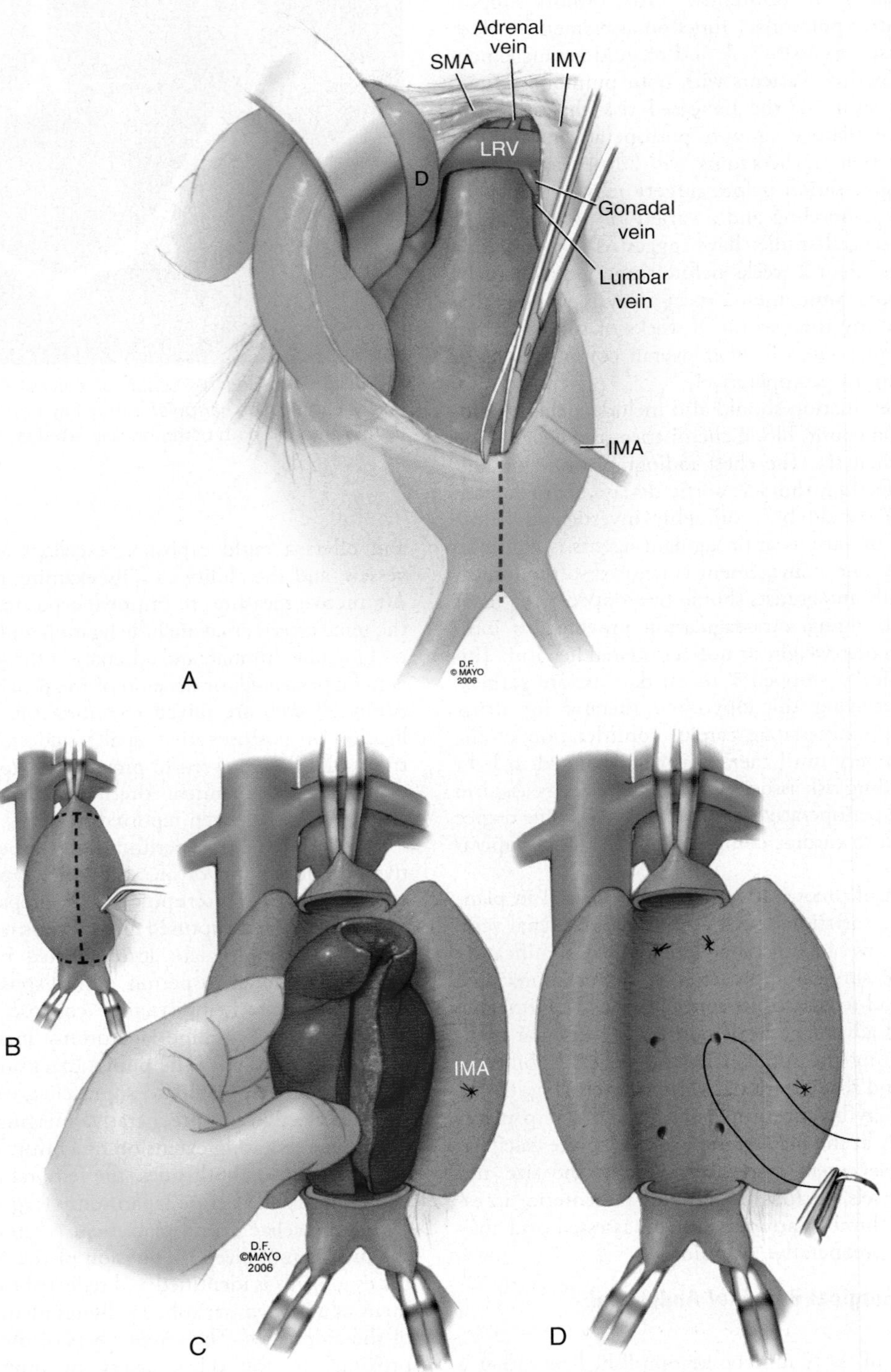

FIGURE 61-6 Technique of open operative repair of an infrarenal abdominal aortic aneurysm using a straight tube graft **(H)** or a bifurcated aortoiliac or aortofemoral **(I)** configuration. Note the attention to closure of the aneurysm sac over the completed repair, with additional closure of retroperitoneal tissues to exclude the duodenum fully **(J)**. *D,* duodenum; *IMA,* inferior mesenteric artery; *IMV,* inferior mesenteric vein; *LRV,* left renal vein; *SMA,* superior mesenteric artery. (Courtesy Mayo Foundation for Medical Education and Research.)

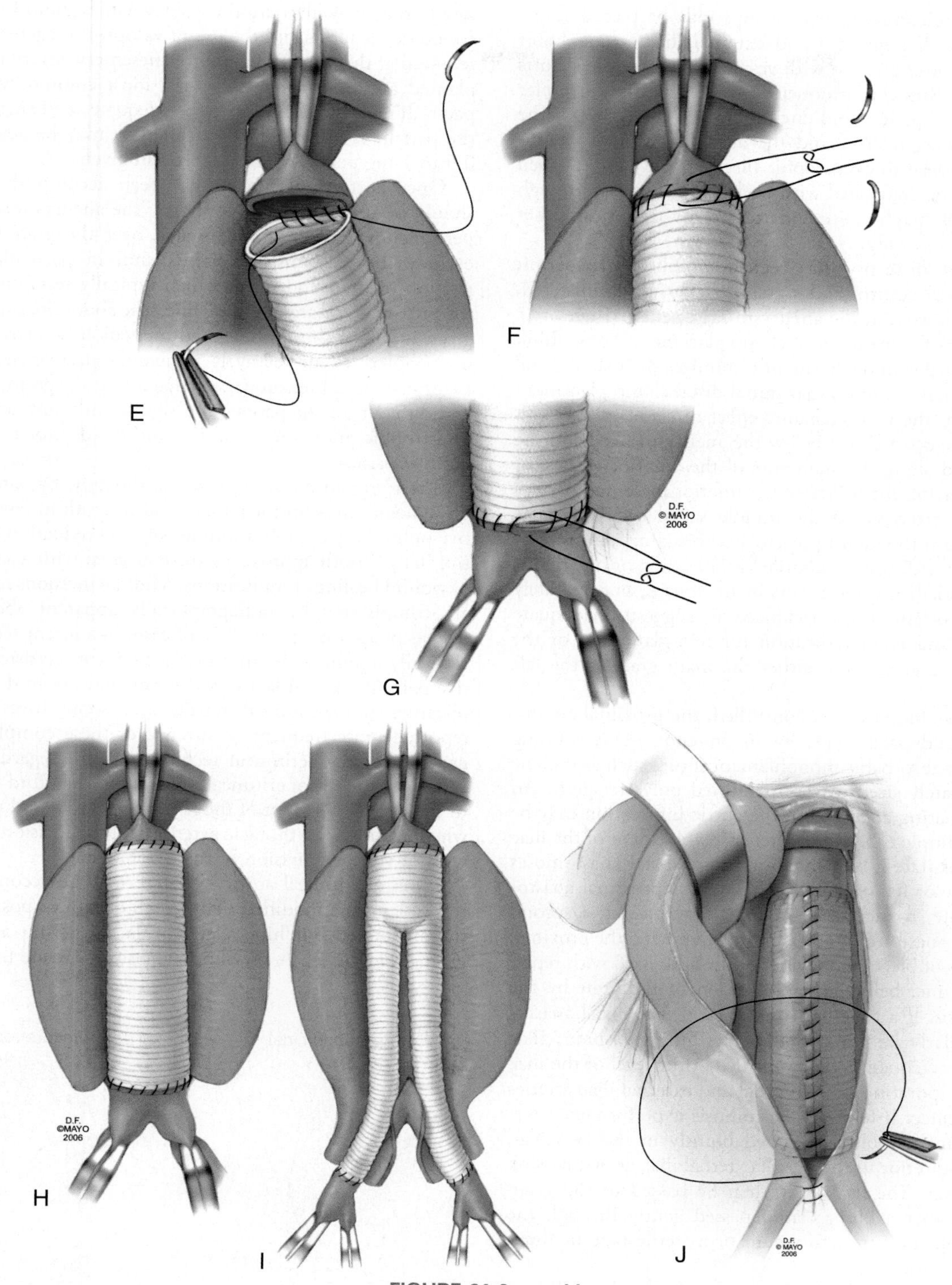

FIGURE 61-6, cont'd

mobilization of the duodenum, distal to the ligament of Treitz, to the patient's right side. The retroperitoneum may then be opened to the level of the iliac bifurcation. Mobilization of the left renal vein facilitates exposure and control of the neck of the aneurysm. At this time, a decision should be made about the necessity of division of either the left renal vein or its tributaries. The iliac arteries may be exposed by careful dissection in the avascular anterior plane, with attention to preservation of the ureter, which will typically cross at the level of the iliac bifurcation, and the pelvic sympathetics, which cross the bifurcation and proximal left common iliac artery. Extensive dissection of the bifurcation and proximal common iliac arteries is not typically necessary as clamp placement in the mid or distal common iliacs is more typical when the aneurysm terminates at or proximal to the aortic bifurcation, permitting repair with a simple tube graft. When aneurysmal or occlusive disease of the iliacs requires replacement of the common iliac, clamps may be placed at the proximal internal (hypogastric) and external iliac arteries. Soft iliac arteries may be controlled with vessel loops placed in a Potts fashion or using a Rumel tourniquet. However, the authors prefer to use vascular clamps to avoid circumferential dissection of the iliac arteries, where possible, and the attendant risk of venous injury, which can lead to catastrophic bleeding. Severely calcified iliac arteries may be controlled with occlusive balloons, although the proximal ends may require endarterectomy to permit either anastomosis or oversewing.

Once adequate dissection has been accomplished to permit proximal and distal control and systemic heparin administered, clamps may be placed and the aneurysm sac opened. There are a variety of opinions for the order of clamp placement. Some think that initial proximal clamp placement minimizes the risk of distal embolization; others maintain that initial distal clamp placement permits staging of the hemodynamic effect of clamp placement. The sac should be opened just below the aneurysm neck and the opening extended along the right side of the anterior surface of the aneurysm, leaving the orifice of the inferior mesenteric artery in situ. Lumbar arteries and the middle sacral artery may be ligated from within the sac to prevent backbleeding. An inferior mesenteric artery with brisk, pulsatile backbleeding or one that is chronically occluded, as often occurs in aneurysms, may be safely oversewn at its origin. Poor backbleeding suggests inadequate collateralization and is an indication for reimplantation of the inferior mesenteric artery into either the main graft or the left iliac limb.

Once backbleeding has been controlled, the proximal anastomosis may be addressed, typically in an end-to-end running fashion using nonabsorbable monofilament suture such as Prolene and an appropriately sized woven or knitted polyester graft. An aneurysm terminating at or before the aortic bifurcation may be repaired with a simple tube graft, whereas involvement of the iliac vessels may necessitate a bifurcated graft and distal anastomoses to either the iliac or femoral arteries. Once the proximal anastomosis is complete, it should be examined by placing a second clamp below the anastomosis and carefully removing the proximal clamp. Any areas of bleeding may be readily addressed with repair sutures at this time, before immobilization of the graft by the distal anastomosis. If a tube graft is sufficient, the distal anastomosis may similarly be completed in a running fashion. Iliac anastomoses may frequently be performed at the level of the iliac bifurcation, incorporating both internal and external iliac arteries as a common orifice. If femoral anastomosis is performed, a retroperitoneal tunnel should be created bluntly in the avascular, anatomic plane anterior to the native external iliac artery, passing beneath the ureter. The limb may then be passed to the groin incision using either a blunt clamp passed gently through the tunnel from groin to retroperitoneum or a sterile tape or drain passed along the same course.

Before completion of the distal anastomosis, the distal iliac or femoral vessels should sequentially be permitted to backbleed to flush out any thrombus or atherosclerotic debris, the proximal clamp briefly removed to flush the graft, and the graft flushed with heparinized saline. The proximal and distal clamps may then be removed. It is imperative that the surgical and anesthesia teams communicate well during this process as clamping and unclamping of the aorta produce profound hemodynamic effects. The patient should be well resuscitated before unclamping as this act is frequently attended by a significant hypotension. Slightly staging release of the iliac arteries or limbs, in the case of a bifurcated graft, may alleviate this somewhat. Sodium bicarbonate to counteract acidosis and the use of vasopressor agents may also be required at this time. The inferior mesenteric artery may be reimplanted at this time, if necessary, most commonly as a Carrel patch. If hemostasis appears to be adequate at all anastomoses and the patient is normotensive, protamine may be administered at 0.5 to 1 mg per 100 units of heparin given.

Once aortic replacement has been accomplished, attention should be turned to graft coverage. The aneurysm sac and retroperitoneum may be approximated over the graft to effectively exclude the abdominal contents and, in particular, the third portion of the duodenum, which typically rests just anterior to the proximal, infrarenal suture line. The abdominal and, if present, groin incisions should be closed meticulously. Hernias, as previously noted, occur relatively frequently after open aneurysmorrhaphy. Wound breakdown, particularly at the groin, can be costly and difficult for the patient and significantly increases the risk of catastrophic graft infection. The authors do not routinely drain groin incisions.

The retroperitoneal approach is thought, by some, to reduce physiologic stress on the patient and to result in fewer postoperative pulmonary complications as well as a reduction of postoperative ileus.[49] Both approaches are associated with a significant rate of wound healing complications. Midline incisions for AAA repair are complicated by radiographically apparent abdominal wall defects in approximately 20% of cases in a recent series, although clinically significant hernias are less frequent. Persistent postoperative pain, flank wall laxity, and hernia have been described complicating retroperitoneal repair, and some investigators have reported more frequent occurrence of these complications with use of the retroperitoneal technique. With regard to operative exposure, the retroperitoneal approach does afford greater access to the visceral segment of the abdominal aorta and may be aided, where required, by thoracic extension of the incision and exposure with or without division of the diaphragm.

A retroperitoneal aortic exposure may be accomplished with the patient in a modified right lateral decubitus position with the thorax rotated but hips relatively flat to permit access to both groins (Fig. 61-7). A curvilinear incision is made from the costal

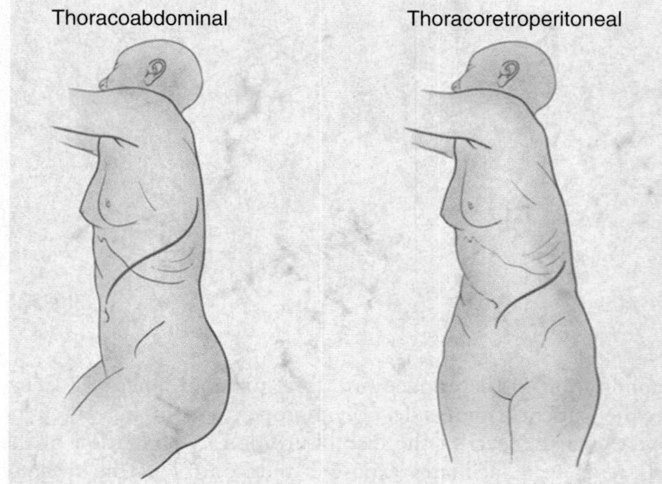

FIGURE 61-7 Patient positioning and incision for thoracoabdominal and thoracoretroperitoneal exposures. Note the open configuration of the hips in the latter, facilitating bilateral access to the iliac and femoral arteries.

margin to below the umbilicus, depending on the extent of exposure required and the patient's habitus. The retroperitoneal plane may be entered at the lateral border of the rectus sheath. The rectus abdominis may be reflected either medially or laterally. Some surgeons prefer lateral reflection as this may result in less difficulty with postoperative body wall laxity. Care is taken to avoid entering the peritoneum. Much of the initial portion of this dissection may be carried out bluntly, with the aid of a tonsil sponge on a ring or Kelly forceps. The abdominal contents, enveloped in peritoneum, may be swept medially. The ureter will be visualized and swept medially. The left kidney may be either elevated or left in situ, although the authors generally prefer to medialize the kidney, which also serves to mobilize the left renal vein. The gonadal tributary, however, must generally be identified, ligated, and divided. Proximally, the spleen is carefully mobilized within its peritoneal covering to expose the underside of the diaphragm. The fibers of the left crus of the diaphragm, when divided, expose the supraceliac and visceral portions of the aorta. The left renal artery should be readily accessible, and the celiac and superior mesenteric arteries may be mobilized by careful dissection. The right renal artery is frequently difficult to isolate before aortotomy. Distally, the iliacs are carefully exposed in the avascular plane by gently mobilizing overlying structures, including the ureters. Again, the full exposure of the right iliac is typically more difficult by this approach, depending on the patient's habitus. The extensive exposure of the supraceliac and visceral portions of the aorta permits full access and nuanced decision making about clamp placement, which may be suprarenal, supramesenteric, or supraceliac. Visceral and renal vessels may be controlled by clamp placement, vessel loops, or, after aortotomy, use of occlusion balloons, with great care taken in handling to avoid dissection or embolization. Occlusive disease or aneurysmal involvement of renal or visceral vessels may be readily addressed by this approach. According to the patient's indications and the surgeon's preference, cardiopulmonary bypass may be used as an adjunct and provides the ability to actively perfuse the renal and visceral vessels should a complex or prolonged reconstruction be anticipated.

Once adequate exposure has been achieved, proximal and distal clamps may be placed. As in the transperitoneal approach, repair is typically accomplished by endoaneurysmorrhaphy, using end-to-end proximal and distal anastomoses to replace the diseased portion of aorta as an interposition. Once again, the aneurysm thrombus is removed at the time of aortotomy, and lumbar arteries are ligated within the sac. The same principles of back-bleeding and flushing of the graft before completion of the distal anastomosis apply. This approach does also permit a variety of approaches to reconstruction of the juxtarenal, pararenal, and paravisceral aorta. Branch vessels may be incorporated together by careful beveling of the graft, reimplanted individually as Carrel patches, or reconstructed using short bypass grafts. In treating thoracoabdominal aneurysms, the incision may be extended into the chest at the appropriate rib space and the diaphragm circumferentially divided to afford enough exposure to extend the repair to virtually any level of the descending aorta. The rib may be circumferentially dissected and divided posteriorly to further improve thoracic exposure as needed. When hemostasis is achieved, the sac may again be closed over the graft, although the retroperitoneally placed graft is not as vulnerable to erosion and aortoduodenal fistula as that placed transperitoneally (Fig. 61-8).

Medial visceral rotation, introduced by Mattox for trauma and adapted to aortic reconstruction by Stoney, is a third technique that may, through an abdominal incision, afford exposure of the entire abdominal aorta. This technique may be used for type IV or high paravisceral aneurysms and is best suited for patients who are not obese or asthenic, with narrow costal margins extending to the iliac crest.

Management of the Ruptured Aneurysm

Patients who survive to present to the hospital with a ruptured AAA may range from relatively stable to circulatory collapse. Optimal outcomes rely on the establishment of an institutional system for management of this critical aortic emergency that facilitates the early notification of the operative team, the availability of appropriate equipment (including an inventory of implants) and staff to support endovascular or open repair, and a system for rapid anatomic assessment. Several key principles of management must be considered. First, the appropriate hemodynamic parameters are those of permissive hypotension, with systolic blood pressures as low as 50 to 70 mm Hg considered adequate in a conscious patient, and avoidance of aggressive volume resuscitation. Management of a hemodynamically unstable patient or one in whom aortic control is expected to be delayed, prolonged, or complex, whether open or endovascular, may use percutaneous balloon control of the proximal aorta.[50] When possible, contrast-enhanced CTA should be performed preoperatively, although techniques that rely exclusively on angiography have been described. This may establish whether endovascular repair is possible or preferred, in addition to delineating anatomy and identifying associated aneurysmal or occlusive disease.

In the operating room, consideration should be given to the method and timing of anesthesia. Endovascular repair may be performed initially or in its entirety under local anesthesia. When open repair and general anesthesia are required, it is prudent to complete positioning, sterile preparation, and draping of the field before induction of anesthesia. In treating a ruptured aneurysm, a supraceliac control clamp should greatly facilitate resuscitation and provide a measure of hemodynamic stability. A formal protocol for resuscitative endovascular balloon occlusion of the aorta has been developed and can be of great utility in the unstable patient with ruptured aneurysm as well as other forms of hemorrhagic shock. This balloon may be placed percutaneously to establish proximal control in anticipation of open or endovascular repair.[51] Initial wire access to the suprarenal aorta should be followed by passage of a stiff guidewire and placement of a sheath of sufficient size (14 Fr) to accommodate a large, compliant occlusion balloon and length (40 cm) to support the inflated balloon in a suprarenal position against aortic pulsation.

Postoperative Management

In the immediate postoperative period, patients are typically admitted to an intensive care unit, with continuous cardiopulmonary monitoring. Adequate pain control, appropriate resuscitation, adequate oxygenation, and heart rate control all serve to minimize the risk of postoperative myocardial infarction. Epidural anesthesia and patient-controlled analgesia are both excellent options for postoperative pain management, and epidural anesthesia may actually decrease postoperative complications.[52] The use of appropriate prophylaxis for deep venous thrombosis is important and is not precluded by the use of an epidural catheter. Attention to early mobilization and nutrition of the patient are also essential to recovery.

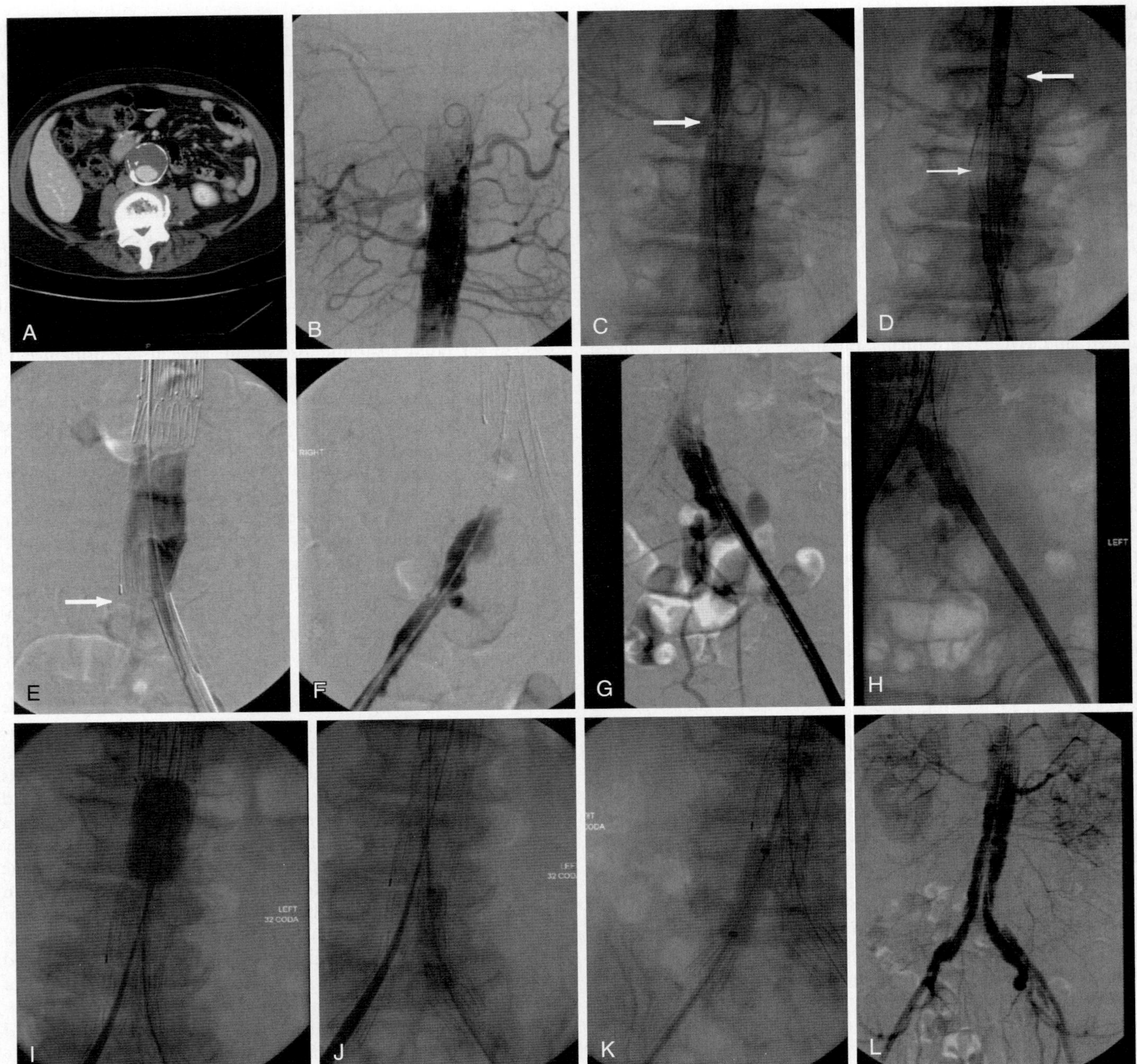

FIGURE 61-8 **Technique of EVAR. A,** Initial aortogram profiling the renal arteries. **B,** Device has been advanced over a stiff wire to the level of the renal arteries. **C,** Note radiopaque markers indicating the beginning of fabric coverage *(arrow).* **D,** Device sheath withdrawn, permitting partial opening of the proximal graft *(thin arrow).* Note that the top cap continues to constrain the suprarenal fixation wires *(thick arrow).* **E,** The contralateral iliac limb gate *(arrow)* has been cannulated; contrast material is introduced with use of a rim catheter to confirm successful cannulation before placement of iliac extension. **F-H,** Angiography of both iliac arteries with marker catheters in place to permit deployment of iliac extensions, with preservation of both internal iliac arteries. **I-K,** Balloon molding of the proximal graft, overlap segments of the main graft and iliac limbs, and distal seal zones of the iliac limbs to facilitate proximal, distal, and intercomponent seals. **L,** Completion aortogram demonstrating successful exclusion of the aneurysm and no evidence of endoleak, which would be manifested as continued filling of the aneurysm sac by contrast material.

Although late events after open surgical repair are relatively rare, a program of surveillance is typical to detect complications such as the formation of anastomotic or para-anastomotic aneurysms, which may occur up to 20% of the time at 15 years after repair.[53,54] The authors typically image patients with CT initially, then at 5-year intervals after repair. Ultrasound may also be used for surveillance but is operator dependent and lacks the sensitivity of CT for detecting anastomotic or para-anastomotic changes.

Ruptured aneurysm may pose a significant challenge in the postoperative period, whether it is approached in an open or endovascular fashion. The incidence of serious complications, such as colon ischemia, renal failure, and spinal cord infarction, is significantly higher than after elective repair and is associated with increased mortality. Surgeons must remain vigilant as colon ischemia may be manifested subtly and must have a low threshold for sigmoidoscopy if it is suspected. Ischemia and reperfusion may also contribute to injury to the lungs, development of lower extremity compartment syndrome with rhabdomyolysis, and abdominal compartment syndrome. The abdominal compartment syndrome may necessitate decompressive laparotomy after successful endovascular repair.

Endovascular Repair

EVAR was first reported by Parodi and colleagues in 1991[55] and has been widely adopted since the first Food and Drug Administration (FDA)–approved devices for EVAR, the AneuRx (Medtronic, Minneapolis, Minn) and the Ancure (Guidant Corporation, Menlo Park, Calif), became available in 1999. In 2006, the Agency for Healthcare Research and Quality published a comparison of EVAR and open surgical repair for AAA that concluded that "EVAR has shorter length of stay, lower 30-day morbidity and mortality but does not improve quality of life beyond 3 months or survival beyond 2 years."[56] These advantages, although limited, have been sufficient to make EVAR more frequently performed in recent years than open surgical repair for aneurysms with suitable anatomy.[57] The advantages of EVAR extend to treatment of ruptured aneurysms, for which multiple studies have confirmed that endovascular repair is associated with lower in-hospital morbidity and mortality.[58] Several anatomic considerations guide patient suitability for EVAR, including the anatomy of the aneurysm neck (size, length, shape, and angulation) and the iliac arteries (caliber, tortuosity, and aneurysmal involvement). The capabilities of currently available devices, as summarized in their approved indications for use, are listed in Table 61-3. The majority of available devices are modular bifurcated grafts consisting of an aortic main body to be used with a variable number of iliac or proximal aortic extension components. Aortouni-iliac devices are also available and may be used, generally in conjunction with femoral-femoral bypass grafting, either primarily or to salvage a failed bifurcated device. Branched devices designed to preserve the hypogastric artery in the setting of an aneurysmal common iliac artery are available in Europe and in clinical trials in the United States.*

Whereas early morbidity and mortality (0.5% to 1.54% versus 3% to 4.8%) are lower with EVAR, there is overall a higher rate of re-intervention (albeit primarily endovascular) after endovascular than after open aneurysm repair and, after 2 to 3 years, no significant difference in the overall mortality rate.[1,59] This relatively new technology has borne an entirely new set of complications. Early, periprocedural complications include endoleak; access-related complications, which occur in up to 3% of cases and include hematoma, pseudoaneurysm, arterial occlusion or dissection, and iliac artery rupture or transection; peripheral embolization; renal insufficiency; local wound complications; inadvertent renal or hypogastric artery occlusion; and rare occurrences, such as colon or spine ischemia. Late complications include rupture, which occurs rarely but at a higher rate than after open repair; graft limb occlusion; endoleak or sac enlargement; and graft infection.[60] Some of these, such as access site complications, have diminished in frequency over time as operator experience has improved and newer generations of devices have incorporated smaller diameters and hydrophilic coatings.

Endoleak is the most common indication for re-intervention after EVAR. Type I endoleak is defined as failure to achieve a satisfactory seal at either the proximal (type Ia) or distal (type Ib) seal zone, representing a failure to exclude the aneurysm sac. In general, a type I endoleak should be addressed at the time of detection. More aggressive balloon inflation within the seal zone, placement of additional graft components to extend the seal zone, and placement of balloon-expandable stents within the seal zone to improve wall apposition through increased radial force are among the most common endovascular therapies for type I endoleak. One FDA-approved device uses helical EndoAnchors (Aptus Endosystems, Sunnyvale, Calif) delivered with a deflectable sheath to address both type I endoleak and migration.[61] Embolization using endovascular coils or liquid embolic agents such as Onyx has also been described.

Type II endoleaks are the most common form and represent continued filling of the aneurysm sac by lumbar branches or the inferior mesenteric artery. Further treatment is indicated if a persistent type II endoleak is accompanied by an increase in sac size. Treatment may include embolization of feeding branches by selective catheterization (transarterial technique) or direct sac puncture (translumbar technique) or laparoscopic or open surgical ligation of these vessels. Efforts have recently focused on identifying preoperative imaging characteristics predictive of persistent type II endoleaks or those that will result in sac enlargement. Aneurysm sac diameter at the level of the inferior mesenteric artery and the number of patent lumbar arteries have been associated with persistent type II endoleak and delayed or recurrent presentation, the presence of inferior mesenteric artery–lumbar artery type of endoleak, and the diameter of the largest feeding or draining artery with sac enlargement.[62-64] Whereas embolization of patent aortic branches at the time of the index procedure seems to decrease the rate of type II endoleak, rupture due to type II endoleak remains rare and difficult to predict; therefore, the role of preemptive branch vessel embolization is controversial.[65,66] Additional techniques, such as perigraft sac embolization, are being investigated.[67]

Type III endoleaks represent failure of an individual component or of the seal between components of a modular graft system. As with type I leaks, all type III endoleaks should be treated, typically by relining the offending area with new graft components. Type IV endoleaks represent seepage through porous graft material and are typically self-limited, resolving when procedural anticoagulation is reversed. Finally, an entity known as endotension is sometimes considered a fifth type of endoleak. This represents persistent growth of the aneurysm sac in the absence of a detectable leak. It is proposed that this phenomenon is due to either the passage of serous ultrafiltrate across an excessively porous fabric or, as some believe, the existence of an undetected endoleak of one of the prior types.

It has also been noted that as operators have gained experience with EVAR, a growing proportion of procedures are performed outside the approved instructions for use. There has, during the same period, been a trend toward treating a greater proportion of patients 80 years of age or older. When demographic and anatomic factors were reviewed, it was noted that only 42% of

*Gore Excluder Iliac Branch Endoprosthesis, Cook Zenith Branch Iliac Endovascular Graft. *http://www.goremedical.com/eu/excluder/, http://zenithglobal.cookmedical.com/zenith-abdominal.html.* Accessed September 29, 2015.

TABLE 61-3 Endovascular Repair Devices: Indications for Use

DEVICE (MANUFACTURER)	STENT OR GRAFT MATERIAL	SHEATH OR DEVICE DIAMETER (MAIN BODY)	AORTIC DIAMETER* (mm)	ILIAC DIAMETER (mm)	MAXIMUM ANGULATION	MINIMUM NECK LENGTH	OTHER
AneuRx (Medtronic)	Nitinol, polyester	21 Fr	20-28 (graft)	12-24 (graft)	45-degree neck	15 mm	Initial FDA approval 1999 No suprarenal fixation or barbs Sheath not required
Talent (Medtronic)	Nitinol, polyester	22 Fr	18-32 (aorta) 22-36 (graft)	8-22 (iliac) 8-24 (graft)	60-degree neck	10 mm	Suprarenal fixation stent Tapered and flared limbs available Uni-iliac Talent Converter device available
Endurant (Medtronic)	Nitinol, polyester	18 Fr, 20 Fr	19-32 (aorta) 23-36 (graft)	8-25 (iliac) 10-28 (graft)	60-degree neck	10 mm	Barbed suprarenal fixation stent Like Talent, approved for 10-mm neck Thin fabric, low delivery profile
Zenith (Cook Medical)	Stainless steel, polyester	18 Fr, 20 Fr, 22 Fr	18-32 (aorta) 22-36 (graft)	7.5-20 (iliac) 9-24 (graft)	60-degree neck	15 mm	Barbed suprarenal fixation stent Tapered limb configurations available Zenith Renu aortouni-iliac graft available Graft sizing based on outer diameter
Excluder (W.L. Gore)	Nitinol, ePTFE	18 Fr, 20 Fr	19-29 (aorta) 23-31 (graft)	8-13.5 (ipsilateral graft) 12-14.5 (ipsilateral graft) 8-18.5 (contralateral graft) 12-20 (contralateral graft) 10-20 (extender)	60-degree neck	15 mm	Available ipsilateral limb sizes vary with size of primary graft Contralateral limb components may be used as iliac extenders Proximal nitinol anchors
Powerlink (Endologix)	Cobalt-chromium, ePTFE	19 Fr, 21 Fr	18-32 (aorta) 22, 25, 28 (graft) 25, 28, 34 (aortic cuff)	10-23 (iliac) 13-16 (graft) 16-25 (extensions)	60-degree neck 90-degree iliac	15 mm	Anatomic fixation on aortic bifurcation Seal achieved with suprarenal or infrarenal proximal aortic cuff IntuiTrak system avoids need to cannulate contralateral gate
AFX (Endologix)	Cobalt-chromium, ePTFE	17 Fr	18-32 (aorta) 22, 25, 28 (graft) 25, 28, 34 (aortic cuff)	10-23 (iliac) 13-16 (graft) 16-25 (extensions)	60-degree neck 90-degree iliac	15 mm	Similar to Powerlink in design Multiple limb configurations Low-profile delivery system for bifurcated graft and proximal cuff
OvationPrime (Trivascular/Endologix)	Cobalt-Chromium/ ePTFE	14 Fr	16-30 (aorta)	8-25 (iliac)	60-degree neck (45-degree if neck <10 mm)	<10 mm†	Uses polymer-filled sealing ring technology for proximal seal Offers integrated crossover lumen as alternative to retrograde cannulation of contralateral gate
Aorfix (Lombard)	Nitinol/woven polyester	22 Fr	19-29 (aorta) 24-31 (graft)	9-19 (iliac) 10-20 (graft)	90-degree neck	20 mm	Combination circular and helical stents to accommodate extreme angulation Proximal fishmouth configuration

*Recommended methods of vessel sizing and guidelines for graft oversizing vary by device.
†Proximal seal based on diameter at 13 mm from lowest renal, as sealing O-ring centered 13 mm from leading edge.

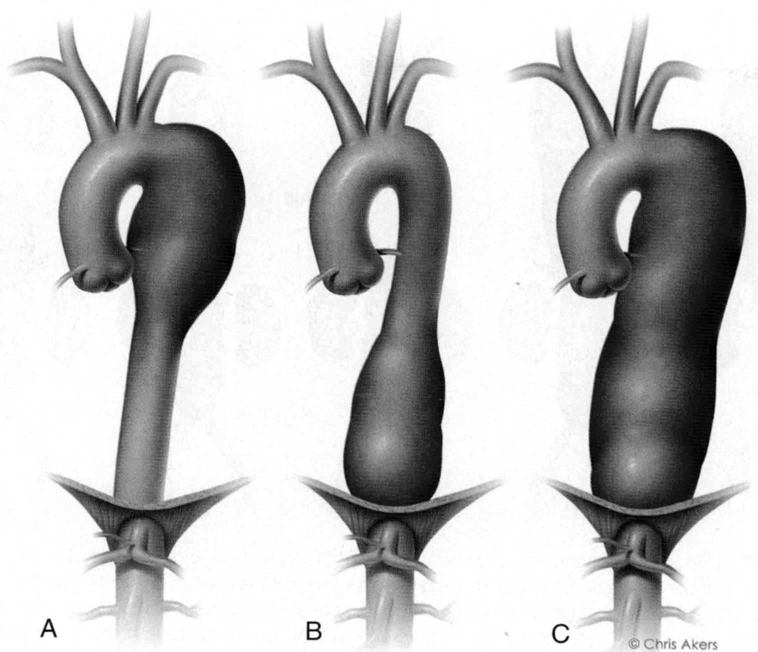

FIGURE 61-9 Classification, descending thoracic aortic aneurysm. **A,** Type A, distal to the left subclavian artery to the sixth intercostal space. **B,** Type B, sixth intercostal space to above the diaphragm (twelfth intercostal space). **C,** Type C, entire descending thoracic aorta, distal to the left subclavian artery to above the diaphragm (twelfth intercostal space). (Courtesy Chris Akers, 2006.)

patients met the conservative definition of instructions for use, whereas 69% met the most liberal definition. Independent predictors of post-EVAR sac enlargement at 5 years were the presence of endoleak, age of 80 years or older, aortic neck diameter of 28 mm or more, aortic neck angulation of 60 degrees or more, and common iliac artery diameter of more than 20 mm, suggesting that factors associated with the gradual liberalization of anatomic criteria over time are associated with sac enlargement and, by implication, worse outcomes.[68] As techniques and devices extend the proximal seal zone into the visceral segment and beyond, one may expect that the trend toward treatment outside instructions for use with infrarenal devices may be reversed.

Device migration, either intraprocedurally or over time, may occur. In the EVAR setting, migration may be facilitated by unfavorable aneurysm neck anatomy. Manufacturers have attempted to address this issue by mechanisms including increased radial force, use of barbs or suprarenal fixation, or use of "anatomic fixation" at the aortic bifurcation. Device failure resulting from fracture of metallic components or fabric failure may also occur. The iliac limbs of these devices are also subject to thrombosis and occlusion, possibly at a higher rate than bifurcated grafts placed during open surgical repair.[69]

It is recommended that contrast CT surveillance be conducted at 1 month, 6 months, and 12 months after graft implantation and annually thereafter. Concern about accumulated lifetime radiation exposure and the use of nephrotoxic contrast agents has driven the expansion of the role of color Doppler and contrast-enhanced duplex ultrasonography in graft surveillance.[70,71] Implantable sensor technology has been approved by the FDA to monitor pressure within the aneurysm sac and may evolve to augment or even to supplant current imaging techniques for postoperative aneurysm surveillance.

Thoracic Aortic Aneurysm

Aneurysms of the descending thoracic aorta may be classified as type A, B, or C, depending on whether the aneurysm involves the proximal, mid, or distal third of the descending aorta, respectively (Fig. 61-9). Thoracoabdominal aneurysms are typically distinguished according to the Crawford classification system (Fig. 61-10). As with aneurysms of the abdominal aorta, rupture risk is closely associated with aneurysm size and, to a lesser extent, female gender. Current guidelines recommend repair of the descending thoracic aorta at 5.5 cm.

Open Repair of Thoracic and Thoracoabdominal Aneurysms

The level of entry into the thoracic cavity for repair of thoracic or thoracoabdominal aneurysm is guided by the proximal extent of the aneurysm. Incision at the fifth or sixth interspace provides excellent exposure of the proximal descending aorta; at the eighth or ninth interspace, the mid-descending aorta; and at the tenth or eleventh interspace, the infradiaphragmatic portion of the aorta. Cardiopulmonary bypass combined with the selective use of distal aortic and visceral perfusion and hypothermic circulatory arrest have yielded exemplary results in experienced hands.[72]

Endovascular Management of Thoracic Aneurysms

In 2005, the FDA approved the GORE TAG Thoracic Endoprosthesis (W.L. Gore & Associates, Flagstaff, Ariz) for treatment of the descending thoracic aorta. Since that time, open surgical therapy for aneurysms of the descending thoracic aorta has largely been supplanted by TEVAR for anatomically suitable lesions.[73]

As with abdominal aortic endografts, initial and subsequent studies have demonstrated a significantly lower rate of short-term morbidity and mortality than with open repair. Unlike EVAR, TEVAR appears to offer a significant, long-term aneurysm-related

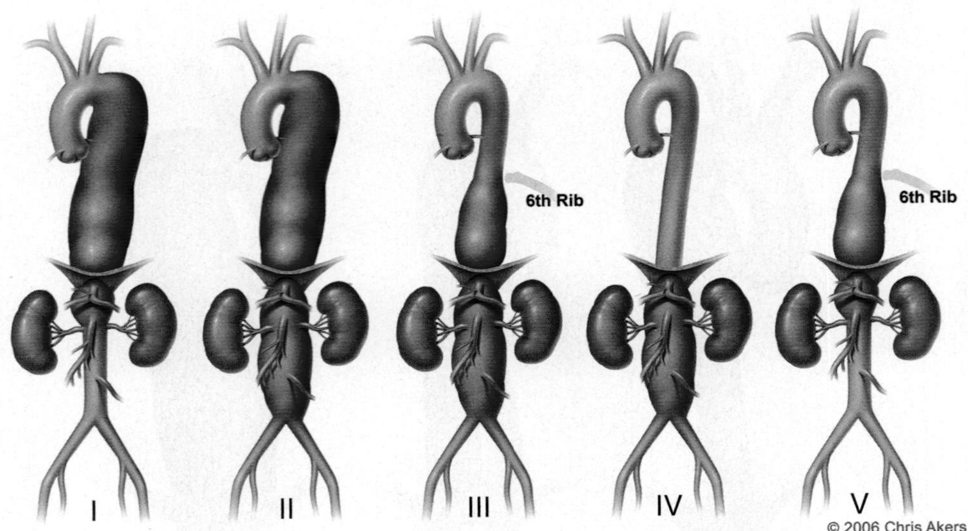

FIGURE 61-10 Normal thoracoabdominal aorta aneurysm classification: extent I, distal to the left subclavian artery to above the renal arteries; extent II, distal to the left subclavian artery to below the renal arteries; extent III, from the sixth intercostal space to below the renal arteries; extent IV, from the twelfth intercostal space to the iliac bifurcation (total abdominal aortic aneurysm); extent V, below the sixth intercostal space to just above the renal arteries (modified Crawford classification). (Courtesy Chris Akers, 2006.)

mortality advantage. The most frequent complications of TEVAR are related to injuries to femoral or iliac access vessels. As the diameters of delivery devices for thoracic endografts may be considerably larger than those required for EVAR, many surgeons have developed a distinctly conservative approach to device access, performing open femoral artery exposure or addressing diminutive iliac vessels through the use of iliac or aortic conduits, open aortic or iliac exposure and direct puncture, or the use of endovascular iliac conduits to prevent injury. Recently, several investigators have pioneered the technique of caval-aortic access for delivery of larger diameter devices to the thoracic aorta or aortic valve.[74] The combination of operator experience and the development of lower profile and hydrophilic delivery systems has, over time, reduced the rate of access-related complications of TEVAR.[75]

Because of the passage of endovascular wires, catheters, and other devices through the aortic arch, TEVAR carries the additional risk of embolic stroke.[76] Nevertheless, TEVAR has consistently yielded lower rates of early mortality and common postoperative complications than in open repair, with Bavaria and colleagues reporting perioperative mortality rates of 2.1% versus 11.7%, spinal cord ischemia rates of 3% versus 14%, respiratory failure rates of 4% versus 20%, and renal insufficiency rates of 1% versus 13% in low-risk patients after endovascular and open repair, respectively.[77]

Several anatomic considerations guide the selection of patients for TEVAR. As with EVAR, the size and configuration of the proximal aneurysm neck must suit the configuration and capabilities of available grafts. Commercially available thoracic endograft diameters currently range from 21 to 46 mm, creating limitations in patients with large proximal necks or small-caliber aortas. Tapered configurations are also available. The radius of the aortic arch and proximal descending aorta can also challenge device conformability and may result in a "bird's beak" deformity on deployment and, potentially, device collapse with consequent compromise of the aortic lumen (Fig. 61-11). In addition, coverage of one or more supra-aortic vessels may be required to achieve an adequate proximal landing and seal zone for the graft, necessitating decisions about extra-anatomic reconstruction. Most commonly, the left subclavian artery origin is covered. Justifications for surgical reconstruction of the subclavian artery, generally by carotid–subclavian artery bypass or subclavian artery transposition, include prevention of arm claudication, preservation of flow to a dominant left vertebral artery, and perhaps most important, maximization of collateral spinal cord perfusion. More recently, endovascular fenestration of the left subclavian artery by a laser technique has been reported. Ultimately, branched devices such as the GORE TAG Thoracic Branch Endoprosthesis are being trialed to extend the proximal seal zone into the aortic arch. Endoleaks, primarily type I, complicate a significant proportion of TEVAR procedures. Some close spontaneously, perhaps because of reversal of intraprocedural heparin anticoagulation. Others require repair by the same techniques used for endoleaks encountered after EVAR.[78]

As with open repair of thoracic and thoracoabdominal aneurysms, prevention of spinal cord ischemia, which may be manifested as temporary or permanent, unilateral or bilateral paraparesis or paraplegia, is of great importance. Delayed rather than immediate postoperative spinal cord ischemia seems to be more common after TEVAR than after open surgical repair, and these patients may be more likely to experience functional improvement after injury.[79] Risk factors for spinal cord ischemia include the length of aortic coverage, coverage of the distal thoracic aorta, compromise of multiple collateral territories, preoperative renal insufficiency, and hypotension.[80] Whereas institutional protocols vary, particularly with regard to selection of patients for cerebrospinal fluid drain placement, the mainstays of prevention of spinal cord ischemia and the treatment of delayed-onset symptoms remain avoidance of hypotension, blood pressure augmentation (target mean arterial pressure > 90 mm Hg), and cerebrospinal fluid drainage to minimize ischemia related to cord compression in the setting of elevated cerebrospinal fluid pressure after ischemia-reperfusion.

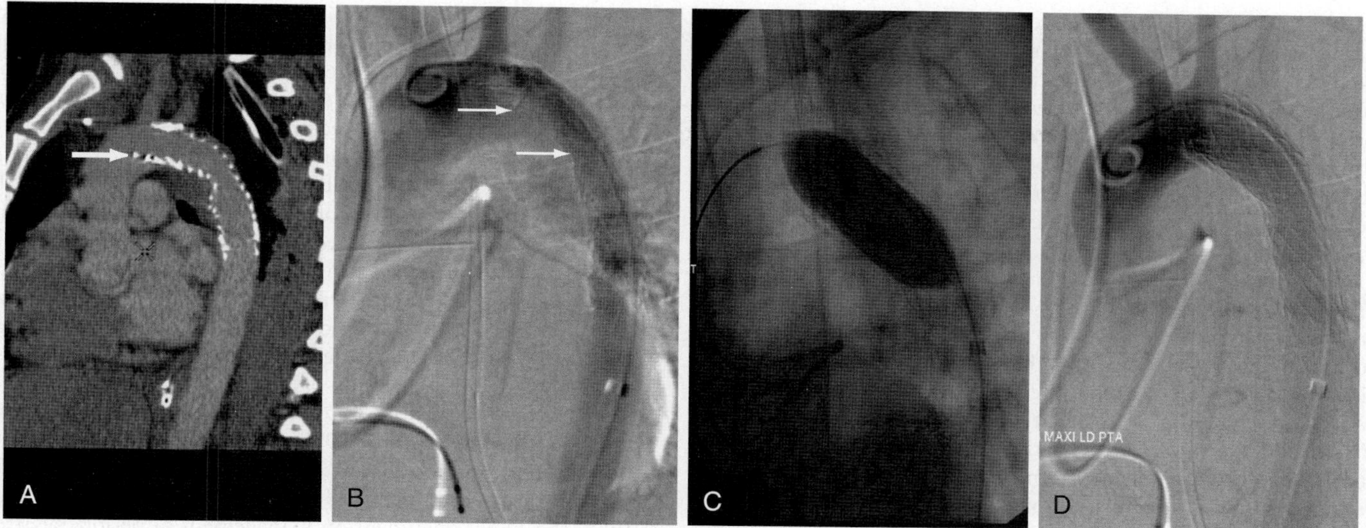

FIGURE 61-11 **A,** CT scan demonstrating thoracic endograft with bird's beak deployment along the lesser curve of the aorta, leaving the leading edge of the endograft projecting into the lumen *(arrow)*. **B,** Thoracic aortogram demonstrating subsequent collapse of the endograft caused by pressure on the protruding proximal portion of the endograft, resulting in distal hypoperfusion *(arrows)*. **C** and **D,** Deployment of a balloon-expandable Palmaz stent to reopen the proximal graft.

Endovascular Repair of Aneurysms Involving the Visceral Segment: Snorkels, Fenestrations, and Branched Grafts

Endovascular therapy for juxtarenal, suprarenal, and thoracoabdominal aneurysms was, until recently, limited to a few centers with access to investigational fenestrated devices or with substantial experience in either creating customized fenestrated devices (Fig. 61-12) or using debranching (antegrade grafts from the thoracic aorta or retrograde iliac grafts to the renovisceral vessels, permitting stent graft coverage of the perivisceral segment) or "snorkel" or "chimney" techniques (use of covered stents extending from the branch vessels beyond the proximal or distal extent of an aortic stent graft) to maintain perfusion to branch vessels.[81,82]

At present, a broader range of centers have gained critical experience in the use of surgeon-modified grafts or snorkel techniques for the treatment of aneurysms involving the visceral segment of the aorta.[83] In 2012, the FDA issued the first U.S. approval for a fenestrated device for the treatment of juxtarenal and pararenal aneurysms, the custom-made Zenith Fenestrated AAA Endovascular Graft (Cook Medical, Bloomington, Ind). This approval mandated a rigorous physician training program including an intensive 2-day training session for the initial group of implanting physicians, selected for their extensive EVAR experience, followed by physician proctoring. Additional branched or fenestrated devices have gained European CE Mark approval or are in investigational stages either in the United States or abroad. There is particular interest in the development of "off-the-shelf" devices that would permit accommodation of the majority of anatomic configurations without the 3- to 4-week manufacturing period required to obtain the custom-manufactured grafts. Devices currently in U.S. clinical trials include the Cook Zenith p-Branch and Endologix (Irvine, Calif) Ventana and the Cook Zenith t-Branch Thoracoabdominal Endovascular Graft, which incorporates four caudally oriented branches into an off-the-shelf design for the treatment of thoracoabdominal aneurysms. The

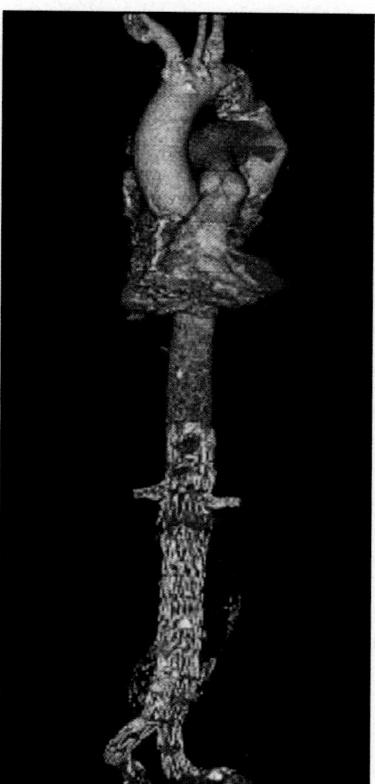

FIGURE 61-12 CT reconstruction demonstrating successful placement of an endovascular graft with fenestrations at the level of the renal arteries, permitting renal stent placement and use of a proximal seal zone above the renal arteries, with preservation of renal perfusion. (Courtesy Dr. Gilbert R. Upchurch, Jr.)

Gore Excluder Thoracoabdominal Branch Endoprosthesis, which began enrolling in clinical trials outside the United States in November 2014 and anticipates initiating enrollment at six U.S. sites in September 2015, includes four visceral branches that are precannulated to facilitate branch vessel selection. The features of the next generation of thoracoabdominal grafts address many of the drawbacks of current custom-made fenestrated grafts and, certainly, of the surgeon-modified branched or fenestrated and various snorkel configurations.

Blunt Thoracic Aortic Injury

In the modern era, the majority of blunt aortic injury is related to motor vehicles and involves the thoracic aorta. True transections are rapidly fatal, generally before arrival at the hospital; some estimates of prehospital mortality are as high as 80% to 90%. Patients may, however, arrive relatively stable with injuries ranging from contained pseudoaneurysms to intramural hematoma to relatively subtle intimal disruptions. The current "gold standard" for imaging of aortic trauma is contrast-enhanced CTA. The most frequent site of injury is the aortic isthmus, and it is typically a transverse tear that can encompass partial or full aortic circumference and may be either partial or transmural. It is thought that injury at this location is a result of rapid deceleration, which creates severe torsion and shearing forces where relatively mobile segments of the aorta become fixed, such as the ligamentum arteriosum, aortic root, and diaphragm.

Particularly in the setting of other distracting or disabling injuries, the history and physical examination may be unrevealing. Chest radiography may demonstrate mediastinal widening, apical pleural cap, loss of the aortopulmonary window, rightward deviation of the mediastinal structures or instrumentation, or depression of the left mainstem bronchus. CT is sensitive and may distinguish between mediastinal hematoma with a preserved periaortic plane and true periaortic hematoma. One must also distinguish between ductus remnants or diverticula and acute injury.

Since the first report of endovascular repair of a traumatic injury to the thoracic aorta in 1997, data have rapidly accumulated to support preferential use of endovascular stent graft over traditional open repair because of consistently reduced rates of mortality (8% to 9% versus 19%), paraplegia (0.5% to 3% versus 3% to 9%), and end-stage renal disease (5% versus 8%) as well as a comparable stroke rate (2.5% versus 1%).[84,85] In practice, endovascular repair was adopted rapidly despite initial concerns about its durability, accounting for 65% of blunt thoracic aortic injury repairs within a decade of the initial publication. During this time, despite technical challenges related to the smaller aortic sizes, endovascular repair offers the additional benefits of reduced hemodynamic impact, lower complication rate, and less overall morbidity. The lower risk nature of the procedure itself may permit earlier aortic repair in patients with significant concurrent injuries.

AORTOILIAC OCCLUSIVE DISEASE

In 1950, the first aortic reconstruction for AIOD (Leriche syndrome) was performed by Jacques Oudot in France. This was performed through a retroperitoneal approach using homograft. Following the investigational and clinical work of Arthur Voorhees at Columbia University, prosthetic grafts of Vinyon-B and nylon were used for reconstruction of aortic occlusive as well as aneurysmal disease. Both of these materials had significant problems associated with them. Wylie introduced aortoiliac endarterectomy to the United States in 1952, and that technique was the most commonly used during the 1950s. In 1958, DeBakey introduced Dacron grafts, and aortofemoral grafting with Dacron became the most widely used technique for open reconstruction, although aortoiliac endarterectomy was still performed at certain centers, notably San Francisco, Boston, and Portland, Oregon. It is still useful for patients with aortoiliac disease confined to the aorta and common iliac arteries, especially those patients with small aortas and iliac arteries, for whom endovascular repair may not be optimal. Axillofemoral artery grafting and femoral-femoral artery grafting were introduced to provide inflow procedures for poor-risk patients and patients with unilateral iliac disease, respectively.

Endovascular repair for occlusive disease of the aorta and iliac arteries was introduced in the 1990s. The use of kissing stents and the size of the common iliac arteries especially have allowed this modality to work extremely well for the majority of patients with AIOD. The TASC document on management of peripheral arterial disease (TASC I) was published in January 2000.[86,87] These guidelines were developed to help in the rational choice of an open or endovascular approach to aortoiliac disease in particular patients. At present, endovascular treatment is the treatment of choice for type A lesions. It is also the most commonly used modality for type B. For type C lesions with more extensive disease of the external iliacs or bilateral occlusions of the common iliacs, surgical treatment has been more often recommended. For type D lesions, that is, extensive disease of the common and external iliac arteries, surgery has been the treatment of choice. Nonetheless, multiple authors have documented good success with endovascular treatment even for TASC C and D lesions.[88-90]

The next iteration of the TASC recommendation is shortly expected, and it is likely that endovascular treatment will be the recommended first-line treatment for all patients. It is difficult, however, to imagine endovascular therapy to be as good or as long lasting for AIOD for these extensive lesions, especially in young patients. It is worth noting the proportion of aortofemoral bypass patients whose concomitant femoral disease requires endarterectomy at the time of the index operation.[91] These patients as well as patients with a significant aortic component of their AIOD may not be well served by endovascular therapy alone. It is also difficult to imagine its utility for juxtarenal aortic occlusion, with its "dunce's cap" of chronic thrombus extending upward between the renal arteries, without a disproportionate increase in renal failure. Hybrid techniques, such as the combination of femoral endarterectomy with the placement of iliac stents, may address some of the limitations of the percutaneous-only approach.

Concomitant with the change in TASC definitions has been a marked increase in the use of endovascular techniques in comparison to open techniques. This increase corresponds to improvements in the delivery systems and stents that are employed as well as to improved skill sets of vascular radiologists, cardiologists, and vascular surgeons. Upchurch and colleagues documented an increase of 850% in endovascular use by 2000 with a concomitant 16% decrease in open cases. There was a 34% increase in treated disease without an increase in the prevalence of the disease.[92] These trends have continued and amplified; endovascular repair for AIOD is performed much more commonly than open repair.

The classic indications for AIOD were claudication, rest pain, and threatened limb viability, manifested by tissue loss, nonhealing ulcers, or frank gangrene. Rest pain and threatened limb viability implied extensive disease of either the deep femoral artery or the femoropopliteal segments in addition to the aortoiliac disease. The advent of endovascular techniques has, as stated before, broadened the indications, with mild claudication being treated much more frequently than in the past. There is certainly more justification for stenting of short-segment iliac stenoses than there is for performing aortofemoral bypass grafting for them.

Nonetheless, open surgery remains the gold standard for long-term patency. Chiu and associates in Birmingham, England, performed a meta-analysis of aortofemoral bypass grafting, iliofemoral bypass grafting, and aortoiliac endarterectomy. Their analysis yielded 29 studies including 5738 patients for aortofemoral bypass grafting, 11 studies incorporating 778 patients for iliofemoral bypass grafting, and 11 studies including 1490 patients for endarterectomy. Operative mortality was 4.1% for aortofemoral bypass grafting, 2.7% for iliofemoral bypass grafting, and 2.7% for aortoiliac endarterectomy. Morbidity was 16%, 18.9%, and 12.5%, respectively. Five-year primary patency rates were 86.3%, 85.3%, and 88.3%, respectively.[93] A meta-analysis published in 2009 suggests that formal aortic reconstruction is still the procedure of choice in terms of long-term patency. That durability may be more appealing to younger, healthier patients than return trips for further endovascular intervention. Similarly, an earlier meta-analysis covering the years 1970 to 1996 showed constant patency rates for aortic bifurcation grafts and declining mortality and morbidity over time. Mortality after 1975 was 3.3%.[94]

Axillofemoral artery bypass grafting is reserved for extremely poor risk patients with rest pain or tissue loss. Its suspect patency makes it a poor choice for claudicants. It is of course used as one of the mainstays of reconstruction for infected aortic grafts or aorta-enteric fistulas. This modality is offered to a different, higher risk group than is aortofemoral bypass grafting. Hertzer reported a 12% mortality compared with 5.6% for femoral-femoral grafting and 2.3% for aortic reconstruction. Within that group, mortality was only 1.2% for aortofemoral bypass grafting but 5.6% for aortoiliac endarterectomy or aortoiliac grafting.[95]

Iliofemoral grafting yields patency rates superior to femoral-femoral bypass in the treatment of unilateral external iliac occlusive disease not amenable to endovascular therapy or when endovascular therapy has failed. Ricco and Probst compared the two operative methods in 143 patients. Primary 5-year patency for iliofemoral grafting was 92.7% versus 73.2% for femoral-femoral grafting.[96]

As in all vascular beds, endovascular repair of the aortoiliac segments requires much more re-intervention than its open counterpart, but the mortality is lower. At some "aortic centers," there is no difference in mortality, but on average, open mortality is about 4%. Hertzer reported mortality of 2.3% for direct aortic reconstructions in an elegant paper.[95] Both Hertzer and Reed and colleagues found increased limb occlusion in patients with small arteries, especially women.[97] Primary assisted and secondary patency rates for endovascular repair nearly equal the primary patency rates of open reconstruction, and this has indeed been the rationale for the widespread application of endovascular techniques for most patients with AIOD, accepting repeated intervention as a necessary component of treatment.

Multiple authors have written about the endovascular treatment of TASC C and D lesions as well as aortic occlusion. Klonaris and colleagues recommended primary stenting for all aortic occlusive disease, including occlusion. Their study, however, did not include juxtarenal aortic occlusions as opposed to more distal aortic obstruction.[98]

Jongkind and colleagues reviewed all published articles of patients undergoing endovascular treatment of TASC C and D lesions from 2000 to 2009. There were 1711 patients identified. Technical success was achieved in 86% to 100% of those studies. Clinical symptoms were improved in 83% to 100%. Mortality ranged from 1.2% to 6.7% and complication rates varied, being reported between 3% and 45%. Primary patency ranged from 60% to 86% and secondary patency from 80% to 98%.[88]

Ichihashi and colleagues reported technical success in 99% of their 125 patients with TASC C and D lesions. Complications were significantly higher than for their TASC A and B patients (9% versus 3%). Their 5-year patency was 83%, among the very highest reported.[89]

Ye and associates performed a meta-analysis of TASC C and D patients undergoing endovascular reconstruction. TASC C patients had a 93.7% technical success rate and a 1-year primary patency of 89.6%. TASC D patients had 90.1% technical success and 87.3% 1-year patency.[90] Indes and colleagues, reviewing the Nationwide Inpatient Sample for 4119 patients, found that endovascular procedures were associated with lower cost, lower complication rates, and shorter length of stay. Mortality was not different statistically, being 1.8% for endovascular procedures and 2.5% for open procedures.[99] There is a third option for aortic reconstruction, and that is laparoscopic aortic surgery. Its greatest proponents have been in Europe, particularly France, and Québec. This has not gained widespread popularity in the United States.[100]

Presentation and Evaluation

Patients with AIOD may present with claudication. It is a much more likely presentation for AIOD than is rest pain or tissue loss. Rest pain or tissue loss, as stated previously, indicates disease of the deep femoral artery or the femoral popliteal segments in addition to the aorta and iliac segments. Physical examination historically has been accurate in these patients. A decreased femoral pulse is indicative of at least common femoral disease or more proximal aortoiliac disease. With the advent of the obesity epidemic in this country, physical examination of femoral pulses is not as accurate as it once was. Consequently, vascular laboratory examination is of even more importance than in the past. Wave patterns as well as ankle-brachial indices are necessary to localize the disease to aortoiliac segments, femoral-popliteal segments, or both. It is also vital in identifying the contribution of AIOD to patients with multiple diseases contributing to their lower extremity problems, including neurogenic claudication, spinal stenosis, and hip arthritis, either alone or in combination with arterial disease.

With a tentative diagnosis of AIOD, the most commonly used modality to visualize the arteries is CTA. There are some patients in whom the calcium load is so great that either MRA or conventional arteriography is necessary to determine whether areas of calcific involvement are highly stenotic. Those surgeons for whom endovascular treatment is uniformly their first choice may proceed directly to conventional arteriography with planned endovascular intervention at the same time.

As with all vascular patients, cardiac risk is the greatest one at operation. Consequently, most authors recommend that all of these patients undergo cardiac function evaluation by stress testing. Those patients with myocardium at risk are usually treated by cardiologists or cardiac surgeons before embarking on an aortic reconstruction in an elective situation. Hertzer showed a marked decrease in cardiac mortality when patients underwent preoperative cardiac evaluation and treatment.[95]

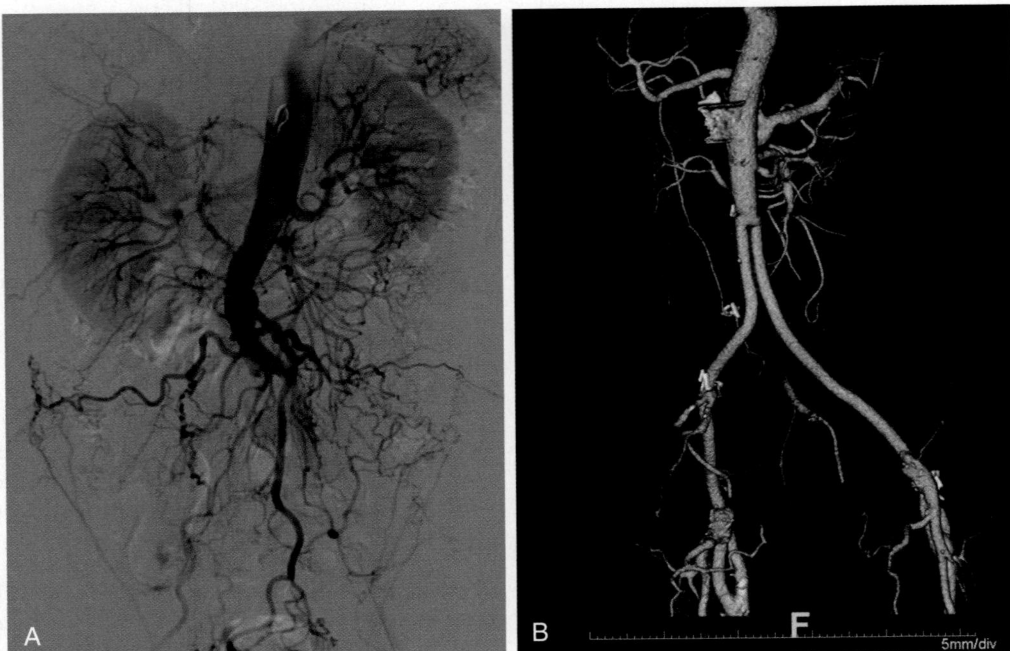

FIGURE 61-13 A, Preoperative aortogram demonstrating occlusion of the distal aorta and iliacs with extensive collateralization. **B,** Postoperative three-dimensional CT reconstruction demonstrating revascularization with an aortofemoral bypass graft.

As endovascular techniques gain wider acceptance, the most common indication for formal aortic reconstruction may be claudication or severe ischemia in the setting of failed multiple attempts at endovascular repair. These occluded stents make the operation more complex, with the need for suprarenal aortic clamping and more extended profundaplasties in many cases.

Technique of Open Reconstruction

Aortofemoral Bypass Grafting

For aortofemoral bypass grafting (Fig. 61-13), the patient is prepared from the nipples to the knees. If concomitant distal bypass grafting will be necessary, the patient is prepared to the toes. This would be done for tissue loss with multilevel disease only. Epidural catheters may be used to alleviate postoperative pain. Bilateral groin incisions are made. These are usually done in a vertical or slight curvilinear fashion. The common, superficial, and deep femoral arteries are dissected free. These need to be dissected distally to where they are soft and suitable for anastomosis. Most surgeons use a midline incision for the aortic exposure, although a transverse incision or a retroperitoneal approach can be used. The authors favor standard midline with infracolic exposure. The abdominal contents are mobilized so that the retroperitoneum can be entered. If the mobilized viscera can be kept inside the abdominal cavity rather than being placed on the abdominal wall, the patient's gastrointestinal functional recovery is usually a bit quicker. The retroperitoneum is entered. Care is taken to stay to the patient's right of the inferior mesenteric vein to avoid violating the left mesocolon. The aorta is dissected free below the renal arteries. The surgeon needs to remember that this disease extends from the renal arteries and not from the lower-lying renal vein level. The vein may be mobilized by division and ligation of its tributaries. In general, the exposure required for occlusive disease is less than is necessary in aneurysmal disease. The aorta is exposed down to the level of the inferior mesenteric artery. Retroperitoneal tunnels connecting this wound with the groin wounds are made. On the left side, a counterincision in the gutter lateral to the white line of Toldt may be necessary. The tunnels should be made posterior to the ureters. It is our habit to create the left tunnel posterior to the inferior mesenteric artery as well to allow the left limb of the graft to be isolated from the gastrointestinal tract by the left mesocolon after completion of reconstruction. The patient is heparinized.

Control is obtained of the aorta below the renal arteries and of the distal aorta. The aorta is divided. Distally, a portion of it is resected on an angular bias and the distal aorta oversewn. That area of excision should be done proximal to the inferior mesenteric artery. This allows comfortable placement of an end-to-end graft. An appropriately chosen graft is fashioned to fit and sewn to the end of the proximal aorta using running 3-0 or 4-0 permanent suture. If one extremity has been less symptomatic that the other, that side is reconstructed first as it is less used to ischemia. The graft is brought through the tunnel into the groin, and control is obtained of the femoral arteries. An arteriotomy is made running from the common femoral artery down to the appropriate level. In many cases, this would be down to a point on the deep femoral artery. If endarterectomy of the common and deep femoral arteries is necessary, it is undertaken at this point. The graft is fashioned to fit and sewn end to side using either running 4-0 or 5-0 permanent suture. Appropriate backbleeding and forward bleeding is allowed before that. The opposite is done in a similar manner. When flow is restored into the limbs, it is restored first to the common, then to the deep, and last to the superficial femoral artery.

In general, end-to-end anastomoses are performed. These may lessen the chance of aortoenteric fistula. They have better flow characteristics than end-to-side proximal anastomoses. If the patient has bilateral external iliac artery occlusions, either a proximal end-to-side aortic anastomosis or a formal reconstruction of one of the internal iliac arteries is necessary to ensure continued blood flood into the pelvis.

The retroperitoneum should be carefully closed in layers to exclude the graft from the gastrointestinal tract. If there is insufficient tissue, an omental flap should be created and placed over the graft to isolate it from the duodenum.

Axillofemoral Bypass Grafting

Axillobifemoral bypass grafting (Fig. 61-14) was introduced in the 1960s to provide inflow to patients who were poor physiologic candidates for aortic reconstruction. Its use has been extended to those patients having aortic graft infections or otherwise hostile abdomens for whom an in-line aortic reconstruction is considered too hazardous.

The patient is prepared from the shoulders down to the knees. It is our practice to extend the upper extremity on the side on which the graft is to be based 90 degrees. This will prevent the graft from being too taut when the patient moves the extremity. Reports of pseudoaneurysms and indeed ruptures secondary to short grafts have been published. A transverse incision is made in the deltopectoral groove. The axillary artery is exposed as medial as is possible. The more medial the anastomosis, the less excursion of the graft with use of the upper extremity. The pectoralis minor tendon may be incised to facilitate this exposure. If the tendon is not incised, the tunnel should be posterior to the tendon and then brought to the midaxillary line. In general, the right side is chosen if at all possible as the right subclavian artery is less prone to atherosclerotic disease than the left. Furthermore, if a later formal aortic reconstruction is planned, a right axillofemoral graft is much less a hindrance than one on the left, especially if a retroperitoneal approach is planned. Bilateral groin incisions are made. If the tunnel connecting the ipsilateral groin incision to the axillary incision can be created without a counterincision, this maneuver should be performed in that manner. If not, a counterincision can be made in the patient's flank. The counterincision seems to be prone to infection, and we try to avoid its use. Grafting is then done in the usual manner. The long portion of the graft should be at least 8 mm and preferably 10 or 12 mm in diameter to prevent a functional aortic stenosis. Mortality figures are higher for these patients than for patients having aortic reconstruction, ranging from 10% to 15%. This is because this is a population of much sicker patients. Five-year primary patencies vary greatly, but approximately 50% failure can be expected during the course of 5 years.

Femoral-Femoral Artery Bypass Grafting

Femoral arteries are exposed in the standard manner. Most surgeons now use a bucket-handle approach rather than trying to create a completely antegrade sigmoid-shaped reconstruction. This is done superior to the pubis at the subcutaneous level. Either polyester or expanded polytetrafluoroethylene can be used. Grafts of at least 7 or 8 mm are usually preferred. Patency of this has not been nearly as good as was first expected, ranging from 60% to 80% at 5 years. See Figure 61-15.

Iliofemoral Artery Bypass Grafting

In-line reconstruction of isolated external iliac artery lesions is preferable to femoral-femoral artery grafting if the patient's physiology and anatomy will allow. A flank incision is made and the retroperitoneal plane developed. The proximal anastomosis is performed to the common iliac artery or to the distal aorta as is necessary and then brought through that tunnel into the groin. Patency rates for this at 5 years are in the 90% range. See Figure 61-16.

Aortoiliac Endarterectomy

This operation is usually done through a midline incision. In contradistinction to exposure for aortic grafting, for endarterectomy, the aorta, the common iliac arteries, and the origins of the internal and external iliac arteries all need to be circumferentially exposed. In addition to the clamping of the aorta and the iliac arteries, it is also best to clamp the lumbar arteries with small clamps to prevent annoying backbleeding, which impedes accurate endarterectomy. The patient is heparinized. Control is obtained of the aorta and the iliac arteries. A vertical aortotomy is made. With use of an elevator, an endarterectomy of the aorta down to the origins of the common iliacs is performed. At this point, either transverse incisions, which is our preference, or vertical incisions may be made at the distal common iliac arteries. The endarterectomy plane is begun here. There may be a tongue of atherosclerosis extending into the origin of the external iliac and the internal iliac. These are elevated. A stripper, such as a Wylie stripper, is used. Classically, this is passed in a retrograde manner. It may be that in some patients with deep pelvises, passing in an antegrade manner is more advantageous. An appropriate-sized stripper is picked, and the endarterectomy of the iliac artery is completed. The atherosclerotic plaque from both the aorta and the iliac arteries may be brought out as a single specimen if retrograde iliac endarterectomy has been performed. The arterial incisions are closed primarily with fine permanent suture after appropriate flushing and ascertainment of good end points. When flow is restored, interestingly enough, the aorta remains essentially the same size and the common iliac arteries balloon up much like pantaloons. The retroperitoneum and abdomen are then closed in standard manner. See Figure 61-17.

Complications of Open Aortic Surgery

A number of complications may arise after operations to repair the aorta, whether for aneurysmal or occlusive disease.[101] These may be site-specific complications, such as wound infection or hematoma, also commonly seen with endograft approaches. Of more concern and major morbidity are the intra-abdominal and systemic complications. Cardiac ischemia is the most frequent complication of open aortic surgery, and in the very best of hands one can expect that 50% of deaths related to aortic reconstruction will be attributable to the heart. Only a minority of patients with occlusive disease have normal coronary arteries. Stress testing, cardiac angiography, and coronary intervention (catheter based or, more rarely, open) have reduced mortality for direct aortic operations. Some specialty centers with aggressive heart evaluation management schemes have reported mortality in the range of 1% to 2.5%.[95]

Renal insufficiency is a common complication and may result from embolization from clamping, prolonged ischemia with suprarenal clamping, intrinsic renal artery disease, hypovolemia, or hypoperfusion. It is exacerbated by paravisceral aortic repair and intraoperative complications. It most probably relates directly to the patient's preoperative renal and cardiac status. Accurate assessment of the patient's anatomy and a precise preoperative plan for clamping site and sequence are necessary to minimize the incidence of perioperative renal insufficiency.

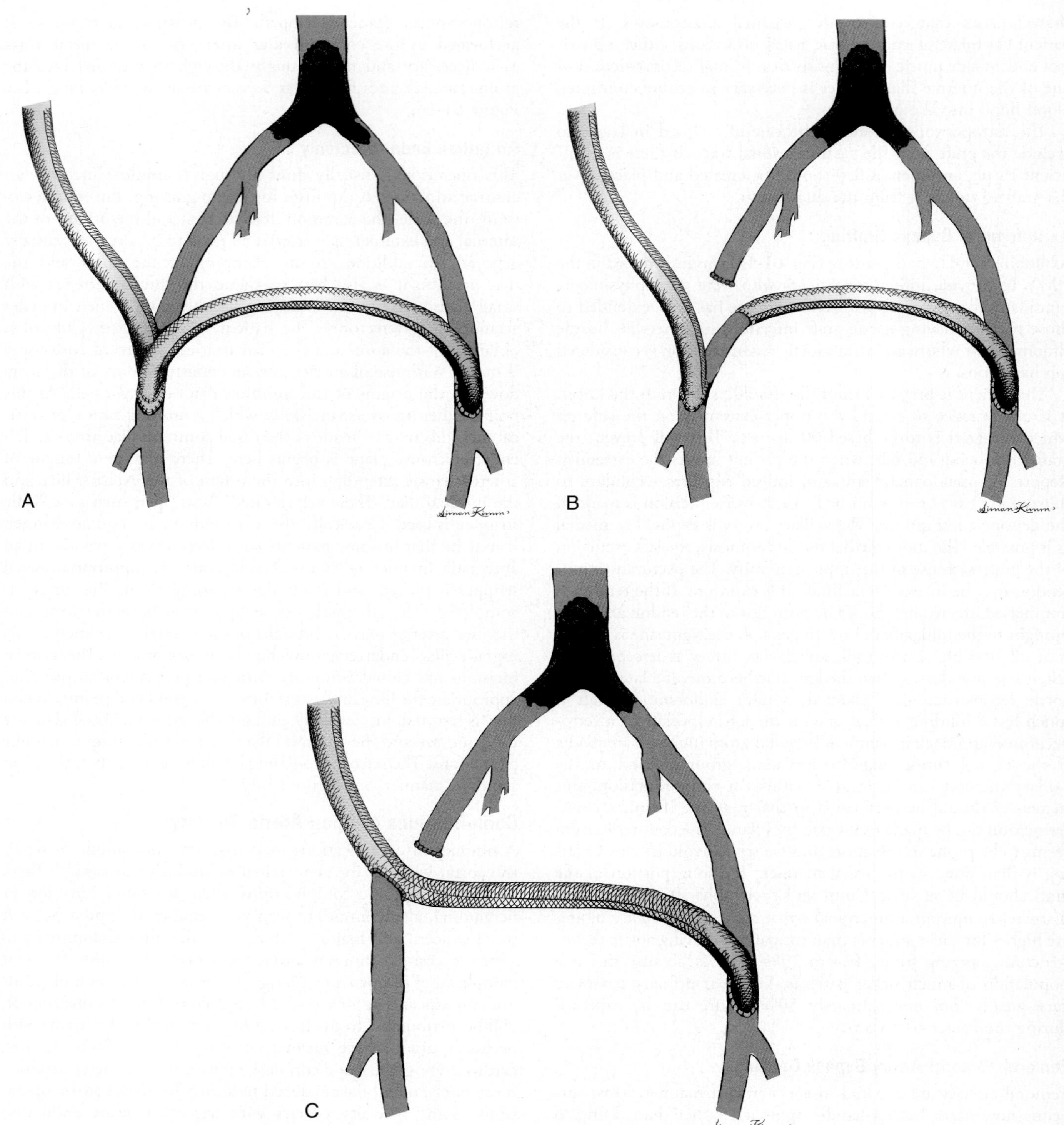

FIGURE 61-14 Three configurations of axillobifemoral bypass grafts. All three are shown with a right-sided axillofemoral graft component. **A,** The most common configuration. **B** and **C,** Modifications described by Blaisdell and associates **(B)** and Rutherford and Rainer **(C),** designed to prevent competitive inflow from a patent ipsilateral iliac system. (From Cronenwett J, Johnston KW, editors: *Rutherford's vascular surgery*, ed 7, Philadelphia, 2011, Elsevier.)

Pulmonary dysfunction is a frequent and serious complication. This, too, is more prevalent with proximal and paravisceral aortic procedures. Transverse abdominal incisions, epidural analgesia, and retroperitoneal approaches may mitigate pulmonary complications.

Abdominal wall hernia is a common late complication of open aneurysm repair, occurring at a much higher rate (10% to 33%) than after other open operations requiring midline laparotomy, suggesting that there are patient factors associated with the pathology of AAA that predispose this population to hernia. However,

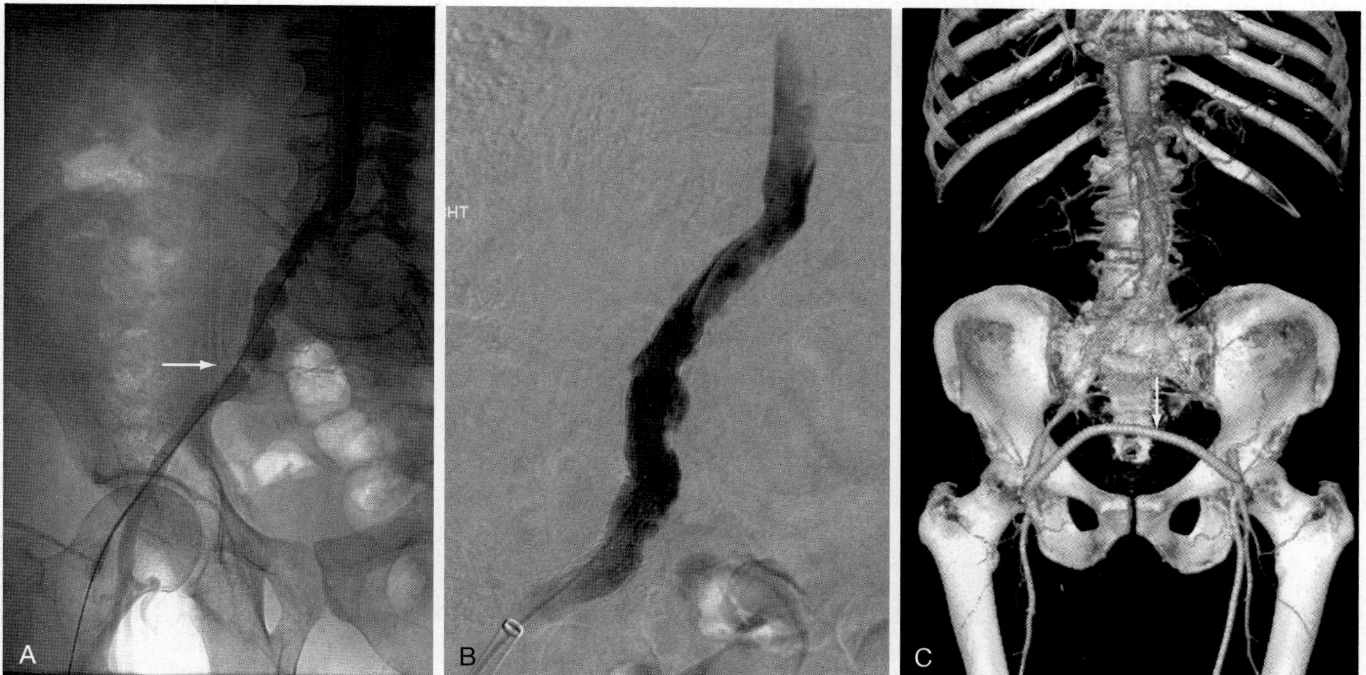

FIGURE 61-15 **A,** Preoperative angiogram demonstrating occlusion of the left iliac system in severe focal atherosclerotic disease of the right iliac artery *(arrow)*. **B,** Magnified view of the right iliac system after angioplasty and stent placement to establish adequate inflow for femoral-femoral bypass graft. **C,** Three-dimensional CT reconstruction demonstrating completed right to left femoral-femoral bypass graft *(arrow)*.

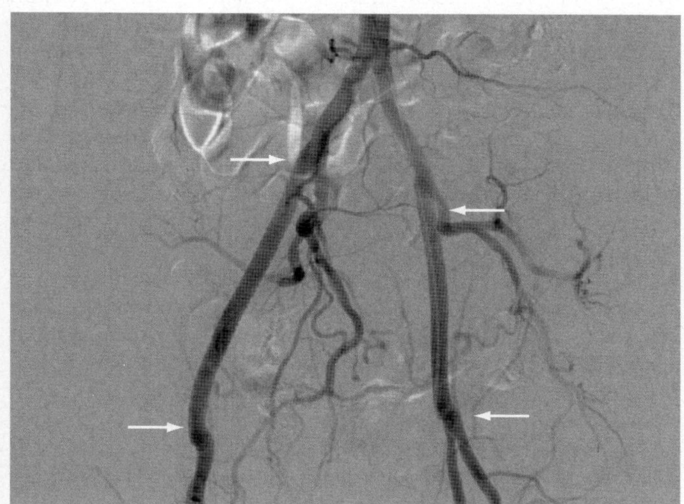

FIGURE 61-16 Arteriogram demonstrating iliofemoral bypasses extending from the bilateral common iliac to common femoral arteries *(arrows)*.

attention to fascial closure remains important to minimize this complication; a prospective study has demonstrated a relatively low 11.6% rate of midline hernia, with a suture length to wound length ratio of less than 4:1 predictive of hernia development. This study, contrary to earlier findings, did not note a statistically significant difference between the aneurysm and occlusive disease groups.[102] Retroperitoneal exposures crossing the flank are prone to subsequent abdominal wall laxity, which is not a true hernia but remains bothersome to patients.

Graft limb thrombosis occurs in 5% to 10% of patients and is associated with female gender, younger patients, and extra-anatomic bypass graft.[96,97]

An anastomotic pseudoaneurysm may be a sterile process or the result of infection. These pseudoaneurysms occur more frequently at the femoral anastomosis than at iliac and aortic anastomoses, which may reflect the higher rate of wound complications and graft infection in this region and the more clinically apparent nature of degeneration at the femoral site. Anastomotic pseudoaneurysms may result from degeneration of the suture line. True aneurysms tend to be para-anastomotic in nature, forming in the aorta proximal to or the iliac or femoral arteries distal to an aortic graft. True aneurysms occur more frequently in patients treated for aneurysmal than occlusive disease. Hypertension, COPD, smoking, hyperlipidemia, suture type, technical failures, and postoperative wound complications may be associated with this phenomenon.

Detection of anastomotic pseudoaneurysms in the iliac or aortic positions is highly reliant on imaging. Prospective studies using routine imaging of arterial grafts in a variety of anatomic positions have demonstrated higher rates of anastomotic pseudoaneurysm than those relying on clinical detection. Routine surveillance with ultrasound, for instance, demonstrated intra-abdominal anastomotic pseudoaneurysms in 10% of patients and 6.3% of aortic anastomoses after abdominal aortic graft placement at a mean interval of 12 years from operation.[54] CT and MRI provide excellent visualization of pseudoaneurysm and aneurysmal degeneration of the para-anastomotic area (Fig. 61-18).

Although some anastomotic pseudoaneurysms are sterile, it is prudent to begin evaluation and treatment with a presumption of infection. Diagnosis should include history (fever, chills, malaise, or weight loss), physical examination (erythema, fluctuant mass,

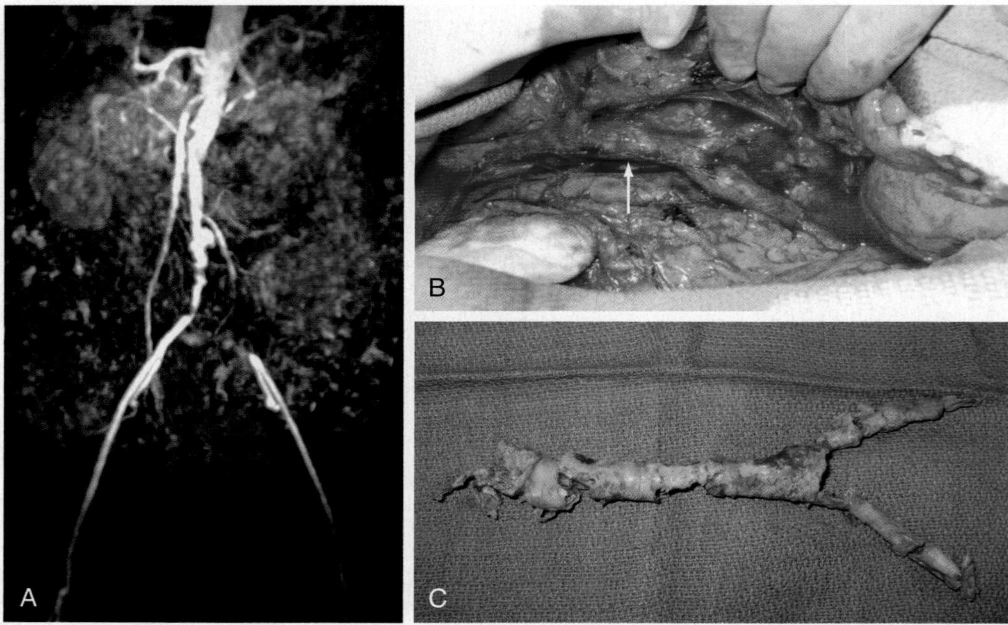

FIGURE 61-17 **A,** Preoperative MRA demonstrating severe atherosclerotic disease involving the infrarenal aorta and both common iliac arteries. **B,** Intraoperative photograph of completed aortoiliac endarterectomy showing suture line of primary closure *(arrow)*. **C,** Photograph of intact specimen demonstrating contiguous near-occlusive plaque.

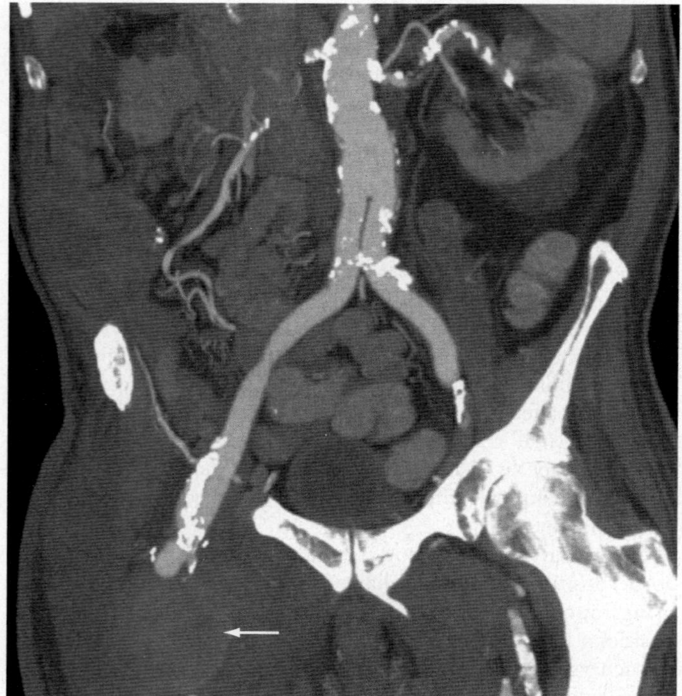

FIGURE 61-18 CT demonstrating large anastomotic pseudoaneurysm arising at the right femoral anastomosis of an aortofemoral graft.

induration, drainage, or tenderness to palpation), and laboratory evaluation (complete blood count, blood and fluid cultures, C-reactive protein level, or erythrocyte sedimentation rate). With regard to imaging, ultrasound may demonstrate the pseudoaneurysm itself as well as perigraft fluid suggestive of infection. CT and MRI may more completely characterize these findings (Fig. 61-19). The use of nuclear medicine modalities, such as indium In 111 or technetium Tc 99m tagged white blood cell scans, has greatly improved the surgeon's ability to evaluate for infection in a noninvasive manner (Fig. 61-20). Whereas positive cultures are definitive, many of the organisms common in graft infections are fastidious and may yield multiple negative cultures despite clear clinical evidence of infection. When diagnostic investigation yields evidence of infection, thorough débridement of infected material accompanied by in situ or extra-anatomic arterial reconstruction is the mainstay of management. Surgical management of anastomotic pseudoaneurysm is dictated by the presence or absence of infection, the nature of presentation, and the surgeon's experience and preference. In an uninfected field, débridement and interposition grafting may suffice. Whereas aneurysmal degeneration at or near the graft anastomoses historically necessitated open repair, a growing proportion are now successfully managed by endovascular techniques.[103] In any event, expeditious treatment is appropriate for a large, enlarging, or symptomatic lesion.

Surgical Treatment of Aortic Graft Infection

Infection should be managed by removal of the entire affected graft with débridement of all infected or devitalized tissue, traditionally accompanied by extra-anatomic reconstruction. Staging of this process by performing the extra-anatomic bypass and then either proceeding to débridement or permitting a recovery interval of up to several days greatly improved the historically substantial morbidity and mortality associated with primary graft resection followed by reconstruction.[104] Further investigation has suggested that in instances of infection limited to a single limb of the graft, satisfactory results may be achieved by limiting resection to the involved limb or limb segment, followed by in situ or extra-anatomic reconstruction and, according to the surgeon's

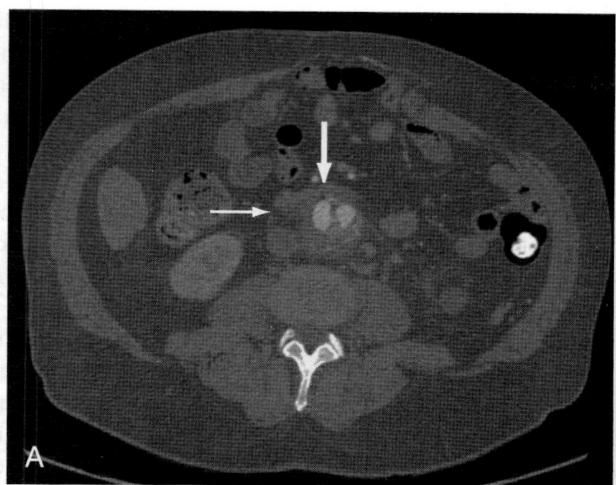

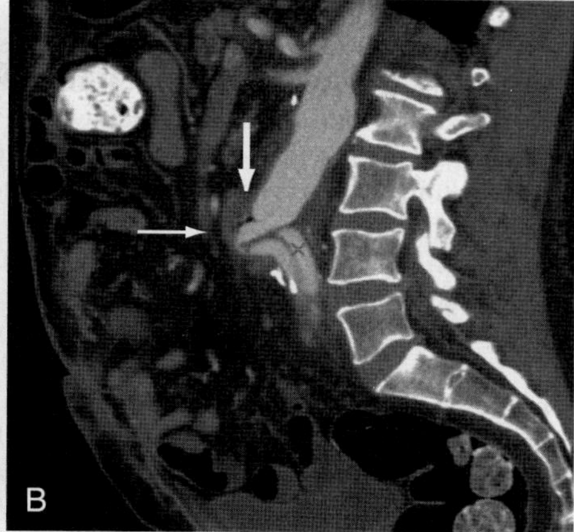

FIGURE 61-19 Axial **(A)** and sagittal **(B)** CT views of an infected aortofemoral graft after repair of an infrarenal aneurysm. Foci of gas *(thick arrows)* and extensive inflammation *(thin arrows)* are visible surrounding the graft. Of note, the tortuosity of the limbs of this graft represents a technical error.

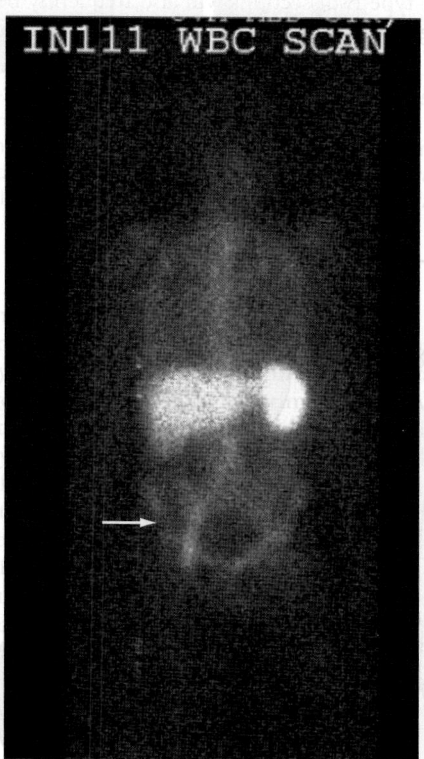

FIGURE 61-20 ^{111}In-tagged white blood cell scan image at 20 hours of delay demonstrates abnormal uptake in the region of the right limb of an aortofemoral graft *(arrow)*.

preference, combined with sterile antibiotic irrigation of the field through operatively placed drains.[105] However, recurrent graft infection, graft thrombosis, and the nearly invariably fatal complication of aortic stump infection or disruption continue to contribute to significant morbidity, mortality, and limb loss after this operation. Thorough débridement, layered closure, and vascularized pedicle flap coverage of the aortic stump are considered of paramount importance in avoiding the last complication.

In situ reconstruction may be accomplished by using rifampin-soaked or silver-coated polyester graft, cryopreserved arterial allograft, or saphenofemoral vein allograft.[106-109] The first of these is the most expeditious but yields a higher rate of reinfection as well as poor results in grossly purulent operative fields. Those espousing its use tend to embrace adjuncts such as wrapping the new graft and anastomoses in vascularized pedicle flaps, antibiotic irrigation therapy, or creation of clean retroperitoneal tunnels. The neoaortoiliac system venous autograft reconstruction described by Clagett is a lengthy procedure that places significant demands on both the patient and the operative team but yields the lowest reported rate of reinfection. Reported results using cryopreserved arterial allograft for in situ reconstruction have been mixed but generally reflect an intermediate rate of reinfection.[106] Endovascular treatment of anastomotic disruptions is generally limited to cases without evidence of infection and may use covered stent exclusion of the pseudoaneurysm or embolization of the pseudoaneurysm, generally with coils or occlusion devices. Aortoenteric fistula represents the most severe manifestation of aortic graft infection. It rarely occurs as a primary process, generally due to erosion of an untreated aneurysm into the duodenum. Most commonly, the lesion is at the point of contact of the third portion of the duodenum with the proximal graft anastomosis. Aortoenteric fistula has been reported in association with aortic stent graft placement. This complication generally is manifested with herald upper or lower gastrointestinal bleeding, which, if left untreated, may be followed by exsanguinating hemorrhage. Aortoenteric fistula should be suspected when gastrointestinal bleeding develops in a patient with a history of abdominal aortic surgery or endograft. Although endoscopy may confirm the diagnosis, demonstrating either an erosion or frank exposure of graft most frequently in the duodenum, CT is a more sensitive diagnostic study. The placement of synthetic or endovascular grafts in the setting of infected pseudoaneurysm, graft infection, primary aortic infection, or aortoenteric fistula is perhaps best viewed as a temporizing measure and is attended by high rates of re-intervention, morbidity, and mortality.[110] Repair of aortoenteric fistula or primary aortic infection follows many of the same principles as for infected graft removal: consideration of staged extra-anatomic bypass, appropriate selection of conduit if in situ reconstruction is elected, establishment of safe proximal control, wide débridement of infected material, coverage of in situ graft with a pedicle flap such as omentum, and appropriate use of antibiotic and antifungal therapy.

in European markets. Another potentially important development in this area is the application of fenestrated and branched graft techniques to address aneurysmal degeneration of the abdominal aorta and even the aortic arch.[122]

Procedural complications of endovascular stent graft therapy for dissection generally parallel those of TEVAR. There are, however, several complications largely specific to the treatment of dissection, including retrograde dissection (converting a type B into a type A dissection), creation or worsening of malperfusion, and continued false lumen filling with inability to induce thrombosis.

REFERENCES

1. Schermerhorn ML, Giles KA, Sachs T, et al: Defining perioperative mortality after open and endovascular aortic aneurysm repair in the US Medicare population. *J Am Coll Surg* 212:349–355, 2011.
2. Deaths: Final data for 2013. NCVR Volume 64, Number 2. CDC. <http://www.cdc.gov/nchs/data/nvsr/nvsr64/nvsr64_02.pdf>. Accessed September 23, 2015.
3. Wassef M, Upchurch GR, Jr, Kuivaniemi H, et al: Challenges and opportunities in abdominal aortic aneurysm research. *J Vasc Surg* 45:192–198, 2007.
4. Chaikof EL, Brewster DC, Dalman RL, et al: The care of patients with an abdominal aortic aneurysm: The Society for Vascular Surgery practice guidelines. *J Vasc Surg* 50:S2–S49, 2009.
5. Allardice JT, Allwright GJ, Wafula JM, et al: High prevalence of abdominal aortic aneurysm in men with peripheral vascular disease: Screening by ultrasonography. *Br J Surg* 75:240–242, 1988.
6. O'Kelly TJ, Heather BP: General practice-based population screening for abdominal aortic aneurysms: A pilot study. *Br J Surg* 76:479–480, 1989.
7. Bengtsson H, Norrgard O, Angquist KA, et al: Ultrasonographic screening of the abdominal aorta among siblings of patients with abdominal aortic aneurysms. *Br J Surg* 76: 589–591, 1989.
8. Shapira OM, Pasik S, Wassermann JP, et al: Ultrasound screening for abdominal aortic aneurysms in patients with atherosclerotic peripheral vascular disease. *J Cardiovasc Surg (Torino)* 31:170–172, 1990.
9. Webster MW, Ferrell RE, St Jean PL, et al: Ultrasound screening of first-degree relatives of patients with an abdominal aortic aneurysm. *J Vasc Surg* 13:9–13, discussion 13-14, 1991.
10. Bengtsson H, Sonesson B, Lanne T, et al: Prevalence of abdominal aortic aneurysm in the offspring of patients dying from aneurysm rupture. *Br J Surg* 79:1142–1143, 1992.
11. MacSweeney ST, O'Meara M, Alexander C, et al: High prevalence of unsuspected abdominal aortic aneurysm in patients with confirmed symptomatic peripheral or cerebral arterial disease. *Br J Surg* 80:582–584, 1993.
12. Lindholt JS, Juul S, Henneberg EW, et al: Is screening for abdominal aortic aneurysm acceptable to the population? Selection and recruitment to hospital-based mass screening for abdominal aortic aneurysm. *J Public Health Med* 20: 211–217, 1998.
13. Lederle FA, Johnson GR, Wilson SE, et al: Prevalence and associations of abdominal aortic aneurysm detected through screening. Aneurysm Detection and Management (ADAM) Veterans Affairs Cooperative Study Group. *Ann Intern Med* 126:441–449, 1997.
14. van der Graaf Y, Akkersdijk GJ, Hak E, et al: Results of aortic screening in the brothers of patients who had elective aortic aneurysm repair. *Br J Surg* 85:778–780, 1998.
15. Lawrence PF, Lorenzo-Rivero S, Lyon JL: The incidence of iliac, femoral, and popliteal artery aneurysms in hospitalized patients. *J Vasc Surg* 22:409–415, discussion 415-416, 1995.
16. Biebl M, Hakaim AG, Hugl B, et al: Endovascular aortic aneurysm repair with the Zenith AAA Endovascular Graft: Does gender affect procedural success, postoperative morbidity, or early survival? *Am Surg* 71:1001–1008, 2005.
17. Velazquez OC, Larson RA, Baum RA, et al: Gender-related differences in infrarenal aortic aneurysm morphologic features: Issues relevant to Ancure and Talent endografts. *J Vasc Surg* 33:S77–S84, 2001.
18. Brown LC, Powell JT, UK Small Aneurysm Trial Participants: Risk factors for aneurysm rupture in patients kept under ultrasound surveillance. *Ann Surg* 230:289–296, discussion 296-297, 1999.
19. Brown PM, Zelt DT, Sobolev B: The risk of rupture in untreated aneurysms: The impact of size, gender, and expansion rate. *J Vasc Surg* 37:280–284, 2003.
20. Cronenwett JL, Murphy TF, Zelenock GB, et al: Actuarial analysis of variables associated with rupture of small abdominal aortic aneurysms. *Surgery* 98:472–483, 1985.
21. Norman PE, Powell JT: Abdominal aortic aneurysm: The prognosis in women is worse than in men. *Circulation* 115:2865–2869, 2007.
22. Englesbe MJ, Wu AH, Clowes AW, et al: The prevalence and natural history of aortic aneurysms in heart and abdominal organ transplant patients. *J Vasc Surg* 37:27–31, 2003.
23. Sonesson B, Sandgren T, Lanne T: Abdominal aortic aneurysm wall mechanics and their relation to risk of rupture. *Eur J Vasc Endovasc Surg* 18:487–493, 1999.
24. Hall AJ, Busse EF, McCarville DJ, et al: Aortic wall tension as a predictive factor for abdominal aortic aneurysm rupture: Improving the selection of patients for abdominal aortic aneurysm repair. *Ann Vasc Surg* 14:152–157, 2000.
25. Fillinger MF, Marra SP, Raghavan ML, et al: Prediction of rupture risk in abdominal aortic aneurysm during observation: Wall stress versus diameter. *J Vasc Surg* 37:724–732, 2003.
26. Fillinger MF, Raghavan ML, Marra SP, et al: In vivo analysis of mechanical wall stress and abdominal aortic aneurysm rupture risk. *J Vasc Surg* 36:589–597, 2002.
27. Lederle FA: Risk of rupture of large abdominal aortic aneurysms. Disagreement among vascular surgeons. *Arch Intern Med* 156:1007–1009, 1996.
28. Parkinson F, Ferguson S, Lewis P, et al: Rupture rates of untreated large abdominal aortic aneurysms in patients unfit for elective repair. *J Vasc Surg* 61:1606–1612, 2015.
29. Darling RC, Messina CR, Brewster DC, et al: Autopsy study of unoperated abdominal aortic aneurysms. The case for early resection. *Circulation* 56:II161–II164, 1977.
30. Engellau L, Albrechtsson U, Dahlstrom N, et al: Measurements before endovascular repair of abdominal aortic aneurysms. MR imaging with MRA vs. angiography and CT. *Acta Radiol* 44:177–184, 2003.

31. U.S. Preventive Services Task Force: Abdominal aortic aneurysm: Screening. <http://www.uspreventiveservicestaskforce.org/uspstf/uspsaneu.htm>. Accessed August 2, 2011.
32. McCarthy RJ, Shaw E, Whyman MR, et al: Recommendations for screening intervals for small aortic aneurysms. *Br J Surg* 90:821–826, 2003.
33. Lederle FA: Abdominal aortic aneurysm: Still no pill. *Ann Intern Med* 159:852–853, 2013.
34. Meijer CA, Stijnen T, Wasser MN, et al: Doxycycline for stabilization of abdominal aortic aneurysms: A randomized trial. *Ann Intern Med* 159:815–823, 2013.
35. Baxter BT, Terrin MC, Dalman RL: Medical management of small abdominal aortic aneurysms. *Circulation* 117:1883–1889, 2008.
36. Sconfienza LM, Santagostino I, Di Leo G, et al: When the diameter of the abdominal aorta should be considered as abnormal? A new ultrasonographic index using the wrist circumference as a body build reference. *Eur J Radiol* 82:e532–e536, 2013.
37. Hannawa KK, Eliason JL, Upchurch GR, Jr: Gender differences in abdominal aortic aneurysms. *Vascular* 17(Suppl 1):S30–S39, 2009.
38. Suckow BD, Schanzer A, Hoel AW, et al: A novel quality of life instrument for patients with an abdominal aortic aneurysm. *J Vasc Surg* 61:43S–44S, 2015.
39. Fleisher LA, Beckman JA, Brown KA, et al: ACC/AHA 2007 guidelines on perioperative cardiovascular evaluation and care for noncardiac surgery: A report of the American College of Cardiology/American Heart Association Task Force on Practice Guidelines (Writing Committee to Revise the 2002 Guidelines on Perioperative Cardiovascular Evaluation for Noncardiac Surgery): Developed in collaboration with the American Society of Echocardiography, American Society of Nuclear Cardiology, Heart Rhythm Society, Society of Cardiovascular Anesthesiologists, Society for Cardiovascular Angiography and Interventions, Society for Vascular Medicine and Biology, and Society for Vascular Surgery. *Circulation* 116:e418–e499, 2007.
40. Shah TR, Veith FJ, Bauer SM: Cardiac evaluation and management before vascular surgery. *Curr Opin Cardiol* 29:499–505, 2014.
41. Fleischmann KE, Beckman JA, Buller CE, et al: 2009 ACCF/AHA focused update on perioperative beta blockade: A report of the American College of Cardiology Foundation/American Heart Association Task Force on Practice Guidelines. *Circulation* 120:2123–2151, 2009.
42. Schouten O, Hoeks SE, Welten GM, et al: Effect of statin withdrawal on frequency of cardiac events after vascular surgery. *Am J Cardiol* 100:316–320, 2007.
43. Corriere M, Edwards M, Hansen KJ: Abdominal aortic aneurysm and renal artery stenosis. *Vasc Dis Manage* 5:16–21, 2008.
44. Lee SM, Takemoto S, Wallace AW: Association between withholding angiotensin receptor blockers in the early postoperative period and 30-day mortality: A cohort study of the Veterans Affairs Healthcare System. *Anesthesiology* 123:288–306, 2015.
45. Hersey P, Poullis M: Does the administration of mannitol prevent renal failure in open abdominal aortic aneurysm surgery? *Interact Cardiovasc Thorac Surg* 7:906–909, 2008.
46. Wijnen MH, Vader HL, Van Den Wall Bake AW, et al: Can renal dysfunction after infra-renal aortic aneurysm repair be modified by multi-antioxidant supplementation? *J Cardiovasc Surg (Torino)* 43:483–488, 2002.
47. Upchurch GR, Jr, Proctor MC, Henke PK, et al: Predictors of severe morbidity and death after elective abdominal aortic aneurysmectomy in patients with chronic obstructive pulmonary disease. *J Vasc Surg* 37:594–599, 2003.
48. Myers K, Hajek P, Hinds C, et al: Stopping smoking shortly before surgery and postoperative complications: A systematic review and meta-analysis. *Arch Intern Med* 171:983–989, 2011.
49. Sicard GA, Toursarkissian B: Midline versus retroperitoneal approach for abdominal aortic aneurysm surgery. In Calligaro KD, Dougherty MJ, Hollier LH, editors: *Diagnosis and treatment of aortic and peripheral arterial aneurysms*, Philadelphia, 1999, WB Saunders, pp 135–148.
50. Berland TL, Veith FJ, Cayne NS, et al: Technique of supraceliac balloon control of the aorta during endovascular repair of ruptured abdominal aortic aneurysms. *J Vasc Surg* 57:272–275, 2013.
51. Stannard A, Eliason JL, Rasmussen TE: Resuscitative endovascular balloon occlusion of the aorta (REBOA) as an adjunct for hemorrhagic shock. *J Trauma* 71:1869–1872, 2011.
52. Nishimori M, Ballantyne JC, Low JH: Epidural pain relief versus systemic opioid-based pain relief for abdominal aortic surgery. *Cochrane Database Syst Rev* (3):CD005059, 2006.
53. Ylonen K, Biancari F, Leo E, et al: Predictors of development of anastomotic femoral pseudoaneurysms after aortobifemoral reconstruction for abdominal aortic aneurysm. *Am J Surg* 187:83–87, 2004.
54. Edwards JM, Teefey SA, Zierler RE, et al: Intraabdominal paraanastomotic aneurysms after aortic bypass grafting. *J Vasc Surg* 15:344–350, discussion 351-353, 1992.
55. Parodi JC, Palmaz JC, Barone HD: Transfemoral intraluminal graft implantation for abdominal aortic aneurysms. *Ann Vasc Surg* 5:491–499, 1991.
56. Wilt TJ, Lederle FA, Macdonald R, et al: Comparison of endovascular and open surgical repairs for abdominal aortic aneurysm. *Evid Rep Technol Assess (Full Rep)* 144:1–113, 2006.
57. Dimick JB, Upchurch GR, Jr: Endovascular technology, hospital volume, and mortality with abdominal aortic aneurysm surgery. *J Vasc Surg* 47:1150–1154, 2008.
58. Ali MM, Flahive J, Schanzer A, et al: In patients stratified by preoperative risk, endovascular repair of ruptured abdominal aortic aneurysms has a lower in-hospital mortality and morbidity than open repair. *J Vasc Surg* 61:1399–1407, 2015.
59. Chang DC, Parina RP, Wilson SE: Survival after endovascular vs open aortic aneurysm repairs. *JAMA Surg* 2015. [Epub ahead of print].
60. Heyer KS, Modi P, Morasch MD, et al: Secondary infections of thoracic and abdominal aortic endografts. *J Vasc Interv Radiol* 20:173–179, 2009.
61. Mehta M, Henretta J, Glickman M, et al: Outcome of the pivotal study of the Aptus endovascular abdominal aortic aneurysms repair system. *J Vasc Surg* 60:275–285, 2014.
62. Muller-Wille R, Schotz S, Zeman F, et al: CT features of early type II endoleaks after endovascular repair of abdominal aortic aneurysms help predict aneurysm sac enlargement. *Radiology* 274:906–916, 2015.

63. Zhou W, Blay E, Jr, Varu V, et al: Outcome and clinical significance of delayed endoleaks after endovascular aneurysm repair. *J Vasc Surg* 59:915–920, 2014.
64. Guntner O, Zeman F, Wohlgemuth WA, et al: Inferior mesenteric arterial type II endoleaks after endovascular repair of abdominal aortic aneurysm: Are they predictable? *Radiology* 270:910–919, 2014.
65. Alerci M, Giamboni A, Wyttenbach R, et al: Endovascular abdominal aneurysm repair and impact of systematic preoperative embolization of collateral arteries: Endoleak analysis and long-term follow-up. *J Endovasc Ther* 20:663–671, 2013.
66. Sidloff DA, Gokani V, Stather PW, et al: Type II endoleak: Conservative management is a safe strategy. *Eur J Vasc Endovasc Surg* 48:391–399, 2014.
67. Quinones-Baldrich W, Levin ES, Lew W, et al: Intraprocedural and postprocedural perigraft arterial sac embolization (PASE) for endoleak treatment. *J Vasc Surg* 59:538–541, 2014.
68. Schanzer A, Greenberg RK, Hevelone N, et al: Predictors of abdominal aortic aneurysm sac enlargement after endovascular repair. *Circulation* 123:2848–2855, 2011.
69. Greenhalgh RM, Brown LC, Powell JT, et al: Endovascular versus open repair of abdominal aortic aneurysm. *N Engl J Med* 362:1863–1871, 2010.
70. Gurtler VM, Sommer WH, Meimarakis G, et al: A comparison between contrast-enhanced ultrasound imaging and multislice computed tomography in detecting and classifying endoleaks in the follow-up after endovascular aneurysm repair. *J Vasc Surg* 58:340–345, 2013.
71. Nagre SB, Taylor SM, Passman MA, et al: Evaluating outcomes of endoleak discrepancies between computed tomography scan and ultrasound imaging after endovascular abdominal aneurysm repair. *Ann Vasc Surg* 25:94–100, 2011.
72. Kouchoukos NT, Masetti P, Murphy SF: Hypothermic cardiopulmonary bypass and circulatory arrest in the management of extensive thoracic and thoracoabdominal aortic aneurysms. *Semin Thorac Cardiovasc Surg* 15:333–339, 2003.
73. Hiratzka LF, Bakris GL, Beckman JA, et al: 2010 ACCF/AHA/AATS/ACR/ASA/SCA/SCAI/SIR/STS/SVM guidelines for the diagnosis and management of patients with Thoracic Aortic Disease: A report of the American College of Cardiology Foundation/American Heart Association Task Force on Practice Guidelines, American Association for Thoracic Surgery, American College of Radiology, American Stroke Association, Society of Cardiovascular Anesthesiologists, Society for Cardiovascular Angiography and Interventions, Society of Interventional Radiology, Society of Thoracic Surgeons, and Society for Vascular Medicine. *Circulation* 121:e266–e369, 2010.
74. Greenbaum AB, O'Neill WW, Paone G, et al: Caval-aortic access to allow transcatheter aortic valve replacement in otherwise ineligible patients: Initial human experience. *J Am Coll Cardiol* 63:2795–2804, 2014.
75. Vandy FC, Girotti M, Williams DM, et al: Iliofemoral complications associated with thoracic endovascular aortic repair: Frequency, risk factors, and early and late outcomes. *J Thorac Cardiovasc Surg* 147:960–965, 2014.
76. Gutsche JT, Cheung AT, McGarvey ML, et al: Risk factors for perioperative stroke after thoracic endovascular aortic repair. *Ann Thorac Surg* 84:1195–1200, discussion 1200, 2007.
77. Bavaria JE, Appoo JJ, Makaroun MS, et al: Endovascular stent grafting versus open surgical repair of descending thoracic aortic aneurysms in low-risk patients: A multicenter comparative trial. *J Thorac Cardiovasc Surg* 133:369–377, 2007.
78. Adams JD, Tracci MC, Sabri S, et al: Real-world experience with type I endoleaks after endovascular repair of the thoracic aorta. *Am Surg* 76:599–605, 2010.
79. DeSart K, Scali ST, Feezor RJ, et al: Fate of patients with spinal cord ischemia complicating thoracic endovascular aortic repair. *J Vasc Surg* 58:635–642.e2, 2013.
80. Czerny M, Eggebrecht H, Sodeck G, et al: Mechanisms of symptomatic spinal cord ischemia after TEVAR: Insights from the European Registry of Endovascular Aortic Repair Complications (EuREC). *J Endovasc Ther* 19:37–43, 2012.
81. Duwayri Y, Jim J, Sanchez L: Alternative techniques to abdominal debranching. *Vasc Dis Manage* 7:E210–E213, 2010.
82. Greenberg R, Eagleton M, Mastracci T: Branched endografts for thoracoabdominal aneurysms. *J Thorac Cardiovasc Surg* 140:S171–S178, 2010.
83. Donas KP, Lee JT, Lachat M, et al: Collected world experience about the performance of the snorkel/chimney endovascular technique in the treatment of complex aortic pathologies: The PERICLES registry. *Ann Surg* 262:546–553, 2015.
84. Fox N, Schwartz D, Salazar JH, et al: Evaluation and management of blunt traumatic aortic injury: A practice management guideline from the Eastern Association for the Surgery of Trauma. *J Trauma Acute Care Surg* 78:136–146, 2015.
85. Murad MH, Rizvi AZ, Malgor R, et al: Comparative effectiveness of the treatments for thoracic aortic transection [corrected]. *J Vasc Surg* 53:193–199.e1–21, 2011.
86. Dormandy JA, Rutherford RB: Management of peripheral arterial disease (PAD). TASC Working Group. TransAtlantic Inter-Society Consensus (TASC). *J Vasc Surg* 31:S1–S296, 2000.
87. Norgren L, Hiatt WR, Dormandy JA, et al: Inter-Society Consensus for the Management of Peripheral Arterial Disease (TASC II). *J Vasc Surg* 45(Suppl S):S5–S67, 2007.
88. Jongkind V, Akkersdijk GJ, Yeung KK, et al: A systematic review of endovascular treatment of extensive aortoiliac occlusive disease. *J Vasc Surg* 52:1376–1383, 2010.
89. Ichihashi S, Higashiura W, Itoh H, et al: Long-term outcomes for systematic primary stent placement in complex iliac artery occlusive disease classified according to Trans-Atlantic Inter-Society Consensus (TASC)-II. *J Vasc Surg* 53:992–999, 2011.
90. Ye W, Liu CW, Ricco JB, et al: Early and late outcomes of percutaneous treatment of TransAtlantic Inter-Society Consensus class C and D aorto-iliac lesions. *J Vasc Surg* 53:1728–1737, 2011.
91. Kashyap VS, Pavkov ML, Bena JF, et al: The management of severe aortoiliac occlusive disease: Endovascular therapy rivals open reconstruction. *J Vasc Surg* 48:1451–1457, 1457.e1-3, 2008.
92. Upchurch GR, Dimick JB, Wainess RM, et al: Diffusion of new technology in health care: The case of aorto-iliac occlusive disease. *Surgery* 136:812–818, 2004.

93. Chiu KW, Davies RS, Nightingale PG, et al: Review of direct anatomical open surgical management of atherosclerotic aorto-iliac occlusive disease. *Eur J Vasc Endovasc Surg* 39:460–471, 2010.
94. de Vries SO, Hunink MG: Results of aortic bifurcation grafts for aortoiliac occlusive disease: A meta-analysis. *J Vasc Surg* 26:558–569, 1997.
95. Hertzer NR, Bena JF, Karafa MT: A personal experience with direct reconstruction and extra-anatomic bypass for aortoiliofemoral occlusive disease. *J Vasc Surg* 45:527–535, discussion 535, 2007.
96. Ricco JB, Probst H: Long-term results of a multicenter randomized study on direct versus crossover bypass for unilateral iliac artery occlusive disease. *J Vasc Surg* 47:45–53, discussion 53-54, 2008.
97. Reed AB, Conte MS, Donaldson MC, et al: The impact of patient age and aortic size on the results of aortobifemoral bypass grafting. *J Vasc Surg* 37:1219–1225, 2003.
98. Klonaris C, Katsargyris A, Tsekouras N, et al: Primary stenting for aortic lesions: From single stenoses to total aortoiliac occlusions. *J Vasc Surg* 47:310–317, 2008.
99. Indes JE, Mandawat A, Tuggle CT, et al: Endovascular procedures for aorto-iliac occlusive disease are associated with superior short-term clinical and economic outcomes compared with open surgery in the inpatient population. *J Vasc Surg* 52:1173–1179, 1179.e1, 2010.
100. Cau J, Ricco JB, Corpataux JM: Laparoscopic aortic surgery: Techniques and results. *J Vasc Surg* 48:37S–44S, discussion 45S, 2008.
101. Cherry KJ: Complications following reconstructions of the pararenal aorta and its branches. In Towne JB, Hollier LH, editors: *Complications in vascular surgery*, ed 2, New York, 2004, Marcel Dekker, pp 275–287.
102. Gruppo M, Mazzalai F, Lorenzetti R, et al: Midline abdominal wall incisional hernia after aortic reconstructive surgery: A prospective study. *Surgery* 151:882–888, 2012.
103. Sachdev U, Baril DT, Morrissey NJ, et al: Endovascular repair of para-anastomotic aortic aneurysms. *J Vasc Surg* 46: 636–641, 2007.
104. Reilly LM, Stoney RJ, Goldstone J, et al: Improved management of aortic graft infection: The influence of operation sequence and staging. *J Vasc Surg* 5:421–431, 1987.
105. Oderich GS, Bower TC, Cherry KJ, Jr, et al: Evolution from axillofemoral to in situ prosthetic reconstruction for the treatment of aortic graft infections at a single center. *J Vasc Surg* 43:1166–1174, 2006.
106. Brown KE, Heyer K, Rodriguez H, et al: Arterial reconstruction with cryopreserved human allografts in the setting of infection: A single-center experience with midterm follow-up. *J Vasc Surg* 49:660–666, 2009.
107. Noel AA, Gloviczki P, Cherry KJ, Jr, et al: Abdominal aortic reconstruction in infected fields: Early results of the United States cryopreserved aortic allograft registry. *J Vasc Surg* 35: 847–852, 2002.
108. Batt M, Magne JL, Alric P, et al: In situ revascularization with silver-coated polyester grafts to treat aortic infection: Early and midterm results. *J Vasc Surg* 38:983–989, 2003.
109. Clagett GP, Bowers BL, Lopez-Viego MA, et al: Creation of a neo-aortoiliac system from lower extremity deep and superficial veins. *Ann Surg* 218:239–248, discussion 248–249, 1993.
110. Lonn L, Dias N, Veith Schroeder T, et al: Is EVAR the treatment of choice for aortoenteric fistula? *J Cardiovasc Surg (Torino)* 51:319–327, 2010.
111. Cherry KJ, Dake MD: Aortic dissection. In Hallett JW, Mills JL, Earnshaw JJ, et al, editors: *Comprehensive vascular and endovascular surgery*, ed 2, Philadelphia, 2009, Mosby, pp 517–531.
112. Swee W, Dake MD: Endovascular management of thoracic dissections. *Circulation* 117:1460–1473, 2008.
113. Estrera AL, Miller CC, 3rd, Safi HJ, et al: Outcomes of medical management of acute type B aortic dissection. *Circulation* 114:I384–I389, 2006.
114. Panneton JM, Teh SH, Cherry KJ, Jr, et al: Aortic fenestration for acute or chronic aortic dissection: An uncommon but effective procedure. *J Vasc Surg* 32:711–721, 2000.
115. Trimarchi S, Nienaber CA, Rampoldi V, et al: Role and results of surgery in acute type B aortic dissection: Insights from the International Registry of Acute Aortic Dissection (IRAD). *Circulation* 114:I357–I364, 2006.
116. Tian DH, De Silva RP, Wang T, et al: Open surgical repair for chronic type B aortic dissection: A systematic review. *Ann Cardiothorac Surg* 3:340–350, 2014.
117. Kouchoukos NT, Kulik A, Castner CF: Open thoracoabdominal aortic repair for chronic type B dissection. *J Thorac Cardiovasc Surg* 149:S125–S129, 2015.
118. Dake MD, Kato N, Mitchell RS, et al: Endovascular stent-graft placement for the treatment of acute aortic dissection. *N Engl J Med* 340:1546–1552, 1999.
119. Durham CA, Cambria RP, Wang LJ, et al: The natural history of medically managed acute type B aortic dissection. *J Vasc Surg* 61:1192–1198, 2015.
120. Nienaber CA, Kische S, Rousseau H, et al: Endovascular repair of type B aortic dissection: Long-term results of the randomized investigation of stent grafts in aortic dissection trial. *Circ Cardiovasc Interv* 6:407–416, 2013.
121. Hofferberth SC, Newcomb AE, Yii MY, et al: Combined proximal stent grafting plus distal bare metal stenting for management of aortic dissection: Superior to standard endovascular repair? *J Thorac Cardiovasc Surg* 144:956–962, discussion 962, 2012.
122. Kitagawa A, Greenberg RK, Eagleton MJ, et al: Fenestrated and branched endovascular aortic repair for chronic type B aortic dissection with thoracoabdominal aneurysms. *J Vasc Surg* 58:625–634, 2013.

62 CHAPTER

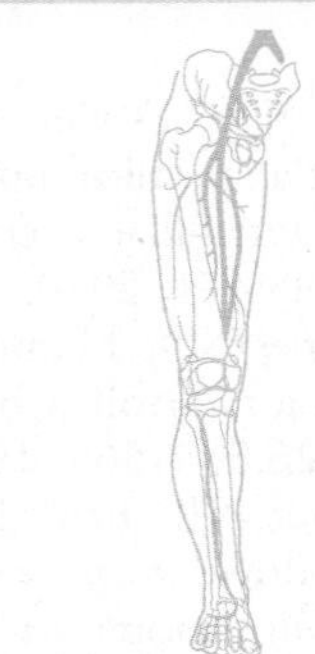

Peripheral Arterial Disease

Charlie C. Cheng, Faisal Cheema, Grant Fankhauser, Michael B. Silva, Jr.

OUTLINE

The specialty of vascular surgery has matured dramatically during the past decade. With the advent of new devices and techniques and the expansion of catheter and guidewire skills, the management of almost all vascular pathologic processes has been undergoing a process of reevaluation. Surgeons have traditionally been called on to make diagnoses and to manage patients with emergent, urgent, and elective vascular surgical conditions. Although other medical disciplines are participating in this process to a greater degree, the surgeon with advanced open skills and complete facility with endovascular techniques is ideally suited to manage these patients. As our population ages and the prevalence of vascular disease increases, along with the growing awareness of potential therapeutic benefits by an educated populace, it is incumbent on the vascular specialist to be facile with a widening set of tools and techniques—medical, surgical, and endovascular—to meet the needs of our patients.

This chapter covers epidemiology, basic science, diagnostic workup, and medical treatment of peripheral vascular disease. Treatments of acute and chronic limb ischemia, open and endovascular, are discussed. Management of the diabetic foot, with an emphasis on amputations, is included. Less common causes of limb ischemia are presented for completion. The rapidly changing treatment paradigm of carotid stenosis is discussed, as is that of renovascular hypertension. Management of peripheral and splanchnic aneurysms is reviewed. Finally, arteriovenous access for the patient with end-stage renal disease is presented in detail because this remains an important component of contemporary general and vascular surgical practice.

EPIDEMIOLOGY

Peripheral artery occlusive disease, commonly referred to as peripheral arterial disease (PAD) or peripheral vascular disease (PVD), refers to the obstruction or deterioration of arteries other than those supplying the heart and within the brain. There are a number of pathologic processes that manifest their effects on the arterial circulation.

The common denominator among these processes is the impairment of circulation and resultant ischemia to the end organ involved. Highly prevalent in our society, arterial occlusive disease, in its myriad iterations, constitutes the leading overall cause of death. In addition to death from myocardial infarction or stroke, significant disability and loss of function from PAD result in an enormous cost in impaired quality of life for our aging population and a direct financial cost to our health care system.

The incidence of symptomatic PAD increases with age, from approximately 0.3%/yr for men aged 40 to 55 years to approximately 1%/yr for men older than 75 years. In the United States, PAD affects 12% to 20% of Americans aged 65 years and older.

PAD is more prevalent in nonwhite populations, and this is not completely explained by an increased incidence of comorbid diseases.[1] An ankle-brachial index (ABI) less than 0.90 is almost twice as common in non-Hispanic blacks as in whites. Risk is increased in smokers and in patients with hypertension, dyslipidemia, hypercoagulable states, renal insufficiency, and diabetes mellitus (Fig. 62-1). The prevalence of PAD is strikingly higher in a younger diabetic population, affecting one in three diabetics older than 50 years. Diagnosis is critical because people with PAD have a risk of heart attack or stroke four to five times higher than that of the age-matched population (Fig. 62-2). The risk of PAD also increases in individuals who are older than 50 years, male, or obese and in those with a family history of vascular disease, heart attack, or stroke. Other risk factors that are being studied include levels of various inflammatory mediators, such as C-reactive protein and homocysteine.

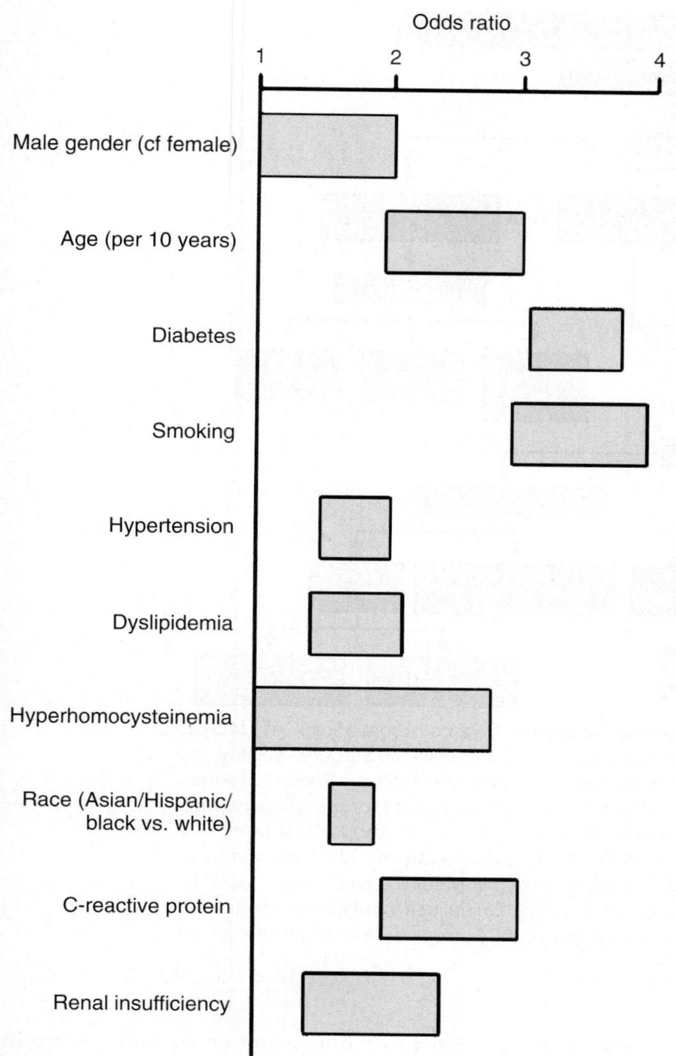

FIGURE 62-1 Risk factors for symptomatic peripheral arterial disease.

BASIC SCIENCE OF VASCULAR DISEASE

Vascular Wall Microanatomy

The arterial wall consists of three concentric layers:

1. The innermost layer is the intima. This is structurally a tube of endothelial cells in which the long axis of each cell is oriented longitudinally. The cells are aligned in a single layer and interface with the blood, providing metabolic reactivity and signaling by transport of mediators through their internal cellular architecture. The intima is separated from the media by the internal elastic membrane.
2. The media is the major structural support for the artery. It is composed predominantly of circumferentially arranged smooth muscle cells, collagen, elastin, and proteoglycans. Proteoglycans are formed of disaccharides bound to protein; they serve as binding or cement material in the interstitial spaces. The blood supply for the inner part of the media is by direct diffusion through the intima, whereas the outer part is supplied by smaller penetrating arteries, known as vasa vasorum. The media is separated from the outermost layer, the adventitia, by the external elastic membrane.
3. The adventitia contains fibroblasts, collagen, and elastic tissue and is the strength layer of the artery.

Atherosclerosis

Atherosclerosis is the most common pathologic change associated with PAD. A number of terms are used to describe this process that are similar and yet distinct in spelling and meaning and are often confused. The principal root, *athera*, is from the Greek word meaning gruel; an atheroma can be translated literally as a lump of gruel. Atherosclerosis is a hardening of an artery specifically caused by an atheromatous plaque. The term *atherogenic* is used for substances or processes that cause atherosclerosis. *Arteriosclerosis* is a general term describing any hardening (and loss of elasticity) of medium or large arteries (from the Greek *arteria*, meaning artery, and *sclerosis*, meaning hardening); arteriolosclerosis is any hardening (and loss of elasticity) of arterioles (small arteries).

A number of causative factors have been identified for atherosclerosis. Hyperlipidemia, hypercholesterolemia, hypertension, diabetes mellitus, and exposure to infectious agents or toxins, such as from cigarette smoking, are all important and independent risk factors. The common mechanism is thought to be endothelial cell injury, smooth muscle cell proliferation, inflammatory reactivity, and plaque deposition.

Several components are found in atherosclerotic plaque—lipids, smooth muscle cells, connective tissue, and inflammatory cells, often macrophages. Lipid accumulation is central to the process and distinguishes atheromas from other arteriopathies. In advanced plaques, calcification is seen and erosive areas or ulcerations can occur, exposing the contents of the plaque to circulating prothrombotic cells. There is an important correlation between plaque morphology and clinical sequelae. The plaque's lipid core may become a necrotic mix of amorphous extracellular lipid, proteins, and prothrombotic factors covered by a layer of smooth muscle cells and connective tissue of variable thickness, the fibrous cap. If the thin fibrous cap ruptures and the contents of the lipid core are exposed to circulating humoral factors, the body, perceiving the ulceration as an injury, may lay down platelets and initiate clot formation. In this manner, a relatively low grade, hemodynamically insignificant narrowing can precipitate an acute thrombosis and result in a dramatically significant ischemic event, such as a myocardial infarction.

Plaque morphology can be evaluated by ultrasound and magnetic resonance imaging (MRI). The heterogeneous plaque with a thin fibrous cap or ulceration, often described as unstable or vulnerable, is more likely to be virulent in nature, with an increased risk for embolization of particulate and thrombotic material. Ischemia, therefore, can result from a number of possible plaque behaviors, such as encroachment on the lumen (stenosis or narrowing) with hypoperfusion, stagnation, and thrombosis; rupture of the fibrous cap inducing thrombus formation in the lumen, with outright occlusion; and embolization of thrombotic debris into the downstream circulation.

Although atherosclerosis is a systemic disorder, there is an interestingly predictable pattern of distribution of atheromatous plaques throughout the arterial tree that is likely a result of consistent hemodynamic stresses associated with human anatomic design. Plaques tend to occur at bifurcations or bends associated with repetitive external stresses. Areas at which shear stress increases from disturbances in flow or turbulence, with lateralizing vectors and eddy formation, are prone to atheromatous degeneration. The infrarenal abdominal aorta, iliac bifurcations, carotid bifurcations, superficial femoral arteries as they exit at Hunter

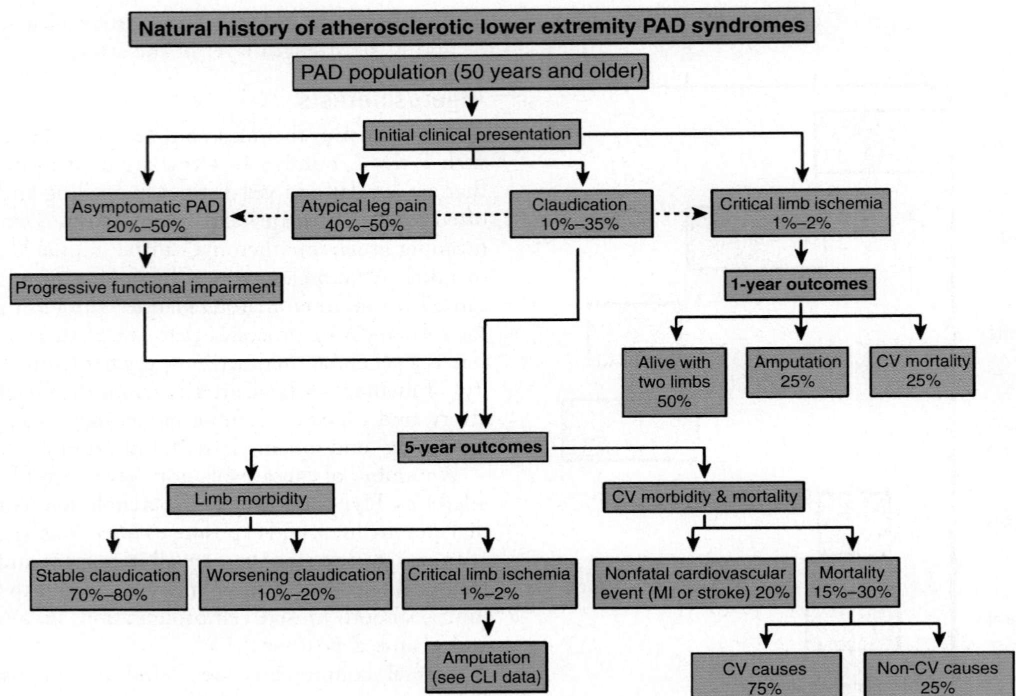

FIGURE 62-2 Outcomes of atherosclerotic peripheral arterial disease at 5 years. (From Hirsch AT, Haskal ZJ, Hertzer NR, et al; American Association for Vascular Surgery/Society for Vascular Surgery; Society for Cardiovascular Angiography and Interventions; Society for Vascular Medicine and Biology; Society of Interventional Radiology; ACC/AHA Task Force on Practice Guidelines: ACC/AHA Guidelines for the Management of Patients with Peripheral Arterial Disease [lower extremity, renal, mesenteric, and abdominal aortic]: A collaborative report from the American Associations for Vascular Surgery/Society for Vascular Surgery, Society for Cardiovascular Angiography and Interventions, Society for Vascular Medicine and Biology, Society of Interventional Radiology, and the ACC/AHA Task Force on Practice Guidelines [writing committee to develop guidelines for the management of patients with peripheral arterial disease]—summary of recommendations. *J Vasc Interv Radiol* 17:1383–1397, 2006.)

canal, and ostia of the coronary, renal, and mesenteric arteries are all common sites of plaque formation. Conversely, the upper extremity arteries and common carotid, renal, and mesenteric arteries, beyond their origins, are often much less involved.

EVALUATING AND TREATING THE PATIENT WITH PERIPHERAL ARTERIAL DISEASE

Patients are typically referred to the vascular specialist for clarification of a diagnosis and determination of a strategy for treatment. The process involves clinical assessment, establishing the particulars of the patient's medical history and performing a physical examination; diagnostic studies to clarify and to localize the problem and potentially to elucidate the functional severity of the condition; and ultimately balancing the severity of the patient's condition with the potential risks and benefits of therapeutic intervention.

History and Physical Examination

Rapidly advancing technology in imaging and endovascular therapies epitomize the cutting edge, the "high-tech" side of vascular surgery, but the foundation of this field is profoundly "low-tech." The history and physical examination process can often identify the location and relative severity of the patient's vascular disease accurately.

The most common presenting symptom in lower extremity vascular disease is pain. Characterizing the pain—location; precipitating, aggravating, and relieving factors; and frequency, duration, and evolution—can allow one to diagnose or to exclude most arterial and venous diseases with a high degree of sensitivity, even before examining the patient. Clarifying the nature of the pain as a starting point allows one to segregate patients into two broad categories of presentation for PAD, chronic arterial insufficiency and acute arterial occlusion.

Chronic Arterial Insufficiency

The clinical presentation ranges from asymptomatic to gangrenous tissue loss. Intermittent claudication is a common presentation in the outpatient setting and usually signifies mild to moderate vascular occlusive disease. Classically, pain occurs with activity or ambulation and is relieved with rest. Because of the frequency of superficial femoral arterial disease, the usual location of the pain is in the calf, but claudication may also involve the thighs or the buttocks because the arterial disease may be located in the aortoiliac segment. The arterial disease is usually one level above the symptomatic muscle group. The differential diagnosis of leg pain is broad, and the treatment modalities are equally disparate. Table 62-1 outlines an approach to the differential diagnosis of claudication.

Patients who are limited in ambulation because of arthritis, severe lung disease, or heart failure or who are diabetic with

TABLE 62-1 Differential Diagnosis of Intermittent Claudication

CONDITION	LOCATION OF PAIN OR DISCOMFORT	CHARACTERISTIC DISCOMFORT	ONSET RELATIVE TO EXERCISE	EFFECT OF REST	EFFECT OF BODY POSITION	OTHER CHARACTERISTICS
Intermittent claudication	Buttock, thigh, or calf muscles and rarely the foot	Cramping, aching, fatigue, weakness, or frank pain	After some degree of exercise	Quickly relieved	None	Reproducible
Nerve root compression (e.g., herniated disc)	Radiates down leg, usually posteriorly	Sharp lancinating pain	Soon, if not immediately after onset	Not quickly relieved (also often present at rest)	Relief may be aided by adjusting back position	History of back problems
Spinal stenosis	Hip, thigh, buttocks (follows dermatome)	Motor weakness more prominent than pain	After walking or standing for variable lengths of time	Relieved by stopping only if position changed	Relief by lumbar spine flexion (sitting or stooping forward)	Frequent history of back problems, provoked by intra-abdominal pressure
Arthritic, inflammatory process	Foot, arch	Aching pain	After variable degree of exercise	Not quickly relieved (and may be present at rest)	May be relieved by not bearing weight	Variable, may relate to activity level
Hip arthritis	Hip, thigh, buttocks	Aching discomfort, usually localized to hip and gluteal region	After variable degree of exercise	Not quickly relieved (and may be present at rest)	More comfortable sitting, weight taken off legs	Variable, may relate to activity level, weather changes
Symptomatic Baker cyst	Behind knee, down calf	Swelling, soreness, tenderness	With exercise	Present at rest	None	Not intermittent
Venous claudication	Entire leg, but usually worse in thigh and groin	Tight, bursting pain	After walking	Subsides slowly	Relief speeded by elevation	History of iliofemoral deep venous thrombosis, signs of venous congestion, edema
Chronic compartment syndrome	Calf muscles	Tight, bursting pain	After much exercise (e.g., jogging)	Subsides very slowly	Relief speeded by elevation	Typically occurs in heavily muscled athletes

Adapted from Dormandy JA, Rutherford RB: Management of peripheral arterial disease (PAD). TASC Working Group. TransAtlantic Inter-Society Consensus (TASC). *J Vasc Surg* 31:S1–S296, 2000.

neuropathy may not experience leg pain and may present initially with advanced disease. Worsening perfusion leads to critical limb ischemia, which may be manifested by rest pain. This is described as pain that occurs at rest; it may wake the patient from sleep. This is usually in the dorsum of the foot and is relieved with dangling the leg over the edge of the bed. The patient may also have tissue loss with ulcerations or nonhealing wounds of the foot (Table 62-2).

Initial evaluation must include a detailed medical history of comorbid conditions. In addition to coronary artery disease, carotid artery stenosis, and prior stroke, risk factors for atherosclerosis (e.g., diabetes, hypertension, dyslipidemia, tobacco abuse, hyperhomocysteinemia) should be queried and their level of optimization understood. Because medical management is a cornerstone of vascular therapy, a review of the patient's medications is imperative, with attention to the potential need for antiplatelet agents, beta blockers, angiotensin-converting enzyme inhibitors, and statins as a matter of course. Previous exposure to heparin, protamine, and NPH insulin should be noted. Allergies to contrast agents or iodine should be documented.

The surgical history and physical examination include details of surgical incisions as indicative of prior surgical intervention. Many patients will have undergone coronary artery bypass grafting; the presence of a left internal mammary–left anterior descending coronary graft and previous great saphenous vein harvest can change the surgical plan for peripheral revascularization. Frequent or recent coronary catheterization (or peripheral angiography) can suggest challenging groin access with significant scar tissue. Procedure reports should be reviewed for details of

TABLE 62-2 Clinical Classification of Peripheral Arterial Disease: Fontaine and Rutherford Systems

FONTAINE CLASSIFICATION		RUTHERFORD CLASSIFICATION	
STAGE	CLINICAL	GRADE	CLINICAL
I	Asymptomatic	0	Asymptomatic
IIa	Mild claudication	1	Mild claudication
IIb	Moderate to severe claudication	2	Moderate claudication
		3	Severe claudication
III	Ischemic rest pain	4	Ischemic rest pain
IV	Ulceration or gangrene	5	Minor tissue loss
		6	Major tissue loss

access closure or incidental findings of peripheral artery stenoses. Previous surgery, whether neck, abdominal, spine, joint, or vascular operations, can affect decision making, and efforts to gain the details of these are important. A family history of a first-degree relative with abdominal aortic aneurysm, stroke, or early myocardial infarction should be sought.

A vascular review of symptoms documents the presence or absence of transient ischemic attack (TIA) or stroke, such as unilateral weakness or sensory deficit, difficulty with speech or swallowing, word-finding difficulties or memory changes, dizziness, drop attacks, blurry vision, arm fatigue, weight loss or pain after eating, renal insufficiency or poorly controlled hypertension, impotence, claudication, rest pain, or tissue loss. As for all patients, a detailed understanding of the patient's functional status helps delineate goals of therapy and perioperative risk. Patients who are limited in their activities of daily living by their vascular disease or other comorbidities cannot provide an accurate picture of their cardiac function and will likely require further cardiac workup. History of tobacco abuse as well as all clinical efforts for encouraging smoking cessation must be documented.

The physical examination begins with vital signs, which often reveal hypertension and tachycardia. Blood pressure in both arms should be documented. The presence or absence of carotid bruits, cardiac murmurs, abdominal bruits, flank bruits, or groin bruits should be noted. The abdomen should be palpated for the aortic pulsation. Incision scars should be noted. Bilateral carotid, radial, ulnar, femoral, popliteal, dorsalis pedis, and posterior tibial pulses should be palpated and characterized. If pulses are not palpable, a continuous-wave Doppler examination can be used to check for signals. Common physical findings of PAD include hair loss and dry, shiny skin with nail hypertrophy. In critical limb ischemia, the classic findings of dependent rubor and pallor with elevation of the limb can be observed. In cases of severe rest pain, patients may have peripheral edema because they are unable to take their legs from the dependent position without pain. The feet should be meticulously inspected for wounds and signs of skin breakdown. A neurologic examination documenting equivalent strength and sensation in the limbs and cranial nerves should be performed.

Routine laboratory work should include a complete blood count, chemistry (to evaluate renal function and glucose concentration), and a lipid panel. An albumin level can be helpful in delineating the adequacy of a patient's nutritional status, if this is in question. The hemoglobin A1c level indicates the patient's level of glycemic control during the previous 120 days.

A baseline electrocardiogram should be obtained. Any previous cardiac testing, including echocardiography, stress echocardiography, dobutamine-adenosine sestamibi scan, and coronary catheterization, should be reviewed and documented.

Physiologic Testing and Imaging

The vascular laboratory is a powerful tool in the armamentarium of the surgeon. Noninvasive testing confirms and localizes disease, provides end points to demonstrate improvement after intervention, enables long-term follow-up of bypass grafts and percutaneous interventions, and can detect silent disease recurrence. Tests commonly performed in the laboratory include the ABI with multisegmental pressures and waveforms, toe-brachial index, pulse volume recording, photoplethysmography, and arterial duplex examination. The vascular laboratory represents one of the last arenas in which a nonimaging indirect measure of physiology is still widely used as a diagnostic tool.

Regardless of plans for intervention, it is recommended that asymptomatic patients at risk for PAD and those with symptoms undergo ABI testing. This examination can be performed simply with a manual blood pressure cuff at the ankle and a continuous-wave Doppler probe. With the patient in a supine position, after several minutes of rest to allow limb pressure to return to baseline, the cuff is inflated at the ankle, with the Doppler probe held at the location of the distal dorsalis pedis or posterior tibial signal. The systolic pressure is recorded as the pressure in the cuff when the Doppler signal returns. This process can be performed with multiple cuffs, allowing segmental pressure determination (Fig. 62-3), which is helpful in localizing the level of the obstructing lesion. The ABI for a limb is calculated using the higher of the two ankle pressures divided by the higher of the two brachial pressures (Tables 62-3 and 62-4). Patients with an ABI of 0.90 or less have a threefold to sixfold increased risk of cardiovascular mortality.

Continuous-wave Doppler analog waveforms can be obtained along with the segmental pressures. Photoplethysmography uses an infrared light–emitting source and a photosensor; it is based on the principle that red light is decreased with increased blood flow in tissues to generate a pressure and waveform within the

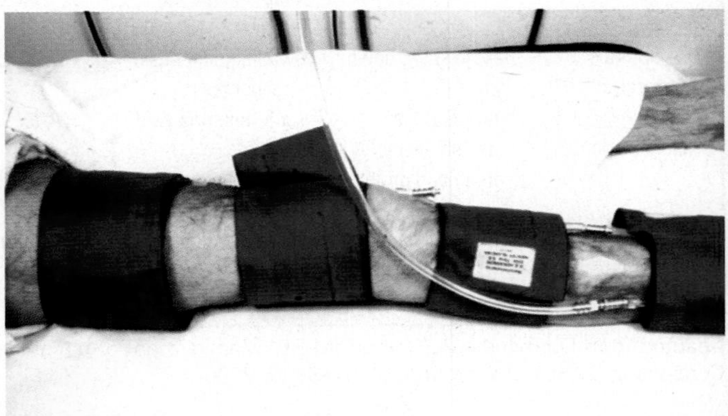

FIGURE 62-3 Segmental pressure is measured with the same technique as ankle pressure, but with cuffs placed at the upper part of the thigh, at the lower part of the thigh, below the knee, and at the ankle. (From Kohler TR, Sumner DS: Vascular laboratory: Arterial physiologic assessment. In Cronenwett JL, Johnston W, editors: *Rutherford's vascular surgery*, ed 7, Philadelphia, 2010, Saunders.)

TABLE 62-3 Clinical Correlation of Different Levels of Ankle-Brachial Index

ABI*	PRESENTATION
1.11 ± 0.10	Normal
0.59 ± 0.15	Intermittent claudication
0.26 ± 0.13	Ischemic rest pain
0.05 ± 0.08	Tissue loss

From Moneta GL, Zaccardi MJ, Olmsted KA: Lower extremity arterial occlusive disease. In Zierler RE, editor: *Strandness's duplex scanning in vascular disorders*, ed 4, Philadelphia, 2010, Lippincott Williams & Wilkins, Wolters Kluwer Health, pp 133–147.

*The diagnosis of peripheral arterial disease is given to ABI < 0.9. ABI > 1.3 is interpreted as abnormal because of incompressible tibial arteries, frequently seen in diabetes and end-stage renal failure.

digit. The data generated from these studies should include bilateral brachial artery, high thigh, low thigh, calf, dorsalis pedis, posterior tibial, and toe pressures with waveforms (Fig. 62-4). A decrease in pressure of 20 to 30 mm Hg between adjacent segments is indicative of a significant lesion. The normal Doppler arterial waveform demonstrates triphasic flow with a sharp systolic upstroke, reversal of flow in early diastole from vessel compliance, and low-amplitude forward flow throughout diastole. With obstructive disease, the initial feature lost is the reversal of the flow component, leading to multiphasic (previously called biphasic) flow. Severe disease leads to blunting of the arterial waveform, with decreased amplitude and decreased slope of the upstroke. With worsening symptoms, there is increased diastolic flow, resulting in monophasic flow. A change in waveform can be interpreted, along with a decrease in pressure, as indicative of disease at that level. Limitations of ABI and segmental pressure determinations include mural calcification, such as in diabetes mellitus and end-stage renal disease, leading to elevated pressures that do not accurately reflect intra-arterial perfusion pressure. With a noncompressible vessel, a toe-brachial index higher than 0.70 with an absolute digit pressure higher than 50 mm Hg, with a normal waveform, is indicative of preserved flow because digit arteries are relatively resistant to the intramural calcification. The high thigh pressure cannot always distinguish among common

TABLE 62-4 Calculation of Ankle-Brachial Index

PARAMETER	RIGHT	LEFT
Brachial blood pressure	150 mm Hg	100 mm Hg
Dorsalis pedis	50 mm Hg	25 mm Hg
Posterior tibia	25 mm Hg	50 mm Hg
ABI	0.30	0.30

Example: The ABI is calculated using the higher of the two ankle pressures (as indicative of limb perfusion) and the higher brachial pressure (as indicative of systemic pressure). In this example, the left and right ABI values are both 0.30.

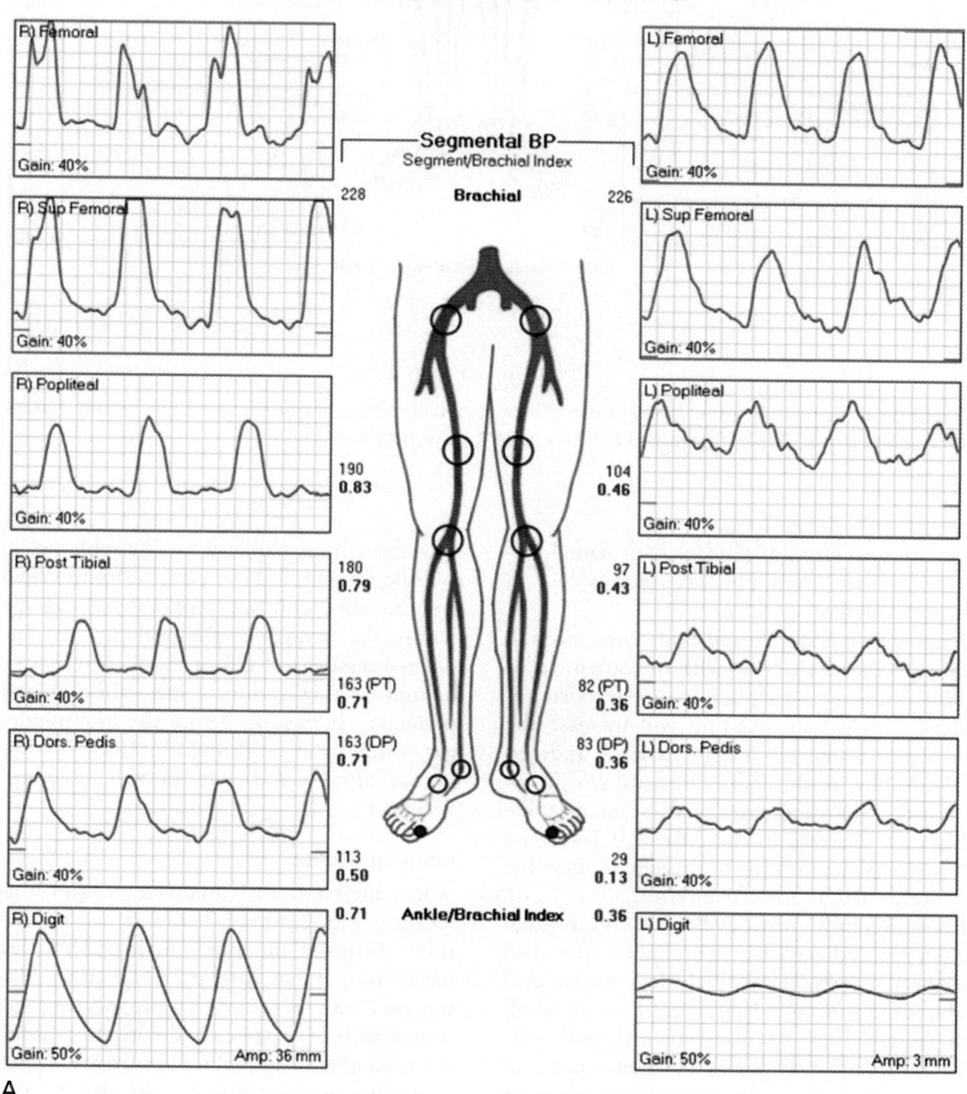

FIGURE 62-4 A, Patient with severe left leg claudication and diabetes. Segmental pressures demonstrate left iliofemoral obstruction.

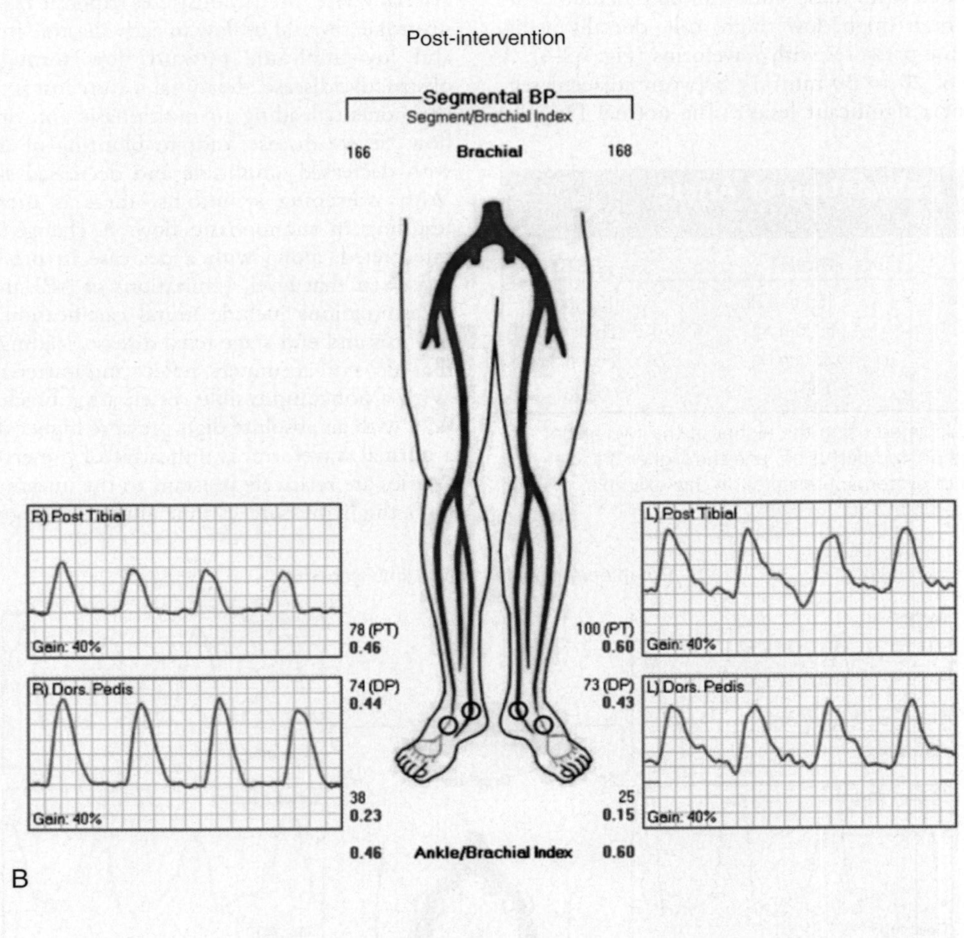

FIGURE 62-4, cont'd B, After left iliofemoral bypass and common iliac artery stent placement, the ankle-brachial index is significantly improved and the patient is asymptomatic.

iliac, external iliac, or common femoral disease. A proximal stenosis can decrease flow to the extent that accuracy is lost in interpreting gradients downstream.

Symptomatic patients with palpable distal pulses or a normal resting ABI should undergo exercise testing with measurement of the postexercise ABI. The decrease in peripheral vascular resistance that occurs with exercise-induced vasodilation will increase the drop in pressure seen across a stenotic lesion. Patients undergo resting ABI testing, followed by treadmill exercise until symptoms occur; repeated ABI testing may then reveal a decrease in ankle pressure of 20 mm Hg or a decrease in the ABI of 0.20. These changes and a failure of the ABI to return to preexercise baseline within 3 minutes are interpreted as a positive result.

Arterial duplex ultrasonography provides B-mode (gray-scale) imaging, pulsed Doppler spectral waveforms, and color flow data for analysis; in experienced hands, it can provide sensitive and specific information about the abdominal aorta and visceral, renal, iliac, and distal limb vessels. Peak systolic velocities and end-diastolic velocities are recorded. Waveforms are generated and analyzed. Color flow is useful for demonstrating patent vessels in low-flow states and for distinguishing antegrade from retrograde flow. As in continuous-flow Doppler analysis, a change in waveform from triphasic to monophasic, or an increase in peak systolic velocity followed by a drop in velocity, indicates a hemodynamically significant lesion. A ratio of the peak systolic velocity within the stenosis to the peak systolic velocity of the proximal normal segment of 2.0 or more correlates with a stenosis of 50% or more. Visualization of intra-abdominal segments requires the patient to be fasting before the examination to eliminate bowel gas; studies can be limited by body habitus. Severe calcification of the distal vessels can impede imaging of flow (Figs. 62-5 and 62-6).

Imaging Studies

When intervention is planned, further imaging to delineate the location and nature of disease is needed. The "gold standard" for these purposes has been angiography. Because of the invasive nature of this test, with attendant risks of complications, imaging was previously reserved as a preoperative study for patients determined to be operative candidates because of the severity of their disease and their suitability for surgery. This algorithm has changed somewhat in contemporary practice. Most angiography is therapeutic rather than diagnostic, with lesions that are deemed amenable for endovascular intervention addressed in the same setting

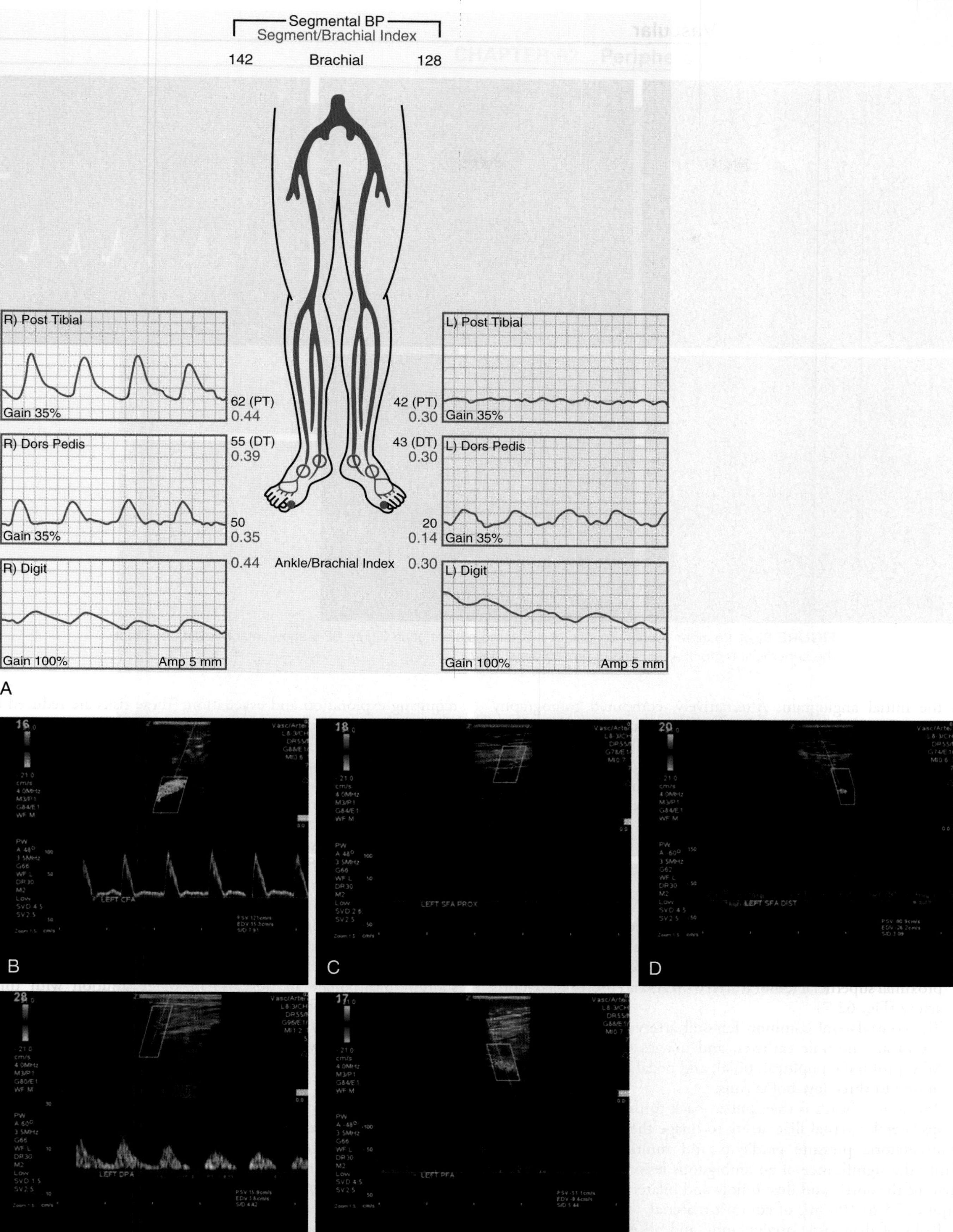

FIGURE 62-5 Arterial duplex scanning, left critical limb ischemia. Although both ankle-brachial indices are abnormal **(A),** the right limb waveforms are multiphasic and the left-sided waveforms are monophasic. Arterial duplex images show normal left common femoral artery **(B)** and no flow in the proximal superficial femoral artery **(C);** however, flow in the distal superficial femoral artery **(D)** and dorsalis pedis artery **(E)** is present because of collateral flow from the profunda femoris **(F).**

TABLE 62-5 Medical Therapy for Peripheral Arterial Disease

DISORDER	RECOMMENDED PHARMACOLOGIC AGENT	PURPOSE OF CARDIOVASCULAR RISK REDUCTION	CLASS OF RECOMMENDATIONS	LEVEL OF EVIDENCE	COMMENTS
Dyslipidemia	Statin	Statin therapy, with target LDL <100 mg/dL	I	B	
		Statin therapy, with target LDL <70 mg/dL	II	B	High-risk patients with multiple and/or poorly controlled risk factors: DM, continued tobacco abuse, metabolic syndrome (TG ≥200 mg/dL + HDL ≤40 mg/dL + non-HDL ≥130 mg/dL), acute coronary syndrome
	Gemfibrozil	May be useful in PAD patients with low HDL, normal LDL, high TG	II	C	Gemfibrozil reduces risk of nonfatal MI or cardiovascular death by 22% in CAD patients with low HDL; effects on PAD unknown
Hypertension		140/90 mm Hg in nondiabetics, 130/80 mm Hg in DM and CRI	I	A	Reduces risk of MI, CHF, cardiovascular death and stroke
	Beta blocker	Effective, not contraindicated	I	A	Reduces risk of MI and death in CAD patients; does not impair walking distance
	ACE inhibitors	Reasonable in symptomatic PAD to decrease risk of cardiovascular events	IIa	B	In patients with symptomatic PAD, ramipril reduces risk of MI, stroke, or vascular death by ≈25%
		May be used in asymptomatic PAD to decrease risk of cardiovascular events	IIb	C	No evidence for efficacy of ACE inhibitors in patients with asymptomatic PAD
Diabetes		Proper foot care; skin lesions, ulcerations should be addressed urgently in all diabetic patients with lower extremity PAD	I	B	
		Hemoglobin A1c <7%	IIa	C	Can be effective to reduce microvascular complications, potentially improve cardiovascular outcome
Atherosclerosis	Aspirin	75-325 mg PO qd; reduces risk of MI, stroke, and vascular death	I	A	Reduces risk of events by 26% to 32%
	Clopidogrel	75 mg PO qd; effective alternative to aspirin to reduce risk of MI, stroke, vascular death	I	B	Reduces risk of events by 23.8%
Smoking		Clinicians to advise smoking cessation, offer medical therapy	I	B	Physician's advice with frequent follow-up: 1-year success rate, 5% Without physician's interventions: 1-year success rate, 0.1% With nicotine replacement: 1-year success rate, 16% With bupropion: 1-year success rate, 30%

Adapted from Hirsch AT, Haskal ZJ, Hertzer NR, et al: ACC/AHA 2005 Practice Guidelines for the management of patients with peripheral arterial disease (lower extremity, renal, mesenteric, and abdominal aortic): A collaborative report from the American Association for Vascular Surgery/Society for Vascular Surgery, Society for Cardiovascular Angiography and Interventions, Society for Vascular Medicine and Biology, Society of Interventional Radiology, and the ACC/AHA Task Force on Practice Guidelines (Writing Committee to Develop Guidelines for the Management of Patients With Peripheral Arterial Disease): Endorsed by the American Association of Cardiovascular and Pulmonary Rehabilitation; National Heart, Lung, and Blood Institute; Society for Vascular Nursing; TransAtlantic Inter-Society Consensus; and Vascular Disease Foundation. *Circulation* 113:e463–e654, 2006.

ACE, angiotensin-converting enzyme; *CAD*, coronary artery disease; *CHF*, congestive heart failure; *CRI*, chronic renal insufficiency; *DM*, diabetes mellitus; *HDL*, high-density lipoprotein; *LDL*, low-density lipoprotein; *MI*, myocardial infarction; *PAD*, peripheral arterial disease; *TG*, triglyceride.

Intermittent claudication patients with an initial ankle pressure of 40 to 60 mm Hg have an annual limb loss rate of 8.5%.

Patients who present initially with low ankle pressures or absent femoral pulses or patients who return with unabated, severe, lifestyle-limiting symptoms that have not adequately responded to nonoperative measures are considered for intervention (Fig. 62-10).

Critical limb ischemia. Patients who present initially with rest pain or who progress from claudication to rest pain undergo the same detailed history and physical examination with risk factor modification as patients presenting with milder disease. However, because rest pain is associated with a significant risk of limb loss without intervention, patients are immediately offered imaging and revascularization if prohibitive perioperative risk does not preclude this.

Similarly, patients who present with nonhealing wounds of the feet, dry gangrene, or necrotizing infection are offered an expeditious workup to plan a revascularization that will reestablish in-line blood flow to the foot. In case of tissue loss with infection, an immediate decision about the need for operative débridement or amputation before revascularization must be made. In case of severe sepsis with hemodynamic instability or evidence of multisystem organ failure, patients may require amputation before revascularization. However, if a patient with systemic toxicity from the infection responds rapidly to IV administration of antibiotics, revascularization before débridement may minimize tissue loss (Fig. 62-11).

Diabetic foot. PVD is common among patients with diabetes (Fig. 62-12). Intermittent claudication is twice as common among diabetic patients as among nondiabetic patients. An increase in hemoglobin A1c by 1% can result in more than a 25% risk of PAD. Major amputation rates are 5 to 10 times higher in diabetics than in nondiabetics. Because of these causal relations, the American Diabetes Association recommends ABI screening every 5 years in patients with diabetes.[2]

The care of diabetic patients should start with preventive measures, and it is important to avoid infections in patients with insensate feet because of neuropathy. These patients need to wear properly fitted shoes at all times for protection. Orthotic inserts should be used to distribute weight evenly to avoid pressure on the metatarsal heads of the foot.

Diabetic patients may be unaware of the presence of infections or ulcerative lesions because of peripheral neuropathy and a decreased ability to sense pain. In this population, infections can progress rapidly, with significant tissue damage from a combination of delayed presentation and compromised immune function.

On presentation, a careful physical examination is important to plan for appropriate treatment. The overlying cellulitis is assessed, and any possible underlying abscess is examined by palpation for crepitus or detection of drainage of purulent fluid. Cellulitis should not be confused with dependent rubor caused by severe ischemia in patients with PAD. The presence of an abscess requires immediate drainage before revascularization.

The status of arterial circulation is documented. The presence or absence of lower extremity pulses in the common femoral, popliteal, and pedal arteries is examined. The pulses may be difficult to palpate because of swelling from foot infection; noninvasive arterial ultrasound can be useful in assessing the extent of arterial disease.

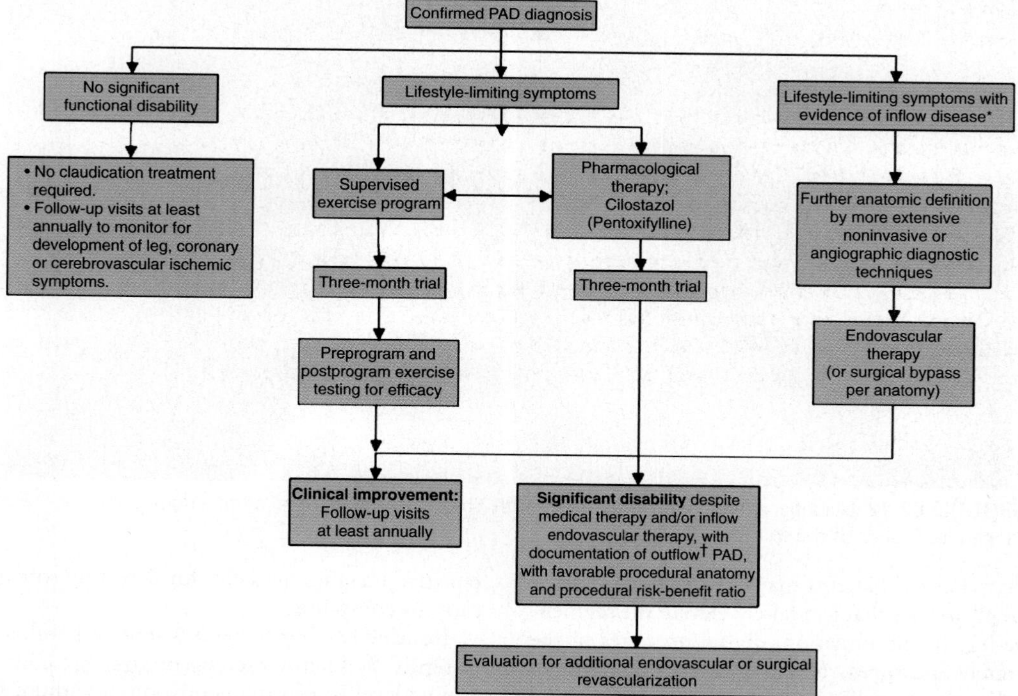

FIGURE 62-10 Treatment Algorithm for Peripheral Arterial Disease. (From Hirsch AT, Haskal ZJ, Hertzer NR, et al: ACC/AHA 2005 Practice Guidelines for the Management of Patients With Peripheral Arterial Disease (Lower Extremity, Renal, Mesenteric, and Abdominal Aortic). *Circ* 113:e463–e654, 2006.) *Inflow disease should be suspected in individuals with gluteal or thigh claudication and femoral pulse diminution or bruit and should be confirmed by noninvasive vascular laboratory diagnostic evidence of aortoiliac stenoses. †Outflow disease represents femoropopliteal and infrapopliteal stenoses, (the presence of occlusive lesions in the lower extremity arterial tree below the inguinal ligament from the common femoral artery to the pedal vessels). PAD indicates peripheral arterial disease.

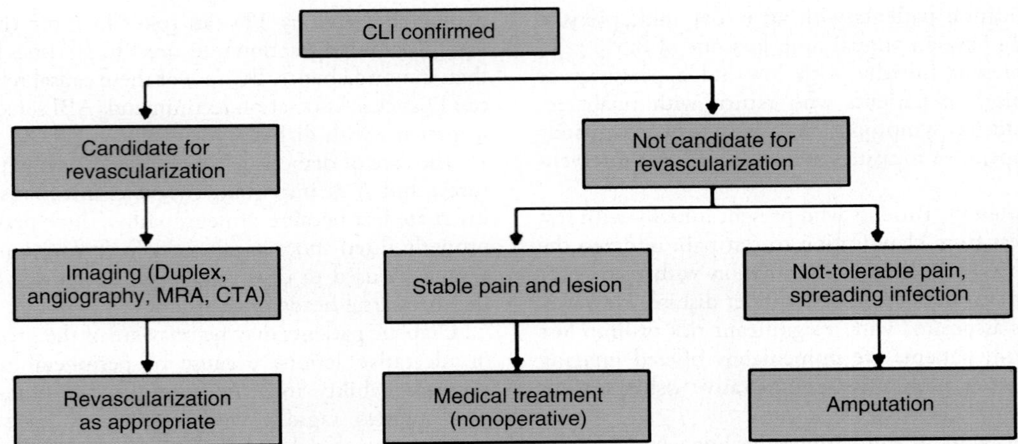

FIGURE 62-11 Algorithm for treatment of the critical limb ischemia (CLI) patient. (From Norgren L, Hiatt WR, Dormandy JA, et al: Inter-Society Consensus for the Management of Peripheral Arterial Disease [TASC II]. *J Vasc Surg* 45[Suppl]:S5–S67, 2007.)

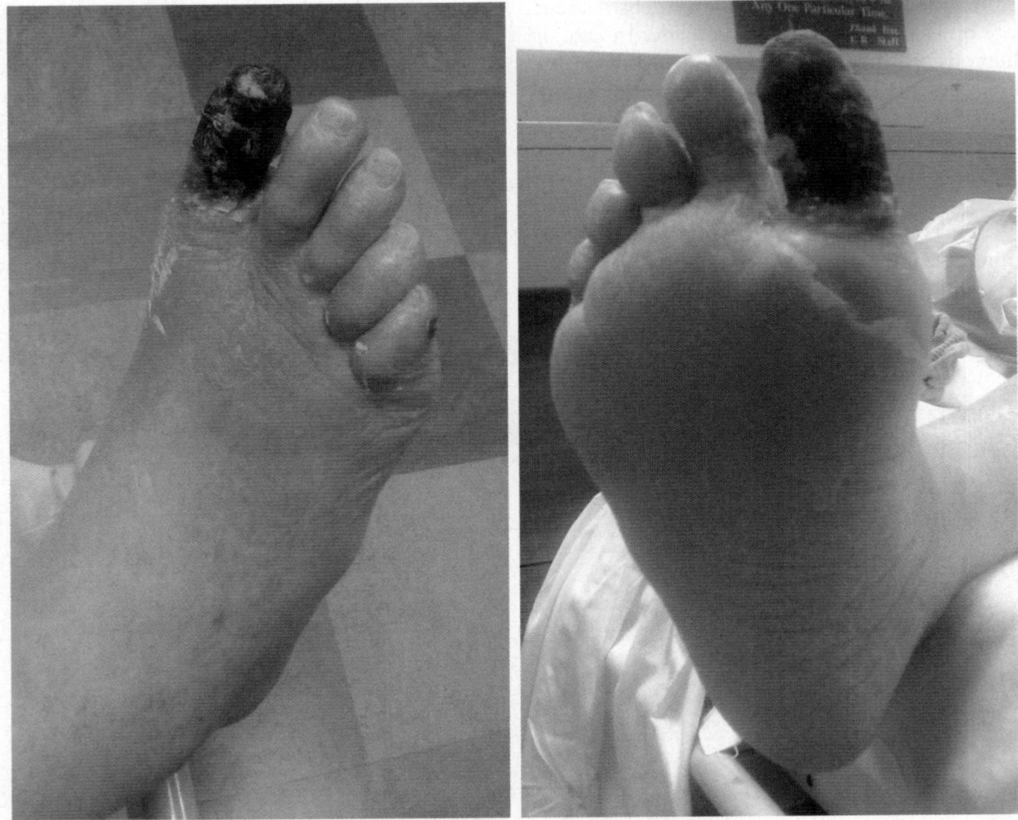

FIGURE 62-12 Diabetic patient who presented with chronic dry gangrene of the right great toe, with dependent rubor of the forefoot.

Insulin-dependent diabetic patients may have calcified walls of the medium and small arteries that can falsely elevate the segmental pressures of the leg. In this situation, digital pressures of the toes can be accurately measured, and a pressure higher than 30 mm Hg is predictive of healing after local amputation and débridement.

Plain radiographs with multiple views of the foot can assist in assessing the extent of foot infection. Gas in soft tissue signifies deep tissue infection and the need for urgent surgical débridement. Advanced osteomyelitis can be detected; however, plain films may not show early bone infection. MRI of the foot is a sensitive imaging modality for detecting soft tissue infection and early osteomyelitis.

Routine laboratory work is sent and evaluated for subtle signs of sepsis. Sudden worsening of glycemic control or a rise in creatinine level is seen frequently, often without leukocytosis.

In infections with only cellulitis and no underlying soft tissue involvement, patients are treated with IV antibiotic therapy. If the cellulitis does not resolve in several days, there may not be adequate antibiotic coverage, and the presence of deep tissue infection is considered. The choice of the antibiotics used and the foot need to be reevaluated; reimaging of the foot may be necessary.

The cause of persistent cellulitis and nonhealing infection is usually underlying deep infection or osteomyelitis. Other patients may present with gangrene, open joint or exposed bone, or abscess. In these patients, surgical débridement is required in addition to antibiotic therapy. Small open wounds can be treated with simple débridement, but often there is deep tissue involvement that is not visible on the surface. For removal of all nonviable tissue and wide drainage, amputation may be required. If there is extensive infection of the foot with gas, calf pain, or systemic sepsis, the patient may require amputation as an initial therapy. After surgical débridement, patients are treated with aggressive wound care by dressing changes and continued, broad-spectrum antibiotic therapy until intraoperative culture sensitivities are finalized and allow the use of targeted antimicrobials. Wounds are evaluated closely for persistent infection that may require additional surgical intervention. In patients with adequate arterial circulation, the wound can be closed secondarily after resolution of the infection.

All patients with evidence of concomitant arterial occlusive disease are considered for lower extremity revascularization with open bypass surgery or endovascular stenting or angioplasty to optimize wound healing and limb salvage.

Lower Extremity Amputations

Amputation, unfortunately, in the minds of most surgeons and their patients, represents a failure of therapy or care. Consent for this operation, regardless of the level, is usually imbued with an emotional gravity that few other, even more complex, dangerous, life-altering procedures carry. Not infrequently, amputations in the vascular patient are prone to breakdown and the need for revision is common, thereby prolonging the patient's time in the hospital, lengthening the recovery process, decreasing the chances of functional recovery, and contributing to a high rate of depression. It is therefore incumbent on the surgeon to ensure that all steps are taken to optimize healing and to minimize the risks of local and systemic complications.

The perioperative mortality rate for below-knee amputation is 5% to 10%, and that of above-knee amputation is even higher, 10% to 15%, testifying to the limited reserves of patients facing these procedures.[3] Wound healing in below-knee amputation is poor; almost one third of patients require débridement or healing by secondary intention or conversion to above-knee amputation (Fig. 62-13). Despite optimistic preoperative counseling, functional recovery with ambulation is poor for above-knee amputation patients.

The determination of the appropriate level for amputation has been studied extensively (Table 62-6). In an effort to preserve limb length and to decrease the metabolic demands of ambulation, toe and transmetatarsal amputations are usually attempted. Aside from clinical judgment, segmental arterial pressures, Doppler waveforms, and toe pressures have been studied. Diabetes, combined with a toe pressure of lower than 30 mm Hg, has been correlated with failure of healing of minor amputations. Transcutaneous oxygen pressure ($TcPO_2$) measurement, easily obtained through a small sensor placed on the skin in the area of proposed amputation, has an accuracy of higher than 87% for predicting

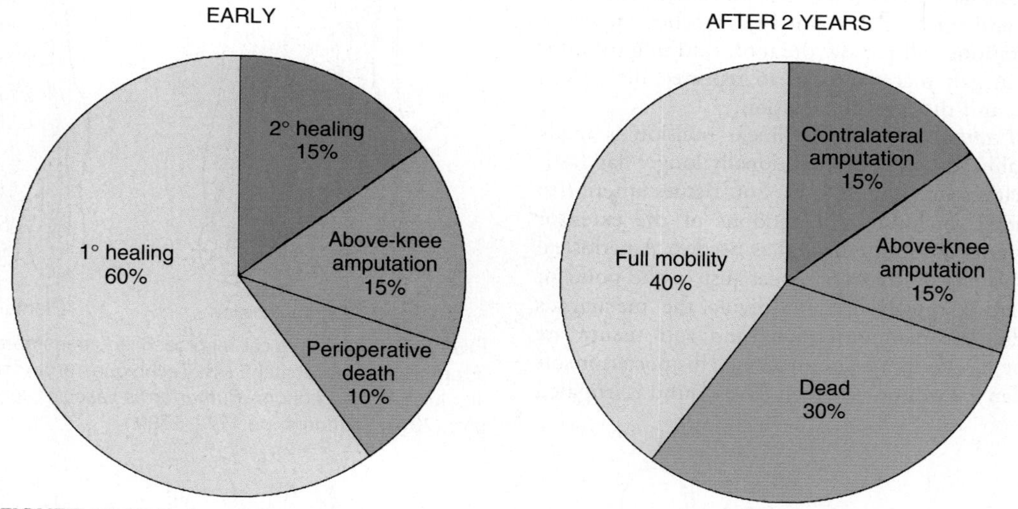

FIGURE 62-13 Early and 2-year outcomes of the below-knee amputation patient. (From Norgren L, Hiatt WR, Dormandy JA, et al: Inter-Society Consensus for the Management of Peripheral Arterial Disease [TASC II]. *J Vasc Surg* 45[Suppl]:S5–S67, 2007.)

TABLE 62-6 Prediction of Wound Healing by Vascular Studies

STUDY	THRESHOLD (mm Hg)	WOUND HEALING (%) BELOW THRESHOLD	WOUND HEALING (%) ABOVE THRESHOLD	SENSITIVITY (%)	SPECIFICITY (%)
SPP	40	10	69	72	88
$TcPO_2$	30	14	63	60	87
TBP	30	12	67	63	90
ABP	80	11	45	74	70

ABP, ankle blood pressure; *SPP*, skin perfusion pressure; *TBP*, toe blood pressure; *$TcPO_2$*, transcutaneous oxygen pressure.

wound healing. A reading higher than 40 mm Hg is associated with successful healing, whereas $TcPO_2$ less than 20 mm Hg is associated with failure. Absolute ankle pressure higher than 60 mm Hg has been shown to predict the healing of below-knee amputations with an accuracy of 50% to 90%.[4]

Ray amputation. For ray amputation, a tennis racquet incision around the base of the affected toe is made. For first toe amputations, the handle of the racquet is oriented along the medial aspect of the metatarsal head; for the fifth toe, it is oriented laterally. For toes 2 to 4, the incision is along the dorsal midline (Fig. 62-14). Neighboring digital vessels are carefully preserved as the soft tissues are divided. The extensor tendons are divided under tension and permitted to retract. The bone is divided proximal to the metatarsal head. If sesamoid bones are encountered, these are removed. Plantar soft tissue is divided; flexor tendons are similarly allowed to retract after being divided under tension. Soft tissue is closed over the metatarsal head with absorbable sutures. Minimal handling of the skin prevents ischemic trauma. The skin is approximated without tension or left open for closure by secondary intention.

The great toe and first metatarsal bone are important for normal gait because weight is transferred from the posterolateral foot during heel strike toward the medial toes, and the transfer of weight forward occurs principally through force transmitted during push off through the first metatarsal and great toe. Because of the significant rate of repeated ulceration and need for revision in up to 60% of patients requiring a great toe ray amputation, some have advocated proceeding directly to transmetatarsal amputation in these patients.

Partial transmetatarsal amputation can be performed when two digits are involved and the foot is deemed salvageable. However, multiple ray amputations will narrow the foot, resulting in instability and change in gait that may lead to repeated ulceration, wound breakdown, and the need for revision.

Transmetatarsal amputation. A curvilinear incision is made above the metatarsal heads, with an intentionally longer flap fashioned on the plantar surface (Fig. 62-15). Soft tissues anterior to the bone are divided, including the tendons of the extensor muscles. Digital arteries are suture ligated as needed. A periosteal elevator is applied to elevate the soft tissues just to the point of division. An oscillating saw is used to divide the metatarsals behind their heads. The plantar tendons and soft tissues are divided distal to the level of bone amputation. This posterior soft tissue is used as a flap for wound coverage. The wound is irrigated with a mechanical lavage system and inspected for hemostasis. The soft tissue is reapproximated over the bone with absorbable sutures. The skin is reapproximated, with minimal manipulation and without tension, with interrupted nylon vertical mattress sutures. Non–weight-bearing status is encouraged for at least 4 weeks. In case of infection, a guillotine procedure may be performed and a vacuum dressing applied, with placement of a split-thickness skin graft after the wound bed has adequately granulated.

Alternatively, more proximal transmetatarsal amputation incisions include the Lisfranc and Chopart amputations (Fig. 62-16). The Syme amputation is rarely used because it is thought to provide the patient with less functional ambulation than a transtibial amputation. There is evidence to support multiple revisions and preservation of length in diabetic patients. In one study, 56% of patients failed to heal their initial transmetatarsal amputations. Of these, 9 of 41 underwent major amputation; 32 underwent midfoot amputations and achieved functional ambulation. Toe pressure higher than 50 mm Hg had a positive predictive value

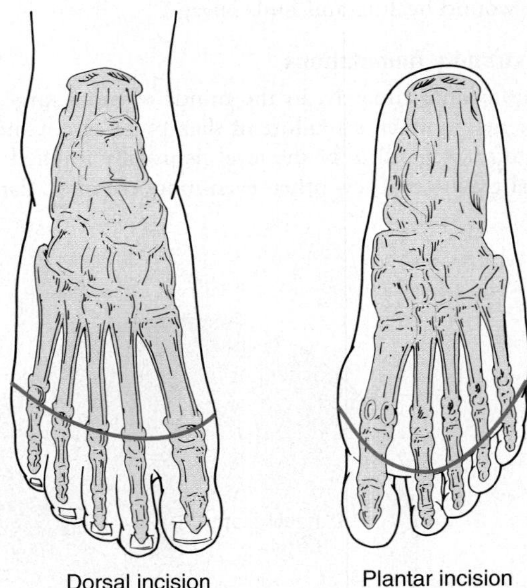

FIGURE 62-15 Surgical approach to transmetatarsal amputation. (From Eidt JF, Kalapatapu VR: Techniques and results. In Cronenwett JL, Johnston W, editors: *Rutherford's vascular surgery*, ed 7, Philadelphia, 2010, Saunders, pp 1772–1790.)

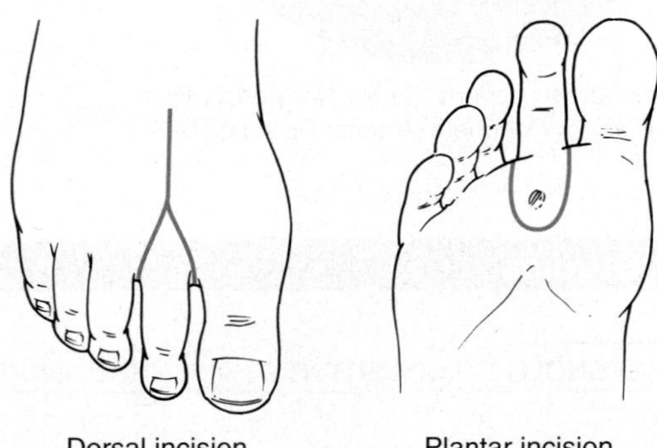

FIGURE 62-14 Surgical approach to ray amputation. (From Eidt JF, Kalapatapu VR: Techniques and results. In Cronenwett JL, Johnston W, editors: *Rutherford's vascular surgery*, ed 7, Philadelphia, 2010, Saunders, pp 1772–1790.)

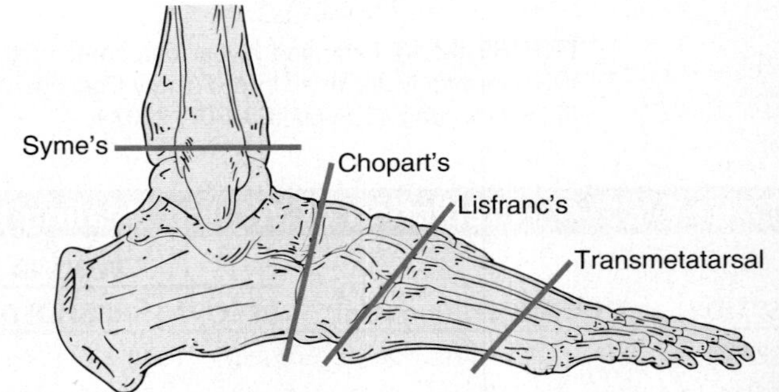

FIGURE 62-16 Alternative distal amputation approaches. (From Eidt JF, Kalapatapu VR: Techniques and results. In Cronenwett JL, Johnston W, editors: *Rutherford's vascular surgery*, ed 7, Philadelphia, 2010, Saunders, pp 1772–1790.)

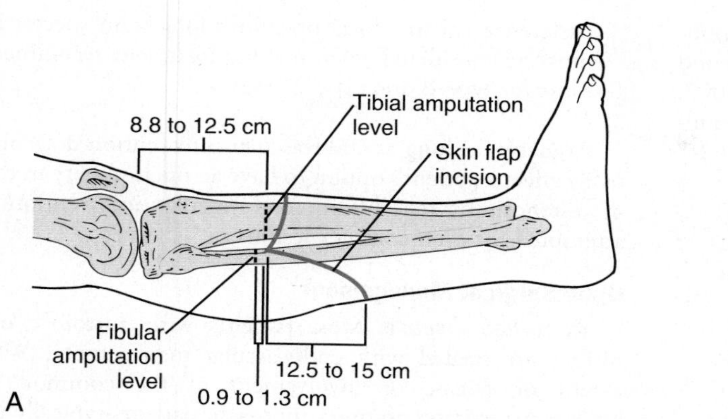

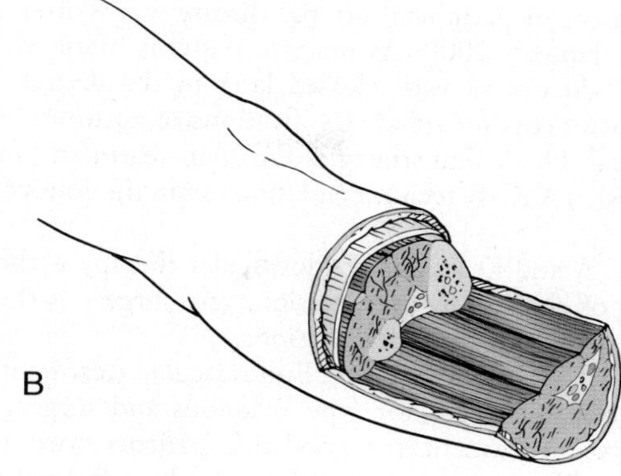

FIGURE 62-17 Surgical approach to posterior flap for below-knee amputation. (From Eidt JF, Kalapatapu VR: Techniques and results. In Cronenwett JL, Johnston W, editors: *Rutherford's vascular surgery*, ed 7, Philadelphia, 2010, Saunders, pp 1772–1790.)

of 91% for determining healing of transmetatarsal-midfoot amputations.[5]

Below-knee amputation. There are multiple skin incisions described for below-knee amputation (Fig. 62-17). The most common is the long posterior flap. A tourniquet may be used to decrease blood loss, which can be substantial, even in the vascular patient. Approximately 10 cm below the tibial tuberosity, an anterior incision of two thirds of the circumference is created. The great saphenous vein is ligated and divided. All muscle and soft tissue structures anterior to the tibia are divided. Vascular bundles are suture ligated with care because they are likely to be extremely calcified. Nerves are tied under tension, divided, and allowed to retract. The tibia is divided with an oscillating saw and beveled anteriorly. The fibula is divided approximately 2 cm proximal to the tibia after detachment of the anterior, lateral, and posterior compartment muscles. The posterior flap incision is created with the length approximately one third of the circumference of the leg. The muscle flap is created just deep to the tibia, including the soleus and gastrocnemius muscles. After irrigation and inspection for hemostasis, the fascia is reapproximated with interrupted absorbable sutures. The skin is reapproximated with monofilament vertical mattress sutures or staples. A dressing of gauze wrap and elastic bandage is applied. A splint is created or a well-padded knee immobilizer is applied to prevent knee contracture.

In case of severe necrotizing foot infection, emergent guillotine transtibial amputation can be performed just proximal to the ankle, followed by formal revision to a below-knee amputation once the infectious process has resolved.[6]

Cryoamputation or physiologic amputation has been described to isolate the infected or acutely ischemic limb and to prevent it from causing systemic effects in an already critically ill individual.

Above-knee amputation. In general, the longer the stump, the better. A fish-mouth incision is created (Fig. 62-18). The great saphenous vein is ligated and divided. The sartorius, rectus femoris, and vastus lateralis are divided. The femoral artery and vein are separately suture ligated and divided. Laterally, the vastus lateralis and intermedius are divided. The periosteal elevator is used to clear the femur at the level of the skin; the bone is divided by use of a pneumatic saw and beveled anteriorly. The profunda femoris artery and vein or their branches are ligated and divided. The sciatic nerve is cut under tension and allowed to retract. After irrigation and inspection of hemostasis, the fascia of the muscles

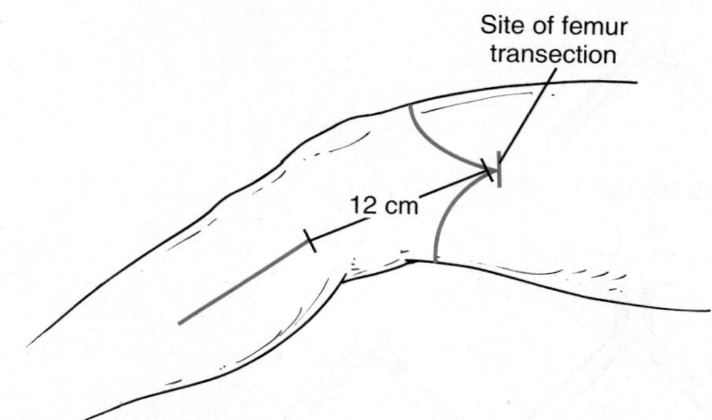

FIGURE 62-18 Surgical approach to fish-mouth incision for transfemoral above-knee amputation. (From Eidt JF, Kalapatapu VR: Techniques and results. In Cronenwett JL, Johnston W, editors: *Rutherford's vascular surgery*, ed 7, Philadelphia, 2010, Saunders, pp 1772–1790.)

is approximated over the bone with absorbable interrupted sutures, and the skin is closed.

Complications of above-knee amputation include hip contracture; this and the poor rates of ambulation are related to unopposed action of the hip flexors. Preservation of adductor function is improved with myodesis; the length of the adductor magnus may be preserved and anchored to the lateral aspect of the femur through drill holes.

Trans-knee amputations may be used as an alternative to above-knee amputation in younger patients for improved functional capability.

Surgical Revascularization Procedures

There are fewer areas in medicine today in which treatment algorithms are changing more rapidly than in arterial occlusive disease. Currently, the decision for revascularization is based on the risks for the surgical intervention balanced against the expected benefits, including the durability of the treatment and options for further intervention if there is recurrence of symptoms. Rapid advances in endovascular techniques and devices have made the therapeutic decision-making process increasingly complex; opinions about which therapies should be used first are varied. In an effort to characterize patients and their lesions and to provide guidance about open versus endovascular alternatives, the TransAtlantic Inter-Society Consensus (TASC) document on management of peripheral arterial disease was written and published in January 2000. As practice patterns matured, a second TASC II document was released later in the decade, in 2007. These documents provided classifications of aortoiliac and femoropopliteal disease and strategies for their treatment (Tables 62-7 and 62-8). TASC II recommendations state the following:

> TASC A and D lesions: Endovascular therapy is the treatment of choice for type A lesions and surgery is the treatment of choice for type D lesions.
>
> TASC B and C lesions: Endovascular treatment is the preferred treatment for type B lesions and surgery is the preferred treatment for good-risk patients with type C lesions. The patient's comorbidities, fully informed patient preference and the local operator's long-term success rates must be considered when making treatment recommendations for type B and type C lesions.

Arguably, as long as endovascular intervention does not negatively affect a patient's option to have an open surgery in the event of restenosis or reocclusion, endovascular intervention can be attempted for even complex lesions.

Open Surgical Management

Aortoiliac disease. Most patients with aortoiliac occlusive disease are treated with endovascular management. When the extent of disease or involvement of the common femoral arteries necessitates an open approach, patients typically undergo

TABLE 62-7 TransAtlantic Inter-Society Consensus (TASC) Classification of Aortoiliac Lesions

Lesion type	Description
Type A lesions 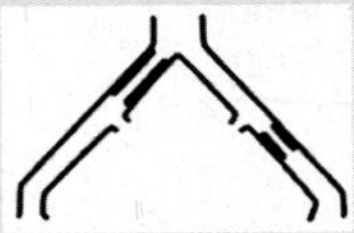	• Unilateral or bilateral stenoses of CIA • Unilateral or bilateral single short (≤3 cm) stenosis of EIA
Type B lesions 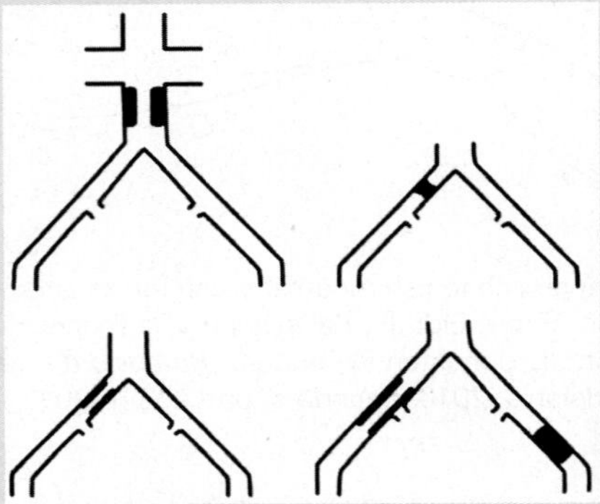	• Short (≤3 cm) stenosis of infrarenal aorta • Unilateral CIA occlusion • Single or multiple stenosis totaling 3-10 cm involving the EIA not extending into the CFA • Unilateral EIA occlusion not involving the origins of internal iliac or CFA
Type C lesions 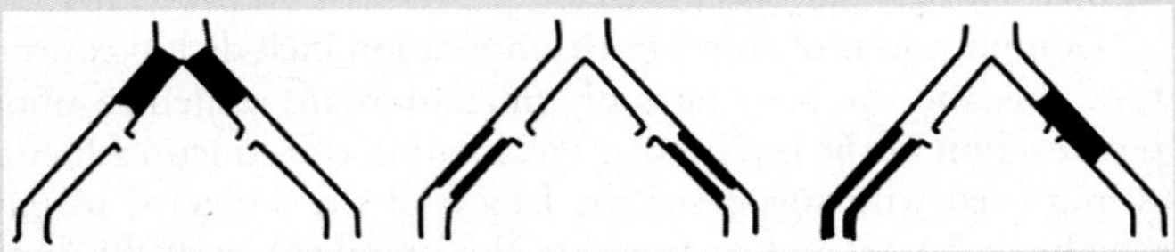	• Bilateral CIA occlusions • Bilateral EIA stenoses 3-10 cm long not extending into the CFA • Unilateral EIA stenosis extending into the CFA • Unilateral EIA occlusion that involves the origins of internal iliac and/or CFA • Heavily calcified unilateral EIA occlusion with or without involvement of origins of internal iliac and/or CFA
Type D lesions 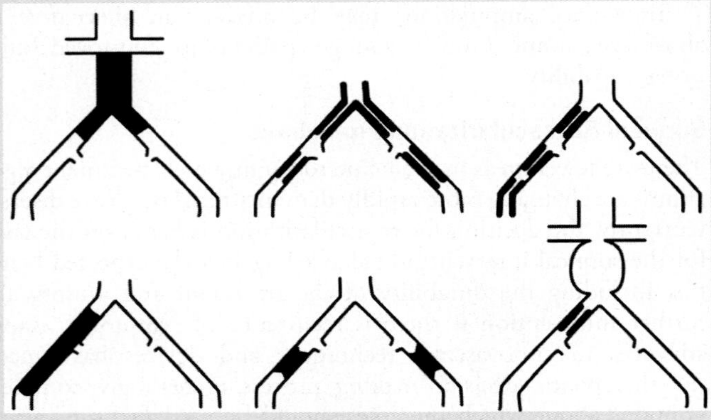	• Infrarenal aortoiliac occlusion • Diffuse disease involving the aorta and both iliac arteries requiring treatment • Diffuse multiple stenoses involving the unilateral CIA, EIA, and CFA • Unilateral occlusions of both CIA and EIA • Bilateral occlusions of EIA • Iliac stenoses in patients with AAA requiring treatment and not amenable to endograft placement or other lesions requiring open aortic or iliac surgery

From Norgren L, Hiatt WR, Dormandy JA, et al: Inter-Society Consensus for the Management of Peripheral Arterial Disease (TASC II). *J Vasc Surg* 45(Suppl S):S5–S67, 2007.

AAA, abdominal aortic aneurysm; *CFA,* common femoral artery; *CIA,* common iliac artery; *EIA,* external iliac artery.

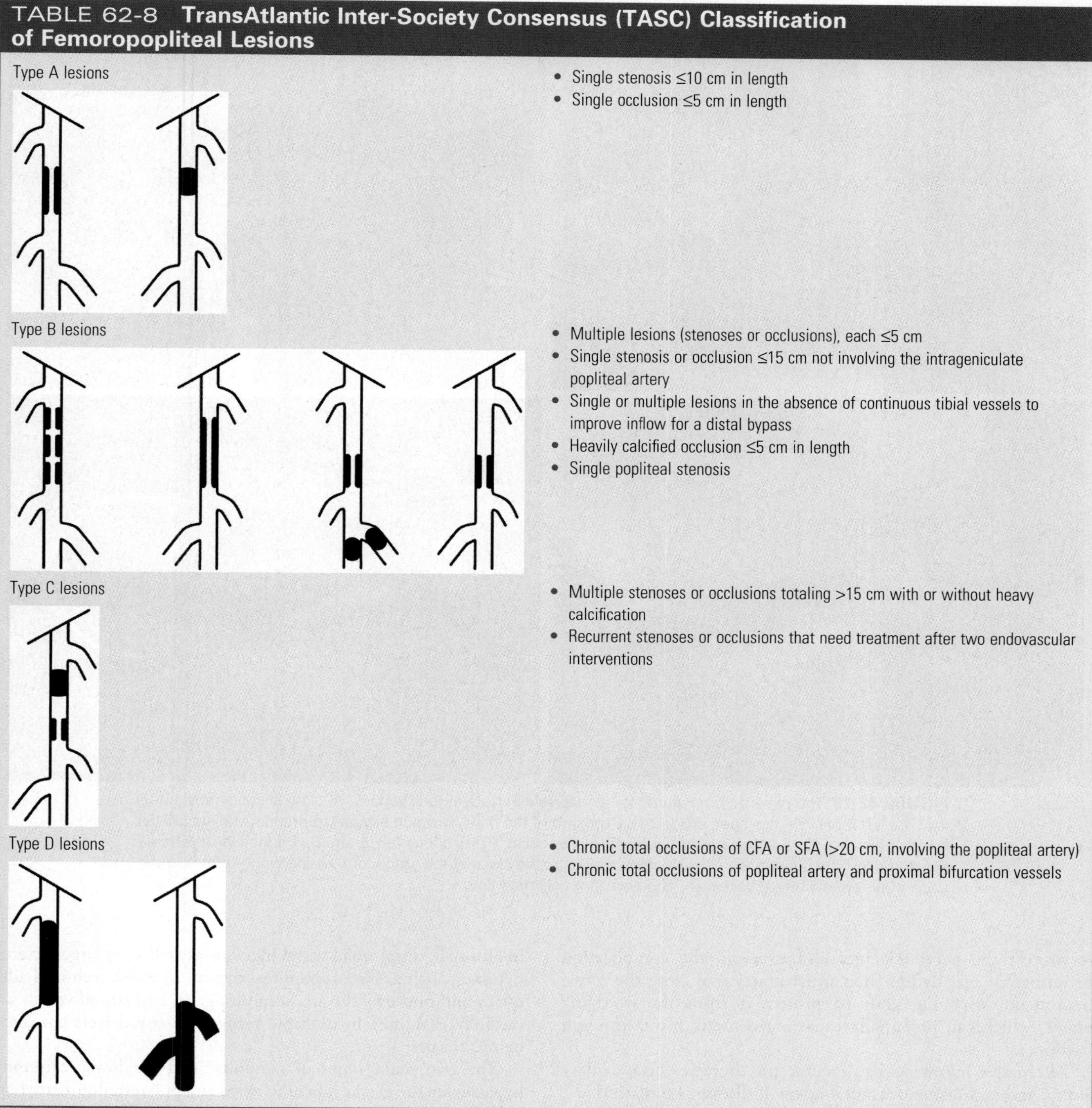

TABLE 62-8 TransAtlantic Inter-Society Consensus (TASC) Classification of Femoropopliteal Lesions

Type A lesions	• Single stenosis ≤10 cm in length • Single occlusion ≤5 cm in length
Type B lesions	• Multiple lesions (stenoses or occlusions), each ≤5 cm • Single stenosis or occlusion ≤15 cm not involving the intrageniculate popliteal artery • Single or multiple lesions in the absence of continuous tibial vessels to improve inflow for a distal bypass • Heavily calcified occlusion ≤5 cm in length • Single popliteal stenosis
Type C lesions	• Multiple stenoses or occlusions totaling >15 cm with or without heavy calcification • Recurrent stenoses or occlusions that need treatment after two endovascular interventions
Type D lesions	• Chronic total occlusions of CFA or SFA (>20 cm, involving the popliteal artery) • Chronic total occlusions of popliteal artery and proximal bifurcation vessels

From Norgren L, Hiatt WR, Dormandy JA, et al: Inter-Society Consensus for the Management of Peripheral Arterial Disease (TASC II). *J Vasc Surg* 45(Suppl S):S5–S67, 2007.
CFA, common femoral artery; *SFA,* superficial femoral artery.

aortobifemoral bypass with a prosthetic graft through the transabdominal or retroperitoneal approach (Fig. 62-19). Preoperative imaging should delineate the target vessels, usually the common femoral or profunda femoris arteries. Proximal anastomoses can be performed in end-to-end or end-to-side configuration. For patients with external iliac occlusive disease, the end-to-side configuration is more commonly used because it may preserve perfusion to the pelvis through the diseased but patent common iliac, sacral, and lumbar collaterals. Arguments for end-to-end anastomosis include improved flow dynamics and the potential for decreased friction between the overlying bowel and graft. In the past, it was common practice to cut the body of the graft to leave minimal redundancy; however, it has become more popular to leave a longer segment of graft body and shorter limbs to ease the endovascular up-and-over approaches in the future. Minimal dissection in the area of the left common iliac artery is performed

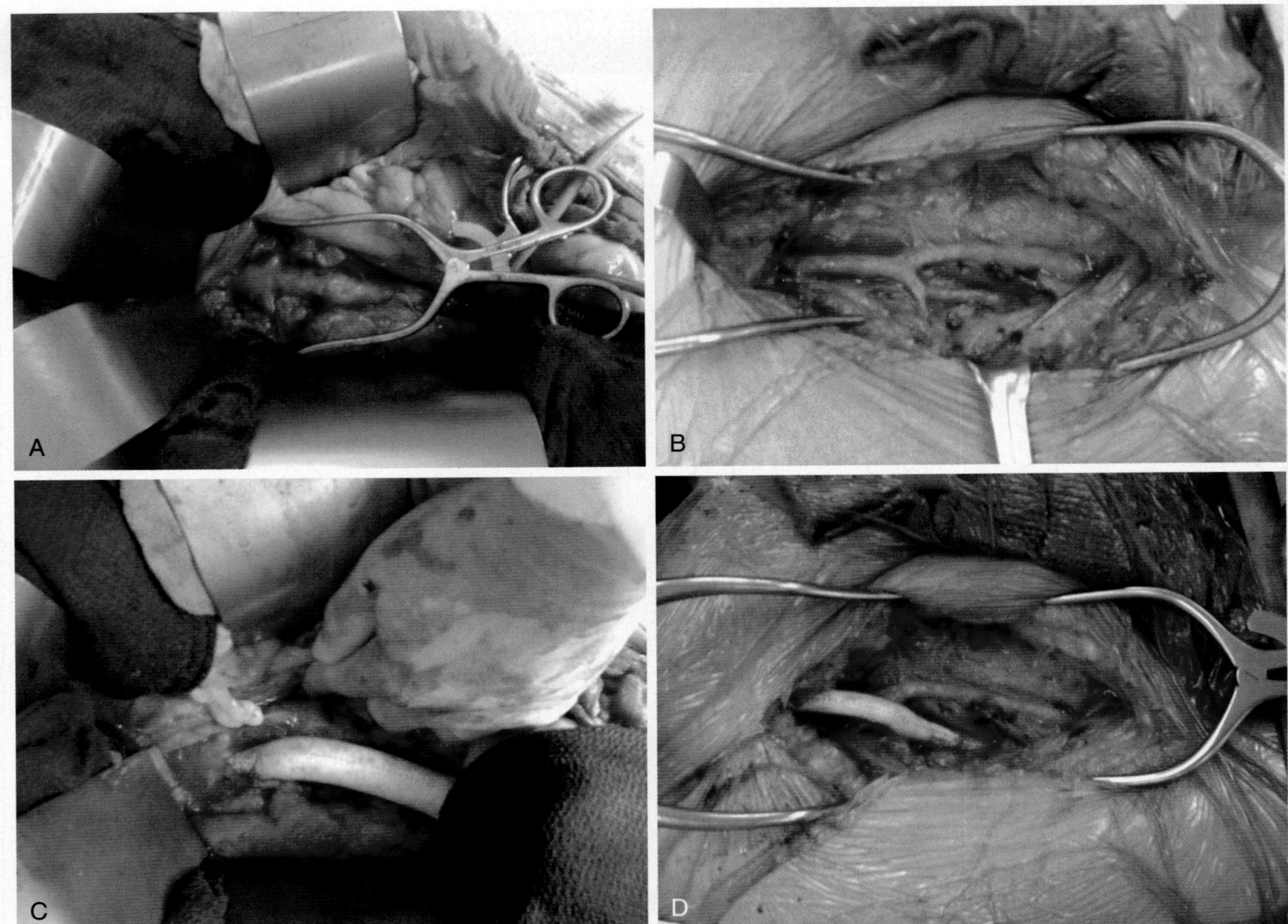

FIGURE 62-19 The patient from Figure 62-7 underwent aortobifemoral bypass. **A,** Note bilateral renal arteries. The left renal vein has been divided. **B,** Exposure of the right common femoral, profunda, and superficial femoral arteries. **C,** End-to-side aortic anastomosis using PTFE bifurcated graft. **D,** End-to-side profunda anastomosis. The patient had palpable distal pulses at the close of the procedure, despite long-term bilateral superficial femoral artery occlusion, and excellent collateral flow.

to protect the nervi erigentes and to avoid the complication of retrograde ejaculation. It is usual practice to close the retroperitoneum over the graft to protect it from the overlying bowel, which can potentially cause aortoenteric fistula through friction.

Alternative inflow sources include the thoracic aorta, axillary artery, and contralateral femoral artery if disease is unilateral.

Lower extremity occlusive disease. Patients with significant lesions involving the common femoral artery and origin of the profunda artery are usually best served with open groin exploration, common femoral artery endarterectomy, and profundaplasty or iliofemoral bypass. If concomitant iliac artery or SFA disease is present, patients may undergo combination procedures with iliac stent placement through open femoral access or SFA revascularization by femoropopliteal bypass or SFA stenting.

Vascular control is achieved with minimal force or traction. Heparin, 80 to 100 units/kg, is given for anticoagulation during periods of vascular occlusion. Anastomoses are constructed with care using small, evenly placed bites to include all layers of the vessel wall. Intraoperative completion arteriography is performed in all small, distal tibial vessel bypasses as well as in larger arterial bypasses, such as femoropopliteal bypass, to assess technical adequacy and outflow. The anastomoses, graft, and runoff vessels are carefully examined in multiple planes and any defects corrected before closure.

The two main types of conduits used for lower extremity bypasses are the great saphenous veins and polytetrafluoroethylene (PTFE) grafts. The great saphenous veins should be used preferentially in all bypasses, especially in those reconstructions using below-knee popliteal and small tibial arteries as the distal target vessels. PTFE grafts can be used for bypasses to above-knee popliteal arterial segments with satisfactory patency rates.

To date, the disappointing patency rates for prosthetic grafts in below-knee and tibial bypasses have discouraged their use. Recently, a new PTFE graft with heparin coating on the luminal surface has been shown to be more resistant to thrombosis. Although these grafts may have an advantage over non–heparin-coated grafts, an adequately sized (4 mm or larger) saphenous vein remains preferable to synthetic conduits because of its innate antithrombotic properties.

The great saphenous vein can be placed in situ or reversed because of the presence of valves. The advantage of the reversed saphenous vein graft is that the valves do not need to be rendered incompetent with the use of a valvulotome. For the in situ vein graft, there is better size match—larger thigh vein for the common femoral artery and smaller leg vein for the tibial artery. Care must be used in passing the valvulotome to avoid tearing of the delicate vein. Neither of these configurations has been shown to be superior and surgeons use both, depending on their personal preference.

In the absence of a usable great saphenous vein, the cephalic and basilic veins from the upper extremities as well as the small saphenous vein of the leg should be evaluated. However, these veins have thinner walls and may have diseased segments that appear normal on external inspection. Furthermore, when several veins are joined to form a composite graft to achieve adequate length, there is the potential for technical complications and reduced overall patency. There is some evidence that the use of a vein patch with a prosthetic femorodistal bypass improves patency. Other conduits include cryopreserved arteries and veins, which have been shown to be more resistant to infection in the setting of gross infection.

For endarterectomy patch angioplasty, there are prosthetic patches of PTFE or Dacron. Bovine pericardial patches are also available. Alternatively, an endarterectomized segment of the native occluded SFA can be used for common femoral or profunda artery patch angioplasty or as a short-segment bypass conduit.

Femoropopliteal bypass. The femoropopliteal bypass is used in patients with superficial femoral and popliteal arterial occlusion with a popliteal artery segment distal to the occlusion that is patent, with luminal continuity with any tibial arterial branches. Bypasses can be performed even if one or more of the tibial arteries are occluded in the leg.

A longitudinal groin incision is used to access the common femoral artery. The popliteal artery is exposed medially from the thigh or the leg. In above-knee popliteal bypasses, an incision is made proximal to the knee for exposure of the artery near the adductor hiatus or Hunter canal, distal to the occlusive disease. In below-knee popliteal bypass, the popliteal space is accessed. The more superficial popliteal vein is retracted with a Silastic loop to assist with dissection of the underlying popliteal artery. If the saphenous vein is to be used, skin incisions are placed directly over the vein. A single long incision or multiple smaller skip incisions can be used. Alternatively, endoscopic vein harvesting can be performed. The graft is tunneled and placed in the anatomic space, under the sartorius muscle, unless an in situ saphenous vein graft is used.

Infrapopliteal bypass. The infrapopliteal bypass is used for arteries beyond the popliteal artery when there is arterial disease that involves the popliteal or proximal tibial artery. The target tibial artery will have luminal continuity to the foot without obstruction. With femoropopliteal and infrapopliteal bypasses, a tibial artery with stenosis of less than 50% distal to the distal anastomosis is acceptable, and neither the absence of a complete plantar arch nor the presence of vascular calcification is considered a contraindication to revascularization. The common femoral artery is generally used as the inflow for these bypasses. Shorter bypasses are preferred because of improved patency, so the SFA or popliteal artery may provide inflow if there is no proximal arterial disease. Bypasses to the arteries near the ankle or the foot can be performed if there is no patent artery more proximally.

Exposure of the posterior tibial artery is through a medial calf incision. The soleus muscle attachments to the tibia are taken down to expose the posterior tibial artery. Division of the overlying tibial veins exposes the tibial peroneal trunk. Further separation of the soleus muscle from the tibia provides access to terminal branches, the peroneal and posterior tibial arteries. For bypass to the anterior tibial artery, an additional anterolateral incision in the leg is made, midway between the tibia and fibula. Separation of the anterior tibial muscle and the extensor longus muscle exposes the neurovascular bundle. Further posterior dissection allows access to the interosseous membrane, and an incision is made to allow tunneling of the bypass graft. Exposure of the peroneal artery can be made through a medial incision, laterally by fibulectomy, or posteriorly by mobilization of the Achilles tendon.

Complications. Complications of surgery include superficial and deep wound infections, including those that involve the graft itself. One of the dreaded complications of aortic bypass is aortoduodenal fistula, which has high mortality rates. The treatment is extra-anatomic bypass and graft removal, with débridement of the retroperitoneal tissues. An alternative to extra-anatomic bypass grafting is in situ bypass using bilateral superficial femoral veins, cryopreserved aortoiliac arteries, or antibiotic-soaked Dacron graft as conduit. In case of severe sepsis, an endograft system can be placed as a temporizing measure, with endograft and graft explantation when the patient is more stable. Other complications include groin hematoma, lymphatic leak or lymphocele, femoral nerve entrapment, limb swelling, and knee contracture.

Endovascular Management

Endovascular techniques require familiarity with a variety of devices, such as wires of varying lengths, thicknesses, and flexibility with hydrophobic or hydrophilic coatings; catheters with differing curves to negotiate angles with varying degrees of flexibility; sheaths to provide scaffolding support; balloons to dilate lesions; and bare-metal and covered stents to provide continuous outward radial force, to prevent arterial recoil, and to manage occlusive disease or dissections (Fig. 62-20).

A multitude of endovascular devices and techniques are available to the surgeon to treat PAD and aneurysmal disease, but there is little consensus about the best choice. The following are all viable alternatives to reestablish continuity of blood flow; each method has its enthusiastic proponents.

Subintimal angioplasty. First described in 1987,[7] the subintimal angioplasty technique involves use of a wire to create an arterial dissection purposely, beginning at the proximal segment of the arterial occlusion. With use of this plane, a chronic total occlusion can be circumvented. Once the wire has passed beyond the lesion, it reenters the true arterial lumen. The false lumen is treated with balloon angioplasty to increase its diameter. Although technical success rates have been favorable, long-term patency and limb salvage rates have not been impressive. In a review of 472 patients treated for principally TASC C and D lesions, 63% of patients presented with critical limb ischemia and the remaining with disabling claudication.[8] Stenotic lesions were not included. The mean increase in ABI was 0.27, from 0.50 ± 0.16 to 0.77 ± 0.23. The primary patency rates were disappointing at 45%, 30%, and 25% at 12, 24, and 36 months, respectively. Patency was higher in limbs treated for claudication, whereas reduced patency was significantly associated with femorotibial occlusions and critical limb ischemia. At 3 years, primary patency was 30% for claudication and 21% for critical limb ischemia.

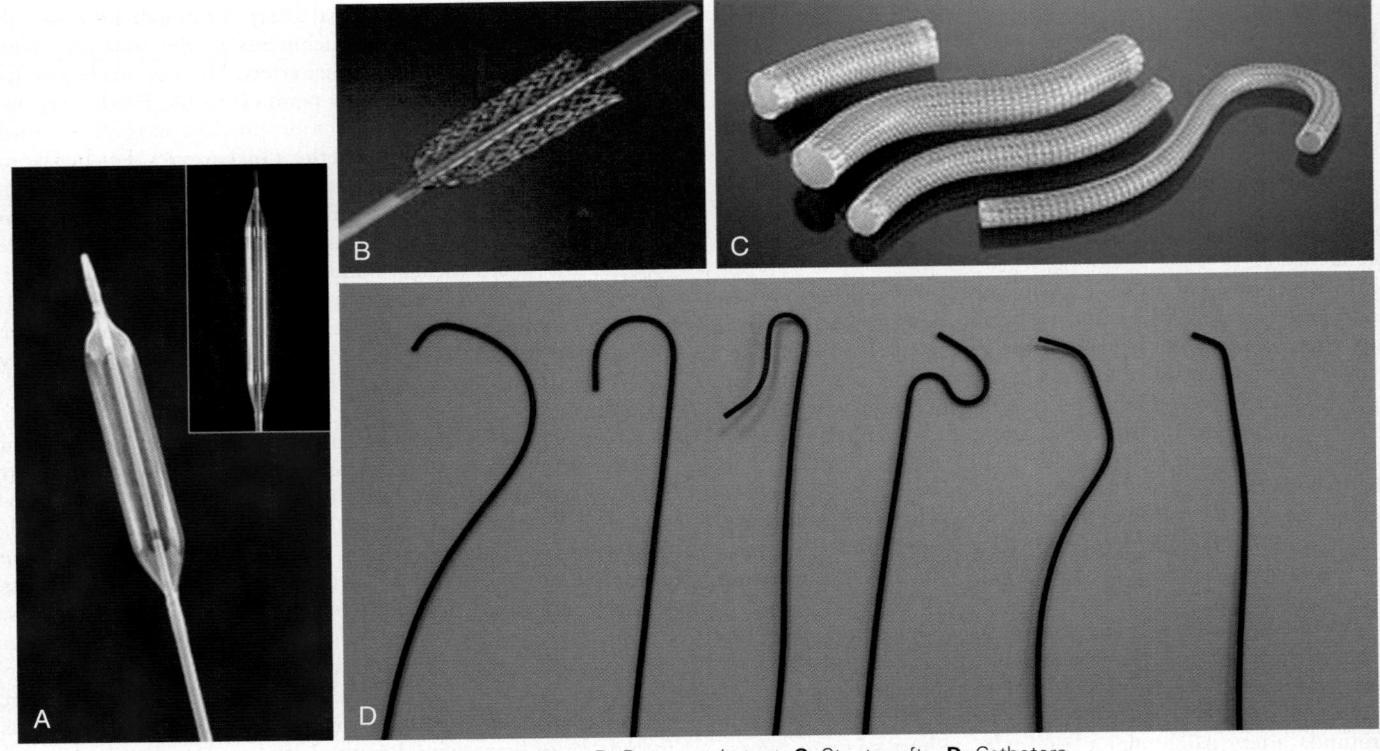

FIGURE 62-20 **A,** Balloon. **B,** Bare-metal stent. **C,** Stent grafts. **D,** Catheters.

Bare-metal stents were used in 20.3% of successful cases, but stent use was not associated with improved patency. Limb salvage for critical limb ischemia was a respectable 88% at 12 months, 81% at 24 months, and 75% at 36 months. Claudication was improved in 96.8% of limbs and sustained in 67% at 36 months. Overall, the results of subintimal angioplasty as a stand-alone procedure for critical limb ischemia have been underwhelming; adjuncts such as stents and stent grafts are often used to increase patency.

Balloon angioplasty. Balloon angioplasty, originally described in 1974, first requires crossing the arterial lesion transluminally with a guidewire and then inflating a balloon advanced over the wire at the location of the lesion. The treatment is considered successful if the residual stenosis is less than 30% or there is no pressure gradient across the area treated.

In the femoropopliteal segments, Clark and colleagues[9] reported a multicenter experience with 219 limbs in 205 patients. Patients were observed prospectively with clinical outcomes as well as objective testing by angiography or duplex ultrasound. The primary patencies at 12, 24, 36, 48, and 60 months for all limbs were 87%, 80%, 69%, 55%, and 55%, respectively. A negative predictor of long-term patency was found to be poor tibial runoff, specifically single tibial vessel runoff with 50% to 99% stenosis or occlusion. Diabetes or renal failure was also associated with lower patency.

In the tibioperoneal segment, Dorros and associates[10] reported a nonrandomized series of 312 patients with 417 vessels and 657 lesions. Overall technical success was 92% (98% in stenotic and 77% in occlusive lesions); 13 patients required stenting for intimal flap or dissection refractory to prolonged inflation. Claudication was relieved in 98% of patients with stenoses and in 86% of patients presenting with occlusions. Resolution of critical limb ischemia was noted in 98% of patients when stenotic lesions were treated and in 77% of patients with occlusions. In a subsequent report of the 5-year experience for the same patients, there were 284 limbs in 235 patients with 529 lesions.[11] Follow-up was obtained in 215 (97%) successfully treated patients; 8% of the limbs required bypass surgery and 9% required amputation, yielding an overall limb salvage rate of 91% at 5 years.

Kudo and associates[12] published a 10-year experience of angioplasty for critical limb ischemia with 138 limbs in 111 patients. The most distal lesions treated were 33% in the iliac, 30% in the femoropopliteal, and 37% in the below-knee group. By Kaplan-Meier analysis, the primary patency and limb salvage rates for the femoropopliteal and below-knee groups at 3 years were 59.4% and 92.7% and 23.5% and 77.3%, respectively. Significant independent risk factors for outcomes included multiple-segment, more distal, and TASC D lesions.

Stenting. Sabeti and colleagues[13] have reported their experience with stainless steel and nitinol self-expanding stents for the treatment of femoropopliteal diseases in a retrospectively reviewed nonrandomized study. In their studies, 175 consecutive patients presented with claudication (150 patients) and critical limb ischemia (25 patients). Stents were placed electively after balloon angioplasty failure caused by residual stenosis or flow-limiting dissection. The cumulative patency rates at 6, 12, and 24 months were 85%, 75%, and 69%, respectively, for nitinol stenting versus 78%, 54%, and 34%, respectively, for stainless steel stenting. The authors noted significantly improved primary patency rates for nitinol stents.

The same authors also reported their early experience with long lesions (median length was 16 cm) in the femoropopliteal segment using only nitinol stents after primary failure of balloon angioplasty. The overall cumulative freedom from restenosis at 6 and 12 months was 79% and 54%, respectively. This was not affected by stent length or the number of stents used.

They later randomly assigned 104 patients with stenotic or occlusive SFA lesions to undergo primary stenting (51 patients) or angioplasty (53 patients), with optional stenting (32% receiving stents).[14] The mean length of the lesions was 13.2 cm for the stent group and 12.7 cm for the angioplasty group. At 6 months, the rate of restenosis was 24% in the stent group and 43% in the angioplasty group. These results were sustained at 2 years; the restenosis rate was 45.7% for the stent group versus 69.2% for the angioplasty group. During this period, re-intervention was also lower in the primary stenting group (37% versus 53.8%).

With advances in technology, angioplasty and stenting of infrapopliteal lesions are gaining acceptance. Kickuth and coworkers[15] reported their initial experience with a low-profile, self-expanding nitinol stent. They treated 35 patients, 19 with lifestyle-limiting claudication and 16 with critical limb ischemia. Selective stenting was performed after failed balloon angioplasty caused by residual stenosis, elastic recoil, or flow-limiting dissections. Stent placement was performed in 22 patients with distal popliteal artery lesions and in 13 patients with tibioperoneal artery lesions. Technical success was achieved in all patients. Follow-up studies were performed with duplex ultrasound and angiography. The 6-month primary patency rate was 82%. The authors noted the feasibility of treating infrapopliteal lesions with the new nitinol stent.

A meta-analysis was reported by Mwipatayi and colleagues[16] comparing balloon angioplasty with stenting for the treatment of femoropopliteal lesions. Seven randomized controlled trials between September 2000 and January 2007 comparing angioplasty with stenting were used for this meta-analysis. Of a total of 934 patients, 482 patients were treated with stenting and the rest (452) with balloon angioplasty. The mean length treated was 4.3 cm in the angioplasty group and 4.6 cm in the stent group. The use of stents did not improve the patency rate at 1 year, which varied from 63% to 90%. However, limitations include length of follow-up, various stents used, and inconsistent use of optimal medical therapy.

Stent graft. One of the most widely used stent grafts (Fig. 62-21) in the treatment of chronic lower extremity ischemia is the Viabahn endoprosthesis (Gore Medical, Flagstaff, Ariz). It is constructed with an expanded PTFE liner attached to an external nitinol stent. The inner surface is bonded with heparin. This stent graft is extremity flexible, allowing it to conform closely to the anatomy of the SFA.

Railo and coworkers[17] first reported preliminary results in 15 patients with femoropopliteal lesions. The clinical presentation varied from claudication to acute leg ischemia as well as one ruptured popliteal artery aneurysm. Primary patency rates at 1 month, 12 months, and 24 months were 100%, 93%, and 84%, respectively. There was no limb loss during the follow-up period.

In a 6-year experience, Fischer and associates[18] evaluated outcomes for 57 patients treated for stenoses (13%) or occlusions (87%) of the SFA. The average length of treated lesions was 10.7 cm; 10% suffered early thrombosis of the graft within 30 days. The mean follow-up was 55 months (range, 8 to 78 months). The primary patency rates for 30 days, 1 year, 3 years, and 5 years were 90%, 67%, 57%, and 45%, respectively. In an earlier long-term study, Bleyn and coworkers[19] treated 67 patients with a mean lesion length of 14.3 cm. The 5-year primary patency rate was 47%.

Comparison of Viabahn treatment with different modalities has been reported by several authors. Saxon and associates[20] compared stent graft with percutaneous transluminal angioplasty alone in a multicenter, prospective randomized study. The stent graft group had a significantly higher technical success rate (95% versus 66%; $P < .0001$) and higher 1-year primary patency rate (65% versus 40% for percutaneous transluminal angioplasty alone).

In a prospective randomized study, Kedora and coworkers[21] compared Viabahn with above-knee surgical bypass with synthetic graft material; 86 patients with 100 limbs were randomized to 50 limbs each for the stent graft and bypass. The mean length of artery stented was 25.6 cm. ABIs and duplex ultrasonography were used for follow-up. At 3, 6, 9, and 12 months, the primary patency rates were 84%, 82%, 75.6%, and 73.5% for stent grafts, respectively; for bypass, they were 90%, 81.8%, 79.7%, and 74.2%, respectively. The authors also noted similar re-intervention and secondary patency rates.

Cutting balloon. The cutting balloon was originally designed for use in the coronary artery for lesions resistant to compliant balloon angioplasty or in-stent restenotic lesions. The balloon features three or four atherotomes, or microsurgical blades, mounted longitudinally on the surface of a noncompliant balloon. The blades score the lesion and dilate the vessels with less force than in conventional balloon angioplasty.

Atherectomy. Endovascular atherectomy allows the physical removal of atherosclerotic plaque material from the blood vessel, with a theoretical benefit of removing the obstructing plaque rather than merely displacing it, as with angioplasty and stenting. Excisional atherectomy catheters remove and collect the atheroma, whereas ablative devices fragment the atheroma into small particles. Rotational cutters turn at speeds up to 8000 rpm, shaving the atherosclerotic plaque material from the luminal surface of the arterial wall and collecting it in a storage chamber. The 1-year patency rates range from 22% to 84%, with limb salvage rates of 62% to 86%.[22]

An example of ablative atherectomy includes the laser atherectomy, a cold-tipped laser that delivers bursts of ultraviolet xenon energy in short pulse durations. Its reported key feature is the ability to debulk tissue without damaging surrounding tissue, minimizing restenosis. Compared with balloon angioplasty alone, no difference was reported in 1-year patency or technical success.[23] The largest trial was the LACI (Laser Angioplasty for Critical Limb Ischemia) phase 2 study that involved 14 sites in the United States and Germany.[24] There were 145 patients with 155 limbs and 423 lesions: 41% SFA, 15% popliteal, 41% infrapopliteal, and 70% a combination of stenoses. Technical success was achieved in 86% of limbs, with most lesions TASC C and D. Limb salvage at 6 months was 93%.

Acute Limb Ischemia

A popular mnemonic for describing the presentation of an acutely ischemic leg is referred to as the five or six *p*'s, depending on one's willingness to include *p*oikilothermia; *p*ain, *p*allor, *p*ulselessness, *p*aresthesias, and *p*aralysis are often cited as indicative of acute arterial ischemia. These symptoms and findings, however, are often variable in degree and not necessarily predictive of the extent of disease or degree of ischemia. A similar presentation may be seen in the setting of blunt or penetrating trauma, in which the native, nondiseased blood supply is suddenly interrupted. It is the acuity of the insult that leads to this constellation of symptoms; the chronically ischemic limb may have become so over a duration of time that allowed collateral flow to develop. The patient with acute ischemia may have less developed collateral circulation and less tolerance to prolonged ischemia.

The cause of acute limb ischemia is usually thromboembolism in the intervention-naïve patient. The source of the embolism can

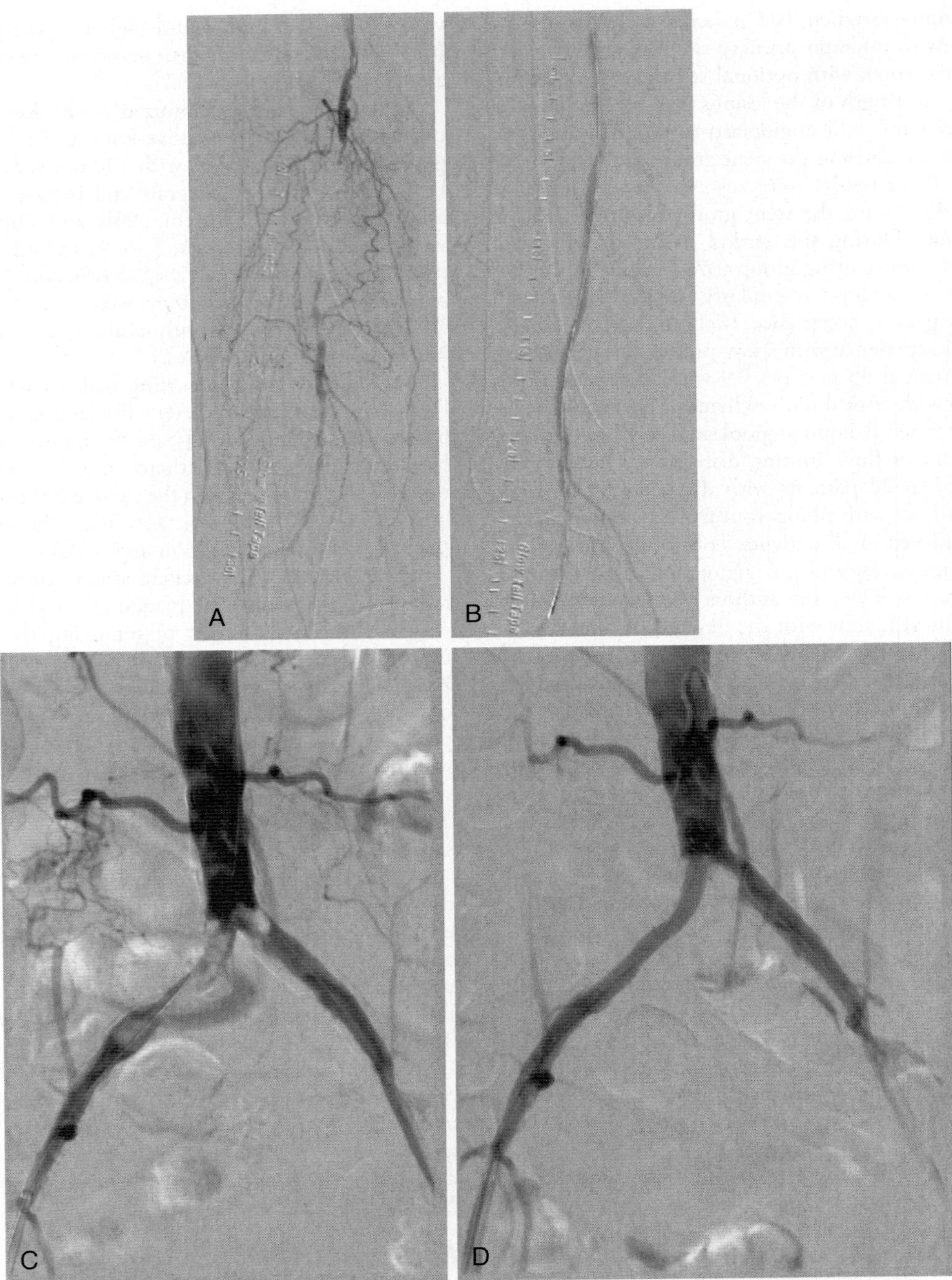

FIGURE 62-21 **A,** Distal superficial femoral to proximal popliteal artery occlusion. **B,** Completion angiogram after recanalization and stent placement. **C,** Bilateral common iliac artery thrombus, acute. **D,** Successful treatment with stent graft. Flow was restored without distal embolization.

be the heart, in which case atrial fibrillation is a commonly observed comorbidity. Alternative embolic sources include the valvular leaflets, and the aorta and iliac arteries may house thrombus, with or without concurrent aneurysmal disease. Patients presenting with a surgical history of previous bypass or stent placement may have an acute occlusion from graft or stent failure or may have disease progression. This history and the location of the occlusive lesion will affect surgical decision making. Acute limb ischemia constitutes a surgical emergency. As in most cases of vascular disease, there are endovascular and open surgical methods for addressing the problem.

As in all cases, a detailed history and physical examination are needed for a clinical diagnosis of the severity of disease:

- Category I limbs are viable and not immediately threatened.
- Category IIa limbs are threatened but salvageable if treated.
- Category IIb limbs are salvageable if treated as an emergency.
- Category III limbs have irreversible ischemia and are not salvageable.

Therefore, patients whose limbs are viable and do not appear immediately threatened (category I) as well as patients whose limbs are threatened but salvageable without paralysis but with mild sensory changes (category IIa) are potential candidates for

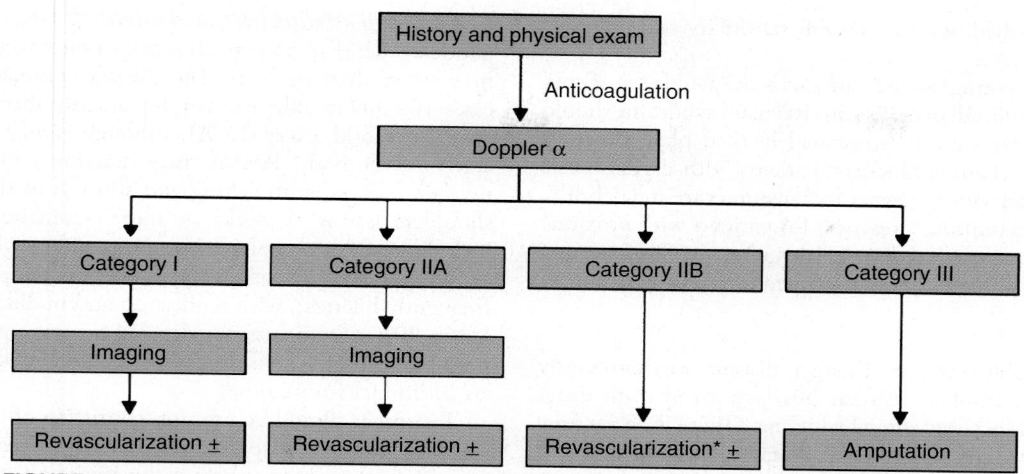

FIGURE 62-22 Treatment Algorithm for Acute Limb Ischemia. (From Norgren L, Hiatt WR, Dormandy JA, et al: Inter-Society Consensus for the Management of Peripheral Arterial Disease [TASC II]. *J Vasc Surg* 45 [Suppl]:S5–S67, 2007.) Category I—Viable; Category IIA—Marginally Threatened; Category IIB—Immediately Threatened; α Confirming either absent or severely diminished ankle pressure/signals; *In some centers imaging would be performed.

thrombolytic therapy. Patients with threatened limbs with more significant neurologic changes (category IIb) require a more urgent intervention and may best be served with an operative intervention. Patients with irreversible ischemia and a nonsalvageable limb usually require primary amputation (Fig. 62-22).

Patients with viable or minimally threatened limbs are candidates for thrombolytic therapy. They must have no contraindication to thrombolysis, which would include an active bleeding diathesis, recent gastrointestinal bleeding (<10 days), intracranial or spinal surgery, and intracranial trauma within the previous 3 months. Also, patients with a recent cerebrovascular accident, within 2 months, represent an absolute contraindication to thrombolysis. Relative major contraindications include major nonvascular surgery or trauma within the previous 10 days, uncontrolled hypertension, puncture of noncompressible vessels, intracranial tumors, and recent eye surgery. Minor contraindications to thrombolysis include hepatic failure, bacterial endocarditis, pregnancy, and diabetic hemorrhagic retinopathy.

An alternative to thrombolysis is open thrombectomy. Patients are begun on heparin on presentation. Proximal and distal control on the femoral versus below-knee popliteal artery is obtained. A longitudinal arteriotomy is created, and the thrombectomy balloon is passed proximally and distally with care until excellent forward bleeding and reasonable backbleeding are seen. Fluoroscopy can be used to assist in the thrombectomy procedure, with contrast material used in the embolectomy balloon and within the artery. Once the clot is successfully removed, the artery is flushed proximally and distally with heparinized saline before the clamps are replaced. Patch angioplasty should be considered to avoid narrowing of the artery. Completion angiography is helpful for confirming removal of most of the thrombus and identifying a culprit lesion. Four-compartment fasciotomy may be necessary, depending on the duration of ischemic insult.

Complications of open thrombectomy include intimal damage and dissection. Complications of thrombolysis include bleeding, which in minor cases is from the arterial access, venipuncture sites, or Foley catheter, but it can be severe and lead to hemothorax, gastrointestinal bleeding, and symptomatic intracranial hemorrhage.

If no culprit lesion is found, the patient should undergo a hypercoagulable workup. Oral anticoagulation should be considered.

OTHER CAUSES OF ACUTE AND CHRONIC LIMB ISCHEMIA

Nonatherosclerotic Arteriopathies

Other causes of arterial occlusive disease, although far less common than atherosclerosis in the West, should be considered for patients who do not fit the risk factor profile outlined earlier.

Raynaud Syndrome

Episodic digital ischemia was first described by Maurice Raynaud in 1862. Raynaud phenomenon is characterized by recurrent episodic vasospasm of the digits precipitated by a stimulus such as environmental cold or emotional stress, manifesting as tricolor changes—white, blue, and red. It initially produces pallor from cold exposure and vasoconstriction, subsequent cyanosis from hypoxia, and then rubor from the hyperemic response associated with rewarming. The digits return to normal 10 to 15 minutes after removal of the stimulus, and the fingers remain normal between ischemic episodes. Fingers of both hands are usually involved, extending to the metacarpophalangeal joint, with sparing of the thumb. The lower extremities are rarely involved. The clinical spectrum is broad, ranging from milder forms managed by avoidance to cold to more severe symptoms of ulceration and tissue loss from vascular occlusions beyond vasospasm. Secondary Raynaud phenomenon can be associated with various connective tissue diseases, such as scleroderma, or exposure to drugs, toxins, or repetitive trauma.

The prevalence of Raynaud syndrome varies with climate, approaching 20% to 25% in cool, damp regions such as Scandinavia and the Pacific Northwest. It usually occurs in young women, with a median age at onset of 14 years, and rarely after the age of 40 years. In these patients, 25% have a family history of Raynaud syndrome in a first-degree relative.

The evaluation of patients for Raynaud syndrome should include complete blood cell count determination of erythrocyte sedimentation rate, antinuclear antibody titer, and rheumatoid factor. Routine vascular laboratory testing with digital photoplethysmography and digital blood pressures can help distinguish patients with obstructive disease from those with an abnormal vasoconstrictive response. A digital hypothermic cold challenge test has been described, with an overall sensitivity and accuracy of approximately 90%.

The hallmark of conservative treatment is the avoidance of cold and emotional stimuli. All patients with Raynaud syndrome should refrain from tobacco use. The most widely used pharmacologic agents are calcium channel blockers. Patients with digital ulcers can usually be healed with aggressive local wound care and débridement. Surgical intervention is reserved for patients with proximal atherosclerotic or aneurysmal disease in an effort to eliminate any embolic source or potential physical impediment to perfusion.

Buerger Disease

Thromboangiitis obliterans, or Buerger disease, predominantly affects young male smokers in their 30s, presenting with distal limb ischemia and localized digital gangrene. There is an increasing incidence in women that likely parallels changes in smoking patterns. There is an increased incidence in patients of eastern European or Japanese heritage. Diagnostic hallmarks include age at onset before 45 years, exposure to tobacco, absence of arterial lesions proximal to the knee or elbow, and absence of other atherosclerotic risk factors.

Thromboangiitis obliterans is a polyarteritis nodosa vasculitis, with surgical specimens showing involvement of arteries and veins. Occlusive lesions are seen typically in small and medium-sized arteries. It usually occurs in the distal portions of the upper and lower extremities distal to the elbow and knee. Patients frequently have rest pain, ulceration, and, often, digital gangrene. Objective confirmation can be obtained with four-limb digital plethysmography, showing obstructive arterial waveforms in all digits. Arteriography typically reveals extensively diseased infrageniculate vessels and diffuse plantar arterial occlusions. The reconstitution of distal arterial segments is provided by tortuous, pathognomonic, corkscrew collaterals.

Treatment requires absolute tobacco cessation, which often results in clinical remission. Finger ulcers can frequently be healed with aggressive local wound care. Up to one third of patients with lower extremity disease will eventually require major amputation. Distal arterial bypass or endovascular intervention should be considered when it is anatomically feasible for critical limb ischemia, but the distal to proximal pattern of disease progression often precludes successful surgical revascularization. Currently, there is no effective pharmacologic treatment.

Vasculitis

The term *vasculitis* refers to a primary inflammatory process involving blood vessels with resultant transmural injury, necrosis, and obstruction or obliteration of the lumen. Vessels of any size and location can be affected. A useful classification system for vasculitis may be based on the size of the vessels involved by the inflammatory process: large-, medium-, or small-vessel vasculitis.

Large-Vessel Vasculitis

The large-vessel vasculitides includes giant cell arteritis (GCA), also referred to as temporal arteritis, and Takayasu arteritis. Although both vasculitides can affect the aorta and its major branches, GCA primarily involves the extracranial branches of the carotid artery. GCA usually occurs in older patients, whereas Takayasu arteritis afflicts younger female patients, with a higher prevalence in those of Asian or eastern European heritage. Both conditions are associated with the development of aneurysms of the thoracic and abdominal aorta and the progression of occlusive disease in the carotid, upper extremity, visceral, and renal arteries.

Giant cell arteritis (temporal arteritis). GCA usually occurs in patients older than 55 years. It is two to three times more common in women than in men. The average annual incidence is 18 cases/100,000 in older women. It primarily affects branches of the external carotid artery (ECA), although it may involve any large artery of the body. Patients may describe a history of a febrile myalgic process, with aching and stiffness of the hip, back, and shoulders lasting 4 weeks or more. Constitutional symptoms include headaches, malaise, anorexia, and weight loss. A characteristic presentation is severe pain over the temporal artery that is frequently bilateral, with tenderness and nodularity of the artery. Up to 20% of patients may develop permanent unilateral blindness; one third of them progress to contralateral blindness within an additional week's time.

Treatment should be prompt, consisting of high-dose corticosteroids. Patients suspected of having GCA should undergo temporal artery biopsy before the initiation of steroid therapy. Bilateral sequential temporal artery biopsies may be needed. The erythrocyte sedimentation rate is elevated in 75% of patients, although the C-reactive protein level may be a more sensitive indicator.

Early initiation of steroid therapy can result in prevention of blindness and restoration of pulses. Revascularization is rarely needed because of the collateral vessels that develop; it is relatively contraindicated during the acute phase of GCA.

Takayasu disease. Takayasu disease most commonly occurs in young, Asian female patients ranging in age from 3 to 35 years (85%). Patients present initially with fever, anorexia, and myalgia, followed by a second stage of multiple arterial occlusive symptoms, depending on the location of disease involvement.

The disease frequently affects the aorta, its major branches, and the pulmonary artery. Lesions are usually stenotic but may also be manifested as aneurysmal degeneration. Four patterns of cardiovascular manifestations have been described. Type I is localized to the arch and the arch vessels. Type II involves the descending thoracic and abdominal aorta. Type III involves the arch vessels and abdominal aorta and its branches. Type IV involves the pulmonary arteries.

Patients are best treated with conservative medical management. Surgical or endovascular intervention is used for symptomatic stenotic disease but is undertaken only when the active inflammatory process has been brought under control.

Medium-Vessel Vasculitis

Polyarteritis nodosa. Polyarteritis nodosa is a disseminated disease with transmural arterial necrosis of the medium-sized arteries. It occurs typically in the fourth to sixth decade and is more common in men than in women by a 2:1 margin. The arteries of the kidney, liver, heart, and gastrointestinal tract are commonly affected. It is characterized by the formation of multiple visceral aneurysms, with attendant risk of rupture. Alternatively, the inflammatory process of polyarteritis nodosa may lead to arterial occlusions, manifesting as enteric perforation, gastrointestinal bleeding, or appendicitis.

Immunosuppressive therapy has greatly improved the 5-year survival from 15% to 80%. Patients with mild symptoms can be treated with steroid therapy alone. However, patients with poor prognostic indicators, such as renal insufficiency, require immunosuppressive therapy in addition to steroids.

Kawasaki disease. Kawasaki disease is an acute vasculitis with a predilection for involving the coronary arteries in children younger than 5 years, with a peak incidence at 1 year of age. Boys are affected more commonly than girls. The distinguishing feature of advanced Kawasaki disease is the formation of diffuse fusiform and saccular coronary artery aneurysms. Systemic arteritis can also occur, commonly affecting the iliac arteries in addition to the coronaries.

Death may result from acute myocardial infarction or arrhythmia following thrombosis of a coronary artery aneurysm. Alternatively, aneurysm rupture may occur. Treatment with aspirin and immune globulin therapy has decreased the mortality during the past 2 decades and reduced the incidence of coronary artery aneurysmal degeneration. If refractory, more complete immunosuppressive therapy should be considered.

Behçet disease. Behçet disease commonly is manifested as iritis associated with oral and genital mucocutaneous ulcerations. It primarily affects patients from the Mediterranean area and Japan. The vasculitis component of Behçet disease involves the venous and arterial systems. Venous thrombosis is the most common vascular disorder with Behçet disease. Arterial lesions, although less frequent, are associated with a higher incidence of mortality. The usual cause of mortality in these patients is aortic aneurysmal degeneration and rupture.

Patients with Behçet disease and venous thrombosis are managed with lifelong oral anticoagulation. Immunosuppressive therapy is used for nonarterial symptoms, such as mucocutaneous lesions and eye disease. Traditional aneurysm repair with interposition grafting has been associated with a high incidence of thrombosis and anastomotic pseudoaneurysms. Endovascular aneurysm repair is emerging as the treatment of choice.

Cogan syndrome. Cogan syndrome is a rare disease consisting of interstitial keratitis and vestibuloauditory symptoms. It may occasionally consist of aortitis, with subsequent aortic valvular insufficiency. Cogan syndrome commonly affects young patients in their third decade. High-dose steroid therapy can be used to reverse visual and auditory complications. Surgical intervention may be needed for aortic valve replacement, mesenteric revascularization, or thoracoabdominal aortic aneurysm repair.

Small-Vessel Vasculitis

Antineutrophil cytoplasmic antibody–associated vasculitides. The major forms of small-vessel vasculitis are associated with the presence of antineutrophil cytoplasmic antibodies, autoantibodies formed against enzymes found in primary granules of neutrophils. Antineutrophil cytoplasmic antibody–associated vasculitides include Wegener granulomatosis, microscopic polyangiitis, and Churg-Strauss syndrome and often have circulating antineutrophil cytoplasmic antibodies. Wegener granulomatosis is the most common form. The overall incidence of antineutrophil cytoplasmic antibody–associated vasculitides in the population is 10 to 20 per million/year, affecting men and women equally, with a peak onset in the 60s. Patients present with constitutional symptoms that include fever and weight loss. Wegener granulomatosis is characterized by renal and respiratory tract involvement. Microscopic polyangiitis is characterized by rapid progressive glomerulonephritis in almost all patients. Churg-Strauss syndrome is characterized by allergic rhinitis and asthma, eosinophilic infiltrative disease, and small-vessel vasculitis. Diagnostic testing should include assessment for inflammatory markers and for liver and renal function as well as assays for antineutrophil cytoplasmic antibodies, antinuclear antibodies, and rheumatoid factor. Small-vessel vasculitis can be documented by microscopic examinations of biopsy specimens from affected tissues, such as skin and kidney. Treatment involves three stages using corticosteroids and immunosuppressive therapy—induction of remission, maintenance of remission, and treatment of relapses.

Vasculitis Associated With Connective Tissue Diseases

Vasculitis is frequently associated with scleroderma, rheumatoid arthritis, and systemic lupus erythematosus. Scleroderma is characterized by small-vessel occlusion within the arterioles of the skin, gastrointestinal tract, kidneys, lung, and heart. Rheumatoid arthritis typically involves digital arteries and small vessels of the vasa nervorum. Lupus patients commonly have Raynaud syndrome but may also have atherosclerosis of large vessels. Treatment consists of steroid and immunosuppressive therapies.

Heritable Arteriopathies

Cystic Medial Necrosis

Cystic medial necrosis, formerly known as medial degeneration, is associated with collagen vascular disorders, Ehlers-Danlos syndrome, and Marfan syndrome, with elastolysis degrading aortic medial collagen and elastin. Aortic dissection is the result. Although it is also seen in normal aging, cystic medial necrosis is accelerated by hypertension and atherosclerosis.

Pseudoxanthoma Elasticum

Pseudoxanthoma elasticum is an inherited disease, with most patients demonstrating an autosomal recessive inheritance. The prevalence is 1 in 70,000 to 160,000. Patients present with baggy skin and yellow-orange cutaneous papules in intertriginous areas. Symptoms may include intermittent claudication, angina, and abdominal pain caused by involvement of cerebral, coronary, visceral, and peripheral vessels. Arterial disease can be seen in young patients (20s to 30s) without risk factors for atherosclerosis. Digital plethysmography shows abnormal pulse waveforms from loss of the elastic recoil of vessels. Arterial stenosis and occlusion with extensive calcification can be seen radiographically. Surgical and endovascular management options are the same as for atherosclerotic occlusive disease.

Arteria Magna Syndrome

Arteria magna syndrome is a disease characterized by arterial elongation, dilation, and tortuosity. It occurs in younger patients with no evidence of atherosclerosis, with a familial incidence in first-degree relatives. There is a propensity for arterial aneurysm formation in multiple sites. Arteriograms show characteristic arterial widening and tortuosity, slow arterial flow velocity, and multiple aneurysms. The low-velocity arterial flow makes arteriography difficult to perform, requiring a large volume of contrast material and multiple injections with delayed timing. These patients should be screened annually for the development of aneurysms in the aorta and iliac, femoral, and popliteal arteries. Symptomatic aneurysms or those whose diameter is 2 to 2.5 times that of the parent arteries should be repaired. Complications of arterial occlusions are almost always caused by thrombosis or embolization. A number of surgical interventions are often needed for aneurysms at multiple sites.

Congenital Conditions Affecting the Arteries

Persistent Sciatic Artery

The sciatic artery in the embryo is a vessel that arises from the umbilical artery and supplies the lower extremity. During development, this artery is replaced by the femoral artery from the external iliac artery, and the remnants of the sciatic artery remain as the inferior gluteal artery, distal popliteal artery, and peroneal artery. Rarely, this sciatic artery persists as a large artery that is located in the posterior thigh, exiting the pelvis to continue as the popliteal artery. The SFA may coexist or be hypoplastic or absent. On occasion, this may be detected in an individual with an absent femoral pulse but palpable distal pulses. However, the persistent sciatic artery usually is not detected until patients are in their 50s and symptoms typical of PVD develop. Up to 25% of patients may present with pulsatile buttock masses caused by aneurysmal degeneration. Surgical intervention is indicated for ischemic and aneurysmal complications. Options include arterial ligation, endovascular coiling for occlusion of an isolated aneurysm, and iliopopliteal or femoropopliteal bypasses.

Popliteal Entrapment Syndromes

This syndrome is based on an anomalous anatomic relationship between the popliteal artery and surrounding gastrocnemius muscle that may occur during embryonic development. The most common variant (50%) is the medial location of the popliteal artery to the normally placed medial head of the gastrocnemius muscle. The second most common variant (25%) is the medial location of the popliteal artery to the abnormally attached medial head of the gastrocnemius muscle. In other variants, the normally located popliteal artery may be compressed by muscle slips of the medial head of the gastrocnemius muscle or fibrous bands. Symptoms are caused by obstruction of the popliteal artery with gastrocnemius contraction. The typical patient is a younger man (younger than 30 years; 90%) without risk factors for PVD; 20% of patients have the disorder bilaterally. Popliteal entrapment syndrome should be suspected in younger patients with calf claudication.

Diagnosis with noninvasive arterial duplex ultrasound and photoplethysmography is difficult and findings are nonspecific. Arteriography may be nonspecific. MRI is the diagnostic modality of choice because it will show the anomalous relationships between the popliteal artery and gastrocnemius muscle. Treatment is indicated for symptomatic patients and requires surgical intervention. Removal of the medial gastrocnemius head may be sufficient for patients with minimal arterial disease. Patients with arterial stenosis or aneurysmal degeneration should be treated with arterial bypass using autogenous veins.

Adventitial Cystic Disease

Adventitial cystic disease is another rare condition that should be considered in younger patients with claudication. The arterial stenosis is caused by compression of the lumen from synovial-like cysts in the subadventitial layer of the arterial wall. It is commonly located in the popliteal artery but may also be found in the iliac and femoral arteries. Patients present in their 40s, and 80% are men. Diagnosis may be made with ultrasonography, CT, or MRI. Arteriography may show a scimitar sign, with luminal compression by the cyst. The artery is normally placed, with no signs of atherosclerotic disease. Treatment with CT- or ultrasound-guided needle aspiration may be used for small cysts, although there may be a 10% rate of recurrence. Arterial bypass with an autogenous vein is used for patients with large cysts causing arterial compression or occlusion.

Peripheral Artery Aneurysms

Femoral and Popliteal Artery Aneurysms

Femoral and popliteal artery aneurysms account for more than 90% of peripheral aneurysms, with popliteal artery aneurysms being the most common (70%). However, they are still relatively uncommon. The estimated incidence of femoral and popliteal aneurysms is approximately 7/100,000 men and 1/100,000 women. Femoral aneurysms usually involve the common femoral artery but may occasionally extend or be limited to the SFA in the midthigh. Femoral and popliteal aneurysms are commonly associated with other aneurysms, with approximately 80% of patients having multiple aneurysms. In patients with common femoral aneurysms, 90% have an aortoiliac aneurysm and 60% have bilateral femoral aneurysms. In patients with popliteal aneurysms, 70% have an aortoiliac aneurysm and 50% have bilateral popliteal aneurysms. Femoral and popliteal aneurysms show a high incidence of thromboembolic complications, which can result in limb loss.

The diagnosis of femoral and popliteal aneurysms is suspected in patients with widened pulses that are easily palpated. These aneurysms should be considered in patients presenting with foot embolization or acute limb ischemia. CT and ultrasonography can accurately diagnose the femoral and popliteal aneurysms. Ultrasonography should be used for patients with aortoiliac aneurysms to search for these peripheral aneurysms. Arteriography is important for visualization of the aneurysms and runoff to plan for surgical intervention.

Femoral and popliteal aneurysms should be considered for treatment when the diagnosis is made. Because of the high incidence of thromboembolic events, these aneurysms are repaired, regardless of size. Even small aneurysms can cause ischemic limb complications. Surgical intervention of the femoral aneurysms consists of resection of the aneurysms with interposition grafts. Treatment of the popliteal aneurysms usually involves bypass using autogenous veins, with exclusion of the aneurysm to prevent embolization. Patients with ischemic limbs from embolic complications may require thrombolytic therapy to establish arterial outflow before bypass surgery. Endovascular repair with covered stents is emerging as the treatment of choice for popliteal aneurysms (Fig. 62-23).

Evaluating the Success of Revascularization Procedures

Although there is a lack of consensus about the best endovascular modality to use for most patients, there is certainly a need for routine follow-up and close involvement of all patients treated for claudication and critical limb ischemia. The ultimate success of any intervention performed, endovascular or open surgical bypass, can be improved by a continued relationship with the patient and regular examination. Smoking cessation counseling and adjuvant techniques, such as medications and nicotine replacement, are used routinely to help patients with this important aspect of their treatment. Lifelong administration of oral antiplatelet agents (81 mg aspirin daily and 75 mg clopidogrel daily) and aggressive lipid modification in all patients who have had a vascular intervention are routine.

Duplex arterial ultrasound has gained wide acceptance as the modality of choice for surgical bypass graft surveillance, and it has become the standard for observing patients treated with endovascular therapy. Contemporary practice guidelines include a baseline duplex ultrasonography scan before intervention, another after the intervention to document improvement (the timing of this scan varies from 1 day to 2 weeks after the intervention), and then additional scans at 3 and 6 months after the procedure to assess for continued efficacy. Duplex ultrasonography is then performed at 6-month intervals thereafter. Evaluation of continued

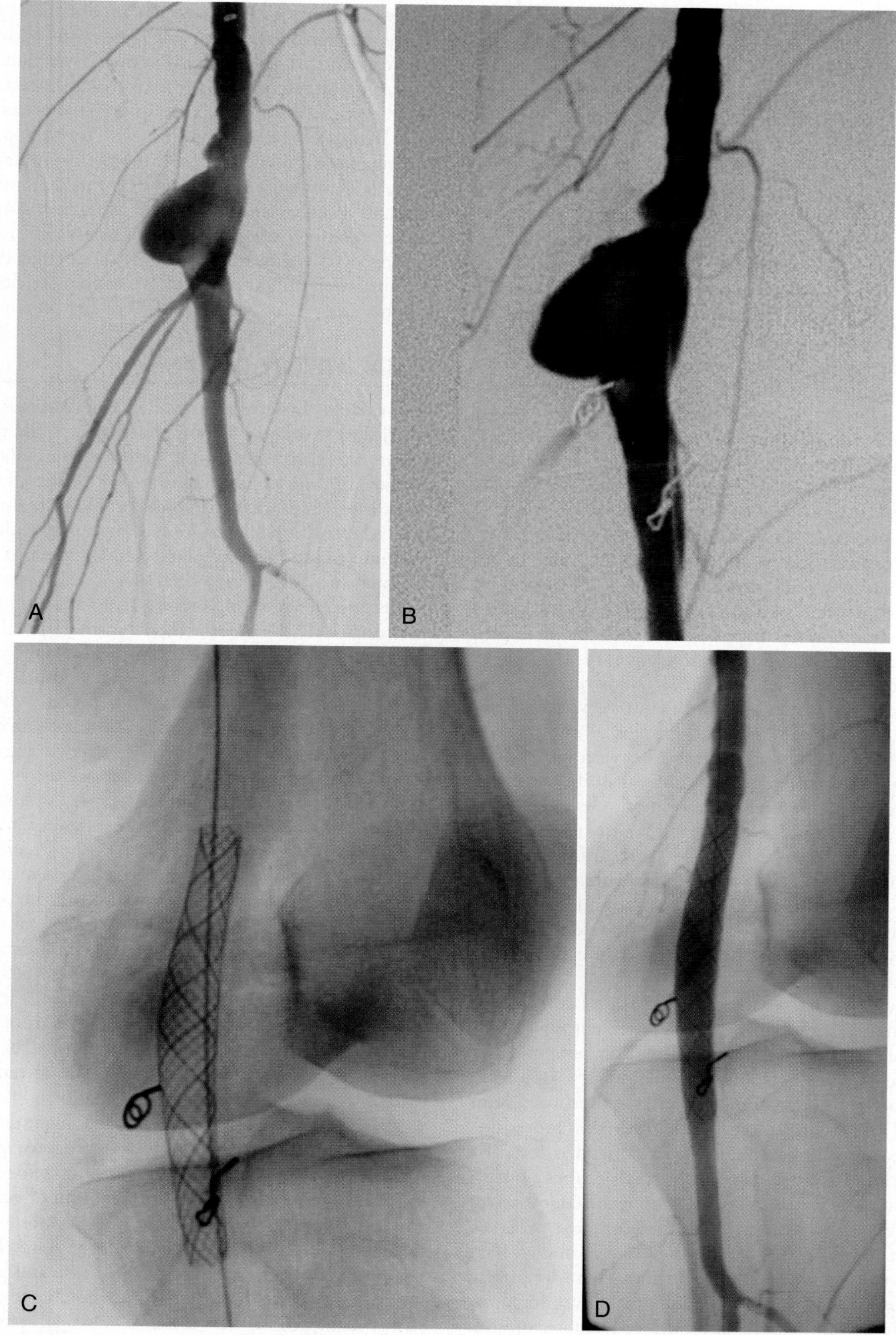

FIGURE 62-23 **A,** Popliteal aneurysm. **B,** Collateral feeding branches treated with coil embolization. **C,** Stent placement to exclude flow into aneurysm sac. **D,** Completion angiogram showing successful repair.

subjective clinical improvement and determination of ABIs are essential and simple adjunctive measures that should be performed at each visit. Most studies discussed earlier used duplex ultrasonography as their method of imaging follow-up. Although very early studies and coronary trials used routine postprocedure contrast angiography (at 6 months and 1 year), the ready availability, lower risk, and proven sensitivity and specificity of duplex ultrasonography have made it the preferred method of follow-up over contrast angiography. Once a problem has been identified, routine surveillance with duplex ultrasonography and selective angiography is the standard for open and endovascular intervention.

The benefit of graft surveillance by duplex ultrasonography in lower extremity bypass has been established. Reports have shown that all vein grafts progress to occlusion when stenosis of more than 70% diameter reduction is detected by ultrasound surveillance. Buth and coworkers further established the duplex criteria needed to identify high-risk lesions: peak systolic velocity at the site of the lesion exceeding 300 to 350 cm/sec or a velocity ratio exceeding 3.5 or 4.[25] The ratio is calculated using the peak systolic velocity at the site of the lesion divided by the peak systolic velocity of a normal graft segment proximal to the lesion.

Using these duplex criteria, Mills and colleagues[26] studied the natural history of autogenous infrainguinal vein grafts with intermediate and critical stenosis. A peak systolic velocity higher than 300 cm/sec or velocity ratio of more than 4 was used to detect critical stenosis. In grafts with the unrevised critical stenosis, almost 80% progressed to occlusion, all within 4 months of ultrasound detection. For grafts with intermediate stenosis, the occlusion rate was no different from that of grafts without stenosis, and serial surveillance was safe and effective.

Calligaro and associates[27] have established the usefulness of surveillance in prosthetic grafts; 85 prosthetic bypasses in 59 patients were studied in a graft surveillance protocol. There were 35 femoropopliteal, 16 femorotibial, 15 iliofemoral, 13 axillofemoral, and 6 femorofemoral bypasses. The benefit of duplex ultrasound was compared with other noninvasive studies, such as changes in symptoms or pulses and ABI. Follow-up was performed 1 week and every 3 months after the initial bypass or after graft revision, for a mean of 11 months. Duplex ultrasound was able to predict 81% of graft failures versus 24% with use of nonultrasound findings. In the presence of a normal study, the likelihood of a graft failure was 7% with use of duplex criteria versus 21% with nonultrasound studies. In contrast, Carter and coworkers[28] concluded that surveillance is a valid method for detecting high-risk lesions in vein grafts but failed in prosthetic and femorocrural grafts. It was noted that prosthetic grafts and femorocrural bypasses tended to occlude without any prior documented stenosis, whereas vein grafts were more likely to develop progressive stenosis before occlusion.

Lesion characteristics detected during ultrasound surveillance may also be used to determine the type of re-intervention needed. Gonsalves and colleagues[29] noted factors based on temporal and duplex data. Percutaneous transluminal angioplasty is recommended for short (<2 cm) stenoses in good-caliber veins (≥3.5 mm) found more than 3 months after the bypass procedure. Direct surgical repair or replacement is recommended for early (<3 months) and long-segment stenoses in small-caliber veins.

Although the use of duplex ultrasonography in endovascular follow-up is intuitive and consistent with the usefulness observed in the management of surgical bypass, few large studies have looked at its ability to predict failure and impact on long-term results. Tielbeek and coworkers[30] used duplex ultrasonography surveillance, clinical examination, and ABI on femoropopliteal lesions successfully treated with endovascular interventions. Impending failure was diagnosed with a peak systolic velocity ratio of more than 2.5. Failure was diagnosed as occlusion or recurrent stenosis requiring intervention for severe symptoms. Treatment failure was predicted by duplex ultrasonography, with a sensitivity of 86% and a specificity of 75%. Interestingly, ABI decrease was even more predictive, with a sensitivity of 93% and specificity of 90%.

Critical limb ischemia is often a hallmark of the beginning of the end game in the battle for survival in patients with diffuse atherosclerotic disease. With a known 5-year survival of less than 50%, this population is extremely disadvantaged. The surgeon's best chance for helping this group of patients lies in providing the least invasive intervention that will provide pain relief, tissue healing, and limb salvage. Close follow-up with appropriate counseling is essential, as is intensive medical management with repeated interventions performed as clinical conditions warrant. These measures offer the best strategy for limb salvage and improved mortality for patients with vascular disease. However, the final determinant of success is the patient's perception of enhancement in the quality of his or her remaining years of life.

RENAL ARTERY DISEASE

Renovascular hypertension occurs as a consequence of decreased blood flow through a stenotic renal artery. The renin-angiotensin system is a potent regulator of blood pressure. Renin is an enzyme produced in the juxtaglomerular cells of the afferent arterioles of the kidney. It is released into the bloodstream in response to reduced renal blood flow. Once it is systemic, renin acts on a plasma substrate to produce angiotensin I. Angiotensin I is converted to angiotensin II in the pulmonary circulation by angiotensin-converting enzyme. Angiotensin II, in addition to being a potent vasoconstrictor of smooth muscle in the arterial walls, stimulates the secretion of aldosterone from the adrenal cortex. Aldosterone enhances sodium absorption in the renal tubules, with an attendant increase in water retention and overall volume expansion. Angiotensin-converting enzyme inhibitors, which prevent the conversion of angiotensin I to the vasoactive angiotensin II, are a commonly used class of antihypertensive drugs.

In patients with unilateral renal artery stenosis, renin is elaborated and the blood pressure rises in response to arterial constriction and volume retention. The opposite unaffected kidney may successfully respond by excreting the excess intravascular volume. This condition, of elevated renin levels in the presence of unilateral renal artery stenosis and the contralateral kidney producing compensatory euvolemia, is known as renin-dependent hypertension. In patients with bilateral renal artery stenosis, renin levels rise and volume expands and is maintained. Elevated renin levels may initiate a negative feedback response from the afferent arteriole endothelium, with a resultant normal or decreased serum renin level but a persistent expansion of intracellular and intravascular volume. Thus, bilateral renal artery stenosis results in what is referred to as volume-dependent hypertension. The natural history of renal artery stenosis is a progressive decline in renal function and worsening hypertension refractory to medical management, presumably from a combination of ischemia and repetitive embolization. Atherosclerosis is the most common cause of renal artery stenosis, and renal atrophy has been observed in patients with atherosclerotic renal disease and progression of stenoses.[31,32] Hypertension directly attributable to renal artery stenosis is identified in less than 5% of all patients treated for hypertension. However, the prevalence of renal artery stenosis increases in certain populations, such as patients with atherosclerotic peripheral or coronary artery disease, young patients presenting with hypertension, and patients with a combination of hypertension refractory to medical management and concomitant renal insufficiency. Renal insufficiency and ischemic nephropathy can be a direct result of renal artery stenoses. As many as 40% of patients with end-stage renal disease requiring dialysis have been found to have a significant renal artery stenosis on evaluation with duplex ultrasound.[33]

Diagnosis

The diagnosis of renal artery stenosis can be made by duplex ultrasonography examination of the renal arteries. Duplex ultrasonography combines direct visualization of the renal arteries (B mode) with hemodynamic measurements in the renal arteries (Doppler-derived velocity). Furthermore, ultrasonography allows direct measurement of renal size. The procedure identifies the abdominal aorta at the level of the renal arteries and records blood velocity at this site, followed by identification and measurement of blood velocity in the renal arteries. Other measurements include those of renal parenchymal velocities from the upper, middle, and lower poles of the kidneys as well as renal size. The important parameter is the ratio of velocity in the renal artery to that of the aorta. If the ratio is more than 3.5, this is likely to be associated with a stenosis of more than 60%. If the renal artery velocity is more than 180 cm/sec, this is also considered abnormal. The test is limited by the experience of the operator and by the patient's habitus (being more difficult in obese patients) and bowel gas. Thus, Doppler ultrasonography of the kidneys is best performed in the early morning, after fasting. Reported sensitivity and specificity range from 90% to 95% and 60% to 90%, respectively. In one study, if renal arteriograms were obtained on all patients with a positive finding on Doppler ultrasound, a 2.7% false-positive rate was found. A further use of Doppler ultrasonography may be in predicting which patients would benefit from revascularization. The renal resistive index (RRI) is obtained from Doppler ultrasonography. It can be expressed by the following:

$$\text{RRI} = 1 - \frac{\text{End-diastolic velocity}}{\text{Maximal systolic velocity}} \times 100$$

The RRI has been predictive in determining the response of blood pressure to revascularization. An RRI higher than 0.80 has identified patients with renal artery stenosis in whom angioplasty or surgery did not improve blood pressure or renal function. Finally, the presence of asymmetrical kidney size may be a clue to underlying renal artery stenosis and renal ischemia.

Magnetic Resonance Angiography

This technique can be used for the diagnosis of proximal (and thus largely atherosclerotic) renal artery stenosis. Gadolinium is used as a contrast agent for patients with a glomerular filtration rate of more than 30 mL/min. Reconstructions of images are used to obtain detailed views of the renal arteries. Limitations include the high cost, limited availability, and substantial expertise needed to analyze images. Results for CTA are similar, again with the disadvantage of requiring contrast material, with the attendant risk of nephropathy.

Other imaging studies in addition to MRA, such as contrast angiography, may also be diagnostic but are associated with increased cost and morbidity. In practice, however, many renal artery stenotic lesions are discovered incidentally during studies performed for other reasons.

Serologic renin measurements of blood obtained by venous sampling were once commonly used to validate the significance of an identified renal artery stenosis. These required that a catheter be inserted into the venous system and blood samples obtained from each renal vein and the vena cava. In patients with unilateral renal artery stenosis, a renin ratio of the affected kidney to the opposite kidney of 1.5 or higher is highly suggestive of the stenosis functionally activating the renin system. In a large series, an abnormal ratio was 92% predictive of curability with revascularization; however, 65% of patients with nonlateralizing renin ratios also had curable disease. In an effort to improve the sensitivity and specificity of the test, the renal-systemic renin index has been used. This allows determination of the functional significance of bilateral lesions. The index is obtained by subtracting the systemic (infrarenal vena cava) plasma renin activity from the plasma renin activity in the renal veins and dividing by the systemic plasma renin activity. An index above 0.24 indicates excessive renin production from that kidney, whereas lower levels are indicative of renin suppression. However, given the invasive nature of these tests and the low specificity, renal vein renin sampling is usually reserved for diagnostic dilemmas.

Treatment

Difficult to control hypertension (e.g., the patient is taking three or more antihypertensive medications) or decreased renal function and a hemodynamically significant stenosis are the most commonly used indications for intervention.

Open Renal Artery Bypass

Open renal artery bypass is rarely performed as an isolated procedure with the advent of renal artery stenting. Surgical procedures used to correct renal artery stenosis included aortorenal bypass with vein grafts, arterial autografts (for children) or prosthetic grafts, aortorenal endarterectomy, hepatic artery–renal artery bypass, gastroduodenal–renal artery bypass, and splenic artery–renal artery bypass. These procedures, although durable and revered by surgeons, are obviously maximally invasive and can be associated with significant morbidity. They have been almost universally supplanted by angioplasty and stenting procedures.

Renal Artery Stenting

Value, limitations, and techniques. Percutaneous therapy for renovascular occlusive disease has become the preferred alternative to open renal revascularization. In the appropriately selected patient, angioplasty and stenting of renal artery stenoses have been shown to be safe and effective options for severe hypertension and ischemic nephropathy. Catheter-based treatment, especially when it is performed with lower profile systems, can be performed with minimal morbidity and a reliably high degree of initial technical success. The long-term beneficial effects on blood pressure control and renal function have been debated but appear to be valid.

Renal angioplasty was first performed in 1978 by Grüntzig and colleagues,[34] and there have been many series demonstrating the success of this interventional procedure. With the advent of the stent, durability, efficacy, and ultimately acceptance of catheter-based management of renal artery lesions have increased. Stents were initially used for cases of immediate technical failure, such as residual anatomic stenoses of more than 30%, residual pressure gradients or postangioplasty dissections, or recurrent stenoses after prior angioplasty. Routine stenting of renal artery stenoses (as an adjunct to balloon angioplasty), especially in treatment of ostial lesions, has become an accepted practice. The incidence of recurrent stenosis has been shown to be significantly decreased with angioplasty and stent placement versus angioplasty alone.[35]

Although the number of patients completely cured of renovascular hypertension after renal artery stenting has been reported to be as low as 5% or less,[36] up to 80% of patients treated demonstrate measurable improvement in blood pressure control.[35-39] Henry and associates[37] have reported a series of 210 patients with chronic hypertension and a diastolic blood pressure higher than 90 mm Hg who underwent renal artery angioplasty and stenting. A favorable response was seen in 80% of patients, with 35% reported as cured of hypertension. In this study, a hypertensive cure was defined as diastolic blood pressure less than 90 mm Hg achieved without the administration of antihypertensive medications. In another series of patients treated with stenting for renal artery stenosis associated with hypertension, impaired renal function, or both, only 4.2% achieved a complete cure, but an additional 79% benefited from an improvement in hypertensive control.[36] A meta-analysis of 14 studies involving renal angioplasty and stenting has found an overall 20% cure rate for hypertension, with 49% of patients experiencing an improvement in hypertensive control.[35] This meta-analysis recognized the variability in reporting criteria for a cure among the different renal angioplasty and stent series.

Improvement in serum creatinine level may be seen in approximately 30% of patients after renal angioplasty and stenting.[37] However, a higher percentage of patients demonstrate a clinical benefit of creatinine stabilization when renal artery stents are placed for ischemic nephropathy.[36,40] Rundback and coworkers[41] have reported a series of 45 patients with azotemia who received a renal stent for treatment of a renal stenosis. A clinical benefit was defined as improvement or stabilization of creatinine levels. Life-table analysis demonstrated a benefit at 12, 24, and 36 months in 72%, 62%, and 54% of patients, respectively. In patients with significant renal artery stenosis and a solitary functioning kidney, renal artery stenting has been shown to be a safe alternative to surgery. Bush and colleagues[42] have reported a series of 27 patients, each with a solitary functioning kidney and azotemia, who underwent endovascular treatment of significant renal artery stenosis. An improvement or stabilization of renal function was seen in 74% of patients.

There is variability among series in terms of renal stent patency rates. The reported incidence of recurrent stenoses of renal stents has ranged from as low as 1.5%[43] to as high as 25%[44] at 6 months. Several series of renal artery stenting have shown a patency of up to 5 years by life-table analysis. Rodriquez-Lopez and associates[45] have performed a life-table analysis of 108 patients undergoing renal angioplasty and primary stent placement and found 74% primary and 85% secondary patency rates. A larger series of patients with renal artery stents placed for failed angioplasty, recurrent stenosis, dissection, or ostial lesions was reported by Henry and colleagues.[37] This series demonstrated a 79% primary and 98% secondary patency at 5 years by life-table analysis.

Duplex surveillance is accurate for identifying recurrent renal artery stenosis.[46] The stenosis within a stent is most often caused by myointimal hyperplasia. Treatment usually consists of repeated angioplasty, and occasionally a new stent is required. Bax and colleagues[47] have reported a series of 15 patients with 20 stents with recurrent stenoses; 18 stents were successfully treated with angioplasty alone, and only two required the placement of a second stent. The 1-year success rate of the repeated interventions was 75%. Balloon-expandable covered stents may be helpful for recurrent in-stent restenosis in the future.

The morbidity and mortality of a major operative procedure can be avoided with endovascular treatment of renal artery stenoses. Mackrell and associates[48] have reported their experience with 165 patients who underwent endovascular or surgical intervention for renal artery stenosis. They noted a shift from open surgical revascularization of renal artery stenosis to endovascular treatment. In comparing endovascular treatment with surgical renal revascularization and combined aortic and renal revascularization, all had excellent technical success rates, but the surgical group had a significantly higher morbidity (5.6% versus 15% and 23%, respectively) and mortality rate (0% versus 9.1% and 8.1%).

With combined aortic and renal open reconstructions, the complexity of surgery is increased. Endovascular repair has become popular for the treatment of abdominal aortic aneurysms with suitable aortic anatomy. A renal artery stenosis in the presence of an abdominal aortic aneurysm can be treated before or after the aortic endograft is placed. A benefit to placing the renal stent before the endograft is to allow the stent to serve as a radiopaque marker for the origin of the renal artery. This may help in positioning and placement of the endograft below the renal arteries. One must be cautious not to entrap the endograft or the delivery system on the stent if it protrudes out into the aortic lumen.

The technical success of renal artery stent placement is high in most of the series, with technical failures usually caused by poor positioning or deployment of the stent. Access to the renal artery is an important consideration for renal artery stenting. The angulation of the renal arteries relative to the aorta and the short distance of the renal artery beyond the stenosis for secure guidewire placement can make renal stenting from a femoral artery access point challenging. A brachial or axillary approach is sometimes required to overcome the angulation of the renal artery or to avoid significant aortic and iliac disease. Radial artery access with angioplasty and stenting of the renal artery has been described.[49]

One early technical limitation of renal artery stenting was the large size of the 0.035-inch guidewire-based balloons and stents. These platforms required a 7 Fr or 8 Fr sheath, and tracking the stent into an angulated renal artery was difficult or sometimes not possible from a femoral approach. Miniaturization of balloons and stents was first shown to be safe and effective in coronary use[50] and, in some cases, resulted in shorter procedural times and use of less contrast material.[51] The required guiding sheath size is reduced with the lower profile balloons and stents that use 0.014- and 0.018-inch guidewire platforms. The lower profile angioplasty balloons and stents have a better ability to negotiate difficult angles. These factors have led to the routine use of 0.014-inch systems for renal artery stenosis. The following is a stepwise guide to our preferred technique for renal artery angioplasty and stenting with use of the lower profile angioplasty balloons and stents.

Renal Angioplasty and Stent Procedure

See Figure 62-24.

Renal artery access and guide sheath positioning. Arterial access, femoral or brachial, is an important initial decision that has been made easier with the lower profile balloon, stent, and sheath systems. Retrograde common femoral access is the first choice, usually secondary to table and patient positioning constraints. Brachial access is used only in certain circumstances, such as severe aortoiliac occlusive disease, aortic aneurysms, and extreme caudal renal artery angulation. In most cases, an anteroposterior aortogram is first obtained, with a pigtail catheter in the suprarenal position. Oblique angulation is sometimes required to better visualize the renal origins. To limit contrast material, a selective catheterization can be made without the aortogram if one has been previously obtained. Alternative contrast agents, such as carbon dioxide and gadolinium, have been successfully used in renal angiography and renal artery interventions.[52,53] Most renal arteries can be accessed simply with an angled catheter; however, some will require a more complex-shaped catheter, such as a cobra, shepherd's hook, or Simmons catheter. A selective renal

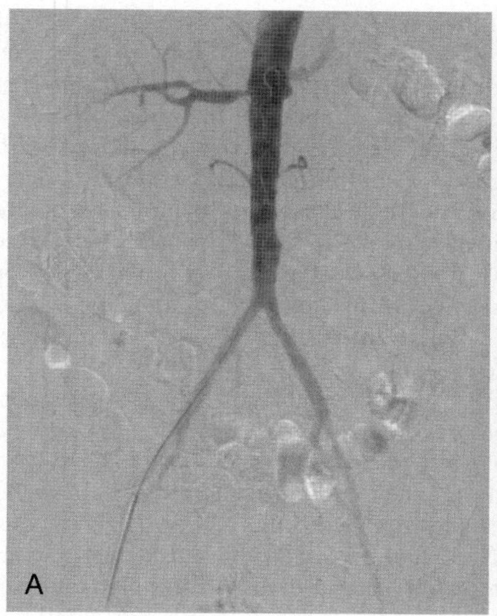

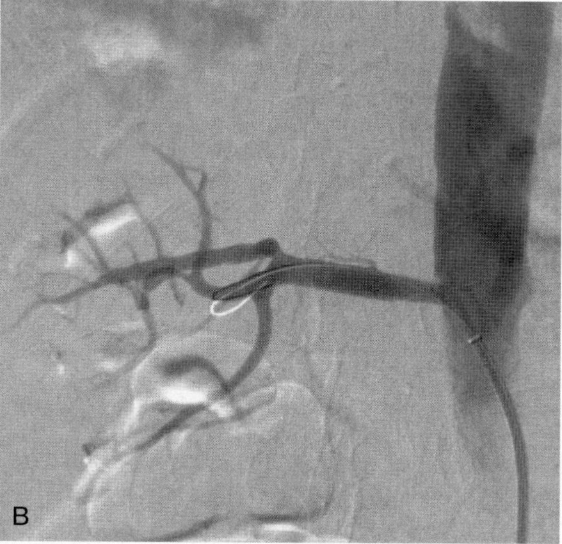

FIGURE 62-24 Renal artery stent. **A,** Right renal artery stenosis. **B,** Lesion improved after stent placement.

angiogram is then obtained with hand injections of contrast material or careful power injections. All phases of the renal circulation are visualized, including the arterial, parenchymal, and venous phases.

A 0.035-inch guidewire is then positioned in the tertiary renal branches. Maintaining guidewire position and stability becomes difficult because of the relatively short length of the renal artery. A 6 Fr guide sheath is advanced into the proximal renal artery. With use of a 4 Fr or 5 Fr glide catheter to help maintain guidewire crossing of the renal stenosis, a 0.035-inch guidewire is then exchanged for a 0.014-inch guidewire.

Renal angioplasty. Over the 0.014-inch guidewire, an angioplasty balloon is advanced across the stenosis. The balloon should be approximately the size of the native normal renal artery beyond the stenosis, not a segment with poststenotic dilation. Typically, the initial angioplasty is performed with a 4-mm semicompliant balloon. The compliant nature of the balloon gives a range of diameters above and below 4 mm, depending on the inflation pressure. While the balloon is inflated, a saved image is obtained to compare the size of the angioplasty balloon with the native artery. This comparison will be taken into account in deciding whether a larger angioplasty balloon is needed and what size stent to choose.

Stent placement. A postangioplasty angiogram is then obtained and the renal artery is assessed for residual stenosis or significant dissection; if this is present, a stent is placed. All renal artery lesions involving the origin will require a stent. A balloon-expandable stent from a low-profile 0.014- and 0.018-inch system is used (0.018-inch balloons and stents can also be delivered over a 0.014-inch guidewire). Contrast material may be puffed through the sheath positioned in the aorta near the ostium of the renal artery to confirm proper positioning of the renal stent. The stent is deployed by expanding the angioplasty balloon to its predetermined deployment pressure. Higher pressures may be required to expand the stent further. However, the rated burst pressure should not be exceeded.

Completion angiography. Before removal of the guidewire and sheath, a completion angiogram with a flush catheter in the aorta is obtained. This presents an interesting question: How can a good-quality completion study be obtained to include the renal artery origin without losing guidewire access? This can easily be done using a tandem wire technique. The sheath is withdrawn into the infrarenal aorta while maintaining guidewire position across the stented segment of renal artery. A second guidewire is advanced into the aorta; a 4 Fr pigtail catheter is placed over this wire and through the same sheath in the suprarenal position to obtain good detail of the renal artery origin.

Technical Tips

- The renal arteries often originate anteriorly or posteriorly, and the initial diagnostic evaluation of the renal artery origins may be improved with oblique image intensifier views.
- Catheter selection for initial access to the renal artery will depend on the patient's anatomy. Although most branch vessels can be accessed with just an angled Glidecath, a formed catheter such as a cobra or Simmons catheter may be required.
- Arterial perforation is possible with inadvertent guidewire advancement into the renal parenchyma; thus, one should be conscious of the tip of the wire throughout the entire procedure.
- The saved image of the fully expanded initial angioplasty balloon will help estimate the native artery diameter and optimal stent size.
- Care must be taken not to overdilate and risk rupture of the renal artery.
- Stents placed for ostial lesions should extend into the aorta by approximately 2 mm.
- Always read the package insert for the balloon and stent system for sheath and guidewire compatibility, balloon compliance, and the nominal deployment and rated burst pressures.

Renal artery stenting may be an effective treatment of renovascular hypertension and ischemic nephropathy that avoids the morbidity and mortality of open surgical treatment. The role of renal stents after angioplasty can be debated; however, there is good evidence for stenting of all ostial lesions. A more traditional approach to stenting may be used for nonostial stenosis, with the stent reserved for angioplasty failures. Lesions caused by fibromuscular dysplasia usually do not require adjuvant stenting because they respond well to primary angioplasty. The technical success of renal stenting is high, with most technical failures caused by imprecise stent placement. A lower profile 0.014- or 0.018-inch platform for percutaneous renal artery interventions will reduce the sheath size necessary for access and has replaced the more cumbersome 0.035-inch platforms.

SPLANCHNIC ANEURYSMS: SPLENIC, MESENTERIC, AND RENAL ARTERY ANEURYMS

The most common splanchnic artery aneurysm (Fig. 62-25) is the splenic artery aneurysm, accounting for 60% of all splanchnic artery aneurysms. However, it is still rare, with an incidence of 0.78% in patients undergoing abdominal arteriography; it is found incidentally in 0.1% to 10% of autopsies. Splenic aneurysms are more common in women than in men, with a ratio of 4:1. Pregnancy is associated with up to 50% of all ruptures. The overall mortality from rupture is approximately 25%. However, rupture during pregnancy is associated with high maternal (80%) and fetal (90%) mortality. The most common risk factors associated with splenic aneurysms are female gender, history of multiple pregnancies, and portal hypertension.

Splenic aneurysms are commonly diagnosed incidentally during arteriographic and CT studies performed for other indications. A signet ring calcification in the left upper quadrant may be seen on plain abdominal radiographs. Ultrasonography, CT, and MRI are useful for aneurysm surveillance in asymptomatic patients.

Patients with splenic aneurysms may report a history of left upper quadrant or epigastric pain. The term *double rupture* has been used to describe these aneurysms, but it is relatively rare. There is initial contained bleeding in the lesser sac, followed by free hemorrhage into the peritoneal cavity, causing hypovolemic shock. Treatment should be considered in aneurysms larger than 2 cm in diameter. Because of the high mortality rate, treatment

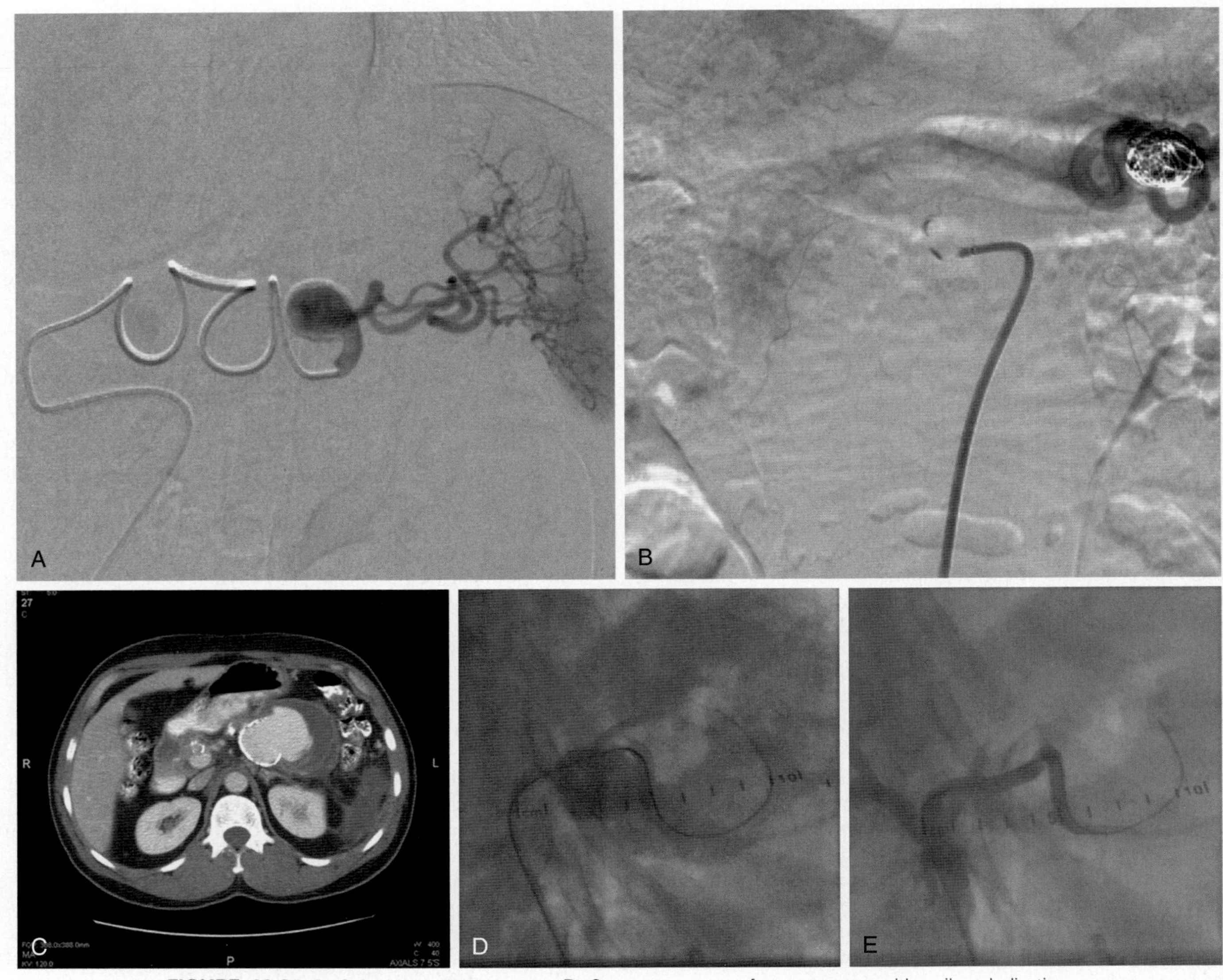

FIGURE 62-25 A, Splenic artery aneurysm. **B,** Same aneurysm after treatment with coil embolization. **C,** CT scan demonstrating ruptured splenic aneurysm. **D,** Arteriogram demonstrates sac with wire passing through aneurysm into intact distal artery. **E,** Flow into sac excluded with stent graft.

is warranted for pregnant women and those of childbearing age. Simple ligation or excision of the aneurysm is preferred to splenectomy. Endovascular repair is emerging as the treatment of choice, with embolization or exclusion with a covered stent.

Hepatic aneurysms are the second most common splanchnic aneurysms, accounting for 20%. These are usually discovered incidentally. Management recommendations are for immediate repair in symptomatic patients or when pseudoaneurysm is suspected, such as those lesions related to iatrogenic injury; otherwise, asymptomatic aneurysms are repaired when the diameter is more than 2 cm. The surgical approach depends on the location of the lesion; options include ligation of common hepatic artery lesions, open aneurysmorrhaphy, and aneurysmectomy with reconstruction. In favorable anatomy, endovascular exclusion can be successful with either covered stents or coil embolization.

Superior mesenteric artery aneurysms account for 5.5% of splanchnic aneurysms; the majority are mycotic and symptomatic, presenting with abdominal pain, nausea, vomiting, or gastrointestinal bleeding. Because of the high mortality risk associated with rupture or intestinal ischemia, superior mesenteric artery aneurysms are repaired regardless of size. Surgical options, which depend on patient factors as well as the anatomy, include ligation, open aneurysmorrhaphy or resection, and endovascular repair with either covered stent grafts or coil embolization.

Celiac axis aneurysms are rarer still and constitute 5% of all splanchnic aneurysms. These are associated with infection, trauma, and dissection as well as with degenerative disease. Similar to splenic lesions, these may initially be manifested with rupture into the lesser sac with epigastric pain and hypotension, followed by shock due to free rupture into the abdominal cavity. Because of the high mortality, all symptomatic lesions as well as asymptomatic lesions larger than 1.5 cm in diameter are repaired immediately. Ligation may be well tolerated. Open or endovascular intervention should be selected on the basis of the patient's anatomy.

The true incidence of renal artery aneurysms is difficult to estimate, ranging from 0.09% to 0.9% on the basis of autopsy studies or radiographic series. Pathogenic contributors include fibromuscular dysplasia, atherosclerotic disease, and trauma. The majority of true aneurysms are saccular and often occur at the main renal artery bifurcation, complicating surgical repair; 10% bilaterality is seen. Fibromuscular dysplasia, particularly medial dysplasia, is known to cause multiple stenoses with poststenotic dilation, effecting the "string of beads" appearance on imaging. The majority are asymptomatic; symptomatic patients present with rupture. Indications for repair include symptomatic lesions, lesions larger than 2 cm, and lesions in women of childbearing age. Options for repair depend on the location of the lesion. Fibromuscular dysplasia is treated with balloon angioplasty alone. The rare aneurysm that occurs along the straight portion of the artery can be treated with either coil embolization or covered stent placement or both. Aneurysms that occur at major branch points, in which one of the branches cannot be sacrificed, require open repair. The complexity of this approach varies from simple aneurysmorrhaphy to resection with reconstruction with inflow from the aorta (or the hepatic, splenic, or iliac arteries), explantation of the kidney for back table repair, and nephrectomy.

CAROTID ARTERY DISEASE

Stroke is the third leading cause of death and is the leading cause of serious disability in the United States. There are about 700,000 strokes per year, with almost 175,000 deaths (25%) occurring within 1 year after the stroke. Approximately 85% of strokes have an ischemic cause; 15% are caused by primary hemorrhage, such as intraparenchymal bleeding from hypertension. Of the ischemic strokes, 20% to 30% are secondary to emboli from atherosclerotic cerebrovascular disease. In patients with greater than 50% stenosis, 20% of patients were shown to have embolic events in transcranial Doppler studies. The incidence and frequency increase with increased stenosis and recent symptomatic neurologic events. The most common location for atherosclerosis in the cerebrovascular circulation is the carotid bifurcation; thus, many strokes are preventable with carotid intervention.

Pathophysiology

The development of atherosclerotic plaque in the extracranial arteries is the leading cause of ischemic stroke in North America and Europe. It accounts for approximately 90% of extracranial cerebrovascular disease; the remaining 10% is caused by disease processes such as fibromuscular dysplasia and arteritis. Atherosclerotic lesions usually occur at the proximal internal carotid artery (ICA) and carotid bifurcation along the wall opposite the origin of the ECA. The enlargement of the carotid bifurcation at the carotid bulb creates a well-defined region of low wall shear stress, flow separation, and loss of unidirectional flow. In this region of low shear stress with sluggish flow, there is prolonged exposure and interaction of plasma lipids and vessel walls, which may account for the localized plaque at the carotid bulb. In contrast, regions with high shear stress, such as the inner border of the carotid sinus, are usually free of atherosclerosis. After the development of a hemodynamically significant stenosis, the atherosclerotic plaque may cause stroke by one of three principal mechanisms: embolization of atherosclerotic particle, thrombotic occlusion, or hypoperfusion.

Clinical Presentation

Symptoms of carotid artery disease include TIAs, amaurosis fugax, and stroke. A TIA is defined as a brief acute loss of focal cerebral function, generally less than 24 hours in duration. There is no persistent deficit after each TIA, but there are often multiple attacks. The loss of function can be localized to a region of brain that is supplied by one vascular system, such as the right or left carotid artery. Most TIAs are brief, lasting 2 to 15 minutes, and are rapid in onset. Symptoms include unilateral motor and sensory loss, aphasia (difficulty finding words), and dysarthria (difficulty speaking because of motor dysfunction). Motor function loss may be manifested as weakness, paralysis, dysarthria, or clumsiness of the upper or lower extremities or face that is contralateral to the affected carotid artery. Sensory function loss may be manifested as numbness or paresthesia of the contralateral upper or lower extremities or face. Aphasia occurs when the speech center, usually located in the dominant hemisphere, is affected. If the neurologic deficit lasts longer than 24 hours but there is return of full neurologic function with 48 to 72 hours, it is termed a reversible ischemic neurologic deficit. A patient with persistent neurologic deficit is considered to have a stroke. In contrast, fleeting episodes lasting only a few seconds are usually not considered to be TIAs.

Amaurosis fugax is the transient unilateral loss of vision. It is caused by an embolus to the ophthalmic artery, the first branch of the ICA. Patients describe the event as a shade descending or ascending over the entire eye, half of the eye, or a quadrant of one eye. The location of the affected visual field depends on whether the embolization is to the superior or inferior retinal artery. If the entire retinal artery is transiently affected, the patient may complain of complete loss of vision in one eye. Similar to TIAs, most incidents of amaurosis fugax are sudden in onset and last for minutes. However, there may be occasional patients with permanent blindness.

A patient may also be asymptomatic when diagnosed with hemodynamically significant carotid artery disease. An audible carotid bruit may be heard in the neck during routine physical examination. It should be noted that severe carotid disease may not have an audible bruit because of markedly reduced blood flow. A screening carotid duplex ultrasound examination should be performed in asymptomatic patients with bruits or high-risk patients without bruits.

Diagnosis

Once a patient is diagnosed with TIA, amaurosis fugax, or stroke, expedient workup with confirmation of carotid artery disease and treatment are needed because the risk of a stroke is greatest within the first 3 months after the initial event. This risk returns to baseline at approximately 6 months. The most useful test for the diagnosis of extracranial carotid artery disease is duplex ultrasound. Carotid duplex ultrasonography (Fig. 62-26) allows accurate indirect determination of the severity of the carotid stenosis by measuring velocity. As the stenosis increases and the lumen narrows, there is an increase in the blood velocity to maintain distal flow. Many studies have confirmed the correlation of increased velocity with severity of disease. CTA and MRA (Fig. 62-27) can also be used to determine the degree of carotid stenosis

	cm/s			
RIGHT	(S)	(D)	Percent	Plaque
ECA	266	0		
DICA	56	24		
MICA	80	28		
PICA	867	443		
DCCA	56	11		
MCCA	62	8		
PCCA	77	12		
SUBCL	155	0		

Max ICA Stenosis 80-99%
ICA/CCA Ratio 11.3

	cm/s			
LEFT	(S)	(D)	Percent	Plaque
ECA	249	0		
DICA	97	28		
MICA	83	31		
PICA	149	37	50-79%	
DCCA	147	36		
MCCA	101	27		
PCCA	103	20		
SUBCL	176	0		

Max ICA Stenosis 50-79%
ICA/CCA Ratio 1.0

A

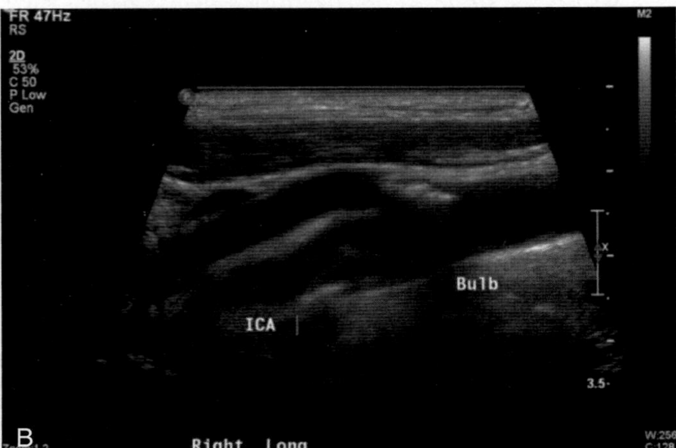

FIGURE 62-26 **A,** Carotid duplex velocities demonstrating severe right internal carotid artery stenosis. **B,** Soft plaque is seen within the right internal carotid artery on gray-scale imaging.

at the bifurcation. In addition, they are useful to study potential tandem lesions that may be present in the proximal supra-aortic trunk or intracranial vessels and to assess the configuration of the aortic arch. These studies are also useful for confirmation of duplex findings and planning of intervention with a carotid endarterectomy (CEA) or stenting. Contrast arteriography (Fig. 62-28) is occasionally performed. It is most useful for patients with normal findings on duplex studies or for whom a noninvasive study is in disagreement with the clinical presentation. In addition to findings similar to those of CTA and MRA, contrast arteriography can be used to identify intracranial vascular disease or unusual nonatherosclerotic arteriopathies, such as fibromuscular dysplasia.

Treatment

Carotid Endarterectomy

Indications. CEA is the removal of the atherosclerotic plaque from the carotid bifurcation. In the North American Symptomatic Carotid Endarterectomy Trial (NASCET), the effectiveness of CEA was evaluated for symptomatic patients with carotid artery stenosis ranging from 30% to 99% in the United States and Canada. Patients with TIA, amaurosis fugax, or nondisabling stroke were randomized to best medical therapy or CEA. In the first study of patients with 70% stenosis or greater, CEA reduced the incidence of ipsilateral stroke from 26% to 9% at 2 years. The incidence of a major or fatal ipsilateral stroke was 13.1% for the medical group and 2.5% for the surgical group. In a subsequent report, the results of patients with symptomatic mild (30% to 49%) and moderate (50% to 69%) ipsilateral stroke were reported. The 5-year risk of ipsilateral stroke in patients with moderate stenosis was 22.2% for the medical group and 15.7% for the surgical group. For patients with mild stenosis, the risk of ipsilateral stroke was equivalent for the medical and surgical groups. The NASCET outcome showed that symptomatic patients with severe stenosis (70% to 99%) gained substantial benefit from surgical intervention during a brief period of less than 2 years. The results also favored surgery in symptomatic patients with 50% to 69% stenosis. The best medical therapy at the time of the NASCET trial did not include clopidogrel (Plavix) or statin anticholesterol agents, both of which have been shown to decrease the risk of stroke.

CEA has also been shown to be effective in asymptomatic patients. The Asymptomatic Carotid Atherosclerosis Study (ACAS) randomized asymptomatic patients with 60% to 99% stenosis to best medical treatment or CEA. The 5-year risk of ipsilateral stroke and any perioperative stroke or death was 11% for the medical group and 5.1% for the surgical group. The perioperative complication rate was low, 2.3%, with approximately 50% of the risk associated with mandatory preoperative contrast arteriography for patients randomized to CEA. Therefore, the actual surgical complication rate was only 1.5%. The largest trial was the Asymptomatic Carotid Surgery Trial (ACST), with equal randomization of 3120 patients to CEA or medical treatment. The results were similar, with a 5-year stroke risk of 11.8% in the medical group and 5.4% in the surgical group. The perioperative complication rate was also low, 3.1%.

The results of landmark studies of CEA have confirmed that surgery provides better protection from ipsilateral stroke in patients with symptomatic or asymptomatic disease. The Stroke Council of the American Heart Association convened a consensus conference on the indications for CEA. The recommendation recognized four categories: (1) proven—the strongest indication,

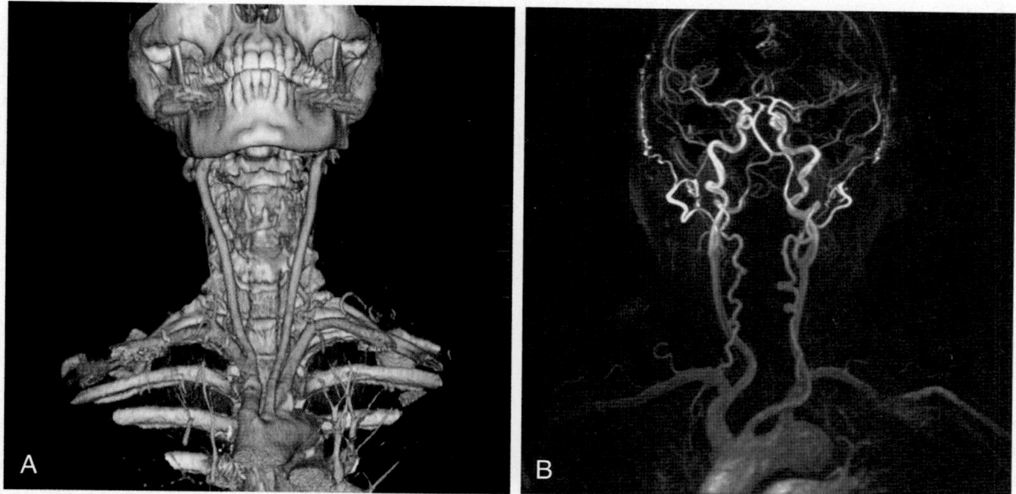

FIGURE 62-27 **A,** Arch and cervical carotid CTA reconstruction. **B,** Arch, cervical, and intracranial MRA scans with gadolinium. (Courtesy Dr. Douglas Hughes, University of Texas Medical Branch at Galveston, Department of Radiology.)

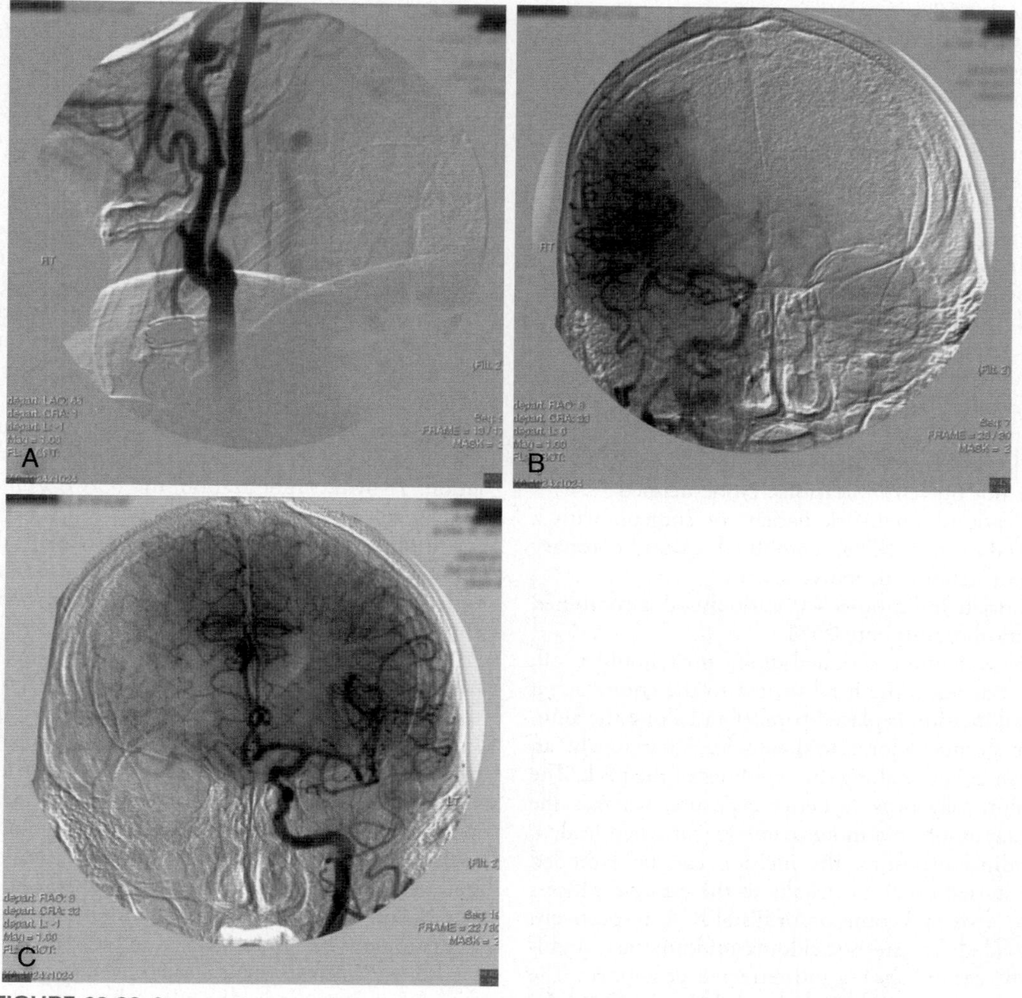

FIGURE 62-28 Same patient as in Figure 62-26. **A,** Severe right internal carotid artery stenosis, correlating with carotid duplex findings. **B,** Intracerebral anteroposterior angiogram of right common carotid artery injections demonstrates no filling of the anterior circulation. **C,** Injection of the left internal carotid artery demonstrates filling of the right anterior circulation.

usually supported by results of prospective, randomized trials; (2) acceptable but not proven—a good indication for operation supported by promising but not scientifically certain data; (3) uncertain—data insufficient to define the risk-benefit ratio; and (4) proven inappropriate—current data adequate to show that the risk of surgery outweighs any benefits. The recommendations are further classified for patients with symptomatic or asymptomatic carotid disease.

For symptomatic good-risk patients treated by a surgeon whose surgical morbidity and mortality rate is less than 6%, the indications for CEA are as follows:

Proven indications

- One or more TIAs in the last 6 months and carotid stenosis ≥70%
- Mild stroke with carotid stenosis ≥70%

Acceptable but not proven indications

- TIAs in the past 6 months and stenosis of 50% to 69%
- Progressive stroke and stenosis ≥70%
- Mild or moderate stroke in the past 6 months and stenosis of 50% to 69%
- CEA ipsilateral to TIAs and stenosis ≥70%, combined with required coronary bypass grafting

Uncertain indications

- TIAs with stenosis ≤50%
- Mild stroke with stenosis ≤50%
- Symptomatic acute carotid thrombosis

Proven inappropriate indications

- Moderate stroke with stenosis ≤50%, not receiving aspirin
- Single TIA, stenosis ≤50%, not receiving aspirin
- High-risk patient with multiple TIAs, stenosis ≤50%, not receiving aspirin
- High-risk patient, mild or moderate stroke, stenosis ≤50%, not receiving aspirin
- Global ischemic symptoms with stenosis ≤50%
- Acute internal carotid dissection, asymptomatic, receiving heparin

For asymptomatic good-risk patients treated by a surgeon whose surgical morbidity and mortality rates are each less than 3%, the indications for CEA are as follows:

- Proven indications: Stenosis ≥60%
- Acceptable but not proven indications: None defined
- Uncertain indications: High-risk patient or surgeon with a morbidity-mortality rate >3%, combined carotid-coronary operation, or nonstenotic ulcerative lesions
- Proven inappropriate indications: Operations with a combined stroke morbidity-mortality rate ≥5%

Technique. The patient is positioned supine on a shoulder roll, with the neck extended and the head turned to the contralateral side. A longitudinal incision is placed parallel and along the anterior border of the sternocleidomastoid muscle. Alternatively, an oblique incision can be made along the skin lines of the neck. The longitudinal incision may provide better exposure, whereas the oblique incision may result in a more cosmetic scar when healed. With the longitudinal exposure, the incision can be extended proximally to the sternal notch or distally to the mastoid process for exposure of the proximal common or distal ICA, respectively. The platysma is divided. The sternocleidomastoid muscle is mobilized away from the carotid sheath and retracted posteriorly. The internal jugular vein may be exposed along the anterior border until the large common facial vein is identified. The common facial vein is divided; the carotid bifurcation is usually located underneath. The internal jugular vein may be mobilized laterally to provide exposure to the carotid bifurcation. The vagus nerve (cranial nerve X) is found posterolateral to the common carotid artery (CCA) in the carotid sheath. Therefore, dissection of the CCA is performed anteriorly to avoid nerve injury. However, care must still be exercised to identify the occasional anomalous anterior course of the vagus nerve and the presence of a rare nonrecurrent laryngeal nerve that branches directly from the vagus to innervate the vocal cord. The nonrecurrent laryngeal nerve usually occurs on the right side of the neck.

Meticulous dissection of the carotid artery is necessary to avoid embolization. Movement of the carotid bulb should be minimized; the initial dissection should be limited to the normal ICA and ECA distal to the diseased segment and the CCA proximal to the diseased segment. During mobilization of the ICA superiorly, the hypoglossal nerve (cranial nerve XII) needs to be identified and protected (Fig. 62-29). Dissection near the carotid bifurcation and carotid body may cause reflex bradycardia and hypotension. This can be prevented with the injection of 1% lidocaine into the carotid body.

On occasion, there may be patients with a high carotid bifurcation or an extensive lesion, and maximum exposure of the ICA may be needed. Several techniques can be used to provide this exposure. The skin incision is first extended all the way superiorly to the mastoid process and the sternocleidomastoid muscle is mobilized to its tendinous insertion on the mastoid process. At this level of dissection, the spinal accessory nerve (cranial nerve XI) is identified and protected. Additional exposure of the ICA can be achieved with the division of the posterior belly of the digastric muscle. If further exposure of the ICA superiorly is necessary, the styloid process can be transected and the mandible displaced anteriorly. At this level of dissection, the glossopharyngeal nerve (cranial nerve IX) crosses the ICA near the base of the skull. Injury to this nerve can be avoided by dissecting close to the anterior surface of this artery. In retracting the wound superiorly, care should also be exercised to avoid other nerve injuries. There can be temporary compression injury to the greater auricular nerve laterally and the marginal mandibular branch of the facial nerve medially.

Once the carotid arteries are fully exposed, vessel loops are placed around the arteries and heparin is given for full anticoagulation. To avoid embolization, the ICA is clamped first, followed by control of the CCA and ECA. The CCA is opened, and a longitudinal arteriotomy is extended through the plaque into the normal ICA distally. If a shunt is to be used, it is inserted at this time. The decision whether to shunt can be made using electroencephalographic or back-pressure criteria. Using back-pressure criteria, an arterial pressure transducer is set up. A 22-gauge needle bent at a 45-degree angle is carefully inserted into the CCA, with the distal needle in the lumen of the ICA. The pressure of the ICA is measured with the ECA and CCA clamped. If the back-pressure is a mean arterial pressure of 65 mm Hg or higher, there is adequate collateral cerebral circulation and a shunt can be avoided. Alternative methods of cerebral blood flow evaluation include intermittent neurologic checks on the awake patient undergoing CEA with local anesthesia only and transcranial duplex or electroencephalographic monitoring of the patient undergoing CEA under general anesthesia.

The endarterectomy is started in the CCA. The optimal plane for endarterectomy is the plane between the inner and outer medial layers. This results in the removal of the intima, the plaque, and a portion of the media. The remaining arterial wall thus consists of the adventitia and residual media. The plaque is divided

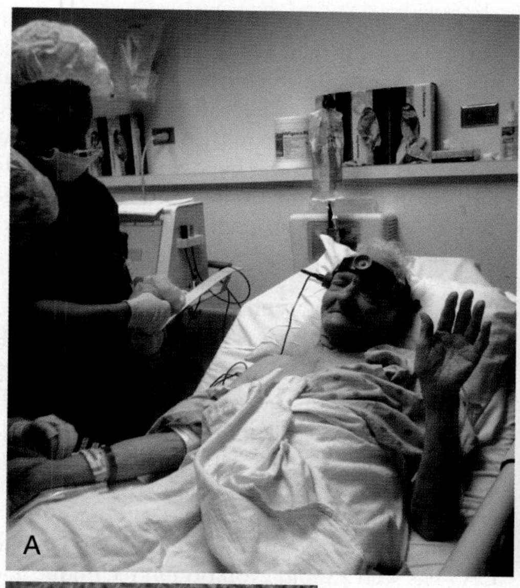

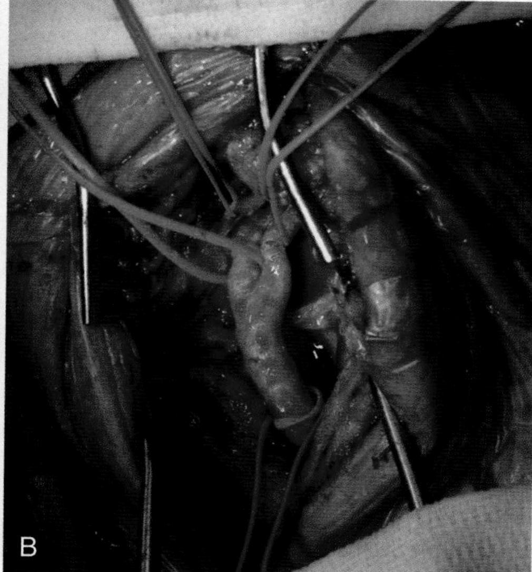

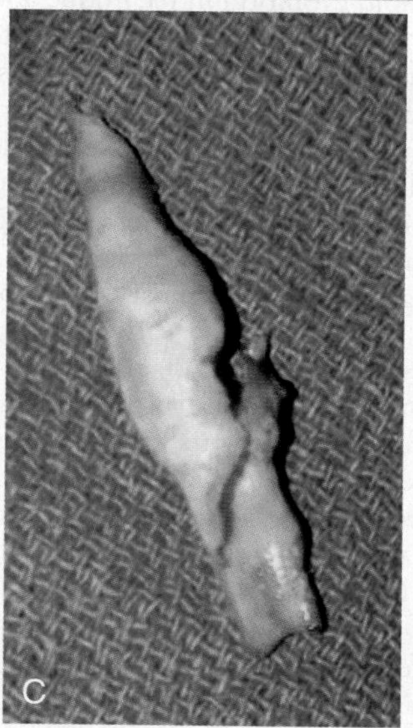

FIGURE 62-29 A, Patient preparing for carotid endarterectomy with intraoperative transcranial duplex monitoring. **B,** Carotid exposure with hypoglossal nerve at top of incision. **C,** Carotid plaque with calcified and friable components.

proximally in the CCA, and the endarterectomy is extended distally into the carotid bulb. The vessel loop around the ECA is loosened, and endarterectomy of the ECA is performed by simple eversion. Removal of the plaque is continued distally into the ICA. Endarterectomy of the distal ICA is feathered to its transition to the normal distal intima. If the distal plaque cannot be feathered, the residual intima is sharply transected and secured in place with tacking sutures. After completion of the endarterectomy, the residual wall is copiously irrigated with heparinized saline solution, and any remaining debris or medial fibers are removed to prevent embolization. The ICA, ECA, and CCA are allowed to backbleed.

The arteriotomy is closed with a patch. There is evidence showing that patch angioplasty has better results with a reduced risk of restenosis, especially in female patients, patients with small ICAs, and patients who continue to smoke. Once the arteriotomy is completed, flow is first established to the ECA with release of clamps to the ECA and CCA. After several heartbeats to flush debris out of the ECA, flow is then reestablished into the ICA.

If desired, heparin reversal is given with protamine.

Postoperative care. At the completion of the endarterectomy, a gross neurologic examination of the patient is performed in the operating room. If no deficit is found, the patient is transferred to the recovery room. Patients are monitored closely during the postoperative period. Although they were formerly cared for in the intensive care unit routinely, most patients now can be transferred to a regular room if they are neurologically intact and hemodynamically normal in the postanesthesia care unit. Usually, patients are discharged safely the next day. Important factors to be monitored are the patient's neurologic status, blood pressure, and incision to evaluate for hematoma.

If, at the completion of the procedure, there is neurologic deficit, the patency of the ICA is evaluated with noninvasive carotid duplex ultrasound. Initial flap or occlusion of the ICA on duplex imaging requires immediate reoperation. If the ICA is patent, arteriography is performed to detect possible clots or defects. Any lesion is treated with reoperation. If there is no lesion on the arteriogram in a patent ICA, the patient is treated conservatively with anticoagulation, antiplatelet agents, or both. However, if the patient continues to have repeated or worsening neurologic events, immediate reoperation may be needed.

Blood pressure monitoring and control during the postoperative period are of paramount importance to prevent stroke. Immediately after CEA, 20% of patients may have significant hypertension and 30% may have hypotension. Up to 9% of these patients were found to have neurologic deficits, whereas there was no neurologic morbidity in normotensive patients. In addition, blood pressure fluctuation has adverse effects on myocardial function. Systolic blood pressure should be kept below 140 mm Hg for normotensive patients and below 160 mm Hg for chronically hypertensive patients. Diastolic pressure is maintained below 100 mm Hg. Hypertension should be treated immediately; sodium nitroprusside can be used. Hypotension is initially treated with fluid to correct the volume deficit; if it is refractory, vasoconstrictors can be initiated.

The use of antiplatelet therapy and intraoperative heparin anticoagulation can cause wound hematoma after endarterectomy; the incidence of reoperation for hematoma drainage is less than 1%. Usually, there is diffuse ooze from the wound rather than bleeding from the suture line. A large hematoma may cause compression on the ICA and adjacent cranial nerves and wound infection. If there is airway compromise, the incision needs to be opened at the bedside for drainage of the hematoma. The incidence may be decreased with the routine use of a Silastic drain.

It is not unusual for patients to complain of headache after CEA; they may complain of these symptoms at approximately 3 to 5 days postoperatively. This is likely caused by reperfusion syndrome from dysfunction in the cerebral circulation autoregulation once the blood flow is restored after endarterectomy. It is usually self-limited and resolves spontaneously. However, if there is associated neurologic deficit, CT should be performed.

Complications. Stroke is the most feared complication of CEA; it occurs in 1% to 3% of patients, depending on the indication for the surgery. Causes include embolization from a friable or ulcerated plaque during carotid dissection, inadequate cerebral perfusion during endarterectomy, thrombosis from a flap or technical error, and reperfusion syndrome. Most of the reported low rates of stroke are from specialized centers, and a more realistic complication rate from the community data for combined stroke morbidity and mortality ranges from 6% to 20%. The Stroke Council of the American Heart Association has set standards for upper acceptable limits of stroke and death as a function of indications for endarterectomy. For patients with asymptomatic carotid disease, the combined operative stroke morbidity and mortality should not be more than 3%; for TIA, 5%; for history of previous stroke, 7%; and for recurrent carotid stenosis, 10%.

Injury to the cranial nerves can cause postoperative morbidity. The incidence has been found to be approximately 16%; incidence increased to 39% if further evaluation was performed by a speech pathologist. Only 60% of these patients were symptomatic, and most of these symptoms were temporary. After 6 weeks, the incidence was between 1% and 4%. Dysfunction of the superior laryngeal and recurrent laryngeal nerves is the most common cranial nerve injury encountered. This is likely caused by retraction injury or direct trauma by forceps during surgery, which can lead to paralysis of the vocal cord in the paramedian position, resulting in hoarseness and loss of an effective cough mechanism. Unilateral injury can be asymptomatic, but airway obstruction can be caused if there is bilateral injury. If staged bilateral CEA is planned, routine direct visualization of the vocal cord by laryngoscopy is recommended after the first endarterectomy. Staged surgery is delayed if there is cord paralysis. Wound retraction can also cause injury to the hypoglossal nerve during superior exposure for high carotid bifurcation. This is manifested by tongue deviation to the ipsilateral side, but it can occasionally cause speech impairment and mastication problems.

Carotid Angioplasty and Stent Procedure

Many randomized trials have shown that CEA is effective in preventing stroke in symptomatic and asymptomatic patients with significant internal carotid stenosis. It has been accepted that CEA is the gold standard of treatment for these patients. However, there remain a group of patients who have been identified as high risk for CEA. Carotid angioplasty with stenting (CAS) has emerged as a safe and effective alternative to CEA for patients with indications for carotid intervention. During the past decade, CAS has seen a rapid evolution in technique and technology with the introduction of self-expanding nitinol stents, smaller delivery systems, and embolic protection devices (EPDs).

Early single-center studies performed from 1990 to 1999 showed significantly higher rates of stroke and death for CAS than for CEA in 30-day outcomes for symptomatic patients. The risk of major stroke or death was 3.9% after CAS and 2.2% after CEA, and the risk of any stroke or death was 7.8% for CAS and 4% for CEA. During these studies, most CAS procedures were performed without an EPD. When early studies were designed to randomize patients between CAS and CEA, many had to be terminated prematurely because of inferior results with CAS. These studies showed that patients with unprotected CAS without EPD had a higher stroke rate than with CEA and protected CAS and that unprotected CAS was not equivalent to CEA. The Stenting and Angioplasty with Protection in Patients at High Risk for Endarterectomy (SAPPHIRE) trial was the first randomized study to show the benefits of using EPD in CAS and that protected CAS was not inferior to CEA in high-risk patients. Most recently, in 2010, preliminary results from the Carotid Revascularization Endarterectomy versus Stent Trial (CREST) became available.[54] This was the first multicenter prospective, randomized clinical trial funded by the National Institutes of Health to compare the safety and efficacy of CAS and CEA in symptomatic and asymptomatic patients. Preliminary end points were any clinical stroke, myocardial infarction, or death and any ipsilateral stroke during the entire follow-up period. There were 2502 patients (asymptomatic, 47%; symptomatic, 53%), with a median follow-up period of 2.5 years. In regard to the primary composite end point, there was no difference between CAS and CEA (7.2% for CAS versus 6.8% for CEA; $P = .51$). There was a statistically significant difference in 30-day stroke rate, 4.1% for CAS and 2.3% for CEA. The risk of myocardial infarction was significantly lower for CAS, 1.1%, compared with CEA, 2.3%. At median follow-up of 2.5 years, there was no difference in stroke rate between CAS and CEA.

The data from CREST have shown similar composite outcomes between the two procedures, which led the investigators to conclude that both CAS and CEA had similar composite outcomes, with differences in periprocedural stroke and myocardial infarction. It is likely that there will be more demand from the public for this less invasive modality for the treatment of high-grade carotid disease. Of note, CAS procedures performed during the second half of this 10-year trial had a significantly lower incidence of complications compared with those CAS procedures performed during the first half of the study. These findings indicate improvements in device design and operator experience over time and suggest that future results may continue to improve with this technique.

Indications and contraindications. CAS is currently indicated for symptomatic high-risk patients. Indications for symptomatic patients with high-grade carotid stenosis were outlined in the consensus conference of the Stroke Council of the American Heart Association (see earlier). At the time of this printing, the Centers for Medicare and Medicaid Services continue to deny coverage for carotid stent procedures for asymptomatic patients as well as for symptomatic patients who are deemed good-risk candidates for CEA.

There is a group of patients who are considered at high risk for open surgical CEA. They can be divided into two main categories: those with anatomic conditions and those with physiologic conditions. High-risk anatomic conditions include the following: restenosis after previous CEA caused by association with higher risk of cranial nerve injury; "hostile" neck from previous neck radiation, radical neck dissection, permanent tracheostomy, or frozen neck; high or low lesions above C2 or below the clavicle, respectively; and other carotid lesions, including tandem lesions within the same carotid artery and contralateral high-grade ICA disease. High-risk physiologic conditions include the following: class III or class IV angina or congestive heart failure; severe chronic obstructive pulmonary disease (forced expiratory volume ≤1 or the need for home oxygen); and cardiac disease necessitating open heart surgery within 4 weeks.

Contraindications to CAS include coils or kinking of the CCA or ICA and excessive calcification of the carotid disease. Difficult access because of iliac disease and a tortuous and calcified arch or tandem CCA stenoses may also contribute to difficulties in stent delivery.

Technique

Carotid artery access and guide sheath positioning. Just as in CEA, patients are medically optimized with antihypertensives, statins, and smoking cessation. Patients who have not been taking clopidogrel are given an oral loading dose of 600 mg and then maintained on 75 mg by mouth daily. Retrograde common femoral artery access is usually the first choice, primarily secondary to table and patient positioning constraints. Brachial access is used only in certain circumstances, such as severe aortoiliac occlusive disease. In most cases, diagnostic arteriography and the intervention are performed at separate times. Diagnostic arch aortography with four-vessel extracranial and bilateral cerebral arteriography is first performed for the evaluation of the carotid disease and cerebral circulation and for procedural planning. The aortogram is obtained with a pigtail catheter in the ascending aorta in left anterior oblique angulation. The bilateral CCAs are then catheterized for arteriograms of the ICA and cerebral circulation. The subclavian arteries are catheterized for the evaluation of vertebral arteries. After diagnostic arteriography, the patient is discharged on the same day.

For patients requiring treatment, the intervention is performed at a later time. Based on the diagnostic arteriogram, appropriately shaped catheters and sheaths are chosen. To limit contrast material, a selective catheterization can be made on the basis of a previous arch aortogram. Most CCAs can be accessed simply with an angled catheter; however, some will require a more complex-shaped catheter, such as a Simmons catheter. Selective carotid angiography is then performed with careful hand injections of contrast material. A 0.035-inch guidewire is positioned in the ECA and catheterized by the angled catheter. An angiogram is used to confirm the location of the ECA. A stiff wire is then placed in this artery, and the catheter and short groin sheath are removed and exchanged for a long 6 Fr sheath. The tip of the sheath is advanced to the distal CCA. The stiff wire is removed from the patient.

Placement of embolic protection device. With the long sheath near the carotid bulb, a careful angiogram with hand injection is obtained to determine the anatomy of the disease and location of the ICA. The wire with the EPD is advanced across the disease and into the distal ICA, just before the horizontal petrous segment. The EPD is deployed. Flow through the EPD and its apposition to the wall are evaluated.

Carotid stent placement. An angiogram is then obtained, noting the location of the carotid disease. The stent is advanced carefully across the disease, and it is deployed from the ICA into the CCA, covering the ECA origin (Fig. 62-30). Prestenting angioplasty is not routinely performed unless it is necessary to create a space needed for placement of the stent in near-occlusive lesions. The self-expanding nitinol stent is typically 8 to 10 mm in diameter by 30 mm in length. It is sized to the largest portion of the vessel, usually the distal CCA. A small stent that does not oppose the carotid wall may become a nidus for thrombus formation. Current stents are designed to be used in small delivery systems with a rapid exchange or monorail platform.

Carotid angioplasty. After stenting, poststenting angioplasty is performed. The patient receives 0.5 mg of atropine or 0.1 mg of glycopyrrolate intravenously immediately before angioplasty to blunt the effect of pressure from the balloon on the carotid bulb. An angioplasty balloon is advanced over the 0.014-inch guidewire across the location of the narrowest area of the stent. The balloon should approximate the size of the native normal ICA beyond the stenosis, not a segment with poststenotic dilation. Typically, the initial angioplasty is performed with a 5-mm semicompliant balloon. The balloon is inflated slowly until apposition is achieved and then deflated slowly. Transcranial Doppler imaging may be used to monitor for embolic debris. Experience with this procedure has shown that the greatest number of emboli are released with balloon deflation.

Completion angiogram. Before removal of the guidewire and sheath, a completion angiogram is obtained to confirm adequate resolution of the carotid disease and to ensure flow through the ICA. Spasm of the ICA distal to the stent can be treated with a vasodilator, such as nitroglycerin or papaverine. However, most spasms resolve with removal of the EPD. Once the EPD is removed, another angiogram is obtained to confirm vasodilation of the vessel and flow. A closure device is then used to close the arteriotomy. If a patient has neurologic functional changes, a cerebral angiogram is obtained and compared with previous diagnostic angiograms. Nonvisualization of cerebral arteries after stenting that were previously seen on a diagnostic angiogram is of concern for an embolic event, and an intervention must be carried out (Fig. 62-31).

Neurologic deficits that occur as a result of stent placement are not the same as those that occur with carotid surgery.[55] Rather than an immediate intraprocedural event, a substantial number of the periprocedural events that occur with CAS occur hours to days after the procedure. In one study, 26% of the periprocedural neurologic events occurred more than 1 day (and up to 14 days) after the procedure and after discharge of the patient.[56] In another

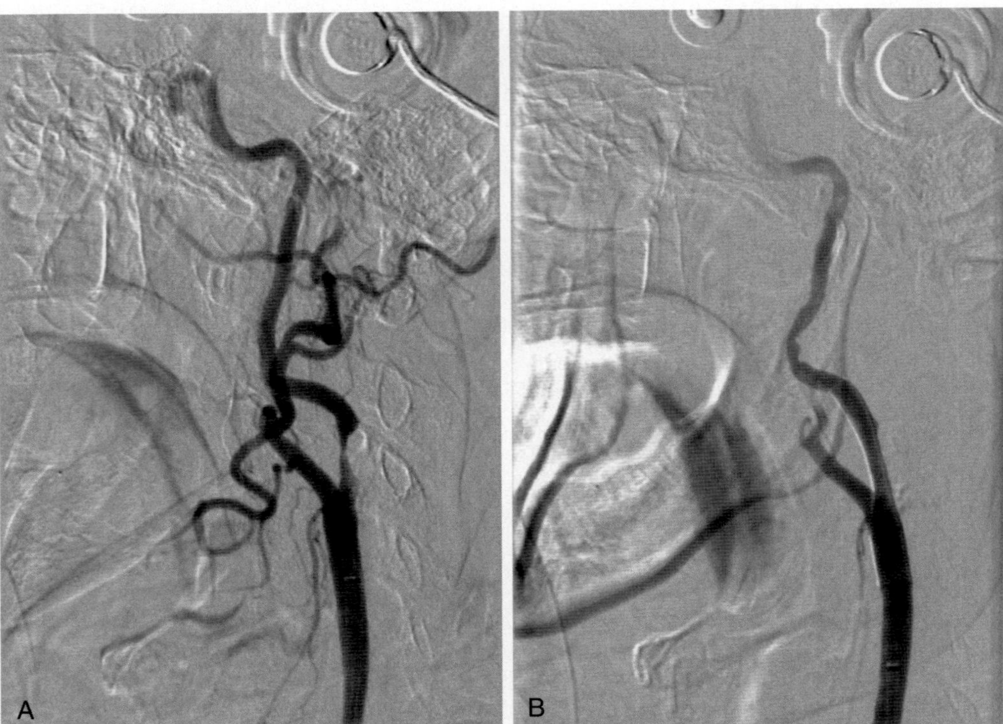

FIGURE 62-30 Carotid stent. A, Severe internal carotid artery stenosis. B, Improved flow after internal carotid artery stent placement.

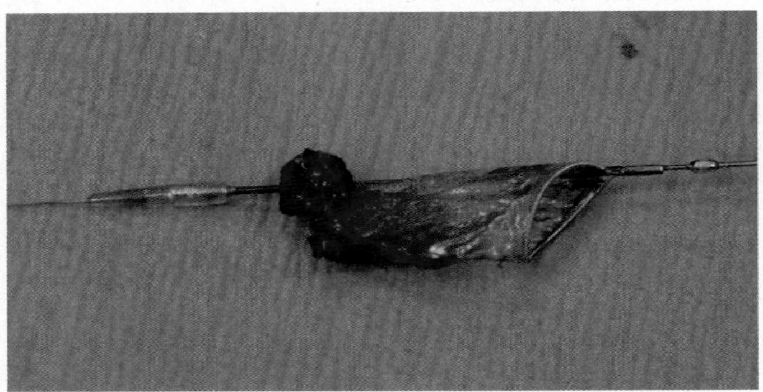

FIGURE 62-31 Embolic protection device; filter with acute thrombus.

study, 71% of the periprocedural deficits (10 of 14) after carotid stent placement in 111 patients occurred after the procedure was completed rather than during the procedure.[57] This presents logistic challenges if intracranial thrombolysis ever becomes the standard method for managing this problem because it often occurs after catheters and intra-arterial access devices have been removed; in some cases, the patient may already have been discharged. The patient would have to return and be treated in a timely manner. The site at which the carotid stent was placed would require repeated instrumentation (crossing with guidewires and catheters), with the attendant added risk of additional embolization.

Conclusions. The CREST trial demonstrated a significant learning curve with CAS. In CAS, selection of patients is the key to early success. Patients who are good stent candidates because of high medical comorbidities may not always have favorable anatomy for stent placement and will likely have an elevated risk of periprocedural complications, even from a percutaneous procedure. Some patients with complex anatomy who are otherwise good candidates for CAS may have to be treated by alternative means if they are seen early in the program's development, while the physician is accumulating experience. The best early candidates for CAS are patients with focal recurrent stenosis. Performance of CAS requires excellent imaging; the procedure is facilitated by the use of a floating radiolucent table. Specific equipment and tools for carotid arteriography, balloon angioplasty, and stent placement differ somewhat from those used for other vascular beds. The components for carotid intervention must be determined, understood, requested, and assembled before proceeding. There is growing consensus that CAS may be an effective alternative treatment for high-grade carotid artery disease that avoids the morbidity and mortality of open surgical treatment. Outside of clinical trials, it is currently indicated for symptomatic high-risk patients. With the results from CREST recently published, it is likely that approved indications will be expanded to include normal-risk, high-grade symptomatic and asymptomatic patients. Vascular surgeons have traditionally assumed a leadership role in the management of carotid disease. If we are to continue to provide our patients with the full breadth of therapeutic alternatives, it is imperative that we develop the necessary skills to perform safe and effective CAS procedures while maintaining our open surgical expertise with CEA. Further rigorous scientific investigation will allow us to elucidate the subtle characteristics of patients and their lesions that may better inform our recommendations for one of these two competing treatment options.

DIALYSIS ACCESS

Dialysis Outcomes Quality Initiative Guidelines

Three types of access are commonly placed for hemodialysis: (1) autogenous fistula (AF); (2) prosthetic bridging graft (BG); and

(3) indwelling central venous catheter. The ideal access delivers a flow rate sufficient for effective dialysis, is easily cannulated, has a long life, and has a low complication rate.

Currently, AFs are preferred to prosthetic grafts and central venous catheters because of their higher primary patency rates and lower frequency of stenosis, thrombosis, and infection.[58] Previously, prosthetic conduit was often used for the initial hemodialysis access. Justification for a preference for prosthetic grafts included technical ease of procedure, avoidance of prolonged maturation times, ease of cannulation, differences in reimbursement, and disbelief in the superiority of AFs.[59] The reluctance to perform native fistulas was also fueled by the wide range of reported rates of patency and maturation to a functional access with traditional single-incision direct arteriovenous fistulas, such as the wrist radiocephalic fistula. Maturation rates of arteriovenous fistulas range from 25% to 90%.[60-62]

The U.S. Renal Data System, which accumulates and reviews data from the nation's dialysis centers, reported in 1995 that the frequency of native AF construction in the United States was less than 30% of total access procedures performed, with some regions having AF placement rates of less than 10%.[63] In 1996, the Dialysis Outcomes Quality Initiative (DOQI) Vascular Access Work Group met at the request of the National Kidney Foundation to address all aspects of current medical and surgical issues associated with hemodialysis and to publish a set of practice guidelines.[64] This was updated in 2000.[58]

To attain the goals recommended by the DOQI, surgeons are expected to increase their rates of autogenous arteriovenous fistulas to at least 50% of all new permanent hemodialysis accesses constructed. An important objective of the DOQI is to have a prevalence of AFs in 40% of all hemodialysis patients.

Nomenclature

In 2002, the Committee on Reporting Standards for Arterio-Venous Accesses of the Society for Vascular Surgery and the American Association for Vascular Surgery published standardized definitions related to arteriovenous access procedures and recommended reporting standards for patency and complications.[65] *Autogenous* refers to the native vein. An autogenous arteriovenous access is an access created by a connection between an artery and vein, and the vein serves as the access site for needle cannulation. A *transposition* is an access performed with a transposed vein. The peripheral portion of the vein is moved from its original position, usually through a superficial subcutaneous tunnel, and connected to the artery. The more central venous segment in a transposed access is left in its anatomic position. In contrast, the term *translocated* is used to describe an access constructed from a segment of vein that has been completely mobilized, disconnected proximally and distally, and placed in a location remote from its origin. The recommended nomenclature for the autogenous transposition procedures can be found in Table 62-9.

Configuration descriptors provide information about the anastomotic connection and course of the conduit. An access has a direct or indirect configuration. A direct access describes the connection between native artery and vein and involves such configurations as end-to-side, side-to-side, and end-to-end anastomoses.[65] In an indirect access, an autogenous or prosthetic graft is interposed between the native artery and vein. Additional descriptors may be used, such as transposed, translocated, straight, and looped.

Primary patency refers to the interval from the time of access placement to the intervention designed to maintain or to reestablish patency or access thrombosis or the time of measurement of patency. *Assisted primary patency* refers to the interval from the time of access placement until access thrombosis or the time of measurement of patency, including interventions designed to maintain the function of a patent access. *Secondary patency* refers to the interval from the time of access placement until access abandonment or thrombosis or the time of patency measurement, including interventions to reestablish function in a thrombosed access.[65]

TABLE 62-9 Recommended Nomenclature for Transposition Access Procedures

RECOMMENDED NOMENCLATURE	TRADITIONAL NOMENCLATURE
Forearm	
Autogenous radial-basilic forearm transposition	Superficial venous transposition in the forearm, basilic vein to radial artery
Autogenous ulnar-basilic forearm transposition	Superficial venous transposition in the forearm, basilic vein to ulnar artery
Autogenous radial-cephalic forearm transposition	Superficial venous transposition in the forearm, cephalic vein to radial artery
Autogenous brachial-cephalic forearm transposition	Superficial venous transposition in the forearm, cephalic vein to brachial artery
Upper Arm	
Autogenous brachial-basilic upper arm transposition	Basilic vein transposition
Lower Extremity	
Autogenous femoral–greater saphenous looped access transposition	Greater saphenous vein end-to-side to femoral artery fistula

Adapted from Sidawy AN, Gray R, Besarab A: Recommended standards for reports dealing with arteriovenous hemodialysis accesses. *J Vasc Surg* 35:603–610, 2002.

Superficial Venous System of the Upper Extremity

An understanding of the venous anatomy of the upper extremity is essential for the planning of permanent hemodialysis access. Although there is an anatomic commonality among patients that represents a starting point for inspection, anatomic variations and segmental venous stenoses and occlusions from previous medical or surgical interventions are important to identify by thorough preoperative assessment.

Cephalic Vein

The cephalic vein arises from the radial aspect of the veins draining the dorsum of the hand and travels around the radial border of the forearm. On the proximal aspect of the volar forearm, the median cubital vein arises. This vein communicates with the deep veins in the forearm and then crosses the antecubital fossa to join the basilic vein. As it crosses the elbow, the cephalic vein is found in an anatomic groove between the brachioradialis and biceps muscles. The cephalic vein travels superficially to the musculocutaneous nerve and then ascends in the groove along the lateral border of the biceps muscle. In the upper third of the arm, the cephalic vein passes between the pectoralis major and deltoid muscles, crosses the axillary artery, and joins the axillary vein just below the clavicle. The accessory cephalic vein arises from the ulnar side of the dorsum of the hand or the posterior aspect of the forearm and usually joins the cephalic vein below the elbow.

Basilic Vein

The basilic vein originates on the ulnar aspect of the dorsum of the hand and travels in the subcutaneous space up the ulnar side of the forearm, shifting from the posterior surface distally toward a more anterior orientation below the elbow. The median antecubital vein joins the basilic vein in the antecubital fossa and then travels in the groove between the biceps and pronator teres muscles to cross the brachial artery. In this region, the vein is crossed anteriorly and posteriorly by branches of the median cutaneous nerve. As it courses proximately along the medial border of the biceps muscle, the basilic vein descends below the deep fascia to travel parallel to the brachial artery and vein. The union of the basilic and brachial veins in the axilla forms the axillary vein.

Median Antebrachial Vein

The median antebrachial vein drains the palmar surface of the hand and is located on the ulnar side of the anterior forearm. In the proximal forearm, it joins the basilic vein or median antecubital vein.

Initial Evaluation for New Access

The first step in establishing hemodialysis access is to select the best available site, based on optimal arterial inflow and venous outflow, observing the preference of an AF over a BG, the forearm over the upper arm, and the nondominant over the dominant upper extremity. Visual inspection and physical examination of the upper extremity are performed but may be inadequate to assess certain factors, especially vein size, quality, and adequacy of central venous outflow. For this reason, duplex ultrasound scanning is used for all patients.

The examination is initiated at the wrist of the nondominant upper extremity, and a tourniquet is placed at the midforearm. After dilation of the superficial veins by gentle tapping and stroking, the veins are insonated with a 5- or 7-MHz scanning probe. They are evaluated for diameter, compressibility, and continuity with upper arm veins. Patency of the deep system and continuity with patent axillary and subclavian veins are also verified. However, central venous stenosis or thrombosis does not preclude the use of that arm; multiple large collateral veins are able to provide outflow and support an AF.

The largest diameter superficial vein of good quality is mapped with skin markings. Suitability criteria for access include the following:

- Target vein diameter of more than 2.5 mm for an AF and more than 4.0 mm for a BG
- Continuity with the deep and central system
- Absence of stenosis in the vein itself

When favorable venous anatomy is found, the arterial system is then evaluated for target artery diameter and patency of the palmar arch. Reduced pressure measurements compared with the other arm or abnormal Doppler waveforms indicate proximal arterial stenosis and preclude use of that arm for access unless the problem is successfully addressed. The basic requirements are as follows:

- An arterial luminal diameter of more than 2.0 mm
- Absence of obliterating calcification
- Palmar arch patency

Evaluation of central venous outflow stenosis or occlusion is an integral part of the duplex ultrasound examination. Central venous stenosis usually results from previous use of central catheters, especially in the subclavian vein.

If a unilateral central vein problem is found, the contralateral extremity becomes the preferred choice regardless of the issue of extremity dominance. If bilateral central vein problems exist but are amenable to endovascular treatment, this should be attempted on the least diseased side.

If a subsequent duplex scan confirms effective treatment of the central vein problem, this arm can be selected for access. If not, the patient may require a nonstandard complex access solution (see later). Patients with multiple large collateral veins from chronic central venous disease can still have AF attempted if a suitable vein is available.

The anticipated duration of dialysis determines the type of catheter access selected.

- Patients expected to require dialysis for less than 3 weeks are candidates for noncuffed central venous catheter access for dialysis; these dual-lumen catheters may be placed at the bedside without fluoroscopic guidance.
- For patients expected to require dialysis for longer than 3 weeks, cuffed tunneled catheters are placed.
- For patients undergoing placement of an AF who require immediate dialysis, a cuffed tunneled catheter is placed concurrently, typically in the contralateral internal jugular vein, to provide access while the AF matures.

The internal jugular vein is preferred to the subclavian vein; the contralateral deep venous system is accessed when possible to avoid catheter obstruction of venous outflow or catheter-induced venous stenosis during the period of AF maturation. Duplex scans aid in the selection of a patent normal vein for catheter placement. Femoral catheters can also be used on a temporary basis if the deep central venous system of the upper extremity is intractably compromised.

Central Venous Catheters

A cuffed central venous catheter is placed in all patients requiring immediate dialysis after AF formation so that adequate maturation time (6 to 12 weeks) can be provided before cannulation of the AF. Because a BG can generally be used within 3 weeks, temporary noncuffed catheters can be used in this group.

The contralateral internal jugular vein is the preferred site, if it is available, because it limits ipsilateral venous outflow obstruction and would not be associated with the development of subclavian vein stenosis. Alternative sites may be used:

- Ipsilateral internal jugular vein. This choice poses some risk of venous outflow obstruction because the catheter physically rests across the confluence of the internal jugular vein and the now high-flow subclavian vein, but it has the benefit of limiting subclavian vein stenosis.
- Contralateral subclavian vein. Perhaps there would be less outflow obstruction but greater potential for negative long-term sequelae if stenosis results.
- Ipsilateral subclavian vein. This is the least attractive alternative, with potential for outflow obstruction and stenosis.

The routine use of upper extremity duplex ultrasound imaging for access planning identifies many patients who have veins suitable for AF formation but that are too deep for successful cannulation or that are too remote from the optimal arterial inflow to allow direct anastomosis without tension. Superficial venous transposition in the forearm increases AF rates in these patients.[66] This technique involves extensive dissection of a vein identified by duplex scan as being suitable in diameter, with ligation of side branches and transposition to a subcutaneous tunnel along the volar aspect of the forearm, bringing the vein to the inflow artery. This position is optimal for comfortable arm positioning during dialysis.

Types of Venous Transpositions

Upper Arm Venous Transposition

The basilic vein in the upper arm is often a good conduit for dialysis access because of its relatively large size and location in the deeper tissue planes. The traumatic consequences of repeated venipunctures observed in more superficial veins are not seen in the basilic vein because of its deeper position. Classically, the brachiobasilic transposition was regarded as a secondary option after a failed forearm fistula or graft.[67] The creation of an access using the proximal basilic vein was devised on the basis of the theoretical benefits of using a superficial vein spared repeated venipunctures, with a relatively large diameter and length. As with all venous transpositions, only one anastomosis is required, and anatomic continuity with the axillary vein is maintained. The transposition of the basilic vein to the brachial artery was described by Dagher in 1976. Four years after the original description of 24 brachiobasilic fistulas, the 5-year follow-up of a series of 90 fistulas was reported, with a 73.5% patency rate. The long-term patency remained good; a 70% functional patency rate at 8 years in 176 fistulas was reported.[68]

In certain subgroups of patients, such as those with small cephalic veins, PVD, and diabetes, the maturation rate of the radiocephalic fistula has been poor. The brachiobasilic transposition has been a good second option for these patients. Hakaim and associates[61] have reported on the superior fistula maturation in brachiobasilic transpositions (73%) compared with primary radiocephalic arteriovenous fistulas (30%). Ascher and coworkers[69] have reviewed their experience using arm veins to create brachiocephalic and brachiobasilic arteriovenous fistulas. They found no significant difference between primary patency rates at 1 year (72% for brachiocephalic versus 70% for brachiobasilic). Because of excellent patency with these fistulas, this group proposed an algorithm for the placement of arteriovenous fistulas. If a radiocephalic fistula is not feasible, a brachiocephalic fistula should first be attempted. If the brachiocephalic fistula fails or is not possible, a brachiobasilic fistula should be placed before an arteriovenous graft. In an attempt to maximize the AF rate, we favor a similar algorithm, with the addition of the superficial venous transposition of the forearm before performance of the brachial artery–based fistulas, that is, radiocephalic fistula, followed by forearm basilic venous transposition, followed by brachiocephalic fistula, followed by brachiobasilic fistula.

Long-term patency with transposed brachiobasilic fistulas that have matured has been good, with reported primary patency rates as high as 90% at 1 year and 86% at 2 years.[70] In 2003, Taghizadeh and associates[71] reported a series of 75 brachiobasilic transpositions performed during 5 years, with a mean follow-up of 14 months. In their series, 92% of fistulas matured to allow hemodialysis access. The cumulative patency was 66% at 1 year, 52% at 2 years, and 43% at 3 years. Overall, complications developed in 55% of fistulas; these included thrombosis (33%), stenosis (11%), local infection (6%), arm edema (5%), hemorrhage (3%), aneurysm (1%), and steal syndrome (1%).

The overall patency rate for autogenous brachial-basilic transpositions is superior to that of PTFE upper arm dialysis grafts. A review of all basilic vein transpositions and brachial PTFE arteriovenous fistulas created during a 5-year period has demonstrated a statistically significant difference in primary patency rate at 1 year (90% versus 70%; $P < .01$) and 2 years (86% versus 49%; $P < .001$).[70] In this study, complications occurred approximately twice as frequently with the PTFE grafts than with the venous transpositions.

Forearm Venous Transpositions

The radiocephalic fistula, performed through a single incision, was initially described in 1966 by Brescia and coworkers.[72] This primary arteriovenous fistula was a dramatic improvement over the other, less durable modes of hemodialysis access available at the time and soon became the preferred approach to long-term dialysis access. The hemodialysis population has changed, and the dialysis patient who has a suitable vein close to the radial artery is becoming uncommon. Therefore, venous transposition procedures in the forearm have become important for enabling these patients to have a primary arteriovenous fistula.

Physical examination and visual inspection alone poorly identify suitable arteries and veins in the upper extremity. Duplex ultrasound examination allows a more thorough evaluation of the superficial venous system, increasing the number of patients who can have a forearm fistula.[66] The duplex scan can identify veins in the forearm that may have been spared repeated venipunctures because of their deeper subcutaneous location. The size of these veins may be suitable for arteriovenous creation, but if left in situ, their position in the deeper subcutaneous tissues and their anatomic position on the forearm make needle cannulation for hemodialysis technically more difficult. These usable veins on the posterior aspect of the forearm, such as the basilic vein, if not transposed, require uncomfortable and awkward positioning of the arm for dialysis. Therefore, once identified by duplex scanning, these veins are mobilized and transposed to a more favorable location on the forearm through a superficial subcutaneous plane.

To increase the number of primary AFs, Silva and colleagues,[66] in 1997, described the routine use of duplex scanning for preoperative access planning for superficial venous transposition of forearm veins for autogenous hemodialysis access. They reported a series of 89 patients in whom arteries and veins were identified with duplex scanning as suitable for primary arteriovenous fistulas. After the superficial venous transposition procedure, 91% of the fistulas matured, to be used for hemodialysis access. The primary patency rate was 84% at 1 year and 69% at 2 years. (The beneficial impact of preoperative duplex ultrasound assessments was reported in 1998.[60]) This group demonstrated a dramatic improvement in their AF rate with the institution of the protocol of routine use of duplex scanning for preoperative access planning. Their AF rate was 14% before the institution of the protocol and 63% after the protocol was established. Table 62-10 demonstrates the three general areas in which the superficial veins are found and the rates at which they were used in the study. Note that the minority (15%) of the transpositions were accomplished through a single incision, with the artery and vein in proximity. Approximately 50% of transposed veins arose from the volar surface of the forearm, and a third were harvested from the dorsal aspect of the forearm.

Lower Extremity Venous Transpositions

The upper extremity is the preferred site for hemodialysis access, with the lower extremity generally being reserved for use once upper extremity options have been exhausted. If the extremity is not suitable for fistula creation, a prosthetic graft can be placed. However, there is a concern about increased thrombosis and

TABLE 62-10 Superficial Venous Transpositions of the Forearm

TRANSPOSITION PERFORMED	% OF TOTAL
Type A	15
Artery and vein in immediate proximity	
Single incision	
Superficial subcutaneous transposition only	
Type B	33
Dorsally located vein transposed to volar surface artery	
Separate incisions	
Superficial subcutaneous transposition	
Type C	52
Volar vein transposed to midforearm volar surface	
Separate incisions	
Superficial subcutaneous transposition	

From Silva MB Jr, Hobson RW 2nd, Pappas PJ, et al: Vein transposition in the forearm for autogenous hemodialysis access. *J Vasc Surg* 26:981–986, 1997.

infection rates in thigh hemodialysis grafts, which have been reported as high as 55% and 35%, respectively. Tashjian and associates,[73] reviewing their experience with 73 femoral artery–based hemodialysis grafts, found a primary patency rate of 71% and a secondary patency rate of 83% at 1 year. The infection rate in this series was 22%.

Venous transpositions in the lower extremity using the great saphenous vein and superficial femoral vein have been described.[74] The transposed great saphenous veins and superficial femoral veins in the leg have theoretical benefits similar to those of venous transpositions in the upper extremity. The venous conduits are long and generally of good caliber and are less prone to infection than prosthetic grafts. Importantly, only one anastomosis is required because the more central venous segment maintains its native connection with the common femoral vein.

The superficial femoral vein, part of the deep venous system, has a diameter in the range of 6 to 10 mm, has relatively thick walls, and has been used for a wide variety of vascular reconstructions.[75] Gradman and coworkers have reported a retrospective analysis of 25 patients who underwent arteriovenous construction with use of superficial femoral veins. Of these patients, 18 underwent superficial femoral vein transposition and 7 were given a composite loop fistula of superficial femoral vein and PTFE. The cumulative primary fistula patency rate was 78% at 6 months and 73% at 1 year. The cumulative secondary patency rate was 91% at 5 months and 86% at 1 year. There were no fistula infections, but the rate of major wound complications was 28%. Eight patients required secondary procedures for symptomatic steal syndrome, and one patient ultimately needed an above-knee amputation after the development of ipsilateral compartment syndrome.[74]

The saphenous vein has been used for arterial reconstructions in almost all vascular beds and in the construction of arteriovenous access in the upper and lower extremities. The great saphenous vein has been used to create an AF in the upper thigh in a looped configuration and an arterial anastomosis with the common femoral artery or SFA.[76]

Techniques of Venous Transposition

Assessment of the Patient and Selection of Optimal Site

The evaluation and preoperative assessment of the patient are the most important steps in the establishment of durable hemodialysis access. First, the best available site is selected on the basis of optimal arterial inflow and venous outflow. According to the DOQI guidelines, the preference is for an AF over a prosthetic graft, for the forearm over the upper arm, and for the nondominant arm over the dominant arm.

Preference for the nondominant arm relates to convenience for the patient, allowing the dominant arm to be used for activity during dialysis. When duplex ultrasound surveillance identifies a suitable vein and artery in the nondominant forearm, an AF constructed between them becomes the procedure of choice. Duplex ultrasonography is also used to select the optimal anastomotic site. If the radial or ulnar arteries are disadvantaged, a suitable vein in the forearm may be dissected and looped back to the brachial artery in the antecubital space. All autogenous forearm possibilities are exhausted before proceeding to autogenous upper arm alternatives because this maximizes future possible sites.

Absence of suitable veins in both forearms necessitates construction of the access in the upper arm. Again, duplex ultrasonography is valuable in identifying a superficial (preferred) or deep (second-choice) arm vein that can be transposed to a volar subcutaneous location for creation of an AF with the brachial artery. The dominant upper arm is used if the arteries and veins in the nondominant upper arm are unsuitable.

If there are no suitable veins for an AF, outflow through the deeper venous system in the arm is examined to identify a possible site of placement of a prosthetic BG. A looped BG configuration is used in the nondominant forearm when an appropriate antecubital vein and brachial artery are present.

The dominant forearm is the next site of choice. If both forearms are unsuitable, the nondominant upper arm, followed by the dominant upper arm, is the next option. To maximize the number of BG possibilities, a prosthetic graft is initially placed between the brachial artery and the brachial vein in the distal upper arm, followed by the vein in the mid arm and the proximal arm, and finally the axillary vein.

Duplex ultrasonography is used to identify and to mark the best possible location for the anastomosis and to confirm adequate central venous runoff. When possible, avoid placement of prosthetic BGs in patients who are significantly immunocompromised because of the significant risk of infection and the complexities involved with removal of the BG and restoration of prograde arterial flow.

Superficial Venous Transposition of the Forearm

The superficial venous transposition of the forearm is performed using local 1% lidocaine infusion supplemented with IV sedation. Lidocaine with epinephrine is avoided because of its vasoconstrictive properties.

A longitudinal incision is made directly over the cephalic or basilic vein, beginning at the distal extent of the previously mapped and marked vein. The incision proceeds toward the antecubital fossa for a distance of at least 15 cm. Multiple short skip incisions can also be used. A 3-0 silk suture ligature is used to ligate the portion of vein remaining in its distal bed, and the vein is transected at the wrist. The vein is dissected free from its surrounding tissue so that it may be completely transposed to a superficial tunnel in the midportion of the volar aspect of the forearm. Most venous branches along the length of the vein are ligated and divided; however, those that will not interfere with transposition are left intact to maximize outflow. Heparinized saline is flushed through the open end of the vein with digital compression for occlusion of outflow at the antecubital fossa; this results in substantial dilation of the freed segment of vein. The vein is wrapped in a heparin- and saline-soaked sponge, and attention is then turned to the arterial dissection.

The segment of artery that has been preoperatively identified as suitable for inflow is exposed. Usually, the radial artery is identified between the brachial radialis and flexor carpi radialis tendons. The superficial branch of the radial nerve is located lateral to the radial artery, and this nerve is separated from the radial artery by the brachial radialis muscle. The nerve is sensory at this level, and care must be taken not to injure it. Concomitant veins run parallel to the artery on either side. These should be carefully dissected free from the artery, facilitating identification of the numerous small arterial branches. Although there are usually no arterial branches on the anterior aspect of the artery, several paired arterial branches usually leave the radial artery on each side, and they must be addressed. These may be ligated, with the ligature placed approximately 2 mm away from the radial artery to avoid impingement once dilation has occurred. Vessel loops are placed proximally and distally along the artery for vascular control.

A tunneling instrument is passed through the subcutaneous tissues to develop a superficial tunnel. The vein is marked on the anterior surface along its length with a sterile marking pen to facilitate passage through the tunnel without twisting or kinking. Once the vein has been passed through the subcutaneous tunnel and hemostasis has been ensured, the patient is typically given 3000 units of heparin intravenously, and a 1- to 2-mm arteriotomy is made with a No. 11 scalpel blade on the volar surface of the artery. The arteriotomy is extended to approximately 15 to 20 mm with fine Potts scissors. With an 18-gauge angiocatheter, the artery is heparinized locally by injection of heparinized saline distally and then proximally while the vessel loops are simultaneously opened.

An end-to-side anastomosis is performed with 7-0 polypropylene or Gore-Tex PTFE suture (Gore Medical). Before completion of the anastomosis, vascular dilators are used to size the vein and radial artery. This step has the benefit of allowing enlargement of blood vessels in spasm from vessel loops and manipulation.

After the anastomosis is constructed, it is essential that a thrill be felt within the vein. Absence of a thrill indicates a probable technical or anatomic defect and requires further investigation, with exploration of the anastomosis. Wounds are closed with a running subcuticular absorbable stitch. Care is taken to maintain strict atraumatic technique during handling of the skin edges to limit wound complications. Adhesive strips and tape applied directly to the skin are not used.

Superficial Venous Transposition of the Arm

The transposition of the cephalic or basilic vein is performed with local anesthesia using 1% lidocaine and IV sedation or regional anesthesia using an interscalene nerve block. The entire arm and ipsilateral axilla and shoulder are prepared in a sterile fashion. For the cephalic vein transposition, the vein is found in an anatomic groove between the brachioradialis and biceps muscles. It travels superficially to the musculocutaneous nerve and then ascends in the groove along the lateral border of the biceps muscle. A longitudinal incision over the cephalic vein is used for exposure. For the basilic vein transposition, the vein is identified anterior to the medial epicondyle of the humerus, and through a longitudinal incision along the medial aspect of the upper arm to the axilla, the basilic vein is exposed. The median cutaneous nerve is close to the basilic vein and should be preserved.

All venous branches are ligated and divided. The cephalic vein is mobilized for at least 15 cm. The basilic vein is mobilized to its junction with the brachial vein. The brachial artery can be exposed through the same incision or through a separate incision. Vessel loops are loosely encircled around the brachial artery proximally and distally.

Next, the cephalic or basilic vein is divided near the antecubital fossa and flushed and distended with heparinized saline. A sterile marking pen is used to mark the vein along its entire length to help avoid twisting during passage through the subcutaneous tunnel created anteriorly between the axilla and antecubital fossa. Approximately 3000 units of heparin is administered intravenously, and proximal and distal control of the brachial artery is obtained with the vessel loops. An end-to-side anastomosis with the brachial artery is constructed with 6-0 polypropylene sutures. After completion of the anastomosis, the fistula is inspected for a thrill. If a thrill is not present, a technical or structural problem is suspected that will require correction. The subcutaneous tissues and skin are closed with absorbable suture.

Follow-Up

Adequate arterialization of the vein usually occurs within 8 to 12 weeks. Hand exercises are advocated to encourage fistula maturation.

The AF access is studied by duplex ultrasound approximately 6 weeks after placement to assess maturation and to mark sites most suitable for initial cannulation by the dialysis center staff. For a new AF, dialysis should be initiated through a 16- or 17-gauge needle and for longer sessions at minimal rates of flow.

At least three successful hemodialysis sessions should be accomplished before removal of the central venous catheter. If flow rates are insufficient for successful dialysis or if follow-up duplex ultrasonography identifies a problem in the access, the access is considered a failure, and the patient is referred for evaluation and treatment (see next section).

Patients With Failing or Failed Access

For patients with a failing or failed access, the first step is a thorough duplex ultrasound evaluation of the access and underlying arterial and venous anatomy to ascertain the cause of failure, correctability, or salvage and alternative sites. In particular, patients with a prosthetic BG should be evaluated for graft salvage and for the identification of a possible site for placement of a new AF in case the BG salvage is not successful.

Patients with a failing dialysis catheter typically present with suboptimal flow on dialysis or, less commonly, upper extremity swelling secondary to pericatheter deep venous thrombosis. A duplex ultrasound scan can easily identify the latter, in which case endovascular treatment to reestablish deep venous outflow after catheter removal is considered. Subsequent imaging is directed at assessing the efficacy of treatment and identifying an alternative insertion site.

In patients with poor catheter flow rates but no evidence of central venous compromise, transcatheter thrombolytic therapy has been effective. Tissue plasminogen activator instilled directly through the catheter access port and allowed to dwell for some time has been effective.

Catheters compromised by malpositioning of the tip or encapsulation in a fibrin sheath can be treated endovascularly. If catheter salvage is unsuccessful, the catheter is exchanged. Over-the-wire techniques may be used for noncuffed catheters but can be challenging with cuffed catheters having exit sites remote from the insertion site. This technique may result in similarly poor flow rates if the problem is a suboptimal subcutaneous tunnel, either acutely angled or compromised by proximity to the clavicle. Usually, a new percutaneous placement is performed at the site identified as optimal by duplex ultrasound scans.

Information available from duplex ultrasound examination of a threatened or failed AF or BG is essential for directing treatment. Results of salvage are significantly worse with fistulas or grafts that have thrombosed than with those that are patent but have an identifiable stenosis. Thrombolytic therapy and surgical thrombectomy have poor 6-month primary efficacy rates. Nonetheless, the value of sustaining each access site in today's dialysis population usually warrants an attempt at salvage.

Thrombolysis and surgical thrombectomy are aimed at removal of the clot as a prerequisite to identifying the underlying anatomic anomaly. Post-thrombectomy access imaging in the surgical suite is imperative. Appropriate adjunctive management of the offending lesion follows—first with endovascular options, if warranted, and surgical revision if this proves unsuccessful.

Prospective monitoring of the access for hemodynamically significant stenoses, combined with correction, improves patency and decreases the incidence of thrombosis. A number of techniques have been proposed to monitor for stenoses. These include intra-access flow, static or dynamic venous pressure measurements, measurements of recirculation using urea concentration or dilution techniques, and observation for changes in characteristics of pulse or thrill in the access and prolongation of bleeding after needle withdrawal. Most of these techniques suggest increasing resistance at the venous anastomosis, which is the most common site of myointimal hyperplastic problems.

The DOQI guidelines suggest that persistent abnormalities in any of these parameters mandate venography. A comprehensive duplex scan can also serve as the initial examination. The decision to proceed with endovascular or surgical treatment is determined by the type of lesion identified and the physician's experience.

In modern vascular practice, endovascular balloon dilation of venous outflow stenoses in a BG or segmental stenoses in an AF is the initial choice of treatment. This must eliminate the hemodynamically significant stenosis and restore normal flow for it to be considered a success (Fig. 62-32).

Postprocedure evaluation by duplex ultrasound scan at 1 month to assess efficacy is recommended. Repeated angioplasty may be performed if indicated. In our practice, two failures of endovascular treatment for the same lesion within a 3-month period prompt open surgical intervention.

Surgical revision can be guided by the duplex scan and by subsequent contrast studies obtained during attempted endovascular revision. Surgical revision is focused on eliminating the causative lesion and preserving the maximal usable segment of vein for future use.

Recalcitrant stenoses in an AF can be treated by patch angioplasty or segmental resection and interposition of a translocated reversed segment of vein or, frequently, by mobilization of the matured vein and primary repair. Arterial or venous stenoses near or involving the anastomosis can be treated with patch angioplasty or, alternatively, with mobilization and formation of a new arteriovenous connection.

For focal defects in a BG, such as midgraft stenosis or pseudoaneurysm, direct excision and interposition of a new segment may be indicated. The BG venous outflow lesion resistant to endovascular treatment may be treated with surgical patch angioplasty or a jump graft to a segment of uninvolved vein with good outflow.

Any failed or failing graft that undergoes successful revision and salvage is reassessed at 1 month by duplex ultrasound examination. To achieve the reported 60% 1-year success rates after endovascular or surgical intervention, further intervention is typically required.

Secondary Interventions in Autogenous Fistulas

Few published series have focused on re-intervention of failing or nonmaturing autogenous arteriovenous fistulas, and most of those that have been reported focused on the traditional radiocephalic arteriovenous fistula. Recognizing this, Hingorani and colleagues[77] have reviewed their experience with salvage procedures in the management of nonfunctioning or nonmaturing arteriovenous fistulas, which included fistulas based in the upper arm. The distribution of fistulas that required salvage procedures was 37% radiocephalic, 47% brachiocephalic, and 16% brachiobasilic. In 46 patients (49 fistulas), 75 procedures, both open and endovascular, were performed; 17 patients underwent 26 balloon angioplasties and 20 patients had vein patch angioplasty. The group performed 12 fistula revisions to a more proximal level and 4 vein interposition grafts. Although the total number of subsequent procedures required for percutaneously treated fistulas was higher than that for open repair, there was no statistical difference

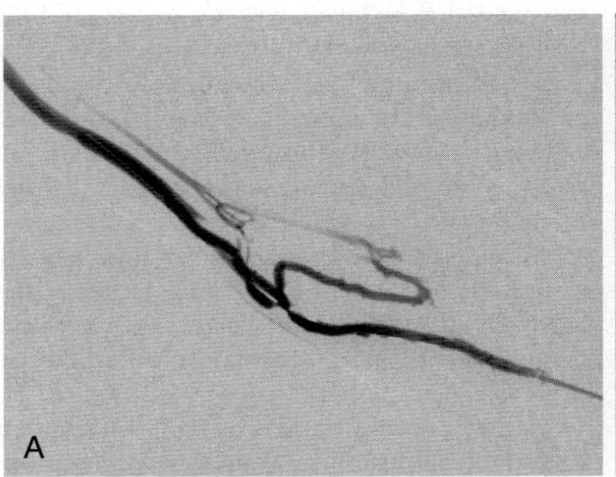

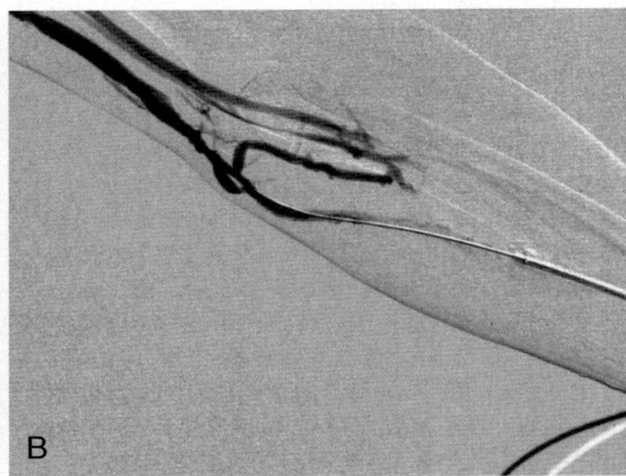

FIGURE 62-32 Endovascular-assisted arteriovenous fistula maturation. **A,** Severe stenosis of radiobasilic arteriovenous fistula. **B,** After balloon angioplasty, flow improved, and the patient was able to undergo dialysis within 2 weeks using the arteriovenous fistula.

between primary patency rates. It was concluded that salvage procedures may allow maturation and extend the life span of arteriovenous fistulas for hemodialysis.

The beneficial effects of secondary interventions on the maturation and maintenance of autogenous arteriovenous fistulas have been demonstrated by Berman and Gentile.[78] They placed 170 AFs in 163 patients (115 brachiocephalic, 47 radiocephalic, and 8 brachiobasilic). Secondary procedures were required for failure to mature in nine patients and for failure of previously functioning fistulas in six patients. A functional access was achieved in 90% of patients; these researchers demonstrated a 10% improvement in accomplishing or maintaining functional autogenous access through secondary procedures.

In the series of 89 patients with superficial venous transposition of forearm veins after duplex mapping for establishment of hemodialysis access, Silva and coworkers[66] reported a total of 18 failed fistulas. With surgical revision, four were successfully salvaged and six were converted to ipsilateral prosthetic grafts (three forearm, three upper arm). In addition, access was established on the other arm in five patients (three AFs, two prosthetic grafts).

Complex Access

Complex access solutions are required when all upper extremity access sites have been exhausted or when extensive central venous obliteration is not responsive to endovascular treatment. If the central venous system is patent, placement of a cuffed catheter is the simplest alternative.

In patients with refractory central subclavian vein occlusion and a patent ipsilateral internal jugular vein, the jugular vein turndown procedure may be performed.[79] The cephalad portion of the jugular vein at the angle of the mandible is divided; after mobilization, the jugular vein is anastomosed to the patent axillary vein segment, just proximal to the subclavian occlusion, to provide runoff for the upper arm. Resection of the central portion of the clavicle may be performed to facilitate a favorable anatomic lie of the vein graft. Other nonstandard access configurations, such as axillary artery to axillary vein body wall prosthetic grafts (loop configuration if ipsilateral, crossover or collar graft if contralateral), may be considered. Axillary arterial to right atrial BGs and axillary arterial to arterial prosthetic configurations have been used when extensive central venous obliteration is encountered, but these options are compromised by their potential for increased morbidity.

If upper extremity options are unsatisfactory and the superior central venous system is occluded, lower extremity access options can be used. Transposition of the saphenous vein in a loop configuration to the SFA or common femoral artery has been performed. Alternatively, a prosthetic BG can be placed in a loop configuration from the common femoral vein to the SFA or common femoral artery. A prosthetic BG can also be created from one femoral artery to a contralateral femoral vein and tunneled subcutaneously across the lower anterior abdominal wall. With a percutaneous approach to the femoral vein, a cuffed catheter can be tunneled into the anterior thigh. In patients with lower extremity venous thrombosis, a translumbar approach to the inferior vena cava has been used with a lateral tunnel for the cuffed catheter.

Vascular Access Complications

Infection is the second leading cause of death in dialysis patients, causing 10% of deaths, exceeded only by cardiovascular disease. Most of the systemic infections are directly related to infections from vascular access. The increased rate of infection in dialysis patients is caused by immunodeficiency and poor wound healing associated with chronic renal failure. *Staphylococcus aureus* is the most common cause of infection, and the use of aseptic technique is the best way to prevent bacterial colonization and vascular access site infection. Infection of an autogenous arteriovenous fistula is rare; it can be treated with appropriate antibiotics and local wound care, with drainage of abscess. Infection of a prosthetic arteriovenous graft is more common and is caused by contamination from skin flora during implantation or direct inoculation of the graft by an access needle from inadequately prepared skin. Treatment is with excision of the prosthetic material. The use of perioperative antibiotics has been shown to be effective in reducing infections. Cephalosporins can significantly decrease postoperative wound infections, and vancomycin can reduce graft infections.

The most common complication of vascular access is thrombosis of the venous fistula or prosthetic graft. The cause of most graft failures is the development of intimal hyperplasia at the venous anastomosis or venous outflow tract. This can account for 85% of graft failures, with 55% of thromboses caused by venous anastomosis and 30% caused by venous outflow occlusion or long-segment stenosis. For venous fistula, the specific offending location is not as clear. The lesion can be located at the arterial anastomosis or within the fistula. Flow in the vascular access can be restored with open surgical thrombectomy or endovascular thrombolysis and angioplasty. Venous outflow or anastomotic lesions need to be treated to prevent a high graft failure rate of 70% at 6 months. An improved patency rate of more than 70% at 6 months can be achieved with surgical anastomotic revision or endovascular stenting.

Aneurysmal degeneration of fistula can develop over time. These massively dilated venous segments can involve the skin, placing the patient at risk of significant bleeding. The low resistance of the enlarged fistula can lead to steal syndrome. Treatment is with interposition grafts and removal of the enlarged portion (Fig. 62-33).

Arterial insufficiency, or steal syndrome, can develop in patients with vascular access. The creation of this access results in a low-resistance circulation that shunts arterial inflow into this

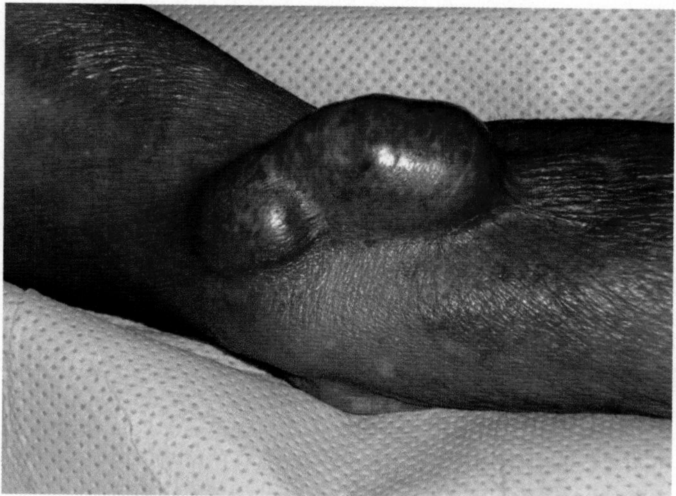

FIGURE 62-33 Fistula aneurysm without evidence of skin involvement.

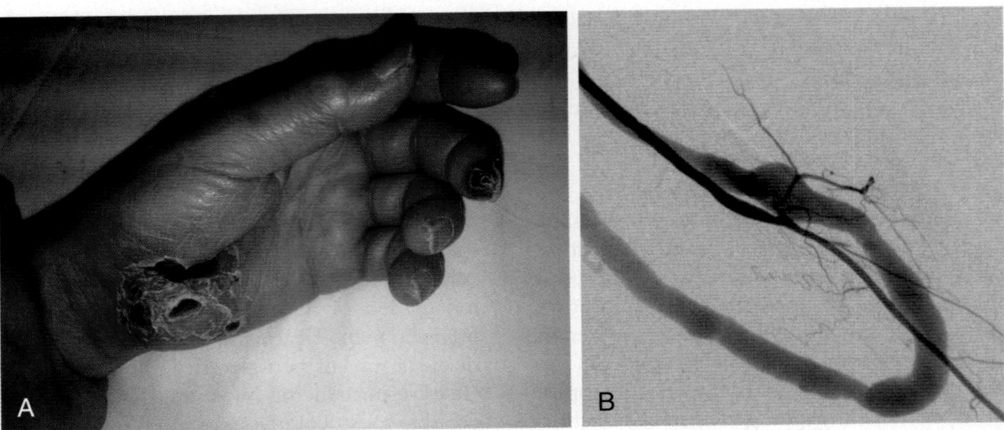

FIGURE 62-34 **A,** Patient with tissue loss of the hand because of steal. He underwent arterial duplex ultrasound examination and angiography before distal revascularization and interval ligation **(B),** with immediate symptomatic improvement.

low-pressure venous outflow. In addition, the flow in the artery distal to the access origin may become retrograde and is no longer antegrade. The effect is that the vascular access steals arterial flow, which may compromise distal limb perfusion. This physiologic steal phenomenon can be demonstrated in 75% to 90% of patients; however, only 1% to 6% are symptomatic. Symptoms may include a cold and painful hand or foot; with significant flow compromise, patients may develop tissue loss in their fingers or toes (Fig. 62-34). In patients with forearm vascular access using radial artery as inflow, such as radiocephalic or radiobasilic fistulas, ligation of the artery just distal to the fistula restores flow in the palmar arch through the ulnar artery. In patients with vascular access in the upper arm, the distal revascularization with interval ligation procedure is used to revascularize the distal limb while preserving the vascular access. The procedure is a bypass from the inflow artery proximal to the access to the artery distal to the access. The arterial segment between the vascular access and distal anastomosis of the bypass is ligated to prevent steal. The low-pressure zone around the access origin may shunt blood flow from the bypass into the access rather than restoring distal flow. An autogenous conduit should be used for this bypass if possible.

CONCLUSION

Ultimately, the goals of the DOQI are to minimize the deep effects on the end-stage renal disease patient's quality of life that hemodialysis dependence entails. Increasing rates of autogenous arteriovenous access increase patency rates, decrease complications, and therefore decrease the number of unplanned interventions and hospitalizations that this population is required to endure. This vision cannot be realized with traditional arteriovenous access alone. Early referral to vascular surgery, institutional strategies of preoperative noninvasive vascular assessments, and use of venous transposition procedures can be effective in increasing autogenous access in the dialysis population. A system of prospective monitoring for the development of hemodynamically significant stenosis can improve long-term assisted patency. A multidisciplinary approach involving the nephrologist, vascular surgeon, and hemodialysis center nurses as well as the patient and the patient's social support system is required to optimize the care of this population of complex patients.

SELECTED REFERENCES

Adam DJ, Beard JD, Cleveland T, et al: Bypass versus angioplasty in severe ischaemia of the leg (BASIL): Multicentre, randomised controlled trial. *Lancet* 366:1925–1934, 2005.

This randomized trial showed that in patients with severe limb ischemia due to infrainguinal disease and who are suitable for surgery and angioplasty, strategies of bypass surgery first and balloon angioplasty first are associated with broadly similar outcomes in terms of amputation-free survival, and in the short-term, surgery was more expensive than angioplasty.

Barnett HJ, Taylor DW, Eliasziw M, et al: Benefit of carotid endarterectomy in patients with symptomatic moderate or severe stenosis. North American Symptomatic Carotid Endarterectomy Trial Collaborators. *N Engl J Med* 339:1415–1425, 1998.

NASCET was a randomized prospective trial confirming the superiority of CEA over medical management for patients with high-grade symptomatic carotid disease.

Brott TG, Hobson RW, 2nd, Howard G, et al: Stenting versus endarterectomy for treatment of carotid-artery stenosis. *N Engl J Med* 363:11–23, 2010.

CREST, the definitive randomized prospective trial comparing carotid stenting and CEA, lasted more than 10 years and produced the best results from both therapies ever reported in such a trial. Results from carotid stenting were dramatically improved during the second half of the trial compared with the first half, suggesting the evolutionary nature of endovascular procedures and an identifiable learning curve for new technologies.

CAPRIE Steering Committee: A randomised, blinded, trial of clopidogrel versus aspirin in patients at risk of ischaemic events (CAPRIE). *Lancet* 348:1329–1339, 1996.

This blinded randomized trial showed clopidogrel to be more effective and safer than aspirin in reducing the combined risk of ischemic stroke, myocardial infarction, or vascular deaths in patients with atherosclerosis.

Endarterectomy for asymptomatic carotid artery stenosis: Executive Committee for the Asymptomatic Carotid Atherosclerosis Study. *JAMA* 273:1421–1428, 1995.

ACAS was a randomized prospective trial confirming the superiority of CEA over medical management for the treatment of asymptomatic carotid disease.

Hirsch AT, Haskal ZJ, Hertzer NR, et al: ACC/AHA 2005 Practice Guidelines for the management of patients with PAD (lower extremity, renal, mesenteric, and abdominal aortic): A collaborative report from the American Association for Vascular Surgery/Society for Vascular Surgery, Society for Cardiovascular Angiography and Interventions, Society for Vascular Medicine and Biology, Society of Interventional Radiology, and the ACC/AHA Task Force on Practice Guidelines (Writing Committee to Develop Guidelines for the Management of Patients With Peripheral Arterial Disease): Endorsed by the American Association of Cardiovascular and Pulmonary Rehabilitation; National Heart, Lung, and Blood Institute; Society for Vascular Nursing; TransAtlantic Inter-Society Consensus; and Vascular Disease Foundation. *Circulation* 113:e463–e654, 2006.

The ACC/AHA guidelines are a consensus document describing targets for medical management of vascular disease, including current thoughts on prevention.

Norgren L, Hiatt WR, Dormandy JA, et al: Inter-Society Consensus for the Management of Peripheral Arterial Disease (TASC II). *J Vasc Surg* 45(Suppl):S5–S67, 2007.

This consensus document describes an approach for choosing open revascularization versus endovascular therapy for patients on the basis of lesion characteristics.

REFERENCES

1. Criqui MH, Vargas V, Denenberg JO, et al: Ethnicity and peripheral arterial disease: The San Diego Population Study. *Circulation* 112:2703–2707, 2005.
2. Norgren L, Hiatt WR, Dormandy JA, et al: Inter-Society Consensus for the Management of Peripheral Arterial Disease (TASC II). *J Vasc Surg* 45(Suppl S):S5–S67, 2007.
3. Feinglass J, Pearce WH, Martin GJ, et al: Postoperative and late survival outcomes after major amputation: Findings from the Department of Veterans Affairs National Surgical Quality Improvement Program. *Surgery* 130:21–29, 2001.
4. Taylor SM, Kalbaugh CA, Blackhurst DW, et al: Preoperative clinical factors predict postoperative functional outcomes after major lower limb amputation: An analysis of 553 consecutive patients. *J Vasc Surg* 42:227–235, 2005.
5. Stone PA, Back MR, Armstrong PA, et al: Midfoot amputations expand limb salvage rates for diabetic foot infections. *Ann Vasc Surg* 19:805–811, 2005.
6. Fisher DF, Jr, Clagett GP, Fry RE, et al: One-stage versus two-stage amputation for wet gangrene of the lower extremity: A randomized study. *J Vasc Surg* 8:428–433, 1988.
7. Bolia A, Sayers RD, Thompson MM, et al: Subintimal and intraluminal recanalisation of occluded crural arteries by percutaneous balloon angioplasty. *Eur J Vasc Surg* 8:214–219, 1994.
8. Scott EC, Biuckians A, Light RE, et al: Subintimal angioplasty: Our experience in the treatment of 506 infrainguinal arterial occlusions. *J Vasc Surg* 48:878–884, 2008.
9. Clark TW, Groffsky JL, Soulen MC: Predictors of long-term patency after femoropopliteal angioplasty: Results from the STAR registry. *J Vasc Interv Radiol* 12:923–933, 2001.
10. Dorros G, Jaff MR, Murphy KJ, et al: The acute outcome of tibioperoneal vessel angioplasty in 417 cases with claudication and critical limb ischemia. *Cathet Cardiovasc Diagn* 45:251–256, 1998.
11. Dorros G, Jaff MR, Dorros AM, et al: Tibioperoneal (outflow lesion) angioplasty can be used as primary treatment in 235 patients with critical limb ischemia: Five-year follow-up. *Circulation* 104:2057–2062, 2001.
12. Kudo T, Chandra FA, Ahn SS: The effectiveness of percutaneous transluminal angioplasty for the treatment of critical limb ischemia: A 10-year experience. *J Vasc Surg* 41:423–435, discussion 435, 2005.
13. Sabeti S, Schillinger M, Amighi J, et al: Primary patency of femoropopliteal arteries treated with nitinol versus stainless steel self-expanding stents: Propensity score–adjusted analysis. *Radiology* 232:516–521, 2004.
14. Schillinger M, Sabeti S, Dick P, et al: Sustained benefit at 2 years of primary femoropopliteal stenting compared with balloon angioplasty with optional stenting. *Circulation* 115:2745–2749, 2007.
15. Kickuth R, Keo HH, Triller J, et al: Initial clinical experience with the 4-F self-expanding XPERT stent system for infrapopliteal treatment of patients with severe claudication and critical limb ischemia. *J Vasc Interv Radiol* 18:703–708, 2007.
16. Mwipatayi BP, Hockings A, Hofmann M, et al: Balloon angioplasty compared with stenting for treatment of femoropopliteal occlusive disease: A meta-analysis. *J Vasc Surg* 47:461–469, 2008.
17. Railo M, Roth WD, Edgren J, et al: Preliminary results with endoluminal femoropopliteal thrupass. *Ann Chir Gynaecol* 90:15–18, 2001.
18. Fischer M, Schwabe C, Schulte KL: Value of the Hemobahn/Viabahn endoprosthesis in the treatment of long chronic lesions of the superficial femoral artery: 6 years of experience. *J Endovasc Ther* 13:281–290, 2006.
19. Bleyn J, Schol F, Vanhandenhove I, et al: Endovascular reconstruction of the superficial femoral artery. In Becquemin JP, Alimi YS, Watelet J, et al, editors: *Controversies and updates in vascular cardiac surgery, 14*, Torino, Italy, 2004, Edizioni Minerva Medica, pp 87–91.
20. Saxon RR, Dake MD, Volgelzang RL, et al: Randomized, multicenter study comparing expanded polytetrafluoroethylene–covered endoprosthesis placement with percutaneous transluminal angioplasty in the treatment of superficial femoral artery occlusive disease. *J Vasc Interv Radiol* 19:823–832, 2008.
21. Kedora J, Hohmann S, Garrett W, et al: Randomized comparison of percutaneous Viabahn stent grafts vs prosthetic femoral-popliteal bypass in the treatment of superficial

femoral arterial occlusive disease. *J Vasc Surg* 45:10–16, discussion 16, 2007.
22. Keeling WB, Shames ML, Stone PA, et al: Plaque excision with the Silverhawk catheter: Early results in patients with claudication or critical limb ischemia. *J Vasc Surg* 45:25–31, 2007.
23. Scheinert D, Laird JR, Jr, Schroder M, et al: Excimer laser–assisted recanalization of long, chronic superficial femoral artery occlusions. *J Endovasc Ther* 8:156–166, 2001.
24. Laird JR, Zeller T, Gray BH, et al: Limb salvage following laser-assisted angioplasty for critical limb ischemia: Results of the LACI multicenter trial. *J Endovasc Ther* 13:1–11, 2006.
25. Buth J, Disselhoff B, Sommeling C, et al: Color-flow duplex criteria for grading stenosis in infrainguinal vein grafts. *J Vasc Surg* 14:716–726, discussion 726–728, 1991.
26. Mills JL, Sr, Wixon CL, James DC, et al: The natural history of intermediate and critical vein graft stenosis: Recommendations for continued surveillance or repair. *J Vasc Surg* 33:273–278, discussion 278–280, 2001.
27. Calligaro KD, Doerr K, McAffee-Bennett S, et al: Should duplex ultrasonography be performed for surveillance of femoropopliteal and femorotibial arterial prosthetic bypasses? *Ann Vasc Surg* 15:520–524, 2001.
28. Carter A, Murphy MO, Halka AT, et al: The natural history of stenoses within lower limb arterial bypass grafts using a graft surveillance program. *Ann Vasc Surg* 21:695–703, 2007.
29. Gonsalves C, Bandyk DF, Avino AJ, et al: Duplex features of vein graft stenosis and the success of percutaneous transluminal angioplasty. *J Endovasc Surg* 6:66–72, 1999.
30. Tielbeek AV, Rietjens E, Buth J, et al: The value of duplex surveillance after endovascular intervention for femoropopliteal obstructive disease. *Eur J Vasc Endovasc Surg* 12:145–150, 1996.
31. Guzman RP, Zierler RE, Isaacson JA, et al: Renal atrophy and arterial stenosis. A prospective study with duplex ultrasound. *Hypertension* 23:346–350, 1994.
32. Caps MT, Zierler RE, Polissar NL, et al: Risk of atrophy in kidneys with atherosclerotic renal artery stenosis. *Kidney Int* 53:735–742, 1998.
33. Mailloux LU, Napolitano B, Bellucci AG, et al: Renal vascular disease causing end-stage renal disease, incidence, clinical correlates, and outcomes: A 20-year clinical experience. *Am J Kidney Dis* 24:622–629, 1994.
34. Grüntzig A, Kuhlmann U, Vetter W, et al: Treatment of renovascular hypertension with percutaneous transluminal dilatation of a renal-artery stenosis. *Lancet* 1:801–802, 1978.
35. Leertouwer TC, Gussenhoven EJ, Bosch JL, et al: Stent placement for renal arterial stenosis: Where do we stand? A meta-analysis. *Radiology* 216:78–85, 2000.
36. Gill KS, Fowler RC: Atherosclerotic renal arterial stenosis: Clinical outcomes of stent placement for hypertension and renal failure. *Radiology* 226:821–826, 2003.
37. Henry M, Amor M, Henry I, et al: Stents in the treatment of renal artery stenosis: Long-term follow-up. *J Endovasc Surg* 6:42–51, 1999.
38. Webster J, Marshall F, Abdalla M, et al: Randomised comparison of percutaneous angioplasty vs continued medical therapy for hypertensive patients with atheromatous renal artery stenosis. Scottish and Newcastle Renal Artery Stenosis Collaborative Group. *J Hum Hypertens* 12:329–335, 1998.
39. van Jaarsveld BC, Krijnen P, Pieterman H, et al: The effect of balloon angioplasty on hypertension in atherosclerotic renal-artery stenosis. Dutch Renal Artery Stenosis Intervention Cooperative Study Group. *N Engl J Med* 342:1007–1014, 2000.
40. Rocha-Singh KJ, Ahuja RK, Sung CH, et al: Long-term renal function preservation after renal artery stenting in patients with progressive ischemic nephropathy. *Catheter Cardiovasc Interv* 57:135–141, 2002.
41. Rundback JH, Gray RJ, Rozenblit G, et al: Renal artery stent placement for the management of ischemic nephropathy. *J Vasc Interv Radiol* 9:413–420, 1998.
42. Bush RL, Martin LG, Lin PH, et al: Endovascular revascularization of renal artery stenosis in the solitary functioning kidney. *Ann Vasc Surg* 15:60–66, 2001.
43. Henry M, Amor M, Henry I, et al: Stent placement in the renal artery: Three-year experience with the Palmaz stent. *J Vasc Interv Radiol* 7:343–350, 1996.
44. Dorros G, Jaff M, Jain A, et al: Follow-up of primary Palmaz-Schatz stent placement for atherosclerotic renal artery stenosis. *Am J Cardiol* 75:1051–1055, 1995.
45. Rodriguez-Lopez JA, Werner A, Ray LI, et al: Renal artery stenosis treated with stent deployment: Indications, technique, and outcome for 108 patients. *J Vasc Surg* 29:617–624, 1999.
46. Zeller T, Frank U, Muller C, et al: Duplex ultrasound for follow-up examination after stent-angioplasty of ostial renal artery stenoses. *Ultraschall Med* 23:315–319, 2002.
47. Bax L, Mali WP, Van De Ven PJ, et al: Repeated intervention for in-stent restenosis of the renal arteries. *J Vasc Interv Radiol* 13:1219–1224, 2002.
48. Mackrell PJ, Langan EM, 3rd, Sullivan TM, et al: Management of renal artery stenosis: Effects of a shift from surgical to percutaneous therapy on indications and outcomes. *Ann Vasc Surg* 17:54–59, 2003.
49. Kessel DO, Robertson I, Taylor EJ, et al: Renal stenting from the radial artery: A novel approach. *Cardiovasc Intervent Radiol* 26:146–149, 2003.
50. Schobel WA, Mauser M: Miniaturization of the equipment for percutaneous coronary interventions: A prospective study in 1,200 patients. *J Invasive Cardiol* 15:6–11, 2003.
51. Rakhit RD, Matter C, Windecker S, et al: Five French versus 6 French PCI: A case control study of efficacy, safety and outcome. *J Invasive Cardiol* 14:670–674, 2002.
52. Spinosa DJ, Matsumoto AH, Angle JF, et al: Renal insufficiency: Usefulness of gadodiamide-enhanced renal angiography to supplement CO_2-enhanced renal angiography for diagnosis and percutaneous treatment. *Radiology* 210:663–672, 1999.
53. Ailawadi G, Stanley JC, Williams DM, et al: Gadolinium as a nonnephrotoxic contrast agent for catheter-based arteriographic evaluation of renal arteries in patients with azotemia. *J Vasc Surg* 37:346–352, 2003.
54. Brott TG, Hobson RW, 2nd, Howard G, et al: Stenting versus endarterectomy for treatment of carotid-artery stenosis. *N Engl J Med* 363:11–23, 2010.
55. Sheehan MK, Baker WH, Littooy FN, et al: Timing of postcarotid complications: A guide to safe discharge planning. *J Vasc Surg* 34:13–16, 2001.
56. Wholey MH, Wholey MH, Tan WA, et al: Management of neurological complications of carotid artery stenting. *J Endovasc Ther* 8:341–353, 2001.
57. Qureshi AI, Luft AR, Janardhan V, et al: Identification of patients at risk for periprocedural neurological deficits

associated with carotid angioplasty and stenting. *Stroke* 31: 376–382, 2000.

58. III. NKF-K/DOQI Clinical Practice Guidelines for Vascular Access: Update 2000. *Am J Kidney Dis* 37:S137–S181, 2001.
59. Huber TS, Ozaki CK, Flynn TC, et al: Prospective validation of an algorithm to maximize native arteriovenous fistulae for chronic hemodialysis access. *J Vasc Surg* 36:452–459, 2002.
60. Silva MB, Jr, Hobson RW, 2nd, Pappas PJ, et al: A strategy for increasing use of autogenous hemodialysis access procedures: Impact of preoperative noninvasive evaluation. *J Vasc Surg* 27:302–307, discussion 307–308, 1998.
61. Hakaim AG, Nalbandian M, Scott T: Superior maturation and patency of primary brachiocephalic and transposed basilic vein arteriovenous fistulae in patients with diabetes. *J Vasc Surg* 27:154–157, 1998.
62. Mendes RR, Farber MA, Marston WA, et al: Prediction of wrist arteriovenous fistula maturation with preoperative vein mapping with ultrasonography. *J Vasc Surg* 36:460–463, 2002.
63. U.S. Renal Data System: USRDS 1995 Annual Data Report. *Am J Kidney Dis* 26:S12–S166, 1995.
64. NKF-DOQI Clinical Practice Guidelines for Vascular Access: National Kidney Foundation–Dialysis Outcomes Quality Initiative. *Am J Kidney Dis* 30:S150–S191, 1997.
65. Sidawy AN, Gray R, Besarab A, et al: Recommended standards for reports dealing with arteriovenous hemodialysis accesses. *J Vasc Surg* 35:603–610, 2002.
66. Silva MB, Jr, Hobson RW, 2nd, Pappas PJ, et al: Vein transposition in the forearm for autogenous hemodialysis access. *J Vasc Surg* 26:981–986, discussion 987–988, 1997.
67. LoGerfo FW, Menzoian JO, Kumaki DJ, et al: Transposed basilic vein–brachial arteriovenous fistula. A reliable secondary-access procedure. *Arch Surg* 113:1008–1010, 1978.
68. Dagher FJ: The upper arm AV hemoaccess: Long term follow-up. *J Cardiovasc Surg (Torino)* 27:447–449, 1986.
69. Ascher E, Hingoran A, Gunduz Y, et al: The value and limitations of the arm cephalic and basilic vein for arteriovenous access. *Ann Vasc Surg* 15:89–97, 2001.
70. Coburn MC, Carney WI, Jr: Comparison of basilic vein and polytetrafluoroethylene for brachial arteriovenous fistula. *J Vasc Surg* 20:896–902, discussion 903–904, 1994.
71. Taghizadeh A, Dasgupta P, Khan MS, et al: Long-term outcomes of brachiobasilic transposition fistula for haemodialysis. *Eur J Vasc Endovasc Surg* 26:670–672, 2003.
72. Brescia MJ, Cimino JE, Appel K, et al: Chronic hemodialysis using venipuncture and a surgically created arteriovenous fistula. *N Engl J Med* 275:1089–1092, 1966.
73. Tashjian DB, Lipkowitz GS, Madden RL, et al: Safety and efficacy of femoral-based hemodialysis access grafts. *J Vasc Surg* 35:691–693, 2002.
74. Gradman WS, Cohen W, Haji-Aghaii M: Arteriovenous fistula construction in the thigh with transposed superficial femoral vein: Our initial experience. *J Vasc Surg* 33:968–975, 2001.
75. Huber TS, Ozaki CK, Flynn TC, et al: Use of superficial femoral vein for hemodialysis arteriovenous access. *J Vasc Surg* 31:1038–1041, 2000.
76. May J, Tiller D, Johnson J, et al: Saphenous-vein arteriovenous fistula in regular dialysis treatment. *N Engl J Med* 280:770, 1969.
77. Hingorani A, Ascher E, Kallakuri S, et al: Impact of reintervention for failing upper-extremity arteriovenous autogenous access for hemodialysis. *J Vasc Surg* 34:1004–1009, 2001.
78. Berman SS, Gentile AT: Impact of secondary procedures in autogenous arteriovenous fistula maturation and maintenance. *J Vasc Surg* 34:866–871, 2001.
79. Puskas JD, Gertler JP: Internal jugular to axillary vein bypass for subclavian vein thrombosis in the setting of brachial arteriovenous fistula. *J Vasc Surg* 19:939–942, 1994.

63 CHAPTER

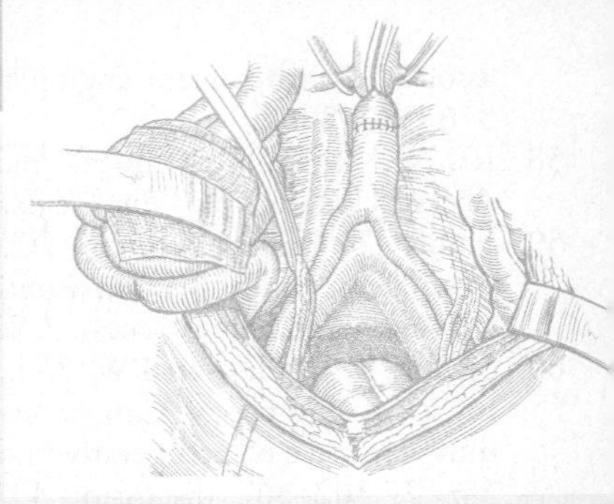

Vascular Trauma

Michael J. Sise, Carlos V.R. Brown, Howard C. Champion

OUTLINE

Despite the widespread implementation of trauma systems with designated trauma centers, the prompt recognition and effective management of vascular trauma still have significant challenges in the care of injured patients. Although the incorporation of lessons learned from combat casualty care in the wars in Afghanistan and Iraq has improved overall outcomes after vascular injury, the risk to life and limb remains significant and the margin for error is very thin. Either delay in recognition of or failure to adequately manage vascular injuries remains alarmingly common in trauma centers. An organized approach with well-planned and implemented practice guidelines is essential to convert an error-prone process into one of prompt diagnosis and safe and effective treatment.

Effective management of vascular injuries requires trauma team members with both skill and experience in open vascular techniques and the capability to perform timely endovascular techniques. These skills cannot be taken for granted and must be carefully managed to provide injured patients timely access to the right physicians with the right skills. The widespread preference for endovascular techniques for elective vascular surgery coupled with fewer and fewer open vascular surgery cases has produced a shortage of surgeons who feel capable of and comfortable in performing open vascular repairs for vascular trauma. The steadily decreasing volume of open vascular procedures in both general surgery residencies and vascular fellowships has significantly eroded the skill level of both trauma surgeons and the vascular surgeons who support them in managing vascular injuries. The need for innovative solutions to restore the skill level among trauma and vascular surgeons is compelling.

This chapter reviews the pathophysiology, clinical presentation, diagnostic workup, management, and outcome of vascular injuries. Education and training solutions to restore the skills required to manage vascular injuries are also presented. The educational objectives of this review are the following: to elucidate the mechanisms of vessel injury and the resulting clinical manifestations; to provide an organized approach to rapid assessment of injured patients for the presence of vascular injuries in the neck, torso, and extremities; to present management guidelines to assist in the decision of which treatment options best apply and how to effectively implement them; to identify the clinically important sequelae of vascular injuries and the appropriate measures required to maximize functional recovery; and to review the available education and training opportunities to maintain the open surgical skills that are essential to effective management of vascular trauma.

MECHANISM OF INJURY AND PATHOPHYSIOLOGY

Vascular injury can be produced by either a blunt or a penetrating mechanism. Penetrating injury tends to be more discrete and to produce focal injuries; blunt trauma is more diffuse, producing injuries not only to the vascular structures but also to the bone, muscle, and nerves. Blunt injury not only affects major arteries, it also disrupts smaller vessels that would normally provide collateral flow. As a result, ischemia may be worsened. Knife wounds produce focal injury along their track. Gunshot wounds produce injury of varying degrees dependent on the characteristics of both the weapon and the projectile.

Penetrating gunshot wound injury is generally classified as low velocity (<2500 ft/sec, typically a handgun wound) or high velocity (>2500 ft/sec, such as a military rifle wound).[1] High-velocity military-style weapons produce significantly more tissue damage than low-velocity weapons because of the high amount of kinetic energy (energy = mass × velocity^2). The bullet creates a cavity by the rapidly expanding and rapidly contracting tissue surrounding the bullet's course that can reach a size equal to 30 times the diameter of the projectile at right angles to the missile track. Tearing of the adjacent tissue can be devastating. Impact with bone can lead to further damage from secondary bullet and bone fragment impact on the adjacent tissue. Civilian gunshot injuries involve predominantly low-velocity projectiles and create more focal injuries with little cavitation.[2]

Shotgun wounds, depending on the proximity to the gun barrel, the gunpowder load, and the size of the shot, cause highly variable injury patterns. The spread and force of the shot determine the extent of injury. Close-range gunshot wounds are defined as within 6 feet; intermediate, 6 to 18 feet; and long range, beyond 18 feet.[3] Close-range injures are devastating and often lethal. Intermediate-range injuries are often severe, and longer range injuries may be mild.

Vascular trauma produces a spectrum of findings from life-threatening hemorrhage from major vessel laceration to no overtly detectable findings in minimal injuries. Hemorrhage is produced when all of the vessel layers (intima, media, and adventitia) are disrupted or lacerated. If the bleeding is controlled locally, a hematoma is produced, which may or may not be pulsatile. If bleeding is not contained, exsanguination can occur. Completely transected extremity vessels often retract and constrict secondary to spasm of the muscular middle layer of the vessel wall. The surrounding adventitia is highly thrombogenic. Subsequently, hemorrhage may cease secondary to thrombosis. Paradoxically, partially transected arteries and veins cannot retract and thrombose and may cause much more extensive hemorrhage.

Arterial thrombosis occurs if there is damage to the intima, exposing the underlying media and causing local thrombus formation, which may propagate and either occlude the lumen or embolize distally. In addition, the injured intima can prolapse into the lumen as a result of blood flow dissecting this layer into the lumen, producing partial or complete obstruction. Trauma to surrounding bone structures may cause external compression of the vessel, interrupting flow and producing thrombosis. Spasm occurs if there is external trauma to the vessel, such as stretching or contusion, which can stimulate the release of mediators (such as hemoglobin) that cause constriction of the vascular smooth muscle. Spasm, by reducing the cross-sectional area of the vessel, reduces flow.

Vascular trauma can produce subacute, chronic, or occult injuries. The most common of these are arteriovenous fistula and pseudoaneurysm. An arteriovenous fistula typically occurs after penetrating trauma that causes injury to both an artery and a vein in proximity. The high-pressure flow from the artery will follow the path of least vascular resistance into the vein, producing local, regional, and systemic signs and symptoms. These include local tenderness and edema, regional ischemia from "steal," and congestive heart failure if the fistula enlarges.[4] A pseudoaneurysm is a result of a puncture or laceration of an artery that bleeds into and is controlled by the surrounding tissue. Pseudoaneurysms can enlarge and produce local compressive symptoms, erode adjacent structures, or, rarely, be a source of distal emboli.[4] They can initially be clinically occult but with time become symptomatic.[4]

CLINICAL PRESENTATION

Vascular injuries have a broad spectrum of clinical manifestations varying from profound hemorrhagic shock to subtle findings, such as an asymptomatic bruit. Patients who present in hemorrhagic shock must be assumed to have a major vascular injury until proven otherwise.[5] There are five anatomic areas to consider, each with specific considerations. In the head and neck, external hemorrhage is required for vascular injuries to result in shock. Relatively small and tightly organized tissue planes preclude significant internal hemorrhage. In the chest, each hemithorax can accommodate lethal amounts of hemorrhage from cardiac, pulmonary, or great vessel arterial and venous injuries. Abdominal and pelvic vascular injuries can also result in lethal hemorrhage, particularly from the aorta and iliac arteries. As in the head and neck, extremity vascular injuries generally cause hemorrhagic shock only if there is significant external hemorrhage. The patient with hypotension and a lack of chest, abdomen, and pelvic findings may have what appears to be a trivial neck or extremity laceration that initially communicated with a major vessel injury. A hemorrhage sufficient to produce hypotension can be followed by thrombosis. It is therefore necessary to obtain a history from the prehospital personnel about the amount of blood at the scene or the initial presence of severe wound hemorrhage. It is also necessary to thoroughly examine the patient for additional wounds and to carefully assess each of them.[5]

Extremity vascular trauma may be immediately apparent on presentation because of external hemorrhage, hematoma, or obvious limb ischemia. A history of penetrating trauma associated with hypotension, pulsatile bleeding, or a large quantity of blood at the scene suggests vascular injury. Blunt trauma is also capable of causing significant vascular injury that can be overlooked when serious head, chest, or abdominal injuries are present. Extremity fractures may result in vascular injury. Supracondylar humerus fracture can be associated with brachial artery injury, and knee dislocation carries a significant risk of popliteal artery injury.[6] Crush injuries of the extremity without fracture may also result in vascular injury.

A relatively small number of vascular injuries are manifested in a delayed fashion without initial findings. These are limited to thrombosis of a previously partially disrupted but initially patent vessel, distal emboli from an intimal tear of the arterial wall with formation of platelet debris, and, least commonly, rupture or expansion of a pseudoaneurysm that was initially small and contained by the outer arterial wall and local tissue.[4] Local signs of hematoma, diminished pulses, and patterns of associated injuries should point to the presence of these vascular injuries. A thorough history and physical examination and appropriate adjunctive imaging studies will result in effective initial diagnosis and a decrease in the frequency of these delayed presentations.

Because such a broad spectrum of clinical findings are associated with vascular trauma, it is best to assume that vascular injury is present until proven otherwise in all patients with hemorrhagic shock and all patients with extremity fractures.[5]

DIAGNOSIS

Physical Examination

Vascular injury can produce systemic symptoms of hypotension, tachycardia, and altered mental status by hypovolemic shock caused by hemorrhage. As a result, vascular injury can be life-threatening, and attention must initially be directed to the primary survey using the principles of advanced trauma life support.[5] The airway must be assessed, adequate oxygenation and ventilation ensured, and intravenous access achieved. Once this is completed and resuscitation is under way, the secondary survey is undertaken. A thorough history and careful physical examination are then performed. This examination must include a careful inspection of the injured sites and wounds, a complete sensory and motor assessment, and a pulse examination of each extremity. The presence of a hematoma, bruit, or thrill must be noted. If distal pulses are diminished or absent, ankle or wrist systolic blood pressure should be determined with a continuous-wave Doppler device and compared with the uninjured side. A significant difference in systolic blood pressure (>10 mm Hg) between extremities may be an indication of vascular injury. Patients with "hard" findings of vascular injury (Table 63-1) should be taken directly to the operating room.

In patients with "soft" findings (Table 63-1), vascular imaging can be used to rule out the need for operation. In addition, patients with hard findings but with multilevel injuries in the same extremity may also need imaging. Catheter arteriography is both sensitive and specific in the diagnosis of extremity vascular injuries (Fig. 63-1). However, computed tomography (CT) angiography with the latest generation scanners is readily available and highly accurate and obviates the delay caused by mobilizing the angiography suite for catheter angiography (Fig. 63-2).[7-9] Although this imaging technique requires an infusion of contrast material, it does not require arterial catheterization, is easily performed, and is less costly and less time-consuming than conventional angiography.[7] The important distinction, however, is the ability to perform endovascular techniques with catheter access in the angiography suite or properly equipped operating room. Therefore, an orchestration of CT imaging and catheter imaging to meet the patient's needs and to manage vascular injuries in a timely and effective manner is essential.

Severely injured patients who must be taken to the operating room for treatment of life-threatening associated injuries, such as penetrating thoracic injury or ruptured spleen, may not be able to undergo CT angiography. In such cases, it is not prudent to delay operative therapy to obtain formal vascular imaging. An arteriogram can be obtained in the operating room by cannulating the artery proximal to the suspected vascular injury, injecting 20 to 25 mL of a full-strength radiographic contrast agent, and taking a radiograph or using fluoroscopy (Fig. 63-3).[10] If doubt remains about the presence of a vascular injury and the imaging studies and other diagnostic tests are inconclusive, there is a role for operative exploration and direct assessment of the artery. Routine operative exploration in the stable patient with soft signs, however, has a 5% to 30% incidence of morbidity, occasional mortality, and low diagnostic yield.[11] These patients are better served with formal vascular imaging.

Duplex color flow imaging is not used for the acute assessment of vascular injury. Wounds, swelling, air in the tissue, and dressings or splints impair the ability to obtain satisfactory images. Duplex imaging does have a role in the follow-up of treated lesions (i.e., to assess patency of bypass grafts or to detect luminal stenosis at an anastomosis) or in the follow-up of nonoperative

TABLE 63-1 History and Physical Examination Findings of Vascular Injury

Hard Findings

Indicate need for immediate intervention for vascular injury

- Pulsatile bleeding
- Expanding hematoma
- Palpable thrill or audible bruit
- Evidence of extremity ischemia
  - Pallor
  - Paresthesia
  - Paralysis
  - Pain
  - Pulselessness
  - Poikilothermia

Soft Findings

Consider further imaging and evaluation for vascular injury

- History of moderate hemorrhage
- Proximity fracture, dislocation, or penetrating wound
- Diminished but palpable pulse
- Level of peripheral nerve deficit in proximity to major vessel
- Wounds in proximity to extremity or neck vessels in patients with unexplained hemorrhagic shock

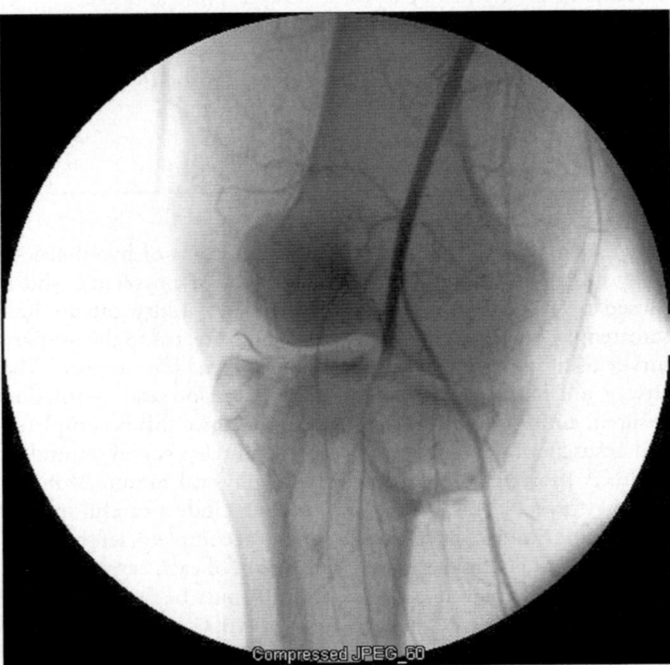

FIGURE 63-1 Catheter arteriogram demonstrating an acute occlusion of right popliteal artery secondary to blunt injury with associated tibial plateau fracture.

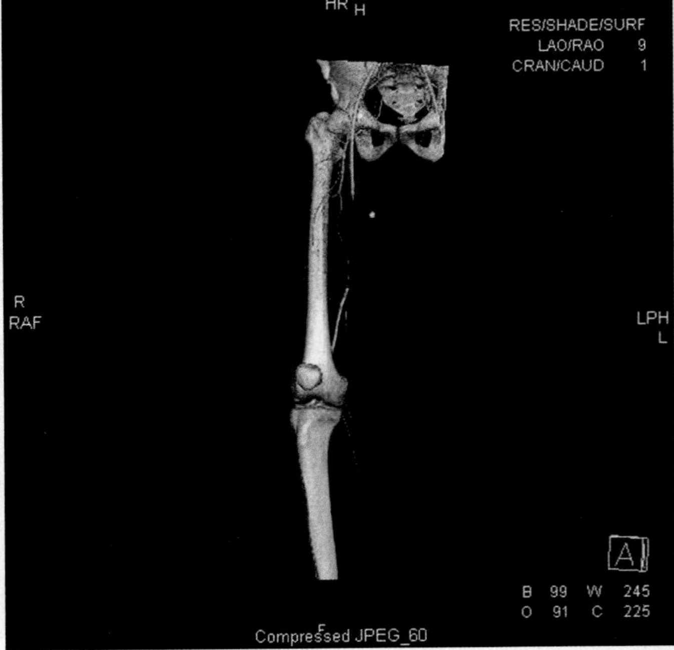

FIGURE 63-2 CT angiogram with VTR view of a gunshot wound to the right superficial femoral artery resulting in segmental thrombosis.

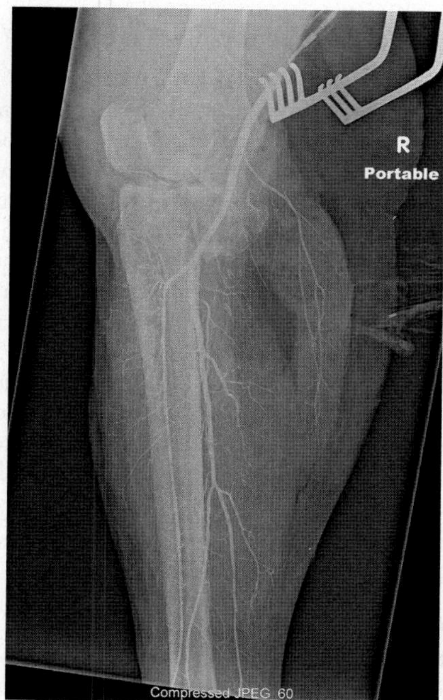

FIGURE 63-3 Intraoperative plain film (direct injection arteriogram) in the patient described in Figure 63-2 with blunt injury of the knee. Exploration of the popliteal artery with fasciotomy of the posterior compartments released compression of the artery with return of flow. This intraoperative arteriogram confirms a normal popliteal artery.

management of minimal vascular injury, such as small pseudoaneurysms or arteriovenous fistulas.

MINIMAL VASCULAR INJURY AND NONOPERATIVE MANAGEMENT

The widespread application of CT angiography in the evaluation of injured extremities results in the detection of clinically insignificant lesions.[12] There is now an extensive body of experience with lesions that are not limb-threatening. These minimal vascular injuries include intimal irregularity, small nonocclusive intimal flaps, focal spasm with minimal narrowing, and small pseudoaneurysms. They are often asymptomatic and usually do not progress.[6,12]

A small, nonocclusive intimal flap is the most commonly encountered clinically insignificant minimal vascular injury. The likelihood that it will progress to cause either occlusion or distal embolization is approximately 10% or less.[6,12] This progression, if it occurs, will be early in the postinjury course. Spasm is another common minimal vascular injury. This finding should resolve promptly after initial discovery. Failure of the return of normal extremity perfusion pressure indicates that a more serious vascular injury is present and intervention is needed. Small pseudoaneurysms are more likely to progress to the point of needing repair and must be actively observed with Duplex color flow imaging. Arteriovenous fistulas always enlarge over time and should be promptly repaired.

There is extensive evidence supporting nonoperative therapy for many asymptomatic lesions. However, successful nonoperative therapy requires continuous surveillance for subsequent progression, occlusion, or hemorrhage. Operative therapy is required for thrombosis, symptoms of chronic ischemia, and failure of small pseudoaneurysms to resolve.[12]

ENDOVASCULAR MANAGEMENT

Endovascular techniques are an important component of effective management of vascular injuries.[13,14] They are, however, one tool among many that are required to manage the full spectrum of these injuries. Endovascular therapy for atherosclerotic arterial disease has become the first choice in management. Endoluminal stent deployment for occlusive lesions and stent graft for aortic aneurysms have become widely accepted. However, there is a strong tendency to generalize from this elective experience in elderly patients with atherosclerosis to the treatment of younger patients with acute vascular injuries. The evidence to support these approaches in preference to traditional open techniques is not well developed, and there have been problems.[6,15] The striking decrease in open vascular surgical experience among general surgeons and vascular surgeons trained in the 21st century creates a lack of comfort and competence in performing open vascular repairs.[16,17] A balanced approach using each of these techniques where they best apply supported by clinical evidence is essential to good outcomes in patients with vascular trauma.

Endovascular Operating Rooms

There is a widespread proliferation of “hybrid” operating rooms. These high-technology suites have both advanced imaging capability and traditional operating room properties. They require a major commitment of resources and personnel to be effective. They are ideal for complex elective endovascular cases. Not all trauma centers have hybrid operating rooms, or if they do, they cannot staff them on an emergency basis for the often after-hours management of vascular trauma.

Many centers create “hybrid operating rooms of opportunity” with high-resolution digital subtraction C-arm fluoroscopy equipment, mobile cabinets with the appropriate catheters and stent grafts, and on-call technical staff. They can create hybrid suite capabilities in an operating room large enough for the C-arm and the rolling cabinets with a standard orthopedic surgery operating table that accommodates fluoroscopy. An unstable trauma patient taken directly to the operating room with a major vascular injury or solid organ hemorrhage can be placed on an orthopedic surgery table and then be managed with all the functionality of a dedicated hybrid operating room. Many trauma centers already provide these mobile capabilities to their vascular surgeons performing elective endovascular abdominal aortic aneurysm repair. All trauma centers need to develop this capacity for their trauma patients.

Endovascular Management of Torso Vascular Injuries

Endovascular techniques offer a variety of options for hemorrhage control in the torso. Intra-arterial catheter-directed embolization has become a mainstay of the management of solid organ hemorrhage in the abdomen.[18,19] Whether it is used as the sole treatment or in combination with open procedures, this approach has been effective in liver, spleen, and kidney injuries. Less commonly used intra-arterial balloon occlusion for proximal control is a promising adjunct to open repair.[20,21] The availability of retrograde endovascular balloon occlusion of the aorta is growing and will soon be common practice in the same clinical setting of exsanguinating abdominal hemorrhage in which an aortic cross-clamp in the chest is needed. In trauma centers with the appropriately trained surgeons and proper equipment, these techniques are quick, accurate, and easily performed. The major obstacle to widespread popularity has been the reluctance of surgeons either to adopt catheter skills or to partner with interventional radiologists to bring these techniques to the trauma operating room. This reluctance to adopt new and promising technology must be avoided, and trauma surgeons need either to add surgeons or radiologists with endovascular capabilities to their specialty physician call panels or to obtain the training themselves.

The early use of catheter-directed control of hemorrhage associated with pelvic fracture is an effective method of limiting blood loss and improving outcome.[22] This approach is well tolerated and has proved superior to open attempts at hemorrhage control by packing in most patients. Unstable patients benefit from an immediate trip to the operating room. If intraoperative endovascular capability is present, a combined approach may offer the best results.

Enthusiasm for stent graft management of great vessel injuries in the chest has steadily grown.[23,24] The success of stent grafts for the treatment of aneurysm disease in the infrarenal aorta has led to the use of similar devices to treat contained thoracic aortic lacerations after blunt trauma. The initial results have been encouraging, but they are not without complications (Table 63-2).[24,25] Lifelong CT imaging is necessary because of the possibility of delayed endoleak and the possible loss of device fixation as the aorta enlarges over time. There is a promising role for covered stents in proximal branches of the aorta in both the thorax and abdomen. In stable injuries at risk for delayed hemorrhage or thrombosis, carefully placed stents have the potential to lower morbidity compared with open procedures that require extensive operative dissection for exposure and control. Endoluminal management with stent grafts appears most effective in those torso injuries that are surgically inaccessible with the potential for significant hemorrhage in stable patients (Fig. 63-4). These techniques should be used only in centers with an active elective endovascular practice that has experience in treating trauma patients.

TABLE 63-2 Comparison of Endovascular and Open Blunt Thoracic Aortic Injury Repairs

	RELATIVE DEGREE OF RISK		
TECHNIQUE	CLAMP AND SEW	PARTIAL BYPASS	ENDOVASCULAR
Complications			
Physiology impact	High	Medium	Low
Blood loss	Medium	Medium	Low
Operative time	Medium	High	Low
Paraplegia	High	Medium	Low
Clinical Variables			
High surgical risk	High	Medium	Low
Severe lung injury	High	Medium	Low
Severe head injury	High	High	Low
Challenging aortic anatomy	Medium	Low	High

From Neschis DG, Scalea TM, Flinn WR, et al: Blunt aortic injury. *N Engl J Med* 359:1708–1716, 2008.

Endovascular Management of Cerebrovascular Vascular Injuries

Endovascular techniques offer advantages in anatomic regions where direct operative control is difficult or impossible. For example, hemorrhage from a penetrating injury at the base of the skull is extremely difficult to control (Fig. 63-5). Catheter-directed placement of coils, balloons, or hemostatic agents in the injured carotid or vertebral artery could be lifesaving. Stent placement initially appeared less effective than anticoagulation in partially occluded injuries without associated hemorrhage.[26] However, the role of stents in cerebrovascular trauma has yet to be defined and may prove safe.[27,28] This use of endoluminal cerebrovascular interventions requires significant expertise and experience. If such experience does not exist at the receiving hospital, consideration should be given to transfer of the patient to a medical center with experience in this mode of therapy.

Endovascular Management of Extremity Vascular Injuries

The use of stent grafts in extremity vascular injuries is becoming more common.[13] The long-term results, however, have not been documented, and caution should be used in considering this type of treatment. In hemodynamically stable patients with contained hemorrhage, difficult to access proximal subclavian or iliac arterial injuries may be effectively treated with covered stents. In the extremities distal to these areas, autologous vein interposition grafts have excellent long-term patency rates and remain the "gold standard" for vascular repairs.

Catheter-directed therapies for controlling hemorrhage from large branch vessels in the extremities are often effective and sufficient to manage these injuries. Endoluminal treatment is used sparingly for pseudoaneurysms of extremity arteries. Small pseudoaneurysms are likely to resolve without any intervention, and large pseudoaneurysms are best treated with open techniques because the risk of arterial thrombosis or distal embolization is high with this endovascular intervention (Fig. 63-6).

Who Should Perform Endovascular Repairs?

Successful management of vascular injuries requires that the most qualified person do the indicated intervention in the appropriate patient in the appropriate place at the appropriate time. Endovascular surgery is an operative procedure and, like all operations, should be performed by readily available trained clinicians who not only are cognizant of the technical aspects of a procedure but are also knowledgeable about the disease for which the procedure is being performed. In many centers, this person is the interventional radiologist. Other centers have catheter-trained vascular surgeons, and a few others have trauma surgeons who are capable of performing endovascular procedures. Catheter skills training is being integrated in many surgical critical care fellowships and may subsequently become more available in the near future at many trauma centers. (See later section on training and preparation.)

Endoluminal management of vascular trauma does not require a full endovascular hybrid operating room, as explained before. Planning and preparation, however, are essential for the endovascular capability, which more often than not is needed in the middle of the night. Preparing a team who can perform these techniques and who can organize the appropriate equipment with brief notice requires commitment, dedication, collaboration, and training.

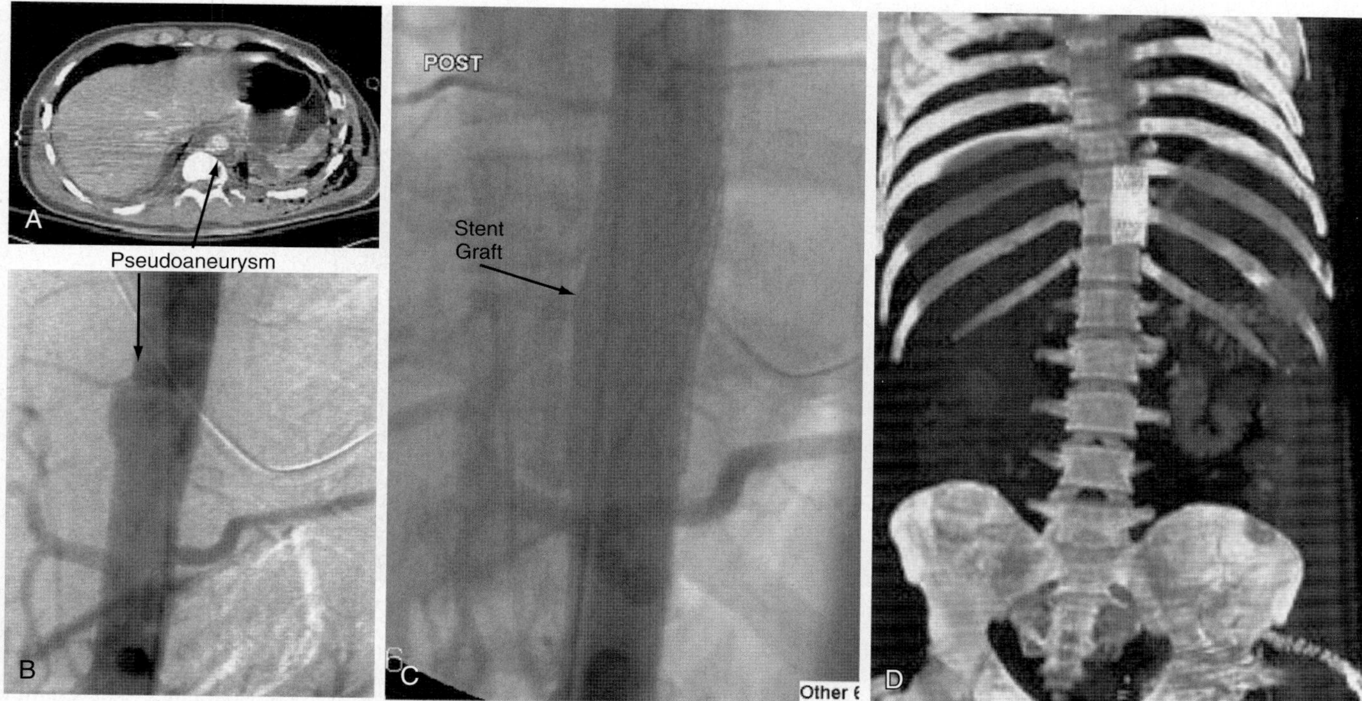

FIGURE 63-4 Endovascular repair of a difficult to expose aortic injury with pseudoaneurysm at the diaphragm from blunt-force trauma. **A,** CT angiogram showing cross-sectional view of pseudoaneurysm and associated thoracic spine fracture. **B,** Catheter arteriogram demonstrating the pseudoaneurysm. **C,** Deployed stent graft. **D,** CT scan of level of aortic stent graft in mid torso (VTR view).

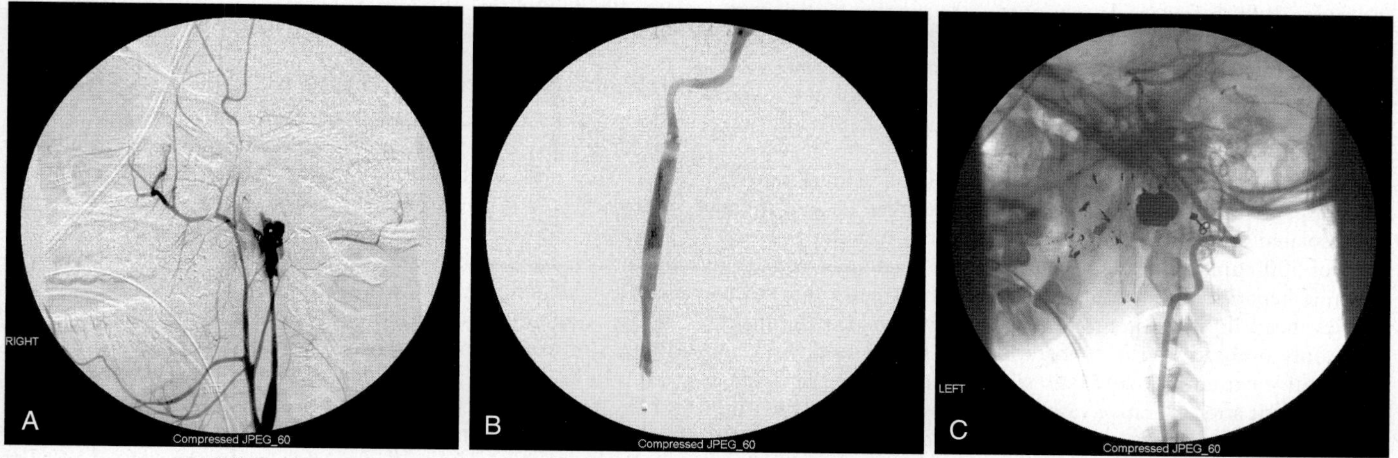

FIGURE 63-5 **A,** Gunshot wound with laceration and hemorrhage of internal carotid artery at the base of the skull. **B,** Covered stent placed at site of internal carotid artery injury. **C,** After placement of a covered stent in the internal carotid artery at base of the skull.

OPEN SURGICAL MANAGEMENT

Preparation for Operative Management

Operative procedures to manage vascular injuries should be limited to those surgeons who are capable, experienced, and qualified. Board certification in vascular surgery is not enough to qualify a surgeon as capable to handle these injuries, just as the lack of certification does not necessarily disqualify a surgeon. Many surgeons who perform elective vascular surgery are not sufficiently experienced in the management of vascular trauma. Conversely, there are many trauma surgeons who are very skilled in vascular technique by virtue of their interest and experience. The results of major open vascular repairs are dependent on the skill level of the vascular trauma–capable surgeon independent of board preparation. In a multicenter review of close to 700 major extremity vascular injuries, board-certified general surgeons and board-certified vascular surgeons had nearly identically high limb salvage rates for major vascular surgical repairs.[29] Every trauma center needs to develop a call panel of surgeons with the skill and knowledge to perform the full spectrum of vascular trauma repairs.

Successful operative management of vascular injuries requires a systematic approach with careful preparation. This begins with

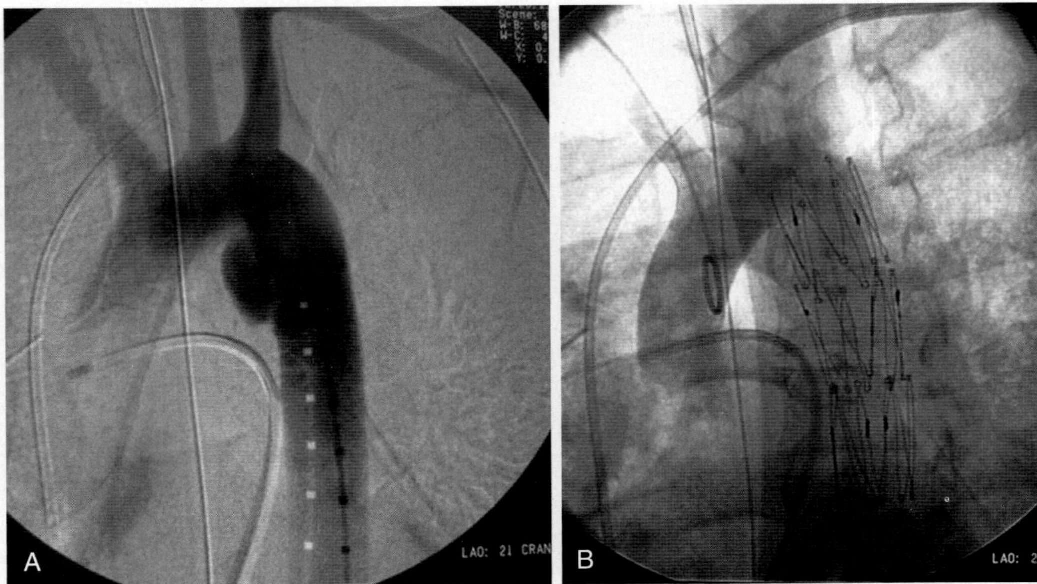

FIGURE 63-6 **A,** Acute traumatic pseudoaneurysm of the thoracic aorta. **B,** Fluoroscopy image after stent graft deployment.

airway control, adequate intravenous access, and availability of blood products. The administration of these blood products, however, should not begin before obtaining control of hemorrhage unless the patient is profoundly hypotensive.[5] If the blood pressure is below 80 to 90 mm Hg, the goal should be to provide adequate volume restoration with type O-negative packed cells and type AB fresh-frozen plasma infusion to support transport to the operating room for definitive hemorrhage control without delay. Volume infusion that raises the blood pressure above a systolic pressure of 90 to 100 mm Hg may increase bleeding and have a negative impact on outcome, particularly if the infusion delays transport to the operating room.[5]

Broad-spectrum preoperative antibiotics (and tetanus toxoid, if it is a penetrating wound) should be administered, and if there is an isolated extremity injury without significant hemorrhage, a bolus of 5000 units of heparin should also be given intravenously. Systemic heparinization should be avoided in patients with torso injuries, head injuries, or multiple extremity injuries. The most commonly omitted step in preparation is a failure to document preoperative extremity neurologic status. The presence of a neurologic deficit after operative vascular repair without knowing the preoperative status presents a difficult management challenge. A new neurologic deficit after vascular repair merits investigation and, possibly, reoperation. Therefore, a thorough preoperative neurologic examination and careful documentation are essential to effective management.

The operative management of extremity vascular injuries must be carefully orchestrated with the overall care of the patient. The choice between definitive repair and damage control should be made as soon as possible in patients with life-threatening torso injuries or severe head injuries. This includes coordinating two surgical teams to work simultaneously to care for the torso injury and the extremity vascular injury at the same time. Associated injuries to the soft tissue and bone require a coordinated assessment and treatment with orthopedic and plastic surgery consultants. These specialists should be involved as early as possible to facilitate any additional imaging or diagnostic procedures before proceeding to the operating room. The conduct of the operation should also be discussed with these colleagues. For example, the use of damage control procedures with shunt placement followed by orthopedic stabilization can remove the sense of urgency to restore blood flow. Extensive soft tissue injuries may compromise the proper coverage of vascular repairs and fracture fixation. The advice and assistance of a plastic and reconstructive surgeon can be helpful in obtaining coverage of exposed grafts and fractures.

Vascular Exposure and Control

Always place the patient with major hemorrhage or suspected vascular injury on a fluoroscopy-capable operating room table to allow the endovascular therapy option for hemorrhage control or vascular repair. A generous sterile field should be prepared to allow adequate exposure of vessels to obtain proximal and distal control. In torso injuries, this includes preparing the chest and abdomen to the table laterally on both sides and both legs in case distal access or an autologous conduit is needed. For proximal vascular injuries of the extremities (at the groin crease or axilla), the chest or abdomen should be prepared to obtain proximal control out of the zone of injury. An uninjured leg should also be prepared for harvesting of autologous venous conduit.

Proximal control is the first priority in the exposure of vascular injuries. In the torso, chest injuries with life-threatening hemorrhage are best approached through a fourth intercostal space anterolateral thoracotomy that can be extended across the sternum into the third intercostal space of the right side of the chest to create a "clamshell" incision.[30] Thoracic outlet and proximal neck vascular injuries may require median sternotomy with extension above the clavicle up along the ipsilateral sternocleidomastoid muscle. For abdominal vascular injury, a generous xiphoid to pubis incision is needed for adequate exposure.[31] Proximal control for aortic injuries can be obtained just below the aortic hiatus of the diaphragm or may require a left anterolateral thoracotomy to clamp the distal thoracic aorta. If retrograde endovascular balloon occlusion of the aorta is available, it should be considered for temporary proximal thoracic aorta occlusion in the presence of high intra-abdominal aortic injury.[21]

In the proximal extremity injuries with active hemorrhage, the first incision site is chosen to give the fastest exposure of inflow vessels for clamping. For proximal upper extremity injuries, this may include incisions over the infraclavicular region of the chest to expose the axillary artery. For injuries in the groin, prepare to enter the lower quadrant of the abdomen for access to the external iliac vessels. In mid and distal extremity vascular injuries associated with active hemorrhage, tourniquets can rapidly obtain control in the trauma resuscitation room. In the operating room, have one team member precisely compress the bleeding site with a gloved hand and a sponge, remove the tourniquet, and prepare the extremity. A 5000-unit heparin bolus is then given, if appropriate, and the extremity is prepared and draped and a sterile tourniquet is placed proximal to the wound and inflated. The injury site can then be explored in a controlled fashion and clamps or vessel loops placed above and below the vascular injury. In certain injuries, distal arterial occlusion and retrograde intraluminal insertion of a Fogarty catheter with a stopcock to maintain balloon inflation will provide rapid hemorrhage control.[6]

Incisions used to manage vascular injuries are often the same as those used to manage elective cases but are generally more generous. The use of smaller incisions may lead to error in identifying the extent of vascular injury, adequately controlling branch vessel hemorrhage, and identifying associated venous lacerations. This is particularly true for popliteal artery and vein injuries. A limited approach with separate medial above- and below-knee incisions will not adequately expose the site of injury. A medial incision from the proximal popliteal space to the distal popliteal space with division of the medial head of the gastrocnemius muscle and the semimembranosus and semitendinosus muscles with full exposure of the popliteal artery and vein and the tibial nerve provides adequate exposure. This ensures adequate vascular control and the opportunity for successful repair. Closure of the wound to include approximation of the divided muscles yields an excellent functional result. Dividing the inguinal ligament in the groin, dividing the pectoralis major in the axilla, and removing the midclavicle may rarely be necessary. In each of these areas, rapid endovascular balloon occlusion offers an excellent adjunct to proximal control. In the presence of life-threatening hemorrhage that cannot be controlled by any other approach, these structures should not stand in the way of adequate exposure and control.

Vascular Damage Control

Damage control has gained wide acceptance in trauma surgery and is directed at rapid control of hemorrhage and closure of enteric wounds so that the patient can be warmed and resuscitated. The choice between definitive time-consuming vascular repair and temporary measures that achieve control must be made early in care of patients with vascular injury and hypovolemic shock. This is particularly important when an extremity vascular injury is associated with major torso injuries. Ligation and placement of intraluminal shunts are the mainstays of vascular damage control.[32,33]

Ligation should be reserved for vessels with adequate distal collateral flow. In the torso, this includes the subclavian and innominate arteries, the celiac artery, and the inferior mesenteric artery. In the upper extremity, proximal injuries of the axillary artery and distal injuries to either the radial or ulnar artery may be ligated, provided there is evidence of adequate distal collateral flow assessed by either physical examination or continuous-wave Doppler interrogation. Similarly, in the lower extremity, ligation of a single tibial artery or the peroneal artery can be performed after a similar assessment. If distal perfusion is compromised, an intraluminal shunt should be inserted, rather than ligating the vessel. Superior mesenteric artery (SMA) ligation is associated with a high risk of bowel necrosis, and damage control is best accomplished with placement of an intraluminal shunt. In the extremities, ligation of the brachial, external iliac, superficial femoral, or popliteal artery has a high likelihood of producing limb-threatening ischemia and should be avoided, if possible.

A variety of commercially available shunts can be used for damage control. If these are not available, sterile intravenous tubing is of adequate size to "shunt" both the artery and the vein, if necessary. Venous shunt placement (instead of ligation) may improve extremity perfusion and lower the risk of compartment syndrome. Damage control shunt placement begins with obtaining adequate proximal and distal control. Thrombus should be cleared with a Fogarty embolectomy catheter, followed by the instillation of regional heparinized saline (5000 units heparin/500 mL saline). The shunt should be placed in a straight line and be long enough to remain safely held in place in the proximal and distal vessel with a tied umbilical tape or 2-0 silk tie at each end. Long, looped shunts run the risk of becoming dislodged during subsequent dressing changes and should be avoided. The ties securing the shunt cause intimal damage, and those portions of the artery must be resected at the time of definitive vascular repair.

The condition of the patient determines the timing of definitive vascular repair after damage control. Hemorrhage must be controlled, coagulopathy and acidosis corrected, and temperature normalized.

Choice of Repair and Graft Material

Vessel injuries that cannot be repaired by primary end-to-end technique will require an interposition graft. The most desirable graft is autologous great saphenous vein harvested from an uninjured leg.[6] Native vein graft is preferable because it has elastic properties that make it compliant with the normal pulsatile flow of an artery; it has a diameter that approximates that of an extremity artery, producing an adequate size match for grafting in the arm and leg; it is not thrombogenic; and it has superior long-term patency in elective vascular surgery compared with prosthetic material when it is used with smaller vessels (popliteal and tibial). Cephalic vein and lesser saphenous vein have been suggested as suitable second choices, but cephalic vein is less muscular than the great saphenous and, like the lesser saphenous, may present problems with harvesting in a trauma patient.[6] Also, upper extremity venous access becomes compromised when the cephalic vein is used.

Saphenous vein may not be suitable in all instances because of inadequate size or because it has been traumatized or harvested previously. In such cases, a prosthetic conduit may be needed. Initial experiences with the use of prosthetic material (Dacron) in traumatic vascular injuries were not good. Rich and Hughes reported a complication rate of 77% (infection and thrombosis were the most common) in 26 patients.[34] However, more recent experience with newer graft material (polytetrafluoroethylene [PTFE]) has shown improved patency (70% to 90% short term) and rare infection (even in contaminated wounds).[35] Early rates of patency with PTFE grafts are equivalent to those with vein for injuries proximal to the popliteal artery and in the brachial artery. Distal to these levels, PTFE is inferior to vein for popliteal and more distal vessels and in the arm and leg. PTFE grafts of less than 6 mm should not be used.[35] PTFE and vein grafts must be covered or there is a significant risk of hemorrhage from desiccation of the vein with subsequent autolysis or breakdown of the anastomosis.[21,35]

Intraoperative Imaging and Noninvasive Evaluation

The successful management of vascular injury requires knowing precisely the status of blood flow in the area of the vessel injury. Preoperative imaging with catheter angiography or CT angiography is not always possible. In addition, when a vascular repair has been completed, the presence of thrombus, kinking, or unexpected technical problems may cause early failure. Intraoperative imaging is therefore an important part of assessing the injured vessels and the repair site.[6] Either single-injection radiography or fluoroscopy is effective in providing images in the operating room (see Fig. 63-6). Intraoperative duplex scanning is also effective but requires significant training and experience for it to be performed adequately. Hand-held continuous-wave Doppler interrogation can be helpful but requires considerable experience to be used effectively. Ankle or wrist pressure measurements may be misleading because of regional vasospasm in the proximal injured extremity, resulting in a reduced distal pressure compared with the uninjured leg. Intraoperative radiographic imaging remains the most accurate and useful method to detect technical problems with a vascular repair or to determine the presence of thrombus in the runoff vessels distal to a repair. Routine completion arteriography after vascular repairs will yield findings of clinical importance in approximately 10% of patients.[6]

Role of Tissue Coverage

All vascular repairs must be covered to prevent desiccation and disruption. In crushed or badly mangled extremities, this can be a difficult challenge. Rotation of regional muscle or skin flaps may be required. The early involvement of a plastic and reconstructive surgeon is essential to obtain tissue coverage when there is extensive soft tissue injury or loss. Local muscle can be advanced into the wound at the initial operation. If there is a large contaminated wound and local muscle viability is questionable, early reexploration and preparation for a free flap should be considered. On occasion, tissue loss may be so extensive that an extra-anatomic course for an interposition graft may be required. Attention to coverage is also essential in damage control procedures to avoid shunt dislodgment during dressing changes.

Role of Fasciotomy

Failure to perform an adequate fasciotomy after revascularization of an acutely ischemic limb is the most common cause of preventable limb loss.[6] Calf compartment syndrome is the most common indication for fasciotomy. Forearm and thigh compartment syndromes are less common. Any muscle group can develop compartment syndrome, including those in the hands and feet.

Compartment syndrome may be manifested immediately or delayed to 12 to 24 hours after reperfusion. If it is not promptly diagnosed and treated, the risk of limb loss or limb dysfunction is high. Calf compartment syndrome most commonly results from prolonged ischemia or a crush injury. Frequent physical examinations augmented with compartment pressure measurements are necessary to detect this complication in its early stage. The first clinical finding is loss of light touch sensation in the distribution of the nerve in the compartment. The diagnosis of compartment syndrome should be suspected in any patient complaining of increasing pain after injury. The physical findings include a tense compartment, pain on passive range of motion, progressive loss of sensation, and weakness. The loss of arterial pulses is a late finding, which usually indicates a poor prognosis. Neurologic signs and symptoms, although helpful, are neither sensitive nor specific in the upper extremity after arterial injury because associated peripheral nerve injury often exists. Early diagnosis must be predicated on measurement of compartment pressures. The normal tissue compartment pressure ranges from 0 to 9 mm Hg. Much controversy exists about what constitutes a pathologic elevation. However, the safest approach is to perform fasciotomy when compartment pressure exceeds 25 mm Hg.[6,36,37]

A compartment syndrome can also develop in either the upper arm (triceps, deltoid, or along the axillary sheath) or the forearm. The forearm compartment syndrome is more common. Increased tissue pressure can follow either blunt or penetrating trauma because of hematoma, post-traumatic transudation of serum into the interstitial space, venous thrombosis, or reperfusion after ischemia.[36] The possibility of a compartment syndrome must always be a consideration in a patient who has been injured, particularly one with prolonged ischemia before reperfusion.

Role of Immediate Amputation

A very limited role for primary amputation exists in the management of complex extremity vascular injuries. Patients with extensive soft tissue loss, neurologic deficit, extensive fractures, and vascular injuries should be evaluated collaboratively with orthopedic, neurosurgical, and plastic and reconstructive surgery colleagues to determine if primary amputation is the best initial management. Scoring systems to predict the need for amputation have not been useful.[38,39] Because of the emotional impact of amputation and because marginally viable tissue often takes hours to demarcate or declare, it may be best to proceed with initial intraoperative evaluation and documentation (pictures, radiographs, and consultation), damage control using intravascular shunts for the vascular injuries, and a second look in 24 hours. The interval of time allows communication with the patient and the family and a more planned approach. Immediate amputation should also be considered in patients with extensive soft tissue, bone, and neurovascular disruption who have life-threatening torso injuries as mentioned earlier in the discussion of damage control techniques. If immediate amputation is required, extensive documentation of the extremity injury with photographs placed in the chart will be helpful in later explaining the decision to the patient and family and will help with their acceptance of this drastic surgical procedure.

Common Errors and Pitfalls

The management of vascular injuries is challenging. An organized approach is necessary to avoid the common errors and pitfalls. One of the most common errors is the lack of recognition of an extremity vascular injury in a patient with multiple torso injuries. Failure to recognize and adequately treat compartment syndrome is another error that is all too common and has devastating consequences. In torso injuries to the great vessels, failure to adequately expose and control the injured site can lead to a rapid death from exsanguination. Finally, failure to recognize the need for damage control techniques and a rapid completion of the operation in an unstable patient can also be deadly. The three most common factors in generating errors in caring for the injured are fatigue, distraction, and familiarity.[40] Each of these factors is inherent to process of care at busy trauma centers. An organized approach mitigates these factors and intercepts errors in progress before they are completed and the patients suffer.

SPECIFIC INJURIES

Head, Neck, and Thoracic Outlet

Vascular injuries of the head, neck, and thoracic outlet are often challenging to manage. Penetrating trauma can injure large vessels, such as the innominate and subclavian arteries, which can lead to exsanguination. Blunt trauma to the carotid and vertebral arteries, collectively known as blunt cerebrovascular injuries, is often occult and, if not diagnosed and treated rapidly, can lead to cerebral ischemia, infarction, and possibly death.

The principles of management of penetrating trauma to this region are based on the location of the injury relative to the three zones of the neck: zone 1, inferior to the cricoid cartilage; zone 2, cricoid cartilage to the angle of the mandible; and zone III, cephalad from the angle of the mandible. In a stable patient with a suspected vascular injury in either zone 1 or zone 3, vascular imaging is mandatory to confirm the suspicion of vascular injury and to plan proximal and distal control.[41] Vascular imaging is also recommended for stable patients with penetrating trauma in zone 2, but exploration should be undertaken expeditiously for patients with an expanding hematoma or impending airway compromise (manifested by hoarseness and tracheal deviation).[41] In the unstable patient, a Foley urinary catheter with the balloon inflated can be inserted into the wound to achieve temporary tamponade of injuries in these regions. Conventional angiography can have a dual role for injuries in zone 1 or zone 3. It not only can provide the diagnosis but also may provide a venue for endoluminal management—coiling of bleeding vessels or pseudoaneurysms in zone 3 or placement of covered stents in zone 1.

Blunt cerebrovascular injuries are often occult and asymptomatic. Therefore, rapid diagnostic screening is essential and provides the underpinning of successful management. Initially, blunt cerebrovascular injuries were thought to be rare, occurring in about 0.1% of patients; but with use of the screening criteria developed by the group at Denver General Hospital, the incidence is actually 10 to 20 times that.[27] Factors associated with these injuries include displaced midface fractures, basilar skull fracture with carotid canal involvement, cervical spine fracture, closed head injury consistent with diffuse axonal injury and Glasgow Coma Scale score below 6, and blunt neck trauma from hanging or seat belt injuries. Both carotid and vertebral artery injuries occur from stretching or tearing of the intima of the vessels produced by rapid extreme extension or flexion of the neck or by direct blunt-force injury. The carotid artery is particularly vulnerable where it lies close to the second and sixth cervical transverse processes. The vertebral artery is also vulnerable to stretch injuries and fractures of the transverse process of the cervical vertebrae that involve the foramen transversarium. Cerebrovascular injuries vary from minor intimal irregularities to arterial rupture and severe hemorrhage (Table 63-3).[27]

Patients who fulfill the Denver criteria should undergo CT angiography of the neck.[26,27] The treatment of blunt carotid and vertebral artery injuries is anticoagulation in patients who do not have a contraindication.[26] Aspirin is the only alternative in patients who cannot be safely anticoagulated. The use of endovascular techniques has a very limited role as discussed before. However, in patients with carotid injuries at the base of the skull or injuries of the vertebral artery, covered stents or embolization offers the best results (see Fig. 63-5).

TABLE 63-3 Spectrum of Severity of Blunt Cerebrovascular Arterial Injury

Grade I	Luminal irregularity with <25% luminal narrowing
Grade II	Dissection of hematoma with ≥25% luminal narrowing
Grade III	Pseudoaneurysm
Grade IV	Occlusion
Grade V	Transection with extravasation

Vascular injuries of the thoracic outlet are challenging because they involve large-caliber vessels that can be difficult to expose and to control. Unstable patients with vascular injury in the region of the thoracic outlet must be expeditiously taken to the operating room. Stable patients should have preoperative imaging with catheter or CT angiography to locate the injury and to determine its extent. This will allow planning for endoluminal treatment or open exposure.[42,43] Operative control may require a simple supraclavicular incision, a sternotomy, or a combination of the two incisions, depending on the location and extent of the injury. Clamp application on the proximal subclavian and carotid arteries must be precise to avoid injury to the vagus, phrenic, or recurrent laryngeal nerves, all of which reside in this anatomic region. Sternotomy is frequently used for proximal innominate, proximal right subclavian, and proximal right carotid arterial injuries. Left subclavian artery proximal control is best obtained through a posterolateral thoracotomy for definitive repair. However, for supraclavicular injuries, a third intercostal space anterolateral thoracotomy provides exposure for proximal control. Distal control of the carotid arteries is obtained by extending the median sternotomy superiorly along the border of the ipsilateral sternocleidomastoid muscle. Distal subclavian arterial control is obtained through a supraclavicular incision. Resection of the clavicle results in little or no morbidity and can be performed quickly to control hemorrhage if needed. Suturing of the subclavian and axillary arteries must be done with extreme caution. Undue tension or traction will result in a tear of these vessels.[44] Endovascular balloon occlusion, when it is rapidly available, is an excellent adjunctive measure for proximal control.

Intrathoracic Great Vessels

Penetrating injuries of the intrathoracic great vessels (aorta, superior and inferior venae cavae, pulmonary arteries and veins) usually cause death at the time of injury from exsanguination. The small number of patients with penetrating injuries of the intrathoracic great vessels who arrive to the trauma center alive often present hemodynamically unstable and require emergent operative intervention. Repair of intrathoracic great vessel injuries may be achieved through sternotomy, left or right anterolateral thoracotomy, or, in many cases, bilateral (or clamshell) anterolateral thoracotomy.[30] Although many of these structures are exposed through a posterolateral thoracotomy in the elective setting, patients who present in hemorrhagic shock and without a distinct diagnosis should be managed with more versatile incisions, such as median sternotomy and anterolateral thoracotomy.

Injuries to the ascending aorta and the superior or inferior vena cava are best exposed and treated through a median sternotomy.[30] These injuries should be controlled with digital pressure and then placement of a side-biting clamp to allow suture repair of the injury and may require cardiopulmonary bypass to achieve repair. Injuries of the descending aorta are ideally approached through a left posterolateral thoracotomy. However, most of these injuries will be discovered during emergent left anterolateral thoracotomy and will need to be quickly repaired. Injuries of the pulmonary arteries and veins can be approached through a sternotomy or anterolateral thoracotomy, depending on their proximity to the heart.[30] If possible, these injuries should be repaired primarily. However, destructive injuries to the pulmonary arteries and veins may necessitate pneumonectomy for definitive control.

Blunt injuries to the intrathoracic great vessels consist primarily of blunt thoracic aortic injury (BTAI). BTAI occurs as a result of high-energy blunt trauma. The most common mechanisms of injury resulting in BTAI are high-speed motor vehicle crashes and falls from a height. The aorta is typically injured in a location where it is relatively fixed (root of the aorta, ligamentum arteriosum, diaphragmatic hiatus), and the majority (85% to 90%) of patients die at the scene. Patients with BTAI who arrive at the hospital alive have typically sustained multisystem associated injuries. BTAI must be ruled out when there is a high-energy mechanism injury or a chest radiograph shows a widened mediastinum. However, definitive diagnosis of BTAI is established with a high-resolution CT scan of the chest. Injuries vary from an intimal injury to pseudoaneurysm or a contained periaortic hematoma just distal to the left subclavian artery.[7,9]

Once the diagnosis of BTAI is confirmed, the initial management is focused on blood pressure control and addressing associated immediately life-threatening injuries. Blood pressure is best controlled with a short-acting intravenous beta blocker (e.g., esmolol) that can be titrated to a systolic blood pressure of less than 110 mm Hg while also keeping heart rate below 100 beats/min.[30] If beta blockade does not achieve blood pressure goals, other intravenous agents, such as calcium channel blockers, nitroglycerin, and nitroprusside, may be used. Whereas some stable minimal BTAIs may be managed nonoperatively, most will require definitive repair through the open or endovascular approach. Regardless of the approach, most BTAIs should be repaired in a delayed fashion after the patient is stable. Early repair of these injuries has been associated with increased mortality.[30]

Open repair of BTAI has been the mainstay of treatment for decades. Open repair is achieved through a left posterolateral thoracotomy, cardiopulmonary bypass, and placement of a synthetic aortic interposition graft. Endovascular repair of BTAI has become increasingly more common during the past decade (Fig. 63-7). Although there are no prospective, randomized trials comparing open versus endovascular management of BTAI, there have been two multicenter American Association for the Surgery of Trauma trials showing lower morbidity (spinal cord ischemia, stroke) and mortality with the endovascular approach.[24,25] However, patients who undergo endovascular repair require lifelong surveillance because there is no information about long-term sequelae of endovascular grafts in the aortic position in young patients. In addition, many young patients do not have favorable anatomy for endovascular repair and still require the open approach. More recent series of open repair with spinal cord protection from partial cardiopulmonary bypass have a competitively low rate of paraplegia.[25] The widespread preference for thoracic endovascular aortic repair may suffer from the famous British thoracic surgeon Ronald Belsey's observation that "the follow-up clinics are the shoals upon which founder many attractive theories in surgery."[45] Late graft failure due to endoleak and possible collapse within aortas susceptible to the elongation and widening that occur with age may be a future source of major morbidity and mortality. As of 2016, there is not conclusive evidence that thoracic endovascular aortic repair in young patients is superior to well-performed open repairs with partial bypass for spinal cord protection.[25]

Abdominal Vascular Injury

Abdominal vascular injury most often results from penetrating trauma, and all are treated through a generous midline laparotomy.[31] Many of these injuries will require supraceliac control of the aorta to achieve adequate visualization to complete exposure and repair. Penetrating injuries to the abdominal aorta are best exposed and repaired with a left medial visceral rotation that exposes the aorta from the diaphragmatic hiatus to the iliac bifurcation (see Fig. 63-7). The injury can typically be controlled with direct digital pressure, which allows time for placement of vascular clamps proximal and distal to the site of injury.[31] Abdominal aortic injuries may be repaired primarily after stab wounds, but gunshot wounds will often require a patch repair or interposition graft. Uncommonly, patients will sustain a blunt abdominal aortic injury without life-threatening hemorrhage, and these injuries are best repaired by endovascular techniques.

The inferior vena cava is exposed with a right medial visceral rotation that exposes the vena cava from iliac vein confluence to inferior edge of the liver (see Fig. 63-7).[31] Injury to the vena cava is best controlled with direct digital pressure, with subsequent proximal and distal control using sponge sticks or vessel loops. Lumbar tributaries and renal veins may also need to be controlled to clearly visualize and repair the injury. Injuries to the anterior or lateral surfaces of the vena cava can most often be repaired primarily as long as the repair does not narrow the lumen more than 50%. Penetrating injuries to the vena cava may be through-and-through and require repair of a posterior injury as well. Injuries to the posterior vena cava may be repaired through the anterior injury, or the vena cava may be mobilized after ligating and dividing lumbar veins. Complex injuries may require patch repair, interposition graft, shunting with delayed reconstruction, or ligation.[31] Complexity of repair will depend on physiologic status of the patient and location of the injury. Hemodynamically unstable patients with ongoing hemorrhage are not candidates for complex repairs and should have the vena cava ligated or shunted. Hemodynamically stable patients with injuries at or above the level of the renal veins may be candidates for complex reconstruction, but ligation is still an option for the exsanguinating patient.[31]

The right common, external, and internal iliac arteries are best exposed by widely mobilizing the cecum, whereas injuries to the left iliac arteries are exposed by completely mobilizing the sigmoid colon.[31] Keep in mind the course of the ureter on both sides as it crosses the iliac vessels. Injuries to the common and external iliac arteries are initially controlled with digital pressure to allow proximal and distal control with vascular clamps or vessel loops. Injuries to the common and external iliac arteries may be repaired primarily but will often require a synthetic interposition graft. The common and external iliac arteries should never be ligated; if a patient is hemodynamically unstable, these injuries should be shunted and repaired in a delayed fashion. However, injuries to the internal iliac artery can be routinely ligated.[31]

Iliac veins are exposed in the same manner as for iliac arteries. Exposure is made more challenging by the location of the confluence of the iliac veins with the inferior vena cava directly posterior to the right common iliac artery. It will need to be widely mobilized to allow access to the confluence of the iliac veins. However, we do not advocate division of the right iliac artery to achieve exposure of the iliac vein confluence. Once the common, external, and internal iliac veins are exposed, the injury is best controlled with direct digital pressure, then proximal and distal control may be achieved with vessel loops. If possible, simple injuries to the iliac veins should be repaired with primary venorrhaphy. However,

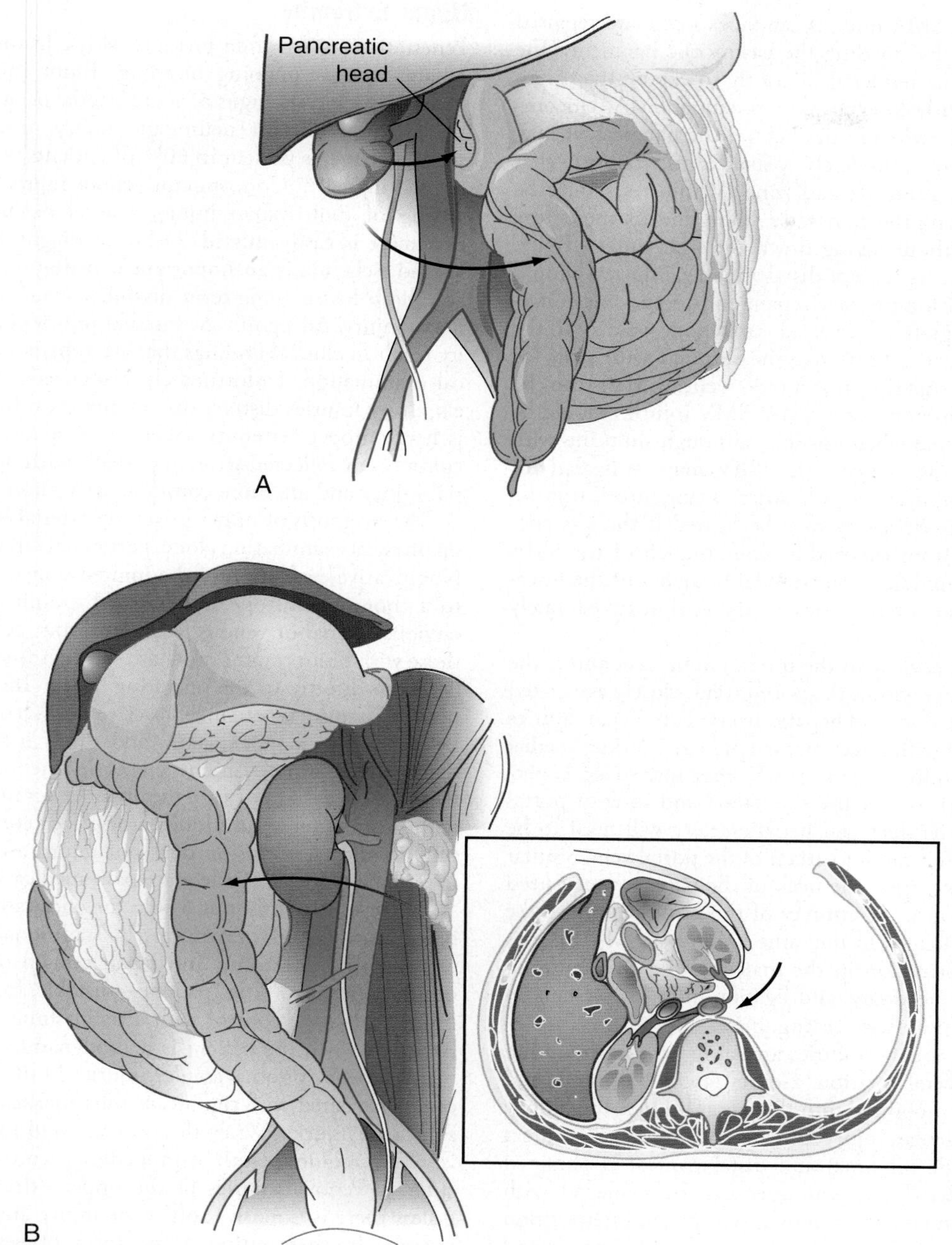

FIGURE 63-7 A, Left-sided medial visceral rotation for exposure of great vessels in the retroperitoneum. **B,** Right-sided medial visceral rotation for exposure of vena cava and renal veins in the retroperitoneum.

complex repairs of destructive injuries to the iliac veins should not be attempted, and these injuries should be ligated.[31]

Injuries to the mesenteric vessels are some of the most challenging injuries to expose and to repair. In the elective setting, the celiac trunk is often approached through the lesser sac; but in the setting of trauma, this may prove difficult because of a large lesser sac hematoma that obscures the usual landmarks. In the setting of trauma, the celiac trunk is best exposed through a wide left medial visceral rotation that mobilizes the spleen and tail of pancreas but leaves the left kidney in situ.[31] Once exposed, most injuries to the celiac trunk should be ligated because repair is difficult and ligation is well tolerated in the majority of patients. Although the SMA and celiac trunk take off from the aorta within 1 to 2 cm of each other, the exposure and treatment algorithm for SMA injuries is different. Management of SMA injuries will depend on location based on the Fullen classification: zone I, beneath the pancreas; zone II, between pancreaticoduodenal and middle colic branches; zone III, beyond middle colic branch; zone IV, enteric branches. Injuries that present with a large contained central hematoma at the root of the mesentery are best approached with a left medial visceral rotation. Active hemorrhage is controlled by manual compression followed by left medial visceral rotation.[31] This will allow exposure and control of the aorta proximal and distal to the SMA or direct clamping of the SMA as it comes off the aorta. Once this control has been achieved, attention is turned anteriorly for definitive exposure and repair of the SMA injury.

Zone I and zone II SMA injuries can be exposed and repaired through the lesser sac by dividing the gastrocolic ligament. The pancreas will need to be retracted inferiorly to expose the origin of the SMA or superiorly to expose the proximal SMA. Uncommonly, in active bleed SMA injuries behind the pancreas, it may need to be divided to completely visualize and control that segment of the SMA. Zone III and zone IV injuries should be approached by reflecting the transverse colon and its mesentery superiorly with or without taking down the ligament of Treitz. All zones of SMA injuries (except distal zone IV injuries) should always be repaired, with a primary repair, end-to-end anastomosis, or interposition graft of reversed saphenous vein.[31] If the patient is in extremis, the SMA may be shunted with plan for delayed repair. The superior mesenteric vein (SMV) can be exposed in the same fashion as the SMA. SMV injuries should be repaired or reconstructed when possible, although shunting with delayed repair is also an option. The SMV may be ligated for patients in extremis who would otherwise exsanguinate. Injuries to the inferior mesenteric artery may be ligated if there is adequate collateral flow from the middle colic branch of the SMA and the inferior and middle hemorrhoidal branches of the internal iliac arteries. The inferior mesenteric vein may be safely ligated if required.

The portal vein runs close to the inferior vena cava and is the most posterior structure within the portal triad, closely associated with the common bile duct and hepatic artery. Portal vein injuries are initially controlled with direct manual pressure. A right medial visceral rotation, including a generous Kocher maneuver, is performed to expose and to visualize the lateral and inferior portal vein. The common bile duct and hepatic artery will need to be mobilized to expose the anterior surface of the portal vein. Similar to SMA and SMV exposure, the neck of the pancreas may need to be divided to visualize the entirety of the portal vein.[31] These injuries should be managed in the same fashion as SMV injuries with repair or reconstruction in the majority of cases, shunting and delayed repair if necessary, and ligation only for patients in extremis who would otherwise exsanguinate.

Penetrating renal vascular injuries are easily exposed on either side after medial visceral rotation. Gerota fascia is opened, and the kidney is bluntly mobilized into the wound. Once the kidney is mobilized, the vascular injury can be controlled with direct manual pressure while proximal and distal control is obtained with vessel loops. Renal artery injuries can be managed with primary repair, end-to-end anastomosis, vein patch, interposition graft, or nephrectomy (after confirming a normal contralateral kidney by palpation). Treatment of renal artery injuries is based on complexity of the injury and physiologic status of the patient. Renal vein injuries can be repaired with primary venorrhaphy or ligation. On the right, ligation of the renal vein will require a nephrectomy, and patch angioplasty or interposition graft should be considered in stable patients. The left renal vein may be safely ligated near the inferior vena cava because of collateral flow through the adrenal, gonadal, and lumbar veins.[31] Combined injuries to the renal artery and vein should be treated with nephrectomy in unstable patients. Renal artery injuries rarely occur after blunt trauma. These injuries may be managed nonoperatively with expected involution of the affected kidney or nephrectomy. It is uncommon to successfully salvage renal function with vascular reconstruction of complete blunt renal artery occlusion. Management must consider several factors, including overall status of the patient, warm ischemia time, and need for laparotomy for associated intra-abdominal injuries.

Upper Extremity

Penetrating injury often presents with a history of either arterial hemorrhage or ongoing bleeding. Blunt injury usually causes thrombosis and the signs of acute arterial occlusion with resultant ischemia. Significant neurologic injury, usually involving the median nerve, is present in 60% of patients with upper extremity arterial injury.[6,46] Concomitant venous injury is common. In the setting of multisystem injury, arterial occlusion in the upper extremity is easily missed. Delay in diagnosis resulting in prolonged ischemia is an important contributing factor to preventable limb loss or long-term disability from irreversible ischemic nerve injury. All significant vascular injuries of the upper extremity result in clinical findings that are apparent on thorough physical examination. Unfortunately, associated severe torso or lower extremity injuries distract the trauma team from the injured and ischemic upper extremity. Delays in diagnosis and treatment are common in collected series of patients with upper extremity arterial injury and are more common after blunt-force trauma.[6,46]

The diagnosis of upper extremity arterial injury is often made on physical examination alone, particularly in penetrating injuries. Noninvasive evaluation of the injured upper extremity adds little to a thorough history and physical examination. Patients with obvious arterial or venous laceration from penetrating trauma or those with blunt trauma and hard findings (see Table 63-1) should be taken directly to the operating room. The arterial bed of the upper extremity is extremely reactive to vasoconstriction produced by hypovolemic shock, pain, and drugs including cocaine and methamphetamine. Absent pulses in the presence of complex fractures or crush injuries of the upper extremity need to be assessed with imaging (either multidetector CT or conventional angiography) if normal perfusion does not return after resuscitation and the administration of adequate pain medications.

There is currently not a role for endovascular therapy in the brachial artery and forearm vessels. Traditional operative exposure, catheter thrombectomy, and repair remain the best approach to optimize results.[6,46] In patients unstable from associated torso injuries, damage control with arterial shunt placement followed by repair when the patient is hemodynamically stable is the best management option. Vascular injuries in the upper extremity are often associated with significant musculoskeletal, neurologic, and soft tissue injuries. When this occurs, a multidisciplinary approach is often required with orthopedics, neurosurgery, and plastic surgery. Venous injuries of the upper extremity can be ligated unless there is extensive soft tissue injury and loss of venous collaterals. In that setting, some form of venous reconstruction should be considered.

On occasion, bleeding from a partially transected arm or forearm vessel can be significant. The senior surgeon should make certain that adequate control is obtained and maintained during resuscitation, transportation to the operating room, and surgical preparation and draping. Although they have proved lifesaving in the field for management of hemorrhage from extremities, tourniquets should be used sparingly in the trauma bay and only placed and carefully monitored for adequacy of compression and duration of application by the senior surgeon present.

The patient should be widely prepared and draped with generous inclusion of the entire upper extremity, the shoulder, and the anterior-superior aspect of the chest to allow incisions for proximal control.[6] An uninjured leg should also be prepared and draped from inguinal region to toes to allow saphenous vein harvest. Adjunctive measures, such as bolus intravenous systemic heparinization, administration of a continuous infusion of low-molecular-weight dextran, and administration of intravenous antibiotics, should be considered and used where appropriate. In patients with multisystem injuries, especially head injury, local or regional infusion of heparin should be used in place of systemic administration. Loupe magnification and coaxial lighting ("headlight") are technical adjuncts that may be useful in suturing small blood vessel with fine suture.

Surgical exposure requires generous incisions placed to maximize exposure and to provide appropriate options for further exploration and repair. The brachial artery is best exposed through a longitudinal incision along the medial aspect of the upper arm over the groove between the triceps and biceps muscles. The incision can be extended distally with an S-shaped extension across the antecubital fossa from ulnar to radial aspect and onto the forearm to expose the origins of the forearm vessels.[6,46] Proximal brachial artery injuries may require control of the infraclavicular axillary artery. Vascular repair requires attention to detail in all phases. Balloon catheter thrombectomy and flushing with heparinized saline followed by débridement of damaged arterial wall are essential to successful repair. Lacerated veins should be ligated unless there is extensive soft tissue injury and collateral venous flow is compromised. In such cases, the vein should be repaired. In repairing both venous and arterial injuries, the vein should be repaired first. If the duration of arterial occlusion and ischemia is a concern, temporary intraluminal shunts may be placed in the artery. Primary arterial repair of undamaged ends of vessel (end-to-end anastomosis) should be performed only if the repair is tension free. Saphenous vein interposition should be chosen whenever vessel injury is extensive or if primary tension-free repair is not possible. PTFE needs to remain a second choice to autologous vein in the management of injuries distal to the axillary artery.[2,6,46]

Forearm fasciotomy, particularly in the setting of prolonged ischemia, must always be considered before completion of the operation, and compartment pressures should be measured at the completion of the operation. If normal pressures are obtained, fasciotomy is not necessary, but pressure measurements should be repeated frequently because compartment syndrome can occur in the postoperative period as a consequence of reperfusion.[37,46]

There is a limited but important role for "primary" or early amputation in the management of upper extremity vascular injuries. Patients with extensive soft tissue loss or with scapulothoracic dissociation who have severe neurologic deficits, extensive fractures, and vascular injuries should be evaluated collaboratively with orthopedic, neurosurgery, and plastic surgery colleagues to determine if early amputation is appropriate. The best approach is intraoperative, multidisciplinary assessment, damage control, and plan for reoperative assessment in 24 to 48 hours. This will allow discussions with the patient and family and a second look.

Combined ulnar and radial artery injury in the forearm requires repair of at least one vessel. The ulnar artery is usually larger in the proximal forearm and is a better target for direct repair or saphenous vein bypass. Distally, the vessel repair should be performed in whichever vessel is largest or amenable to simple repair.[6,46]

Isolated ulnar or radial artery injuries can be managed with simple ligation only if there is absolute certainty that flow through the remaining vessel is adequate. Close inspection of the forearm and hand with palpation of pulses augmented by continuous-wave (hand-held) Doppler interrogation is essential.[6]

Lower Extremity

Vascular injuries in the legs are more common in military series (30% to 40%) than in civilian practice (20%).[2,47] Although penetrating injuries are more common, blunt vascular trauma in the lower extremity remains a significant challenge. In the thigh and the leg, fractures and dislocations can be associated with vascular injuries. The popliteal artery is at particularly high risk of injury after dislocation of the knee.[2,47]

Findings at presentation vary from significant hemorrhage from a wound (i.e., open fracture, stab, or gunshot) to occult arterial occlusion from blunt injury. A systematic approach with a thorough extremity vascular examination is essential to avoid errors in recognition and delays in treatment.

Exposure is obtained with incisions used for elective surgical procedures. The common femoral artery is best exposed through a longitudinal incision overlying its course from the inguinal ligament inferiorly for 8 to 12 cm. Proximal control may require exposure of the external iliac artery, best accomplished through an oblique muscle-splitting lower quadrant abdominal incision carried into retroperitoneum, where the artery and vein can be controlled. Superficial femoral artery (SFA) injuries are best exposed through a longitudinal groin incision similar to that used for femoral bifurcation exposure for the proximal portion. The mid-SFA is approached through an oblique incision over the sartorius muscle. The junction of the SFA and popliteal can be exposed by extending this incision, dividing the adductor tendon.

Popliteal injuries are exposed through a generous medial incision. Exposure of the artery in the area at the knee joint requires division of the medial head of the gastrocnemius muscle and the semimembranosus and semitendinosus muscles. The distal popliteal artery is exposed with an incision along the posterior margin of the tibia.

Repair of lower extremity vascular injuries usually requires an interposition graft. This is particularly true in the popliteal artery. Reverse saphenous vein from the contralateral extremity is the first choice for interposition grafts. In the common femoral artery, PTFE is an acceptable choice for interposition if the saphenous vein is not of sufficient size, but it should not be used in the below-knee popliteal arteries.[35]

Injuries below the popliteal artery at the level of the tibial vessels are best managed by ligation if two of the three calf vessels are patent and there is adequate collateral flow. In the presence of both anterior and posterior tibial vessel occlusion, the peroneal artery is usually not sufficiently connected to the distal arterial bed by collaterals, and repair of one of the injured vessels should be performed. The choice of which vessel to repair is based on both the extent of associated soft tissue injury and the patency of the distal segments of those vessels.

Damage control techniques with arterial and venous shunt placement with delayed definitive repair are an important part of managing lower extremity vascular injury associated with major torso injuries and hemodynamic instability (Fig. 63-8). All efforts should be made early postoperatively to achieve adequate stability as rapidly as possible to allow a timely return to the operating room for definitive vascular repair before shunt thrombosis and prolonged ischemia.

Operative Techniques for Extremity Fasciotomy

Fasciotomy of the forearm compartments requires release of individual muscle bundles. Generous incisions are required to release the dorsal and volar compartments and the mobile wad. Fasciotomy in the leg requires release of the anterior and lateral compartments on the anterior lateral aspect of the calf and the deep and superficial posterior compartments through incisions on the lateral and medial aspects of the calf (Fig. 63-9). These incisions should be generous in their length to accommodate subsequent muscle swelling and to avoid further compression.[6]

Thigh compartment syndrome is uncommon. The most common cause is thigh crush injury associated with femur fracture. Fasciotomy should release the three compartments: lateral, medial, and posterior. Two incisions, one lateral for the lateral compartment and one medial for the other two compartments, are sufficient. These need to be generous in their length. Compartment syndromes occur in the hands and feet, and these are best managed by orthopedic surgeons or hand surgeons.[6]

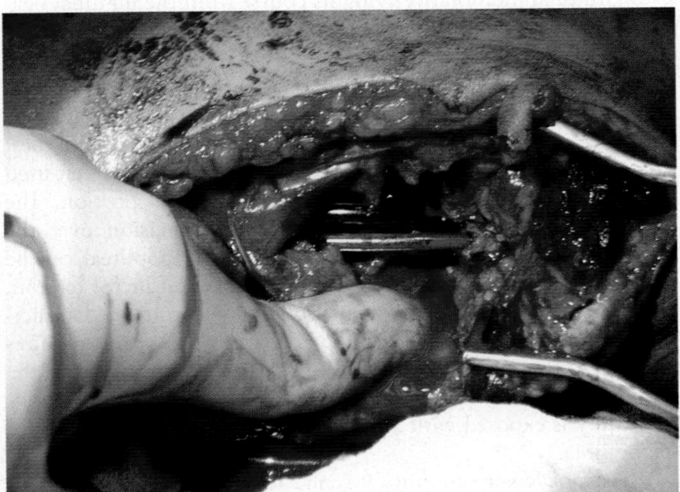

FIGURE 63-8 Damage control for multiple gunshot wounds with shunt placement in the popliteal artery and vein in a patient with associated major torso hemorrhage.

POSTOPERATIVE MANAGEMENT

The cornerstone of postoperative management is close follow-up to detect a change in the vascular examination findings. This includes frequent assessment of the vital signs, the distal extremity pulse, the continuous-wave Doppler signal, the capillary refill, and the neurologic examination findings of the injured extremity. If there is concern about any portion of the examination, an immediate return to the operating room may avert a potentially limb-threatening problem. Because failure of a vascular repair due to thrombosis can occur during the first 48 hours after the repair, careful follow-up with frequent examinations should continue for at least that length of time.

Reperfusion edema or intracompartmental hemorrhage can lead to a delayed onset of a compartment syndrome.[37] Physical examination alone may not detect the presence of compartment syndrome. Frequent postoperative compartment pressure measurements are the only way to accurately assess the injured extremity in patients who are not conscious and cooperative. The presence of a new postoperative extremity neurologic deficit is an important indicator of ongoing ischemia and should prompt assessment of both the patency of the vascular repair and the pressure within muscle compartments.

OUTCOMES AND FOLLOW-UP

The most common cause of amputation after vascular injury is the neurologic insult from either direct trauma to the nerve or ischemia. This should be remembered as one contemplates repair of a vascular injury in a "flail extremity" (permanently denervated secondary to irreversible neurologic injury).[38,39] Functional outcome after vascular repair is related to the severity of the associated injuries of muscle, bone, and nerve. Regular follow-up of patients with vascular repairs should continue to assess patency of the repair and to determine the presence of late complications.

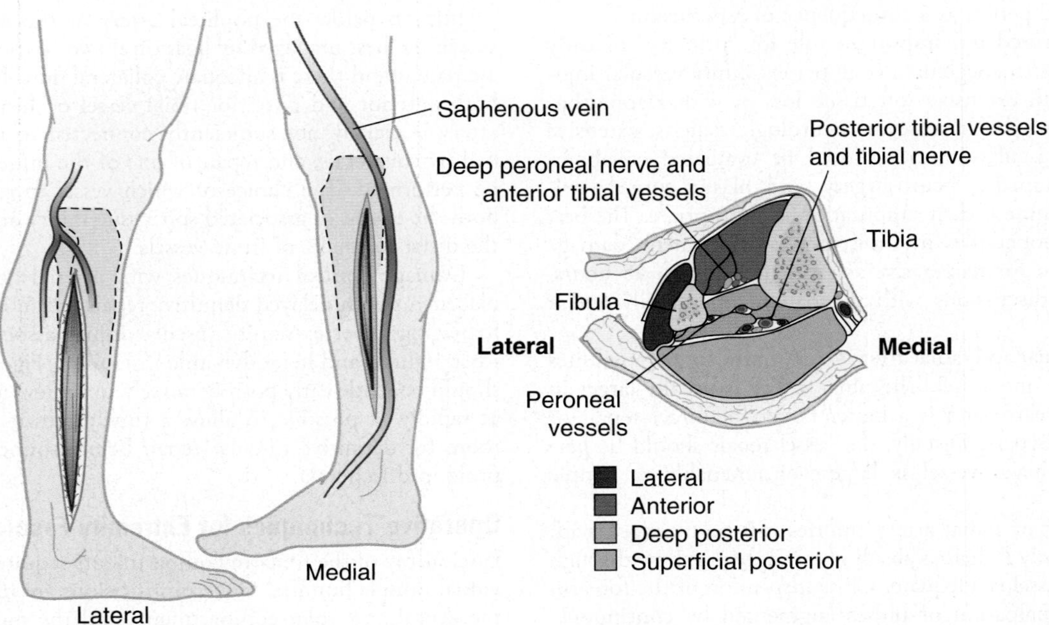

FIGURE 63-9 Calf muscle compartments and incisions for fasciotomy.

These include aneurysmal dilation or segmental stenosis of vein grafts, venous insufficiency from venous ligation, thrombosis of a pseudoaneurysm, and arteriovenous fistula. Ideally, these patients should be seen in yearly follow-up. Pulse examination and, if indicated, noninvasive imaging should be performed on a regular basis. Imaging with CT angiography or catheter angiography should be used if there is a suspicion of a complication.

Torso vascular injuries have relatively few late complications. Venous interposition grafts, when used, should be observed with periodic noninvasive imaging and, if indicated, CT angiography. Aortic and iliac arterial repairs should be observed similarly, and surveillance should ascertain signs and symptoms of arterial occlusive disease, such as upper or lower extremity claudication. Patients with synthetic interposition grafts should be counseled on the need for antibiotic prophylaxis during subsequent dental work or invasive procedures. Although late infections are uncommon, patients should be made aware of this possibility and counseled to notify all of their health care providers of the presence of a vascular prosthesis.

TRAINING AND PREPARATION FOR SUCCESSFUL MANAGEMENT

Vascular surgery carries a high risk of technical surgical error compared with many other areas of surgery. The optimal treatment of vascular trauma remains challenging and is rapidly evolving. Establishing goals for training in vascular trauma cannot be discussed without understanding the trends of increasing endovascular approaches and declining numbers of open repairs. Although one can acquire the didactic knowledge base from reading chapters such as this, the acquisition of decision-making abilities and surgical skills is based on experience that is becoming more and more difficult to obtain during surgical training. The average general surgical resident completes surgical residency having managed less than one vascular trauma case.[48,49] The average high-volume major trauma center in the United States manages approximately 10 to 15 vascular training cases a year. Fellowship-trained vascular surgeons receive vastly more exposure to chronic vascular disease and endovascular techniques than training in the rapid exposure of major vessels for proximal and distal control, let alone their open surgical management. The number of trauma surgeons contemporarily trained in endovascular techniques is extremely low. Many military general surgeons deployed to Afghanistan and Iraq for combat surgical care of wounded warriors site deficiencies in open vascular surgeries as their number one concern (personal communication to the authors).

General Surgery Training

The shrinking volume of open elective and emergency vascular surgery operations combined with resident work hour limitations has created significant obstacles to obtaining adequate experience in vascular surgical technique.[48] As opposed to residents graduating 2 decades ago, today's general surgeons rarely have enough experience to make them competent and capable of independently performing vascular surgery. Currently, there are a significant number of general surgeons who include vascular surgical cases in their practices. However, almost all completed their training before 2000 and the advent of the extensive use of endovascular techniques. These surgeons honed skills on open aortic aneurysm repairs, aortobifemoral bypass, and femoral popliteal bypass procedures.

The numbers of vascular surgery cases done by residents appears to be rising according to the Residency Review Committee. However, a closer look reveals the harsh reality that the case logs include a growing number of endovascular and venous procedures and an alarming decrease in open arterial procedures.[48-50] There has been as much as a 65% decrease in open arterial reconstruction case volume for graduate general surgery residents.[48,49] Open aortic surgery experience is much more uncommon, with many residents participating in five or fewer open aortic cases. Most surgery residents, however, claim endovascular aortic aneurysm repair (EVAR) among their vascular surgery numbers. Dialysis access cases have ironically become one of the last bastions of giving residents training in vascular techniques. The above-knee elective femoral popliteal bypass on mildly or moderately diseased vessels has all but disappeared. Most lower extremity bypasses are performed to very small distal vessels, and residents are often not able to perform these anastomoses.

Vascular Fellowship Training

The shrinking volume of open cases has also had an impact on vascular fellowship training. EVAR has become the treatment of choice for elective aneurysm repair, and emergency EVAR capabilities for ruptured abdominal aortic aneurysm have become a widespread practice. Consequently, there is real concern about the lack of open aortic cases available for training vascular surgery fellows. A conservative estimate of the number of cases required to give a surgeon adequate experience to competently handle the difficult ruptured aorta is well above 20 to 30 cases. The old saying that it takes up to 50 to 100 aortic repairs before the surgeon's fear transforms to profound respect for the aorta is probably accurate. Very few training programs come close to that volume. In reality, with widespread use of EVAR as the first-line therapy for elective abdominal aortic aneurysm repair, most graduating fellows will not see 100 open cases in the first 10 to 15 years of practice. The "fear factor" remains a considerable issue for these surgeons to contend with.

The decrease in open case volume during training and the significant rise in endovascular experience have produced a generation of vascular fellowship graduates who are more comfortable with closed techniques versus open techniques in many areas. This translates to a reluctance to convert to open technique and a discomfort with situations such as vascular trauma in which endovascular techniques may not be an option.

Vascular Trauma Realities

In a multi-institutional study presented in September 2012 at the annual meeting of the American Association for the Surgery of Trauma, Shackford and colleagues reported that more than 60% of complex extremity vascular reconstructions performed at 12 trauma centers across the country between 1995 and 2010 were performed by general surgeons.[29] The outcome of these repairs by general surgeons was not significantly different from the outcome of repairs performed by fellowship-trained cardiac and vascular surgeons. The overall amputation rate was low. All 12 hospitals were mature trauma centers with well-organized surgical specialty support. The average age of the surgeons who performed these repairs suggested that they all had adequate exposure during their surgical residency. What all the surgeons from the centers in this study had in common was a commitment to maintaining the skills needed to manage vascular injuries. The results of this approach were successful management of these complex injuries.

The conventional wisdom at successful trauma centers has always been to have the right surgeon available to do the right operation in a timely fashion. This has been especially important in repair of vascular injuries. Whether this capability will continue to be widely available remains to be seen. Few recent graduates of general surgery residencies feel confident in managing vascular injuries or other vascular emergencies. The alarming lack of open abdominal vascular procedures in most fellowship training programs has similarly eroded the confidence and competence of recently trained vascular surgeons. The paucity of capable vascular surgical emergency backup represents a threat to most of our trauma and emergency centers.

Need for Remedial Training and Review

We cannot expect the current general surgery and vascular surgery training programs to mitigate this lack of technical and cognitive competence without adding additional educational content focusing on areas of limited experience. The alternatives to hands-on operative experience remain limited. Simulation, although promising, has yet to accomplish the vision that it can replace actual experience as an adequate teaching opportunity. Maximizing open experience by resident participation in abdominal organ harvest by the transplantation team has been somewhat helpful.

There are two approaches in residency and fellowship training programs that hold promise. One is to actively audit general surgery and vascular fellowship trainee case logs to detect which resident should be the next participant in a major abdominal vascular procedure. These cases are precious training opportunities and should be shared evenly with all trainees. At this operation, the resident must be taught by actually performing the procedure, not simply watching. Attending surgeons must have the patience and forbearance to actually allow the trainee to perform the operation. Preparation with thoughtful didactic material focusing on these key operations should occur early in the trainee's rotation so that the operative experience has maximum educational impact. Postprocedure debriefing with a thorough discussion of decision points, troubleshooting, and management of different versions of the anatomy and pathologic findings needs to be rigorously performed.

The second important educational opportunity is participation in courses such as the American College of Surgeons–sponsored Advanced Surgical Skills for Exposure in Trauma (ASSET) and Advanced Trauma Operative Management (ATOM). These courses combine appropriate focused didactic material with either cadaver or live animal dissection. They are highly successful in improving both the knowledge and skill set of the participants. Equally important is the increase in confidence all participants report.

Additional courses developed through international cooperation are extremely promising. The Definitive Surgical Trauma Care course was developed by the International Association for Trauma and Surgical Intensive Care. The Definitive Surgical Trauma Skills course was developed by the Royal College of Surgeons of England with the Royal Defence Medical College and the Uniformed Services University of the Health Sciences in the United States. Completing either of these two courses provides excellent surgical training in trauma surgery decision making, vascular exposures, and vascular repairs.

The Need for Action

The rapidly disappearing knowledge and experience base of major open vascular surgical technique threatens all trauma centers' ability to provide effective care for patients with major vascular injury and other vascular emergencies. Not taking action ensures a crisis in the near future that will result in poor outcomes. New education strategies are called for. Combining the maximal education value of a decreasing number of key open cases with appropriate courses that use cadaver and live animal operative experience will partially mitigate this looming deficit of open operative cases. Simulation is a cornerstone of training and maintenance of competence in commercial aviation. Simulation in surgery has yet to achieve its promise to augment real operative experience. However, in the future, it may become an important method for both acquiring and maintaining skills.

SELECTED REFERENCES

Biffl WL, Cothren CC, Moore EE, et al: Western Trauma Association critical decisions in trauma: Screening for and treatment of blunt cerebrovascular injuries. *J Trauma* 67:1150–1153, 2009.

This practice recommendation from the Western Trauma Association offers an evidence-based approach to the diagnosis of blunt cerebrovascular injuries.

Feliciano DV, Mattox KL, Graham JM, et al: Five-year experience with PTFE grafts in vascular wounds. *J Trauma* 25:71–82, 1985.

This is a landmark report establishing the acceptability of PTFE in vascular trauma repairs. It remains the best work in this area.

Gilani R, Tsai PI, Wall MJ, Jr, et al: Overcoming challenges of endovascular treatment of complex subclavian and axillary artery injuries in hypotensive patients. *J Trauma Acute Care Surg* 73:771–773, 2012.

This report of eight patients, the majority of whom were hypotensive from major upper torso injuries, has major ramifications for the ability to use emergency endovascular techniques to control hemorrhage and to repair significant vascular injuries. This approach represents a promising future of a blended open and endovascular approach to vascular injuries.

Mattox KL, Feliciano DV, Burch J, et al: Five thousand seven hundred sixty cardiovascular injuries in 4459 patients. Epidemiologic evolution 1958 to 1987. *Ann Surg* 209:698–705, 1989.

This is the largest epidemiologic study in the literature on civilian vascular injuries, and it remains the best work on the subject.

Neschis DG, Scalea TM, Flinn WR, et al: Blunt aortic injury. *N Engl J Med* 359:1708–1716, 2008.

This review of series of both open and endovascular repairs of blunt thoracic injury provides a valuable overview of the risks versus benefits of each technique.

Patel MB, Guillamondegui OD, May AK, et al: Twenty-year analysis of surgical resident operative trauma experiences. *J Surg Res* 180:191–195, 2013.

This report gives a sobering perspective on the dwindling open surgical experience for surgical residents and highlights the need for alternative training modalities.

Patterson BO, Holt PJ, Cleanthis M, et al: Imaging vascular trauma. *Br J Surg* 99:494–505, 2012.

This systematic review was performed of literature relating to radiologic diagnosis of vascular trauma from 2000 to 2010. This excellent review conclusively established the superiority of CT angiography for the diagnosis of vascular injuries.

Reuben BC, Whitten MG, Sarfati M, et al: Increasing use of endovascular therapy in acute arterial injuries: Analysis of the National Trauma Data Bank. *J Vasc Surg* 46:1222–1226, 2007.

This report was a harbinger of the shift away from open vascular repairs and, from the perspective of 2016, was a predictor of the loss of open surgical experience and skills in the management of vascular injuries.

Sirinek KR, Levine BA, Gaskill HV, 3rd, et al: Reassessment of the role of routine operative exploration in vascular trauma. *J Trauma* 21:339–344, 1981.

This report was the basis for the cessation of operative exploration in stable patients in favor of angiography. In its time, it was a landmark paper and vastly improved the workup of patients with suspected vascular injury.

Stannard A, Eliason JL, Rasmussen TE: Resuscitative endovascular balloon occlusion of the aorta (REBOA) as an adjunct for hemorrhagic shock. *J Trauma* 71:1869–1872, 2011.

This report on the use of REBOA serves as a thorough update on the current practice and points out future directions in the development of this important aid for hemorrhage control.

REFERENCES

1. Amato JJ, Rich NM, Billy LJ, et al: High-velocity arterial injury: A study of the mechanism of injury. *J Trauma* 11:412–416, 1971.
2. Mattox KL, Feliciano DV, Burch J, et al: Five thousand seven hundred sixty vascular injuries in 4459 patients. Epidemiologic evolution 1958 to 1987. *Ann Surg* 209:698–707, 1989.
3. *Prehospital trauma life support*, ed 7, Chicago, 2012, American College of Surgeons.
4. Rich NM: Historic review of arteriovenous fistulas and traumatic false aneurysms. In Rich NM, Mattox KL, Hirshberg A, editors: *Vascular trauma*, Philadelphia, 2004, Elsevier Saunders, pp 457–524.
5. *Advanced trauma life support for doctors*, ed 9, Chicago, 2012, American College of Surgeons.
6. Sise MJ, Shackford SR: Peripheral vascular injury. In Mattox KL, Moore EE, Feliciano DV, editors: *Trauma*, ed 7, New York, 2013, McGraw-Hill, pp 817–847.
7. Patterson BO, Holt PJ, Cleanthis M, et al: Imaging vascular trauma. *Br J Surg* 99:494–505, 2012.
8. Seamon MJ, Smoger D, Torres DM, et al: A prospective validation of a current practice: The detection of extremity vascular injury with CT angiography. *J Trauma* 67:238–244, 2009.
9. White PW, Gillespie DL, Feurstein I, et al: Sixty-four slice multidetector computed tomographic angiography in the evaluation of vascular trauma. *J Trauma* 68:96–102, 2009.
10. O'Gorman RB, Feliciano DV, Bitondo CG, et al: Emergency center arteriography in the evaluation of suspected peripheral vascular injuries. *Arch Surg* 152:323–325, 1984.
11. Sirinek KR, Levine BA, Goskill HV, et al: Reassessment of the role of routine operative exploration in vascular trauma. *J Trauma* 21:339–344, 1981.
12. Dennis JW: Minimal vascular injury. In Rich NM, Mattox KL, Hirshberg A, editors: *Vascular trauma*, ed 2, Philadelphia, 2004, Elsevier Saunders, pp 85–96.
13. Reuben BC, Whitten MG, Sarfati M, et al: Increasing use of endovascular therapy in acute arterial injuries: Analysis of the National Trauma Data Bank. *J Vasc Surg* 46:1222–1226, 2007.
14. Worni M, Scarborough JE, Gandhi M, et al: Use of endovascular therapy for peripheral arterial lesions: An analysis of the National Trauma Data Bank from 2007 to 2009. *Ann Vasc Surg* 27:299–305, 2013.
15. Cothren CC, Moore EE, Ray CE, Jr, et al: Carotid artery stents for blunt cerebrovascular injury: Risks exceed benefits. *Arch Surg* 140:480–486, 2005.
16. Patel MB, Guillamondegui OD, May AK, et al: Twenty-year analysis of surgical resident operative trauma experiences. *J Surg Res* 180:191–195, 2013.
17. Schanzer A, Steppacher R, Eslami MH, et al: Vascular surgery training trends from 2001-2007: A substantial increase in total procedure volume is driven by escalating endovascular procedure volume and stable open procedure volume. *Vasc Surg* 49:1330–1344, 2009.
18. Richardson JD, Franklin GA, Lukan JK, et al: Evolution in the management of hepatic trauma: A 25 year perspective. *Ann Surg* 232:324–330, 2000.
19. Dent D, Alsabrook G, Erikson BA, et al: Blunt splenic injuries: High non-operative management rate can be achieved with selective embolization. *J Trauma* 56:1063–1067, 2004.
20. Martinelli T, Thony F, Decléty P, et al: Intra-aortic balloon occlusion to salvage patients with life-threatening hemorrhagic shocks from pelvic fractures. *J Trauma* 68:942–948, 2010.
21. Stannard A, Eliason JL, Rasmussen TE: Resuscitative endovascular balloon occlusion of the aorta (REBOA) as an adjunct for hemorrhagic shock. *J Trauma Acute Care Surg* 71:1869–1872, 2011.
22. Velmahos GC: Pelvis. In Mattox KL, Moore EE, Feliciano DV, editors: *Trauma*, ed 7, New York, 2013, McGraw-Hill, pp 655–668.
23. Mattox KL, Whigham C, Fisher RG, et al: Blunt trauma to the thoracic aorta: Current challenges. In Lumsden AB, Lin PH, Chen C, et al, editors: *Advanced endovascular therapy of aortic disease*, London, 2007, Blackwell Publishing, pp 127–133.
24. Demetriades D, Velmahos GC, Scalea TM, et al; American Association for the Surgery of Trauma Thoracic Aortic Injury Study Group: Operative repair or endovascular stent graft in blunt traumatic thoracic aortic injuries: Results of an

American Association for the Surgery of Trauma Multicenter Study. *J Trauma* 64:561–570, 2008.
25. Neschis DG, Scalea TM, Flinn WR, et al: Blunt aortic injury. *N Engl J Med* 359:1708–1716, 2008.
26. Cothren CC, Biffl WL, Moore EE, et al: Treatment for blunt cerebrovascular injuries: Equivalence of anticoagulation and antiplatelet agents. *Arch Surg* 144:685–690, 2009.
27. Biffl WL, Cothren CC, Moore EE, et al: Western Trauma Association critical decisions in trauma: Screening for and treatment of blunt cerebrovascular injuries. *J Trauma* 67:1150–1153, 2009.
28. DuBose J, Recinos G, Teixeira PG, et al: Endovascular stenting for the treatment of traumatic internal carotid injuries: Expanding experience. *J Trauma* 65:1561–1566, 2008.
29. Shackford SR, Kahl JE, Calvo RY, et al: Limb salvage after complex repairs of extremity arterial injuries is independent of surgical specialty training. *J Trauma Acute Care Surg* 74:716–724, 2013.
30. Wall MJ, Tsai P, Mattox KL: Heart and thoracic vascular injuries. In Mattox KL, Moore EE, Feliciano DV, editors: *Trauma*, ed 7, New York, 2013, McGraw-Hill, pp 485–511.
31. Dente CJ, Feliciano DV: Abdominal vascular injury. In Mattox KL, Moore EE, Feliciano DV, editors: *Trauma*, ed 7, New York, 2013, McGraw-Hill, pp 633–654.
32. Ding W, Wu X, Li J: Temporary intravascular shunts used as a damage control surgery adjunct in complex vascular injury: Collective review. *Injury* 39:970–977, 2008.
33. Subramanian A, Vercruysse G, Dente C, et al: A decade's experience with temporary intravascular shunts at a civilian level I trauma center. *J Trauma* 65:316–324, 2008.
34. Rich NM, Hughes CW: The fate of prosthetic material used to repair vascular injuries in contaminated wounds. *J Trauma* 12:459–467, 1972.
35. Feliciano DV, Mattox KL, Graham JM, et al: Five-year experience with PTFE grafts in vascular wounds. *J Trauma* 25:71–82, 1985.
36. Kim JY, Buck DW, Forte AJ, et al: Risk factors for compartment syndrome in traumatic brachial artery injuries: An institutional experience in 139 patients. *J Trauma* 67:1339–1344, 2009.
37. Branco BC, Inaba K, Barmparas G, et al: Incidence and predictors for the need for fasciotomy after extremity trauma: A 10-year review in a mature level I trauma center. *Injury* 42:1157–1163, 2011.
38. Ly TV, Travison TG, Castillo RC, et al: Ability of lower-extremity injury severity scores to predict functional outcome after limb salvage. *J Bone Joint Surg Am* 90:1738–1743, 2008.
39. Busse JW, Jacobs CL, Swiontkowski MF, et al: Complex limb salvage or early amputation for severe lower-limb injury: A meta-analysis of observational studies. *J Orthop Trauma* 21:70–76, 2007.
40. Dekker S: *The field guide to understanding human error*, Hampshire, UK, 2006, Ashgate Publishing Ltd.
41. Feliciano DV, Vercruysse GA: Neck. In Mattox KL, Moore EE, Feliciano DV, editors: *Trauma*, ed 7, New York, 2013, McGraw-Hill, pp 414–442.
42. Du Toit DF, Lambrechts AV, Stark H, et al: Long-term results of stent graft treatment of subclavian artery injuries: Management of choice for stable patients? *J Vasc Surg* 47:739–743, 2008.
43. Gilani R, Tsai P, Wall MJ: Overcoming challenges of endovascular treatment of complex subclavian and axillary artery injuries in hypotensive patients. *J Trauma Acute Care Surg* 73:771–773, 2012.
44. Carrick MM, Morrison CA, Pham HQ: Modern management of traumatic subclavian artery injuries: A single institution's experience in the evolution of endovascular repair. *Am J Surg* 199:28–34, 2010.
45. Cooper JD: The history of surgical procedures for emphysema. *Ann Thorac Surg* 63:312–319, 1997.
46. Franz RW, Goodwin RB, Hartman JF, et al: Management of upper extremity arterial injuries at an urban level I trauma center. *Ann Vasc Surg* 23:8–16, 2009.
47. Franz RW, Shah KJ, Halaharvi D, et al: A 5-year review of management of lower extremity arterial injuries at an urban level I trauma center. *J Vasc Surg* 53:1604–1610, 2011.
48. Keir J: Changes in caseload and the potential impact on surgical training: A retrospective review of one hospital's experience. *BMC Med Ed* 6:6–10, 2006.
49. Kairys JC, McGuire K, Crawford AG, et al: Cumulative operative experience is decreasing during general surgery residency: A worrisome trend for surgical trainees? *J Am Coll Surg* 206:804–811, 2008.
50. Grabo DJ, DiMuzio PJ, Kairys JC, et al: Have endovascular procedures negatively impacted general surgery training? *Semin Vasc Surg* 19:168–171, 2006.

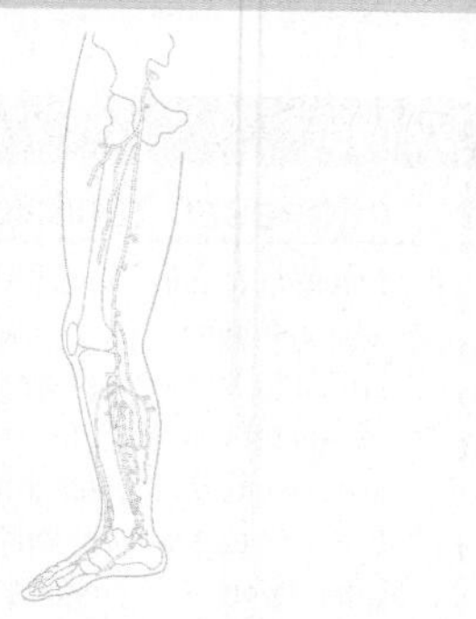

CHAPTER 64

Venous Disease

Julie A. Freischlag, Jennifer A. Heller

OUTLINE

Please access ExpertConsult.com to view the corresponding videos for this chapter.

An understanding of venous physiology provides the surgeon with valuable information with which to formulate a diagnostic and treatment plan. Technologic advances have broadened the therapeutic armamentarium. This chapter provides the reader with a thorough overview of the physiology and pathophysiology of the venous system. Pathognomonic features of superficial and deep venous disorders are described with discussion of appropriate diagnostic modalities and therapeutic interventions.

ANATOMY

To determine whether a pathophysiologic process is present, knowledge of venous anatomy is essential. Venous drainage of the legs is the function of two parallel and associated units, the deep and superficial veins. A third system, the perforating veins, interconnects the superficial and deep veins. The nomenclature of the venous system of the lower limb was revised in 2002, and the most relevant changes are addressed here.[1] The revised nomenclature is delineated in Tables 64-1 and 64-2.

Superficial Venous System

The superficial veins of the lower extremity form a network that connects the superficial dorsal veins of the foot and deep plantar veins. The dorsal venous arch, into which empty the dorsal metatarsal veins, is continuous with the great saphenous vein medially and the small saphenous vein laterally (Fig. 64-1).

The great saphenous vein arises from dorsal veins of the foot. The great saphenous vein extends cephalad and travels over the medial aspect of the tibia and in parallel to the saphenous nerve. As the great saphenous vein ascends through the thigh, multiple accessory branches are demonstrated, and variability of the number and location of these branches is the norm. The great saphenous vein travels within its own fascia, called the saphenous sheath. This structure is superior to the deep fascia of the leg. Although a classic feature, the great saphenous vein can be contained completely within the saphenous sheath or exit the fascia and reenter at another point in its course along the extremity. In some cases, patients exhibit an incomplete saphenous sheath, which makes identification of the great saphenous vein difficult. The great saphenous vein terminates into the saphenofemoral junction, where it is joined by the confluence of the superficial circumflex iliac veins, the external pudendal veins, and the superficial epigastric veins. It then ascends in the superficial compartment and empties into the common femoral vein after entering the fossa ovalis (Fig. 64-2).

The small saphenous vein arises from the dorsal venous arch at the lateral aspect of the foot and ascends posterior to the lateral malleolus, rising cephalad in the midposterior calf. The small saphenous vein continues to ascend, penetrates the superficial fascia of the calf, and then terminates into the popliteal vein. However, this anatomy is extremely variable. Most commonly, the small saphenous vein terminates within a lateral branch of the thigh, bypassing the classic saphenopopliteal junction. The sural nerve lies parallel to the small saphenous vein. This relationship becomes more intimate at the distal calf. A common vein branch, the vein of Giacomini, connects the small saphenous vein with the great saphenous vein.

Deep Venous System

The plantar digital veins in the foot empty into a network of metatarsal veins that compose the deep plantar venous arch. This continues into the medial and lateral plantar veins, which then drain into the posterior tibial veins. The dorsalis pedis veins on the dorsum of the foot form the paired anterior tibial veins at the ankle.

The paired posterior tibial veins, adjacent to and flanking the posterior tibial artery, run under the fascia of the deep posterior compartment. These veins enter the soleus and join the popliteal vein, after joining with the paired peroneal and anterior tibial veins. There are large venous sinuses within the soleus muscle—soleal sinuses—that empty into the posterior tibial and peroneal veins. Bilateral gastrocnemius veins empty into the popliteal vein distal to the point of entry of the small saphenous vein into the popliteal vein.

TABLE 64-1 Superficial Veins

ANATOMIC TERMINOLOGY	PROPOSED TERMINOLOGY
Greater or long saphenous vein	Great saphenous vein
	Superficial inguinal veins
External pudendal vein	External pudendal vein
Superficial circumflex vein	Superficial circumflex iliac vein
Superficial epigastric vein	Superficial epigastric vein
Superficial dorsal vein of clitoris or penis	Superficial dorsal vein of clitoris or penis
Anterior labial veins	Anterior labial veins
Anterior scrotal veins	Anterior scrotal veins
Accessory saphenous vein	Anterior accessory great saphenous vein
	Posterior accessory great saphenous vein
	Superficial accessory great saphenous vein
Smaller or short saphenous vein	Small saphenous vein
	Cranial extension of small saphenous vein
	Superficial accessory small saphenous vein
	Anterior thigh circumflex vein
	Posterior thigh circumflex vein
	Intersaphenous veins
	Lateral venous system
Dorsal venous network of the foot	Dorsal venous network of the foot
Dorsal venous arch of the foot	Dorsal venous arch of the foot
Dorsal metatarsal veins	Superficial metatarsal veins (dorsal and plantar)
Plantar venous network	Plantar venous subcutaneous network
Plantar venous arch	
Plantar metatarsal veins	Superficial digital veins (dorsal and plantar)
Lateral marginal vein	Lateral marginal vein
Medial marginal vein	Medial marginal vein

TABLE 64-2 Deep Veins

ANATOMIC TERMINOLOGY	PROPOSED TERMINOLOGY
Femoral vein	Common femoral vein
	Femoral vein
Profunda femoris vein or deep vein of thigh	Profunda femoris vein or deep femoral vein
Medial circumflex femoral vein	Medial circumflex femoral vein
Lateral circumflex femoral vein	Lateral circumflex femoral vein
Perforating veins	Deep femoral communicating veins (accompanying veins of perforating arteries)
	Sciatic vein
Popliteal vein	Popliteal vein
	Sural veins
	Soleal veins
	Gastrocnemius veins
	Medial gastrocnemius veins
	Lateral gastrocnemius veins
	Intergemellar vein
Genicular veins	Genicular venous plexus
Anterior tibial veins	Anterior tibial veins
Posterior tibial veins	Posterior tibial veins
Fibular or peroneal veins	Fibular or peroneal veins
	Medial plantar veins
	Lateral plantar veins
	Deep plantar venous arch
	Deep metatarsal veins (plantar and dorsal)
	Deep digital veins (plantar and dorsal)
	Pedal vein

The popliteal vein enters a window in the adductor magnus, at which point it is termed the femoral vein, previously known as the superficial femoral vein. The femoral vein ascends and receives venous drainage from the profunda femoris vein, or deep femoral vein, and after this confluence, it is the common femoral vein. As the common femoral vein crosses the inguinal ligament, it becomes the external iliac vein.

Venous System Perforators

Perforating veins connect the superficial venous system to the deep venous system by penetrating the fascial layers of the lower extremity. These perforators run in a perpendicular fashion to the axial veins previously described. Although the total number of perforator veins is variable, up to 100 have been documented. The perforators enter at various points in the leg—the foot, medial and lateral calf, and mid and distal thigh (Fig. 64-3). Some have been named by the surgeons who first identified them: Crockett perforators, which connect the posterior arch and posterior tibial veins; Boyd perforators, which connect the great saphenous and gastrocnemius veins; and hunterian and Dodd perforators, which connect the great saphenous and superficial femoral veins. The perforator veins have an important function. Their valve system aids in preventing reflux from the deep to the superficial system, particularly during periods of standing and ambulation.

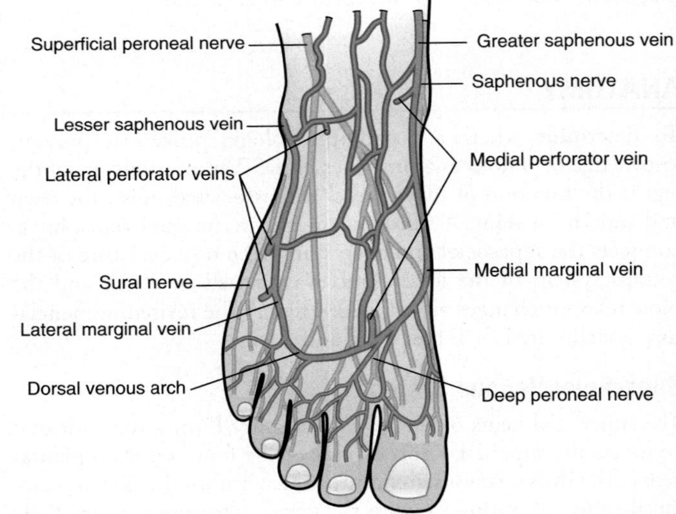

FIGURE 64-1 Venous drainage of the foot.

Normal Venous Histology and Function

The venous wall is composed of three layers, the intima, media, and adventitia. Vein walls have less smooth muscle and elastin

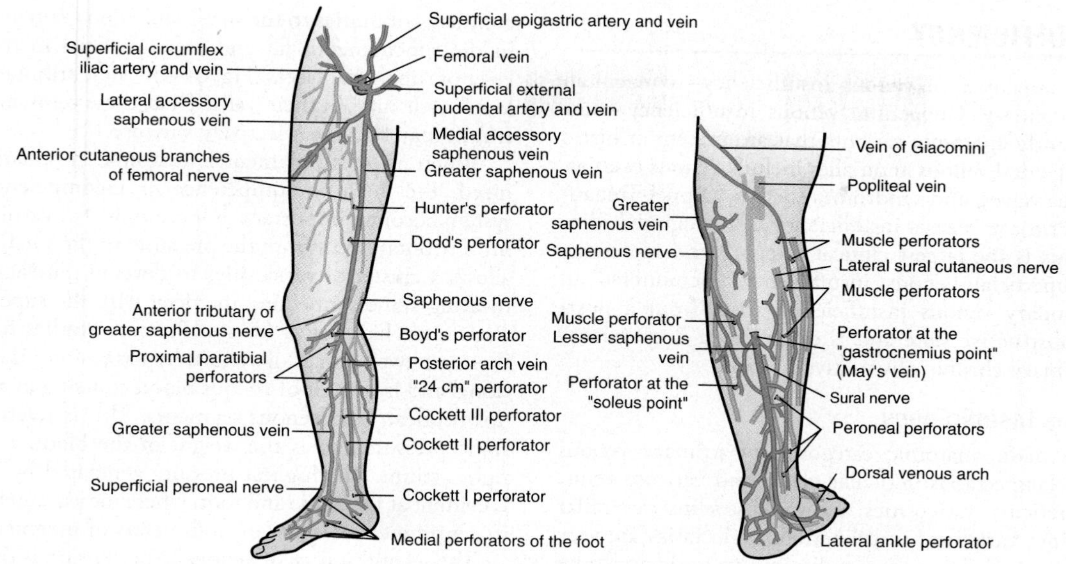

FIGURE 64-2 Venous drainage of the lower limb.

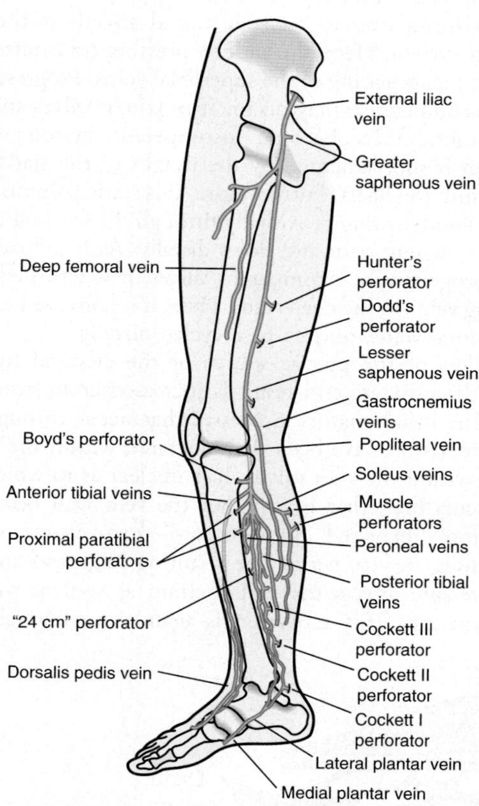

FIGURE 64-3 Perforating veins of the lower limb.

than their arterial counterparts. The venous intima has an endothelial cell layer resting on a basement membrane. The media is composed of smooth muscle cells and elastin connective tissue. The adventitia of the venous wall contains adrenergic fibers, particularly in the cutaneous veins. Central sympathetic discharge and brainstem thermoregulatory centers can alter venous tone, as can other stimuli, such as temperature changes, pain, emotional stimuli, and volume changes.

The histologic features of veins vary, depending on the caliber of the veins. The venules, the smallest veins, range from 0.1 to 1 mm and contain mostly smooth muscle cells, whereas the larger extremity veins contain relatively few smooth muscle cells. These larger caliber veins have limited contractile capacity in comparison to the thicker walled great saphenous vein. The venous valves prevent retrograde flow; it is their failure or valvular incompetence that leads to reflux and its associated symptoms. Venous valves are most prevalent in the distal lower extremity, whereas as one proceeds proximally, the number of valves decreases to the point that no valves are present in the superior vena cava and inferior vena cava (IVC).

Most of the capacitance of the vascular tree is in the venous system. Because veins do not have significant amounts of elastin, veins can withstand large volume shifts with comparatively small changes in pressure. A vein has a normal elliptical configuration until the limit of its capacitance is reached, at which point the vein assumes a round configuration.

The calf muscles augment venous return by functioning as a pump. In the supine state, the resting venous pressure in the foot is the sum of the residual kinetic energy minus the resistance in the arterioles and precapillary sphincters. Thus, a pressure gradient is generated to the right atrium of approximately 10 to 12 mm Hg. In the upright position, the resting venous pressure of the foot is a reflection of the hydrostatic pressure from the upright column of blood extending from the right atrium to the foot.

The return of the blood to the heart from the lower extremity is facilitated by the muscle pump function of the calf, a mechanism whereby the calf muscle, functioning as a bellows during exercise, compresses the gastrocnemius and soleal sinuses and propels the blood toward the heart. The normally functioning valves in the venous system prevent retrograde flow; when one or more of these valves become incompetent, symptoms of venous insufficiency can develop. During calf muscle contraction, the venous pressure of the foot and ankle drops dramatically. The pressures developing in the muscle compartments during exercise range from 150 to 200 mm Hg, and when there is failure of perforating veins, these high pressures are transmitted to the superficial system.

VENOUS INSUFFICIENCY

There are three categories of venous insufficiency—congenital, primary, and secondary. Congenital venous insufficiency comprises predominantly anatomic variants that are present at birth. Examples of congenital venous anomalies include venous ectasias, absence of venous valves, and syndromes such as Klippel-Trénaunay syndrome. Primary venous insufficiency is an acquired idiopathic entity. This is the largest clinical category and represents most of the superficial venous insufficiency encountered in the office. Secondary venous insufficiency arises from a postthrombotic or obstructive state and is caused by a deep venous thrombus or primary chronic obstructive process.

Primary Venous Insufficiency

There are three main anatomic categories of primary venous insufficiency—telangiectasias, reticular veins, and varicose veins. Telangiectasias, reticular varicosities, and varicose veins are similar but exhibit distinct variations in caliber. Telangiectasias are very small intradermal venules that are too diminutive to demonstrate reflux. These structures measure less than 3 mm. Without associated symptoms and stigmata of other venous disease, they are idiopathic in nature and are not medically necessary to treat. However, although not of concern from a venous standpoint, leg telangiectasias of multiple causes may be a manifestation of a systemic disease. Some of these disorders include autoimmune diseases (such as lupus erythematosus and dermatomyositis), exogenous causes, and xeroderma pigmentosum. Reticular veins are vein branches that enter the tributaries of the main axial, perforating, or deep veins. The axial veins, the great and small saphenous veins, represent the largest caliber veins of the superficial venous system.

Pathology

The precise pathophysiologic mechanism of venous insufficiency has yet to be elucidated. This describes some of the areas in which research has started to reveal its multifactorial pathogenesis.

Mechanical abnormalities. Anatomic differences in the location of the superficial veins of the lower extremities may contribute to the pathogenesis. Primary venous insufficiency may involve both the axial veins (great and small saphenous), either vein, or neither vein. Perforating veins may be the sole source of venous pathophysiologic changes, perhaps because the great saphenous vein is supported by a well-developed medial fibromuscular layer and fibrous connective tissue that bind it to the deep fascia. In contrast, tributaries to the small saphenous vein are less supported in the subcutaneous fat and are superficial to the membranous layer of superficial fascia (Fig. 64-4). These tributaries also contain less muscle mass in their walls. Thus, these veins, and not the main trunk, may become selectively varicose.

When these fundamental anatomic peculiarities are recognized, the intrinsic competence or incompetence of the valve system becomes important. For example, failure of a valve protecting a tributary vein from the pressures of the small saphenous vein allows a cluster of varicosities to develop. Furthermore, communicating veins connecting the deep with the superficial compartment may have valve failure. Pressure studies have shown that there are two sources of venous hypertension. The first is gravitational and is a result of venous blood coursing in a distal direction down linear axial venous segments. This is referred to as hydrostatic pressure and is the weight of the blood column from the right atrium. The highest pressure generated by this mechanism is evident at the ankle and foot, where measurements are expressed in centimeters of water or millimeters of mercury.

The second source of venous hypertension is dynamic. It is the force of muscle contraction, usually contained within the compartments of the leg. If a perforating vein fails, high pressures (range, 150 to 200 mm Hg) developed within the muscular compartments during exercise are transmitted directly to the superficial venous system. Here, the sudden pressure transmitted causes dilation and lengthening of the superficial veins. Progressive distal valvular incompetence may occur. If proximal valves such as the saphenofemoral valve become incompetent, systolic muscular contraction is supplemented by the weight of the static column of blood from the heart. Furthermore, this static column becomes a barrier. Blood flowing proximally through the femoral vein spills into the saphenous vein and flows distally. As it refluxes distally through progressively incompetent valves, it is returned through perforating veins to the deep veins. Here, it is conveyed once again to the femoral veins, only to be recycled distally.

Regardless of the precise source of the elevated hydrostatic pressure, the ultimate end result is increased ambulatory hypertension. The inflammatory processes that occur throughout the venous circulation have been demonstrated within the vein wall as well as within the vein valves. It is unclear as to which abnormality occurs first, that is, whether the vein wall becomes distended from increased pressure and then causes vein wall abnormalities, or vice versa. The resulting increased ambulatory venous pressure affects the endothelium as well as the venous microcirculation. This activation is again caused by changes in

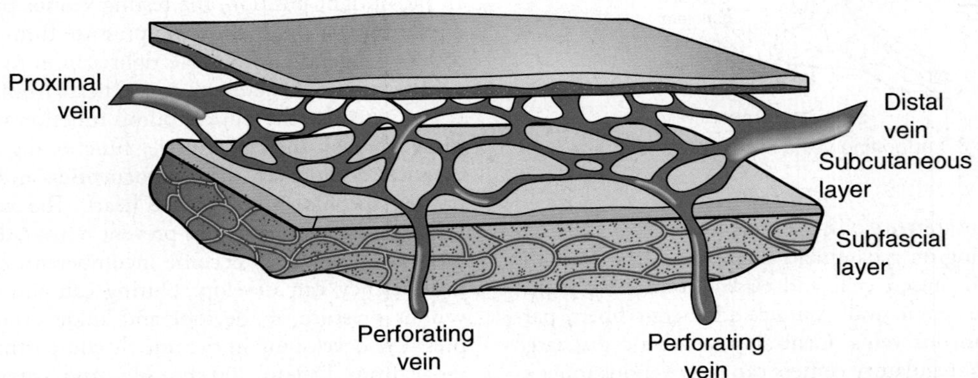

FIGURE 64-4 Dilation of superficial venous tributaries caused by increased transmission of pressure by the perforating veins.

shear stress and mechanical stress of the vein wall and vein valves. Altered shear stress causes the endothelial cells to release a variety of agents, including chemokines and inflammatory molecules, which precipitates the inflammatory cascade. In particular, cytokines and metalloproteinases play a prominent role in the mechanical and inflammatory process of venous hypertension. The inflammatory process involves many different pathways that result in elevations of inflammatory modulators and cytokines, growth factors, and metalloproteinase activity.[2] Fundamental defects in the strength and characteristics of the venous wall have been identified. Varicose vein walls demonstrate decreased amounts of elastin and collagen, suggesting a contributing role toward venous pathophysiology.[3]

Risk Factors

Risk factors for the development of varicose veins include advancing age, female gender, multiparity, heredity, and history of trauma to the extremity. Additional risk factors include obesity and a positive family history. Advancing age appears to be the most significant risk factor. Venous function is undoubtedly influenced by hormonal changes. In particular, progesterone liberated by the corpus luteum stabilizes the uterus by causing the relaxation of smooth muscle fibers.[4] This directly influences venous function. The result is passive venous dilation, which in many cases causes valvular dysfunction. Although progesterone is implicated in the first appearance of varicosities in pregnancy, estrogen also has profound effects. It produces the relaxation of smooth muscle and a softening of collagen fibers. Furthermore, the estrogen-to-progesterone ratio influences venous distensibility. This ratio may explain the predominance of venous insufficiency symptoms on the first day of a menstrual period, when a profound shift occurs from the progesterone phase of the menstrual cycle to the estrogen phase. Autosomal dominant penetrance has been identified as the underlying genetic risk factor for subsequent development of varicose veins.

Symptoms

Venous valvular dysfunction causes venous hypertension, and as such, patients' symptoms are attributed to excess venous pooling. The patient with symptomatic varicose veins commonly reports heaviness, discomfort, and extremity fatigue. The pain is characteristically dull, does not usually occur during recumbency or early in the morning, and is exacerbated in the afternoon, especially after periods of prolonged standing. Swelling is commonly described. The discomforts of aching, heaviness, and fatigue are usually relieved by leg elevation or elastic support. Cutaneous burning, termed venous neuropathy, can also occur in patients with advanced venous insufficiency. Pruritus occurs from excess hemosiderin deposition and tends to be located at the distal calf or in areas of phlebitic varicose branch segments. Patients may report cramping pain that occurs during or after exercise and is relieved with rest and leg elevation. This syndrome is termed venous claudication and is a clinical manifestation of venous outflow obstruction, secondary venous insufficiency. Predominant causes of venous claudication include a prior deep venous thrombosis (DVT) and May-Thurner syndrome.

Multiparous female patients in their childbearing years may report a constellation of symptoms that involve varicosities of the leg in conjunction with chronic pelvic pain. The lower extremity symptoms may or may not be present. Additional symptoms include a feeling of bladder fullness with standing, dyspareunia, and chronic pelvic pain. This clinical picture suggests pelvic congestion syndrome. As the differential diagnosis for pelvic pain is extensive, the diagnosis of pelvic venous congestion tends to be one of exclusion; diagnostic modalities to confirm its presence include magnetic resonance venous imaging (MRVI) of the pelvis and conventional pelvic venography, which can be both diagnostic and therapeutic.

Physical Examination

A comprehensive examination includes assessment of the arterial circulation. Briefly, palpation of the femoral, popliteal, dorsalis pedis, and posterior tibialis pulses is performed. Nonpalpable pulses necessitate further evaluation. Auscultation of pulse flow is indicated when a thrill or widened pulse is appreciated. Decreased hair, dependent rubor, pallor on elevation, and tissue loss are all indicative of advanced arterial ischemia.

The venous examination includes assessment of the patient in the standing and supine positions. The examination room must be well lighted and warm so that vasospasm does not occur, limiting a comprehensive evaluation. Standing increases venous hypertension and dilates veins, thereby facilitating examination. Patients with superficial axial incompetence commonly exhibit palpable great saphenous veins (Fig. 64-5).

Visual inspection is critical. Location of varicosities can commonly identify a "blown valve" or the axial vein from which the varicosities developed. For example, medial thigh varicose veins are likely to develop from an incompetent great saphenous vein, whereas posterior calf or lateral calf varicose veins tend to originate from the small saphenous vein. In addition, the location of varicose veins can be a diagnostic predictor of a larger process. Varicosities of the scrotum can be associated with gonadal vein incompetence, otherwise termed the nutcracker syndrome (compression of the left renal vein between the aorta and the superior mesenteric artery). Perineal or vulvar varicosities can be a sign of ovarian or pelvic venous insufficiency, or iliac vein obstruction.

The physical examination can provide the physician with important information on the history of the venous disease that the patient might have neglected or forgotten to mention during

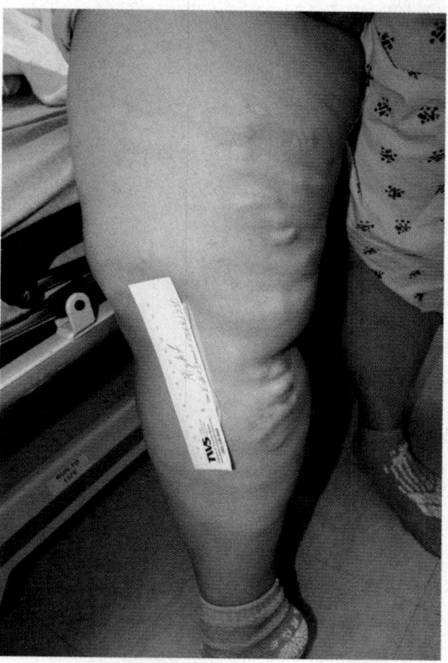

FIGURE 64-5 Varicose veins.

the history. For example, signs of a chronic or resolved thrombophlebitis may include a partially thrombosed varicosity; a brownish discoloration around a varicosity or along a palpable segment of the axial veins, consistent with hemosiderin deposition; and palpable segments of axial vein, suggesting partially or completely occluded axial vein segments.

Signs of advanced venous insufficiency include hyperpigmentation in the distal calf or gaiter distribution, secondary to hemosiderin deposition, and lipodermatosclerosis. Lipodermatosclerosis develops over time because of prolonged ambulatory venous hypertension and chronic inflammation. Physical examination findings that reflect lipodermatosclerosis are brawny edema of the distal calf, "champagne bottle leg," fibrotic and hypertrophic skin, and hyperpigmentation. Advanced lipodermatosclerosis may involve fibrosis of the Achilles tendon, impairing motor function of the extremity. Therefore, examination should include motor function at the ankle. Atrophie blanche is an area of pale hue, visualized around the medial malleolus; it is commonly mistaken for a healed ulcer because of its lighter pigmentation (Fig. 64-6). Corona phlebectatica is a term used to describe an accumulation of tiny telangiectasias or venous flare, usually located at the medial malleolus or the dorsum of the foot. Skin changes from chronic venous insufficiency (CVI) can mimic other dermatologic phenomena; both dermatitis and eczematous changes can be seen from venous disease.

Venous stasis ulcers exhibit pathognomonic features that distinguish them from their arterial or neuropathic counterparts. Venous ulcers are not generally painful and appear at the medial malleolus, not in the mid to distal foot. Lack of arterial pulses in patients with a venous ulcer is unusual.

Venous stasis dermatitis is visualized at the distal ankle and can mimic eczema or dermatitis of another cause. It is this important attention to supporting features of the physical examination and history as well as confirmation with duplex reflux examination that will distinguish advanced venous stasis disease from dermatologic conditions.

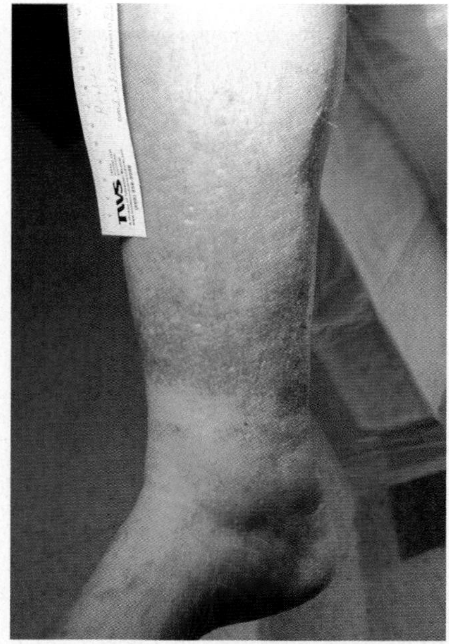

FIGURE 64-6 Lipodermatosclerosis, atrophie blanche, and brawny edema.

Diagnostic Evaluation of Venous Dysfunction

The Perthes test for deep venous occlusion and the Brodie-Trendelenburg test of axial reflux have been replaced by in-office use of the continuous-wave, hand-held Doppler instrument supplemented by duplex ultrasound evaluation. The hand-held Doppler instrument can confirm an impression of saphenous reflux, which in turn dictates the operative procedure to be performed in a given patient. A common misconception is the belief that the Doppler instrument is used to locate perforating veins. Instead, it is used in specific locations to determine incompetent valves, for example, the hand-held, continuous-wave, 8-MHz flow detector placed over the great and small saphenous veins near their terminations. With distal augmentation of flow and release, normal deep breathing, and performance of a Valsalva maneuver, valve reflux is accurately identified. Formerly, the Doppler examination was supplemented by other objective studies, including photoplethysmography, mercury strain-gauge plethysmography, and photorheography. These are no longer in common use.

Another instrument reintroduced to assess physiologic function of the muscle pump and venous valves is air displacement plethysmography.[5] Its use was discontinued after the 1960s because of its cumbersome nature. Computer technology has now allowed its reintroduction, as championed by Christopoulos and colleagues.[6] It consists of an air chamber that surrounds the leg from knee to ankle. During calibration, leg veins are emptied by leg elevation, and the patient is then asked to stand so that leg venous volume can be quantitated and the time for filling recorded. The filling rate is then expressed in milliliters per second, thus giving readings similar to those obtained with the mercury strain-gauge technique.

Today, duplex imaging is the first and best modality to assess for the normal function and presence of venous insufficiency of the lower extremities. Duplex technology more precisely defines which veins are refluxing by imaging the superficial and deep veins. The duplex examination is commonly done with the patient supine, but this yields an erroneous evaluation of reflux. In the supine position, even when no flow is present, the valves remain open. Valve closure requires a reversal of flow with a pressure gradient that is higher proximally than distally. Thus, the duplex examination needs to be done with the patient standing or in the markedly trunk-elevated position.[7]

There are many advantages of ultrasound imaging. The ultrasound examination is noninvasive, requires no contrast material, and can be performed in the office as well as in the hospital. Drawbacks to the modality include interobserver variability and limitations in imaging in patients with an elevated body mass index and extensive dressings. Imaging is obtained with a 7.5- or 10-MHz probe; the pulsed Doppler consists of a 3.0-MHz probe. The examination begins with the probe placed longitudinally on the groin. First, all of the deep veins are examined. Next, the superficial veins are evaluated. There are four basic components of the examination that should be included to complete a comprehensive venous evaluation of the lower extremity veins: compressibility, venous flow, augmentation after reflux, and visibility. Reflux can be demonstrated with the patient performing a Valsalva maneuver or by manual compression and release of the extremity distal to the point of the examination. A Valsalva maneuver is performed for the proximal extremity, that is, the thigh and groin, whereas compression is used for the calf. Reflux times of 500 milliseconds or longer are considered significant. Perforator veins can be visualized well with the duplex examination. Significant perforator reflux is defined as a diameter of more than 3.5 mm and a reflux time of 500 milliseconds or longer. Demonstration on duplex images of to-and-fro flow, with the presence of dilated segments, constitutes findings compatible with a refluxing perforator. In addition, Doppler studies can provide the clinician with information about the deep system. Widespread use of duplex scanning has allowed a comparison of findings between standard clinical examinations and duplex Doppler studies.[8,9]

Phlebography and venography. In general, phlebography is unnecessary in the diagnosis and treatment of primary venous insufficiency. In cases of secondary CVI, phlebography has specific usefulness. Ascending phlebography is performed by injection of contrast material into a superficial pedal vein after a tourniquet is applied at the ankle to prevent flow into the superficial venous system. Observation of flow defines anatomy and regions of thrombus or obstruction. Therefore, ascending phlebology differentiates primary from secondary venous insufficiency. Descending phlebography is performed with retrograde injection of contrast material into the deep venous system at the groin or popliteal fossa (femoral vein or popliteal vein). This diagnostic modality identifies specific valvular incompetence suspected on B-mode scanning and clinical examination. These studies are performed only as preoperative adjuncts when deep venous reconstruction is being planned.

Magnetic resonance venous imaging. MRVI is a diagnostic imaging modality reserved for evaluation of the abdominal and pelvic venous vasculature. MRVI, unlike venography, is noninvasive and does not require intravenous (IV) administration of contrast material. Studies have documented similar rates of specificity and sensitivity compared with venography. MRVI is used to evaluate pelvic venous outflow obstruction, providing information from the IVC through the iliac venous system. Furthermore, it is an excellent test to evaluate for pelvic congestion syndrome. In some institutions, the computed tomography scan has applications that can be used similar to the MRVI scan.

Classification Systems

In 1994, the American Venous Forum devised the CEAP classification system, which is a scoring system that stratifies venous disease on the basis of clinical presentation, etiology, anatomy, and pathophysiology (Table 64-3). It is useful in helping the physician assess a limb afflicted with venous insufficiency and then arrive at an appropriate treatment plan. A revised CEAP classification was introduced in 2004 that included a Venous Disability Score to document a patient's ability to perform activities of daily living.[10] Although the CEAP classification is a valuable tool to grade venous disease, assessment of outcomes after intervention cannot be realized. As a result, two additional scoring systems, the Venous Clinical Severity Score and the Venous Segmental Disease Score, enhance the CEAP score with the increased ability to plot outcome. These three classification modalities now provide clinical researchers with invaluable tools to study treatment outcomes.[11]

Treatment of Superficial Venous Insufficiency

Nonoperative management. Symptoms of primary venous insufficiency are manifestations of valvular incompetence. Therefore, the objective of conservative management is to improve the symptoms caused by venous hypertension. The first measure is external compression using elastic hose, 20 to 30 mm Hg, to be worn during the daytime hours. Although the exact mechanism whereby compression is of benefit is not entirely known, a number of physiologic alterations have been observed with compression. These include reduction in ambulatory venous pressure, improvement in skin microcirculation, and increase in subcutaneous pressure, which counters transcapillary fluid leakage. Patients are instructed to wear the hose during the day only, but to put the stockings on as soon as the day begins; swelling with standing will make stocking placement difficult. Care must be taken with patients who have concomitant arterial insufficiency because the compression stockings may exacerbate arterial outflow to the foot. Therefore, these patients require less compression—in some cases, no compression whatsoever—depending on the severity of the arterial disease. In general, an ankle-brachial index of less than 0.7 contraindicates the use of 20 to 30 mm Hg compression stockings.

The second part of conservative therapy is to practice lower extremity elevation for two brief periods during the day, instructing the patient that the feet must be above the level of the heart, or "toes above the nose." With good compliance, these measures may ameliorate symptoms so that patients may not require further intervention. Third, patients are encouraged to participate in activities that activate the calf musculovenous pump, thereby decreasing ambulatory venous hypertension. These activities include frequent ambulation and exercise.

Patients who exhibit venous stasis ulceration will require local wound care (Fig. 64-7). A triple-layer compression dressing, with a zinc oxide paste gauze wrap in contact with the skin, is used most commonly, from the base of the toes to the anterior tibial tubercle with snug graded compression. This is an example of what is generally known as an Unna boot. A 15-year review of 998 patients with one or more venous ulcers treated with a similar compression bandage demonstrated that 73% of the ulcers healed in patients who returned for care (Fig. 64-8). The median time to healing for individual ulcers was 9 weeks. In general, snug, graded-pressure, triple-layer compression dressings result in more rapid healing than with compression stockings alone.

For most patients, well-applied, sustained compression therapy offers the most cost-effective and efficacious therapy in the healing of venous ulcers. After healing, most cases of CVI are controlled with elastic compression stockings to be worn during waking hours. On occasion, older patients and those with arthritic conditions cannot apply the compression stocking required, and control must be maintained by triple-layer zinc oxide compression dressings, which can usually be left in place and changed once a week. In addition to compression, wound care, and surgery, large chronic venous ulcers may benefit from venoactive medications, in particular, pentoxifylline and micronized purified flavonoid fraction.

Indications for interventional treatment are symptoms refractory to conservative therapy, recurrent superficial thrombophlebitis, variceal bleeding, and venous stasis ulceration. After clinical and objective criteria have established the presence of symptomatic varicose veins, the next step is to plan a course of therapy.

The efficacy of conservative versus surgical treatment for varicose veins was studied in the Randomised Clinical Trial, Observational Study and Assessment of Cost-Effectiveness of the Treatment of Varicose veins (REACTIV) trial. The authors concluded that surgical treatment was more cost-effective and patients had a higher quality of life benefit than the group who had maintained conservative management alone with compression therapy.[12,13]

Treatment options for telangiectasias. By definition, telangiectasias, as they are structures with diameters smaller than 3 mm,

TABLE 64-3 Classification of Chronic Lower Extremity Venous Disease

C	Clinical signs (grade$_{0-6}$), supplemented by A for asymptomatic and S for symptomatic presentation
E	Classification by cause (etiology)—*c*ongenital, *p*rimary, *s*econdary
A	Anatomic distribution—*s*uperficial, *d*eep, or *p*erforator, alone or in combination
P	Pathophysiologic dysfunction—*r*eflux or *o*bstruction, alone or in combination

Clinical Classification (C_{0-6})

Any limb with possible chronic venous disease is first placed into one of seven clinical classes (C_{0-6}), according to the objective signs of disease.

Clinical Classification of Chronic Lower Extremity Venous Disease*

CLASS	FEATURES
0	No visible or palpable signs of venous disease
1	Telangiectasia, reticular veins, malleolar flare
2	Varicose veins
3	Edema without skin changes
4	Skin changes ascribed to venous disease (e.g., pigmentation, venous eczema, lipodermatosclerosis)
5	Skin changes as defined above with healed ulceration
6	Skin changes as defined above with active ulceration

*Limbs in higher categories have more severe signs of chronic venous disease and may have some or all of the findings defining a less severe clinical category. Each limb is further characterized as asymptomatic (A)—for example, $C_{0-6,A}$—or symptomatic (S)—for example, $C_{0-6,S}$. Symptoms that may be associated with telangiectatic, reticular, or varicose veins include lower extremity aching, pain, and skin irritation. Therapy may alter the clinical category of chronic venous disease. Limbs should therefore be reclassified after any form of medical or surgical treatment.

Classification by Cause (E_c, E_p, or E_s)

Venous dysfunction may be congenital, primary, or secondary. These categories are mutually exclusive. Congenital venous disorders are present at birth but may not be recognized until later. The method of diagnosis of congenital abnormalities must be described. Primary venous dysfunction is defined as venous dysfunction of unknown cause but not of congenital origin. Secondary venous dysfunction denotes an acquired condition resulting in chronic venous disease—for example, deep venous thrombosis.

Classification by Cause of Chronic Lower Extremity Venous Disease

Congenital (E_c)	Cause of the chronic venous disease present since birth
Primary (E_p)	Chronic venous disease of undetermined cause
Secondary (E_s)	Chronic venous disease with an associated known cause (e.g., post-thrombotic, post-traumatic, other)

Anatomic Classification (A_s, A_d, or A_p)

The anatomic site(s) of the venous disease should be described as superficial (A_s), deep (A_d), or perforating (A_p) vein(s). One, two, or three systems may be involved in any combination. For reports requiring greater detail, the involvement of the superficial, deep, and perforating veins may be localized by use of the anatomic segments.

Segmental Localization of Chronic Lower Extremity Venous Disease

SEGMENT NO.	VEINS
Superficial veins (A_{s1-5})	
1	Telangiectasia/reticular veins
	Greater (long) saphenous vein
2	Above knee
3	Below knee
4	Lesser (short) saphenous vein
5	Nonsaphenous
Deep veins (A_{d6-16})	
6	Inferior vena cava
	Iliac
7	Common
8	Internal
9	External
10	Pelvic: gonadal, broad ligament
	Femoral
11	Common
12	Deep
13	Superficial

TABLE 64-3 Classification of Chronic Lower Extremity Venous Disease—cont'd

14	Popliteal
15	Tibial (anterior, posterior, or peroneal)
16	Muscular (gastrointestinal, soleal, other)
17	Thigh
18	Calf
Pathophysiologic Classification ($P_{r,o}$)	
Clinical signs or symptoms of chronic venous disease result from reflux (P_r), obstruction (P_o), or both ($P_{r,o}$).	
Pathophysiologic Classification of Chronic Lower Extremity Venous Disease	
Reflux (P_r)	
Obstruction (P_o)	
Reflux and obstruction ($P_{r,o}$)	

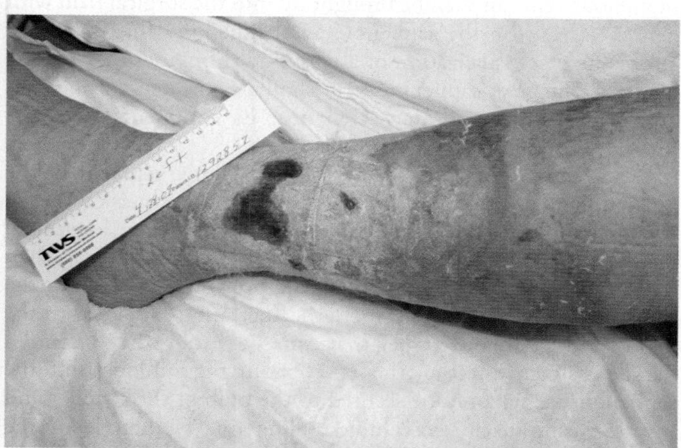

FIGURE 64-7 Venous stasis ulcer.

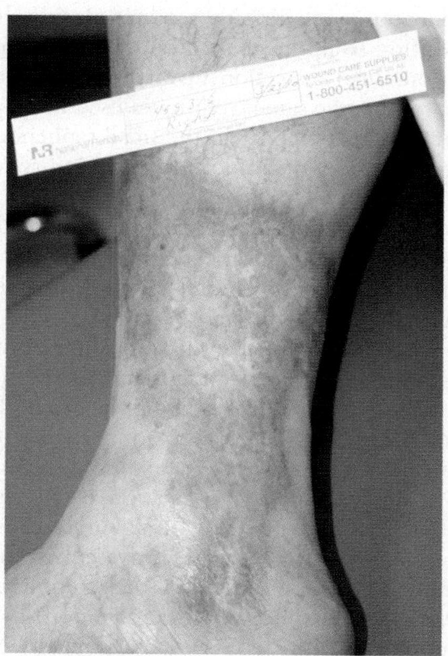

FIGURE 64-8 Healed venous stasis ulcer.

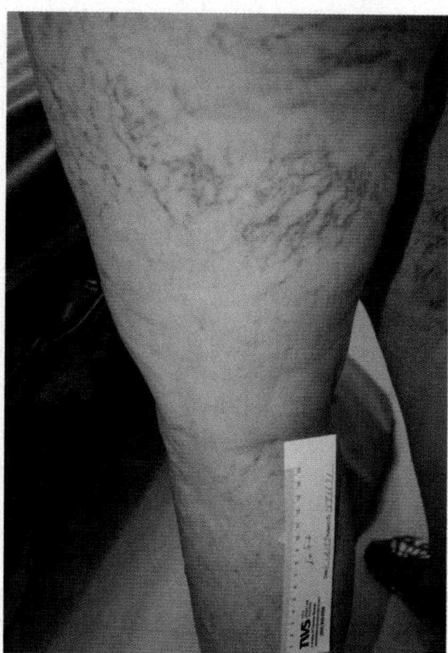

FIGURE 64-9 Spider telangiectasias.

are not appropriate for surgical treatment. Asymptomatic telangiectasias are of cosmetic concern only. In these asymptomatic patients with only C_1 disease, a reflux examination is not indicated. However, if the patient describes symptoms consistent with possible venous insufficiency or has concomitant varicosities or more advanced disease on physical examination, a reflux examination is indicated. Treatment options for telangiectasias (spider veins and reticular veins) include injection sclerotherapy and transdermal laser treatment (Fig. 64-9).

Injection sclerotherapy is a technique that involves direct injection of a sclerosant agent into the feeding vein (reticular vein) or spider vein. This procedure is performed in the office setting. There is no preprocedural preparation of the patient. However, patients are asked not to shave or to apply lotions to the extremity before the treatment. Patients leave the office and are able to perform regular activities immediately. Direct sunlight exposure to the treatment area is avoided for a few weeks after the injection. Although it is a safe technique, injection sclerotherapy is contraindicated in the following situations: pregnancy, patients receiving anticoagulation, patients with acute superficial thrombophlebitis, patients with acute DVT, and patients with a history of severe allergy or severe asthma.

Sclerosants act to disrupt the venous endothelium, causing a periphlebitic reaction, which acts to obliterate the vein segment. There are many sclerosants available, and there are particular categories of sclerosants. They include osmotic, detergent, chemical, and corrosive. Hypertonic saline, in various concentrations, was long considered the agent of choice; however, it can be painful with injection (despite the addition of lidocaine) and appears to exhibit a higher incidence of hyperpigmentation after treatment. Therefore, varying concentrations of sodium tetradecyl sulfate (Sotradecol) and polidocanol (Aethoxysklerol) are now the preferred agents.

The procedure should be performed in a well-lit room. Dilute solutions of sclerosant (e.g., 1% to 3% sodium tetradecyl sulfate; polidocanol 0.5%, 1%, 1.5%) can be injected directly into the venules. Care must be taken to ensure that no single injection dose exceeds 0.1 mL but that multiple injections completely fill all feeding vessels. Larger spider veins should be injected first. Injection should begin proximally and proceed distally. When the session is complete, a pressure dressing is applied, consisting of cotton balls at each injection site, and then covered with compression stockings. Patients are advised to ambulate frequently during the first 24 hours and to abstain from direct sun exposure and airline travel for 2 weeks. On occasion, entrapped blood may form, and patients report significant discomfort. Needle drainage is performed at the site, which facilitates healing and cosmesis and rapidly improves discomfort. This liberation of entrapped blood is as important to success as the primary injection. This therapy is remarkably successful in achieving an excellent cosmetic result. C_1 larger than 1 mm and smaller than 3 mm can also be injected with a sclerosant of slightly greater concentration, but the amount injected at one site needs to be limited to less than 0.5 mL. A total volume of sclerosant should not exceed 4 mL during a treatment session. If one is using hypertonic saline, maximum treatment volume can be 10 mL. Although injection sclerotherapy has met with significant success, complications do occur. They include hyperpigmentation, venous matting, postsclerotherapy necrosis, and an allergic reaction to the sclerosant. In addition, telangiectasia formation after injection sclerotherapy treatment tends to occur. Patients will commonly observe return of spider veins 8 to 12 months after treatment. Although patients may report localized discomfort, sclerotherapy of telangiectasias is considered cosmetic and does not influence the venous circulation of the extremity.[14]

Laser treatment of spider telangiectasias has been performed with a variety of wavelengths and varying techniques, such as high-intensity pulsed light, fiber-guided laser coagulation, and neodymium:yttrium-aluminium-garnet (Nd:YAG) laser with a wavelength of 1064 nm. Evaluation of all existing laser modalities has suggested that the Nd:YAG laser has the most success. However, to date, there have not been any prospective randomized trials to support this presumption. Laser treatment does tend to be more painful. Laser treatment in most centers will be used in conjunction with injection sclerotherapy, that is, injection treats the feeding venules; laser treatment will be used to treat the extremely small branches not adequately addressed with the injection technique. Most patients are satisfied with the injection-only method.

Surgery for axial venous incompetence

Vein stripping. It has been more than a century since surgeons began to develop techniques to treat superficial axial venous reflux. Keller introduced saphenous vein invagination and stripping, and Mayo pioneered use of an external stripper to remove the saphenous vein. Babcock described stripping the saphenous vein intraluminally from the ankle to groin. High ligation of the great saphenous vein briefly gained popularity as a method for treating venous reflux without removing the great saphenous vein. Enthusiasm for high ligation of the great saphenous vein quickly faded as it proved to be ineffective because the reflux in the axial vein was not eliminated. Today, traditional surgical treatment of superficial venous reflux involves high ligation as well as stripping of the great saphenous vein from the knee to the groin. Stripping at the ankle has been largely abandoned because of a high incidence of saphenous nerve injury.

High ligation and vein stripping usually require general or spinal anesthesia. A transverse or oblique groin incision is made just medial to the femoral artery pulse and inferior to the inguinal crease. Sharp dissection allows identification of the proximal great saphenous vein and other venous tributaries that can be ligated and divided. A brief exploration to identify the presence of a duplicate saphenous system should be performed. The great saphenous vein can then be brought up into the surgical field with gentle traction on the saphenofemoral junction. This maneuver affords further visualization of any missed tributaries that require ligation. The great saphenous vein should be ligated with a nonabsorbable suture and transected near its confluence with the femoral vein.

Attention is then directed to the below-knee segment of the great saphenous vein by making a small transverse incision on the proximal, medial calf. The great saphenous vein is identified, ligated distally, and transected. The Codman stripper is then advanced proximally through the great saphenous vein to exit the transected vein in the groin incision. The bulb is attached to the end of the Codman stripper that exits the groin incision, and a handle is attached to the other end (exiting the calf incision). The saphenous vein should be secured to the bulb of the stripper and inverted onto itself. Forcefully pulling on the handle of the Codman stripper removes the great saphenous vein from the groin to the knee. Before stripping, the lower extremity should be wrapped circumferentially to aid in hemostasis and to prevent postoperative edema and permanent hyperpigmentation due to blood extravasation.

Small saphenous vein stripping requires placing the patient in the prone position to optimize surgical exposure. The procedure starts with a proximal dissection involving the saphenopopliteal junction and follows the same techniques used in stripping of the great saphenous vein. Stripping of the small saphenous should be done only to the level of the midcalf to avoid injury to the closely aligned sural nerve.

Complications. Neovascularization refers to the development of new venous tributaries and varicose veins around the previously ligated and divided saphenofemoral junction. The incidence of neovascularization after high ligation and stripping of the great saphenous vein exceeds 30% according to some reports. Interestingly, neovascularization does not occur after endovenous ablation procedures, which obviate the need for a groin dissection or venous tributary ligation. This observation challenges the long-held tenet of varicose vein surgery that stressed the importance of a thorough groin dissection with ligation of all visible venous tributaries. Rather than being beneficial, surgical dissection and tributary ligation may actually trigger neovascularization and varicose vein recurrence. Monitoring for this complication usually involves periodic duplex ultrasound examination.

Saphenous nerve injury is a well-documented complication that occurs more frequently when the great saphenous vein is

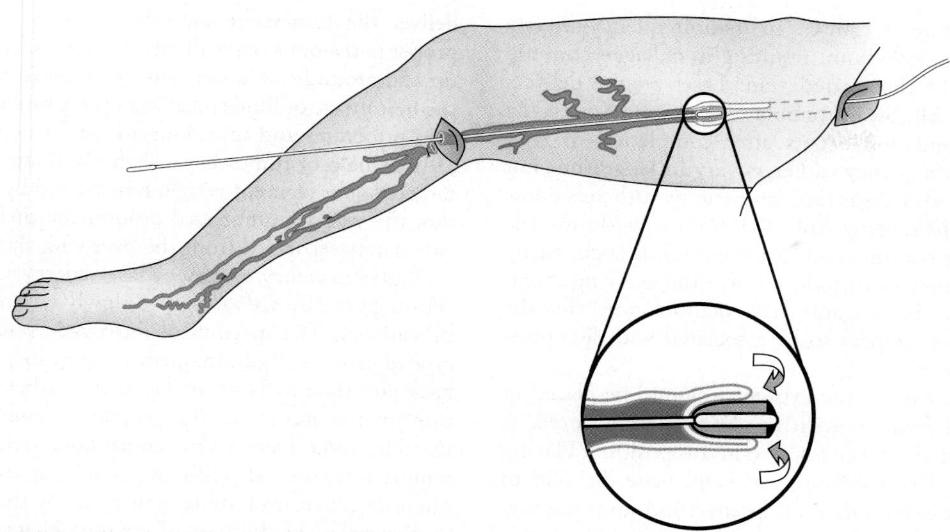

FIGURE 64-10 Inversion stripping of the saphenous vein for superficial venous reflux caused by an incompetent saphenofemoral junction.

stripped from the ankle to the groin. The saphenous nerve runs close to the great saphenous vein in the calf compared with the thigh, where the nerve and vein have more separation. This anatomic detail may explain why stripping from the knee to the thigh only reduces the risk of nerve injury (Fig. 64-10).[15]

Although axial venous stripping was considered the "gold standard" of therapy for several decades, several disadvantages to the technique have been realized. Patients required general anesthesia and a hospitalization. In addition, once discharged, patients experienced a prolonged convalescence before resuming baseline activity. Also, the problems of nerve injury and neovascularization were frustrating to surgeons and patients.

In an effort to address and to correct these limitations, endovenous techniques have been developed. They are discussed in the next section. As a result of their efficacy, stripping is now considered only in select cases.

Endovenous thermal ablation

Percutaneous vein ablation. Percutaneous endovenous ablation of the superficial axial veins revolutionized the treatment of superficial venous insufficiency. As a minimally invasive alternative to surgical vein stripping, percutaneous endovenous ablation can be performed on an outpatient basis with local anesthesia. Advantages of this technique include less discomfort of the patient and a more rapid recovery. Patients now actively seek treatment for varicose veins, prompting the proliferation of outpatient vein treatment centers. There are three types of endovenous thermal therapy for the superficial axial veins: radiofrequency ablation, laser ablation, and ultrasound-guided sclerotherapy (UGS).

Endovenous thermal ablation requires minimal preprocedure preparation. Healthy patients with no medical history do not require laboratory work, whereas standard laboratory evaluation is usually obtained for patients with significant medical comorbidities. Patients who are receiving anticoagulation should remain on their standard regimen. The risk of bridging therapy is greater than the risk of keeping patients on their baseline anticoagulation as long as the international normalized ratio (INR) is 3 or less. Guidelines for periprocedural DVT prophylaxis remain unclear. The author gives a single preprocedure dose of low-molecular-weight heparin (LMWH) to patients with two or more risk factors for DVT. All antiplatelet medications can be continued throughout the procedural course. The author does not routinely administer prophylactic antibiotics. Patients with advanced CVI and skin changes usually receive a preprocedure dose of cefazolin.

Anesthesia for endovenous thermal ablation procedures can range from local injections to conscious sedation. Many patients tolerate the procedure with minimal anesthesia consisting only of tumescent infusion of dilute lidocaine around the great saphenous vein. Ideally, these patients can be treated in an office setting. Moderate sedation requires hemodynamic monitoring equipment and is more suited for an outpatient surgical center. The choice of anesthesia ultimately depends on the preferences of the patient and physician as well as the available resources and practice environments.

The venous duplex ultrasound examination plays an essential role in planning of endovenous thermal ablation procedures. The ultrasound examination should provide the treating physician with the following information: patency of the deep venous system, location of normal and refluxing axial veins, areas of communication between the varicosities and the axial vein, and presence of duplicate or accessory refluxing vein segments.

An acute occlusive DVT is an absolute contraindication to endovenous thermal ablation, whereas a chronically recanalized deep venous system in the extremity to be treated is a relative contraindication. In patients who harbor secondary venous insufficiency, the superficial veins play a more important role in venous drainage compared with patients with a pristine deep venous system and primary venous insufficiency. Care must be taken to ensure that superficial venous ablation will not compromise the venous outflow of the post-thrombotic limb.

The site of percutaneous access depends on the patient's symptoms and the location of the varicose vein tributaries. If endovenous thermal ablation of the great saphenous vein is planned in a patient with painful varicosities on the proximal calf, it is helpful to evaluate these branches with ultrasound. Percutaneous access on the distal calf just inferior to the varicose veins will ensure that maximum resolution of the tributary branches is achieved with endovenous thermal treatment.

Radiofrequency ablation and laser energy deliver two different types of energy to the vein lumen. Radiofrequency heat is delivered at a temperature of 120° C. The radiofrequency directly injures the vein wall endothelium, resulting in collagen contraction and thrombosis of the treated vein. Laser energy delivers energy to the blood itself. Steam bubbles are generated with the laser energy, and coagulation occurs after completion of laser energy delivery. Radiofrequency catheters vary in length but not in temperature delivered. In contrast, laser energy catheters come in different wavelengths ranging from 810 nm to 1470 nm. The type of laser catheters continues to develop, and as such, many laser catheters are frequently introduced into the evolving therapeutic armamentarium. Investigators have demonstrated that the higher wavelength fibers appear to be associated with less postprocedural discomfort.

Technique. In most cases, the extremity should be placed in a position of external rotation with the knee slightly flexed. A sheet "bump" may help the patient maintain this position. Placing the patient in reverse Trendelenburg can help dilate the vein to be accessed. After the standard sterile preparation and draping, the ultrasound probe is brought onto the field in a sterile transducer cover. The author reexamines the vein to be treated along its entire course, noting areas of aneurysmal dilation or tortuosity that may affect catheter placement. Ideally, the puncture site should be distal to the lowest level of truncal reflux and provide unobstructed access to the refluxing vein segment.

At the chosen site of percutaneous access, the ultrasound probe is positioned to obtain a stable gray-scale image of the vein in either the transverse or sagittal plane. After puncture of the skin, limited, small movements of the 21-gauge needle help identify its tip on the ultrasound image. On real-time imaging, the needle is guided into the vein lumen and exchanged over a wire for a 6 Fr or 7 Fr sheath using the modified Seldinger technique. With ultrasound guidance, the radiofrequency catheter or laser catheter is then advanced through the sheath, and the ultrasound probe is positioned in the groin to visualize the catheter tip, the saphenofemoral junction, and the deep system. Using ultrasound guidance, the tip of the ablation catheter is placed 2 to 3 cm distal to the saphenofemoral junction to minimize the chance of heat transmission into the femoral vein. Definitive positioning of the therapeutic catheter must be completed at this point, before the administration of local anesthesia during the next stage of the procedure. Imaging artifacts from the tumescent anesthesia tend to impede visualization of the catheter tip, making it difficult to adjust its position.

Before tumescent anesthesia is begun, the patient should be placed in the Trendelenburg position to help empty the vein. Tumescent anesthesia is the infusion of a large volume of dilute local anesthetic. Although there are many recipes for tumescent solution, the main components are lidocaine, epinephrine, and sodium bicarbonate diluted with lactated Ringer solution or normal saline. During laser treatment and radiofrequency ablation procedures, tumescent anesthesia performs three functions: it provides anesthesia over a large area; it compresses the vein around the therapeutic catheter; and it acts as a protective barrier to prevent heating of nontarget tissues, including skin, nerves, arteries, and the deep veins.

For great saphenous vein procedures, the target of tumescent anesthesia is the saphenous sheath. When it is viewed in the transverse plane, the saphenous canal resembles an eye, and the ultrasound image is often referred to as the "saphenous eye." Administration of tumescent anesthesia starts distally on the lower extremity and progresses proximally. Real-time ultrasound imaging guides a 21- to 25-gauge needle into the saphenous canal to deliver the tumescent anesthesia. When it is injected into the proper perivenous tissue plane, the tumescent anesthesia will track up and around the target vein. A long-axis ultrasound view gives the best image of fluid spreading up the saphenous canal. Multiple skin punctures and injections are performed until the vein has a 10-mm halo of tumescent anesthesia along its entire course. The targeted vein segment is then reinspected by ultrasound to ensure that the vein is compressed around the therapeutic catheter and adequately separated from the overlying skin.

Radiofrequency energy or laser energy is then applied to the vein segment by activating and slowly withdrawing the therapeutic catheter. The specifics of retrograde pullback depend on the type of catheter. Radiofrequency energy involves a segmental pullback governed by hash marks on the catheter and a timed activation on the accompanying generator. Laser energy catheters are variable; some have a slow continuous pullback, whereas others require a segmental pullback. Gray-scale ultrasound images can often detect steam bubbles generated by the laser fiber.

Regardless of the type of energy delivered, once the vein has been completely treated, the sheath and accompanying catheter are removed. Ultrasound imaging resumes, confirming the patency of the femoral vein as well as successful occlusion of the great saphenous vein. Color Doppler imaging is often the only way to assess patency at this point because of the distortion caused by the ablation and the surrounding tumescent anesthesia. It is also important to verify retrograde epigastric venous flow into the proximal segment of the great saphenous vein. This provides a "protective flush" of the great saphenous vein. It is believed by many venous experts that this flow pattern prevents postprocedural development of endovenous heat-induced thrombus.

Postprocedural instructions vary by practitioner. The patient's extremity is usually wrapped in a layered compression dressing, or a 20 to 30 mm Hg compression stocking is applied. The patient is instructed to walk every hour until bed. Regular activity except for vigorous cardiovascular exercise can be resumed the following day. After a satisfactory postprocedural duplex examination, all activity restrictions are lifted.

All follow-up protocols should include a duplex ultrasound examination 2 to 5 days after the procedure. The duplex ultrasound examination ensures that the deep venous system remains patent and confirms the ablation of the great saphenous vein. Reported rates of DVT after endovenous ablation range from 0% to 16% after radiofrequency ablation and 0% to 7.7% after laser ablation. Although the incidence of postablation DVT is extremely low, duplex ultrasound examination can detect thrombus in the proximal great saphenous vein that can extend into the common femoral vein. Lowell Kabnick coined the term *endovenous heat-induced thrombus* (EHIT) to describe this ultrasound finding. He classified EHIT into four different levels based on of the size of the thrombus and its extension into the deep venous system.

The mechanism of EHIT formation remains unclear. General consensus assumes that heat-triggered thrombus in the great saphenous vein propagates into the saphenofemoral junction and encroaches on the deep venous system. EHIT and acute DVT differ in their sonographic characteristics and natural history. EHIT becomes sonographically echogenic quickly (<24 hours), whereas acute DVT usually remains hypoechoic for several days after its initial detection. Although EHIT appears to have a low propensity to propagate or to embolize, pulmonary embolism has been reported after venous ablation procedures. Follow-up ultrasound examinations usually demonstrate retraction or complete resolution of EHIT within 7 to 10 days. Given this benign natural history, most practitioners do not treat class 1 and class 2 EHIT. Class 3 EHIT, which involves partial, nonocclusive extension into the deep venous system, usually warrants anticoagulation therapy, the duration of which can vary on the basis of the physician's discretion. Because class 4 EHIT represents occlusive DVT, it requires a 3-month course of anticoagulation.

The choice of whether to use radiofrequency ablation or laser as the energy source for venous ablation procedures remains a matter of the physician's preference. Randomized prospective studies comparing the two techniques have detected few differences. Patients treated with laser ablation tended to have more discomfort in the very early postprocedural period; however, all other outcome variables were similar.[16,17]

Ultrasound-guided sclerotherapy. UGS was first described in 1989 as a treatment for the superficial axial system. Since then, the use of UGS has expanded to treatment of incompetent perforator branches and large venous tributaries caused by neovascularization. UGS gained popularity as a simple, minimally invasive technique that allows patients to rapidly return to their baseline activity level. Preparation for UGS requires a comprehensive duplex examination.

The closed needle technique is the most common method for performing UGS. A 25-gauge needle is used as this is the smallest caliber needle that can be visualized with gray-scale ultrasound. The needle is attached to a syringe containing the sclerosant. The vein can be sonographically visualized in a transverse or longitudinal plane, depending on the operator's preference. The frequency of the transducer depends on the depth of the vein to be treated. High-frequency transducers visualize superficial veins better, whereas deeper veins require lower frequency transducers. The needle tip must be visualized immediately as it penetrates the dermis. After entering the vein, the needle should be aspirated to confirm its position within the vein lumen. Injecting a small test dose of sclerosant provides further confirmation of the needle's position. An alternative method of UGS uses a butterfly needle instead of the needle attached to a syringe.

Volumes and concentrations of sclerosant are dependent on the size and length of vein to be treated. In general, UGS requires high concentrations of sclerosant because of the large caliber of the targeted veins. Specific details about sclerosant preparation are outside the scope of this chapter. Early investigational studies reported promising results. Further study using randomized prospective trials with all modalities is necessary before true standards of practice can be formalized.

Nontumescent ablation and future modalities for axial vein incompetence. In addition to the ultrasound-guided foam sclerotherapy, many other newer techniques have been recently introduced into the therapeutic armamentarium. One device is mechanical chemical ablation. The catheter device is composed of two components. A mechanical portion rotates inside the vein lumen and denudes the venous endothelium. The second component is the chemical portion, which involves concomitant injection of a liquid sclerosant as the mechanical rotation inside the vein is taking place. Potential advantages over the endothermal devices are the lack of tumescence because no heat is required and the small profile of the catheter. Access of the vein is similar. The glue and foam injectable category comprises another group of devices that are also "tumescent free." Time will tell as further data are obtained to determine the role of each therapy in superficial axial insufficiency.

Treatment of branch varicosities. There are three techniques to treat secondary branch varicosities: conventional stab phlebectomy, powered phlebectomy (TriVex; InaVein, Lexington, Mass), and foam sclerotherapy. Ambulatory phlebectomy is performed by the stab avulsion technique (Fig. 64-11). The patient's varicosities are marked after standing to allow optimal dilation and visualization of affected veins. A variety of anesthetic methods are used successfully, including local anesthesia with tumescence and IV sedation. First, 1-mm incisions are made along Langer skin lines, and the vein is retrieved with a hook. Continuous retraction of the vein segment affords maximal removal of the vein, and direct pressure is applied over the site. Incisions are made at approximately 2-cm intervals. The extremity is wrapped with a layered compression dressing, and patients are instructed to ambulate on the day of surgery. The postoperative course is brief, and rarely do patients require more than acetaminophen or nonsteroidal anti-inflammatory drugs for discomfort. Compression stockings are worn for 2 weeks after the procedure. Complications are unusual but include bleeding, infection, temporary or permanent paresthesias, and phlebitis from retained vein segments. There can be recurrence.

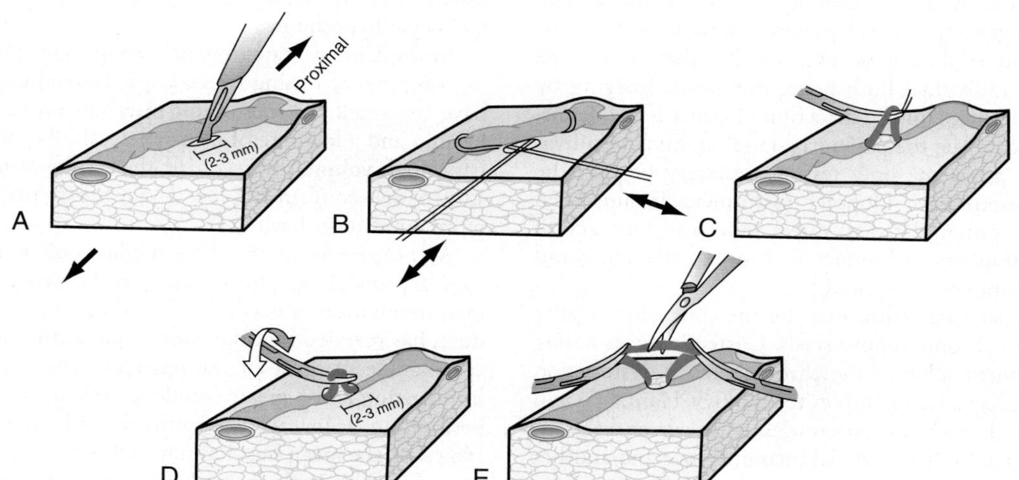

FIGURE 64-11 A-E, Technique of ambulatory phlebectomy (otherwise known as stab avulsions of varicosities).

Powered phlebectomy (TriVex) is a modality that can be used to treat extensive secondary branch varicosities. The patient's varicosities are circumferentially marked preoperatively; in the operating room, 2-mm incisions are made at these boundary sites. These incisions permit placement of a transilluminator and resection device. The instruments are inserted through a subcutaneous plane, just deep to the varicosities. The transilluminator not only provides visualization of the veins but also administers tumescent anesthesia. The resector is a rotating blade that transects the veins and then removes them through a high-suction tubing system. The extremity is wrapped with a multilayer compression dressing, and the patient is discharged with instructions to ambulate hourly. The patient returns to the office for a dressing change within 48 hours and usually is changed to standard compression hose. Discomfort is minimal, and over-the-counter analgesia is sufficient. A second-generation TriVex device has been developed; technical issues with the first-generation instrument were revised, and studies now focus on methods to use the TriVex system in an outpatient setting. A steep learning curve occurs with this device, but once it is achieved, experienced physicians can perform most TriVex procedures within 30 minutes. Complications are unusual but can include contained hematoma, bleeding, temporary or permanent paresthesias, and phlebitis.[18]

Secondary Venous Insufficiency

Secondary venous insufficiency is usually caused by a deep venous thrombus. Clinical manifestations of secondary venous insufficiency usually present in a more advanced stage than their primary counterparts. In addition, patients may describe venous claudication, or a bursting pain in the calf, that is classic for secondary venous insufficiency. Conservative treatment regimens are similar to those described in the preceding section for primary insufficiency; however, these patients require a higher grade of compression for efficacy (30 to 40 mm Hg). Interventional treatment focuses on the superficial and deep systems. Diagnostic interrogation of the deep venous system must be more comprehensive in these patients to determine whether they are candidates for deep surgical or endovenous reconstruction.

Treatment

Surgery for deep venous insufficiency. While conservative therapy is being pursued or ulcer healing is achieved, appropriate diagnostic studies generally reveal patterns of venous reflux or segments of venous occlusion so that specific therapy can be prescribed for the individual limb being evaluated. Imaging by duplex ultrasound suffices for the detection of reflux if the examination is carried out while the patient is standing. Such noninvasive imaging may prove the only testing necessary beyond the hand-held, continuous-wave Doppler instrument if superficial venous ablation is contemplated. If direct venous reconstruction by bypass or valvuloplasty techniques is planned, ascending and descending phlebography is required.[19]

Surprisingly, superficial reflux may be the only abnormality present in advanced chronic venous stasis. Correction goes a long way toward permanent relief of the chronic venous dysfunction and its cutaneous effects. Using duplex technology, Hanrahan and associates[20] found that in 95 extremities with current venous ulceration, 16.8% had only superficial incompetence and another 19% showed superficial incompetence combined with perforator incompetence. Another study has demonstrated ulcer healing and decreased ulcer recurrence with perforator reconstruction.[21]

A significant proportion of patients with venous ulceration have normal function in the deep veins, and surgical treatment is a useful option that can definitively address the hemodynamic derangements. Maintaining that all venous ulcers are surgically incurable is not reasonable when data suggest that superficial vein surgery holds the potential for ameliorating the venous hypertension. A randomized controlled trial comparing compression therapy and surgery for superficial reflux versus conservative management alone has revealed significant improvement in patients who had been treated by the surgical component.[21] Early success in patients with CVI, superficial valvular incompetence, and venous ulceration has been obtained with endovenous radiofrequency and laser therapies.

In the 1938, Linton[22] emphasized the importance of perforating veins, and their direct surgical interruption was advocated. This has fallen into disfavor because of a high incidence of postoperative wound healing complications. However, video techniques that allow direct visualization through small-diameter endoscopes have made endoscopic subfascial exploration and perforator vein interruption the desirable alternative to the Linton technique, minimizing morbidity and wound complications. The connective tissue between the fascia cruris and underlying flexor muscles is so loose that this potential space can be opened up easily and dissected with the endoscope. This operation, done with a vertical proximal incision, accomplishes the objective of perforator vein interruption on an outpatient basis.

The availability of subfascial endoscopic perforator vein surgery has had an impact on the care of venous ulcers in Western countries, albeit not as dramatic as its proponents had hoped. As the limbs of patients with severe CVI were studied accurately, the term *post-thrombotic syndrome* (PTS) had to give way to the term *chronic venous insufficiency;* a link to platelet and monocyte aggregates in the circulation reflected the leukocytic infiltrate of the ankle skin, with its lipodermatosclerosis and healed and open ulcerations.[23]

Data regarding leukocytes in CVI accumulated and were consistent, showing that the activation of leukocytes sequestered in the cutaneous microcirculation during venous stasis was important to the development of the skin changes of CVI. This is reflected in the finding of adhesion markers between leukocytes and endothelial cells and increased production of leukocyte degranulation enzymes and oxygen free radicals. Nevertheless, experimental evidence was still required for decisive proof of the leukocyte hypothesis.

In the United States, several groups have performed perforating vein division using laparoscopic instrumentation. Initial data have suggested that perforator interruption produces rapid ulcer healing and a low rate of recurrence. The North American Registry, which voluntarily recorded the results of perforating venous surgery, has confirmed a low 2-year recurrence rate of ulcers and more rapid ulcer healing.[24]

A comparison of the three methods of perforator vein interruption, including the classic Linton procedure, laparoscopic instrumentation procedure, and single open-endoscope procedure, has revealed that the endoscopic technique produces results comparable to those of the open Linton operation, with much less scarring and a greater tendency toward a fast recovery. More perforating veins were identified with the open technique. However, the mean hospital stay and period of convalescence were more favorable with the endoscope procedures.[25]

In general, registry reports and individual institution clinical experience have shown that patients with true post-thrombotic limbs are disadvantaged by the procedure, enough so that at Leicester (England), the students of the procedure said, "We conclude that perforating vein surgery is not indicated for the treatment of venous ulceration in limbs with primary deep venous incompetence."[25] Nevertheless, studies were reported in which previous superficial reflux was corrected with failures of such treatment. Rescue of these limbs with perforating vein division produced satisfactory results and verified that perforating veins are important in the genesis of venous ulceration and that their division accelerates healing and may reduce recurrence of ulceration.

Part of the difficulty in understanding the need for perforating vein division is the disparity between venous hemodynamics and the severity of cutaneous changes. This is not surprising because the cutaneous changes of CVI are dependent on leukocyte-endothelium interactions, which may not be directly related to venous hemodynamics. However, endoscopic perforator vein division has improved venous hemodynamics in some limbs, as would be expected, by removing superficial reflux and perforating vein outflow. In an effort to eliminate incompetent perforator veins without the associated morbidity described earlier, UGS has been developed as an alternative technique. Early study results are promising and have revealed improved wound healing rates compared with the subfascial endoscopic perforator surgery.[26]

Percutaneous endovenous techniques are also now commonly used modalities to treat incompetent perforator veins. These therapies consist of the same treatments described in the percutaneous vein ablation section. Further study is required to determine the safest and most efficacious technique. For now, the physician has a wealth of varying modalities from which to treat. Interestingly, this may serve the field well; there may be a unique role for each of these techniques.

Direct venous reconstruction. Radiofrequency ablation, laser ablation, and UGS are all commonly used modalities. Historically, the first successful procedures done to reconstruct major veins were the femorofemoral crossover graft of Eduardo Palma and the saphenopopliteal bypass he described, also used by Richard Warren of Boston. These operations were elegant in their simplicity, use of autogenous tissue, and reconstruction by a single venovenous anastomosis.

With regard to femorofemoral crossover grafts, the only group to provide long-term physiologic data on a large number of patients has been Halliday and coworkers from Sydney, Australia. Although phlebography was used in selecting patients for surgery, no other details of preoperative indications were given. These investigators documented that 34 of 50 grafts remained patent in the long term, as assessed by postoperative phlebography. They believed that the best clinical results were achieved in relief of postexercise calf pain but thought that a patent graft also slowed the progression of distal liposclerosis and controlled recurrent ulceration. No proof of this was given in their report. The history of application of bypass procedures for venous obstruction is a fascinating one. Nevertheless, the advent of endovascular techniques has made those operations almost obsolete.[27]

Perforator interruption, combined with superficial venous ablation, has been effective in controlling venous ulceration in 75% to 85% of patients. However, emphasis on failures of this technique led to Masuda and Kistner's[28] significant breakthrough in direct venous reconstruction with valvuloplasty in 1968 and the general recognition of this procedure after 1975. Late evaluations of direct valve reconstruction have indicated good to excellent long-term results in more than 80% of patients.[29] One cannot overestimate Kistner's contributions. The technique of directing the incompetent venous stream through a competent proximal valve by venous segment transfer was his next achievement. After Kistner's studies, surgeons were provided with an armamentarium that included Palma's venous bypass, direct valvuloplasty (of Kistner), and venous segment transfer (of Kistner). Moreover, external valvular reconstruction, as performed by various techniques, including monitoring by endoscopy, has led to renewed interest in this form of treatment of venous insufficiency. Axillary to popliteal autotransplantation of valve-containing venous segments has been considered since the early observations of Taheri and colleagues.[30] However, long-term verification of the preliminary excellent results has not been accomplished.

DEEP VENOUS THROMBOSIS

Lower Extremity Deep Venous Thrombosis

Acute DVT is a major cause of morbidity and mortality in the hospitalized patient, particularly in the surgical patient. The triad of venous stasis, endothelial injury, and hypercoagulable state, first posited by Virchow in 1856, has held true more than a century and a half later.

Acute DVT poses several risks and has significant morbid consequences. The thrombotic process initiated in a venous segment, in the absence of anticoagulation or in the presence of inadequate anticoagulation, can propagate to involve more proximal segments of the deep venous system, thus resulting in edema, pain, and immobility. The most dreaded sequel to acute DVT is that of pulmonary embolism, a condition of potentially lethal consequence. The late consequence of DVT, particularly of the iliofemoral veins, can be CVI and ultimately PTS as a result of valvular dysfunction in the presence of luminal obstruction.

Thus, understanding the pathophysiology, standardizing protocols to prevent or to reduce DVT, and instituting optimal treatment promptly are critical to reducing the incidence and morbidity of this unfortunately common condition.

Causes

The triad of stasis, hypercoagulable state, and vessel injury is present in most surgical patients. It is also clear that increasing age places a patient at a greater risk, with those older than 65 years representing a higher risk population. In addition, many epidemiologic studies have reviewed additional factors that place patients at risk for the development of deep venous thrombus, including malignant disease, increased body mass index, increasing age (especially >60 years), pregnancy, prolonged immobilization, tobacco use, and prior deep vein thrombus.[31]

Stasis. Labeled fibrinogen studies in patients as well as in autopsy studies have demonstrated convincingly that the soleal sinuses are the most common sites of initiation of venous thrombosis. The stasis may contribute to the endothelial cellular layer contacting activated platelets and procoagulant factors, thereby leading to DVT. Stasis, in and of itself, has never been shown to be a causative factor for DVT.

Hypercoagulable state. Our knowledge of hypercoagulable conditions continues to improve, but it is still in its early stages. The standard array of conditions screened for in searching for a hypercoagulable state is listed in Box 64-1. If any of these conditions is identified, a treatment regimen of anticoagulation is instituted for life, unless specific contraindications exist. It is generally appreciated that the postoperative patient, after major surgery, is predisposed to the formation of DVT. After major operations,

BOX 64-1 Hypercoagulable States

Factor V Leiden mutation
Prothrombin gene mutation
Protein C deficiency
Protein S deficiency
Antithrombin III deficiency
Homocysteinemia
Antiphospholipid syndrome
Lupus antibody
Anticardiolipin antibody

large amounts of tissue factor may be released into the bloodstream from damaged tissues. Tissue factor is a potent procoagulant expressed on the leukocyte cell surface as well as in a soluble form in the bloodstream. Increases in platelet count, adhesiveness, changes in coagulation cascade, and endogenous fibrinolytic activity result from physiologic stress, such as major operation or trauma, and have been associated with an increased risk for thrombosis.

Venous injury. It has been clearly established that venous thrombosis occurs in veins that are distant from the site of operation; for example, it is well known that patients undergoing total hip replacement frequently develop contralateral lower extremity DVT.

In a series of experiments, animal models of abdominal and total hip operations were used to study the possibility of venous endothelial damage distant from the operative site. In these studies, jugular veins were excised after the animals were perfusion fixed. These experiments demonstrated that endothelial damage occurred after abdominal operations and was more severe after hip operations. There were multiple microtears noted within the valve cusps that resulted in exposure of the subendothelial matrix. The exact mechanisms whereby this injury at a distant site occurs and which mediators, cellular or humoral, are responsible are not clearly understood, but that the injury occurs is evident from these and other studies.

Diagnostic Considerations

Incidence. Venous thromboembolism occurs for the first time in approximately 100 persons/100,000 each year in the United States. This incidence increases with increasing age, with an incidence of 0.5%/100,000 at 80 years of age. More than two thirds of these patients have DVT alone, and the rest have evidence of pulmonary embolism. The recurrence rate with anticoagulation has been noted to be 6% to 7% in the ensuing 6 months.

In the United States, pulmonary embolism causes 50,000 to 200,000 deaths annually. A 28-day case-fatality rate of 9.4% after first-time DVT and of 15.1% after first-time pulmonary thromboembolism has been observed. Aside from pulmonary embolism, secondary CVI (resulting from DVT) is significant in terms of cost, morbidity, and lifestyle limitations.

If the consequences of DVT, in terms of pulmonary embolism and CVI, are to be prevented, the prevention, diagnosis, and treatment of DVT must be optimized.

Clinical diagnosis. The diagnosis of DVT requires a high index of suspicion. Most are familiar with Homan sign, which refers to pain in the calf on dorsiflexion of the foot. Although the absence of this sign is not a reliable indicator of the absence of venous thrombus, the presence of Homan sign should prompt one to attempt to confirm the diagnosis. The extent of venous thrombosis in the lower extremity is an important factor in the manifestation of symptoms. For example, most calf thrombi may be asymptomatic unless there is proximal propagation. This is one reason that radiolabeled fibrinogen testing demonstrates a higher incidence of DVT than studies using imaging modalities. Only 40% of patients with venous thrombosis have any clinical manifestations of the condition.

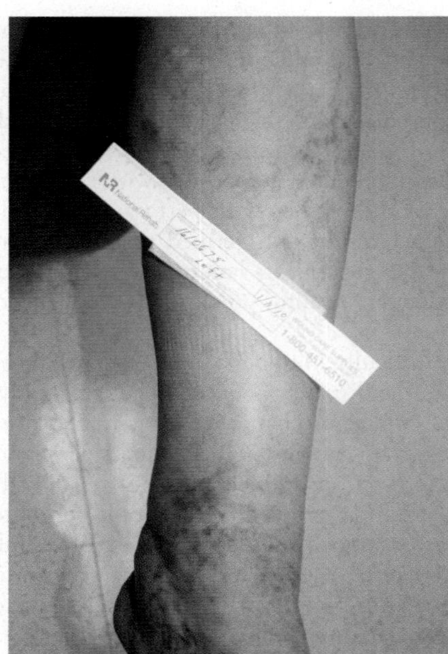

FIGURE 64-12 Edema. Note the loss of ankle definition.

Major venous thrombosis involving the iliofemoral venous system results in a massively swollen leg, with pitting edema (Fig. 64-12), pain, and blanching, a condition known as phlegmasia alba dolens. With further progression of disease, there may be such massive edema that arterial inflow can be compromised. This condition results in a painful blue leg, a condition called phlegmasia cerulea dolens. With this evolution of the condition, venous gangrene can develop unless flow is restored.

PTS is a common and unfortunate manifestation of deep venous thrombus. It occurs in 20% to 50% of patients after a documented episode of DVT. The clinical presentation includes chronic edema, pain, and venous claudication. Venous ulcerations occur. Risk factors for the development of PTS include persistent leg symptoms for months after the acute episode of DVT, an anatomically extensive DVT involving the iliofemoral system, recurrent ipsilateral DVTs, and a prolonged state of subtherapeutic anticoagulation for DVT. Unfortunately, treatment of PTS remains supportive, and compression therapy remains the mainstay of treatment for PTS. Some investigators have advocated the early use of thrombolysis to prevent PTS, but that has not been consistently proven.

Imaging Studies and Laboratory Tests

Venography. Injection of contrast material into the venous system has been long considered the most accurate method of confirming DVT and its location. The superficial venous system has to be occluded with a tourniquet, and the veins in the foot are injected for visualization of the deep venous system. Although this is a good test for finding occlusive and nonocclusive thrombus, it is also invasive, subject to risks of IV administration of contrast material. As a result, this technique has been replaced by less invasive modalities.

Impedance plethysmography. Impedance plethysmography measures the change in venous capacitance and rate of emptying of the venous volume on temporary occlusion and release of the occlusion of the venous system. A cuff is inflated around the upper thigh until the electrical signal has plateaued. When the cuff is deflated, there is usually rapid outflow and reduction of volume. With a venous thrombosis, one notes a prolongation of the outflow wave. It is not useful clinically for the detection of calf venous thrombosis and of patients with prior venous thrombosis.

Fibrin and fibrinogen assays. Fibrin and fibrinogen levels can be determined by measuring the degradation of intravascular fibrin. The D-dimer test measures cross-linked degradation products, which is a surrogate of plasmin's activity on fibrin. In combination with clinical evaluation and assessment, the sensitivity exceeds 90% to 95%. The negative predictive value is 99.3% for proximal evaluation and 98.6% for distal evaluation. In the postoperative patient, D-dimer is causally elevated because of surgery, and as such, a positive result of the D-dimer assay for evaluating for DVT is not useful. However, a negative D-dimer test result in patients with suspected DVT has a high negative predictive value, ranging from 97% to 99%.[32]

Duplex ultrasound. The current test of choice for the diagnosis of DVT is duplex ultrasound, a modality that combines Doppler ultrasound and color flow imaging. The advantage of this test is that it is noninvasive, comprehensive, and without any risk of reaction to contrast angiography. This test is also highly operator dependent, which is one of its potential drawbacks.

Doppler ultrasound is based on the principle of the impairment of an accelerated flow signal caused by an intraluminal thrombus. A detailed interrogation begins at the calf with imaging of the tibial veins and then proximally over the popliteal and femoral veins. A properly done examination evaluates flow with distal compression, which results in augmentation of flow, and with proximal compression, which should interrupt flow. If any segment of the venous system being examined fails to demonstrate augmentation on compression, venous thrombosis is suspected.

Real-time B-mode ultrasonography with color flow imaging has improved the sensitivity and specificity of ultrasound scanning. With color flow duplex imaging, blood flow can be imaged in the presence of a partially occluding thrombus. The probe is also used to compress the vein. A normal vein is easily compressed, whereas in the presence of a thrombus, there is resistance to compression. In addition, the chronicity of the thrombus can be evaluated on the basis of its imaging characteristics, namely, increased echogenicity and heterogeneity. Duplex imaging is significantly more sensitive than indirect physiologic testing. There are many advantages associated with duplex ultrasound: noninvasiveness, portability, and no need for a contrast agent. However, there are significant disadvantages as well; these include interuser variability and skill, body habitus, and suboptimal visualization in regions such as the lower pelvis.

Magnetic resonance venous imaging. With major advances in imaging technology, MRVI has come to the forefront of imaging for proximal venous disease. The cost and the issue of patient tolerance because of claustrophobia limit its widespread application, but this has been changing. It is a useful test for imaging the iliac veins and IVC, an area where the use of duplex ultrasound is limited. MRVI is less invasive than conventional venography and is able to directly visualize the thrombus.

Prophylaxis

The patient who has undergone major abdominal or orthopedic surgery, has sustained major trauma, or has prolonged immobility (>3 days) represents an elevated risk for the development of venous thromboembolism. The specific risk factor analysis and epidemiologic studies detailing the causes of venous thromboembolism are beyond the scope of this chapter. The reader is referred to a more extensive analysis of this problem.[31]

The methods of prophylaxis can be mechanical or pharmacologic. The simplest method is for the patient to walk. Activation of the calf pump mechanism is an effective means of prophylaxis, as evidenced by the fact that few active people without underlying risk factors develop venous thrombosis. A patient who is expected to be up and walking within 24 to 48 hours is at low risk for development of venous thrombosis. The practice of having a patient out of bed into a chair is one of the most thrombogenic positions that could be ordered for a patient. Sitting in a chair, with the legs in a dependent position, causes venous pooling, which in the postoperative milieu could easily be a predisposing factor for the development of thromboembolism.

The most common method of surgical prophylaxis has traditionally revolved around sequential compression devices, which periodically compress the calves and essentially replicate the calf bellows mechanism. This has clearly reduced the incidence of venous thromboembolism in the surgical patient. The most likely mechanism for the efficacy of this device is prevention of venous stasis. Some studies have suggested that fibrinolytic activity systemically is enhanced by a sequential compression device. However, this has not been definitively established because a considerable number of studies have demonstrated no enhancement of fibrinolytic activity.[33]

Another traditional method of thromboprophylaxis has been the use of low-dose unfractionated heparin. The dosage traditionally used was 5000 units of unfractionated heparin every 12 hours. However, analyses of trials comparing placebo versus fixed-dose heparin have shown that the stated dose of 5000 units subcutaneously every 12 hours is no more effective than placebo. When subcutaneous heparin is used on a dosing regimen of every 8 hours rather than every 12 hours, there is a reduction in the development of venous thromboembolism.

More recently, a number of studies have revealed the efficacy of fractionated LMWH for the prophylaxis and treatment of venous thromboembolism. LMWH inhibits factor Xa and IIa activity, with the ratio of anti–factor Xa to anti–factor IIa activity ranging from 1 : 1 to 4 : 1. LMWH has a longer plasma half-life and significantly higher bioavailability. The consistent bioavailability and clearance of LMWH do not require monitoring of factor Xa levels, which facilitates use by the patient. Dosing is merely based on the patient's weight. There is a more predictable anticoagulant response than with unfractionated heparin. No laboratory monitoring is necessary because the partial thromboplastin time (PTT) is unaffected. Various analyses, including a major meta-analysis, have shown that LMWH results in equivalent if not better efficacy, with significantly fewer bleeding complications. It was first thought that LMWH results in less bleeding than unfractionated heparin, but no clinical observations have confirmed this. This property may be more a function of dose than an intrinsic drug action.

Comparison of LMWH with mechanical prophylaxis has demonstrated the superiority of LMWH for reduction of the development of venous thromboembolic disease.[34-36] Prospective trials evaluating LMWH in head-injured and trauma patients have also proved the safety of LMWH, with no increase in intracranial bleeding or major bleeding at other sites.[37] In addition, LMWH shows a significant reduction in the development of venous thromboembolism compared with other methods.

Thus, LMWH is considered the optimal method of prophylaxis for moderate- and high-risk patients. Even the traditional reluctance to use heparin in high-risk groups, such as the multiply injured trauma patient and head-injured patient, must be reexamined, given the efficacy and safety profile of LMWH in multiple prospective trials.

Treatment

After a diagnosis of venous thrombosis has been made, a treatment plan must be instituted. Complications of calf DVT include proximal propagation of thrombus in up to one third of hospitalized patients and PTS. In addition, untreated lower extremity DVT carries a 30% recurrence rate.

Any venous thrombosis involving the femoropopliteal system is treated with full anticoagulation. Traditionally, the treatment of DVT has centered around heparin treatment to maintain the PTT at 60 to 80 seconds, followed by warfarin therapy to obtain an INR of 2.5 to 3.0. If unfractionated heparin is used, it is important to use a nomogram-based dosing therapy. The incidence of recurrent venous thromboembolism increases if the time to therapeutic anticoagulation is prolonged. Therefore, it is important to reach therapeutic levels within 24 hours. An initial bolus of 80 units/kg or 5000 units IV bolus is administered, followed by 18 units/kg/hr. The rate is dependent on a target PTT corresponding to an anti–factor Xa level of 0.3 to 0.7 unit/mL.[38] The PTT needs to be checked 6 hours after any change in heparin dosing. Warfarin is started on the same day. If warfarin is initiated without heparin, the risk for a transient hypercoagulable state exists because protein C and protein S levels fall before the other vitamin K–dependent factors are depleted. With the advent of LMWH, it is no longer necessary to admit the patient for IV heparin therapy. It is now accepted practice to administer LMWH on an outpatient basis, as a bridge to warfarin therapy, which is also monitored on an outpatient basis.

The recommended duration of anticoagulant therapy continues to evolve. A minimum treatment time of 3 months is advocated in most cases. The recurrence rate is the same with 3 months versus 6 months of warfarin therapy. If the patient has a known hypercoagulable state or has experienced episodes of venous thrombosis, however, lifetime anticoagulation is required in the absence of contraindications. The accepted INR range is 2.0 to 3.0; a randomized double-blind study has confirmed that a goal INR of 2.0 to 3.0 is more effective in preventing recurrent venous thromboembolism than a low-intensity regimen with a goal INR of 1.0 to 1.9.[39] In addition, the low-intensity regimen did not reduce the risk for clinically important bleeding.

Oral anticoagulants are teratogenic and thus cannot be used during pregnancy. In the case of the pregnant patient with venous thrombosis, LMWH is the treatment of choice; this is continued through delivery and can be continued postpartum, as indicated.

Thrombolysis. The advent of thrombolysis has resulted in increased interest in thrombolysis for DVT. The purported benefit is preservation of valve function, with a subsequently lesser chance for development of CVI. However, there have been few definitive convincing studies to support the use of thrombolytic therapy for DVT.

One exception is the patient with phlegmasia, for whom thrombolysis is advocated for relief of significant venous obstruction. In this condition, thrombolytic therapy probably results in better relief of symptoms and fewer long-term sequelae than heparin anticoagulation alone. The alternative for this condition is surgical venous thrombectomy. No matter which treatment is chosen, long-term anticoagulation is indicated. The incidence of major bleeding is higher with lytic therapy.[27]

Endovascular reconstruction. Chronic proximal venous occlusion of the iliofemoral system is a challenging clinical problem. The presentation is variable, and there is no reliable diagnostic modality to measure proximal iliofemoral venous stenosis and to assess outflow obstruction accurately. The pathophysiologic mechanism is often a combination of primary and secondary venous insufficiency. Therefore, evaluation and treatment can be challenging. Endovascular reconstruction removes the need for surgical bypass and has been used successfully. Recanalization of the occluded iliac vein is performed endovascularly. Balloon dilation of the lesion is then performed, and a stent is placed across the dilated segment. Excellent results have been achieved, thereby obviating an open surgical procedure. Endovascular iliac therapy has evolved to become first-line therapy for iliac occlusions.

Upper Extremity Deep Venous Thrombosis

Upper extremity DVT is much less common than its lower extremity counterpart, constituting only approximately 5% of all documented DVTs. Although not as common, it is a serious problem; pulmonary embolism occurs in up to one third of all patients with an upper extremity DVT. Upper extremity DVT usually refers to thrombosis of the axillary or subclavian veins. The syndrome can be divided into two categories, primary idiopathic and secondary.

Primary causes include Paget-Schroetter syndrome and idiopathic upper extremity DVT. Patients with Paget-Schroetter syndrome develop effort thrombosis of the extremity caused by compression of the subclavian vein, the venous component of thoracic outlet syndrome. A classic presentation involves a young athlete who uses the upper extremity in a repetitive motion, such as swimming, which causes repetitive extrinsic compression of the subclavian vein. In these patients, anatomic anomalies such as a cervical rib or myofascial bands cause the venous compression. Plain films are one of the first diagnostic tests used to confirm thoracic outlet syndrome. Treatment with initial thrombolysis followed by first rib resection is the standard of care. Idiopathic upper extremity DVT is sometimes eventually attributed to an occult malignant neoplasm, and therefore a diagnosis of idiopathic upper extremity DVT warrants evaluation for an undetected malignant neoplasm.

Secondary causes of upper extremity DVT are more common. These include an indwelling central venous catheter, pacemaker, thrombophilia, and malignant disease.

Classic findings on physical examination include unilateral swelling, pain, extremity discomfort, erythema, and a palpable cord. Diagnosis is confirmed by duplex ultrasonography. Because the clavicle obscures the midportion of the subclavian vein, venography or magnetic resonance venography may be required; these are second-line imaging modalities.

Treatment

Treatment of upper extremity DVT involves anticoagulation therapy. Therapeutic dosing parameters are the same as for lower extremity DVT. Treatment should be for 3 months and consist of heparin or LMWH plus warfarin for at least 3 months. Long-term complications of upper extremity DVT include recurrence and

BOX 64-2 Indications for a Vena Cava Filter

Recurrent thromboembolism despite adequate anticoagulation
Deep venous thrombosis in a patient with contraindications to anticoagulation
Chronic pulmonary embolism and resultant pulmonary hypertension
Complications of anticoagulation
Propagating iliofemoral venous thrombus in anticoagulation

BOX 64-3 Indications for Placement of a Retrievable Inferior Vena Cava Filter

Prophylactic placement in a high-risk trauma patient (orthopedic, spinal cord patients)
Short-term duration, contraindication to anticoagulation therapy
Protection during venous thrombolytic therapy
Extensive iliocaval thrombosis

PTS. Thrombolysis has not been shown to decrease long-term manifestations from upper extremity DVT and thus PTS. PTS is treated with extremity elevation and graduated elastic compression.[40,41]

Vena cava filter. The most worrisome and potentially lethal complication of DVT is pulmonary embolism. The symptoms of pulmonary embolism, ranging from dyspnea, chest pain, and hypoxia to acute cor pulmonale, are nonspecific and require a high index of suspicion. The gold standard remains pulmonary angiography, but increasingly, this has been displaced by computed tomography angiography.

Adequate anticoagulation is usually effective for stabilizing venous thrombosis, but if a patient develops a pulmonary embolism in the presence of adequate anticoagulation, a vena cava filter is indicated. The general indications for a vena cava filter are listed in Box 64-2. Modern filters are placed percutaneously over a guidewire. The Greenfield filter, most extensively used and studied, has a 95% patency rate and a 4% recurrent embolism rate. This high patency rate allows safe suprarenal placement if there is involvement of the IVC up to the renal veins or if it is placed in a woman in her childbearing years.

Device-related complications are wound hematoma, migration of the device into the pulmonary artery, and caval occlusion caused by trapping of a large embolus. In the last situation, the dramatic hypotension that accompanies acute caval occlusion can be mistaken for a massive pulmonary embolism. The distinction between the hypovolemia of caval occlusion and the right-sided heart failure from pulmonary embolism can be made by measuring filling pressures of the right side of the heart. The treatment of caval occlusion is volume resuscitation.

Retrievable vena cava filters. Although they are generally safe, IVC filters are not without risk and significant morbidity. Therefore, permanent placement of a caval filter, particularly in a young patient who may require only short-term caval protection, is not generally accepted. Retrievable filters entered the field as a potential solution for the patient with temporary indications for pulmonary embolus prophylaxis. There are three retrievable IVC filters that have U.S. Food and Drug Administration approval: the Recovery filter (Bard, Helsingborg, Sweden), OptEase filter (Cordis, Johnson & Johnson Gateway, Piscataway, NJ), and Gunther-Tulip filter (Cook Medical, Bloomington, Ind). These filters vary slightly with respect to shape and length. All can be deployed from the internal jugular vein or femoral vein and retrieved from the right jugular vein (Gunther-Tulip and Recovery) or right femoral vein (OptEase). Before retrieval, venography is performed to ensure that there is no nidus of IVC thrombus in the filter. These filters can be placed in an angiography suite or at the bedside using intravascular ultrasound. A major advantage to retrievable filters is that they may be removed when the patient no longer requires pulmonary embolism protection or can undergo anticoagulation. Patient groups that may benefit from retrievable filters include multiple-trauma patients and high-risk surgical patients. Insertion complications reported include vena cava perforation, filter migration, and venous thrombosis at the insertion site. Retrieval complications include failure to retrieve the filter, thrombus embolization from the filter, vein retrieval site thrombus, and groin hematoma. However, the role of retrievable filters continues to be a work in progress. Further investigation is required before definitive practice guidelines can be established (Box 64-3).[42,43]

SUPERFICIAL THROMBOPHLEBITIS

Superficial thrombophlebitis is a common disorder, diagnosed in the hospital and outpatient setting. In hospitalized patients, superficial thrombophlebitis is usually caused by an indwelling catheter. In the clinic, patients with thrombophlebitis report common predisposing risk factors, such as recent surgery, recent childbirth, venous stasis, varicose veins, or IV drug use. Patients who deny any of these factors may be classified with idiopathic thrombophlebitis. In these cases, care must be taken to ensure that the patient does not harbor an occult hypercoagulable state or occult malignant disease. In 1876, Trousseau identified the phenomenon of migratory thrombophlebitis and malignant disease, particularly involving the tail of the pancreas. Mondor disease involves superficial thrombophlebitis of the superficial veins of the breast. Diagnosis of superficial thrombophlebitis can be easily made by physical examination of an erythematous palpable cord coursing along a superficial vein, usually located along the lower extremities. Duplex ultrasonography is used if there is suspicion of proximal propagation into the deep venous system. With this diagnosis of DVT, anticoagulation is indicated. If, however, thrombus abuts the saphenofemoral junction, treatment of this more elusive condition is controversial. Some authors recommend serial ultrasound examinations and others anticoagulation; another alternative is operative ligation at the junction.

The treatment of localized noncomplicated thrombophlebitis involves conservative therapy, which consists of anti-inflammatory medication and compression stockings. When the thrombophlebitis involves clusters of varicosities, particularly in the lower extremities, excision is indicated. Selective removal of the entire vein along its course is indicated only in the rare case of suppurative septic thrombophlebitis after all other sources of sepsis have been excluded.

CONCLUSION

The spectrum of venous disease is widespread and diverse, providing surgeons who fully understand the unique physiology of veins a rewarding and rich arena for future investigation.

SELECTED REFERENCES

Bergan JJ, Pascarella L, Schmid-Schönbein GW: Pathogenesis of primary chronic venous disease: Insights from animal models of venous hypertension. *J Vasc Surg* 47:183–192, 2008.

This article provides a comprehensive review of the known aspects of venous hypertension pathophysiology.

Caggiati A, Bergan JJ, Gloviczki P, et al: Nomenclature of the veins of the lower limbs: An international interdisciplinary consensus statement. *J Vasc Surg* 36:416–422, 2002.

Revised terminology for the venous anatomy of the lower extremity is outlined.

Eklöf B, Rutherford RB, Bergan JJ, et al: American Venous Forum International Ad Hoc Committee for Revision of the CEAP Classification: Revision of the CEAP classification for chronic venous disorders: Consensus statement. *J Vasc Surg* 40:1248–1252, 2004.

Essential adjunct to the original CEAP document.

Leopardi D, Hoggan BL, Fitridge RA, et al: Systematic review of treatments for varicose veins. *Ann Vasc Surg* 23:264–276, 2009.

Systematic overview of current treatment modalities for superficial venous disease.

Meissner MH, Eklof B, Smith PC, et al: Secondary chronic venous disorders. *J Vasc Surg* 46(Suppl):68S–83S, 2007.

Meissner MH, Gloviczki P, Bergan J, et al: Primary chronic venous disorders. *J Vasc Surg* 46(Suppl):54S–67S, 2007.

These two supplements provide an extremely comprehensive evaluation of venous insufficiency, including pathophysiology, medical and surgical management, and outstanding references.

Wakefield TW, Caprini J, Comerota AJ: Thromboembolic diseases. *Curr Probl Surg* 45:844–899, 2008.

Excellent review of secondary venous disorders.

REFERENCES

1. Caggiati A, Bergan JJ, Gloviczki P, et al: Nomenclature of the veins of the lower limbs: An international interdisciplinary consensus statement. *J Vasc Surg* 36:416–422, 2002.
2. Raffetto JD: Inflammation in chronic venous ulcers. *Phlebology* 28(Suppl 1):61–67, 2013.
3. Kowalewski R, Malkowski A, Sobolewski K, et al: Evaluation of transforming growth factor-β signaling pathway in the wall of normal and varicose veins. *Pathobiology* 77:1–6, 2010.
4. Pascarella L, Schonbein GW, Bergan JJ: Microcirculation and venous ulcers: A review. *Ann Vasc Surg* 19:921–927, 2005.
5. Neglen P, Raju S: A rational approach to detection of significant reflux with duplex Doppler scanning and air plethysmography. *J Vasc Surg* 17:590–595, 1993.
6. Christopoulos D, Nicolaides AN, Szendro G: Venous reflux: Quantification and correlation with the clinical severity of chronic venous disease. *Br J Surg* 75:352–356, 1988.
7. van Bemmelen PS, Bedford G, Beach K, et al: Quantitative segmental evaluation of venous valvular reflux with duplex ultrasound scanning. *J Vasc Surg* 10:425–431, 1989.
8. Gloviczki P, Comerota AJ, Dalsing MC, et al: The care of patients with varicose veins and associated chronic venous diseases: Clinical practice guidelines of the Society for Vascular Surgery and the American Venous Forum. *J Vasc Surg* 53:2S–48S, 2011.
9. Singh S, Lees TA, Donlon M, et al: Improving the preoperative assessment of varicose veins. *Br J Surg* 84:801–802, 1997.
10. Eklof B, Rutherford RB, Bergan JJ, et al: Revision of the CEAP classification for chronic venous disorders: Consensus statement. *J Vasc Surg* 40:1248–1252, 2004.
11. Rutherford RB, Padberg FT, Jr, Comerota AJ, et al: Venous severity scoring: An adjunct to venous outcome assessment. *J Vasc Surg* 31:1307–1312, 2000.
12. Michaels JA, Brazier JE, Campbell WB, et al: Randomized clinical trial comparing surgery with conservative treatment for uncomplicated varicose veins. *Br J Surg* 93:175–181, 2006.
13. Heller JA: Varicose veins. In Gahtan V, Costanza MJ, editors: *Essentials of vascular surgery for the general surgeon*, New York, 2014, Springer, pp 167–183.
14. Franz RW, Knapp ED: Transilluminated powered phlebectomy surgery for varicose veins: A review of 339 consecutive patients. *Ann Vasc Surg* 23:303–309, 2009.
15. Dwerryhouse S, Davies B, Harradine K, et al: Stripping the long saphenous vein reduces the rate of reoperation for recurrent varicose veins: Five-year results of a randomized trial. *J Vasc Surg* 29:589–592, 1999.
16. Raju S, Hollis K, Neglen P: Use of compression stockings in chronic venous disease: Patient compliance and efficacy. *Ann Vasc Surg* 21:790–795, 2007.
17. van den Bos R, Arends L, Kockaert M, et al: Endovenous therapies of lower extremity varicosities: A meta-analysis. *J Vasc Surg* 49:230–239, 2009.
18. Marston WA, Owens LV, Davies S, et al: Endovenous saphenous ablation corrects the hemodynamic abnormality in patients with CEAP clinical class 3-6 CVI due to superficial reflux. *Vasc Endovascular Surg* 40:125–130, 2006.
19. Neglen P, Hollis KC, Olivier J, et al: Stenting of the venous outflow in chronic venous disease: Long-term stent-related outcome, clinical, and hemodynamic result. *J Vasc Surg* 46:979–990, 2007.
20. Hanrahan LM, Araki CT, Rodriguez AA, et al: Distribution of valvular incompetence in patients with venous stasis ulceration. *J Vasc Surg* 13:805–811, 1991.
21. O'Donnell TF, Jr: The present status of surgery of the superficial venous system in the management of venous ulcer and the evidence for the role of perforator interruption. *J Vasc Surg* 48:1044–1052, 2008.
22. Linton RR: The communicating veins of the lower leg and the operative technic for their ligation. *Ann Surg* 107:582–593, 1938.
23. Powell CC, Rohrer MJ, Barnard MR, et al: Chronic venous insufficiency is associated with increased platelet and monocyte activation and aggregation. *J Vasc Surg* 30:844–851, 1999.

24. Gloviczki P, Bergan JJ, Rhodes JM, et al: Mid-term results of endoscopic perforator vein interruption for chronic venous insufficiency: Lessons learned from the North American subfascial endoscopic perforator surgery registry. The North American Study Group. *J Vasc Surg* 29:489–502, 1999.
25. Murray JD, Bergan JJ, Riffenburgh RH: Development of open-scope subfascial perforating vein surgery: Lessons learned from the first 67 cases. *Ann Vasc Surg* 13:372–377, 1999.
26. Masuda EM, Kessler DM, Lurie F, et al: The effect of ultrasound-guided sclerotherapy of incompetent perforator veins on venous clinical severity and disability scores. *J Vasc Surg* 43:551–556, 2006.
27. Sillesen H, Just S, Jorgensen M, et al: Catheter directed thrombolysis for treatment of ilio-femoral deep venous thrombosis is durable, preserves venous valve function and may prevent chronic venous insufficiency. *Eur J Vasc Endovasc Surg* 30:556–562, 2005.
28. Kistner RL: Surgical repair of the incompetent femoral vein valve. *Arch Surg* 110:1336–1342, 1975.
29. Masuda EM, Kistner RL: Long-term results of venous valve reconstruction: A four- to twenty-one-year follow-up. *J Vasc Surg* 19:391–403, 1994.
30. Taheri SA, Lazar L, Elias S, et al: Surgical treatment of postphlebitic syndrome with vein valve transplant. *Am J Surg* 144:221–224, 1982.
31. Anderson FA, Jr, Spencer FA: Risk factors for venous thromboembolism. *Circulation* 107:I9–I16, 2003.
32. Kovacs MJ, MacKinnon KM, Anderson D, et al: A comparison of three rapid D-dimer methods for the diagnosis of venous thromboembolism. *Br J Haematol* 115:140–144, 2001.
33. Killewich LA, Cahan MA, Hanna DJ, et al: The effect of external pneumatic compression on regional fibrinolysis in a prospective randomized trial. *J Vasc Surg* 36:953–958, 2002.
34. Bernardi E, Prandoni P: Safety of low molecular weight heparins in the treatment of venous thromboembolism. *Expert Opin Drug Saf* 2:87–94, 2003.
35. Couturaud F, Julian JA, Kearon C: Low molecular weight heparin administered once versus twice daily in patients with venous thromboembolism: A meta-analysis. *Thromb Haemost* 86:980–984, 2001.
36. Offner PJ, Hawkes A, Madayag R, et al: The role of temporary inferior vena cava filters in critically ill surgical patients. *Arch Surg* 138:591–594, discussion 594-595, 2003.
37. Mismetti P, Laporte S, Darmon JY, et al: Meta-analysis of low molecular weight heparin in the prevention of venous thromboembolism in general surgery. *Br J Surg* 88:913–930, 2001.
38. Norwood SH, McAuley CE, Berne JD, et al: Prospective evaluation of the safety of enoxaparin prophylaxis for venous thromboembolism in patients with intracranial hemorrhagic injuries. *Arch Surg* 137:696–701, 2002.
39. Kearon C, Ginsberg JS, Kovacs MJ, et al: Comparison of low-intensity warfarin therapy with conventional-intensity warfarin therapy for long-term prevention of recurrent venous thromboembolism. *N Engl J Med* 349:631–639, 2003.
40. Joffe HV, Goldhaber SZ: Upper-extremity deep vein thrombosis. *Circulation* 106:1874–1880, 2002.
41. Martinelli I, Battaglioli T, Bucciarelli P, et al: Risk factors and recurrence rate of primary deep vein thrombosis of the upper extremities. *Circulation* 110:566–570, 2004.
42. Rosenthal D, Wellons ED, Lai KM, et al: Retrievable inferior vena cava filters: Initial clinical results. *Ann Vasc Surg* 20:157–165, 2006.
43. Kearon C, Kahn SR, Agnelli G, et al: Antithrombotic therapy for venous thromboembolic disease: American College of Chest Physicians Evidence-Based Clinical Practice Guidelines (8th Edition). *Chest* 133:454S–545S, 2008.

65 CHAPTER

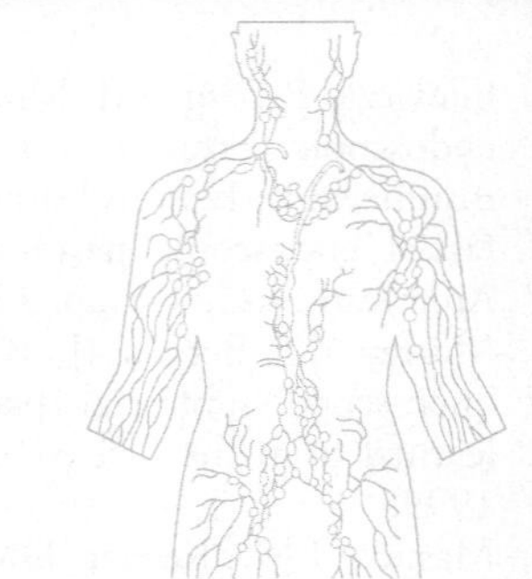

The Lymphatics

Iraklis I. Pipinos, B. Timothy Baxter

OUTLINE

EMBRYOLOGY AND ANATOMY

The primordial lymphatic system is first seen during the sixth week of development in the form of lymph sacs located next to the jugular veins. During the eighth week, the cisterna chyli forms just dorsal to the aorta, and at the same time, two additional lymphatic sacs corresponding to the iliofemoral vascular pedicles begin forming. Communicating channels connecting the lymph sacs, which will become the thoracic duct, develop during the ninth week.

From this primordial lymphatic system sprout endothelial buds that grow with the venous system to form the peripheral lymphatic plexus (Fig. 65-1). Failure of one of the initial jugular lymphatic sacs to develop proper connections and drainage with the lymphatic system and, subsequently, the venous system may produce focal lymph cysts (cavernous lymphangiomas), also known as cystic hygromas.[1] Similarly, failure of embryologic remnants of lymphatic tissues to connect to efferent channels leads to the development of cystic lymphatic formations (simple capillary lymphangiomas) that, depending on their location, are classified as truncal, mesenteric, intestinal, and retroperitoneal lymphangiomas. Hypoplasia or failure of development of drainage channels connecting the lymphatic systems of extremities to the main primordial lymphatic system of the torso may result in primary lymphedema of the extremities.

Lymphangiogenesis appears to be regulated by the vascular endothelial growth factors C and D (VEGF-C, VEGF-D); their receptor, VEGFR-3; and their binding protein, neuropilin 2 (Nrp2). Consistent with these findings, Nrp2-deficient mice have lymphatic hypoplasia, and heterozygous inactivating mutation of VEGFR-3 is found in Chy mice, an animal model of primary lymphedema, which appears to be the underlying problem in patients with Milroy disease (congenital familial lymphedema).[2] A number of additional genes have recently been found to be related to lymphatic disorders.[3] The best studied at this point are the gene for the forkhead family transcription factor FOXC2 (responsible for the hereditary lymphedema-distichiasis syndrome) and the gene for the transcription factor SOX18 (related to recessive and dominant forms of hypotrichosis-lymphedema-telangiectasia). As more causal genes are identified, the possibility arises for a classification built on patient phenotypes for which the gene is known.[4]

FUNCTION AND STRUCTURE

The lymphatic system is composed of three elements: (1) the initial or terminal lymphatic capillaries, which absorb lymph; (2) the collecting vessels, which serve primarily as conduits for lymph transport; and (3) the lymph nodes, which are interposed in the pathway of the conducting vessels, filtering the lymph and serving a primary immunologic role.

The terminal lymphatics have special structural characteristics that allow entry not only of large macromolecules but even of cells and microbes. Their most important structural feature is a high porosity resulting from a very small number of tight junctions between endothelial cells, a limited and incomplete basement membrane, and anchoring filaments (4 to 10 nm) tethering the interstitial matrix to the endothelial cells. These filaments, once the turgor of the tissue increases, are able to pull on the endothelial cells and essentially introduce large gaps between them, which then allow very low resistance influx of interstitial fluid and macromolecules in the lymphatic channels. The collecting vessels ascend alongside the primary blood vessels of the organ or limb, pass through the regional lymph nodes, and drain into the main lymph channels of the torso. These channels eventually empty into the venous system through the thoracic duct. There are additional communications between the lymphatic and the venous systems. These smaller lymphovenous shunts mostly occur at the level of lymph nodes and around major venous structures, such as the jugular, subclavian, and iliac veins. Several structures in the body contain no lymphatics. Specifically, lymphatics have not been found in the epidermis, cornea, central nervous system, cartilage, tendon, and muscle.

The lymphatic system has three main functions. First, tissue fluid and macromolecules that undergo ultrafiltration at the level of the arterial capillaries are reabsorbed and returned to the

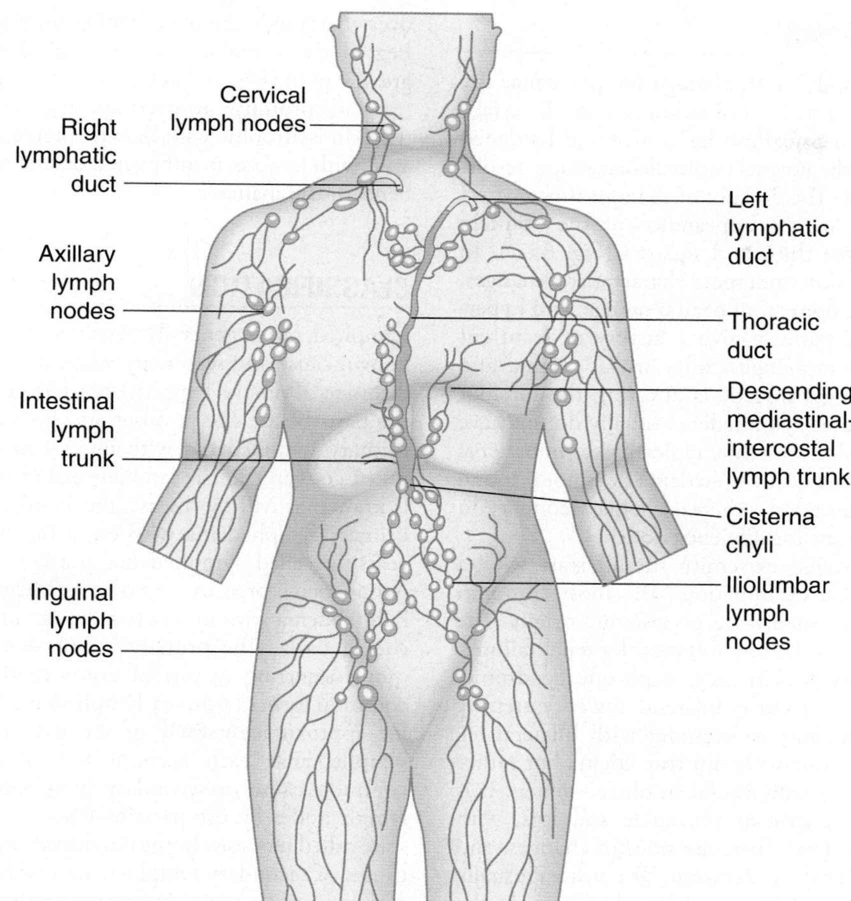

FIGURE 65-1 Major anatomic pathways and lymph node groups of the lymphatic system.

circulation through the lymphatic system. Every day, 50% to 100% of the intravascular proteins are filtered this way in the interstitial space. Normally, they then enter the terminal lymphatics and are transported through the collecting lymphatics back into the venous circulation. Second, antigens, immune cells, microbes, and mutant cells arriving in the interstitial space enter the lymphatic system and are presented to the lymph nodes, which represent the first line of the immune system. Last, at the level of the gastrointestinal tract, lymph vessels are responsible for the uptake and transport of most of the fat absorbed from the bowel. Recent data suggest that a relationship between fat and lymphatics may exist well beyond the gut alone. It appears that peripheral tissue lipid transport and homeostasis may be, in part, determined by lymphatic function, hence the increased fat deposition seen in lymphedema.[3,5]

In contrast to what happens with venous forward flow, lymph's centripetal transport occurs mainly through intrinsic contractility of the individual lymphatic vessels, which in concert with competent valvular mechanisms is effective in establishing constant forward flow of lymph. In addition to the intrinsic contractility, other factors, such as surrounding muscle activity, negative pressure secondary to breathing, and transmitted arterial pulsations, have a lesser role in the forward lymph flow. These secondary factors appear to become more important under conditions of lymph stasis and congestion of the lymphatic vessels.

PATHOPHYSIOLOGY AND STAGING

Lymphedema is the result of an inability of the existing lymphatic system to accommodate the protein and fluid entering the interstitial compartment at the tissue level.[6] In the first stage of lymphedema, impaired lymphatic drainage results in protein-rich fluid accumulation in the interstitial compartment. Clinically, this is manifested as soft pitting edema. In the second stage of lymphedema, the clinical condition is further exacerbated by accumulation of fibroblasts, adipocytes, and, perhaps most important, macrophages in the affected tissues, which culminates in a local inflammatory response. This results in important structural changes from the deposition of connective tissue and adipose elements at the skin and subcutaneous level. In the second stage of lymphedema, tissue edema is more pronounced, is nonpitting, and has a spongy consistency. In the third and most advanced stage of lymphedema, the affected tissues sustain further injury as a result of both the local inflammatory response and recurrent infectious episodes that typically result from minimal subclinical breaks in the skin. Such repeated episodes injure the incompetent, remaining lymphatic channels, progressively worsening the underlying insufficiency of the lymphatic system. This eventually results in excessive subcutaneous fibrosis and scarring with associated severe skin changes characteristic of lymphostatic elephantiasis.

DIFFERENTIAL DIAGNOSIS

In most patients with second- or third-stage lymphedema, the characteristic findings on physical examination can usually establish the diagnosis. The edematous limb has a firm and hardened consistency. There is loss of the normal perimalleolar shape, resulting in a "tree trunk" pattern. The dorsum of the foot is characteristically swollen, resulting in the appearance of the "buffalo hump," and the toes become thick and squared (Fig. 65-2). In advanced lymphedema, the skin undergoes characteristic changes, such as lichenification, development of peau d'orange, and hyperkeratosis.[6] In addition, the patients give a history of recurrent episodes of cellulitis and lymphangitis after trivial trauma and frequently present with fungal infections affecting the forefoot and toes. Patients with isolated lymphedema usually do not have the hyperpigmentation or ulceration one typically sees in patients with chronic venous insufficiency. Lymphedema does not respond significantly to overnight elevation, whereas edema secondary to central organ failure or venous insufficiency does.

The evaluation of a swollen extremity should start with a detailed history and physical examination. The most common causes of bilateral extremity edema are of systemic origin. The most common cause is cardiac failure, followed by renal failure.[7] Hypoproteinemia secondary to cirrhosis, nephrotic syndrome, and malnutrition can also produce bilateral lower extremity edema. Another important cause to consider with bilateral leg enlargement is lipedema. Lipedema is not true edema but rather excessive subcutaneous fat typically found in obese women. It is bilateral, nonpitting, and greatest at the ankle and legs, with characteristic sparing of the feet. There are no skin changes, and the enlargement is not affected by elevation. The history usually indicates that this has been a lifelong problem that "runs in the family."

Once the systemic causes of edema are excluded in the patient with unilateral extremity involvement, edema secondary to venous and lymphatic disease should be entertained. Venous disease is overwhelmingly the most common cause of unilateral leg edema. Leg edema secondary to venous disease is usually pitting and is greatest at the legs and ankles with a sparing of the feet. The edema responds promptly to overnight leg elevation. In the later stages, the skin is atrophic with brawny pigmentation. Ulceration associated with venous insufficiency occurs above or posterior to and beneath the malleoli.

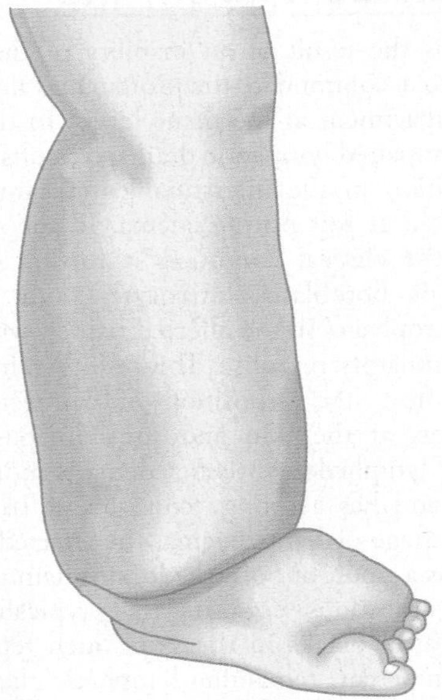

FIGURE 65-2 Lymphedema with characteristic loss of the normal perimalleolar shape, resulting in a "tree trunk" pattern. Dorsum of the foot is characteristically swollen, resulting in the appearance of the "buffalo hump."

CLASSIFICATION

Lymphedema is generally classified as primary when there is no known cause and secondary when its cause is a known disease or disorder.[8] Primary lymphedema has generally been classified on the basis of the age at onset and presence of familial clustering. Primary lymphedema with onset before the first year of life is called congenital. The familial version of congenital lymphedema is known as Milroy disease and is inherited as a dominant trait. Primary lymphedema with onset between the ages of 1 and 35 years is called lymphedema praecox. The familial version of lymphedema praecox is known as Meige disease. Finally, primary lymphedema with onset after the age of 35 years is called lymphedema tarda. The primary lymphedemas are relatively uncommon, occurring in one of every 10,000 individuals. The most common form of primary lymphedema is praecox, which accounts for approximately 80% of the patients. Congenital and tarda lymphedemas each account for 10%. Worldwide, the most common cause of secondary lymphedema is infestation of the lymph nodes by the parasite *Wuchereria bancrofti* in the disease state called filariasis. In the developed countries, the most common causes of secondary lymphedema involve resection or ablation of regional lymph nodes by surgery, radiation therapy, tumor invasion, direct trauma, or, less commonly, an infectious process.

DIAGNOSTIC TESTS

The diagnosis of lymphedema is relatively easy in the patient who presents in the second and third stages of the disease. It can, however, be a difficult diagnosis to make in the first stage, particularly when the edema is mild, pitting, and relieved with simple maneuvers such as elevation.[8,9] For patients with suspected secondary forms of lymphedema, computed tomography and magnetic resonance imaging are valuable and indeed essential for exclusion of underlying oncologic disease states.[10] In patients with known lymph node excision and radiation treatment as the underlying problem of their lymphedema, additional diagnostic studies are rarely needed except as these studies relate to follow-up of an underlying malignant disease. For patients with edema of unknown cause and a suspicion for lymphedema, lymphoscintigraphy is the diagnostic test of choice. When lymphoscintigraphy confirms that lymphatic drainage is delayed, the diagnosis of primary lymphedema should never be made until neoplasia involving the regional and central lymphatic drainage of the limb has been excluded through computed tomography or magnetic resonance imaging. If a more detailed diagnostic interpretation of lymphatic channels is needed for operative planning, contrast lymphangiography may be considered.

Lymphoscintigraphy (or isotope lymphography) has emerged as the test of choice in patients with suspected lymphedema.[10,11] It cannot differentiate between primary and secondary lymphedemas; however, it has a sensitivity of 70% to 90% and a specificity

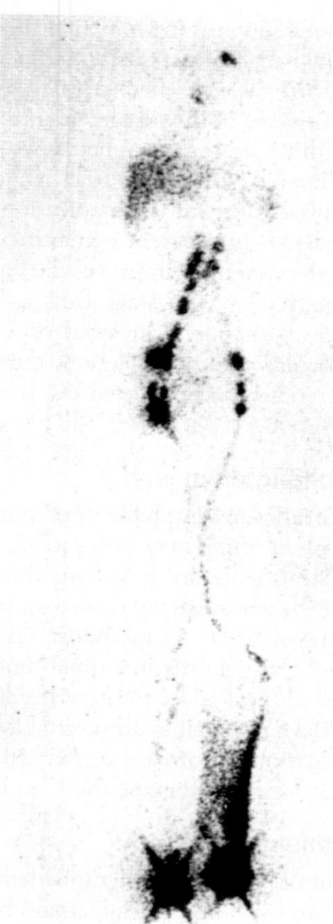

FIGURE 65-3 Lymphoscintigraphic pattern in primary lymphedema. Note area of dermal backflow on the left and diminished number of lymph nodes in the groin. (From Cambria RA, Gloviczki P, Naessens JM, et al: Noninvasive evaluation of the lymphatic system with lymphoscintigraphy: A prospective, semiquantitative analysis in 386 extremities. *J Vasc Surg* 18:773–782, 1993.)

of nearly 100% in differentiating lymphedema from other causes of limb swelling. The test assesses lymphatic function by quantitating the rate of clearance of a radiolabeled macromolecular tracer (Fig. 65-3). The advantages of the technique are that it is simple, safe, and reproducible, with small exposure to radioactivity (approximately 5 mCi). It involves the injection of a small amount of radioiodinated human albumin or technetium Tc 99m–labeled sulfur colloid into the first interdigital space of the foot or hand. Migration of the radiotracer within the skin and subcutaneous lymphatics is easily monitored with a whole body gamma camera, thus producing clear images of the major lymphatic channels in the leg as well as measuring the amount of radioactivity at the inguinal nodes 30 and 60 minutes after injection of the radiolabeled substance in the feet. An uptake value that is less than 0.3% of the total injected dose at 30 minutes is diagnostic of lymphedema. The normal range of uptake is between 0.6% and 1.6%. In patients with edema secondary to venous disease, isotope clearance is usually abnormally rapid, resulting in more than 2% ilioinguinal uptake. Importantly, variation in the degree of edema involving the lower extremity does not appear to significantly change the rate of clearance of the isotope.

Direct contrast lymphangiography provides the finest details of the lymphatic anatomy.[12] However, it is an invasive study that involves exposure and cannulation of lymphatics at the dorsum of the forefoot, followed by slow injection of contrast medium (ethiodized oil). The procedure is tedious, the cannulation often necessitates aid of magnification optics (frequently an operating microscope is needed), and the dissection requires some form of anesthetic. After cannulation of a superficial lymph vessel, contrast material is slowly injected into the lymphatic system. A total of 7 to 10 mL of contrast material is ideal for lower extremity and 4 to 5 mL for upper extremity evaluation. Potential complications include damage of the visualized lymphatics, allergic reactions, and pulmonary embolism if the oil-based contrast agent enters the venous system through lymphovenous anastomoses. Lymphangiography in the present practice of vascular surgery is used infrequently and reserved for the preoperative evaluation of selected patients who are candidates for direct operations on their lymphatic vessels.

New Diagnostic Tests

The field of lymphatic imaging is ever evolving, and we can expect that technologic advances, combined with the development of new contrast agents, will continue to improve diagnostic accuracy.[10] The most promising new test appears to be contrast magnetic resonance lymphangiography.[10,13] The test is performed after intracutaneous injection of gadobenate dimeglumine into the interdigital webs of the dorsal foot. Reported data suggest that the new test is capable of visualizing the anatomy and functional status of lymph flow transport of lymphatic vessels and lymph nodes of lymphedematous limbs.

THERAPY

The majority of lymphedema patients can be treated with a combination of limb elevation, a high-quality compression garment, complex decongestive physical therapy, and compression pump therapy. We currently have no effective medications for the treatment of lymphedema. Operative treatment may be considered for patients with advanced complicated lymphedema for whom management with nonoperative means has failed.

General Therapeutic Measures

All patients with lymphedema should be educated in meticulous skin care and avoidance of injuries.[9,14,15] The patients should always be instructed to see their physicians early for signs of infections because these may progress rapidly to serious systemic infections. Infections should be aggressively and promptly treated with appropriate antibiotics directed at gram-positive cocci. Eczema at the level of the forefoot and toes requires treatment, and hydrocortisone-based creams may be considered. In addition, basic range of motion exercises for the extremities have been shown to be of value in the management of lymphedema in the long term. Finally, the patients should make every effort to maintain ideal body weight.

Elevation and Compression Garments

For lymphedema patients in all stages of disease, management with high-quality elastic garments is necessary at all times except when the legs are elevated above the heart.[16,17] The ideal compression garment is custom fitted and delivers pressures in the range of 30 to 60 mm Hg. Such garments may have the additional benefit of protecting the extremity from injuries, such as burns, lacerations, and insect bites. The patients should avoid standing for prolonged periods and should elevate their legs at night by supporting the foot of the bed on 15-cm blocks.

Complex Decongestive Physical Therapy

This specialized massage technique for patients with lymphedema is designed to stimulate the still functioning lymph vessels, to evacuate stagnant protein-rich fluid by breaking up subcutaneous deposits of fibrous tissue, and to redirect lymph fluid to areas of the body where lymph flow is normal.[18] The technique is initiated on the normal contralateral side of the body, evacuating excessive fluid and preparing first the lymphatic zones of the nonaffected extremity, followed by the zones in the trunk quadrant adjacent to the affected limb, before attention is turned to the swollen extremity. The affected extremity is massaged in a segmental fashion, with the proximal zones being massaged first, proceeding to the distal limb. The technique is time-consuming but effective in reducing the volume of the lymphedematous limbs.[18] After the massage session is complete, the extremity is wrapped with a low-stretch wrap, and then the limb is placed in the custom-fitted garment to maintain the decreased girth obtained with the massage therapy. This kind of therapy is appropriate for patients with all stages of lymphedema.

When the patient is first referred for complex decongestive physical therapy, the patient undergoes daily to weekly massage sessions for up to 8 to 12 weeks. Limb elevation and elastic stockings are a necessary adjunct in this phase. After maximal volume reduction is achieved, the patient returns for maintenance massage treatments every 2 to 3 months.

Compression Pump Therapy

Pneumatic compression pump therapy is another effective method of reducing the volume of the lymphedematous limb by a similar principle to massage therapy. The device consists of a sleeve containing several compartments. The lymphedematous limb is positioned inside the sleeve, and the compartments are serially inflated to milk the stagnant fluid out of the extremity.[19]

When a patient with advanced lymphedema is first referred for therapy, an initial approach with hospitalization for 3 or 4 days involving strict limb elevation, daily complex decongestive physical therapy, and compression pump treatments may be necessary to achieve optimal control of the lymphedema. Patients with cardiac or renal dysfunction should be monitored for fluid overload. After this initial period of intensive therapy, the patients are fitted with high-quality compression garments to maintain the limb volume. Maintenance sessions are then prescribed for the patients on an as-needed basis.

Drug Therapy

Benzopyrones have attracted interest as potentially effective agents in the treatment of lymphedema. This class of medications including coumarin (1,2-benzopyrone) is thought to reduce lymphedema through stimulation of proteolysis by tissue macrophages and stimulation of the peristalsis and pumping action of the collecting lymphatics. Benzopyrones have no anticoagulant activity. The first randomized, crossover trial of coumarin in patients with lymphedema of the arms and legs was reported in 1993.[20] The study concluded that coumarin was more effective than placebo in reducing not only volume but other important parameters, including skin temperature, attacks of secondary acute inflammation, and discomfort of the lymphedematous extremities; skin turgor and suppleness were improved with coumarin. A second randomized, crossover trial was reported in 1999.[21] This study focused on effects of coumarin in women with secondary lymphedema after treatment of breast cancer. The trial investigators found that coumarin was not effective therapy for the specific group of women. Because of the disagreement between these two major trials, the enthusiasm for use of benzopyrones in the United States has been tempered. Additional trials should be undertaken to clarify the potential effects of the medications on primary and secondary lymphedemas in different extremities and stages.

Diuretics may temporarily improve the appearance of the lymphedematous extremity with stage I disease, leading patients to request continuous therapy. However, other than producing temporary intravascular volume depletion, there is no long-term benefit. Thus, diuretics have no role in the treatment of lymphedema at any stage.

Molecular Lymphangiogenesis

Fundamental discoveries in lymphatic development have pointed to the potential of exciting new treatments for lymphedema. These molecular treatments are based on the activation of the VEGFR-3 pathway by administration of cognate ligands VEGF-C and VEGF-D using a variety of methods.[22] At this point, these treatments have been tested only in animal models, with promising results. Formal clinical trials are now needed to evaluate the therapeutic potential and possible untoward effects (including the possibility of stimulation of dormant tumor cells as a consequence of increased angiogenesis) of therapeutic lymphangiogenesis.[23]

Operative Treatment

Ninety-five percent of patients with lymphedema can be managed nonoperatively. Surgical intervention may be considered for patients with stage II and stage III lymphedema who have severe functional impairment, recurrent episodes of lymphangitis, and severe pain despite optimal medical therapy. Two main categories of operations are available for the care of patients with lymphedema: reconstructive and excisional.

Reconstructive operations[24,25] should be considered for those patients with proximal (either primary or secondary) obstruction of the extremity lymphatic circulation with preserved, dilated lymphatics peripheral to the obstruction. In these patients, the residual dilated lymphatics can be anastomosed either to nearby veins or to transposed healthy lymphatic channels (usually mobilized or harvested from the healthy lower extremity) in an attempt to restore effective drainage of the lymphedematous extremity. Some of the most common candidates for reconstructive procedures are patients with upper extremity lymphedema secondary to axillary lymphadenectomy or patients with leg lymphedema secondary to inguinal or pelvic lymphadenectomy. Treatment of selected lymphedema patients with lymphovenous anastomoses or lymphovenous bypass or lymphaticolymphatic bypass has resulted in objective improvement in 30% to 80% of the patients, with an average initial reduction in the excess limb volume of 30% to 84%.[26-29]

For those patients with primary lymphedema who have hypoplastic and fibrotic distal lymphatic vessels, such reconstructions are not an option. For such patients, a surgical strategy involving transfer of lymphatic-bearing tissue (portion of the greater omentum) into the affected limb has been attempted. This is intended to connect the residual hypoplastic lymphatic channels of the leg to competent lymphatics in the transferred tissue. Omental flap operations have been found to have poor results.[30] Alternatively, a segment of the ileum can be disconnected from the rest of the bowel, stripped of its mucosa, and mobilized to be

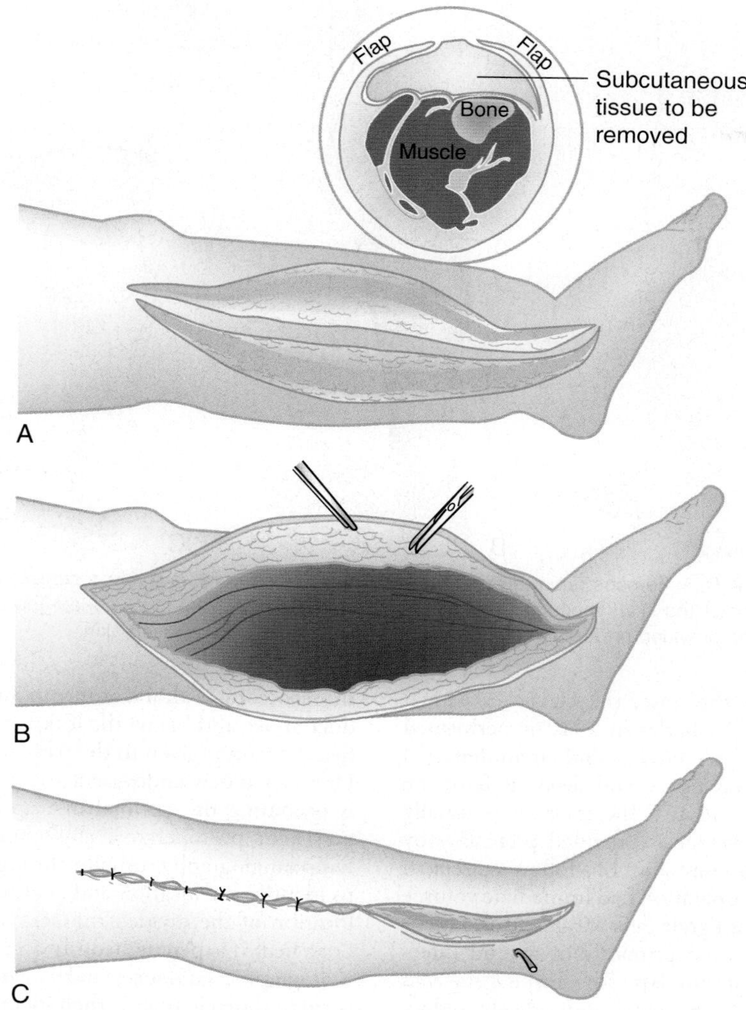

FIGURE 65-4 A-C, Schematic representation of the Kontoleon or Homan procedure. Relatively thick skin flaps are raised anteriorly and posteriorly, and all subcutaneous tissue beneath the flaps and the underlying medial calf deep fascia are removed along with the necessary redundant skin.

sewn onto the cut surface of residual ilioinguinal nodes in an attempt to bridge the lower extremity with mesenteric lymphatics. When this enteromesenteric bridge procedure was applied to a group of eight carefully selected patients, the outcomes were promising, with six patients showing sustained clinical improvement in long follow-up.[31]

Excisional operations are essentially the only viable option for patients without residual lymphatics of adequate size for reconstructive procedures. For patients with recalcitrant stage II and early stage III lymphedema in whom the edema is moderate and the skin is relatively healthy, an excisional procedure that removes a large segment of the lymphedematous subcutaneous tissues and overlying skin is the procedure of choice. This palliative procedure was introduced by Kontoleon in 1918 and was later popularized by Homan as "staged subcutaneous excision underneath flaps" (Fig. 65-4). The operative approach starts with a medial incision extending from the level of the medial malleolus through the calf into the midthigh.[32,33] Flaps about 1 to 2 cm thick are elevated anteriorly and posteriorly, and all subcutaneous tissue beneath the flaps along with the underlying medial calf deep fascia is removed with the redundant skin. The sural nerve is preserved. After the first-stage procedure is completed and if additional lymphedematous tissue removal is necessary, a second operation is performed usually 3 to 6 months later. The second-stage operation is performed by similar techniques through an incision on the lateral aspect of the limb. In a recent long-term follow-up study, 80% of patients undergoing staged subcutaneous excision underneath flaps had significant and long-lasting reduction in extremity size associated with improved function and extremity contour. Wound complications were encountered in 10% of the patients.[32]

A minimally invasive version of the Kontoleon procedure is gaining increasing support among lymphedema experts.[34,35] A number of reports have demonstrated that use of liposuction through small incisions is safe and is able to achieve control, at least on a short-term basis, of clinically disabling conditions associated with advanced stages of lymphedema. Surgeons with experience in this technique recommend initial conservative treatment of pitting lymphedema to remove excess fluid, followed by liposuction to remove remaining excess volume bothersome to the patient.[35]

When the lymphedema is extremely pronounced and the skin is unhealthy and infected, the simple reducing operation of

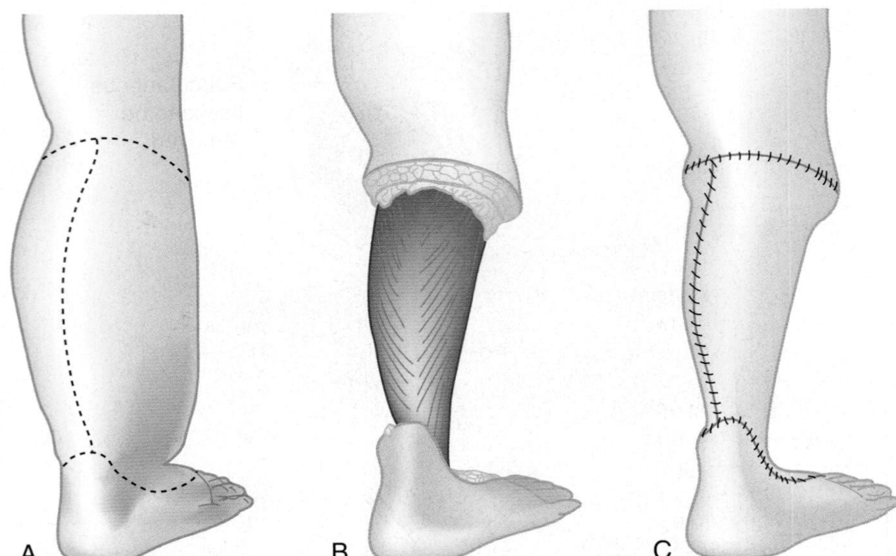

FIGURE 65-5 A-C, Schematic representation of the Charles procedure. It involves complete and circumferential excision of the skin, subcutaneous tissue, and deep fascia of the involved leg and dorsum of the foot. Coverage is provided preferably by full-thickness grafting from the excised skin.

Kontoleon is not adequate. In this case, the classic excisional operation originally described by Charles in 1912 is performed (Fig. 65-5). The procedure involves complete and circumferential excision of the skin, subcutaneous tissue, and deep fascia of the involved leg and dorsum of the foot.[36] The excision is usually performed in one stage, and coverage is provided preferably by full-thickness grafting from the excised skin. In a follow-up report, patients subjected to the Charles operation had immediate volume and circumference reduction. Skin graft take was 88%, and complications of the operation consisted primarily of wound infections, hematomas, and necrosis of skin flaps. The hospital stay was 21 to 36 days.[37] Although this is a successful and radically reducing operation, the behavior in the healing skin graft is unpredictable. Between 10% and 15% of the grafted segments do not take and can be difficult to manage because of frequent localized sloughing, excessive scarring, focal recurrent infections, and hyperkeratosis or dermatitis. These complications seem to be worse in patients in whom leg resurfacing is performed with split-thickness grafts from the opposite extremity. In advanced cases, the exophytic changes within the grafted skin, chronic cellulitis, and skin breakdown may eventually lead to leg amputation.[38]

CHYLOTHORAX

Chylous pleural effusion is usually secondary to thoracic duct trauma (usually iatrogenic after chest surgery) and rarely a manifestation of advanced malignant disease with lymphatic metastasis.[39] Presence of chylomicrons on lipoprotein analysis and a triglyceride level of more than 110 mg/dL in the pleural fluid are diagnostic. Initially, patients can be treated nonoperatively with tube thoracostomy, medium-chain triglyceride diet or total parenteral nutrition, and octreotide/somatostatin therapy.[40] For patients with thoracic duct injury and an effusion that persists after 1 week of treatment with appropriate diet, octreotide, and thoracostomy drainage, an intervention should be considered to identify and to occlude the thoracic duct above and below the leak. The operative approach of choice has been video-assisted thoracoscopy or thoracotomy to identify and to ligate the thoracic duct above and below the leak (the site of the leak can be identified if cream is given to the patient a few hours before operation). However, a new endovascular technique has been introduced and is becoming the optimal first approach for the management of persistent postoperative chylothorax. The approach starts with lymphangiography, usually through a groin lymph node access, to identify the location and anatomy of the cisterna chyli and the location of the divided thoracic duct. Once the cisterna chyli is opacified, it is percutaneously accessed with a spinal needle, using radiographic guidance, and is catheterized. The location of the divided thoracic duct is then identified with repeated lymphangiography, and the duct is embolized. In expert hands, this technique has a more than 50% success rate.[41,42] For patients with cancer-related chylothorax and persistent drainage despite optimal chemotherapy and radiation therapy, pleurodesis is highly successful in preventing recurrences.

CHYLOPERITONEUM

In contrast to chylothorax, the most common cause of chylous ascites is congenital lymphatic abnormalities in children and malignant disease involving the abdominal lymph nodes in adults. Postoperative injury to abdominal lymphatics resulting in chylous ascites is rare.[43] Presence of chylomicrons on lipoprotein analysis and a triglyceride level of more than 110 mg/dL are diagnostic. Initial treatment includes paracentesis followed by medium-chain triglyceride diet or total parenteral nutrition. In patients with postoperative chyloperitoneum, if ascites does not respond after 1 to 2 weeks of nonoperative management, percutaneous embolization[41,42] or surgical exploration should be employed to identify and to occlude or ligate the leaking lymphatic duct. Congenital and malignant causes should be given longer periods (up to 4 to 6 weeks) of nonoperative management. If ascites persists in patients with congenital ascites, lymphoscintigraphy or lymphangiography is performed before an attempt is made to control the leak with celiotomy. At the time of exploration, control of the leak can be achieved by ligation of leaking lymphatic vessels or resection of the bowel associated with the leak. Patients with malignant neoplasms should receive aggressive management for their underlying disease, which generally is effective at controlling the chyloperitoneum.

TUMORS OF THE LYMPHATICS

Lymphangiomas are the lymphatic analogue of the hemangiomas of blood vessels. They are generally divided into two types, (1) simple or capillary lymphangioma and (2) cavernous lymphangioma or cystic hygroma.[44] They are thought to represent isolated and sequestered segments of the lymphatic system that retain the ability to produce lymph. As the volume of lymph inside the cystic tumor increases, it grows larger within the surrounding tissues. The majority of these benign tumors are present at birth, and 90% of them can be identified by the end of the first year of life. The cavernous lymphangiomas almost invariably occur in the neck or the axilla and very rarely in the retroperitoneum. The simple capillary lymphangiomas also tend to occur subcutaneously in the head and neck region as well as in the axilla. Rarely, however, they can be found in the trunk within the internal organs or the connective tissue in and about the abdominal or thoracic cavities. The treatment of lymphangiomas should be surgical excision, with care taken to preserve all normal surrounding infiltrated structures.

Lymphangiosarcoma is a rare tumor that develops as a complication of long-standing (usually more than 10 years) lymphedema.[45] Clinically, the patients present with acute worsening of the edema and appearance of subcutaneous nodules that have a propensity toward hemorrhage and ulceration. The tumor can be treated, like other sarcomas, with preoperative chemotherapy and radiation followed by surgical excision, which usually may take the form of radical amputation. Overall, the tumor has a very poor prognosis.[46]

SELECTED REFERENCES

Baumeister RGH: Lymphedema. In Cronenwett JL, Johnston KW, editors: *Rutherford's vascular surgery*, ed 8, Philadelphia, 2014, Elsevier Saunders, pp 1028–1042.

This authoritative treatise provides a succinct summary of the treatment of lymphatic disorders.

Campisi CC, Ryan M, Boccardo F, et al: A single-site technique of multiple lymphatic-venous anastomoses for the treatment of peripheral lymphedema: Long-term clinical outcome. *J Reconstr Microsurg* 2015. [Epub ahead of print].

Granzow JW, Soderberg JM, Kaji AH, et al: Review of current surgical treatments for lymphedema. *Ann Surg Oncol* 21:1195–1201, 2014.

These comprehensive reviews summarize the important elements in the management of patients with lymphedema.

Rockson SG: Diagnosis and management of lymphatic vascular disease. *J Am Coll Cardiol* 52:799–806, 2008.

The diagnosis and treatment of peripheral lymphedema. 2009 Consensus Document of the International Society of Lymphology. *Lymphology* 42:51–60, 2009.

These two reviews illustrate the current knowledge and controversies in the pathophysiology, classification, natural history, differential diagnosis, and treatment of lymphedema.

REFERENCES

1. Levine C: Primary disorders of the lymphatic vessels—a unified concept. *J Pediatr Surg* 24:233–240, 1989.
2. Alitalo K, Tammela T, Petrova TV: Lymphangiogenesis in development and human disease. *Nature* 438:946–953, 2005.
3. Mortimer PS, Rockson SG: New developments in clinical aspects of lymphatic disease. *J Clin Invest* 124:915–921, 2014.
4. Connell FC, Gordon K, Brice G, et al: The classification and diagnostic algorithm for primary lymphatic dysplasia: an update from 2010 to include molecular findings. *Clin Genet* 84:303–314, 2013.
5. Dixon JB: Lymphatic lipid transport: Sewer or subway? *Trends Endocrinol Metab* 21:480–487, 2010.
6. Browse NL, Stewart G: Lymphoedema: Pathophysiology and classification. *J Cardiovasc Surg (Torino)* 26:91–106, 1985.
7. Cho S, Atwood JE: Peripheral edema. *Am J Med* 113:580–586, 2002.
8. Radhakrishnan K, Rockson SG: The clinical spectrum of lymphatic disease. *Ann N Y Acad Sci* 1131:155–184, 2008.
9. Rockson SG: Diagnosis and management of lymphatic vascular disease. *J Am Coll Cardiol* 52:799–806, 2008.
10. Barrett T, Choyke PL, Kobayashi H: Imaging of the lymphatic system: New horizons. *Contrast Media Mol Imaging* 1:230–245, 2006.
11. Szuba A, Shin WS, Strauss HW, et al: The third circulation: Radionuclide lymphoscintigraphy in the evaluation of lymphedema. *J Nucl Med* 44:43–57, 2003.
12. Weissleder H, Weissleder R: Interstitial lymphangiography: Initial clinical experience with a dimeric nonionic contrast agent. *Radiology* 170:371–374, 1989.
13. Liu NF, Lu Q, Jiang ZH, et al: Anatomic and functional evaluation of the lymphatics and lymph nodes in diagnosis of lymphatic circulation disorders with contrast magnetic resonance lymphangiography. *J Vasc Surg* 49:980–987, 2009.
14. The diagnosis and treatment of peripheral lymphedema. 2009 Consensus Document of the International Society of Lymphology. *Lymphology* 42:51–60, 2009.
15. Kerchner K, Fleischer A, Yosipovitch G: Lower extremity lymphedema update: Pathophysiology, diagnosis, and treatment guidelines. *J Am Acad Dermatol* 59:324–331, 2008.
16. Yasuhara H, Shigematsu H, Muto T: A study of the advantages of elastic stockings for leg lymphedema. *Int Angiol* 15:272–277, 1996.
17. Badger CM, Peacock JL, Mortimer PS: A randomized, controlled, parallel-group clinical trial comparing multilayer bandaging followed by hosiery versus hosiery alone in the treatment of patients with lymphedema of the limb. *Cancer* 88:2832–2837, 2000.
18. Franzeck UK, Spiegel I, Fischer M, et al: Combined physical therapy for lymphedema evaluated by fluorescence microlymphography and lymph capillary pressure measurements. *J Vasc Res* 34:306–311, 1997.

19. Richmand DM, O'Donnell TF, Jr, Zelikovski A: Sequential pneumatic compression for lymphedema. A controlled trial. *Arch Surg* 120:1116–1119, 1985.
20. Casley-Smith JR, Morgan RG, Piller NB: Treatment of lymphedema of the arms and legs with 5,6-benzo-[alpha]-pyrone. *N Engl J Med* 329:1158–1163, 1993.
21. Loprinzi CL, Kugler JW, Sloan JA, et al: Lack of effect of coumarin in women with lymphedema after treatment for breast cancer. *N Engl J Med* 340:346–350, 1999.
22. Nakamura K, Rockson SG: Molecular targets for therapeutic lymphangiogenesis in lymphatic dysfunction and disease. *Lymphat Res Biol* 6:181–189, 2008.
23. Tervala T, Suominen E, Saaristo A: Targeted treatment for lymphedema and lymphatic metastasis. *Ann N Y Acad Sci* 1131:215–224, 2008.
24. Campisi C, Boccardo F: Lymphedema and microsurgery. *Microsurgery* 22:74–80, 2002.
25. Gloviczki P: Principles of surgical treatment of chronic lymphoedema. *Int Angiol* 18:42–46, 1999.
26. Damstra RJ, Voesten HG, van Schelven WD, et al: Lymphatic venous anastomosis (LVA) for treatment of secondary arm lymphedema. A prospective study of 11 LVA procedures in 10 patients with breast cancer related lymphedema and a critical review of the literature. *Breast Cancer Res Treat* 113:199–206, 2009.
27. Nagase T, Gonda K, Inoue K, et al: Treatment of lymphedema with lymphaticovenular anastomoses. *Int J Clin Oncol* 10:304–310, 2005.
28. Baumeister RG, Frick A: [The microsurgical lymph vessel transplantation]. *Handchir Mikrochir Plast Chir* 35:202–209, 2003.
29. Campisi CC, Ryan M, Boccardo F, et al: A single-site technique of multiple lymphatic-venous anastomoses for the treatment of peripheral lymphedema: Long-term clinical outcome. *J Reconstr Microsurg* 2015. [Epub ahead of print].
30. Goldsmith HS: Long term evaluation of omental transposition for chronic lymphedema. *Ann Surg* 180:847–849, 1974.
31. Hurst PA, Stewart G, Kinmonth JB, et al: Long term results of the enteromesenteric bridge operation in the treatment of primary lymphoedema. *Br J Surg* 72:272–274, 1985.
32. Miller TA, Wyatt LE, Rudkin GH: Staged skin and subcutaneous excision for lymphedema: A favorable report of long-term results. *Plast Reconstr Surg* 102:1486–1498, discussion 1499-1501, 1998.
33. Wyatt LE, Miller TA: Lymphedema and tumors of the lymphatics. In Moore W, editor: *Vascular surgery, a comprehensive review*, Philadelphia, 1998, WB Saunders, pp 829–843.
34. Espinosa-de-Los-Monteros A, Hinojosa CA, Abarca L, et al: Compression therapy and liposuction of lower legs for bilateral hereditary primary lymphedema praecox. *J Vasc Surg* 49:222–224, 2009.
35. Brorson H, Ohlin K, Olsson G, et al: Controlled compression and liposuction treatment for lower extremity lymphedema. *Lymphology* 41:52–63, 2008.
36. Dellon AL, Hoopes JE: The Charles procedure for primary lymphedema. Long-term clinical results. *Plast Reconstr Surg* 60:589–595, 1977.
37. Dandapat MC, Mohapatro SK, Mohanty SS: Filarial lymphoedema and elephantiasis of lower limb: A review of 44 cases. *Br J Surg* 73:451–453, 1986.
38. Miller TA: Charles procedure for lymphedema: A warning. *Am J Surg* 139:290–292, 1980.
39. Platis IE, Nwogu CE: Chylothorax. *Thorac Surg Clin* 16:209–214, 2006.
40. Bender B, Murthy V, Chamberlain RS: The changing management of chylothorax in the modern era. *Eur J Cardiothorac Surg* 49:18–24, 2016.
41. Lee EW, Shin JH, Ko HK, et al: Lymphangiography to treat postoperative lymphatic leakage: A technical review. *Korean J Radiol* 15:724–732, 2014.
42. Lyon S, Mott N, Koukounaras J, et al: Role of interventional radiology in the management of chylothorax: A review of the current management of high output chylothorax. *Cardiovasc Intervent Radiol* 36:599–607, 2013.
43. Aalami OO, Allen DB, Organ CH, Jr: Chylous ascites: A collective review. *Surgery* 128:761–778, 2000.
44. Ha J, Yu YC, Lannigan F: A review of the management of lymphangiomas. *Curr Pediatr Rev* 10:238–248, 2014.
45. Nakazono T, Kudo S, Matsuo Y, et al: Angiosarcoma associated with chronic lymphedema (Stewart-Treves syndrome) of the leg: MR imaging. *Skeletal Radiol* 29:413–416, 2000.
46. Sordillo PP, Chapman R, Hajdu SI, et al: Lymphangiosarcoma. *Cancer* 48:1674–1679, 1981.

SECTION XIII

Specialties in General Surgery

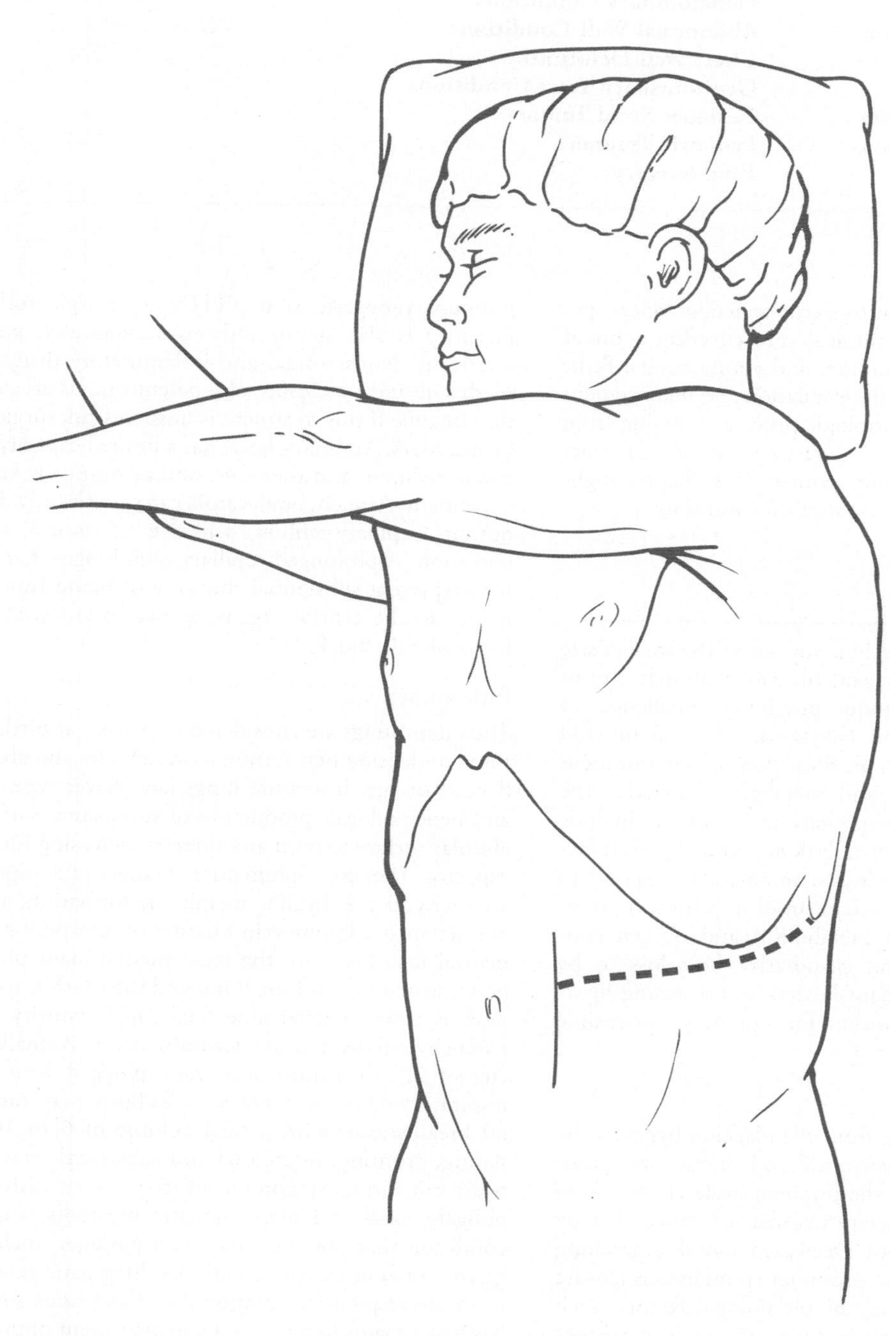

66 CHAPTER

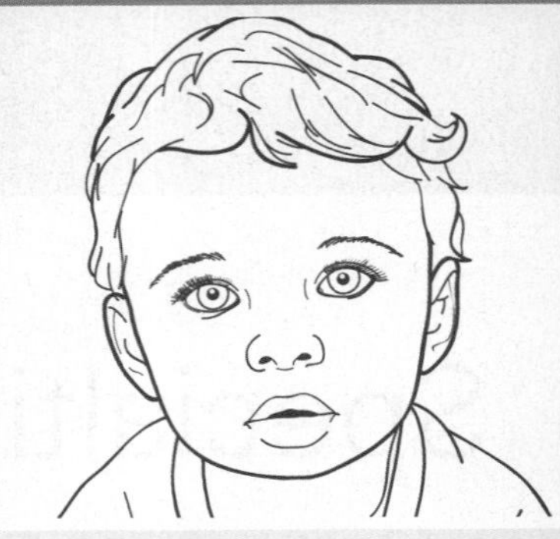

Pediatric Surgery

Dai H. Chung

OUTLINE

Pediatric surgery is the last bastion of a true general surgical specialty, delivering comprehensive surgical care covering a broad scope of conditions in infants, children, and young adults. Pediatric surgeons are challenged with the evaluation and management of a wide spectrum of surgical pathologic processes ranging from head and neck lesions to thoracic and gastrointestinal (GI) tract anomalies, oncologic disorders, and trauma. This chapter highlights common and unique pediatric surgical conditions.

NEWBORN PHYSIOLOGY

The newborn physiology is unique in many ways. The smaller size of the patient, volume capacities, and functional immaturity of various organ systems present unique physiologic challenges in the management of surgical disease. Newborns are at risk for cold stress and must be maintained in an ideal thermal environment to reduce oxygen consumption and metabolic demands. The major contributing factors for hypothermia in infants include their relatively large body surface area, lack of hair and subcutaneous tissue, and greater insensible losses. Infants also respond to cold ambient temperature by a mechanism of nonshivering thermogenesis, whereby increases in metabolism and oxygen consumption occur. For radiant and evaporative heat loss to be avoided, the use of overhead radiant heaters and warming lights is a common practice, but a caution for significant insensible water losses should be made.

Cardiovascular

In fetal circulation, arterial blood from the placenta bypasses the lungs through the patent foramen ovale and ductus arteriosus. With the newborn's first breath, the foramen ovale closes, along with a precipitous drop in pulmonary vascular resistance, thereby increasing pulmonary blood flow. Decreased blood flow along with a higher oxygen content also promotes spontaneous closure of the ductus arteriosus. A variety of physiologic factors, such as hypoxemia, acidosis, and sepsis, can contribute to persistent pulmonary hypertension (PPHN) with right-to-left shunt. Prematurity is also significantly associated with persistent ductus arteriosus. Nonsteroidal anti-inflammatory drugs, such as indomethacin, induce closure of a patent ductus arteriosus in premature infants. If this treatment is unsuccessful, surgical ligation may be necessary. An infant heart has a limited capacity to increase the stroke volume, and therefore cardiac output is largely heart rate dependent. As such, bradycardia can significantly diminish cardiac output. Capillary refill is a sensitive indicator of adequate cardiac perfusion. A prolonged capillary refill longer than 1 to 2 seconds may represent substantial shunting of blood from the peripheral tissues to the central organs, as may occur with cardiogenic or hypovolemic shock.

Pulmonary

The infant lungs are considered immature at birth, and they continue to develop new terminal bronchioles and alveoli until about 8 years of age. Immature lungs have fewer type II pneumocytes and hence a lower production of surfactant. Surfactant regulates alveolar surface tension and thereby increasing functional residual capacity. Therefore, premature infants are at significant risk for alveolar collapse, hyaline membrane formation, and barotrauma. Surfactant is a lipoprotein mixture of phospholipid, protein, and neutral fats. Lecithin, the most predominant phospholipid, can be measured in amniotic fluid, and the lecithin-to-sphingomyelin ratio is used to determine fetal lung maturity. In addition to parenchymal disease, the newborn airway is small (tracheal diameter of 2.5 to 4 mm) and easily plugged with secretions. The respiratory rate for a normal newborn may range from 40 to 60 breaths/min, with a tidal volume of 6 to 10 mL/kg. Nasal flaring, grunting, intercostal and substernal retractions, and cyanosis constitute symptoms of respiratory distress. Infants are obligate nasal and diaphragmatic breathers, and therefore any condition that obstructs the nasal passages (including the nasogastric tube) or interferes with diaphragmatic function may result in severe respiratory compromise. Exogenous surfactant therapy has had a major impact on the management of premature infants.

This has resulted in improved survival and decreased incidence of bronchopulmonary dysplasia, a condition characterized by oxygen dependence, radiologic abnormality, and chronic respiratory symptoms beyond the first 28 days of life. The administration of nitric oxide gas, a potent inducer of vascular smooth muscle relaxation, has also proved useful in infants with PPHN.

Immunology

Infants have lower levels of immunoglobulins (A, G, and M) and of the C3b component of complement at birth. As such, premature infants are at higher risk for systemic infection. The evaluation of sepsis in neonates requires an extensive workup of surveillance cultures of blood, urine, and cerebrospinal fluid as well as a complete blood count with platelet count, differential smear, and plain radiography. Sepsis may result from various invasive devices and therapies that are essential to the care of premature infants, such as prolonged endotracheal intubation, umbilical catheters, and bladder catheterization. Based on subtle clinical changes (e.g., decreased tolerance of enteral feeding, temperature instability, reduced capillary refill, tachypnea, irritability), implementation of empirical antibiotic therapy targeted at common bacterial pathogens, such as group B beta-hemolytic streptococcus, methicillin-resistant *Staphylococcus aureus,* and *Escherichia coli,* may be lifesaving.

FLUIDS, ELECTROLYTES, AND NUTRITION

Fluid and Electrolytes

Fluid and electrolyte therapy requires careful assessment of total fluid intake and losses and electrolyte imbalances before initiation of fluid administration. It also requires frequent monitoring during the course of therapy to ensure the proper response. Accurate estimation of intravenous (IV) fluid and electrolytes is critical, especially in small infants with a narrow margin for error. Because of higher insensible water losses through a thin immature skin barrier, fluid requirements for premature infants are substantial. Insensible water losses are directly related to gestational age, ranging from 45 to 60 mL/kg/day for premature infants weighing less than 1500 g to 30 to 35 mL/kg/day for term infants. Radiant heat warmers, phototherapy for hyperbilirubinemia, and respiratory distress can result in additional fluid loss. In the first 3 to 5 days of life, there is a physiologic water loss of up to 10% of the body weight of the infant. As such, fluid replacement volumes are less during the first several days of life. These fluid volumes are regarded as estimates and may change according to differing clinical conditions.

Fluid requirements are calculated according to body weight (Table 66-1). During the first few days of life, the fluid recommendations are conservative; however, infants require 100 to 130 mL/kg/day for maintenance fluids by the fourth day of life. Infants with conditions that are associated with excessive fluid losses (e.g., gastroschisis) can require as much as 1.5 times maintenance volume. The best indicators of sufficient fluid intake are urine output and osmolarity. The minimum urine output in a newborn and young child is 1 to 2 mL/kg/day. Although adults can concentrate urine in the range of 1200 mOsm/kg, an infant responding to water deprivation is able to concentrate urine only up to approximately 700 mOsm/kg. Clinically, this indicates that greater fluid intake and urine output are necessary to excrete the solute load presented to the kidney during normal metabolism. In general, the daily requirements for sodium and potassium are 2 to 4 and 1 to 2 mEq/kg, respectively. These requirements are usually met with 5% dextrose in 0.45% normal saline with 20 mEq/liter of potassium at the calculated maintenance rate. Fluid losses from gastric drainage, ostomy output, or diarrhea should also be carefully assessed and replaced with an appropriate solution. Gastric losses should be replaced in equal volumes with 0.45% normal saline with 20 mEq/liter of potassium. Diarrheal, pancreatic, and biliary losses are replaced with isotonic lactated Ringer solution. Hypovolemia due to acute hemorrhage should be corrected with rapid transfusion of blood products at a bolus of 10 to 20 mL/kg of packed red blood cells, plasma, or 5% albumin.

Nutrition

Calorie Requirements

Energy requirements vary significantly from birth to childhood and also under different clinical conditions (Table 66-2). The parameter that is most indicative of sufficient delivery of calories in neonates is appropriate weight gain. Total daily calorie requirements and the weight growth curve plateau with age. Nearly 50% of the energy used in term infants younger than 2 weeks and 60% of energy intake in premature infants weighing less than 1200 g is devoted to growth. A general guideline for the enteral calorie requirement of infants is 120 calories/kg/day to achieve an ideal weight gain on average of about 1% of body weight/day. The standard infant formulas as well as breast milk contain 20 calories/ounce. Formulas with higher calorie density are available for those who are unable to consume sufficient volumes to meet their calorie requirements or require fluid restriction. Breast milk or a protein hydrolysate formula (e.g., Pregestimil, Alimentum) should be considered when initiating enteral feedings in infants with compromised gut functions, such as necrotizing enterocolitis or short bowel syndrome. In general, continuous feedings are initiated for infants with a stressed gut and later transitioned to bolus feedings. The enteral feeding tolerance is carefully monitored by assessing for abdominal girth, gastric residuals, and stool output.

TABLE 66-1 Daily Fluid Requirements

WEIGHT	VOLUME
Premature infants <2 kg	140-150 mL/kg/day
Infants, 2-10 kg	100 mL/kg/day
Toddler, 10-20 kg	1000 mL + 50 mL/kg/day for weight 10-20 kg
Children >20 kg	1500 mL + 20 mL/kg/day for weight >20 kg

TABLE 66-2 Average Calorie and Protein Requirements

AGE	CALORIES (kcal/kg/day)	PROTEIN (g/kg/day)
0-1 year	90-120	2.0-3.5
1-7 years	75-90	2.0-2.5
7-12 years	60-75	2.0
12-18 years	30-60	1.5
>18 years	25-30	1.0

Carbohydrate

Carbohydrates are stored mainly as glycogen in the liver and muscles. Because newborn liver and muscle masses are disproportionately smaller than those of the adult, infants are susceptible to hypoglycemia with risks for seizure and neurologic impairment. The minimum glucose infusion rate for neonates is 4 to 6 mg/kg/min. This rate must be calculated daily while the infant is receiving parenteral nutrition. For total parenteral nutrition (TPN), the glucose infusion rate is increased in daily increments of 1 to 2 mg/kg/min to a maximum of 10 to 12 mg/kg/min. Ultimately, the amount of weight gain should dictate the need to continue advancing glucose calories. Furthermore, hyperglycemia from too rapid advancement or underlying sepsis should be avoided because it can lead to rapid hyperosmolarity and dehydration.

Protein

The average intake of protein represents approximately 15% of the total daily calories and ranges from 2 to 3.5 g/kg/day in infants. This protein requirement is reduced in half by the age of 12 years and approaches the adult requirement (1 g/kg/day) by 18 years of age (see Table 66-2). The provision of greater amounts of protein relative to nonprotein calories will result in rising blood urea nitrogen levels. The nonprotein calorie (carbohydrate plus fat calories)–to–protein calorie ratio (when expressed in grams of nitrogen) is therefore not less than 150 to 1. For infants receiving parenteral nutrition, protein administration usually starts at 0.5 g/kg/day and advances in daily increments of 0.5 g/kg/day to the target goal of approximately 3.5 g/kg/day.

Fat

Fat is the other major source of nonprotein calories. Linoleic acid, an 18-carbon chain with two double bonds, is considered an essential fatty acid; its deficiency results in dryness, rash, and desquamation of skin. In pediatric patients, fat is provided as a major source of calories to prevent the development of essential fatty acid deficiency. The lipid requirements for growth are significant, and fat is a robust calorie source. Similar to protein, fat infusions are started at 0.5 g/kg/day and advanced up to 2.5 to 3.5 g/kg/day. In infants with unconjugated hyperbilirubinemia, fat is administered with caution because fatty acids may displace bilirubin from albumin. The free unconjugated bilirubin may then cross the blood-brain barrier and can lead to kernicterus, resulting in mental retardation.

Total Parenteral Nutrition

TPN is reserved for infants for whom GI delivery of adequate daily calories is not feasible for various reasons. Deposition of body fat occurs in the later stages of fetal development, leaving premature infants poorly equipped to deal with periods of starvation as rapid as 2 to 3 days. Thus, an infant's need for parenteral nutrition should be addressed early. Unlike in adults, the key to prescribing pediatric TPN is that the IV infusion rate remains the same, whereas the concentration of nutrients is gradually increased daily until nutritional goals are met. Infants with surgical conditions often become cholestatic, usually caused by prolonged TPN support; however, other causes should be ruled out. Serum bile acid levels are usually elevated first, then direct bilirubin concentration, followed by liver enzyme levels. The ideal treatment for TPN-associated cholestasis is enteral feeding. The use of omega-3 fat emulsion (Omegaven) has helped infants with TPN-induced cholestasis. A medium-chain triglyceride–containing formula is used, and if an infant is receiving total enteral nutrition, fat-soluble vitamins should be supplemented.

HEAD AND NECK LESIONS

Dermoid and Epidermoid Cysts

Dermoid and epidermoid cysts are slow-growing benign lesions that typically occur in the scalp and the skull of infants and children. These cysts usually arise from part of the dermal or epidermal tissues, forming a small cyst filled with normal skin components. Dermoids may contain hair, teeth, and skin glands. Epidermoids typically contain only epidermal tissue and keratin debris. They commonly occur on the forehead, lateral corner of the eyebrow, or anterior fontanelle or in the postauricular space. They are generally asymptomatic but may slowly increase in size over time. Cysts may erode into the skull and in the extremely rare situation may even penetrate into the brain. Most scalp lesions can be accurately diagnosed by physical examination alone. However, imaging studies may be important for those at midline to rule out a communicating cephalocele. Surgical excision is recommended.

Lymphadenopathy

Enlarged lymph nodes are one of the most common pediatric conditions resulting in referral to a pediatric surgeon for evaluation, biopsy, or excision. They occur usually along the sternocleidomastoid muscle border, often in clusters. The cause is unknown but thought to be multifocal. A detailed history and physical examination are sufficient to determine surgical indications. The use of ultrasound has become prevalent recently. In most healthy children, cervical lymphadenopathy presents as a small, mobile, rubbery, palpable mass in the anterior cervical triangle. However, relatively fixed, nontender, progressively enlarging nodes in the supraclavicular region should raise suspicion for more serious underlying conditions. Other symptoms, such as night sweats and recent weight loss, should also prompt a thorough investigation. Chest radiography can be a helpful screening modality to detect mediastinal adenopathy. Patients with acute, bilateral cervical lymphadenitis from respiratory viral infectious causes (e.g., adenovirus, influenza virus, respiratory syncytial virus) are observed alone. *S. aureus* and group A streptococcus are responsible for the majority of acute pyogenic lymphadenitis. When nodes become fluctuant because of central areas of liquefying necrosis, a needle aspiration or incision and drainage should be performed.

Cat-scratch disease is a self-limited infectious condition characterized by painful regional lymphadenopathy. *Bartonella henselae,* a gram-negative bacillus, is responsible for most cases. A history of exposure to cats is helpful but not always present. Indirect immunofluorescent antibody testing has only moderate specificity, and therefore polymerase chain reaction assay of a lymph node biopsy specimen is more useful for diagnosis. There is no specific treatment for cat-scratch disease because it is usually self-limited. A less common infectious cause of cervical lymphadenitis is nontuberculous mycobacterial infection. The nodes are fluctuant, with a violaceous appearance of the overlying skin. The diagnosis is made by positive cultures for nontuberculous acid-fast bacilli along with a tuberculin skin test. Surgical excision is usually indicated because most nontuberculous mycobacteria are resistant to conventional chemotherapy.

Cystic Hygroma

Cystic hygroma is a multiloculated cystic space lined by endothelial cells occurring as a result of lymphatic malformation. Most cystic hygromas involve the lymphatic jugular sacs and present in the posterior neck region. The other common sites are the axillary, mediastinal, inguinal, and retroperitoneal regions, and approximately 50% of these cystic lesions are present at birth. Cystic hygromas are soft cystic masses that distort the surrounding anatomy, including the airway. A large cystic mass of the neck in the fetus can impose a significant risk to the airway at birth and may be associated with chromosomal abnormalities. Prenatal ultrasound and fetal magnetic resonance imaging (MRI) studies allow careful coordination of surgical intervention at the time of delivery. Cystic hygromas are prone to infection and hemorrhage within the mass. MRI can be helpful in preoperative planning. In general, complete surgical excision is the preferred treatment. However, this may be difficult because of the intimate involvement with surrounding vital structures. Surgical resections are generally tedious, requiring careful isolation and ligation of lymphatic branches. Aggressive blunt and electrocautery dissections can result in incomplete control of lymphatics, leading to recurrence or infection caused by accumulation of the lymphatic leak. Radical resection with sacrifice of vital structures must be avoided. Injection of sclerosing agents, such as bleomycin, doxycycline, or OK-432 derived from *Streptococcus pyogenes,* has been reported to be effective in the nonoperative management of cystic hygromas.[1]

Thyroglossal Duct Cyst

A thyroglossal duct cyst is a midline neck lesion that originates at the base of the tongue at the foramen cecum and descends through the central portion of the hyoid bone. Although thyroglossal duct cysts may occur anywhere from the base of the tongue to the thyroid gland, most are found at or just below the hyoid bone (Fig. 66-1*A*). A thyroid diverticulum develops as a median endodermal thickening at the foramen cecum in the embryonic stage of development. The thyroid diverticulum descends in the neck and remains attached to the base of the tongue by the thyroglossal duct. Also, as the thyroid gland descends to its normal pretracheal position, the ventral cartilages of the second and third branchial arches form the hyoid bone—hence the intimate anatomic relationship of the thyroglossal duct remnant with the central portion of the hyoid bone. The thyroglossal duct normally regresses by the time the thyroid gland reaches its final position. When the elements of the duct persist despite complete thyroid descent, a thyroglossal duct cyst may develop. Failure of normal caudal migration of the thyroid gland results in a lingual thyroid, in which no other thyroid tissue is present in the neck. Ultrasound or radionuclide imaging may provide useful information to identify the presence of an ectopic thyroid gland in the neck. The standard operation for thyroglossal duct cysts has remained unchanged since it was described by Sistrunk in 1928, which involves complete excision of the cyst in continuity with its tract, the central portion of the hyoid bone, and the tract interior to the hyoid bone extending to the base of the tongue (Fig. 66-1*B*). Failure to remove these tissues entirely will likely result in recurrence because multiple sinuses have been histologically identified in these locations.

Branchial Cleft Remnants

The branchial cleft remnants typically present as a lateral neck mass on a toddler. The structures of the head and neck are derived from six pairs of branchial arches, their intervening clefts, and pouches. Congenital cysts, sinuses, or fistulas result from failure of these structures to regress, persisting in an aberrant location. The location of these remnants generally dictates their embryologic origin and guides the subsequent operative approach. Failure to understand the embryology may result in incomplete resection or injury to adjacent structures. All branchial remnants are present at the time of birth; however, they are often not recognized until later in life. These lesions can be manifested as sinuses, fistulas, or cartilaginous rests in infants (Fig. 66-2). However, they present more commonly as cysts in toddlers and older children. The clinical presentation ranges from a continuous mucoid drainage from a fistula or sinus to the development of a cystic mass that may become infected. Branchial remnants may also be palpable as cartilaginous lumps or cords corresponding with a fistulous track. Dermal pits or skin tags may also be present.

First branchial remnants are typically located in the front or back of the ear or in the upper neck near the mandible. Fistulas typically course through the parotid gland, deep or through

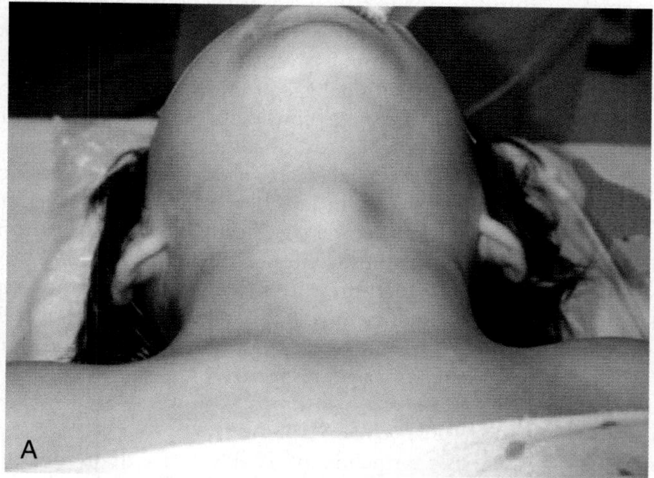

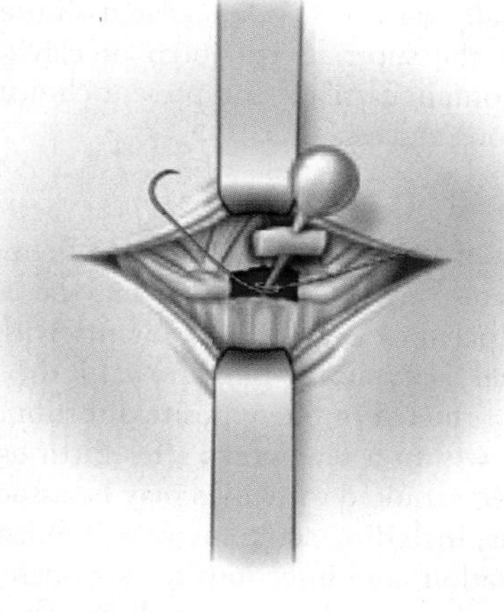

FIGURE 66-1 A, Thyroglossal duct cyst presents as a midline neck mass. **B,** Sistrunk procedure consists of excision of the thyroglossal duct cyst up to its origin at the foramen cecum, including the central portion of hyoid bone. (From Josephs MD: Thyroglossal duct cyst. In Chung DH, Chen MK, editors: *Atlas of pediatric surgical techniques,* Philadelphia, 2010, Elsevier Saunders, pp 28–33.)

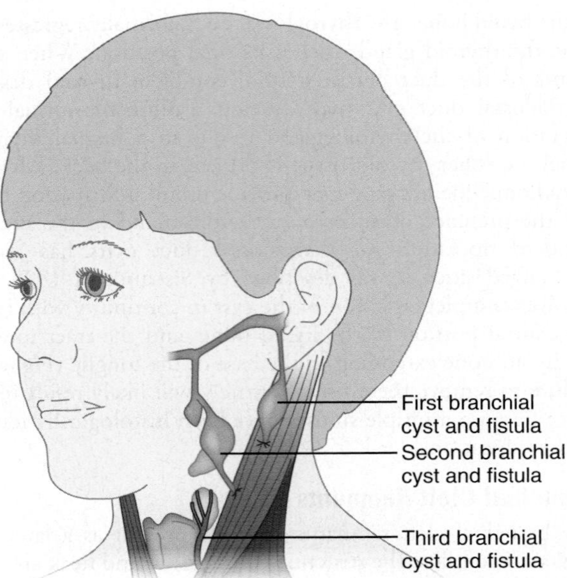

FIGURE 66-2 Branchial cleft cyst and fistula. First branchial cleft sinus occurs along the line extending from the auditory canal to the angle of the mandible. Second branchial cleft sinus is the more common type, typically along the anterior border of the sternocleidomastoid muscle. Third and fourth branchial cleft sinuses are rare in the more inferior aspect of the neck. (From Wesley JR: Branchial cysts, sinuses, and fistulas. In Spitz LS, Coran AG, editors: *Operative pediatric surgery*, London, 2006, Edward Arnold Ltd, p 60.)

branches of the facial nerve, and end in the external auditory canal. The second branchial cleft remnants are the most common type. The external ostium of these remnants is located along the anterior border of the sternocleidomastoid muscle, usually in the vicinity of the upper half to lower third of the muscle. The course of the fistula must be anticipated preoperatively because stepladder counterincisions are often necessary to excise the fistula track completely. Typically, the fistula penetrates the platysma, ascends along the carotid sheath to the level of the hyoid bone, and turns medially to extend between the carotid artery bifurcations. The fistula then courses behind the posterior belly of the digastric and stylohyoid muscles to end in the tonsillar fossa. Third branchial cleft remnants usually do not have associated sinuses or fistulas and are located in the suprasternal notch or clavicular region. These most often contain cartilage and present clinically as a firm mass or subcutaneous abscess.

Torticollis

Torticollis is a state of abnormal muscle tone in the neck, causing the head to twist and turn to one side. It may be congenital or acquired and can occur at any age. In infants with congenital torticollis, the head is typically tilted toward the side of the affected muscle and rotated in the opposite direction. Congenital torticollis presents within a few weeks after birth as an isolated condition. However, acquired torticollis may be associated with a range of conditions, including acute myositis, brainstem tumors, atlantoaxial subluxation, and infectious causes, such as retropharyngeal abscess, cervical adenitis, or tonsillitis. The diagnosis is typically based solely on the clinical examination findings. Treatment is physical therapy involving passive range of motion stretching of the affected muscle for several months. Surgical resection or division of the involved muscle is rarely indicated.

EXTRACORPOREAL LIFE SUPPORT

Extracorporeal life support (ECLS) is a cardiopulmonary bypass that provides temporary support for the critically ill patient with acute refractory respiratory or cardiac failure. In general, ECLS delivers sufficient gas exchange and maintains circulatory support, thus allowing physiologic recovery. The largest experience with ECLS has been for respiratory failure in newborns. Since its first reported neonatal case in 1976, ECLS has become a standard therapeutic option for refractory cardiopulmonary failure in infants and children. There are 226 centers around the world contributing registry data to the Extracorporeal Life Support Organization database (ELSO registry data; July 2015). In 2014 alone, 6510 pediatric and adult patients were supported on ECLS.

Indications

The major indications for neonatal extracorporeal membrane oxygenation (ECMO) include meconium aspiration, respiratory distress syndrome, PPHN, sepsis, and congenital diaphragmatic hernia. Neonates with complex congenital cardiac defects may be supported with ECMO perioperatively. Meconium aspiration is the most common application for neonatal ECMO with the highest survival rate (>90%) among all conditions. Inclusion criteria for the neonatal ECMO vary somewhat among institutions. In general, ECMO is justified when an infant's overall condition deteriorates to a point of roughly 80% predicted mortality. Two guidelines have been historically used as a means to predict survival without ECMO. The alveolar-arterial difference in the partial pressure of oxygen ($PAO_2 - PaO_2$ [also known as $AaDO_2$]) is calculated as

$$AaDo_2 = (\text{atmospheric pressure} - 47) - (Pao_2 + Paco_2)$$

$AaDO_2$ above 610 for longer than 8 to 12 hours and $AaDO_2$ above 620 for 6 hours, associated with extensive barotrauma and severe hypotension requiring inotropic support, are considered to be criteria for ECMO. The oxygen index is calculated as the fraction of inspired oxygen (usually 1.0) multiplied by the mean airway pressure × 100 divided by PaO_2. An 80% mortality is observed with an oxygen index above 40. Exclusion criteria include gestational age of less than 34 weeks, birth weight of less than 2 kg, intracranial hemorrhage, and a nonreversible pulmonary disease such as congenital alveolar dysplasia. However, with recent advances, gestational age of less than 34 weeks and weight of less than 2 kg are now considered only relative contraindications at many centers. Additional exclusion criteria are presence of cyanotic congenital heart disease or major genetic defects that preclude survival, intractable coagulopathy or hemorrhage, sonographic evidence of a significant intracranial hemorrhage (higher than a grade I intraventricular hemorrhage), and more than 10 to 14 days of high-pressure mechanical ventilatory support. Before ECMO, infants must be evaluated with echocardiography and cranial ultrasound for cyanotic heart defect and significant intracranial hemorrhage, respectively.

Physiology

The basic principle of ECLS is to drain desaturated venous blood, to exchange carbon dioxide and oxygen through the membrane oxygenator, and then to return oxygenated warmed blood into the circulation. Venoarterial bypass is used most commonly for full cardiopulmonary support. The right internal

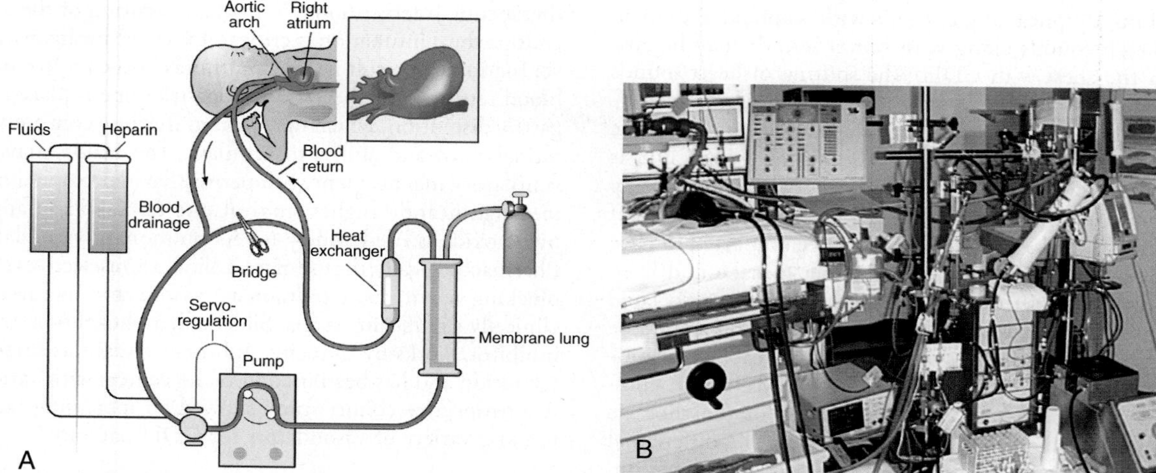

FIGURE 66-3 A, Extracorporeal life support circuit. A venoarterial circuit diagram is shown here. (From Shanley CJ, Bartlett RH: Extracorporeal life support: Techniques, indications, and results. In Cameron JL, editor: *Current surgical therapy*, ed 4, St. Louis, 1992, Mosby Year Book, pp 1062–1066.) **B,** A photograph of ECMO circuit supporting an infant with congenital diaphragmatic hernia.

jugular vein and common carotid artery are typically chosen for cannulation because of their vessel sizes, accessibility, and collateral circulation. The ECLS circuit is composed of a silicone rubber bladder that collapses when venous return is diminished, roller pump, membrane oxygenator, heat exchanger, tubing, and connectors. Venous blood from the right atrium drains through the venous cannula to the bladder and is pumped to the membrane oxygenator, where carbon dioxide is removed and oxygen is added (Fig. 66-3). The oxygenated blood then passes through the heat exchanger and is returned to the patient through the arterial cannula. Systemic anticoagulation to prevent clotting of the ECLS circuit puts patients at risk for bleeding complications. Hematocrit, platelet counts, and fibrinogen levels are closely monitored and maintained within acceptable parameters. An ultrasound examination of the head is performed for the first few days of ECLS to monitor for onset of intracranial hemorrhage. Extracorporeal flow is gradually weaned as native cardiac or pulmonary function improves. Indicators of lung recovery include an increasing PaO_2, improved lung compliance, and clearing of the chest radiograph. Once the extracorporeal flow rate reaches minimal levels, the patient is trialed off bypass by temporary clamping of the cannulas. If this is tolerated, the patient is taken off ECLS on moderate conventional ventilatory settings. Venovenous bypass support by a double-lumen cannula has the advantages of avoiding carotid arterial cannulation. Often, perfusion of well-oxygenated blood through venovenous ECMO restores hemodynamic stability.

Complications

Bleeding, the most common complication of ECLS, can occur at any invasive catheter sites, such as cannulas in the neck or an arterial line, and in the head, leading to devastating intracranial hemorrhage. Birth weight and gestational age are the most significant correlates of intracranial hemorrhage on ECLS; infants weighing less than 2 kg and younger than 34 weeks of gestational age are at highest risk. Other complications associated with ECLS include seizures, neurologic impairment, renal failure requiring hemofiltration or hemodialysis, hypertension, infection, and mechanical malfunction (e.g., failure of the membrane oxygenator, pump, and heat exchanger).

CONGENITAL DIAPHRAGMATIC HERNIA

Congenital diaphragmatic hernia (CDH) remains one of the most challenging conditions to treat in pediatric surgery. The overall incidence is 1 in 2000 to 5000 live births. Most CDH defects occur on the left side (80%); bilateral defects are extremely rare. A hernia sac is present 20% of the time. Despite recent innovative treatment strategies, such as fetal tracheal occlusion, ECMO, inhaled nitric oxide, and permissive hypercapnic management protocol, the overall survival rates have not changed significantly and remain in the 70% to 90% range. Accurate determination of true survival rate is distorted by the fact that many infants with CDH are stillborn, and many reports tend to exclude infants with complex associated anomalies from survival calculations.

Pathogenesis

CDH is thought to result from failure of closure of the pleuroperitoneal canal in the developing fetus. Normally, the pleuroperitoneal cavities become separated by the developing membrane during weeks 8 to 10 of gestation. When this process fails, the pleuroperitoneal canal does not close, and a posterolateral diaphragmatic defect results. The posterolateral location of this hernia is known as Bochdalek hernia; it is distinguished from a CDH of the anteromedial location known as Morgagni hernia. As a result of the defect, abdominal contents herniate into the thoracic cavity, compressing the ipsilateral developing lung. These lungs have smaller bronchi, with less bronchial branching and less alveolar surface area than lungs in normal infants. The ipsilateral lung is affected more severely; however, both lungs are affected by pulmonary hypoplasia. In addition to the abnormal airway development, the pulmonary vasculature is also significantly affected by increased thickness of arteriolar smooth muscle. Also, arteriolar vasculature is extremely sensitive to the multiple local and systemic vasoactive factors. Hence, the severity of pulmonary hypoplasia and pulmonary hypertension significantly affect the overall morbidity and mortality in CDH infants.

Clinical Presentation and Diagnosis

Most infants with CDH experience respiratory distress at birth. The initial symptoms and signs may include grunting respiration, chest retractions, dyspnea, and cyanosis with scaphoid abdomen. Decreased breath sounds along with bowel sounds may be auscultated over the chest with CDH. The shifting of heart sounds to the right (for left-sided CDH) is common. A significant differential of preductal and postductal pulse oximetry indicates the right-to-left shunting due to PPHN. The diagnosis of CDH is frequently made prenatally as early as 15 weeks of gestation during a routine ultrasound evaluation. Infants who have a late onset of CDH (beyond 25 weeks of gestation) have been reported to have better overall survival. The herniation of the stomach and liver, polyhydramnios, and associated anomalies have been associated with poor outcome. The delivery of a fetus with CDH should be carefully planned and take place at an institution capable of providing advanced neonatal care, including ECMO. The chest radiograph demonstrates multiple bowel loops in the thoracic cavity along with mediastinal shift (Fig. 66-4*A*). The differential diagnosis includes congenital cystic adenomatoid malformation, bronchogenic cyst, diaphragmatic eventration, and cystic teratoma. In Morgagni hernia, the diagnosis is often delayed until childhood because most infants are asymptomatic. Typically, the infant does well for several hours after delivery during the so-called honeymoon period and then begins to demonstrate worsening respiratory function. Therapeutic interventions are aimed at stabilizing and treating PPHN. In approximately 10% to 20% of cases, CDH is diagnosed beyond the first 24 hours of life, at which time infants present with various symptoms of feeding difficulties, respiratory distress, and pneumonia.

Treatment

The open fetal surgery for CDH failed to show an overall survival advantage and therefore has been abandoned. However, laparoscopic occlusion of the fetal trachea, resulting in accumulation of lung fluid to stimulate lung growth, has gained increasing interest. External tracheal clips or endotracheal balloons can be placed laparoscopically (often referred to as fetoscopy) to occlude the fetal trachea. The Tracheal Occlusion To Accelerate Lung growth (TOTAL) trial is led by several European centers.[2] However, this intervention is not available in the United States because of lack of a Food and Drug Administration–approved device. The postnatal management of CDH is directed toward stabilization of the cardiorespiratory status while minimizing iatrogenic injury from therapeutic interventions. Immediate securing of the airway with endotracheal intubation is critical. Excessive mean airway pressure ventilation can result in pneumothorax and compromised venous blood return to the heart. An orogastric tube is placed to prevent gastric distention, which may worsen the lung compression, mediastinal shift, and ability to ventilate. The major focus in gentler ventilatory management with permissive hypercapnia has resulted in a significantly higher survival rate for CDH infants. Inhaled nitric oxide is used widely for its pulmonary vasodilatory effect. Pharmacologically, the use of tolazoline, a nonselective α-adrenergic blocking agent, as a pulmonary vasodilator has not produced clinically significant results. Sildenafil, a phosphodiesterase type 5 inhibitor, works by inducing pulmonary vascular smooth muscle relaxation and has been used in many centers with various results. A retrospective cohort study showed an increasing trend for the use of a variety of vasodilators for CDH patients.[3]

Surgical Repair

For infants with relatively stable pulmonary status, CDH repair can be safely performed on the second to fourth day of life after the potential honeymoon period. However, the ideal timing of CDH repair on ECMO remains controversial and highly debated; some advocate early operative repair on ECMO, whereas others recommend repair at the time of weaning from ECMO or even after decannulation. There are no clear prospective data to endorse an exact timing of CDH repair for those requiring ECMO support. However, recent reports suggest that CDH repair after ECMO is associated with improved survival compared with repair while on ECMO.[4] At operation, the preferred approach for a posterolateral CDH is through a subcostal abdominal incision. The viscera are reduced into the abdominal cavity, and the posterolateral defect in the diaphragm is approximated with interrupted nonabsorbable sutures. When present (10% to 15% of cases), a hernia sac should be excised. Typically, the hernia defect is large, with only a small leaflet of diaphragmatic tissue present anteromedially. Although primary repair of the defect is ideal, closure with excessive tension must be avoided to prevent hernia recurrence. Some surgeons advocate the use of pledgeted sutures. A number of reconstructive techniques and materials are available for the repair of large hernia defects. The surgical technique of abdominal or thoracic muscle flaps can be considered, but the use

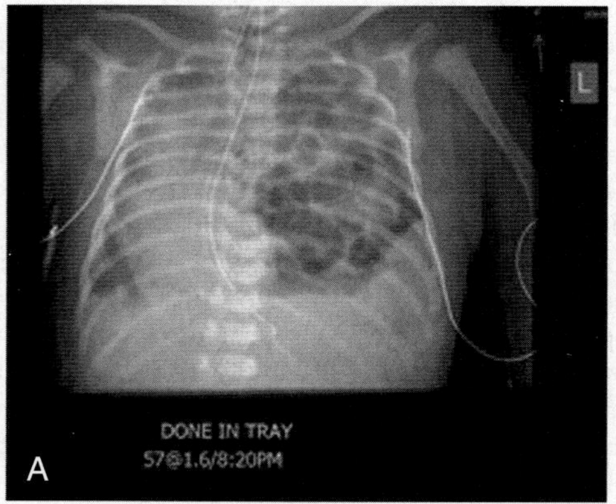

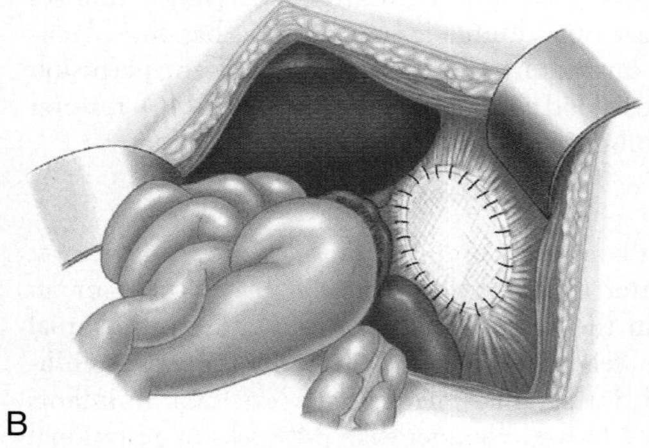

FIGURE 66-4 A, Congenital diaphragmatic hernia. Multiple gas-filled bowel loops are located in the left hemithorax, and the mediastinum is shifted to the right. **B,** Diagram depicting repair of a left congenital diaphragmatic hernia with Gore-Tex patch graft. (From Frischer JS: Congenital diaphragmatic hernia and eventration of the diaphragm. In Chung DH, Chen MK, editors: *Atlas of pediatric surgical techniques*, Philadelphia, 2010, Elsevier Saunders, pp 83–96.)

of prosthetic material, most commonly Gore-Tex patch, has become widespread (Fig. 66-4*B*). The advantages of a prosthetic patch are shorter operative time and a tension-free repair. However, the major potential problems with prosthetic patches are the risks of infection and recurrence of the hernia. Recently, the use of regenerative extracellular matrix biomaterials has garnered significant interest as an ideal biodegradable patch (e.g., Surgisis [Cook Medical Bloomington, Ind]; AlloDerm [LifeCell, Branchburg, NJ]) to repair diaphragmatic hernia defects. At times, the abdominal cavity may be too small to accommodate the reduced viscera from the thoracic cavity. A temporary abdominal silo may be considered, but allowing an incisional hernia with skin-only closure until the definitive fascia closure can be performed is an alternative surgical option. When CDH is repaired on ECMO, particular attention must be paid to achieve hemostasis. However, despite the use of careful surgical techniques with diligent hemostasis, postoperative bleeding is a common major complication. Beyond the immediate postoperative period, many infants with CDH experience significant morbidity because of PPHN and respiratory dysfunction. For example, infants who survive aggressive management of severe respiratory failure may manifest neurologic problems, such as motor and cognitive deficits, developmental delay, seizures, and hearing loss. Other problems include gastroesophageal reflux (GER) disease and foregut dysmotility. Other morbidities associated with CDH survivors include chronic lung disease, scoliosis, growth retardation, and pectus excavatum deformities.

BRONCHOPULMONARY MALFORMATIONS

Bronchopulmonary malformations are congenital abnormalities of the airway, such as bronchogenic cysts, intralobar and extralobar sequestrations, congenital pulmonary airway malformations, and congenital lobar emphysema.[5] Their natural histories vary widely. In the perinatal period, these lung lesions can result in pleural effusions, polyhydramnios, hydrops, and pulmonary hypoplasia with subsequent respiratory distress and airway obstruction. If severe enough, fetal demise can ensue. With increasing importance placed on prenatal care, many of these lesions are being diagnosed prenatally with imaging. Fetal surgery has been pursued when fetal viability is at risk. Although these congenital abnormalities are often asymptomatic and may even spontaneously regress, there is concern that these anomalies may cause recurrent infections and exhibit long-term malignant potential.

Bronchogenic Cyst

Bronchogenic cyst is the most common cystic lesion of the mediastinum. The cyst wall consists of fibroelastic tissue, smooth muscle, and cartilage, whereas the cyst itself is lined with respiratory tract epithelia (ciliated columnar cells). It can also contain mucus-producing cuboidal cells, which contribute to enlargement of the cyst with mucus. They may occur anywhere along the tracheobronchial tree but are usually found near the carina and right hilum. Less frequently, they present in the neck, lung, pleura, or pericardium or below the diaphragm. When the cysts are large, they can compress the airway or other vital structures. Infants are particularly at risk because of their narrow, easily compressible trachea and bronchus. Cysts can also cause dysphagia, pneumothorax, cough, and hemoptysis or become infected, especially when presenting later in life. Often identified on a routine chest radiograph, the diagnosis is confirmed by computed tomography (CT) as a spherical nonenhancing, mucus-filled cystic mass, although an air-fluid level can be seen if the cyst communicates with the airway. Cysts within the pulmonary parenchyma typically communicate with a bronchus, whereas those in the mediastinum usually do not. Bronchogenic cysts are resected even if asymptomatic, although some argue otherwise. Rare cases of malignant transformation have been reported. Resection can be performed either thoracoscopically (i.e., by video-assisted thoracic surgery) or open (by minithoracotomy).

Congenital Pulmonary Airway Malformation

Congenital pulmonary airway malformations (CPAMs) have been described as hamartomatous lesions in which a multicystic mass replaces normal lung tissue. They are connected to the tracheobronchial tree, and the blood supply is pulmonary. Although they are usually unilateral and unilobar, they can present in the immediate perinatal period with life-threatening respiratory distress. The majority of CPAMs are asymptomatic at infancy; however, unrecognized CPAMs can present with chronic cough or recurrent pneumonia at a later time. CPAMs can undergo malignant transformation; rhabdomyosarcoma has been reported. They are classified on the basis of their appearance on imaging, and confirmation is made by pathologic examination. According to the Stocker classification, type I lesions account for almost 75% of all cases and consist of a small number of large, 2- to 10-cm cysts that can compress normal lung parenchyma. Type II lesions have numerous cysts, usually measuring less than 1 cm in diameter. Type III lesions are rare and appear to be only a few millimeters in diameter.[6] However, they are associated with mediastinal shift, hydrops, and a poor prognosis.

Prenatal fetal MRI can be used to differentiate CPAM from other congenital thoracic abnormalities. When fetal distress occurs in utero, options include fetal thoracotomy and thoracoamniotic shunting (if the fetus is <32 weeks), but this is extremely rare. Most fetuses with a prenatally diagnosed CPAM experience partial regression in the third trimester and can be treated with expectant management.[5] Some report favorable outcomes with the use of steroids prenatally, which may help promote spontaneous regression or stabilize disease progression in utero.[7] CPAM is generally asymptomatic at birth. However, on rare occasion, infants present with acute respiratory distress requiring emergent open resection. A chest radiograph is usually diagnostic, revealing a cystic thoracic mass with air-fluid levels occasionally; however, ultrasound and CT examinations are frequently obtained for confirmation (Fig. 66-5*A*). The management of asymptomatic patients is somewhat controversial with respect to ideal timing of the operation. It is generally agreed that they should be resected, given the risk of infection and malignant transformation, such as pleuropulmonary blastoma. Most advocate surgical resection around 6 months of age.

Pulmonary Sequestration

Bronchopulmonary sequestrations (BPSs) are nonfunctional nests of microcystic pulmonary tissue that have no connection to the tracheobronchial tree but are fed by an aberrant systemic artery. There are two types, intralobar and extralobar; the intralobar type is contained within normal lung parenchyma, and the extralobar type is separate and encased by its own pleura.[5] Extralobar sequestrations (ELSs) occur predominantly in males, and in 40% of cases, other congenital anomalies, such as posterolateral diaphragmatic hernia, pectus excavatum and carinatum, and enteric duplication cysts, can be found.

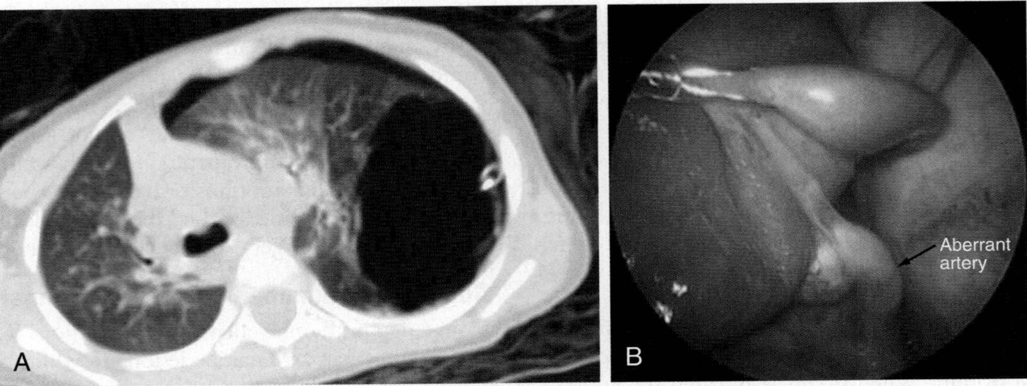

FIGURE 66-5 **A,** CT scan demonstrating a large left lung CPAM lesion. **B,** Anomalous arterial vascular pedicle to extralobar pulmonary sequestration. The arterial branch comes directly off the thoracic aorta.

Lacking a communication to the airway, sequestrations do not form enlarged cysts or cause spontaneous pneumothoraces. They can, however, infarct, become infected, and cause hemoptysis. It has been reported that ELSs can undergo torsion as well. Because of their aberrant systemic vascular supply (Fig. 66-5*B*), BPSs can result in significant left-to-right shunting in infants, who are then susceptible to high-output cardiac failure. For an initial evaluation, Doppler ultrasound may reveal a systemic arterial supply from the infradiaphragmatic or thoracic aorta. The lesion itself may appear solid, but it can also be cystic. CT or MRI can aid in further defining the vascular anatomy. Accounting for 75% of all BPSs, intralobar sequestrations (ILSs) are found within the medial or posterior segments of the lower lobes, more on the left side. Most ELSs are found posteromedially in the left lower chest but can occur within or below the diaphragm. Air within an ILS usually signifies infection, whereas the same finding in an ELS suggests the presence of a fistulous connection with the esophagus.[5]

If a BPS is identified on prenatal ultrasound, the fetus is observed with serial ultrasound monitoring for enlargement and potential pleural effusion, polyhydramnios, or hydrops. BPS has been reported to spontaneously regress. In fact, it is estimated that 68% of BPSs undergo spontaneous regression in utero as they become isodense with the surrounding lung. The involution may occur as the lesion outgrows its blood supply. Because of the risk for infection and bleeding, ILSs are usually resected by segmentectomy or lobectomy. ELSs are usually asymptomatic, and because there is generally no tracheobronchial communication, the risk of infection is low. As such, many of these lesions can be observed.

Congenital Lobar Emphysema

Congenital lobar emphysema (CLE) describes a progressively distended, hyperlucent lobe caused by abnormal bronchopulmonary development. Air trapping in the emphysematous lobes occurs with intrinsic or extrinsic obstruction, which includes endobronchial obstruction from mucosal proliferation and extrinsic compression from vascular anomalies. In more than 90% of cases, it involves the left upper or right middle lobe. CLE is rarely diagnosed prenatally, and its prevalence is only 1 in every 20,000 to 30,000 deliveries. It tends to be manifested in the first few days of life and as late as 6 months after birth. On ultrasound examination, CLE appears as an echogenic homogeneous lung mass. When CLE is discovered incidentally, observation is recommended because these lesions can regress spontaneously. A chest radiograph is customarily diagnostic, revealing overdistention of the involved lobe. Importantly, the lucency should not be mistaken for a pneumothorax, and positive pressure ventilation should be used with caution because of the propensity of these patients to undergo auto–positive end-expiratory pressure; auto–positive end-expiratory pressure is defined as the end-expiratory intrapulmonary pressure that develops as a result of dynamic airflow resistance during mechanical ventilation. When the CLE progresses to cause mediastinal shift and worsening symptoms, an open lobectomy is indicated.

ALIMENTARY TRACT CONDITIONS

Esophageal Atresia and Tracheoesophageal Fistula

Esophageal atresia is a congenital condition of esophageal discontinuity that results in proximal esophageal obstruction. A tracheoesophageal fistula (TEF) is an abnormal fistula communication between the esophagus and trachea. Esophageal atresia and TEF can occur alone or in combination. The incidence of this anomaly is 1 in 1500 to 3000 live births, with a slight male predominance. Approximately one third of infants are born with low birth weight, and 60% to 70% have associated anomalies. During the fourth week of gestation, the esophagotracheal diverticulum of the foregut fails to divide completely to form the esophagus and trachea. In 10% of patients, there is a nonrandom, nonhereditary association of anomalies referred to by the acronym VATER (vertebral, anorectal, tracheal, esophageal, renal or radial limb); an alternative acronym is VACTERL (vertebral, anorectal, cardiac, tracheal, esophageal, renal, and limb). Five anatomic variants of esophageal atresia are depicted in Figure 66-6. In the most common type (C lesion) of proximal esophageal atresia with distal TEF, the proximal blind pouch ends approximately the distance of one or two vertebral bodies from the distal TEF. The distal TEF is typically located approximately 1 cm above the carina in the membranous portion of the trachea.

Clinical Presentation and Diagnosis

The diagnosis of esophageal atresia is considered in an infant with excessive salivation along with coughing or choking experienced at the first oral feeding. A maternal history of polyhydramnios is common, more often in isolated proximal atresia (86%). In an infant with proximal esophageal atresia with distal TEF, acute gastric distention may occur as a result of air entering the distal esophagus and stomach with each inspired breath. Reflux of gastric contents into the distal esophagus will traverse the TEF

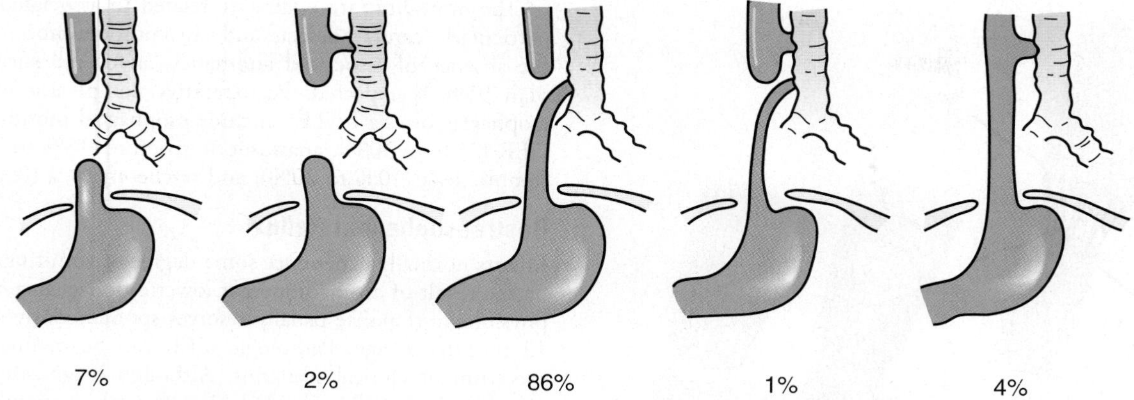

FIGURE 66-6 Anatomic variants and incidence of esophageal atresia with tracheoesophageal fistula.

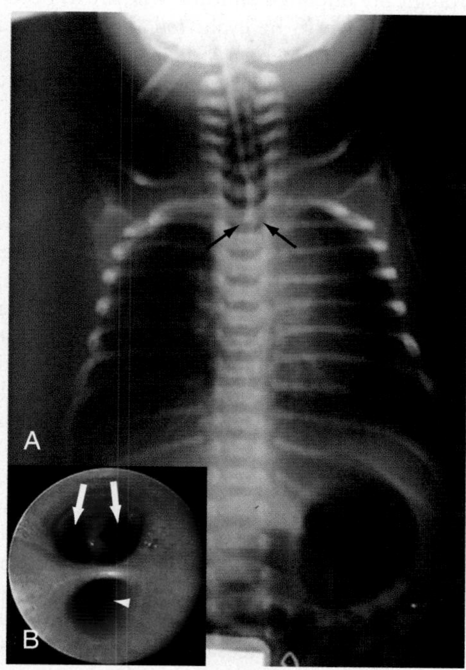

FIGURE 66-7 A, Plain chest radiograph of infant with proximal esophageal atresia with distal tracheoesophageal fistula. The distal tip of the orogastric tube is noted, with a surrounding gas-filled proximal esophagus *(arrows)*. The distal tracheoesophageal fistula is indicated by the presence of gastric air. **B,** Rigid bronchoscopy inspection of distal tracheoesophageal fistula. The luminal size of the fistula *(arrowhead)* is equal to that of either main bronchus *(arrows)*.

and spill into the trachea, resulting in cough, tachypnea, apnea, or cyanosis. The clinical presentation of isolated TEF without esophageal atresia may be subtle, often beyond the newborn period. In general, these infants experience choking and coughing associated with feedings. The inability to pass a nasogastric tube into the stomach is a cardinal feature for the diagnosis of esophageal atresia. If gas is present below the diaphragm, an associated TEF is confirmed (Fig. 66-7*A*). Conversely, the inability to pass a nasogastric tube in an infant with absent radiographic evidence of air in the GI tract is virtually diagnostic of an isolated esophageal atresia. The use of isotonic contrast medium to demonstrate the presence or level of the proximal esophageal atresia is strongly discouraged because of risk for aspiration. The diagnostic evaluation includes screening for other associated anomalies. Echocardiography and renal ultrasound are routinely performed to evaluate for congenital heart defects (including aortic arch anomaly) and genitourinary malformations.

Management

Initial management includes decompression of the proximal esophageal pouch with a sump tube (e.g., Replogle tube) placed on continuous suction. The infant is positioned in an upright prone position to minimize GER and to prevent aspiration. Broad-spectrum IV antibiotic coverage is started empirically. Routine endotracheal intubation is avoided because positive pressure ventilation may be inadequate to inflate the lungs as air is directed into the TEF through the path of least resistance (Fig. 66-7*B*). Ventilation may be compounded further by the resultant gastric distention. Gastrostomy to decompress the distended stomach should be avoided because it may abruptly worsen the ability to ventilate the patient. In these circumstances, manipulation of the endotracheal tube advanced distal to the TEF (e.g., right mainstem intubation) may minimize the leak and permit adequate ventilation. The placement of an occlusive balloon (Fogarty) catheter into the fistula through a rigid bronchoscope may also be useful. As a last resort, emergent thoracotomy with ligation of the fistula alone may be required. A preoperative chest radiograph and echocardiogram provide sufficient information to determine the aortic arch anatomy. A right thoracotomy is performed for the operative repair in patients with a normal left-sided aortic arch. However, for infants with a right-sided arch, a left thoracotomy would be preferred. A higher incidence of aortic arch anomalies (e.g., vascular rings) and postoperative complications has been reported with a right-sided aortic arch.[8]

The surgical approach for the most common type of proximal esophageal atresia with distal TEF is an open thoracotomy with an extrapleural dissection. Recently, thoracoscopic repair has been described by several pediatric surgical centers. Some advocate routine rigid bronchoscopy at the start of the operation to exclude the presence of a second fistula or placement of a catheter through the fistula to aid in identifying TEF. However, this technique may be more useful for recurrent fistula repairs. After exposure of the posterior mediastinum, the azygos vein is divided to reveal the underlying TEF. The TEF is dissected circumferentially, and its attachment to the membranous portion of trachea is taken down. The tracheal opening is approximated with interrupted nonabsorbable sutures. The proximal esophageal pouch is then mobilized as high as possible to facilitate a tension-free esophageal

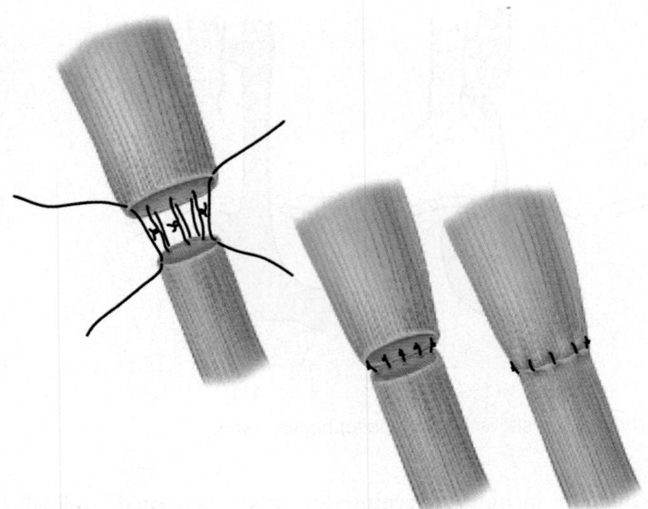

FIGURE 66-8 A single-layer end-to-end anastomosis is performed with nonabsorbable sutures. Two corner stitches are placed, and a back row anastomosis is completed first. Just before completion of the anterior row of the anastomosis, a nasogastric tube is placed across it.

anastomosis. The blood supply to the upper esophageal pouch is generally robust from arteries derived from the thyrocervical trunk. However, the lower esophageal vasculature is more tenuous and segmental, originating from intercostal vessels. As such, extensive mobilization of the lower esophagus should be avoided to prevent ischemia. The esophageal anastomosis is performed with a single- or double-layer technique (Fig. 66-8). The anastomotic leak rates are slightly higher with the single-layer anastomosis, whereas the esophageal stricture rates are higher with the double-layer technique.

In case of a long gap between the two ends of the esophagus, there are several options. A circular or spiral esophagomyotomy of the upper pouch can be performed to gain additional length for a primary anastomosis. Another option is to suture the divided closed end of the distal esophagus to the prevertebral fascia and mark the area with a hemoclip. Over time, the proximal esophageal pouch will lengthen so that a subsequent primary esophageal anastomosis can be considered. In infants with pure esophageal atresia, primary anastomosis in the newborn period is not feasible because of a long gap between the esophageal stumps. Gastrostomy is initially placed for enteral feeding access. Traditionally, a cervical esophagostomy is performed for drainage of oral secretions, and then an esophageal replacement operation using either right or left colon is carried out at approximately 1 year of age. Alternatively, proximal esophageal pouch secretion can be managed with an indwelling orogastric tube (Replogle tube) without cervical esophagostomy until adequate esophageal lengthening takes place, as assessed by a fluoroscopic study. Then, a primary intrathoracic segmental esophageal replacement using a colonic segment can be performed around 4 to 6 months of age. The stomach has also been used as an esophageal replacement but with much less frequency. Small intestinal free graft is another option, but this requires microvascular anastomosis and has poor results. In patients with pure TEF, without esophageal atresia, the TEF is usually near the thoracic inlet. In this case, the surgical approach is made through a cervical incision. At operation, rigid bronchoscopy and cannulation of the TEF with a guidewire can be helpful.

The mortality rate is directly related to associated anomalies, particularly cardiac defects and chromosomal abnormalities. In the absence of associated anomalies, an overall survival greater than 95% is expected. Postoperative complications unique to esophageal atresia or TEF include esophageal motility disorders, GER (25% to 50%), anastomotic stricture (15% to 30%), anastomotic leak (10% to 20%), and tracheomalacia (8% to 15%).

Gastroesophageal Reflux

Infants normally experience some degree of vomiting, thought to be the result of an incompetent lower esophageal sphincter. This physiologic response usually resolves spontaneously around 6 to 12 months of age. Pathologic GER can be manifested with a spectrum of clinical scenarios. Although diagnostic studies are valuable in identifying pathologic reflux, the patient's symptoms remain equally important in deciding the surgical treatment of GER. Neurologically impaired children who are in need of enteral feeding access also have to be evaluated for concomitant reflux before gastrostomy placement. A laparoscopic approach has become a standard for fundoplication with gastrostomy in pediatric patients.

Clinical Presentation

The symptoms of pathologic GER vary considerably, depending on the age of the patient and underlying associated medical conditions. Although vomiting is a common feature, failure to thrive from calorie deprivation is one of the most serious complications of persistent GER. Aspiration of gastric contents can also result in recurrent bronchitis or pneumonia, leading to chronic cough or wheezing. Reflux may stimulate vagal reflex, producing laryngospasm or bronchospasm and leading to an asthma-like clinical presentation.[9] The significant airway spasm caused by reflux can result in apnea or choking spells and may contribute to near-miss sudden infant death syndrome (SIDS). Irritability and crying in infants may also represent pain because of esophagitis induced by chronic reflux. Chronic acid insult to the lower esophagus can progress to the formation of stricture from chronic scarring and produce obstructive symptoms. Although it is rare in pediatric patients, chronic progressive esophagitis can lead to metaplasia of lower esophageal squamous mucosa to columnar epithelium. This condition, known as Barrett esophagus, requires close surveillance to detect the progression of premalignant dysplastic changes.

Many infants and children with neurodevelopmental disabilities require permanent feeding access, such as a gastrostomy. Hence, some are also considered for antireflux surgery at the time of the gastrostomy placement, especially patients who are unable to protect their airway reliably or who already have significant vomiting associated with intragastric tube feeding. However, prophylactic fundoplication in neurologically impaired children is no longer a routine procedure at the time of gastrostomy placement. Some surgeons advocate studies to evaluate for GER disease before gastrostomy, but others rely on clinical judgment, such as tolerance of enteral feeding through an indwelling nasogastric tube. These patients are also at high risk for delayed gastric emptying because of upper gastroduodenal dysmotility. However, fundoplication alone may result in enhanced gastric emptying function, and a gastric emptying procedure is rarely indicated.

Diagnosis

A detailed clinical history will provide valuable information to determine the severity of GER. A near-miss SIDS episode or progressive neurologic disorders may indicate the desirability of an antireflux procedure, regardless of diagnostic study results. There are various diagnostic tools to objectively assess the presence of pathologic GER. Contrast esophagography is used most frequently to acquire anatomic and functional data. Esophageal stricture or mechanical evidence of gastric outlet obstruction, such as antral, duodenal web, or intestinal malrotation, can also be identified. In addition, motility of the esophagus and gastric emptying function can be estimated. However, one drawback is the lack of specificity. A 24-hour esophageal pH probe study remains the "gold standard" for diagnosis of GER. It can measure the frequency and duration of acid reflux episodes along with reflux patterns, such as the total length of acid ($pH < 4$) reflux, duration of each episode, and longest continuous period of acid reflux. A combined multichannel intraluminal impedance pH test, in which reflux is detected by changes in intraluminal resistance determined by the presence of liquid or gas and pH changes, has become a more reliable comprehensive diagnostic modality. A gastric emptying scan is obtained when a radionuclide-labeled (technetium Tc 99m sulfur colloid) liquid or semisolid food is used to quantitatively assess gastric emptying. In general, approximately 50% of the isotope-labeled meal is normally emptied from the stomach within 60 minutes and approximately 80% by 90 minutes. Delayed gastric emptying may improve simply after an antireflux procedure alone.

Esophageal manometry measures the esophageal body and lower esophageal sphincter pressures and helps identify abnormal esophageal motility. Although it is relatively simple to perform, manometry is infrequently used to evaluate GER disorders in pediatrics. The severity of GER in infants does not always correlate with an incompetent lower esophageal sphincter mechanism. There is also considerably less experience with manometric studies in pediatric patients. However, identifying esophageal dysmotility may be important for choosing the appropriate antireflux procedure. Children with poor esophageal motility are prone to development of refractory dysphagia after complete wrap fundoplication. Endoscopic evaluation of the esophageal mucosa provides a gross and microscopic assessment of mucosal injury secondary to GER. Patients who present with hematemesis or dysphagia may have significant underlying esophagitis. Esophagoscopy can determine the spectrum of esophagitis, from inflammation to ulceration to stricture, and is also helpful in identifying Barrett esophagus. The prevalence of eosinophilic esophagitis in the pediatric population has become more recognized in recent years.[10] Because of inflammation and edema, patients with eosinophilic esophagitis can often present with dysphagia and pain mimicking GER disease. The diagnosis of eosinophilic esophagitis can be made by histologic evaluation of esophageal biopsy specimens obtained at the time of endoscopic evaluation.

Treatment

Conservative management of significant GER includes thickening of formula with cereal, reducing the volume of feeding, and postural maneuvers. In addition, pharmacologic acid suppression may be useful. Indications for surgical intervention include severe GER that is unresponsive to aggressive medical management. Surgery is generally warranted for patients with life-threatening near-miss SIDS episodes, failure to thrive, or esophageal stricture. Other relative indications include those requiring complex surgical airway reconstruction, neurologic impairment requiring permanent feeding access, and a history of recurrent pneumonias or persistent asthma. The gold standard surgical procedure for infants and children with pathologic GER is Nissen fundoplication (360-degree esophageal wrap). It is the most effective method to control the symptoms of GER; however, the undesirable side effect of gas bloat or dysphagia is more likely to occur after a full fundic wrap than after a partial one. A partial wrap (e.g., Toupet, 270 degrees; Thal, 180 degrees) has been reported to produce fewer complications of dysphagia but is less effective in controlling the reflux symptoms as well. Regardless of which type of fundoplication is performed, a laparoscopic approach has become the standard technique.

Hypertrophic Pyloric Stenosis

Hypertrophic pyloric stenosis (HPS) is a disease of newborns, with an incidence of 1 in 300 to 900 live births. It is most common between the ages of 2 and 8 weeks. Boys are affected four times more often than girls, with first-born male infants being at highest risk. Hypertrophy of the circular muscle of the pylorus results in constriction and obstruction of the gastric outlet, leading to nonbilious, projectile emesis, loss of hydrochloric acid with the onset of hypokalemic hypochloremic metabolic alkalosis, and dehydration. Although the exact cause of HPS remains unknown, a lack of nitric oxide synthase in pyloric tissue has been implicated.

Clinical Presentation

Infants with HPS generally present with progressively worsening nonbilious emesis. Over time, the emesis becomes more frequent, forceful, and projectile in nature. On occasion, visible gastric peristalsis may be observed as a wave of contractions from the left upper quadrant to the epigastrium. Shortly after emesis, infants usually crave additional feedings. A plain abdominal radiograph can show an enlarged gastric gas bubble. Palpation of the pyloric "olive" tumor in the epigastrium by an experienced examiner is pathognomonic for HPS. If the olive is confirmed, no additional diagnostic testing is necessary. When the olive is not appreciated, an ultrasound study should be obtained. Pyloric muscle thickness of more than 3 to 4 mm or a pyloric length greater than 15 to 18 mm in the presence of functional gastric outlet obstruction is diagnostic. With an equivocal clinical presentation, an upper GI contrast study may be useful to evaluate for other causes of vomiting.

Management

The Ramstedt pyloromyotomy remains the standard operation for HPS. Preoperatively, it is imperative that the infant be fully resuscitated with IV fluids to establish an adequate urine output and to restore normal electrolyte balance. If not, there is a high risk for postoperative apnea because the infant with metabolic alkalosis has a propensity to compensate by retaining respiratory carbon dioxide. Thus, the serum bicarbonate level needs to be normalized before surgery, at least to a value of less than 30 mEq/L. Pyloromyotomy involves incising the thickened pyloric musculature while preserving the underlying mucosa. This is performed through a right upper quadrant or periumbilical incision. A laparoscopic approach (Fig. 66-9) has gained popularity because of its smaller incision. However, the general principle of pyloromyotomy is the same regardless of laparoscopic or open procedures, with equivalent outcomes.[11] Postoperatively, infants are allowed to resume enteral feedings gradually. There are various feeding protocols, which range from immediate full ad lib feedings to volume-based incremental advancement. Vomiting after surgery occurs frequently but is generally self-limited. Potential complications include incomplete myotomy and mucosal perforation.

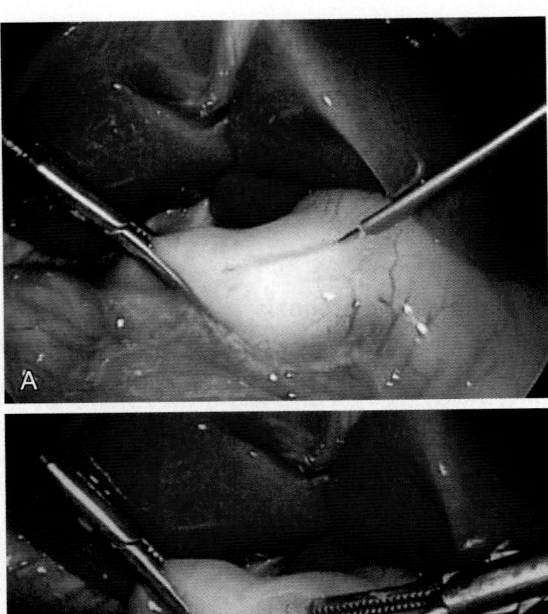

FIGURE 66-9 A, Laparoscopic Ramstedt pyloromyotomy is started with a retractable blade. **B,** A spreader with grooves on the outer surface is used to complete the pyloromyotomy. Intact mucosal bulging along with independent muscle wall motion is confirmed. (From St. Peter SD, Ostlie DJ: Laparoscopic and open pyloromyotomy. In Chung DH, Chen MK, editors: *Atlas of pediatric surgical techniques*, Philadelphia, 2010, Elsevier Saunders, pp 253–265.)

Intestinal Atresia

Duodenal atresia is thought to result from failure of vacuolization of the duodenum from its solid cord stage. The range of anatomic variants includes duodenal stenosis, mucosal web with intact muscle wall (so-called windsock deformity), two ends separated by a fibrous cord, and complete separation with a gap within the duodenum. It is associated with several conditions, including prematurity, Down syndrome, maternal polyhydramnios, malrotation, annular pancreas, and biliary atresia. Other anomalies, such as cardiac, renal, esophageal, and anorectal anomalies, are also common. In most cases, the duodenal obstruction is distal to the ampulla of Vater (85%); therefore, infants present with bilious emesis. In patients with a mucosal web, the symptoms of postprandial emesis may occur later in life.

Infants with duodenal obstruction are generally first detected during a prenatal ultrasound evaluation. Immediately after birth, a plain abdominal radiograph shows a typical double-bubble sign if it is obtained before orogastric tube decompression of swallowed gastric air (Fig. 66-10*A*). If distal air is present, an upper GI contrast study should be considered not only to confirm the diagnosis of duodenal stenosis or atresia but also to exclude midgut volvulus, which would constitute a surgical emergency.

The management is by surgical bypass of the duodenal obstruction as a side-to-side or proximal transverse to distal longitudinal (diamond-shaped) duodenoduodenostomy (Fig. 66-10*B*). At the time of anastomosis, additional intestinal atresia should be ruled out by injecting saline into a distal limb using a soft red rubber catheter. When the proximal duodenum is markedly dilated, a tapering duodenoplasty with staples or sutures should be considered to narrow the duodenal caliber to lessen dysmotility. In patients with a duodenal mucosal web, the web is excised transduodenally; caution must be exercised to avoid injury to the ampulla.

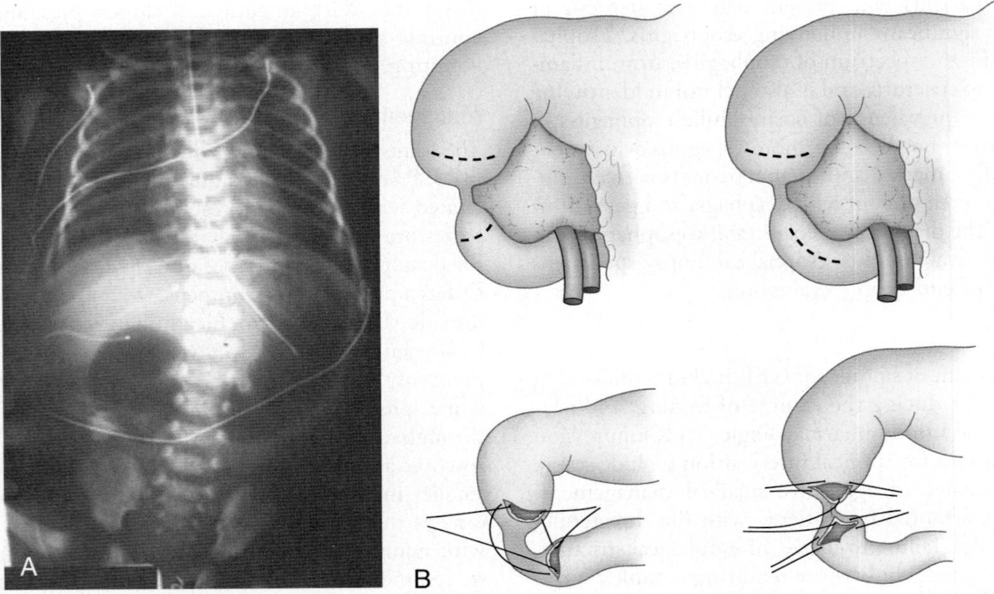

FIGURE 66-10 A, Plain abdominal radiograph shows double-bubble appearance of duodenal atresia. **B,** Proximal transverse to distal longitudinal (diamond-shaped) or side-to-side duodenoduodenostomy is performed for congenital duodenal obstruction. (From Duodenal obstruction. In O'Neill JA Jr, Grosfeld JL, Fonkalsrud EW, et al, editors: *Principles of pediatric surgery*, ed 2, St. Louis, 2003, Mosby, p 474.)

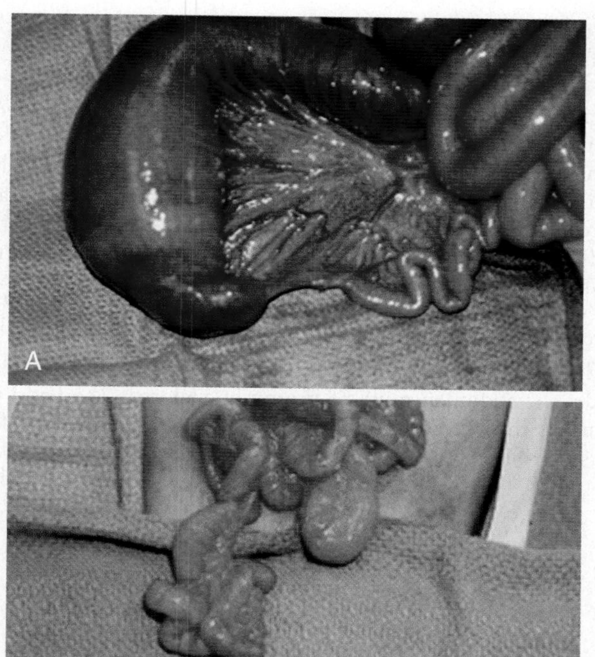

FIGURE 66-11 Jejunoileal Atresia. A, Massively dilated jejunum with narrow distal bowel segment. **B,** Apple peel type of atresia with a large mesenteric gap.

Jejunoileal atresia is the most common GI atresia; it occurs in 1 in 2000 live births. It is thought to result from an intrauterine mesenteric vascular accident. Atresias are slightly more common in the jejunum than in the ileum. Jejunoileal atresias are classified as type I, a mucosal web or diaphragm (Fig. 66-11*A*); type II, with an atretic cord between two blind ends of bowel with intact mesentery; type IIIa, a complete separation of the blind ends of the bowel by a V-shaped mesenteric gap; and type IIIb, an apple peel or Christmas tree deformity with a large mesenteric gap (Fig. 66-11*B*), in which the distal bowel receives a retrograde blood supply from the ileocolic or right colic artery. This tenuous blood supply has implications for anastomotic failures and the potential for ischemic necrosis from volvulus. Thus, many of these infants with this type of atresia are born with reduced intestinal length. In type IV, there are multiple atresias, with a string of sausage appearance.

Infants present with bilious emesis, abdominal distention, and failure to pass meconium. The clinical presentation varies by the location of the atretic obstruction. In proximal atresia, abdominal distention is less, but significant bilious emesis is present. Abdominal radiographs can show air-fluid levels with absent distal gas. In distal atresias, abdominal distention is more common. A contrast enema study can demonstrate a narrow caliber of colon and may also be useful to exclude multiple atresias, which may be present in 10% to 15% of cases. Jejunoileal atresia is generally not associated with other anomalies except cystic fibrosis in approximately 10% of patients.

Infants are managed for neonatal bowel obstruction. An orogastric tube is placed, and appropriate IV fluid resuscitation is implemented. At operation, the main objective is to establish intestinal continuity while preserving as much intestinal length as possible. In multiple atresias, multiple anastomoses over an endoluminal stent may be necessary. If the proximal intestine is significantly dilated, prolonged dysmotility may persist, and therefore a tapering enteroplasty of the dilated segment should be considered. However, in cases of adequate bowel length, resection of the dilated segment can result in faster recovery. The overall survival for infants with jejunoileal atresia is more than 90%.

Colonic atresia is the least common, accounting for only 5% to 10% of intestinal atresia; the incidence is 1 in 20,000 live births. Infants usually present with failure to pass meconium, abdominal distention, and bilious vomiting. A plain radiograph shows multiple dilated bowel loops, but differentiation between small and large bowel is not feasible in this age group because of lack of well-developed haustra and semicircularis landmarks. Contrast enema study can confirm the diagnosis, but the clinical picture of bowel obstruction may be enough evidence to proceed with operative intervention of diverting end colostomy.

Intestinal Malrotation and Midgut Volvulus

The actual incidence of rotational anomalies of the midgut is difficult to determine but is estimated to be 1 in 6000 live births. The midgut normally herniates out of the coelomic cavity through the umbilical ring at approximately the fourth week of fetal development. By the tenth week of gestation, the intestine begins to migrate back into the abdominal cavity in a counterclockwise rotation around the axis of the superior mesenteric artery (SMA) for 270 degrees. The duodenojejunal segment returns first and rotates beneath and to the right of the SMA to fix in the left upper quadrant at the ligament of Treitz. The cecocolic segment also rotates counterclockwise around the SMA to rest in its final position in the right lower quadrant. By week 12, this process of intestinal rotation is complete, and the colon becomes fixed to the retroperitoneum. An interruption or reversal of any of these coordinated movements implies an embryologic explanation for the range of anomalies seen.

Abnormal Intestinal Rotation

Complete nonrotation of the midgut is the most common anomaly and occurs when neither the duodenojejunal nor the cecocolic limb undergoes correct rotation. Consequently, duodenojejunal and ileocecal junctions lie close together and the midgut is suspended on a narrow SMA stalk, which can twist in a clockwise fashion to result in midgut volvulus. Nonrotation of the duodenojejunal limb, followed by normal rotation and fixation of the cecocolic limb, results in duodenal obstruction by abnormal mesenteric bands (Ladd bands) that extend from the colon across the anterior duodenum. In this anomaly, the risk of midgut volvulus is low because there is a relatively broad mesenteric base between the duodenojejunal junction and cecum. Normal rotation of the duodenojejunal limb with nonrotation of the cecocolic segment carries the same risk for midgut volvulus as a complete nonrotation anomaly. In this case, the risks for volvulus are high because of a narrow mesenteric base.

Clinical Presentation

The clinical presentation varies, depending on the specific mechanism of obstruction and whether it involves compromised bowel. The major symptoms are related to the presence of midgut volvulus, duodenal obstruction, or intermittent or chronic abdominal pain, or it is an incidental finding in an otherwise asymptomatic patient. Most patients develop symptoms during the first month of life. Midgut volvulus is a true surgical emergency because of evolving ischemic bowel loops. The acute onset of bilious emesis in a particularly somnolent or lethargic newborn is an ominous sign. Midgut volvulus may also be incomplete or intermittent. Toddlers and children may present with chronic abdominal pain, intermittent episodes of emesis (which may be nonbilious), early satiety, weight loss, failure to thrive, or malabsorption and diarrhea. With partial volvulus, the resultant mesenteric venous and lymphatic obstruction may impair nutrient absorption and produce protein loss into the gut lumen as well as mucosal ischemia and melena as a result of arterial insufficiency.

Diagnosis

Abdominal radiographs may demonstrate upper intestinal obstruction or a gasless abdomen; however, these findings are nonspecific. The upper GI contrast series remains the diagnostic study of choice; it demonstrates an abnormal position of the ligament of Treitz along with the appearance of a bird's beak in the third portion of the duodenum, which indicates an obstruction. The ultrasound examination has proved to be a useful tool for the diagnosis of intestinal malrotation with midgut volvulus, in which the normal relationship of the superior mesenteric vessels (the vein is to the right of artery) is reversed or altered.[12] In the acutely ill child with midgut volvulus and obstruction, immediate operative correction is indicated, and little time is available for IV fluid resuscitation, catheterization, or administration of broad-spectrum antibiotics. Time is critical if intestinal salvage is to be achieved.

Surgical Management

Midgut volvulus is a surgical emergency. Once the diagnosis is made, the abdomen must be promptly explored. The Ladd procedure is the operation of choice for rotational anomalies of the intestine (Fig. 66-12). On entering the peritoneal cavity, chylous

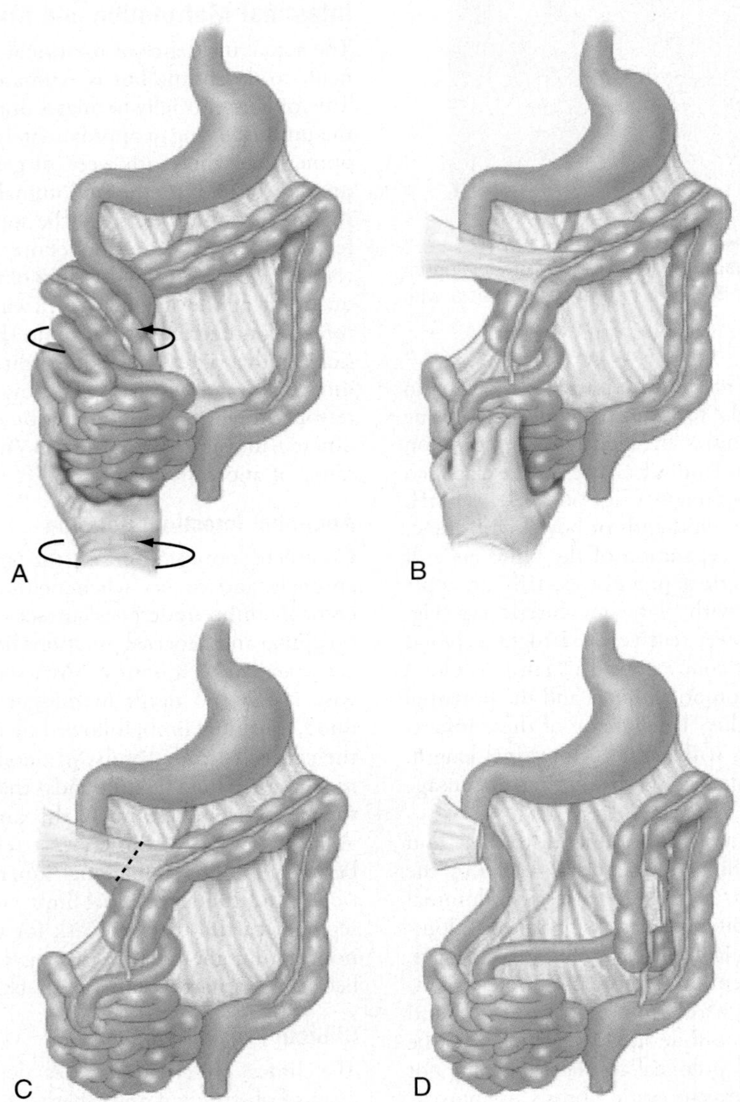

FIGURE 66-12 Ladd Procedure. A, Twisted bowel is eviscerated. **B,** The bowel is derotated in a counterclockwise fashion. **C,** The peritoneal attachment between the cecum and retroperitoneum (Ladd band) is divided. **D,** The base of the mesentery is widened, and an appendectomy is performed. (From Warner BW: Imperforate anus. In Chung DH, Chen MK, editors: *Atlas of pediatric surgical techniques*, Philadelphia, 2010, Elsevier Saunders, pp 138–142.)

ascites from obstructive lymphatics is frequently seen. The volvulus is untwisted in a counterclockwise fashion. After detorsion, the intestine may be congested and edematous, and some areas may appear necrotic. Placement of warm sponges and observation for a time may improve the appearance of the intestine when the vascular integrity has been compromised. Necrotic segments are resected; however, marginally ischemic segments may be left in place and a second-look laparotomy performed after 24 to 36 hours. Ladd bands are divided as they extend from the ascending colon across the duodenum to the posterior aspect of the right upper quadrant. In dividing the medial bands, the cecum is mobilized and the mesenteric base is broadened to prevent recurrent volvulus. Securing the cecum or duodenum to the abdominal wall by sutures has no proven benefit. In addition, an intraluminal duodenal obstruction may coexist, and therefore an orogastric tube may be advanced into the distal duodenum to exclude any associated anomaly. An incidental appendectomy is performed because the cecum will ultimately lie on the left side of the abdomen after the Ladd procedure. The intestine is replaced into the abdominal cavity with the small bowel loops on the right side; the colon is positioned on the left. Recurrent volvulus has been reported in up to 10% after the Ladd procedure. The more common cause of postoperative obstruction is adhesive bands. Prolonged ileus is common, particularly if a volvulus has progressed to necrosis, requiring extensive resection. Midgut volvulus accounts for approximately 18% of cases of short gut syndrome in the pediatric population. Urgent recognition and treatment are the most important factors in preventing this complication.

Necrotizing Enterocolitis

Necrotizing enterocolitis (NEC) is the most common GI surgical emergency in the neonatal period. Although several contributing factors, such as ischemia, bacteria, cytokines, and enteral feeding, have been established, prematurity is the single most important risk factor. Recent medical advances in the management of premature infants have led to improved overall survival, hence resulting in more premature infants at risk for development of NEC. However, the overall incidence appears to have decreased because of implementation of a gradual feeding regimen as well as promotion of the use of breast milk. Yet, the exact cause of NEC remains unknown, and research advances have been hampered by the fact that a correlative animal model for NEC does not exist.

Clinical Presentation and Diagnosis

The clinical presentation of NEC can be variable and unpredictable. Acute abdominal distention, tenderness, and feeding intolerance with gross or occult blood in the stool are hallmark features for NEC. Other nonspecific signs include irritability, temperature instability, and episodes of apnea or bradycardia. NEC typically occurs in the first few days of life with the initiation of enteral feedings. In approximately 80% of cases, however, it occurs within the first month of life. As NEC progresses, sepsis develops with hemodynamic deterioration and coagulopathy. The pathognomonic radiographic feature of NEC is pneumatosis intestinalis (Fig. 66-13*A*). Pneumatosis is composed of hydrogen gas generated by the bacterial fermentation of luminal substrates. Other radiographic findings may include portal venous gas, ascites, fixed loops of small bowel, and free air. The distal ileum and ascending colon are the usual affected areas, although the entire GI tract can be affected as in NEC totalis.

Medical Management

Initial medical management consists of orogastric tube decompression, fluid resuscitation, blood product transfusion, and broad-spectrum antibiotics. NEC can be successfully treated medically in approximately 50% of cases with a 10- to 14-day course of an IV antibiotic regimen and bowel rest. Serial abdominal examinations are performed to closely monitor for any subtle signs for surgical abdomen. The absolute indication for operative management of NEC is the presence of intestinal perforation, as revealed by free air on plain abdominal radiographs (Fig. 66-13*B*). Other relative indications for surgery include clinical deterioration, abdominal wall cellulitis, palpable abdominal mass, and a persistent fixed radiographic bowel loop.

Surgical Management

The general principles of surgical management of NEC include resection of all nonviable intestinal segments with ostomy diversion. Every effort must be made to preserve maximum intestinal length. Thus, it may be necessary to resect multiple intervening necrotic segments of bowel, preserving all viable intestine. In cases in which the bowel is ischemic but not frankly necrotic, a second-look operation may be performed after 24 to 48 hours. Bowel resection with primary anastomosis may be considered in the rare stable infant with a focal isolated perforation and minimal

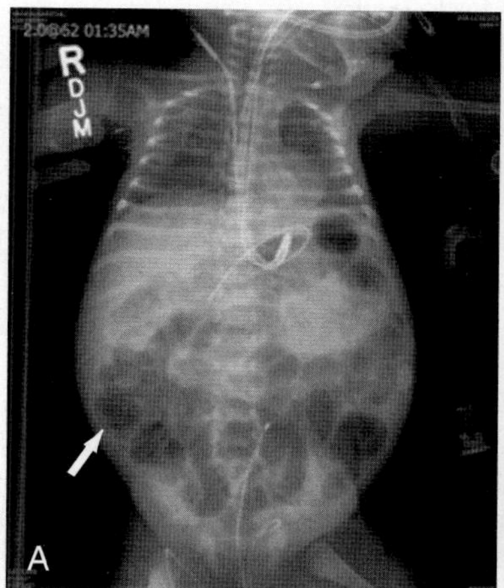

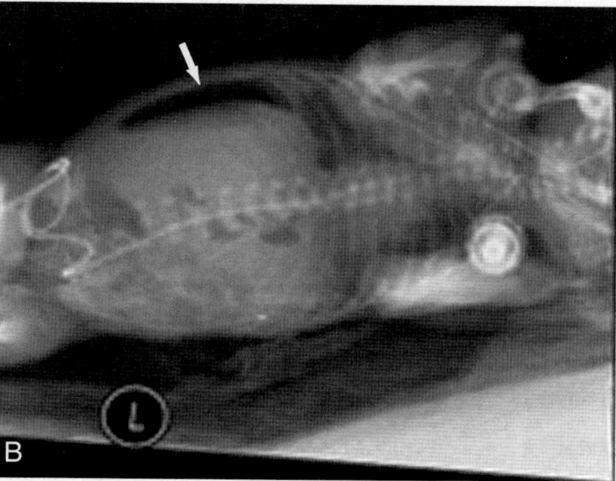

FIGURE 66-13 A, Pneumatosis intestinalis *(arrow),* a pathognomonic radiographic sign for necrotizing enterocolitis. **B,** Pneumoperitoneum *(arrow)* on lateral decubitus radiograph.

peritoneal contamination; however, the serious risks for anastomotic leak and stricture have tempered enthusiasm for this approach.

For infants of extremely low birth weight with perforated NEC, a bedside peritoneal drain placement is an alternative temporizing measure. Drainage of the contaminated peritoneal fluid may improve ventilation and halt the progression of sepsis in select critically ill preterm infants. Surprisingly, drain placement turned out to be the only intervention in some infants. However, percutaneous drain was reported to have poor outcomes in infants of extremely low birth weight (<1000 g). Evidence to support peritoneal drainage as an accepted mode of treatment for NEC was established in a multicenter, randomized prospective clinical trial.[13] In this study, survival, need for parenteral nutrition, and length of hospital stay were similar for NEC infants weighing less than 1500 g treated by peritoneal drainage or laparotomy. The overall mortality rate for surgically managed NEC ranges from 10% to 50%. NEC remains the most common cause of short gut syndrome. Intestinal strictures may develop after medical or surgical management of NEC in approximately 10% of infants. Because of the risk for post-NEC stricture, most notably in splenic flexure of the colon, a contrast enema study is done routinely before stoma reversal. Neurodevelopmental delay is also a frequent long-term complication.

Short Bowel Syndrome

Short bowel syndrome (SBS) is a clinical condition in which there is inadequate length of functional intestine to sustain normal enteral nutrition as a result of massive small bowel resection. Common conditions that can lead to SBS are intestinal atresia, midgut volvulus, NEC, and gastroschisis. In SBS, intestinal function depends on a number of factors, such as total bowel length, presence of the ileocecal valve, and residual segments of intestine. The jejunum is the site of absorption of most macronutrients and minerals. GI hormones that are critical for gut function, such as cholecystokinin and secretin, are produced in the jejunum. The ileum is essential for the absorption of carbohydrates, proteins, fluids, and electrolytes. Bile acids, vitamin B_{12}, and the fat-soluble vitamins (A, D, E, K) are primarily absorbed in the ileum. Ileocecal valve function is particularly important in SBS, in which intestinal transit time can be significantly altered. The colon is important in SBS patients for absorption of water and electrolytes. After massive small bowel resection, a physiologic process known as intestinal adaptation occurs to compensate for the loss of intestinal length. Many factors are involved in this adaptive process to enhance the absorptive function of the residual intestine. Medical treatment of SBS includes the use of an elemental diet, glutamine and various growth factors, and careful delivery of TPN.[12] Several surgical techniques (excluding small bowel transplantation) aimed at slowing intestinal transit time or increasing the mucosal surface area for enhanced absorption have been described.[14] These include reversed intestinal segment, recirculating loop, artificial intestinal valve, colon interposition, and intestinal pacing. Two procedures that are generally used are the Bianchi procedure and serial transverse enteroplasty (STEP).

Surgical Management

Bianchi procedure. Bianchi[15] originally described an intestinal lengthening procedure in which the mesenteric vascular bed is separated into two systems; the dilated small intestine is split into two parallel segments, each with its own blood supply, and the ends are approximated (Fig. 66-14*A*). This resulted in a 50%

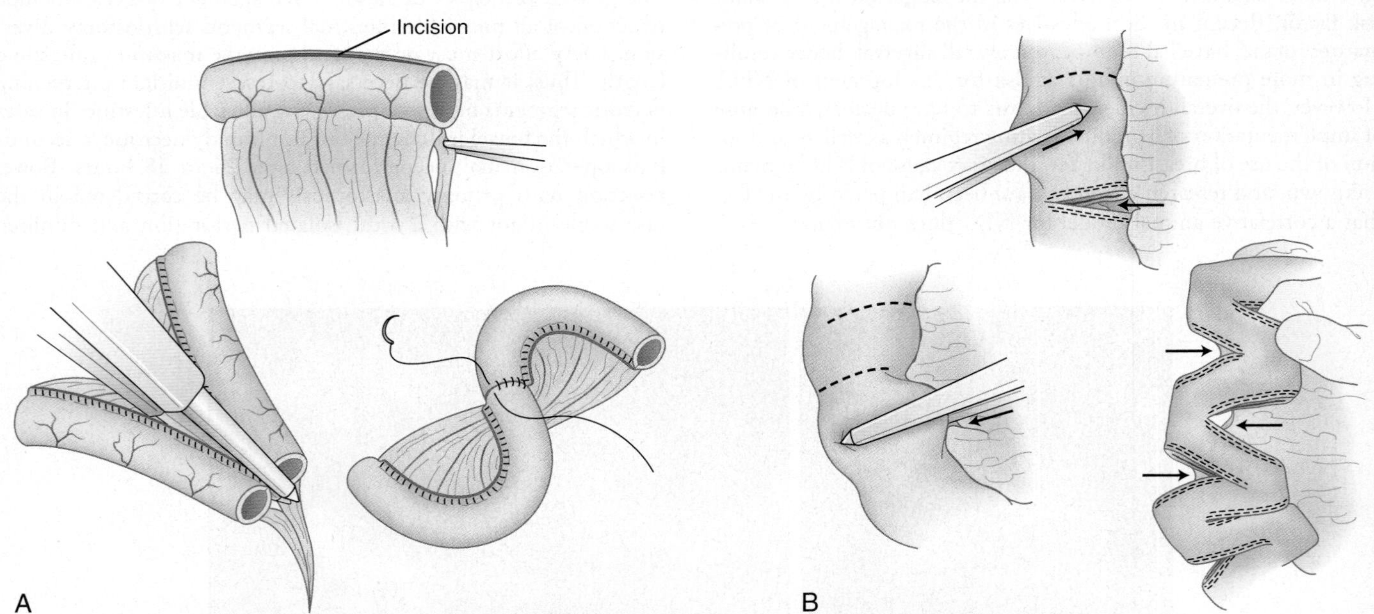

FIGURE 66-14 Bowel-Lengthening Procedures. A, Bianchi technique separates two mesenteric planes. A dilated segment of bowel is stapled longitudinally to create two narrower segments for sequential anastomosis. **B,** Serial transverse enteroplasty (STEP) involves stapling a dilated bowel into V shapes on alternating sides, decreasing width and increasing length. (**A** adapted from Abu-Elmagd KM, Bond G, Costa G, et al: Gut rehabilitation and intestinal transplantation. *Therapy* 2:853–864, 2005. **B** from Kim HB, Fauza D, Garza J, et al: Serial transverse enteroplasty [STEP]: A novel bowel-lengthening procedure. *J Pediatr Surg* 38:425–429, 2003.)

decreased diameter of the small intestine and increased length by 200%. The Bianchi procedure has been shown to be an effective surgical option for treating patients with SBS.

Serial transverse enteroplasty. Since its description in 2003,[16] the STEP procedure has garnered significant interest by the pediatric surgical community. In contrast to the Bianchi procedure, dilated small intestine is serially stapled in a transverse fashion to create a narrower lumen and longer intestinal length (Fig. 66-14*B*). The STEP procedure improved enteral feeding tolerance, resulting in significant catch-up growth, and was not associated with increased mortality.[17] A recent study reported improved enteral tolerance in the majority of 20 patients observed for more than a 7-year period after STEP procedures.[18]

Meconium Ileus

Meconium ileus is a unique form of neonatal obstruction that occurs in infants with cystic fibrosis (CF), an autosomal recessive disorder resulting from a mutation in the CF transmembrane regulator gene *(CFTR)*. It is estimated that 3.3% of the white population in the United States are asymptomatic carriers of the mutated *CFTR* gene. The abnormal chloride transport in patients with CF results in tenacious viscous secretions with a protein concentration of almost 80% to 90%. It affects a wide variety of organs, including the intestine, pancreas, lungs, salivary glands, reproductive organs, and biliary tract. Meconium ileus is classified as simple or complicated.

Clinical Presentation

Meconium ileus in the newborn represents the earliest clinical manifestation of CF; it affects approximately 10% to 15% of patients with this inherited disease. The incidence of CF ranges from 1 in 1000 to 2000 live births. Infants present with three cardinal signs in the first 24 to 48 hours of life: (1) generalized abdominal distention; (2) bilious emesis; and (3) failure to pass meconium. Maternal polyhydramnios occurs in approximately 20% of cases. In simple meconium ileus, the terminal ileum is dilated and filled with thick, tarlike, inspissated meconium. Smaller pellets of meconium are found in the more distal ileum, leading into a relatively small colon. In patients with simple meconium ileus, important plain abdominal radiographic findings include dilated and gas-filled loops of small bowel, absence of air-fluid levels, and a mass of meconium in the right side of the abdomen mixed with gas to give a ground-glass or soap bubble appearance.

Simple Meconium Ileus

Abdominal radiographs show dilated bowel loops with relatively absent air-fluid levels because of thick viscous meconium. A ground-glass appearance is noted in the right lower quadrant corresponding to bowel loops filled with thick meconium mixed with air. The initial diagnostic study of choice is contrast enema using a water-soluble ionic solution. In simple meconium ileus, a Gastrografin contrast enema study can demonstrate a small narrow-caliber colon and inspissated meconium pellets in the terminal ileum (Fig. 66-15*A*). Gastrografin is a hypertonic solution that can aid in the evacuation of meconium. However, it is imperative that the infant be well hydrated and vital signs carefully monitored after the Gastrografin study. Contrast enema is successful in relieving the obstruction in up to 75% of cases, with a bowel perforation rate of less than 3%. The pilocarpine iontophoresis sweat test revealing a chloride concentration higher than 60 mEq/L is the most reliable and definitive method to confirm the diagnosis of CF. A more immediate test is detection of the mutated *CFTR* gene.

Surgical management. Operative management of simple meconium ileus is required when the obstruction is persistent despite contrast enema, along with 5 mL of 10% *N*-acetylcysteine (Mucomyst) solution administered every 6 hours through a nasogastric tube. Historically, the dilated terminal ileum was resected and various types of stomas were created, allowing intestinal

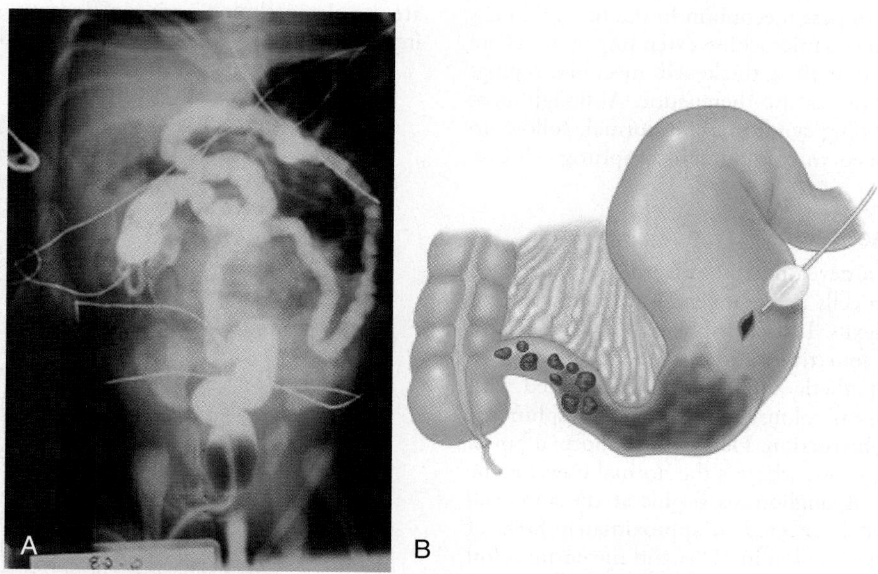

FIGURE 66-15 Surgical management of simple meconium ileus. **A,** Contrast enema study shows microcolon with soap bubble appearance in the right lower quadrant. **B,** Removal of meconium can be facilitated by gentle use of a catheter along with a 2% to 4% *N*-acetylcysteine solution. (From Brandt ML: Meconium disease. In Chung DH, Chen MK, editors: *Atlas of pediatric surgical techniques*, Philadelphia, 2010, Elsevier Saunders, pp 44–53.)

decompression and recovery. However, enterotomy, irrigation with warmed saline solution or 4% *N*-acetylcysteine, and simple evacuation of the luminal meconium without a stoma has also been advocated (Fig. 66-15*B*). *N*-Acetylcysteine serves to break the disulfide bonds in the meconium to facilitate separation from the bowel mucosa. The meconium is manipulated into the distal colon or removed through the enterotomy. After the obstruction is relieved, the enterotomy is closed in standard fashion. If meconium evacuation is incomplete, a T tube may be left in place in the ileum to facilitate continued postoperative irrigation.

Complicated Meconium Ileus

Meconium ileus is considered complicated when perforation of the intestine has taken place in utero or in the early neonatal period. Extravasation of meconium can result in severe peritonitis, with a dense inflammatory response and calcification. The variable clinical presentation includes a meconium pseudocyst, adhesive peritonitis with or without secondary bacterial infection, and ascites. Abdominal radiographs can demonstrate calcifications, bowel dilation, mass effect, and ascites. A distal ileal obstructive syndrome, formerly known as meconium ileus equivalent, may develop as a consequence of noncompliance with oral enzyme replacement therapy or bouts of dehydration. This is managed nonoperatively in most patients with enemas or oral polyethylene glycol purging solutions. Other diagnoses must also be considered, including simple adhesive intestinal obstruction. Furthermore, with the introduction of enteric-coated, high-strength pancreatic enzyme replacement therapy, a fibrosing cholangiopathy has been described. Resection of the inflammatory colon stricture may be necessary.

Meconium Plug Syndrome

Meconium plug syndrome is unrelated to meconium ileus and in most cases is not a sequela of CF. However, it is a frequent cause of neonatal intestinal obstruction and is associated with a number of conditions, including Hirschsprung's disease, maternal diabetes, and hypothyroidism. Infants present with significant abdominal distention and failure to pass meconium in the first 24 hours of life. Contrast enema shows a microcolon extending up to where the colon is dilated, filled with a thickened meconium plug. Often, a contrast enema study is also therapeutic. Although most children with meconium plug syndrome are normal, follow-up studies should be performed to rule out Hirschsprung's disease and CF.

Hirschsprung's Disease

Hirschsprung's disease is a developmental disorder characterized by an absence of ganglion cells in the myenteric (Auerbach) and submucosal (Meissner) plexus. It occurs in 1 in 5000 live births, with boys being affected four times more frequently than girls. This neurogenic parasympathetic abnormality is associated with muscular spasm of the distal colon and internal anal sphincter, resulting in a functional obstruction. Hence, the abnormal bowel is the contracted distal segment, whereas the normal bowel is the proximal dilated portion. Aganglionosis begins at the anorectal line, and the rectosigmoid is affected in approximately 80% of cases, the splenic or transverse colon in 17%, and the entire colon in 8%. The area between the dilated and contracted segments is referred to as the transition zone. Here, ganglion cells begin to appear, but in reduced numbers. Of these patients, 3% to 5% have Down syndrome, and the risk for Hirschsprung's disease is greater if there is a family history. An abnormal locus on chromosome 10 has been identified in some families and is associated with the *RET* oncogene.[19]

Clinical Presentation

Most infants (>90%) present with abdominal distention and bilious emesis with failure to pass meconium within the first 24 hours of life. Infants whose Hirschsprung's disease is not recognized early may present with a chronic history of poor feeding, abdominal distention, and significant constipation. Enterocolitis is the most common cause of death in patients with uncorrected Hirschsprung's disease and may be manifested as diarrhea alternating with periods of obstipation, abdominal distention, fever, hematochezia, and peritonitis.

Diagnosis

The diagnostic test of choice in a newborn with radiographic evidence of a distal bowel obstruction is a contrast enema study. In a study with normal findings, the rectum is wider than the sigmoid colon. In patients with Hirschsprung's disease, spasm of the distal rectum usually results in a narrow caliber with a transition zone and dilated proximal sigmoid colon (Fig. 66-16). Failure to evacuate the instilled contrast medium completely after 24 hours strongly suggests Hirschsprung's disease. An important goal of the study is to exclude other causes of constipation, such as meconium plug, small left colon syndrome, and atresia. The manometric finding of high internal sphincter pressure when the rectum is distended with a balloon can also be useful information in older children, but this is rarely performed. A rectal biopsy is the gold standard for the diagnosis of Hirschsprung's disease. In the newborn period, this is performed at the bedside using a suction rectal biopsy kit. It is important to obtain biopsy specimens at least 2 cm above the dentate line to avoid sampling the normal aganglionated region of the internal sphincter. In older children, a full-thickness biopsy specimen is obtained under general anesthesia because the thicker rectal mucosa is not amenable to suction biopsy technique. Absent ganglia, hypertrophied nerve trunks, and robust immunostaining for acetylcholinesterase are the histopathologic criteria. Recently, calretinin immunostaining has become more widely used and is considered superior

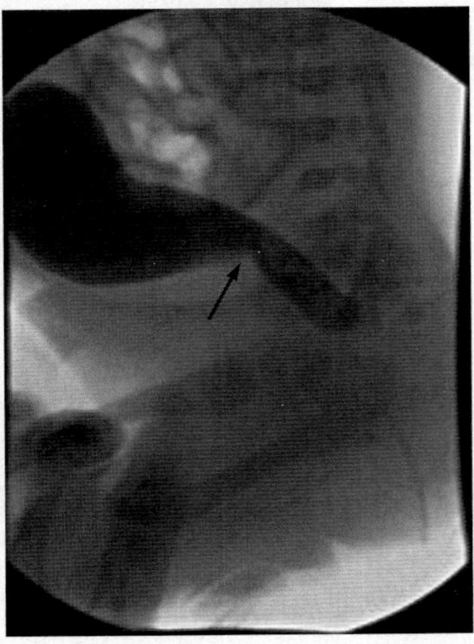

FIGURE 66-16 Contrast enema demonstrating transition point *(arrow)* in Hirschsprung's disease.

to acetylcholinesterase staining to confirm the diagnosis of Hirschsprung's disease.[20]

Surgical Management

Historically, a leveling colostomy was performed initially through a left lower quadrant surgical incision. The location of the transition zone is confirmed by frozen section evaluation of multiple seromuscular biopsy specimens. A diverting colostomy (end or loop) is then performed in the region of normal ganglionated bowel, and a definitive procedure is performed at a later age. There are definitive surgical options for Hirschsprung's disease. In the Swenson procedure, the aganglionic bowel is removed down to the level of the internal sphincters and a coloanal anastomosis is performed. In the Duhamel procedure, the aganglionic rectal stump is left in place and the ganglionated normal colon is pulled behind the stump. A stapler is then inserted through the anus, with one arm within the normal ganglionated bowel posteriorly and the other in the aganglionic rectum anteriorly. Stapling results in the formation of a neorectum that empties normally because of the posterior patch of ganglionated bowel. The Soave technique involves an endorectal mucosal dissection within the aganglionic distal rectum. The ganglionated normal colon is then pulled through the remnant muscular cuff, and a coloanal anastomosis is performed. The laparoscopy-assisted Soave procedure has become popular; it is performed on newborns and has the advantages of primary definitive operation without an initial colostomy. The Soave procedure is also performed entirely through a transanal approach. Postoperatively, the stool dysfunction can persist and be difficult to manage, requiring intermittent rectal decompression in some cases. Constipation is a common postoperative problem along with frequent soiling, incontinence, and postoperative enterocolitis.

Anorectal Malformation

The incidence of imperforate anus is 1 in 5000 live births, and boys are more affected (58%). The spectrum of anorectal malformations ranges from simple anal stenosis to the persistence of a cloaca. The most common defect is an imperforate anus with a fistula between the distal colon and urethra in boys or the vestibule of the vagina in girls.

Embryology

By the sixth week of gestation, the urorectal septum moves caudally to divide the cloaca into the anterior urogenital sinus and posterior anorectal canal. Failure of this septum to form results in a fistula between the bowel and urinary tract (in boys) or vagina (in girls). Complete or partial failure of the anal membrane to resorb results in an anal membrane or stenosis. The perineum also contributes to the development of the external anal opening and genitalia by the formation of cloacal folds, which extend from the anterior genital tubercle to the anus. The perineal body is formed by fusion of the cloacal folds between the anal and urogenital membranes. Breakdown of the cloacal membrane anywhere along its course results in the external anal opening being anterior to the external sphincter (i.e., anteriorly displaced anus).

Classification

An anatomic classification of anorectal anomalies is based on the level at which the blind-ending rectal pouch ends—low, intermediate, or high in relationship to the levator ani musculature. A more therapeutic and prognostic classification is depicted in Box 66-1. An invertogram, a lateral pelvic radiograph taken after the infant is held upside-down for several minutes, was used in the past to determine the most distal point of the rectal pouch. In most cases, a careful inspection of the perineum alone can predict the pouch level. If an anocutaneous fistula is observed anywhere on the perineal skin of a boy or external to the hymen of a girl, a low lesion can be assumed. Most other types of lesions are high or intermediate. Rectal atresia refers to an unusual lesion in which the lumen of the rectum is completely or partially interrupted, with the upper rectum being dilated and the lower rectum consisting of a small anal canal. A persistent cloaca is defined as a defect in which the rectum, vagina, and urethra all fuse to form a single common channel. In girls, a single orifice in the perineum indicates a cloaca. If two perineal orifices are seen (i.e., urethra and vagina), the defect represents a high imperforate anus or, less commonly, a persistent urogenital sinus comprising one orifice and a normal anus as the other orifice. Anorectal malformation often coexists with other lesions, and the VACTERL association must be considered during evaluation. Bone abnormalities of the sacrum and spine, such as absent vertebrae, accessory vertebrae, or hemivertebrae or an asymmetrical or short sacrum, can occur in approximately one third of patients. Absence of two or more vertebrae is associated with a poor prognosis for bowel and bladder continence. Occult dysraphism of the spinal cord may also be present; this consists of a tethered cord, lipomeningocele, or fat within the filum terminale.

BOX 66-1 Classification of Congenital Anomalies of the Anorectum

Female	Male
Cutaneous (perineal fistula)	Cutaneous (perineal fistula)
Vestibular fistula	Rectourethral fistula
Imperforate anus without fistula	Bulbar
Rectal atresia	Prostatic
Cloaca	Recto–bladder neck fistula
Complex malformation	Imperforate anus without fistula
	Rectal atresia

Evaluation

Aside from physical examination, plain radiography of the spine and ultrasound of the spinal cord are performed. Genitourinary abnormalities other than the rectourinary fistula occur in 25% to 60% of patients. Vesicoureteral reflux and hydronephrosis are the most common, but other conditions, such as horseshoe, dysplastic, or absent kidney as well as hypospadias or cryptorchidism, must be considered. In general, the higher the anorectal malformation, the greater the frequency of associated urologic abnormalities. In patients with a persistent cloaca or rectovesical fistula, the likelihood of a genitourinary abnormality is approximately 90%. In contrast, the frequency is only 10% with low defects (e.g., perineal fistula). Renal ultrasound and voiding cystourethrography are obtained to assess the urinary tract. If a cardiac defect is suspected, echocardiography is performed before any surgical procedure. Esophageal atresia can also be ruled out with an orogastric tube placement. The decision algorithms for the management of male and female newborns with anorectal malformation are shown in Figures 66-17 and 66-18.

Surgical Management

Low lesions. A newborn with a low lesion can undergo a primary single-stage repair without colostomy. For anal stenosis

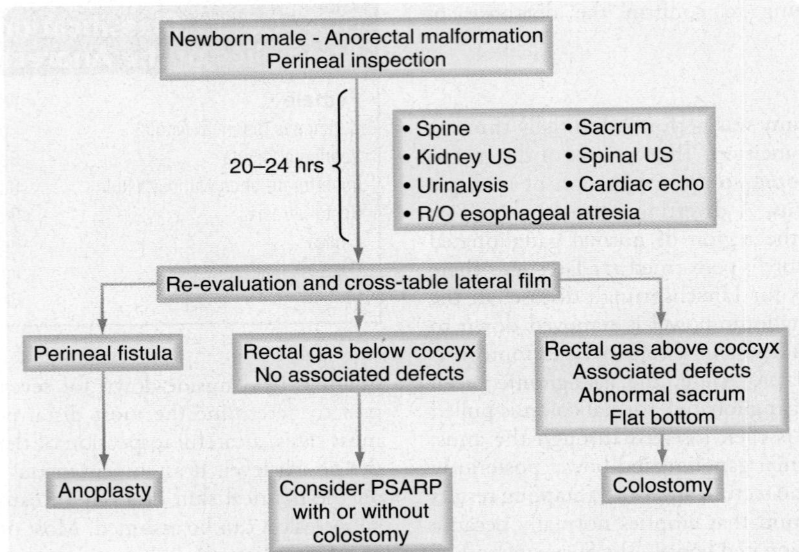

FIGURE 66-17 Decision algorithm for the management of male patients with anorectal malformation. *PSARP,* Posterior sagittal anorectoplasty. (From Levitt M, Peña A: Imperforate anus. In Chung DH, Chen MK, editors: *Atlas of pediatric surgical techniques*, Philadelphia, 2010, Elsevier Saunders, pp 185–205.)

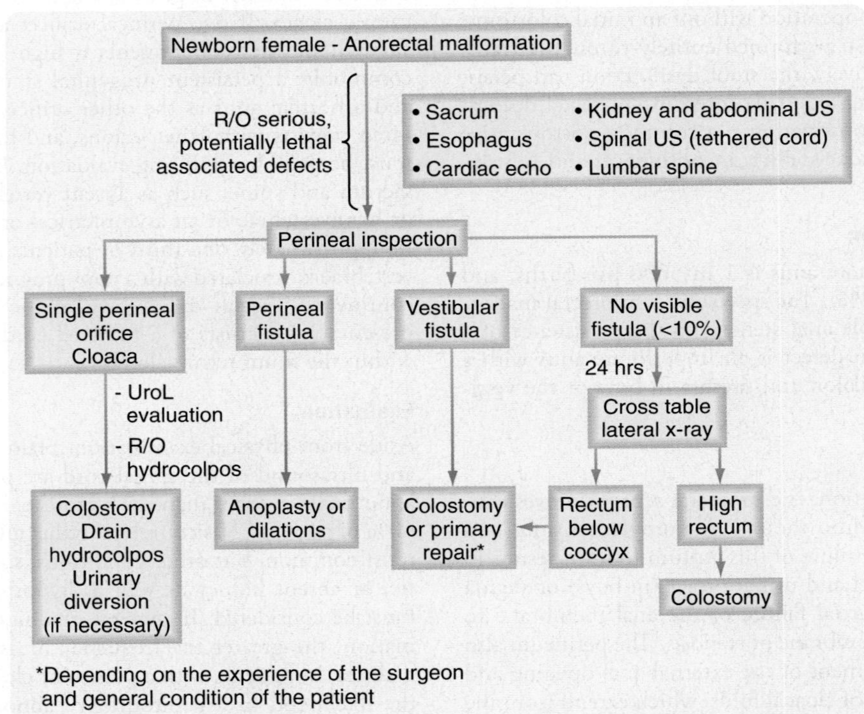

FIGURE 66-18 Decision algorithm for the management of female patients with anorectal malformation. (From Levitt M, Peña A: Imperforate anus. In Chung DH, Chen MK, editors: *Atlas of pediatric surgical techniques*, Philadelphia, 2010, Elsevier Saunders, pp 185–205.)

in which the anal opening is in a normal location, serial dilation alone is usually sufficient. Dilations are performed daily with gradual size increase over time. If the anal opening is anterior to the external sphincter (i.e., anteriorly displaced anus), with a small distance between the opening and the center of the external sphincter, and the perineal body is intact, a cutback anoplasty may be performed. This consists of an incision extending from the ectopic anal orifice to the central part of the anal sphincter, thus enlarging the anal opening. Alternatively, if there is a significant distance between the anal opening and central portion of the external anal sphincter, a transposition anoplasty is performed in which the aberrant anal opening is transposed to the normal position within the center of the sphincter muscles, and the perineal body is reconstructed.

Intermediate or high lesions. Newborns with intermediate or high lesions generally require a diverting colostomy as the first part of a three-stage reconstruction. The colon is completely divided, and an end sigmoid colostomy with a mucous fistula is constructed to minimize fecal contamination into the area of a rectourinary fistula. Furthermore, the distal mucous fistula limb can be used later for a contrast study to determine the rectourinary fistula. The second-stage procedure usually is performed at 3 to 6 months of age. The operation consists of dividing the rectourinary or rectovaginal fistula with a pull-through of the terminal rectal pouch into the normal anal position. A posterior sagittal anorectoplasty, as first described by deVries and Peña, is the procedure of choice.[21] This consists of determining the location of the central position of the anal sphincter by electrical stimulation of the perineum. An incision is then made in the midline, extending from the coccyx to the anterior perineum and through the sphincter and levator musculature until the rectum is identified. The fistula from the rectum to the vagina or urinary tract is divided. The rectum is mobilized and the perineal musculature reconstructed. The third and final stage is colostomy reversal, which is performed several weeks later. Anal dilations begin 2 weeks after the anorectoplasty and continue for several months after the colostomy closure.

A laparoscopically assisted posterior sagittal anorectoplasty has significant advantages as a minimally invasive approach for anorectal malformation with good outcomes.[22] This technique offers the theoretical advantages of placing the neorectum within the central position of the sphincter and levator muscle complex under direct vision and avoids the need to cut across these structures. The long-term outcome of this new approach compared with the standard posterior sagittal method is presently unknown.

Morbidity in patients with anorectal malformations relates to associated anomalies. Fecal continence is the major goal regarding correction of the defect. Prognostic factors for continence include the level of the pouch and whether the sacrum is normal. In general, 75% of patients have voluntary bowel movements. However, 50% of this group still soils their underwear occasionally; the other 50% is considered totally continent. Constipation is the most common sequela. A bowel management program consisting of daily enemas is an important postoperative plan to reduce the frequency of soilage and to improve the quality of life for these patients.

Intussusception

Intussusception is a telescoping of one portion of the intestine into the other; it is usually idiopathic, without an obvious anatomic lead point. It occurs predominantly at the ileocecal junction. Invariably, there is marked swelling of the lymphoid tissue in the region of the ileocecal valve. It is unknown whether this represents the cause or effect of the ileocolic intussusception. The incidence of intussusception is associated with a history of recent episodes of viral gastroenteritis, upper respiratory infections, and even administration of rotavirus vaccine, implying lymphoid swelling in the pathogenesis of intussusception. In older children, the incidence of a pathologic lead point is up to 12%, and Meckel's diverticulum is found to be the most common lead point for intussusception. However, other causes, such as intestinal polyps, inflamed appendix, submucosal hemorrhage associated with Henoch-Schönlein purpura, foreign body, ectopic pancreatic or gastric tissue, and intestinal duplication, must also be considered. Postoperative small bowel intussusception in the absence of a lead point can also occur; this represents up to 5% of all pediatric cases of intussusception.

Clinical Presentation and Diagnosis

Intussusception produces severe cramping abdominal pain in an otherwise healthy child from 3 months to 3 years. Two thirds of children presenting with intussusception are younger than 1 year. The child often draws the legs up during the pain episodes and is usually quiet during the intervening periods. Other symptoms include vomiting, passage of bloody mucus (currant jelly stool), and a palpable abdominal mass. In approximately 50% of cases, the diagnosis of ileocolic intussusception can be suspected on plain abdominal radiographs by the presence of a mass, sparse colonic gas, or complete distal small bowel obstruction. Currently, abdominal ultrasound is used as an initial diagnostic test. The characteristic sonographic findings of the "target sign" of the intussuscepted layers of bowel on a transverse view or the "pseudokidney sign" when seen longitudinally should prompt air-contrast enema study.

Management

Hydrostatic reduction by enema using contrast material or air is the therapeutic procedure of choice. Contraindications to this approach include the presence of peritonitis and hemodynamic instability. Furthermore, an intussusception located entirely within the small intestine is unlikely to be reduced by an enema and more likely to have an associated lead point. Hydrostatic reduction by air enema is the standard modality. Successful reduction is accomplished in more than 80% of cases and confirmed by resolution of the mass, along with reflux of air into the terminal ileum. For those refractory to air enema attempts, many centers will try a delayed, repeated air enema study a few hours later with some success.[23] The recurrence rate after hydrostatic reduction is approximately 11%, and it usually occurs within the 24 hours after the reduction. When it recurs, it is usually managed by another air enema reduction. A third recurrence is an indication for operative management.

Surgical management. The operative indications with intussusception include peritonitis or bowel obstruction at initial presentation and failed hydrostatic enema reduction or multiple recurrences. The intussusceptum is delivered through a transverse incision in the right side of the abdomen and reduced in a retrograde fashion by pushing the mass proximally. Once it is reduced, warm lap pads may be placed over the bowel, and a period of observation may be warranted in cases of questionable bowel viability. The lymphoid tissue in the ileocecal region is thickened and edematous and may be mistaken for a tumor within the small bowel; therefore, great caution should be exercised before committing to surgical resection. Recurrence rates are extremely low after surgical reduction. Bowel resection is required in cases in which the intussusception cannot be reduced, the viability of the bowel is uncertain, or a lead point is identified. An ileocolectomy with primary anastomosis is usually performed. An appendectomy is an essential component, irrespective of bowel resection. Laparoscopic reduction of intussusception has recently gained some popularity.

Meckel's Diverticulum

Meckel's diverticulum is the most common congenital anomaly of the GI tract and occurs in approximately 2% of the population. More than 70% of symptomatic patients have heterotopic gastric mucosa and another 5% have pancreatic tissue. The rule of 2s is often cited in association with Meckel's diverticulum. Aside from its 2% incidence and two types of heterotopic mucosa, it is located within 2 feet of the ileocecal valve, approximately 2 inches in length, and usually symptomatic by 2 years of age. Meckel's diverticulum is caused by a failure of normal regression of the vitelline duct that occurs during weeks 5 to 7 of gestation. Meckel's diverticulum is a true diverticulum containing all normal intestinal layers.

Diagnosis

The clinical symptoms are related to hemorrhage, obstruction, or inflammation; the most common presenting symptom is a painless, massive, lower GI bleeding in children younger than 5 years. Diagnosis of a persistent vitelline duct remnant may be established by umbilical ultrasound or lateral contrast radiography. Bleeding Meckel's diverticulum may be confirmed by a ^{99m}Tc-pertechnetate isotope scan to detect gastric mucosa. Of note, ectopic gastric mucosa can also be present in patients with intestinal duplication.

Surgical Management

Surgical resection is the definitive therapy for Meckel's diverticulum. A simple V-shaped diverticulectomy with transverse closure of the ileum is an acceptable technique. In patients in whom there is ulceration or inflammation at the base of the diverticulum, a segmental resection of the involved ileum with a primary end-to-end anastomosis is preferred.

HEPATOBILIARY CONDITIONS

Extrahepatic Biliary Atresia

Biliary atresia (BA) is a rare disease of neonates characterized by the inflammatory obliteration of intrahepatic and extrahepatic bile ducts. The incidence is estimated to be 1 in 5000 to 12,000 infants, depending on region. It may be associated with other congenital malformations, particularly splenic abnormalities (e.g., asplenia, double spleen), absence of the inferior vena cava (IVC), and intestinal malformation. If BA is left untreated, progressive cirrhosis and death occur by 2 years of age.

Pathophysiology

The exact mechanism whereby BA develops is unknown, but several theories exist. One theory suggests that the ductal injury is immune mediated—inflammatory cells infiltrate and obliterate the bile ducts. Proinflammatory cytokines, such as interleukin-2, interferon-γ, and tumor necrosis factor, are present. $CD4^+/CD8^+$ T cells and natural killer cells are also prominent.[24] However, it remains unclear how the inflammatory process is initiated and progresses. Another theory is that a viral insult, group C rotavirus infection, triggers the immune-mediated fibrosclerosis and obstruction of the extrahepatic bile ducts. Interestingly, animal studies have shown that infection of newborn mice with rotavirus leads to a similar presentation as in infants, with the onset of hyperbilirubinemia, jaundice, and acholic stools. On histologic examination, inflammation and obstruction of the extrahepatic bile ducts are observed. However, this theory has yet to be proven in human newborns because many lack serologic evidence of viral infection. Another hypothesis is that there are genetic components that contribute to the development of BA. There may be an association with human leukocyte antigen (HLA) type. Patients with BA have a significantly high frequency of HLA-B12. It is unclear whether this is causal, but some have argued that abnormal expression of HLA makes biliary ductal epithelial cells a susceptible target for immunologic assault. Another putative gene, *CFC1*, encodes a protein important in the embryonic differentiation of the left-right axis; when mutated, it is thought to predispose to the development of BA. On histopathologic evaluation, there is significant extrahepatic biliary obstruction with portal tract fibrosis, inflammatory cell infiltration, bile duct proliferation, and cholestasis with bile plugging.

Clinical Presentation and Diagnosis

The disease is classified according to the level of the most proximal biliary obstruction. Type 1 BA has patency to the level of the common bile duct; type 2 has patency to the level of the common hepatic duct; and type 3, which accounts for more than 90% of cases, occurs when the left and right hepatic ducts at the level of the porta hepatis are involved. This aids in the differentiation between correctable BA and others. Correctable BA requires that patent hepatic ducts exist to the porta hepatis. Types 1 and 2 may be amenable to a direct extrahepatic biliary duct–intestinal anastomosis.

Infants present shortly after birth with jaundice, pale stools, and dark urine. Older infants may have failure to thrive and present with hepatomegaly and ascites suggestive of cirrhosis. If, in the postnatal period, the jaundice persists after 14 days in a term infant, an evaluation for liver disease should be initiated. This consists of determining direct or conjugated bilirubin level, which will be elevated (>2.0 mg/dL) in those with liver disease. Liver function test results should also be monitored because derangements are typically seen. Coagulopathy is not generally encountered early because hepatic synthetic function is relatively intact. Other exclusion studies include serologic testing for TORCH (toxoplasmosis, rubella, cytomegalovirus, and herpes) and hepatitis B and C infections, α_1-antitrypsin, and CF. Metabolic disorders, such as galactosemia and tyrosinemia, and endocrine abnormalities must also be ruled out.

Evaluation of the biliary anatomy often begins with ultrasound. The gallbladder may be atrophic or absent, and intrahepatic ducts may also be notably absent. The liver may appear echogenic. Other imaging modalities, such as hepatobiliary iminodiacetic acid (HIDA) scintigraphy, magnetic resonance cholangiopancreatography (MRCP), and endoscopic retrograde cholangiopancreatography (ERCP), have been used, with varying success. An HIDA scan would reveal uptake of the technetium isotope but an absence of emptying into the duodenum. MRCP or ERCP can better define the biliary anatomy, but because of the relatively small size of the ducts, it is difficult from a technical and resolution standpoint. Although these are useful adjuncts, liver biopsy is the gold standard for the diagnosis of BA and can safely be done percutaneously.

Surgical Management

Once the diagnosis is suspected, an operative exploration is warranted along with intraoperative cholangiography. Once the diagnosis is confirmed, a Kasai hepatoportoenterostomy is the surgical procedure of choice. Here, the extrahepatic biliary tree is dissected proximally to the level of the liver capsule, where the porta hepatis (portal plate) is transected. The reconstruction is performed by a Roux-en-Y hepaticojejunostomy (Fig. 66-19). Some advocate the use of ursodeoxycholic acid and phenobarbital to promote biliary drainage, but it is uncertain whether these actually improve outcomes. The use of steroids after the Kasai procedure has been advocated by many and thought to promote biliary drainage with

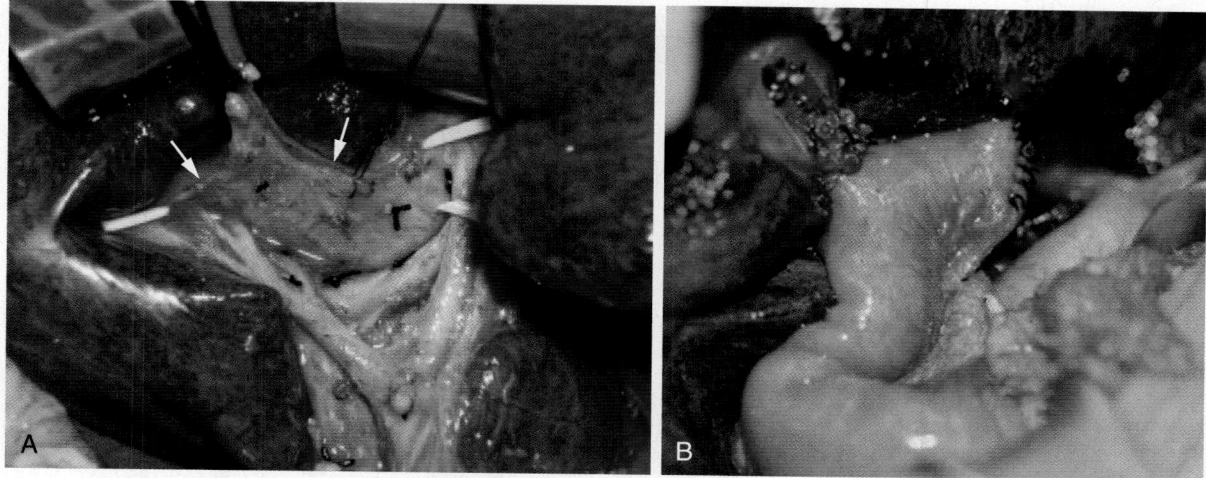

FIGURE 66-19 Kasai Portoenterostomy. A, The dissection of fibrous extrahepatic biliary remnant is continued up to the capsular surface of the liver within the bifurcation of the portal vein (*arrows* indicate fibrous portal plate; yellow vessel loops mark lateral dissection margins). **B,** Completed Roux-en-Y portoenterostomy. (From Nathan JD, Ryckman FC: Biliary atresia. In Chung DH, Chen MK, editors: *Atlas of pediatric surgical techniques*, Philadelphia, 2010, Elsevier Saunders, pp 220–231.)

shorter hospital stay.[25] However, the Biliary Atresia Clinical Research Consortium's recent randomized, double-blinded, placebo-controlled trial of steroid therapy (the START trial) after the Kasai procedure demonstrated that high-dose steroid therapy after the procedure did not result in significant treatment differences in bile drainage at 6 months.[26] Furthermore, steroid treatment was associated with earlier onset of serious adverse events.[26] However, steroid pulse therapy remains a treatment option for post-Kasai cholangitis. Antibiotics are also continued postoperatively because the risk of cholangitis is high (45% to 60%) as a result of the ease with which intestinal bacteria can ascend and colonize the bile ducts. Unfortunately, if the Kasai procedure is unable to reestablish bile flow and liver failure or cirrhosis ensues, liver transplantation is indicated.

Kasai hepatoportoenterostomy does not cure BA, which will inevitably progress in more than 70% of infants who undergo this procedure. The rate with which the disease progresses, as evidenced by cirrhosis and portal hypertension, is variable, but it may be expedited by recurrent cholangitis. It is estimated, however, that 80% of those who have successfully undergone a Kasai procedure can live up to 10 years before liver transplantation is needed. In those infants who undergo transplantation, outcomes are good, with 10-year graft survival and overall patient survival of 73% and 86%, respectively.[27]

Choledochal Cyst

Choledochal cysts are cystic dilations of the common bile duct (CBD). They have an incidence of 1 in 100,000 to 150,000 live births, with a 3 to 4 : 1 female-to-male preponderance. They are classified on the basis of location, and their frequency varies (Fig. 66-20). Type I (50% to 80%) is a simple cyst that can involve any portion of the CBD, and type II (2%) describes a diverticulum arising off the CBD. Choledochoceles represent type III cysts (1.4% to 4.5%), consisting of dilation confined to the distal intrapancreatic portion of the CBD. Although type IV (15% to 35%) involves intrahepatic and extrahepatic bile ducts, type V (20%) is limited to the intrahepatic ducts only. Choledochal cysts can be associated with other congenital anomalies, including duodenal and colonic atresia, imperforate anus, pancreatic arteriovenous malformation, and pancreatic divisum.[28] Moreover, choledochal cysts are considered premalignant lesions.

Pathogenesis

The pathogenesis of choledochal cysts remains unknown, but one hypothesis is that pancreaticobiliary reflux allows the activation of pancreatic enzymes within the duct. The subsequent inflammatory response compromises the integrity of the duct wall, which eventually results in dilation. In support of this theory, amylase and trypsinogen levels in the bile from patients with choledochal cysts are often elevated.[28] Another theory is that these cysts arise from CBD obstruction, which can occur with functional obstruction at the sphincter of Oddi.

Clinical Presentation and Diagnosis

The classic triad of jaundice, a palpable right upper quadrant mass, and abdominal pain is seen in less than 20% of patients, but 85% of children have at least two of these symptoms on presentation. Patients younger than 12 months generally present with obstructive jaundice and abdominal masses, whereas older patients complain of pain, fever, nausea with vomiting, and jaundice. Common complications include cholangitis, pancreatitis, and bile peritonitis secondary to cyst rupture.[28] Abdominal ultrasound can reveal a cystic mass that is separate from the gallbladder and also allows anatomic assessment of the biliary tree. When a diagnosis is uncertain, an HIDA scan should be considered, demonstrating absent filling of the cyst initially, followed by uptake in the cyst and finally delayed emptying into the duodenum. CT is a useful modality for defining the intrahepatic biliary anatomy and evaluating the distal CBD and pancreatic head. Moreover, it has better resolution with regard to confirming continuity of the cyst with the CBD. MRCP is obtained with increasing frequency and can be helpful. However, ERCP is rarely indicated.

Treatment

Prompt excision of the cysts is recommended. After cyst excision, a Roux-en-Y hepaticojejunostomy is performed for

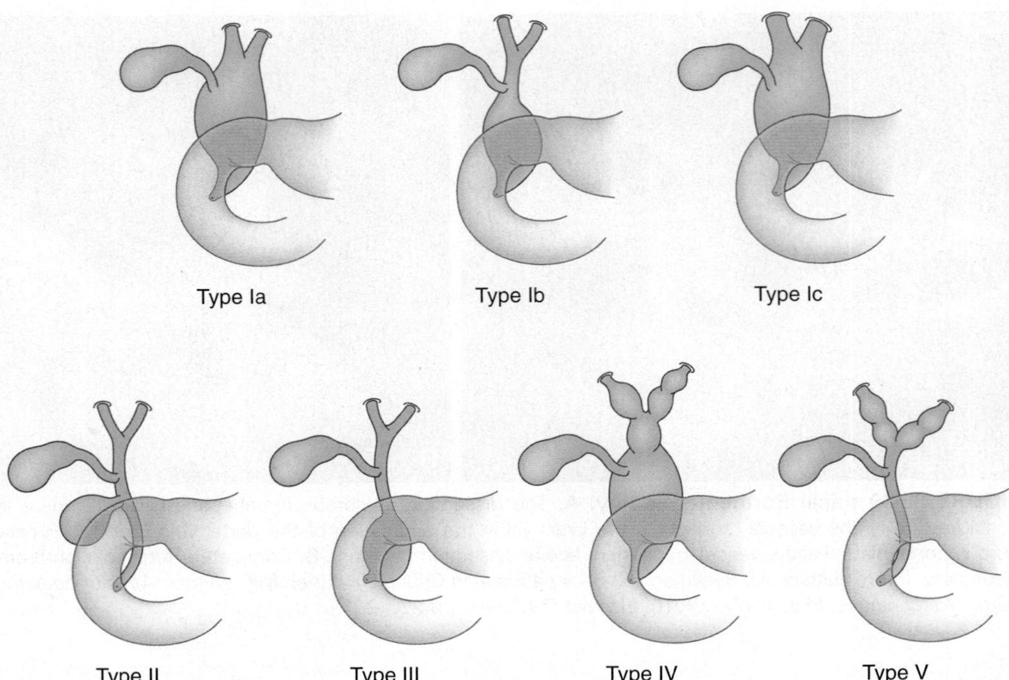

FIGURE 66-20 Classification of choledochal cyst. (From O'Neill JA: Choledochal cyst. In Grosfeld JL, O'Neill JA, Fonkalsrud EW, et al, editors: *Pediatric surgery*, ed 6, Philadelphia, 2006, Mosby Elsevier, pp 16–21.)

reconstruction. Complete excision is important because the risk of a primary malignant neoplasm is as high as 6% with a retained choledochal cyst. If the cyst cannot be completely excised because of scarring from chronic inflammation, the cyst should be enucleated. These patients should be monitored by ultrasound examination. Postoperative anastomotic strictures are a common complication and probably arise from chronic intrahepatic cholelithiasis and recurrent cholangitis. Aside from this, outcomes are generally good.

Hereditary Pancreatitis and Pancreas Divisum

Hereditary pancreatitis is an autosomal dominant disorder with a high degree of penetrance. It is rare, representing less than 1% of instances of chronic pancreatitis. The disease results from a mutation in the cationic trypsinogen gene *(PRSS1),* which leads to an increase in the autoactivation of trypsin and resistance to deactivation.[29] The gene has been mapped to chromosome 7q35; the two most common allelic mutations are *R122H* and *N29I.*[29] Recurrent bouts of pancreatitis usually begin in childhood, between 5 and 10 years of age, with no identifiable cause. Aside from the age at onset, the presentation, natural history, diagnosis, and treatment of this disease are similar to those for other causes of pancreatitis.

Hereditary pancreatitis should be suspected in any patient who experiences at least two bouts of acute pancreatitis without obvious risk factors, such as trauma, hyperlipidemia, gallstones, or pancreas divisum. It should also be considered in any child with acute pancreatitis and a family history of this disease and in children. Making the correct diagnosis is important because there is an extremely high lifetime risk of malignant transformation. It is estimated that these patients have a 50- to 70-fold increase in the risk for development of pancreatic adenocarcinoma within 7 to 30 years of disease onset. The cumulative lifetime risk is estimated to be 40% by the age of 70 years. Therefore, screening by endoscopic ultrasound is recommended, starting at the age of 30 years.

Pancreas divisum is a congenital anatomic anomaly in which the ventral pancreas and dorsal pancreas fail to fuse. The resultant pancreas has dual drainage, with the dorsal pancreas draining through the duct of Santorini and the ventral pancreas (head and uncinate process) draining through the duct of Wirsung. The onset of symptoms is variable, ranging from early childhood to adulthood. Although ultrasound and CT are usually performed, ERCP is frequently used to confirm the diagnosis. However, MCRP has been touted as more advantageous because it can delineate the dorsal pancreatic duct in its entirety, as opposed to ERCP, which can assess only the ventral duct on cannulation of the major duodenal papilla. The significance of pancreas divisum and its predisposition to chronic pancreatitis remains controversial. Some have suggested that it may result in pancreatitis because all pancreatic output is forced to empty through the smaller lesser papilla. The result is an outflow obstruction that leads to ductal dilation. Treatment consists of transduodenal sphincteroplasty or a Puestow procedure (pancreaticojejunostomy); a Puestow procedure is preferred if the dorsal pancreatic duct is dilated or obstructed.

Biliary Dyskinesia

Obesity has also become a major health problem for adolescents. Along with that, we are seeing an increasing number of pediatric patients with cholelithiasis and biliary colic due to dyskinesia of the gallbladder. Biliary dyskinesia has become more prevalent and should be considered on evaluation of a teenager with epigastric pain. Pediatric surgeons are often consulted to evaluate for the appropriateness of performing a cholecystectomy based on a low ejection fraction from a cholecystokinin-stimulated HIDA scan. When an ejection fraction of less than 35% to 40% correlates with characteristic biliary colic, a cholecystectomy can be therapeutic.[30] However, in patients with vague symptoms, inconsistent with biliary colic, the beneficial role of cholecystectomy is seriously questioned.

ABDOMINAL WALL CONDITIONS

Abdominal Wall Defects

Anterior abdominal wall defects are a relatively frequent neonatal surgical condition in pediatric surgery. During normal development of the human embryo, the midgut herniates outward through the umbilical ring and continues to grow. By the eleventh week of gestation, the midgut returns to the coelomic cavity and undergoes proper rotation and fixation, along with closure of the umbilical ring. If the intestine fails to return, the infant is born with the abdominal contents protruding directly through the umbilical ring, with an intact sac covering the abdominal viscera, termed an omphalocele (Fig. 66-21*A*). In contrast, gastroschisis represents the abdominal wall defect, which is always to the right of an intact umbilical cord, without sac covering the abdominal viscera (Fig. 66-21*B*).

Omphalocele

Omphalocele is recognized as a central defect of the abdominal wall. Its defect is generally more than 4 cm in diameter with an intact membranous sac, which is composed of an outer layer of amnion and an inner layer of peritoneum. Defects less than 4 cm in diameter are arbitrarily designated hernias of the cord. Infants with an omphalocele have an approximately 50% incidence of associated anomalies. Beckwith-Wiedemann syndrome is a combination of gigantism, macroglossia, and an umbilical defect, either hernia or omphalocele. Chromosomal abnormalities, trisomies 13, 15, 18, and 21, have also been associated with omphalocele. Other major associated anomalies include exstrophy of the bladder or cloaca and the pentalogy of Cantrell—omphalocele, anterior diaphragmatic hernia, sternal cleft, ectopia cordis, and intracardiac defect, such as ventricular septal defect.

The treatment of omphalocele begins with the preservation of the intact sac with sterile, moistened, saline gauze or transparent bowel bag. IV fluid should be promptly started, along with gastric tube decompression and IV antibiotics. Great care should be taken to prevent hypothermia. A thorough diagnostic workup should be performed to identify associated anomalies. Primary surgical closure of the small to medium-sized defect is preferred. Alternative options to primary closure include prosthetic patch closure (e.g., Gore-Tex), porcine small intestinal submucosa–derived biomaterial (e.g., Surgisis), skin flap closure, and placement of a silo for sequential reduction and staged closure. Giant omphaloceles may be treated by topical application of escharotic agents such as povidone-iodine (Betadine) ointment, merbromin (Mercurochrome), or silver nitrate, allowing the sac to thicken and to epithelialize gradually. The overall survival for infants with omphalocele depends on the size of the defect and the severity of associated anomalies.

Gastroschisis

The gastroschisis defect is usually just to the right of the umbilical cord, at the site of the obliterated right umbilical vein. The fascial defect is typically approximately 4 cm in diameter. Because of the absence of a sac and direct exposure of the intestine to amniotic fluid in utero, the intestine is often thickened, edematous, and foreshortened. Associated anomalies are rare, but intestinal atresia is present in up to 15% of cases. Infants born with gastroschisis should be carefully handled to avoid injury to exposed bowel loops and to minimize fluid losses. In general, infants are placed in a warm, saline-filled plastic organ bag up to the nipple line. This allows gross inspection of eviscerated bowel at all times and also lessens fluid losses. One should be cautious for potential volvulus of eviscerated malrotated intestine. IV fluids are started at 1.5 times maintenance along with IV antibiotics. In general, fluid requirements are greater than those required for omphalocele because of increased fluid losses. An orogastric tube is placed to decompress the stomach.

For primary closure, bowel loops are reduced, and the fascia and skin are approximated. For defects requiring a prosthetic patch closure, a Gore-Tex patch can be used and the skin closed over it. Other biomaterial substitutes (e.g., AlloDerm, Surgisis) have been used with variable success.[31] If the viscera cannot be reduced into the abdomen, a silo is placed at the bedside and the eviscerated intestines are reduced serially during 5 to 7 days, followed by operative fascial closure. During the immediate postoperative period, if the abdominal wall closure is tight, patients may require aggressive fluid resuscitation to maintain adequate tissue perfusion and to prevent metabolic acidosis. Patients are maintained on TPN until they gain bowel function. In cases of associated intestinal atresia or stenosis, inflammation of the bowel may preclude an immediate repair. Then, the abdominal wall is repaired in a usual fashion and intestinal atresia is addressed in 6 to 8 weeks, when the inflammation resolves. Late occurrence of NEC has been reported in up to 20% of patients after gastroschisis

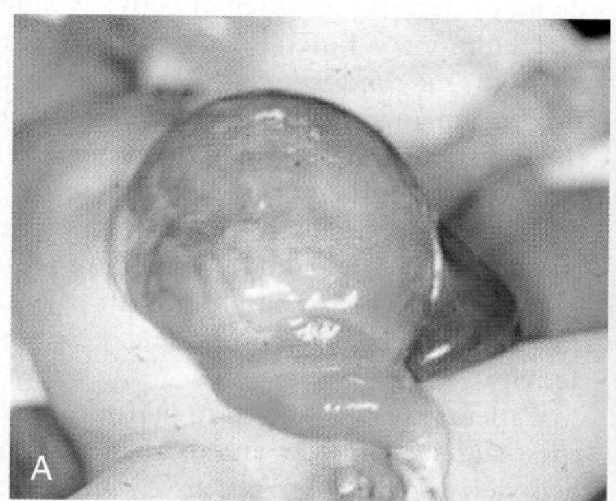

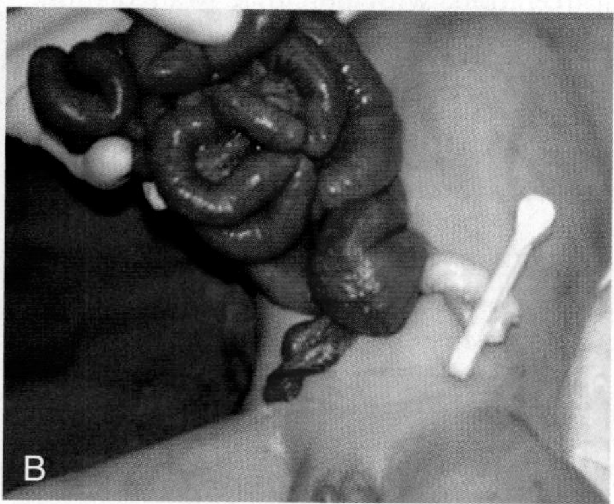

FIGURE 66-21 **Abdominal Wall Defects. A,** Omphalocele with intact sac. **B,** Gastroschisis with eviscerated multiple bowel loops to the right of the umbilical cord.

repair.[32] Undescended testes are also present in 10% to 20% of infants born with gastroschisis. When found outside the coelomic cavity, the testes should be placed into the abdominal cavity at the time of abdominal wall closure or silo bag placement. They are observed for a time to assess for spontaneous descent into the scrotum. If not, orchidopexy is performed. The majority of infants have prolonged ileus. Although TPN has been a lifesaving maneuver, it is associated with a high incidence of cholestasis and cirrhosis. One of the most difficult challenges in the management of gastroschisis remains managing dysfunctional intestine or short gut syndrome.

Hernias

Inguinal Hernia

Inguinal hernia repair is one of the most common surgical procedures in pediatric surgery. The incidence of inguinal hernia, which is almost all indirect and congenital in nature, is approximately 3% to 5% in term infants and 9% to 11% in premature infants. It affects boys approximately six times more often than girls. Sixty percent of inguinal hernias occur on the right side, 30% are on the left side, and 10% are bilateral. The processus vaginalis is an elongated diverticulum of the peritoneum that accompanies the testicle on its descent into the scrotum; it generally is obliterated during the ninth month of gestation or soon after birth. The variable persistence of the processus vaginalis results in a spectrum of clinical presentations, including a scrotal hernia with protrusion of intestine, ovaries, omentum, or communicating hydrocele, with intermittent accumulation of peritoneal fluid. All communicating hydroceles are repaired in the same manner as an indirect inguinal hernia.

Clinical presentation. Diagnosis is established by clinical history and examination alone, especially when the contents of the hernia reduce into the peritoneal cavity. Communicating hydroceles can be difficult to reduce at times and therefore can be misdiagnosed as simple hydroceles. Transillumination of the scrotum to differentiate a hydrocele from a hernia can be misleading because a herniated, thin-walled bowel loop can easily be transilluminated. Palpation of the cord may elicit a "silk glove sign," which is produced by rubbing the opposing peritoneal membranes of the empty sac. At times, palpation of a thickened cord in comparison to the contralateral side and a reliable history are sufficient to derive a diagnosis. The acute development of hydrocele may also be associated with the onset of other conditions, such as epididymitis, testicular torsion, and torsion of testicular appendage. In these clinical settings, ultrasound may be helpful to determine the diagnosis. The major risk factor of inguinal hernia is bowel incarceration, with potential strangulation. The incidence of incarceration is higher in premature infants in the first year of life.

Surgical management. Although early hernia repair may be associated with a higher risk for injury to the cord structures, recurrence rate, and postoperative apneic episodes, most pediatric surgeons advocate operative repair before discharge from the hospital for premature infants because of their significant risks for incarceration. However, for those infants diagnosed after hospital discharge, elective hernia repair may be deferred until the infant is beyond a safe postconceptional age of 52 to 55 weeks, when postoperative apnea risk decreases. In patients presenting with incarcerated inguinal hernia, unless there is clinical evidence of peritonitis, attempts are made to reduce the hernia. Manual reduction is successful in up to 70% of cases. Once the hernia is reduced, the patient is admitted for observation, and hernia repair is performed at 24 to 48 hours, when local tissue edema resolves. A nonreducible incarcerated hernia should be promptly explored in the operating room. Routine contralateral inguinal exploration at the time of symptomatic hernia repair for infants is standard practice based on the high incidence of contralateral patent processus vaginalis (4% to 65%). However, the issue regarding the routine exploration of the asymptomatic contralateral side in toddlers remains unresolved. Most pediatric surgeons routinely explore the asymptomatic contralateral side in children 2 years of age or younger; some surgeons extend the routine contralateral exploration criteria to those up to 5 years of age.

Umbilical Hernia

In general, umbilical hernia has a tendency to close on its own in approximately 80% of cases, and therefore elective repair should be deferred until approximately 5 years of age. The umbilical hernia rarely presents with complications, but there are unique exceptions to this general rule for which an earlier elective repair should be considered. Although rare, a history of incarceration clearly warrants prompt surgical repair, irrespective of age. Enlarging umbilical hernia over time, in particular with a large skin proboscis more than 3 cm or a significantly large umbilical fascial defect (>2 cm), is unlikely to resolve spontaneously; therefore, surgical repair should be considered at an early age.

CHEST WALL DEFORMITIES

The two major types of congenital chest wall deformities are pectus excavatum and pectus carinatum. Pectus excavatum is more prevalent, five times more common than pectus carinatum (Fig. 66-22*A*). Its incidence is estimated at approximately 1 in 100 children, with a male-to-female ratio of 3 to 4 : 1. The deformity is usually present at birth and steadily becomes more prominent. It can become more pronounced between 8 and 10 years of age and later again during puberty. It is also common to have associated kyphosis and scoliosis. Although the exact cause is unknown, abnormalities of costal cartilage development have been implicated. Pectus excavatum can be associated with congenital heart disease, including mitral valve prolapse, Ehlers-Danlos syndrome, and Marfan syndrome, and therefore thorough preoperative evaluation, such as ophthalmologic evaluation and echocardiography, should be considered.

To determine the severity of pectus excavatum and to assess the indications for surgery, two or more of the following criteria should be met: (1) Haller index (ratio of width of chest wall to depth of sternum to vertebral body) of more than 3.2; (2) abnormal pulmonary function test result; (3) mitral valve prolapse, murmurs, or conduction abnormalities on echocardiography; and (4) documentation of progression of deformity. Regardless of these objective measurements, one must carefully assess for the psychosocial burden caused by the pectus deformities. This is a critical issue, particularly for adolescents with significant concerns about body image and development of self-esteem. A multicenter study has shown that surgical repair of pectus excavatum significantly improves body image and perceived ability for physical activity.[33]

Patients are encouraged to perform exercises to strengthen the chest and back muscles and to maintain proper posture. Standard two-view chest radiographs are essential to assess for Haller index and to detect the presence of thoracic scoliosis. Pulmonary function tests may be indicated to document restrictive or obstructive

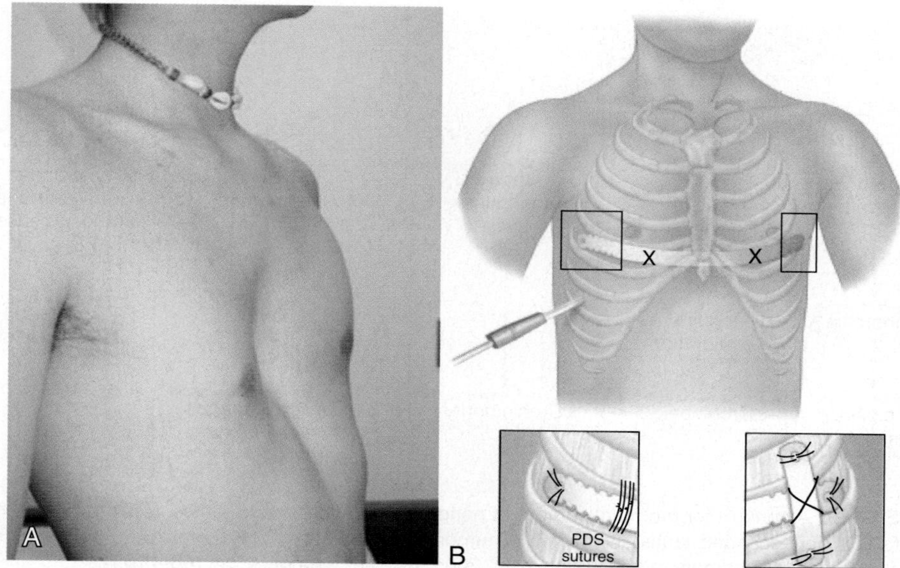

FIGURE 66-22 **A,** Pectus excavatum. **B,** A bar is placed beneath the sternum and secured onto the chest wall with stabilizers. (From Goretsky MJ, Nuss D: Surgical treatment of chest wall deformities: Nuss procedure. In Chung DH, Chen MK, editors: *Atlas of pediatric surgical techniques*, Philadelphia, 2010, Elsevier Saunders, pp 97–103.)

abnormalities. Aside from plain chest radiographs, a limited CT scan has been used to determine Haller index.

Surgical Management

The optimal age for pectus excavatum repair is 10 to 14 years because the chest wall is still soft and malleable. Also, recovery seems faster in this age group. After puberty, the chest wall is more rigid, thus requiring a longer period of bar support, even with the insertion of two bars. The Ravitch procedure, originally described in 1949, can be performed for pectus excavatum or carinatum deformities. It consists of a transverse inframammary skin incision overlying the deformity, bilateral subchondral resection of abnormal costal cartilages, sternal osteotomy, and anterior fixation of the sternum with a temporary retrosternal stainless metal bar, which is removed at a later time.

In the Nuss procedure, which was developed for pectus excavatum, a curved metal bar, contoured to elevate the sternum, is passed in a retrosternal plane from one hemithorax into the other through two lateral intercostal incisions (Fig. 66-22*B*). The Nuss bar is then flipped so that the convexity is outward, and the chest wall defect is immediately corrected. The bar is left in place for approximately 2 years. In contrast to the Ravitch procedure, a minimally invasive Nuss procedure involves less surgical tissue trauma and thus significantly less surgical morbidity. A multicenter prospective study has demonstrated that surgical repair for pectus excavatum can be performed safely with adequate pain management.[33]

Pectus carinatum occurs less frequently than pectus excavatum. Preoperative considerations are similar to those for pectus excavatum. Despite some compliance issues, a reasonably good outcome can be expected with the use of an external chest brace, especially when patients wear the brace for 14 to 16 hours daily.[34] It can also be surgically repaired by costal cartilage resection and sternal fixation, similar to that for pectus excavatum. However, this operation is becoming obsolete.

GENITOURINARY TRACT CONDITIONS

Cryptorchidism

Cryptorchidism is a condition in which one testis or both testes fail to descend into the scrotum before birth. Up to 30% of preterm infants can present with an undescended testis, but it also occurs in approximately 3% of full-term infants. Some undescended testes eventually descend by 1 year of age, but they are unlikely to descend after this time. The undescended testis is associated with histologic and morphologic changes as early as 6 months of age; atrophy of Leydig cells, decrease in tubular diameter, and impaired spermatogenesis can occur by 2 years of age. An undescended testis has had its descent halted somewhere along the path of normal descent and is most commonly located in the inguinal canal. A retractile testis is a normally descended testis that retracts into the inguinal canal but can be brought down into the scrotal sac during the examination. It is thought to result from a hyperreflexive cremasteric muscle contraction and does not require operative intervention. Nonpalpable testes may include an intra-abdominal, absent, or vanishing testis. Ectopic testes have had an aberrant path of descent; these can be found in perineal, femoral canal, and suprapubic regions.

Diagnosis and Treatment

Although ultrasound has been used increasingly to evaluate for undescended testes, an examination by an experienced surgeon has a higher sensitivity for locating an undescended testis in the inguinal canal. For a unilateral palpable testis in the inguinal canal, standard dartos pouch orchidopexy is performed. The recommended timing for this procedure is 6 months to 1 year of age. A general management algorithm for nonpalpable testes is shown in Figure 66-23. When an undescended testis is not palpable in the inguinal canal, a diagnostic laparoscopy is useful. If the testicular vessels are seen exiting the internal ring, an open inguinal orchidopexy is performed. For an intra-abdominal testis, a

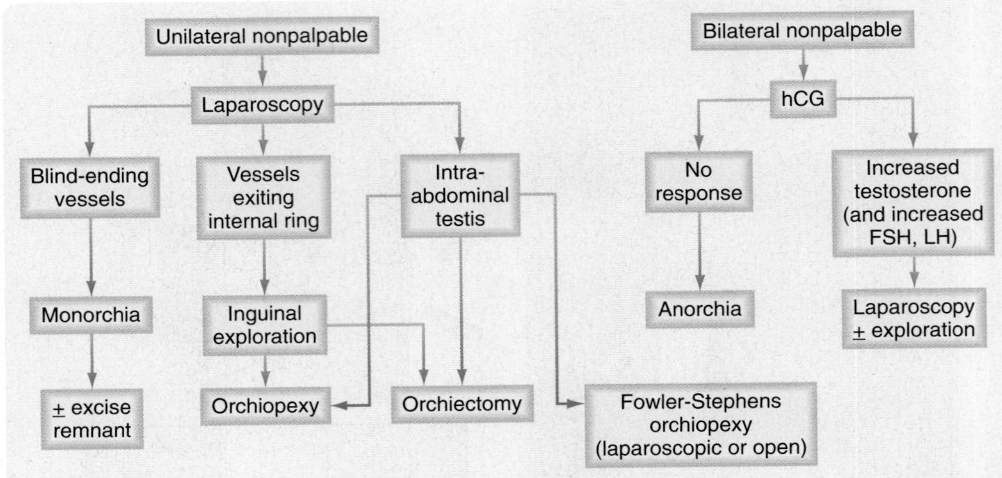

FIGURE 66-23 Algorithm for the management of nonpalpable undescended testes. (Adapted from Lee KL, Shortliffe LD: Undescended testis and testicular tumors. In Ashcraft KW, Holcomb GW, Holcomb GW III, et al, editors: *Pediatric surgery*, ed 4, Philadelphia, 2005, Elsevier Saunders, pp 706–716.)

two-stage Fowler-Stephens orchidopexy can be considered, in which testicular vessels are ligated as a first stage to allow collateral circulation to develop for 6 months before orchidopexy is performed as a second stage of the procedure. However, single-stage laparoscopic orchidopexy is also an ideal option for intra-abdominal testes. If both testes are nonpalpable, a human chorionic gonadotropin (hCG) stimulation test is carried out to confirm the presence of functioning testes. If present, diagnostic laparoscopy is performed to identify the testes and to determine surgical therapy. The risk of malignant transformation has been reported to be significantly greater for men with a history of undescended testes. Although orchidopexy does not decrease the malignancy risk associated with undescended testes, it allows earlier detection. Nonseminomatous germ cell tumors are usually associated with undescended testes.

Testicular Torsion

Torsion of the testis is the most common genitourinary tract emergency of childhood. On diagnosis, a prompt surgical detorsion with testicular fixation should be performed to relieve acute testicular ischemia. Extravaginal torsion is more common in neonates, in whom there can be torsion of the spermatic cord along its course outside the tunica vaginalis. Intravaginal torsion is associated with bell clapper deformity, in which the suspended testis can twist to torsion. Torsion of the testis occurs most frequently in early adolescence with a peak incidence at 14 years of age. Scrotal pain that is abrupt or gradual in nature is the primary symptom. On examination, the testis that has undergone torsion may be high-riding, edematous, and significantly tender. Urinary tract symptoms, such as frequency, urgency, dysuria, and fever, tend to occur more frequently with infectious or inflammatory conditions, such as epididymitis; however, in no way does this rule out testicular torsion. In most cases, a careful history and examination are sufficient to confirm the diagnosis of testicular torsion. However, if the diagnosis is uncertain, prompt ultrasonography may be helpful to determine vascular flow to the testicles. Radioisotope scanning is the most specific diagnostic test, but it can be time-consuming to obtain. The time for diagnosis and surgical repair directly correlates with the testicular salvage rate. Immediate surgical detorsion through a scrotal medial raphe approach is the appropriate treatment. After detorsion of the affected testis, it is assessed for viability and fixed to the scrotum. In all cases, the contralateral testis should also be fixed in the scrotum. For torsion of less than 6 hours, 90% of testes can be salvaged. However, this salvage rate significantly decreases to less than 10% with more than 24 hours of symptoms.

Testicular Tumors

Testicular cancer accounts for less than 2% of all pediatric solid tumors. The peak incidence is 2 years of age, with a second peak during puberty. These tumors typically are manifested as a painless scrotal mass, often discovered incidentally. An ultrasound examination is useful, but CT scan is critical to evaluate for retroperitoneal lymphadenopathy as well as potential metastatic disease. Serum tumor markers are useful for diagnosis and for follow-up. α-Fetoprotein (AFP) is a glycoprotein produced by the fetal yolk sac, and its level is elevated in yolk sac tumors of the testes; β-hCG is produced by embryonal carcinomas and mixed teratomas. The most common prepubertal testicular cancer is of germ cell origin; yolk sac tumor, also known as endodermal sinus tumor, and embryonal carcinomas account for almost 40%. Children with yolk sac tumors present with elevated serum AFP levels, and tumors are typically localized to the testis. The standard surgical approach is radical inguinal orchiectomy. The role of retroperitoneal lymph node dissection with yolk sac tumor is controversial. Tumors with microscopic node involvement or nodal disease require systemic chemotherapy, with modified retroperitoneal lymphadenectomy. The overall survival from yolk sac tumors is approximately 70% to 90%.

PEDIATRIC SOLID TUMORS

Solid tumors in infants and children represent a challenging therapeutic problem, but with advances in diagnosis, staging, and treatment, outcomes are steadily improving. However, those with advanced-stage disease remain difficult to cure despite multimodality therapy. It is this population of patients that stands to gain the most with cancer biology discoveries.

Neuroblastoma

Neuroblastoma is the most common extracranial solid tumor in infants and children, accounting for 8% to 10% of all childhood cancers and 15% of all cancer-related deaths in the pediatric population.[35] There are approximately 600 new diagnoses reported annually. Although 90% of cases are diagnosed before the age of 5 years, 30% of those are diagnosed in the first year of life. The median age at diagnosis is 22 months.

Clinical Presentation

Arising from neural crest cells, neuroblastoma is a malignant neoplasm of the sympathetic nervous system and therefore occurs in sympathetic ganglia. Approximately 65% are found in the abdomen, with 50% localized to the adrenal medulla. They can also occur in the neck (5%), chest (20%), or pelvis (5%), and 1% of patients have no detectable primary. A patient's clinical presentation is dictated by tumor location, size, extent of invasion, and metabolic activity and presence of paraneoplastic symptoms. Many patients are asymptomatic, although it is not uncommon for some to present with constitutional symptoms (e.g., malaise, fevers, weight loss), an enlarging mass, pain, abdominal distention, lymphadenopathy, or respiratory distress. Pelvic masses may cause constipation or bladder dysfunction, whereas thoracic lesions can cause dysphagia or dyspnea. For cervical tumors, a patient may develop Horner syndrome or stridor, and in up to 15% of patients, epidural involvement may result in neurologic deficits, which, when progressive, can lead to paralysis.

At diagnosis, 50% of patients have localized disease and 35% have regional lymph node involvement. Metastasis to distant organs (e.g., liver, bone, skin) occurs by hematogenous and lymphatic routes. For bone marrow invasion, patients may become anemic, bruise easily, and complain of weakness. Bone metastasis can result in pain, swelling, limp, and pathologic fractures. The orbits are frequently involved, which is manifested as periorbital swelling and proptosis (raccoon eyes). Blue subcutaneous nodules represent skin dissemination of tumor associated with the blueberry muffin syndrome. Neuroblastomas can secrete catecholamines, resulting in early-onset hypertension and tachycardia. Patients may also experience paraneoplastic syndromes, which include intractable diarrhea caused by vasoactive intestinal peptide secretion, encephalomyelitis, and neuropathy. Opsoclonus-myoclonus syndrome—rapid, conjugate eye nystagmus with involuntary spasms of the limbs—although rare, occurs when antibodies cross-react with cerebellar tissue.

Genomics

Neuroblastoma occurs as whole chromosome gains, which result in hyperdiploidy and are associated with a favorable prognosis, or segmental chromosomal aberrations, which encompass *MYCN* amplification and gains or losses that tend to be associated with worse outcomes. The *MYCN* oncogene, which is amplified at chromosome 2p24 in 25% of cases, is overexpressed in 30% to 40% of stage 3 and stage 4 neuroblastomas but only in 5% of localized or stage 4S tumors. Therefore, it is used as a biomarker for disease stratification. It has been shown that deletion of the 1p36 region occurs in 70% of tumors and is usually associated with *MYCN*-amplified, high-stage tumors that confer a poor prognosis.[36] Conversely, a whole chromosome 17 gain is associated with a good prognosis. Deletions of chromosome 11q have been identified in 15% to 22% of neuroblastomas and are also associated with unfavorable patient outcomes and a reduced time of progression-free survival.

Diagnosis

An initial workup includes basic serum tests, imaging, and determination of urine levels of catecholamines or their metabolites (e.g., dopamine, vanillylmandelic acid, homovanillic acid). Patients may have elevated levels of nonspecific biomarkers, such as lactate dehydrogenase (>1500 U/mL), ferritin (>142 ng/mL), and neuron-specific enolase (>100 ng/mL), which are associated with advanced stage or relapse. Ultrasonography may be used to initially characterize the mass, but CT scan is essential to localize the tumor and to determine the degree of involvement (Fig. 66-24*A*). MRI may have advantages if there is concern for spinal extension. Although it is not routinely used, a ^{131}I- metaiodobenzylguanidine (MIBG) scan is valuable in the detection of primary tumor and metastases because a norepinephrine analogue is selectively concentrated in sympathetic tissue. The ^{131}I-MIBG scan is also used for the surveillance of treatment response and recurrence. The diagnosis is confirmed by demonstrating undifferentiated small round blue cells on histologic section (Fig. 66-24*B*).

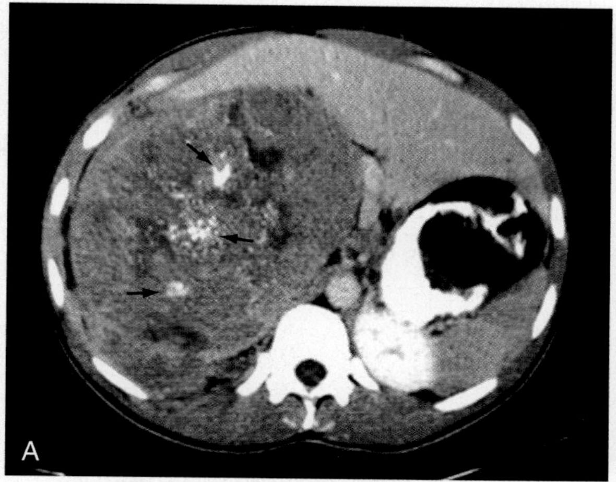

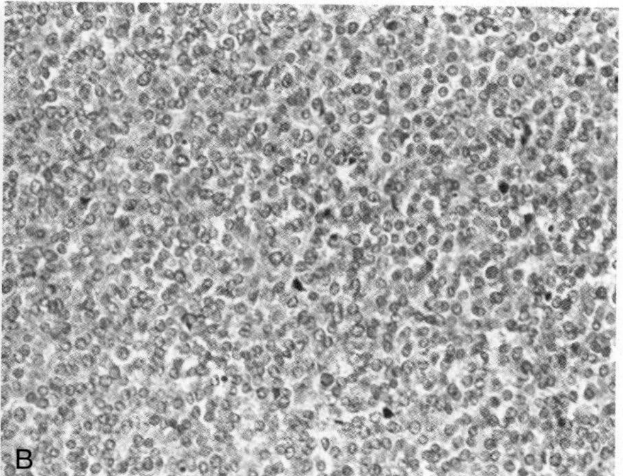

FIGURE 66-24 A, CT scan of neuroblastoma demonstrating areas of calcification *(arrows)*. **B,** Small blue round cells of undifferentiated hyperchromatic neuroblasts. (From Kim S, Chung DH: Pediatric solid malignancies: Neuroblastoma and Wilms' tumor. *Surg Clin North Am* 86:469–487, 2006.)

Stage 1 or stage 2 disease can be resected primarily, but advanced-stage neuroblastomas generally require a tissue biopsy specimen from the unresectable tumor first or bone marrow. Molecular studies, such as fluorescent in situ hybridization, can be performed on tissue specimens to assess ploidy, *MYCN* amplification, and other chromosomal abnormalities. This information is required to outline specific risk category–based therapy for individual patients.

Staging

Neuroblastoma can be classified on the basis of the degree of neuroblastic differentiation and mitosis-karyorrhexis index (low, intermediate, or high). On histologic evaluation, neuroblastoma has limited Schwann cell production, is stroma poor, and has abundant neuroblasts.[37] The modified Shimada classification, on which the International Neuroblastoma Staging System (INSS; Table 66-3) is based, has been used to predict prognosis by the histopathologic features of the tumor and age of the patient. This system takes into account the degree of cell differentiation, mitosis-karyorrhexis index, and presence of Schwann cells. The Children's Oncology Group currently stratifies patients into low-, intermediate-, or high-risk categories on the basis of the patient's age at diagnosis, INSS stage, tumor histopathology, DNA index, and *MYCN* amplification status.[38] Thus, treatment recommendations depend on the stage to which the patient is assigned.

Treatment

The standard multimodality therapy is based on disease risk classification and treatment stratification (Table 66-4). Induction chemotherapy consists of a multidrug regimen, including but not limited to cyclophosphamide, doxorubicin, cisplatin, carboplatin, etoposide, and vincristine. However, high-risk group neuroblastomas frequently acquire resistance to chemotherapeutics and thus have high disease relapse. This usually necessitates autologous hematopoietic stem cell transplantation. Complete surgical resection correlates with a lower local recurrence, especially in combination with induction chemotherapy and local radiation therapy. Thus, some advocate that surgical resection should be considered only after adjuvant therapy. Primary surgical resection is recommended for stages 1 to 2B tumors. For more advanced stages 3 and 4, only the incisional biopsy specimen is obtained initially for tumor biology studies. The role of aggressive surgical resection of the primary tumor site for metastatic stage 4 neuroblastoma in patients 18 months or older has recently been questioned.[39] For infants with stage 4S disease, surgical resection is not recommended because of the high rate of spontaneous differentiation and regression.

For high-risk patients, radiation therapy is often needed for local and metastatic control. Radiation is contraindicated for intraspinal tumors because it can lead to vertebral damage, growth arrest, and scoliosis. However, it may be necessary for palliation in the setting of pain, hepatomegaly with respiratory compromise, or acute neurologic symptoms caused by tumor compression of the cord. It is further indicated when there is minimal residual disease after induction chemotherapy and resection. The overall outcomes in patients with neuroblastoma have improved steadily during the past decades, with 5-year survival rates rising from 52% to 74%.[38] The low-risk group has shown significant improvement in survival rates of up to 92%. It is estimated that 50% to 60% of the high-risk group relapse after standard therapy. However, immunotherapy with granulocyte-macrophage colony-stimulating factor and interleukin-2 improved survival in children with high-risk disease in remission after myeloablative therapy and stem cell rescue.[40]

Wilms Tumor

Wilms tumor (WT), also known as nephroblastoma, is an embryonal renal neoplasm consisting of metanephric blastema; it accounts for 85% of cases.[41] It represents 5.9% of all pediatric malignant tumors and has an annual incidence of 7.6 cases/million children younger than 15 years. There are 500 reported new cases annually, and approximately 75% of WT cases are diagnosed in children younger than 5 years. The peak incidence

TABLE 66-3 International Neuroblastoma Staging System

STAGE	DEFINITION
1	Localized tumor with complete gross excision, with or without microscopic residual disease; representative ipsilateral lymph nodes negative for tumor microscopically (nodes attached to and removed with the primary tumor may be positive)
2A	Localized tumor with incomplete gross excision; representative ipsilateral nonadherent lymph nodes negative for tumor microscopically
2B	Localized tumor with or without complete gross excision, with ipsilateral nonadherent lymph nodes positive for tumor; enlarged contralateral lymph nodes must be negative microscopically
3	Unresectable unilateral tumor with contralateral regional lymph node involvement or midline tumor with bilateral extension by infiltration (unresectable) or by lymph node involvement
4	Any primary tumor with dissemination to distant lymph nodes, bone, bone marrow, liver, skin, or other organs (except as defined for stage 4S)
4S	Localized primary tumor (as defined for stage 1, 2A, or 2B), with dissemination limited to skin, liver, or bone marrow (limited to infant <1 year of age)

TABLE 66-4 Risk Group Categories for Neuroblastoma

RISK GROUP	STAGE	FACTORS
Low	1	
	2	<1 yr
		>1 yr, low N-*myc*
		>1 yr, amplified N-*myc;* favorable histology
	4S	Favorable biology*
Intermediate	3	<1 yr, low N-*myc*
		>1 yr, favorable biology*
	4	<1 yr, low N-*myc*
	4S	Low N-*myc*
High	2	>1 yr, all unfavorable biology*
	3	<1 yr, amplified N-*myc*
		>1 yr, any unfavorable biology*
	4	<1 yr, amplified N-*myc*
		>1 yr
	4S	Amplified N-*myc*

*Favorable biology denotes low N-*myc,* favorable histology, and hyperdiploidy (infants).

occurs at 2 to 3 years. Of all patients, 13% can present with a bilateral tumor, which is usually synchronous in 60% of cases.

Genomics

Divided into overgrowth and nonovergrowth disorders, a number of syndromes can predispose to the development of WT. These include Beckwith-Wiedemann (macroglossia, macrosomia, midline abdominal wall defects, and neonatal hypoglycemia), Li-Fraumeni (*p53* germline mutation with predisposition to various cancers), and Denys-Drash (gonadal dysgenesis, nephropathy, and WT) syndromes and neurofibromatosis. In 10% of patients, WT can be associated with other congenital anomalies, collectively known as WAGR syndrome (aniridia, hemihypertrophy, genitourinary malformations, and mental retardation).[42]

The WT suppressor gene *WT1* is located on chromosome 11p13, which contains genes responsible for the development of the kidney, genitourinary tract, and eyes. Mutations in *WT1* result in genitourinary abnormalities, such as cryptorchidism and hypospadias, but also increase the risk for development of WT. Aniridia is found in 1.1% of WT patients, and when *WT1* deletions are found in these patients, there is a 40% rate of WT development. Moreover, mutations in *WT2*, located at 11p15, have been linked to Beckwith-Wiedemann syndrome, and there is a 4% to 10% risk for development of WT in those who also have hemihypertrophy. A study has determined that the X-linked tumor suppressor gene *WTX* can be inactivated in up to one third of WT cases.

Clinical Presentation

WT is typically discovered incidentally during a physical examination or because parents palpate an abdominal mass. Other presenting symptoms include abdominal pain and hematuria, which may signify tumor invasion into the collecting system or ureter. Another 25% develop hypertension, which is thought to occur secondary to disturbances in the renin-angiotensin feedback loop. Less than 10% of patients have atypical presentations; these include varicocele, hepatomegaly caused by hepatic vein obstruction, ascites, and congestive heart failure. WT may also be associated with predisposing syndromes, and the index of suspicion in these cases should be high, with a low threshold to obtain a screening ultrasound study.

Diagnosis

Ultrasonography is initially performed to determine whether the tumor is actually of renal origin, is cystic or solid, or extends into the renal vein or IVC. A CT scan is useful to delineate WT from neuroblastoma (Fig. 66-25) and also to evaluate for regional adenopathy, contralateral kidney involvement, and distant metastasis. MRI is also a useful adjunct for evaluating intravascular invasion; however, an ultrasound study may be preferred. Lung metastases, which are present in 8% at the time of diagnosis, can be identified on an initial chest radiograph, but CT scan is obtained routinely.

Pathology

The histology of WT is categorized as favorable or unfavorable. Favorable histology is more common, characterized by the presence of three elements—blastemal, stromal, and epithelial cells. WT with predominantly epithelial differentiation behaves less aggressively and tends to be stage I when it is diagnosed early. Blastemal-predominant tumors tend to be clinically aggressive and are associated with advanced disease. Outcomes are correlated with histopathologic features and tumor stage. Unfavorable histology is defined by the presence of anaplasia, clear cell sarcoma, or rhabdoid tumor. Anaplastic WT can be focal or diffuse and is synonymous with unfavorable histology whenever it is encountered; it is associated with an increased risk of tumor recurrence and resistance to standard chemotherapy. Nephrogenic rests are precursor lesions found in 25% to 40% of kidneys with WT but do not have oncologic potential. Instead, they can undergo differentiation and spontaneously regress through unclear mechanisms.

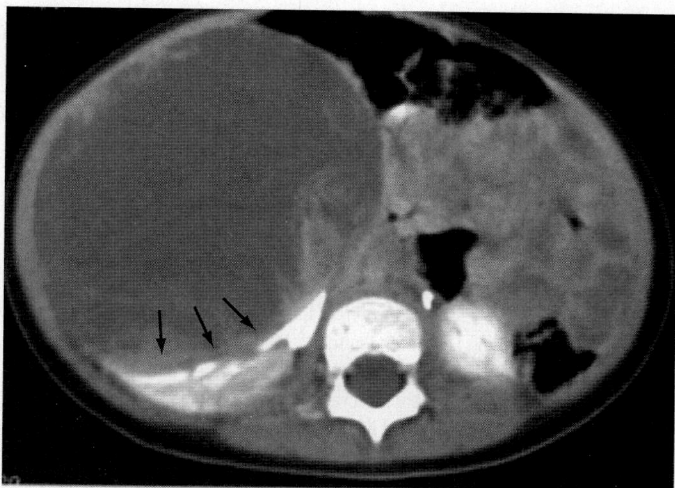

FIGURE 66-25 CT image of Wilms tumor with a claw sign *(arrows)*. (From Kim S, Chung DH: Pediatric solid malignancies: Neuroblastoma and Wilms' tumor. *Surg Clin North Am* 86:469–487, 2006.)

Staging

Tumor staging is one of the most important criteria in the therapeutic and prognostic consideration of WT. The International Society of Pediatric Oncology (SIOP) staging system is based on preoperative chemotherapy but is applied after resection. The presence of metastases is evaluated at presentation, relying on imaging studies, and chemotherapy is instituted before operative intervention. The National Wilms Tumor Study Group (NWTSG) has also developed a staging system that incorporates the clinical, surgical, and pathologic information that was obtained at the time of resection but stratifies patients before the initiation of chemotherapy (Table 66-5). The advantage of this system is that it favors stage-based therapy, thereby avoiding unnecessary chemotherapy in patients who might not otherwise benefit from it.[43]

Treatment

The mainstay of therapy for WT is surgery and chemotherapy. Surgical exploration is necessary for formal staging, and a radical nephrectomy is the standard. Utmost care must be taken to ensure en bloc resection with tumor-free margins because contamination and tumor spillage result in local recurrence. Vascular tumor extension into the IVC constitutes stage III disease and is managed accordingly. Sampling of the hilar, para-aortic, and paracaval lymph nodes is critical. Nephron-sparing surgery is usually reserved for children with a solitary kidney or bilateral WT. In these patients, preoperative chemotherapy may be used to induce tumor shrinkage to allow a more complete resection. However, there is an increased risk of positive surgical margins and local tumor recurrence. Partial nephrectomy may be considered if the tumor involves only one pole of the kidney, there is no evidence

TABLE 66-5 National Wilms Tumor Study Group Staging System

STAGE	DEFINITION
I	Tumor limited to the kidney and completely excised without rupture or biopsy. Surface of the renal capsule is intact.
II	Tumor extends through the renal capsule but is completely removed, with no microscopic involvement of the margins. Vessels outside the kidney contain tumor. Also placed in stage II are cases in which the kidney has undergone biopsy before removal or where there is local spillage of tumor (during resection) limited to the tumor bed.
III	Residual tumor is confined to the abdomen and of nonhematogenous spread. Includes tumors with involvement of the abdominal lymph nodes, diffuse peritoneal contamination by rupture of the tumor extending beyond the tumor bed, peritoneal implants, and microscopic or grossly positive resection margins.
IV	Hematogenous metastases at any site
V	Bilateral renal involvement

BOX 66-2 Treatment Regimens for Wilms Tumor*

- Stage I (FH, focal anaplasia): Surgery, VA × 18 wk, no XRT
- Stage II (FH): Surgery, VA × 18 wk, no XRT
- Stage II (focal anaplasia): Surgery, VDA × 24 wk, XRT to tumor bed
- Stage III (FH, focal anaplasia): Surgery, VDA × 24 wk, XRT to tumor bed
- Stage III (focal anaplasia): Surgery, VDA × 24 wk, XRT to tumor bed
- Stage IV (FH; focal anaplasia): Surgery, VDA × 24 wk, XRT to tumor bed according to local tumor stage and lung or other metastatic sites
- Stages II-IV (diffuse anaplasia): Surgery, VDEC × 24 wk, XRT to whole lung and abdomen
- Stages I-IV (clear cell sarcoma): Surgery, VDEC × 24 wk, XRT to abdomen; XRT to whole lung for stage IV only
- Stages I-IV (rhabdoid tumor): Surgery, ECCa × 24 wk, XRT

A, Dactinomycin; *C,* cyclophosphamide; *Ca,* carboplatin; *D,* doxorubicin; *E,* etoposide; *FH,* favorable histology; *V,* vincristine; *XRT,* radiation therapy.

*National Wilms Tumor Study. Infants younger than 11 months are given half the recommended dose of all drugs.

of collecting system or vascular involvement, clear margins exist between the tumor and surrounding structures, and the involved kidney demonstrates appreciable function. Unfortunately, less than 5% of patients meet these criteria, and it is uncertain whether this approach provides any long-term benefit. According to NWTSG recommendations (Box 66-2), the typical chemotherapy regimen consists of vincristine and dactinomycin, with the addition of doxorubicin (Adriamycin) or radiation therapy based on tumor stage and histologic favorability. The SIOP advocated the use of preoperative chemotherapy to improve cure and disease-free survival rates at 5 years. The overall survival for children with WT has improved from 30% to almost 90% 5- to 7-year survival. Stage I or stage II favorable histology or stage I unfavorable histology has nearly 95% survival rate. For WT with unfavorable histology, stages II, III, and IV are associated with 70%, 56%, and 17% 4-year survival rates, respectively.

Rhabdomyosarcoma

Derived from embryonic mesenchymal cells that can later differentiate into skeletal muscle, rhabdomyosarcoma is a soft tissue malignant neoplasm that accounts for approximately 4% of all pediatric cancer. The incidence is 4.3 cases/million children, with approximately 350 new cases diagnosed annually.[44] With a bimodal peak incidence, children are affected between the ages of 2 and 5 years and again from 15 to 19 years. Almost 50% are diagnosed before the age of 5 years. Most cases occur sporadically, with no recognizable risk factors, although rhabdomyosarcoma is known to occur with increased frequency in patients with neurofibromatosis type 1 and Li-Fraumeni and Beckwith-Wiedemann syndromes.

Pathology

Rhabdomyosarcoma has been pathologically classified into three types: embryonal, alveolar, and pleomorphic. Embryonal rhabdomyosarcoma is the most common, accounting for more than two thirds of all rhabdomyosarcomas. Two subtypes of embryonal rhabdomyosarcoma, botryoid and spindle cell, appear to be associated with a better prognosis than others of similar histology. On examination of a sample, characteristic rhabdomyoblasts may be present; immunohistochemical staining for muscle-specific proteins, such as myosin and actin, desmin, and myoglobin, can bolster the diagnosis.

Clinical Presentation

Rhabdomyosarcoma can appear at any site in the body, including those that do not typically contain skeletal muscle. The most common sites in children are the head and neck (35%), genitourinary tract (25%), and extremities (20%). Less common primary sites are the trunk, GI tract, and intrathoracic and perineal regions. Head and neck lesions tend to occur in the parameningeal region, orbits, and pharynx. Other specific sites include the bladder, prostate, vagina, uterus, liver, biliary tract, paraspinal region, and chest wall. These tumors are typically asymptomatic, although most symptoms are related to compressive effects and can result in pain. Orbital tumors can produce proptosis, decreased visual acuity, and ophthalmoplegia. Those arising from parameningeal sites frequently produce headaches and nasal or sinus obstruction that can be accompanied by a mucopurulent or bloody discharge. Moreover, these tumors can invade intracranially to produce cranial nerve palsies. For genitourinary rhabdomyosarcoma, paratesticular tumors may present as painless swelling in the scrotum, which may be confused with a hernia, hydrocele, or varicocele. Bladder tumors, commonly located at the base and trigone, result in hematuria and urinary obstruction. Vaginal tumors in girls present with a protruding mass or vaginal bleeding and discharge. Biliary tract tumors represent 0.8% of all rhabdomyosarcomas, and as with other causes of biliary obstruction, patients present with jaundice, abdominal swelling, fever, and loss of appetite. In the extremities, rhabdomyosarcomas involve the distal limb more commonly, and the lower extremities are affected more often. At the time of diagnosis, almost 50% of patients have regional lymph node metastasis. Retroperitoneal tumors can be quite large at presentation. Symptoms arise secondary to invasion of adjacent structures, and the associated pain and distention are typical late features of disease.

Diagnosis and Staging

There are no specific serum tumor markers for diagnosis. Depending on tumor location, MRI or CT should be used to characterize

BOX 66-3 Staging for Rhabdomyosarcoma

Group I: Localized disease that is completely resected, with no regional node involvement

Group II

A. Localized, grossly resected tumor with microscopic residual disease but no regional nodal involvement
B. Locoregional disease with tumor-involved lymph nodes with complete resection and no residual disease
C. Locoregional disease with involved nodes, grossly resected, but with evidence of microscopic residual tumor at the primary site and/or histologic involvement of the most distal regional node (from the primary site)

Group III: Localized, gross residual disease including incomplete resection or biopsy only of the primary site

Group IV: Distant metastatic disease present at time of diagnosis

the mass and to evaluate for adjacent structural invasion, vessel encasement, metastasis, and adenopathy. One of the most critical aspects of the diagnostic evaluation is obtaining tissue samples for histologic confirmation, which is usually accomplished by an incisional or core needle biopsy. A complete surgical resection is ideal, but a large tumor may necessitate preoperative chemotherapy for preoperative tumor shrinkage. Botryoid (cluster of grapes) and spindle cell rhabdomyosarcomas are noted to have a favorable prognosis, whereas embryonal and pleomorphic histology confers an intermediate prognosis, and alveolar and undifferentiated histology exhibits a poor prognosis.

Pretreatment staging serves to stratify patients, to determine the most appropriate treatment regimen, and to compare outcomes. Because it relies on preoperative imaging, this is technically clinical staging, although it is still based on TNM criteria (Box 66-3). Intraoperative or pathologic results from resected samples should have no bearing on stage. This is reserved for what is known as clinical grouping, which consists of selection into a group depending on operative findings, pathology, margins, and node status. Taken together, clinical grouping and pretreatment staging have been shown to correlate with outcomes. For example, low-risk patients have an estimated 3-year failure-free survival rate of 88%, intermediate-risk patients have an estimated 3-year failure-free survival rate of 55% to 76%, and high-risk patients have a 3-year failure-free survival rate of less than 30%.

Treatment

The main goal of multimodality therapy is to achieve cure or, at a minimum, to obtain local control. Equally important is the need to minimize the short- and long-term effects of therapy. Currently, all patients with rhabdomyosarcoma receive some combination chemotherapy because it improves progression-free and overall survival. The recommended regimen depends on the risk stratification, with low-risk patients in subgroup A receiving vincristine and dactinomycin. For patients in the low-risk subgroup B and higher, cyclophosphamide is added to this therapy. Radiation therapy has been found to be effective for the local control of rhabdomyosarcoma, especially in patients who have microscopic disease after resection. It has also been successfully used in patients in whom surgery could result in significant disfigurement, such as with head and neck lesions. However, complications of radiation therapy are not negligible, including the potential development of secondary malignant neoplasms.

As is the case with most surgical approaches, a complete resection with negative margins and nodal sampling is the mainstay of treatment. The specific operative guidelines depend on the location of the tumor. For example, for head and neck tumors that are superficial and nonorbital, wide excision of the primary tumor with sampling of ipsilateral cervical lymph nodes is acceptable. Parameningeal lesions are particularly difficult to resect completely, given their degree of extension into critical structures. In these patients and in patients with tumors that are considered unresectable, chemotherapy and radiation therapy are first-line treatment. For extremity lesions, it is imperative to achieve complete wide local excision. Amputation is rarely necessary, except for distal tumors in the hand or foot that involve neurovascular structures. Given that trunk and extremity lesions have a high incidence of lymph node metastasis, sentinel lymph node mapping is being increasingly used. Re-excision may also be considered with evidence of minimal residual disease after initial resection. Patients with extremity tumors receive combination chemotherapy, but because of the high incidence of the alveolar histology, radiation therapy is also often used. For genitourinary tumors, preservation of bladder function is the key in resection of tumors involving the bladder or prostate. If this goal cannot be met, preoperative chemoradiation is usually recommended. If residual disease remains despite this, more aggressive measures can be considered, including a partial cystectomy, prostatectomy, or anterior (rectum-sparing) exenteration. Patients with paratesticular rhabdomyosarcoma should undergo a radical inguinal orchiectomy, with a retroperitoneal lymph node dissection in boys younger than 10 years because of the frequent prevalence of metastasis. When the tumor is clearly fixed to scrotal skin, resection is required. Chemotherapy is standard, whereas radiation therapy is indicated only with positive nodes. For patients with vaginal or vulvar rhabdomyosarcoma, vaginectomy and wide local excision, respectively, and multiagent chemotherapy are recommended. Approximately 15% of children present with metastatic disease, and their prognosis remains poor. Nearly 30% will experience disease relapse, and 50% to 95% of them will die as the disease progresses. Median survival from the first recurrence is 0.8 year, with an estimated 5-year survival rate of only 17%. Despite these harrowing data, however, rhabdomyosarcoma is a curable disease in most children, with more than 60% surviving 5 years after diagnosis. Survival for children with this malignant neoplasm has improved secondary to a number of factors, including better imaging and pathologic classification, use of multiagent chemotherapy, and appropriate use of radiotherapy.

Liver Tumors

Primary tumors of the liver are rare in the pediatric population but are malignant in approximately 60% of cases. The two most common tumors are hepatoblastoma and hepatocellular carcinoma (HCC). Hepatoblastoma represents 80% of all malignant liver tumors and 1% of all pediatric cancer. The peak incidence of hepatoblastoma is at 3 years of age; the median age for children with HCC is 10 to 11.2 years. More than 90% of patients younger than 5 years with primary liver tumors have hepatoblastoma, whereas 87% of those between 15 and 19 years have HCC.[45] Patients with familial adenomatous polyposis, Gardner, and Beckwith-Wiedemann syndromes are at increased risk for development of hepatoblastoma. HCC is associated with acquired hepatitis B and C and has been observed in children with several types of congenital diseases, including tyrosinemia, glycogen storage disease type I, α_1-antitrypsin deficiency, and cholestasis caused by biliary atresia.

Clinical Presentation

Hepatoblastoma typically is manifested as a painless palpable abdominal mass. Other symptoms are nonspecific and include anorexia, weight loss and failure to thrive, abdominal pain, anemia, and abdominal distention. Jaundice is not commonly encountered because liver function remains relatively normal except in a very advanced tumor. Some patients present with tumor rupture, resulting in intra-abdominal bleeding and peritonitis. HCC is manifested similarly, although stigmata of cirrhosis, such as jaundice, spider angiomas, ascites, and splenomegaly, may be encountered. Almost 25% of patients have metastatic spread to abdominal and mediastinal lymph nodes, lung, bone marrow, and brain.

Diagnosis and Staging

Basic blood tests usually reveal normal liver function in hepatoblastoma, whereas there will be abnormalities in HCC. Anemia, thrombocytopenia, or pancytopenia can be found with splenomegaly caused by sequestration. AFP levels are elevated in more than 70% of hepatoblastoma patients. However, an elevated AFP level is not pathognomonic, and depending on the age of the patient, other disease processes must be ruled out. For example, in infants younger than 6 months, elevated AFP levels may also be seen in sarcomas, yolk sac tumors, and hamartomas. All children being evaluated for HCC should be tested for exposure to hepatitis B and C viruses.

Abdominal ultrasonography is an excellent initial diagnostic study. Doppler ultrasound can also detect the presence of tumor extension into or thrombosis of major vessels, namely, the hepatic veins, IVC, and portal vein. A CT scan is essential in assessing the relationship of the tumor to adjacent vital structures, such as bile ducts and vessels, and excluding intra-abdominal tumor extension beyond the liver. MRI can similarly be used in this setting but does not necessarily provide significant advantages over CT. Because hepatoblastoma frequently spreads hematologically to the lungs, chest CT should also be performed. Bone scintigraphy is recommended for staging in children with HCC because of the high incidence of bone metastases. Hepatoblastoma characteristically appears as a unifocal mass surrounded by a pseudocapsule; it may be a pure epithelial type that contains fetal or embryonal cells or a mixture of the two histologic subtypes, which contains mesenchymal tissue in addition to epithelial components. On the other hand, HCC is characterized by large, pleomorphic epithelial cells that appear much like mature hepatocytes. In gross appearance, HCC forms multifocal nodules that lack a fibrous tumor and often lead to diffuse intrahepatic involvement. Unlike in adults, there has been no indisputable evidence that histopathologic type has any bearing on prognosis.

A standard TNM system has been used for staging purposes, but much effort has been put into the development of a pretreatment staging system, known as the PRE-Treatment EXTent of disease (PRETEXT) definition system (Table 66-6).[46] The PRETEXT system was developed by the International Childhood Liver Tumor Strategy Group (SIOPEL) for staging and risk stratification of liver tumors. It divides the liver into four sections based on segmental anatomy of the liver, and the tumor is subsequently classified by the number of tumor-free sections of liver (Fig. 66-26). This system takes caudate lobe involvement, tumor rupture, ascites, extension into the stomach or diaphragm, tumor focality, lymph node involvement, presence of distant metastases, and vascular involvement into further consideration. Patients are considered at high risk if they have a serum AFP level above 100 ng/mL, extension beyond the liver, distant metastases, intraperitoneal hemorrhage, and invasion of the hepatic veins, IVC, or portal vein. For PRETEXT I and II, hepatoblastoma may be resected by segmentectomy or anatomic lobectomy.

TABLE 66-6 PRETEXT Definition for Hepatoblastoma

PRETEXT GROUP	DEFINITION
I	One section involved; three adjoining sections are tumor free
II	One or two sections involved; two adjoining sections are tumor free
III	Two or three sections involved; one adjoining section is tumor free
IV	Four sections involved

Treatment

Liver transplantation is a potential surgical option for patients with a massive unresectable tumor. Neoadjuvant chemotherapy is used for tumor shrinkage and potential complete resection. Interestingly, some advocate the use of preoperative chemotherapy to treat what would otherwise be residual microscopic disease left behind after resection. They argue that doing so eliminates tumor cells that could respond to hepatotrophic factors during liver regeneration, thereby decreasing the risk of recurrence. There are two current approaches to hepatoblastoma: (1) tumor resection followed by chemotherapy and (2) tumor biopsy followed by chemotherapy and delayed resection. Patients with stage I tumors with pure fetal histology usually do not require postoperative chemotherapy. However, patients with stage II or higher tumors and tumors of any other type of histology do require chemotherapy consisting of cisplatin, 5-fluorouracil, and vincristine. For patients with residual tumor after resection, chemotherapy should be coupled with an evaluation for transplantation.[45] Criteria for transplantation include having no more than three tumors smaller than 3 cm in diameter and no evidence of extrahepatic disease or vascular invasion. When relapses occur, doxorubicin, irinotecan, and ifosfamide have been used, often with some success. Another modality being used with variable success in children whose tumors are unresponsive to systemic chemotherapy is direct arterial chemotherapy or chemoembolization. Long-term outcomes have yet to be determined. Long-term disease-free survival of more than 85% to 90% can be achieved for resectable hepatoblastoma, although similar estimates have been noted for patients with unresectable hepatoblastoma treated by liver transplantation. The same cannot be said for HCC, in which survival rates with partial hepatectomy remain poor because of relapse. In the past decade, early transplantation has been shown to result in better outcomes in some centers.

Teratoma

Teratomas are typically benign neoplasms that contain elements derived from more than one of the three embryonic germ layers, endoderm, mesoderm, and ectoderm. They are composed of tissue that is foreign to the anatomic site in which they are found. Although teratomas may occur anywhere along the midline, they

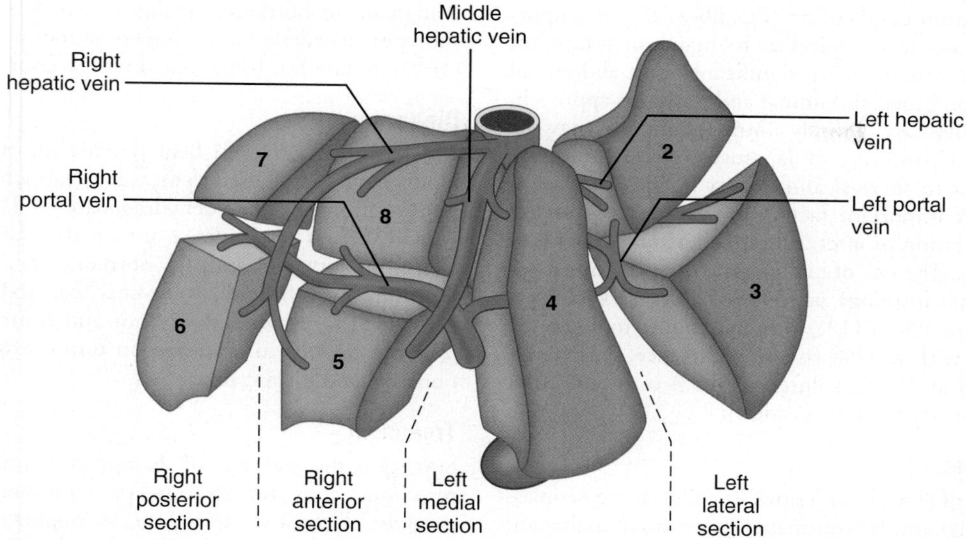

FIGURE 66-26 A diagram of PRETEXT definition system for hepatoblastoma. The liver is divided into four sections based on segmental anatomy of the liver, and the tumor is subsequently classified by the number of tumor-free sections of liver. (From Roebuck DJ, Aronson D, Clapuyt P, et al: 2005 PRETEXT: A revised staging system for primary malignant liver tumors of childhood developed by the SIOPEL group. *Pediatr Radiol* 37:123–132, 2007.)

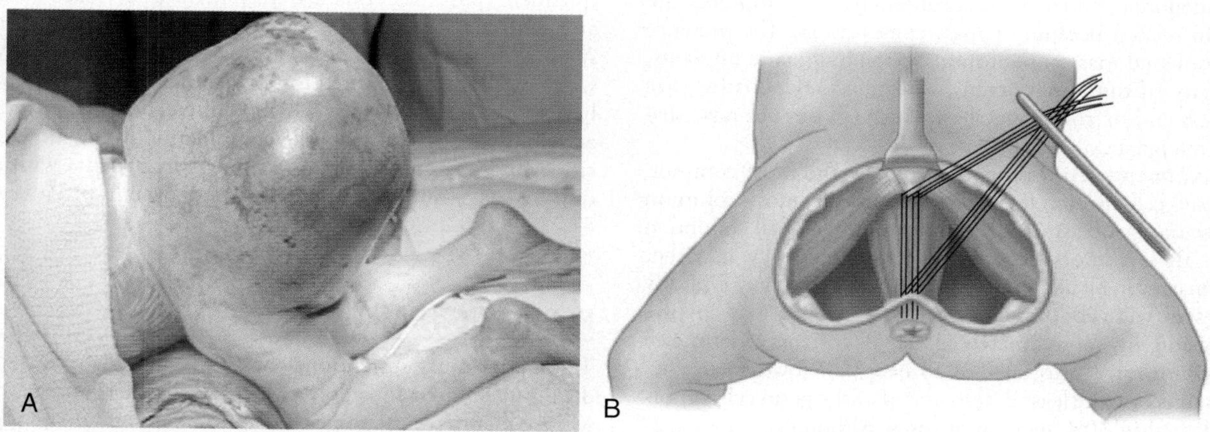

FIGURE 66-27 A, Sacrococcygeal teratoma. **B,** Levator ani and gluteal muscles are reconstructed and a drain is left in place. (**B** from Dicken BJ, Rescorla FJ: Sacrococcygeal teratoma. In Chung DH, Chen MK, editors: *Atlas of pediatric surgical techniques*, Philadelphia, 2010, Elsevier Saunders, pp 364–373.)

are usually found in sacrococcygeal, mediastinal, retroperitoneal, and gonadal locations. Teratomas may be solid, cystic, or mixed and are classified as mature or immature. Although immature teratomas can be potentially malignant, the incidence of malignant transformation in mature teratomas is low. There is a preponderance based on gender; almost 80% of all teratomas occur in females. Moreover, location has been associated with age, as evidenced by the fact that extragonadal tumors occur primarily in neonates and young children, whereas gonadal tumors are more commonly noted in adolescents.

Sacrococcygeal Teratomas

Sacrococcygeal teratomas (SCTs) account for 60% of all teratomas and can be manifested as large exophytic masses in utero. In such cases, they are detected on prenatal ultrasound. Complications include polyhydramnios and fetal hydrops, which can result in fetal demise caused by a tumor-induced vascular steal syndrome that leads to high-output heart failure. Symptoms can include weakness, paralysis, bowel or bladder dysfunction, and other neurologic symptoms that may indicate intradural spinal extension. The diagnosis can be made clinically, especially with exophytic SCTs (Fig. 66-27*A*). If the AFP or β-hCG level is elevated, yolk sac or choriocarcinoma components, respectively, make up the teratoma. Ultrasonography, CT, or MRI may be necessary to detect intra-abdominal lesions or to determine whether there is pelvic or abdominal extension.

Surgical resection is the standard of care and should be performed promptly because of the risk of hemorrhage and tumor rupture. Operative planning must take into account the degree of intra-abdominal extension. Most tumors can be resected by a posterior approach, in which a chevron incision allows the division of the gluteal muscles, ligation of the blood supply, and en bloc resection of the tumor and coccyx (Fig. 66-27*B*). It is important to preserve the anorectal complex to maintain long-term continence. External tumors with significant intra-abdominal extension require a combined abdominal and posterior approach, whereas teratomas that are entirely intra-abdominal may be approached through laparotomy or laparoscopy. Outcomes are favorable with respect to survival and quality of life. The age at diagnosis is the most important factor; those diagnosed at less than 30 weeks of gestation or after 2 months postnatally tend to have a poor prognosis. The risk of malignant transformation associated with embryonal histology is 15% to 20%. Risk of local recurrence ranges from 4% to 11%, although failure to resect the coccyx is associated with a 37% risk of recurrence. AFP levels should be monitored at 3-month intervals for 3 to 4 years. For recurrence, re-excision should be considered.

Ovarian Neoplasms

Approximately 50% of all ovarian lesions in children are neoplastic but are rarely malignant. It is estimated that ovarian malignant neoplasms represent 10% of all ovarian masses but only 1% of childhood cancers. Primary ovarian malignant neoplasms can be classified as germ cell, epithelial cell, and sex cord stromal tumors. Germ cell tumors include teratomas and choriocarcinoma; sex cord stromal tumors consist of granulosa (thecal) and Sertoli (Leydig) cells. Epithelial cell tumors encompass serous and mucinous cystadenomas and cystadenocarcinomas.[47] Symptoms are usually pain related because of mass compression. The presence of ascites, omental masses, peritoneal or diaphragmatic implants, adherence to surrounding organs, aortoiliac adenopathy, size larger than 8 cm, or contralateral ovarian mass should raise suspicion for malignancy.

Germ cell tumors. An ovarian teratoma is the most common ovarian germ cell tumor. It also represents the most common pediatric ovarian neoplasm and accounts for 25% of all childhood teratomas. These tumors occur with equal frequency in either ovary and may even be bilateral in 10% of patients. They typically are manifested with abdominal or pelvic pain and may involve ovarian torsion in approximately 25% of patients. Germ cell tumors account for 7% to 80% of all neoplastic ovarian masses. Dysgerminomas are the least differentiated of the germ cell tumors and are bilateral in 10% to 15% of cases. Although pure dysgerminomas are malignant, they tend to present while still localized and are highly responsive to chemoradiation. Survival is almost 90% with complete surgical resection.

Sex cord tumors. Sex cord tumors arise from the stromal elements of the ovary, producing hormones that may result in precocious puberty. Interestingly, these tumors have been associated with Peutz-Jeghers syndrome. Abnormal menstruation, swelling, and pain are common chief complaints. Outcomes after resection are good in this group because most lesions are still limited to the ovary. Advanced-stage tumors are responsive to platinum-based chemotherapy. Granulosa cell tumors account for 1% to 10% of ovarian malignant neoplasms in females younger than 20 years, whereas Sertoli-Leydig cell tumors account for 20% of ovarian sex cord stromal tumors. Because they are androgenic, serum testosterone metabolite levels can be elevated. With estrogen excess, patients develop early sexual characteristics, such as breast or labial enlargement, axillary and pubic hair growth, and galactorrhea.

Epithelial tumors. Less than 20% of ovarian tumors in childhood are epithelial in nature, given that they are rare before menarche. The two main histologic subtypes are serous and mucinous tumors, which can be further described as benign, malignant, or borderline malignant. It is possible to classify the subtypes as adenoma or adenocarcinoma; adenocarcinoma is extremely rare but is associated with a poor prognosis.

Diagnosis

AFP and β-hCG levels help provide information about tumor biology and can be used to measure treatment response. Although nonspecific, the lactate dehydrogenase level may also be elevated. Also, if there is any evidence of menstrual abnormalities or precocious puberty, luteinizing hormone and follicle-stimulating hormone levels should also be checked. Abdominal ultrasound is performed to evaluate the tumor and contralateral ovary. A CT scan can provide information on tumor extension, regional adenopathy, and distant metastasis.

Treatment

Surgery is the mainstay of therapy and aims to ensure complete resection, with preservation of reproductive function when possible. Definitive treatment is oophorectomy or salpingo-oophorectomy. Care should be taken to resect the tumor without disrupting the capsule or spilling tumor contents to avoid upstaging of malignant lesions. Ascites, if present, should be tested for cytology evidence of tumor. At operation, liver, diaphragm and peritoneal surfaces, and omentum are examined for ovarian implants, which, when present, should be biopsied for staging and treatment purposes. Bilateral retroperitoneal, iliac, para-aortic, and perirenal lymph nodes should be sampled for appropriate staging. Ascites or peritoneal washings should be sent for cytology. Chemotherapy is indicated for any ovarian tumor with extension beyond the affected ovary, which is often the case with germ cell and epithelial cell tumors. The combination of low-dose bleomycin, etoposide, and cisplatin treatment in patients with stage II disease has resulted in event-free and overall survival rates of 87.5% and 93.8%, respectively.

PEDIATRIC TRAUMA

Traumatic injury, intentional or unintentional, results in more deaths in children and adolescents than all other causes combined. Most pediatric trauma is a result of blunt trauma, although penetrating injury accounts for 10% to 20% of all pediatric trauma admissions with the increase in violence among 13- to 18-year-olds. It must be stressed that the pediatric patient is different physiologically from an adult counterpart, but the basic principles remain the same.

ABCs of Trauma

Evaluation of the pediatric patient's airway is of utmost importance. A child who is crying or able to verbalize is able to protect his or her airway. If a patient is drooling, gurgling, or wheezing, one must rule out correctable causes of airway obstruction, such as a retrievable foreign object in the oropharynx. The threshold for endotracheal intubation, especially with excessive sedation, should be low. The appropriate endotracheal tube size can be estimated as being equivalent to the diameter of the child's fifth digit. Alternatively, the endotracheal tube inner diameter can be calculated (4 + the patient's age in years divided by 4). The trachea is also shorter and narrower in children.

After the airway is secured, a rapid assessment should be made of the respiratory status by determining the presence of flail chest, dyspnea, tachypnea, or unequal breath sounds. Caution should be exercised in using pulse oximetry because it does not reflect proper ventilation. Next, circulation should be assessed to ensure adequate oxygen delivery. The patient should be examined for general color, capillary refill, and presence of peripheral pulses. A weak and thready pulse along with hypotension indicates hypovolemic shock. Blood transfusion should be considered in those with hypovolemic shock unresponsive to two boluses of 20 mL/kg crystalloid. In children younger than 6 years, intraosseous access may be considered when it is difficult to establish peripheral IV lines. After the initial ABCs, a secondary survey should be performed. Hypothermia must be avoided to prevent complications of coagulopathy and acidosis. A detailed examination should be performed of the head and neck, including palpation of the posterior neck beneath the C-collar, and of the torso, back, and extremities.

Head and Spine Injuries

Traumatic brain injury (TBI) is the leading cause of death among injured children. In toddlers 2 years or younger, physical abuse, such as that seen in shaken baby syndrome, is the most common cause of serious head injury. This may be manifested as retinal, subdural, or subarachnoid hemorrhages. In children aged 3 years and older, falls and motor vehicle, bicycle, and pedestrian accidents are responsible for most TBIs. The initial CT scan may demonstrate diffuse edema, and with time, the brain injury may evolve with evidence of diffuse axonal injury, hemorrhage, or parenchymal damage. Children with a mild head injury usually complain of headache and nausea or exhibit amnesia, impaired concentration, and behavior disturbances. Up to 20% of children who sustain mild TBIs can have an intracranial hemorrhage, and approximately 3% will eventually require operative intervention. There is no consensus on how to approach the child with a mild TBI; many advocate the use of a screening head CT scan with close clinical examination. When appropriate, cerebral perfusion pressure must be monitored. Because of its transient effect and propensity to induce vasospasm, prophylactic hyperventilation should be avoided unless there is imminent concern for herniation. Aside from diuretics and hypertonic saline, a barbiturate-induced coma and hypothermia are other maneuvers that can be used to lower the intracranial pressure. Intracranial bleeding causing focal neurologic symptoms or mass effect should be surgically addressed.

Although relatively infrequent, motor vehicle accidents account for most traumatic spinal cord injuries in children. Fractures of the C1 and C2 vertebrae are commonly seen in younger children, whereas compression and chance fractures, frequently associated with improper seat belt use, are seen in older children. Spinal cord injury without radiologic abnormality is a clinical condition in which a child (<8 years of age) can present with transient neurologic deficits. It is thought to occur because incomplete vertebral ossification and ligament laxity allow the cord and nerve roots to stretch or to impact on the opposing bone surfaces of the spinal canal.

Thoracic Trauma

Thoracic injury is the second leading cause of death in pediatric trauma and accounts for 5% of trauma-related hospital admissions. Blunt trauma, particularly from motor vehicle accidents, is responsible for most thoracic injuries. Rib cages in children are primarily cartilaginous and therefore more pliable. Thus, a child may present with a significant intrathoracic injury (e.g., pulmonary contusion, pneumothorax, hemothorax) without obvious evidence of rib fractures. Pulmonary contusions result in an inflammatory response with edema, atelectasis, and subsequent consolidation. Hypoxemia, hypercarbia, and tachypnea can be significant and necessitate intubation. Radiographic findings are variable and unreliable. Nonetheless, most patients respond to conservative management without long-term sequelae. Traumatic asphyxia is a rare presentation after blunt trauma, but sudden compression or crushing of the thorax can result in airway obstruction and retrograde high-pressure flow in the superior vena cava. When this occurs, patients present dramatically with head and neck cyanosis, subconjunctival hemorrhaging, and petechiae. Rib fractures in children younger than 3 years should be approached with a high index of suspicion for child abuse. Surgical exploration of the chest may be indicated for an acute bloody chest tube output of more than 20% of the patient's blood volume or chest tube blood drainage of 2 mL/kg/hr. Intercostal artery bleeding is a common cause.

Tracheobronchial injuries usually occur near the carina and are thought to result from anteroposterior compression of the pliable pediatric chest. The patient can present with pneumothorax, pneumomediastinum, and subcutaneous emphysema. Tracheobronchial disruption results in massive air leak with potential tension pneumothorax, compromising respiratory function and venous return. Aside from hemodynamic instability, primary repair is indicated if the injury involves more than one third of the diameter of the bronchus or if nonoperative management fails. A widened mediastinum on the chest radiograph is rare in children. Most of these injuries result from blunt trauma and are found at the ligamentum arteriosum. Traumatic diaphragmatic rupture with herniation of the stomach and bowel occurs in approximately 1% of children with blunt chest trauma. Left-sided rupture is more common because the liver protects against right-sided rupture.

Abdominal Trauma

When a seat belt sign, a bruising of the midanterior abdominal wall after a motor vehicle accident, is present on a child, the CT scan should be reviewed for any subtle signs of bowel injury or presence of free peritoneal fluid. Intra-abdominal fluid on a CT scan without a solid organ injury should raise the index of suspicion for a hollow viscus injury. Blunt injuries to the stomach are generally seen in children who are struck by a vehicle or who fall across bicycle handlebars and present as blowout or perforation of the greater curvature. Usually seen in restrained children involved in motor vehicle accidents, intestinal injury secondary to blunt trauma is estimated to be less than 15%. Several mechanisms can explain the injury pattern, such as rapid deceleration causing the lap belt to compress the intestines against the spine. The increase in intraluminal pressure may predispose to perforation or rupture. Small intestinal injuries occur predominantly in areas of fixation, such as at the ligament of Treitz or ileocecal valve. A duodenal or mesenteric hematoma may ensue and cause obstruction, with subsequent nausea and bilious emesis. It is not uncommon to encounter retroperitoneal injuries as well.

Treatment of Solid Organ Injuries

The intra-abdominal solid organs are particularly vulnerable to blunt trauma in children. Nonoperative management is the standard therapy for hemodynamically stable children with blunt solid organ injury. Those who fail to respond to nonoperative management usually do so within the first 12 hours. The American Pediatric Surgical Association has detailed guidelines regarding the

TABLE 66-7 Classification of Intra-abdominal Solid Organ Injuries

GRADE	LIVER	SPLEEN	KIDNEY
I	Hematoma: <10% subcapsular surface area Laceration: capsular tear <1 cm	Hematoma: <10% subcapsular Laceration: capsular tear <1 cm	Contusion: microscopic or gross hematuria Hematoma: subcapsular, nonexpanding, no parenchymal tear
II	Hematoma: 10%-50% subcapsular surface area, <10 cm intraparenchymal hemorrhage Laceration: capsular tear 1-3 cm deep, <10 cm length	Hematoma: 10%-50% subcapsular surface area, <5 cm intraparenchymal hemorrhage Laceration: capsular tear, 1-3 cm parenchymal depth not involving a trabecular vessel	Hematoma: nonexpanding perirenal hematoma confined to retroperitoneum Laceration: <1 cm parenchymal depth of renal cortex without collecting system rupture or urinary extravasation
III	Hematoma: >50% expanding subcapsular surface area, ruptured subcapsular hematoma with active bleeding, or intraparenchymal hematoma ≥2 cm or expanding Laceration: >3 cm parenchymal depth	Hematoma: ruptured subcapsular or parenchymal hematoma; intraparenchymal hematoma >5 cm or expanding Laceration: >3 cm parenchymal depth involving trabecular vessels	Laceration: >1 cm parenchymal depth of renal cortex without collecting system rupture or urinary extravasation
IV	Hematoma: ruptured parenchyma with active bleeding Laceration: parenchymal disruption involving 25%-75% of hepatic lobe	Hematoma: ruptured parenchyma with active bleeding Laceration: hilar vessels with major devascularization (>25% of spleen)	Laceration: parenchymal laceration extending through the renal cortex, medulla, and collecting system Vascular: main renal artery or vein injury with contained hemorrhage
V	Laceration: parenchymal disruption involving >50% of hepatic lobe Vascular: juxtahepatic venous injuries (retrohepatic vena cava, central major hepatic veins)	Laceration: completely shattered spleen Vascular: hilar vascular injury with total devascularization	Laceration: completely shattered kidney Vascular: avulsion of renal hilum with devascularization of kidney
VI	Vascular: hepatic avulsion		

management of isolated liver and spleen injuries based on initial CT findings; these have been shown to reduce the length of hospital stay significantly, without adverse outcomes (Table 66-7). Splenic injuries are relatively common in pediatric trauma. Splenic injuries are managed conservatively unless there is evidence of hemodynamic instability. CT scan can delineate the extent of splenic injury. The role of splenic artery embolization in the treatment of pediatric blunt splenic injury remains uncertain, unlike in adult patients. An isolated hepatic injury without involvement of the hepatic vein, IVC, or portal vein can also be managed conservatively. Some have reported that 85% to 90% of patients can successfully be treated with nonoperative management. However, those who fail to respond do so because of hemodynamic instability, changes in clinical examination findings, or transfusion requirements of more than half of blood volume (roughly 40 mL/kg/day). Delayed bleeding after liver injury has been reported as late as 6 weeks after injury and may be seen in 1% to 3% of patients. As is the case with splenic lacerations, one should proceed with definitive surgical treatment whenever there is hemodynamic instability despite adequate resuscitation.

Pancreatic Injury

Pancreatic injuries occur from blunt trauma, such as falling into bicycle handlebars. An elevated amylase or lipase level is present. CT scan is a useful diagnostic modality for evaluation of most pancreatic trauma, although it is not as sensitive or specific for determination of pancreatic ductal injuries. There is little role for ERCP in acute settings of pediatric pancreatic injury. When presented acutely, transection of pancreas from blunt trauma is best managed with operative intervention of distal pancreatectomy. For those with delayed presentation, a conservative management is more appropriate. This may include TPN and bowel rest. ERCP is considered to evaluate for ductal injuries. External drainage procedure may be required.

Renal Injury

The nonoperative management of organ injury also applies to renal injuries. Retroperitoneal injuries are frequently seen with direct blows to the back or flank, and the kidney is involved in 10% to 20% of cases. In children, there is a lack of perinephric fat, which makes the kidney a susceptible target. Contusion is the most common renal injury encountered in children, whereas fracture of the renal pelvis occurs in children who have congenital renal abnormalities. Interestingly, the presence of hematuria does not correlate with the severity of renal injury. Conservative management is standard for low-grade renal injuries (grades I to III), and there is no consensus on the controversial management of high-grade renal injuries (grades IV and V). An absolute indication for renal exploration is an expanding or pulsatile hematoma. Relative indications include urinary extravasation, necrosis, and arterial injury. In the case of urinary extravasation, ureteral stenting can be attempted. Grade V injuries usually require operative management, but the salvage rate is poor.

FETAL SURGERY

With modern prenatal care, many congenital conditions are diagnosed before birth. Although these anomalies rarely progress in such a way that fetal survival is threatened, there are cases in which an intervention is warranted. Fetal surgery is a progressive field that aims to alter the natural progression of congenital disease in utero. Many of these anomalies have severe complications associated with fetal demise if they are left untreated. However, given the high-risk nature of the procedures themselves, selection of which patients would benefit most and how best to manage them is the key. Indications for fetal surgery include myelomeningocele, hydrops caused by CPAM, steal syndrome and cardiac failure from SCTs, and oligohydramnios with renal failure from lower urinary tract obstruction. Although initial outcomes were disappointing, recent improvements have been made in selection criteria based on outcomes research, which aims to identify patients with malformations who would see reasonable benefit from prenatal intervention. Ultrasonography continues to be the primary prenatal imaging modality because it is noninvasive and without radiation exposure. However, ultrafast MRI has become a useful imaging adjunct, particularly when the diagnosis is unclear or needs further evaluation.

One of the most significant advances in fetal surgery was made in the treatment of myelomeningocele, the most common form of spina bifida. In a multicenter randomized trial, prenatal surgical repair for myelomeningocele was shown to reduce the need for shunting by the age of 12 months and improved motor outcomes at 30 months compared with standard postnatal surgical repair.[48] Several fetal centers have continued to experience successful outcomes with prenatal repair for myelomeningocele. In contrast, fetal surgery was attempted in the treatment of CDH, but with dismal results because of premature births and other complications. In high-risk fetuses with CDH complicated by thoracic herniation of the liver, reduction of the liver back into the abdomen was associated with kinking of the umbilical vein and subsequent fetal demise. In recent years, the fetal intervention for CDH has focused on reversible tracheal occlusion with clips or endoluminal balloons to induce intrauterine lung growth. Initial outcome data have been variable without significant improvement in survival, with premature rupture of membranes being a frequent complication of the procedure itself.[49] However, the TOTAL trial led by several European centers showed some promising results.[2]

Procedures involving tracheal occlusion have led to the development of the ex utero intrapartum treatment (EXIT) procedure, which is a delivery technique used for fetuses with airway compression that may be caused by the presence of a thoracic mass. To secure the fetus' airway during delivery, the mother is given tocolytics and anesthesia to induce maximal uterine relaxation while maintaining uteroplacental circulation. This allows an airway to be established by endotracheal intubation before the umbilical cord is clamped. After delivery, the newborn can be stabilized for postnatal interventions, when indicated.

SCT is another condition for which fetal surgery may be indicated, but reports of in utero resection are rare. The development of hydrops in a fetus with SCT is caused by high-output cardiac failure from arteriovenous shunting through the tumor. To reduce blood flow to the tumor, coagulation of the arteriovenous shunt, laser photocoagulation, and radiofrequency ablation of the feeding vessels have been used with some success in small studies. Open fetal surgery for SCT is controversial. Because most fetuses with SCT undergo postnatal resection without complication, intrauterine intervention is advocated only for those patients with symptoms related to hydrops. It is unclear whether these interventions change overall survival, given the poor prognosis associated with the development of these symptoms.

CPAM can result in hydrops and pulmonary hypoplasia when it is large enough. One study has found a correlation between the volume of the CPAM and head circumference, which indicated that when the ratio is more than 1.6, the risk for development of hydrops was found to be 80%. It is this subset of patients that benefits from in utero intervention. Typically, microcystic lesions can be resected with a lobectomy and macrocystic masses can be aspirated or shunted. Outcomes are good; these interventions reverse hydropic symptoms and result in a survival rate of more than 70%.[50]

The application of minimally invasive techniques has been increasing, and its role in fetal surgery is still being explored. It is used for lower urinary tract obstructions, in which oligohydramnios causes pulmonary insufficiency and compression deformities of the face and limbs. These patients may benefit from vesicoamniotic shunting and ablation of posterior valves. Fetoscopic surgery has also been successfully used in the laser ablation of the communicating placental blood vessels in twin-twin transfusion syndrome, characterized by hypovolemia, oliguria, and oligohydramnios in the donor twin and hypervolemia, polyuria, and polyhydramnios in the recipient twin. The procedure is associated with a 75% survival rate of at least one twin.

SELECTED REFERENCES

Adzick S, Thom EA, Spong CY, et al: A randomized trial of prenatal versus postnatal repair of myelomeningocele. *N Engl J Med* 364:993–1004, 2011.

This report details results of a multicenter randomized trial of fetal intervention for myelomeningocele.

Coran AG, Adzick NS, Krummel TM, et al, editors: *Pediatric surgery*, ed 7, Philadelphia, 2012, Elsevier Saunders.

This two-volume set is a comprehensive textbook on pediatric surgery, considered to be the most authoritative textbook for pediatric surgeons.

Holcomb GW, III, Murphy JP, Ostlie DJ, et al, editors: *Ashcraft's pediatric surgery*, ed 6, Philadelphia, 2014, Elsevier Saunders.

This is an excellent single-volume reference. This textbook is easy to read and serves as a good practical resource, especially for young surgical residents, fellows, and medical students.

O'Neill JA, Grosfeld JL, Fonkalsrud EW, et al, editors: *Principles of pediatric surgery*, ed 2, St. Louis, 2004, Mosby.

This is an outstanding textbook for medical students, surgical residents, and pediatric surgical fellows. It is comprehensive yet concisely highlights core elements of pediatric surgical knowledge written by 5 editors and 10 associate editors.

Vandenplas Y: Management of paediatric GERD. *Nat Rev Gastroenterol Hepatol* 11:147–157, 2014.

This is an excellent review for the management of pediatric gastroesophageal reflux disorders.

REFERENCES

1. Perkins JA, Manning SC, Tempero RM, et al: Lymphatic malformations: Review of current treatment. *Otolaryngol Head Neck Surg* 142:795–803, 803.e1, 2010.

2. Deprest J, Brady P, Nicolaides K, et al: Prenatal management of the fetus with isolated congenital diaphragmatic hernia in the era of the TOTAL trial. *Semin Fetal Neonatal Med* 19:338–348, 2014.
3. Hagadorn JI, Brownell EA, Herbst KW, et al: Trends in treatment and in-hospital mortality for neonates with congenital diaphragmatic hernia. *J Perinatol* 35:748–754, 2015.
4. Partridge EA, Peranteau WH, Rintoul NE, et al: Timing of repair of congenital diaphragmatic hernia in patients supported by extracorporeal membrane oxygenation (ECMO). *J Pediatr Surg* 50:260–262, 2015.
5. Parikh DH, Rasiah SV: Congenital lung lesions: Postnatal management and outcome. *Semin Pediatr Surg* 24:160–167, 2015.
6. Masters IB: Congenital airway lesions and lung disease. *Pediatr Clin North Am* 56:227–242, xii, 2009.
7. Derderian SC, Coleman AM, Jeanty C, et al: Favorable outcomes in high-risk congenital pulmonary airway malformations treated with multiple courses of maternal betamethasone. *J Pediatr Surg* 50:515–518, 2015.
8. Berthet S, Tenisch E, Miron MC, et al: Vascular anomalies associated with esophageal atresia and tracheoesophageal fistula. *J Pediatr* 166:1140–1144.e2, 2015.
9. Vandenplas Y: Management of paediatric GERD. *Nat Rev Gastroenterol Hepatol* 11:147–157, 2014.
10. Papadopoulou A, Koletzko S, Heuschkel R, et al: Management guidelines of eosinophilic esophagitis in childhood. *J Pediatr Gastroenterol Nutr* 58:107–118, 2014.
11. Oomen MW, Hoekstra LT, Bakx R, et al: Open versus laparoscopic pyloromyotomy for hypertrophic pyloric stenosis: A systematic review and meta-analysis focusing on major complications. *Surg Endosc* 26:2104–2110, 2012.
12. McMellen ME, Wakeman D, Longshore SW, et al: Growth factors: Possible roles for clinical management of the short bowel syndrome. *Semin Pediatr Surg* 19:35–43, 2010.
13. Moss RL, Dimmitt RA, Barnhart DC, et al: Laparotomy versus peritoneal drainage for necrotizing enterocolitis and perforation. *N Engl J Med* 354:2225–2234, 2006.
14. Jones BA, Hull MA, McGuire MM, et al: Autologous intestinal reconstruction surgery. *Semin Pediatr Surg* 19:59–67, 2010.
15. Bianchi A: Intestinal loop lengthening—a technique for increasing small intestinal length. *J Pediatr Surg* 15:145–151, 1980.
16. Kim HB, Fauza D, Garza J, et al: Serial transverse enteroplasty (STEP): A novel bowel lengthening procedure. *J Pediatr Surg* 38:425–429, 2003.
17. Ching YA, Fitzgibbons S, Valim C, et al: Long-term nutritional and clinical outcomes after serial transverse enteroplasty at a single institution. *J Pediatr Surg* 44:939–943, 2009.
18. Oh PS, Fingeret AL, Shah MY, et al: Improved tolerance for enteral nutrition after serial transverse enteroplasty (STEP) in infants and children with short bowel syndrome—a seven-year single-center experience. *J Pediatr Surg* 49:1589–1592, 2014.
19. Sanchez-Mejias A, Fernandez RM, Lopez-Alonso M, et al: Contribution of RET, NTRK3 and EDN3 to the expression of Hirschsprung disease in a multiplex family. *J Med Genet* 46:862–864, 2009.
20. Kapur RP, Reed RC, Finn LS, et al: Calretinin immunohistochemistry versus acetylcholinesterase histochemistry in the evaluation of suction rectal biopsies for Hirschsprung disease. *Pediatr Dev Pathol* 12:6–15, 2009.
21. Keckler SJ, Yang JC, Fraser JD, et al: Contemporary practice patterns in the surgical management of Hirschsprung's disease. *J Pediatr Surg* 44:1257–1260, discussion 1260, 2009.
22. Bischoff A, Pena A, Levitt MA: Laparoscopic-assisted PSARP—the advantages of combining both techniques for the treatment of anorectal malformations with recto-bladderneck or high prostatic fistulas. *J Pediatr Surg* 48:367–371, 2013.
23. Lautz TB, Thurm CW, Rothstein DH: Delayed repeat enemas are safe and cost-effective in the management of pediatric intussusception. *J Pediatr Surg* 50:423–427, 2015.
24. Bassett MD, Murray KF: Biliary atresia: Recent progress. *J Clin Gastroenterol* 42:720–729, 2008.
25. Lao OB, Larison C, Garrison M, et al: Steroid use after the Kasai procedure for biliary atresia. *Am J Surg* 199:680–684, 2010.
26. Bezerra JA, Spino C, Magee JC, et al: Use of corticosteroids after hepatoportoenterostomy for bile drainage in infants with biliary atresia: The START randomized clinical trial. *JAMA* 311:1750–1759, 2014.
27. Hartley JL, Davenport M, Kelly DA: Biliary atresia. *Lancet* 374:1704–1713, 2009.
28. Singham J, Yoshida EM, Scudamore CH: Choledochal cysts: Part 1 of 3: Classification and pathogenesis. *Can J Surg* 52:434–440, 2009.
29. Rygiel AM, Beer S, Simon P, et al: Gene conversion between cationic trypsinogen (PRSS1) and the pseudogene trypsinogen 6 (PRSS3P2) in patients with chronic pancreatitis. *Hum Mutat* 36:350–356, 2015.
30. Srinath AI, Youk AO, Bielefeldt K: Biliary dyskinesia and symptomatic gallstone disease in children: Two sides of the same coin? *Dig Dis Sci* 59:1307–1315, 2014.
31. Beres A, Christison-Lagay ER, Romao RL, et al: Evaluation of Surgisis for patch repair of abdominal wall defects in children. *J Pediatr Surg* 47:917–919, 2012.
32. Lao OB, Larison C, Garrison MM, et al: Outcomes in neonates with gastroschisis in U.S. children's hospitals. *Am J Perinatol* 27:97–101, 2010.
33. Kelly RE, Jr, Mellins RB, Shamberger RC, et al: Multicenter study of pectus excavatum, final report: Complications, static/exercise pulmonary function, and anatomic outcomes. *J Am Coll Surg* 217:1080–1089, 2013.
34. Colozza S, Bütter A: Bracing in pediatric patients with pectus carinatum is effective and improves quality of life. *J Pediatr Surg* 48:1055–1059, 2013.
35. Irwin MS, Park JR: Neuroblastoma: Paradigm for precision medicine. *Pediatr Clin North Am* 62:225–256, 2015.
36. Brodeur GM: Neuroblastoma: Biological insights into a clinical enigma. *Nat Rev Cancer* 3:203–216, 2003.
37. Ishola TA, Chung DH: Neuroblastoma. *Surg Oncol* 16:149–156, 2007.
38. Maris JM: Recent advances in neuroblastoma. *N Engl J Med* 362:2202–2211, 2010.
39. Simon T, Haberle B, Hero B, et al: Role of surgery in the treatment of patients with stage 4 neuroblastoma age 18 months or older at diagnosis. *J Clin Oncol* 31:752–758, 2013.
40. Yu AL, Gilman AL, Ozkaynak MF, et al: Anti-GD2 antibody with GM-CSF, interleukin-2, and isotretinoin for neuroblastoma. *N Engl J Med* 363:1324–1334, 2010.

41. Vujanic GM, Sandstedt B: The pathology of Wilms' tumour (nephroblastoma): The International Society of Paediatric Oncology approach. *J Clin Pathol* 63:102–109, 2010.
42. Dumoucel S, Gauthier-Villars M, Stoppa-Lyonnet D, et al: Malformations, genetic abnormalities, and Wilms tumor. *Pediatr Blood Cancer* 61:140–144, 2014.
43. Kaste SC, Dome JS, Babyn PS, et al: Wilms tumour: Prognostic factors, staging, therapy and late effects. *Pediatr Radiol* 38:2–17, 2008.
44. Paulino AC, Okcu MF: Rhabdomyosarcoma. *Curr Probl Cancer* 32:7–34, 2008.
45. Otte JB: Progress in the surgical treatment of malignant liver tumors in children. *Cancer Treat Rev* 36:360–371, 2010.
46. Meyers RL, Czauderna P, Otte JB: Surgical treatment of hepatoblastoma. *Pediatr Blood Cancer* 59:800–808, 2012.
47. Kelleher CM, Goldstein AM: Adnexal masses in children and adolescents. *Clin Obstet Gynecol* 58:76–92, 2015.
48. Adzick NS, Thom EA, Spong CY, et al: A randomized trial of prenatal versus postnatal repair of myelomeningocele. *N Engl J Med* 364:993–1004, 2011.
49. Rossi AC: Indications and outcomes of intrauterine surgery for fetal malformations. *Curr Opin Obstet Gynecol* 22:159–165, 2010.
50. Deprest JA, Flake AW, Gratacos E, et al: The making of fetal surgery. *Prenat Diagn* 30:653–667, 2010.

67 CHAPTER

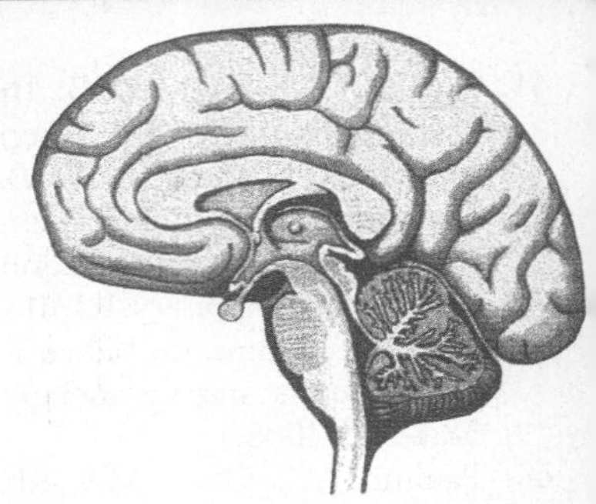

Neurosurgery

Juan Ortega-Barnett, Aaron Mohanty, Sohum K. Desai, Joel T. Patterson

OUTLINE

Neurosurgery is surgery of the brain, spinal cord, peripheral nerves, and their supporting structures, including the blood supply, protective elements, spinal fluid spaces, bony cranium, and spine. This chapter is intended for non-neurosurgeons who want to initiate a framework on which to add further knowledge and experience. It is hoped that it will also help personnel in a community hospital emergency department or a medical student on the ward for the first time communicate patient problems efficiently to neurosurgeons. The chapter first provides an overview of the underlying principles of neurosurgery, with a focus on intracranial dynamics. The remaining sections include a discussion of the following: cerebrovascular disorders, which include subarachnoid hemorrhage, intracerebral hemorrhage, aneurysm, and arteriovenous malformation (AVM); central nervous system (CNS) tumors, which include neoplasms of the brain, skull base, cranial nerves, spinal cord, meninges, and peripheral nerves; traumatic brain injury; degenerative diseases of the spine; functional neurosurgery, which includes stereotactic radiosurgery (SRS), epilepsy surgery, and surgery for the management of pain and movement disorders; hydrocephalus; pediatric neurosurgery; and neurosurgical management of CNS infections. The field of neurosurgery is simply too broad to make a detailed encyclopedic overview realistic, but some introduction to these issues will be useful to the reader.

INTRACRANIAL DYNAMICS

It is essential at the outset to grasp a few basic principles concerning intracranial dynamics, cerebrospinal fluid (CSF), cerebral blood flow (CBF), and intracranial pressure (ICP), and these are summarized here for quick review. Some of these principles are obvious, whereas others might be considered counterintuitive.

The first principle is obvious. The cranial cavity has a fixed volume composed of brain tissue (parenchyma), CSF, and blood vessels and intravascular blood. According to the Monro-Kellie doctrine, the sum of these components within the fixed volume of the cranial cavity implies that an increase in one component must be accompanied by an equal and opposite decrease in one or both of the remaining components.[1] If this does not occur, the ICP will rise, and at some point, the increase in pressure per unit increase in volume becomes asymptotic, approaching levels close to the systemic blood pressure, producing a reverberating blood flow pattern with no net flow. As a consequence, if there is an elevation in the volume of any one compartment, there is a stage of compensation in which the volume of one or more of the other compartments can be reduced to avoid elevations in the ICP. Table 67-1 summarizes and simplifies some of the excess volume syndromes and specific treatment for each.

The second principle is not obvious and may seem counterintuitive. Spinal fluid is produced at a constant rate (≈15 to 20 mL/hr), by an energy-dependent, physicochemical process, mainly by the choroid plexus of the ventricles. It is essential to understand that production is little affected by any intracranial backpressure; thus, CSF production continues unabated, even to lethal elevations of ICP. Because production is almost always constant, it follows that derangement of CSF dynamics almost always involves some aspect of impeding CSF absorption through obstruction along the CSF pathways inside the brain, subarachnoid spaces at the basal cisterns or cerebral convexity, or arachnoid granulations from which most absorption occurs. In the following discussions on tumors, infection, intracranial hemorrhage, and trauma, many examples will become apparent whereby impaired CSF absorption contributes to the pathologic condition. The only exceptions to the almost constant CSF production are the excess production associated with the rare choroid plexus papilloma tumor and the occasional decreased CSF production seen with some gram-negative bacterial meningitis with ventriculitis.

The third basic principle is that the CBF normally varies over a wide range (30 to 100 mL/100 g of brain tissue per minute), depending on metabolic demand from neuronal activity within a particular area of the brain. The blood flow to any brain area is generally abundant, exceeding demand by a wide margin, so that oxygen extraction ratios are often low. The brain vasculature

TABLE 67-1 Intracranial Excess Volume Syndromes and Therapy

COMPONENT	EXCESS VOLUME SYNDROME	SPECIFIC TREATMENT
Brain tissue	Edema: cytotoxic, vasogenic, perineoplastic, inflammatory	Diuretics: mannitol, furosemide, hypertonic saline; steroids for perineoplastic and inflammatory vasogenic edema
Vascular	Elevated P_{CO_2}: hyperperfusion state with loss of autoregulation as in severe hypertension, after trauma or AVM removal; relative venous obstruction	Increased ventilation; diuretics (in hyperperfusion state, avoid mannitol), barbiturates; clear venous obstruction; elevate head of bed (to reduce venous volume)
Cerebrospinal fluid	Impaired absorption with congenital, posthemorrhagic, or postinfectious hydrocephalus, communicating or obstructive; loculations; arachnoid or periventricular cysts; rare increased production of CSF with choroid plexus papilloma	Ventricular external drainage (or lumbar drainage only if no threat of herniation) or shunt; with flocculation, or with some types of obstructive hydrocephalus, endoscopic fenestration or third ventriculostomy may be possible; acetazolamide and steroids may temporarily decrease CSF production
Mass lesion	Tumor, cyst, abscess, hematoma, radiation necrosis, or cerebral infarction necrosis	Remove, fenestrate, aspirate lesion (often with stereotactic guidance); less commonly, it might be useful to enlarge intracranial volume by decompression

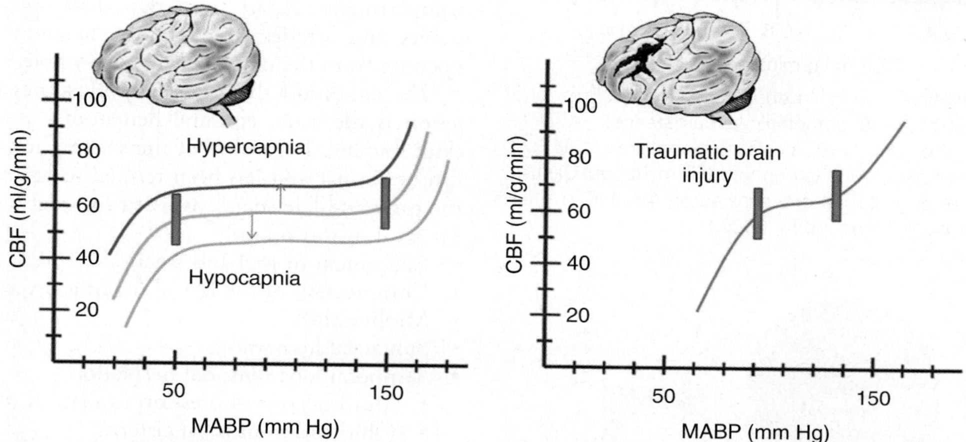

FIGURE 67-1 Cerebral blood flow (CBF) as a function of mean arterial blood pressure (MABP). Note the upward and downward shifts with hypercapnia and hypocapnia, respectively. In traumatic brain injury, the curve is steeper, with large CBF changes occurring with small pressure changes. (Adapted from Rangel-Castilla L, Gasco J, Nauta HJ, et al: Cerebral pressure autoregulation in traumatic brain injury. *Neurosurg Focus* 25:E7, 2008.)

matches the blood flow to tissue metabolic demand, and the CBF generally maintains what is needed, despite wide variations in systemic blood pressure, by a phenomenon known as autoregulation. Factors such as an elevated or decreased arterial P_{CO_2} shift the curve as indicated. In the setting of traumatic brain injury, the curve becomes more pronounced (i.e., smaller changes in blood pressure or P_{CO_2}) and affects the CBF dramatically (Fig. 67-1). If tissue demand exceeds autoregulation, or if CBF declines for pathologic reasons, the first defense is that the oxygen extraction will increase (i.e., arteriovenous oxygen difference). The tissue begins to experience dysfunction at levels below 0.25 mL per gram of brain tissue per minute. With levels between 0.15 and 0.20, the brain tissue may undergo reversible ischemia; however, infarction will occur when levels range between 0.10 and 0.15 (Fig. 67-2). The metabolic consumption of oxygen in the brain is decreased after traumatic brain injury to levels between 0.6 and 1.2 μmol/mg/min. Complete loss of blood flow to any brain area results in infarction (irreversible damage) within a few minutes. Swelling of the infarcted tissue takes days to peak and weeks to resolve.[2]

An important implication is that if brain dysfunction is occurring clinically because compensatory mechanisms (e.g., autoregulation changing the vascular resistance, capacity to elevate mean systemic arterial pressure, ability to increase oxygen extraction) have been exceeded, the tolerance for further decline in blood flow is low, and there is a serious threat for tissue damage. Therapy to increase blood pressure or to decrease ICP may be urgently needed. When time permits because the dysfunction fluctuates chronically, it may sometimes be appropriate to measure oxygen extraction ratios as one index of the overall adequacy of the CBF. At a low CBF, oxygen extraction is increased with a lower venous P_{O_2}. The variations in CBF and extraction ratios related to neuronal activity are said to underlie the ability to image function by functional magnetic resonance imaging (MRI), a technique that is finding wider use in the clinical neurosciences.

A fourth principle derives from the other three and the fact that injured tissue swells, making obvious the potential for a cascading injury by a vicious circle mechanism (Fig. 67-3). If the stage of compensation (see earlier), even with therapy, is exceeded, and ICP is elevated high enough by some mechanism so that cerebral perfusion pressure (CPP) declines, CBF can decline to levels at which tissue injury occurs.

$$CPP = \text{mean arterial pressure (MAP)} - ICP$$

Brain edema (swelling) within the closed cranium will lead to further increases in ICP with even further decreases in CPP in a

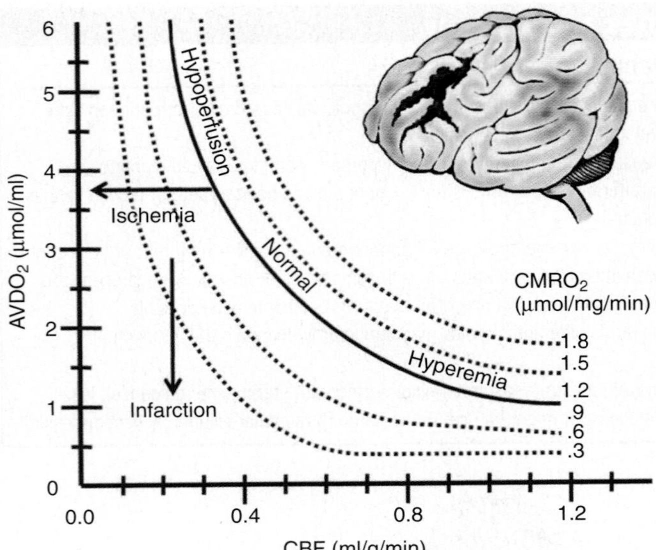

FIGURE 67-2 Relationships among cerebral flow, metabolism, and oxygen extraction in normal and pathologic circumstances. *$AVDO_2$,* arteriovenous oxygen difference; *CBF,* cerebral blood flow; *$CMRO_2$,* cerebral metabolic rate of oxygen consumption. (From Rangel-Castilla L, Gasco J, Nauta HJ, et al: Cerebral pressure autoregulation in traumatic brain injury. *Neurosurg Focus* 25:E7, 2008.)

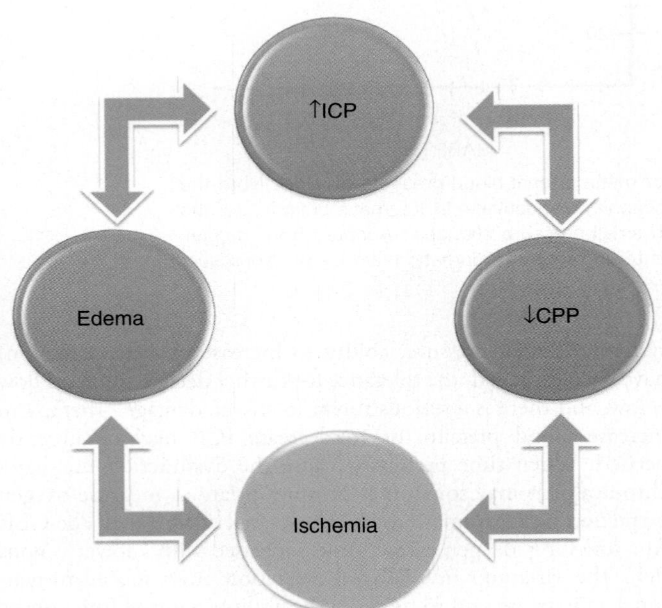

FIGURE 67-3 Relationship among increased intracranial pressure (ICP), reduced cerebral perfusion pressure (CPP), development of ischemia and infarction, and cerebral edema.

stage of decompensation. When the capacity for autoregulation is exceeded or damaged so that it can no longer play a role, CBF is linked directly to the CPP.

In the management of intracranial disease, ICP and CPP are easy to measure continuously and thus serve as highly practical surrogates for the more fundamental but much more difficult to measure CBF. However, these are not equivalent, and the limitations of these parameters for guiding therapy need to be remembered. Regardless of causation, when concern arises about the possibility of cascading injury, every effort is made to keep the CPP in the realm of 60 mm Hg (range, 50 to 70 mm Hg) and ICP below 20 mm Hg if possible. Routinely using pressors and volume expansion to maintain CPP higher than 70 mm Hg is not supported on the basis of systemic complications.[3]

A fifth principle concerns focal mass effect and its progression in regard to the complex anatomy of the cranial cavity. The cranial cavity is not just a hollow spherical space but contains several almost knifelike projections of folded dura, the falx and tentorium, which divide the cavity into a right and left supratentorial compartment and an infratentorial compartment, the posterior fossa. The sphenoid wing is a prominent, mostly bony ridge that separates the anterior fossa containing the frontal lobe from the middle fossa containing the temporal lobe. A narrow opening, the incisura, edged by the tentorium, surrounds the midbrain and is the only passage between the supratentorial and infratentorial compartments. Apart from the small openings for the cranial nerves and arteries, the foramen magnum is the only sizable opening from the cranial cavity as a whole.

The condition that classically illustrates the expanding mass lesion is the acute epidural hematoma, seen after trauma with skull fracture. Regardless of the source, however, the progression can be similar and has been termed rostrocaudal decay to reflect the early and late stages, as listed in order here:

- Focal distortion only
- Effacement of gyri and sulci
- Compression of the lateral (or other) ventricle
- Midline shift
- Subfalcial herniation
- Temporal lobe tentorial herniation
    - Third nerve compression (unilateral dilated pupil)
    - Obliteration of basal cisterns
    - Midbrain compression
    - Midbrain infarction, Duret hemorrhages (both pupils dilate, with irreversible damage to midbrain)
- Further brainstem compression
    - Loss of brainstem reflexes: progression from flexor posturing to extensor posturing; vestibulo-ocular and oculocephalic reflexes; corneal reflexes
    - Medullary compression syndrome: respiratory reflexes; vasomotor reflexes, Cushing reflex with elevation of the systolic blood pressure, widening of the pulse pressure, bradycardia
- Foramen magnum herniation

At stages beyond tentorial herniation, it is unusual for focal mass effects not to be accompanied by an overall increase in ICP. The point at which focal mass effect evolves to include a rise in overall ICP depends largely on the compliance within the cranial cavity. Young patients with so-called tight brains can develop raised ICP, even with relatively small volumes of mass that produce only effacement of the cortical gyri. On the other hand, patients with advanced cerebral atrophy can, for example, tolerate large frontal intracerebral hematomas or chronic subdural hematomas with compression of the lateral ventricle and midline shift while maintaining a tolerable ICP and a surprising degree of intact neurologic function.

Normal ICP varies over a wide range, with generally accepted values between 0 and 20 mm Hg. Diffuse raised ICP, in the fully evolved pure form, results in a clinical picture that may include symptoms of headache, nausea and vomiting, double vision, and obscuration of vision. The accompanying clinical signs may include papilledema and sixth cranial nerve palsy with lateral rectus weakness and side-by-side diplopia, initially worse on far vision or gaze directed toward the side of the palsy. The papilledema is a mostly chronic phenomenon and is not seen acutely. The sixth nerve palsy of raised ICP can occur regardless of its cause and does not imply direct involvement by a mass lesion, large or small, on the sixth nerve. In this situation, the sixth nerve palsy is a false localizing sign. With raised ICP, there may also be obscurations of vision, in which patients report that their vision temporarily fades or becomes gray, in combination with headache. Again, these obscurations are caused by the effect of diffusely increased ICP on the sensitive optic nerves. They do not imply the presence of a focal mass lesion directly affecting the optic nerves or pathways. Intuitively, it seems that if there is a slow increase in a process raising ICP, the pressure would also rise slowly and evenly, in pace with the evolving process. However, as first shown by Lundberg in 1960,[4] the intermediate stages of decompensation are characterized by transient pronounced elevations in ICP (to 60 mm Hg) that characteristically plateau for up to 45 minutes and then transiently cycle down again to a more normal range.

CEREBROVASCULAR DISORDERS

Cerebrovascular disorders encompass a host of disorders: congenital, acquired, and idiopathic (Box 67-1).

Arteriovenous Malformations

An AVM is an abnormal collection of blood vessels wherein arterial blood flows directly into draining veins without the normal interposed capillary beds. AVMs are congenital lesions that can enlarge somewhat with age, recruiting new vascular supply, and often progress from low-flow lesions at birth to higher flow lesions in adulthood. They present with hemorrhage, ischemia of the brain parenchyma around the lesion due to a vascular "steal" phenomenon, or seizures. They have a prevalence of 15 to 18/100,000 and typically are manifested before the age of 40 years. The risk of hemorrhage rate is up to 4% per year,[5] and once they bleed, they may be even more prone to hemorrhage. They are typically composed of one or more feeding arteries; a nidus of varying size, shape, and compactness that is composed of abnormal vessels; and draining veins. They are sometimes associated with high-flow related aneurysms of the feeding arteries.

Patients typically present with headaches, neurologic deficit, seizures, or varying combinations of the three. Workup generally includes computed tomography (CT) and MRI, demonstrating the lesion (Fig. 67-4). Catheter angiography is then performed to define the vascular anatomy of the lesion and is used for treatment planning.

BOX 67-1 Cerebral Vascular Disease

Congenital
Arteriovenous malformation and fistula
Cavernous malformation
Telangiectasis
Venous anomaly (angioma)

Acquired
Traumatic
- Some arteriovenous fistulas (type I carotid-cavernous fistula)
- Traumatic aneurysm

Degenerative
- Atherosclerotic, occlusive disease
- Most cerebral (berry) aneurysms
- Some arterial dissections
- Spontaneous intracerebral hemorrhage

Infectious
- Mycotic aneurysms

Idiopathic
Moyamoya
Some arteriovenous fistulas: dural AVM–like or type II carotid-cavernous fistulas

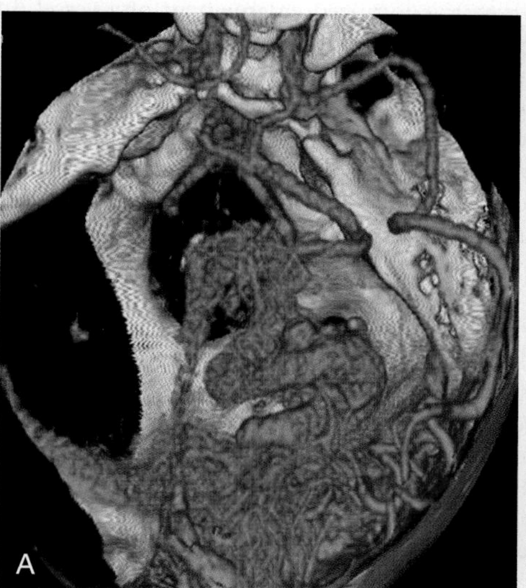

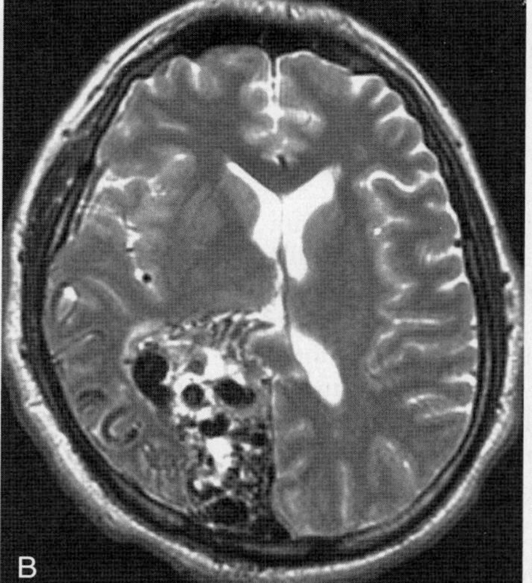

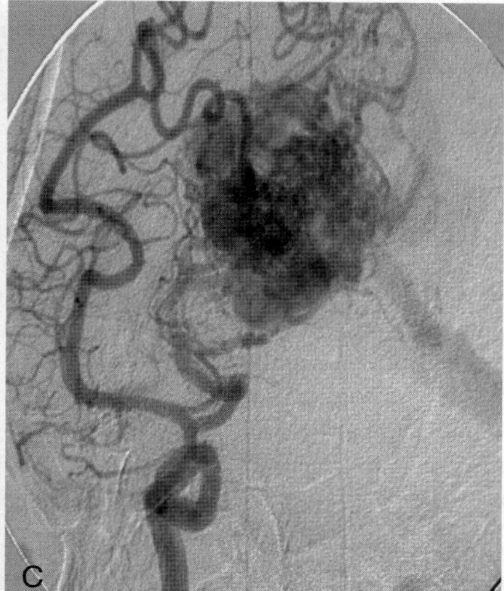

FIGURE 67-4 CT angiography with three-dimensional reconstruction **(A)**, MRI **(B)**, and conventional angiogram **(C)** of a large AVM with supply from the middle and posterior cerebral arteries and ill-defined nidus. Complex deep and superficial venous drainage is present.

TABLE 67-2 Spetzler-Martin Grading System

FEATURE	POINTS
Nidus size (cm)	
Small (<3)	1
Medium (3-6)	2
Large (>6)	3
Eloquence of adjacent brain	
Noneloquent	0
Eloquent (sensorimotor, language, visual, thalamus, hypothalamus, internal capsule, brainstem, cerebellar peduncles, deep cerebellar nuclei)	1
Pattern of venous drainage	
Superficially only	0
Deep	1

Treatment options include craniotomy with surgical resection of the lesion, embolization, and SRS. Commonly, more than one modality is used. SRS is usually reserved for compact lesions less the 2.5 cm in diameter. It can take up to 3 years for irradiated AVMs to shut down after SRS. The Spetzler-Martin grading system was developed 30 years ago and continues to be used to help make treatment decisions (Table 67-2).[6]

Cavernous Malformations

A cavernous malformation is a well-circumscribed, benign vascular lesion consisting of irregular thin-walled sinusoidal vascular channels located within the brain but lacking intervening neural parenchyma, large feeding arteries, or large draining veins. Characterized by McCormick in an autopsy series,[7] these lesions have a prevalence of approximately 0.5%. There are three familial forms described. Because these are low-pressure, low-flow lesions, hemorrhage is typically not catastrophic unless it is in a highly eloquent area of the brain.

Patients usually present with hemorrhage or headaches with or without a history of new-onset seizures. Although it is often evident on CT, MRI is the imaging modality of choice and demonstrates a characteristic dark hemosiderin ring. Treatment for symptomatic lesions includes seizure control and surgical excision. Radiosurgery has not been shown to significantly alter the natural history of these lesions.

Capillary Telangiectasia

This lesion is composed of vascular channels with extremely thin walls similar to those of dilated capillaries. These are usually grouped in small clusters, generally with prominent intervening brain tissue. They are often clinically silent and generally do not appear on imaging studies. They are not evident on conventional catheter angiography unless they are large, and then only in the capillary venous phase. They clearly differ from an AVM in that flow through the lesion is not fast enough to demonstrate arteries and veins in the same conventional angiographic image. These lesions are typically not treated surgically.

Developmental Venous Anomaly: Venous Angioma

These lesions are composed of an abnormally configured venous drainage system converging on a single, enlarged venous outflow channel. The typical appearance is that of a hydra, with radially converging veins. A characteristic feature of this lesion appears to be that the abnormal venous bed is poorly collateralized. The abnormal venous drainage may or may not be fully adequate to the needs of the brain tissue supplied. Slowly evolving degenerative changes in the brain tissue supplied can occur as a result, but unfortunately, this is not helped by any known intervention. However inadequate, the venous anomaly represents the only venous drainage available to that area of brain, and therefore removal of the venous anomaly is not recommended. Doing so could lead to a venous infarction with swelling and hemorrhage, the consequences of which are particularly dangerous in the posterior fossa.

Traumatic Fistula

Both the internal carotid artery and vertebral artery enter the cranial cavity immediately after passing through a venous network. The internal carotid artery passes through the cavernous sinus, which communicates with the superior ophthalmic vein, petrosal sinus, and sphenoparietal sinus. The vertebral artery passes through a venous plexus at the occipital-C1 epidural space, which communicates with the jugular vein, epidural venous plexus, and paraspinal venous plexus. Trauma leading to a tear in the carotid or vertebral artery at its tether point passing through the skull base can lead to fistula with the surrounding venous plexus. The consequences may vary in severity and suddenness but typically include periorbital swelling, with proptosis and scleral edema in the case of the carotid-cavernous fistula (CCF) and prominent pulsatile bruit in the case of the vertebral-jugular fistula. Intraocular pressure measurement by tonometry can guide the urgency in treating CCF. On radiologic examination, dilation of the superior ophthalmic vein is characteristic (Fig. 67-5). These lesions are usually treated by endovascular techniques. A catheter is advanced through the tear in the artery into the venous side of the fistula. The high flow and large fistulous channel facilitate this process. Embolic material, a coil, or a detachable balloon is then used to occlude the venous side of the fistula. When conventional transvenous routes fail, a direct approach through transorbital puncture may be required to provide endovascular therapy.[8]

Aneurysms

Aneurysms are an excessive localized enlargement of a vessel due to a weakening and subsequent defect in the wall of the artery. There is an adult prevalence of 2% (this varies according to the study) with an annual incidence of aneurysmal subarachnoid hemorrhage of 6 to 8/100,000 with peak age at 50 years. Modifiable risk factors for subarachnoid hemorrhage include hypertension, smoking, and excessive alcohol. Aneurysms may be further divided into saccular, fusiform, dissecting, infectious, and traumatic aneurysms.

Saccular Aneurysms

As the name implies, these aneurysms, also referred to as berry aneurysms, are usually saccular in form and come off the vessel wall or at a bifurcation. Many of these are found incidentally, given the frequency of neuroimaging, but many present with hemorrhage.[9] The classic presentation of subarachnoid hemorrhage due to a cerebral aneurysm is that of sudden onset of a headache, described as the "worst headache of my life." Workup typically includes a CT scan, demonstrating a typical distribution of blood (Fig. 67-6). Between 10% and 15% of subarachnoid hemorrhages from saccular aneurysms are fatal before the hospital is even reached. Of those individuals who reach a medical facility,

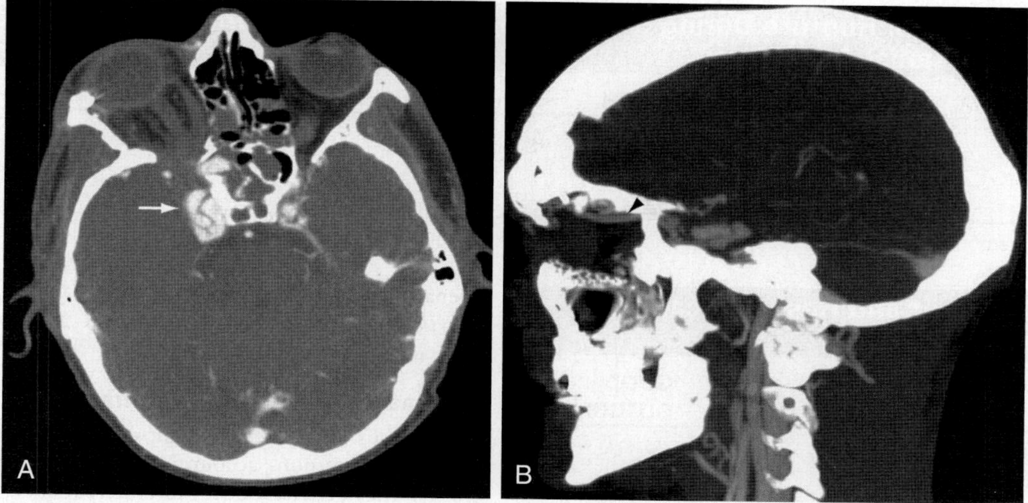

FIGURE 67-5 Right internal carotid–cavernous sinus fistula (**A,** *arrow*) with dilation of the superior ophthalmic drain (**B,** *arrowhead*), a typical imaging finding of this pathologic process.

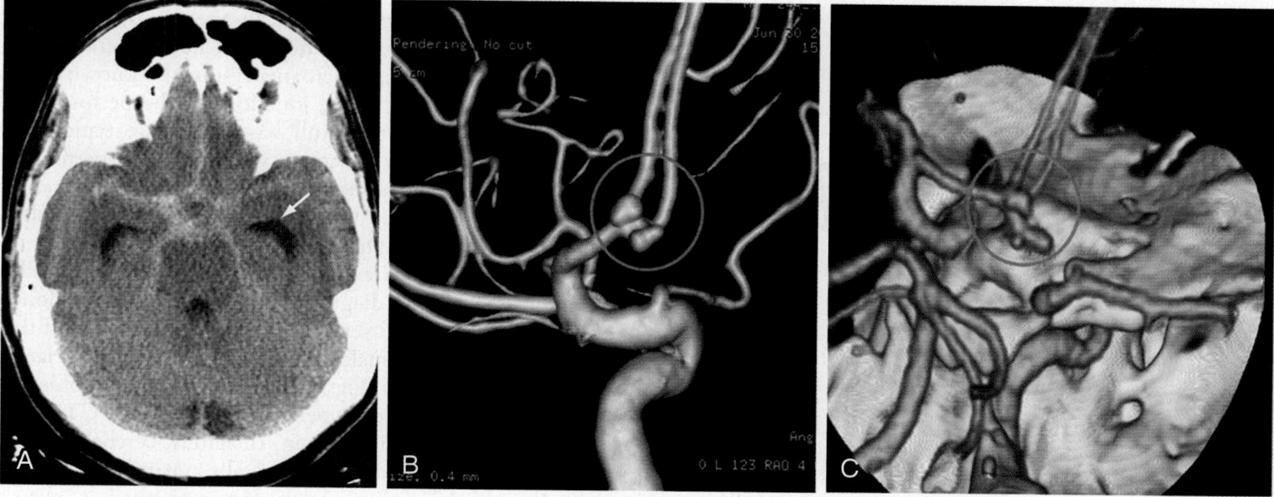

FIGURE 67-6 **A,** CT scan of brain showing subarachnoid blood in the basal cisterns. Dilated temporal horns (*arrow*) indicate the presence of hydrocephalus. **B,** Cerebral angiogram shows two aneurysms located at the junction of the A1 and A2 segments of the anterior cerebral artery (*circle*). **C,** CT angiography with three-dimensional reconstruction showing the relationship of the aneurysms (*circle*) with the skull base.

one third do not survive (usually because of rebleeding), one third will survive with varying degrees of neurologic disability, and one third return to their baseline level.

The major complications of subarachnoid hemorrhage include rebleeding, hydrocephalus (which is observed in around 15% to 20% of cases), cardiac events in around 50% of patients, vasospasm, hyponatremia, and seizures. Rebleeding is a major cause of death in patients who reach medical care after their initial episode of bleeding. Hydrocephalus is caused by disruption in the function of the arachnoid granulations and is commonly treated with an external ventricular drain. Vasospasm is a narrowing of the cerebral arteries thought to be caused by smooth muscle dysfunction related to blood breakdown products in the spinal fluid. When present, it can contribute to significant ischemia of the brain and, as such, be a significant cause of morbidity. Treatment of symptomatic vasospasm is typically multimodality and includes the use of hypervolemia and induced hypertension, endovascular procedures, and a variety of pharmacologic agents (Box 67-2).[10-12]

BOX 67-2 Treatment of Vasospasm

Prevention of Arterial Narrowing

Subarachnoid blood removal
Prevention of dehydration and hypotension
Calcium channel blockers (nimodipine)

Reversal of Arterial Narrowing

Intra-arterial calcium channel blockers
Transluminal balloon angioplasty

Prevention and Reversal of Ischemic Neurologic Deficit

Hypertension, hypervolemia, hemodilution

A classic study of cerebral aneurysms and their treatment documents the risk for rupture according to size and location as demonstrated in Table 67-3.[13] As a means of predicting possible vasospasm and overall outcomes, the Hunt and Hess clinical grading scale[14] and the World Federation of Neurological

TABLE 67-3 Risk of Rupture During 5 Years (%) According to International Study of Unruptured Intracranial Aneurysms

TYPE OF ANEURYSM	<7 mm AND NO PRIOR SAH	<7 mm AND PRIOR SAH	7-12 mm	13-24 mm	>24 mm
Carotid-cavernous	0	0	0	3.0	6.4
Anterior circulation	0	1.5	2.6	14.5	40.0
Posterior circulation	2.5	3.4	14.5	18.4	50.0

SAH, subarachnoid hemorrhage.

TABLE 67-4 Hunt and Hess Clinical Grading Scale

DESCRIPTION	GRADE	GOOD OUTCOME
Asymptomatic or minimal headache and slight nuchal rigidity	1	≈70
Moderate to severe headache, nuchal rigidity, ± cranial nerve palsy only	2	≈70
Drowsy, confusion, or mild focal deficit	3	≈15
Stupor, moderate to severe hemiparesis, possibly early decerebrate rigidity	4	≈15
Deep coma, decerebrate rigidity, moribund appearance	5	≈0

TABLE 67-5 World Federation of Neurological Surgeons Clinical Grading Scale

GRADE	GCS SCORE	MOTOR DEFICIT
I	15	No
II	13-14	No
III	13-14	Yes
IV	7-12	Yes or no
V	3-6	Yes or no

GCS, Glasgow Coma Scale.

TABLE 67-6 Fisher Grading for Appearance of SAH on Computed Tomography

GRADE	CT FINDINGS
I	No hemorrhage evident
II	Diffuse SAH with vertical layers < 1 mm thick
III	Localized clots and/or vertical layers of SAH > 1 mm thick
IV	Diffuse or no SAH, but with intracerebral or intraventricular hemorrhage

SAH, subarachnoid hemorrhage.

Surgeons clinical grading scale[15] were developed (Tables 67-4 and 67-5). Another method of classifying subarachnoid hemorrhage is described by Fisher and colleagues[16] and is based on CT scan imaging (Table 67-6).

Treatment of saccular aneurysms consists of coiling, coiling through a stent, or surgical clipping (Figs. 67-7 and 67-8) with subsequent intensive critical care unit management of potential vasospasm and comorbidities. Once the standard of care in the treatment of cerebral aneurysms, open craniotomy and clipping is now typically reserved for those lesions believed not to be amenable to endovascular techniques.[13,17,18] It is generally believed that treatment of ruptured aneurysms is best accomplished as soon as possible after the initial hemorrhage.

Spontaneous Intracerebral Hemorrhage

Spontaneous intracerebral hemorrhages into the brain parenchyma are common, accounting for approximately 10% of all strokes. They generally occur in older patients, usually because of degenerative changes in the cerebral vessels that are often associated with chronic hypertension (Box 67-3). In younger patients, they are more likely related to drug abuse or vascular malformation. They can occur anywhere in the cerebral circulation or brainstem but are classically described in association with small degenerative aneurysms (microaneurysms; also known as Charcot-Bouchard aneurysms) at the junctions of the perforating vessels and larger vessels at the skull base. They are typically on the middle cerebral artery junctions with the small perforating lenticulostriate vessels, leading to hemorrhage into the putamen. The clinical presentation is with a stroke pattern of sudden-onset neurologic signs and symptoms that depend on the area of brain affected. Symptoms are more likely to include headache than ischemic stroke. The diagnosis is with CT, usually done in an emergency department setting. The size and location of the acute hematoma are well visualized with CT, as is any associated brain shift or hydrocephalus (Figs. 67-9*A* and 67-10). In older patients with a known history of hypertension and classic CT appearance of a hematoma in the putamen, thalamus, cerebellum, or pons, further diagnostic studies are generally not indicated. Rehemorrhage is unlikely in that setting. However, further investigation might be warranted with an atypical hematoma location or appearance, especially if there is any component of subarachnoid blood. Also, investigation is usually recommended for younger patients without known hypertension and those with a potential underlying cause for hemorrhage (e.g., history of neoplasm, blood dyscrasias, bacterial endocarditis).

Further investigation is generally done with contrast MRI or magnetic resonance angiography. Any suggestion of aneurysm or AVM is followed by conventional catheter angiography. In older patients with a history of early dementia and multiple episodes of more peripherally located intracerebral hematomas, the diagnosis of amyloid angiopathy needs to be considered.

Most cases of spontaneous intracerebral hemorrhage do not require an operative procedure. Many hemorrhages are small enough to be well tolerated and do not require surgery. Others are so large at the outset that surgery is of little benefit. Relief of any obstructive hydrocephalus by ventricular drainage is usually offered, except in the most impossible cases. Patients who obey commands and can be monitored by changes in their neurologic examination can generally be managed conservatively with hospital observation for at least 5 to 7 days. Peak swelling and decompensation are probably most likely to occur within that time frame. Surgery for evacuation of the hematoma may be

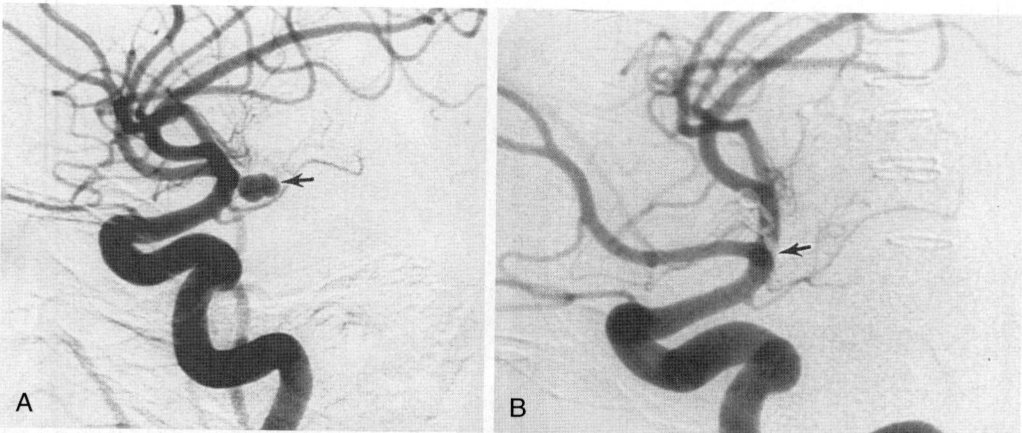

FIGURE 67-7 **A,** Subtraction carotid angiogram shows a 4 × 6-mm berry aneurysm *(arrow)* originating from the distal internal carotid artery. **B,** Postoperative carotid angiogram shows clip placement *(arrow),* with total obliteration of the aneurysm.

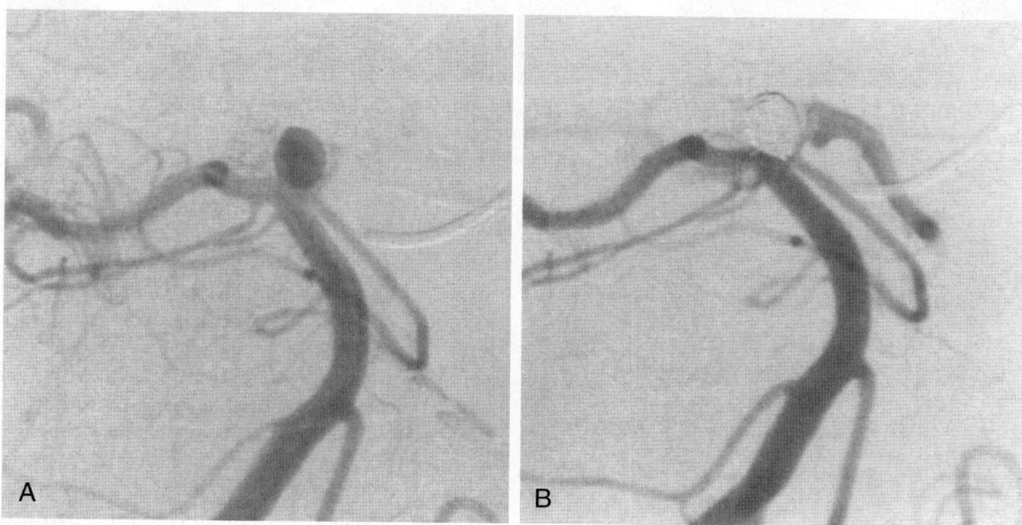

FIGURE 67-8 **A,** Subtraction vertebral angiogram shows a basilar tip aneurysm. **B,** Subtracted vertebral angiogram after the placement of coils demonstrates excellent obliteration of the aneurysm and preservation of adjacent vessels.

BOX 67-3 Causes of Spontaneous Intracerebral Hemorrhage

Hypertension	Cerebral amyloid angiopathy
Vascular anomaly	Coagulopathy
Cerebral aneurysm	Tumors
Arteriovenous malformation	Drug abuse
Cavernous malformation	Other
Cerebral infarction (stroke) transformation	

appropriate in a small group of patients with intermediate-sized hemorrhages in accessible locations who appear to tolerate the hematoma initially but then deteriorate in a delayed fashion with edema, despite medical therapy. Steroids have not demonstrated benefit. Attempts to predict which patients will deteriorate solely on the basis of hematoma volume have been frustrated by the broad spectrum of intracranial compliance exhibited by different patients. In general, younger patients with smaller ventricles and small subarachnoid spaces have a lower compliance, with lower tolerance, than older patients with cerebral atrophy and generous ventricles and subarachnoid spaces.

The Surgical Trial in Intracerebral Hemorrhage has noted a lack of clinical outcome difference in comparing early surgery with conservative management.[19] If indicated, surgical evacuation is usually done by craniotomy over the most accessible part of the hematoma (Fig. 67-9*B*). Intraoperative ultrasound is often helpful in finding hematomas that do not quite come to the cortical surface and in monitoring the progress of the evacuation. The goal of surgery is decompression more than complete removal, but it is generally done as far as safely practical. The wall of the hematoma cavity is inspected for any underlying cause, and a biopsy specimen is taken, if indicated. Putamen hemorrhage can sometimes be evacuated with minimal surgical damage to the overlying brain by a trans–sylvian fissure–transinsular approach. Stereotactic aspiration and methods with fibrinolytic agents are being developed and may be a consideration for patients with hematomas in deep locations that are otherwise difficult to access.

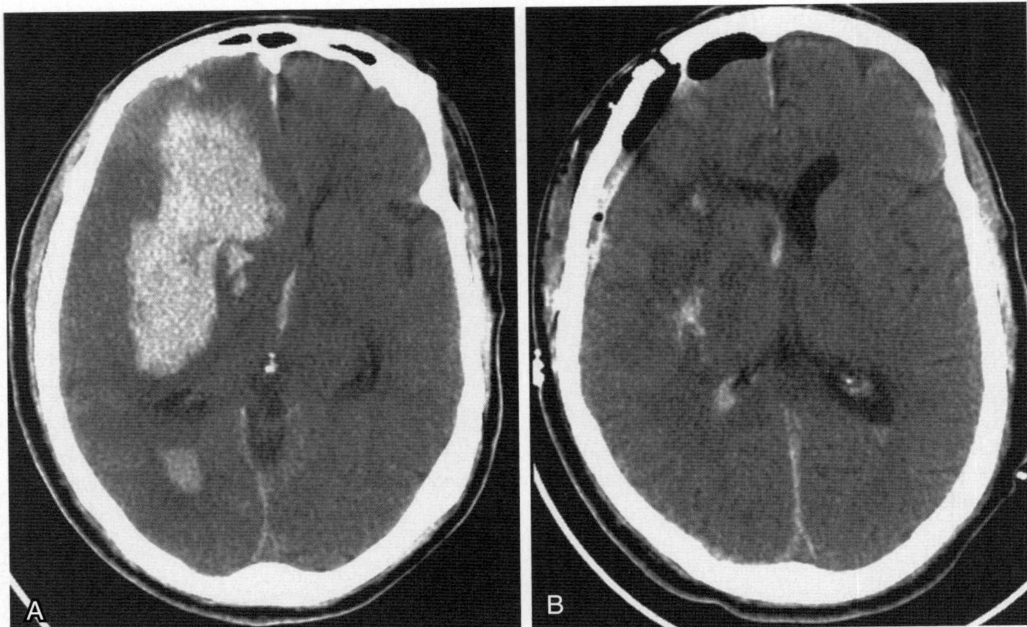

FIGURE 67-9 Nonenhanced CT scan of the head. **A,** Spontaneous hypertensive intracerebral hematoma in the right basal ganglia, with extension to the frontal and temporal lobes. **B,** Immediate postoperative CT scan shows near-total removal of the intracerebral hematoma.

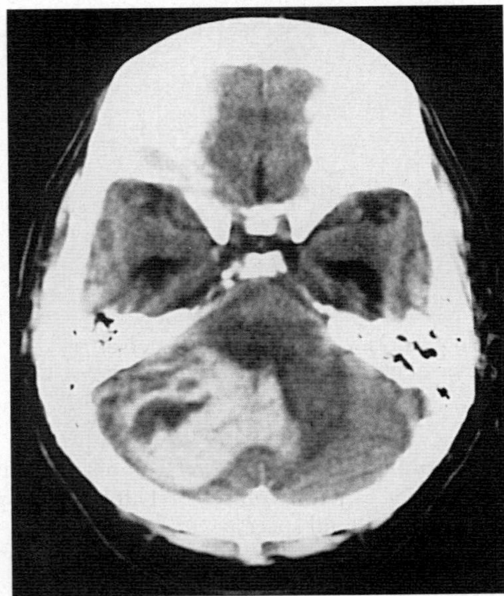

FIGURE 67-10 Nonenhanced CT scan of the brain shows a large, hypertensive, intracerebellar hematoma with obstruction of the fourth ventricle and enlargement of the temporal horns, indicating obstructive hydrocephalus.

A special situation to consider is the patient with cerebellar hemorrhage (Fig. 67-10). Surgery is offered more readily in these cases because the danger of sudden deterioration from brainstem compression is more of a concern and because even extensive damage to the cerebellum itself is generally survivable, with good functional outcome. Patients with fourth ventricular obstruction and hydrocephalus from cerebellar hemorrhage can sometimes be treated with ventricular drainage alone but are usually offered surgical evacuation of the hematoma by suboccipital craniotomy because of the risk for brainstem compression.

Mycotic Aneurysms

These aneurysms are associated with a systemic infection capable of showering small particles of bacteria-infected material into the cerebral vascular bed. Subacute bacterial endocarditis and some pulmonary infections can do this. A distinguishing feature of these aneurysms is that they are generally found more distal in the cerebral vascular bed, as opposed to berry aneurysms, which are usually found on larger vessels near the circle of Willis. There can also be many of them. When the bacterial emboli lodge in distal cerebral arterial branches, they can erode through the wall of these smaller vessels, often creating a hemorrhage contained by the perivascular tissue. Maximal antibiotic treatment is essential at the outset. The presence of an intracerebral hematoma may force immediate craniotomy for evacuation. Operation on the aneurysm at this early stage often reveals a component of subarachnoid hemorrhage and an early inflammatory reaction in the subarachnoid space, with only a blood collection covering the erosion defect in the wall of the small artery. Attempts to dissect and to define a neck are frustrated by a lack of developed fibrous tissues, and intraoperative hemorrhage is then common. Typically, the diseased arterial segment must be occluded and resected when it is operated on in this early stage. The need for arterial bypass to maintain blood flow to critical cerebral areas should be anticipated, but this is not always possible.

If the mycotic aneurysms are discovered or treated at some later stage, a fibrous wall to the aneurysm may have had time to develop, and clipping can then be a possibility. However, the surgeon needs to be forewarned that it may be difficult to find the aneurysm in a distal location, often buried deep in a cerebral sulcus thickened with reactive fibrous scar tissue.

Moyamoya Disease

Moyamoya disease is a cerebrovascular disorder that is characterized by an idiopathic nonatherosclerotic narrowing or occlusion of major intracranial blood vessels with the development of a conspicuous compensatory collateral rete vessel network, which allows continued cerebral perfusion around the occluded or severely narrowed segment. The disorder is usually bilateral, although not necessarily exactly symmetrical. Although generally rare, the disease is more common in persons of Asian ancestry and was first recognized from cases studied with angiography in Japan before the advent of CT and MRI. The term *moyamoya* comes from the Japanese word for "puff of smoke" or mist. The actual disease is sometimes confused with the less conspicuous collateral vascular networks seen around severe narrowing of common atherosclerotic origin in persons of Western origin. In the juvenile form, moyamoya typically is manifested as cognitive decline, with deteriorating school performance and evidence of multiple infarcts. Angiography reveals the internal carotid artery, proximal middle cerebral artery, or proximal anterior cerebral artery with severe narrowing or occlusion and, generally, multiple clusters of fine collateral vessels. In the adult form of moyamoya disease, the rete vessels cause subarachnoid or basal ganglia hemorrhage, the most common presentations. The hemorrhage can usually be treated conservatively. Some form of extracranial to intracranial bypass is generally attempted to take the load off the collateral vascular network. In younger patients, the results are good, with an onlay interposition of the superficial temporal artery sewed into the dura after a strip craniotomy. A feature of the disorder is the vigor with which collaterals form from the onlay transposed vessel. In the adult form, a microvascular anastomosis with the superficial temporal artery or grafted vessel may be preferred.

Dural Arteriovenous Malformations

Dural AVMs (type II CCF is a subtype) are not often seen in younger patients. The lesions seem to occur only in adults and are probably acquired lesions that follow a dural sinus thrombosis, usually of the cavernous sinus or sigmoid-transverse sinus junction area. With subsequent healing, the thrombosed segment triggers a neovascular response that evolves to an AVM configuration with fistulous channels that can gradually enlarge. Usually, there is associated stenosis of the affected dural segment, suggesting the earlier thrombosis. The lesions are generally not dangerous unless they cause retrograde venous drainage into the cerebral circulation. The risk for intracranial hemorrhage is then fairly high; it is important at least to separate the dural AVM drainage from the cerebral circulation when that occurs. In the case of transverse-sigmoid sinus dural AVM, the patient usually complains of a bruit, and embolization or resection is optional, depending on symptom tolerance. In the case of type II CCF, the problem is usually intraocular and intraorbital venous hypertension, with proptosis, chemosis, and sometimes threatened vision. Ocular tonometry can help determine the extent of the threat to vision. Treatment of type II CCF involves endovascular embolization of prominent feeders, followed by occlusion of the affected venous dural sinus. As long as the dural AVM drainage is separated from the cerebral circulation, occlusion of the affected venous drainage is safe and curative. The affected stenotic transverse-sigmoid sinus segment can be reached by endovascular techniques through the jugular vein. The cavernous sinus can be reached by the petrosal sinus or, with neurosurgical assistance, through the superior orbital vein.

CENTRAL NERVOUS SYSTEM TUMORS

Intracranial Tumors

Intracranial tumors can be classified as primary versus secondary, as pediatric versus adult, by cell of origin, or by location in the nervous system. Primary tumors arise from tissues in the nervous system, whereas secondary tumors originate from tissues outside the nervous system and metastasize secondarily to the brain. They may represent local extension of regional tumors, such as chordoma or scalp cancer, but usually reach the nervous system through the hematogenous route.

In general, the incidence of primary brain tumors is higher in whites than in blacks, and mortality is higher in males than in females. According to the Central Brain Tumor Registry of the United States (CBTRUS), the overall incidence of primary brain tumors was 14.8/100,000 person-years between 1998 and 2002 (CBTRUS statistical report, 2005-2006). On the other hand, secondary tumors outnumber primary brain tumors by 10:1 and occur in 20% to 40% of cancer patients.[20] Because no national cancer registry documents brain metastases, the exact incidence is unknown, but it has been estimated that 98,000 to 170,000 new cases are diagnosed in the United States each year.[21]

Clinical Presentation

The clinical manifestations of various brain tumors can be divided into those caused by focal compression and irritation by the tumor itself and those attributed to secondary consequences, namely, increased ICP, peritumoral edema, and hydrocephalus. Usually, symptoms are caused by a combination of these factors.

The clinical presentation does not differ much by tumor histology; rather, rate of growth and location of the tumor contribute to the clinical features. A meningioma peripherally located in a relatively silent area of the brain, with a slow rate of growth, may enlarge to a significant size in a neurologically intact patient because the brain can accommodate to a slowly growing lesion. On the other hand, a small metastatic lesion at the foramen of Monro or in the sensorimotor strip can cause acute hydrocephalus or seizures, respectively.

Headache occurs in 50% to 60% of primary brain tumors and in 35% to 50% of metastatic tumors. It is classically described as being worse in the morning, probably because of hypoventilation during sleep, with consequent elevation of the PCO_2 and cerebrovascular dilation. The headache is associated with nausea and vomiting in 40% of patients and may be temporarily relieved by vomiting as a result of hyperventilation. Seizures may be the first symptom of a brain tumor. Patients older than 20 years presenting with a new-onset seizure are aggressively investigated for a brain tumor.

Infratentorial lesions may be manifested with headache, nausea and vomiting, gait disturbance and ataxia, vertigo, cranial nerve deficits leading to diplopia (abducens nerve), facial numbness and pain (trigeminal nerve), unilateral hearing deficit and tinnitus (vestibulocochlear nerve), facial weakness (facial nerve), dysphagia (glossopharyngeal and vagus nerves), and CSF obstruction causing hydrocephalus and papilledema. Supratentorial lesions may be manifested with different symptoms, depending on the location. Frontal lobe lesions are manifested as personality changes, dementia, hemiparesis, or dysphasia. Temporal lobe lesions may be manifested with memory changes, auditory or olfactory hallucinations, or contralateral quadrantanopia. Patients with parietal lobe lesions may develop contralateral motor or sensory impairment, apraxia, and homonymous hemianopia, whereas those with occipital lobe lesions may show contralateral visual field deficits and alexia.

Imaging Studies

The initial workup generally involves a relatively inexpensive diagnostic tool, a CT scan of the brain. CT provides a rapid means of evaluating changes in brain density, such as calcifications, hyperacute hemorrhages (<24 hours old), and skull lesions. MRI of the brain, however, is the "gold standard" modality for diagnosis, presurgical planning, and post-therapeutic monitoring of brain tumors. Gadolinium contrast enhancement with MRI is more sensitive in demonstrating defects in the blood-brain barrier and localizing small metastases (up to 5 mm). It can be used in patients allergic to iodine and those with renal failure. Advances in MRI techniques have evolved from strictly morphology-based imaging to a modality that encompasses function, physiology, and anatomy. Diffusion-weighted imaging can help distinguish between gliomas and abscesses, and perfusion-weighted imaging can predict response to radiotherapy in low-grade gliomas. Functional MRI can be used in planning of surgery for tumors in eloquent areas of the brain to enable radical resection with less morbidity. Diffusion tensor imaging can demonstrate the effect of a tumor on white matter tracts. Magnetic resonance angiography is used more routinely as a noninvasive modality to evaluate the vascularity of a tumor or anatomic relationship of a tumor to normal cerebral vasculature.[22]

Surgery

Dexamethasone is recommended for the management of brain tumors because of its propensity to reduce peritumoral edema by stabilizing the cell membrane. An antiepileptic drug is also recommended for tumors close to the sensorimotor strip. Mannitol is often administered before dural opening and operative resection.

Technical advances have made tumor surgery safer and more effective. The intraoperative microscope provides superior illumination and magnification, thereby allowing the surgeon to resect tumors from critical areas through small cranial openings. The cavitational ultrasonic surgical aspirator simultaneously breaks up and sucks away firm tumors while protecting vital neural and vascular structures. Intraoperative ultrasonography provides real-time imaging of tumors and cysts in subcortical and deep areas of the brain. Intraoperative CT or MRI is standard practice in some centers, enabling on-table imaging of the extent of resection (Fig. 67-11*A*). CT and MRI also allow real-time visualization of a biopsy needle within a target. Image-guided (CT or MRI) frameless surgical navigation allows instant and accurate localization of the tip of a probe during a craniotomy by displaying that point on a preoperative CT or MRI scan (Fig. 67-11*B*).

The primary goals of surgery include histologic diagnosis and reduction of mass effect by removal of as much tumor as is safely possible to preserve neurologic function. The decision between a needle biopsy and more radical surgical resection depends on the location and size of the tumor, its sensitivity to radiation or chemotherapy, the preoperative Karnofsky performance score of the patient, and the systemic status of the primary cancer in case of metastatic brain lesions.

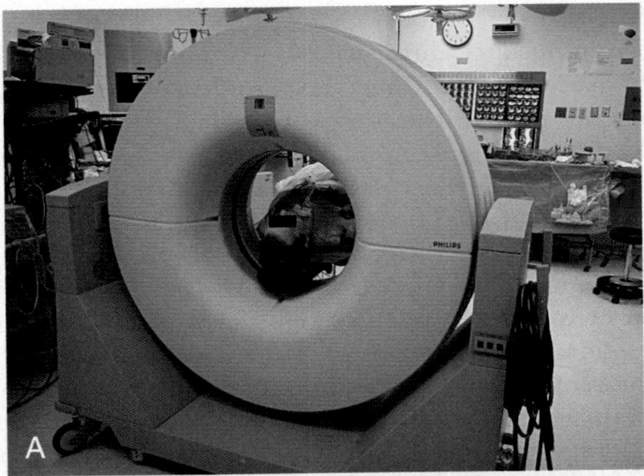

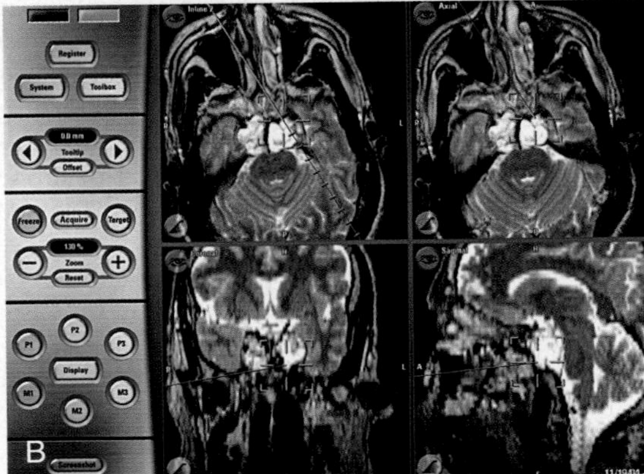

FIGURE 67-11 Technologic advances in the operating room. **A,** Intraoperative CT scanner. **B,** Computer-guided surgical navigation showing real-time location of a surgical probe tip on the preoperative MRI study during resection of clival chordoma.

PRIMARY BRAIN TUMORS

Primary tumors of the brain are divided into intra-axial (those arising from within the brain parenchyma) and extra-axial (those arising from outside the brain parenchyma).

Intra-Axial Brain Tumors

Intra-axial brain tumors develop from the glia, or supportive structures, of the neurons and are collectively called gliomas. Total surgical resection of gliomas is extremely rare because of their ability to infiltrate widely along the white matter tracts and to cross the corpus callosum into the contralateral hemisphere. Radiation therapy and chemotherapy options vary according to the histology of the brain tumor. Therapy involving surgically implanted carmustine-impregnated polymer combined with postoperative radiation therapy has a role in the treatment of de novo and recurrent high-grade gliomas. Biologic therapies are currently under evaluation for patients with brain tumors and include dendritic cell vaccination, tyrosine kinase receptor inhibitors, farnesyltransferase inhibitors, virus-based gene therapy, and oncolytic viruses. An ideal therapy will target rapidly growing malignant glioma cells along with infiltrating tumor cells, with minimal toxicity to normal cells. This requires that the therapeutic vehicle of choice have access to all cells in the brain and be able to distinguish invasive or quiescent tumor cells from normal cells.[23]

The current histopathologic classification of brain tumors was recently updated by the World Health Organization (WHO).[24] WHO classifies intra-axial brain tumors by cell type and grades them on a scale of I to IV based on light microscopy characteristics that include the degree of cellularity, pleomorphism, mitotic figures, endothelial proliferation, and necrosis. The higher the grade, the more aggressive and malignant is the tumor.

An exhaustive review of neuro-oncology is beyond the scope of this chapter. What follows is an overview of the most commonly encountered and unique tumors of the central and peripheral nervous systems.

Astrocytic Tumors

Glioblastoma multiforme. A WHO grade IV tumor, this is the most commonly encountered primary brain tumor in adults. Presentation can include headache, seizures, focal deficits, and personality changes. Imaging usually demonstrates a ring enhancing lesion with surrounding edema and mass effect (Fig. 67-12). Treatment of accessible lesions involves attempted gross total resection and postoperative radiation therapy and chemotherapy. Temozolomide is the current drug of choice and has been shown to improve both survival and quality of life. Recurrence is common, and repeated surgical resection is often deemed reasonable.

Anaplastic astrocytoma. A WHO grade III tumor, this presents much the same as glioblastoma multiforme, with similar treatment but slightly better long-term prognosis (Fig. 67-13).

Pilocytic astrocytoma. Pilocytic astrocytomas are typically classified as WHO grade I gliomas. When arising in the posterior fossa, they can cause obstructive hydrocephalus and cerebellar signs on examination. Surgical resection is the treatment of choice for these posterior fossa lesions. However, for lesions in the hypothalamus or optic tract, biopsy and chemotherapy or radiation therapy should be considered.

Oligodendroglioma

These tumors originate from oligodendroglial cells and represent 25% of all glial tumors; they occur with a male to female predominance of 3:2, observed at an average age of 40 years. They often present clinically with seizures or hemorrhage and nonspecific mass effect. A 5-year survival rate can be observed between 40% and 70%, depending on the grade, with an overall median survival of 3 years. Another form known as oligoastrocytoma

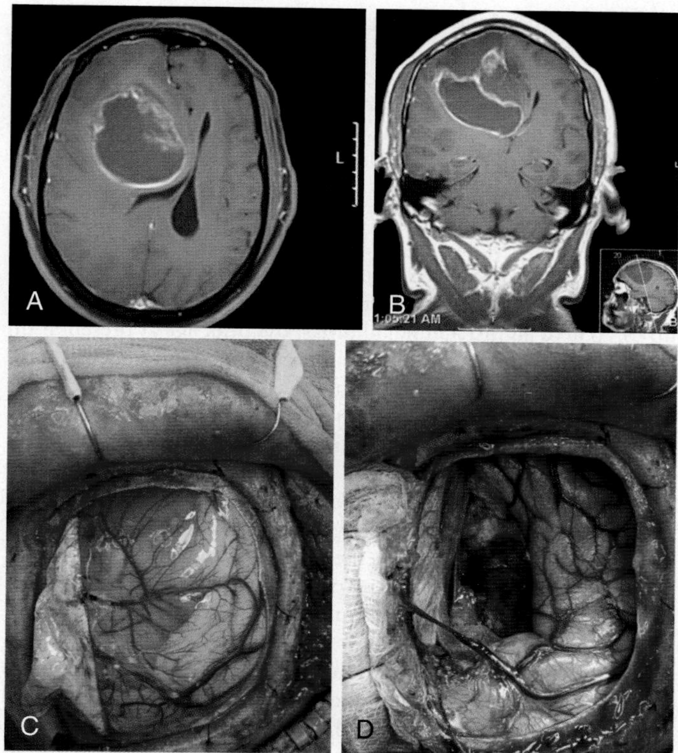

FIGURE 67-12 MRI and intraoperative pictures of a patient with a glioblastoma multiforme. Gadolinium-enhanced axial **(A)** and coronal **(B)** MRI scans show a large tumor with ring enhancement causing a 1-cm subfalcine shift of midline structures. Intraoperative pictures show the yellowish tumor surrounded by normal brain gyri **(C)** and the surgical field after resection of the tumor **(D)**.

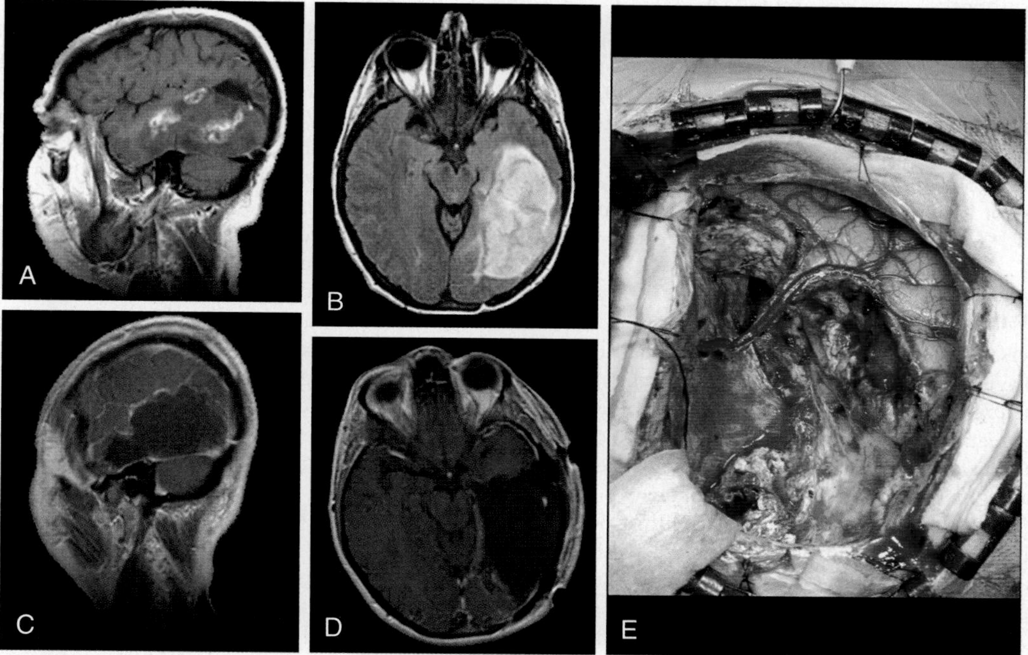

FIGURE 67-13 Radiographic and intraoperative images of a patient with a left temporal anaplastic astrocytoma. **A,** A partially enhancing tumor is noted in the left temporal lobe on this gadolinium-enhanced sagittal MRI study. **B,** Fluid-attenuated inversion recovery sequence axial MRI shows the extent of the tumor. The postoperative gadolinium-enhanced sagittal **(C)** and axial **(D)** MRI scans show near-total resection of the tumor. **E,** Intraoperative illustration of the surgical field after resection of the tumor.

behaves like oligodendroglioma, and both have aggressive anaplastic forms.

Treatment consists of surgical resection followed by chemotherapy. A particularly favorable response rate is associated with tumors that show allelic losses of chromosomes 1p and 19q. Radiation therapy is considered for tumors with anaplastic transformation.

Ependymoma

These tumors constitute around 5% of all intracranial gliomas across all ages. In the pediatric population, they may constitute up to 70% of all intracranial gliomas; the peak age at presentation is between 10 and 15 years. In children, ependymomas will typically be found in the fourth ventricle floor. A variant known as subependymoma is a rare form that is generally found incidentally in older patients and rarely requires surgical excision.

An ependymoma typically is manifested as a slowly growing posterior fossa mass that may cause obstruction of CSF flow, leading to hydrocephalus and symptoms of increased ICP with nausea, vomiting, and intense headaches. Up to 80% will have a 5-year survival in treated young patients; however, in the anaplastic variety, the presentation is much more aggressive and outcome is poor.

Treatment consists of maximal possible resection because extent does affect survival, followed by fractionated radiation. Recommendations for spinal MRI plus a lumbar puncture for cytology to rule out subarachnoid drop metastases are required for possible spinal radiation should these be positive.

Ependymomas of the spinal cord and cauda equina are also infrequently seen. Cauda equina lesions are of the myxopapillary variant.

Choroid Plexus Papilloma and Carcinoma

These intraventricular tumors represent 1% of all intracranial tumors, and up to 70% are seen in children 2 years of age or younger. The majority are benign papillomas. They typically are manifested with hydrocephalus. The 5-year survival rate is around 85% with benign lesions; however, only 40% of patients with choroid plexus carcinoma survive 5 years or more. The atypical papilloma variant has an intermediate prognosis.

Treatment entails total surgical excision and adjuvant chemotherapy in the case of benign lesions. Radiation therapy, in addition to gross total resection, should be used when carcinoma is observed.

Pediatric Brainstem Gliomas

These tumors represent around 10% to 20% of all pediatric brain tumors; the mean age at presentation is 7 years. Midbrain gliomas (tectal and tegmental) usually have better survival rates than pontine gliomas. Tectal gliomas typically are manifested with hydrocephalus but have up to an 80% 5-year progression-free survival rate. Focal tegmental mesencephalic tumors may be manifested with hemiparesis that slowly progresses. The diffuse pontine glioma will usually present with multiple cranial nerve palsies and ataxia with increased ICP and have a poor overall median survival of less than 1 year.

Treatment of tectal gliomas requires vigilant follow-up and frequently CSF diversion or shunting. Focal tegmental mesencephalic tumors might be surgically resected and require adjuvant chemotherapy and radiation therapy if they recur. In the case of diffuse pontine gliomas, treatment is with radiation with or without experimental chemotherapy or palliative care.

Neuronal and Mixed Neuronal-Glial Tumors

Ganglioglioma and Gangliocytoma

These represent less than 12% of all intracranial tumors; presentation is generally before the age of 30 years, with a peak at 11 years. They typically are manifested with seizures and are benign and slow growing. With treatment, the survival rate between 5 and 10 years is 80% to 90%. Treatment should include complete resection when possible, and radiation therapy should be considered for rare anaplastic ganglioglioma.

Central Neurocytoma

These tumors are rare and represent around 10% of all intraventricular tumors and are rarely found extraventricularly. Most cases, around 75%, are found between the ages of 20 and 40 years and present typically with hydrocephalus, increased ICP, and seizures. They are usually slow growing and benign and rarely hemorrhage; they have a survival rate of more than 80%. Treatment with complete resection usually cures, requiring only SRS or chemotherapy should a rare recurrence happen.

Dysembryoplastic Neuroepithelial Tumor

Typically, dysembryoplastic neuroepithelial tumors represent less than 1% of all primary brain tumors, affecting primarily children and young adults younger than 20 years. Patients also typically present with history of seizures, and these tumors are generally benign with very slow or even no growth. Treatment consists of surgical resection of tumor and possible neighboring epileptogenic foci.

Paraganglioma

This tumor is manifested as a slow-growing mass with systemic features of catecholamine release and carcinoid-like syndrome with cranial nerve palsies related to its location. These tumors are commonly slow growing and benign, with a 5-year survival rate of around 90%; they rarely bleed.

Depending on their location, paragangliomas can be named. When the paraganglioma is located at the carotid bifurcation, it is designated a carotid body tumor; at the superior vagal ganglion, glomus jugulare tumor; at the auricular branch of the vagus, glomus tympanicum; at the inferior vagal ganglion, glomus intravagale; and finally, in the adrenal medulla and sympathetic chain, pheochromocytoma. Treatment includes medical therapy to prevent blood pressure lability and arrhythmias with alpha and beta blockers. Surgical resection is preferred, and embolization before resection can sometimes reduce the intraoperative blood loss. When surgery is not possible, radiation therapy will be used.

Other neuronal and mixed neuronal-glial tumors include dysplastic cerebellar gangliocytoma (also known as Lhermitte-Duclos disease), desmoplastic infantile ganglioglioma, cerebellar liponeurocytoma, papillary glioneuronal tumor, and rosette-forming glioneuronal tumor of the fourth ventricle.

Pineal Region Tumors

Pineocytoma

These represent less than 1% of all primary brain tumors; they are observed mainly in children and young adults with a peak incidence between 10 and 20 years of age. As the tumors enlarge, they will typically present with hydrocephalus, increased ICP, and Parinaud syndrome (which is a supranuclear vertical gaze disturbance caused by compression of the tectal plate). Pineocytomas are usually stable and slow growing, with a 5-year survival rate of around 90%, and they rarely hemorrhage. When they are symptomatic or enlarging, the treatment is surgical. Stereotactic biopsy is considered by many to be high risk because of the surrounding venous vasculature.

Pineoblastoma

This tumor also represents less than 1% of all brain tumors. All pineocytomas, pineoblastomas, and those tumors that are intermediate of both (that have features of both) account for 15% of the pineal region tumors. Most are seen in children at a peak age of 3 years and predominantly in females with a ratio of 2:1. Like pineocytomas, pineoblastomas present with increased ICP, hydrocephalus, and Parinaud syndrome. Up to 50% will have CSF seeding, giving a median survival of 2 years from the time of diagnosis. Treatment should consist of surgical resection plus irradiation of the cranial vault and entire spinal axis. If the patient is older than 3 years, chemotherapy should also be considered.

Papillary Tumor of the Pineal Region

This is a rare tumor of children and young adults. It will typically be manifested with hydrocephalus and will behave like a grade II or grade III tumor according to the WHO classification. It can recur and require surgical resection followed by focal irradiation.

Primitive Neuroectodermal Tumors

Medulloblastomas are found to be 15% to 20% of all brain masses and up to one third of all posterior fossa tumors in the pediatric population. They are rarely seen in adults; most are diagnosed by the age of 5 years, with a male to female ratio of 3:1. They tend to have a rapid presentation with hydrocephalus, increased ICP, and cerebellar signs. These tumors tend to disseminate through the CSF and are often found to involve the spinal subarachnoid space in a sizable number of patients at the time of diagnosis. Treatment consists of attempted gross total resection followed by adjuvant chemotherapy and radiation therapy if the child is older than 3 years.

Tumors of Cranial and Spinal Nerves

Schwannoma

Schwannomas make up around 8% of all intracranial tumors. When located within the parenchymal region, they will clinically be manifested with seizures or focal deficit before the age of 30 years. Vestibular schwannomas will usually have sensorineural hearing loss with tinnitus and dizziness and typically present at an age older than 30 years. They are usually slow growing, with an average of 10% recurrence after total resection. When vestibular schwannomas are present bilaterally, the diagnosis of neurofibromatosis type 2 should be ruled out.

Treatment should entail audiology assessment to determine baseline status. Lesions less than 3 cm can be observed with clinical examinations, symptoms, radiographic evaluations, and audiology every 6 months. Some authors will recommend SRS for growing tumors less than 3 cm in diameter; 90% of tumor control is possible with rare facial palsy, and up to 50% to 90% hearing preservation is obtained. When surgical resection is performed on tumors less than 3 cm, this adds the benefit of tumor removal with 80% normal or near-normal facial nerve preservation and between 40% and 80% hearing preservation overall, depending on literature reviewed. When tumors are larger than 3 cm, surgical resection is always recommended, but it is usually accompanied with total loss of hearing and a greater risk of facial palsy.

Neurofibroma

Neurofibromas are rarely found intracranially and can be associated with neurofibromatosis type 1. When located in the head, they can be found as plexiform neurofibromas often in the orbit from cranial nerve V1, scalp, or parotid (cranial nerve VII). Along the spinal canal, they can develop into dumbbell-shaped masses as they exit the neuroforamina or on occasion into large peripheral nerve sheath tumors. They typically are manifested as a painless mass with slow growth that is histologically benign, but between 2% and 12% can degenerate into malignant peripheral nerve sheath tumor with a high recurrence rate. Treatment consists of surgical resection; however, most neurofibromas will encompass nerve fibers, and total resection results in nerve sacrifice as opposed to schwannoma resection, which usually can be achieved without nerve sacrifice.

Tumors of the Meninges

Meningiomas

Meningiomas are observed in between 15% and 20% of all primary intracranial tumors, second only to glioblastoma multiforme. The prevalence is in females (2:1), and it is rare in childhood unless it is associated with neurofibromatosis type 1. The presentation is usually incidental in up to 50% of cases; they are typically slow growing, and overall 5-year survival is greater than 90%.[25] Meningiomas can recur, depending on the resection obtained at surgery as described on the Simpson grading system for meningioma resection (Table 67-7) as well as the atypical histology. Overall, less than 1% will have malignant histology. Surgical resection is the treatment of choice if the patient is neurologically symptomatic. Many small, asymptomatic tumors can be observed.

Hemangioblastoma

Hemangioblastomas are observed in 1% to 2% of all primary intracranial tumors; between 25% and 40% are associated with von Hippel–Lindau syndrome (VHL). When they are associated with VHL, hemangioblastomas typically occur in young adults with a slight male predominance. However, in general, hemangioblastomas make up around 10% of posterior fossa tumors; when they are not associated with VHL, they have a sporadic peak at the age of 50 years. They tend to present with mass effect because of cyst expansion and typically are slow growing and histologically benign. They have an 85% 10-year survival postresection rate with a 15% recurrence.

TABLE 67-7 Simpson Grading System for Meningioma Resection

GRADE	EXTENT OF RESECTION	RECURRENCE RATE*
I	Complete including dural attachment and abnormal bone	10%
II	Complete with cauterization of dural attachment	15%
III	Complete without dural attachment	30%
IV	Incomplete resection	Up to 85%
V	Biopsy	100%

*Length of follow-up varies around 5 years; numbers may increase with longer follow-up.

Lymphomas and Hematopoietic Tumors

Primary Central Nervous System Lymphoma

The incidence of primary CNS lymphomas has increased to 10% of all primary intracranial tumors, and they are observed in 2% to 6% of patients with AIDS. The mean age at presentation is 60 years in immunocompetent patients and 35 years in patients with acquired immunodeficiency with a slight male predominance. The presentation can be with symptoms from a mass effect and, depending on location, sometimes with neuropsychiatric changes. The median survival is 1 to 4 months without treatment, 1 to 4 years when the patient is treated, and 2 to 6 months in patients with AIDS. There is a dramatic but short-lived response to steroids. Treatment consists of stereotactic biopsy followed by radiation therapy and chemotherapy because of their chemosensitivity to methotrexate. Intrathecal methotrexate will usually be advised for young patients.

Plasmacytoma

Plasmacytoma will usually involve the skull when it is found intracranially. It will often mimic meningioma and is considered at high risk for development of multiple myeloma within 10 years of diagnosis. Treatment consists of ruling out systemic multiple myeloma with urinalysis for protein and serum protein electrophoresis. Complete surgical excision should be followed by radiation therapy.

Germ Cell Tumors

Germinomas compose 1% to 2% of all primary CNS tumors; 50% are found in the pineal region and have most frequently been described in the Japanese population. The peak age at presentation is around 10 years, with more than 90% being found in the population younger than 20 years. The male to female ratio is 10:1 for the pineal region, whereas suprasellar germinomas are more common in females.

When located in the pineal region, they can become large and are present with hydrocephalus and Parinaud syndrome. This consists of paralysis of upward gaze, convergence, and accommodation and is associated with lid retraction, creating the so-called setting sun sign.

When located in the suprasellar region, they may produce compression of the hypothalamus and cause hypothalamic-pituitary dysfunction with diabetes insipidus and visual decline from compression of the optic tracts. Tumor markers help confirm diagnosis and a favorable prognosis when low secretion of human chorionic gonadotropin is observed. There is a 5-year survival rate greater than 90%, and they are usually sensitive and responsive to radiation therapy and chemotherapy. The first line of treatment consists of biopsy, then radiation therapy plus chemotherapy and treatment of hydrocephalus with either placement of a ventricular peritoneal shunt or a third ventriculostomy.

Nongerminomatous germ cell tumor is found most frequently between the ages of 0 and 3 years. These tumors are generally associated with a worse prognosis than germinomas are, with a 5-year survival rate of less than 50%. Embryonal carcinoma (malignant germ cell tumor) represents less than 1% of all CNS tumors and affects prepubertal children but is rarely found in children younger than 4 years; it is associated with Klinefelter syndrome and is considered malignant and invasive. Yolk sac tumors are also known as endodermal sinus tumors; they are usually found in infants or adolescents and are aggressive and malignant. Choriocarcinomas, which are also malignant and highly hemorrhagic, are another variety. Teratomas can be subdivided into mature and immature. The mature variety can be curable when complete resection is obtained. However, in the subtypes, the treatment algorithms, which include attempted resection plus chemotherapy and radiation therapy versus primary chemotherapy plus radiation therapy, are unclear; none of these has shown any significant survival difference. Mixed germ cell tumor is also a variety of the nongerminomatous germ cell tumors.

Tumors of the Sellar Region

Pituitary adenomas (Fig. 67-14) make up 10% of all intracranial tumors, with an equal male to female incidence; the peak incidence is in the third and fourth decades. The tumors can be associated with multiple endocrine neoplasia syndromes. Around 50% present as macroadenomas that are larger than 1 cm in diameter. Symptoms develop from mass effect on the optic tract or hypothalamic-pituitary disturbance with endocrine abnormalities and rarely apoplexy. Typically, when it is a hormone-producing tumor, symptoms will appear at earlier stages in tumor growth than when nonfunctioning adenomas are found.

Treatment consists of endocrine laboratory workup and evaluation with ophthalmology and visual fields. Prolactin levels of 25 ng/mL or less are considered normal; if the prolactin level is between 25 and 150 ng/mL, it is generally considered "stalk effect," although levels above 100 ng/mL should be considered suspicious. However, when the level is higher than 150 ng/mL, it is considered diagnostic for prolactinoma. In the case of apoplexy presentation, rapid administration of corticosteroid and possible surgical decompression must be considered. Surgical options include a trans-sphenoidal approach with microscope or endoscope, open craniotomy, and combination of these two procedures, which would be the case in large extensive suprasellar lesions. Focal or stereotactic radiation is usually reserved for refractory cases. It is always important for an endocrinologic follow-up.

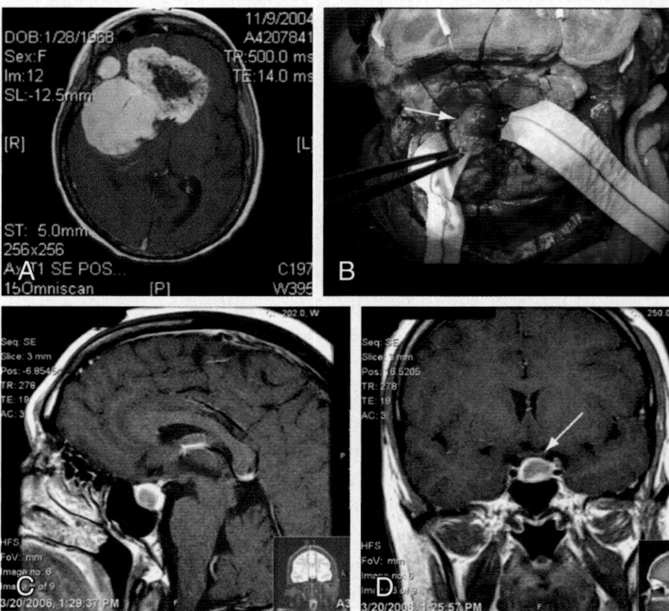

FIGURE 67-14 **A,** A large enhancing meningioma can be seen in this gadolinium-enhanced axial MRI study. **B,** Intraoperative picture showing dissection of the meningioma *(arrow)* from the surrounding gyri. Gadolinium-enhanced sagittal **(C)** and coronal **(D)** MRI scans of a patient with a pituitary macroadenoma show impingement on the optic chiasm *(arrow)*.

The classic presentation and associated treatment for pituitary adenomas are as follows.

Prolactinoma will be manifested with amenorrhea and galactorrhea in females and impotence in males. Infertility will be present in both. The treatment consists of dopamine agonist (e.g., bromocriptine) and generally provides complete control.

Adrenocorticotropin adenoma will be manifested as Cushing disease and classic hyperpigmentation of the skin and mucous membranes, ecchymoses, and purple striae, especially in the flanks, breast, and lower abdomen. Generalized muscle wasting with complaints of easy fatigability are among the other well documented signs and symptoms. The first line of treatment is surgery.

Growth hormone secreting tumors will produce acromegaly in adults and gigantism in prepubertal children. Surgery is the first line of treatment. Some patients may respond to octreotide, and others may show improvement with dopamine agonist.

Thyroid-stimulating hormone secreting tumors may present as hyperthyroidism, anxiety, and palpitations (due to atrial fibrillation). Patients have heat intolerance, hyperhidrosis, and thyrotoxicosis, for which the treatment will require surgery.

For both gonadotropin-secreting and nonfunctional adenomas, clinical presentations will be due to mass effect and stalk compression. If the tumor extends to the suprasellar region and compresses the optic chiasm, this will cause bitemporal hemianopia and may also have cranial nerve deficits. Treatment for these last two is also surgical resection.

Craniopharyngiomas are tumors that represent between 2% and 5% of all intracranial tumors; 50% are in children, with a peak incidence between 5 and 10 years of age. Their clinical presentation is similar to that of suprasellar masses with compression of the surrounding structures. The tumor is histologically benign but may sometimes have local aggressive and relentless behavior. Craniopharyngiomas have a 5-year survival rate of 55% to 85%, but recurrences typically happen within 1 year from surgery. The most frequent postoperative complications include diabetes insipidus and hypothalamic injury with 5% to 10% mortality. Treatment requires medical optimization before surgical resection because if there is adrenal cortical insufficiency, hydrocortisone coverage will often be needed perioperatively. Attempts to obtain total gross resection should be sought if appropriate. It is when subtotal resection is encountered that possible postoperative radiation therapy might be beneficial, but it does add to the morbidity.

Central Nervous System Metastasis

Cerebral metastases are the most common brain tumor in adults and make up more than 50% of all brain tumors across all ages. However, they account for only 6% of all pediatric brain tumor cases.[26] Approximately 20% to 40% of patients with cancer develop brain metastases during the course of their illness.[27] More than 550,000 patients die of cancer in the United States each year, and around 20% of these patients will have brain metastasis.[26,27] It is well known that most brain metastases arise from lung, breast, and renal cell tumors; however, melanoma, followed by lung, breast, and renal cell carcinoma, has the greatest propensity to develop brain metastasis. What is observed frequently is that breast and renal cell carcinoma tends to present as a single metastasis within the brain, whereas melanoma and lung cancers have an increased incidence of multiplicity.[27] The highest incidence of brain metastasis is seen in the fifth to seventh decades of life, and it is equally common among men and women. Lung cancer is the most common source of brain metastasis in men, and breast carcinomas are the most common source of metastases in women. Men with melanoma are more likely to develop brain metastasis than are women. The interval or time period between the diagnosis of the primary cancer and the development of brain metastasis depends on the histology of the primary cancer; breast cancer generally exhibits the longest interval (mean, 3 years) and lung cancer the shortest (mean, 4 to 10 months).[28]

Metastatic lesions tend to cause significant brain edema that initially will respond well to steroids. Typically, dexamethasone is used and will reduce the vasogenic edema. Anticonvulsants are used to reduce the likelihood of seizure but are generally given if the patient has had a seizure. When the lesion is initially encountered and no primary tumor is known, recommendations for stereotactic biopsy or excision should be given. However, if the disease is widespread, with a short life expectancy, and the patient has a poor preoperative status, consideration should be given to possible biopsy or radiotherapy and palliation.[29,30] If, on the other hand, a solitary metastasis is encountered, total surgical excision should be attempted, followed by whole brain radiotherapy. SRS generally will be recommended if surgery is not feasible.[31] When multiple metastases are encountered, consideration should be given to excision of the symptomatic lesion or multiple lesions (but this is controversial), followed by brain therapy or radiotherapy alone, and SRS will usually be considered if surgery is not feasible[32,33] (Fig. 67-15).

TRAUMATIC BRAIN INJURY

The goal of this section on traumatic brain injury is not to present a comprehensive review of the epidemiology, basic science research, and outcome studies on brain injury but to give a practical, common-sense approach to the management of injuries of the brain. There is bound to be overlap between this section and other parts of this text. Guidelines for the management of severe head injury were first published by the Brain Trauma Foundation in 1995 and last reviewed in 2007.[34] These evidence-based guidelines have been a tremendous aid to the physician caring for brain-injured patients. The following discussion on the management of severe traumatic brain injury is based largely on these guidelines. As with all practice guidelines, they can and need to be modified, as dictated by the experience of the treating physician and in accordance with the needs of the patient. This report and the protocols laid out in the advanced trauma life support guidelines, published by the American College of Surgeons Committee on Trauma, are also invaluable resources for the student and physician.

We first present the epidemiology, pathophysiology, prehospital and emergency management, and definitive treatment of severe traumatic brain injury.

Epidemiology

Depending on the source of information, it is estimated that there are anywhere from 500,000 to well above 1 million cases of head injury every year. Most of these are classified as mild injuries, with approximately 20% classified as moderate to severe. Approximately 50% of the 150,000 trauma deaths every year are caused by head injury. The social, medical, and economic implications are profound. Fortunately, prevention programs appear to be decreasing the incidence of severe traumatic brain injury.

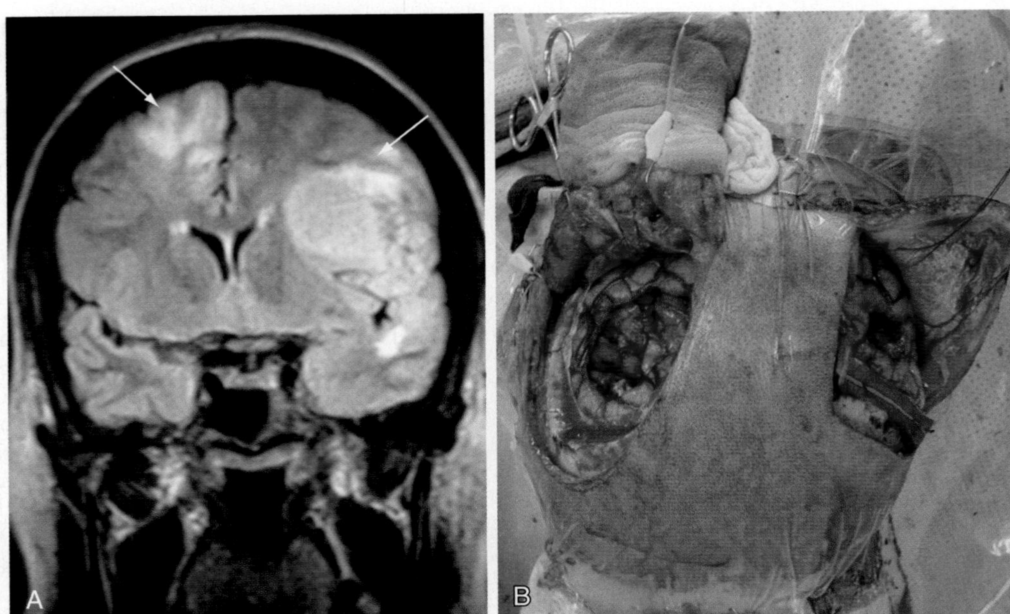

FIGURE 67-15 **A,** Fluid-attenuated inversion recovery sequence coronal MRI of a patient with two simultaneous metastatic tumors along the right and left frontal lobes *(arrows)*. **B,** Simultaneous right and left frontal craniotomies for resection of both metastatic lesions.

Pathophysiology

Traumatic brain injury can be classified into primary and secondary injuries. Primary injury occurs at impact and is considered first. It includes bone fracture, intracranial hemorrhage, and diffuse axonal injury (DAI). Fractures of the cranial vault and skull base are indicative of the forces applied to the skull at the time of impact. Fractures of the skull base may be associated with cranial nerve deficit, arterial dissection, and CSF fistula formation. Fractures of the cranial vault are classified as follows:

Open or closed
Depressed or nondepressed
Linear or comminuted

Any fracture of the cranial vault can cause disruption of the underlying meningeal arteries or dural venous sinuses, which can lead to intracranial bleeding. Intracranial hemorrhage can be classified as epidural, subdural, subarachnoid, and intraparenchymal or intracerebral. Epidural hemorrhage occurs between the dura and skull and is usually the result of a skull fracture causing the laceration of a meningeal artery.

Rarely, a fracture crossing a dural venous sinus can cause a venous epidural hematoma, especially in children. Subdural hemorrhage occurs in the potential space between the dura and arachnoid. This is often the result of shearing of the bridging veins between the brain and the dural venous sinuses. Sometimes, it comes from injury to cortical vessels, which then bleed into the subdural space. Subarachnoid hemorrhage from trauma consists of bleeding into the spinal fluid spaces surrounding the blood vessels feeding the cerebral cortex. Trauma is the most common cause of subarachnoid hemorrhage. Rupture of an intracranial aneurysm is the second most common cause of subarachnoid hemorrhage and is generally distinguished from traumatic subarachnoid hemorrhage by history and sometimes by the distribution of blood on a CT scan. Intraparenchymal or intracerebral hemorrhage is bleeding into the brain itself. This can run the spectrum from small contusions (bruises of the brain) to large intracerebral clots (which usually are the result of coup and contrecoup injuries) that require emergent surgical evacuation. Although often small and nonsurgical at first, these can blossom and become life-threatening during a period of hours to days. DAI is a rotational acceleration-deceleration injury to the white matter pathways of the brain. This results in a functional or anatomic disruption of these pathways and is cited as the cause of loss of consciousness in patients without mass lesions. DAI can occur with or without other primary injuries, such as an epidural or subdural hematoma (Fig. 67-16). In addition to being one of the many primary injuries seen in severe traumatic brain injury, DAI can also be considered a secondary injury.

Secondary injury to the brain occurs as a result of decreased oxygen delivery to the brain, which in turn sets off a cascade of events that causes even more damage than the initial injury. With severe traumatic brain injury, there can be an alteration in cerebral vessel autoregulation. Systemic hypotension in the presence of this altered autoregulation results in decreased CBF and decreased oxygen delivery. This ischemia is exacerbated even further by systemic hypoxemia; intracranial hypertension, which decreases CBF even further, and a cascade of events involving mediators of inflammation, excitotoxicity, calcium influx, and Na^+,K^+-ATPase dysfunction lead to neuronal cell dysfunction and death. The prevention of secondary injury is therefore thought to lead to increased cell survival and improved outcome. This is achieved by preventing hypotension and hypoxia while taking measures to control ICP and to maintain CPP.

Prehospital and Emergency Department Management

The prehospital and emergency department management of the traumatized patient is reviewed elsewhere in this and other texts. Here we deal more specifically with issues critical to the patient with severe brain injury. The ABCs must always be addressed first, regardless of the severity of the patient's injury. Attention is first

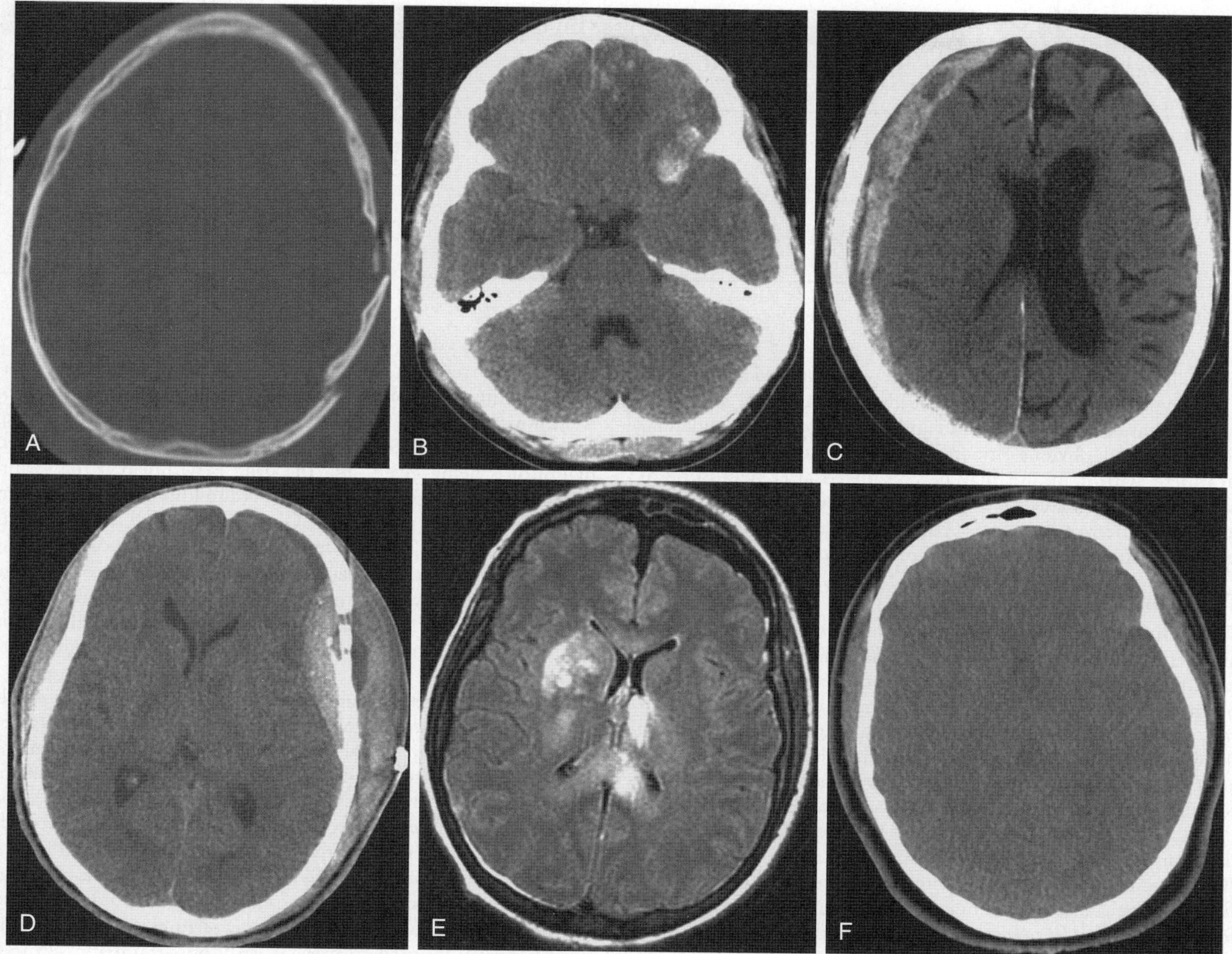

FIGURE 67-16 Typical radiologic findings in traumatic brain injury. **A,** Skull fracture shown on CT. **B,** Intraparenchymal contusions. **C,** Subdural hematoma. **D,** Epidural hematoma. **E,** Diffuse axonal injury. **F,** Intracranial hypertension. Note the effacement of sulci and gray-white matter differentiation.

paid to securing a patent airway, establishing adequate ventilation and oxygenation, and maintaining adequate circulation. By doing this, one may avoid hypotension and hypoxia and, in so doing, avoid or minimize secondary brain injury. In patients with severe traumatic brain injury, a systolic blood pressure less than 90 mm Hg or a PaO_2 less than 60 mm Hg is a predictor of poor outcome. Appropriate spine precautions are observed in the initial resuscitation of the patient with a severe traumatic brain injury.

Once airway, breathing, and circulation have been addressed, neurologic evaluation may proceed. The Glasgow Coma Scale (GCS) is a simple and reproducible method of neurologic assessment. It is also used to grade traumatic brain injury as mild, moderate, or severe. The GCS consists of three components—intensity of stimulus required to cause eye opening, verbal response, and motor response (Table 67-8). Pupillary size and reactivity are also essential components of the initial neurologic examination. Hypoxia, hypotension, alcohol, and drugs may all contribute to abnormal findings on the neurologic examination. In the absence of hypotension and hypoxia, an abnormal finding on examination is considered to be a primary brain injury until proven otherwise. Once all life-threatening injuries have been addressed and stabilized, the patient with a suspected traumatic brain injury undergoes CT. The CT scan is used to evaluate the presence or absence of fracture, epidural and subdural hematomas, intracerebral hematomas and contusions, shift of the midline structures, and appearance of the basal and perimesencephalic cisterns. In many centers with multislice scanners, routine scanning of the cervical spine is also performed to rule out acute fractures or traumatic dislocations. If life-threatening injuries elsewhere necessitate immediate transport of the patient to the operating room and the patient has a suspected intracranial hematoma (e.g., unilateral fixed and dilated pupil on one side, with a contralateral hemiparesis), exploratory burr holes may be performed in the operating room concurrently with the laparotomy or thoracotomy.

Not infrequently, trauma patients with brain injury will require transfer to a hospital equipped to provide those patients with a higher level of care. In preparing these patients for transfer, the physician needs to follow the advanced trauma life support guidelines and secure the airway, ensure adequate ventilation, and

TABLE 67-8 **Neurologic Assessment Using the Glasgow Coma Scale**

EYE OPENING RESPONSE		VERBAL RESPONSE		MOTOR RESPONSE	
SCORE	RESPONSE	SCORE	RESPONSE	SCORE	RESPONSE
4	Spontaneous	5	Oriented	6	Obeys commands
3	To speech	4	Confused	5	Localizes to painful stimulus
2	To pain	3	Inappropriate responses	4	Withdraws to painful stimulus
1	No response	2	Incomprehensible responses	3	Flexion to painful stimulus
		1	No response	2	Extension to painful stimulus
				1	No response

maintain circulation. Anemia is treated with transfusion, as necessary. Hypoxia and hypotension need to be avoided. Adequate immobilization with a backboard and cervical collar is mandatory. In patients with obvious intracranial hypertension or mass lesions, treatment with mannitol may be considered after neurosurgical consultation. Vigilance and attention to detail as well as communication between the transferring and accepting physicians are key to the successful transfer and treatment of these patients.

Treatment

When the workup of a patient reveals an intracranial mass lesion and deficits thought to be related to that lesion, operative intervention is indicated. In general, any clot or contusion more than 30 mL is thought to be operable. Epidural and subdural hematomas (Fig. 67-16) are addressed with similar approaches, with the craniotomy centered on the clot. Intracerebral hematomas are addressed through appropriately located craniotomies. ICP monitors are often placed at operation. These can be intraventricular drains, intraparenchymal monitors, or devices placed in the epidural or subdural spaces. The decision about when to place an ICP monitor depends on the patient's preoperative examination findings, appearance of the brain at operation, and potential risk for deterioration. In general, all patients with a GCS score of 8 or less have ICP monitors placed. Some patients with moderate traumatic brain injury may also benefit from ICP monitoring. Postoperatively, the patient is managed similarly to those with nonoperable traumatic brain injury.

The following is a simplified algorithm for the management of intracranial hypertension in the intensive care setting. The head of the bed is elevated to 30 degrees, with the head placed in a neutral position. Care is taken to ensure that any cervical spine immobilization device is not obstructing jugular venous flow because this can increase ICP. The goal of treatment is to try to keep the ICP below 20 mm Hg and to maintain CPP at or above 70 mm Hg (remember that CPP is MAP minus ICP). If the ICP is persistently elevated above 20 mm Hg, it is treated. CSF drainage is now the first line of therapy in decreasing ICP. This is accomplished by an external ventricular drain, or ventriculostomy, which is a drain placed in the operating room or at bedside in the intensive care unit in an appropriately monitored patient. If ICP remains persistently elevated despite CSF drainage, the patient can be sedated and even paralyzed pharmacologically to keep the ICP down. The physician is dependent on the pupillary examination and ICP reading in this situation. If the ICP changes rapidly or the pupillary examination findings change (i.e., blown pupil), emergent CT of the head is indicated. Sedation and paralysis can occasionally be discontinued to allow an adequate neurologic evaluation in this situation.

If the ICP remains persistently elevated despite these interventions, mannitol and other diuretic agents may be used. Mannitol is administered as an intravenous (IV) bolus of 0.25 to 1 g/kg every 4 to 6 hours. Serum osmolality is followed closely when mannitol is being given, and the drug is withheld if the serum osmolality exceeds 320 mOsm/kg. It is also important to maintain euvolemia in these patients. If ICP is still elevated, hyperventilation to a $PaCO_2$ of 30 to 35 mm Hg may be used judiciously. At this point, second-tier therapeutic interventions (e.g., hypertonic saline, high-dose barbiturate therapy, decompressive craniectomy) may be considered.[35,36] Serial CT scans are critical throughout this treatment algorithm, and their use is tailored to the individual patient.

Several comments regarding nutrition, steroids, anticonvulsants, and $PaCO_2$ are appropriate here. Energy requirements after traumatic brain injury are increased. The nonparalyzed patient requires replacement of 140% of his or her resting metabolism expenditure, and the paralyzed patient requires 100%. Of this, 15% is protein. Feeding begins within 7 days of injury. Steroids have no proven benefit in the management of traumatic brain injury and are not used. Prophylactic use of anticonvulsant drugs (e.g., phenytoin, carbamazepine, phenobarbital) is not indicated for the prevention of late post-traumatic seizures. Anticonvulsants may, however, be used to prevent early post-traumatic seizures, primarily in patients at high risk for early seizures who may suffer adverse effects if they were to seize early in their hospital course. These can usually be tapered after 1 week of therapy. Hyperventilation causes a decrease in ICP by lowering $PaCO_2$, which causes vasoconstriction and decreases intracranial blood volume. Unfortunately, it also causes decreased CBF. If hyperventilation to a $PaCO_2$ of less than 30 mm Hg is required for the maintenance of an acceptable ICP and CPP, monitoring of CBF is strongly recommended by some. Jugular venous oxygen saturation and cerebral oxygen extraction may also be useful in this clinical scenario. Table 67-9 presents a summary of the recommendations of the 2007 guidelines provided by the Brain Trauma Foundation for traumatic brain injury.

DEGENERATIVE DISORDERS OF THE SPINE

Relevant Spinal Anatomy

In adults, the spinal cord terminates at the lower border of L1. The filum terminale, a relatively fibrous structure, extends from the lower border of the spinal cord to attach at the S2 level. On both sides at each level, anterior and posterior nerve roots exit and traverse toward the nerve root foramen and enter the root canal to join and form the spinal nerve. The first spinal nerve roots (C1) exit above the atlas, the C2 roots exit between C1 and C2, and

TABLE 67-9 Brain Trauma Foundation Recommendations for Traumatic Brain Injury

PARAMETER	GUIDELINE
Hyperosmolar therapy	Mannitol effective for control of raised ICP (0.25-1 g/kg)
Prophylactic hypothermia	Preliminary data suggest that mortality could be decreased when target temperatures are maintained >48 hours
Infection prophylaxis	Routine external ventricular catheter exchange not recommended; indicated if GCS score = 3-8 on admission and abnormal CT; in severe traumatic brain injury and normal CT, indicated with two or more of the following: age >40 years, unilateral posturing, hypotension with systolic blood pressure <90 mm Hg
ICP monitoring	Ventricular catheters are most reliable and cost-effective method; ICP should be kept <20 mm Hg
CPP threshold	CPP <50 mm Hg should be avoided; aggressive interventions to maintain it above 70 mm Hg have a considerable risk of acute respiratory distress syndrome
Brain oxygen monitoring and thresholds	Jugular venous saturation (50%) and brain tissue oxygen tension (15 mm Hg) are treatment thresholds
Blood pressure and oxygenation	Blood pressure should be monitored, hypotension (systolic blood pressure = 90 mm Hg) avoided; hypoxia (saturation <90% or Po_2 <60 mm Hg) should be avoided
Nutrition	Should be initiated within 7 days of injury
Sedatives	High-dose barbiturates recommended to control refractory ICP in the hemodynamically stable patient; propofol recommended for ICP control but does not improve mortality
Seizure prophylaxis	Decreases early post-traumatic seizures (<7 days after injury)
Hyperventilation	Recommended as temporizing measure; Pco_2 below 25 mm Hg not recommended; avoid in first 24 hours after injury
Steroids	Not recommended, contraindicated

TABLE 67-10 Clinical Findings in Common Lumbar Disc Herniations

DISC	INCIDENCE (%)	ROOT	PAIN DISTRIBUTION	MUSCLE INVOLVED	SENSORY DEFICITS	REFLEX LOSS
L3-4	3-10	L4	Anterior thigh	Quadriceps femoris	Medial malleolus and medial foot	Knee jerk
L4-5	40-45	L5	Posterolateral thigh and leg	Tibialis anterior; extensor hallucis longus	Large toe web, dorsum of foot	None
L5-S1	45-50	S1	Posterolateral thigh and leg down to ankle	Gastrocnemius	Lateral malleolus, lateral foot	Ankle jerk

TABLE 67-11 Clinical Findings in Common Cervical Disc Herniations

DISC	INCIDENCE (%)	ROOT	PAIN DISTRIBUTION	MUSCLE INVOLVED	REFLEX LOSS
C4-5	2	C5	Shoulder	Deltoid	Deltoid
C5-6	19	C6	Upper arm, thumb, radial forearm	Biceps, extensor carpi radialis	Biceps, brachioradialis
C6-7	69	C7	Fingers 2 and 3, all fingertips	Triceps	Triceps
C7-T1	10	C8	Fingers 4 and 5	Hand intrinsics	Finger jerk

the C8 nerve exists between C7 and T1 (thus, there are only seven cervical vertebrae, whereas there are eight pairs of cervical nerve roots). This is significant in localization of the spinal nerve involvement by a prolapsed disc as a C5-6 disc will involve the C6 nerve root. In the thoracic and lumbar region, the corresponding thoracic nerve root exits below the corresponding vertebra; thus, the L4 nerve root exits between the L4 and L5. However, in the lumbar region, an extreme lateral course of the nerve root while exiting predisposes the next root to be involved in disc prolapse at the corresponding level. For example, in L4-5 disc prolapse, the L5 nerve root is commonly involved as the L4 root crosses the L4-5 disc space at the extreme lateral edge, thus escaping compression. The L5 root courses across the L4-5 disc space more medially, thus being involved in the process. Hence, although prolapsed discs commonly involve the lower level root in both the cervical and lumbar regions, the causes are different in both regions. The motor, sensory, and reflex distribution of the nerve roots are summarized in Tables 67-10 and 67-11.

Pathophysiology of the Degenerative Diseases of the Spine

The intervertebral disc essentially consists of three parts: the annulus fibrosus, which is the tough outer ring composed of 10 to 12 layers of fibrous tissue and fibrocartilage; the central nucleus pulposus, which is initially gelatinous but becomes more fibrous with advancing age; and end plates, which are thin plates of hyaline cartilage attaching the disc to the upper and lower vertebral body. Although the nucleus pulposus can herniate in any direction, posterior and posterolateral herniations cause compression of the adjacent nerve roots and give rise to clinical symptoms. Superior and inferior herniations into the vertebral body are known as Schmorl nodes and are incidental findings. The intervertebral disc herniation is most common in the lower cervical and lower lumbar levels, although it can occur at any level from C2 to L5.

Apart from the soft disc herniations as mentioned before, degeneration of the disc results in small annular tears and mild protrusion of the fragments outside the confines of the disc. This, during a prolonged period, leads to hypertrophy of the adjacent bone edges known as osteophytes. The osteophytes projecting posteriorly can compress on the adjacent nerve root or the spinal cord. Associated hypertrophy and infolding of the ligamentum flavum can cause reduction in the intraspinal space with predominant posterior compression. Facet hypertrophy can result in reduction in the lateral recess of the spinal canal, causing lateral recess stenosis. Most often, these coexist with compression of the neural structures from multiple directions. Severe degeneration of the facets and laxity of the ligaments result in degenerative spondylolisthesis, which is common at L4-5 and L5-S1 levels in the lumbar region and C3-4 and C4-5 levels in the cervical region. This listhesis can result in compression of the spinal cord and adjacent roots.

Cervical Disc Prolapse, Cervical Spondylosis, and Cervical Stenosis

Approximately 90% of the herniated discs in the neck are located at C5-6 and C6-7 levels. An acutely herniated disc (soft disc; Fig. 67-17) typically presents with local pain and tenderness, with the pain radiating in the distribution of the affected nerve root. The symptoms may be precipitated by a minor trauma. Initial local pain often precedes the radiating pain by several weeks. Movement of the cervical spine usually aggravates the pain. Features of nerve root dysfunction in the form of motor weakness or sensory numbness usually follow the initial pain. Large disc prolapse can cause spinal cord compression, resulting in spasticity and weakness of the lower limbs. In severe cases, there may be accompanying urinary retention.

On the other hand, the presentation of the cervical spondylosis (hard disc) is usually more subtle, with waxing and waning neck pain and paresthesias in the upper limbs. Spondylotic lesions compressing the spinal cord can result in progressive spasticity and weakness of the lower limbs (spondylotic myelopathy) apart from the radiculopathic changes in the upper limbs. The presence of myelopathy is of considerable clinical significance as it usually necessitates a surgical intervention for the patient.

Stenosis of the cervical spinal canal may be either congenital or acquired. Congenital stenosis often presents in young adults with progressive myelopathy and gait disturbances. Acquired stenosis is most commonly due to cervical spondylosis with hypertrophy of the ligamentum flavum (Fig. 67-17).

Diagnosis

The symptoms of acutely herniated disc are so characteristic that the diagnosis is apparent during the clinical evaluation. The

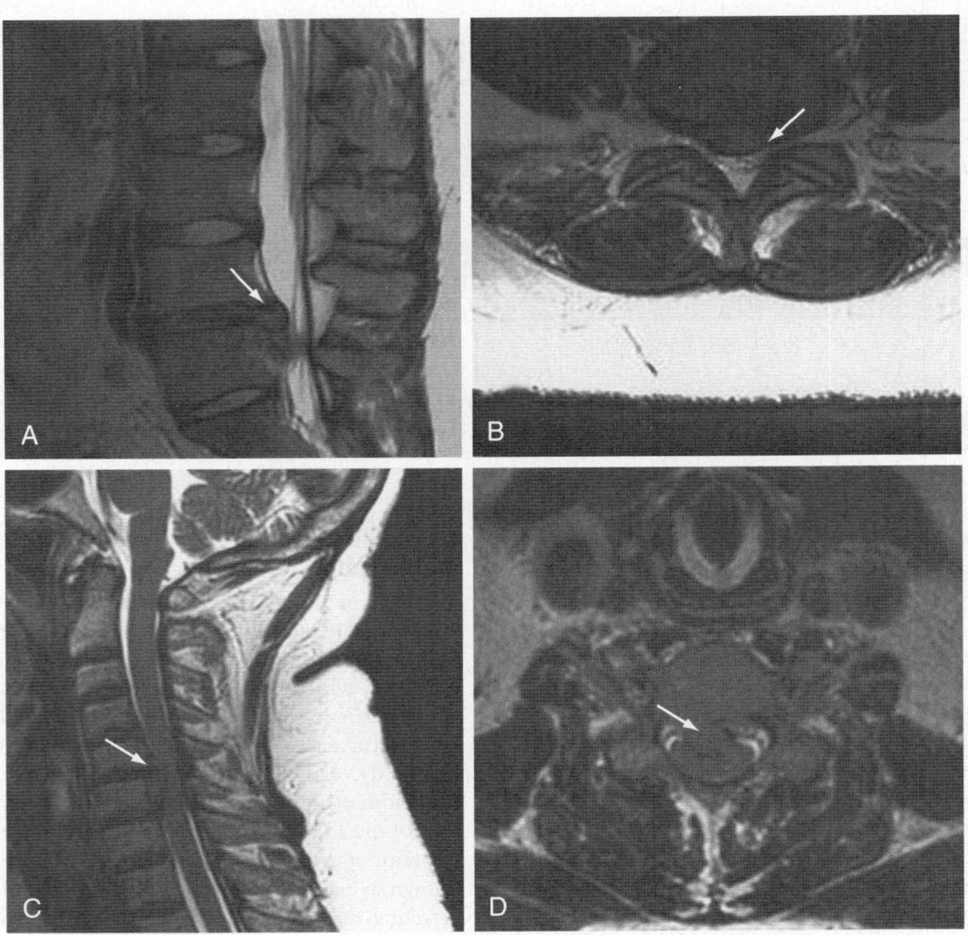

FIGURE 67-17 A, T2-weighted sagittal MRI study showing a herniated lumbar disc fragment *(arrow)* at the L4-5 level. **B,** T2-weighted axial MRI showing the same fragment *(arrow)* compressing the thecal sac. **C,** T2-weighted sagittal MRI of a patient with a large anterior disc prolapse at C5-6 level *(arrow)*. **D,** Axial images showing the disc compressing the spinal cord *(arrow)*.

diagnostic studies confirm the level and the nature of the disc prolapse. On occasion, nerve root tumors (schwannoma) may present similarly. MRI of the cervical spine will demonstrate the location and extent of the disc bulge as well as if there are any signal changes in the spinal cord. Myelomalacia of the cord suggests chronic significant spinal cord compression and often is prognostic of potential residual deficits after adequate decompression of the spinal cord. In patients with spondylotic changes, MRI demonstrates the degree of osteophyte formation, associated ligamentous hypertrophy, and number of segments involved. Associated cervical spinal stenosis is also identified. CT myelography is often indicated in patients who cannot have MRI scans or when anatomic bone details are essential in making a management decision. Electromyography and nerve conduction studies are sometimes required to exclude other causes like plexopathies and peripheral nerve involvement.

Management Options

Acute *cervical radiculopathy* is often well managed conservatively with rest, analgesics, muscle relaxants, and a short course of steroids. Surgery is considered in patients with persistent pain and persistent neurologic deficits while they are receiving conservative therapy. The aim of the surgery is nerve root decompression. However, with presence of *cervical myelopathy* suggesting spinal cord compression, surgery is indicated to decompress the spinal canal and to relieve the compression on the spinal cord. Although improvement can be anticipated, an arrest of the progression of the myelopathy is often achieved (Fig. 67-18).

With a predominant anterior pathologic process and compression of the neural structures (e.g., compression from bulging disc, osteophytes, or spondylotic bars), the anterior cervical approach with discectomy is usually considered (Fig. 67-19). The osteophytes can be drilled out to decompress the spinal cord and the nerve roots. For a single-level discectomy, an interbody fusion with bone graft may or may not be considered. However, for multilevel discectomies, anterior interbody fusion with bone graft and instrumentation is considered the standard of care. Often with extensive pathologic processes across the vertebral body, the surgeon considers drilling out the vertebral body and replacing it with an iliac crest bone graft or a metallic/synthetic cage. Although the anterior approach is relatively safe and has a quick recovery period, injuries to the adjacent structures like esophagus and recurrent laryngeal nerve are the unique complications.

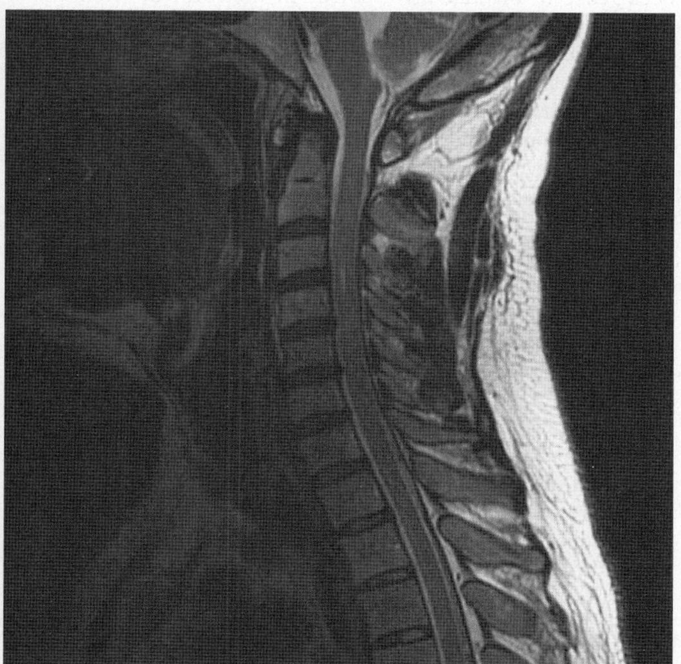

FIGURE 67-18 T2-weighted sagittal MRI scan of a patient with significant cervical canal stenosis. Note the hyperintensity in the cervical spinal cord at the C3-4 level, suggesting myelomalacic changes. This may be indicative of permanent residual deficits.

The posterior approaches to the cervical spine include foraminotomy and decompression, decompressive laminectomy, decompressive laminectomy with fusion, and cervical laminoplasty. *Cervical foraminotomy* is usually indicated for cervical radiculopathy with a lateral osteophyte or a soft disc. The other three approaches are usually considered for patients with a predominant posterior compression of the spinal cord (e.g., ligamentum flavum hypertrophy, degenerative canal stenosis with facet hypertrophy, congenital canal stenosis). *Cervical decompressive laminectomy* during a prolonged follow-up period often predisposes to kyphotic deformity (swan neck deformity) of the cervical spine and is often avoided in younger patients. In these patients, cervical decompressive laminectomy is usually combined with *posterior fusion with instrumentation* and bone graft. In *cervical laminoplasty*, the cervical laminae are fractured and displaced outward by spacers to increase the spinal canal diameter in the anterior-posterior plane. In patients with complex pathologic processes due to chronic spondylotic changes, an anterior and posterior approach can be combined in a single or staged manner.

Lumbar Disc Prolapse and Lumbar Degenerative Conditions

Lumbar Disc Prolapse

Like cervical disc prolapse, approximately 90% of the lumbar disc prolapse occurs at either the L4-5 or L5-S1 level, with the remainder at the L3-4 level. Lumbar disc prolapse at other levels is distinctly uncommon. There are two common presentations of the lumbar disc prolapse: acute radiculopathy and chronic low back pain. The first presentation, acute radiculopathy, usually involves a patient with a prior history of back discomfort manifested with acute back pain precipitated by an episode of lumbar strain, such as bending forward and lifting heavy objects. The pain is usually in the low back region and often radiates to one of the lower limbs aggravated by coughing or straining. These patients will have restricted straight leg raising; they may have numbness in the dermatomal distribution and associated weakness that may appear a few days later. In severe cases, there may be bladder dysfunction. These patients usually have an annular rupture with herniation of the disc material into the spinal canal compressing the nerve root (see Fig. 67-17). The second category of patients have a long history of chronic backache with intermittent aggravations and remissions, with recent occurrence of leg pain and intermittent paresthesias in the lower limbs that are often poorly localized.

Lumbar Canal Stenosis

Narrowing of the canal diameter can be present congenitally (primary lumbar canal stenosis, congenital lumbar canal stenosis) or be secondary to degenerative changes (secondary lumbar canal stenosis). Advanced degenerative changes leading to arthrosis,

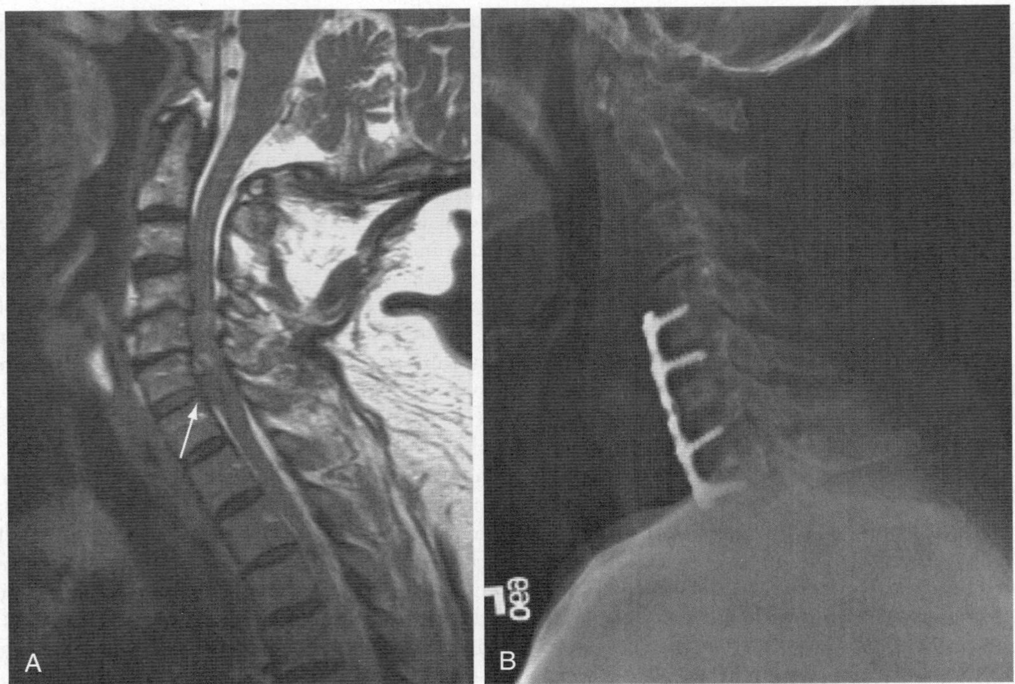

FIGURE 67-19 **A,** T2-weighted sagittal MRI study of a patient with advanced cervical spondylosis and stenosis from C3-4 down to C6-7 with an acute herniated disc fragment at C6-7 *(arrow)* after cervical spine manipulation. **B,** Postoperative lateral radiograph showing C4-5, C5-6, and C6-7 anterior cervical discectomy and fusion using a bone allograft and titanium plate and screws.

facet hypertrophy, and ligamentum hypertrophy result in canal stenosis. Apart from stenosis of the thecal sac, foraminal stenosis can be due to extension of the stenosis to the neural foramen causing radiculopathic changes. Lumbar canal stenosis classically presents as claudication pain in both the legs that is precipitated by walking and occasionally even by standing for a prolonged period. This neurogenic claudication is relieved by maneuvers causing flexion of the spine (e.g., sitting down or bending forward) in addition to stopping the activity, as opposed to vascular claudication, which is relieved by stopping of the activity. The neurologic evaluation often does not elicit any gross deficits unless coexistent pathologic changes are present.

Localization and Diagnosis

The clinical localization is well apparent in the patients who present with radicular pain as the dermatomal distribution of the pain suggests the involved nerve root (Tables 67-10 and 67-11). The radiologic evaluation, in addition to confirming the disc bulge, demonstrates the degree of the bulge and associated additional pathologic change (canal stenosis, adjacent level disc disease, and spondylolisthesis).

Management

The initial management usually involves adequate bed rest, analgesics, muscle relaxants, and minor tranquilizers like diazepam. Most patients will experience benefit with this regimen and will be able to resume activity in a reduced capacity in a few weeks. The second line of treatment is by oral steroids and epidural steroid injection, which often reduces pain. Physical therapy is also useful during the recovery phase.

Certain symptoms and signs indicate the need for hospitalization. Presence of significant motor deficits (e.g., footdrop or occurrence of bladder involvement in the form of retention or urgency) is usually an indication for hospitalization. Surgical intervention is usually considered under these circumstances. The conventional surgical treatment includes a midline approach, partial laminectomy, and excision of the protruded disc with decompression of the nerve root. Radiographic identification of the correct level is essential. The herniated fragment is removed, and the nerve root is traced to the neural foramen to exclude associated foraminal stenosis, which if present would require foraminal decompression. A minimally invasive microscopic approach and an endoscopic approach using paramedian incisions have also been used. The recovery is usually quick, and patients are often discharged on the same evening or the next day. A 10% recurrence rate at the same level is reported with microsurgical discectomy.

The surgical approach is often tailored to the associated conditions. Associated canal stenosis requires a decompressive laminectomy and decompression of the neural foramen. Lumbar fusion and instrumentation are considered for failed surgery, associated spondylolisthesis, or extensive decompression, which can precipitate future instability. Some of the common lumbar fusion techniques include posterolateral fusion with pedicle screws, posterior lumbar interbody fusion, and anterior lumbar interbody fusion. A bone fusion between the adjacent segments is ideally achieved by interposition of cadaveric or autologous bone graft aided with additions like demineralized bone matrix or recombinant bone morphogenic protein. Instrumentation of the adjacent segments helps keep the ends apposed and immobilized.

FUNCTIONAL AND STEREOTACTIC NEUROSURGERY

Functional neurosurgery is concerned with the anatomic or physiologic alteration of the nervous system to achieve a desired effect. This can be done with focal electrical stimulation procedures, ablative procedures, or implantation of pumps to deliver drugs, usually to the CSF but possibly also to the parenchyma. The field of functional neurosurgery deals primarily with the treatment of pain, movement disorders, epilepsy, and some psychiatric disorders when they are refractory to conventional treatments. These disorders all have in common hyperfunction or deranged function of some part of the CNS. Sometimes, the hyperfunction results from a loss of function in some other part of the brain, such as in the output pathways of the globus pallidus when the dopamine system in the brain degenerates, as in Parkinson disease. The transmitter of the overactive globus pallidus output system is inhibitory; the overall effect on the motor system is also inhibitory. The physiology of each functional disorder is often complex and only partly understood. It is not our focus here to detail what is known about the mechanism underlying each of these disorders; we focus on the surgery, especially the stereotactic techniques and possible interventions at the target site. This section also discusses SRS in general terms.

In considering brain stimulation, if the reader could image the consequences of placing two electrodes on the central processing unit of a computer and running a pulsatile stimulating current across it, not many would expect that the functioning of the computer would be enhanced. Rather, we would expect part of the computer not to work at all as a result. Although we talk about neuroaugmentation as if it were always adding something to the function of the nervous system, most of the interventions are actually effective because they stop certain unwanted activity in the brain. It may be a surprise to many, but in most situations, brain stimulation results in a temporary lesion of the stimulated structure. In almost all cases in the older neurosurgical literature in which a focal lesion was found to be effective, modern stimulation of that same structure is also effective. The difference is that a lesion is permanent and static in size and location. The advantage of stimulation is that it can be turned on or off, increased or decreased, and, in the case of an implanted electrode array, changed in location, depending somewhat on which of the several contacts are activated. Thus, stimulation provides a reversible, scalable, and somewhat movable functional lesion.

There are exceptions to the concept that stimulation is equivalent to a functional lesion. The frequency of stimulation can determine its overall effect, and the neurotransmitters at the site of stimulation can also have an effect. The cerebral cortex, with its high concentrations of excitatory neurotransmitters, may actually be turned on with stimulation. Thus, certain crude visual prostheses may be effective on that basis.

Stereotaxis, as applied to neurosurgery, is concerned with the localization of a target in three-dimensional space. The target deep in the brain is not seen directly at surgery. This can be a tumor, white matter pathway, cranial nerve, vascular malformation, or nucleus deep within the brain. The field has evolved using frame-based and frameless systems, but in each case, a calculated inference is used to reach the target accurately.

Frame-based systems use a rigid frame attached to the skull by pins that penetrate the outer table of the skull (Fig. 67-20). This can easily be done under local anesthesia, with the patient wide awake. The patient is then taken for CT or MRI with a localizer on the frame. Using cartesian coordinates, the x, y, and z coordinates of the target can then be determined. In other words, the position of the target in relation to the frame is known. Using an arc system, which is mounted on the frame, the target can be accessed by different trajectories. When the target is a vascular lesion, arteriography can be performed with a localizing frame, and the position of the vascular lesion in three-dimensional space can be determined. Frame-based systems are used for brain biopsies, deep brain stimulation, ablative procedures, and SRS.

SRS involves the delivery of a concentrated dose of radiation to a defined volume in the brain. The dose of radiation delivered would be toxic if given in a broad field to the entire brain. When it is delivered in multiple collimated beams from numerous different angles or in arcs at different angles, the effect on the surrounding brain is minimized. Two methods of frame-based SRS are currently used widely. The gamma knife uses cobalt-201 radiation sources focused on one point. Once the target is localized in three dimensions, it is placed at this point, and different collimators are used to focus the radiation. Modified linear accelerators deliver the radiation dose in multiple arcs, thereby minimizing

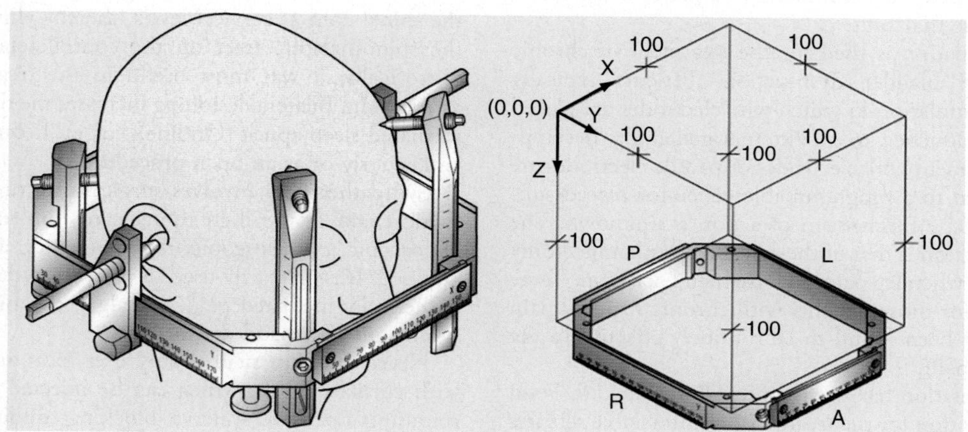

FIGURE 67-20 The Leksell stereotactic coordinate frame is rigidly attached to the head by four threaded pins. The fiducial box is mounted on the frame during the imaging study (MRI or CT). The x, y, and z coordinates are determined directly from the imaging study. The center of the frame is arbitrarily given the coordinates 100, 100, 100. (Courtesy Elekta, Stockholm, Sweden.)

the effect on surrounding brain tissue. Both systems use multiple isocenters for the treatment of irregularly shaped lesions. SRS has been used in the treatment of almost every intracranial lesion but is commonly used in the treatment of metastatic tumors, benign lesions of the cranial nerves, AVMs, and trigeminal neuralgia.[37-41] The primary risks of SRS are radiation necrosis and radiation injury to surrounding structures.

Frameless stereotactic techniques use advanced imaging techniques, fiducials, and reference markers in place of a fixed frame. Robotic arms, infrared reflectors, and light-emitting diodes provide the surgeon with real-time information about the anatomy at hand. This technology can also be fused with a display from the operating microscope, aiding in the operative dissection. It is useful for the planning of incisions and craniotomies and, when combined with intraoperative ultrasound, may be of use in determining the extent of tumor resection. Frameless stereotactic radiosurgical devices are commercially available.[37-41]

Brain Stimulation

Electrical stimulation of the nervous system is used in the treatment of movement disorders, pain, and epilepsy. Stimulation involves placement of an electrode, which is then connected to a subcutaneously placed generator. Here we discuss neurostimulation as it applies to the treatment of movement disorders, chronic pain states, and epilepsy.

Parkinson disease is the most common movement disorder for which patients have surgery. Stereotactic techniques developed in the 1950s were used to create lesions in the pallidum and thalamus. These ablative procedures fell by the wayside for a time with the introduction and widespread use of L-dopa (L-3,4-dihydroxyphenylalanine). In the early 1990s, there was a renewed interest in the use of surgical techniques for Parkinson patients who had become unresponsive to pharmacologic agents or intolerant of their side effects. Lesions of the internal segment of the globus pallidus saw a tremendous resurgence. With improvements in imaging and intraoperative microelectrode recording, deep brain stimulation soon replaced ablative procedures in the surgical treatment of these patients. Stimulation induces a reversible inhibition of neuronal activity, which can be adjusted as the clinical situation demands. The subthalamic nucleus has replaced the globus pallidus as the target of choice. Subthalamic nucleus stimulation is most effective for the treatment of rigidity and akinesia. Tremor is best addressed with stimulation of the ventralis intermedius nucleus of the thalamus.

Spinal cord stimulation is used for the treatment of chronic pain, dystonia, and bladder dysfunction. Patients typically undergo a trial of stimulation in which wire electrodes are placed percutaneously and attached to an external generator. If symptoms improve, permanent wire electrodes or paddle electrodes are placed and connected to a programmable generator placed subcutaneously. The precise mechanism of action is unknown. The most common indication is that of the so-called postlaminectomy syndrome, especially when leg pain is worse than back pain. There is also some benefit for those patients with chronic regional pain syndrome. It has not been found to be routinely effective in the treatment of cancer pain.

Vagal nerve stimulation has been approved by the U.S. Food and Drug Administration for the treatment of intractable seizures and severe depression. The mechanism of action is not clear but is thought to be the result of afferent stimulation of higher cortical centers in the hypothalamus, amygdala, insular cortex, and cerebral cortex through the nucleus of the solitary tract. Stimulation of the left vagus nerve decreases seizure frequency by approximately 50% but rarely makes patients seizure free.[42]

Implantable Pumps

Implantable pumps are used for the treatment of chronic pain and spasticity. An intrathecal catheter is inserted into the lumber spinal canal and a trial infusion used to gauge response. Many patients with cancer pain will respond favorably to intrathecal administration of narcotics through a programmable pump. Baclofen is the agent of choice for the treatment of spasticity with this modality.

Destructive Lesions

Ablative lesioning of the CNS for the treatment of pain, movement disorders, epilepsy, and psychiatric diseases has a long history. Before the advent of antipsychotic drugs, the most efficient way of curing and controlling some patients with severe psychiatric disease was thought to be institutionalization and psychosurgery. Before the development of the technologies described earlier, lesioning of different pathways in the brain and spinal cord was the only method for treating patients with chronic pain and movement disorders. Even though neuroaugmentive procedures and drug infusion technology have replaced many of the neuroablative procedures formerly in widespread use, a few ablative procedures still retain their clinical usefulness.

Dorsal root entry zone lesions are particularly useful for patients with deafferentation pain related to brachial plexus injury and, to a lesser extent, patients with spinal cord injury who have so-called end zone pain. In these conditions, deafferentation of the spinothalamic tract neurons results in spontaneous firing and the sensation of pain. The procedure creates lesions of the dorsal horn of the affected levels using a thermocouple probe. Extension of this concept has been applied to the caudal nucleus of the trigeminal nerve for the treatment of facial pain syndromes.

Myelotomy has traditionally been used in the treatment of bilateral cancer pain. It involves sectioning of the anterior commissure at and above the involved levels, which interrupts pain fibers on their way to the contralateral spinothalamic tract. A modified technique that interrupts only the median raphe of the dorsal columns has been described.[43] This presumably interrupts the second-order visceral pain pathway demonstrated to travel up the mammalian dorsal funiculus.[44]

Cordotomy involves lesioning of the anterolateral quadrant of the spinal cord at cervical levels, thereby eliminating input from the spinothalamic tract on the contralateral side of the body. Historically, it was most useful in the treatment of unilateral cancer pain. Bilateral lesioning increases the risk for neurologically mediated sleep apnea (Ondine's curse). It can be performed percutaneously or as an open procedure.

Sympathectomy involves surgical interruption of the sympathetic chain at the high thoracic or lumbar level. A variety of endoscopic, thoracoscopic, radiofrequency, and open techniques are used. It is primarily used in patients with hyperhidrosis, sympathetically mediated pain, causalgia, chronic regional pain syndrome, and Raynaud disease.

Nerve block or neurectomy uses local anesthetic, sometimes with corticosteroids, which can be injected into the tissues surrounding a peripheral nerve, blocking conductivity and relieving pain. This can result in a long-lasting effect but typically is short-lived. Neurolytic agents (phenol or absolute alcohol) can also be used. Nerves can also be surgically divided or interrupted by radiofrequency techniques. There is a significant risk for recurrence with ablative neurectomy. Local nerve blocks are generally used in diagnostic procedures but can be repeated as necessary for the relief of pain. Ablative neurectomy is usually reserved for short-term relief in patients with a poor prognosis and short life expectancy.

Epilepsy

Epilepsy is not a distinct clinical entity with an identifiable cause but rather a complex collection of disorders of the brain that all share seizures as part of the complex. Seizures are classified as partial, generalized, or unclassified. Partial seizures are simple (consciousness not impaired) or complex (consciousness impaired). Generalized seizures are convulsive or nonconvulsive. Incidence rates in developed countries (40 to 70/100,000) are lower than those in developing countries (100 to 190/100,000). Approximately 20% to 40% of patients with seizures do not respond to anticonvulsant therapy. Failure to respond to three anticonvulsant medications prompts referral to a center specializing in epilepsy evaluation and treatment, and approximately 1.33% to 4.50% of those patients are candidates for surgical intervention.[45]

The goal of the workup of the patient who is a potential candidate for the surgical treatment of epilepsy is to identify the cortical area responsible for the onset of the seizure. When the radiographic workup (MRI, CT, or both) reveals an obvious lesion causing the seizure (e.g., tumor, vascular malformation), the treatment is relatively straightforward and involves removal of the lesion. In other cases, the offending lesion is not as obvious on imaging, and intensive and often invasive monitoring is necessary to determine the epileptogenic focus. It is also important to determine language dominance and areas of the brain that are functionally abnormal during the interictal period. Noninvasive techniques that have become more widely available and better characterized include magnetoencephalography, positron emission tomography, single-photon emission CT, and functional MRI. Invasive modalities used in the evaluation of patients for seizure surgery include the Wada test for language dominance, stereotactically implanted depth electrodes, implanted strip electrodes, and implanted grid electrodes (Fig. 67-21). Any or all of these techniques may be useful in brain mapping. It has long been possible to map critical speech and limb movement areas in awake, locally anesthetized craniotomy patients at the time of seizure focus resection.

On the basis of the information obtained in a noninvasive workup, the patient may be taken to surgery. Dominant hemisphere lesions are often operated on with the patient awake to allow intraoperative confirmatory brain mapping. This is accomplished by stimulating the cortex and observing and monitoring the patient's response, looking for speech arrest, anomia, or limb weakness or numbness. The most common surgical procedures performed for epilepsy are anterior temporal lobectomy, focal cortical resection, multiple subpial transection, hemispherectomy, and corpus callosotomy.

Anterior temporal lobectomy is the most common operation for seizures. An entirely unilateral interictal focus is the ideal indication (Fig. 67-22). The anterior temporal lobe, anterior hippocampus, and amygdala are excised. If the epileptogenic focus is not completely excised, the patient may continue to experience intractable seizures. If too much temporal lobe is resected, it can result in a contralateral superior quadrantanopia or, in dominant hemisphere lesions, speech and language dysfunction.

Focal cortical resection is usually performed in the frontal cortex. The results are more variable than those with temporal lobectomy.

Multiple subpial transection is used in more eloquent areas of the brain and involves making cortical incisions perpendicular to the surface of the gyrus in question. This presumably preserves descending fibers and function while interrupting spread of any epileptogenic activity within the cortical mantel itself.

Corpus callosotomy is used to prevent the rapid spread of seizures rather than to eliminate the focus. It is primarily useful in seizures that suddenly generalize, resulting in atonic drop attacks, as in Lennox-Gastaut syndrome.

Hemispherectomy is usually reserved for young children with seizures restricted to one hemisphere but threatening the good hemisphere by secondary effects of repeated seizures, as in Rasmussen syndrome. There is usually some abnormality of cellular migration. In the past, the entire cortex was removed, leaving the

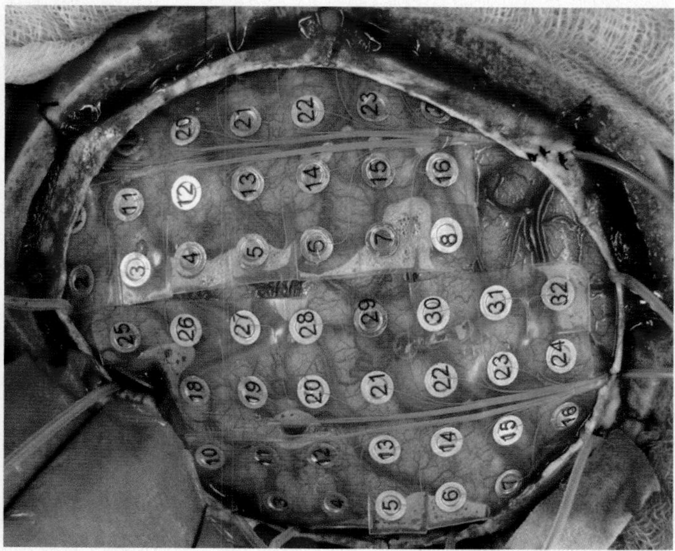

FIGURE 67-21 Intraoperative view of grid electrode placement for epilepsy surgery. (Courtesy Dr. Nitin Tandon, University of Texas, Houston.)

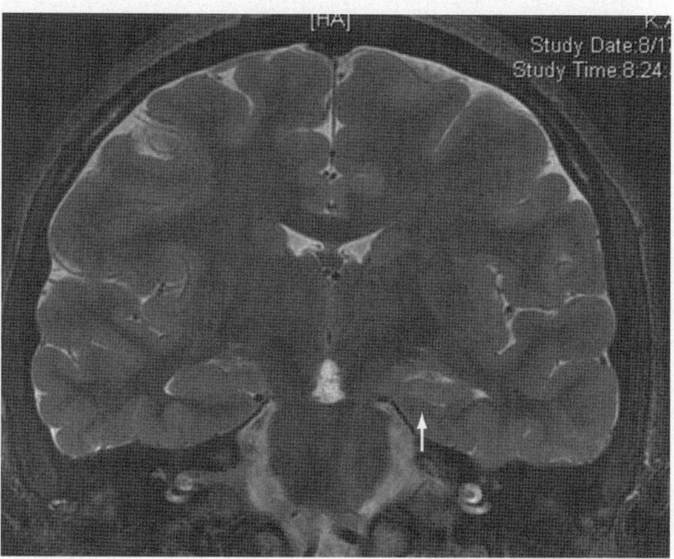

FIGURE 67-22 T2-weighted coronal MRI study shows gliosis and atrophy of the left mesial temporal structure *(arrow)*.

basal ganglia intact. Even though there was a significant decrease in seizure activity, the procedure led to a high complication rate, with ex vacuo brain shifts. A newer technique now involves preservation of portions of the cortex and its blood supply while disconnecting them from the rest of the brain by extensive undercutting of the adjacent white matter.[46]

Trigeminal Neuralgia

Trigeminal neuralgia affects approximately 4 in 100,000 individuals and is characterized by brief episodes of severe, lancinating pain in one or more of the three divisions of the trigeminal nerve, usually V2 and V3. Patients often describe that it is precipitated by touch or extremes of temperature. In extreme cases, a patient may refuse to eat or shave to avoid triggering the severe jolts of pain. Sensation usually remains intact, and significant numbness or jaw weakness leads to suspicion of a compressive mass lesion, such as tumor. Often, patients are referred with an already established diagnosis. It is reassuring if the patient has responded at some point to carbamazepine or an appropriate medication. MRI is used to rule out posterior fossa tumors and multiple sclerosis, which can present with related symptoms. Most patients respond to the oral administration of carbamazepine. Baclofen and gabapentin also have some clinical usefulness in medical treatment. The most common mechanism is presumed to be related to vascular compression of the fifth cranial nerve as it enters the brainstem (Fig. 67-23). With aging, the arteries elongate and can then begin to loop against the cranial nerves. At its entry to the pons, the fifth nerve has lost its peripheral nerve supportive architecture, the reticulin and mesenchymal elements that toughen the nerve more peripherally. Focal pulsatile pressure of the artery against this vulnerable part of the nerve results in ephaptic transmission from large myelinated fibers to small myelinated (A delta) and unmyelinated fibers.

Surgical therapy is usually reserved for patients who fail to respond to medical treatment. Microvascular decompression involves a small suboccipital craniotomy for microsurgical exploration of the dorsal root entry zone of the trigeminal nerve on the affected side. The offending vessel, usually the superior cerebellar artery, is then dissected off the nerve, and a barrier (Teflon or polyvinyl alcohol sponge) is placed between the vessel and nerve to prevent continued pulsatile focal compression. In especially favorable situations, the offending artery can be dissected free to loop away from the nerve, without the need for padding. A small sling of arterial patch graft material can also be sewn to hold the artery loop away from the nerve.

Percutaneous trigeminal rhizotomy techniques generally involve radiofrequency heat lesioning of the trigeminal ganglion, glycerol injection (Fig. 67-24) into the spinal fluid of Meckel cave (which causes an osmotic damage preferentially to the smaller pain-carrying nerve fibers), or mechanical trauma to the nerve or ganglion by transient inflation of a No. 4 Fogarty catheter balloon. Each method has its proponents along with advantages and disadvantages.

SRS has been described for the treatment of trigeminal neuralgia.[37] Although initial results have been encouraging, long-term efficacy has yet to be determined.

HYDROCEPHALUS

Hydrocephalus denotes an excessive accumulation of the CSF in the intracranial compartment. The accumulation of fluid can be in either the intracerebral (ventricular) or extracerebral (subarachnoid spaces and cisterns) compartment.

Normally there exists a fine balance between the CSF production by the choroid plexus and the absorption at the arachnoid villi along the superior sagittal sinuses. The CSF production has been found to be 0.33 mL/kg/hr (20 mL/hr). Almost all the fluid produced is absorbed within 8 hours. Any imbalance in this will lead to excessive accumulation of CSF, causing hydrocephalus. Thus, it can be due to excessive production, decreased absorption, or obstruction anywhere in the pathways.

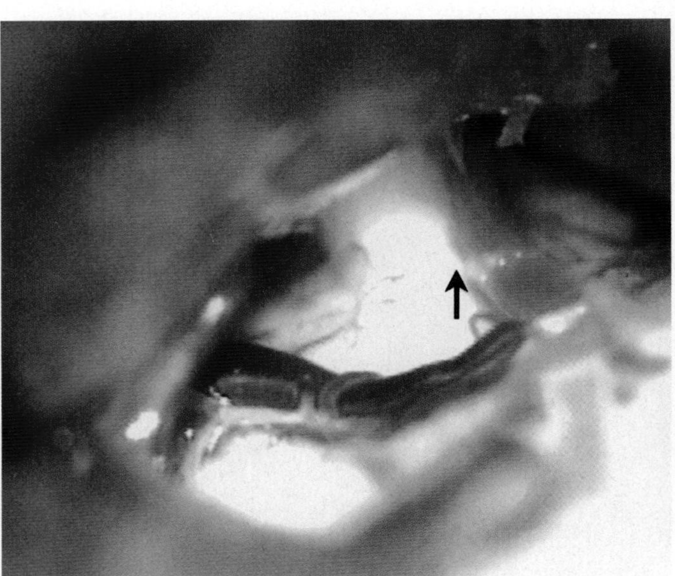

FIGURE 67-23 Intraoperative photograph of a patient with typical trigeminal neuralgia. The left trigeminal nerve is compressed superiorly by an arterial branch of the superior cerebellar artery *(arrow)*.

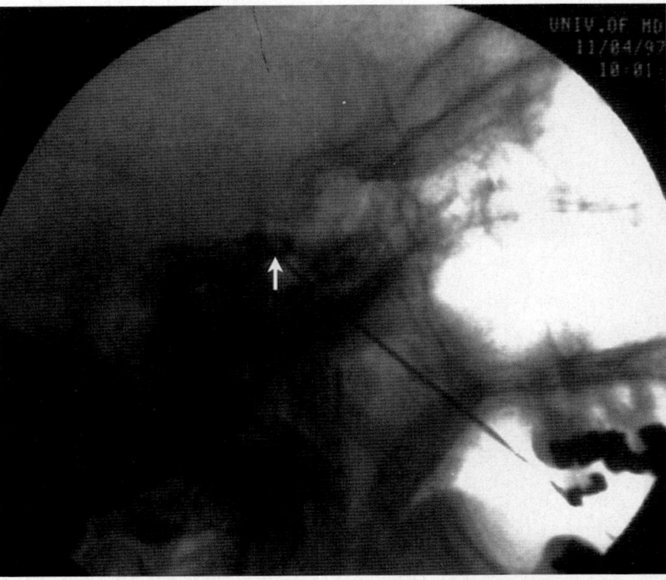

FIGURE 67-24 Lateral skull film in a patient undergoing glycerol rhizotomy for typical trigeminal neuralgia. A 20-gauge spinal needle is directed to the foramen ovale and nonionic contrast agent is injected to outline the trigeminal ganglion *(arrow)*.

Communicating and obstructive hydrocephalus. This distinction was made several decades ago to explain whether the obstructed ventricular CSF communicated with the subarachnoid CSF. In obstructive hydrocephalus, the obstruction is at or proximal to the fourth ventricular outlet foramina (foramen of Magendie and Luschka). However, if the obstruction is beyond the fourth ventricular outlet foramina (cisterns or arachnoid granulations), it is classified as communicating hydrocephalus. Common examples of obstructive hydrocephalus are aqueductal stenosis and hydrocephalus associated with tumors. When the term was initially coined, it took into account the findings of the ventriculogram and pneumoencephalogram. However, with the arrival of CT and MRI, in most cases, these investigations are no longer necessary, and the terms *communicating* and *obstructive* were no longer clinically important. However, as we will see later, the advent of endoscopic third ventriculostomy has generated renewed interest in these terms.

Acute and chronic hydrocephalus. Hydrocephalus developing within days or a few weeks (e.g., hydrocephalus due to tumor) is manifested with rapid progression of symptoms known as acute hydrocephalus. It requires early attention and treatment. On the other hand, CSF accumulation during months (or even years) presents with subtle signs of memory impairment, walking difficulty, or urinary incontinence and is termed chronic hydrocephalus. A classic example of chronic hydrocephalus is normal-pressure hydrocephalus, which is seen usually in the geriatric population. At times, chronic hydrocephalus can present acutely because of a change in the pathophysiologic mechanism of the CSF absorption or flow.

Congenital and acquired hydrocephalus. Hydrocephalus present at birth is known as congenital hydrocephalus. At times, congenital hydrocephalus is apparent a few weeks or months after birth, even though the process started while the child was in utero. Although congenital hydrocephalus is commonly obstructive in nature, it can be communicating, as seen in intrauterine toxoplasmosis or cytomegalovirus infections. In acquired hydrocephalus, the pathologic process starts after birth and includes post-traumatic hydrocephalus, hydrocephalus associated with tumors, and normal-pressure hydrocephalus.

Hydrocephalus ex vacuo or compensatory hydrocephalus. Here the ventricles enlarge compensatory to overall shrinking of the brain tissue. This can mislead an inexperienced physician to diagnose hydrocephalus, whereas really the enlargement of the ventricles is due to the shrinkage of the brain tissue. This is commonly seen in advanced age with brain atrophy, after diffuse head injury or stroke, and with various neurodegenerative conditions. The most important condition that is usually confused with hydrocephalus ex vacuo is normal-pressure hydrocephalus, unfortunately also seen in the geriatric age group.

Porencephaly. Porencephaly (or porencephalic cyst) commonly refers to a condition in which a focal brain substance has suffered some loss of volume (e.g., stroke, postsurgical change in volume) leading to collection of CSF in the cavity. Porencephalic cyst is usually differentiated from hydrocephalus ex vacuo by its localized nature.

Arrested hydrocephalus. This represents a condition in which the ventricles are large with the patient having no significant symptoms to require a surgical procedure. However, this term should be used with caution as it is well known that these patients may develop symptoms during a prolonged period or may present acutely after a precipitating event like minor trauma or infection that alters the CSF dynamics.

Clinical Features of Hydrocephalus

In hydrocephalus, CSF retained inside the cranial compartment results in increased ICP and dilation of ventricles, causing compression of the adjacent brain. The symptoms differ considerably in different age groups. In infants, a thin and relatively nonrigid skull allows an overall cranial expansion, whereas in older children and adults, the rigid fused skull prevents its enlargement. Considering this, in *infantile hydrocephalus,* either the infant is born with a large head or the head abnormally grows during the first few months of life. The anterior fontanelle is usually full; it may or may not be bulging. In extreme cases, a relatively higher ICP causes the blood to be diverted from the intracranial to the extracranial compartment, resulting is prominent and dilated scalp veins. A late feature is the classic "sunset sign" manifested with downward deviation of the eyeballs (like a setting sun). This is due to compression of the midbrain tectum by the posterior part of the dilated third ventricle. In later stages, the child will be irritable and fussy and may not accept feeds. There may be associated vomiting. There usually is no associated fever or diarrhea. Lethargy, drowsiness, and, in extreme cases, lapsing into the comatose state will follow if the child remains untreated.

In *older children and adults,* fusion of the skull bones no longer permits the cranium to enlarge. The enlarging ventricles result in raised ICP and cause compression of the adjacent brain. There are two common modes of presentation: rapidly progressive hydrocephalus and chronic hydrocephalus. In *rapidly progressive hydrocephalus,* the increasing accumulation of CSF increases the ICP, presenting with new-onset headache and vomiting. These are commonly known as features of raised ICP. If untreated, these symptoms worsen and blurring of vision is often experienced. In patients with long-standing raised pressure, papilledema can result in secondary optic atrophy. If still untreated, drowsiness and progression to coma follow. Focal neurologic deficits are not experienced, although walking difficulty or the sensation of "giving away" at the knees can happen.

In *chronic hydrocephalus,* the CSF accumulates more slowly, thus gradually compressing the brain. This type of presentation is predominantly seen in the elderly age group, although it can happen in younger age. The patient becomes progressively dull, apathetic, and uninvolved with the surroundings. Memory impairment for recent events is commonly seen; the remote memory is usually well preserved. A short stepped gait with a wide stance with unsteadiness is evident. Urinary incontinence and urgency are also common findings. Although it is uncertain why most of these patients do not have significant headache, it is assumed that slow dilation of the ventricles compresses the adjacent brain to accommodate the CSF without causing raised pressure.

Although seizures due to hydrocephalus are uncommon, they may be caused by the process that initiates the hydrocephalus. A phenomenon seen in late stages of untreated hydrocephalus is known as cerebellar fits or hydrocephalic attacks. Preceded by progressively severe headache, the patient lapses into transient sudden unconsciousness associated with decerebrate or decorticate response, downward deviation of the eyeballs, and respiratory distress. The recovery is usually spontaneous. These episodes recur until CSF diversion is instituted. This is due to acute transtentorial herniation resulting in compression of brainstem. The condition is associated with significant morbidity and can be uniformly fatal unless prompt CSF drainage is instituted. This is a true medical emergency, and under no circumstances should the treatment be delayed. The survivors often develop permanent hemianopia due to occipital infarcts resulting from compression of the posterior cerebral arteries against the tentorial edge during the herniation.

Investigations

The common investigation used for diagnosis of hydrocephalus is a CT scan often accompanied by an MRI scan. Cranial ultrasound evaluation has been used predominantly in the newborn and infants with open fontanelle. The CT scan shows dilated ventricles and often indicates the pathologic process and the site of obstruction. The ventricular system dilates proximal to the obstruction, whereas the CSF pathways distal to the obstruction are not visualized well. As all the ventricles are usually well visualized on the CT scan, one can infer the level of obstruction from the CT scan. Most tumor disease can be well visualized also on the CT scan. However, the CT scan cannot delineate the exact site or nature of the obstruction. Probably the greatest utility of the CT scan in managing hydrocephalus has been in assessing patients with shunt malfunction. An obstructed shunt commonly *but not always* leads to dilation of the ventricles, which can be easily identified on the CT scan. In addition, the radiopaque shunt tube is well visualized on the CT scan.

MRI has been the imaging modality of choice in newly diagnosed hydrocephalus. The ability of MRI to obtain images in three different planes (coronal, sagittal, and axial) has been of considerable value in diagnosing the exact cause of hydrocephalus and the site of obstruction. With a properly done MRI study, the site of obstruction can be well visualized in most patients with obstructive hydrocephalus (Fig. 67-25). This is of considerable importance as small tumors or cysts causing hydrocephalus can be visualized, and when these are removed, the hydrocephalus can be relieved. Also, MRI is considered essential before considering endoscopic third ventriculostomy and aqueductoplasty, which are exciting alternatives in the management of hydrocephalus, and in assessing the effectiveness of endoscopic third ventriculostomy during the follow-up.

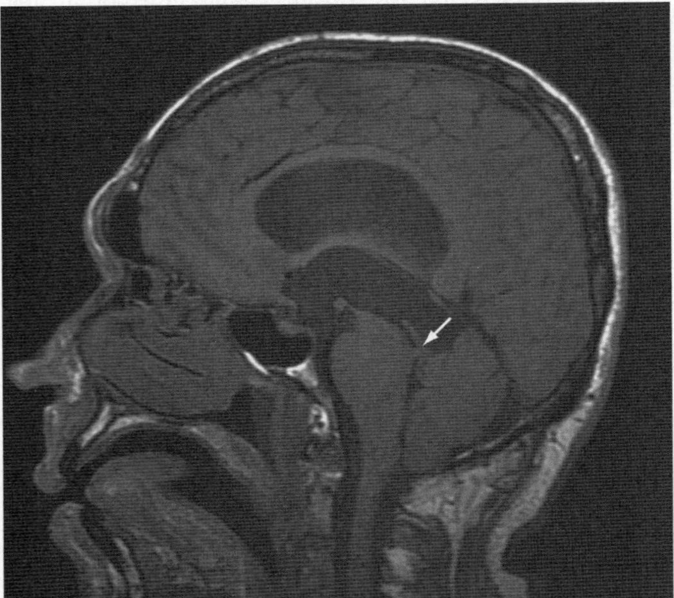

FIGURE 67-25 T1-weighted sagittal MRI scan of patient with gross obstructive hydrocephalus caused by aqueductal stenosis *(arrow)*.

Treatment

The ultimate goal in the treatment of hydrocephalus is to reverse the neurologic damage caused by the raised ICP. Reconstitution of the cerebral mantle to allow normal intellectual development and avoidance of shunt dependency should be considered additional goals in management. In a previous study, cerebral mantle thickness of 2.8 cm or more was found to be associated with good outcome. It was also found that the cortical mantle reconstitution was not satisfactory if the treatment was delayed for more than 5 months.

Surgery for hydrocephalus involves diversion of the accumulated CSF by reopening the obstruction to allow the CSF to flow in its natural pathway, creation of a diversion before the obstruction to let the CSF drain into the intracranial pathways distal to the block, or diversion of the CSF into another cavity to have it absorbed into the bloodstream. Examples of reopening of the obstructed pathway include endoscopic aqueductoplasty and excision of the tumor causing hydrocephalus, whereas endoscopic third ventriculostomy falls into the second category. Ventriculoperitoneal shunts, which have been the mainstay of treatment in hydrocephalus, belong to the third group.

Although shunts have been the mainstay of treatment for several decades, endoscopic procedures have become more popular. These include endoscopic third ventriculostomy, endoscopic aqueductoplasty, and endoscopic aqueductal stenting. Although these alternative procedures appear exciting, strict criteria for selection of patients are required.

It is often difficult for a pediatric neurosurgeon to decide if the patient with ventriculomegaly needs a CSF diversion procedure. Imaging studies and invasive procedures like ICP monitoring have not been able to reliably predict the patients who are likely to develop intellectual deterioration as a result of hydrocephalus. Children younger than 5 years with moderate to severe hydrocephalus without any symptoms often are considered for a CSF diversion procedure as it is often difficult to assess the intellectual development in this age group. It is also considered that mere attainment of developmental milestones is not indicative of adequate development of intellectual function. Insertion of a shunt protects these children against effects of persistent ventriculomegaly and ascertains an optimal environment for future intellectual development. However, children older than 5 years and adults with asymptomatic ventriculomegaly often are closely watched with frequent assessment of intellectual development before a shunt insertion is considered.

Medical management has not proved to be very useful in hydrocephalus. It is often used as a temporary measure and in conjunction with the surgical management. Acetazolamide has been commonly used as it has been found to reduce the CSF production. However, the benefits are minimal, and high doses of the drug causing metabolic acidosis are required to achieve the effect.

Cerebrospinal Fluid Shunts

Although initially the concept of shunt appeared to be simple, it has proved to be more complex over the years. Being purely mechanical devices, shunts have not been able to effectively manage the complexity of the CSF dynamics associated with hydrocephalus. Basically, CSF shunts are tubes with valves that drain the CSF out from one compartment to another. The shunt contains three parts: the ventricular end, the valve complex, and the distal end. The distal end is usually named after the organ where it is inserted (e.g., in ventriculoperitoneal shunts, it is known as the peritoneal end; in ventriculoatrial shunts, the atrial end). Antisiphon devices preventing the CSF siphoning effect (which can result in overdrainage when the person is erect) are often included in the valve complex.

Shunt malfunction, infection, overdrainage, brain injury, seizures, and distal complications are the major complications associated with shunts. Of these, shunt malfunction is the predominant complication of shunt procedures. The malfunction is so common that sometimes it is not considered a complication but a part of natural history of shunt surgery. Of the several predisposing factors for shunt malfunction, age has been found to be a significant factor. In a multicenter study involving 38 neurosurgical centers and 773 patients, 29% of the shunts failed in the first year, requiring reoperation. About half of the shunts (47%) inserted in children younger than 6 months failed compared with 14% of shunts that failed in children older than 6 months. It was also found that shunts placed as emergency procedures failed more often (34%) than shunts placed electively (29%).[47] Shunt components also can become disconnected at the junctions and migrate to either of the cavities. In the event that the distal end of the tube migrates into the abdominal cavity, the tube is usually left behind. It usually freely floats in the abdominal cavity and does not precipitate bowel obstruction. Some neurosurgeons, however, would prefer to remove the abdominal catheter with laparoscopic devices. As in the subcutaneous tissue, the catheter has to be removed if the shunt is infected or with other abdominal infection.

The incidence of shunt infection, the second significant complication, ranges between 4% and 7%. The common organisms include *Staphylococcus epidermidis* (50% to 60%), *Staphylococcus aureus* (20% to 30%), gram-negative bacilli, and *Propionibacterium* species. Most of the shunt infections occur within 3 months of insertion, with a small percentage occurring as late as 6 months. Most of the shunts are inoculated at the time of insertion, although uncommonly it can be a hematogenous spread. *S. epidermidis* forms a biofilm and adheres to the shunt tube, which protects the bacteria against orally or intravenously administered antibiotics. The colonization permits the bacteria to stay quiescent for weeks or sometimes a few months before the infection is manifested. The clinical picture depends on the severity of the infection, the time of diagnosis, and the site of infection. Shunt infections can be infection of the shunt tube either in its subcutaneous track or in the wound (wound infection), infection of the CSF spaces (meningitis) or ventricles (ventriculitis), or infection of the abdominal space (peritonitis). Early subcutaneous infections are manifested with low-grade fever, redness along the shunt tube, and purulent discharge from the incision. Wound breakage and exposure of the shunt tube can occur. Later, as the infection involves the CSF and ventricles, it may be associated with decreased sensorium, seizures, and neurologic deficits. If the infection involves the abdominal cavity, it can present with features of peritonitis. A high degree of suspicion for infection in the postoperative period is the key for an early diagnosis. The possibility of a shunt infection should be considered in any patient with a shunt; however, on the contrary, occasionally only the shunt is related to the fever. The diagnosis is confirmed by shunt tap and CSF culture. Complete removal of the shunt tube is recommended with reinsertion of a new shunt once the infection clears. The incidence of shunt infection is reduced by use of catheters impregnated with rifampicin and clindamycin, which are effective against the gram-positive bacteria.

It is imperative that the general surgeon be acquainted with the *distal complications of ventriculoperitoneal shunts* as they may be encountered not infrequently in general surgical practice. The two common distal complications are ascites and pseudoperitoneal cyst. Reduction in the absorption of the CSF causing generalized fluid accumulation in the peritoneal cavity results in *ascites.* The common causes include reduced absorbing surface (premature infants), high protein content of the CSF, peritoneal scarring from previous infections, and elevated venous pressure. Although usually sterile, ascites can be infected in as high as 15% of cases. Not uncommonly, ascites can present as shunt malfunction due to backpressure and reduction in CSF drainage from the intracranial compartment. In infected ascites, there will be associated signs of local and systemic infection. The shunt is usually removed and placed in another cavity like the atrium. In infected ascites, the shunt is externalized and is replaced into an alternative site (atrium, pleura) after the infection is cleared. In premature infants with a reduced absorptive surface, it is not uncommon to find that the peritoneum often functions satisfactorily after a few years.

In *pseudoperitoneal cyst,* there is a loculated pocket of CSF in the peritoneal cavity walled off by bowel and omental tissue. This results in a cystic fluid collection, which often presents as a mass in the abdomen. Most of the time, this is associated with a low-grade infection of either the shunt tube or the abdomen or a previous infection or surgery of the abdominal cavity that has resulted in scarring and reduced absorption. This is usually easy to diagnose as the shunt tube is seen lying inside a fluid filled cavity in the abdomen. The occurrence of pseudoperitoneal cyst often presents with shunt malfunction with abdominal distention. The surgery involves exteriorizing the shunt tube, treating the infection if present, and then reinserting the shunt either in another compartment (i.e., converting it into a ventriculoatrial shunt) or in another place in the abdominal cavity. Surprisingly, the second approach works in most of the patients.

The distinction between ascites and pseudoperitoneal cyst is significant as pseudoperitoneal cyst is associated with a higher infection rate than ascites. In addition, in ascites, the shunt needs to be removed from the peritoneal cavity as the entire peritoneal cavity has not been able to absorb fluid; in pseudoperitoneal cyst, it usually suffices to remove the shunt and to replace it in another region of the peritoneal cavity.

Alternatives to Shunting

Advances in endoscopic neurosurgery have opened several alternative options to placement of shunts. Endoscopic third ventriculostomy, endoscopic aqueductoplasty, endoscopic aqueductal stenting, and endoscopic septostomy are available as alternatives to shunt procedures. However, all these alternative procedures are currently effective only in certain types of obstructive hydrocephalus, and not all procedures are effective in all types of obstructive hydrocephalus. In *aqueductoplasty,* the obstructed aqueduct is recanalized with the help of a 3 Fr Fogarty catheter under direct endoscopic vision, whereas *in aqueductal stenting,* a stent is placed in the aqueduct to prevent further reclosure. The stent is usually attached to a subcutaneous reservoir to prevent its migration. Both these procedures are indicated only in obstructive hydrocephalus with short-segment aqueductal stenosis where an adequate reopening can be performed without risking injury to the adjacent midbrain. *Endoscopic third ventriculostomy* involves creation of a fenestration in the floor of the third ventricle to bypass the obstructed CSF into the basal cisterns. Endoscopic third ventriculostomy (Fig. 67-26) is effective in obstructive hydrocephalus associated with obstruction at or beyond the aqueduct (aqueductal stenosis, tumors of fourth ventricle, and

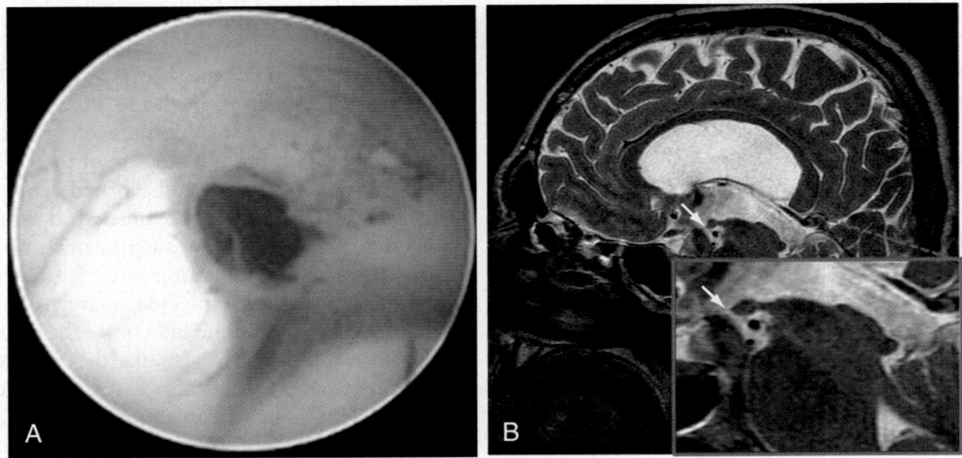

FIGURE 67-26 **A,** Endoscopic view of the third ventricular floor after the third ventriculostomy. **B,** Follow-up MRI scan 4 years later demonstrating good flow at the fenestration site *(arrow)*.

fourth ventricular outlet obstruction). However, the effectiveness of these alternative procedures varies with age; the procedure is least efficacious in neonates (20% to 40% success rate) and 80% effective in older children and adults. Although the cause for this is uncertain, failure of absorption of CSF by the normal absorptive process (arachnoid granulations) has been the most common explanation.

Special Types of Hydrocephalus

Two common but distinct types of hydrocephalus seen in two very different age groups need further mention: benign external hydrocephalus, seen in infants; and normal-pressure hydrocephalus, seen in the geriatric population.

Benign external hydrocephalus. Seen exclusively in children, this is often mistaken for subdural hematoma or hygromas in infants. A relative immaturity of the arachnoid villi, which fail to absorb the required amount of CSF into the bloodstream, is postulated as the cause. With the obstruction at the level of the arachnoid villi, a communicating type of hydrocephalus develops. The child usually presents with a macrocrania with mild delayed milestones. The CT or the MRI scan usually reveals evidence of a prominent ventricular system with prominent subarachnoid spaces. Usually a self-limited condition, this is corrected by 2 years of age and uncommonly may require a subduroperitoneal shunt.

Normal-pressure hydrocephalus. This is another form of communicating hydrocephalus seen in elderly patients, with excessive accumulation of the CSF in the intracranial compartment leading to dilation of ventricles and the subarachnoid spaces. The clinical picture is classic of an elderly patient who presents with the triad of gait ataxia, dementia, and urinary incontinence.

Unfortunately, most of the patients with normal-pressure hydrocephalus are either underdiagnosed or misdiagnosed in clinical practice. Although the exact cause is not known, reduction in absorption of CSF by the arachnoid granulations has been postulated. It is also known in these patients that the brain parenchyma is less stiff (more compliant) to allow it to be compressed by the developing ventriculomegaly and thus does not result in increased ICP; but this is not always true as intermittent increases in ICP have been detected by several investigators. However, hydrocephalus developing after several primary insults (trauma, infection, and previous neurosurgical procedures) can present as normal-pressure hydrocephalus. The diagnosis is usually a combination of clinical features associated with prominent ventricles seen on CT and MRI with no other abnormalities. A therapeutic trial of CSF drainage has been used in patients suspected of normal-pressure hydrocephalus to predict response to treatment. Diversion of CSF, commonly by a ventriculoperitoneal shunt or from the lumbar space by a lumboperitoneal shunt, has been the mainstay of treatment. Variable pressure programmable shunt valves have been found to be extremely useful in regulating the flow to avoid complications of overdrainage while optimizing the overall outcome. An early diagnosis and treatment are associated with higher success rates, justifying an early recognition of this treatable form of dementia.

Shunts and Intra-Abdominal Surgeries

Patients with ventriculoperitoneal shunts often require other surgical procedures. It is not uncommon for the neurosurgeon to be asked about the safety of the procedure before it is contemplated. The circumstances can be broadly divided into the following: surgeries on patients in whom the shunt tube is not exposed; and surgeries on patients in whom the shunt tube will be exposed or may be exposed.

Surgeries on patients in whom the shunt tube is not exposed. These procedures should not cause any mechanical obstruction to the shunt. However, the risk of shunt infection is a potential concern, and the risk is higher if the surgery is performed through a contaminated field with a predisposition to bacterial dissemination (lower gastrointestinal tract; e.g., colonoscopy, colorectal biopsy).

Surgeries on patients in whom the shunt tube will be exposed or may be exposed. This group presents some concerns for the functioning of the shunt in the postoperative period as the shunt tube is expected to be exposed during the procedure. Exposure of the shunt tube also increases the likelihood of shunt infection due to either direct contamination or dissemination during the surgery. Such procedures include abdominal surgeries with an indwelling ventriculoperitoneal shunt and thoracic surgeries with a ventriculopleural shunt. Preoperative discussion with a neurosurgeon and the presence of the neurosurgeon in the operating room is considered ideal under such circumstances.

Shunts and Appendicitis

Appendicitis is a common condition in the general population and it is not uncommon to find patients with shunts attending the emergency department with a diagnosis of appendicitis. Diagnostic errors are not uncommon and often can cause delay in initiating appropriate treatment. Uncomplicated appendicitis often can be effectively managed by the protocols followed conventionally. If the shunt tube is seen during the appendectomy, this often can be managed by replacing the catheter away from the operative site. These patients need to be followed up closely to assess for any chronic abdominal infection that may present several weeks after the initial surgery. Patients with ruptured appendicitis most often need their shunt to be externalized with intravenous antibiotics, and once the peritoneal infection is settled, another site in the peritoneal cavity can be chosen to insert the shunt. Alternatively, a ventriculoatrial or a ventriculopleural shunt can be considered.

Hernia, Hydrocele, and Shunts

It is not uncommon to see an infant with a shunt developing hydrocele or hernia a few months after insertion of the shunt. A prior study reported 15% of shunted children developing inguinal hernias, and hydroceles were seen in another 6% of boys. Persistence of the peritoneovaginal canal causes the CSF to track from the peritoneal cavity into the scrotum, thus causing hydrocele. If the communication is large, bowel loops can migrate into the scrotal sac, which results in inguinal hernia. The collection is usually lax and supple. Uncommonly, the distal end of the shunt tube can migrate into the sac. In most cases, these spontaneously reduce in size and do not need any surgical intervention. However, tense or growing collections need a repositioning of the catheter with correction of the defect.

PEDIATRIC NEUROSURGERY

Neurosurgical conditions in infants and children are significantly different from those in adults. Congenital malformations, hydrocephalus, neoplasms, and pediatric trauma are the major neurosurgical disorders commonly encountered by a pediatric neurosurgeon. Hydrocephalus, pediatric brain tumors, and pediatric trauma have been discussed earlier. Here, we discuss the following congenital malformations: spinal and cranial dysraphism, Chiari malformation, and craniosynostosis.

Spinal Dysraphism

Of the three embryonic layers (ectoderm, mesoderm, and endoderm), the neural structures develop from the ectoderm. The neural tube forms from the neural placode at approximately 21 days of gestation. Failure of the neural tube to form results in neural tube defects, such as spinal dysraphism. Neural tube defects have already formed by the time pregnancy is diagnosed; thus, prevention of these defects by the administration of folic acid has to commence before 21 days of gestation.

The spinal dysraphic state can be classified as spina bifida aperta (open defects, usually apparent) and spina bifida occulta (closed defects, commonly missed by an untrained observer; Fig. 67-27). The most common forms of spina bifida aperta are myelomeningocele and meningocele. The common forms of the spinal bifida occulta include simple spina bifida occulta, spinal dermal sinus, lipomyelomeningocele, diastematomyelia, and tethered spinal cord. Some of these may coexist with each other.

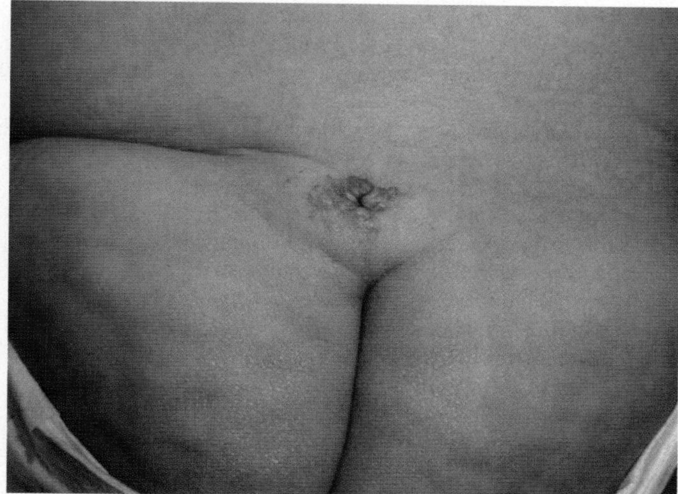

FIGURE 67-27 Child with lumbar cutaneous hemangioma. This often accompanies an underlying spina bifida (spina bifida occulta) during the clinical evaluation.

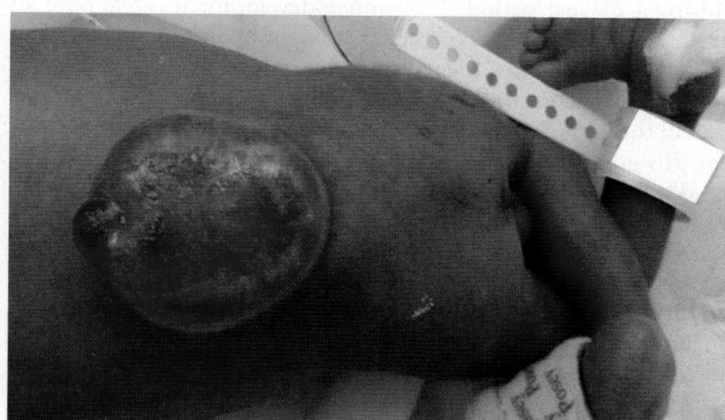

FIGURE 67-28 Myelomeningocele in a neonate. Note the deformity of the lower limbs.

Spina Bifida Aperta

Myelomeningocele. Myelomeningocele, the most common type of spina bifida aperta, has an average incidence of 1/1000 live births. In this disorder, there is protrusion of a varying amount of spinal neural tissue outside the spinal canal confines. It has been associated with folate deficiency in the mother; intake of folate during pregnancy has reduced the incidence considerably. There is a deficiency of the skin, muscle, and bone elements, with the open neural placode exposed anywhere from the thoracic to the sacral level (Fig. 67-28). Varying degrees of motor and sensory deficits with autonomic (bladder and bowel) dysfunction accompany this defect. The degree of the deficit is directly related to the level of the defect, which often determines the child's ability to ambulate in the future. Hence, thoracic defects have the highest incidence of weakness, and sacral defects often have only bladder involvement. Hydrocephalus is also present in 80% of patients and sometimes is manifested after surgical closure of the defect. The incidence of hydrocephalus is also directly related to the level of the defect; thus, thoracic defects have the highest incidence and low sacral defects the lowest. The other significant association is the Chiari II malformation, which occurs in 90% to 95% of cases.

Associated brain anomalies include corpus callosal anomalies, fused tectal plates, and thalamic fusion.

Surgical closure of the myelomeningocele is undertaken within 24 to 48 hours of birth to avoid CNS infection (e.g., meningitis, ventriculitis). Before the closure, the child is usually nursed prone, with the defect covered by moist sterile dressings, and given prophylactic antibiotics. All exposed neural tissue is considered viable unless otherwise proven. During the closure, adequate care is taken to separate the neural tissue (placode) from the cutaneous element to prevent an inclusion dermoid. The dura is closed in a watertight fashion and is supplemented by myofascial closure. Skin grafts often are required for large defects. The child is usually also nursed in the prone position in the postoperative period. Ventricular shunts, if indicated, are placed concurrently with myelomeningocele closure or at a later date. Of children with myelomeningocele, 60% to 70% will ultimately require a shunt insertion, whereas only 15% to 30% of children will require a Chiari decompression.

Serum and amniotic fluid α-fetoprotein screening and prenatal ultrasound have been significantly helpful in diagnosing open neural tube defects in the prenatal period. Prenatal counseling should include a discussion of overall long-term mortality (24% during a 25-year period),[48] cognitive development (75% have an IQ higher than 80 if adequately treated for hydrocephalus), future ambulatory assistance (depending on the level of the defect), and presence of incontinence. A 20% to 65% incidence of latex allergies in this population has led to universal latex allergy precautions for this group of children.

Meningocele. Here, there is a protrusion of dura and arachnoid outside the confines of the spinal canal, with neural tissue remaining within the spinal canal confines. Because no neural elements are present, there are no associated neural deficits and repair is simpler. Meningoceles occur less commonly than myelomeningoceles and can be at any location in the spine, although they are most common in the lumbar region.

Spinal Bifida Occulta

Simple spina bifida occulta. A posterior lumbar bone defect is often present in 5% to 10% of the normal population, without any symptoms or deficits. However, association of other markers, such as a tuft of hair, cutaneous hemangioma, or sinus track, should be viewed with suspicion and warrants further investigation.

Dermal sinus. Occurrence of a dermal sinus track from the skin to the spinal subarachnoid space is often associated with a cutaneous dimple or pit. These are most common in the lumbosacral region but can be seen in the cervical and thoracic regions. Although initially asymptomatic, it can cause ascending infection or be symptomatic, with tethering of the cord. It may be associated with intraspinal inclusion tumors, such as dermoids. MRI is helpful for assessing the course of the track and its termination. The track is usually excised surgically, with care taken to untether the cord.

Diastematomyelia. In diastematomyelia, the spinal cord is split into two hemicords, often by a bone or fibrous band that tethers the cord, preventing its free movement and ascent. It is often associated with a hairy patch on the back at the defect level. This needs to be repaired surgically.

Lipomyelomeningocele. In lipomyelomeningocele, there is a varying amount of fatty tissue in the spinal cord and in the spinal canal tethering the cord. Often associated with a large dural defect, these are complex congenital anomalies. Associated neurologic deficits, although uncommon at birth, usually develop later because of the tethering. Almost all lipomyelomeningoceles have a well-developed skin cover, which allows these children to be operated on electively at a later date. The relatively high incidence of postsurgical neurologic deficits (16% to 47%) in otherwise neurologically intact patients has triggered a controversy about the appropriate timing for the surgery; some favor early surgery, and others consider surgery only when the child has developed deficits.

Cranial Dysraphism

Cranial dysraphism includes encephalocele, meningocele, and cranial dermal sinus. The encephalocele can be in the cranial vault or cranial base. The occipital encephalocele is the most common, followed by anterior encephalocele and then basal encephalocele. Encephaloceles may be associated with other developmental anomalies, such as polydactyly, retinal dysplasia, microphthalmia, and orofacial clefts. Cranial vault encephaloceles present with an observable swelling at birth and have brain tissue and blood vessels contained in the sac. Although the brain tissue is thought to be dysplastic, large encephaloceles often contain functional brain. The usual surgical treatment is excision and repair of the defect in the first few days of life. Cranial expansion may be required for patients with functional brain tissue in the sac. The outcome is generally directly proportional to the amount of neural tissue in the sac, with poorer outcomes seen in encephaloceles with a large amount of brain tissue. Basal encephaloceles present with a CSF leak from the nose or ear or as a polyp.

Chiari Malformation

Abnormal descent of the cerebellar tonsils below the level of the foramen magnum is known as a Chiari malformation. A descent of one tonsil of more than 5 mm or a 3-mm descent with associated syringohydromyelia is suggestive of Chiari malformation. Often, the tonsils are peg shaped and associated with crowding of the craniocervical subarachnoid space. Usually, they are classified as Chiari I, II, and III malformations. These are grouped together, but there is a significant difference in cause among these three types. An isolated descent of the tonsils below the rim of the foramen magnum without any spina bifida is known as Chiari I malformation. Chiari II is invariably associated with open spina bifida and has several other diagnostic features, such as descent of the brainstem and fourth ventricle into the upper spinal canal. In the uncommon Chiari type III malformation, there is an associated high cervical encephalocele containing herniated cerebellar and brainstem tissue. We limit the discussion here to the most common types, Chiari I and II malformations.

Chiari I Malformation

Descent of the cerebellar tonsils more than 5 mm below the rim of the foramen magnum is considered Chiari malformation. The 5-mm classification is somewhat arbitrary because many have tonsillar descent and are asymptomatic. The descended tonsils are usually peg shaped, and the descent is associated with crowding of the soft tissue, obstructing CSF flow (Fig. 67-29). There may or may not be associated syringomyelia. Occipital headache, precipitated or aggravated by maneuvers that increase the intrathoracic pressure (e.g., cough, headaches), is typical. There may be associated tingling or numbness in the extremities and impairment of joint position. In patients with advanced compression, cavitation of the spinal cord (syringomyelia) can occur and can be associated with wasting and weakness of the extremities, scolio-

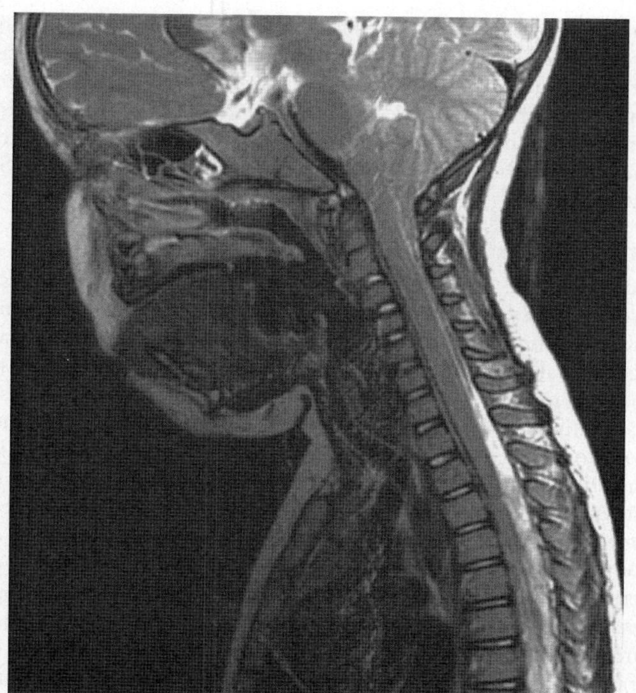

FIGURE 67-29 T2-weighted sagittal MRI scan of a child with a significant type I Chiari malformation. Note the tonsillar descent below the rim of foramen magnum.

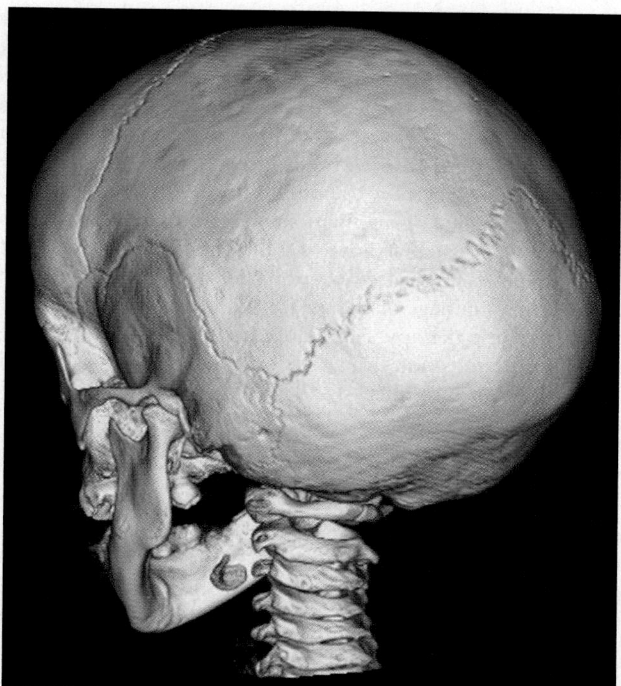

FIGURE 67-30 Three-dimensional reconstruction CT scan of a child with sagittal synostosis. The coronal and lambdoid sutures are well visualized.

sis, and varying degrees of sensory impairment. Coexistent hydrocephalus is seen in 10% of cases.

The aim of surgery is to decompress the region of the foramen magnum and to establish CSF flow. Removal of the rim of the foramen magnum and posterior arch of C1 and duraplasty are the most commonly performed procedures. Some also decompress the cerebellar tonsils. Associated hydrocephalus requires ventriculoperitoneal shunt placement or an endoscopic third ventriculostomy. Rescarring is a concern during follow-up and may require repeated surgery.

Chiari II Malformation

Chiari II malformation is characterized by elongation and caudal displacement of the brainstem and cerebellar tonsils and by association with myelomeningocele. Hydrocephalus is common and syrinx occurs frequently. Although it is a common accompaniment of myelomeningocele, surgery is reserved for children who are symptomatic with lower cranial nerve paresis, weakness, respiratory distress, or syrinx.

Craniosynostosis

Craniosynostosis involves premature fusion of the cranial sutures. This results in restricted growth of the skull bones at the involved suture and compensatory growth at the adjacent patent sutures, causing disfigurement of the cranial shape. In multisutural synostosis, restriction of the cranial growth at various sutures can cause impairment of growth of the developing brain. The incidence of nonsyndromic craniosynostosis varies from 0.25 to 0.6/1000 live births. The most common suture involved is sagittal suture (50% to 60%), followed by coronal suture (30% to 35%), metopic suture (5%), and lambdoid suture (2%). Lambdoid suture synostosis has to be distinguished from positional plagiocephaly, which is common and does not require surgical intervention. Genetic patterns are found in 8% of patients with isolated coronal synostosis and 2% of those with sagittal synostosis. However, more complex disorders, such as Crouzon, Apert, and Pfeiffer syndromes, have a genetic predisposition. The clinical picture is recognized by the abnormal skull shape associated with each sutural fusion—sagittal, elongated skull, or scaphocephaly; coronal, brachycephaly; and metopic, trigonocephaly—and is confirmed by skull radiographs and CT scans. Three-dimensional reconstruction of the calvaria is often beneficial (Fig. 67-30). Surgical correction involves a wide suturectomy and placement in a cranial remodeling helmet in children younger than 4 months and a craniotomy and cranial vault reconstruction in older children. In recent years, simple suturectomies have been performed in children younger than 6 months under endoscopic guidance with a small incision.[49] Patients with coronal craniosynostosis will usually require advancement of the orbital rim in addition to the cranial remodeling.

CENTRAL NERVOUS SYSTEM INFECTIONS

Broadly, CNS infections can be grouped as intracranial infections and spinal infections. The intracranial infections can occur in the epidural space (epidural abscess), in the subdural space (subdural empyema), in the subarachnoid space (meningitis), intracerebrally (cerebral abscess), or in the ventricles (ventriculitis).

Intracranial Infections

Cranial Epidural Abscess

As there is no preexisting epidural space, in epidural abscess, the pus essentially dissects itself in the potential epidural space between the dura and the bone. Cranial epidural abscess accounts for about 2% of all intracranial infections. Epidural abscess is commonly located either in the frontal region associated with frontal sinusitis and osteomyelitis or in the temporal region associated with mastoiditis and chronic ear infection. It can also be seen with nontreated or poorly treated compound depressed skull fractures. Clinically, there is associated local swelling, erythema, and tenderness with signs of localized or systemic infection. The infection, which is contained by the dura if it extends intradurally, can lead to development of meningitis and neurologic deterioration. Cranial CT scan usually shows the infection with osteomyelitis. The treatment is surgical evacuation, débridement of the osteomyelitic bone, drainage of the adjacent infected sinuses, and prolonged antibiotic therapy. A cranioplasty may be required in the future after the infection heals. The outcome is usually good with low morbidity or mortality.

Subdural Empyema

Collection of pus in the subdural space is termed subdural empyema. Usually seen in older children and young adults, it is most commonly related to contiguous spread from the paranasal sinuses or ear infection. Alternatively, infection can enter by retrograde thrombophlebitis of the veins communicating between the mucosal veins of the infected sinuses and dural venous sinuses or by hematogenous spread. About 60% of subdural empyemas occur from the frontal or ethmoid sinuses and about 20% from the inner ear infections. The infection can be on the cerebral convexities, in the hemispheric fissure, or over the tentorium.

Patients with subdural empyema can present with fever, meningeal signs, headache, seizures, focal neurologic deficits, and altered mental status. The most significant complication is cortical venous thrombosis leading to cerebral infarction. It is often heralded by seizures and rapid clinical deterioration. Diagnosis is made by noting presence of a subdural fluid collection adjacent to a known focus of sinus infection. The margins of the collection often enhance with contrast material. Appropriate treatment includes prompt institution of surgical drainage with antibiotic therapy. Anticonvulsants are indicated even in the absence of seizures as there is high risk of seizures. Steroids are often administered with antibiotic to cover life-threatening situations. The overall prognosis depends on the extent of infection, the neurologic status at the time of diagnosis, the association of cortical venous thrombosis, and the response of infection to treatment. The overall outcome has been as high as 82% of patients who underwent combined medical and surgical management. Craniotomy with evacuation of the pus has better overall outcome than burr hole evacuation.

Meningitis

Acute bacterial meningitis is an infection of the subarachnoid spaces and meninges. Symptoms and signs include fever, malaise, altered mental status, neck stiffness, and headache. These result from leptomeningeal irritation and increased ICP. The causative organism varies with the patient's age. Neonatal meningitis is caused by group B streptococcus, *Escherichia coli,* or *Listeria* spp. infection. Late neonatal meningitis can be caused by any of these organisms as well as by staphylococci or *Pseudomonas aeruginosa.* In children, *Streptococcus pneumoniae* (pneumococcus) and *Neisseria meningitidis* (meningococcus) are the most common causative organisms. In the past, *Haemophilus influenzae* was a common cause of meningitis in children, but its prevalence has decreased secondary to vaccination. Pneumococci and meningococci are the most common causative organisms in adults. Treatment consists of prompt CSF culture and immediate IV administration of antibiotics. Altered mental status secondary to communicating hydrocephalus may necessitate placement of an external ventricular drain and eventual placement of a ventriculoperitoneal shunt once the CSF is sterilized. Recurrent episodes of bacterial meningitis prompt investigation into abnormal communication between the CNS and the exterior environment (dermal sinus or CSF fistula).

Brain Abscess

Accumulation of pus in the cerebral tissue (cerebral abscess) usually is seen in children and young adults. About 25% of children with brain abscess have congenital heart disease with tetralogy of Fallot. Contiguous spread of infection from paranasal sinuses, middle ear, or mastoid is the most common cause, accounting for about 50% of all cases. Hematogenous dissemination from lungs or other parts of the body (dental caries, subacute bacterial endocarditis, diverticulitis) accounts for about 25% of patients. In about 20% of cases, the cause is undetermined. Frontal abscesses along the orbital base are often the result of contiguous spread from the frontal sinuses, whereas temporal or cerebellar abscesses are otogenic in origin. Cardiac malformations with polycythemia resulting in increased blood viscosity, sluggish circulation, and cerebral infarction predispose to development of brain abscess. Brain abscesses can be solitary or multiple. Causative organisms are extremely varied and include aerobic and anaerobic organisms, fungi, and uncommonly parasites.

Abscesses are manifested with signs and symptoms related to a rapidly expanding mass lesion with often subtle signs of infection. Patients can present with headache, nausea and vomiting, seizures, focal neurologic deficit, and altered mental status. Features of infection are present in around 60% of patients. Contrast-enhanced CT and MRI reveal a ring enhancing lesion, usually at the gray-white interface, with surrounding edema (Fig. 67-31).

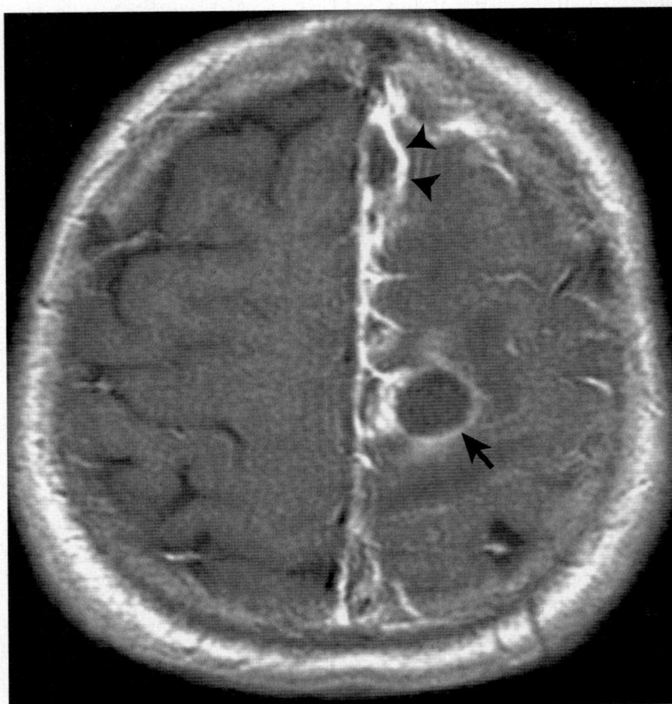

FIGURE 67-31 Brain abscess *(arrow)*, with an area of frontal subdural empyema in the convexity *(arrowheads)*.

This can be confused with glioblastoma multiforme or metastatic tumor. Diffusion-weighted imaging (abscesses are hyperintense) and magnetic resonance spectroscopy (elevated lactate, low choline peaks) can distinguish between the abscess and tumor disease. Acute deterioration of patients can occur when the abscess ruptures into the ventricle or subarachnoid space, with resultant ventriculitis or meningitis. Principles of treatment revolve around accurate identification of the causative organism, relief of mass effect, administration of appropriate antibiotic therapy, and treatment of the underlying cause. Prophylactic anticonvulsants are usually indicated, and steroids often can be given with antibiotic cover. Controversy exists as to whether surgical excision or aspiration of the abscess yields better results. The overall morbidity and mortality depend on the neurologic status at the time of diagnosis.

Ventriculitis

Infection of the ventricles is usually a result of spread of infection from either a ruptured cerebral abscess or other intracranial infection. Shunt infections are the most common cause of ventriculitis. Systemically administered antibiotics often do not penetrate significantly into the ventricle spaces. Drainage of infected CSF with intraventricular instillation of vancomycin, gentamicin, or amikacin (depending on the organisms and sensitivity) is often necessary for adequate treatment of the infection.

Postoperative Infections

Infections of the CNS occurring after neurosurgical procedures are typically caused by staphylococci. Enteric organisms and pseudomonal and streptococcal pathogens can also be problematic. As with any infection, treatment involves identification of the causative organism and appropriate antibiotic administration. Postoperative abscesses are addressed with drainage, surgery, or both, as dictated by the clinical situation.

Post-Traumatic Meningitis

Meningeal infection after head injury is typically related to CSF fistula. Most post-traumatic fistulas stop spontaneously within days of injury. The incidence of meningitis increases if a leak persists for longer than 7 days. Clinically obvious leaks are manifested as CSF rhinorrhea or otorrhea. The prophylactic antibiotic treatment of CSF fistula is controversial and needs to be tailored to the clinical situation. A persistent post-traumatic CSF fistula is addressed surgically to prevent the risks associated with recurrent bouts of meningitis.

Spinal Infections

Spinal infections can be grouped into those affecting the bone (vertebral osteomyelitis), disc space (discitis), and epidural space (spinal epidural abscess). On occasion, infectious processes can involve more than one or even all three.

Vertebral Osteomyelitis

Osteomyelitis of the bone is generally seen in IV drug users, diabetic patients, hemodialysis patients, and older adults. The causative organism is usually *S. aureus,* and spread is hematogenous, although postoperative infections are also seen. These infections can and do affect the integrity of the bone, resulting in collapse. This in turn can result in pain and neurologic compromise. Treatment consists of organism identification, appropriate long-term antibiotics, and maintenance of anatomic spinal alignment, with or without surgical intervention.

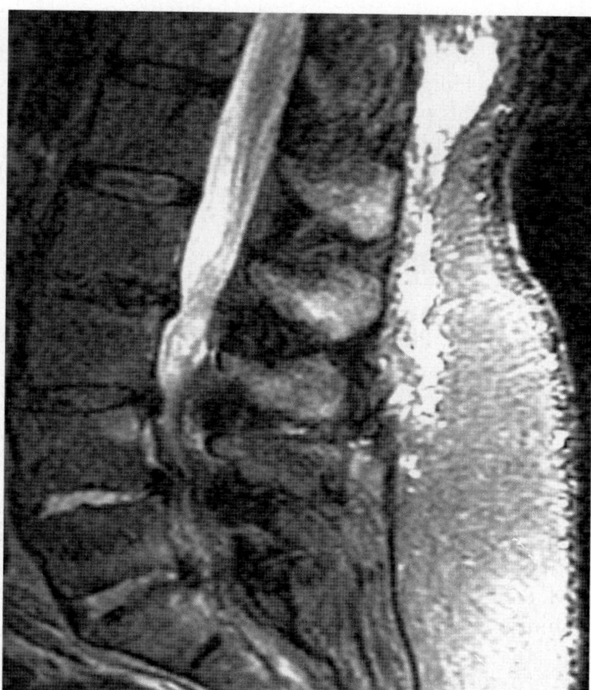

FIGURE 67-32 MRI with gadolinium short T1 inversion recovery sequence revealing disc osteomyelitis in the L4-5 and L5-S1 interspaces suggestive of an infectious process.

Discitis

Infection of the disc (discitis) often occurs concomitantly with osteomyelitis and is seen in the same population of patients. Fever, back pain, and an elevated sedimentation rate or C-reactive protein level are often seen. The white blood cell count may or may not be elevated. It may occur spontaneously or postoperatively. Treatment may or may not be surgical. Long-term antibiotic therapy is usually indicated (Fig. 67-32).

Spinal Epidural Abscess

This usually occurs in the setting of an infectious process elsewhere in the body. Spread occurs hematogenously or by direct extension. Patients present initially with localized back pain and possible radiculopathy. Spinal cord compromise can follow rapidly, with paraplegia or quadriplegia. Predisposing factors are the same as those for osteomyelitis and discitis. Diagnosis is made with contrast-enhanced MRI. When spinal cord compression is evident, surgery is usually performed for decompression and diagnosis. Spinal epidural abscess can sometimes be managed medically, with close neurologic observation and imaging studies. This is usually reserved for cases in which the causative organism is known, the abscess is small, and there is no neurologic compromise. As in all fields of medicine, treatment must be tailored to the individual patient.

Acquired Immunodeficiency Syndrome

The most common CNS opportunistic infection in patients with AIDS is toxoplasmosis caused by *Toxoplasma gondii.* The lesions usually present with ring enhancement on contrast-enhanced imaging studies and are usually in the basal ganglia. They may be solitary or multiple. Primary CNS lymphoma occurs in approximately 10% of AIDS patients and presents as an irregularly enhancing mass (target lesion). Progressive multifocal leukoencephalopathy presents with hypodense, nonenhancing white matter lesions. Fungal abscess and viral encephalopathy are not uncommon in this population of patients. Even though the incidence of CNS opportunistic infections has decreased with the widespread use of highly active antiretroviral therapy, the treatment of these problems remains a challenge.

SELECTED REFERENCES

Benzel EC: *Spine surgery: Techniques, complication avoidance, and management*, ed 2, Philadelphia, 2004, Churchill Livingstone.

A nice review of spine surgery and biomechanics in two volumes; thorough explanation and details from an authority in the field.

Brain Trauma Foundation; American Association of Neurological Surgeons; Congress of Neurological Surgeons; Joint Section on Neurotrauma and Critical Care, AANS/CNS, Bratton SL, Chestnut RM, et al: Guidelines for the management of severe traumatic brain injury. *J Neurotrauma* 24:S1–S106, 2007.

Accepted guidelines commonly used in the management of patients with traumatic brain injury.

Guidelines for the management of acute cervical spine and spinal cord injuries. *Neurosurgery* 72:S1–S259, 2013.

Recently published guidelines concerning the care and management of patients with traumatic injuries of the cervical spine and spinal cord.

Quinones-Hinojosa A: *Schmidek and Sweet: Operative neurosurgical techniques*, ed 6, Philadelphia, 2012, Elsevier Saunders.

Atlas of neurosurgical techniques.

Winn RH, editor: *Youmans neurological surgery*, ed 6, Philadelphia, 2011, Elsevier Saunders.

A traditional resource for neurosurgery residents and faculty.

REFERENCES

1. Stern WE: Intracranial fluid dynamics: The relationship of intracranial pressure to the Monro-Kellie doctrine and the reliability of pressure assessment. *J R Coll Surg Edinb* 9:18–36, 1963.
2. Rangel-Castilla L, Gasco J, Nauta HJ, et al: Cerebral pressure autoregulation in traumatic brain injury. *Neurosurg Focus* 25:E7, 2008.
3. Bratton SL, Chestnut RM, Ghajar J, et al: Guidelines for the management of severe traumatic brain injury. IX. Cerebral perfusion thresholds. *J Neurotrauma* 24(Suppl 1):S59–S64, 2007.
4. Lundberg N: Continuous recording and control of ventricular fluid pressure in neurosurgical practice. *Acta Psychiatr Scand Suppl* 36:1–193, 1960.
5. Ondra SL, Troupp H, George ED, et al: The natural history of symptomatic arteriovenous malformations of the brain: A 24-year follow-up assessment. *J Neurosurg* 73:387–391, 1990.
6. Spetzler RF, Martin NA: A proposed grading system for arteriovenous malformations. *J Neurosurg* 65:476–483, 1986.
7. McCormick WF, Hardman JM, Boulter TR: Vascular malformations ("angiomas") of the brain, with special reference to those occurring in the posterior fossa. *J Neurosurg* 28:241–251, 1968.
8. Ong CK, Wang LL, Parkinson RJ, et al: Onyx embolisation of cavernous sinus dural arteriovenous fistula via direct percutaneous transorbital puncture. *J Med Imaging Radiat Oncol* 53:291–295, 2009.
9. Winn HR, Richardson AE, Jane JA: The long-term prognosis in untreated cerebral aneurysms: I. The incidence of late hemorrhage in cerebral aneurysm: A 10-year evaluation of 364 patients. *Ann Neurol* 1:358–370, 1977.
10. Vajkoczy P, Meyer B, Weidauer S, et al: Clazosentan (AXV-034343), a selective endothelin A receptor antagonist, in the prevention of cerebral vasospasm following severe aneurysmal subarachnoid hemorrhage: Results of a randomized, double-blind, placebo-controlled, multicenter phase IIa study. *J Neurosurg* 103:9–17, 2005.
11. Kern M, Lam MM, Knuckey NW, et al: Statins may not protect against vasospasm in subarachnoid haemorrhage. *J Clin Neurosci* 16:527–530, 2009.
12. Wong GK, Poon WS, Chan MT, et al: Intravenous magnesium sulphate for aneurysmal subarachnoid hemorrhage (IMASH): A randomized, double-blinded, placebo-controlled, multicenter phase III trial. *Stroke* 41:921–926, 2010.
13. Molyneux A, Kerr R, Stratton I, et al: International Subarachnoid Aneurysm Trial (ISAT) of neurosurgical clipping versus endovascular coiling in 2143 patients with ruptured intracranial aneurysms: A randomised trial. *Lancet* 360:1267–1274, 2002.
14. Hunt WE, Hess RM: Surgical risk as related to time of intervention in the repair of intracranial aneurysms. *J Neurosurg* 28:14–20, 1968.
15. Report of World Federation of Neurological Surgeons Committee on a universal subarachnoid hemorrhage grading scale. *J Neurosurg* 68:985–986, 1988.
16. Fisher CM, Kistler JP, Davis JM: Relation of cerebral vasospasm to subarachnoid hemorrhage visualized by computerized tomographic scanning. *Neurosurgery* 6:1–9, 1980.
17. Kulcsar Z, Wetzel SG, Augsburger L, et al: Effect of flow diversion treatment on very small ruptured aneurysms. *Neurosurgery* 67:789–793, 2010.
18. Szikora I, Berentei Z, Kulcsar Z, et al: Treatment of intracranial aneurysms by functional reconstruction of the parent artery: The Budapest experience with the pipeline embolization device. *AJNR Am J Neuroradiol* 31:1139–1147, 2010.
19. Mendelow AD, Gregson BA, Fernandes HM, et al: Early surgery versus initial conservative treatment in patients with spontaneous supratentorial intracerebral haematomas in the International Surgical Trial in Intracerebral Haemorrhage (STICH): A randomised trial. *Lancet* 365:387–397, 2005.
20. Patchell RA: The management of brain metastases. *Cancer Treat Rev* 29:533–540, 2003.
21. Levin VA, Leibel SA, Gutin PH: Neoplasms of the central nervous system. In De Vita VT, Jr, Hellman S, Rosenberg SA, editors: *Cancer: Principles and practice of oncology,*

Philadelphia, 2001, Lippincott Williams & Wilkins, pp 2100–2160.
22. Gupta A, Shah A, Young RJ, et al: Imaging of brain tumors: Functional magnetic resonance imaging and diffusion tensor imaging. *Neuroimaging Clin N Am* 20:379–400, 2010.
23. Kew Y, Levin VA: Advances in gene therapy and immunotherapy for brain tumors. *Curr Opin Neurol* 16:665–670, 2003.
24. Louis DN, Ohgaki H, Wiestler OD, et al: The 2007 WHO classification of tumours of the central nervous system. *Acta Neuropathol* 114:97–109, 2007.
25. Simpson D: The recurrence of intracranial meningiomas after surgical treatment. *J Neurol Neurosurg Psychiatry* 20:22–39, 1957.
26. Jemal A, Tiwari RC, Murray T, et al: Cancer statistics, 2004. *CA Cancer J Clin* 54:8–29, 2004.
27. Gavrilovic IT, Posner JB: Brain metastases: Epidemiology and pathophysiology. *J Neurooncol* 75:5–14, 2005.
28. Sawaya R, Bindal R, Lang FE: Metastatic brain tumors. In Kaye AH, Laws ER, editors: *Brain tumors: An encyclopedic approach*, New York, 2001, Churchill Livingstone, pp 999–1026.
29. Hart MG, Grant R, Walker M, et al: Surgical resection and whole brain radiation therapy versus whole brain radiation therapy alone for single brain metastases. *Cochrane Database Syst Rev* (1):CD003292, 2005.
30. Kalkanis SN, Kondziolka D, Gaspar LE, et al: The role of surgical resection in the management of newly diagnosed brain metastases: A systematic review and evidence-based clinical practice guideline. *J Neurooncol* 96:33–43, 2010.
31. Iwadate Y, Namba H, Yamaura A: Significance of surgical resection for the treatment of multiple brain metastases. *Anticancer Res* 20:573–577, 2000.
32. Paek SH, Audu PB, Sperling MR, et al: Reevaluation of surgery for the treatment of brain metastases: Review of 208 patients with single or multiple brain metastases treated at one institution with modern neurosurgical techniques. *Neurosurgery* 56:1021–1034, discussion 1021-1034, 2005.
33. Muacevic A, Wowra B, Siefert A, et al: Microsurgery plus whole brain irradiation versus Gamma Knife surgery alone for treatment of single metastases to the brain: A randomized controlled multicentre phase III trial. *J Neurooncol* 87:299–307, 2008.
34. Brain Trauma Foundation; American Association of Neurological Surgeons; Congress of Neurological Surgeons; Joint Section on Neurotrauma and Critical Care, AANS/CNS, Bratton SL, Chestnut RM, et al: Guidelines for the management of severe traumatic brain injury. *J Neurotrauma* 24(Suppl 1):S1–S106, 2007.
35. Ogden AT, Mayer SA, Connolly ES, Jr: Hyperosmolar agents in neurosurgical practice: The evolving role of hypertonic saline. *Neurosurgery* 57:207–215, discussion 207–215, 2005.
36. Kakar V, Nagaria J, John Kirkpatrick P: The current status of decompressive craniectomy. *Br J Neurosurg* 23:147–157, 2009.
37. Kondziolka D, Lunsford LD, Flickinger JC, et al: Emerging indications in stereotactic radiosurgery. *Clin Neurosurg* 52:229–233, 2005.
38. Chang SD, Adler JR, Jr: Current treatment of patients with multiple brain metastases. *Neurosurg Focus* 9:e5, 2000.
39. Flickinger JC, Barker FG, 2nd: Clinical results: Radiosurgery and radiotherapy of cranial nerve schwannomas. *Neurosurg Clin N Am* 17:121–128, vi, 2006.
40. Kuo JS, Yu C, Petrovich Z, et al: The CyberKnife stereotactic radiosurgery system: Description, installation, and an initial evaluation of use and functionality. *Neurosurgery* 62(Suppl 2):785–789, 2008.
41. Romanelli P, Schaal DW, Adler JR: Image-guided radiosurgical ablation of intra- and extra-cranial lesions. *Technol Cancer Res Treat* 5:421–428, 2006.
42. Groves DA, Brown VJ: Vagal nerve stimulation: A review of its applications and potential mechanisms that mediate its clinical effects. *Neurosci Biobehav Rev* 29:493–500, 2005.
43. Nauta HJ, Soukup VM, Fabian RH, et al: Punctate midline myelotomy for the relief of visceral cancer pain. *J Neurosurg* 92:125–130, 2000.
44. Willis WD, Jr, Westlund KN: The role of the dorsal column pathway in visceral nociception. *Curr Pain Headache Rep* 5:20–26, 2001.
45. Zimmerman RS, Sirven JI: An overview of surgery for chronic seizures. *Mayo Clin Proc* 78:109–117, 2003.
46. Devlin AM, Cross JH, Harkness W, et al: Clinical outcomes of hemispherectomy for epilepsy in childhood and adolescence. *Brain* 126:556–566, 2003.
47. Di Rocco C, Marchese E, Velardi F: A survey of the first complication of newly implanted CSF shunt devices for the treatment of nontumoral hydrocephalus. Cooperative survey of the 1991-1992 Education Committee of the ISPN. *Childs Nerv Syst* 10:321–327, 1994.
48. Bowman RM, McLone DG, Grant JA, et al: Spina bifida outcome: A 25-year prospective. *Pediatr Neurosurg* 34:114–120, 2001.
49. Jimenez DF, Barone CM: Multiple-suture nonsyndromic craniosynostosis: Early and effective management using endoscopic techniques. *J Neurosurg Pediatr* 5:223–231, 2010.

68 CHAPTER

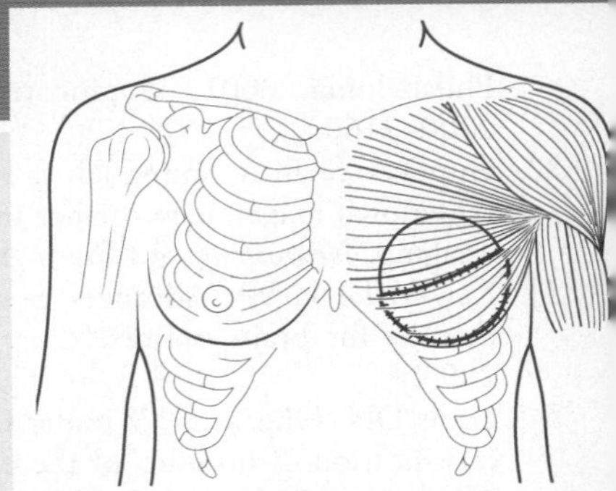

Plastic Surgery

Mary H. McGrath, Jason H. Pomerantz

OUTLINE

Challenged by complex clinical problems, the pace of innovation in plastic surgery has accelerated steadily during the past 30 years. The specialty benefits from the absence of anatomic or organ system boundaries and from the collaboration with other surgical specialists who discover new reconstructive and aesthetic challenges even as they make medical progress. With growing sophistication, plastic surgery has matured into areas of specialization, including surgery for congenital abnormalities, maxillofacial surgery, breast surgery, hand surgery, head and neck surgery, skin and soft tissue surgery, aesthetic surgery, body contouring, wound care, microsurgery, and burn care. Plastic surgeons, in a relatively small specialty, stay aware of innovations in each of these areas and are quick to adopt new ideas developed through the clinical and research experience of other plastic surgeons. With the breadth of exposure that this collaboration brings, it is not surprising that unique solutions for perplexing clinical problems sustain the momentum of innovation.

RECONSTRUCTIVE TECHNIQUES

The concept of a reconstructive ladder is used to guide surgical reconstruction. Ascending the rungs of the ladder represents moving from simple to complex reconstructive techniques in a systemized way that considers the requirements of the defect to be repaired. Direct closure is the simplest and most straightforward technique. This may be precluded by the size of the wound or consequences of wound tension at the closure site, including distortion of the surrounding tissue. In this case, a more complex closure technique, such as a skin graft that brings in additional tissue from a distant site, is required. A wound with exposed structures that do not accept a skin graft mandates a step up to a local flap for coverage. A local flap with no distant donor site may not be an option if the surrounding area is within the zone of injury, in which case a regional flap from an adjacent body region is needed. Microvascular free tissue transfer represents the most complex flap option and is usually the top rung on the reconstructive ladder.

When the concept of the reconstructive ladder is used, the triad of form, function, and safety is the basis for setting the reconstructive goals for any given defect. For example, in reconstructing the face, awareness of form would suggest a more complex technique, such as tissue expansion, instead of the simpler technique of skin grafting because it is optimal to restore with skin and soft tissue of the same thickness, texture, and color. For any specific reconstructive situation, this matrix of going from simple to complex, considering form and function and keeping safety paramount, provides direction.

Primary Wound Closure

Good suture technique starts with an incision with the scalpel at right angles to the skin and continues with careful handling of tissue to avoid devitalizing the skin margins, débridement of skin edges if needed, eversion of the wound margin, and precise approximation without tension. The skin edges need to be lined up at the same level, and wound edges should just touch each other. Postoperative edema is predictable and will create additional tension.

Minimizing tension is essential to reduce scarring. This can be done by using buried deep dermal and subdermal sutures to lessen tension on the skin sutures. It is also accomplished by aligning skin incisions along relaxed skin tension lines. These lines of minimal tension, also called natural skin lines, wrinkle lines, or lines of facial expression, run at right angles to the long axis of the underlying muscles. When underlying muscles contract, the lines of facial expression deepen. For example, transverse forehead furrows appear when the eyebrows are raised by the frontalis muscle, and if an incision is placed in one of these furrows, it will be under minimal tension and will heal with minimal scarring.

Skin Grafts

A skin graft is a segment of dermis and epidermis that is separated from its blood supply and donor site and transplanted to another recipient site on the body. Survival of the skin graft in the new site requires a vascularized wound recipient bed. Graftable beds with adequate blood supply include healthy soft tissues, periosteum, perichondrium, paratenon, and bone surface that is perforated to encourage granulation tissue growth. Poor graft surfaces with inadequate blood supply include exposed bone, cartilage, and tendon and fibrotic chronic granulation tissue. The wound must be free of infection and debris interposed as a barrier between the graft and bed.

Skin grafts are classified in the following manner: autograft, self; allograft, other person; homograft, same species; heterograft, different species. Partial-thickness skin grafts consist of the epidermis and a portion of the dermis and are called split-thickness skin grafts (STSGs). Full-thickness skin grafts (FTSGs) include the epidermis and entire dermis, with portions of the sweat glands, sebaceous glands, and hair follicles. The STSG is harvested with a dermatome, which is an air- or electric-powered instrument that can be adjusted for width and depth to cut uniformly thick grafts, usually in strips of 0.006 to 0.024 inch in thickness. The STSG can be meshed by cutting slits into the sheet of graft and expanding it, usually in a 1:1.5 or 1:2 ratio. Meshed grafts are useful when there is a paucity of available donor skin, the recipient bed is bumpy or convoluted, or the recipient bed is suboptimal, as with exudate. An STSG can be taken from anywhere on the body; donor site considerations include color, texture, thickness, amount of skin required, and scar visibility. The STSG takes readily on the recipient site, and the donor site reepithelializes quickly. Its disadvantages are contracture over time, abnormal pigmentation, and poor durability if subject to trauma. The FTSG is removed with a scalpel and is necessarily small in size because the donor site must be sutured closed. Containing skin appendages, the FTSG can grow hair and secrete sebum to lubricate the skin, has the color and texture of normal skin, and has the potential for growth. In general, FTSGs are taken from areas at which the skin is thin and can be spared without deformity, such as the upper eyelids, postauricular crease, supraclavicular area, hairless groin, or elbow crease. The greater thickness makes the FTSG more durable than the STSG, but this thickness also means that the graft take is not as predictable because more tissue must be revascularized from the recipient bed.

The take of either type of skin graft occurs in three phases:

Plasmatic circulation, also called serum imbibition, during the first 48 hours nourishes the graft with plasma exudate from host bed capillaries.

Revascularization starts after 48 hours with two processes. The primary is neovascularization, in which blood vessels grow from the recipient bed into the graft; and the secondary is inosculation, in which graft and host vessels form anastomoses.

Organization begins immediately after grafting with a fibrin layer at the graft-bed interface holding the graft in place. This is replaced by postgraft day 7 with fibroblasts; in general, grafts are securely adherent to the bed by days 10 to 14.

Sensibility returns to the graft over time, with reinnervation beginning at approximately 4 to 5 weeks and being completed by 12 to 24 months. Pain returns first, with light touch and temperature returning later.

The most common cause of skin graft failure is hematoma under the graft, where the blood clot is a barrier to contact of the graft and bed for revascularization. Similarly, shearing or movement of the graft on the bed will preclude revascularization and cause graft loss. Additional causes are infection, poor quality of the recipient bed, and characteristics of the graft itself, such as thickness or vascularity of the donor site. Dressings can prevent some impediments to graft take. A light pressure dressing minimizes the risk of fluid accumulation. A bolster or tie-over dressing left in place for 4 or 5 days improves survival by maintaining adherence of the graft to the bed, minimizing shearing, and preventing hematoma or seroma. A vacuum-assisted compression device can be placed on the grafted surface to stabilize the graft in place; this is especially useful for larger wounds with an irregular three-dimensional surface.

Skin grafts composed of tissue-cultured skin cells are used for the treatment of burns or other extensive skin wounds. Human epidermal cells in a single-cell suspension are grown in monolayers in vitro during a period of 3 to 6 weeks. Concerns with tissue-cultured skin are fragility, sensitivity to infection, length of time for cultivation, and potential risk of malignancy caused by mitogens present during culturing.

Skin Flap Surgery

A surgical flap consists of tissue that is moved from one part of the body to another with a vascular pedicle to maintain blood supply. The vascular pedicle may be kept intact, or it can be transected for microvascular anastomosis of the flap vessels to vessels at another site. Flap defines the tongue of tissue; pedicle is used to describe the base or stem with the vascular supply.

Skin-bearing flaps are classified according to three basic characteristics—composition, method of movement, and blood supply. Composition refers to the tissue contained within the flap, such as cutaneous, musculocutaneous, fasciocutaneous, osseocutaneous, and sensory flaps. The method of movement is local transfer, as with advancement or rotation flaps, or distant transfer, as with pedicle flaps from the abdomen to the perineum or microvascular free flaps.

With regard to blood supply, arteries perfusing the surgical flap reach the skin component in two basic ways. Musculocutaneous arteries travel perpendicularly through muscle to the overlying skin. Septocutaneous arteries arising from segmental or musculocutaneous vessels travel with intermuscular fascial septa to supply the overlying skin. With either of these patterns, the flap can have a random pattern, which means that it derives its blood supply from the dermal and subdermal vascular plexus of vessels supplied by perforating arteries. Alternatively, it can be an axial flap designed to include a named musculocutaneous or septocutaneous vessel running longitudinally along the axis of the flap to penetrate the overlying cutaneous circulation at multiple points along the course of the flap's length to provide greater length and reliability.

Skin Flaps

Local skin flaps contain tissue lying adjacent to the defect that usually matches the skin at the recipient site in color, texture, hair, and thickness. Flaps should be the same size and thickness as the defect and be designed to avoid distortion of local anatomic landmarks, such as the eyebrow or hairline. They can be planned so that the donor site can be closed directly and usually are elevated with incision lines placed in relaxed skin tension lines. Local flaps rely on the inherent elasticity of skin and are most useful in the older patient whose skin is looser. In some cases, the site from which the flap is raised is closed with a skin graft. Commonly used local skin flaps include the following:

Rotation flaps are semicircular flaps of skin and subcutaneous tissue that revolve in an arc around a pivot point to shift tissue in a circle.

Transposition flaps are rectangular or square and turn laterally to reach the defect.

Advancement flaps move directly forward and rely on skin elasticity to stretch and to fill a defect.

V-Y advancement flaps advance skin on each side of a V-shaped incision to close the wound with a Y-shaped closure.

Rhomboid flaps rely on the looseness of adjacent skin to transfer a rhomboid-shaped flap into a defect that has been converted into a similar rhomboid shape.

Z-plasty transposes two interdigitating triangular flaps without tension to use lateral skin to produce a gain in length along the direction of the common limb of the Z.

Failure of a skin flap usually involves necrosis of the most distal portion of the transferred tissue. This could be caused by a flap design in which the size of the flap exceeds its inherent vascular supply, or it could be a result of extrinsic mechanical compromise of the flap pedicle by pressure from a hematoma, compressive dressings, or twisting or kinking of the flap. Measures to optimize viability include proper flap design and avoidance of extrinsic pedicle compression, undue tension with wound closure, and venous congestion caused by excessive flap dependency.

Muscle and Musculocutaneous Flaps

Consideration of a muscle as a potential flap is possible because muscles have independent, intrinsic blood supply. The motor nerves of a muscle are accompanied by an arteriovenous system that often is the major source of blood supply to that muscle. This vascular pedicle may be a dominant one, capable of sustaining the entire muscle independently. A minor pedicle, regardless of the size of the vessel, is defined as one that maintains only a lesser portion of the muscle. Many muscles have multiple unrelated sources of blood supply so that each nourishes only a segment of the muscle, thus called segmental pedicles. Some muscles have both a dominant pedicle and segmental blood supply. One example is the latissimus dorsi muscle with a dominant pedicle, the thoracodorsal artery in the axilla, and additional segmental perforating branches from the intercostal and lumbar vessels posteriorly. In these muscles, the dominant pedicle can be ligated and the muscle moved on the secondary vessels as a reverse muscle flap.

Muscle flaps are classified according to their principal means of blood supply and the patterns of vascular anatomy (Fig. 68-1):

Type I: Single pedicle (e.g., gastrocnemius, tensor fascia lata)

Type II: Dominant pedicle with minor pedicles (e.g., gracilis, trapezius)

Type III: Dual dominant pedicles (e.g., gluteus maximus, serratus anterior)

Type IV: Segmental pedicles (e.g., sartorius, tibialis anterior)

Type V: Dominant pedicle, with secondary segmental pedicles (e.g., latissimus dorsi)

In terms of reliability of the vascular anatomy and usefulness as a flap, large muscles with a recognized dominant pedicle supplying most of a flap (types I, III, and V) are most useful. The territory of the pedicles in type II muscles may vary, and type IV muscles are useful only when smaller flaps are needed. Connections between regions within a given muscle supplied by more than one pedicle are through small-caliber choke vessels with bidirectional flow. An example of a flap depending on these choke vessels is the transverse rectus abdominis musculocutaneous (TRAM) flap, in which the superior epigastric pedicle alone can support the lower half of the muscle normally supplied by the inferior epigastric vessels below the watershed level at the umbilicus. In muscle, venous territories are in parallel with arterial vessels. This means that venous outflow is adjacent to and in a direction opposite from flow in the major arterial pedicles. In a pattern analogous to that of the bidirectional choke vessels, venous flow from one territory to another occurs through oscillating veins that are devoid of valves.

Compared with skin flaps, muscle flaps are less bulky, less stiff, and more malleable to conform to wounds with irregular three-dimensional contours. They have more robust blood supply and

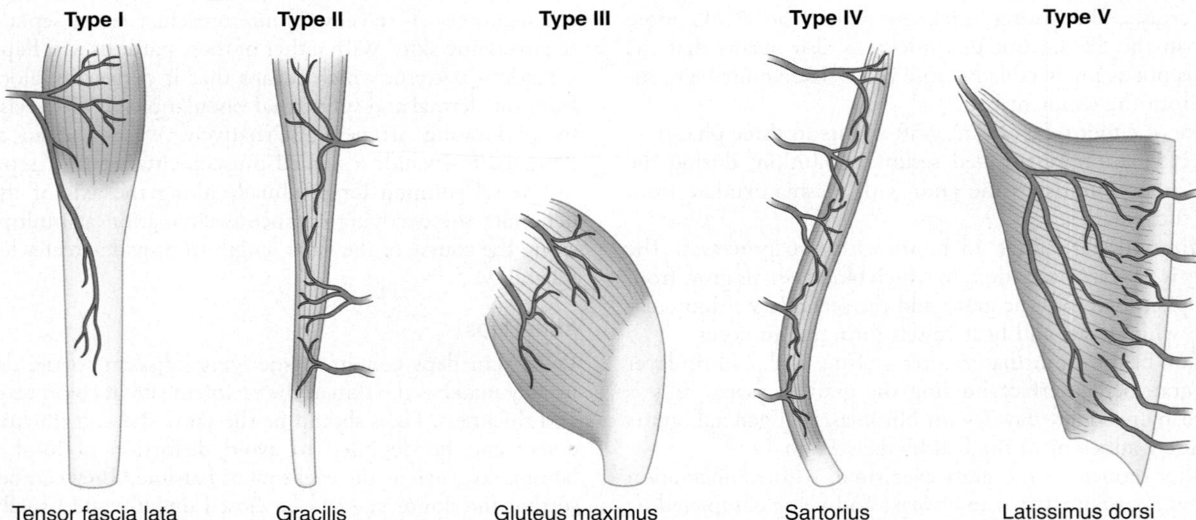

FIGURE 68-1 Classification of muscle and musculocutaneous flaps according to their vascular supply: type I, one vascular pedicle; type II, dominant pedicle and minor pedicles; type III, two dominant pedicles; type IV, segmental vascular pedicles; type V, one dominant pedicle and secondary segmental pedicles. (From Mathes SJ, Nahai F: Classification of the vascular anatomy of muscles: Experimental and clinical correlation. *Plast Reconstr Surg* 67:177–187, 1981.)

demonstrate superiority in wounds compromised by irradiation or infection. The vascular anatomy is predictable and easily identifiable, and the muscle can be put into use as a functional unit for a dynamic tissue transfer. A major consideration with muscle flaps is whether the loss of function is acceptable. In an effort to limit the functional loss associated with use of an entire muscle, methods of functional preservation have been devised. If some portion of the muscle chosen as the flap is left innervated and attached at its insertion and origin, function is preserved after transfer of the remainder of the muscle. This can be done by splitting the muscle into segments, provided each is supplied by a different dominant pedicle. An example is the gluteus maximus, which extends and rotates the thigh laterally. This is not an expendable muscle, but the superior or inferior half of the muscle can be elevated as a flap, with function of the intact half of the muscle preserved.

A musculocutaneous flap, also called a myocutaneous flap, is a muscle flap designed with an attached skin paddle. Each superficial skeletal muscle carries blood supply to the skin lying directly over it through musculocutaneous perforators. The number and pattern of these musculocutaneous perforators vary with each specific muscle; this means that the extent of the skin territory is different for each muscle unit. Through dissection of injected cadaver specimens, the number, size, and location of musculocutaneous perforators have been described; this information, combined with clinical experience, is used to predict the cutaneous territories on the superficial muscles.

In addition to the musculocutaneous branches supplying the overlying skin, source vessels, also called mother vessels, branch within muscle into channels that perforate the deep fascia to anastomose within the subdermal plexus and nourish the skin. The source vessel and its perforating muscular branches can be dissected out of the muscle without jeopardizing skin perfusion. This requires intramuscular dissection to separate the perforators from the muscle and is the basis for the development of muscle perforator flaps. This makes the retention of muscle unnecessary for the survival of the skin paddle; thus, its inclusion serves a passive role, primarily to avoid tedious intramuscular dissection of the vascular tree. To spare the muscle unit, a growing number of muscle perforator flaps have been described, including the deep inferior epigastric perforator flap, which carries the same skin and subcutaneous tissue as the TRAM flap for breast reconstruction. By sparing of the rectus muscle, abdominal wall bulging and other complications are less likely. The superior gluteal artery perforator flap carries the skin territory of the gluteus maximus musculocutaneous flap and preserves the muscle.

Fascia and Fasciocutaneous Flaps

Growing knowledge about musculocutaneous skin circulation has led to the identification of vascular pedicles emerging between muscles, traveling in the intermuscular septum, and entering the deep fascia. Termed septocutaneous perforators, these vessels supply the fascial plexus, which gives off branches to an overlying cutaneous territory. Some state that a fasciocutaneous flap, by definition, should include a specific known septocutaneous perforator. Others accept a less strict definition of a fasciocutaneous flap as a skin flap including the deep fascia.

The anatomic features of a fasciocutaneous flap are the fascial feeder vessels, also called the fascial perforators, which are branches of source vessels to a given angiosome. An angiosome is the three-dimensional block of tissue supplied by a source artery; the entire surface of the body is composed of a multitude of angiosome units. The fascial feeder vessels do not perforate the deep fascia but terminate within the fascial plexus. The fascial plexus is not a structure but a confluence of multiple adjacent vascular intercommunications that exist at the subfascial, fascial, suprafascial, subcutaneous, and subdermal levels (Fig. 68-2).

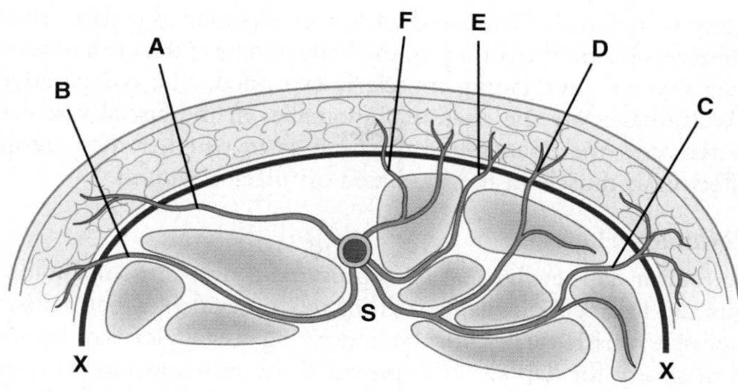

A Direct cutaneous
B Direct septocutaneous
C Direct cutaneous branch of muscular vessel
D Perforating cutaneous branch of muscular vessel
E Septocutaneous perforator
F Musculocutaneous perforator
S Source vessel
X Deep fascia

FIGURE 68-2 Pathways of the various known cutaneous perforators that pierce the deep fascia to supply the fascial plexus. (From Hallock GG: Direct and indirect perforator flaps: The history and the controversy. *Plast Reconstr Surg* 111:855–865, 2003.)

The concept of fasciocutaneous flaps arose from the observation that the size of a skin flap could be increased if it were oriented along a longitudinal axis on the extremity and if the deep fascia were included. Subsequent anatomic studies have confirmed the presence of septocutaneous pedicles supplying a regional fascial vascular system. The larger septocutaneous pedicles tend to be fairly constant in location, and a number of specific fasciocutaneous flaps have come into wide use (e.g., anterior lateral thigh flap, radial forearm flap, scapular flap).

The design of fasciocutaneous flaps has been learned by experience, and the limits of these flaps still remain to be discovered. There are no set rules because deep fascial perforators are frequently anomalous in caliber and location, not only among individuals but also on opposite sides of the same person. The expected range of flap size is learned through the experience of other surgeons.[1,2]

One of the most useful features of a fasciocutaneous flap is that it can be distally based. Unlike in a muscle flap, in which the dominant pedicle is closest to the heart, blood flow in the fascial plexus is multidirectional. The flow to the corresponding angiosome is equivalent for a distal fascial perforator and proximal fascial perforator. This means that a flap pedicle can be distally based with a reliable skin territory and transposed to cover a defect located at the end of an extremity. For example, the distal-based sural flap uses the skin of the calf, based on a distal perforator of the peroneal artery, for transfer to cover the foot and ankle. Obviating the need for a free microvascular transfer, this has become a standard for foot coverage.

In addition to the advantages provided by a distally based flap design, a fasciocutaneous flap can confer sensibility if a sensory nerve is included. Compared with musculocutaneous flaps, they are accessible on the surface of the body and have the great advantage that no functioning muscle is expended. The comparative disadvantages are the anatomic anomalies in the fascial vascular system and the unanswered question as to whether they are as effective as muscle in the irradiated or infected wound.

Perforator Flaps

Perforator flaps evolved as an improvement over musculocutaneous and fasciocutaneous flaps. They rely on evidence that neither a passive muscle carrier nor the underlying fascial plexus of vessels is necessary for flap survival, provided the musculocutaneous or fasciocutaneous vessel is carefully dissected out and preserved. Advantages of perforator flaps include preservation of functional muscle and fascia at the donor site and versatility of flap design with regard to including as little or as much bulk tissue as required. Disadvantages are the difficult dissection needed to isolate the perforator vessels, longer operating time associated with this dissection, anatomic variability of position and size of perforator vessels, short pedicle length available, and fragile nature of these small blood vessels.

A perforator is a blood vessel passing through the deep fascia and contributing blood supply to the fascial plexus. Perforators arise from a source or mother vessel to a given angiosome. There are direct and indirect perforators. Direct perforators are those that travel directly from the mother vessel to the plexus; these include septocutaneous and direct cutaneous branches. Indirect perforators supply other deep structures on their route from the mother vessel to the plexus (e.g., the musculocutaneous perforator passing through muscle).

The nomenclature of perforator flaps is not yet standardized. They are named variably by location (anterolateral thigh flap), arterial supply (deep inferior epigastric artery perforator flap), and muscle of origin (gastrocnemius perforator flap). They are described as cutaneous, musculocutaneous, septocutaneous, fasciocutaneous, composite, and chimeric; the last is a perforator flap with two separate muscular components with a common vascular source. Several suggestions for an ordering nomenclature have been made.

Because of the small size of the vessels and their anatomic variability, Doppler ultrasound is used routinely to locate the perforators before perforator flap elevation. This is not highly accurate, and other technologies, such as color flow duplex scanning and thermography, may be useful in the future. Technical recommendations for harvesting of a perforator flap include identification of at least one vessel with a diameter of 0.5 mm or more, inclusion of at least two or more perforators, sufficient pedicle length for the procedure, and preservation of a subcutaneous vein to use for venous outflow in situations in which the deep system of perforator veins proves anomalous.

The use of perforator flaps continues to evolve. Current work includes flap thinning, a technique for removing excess adipose tissue from the perforator flap as it is raised. This would provide a large delicate segment of vascularized skin for reconstruction in areas such as the ear, in which contour is important. Another innovation is the discovery of new flaps based on perforators smaller than 0.8 mm in diameter found superficial to the fascial plane. By eliminating the dissection needed to trace a perforator through the muscle, operating time is shortened and there is potential for developing a much larger number of suitable flaps. The challenge with these suprafascial free flaps is the supermicrosurgery needed for anastomoses in such small vessels.[3]

Microvascular Free Tissue Transfer

A microvascular free tissue transfer, also called a free flap, brings distant tissue with a pedicled arterial and venous supply from another part of the body to be anastomosed to vessels at the recipient site to reestablish blood flow. The transferred tissue may be skin, fat, muscle, fascia, bone, nerves, small bowel, large bowel, or omentum as needed to reconstruct a given defect. Selection of tissue for transfer depends on the size, composition, and functional capabilities of the tissue needed; technical considerations, such as vessel size and pedicle length; and donor site deformity that will be created with regard to function and aesthetic appearance.

Preoperative planning starts with selection of the patient and analysis of the defect. Environmental factors, such as previous surgery and prior irradiation, which impair the quality of tissue and vessels, may be an indication for angiography to assess the available vasculature. Muscle does not tolerate warm ischemia for longer than 2 hours; skin and fasciocutaneous flaps can tolerate ischemia times of 4 to 6 hours. Planning is the most important factor to minimize the effects of ischemia, and all structures at the recipient site should be ready for the tissue transfer when the donor pedicle is divided. Sound technique requires healthy vessels of reasonable size with good outflow for the anastomosis, which must be made without tension. This may require mobilization of the vessels to gain more length. Vein grafts have been shown to reduce the success rate and are not a primary choice but may be needed if the pedicle is short or the vessels in the field are damaged. Vein grafts can be obtained from the saphenous vein, dorsum of the foot, volar forearm, or donor site. Adventitia is removed from the vessel ends to improve visualization of the vessel walls for accurate suture placement. Both end-to-end and end-to-side arterial anastomoses have similar patency rates, although end-to-side anastomosis is preferred if there is vessel size or wall thickness discrepancy or the continuity of the recipient vessel must be preserved. Dissection and manipulation of the microvessels frequently cause vasospasm. This can be relieved with topical lidocaine or papaverine, stripping the adventitia to remove sympathetic nerve fibers, or mechanical dilation of the vessels. Failure of reperfusion in an ischemic organ after reestablishment of blood supply is termed the no-reflow phenomenon. The causative mechanism is thought to be endothelial injury, platelet aggregation, and leakage of intravascular fluid. The severity of this effect correlates with ischemia time.

Postoperative anticoagulation is not a uniform practice for elective microvascular transfers. If pharmacologic agents are part of postoperative care, aspirin is generally used, followed by dextran and low-molecular-weight heparin. Surveys of microsurgical centers have shown equal success rates for transplants with and without anticoagulation; the concern with the use of anticoagulants is an increased chance of hematoma at donor and recipient sites. Postoperative monitoring of free tissue transfers is critical because rapid identification of postoperative free flap ischemia permits intervention and flap salvage. Most free flap thromboses occur in the first 48 hours after surgery, and salvage rates are high. Clinical evaluation includes observation of skin color, capillary refill, fullness, and color of capillary bleeding, which can be determined by pinprick testing of the flap. If a flap is buried, a temporary skin island can be added for monitoring purposes, or an implantable monitoring device can be used. Many devices are available for flap monitoring, including temperature probes, pulse oximetry, photoplethysmography, hand-held pencil Doppler probes (low-frequency continuous ultrasonography), and implantable Doppler probes.

Tissue survival rates for free tissue transfers exceed 95%. Reexploration rates range from 6% to 25%, and thrombosis of the arterial anastomosis is the most common finding at reoperation. This is termed primary thrombosis when technical faults lead to anastomotic failure. These faults include narrowing of the lumen; sutures tied too loosely so that media of the vessel is exposed in the gap and clot forms; sutures tied too tightly that tear through the vessel; too many sutures with subendothelial exposure and clot formation; and sutures that inadvertently take a bite of the back wall of the vessel, which obstructs the lumen. Secondary thrombosis refers to kinking or compression of vessels by hematoma or edema, which leads to decreased inflow. With reexploration, salvage rates have been seen to vary from 54% to 100% in different series.[4]

The principles and techniques of microvascular surgery are under continual refinement. An area of current emphasis is the identification of tissue transfers that better suit the needs of the recipient site and minimize donor site sequelae, which has led to minimally invasive and endoscopic techniques for harvesting of flap tissue through smaller incisions. It has also led to the development of tissue transfers such as perforator flaps, which preserve functional muscle and fascia at the donor site, and suprafascial free flaps, which require supermicrosurgery techniques.

Supermicrosurgery

The introduction of supermicrosurgery, which allows the anastomosis of smaller caliber vessels and microvascular dissection of vessels ranging from 0.3 to 0.8 mm in diameter, has led to the development of new reconstructive techniques. Free perforator-to-perforator flaps using suprafascial vessels can be transferred more quickly and the tissue can be obtained from better concealed parts of the body.[5] If a discrete perforator can be identified anywhere on the body, a flap can be designed around it. This has been called a freestyle flap. The constraints of using only described territories can be disregarded and the donor site selected solely on the basis of the best possible match for color, contour, and texture at the recipient site. Disadvantages are the anatomic variation of the perforators and the need for supermicrosurgical technique. The supermicrosurgical technique includes the use of 12-0 nylon sutures with 50- to 30-μm needles; the surgeons who pioneered "freestyle reconstruction" have noted that it is difficult to learn and can be tedious.[6]

Tissue Expansion

Tissue expansion is a technique that uses a mechanical stimulus to induce tissue growth so as to generate soft tissue for reconstructive use. It involves placing a prosthesis that is gradually enlarged by the addition of saline, which causes an increase in the surface area of the overlying soft tissue. Initially, the expanded skin is the result of stretching as interstitial fluid is forced out of the tissue, elastic fibers are fragmented, viscoelastic changes (termed creep) occur in the collagen, and adjacent mobile soft tissue is recruited. Over time, it is not just stretching but actual growth of the skin flap that creates an increase in the surface area, with accompanying increases in collagen and ground substance. Histologic changes in the skin include dermal thinning, epidermal thickening, subcutaneous fat atrophy, and no effect on the skin appendages.

Tissue undergoing expansion must have the capacity for growth. Prior irradiation or scar formation may slow the rate of expansion or make it impossible. Expanders perform poorly under skin grafts, under very tight tissue, and in the hands and feet. Contraindications include expansion near a malignant neoplasm, hemangioma, or open leg wound.

Expanders come in various styles, and sizes range from a few cubic centimeters to 1 liter or more. They can be round, square, rectangular, or horseshoe shaped. The injection ports can be remote or integrated into the wall of the expander so that no dissection of a pocket for the remote port is required. The envelope can be smooth or textured for better stabilization at one location in the tissue pocket.

Expanders should be placed under tissue that best matches the lost tissue (Fig. 68-3). Normal landmarks, such as the eyebrow or hairline, should not be distorted. The incision to insert the expander can be placed at the edge of the defect that later will be excised because a scar in this position will be removed at the time of the next surgery. The most common reason for expander failure is construction of a pocket that is too small for the device. An expander with a curled edge may later protrude through the incision or erode through the overlying tissue. Filling of the expander is initiated approximately 2 weeks after surgery and continued at weekly or biweekly intervals. The rate of expansion is limited by the relaxation and growth of the tissue overlying the expander. Pain and palpable tightness over the expander are clinical indicators that guide the rate of expansion. The patient is ready for the second surgical procedure when the expanded tissue is adequate to produce the desired effect. If the flap is to be advanced, it must be measured to ensure that it is large enough and has the correct geometry to cover the defect. At the second surgery, the skin is incised through the old scar, the capsule around the expander is opened, the expander is removed, and the expanded flap is advanced over the defect. It is important to confirm that the expanded tissue will replace the defect before the defect is excised. If it is not sufficient, this is handled by subtotal resection of the defect and leaving the expander in place for a second round of expansion.[7]

Tissue expansion can be combined with other reconstructive techniques. Expander placement in the subcutaneous or submuscular plane can facilitate later repair of abdominal wall hernias. Preexpansion of transposition or rotation flaps increases the amount of tissue, enhances the flap's blood supply, and lessens donor site morbidity. Preexpansion of free flaps increases the surface area and augments the blood supply of the future flap, may make primary closure of the free flap donor site possible, and thins the flap, which may be desirable for reconstructions calling for thinner and more pliable coverage. A disadvantage of the preexpansion of free flaps is the time needed for the expansion process because delay may not be acceptable for oncologic defects and complex wounds. In addition, the preexpanded free flap procedure is technically more difficult because of distortion of the vascular pedicle.

The advantages of expansion are the provision of matching tissue for reconstruction, normal sensibility of the transferred tissue, negligible donor defect, and enhanced success of preexpanded traditional flaps because of enhanced vascularity.

Alloplastic Materials

An alloplastic material is a synthetic substance implanted in living tissue. Its advantages are availability when autologous tissue is not available and the absence of donor site morbidity or scarring. Nonbiodegradable alloplastic materials do not undergo resorption, as do bone or cartilage grafts. In addition, the implant can be manufactured to meet special needs, such as for controlled-release drug delivery systems.

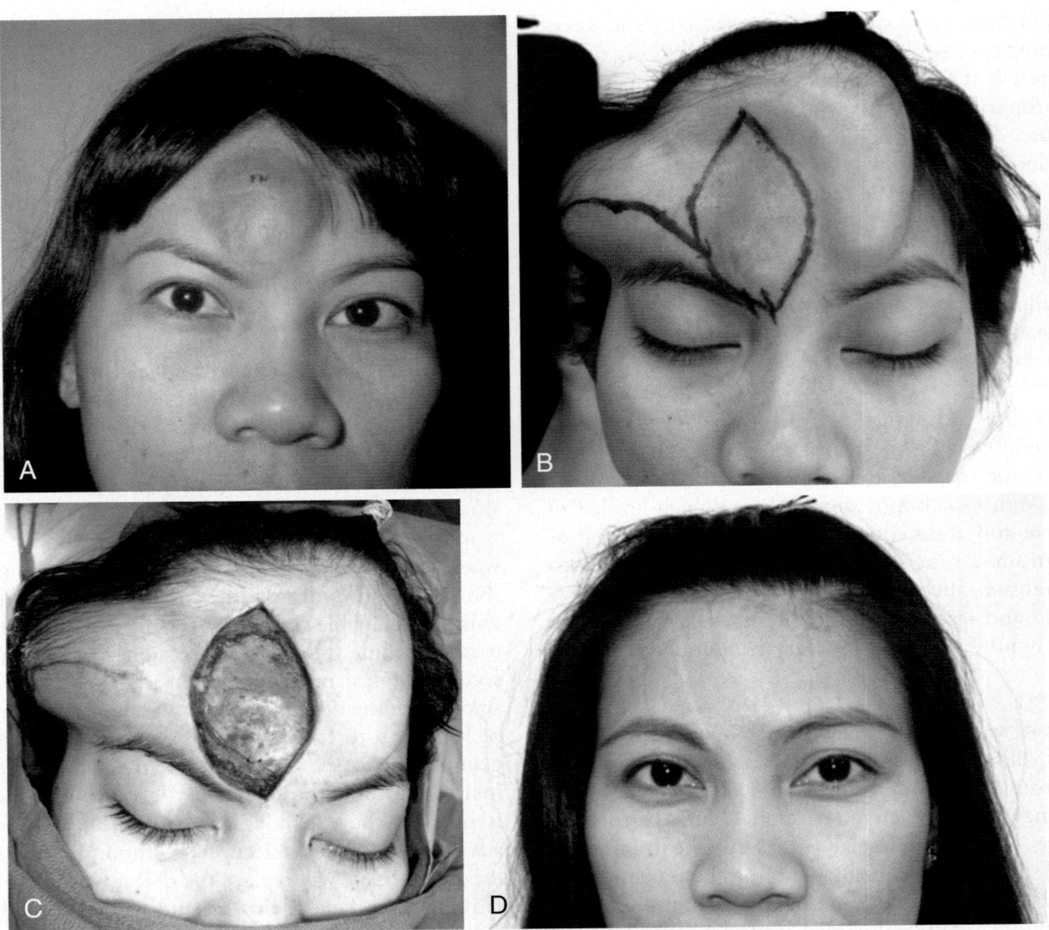

FIGURE 68-3 The use of tissue expansion to generate new soft tissue to restore the forehead and hairline. The expanders are placed under tissue that best matches the lost tissue. **A,** Young woman with an arteriovenous malformation. **B,** Crescent-shaped expander in the central forehead and rectangular expander in the right forehead were expanded gradually with saline during 1 month. **C,** The vascular lesion is excised, and the expanders will be removed with mobilization of the forehead to close the defect. **D,** Postoperative result 1 year after surgery.

The tissue response to different implants varies with the chemical composition and the microstructure and macrostructure of the synthetic material; these differences are used clinically. For example, the vigorous tissue ingrowth with polypropylene mesh in a hernia repair provides strong and lasting support, whereas the fibrous encapsulation around a silicone tendon prosthesis ensures free gliding of a tendon graft. However, certain properties (noncarcinogenic, nontoxic, nonallergenic, nonimmunogenic) and concerns (mechanical reliability, biocompatibility) are common to all implants.

Categorization by chemical composition is the most useful framework for the description and comparison of surgical implants. This materials science approach recognizes that the commonality of different groups of materials arises more from their composition than from the organ systems in which they are used. Chemically, there are three major classes of biomaterials: metallic, ceramic, and polymeric. Although they are polymers, biologic materials such as collagen need to be classified separately because they introduce new considerations of protein antigenicity.

Metals in clinical use are stainless steel, Vitallium (cobalt-chromium-molybdenum alloy), and titanium. The general requirements for a metal device are mechanical strength, suitable elastic modulus, density and weight comparable to those of the surrounding tissue, and resistance to corrosion. Very few metals have sufficient corrosion resistance to be used in the hostile environment of the living organism. Corrosion results from the electrochemical activity of unstable metal ions and electrons in physiologic salt solutions; corrosion products can be cytotoxic, leading to pain, inflammation, allergic reactions, and loosening of the device.

Ceramic materials have high stability and resistance to chemical alteration and include carbon compounds such as hydroxyapatite, which is capable of bonding strongly to adjacent bone. Used to augment the facial skeleton or as a bone graft substitute, it is a permanent microporous implant that undergoes osseointegration by providing a matrix for the deposition of new bone from adjacent living bone.

Polymers are large, long-chain, high-molecular-weight macromolecules made up of repeated units, or mers. There are a vast number of these synthetic implants in surgical use. To a large extent, this is because of the ease and low cost of fabrication and because they can be processed easily into tubes, fibers, fabrics, meshes, films, and foams. Polymers vary across an enormous range of chemical compositions, degree of polymerization, cross-linking between chains, and presence of chemical additives such as plasticizers to increase flexibility or resins to catalyze polymerization.

With the exception of resorbable polymers, most surgical polymers are relatively inert and stimulate fibrous encapsulation. The physical form of the implant, solid versus mesh or smooth versus rough, will determine whether the entire structure is encapsulated as a whole or whether fibrous tissue will penetrate the interstices. Tissue reaction to the implant is influenced also by the chemical composition, factors such as hydrophilicity and ionic charge, and the chemical durability of the polymer. Silicone rubber, polytetrafluoroethylene, and polyethylene terephthalate polyester (Dacron) are among the most stable of polymers, whereas polyamide (nylon) is vulnerable to hydrolytic reaction and undergoes substantial degradation.

PEDIATRIC PLASTIC SURGERY

Craniofacial Surgery

Craniosynostosis refers to the premature fusion of one or more of the cranial sutures, leading to characteristic deformities of the skull and face. It occurs at an overall frequency of approximately 1 in 2500 live births and is usually sporadic. Any suture may be involved in craniosynostosis, and skull growth is restricted perpendicular to the affected suture. Treatment of craniosynostosis is indicated to correct the deformity and to normalize the shape of the head, to protect the eyes by restoring brow projection, and to minimize the risk for development of increased intracranial pressure and associated developmental and visual sequelae. The timing of treatment is based on which suture is fused and on the protocol at a given center, but correction during the first 6 months of life appears to be associated with better neurodevelopmental outcomes.

Surgical treatment of craniosynostosis is generally done with a coronal approach; techniques differ, but all involve release or excision of the fused suture. The cranium then expands and remodels. Residual bone defects reossify secondarily, a process that is robust in the infant up to 2 years of age (Fig. 68-4).

Other less common congenital abnormalities of the head include agenesis of one or a number of layers of scalp or cranium.

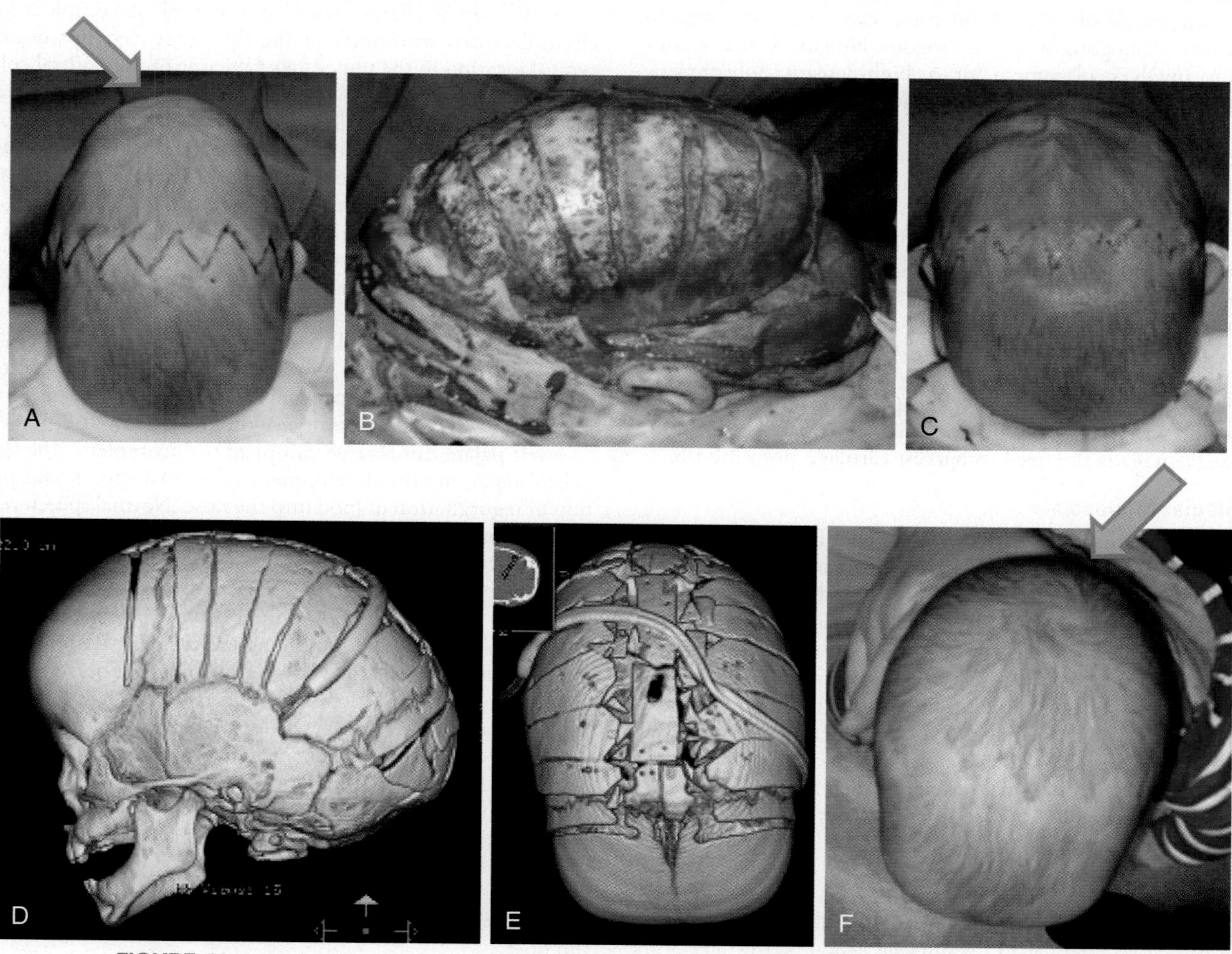

FIGURE 68-4 Infant with sagittal suture craniosynostosis. **A,** Preoperative view showing scaphocephalic head shape. The baby is in a prone position with the face resting on foam. Note the narrow biparietal dimension of the head, typical for this condition *(arrow)*. A zigzag coronal incision is designed to be better hidden once hair grows. **B,** Intraoperative lateral view. The sagittal suture has been removed and reshaped, and lateral barrel stave osteotomies are created to reshape the cranial vault and to relieve growth restriction. **C,** On-table view immediately after the procedure. The biparietal area is widened. **D** and **E,** Lateral and superior views of the postoperative CT scan. **F,** One month after surgery, the skull continues to remodel and the head shape normalizes *(arrow)*.

Aplasia cutis congenita usually refers to a focal defect of skin on the vertex. The defect may include any proportion of skin, bone, or dura. Treatment depends on the size of the defect and layers involved and may encompass local wound care or surgical reconstruction with flaps or grafts in infancy. The cause of this rare condition is unknown and likely varies from case to case. A classification system for aplasia cutis congenita has been developed and is related to the presence of other associated anomalies.

Congenital Ear Deformities

Congenital anomalies of the external ear may occur in isolation or as part of craniofacial microsomia. Common external ear deformities include prominent ears, constricted ears, cryptotia (failure of the upper pole of the ear to stand out from the head), and microtia (a small or abnormally formed outer ear). The most common type of microtia is a malformed vestigial cartilaginous structure associated with a soft tissue component of lobule. In cases of isolated microtia, there is often conductive hearing loss associated with absence of the external auditory canal. This is most important in bilateral cases in which a bone-anchored hearing aid is required.

Reconstruction of typical microtia can take two general approaches, autologous or nonautologous. Nonautologous reconstruction involves placement of a high-density polyethylene implant under the skin. This approach results in good form without the need to harvest tissue from another site or the requirement of shaping a framework. Disadvantages include the presence of a foreign body that may become exposed through the thin skin envelope, is susceptible to infection, and is difficult to salvage in case of complications. The second approach is preferred. This involves the use of autologous tissue (rib cartilage) to shape an ear framework, which is then buried in a subcutaneous pocket. The meticulous shaping of the framework, creation of a thin skin pocket, and use of drains allow the skin to contour around the intricate framework. The procedure requires multiple stages but results in a reconstructed ear that has good form and is capable of responding to trauma and infection like other parts of the body. The disadvantage is the need to harvest cartilage from the rib.

Craniofacial Microsomia

Craniofacial microsomia, also known as hemifacial microsomia, is a constellation of abnormalities involving deficient development of parts of the face related to the first and second branchial arches.[8] Deformity can be unilateral or bilateral and can involve the orbit, mandible, external ear, facial nerve, and facial soft tissue. Each or all of the structures may be involved and to varying degrees. The cause is unknown but is thought to be related to in utero vascular compromise of the stapedial artery. Treatment of craniofacial microsomia is complex, and the approach has to be tailored for individual patients. Functional problems, such as airway compromise or eye exposure, are treated in childhood; reconstruction of other structural defects is delayed until the patient is almost full-grown.

For patients with craniofacial anomalies such as those described as well as for those with cleft lip and palate, the current standard is team care at an established craniofacial center. With referral to a craniofacial center at birth, the craniofacial team can make a diagnosis, carry out genetic testing, educate the family, and outline short- and long-term plans in a coordinated manner, bringing in multiple specialists (e.g., plastic surgeons, neurosurgeons, oral surgeons, orthodontists, speech pathologists, otolaryngologists, ophthalmologists, social workers, nurse practitioners, developmental psychologists, and pediatricians).

Cleft Lip and Palate

Cleft lip and palate are relatively common congenital anomalies. They may be unilateral or bilateral. Most are isolated anomalies, but many syndromes have clefts as one of the features. The genetics of cleft lip and palate is complex, and the condition is multifactorial. The pathophysiologic mechanism of cleft lip and palate is incompletely understood, but the deformity and its variations are well described. A minimum of three operations, and usually four, will be required to correct the deformity. These are performed at specific times corresponding to the developmental stage of the patient:

- Cleft lip repair at 3 months
- Cleft palate repair before 1 year or before speech development begins
- Alveolar bone graft when permanent dentition begins and after orthodontic preparation
- Possible septorhinoplasty in the late teenage years
- Possible lip and nose revision
- LeFort I maxillary advancement, if indicated
- Secondary procedures for speech improvement in 15% of cases

A cleft lip is characterized by a partial or complete lack of circumferential continuity of the lip. Most cleft lips occur at a typical location in the upper lip where one of the philtral columns normally lies, and they extend into the nose. The deformity involves the mucosa, orbicularis oris muscle, and skin. The nasal deformity is characterized by a slumped and widened ala (nostril) that is posteriorly misplaced at its base. The nasal floor is nonexistent in complete clefts and the nasal septum is deviated.

There are many techniques for repair of a cleft lip, but most are a variation of the rotation-advancement repair. Millard introduced this technique of downward rotation of the medial portion of the lip and advancement of the lateral portion into the defect created by the rotation. The repair is based on the principle that existing elements need to be returned to their normal position to restore the normal anatomy while remaining cognizant of future growth and the effects of surgery on growth (Fig. 68-5).[9]

Cleft palate can also be complete or incomplete. The goals of palatal repair are the development of normal speech and prevention of regurgitation of food into the nose. Normal speech requires velopharyngeal competence to close the oral cavity off from the nasal cavity to produce pressure consonants. This requires static physical separation of the two cavities in the region of the hard palate and dynamic closure of the soft palate against the posterior pharyngeal wall with a functioning levator veli palatini muscle. In a cleft palate, the levator veli palatini muscle fibers are oriented abnormally along the cleft. Thus, all modern techniques of cleft palate repair involve repair of the nasal lining and oral mucosa and reorientation and repair of the levator veli palatini muscle. The primary measure of outcome of cleft palate repair is normal speech. The third procedure necessary in most cases is alveolar bone grafting. Cancellous bone, usually from the ilium, is used to restore bone continuity along the dental arch as a foundation for dental implants for missing teeth associated with the cleft, to close a nasolabial fistula (if present), and to produce support for the nose.

Other procedures are indicated for some patients, but this generally cannot be predicted in infancy. Approximately 15% of patients will continue to demonstrate velopharyngeal insufficiency after initial palate repair, and secondary palatal lengthening or other approaches to promote velopharyngeal closure are indicated, typically after 3 years of age.[10] Septorhinoplasty is usually necessary to correct residual nasal deformity in the teenage years

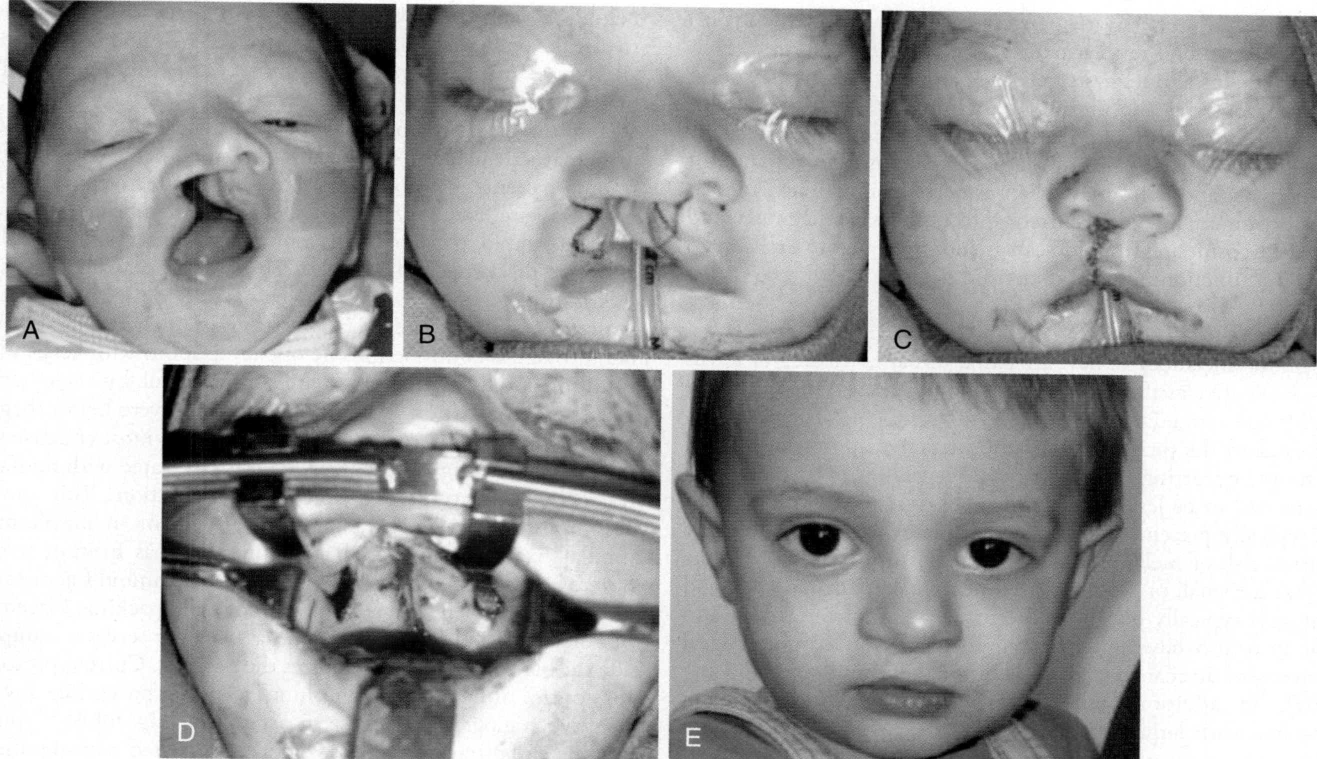

FIGURE 68-5 Infant boy with a wide right-sided unilateral complete cleft lip and palate. **A,** There is a wide cleft with absence of the nasal floor, malrotated central lip element, twisted premaxilla, and severe nasal deformity. **B,** Intraoperative markings for rotation-advancement cleft lip repair at age 3 months. **C,** Immediate postoperative view. **D,** Postoperative views at 11 months of age taken at the time of cleft palate repair. **E,** After primary repair of cleft lip, nose, and palate.

after final dental restoration and orthodontics. A subset of unilateral cleft lip and palate patients will develop maxillary hypoplasia that is iatrogenic and related to scarring and growth retardation from lip and palate surgery. Depending on the degree of maxillary hypoplasia, LeFort I maxillary advancement in the teenage years may be indicated. In sum, treatment of a child born with a cleft lip and palate does not end after palate repair but rather requires observation by a craniofacial team throughout development into adulthood and must be tailored for each individual.

Vascular Anomalies

Vascular anomalies are divided into two major groups, tumors and malformations. Vascular tumors are characterized by increased abnormal proliferation of endothelium. Hemangioma is the most common vascular tumor; others include hemangioendotheliomas, tufted angiomas, hemangiopericytomas, and malignant tumors, such as angiosarcoma. Vascular malformations are the result of abnormal development of arterial, capillary, venous, or lymphatic components of the vascular system. They may involve only one component or may be mixed and are named for the component vessels. They can be high flow, low flow, or mixed. Correct diagnosis depends on the history (e.g., hemangiomas develop in infancy and are usually not visible at birth), physical examination (e.g., malformations with an arterial component may have a palpable pulse or thrill), and imaging to determine the extent of disease and to assist with making the diagnosis.

The natural histories of the different anomalies are diverse. Hemangiomas typically involute spontaneously; 50% involute completely by the age of 5 years. This natural history reduces the indications for surgery to those lesions that are affecting vision or the airway or are large enough that even after involution, the abnormal remaining skin will require surgical modification. In contrast, capillary malformations start as patches, but over time, they typically enlarge and become thick and verrucous; for these lesions, early treatment is indicated. Some vascular malformations or tumors have systemic effects, depending on their mass, status as high or low flow, and thrombosis and consumption of coagulation factors. Treatment of these lesions involves complete resection, when feasible, or debulking if complete resection is not possible. Sclerotherapy is the mainstay of treatment of venous malformations. For arteriovenous malformations, sclerotherapy is useful as an adjunct to surgery but insufficient alone because of the development of collaterals. For these malformations, sclerotherapy and embolization are followed immediately by surgical resection.

Pediatric Neck Masses

Neck masses in the pediatric patient are most likely infectious or congenital noncancerous lesions. In addition to vascular malformations, other common pediatric neck masses include dermoid cysts, teratomas, branchial cleft anomalies, thyroglossal duct cysts, thymic cysts, ranulas, cartilaginous rests, heterotopic neuroectodermal tissue, neurofibromas, ectopic salivary tissue, lymphadenopathy, and malignant tumors. Branchial cleft anomalies may be cysts, sinuses, or fistulas. Cysts and sinuses are located in the anterior cervical triangle and are derived from the first cleft (near the external auditory meatus) and second cleft (below the hyoid) 98% of the time. The treatment of these lesions is surgical excision. Thyroglossal duct cysts may arise anywhere along the course of the thyroglossal duct, from the foramen cecum at the base of the tongue to the thyroid gland. Thyroglossal duct cysts usually present in the first or second decade of life as painless anterior neck masses, and there may be an associated sinus track. Indications for surgery include recurrent infection, tissue diagnosis, and improved cosmesis. Thyroid scan is indicated before excision to rule out a functioning ectopic thyroid gland.

Melanocytic Nevi

Congenital melanocytic nevi are hamartomas consisting of nevus cells. Nevi are classified by size as small (<1.5 cm), medium (1.5 to 19.9 cm), large (>20 cm), and giant (>50 cm). The classification dictates the prognosis and reconstructive approach. Risk of melanoma occurring in a melanocytic nevus varies by report but is estimated to be less than 5% in small or medium-sized lesions and typically presents after puberty. In large and giant nevi, the reported risk of melanoma development is up to 10%.[11] Unlike the case for small or medium-sized nevi, malignancy in large and giant nevi typically occurs in the first 3 years of life. Large and giant nevi also have an increased incidence of leptomeningeal involvement that can be diagnosed by magnetic resonance imaging (MRI). In addition, psychosocial and developmental issues associated with larger nevi are significant, so early excision and reconstruction are recommended for large and giant nevi.

Options for removal of larger nevi include serial excision, excision and grafting, excision and closure with distant flaps, and tissue expansion. Replacement with like tissue is the goal, and therefore tissue expansion is the mainstay approach.

PLASTIC SURGERY OF THE HEAD AND NECK

Maxillofacial Trauma

Facial trauma has decreased in frequency in the United States, and this is attributed in part to the advent of seat belt laws and improved collision safety. However, it remains part of multisystem trauma from motor vehicle accidents, assaults, and combat injuries. Improvements in body armor have resulted in better survival of combat injuries but proportionally more facial injuries.

Emergent Management

Surgical emergencies in the facial trauma patient include airway compromise, life-threatening hemorrhage, and reversible structural injury to the eye or optic nerve. Other injuries, such as lacerations or extraocular muscle entrapment, are treated within the first 24 hours. Fractures are treated within the first 2 weeks. Evaluation of the facial trauma patient follows the advanced trauma life support protocol and includes looking for intracranial trauma and cervical spine injury. Acute airway compromise usually occurs in the setting of combined mandibular-maxillary trauma, with hemorrhage and soft tissue swelling. Endotracheal intubation should be attempted and need not be avoided because of concern about the facial injury. Nasotracheal intubation is contraindicated in the case of severe naso-orbitoethmoid and skull base fractures. Cricothyroidotomy is performed if oral or nasal endotracheal intubation is unsuccessful and should be converted to tracheostomy after the patient has been stabilized. Maxillomandibular fixation by itself is not an indication for tracheostomy because endotracheal intubation may be maintained through the nasal or oral route using an armored tube that can be routed behind the molars without kinking. An alternative technique is to exit the endotracheal tube through a submental incision, which alleviates some of the practical difficulties of working around an oral tube.

Life-threatening hemorrhage, defined as 3 units of blood loss or hematocrit below 29%, occurs in a small percentage of facial trauma patients. In most cases, bleeding is effectively controlled with pressure, packing, and, in the case of significant soft tissue avulsion, rapid placement of temporary bolster sutures. Blind attempts to clamp and ligate vessels should be avoided because this is usually unnecessary and may result in injury to critical structures, such as the facial nerve. With penetrating trauma, hemorrhage is controlled in the operating room with vessel identification and ligation and, if that is unsuccessful, by angiographic selective embolization. With blunt trauma, severe hemorrhage is usually from the internal maxillary artery. The most effective way to control bleeding, especially when it is associated with midfacial fractures, is fracture reduction and stabilization. This can be accomplished quickly by temporary placement in maxillomandibular fixation using rapid techniques such as fixation screws. Severe hemorrhage from skull base and nasoethmoid fractures can often be controlled with anteroposterior nasal packing. Placement of Foley balloon catheters in each nasal airway serves to tamponade the bleeding and also stabilizes the packing. Current protocols for control of hemorrhage in blunt facial trauma settings involve selective angiography if these measures fail (Fig. 68-6).[12] Angiographic embolization is effective but is associated with significant morbidity, including the possibility of stroke or necrosis of midfacial structures, such as the palate. In unstable patients, fracture reduction and nasal packing may be attempted on the angiography table to be followed immediately with embolization, if necessary.

Injuries to the orbit and contents can result in blindness; it is critical to recognize promptly and to treat reversible injuries that

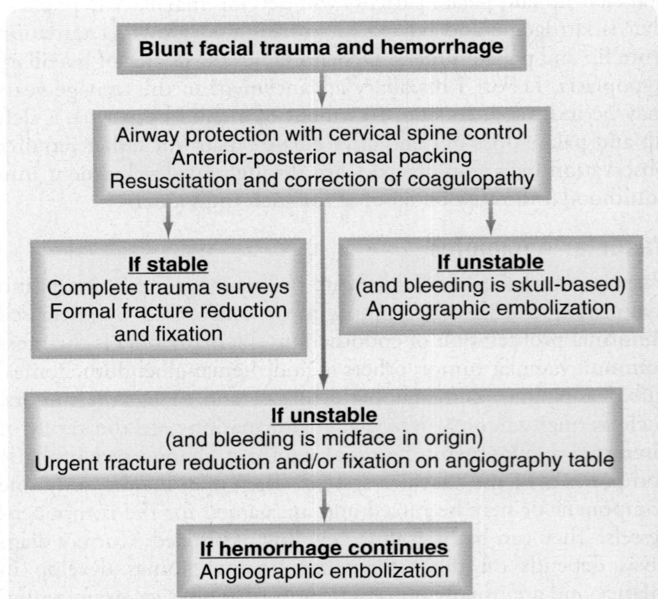

FIGURE 68-6 Algorithm for the management of life-threatening hemorrhage in the setting of blunt facial trauma. (Adapted from Ho K, Hutter JJ, Eskridge J, et al: The management of life-threatening haemorrhage following blunt facial trauma. *J Plast Reconstr Aesthet Surg* 59:1257–1262, 2006.)

are vision threatening. Conditions that require emergent intervention include increased intraocular pressure, globe rupture, and optic nerve impingement. Acute increased intracranial pressure is manifested by pain and vision loss and can result from causes such as hematoma or decreased orbital volume because of fracture or a foreign body. Treatment involves rapid alleviation of intraocular hypertension by lateral canthotomy and administration of mannitol, acetazolamide (Diamox), and steroids. Urgent ophthalmology consultation is indicated. Vision loss may result from mechanical compression of the optic nerve. Computed tomography (CT) will diagnose the presence of a bone fragment or foreign body; such a finding should prompt emergent surgical decompression to preserve vision. Extraocular muscle entrapment presents as the inability to move the eye on the trajectory controlled by the entrapped muscle and is associated with pain on attempted motion. Especially in children, the pain may be severe and accompanied by nausea or vomiting. Muscle entrapment should be treated by surgical release of the entrapped contents. This should be done fairly soon after injury because delaying the treatment of entrapment for 1 week or longer after injury typically results in failure of the entrapped muscle to regain excursion.

Evaluation and Diagnosis

The primary diagnostic studies for facial injury are physical examination and CT. Systematic physical examination can detect deformity, soft tissue injury, cerebrospinal fluid leak, and facial nerve injury. Palpation is used to identify bony stepoffs or midface instability. The eyes are examined for proptosis or enophthalmos, extraocular muscle function, and visual acuity. In patients who cannot cooperate with a physical examination and for whom there is reasonable suspicion of periorbital injury, a forced duction test should be performed. The occlusion is evaluated for subjective or objective malocclusion. Extraocular muscle entrapment, acute enophthalmos, and malocclusion are indications that surgical treatment of facial fractures will be required. Fine-cut CT of the face with direct or reformatted coronal and sagittal views is used to diagnose facial trauma and to direct nonsurgical and surgical treatment. With current CT scanning technology, plain films are not necessary and provide less information. An exception is the Panorex, which is used by many physicians as an adjunct or primary study for mandible fractures and to assess teeth and their roots in particular.

Soft Tissue Injuries

Because of its rich blood supply, even questionable tissue should be salvaged in treating facial lacerations and avulsions. The robust perfusion of facial tissue provides resistance to infection, and repair can be done after a longer delay than would be safe elsewhere on the body. Although there is no strict cutoff, primary repair is generally done up to 24 hours after injury. Even grossly contaminated wounds or those from animal bites are irrigated extensively, débrided, and closed primarily. If there is the possibility of facial nerve injury, this is confirmed by the physical examination finding of weakness or absence of function of a portion of the muscles of facial expression. It is important to recognize a facial nerve laceration so that the distal cut ends can be identified with a nerve stimulator and tagged if they are not to be repaired immediately. Identification of distal stumps by nerve stimulation is not possible after a few days because conduction ceases. Parotid duct injuries should be identified and treated acutely to prevent the formation of sialocele or salivary fistula. In a sharp laceration or penetrating injury to the cheek, a parotid duct injury can be confirmed by direct visualization or injection of dye. This is done by cannulating Stensen duct on the mucosal surface of the cheek and injecting a small amount of methylene blue dye. Extravasation of the dye into the wound indicates a parotid duct laceration, and repair over a stent should be done in the operating room.

Craniofacial Fractures

Current concepts in facial fracture treatment rest on craniofacial techniques to provide surgical exposure of the craniofacial skeleton, anatomic reduction of fractures, and rigid bone fixation with low-profile titanium plates and bone grafting techniques. Failure to reconstruct the bony facial skeleton invariably results in shrinkage and tightening of the facial soft tissue envelope, a sequela that is almost impossible to correct secondarily.

Treatment of forehead fractures involves assessment of the frontal sinus and cranial base. The approach is dictated by injury to the anterior or posterior table of the frontal bone or skull base and whether there is a dural injury or injury to the nasofrontal ducts that drain the frontal sinuses into the nose. Fractures of the upper midface include malar (zygoma) fractures, nasoorbitoethmoid fractures, and orbital fractures. There is considerable overlap in this region. For example, malar fractures occur in association with orbital fractures to a varying degree because the zygoma, in addition to producing cheek projection and determining facial width, is also part of the orbit. Treatment of fractures of the lower midface, the maxilla, focuses on the restoration of the preinjury dental occlusion. It is important to determine the patient's preoperative occlusion; the relationship of the upper and lower teeth is described by the Angle classification.

Maxillary fractures are classified using the LeFort system based on the level at which the midface is separated from the rest of the craniofacial skeleton. Repairs focus on the restoration of facial height and projection. With significant comminution or bone loss, bone grafting may be required to maintain the appropriate position of the maxilla in space. Rigid plate and screw fixation obviates the need for prolonged maxillomandibular fixation. Fractures of the mandible are treated by reduction and rigid fixation using restoration of occlusion as the principle intraoperative and postoperative goal. Many mandibular fractures are treated with open reduction and internal fixation, which may make maxillomandibular fixation unnecessary.[13] Certain fractures, however, are best treated closed, and the decision to pursue an open or closed approach depends on the fracture location and orientation.

The same principles of fracture repair apply in the pediatric patient, with some differences. Early treatment within 1 week is necessary, given the rapid healing in children, and fixation is complicated by the presence of permanent teeth embedded in the maxilla and mandible that are easily damaged by hardware. Resorbable hardware is frequently used for children but does not have the mechanical strength required for most adult fractures.

Scalp Reconstruction

The scalp is composed of skin, subcutaneous tissue, an aponeurotic fascial layer continuous with the frontalis and occipital muscles, a loose areolar layer, and periosteum. Small defects up to a few centimeters in size may be closed primarily, depending on location of the defect and mobility of the surrounding scalp. A skin graft can be placed on intact periosteum. If periosteum is absent, the outer calvarial table can be opened with a burr to expose the diploic space, from which granulation tissue will develop to support a skin graft. In the irradiated scalp or in the case of an open wound with alloplastic material at the base, secondary healing or grafting will not provide stable, durable coverage and a flap will be needed.

Scalp flaps are elevated at the subgaleal level, and many possible designs exist. In theory, defects as large as 30% of the scalp can be closed with scalp flaps elevated on major vessels. Incising, or scoring, the inelastic galea can extend the reach of a scalp flap. Tissue expansion also can be used for the reconstruction of larger defects with hair-bearing tissue.

For large scalp defects not amenable to closure by local remaining scalp, distant flaps may be used. Pedicled flaps with usefulness for scalp coverage include the trapezius, latissimus, and pectoralis major muscle flaps. Pedicled flaps are limited by their arc of rotation, so free microvascular tissue transfer offers more flexibility. The free latissimus dorsi muscle flap is preferred for coverage of near-total or total scalp defects because of its flat contour and ability to cover a large surface area. Traumatic scalp avulsions occur in the subgaleal plane and replantation may be based on a single dominant vessel, with good results.

Facial Reconstruction

Defects of the face are usually the result of tumor resection or trauma. STSG coverage of facial defects has limited application because the tissue match is imperfect. FTSGs are taken from donor sites in the preauricular, postauricular, and supraclavicular areas for the best color match. Local flaps provide tissue of appropriate thickness and have the color and texture of the defect.

Nasal defects up to approximately 1.5 cm in size can be closed with local nasal flaps. For larger defects, the forehead flap is preferred. The forehead flap is based on the supratrochlear vessels, and the reconstruction is performed in a staged fashion. The forehead may be expanded before elevation for closure of larger defects and to assist with primary closure of the donor defect. With nasal defects, different components may be lost, and restoration of skin, mucosal lining, and cartilage may be required. Composite grafts from the ear that contain skin and cartilage are useful for defects of the nasal ala. Reconstruction of total nasal defects is complex and may require bone grafting and free tissue transfer (Fig. 68-7).

In the eyelid, FTSGs are a good option for skin loss alone. For a small, full-thickness lid defect, creating a V-shaped wedge can permit primary closure in layers. Adding a lateral canthotomy helps mobilize the lid margin for closure of larger defects, and in some cases, the incision can be carried out into the temporal skin to mobilize the lid further. Eyelid defects can be repaired with flaps rotated from the other lid; this is useful to provide similar tissue. Extensive eyelid defects require support, typically in the form of a chondromucosal graft obtained from the nasal septum or external ear. The graft is placed and covered with a regional skin flap.

For reconstruction of the cheek, a number of different, smaller local flaps can be designed. For larger defects, cervicofacial rotation flaps mobilize skin from the neck and side of the face for transposition to the more central areas of the face.

In the lip, precise alignment of the vermilion border is critical, as is repair of the orbicularis oris muscle to maintain lip competence. Defects are closed in layers, and direct closure is possible for defects up to one third of the transverse width of the lip. Repair of larger defects requires mobilization of the surrounding tissue to reconstruct the oral sphincter. Central defects of the upper lip are best reconstructed using an Abbe flap, which is a mucosal musculocutaneous flap from the lower lip based on the labial artery. The flap is transferred in a staged fashion, with the donor pedicle divided 2 to 3 weeks after flap inset. Large defects of the lower lip are reconstructed with mucosal musculocutaneous flaps from the surrounding area. These reconstructions should preserve motor function of the orbicularis muscle, thus ensuring oral competence. Microstomia may be produced but is often temporary because the tissues will stretch over time.

Facial Transplantation

The first successful face transplantation was done in November 2005 in Amiens, France. Since then, there have been more than 28 additional reports of successful facial composite tissue transplantation. All were done for devastating defects and were complex three-dimensional reconstructions, with variable amounts of skin, muscle, nerve, bone, and parts, such as eyelids, noses, and lips. As of early 2015, all the recipients had experienced at least one episode of acute graft rejection of variable severity within the first year of transplantation, and three of the recipients have died—one from sepsis, a second after noncompliance with his immunosuppressive program, and a third with tumor recurrence in an HIV-positive person who had previously had cancer resection. Functional recovery in the faces has been satisfactory in the long-term cases, with sensory function recovering at 3 to 8 months and acceptable motor recovery between 9 and 12 months with ongoing improvement over the years. Psychological outcomes have been positive, and this is related to the psychosocial support provided for these patients. Aesthetic outcomes have been variable.[14]

The benefit of facial transplantation is that for a select number of severely disfigured individuals, it can provide a better functional and aesthetic outcome than conventional reconstructive methods and, in doing so, improve their quality of life. The immediate risks associated with surgery to transplant facial tissues are essentially the same as those for conventional reconstructive procedures. The important difference is the risk posed by the lifelong, multidrug immunosuppression required to prevent rejection of the transplanted facial tissue. It is also assumed that there would be risks associated with the process of facial tissue rejection itself should that occur in any of these patients. At present, no cases of chronic rejection have been reported.

Facial Aesthetic Surgery

Aesthetic surgery starts with an initial patient consultation for discussion and evaluation of the patient's perceptions and wishes, current health and past medical history, and realistic assessment of the benefits and risks of surgery to change appearance. The motivation to have aesthetic surgery is often psychological and involves body image, so the key to achieving success is selection of patients. The core value of the surgery lies not in the objective beauty of the visible result but in the patient's opinion of and response to the change. Thus, being able to predict the likelihood that a patient will be satisfied with the surgical result is critical. Persons who consider their deformities greater than they actually are, who harbor unrealistic expectations, or who have substance abuse or mental health problems are not good candidates for aesthetic surgery because the surgery is unlikely to meet their needs.

Forehead and Brow Lift

With aging, the eyebrow descends below its youthful location at or above the superior orbital rim. This ptosis is accompanied by a wrinkled brow, excess tissue hooding of the upper eyelids (especially in the temporal brow area), and creasing at the outer canthi (crow's feet) and over the dorsum of the upper nose. These changes

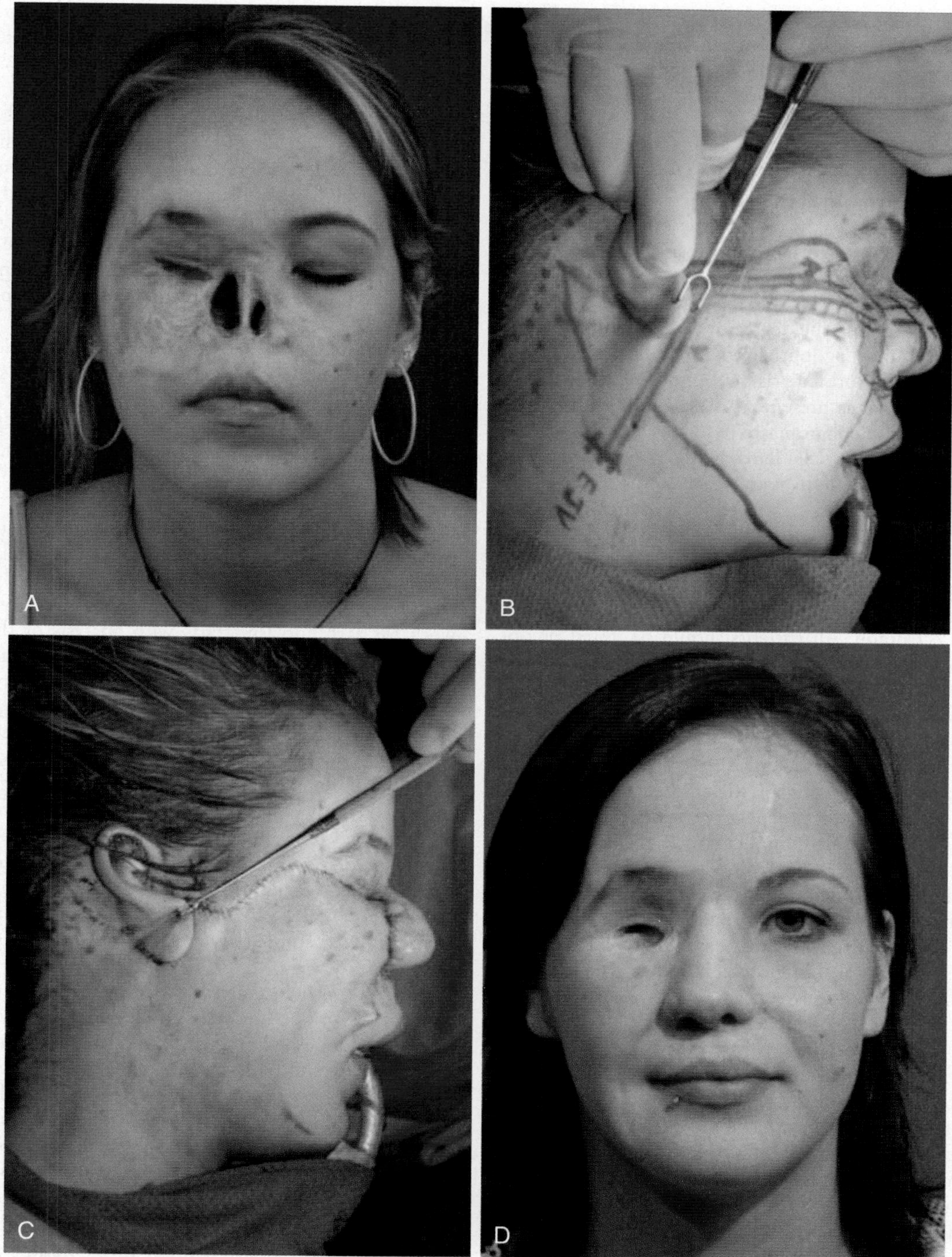

FIGURE 68-7 A, This teenager's nose, orbit, and right cheek were obliterated by a shotgun blast. **B,** A cheek flap with a triangular cervical extension is designed. **C,** The cheek skin component is advanced to resurface the anterior cheek. **D,** The result after facial and nasal repair. Surgical procedures included skin grafting of the right cheek and eyelids, a radial forearm microsurgical free tissue transfer for nasal lining, rib grafts to provide nasal skeletal structure, a three-stage pedicle forehead flap for total external nasal reconstruction, and two cheek skin flaps. (From Menick FJ: Discussion: Simplifying cheek reconstruction: A review of over 400 cases. *Plast Reconstr Surg* 129:1300–1303, 2012.)

can be corrected with a forehead or brow lift done as an open or endoscopic procedure. With an open lift, a bicoronal or modified anterior hairline incision is made. The forehead is elevated as a flap with the plane of dissection between the galea and pericranium and drawn taut, and the excess tissue in the frontal scalp is excised. An endoscopic forehead lift is done through several small incisions within the hairline, extensive subperiosteal dissection to include the orbital rim and root of the nose, release and resection of the corrugator and procerus muscles, preservation of the supratrochlear and supraorbital nerves, and forehead elevation and fixation with percutaneous screws or other devices to reattach it in a higher position. The advantages of an endoscopic forehead lift are minimal scarring and no scalp resection; it is especially useful for patients with frontal baldness.

Blepharoplasty

Blepharoplasty, derived from the Greek *blepharon,* meaning "eyelid," is done for dermatochalasis and corrects bagginess, fatty protrusions, and lax hanging skin around the eyes. If the eyelid itself is drooping, this is termed blepharoptosis and is corrected with a different procedure, a ptosis repair.

Upper eyelid blepharoplasty is done through an incision in the crease of the lid after marking the degree of excess skin to prevent overresection and resultant lagophthalmos (inability to close the eye completely). A strip of orbicularis oculi muscle can be taken, and if excess postseptal fat is present, this protruding orbital fat is resected. Lower eyelid blepharoplasty requires elevation of skin or skin–orbicularis oculi muscle flaps, with removal of skin, muscle, and fat. A transconjunctival approach to the lower eyelid is used for removal of lower lid fat or orbital septum tightening, with little or no skin resection. If the lower lid is lax and poorly adherent to the globe, a lateral canthopexy is done for mild laxity and a lateral canthoplasty is performed for significant laxity.

Complications after blepharoplasty include dry eye syndrome, scleral show, and ectropion. All patients should be tested preoperatively for preexisting dry eye, and a Schirmer test may be predictive of this outcome in those who are prone to this. Scleral show is a complication after lower eyelid blepharoplasty in which the white sclera below the colored iris of the globe is exposed when the patient is in forward gaze. Scleral show is caused by lower eyelid retraction, with shortening of the middle lamella of the orbital septum; patients with preoperative laxity of the lower eyelids are predisposed to this complication if the laxity is not addressed at the time of surgery. Ectropion is eversion of the eyelid with exposure of the conjunctiva and is fairly common in the postoperative period, when the lower eyelid is edematous. Persistent ectropion requires surgery to increase lower lid support, possibly with the addition of skin grafts to augment the lower lid tissue.

Facelift

A facelift, or rhytidectomy, derived from the Greek *rhytis,* meaning "wrinkle," is designed to correct the appearance of facial aging by removing lax, redundant facial and neck tissues. Facial aging is characterized by midface infraorbital flattening, prominent nasolabial folds, deepening of the labiomental crease, downturn of the lateral commissures of the mouth, deepening grooves at the outer corners of the mouth (marionette lines), jowl formation, vertical banding of the platysma muscles in the neck, and laxity of the neck skin. The traditional facelift is a subcutaneous dissection to elevate and to redrape the skin of the face and neck. This has been eclipsed by procedures that also correct the effects of aging and gravity on the deeper tissues and structures of the face.

In addition to skin undermining and redraping, the superficial musculoaponeurotic system (SMAS) of the facial and neck fascia can be tightened by plication. With a lateral SMASectomy, a strip of SMAS is excised along the anterior border of the parotid and the mobile SMAS is brought up and sutured to the fixed SMAS at the malar prominence, which produces durable elevation of the superficial fascia and facial fat. It is effective for patients with a wide variety of anatomic differences and is reproducible and safe. With deep plane rhytidectomy, the facelift flap includes everything down to the fat over the zygomaticus muscles. This procedure corrects midface descent and ptosis but is associated with prolonged facial edema and long recovery.

A number of ancillary procedures are available to enhance the outcome with facelift. Submental lipectomy removes the subcutaneous fat under the chin to improve the contour of the cervical portion of the facelift. Platysmaplasty corrects vertical banding by incising the platysma muscles at the level of the thyroid cartilage and suturing them together in the midline of the upper neck. Fat injection to selected areas under the facelift flaps before closure can fill hollows caused by subcutaneous fat atrophy in areas such as the temple.

Hematoma is the most common complication after facelift; other complications include scarring, alopecia, skin slough, and nerve injury. The most common nerve injury during facelift, occurring at a rate of 3% to 5%, involves the greater auricular nerve, which provides sensation to the lower ear.

Rhinoplasty

Rhinoplasty is a difficult operation because it is a composite of procedures on a number of anatomic structures. When a patient describes a large nose or a long nose, this global description may encompass a dozen contributing structures. Laying the groundwork for a rhinoplasty starts with analysis of the facial proportions, followed by systematic analysis of the nasal components. Starting superiorly, the nasal frontal angle height and depth are noted. The bony pyramid, upper lateral cartilages, and supratip are evaluated for their height, width, and symmetry. The nasal tip is analyzed in terms of its projection, rotation, symmetry, and position of the tip-defining points. The alae are inspected for increased width, collapse, or retraction. The columella is examined for increased or decreased show, and the columellar-labial angle is measured. An internal nasal examination determines whether there is functional deformity by evaluating the septum, turbinates, and internal nasal valves. The soft tissue envelope and thickness of the skin are studied so the effect of underlying changes can be predicted.

Once thorough analysis is complete, this is converted into a surgical plan of action. The initial decision is whether to use an open or endonasal approach. The open rhinoplasty affords excellent exposure and makes it possible to manipulate the osteocartilaginous framework under direct vision. The closed rhinoplasty avoids a visible scar. After the surgical approach is decided on, the rest of the strategy involves choosing techniques based on location-specific criteria. These could include an osteotomy for changing the bony contour of the upper third of the nose, spreader grafts and dorsal resection of the upper lateral cartilages for internal valve collapse and dorsal contour in the middle third of the nose, resection and interdomal sutures for tip refinement and symmetry in the lower third of the nose, and columellar resection or a strut graft for overprojection or loss of tip support at the base of the nose.

The most common surgical complication with rhinoplasty is bleeding, which occurs in up to 3.6% of patients. A more challenging issue is that approximately 5% to 10% of patients require revision or a secondary rhinoplasty for aesthetic or functional reasons. The goal in rhinoplasty is to produce reliable, long-lasting, and natural-appearing results with consistency. It is thought that the key to achieving this goal is component analysis and management of the dorsal, tip, base, and internal nasal structures.[15]

Skin Resurfacing

Several modalities are available to improve the texture, tone, and color of the skin. These include chemical peeling and dermabrasion, but the most rapidly growing technique for skin rejuvenation is laser technology. The use of light as a medical treatment was introduced in the 1960s with the development of the laser (light amplification by stimulated emission of radiation). Ablative lasers (CO_2 and erbium:YAG) have proved highly effective for skin treatment. Removing the epidermis and upper layers of the dermis, this ablation, combined with thermal coagulation of the dermis, heals with robust dermal remodeling that translates into clinical improvement. The problem was resultant scarring in some patients, prolonged edema and erythema, permanent pigmentation abnormalities, and increased risk of infection. Thus, a new concept of fractional photothermolysis was introduced in 2003, which has revolutionized laser surgery. Fractional CO_2 laser resurfacing represents a new class of therapy by delivering dermal coagulative injury without confluent epidermal damage. Distinct lesions of thermal damage are surrounded by larger zones of undisturbed normal skin; this combination allows complete reepithelialization within 24 to 48 hours while producing enough coagulation of the dermal collagen to stimulate connective tissue synthesis and to produce skin tightening. With the fractional approach, results are comparable to those with full-surface ablative lasers without the associated side effects.[16]

The indications for laser resurfacing are facial rhytides, sun-damaged skin, and acne scarring. Benefits of treatment include softening or disappearance of mild to moderate wrinkles, improved skin texture and tone, decreased pore size, and reduction of skin laxity. The entire face, neck, and chest can be treated. Clinical improvement is seen with one or two treatments, scarring and hypopigmentation are rare, and the risk of infection in patients given prophylactic antiviral and antibiotic medications is low because the epidermal layer is restored promptly. When used to treat scars, fractional photothermolysis can flatten out and smooth hypertrophic scars and increases collagen production beneath depressed, atrophic scars, which summate in smoothing of the skin topography. For scarring, a series of treatments at 6- to 12-week intervals may be needed.

Injectable Fillers

In the last few years, there has been more appreciation for the role that loss of volume plays in the contours of the aging face. Contrasting the youthful and aging face shows that areas such as the upper and lateral cheek, temple, nasojugal groove under the eye, and perioral area become atrophic, flat, and hollow in appearance. Restoring volume to reverse the atrophic changes in these areas produces a surprising rejuvenative change.

Volume restoration procedures can include lipotransfer of autologous fat or the use of an increasing number of materials, temporary or permanent, for soft tissue augmentation. Fat grafting is a technique-dependent procedure in which atraumatic handling and methodic layering of the autologous fat is emphasized for long-lasting results. An unexpected finding is that in addition to the volume restoration, fat grafting appears to have rejuvenative effects on the skin itself. The quality of the skin appears to be improved, with softening of wrinkles, decreased pore size, and more even pigmentation.[17] Similar observations are made when fat is injected beneath depressed scars; not only the indentation but the character of the skin itself appears to improve. With reports of the transformative power of fat grafted in areas of radiation damage, chronic ulcers, and other defects, there is much interest in documenting the extent and identifying the mechanism of these effects.[18]

In addition to autologous material, a number of biologic and synthetic products are available for use as soft tissue fillers. Biologic materials derived from organic sources offer the benefits of ready off-the-shelf availability and ease of use but introduce issues of sensitization to foreign animal or human proteins, transmission of disease, and immunogenicity. Also, as the tissue is processed to reduce these untoward side effects, the molecular structure is destabilized so that lack of persistence at the recipient site becomes the rule. The search during the last few years has been for new materials that are better tolerated and have greater longevity. The two major types of biologic tissue fillers are collagen products and hyaluronic acid products.[19]

Synthetic materials can offer permanence. Many injectable and surgically implantable synthetic products have been used over the years, and many have been condemned for complications such as granulomas, acute and delayed infections, migration or displacement, and deformity, which can result from complications or if the material is removed. Thus, only a limited number of synthetic materials are marketed in the United States for facial augmentation.

PLASTIC SURGERY OF THE TRUNK

Reconstruction of the Chest Wall

New techniques for repair of increasingly complex chest wall defects have accompanied advances in surgical and medical treatment of thoracic disease. Indications for chest wall reconstruction include defects arising from oncologic resection, irradiation ulceration, infection, trauma, and congenital defects. Considerations with reconstruction are the status of the pleural cavity, requirement for skeletal support, and provision of soft tissue coverage.

For management of the pleural cavity, principles include adequate débridement and the introduction of well-vascularized tissue to obliterate intrathoracic dead space. Extrathoracic muscles can be transposed to obliterate empyema spaces after pneumonectomy and to close bronchopleural or tracheoesophageal fistulas. Combined with adequate débridement and resection of poorly vascularized tissue, these muscle flaps can be passed through a thoracotomy incision with a two-rib resection and sutured into the defect, with thoracostomy drainage. The choice of muscle depends on the location of the defect; options include the latissimus dorsi, serratus anterior, and pectoralis major muscle flaps. Other muscle flaps with limited but specific uses are the trapezius and superiorly based rectus abdominis. The greater omentum can be transposed on the right gastroepiploic artery as a pedicle flap to provide well-vascularized tissue with the bulk and pliability to obliterate dead space, but it is a secondary choice because of the risks of intra-abdominal complications.

In evaluation of a chest wall defect, a number of variables influence the decision about whether skeletal reconstruction or stabilization is required. These include the site of the chest wall defect, number of ribs resected, extent of resection of other bony structures of the chest wall, history of irradiation, and whether there is wound contamination or infection. The goals of skeletal reconstruction are protection of underlying vital structures, chest wall stability to preserve pulmonary function, and structural support for shoulder and upper limb function.

The number of resected ribs is accepted as the primary clinical determinant of the need for skeletal reconstruction. Stabilization is recommended with resection of four or more consecutive ribs, or 5 cm or more of lateral chest wall, because the resulting flail segment may impair respiratory mechanics. However, there are no conclusive data about the critical size for flail segment reconstruction, and studies of pulmonary ventilation deficits from skeletal chest resection are controversial, particularly in the case of sternal resection.[20] Some of this lack of clarity may be caused by the presence of other factors that influence chest wall stability. Prior irradiation changes affect chest wall stability because soft tissues with radiation fibrosis have the rigidity and stiffness to limit chest wall motion. Location of the defect is relevant because lateral defects are more prone to flail chest deformity than those stabilized by proximity to the sternum or spine. Pancoast tumor resections are stabilized by scapular support, and upper chest wall defects above the fourth rib generally can be closed with soft tissue only.

In the past, reconstruction of the chest skeleton with rib bone grafts or fascia lata was constrained by the limited availability of autologous tissue. One of the important advances in chest wall reconstruction has been the availability of suitable synthetic materials. The ideal characteristics of prosthetic material for chest wall reconstruction are semirigidity, flexibility, biocompatibility, and radiolucency. Several mesh materials are available, including polypropylene (Prolene), crystalline polypropylene and high-density polyethylene (Marlex), and polytetrafluoroethylene (Gore-Tex). Manufactured in a thick sheet, or doubled by folding, these materials provide support and malleability when sutured under tension. If additional rigidity is desired, methyl methacrylate glue can be sandwiched between sheets of mesh and allowed to harden into a rigid shell incorporated within the mesh. These synthetic materials provide good support and stability and perform well, provided they are covered with well-vascularized tissue to prevent infection. Chest wall infections in the presence of synthetic materials can be managed with drainage and antibiotic therapy; if removal of the foreign material can be delayed, a thickened fibrous layer will form to furnish some chest wall stability. In situations in which a chest defect is contaminated or infected at the outset, consideration can be given to the use of a temporary absorbable mesh, but this may have to be replaced when the infection has cleared.

Soft tissue coverage is the final stage of chest wall reconstruction. If a chest wall defect is limited to the skin and subcutaneous tissues, a skin graft is a reconstructive option. Its drawbacks are the eventual contraction that makes it a less attractive form of coverage than a flap and the poor success with graft healing on an irradiated bed. Thus, for chest wall defects with a radiation ulcer or osteoradionecrosis, there is little indication for a skin graft. The healing of skin grafts on the chest wall has been enhanced by the use of the vacuum-assisted closure device, which improves graft stabilization on a bed that is in motion with respiration.

In chest wall reconstruction, vascularized soft tissue flaps are used to close larger defects, to control infection, to obliterate dead space, to cover synthetic materials, and to close wounds with radiation necrosis. Although skin flaps or fasciocutaneous flaps are of some use, the muscle or musculocutaneous pedicle flap is preferred for its robust blood supply. The latissimus dorsi muscle is used frequently for its reliability, large area, and ability to reach almost any chest wall defect on the ipsilateral thorax. Other muscle flaps used for anterolateral soft tissue reconstruction include rectus abdominis, pectoralis major, external oblique, and serratus anterior. Trapezius muscle flaps are useful for defects of the upper third of the back, midback, and shoulders. Free flaps that transfer distant tissue with microvascular anastomoses are not often used and are reserved for situations in which regional flaps are unavailable or have failed or for very large defects. In one series in which aggressive resections of oncologic disease left chest wall defects as large as 300 to 400 cm^2, up to four muscle flaps and free flaps were required to achieve wound closure.[21]

One series of 200 chest wall reconstructions reported a mortality of 6%, with complete or partial flap loss in 5% of patients and pneumonia, respiratory distress, infection, hematoma, and delayed wound healing in 27% of patients. Results were better in patients having immediate reconstruction at the time of resection than in those having delayed reconstruction.[22]

Sternotomy Wounds: Treatment and Prevention

Sternal wound infection and mediastinitis after median sternotomy often require reoperation for débridement and reconstruction. Risk factors include diabetes, smoking, chronic obstructive pulmonary disease, immunosuppression, harvest of internal mammary artery grafts, and use of assist devices. Primary rigid plate fixation of the sternum decreases the incidence of serious complications, and there is current enthusiasm for introducing this surgical method for prevention in high-risk situations.

For sternal instability or infection, débridement, use of wound vacuum-assisted closure devices, muscle and omental flaps, and fixation of the sternum have been described. Although minimal débridement may be needed in the wounds without costochondritis or osteomyelitis, single-stage or serial débridement bridged by vacuum-assisted closure as a sole or adjunct measure for definitive closure of the sternum may be required.[23] Fixation of the separated remaining sternal bone with plates before soft tissue coverage is advocated for earlier extubation, shorter length of stay, a more stable base for an overlying flap, and less long-term chest or shoulder pain. The pectoralis major muscle is the flap of choice for reconstruction of median sternotomy wounds. It is mobilized through the midline incision by detaching it from the sternum, ribs, clavicle, and humeral insertion while preserving the thoracoacromial pedicle (Fig. 68-8). It is advanced medially and, because of its size and arc of rotation, can cover almost the entire sternum. If an aortic vascular graft is exposed, the muscle is mobile enough to wrap around the graft and fill the mediastinum. Another option with the pectoralis major muscle is a turnover flap, in which one or both muscles are left attached on either side of the midline on the perforating branches of the internal mammary artery, dissected free from the remainder of the chest wall, and turned over like a book page to cover the sternum. If the pectoralis muscles are not sufficient, which is sometimes the case over the lower third of the sternum, the rectus abdominis muscle can be mobilized. This is based on the superior epigastric artery and rotated 180 degrees to cover the sternum. If this is done in a patient in whom the ipsilateral internal mammary artery has been harvested for bypass grafting, the rectus abdominis muscle flap can be based on the eighth intercostal vessel; but with this as the pedicle, the distal third may be poorly vascularized. With muscle flap reconstruction, the rates of successful sternal closure are approximately 85%.[24]

The greater omentum has been used for 40 years for the closure of sternal defects and provides reliable coverage. It has been claimed that omentum controls median sternotomy infection more successfully than pedicle muscle flaps, but it has been less commonly used because of exposure of the peritoneal cavity to infection, possibility of later intraperitoneal adhesions, and unavailability of omentum in some patients with previous abdominal surgery. Bringing the omentum into the anterior

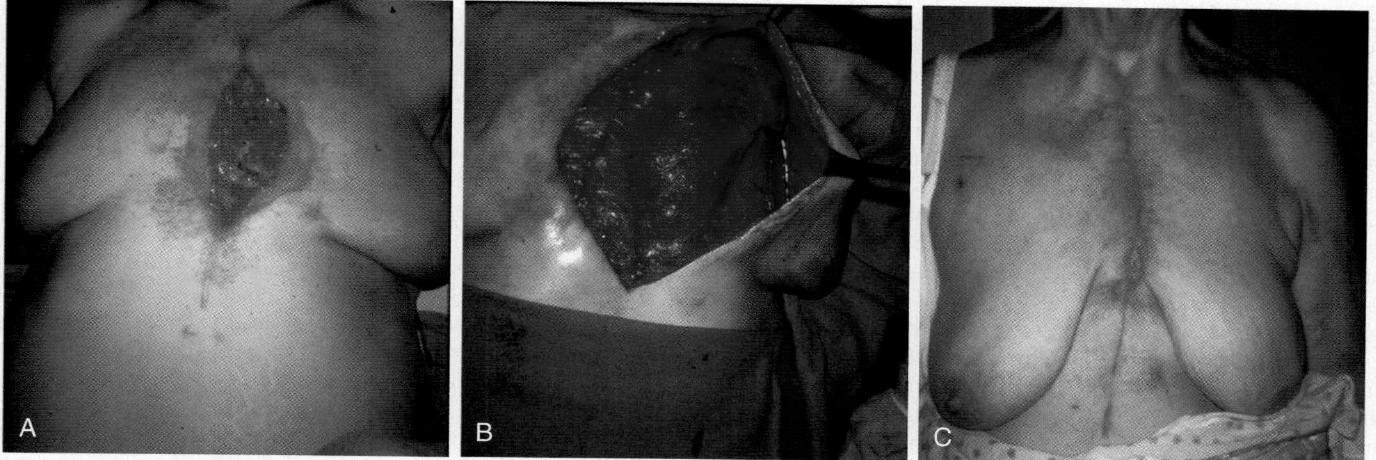

FIGURE 68-8 **A,** 62-year-old woman 1 month after coronary artery bypass procedure with an open infected median sternotomy incision. **B,** The sternal wound was extensively débrided and covered with bilateral pectoralis major muscle flaps. Because the blood supply to the internal mammary perforators was damaged, each pectoralis major muscle was based on its thoracoacromial vascular pedicle after the insertion on the humerus and origin from the ribs was divided to permit muscle transposition. **C,** Postoperative result at 3 months.

mediastinum through a transdiaphragmatic opening has been recently described.[25]

Breast Surgery

Reduction Mammaplasty

Hypertrophy or overgrowth of the breast is excessive development without any pathologic process. It can be familial, with a typical onset during puberty and pregnancy, when hormonal changes exert an abnormal influence on growth in some individuals. Reduction mammaplasty is the resection of excess fat, breast tissue, and skin to achieve a breast size proportional to the body. The principles guiding reduction mammaplasty for breast hypertrophy are to improve the patient's symptoms, to decrease the volume of the breast, to reshape the breast to correct ptosis, to elevate the breast tissue to an anatomically correct position on the chest wall, to reposition the nipple and areola on the reduced and reshaped breast, to preserve the nerve supply to the skin and nipple-areola complex, to maintain blood supply to the breast tissue, and to minimize scars. Surgical techniques are described by the location of the block of tissue to which the nipple and areola are left attached and by the pattern of incisions and subsequent scars.

The pedicle is the portion of the breast tissue preserved with its blood and nerve supply while the surrounding breast tissue is removed. An inferior pedicle technique is used most often, but there are central, superior, medial, lateral, and doubly attached vertical and horizontal pedicles. All variants are designed to maximize blood supply while allowing adequate tissue removal. Suction-assisted lipectomy is used with excision techniques to remove excess fat laterally, and there are a small number of patients with mild to moderate hypertrophy, fatty breasts, good skin tone, no ptosis, and good breast shape for whom liposuction alone will reduce volume, with small scars. In the very large pendulous breast, in which the pedicle would be exceptionally long, the nipple-areola complex is removed and transplanted as a graft. This technique is useful also for patients with vascular disorders or impaired wound healing.

Before reduction mammaplasty, breast cancer screening with examination and mammography usually is done in patients 35 years of age and older. A small number of breast cancers are discovered at the time of reduction by identifying a suspicious area or during routine pathologic study of the tissue; all breast tissue removed surgically should be sent for histopathologic study. There is no set lower age limit, but for the adolescent with breast hypertrophy, reduction is deferred until the breasts have stopped growing and are stable in size for at least 12 months before surgery. Secondary or repeated breast reduction has a higher complication rate because problems associated with a damaged blood supply, such as delayed wound healing, fat necrosis, and loss of the nipple and areola, are seen when a pedicle is developed again in a previously reduced breast. Wound healing is impaired in the previously irradiated breast because of radiation-induced vascular changes. Recommendations in these patients include the following: delay between radiation and mammaplasty to allow some of the vascular changes to subside; and technical modifications using pedicles that are broader and shorter than usual and minimizing adjustments to the breast tissue. Obese patients are poor candidates for breast reductions, with more local and systemic complications. Smoking is a contraindication to breast reduction.

Sequelae of reduction mammaplasty include changes in the sensibility of the nipple and areola in 20% to 25% of cases, usually a decrease but occasionally an increase in sensation. Lactation and breastfeeding are not always possible after breast reduction. Complications with reduction mammaplasty include wound dehiscence, skin slough, loss of tissue, hematoma, infection, and fat necrosis with palpable nodules of poorly vascularized fat. Fat necrosis may prompt later investigation or biopsy to distinguish these lumps from breast neoplasms.

Outcome studies after reduction mammaplasty have shown that patients gain relief from symptoms, can engage more in activities of daily life, and are happy with the results. In one study of 185 women, 97% reported improvement in back, shoulder, and neck pain; 95% said they were happy or very happy with the results of surgery, and 98% said they would recommend it to others.[26]

Breast Augmentation

Augmentation mammaplasty is a cosmetic procedure done to resolve the dissatisfaction that some women feel with small breasts, either because their breasts never developed to a desired size or because their breasts lost volume after pregnancy or weight loss or with aging. With the development of the sealed silicone gel breast implant in 1962, breast augmentation became widely accepted. All U.S. Food and Drug Administration–approved breast implants, regardless of filling material, have an outer shell or envelope constructed of silicone elastomer. Silicone gel–filled implants are polymerized to a consistency similar to that of breast tissue. Newer gel implants have a thicker, more viscous gel than previous generations of these devices. Called cohesive gel, the material tends to stay in place, even if the shell of the implant is damaged. Gel implants are prefilled and sealed and cannot be adjusted in size in the operating room. Saline-filled implants are silicone rubber shells filled in the operating room. Advantages of the saline implants are the benign nature of saline, some flexibility in adjusting size by varying the amount of fluid put in the implant, and smaller incisions because the implants are inserted while empty. The primary disadvantage is a higher incidence of visible rippling or wrinkling of the implant under the skin, particularly in thin patients.

Breast augmentation requires an incision in the skin and subcutaneous tissue, with creation of a pocket in which a breast implant is placed and positioned. There are a number of technical variations. One of three incisions can be used, each with advantages and drawbacks. The inframammary incision provides excellent access and does not require dissection within the breast parenchyma; the disadvantage is a scar that may be noticeable in the smaller breast. A periareolar incision is camouflaged in the areola and heals with little visible scarring but has the disadvantage of possible changes in sensation in the nipple-areola area. An axillary incision leaves no scars on the breast, but it is more difficult to create the pocket with this approach. The pocket into which the implant will be placed can be in one of two positions relative to the breast tissue and pectoralis major muscle. Subglandular placement superficial to the pectoralis muscle fascia provides more ability to control the shape of the breast and is associated with a more rapid postoperative recovery. With submuscular placement of the implant, the contour of the breast may be smoother because the edges of the implant are blunted by the muscle, there is less chance for development of capsular contracture (hardened scar around the implant), nipple sensation is protected, and mammogram interpretation may be more accurate when the breast tissue is lifted up and away from the implant by the muscle. Disadvantages include more postoperative discomfort and longer recovery, movement of the implant when the muscle is flexed, and less ability to lift the parenchyma in a breast with some degree of ptosis.

In considering potential problems that can develop after augmentation mammaplasty, it is useful to distinguish between operative complications and implant concerns. Perioperative complications are relatively low, with bleeding or hematoma in 1% to 3%, wound infections in 1% to 2%, and some degree of diminished sensibility of the nipple-areola complex in approximately 15% of patients, depending on the incision used and position of the implant relative to the muscle. More numerous and more serious are the sequelae presenting weeks or years after the surgery. These include capsular contracture, implant deflation, implant rupture, and implant displacement.

Capsular contraction occurs when the normal envelope of fibrous tissue around an implant becomes thicker or tighter so that the implant no longer feels soft and pliant. If the degree of capsular contracture is great, there can be pain, distortion, and palpability or distortion of the implant. Capsular contracture occurs in approximately 15% of patients, and it is not possible to predict who will develop it or to take preventive measures. Treatment involves removing the fibrous capsule surgically and replacing the implant, but this often results in recurrence of the capsular contracture. The only permanent correction is removal of the implant.

Saline-filled implants can deflate when the fluid leaks out of the implant through the valve or implant shell. This occurs in approximately 7% of patients within the first 5 years after surgery. Causes include damage from handling at the time of surgery, pressure from capsular contracture, compression of the implant due to trauma, and other reasons that remain unknown.

Silicone gel implants can rupture, releasing the gel material; its frequency is similar to that of deflation of saline implants. However, there is an important difference in how the rupture is detected. When a gel implant ruptures, the breast volume will not change because the gel remains in the area; in many cases, the rupture remains undiagnosed—a silent rupture. Thus, it is recommended that gel implants be studied by MRI at intervals of 3 to 5 years so that silent ruptures can be detected and treated. Mammography is not a reliable diagnostic tool for rupture, and surveillance with MRI is the standard.[27]

Three areas of extensive study have been the questions of whether breast implants are associated with breast cancer, whether a type of anaplastic large cell lymphoma (ALCL) is associated with breast implants, and whether the silicone material in breast implants is associated with connective tissue disease. No study has ever suggested that the presence of a breast implant is a cause of breast cancer. The primary question has been whether the presence of an implant is responsible for delayed detection or poorer prognosis because of compromise of screening mammography. Standard mammograms in a woman with breast implants show only approximately 75% of the breast tissue because the remainder is obscured by the implant. Displacement techniques are used to address this, and additional views are needed. Studies have shown no significant difference between women with and without implants who develop breast cancer in terms of the size or stage of the tumor when it is diagnosed. One series of 3182 women observed for 18.7 years after breast augmentation has shown no increased risk, no delay in diagnosis, and no worse prognosis for these patients compared with a comparable group of women without implants.[28]

There is substantial evidence that a type of ALCL is associated with breast implants. As of 2015, there are reports of 173 patients with breast implants who developed ALCL in the breast. The clinical course seems to be unusually benign compared with other systemic ALCL, but many of the patients are treated with radiation therapy or chemotherapy.[29] Work to standardize an approach to diagnosis, staging, and treatment is currently under way.

Concern about the association of breast implants with the development of autoimmune or connective tissue diseases, such as lupus, scleroderma, or rheumatoid arthritis, arose because of cases reported in the literature in the early 1980s. A number of subsequent epidemiologic analyses failed to support this association, and a committee of the Institute of Medicine of the National Academy of Sciences reviewed more than 2000 peer-reviewed studies and 1200 data sets. In 1999, the Institute of Medicine concluded that there was no definitive evidence linking breast implants to cancer, immunologic disease, or neurologic disease and that women with breast implants were no more likely to develop these disorders than those in the rest of the population.

Breast Ptosis and Mastopexy

Breast ptosis describes the downward displacement of the glandular tissue of the breast. Sagging and drooping develop when lax skin with poor elasticity cannot support and shape the underlying breast parenchyma and the fascial attachments, the suspensory ligaments of Cooper, lose elasticity and become attenuated. These changes are seen with significant weight loss, postpartum atrophy, postmenopausal involution, and the continual gravitational pull associated with aging. Breast ptosis is classified by the position of the nipple-areola complex relative to the inframammary fold and breast mound; the degree of ptosis is considered in choosing the technique for surgical correction. There are numerous options for mastopexy, and these draw on both breast reduction and breast augmentation techniques. The key elements are the removal and tightening of redundant skin and breast tissue and the possible addition of a breast implant. The primary intention when introducing a breast implant is not increased size; rather, the implant adds volume to the flattened upper pole of the breast and provides support and lift for a soft, involuted breast with thin, inelastic skin. The challenge with mastopexy is balancing tightening with restoration of volume. The effects of surgery are only temporary, and ptosis recurs with the passage of time, depending on the age of the patient, the cause of the ptosis, the size of the breast, and whether an implant was used.

Fat Grafting to the Breast

Autologous fat injection into the breast has been used successfully for breast enlargement, correction of breast deformities, additional coverage to disguise breast implants, and treatment of radiation damage to the chest. Historically, there was concern that injected fat would not survive and fat necrosis or calcification might impede breast cancer screening. However, drawing on experience with fat grafting in the face, techniques for harvesting fat with minimal trauma and injecting it into the breast in small aliquots were described. By taking care to avoid placing large amounts of fat at one site, the incidence of fat necrosis is lower, and lipografting in the breast is being done much more commonly. Adjunctive techniques include expanding the skin envelope and generating a recipient matrix before serial seeding with micrografts, placing the grafts outside the breast parenchyma itself, and layering the fat into different levels. With evidence that technical performance is critical, excellent long-lasting results are being reported.[30] An area of intense interest and scrutiny is the use of adipose stem cells in fat grafting for breast enlargement. Still largely theoretical in clinical practice, the possibility of stimulating permanent fat survival in the breast is being weighed against the risk of introducing growing cell lines into tissue that will develop malignancy in some percentage of the treated population.

Gynecomastia

Male breast enlargement occurs bilaterally in 50% to 55% of cases; most patients are asymptomatic or report some tenderness, soreness, or sensitivity. Caused by an increased estrogen to androgen ratio, the incidence is increased with generalized obesity because of increased conversion of testosterone to estradiol in adipose tissue. On histologic evaluation, variable degrees of ductal proliferation and stromal hyperplasia present in three patterns, described as florid, intermediate, or fibrous. The florid pattern shows ductal hyperplasia surrounded by loose cellular connective tissue. The fibrous pattern has extensive fibrosis of the stroma with little ductal proliferation and is seen with gynecomastia longer than 1 year in duration. The intermediate pattern represents a transition between the florid and fibrous types.

There are physiologic, pathologic, and pharmacologic causes. Physiologic or idiopathic gynecomastia, with no pathologic basis, develops transiently in more than 60% of newborns because of exposure to transplacental estrogens. During puberty, estrogen and testosterone shifts result in a prevalence of 50% to 60%, with presentation during midpuberty (14 years) and a self-limited average duration of 1 to 2 years. With increasing age, the prevalence gradually increases to more than 70% in the seventh decade. Pathologic gynecomastia is associated with cirrhosis, malnutrition, hypogonadism, Klinefelter syndrome, renal disease, hyperthyroidism, hypothyroidism, and neoplastic disease. Tumors that may lead to gynecomastia are testicular tumors (e.g., Leydig cell and Sertoli cell tumors, choriocarcinomas), adrenal tumors, pituitary adenomas, and lung carcinoma. Gynecomastia is not associated with male breast cancer except in patients with Klinefelter syndrome, in whom the incidence of mammary carcinoma is 20 to 60 times greater than in men without this chromosomal aberration. Pharmacologic gynecomastia is caused by drugs from a number of classes, including antiandrogens, antibiotics, chemotherapeutic agents, cardiovascular disease drugs, and drugs of abuse (e.g., alcohol, heroin, amphetamines, marijuana).

For the patient presenting with gynecomastia, pertinent history includes duration, concomitant disease, and medication use. The breasts, thyroid, abdomen, testes, and overall degree of virilization are examined. Laboratory studies include determinations of hormone levels and, as indicated, additional selected studies, such as checking karyotype, testicular ultrasound, hepatic or renal function tests, mammography, and imaging studies of the chest or adrenals. Treatment of an underlying disorder may lead to regression of gynecomastia, especially when an offending medication can be identified and withdrawn in drug-related cases or when testosterone is administered for testicular failure. However, gynecomastia of long duration, with a fibrous pattern, is unlikely to resolve spontaneously.

Indications for surgery include symptomatic gynecomastia, enlargement persisting for more than 18 to 24 months in adolescent boys, gynecomastia of long duration that has progressed to fibrosis, and gynecomastia in patients at risk for breast cancer (e.g., those with Klinefelter syndrome). Surgical approaches depend on the degree of enlargement and whether there is associated ptosis (drooping) of the breasts. For patients with mild to moderate gynecomastia with minimal drooping, there are several options, including suction-assisted liposuction, ultrasound-assisted liposuction, direct excision through a small incision confined to the areola, and a combination of these techniques. For the patient with moderate to large gynecomastia and associated laxity and descent of the breast, skin resection and transposition of the nipple-areola complex superiorly to an appropriate position on the chest wall are required. This necessitates additional incisions, with resultant scarring; there are various techniques to minimize the appearance of these scars. For the patient with massive gynecomastia, an en bloc resection of excessive skin and breast tissue is needed, with free nipple grafting or repositioning of the nipple-areola complex on a pedicle flap.[31]

The challenge with surgical excision of gynecomastia is achieving perfect symmetry of the two breasts and producing a smooth contour, without indentations or irregularities. Suction-assisted lipectomy is helpful to smooth the contours and to taper the area of resection into the surrounding subcutaneous tissue on the chest wall to make it undetectable. Postoperative complications include hematoma or seroma caused by the extensive dissection and undermining of the skin through a small incision; these can be mitigated with good hemostasis and the use of drains and compression garments. Less common complications include infection and tissue loss, including loss of a portion of the nipple-areola complex.

Congenital and Developmental Deformities

Breast and chest wall deformities range from hyperplastic anomalies, such as polymastia and polythelia, to hypoplastic deformational anomalies characterized by a paucity of breast tissue, as seen in Poland syndrome. Described by Alfred Poland in 1841, this syndrome is a severe form of chest wall and breast hypoplasia that occurs in approximately 1 in 25,000 live births. It occurs sporadically, is generally unilateral, and affects males more frequently than females (3 : 1). The syndrome includes a spectrum of deformities, the most consistent of which is absence of the sternocostal head of the pectoralis major muscle. Other features can include absence of the ipsilateral pectoralis major and minor muscles, absence of the anterior portions of ribs 2 to 5, loss of the latissimus dorsi and serratus anterior muscles, absence of axillary hair, limited subcutaneous chest wall fat, and brachysyndactyly of the ipsilateral hand. There can be absence of the breast or a varying degree of hypoplasia, and the nipple can be absent or displaced.

Treatment options for Poland syndrome include autologous tissue, alone or in combination with synthetic implant materials, to correct the contour deformity of the chest wall and to reconstruct the breast. Because of its proximity, a pedicled latissimus dorsi muscle flap is preferred if the muscle itself is not involved; as an alternative, the rectus abdominis muscle can be introduced as a pedicle or free flap. The timing of surgery requires careful consideration. In general, reconstruction is deferred until late adolescence to avoid the risk of growth inhibition with early operative trauma and to minimize the need for multiple revisions to keep pace with chest wall and breast growth.

Abdominal Wall Surgery

Components Separation and Flap Coverage

Acquired abdominal wall defects are caused by incisional hernia, tumor resection, infection, irradiation, and trauma. The goals of abdominal wall reconstruction are protection of the abdominal contents, restoration of the integrity of the musculofascial wall, and provision of dynamic muscle support. Treatment is selected on the basis of a number of factors, including the medical status of the patient, wound bed preparedness, size of the defect, position of the defect, and whether there is loss of stable skin and subcutaneous tissue or loss of myofascial tissue. If skin coverage and myofascial continuity are absent, the defect is a complete, full-thickness loss, and both layers will have to be restored by more complex approaches.

The timing of immediate versus delayed reconstruction depends on the clinical situation. Assessment of the patient includes body mass index and pulmonary evaluation because postoperative loss of domain may decrease vital capacity, total lung capacity, and functional residual capacity.[32] Nutritional status, tobacco use, and fluid and electrolyte imbalance are corrected. Assessment of the wound bed includes identification of bacterial contamination, exposed viscera, adherent bowel, enterocutaneous fistulas, previous irradiation, prosthetic material used in previous operations, and previous incisions or scars that interrupt the abdominal circulation. The presence of inflammation and edema, even in a clean wound, limits local tissue advancement; significant inflammation may be present after dehiscence, traumatic defects, fistulas, or recent infection.

Immediate and one-stage reconstruction of a wall defect is the approach of choice for a patient who is medically stable, with a clean wound bed and reliable reconstructive options. This approach is suitable for patients having ventral herniorrhaphy or tumor extirpation requiring concomitant reconstruction. Definitive repair is delayed if the patient is unstable, the wound is contaminated, further explorations are planned, or there is abdominal distention or inflammation. In these cases, the wound is managed with skin grafts, prosthetic mesh, or vacuum-assisted closure device as a temporary measure until reconstruction can be done.

STSGs have a high rate of success (even in colonized wounds), provide stable coverage to protect from infection, and prevent continued fluid and protein loss from granulation tissue. In addition, they aid in eventual closure by reducing the size of the wound through contracture. The problem is that STSGs become fixed to the viscera on which they are placed; the consequences of skin grafting include hernia, abdominal wall bulge, and possible trauma to the viscera. Later reconstruction involving removal of the skin grafts should be delayed for a minimum of 6 months, until the wound has matured. This will decrease the density of the adhesions and scar tissue and help control the rate of inadvertent enterotomy, which converts a clean case in which prosthetic mesh could be used into a contaminated one.

If temporary fascial support of a contaminated wound is needed to prevent evisceration and to maintain domain, an absorbable mesh can be used while the acute problems are addressed. Absorbable mesh made from polyglycolic acid can remain in place for 3 to 4 months, protecting the intra-abdominal contents and providing support while granulation tissue develops and is skin grafted. This type of mesh undergoes hydrolytic degradation, so its usefulness is temporally limited because of loss of structural strength, with ulceration and delayed hernia formation. If it is left in place, there will be eventual loss of support, but there will be no difficulty in removing the prosthetic material 6 to 12 months later in a patient undergoing definitive repair of the defect.

The vacuum-assisted closure device is effective for temporary closure of an abdominal wall defect by providing the support of a nondistensible dressing, limiting fascial retraction by applying constant medial tension, and stimulating granulation tissue growth. With modification of the standard vacuum pack dressing, visceral adherence to the abdominal wall can be limited, whereas fascial closure is encouraged. Studies in a laboratory model have shown that the vacuum-assisted closure device results in a fourfold increase in vascularization to the wound, decreased bacterial colonization, increased formation of granulation tissue by 103%, and increased flap survival by 21% compared with controls.[33]

In planning of definitive repair, reconstructive options are considered in terms of the type of abdominal wall defect, which can be broadly classified into one of three categories:

Loss of skin and subcutaneous tissue only. These partial defects are closed primarily if small, with skin grafting, random or local flaps, fasciocutaneous flaps, vacuum-assisted closure device, or tissue expander before primary closure.

Loss of musculofascial tissue, with intact skin coverage. These partial defects are repaired with prosthetic mesh or with

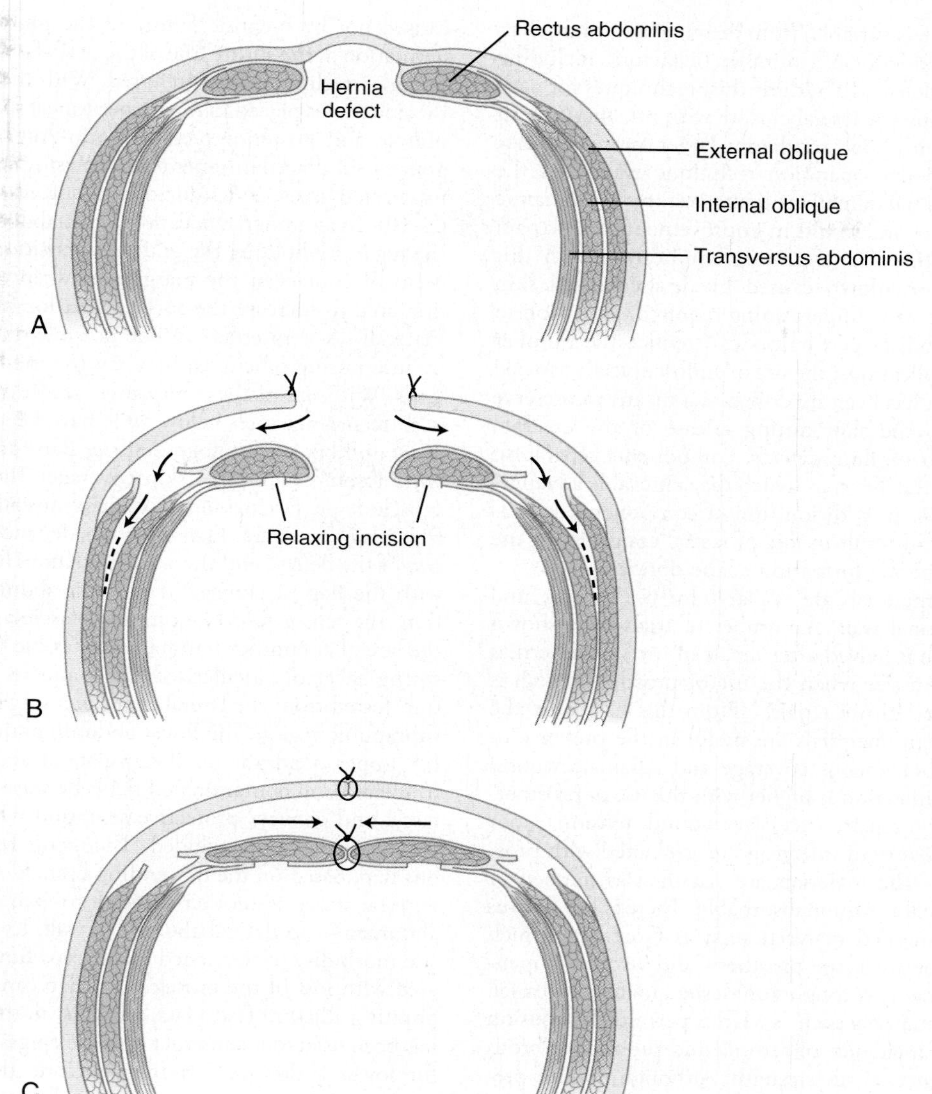

FIGURE 68-9 Components separation to mobilize the musculofascial tissue for closure of a midline abdominal wall defect. **A,** Anterior midline abdominal wall defect. **B,** Anterior rectus sheath separated from the external oblique aponeurosis. Longitudinal relaxing incisions are made anteriorly along the linea semilunaris and posteriorly in the posterior rectus sheath. **C,** Relaxing incisions in anterior and posterior rectus sheath. These allow stretching of the rectus muscle as the anterior rectus wall is pulled medially to correct the defect. (From Nozaki M, Sasaki K, Huang TT: Reconstruction of the abdominal wall. In Mathes SJ, editor: *Plastic surgery*, ed 2, Philadelphia, 2006, Saunders Elsevier, p 1182.)

autologous tissue reconstruction. Autologous techniques include primary repair, open or endoscopically assisted components separation, or local flap and distant flaps selected on the basis of the location of the fascial defect on the trunk.

Loss of both the skin and fascial layers, with a full-thickness open defect. These complete defects can be approached with staged reconstruction to close the skin and return later to provide fascial replacement. Alternatively, a local or distant muscle flap, musculocutaneous flap, fasciocutaneous flap, or free tissue transfer can supply well-vascularized tissue with the use of prosthetic material for fascial support as needed.

Components separation is a technique in which a series of fascial incisions are used to separate the structural components of the abdominal wall and to mobilize the musculofascial tissue for closure of a midline abdominal wall defect (Fig. 68-9). The anterior rectus sheath is separated from the external oblique aponeurosis by making a longitudinal relaxing incision along the linea semilunaris. This allows the anterior rectus sheath and muscle to move medially while maintaining its neurovascular supply, which comes from between the internal oblique and transversus abdominis in a segmental fashion. Posteriorly, the rectus muscle is released from its posterior sheath with medial advancement of 5 cm in the epigastric region, 10 cm at the umbilicus, and 3 cm in the suprapubic region. With the modification of also dividing the internal oblique component of the anterior rectus sheath, unilateral advancement increases to 8 to 10 cm in the epigastrium, 10 to 15 cm in the midabdomen, and 6 to 8 cm in the suprapubic region. With the components separation technique, the reported rate of hernia recurrence is variable, from below 5% to more than 30%, presumably dependent on a number of factors, including the dimensions of the defect. To address this, techniques for augmenting but not bridging the fascial closure with prosthetic mesh have been described, with good results for larger, more complex hernias.[34] The components separation technique eliminates the need for prosthetic material in many patients, restores the dynamic abdominal wall function, and results in improvement in back pain and postural abnormalities. A common complication with this technique is wound breakdown caused by devascularized skin flaps consequent to the wide undermining required. Attention to preserving the periumbilical perforators can reduce the number of wound healing complications; the use of endoscopically assisted components separation has been described as a means to preserve midline perforators to the skin during release of the external oblique. In contrast to midline defects, components separation has limited use in lateral defects, in which the achievable advancement decreases by 50%. In addition, use of components separation in lateral repairs can result in loss of fascial congruity of the abdominal wall, with hernia formation at the donor site.

Various prosthetic materials are available for use as structural support of the abdominal wall. A number of trials have shown that the recurrence rate is halved after repair of incisional hernias more than 5 to 6 cm in size when the use of prosthetic mesh is compared with primary suture repair.[35] From this has come the consensus that prosthetic materials are useful in the presence of adequate skin and subcutaneous coverage and adequate wound bed. The incidence of infection is higher with the use of prosthetics than with primary repair; excessive wound tension, poor wound status, and a history of infection are associated with prosthetic material failure. The materials are classified as meshed or nonmeshed and absorbable or nonabsorbable. There is less fibrous ingrowth with a nonmeshed material such as Gore-Tex, which minimizes adhesions between the prosthesis and viscera; reopening of the abdominal cavity through nonmeshed material is easier. Alternatively, meshed material such as Marlex permits the effusion of fluid for a reduced incidence of seroma and promotes fibrous ingrowth, which enhances tissue strength. Although mesh is preferred, complications can include infection, extrusion of the prosthetic material, and bowel erosion when folds and wrinkles in the mesh exert pressure against the bowel wall. Softer, smoother mesh, made from Prolene, is more pliable, and erosion into bowel is less common. In an effort to avoid these complications of infection, extrusion, abdominal wall stiffness, pain, and fistula formation that are associated with nonabsorbable materials, biomaterials derived from human and animal sources have been developed. These bioprostheses are absorbable; they include human acellular dermis (AlloDerm), porcine acellular dermis (Permacol), and porcine small intestinal submucosa (Surgisis). These materials have an acellular collagen matrix that promotes host tissue remodeling and replacement. Although they are resistant to infection, biocompatible, and mechanically stable over the short term, their disadvantages are high cost and few long-term studies establishing outcomes with regard to hernia recurrence.

Several techniques are used to place prosthetic material—mesh onlay, mesh inlay, retrorectus placement, and intraperitoneal underlay. For onlay grafts, the material is cut larger than the fascial defect, placed superficially to the anterior rectus sheath, and anchored at its margins with sutures. With inlay grafts, the prosthetic material is cut to the same size as the fascial defect, placed in the defect, and anchored to the edges with sutures. With these techniques for mesh repair, recurrence is not uncommon. This is caused not by intrinsic failure of the prosthetic material but by herniation at the suture line of the graft-fascia interface. Therefore, underlay techniques are preferred. With the retrorectus approach, the material is placed in the preperitoneal space between the rectus muscle and posterior rectus sheath. Alternatively, the underlay graft can be placed intraperitoneally, using an endoscopic approach in selected cases, and secured with sutures, tacks, or staples (Fig. 68-10). In an underlay location, intra-abdominal pressure bolsters the repair by holding the graft in apposition to the fascia; at least 4 cm of contact at the margins between the mesh and fascia is desirable to increase the surface area for fibrous ingrowth at the material-fascia interface. When possible, the viscera are protected by interposing omentum between the mesh and abdominal contents. With use of these measures, secure and physiologic repairs with recurrence rates below 10% have been reported.

A number of autologous tissue flaps are available for defects with absent or unstable skin coverage. These include skin flaps, muscle flaps, fasciocutaneous flaps, musculocutaneous flaps, and free tissue transfers. Flap selection depends on the location and size of the defect, and there are guidelines for matching the defect with the flap of choice.[36] For lower abdominal wall reconstruction, the tensor fascia lata musculofasciocutaneous flap based on the lateral circumflex femoral artery is the flap of choice. A dense, strong sheet of vascularized fascia and its overlying skin can be transferred from the lateral thigh in a single stage to resurface the suprapubic region, the lower abdominal quadrants, or as high as the upper quadrant on the ipsilateral abdomen. It is useful in irradiated and contaminated fields because it provides autologous fascia and conveys protective sensation when the lateral femoral cutaneous nerve is included. The rectus femoris musculocutaneous flap, based on the descending branch of the lateral circumflex femoral artery, is another choice for repair of the lower half of the abdomen or ipsilateral abdominal wall. Its drawback is the donor site morbidity of weakened quadriceps function in the leg associated with loss of the muscle. This flap can be extended by incorporating adjacent fascia lata, and this "mutton chop" modification has been used to reconstruct into the epigastrium. Additional flaps for lower abdominal coverage include the anterior thigh flap, external oblique muscle, and rectus abdominis musculocutaneous flap, based inferiorly on the inferior epigastric vessels, which is also the flap of choice for lateral defects of the lower two thirds of the abdomen. In the upper half of the abdomen, the superiorly based vertical or transverse abdominis musculocutaneous flap, based on the superior epigastric artery, is useful for central defects, and the latissimus dorsi musculocutaneous flap, based on the thoracodorsal vessels, is suitable for reconstruction of the lateral parts of the upper abdomen. Free flaps are considered when local tissues are not available or when a pedicle flap cannot reach or is too small to cover a defect. In the case of a free tissue transfer to the abdomen, suitable recipient vessels are required. Usually, the inferior epigastric, deep circumflex iliac, superior epigastric, internal thoracic, or saphenous vein graft may be used. Because it contains fascia, the tensor fascia lata flap is the most commonly used free flap, but use of an innervated free latissimus dorsi flap has been described as a means to bring contractile function and strength to the lost abdominal wall.

Abdominoplasty

Abdominoplasty removes fat and skin from the abdominal wall and repairs fascial laxity or dehiscence to produce an abdominal profile that is smoother and firmer. It is most effective in persons of normal weight who have loose, sagging skin because of heredity,

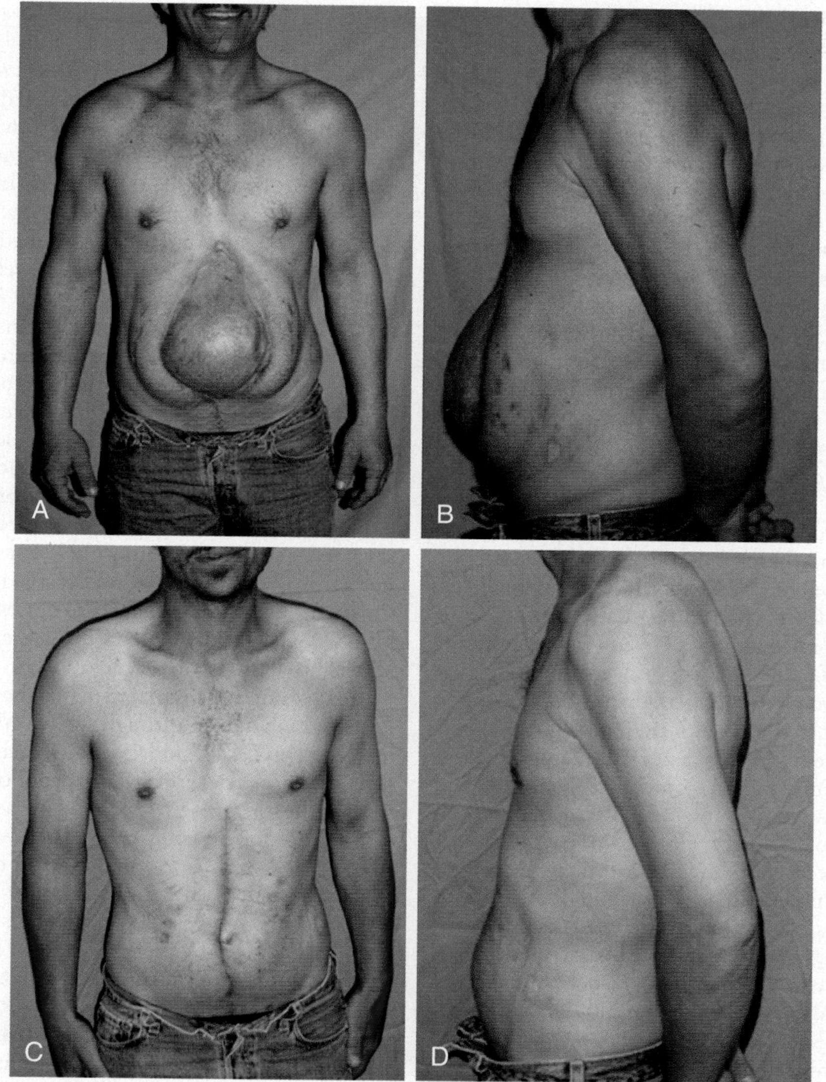

FIGURE 68-10 Abdominal defect with skin graft coverage in a man who sustained major visceral injuries in a motor vehicle accident. **A,** Abdominal compartment syndrome required release of the abdominal closure and split-thickness skin grafts for coverage. **B,** Lateral view of ventral hernia with skin grafts on viscera. **C** and **D,** Postoperative view 1 year after peritoneal mesh reconstruction of abdominal wall.

multiple pregnancies, fluctuations in weight, or significant weight loss. The basic technique includes a horizontal skin incision low on the abdominal wall between the umbilicus and pubic hairline; elevation of the skin and subcutaneous tissue from the deep fascia up to the level of the xiphoid and costal margins; incision around the umbilicus, leaving it attached to the underlying fascia as an isolated island; repair of a diastasis or plication of the muscle fascia; drawing of the flap inferiorly under mild tension; excision of excess skin and subcutaneous tissue; securing of the flap inferiorly to Scarpa or deep fascia; creation of a new opening in the flap for exteriorization of the umbilicus; and placement of multiple drains under the abdominal flap.

In addition to the traditional abdominoplasty, there are several variations. A miniabdominoplasty is a limited abdominoplasty, useful when the excess skin and fat are primarily below the umbilicus. Fleur-de-lis abdominoplasty refers to an inverted T type of abdominoplasty, which is useful for individuals with large amounts of excess skin. An umbilical float may be used in conjunction with a miniabdominoplasty to avoid the incision and scarring around the umbilicus. Here, the umbilicus is left attached to the skin, cut loose from the underlying abdominal fascia, and allowed to descend or float toward the pubic area as the skin is tightened. This shortens the distance between the umbilicus and pubic bone, so it is not suitable if the distance will be shortened greatly.

Complications, most frequently surgical site infection, hematoma, seroma, marginal skin loss, and minor wound separation, occur in 12% to 32% of abdominoplasty patients.[37] Major complications are reported in 1.4% of cases and include major skin loss, deep venous thrombosis, and pulmonary embolus. Risk factors include diabetes, hypertension, and smoking. Complications are magnified dramatically in obese patients, with reports of complications in 80% of obese patients. Adherence to the guideline that a patient should be at or near his or her ideal body mass index results in fewer serious complications and higher patient satisfaction. Preoperative smoking cessation is mandatory.

Reconstruction of the Perineum

The indications for perineal wound reconstruction have escalated rapidly in the last few years. This is a consequence of more radical surgical resections, in which abdominoperineal resection (APR) may be combined with vaginectomy, sacrectomy, or exenteration of pelvic organs, and of the expanded role for adjuvant radiotherapy in the treatment of rectal cancer. When APR follows chemoradiotherapy, perineal wound complications, including nonhealing wounds, abscess, dehiscence, and fistula, have been reported in 41% of primary perineal wound closures.[38] These complications are caused by the presence of a wide cavity with dead space, poor vascularity of the surrounding tissue, use of irradiated skin in the closure, and bacterial contamination with bowel resection. Musculocutaneous flap reconstruction of a pelvic soft tissue defect introduces well-vascularized nonirradiated tissue with enough bulk to obliterate dead space, brings in a skin paddle for cutaneous wound closure, and provides functional restoration after vaginectomy.

Immediate flap reconstruction has been readily accepted for large perineal defects when the skin cannot be closed primarily or a massive dead space is present. More recently, there has been interest in extending the role of a flap into situations in which a skin paddle is not essential for cutaneous closure of the perineal wound or a large amount of tissue bulk is not needed to fill pelvic dead space. Early results using a musculocutaneous flap to reconstruct irradiated APR defects that could alternatively be closed primarily have shown a reduced incidence of major perineal wound complications. Comparing the outcomes of immediate vertical rectus abdominis musculocutaneous (VRAM) flap reconstruction with outcomes of primary closure in patients with similar irradiated APR defects has shown a 4-fold reduction in major perineal wound dehiscence and a 10-fold reduction in perineal abscess formation associated with flap use.[39]

Flap reconstruction is preferably accomplished at the time of the original extirpative procedure rather than in a delayed manner. Functional issues can be addressed at the same time; in the pelvic area, this typically involves vaginal or penile reconstruction, ideally using the same flap for reparative and functional purposes. Clinical indications for flap reconstruction of the perineum include the following:

- Repair after APR with extensive skin resection
- Repair after APR following chemoradiation of the pelvis to bring in well-vascularized tissue, even when skin is sufficient
- Repair after extended APR with wide tissue resection
- Repair after pelvic exenteration for urologic and gynecologic cancer
- Reconstruction after partial or complete vaginectomy
- Repair of a radical sacrectomy defect
- Repair of the perineum in severe, perianal Crohn's disease
- Neovaginal reconstruction in congenital absence of the vagina
- Repair of postirradiation ulcerated wounds of the perineum
- Pelvic excisions with intraoperative radiation therapy

Commonly used flaps for perineal reconstruction include the rectus abdominis musculocutaneous, gracilis musculocutaneous, posterior thigh fasciocutaneous, and gluteus maximus musculocutaneous flaps. An omental flap is an option in select cases. In the past, thigh-based flaps were regarded as most useful, and unilateral or bilateral gracilis musculocutaneous flaps were preferred for many applications. Today, an abdominal musculocutaneous flap has become the technique of choice.

A pedicled rectus abdominis flap based inferiorly on the inferior epigastric vessels can be designed with a skin paddle oriented obliquely (Taylor flap), horizontally (TRAM flap), or vertically (VRAM flap) along the muscle. This last design, the VRAM flap, is particularly well suited for perineal reconstruction (Fig. 68-11). The VRAM flap has bulk for filling dead space, adequate length to reach to the perineum and sacrum, reliable blood supply, and consistent anatomy and can be designed with a large, sturdy skin paddle 5 to 10 cm wide for perineal skin reconstruction or vaginal reconstruction. In one study of surgical outcomes and complications in patients undergoing immediate reconstruction of the perineum, VRAM flaps performed well, with a 15% rate of major complications versus 42% with thigh flaps.[40] Although harvesting of a VRAM flap results in greater tension on the abdominal wall fascial closure, higher rates of abdominal wound separation and incisional hernias have not been reported. Reinforcement of the donor site with synthetic mesh material is helpful, but other options include using a components separation technique to close the abdominal wall on the donor side and the development of perforator flaps to spare the muscle and fascia.

Use of the VRAM flap requires careful planning because taking one of the rectus abdominis muscles with the flap has implications for ostomy placement. If one rectus muscle is used, a colostomy can be brought out through the opposite rectus muscle. However, if a second ostomy is required for an ileal conduit for urinary diversion after pelvic exenteration or for colostomy relocation to treat a parastomal hernia, there will be no intact, untouched rectus muscle remaining through which the second ostomy can be placed. This can be addressed by placing the new ostomy through the abdominal wall on the flap donor side, lateral to the empty rectus sheath. This is successful in some series, but others have found it problematic, with localized wound infections, abdominal wound dehiscence, and malposition of the associated stoma.

There may be situations encountered that limit the use of a VRAM flap. These include situations in which the rectus muscle or inferior epigastric pedicle has been divided by previous abdominal incisions and scarring, prior elevation of an abdominal flap (as with ventral hernia repair or cosmetic abdominoplasty), and preexisting stomas for fecal and urinary diversion exiting through the rectus muscles. In addition, transfer of the VRAM flap into the pelvis typically requires a laparotomy. Therefore, in cases that can be approached from the perineum alone, a thigh-based flap might be preferable to avoid a transabdominal procedure.[41]

The pedicled gracilis muscle or musculocutaneous flap is a suitable alternative if the need to fill dead space is relatively small. The gracilis muscle originates from the pubis symphysis and inserts on the medial tibial condyle. Its blood supply is from the medial circumflex branch of the profunda femoris vessel and can be found 8 to 10 cm from its origin. This distal location of the dominant vascular pedicle, at the junction of the proximal and middle thirds of the thigh, means a restricted arc of rotation and limits how far the flap can reach onto the perineum and into the pelvis. When gracilis flaps are used for vaginal reconstruction, the depth of the reconstructed vault may be limited. In addition, the skin paddle is smaller and less reliable than the VRAM flap, and flap-specific complications, with wound healing and flap loss, are significantly higher with the gracilis flap.

Another alternative is the posterior thigh flap, a fasciocutaneous flap based on the descending branch of the inferior gluteal artery. This flap can provide an abundant and reliable amount of soft tissue for transfer from the posterior thigh, and because the vascular pedicle is proximal, the flap can easily reach high into the pelvis. The skin is innervated by the posterior femoral cutaneous nerve (S1-3), so the flap can provide sensate soft tissue for perineal

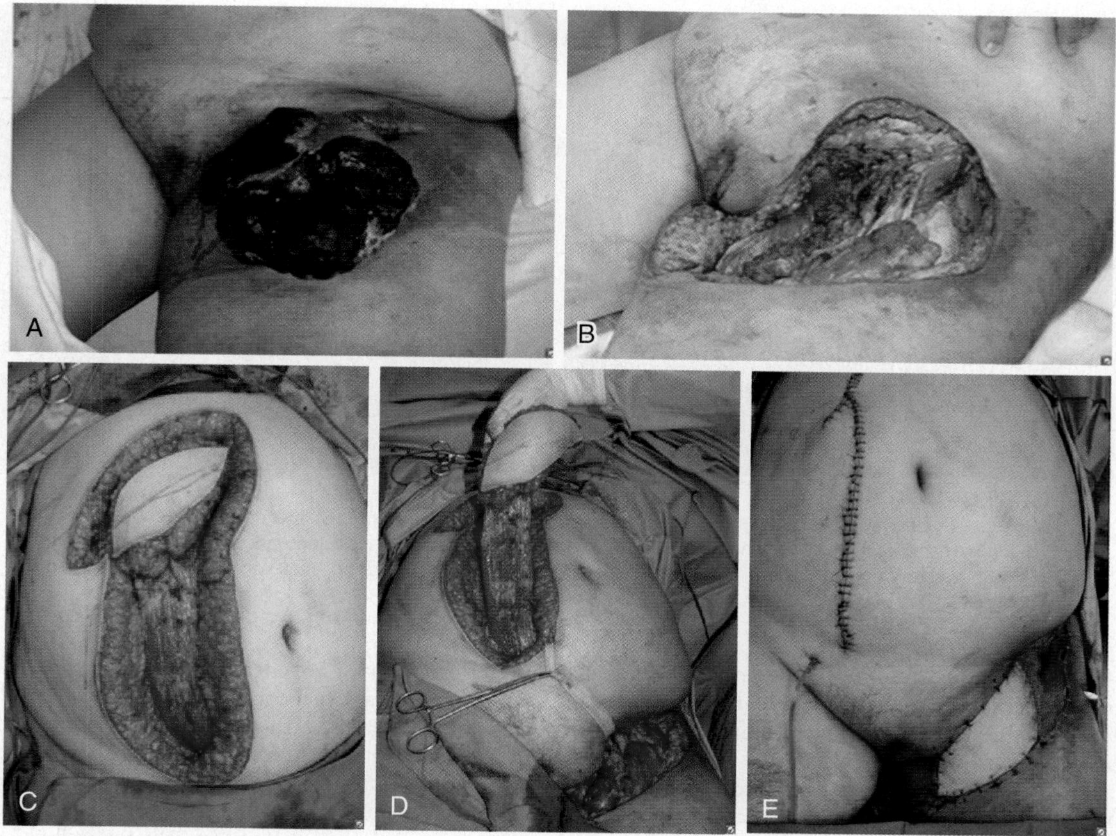

FIGURE 68-11 **A** and **B,** Extensive recurrent melanoma in the groin of a patient previously treated with surgery and irradiation. Resection of the tumor left a large defect with exposed femoral vessels. **C,** An obliquely oriented VRAM flap is elevated on the contralateral side of the abdomen. **D** and **E,** The flap is passed through a subcutaneous tunnel into the groin and used to cover the femoral triangle. A skin graft is placed on the lateral portion of the groin wound where the fascia lata was intact and there were no exposed neurovascular structures.

or vaginal reconstruction, although this is dysesthetic in some patients. There is a relatively high rate of wound healing complications with this flap, but it is a suitable choice when other flaps are unavailable or unsuitable for an individual patient.[42]

A pedicled gluteus maximus musculocutaneous flap based on the inferior gluteal artery has application for some anorectal wounds but will not reach deep into the pelvis. Similarly, flaps of the greater omentum can protect abdominal contents and reach the sacrum but do not provide vascularized skin for tension-free perineal wound closure. However, both these flaps have been shown to improve perineal healing in certain settings. This highlights the importance of preoperative planning for flap selection in clinical practice. Flap choice depends on previous scars, where new incisions will be made, planned location of stomas, vascular patency, and availability of donor sites. Whichever flap is preferred, comparative studies have shown that immediate reconstruction can result in significant improvements in wound healing after radical perineal surgery.

Surgery of Back Defects

Posterior trunk defects result from traumatic wounds; defects after oncologic resection, with or without radiation necrosis; wound breakdown or infection after spinal surgery, with or without exposed orthopedic hardware; and congenital deformities (e.g., spina bifida with myelomeningocele). Posterior trunk reconstruction must provide coverage for exposed major neurovascular structures; coverage for exposed bone and skeletal prostheses; and stable soft tissue to obliterate dead space, to protect dura, to control infection, and to permit tension-free wound closure. To meet these needs, reconstruction generally involves muscle or musculocutaneous flaps to provide bulky, durable, well-vascularized tissue. Depth and location are the two wound parameters that determine flap selection. Deep wounds of the spine can be repaired with paraspinal muscle flaps, whereas more superficial wounds are treated with surface muscle flaps. The length of the back means that various regional muscle units can treat different areas of the posterior trunk.

Preparation for surgical coverage depends on the pathogenesis of the defect. Although exposed meninges must be covered promptly, necrotic or infected tissue may require débridement over time, treatment with antibiotic-impregnated materials for exposed hardware, and negative pressure wound therapy to promote granulation tissue. As spine surgery has become more sophisticated, the need has grown for immediate, complex, soft tissue coverage and for strategies for salvage of postoperative complications. Techniques for covering the spine, exposed dura, and any exposed implants rely on mobilization, advancement, and midline closure of the bilateral paraspinous muscles that run the

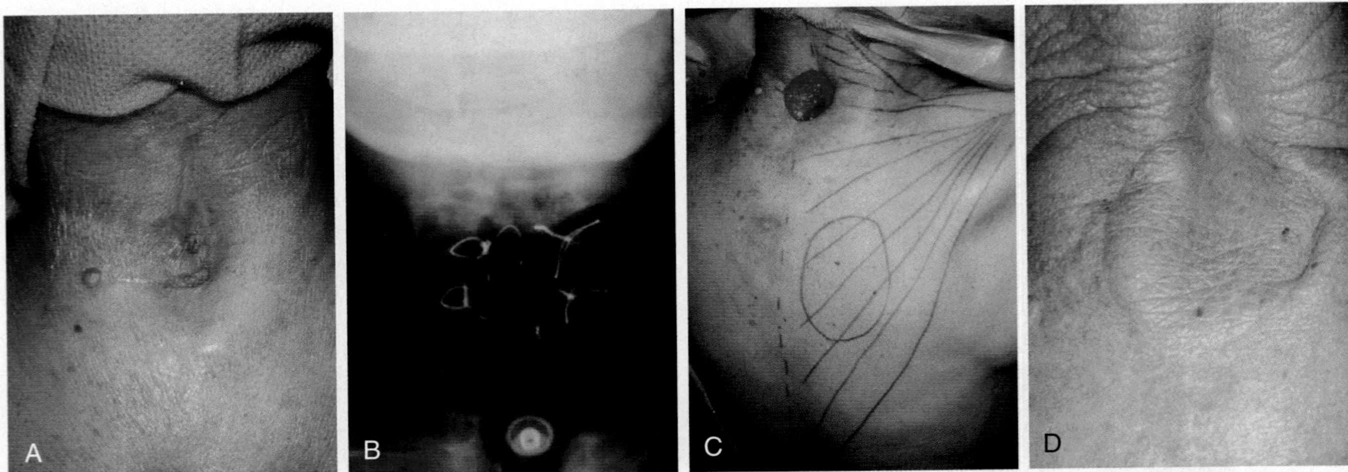

FIGURE 68-12 **A,** Posterior neck with a chronic open wound, with exposed bone and unstable surrounding soft tissue. **B,** Radiographs show surgical hardware in the cervical vertebrae. **C,** The defect is débrided back to healthy margins, and the skin paddle on the posterior trapezius musculocutaneous flap is planned. **D,** Postoperative view at 6 months with the healed flap in place. The donor site for the flap was closed primarily.

length of the vertebral column deep to the thoracolumbar fascia. This is done as a precautionary measure in patients with multiple previous operations, irradiation, attenuated skin, or stiff and heavily scarred soft tissue.

Conceptually, the posterior trunk is divided into upper, middle, and lower thirds. Each has muscle flap options that are best suited for that part of the posterior trunk. Posterior cervical and upper back defects are reconstructed with the pedicled trapezius muscle or musculocutaneous flap or with the dorsal scapular artery perforator flap (Fig. 68-12). The trapezius flap is reliable and versatile and can include a large skin paddle. It is based on the transverse cervical artery, which has two major branches. The trapezius thus offers two separate muscular territories; the lower portion of the muscle can be elevated and transposed superiorly to cover the cervical spine. Alternatively, a trapezius turnover flap is an easily elevated, reliable solution for cervicothoracic wounds. For the midback, latissimus dorsi muscle and musculocutaneous flaps can be mobilized on the thoracodorsal branch of the subscapular vessels to be rotated for broad, reliable coverage. To extend coverage to the midline farther inferiorly, the latissimus flap can be raised as a reverse turnover flap based on secondary segmental intercostal and lumbar artery perforators. The upper portion of the lower third of the back is the most difficult to cover. More inferiorly on the back, the gluteus maximus muscles provide excellent coverage for the sacrum (see later, "Pressure Sores"). However, in the lumbar area, where it is difficult for the more conventional muscle flaps to reach, perforator flaps, latissimus dorsi with a thoracolumbar fasciocutaneous extension, or vein grafting to the thoracodorsal vessels may be required. The pedicled omental flap also is used for the coverage of lumbar defects. The omentum can be transferred, based on the right or left gastroepiploic artery, by dividing attachments to the transverse colon, ligating one gastroepiploic artery, mobilizing the omentum off the greater curvature of the stomach, and passing it through the retroperitoneum and lumbar fascia to cover the spinal column while the back wound is closed with cutaneous advancement flaps.[43]

With partial or total sacrectomy, extensive soft tissue defects are created by oncologic ablation for chordoma, osteogenic sarcoma, or extension of pelvic carcinoma. An anterior and posterior approach is generally used for resection of the tumor, which creates a large communication between the abdominal cavity and gluteal area. These ablations often require large amounts of hardware for bone repair by the orthopedic surgeon; the hypogastric and gluteal vessels are divided during resection, which eliminates the use of potential local back flaps for repair. Successful reconstruction in these cases calls for well-vascularized tissue to fill the defect, to cover the orthopedic appliances, to close the abdominal cavity to prevent herniation, and to close the skin on the posterior trunk. Initial efforts with gluteal flaps and omentum and the placement of synthetic mesh to prevent herniation had some usefulness. More recently, an inferiorly based, pedicled VRAM flap passed transabdominally has proven effective. With no need for mesh, the VRAM flap has a high success rate, with a low incidence of complications and low morbidity.[44]

Meningomyelocele

Meningomyelocele is a congenital spinal malformation that results from failure of the neural tube to close during the first month of gestation. The most common of the four types of spina bifida, meningomyelocele is a cystic herniation of the meninges and neural tissue that presents as a defect on the surface of the lumbosacral skin. The open meningomyelocele defect should be closed soon after birth to prevent meningitis and to protect the exposed neural structure from desiccation and further damage. Early closure has been shown to be a determinant in the neurosurgical outcome. Approximately 75% of meningomyelocele defects are small enough that soft tissue closure can be achieved by simple undermining of the skin edges and tension-free closure in the midline after dural repair. For defects larger than 5 to 8 cm in diameter, a number of techniques have been described.

The surgical options for closing a meningomyelocele defect include skin grafting, local flaps, musculocutaneous flaps, and fasciocutaneous flaps. Local skin flaps including advancement flaps, bipedicle flaps, transposition flaps, double Z-plasty, bilobed flaps, rhomboid flaps, and V-Y advancement flaps have all been used successfully. For larger defects, latissimus dorsi and gluteus maximus musculocutaneous flaps have been described.[45] For all of these, the first criterion is reliable wound healing so that the defect is closed securely and definitively to avoid cerebrospinal fluid leakage and its accompanying morbidity. (See "Pediatric Neurosurgery" in Chapter 67.)

PRESSURE SORES

Prolonged weight bearing, as in an immobilized or paralyzed patient, can elevate tissue pressure above arterial capillary perfusion pressure (32 mm Hg) and result in compromised oxygenation, ischemia, and eventual tissue necrosis. In models of ischemia, external pressure higher than 60 mm Hg for 2 hours leads to irreversible tissue damage, and clinical studies have confirmed this. The clinical sequelae of this damage are pressure sores with ulceration, infection, and exposure of bone. In order of occurrence, the surfaces most commonly involved are those over the sacrum, calcaneus, ischium, and greater trochanter (Fig. 68-13).

Extrinsic and intrinsic factors contribute to the pathogenesis of pressure ulcers. Extrinsic factors include unrelieved pressure seen in debilitated or spinal cord injury patients and factors that worsen the local wound environment, such as moisture in the perineal area, incontinence, and shearing forces from repositioning of the patient. Intrinsic factors include underlying conditions that lead to poor wound healing, such as advanced age, diabetes, malnutrition, and edema. The Braden Scale for Predicting Pressure Sore Risk is a widely used nursing assessment tool to help predict patients' risk for development of pressure sores. Although there is no clear evidence that using risk assessment scales decreases the incidence of pressure ulcers, the Braden Scale has reasonable predictive capacity, with high interrater reliability. This scale accounts for several extrinsic and intrinsic causative factors by scoring six subscales—sensory perception, moisture, activity, mobility, nutrition, and friction and shear.

Stages of Pressure Ulcers

The National Pressure Ulcer Advisory Panel has defined the stages of pressure ulcers, including an original four stages and adding two stages in 2007:

Stage I: Skin intact but reddened for longer than 1 hour after relief of pressure. This stage represents intact skin with various degrees of erythema that does not blanch when it is compressed. This wound is potentially reversible if extrinsic forces and intrinsic wound healing factors are optimized.

Stage II: Blister or other break in the dermis with or without infection. Here, the skin has broken down, with a partial-thickness loss of dermis. By maintenance of coverage over the wound, these wounds often can generate granulation tissue and undergo wound contraction to heal by secondary intention. Because there is violation of skin, the local environment must be monitored carefully for moisture and soiling to allow this stage to heal. Stage I and stage II pressure ulcers are the most prevalent.

Stage III: Full-thickness tissue loss with visible subcutaneous fat but no exposed bone, tendon, or muscle. In the absence of bone exposure, these sores can heal and contract over a bone prominence. However, this is usually a temporally brief stage because muscle is the most oxygen-sensitive tissue and is most sensitive to ischemic necrosis, quickly reaching the final stage of exposed bone.

Stage IV: Exposed bone, joint, muscle, or tendon, with or without infection, often including undermining and tunneling. This is the most common stage that prompts a surgical consultation because the ulcer is down to the causative bone prominence.

Suspected deep tissue injury: Purple or maroon localized area of discolored intact skin or blood-filled blister caused by damage of underlying soft tissue from pressure or shear. This stage identifies clinically suspicious deep tissue injury.

Unstageable: Full-thickness tissue loss in which the base of the ulcer is covered by slough (yellow, tan, gray, green, or brown) or eschar (tan, brown, or black) in the wound bed. Until enough slough or eschar is removed to expose the base of the wound, the true depth and stage cannot be determined.

Swab cultures of the surface of a pressure sore invariably are positive because of local contamination, so culture samples must be taken from biopsy specimens of soft tissue and bone deep to the surface. Infections generally are polymicrobial, with *Proteus, Bacteroides, Pseudomonas,* and *Escherichia coli* accompanying staphylococcal and streptococcal species. More than 50% of long-term care patients harbor methicillin-resistant *Staphylococcus aureus* organisms. In stage IV pressure ulcers with bone exposure, the desiccation and bacterial colonization of the surface of the bone is termed osteitis. If the deep bone has good blood supply and the patient is not immunocompromised, the bone inflammation of osteitis can be tolerated for protracted periods as long as wound care can contain the zone of injury. Osteomyelitis is infection of the bone requiring long-term systemic antibiotics; definitive diagnosis is made with bone biopsy and bacterial culture. Imaging modalities to diagnose osteomyelitis include radiography, tagged white blood cell scans, and MRI. Appropriate imaging is useful to evaluate the extent of bone involvement and to identify the source of infection in pressure sores associated with perianal fistulas or spinal hardware abscesses.

The management of a pressure sore starts with the correction of causative factors. Surgical interventions will not heal and the sores will recur unless the cause is addressed with pressure-relieving cushions and beds, relief of spasticity, correction of joint contractures, incontinence aids, nutritional support, and infection control.[46] Surgical treatment involves drainage of collections, wide débridement of devitalized and scarred soft tissue, excision of sinus tracks and the bursa-like lining of the chronic wound, ostectomy of involved bone, hemostasis with suction drainage, and obliteration of all residual dead space with well-vascularized tissue introduced to cover bone, to provide padding, and to close the open wound without tension.

Intraoperative débridement of superficial bone is carried out by visual assessment of avascular bone versus bleeding bone. Using rongeurs and rasps to smooth jutting prominences or to excise heterotopic bone accomplishes the second purpose of bone resection, reducing the physical prominence of bone that causes pressure and predisposes to recurrence of the sore. After adequate bone débridement, a biopsy specimen of the deeper, healthy-appearing bone is sent for bone culture. If the culture is positive, the remaining bone is still infected and the patient will need a long-term course of intravenous antibiotics to treat the osteomyelitis. Bone resection must be approached thoughtfully because resecting one of a paired set of pressure points, such as the ischia, shifts the patient's weight to the contralateral side, increasing the risk of a new pressure sore on the second side.

Reconstruction with a flap is necessary for most pressure sores because less complex options, such as primary closure or skin grafting, have limited usefulness. Primary closure places the surgical suture line directly over the area of pressure, whereas a flap shifts the closure and scar away from the pressure point. A skin

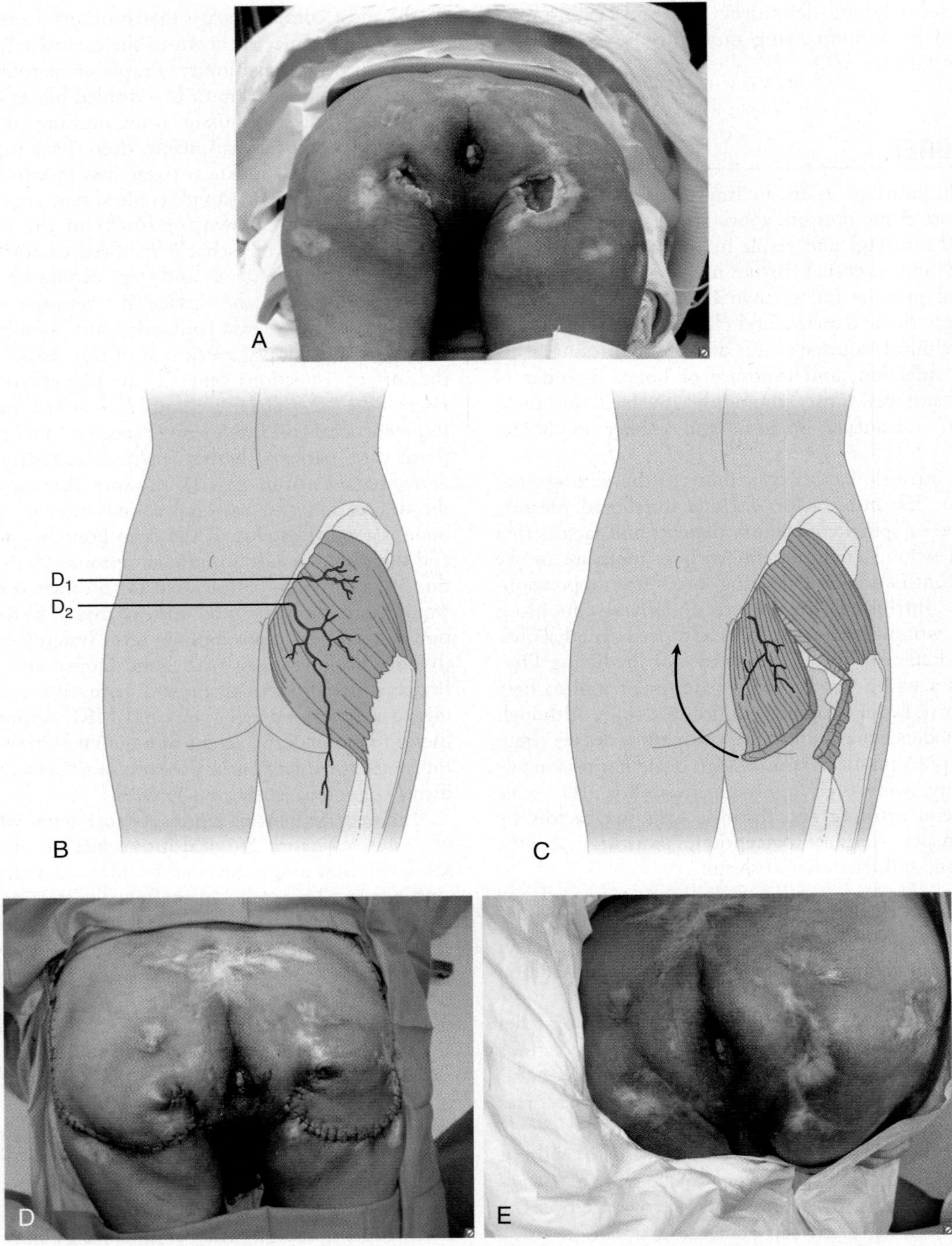

FIGURE 68-13 A 51-year-old paraplegic patient has bilateral stage IV ischial pressure sores with bone exposure in the wounds. **A,** Preoperative view shows bilateral defects and scarring of the surrounding tissue from previous pressure sores and surgical repairs. After débridement and bilateral ischiectomy, well-vascularized tissue will be needed to cover bone, to provide padding, and to close the wound without tension. **B,** The gluteus maximus muscle has blood supply from two branches of the hypogastric artery—the superior gluteal artery to the upper half and the inferior gluteal artery to the lower half. **C,** Based on these two separate upper and lower pedicles, the muscle can be divided into upper and lower halves. **D,** The lower half of the gluteus muscle on each side is detached from the greater tuberosity of the femur and transposed inferiorly with the overlying buttock skin to fill the ischial defects. **E,** Three-month postoperative view shows coverage of both defects. The superior half of the gluteus maximus muscle is preserved.

graft is a thin and fragile coverage option, subject to the shearing forces that created the ulcer in the first place. In addition, a skin graft requires a clean, healthy recipient site, with good blood supply and no exposed bone. Only the most superficial of pressure sores meets these requirements for a base that can be covered successfully with a skin graft. Transferring healthy tissue with its own blood supply to fill the pressure sore can be accomplished with cutaneous, fasciocutaneous, musculocutaneous, muscle-only, and free microvascular flaps.

Sacral pressure sores develop in supine or semireclining patients, and because of the broad pointed shape of the sacrum and thinness of the overlying soft tissue, most ulcers have exposed bone. The soft tissues surrounding the sacrum receive their blood supply from perforators from the superior and inferior gluteal arteries, which are also the arteries supplying the gluteus maximus muscle. This muscle extends and rotates the thigh laterally and is required for ambulation, so the gluteus maximus is not considered expendable except in the spinal cord injury patient. However, the gluteus maximus can survive on either vascular pedicle alone, and using only the superior or inferior half of the muscle will preserve function. Muscle or musculocutaneous flaps of the superior half of the muscle are constructed and moved in two primary ways, a rotational flap or V-Y advancement flap. A rotational flap can be an advancement or with a musculocutaneous skin island. The V-Y advancement technique involves creating a triangular skin island over the muscle, with one side being the defect and the other two sides forming a V. The central V is shifted into the open wound, and the defect is closed in a Y configuration. To get extended coverage of the sacrum, bilateral V-Y advancement flaps can be used, one based on the right and one based on the left gluteal area.

The ischial tuberosities are under high pressure in a seated patient. Unilateral or bilateral ischial sores develop in individuals who are seated for protracted periods without adjusting their position and weight distribution. Ischial ulcers are challenging for several reasons. The pressure points are bilateral, which means that unweighting one side for pressure-reducing purposes shifts increased pressure onto the contralateral ischium. Resecting bone on both sides runs the risk of shifting weight bearing onto the perineal soft tissues, which can cause later scrotal or urethral sores. There can be fistulas involving the rectum or urethra; these may require diversion and control before the ischial ulcers are addressed. Finally, because of the strong hip flexors, there can be flexion contractures with varying degrees of deformity, which reduce mobility and the capacity for normal weight distribution in the sitting or lying position. Because the ischium has a number of surrounding muscles, various flaps suitable for coverage have been described. These include the inferior gluteus maximus rotational, inferior gluteal fasciocutaneous thigh, V-Y hamstring advancement, gracilis muscle, tensor fascia lata rotational, and rectus abdominis rotational flaps.

Because of the mobility of the hip, pressure sores over the greater trochanter characteristically have extensive bursa formation with smaller areas of skin loss. After resection of the trochanter, flaps available for the repair of trochanteric pressure sores include local fasciocutaneous rotational, tensor fascia lata musculocutaneous, and inferior gluteal thigh fasciocutaneous flaps and muscle flaps incorporating the vastus lateralis, rectus femoris, or rectus abdominis muscles.

On the feet, pressure sores can present over the heels, malleoli, and plantar surfaces. Unlike other pressure sores, foot ulcers lack a thick subcutaneous layer, are often modest in size and depth, and may respond favorably to conservative treatment. Stable (dry, adherent, intact, without erythema or fluctuance) eschar on the heels acts as a biologic dressing and need not be removed. In non–weight-bearing areas requiring a less durable surface, pressure sores may be treated conservatively because a scar left by wound contraction and epithelialization may suffice. For larger wounds, débridement and STSG may be useful. If the ulceration involves a large portion of the weight-bearing surface or if osteomyelitis of the calcaneus is present, débridement of devitalized bone with flap coverage is needed. Muscle flaps of the abductor digiti minimi, abductor hallucis, and flexor digitorum brevis have been described. Fasciocutaneous flaps based on the dorsalis pedis, medial plantar, and lateral plantar arteries can also provide coverage.

Postoperative protocols call for 2 to 6 weeks of strict pressure precautions because a newly transferred flap is vulnerable to pressure necrosis. When weight bearing is resumed in the area of the previous pressure sore, the transition is planned with progressive increases in time each day and frequent wound checks.

RECONSTRUCTION OF THE LOWER EXTREMITY

The goal of lower extremity reconstruction is restoration or maintenance of function. For functionality, there must be a stable skeleton to support weight, muscle to power motion and joint movement, neural supply for proprioception and plantar sensibility, blood supply to sustain the underlying structures, and soft tissue to provide a stable skin envelope. Based on these needs, reconstruction may be needed for open fractures, defects from sarcoma resections, radiation wounds, chronic traumatic wounds of the distal third of the leg, diabetic ulcers, venous ulcers, osteomyelitis of the tibia, unstable scars, and infected vascular grafts. Many reconstructions are complex because they need to contribute more than one element, such as vascularized bone grafts or composite flaps with sensory potential, and many require a multidisciplinary surgical team.

Soft Tissue Coverage of Traumatic Wounds

The loss of soft tissue cover over a fracture, particularly when interrupted endosteal blood supply is combined with periosteal damage, demands coverage of the exposed bone with vascularized tissue after thorough débridement of devitalized tissue (Fig. 68-14). Determinants of outcome after open fractures are wound size, degree of soft tissue injury, and amount of contamination. The Gustilo classification system is used to categorize open fractures of the leg into subtypes predictive of prognosis:

Gustilo I: Open fractures with wound <1 cm
Gustilo II: Open fractures with wound 1-10 cm with moderate tissue damage
Gustilo III: Open fractures with wound >10 cm and extensive tissue damage, making it difficult to cover bone or hardware
Gustilo IIIA: Adequate soft tissue coverage of bone with extensive soft tissue laceration or flaps
Gustilo IIIB: Inadequate soft tissue with periosteal stripping and bone exposure
Gustilo IIIC: As above, with vascular injury and ischemia requiring repair

Gustilo grade I and most grade II fractures can be closed primarily after débridement and orthopedic fixation are applied. However, larger grade II and most grade III fractures require advanced reconstructive techniques. When flap coverage is required, it can be done at the time of fracture stabilization or as

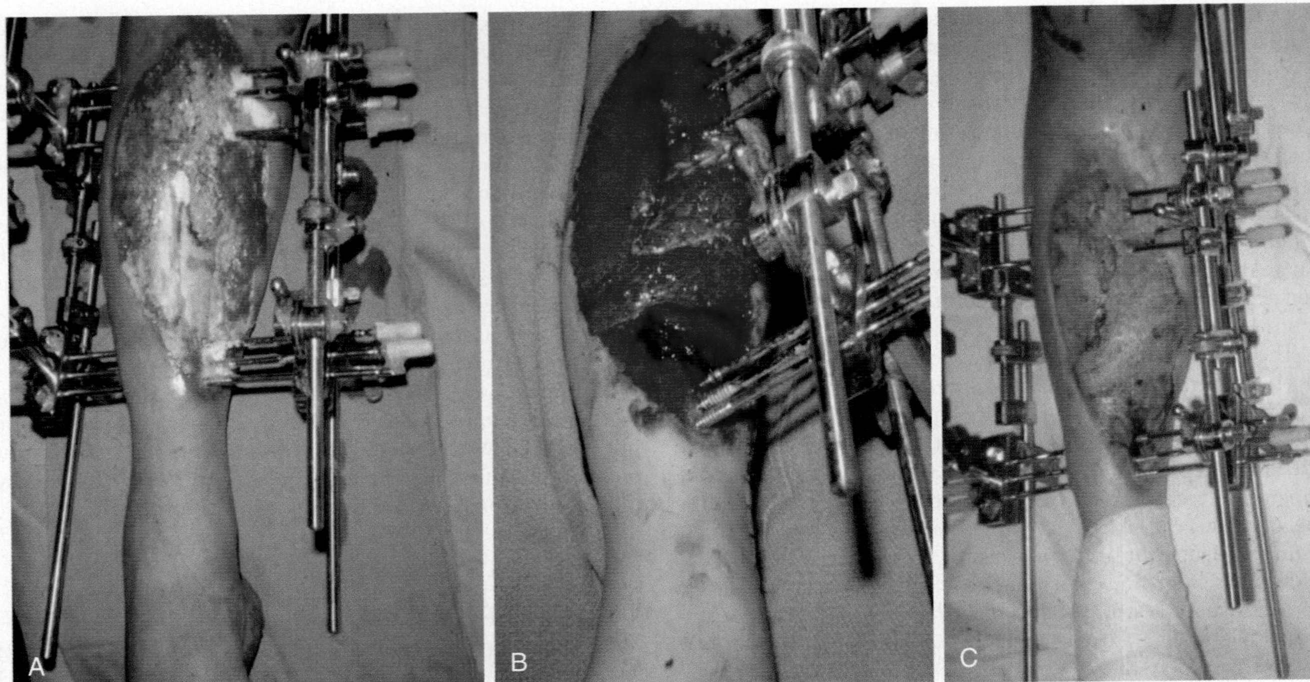

FIGURE 68-14 Soleus muscle flap for coverage of traumatic open fracture of the tibia in the middle third of the leg. **A,** Soft tissue defect with 10 cm of exposed bone after fracture fixation. **B,** The broad flat muscle deep to the gastrocnemius muscle has been mobilized on its proximal pedicles from the posterior tibial and peroneal arteries. It is transposed medially to cover the middle third of the tibia. **C,** Postoperative result. The muscle flap has been covered with a split-thickness skin graft to provide stable wound coverage.

a secondary procedure. Early coverage of exposed bone, tendons, and neurovascular structures decreases the risk of infection, osteomyelitis, nonunion, and ongoing tissue loss. Although the advantages of radical débridement and early wound closure have been accepted, the definition of the duration of the early phase varies. Earlier bone healing and reduced infection rates have been demonstrated if coverage is completed within 72 hours of fracture stabilization; others have shown comparable results when the wounds are closed within the first 6 days after injury. Early reconstruction may be precluded by other injuries or when severely contaminated wounds require serial débridement before delayed reconstruction.[47]

For many years, muscle flaps have been the choice for traumatic lower limb defects. The gastrocnemius and soleus are accessible as local flaps to cover the upper and middle thirds of the leg, and smaller muscles such as the tibialis anterior, extensor digitorum longus, and peroneus brevis can be used for more distal small defects. For larger defects of the distal third of the leg, ankle, and foot, microvascular free tissue transfers of muscles such as the latissimus dorsi, gracilis, serratus anterior, or rectus abdominis are preferred. These free tissue transfers provide more bulk, have longer pedicles for greater flexibility in positioning, and are not dependent on blood supply within the injured area. Most series of lower extremity reconstructions have reported flap failure rates just below 10%. This is higher than at other sites on the body because of associated vascular injuries and preexisting vascular disease in these patients.

More recently, novel wound technologies, combined with growing experience with local fasciocutaneous flaps, are creating new options for reconstruction. Use of the vacuum-assisted closure device reduces edema, decreases wound area, and stimulates granulation tissue, making it possible in some cases to close previously large wounds with local or regional flaps. Fasciocutaneous flaps can cover small to moderate-sized defects, and use of the reverse sural, perforator, and bipedicle flaps is decreasing the need for free microvascular transfers. Clinical advantages of this shift from free flaps to a wider use of skin grafts and local flaps include shorter operations in the trauma patient and elimination of the need for anastomosis to a major leg artery, which may not be available in some traumatic cases.

In injuries with bone loss and a soft tissue defect, the options for skeletal reconstruction include autogenous bone grafts, vascularized bone transfer (pedicle or free), and the Ilizarov technique for osteosynthesis. Bone grafts generally are delayed for approximately 6 weeks after soft tissue reconstruction while orthopedic hardware holds the fracture fragments at length across the gap. The size and location of the bone defect will determine bone graft technique, with a vascularized procedure preferred for larger losses. An alternative to delayed bone grafting is immediate one-stage reconstruction of the bone and soft tissue with an osteocutaneous free tissue transfer.

There are contraindications to salvage of a Gustilo grade IIIC injury of the lower extremity. The most important element in considering primary amputation is disruption of the sciatic or posterior tibial nerve. With laceration of the posterior tibial nerve, the plantar surface is insensate, which results predictably in recurrent ulceration, infection, and osteomyelitis. Other elements include severe infection or contamination, tibial bone loss of more than 8 cm, multilevel severe injury, ischemia time longer than 6 hours, and preexisting severe medical illness. There are several scoring systems to assist in making a decision about limb salvage versus amputation, but these tend to identify patients with good potential for salvage rather than those who will need eventual amputation. The Mangled Extremity Severity Score is used widely but should not be the sole criterion on which an amputation decision is made.[48] Replantation of a severed lower limb is rarely done in the adult because of the inability to restore neurologic function to the foot. A nonfunctional or marginally functional lower extremity is a greater liability than a prosthetic limb capable of allowing high-level function. Absolute contraindications to replantation are older age, poor baseline health, multilevel injury that results in immobility of the knee or ankle, and warm ischemia time longer than 6 hours.

Soft Tissue Reconstruction in the Groin and Thigh

The groin is the most common site of distal extremity prosthetic graft infections. Traditional treatment included removal of the graft material or a salvage attempt at graft preservation with secondary intention healing and its attendant risks of thrombosis, superinfection, and anastomotic disruption. Today, muscle flaps are the mainstay for managing vascular graft infections. Healthy muscle increases tissue oxygen tension in the wound, augments the delivery of antibiotics to the site, and eliminates dead space. Muscle flaps are useful to aid graft salvage in the presence of established infection, when there is increased dead space after drainage of a seroma or hematoma, or in situations in which the tissue bed is compromised by previous surgeries and scarring.

Several muscle flaps are useful for coverage of the femoral vessels. The sartorius muscle is used as first-line treatment because of its proximity, expendability, and relative ease of elevation. The muscle originates on the anterior superior iliac spine, inserts at the medial tibial condyle, and has a segmental blood supply with five or six direct branches from the superficial femoral artery. The muscle is mobilized by dividing the origin and two proximal vascular pedicles, which frees the proximal end of the muscle to be transposed medially and sutured to the inguinal ligament to provide vascularized muscle coverage of the femoral vessels. Disadvantages of the sartorius flap are that it is divided by some surgical incisions in the groin and that division of more than two adjacent pedicles results in devascularization of the muscle. Another local flap option is the rectus femoris muscle; distant pedicled muscle flaps for groin coverage are the gracilis and rectus abdominis.

Defects after oncologic surgery in the thigh and groin are distinctive because extirpation of lower extremity tumors, typically sarcomas, often necessitates wide or radical margins combined with adjuvant radiation therapy. There is a higher incidence of infection and dehiscence after limb-sparing surgery in the thigh and groin than in more distal parts of the lower extremity because of greater dead space, exposure of neurovascular structures, difficulty in keeping the wound clean and dry, and tension with ambulation and hip abduction. For these larger irradiated defects, flap reconstruction is necessary. A number of thigh muscles can be used as a local flap, with or without skin grafts or a skin paddle; these include gracilis, tensor fascia lata, and vastus lateralis flaps. Fasciocutaneous flaps, such as the medial thigh, lateral posterior thigh, and anterior lateral thigh, are also available. In some cases, these local options are no longer useful because of inclusion in the field of radiation, so distant or free flaps are needed for coverage. Reported outcomes after reconstruction of these difficult wounds with a VRAM flap have been promising, with a 9.4% incidence of postoperative wound complications with immediate reconstruction but a significantly higher incidence of 47% in patients with delayed reconstruction.[49]

Soft Tissue Coverage of the Knee, Leg, and Foot

Wounds around the knee can result from trauma, tumor extirpation, or exposure of an infected knee endoprosthesis after total knee replacement. For each of these defects, durable soft tissue coverage is required; a pedicled medial gastrocnemius muscle or musculocutaneous flap based on the medial sural artery is preferred for genicular soft tissue reconstruction. The gastrocnemius muscle has a medial head and lateral head originating from the medial and lateral condyles of the femur, respectively; the two heads share a common insertion on the calcaneus through the Achilles tendon. As a result, one head can be detached from the Achilles tendon independently and transposed with its robust blood supply and vascular drainage without impairing foot dorsiflexion. Because the medial head is longer, it is preferred for knee wounds and can be transposed with or without a skin paddle. In situations in which a pedicled gastrocnemius flap has failed or is unavailable, free tissue transfer of a latissimus dorsi or rectus abdominis muscle flap has led to a high rate of salvage of limbs and knee prostheses.

Options for soft tissue coverage of the leg are determined by the position of the defect relative to the tibia:

Proximal tibia: medial gastrocnemius, lateral gastrocnemius, fasciocutaneous flap

Middle tibia: soleus, gastrocnemius, extensor digitorum longus, tibialis anterior, fasciocutaneous flap

Distal tibia: peroneus brevis, extensor brevis, distal-based soleus, reverse sural artery flap, lateral supramalleolar flap, dorsalis pedis fasciocutaneous flap, free flap

Foot: flexor digitorum brevis, abductor hallucis, abductor digiti minimi, reverse sural flap, medial plantar artery flap, lateral calcaneal artery flap, V-Y advancement, free flap

Muscle flaps are often unreliable in treating distal-third leg wounds. Except for the soleus and gastrocnemius muscles, local muscles on the lower leg are only adequate to cover small defects. This, along with several other factors, means that treatment of the distal tibia, ankle, and foot is difficult. The area is vulnerable to injury because the distal portion of the leg has poor skin elasticity, has bone lying in the subcutaneous space, and may be edematous. The distal third of the leg has little muscle but many tendinous structures, and they support skin grafts poorly. Finally, the foot and ankle require especially durable integument because they are exposed continually to friction and shear with walking and footwear. Any transferred flap may slip or slide at the interface with the underlying structures because the transferred tissue lacks the glabrous quality of the native plantar skin. If the transferred tissue is insensate, it will be at significant risk for eventual breakdown.

For larger defects, reconstruction in the distal third of the leg relies on free tissue transfer techniques. The vascular status of the extremity and recipient vessel selection are key factors for success. Guidelines for the use of free flaps in the lower extremity include making anastomoses to healthy recipient vessels outside the zone of injury and using end-to-side arterial anastomoses, whereas venous anastomoses can be end to side or end to end. Free tissue transfer remains the best option for large defects, for wounds with trauma (e.g., crush injury to the surrounding vicinity that damages blood supply to all local tissues), and when the transfer of vascularized bone with the free flap is desirable. Free fibula flaps with skin paddles are preferred for lower extremity wounds with bone and soft tissue deficits.

More recently, the advent of local fasciocutaneous flaps has begun to change the treatment of difficult lower leg wounds.

Recognition that the vascular plexus accompanying cutaneous sensory nerves can supply overlying skin and soft tissue has allowed the development of many useful, axial pattern fasciocutaneous flaps.[50] Currently, one of the most versatile of these is the distally based, or reverse, sural fasciocutaneous flap. One to three arteries accompany the sural nerve as it travels subcutaneously in the posterior calf. A skin paddle as large as 14 cm in diameter can be elevated on the proximal posterior calf as part of a distally based sural nerve flap; this tissue may be transposed to cover distal leg and foot wounds. Because the sural nerve flap is supported by perforators from the peroneal artery, the patency of this vessel must be ensured for flap success.

BODY CONTOURING

Body Contouring After Bariatric Surgery

With the advent of bariatric surgery and successful treatment of severe obesity, a new deformity has emerged. After massive weight loss, the patient is left with excess skin and subcutaneous tissue that fails to retract and hangs from the torso, abdomen, and extremities. More than a cosmetic issue, this extreme skin redundancy can be painful, limits mobility, and is susceptible to recurrent infection in the intertriginous areas hooded by overhanging tissue. Patients seek body contouring surgery because many are deeply distressed by their appearance. These patients should be no less than 12 to 18 months after bariatric surgery, be stable in weight for 3 to 4 months, have a body mass index of less than 30, and be well-nourished, with no protein or vitamin deficiencies. Proceeding before these criteria are met can result in recurrent skin laxity and delayed wound healing and may be inconsistent with the patient's health insurer's requirements.

Body contouring after bariatric surgery is different from similar procedures in those who have not been obese. The deformity after bariatric surgery is more severe because the skin damage and associated loss of tone and elasticity do not recover, and the laxity is global. A number of procedures may be required; some of these involve restoring volume to areas of deficiency rather than removing tissue. When surgery is done in multiple stages, the procedures are separated by 4 to 6 months to optimize wound healing. The procedures are lengthy, and deep venous thrombosis prophylaxis is required. Abdominal wall hernias, particularly at surgical port sites, are found frequently and are repaired during the course of abdominal contouring. Except for large ventral hernias, these repairs are accomplished easily because the fascia can be approximated readily after massive weight loss (Fig. 68-15). Various techniques are used for contouring:

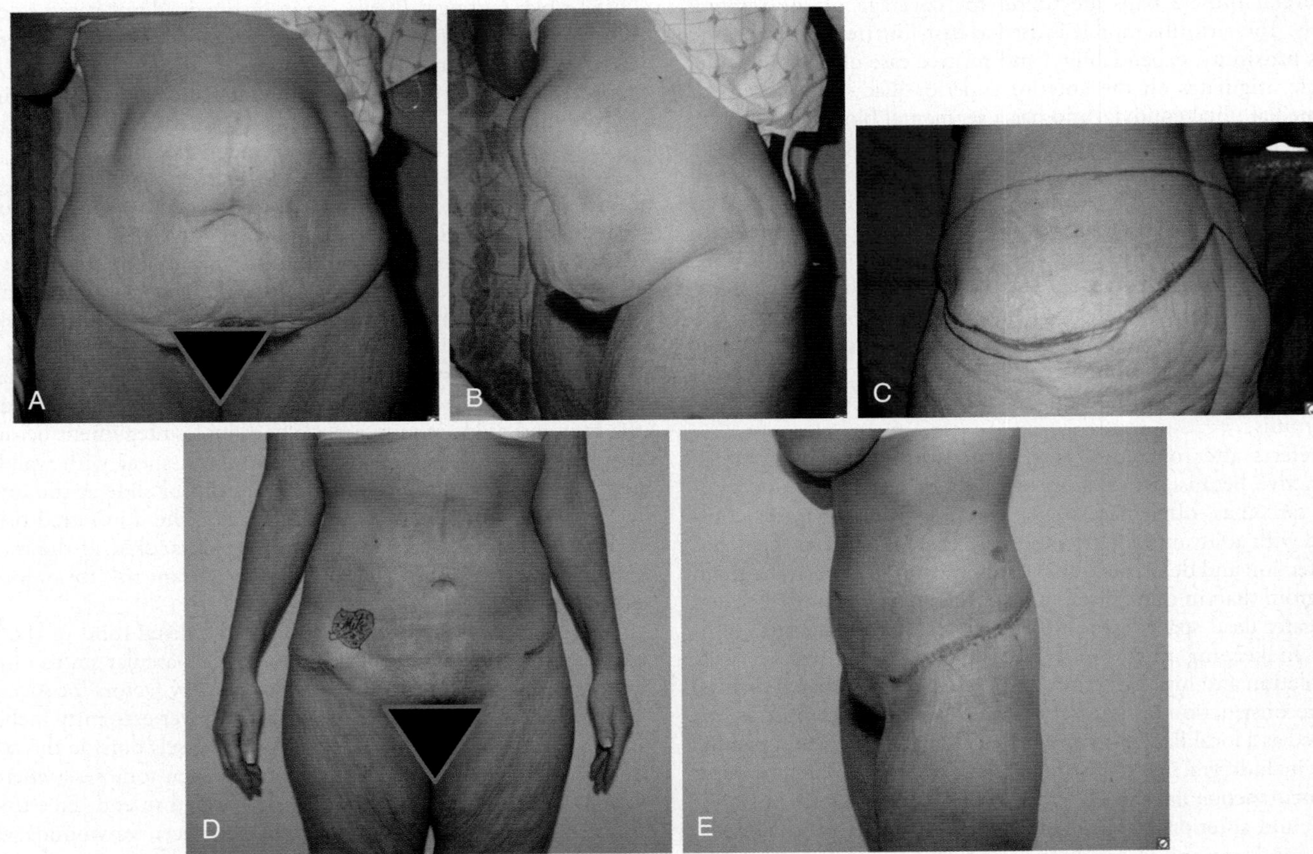

FIGURE 68-15 After gastric bypass, this 40-year-old woman lost 195 pounds. **A** and **B,** The patient presented with a 10-cm ventral hernia, a 2-cm umbilical hernia, and redundant soft tissue. Hernia repair, abdominoplasty, and belt lipectomy were planned. **C,** The planned excision of the redundant soft tissue over the sides and back is shown. **D** and **E,** The postoperative result after primary repair of the ventral hernia in a vertical direction, plication of the rectus fascia inferior to the herniorrhaphy for contour improvement, umbilical hernia repair, modified vertical abdominoplasty, and circumferential resection of soft tissue. A total of 3733 g of soft tissue was resected.

Panniculectomy is removal of excess skin and soft tissue from the abdominal wall without umbilical transposition. It is limited to removal of the overhanging pannus without mobilizing surrounding soft tissue.

Abdominoplasty includes panniculectomy with wide undermining of the upper abdominal flap and umbilical transposition. Unlike in a traditional abdominoplasty, a vertical ellipse or fleur-de-lis pattern of excision often is necessary to remove significant excess skin in the horizontal dimension superior to the umbilicus.

Reverse abdominoplasty uses incisions in the inframammary crease to remove rolls of excess skin from the upper quadrants of the abdomen.

Belt lipectomy is also termed a lower body lift; it corrects the circumferential roll of excess tissue found in most patients by extending the abdominal resection around the sides of the abdomen to include the lower back. In the course of resecting this circumferential ring of tissue, the lateral thighs and buttocks are also lifted.

An upper body lift removes excess skin from the lateral sides of the chest and upper back through a horizontal incision across the back.

A medial thigh lift is excision of a long ellipse of excess tissue parallel to the long axis of the thigh to remove hanging skin on the inner thigh.

A mastopexy is a breast lift for ptosis. No breast tissue is removed because the volume of breast tissue may be small in the drooping, deflated, pancake breast after massive weight loss. The breast skin is resected as the breast is reshaped, and the nipple-areola complex is elevated and centralized. In some cases, augmentation with breast implants is done to restore volume. Alternatively, excess folds of skin under the arms can be deepithelialized and rotated anteriorly to augment the volume of the breast.

Male mastopexy removes excess drooping skin to reduce fullness, with superior elevation of the nipple-areola complex as a flap or with free nipple grafting.

Brachioplasty is the excision of a long ellipse of excess tissue parallel to the long axis of the arm to correct the excess skin, or "bat wing," hanging from the proximal half of the arm.

A minibrachioplasty excises an ellipse of tissue just distal to the axilla perpendicular to the long axis of the arm to remove a mild excess of tissue. The scar is placed in the axilla.

Body contouring after bariatric surgery is a component in the treatment of the obese patient and is well accepted by patients, despite the extensive scarring with all of the surgical procedures. There is evidence that post–bariatric surgery patients who have subsequent body contouring surgery maintain their weight loss. This could merely be a reflection of the motivation of this cohort of patients, but ongoing work is focused on better understanding of the psychological impact of extreme body contouring.

Suction-Assisted Lipectomy

Suction-assisted lipectomy, also termed liposuction, lipoplasty, or liposculpture, was introduced in the late 1970s and early 1980s when plastic surgeons developed the concept of inserting a blunt-ended hollow cannula under the skin and connecting it to a vacuum pump, which generates negative pressure to aspirate the fatty tissue. Before a small opening is made in the skin to introduce the cannula, the area to be treated is injected with a wetting solution, which is saline supplemented with local anesthetic and low concentrations of epinephrine. Terms used to describe variations in this fluid infiltrate are based on the amount of fluid used; these are *dry, wet, superwet,* and *tumescent.* Although the more generous use of saline, lidocaine, and epinephrine results in less blood loss, greater ease of fat removal, and decreased postoperative pain, it also raises concerns about fluid overload and drug toxicity, which call for close intraoperative monitoring of ventilation, circulation, and cardiac function.

The areas usually treated with liposuction are the neck, abdomen and waist, back, and hips and thighs. Good results can be obtained, provided the volume of fat is not too great and there is good skin elasticity. Large-volume liposuction is associated with hemodynamic instability and a risk of damaging the blood supply to the overlying skin, causing skin necrosis. Elastic rebound of the skin after the underlying fat is removed is essential to the success of liposuction. In general, even when large amounts of fat are removed, skin has good elasticity and will conform to the new underlying volume. However, skin that is flaccid or sagging will not retract, and therefore good results are more difficult to achieve in areas such as the face, arms, and inner thighs. The looseness of the skin and the likelihood that it will exhibit poor adaptability means that liposuction will exacerbate the drooping and leave significant surface irregularities.

Suction-assisted lipectomy is a useful surgical treatment for several medical disorders. It is a treatment of choice for gynecomastia when combined, as needed, with resection of any glandular tissue. The skin of the chest wall tends to retract well, and liposuction is particularly useful for tapering the boundaries of the treated area for a smooth contour. Liposuction alone is less often useful to reduce the size of the female breast because the large breast will become droopy if volume is removed without lifting and tightening the skin. The greater benefit of liposuction is in combination with surgical breast reduction techniques, in which it is used to smooth the contours under the arms and at the margins of the breast. For patients with a buffalo hump, liposuction makes it possible to reduce fat deposits on the upper back and lower neck that previously could not be removed without extensive surgery. For patients with HIV infection, lipodystrophy is a syndrome of abnormal fat distribution associated with the therapeutic use of protease inhibitors. The lipodystrophy may be in the form of a neck and upper back fat pad, fat deposition in the trunk and lower face, or increase in the adipose tissue of the breasts. All these respond well to treatment with liposuction.

The most common complications with suction-assisted lipectomy are contour deformity, excessive blood loss, hematoma, seroma, fluid overload, and asymmetry. Less commonly, overlying skin loss, skin burns, deep venous thrombosis, and pulmonary embolus are seen. There have been infrequent reports of fat embolus, cannula penetration of the abdominal cavity, lidocaine toxicity, and surgical shock. A national survey conducted in 2001 found that combining liposuction with other procedures such as abdominoplasty increased the mortality risk almost fivefold. This is presumably related to the longer length of the surgery, greater blood loss, and larger fluid shifts. On the basis of this information, subsequent technical and practice guidelines include limiting of concomitant procedures performed at the time of liposuction, stricter criteria for selection of patients with regard to obesity and general health factors, removal of less fat in one operative session, placement of limits on the length of the surgery, modifications in anesthetic techniques, and additional patient monitoring.

CONCLUSIONS

Plastic surgery continues to evolve with the development of new approaches for the care of people with congenital and acquired deformities. With therapeutic advances in medicine and surgery, new problems have emerged that call for novel reconstructive techniques. Challenged by these difficult problems, plastic surgery continues to look for ways to treat life- and limb-threatening problems and, at the same time, to restore form and function. Chest wall, abdominal wall, and perineal reconstruction are progressing rapidly, and defects that were incapacitating a decade ago are now correctable. Lower extremity salvage after devastating injury is now commonplace. With advances in other surgical specialties such as bariatric surgery, entirely new areas requiring plastic surgery have emerged. Old techniques, such as perforator flaps, continue to evolve and supply better ways to reconstruct defects. New techniques, such as fat grafting, which may revolutionize clinical practice, have come from empirical observations. Developed from new research studies, tissue engineering, gene therapy, and stem cell work will change reconstruction in unforeseeable ways in the future. The search continues for the most reliable, durable, and aesthetic ways to "restore, repair, and make whole those parts … which fortune has taken away" (Gaspare Tagliacozzi [Italian surgeon who became famous for his skill in reconstructive surgery], *De Curtorum Chirurgia per Insitionem*, Venice, 1579).

SELECTED REFERENCES

Hashim PW, Patel A, Yang JF, et al: The effects of whole-vault cranioplasty versus strip craniectomy on long-term neuropsychological outcomes in sagittal craniosynostosis. *Plast Reconstr Surg* 134:491–501, 2014.

This multicenter study compares long-term cognitive outcomes in children with sagittal craniosynostosis treated with either total cranial vault reconstruction or endoscopic sagittal suturectomy. It shows that children having early (before 6 months of age) whole vault cranioplasty attain higher intelligence quotients and achievement scores. It is the first comparative analysis establishing the effects of technique and timing on long-term intellectual functioning in these children.

Kiwanuka H, Bueno EM, Diaz-Siso JR, et al: Evolution of ethical debate on face transplantation. *Plast Reconstr Surg* 132:1558–1568, 2013.

This article examines the evolution of the debate in the scientific literature about the ethics of face transplantation. It notes changes in the dialogue since 2002 as experience-based practical issues have arisen and outlines 15 major ethical concerns that need to be considered to ethically advance the field of face transplantation.

Koshima I, Yamamoto T, Narushima M, et al: Perforator flaps and supermicrosurgery. *Clin Plast Surg* 37:683–689, 2010.

The introduction of supermicrosurgery, the microvascular anastomosis of vessels ranging from 0.3 to 0.8 mm in diameter, opens up a wide array of new reconstructive options. Free perforator flaps can be obtained from anywhere on the body and provide thinner, more pliant tissue for repair of extremity and facial defects. This paper reviews these new options as well as the technical challenges of supermicrosurgery.

Pannucci CJ, Bailey SH, Dreszer G, et al: Validation of the Caprini risk assessment model in plastic and reconstructive surgery patients. *J Am Coll Surg* 212:105–112, 2011.

This study of the incidence of venous thromboembolism (VTE) in 1126 plastic surgery patients at five tertiary referral centers found that the Caprini Risk Assessment Model effectively risk stratifies plastic and reconstructive surgery patients for VTE risk. Among patients with Caprini score higher than 8, 11.3% have a postoperative VTE when chemoprophylaxis is not provided. In higher risk patients, there was no evidence that VTE risk is limited to the immediate postoperative period.

Walmsley GG, Maan ZN, Wong VW, et al: Scarless wound healing: Chasing the holy grail. *Plast Reconstr Surg* 135:907–917, 2015.

This article on regenerative medicine reviews the stages of wound healing, the differences between adult and fetal wound healing, and the various mechanical, genetic, and pharmacologic strategies to reduce scarring. It discusses the biology of skin stem/progenitor cells that may hold the key to scarless regeneration and concludes that the characterization of functional cell lineages in the integument will follow from increased understanding of signaling molecules, growth factors, and lineage-specific cell origin and function.

REFERENCES

1. Tamai M, Nagasao T, Miki T, et al: Rotation arc of pedicled anterolateral thigh flap for abdominal wall reconstruction: How far can it reach? *J Plast Reconstr Aesthet Surg* 68:1417–1424, 2015.
2. Buchanan PJ, Kung TA, Cederna PS: Evidence-based medicine: Wound closure. *Plast Reconstr Surg* 134:1391–1404, 2014.
3. Hong JP, Koshima I: Using perforators as recipient vessels (supermicrosurgery) for free flap reconstruction of the knee region. *Ann Plast Surg* 64:291–293, 2010.
4. Wei F, Tay SKL: Principles and techniques of microvascular surgery. In Nelligan PC, editor: *Plastic surgery*, ed 3, London, 2013, Elsevier Saunders, pp 587–621.
5. Koshima I, Yamamoto T, Narushima M, et al: Perforator flaps and supermicrosurgery. *Clin Plast Surg* 37:683–689, 2010.
6. Hong JP: The use of supermicrosurgery in lower extremity reconstruction: The next step in evolution. *Plast Reconstr Surg* 123:230–235, 2009.
7. Marks MW, Argenta LC: Principles and applications of tissue expansion. In Nelligan PC, editor: *Plastic surgery*, ed 3, London, 2013, Elsevier Saunders, pp 622–653.
8. Gougoutas AJ, Singh DJ, Low DW, et al: Hemifacial microsomia: Clinical features and pictographic representations of the OMENS classification system. *Plast Reconstr Surg* 120:112e–120e, 2007.

9. Stal S, Brown RH, Higuera S, et al: Fifty years of the Millard rotation-advancement: Looking back and moving forward. *Plast Reconstr Surg* 123:1364–1377, 2009.
10. Sullivan SR, Marrinan EM, LaBrie RA, et al: Palatoplasty outcomes in nonsyndromic patients with cleft palate: A 29-year assessment of one surgeon's experience. *J Craniofac Surg* 20(Suppl 1):612–616, 2009.
11. Tromberg J, Bauer B, Benvenuto-Andrade C, et al: Congenital melanocytic nevi needing treatment. *Dermatol Ther* 18:136–150, 2005.
12. Ho K, Hutter JJ, Eskridge J, et al: The management of life-threatening haemorrhage following blunt facial trauma. *J Plast Reconstr Aesthet Surg* 59:1257–1262, 2006.
13. Ellis E, 3rd, Miles BA: Fractures of the mandible: A technical perspective. *Plast Reconstr Surg* 120:76S–89S, 2007.
14. Khalifian S, Brazio PS, Mohan R, et al: Facial transplantation: The first 9 years. *Lancet* 384:2153–2163, 2014.
15. Janis JE, Rohrich RJ: Clinical decision-making in rhinoplasty. In Nahai F, editor: *The art of aesthetic surgery: Principles and techniques*, St. Louis, 2005, Quality Medical, pp 1515–1533.
16. Carniol PJ, Hamilton MM, Carniol ET: Current status of fractional laser resurfacing. *JAMA Facial Plast Surg* 17:360–366, 2015.
17. Mojallal A, Lequeux C, Shipkov C, et al: Improvement of skin quality after fat grafting: Clinical observation and an animal study. *Plast Reconstr Surg* 124:765–774, 2009.
18. Marino G, Moraci M, Armenia E, et al: Therapy with autologous adipose-derived regenerative cells for the care of chronic ulcer of lower limbs in patients with peripheral arterial disease. *J Surg Res* 185:36–44, 2013.
19. Carruthers JD, Glogau RG, Blitzer A: Advances in facial rejuvenation: Botulinum toxin type A, hyaluronic acid dermal fillers, and combination therapies—consensus recommendations. *Plast Reconstr Surg* 121:5S–30S, 2008.
20. Netscher DT, Baumholtz MA: Chest reconstruction: I. Anterior and anterolateral chest wall and wounds affecting respiratory function. *Plast Reconstr Surg* 124:240e–252e, 2009.
21. Chang RR, Mehrara BJ, Hu QY, et al: Reconstruction of complex oncologic chest wall defects: A 10-year experience. *Ann Plast Surg* 52:471–479, 2004.
22. Losken A, Thourani VH, Carlson GW, et al: A reconstructive algorithm for plastic surgery following extensive chest wall resection. *Br J Plast Surg* 57:295–302, 2004.
23. Preminger BA, Yaghoobzadeh Y, Ascherman JA: Management of sternal wounds by limited debridement and partial bilateral pectoralis major myocutaneous advancement flaps in 25 patients: A less invasive approach. *Ann Plast Surg* 72:446–450, 2014.
24. Davison SP, Clemens MW, Armstrong D, et al: Sternotomy wounds: Rectus flap versus modified pectoral reconstruction. *Plast Reconstr Surg* 120:929–934, 2007.
25. Vyas RM, Prsic A, Orgill DP: Transdiaphragmatic omental harvest: A simple, efficient method for sternal wound coverage. *Plast Reconstr Surg* 131:544–552, 2013.
26. Dabbah A, Lehman JA, Jr, Parker MG, et al: Reduction mammoplasty: An outcome analysis. *Ann Plast Surg* 35:337–341, 1995.
27. Handel N, Garcia ME, Wixtrom R: Breast implant rupture: Causes, incidence, clinical impact, and management. *Plast Reconstr Surg* 132:1128–1137, 2013.
28. Deapen D, Hamilton A, Bernstein L, et al: Breast cancer stage at diagnosis and survival among patients with prior breast implants. *Plast Reconstr Surg* 105:535–540, 2000.
29. Gidengil CA, Predmore Z, Mattke S, et al: Breast implant–associated anaplastic large cell lymphoma: A systematic review. *Plast Reconstr Surg* 135:713–720, 2015.
30. Largo RD, Tchang LA, Mele V, et al: Efficacy, safety and complications of autologous fat grafting to healthy breast tissue: A systematic review. *J Plast Reconstr Aesthet Surg* 64:437–448, 2014.
31. Petty PM, Solomon M, Buchel EW, et al: Gynecomastia: Evolving paradigm of management and comparison of techniques. *Plast Reconstr Surg* 125:1301–1308, 2011.
32. Agnew SP, Small W, Jr, Wang E, et al: Prospective measurements of intra-abdominal volume and pulmonary function after repair of massive ventral hernias with the components separation technique. *Ann Surg* 251:981–988, 2010.
33. Morykwas MJ, Argenta LC, Shelton-Brown EI, et al: Vacuum-assisted closure: A new method for wound control and treatment: Animal studies and basic foundation. *Ann Plast Surg* 38:553–562, 1997.
34. Butler CE, Campbell KT: Minimally invasive component separation with inlay bioprosthetic mesh (MICSIB) for complex abdominal wall reconstruction. *Plast Reconstr Surg* 128:698–709, 2011.
35. den Hartog D, Dur AH, Tuinebreijer WE, et al: Open surgical procedures for incisional hernias. *Cochrane Database Syst Rev* (3):CD006438, 2008.
36. Althubaiti G, Butler CE: Abdominal wall and chest wall reconstruction. *Plast Reconstr Surg* 133:688e–701e, 2014.
37. Hurvitz KA, Olaya WA, Nguyen A, et al: Evidence-based medicine: Abdominoplasty. *Plast Reconstr Surg* 133:1214–1221, 2014.
38. Bullard KM, Trudel JL, Baxter NN, et al: Primary perineal wound closure after preoperative radiotherapy and abdominoperineal resection has a high incidence of wound failure. *Dis Colon Rectum* 48:438–443, 2005.
39. Butler CE, Gundeslioglu AO, Rodriguez-Bigas MA: Outcomes of immediate vertical rectus abdominis myocutaneous flap reconstruction for irradiated abdominoperineal resection defects. *J Am Coll Surg* 206:694–703, 2008.
40. Nelson RA, Butler CE: Surgical outcomes of VRAM versus thigh flaps for immediate reconstruction of pelvic and perineal cancer resection defects. *Plast Reconstr Surg* 123:175–183, 2009.
41. Wong DS: Reconstruction of the perineum. *Ann Plast Surg* 73(Suppl 1):S74–S81, 2014.
42. Friedman JD, Reece GR, Eldor L: The utility of the posterior thigh flap for complex pelvic and perineal reconstruction. *Plast Reconstr Surg* 126:146–155, 2010.
43. O'Shaughnessy BA, Dumanian GA, Liu JC, et al: Pedicled omental flaps as an adjunct in the closure of complex spinal wounds. *Spine (Phila Pa 1976)* 32:3074–3080, 2007.
44. Glatt BS, Disa JJ, Mehrara BJ, et al: Reconstruction of extensive partial or total sacrectomy defects with a transabdominal vertical rectus abdominis myocutaneous flap. *Ann Plast Surg* 56:526–530, discussion 530–531, 2006.
45. Zakaria Y, Hasan EA: Reversed turnover latissimus dorsi muscle flap for closure of large myelomeningocele defects. *J Plast Reconstr Aesthet Surg* 63:1513–1518, 2010.

46. Cushing CA, Phillips LG: Evidence-based medicine: Pressure sores. *Plast Reconstr Surg* 132:1720–1732, 2013.
47. Ong YS, Levin LS: Lower limb salvage in trauma. *Plast Reconstr Surg* 125:582–588, 2010.
48. Shawen SB, Keeling JJ, Branstetter J, et al: The mangled foot and leg: Salvage versus amputation. *Foot Ankle Clin* 15:63–75, 2010.
49. Parrett BM, Winograd JM, Garfein ES, et al: The vertical and extended rectus abdominis myocutaneous flap for irradiated thigh and groin defects. *Plast Reconstr Surg* 122:171–177, 2008.
50. Parrett BM, Talbot SG, Pribaz JJ, et al: A review of local and regional flaps for distal leg reconstruction. *J Reconstr Microsurg* 25:445–455, 2009.

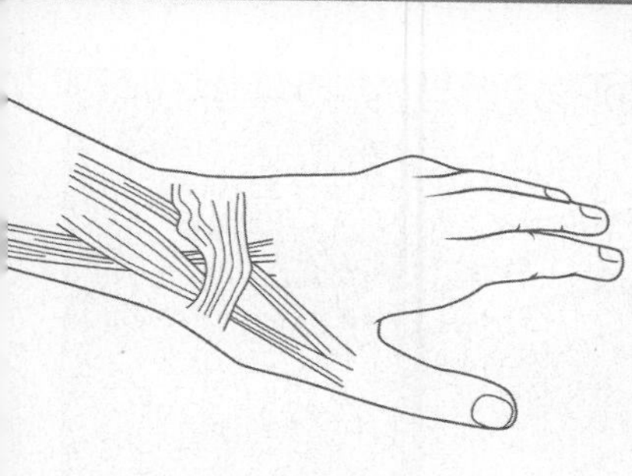

CHAPTER 69

Hand Surgery

David Netscher, Kevin D. Murphy, Nicholas A. Fiore II

OUTLINE

Although hand surgery fellowships traditionally receive trainees primarily with backgrounds in orthopedic surgery or plastic surgery, fellowship training in hand surgery may also be undertaken by those having completed a residency in general surgery. Basic tenets of hand surgery must be acquired by all general surgeons. Depending on the practice locale (rural or urban), type of hospital, and residency rotations (e.g., surgical intern covering the emergency department) or even for the purposes of board examinations, the ability to evaluate and to manage hand injuries and problems is a necessary skill for the general surgeon. The purpose of this chapter is not to provide the general surgeon with an exhaustive study of hand surgery, because specialty texts are more appropriate, but to provide an overview of pathologic processes of the hand encountered more commonly by the general surgeon and especially to emphasize basics in anatomy, physical examination, and treatment of common hand and upper extremity emergencies.

Interestingly, there is a modest amount of recent literature on the quality and duration of hand fellowship training. In a recent survey to which 80% of program directors responded, the majority thought that a 1-year fellowship was still sufficient training despite the increasing breadth of knowledge in the field and new technologic developments.[1] However, programs needed to evaluate their own training to highlight areas that may need enhancement. Nonetheless, many training programs admittedly remain deficient in areas, especially shoulder and elbow, replantation, brachial plexus, congenital, and flap surgery.[2]

BASIC ANATOMY

The arm and hand are divided into volar or palmar and dorsal aspects. Distal to the elbow, structures are termed radial or ulnar to the middle finger axis rather than lateral and medial, respectively, because with forearm pronation and supination, the latter terms become confusing. The nomenclature of digits has become standardized. The hand has five digits, namely, the thumb and four fingers (the thumb is not called a finger). The four fingers are respectively termed the index, long (middle), ring, and small (little) fingers. The use of numbers to designate digits is no longer accepted (Fig. 69-1). Within the hand, those structures close to the fingertips are termed distal, whereas those farther up toward the wrist are termed proximal. Motion in a palmar direction is flexion, whereas dorsal motion is termed extension. Finger motion away from the long finger axis is termed abduction, whereas motion toward the axis of the long finger is termed adduction. The description of the motion of the thumb is sometimes confusing. Extension of the thumb is in the plane of the palm of the hand, whereas palmar abduction of the thumb is the motion that occurs at 90 degrees away from the plane of the palm. Finally, side to side motion of the wrist is termed radial and ulnar deviation.

Intrinsic muscles of the hand are those that have their origins and insertions in the hand, whereas the extrinsic muscles have their muscle bellies in the forearm and their tendon insertions in the hand. The intrinsic muscles that make up the thenar eminence are the abductor pollicis brevis, flexor pollicis brevis, opponens pollicis, and adductor pollicis. There are four dorsal interossei that arise from adjacent sides of each metacarpal and provide abduction of the metacarpophalangeal (MP) joints of the index, middle, and ring fingers. There are three palmar interossei that adduct the index, ring, and little fingers toward the middle finger. Four lumbricals originate on the flexor digitorum profundus (FDP) tendons in the palm and insert on the radial sides of the extensor mechanisms of the four fingers. Together with the interossei, these bring about flexion of the MP joints and extension of the interphalangeal (IP) joints of the fingers (Fig. 69-2). The flexor pollicis brevis flexes the thumb at the MP joint, in contrast with the extrinsic flexor pollicis longus (FPL), which flexes the thumb IP joint.

The hypothenar muscles consist of the flexor digiti minimi, which flexes the little finger at the MP joint, and the abductor digiti minimi and opponens digiti minimi. A small muscle called the palmaris brevis is located transversally in the subcutaneous tissue at the base of the hypothenar eminence. It is innervated by the ulnar nerve, puckers the skin, and helps in cupping the skin of the palm during grip (Table 69-1).

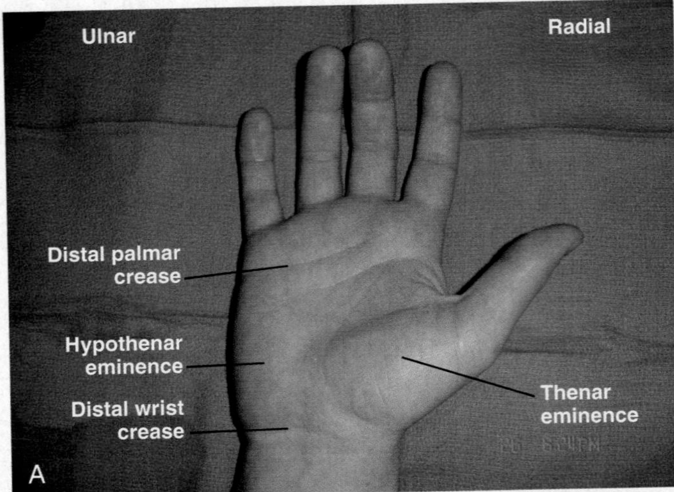

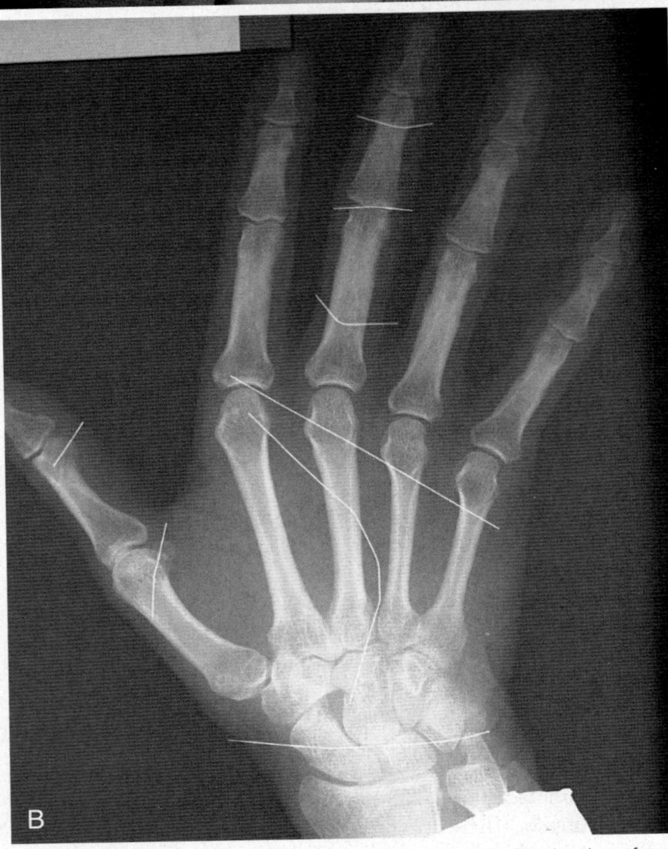

FIGURE 69-1 Surface Anatomy of the Hand. A, Hand surfaces and nomenclature. **B,** Skin creases of the hand superimposed on the skeletal structures.

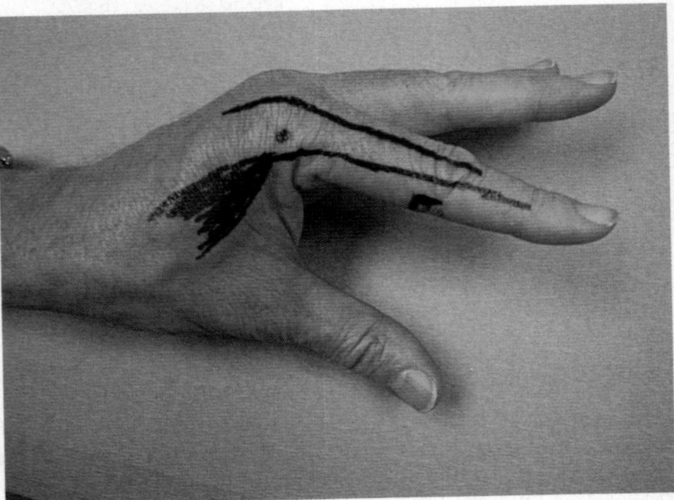

FIGURE 69-2 Outline of first dorsal interosseous muscle on the index finger shows how it passes volar to the fulcrum of flexion of the metacarpophalangeal joint and dorsal to the interphalangeal joints. Interossei flex metacarpophalangeal joints and extend proximal and distal interphalangeal joints. The long extrinsic extensor tendon passes dorsal to all joints.

TABLE 69-1 Intrinsic Muscles of the Hand

MUSCLE	INNERVATION*	FUNCTION
Abductor pollicis brevis	Median	Abducts the thumb
Flexor pollicis brevis	Median	Flexes the thumb
Opponens pollicis	Median	Opposes the thumb
Lumbricals	Median and ulnar	Flex MP joints and extend IP joints
Palmaris brevis	Ulnar	Wrinkles the skin on the medial (ulnar) side of the palm
Adductor pollicis	Ulnar	Adducts the thumb
Abductor digiti minimi	Ulnar	Abducts the small finger
Flexor digiti minimi	Ulnar	Flexes the small digit
Opponens digiti minimi	Ulnar	Opposes the small finger
Dorsal interossei	Ulnar	Abduct the fingers; flex MP joints and extend the IP joints
Palmar interossei	Ulnar	Adduct the fingers; flex MP joints and extend the IP joints

IP, interphalangeal; *MP*, metacarpophalangeal.
*All the thenar intrinsic muscles are supplied by the median nerve except the adductor pollicis; all the remaining intrinsic muscles are supplied by the ulnar nerve except the two radial lumbricals.

The extrinsic muscles originate proximal to the wrist and comprise the long flexors and extensors of the wrist and digits. The extensors are located dorsally and are divided into three subgroups. The radialmost subgroup is termed the mobile wad and comprises the brachioradialis, extensor carpi radialis longus (ECRL), and extensor carpi radialis brevis (ECRB). The ECRL and ECRB extend the wrist and deviate it radially. The second group is located in a more superficial layer and comprises three muscles, namely, the extensor carpi ulnaris (ECU), extensor digiti minimi (EDM), and extensor digitorum communis (EDC). The ECU deviates the wrist in an ulnar direction and extends the wrist, whereas the EDM and EDC extend the MP joints of the fingers. The third and deeper subgroup comprises four muscles, three of which act on the thumb; the remaining muscle influences the index finger. The abductor pollicis longus (APL), extensor pollicis longus (EPL), and extensor pollicis brevis (EPB) provide function to the thumb, and the extensor indicis proprius (EIP) extends the MP joint to the index finger. Last of the deep muscles is the supinator, which is located proximally in the forearm (Table 69-2).

The extensor tendons pass through six compartments deep to the extensor retinaculum at the dorsum of the wrist. From radial to ulnar side, these tendons and compartments are arranged as follows. The first compartment contains the APL and EPB, which also forms the radial boundary of the so-called anatomic snuffbox. The second compartment consists of the ECRL and ECRB, and the third compartment (which also forms the ulnar boundary of the anatomic snuffbox) contains the EPL. The EIP and EDC pass through the fourth compartment and the EDM passes through the fifth compartment, where they overlie the distal radioulnar joint. The sixth compartment contains the ECU (Fig. 69-3).

At the level of the MP joints, the long extrinsic extensor tendons broaden out to form the extensor hood. The proximal part of the hood at this level is called the sagittal band. It loops around the MP joint and blends into the volar plate, thus forming a lasso around the base of the proximal phalanx, through which it extends the MP joint. The insertions of the interossei and lumbricals enter into the extensor hood as the lateral bands. These lateral bands insert distally and dorsally to the axis of the proximal interphalangeal (PIP) joint, and it is through this distal insertion that the intrinsic muscles (the interossei and lumbricals) are flexors of the MP joints and yet extensors of the IP joints. The extensor hood inserts to the base of the middle phalanx, which is termed the central slip, and finally proceeds on to the base of the distal phalanx, where it inserts through the terminal slip, thus extending the distal interphalangeal (DIP) joint (Fig. 69-4).

TABLE 69-2 Extrinsic Muscles of the Dorsal Forearm

MUSCLE	INNERVATION*	FUNCTION
Extensor pollicis brevis	Radial	Abducts the hand and extends the thumb at the proximal phalanx
Abductor pollicis longus	Radial	Abducts the hand and thumb
Extensor carpi radialis longus	Radial	Extends and radially deviates the hand
Extensor carpi radialis brevis	Radial	Extends and radially deviates the hand
Extensor pollicis longus	Radial	Extends the distal phalanx of the thumb
Extensor digitorum communis	Radial	Extends the fingers and the hand
Extensor indicis proprius	Radial	Extends the index finger
Extensor digiti minimi/quinti	Radial	Extends the small finger
Extensor carpi ulnaris	Radial	Extends and ulnarly deviates the wrist
Supinator	Radial	Supination
Brachioradialis	Radial	Flexes the forearm

*All muscles of the dorsal forearm are innervated by the radial nerve and its respective branches.

The extrinsic flexor muscles are located on the volar aspect of the forearm and are arranged in three layers. The superficial layer comprises four muscles—pronator teres, flexor carpi radialis (FCR), flexor carpi ulnaris (FCU), and palmaris longus. The palmaris longus muscle may be absent in as many as 10% to 12% of individuals. These muscles originate from the medial humeral epicondyle in the proximal forearm and function to flex the wrist and to pronate the forearm. The intermediate layer consists of the flexor digitorum superficialis (FDS), which allows independent flexion of the PIP joints of the fingers. In the deep layer, there are three muscles: the FPL, which flexes the IP joint to the thumb; the FDP, which flexes the DIP joints of the fingers; and a distal quadrangular muscle that spans between the radius and ulna, termed the pronator quadratus, which helps in pronation of the forearm (Table 69-3).

Nerve supply to the hand is by three nerves, the median, ulnar, and radial nerves. A knowledge of the surface anatomy of nerves helps in evaluation of specific lacerating injuries (Fig. 69-5). The ulnar attachment to the flexor retinaculum is to the pisiform and hook of the hamate, and the radial attachment is to the scaphoid and ridge of the trapezium. The median nerve passes through the carpal tunnel between these landmarks. It gives sensation to the thumb, index finger, middle finger, and radial half of the ring finger. The palmar cutaneous branch of the median nerve originates from its radial side 5 to 6 cm proximal to the wrist, providing sensation to the palmar triangle. The ulnar nerve travels to the radial side of the pisiform and passes to the ulnar side of the hook

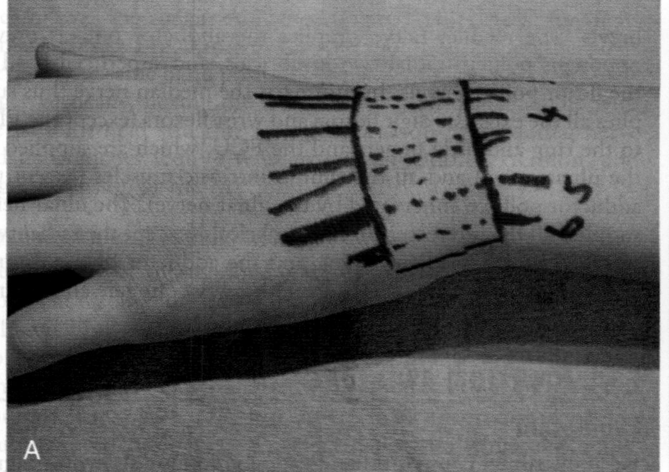

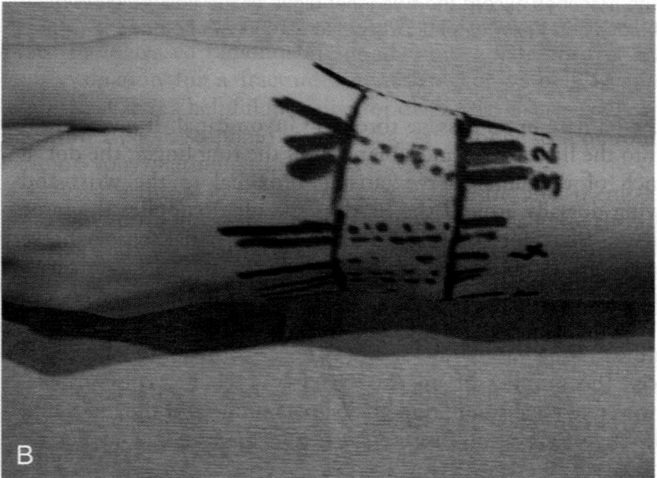

FIGURE 69-3 **A** and **B,** Surface anatomy of the six dorsal extensor compartments at the wrist. Note that the first (abductor pollicis longus and extensor pollicis brevis) and third (extensor pollicis longus) compartments form the radial and ulnar boundaries, respectively, of the anatomic snuffbox.

extensors (EPL and EPB) and long abductor of the thumb are tested by asking the patient to extend his or her thumb against resistance while these tendons are individually palpated. Long extensors of the fingers are tested by asking the patient to extend them against resistance applied to the dorsum of the proximal phalanx.

A closed boutonnière jamming injury may be difficult to initially diagnose. In this type of injury, the central slip insertion is disrupted from the middle phalanx and the triangular ligament on each side of the central slip is stretched or disrupted. The lateral

In the case of injuries, treatment is directed at the specific structures damaged—skeletal, tendon, nerve, vessel, integument.[3,4] In emergency situations, the goals of treatment are to maintain or to restore distal circulation, to obtain a healed wound, to preserve motion, and to retain distal sensation. Stable skeletal architecture is established in the primary phase of care because skeletal stability is essential for effective motion and function of the extremity. This also reestablishes skeletal length, straightens deformities, and corrects the compression or kinking of nerves and vessels. Arteries

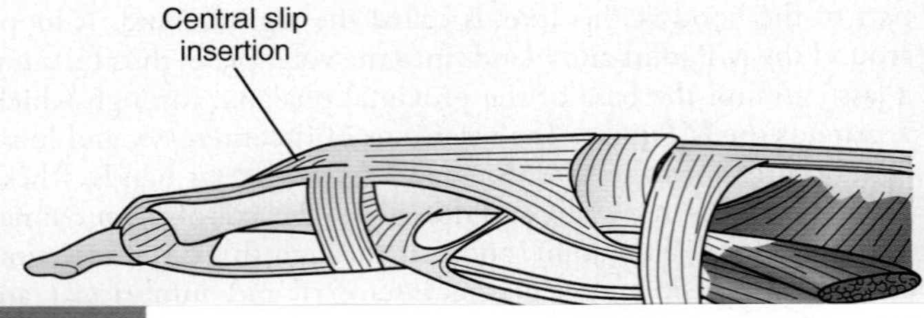

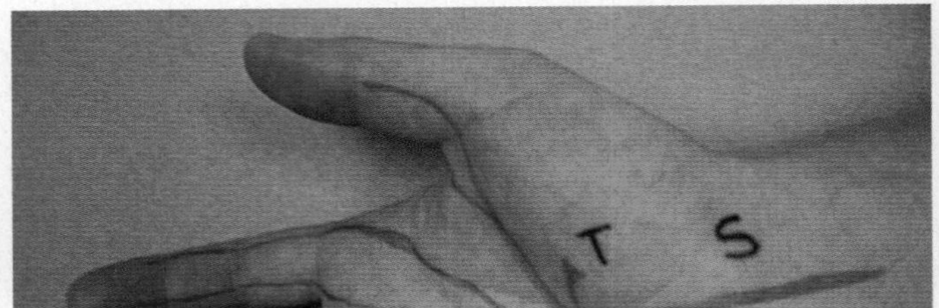

been controlled, and hematoma has been evacuated, the distal extremity can be assessed more adequately. At this time, lacerated vessel ends are controlled by atraumatic vascular clamps and a tourniquet can be released. Capillary refill and perfusion of the distal extremity can then be assessed, as can backflow from the distal lacerated vessel ends. Digital blood pressure can be quantified with a sterile Doppler probe and cuff; a digital brachial index of 0.7 or greater suggests adequate perfusion. If there is poor collateral flow, arterial reconstruction is performed. At this time, standard of care does not require arterial repair of isolated noncritical vessels. In combined radial and ulnar artery injuries, one or both vessels are reconstructed. If possible, both vessels are repaired.[18]

Muscles often swell after prolonged periods of ischemia. This can lead to an increase of pressure within the closed compartment of the forearm, resulting in a compartment syndrome. It is thus the practice of most surgeons to perform a routine fasciotomy to decompress the forearm compartment after a true revascularization procedure has been performed. During the period of ischemia to the muscles, there may be a buildup of lactic acid. Furthermore, myonecrosis might occur. Restoration of circulation to such a limb can cause a sudden flooding of the circulation with myoglobin, lactic acid, and other toxic substances. This is called reperfusion syndrome and can lead to multiorgan failure, especially affecting the renal and cardiac systems.

Replantation and Amputations

It can often be frustrating for the novice general surgeon to be told by a replantation surgeon in the middle of the night that a consultation was obtained inappropriately or not soon enough. There are general indications for the replantation of amputated parts, but the overriding decision is still to save life before limb. Although patients and family members may desire replantation, and in some cases have even been promised it by members of the primary team, it is not performed in patients with severe associated medical problems or injuries. Replantation is also generally not considered under the following circumstances[4,19]:

- Severe crush or multilevel injury of the amputated part
- A psychotic patient who has willfully self-amputated the part
- Amputation of a single digit proximal to the FDS distal insertion (zone 2), except for single-digit amputations in children or those with a demanding profession (e.g., a musician)
- Amputation in patients with severely atherosclerotic arteries (sometimes this can be determined only when the vessels are explored in the operating room)

Indications for replantation of amputated parts are as follows:

- Whenever possible, for a thumb amputation (it provides >40% of the overall hand function)[19]
- Single digits that have been amputated distal to the FDS insertion (e.g., a manual worker may likely desire revision of amputation and desires to return to work quickly)
- Multiple injured digits
- Most amputations in children, including single-digit amputations
- Guillotine-sharp clean amputations at the hand, wrist, or distal forearm

Replantation is the reattachment of the part that has been completely amputated. Revascularization requires reconstruction of vessels in a limb that has been severely injured or incompletely severed in such a way that vascular repair is necessary to prevent distal necrosis, but some soft tissue (e.g., skin, tendon, nerve) is still intact. Revascularization generally has a better success rate than replantation because venous and lymphatic drainage may be intact.

Minor replantation is a reattachment at the wrist, hand, or digital level, whereas major replantation is performed proximal to the wrist. This clinical distinction exists because in the case of a major replantation, ischemic time is crucial to the viability of muscle and to functional outcome. Ischemic muscle may result in myonecrosis, myoglobinemia, and infection, which may threaten the patient's life (as well as limb). There are three types of amputations:

- Guillotine amputation, whereby the tissue is cut with a sharp object and is minimally damaged
- Crush amputation, in which a local crushing injury can be converted into a guillotine injury simply by débriding back the edges, although this may not be possible in a diffusely crushing amputation
- Avulsion amputation, which is the most unfavorable type for replantation because structures are injured at different levels

Avulsion amputation may occur, for example, with a so-called ring avulsion injury. The extensor tendons are shredded, flexor tendons are often avulsed at the musculotendinous junctions, and nerves are stretched and may be ripped from end organs.

Ischemia time is also an important consideration in evaluating a patient for replantation. For amputated digits, more than 12 hours of warm ischemia is a relative contraindication. Promptly cooling the part to 4° C dramatically alters the ischemia factor, but even ischemia exceeding 24 hours does not necessarily preclude successful digital replantation. Ischemia time is more crucial for replantation above the proximal forearm, and reimplantation is not considered after more than 6 to 10 hours of warm ischemia time. Single digits in adults, other than the thumb in zone 2, are generally not reattached because of the consequent adverse overall functional result on the hand, with a single stiff finger.[19]

Amputation is not an outmoded operation; rather, it is necessary in a patient in whom replantation might not be indicated. When primary amputation is performed, the stump is preserved with as much length as possible. An exception might be made if there is only a very short segment of proximal phalanx. A short proximal phalangeal remnant at the index finger position may serve as an impediment for thumb to middle finger prehension, and one might consider a formal ray amputation in this case to improve overall hand function. The ends of the cut nerve are cut sharply and allowed to retract to minimize the occurrence of painful neuromas at the amputation tip. Tendons are also divided sharply and allowed to retract. The practice of suturing flexor and extensor tendons over the ends of the middle, ring, or small finger stump seriously impairs the motion of the uninjured fingers because of the common origin of the flexors. There will be an active flexion deficit in the uninjured digits, the quadriga syndrome; this is corrected simply by release of the flexor tendon remnant at the injured amputated digit.

If it is anticipated that the amputated part will be considered for replantation, it is critical to transport the patient and the part in an appropriate manner. The amputated part is placed in a clean, dry, plastic bag, which is sealed and placed on top of ice in a Styrofoam container. This keeps the part sufficiently cool at 4° C to 10° C without freezing. The amputated part is wrapped in a lightly moistened saline gauze to prevent tissue drying.

With only a few minor variations, the sequence of replantation has been standardized. Preliminary exploration of the distal amputated part under a microscope by an initial surgical team not only determines whether a replantation is technically feasible but also can be started while the patient is being prepared for the operating room. Bone shortening allows skin to be débrided back to where it is free of contusion and direct tension-free closure can be achieved. In the thumb, bone shortening is minimized to less than 10 mm. The order of repair is usually bone, tendons, muscle units, arteries, nerves, and finally veins. Establishment of arterial flow before venous flow clears lactic acid from the replanted part. The functional veins can now also be detected by spurting bleeding. However, blood loss must be closely monitored.

For major replantations, reestablishing arterial circulation as rapidly as possible is crucial to limiting ischemia time. A dialysis shunt or carotid shunt may be placed between the arterial ends. Intermittent clamping of the shunt may be necessary to restrict blood loss. In the upper extremity, bone shortening can be aggressive to achieve primary skin closure and primary nerve repair. Judicious use of anticoagulants may enhance the success of replantation. Topical application of 2% lidocaine or papaverine may help relieve vasospasm. Postoperative dressings consist of nonadherent mesh gauze, loose flap gauze, and a plaster splint, with postoperative elevation to minimize edema and venous congestion. The patient's room must be kept warm, and smoking is forbidden postoperatively. Aside from antibiotics and analgesics, one aspirin tablet daily for its retarding effect on platelet aggregation is suggested. Postoperative monitoring is done hourly to assess color, pulp turgor, capillary refill, and digital temperature.

Fractures and Dislocations

Pain, swelling, limited motion, and deformities suggest the presence of a fracture or dislocation. Standard anteroposterior and lateral radiographs may miss some fractures and dislocations, and multiple views may be necessary to establish the exact diagnosis. Fractures may be rotated, angulated, telescoped, or displaced. Angulation is described by the direction in which the apex of the fracture is pointing, and displacement is described by the direction of the distal fragment. Fractures may be open or closed, depending on whether a wound is involved. They may also be complete, incomplete, or comminuted (more than two pieces). Fractures are also described by their pattern; they may be transverse, longitudinal, oblique, or spiral. Open fractures need to be thoroughly irrigated and débrided urgently. Displaced fractures or dislocations are repositioned as soon as possible. A dislocation is described according to the direction of displacement of the distal bone in the involved joint. The separation of joints may be complete or incomplete (subluxed), depending on the severity of the capsular injury.[6,20,21]

Displaced fractures or dislocations are repositioned as soon as possible to decrease soft tissue injury, to decompress nerves that might be stretched, and to relieve kinking of blood vessels. Good bone contact and stability are necessary for fractures to heal. Some fractures are stable and require only external support in a splint or cast, whereas others are unstable and require internal support, which can be provided by Kirschner wires, internal wire sutures through drill holes in the fracture fragments, screws, plates, or even external fixation devices (Table 69-4). The more complicated the fixation, the more dissection is required to apply that fixation and therefore the greater the potential for scarring around adjacent tendons and consequential stiffness. Plates and screws, however, can nonetheless establish a degree of rigid fixation that allows early motion of the part and thus potentially reduces the risk for cicatricial stiffness. Intra-articular fractures require accurate reduction to preserve motion and to minimize the risk for later development of arthrosis. Persistent rotational and significant lateral angular deformities generally do not remodel with time; these can be avoided by observing the alignment of the injured fingers compared with adjacent digits while passively and gently flexing them into a fist after reduction is attained. If they do not fit comfortably adjacent to each other and do not point toward the distal pole of the scaphoid, a fresh attempt at reduction must be performed. A thorough neurovascular examination is always performed before and after fracture reduction has been completed.

Distal Phalangeal Fractures

Fractures of the distal phalanx are the most frequent hand fractures, representing 50% of all hand fractures. Most result from crush injuries with associated nail bed injuries. Precise reduction is generally not required, and treatment typically consists of splinting alone. However, unstable shaft fractures with overriding fragments are indications for reduction and longitudinal Kirschner wire fixation.

Most closed mallet fractures can be managed by splinting the DIP joint in extension, provided the fracture involves less than 50% of the joint surface and is not associated with DIP joint subluxation. If fixation is required, the fracture fragment is held in place with a monofilament wire or nonabsorbable suture passed through to the palmar aspect of the finger through the distal phalanx. A transarticular longitudinal Kirschner wire is used to keep the joint in neutral position. A so-called jersey finger is an avulsion fracture of the insertion of the FDP tendon into the distal phalanx. It occurs after a pull of the FDP against resistance,

TABLE 69-4 Comparison of Methods of Skeletal Fixation

METHOD OF FIXATION	ADVANTAGES	DISADVANTAGES
Kirschner wires	Come in varying diameters	Pins can loosen
	Can be applied percutaneously or open	Cannot provide rigid fixation
	Second surgery not required for removal	Soft tissue may be transfixed (but can be avoided by careful placement)
	Require less soft tissue dissection than plates and screws	Infection can occur along pin tracks
Screws	Have high stability	Frequently require open approach (although not always)
	Allow early finger mobilization	
Plates	Can be used when fracture line is not oblique enough for screws	Require open approach
		Require extensive soft tissue dissection
	Allow early finger mobilization	Have relatively high profile and may be palpable through the dorsum of fingers and hand
		May promote extensor tendon adhesions by their relative bulk and dissection required for placement

as can occur when a footballer catches onto the jersey of an opponent. On occasion, the avulsed fragment may lie as far proximally as the palm. This fracture fragment generally requires open reduction and internal fixation.[6]

Middle Phalanx and Proximal Phalanx Fractures

Fractures may involve the head, neck, shaft, or base of the respective bone. Head and base fractures may be intra-articular. A middle phalangeal shaft fracture is displaced according to the forces exerted by the insertions of the FDS and central slip mechanism. If the fracture lies distal to the FDS insertion, the proximal fragment is flexed by this muscle, resulting in a volar angulation. In contrast, if the fracture is proximal to the FDS insertion, the proximal fragment is extended by the central slip, whereas the distal part is flexed by the FDS. This results in a dorsal angulation. Most shaft fractures of the proximal phalanx tend to angulate volarward because the interossei reflect the proximal fragment and the central slip, through the PIP joint, extends the distal fragment. Displaced and unstable shaft fractures require open reduction followed by fixation with Kirschner wires, plates, or screws.

Metacarpal Fractures

Stable metacarpal fractures may be treated with splinting alone. Fractures with dorsal or volar angulation can be stabilized by percutaneous insertion of intramedullary fixation pins. If they are displaced or unstable, such as oblique, spiral, or multiple metacarpal fractures, open reduction and internal fixation of these metacarpal fractures are performed. The internal fixation can be achieved with Kirschner wires, lag screws, or plate and screws, depending on the fracture pattern configuration. Dorsally angulated fractures at the neck of the little finger metacarpal, the so-called boxer fracture, do not require reduction if the dorsal angulation is less than 30 degrees. The mobility of the carpometacarpal joint will compensate for this degree of angulation. The index and middle finger metacarpals are less mobile than the ring and little finger metacarpals. Therefore, a maximum of 15 degrees of angular deformity can be tolerated in the index and middle finger metacarpals.

Oblique fractures at the base of the thumb metacarpal (Bennett fracture) result in the small proximal fragment's being held in position by the volar oblique ligament to the trapezium. The remaining portion of the thumb metacarpal is displaced dorsally and radially because of the pull of the APL tendon (Fig. 69-31). These fracture fragments must be properly reduced and secured with internal fixation with Kirschner wires or a screw. Comminuted fractures at the base of the thumb metacarpal (Rolando fracture) are infrequently treated by closed reduction. If the fragments are large and badly displaced, an open reduction is indicated to ensure accurate restoration of the joint surface at the base of the thumb metacarpal. Fractures of the shaft of the thumb metacarpal tend to become displaced by the opposing muscle forces of the abductor and adductor on the proximal and distal fragments, respectively. Even undisplaced fractures may become progressively more displaced and angulated over time, necessitating an internal fixation. If initial splint immobilization is chosen for an undisplaced thumb metacarpal fracture, close follow-up is required to detect the earliest signs of displacement and instability. Fracture at the base of the little finger metacarpal is analogous to Bennett fracture of the thumb and is sometimes called a reverse Bennett fracture. This results in a fracture-dislocation, with the deforming force being the insertion of the extensor carpi ulnaris tendon.

Scaphoid Fractures

The scaphoid is the most common carpal bone fracture and accounts for approximately 60% of all carpal injuries. Clinical examination shows tenderness over the anatomic snuffbox and over the scaphoid tubercle. If a scaphoid fracture is suspected, the initial radiographic examination includes not only the standard three views of the wrist but also a scaphoid view, which is a posteroanterior image with the wrist in full ulnar deviation (Fig. 69-32). Frequently, immediate postinjury radiographs may not reveal a fracture. CT or MRI may help in these cases, or one may elect to apply a splint and to repeat the radiographs in 2 weeks.[22]

Treatment of a nondisplaced scaphoid fracture is with a long arm cast that includes the thumb. The thumb spica cast is maintained for 6 weeks, followed by a short arm cast until radiographic healing has occurred. There has been a trend toward percutaneous screw fixation of even, undisplaced scaphoid fractures.

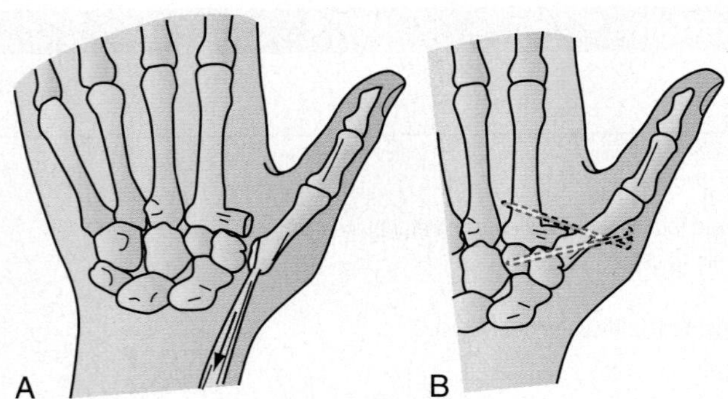

FIGURE 69-31 **A,** Fracture-dislocation at the base of the thumb metacarpal is called Bennett fracture. The deforming force is produced by the pull of the abductor pollicis longus muscle. **B,** Open reduction and pinning of the fracture are frequently required.

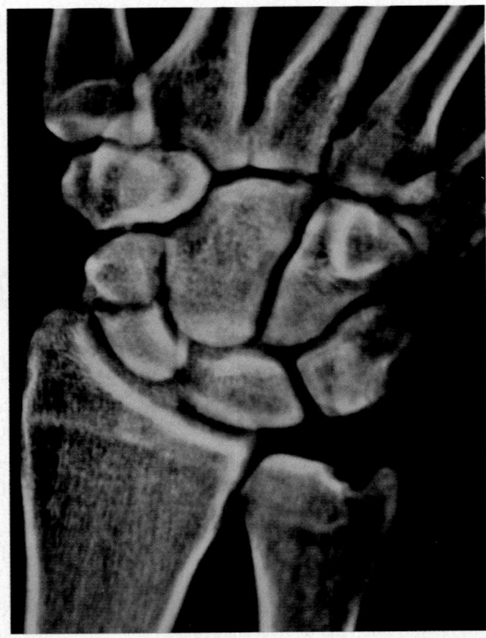
FIGURE 69-32 Anteroposterior radiograph of the wrist demonstrating a fracture of the waist of the scaphoid, the bone in the hand that is usually fractured.

Displaced scaphoid fractures require open reduction with internal fixation, generally using a compression screw. Complications with inadequately treated scaphoid fractures are notorious. The blood vessels enter the scaphoid mainly through its distal half, and fractures through the waist of the scaphoid may deprive the proximal half of its blood supply, leading to avascular necrosis of the proximal pole of the scaphoid. Nonunion also occurs with relative frequency, and these cases need to be treated with cancellous bone grafting or even a pedicle vascularized bone graft. Early diagnosis of scaphoid fractures is essential so that appropriate treatment can be instituted to reduce the risks for these complications. Modern cannulated compression screws, intraoperative fluoroscopy, and arthroscopy have allowed minimally invasive percutaneous fixation of some of these scaphoid fractures, resulting in a trend toward more aggressive surgical treatment of these fractures.

Fractures in Children

The Salter-Harris classification describes five types of epiphyseal injuries (Fig. 69-33). Pediatric bones are still growing and thus permit a greater degree of remodeling. Hence, moderate angular and translational displacement of fractures tends to correct with age. However, rotational deformities never correct in the hand and are totally unacceptable, even in children. Implants that cross the epiphysis must have minimal potential for damage. Hence, smooth Kirschner wires are generally used for the fixation of pediatric skeletal injuries, and threaded screws are usually avoided.

Dislocations

Dislocations are more frequently seen at the PIP joint. A closed dislocation of the PIP joint can frequently be managed by closed reduction and splinting. If the joint is unstable after reduction, it needs exploration for collateral ligament repair. The most common type of PIP joint dislocation is a dorsal dislocation. A PIP joint volar dislocation is often associated with a tear in the triangular ligament of the extensor mechanism through which the head of the proximal phalanx protrudes and becomes trapped. Attempts at closed reduction fail because they tighten the fibers of the lateral bands and central slip around each side of the protruding proximal phalangeal neck; these injuries often require open reduction with repair of the extensor tear.

Palmar dislocations of the head of the index finger metacarpal often require open reduction. The head of the metacarpal becomes trapped between the superficial transverse metacarpal ligament, flexor tendons, and lumbrical muscles, whereas the volar plate becomes trapped between the metacarpal head and base of the proximal phalanx. Attempts at closed reduction are fruitless because of the entrapment resulting from this arrangement.

MP joint dislocation of the thumb often results from jamming it in a radial direction, thus tearing the ulnar collateral ligament. The ulnar collateral ligament may pull proximally and come to rest dorsal to the extensor hood (Stener lesion; Fig. 69-34). It cannot heal spontaneously because the ulnar collateral ligament is prevented from reattaching to bone. This so-called ski pole injury may then require operative repair. Stress radiography, sometimes able to be performed only after the digit is anesthetized with a metacarpal block, may be required to facilitate diagnosis of a complete ulnar collateral ligament injury of the thumb metacarpal joint.

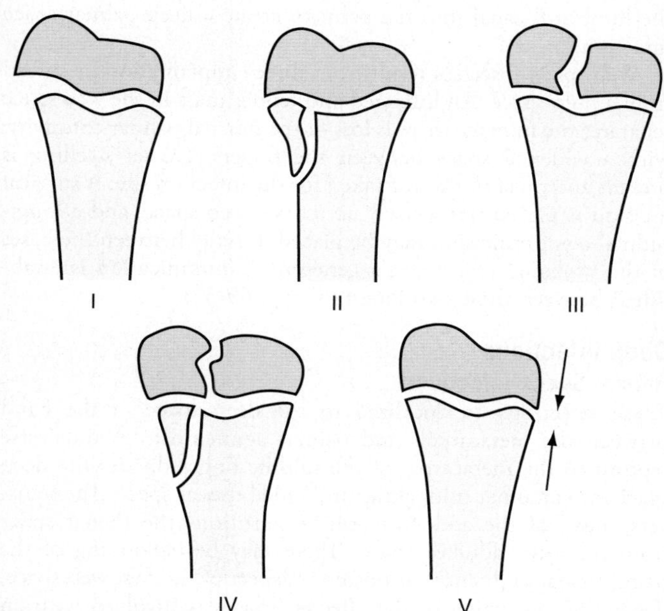

FIGURE 69-33 Salter-Harris fracture patterns involving the epiphysis in children.

INFECTIONS

Hand infections commonly present to the surgical resident covering the emergency department. When the infection is diagnosed

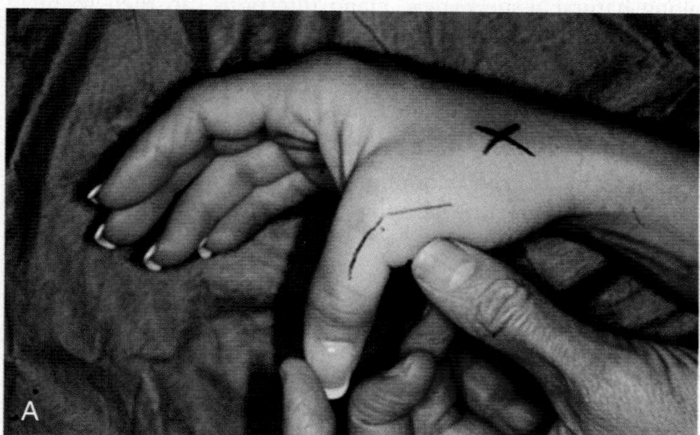

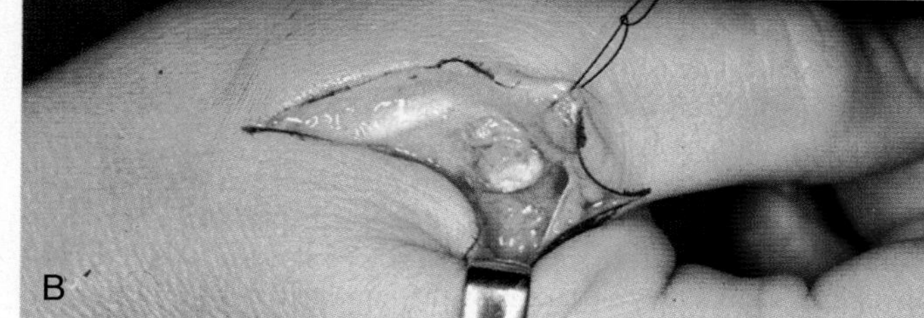

FIGURE 69-34 **A,** Instability of the ulnar collateral ligament of the metacarpophalangeal joint of the thumb. **B,** Stener lesion shows that the distal insertion of the collateral ligament has avulsed proximal to the extensor hood and is thus blocked from spontaneous reattachment. Open operation is required to reanchor the collateral ligament insertion to the base of the proximal phalanx.

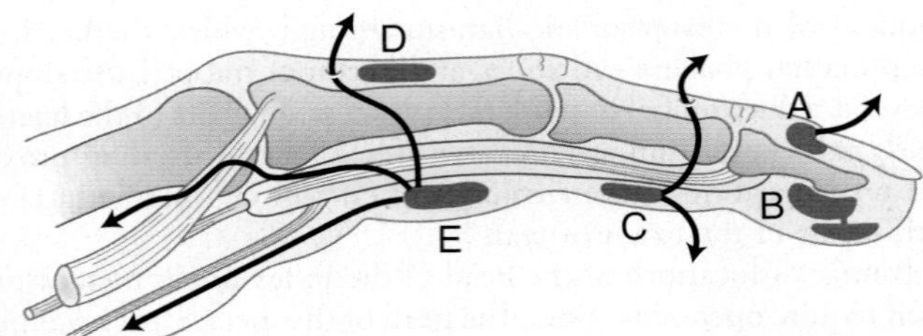

FIGURE 69-35 Spread of soft tissue infections in the hand occurs through loss of containment from the original site and erosion into and spread through contiguous anatomic compartments. **A,** Paronychium. Infecting organisms access periungual tissues through fissures in the eponychial or paronychial tissues and often are discharged spontaneously in these areas. **B,** Infection of pulp tissues (felon). Fibrous septa within the pulp create collar stud abscesses within the pulp. **C,** Volar subcutaneous infections in the digit may be discharged percutaneously on either surface of the digit or penetrate dorsally and spread along the sheaths of the flexor or extensor tendons. **D,** Subcutaneous infections on the dorsum of the digit are usually discharged percutaneously because of the thin and areolar nature of the soft tissues. **E,** Proximally located digital infections or web space infections may rupture into the palmar spaces by tracking along tendon sheaths, palmar fascia, or lumbrical canal. The continuous sheaths of the thumb and little fingers (radial and ulnar bursae) are continuous with the carpal tunnel and space of Parona at the wrist.

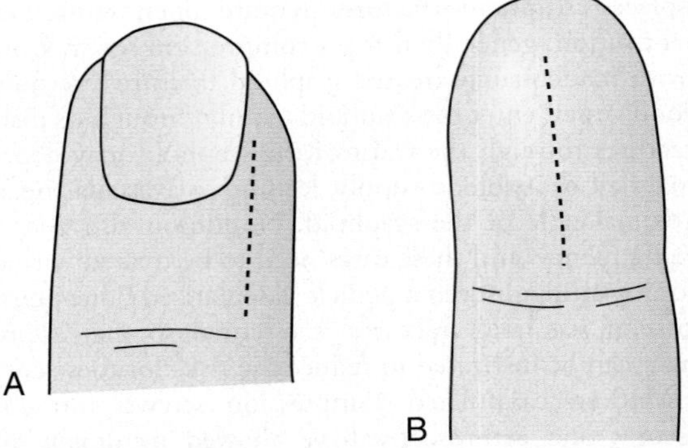

FIGURE 69-36 Incisions for paronychia **(A)** and felon **(B)**.

and treated properly initially, most patients do well. The extent of deep palmar infections may often be underestimated during the early phases because the volar aspect of the hand does not show edema as readily as the dorsal aspect of the hand. Thus, if infections in the hand are not diagnosed at an early stage, infections may spread from one anatomic compartment to another along natural tissue planes. Hand infections can then result in significant morbidity and severe functional compromise if they are not appropriately diagnosed and treated (Fig. 69-35). Some of the more common types of infections are discussed here.

Superficial Paronychial Infections

Paronychia is the most common infection of the hand; it usually results from trauma to the eponychial or paronychial region. The infection localizes around the nail base, advances around the nail fold, and burrows beneath the base of the nail. If pus is trapped beneath the nail, pressure on the nail evokes exquisite pain. The most common causative organism is *Staphylococcus aureus.* Early treatment is with antibiotics, preferably penicillin in combination with a β-lactamase inhibitor such as sulbactam or clavulanic acid. However, there has now been an increasing incidence of methicillin-resistant *S. aureus* in community-acquired infections. After an abscess develops, surgical drainage is required. The surgical approach to an acute paronychia depends on the extent of the infection. Incisions may not be necessary. A Freer elevator is used to lift approximately 25% of the nail adjacent to the infected perionychium, extending proximally to the edge of the nail. This portion of the nail is transected, and gauze packing is inserted beneath the nail fold. A single incision to drain the affected perionychium also allows elevation of the eponychial fold when both eponychium and paronychium are involved (Fig. 69-36).[23-25]

Infections of Intermediate-Depth Spaces

Infections of intermediate-depth spaces are pulp space infections (felons) and deep web space infections. The pulp space infections may involve the terminal, middle, or proximal volar pulp spaces and may result from direct implantation with a penetrating injury or may represent spread from a more superficial subcutaneous infection. The volar pulp of the distal digital segment is a fascial space closed proximally by a septum joining the distal flexion crease to the periosteum, where the long flexor tendon is inserted. This space is also partitioned by fibrous septa. Tension in the distal digital segment can become so great that the arteries to the bone are compressed, resulting in gangrene of the fingertip and necrosis of the distal 75% of the terminal phalanx. With infection of the digital pulp space, one must not wait for fluctuance before making the decision for surgery because of the danger of ischemic necrosis of the skin and bone. Clinical diagnosis is made by the rapid onset of throbbing pain, swelling, and exquisite tenderness of the affected pulp space. Surgical drainage is required. A single volar or unilateral longitudinal incision may be used (Fig. 69-36). Postoperative care includes packing of the wound and elevation of the extremity. Use of antibiotics is guided by the results of Gram staining. Similar to a paronychia, *S. aureus* is the most common causative agent. Spread from a pulp space infection may move into a joint space or underlying bone or burst through the septum proximally to involve the rest of the finger. More proximally, a pulp space infection at the base of the finger can travel through the lumbrical canal into the palm to create a deep palmar space infection.[25]

Web space abscesses result from direct implantation or spread from a pulp space. An inflamed and tender mass in the web space separates the fingers. There is loss of the normal palmar concavity, with a widened space between the fingers. Dorsal swelling is present and must not be mistaken for the infection site. A surgical incision is placed transversely across the web space, and a longitudinal counterincision may be placed dorsally between the bases of the proximal phalanges; a generous communication is established between these two incisions (Fig. 69-37).

Deep Infections

Palmar Space Infections

These infections are localized to the deep space of the hand between the metacarpals and palmar aponeurosis. A transverse septum to the metacarpal of the middle finger divides the deep space into an ulnar midpalmar and radial thenar space. The transverse head of the adductor pollicis partitions the thenar space from the retroadductor space. There may be ballooning of the palm, thenar eminence, or posterior aspect of the first web space, depending on which of the affected spaces is involved with an abscess. The dorsal subaponeurotic space of the hand deep to the extensor tendons may also be affected by an isolated infection,

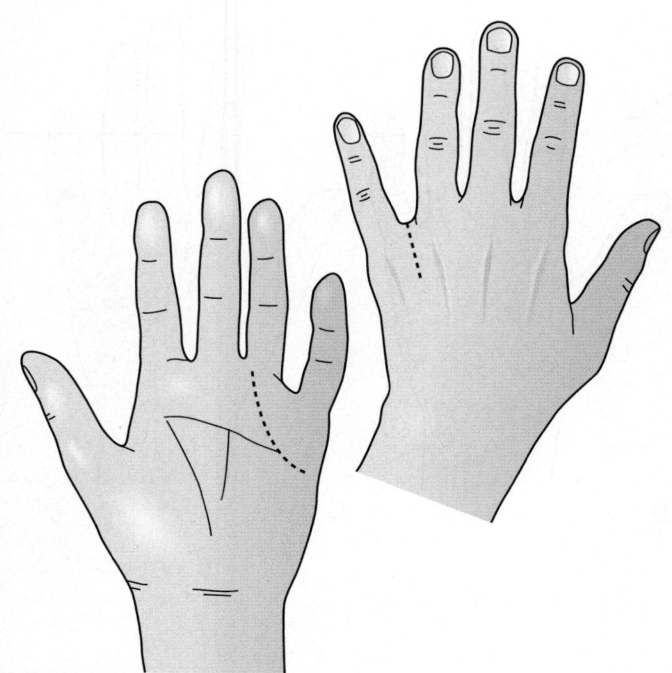

FIGURE 69-37 Incisions for web space abscess between the little and ring fingers.

generally as the result of direct implantation (Fig. 69-38*A*). For a thenar space infection, the preferred approach to surgical drainage is a dual volar and dorsal incision (Fig. 69-38*B*). On the volar side, an incision is made adjacent and parallel to the thenar crease. Great care is taken to avoid injury to the palmar cutaneous branch of the median nerve in the proximal part of the incision and the motor branch of the median nerve in a deeper plane. A second, slightly curved longitudinal incision is made on the dorsum of the first web space. Dissection is continued more deeply into this area between the first dorsal interosseous muscle and adductor pollicis. A drain is placed in the incision after thorough exploration of the respective spaces. With midpalmar space infections, dorsal swelling of the hand will be present, as is the case with all palmar infections, and must not be mistaken for the infection site. Motion of the middle and ring fingers is limited and painful. A longitudinal curvilinear incision is the preferred approach for drainage of this space (Fig. 69-38*C*).

Infection of Parona space occurs in the potential space deep to the flexor tendons in the distal forearm and superficial to the pronator quadratus muscle. It is usually the result of spread from the adjacent contiguous midpalmar space or from the radial or ulnar bursa. Swelling, tenderness, and fluctuation will be present in the distal volar forearm. A midpalmar infection may be associated. Active digital flexion is painful, as is passive finger extension. A surgical incision must be planned to leave the median nerve adequately covered with soft tissue.

Pyogenic Flexor Tenosynovitis

Kanavel's four cardinal signs include the following: (1) the finger is held flexed because this position allows the synovial sheath its maximum volume and eases pain; (2) symmetrical fusiform swelling of the entire finger is present, with edema of the back of the hand; (3) the slightest attempt at passive extension of the affected digit produces exquisite pain; and (4) the site of maximum tenderness is at the proximal cul-de-sac of the index, middle, and ring finger synovial sheaths in the distal palm or, in the case of infection of the sheaths of the thumb and little finger, more proximally in the palm (Fig. 69-38). The radial and ulnar bursae communicate in approximately 80% of cases and may be simultaneously infected. Bursal infections may spread into the forearm space of Parona, deep to the flexor tendons in the distal part of the forearm, creating a horseshoe abscess.

Pyogenic flexor tenosynovitis may be aborted with parenteral antibiotics, extremity elevation, and hand immobilization if the patient is seen within the first 24 hours of onset of infection. If this course is unsuccessful or if the patient is seen more than 48 hours after onset of infection, surgical drainage is undertaken. The preferred surgical approach is through two separate incisions. The first incision is a midaxial incision made on the finger, usually on the ulnar side of the digit (on the radial side of the thumb or little finger); the digital artery and nerve remain in the volar flap, with the dissection proceeding directly to the tendon sheath. The synovium between the A3 and A4 pulleys is incised, and cloudy fluid is encountered. A second incision is made in the palm over the tendon to drain the cul-de-sac. A 16-gauge polyethylene catheter is inserted beneath the A1 pulley into the sheath, and the sheath is flushed manually with sterile saline every 2 hours after surgery. A bulky hand dressing absorbs the drainage. Studies have found that postoperative catheter drainage may not always be necessary.[26,27]

Chronic and Atypical Infections

Chronic paronychia is generally the result of *Candida albicans* (>95%) infection and is not bacterial. When bacteria are involved, they are more commonly atypical mycobacteria or gram-negative organisms. Chronic paronychia generally responds to treatment with topical antifungal agents, although oral antifungal agents are sometimes used. On occasion, surgical treatment by means of marsupialization of the eponychial fold is required. If the lesion is refractory to treatment, the possibility of a malignant neoplasm is entertained.

Chronic tenosynovitis can occur in the flexor tendons or in the dorsum of the wrist and extensor tendons. It is usually of a granulomatous type and is caused by mycobacteria or fungi. Treatment includes surgical excision of the involved synovium and prolonged treatment with the appropriate antimicrobial agents. Chronic infected tenosynovitis must be differentiated from other causes of chronic granulomatous synovitis, such as sarcoidosis, amyloidosis, gout, and rheumatoid arthritis.

Herpetic Whitlow

Herpetic whitlow is caused by type 1 or type 2 herpes simplex virus and may be confused with a paronychia. Infection begins with the appearance of small clear vesicles with localized swelling, erythema, and intense pain. The vesicles may subsequently appear turbid and coalesce over the next few days before ulcerating. Diagnosis is confirmed by culturing the virus from the vesicular fluid, assessing immunofluorescent serum antibody titers, or performing a Tzanck smear. However, these measures are rarely required because clinical diagnosis is usually sufficient. Infection can occur from autoinoculation from an oral or genital lesion or exposure as a health care worker. Pain is often out of proportion to the physical findings. Treatment is generally nonoperative because this infection is usually self-limited. Antivirals such as acyclovir or famciclovir may be of some benefit if started within the first 48 hours of symptom onset. Surgical incision and

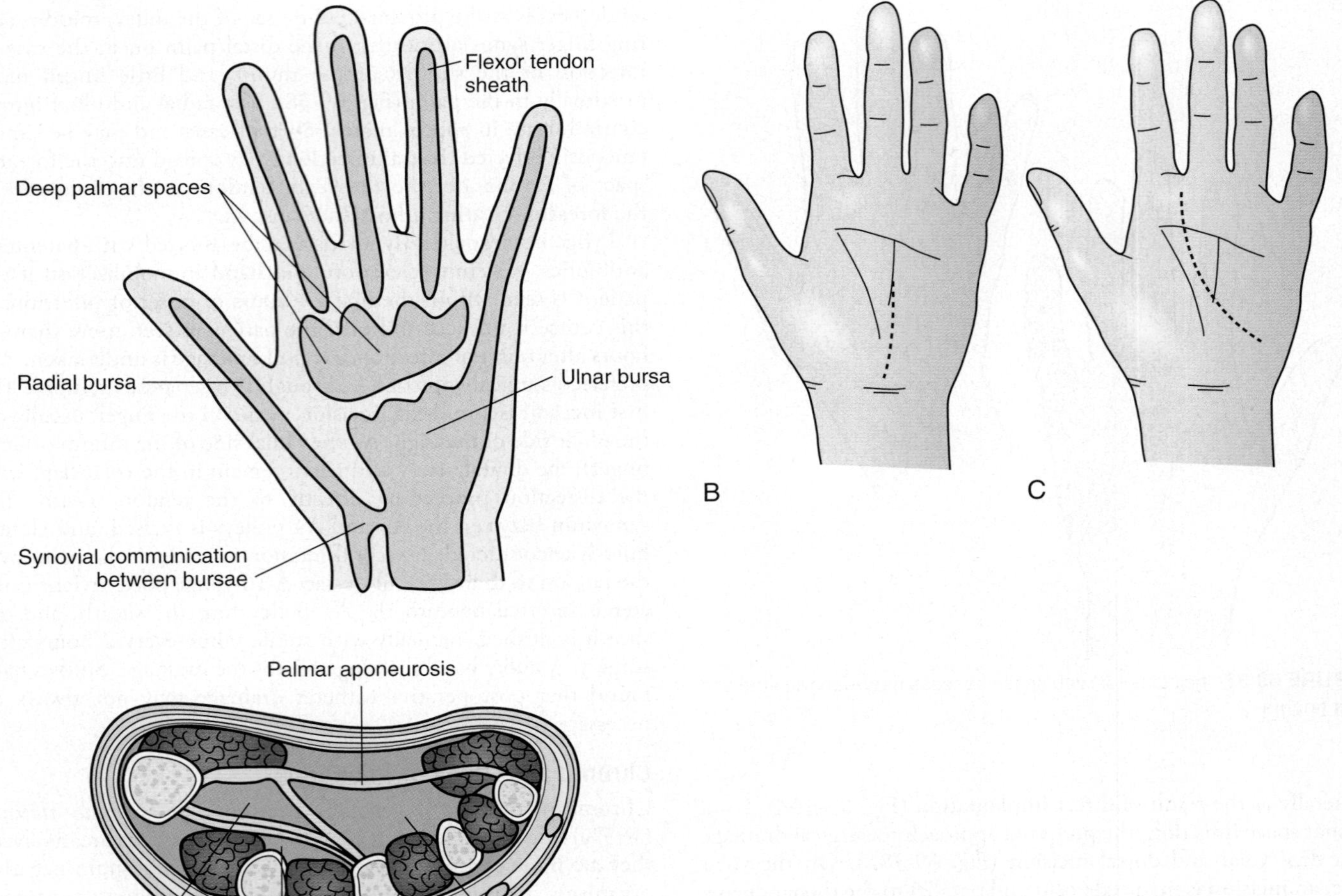

FIGURE 69-38 **A,** Deep spaces of the hand and synovial bursae. Infections may be bound by these spaces or may track along anatomic dissection planes between these spaces. **B,** Incision for thenar space infection. A dorsal first web space incision is also often required. **C,** Incision for midpalmar space abscess.

drainage can lead to systemic involvement and possible viral encephalitis.

Animal and Human Bites

The most striking difference in the microbial flora of human and animal bite wounds is the higher number of bacterial isolates per wound in human bites, the difference being mostly caused by the presence of anaerobic bacteria. Human bites can occasionally transmit other infectious diseases, such as hepatitis B, tuberculosis, syphilis, or actinomycosis. The incidence of *Eikenella corrodens* in human bite infections of the hand has been reported to vary between 7% and 29%. Usually, isolated organisms from infected human bite wounds are, as in animal bites, alpha-hemolytic streptococci and *S. aureus,* β-lactamase–producing strains of *S. aureus,* and *Bacteroides* spp. Anaerobic bacteria, including *Bacteroides, Clostridium, Peptococcus,* and *Veillonella,* are more prevalent in human bite infections than previously recognized. Most studies of animal bite wounds have focused on the isolation of *Pasteurella multocida,* disregarding the role of anaerobes. However, more recent studies have shown that dog bite wounds indicate multiple organisms, with *P. multocida* being isolated from only 26% of dog bite wounds in adults. Most animal bites cause mixed infections of aerobic and anaerobic bacteria.

Pyogenic joint infections usually result from trauma, such as a bite wound from a tooth when the assailant's hand strikes the jaw. A tooth struck by the clenched fist of an attacker penetrates the skin, tendon, joint capsule, and metacarpal head. Once the finger is extended, the four puncture wounds separate from each other to create a closed space within the joint. All these so-called fight bite wounds of the MP joint need to be explored surgically, débrided, and thoroughly lavaged. Human bite wounds are not closed primarily and are treated with appropriate antibiotics.

COMPARTMENT SYNDROME, HIGH-PRESSURE INJECTION INJURIES, AND EXTRAVASATION INJURIES

High-Pressure Injection Injuries

High-pressure injection injuries to the hand are relatively uncommon, but consequences of a misdiagnosis are serious. Urgent treatment is required. High-pressure injection guns are used for painting, lubricating, cleaning, and farm animal vaccinations. Materials that may be injected with these devices include paint, paint thinners, oil, grease, water, plastic, vaccines, and cement. These high-pressure injection guns may generate pressures ranging between 3000 and 12,000 psi. Injection injuries can also be caused by other sources, such as defective lines and valves, pneumatic hoses, and hydraulic lines. The type of material injected is the most important prognostic factor. Oil-based paints and paint thinners can generate significant early inflammation, leading to severe fibrosis. Because tendon sheaths at the index, middle, and ring fingers end at the level of the MP joints, material injected at the DIP or PIP flexion creases will remain within these digits. However, tendon sheaths at the thumb and little finger extend all the way into the radial and ulnar bursae. Thus, material injected at the little finger or at the IP flexion crease of the thumb may potentially extend all the way into the forearm and even cause a compartment syndrome.

Initial presentation of a patient with a high-pressure injection may be benign and subtle. This may result in mismanagement by minimizing the patient's complaints. The break in the skin may be a benign-looking, pinhole-sized puncture site. However, within several hours, the digit becomes increasingly more painful, swollen, and pale. Prompt recognition and realization of the severity of injury are paramount. Radiographs may help determine the extent and dispersion of the injected material, either in the form of subcutaneous emphysema or, with lead-based paints, appearing as radiopaque soft tissue densities. The entire digit must be surgically decompressed and all foreign material and necrotic tissue débrided (Fig. 69-39). Wounds are closed loosely over Penrose drains or in a delayed manner. Appropriate antibiotics must be administered. Despite prompt recognition and

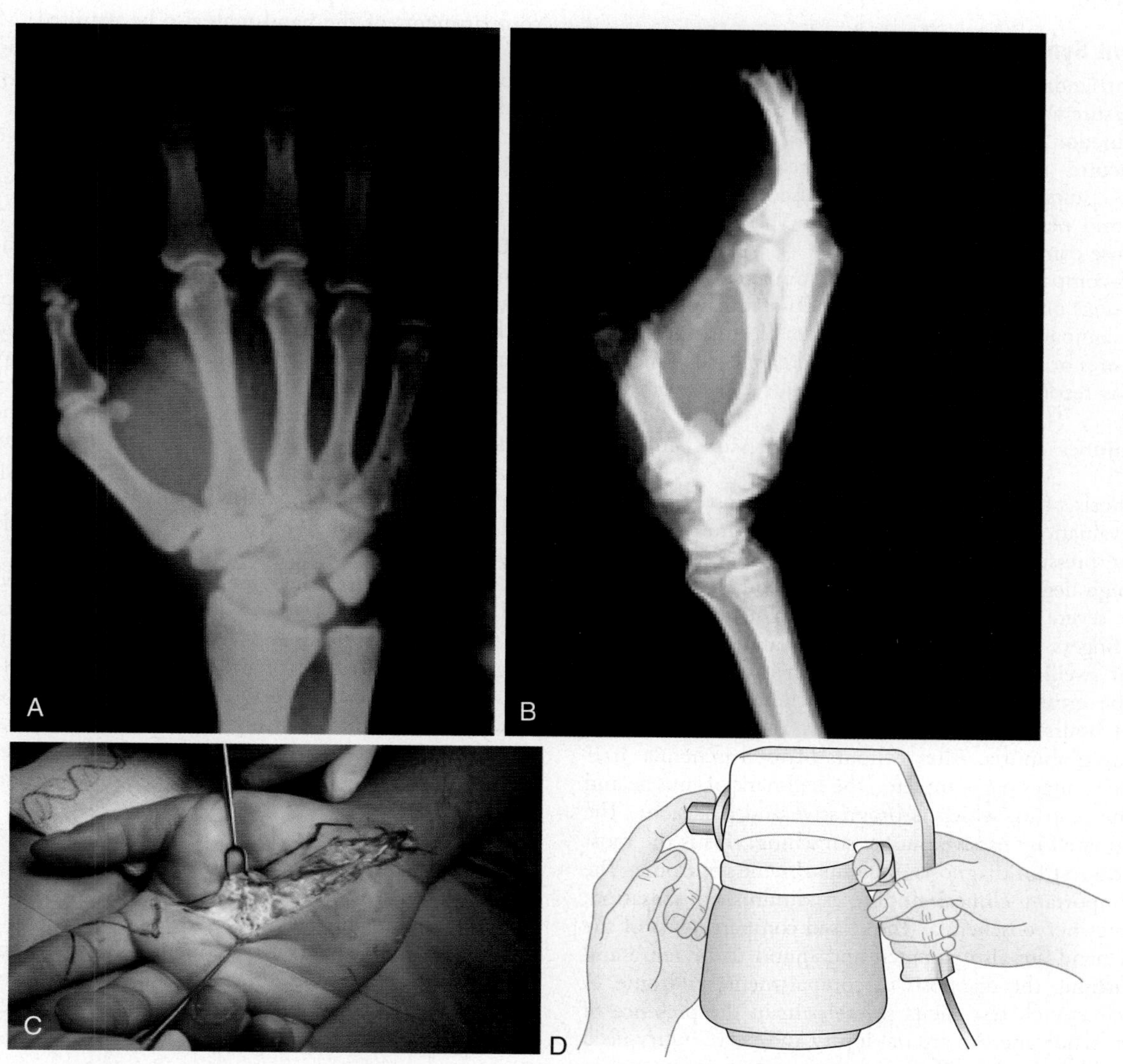

FIGURE 69-39 High-pressure injection injury from paint gun appears completely innocuous, with tiny puncture wound on presentation. **A** and **B,** Anteroposterior and lateral radiographs of the right hand show widely disseminated radiopaque foreign material in soft tissues of the palm and thenar eminence. **C,** Intraoperative photograph of left-handed man with palmar high-pressure injection injury from a paint gun on the nondominant palm. The tissues are extensively infiltrated by paint from the base of the finger to the wrist and require urgent débridement and decompression. **D,** Removal of the guard allows the nozzle to come into close contact, exponentially increasing the pressure delivered to soft tissues.

treatment, many such injuries ultimately result in surgical amputation of the digits.

Extravasation Injuries

In the past, extravasation injuries of chemotherapeutic agents frequently affected the upper extremity. However, subcutaneously tunneled central lines have now reduced the incidence of these injuries. If extravasation is suspected, infusion must be stopped immediately. Cold packs are applied for 15 minutes four times a day, and the extremity is elevated during the next 48 hours. This treatment is generally effective for most extravasation injuries. However, if blistering, ulceration, and pain occur in the damaged tissue, progressive necrosis to the limits of the extravasation will follow, and surgical excision of all damaged tissue is necessary. Most subsequent wounds can generally be treated with delayed split-thickness skin grafting, although the options for wound coverage after débridement depend on the extent of the débridement that was required.

Compartment Syndrome

Compartment syndrome results in symptoms and signs caused by increased pressure within a limited space that compromises circulation and function of the tissues in that space. Volkmann ischemic contracture is the sequel of untreated compartment syndrome; it results in muscle that is fibrosed, contracted, and functionless and nerves that are insensible. Various injuries are known to cause compartment syndrome:

- Decreased compartment volume (e.g., from externally applied tight dressings or casts, lying on a limb in a comatose state)
- Increased compartment content (e.g., from bleeding or trauma with fractures or finger injuries; increased capillary permeability, such as reperfusion after ischemic injury; electrical burn injuries)
- Other injuries (e.g., snakebites, high-pressure injection injuries)[28]

The diagnosis of compartment syndrome is based primarily on clinical evaluation. Although it is possible to measure intracompartment pressure, the decision to perform fasciotomy is based on a high degree of clinical suspicion. Compartment ischemia may be severe and still not affect the color or temperature of the distal fingers, and the distal pulses are rarely obliterated by compartment swelling. However, circulation in the muscle and nerve may be greatly reduced. Muscle ischemia that lasts for more than 4 hours leads to muscle death and may also cause significant myoglobinuria. After 8 hours of total ischemia, irreversible nerve changes are complete. The hallmark of muscle and nerve ischemia is pain, which is progressive and persistent. The pain is accentuated by passive muscle stretching; this is the most reliable clinical test for diagnosis of compartment syndrome. The next most important clinical finding is diminished sensation, which indicates nerve ischemia. The closed compartments of the forearm and hand are also palpated and found to be tense and tender, confirming the diagnosis of compartment syndrome. A passive muscle stretch test elicits severe pain in the presence of compartment syndrome. An arterial injury and nerve injury need to be distinguished in the differential diagnosis of compartment syndrome. All three of these injuries produce paresthesias and paresis; pain with passive stretch is present in compartment syndrome and arterial occlusion, but not in neurapraxia; and pulses are intact in compartment syndrome and neurapraxia, but not with arterial occlusion. In situations in which the patient cannot cooperate because of inebriation or unconsciousness and the clinical diagnosis is difficult, compartment pressure can be measured.

Release of a forearm compartment syndrome always requires carpal tunnel release (Fig. 69-40). The palmar incision starts in the valley between the thenar and hypothenar muscles, and the incision then curves transversely across the flexion crease of the wrist at the ulnar border. This incision must avoid the palmar cutaneous branch of the median nerve and prevent flexion contracture across the wrist crease. It also provides an opportunity to release Guyon canal. The incision then extends proximally up the forearm before curving back in a radial direction so as to have a large skin flap that will cover the median nerve and distal forearm tendons. At the elbow, the incision for the flap then curves again across the antecubital fossa, providing cover for the brachial artery and median nerve and preventing linear contracture across the antecubital fossa. The dorsal and so-called mobile wad compartments of the forearm are readily released through a straight incision, as needed. Appropriate release of the various intrinsic compartments of the hand may also be required. Most wounds can be partially closed at 5 days. If the skin cannot be closed secondarily within 10 days, a split-thickness skin graft can be applied.

TENOSYNOVITIS

de Quervain Disease

de Quervain disease is a stenosing tenosynovitis of the first dorsal compartment of the wrist and is a common cause of pain and disability. Diagnosis is easily made from a history of pain localized to the radial side of the wrist and aggravated by movement of the thumb. There is frequently a history of chronic overuse of the wrist and hand. Other features are local tenderness and swelling over the first dorsal compartment of the wrist and a positive Finkelstein test result—the patient clasps the thumb and brisk ulnar deviation to the hand elicits extreme pain. Crepitus may be palpable. This condition must be differentiated by radiographic and physical examination from arthritis of the thumb carpometacarpal joint.

Nonoperative treatment includes local steroid injection, thumb and wrist immobilization, local heat, and systemic anti-inflammatory medications. If these nonoperative measures fail, surgical decompression of the first dorsal compartment at the wrist is performed. Care must be taken to protect the radial sensory nerve branches during the course of the operation because these branches traverse just under the skin in this area, and trauma or transection may lead to painful disabling neuromas.

Intersection Syndrome

This condition is not well understood but is characterized by pain and crepitus at the point at which the APL and EPB tendons cross over the tendons of the second dorsal compartment (ECRL and ECRB; Fig. 69-41). Initial treatment is by splinting, local corticosteroid injection, and anti-inflammatory medications. Refractory cases require surgical release at the second dorsal compartment and excision of involved tenosynovial membranes.

Trigger Thumb and Fingers

Trigger finger is a constricting tenosynovitis of the flexor tendons, generally at the level of the A1 pulley. The patient can flex the digit, but an apparent nodule catches at the proximal edge of the A1 pulley, locking the PIP joint (or the IP joint of the thumb) in this flexed position. Attempts at extending the digit cause it to

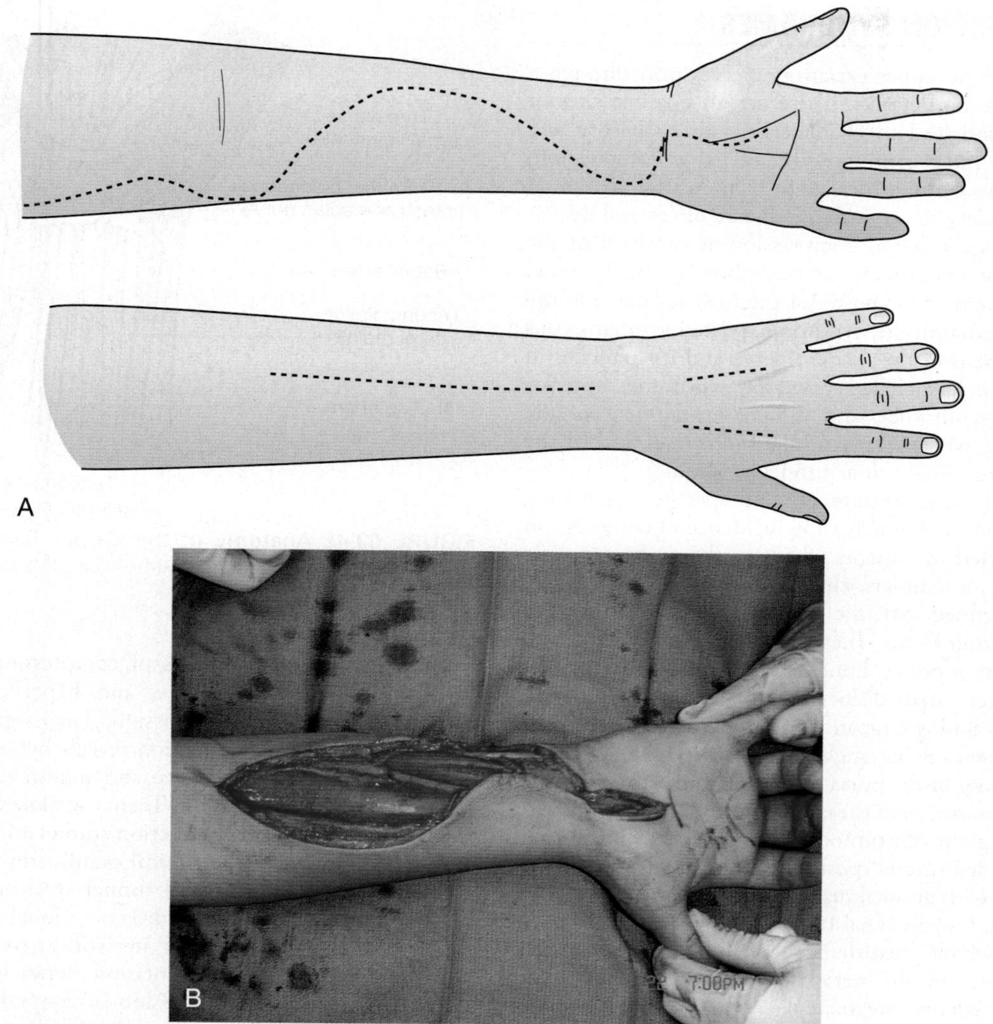

FIGURE 69-40 A, Incisions for forearm fasciotomy. **B,** Fasciotomy in a child for compartment syndrome after a snakebite.

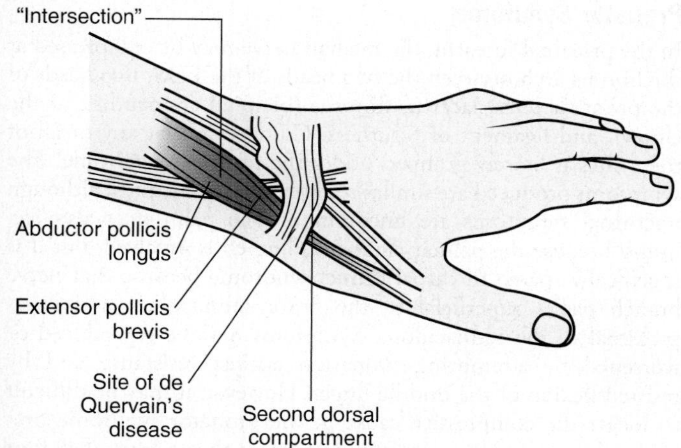

FIGURE 69-41 Anatomic locations for de Quervain stenosing tenosynovitis and intersection syndrome.

snap back suddenly, much like the trigger of a gun. Often, the patient needs to use the opposite hand to unlock and to extend the digit. In its most severe form, the constriction is so tight that the patient cannot flex the digit or it becomes fixed in a flexed position and can no longer be fully extended. A congenital form of trigger thumb or finger presents in infants, but most cases resolve by the time the child reaches 1 year of age; if not, an operation is indicated.

Nonoperative treatment in adults includes local injection of corticosteroids. If this regimen fails, the A1 pulley is longitudinally divided by surgery.[29]

Other Sites of Tenosynovitis

Other sites include the FCR and FCU tendons. They can frequently be treated by splinting and local corticosteroid injection, although surgery occasionally may be required. Inflammation of the ECU may also be an enigmatic cause of ulnar-sided wrist pain. Diagnosis is made by eliciting tenderness along the ECU tendon, pain on active resisted extension, and ulnar deviation of the wrist.

NERVE COMPRESSION SYNDROMES

Along the length of the upper extremity, nerves pass through a number of anatomic bottlenecks. These are all possible sites of nerve entrapment and lead to characteristic distal sensory and motor deficits. The most common sites of nerve compression, from proximal to distal along the length of the extremity, are at the nerve root secondary to cervical disc disease or cervical degenerative arthritis, thoracic outlet compression at the level of the clavicle, ulnar nerve entrapment at the elbow (cubital tunnel syndrome), entrapment of the posterior interosseous nerve in the proximal forearm (radial tunnel syndrome, posterior interosseous syndrome), entrapment of the median nerve and its branches in the proximal forearm (so-called pronator syndrome, anterior interosseous nerve syndrome), and, finally, entrapment of the median nerve at the wrist (carpal tunnel syndrome) and of the ulnar nerve in Guyon canal (ulnar tunnel syndrome).

In most cases of nerve entrapment, no specific aggravating causative factor is found. An increasing incidence of compression neuropathy is reported in patients whose work involves chronic repetitive stress (e.g., assemblers, chicken cutters). In some, there may be a clearly defined extrinsic compressive problem on the nerve or an aggravating factor. These include the following:

- Trauma that can produce bone compression, for example, carpal tunnel after carpal dislocations or a distal radius malunion (median) and supracondylar humerus fractures that increase the elbow carrying angle (ulnar nerve at the elbow)
- Synovial thickening of the bursa in rheumatoid arthritis in the carpal tunnel (median) or at the elbow (posterior interosseous)
- Tumors such as giant cell tumor in Guyon canal (ulnar) or a lipoma in the radial tunnel (posterior interosseous)
- Developmental, with anomalous muscles present in the carpal tunnel (median), Guyon canal (ulnar), or forearm (median)
- Metabolic, in which disturbances of fluid balance cause increased pressure on the nerve, particularly at the carpal tunnel (e.g., myxedema, pregnancy)

Carpal tunnel syndrome is the most common peripheral nerve entrapment syndrome, followed by ulnar nerve entrapment at the elbow.[30] The other entrapment syndromes are less common.

Diabetes mellitus is recognized as a risk factor for carpal tunnel syndrome, and the response to treatment has previously been unclear. However, studies suggest that patients with diabetes do similarly well to normoglycemic patients after carpal tunnel release.

Carpal Tunnel Syndrome

The carpal tunnel is a packed fibro-osseous tunnel at the wrist that is traversed by the median nerve and nine long extrinsic digital flexor tendons (Fig. 69-42). Its floor is formed by the carpal bones and roofed by the flexor retinaculum (transverse carpal ligament). Normal pressures in this tunnel are 20 to 30 mm Hg. A rise in pressure above this causes a chronic compressive ischemic injury to the nerve segment, resulting first in demyelination and eventually in axonal death. There is progressive conduction block in the nerve, with subsequent sensory and motor dysfunction. The earliest symptoms are pain and paresthesias, which are characteristically more obvious at night, after prolonged activity, and with positional postural changes at the wrist, such as when driving, using a hand-held hair dryer, or reading a book. The patient may complain of clumsiness and a tendency to drop objects. The paresthesias characteristically follow the distribution of the median nerve, including the thumb and index and middle fingers.

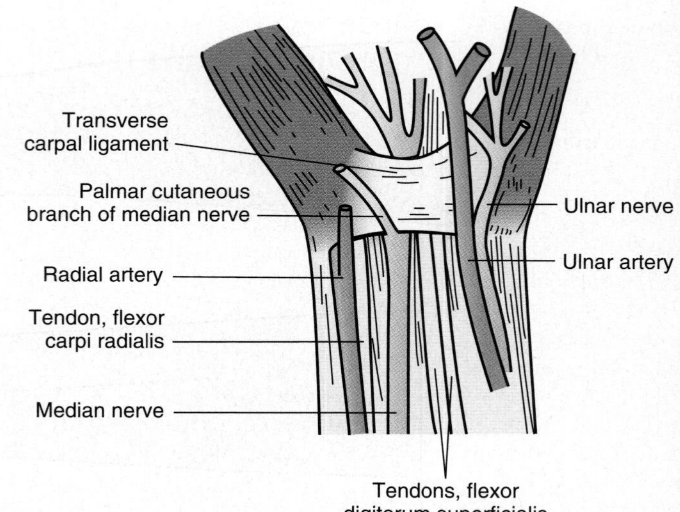

FIGURE 69-42 Anatomy of the Carpal Tunnel. The transverse carpal ligament (flexor retinaculum) is divided longitudinally during a carpal tunnel release.

Physical examination consists of compressing the carpal canal, percussing the median nerve, and hyperflexing the wrist to produce paresthesias (Durkan sign, Tinel sign, and Phalen test, respectively). Sensory evaluation reveals hypoesthesia in the distribution of the median nerve and may reveal a widened two-point sensory discrimination. Thenar weakness or muscle wasting is a late finding. Nerve conduction studies and electromyography are useful adjuncts to the clinical examination.

Initial treatment of carpal tunnel syndrome includes use of wrist splints (especially at night), occasional local corticosteroid injections, and modification in work patterns. If symptoms persist, or if the initial presentation shows severe carpal tunnel syndrome, surgical decompression is required. This is performed by longitudinally dividing the flexor retinaculum by open or endoscopic means. Both the Agee (single-portal) and Chow (two-portal) procedures have shown similar efficacy to the open approach.[31] Synovectomy and removal of any mass lesion may also be required if that is the cause of the problem.[32]

Pronator Syndrome

In the proximal forearm, the median nerve may be compressed at the fibrous arch between the two heads of the FDS, two heads of the pronator teres, lacertus fibrosus (bicipital aponeurosis at the elbow), and ligament of Struthers. Compression at any or all of these sites is loosely grouped under the pronator syndrome. The symptoms produced are similar to those of carpal tunnel, although nocturnal symptoms are uncommon. The palm may also feel numb because the palmar cutaneous branch is involved, but it is specifically spared in carpal tunnel syndrome because that nerve branch passes superficial to the flexor retinaculum and arises proximal to the retinaculum. Symptoms may be reproduced or worsened by attempting pronation against resistance and by resisted flexion of the middle finger. However, it may be difficult to locate the compressive cause in the pronator syndrome precisely, and surgical decompression often involves release of all four potential sites of compression.

The anterior interosseous nerve branch of the median nerve may occasionally be compressed in isolation. This does not produce any sensory symptoms but specifically targets the three muscles innervated by the anterior interosseous nerve—FPL, FDP to the index and middle fingers, and pronator quadratus.

Ulnar Nerve Compression

The ulnar nerve may be compressed in Guyon canal at the wrist or in the so-called cubital tunnel at the elbow and distal upper arm.

Guyon Canal Compression

This canal is bounded by the hook of the hamate, pisiform, piso-hamate ligament, and palmar carpal ligament. Compression by mass lesions may occur at this site, including a ganglion, giant cell tumor, ulnar artery thrombosis, and ulnar artery aneurysm, as in the hypothenar hammer syndrome. Compression at this site may also be idiopathic. Distal ulnar deficits may be in the motor or sensory distribution or both, depending on where in the canal the compression occurs relative to the takeoff of the deep motor branch of the ulnar nerve. Tinel sign may be present, and there may be worsening of symptoms by direct compression over Guyon canal. Treatment is surgical; it consists of dividing the palmaris brevis muscle and palmar carpal ligament as well as removing any offending mass in this region.

Cubital Tunnel Syndrome

The cubital tunnel is a long tunnel starting in the distal upper arm and extending into the proximal forearm. As the ulnar nerve passes into the forearm, it curves tightly around the grooved posterior and inferior surfaces of the medial epicondyle of the humerus. This groove is bridged by the aponeurosis between the two heads of the FCU, the leading edge of which may be thickened and fibrosed, called Osborne ligament. More proximally, the ulnar nerve passes from the anterior compartment of the arm into the posterior compartment, which may be bridged by a long tunnel called the arcade of Struthers. The medial intermuscular septum in the upper arm may also cause ulnar nerve compression. The most distal fibro-osseous tunnel is more accurately termed the cubital tunnel. However, compression on the ulnar nerve can occur at any of these sites, proximal to distal, starting in the upper arm and extending into the forearm. Motor and sensory symptoms develop in the distribution of the ulnar nerve and are worsened by adopting a flexed position at the elbow. Examination reveals Tinel sign over the tunnel. Paresthesias are described in the distribution of the ulnar nerve to the little and ring fingers and ulnar border of the hand. A differential diagnosis includes thoracic outlet syndrome, compression of the ulnar nerve in Guyon canal, and nerve root compression in the neck.

Initial treatment consists of splinting the elbow in extension at night. Use of soft extension elbow pads prevents elbow flexion and direct pressure on the nerve. Failure of nonoperative measures and significant changes in electrodiagnostic studies are indications for surgical decompression. Usually, all the fibrous restraints on the ulnar nerve around the elbow are released, and the nerve is transposed anteriorly to the medial epicondyle into a subcutaneous or submuscular position. There have been preliminary reports of success with endoscopic in situ decompression of the ulnar nerve at the elbow.

Radial Nerve Compression

The radial nerve may be compressed proximally in the triangular space in the axilla (specifically involving the axillary branch), spiral groove posterior to the humerus in the arm, and lateral intermuscular septum proximal to the elbow. More distally in the forearm, the posterior interosseous nerve, the principal motor division of the radial nerve, can be compressed in the so-called radial tunnel, starting at the leading fibrous edge of the supinator (ligament of Frohse). There may be a variable degree of interosseous nerve paresis, or there may be pain radiating down the dorsoradial aspect of the forearm (called radial tunnel syndrome). Initial treatment is nonoperative with splinting, but if this fails, surgical decompression may occasionally be required.

Thoracic Outlet Compression

The thoracic outlet is a narrow space at the base of the neck bounded by the first rib medially, scalenus anterior muscle and clavicle anteriorly, and scalenus medius muscle posteriorly. All elements of the brachial plexus as well as the subclavian artery and vein pass through this narrow space and can be potentially compressed at this site. A Tinel sign can often be elicited at the supraclavicular and infraclavicular regions. A Roos test is performed by asking the patient to hold both arms overhead in a surrender position while opening and closing the fists. This reproduces symptoms within 1 minute and, if continued, the arm collapses at the side. Adson test involves palpating the radial pulse while the patient turns the chin toward the same side, inhales deeply, and holds his or her breath. The radial pulse disappears or diminishes. The costoclavicular compression test involves sustained downward pressure on the clavicle, and the symptoms are reproduced. Radiographic evaluation may reveal a cervical rib. Results of nerve conduction studies are often normal.

Thoracic outlet compression may occur in association with other peripheral sites of nerve compression, a condition termed double-crush syndrome. Treatment is primarily nonoperative, involving posture-improving exercises and avoidance of aggravating activities. If symptoms persist, especially if they are associated with vascular compression, the thoracic outlet may be surgically decompressed. This is accomplished by a transcervical or transaxillary resection of the first rib, often with release of the scalene muscles.

TUMORS

Ganglions and mucous cysts represent 60% to 70% of hand tumors, followed in frequency by inclusion cysts, warts (verrucae), giant cell tumors in tendon sheaths, foreign body granulomas, lipomas, hemangiomas, and pyogenic granulomas (Table 69-5). Benign tumors account for 95% of hand neoplasms. Squamous cell carcinoma is the most frequent primary malignant neoplasm of the hand, basal cell carcinoma is rare, and melanoma is relatively uncommon in the upper extremity. Acral lentiginous melanoma (e.g., in the palm, sole, nail bed) has a tendency for early metastasis. Primary bone tumors of the hand are generally benign; the most common are enchondromas and osteochondromas. Giant cell tumors of bone are rare in the hand, occurring usually in the distal radius. They are locally aggressive and may occasionally metastasize. Of malignant bone tumors, only 1.2% affect the hand. Although bone metastases in other parts of the body are relatively common, bones of the hand are rarely affected by metastases from other sites.[33,34]

Soft tissue sarcomas are rare, representing 1% of all malignant neoplasms of the body, excluding skin tumors. Although uncommon, certain types predominate in the hand. Epithelioid, synovial, and clear cell sarcomas are relatively rare in other sites but by comparison are more common in the hand.

TABLE 69-5 Benign Connective Tissue Tumors of the Hand

SOFT TISSUE TUMORS	PRESENTATION	MOST COMMON LOCATIONS	TISSUE OF ORIGIN AND APPEARANCE	TREATMENT	RADIOGRAPHIC APPEARANCE
Ganglion	Swelling, sometimes painful; DIP mucous cyst may spontaneously drain clear gelatinous fluid; 70% of hand swellings	Volar and dorsal wrist, flexor tendon sheath, dorsum of DIP joint	Synovial cyst containing thick gelatinous fluid	No treatment versus aspiration versus excision	No radiographic alterations; mucous cyst at DIP joint may have osteophytes associated with osteoarthritis
Giant cell tumor of tendon sheath	Progressive enlargement, painless, deeply adherent; potential recurrence after excision; second most common hand tumor	Any synovial site, including tendon sheath, joint, palmar plate, usually in a digit	Synovium and histiocytes; bosselated and yellow-brown color from hemosiderin pigmentation	Excision	Pressure resorption of bone
Lipoma	Painless enlarging mass, usually on volar surface of hand or finger; may reach very large size; seldom nerve compression symptoms	Volar hand and finger	Mature fat cells	Excision (shell out)	Characteristic water-clear appearance on radiograph
Inclusion cyst (implantation dermoid)	Painless, enlarging lesion, adherent to overlying dermis; more common in laborers and those subject to minor hand trauma; may become infected	Palm and fingertips	Implanted epidermis cyst containing keratinous debris	Excision of entire epithelium-lined sac	May cause pressure resorption of bone
Neurofibroma	May be localized, diffuse, or plexiform; may be associated with von Recklinghausen disease; painless enlargement, but pain arouses suspicion of malignant change	Less common on hand than elsewhere; seen more frequently on palm	Perineurial fibroblasts	Excision if noncritical nerve; biopsy if malignancy suspected; possible nerve grafting	Characteristic MRI lobulated appearance
Schwannoma	Painless small mass in a peripheral nerve that is laterally mobile; may be an incidental finding at time of carpal tunnel surgery; occasional distal dysesthesias	Median and digital nerves	Schwann cells	Microneural surgery can shell the tumor out of the nerve without leaving neurologic deficit	No changes on plain radiograph
Pyogenic granuloma	Often at site of previous trivial skin injury on the fingers; friable and bleeds easily; grows rapidly	Fingers	Granulation tissue	Small lesions can be cauterized; excise larger lesions	No radiographic changes
Glomus tumor	Very small lesions; exquisitely painful, localized tenderness, cold sensitive; patients sometimes labeled as malingering	Subungual or volar fingertip; may be multiple	Neuromyoarterial apparatus	Excision; repair nail bed if subungual	May show indentation of distal phalanx

Within the spectrum of benign and malignant tumors, there is a group with intermediate malignancy. Giant cell and desmoid tumors (of soft tissue) have a propensity for local recurrence after surgical excision. Their histologic patterns may belie their behavior. Juvenile aponeurotic fibroma and nodular fasciitis may appear histologically more aggressive than desmoid tumors but are self-limited. The tiny glomus tumor is uncommon but has a propensity for the fingertips and subungual regions. It may be an enigmatic cause of severe and exquisite pain at the fingertips and can be recognized by a pinpoint site of extreme local tenderness and a violaceous hue deep to the nail plate. MRI may occasionally detect these tiny lesions at the fingertip.

If a lesion is thought to be benign, excision without further workup, except perhaps for routine radiographs, is appropriate. However, if a primary malignant neoplasm of bone or soft tissue is suspected, additional studies must be undertaken before biopsy. CT may help delineate tumor boundaries. Desmoid tumors have radiographic density identical to that of muscle and are better demonstrated by MRI.

Soft Tissue Tumors

Ganglion Cysts

Ganglions are formed by an outpouching of the synovial membrane from a joint or tendon sheath and contain thick, jelly-like, mucinous material similar in composition to synovial fluid (Fig. 69-43). Of ganglions, 60% occur on the dorsal aspect of the wrist, arising in the region of the scapholunate ligament. Other sites for ganglions in the hand are at the volar wrist, arising from one of the scaphoid articulations; at the flexor tendon sheath at the area of the A1 pulley; and at the dorsum of the DIP joint, called a mucous cyst, where they are often associated with osteoarthritis of that DIP joint. In the last location, the ganglion cyst can exert pressure on the germinal matrix of the nail bed, resulting in a deformed or grooved nail.

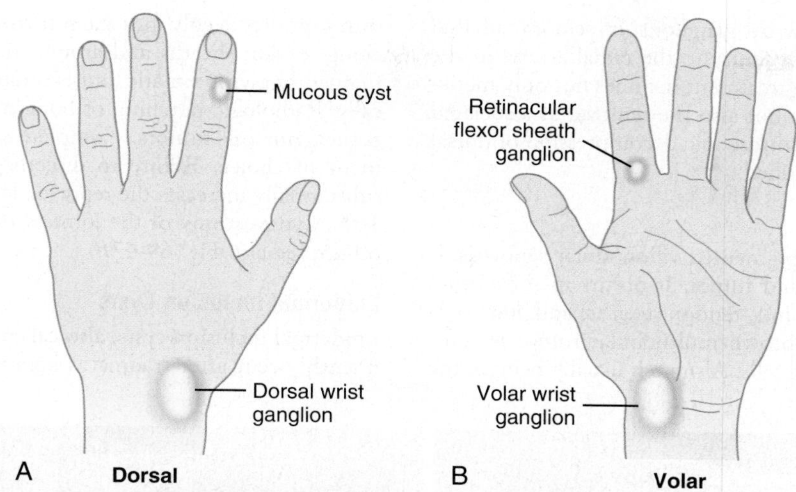

FIGURE 69-43 Dorsal (**A**) and volar (**B**) aspects of the hand and wrist showing common types of ganglions, including the dorsal wrist ganglion, volar wrist ganglion, flexor sheath ganglion (volar retinacular cyst), and mucous cyst.

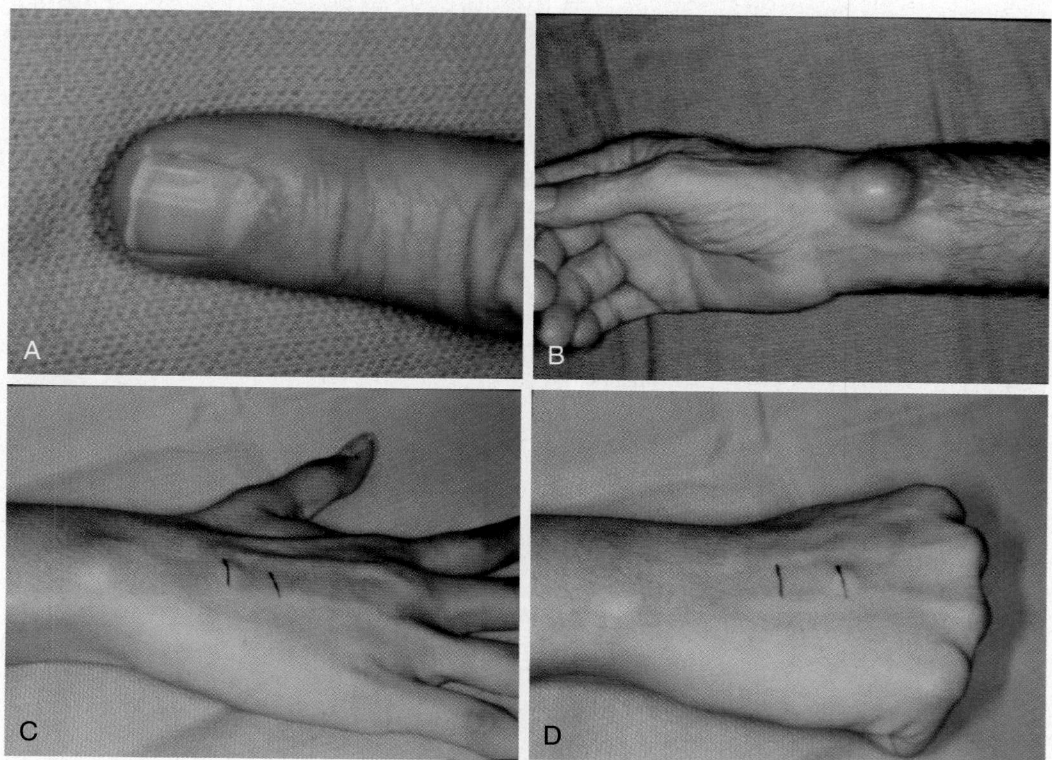

FIGURE 69-44 Ganglions in the Hand. A, Ganglion associated with osteoarthritis of the distal interphalangeal joint (mucous cyst), causing longitudinal linear groove in the nail plate from pressure on the germinal matrix. **B,** Volar wrist ganglion on the radial side of the flexor carpi radialis tendon is closely related to the radial artery and should not be aspirated. **C,** Ganglion arising from the extensor digitorum communis tendon of the ring finger located at the level of the proximal skin marking with fingers extended. **D,** Movement of ganglion 2 cm to the level of the more distal skin marking when the fist is clenched. Distal movement of the swelling with the gliding extensor tendon confirms its attachment to the tendon.

Ganglions are most common in women in the third decade of life. They are innocuous and can often be left alone. However, treatment may be required for cosmetic purposes or to relieve pressure effects on adjacent structures (Fig. 69-44). The dorsal wrist ganglion can sometimes be painful as a result of pressure on the posterior interosseous nerve at that location. A very small impalpable dorsal wrist ganglion can become quite painful, the so-called occult ganglion, and on occasion may best be diagnosed by MRI. Treatment of a dorsal wrist ganglion may be performed by aspiration of the mucinous substance with a large-bore needle. If this fails, the ganglion can then be surgically excised. Care must be taken to trace and to resect the pedicle of the ganglion all the way down to the joint or tendon sheath from which it arises.[35] A volar wrist ganglion may often be closely related to the radial artery. Aspiration of volar wrist ganglions is seldom advised because of the potential risk of injury to the radial artery. At the level of the DIP joint, optimal treatment includes not only meticulous excision of the ganglion but also the removal of associated osteophytes from the joint. Arthroscopic decompression of dorsal wrist ganglions has been described.

Giant Cell Tumor

Giant cell tumor, also called pigmented villonodular synovitis, is the second most common hand tumor. It occurs in soft tissues (e.g., synovial membrane of joints, tendon sheaths) and, less commonly, in bone. This yellow-brown multilobular tumor is composed of multinucleated giant cells. Although usually benign, the tumor pushes deeply into the soft tissues of the digits and extends along tendon sheaths and around neurovascular structures. It is frequently asymptomatic and is often larger than suspected clinically. Radiologic notching of bone may be evident in larger, soft tissue giant cell tumors. Complete surgical excision is the treatment of choice. Failure to discern and to remove each lobule substantially increases the reported local recurrence rate of almost 10%. Synovectomy of the joint of origin may be necessary (Fig. 69-45; see also Fig. 69-47*B*).

Epidermal Inclusion Cysts

Epidermal inclusion cysts, also called implantation dermoids, frequently occur after trauma as keratin-producing epidermal cells

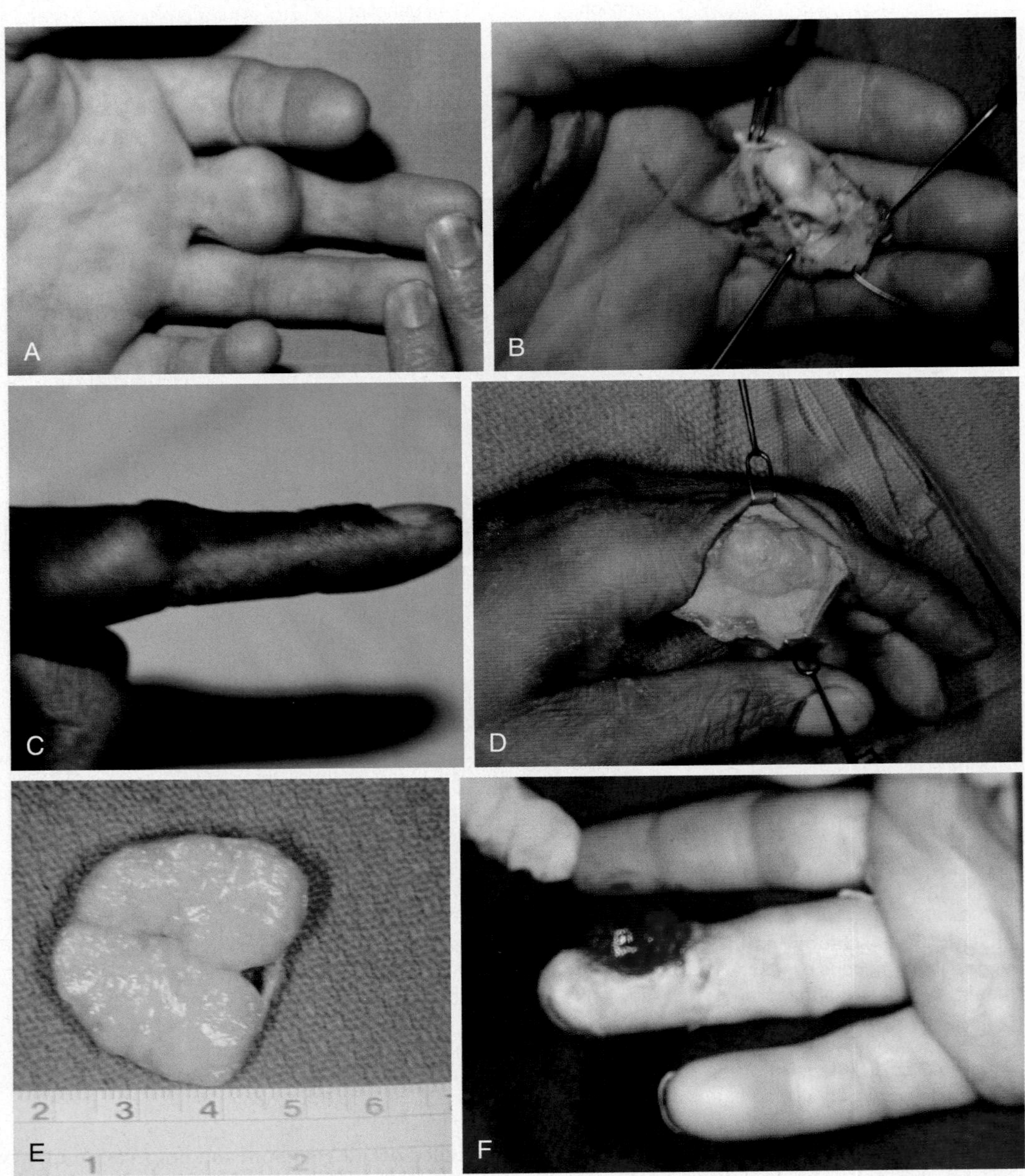

FIGURE 69-45 **Soft Tissue Tumors of the Hand. A,** Traumatically induced inclusion cyst on the palmar aspect of the middle finger in a manual worker. **B,** Intraoperative photograph demonstrates cyst filled with toothpaste-like gel derived from keratin. **C,** Firm, progressively enlarging swelling on the radial side of the left index finger. **D,** Firm, lobulated, yellow-brown giant cell tumor insinuating onto the dorsal and volar aspects of the finger is noted intraoperatively. **E,** Giant cell tumor is the most common solid soft tissue tumor encountered in the hand. **F,** Fleshy friable pyogenic granuloma bleeds easily on contact.

become lodged in the subcutaneous tissues (Fig. 69-45). The resulting cystic mass contains a thick toothpaste-like material. They occur more commonly in men, especially in manual laborers, and most frequently involve the palm of the hand and fingertips. They may also occur in previous surgical scars. Treatment is surgical excision, and recurrence is rare.

Lipoma

Lipomas are small, benign, soft, fluctuant, fatty tumors (Fig. 69-46). In the hand, they usually occur on the thenar eminence. Although generally painless, they may enlarge significantly, insinuating into deep palmar spaces and causing pain by compression on adjacent nerves. Intracarpal lipoma is a rarer cause of carpal

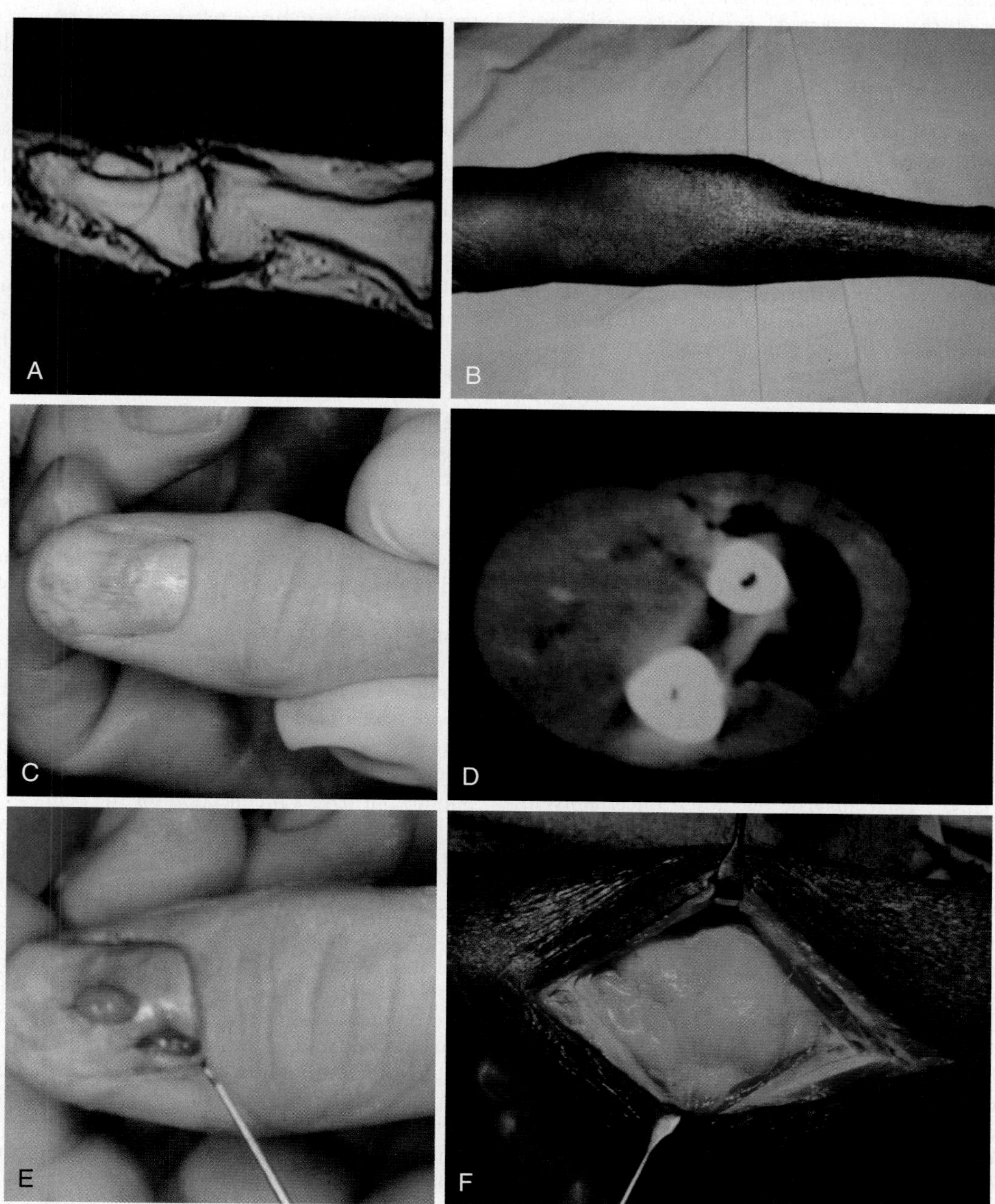

FIGURE 69-46 Soft Tissue Tumors of the Hand. A, Patient presenting with pain in tip of thumb, exacerbated in cold weather. Exquisite pain on palpation of the thumb nail plate is typical of a subungual glomus tumor that can be demonstrated by MRI. **B,** Occult subungual glomus tumor may be difficult to appreciate, even after removal of the nail plate, but it can often be identified by a surface bulge of the nail bed. **C,** Excised glomus tumor sitting on nail bed. A nail bed defect requires repair with fine absorbable sutures. **D,** Man with swelling of left dorsoradial forearm and weakness of finger and thumb extension. **E,** MRI reveals a dorsal forearm mass compressing the posterior interosseous nerve. **F,** Dorsal approach over the mass reveals intramuscular benign lipoma when extensor muscles are split.

tunnel syndrome. Resection of symptomatic lipomas is curative, although 1% to 2% may recur.

Pyogenic Granuloma

Pyogenic granuloma is a misnomer for an exuberant outburst of highly vascular granulation tissue at the site of previous relatively trivial trauma. These lesions are friable, bleed easily, and may grow rapidly. They respond to curettage or simple excision. They usually occur on the fingertips. Histologic confirmation of the diagnosis is necessary because of occasional confusion with aggressive malignant lesions, such as ulcerated, amelanotic, malignant melanomas.

Verruca Vulgaris

Verrucae vulgaris are common contagious warts associated with human papillomavirus type 1. They occur usually as hyperkeratotic filiform lesions on the digits or about the nail bed. The most effective topical treatments are salicylates, liquid nitrogen cryotherapy, and especially curettage. Recalcitrant lesions respond to oral cimetidine given for 6 to 8 weeks and to imiquimod, an immunomodulator that increases interferon production.[36] Their incidence, like that of squamous cell carcinomas, is increased in immunocompromised patients, such as in those after transplantation. Recurrence is relatively common.[37]

Seborrheic Keratoses

Seborrheic keratoses are benign, hyperkeratotic, scaly lesions. They are frequently pigmented and common on the dorsum of the hand in older adults. Occasional confusion occurs with pigmented basal cell carcinomas. When necessary, these superficial scaly lesions are best treated by shave excision, and sutures are unnecessary. Rapid reepithelialization occurs.

Keratoacanthoma

Keratoacanthoma occurs on exposed body parts such as the dorsum of the hand. It grows rapidly during approximately 3 weeks into a nodule with a central umbilicated keratotic plug, often followed by spontaneous resolution in many weeks or months. The resulting scar is often worse than if the lesion had been excised initially.[38] There may be diagnostic uncertainty in regard to well-differentiated squamous cell carcinomas. Hence, most authors recommend surgical excision.

Dermatofibroma

A dermatofibroma arises from fibrous dermal tissue as a firm erythematous plaque, sometimes having central umbilication. It is often adherent to the overlying epidermis. Surgery is required primarily for diagnosis.

Vascular Malformations and Hemangiomas

Hemangiomas are hamartomas that are rarely visible at birth and are usually noticed weeks to months later. Rapid proliferation occurs in the first year of life. On histologic evaluation, proliferation of endothelial cells with increased mitotic activity is seen in conjunction with pericytes and dendritic and mast cells. Hemangiomas occur 10 times more commonly than vascular malformations, and approximately 70% involute by the age of 7 years, leaving a fibrofatty scar with redundant skin. Excision is seldom required and, after involution, is usually cosmetic. On occasion, oral or injectable steroids may be necessary to control rapidly proliferating lesions that cause pain or interfere with function. Propranolol, which reduces basic fibroblast growth factor and vascular endothelial growth factor expression, is sometimes added in conjunction with steroids for problematic hemangiomas.[39]

By contrast, vascular malformations show normal endothelial growth characteristics and normal mast cell counts. They are often noted at birth, and growth is usually commensurate with the child for low-flow lesions. They do not undergo spontaneous involution.

Vascular malformations are subclassified into low-flow lesions; capillary, venous, and lymphatic lesions predominate. Arterial and arteriovenous fistulas predominate in high-flow lesions, and accelerated growth may occur relative to the patient. Pressure effects, ulceration, bleeding, and high-output cardiac failure can occur in severe cases. Enlarging lesions hinder hand function. Compression garments can provide symptomatic relief in some cases. Pain is often caused by vascular engorgement, phlebitis, or intralesional coagulation. D-dimer levels may be elevated, and some patients obtain relief from aspirin. Combined surgical excision[40] and radiologic embolization[41] are most effective in preventing recurrence caused by dilation of collateral vascular channels after simple excision.

Lymphaticovenous malformations may also be associated with generalized hypertrophy of an extremity. Vascular malformations and isolated macrodactyly are seen in Klippel-Trénaunay syndrome.

Malignant Skin Tumors

Basal Cell Carcinoma

Basal cell carcinoma is rare on the hand and is generally located on the dorsum. It is usually an ulcer with raised pearly edges. Treatment consists of excision with a margin of normal adjacent tissue. Nail bed lesions can be mistaken for paronychial infection, and amputation at the DIP joint may be required.[42]

Squamous Cell Carcinoma

Squamous cell carcinoma may arise de novo from ultraviolet light exposure because of occupation or climate, usually on the sun-exposed dorsum of the hand. Approximately 16% of actinic keratoses may progress to squamous cell carcinoma. Arsenical keratoses may develop secondary to exposure to inorganic arsenic compounds but have a predilection for the palm.

Bowen disease is an intraepidermal squamous cell carcinoma (carcinoma in situ).[43] It is a plaquelike lesion with crusting. Complete surgical excision with a margin of normal tissue is curative. When the nail matrix is involved, amputation at the DIP joint may be necessary.

For squamous cell carcinoma lesions smaller than 2.5 cm in diameter, wide excision with approximately a 6-mm clear margin is recommended. However, for larger lesions, more radical excision may be required, which may even include ray or segmental amputation for deeply adherent and invasive lesions. Mohs micrographic surgery and three-dimensional histologic reconstruction with a pathologist at the time of radical resection help ensure complete excision. Routine prophylactic lymphadenectomy is not beneficial.[44] However, lymphadenectomy may be advised for recurrent tumors, even though lymph nodes may not be clinically palpable. Malignant degeneration may occur in cicatricial tissue and chronic ulcers (e.g., Marjolin ulcer) and, in particular, in burn scars. Prognosis tends to be poorer.[45]

Malignant Melanomas

Melanoma of the hand is cutaneous or subungual. There is an almost equal distribution of cases between the two types.[46]

Frequently, there is a delay in treatment, particularly with subungual melanomas. Suspicious lesions should be biopsied.

Any subungual pigmented lesions should generally be biopsied. Under tourniquet control and with loupe magnification, the nail plate is atraumatically removed, and a longitudinal, elliptical, full-thickness excision of the lesion is performed. Careful nail bed repair is done after biopsy by the advancement of adjacent tissues and using fine absorbable sutures. The nail plate is then reapplied to act as a splint.

Benign melanocytic hyperplasia, without evidence of atypia, is completely treated by this form of biopsy. If there is any evidence of melanocytic atypia, absolute confirmation of complete excision is required. In the absence of a clear margin or with recurrence of such a lesion, total nail bed excision and reconstruction with a full-thickness skin graft are required. Melanoma in situ is similarly treated. Invasive melanoma of the nail bed is treated by amputation at the next most proximal joint. Acral lentiginous melanoma of the palm may sometimes be mistaken for a wart, which may also delay diagnosis. These tumors are aggressively treated with wide local excision and potential sentinel node biopsy, as they might be treated anywhere else on the body.

Bone Tumors

Osteoid Osteoma

This may occur in the hand and classically causes pain that is worse at night and unrelated to use or motion of the hand (Table 69-6). Osteoid osteomas produce prostaglandins; symptoms are relieved by nonsteroidal anti-inflammatory drugs (NSAIDs). On radiologic examination, a round lucent tumor with sclerotic edges is seen (Fig. 69-47*A*). Conservative treatment with NSAIDs may be considered, but definitive treatment is surgical.

Aneurysmal Bone Cyst

This is an expansile osteolytic bone lesion with a thin wall. It is usually derived from a preexisting bone tumor, usually a giant cell tumor (20% to 40% of cases). Of these, 25% occur in the upper extremity, causing pain that peaks during 2 to 3 months. A bone swelling may be detectable, with increased overlying skin temperature.

Enchondroma

Enchondromas usually occur in the hand and are the most common bone tumor of the hand. Peak incidence is in the second decade, with equal gender distribution. They are frequently asymptomatic and noted incidentally as lytic lesions on plain radiology. Pain, bone swelling, or pathologic fracture may occur as these cartilaginous intraosseous cysts compromise bone structural integrity (Fig. 69-47*D*). Treatment is by curettage and bone grafting of the osseous defect. Multiple enchondromatosis occurs in Ollier disease and is associated with angiomas in Maffucci syndrome.

Primary Bone Sarcomas

These malignant tumors are rare in the hand.

Secondary (Metastatic) Bone Tumors

Metastatic tumors, even those with a tendency to metastasize to bone, usually occur in the axial skeleton and long bones. They are very rare in the hand.

CONGENITAL ANOMALIES

The causes of congenital hand anomalies may be genetic, teratogenic, or idiopathic and may also have a syndromic association

TABLE 69-6 Bone Tumors of the Hand

TUMOR	PRESENTATION	MOST COMMON LOCATIONS	TISSUE OF ORIGIN AND APPEARANCE	TREATMENT	RADIOGRAPHIC APPEARANCE
Enchondroma	Often incidental finding on routine hand radiograph; presents as pain secondary to pathologic fracture; most common bone tumor of hand	Proximal and middle phalanges and metacarpals	Fragments of cartilage nests; multiple (Ollier disease); when associated with hemangiomas (Maffucci syndrome), may undergo malignant change	Curettage, filling of defect with cancellous bone if structural bone integrity is compromised	Lesion eccentric in bone shaft with calcific stippling
Osteochondroma	Benign bone prominence (capped with cartilage); rare in hand; may cause angular growth and interfere with joint motion	Fingers and wrist; growth stops after skeletal maturity reached	Aberrant focus of cartilage; multiple osteochondromatosis is autosomal dominant; malignant change may occur	Surgery may be necessary, generally after epiphyseal closure	Exostosis, often at base of proximal phalanx; often shortening of parent bone
Osteoid osteoma	Aching pain, greatest at night, sometimes responding specifically to aspirin; patient may be labeled as malingerer	Phalanges, metacarpals, carpals	Nidus composed of loose fibrovascular connective tissue between bars of osteoid and bone trabeculae	Surgical excision to include the nidus	Very small lesion; some not seen on plain radiographs and require CT scan; cortical sclerosis surrounding a radiolucent area of nidus
Giant cell tumor of bone	Expansile bone swelling at distal radius or in phalanx	Distal radius most common site	May be locally aggressive and even metastasize	Curettage for low-grade lesions, but en bloc resection for high-grade lesions; do not irradiate because it could induce sarcomatous change	Expansile soap bubble lesion in bone; high-grade lesions break through cortex

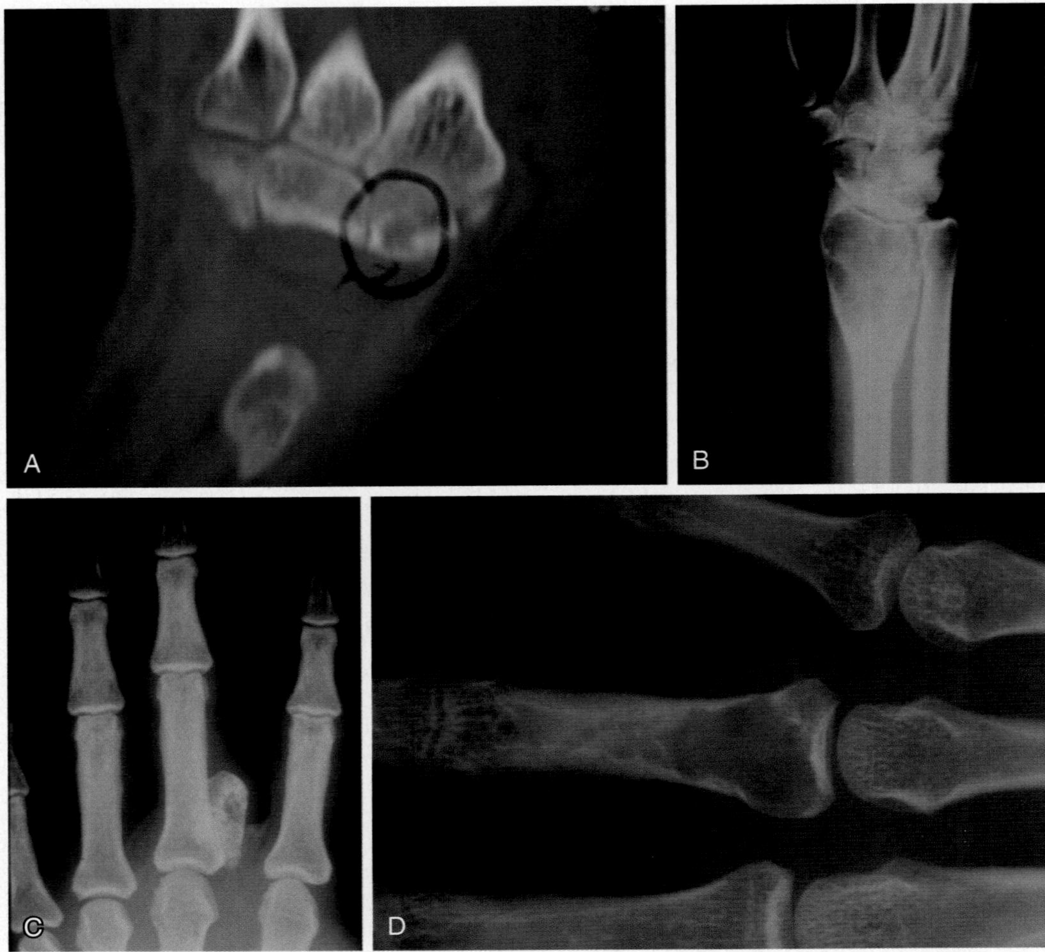

FIGURE 69-47 Plain radiographs of the upper extremity. **A,** Osteoid osteoma of carpus. **B,** Soap bubble appearance of giant cell tumor expanding the metaphysis of the distal radius. **C,** Osteochondroma of proximal phalanx of middle (long) finger. **D,** Patient with finger pain after trivial injury. This is a pathologic fracture of the base of the proximal phalanx through an enchondroma that has replaced most of proximal metaphysis and medulla.

with anomalies elsewhere in the body. Knowledge of these associations is important because the more life-threatening associated problems frequently need to be treated first, before the hand and upper extremity reconstruction can be performed. Such an association is found in a constellation of problems that occur in the VACTERL association of congenital defects (vertebral anomalies, anal atresia, cardiac abnormalities, tracheoesophageal fistula, renal agenesis, and limb anomalies). A number of factors must be considered in optimizing the timing of each surgical procedure to the upper extremity, including the psychosocial development of the child, presence of other illnesses, size of the structures to be operated on, and normal growth and development of the hand. Modern technologic advances have allowed us to operate on smaller structures; the timing of the procedure can now be guided by knowledge of the anatomy and development of the growing hand. Optimal function is the primary goal of surgery. Principles of treatment of congenital hand anomalies recognize that an infant's immunity to infection develops over time, early surgery prevents the emotional scarring associated with a child's awareness of the deformity, and some congenital problems may not be apparent in the neonate. The hand surgeon must work closely with the pediatrician to identify general conditions that may affect the child's health. Some congenital anomalies of the extremities, especially those with the radial ray, may be associated with bone marrow failure (Fanconi syndrome) or heart defects that may not be immediately apparent in the neonate. Children with congenital anomalies will attempt to keep up with their peers and often develop successful hand substitution techniques. However, once a child experiences the cruel ridicule of playmates or the unintentional but sometimes overly solicitous supervision of a teacher, his or her deformity becomes important. In general, plans for surgical reconstruction are designed to be completed by school age, so that the child may adapt to and fully use the reconstructed limb.[47]

The rationale for early surgery includes the avoidance of deformity and malfunction and optimal use of infantile tissue plasticity. Because hand length almost doubles during the first 2 years of life, a digit tethered to another digit that fails to grow can produce a major deformity during the early growth spurt. For example, with separation of syndactyly that involves the border digits of the hand, because of adjacent tethering to a digit of unequal length, surgical separation of the syndactyly is required at an early age, as early as 6 months, to avoid secondary angular deformity of the digits.

In rare circumstances, urgent treatment in the neonate is required. The distal lymphedema of a severe constriction band syndrome may be so marked as to inhibit function totally or even to threaten distal viability. This may require urgent release. The unusual clinical entity of aplasia cutis may result in exposure of vital structures, requiring urgent soft tissue coverage, even in the neonatal period.

Early operation, although not urgent, may be required not only because of the rapid growth that occurs in the first 2 years of life but also because of functional consequences. Surgery at a young age is considered mandatory in children with malformations in which hand function may be altered by surgery or in those who are at risk for development of certain grasping habits that would have to be unlearned after corrective surgery. An older child, 12 to 14 years of age, has developed grasp patterns that would have to be altered by prolonged periods of physical therapy after corrective surgery.[47,48]

The ability to place the upper limbs in space (a cortical function) and development of a strong grasp are established by 1 year of age, as are grasp and pinch maneuvers between the thumb and fingers. Accuracy of prehension and refinement of coordination continue until 3 years of age. Surgery must be performed early to allow the affected parts to develop differently when the function of the parts of the hand is altered by transposition (e.g., pollicization of an index finger for thumb aplasia). Duplicated thumb correction is carried out before 1 year of age, well in advance of the development of integrated thumb grasp patterns.

Finally, the physical ability of infant bone and soft tissues to adapt to change produced by surgery is also a key factor in deciding when to operate. In the early pollicization of the index finger, the first dorsal interosseous muscle hypertrophies to form a thenar eminence and the first metacarpal (formerly known as the proximal phalanx of the index finger) broadens. If centralization of the wrist for radial dysplasia (formerly known as radial club hand) has been undertaken early, the head of the ulna broadens to resemble the distal end of the radius.

Thus, a number of issues are taken into consideration when deciding on the optimum time for surgical reconstruction of congenital hand and upper extremity anomalies. The more common hand anomalies include syndactyly, polydactyly, constriction band syndrome, and absent or hypoplastic thumb.

Syndactyly results from the failure of programmed cell death (apoptosis) between the individual finger rays. Consequently, there is a resulting fusion of adjacent digits. It can involve part or all of the length of the digits (incomplete or complete) and may be limited to skin and soft tissue only (simple syndactyly) or can also involve skeletal fusion (complex syndactyly). Apert syndrome also involves craniofacial anomalies and is a severe form of bilaterally symmetrical complex syndactyly. Surgical treatment involves digit separation using a local flap to reconstruct the depths of the commissure between the fingers and release of the finger borders with zigzag incisions and the use of full-thickness skin grafts (Fig. 69-48*A*).

Polydactyly is the presence of extranumerary digits on the hand. Preaxial (radial) polydactyly involves the thumb. It is not as common as postaxial (ulnar) polydactyly, which is the most frequent congenital hand anomaly in African Americans. Polydactyly can be as simple as the presence of a skin tag–like structure or may have a complex arrangement of shared vessels, nerves, and bones. Thumb polydactyly is not merely a duplication but a splitting of a single digit, with variable degrees of development in each of the separate parts. It is typically classified into seven subtypes by the Wassel classification, which is based on the specific duplication, progressing from distal to proximal in which the odd numbers are at distal and proximal phalanx and metacarpal, and even numbers are at IP, MP and CMC joints respectively. Type IV is the most common type, with total duplication of proximal and distal phalanges and a shared MP joint. Type VII refers to associated triphalangia with a duplication. Reconstructive goals include stabilization without sacrificing mobility, proper alignment of joints along the longitudinal axis of the thumb, balanced motor units, and a cosmetically acceptable nail plate (Fig. 69-48*B* and *C*).

The Blauth classification categorizes thumb hypoplasia from type I, which represents minor hypoplasia, to type V, which is a total thumb absence. Surgical correction ranges from reconstruction of the existing hypoplastic thumb to pollicization (creating a thumb from the index finger) for complete absence or for the more severe types of hypoplasia (Fig. 69-49).

Clinodactyly is a curving of the digits in a radial or ulnar direction. It is common, particularly involving the little finger in many individuals, but a curvature of more than 10 degrees is considered abnormal. The distal phalanx is usually affected and a delta phalanx may be associated. A delta phalanx occurs when the epiphysis forms a C shape around the metaphyseal core in the middle phalanx. Most patients present with little or no functional or cosmetic deformity, and operative intervention is seldom required. If there is a functionally impairing deviation of the finger, corrective osteotomy can be done.

Camptodactyly is a congenital flexion deformity of digits. It usually occurs in the little finger PIP joint. The exact cause is unclear, but it has been attributed to a variety of different structures around the PIP joint, including a skin pterygium, collateral ligaments, volar plate, flexor tendon, abnormal insertions of lumbrical or interosseous muscles, and size and shape of the head of the proximal phalanx. Treatment is generally nonoperative and may involve serial splinting. If no improvement occurs and the flexion deformity is sufficient to cause a functional problem, surgical intervention may be required; this includes correction of the deformity with Z-plasty and possibly grafts. One author has reported that all his patients who had reconstructive surgery on one hand did not ask for corrective surgery on the opposite affected hand.

Constriction band syndrome is secondary to intrauterine amniotic bands (Fig. 69-48*D*). These can act like tourniquets and threaten the viability of digits and even limbs, resulting in congenital amputation. Infants may suffer from a similar problem from the external ligature effect of cotton strands coming off protective booties and even from a human hair, termed the hair-thread tourniquet syndrome.

OSTEOARTHRITIS AND RHEUMATOID ARTHRITIS

Osteoarthritis may be primary or post-traumatic (secondary). Primary osteoarthritis is a degenerative joint disease occurring in later life. An injury that leaves articular surfaces of a joint incongruous can precipitate secondary osteoarthritis. Osteoarthritis begins with biochemical alteration of the water content of articular cartilage. The cartilage weakens and develops cracks, called fibrillation. Progressive erosion and thinning of the cartilage result, and the subchondral bone becomes sclerotic, termed eburnation. New bone forms around the edges of the articular cartilage, and these outcroppings are called osteophytes (Fig. 69-50).

The joints usually affected in the hand are the DIP and PIP joints of the fingers and carpometacarpal joint at the base of the thumb. Osteophytes at the DIP joint are called Heberden nodes,

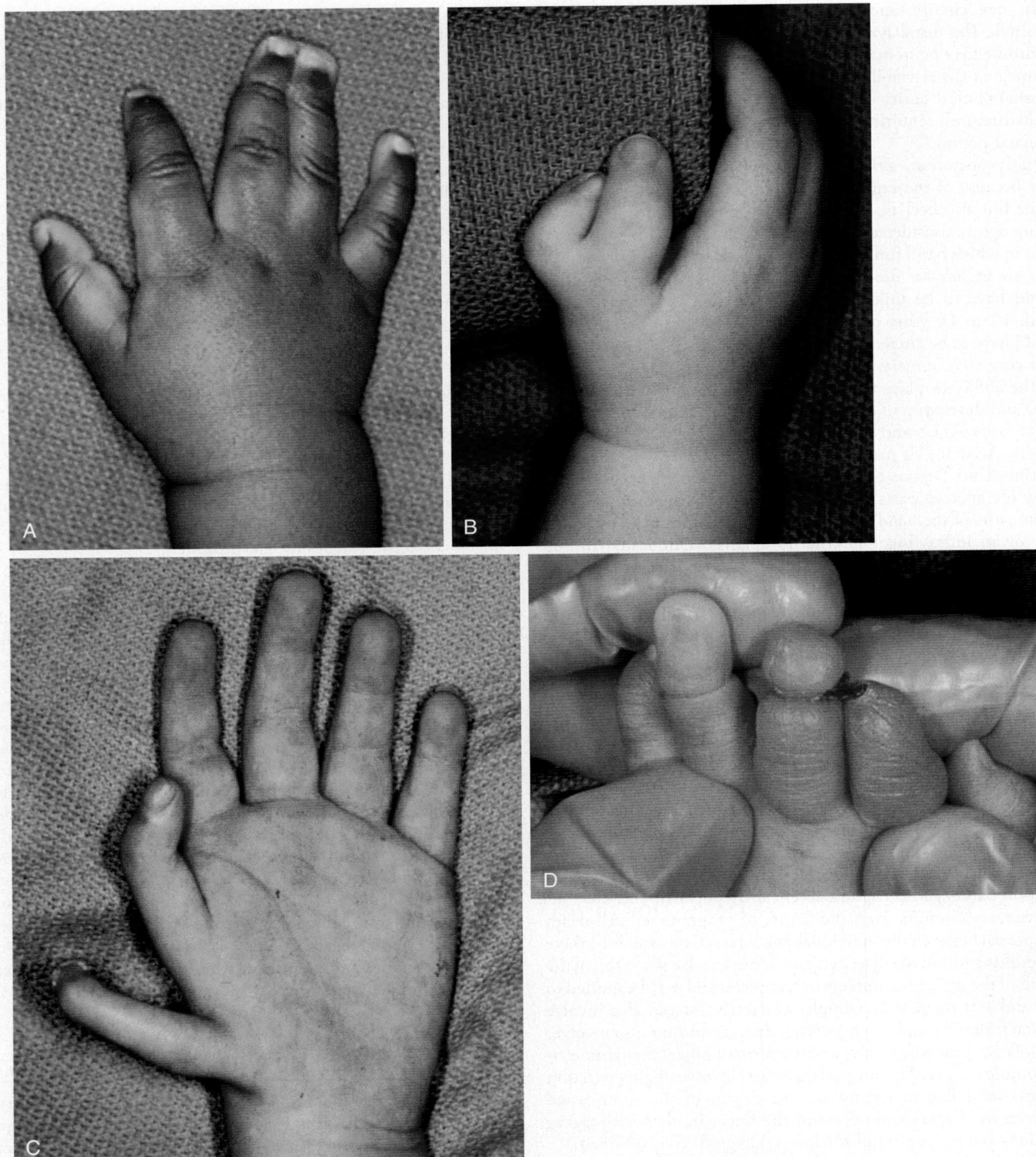

FIGURE 69-48 Congenital hand anomalies include syndactyly **(A)**, Wassel type IV thumb polydactyly **(B)**, Wassel type VI polydactyly **(C)**, and constriction band **(D)**.

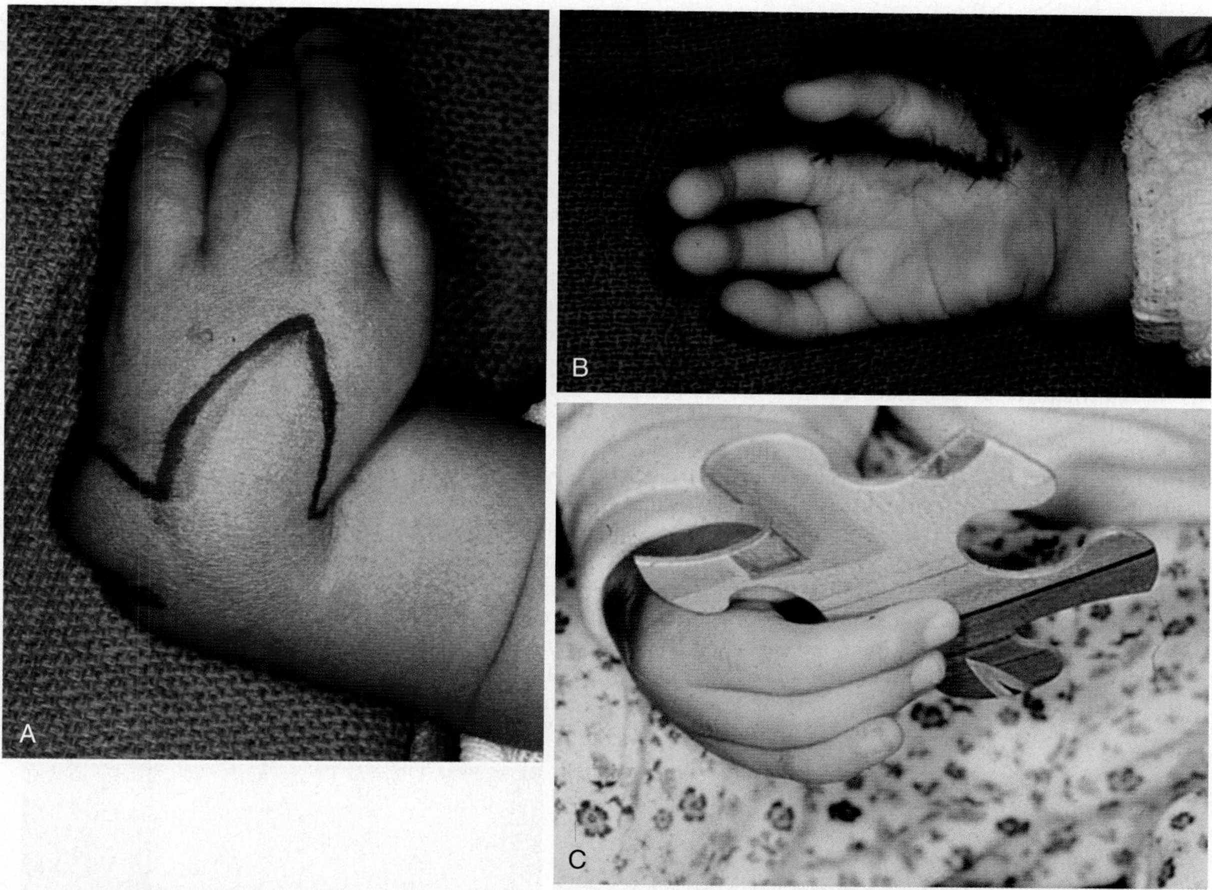

FIGURE 69-49 **A,** Patient with radial dysplasia and absent thumb. **B,** After centralization of the wrist on the distal ulna, pollicization of the index finger is performed. **C,** Natural prehension has been restored to this three-finger hand with a reconstructed wrist and thumb.

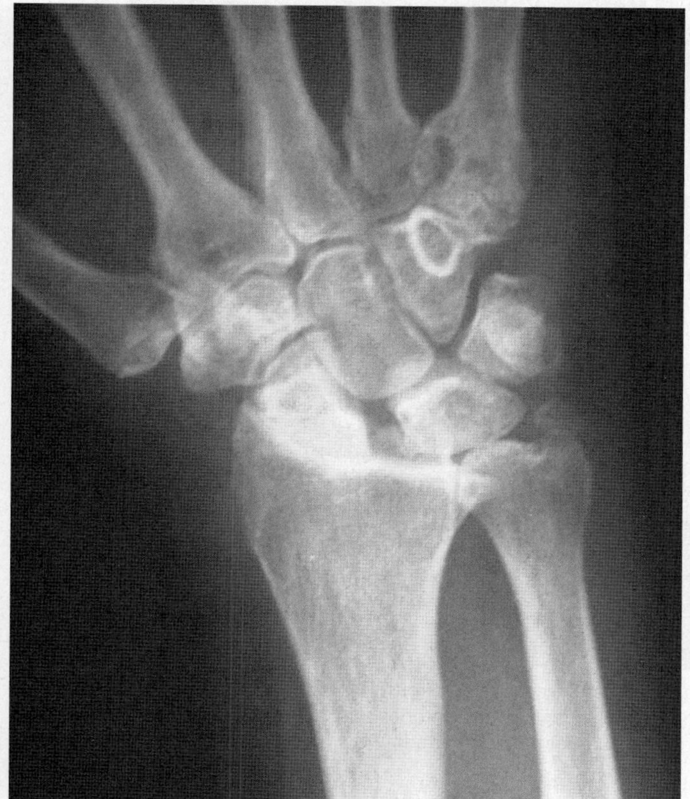

FIGURE 69-50 Radiograph of a hand with a scapholunate advanced collapse wrist showing post-traumatic osteoarthritis at the radioscaphoid junction. This is many years after a wrist sprain in which the scapholunate ligament was torn; a wide scapholunate gap is visible on the radiograph.

and those at the PIP joint are known as Bouchard nodes. The involved joints may be painful, stiff, deformed, or subluxated. Radiographs reveal narrowing of the joint space, sclerosis of subchondral bone, and presence of osteophytes.

Initial treatment may be symptomatic and may include splinting and even local corticosteroid injections. NSAIDs may be helpful, and chondroprotective medications such as glucosamine and chondroitin sulfate can reduce symptoms. In advanced cases, the DIP joints respond best to arthrodesis. The PIP joints may be surgically treated by replacement arthroplasty or by arthrodesis (Fig. 69-51). The thumb carpometacarpal joint may be treated by arthrodesis, which is favored particularly for the young patient who might have post-traumatic arthritis after, for example, an improperly treated Bennett or Orlando fracture. In an older patient with primary osteoarthritis at the thumb base, excision of the trapezium followed by tendon suspension (interposition) arthroplasty may be preferred. This uses local tendons for construction of a sling arthroplasty, with interposition of tendon material.

Rheumatoid arthritis is an autoimmune process whereby destruction of the musculoskeletal system may occur. Synovial inflammation results in pain, joint destruction, tendon ruptures, and characteristic deformities. Some of the more common deformities associated with rheumatoid arthritis include a swan neck deformity (hyperextension of the PIP joint with concurrent flexion at the DIP joint), boutonnière deformity (flexion at the PIP joint, with concurrent hyperextension at the DIP joint), joint subluxation, radial deviation of the wrist, and ulnar deviation and flexion of the fingers (Fig. 69-52). Rheumatoid arthritis is primarily a medical illness for which a number of medications are currently available. Thus, there must be excellent lines of communication between the rheumatologist and surgeon. NSAIDs as well as disease-modifying antirheumatoid drugs are used. Rheumatoid arthritis is a progressive disorder, and ongoing slow destruction may be anticipated despite surgery (Fig. 69-53). Some of the more common surgical procedures include joint synovectomy, tenosynovectomy, tendon transfers, joint replacements (especially at the MP and PIP joints), and arthrodesis (more commonly at the wrist and thumb MP joint).[49]

CONTRACTURES

Volkmann ischemic contracture develops as a result of myofascial contractures in response to prolonged ischemia. This most common contracture results from untreated compartment syndrome of the forearm and hand. Muscle necrosis occurs, and the muscles become replaced by fibrous scar tissue. The FDP and FPL muscles are usually affected, being in the deepest forearm volar compartment, and digits are characteristically flexed, with passive

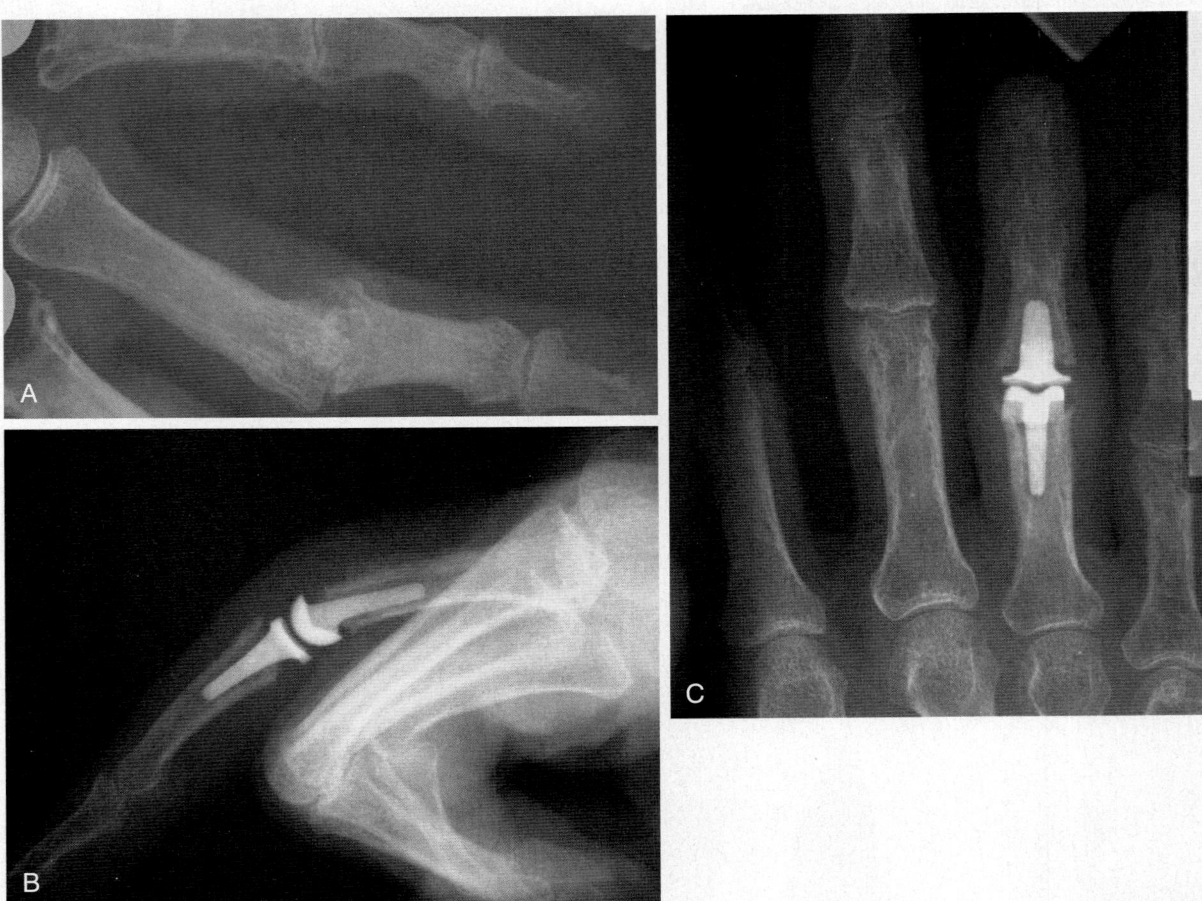

FIGURE 69-51 **A,** Patient with painful and unstable proximal interphalangeal joint from osteoarthritis. **B** and **C,** Reconstruction is performed by implant arthroplasty. An advantage over arthrodesis is that motion is retained, although there remains the potential for future recurrent joint instability and wear of the artificial joint.

extension of the wrist worsening the flexion deformity of the digits. Intrinsic contractures can occur in the hand; these can be investigated using Bunnell test, in which passive extension of the MP joint makes passive flexion of the PIP joint more difficult.

In the milder forms of Volkmann ischemic contracture, serial splinting and passive stretching exercises may resolve the problem. In more severe contractures, Z-type lengthening of tendons may be required. A flexor pronator muscle slide—subperiosteal elevation of the common flexor origin from the medial epicondyle of the humerus and from the ulna—allows the muscles to slide distally until the contracture is corrected. In the most severe form, all the muscles of the volar forearm may be affected, requiring tendon transfers, even microvascular functional muscle transfers to provide some functional return.

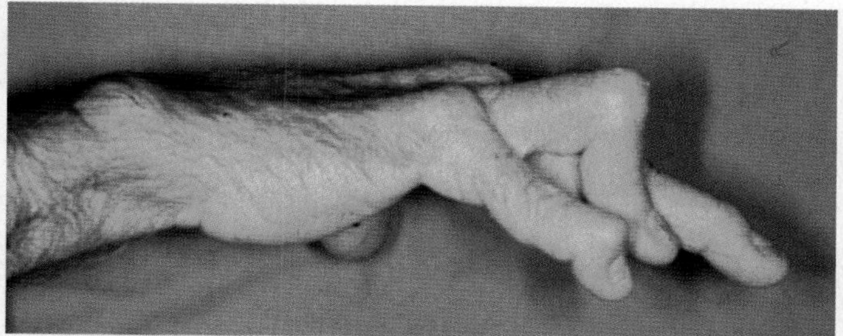

FIGURE 69-52 Patient with inflammatory arthritis has both boutonnière deformity and swan neck deformity on the same hand.

Post-traumatic contractures are the most common type of contracture. These can be prevented by appropriate treatment of the primary injury, especially with attention to detail in how the hand and upper extremity are splinted and immobilized. Once contractures have developed, if they are mild, they may be able to be stretched out by exercises and hand therapy. If these contractures are severe and functionally deforming, surgical release of joint contractures and release of tendon adhesions may be required.

Dupuytren contracture is a disease process of contracting collagen affecting the palmar fascia; it can also affect the dorsum of the fingers (knuckle pads), soles of the feet, and penis (Peyronie disease). It is thought to be a hereditary mendelian dominant disorder and is bilateral in 65% of cases. It is six times more frequent in males and predominantly involves the ring and little fingers (Fig. 69-54).

The process of Dupuytren contracture occurs in the normal bands of collagen tissue that form the palmar fascia, natatory ligaments, and digital sheaths. Nodules containing myofibroblasts and immature collagen (type III) develop in these tissues or in the dermis. The nodules progressively increase in size, leading to thickened contractures and shortened fascial bands that develop into cords extending up the digits. Treatment is surgical excision; it is indicated in MP contractures of 30 degrees or more, when the patient fails the so-called tabletop test and cannot place the palm of the hand flat on a surface, and whenever there is a PIP joint contracture. Careful surgical technique is necessary to avoid complications such as skin necrosis, hematoma, and digital nerve

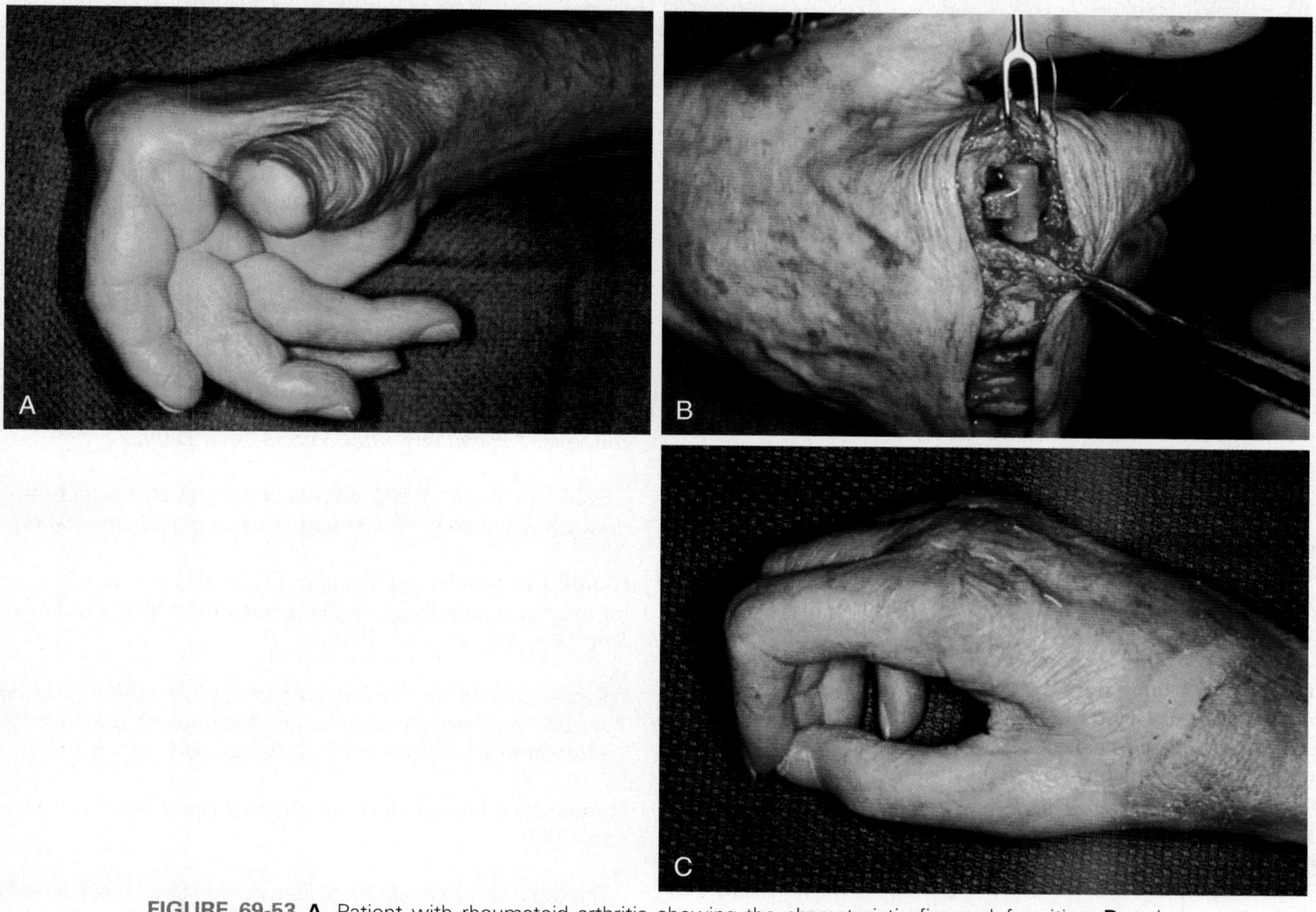

FIGURE 69-53 **A,** Patient with rheumatoid arthritis showing the characteristic finger deformities. **B** and **C,** Implant arthroplasty at the metacarpophalangeal joints restores function and aesthetics to the hand

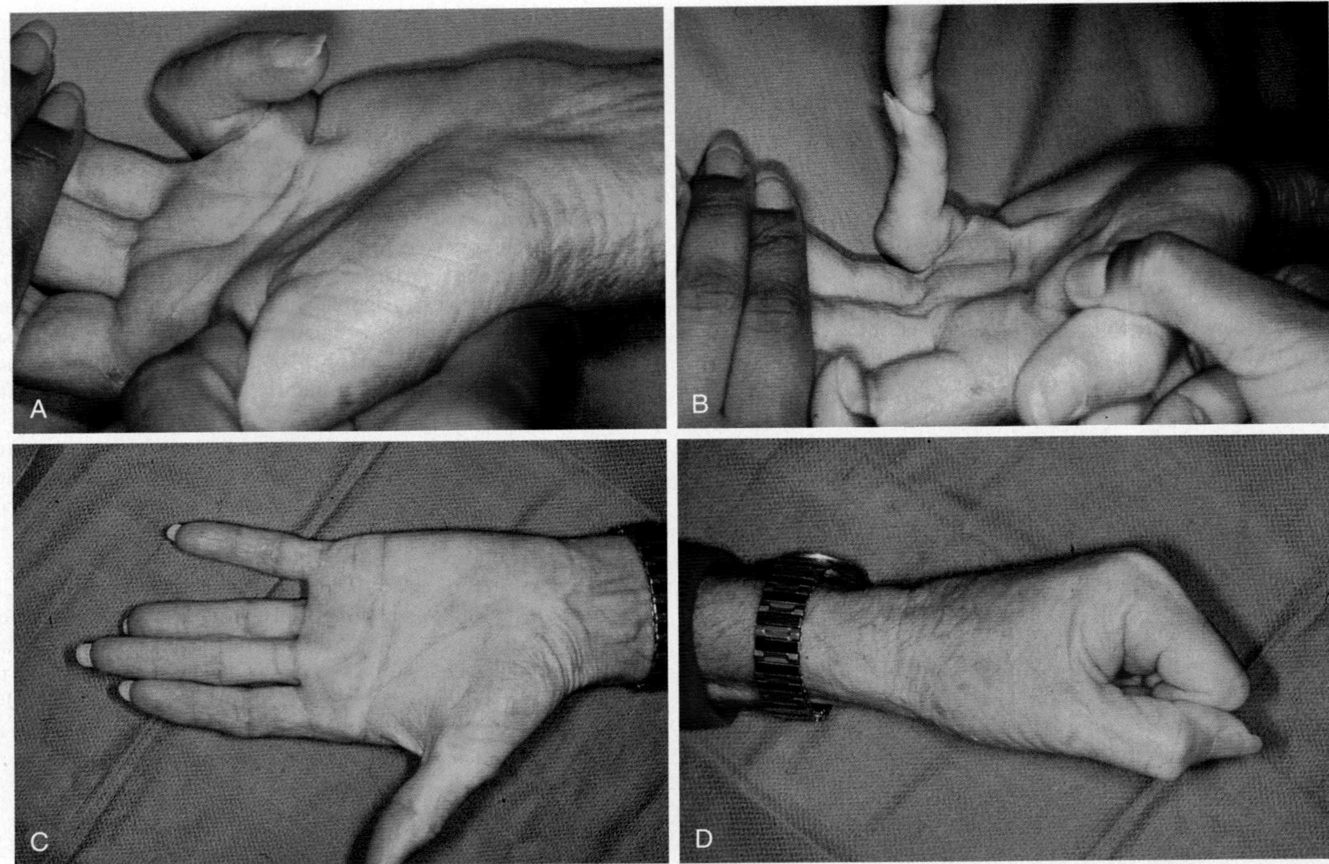

FIGURE 69-54 A-D, Patient with Dupuytren contracture is treated by regional palmar and digital fasciectomy, and good hand function is restored.

injuries. Collagenase injections using enzyme derived from *Clostridium histolyticum* have been attempted and have shown some promise in the treatment of Dupuytren contracture. However, long-term follow-up in patients who had these injections is still necessary.[50-52]

Percutaneous needle fasciotomy is also a reasonable option for treatment of Dupuytren disease and seems to be effective for MP joint contractures but less effective for the PIP joint.[53] An extension external fixation torque device may also preliminarily reverse the PIP contracture before excision of the diseased tissue.[54]

CONCLUSION

The specialty of hand surgery is exhaustive, and a number of specialty textbooks are available. Although general surgeons may be responsible for the basic tenets of hand surgery, knowledge of minute details is often not necessary; thus, most details have been omitted from this chapter because its purpose has been to see the big picture in regard to hand surgery. Those topics of hand surgery that the general surgeon is most likely to encounter have been emphasized, particularly with regard to principles of anatomy, physical examination, and emergency treatments. Taking this into consideration, Table 69-7 includes some high-yield facts relevant to hand surgery that have been compiled from various general surgery review books as well as topics discussed in the American Board of Surgery In-Training Examination (ABSITE).[55,56] This list is provided for the convenience of general surgeons preparing for ABSITE or board examinations.

SELECTED REFERENCES

General

Bruen KJ, Gowski WF: Treatment of digital frostbite: Current concepts. *J Hand Surg [Am]* 34:553–554, 2009.

Experience with tissue plasminogen activator is reported. It shows promise in decreasing rates of digital amputation.

Cordill LL, Schubkegel T, Light TR, et al: Lipid infusion rescue for bupivacaine-induced cardiac arrest after axillary block. *J Hand Surg [Am]* 35:144–146, 2010.

Successful resuscitation of a hand surgery patient after inadvertent intravascular injection of bupivacaine during administration of an axillary block is discussed.

Harness NG: Digital block anesthesia. *J Hand Surg [Am]* 34:142–145, 2009.

The optimum techniques for providing digital block anesthesia are discussed.

TABLE 69-7 American Board of Surgery Review Topics

TOPIC	ANSWER
Fracture of the distal radius	Injury to the median nerve
Innervation of flexor digitorum profundus to the ring and small fingers	Ulnar nerve
Injury to the ulnar nerve at the elbow	Weakness in abduction and adduction of the index finger through small digits
Midshaft humeral fracture	Associated with radial nerve injury
Distal phalanx fractures	>50% of all hand fractures
Joint involved in Bennett fracture	Carpometacarpal joint of the thumb
Common name for metacarpal fracture of the small finger	Boxer fracture
Most frequently fractured carpal bone	Scaphoid
Complications associated with displaced fractures	Avascular necrosis and nonunion of the scaphoid
Axonal nerve growth rate	1 mm/day
Common maximum intraoperative tourniquet time in hand surgery	2 hours
Single digits that are primarily replanted	Thumbs in adults and children, all digits whenever possible in children
Maximal period of anoxia compatible with replantation	Finger—8 hours (warm ischemia), but longer times have been anecdotally reported; upper and lower extremity—6 hours
Proper method for transportation of an amputated body part to maximize replantation success	Cleaned of debris, wrapped in sterile towel or gauze, moistened with sterile lactated Ringer solution, placed in sterile plastic bag, transported in insulated cooler with ice water (ideal temperature, 4° C)
Complications if nerve repair is delayed >2 weeks	Retraction of nerve's ends resulting in need for nerve grafting
Zone 2, no man's land	Area of flexor tendon injury between metacarpophalangeal joint and flexor digitorum superficialis insertion
Mallet finger	Injury to extensor mechanism at level of distal interphalangeal joint
Gamekeeper thumb	Rupture of ulnar collateral ligament of thumb metacarpophalangeal joint, with resultant instability of the joint to radial-directed force
Most common organism causing hand infections	*Staphylococcus aureus*
Classic symptoms of carpal tunnel syndrome	Paresthesias in median nerve distribution, often waking the patient at night
Most effective therapy for full-thickness burns of the hand	Early excision and grafting
Most common location of ganglion cysts	Scapholunate interosseous ligament at the dorsal wrist
Treatment of de Quervain stenosing tenosynovitis after failed nonoperative management	Surgical release of first extensor compartment
Cause of trigger finger	Stenosing tenosynovitis in the region of the metacarpophalangeal joint, A1 pulley
Late findings of rheumatoid arthritis	Subluxation of involved joints resulting in deformity
Swan neck deformity	Hyperextension of proximal interphalangeal joint with flexion of distal interphalangeal joint
Boutonnière deformity	Flexion of proximal interphalangeal joint with hyperextension of distal interphalangeal joint
Nonoperative measures for Dupuytren contracture	Exercise, local steroid injections, collagenase injections, radiotherapy
Digits usually affected in Dupuytren contracture	Ring and small fingers
Cause of Dupuytren contracture	Proliferation and fibrosis of the palmar fascia
Fractures likely to cause compartment syndrome, Volkmann ischemic contracture	Supracondylar fracture of the humerus
Artery and nerve compromised in Volkmann ischemic contracture	Median nerve and anterior interosseous artery
Complication of cast placement for supracondylar fractures of the humerus	Volkmann ischemic contracture

Omer GE: Development of hand surgery: Education of hand surgeons. *J Hand Surg [Am]* 25:616–628, 2000.

This article traces the development of hand surgery from the publication, in 1916, of Kanavel's classic book on infections of the hand, through the recognition of the specialty of hand surgery, to the training of modern-day hand surgeons and their educational requirements. The article contains historical vignettes and mentions many giants in hand surgery.

Patel MM, Catalano LW: Bone graft substitutes: Current uses in hand surgery. *J Hand Surg [Am]* 34:555–556, 2009.

Bone grafts are used for structural support and biologic properties. The use of bone graft substitutes limits donor morbidity and also shortens operative time.

Slutsky DJ, Nagle DJ: Wrist arthroscopy: Current concepts. *J Hand Surg [Am]* 33:1228–1244, 2008.

Wrist arthroscopy has grown from a diagnostic procedure to a valuable treatment modality for a variety of wrist disorders, such as degenerative arthritis, acute carpal and metacarpal fractures, wrist instability, and ganglions.

Soft Tissue

Foucher G, Khouri RK: Digital reconstruction with island flaps. *Clin Plast Surg* 24:1–32, 1997.

New information of the intrinsic flaps of the hand enables ingenious soft tissue reconstructions using local tissues from the hand and fingers as pedicled, vascularized, island flaps. A thorough knowledge of the vasculature of the hand is required in addition to that in standard anatomy texts.

Godina M: Early microsurgical reconstruction of complex trauma of the extremities. *Plast Reconstr Surg* 78:285–292, 1986.

This paper emphasizes the concept of primary repair and reconstruction of all damaged tissues (including microvascular soft tissue coverage) acutely after major trauma.

Martin D, Bakhach J, Casoli V, et al: Reconstruction of the hand with forearm island flaps. *Clin Plast Surg* 24:33–48, 1997.

Knowledge of the vascular anatomy of the forearm enables an array of pedicled flaps to be used for soft tissue reconstruction of the hand, thus avoiding the need to use microvascular anastomoses.

Flexor Tendons

Hunter JM, Salisbury RE: Flexor tendon reconstruction in severely damaged hands: A two-stage procedure using a silicone-Dacron reinforced gliding prosthesis prior to tendon grafting. *J Bone Joint Surg Am* 53:829–858, 1971.

This paper introduces the concept of two-stage flexor tendon repair in patients in whom the flexor tendon sheath is scarred in a late repair. A tendon spacer is placed as a preliminary procedure to later tendon grafting. This remains a time-honored way of dealing with late flexor tendon reconstructions.

Kim HM, Nelson G, Thomopoulos S, et al: Technical and biological modifications for enhanced flexor tendon repair. *J Hand Surg [Am]* 35:1031–1037, 2010.

An up-to-date current concept on technical essentials to enhance outcome and the potential for future biologic manipulation of the tendon repair site.

Kleinert H, Kutz JE, Atasoy E, et al: Primary repair of flexor tendons. *Orthop Clin North Am* 4:865–876, 1973.

This article was the first substantive evidence that flexor tendons could be safely and effectively repaired in no man's land, emphasizing the importance of postoperative controlled mobilization of the fingers.

Strickland JW: Development of flexor tendon surgery: Twenty-five years of progress. *J Hand Surg [Am]* 25:214–235, 2000.

This excellent review article describes the current state of the art for treatment of flexor tendon injuries.

Extensor Tendons

Merritt WH: Relative motion splint: Active motion after extensor tendon injury and repair. *J Hand Surg [Am]* 39:1187–1194, 2014.

This publication has excellent accompanying videos that demonstrate how this very practical splinting technique can be used for rehabilitation of extensor tendon lacerations, boutonnière deformity, and sagittal band injury.

Nerve Injuries

Cho MS, Rinker BD, Weber RV, et al: Functional outcome following nerve repair in the upper extremity using processed nerve allograft. *J Hand Surg [Am]* 37:2340–2349, 2012.

Nerve repair using decellularized allograft for a nerve gap gives results comparable to nerve autograft for median and ulnar nerve. Off-the-shelf nerve allografts have become a helpful addition to nerve repair.

Isaacs T: Treatment of acute peripheral nerve injures: Current concepts. *J Hand Surg [Am]* 35:491–497, 2010.

Although outcomes after nerve repair are not always excellent, this article assesses well-established basic principles and also includes a number of strategies for repair techniques for small and large traumatic nerve gaps.

Lundborg G: A 25-year perspective of peripheral nerve surgery: Evolving neuroscientific concepts and classical significance. *J Hand Surg [Am]* 25:391–414, 2000.

This excellent article establishes the experimental basis and neuroscience behind nerve repair and nerve regeneration. The rationale for nerve conduits is discussed.

Millesi H, Meissl G, Berger A: The interfascicular nerve-grafting of the median and ulnar nerves. *J Bone Joint Surg* 54:727–750, 1972.

This landmark article emphasizes the importance of tension-free nerve repair, matching of proximal and distal fascicular groups, and use of nerve grafts in cases of a large nerve gap injury.

Weber RV, Mackinnon S: Nerve transfers in the upper extremity. *J Am Soc Surg Hand* 4:200–213, 2004.

The innovative use of nerve transfers is described to bypass and to overcome long nerve gaps after nerve injury to hasten and to improve functional recovery.

Replantation

Buncke HJ: Microvascular hand surgery—transplants and replants—over the past 25 years. *J Hand Surg [Am]* 25:415–428, 2000.

This article traces the history of microvascular surgery as it applies to the upper extremities and of the milestones achieved. It discusses the many microvascular reconstructive options available for free tissue transfer and microvascular toe to hand transfers and also evaluates anticipated survival and functional outcomes for replantation surgery.

Fractures

Carlsen BT, Moran SL: Thumb trauma: Bennett fractures, Rolando fractures and ulnar collateral ligament injuries. *J Hand Surg [Am]* 34:945–952, 2009.

Recent advancements for the treatment of these common injuries are discussed.

Kawamura K, Chung KC: Treatment of scaphoid fractures and non-unions. *J Hand Surg [Am]* 33:938–997, 2008.

Scaphoid fractures are a common injury presenting with unique challenges because of a tenuous scaphoid blood supply. This article updates the reader about diagnostic imaging and current treatment strategies for displaced and nondisplaced acute scaphoid fractures, scaphoid nonunions, and avascular necrosis.

Russe O: Fracture of the carpal navicular: Diagnosis, non-operative, and operative treatment. *J Bone Joint Surg Am* 42:759–768, 1960.

Although new innovations of cannulated compression screw and minimally invasive surgery have changed the management of scaphoid fractures, this article is still relevant in regard to understanding and treatment of scaphoid fractures and their complications.

Stern PJ: Management of fractures of the hand over the last 25 years. *J Hand Surg [Am]* 25:817–823, 2000.

Fluoroscopic imaging has greatly facilitated the operative management of hand fractures. The evolution from Kirschner wires to plates and screws is discussed. Innovations included self-tapping screws, low-profile plates, and cannulated screws, with the goal of achieving rigid bone fixation to enable restoration of early digital motion to minimize the risk for tendon adhesions and joint contractures.

Infections

Kanavel AB: An anatomical, experimental, and clinical study of acute phlegmons of the hand. *Surg Gynecol Obstet* 1:221–259, 1905.

This classic paper described the anatomic spaces of the hand. It changed the course of infection treatment and also saw the origins of hand surgery. The clinical outcome was changed from amputation to surgical management, which preserved the function of structures, emphasizing that hand surgery is founded on a sound knowledge of anatomy. The basic principles of this article, written in the preantibiotic era, still remain true.

Compartment Syndrome

Mubarak SJ, Hargens AR: Acute compartment syndromes. *Surg Clin North Am* 63:539–565, 1983.

This excellent article describes the pathogenesis of acute compartment syndrome, including the diagnosis and surgical management in the upper extremity.

Entrapment Neuropathy

Bickel KD: Carpal tunnel syndrome. *J Hand Surg [Am]* 35:147–152, 2010.

This is the most common compressive neuropathy in the upper extremity. Evidence-based guidelines for diagnosis and treatment are provided.

Koo JT, Szabo RM: Compression neuropathies of the median nerve. *J Am Soc Surg Hand* 4:156–175, 2004.

This comprehensive article gives excellent anatomic descriptions of all the anatomic sites in the upper extremity in which chronic compression of the median nerve can occur. Nonsurgical and surgical management guidelines are outlined for each.

Palmer BA, Hughes TB: Cubital tunnel syndrome. *J Hand Surg [Am]* 35:153–163, 2010.

This up to date article provides current concepts in diagnosis and treatment strategies for cubital tunnel syndrome.

Phalen GS: The carpal-tunnel syndrome: Seventeen years' experience in diagnosis and treatment of six hundred fifty-four hands. *J Bone Joint Surg Am* 48:211–228, 1966.

This is a classic paper written by a founder and past president of the American Society for Surgery of the Hand. It presents an understanding of median nerve compression at the wrist that is surgically treated by decompression and release of the transverse carpal ligament. The most common procedure performed by hand surgeons today is median nerve decompression.

Vascular Tumors

Mulliken JB, Glowacki J: Hemangioma and vascular malformations in infants and children: A classification based on endothelial characteristics. *Plast Reconstr Surg* 69:412–422, 1982.

The authors attempted to unify the classification of hemangiomas and vascular malformations. Suggested classifications fall into six broad categories—embryology, histology, clinical features, dynamics of growth, hemodynamic patterns, and cell biology. A classification is useful only if it has diagnostic applicability and aids in planning therapy and understanding pathogenesis.

Congenital Anomalies

McCarroll HR: Congenital anomalies: A 25-year overview. *J Hand Surg [Am]* 25:1007–1037, 2000.

This excellent review discusses the more commonly treated congenital hand anomalies. It also identifies some of the newer (at that time) developments in surgical treatment, which include distraction lengthening, pollicization, microvascular surgery, and potential for in utero interventions. Useful classifications for treatment management are provided.

Netscher DT, Scheker LR: Timing and decision making in the treatment of congenital upper extremity deformities. *Clin Plast Surg* 17:113–131, 1990.

This review describes commonly treated congenital hand anomalies and provides a rational basis for timing surgical interventions to meet critical hand functional milestones.

Osteoarthritis

Burton RI, Pellegrini VD: Surgical management of basal joint arthritis of the thumb. Part II. Ligament reconstruction with tendon interposition arthroplasty. *J Hand Surg [Am]* 11:324–332, 1986.

An excellent description of the pathogenesis and surgical management of basilar joint osteoarthritis of the thumb. This is the usually performed surgical procedure for carpometacarpal joint osteoarthritis of the thumb.

Eaton RG, Littler JW: Ligament reconstruction for the painful thumb carpometacarpal joint. *J Bone Joint Surg Am* 55:1655–1666, 1973.

One of the most common joints affected by osteoarthritis is at the base of the thumb. This operation, originally described by these authors for surgical management, still forms the basis of surgical treatment today, with few modifications in technique.

Rheumatoid Arthritis

Brasington R: TNF-α antagonists and other recombinant proteins for treatment of rheumatoid arthritis. *J Hand Surg Am* 34:349–350, 2009.

Disease-modifying antirheumatic drugs are discussed that specifically target individual molecules. Medical treatment of rheumatoid conditions has changed dramatically in recent years.

Swanson AB: Flexible implant arthroplasty for arthritic finger joints: Rationale, technique, and results of treatment. *J Bone Joint Surg Am* 54:435–455, 1972.

A landmark article that changed the course of treatment for rheumatoid arthritis. In this paper, Swanson introduced small joint arthroplasty.

Contractures

Curtis RM: Capsulectomy of the interphalangeal joints of the fingers. *J Bone Joint Surg Am* 36:1219–1232, 1954.

This classic article changed the course of treatment of the stiff hand and promoted interest in the complex anatomy of the proximal interphalangeal joint. The author was meticulous in technique and insisted on rigid postoperative therapy.

Eaton C: Percutaneous fasciotomy for Dupuytren's contracture. *J Hand Surg Am* 36:910–915, 2011.

Percutaneous needle fasciotomy is a less invasive treatment than surgery. This article describes that technique.

McFarlane RM: Patterns of the diseased fascia in the fingers in Dupuytren's contracture: Displacement of the neurovascular bundle. *Plast Reconstr Surg* 54:31–44, 1974.

This article clearly outlines the pathology, anatomy, and proposed surgical treatment of Dupuytren's contracture. The author describes the patterns of diseased fascia in the palm and fingers and how displacement of the digital neurovascular bundle may occur.

Meals RA, Hentz VR: Technical tips for collagenase injection treatment for Dupuytren contracture. *J Hand Surg Am* 39:1195–1200, e2, 2014.

Collagenase injection has become an increasingly popular method of treating Dupuytren contracture. This article outlines the technique involved for this seemingly less invasive treatment.

REFERENCES

1. Kakar S, Bakri K, Shin AY: Survey of hand surgeons regarding their perceived needs for an expanded upper extremity fellowship. *J Hand Surg [Am]* 37:2374–2380, e1-3, 2012.
2. Sears ED, Larson BP, Chung KC: A national survey of program director opinions of core competencies and structure of hand surgery fellowship training. *J Hand Surg [Am]* 37:1971–1977, e7, 2012.
3. Green DP: General principles. In Hotchkiss RN, Pederson WC, Wolfe SW, et al, editors: *Green's operative hand surgery*, ed 5, Philadelphia, 2005, Elsevier, pp 3–24.
4. Idler RS, Manktelow RT: *The hand: Primary care of common problems*, ed 2, Philadelphia, 1990, Churchill Livingstone.
5. Klenerman L: Tourniquet time—how long? *Hand* 12:231–234, 1980.
6. Netscher DT, Cohen V: Phalangeal fractures. In Evans GRD, editor: *Operative plastic surgery*, New York, 2000, McGraw-Hill, pp 979–991.
7. Hunter JM, Salisbury RE: Flexor-tendon reconstruction in severely damaged hands. A two-stage procedure using a silicone-Dacron reinforced gliding prosthesis prior to tendon grafting. *J Bone Joint Surg Am* 53:829–858, 1971.
8. Tomaino M, Mitsionis G, Basitidas J, et al: The effect of partial excision of the A2 and A4 pulleys on the biomechanics of finger flexion. *J Hand Surg [Br]* 23:50–52, 1998.
9. Tang JB: Indications, methods, postoperative motion and outcome evaluation of primary flexor tendon repairs in zone 2. *J Hand Surg Eur Vol* 32:118–129, 2007.
10. Lalonde DH: Wide-awake flexor tendon repair. *Plast Reconstr Surg* 123:623–625, 2009.
11. Tang JB, Zhang Y, Cao Y, et al: Core suture purchase affects strength of tendon repairs. *J Hand Surg [Am]* 30:1262–1266, 2005.
12. Williamson DT, Richards RS: Flexor tendon injuries and reconstruction. In Mathes SJ, Hentz VR, editors:

Plastic surgery, ed 2, Philadelphia, 2006, Elsevier, pp 351–391.
13. Matarrese MR, Hammert WC: Flexor tendon rehabilitation. *J Hand Surg [Am]* 37:2386–2388, 2012.
14. Ahmad Z, Wardale J, Brooks R, et al: Exploring the application of stem cells in tendon repair and regeneration. *Arthroscopy* 28:1018–1029, 2012.
15. Netscher DT: Extensor tendon injuries. In Goldwyn RM, Cohen MN, editors: *The unfavorable result in plastic surgery*, Philadelphia, 2001, Lippincott Williams & Wilkins, pp 751–770.
16. Cheng CJ: Synthetic nerve conduits for digital nerve reconstruction. *J Hand Surg [Am]* 34:1718–1721, 2009.
17. Oberlin C, Beal D, Leechavengvongs S, et al: Nerve transfer to biceps muscle using a part of ulnar nerve for C5-C6 avulsion of the brachial plexus: Anatomical study and report of four cases. *J Hand Surg [Am]* 19:232–237, 1994.
18. McClinton MA, Wilgis EFS: Ischemic conditions of the hand. In Mathes SJ, Hentz VR, editors: *Plastic surgery*, ed 2, Philadelphia, 2006, Elsevier, pp 791–822.
19. Soucacos PN: Indications and selection for digital amputation and replantation. *J Hand Surg [Br]* 26:572–581, 2001.
20. Netscher DT, Cohen MN: Metacarpals and phalanges. In Evans GRD, editor: *Operative plastic surgery*, New York, 2000, McGraw-Hill, pp 959–978.
21. Stern PJ: Fractures of the metacarpals and phalanges. In Hotchkiss RN, Pederson WC, Wolfe SW, et al, editors: *Green's operative hand surgery*, ed 5, Philadelphia, 2005, Elsevier, pp 277–342.
22. Kumar S, O'Connor A, Despois M, et al: Use of early magnetic resonance imaging in the diagnosis of occult scaphoid fractures: The CAST Study (Canberra Area Scaphoid Trial). *N Z Med J* 118:U1296, 2005.
23. Clark DC: Common acute hand infections. *Am Fam Physician* 68:2167–2176, 2003.
24. Rockwell PG: Acute and chronic paronychia. *Am Fam Physician* 63:1113–1116, 2001.
25. Stevanovic MV, Sharpe F: Acute infections in the hand. In Hotchkiss RN, Pederson WC, Wolfe SW, et al, editors: *Green's operative hand surgery*, ed 5, Philadelphia, 2005, Elsevier, pp 55–93.
26. Lille S, Hayakawa T, Neumeister MW, et al: Continuous postoperative catheter irrigation is not necessary for the treatment of suppurative flexor tenosynovitis. *J Hand Surg [Br]* 25:304–307, 2000.
27. Mollitt DL: Infection control: Avoiding the inevitable. *Surg Clin North Am* 82:365–378, 2002.
28. Kare JA: *Volkmann contracture*, 2010. Available at: <http://emedicine.medscape.com/article/1270462-overview>.
29. Patel MR, Bassini L: Trigger fingers and thumb: When to splint, inject, or operate. *J Hand Surg [Am]* 17:110–113, 1992.
30. Trumble TE: Compressive neuropathies. In Trumble TE, editor: *Principles of hand surgery and therapy*, Philadelphia, 2000, WB Saunders, pp 324–342.
31. Trumble TE, Diao E, Abrams RA, et al: Single-portal endoscopic carpal tunnel release compared with open release: A prospective, randomized trial. *J Bone Joint Surg Am* 84-A:1107–1115, 2002.
32. Mackinnon SE, Novak CB: Compression neuropathies. In Hotchkiss RN, Pederson WC, Wolfe SW, et al, editors: *Green's operative hand surgery*, ed 5, Philadelphia, 2005, Elsevier, pp 999–1046.
33. Athanasian EA: Bone and soft tissue tumors. In Hotchkiss RN, Pederson WC, Wolfe SW, et al, editors: *Green's operative hand surgery*, ed 5, Philadelphia, 2005, Elsevier, pp 2211–2265.
34. Netscher DT, Hildreth DH, Kleinert HE: Tumors of the hand. In Georgiade GS, Riefkohl R, Levin LS, editors: *Plastic, maxillofacial, and reconstructive surgery*, Baltimore, 1997, Williams & Wilkins, pp 1046–1070.
35. Cohen V, Netscher DT: Excision of ganglion cysts. In Evans GRD, editor: *Operative plastic surgery*, New York, 2000, McGraw-Hill, pp 924–935.
36. Glass AT, Solomon BA: Cimetidine therapy for recalcitrant warts in adults. *Arch Dermatol* 132:680–682, 1996.
37. Shenefelt PD: *Warts, nongenital*, 2010. Available at: <http://emedicine.medscape.com/article/1133317-overview>.
38. Kopf AW: Keratoacanthoma: Clinical aspects. In Andrade R, Gumport SL, Popkin GL, et al, editors: *Cancer of the skin*, Philadelphia, 1976, WB Saunders, pp 755–781.
39. Buckmiller LM, Munson PD, Dyamenahalli U, et al: Propranolol for infantile hemangiomas: Early experience at a tertiary vascular anomalies center. *Laryngoscope* 120:676–681, 2010.
40. Sofocleous CT, Rosen RJ, Raskin K, et al: Congenital vascular malformations in the hand and forearm. *J Endovasc Ther* 8:484–494, 2001.
41. Koman LA, Ruch DS, Paterson SB: Vascular disorders. In Hotchkiss RN, Pederson WC, Wolfe SW, et al, editors: *Green's operative hand surgery*, ed 5, Philadelphia, 2005, Elsevier, pp 2265–2313.
42. Butler ED, Hamill JP, Seipel RS, et al: Tumors of the hand. A ten-year survey and report of 437 cases. *Am J Surg* 100:293–302, 1960.
43. Bowen JT: Pre-cancerous dermatosis. *J Cutan Dis* 33:787–802, 1915.
44. Johnson RE, Ackerman LV: Epidermoid carcinoma of the hand. *Cancer* 3:657–666, 1950.
45. Novick M, Gard DA, Hardy SB, et al: Burn scar carcinoma: A review and analysis of 46 cases. *J Trauma* 17:809–817, 1977.
46. Glat PM, Shapiro RL, Roses DF, et al: Management considerations for melanonychia striata and melanoma of the hand. *Hand Clin* 11:183–189, 1995.
47. Netscher DT: Congenital hand problems. Terminology, cause, and management. *Clin Plast Surg* 25:537–552, 1998.
48. McCarroll HR: Congenital anomalies: A 25-year overview. *J Hand Surg [Am]* 25:1007–1037, 2000.
49. Feldon P, Terrono AL, Nalebluff EA: Rheumatoid arthritis and other connective tissue diseases. In Hotchkiss RN, Pederson WC, Wolfe SW, et al, editors: *Green's operative hand surgery*, ed 5, Philadelphia, 2005, Elsevier, pp 2049–2136.
50. Hurst LC, Badalamente MA: Nonoperative treatment of Dupuytren's disease. *Hand Clin* 15:97–107, vii, 1999.
51. Reilly RM, Stern PJ, Goldfarb CA: A retrospective review of the management of Dupuytren's nodules. *J Hand Surg [Am]* 30:1014–1018, 2005.
52. Saar JD, Grothaus PC: Dupuytren's disease: An overview. *Plast Reconstr Surg* 106:125–134, 2000.
53. van Rijssen AL, Werker PM: Percutaneous needle fasciotomy for recurrent Dupuytren disease. *J Hand Surg [Am]* 37:1820–1823, 2012.

54. Agee JM, Goss BC: The use of skeletal extension torque in reversing Dupuytren contractures of the proximal interphalangeal joint. *J Hand Surg [Am]* 37:1467–1474, 2012.
55. Blecha M, Brown A: Orthopedic and hand surgery pearls. In Blecha M, Brown A, editors: *General surgery: Pearls of wisdom*, Lincoln, Mass, 2004, Boston Medical, pp 217–224.
56. Deziel DJ, Witt TR, Bines SD: Hand surgery. In Deziel DJ, Witt TR, Bines SD, et al, editors: *Rush University review of surgery*, ed 3, Philadelphia, 2000, WB Saunders, pp 579–589.

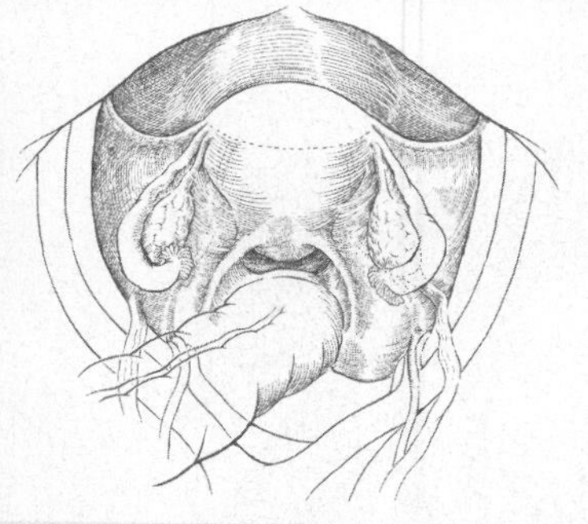

CHAPTER 70

Gynecologic Surgery

Howard W. Jones III

OUTLINE

Please access ExpertConsult.com to view the corresponding videos for this chapter.

Gynecologic surgery involves the operative treatment of benign and malignant conditions of the female genital tract. Because of the hormonal responsiveness of these tissues and organs during the menstrual cycle and during the premenarchal, reproductive, and postmenopausal periods of life, the diagnosis, management, and even surgical approach may differ because of the hormonal milieu and the patient's desire for future fertility. All these factors may be even further complicated in pregnant women, in whom the surgical and anesthetic approach must consider the pregnant uterus and fetus. The surgeon who understands and is able to consider the physiology, endocrinology, and anatomy of the female pelvis is most prepared to select the most appropriate and successful operative procedure. In addition, by knowing the alternatives to surgery and risks and advantages of several possible management approaches, a treatment most likely to correct the problem and to be consistent with the patient's desires for fertility preservation, a minimally invasive surgical approach, or even no surgery at all can be accomplished with the best opportunity for a good outcome.

The general surgeon may be called on to assist the gynecologic surgeon when endometriosis or ovarian cancer involves the sigmoid colon, when a diverticular abscess or carcinoma of the colon involves the ovary, in the pregnant woman with acute appendicitis or cholecystitis, or in smaller communities in which there is no gynecologist at all.

A full discussion of gynecologic surgery is beyond the scope of a single chapter. I address the basics of pelvic anatomy, reproductive physiology, clinical evaluation of common gynecologic symptoms, surgical technique for several common operations, and surgical approach to the pregnant patient.

PELVIC EMBRYOLOGY AND ANATOMY

Embryology

The female external genitalia are derived embryologically from the genital tubercle, which, in the absence of testosterone, fails to undergo fusion and devolves to the vulvar structures. The labial structures are of ectodermal origin. The urethra, vaginal introitus, and vulvar vestibule are derived from uroepithelial entoderm. The lower third of the vagina develops from the invagination of the urogenital sinus.

The internal genitalia are derived from the genital ridge. The ovaries develop from the incorporation of primordial germ cells into coelomic epithelium of the mesonephric (wolffian) duct, and the tubes, uterus, cervix, and upper two thirds of the vagina develop from the paramesonephric (müllerian) duct. The embryologic ovaries migrate caudad to the true pelvis. Primordial ovarian follicles develop but remain dormant until stimulation in adolescence by gonadotropins. The paired müllerian ducts migrate caudad and medially to form the fallopian tubes and fuse in the midline to form the uterus, cervix, and upper vagina. The wolffian ducts regress. Failure or partial failure of these processes can result in distortions of anatomy and potential diagnostic dilemmas (Table 70-1).

Anatomy

External Genitalia

The external genitalia consist of the mons veneris, labia majora, labia minora, clitoris, vulvar vestibule, urethral meatus, and ostia of the accessory glandular structures (Fig. 70-1). These structures overlie the fascial and muscle layers of the perineum. The perineum is the most caudal region of the trunk; it includes the pelvic floor and those structures occupying the pelvic outlet. It is bounded superiorly by the funnel-shaped pelvic diaphragm and inferiorly

TABLE 70-1 Selected Anatomic Abnormalities as a Result of Disrupted Embryogenesis

ORGAN	ABNORMALITY
Ovary	Duplication of ovary; secondary ovarian rests; paraovarian cysts (wolffian remnants)
Tube	Congenital absence; paratubal cyst (hydatid of Morgagni)
Uterus	Agenesis; complete or partial duplication of the uterine fundus
Cervix	Agenesis; complete or partial duplication of the cervix
Vagina	Agenesis; transverse or longitudinal septum; paravaginal (Gartner duct) cyst
Vulva	Fusion; hermaphroditism; cyst of the canal of Nuck (round ligament cyst)

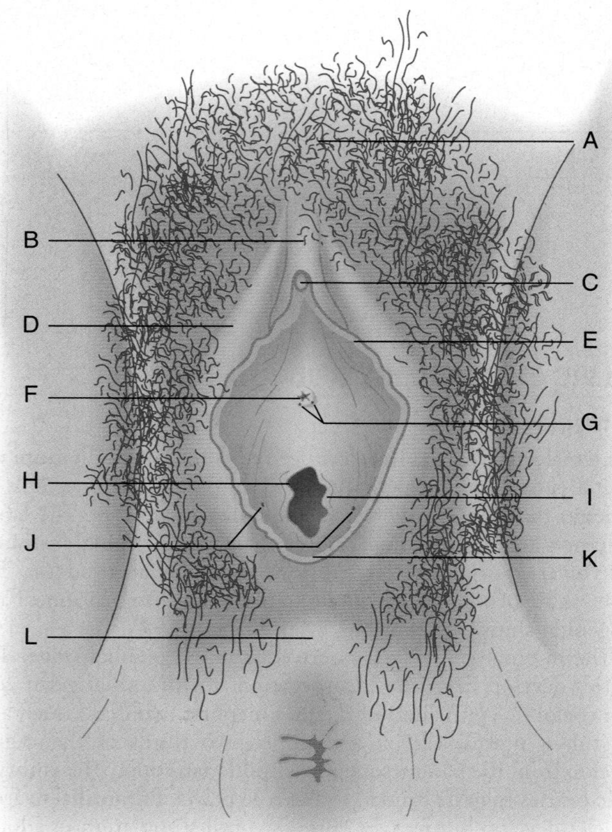

FIGURE 70-1 The External Genitalia. A, Mons pubis; B, prepuce; C, clitoris; D, labia majora; E, labia minora; F, urethral meatus; G, Skene ducts; H, vagina; I, hymen; J, Bartholin glands; K, posterior fourchette; L, perineal body.

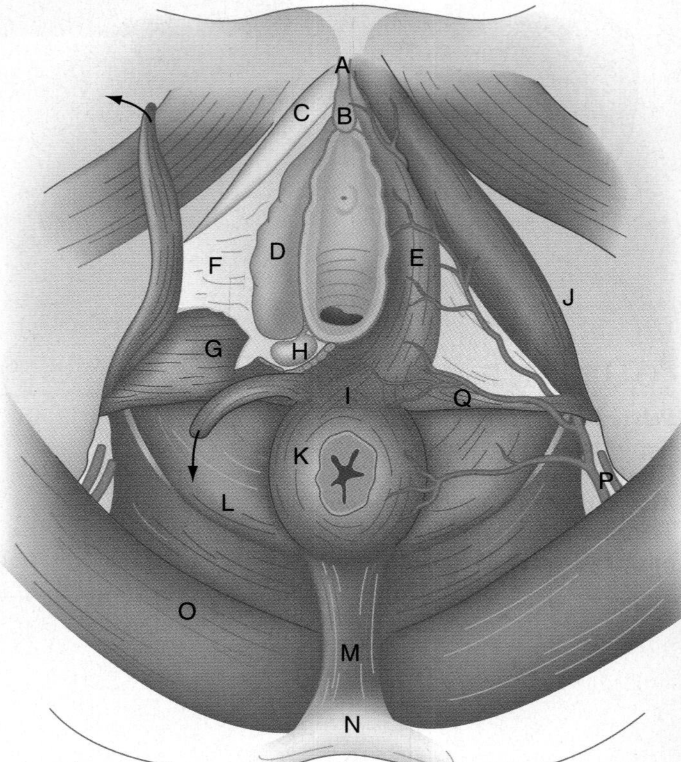

FIGURE 70-2 The Muscles and Fascia of the Perineum. A, Suspensory ligament of clitoris; B, clitoris; C, crus of clitoris; D, vestibular bulb; E, bulbocavernosus muscle; F, inferior fascia of urogenital diaphragm; G, deep transverse perineal muscle; H, Bartholin gland; I, perineal body; J, ischiocavernosus muscle; K, external anal sphincter; L, levator ani muscle; M, anococcygeal body; N, coccyx; O, gluteus maximus muscle; P, pudendal artery and vein; Q, superficial transverse perineal muscle.

by the skin covering the external genitalia, anus, and adjacent structures. Laterally, the perineum is bounded by the medial surface of the inferior pubic rami, obturator internus muscle below the origin of the levator ani muscle, coccygeus muscle, medial surface of the sacrotuberous ligaments, and overlapping margins of the gluteus maximus muscles (Fig. 70-2).

The pelvic outlet can be divided into two triangles separated by a line drawn between the ischial tuberosities. The anterior or urogenital triangle has its apex anteriorly at the symphysis pubis, and the posterior or anal triangle has its apex at the coccyx.

The urogenital triangle contains the urogenital diaphragm, a muscular shelf extending between the pubic rami and penetrated by the urethra and vagina, and the external genitalia, consisting of the mons pubis, labia majora and minora, clitoris, and vestibule. The mons pubis is a suprapubic fat pad covered by dense skin appendages. The labia majora extend posteriorly from the mons, forming the lateral borders of the vulva. They have a keratinized, stratified squamous epithelium with all the normal skin appendages and extend posteriorly to the lateral perineum. Within the confines of the labium are fat and the insertion of the round ligament. Medial to the labia majora are interlabial grooves and the labia minora, of similar cutaneous origin but devoid of hair follicles. The labia minora are richly vascularized, with an erectile venous plexus. The bilateral roots of the clitoris fuse in the midline to form the glans at the lower edge of the pubic symphysis. The labia minora fuse over the clitoris to form the hood and, to a variable degree, below to create the clitoral frenulum.

Contiguous to the medial aspect of the labia minora, demarcated by Hart line, is the vulvar vestibule, extending to the hymenal sulcus. The vestibular surface is a stratified, squamous mucous membrane that shares embryology with and has similar characteristics to the distal urethra and urethral meatus. Bartholin glands at 5 and 7 o'clock, the paraurethral Skene glands, and minor vestibular glands positioned around the lateral vestibule are all under the vestibular bulb, subjacent to the bulbocavernosus muscle. The ostia of these glands pass through the vestibular mucosa, directly adjacent to the hymenal ring.

The muscles of the external genitalia consist of the deep and superficial transverse perineal muscles; paired ischiocavernosus muscles that cover the crura of the clitoris; and bulbocavernosus muscles lying on either side of the vagina, covering the vestibular bulbs.

The anal triangle contains the anal canal, with surrounding internal and external sphincters; ischiorectal fossa, filled with fatty tissue; median raphe; and overlying skin.

Blood supply to the perineum is predominantly from a posterior direction from the internal pudendal artery, which, after arising from the internal iliac artery, passes through Alcock canal, a fascial tunnel along the obturator internus muscle below the origin of the levator ani muscle. On emerging from Alcock canal, the internal pudendal artery sends branches to the urogenital triangle anteriorly and to the anal triangle posteriorly. Anteriorly, there is blood supply to the mons pubis from the inferior epigastric artery, a branch of the femoral artery. Laterally, the external pudendal artery arises from the femoral artery and supplies the lateral aspect of the vulva. Venous return from the perineum accompanies the arterial supply and therefore drains into the internal iliac and femoral veins. It is important for the surgeon dissecting the external genitalia to be cognizant of the variability of direction from which the blood supply of the operative field is derived.

The major nerve supply to the perineum comes from the internal pudendal nerve, which originates from the S2 to S4 anterior rami of the sacral plexus and travels through Alcock canal, along with the internal pudendal artery and vein. Anterior branches supply the urogenital diaphragm and external genitalia, whereas posterior branches, the inferior rectal nerve, supply the anus, anal canal, ischiorectal fossa, and adjacent skin. Branches of the posterior femoral cutaneous nerve from the sacral plexus innervate the lateral aspects of the ischiorectal fossa and adjacent structures. The mons pubis and anterior labia are supplied by the ilioinguinal and genitofemoral nerves from the lumbar plexus; they travel through the inguinal canal and exit through the superficial inguinal ring. All these paired nerves routinely cross the midline for partial innervation of the contralateral side. The visceral efferent nerves responsible for clitoral erection are derived from the pelvic splanchnic nerves and reach the external genitalia along with the urethra and vagina as they pass through the urogenital diaphragm.

Surgical injury to the pelvic nerve plexus can result in neuropathic pain and diminished sexual, voiding, and excretory function.

The lymphatic drainage of the perineum, including the urogenital and anogenital triangles, travels for the most part with the external pudendal vessels to the superficial inguinal nodes. The deep parts of the perineum, including the urethra, vagina, and anal canal, drain in part through the lymphatics that accompany the internal pudendal vessels and into the internal iliac lymph nodes.

The fascia and fascial spaces of the perineum are important in the spread of extravasated fluids and superficial and deep infections. Fascia covers each of the muscles bounding the perineum, including the deep surface of the levator ani, obturator internus, and coccygeus, as well as other perineal muscles, such as the urogenital diaphragm. The fascia of the levator ani muscles fuses with the obturator internus fascia and pubic rami, creating well-defined fascial spaces, the ischiorectal fossae. Beneath the skin of the external genitalia is a layer of fat; deep to this is Colles fascia, which is attached to the ischiopubic rami laterally and the posterior edge of the urogenital diaphragm. Anteriorly, Colles fascia of the vulva is continuous with Colles fascia of the anterior abdominal wall.

Infections or collections of extravasated urine deep to the urogenital diaphragm are usually confined to the ischiorectal fossa, including the anterior recess, which is superior to the urogenital diaphragm. Collections of fluid or infections superficial to the urogenital diaphragm may pass to the abdominal wall deep to Colles fascia. Because of various fascial fusions, infections spreading from the vulva to the anterior abdominal wall do not spread into the inguinal regions or the thigh.

Internal Genitalia

The internal genitalia consist of the ovaries, fallopian tubes, uterus, cervix, and vagina, with associated blood supply and lymphatic drainage (Figs. 70-3 to 70-5).

Ovary. The oblong ovaries, glistening white in color, vary in size, which is dependent on age and status of the ovulatory cycle. In the prepubescent girl, the ovary will appear as a white sliver of tissue smaller than 1 cm in any dimension. The ovary of a woman during her reproductive years will vary in size and shape. The size of the nonovulating ovary will typically be in the range of 3 × 2 × 1 cm. When a follicular or corpus luteum cyst is present, the size may extend up to 5 to 6 cm. A follicular cyst is an asymmetrical, translucent, clear structure. A corpus luteum cyst will generally be characterized by areas of golden yellow and, occasionally, by hematoma. The ovaries are suspended from the lateral side wall of the pelvis below the pelvic brim by the infundibulopelvic ligament and attach to the superolateral aspect of the uterine fundus by the utero-ovarian ligament.

The primary blood supply to the ovary is the ovarian artery. It arises directly from the aorta and courses with the vein through the infundibulopelvic ligament into the medulla on the lateral aspect of the ovary. The right ovarian vein generally drains to the inferior vena cava, and the left ovarian vein drains to the common iliac vein; however, variations commonly occur. There is a rich anastomotic arterial complex arising from the uterine artery that spreads across the broad ligament and mesosalpinx. The venous return accompanies that arterial supply. There is no somatic innervation to the ovary, but the autonomic fibers arise from the lumbar sympathetic and sacral parasympathetic plexuses. Lymphatic drainage parallels the iliac and aortic arteries.

There are three important relationships to be considered in carrying out surgical dissection. The infundibulopelvic ligament, with the ovarian blood supply, crosses over the ureter as it descends into the pelvis. As the surgeon divides and ligates the ovarian vessels, it is critical that this relationship be identified to avoid transecting, ligating, or kinking the ureter. The risk for ureteral injury is greater with a more proximal dissection of the ligament. Also, in its natural position, the suspended ovary drops along the pelvic side wall along the course of the midureter. If there are adhesions between the ovary and peritoneum of the pelvic side wall, careful dissection is necessary to avoid tenting the peritoneum with the attached ureter and causing injury. The third surgical relationship is the complex of external iliac vessels and femoral nerve, which course along the iliopsoas muscle, directly below the course of the ovarian vessels; with anterior adhesions of an ovary, these structures may be subjacent to the malpositioned ovary.

Fallopian tubes. The fallopian tubes are cylindrical structures approximately 8 cm in length. They originate at the uterine cavity

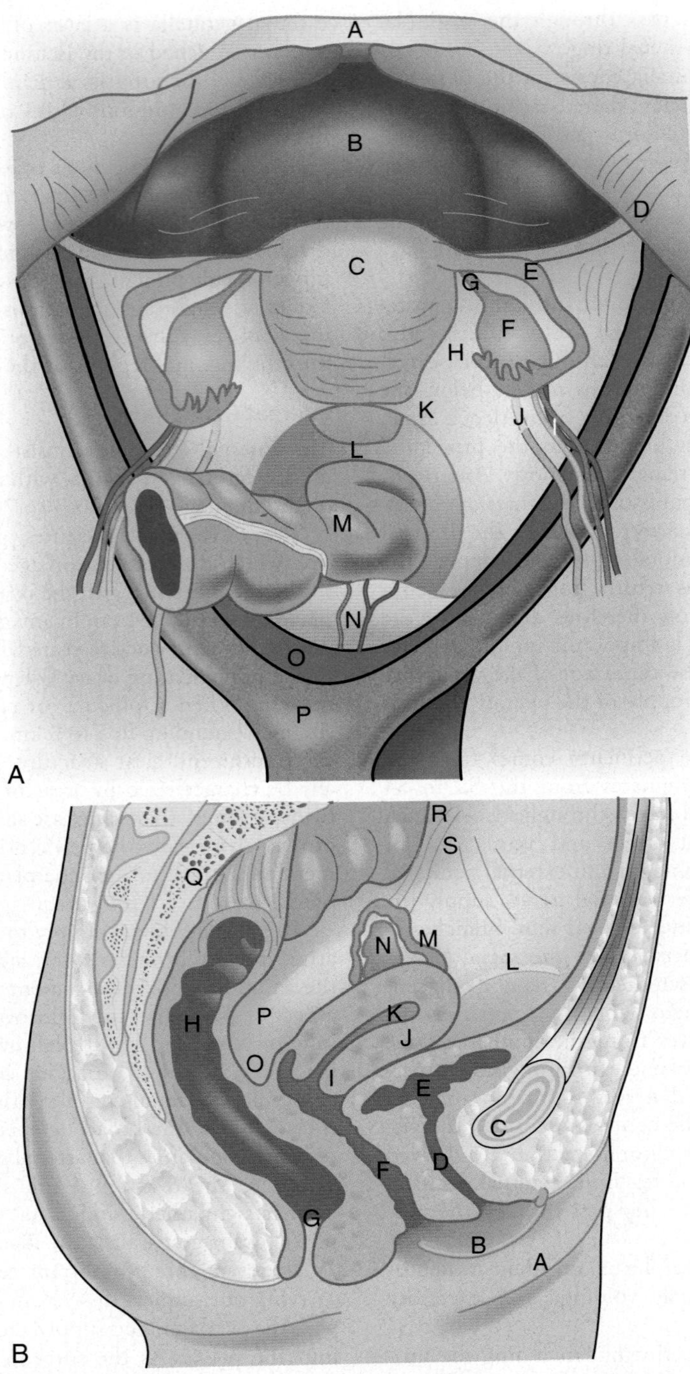

FIGURE 70-3 The Internal Genitalia. A, A, Symphysis pubis; B, bladder; C, corpus uteri; D, round ligament; E, fallopian tube; F, ovary; G, utero-ovarian ligament; H, broad ligament; I, ovarian artery and vein; J, ureter; K, uterosacral ligament; L, cul-de-sac; M, rectum; N, middle sacral artery and vein; O, vena cava; P, aorta. **B,** A, Labium majus; B, labium minus; C, symphysis pubis, D, urethra; E, bladder; F, vagina; G, anus; H, rectum; I, cervix uteri; J, corpus uteri; K, endometrial cavity; L, round ligament; M, fallopian tube; N, ovary; O, cul-de-sac; P, uterosacral ligament; Q, sacrum; R, ureter; S, ovarian artery and vein.

in the uterine cornua, with an intramural segment of 1 to 2 cm and a narrow isthmic segment of 4 to 5 cm, flaring over 2 to 3 cm to the funnel of the infundibular segment and terminating in the fimbriated end of the tube. The fimbriae are fine, delicate mucosal projections that are positioned to allow capture of the extruded oocyte to promote the potential for fertilization. The blood supply to the tube is derived primarily from branches of the uterine artery, with a delicate cascade of vessels in the mesosalpinx. There is a secondary supply from the anastomosis with the ovarian vessels.

The surgeon must be aware of the fragility of the fallopian tube and handle this structure delicately, especially in women wishing

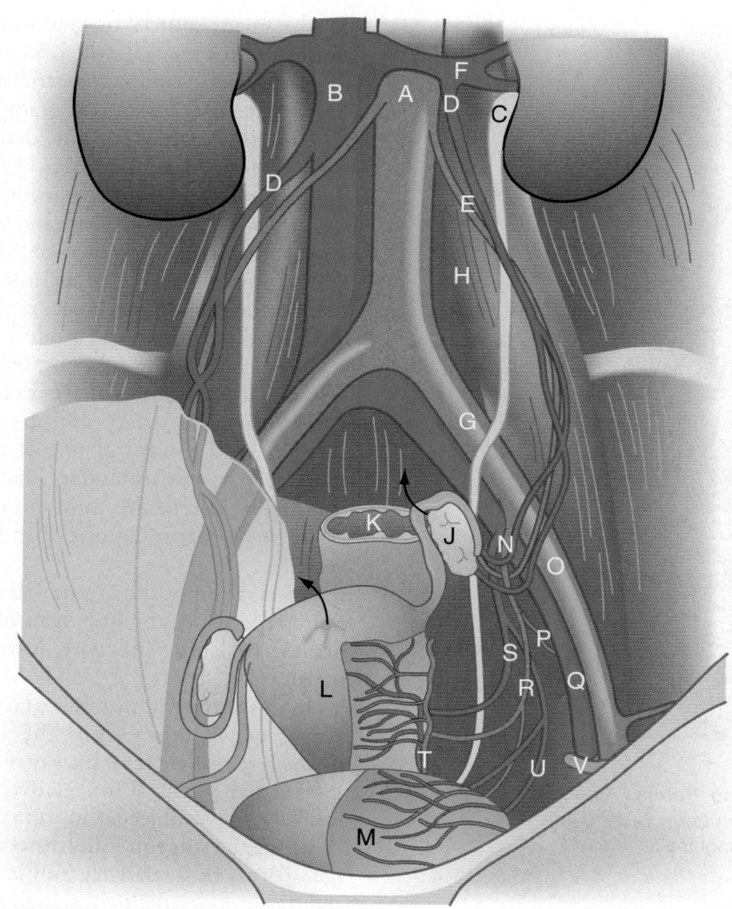

FIGURE 70-4 Blood Supply of the Pelvis. A, Aorta; B, inferior vena cava; C, ureter; D, ovarian vein; E, ovarian artery; F, renal vein; G, common iliac artery; H, psoas muscle; J, ovary; K, rectum; L, corpus uteri; M, bladder; N, internal iliac (hypogastric) artery, anterior branch; O, external iliac artery; P, obturator artery; Q, external iliac vein; R, uterine artery; S, uterine vein; T, vaginal artery; U, superior vesical artery; V, inferior epigastric artery.

to preserve their fertility. The mucosa lining the tubal lumen, especially at the fimbriated end, is highly specialized to facilitate transport of the oocyte and fertilized zygote. Traumatic manipulation of the tube can induce tubal infertility or predispose to later tubal pregnancy through damage to the mucosa or distortion of the tubal position by adhesions, thereby interfering with the access or transport mechanisms.

Uterus and cervix. The uterus, with the cervix, is a midline, pear-shaped organ suspended in the midplane of the pelvis by the cardinal and uterosacral ligaments. The cardinal ligaments are dense fibrous condensations arising from the fascial covering of the levator ani muscles of the pelvic floor and inserting into the lateral portions of the uterocervical junction. The uterosacral ligaments arise posterolaterally from the uterocervical junction and course obliquely in a posterolateral direction to insert into the parietal fascia of the pelvic floor at the sacroiliac joint. The round ligaments of the uterus arise from the anterolateral superior aspect of the uterine fundus, course anterolaterally to the internal inguinal ring, and insert into the labia majora. The round ligaments are highly stretchable and serve no function in pelvic organ support. The broad ligaments are composed of a visceral peritoneal surface containing loose adventitious tissue. These ligaments also provide no pelvic organ support but do allow access to an avascular plane of the pelvis through which the retroperitoneal vasculature and ureter can be exposed.

The size of the uterus is influenced by age, hormonal status, prior pregnancy, and common benign neoplasms. The normal uterus during the reproductive years is approximately 8 × 6 × 4 cm and weighs approximately 100 g. The prepubertal or postmenopausal uterus is substantially smaller. The mass of the uterus is almost exclusively made up of myometrium, a complex of interlacing bundles of smooth muscle. The uterine cavity is 4 to 6 cm from the internal cervical os to the uterine fundus, shaped as an inverted triangle 2 to 3 mm wide at the cervix and 3 to 4 cm across the fundus, extending from cornua to cornua. It is only a few millimeters deep between the anterior and posterior walls, with no defined lateral walls in the nonpregnant state. The most common reason for variation in size is current pregnancy, followed by uterine fibroids.

If, during a surgical procedure, the surgeon encounters an enlarged uterus, undiagnosed pregnancy must be considered. The morphologic differences between a uterus enlarged by a pregnancy and one enlarged by fibroid include symmetrical enlargement in pregnancy and generally asymmetrical enlargement with fibroids. If enlargement is symmetrical, consider the origin of the round ligaments. With pregnancy, the round ligaments stretch as the

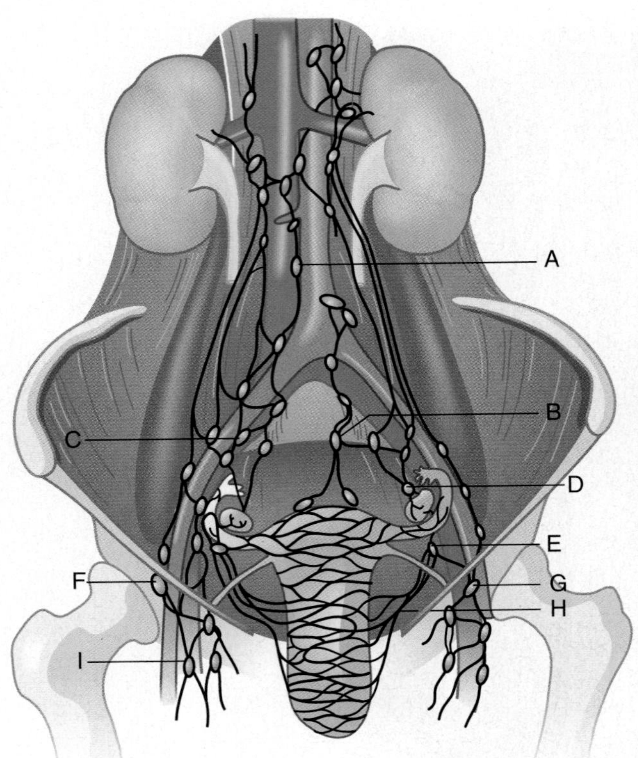

FIGURE 70-5 Lymphatics of the Pelvis. A, Aortic; B, sacral; C, common iliac; D, hypogastric; E, obturator; F, deep inguinal; G, Cloquet node; H, parametrial; I, superficial inguinal.

uterus grows and continue to originate from the normal site; even with an apparently symmetrical fibroid uterus, the origin of the round ligaments is frequently displaced from the top of the uterine fundus or in an asymmetrical course through the pelvis. Finally, the pregnant uterus is usually dusky and soft; fibroids, generally firm and nodular masses, can be palpated in the myometrial wall.

The uterine cavity is lined by the endometrium, a complex epithelial-stromal-vascular secretory tissue. The arterial supply to the endometrium is derived from branches of the uterine artery that perforate the myometrium to the inactive basalis layer. There, they form the arcuate vessels, which produce radial branches extending through the functional layer toward the compacted surface layer. There will be further description of the menstrual cycle here, but during the postovulatory phase, these vessels differentiate into spiral arteries, uniquely suited to allow menstruation and subsequent hemostasis.

The uterine cervix is histologically dynamic, with changes in cervical mucus production during the ovarian cycle. In the follicular phase, under estrogen stimulation, copious clear mucus is produced that facilitates the transport of sperm through the cervical canal to ascend through the uterine cavity to the fallopian tubes. During progesterone-dominant states, either luteal phase or with exogenous hormones, the mucus becomes viscous and plugs the cervix. The secretory epithelium of the endocervical canal has a dynamic metaplastic interaction with the stratified squamous epithelium of the portio vaginalis of the ectocervix under hormonal stimulation. Because the cervical canal is continuous with the vagina, surgical procedures involving the uterus and tubes are considered to be clean-contaminated cases.

The major sources of blood supply for the uterus and cervix are the uterine arteries, which are branches of the anterior division of the internal iliac (hypogastric) arteries. Although the origin of the uterine artery is usually a single identifiable vessel, it divides into multiple ascending and descending branches as it courses medially to the lateral margins of the cervicouterine junction. The distance from the uterus at which this division occurs is highly variable. Venous return from the uterus flows into the companion internal iliac vein. Lymphatics from the cervix and upper vagina drain primarily through the internal iliac nodes; but from the uterine fundus, drainage occurs primarily along a presacral path directly to the para-aortic nodes.

The primary surgical consideration for managing the uterine vessels is the proximity of the ureter, which courses approximately 1 cm below the artery and 1 cm lateral to the cervix. If the surgeon loses control of one of the branches of the vessel, it is important to use techniques that avoid clamping or kinking of the ureter. Often, the most prudent way to secure the uterine artery is to expose its origin and place hemostatic clips on the vessel.

Innervation of the uterus and cervix is derived from the autonomic plexus. Autonomic pain fibers are activated with dysmenorrhea, in labor, and with instrumentation of the cervix and uterus.

In the retroperitoneal space lateral to the uterus is the obturator nerve, which arises from the lumbosacral plexus and passes through the pelvic floor by way of the obturator canal to innervate the medial thigh. With relatively normal pelvic anatomy, it is unlikely to be subjected to injury; however, under circumstances in which the surgeon must dissect the retroperitoneal or paravaginal spaces, this relatively subtle structure can be injured, with significant neuropathic residual.

Vagina. The vagina originates at the cervix and terminates at the hymenal ring. The anatomic axis of the upper vagina is posterior to anterior in a caudad direction. The anterior and posterior walls of the upper two thirds of the vagina are normally opposed to each other to create a transverse potential space, distensible through pliability of the lateral sulci. The lower third of the vagina has a relatively vertically oriented caudad lumen. The mucosa of the vagina is nonkeratinized, stratified, squamous epithelium that responds to estrogen stimulation.

The blood supply to the vagina is provided by descending branches of the uterine artery and vein and ascending branches of the internal pudendal artery and its companion vein. These vessels course along the lateral walls of the vagina. Innervation is derived from the autonomic plexus and pudendal nerve, which track with the vessels.

Traumatic lacerations of the vagina are usually located along the lateral side walls, and the degree to which there is major injury to the vessels can be associated not only with significant evident hemorrhage but also with concealed hemorrhage. Spaces in which a hematoma can be concealed are the retroperitoneum of the broad ligaments, paravesical and pararectal spaces, and ischiorectal fossa. Because of the proximity of the pudendal nerve, attempts to ligate the vessels require maintaining orientation to the location of Alcock canal to avoid creating neuropathic injury. In the absence of an accumulating hematoma, the best approach to management is often a bulk vaginal pack to achieve tamponade. To accomplish this requires significant sedation or anesthesia and an indwelling urinary catheter.

The uterus, cervix, and vagina, with their fascial investments, compose the middle compartment of the pelvis. The structures of the anterior compartment, the bladder and urethra, and of the posterior compartment, the rectum, are each invested with a fascial layer. Avascular planes of loose areolar tissue separate the posterior fascia of the bladder and anterior fascia of the vagina and the anterior fascia of the rectum and posterior fascia of the vagina. Anteriorly, the bladder is attached to the lower uterine segment by the continuous visceral peritoneum. This vesicouterine fold can be incised transversely with minimal difficulty to expose the plane and to allow dissection of the bladder from the cervix and vagina. Posteriorly, the proximity of the rectum to the posterior vagina is significant only below the peritoneum of the cul-de-sac of Douglas, unless the cul-de-sac anatomy is distorted by dense adhesions.

Operative techniques for gynecologic procedures are optimized by careful identification of these planes to separate and to protect the adjacent organs from operative injury. The surgeon can create an incidental cystotomy, which may or may not be recognized, or devitalize the bladder wall with a crush or stitch, with delayed development of a vesicovaginal fistula.

In the lower pelvis, the ureter courses anteromedially after it passes under the uterine vessels and progresses toward the trigone of the bladder through a fascial tunnel on the anterior vaginal wall. The fixation of the ureter by the tunnel precludes effective displacement from the operative site by retracting. Although the location of the fascial tunnel is generally 1 to 2 cm safely below the usual site for vaginotomy during hysterectomy, in patients with a large cervix, distorting uterine myoma, prior cesarean birth, or bleeding from the bladder base or vaginal wall, the ureter can be transected, crushed, or kinked with a stitch.

The rectovaginal septum is surgically relevant during the repair of an episiotomy or obstetric laceration, repair of rectovaginal fistula, or pelvic support procedures. Identification of the fascial layers investing the subjacent structures and use of the tissue strength are critical to an optimal repair.

REPRODUCTIVE PHYSIOLOGY

The development of a differential diagnosis of gynecologic complaints is facilitated by an understanding of the reproductive cycle and elicitation of a careful menstrual history. Many conditions are a direct consequence of aberrations in the hypothalamic-pituitary-ovarian cycle and the effects of the hormonal milieu on the endometrium. Others tend to be mere variations in the presentation of different phases of the cycle. A detailed description of the cycle is beyond our scope here, but the surgeon needs to have a basic understanding of the relationships in this complex process to elicit an adequate history, to interpret the findings on physical examination, to use ancillary tests appropriately, and to formulate the differential diagnosis (Fig. 70-6).

Ovarian Cycle

Under the stimulus of hypothalamic secretion of gonadotropin-releasing hormone (GnRH) to the pituitary gland, follicle-stimulating hormone (FSH) is released into the systemic circulation. During this secretory phase of the ovarian cycle, the primordial follicles of the ovary are targeted and stimulated toward growth and maturity. Multiple follicles are recruited each cycle, but generally only one follicle becomes dominant, destined to reach maturity and extrusion at ovulation. The effects of the maturation process include not only the completion of meiotic germ cell development but also the stimulation of the granulosa

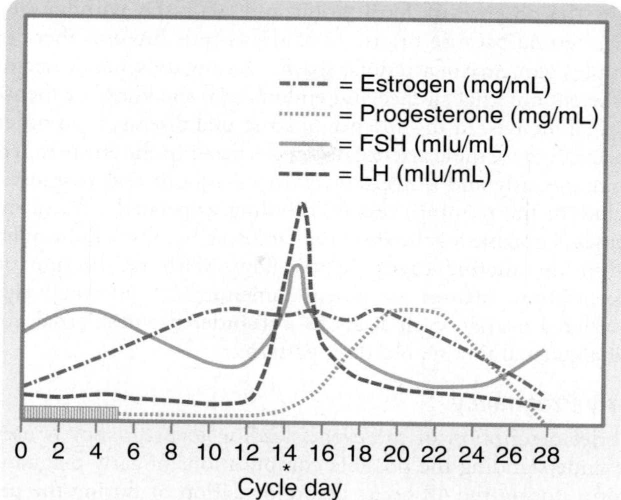

FIGURE 70-6 Hormonal changes during the menstrual cycle. Menses, days 0 to 5; ovulation, day 14.

cells that surround the follicle to secrete estradiol, other estrogenic compounds, and inhibin. As the estradiol level increases in the circulation, it has a positive regulatory effect on GnRH, which in turn stimulates the pituitary gland to release a surge of luteinizing hormone (LH). The LH surge stimulates the release of the oocyte from the follicle. After release, the follicle site converts to the corpus luteum; the dominant hormone secreted during this luteal phase is progesterone. This sequence of hormonal events prepares the cervix, uterus, and tubes for sperm transport into the upper genital tract, fertilization, implantation, and support of the early gestation. In the absence of conception, the corpus luteum undergoes atresia, and the next ovarian cycle begins.

Endometrial Cycle

The hormonal sequence of the ovarian cycle controls the physiologic changes in the endometrium. By convention, each endometrial cycle begins on day 1, defined as the onset of menses. In an idealized cycle, the LH surge and ovulation occur on day 14. Atresia of the corpus luteum occurs on day 28, and menses begin the next day, day 1 of the new cycle.

During the follicular phase of the ovarian cycle, estrogen exerts a stimulatory effect on the endometrium, producing the proliferative phase of the endometrial cycle. The endometrial tissues that are affected include the surface and glandular epithelium, stromal matrix, and vascular bed. The stromal layer thickens, the glandular elements elongate, and the terminal arterioles of the endometrial circulation extend from the basalis toward the endometrial surface. The mucous secretions of the glands of the endometrium and the endocervix become profuse and watery, facilitating the ascent of spermatozoa for potential fertilization.

During the luteal phase of the ovarian cycle, corresponding to the secretory phase of the endometrial cycle, progesterone domination converts the endometrium toward receptivity for implantation of the fertilized oocyte. Several endometrial changes occur under progesterone stimulation. The growth of the endometrial stroma is terminated, the surface layer of the endometrium becomes compacted, the glandular secretions become more viscous, and the terminal arterioles become coiled, creating the spiral arterioles. Cervical mucus similarly becomes more viscous and tenacious, creating a relative barrier between the vagina and uterine cavity.

In the absence of fertilization and with the withdrawal of progesterone because of atresia of the corpus luteum, there is a complex sequence of arteriolar spasm, leading to ischemic necrosis of the endometrial surface and endometrial shedding, or menses. Normal menses, in the absence of structural disease, is an orderly process because these arteriolar changes occur in the entire mucosa simultaneously and universally, with vasospasm and coagulation occluding the terminal vessels. Bleeding associated with normal menses is notable for the absence of clotting because of fibrinolysis within the uterine cavity before flow. With fertilization and implantation, menses are absent (amenorrhea). Alternatively, a disordered ovarian cycle leads to a disordered endometrial cycle and abnormal uterine bleeding patterns.

Early Pregnancy

A brief description of the events leading to pregnancy is useful for understanding the possible complications of early pregnancy. Coitus during the 48 hours before ovulation or during the periovulatory period establishes the conditions for fertilization. As noted, sperm transport is facilitated by the estrogenic environment; the spermatozoa ascend through the cervix and uterine cavity to the fallopian tube. When a mature oocyte and spermatozoa come into contact in the distal fallopian tube, fertilization can occur, usually 3 to 5 days after ovulation. During tubal transport, the zygote undergoes multiple divisions to reach the stage of the morula by the time it reaches the cavity. Implantation generally occurs approximately 5 to 7 days after fertilization.

There are two significant clinical implications to delay in the fertilization-transport sequence. If the zygote has not matured adequately before reaching the endometrial cavity, implantation will not occur, and a preclinical unrecognized pregnancy will be lost. If there is delay in the fertilization-transport sequence, either because of the randomness of coital timing or because of altered tubal structure or function, the zygote can reach the stage at which it is programmed to adhere to genital mucosa while still in the fallopian tube, resulting in an ectopic pregnancy.

Amenorrhea and Abnormal Menses

A disrupted sequence of the hypothalamic-pituitary-ovarian interaction has a profound effect on the endometrium and menses. There are two broad classes of amenorrheic disorders, hypogonadotropic and anovulatory. Although the details of the pathology and evaluation are beyond our scope of this text, hypogonadotropic conditions result from central disruption of the hypothalamic-pituitary axis. Common causes for this condition include stress, hyperprolactinemia, and low body mass (e.g., those with anorexia nervosa, athletes [distance runners, gymnasts, ballerinas]). Because of the hypogonadotropic state, follicles are not stimulated, estrogen is not secreted, and endometrial proliferation does not occur. The result is an atrophic endometrium.

An atrophic endometrium can be identified with ultrasound, measuring the endometrial bilayer. Although local equipment and operator experience will vary, an endometrial bilayer less than 5 mm in a young amenorrheic woman is highly supportive of the diagnosis. This must be followed by a thorough investigation of the entire axis.

Anovulation results from a disrupted sequence of the axis from failure of the feedback loop to trigger the LH surge. The patient may have normal or elevated FSH levels, but FSH continues to stimulate the continuous production of estrogen from the granulosa cells. The chronic unopposed estrogen promotes continuous proliferation of the endometrium, without the maturing sequence induced by progesterone. The proliferation of the endometrium results in excessive thickness. This becomes clinically manifested by prolonged amenorrhea, often followed by prolonged and profuse uterine bleeding (hypermenorrhea, menorrhagia). The most common cause for this presentation is polycystic ovarian disease, but physiologic or social stress can produce a similar clinical scenario.

Ultrasound measurement of the endometrial bilayer can exceed 20 mm. Patients with chronic anovulation with chronic unopposed estrogen are at risk for endometrial hyperplasia and even endometrial cancer. The evaluation of the patient must address the cause for the chronic anovulation and the endometrial consequences. Histologic diagnosis requires an endometrial biopsy or curettage.

After prolonged amenorrhea with excessive proliferation of the endometrial lining, hypermenorrhea and menorrhagia may occur as a result of four parallel mechanisms. The growth of tissue from the basalis to the surface extends beyond the terminal branches of the arterioles, resulting in surface ischemia and necrosis. The volume of endometrial tissue is obviously increased. The normal hemostatic mechanisms of the spiral arterioles in the menstrual cycle are absent. Finally, the shedding of the endometrial surface is not a universal event but is random and leads to multiple foci of bleeding that are dyssynchronous and occur over a prolonged time. Frequently, the rate of bleeding exceeds the capacity of the normal intracavitary fibrinolytic processes, and blood clots are common in the flow.

CLINICAL EVALUATION

Acute life-threatening conditions frequently involve pregnancy, such as a ruptured ectopic pregnancy and heavy vaginal bleeding associated with miscarriage. Therefore, in the acute setting, the possibility of pregnancy must be considered and history focused on this area. It is immediately apparent that many questions in a gynecologic or obstetric history are personal and sensitive, so it may be helpful to conduct the interview or at least part of it in private, without the presence of family members and after attempting to gain the patient's trust and understanding.

Patients will typically present with aberrant bleeding patterns, pelvic-abdominal pain or ill-defined discomfort, or a combination of these symptoms. With a focused history, the differential diagnosis can be constructed with further refinement from physical findings and ancillary tests. The key elements to be elicited are age, pregnancy history, recent and past menstrual history, sexual history, contraception, prior gynecologic disease and procedures, and evolution of the current complaints.

Diagnostic Considerations

Although there are always atypical crossover presentations for any of the possible diagnoses, the most common considerations for the differential diagnosis of symptom complexes are as presented here.

Bleeding Without Pain

- Anovulatory cycle
- Threatened or spontaneous abortion (miscarriage of intrauterine pregnancy)
- Vaginal laceration
- Vaginal or cervical neoplasm

Bleeding Associated With Midline Suprapubic Pain

- Dysmenorrhea
- Threatened or spontaneous abortion (miscarriage of intrauterine pregnancy)
- Endometritis associated with pelvic infection
- Uterine fibroids
- Early presentation of a complication of extrauterine pregnancy
- Vaginal laceration

Bleeding Associated With Lateralized Pelvic Pain

- Extrauterine pregnancy, before rupture
- Functional ovarian cyst
- Ruptured functional ovarian cyst
- Ruptured corpus luteum, with or without an intrauterine pregnancy
- Vaginal trauma

Bleeding Associated With Generalized Pelvic Pain

- Ruptured extrauterine pregnancy
- Ruptured corpus luteum, with or without an intrauterine pregnancy
- Septic spontaneous or induced abortion
- Vaginal trauma

Midline Pelvic Pain Without Bleeding

- Endometritis or pelvic inflammatory disease (PID)
- Endometriosis
- Pelvic neoplasm
- Urinary tract infection
- Constipation

Lateralized Pelvic Pain Without Bleeding

- Extrauterine pregnancy
- Functional ovarian cyst, with or without intraparenchymal hemorrhage
- Functional ovarian cyst with rupture
- Functional or neoplastic ovarian cyst with intermittent torsion
- Pedunculated paratubal or paraovarian cyst with intermittent torsion
- Endometriosis
- Ovarian remnant syndrome
- Ureteritis
- Constipation

Generalized Abdominal Pain Without Bleeding

- Ruptured extrauterine pregnancy
- Ruptured ovarian cyst
- PID with pelvic peritonitis
- Endometriosis

Obstipation

- Cul-de-sac hematoma
- Cul-de-sac adnexal mass
- Posterior uterine fibroid
- Pelvic abscess
- Endometriosis

Flank Pain

- Pyelonephritis
- Ureteral obstruction
- Ovarian remnant syndrome, with or without ureteral obstruction

Other Acute Clinical Presentations

Acute Vulvovaginitis

Acute vulvovaginitis is a common presenting emergency complaint. Presenting symptoms are intense pruritus or cutaneous pain with discharge. The most frequent pathogens are mycotic or herpetic infections. Mycotic infections are generally characterized by a thick, white, cottage cheese–like discharge. Primary herpetic infections often present with profuse watery discharge, inguinal adenopathy, and signs of a viremia. In contrast, other common vaginal infections, such as bacterial vaginosis and trichomoniasis, may cause irritative symptoms and malodorous discharge but rarely cause pain.

Common acute vulvar complaints include infection of skin appendages—folliculitis, furunculosis, and cellulitis. The ostium of the Bartholin gland may become occluded, with or without infection. Sterile cysts are only minimally uncomfortable, but a Bartholin cyst abscess is exquisitely painful.

Necrotizing Fasciitis

Necrotizing fasciitis is a life-threatening infection that can occur in the vulva. It can begin as a cellulitis, from infected skin appendages, or follow biopsy or episiotomy. Once established, it can quickly extend through the fascial planes. Women at risk are patients with obesity, diabetes, and steroid or other immunosuppressive drug use. Treatment is immediate surgical débridement. Patients may require several débridements to determine the extent of the fascial involvement. Skin grafts are often needed to repair large defects. It is important that women with risk factors for necrotizing fasciitis who present with a vulvar cellulitis be admitted for treatment with intravenous (IV) antibiotics and possible surgery.

Pelvic Masses

Masses identified in the pelvis can be functional, congenital, neoplastic, hemorrhagic, or inflammatory and can arise from the ovary or the uterus. Also, the anatomy of the cul-de-sac of Douglas in its dependent position in the pelvis facilitates restriction of pelvic infection as collections or abscesses to that location.

Common ovarian masses include functional cysts, hemorrhagic cysts, paraovarian or paratubal wolffian remnants, endometrioma, and benign or malignant tumors (e.g., epithelial, germ cell, stromal). The most common neoplastic mass in young women is the benign cystic teratoma. Because of the sebaceous content of these lesions, they frequently float to the anterior cul-de-sac between the uterus and bladder. Diagnostic considerations for differentiating among ovarian masses of various causes are discussed in detail in the later section on ovarian cancer.

Common uterine masses include leiomyoma, adenomyoma, and bicornuate uterus. Common inflammatory masses are tubo-ovarian abscesses (TOAs), pelvic collection, and appendiceal or diverticular abscesses.

Inflammatory masses in the anterior cul-de-sac most commonly originate from sigmoid diverticular disease.

History

Age

The patient's age is relevant primarily because of the phases of the reproductive life cycle—menarche at adolescence, perimenopause in middle age, and menopause.

At the time of menarche, the synchrony of the hypothalamic-pituitary-ovarian axis is immature, and the sequence of hypergonadotropic, anovulatory, amenorrhea-hypermenorrhea is common.

Similarly, this is the age group in which emotional stress, anorexia nervosa, and excessive athleticism commonly occur, and the amenorrheic patient may have hypogonadotropic amenorrhea. Finally, however, the young patient may be fertile and sexually active, so pregnancy with complications must always be considered.

In the perimenopausal years, the ovary is less responsive to the gonadotropic stimulus, and anovulation with the amenorrhea-hypermenorrhea sequence is common. In this age group, however, anatomic abnormalities, such as uterine leiomyomas or endometrial polyps, may confound the presentation.

Menopause is defined as cessation of menses for 1 year or more. Any postmenopausal woman who presents with uterine bleeding must be presumed to have uterine disease and needs to undergo an appropriate evaluation for a possible hyperplastic or neoplastic endometrial pathologic process.

Pregnancy History

The commonly used notation for describing pregnancy history is G, T, P, A, L—gravidity (number of pregnancies), term births, preterm births, abortions (spontaneous, induced, or ectopic), and living children. Additional comment is made if there have been recurring spontaneous abortions, ectopic pregnancies, or multiple gestations.

Although any pregnancy can develop complications, the patient with a history of poor outcomes in prior pregnancies will be at higher risk for another adverse outcome. In the acute setting, with pain or bleeding, pregnancy complications must be considered.

Menstrual History

The date of the last menstrual period and the prior menstrual period must be determined as accurately as possible. It is often necessary to elicit menstrual events over several prior months to establish a pattern. In addition, it is important to obtain a description of any variation from the patient's normal pattern of quantity and duration of menstrual flow. One can place the current complaints of bleeding and pain in perspective in the context of this menstrual history.

The amenorrhea-hypermenorrhea sequence has been described earlier. The patient who describes "two periods this month" may merely be describing a normal 28-day cycle beginning early and then late in the same calendar month. Alternating episodes of light bleeding with normal flow may suggest breakthrough bleeding at the time of ovulation or when the patient is taking oral contraceptives. Excessive flow (menorrhagia) associated with regular cycles at normal intervals suggests structural abnormalities of the endometrial cavity, usually submucous leiomyomas or endometrial polyps. Random or intermittent bleeding episodes during the cycle prompt consideration of a lesion of the cervix, endometrial hyperplasia, or, occasionally, adenocarcinoma of the endometrium.

Dysmenorrhea (menstrual cramps) is generally considered to occur only with ovulatory cycles. The patient who typically has dysmenorrhea but who currently denies cramps, even with a current episode of heavy flow, may be having an anovulatory bleeding episode, regardless of the interval between periods. Patients with high-volume flow, with insufficient intracavitary fibrinolysis, may experience cramps as the uterus contracts to expel the clot. Bleeding associated with threatened pregnancy loss or from an extrauterine pregnancy must be considered, whether heavy or light flow, continuous or episodic, preceded by reported normal cycles, or occurring after amenorrhea. Bleeding after menopause demands consideration of endometrial disease and appropriate workup to rule out hyperplasia or carcinoma. Postcoital bleeding suggests cervical lesions, including cervicitis, polyps, and neoplasia.

Sexual History

Sexual activity, a sensitive and personal subject that is often difficult to elicit reliably in the acute setting, may significantly influence the formulation of the differential diagnosis. Beyond the possibility of pregnancy, the patient who will acknowledge unprotected coitus with casual sexual partners is considered to be at high risk for sexually transmitted infections. Reliable reports of the use of barrier contraception reduce but do not eliminate the possibility of a sexually transmitted infection.

Pregnancy must be ruled out in any circumstance in which there is a clinical presentation that is not inconsistent with complications of pregnancy.

Contraception

Reliable use of contraception does not totally preclude the possibility of pregnancy but raises other possible diagnoses to a higher level in the differential diagnosis. Breakthrough bleeding on hormonal contraception is typically low volume and is rarely associated with cramps or pain. In the presence of other symptoms, however, pregnancy complications and genital tract infections need to be considered. Patients with an intrauterine contraceptive device (IUD) may have spotting and cramping, but because use of an IUD increases the risk for endometrial infection and because a disproportionate percentage of pregnancies that are conceived with an IUD are extrauterine, these patients need careful evaluation.

Patients with previous tubal sterilization have a 1% to 3% lifetime risk for pregnancy, with a disproportionate number of extrauterine pregnancies. Irregular bleeding associated with pain mandates careful evaluation.

Prior Gynecologic Diseases and Procedures

The past gynecologic history may indicate recurring conditions suggesting lifestyle issues that create risk for recurrence or raise consideration for complications of previous interventions. Tubal ligation, prior tubal injury from an ectopic pregnancy, endometriosis, and PID all increase the risk for extrauterine pregnancy. Endometriosis with an intraperitoneal inflammatory response may cause significant pain. Patients with a history of functional ovarian cysts, with or without intraparenchymal hemorrhage, have a higher risk for recurrence. Previous pelvic surgery with periovarian adhesions can cause significant pain, even with benign, self-limited ovarian cyst accidents, but it also may predispose to ovarian torsion.

The ovarian remnant syndrome is an interesting and confusing entity. It can cause pelvic pain in ill-defined patterns. The cause of the syndrome is a retained fragment of ovarian capsule after previous ovarian surgery. The fragment is adherent to the peritoneum and remains viable through a parasitic blood supply. Active follicles can be recruited through gonadotropin stimulation, and the dynamics of peritoneal inflammation can be severely symptomatic. These remnants are usually found after resection of a densely adherent ovary with endometriosis or purulent infection of the pelvis. They are frequently located along the course of the ureter and may present with flank pain from urinary obstruction.

History of Present Illness

The surgeon elicits the elements of the history, as described, to determine the evolution of the presenting complaint and to formulate a plan for further evaluation and treatment. This section focuses on the most common emergency presentations, bleeding and pain.

Bleeding

- When did bleeding begin?
- How does the current flow compare with normal? Are there clots in the menstrual flow normally? Currently?
- How did the timing of onset relate to previous menses? Was there any prolongation of the interval between the last period and the onset of the current bleeding event?
- Were recent menses normal? Expected timing, flow, duration?
- Are menstrual periods normally associated with menstrual cramps? Is the current episode associated with similar cramps? No cramps, more intense discomfort?

Pain

- When did the pain begin? Relationship to last menses, ovulatory?
- What is the character of the pain—cramping, sharp, pressure, stabbing, colicky?
- What is the pattern of the pain—constant, intermittent, episodic?
- Where is the pain located—generalized, midline suprapubic, lateralized?
- Does the pain radiate—vagina, rectum, legs, back, upper abdomen, shoulder?
- Were there changes in the character, pattern, or location of the pain over time? For example, did cramping midline pain become acute sharp lateralized pain, followed by relief, evolving to generalized abdominal pain radiating to the shoulder? Did lateralized constant intense pressure evolve to acute sharp pain or intermittent colicky pain?
- Is there exacerbation of the pain with movement, intercourse, coughing?
- Are there any urinary tract symptoms, dysuria?
- Are there any intestinal symptoms, constipation, obstipation, diarrhea?

Physical Examination

The approach to the physical examination of the gynecologic patient must account for the threat to dignity and modesty that a genital examination poses. In the emergency setting, against a background of fear or pain, and especially in young and older patients, the patient must be afforded maximum comfort. This includes an adequate sense of physical privacy, continuous presence of a chaperone, comfortable examination table on which to assume the lithotomy position, and patience by the examiner.

Although the chief complaint might suggest that only a focused pelvic examination is necessary, the examiner will enhance comfort and trust by a more general examination before the pelvic examination. The examiner must remember that the patient cannot see and cannot anticipate what she will experience next; the examiner or assistant informs the patient at every step in the process what the next sensation will be.

At the beginning of the pelvic examination, the examiner encourages relaxation and exposure by having the patient relax her medial thighs to allow the knees to drop out toward laterally placed hands. The knees must never be pushed apart by the examiner. Before contacting the genitalia, gentle touch of the gloved hand on the medial thigh, with gentle pressure and movement toward the vulva, will orient the patient to the progress of the examination. The external genitalia are inspected for lesions and evidence of trauma. This is followed by the insertion of a properly sized, lubricated vaginal speculum. The patient needs to be prepared for the speculum by the examiner's placing a finger on the perineum and exerting gentle pressure with encouragement to relax the introital muscles. The speculum is placed at the hymenal ring at a 30-degree angle from the vertical to minimize lateral or urethral pressure. After the leading edge is through the introitus, the speculum is rotated to the horizontal plane as it is advanced toward the apex of the vagina. The blades are gently separated as the midvagina is approached so that the cervix can be visualized and the blades are spread to surround the cervix. During the advancement and subsequent withdrawal, the walls of the vagina are visualized for lesions or trauma. The cervix is inspected for lesions, lacerations, dilation, products of conception, and purulent discharge. Support of the pelvic structures in the anterior, posterior, and superior compartments is evaluated. Vaginal swabs for microscopic wet mount examination of the vaginal environment, for gonorrhea and chlamydia, and for a Papanicolaou (Pap) test are obtained as indicated.

After the speculum examination, the index and middle fingers of the examiner's dominant hand are inserted into the vagina. Before placing his or her abdominal hand, the examiner's fingers gently palpate the vaginal walls to elicit tenderness or to detect fullness or mass. The cervix is palpated for size and consistency. The examiner's fingers are placed sequentially along the side in all four quadrants of the cervix, and gentle pressure is exerted to move the cervix in the opposite direction to elicit cervical motion tenderness.

Because the major supporting structures for the uterus are the cardinal and uterosacral ligaments that insert at the cervicouterine junction, the junction serves as the fulcrum for leverage. As the cervix is moved in one direction, it is likely that the uterine fundus is being displaced in the opposite direction. Tenderness with cervical motion may be related to traction on the ligamentous attachments, collision of the cervix against a structure in the direction to which the cervix is being displaced, or collision of the fundus against a structure on the opposite side.

The bimanual examination is performed with gentle pressure from the examiner's nondominant hand systematically mobilizing pelvic contents against the vaginal fingers. Except for large masses that are palpable on abdominal examination, the primary information gathered is detected by the examiner's vaginal fingers. The examiner should specifically note lateralized tenderness and masses. The rectovaginal examination provides additional perspective, especially for the cul-de-sac and adnexal structures.

Very young women and some older women will not tolerate the insertion of two fingers or occasionally even one. Under these circumstances, a rectal finger along with the abdominal placement of the other hand can simulate a bimanual examination.

Ancillary Tests

Imaging

The single most effective and efficient modality for assessing pelvic anatomy and pathology is real-time ultrasound, especially with a transvaginal transducer. This technique not only allows assessment of the size and relationship of the pelvic structures but also, by clear delineation of echogenicity, can provide strong suggestion of the nature of the pathologic process. With real-time Doppler flow assessment, blood flow to an organ or mass and fetal heart motion are readily apparent.

Axial tomography and magnetic resonance imaging (MRI) rarely provide additional information for benign pelvic disease but are valuable techniques for assessing malignant neoplasms. IV pyelography may be useful if ultrasound assessment of the urinary tract is inadequate to delineate obstruction or anatomic distortion.

Pregnancy Tests

There are two useful endocrine tests for determining the presence and health of a pregnancy, the β subunit of human chorionic gonadotropin (β-hCG) and progesterone.

Pregnancy tests measure the β-hCG level; the value obtained by the qualitative urine assay can be as low as 20 mIU/mL. This is sufficiently low as almost to exclude all but the earliest of gestations. Unless a viable fetus can be detected clinically or by ultrasound, a positive urine test result in the clinical setting that might suggest an ectopic pregnancy must be followed with a quantitative serum radioimmunoassay. A value lower than 5 mIU/mL is a negative test result. In most laboratories and depending on the quality of the ultrasound equipment and experience of the sonographer, a healthy intrauterine pregnancy that has produced 2000 mIU/mL of β-hCG is generally visualized. In the absence of that threshold, serial β-hCG tests are scheduled at 2-day intervals.[1]

In the so-called typical healthy intrauterine pregnancy, serum β-hCG levels double every 48 hours. However, this description is based on pooled aggregated data; within data sets, there are many patients with successful pregnancies who will have intervals with a lower slope of increase followed by an interval with a steep increase. A decline in value during a 2-day period is always ominous and therefore demands a clinical decision about an intrauterine versus extrauterine failed pregnancy. The greater challenge occurs when the rate of increase is less than 60% during 48 hours. This is ambiguous; if the β-hCG level is below the discriminatory value of 2000 mIU/mL, clinical presentation and clinical judgment are vital to determine whether continued observation or intervention is the appropriate course.[2]

Note that there are three commonly used reference standards for β-hCG as well as significant interlaboratory variation in test results. It is critical to understand the standard used and to be certain that sequential tests are performed in the same laboratory. If a change in laboratories is necessary, repeated parallel testing in the new laboratory using the residual serum from the original sample will resolve the question. Significantly elevated β-hCG levels raise suspicion of a hydatidiform mole or germ cell tumor.

Determining the serum progesterone level can be a useful adjunct in assessing the viability of a pregnancy. The quantitative relationship with pregnancy status is not as discrete, and cutoff values must be established in each laboratory. Progesterone levels lower than 5 ng/mL are rarely associated with successful pregnancies. Studies have demonstrated 100% sensitivity for ectopic pregnancy and 100% negative predictive value for a progesterone level cutoff of 22 ng/mL, but specificity and positive predictive value were poor. The role of the progesterone assay results in the clinical management of the acute patient is not yet clear.

Serum Hormone Assays

Other than the assessment of pregnancy, there is relatively little value to ordering the determination of reproductive hormone levels in the acute setting. These tests are relatively expensive, and the sequence of ordering them is determined by the clinical findings. The laboratory turnaround time is rarely less than 1 day.

Cervicovaginal Cultures, Gram Staining, and Vaginal Wet Mount

Because the healthy vagina is a polymicrobial environment, there are only four organisms for which cervicovaginal cultures are clinically useful—gonococcus, *Chlamydia trachomatis,* herpes simplex, and, in pregnancy, group B beta-hemolytic streptococci. The tests for gonococcus and chlamydia can be combined in a single-swab medium kit for their molecular analysis.

Gram staining of purulent cervical discharge is useful in the emergency setting for identification of the gram-negative intracellular diplococci, diagnostic of gonococcus. The test may also be useful in helping identify *Trichomonas vaginalis.* Culture and Gram staining of purulent material from an abscess of Bartholin gland may allow the physician to select a narrow-spectrum antibiotic as an adjunct to drainage.

The vaginal wet mount (wet preparation) is useful for diagnosis of the offending organism in acute vaginitis. A sample of discharge is taken from the vaginal pool and by rubbing the vaginal walls with a cotton swab. The swab is placed in 1 to 2 mm of saline in a tube to create a slurry. One drop of the slurry is placed on a slide with a cover slip and examined by low- and high-power light microscopy for polymorphonuclear leukocytes, clue cells, trichomonads, hyphae, and budding yeast forms. If hyphae and budding yeast forms are not identified, a second slide is prepared by mixing one drop of the slurry with one drop of potassium hydroxide, which will lyse the epithelial cells and highlight the fungal organisms.

The clue cell is an epithelial cell with densely adherent bacteria, creating a stippled effect. To make this diagnosis, the density of bacteria must obscure cell margins in a substantial percentage of the cells. These, along with a strong amine (fishy) odor, are diagnostic of bacterial vaginosis. There is rarely a significant white cell response to this condition because it is not an infection but a shift in the normal vaginal ecosystem.

Trichomonads are often obvious as flagellated motile organisms similar in size to white blood cells. The organism is fragile, however, and motility can be inhibited by severe infection or cooling of the specimen during a delay before inspection.

Lower Genital Cytology

The Pap cytology technique has had significant public health impact, reducing the incidence of invasive cervical cancer. Although the processing time for the smear limits usefulness in the acute setting, there are two important reasons to consider obtaining the sample. The first is to take the opportunity of the visit to test a previously noncompliant patient. The second is to satisfy any significant concern about a high-grade cervical lesion before surgical manipulation of the cervix.

There are two fundamental approaches for obtaining and preparing the specimen. In the older technique, a cervical spatula is placed in the cervical os and rotated circumferentially against the cervical epithelium. This is followed by a cotton swab placed in the cervical canal and rotated on its long axis. As each step is completed, the instrument is wiped across a glass slide and spray fixative is applied. In the more recent technique, the specimen from the instrument is swirled in a fluid-based preservative, which is processed to provide a more homogeneous slide for Pap staining. Although the cost of the fluid-based technique is higher, the improved accuracy and reduction of false-positive and false-negative results make this more cost-effective.

ALTERNATIVES TO SURGICAL INTERVENTION

There are valid indications for medical or observational management of many acute gynecologic conditions, even if there is also a surgical option available. Because acute pelvic disease is often accompanied by severe pain or bleeding to a degree that the general surgeon would consider it a surgical emergency in the upper abdomen, some guidance is provided here about the clinical judgment to allow the surgeon to avoid or to defer surgery. Also provided is an overview approach to medical treatment and the points to observe during follow-up observation.

Dysfunctional Uterine Bleeding

Dysfunctional uterine bleeding is uterine bleeding that occurs as a result of abnormal or dyssynchronous pituitary hormonal stimulation of the ovary, abnormal ovarian hormone production, or abnormal response of the endometrium to normal hormonal stimulation.[1-3] If a pregnancy-related condition has been ruled out and the bleeding is not too severe, medical treatment does not require a tissue or even ultrasound diagnosis. Emergency implementation of dilation and curettage is not necessary. The episode can be truncated by inducing acute proliferation and regeneration of the endometrium with high-dose estrogens, followed by induction of a secretory endometrium with a progestin.

An oral or IV bolus of estrogens (e.g., conjugated estrogens, 5 mg orally every 6 hours for four to six doses, or 25 mg IV in two doses 6 hours apart) with simultaneous administration of an active progestin (micronized progesterone, 100 mg orally twice daily, or medroxyprogesterone, 10 mg four times daily) will stabilize the endometrium. The progestin must be continued for at least 7 days and then withdrawn to simulate atresia of the corpus luteum. This will mimic the orderly menses of an ovulatory cycle, although perhaps with heavy bleeding. The patient receives oral contraceptives for several months to stabilize iron stores, to allow orderly evaluation of structural disease, and to initiate a plan to assess underlying hypothalamic-pituitary-ovarian cycle disease.

Spontaneous Abortion

First-trimester pregnancies fail 10% to 15% of the time, often with minimal symptoms. For the patient who presents with pain or bleeding, confirm that this is an early gestation. On inspection of the cervix, observe whether there is placental tissue in the dilated cervical os; if so, it can often be removed with a sponge forceps, which will often resolve the event. The need for acute surgical intervention with curettage is wholly dependent on the amount of blood loss and intensity of pain. The patient who is hemodynamically stable and has pain control may spontaneously complete her miscarriage without any procedural intervention.

Ectopic Pregnancy

Ruptured ectopic pregnancy is a surgical emergency, but there are two other tubal pregnancy scenarios that are amenable to less aggressive treatment for the patient who is hemodynamically stable and has limited intraperitoneal blood loss, tubal abortion and unruptured ectopic pregnancy. A tubal abortion results when the pregnancy is extruded from the fimbriated end of the tube. Pain is often described as lateralized cramping, and the volume of blood identified in the cul-de-sac is approximately 100 mL. These events may be self-limited, and if pain and hemodynamic status are under control during observation, surgery may be avoided.

A patient may present with pain and vaginal bleeding; an intact tubal pregnancy is identified by ultrasound. There are varying sets of criteria for medical management of the unruptured tubal pregnancy, based on gestational size (<3 to 5 cm) and the presence of fetal cardiac activity, but the physician must actively consider medical rather than surgical management.[4]

Surgical procedures for managing an ectopic pregnancy include salpingectomy, salpingostomy, and segmental resection.[5] For the patient desiring to maintain maximal future fertility, preservation of the tube is preferable.

The medical treatment of tubal pregnancy relies on the cytotoxic effect of methotrexate. There are several protocols for dosage (e.g., 1 mg/kg) and follow-up. Consultation with an experienced gynecologist before initiation is advisable.

Pelvic Infection

The diagnosis of PID can be challenging. The differential diagnosis usually includes appendicitis, urinary tract infection, ruptured ovarian cyst, and ectopic pregnancy, all of which share some of the signs and symptoms of PID. The diagnosis of PID is made only when the patient has fever, leukocytosis, purulent discharge from the cervix, bilateral adnexal tenderness on gentle palpation, and peritoneal signs limited to the pelvis. Appendicitis is differentiated by antecedent gastrointestinal symptoms, evolving pain pattern, absence of cervical discharge, and generalized peritonitis. Lower urinary tract infection is distinguished by dysuria and obvious pyuria. Rarely do ovarian cysts or ectopic pregnancy present with significant fever or leukocytosis. In a classic study, Wølner-Hanssen and associates[6] concluded that the sensitivity and specificity of clinical assessment for PID were so poor that laparoscopic inspection of the pelvis is necessary to make a firm diagnosis. Although that may be unduly aggressive in many cases, this diagnosis must be applied cautiously because it is stigmatizing and labels the patient, disproportionately a woman of color, from lower socioeconomic status, or with a counterculture lifestyle.

Acute PID, as a polymicrobial infection, is a medical, not a surgical, disease. The major acute complication of this disease is a TOA. In contrast to abscesses related to the intestine, however, initial management of a TOA is with broad-spectrum IV antibiotics. Indications for surgical intervention are a ruptured TOA with generalized peritonitis and failure to respond to medical therapy.

A pelvic inflammatory collection is a clinical variant of a TOA. Whereas an abscess is an infectious process bounded by an inflammatory response across natural tissue planes, the collection, which may be indistinguishable on ultrasound or computed tomography scan, is bounded by anatomic surfaces of the posterior cul-de-sac, rectum, uterus, and intestine. Pelvic collections are more common than true abscesses and are much more likely to respond to medical therapy than abscesses are.

Functional Ovarian Cysts

Rupture of a follicle or corpus luteum cyst, or intraparenchymal hemorrhage in the corpus luteum, can result in extreme pain, with signs of localized peritoneal irritation. If ultrasound evaluation reveals a simple cyst and does not demonstrate significant intraperitoneal bleeding, and if Doppler flow rules out an ovarian torsion, this acute condition will resolve in 12 to 24 hours. Fluids and analgesic support are all that is necessary.

If the right ovary is affected, the acuity clearly will force the consideration of appendicitis, but prior gastrointestinal symptoms, fever, and leukocytosis are rarely present.

Ovarian torsion is a surgical emergency and sometimes mandates oophorectomy. However, unless the ovary is obviously necrotic at the time of laparoscopic inspection, the surgeon needs to untwist the ovarian pedicle and directly observe for return of blood flow before considering removal.

Uterine Leiomyomas

Uterine leiomyomas are benign myometrial tumors present in up to 40% of women, more prevalent in African American women. With clinical or ultrasound confirmation of the diagnosis, observation for stability over time is indicated. Surgical intervention is warranted if the patient has unresponsive menorrhagia, intolerable pressure symptoms, rapid growth, or change in consistency of palpable masses. Leiomyosarcoma is sufficiently rare that hysterectomy or myomectomy to rule out malignant disease carries a greater statistical risk than the lesion itself.

Observational management is especially valid in women who are approaching menopause because leiomyomas are estrogen dependent, and with the decline in estrogen production, the lesions will typically decrease in size. Continued observation is important after menopause because progressive growth during this period may reflect malignant transformation.

Endometriosis and Endometriomas

Endometriosis is a complex disease created by the presence of ectopic endometrial tissue in the peritoneal cavity or adnexa. The endometrial tissue transforms and bleeds with the ovarian cycle. This process induces a sterile inflammatory response, resulting in pain, pelvic adhesions, and, when it is located in the ovary, a complex hemorrhagic mass known as an endometrioma. First-line therapy for this disease is medical induction of temporary menopause and suppression of ovarian estrogen. Surgical treatment for younger women is conservative, with local destruction of lesions and maximum conservation of reproductive organs. Women who have completed their reproductive plans will benefit from hysterectomy and oophorectomy.

TECHNICAL ASPECTS OF SURGICAL OPTIONS

Surgical Approaches

Similar to all the surgical specialties, minimally invasive surgical approaches have become increasingly adopted in gynecologic surgery during the past decade. Laparoscopy and, more recently, robotically assisted surgery have become more widely used for benign and malignant gynecologic conditions.[7-9] These minimally invasive techniques offer fewer postoperative complications and a shorter postoperative recovery. Postoperative adhesions are markedly reduced in many studies; this translates to a lower risk of infertility, which can be an important consideration after pelvic surgery. Shorter hospitalization and rapid recovery to full function are also major advantages to many patients. Today, most patients are discharged the morning after their hysterectomy if laparoscopy or robotic surgery is used; a 5-day hospitalization with slow return of bowel function is typical for patients managed by a traditional open abdominal hysterectomy.

Although these minimally invasive approaches are popular with patients and surgeons, they often require a longer operative time and definitely require advanced surgical training and skills. They also require significant specialized instrumentation and a well-trained and experienced surgical team. Because of their complexity and special instrumentation required for these approaches, they are not discussed in detail in this chapter. The transvaginal approach is commonly used by gynecologic surgeons and is also highly effective for pelvic disease, especially for the correction of pelvic organ prolapse and various urogynecologic conditions. These techniques also require special training and experience and are not discussed in this chapter, although they are commonly used by gynecologic surgeons.

Surgery for Menorrhagia or Abnormal Uterine Bleeding

The classic gynecologic procedure for the evaluation and possible therapeutic treatment of menorrhagia, menometrorrhagia, and abnormal uterine bleeding is dilation and curettage. It is now understood that its therapeutic success is 25% or less and is usually temporary. Because it is a blind procedure, it is difficult to ensure that the entire endometrium is curetted uniformly, much like attempting to scoop cake batter out of a bowl with a spoon. Therefore, more commonly now, hysteroscopy is used in conjunction with dilation and curettage so that the cavity can be visualized and any pathologic change seen can be directly resected or removed. The combination of the two adds to the evaluation and therapeutic success.

In addition, ablative techniques are being used for improved therapy for nonstructural bleeding abnormalities. These ablative techniques (e.g., rollerball, thermal balloon, hydrotherapy, cryotherapy, microwave) are advanced techniques best reserved for a surgeon with extensive experience in hysteroscopy and the evaluation and manipulation of the endometrial cavity.

Technique: Dilation and Curettage

A weighted speculum and anterior retracting blade or a bivalve Graves speculum is used in the vagina to visualize the cervix. The cervix is grasped transversely on the anterior lip with a single-toothed tenaculum. A Kevorkian curet is used to curet the endocervix for a specimen. A sound is placed through the cervix and into the uterus and gently tapped on the fundus of the uterus to measure the depth of the cavity. This step is important to help prevent or to recognize uterine perforation for the remainder of the procedure. The cervix is dilated with graduated dilators of increasing diameter. At this time, if hysteroscopy is going to be performed, the hysteroscope is introduced through the cervix and into the uterus for visualization of the endometrial cavity; glycine or saline is commonly used as a distention medium. The curettage phase is performed. A sharp curet, the largest diameter that will easily fit through the cervix, is introduced gently into the cervix and endometrial cavity. This is done without excessive pressure or undue force. The fundus is found, and a firm withdrawal stroke is applied until the curet reaches the cervicouterine junction. This is repeated while moving circumferentially around the uterine cavity, attempting to curet as much of the endometrial cavity as possible. The procedure is then terminated; the instruments are removed with careful attention to the cervix, which may bleed when the tenaculum is removed. The bleeding usually stops with pressure, silver nitrate, or Monsel solution.

Potential Complications

As with any surgical procedure, infection from instrumenting the cavity or bleeding from the denuded endometrial lining can occur. In addition, perforation of the uterine cavity is possible and can occur during any phase of the procedure. However, it usually occurs during the sounding of the uterus, and bleeding from the perforated area can result. The perforation is usually midline and self-limited. In general, observation for 24 hours is all that is required. If there is continued bleeding, as evidenced by a decreasing hemoglobin level or increased abdominal pain, or if other symptoms are present, exploration by laparoscopy or laparotomy may be required. Injury to the bowel is possible, although rare, with perforation.

Treatment of Bartholin Gland Cyst or Abscess

Large, symptomatic Bartholin gland cysts or painful abscesses may not respond to conservative treatment. Surgical treatment options are incision and drainage with Word catheter placement, marsupialization, and excision of the gland itself.

Excision of the gland is rarely indicated. Typically, all that is needed to treat this condition is incision and drainage with appropriate follow-up, with or without marsupialization.

Incision and drainage are generally done on the vestibular side at the hymenal ring in a lower dependent portion of the cyst or abscess using a sharp knife. The cyst is stabilized, and an incision is made into the cyst itself. A small Word catheter is placed into the cyst for drainage and is reevaluated on a weekly basis. Patients with abscesses are pretreated with antibiotics.

To perform a marsupialization, an elliptical incision is made in the vestibular mucosa down to the wall of the gland. The wall of the gland is incised along the entire length of the ellipse. The contents are evacuated, and the wall of the cyst is sutured to the vestibular mucosa with 3-0 synthetic absorbable sutures in an interrupted fashion or using a baseball stitch (Fig. 70-7). The patient is prescribed a regimen of hot sitz baths. If the lesion is an abscess, the patient is given antibiotics. Whether marsupialization or incision and drainage have been performed, sexual intercourse is avoided until the area has completely healed.

Cone Procedure

Conization can be performed with a cold knife or a LEEP. A LEEP (loop electrosurgical excision procedure) conization entails removal of the transformation zone with an ectocervical loop, followed by removal of an endocervical specimen with an endocervical loop. This is called a top hat procedure and allows

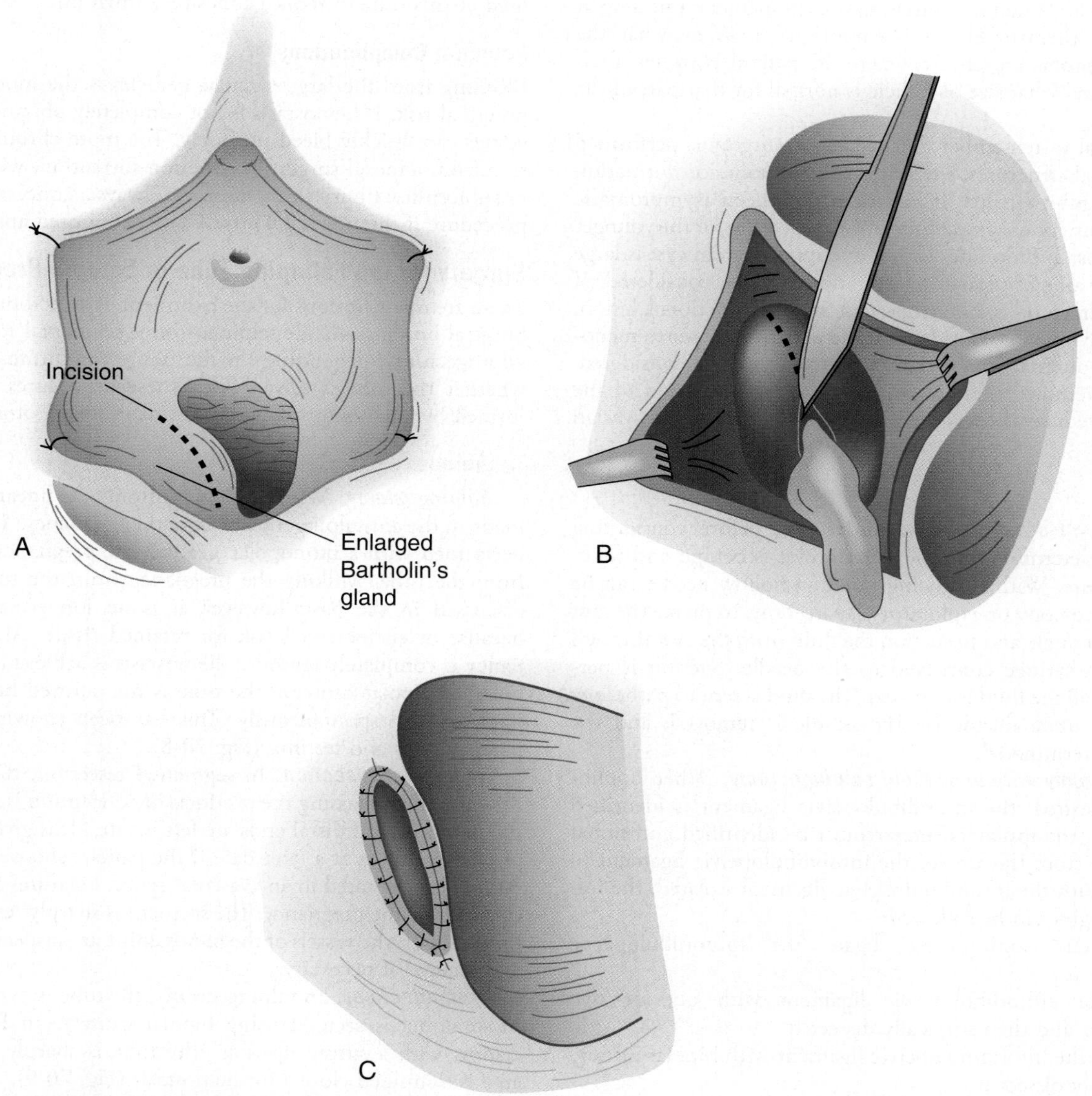

FIGURE 70-7 Bartholin Gland Marsupialization. A, Retraction of the labia and incision over the mucosa of the vagina. **B,** Wall of the gland is excised. **C,** Completed marsupialization. (Adapted from Mitchell CW, Wheeless CR: *Atlas of pelvic surgery*, ed 3, Philadelphia, 1997, Lippincott Williams & Wilkins.)

sampling of the canal. If a cold knife conization is done in the operating room, a single-toothed tenaculum is placed on the anterior lip of the cervix. Figure-of-eight retention sutures of 0-0 Vicryl are placed at 3 and 9 o'clock. A circumferential incision is made around the transformation zone and lesion. The specimen is grasped with Allis clamps to maintain orientation, and a deeper circumferential incision is made in the cervix. The specimen is removed with a scalpel or Mayo scissors. A marking stitch is placed at 12 o'clock on the specimen, and an endocervical curetting is performed above the cone biopsy. Risk for recurrence of dysplasia is dependent on the status of the endocervical and ectocervical margins as well as on whether the endocervical curetting is positive for dysplasia.

Surgery for Ovarian Cysts

Ovarian cysts are common, especially functional cysts. Benign ovarian cysts have been discussed previously. When a cyst is found, it is necessary to determine which type of treatment is most appropriate. It is individualized to each patient, depending on the clinical scenario. When an ovarian cyst is an incidental finding at the time of other surgery, it is important to know what the patient's symptoms are, if any; where the patient is in her menstrual cycle; and what size of follicle is normal for that part of the cycle.

It is critical to remember that whenever surgery is performed on the adnexal structures, there is a risk for adhesion formation that might inhibit fertility. If the patient has been asymptomatic with a small functional cyst, observation, especially for the younger patient, is most appropriate. If the functional ovarian cyst is large (>5 to 6 cm) or symptomatic, aspiration may be considered. If the cyst is larger or is not consistent with a functional lesion, oophorectomy may be considered if the patient is closer to menopause. As an alternative, ovarian cystectomy may be considered. This option removes the cyst but preserves the function of the ovary. It also reduces the risk for recurrence compared with ovarian cyst drainage.

Technique

Ovarian cyst drainage. It is imperative, before considering drainage, to determine that the ovarian cyst is benign and functional in nature. With this being noted, a hollow needle can be used, by laparoscopy or exploratory laparotomy, to pierce the cyst at a 90-degree angle and to suction the fluid from the cyst through tubing and a syringe connected to the needle. Suction is performed until all the fluid is removed. The fluid is sent to pathology to ensure accurate diagnosis. The needle is removed, and the procedure is terminated.

Oophorectomy with or without salpingectomy. When oophorectomy is desired, the infundibulopelvic ligament is identified and isolated. The ipsilateral ureter must be identified and noted to be remote from the area of the infundibulopelvic ligament to be ligated. With the infundibulopelvic ligament isolated, the following strategies can be followed:

1. Clamp, cut, and suture ligate the infundibulopelvic ligament.
2. Ligate the infundibulopelvic ligament with one or two Endoloops and then surgically dissect it.
3. Cauterize the infundibulopelvic ligament with bipolar cautery and sharply dissect it.

If the ipsilateral tube is to be removed, dissection across the mesosalpinx is performed with clamp, sharp dissection, and suture ligation or with bipolar coagulation and sharp dissection. If the uterus is present, attention is directed to the utero-ovarian ligament. This ligament is dissected in a similar fashion, as described, through bipolar cautery or the clamping technique. The ovary, completely dissected, possibly in conjunction with the fallopian tube, can be removed.

Ovarian cystectomy. To begin an ovarian cystectomy, a surgical line into the ovarian capsule is developed sharply over the area of the cyst, on the antimesovarian side of the ovary. After the incision into the capsule, the cyst is dissected away from the capsule using sharp or blunt dissection. Scissors, knife, Kitner, hydrodissection, or a combination of these may be used for this dissection, taking care to avoid rupture of the cyst. After the cyst is completely removed, the base of the ovarian capsule usually has some bleeding. Hemostasis can be obtained at the base with electrocautery or by suturing. After hemostasis is obtained, most surgeons do not suture the capsule but approximate the edges loosely together to heal spontaneously. It is believed that this reduces the risk for adhesion formation. A Gynecare Interceed absorbable adhesion barrier or another adhesion barrier can be used at this time to reduce adhesion formation.

Potential Complications

Bleeding from the large vascular pedicles is the most dangerous potential risk. If hemostasis is not completely obtained, the large vessels can quickly bleed profusely. The more chronic complication from adnexal surgery is adhesion formation, with infertility or subfertility. Injury to the ureter is always a concern during this procedure if the ureteral course is not monitored appropriately.

Surgery for the Fallopian Tube or Ectopic Pregnancy

There are many options for the treatment of an ectopic pregnancy. Surgical options include salpingostomy, segmental resection, and salpingectomy, depending on the desire for future fertility and whether the tube is salvageable. These procedures can be performed by laparoscopy, laparotomy, or minilaparotomy.

Technique

Salpingostomy. With a salpingostomy, a linear incision is made in the antisalpingetic line over the pregnancy. This is usually performed with a monopolar needle. The pregnancy is removed from the tube. Milking the pregnancy from the tube has been discussed in the past; however, it is no longer recommended because of an increased risk for retained tissue. After the pregnancy is completely removed, hemostasis is achieved with monopolar or bipolar cautery. The tube is not sutured but rather left open to heal spontaneously. This has been shown to improve patency rates and fertility (Fig. 70-8).

Segmental resection. In segmental resection, the portion of the tube encompassing the products of conception is resected, and the proximal and distal ends are left in situ. This gives the option of reanastomosis at a later date if the patient chooses. The mesosalpinx is perforated in an avascular space. Ligatures are placed on each side of the pregnancy. The segment is sharply resected within the ligatures; the vessels of the mesosalpinx are inspected for injury and secured if necessary.

Salpingectomy. In salpingectomy, the tube is grasped and the mesosalpinx is secured using bipolar cautery, an Endoloop, or clamps with a suture ligation. The tube is sharply excised. The area is examined closely for hemostasis (Fig. 70-9).

In rare cases, the ectopic pregnancy is in the abdomen and not in the fallopian tube. In these situations, the fetus is removed with ligation of the umbilical cord near its insertion into the placenta.

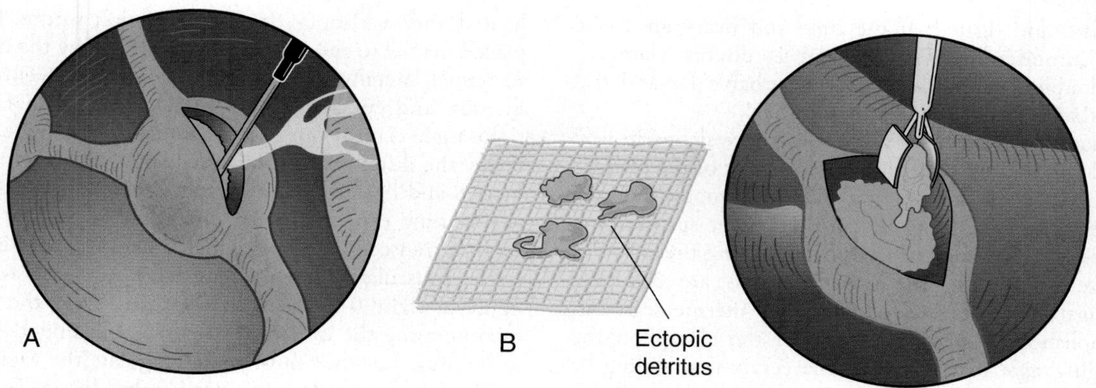

FIGURE 70-8 Salpingostomy. **A,** Fallopian tube is opened in a longitudinal manner. **B,** Trophoblastic tissue is removed in pieces. (Adapted from Mitchell CW, Wheeless CR: *Atlas of pelvic surgery*, ed 3, Philadelphia, 1997, Lippincott Williams & Wilkins.)

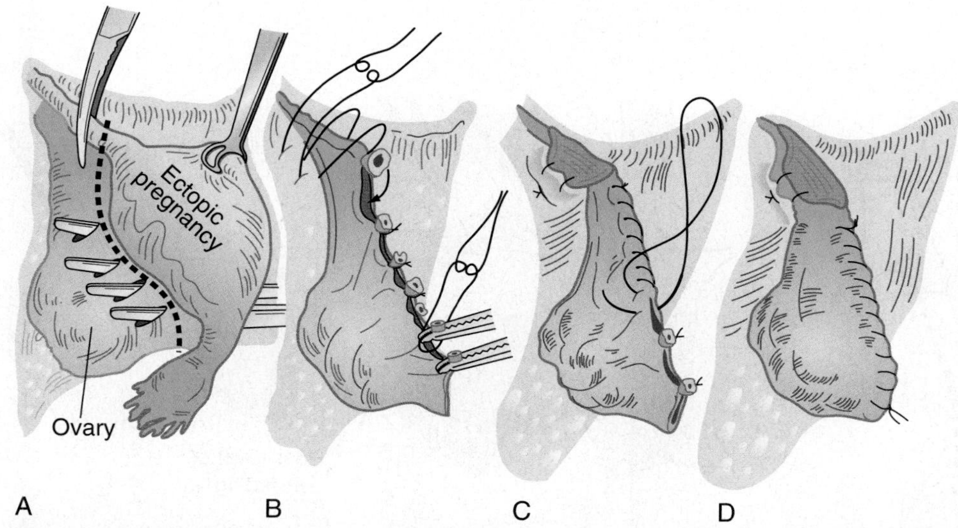

FIGURE 70-9 Salpingectomy. **A,** Tube is excised from the cornual portion across the mesosalpinx to the fimbria. **B,** Pedicles are tied, peritoneal lining is reestablished, and cornual portion of the tube is buried into the posterior segment of the uterine cornu. **C,** Mesosalpinx is reperitonealized. **D,** Mesosalpinx is closed and the procedure completed. (Adapted from Mitchell CW, Wheeless CR: *Atlas of pelvic surgery*, ed 3, Philadelphia, 1997, Lippincott Williams & Wilkins.)

Because of the vascularity of the placenta, the placenta is left in situ, with subsequent medical therapy with methotrexate.

Potential Complications

The vascular supply of the tube in pregnancy is markedly increased; therefore, bleeding is a risk during the surgery and after it is completed. If the tube is preserved, there is a risk for subsequent recurrent ectopic pregnancy. Also, there is a risk for retained placental tissue in the tube and persistent ectopic pregnancy. Adhesions of the affected adnexa are also a significant risk, whether the tube is preserved or removed.

Hysterectomy

Hysterectomy is one of the most common gynecologic procedures performed. The route of hysterectomy depends on the indication for surgery, size of the uterus, descent of the cervix and uterus, shape of the vagina, size of the patient, and skill and preference of the surgeon. Surgical routes for hysterectomy include total abdominal hysterectomy, total vaginal hysterectomy, laparoscopically assisted vaginal hysterectomy, and two more recent techniques—total laparoscopic hysterectomy and laparoscopic supracervical hysterectomy. Robotically assisted total laparoscopic hysterectomy is a popular variation of total laparoscopic hysterectomy.

Because of the significant impact of the transvaginal approach on appreciating anatomic relationships, vaginal hysterectomy and laparoscopically assisted hysterectomy must be performed only by an experienced vaginal surgeon.

Technique

Any lower abdominal incision (vertical, Pfannenstiel, Maylard, Cherney) can be used. The bowel is packed from the pelvis, and the patient is placed in the Trendelenburg position. The ureters are identified, and the following steps are performed bilaterally (Fig. 70-10).

The round ligament is identified, incised between clamps, and ligated with 0-0 absorbable suture. The leaves of the broad ligament are sharply opened anteriorly and posteriorly, with the anterior leaf open to the vesicouterine fold. If the ovary is to be preserved, the proximal tube and utero-ovarian ligament are clamped, incised, and ligated. If the tube and ovary are to be removed, the infundibulopelvic ligament is doubly clamped, incised, and double-ligated with a 0-0 absorbable tie and 0-0 synthetic absorbable suture, as described earlier.

After this has been performed bilaterally, the vesicoperitoneal fold is elevated and incised. The filmy attachments of the bladder to the pubovesical fascia are sharply dissected, mobilizing the bladder off the cervix. The filmy adventitious tissue surrounding the uterine vessels is skeletonized sharply, dissecting the tissue to expose the uterine vessels. The uterine vessels are clamped, incised, and ligated at the level of the lower uterine segment. This is accomplished by placing the tip of the clamp on the uterus at a right angle to the axis of the cervix and sliding or stepping off the uterus. The pedicle is incised, and a simple absorbable 0-0 suture ligature is placed. The cardinal and uterosacral ligaments are sequentially clamped, incised, and suture ligated with a Heaney double transfixion suture. Each clamp is placed medial to the previous pedicle to allow the ureter passively to retract laterally. The anterior vagina can be entered by a stab incision and cut across with a scalpel or scissors. Alternatively, right-angle clamps can be used to clamp the angle of the vagina, below the distal cervix. The tissue above this angle clamp is then incised and ligated with a Heaney stitch. With the lumen of the vagina now exposed, sharp dissection is used to complete the vaginal transection. The vaginal wall, incorporating perivaginal fascia, muscularis, and mucosal edge, is closed with a series of figure-of-eight 0-0 absorbable sutures, with the angle stitches incorporating the ipsilateral uterosacral ligament. Ligatures need to be snug, but they must not strangulate the vaginal edges. The pelvic peritoneum does not need to be closed. The pelvis is irrigated, hemostasis is ensured, and the abdominal incision is closed routinely.

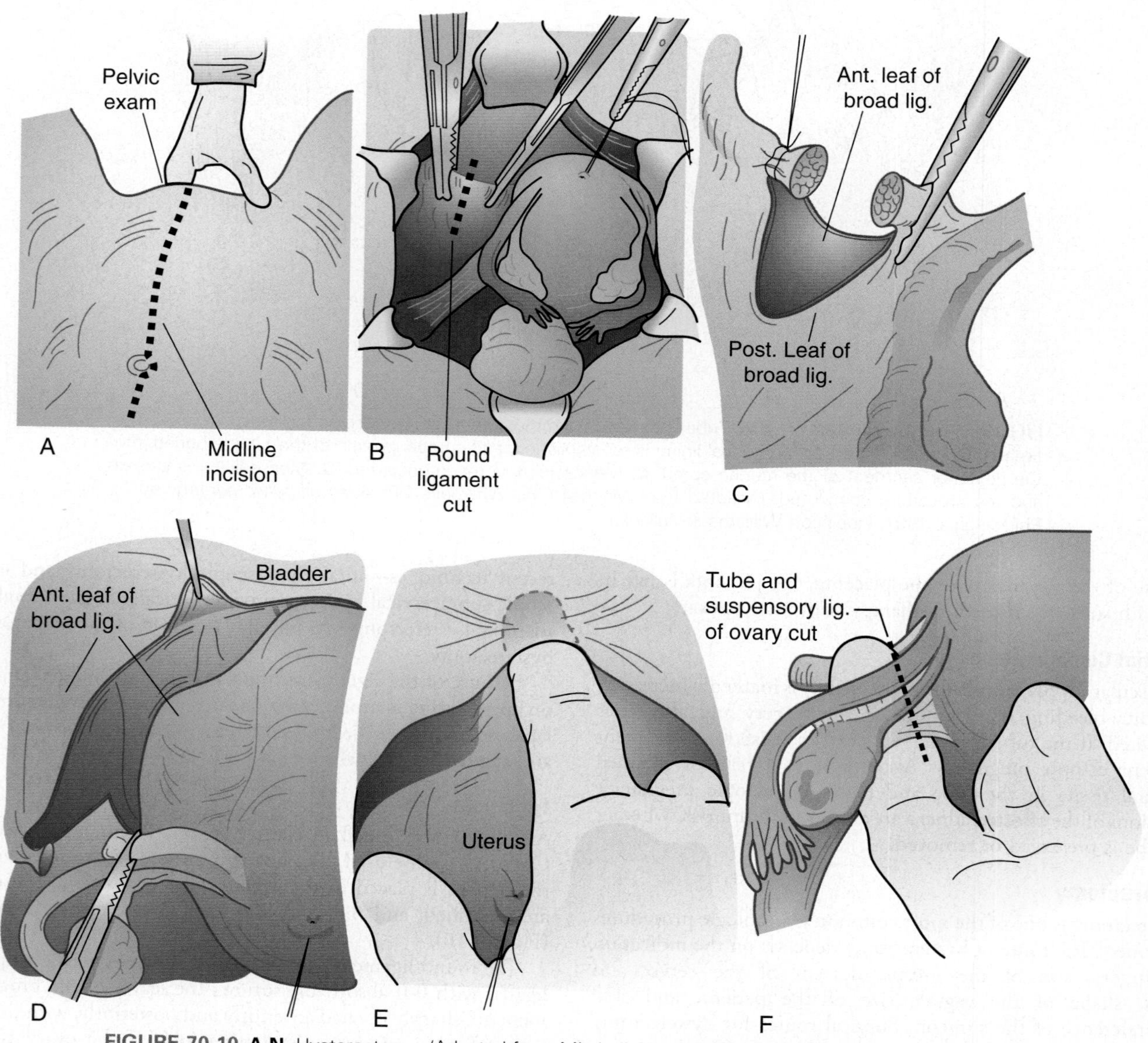

FIGURE 70-10 A-N, Hysterectomy. (Adapted from Mitchell CW, Wheeless CR: *Atlas of pelvic surgery*, ed 3, Philadelphia, 1997, Lippincott Williams & Wilkins.)

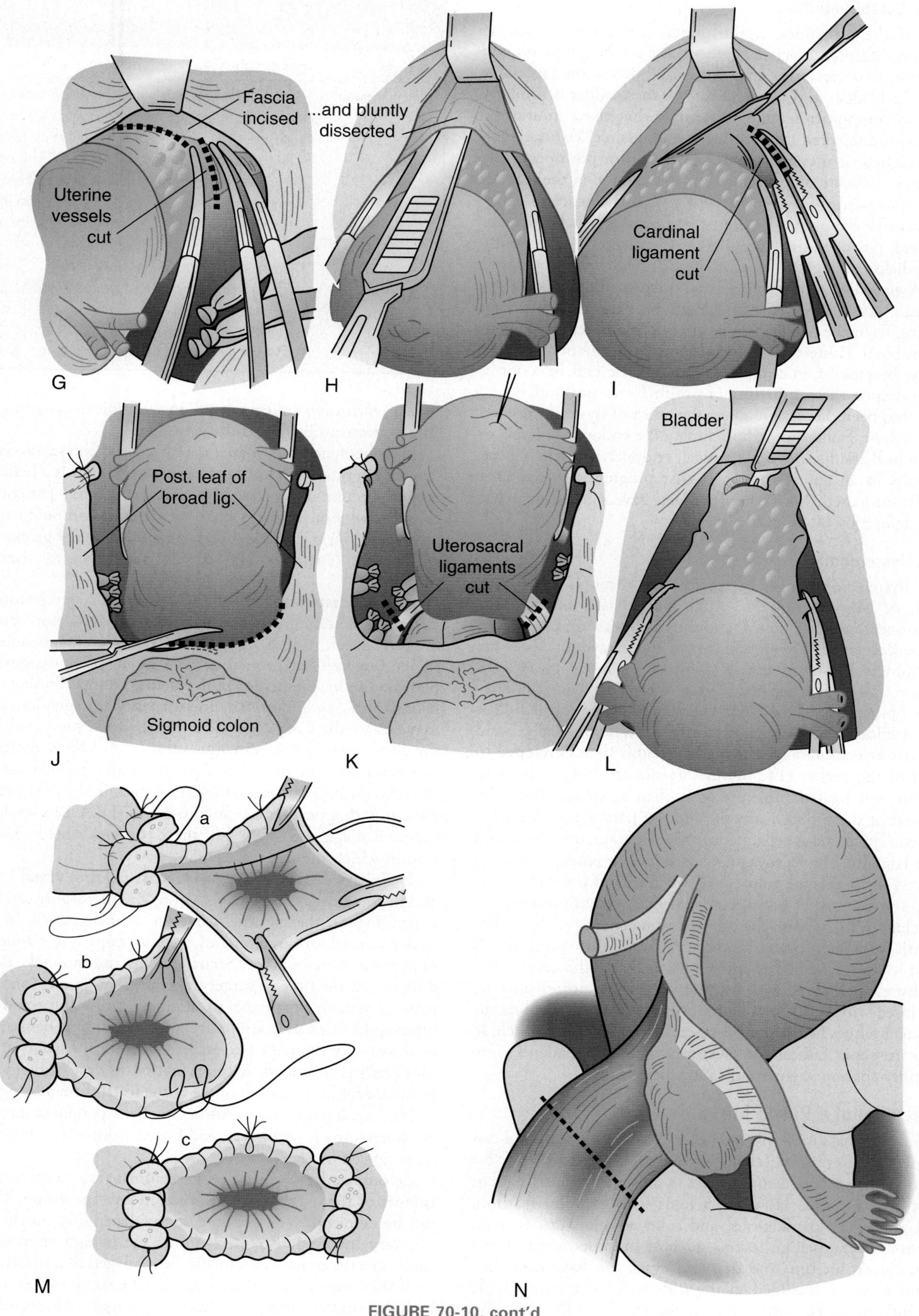

FIGURE 70-10, cont'd

Potential Complications

Because of the proximity of the ureter to the cervix, uterine vessels, and infundibulopelvic ligament, the ureter can be injured during the hysterectomy, and with the dissection necessary between the bladder and cervix, injury to the bladder is similarly a common complication. It is imperative that these injuries be recognized and repaired intraoperatively, if possible. Fistulas, such as vesicovaginal or ureterovaginal, can also form postoperatively secondary to ischemic injury caused by denudation of the bladder muscularis or partial entrapment with a vaginal closure stitch.

The vascular supply to the uterus and ovaries is rich. Intraoperative and postoperative bleeding is a concern. A previously secure pedicle can begin to bleed acutely during the postoperative period. A vaginal stump vessel, missed because of operative vasospasm, can cause a pelvic cuff hematoma. Thromboembolism originating from the pelvic vasculature is also a potential postoperative problem. Hysterectomy is considered a clean-contaminated procedure because of entering the vagina. Pelvic cuff infection is common despite the routine use of prophylactic antibiotics.

There has been discussion about the effect of hysterectomy on the pelvic floor. Failure to reapproximate the endopelvic fascia or failure to heal results in a large, apical, endopelvic fascial defect. This results in an apical enterocele that progresses in size over time. It is estimated that 60% of women have significant pelvic support defects by 60 years of age.

Radical Hysterectomy

Radical hysterectomy can be performed through a vertical, Cherney, or Maylard incision. After the pelvis is entered, the retroperitoneal space is opened, and the paravesical and pararectal spaces are developed. The boundaries of the paravesical space are the symphysis pubis anteriorly, cardinal ligament posteriorly, obliterated umbilical artery medially, and external iliac vein laterally. The boundaries of the pararectal space are the cardinal ligament anteriorly, sacrum posteriorly, ureter medially, and hypogastric artery laterally. The bladder flap is then developed to the level of the vagina. The uterine arteries are isolated back to the origin and ligated. The ureter is then separated from the medial leaf of the broad ligament, and the parametrial tunnel is developed. The ureter is separated from the parametrial tissue and is rolled laterally. The rectovaginal space is then entered, and the uterosacral ligaments are transected two thirds of the way to the sacrum. The amount of postoperative urinary retention is related to how close to the sacrum the uterosacral ligament is ligated. The parametria are then taken at the side wall. The specimen is removed when the vagina is entered 1 cm below the cervix. The angle sutures are secured with 0-0 Vicryl Heaney sutures, and the cuff is closed with 0-0 Vicryl figure-of-eight sutures. More recent surgical techniques for the management of cervical cancer include total laparoscopic radical hysterectomy with lymphadenectomy and fertility-sparing vaginal radical trachelectomy.

Management of a Pelvic Mass

When a pelvic mass is discovered on examination, ultrasound can be helpful in determining characteristics that are worrisome for malignancy. In general, a simple cyst in a premenopausal patient will not be cancerous. However, a mass with complex features, such as septations, papillations, and solid components, is more worrisome. Several benign lesions, such as endometriomas, hemorrhagic corpus luteum, and dermoid cysts, can have these features and must be included in the differential diagnosis (Table 70-2). Inflammatory conditions, including a TOA, can also appear worrisome on ultrasound, so the clinical scenario is important in determining the treatment plan.

TABLE 70-2 Differential Diagnosis of Ovarian Masses

MASS	DIFFERENTIAL DIAGNOSIS
Benign disease	Hemorrhagic corpus luteum, endometrioma, tubo-ovarian abscess, ectopic pregnancy, serous or mucinous cystadenoma, cystadenofibroma, fibroma, Brenner tumor, dermoid
Malignant disease	Serous borderline tumor, mucinous epithelial borderline tumor, invasive cancer (papillary serous, endometrioid, transitional cell, clear cell, neuroendocrine or small cell, malignant mixed müllerian tumor)
Germ cell	Dysgerminoma, endodermal sinus tumor, choriocarcinoma, immature teratoma, embryonal carcinoma, polyembryoma
Stromal	Sertoli-Leydig cell tumor, granulosa cell tumor
Metastasis	Colon cancer, stomach cancer, breast cancer, lymphoma

In a premenopausal patient with a simple cyst, ultrasound is repeated in 6 to 8 weeks to determine whether it is a hemorrhagic corpus luteum. However, in a postmenopausal patient with a complex adnexal mass, evaluation includes computed tomography to rule out metastatic disease or another site of primary tumor and barium enema study to rule out colon involvement or primary.[10]

Carbohydrate antigen 125 (CA 125) is a glycoprotein produced by certain tumors. Unfortunately, it is not specific for ovarian cancer; its level may be elevated in lung, appendiceal, and signet ring cell carcinomas as well as in other malignant neoplasms. In the premenopausal patient, benign findings such as leiomyomas, endometriosis, menstruation, pregnancy, and PID may elevate the CA 125 level. Other diseases, such as cirrhosis of the liver, may also elevate the value. CA 125 is therefore not checked in the premenopausal patient with a pelvic mass because the false-positive rate is too high. However, in the postmenopausal patient with a pelvic mass and an elevated CA 125 level, ovarian cancer is diagnosed in 80% of these patients. This is the population in which the test is helpful.

Definitive diagnosis of a pelvic mass requires visual inspection and histologic diagnosis. Laparoscopy or laparotomy can be done, depending on the clinical suspicion of malignancy. In patients with potential for carcinomatosis, laparoscopy is not done because of port site metastasis that occurs quickly and can make debulking difficult. At the time of surgery, pelvic washings are done, and the mass is visually inspected to augment prior information from ultrasound. If all indications are that the lesion is benign, ovarian cystectomy or drainage (see earlier, "Technical Aspects of Surgical Options") is indicated, with evaluation of cyst cytology or gross or microscopic evaluation of the tissue to confirm a benign lesion. If there is a higher level of suspicion or the patient is menopausal, oophorectomy is performed and frozen section histologic diagnosis is carried out.[11-13]

Serous and mucinous cystadenomas are common benign tumors of the ovary that can occur in any age group. Treatment can be cystectomy or oophorectomy, depending on the amount of ovary involved. Brenner tumors are benign transitional cell tumors of the ovary that can also be managed in a similar fashion.

If the lesion is an invasive, epithelial ovarian cancer, treatment includes hysterectomy, bilateral salpingo-oophorectomy, and omentectomy, with peritoneal biopsy specimens of the diaphragm, bilateral paracolic gutters, bilateral pelvis, and cul-de-sac and lymph node sampling. If the cell type is mucinous, an appendectomy is also performed to rule out metastasis from the appendix. Attention has turned toward minimally invasive (laparoscopic) and fertility-sparing surgical approaches. Interval laparoscopic staging of newly diagnosed ovarian tumors, with no suspicion of carcinomatosis, may be performed in selected patients.[8]

Extensive disease mandates tumor debulking to remove all possible tumor. Patients who undergo optimal tumor reductive surgery (<2 cm of visible disease) have a survival advantage over patients who cannot be or are not optimally debulked. Complete staging is important because patients who have a grade 1 or grade 2 stage IA ovarian cancer do not require chemotherapy. With other stages, surgery is followed by chemotherapy.

Borderline tumors do not behave like invasive ovarian cancers. Typically, they are treated with surgery alone and do not require chemotherapy. They tend to occur in younger women. If it is found at frozen section and the patient is finished with childbearing, pelvic washings, hysterectomy, bilateral salpingo-oophorectomy, omentectomy, peritoneal biopsies, and lymph node biopsies are performed. If the patient desires future fertility, a unilateral oophorectomy, omentectomy, peritoneal biopsies, and lymph node biopsies on the side of the tumor can be performed. The other ovary can then be monitored with ultrasound. Staging is done in case an invasive ovarian cancer is found at the time of final pathology. Mucinous borderline tumors have also been associated with abnormalities in the appendix. Therefore, an appendectomy is performed in conjunction with other staging.

Other types of ovarian tumors include sex cord stromal tumors, such as granulosa cell and Sertoli-Leydig cell tumors. These typically appear solid but occasionally have a cystic appearance. Hysterectomy, bilateral salpingo-oophorectomy, and staging are performed. For stage I tumors of the adult type, no further therapy is needed. For patients with a higher stage, postoperative chemotherapy or radiation therapy is added.

Germ cell tumors must be considered in girls and young women. The most common cell type is a dysgerminoma; 90% of these are diagnosed at stage I. Conservative surgery with unilateral oophorectomy and staging can be performed, leaving the uterus and other tube and ovary in place. No further treatment is needed.[14] Other germ cell tumors include endodermal sinus tumor, choriocarcinoma, immature teratoma, and embryonal carcinoma. A mixture of these cancers can be present. Tumor markers such as β-hCG, α-fetoprotein, and lactate dehydrogenase may be detected in certain germ cell tumors. Patients who have a gonadoblastoma must be tested by chromosome evaluation. If XY chromosomes are discovered, the gonads are removed to prevent the development of dysgerminoma. This may occur in 20% of patients with gonadoblastoma.

Because these are potentially aggressive tumors, postoperative chemotherapy is implemented with the diagnoses of teratoma (stage IA, grade 2 or grade 3 immature teratoma, or any higher stage), dysgerminoma (stage II and above), any endodermal sinus tumor, or choriocarcinoma.

SURGERY DURING PREGNANCY

Approximately 0.1% to 2.2% of pregnant women require surgery during pregnancy. Changes in maternal-fetal physiology, enlarging gestation, and changes in maternal organ placement can make diagnosis and treatment challenging. This section addresses important issues for the surgeon to consider before proceeding to the operating room.

Physiologic Changes

During pregnancy, multisystem adaptations result in altered physiology.

Cardiovascular System

Blood volume increases by 45% to 50% at term. Placental hormone production stimulates maternal erythropoiesis, which increases red cell mass by approximately 20%. This results in a functional hemodilution manifested by a physiologic anemia. Therefore, pregnancy needs to be considered a hypervolemic state.

The maternal heart rate increases as early as 7 weeks' gestation. In late pregnancy, the maternal heart rate is increased by approximately 20% over antepartum values. Systemic vascular resistance decreases by 20% but gradually increases near term. This results in a decrease in systolic and diastolic blood pressure during pregnancy, with a gradual recovery to nonpregnant values by term. Because there is increased pressure in the venous system, there is decreased return from the lower extremities, resulting in dependent edema.

Respiratory System

In pregnancy, minute volume is increased, whereas functional residual volume is decreased (Table 70-3). Although it seems intuitive that lung volume would decrease during pregnancy, an increase in minute volume in association with an expansion of the anterior and posterior diameter of the chest results in increased tidal volume, thereby also increasing minute ventilation. These changes result in a compensated respiratory alkalosis. Normal PCO_2 values in pregnancy range from 28 to 35 mm Hg. The PO_2

TABLE 70-3 Physiologic Changes of Pregnancy

SYSTEM	CHANGES	RESULT
Cardiovascular, hemodynamic	Blood volume increased by 50%; red cell mass increased by 20%; cardiac output increased by 50%; heart rate increased by 20%; systemic vascular resistance decreased by 20%	High-output cardiac state with a hemodilutional anemia
Respiratory	Minute volume increased by 20%; functional residual capacity decreased by 15%; tidal volume increased by 20% to 30%; oxygen consumption increased by 20%	Compensated respiratory alkalosis
Gastrointestinal	Smooth muscle relaxation; delayed gastrointestinal emptying	Full stomach; constipation
Coagulation	Fibrinogen increased by 30%; protein S decreased by 30% to 40%	Hypercoagulable state regardless of risk factors
Renal	Glomerular filtration rate increased by 50%; serum creatinine decreased by 40%; physiologic hydronephrosis	Increased urination; increased risk for upper tract infection

value is usually 100 mm Hg or higher. Oxygen consumption and basal metabolic rate are also increased during pregnancy by approximately 20%.

These physiologic changes result in less pulmonary reserve for the acutely ill pregnant patient, reducing the time needed for the deterioration of respiratory distress to respiratory failure. Early intervention is mandatory.

Gastrointestinal Tract

During pregnancy, there is a decrease in gastrointestinal motility caused by mechanical changes in the abdomen, with the enlarging uterus and smooth muscle relaxation resulting from the increased production of progesterone in pregnancy. Gastric emptying may be delayed for up to 8 hours. Pregnant women are considered to have a functionally full stomach at all times. In addition, a decrease in large intestine motility may result in constipation severe enough to cause significant abdominal pain.

Coagulation Changes

Pregnancy is a hypercoagulable state. Fibrinogen is increased approximately 30% over baseline values. The hypercoagulable state of pregnancy is associated with an increased risk for deep venous thrombosis and pulmonary embolus. This is particularly compounded when bed rest or immobilization occurs during the gestational period.

Renal Changes

Pregnancy increases blood flow to the renal pelvis by approximately 50%. This results in an increased glomerular filtration rate. Frequent urination is common. The serum creatinine level is approximately 40% less than in a nonpregnant state. Therefore, a creatinine level of 1 mg/dL during gestation is considered abnormal.

Ureteral diameter increases in pregnancy secondary to compression and smooth muscle relaxation. Peristalsis is delayed, and reflux occurs freely from the bladder into the lower ureteral segment. This results in an increased incidence of pyelonephritis during pregnancy. Therefore, asymptomatic bacteriuria must be aggressively treated.

Diagnostic Considerations and Evaluation

Imaging Techniques

The most common imaging technique used during pregnancy is ultrasound, which is considered the safest modality and is used for fetal assessment. In patients with abdominal pain, ultrasound is considered the first-line diagnostic test. During ultrasound, the presence of an intrauterine pregnancy needs to be documented, if possible. In addition, evaluation of the cul-de-sac for fluid, the ureter for dilation or stones, the gallbladder for the presence of gallstones, and the placenta for abnormalities can be carried out.

MRI also can be used during pregnancy. To date, no evidence has suggested an increased risk from this modality; in fact, MRI is used to diagnose fetal abnormalities, especially abnormalities of the central nervous system.

Although there are theoretical risks associated with ionizing radiation, most diagnostic x-ray procedures are associated with minimal or no risk to the fetus. Evidence suggests that there is no increased risk to the fetus with regard to congenital malformations, growth restriction, or abortion from x-ray procedures that expose the fetus to doses of 5 cGy or less. In 1995, the American College of Obstetrics and Gynecology published guidelines regarding diagnostic imaging during pregnancy. Women need to be reassured that concern about radiation exposure must not prevent medically indicated diagnostic procedures. It cannot be stressed enough that maternal well-being is of the utmost importance, and appropriate diagnostic procedures need to be performed to facilitate a rapid diagnosis.

Clinical Evaluation

Abdominal pain during pregnancy can be confusing to the clinician. It is natural for the clinician to attribute most abdominal pain to the pregnancy; however, other organ systems are affected during pregnancy at the rate of the general population. In addition to these diagnoses, diagnosis specific to pregnancy also needs to be considered.

Common Surgical Complications of Pregnancy

Appendicitis

Appendicitis is one of the most common surgical complications of pregnancy, with an incidence of approximately 2/1000 pregnant women. This incidence is no higher than that of the general population; however, appendiceal location during pregnancy changes with the upward displacement of the appendix with advancing gestation (Fig. 70-11). Nevertheless, the most common presenting symptom is pain in the right lower quadrant, which is manifested regardless of gestational age. The diagnosis of appendicitis in pregnancy may be difficult because many of the symptoms of appendicitis are seen during pregnancy. Pain in the right lower quadrant may be mistaken for round ligament pain, and nausea, vomiting, and abdominal discomfort may be mistaken for hyperemesis gravidarum. Because mild leukocytosis is commonly seen in pregnancy, it may confound the diagnosis. However, other symptoms, such as fever and anorexia, can help the clinician establish the diagnosis. Ultrasonography may be used but is of limited value if bowel loops are distended. Computed tomography without contrast enhancement can be used, if needed, to assist in the diagnosis.

Rupture of the appendix during pregnancy increases perinatal morbidity and mortality. This is particularly true when rupture occurs after 20 weeks' gestation. Peritonitis increases the risk for preterm labor and preterm delivery. Therefore, it is prudent that the clinician make an early diagnosis and proceed immediately with surgical intervention.

Cholelithiasis

After appendicitis, biliary tract disease is the second most common general surgical condition encountered during pregnancy. Cholelithiasis of pregnancy usually develops from obstruction of the cystic duct. The clinical presentation ranges from intermittent attacks of biliary colic to persistent pain radiating into the subcapsular area in patients in whom the common bile duct is obstructed by a stone. Ultrasound is helpful for detecting the presence of stones. The differential diagnosis of acute cholelithiasis includes acute pain in the liver of pregnancy, the HELLP (hemolysis, elevated liver enzymes, low platelets) syndrome, and severe preeclampsia. Initial attacks may be treated conservatively with IV fluids, antibiotics, and antispasmodics; however, without prompt resolution of symptoms, surgery needs to be considered. Delay of surgery in a patient with cholecystitis may increase perinatal morbidity. Despite the potential difficulty of operating on a pregnant woman, lower morbidity has been shown in patients managed surgically, particularly in cases involving obstruction. In early gestation, laparoscopic cholecystectomy can be considered.

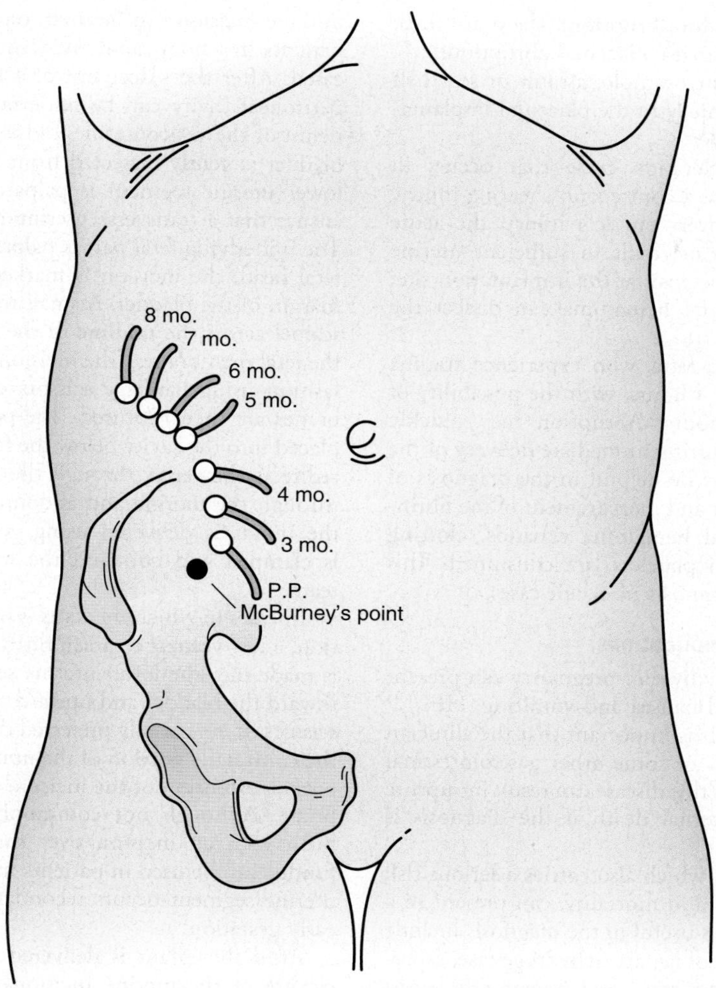

FIGURE 70-11 The approximate location of the appendix during succeeding months of pregnancy is illustrated. In planning an operation, it is better to make the abdominal incision over the point of maximum tenderness unless there is a great disparity between that point and the theoretical location of the appendix. (From Ludmir J, Stubblefield PG: Surgical procedures in pregnancy. In Gabbe S, Neibyl JR, Simpson JL, editors: *Obstetrics: Normal and problem pregnancies*, ed 4, Philadelphia, 2002, Churchill Livingstone, p 617.)

Although rare, pancreatitis may present during pregnancy. The most common cause of pancreatitis in pregnant women is cholelithiasis. However, pancreatitis can be a complication of severe preeclampsia or HELLP syndrome. Pancreatitis caused by milk-alkali toxicity may be seen in patients with an excessive intake of antacids.[15]

Intestinal Obstruction

The incidence of intestinal obstruction in pregnant women is similar to that of the general population. Patients present with classic symptoms of the abdominal colicky pain associated with hyperactive peristalsis. Nausea and vomiting are present in approximately 80% of cases. Bowel distention is marked. Laparotomy needs to be performed before bowel necrosis and perforation occur. If perforation occurs during pregnancy, there is a significant increase in maternal and perinatal morbidity and mortality.

Ovarian Masses

With the frequent use of ultrasound in early pregnancy, the corpus luteum cyst of pregnancy is frequently identified. This is physiologic and, in the absence of symptoms of torsion, requires only follow-up to ensure the diagnosis. The progesterone produced in the first 14 weeks of gestation is necessary to support the pregnancy until placental production of progesterone replaces it. Therefore, if surgery is required for symptoms of torsion or bleeding, every effort must be made to preserve the corpus luteum in the first trimester.[16]

Obstetric Complications Resulting in Abdominal Pain

Placental Abruption

Placental abruption usually occurs in the third trimester and may be associated with excruciating abdominal pain. Contrary to popular belief, overt vaginal bleeding does not need to be present in order for the diagnosis to be made. Ultrasonography is of little use because only 5% to 10% of abruptions can be seen. Therefore, the diagnosis of abruption is clinical. Abruptions are usually associated with uterine hypertonicity, resulting in fetal heart rate abnormalities. It is important for the clinician to diagnose abruption rapidly.

Trauma may increase the risk for abruption. There are three distinct mechanisms for post-traumatic placental abruption:

1. Blunt trauma to the uterus; for example, assault or seat belt placement can cause a direct injury to the placental implantation site.
2. The sudden acceleration-deceleration cycle that occurs in motor vehicle crashes can cause a contrecoup shearing injury.
3. Even in the absence of any overt physical injury, the acute adrenergic reaction to stress can result in sufficient uterine vasospasm to create ischemic necrosis at the implantation site; with reperfusion, a subplacental hematoma can dissect the plane of the implantation site.

The pregnant patient and her fetus who experience trauma need to be monitored for at least 4 hours, with the possibility of prolonged monitoring for 24 hours. Abruption may quickly become a surgical emergency, requiring immediate delivery of the fetus. Laboratory studies that may be helpful in the diagnosis of abruption include a platelet count and measurement of the fibrinogen level. As the retroplacental hematoma expands, clotting factors, especially fibrinogen and platelets, are consumed. This may assist the clinician in the diagnosis in occult cases.

Pregnancy-Related Hepatic Complications

HELLP syndrome and acute fatty liver of pregnancy can present as right upper quadrant pain and nausea and vomiting. HELLP is a form of severe preeclampsia. It is important that the clinician not mistake this for cholelithiasis or some other gastrointestinal pathologic process. Progression of this disease can result in rupture of the hepatic capsule and maternal death if the diagnosis is missed.

Acute fatty liver of pregnancy, which also carries a serious risk for maternal and fetal morbidity and mortality, can present in a similar fashion. Laboratory studies useful in the diagnosis include platelet count and determination of lactate dehydrogenase, aspartate transaminase, creatinine, uric acid, and hematocrit levels. Aspartate transaminase and lactate dehydrogenase levels will be elevated, platelets will be decreased, and the hematocrit value may be increased, especially in association with intravascular volume depletion. In patients with acute fatty liver, the glucose level may also be decreased. It is important that the clinician remember the physiologic changes when interpreting values discussed at the beginning of this chapter.

Trauma

Trauma from accidental injuries occurs in 6% to 7% of all pregnancies. In addition to the risk for placental abruption noted, blunt trauma may increase the risk for preterm labor and preterm rupture of the membranes. It is important that pregnant trauma patients be assessed for the same spectrum of injuries as nonpregnant patients. A number of studies have established that fetal-maternal hemorrhage is increased in women who have suffered trauma. Women who are RhD negative need to have a quantitative assessment of the volume of fetal cells in maternal circulation and an appropriate dose of anti-D immune globulin administered. Peritoneal lavage is not contraindicated in pregnancy and can be performed safely in those patients in whom the possibility of a ruptured viscus is suspected.

Common Obstetric Surgical Procedures

The most common obstetric procedure that the surgeon will perform is cesarean delivery. Most cesarean births are performed through a Pfannenstiel incision; however, a vertical subumbilical midline incision can be used, especially in obese patients and in patients in whom rapid entry into the abdominal cavity is indicated. After the placement of a bladder catheter, entry into the peritoneal cavity can be undertaken. In most cases, the peritoneum of the vesicouterine fold is transected transversely, and the bladder is gently dissected from the lower uterine segment. The lower uterine segment is palpated to check for malrotation to ensure that a transverse uterine incision centers on the midline. The underlying fetal part is palpated. If the presenting part is the fetal head, the incision is marked 1 to 2 cm above the original margin of the bladder. A small transverse incision is made with a scalpel across the midline of the lower uterine segment down to the fetal membranes. The incision may be extended in a transverse fashion using bandage scissors or in blunt fashion. The membranes are then ruptured. The physician's nondominant hand is placed into the cavity below the fetal head to provide leverage that redirects the vertex through the incision. The vertex is delivered through the uterine and abdominal incisions. The remainder of the infant is delivered using gentle fundal pressure. The cord is clamped and cut, and the fetus is handed to the receiving team.

In cases in which the fetus is in a transverse or breech presentation, a low vertical cesarean birth is performed. A vertical incision is made into the lower uterine segment and extended downward toward the bladder and upward toward the fundus using bandage scissors. It is generally preferred that the incision not be taken into the contractile portion of the uterus; however, if head entrapment occurs, extension of the incision in a cephalad direction is appropriate. Although not commonly performed, a classic cesarean birth with an incision over the anterior and superior uterine fundus can be used in patients in whom obstruction of the lower uterine segment occurs secondary to uterine fibroids or in very early gestation.

After the infant is delivered through the incision of choice, closure of the uterine incision may be aided by removing the uterine fundus through the abdominal incision. Delivery of the fundus also facilitates uterine massage. Oxytocin is administered through an IV line. It is recommended that 20 units of oxytocin be placed into a 1-liter bag of IV fluid, with care taken not to run the fluids at a rate of more than 200 mL/hr in most cases. The uterine incision is closed using an interlocking suture of 1-0 Vicryl or a chromic suture. A second imbricating layer may be used to achieve hemostasis. After the uterus incision is reapproximated and completed, care is taken to investigate for bleeding. The abdomen may be irrigated if there is spillage of meconium or vernix outside the operative field. There is no need to reapproximate the peritoneum or rectus muscles. The abdominal wall is closed in the usual fashion with absorbable suture.

It is possible that the surgeon may be called to assist a patient with postpartum hemorrhage. Therefore, it is important to recognize factors that may be unique to pregnancy. As noted at the beginning of the chapter, blood volume is increased during pregnancy. Hemorrhage in pregnancy is defined as blood loss in excess of 1000 mL. Because of the increase in blood volume by term, however, the patient may lose 1500 to 2000 mL of blood before symptoms are manifested. The most common cause of postpartum hemorrhage is uterine atony. Risk factors for uterine atony include prolonged labor, uterine infection, cesarean birth, and overdistention of the uterus. Hemorrhage can also be seen in abruption of the placenta and in patients with placenta previa, before or after delivery. It is recommended that therapy be initiated after the loss of 600 mL.[15,17]

The first step is to assess for vaginal, cervical, or uterine lacerations. If this assessment is negative and uterine atony is the mechanism, manual exploration of the uterus is initiated to ensure complete removal of the placenta, and aggressive fundal massage is begun. If this is unsuccessful, the administration of a solution of oxytocin, 20 units/liter of physiologic saline solution at a rate of 200 mL/hr, may assist with uterine contractility. A rate of as high as 500 mL in 10 minutes can be administered without significant cardiovascular complications; however, maternal hypotension may occur with an IV bolus injection of as low as 5 units.

When oxytocin fails to provide an adequate response, a synthetic 15-methyl prostaglandin $F_{2\alpha}$ (carboprost) is administered intramuscularly or in the uterine wall. In addition, methylergonovine maleate (Methergine), 0.2 mg given intramuscularly, may be administered. Methergine is contraindicated in patients with hypertension. Prostaglandin $F_{2\alpha}$ is contraindicated in patients with asthma. Misoprostol (Cytotec) also has uterotonic properties and can be used at a dose of 1000 μg per rectum.

When pharmacologic measures fail to control hemorrhage, surgical measures are undertaken. If the hemorrhage is secondary to uterine atony, ligation of the uterine vessels may be successful. The first step in ligating the uterine arteries is at the anastomosis of the uterine and ovarian artery high on the fundus, just below the utero-ovarian ligament. A large suture on the atraumatic needle can be passed from the uterus around the vessel and tied. If bilateral utero-ovarian vessel ligation does not stop the bleeding, temporary atraumatic occlusion of the ovarian arteries in the infundibulopelvic ligaments may be attempted. By decreasing perfusion pressure, thrombosis in the vascular bed may produce hemostasis.

If conservative measures are unsuccessful, a cesarean hysterectomy may need to be performed before sequelae of coagulopathy and hemorrhagic shock occur. In the case of postpartum hemorrhage, supracervical hysterectomy is often the procedure of choice. As for the gynecologic hysterectomy described earlier, the superior attachments of the uterus are separated, but after ligation of the uterine arteries, the fundus of the uterus is amputated from the cervix, which is closed with figure-of-eight sutures. This procedure also maintains the integrity of the uterosacral ligaments.

It is difficult to remove the cervix, especially after a vaginal delivery, secondary to dilation of the lower uterine segment. Only surgeons who are skilled in this procedure can proceed without consultation.

Other Procedures

On rare occasions, the surgeon may be consulted to assist with the repair of an episiotomy and extension. Episiotomy is an incision into the perineal body made to help facilitate delivery. Most episiotomies are cut in the midline from the posterior fourchette toward the rectum. Although more comfortable for the patient, these incisions may extend through the anal sphincter (third degree) or through the rectal wall (fourth degree). An inappropriate repair may result in a rectovaginal fistula. These fistulas present with the same symptoms as those seen in other rectal fistulas associated with Crohn's disease but are much easier to repair and have a lower rate of recurrence.

Repair of an episiotomy requires reapproximation of the vaginal tissue and perineal body. Repair of the anal sphincter requires that the fascial capsule that usually retracts posteriorly be identified and reapproximated. If the rectal wall has been compromised, a multilayer closure of mucosa, muscularis, rectovaginal fascia, anal sphincter, vaginal muscularis, and vaginal mucosa using 2-0 or 3-0 absorbable sutures will provide the best opportunity to avoid a fistula. Because of the increased vascularity associated with pregnancy, with an adequate closure without stitch-induced tissue necrosis, healing is not usually a problem.

ACKNOWLEDGMENT

This chapter is a revision of the chapter written by Stephen S. Entman, Cornelia R. Graves, Barry K. Jarnagin, and Gautam G. Rao for the 18th edition of *Sabiston Textbook of Surgery*. I gratefully acknowledge their contribution and am honored to build on their work.

SELECTED REFERENCES

Baggish MS, Karram MM, editors: *Atlas of pelvic anatomy and gynecologic surgery*, ed 3, Philadelphia, 2011, WB Saunders.

Detailed pelvic anatomy and comprehensive coverage of gynecologic procedures with excellent illustrations are presented.

Edge SB, Byrd DR, Compton CC, et al: *AJCC cancer staging handbook*, ed 7, Philadelphia, 2010, Springer.

Comprehensive staging handbook for gynecologic and other cancers.

Fritz MA, Speroff L: *Clinical gynecologic endocrinology and infertility*, ed 8, Philadelphia, 2011, Lippincott Williams & Wilkins.

This is the classic text that explains the pathophysiology and endocrinology of menstrual abnormalities in practical clinical terms.

Hacker NF, Gambone JC, Hobel CJ, editors: *Hacker and Moore's essential of obstetrics and gynecology*, ed 5, Philadelphia, 2010, WB Saunders.

Excellent coverage of obstetrics and gynecology, with color illustrations and photographs.

Rock JA, Jones HW III, editors: *TeLinde's operative gynecology*, ed 10, Philadephia, 2003, Lippincott Williams & Wilkins.

Encyclopedic coverage addresses all areas of gynecologic surgery, with an expanded oncology section.

REFERENCES

1. Espindola D, Kennedy KA, Fischer EG: Management of abnormal uterine bleeding and the pathology of endometrial hyperplasia. *Obstet Gynecol Clin North Am* 34:717–737, 2007.
2. Goldstein SR: Abnormal uterine bleeding: The role of ultrasound. *Radiol Clin North Am* 44:901–910, 2006.
3. Dimitraki M, Tsikouras P, Bouchlariotou S, et al: Clinical evaluation of women with PMB. Is it always necessary an endometrial biopsy to be performed? A review of the literature. *Arch Gynecol Obstet* 283:261–266, 2011.

4. Barnhart KT: Clinical practice. Ectopic pregnancy. *N Engl J Med* 361:379–387, 2009.
5. Ehrenberg-Buchner S, Sandadi S, Moawad NS, et al: Ectopic pregnancy: Role of laparoscopic treatment. *Clin Obstet Gynecol* 52:372–379, 2009.
6. Wølner-Hanssen P, Mårdh PA, Svensson L, et al: Laparoscopy in women with chlamydial infection and pelvic pain: A comparison of patients with and without salpingitis. *Obstet Gynecol* 61:299–303, 1983.
7. Jonsdottir GM, Jorgensen S, Cohen SL, et al: Increasing minimally invasive hysterectomy: Effect on cost and complications. *Obstet Gynecol* 117:1142–1149, 2011.
8. Subramaniam A, Kim KH, Bryant SA, et al: A cohort study evaluating robotic versus laparotomy surgical outcomes of obese women with endometrial carcinoma. *Gynecol Oncol* 122:604–607, 2011.
9. Paley PJ, Veljovich DS, Shah CA, et al: Surgical outcomes in gynecologic oncology in the era of robotics: Analysis of first 1000 cases. *Am J Obstet Gynecol* 204:551.e1–551.e9, 2011.
10. Guzel AI, Kuyumcuoglu U, Erdemoglu M: Adnexal masses in postmenopausal and reproductive age women. *J Exp Ther Oncol* 9:167–169, 2011.
11. Liu JH, Zanotti KM: Management of the adnexal mass. *Obstet Gynecol* 117:1413–1428, 2011.
12. Gad MS, El Khouly NI, Soto E, et al: Differences in perioperative outcomes after laparoscopic management of benign and malignant adnexal masses. *J Gynecol Oncol* 22:18–24, 2011.
13. Perutelli A, Garibaldi S, Basile S, et al: Laparoscopic adnexectomy of suspect ovarian masses: Surgical technique used to avert spillage. *J Minim Invasive Gynecol* 18:372–377, 2011.
14. Eskander RN, Bristow RE, Saenz NC, et al: A retrospective review of the effect of surgeon specialty on the management of 190 benign and malignant pediatric and adolescent adnexal masses. *J Pediatr Adolesc Gynecol* 24:282–285, 2011.
15. Hull AD, Resnik R: Placenta accreta and postpartum hemorrhage. *Clin Obstet Gynecol* 53:228–236, 2010.
16. Hoover K, Jenkins TR: Evaluation and management of adnexal mass in pregnancy. *Am J Obstet Gynecol* 205:97–102, 2011.
17. Gonsalves M, Belli A: The role of interventional radiology in obstetric hemorrhage. *Cardiovasc Intervent Radiol* 33:887–895, 2010.

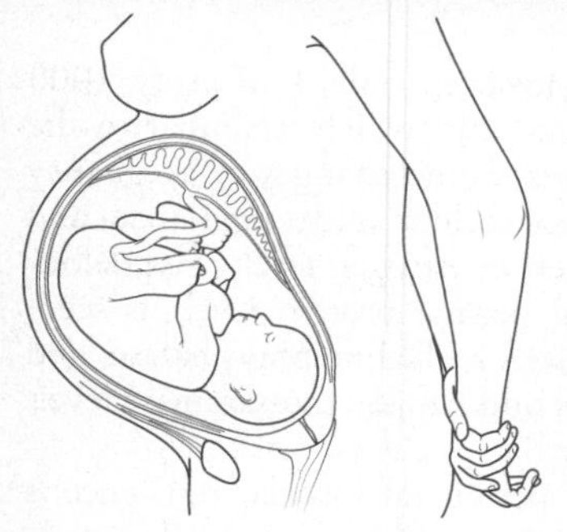

CHAPTER 71

Surgery in the Pregnant Patient

Dean J. Mikami, Jon C. Henry, E. Christopher Ellison

OUTLINE

The pregnant patient presents a complex clinical challenge. An estimated 1% to 2% of pregnant women require surgical procedures, and nonobstetric surgery is necessary in up to 1% of pregnancies in the United States each year. A review by Cohen-Kerem and colleagues[1] evaluated the effects of nonobstetric surgical procedures on maternal and fetal outcomes. These authors reviewed 44 articles and 12,452 patients and reported a maternal death rate of 0.006% and a miscarriage rate of 5.8%. Most indications for surgical intervention are conditions that are common for the patient's age group and unrelated to pregnancy, such as acute appendicitis, symptomatic cholelithiasis, breast masses, or trauma. Changes in maternal anatomy and physiology and safety of the fetus are among the most important issues of which the surgeon must be cognizant. The presentation of surgical diseases in a pregnant patient may be atypical or may mimic signs and symptoms associated with a normal pregnancy, and a standard evaluation may be unreliable because of pregnancy-associated changes in diagnostic tests or laboratory values. Finally, many physicians may be more conservative in diagnostic evaluation and treatment. Any of these factors may result in a delay in diagnosis and treatment, adversely affecting maternal and fetal outcome. Although consultation with an obstetrician is ideal when caring for a pregnant patient, the surgeon needs to be aware of certain fundamental principles when such a consultation is unavailable. This chapter discusses the key points in caring for a pregnant patient who presents with nonobstetric surgical disease.

PHYSIOLOGIC CHANGES OF PREGNANCY

Pregnancy induces many changes to the maternal body through hormonal and mechanical alterations. Normal laboratory and vital sign values differ in the pregnant versus the nonpregnant patient (Table 71-1). Progesterone and estrogen, two of the principal hormones of pregnancy, mediate many of the maternal physiologic changes in pregnancy. Perhaps the greatest hormonal change is seen in smooth muscle tone; elevated progesterone levels and decreased motilin levels lead to relaxation of smooth muscle, which has effects on several body systems. The growing gravid uterus has increasing effects on adjacent maternal organs simply as a result of compression. These changes may also mimic similar pathophysiology that occurs in nonpregnant patients who have cardiac or liver diseases that increase intra-abdominal volumes.

Pregnancy induces multiple changes in the maternal gastrointestinal tract. The gravid uterus expands and displaces the stomach and intestines, which may lead to confusion in diagnoses of intra-abdominal pathology. In the stomach, decreased smooth muscle tone results in diminished gastric tone and motility leading to delayed gastric emptying.[2] The lower esophageal sphincter tone is also decreased; when combined with increased intra-abdominal pressure, this results in an increase in the incidence of gastroesophageal reflux, which may be seen in 80% of pregnant women.[3] Small bowel motility is reduced, increasing small bowel transit time because of compression and decreased smooth muscle tone. However, absorption of nutrients remains unchanged with the exception of iron absorption, which is increased because of increased iron requirements. In women with hyperemesis gravidarum, the severe nausea and vomiting may lead to significant nutrient and electrolyte abnormalities.[4] In the colon, pregnancy-related changes usually manifest as constipation, which is due to a combination of increased colonic sodium and water absorption, decreased motility, and mechanical obstruction by the gravid uterus. An increase in portal venous pressure and in the pressure in the collateral venous circulation results in dilation of the veins at the gastroesophageal junction and in the hemorrhoidal veins leading to hemorrhoids, which are common in many pregnant women.

The liver and biliary systems are also affected by pregnancy. The motility of the gallbladder is decreased, as the chemical composition of bile is altered with increased cholesterol saturation, which leads to more stone and sludge formation during pregnancy. The risk of stones increases with multiple pregnancies. During the second and third trimesters, the volume of the gallbladder may be twice that found in the nonpregnant state, and gallbladder emptying is markedly slower. Up to 11% of pregnant patients have gallstones on routine obstetric ultrasound scans, and

TABLE 71-1 System-Based Physiologic Changes of Pregnancy

Gastrointestinal Tract	
Gastric emptying	Decreased
Gastroesophageal reflux	Increased
Small bowel motility	Decreased
Absorption of iron	Increased
Absorption of all other nutrients	Unchanged
Colonic motility	Decreased
Colonic sodium and water absorption	Increased
Portal venous pressure	Increased
Hepatobiliary System	
Biliary stasis	Increased
Biliary stone production	Increased
Biliary sludge	Increased
Cholecystitis	Unchanged
Albumin levels	Decreased
Alkaline phosphatase levels	Increased
Bilirubin and hepatic transaminase levels	Unchanged
Cardiovascular System	
Heart rate	Increased
Stroke volume	Increased
Mean arterial pressure	Decreased
Vascular resistance	Decreased
Left ventricular mass	Increased
Hematologic System	
Plasma volume	Increased
Red blood cell mass	Increased
Hemoglobin/hematocrit	Decreased
White blood cell mass	Increased
Platelet number	Decreased
Coagulation	Increased
Respiratory System	
Total lung capacity	Decreased
Functional residual capacity	Decreased
Residual capacity	Decreased
Expiratory reserve capacity	Decreased
Inspiratory capacity	Increased
Vital capacity	Unchanged
Oxygen consumption	Increased
PaO_2	Increased
$PaCO_2$	Decreased
Renal System	
Glomerular filtration rate	Increased
Creatinine levels	Decreased
Serum osmolality	Decreased
Endocrine System	
Cortisol levels	Increased
T_4	Increased
TSH	Decreased

$PaCO_2$, Partial arterial carbon dioxide tension; *PaO_2,* partial arterial oxygen tension; *TSH,* thyroid-stimulating hormone; *T_4,* thyroxine.

one third have biliary sludge. However, only 1 of every 1000 pregnant patients develops cholecystitis, which is similar to the incidence in nonpregnant patients. Some changes of pregnancy closely resemble liver disease. These include spider angiomata and palmar erythema from elevated serum estrogen levels. Hypoalbuminemia with decreases in total plasma protein levels is seen, along with elevated serum cholesterol, alkaline phosphatase, and fibrinogen levels. Serum bilirubin and hepatic transaminase levels are unchanged during pregnancy.[3]

In the cardiovascular system, peripheral vascular resistance is decreased by 30% because of diminished vascular smooth muscle tone.[5] Cardiac output increases by 50% during the first trimester of pregnancy and is induced by several factors.[4] There is a gradual increase in maternal heart rate that peaks at 15% to 25% higher in the third trimester. Stroke volume, or the amount of blood pumped during each cardiac cycle, increases 20% to 30% during pregnancy. To accommodate the increased work on the heart, the mass of the left ventricle increases during pregnancy and is 50% larger at term. Despite the decrease in vascular resistance, systolic blood pressure is maintained during pregnancy often with a decrease in diastolic blood pressure, which leads to a slightly lower mean arterial pressure during most of pregnancy.[5]

During the third trimester, cardiac output is dramatically decreased when the mother is lying supine as a result of compromised venous return from compression of the inferior vena cava and impaired arterial perfusion from aortic compression by the gravid uterus.[2] With this decrease in preload, an increase in sympathetic tone usually maintains peripheral vascular resistance and blood pressure. However, 10% of patients may experience supine hypotensive syndrome, in which the sympathetic response is inadequate to maintain blood pressure. During anesthesia induction in the operating room, anesthetic agents may inhibit the compensatory sympathetic response, causing a more precipitous fall in blood pressure. From a surgeon's perspective, it may be necessary to place the patient in a 30-degree left lateral decubitus position during procedures performed during the third trimester, relieving compression on the inferior vena cava by the enlarged uterus.

Venous compression by the gravid uterus has significant effects on the maternal venous system. Compression of the inferior vena cava and iliac veins increases venous pressure to the lower extremities, which leads to increased varicose veins and venous claudication during pregnancy. Inguinal swelling secondary to varicosities of the round ligament also occurs during pregnancy. This swelling is often mistaken for an inguinal or femoral hernia. Appropriate management includes careful physical examination and ultrasound if needed. The varicosities of the round ligament should resolve postpartum, but the lifetime risk of lower extremity varicose veins is increased proportionally to the number of pregnancies for a woman.[6]

Throughout pregnancy, there is a 40% to 50% increase in plasma volume secondary to increased sodium and water retention. There is an increase in red blood cell mass of 30% despite a hemodilutional anemia in pregnancy from the increased plasma volume. Leukocytes progressively increase during pregnancy to 6000 to 16,000 cells/mm^3 in the second and third trimesters. Platelet count progressively declines throughout pregnancy, whereas the mean platelet volume tends to increase after 28 weeks of gestation.[4] There is an increase in clotting factors during pregnancy. Fibrinogen levels are elevated to 400 to 500 mg/dL. Plasma levels of factors V, VII, VIII, IX, X, and XII and von Willebrand antigen also progressively increase, whereas levels of factors XI and

XII and protein S decline, and an acquired resistance develops to protein C. Increased venous stasis and a hypercoagulable state lead to a fivefold increase in the rate of venous thromboembolism events during pregnancy.[7]

The respiratory system is affected by both the mechanical and the hormonal changes of pregnancy. The diaphragm can be elevated in pregnancy up to 4 cm by the gravid uterus, and the circumference of the lower chest wall can widen up to 7 cm as a result of ligamentous relaxation of the rib cage. Lung volume changes are also seen with pregnancy. Total lung capacity decreases 5%, but vital capacity is unchanged because the reduction is the functional residual capacity, which is reduced up to 25%. Because of the decrease in functional residual volume, there is a decrease in volume in both the residual and the expiratory reserve volumes. During pregnancy, inspiratory capacity may be increased 10%.[2] Oxygen consumption increases by 30% with a 15% increase in metabolic rate; this leaves pregnant women with smaller oxygen reserves and they are more susceptible to hypoxia. Minute ventilation increases by 50% as a result of an increase in tidal volume and respiratory rate, which appears to be a result of elevated serum progesterone level. The elevated progesterone not only increases the sensitivity of the respiratory centers to carbon dioxide (CO_2) but also acts as a direct stimulant to the respiratory centers. As a consequence of the increased minute ventilation, maternal partial arterial oxygen tension (PaO_2) levels during late pregnancy are 101 to 105 mm Hg, and maternal partial arterial carbon dioxide tension ($PaCO_2$) is 28 to 31 mm Hg. The decreased $PaCO_2$ increases the CO_2 gradient from the fetus to the mother, facilitating CO_2 transfer from the fetus to the mother. The oxygen-hemoglobin dissociation curve of maternal blood is shifted to the right; this, coupled with the increased affinity for oxygen of fetal hemoglobin, results in increased oxygen transfer to the fetus.[4]

In the kidney, the increased systemic vasodilation and increased plasma volume lead to an increase in the glomerular filtration rate of 50%. Urinary glucose excretion increases as a direct consequence of the increased glomerular filtration rate. Blood urea nitrogen decreases by 25% during the first trimester and stays at that level for the remainder of pregnancy. Serum creatinine also decreases by the end of the first trimester from a nonpregnant value of 0.8 mg/dL to 0.7 mg/dL and may be 0.5 mg/dL by term.[2,4] A 5- to 10-fold increase in serum renin occurs with a subsequent 4- to 5-fold increase in angiotensin. Although a pregnant patient is apparently less sensitive to the hypertensive effects of the increased angiotensin, elevated aldosterone levels result in an increase in sodium reabsorption, overcoming the natriuresis produced by elevated progesterone. However, serum sodium levels are decreased because the increase in sodium reabsorption is less than the increase in plasma volume. Serum osmolality is decreased to 270 to 280 mOsm/kg.

Pregnancy has a significant effect on endocrine physiology. Cortisol levels increase to threefold above nonpregnancy levels as a result of estrogen stimulation of corticosteroid-binding globulin release of free cortisol and placental release of corticotropin-releasing hormone.[8] Early in pregnancy, high levels of human chorionic gonadotropin (hCG) stimulate thyroid production and release, causing levels of thyroxine (T_4) to increase and thyroid-stimulating hormone (TSH) to decrease. Estrogen also increases the production of thyroid-binding globulin leading to more T_4 binding and inducing more thyroid hormone production. These factors lead to a 50% increase in overall serum T_4 concentrations. As hCG decreases later in pregnancy, levels of T_4 decrease, and TSH levels increase.[9]

DIAGNOSTIC IMAGING CONSIDERATIONS

Imaging is paramount in diagnosis of many surgical conditions, including in pregnant patients. The use of radiation is a concern in this patient population because of the teratogenic and carcinogenic risk to the fetus from radiation exposure. The consensus acceptable maximum dose of ionizing radiation during the entire pregnancy is 5 rads (0.05 Gy). The fetus is at the highest risk from radiation exposure from the preimplantation period to approximately 15 weeks of gestation; spontaneous abortions and decreased intelligence have been documented at radiation exposures greater than 10 rads. Primary organogenesis occurs during this time, and the teratogenic effects of radiation, particularly to the developing central nervous system, are at their highest. Perinatal radiation exposure has also been associated with childhood leukemia and certain childhood malignancies, especially when the radiation exposure occurs during the first trimester.[10] As shown in Table 71-2, radiation exposure to the fetus with the doses from the more common radiology procedures is well below the maximum threshold of greater than 5 rads. With the increased use of computed tomography (CT) scans to aid in surgical diagnoses, many medical centers are developing pregnancy protocols that use lower doses of radiation with the tradeoff of decreased imaging quality. Fluoroscopic studies may also be used in pregnant patients, but

TABLE 71-2 Fetal Radiation Exposure With Radiographic Imaging

EXAMINATION	FETAL RADIATION EXPOSURE (mGy)
Plain Film Radiographs	
Cervical spine (2-view)	<0.001
Extremities	<0.001
Chest (2-view)	0.002
Thoracic spine (2-view)	0.003
Abdomen (1 view)	1-3
Lumbar spine (2-view)	1
Mammography	0.4
Pelvic	0.6
Fluoroscopy	
Pyelogram	6
Upper GI series	0.05
Barium enema	7
Angiography and interventions	10-60
CT Scans	
Head	0
Chest (PE)	0.2
CT angiography of the aorta	34
Abdomen/pelvis	25
Other Examinations	
Bone scan	6
PET scan	14
MRI	0
U/S	0
HIDA	0.15

CT, Computed tomography; *GI,* gastrointestinal; *HIDA,* hepatobiliary iminodiacetic acid scan; *MRI,* magnetic resonance imaging; *PE,* pulmonary embolism; *U/S,* ultrasound.

attempts must be made to use the minimal amount of radiation possible by using lower doses for shorter periods of time, and the fluoroscopy machine should be set with an alarm when a certain radiation usage threshold is set.[11] Nonetheless, prudence on the part of the clinician is required to avoid unnecessary fetal exposure to ionizing radiation, especially during the first trimester and early second trimester when the risk from exposure is greatest.

Magnetic resonance imaging (MRI) avoids exposure to ionizing radiation but poses an unknown risk to the fetus. Theoretically, the gradient magnetic fields may produce electric currents within the patient, and the high-frequency currents induced by radiofrequency fields may cause local generation of heat. The long-term effect of exposure is unknown. At the present time, the National Radiological Protection Board advises against the use of MRI during the first trimester of pregnancy.[10]

Contrast agents to enhance imaging modalities have been shown to be safe in pregnancy but should be used with extreme care. Iodine-based agents have a theoretical risk of neonatal hypothyroidism that has not been established in the literature. Gadolinium crosses the placental and can stay in the amniotic fluid for a prolonged time, which has led to its use only in extreme conditions for the mother's safety.[10]

Ultrasonography is routinely used by obstetricians during pregnancy. Although tissue heating and mechanical injuries are theoretical effects of ultrasound exposure, such effects have never been reported.[12] Ultrasound may be a helpful alternative diagnostic tool when trying to avoid exposure to ionizing radiation, but it has some limitations: Deeper structures are difficult to visualize, the ultrasound field is limited, and ultrasound is highly operator dependent.

Endoscopy is a commonly used diagnostic modality in pregnant women. Esophagogastroduodenoscopy is the most commonly used endoscopic therapy in pregnancy and has been shown to be safe with very little risk to the fetus. Sigmoidoscopy has been used successfully with little risk to the fetus. An entire colonoscopy is technically very difficult but if necessary can be done safely. Strong indications for the use of endoscopy in pregnancy are upper gastrointestinal bleed, dysphagia for more than 1 week, and possible malignancy. Finally, endoscopic retrograde cholangiopancreatography (ERCP) has been shown to be successful and safe with very few pregnancy complications, although maternal pancreatitis rates of 15% have been reported when ERCP was performed for obstructive jaundice or cholangitis from choledocholithiasis. Therefore, ERCP has been deemed safe as opposed to surgical intervention for obstructive jaundice, which would carry greater risk for the mother and fetus.[13]

ANESTHESIA SAFETY CONCERNS

Anesthesia concerns during pregnancy include the safety of both the mother and the fetus. The primary concerns for the mother during general anesthesia are hypotension, hypoxia, and airway. The airway of the pregnant woman is generally swollen, reducing the glottis opening and making intubation more difficult. These patients are also more prone to aspiration with anesthesia induction because of increased intra-abdominal pressure. The pulmonary reserve is also greatly reduced, so the pregnant patient may become acutely hypoxic very quickly during induction.[14]

The effects of anesthesia on the fetus during pregnancy can be divided into direct, or active, and indirect, or passive, effects. Direct effects are effects that relate to the possible teratogenic or embryotoxic properties of the drugs used for anesthesia, some of which do cross the placenta. Indirect effects are mechanisms by which an anesthetic agent or surgical procedure may interfere with maternal or fetal physiology, such as inducing hypotension, inducing hypoxia, or altering the acid-base balance, and in doing so may potentially harm the fetus. For the most part, the fetus experiences indirect effects as a consequence of anesthetic agents administered to the mother or the effect on the mother of the underlying disease process. The most profound effects on the fetus are related to decreased uterine blood flow or decreased oxygen content of uterine blood. In contrast to circulation to other vital organs, most notably the brain, the uterine circulation is not autoregulated. During the third trimester, uterine circulation represents nearly 10% of cardiac output. When treating maternal hypotension brought about by general anesthesia, pure α-agonists, such as phenylephrine and metaraminol, are most effective at maintaining maternal blood pressure and promoting continuous perfusion to the gravid uterus. Multiple studies support the use of these vasopressor agents in pregnant women during surgery.[14] Other maneuvers, such as fluid bolus, Trendelenburg and left-lateral positions, compression stockings, and leg elevation, have an impact on increasing uterine blood flow.

In addition to the risks related to maternal hypoxia or hypotension, the risks of spontaneous abortion and teratogenesis related to anesthetic agents are of major concern. Labor induction occurs in 5% of all surgical procedures in pregnant women. Many nonhuman studies demonstrated potential teratogenic effects with anesthetic agents, but human studies have not demonstrated such significant effects.

Because of the risks of anesthesia on the fetus and the mother's physiology, elective surgical procedures should be delayed until at least 6 weeks after delivery, when maternal physiology has returned to the nonpregnant state and when the impact on the fetus is no longer a concern. When emergent procedures are required, the life of the mother takes priority, although the anesthesia administered should be altered to optimize fetal well-being. Elective surgery during the first trimester is often avoided because of the potential teratogenic effects of the anesthesia on the developing fetus during organogenesis. However, multiple studies have shown a single exposure to anesthesia during the first trimester to be safe and associated with the same rate of major birth defects as in the population without surgical anesthesia exposure. It is still advisable to limit surgical intervention during the first trimester. The second trimester has classically been assumed safer for nonobstetric surgeries in pregnant patients, but studies have shown that anesthesia may have effects on neuronal development during this trimester, as this is a major period of neural development in the fetus. Although surgery can be performed during this time, it should be done only if necessary. General anesthesia in the third trimester has been studied less frequently but generally has been accepted as safe if surgery is necessary, although it carries a risk for preterm labor induction.[15]

When a pregnant patient requires surgical intervention, consultation with the obstetrician and possibly a perinatologist is essential. These specialists are helpful in determining the optimal technique to monitor fetal status and are able to assist with perioperative management and diagnose and manage preterm labor. Typically, when emergent surgery is performed during the first trimester or early second trimester, fetal heart tones and tachymeter monitoring should be obtained before and after anesthesia exposure. During the late second trimester and third trimester, when the fetus is of viable age, continuous intraoperative monitoring should be performed when possible with electronic fetal monitoring, fetal pulse oximetry, or possibly transvaginal ultrasound when the surgery is on the abdomen.[16] If any signs of fetal distress occur, the team should be prepared for an emergent cesarean section in fetuses who are past 24 weeks. Continuous monitoring should be used to assess fetal well-being if a significant blood loss is possible or anticipated.

Postoperative pain control in pregnant patients should be monitored closely. Nonsteroidal anti-inflammatory drugs should not be used in pregnancy because of the risk of premature labor, fetal renal injury, and premature closure of the ductus arteriosus.[17] Acetaminophen and opioids are the preferred perioperative analgesic choices for pregnant women. Narcotic analgesics have not been found to cause birth defects in humans in normal dosages. A patient-controlled analgesia pump postoperatively may be the best choice because of the low incidence of maternal respiratory depression and drug transfer to the fetus. Postoperative oral narcotic use is generally considered safe in pregnant patients. Long-term use of narcotics during pregnancy may cause fetal dependency at delivery. It is recommended that a pregnant postsurgical patient be weaned off narcotic use as soon as possible.

PREVENTION OF PRETERM LABOR

The incidence of preterm labor associated with nonobstetric surgery is related to both gestational age and the indication for surgery. Studies have suggested the rate of premature labor induced by nonobstetric elective surgical intervention to approach 5%.[18] Elective procedures are usually delayed until later in the postpartum period when the mother is fully recovered from the pregnancy. An exception may be a patient with cancer diagnosed during pregnancy that warrants an earlier surgery. Gestational age at treatment and severity of the underlying disease are the most predictive indicators of patients at risk for preterm labor. The risk of preterm contractions or preterm labor is higher later in gestation. Intraperitoneal operations and disease processes with intraperitoneal inflammation are the most likely to have postoperative courses complicated by preterm contractions and preterm labor. Laparoscopic and open techniques have an equal incidence of preterm labor.

If surgical intervention is necessary, an obstetrician should be consulted. During surgery, measures to avoid maternal hypotension and hypoxia are thought to mitigate against preterm labor. There is no consensus on the use of prophylactic tocolytics after nonobstetric surgery during pregnancy. Tocolytic use varies widely among centers and physicians. Most studies suggest that tocolytics should be used only if contractions are noted during postoperative monitoring or are felt by the patient. Tocolytics used as needed are generally successful at preventing preterm labor and preterm delivery when postoperative contractions are detected. Terbutaline, magnesium, and indomethacin (Indocin) all have been used in different studies with equivalent results. In general, for patients with postoperative contractions before 32 weeks, indomethacin would be a reasonable treatment, whereas terbutaline could be used as a first-line treatment for patients at greater than 32 weeks' gestation. The use of prophylactic tocolytics should be individualized, depending on the patient's gestational age and the underlying disease process and chosen in consultations with the obstetricians. Tocolytics used for postoperative preterm labor are generally successful when used selectively but should not be used as prophylaxis.

ABDOMINAL PAIN AND THE ACUTE ABDOMEN

When a pregnant patient presents with abdominal pain, it may be difficult to distinguish a pathophysiologic cause from normal pregnancy-associated symptoms. Changes in the position and orientation of abdominal viscera from the enlarging uterus as well as alterations in physiology already described may modify the perception or manifestation of an intra-abdominal process. If early in the pregnancy, the woman may not know that she is pregnant. Additionally, some intra-abdominal processes are exclusive to pregnancy, such as ectopic pregnancy, HELLP (*h*emolysis, *e*levated *l*iver enzymes, *l*ow *p*latelets) syndrome, or acute fatty liver of pregnancy. Moreover, both the patient and the physician may attribute the patient's complaints to normal pregnancy, resulting in a delay in evaluation and treatment. These delays in diagnosis and definitive intervention are the most serious adverse event affecting maternal and fetal outcome. It is usually not the treatment but the delay in diagnosis and severity of the primary disease process that adversely impact outcomes.[3,18] Box 71-1 lists common causes of abdominal pain in pregnant patients, classified according to location. Prompt evaluation and treatment are necessary to avoid maternal and fetal complications.

MINIMALLY INVASIVE SURGERY: SPECIAL CONSIDERATIONS IN PREGNANCY

The field of minimally invasive surgery has advanced tremendously over the last 20 years. The laparoscopic approach, which was previously considered contraindicated in pregnancy, is now

BOX 71-1 Common Causes of Abdominal Pain in Pregnant Patients

Right Upper Quadrant
- Gastroesophageal reflux
- Peptic ulcer disease
- Acute cholecystitis
- Biliary colic
- Acute pancreatitis
- Hepatitis
- Acute fatty liver of pregnancy
- HELLP syndrome
- Preeclampsia
- Pneumothorax
- Pneumonia
- Acute appendicitis
- Hepatic adenoma
- Hemangioma

Right Lower Quadrant
- Acute appendicitis
- Ectopic pregnancy
- Renal or ureteral colic
- Pelvic inflammatory disease
- Tubo-ovarian abscess
- Endometriosis
- Adnexal torsion
- Ruptured ovarian cyst
- Ruptured corpus luteum

Lower Abdomen
- Threatened, incomplete, or complete abortion
- Abruptio placentae
- Preterm labor
- Pelvic inflammatory disease
- Tubo-ovarian abscess
- Inflammatory bowel disease
- Irritable bowel syndrome
- Pyelonephritis

Flank
- Pyelonephritis
- Hydronephrosis of pregnancy
- Acute appendicitis (retrocecal appendix)

Diffuse Abdominal Pain
- Early acute appendicitis
- Small bowel obstruction
- Acute intermittent porphyria
- Sickle cell crisis

HELLP, Hemolysis, elevated liver enzymes, low platelets.

considered a standard approach to many operations done in pregnant patients. Effects of CO_2 pneumoperitoneum on venous return and cardiac output, uterine perfusion, and fetal acid-base status were unknown. Laparoscopy was safely used in several series where the technique was used to evaluate pregnant patients for ectopic pregnancy. Patients with an intrauterine pregnancy had no increase in fetal loss or observed negative effect on long-term outcome.[19] When comparing laparoscopic and open techniques in nonpregnant patients, patients who underwent laparoscopic procedures had decreased postoperative pain, shorter hospital stays, and a quicker return to normal activity.[19,20]

Major concerns of laparoscopy during pregnancy include injury to the uterus, decreased uterine blood flow, fetal acidosis, and preterm labor from increased intra-abdominal pressure. During the second trimester, the uterus is no longer contained within the pelvis. The open technique for abdominal access reduces the risk of injury. Decreased uterine blood flow from pneumoperitoneum remains theoretical because of the significant changes in intra-abdominal pressure that occur normally during pregnancy and during maternal Valsalva maneuvers. The risk of pneumoperitoneum may also be less than the risk of direct uterine manipulation that occurs with laparotomy. Additionally, when comparing laparoscopy and open techniques, no significant difference in preterm labor or delivery-related side effects was observed.[20] Box 71-2 illustrates the general comparison between laparoscopic and open technique.

The Society of American Gastrointestinal Endoscopic Surgeons recommends 23 guidelines for laparoscopic surgery during pregnancy.[21] The guidelines that pertain to laparoscopic surgery are as follows:

- Intraoperative and endoscopic cholangiography exposes the mother and fetus to minimal radiation and may be used selectively during pregnancy. The lower abdomen should be shielded when performing cholangiography during pregnancy to decrease the radiation exposure to the fetus.
- Diagnostic laparoscopy is safe and effective when used selectively in the workup and treatment of acute abdominal processes in pregnancy.
- Laparoscopic treatment of acute abdominal disease has the same indications in pregnant and nonpregnant patients.
- Laparoscopy can be safely performed during any trimester of pregnancy.
- Gravid patients should be placed in the left lateral decubitus position to minimize compression of the vena cava.
- Initial abdominal access can be safely accomplished with an open (Hasson) technique, Veress needle, or optical trocar if the location is adjusted according to fundal height and previous incisions.
- CO_2 insufflation of 10 to 15 mm Hg can be safely used for laparoscopy in pregnant patients.
- Intraoperative CO_2 monitoring by capnography should be used during laparoscopy in pregnant patients.
- Intraoperative and postoperative pneumatic compression devices and early postoperative ambulation are recommended prophylaxis for deep venous thrombosis in gravid patients.
- Laparoscopic cholecystectomy is the treatment of choice in pregnant patients with gallbladder disease, regardless of trimester.
- Choledocholithiasis during pregnancy may be managed with preoperative ERCP with sphincterotomy followed by laparoscopic cholecystectomy, laparoscopic common bile duct exploration, or postoperative ERCP.
- Laparoscopic appendectomy may be performed safely in pregnant patients with appendicitis.
- Laparoscopic adrenalectomy, nephrectomy, and splenectomy are safe procedures in pregnant patients.
- Laparoscopy is safe and effective treatment in pregnant patients with symptomatic ovarian cystic masses. Observation is acceptable for all other cystic lesions, provided that ultrasound is not concerning for malignancy and tumor markers are normal. Initial observation is warranted for most cystic lesions less than 6 cm in size.
- Laparoscopy is recommended for diagnosis and treatment of adnexal torsion unless clinical severity warrants laparotomy.
- Fetal heart monitoring should occur preoperatively and postoperatively in the setting of urgent abdominal surgery during pregnancy.
- Obstetric consultation can be obtained preoperatively or postoperatively based on the severity of the patient's disease, gestational age, and availability of the consultant.

BOX 71-2 Advantages and Disadvantages of Laparoscopy Instead of Laparotomy in Pregnancy

Advantages

Decreased fetal depression secondary to decreased narcotic requirement
Lower rates of wound infections and incisional hernias
Diminished postoperative maternal hypoventilation
Decreased manipulation of the uterus
Faster recovery with early return to normal function
Decreased risk of ileus

Disadvantages

Possible uterine injury during trocar placement
Decreased uterine blood flow
Preterm labor risk secondary to increased intra-abdominal pressure
Increased risk of fetal acidosis and unknown effects of CO_2 pneumoperitoneum
Decreased visualization with gravid uterus

CO_2, Carbon dioxide.

Trocar placement early in pregnancy in a pregnant patient should not differ radically from placement in a nonpregnant patient. Later in pregnancy, the camera port must be placed in a supraumbilical location, and the remaining ports are placed under direct camera visualization. The gravid uterus enlarges superiorly (Fig. 71-1); adjustments in trocar placement must be made to avoid uterine injury and to improve visualization, and an angled scope may aid in viewing over or around the uterus. The uterus should be manipulated as little as possible.

BREAST MASSES

Pregnancy-associated breast cancer is defined as breast cancer that is diagnosed during pregnancy or within 1 year after pregnancy. It has become increasingly more prominent as more women delay childbearing until they are in their 30s and 40s.[22] Overall, pregnancy-associated breast cancer is the most common nongynecologic malignancy associated with pregnancy and has been reported to occur in 1 in 3000 pregnancies; 10% of women with breast cancer younger than 40 years old are pregnant at the time of diagnosis.[22,23] Because pregnancy-related breast cancers occur

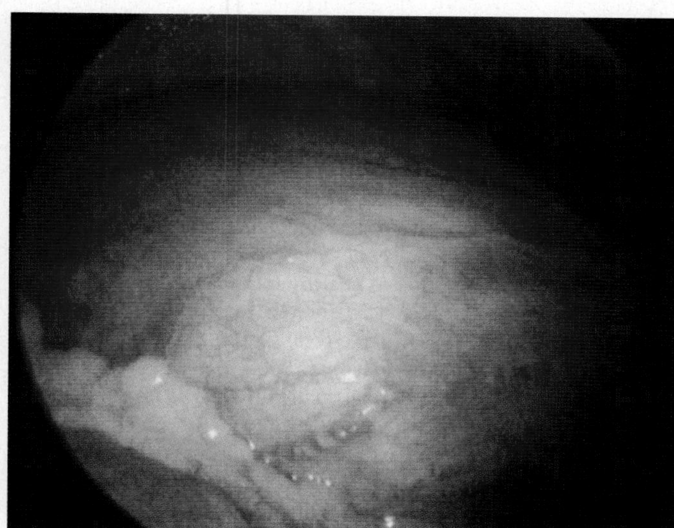

FIGURE 71-1 Intraoperative image of a 24-week gravid uterus taken with a 5-mm, 30-degree, high-definition camera.

at a young age, these women are more apt to have genetic predisposition to breast cancers resulting from *BRAC1* or *BRAC2* mutations. Several studies have demonstrated that pregnancy-associated breast cancer may be more common in women with a genetic predisposition to breast cancer. Patients with *BRCA1*, more than patients with *BRCA2*, were three to four times more likely to develop breast cancer during pregnancy.[24]

Delays in diagnosis and treatment are common. Physiologic changes of breast engorgement, rapid cellular proliferation, and increased vascularity make a reliable physical examination difficult; masses of similar size that would be easily palpable in the nonpregnant state may be obscured, or palpable masses may be attributed to normal pregnancy-related changes. Benign breast lesions, such as galactoceles, mastitis, abscesses, lipomas, fibroadenomas, lobular hyperplasia, and lactational adenomas, account for 80% of breast masses that occur during pregnancy or during lactation. However, any palpable mass that persists for 4 weeks or longer should be evaluated.[23] Most pregnancy-related breast cancers manifest with a painless mass with or without bloody nipple discharge that is often interpreted as a normal pregnancy-related change. Studies have shown that the mean delay of 1 to 2 months in the diagnosis of a breast mass as cancer in a pregnant patient can increase the chance of nodal metastasis from 0.9% to 1.8%.[25]

Compared with age-matched nonpregnant control subjects, women with pregnancy-associated breast cancer are more likely to present with larger primary tumors, increased nodal involvement, and increased inflammatory breast cancer and are more likely to have metastatic disease.[23,26] Most pregnancy-associated breast cancers are poorly differentiated infiltrating ductal carcinomas. Pregnancy-associated breast cancers have estrogen receptor or progesterone receptor expression 25% of the time as opposed to 55% to 60% seen in nonpregnant breast cancers. Her-2 overexpression is seen in 28% to 58% of pregnancy-associated breast cancers, which is slightly higher than in breast cancers with no pregnancy. The pathologic type of breast cancer seen during pregnancy appears to be more aggressive and typically associated with poorer prognosis.[26]

Young age, which would include most pregnant women, has been shown to be an independent risk factor for a worse prognosis and for increased breast cancer–related mortality.[27] There have been several conflicting studies in regard to the effects of pregnancy on breast cancer and the patient's prognosis. A large meta-analysis of 30 published studies of pregnancy-associated breast cancer demonstrated a clear trend of poorer outcomes in patients with pregnancy-associated breast cancer. The group with the worst prognosis included patients diagnosed immediately postpartum, but patients with breast cancer during pregnancy also had a worse prognosis than similar nonpregnant patients.[22]

Imaging of breast masses in pregnant women is often difficult because pregnancy-related changes result in denser breast tissue. Ultrasound should be the first imaging modality used for the workup of a breast mass in a pregnant woman.[27] The ultrasound scan is able to distinguish solid from cystic lesions in greater than 93% of patients and can be used to evaluate for abnormal axillary lymph nodes. Mammography generally has a high false-negative rate during pregnancy secondary to the increased breast density; this decreases mammographic sensitivity from 63% to 78% for detecting breast cancer in a pregnant woman.[26] Despite the use of radiation, if used with appropriate shielding, mammography carries a limited risk to the fetus and is generally considered safe with 0.02 mGy of radiation exposure. If a lesion is suggestive of cancer by ultrasound, mammography is recommended to rule out multiple lesions or bilateral breast cancers.[27] MRI is a third imaging modality commonly used in young women with breast cancer, but its safety in pregnant patients has not been studied. MRI is a tempting option because it does not use radiation, but MRI requires the use of gadolinium for detection of breast cancer, and gadolinium is listed as a pregnancy category C drug because animal studies have shown that it crosses the placenta and causes fetal abnormalities. Breast MRI is not recommended in pregnancy unless it is necessary for treatment planning. If metastatic disease is suspected, low-dose bone scans or noncontrast MRI scans may be used.[26]

When a suspicious lesion is identified, tissue diagnosis is essential. Core-needle biopsy under local anesthesia with or without ultrasound guidance is a safe and reliable method for obtaining tissue that has a sensitivity rate up to 90%.[23] The major risks are hematoma formation and milk fistula development. A pressure dressing should be applied after the biopsy to minimize the risk of hematoma from the hypervascularity of the breasts. The risk of milk fistula may be reduced by stopping lactation for several days before biopsy and by emptying the breast of milk just before the procedure. If the biopsy is done postpartum, a 1-week course of bromocriptine may also be given before biopsy.[26] Fine-needle aspiration is generally not recommended in pregnant women because hormonal changes of the breast that may lead to cellular proliferation may give false-positive results, as the cellular proliferation is hard to distinguish from cancer. If a core-needle biopsy is not definitive, excisional biopsy of the breast lump should be considered, as this can be done safely and provides adequate tissue.

Treatment of pregnant patients with breast cancer requires a multimodality team comprising a surgeon, oncologist, obstetrician, and perinatologist. The mainstay of therapy for pregnancy-associated breast cancer is surgical resection, and resection can be offered during every trimester. Modified radical mastectomy classically has been the first choice for local control of breast cancer because it eliminates the need for adjuvant radiation and its risk to the fetus, but it is not mandatory especially when performed later in pregnancy. The combination of local control and adjuvant therapy may be tailored to the patient according to the stage of pregnancy as well as the stage of the cancer. Classically, in early pregnancy, mastectomy with axillary dissection is preferred for control and appropriate staging. However, at the present time, most breast surgeons avoid axillary dissection unless there are clinically positive nodes. After the first trimester, sentinel node biopsy poses potential risk to the fetus, but more recently it has been shown to be potentially safe. Supravital dyes, such as isosulfan blue dye, can potentially be used in the first trimester but should be used with extreme caution in pregnancy because of the potential for maternal anaphylaxis and pregnancy compromise.[26] Several studies on the use of technetium sulfur colloid for sentinel lymph node detection have been safely performed in pregnant women. Axillary lymph node dissection can be avoided in most pregnant women, especially after the first trimester, as a sentinel lymph node biopsy using technetium sulfur colloid can be recommended.[23]

Breast-conserving therapy is becoming an option for pregnant patients. In patients in whom breast cancer is diagnosed during the late second trimester or later, immediate breast-conserving lumpectomy and axillary dissection followed with radiation postpartum is a treatment option. If the diagnosis of breast cancer is made in the first or early second trimester of pregnancy, lumpectomy and axillary dissection can be followed by chemotherapy after the first trimester and radiation after delivery. Chemotherapy is indicated for node-positive cancers or node-negative tumors greater than 1 cm. Current chemotherapeutic regimens are relatively safe after the first trimester, when the teratogenic risk is greatest. Generally, treatment regimens are the same as for nonpregnant patients with dose alterations because the increased plasma volume, the hypoalbuminemia, and the fact that almost all chemotherapeutic agents cross the placenta change the pharmacokinetics of the drugs. Cytotoxic chemotherapy in the first 4 weeks of gestation results in no detrimental effect on the fetus or loss of the pregnancy. For the rest of the first trimester, at which time organogenesis is occurring, chemotherapy is thought to have a high risk for fetal malformation and is not recommended during this time. The risk of mutations appears to be worsened with the number of agents from 10% with single agents to 25% with multiagent regimens. During the second and third trimesters, chemotherapy has generally been shown to be safe with the risk of fetal malformations being 1.3%. However, chemotherapy during the last two trimesters is not benign, in that almost half of infants born to mothers undergoing chemotherapy have intrauterine growth retardation, prematurity, and low birth weight. Chemotherapy is generally not recommended after 35 weeks so as to reduce the likelihood of myelosuppression in the newborn after delivery.[24] Antimetabolites such as methotrexate should be avoided because of the high risk of spontaneous abortion even after the first trimester. Multiple studies have demonstrated treatment with fluorouracil, doxorubicin (Adriamycin), and cyclophosphamide to be safe. In general, most systemic chemotherapy regimens have been shown to be safe in pregnant women when administered after the first trimester, but patients with early-stage cancer have been shown to have no adverse outcome in delaying therapy until after birth to prevent the low-birth-weight effects on the fetus. Trastuzumab is not recommended during pregnancy because of increased neonatal death. Tamoxifen has shown increased rates of genital abnormalities in newborns and is not recommended in pregnancy.[23,26]

Radiation is typically not offered during pregnancy because of its teratogenic risk and its risk of induction of childhood malignancies. Although the fetal radiation exposure would be relatively low, there is a potential for adverse outcomes. The risk is directly related to dose and developmental stage. During the preimplantation stage and continuing to 15 weeks after conception, during organogenesis, the rapidly proliferating cells of the fetus are most sensitive to radiation, and exposure greater than 1 Gy during this period has a high likelihood of causing fetal death. The standard therapeutic course of 5000 rads (50 Gy) results in a varying exposure to the fetus, depending on the gestational age and proximity of the gravid uterus to the radiation bed. Even with abdominal shielding, the greatest fetal exposure is due to scatter. Although there are several case reports of healthy infants born after maternal radiation exposure, radiation is not recommended during pregnancy because of the risks to the fetus.[23,26]

Elective termination of the pregnancy to receive appropriate therapy without the risk of fetal malformation is no longer routinely recommended because no improvement in survival has been demonstrated. With the treatment options available to the pregnant patient with breast cancer, a combined approach involving the input of the patient, surgeon, oncologist, and maternal-fetal medicine specialist should ensure optimal treatment of the disease, while minimizing risk to the patient and the fetus. A suggested algorithm for the management of breast masses in pregnancy is shown in Figure 71-2.

HEPATOBILIARY DISEASE

Cholelithiasis

Most pregnant women with gallstones are asymptomatic. Although an estimated 2% to 4% of pregnant women may be found to have gallstones by ultrasound, only 0.05% to 0.1% of those women are symptomatic. The symptoms of biliary colic are the same in pregnant and nonpregnant patients. In patients with symptoms consistent with cholelithiasis, ultrasound is the diagnostic examination of choice. Ultrasound is as accurate in identifying gallstones and signs of inflammation in pregnant patients as it is in nonpregnant patients. Jaundice in pregnancy is usually not related to gallstones; it is associated with hepatitis in 45% of cases, benign cholestasis in 20% of cases, and choledocholithiasis in 7% of cases.[3,18]

Cholecystectomy for symptomatic cholelithiasis is second to appendectomy as the most common nonobstetric surgical procedure performed during pregnancy. Historically, pregnant patients with a clear operative indication, such as obstructive jaundice, gallstone pancreatitis, and choledocholithiasis, underwent cholecystectomy regardless of gestational age. Patients with recurrent biliary colic or acute cholecystitis that responded to medical management were treated expectantly until after delivery, at which time they underwent cholecystectomy. As it has become understood that adverse maternal and fetal outcomes are related more to the disease process and not the surgical intervention, management patterns have changed. Additionally, complications from nonoperative management of gallstone disease result in an increase in maternal and fetal mortality. With gallstone pancreatitis during pregnancy, maternal mortality of 15% and fetal mortality of 60% have been reported. In a study of 63 patients who were admitted with symptomatic cholelithiasis, surgical management reduced the need for labor induction, rate of preterm deliveries, and fetal mortality.[28] Surgical intervention should be considered as primary management of gallstones in pregnancy.

The timing of cholecystectomy for biliary colic depends on the gestational age and the severity of symptoms. A spontaneous abortion rate of 12% with open cholecystectomy during the first trimester decreases to 5.6% and 0% during the second and third

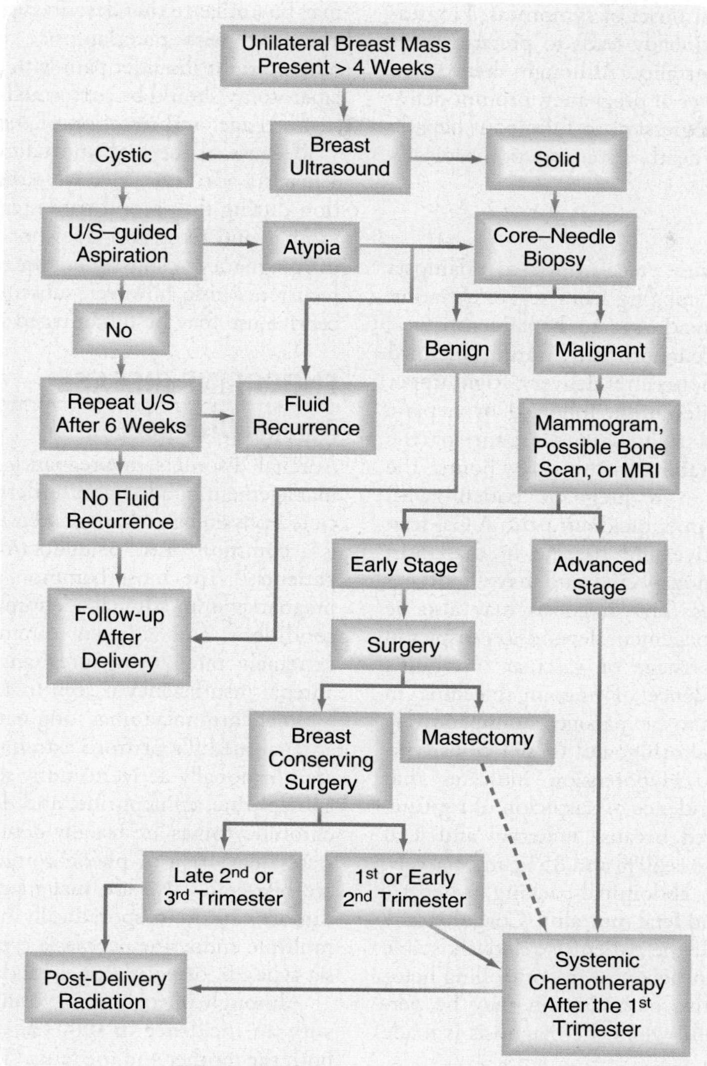

FIGURE 71-2 Algorithm for the management of a breast mass during pregnancy. *MRI,* Magnetic resonance imaging; *U/S,* ultrasound.

trimesters, respectively. The risk of preterm labor is nearly zero during the second trimester and 40% during the third trimester. The optimal time for cholecystectomy is the second trimester, when the risk of spontaneous abortion and preterm labor are the least, unless the patient develops a complication of cholelithiasis.[3]

Acute Pancreatitis

Acute pancreatitis occurs in 3 per 10,000 pregnancies. Gallstone pancreatitis has better outcomes than other causes. Gallstone pancreatitis is managed successfully with the same techniques as in nonpregnant patients, including ERCP with endoscopic sphincterotomy. Cholecystectomy is indicated in the presence of gallstones. The timing of operative intervention for complicated pancreatitis should follow the same guidelines used for nonpregnant patients.[3]

Liver

Liver abnormalities during pregnancy can be classified as occurring exclusively during pregnancy as a direct result of conditions during pregnancy, occurring simultaneously but not exclusively during pregnancy, or developing before the pregnancy. Examples of liver disorders unique to pregnancy include acute fatty liver of pregnancy; intrahepatic cholestasis of pregnancy; and liver disease related to preeclampsia or eclampsia, specifically HELLP syndrome and spontaneous hepatic hemorrhage or rupture. Preexisting liver disorders that may manifest with complications during pregnancy include hepatic adenoma and hepatocellular carcinoma.

Acute Fatty Liver of Pregnancy

The cause of acute fatty liver of pregnancy is unknown, although it is more common in women with first pregnancies, women with twin pregnancies, and women who are pregnant with a male fetus. Although acute fatty liver of pregnancy has been diagnosed at 26 weeks of gestation, it usually occurs during the third trimester, typically at approximately 35 weeks of gestation. Acute fatty liver of pregnancy carries a 20% maternal and fetal mortality rate. Initial nonspecific symptoms, such as malaise, nausea, vomiting, and right upper quadrant pain, are followed by signs of significant liver dysfunction within 2 weeks of onset of symptoms. Progression to fulminant hepatic failure quickly leads to preterm labor and an increased risk of fetal mortality. Although there is no specific treatment for acute fatty liver of pregnancy, prompt delivery after diagnosis may prevent progression to fulminant hepatic failure and reduce the risk of fetal death. Liver function typically returns to normal after delivery.[3,29]

HELLP Syndrome

Approximately 10% of women with preeclampsia or eclampsia have associated liver involvement, ranging from severe elevation of hepatic enzymes to HELLP syndrome to hepatic rupture.[3] Hepatic hemorrhage or rupture occurs primarily during the third trimester or can develop up to 48 hours after delivery. Right upper quadrant pain is the initial manifestation, followed by hepatic tenderness, peritonitis, chest and right shoulder pain, or the development of hemodynamic instability within a few hours. The diagnosis should be suspected in a pregnant patient with preeclampsia who develops right upper quadrant pain. A CT scan of the abdomen is highly sensitive and specific in diagnosis; ultrasound findings are usually nonspecific and have a higher incidence of false-negative studies. The diagnosis may also be made during cesarean section. Management depends on suspicion of ongoing intraperitoneal hemorrhage or vascular instability. Hepatic hematomas without evidence of ongoing bleeding in hemodynamically stable patients may be managed nonoperatively with serial imaging and close monitoring, and these lesions typically heal without intervention. Hypotension indicates that rupture has occurred. If there is evidence or suspicion of rupture, immediate intervention is required because maternal and fetal mortality from hepatic hemorrhage is 60% and 85%, respectively. Immediate laparotomy with either abdominal packing or hepatic artery ligation reduces maternal and fetal mortality. Coagulopathy should be corrected aggressively. If the patient is relatively stable or abdominal packing has been unsuccessful in controlling hemorrhage, angiography with selective embolization may be performed. Angiography is most useful when the diagnosis is made postpartum.[29]

Hepatic Adenomas

Hepatic adenomas are uncommon, benign lesions that are usually associated with oral contraceptive use in young women.[26] Hepatic adenomas are also associated with glycogen storage disease, diabetes, exogenous steroids, and pregnancy. They are usually solitary lesions but may be multifocal, and they have a low potential for malignant transformation. Although the specific cause is unknown, it has been hypothesized that a change in hormone levels, specifically the sex steroids, leads to hepatotoxicity or exposes a hereditary defect in carbohydrate metabolism that results in hepatocyte hyperplasia and adenoma formation. The observation that adenomas may resolve after cessation of exogenous steroid or oral contraceptive use supports this hypothesis. The association of hepatic adenomas with pregnancy supports the hypothesis that elevated levels of endogenous hormones may contribute to adenoma formation, although no data exist showing regression of a hepatic adenoma after pregnancy. Similarly, the true incidence of hepatic adenomas during pregnancy is unknown. Diagnosis is best made with CT or MRI of the liver.

The major risk of a hepatic adenoma during pregnancy is spontaneous rupture, which carries a mortality rate of approximately 45% for both mother and fetus, even with operative intervention. When spontaneous rupture does occur, the presentation may be similar to that described previously for hepatic hemorrhage associated with preeclampsia: right upper quadrant pain with referred right shoulder pain with progression to shock. Immediate laparotomy should be performed with cesarean section, control of hemorrhage, and resection of the adenoma if possible.[30]

Because of the high mortality rate associated with rupture of a hepatic adenoma, elective resection may be performed. Resection during the second trimester minimizes operative risk to the mother and fetus and does not interfere with the remainder of the pregnancy or subsequent pregnancies. Because of the unknown recurrence risk; however, subsequent pregnancy and oral contraceptive use may be discouraged in these patients.

ENDOCRINE DISEASE

Adrenal Disorders

Adrenal disorders in pregnancy are uncommon. Diagnosis and management of adrenal disorders are difficult because of the associated physiologic changes seen in pregnancy. Cushing syndrome is a common cause of endocrine dysfunction seen in pregnant patients.[31] The most common cause of Cushing syndrome in pregnancy is an adrenal adenoma. Other causes include pituitary conditions and adrenal carcinoma. Adrenal insufficiency is extremely rare during pregnancy. It is estimated that primary adrenal insufficiency is seen in 1 of 3000 pregnancies.[31]

Pheochromocytomas originate from chromaffin cells in the adrenal medulla or from extramedullary paraganglion cells. They are hormonally active tumors, secreting the catecholamines norepinephrine, epinephrine, and, less commonly, dopamine. Pheochromocytomas are usually described by the "rule of 10," which states that 10% of pheochromocytomas are extra-adrenal, 10% are bilateral, 10% are malignant, and 10% are familial. These tumors can occur sporadically or as part of a syndrome, such as multiple endocrine neoplasia type 2a, multiple endocrine neoplasia type 2b, or von Hippel-Lindau disease.

Although pheochromocytomas are uncommon in pregnancy with an incidence of 0.007%, they have devastating effects for both the mother and the fetus.[32] Pheochromocytomas that remain undiagnosed during pregnancy have a postpartum maternal mortality rate of 15%, with fetal mortality also exceeding 25%. The greatest risk occurs from the onset of labor to 48 hours after delivery. The index of suspicion should be high in any patient with preeclampsia, paroxysmal hypertension, or unexplained fever after delivery. With diagnosis and appropriate treatment, maternal mortality is reduced to nearly 0%, and fetal mortality is decreased to 15%.[32] The diagnosis is made by elevated urine catecholamines; urinary catecholamines in a pregnant patient without a pheochromocytoma are the same as in a nonpregnant patient. Lack of proteinuria also helps eliminate preeclampsia as a cause of hypertension. Metaiodobenzylguanidine imaging is not recommended during pregnancy because the small molecule may cross the placenta; use of metaiodobenzylguanidine imaging has not been evaluated in pregnancy.

Surgical resection should be performed before 20 weeks of gestation, when spontaneous abortion is less likely and the size of the gravid uterus does not interfere with the procedure. If the diagnosis is made late in the second trimester or during the third trimester, medical management followed by combined cesarean section and resection of the pheochromocytoma may be an option. It is unknown if the standard preoperative management in nonpregnant patients with alpha blockade or calcium channel blockade followed by perioperative beta blockade is safe during pregnancy. The long-term effects of the alpha blocker phenoxybenzamine on the fetus have not been determined, although calcium channel blockers are safe to use during pregnancy. Beta blockers are frequently used during pregnancy with close monitoring for intrauterine growth retardation. Consultation with a maternal-fetal medicine specialist is essential to determine the preoperative management that will ensure the optimal postoperative result for the patient and the fetus. In nonpregnant patients, the management approach depends on suspected malignancy, unilateral versus bilateral tumors, extra-adrenal location, size of the tumor, and surgeon's preference and experience. In all series comparing the different approaches, including open versus laparoscopic technique, pregnant patients were not included.

Thyroid

Thyroid diseases during pregnancy can be categorized into three groups: hypothyroidism, hyperthyroidism, and thyroid cancer. Hypothyroidism is found in 3% to 15% of pregnancies.[33] Of these, only 20% to 30% of patients develop symptoms. The first step is to obtain a serum TSH concentration to help categorize primary hypothyroidism versus hypothyroidism resulting from pituitary or hypothalamic causes. Current guidelines from Lebeau and Mandel for treatment of hypothyroidism during pregnancy are as follows:

1. Check serum TSH.
2. Initial levothyroxine dosage is based on severity of symptoms. Levothyroxine should be started at 1.2 mcg/kg/day for subclinical hypothyroidism with TSH less than 4.2 mIIU/L, 1.42 mcg/kg/day with TSH greater than 4.2 to 10, and 2.33 mcg/kg/day for overt hypothyroidism.[33a]
3. For previously diagnosed hypothyroidism, monitor TSH every 3 to 4 weeks.
4. Goal TSH level is less than 2.5 mU/liter.
5. Monitor serum TSH and total every 3 to 4 weeks with each dose change.

The incidence of hyperthyroidism during pregnancy is less than 0.5%.[34] Gestational thyrotoxicosis is a multifactorial phenomenon. High serum concentrations of hCG during pregnancy activate the TSH receptors. Elevated serum-free T_4 and low-serum TSH levels are seen with this form of thyrotoxicosis. Gestational thyrotoxicosis is usually self-limiting and spontaneously resolves by 20 weeks of gestation, when the hCG level declines. Repeat evaluation is warranted if thyrotoxicosis persists. Most cases of hyperthyroidism are a result of Graves disease. When the diagnosis is made, medical treatment with thionamides (propylthiouracil and methimazole) is the mainstay of treatment. Iodides should be avoided except in patients preparing for thyroidectomy during pregnancy. The dosage of methimazole sufficient to control hyperthyroidism is 15-100 mg daily, administered as divided doses 3 times daily. The appropriate dosage of PTU can range from 300 mg daily to a maximum dose of 1200 mg daily in divided doses 3 times daily. Once serum thyroid hormone levels return to normal, it is necessary to decrease the dosage to 5-20 mg daily of methimazole or 50-300 mg daily for PTU in divided doses. When doses of PTU are >300 mg/day or >20 mg/day for methimazole are taken long term, fetal goiter and hypothyroidism may result. Subtotal thyroidectomy for Graves disease should be reserved for patients who are consistently receiving high-dose propylthiouracil (>600 mg/day) or methimazole (>40 mg/day), are allergic to thionamides, are noncompliant, or experiencing compressive symptoms as a result of goiter size. Surgery should be performed during the second trimester before 24 weeks to minimize the risk of miscarriage. A 2-week course of a β-adrenergic agent, along with potassium iodide, should be implemented before surgery to minimize perioperative complications. Radioactive iodine therapy is contraindicated during pregnancy.

Thyroid nodules may have a higher prevalence during pregnancy as a result of hormonal changes, but thyroid cancers do not. Traditional workup of thyroid cancers should be done during pregnancy. Fine-needle aspiration, along with ultrasound evaluation, remains the cornerstone of diagnosis. If cytology shows thyroid cancer, surgery is recommended during the second trimester, before 24 weeks. If thyroid cancer is found after the second half of pregnancy, surgery can be performed after delivery. Postoperative radioactive iodine therapy should also be delayed until after delivery.

SMALL BOWEL OBSTRUCTION

Intestinal obstruction is the third most common nonobstetric surgical emergency condition in pregnancy, after acute appendicitis and acute cholecystitis. The incidence of small bowel obstruction during pregnancy is estimated at 1 in 4000 live births.[35] Small bowel obstructions usually occur during the second and third trimesters. Adhesions resulting from prior abdominal and pelvic surgeries are the most frequent causes for intestinal obstruction in pregnancy, accounting for 53% to 59% of cases. Other causes of small bowel obstruction in pregnant patients include volvulus, intussusception, malignancy, and hernia, although the displacement of the small bowel out of the pelvis by the enlarging uterus makes this a rare cause.

The symptoms of an obstruction are identical to symptoms i n nonpregnant patients and consist of the triad of abdominal pain, vomiting, and obstipation. Pain, present in 85% to 98% of cases, is usually colicky in nature and located in the midabdomen, although the character and duration are highly variable. Nausea and vomiting are seen in 80% of pregnant patients with small bowel obstruction; however, nausea and vomiting are common during the first trimester of normal pregnancy. Nausea and vomiting that persist or begin later in pregnancy should arouse suspicion and be evaluated. Bowel distention may be marked but difficult to assess because of the gravid uterus. The diagnosis is made by serial examination and plain abdominal radiograph.

Treatment for small bowel obstruction in pregnancy is identical to treatment in a nonpregnant patient. Therapy consists of nasogastric decompression and intravenous fluids. However, a lower threshold for operative management is necessary. If there is no satisfactory patient response after 6 to 8 hours of nonoperative treatment, a laparotomy should be performed before perforation or bowel necrosis occurs. Maternal mortality ranges from 6% to 20% because of sepsis and multisystem organ failure, and fetal loss is 26% to 50%.[35] To avoid the risk to the mother and fetus, a more aggressive approach should be used.

Midgut volvulus accounts for 25% of small bowel obstructions in pregnancy, and it is a difficult diagnosis. It should be treated during the postpartum period. Midgut volvulus is usually more common in a pregnant patient if she has undergone previous abdominal surgery; however, spontaneous midgut volvulus may occur. A case of maternal death caused by midgut volvulus after bariatric surgery was reported.[36] The key is increased vigilance for all the individuals involved in the patient's care. Early exploration is warranted if the diagnosis is unclear.

INFLAMMATORY BOWEL DISEASE

Although some studies report adverse obstetric outcomes with inflammatory bowel disease, the effect of ulcerative colitis or Crohn's disease on pregnancy characteristically depends on the severity of the disease at the time of conception. Management differs in pregnancy.[37]

Ulcerative Colitis

Patients in remission at conception are likely to remain so during the pregnancy. Relapse occurs in up to one third of patients usually in the first trimester. Because of the potential for pregnancy-induced exacerbation, pregnancy should be delayed in patients with active disease until they are in remission.

Crohn's Disease

Crohn's disease follows a course similar to ulcerative colitis. Complications are similar to complications in a nonpregnant patient with the exception of the unusual occurrence of an enterouterine fistula. If there is active Crohn's disease, pregnant patients have an increased incidence of premature delivery and infants with low birth weight. Extensive perianal involvement may warrant a cesarean section to avoid a complicated perineal fistula.

Surgery

If there is a significant exacerbation of the disease, surgery may be necessary. The indications for surgery are the same as in nonpregnant patients. Surgery in the second trimester is preferred. If fulminant colitis develops, a proctocolectomy with end ileostomy is preferred. Ileostomy issues may evolve as the patient gains weight, including stomal retraction, prolapse, or hernia. Preoperative consultation with an enterostomal therapist is advisable.

COLON AND RECTUM

Appendicitis

Acute appendicitis is the most common nonobstetric surgical emergency in pregnant patients, occurring in 1 in 1500 pregnancies.[35] Acute appendicitis is more common in the first two trimesters with an incidence of 32%, 42%, and 26% in the first, second, and third trimesters.[38] Timely and accurate diagnosis is challenging because the typical clinical findings of nausea, vomiting, abdominal pain, and mild leukocytosis may be findings in a normal pregnancy. Delay in diagnosis results in an increased perforation rate of 10%; this has significant consequences for the patient and fetus. Fetal mortality increases from 1.5% in acute appendicitis to 35% in perforated appendicitis.[38] Preterm labor and premature delivery rates are 40% in cases of perforated appendicitis compared with a 13% rate of preterm labor and 4% rate of premature delivery in cases of acute appendicitis.[38,39]

In 1932, Baer studied 78 normal pregnant women with radiographic studies at regular intervals from the second month of pregnancy to 10 days postpartum. As the uterus enlarges, the appendix is driven upward with a counterclockwise rotation. Baer concluded that early in pregnancy, pain is low, and that as the gestation progresses, pain is located higher in the abdomen.[40] A review of 45 pregnant patients with acute appendicitis demonstrated that pain in the right lower quadrant is the most common symptom, regardless of gestational age (first trimester, 86%; second trimester, 83%; third trimester, 85%).[39] Despite the inconsistency, acute appendicitis should be included in the differential diagnosis of every pregnant woman who presents with right-sided abdominal pain. The treatment for suspected acute appendicitis in the pregnant patient is emergent appendectomy. Although helical CT scans have demonstrated greater than 90% sensitivity and specificity in the diagnosis of acute appendicitis, few data are available in pregnant patients. In nonpregnant patients, a 10% to 15% negative laparotomy rate is considered acceptable. Because of the increased risk to both the mother and the fetus with appendiceal perforation, a negative rate of 30% to 33% is acceptable during pregnancy. The debate is then between open versus laparoscopic technique. The argument for open appendectomy is that the laparoscopic approach exposes the fetus to the risks of pneumoperitoneum and trocar placement without the benefit of a significantly smaller incision. The laparoscopic technique enables examination of a larger portion of the abdomen with less uterine manipulation and allows localization of the appendix as it is pushed into the right upper quadrant by the enlarging uterus.

Colonic Pseudo-obstruction

Colonic pseudo-obstruction, or Ogilvie syndrome, is a functional obstruction, or adynamic ileus, without a mechanical cause. Postpartum patients account for 10% of all cases of Ogilvie syndrome. It is characterized by massive abdominal distention with cecal dilation. Although neostigmine is an effective first-line therapy in nonpregnant patients, its safety in pregnancy is unknown. It can be used safely in the postpartum period. Colonoscopic decompression has been described in postpartum patients, with laparotomy indicated only in suspected perforation.[41]

Colon Cancer

The incidence of colon cancer is 1 in 50,000 pregnancies. The diagnosis is often delayed. Treatment follows similar guidelines as treatment in nonpregnant patients with the following exceptions. Carcinoembryonic antigen is not helpful. Neoadjuvant treatment of rectal cancer is avoided. In the presence of a large rectal lesion, cesarean section is advisable. Pregnancy does not in itself alter the maternal prognosis of colorectal cancer.[42]

VASCULAR DISEASE

Ruptured splenic artery aneurysm in a pregnant patient is rare, but the rate of maternal and fetal survival is very poor.[43] Ruptures usually occur during the third trimester, and it is typically misdiagnosed as splenic rupture or uterine rupture. Maternal mortality can be 75% with a fetal mortality of 95%. Increased portal pressures, high splenic artery flow as a result of distal aortic compression, and progressive arterial wall weakening are contributing factors. Multiparity may increase the risk. Most patients who survive a rupture experience a "two-stage rupture," in which the lesser sac temporarily tamponades the bleeding aneurysm.

When ruptured splenic artery aneurysm is treated electively in nonpregnant patients, mortality is only 0.5% to 1.3%. When the diagnosis is made in a woman of childbearing age or in a pregnant patient, a splenic artery aneurysm of 2 cm or larger should be treated electively because of the increased risk of rupture during pregnancy.[44]

Acute iliofemoral venous thrombosis is six times more frequent among pregnant patients compared with nonpregnant patients. Pregnancy may increase the risk of thrombosis through many factors, including mechanical obstruction of venous drainage by the enlarging uterus, decreased activity in late pregnancy and at time of delivery, intimal injury from vascular distention or surgical manipulation during cesarean section, and abnormal levels of coagulation factors already described.[45] Additionally, a wide spectrum of pathologic abnormalities, such as the presence of lupus anticoagulant antibodies and deficiencies of proteins C and S, may further increase the risk of thrombotic disease. Protein S serves as a cofactor for activated protein C, which has anticoagulant activity. A deficiency of protein S leads to spontaneous, recurrent thromboembolic complications in nonpregnant adults. Even in normal individuals, protein S levels are substantially reduced during pregnancy.

The management of acute iliofemoral venous thrombosis during pregnancy is controversial because thrombolytic therapy poses hazards to the fetus. The risk of pulmonary thromboembolism with manipulation of the clot during thrombectomy would have catastrophic effects on both the mother and the fetus. Techniques that have been described include interruption of the inferior vena cava via a right retroperitoneal approach or interruption of the inferior vena cava by passage of a Fogarty catheter through the unaffected contralateral femoral vein. The disadvantage of the retroperitoneal approach is that an extensive dissection is required. The disadvantages of the Fogarty catheter are that the catheter may still dislodge clots that have extended into the vena cava and that once the catheter is removed, an inferior vena cava filter must still be placed. However, the most effective technique is filter placement in the inferior vena cava via the internal jugular vein using ultrasound guidance, followed by thrombectomy.[46]

TRAUMA IN PREGNANCY

Trauma is the leading nonobstetric cause of maternal mortality and occurs in approximately 1 in 12 pregnancies.[47] The most common mechanisms of injury are from falls or from motor vehicle crashes.[45] Compared with age-matched pregnant controls, pregnant women who sustained trauma had a higher incidence of spontaneous abortion, preterm labor, fetomaternal hemorrhage, abruptio placentae, and uterine rupture.[48] Multiple studies have attempted to identify risk factors that predict morbidity and mortality in the pregnant trauma patient. The maternal Injury Severity Score, mechanism of injury, and physical findings are unable to adequately predict adverse outcomes such as abruptio placentae and fetal loss. Early involvement of an obstetrician in the care of an injured pregnant patient is important to evaluate both maternal and fetal well-being.

In the management of a pregnant trauma patient, the critical point is that resuscitation of the fetus is accomplished by resuscitation of the mother. Fetal outcomes are directly related and correlate with the state of maternal resuscitation. Therefore, the initial evaluation and treatment of an injured pregnant patient is identical to that of a nonpregnant patient. Maternal and fetal hypoxia is avoided through rapid assessment and a precise primary survey that includes the maternal airway, breathing, and circulation and ensuring an adequate airway. In the later stages of pregnancy, as already described, uterine compression of the vena cava may result in hypotension from diminished venous return, so a pregnant trauma patient should be placed in left lateral decubitus position. Women in late pregnancy may have difficult airways. Prolonged ventilation can significantly increase the risk of aspiration.[45] If spinal cord injury is suspected, the patient may be secured to a backboard and then tilted to the left.

The increased blood volume associated with pregnancy has important implications in a trauma patient. Signs of blood loss such as tachycardia and hypotension may be delayed until the patient loses nearly 30% of her blood volume. As a result, the fetus may be experiencing hypoperfusion long before the mother manifests any signs. Early and rapid fluid resuscitation should be administered even in a pregnant patient who is normotensive. If an emergent blood transfusion is warranted, Rh-negative blood should be administered.[45]

Along with the primary survey, the secondary survey should proceed in a similar fashion as in a nonpregnant patient. Special attention should be given to the abdominal examination. The uterus remains protected by the pelvis until approximately 12 weeks of gestation and is relatively well sheltered from abdominal injury until that time. As the uterus grows, it becomes more prominent and more vulnerable to injury. Measurement of fundal height provides a rapid approximation of gestational age. At 20 weeks of gestation, the fundal height should be at the level of the umbilicus and should be approximately 1 cm above the umbilicus per week of gestation. Intrauterine hemorrhage or uterine rupture may result in a discrepancy in measurement. Fetal monitoring should be done as soon as the primary survey is complete. A pelvic examination should be performed, by an obstetrician if possible to evaluate for vaginal bleeding, ruptured membranes, or a bulging perineum. Vaginal bleeding may indicate abruptio placentae, placenta previa, or preterm labor. Rupture of the amniotic fluid may result in umbilical cord prolapse, which compresses the umbilical vessels and compromises fetal blood flow. Immediate cesarean section is required. If cloudy white or greenish fluid is seen from the cervical os or perineum, the presence of amniotic fluid is confirmed by Nitrazine paper, which changes from green to blue.

The Kleihauer-Betke test for the assessment of fetomaternal transfusion is useful after maternal trauma and should be ordered with the initial laboratory studies that include a type and crossmatch. Because of the sensitivity of the Kleihauer-Betke test, a small amount of fetomaternal transfusion may be undetected. Therefore, all Rh-negative pregnant trauma patients should be considered for Rh immunoglobulin (RhoGAM) therapy.

Diagnostic radiologic testing in a pregnant patient should be completed if clinically indicated. Ultrasound should be the first imaging modality, followed by judicial use of x-rays and CT scans. CT scan should be considered if there are no other modalities to diagnose a suspected injury.

The most common cause of fetal death after blunt injury is abruptio placentae. Deceleration of the fetal heart rate may be the earliest sign of abruption. The uterus should be evaluated for contractions, rupture, or abruptio placentae. Early initiation of cardiotocographic fetal monitoring adequately warns of deterioration in the condition of the fetus.

SUMMARY

Pregnant patients are susceptible to the same surgical diseases as nonpregnant patients of similar age. Maternal physiologic changes and the enlarging uterus may result in atypical presentation of surgical disease, or symptoms may be attributed to normal pregnancy. A delay in diagnosis and treatment of surgical illnesses in pregnancy poses a greater risk to maternal and fetal well-being than the risks of anesthesia or of surgical intervention. Early consultation with an obstetrician, maternal-fetal medicine specialist, and perinatologist can ensure optimal outcomes and avoid pitfalls. Laparoscopy is becoming increasingly accepted in pregnant patients, and it is hoped that future advances will make it even safer for obstetric patients. Prevention of preterm labor should be individualized based on the patient's gestational age and underlying disease process.

SELECTED REFERENCES

Amant F, Loibl S, Neven P, et al: Breast cancer in pregnancy. *Lancet* 379:570–579, 2012.

This current and comprehensive review of breast cancer in pregnancy includes ongoing trends in treatment.

Babler EA: Perforative appendicitis complicating pregnancy. *JAMA* 51:1310, 1908.

This landmark article contains the first description of appendicitis in pregnancy.

Baer JL: Appendicitis in pregnancy. *JAMA* 98:1359, 1932.

This landmark article illustrates the change in appendiceal location during pregnancy.

Brodsky JB, Cohen EN, Brown BW, Jr, et al: Surgery during pregnancy and fetal outcome. *Am J Obstet Gynecol* 138:1165, 1980.

This large series was the first to look at fetal outcomes in nonobstetric surgery.

Cohen-Kerem R, Railton C, Oren D, et al: Pregnancy outcome following non-obstetric surgical intervention. *Am J Surg* 190:3, 2005.

This large series looked at nonobstetric surgical pregnancy outcomes in 12,452 patients reported in 44 articles. The maternal death rate was 0.006%, and the miscarriage rate was 5.8%.

LeBeau SO, Mandel SJ: Thyroid disorders during pregnancy. *Endocrinol Metab Clin North Am* 35:117–136, 2006.

This article is a comprehensive review of all the major thyroid abnormalities that occur during pregnancy.

Mourad J, Elliott JP, Erickson L, et al: Appendicitis in pregnancy: New information that contradicts longheld clinical beliefs. *Am J Obstet Gynecol* 182:1027, 2000.

This article, which retrospectively reviewed more than 66,000 deliveries and found 45 pregnant patients with appendicitis, challenged the original landmark paper by Baer regarding the presentation of acute appendicitis in pregnant patients.

Pearl J, Price R, Richardson W, et al: Guidelines for diagnosis, treatment, and use of laparoscopy for surgical problems during pregnancy. *Surg Endosc* 25:3479–3492, 2011.

This article presents current guidelines from the Society of American Gastrointestinal Endoscopic Surgeons regarding laparoscopy in pregnancy.

Tarraza HM, Moore RD: Gynecologic causes of the acute abdomen and the acute abdomen in pregnancy. *Surg Clin North Am* 77:1371, 1997.

This review accurately describes the increased risk to the mother and fetus resulting from the underlying pathology as opposed to the risk imposed by surgical intervention.

REFERENCES

1. Cohen-Kerem R, Railton C, Oren D, et al: Pregnancy outcome following non-obstetric surgical intervention. *Am J Surg* 190:467–473, 2005.
2. Tan EK, Tan EL: Alterations in physiology and anatomy during pregnancy. *Best Pract Res Clin Obstet Gynaecol* 27:791–802, 2013.
3. Boregowda G, Shehata HA: Gastrointestinal and liver disease in pregnancy. *Best Pract Res Clin Obstet Gynaecol* 27:835–853, 2013.
4. Costantine MM: Physiologic and pharmacokinetic changes in pregnancy. *Front Pharmacol* 5:65, 2014.
5. Melchiorre K, Sharma R, Thilaganathan B: Cardiac structure and function in normal pregnancy. *Curr Opin Obstet Gynecol* 24:413–421, 2012.
6. Lohr JM, Bush RL: Venous disease in women: Epidemiology, manifestations, and treatment. *J Vasc Surg* 57:37S–45S, 2013.
7. ESHRE Capri Workshop Group: Venous thromboembolism in women: A specific reproductive health risk. *Hum Reprod Update* 19:471–482, 2013.
8. Duthie L, Reynolds RM: Changes in the maternal hypothalamic-pituitary-adrenal axis in pregnancy and postpartum: Influences on maternal and fetal outcomes. *Neuroendocrinology* 98:106–115, 2013.
9. Budenhofer BK, Ditsch N, Jeschke U, et al: Thyroid (dys-) function in normal and disturbed pregnancy. *Arch Gynecol Obstet* 287:1–7, 2013.
10. Wang PI, Chong ST, Kielar AZ, et al: Imaging of pregnant and lactating patients: Part 1, evidence-based review and recommendations. *AJR Am J Roentgenol* 198:778–784, 2012.
11. Goodman TR, Amurao M: Medical imaging radiation safety for the female patient: Rationale and implementation. *Radiographics* 32:1829–1837, 2012.
12. Abramowicz JS: Benefits and risks of ultrasound in pregnancy. *Semin Perinatol* 37:295–300, 2013.
13. Friedel D, Stavropoulos S, Iqbal S, et al: Gastrointestinal endoscopy in the pregnant woman. *World J Gastrointest Endosc* 6:156–167, 2014.
14. Reitman E, Flood P: Anaesthetic considerations for non-obstetric surgery during pregnancy. *Br J Anaesth* 107(Suppl 1):i72–i78, 2011.
15. Palanisamy A: Maternal anesthesia and fetal neurodevelopment. *Int J Obstet Anesth* 21:152–162, 2012.
16. Moaveni DM, Birnbach DJ, Ranasinghe JS, et al: Fetal assessment for anesthesiologists: Are you evaluating the other patient? *Anesth Analg* 116:1278–1292, 2013.

17. Bloor M, Paech M: Nonsteroidal anti-inflammatory drugs during pregnancy and the initiation of lactation. *Anesth Analg* 116:1063–1075, 2013.
18. Evans SR, Sarani B, Bhanot P, et al: Surgery in pregnancy. *Curr Probl Surg* 49:333–388, 2012.
19. Corneille MG, Gallup TM, Bening T, et al: The use of laparoscopic surgery in pregnancy: Evaluation of safety and efficacy. *Am J Surg* 200:363–367, 2010.
20. Germain A, Brunaud L: Visceral surgery and pregnancy. *J Visc Surg* 147:e129–e135, 2010.
21. Pearl J, Price R, Richardson W, et al: Guidelines for diagnosis, treatment, and use of laparoscopy for surgical problems during pregnancy. *Surg Endosc* 25:3479–3492, 2011.
22. Azim HA, Jr, Santoro L, Russell-Edu W, et al: Prognosis of pregnancy-associated breast cancer: A meta-analysis of 30 studies. *Cancer Treat Rev* 38:834–842, 2012.
23. Amant F, Loibl S, Neven P, et al: Breast cancer in pregnancy. *Lancet* 379:570–579, 2012.
24. Brewer M, Kueck A, Runowicz CD: Chemotherapy in pregnancy. *Clin Obstet Gynecol* 54:602–618, 2011.
25. Woo JC, Yu T, Hurd TC: Breast cancer in pregnancy: A literature review. *Arch Surg* 138:91–98; discussion 99, 2003.
26. Viswanathan S, Ramaswamy B: Pregnancy-associated breast cancer. *Clin Obstet Gynecol* 54:546–555, 2011.
27. Cardoso F, Loibl S, Pagani O, et al: The European Society of Breast Cancer Specialists recommendations for the management of young women with breast cancer. *Eur J Cancer* 48:3355–3377, 2012.
28. Lu EJ, Curet MJ, El-Sayed YY, et al: Medical versus surgical management of biliary tract disease in pregnancy. *Am J Surg* 188:755–759, 2004.
29. Joshi D, James A, Quaglia A, et al: Liver disease in pregnancy. *Lancet* 375:594–605, 2010.
30. Almashhrawi AA, Ahmed KT, Rahman RN, et al: Liver diseases in pregnancy: Diseases not unique to pregnancy. *World J Gastroenterol* 19:7630–7638, 2013.
31. Lekarev O, New MI: Adrenal disease in pregnancy. *Best Pract Res Clin Endocrinol Metab* 25:959–973, 2011.
32. Abdelmannan D, Aron DC: Adrenal disorders in pregnancy. *Endocrinol Metab Clin North Am* 40:779–794, 2011.
33. Negro R, Stagnaro-Green A: Diagnosis and management of subclinical hypothyroidism in pregnancy. *BMJ* 349:g4929, 2014.
33a. Abalovich M, Vázquez A, Alcaraz G, et al: Adequate levothyroxine doses for the treatment of hypothyroidism newly discovered during pregnancy. *Thyroid* 23:1479–1483, 2013. doi: 10.1089/thy.2013.0024.
34. Lazarus JH: Management of hyperthyroidism in pregnancy. *Endocrine* 45:190–194, 2014.
35. Miloudi N, Brahem M, Ben Abid S, et al: Acute appendicitis in pregnancy: Specific features of diagnosis and treatment. *J Visc Surg* 149:e275–e279, 2012.
36. Loar PV, 3rd, Sanchez-Ramos L, Kaunitz AM, et al: Maternal death caused by midgut volvulus after bariatric surgery. *Am J Obstet Gynecol* 193:1748–1749, 2005.
37. Friedman S, McElrath TF, Wolf JL: Management of fertility and pregnancy in women with inflammatory bowel disease: A practical guide. *Inflamm Bowel Dis* 19:2937–2948, 2013.
38. Gilo NB, Amini D, Landy HJ: Appendicitis and cholecystitis in pregnancy. *Clin Obstet Gynecol* 52:586–596, 2009.
39. Walker HG, Al Samaraee A, Mills SJ, et al: Laparoscopic appendicectomy in pregnancy: A systematic review of the published evidence. *Int J Surg* 12:1235–1241, 2014.
40. Baer JL: Appendicitis in pregnancy. *JAMA* 98:1359, 1932.
41. Kim TH, Lee HH, Chung SH: Constipation during pregnancy: When a typical symptom heralds a serious disease. *Obstet Gynecol* 119:374–378, 2012.
42. Saif MW: Management of colorectal cancer in pregnancy: A multimodality approach. *Clin Colorectal Cancer* 5:247–256, 2005.
43. Nanez L, Knowles M, Modrall JG, et al: Ruptured splenic artery aneurysms are exceedingly rare in pregnant women. *J Vasc Surg* 60:1520–1523, 2014.
44. Aubrey-Bassler FK, Sowers N: 613 cases of splenic rupture without risk factors or previously diagnosed disease: A systematic review. *BMC Emerg Med* 12:11, 2012.
45. Raja AS, Zabbo CP: Trauma in pregnancy. *Emerg Med Clin North Am* 30:937–948, 2012.
46. Koh MB, Lao ZT, Rhodes E: Managing haematological disorders during pregnancy. *Best Pract Res Clin Obstet Gynaecol* 27:855–865, 2013.
47. Mendez-Figueroa H, Dahlke JD, Vrees RA, et al: Trauma in pregnancy: An updated systematic review. *Am J Obstet Gynecol* 209:1–10, 2013.
48. John PR, Shiozawa A, Haut ER, et al: An assessment of the impact of pregnancy on trauma mortality. *Surgery* 149:94–98, 2011.

72 CHAPTER

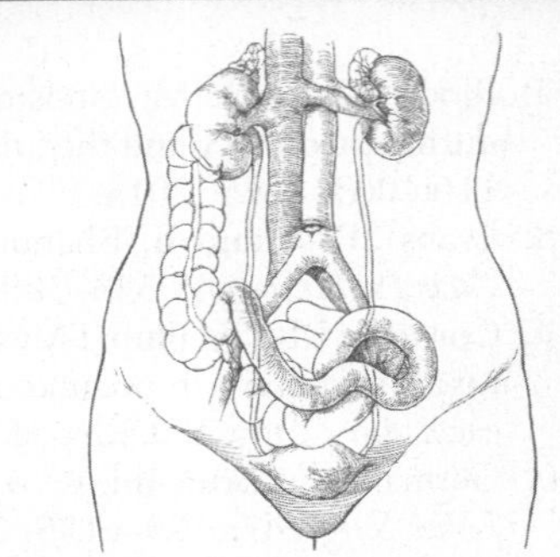

Urologic Surgery

Thomas Gillispie Smith III, Michael Coburn

OUTLINE

Urology is the study, treatment, and surgery of diseases of the retroperitoneum, pelvis, and male genitalia. Of the subspecialties, urology shares the most in common with general surgery because of our operative approaches and techniques (both open and minimally invasive) in the abdomen, retroperitoneum, and pelvis. Like general surgeons, urologists treat patients with open, laparoscopic, robotic, and endoscopic techniques. Frequently, urologists and general surgeons collaborate in care of patients across our many interdisciplinary subspecialties. Examples of this include the stress of major trauma surgery, complexity of exenterative surgery for advanced pelvic malignant neoplasms, management of iatrogenic urologic and surgical injury, and challenges of necrotizing infections of the genitalia and perineum.

General surgeons will encounter patients with urologic conditions as either presenting symptoms of or comorbidities to their general surgical diseases. Urology itself has multiple subspecialties and treats a wide range of patients and diseases spanning pediatrics, stone disease, and oncology. The intent of this chapter is to give the practicing surgeon and trainee a broad overview of the field of urology and to impart a fundamental knowledge of our field to assist in our common goal of surgical care of the patient.

UROLOGIC ANATOMY FOR THE GENERAL SURGEON

The organs of the genitourinary system span the entire retroperitoneum, pelvis, inguinal region, and genital region. Because of the close anatomic relationships of the organs in the abdomen and retroperitoneum, general surgeons must be familiar with all of the urologic organ systems to prevent iatrogenic injury and to deal with variations in normal anatomy. These challenges arise in many fields of surgery, including vascular, oncology, and colorectal surgery.

Upper Abdomen and Retroperitoneum

Adrenal

Beginning at the most superior aspect of the retroperitoneum lie the adrenal glands. These small, paired organs have two different embryologic origins and serve a primary endocrine function. The adrenal glands are composed of the cortex and medulla and are fused after development. The cortex is the outer layer of the adrenal gland and is derived from mesoderm.[1] On cross section, the layers, from external to internal, are the zona glomerulosa, zona fasciculata, and zona reticularis. The different zones secrete various steroid-derived hormones including mineralocorticoids (glomerulosa), glucocorticoids (fasciculata), and sex steroids (reticularis).[2] The adrenal medulla is derived from neural crest cells and is directly innervated by presynaptic sympathetic fibers.[1] The medulla is responsible for secreting catecholamines in response to sympathetic stimulation. The adrenal glands lie within Gerota fascia and have an orange-yellow appearance and an area of usually 3 to 5 cm in transverse diameter.[1] The arterial supply is through three sources: superior—inferior phrenic; medial—abdominal aorta; and inferior—ipsilateral renal artery. The venous drainage does not mirror the arterial supply; on the right, the single adrenal vein drains to the vena cava, whereas on the left, the adrenal vein drains into the left renal vein. Supernumerary veins can exist on either side because of anatomic variation. The adrenal glands are anatomically distinct from the kidney, although there are ventral and dorsal fascial investments that connect it to the kidney. The anatomic relations to the right adrenal gland are the vena cava on the anteromedial aspect and the liver and duodenum on the anterior aspect of portions of the adrenal gland. On the left, the pancreas and splenic vein are anterior to the cortical surface.

Kidney

The kidneys are the next paired organs just inferior to the adrenal glands. These organs are completely enveloped within the perirenal fascia (Gerota fascia) and are mobile structures supported only by the perirenal fat, renal vasculature, and abdominal muscles and viscera. Although Gerota fascia separates the kidney capsule and parenchyma from these adjacent organs and reduces the risk of renal injury with local dissection, renal parenchymal injury is possible with abnormal anatomy. The kidneys are approximately the size of a closed fist, measuring 10 to 12 cm in length and 5 to 7 cm in width. The right kidney lies more inferiorly than the left kidney because of the liver. Despite being located in the retroperitoneum, the kidney is well protected from external injury. Posteriorly, each kidney is covered by the diaphragm on the upper third of its surface and is crossed by the twelfth rib. The inferior aspect of the kidney is adjacent to the psoas muscle medially and the quadratus lumborum and transversus abdominis laterally.[1] The anterior surfaces of the kidneys are intimately related to several intraperitoneal structures. On the right, the liver is attached to the kidney by the hepatorenal ligament, and the anterior upper pole is adjacent to the peritoneal surface of the liver.[1] The duodenum lies on the medial aspect of the anterior right kidney, typically on the hilar structures. The hepatic flexure of the colon crosses anterior to the inferior pole of the right kidney. On the left, the superior pole of the kidney lies posterior to the tail of the pancreas and the splenic vessels and hilum. The spleen is situated anteromedial to the kidney and is directly attached to the kidney by the lienorenal ligament. The splenic flexure of the colon is draped over the caudal aspect of the anterior left kidney.

The renal vasculature has significant variability occurring in 25% to 40% of kidneys.[3] The typical vasculature is based on a paired artery and vein supplying the kidney as direct branches of the aorta and vena cava, respectively. The renal artery branches from the aorta inferior to the superior mesenteric artery at the level of the second lumbar vertebra. The renal artery then branches into four or five segments, each being an end artery.[3] The renal arteries are located posterior and slightly superior to the renal veins. The artery initially branches posteriorly into the posterior segmental artery. The anterior branches are variable but include the apical, upper, middle, and lower segmental arteries. These arteries branch multiple times within the cortical kidney, creating a complex filtration mechanism at the capillary level. The venous capillary branches coalesce to mirror the parenchymal arterial system. Renal segmental veins are not end vascular structures and collateralize extensively. The renal vein on the right is short, typically 2 to 4 cm in length, and enters the posterolateral inferior vena cava.[3] The left renal vein is longer, 6 to 10 cm, and travels anterior to the aorta and inferior to the superior mesenteric artery and enters the left lateral vena cava.[3] The left renal vein also is the common entry point for the left adrenal vein, gonadal vein, and a lumbar vein. Renal ectopia is accompanied by markedly variable and unpredictable renal vasculature, with multiple branches arising from the iliac arteries or aortic bifurcation.

Ureter

The upper collecting system begins within the renal parenchyma at the level of the papilla. The papillae coalesce to become the minor calyces which, in turn, become the major calyces. The major calyces converge to form the renal pelvis. The ureter begins at the inferior aspect of the renal pelvis, where it narrows to become the ureteropelvic junction posterior to the renal artery.[2] Each ureter is typically 22 to 30 cm in length, depending on height, and courses through the retroperitoneum into the pelvis, where it connects to the urinary bladder at the ureterovesical junction.[4] At its origin, the ureter courses along the anterior psoas major muscle and is crossed by the gonadal vessels bilaterally. The ureters cross over the iliac vessels to enter the pelvis, just superior to the bifurcation of the iliac vessels into the internal and external segments. Once in the pelvis, the ureters course medially to enter the bladder. The ureters are divided into three segments, upper, middle, and lower, using this anatomic landmark as a junction point.[4] The upper segment runs from the ureteropelvic junction to the superior margin of the sacrum. The middle segment runs over the bony pelvis. The lower segment begins at the inferior margin of the sacrum and continues into the bladder. The ureteral lumen is not uniform throughout its length and has three distinct narrowing points: the ureteropelvic junction, crossing the iliac vessels, and the ureterovesical junction. The right and left ureters have separate anatomic relationships (peritoneal and retroperitoneal structures). On the right, the ureter is posterior to the ascending colon, cecum, and appendix. The left ureter is posterior to the descending and sigmoid colon. In the male, the ureters are crossed by the vasa deferentia as they emerge from the internal ring before turning medially to join the prostate. The ureteral blood is drawn from multiple vessels throughout its course and within the adventitia; the arterial vessels create an anastomosing plexus. In general, the upper ureteral segments have a medial vascular supply (i.e., renal artery and aorta), and the lower ureteral segments have a lateral vascular supply (i.e., internal iliac and various branches). This unique collateral blood flow allows extensive mobilization of the ureter, outside of its adventitia, without loss of its blood supply.[4]

The ureter is best identified, intraoperatively, in an area of normal anatomy and then followed to the area of concern. This is readily accomplished medial to the lower pole of the kidney or at the iliac bifurcation. After prior surgery or retroperitoneal disease processes, any of these rich collateral blood supply sources may not be contributory; thus, it is critical to avoid unnecessary extensive circumferential dissection of the ureter.

Pelvis

Bladder and Prostate

The bladder, the end reservoir for urine, is located within the inferior pelvis. The bladder, when empty, is located behind the pubic rami; but as the bladder becomes distended, the superior aspect of the bladder extends out of the pelvis and into the lower anterior abdomen.[5] The bladder can be injured on entering of the abdomen through a midline incision in the retropubic space (of Retzius) if the bladder is not displaced posteriorly when the midline rectus fascial incision is extended to the pubis. Superiorly, the bladder is covered by the parietal peritoneum of the pelvis as the peritoneum reflects off the anterior and lateral abdominal walls. The anterior and lateral bladder walls do not have a peritoneal surface but reside within pelvic fat and lie along the musculature of the pelvic side wall or pubis anteriorly. Prior lower abdominal or pelvic surgery can change the anatomic relations of the bladder and cause it to be affixed abnormally within the pelvis. The bladder has a unique cross section with a urothelial lining creating a tight barrier from urine and a central muscular detrusor layer involved in the excretory function of the bladder.[6] Branches of the internal iliac artery, the superior and inferior vesical arteries, supply blood to the bladder. Similar to the ureter, the bladder has a rich collateral vascular network, so ligation or damage to an artery is not detrimental to the bladder. The innervation of the bladder is important because of the excretory function of the bladder. The bladder has autonomic and somatic innervation with a dense neural network to the brain. The sympathetic innervation to the bladder is through the hypogastric nerve, and the parasympathetic supply is through the sacral cord and pelvic nerve.[5] The anatomic relationships of the bladder differ between male and female patients. In the male patient, the posterior bladder wall is adjacent to the anterior sigmoid colon and rectum. Prior pelvic surgery, irradiation, or pelvic trauma can make the plane between these structures difficult to define, resulting in inadvertent injury. In the female patient, the parietal peritoneum becomes contiguous with the anterior uterus, and the superior bladder lies against the lower uterus while the bladder base sits adjacent to the anterior vaginal wall. The spherical bladder funnels caudally into the bladder neck, and this becomes the tubular urethra inferiorly.

In the male patient, the first segment of the urethra is surrounded by and integrated into the prostate. The prostate, an endocrine gland involved with male reproductive function, is located immediately inferior to the bladder and invested in the circular fibers of the bladder neck. The prostate is surrounded by the lateral pelvic fascia on its anterior surface, by endopelvic fascia on its lateral surface, and by Denonvilliers fascia posteriorly.[7] The rectum sits immediately posterior to the prostate and is separated by a second layer of Denonvilliers fascia. This fascia also extends superiorly on the posterior prostate to encompass the seminal vesicles. The seminal vesicles are the reservoirs for seminal fluid that makes up the majority of the ejaculatory fluid. The arterial supply to both structures is through branches of the inferior vesical artery. The venous drainage mirrors the arterial supply, draining through the inferior vesical veins and subsequently into the internal iliac veins. In addition to the rectum, the other major anatomic relationship of the prostate is Santorini plexus, a network of veins derived from the dorsal venous complex of the penis.[7]

Urethra, Male Genitalia, and Perineum

The drainage of urine from the bladder is through the tubular urethra, which begins at the level of the bladder neck. In male patients, the urethra has five distinct segments: prostatic, membranous, penile, bulbar, and glandular (also known as the fossa navicularis). The prostatic and membranous urethra is surrounded by striated muscle, and when the urethra penetrates the genitourinary diaphragm in the perineum, the outer layer becomes spongy vascular tissue. Within the prostate, the ejaculatory duct opens into the urethra and serves as the exit point for seminal emission. The blood supply of the extraprostatic urethra is through the common penile artery, which is a branch of the internal pudendal artery.[5] The venous drainage of the urethra is through the circumflex penile veins and ultimately into the deep dorsal vein of the penis. The major surrounding structure in the proximal male urethra is the rectum, which sits posterior to the proximal bulbar segment. The female urethra is more regular in length and is approximately 4 cm long.[5] The female urethra contains three distinct layers as opposed to the male urethra. The proximal urethra is surrounded by smooth and striated musculature, which forms the urinary sphincter. The arterial and venous blood supply are through the internal pudendal, vaginal, and inferior vesical veins. The only structure adjacent to the female urethra is the anterior vaginal wall.

The male external genitalia consist of the penis, scrotum, and paired testes. The penis consists of three circular erectile bodies: the two dorsal corpora cavernosa and the ventral corpus spongiosum. The corpora cavernosa are responsible for penile erection; the corpus spongiosum provides support and structure to the urethra. Blood supply of the penis is through the external and internal pudendal arteries. The external pudendal artery supplies the penile skin; the internal pudendal artery supplies the urethra and the paired erectile bodies. The venous drainage of the penis is through the superficial and deep dorsal veins and the cavernosal veins. The penis is entirely an external structure, with all three erectile bodies terminating in the perineum. The scrotum is a surprisingly complex structure consisting of a muscular sac covered with a unique epidermal layer with no fat but many sebaceous and sweat glands. The sac is divided into two halves by a midline septum of dartos muscle. The blood supply to the scrotum is through the external pudendal arteries anteriorly and branches of perineal vessels posteriorly. Within the scrotum are the right and left testicles. The testicles have both endocrine and reproductive function in men. Typically, the testes are 4 to 5 cm long and 3 cm wide.[5] The vascular and genital ductal structures leave the testis from the mediastinum in the posterosuperior portion and travel through the scrotal neck into the inguinal canal. The spermatic cord is invested by the internal spermatic fascia, cremaster muscle, and external spermatic fascia, which are derived from the transversalis fascia, internal oblique, and external oblique, respectively. Arterial blood supply is primarily through the testicular or gonadal artery, which is a direct branch from the aorta inferior to the renal artery. Secondary blood supply to the testicle is through the cremasteric and vasal arteries. The venous drainage of the testicle initially begins as a pampiniform plexus coalescing into the gonadal or testicular veins. On the right, the vein drains directly into the vena cava; on the left, the vein drains into the left renal vein. The testicles are also responsible for spermatogenesis. After production, the spermatozoa exit through a series of ductal structures that emerge into the epididymis and ultimately the vas deferens. The epididymis is located posteriorly and slightly lateral to the testis. The spermatic artery, vein, and vas deferens are invested together in the fascial structures of the spermatic cord. The spermatic cord travels through the external inguinal ring through the inguinal canal and then into the pelvis through the internal inguinal ring. The spermatic cord is susceptible to injury during inguinal dissection for hernia repair, especially in redo cases, when it may be encased in fibrosis and injured without recognition. Significant injury to the spermatic cord may put the viability of the testis at risk, even though it is supported by three collateral arteries. The perineum is divided into an anterior and posterior triangle in the male by a line connecting the ischial tuberosities.[5] The posterior perineal triangle contains the anus and internal and external sphincters. The anterior triangle (or urogenital triangle) contains the corpus spongiosum and proximal aspect of the paired erectile bodies, the corpora cavernosa. The layers to the corpus spongiosum consist of the skin, subcutaneous fat, Colles fascia, and bulbospongiosus muscle (surrounding the corpus spongiosum) and ischiocavernosus muscles (surrounding the corpora cavernosa). The blood supply to this region is based on branches of the internal pudendal artery, and drainage is through the internal pudendal vein. The presence of a urethral catheter is helpful in palpating the location of the urethra, but the corpus spongiosum surrounding the bulbar urethra is still vulnerable to injury with dissection in an inflamed or obliterated anatomic plane.

ENDOSCOPIC UROLOGIC SURGERY

Urologists were early adopters of endoscopic surgery and began evaluating the urethra and bladder with cystoscopy in the early part of the 20th century. The first diagnostic and therapeutic endoscopic procedures were performed for treatment of urologic disease processes. Endoscopic procedures are divided on the basis of intervention or evaluation of the lower or upper urinary tract as each has specialized procedure-specific equipment.

Cystoscopy, or cystourethroscopy as it is formally called, is used for evaluation of the urethra, both anteriorly and posteriorly, and the bladder. Cystoscopic procedures are typically performed to evaluate the lower urinary tract in the setting of hematuria, voiding symptoms, or bladder obstruction; for surveillance in the setting of malignant neoplasms; and for removal of genitourinary foreign bodies. Furthermore, cystoscopy can be used to perform diagnostic evaluation of the upper urinary tract with use of ureteral catheters and instillation of contrast material, which is visualized within the collecting system by fluoroscopy. Cystoscopy can be performed with both rigid and flexible endoscopes, each with certain benefits and advantages. Endoscopes are sized with the French size system, which refers to the outer circumference of the instrument in millimeters. The rigid endoscope uses optical lens systems, similar to laparoscopes, and has excellent resolution. The inflexible structure is intuitive and easy to orient. Rigid cystoscopes have a range of sizes typically from 16 Fr to 26 Fr; surgical endoscopes, or resectoscopes, have the largest size of 25 Fr or 26 Fr.[8] Rigid endoscopes have larger luminal diameter, which allows greater irrigation flow, improving visualization, and passage of a number of working instruments. Rigid lower tract endoscopy is more difficult to perform in the awake patient, although it is much better tolerated in the female patient than in the male patient because of the short, straight female urethra. Flexible endoscopes are smaller, 15 Fr or 16 Fr, and better tolerated by patients for examination. Both male and female patients can be examined with local anesthetic. The flexible endoscope does not require any specific patient positioning and can be used supine and at the bedside. Finally, because of the large deflection radius, the bladder is easily evaluated without changing lens or patient position. The optics of flexible endoscopes continue to improve by advancements in camera chip capability, with new digital platforms approaching the resolution of optical lens systems. Pediatric endoscopes are smaller, 8 Fr to 12 Fr, and are typically used in the operating room.

Upper tract evaluation is performed with either a ureteroscope or a nephroscope. The most common reason for either procedure is management of calculous disease, both ureteral and renal. Ureteroscopy can also be used to visualize and to inspect the upper collecting system, ureter, and renal pelvis; for hematuria originating from the upper urinary tract; for surveillance of urothelial carcinoma; and for treatment or biopsy of abnormal findings. Ureteroscopy is performed with both flexible and semirigid endoscopes, each with different benefits and purposes. Semirigid endoscopes are 6 Fr to 7.5 Fr at the tip and gradually enlarge to 8 Fr to 9.5 Fr.[8] The taper at the tip allows introduction into the ureteral orifice at the trigone of the bladder. These endoscopes have larger working channels that allow greater irrigation flow and a larger field of view. Because semirigid ureteroscopes are fairly inflexible, they are used to evaluate and to treat conditions below the level of iliac vessels and mid and distal ureter. Flexible ureteroscopes are 5.3 Fr to 8.5 Fr at the tip and gradually enlarge to 8.4 Fr to 10.1 Fr.[8] The major advantage of flexible ureteroscopes is the deflection of the tip, which ranges from 130 to 250 degrees in one direction and 160 to 275 degrees in the opposite direction, with newer endoscopes approaching 360-degree deflection. In addition, these endoscopes can be advanced through ureteral tortuosity and over external compression, such as the psoas muscle. The working channel on the flexible ureteroscope is typically smaller because of the fiberoptic system, and introduction of instruments, such as baskets or laser fibers, reduces irrigation flow. These flexible endoscopes can be used throughout the upper urinary tract but are most useful in the proximal ureter and renal pelvis and calyceal system.

The other method of upper tract endoscopy is through direct percutaneous access into the renal collecting system. Similar to retrograde ureteroscopy, nephroscopy is most commonly used to treat large renal calculi. More recently, consideration has been given to management of upper tract urothelial tumors with fulguration and resection. Nephroscopy is performed with both rigid and flexible nephroscopes; however, most intervention is performed with the rigid system. The rigid nephroscope is placed through a percutaneous working access sheath, similar to a laparoscopic trocar, to visualize the stone or tumor. Rigid nephroscopes are usually 25 Fr to 28 Fr, and their appearance is similar to a rigid cystoscope, although they have a fixed lens system rather than an exchangeable lens. Newer rigid nephroscopes are built on a digital platform that allows a larger working channel with comparable optics to a standard endoscope. Various intracorporeal lithotripters are placed through the working channel to fragment large stones into manageable pieces. Flexible nephroscopes are essentially flexible cystoscopes that are dual purposed for evaluation of the kidney. Flexible endoscopy of the upper tract is advantageous because all areas of the upper collecting system (upper, mid, and lower pole calyces) can be inspected regardless of angle or direction of the internal infundibula.

Numerous working elements are used in both upper and lower tract endoscopy. Guidewires are commonly used to access the upper urinary tract collecting system or the bladder and serve as guides to pass catheters, stents, and sheaths. Most guidewires have a flexible tip and a rigid shaft and are constructed of inner core and outer covering, which may hydrophilic or neutral (polytetrafluoroethylene). Guidewires range in size from 0.018 to 0.038 inch and have various lengths. Urethral catheters and ureteral catheters may be placed over wires to assist with direct placement into the lower or upper urinary system, respectively. Ureteral stents are hollow catheters with flexible ends that form a coil on the proximal and distal ends to maintain position within the collecting systems. Stents are placed to ensure drainage of the kidney and to bypass blockages of the ureter from inflammation, stones, or tumors. Most stents are composed of thermodynamic material, which becomes softer at higher body temperatures. Stents range in size from 4.8 Fr to 10 Fr and have various lengths to accommodate variable ureteral lengths. Ureteroscopic baskets are used to remove ureteral and renal calculi and to perform extraction and biopsy of tumors. These range in size from 1.3 Fr to 3.2 Fr and are constructed of flexible material to allow placement into various calyceal locations within the kidney.

UROLOGIC INFECTIOUS DISEASE

Urinary tract infections (UTIs) are a common medical problem, although patients with UTI evaluated and treated by urologists have a complicated or unusual element to their diagnosis. Other infections treated by urologists include infections of the genital skin, a spectrum of disease from cellulitis to necrotizing fasciitis, and reproduction organs in men (i.e., orchitis, epididymitis, or prostatitis). Furthermore, these infections may require simple antibiotic therapy or multimodal treatment with surgical drainage or débridement and management in an intensive care setting.

Urinary tract obstruction with proximal infection may result in sepsis, challenging the skills of the urologist and surgical critical care specialist.

Uncomplicated Urinary Tract Infection

Between the years of 2002 and 2007, UTIs in adult women and men accounted for 39 million office visits and 6 million emergency department visits.[9] In adult patients, more than 50% of women and 12% of men will develop a UTI during their lifetime.[9] Urinary infection is considered uncomplicated when it occurs in the immunocompetent host, without underlying anatomic or physiologic abnormalities of the urinary tract in women. UTI diagnosed in men is always considered complicated. For diagnosis of a UTI, a clean catch, midstream urine specimen is preferred, and on culture, 10^5 colony-forming units must be demonstrated. In catheterized specimens, UTI can be diagnosed with as little as 10^3 colony-forming units. The typical symptoms associated with UTI are dysuria, frequency, urgency to void, and malodorous urine. Because of the inherent differences in etiology, evaluation, and treatment, uncomplicated UTIs are divided into those occurring in premenopausal and postmenopausal women. A third category of uncomplicated UTI, that occurring in pregnant patients, is beyond the scope of this overview. In general, risk factors include genetic, biologic, and behavioral; specific aspects are discussed with each group.

Premenopausal Patients

History and physical examination of patients in this age group presenting with symptoms of UTI are particularly important because of overlapping disease processes. In patients without vaginal discharge, the majority can be expected to have a UTI as the diagnosis. However, in sexually active women, sexually transmitted infections (STIs) must be considered, especially in the setting of a negative urine culture. Furthermore, in patients with vaginal discharge, vaginitis caused by yeast, trichomoniasis, and bacterial vaginosis are possible causes. Risk factors for UTI in this population of patients include frequent sexual intercourse, initial UTI at a young age, maternal history of UTI, and number of pregnancies and deliveries.[10] Important aspects of the physical examination in these patients include palpation of costovertebral tenderness (assessing for ascending infection) and pelvic examination to evaluate for STI. The most common cause of infection in these patients is *Escherichia coli* (80% to 85%), followed by *Staphylococcus saprophyticus* (10% to 15%) and *Klebsiella pneumoniae* and *Proteus mirabilis* (4% each).[10] Empirical therapy is acceptable, although confirmatory urine cultures are useful as the incidence of antibiotic resistance continues to rise. Prevention includes increased hydration and evaluation of hygiene practices.

Postmenopausal Patients

As in younger patients, history and physical examination are important aspects of UTI evaluation in this group of patients. Presenting symptoms are similar in this group, although some elderly patients may simply present with altered mental status. Furthermore, an important component in diagnosis and treatment of postmenopausal women is the change in the vaginal pH levels and change or reduction in lactobacillus in the vaginal flora. The physical examination findings may differ in these patients as STIs are less likely but physical changes, such as pelvic organ prolapse and incomplete bladder emptying, become causative factors. In addition, the pathologic bacterial species are different. *E. coli* continues to be the predominant organism but in this age group, *P. mirabilis, K. pneumoniae*, and *Enterobacter* species become more prevalent pathogens.[10] Again, empirical therapy is acceptable, but urine cultures are important because of increasing antibiotic resistance patterns and differing organisms. Prevention includes increased hydration and evaluation of hygiene practices.

Complicated Urinary Tract Infection

Complicated UTIs require more vigilance on the part of the treating physician because of patient factors that may lead to a more rapid progression or worsening of the infection. By definition, complicated UTIs occur in men and in patients with diabetes, immunosuppression, upper tract infection, resistant organisms, urinary tract anatomic abnormalities, prior surgery, calculous disease, spinal cord injury, or recent or current indwelling Foley catheter. In these patients, similar evaluation is warranted, but the evaluation should not be limited to simply history and physical examination. Empirical treatment of complicated UTI alone is not appropriate, and urine cultures should be performed on all patients with suspected complicated UTI before initiation of antibiotic therapy. In addition, imaging is indicated in these patients because of concern for calculous disease and urinary stasis, so at a minimum, a kidney, ureter, and bladder study and renal ultrasound with cross-sectional imaging should be performed in all patients with equivocal or concerning findings. Finally, antibiotic therapy alone may not be adequate, and these patients may require surgical drainage of obstructed urinary systems or later surgical correction of anatomic abnormalities or removal of urinary stones (once infections are treated) to prevent recurrent UTIs. Consultation with infectious disease specialists may also be indicated in patients with urologic anatomic abnormalities and recurrent UTIs with resistant organisms.

Urinary Tract Infection in Men

Because of the lower incidence of UTI in men, when men present with symptoms of infection, it is always considered complicated, regardless of other patient factors. As in women, younger men (younger than 50 years) and older men (older than 50 years) have different causes of their UTI and symptoms. Common presenting symptoms are urethritis, dysuria, hesitancy, frequency, and urgency of urination. A history and physical examination in these patients are important to delineate different sources of symptoms or UTI. Men can present with these symptoms and have different diagnoses, including UTI, STI, urethritis, and chronic pelvic pain. Furthermore, bacterial infections can extend to other proximal areas of the genitourinary system, such as the prostate and testicle. Men younger than 50 years are more likely to have STI as the cause rather than UTI. These men should have a thorough sexual history, genital examination, and microscopic urinalysis performed. Urethral swab or urine tests for STI should be performed as well. Men older than 50 years often have underlying lower urinary tract symptoms (LUTS), and this can be a contributing factor. Men in this age group more frequently will have UTI as a source of their symptoms, and common urinary pathogens, as in women, should be considered. Furthermore, older men should be questioned about recent surgical procedures, catheterization, or hospitalization. Elderly men can also present with mental status changes as their only symptom of UTI, and this diagnosis must be ruled out in these patients. A lower threshold for imaging and hospital admission is necessary in men with UTI as they may present with more systemic symptoms. Patients who cannot tolerate oral intake, are immunocompromised, or have medical comorbidities should be admitted with cross-sectional imaging performed. Broad-spectrum intravenous antibiotics, based on local resistance patterns, and fluid resuscitation should be initiated in these patients while the initial workup and evaluation are completed. Urinary obstruction or stone disease in these patients constitutes a urologic emergency and must be addressed rapidly.

Specific Complicated Genitourinary Infectious States

Pyelonephritis

Pyelonephritis is a spectrum of infectious or inflammatory processes that involve the kidney collecting system or parenchyma. Pyelonephritis results from a UTI moving proximally upward from the lower urinary tract. In the simple form, pyelonephritis may be treated on an outpatient basis with oral antibiotics for 1 to 2 weeks. In this group of patients, urine culture is necessary to identify the causative organism. If the patient appears more acutely infected, hospitalization may be warranted for broad-spectrum intravenous antibiotic therapy, fluid resuscitation, and cross-sectional imaging. *Emphysematous pyelonephritis* represents an advanced form of pyelonephritis and is considered a urologic emergency. These patients have a significant necrotizing infection of the kidney with gas-forming organisms, with pockets of gas within the parenchyma apparent on imaging (Fig. 72-1). The common bacterial pathogens include *E. coli, P. mirabilis,* and *K. pneumoniae.*[11] These patients require either prompt percutaneous drainage of the infection or rapid nephrectomy. Most patients who present with this condition are diabetic or have significant medical comorbidities, and control of the metabolic abnormalities, aggressive broad-spectrum antibiotic therapy, and supportive critical care are essential. *Xanthogranulomatous pyelonephritis* is a chronic infectious process resulting from renal obstruction, recurrent infection, and renal calculous disease. The disease presents in three forms, focal, segmental, or diffuse, and each is treated in a different manner. The underlying histologic process involves a foamy, lipid-laden, macrophage infiltrate in the renal parenchyma, with extensive inflammation, fibrosis, and loss of renal function. On imaging, there may be indications of collecting system dilation; however, drainage attempts often are unproductive because the material is often solid or too viscous to drain. Patients with focal or segmental disease may be treated with antibiotics, but those with diffuse disease frequently require nephrectomy. The risk of iatrogenic adjacent organ injury is high in these nephrectomies, and the renal hilum may be so inflamed and fibrotic that the renal vessels cannot be individually dissected. These cases may require placement of a vascular pedicle clamp with renal excision and oversewing of the pedicle.

Male Genital Organ Infection

UTIs may ascend into the genital ducts, resulting in infection of the prostate, epididymis, or testicle. Beginning in the urethra, the verumontanum is the exit point of the seminal vesicles and vas deferens into the urinary tract. Prostatitis refers to any inflammatory process affecting the prostate, but the general surgeon more commonly may encounter acute bacterial prostatitis, which results

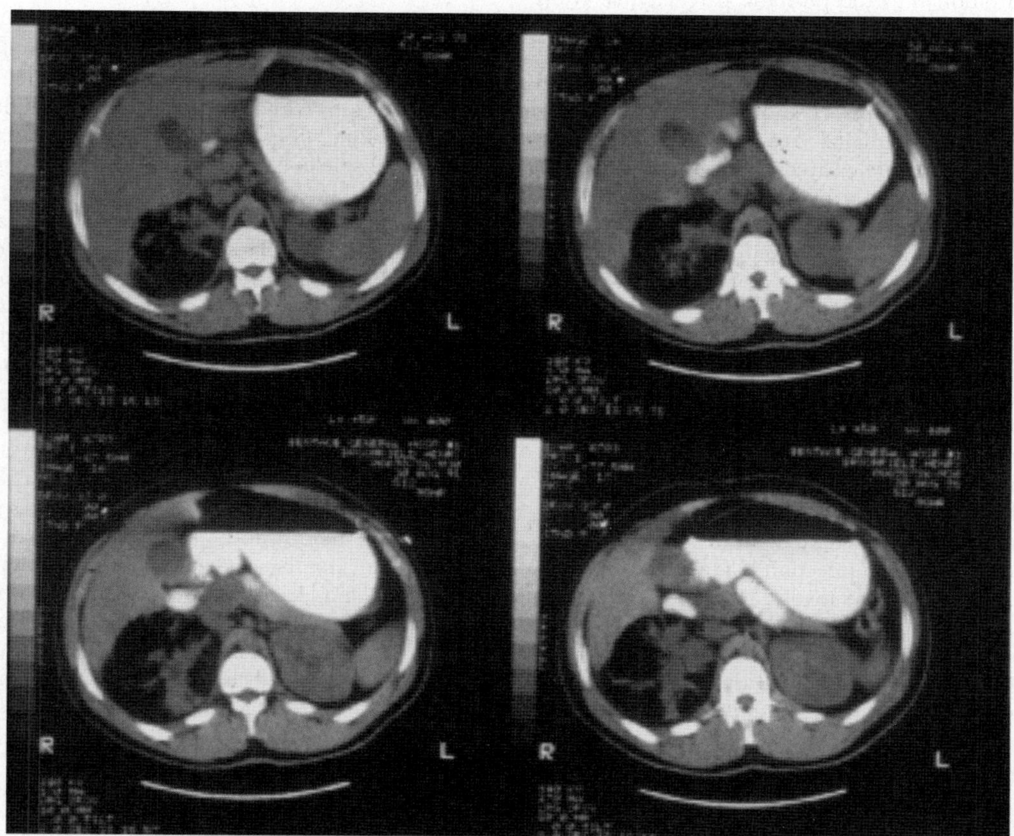

FIGURE 72-1 Emphysematous Pyelonephritis. This CT scan demonstrates extensive destruction of the right kidney with intraparenchymal gas on the right, obliterating the renal architecture. The left kidney is normal.

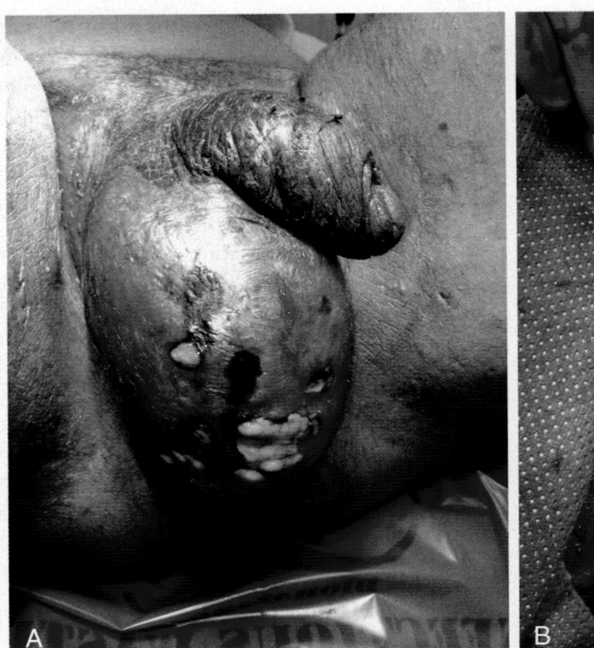

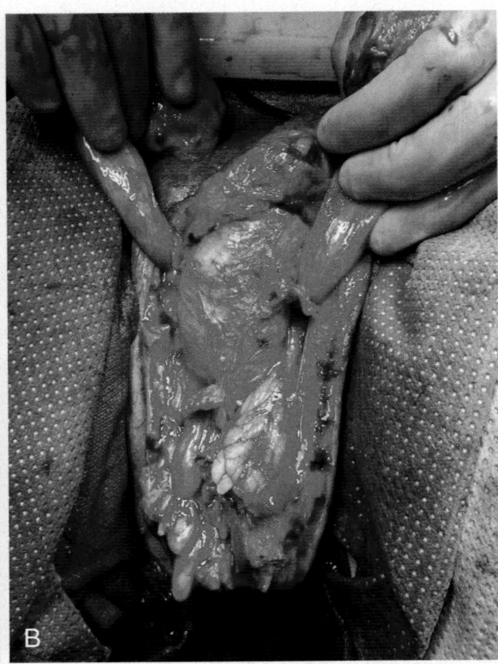

FIGURE 72-2 Fournier Gangrene. **A,** Skin necrosis, purulence, and edema of the scrotum. The skin can also appear normal, with much more subtle physical findings in some cases. **B,** Appearance after extensive débridement of scrotal skin and underlying tissues. The base of the penis is visible centrally; the testes are elevated out of the field, and the spermatic cords are visible anteriorly.

from bacterial infiltration into the prostatic parenchyma. Most infections of the prostate are secondary to gram-negative bacterial infection and typically are associated with UTI. Two important considerations in these patients are physical examination and disease extent. Although a full history and physical examination are warranted, elimination of digital rectal examination (DRE) should be considered as pressure exerted on an infected prostate may lead to hematogenous spread of the bacteria. In addition, patients who do not have reasonably rapid resolution of their symptoms should be evaluated for prostatic abscess. Prostatic abscesses typically do not respond to antibiotic therapy and require transurethral unroofing to allow adequate drainage.

Epididymitis-orchitis results when the UTI ascends through the vas deferens into the epididymis or testicle. Again, the cause is different according to the patient's age; men younger than 35 years typically have an STI as a source, commonly *Chlamydia trachomatis,* whereas men older than 35 years will often have infections related to *E. coli*. Examination of these patients is often difficult because of significant swelling of the affected epididymis or testicle; scrotal ultrasound is useful diagnostically, especially to rule out associated abscess. When infection is advanced, the entire ipsilateral scrotal contents become involved, with overlying skin fixation and edema. It may be difficult to distinguish this entity from late torsion, incarcerated inguinal hernia, or testicular tumor with necrosis and inflammation. Patients without abscess may be managed with antibiotic therapy, rest, and scrotal elevation; however, recovery is slow, with eventual resolution of edema and discomfort. If abscess is present, surgical drainage and often orchiectomy are indicated. A subset of patients may have persistent pain or mass, and on repeated Doppler imaging, signs of testicular ischemia or persistent inflammation may be noted. These patients require exploration and possible orchiectomy to resolve the process.

Fournier Gangrene

Fournier gangrene is a necrotizing infection of the male genitalia and perineum similar to other progressive fasciitis and soft tissue infections (Fig. 72-2). When the genitalia are involved, patients typically present with significant pain and tenderness, scrotal and genital swelling, discoloration or frank necrosis, crepitus, and, at times, foul-smelling discharge. Fournier gangrene is usually a polymicrobial infection with microaerobes, anaerobes, and gram-positive and gram-negative organisms.[12] Risk factors for development include peripheral vascular disease, diabetes mellitus, malnutrition, alcoholism, and other immunocompromised states. This disease represents a urologic emergency. Treatment requires urgent surgical drainage with aggressive débridement of the necrotic tissue, broad-spectrum intravenous antibiotics, and intensive monitoring with supportive care. The magnitude of the débridement depends entirely on the degree of progression of the process. It is rare for the process to involve the testicles or deep tissues of the penis because of the tunica vaginalis and Buck fascia, respectively, so these structures should be preserved. It is uncommon for the urethra to be involved, although a defined urinary tract source may be evident, such as a urethral stricture, with perforation and local infection. Suprapubic tube diversion is generally not necessary; urethral catheter drainage is generally sufficient. Once the active infection is controlled, the predominant management issues become wound care and reconstruction, which may require delayed skin grafting for tissue coverage.

Atypical Urinary Tract Infections

Fungal Infection

Fungal infections in the urinary system are most common in specific populations of patients: diabetics, immunocompromised patients, and the elderly. Fungal infections may not be symptomatic and in an outpatient setting may not require therapy. Most fungal infections are related to the *Candida* species, and it is incumbent on the treating physician to determine which infections require treatment and which represent contamination. Patients who require careful evaluation and treatment include neutropenic patients and intensive care patients, who may need evaluation for an internal source, such as a fungus deposit (ball) in the bladder or kidney. Infectious disease consultation is valuable in these cases because the organisms are atypical and selection of treatment agents may not be straightforward. Renal and bladder imaging with ultrasound may demonstrate a treatable source. These patients may need antifungal bladder or kidney irrigation or occasionally endoscopic removal.

Tuberculosis

The genitourinary tract is the third most common extrapulmonary site for tuberculosis infection. This disease is spread hematogenously from the lungs and into the affected organ system. Most patients with genitourinary tuberculosis are immunocompromised, so assessment of HIV infection status is important. Patients present with various symptoms that include voiding symptoms, sterile pyuria or hematuria, and chronic kidney disease. Not all patients will have a positive PPD test result, and diagnosis is confirmed with acid-fast bacilli smears of urine and mycobacterial culture with sterile pyuria, chest radiograph, and imaging of the genitourinary system to look for anatomic abnormalities. Tuberculosis affecting the kidney may result in segmental or global glomerular dysfunction, and progression antegrade down the urinary system may result in ureteral strictures. Tuberculosis of the epididymis may result in chronic epididymitis or mass. Antibiotic therapy consists of 2 months of a four-drug regimen with a subsequent 7-month treatment with isoniazid and rifampin. Infectious disease consultation is mandatory in treating these patients because of public health concerns. Significant anatomic infection or functional change or loss may ultimately require surgical excision.

Parasitic Infection

With the ease of global transportation and a mobile global population, parasitic infections are considerations in patients with recent travel histories. The main parasitic infections of the genitourinary system are schistosomiasis, echinococcal infection, and filariasis. Each parasite has a different point of entry, systemic spread, and organ infestation. Typically, in schistosomiasis, the parasite enters the body percutaneously and spreads through the venous and lymphatic system. Most infestations affect the bladder, resulting in chronic inflammation and granulomas. These patients present with LUTS or hematuria. Medical therapy (praziquantel) can be used to treat granulomatous disease; however, untreated infections can result in squamous cell carcinoma of the bladder. Echinococcal infections are spread through ingestion of contaminated food, and the parasite penetrates the intestinal walls and infests the liver. On occasion, renal infestation can occur, with the parasite becoming encysted in the parenchyma. Medical therapy can shrink the cysts, but surgical removal by partial or total nephrectomy is required for cure. These cysts must be removed intact as rupture or spillage of internal contents can result in severe anaphylaxis. Filariasis results from direct infection of the lymphatic system through percutaneous entry. The parasite creates noticeable symptoms when it dies, resulting in obstruction of the lymphatics. Only mild infestation can be treated with oral therapy (albendazole); advanced disease requires excision and reconstruction.

VOIDING DYSFUNCTION, NEUROGENIC BLADDER, INCONTINENCE, AND BENIGN PROSTATIC HYPERPLASIA

A central aspect of urology is management of bladder function and evaluation and treatment of bladder dysfunction. The bladder is a large muscular sac responsible for storing and eliminating urine. Common dysfunctions of the bladder include neurogenic problems with bladder function, storage problems, incontinence, and outflow issues related to benign prostatic hyperplasia (BPH) or enlargement. Changes in these functional areas are one of the most common reasons for urologic consultation. Although this is a broad area of urology, concentrating on these core divisions will give the general surgeon an understanding of the complex dynamics of bladder function.

Neurogenic Bladder

Patients with neurogenic bladder dysfunction present with a wide spectrum of neurologic diseases or injuries that affect bladder function on the basis of the location of the injury or disease process. There is a complex interaction between the bladder and brain that primarily regulates bladder storage and bladder emptying. Bladder storage is driven by the sympathetic nervous system, specifically at the level of the adrenergic receptor. α-Adrenergic receptors are the most common adrenergic receptors in the bladder, prostate, and urethra; most are α_1 and α_2, with three subtypes of α_1 identified: α_{1a}, α_{1b}, and α_{1d}.[13] The α_1 receptor is the most common subtype in the lower urinary system. Bladder emptying is driven by the parasympathetic stimulation of cholinergic receptors, specifically the muscarinic receptors. The predominant muscarinic receptors in the bladder are M_2 and M_3.[13] Sensory information is carried away from the bladder by myelinated and unmyelinated afferent nerve fibers traveling through the pelvic and pudendal nerves. Any interruption in the sympathetic or parasympathetic nervous system and its communication with the bladder can result in neurogenic dysfunction. In addition, several centers within the pons, midbrain, and cerebral cortex have direct effect on the storage and emptying of the bladder.[13] Voiding is initiated at the level of the pontine micturition center, which sends out a parasympathetic signal to the bladder to initiate voiding. The pontine micturition center is inhibited by the periaqueductal gray located in the midbrain, and this is connected to the afferent signaling pathways from the bladder. Based on this standard sensory function, specific voiding symptoms or LUTS can be predicted by the location of neurologic disease or injury.

Basic evaluation of these patients includes a through history with neurologic and urologic historical focus, physical examination (focusing on the abdomen, pelvis, and peripheral and central nervous system), and urinalysis. Additional evaluation is tailored to location of injury. Cortical brain disease and injury, such as cerebrovascular accident, are evaluated by history, physical examination, and urinalysis. These disease processes do not directly affect the bladder function, and patients are treated on the basis of symptoms alone. Spinal cord lesions are divided into suprasacral spinal lesions (spinal cord injury, infarcts) and sacral or peripheral spinal cord lesions (pelvic plexus damage from surgery, diabetic neuropathy). Patients with lesions of the suprasacral spinal cord tend to have increased bladder muscle tension, which results in abnormal elasticity of the bladder (poor bladder compliance).[14] In addition, these patients have incoordination of the bladder and urinary sphincter, resulting in detrusor-sphincter dyssynergia. Patients with sacral or peripheral nerve lesions tend to have variable LUTS but typically do not have changes in bladder elasticity.[14] The detrusor muscle is often partially or completely nonfunctional, and the urinary sphincter remains closed. Specialized evaluation of the patients with spinal cord lesions includes upper tract ultrasonography to monitor for evidence of hydronephrosis and urodynamic evaluation. Urodynamic evaluation involves measuring the elasticity of the bladder on filling (compliance), the pressure generated on emptying (detrusor function) by recording the abdominal pressure, and the intraluminal bladder pressure with specialized catheters. Surveillance cystoscopy is indicated in chronic patients to rule out the development of intravesical disease. Treatment for neurogenic bladder has recently been revolutionized by the introduction of onabotulinum toxin. In the past, these patients required complex regimens of antimuscarinic agents and reconstructive surgery. Now, with the use of onabotulinum toxin, most patients are treated with periodic cystoscopic injections and intermittent catheterization.

Problems With Bladder Storage

Overactive bladder (OAB) is the most common storage-related problem of the bladder. It is defined as urinary urgency with or without urgency urinary incontinence in the absence of UTI or other obvious disease.[15] Typical symptoms of this problem include urgency, urinary frequency, nocturia, and urgency urinary incontinence. Urgency refers to the sudden, compelling desire to pass urine that is difficult to defer and replaces the normal urge.[15] Urinary frequency is the complaint of micturition occurring more frequently than previously deemed normal and characterized by daytime and nocturnal voids.[15] Nocturia is the complaint of interruption of sleep one or more times because of the need to urinate.[15] Finally, urgency urinary incontinence is the involuntary loss of urine associated with urgency.[15] A difficult aspect of this disease process is that it occurs in the spectrum of other LUTS and may be the result of long-term bladder outflow obstruction. Other conditions to consider in patients who present with OAB and LUTS are UTI, urinary calculi, diabetes, polydipsia, neurogenic bladder, and malignant disease. OAB has a worldwide prevalence of 11%, and with the aging population, this is presumed to increase over time.[16]

All patients who present with OAB should undergo a thorough evaluation. At the basic level, this includes a thorough history to fully disclose the symptoms and to rule out other causes. Historical elements that may be contributory include caffeine intake, constipation, recurrent UTI, pelvic organ prolapse in women and prostatic enlargement in men, and excessive fluid intake. Physical examination should be directed toward evaluation of the abdomen, pelvis, and neurologic systems. Other findings may include decreased mental status or cognitive function and peripheral edema. The last absolute examination element is urinalysis, which can reveal infection, inflammation, or hematuria that may indicate more serious disease. Simple adjunctive tests that can be performed in the office include measurement of post-void residual urine volume, noninvasive flow test, validated symptom questionnaires, and voiding diaries. Specialized tests and evaluation performed by the urologist may include cystoscopy, ultrasound, and urodynamic testing as appropriate. However, current guidelines do not require any of these specialized tests for initiation of treatment.[17]

Treatment of OAB is directed toward therapy, symptoms, and motivation of the individual patient (Fig. 72-3). As many patients suffering from this problem take multiple medications, pharmacologic therapy is not always offered as an initial treatment. Behavioral therapies are the first-line treatment for all patients. Behavioral therapies may include lifestyle modifications or specific physical therapies. Typically, this includes fluid intake management and modification with particular attention paid to timing of fluid intake and amounts. For example, in patients who complain of nocturia, limiting nighttime fluid intake can be beneficial. Bladder training is a noninvasive method of physical therapy whereby the patient postpones voiding to lengthen the time intervals between voids. This may be coupled with urgency suppression and timed voids to reinforce retraining of the sensory output from the bladder. Finally, voiding diaries are important to help the patient and urologist quantify the number of voids and voided amount to better target improvement goals and to tailor therapy. Pharmacologic management continues to be a mainstay of treatment and is indicated for patients as an adjunct to behavior therapies or for patients unresponsive to first-line therapy. Classic pharmacologic therapy is antimuscarinic agents that target the parasympathetic muscarinic cholinergic receptors, primarily M_2 and M_3, and block the action of these receptors. Most of the drugs in this category are administered daily and have the common side effects of dry mouth, dry eyes, and constipation. A newer pharmacologic agent, beta agonists (β_3), targets receptors in the detrusor muscle to stimulate bladder relaxation. Treatment options for patients who fail to respond to these therapies fall into the specialized third-line treatments, which include neuromodulation (either peripheral or central), onabotulinum toxin, chronic indwelling catheters, and augmentation cystoplasty.

Urinary Incontinence

Urinary incontinence is the involuntary loss of urine; it can be divided into stress urinary incontinence, urge urinary incontinence, and mixed urinary incontinence.[15] National data indicate that the prevalence of urinary incontinence in America is 49.6% in women older than 20 years.[18] Men are typically affected after the age of 50 years, and incontinence develops as a symptom of LUTS or other problems rather than as a primary complaint as in women. Stress urinary incontinence is defined as the involuntary loss of urine with Valsalva maneuver.[15] Urge urinary incontinence is the involuntary loss of urine associated with a strong urge to void.[15] Mixed urinary incontinence is any combination of these two causes.

Evaluation of these patients includes history, physical examination (including pelvic examination), urinalysis, post-void residual volume measurement, and voiding diaries. The history and physical examination are important to rule out any complicating factors including neurogenic source, anatomic changes (pelvic organ prolapse in the female patient and prostatic enlargement in the male patient), and prior surgical intervention (radical prostatectomy in the male patient or hysterectomy in the female patient) that might affect evaluation and the treatment decision. In the neurologically normal patient with no confounding factors, nonsurgical management is the first step in treatment before any surgical intervention. As with OAB, behavior modification and bladder training are the initial steps. Dietary modification is important for management of urinary incontinence. Patients are counseled to limit fluid intake to around 2 liters per day, depending on body size and activity level. In addition, patients should limit caffeine intake and other bladder irritants including alcohol, carbonated beverages, spicy foods, and citrus juices and fruits. Furthermore, bowel programs should be initiated to ensure that the patient has normal bowel function and is not constipated. Other nonsurgical treatment includes weight loss to a normal body mass index and

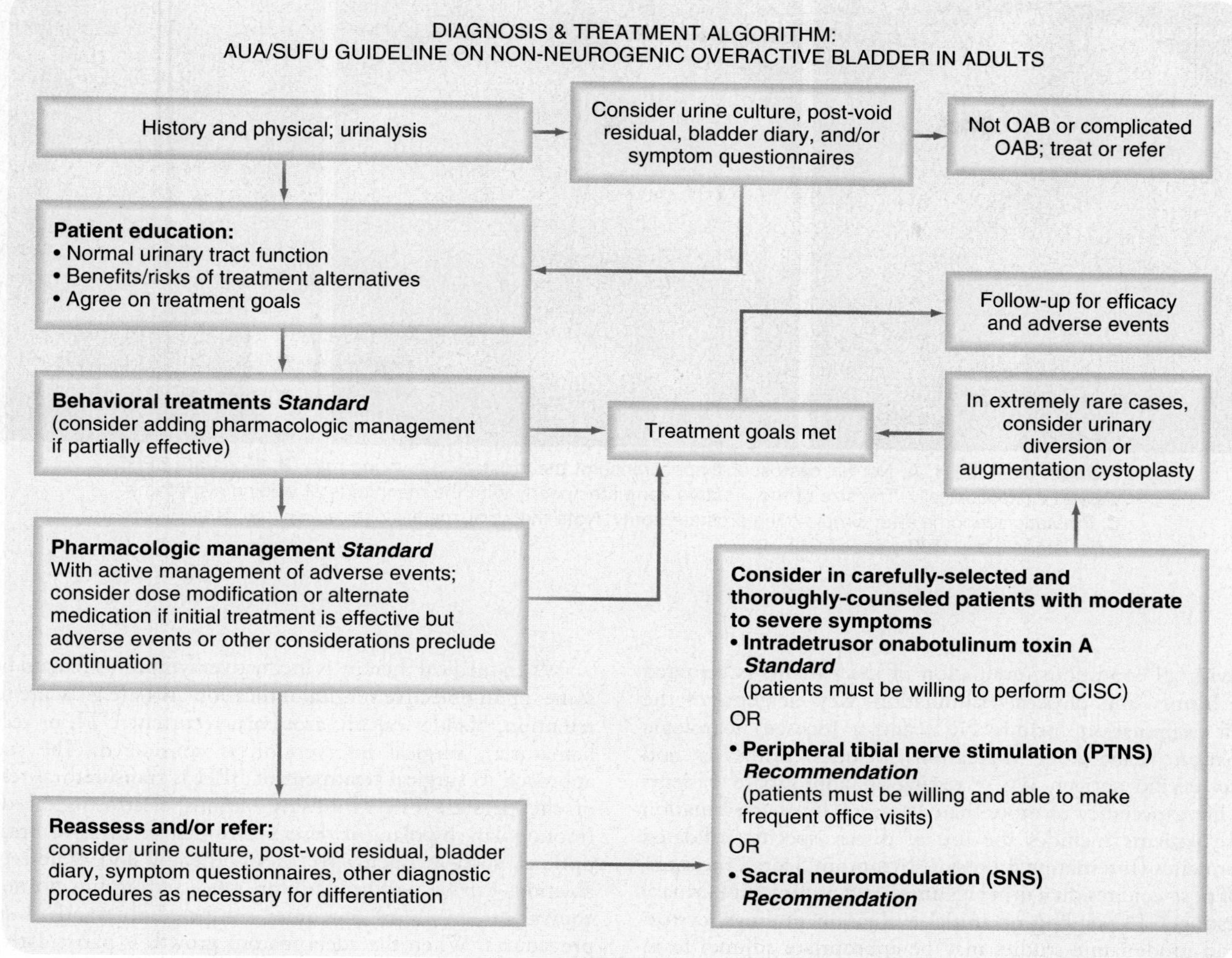

FIGURE 72-3 Algorithm for diagnosis and management of overactive bladder (OAB). (Adapted from Gormley EA, Lightner DJ, Burgio KL, et al: Diagnosis and treatment of overactive bladder [non-neurogenic] in adults: AUA/SUFU guideline. *J Urol* 188:2455–2463, 2012.)

exercise, particularly core muscle exercises. Pelvic floor muscle training and biofeedback have been shown to have acceptable rates in helping patients achieve satisfactory management of their urinary incontinence.

Surgical treatment options for women and men differ because of the inherent mechanism causing the incontinence, typically poor pelvic anatomic support in women and sphincteric in men. In women, treatment options progress from less to more invasive. The simplest treatment is injection of a urethral bulking agent through a cystoscopy. The objective of this treatment is to improve coaptation of the urinary sphincter and to increase the urethral wall volume. Unfortunately, this treatment is not likely to produce long-term cure, and re-treatment or progression to other options is often necessary. The next option is placement of a midurethral sling to resupport the central hammock of the urethra and to provide backing to the urethra during stress maneuvers. These approaches have a higher success rate, and long-term data show cure rates of approximately 90%.[19] With the success and ease of the midurethral sling, fewer open retropubic suspensions are performed. These procedures also work to improve the support of the urethra and to reduce urethral hypermobility. In men, surgical therapy is designed to reinforce the urinary sphincter to increase bladder outlet resistance. Typically, treatments are divided into male urethral slings, which have a larger surface area for the mesh suspension material, and artificial urinary sphincters. An artificial sphincter is a complex device that is implanted in the patient and opened through a one-way valve contained in the scrotum.

Benign Prostatic Hyperplasia

BPH is the development of nodules within the prostate gland as a result of enlargement of the stromal and epithelial components of the gland.[20] As the BPH progresses, the entire prostate enlarges in a process called benign prostatic enlargement, resulting in compression of the prostatic urethra and development of bladder outflow obstruction (Fig. 72-4).[20] As part of the bladder outflow obstruction, patients can develop LUTS requiring evaluation and treatment by a urologist. BPH is prevalent, affecting approximately 70% of men between the ages of 60 and 69 years, making it one of the most common conditions treated by urologists.[20] The LUTS that result from BPH can be divided into storage, voiding, and post-void symptoms. Interestingly, there is little correlation between the measured volume of the prostate and the symptoms that result. In addition, the degree of bladder outflow obstruction does not necessarily correlate with the severity of LUTS.

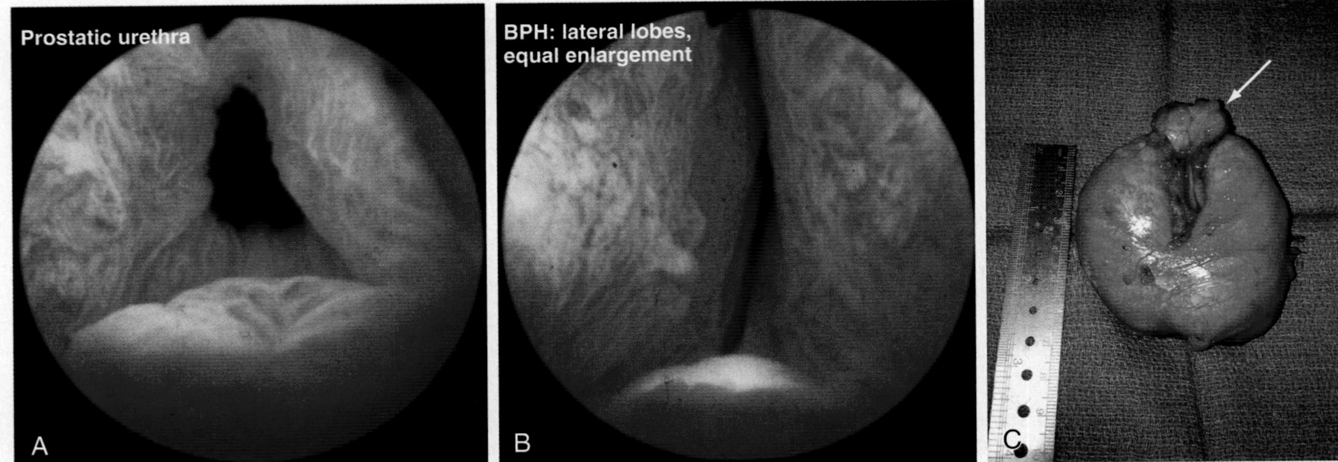

FIGURE 72-4 BPH. **A,** Normal cystoscopic appearance of the prostate in a young man. **B,** Moderate BPH, viewed cystoscopically. The size of the prostate correlates poorly with the magnitude of voiding symptoms. **C,** Prostatic adenoma after simple open prostatectomy. Note the small medial lobe *(arrow, top center),* with large lateral lobes (130-g specimen).

As with all conditions, evaluation of the patients is centered on the history and physical examination. Key elements of the physical examination include DRE and a focused neurologic examination. Laboratory evaluation includes urinalysis and prostate-specific antigen (PSA) testing in appropriate patients with a life expectancy of more than 10 years. Further evaluation of these patients includes the use of disease-specific validated questionnaires (International Prostate Symptom Score), measurement of post-void residual urine volumes, and noninvasive urinary flow testing.[20] Depending on initial evaluation findings, cystoscopy and urodynamic studies may be appropriate adjunct tests. Practice guidelines for BPH have been produced by the American Urological Association (AUA) to guide providers in the diagnosis and management of BPH (Figs. 72-5 and 72-6).[20] Similar to all voiding-related conditions, behavior and dietary modifications are appropriate first-step treatment measures in all patients. Medical therapy can be used in conjunction with the initial behavior modifications or added subsequently.

The mainstay of treatment for LUTS due to BPH is α_1-adrenergic receptor blockers.[20] As previously discussed, α-adrenergic receptors are the most common adrenergic receptors in the bladder, and α_1 is the most common subtype in the lower urinary system, prostate, and urethra. The action of α_1 blockers is to relax the smooth muscle in the bladder neck and prostate and to reduce outflow resistance. This class of drugs has become progressively more selective to the α_1 subtypes, and many now target the α_{1a} subtype receptor specifically. The most common side effects of these drugs are dizziness related to orthostasis, retrograde ejaculation, and rhinitis. A second category of pharmacologic therapy is the 5α-reductase inhibitors that target the glandular component of the prostate. These drugs block the conversion of testosterone to dihydrotestosterone in the prostate and subsequently reduce the prostate volume, thereby reducing outflow resistance. This class of drugs also alters the serum PSA level (reduces it about 50%), which must be kept in mind with regard to prostate cancer screening. In addition, these drugs can be used in combination because of their differing mechanism of action, and studies show superior results to either drug used independently.

When medical therapy is ineffective, symptoms remain bothersome, or an objective surgical indication arises (e.g., acute urinary retention, bladder calculi, azotemia, recurrent UTI, or recurrent hematuria), surgical intervention is considered. The standard approach to surgical treatment of BPH is transurethral resection of the prostate (TURP) using various electrosurgical options (monopolar, bipolar, or laser). Minimally invasive treatment options, such as microwave thermotherapy and radiofrequency ablation, can be performed in an office setting but do not have equivalent long term outcomes compared to standard surgical procedures. When the adenomatous growth is particularly large, open simple prostatectomy is performed to enucleate the adenoma surgically. Outcomes of the transurethral procedures show dramatic improvement in International Prostate Symptom Score numbers, urinary flow rates, and post-void residual volumes. Procedures such as simple prostatectomy have such a long historical use that objective data have not been measured or compiled, but outcomes are similar to those of TURP. Complications of TURP procedures include persistent bleeding, dilutional hyponatremia from fluid absorption of the glycine irrigation, UTI, urinary incontinence, and urethral stricture. With newer electrosurgical systems (bipolar and laser), normal saline irrigation is used and dilutional hyponatremia has been eliminated. In addition, visualization is improved, with a significant reduction in bleeding complications and a lower incidence of urinary incontinence.

MALE REPRODUCTIVE MEDICINE AND SEXUAL DYSFUNCTION

Male infertility and sexual dysfunction are a specialized area of urologic practice. Diagnostic evaluation, medical treatment, and surgical therapy of male infertility represent sophisticated aspects of urologic care. Male sexual dysfunction is becoming more prominent as the field of men's health continues to evolve. Many patients seen and evaluated by general surgeons may be receiving specific medical therapy or have undergone prosthetic surgical implants for sexual dysfunction management. A basic familiarity

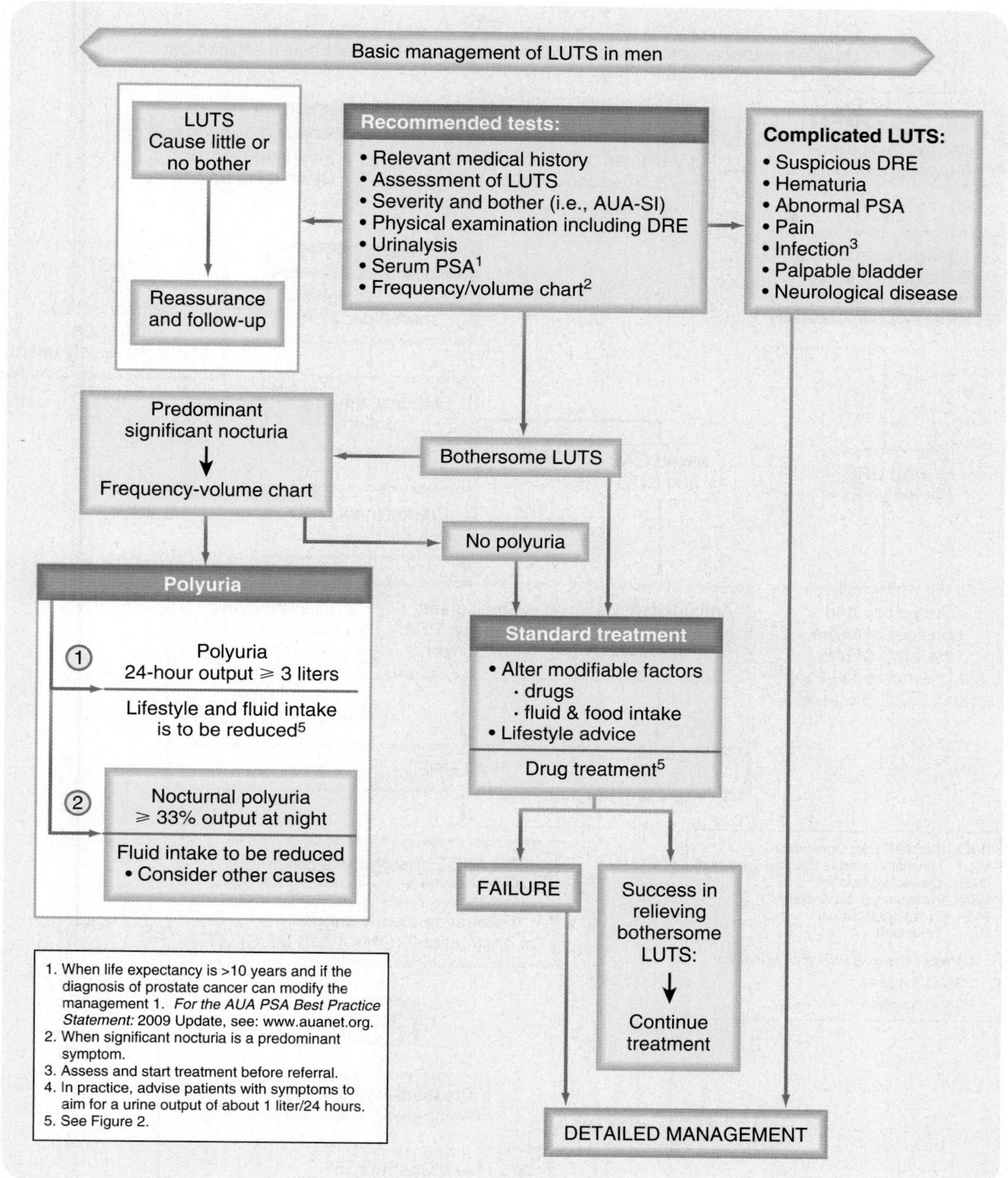

FIGURE 72-5 Algorithm for initial diagnosis and management of BPH. (Adapted from McVary KT, Roehrborn CG, Avins AL, et al: Update on AUA guideline on the management of benign prostatic hyperplasia. *J Urol* 185:1793–1803, 2011.)

with these specialized areas is beneficial to general surgeons in their surgical practice.

Male Infertility: Evaluation and Treatment

Infertility affects approximately 8% to 14% of couples; the male factor is the primary or sole factor in 36% to 75% of these cases.[21] Couples are often referred to the urologist after a period of infertility, and referrals are generally from a primary care physician or from the evaluating gynecologic reproductive endocrinologist. Infertility is defined as a couple's inability to achieve pregnancy after 1 year of unprotected intercourse.[21]

The standard male factor evaluation involves a detailed history, physical examination, and basic laboratory and imaging evaluation. The AUA has produced a series of best practice statements on the evaluation of the infertile man with the following objectives: to recognize and to treat reversible conditions, to categorize disorders potentially amenable to assisted reproductive techniques, to identify syndromes and conditions that may be detrimental to the patient's health, and to distinguish genetic abnormalities that can be transmitted to or affect the health of offspring.[22]

The causes of infertility can be divided into anatomic, behavioral and environmental, and iatrogenic. Anatomic causes of male

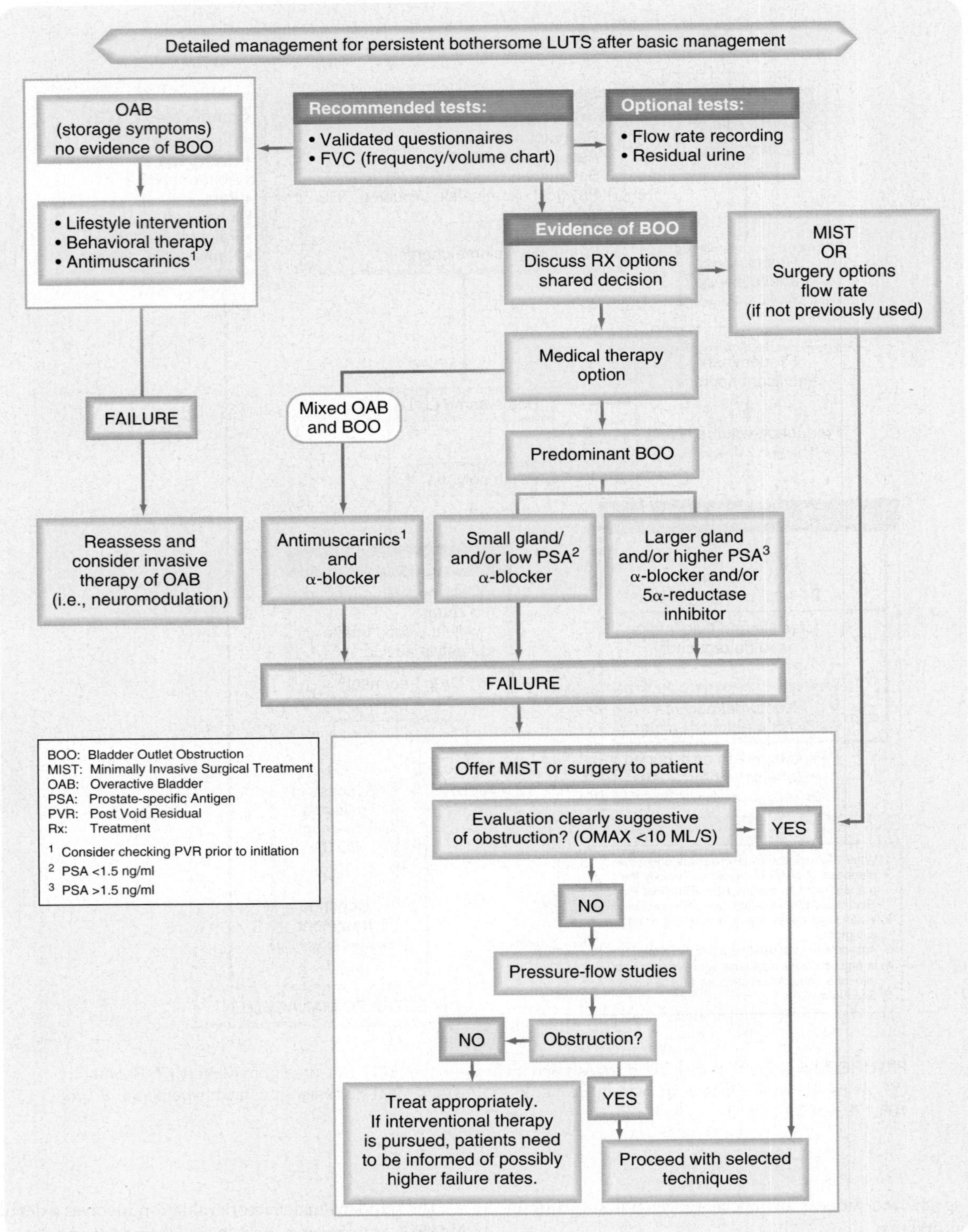

FIGURE 72-6 Algorithm for secondary management of BPH. (Adapted from McVary KT, Roehrborn CG, Avins AL, et al: Update on AUA guideline on the management of benign prostatic hyperplasia. *J Urol* 185:1793–1803, 2011.)

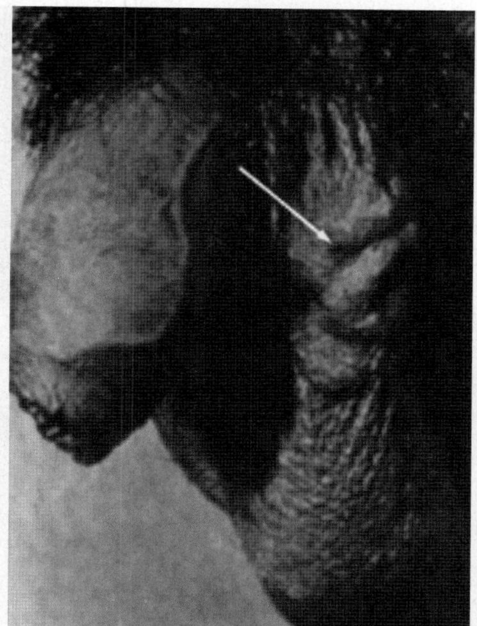

FIGURE 72-7 Varicocele. The bag of worms appearance is visible and palpable through the scrotal skin, representing the dilated branches of the internal spermatic venous system.

infertility are either congenital or acquired.[21] The most significant anatomic cause is congenital absence of the vas deferens, which is a partial or complete agenesis of the vas deferens. Although uncommon, the finding is associated with a cystic fibrosis transmembrane conductance regulator *(CFTR)* gene mutation, making these patients carriers for cystic fibrosis.[22] Other anatomic findings include cryptorchidism, ejaculatory duct obstruction (at the level of the prostate), and varicocele (Fig. 72-7). Behavioral and environmental sources of infertility are more common and easier to reverse than anatomic causes of male infertility. These include obesity, environmental exposures, substance abuse (including exogenous testosterone), and vitamin deficiency. Finally, iatrogenic causes to be considered include prior chemotherapy or radiation therapy, prior inguinal or genital surgery, and current medical treatments. Surgeons must be aware of iatrogenic causes of infertility in groin and pelvic surgical procedures from damage to the spermatic cord vasculature, vas deferens, and ejaculatory duct region or vasal entrapment from mesh used for inguinal hernia repair. The blood supply to the vas deferens or testicle is vulnerable to injury when the groin is explored in reoperative surgery or when the anatomy is obscured because of inguinal trauma as identification of these structures is challenging.

The history should include a discussion of sexual and reproductive history. This includes potential gonadotoxic exposure; urologic infections and STIs; trauma and prior surgery involving the pelvis, groin, and genitalia; and family history of infertility. Physical assessment should include a general evaluation of masculinization and genital findings, including normal meatal location, testicular size and consistency, presence and normalcy of the epididymis and vas deferens, and possible presence of a varicocele. Perineal and rectal examinations are routine parts of this assessment.

Basic Laboratory Assessment

Laboratory evaluation of these patients includes two semen analyses and serum hormone studies. The semen analyses should be separated by 1 month and preceded by 2 to 3 days of abstinence. Semen analysis parameters of importance include semen volume, pH, sperm concentration and total count, total motility, progressive motility, quality of sperm movement, morphology, and presence of red and white blood cells or bacteria.[21] The World Health Organization has defined parameters of normal for routine semen analyses.[21] Semen analysis abnormalities fall into two main categories: azoospermia—the complete absence of sperm from the semen; and abnormal semen parameters—reduced concentration, motility, or morphology and abnormal function. Azoospermia can roughly be divided into three categories: pretesticular, testicular, and post-testicular. Pretesticular azoospermia results from endocrine causes, such as hypogonadotropic hypogonadism, or congenital causes. Testicular causes are the result of primary testicular failure of germinal epithelium of the testis to produce mature sperm. This is often accompanied by normal semen volume and by a markedly elevated serum follicle-stimulating hormone (FSH) level. Post-testicular causes, such as ejaculatory dysfunction and obstruction, account for 40% of cases of azoospermia.[22] Abnormal semen parameters may be indicative of a wide range of disorders that may cause reduced sperm numbers, motility, or morphology, including varicocele, antisperm antibodies, genital duct infection with pyospermia, and prior or current gonadotoxic exposure. Reduced semen volume may be artifactual, indicating incomplete ejaculation or specimen collection, or it may represent true disease, including, for example, congenital absence of the seminal vesicle, ejaculatory duct obstruction, or retrograde ejaculation caused by diabetes or neurologic injury or prior bladder neck surgery or medications.

Serum hormone testing includes determination of levels of FSH, luteinizing hormone, testosterone, free testosterone, and prolactin. Hypogonadotropic hypogonadism may be diagnosed on the basis of serum hormone studies or elevation in the FSH level. A patient with a low testosterone level should have follow-up prolactin levels measured to rule out a prolactinoma of the pituitary gland.

Ultrasound of the scrotum is useful to measure testicular volume and symmetry, to exclude the possibility of testicular neoplasm, to identify epididymal anatomy, and to define or to confirm the presence of a varicocele, which is an abnormal dilation of the pampiniform venous plexus of the internal spermatic venous system (Fig. 72-7). Transrectal ultrasound (TRUS) of the prostate may provide evidence of ejaculatory duct obstruction with seminal vesicle dilation or congenital absence of the seminal vesicle, which may accompany congenital absence of the vas deferens.

Treatment

Treatment of male infertility depends on the identified cause and on the availability and affordability of assisted reproductive technology support options for specific or empirical treatment of failure to conceive. Medical therapy is used to treat hormone deficiencies, hormone excess, thyroid hormone excess, and prolactin excess. The most common medical therapies include hormonal stimulation of spermatogenesis, such as gonadotropin agents and antiestrogen agents, which have been met with mixed results. Anti-inflammatory or antibiotic therapy can be used in patients with findings of pyospermia or concern for genital duct infection. Surgical therapies may include microsurgical reconstruction for vasal or epididymal occlusion (including vasectomy reversal), transurethral resection of the ejaculatory duct for obstructive lesions, and varicocele repair.

Male Sexual Dysfunction and Treatment

Sexual dysfunction in men refers to a range of disorders, including erectile dysfunction (ED), diminished libido, hypogonadism, and ejaculatory dysfunction. Because of the numerous organ system interactions, patients with these conditions may have associated neuropathy, endocrinopathy, vasculopathy, and psychological disorders, and these abnormalities may affect nonurologic patient management and surgery.

Normal erectile function is a complex interaction between the nervous and vascular systems, with unique molecular actions occurring in penile vascular structures. Many medical comorbidities and lifestyle choices can contribute to ED, including age, coronary artery disease, smoking, hypertension, dyslipidemia, atherosclerosis, peripheral vascular disease, obesity, diabetes, spinal cord injury and degenerative neurologic conditions, treatment of pelvic malignant neoplasms, and chronic kidney disease.[23] The causes of ED can be divided into neurologic, vascular, metabolic, medication induced, endocrine, and psychological; importantly, it can be an early marker for coronary artery disease.[23] The initial evaluation of the ED patient centers on the history and physical examination. The history is focused on sexual performance and erectile function; the nonsexual historical aspects center on possible medical and surgical conditions. Social aspects, such as smoking, recreational drug use, and diet, are also important considerations. Validated questionnaires provide objective historical data both for initial treatment and for evaluation of therapy outcomes. The physical examination centers on the genitalia and evaluation of male secondary sexual characteristics. Basic laboratory studies in these patients include morning total testosterone concentration, fasting lipid levels, and hemoglobin A1c level. Important consideration should be given to assessment of cardiovascular function in younger patients because this disease process is considered an early marker for cardiovascular disease, especially in younger patients. Further evaluation is specialized but may include neurologic testing (e.g., biothesiometry) and vascular testing (e.g., penile duplex Doppler ultrasound studies).

Most treatments of ED are based on restoring penile arterial blood flow to achieve or to maintain a satisfactory erection. Lifestyle modifications are an important component of this, and dietary changes and increased regular cardiovascular exercise have been shown to independently improve erectile function. Evaluation and adjustment of offending medications should be considered as well. The basis of medical therapy for ED is phosphodiesterase type 5 inhibitors. These medications improve penile blood flow by limiting the breakdown of cyclic guanosine monophosphate and potentiating penile blood flow. These drugs should be limited in their use in men with known cardiovascular disease, especially those taking oral nitrates. Other forms of nonsurgical treatment include vacuum erection devices, intraurethral suppository therapy with prostaglandin compounds, intracavernosal self-injection, and occasionally psychotherapy. Surgery for ED includes primarily placement of a penile prosthesis and limited vascular reconstruction. Penile implant surgery may involve malleable implants, which have a flexible wire core inside a silicone sleeve, implanted bilaterally in the corpora, or, more commonly, inflatable penile implants. These are fluid-containing, completely internalized systems that may include paired corporal cylinders, a scrotal pumping device, and a fluid reservoir, which is typically positioned in the retropubic space or extraperitoneal lower abdominal quadrant (Fig. 72-8). The general surgeon should be aware that intraperitoneal positioning may also occur, intentionally or through erosion through the peritoneal membrane, and the reservoir or system tubing may be encountered during nonurologic abdominopelvic surgery. Care should be taken not to contaminate any of the implant components or inadvertently injure the tubing or device components. If it is known that an implant is in place and pelvic or inguinal surgery is planned, urologic consultation may be helpful in handling any issues that arise with the implant. Revascularization of the penis to restore erectile function, following arteriography for anatomic documentation, is usually achieved using an inferior epigastric artery pedicle flap, whereby new arterial inflow is brought to the corpora cavernosa. This has limited indications, most relevant in younger patients with traumatic injury to the pelvic blood supply, and national practice guidelines consider this to be controversial.

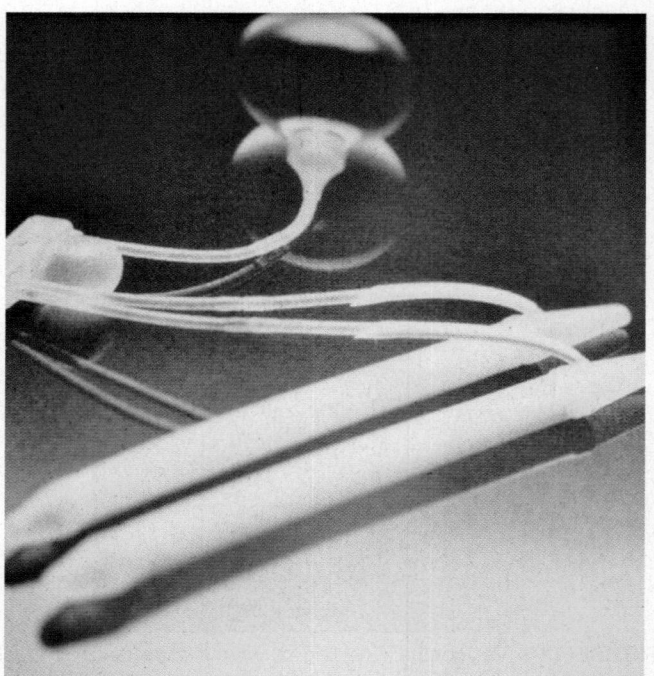

FIGURE 72-8 Inflatable Penile Prosthesis. A three-component device is shown. The reservoir *(top)* is placed retropubically in an extraperitoneal position. The paired cylinders *(right)* are placed within the corpora cavernosa. The pump *(left)* is placed in the scrotum, adjacent to the testes.

The other area of male sexual medicine affecting a significant number of patients is testosterone deficiency or hypogonadism. Serum testosterone is produced in the Leydig cells of the testes (90%) and adrenal glands (10%). Testicular synthesis of testosterone is controlled by the hypothalamus and anterior pituitary. This is a condition in which serum testosterone levels decline and are associated with symptoms of fatigue, lack of energy, depressed mood, irritability, reduced motivation, decreased cognitive acuity, decreased strength and stamina, reduced muscle mass and increased fat, and sexual side effects including decreased libido and ED. There is a normal age-related decline in testosterone as men age, and total testosterone declines by 1%, on average, each year after the age of 40 years. The prevalence of this condition is between 2.1% and 39% of men older than 40 years, depending on the criteria used and association of symptoms.[24] The patient's history should elicit information on the specific symptoms of testosterone deficiency, and physical examination is similar to that for ED with evaluation of the genitalia and secondary sexual characteristics. Validated questionnaires are useful to assess and to monitor therapy. Laboratory studies should include free and total morning testosterone, luteinizing hormone, prolactin, hematocrit, and hemoglobin levels.[25] Therapy for testosterone deficiency is based on lifestyle modifications and testosterone supplementation.[25] Many men who suffer from this condition are either obese or have metabolic syndrome. Dietary changes to improve nutritional status and to result in weight loss have been shown to improve not only baseline medical conditions but also serum testosterone levels. Furthermore, moderate-intensity exercise has been shown to improve serum testosterone levels. In addition to lifestyle modifications, many patients are treated with supplemental testosterone. Synthetic testosterone may be administered orally, transdermally, through intramuscular injections, and by subcutaneous pellets. The goal of therapy is maintenance of testosterone levels between 400 and 700 ng/dL and resolution or improvement of presenting symptoms.[25] Whereas there are few absolute contraindications to testosterone administration, many potential adverse side effects exist and should be discussed before administration of these medications as this is the area of greatest controversy with testosterone supplementation. Potential adverse effects include cardiovascular events and mortality, dermatologic changes, polycythemia, diminished spermatogenesis, gynecomastia, LUTS, prostate cancer, and sleep apnea.[25]

UROLITHIASIS

Urinary tract stones are a common cause of visits to the emergency department. The prevalence of renal calculous disease in the United States is increasing, with a lifetime risk of forming a renal stone at 5% in 1994 and 9% in 2010.[26] The incidence of stone disease peaks in the fourth to sixth decades of life and is more common in men than in women by a 2:1 margin.[26] Renal calculous disease has several aspects of management and evaluation, including acute stone presentation, metabolic evaluation, and medical and surgical therapy. As most general surgeons will encounter patients either in the acute presentation or around the time of surgical intervention, this section focuses on these areas.

Background

The pathogenesis of calculus formation is governed by the physical chemistry characteristics of the urine in the upper collecting system. Most stones are formed by minerals or stone-forming salts and begin to crystallize when their concentration becomes supersaturated in the urine. Just as certain minerals or salts promote calculus formation, there are many inhibitors of calculus formation, including citrate, phosphate, and magnesium. There are many theories to stone formation, none of which are definitively proven, such as Randall plaque formation, stasis, bacteria, and reactive oxygen species from oxalate excretion.[27] Kidney stones are classified by the stone composition, and the mineral composition directs evaluation, treatment, and nonsurgical management. Kidney stones can be generally classified as calcium based, uric acid stones, struvite stones, and cystine stones.[27] Calcium stones are usually composed of two calcium salts, calcium phosphate and calcium oxalate, and are the most common renal calculi. Risk factors for calcium stone formation include abnormal urine pH; high urine concentration of calcium, oxalate, or uric acid; and low urine concentration of the stone inhibitor citrate. Uric acid stones form in a low pH urine in patients with hyperuricosuria and can be the result of purine metabolism from cellular breakdown (tumor lysis) or excessive protein intake. These stones are often radiolucent. Struvite stones, also called infection stones or magnesium ammonium phosphate, result from specific bacterial infections (*P. mirabilis, K. pneumoniae, Staphylococcus aureus,* and *Staphylococcus epidermidis*) that contain urease, which converts urea into ammonia. The base properties of ammonia lead to higher urine pH and crystallization with phosphate. Cystine stones are formed from an autosomal recessive defect in the metabolism of the COLA amino acids (cystine, ornithine, lysine, and arginine), which results in elevated urine cystine levels.[27] The other rare cause of calculi is pharmacologically induced, resulting from poor drug metabolite urine solubility and precipitation in the urine. The most notable of these are protease inhibitors (indinavir and ritonavir), which are not visible on noncontrast computed tomography (CT) scans.

Acute Presentation and Management

Patients presenting with an acute stone episode or renal colic typically have characteristic complaints of abdominal, flank, or back pain that waxes and wanes but cannot be resolved with position changes. Often, these patients can localize the most intense center of the pain, giving some indication of stone location. When the ureter is obstructed by a stone, the pressure in the proximal collecting system rises, and with progressive distention, the patient may experience visceral symptoms, including nausea, vomiting, and ileus. Physical examination in these patients should be focused on the back, flank, abdomen, and genitalia. Patients who have specific vital sign findings in combination (temperature higher than 101.5° F, hypotension, or tachycardia) should be assessed for obstructive upper tract UTI with the potential for sepsis. Basic laboratory evaluation should include complete blood count, metabolic panel, and urinalysis with microscopy. Significant findings of leukocytosis or acute kidney injury may direct urgency of therapy and type of intervention. A non–contrast-enhanced CT scan of the abdomen and pelvis is the preferred imaging study because of its superior sensitivity and specificity compared with intravenous urography and plain radiography. Patients with ureteral calculi may benefit from a plain radiograph, as 85% of calculi are radiopaque, to observe for stone passage.

Once the stone is identified and the location established, pain management is the next step. Patients who are diagnosed with renal or ureteral calculi should receive intravenous nonsteroidal anti-inflammatory drugs (ketorolac) or opioid analgesics as initial therapy. A successful attempt at pain control with oral agents determines if the otherwise hemodynamically stable patient can be discharged or requires inpatient treatment for the stone. Those patients who present with upper tract UTI and obstruction should undergo expeditious drainage with either cystoscopic ureteral stent placement or percutaneous nephrostomy tube placement. If one upper tract is totally obstructed by stone, the patient could have a serious infection with pyonephrosis, and the voided urine would be deceptively normal. Patients who are suitable for hospital discharge include those with no evidence of UTI, hemodynamic stability, good oral intake, pain well controlled on oral analgesics, and a stone size with reasonable chance of spontaneous passage. In patients who are discharged from the hospital, medical expulsive therapy, with agents to promote spontaneous stone passage, is the recommended management.[28] The most common drug used is tamsulosin, the α_{1a} blocker that relaxes ureteral smooth muscle.[28] If a patient is discharged for outpatient management, she or he should be observed closely to determine whether the stone has passed. It should not be assumed that because the pain has resolved, the stone has passed. With persistent upper tract obstruction, the pressure in the collecting system eventually declines as renal blood flow diminishes and urine output drops. The patient's pain can disappear and the kidney can remain obstructed, undergoing silent destruction in the weeks and months that follow. Reimaging is necessary if there is no definitive evidence that the stone has been passed (e.g., the patient brings it in for analysis).

Elective Diagnostic Evaluation and Management

Patients who are diagnosed with asymptomatic renal calculi, such as nonobstructing renal calyceal stones found incidentally during a hematuria evaluation, and patients who have convalesced after an acute presentation undergo a basic metabolic screening evaluation. Important historical aspects to obtain include prior stone passage or treatment, family history, bowel disease or malabsorption, gout, hyperthyroidism, obesity, and dietary supplements.[29] Routine laboratory work includes urinalysis, basic metabolic panel with determination of calcium and uric acid levels, urine culture, and stone analysis (if available). A 24-hour urine specimen is also collected to evaluate the urine for specific chemical and mineral content: volume, pH, creatinine, calcium, oxalate, uric acid, citrate, sodium, and potassium.[29] Specific dietary changes and medical therapy can be used for prevention of stone formation in specific populations. These dietary modifications and pharmacologic treatments are based on stone composition and findings on 24-hour urinalysis. The two most common stone types, calcium and uric acid, are discussed.

In patients with calcium-based stone disease (oxalate or phosphate), the single most important treatment or dietary modification is increased fluid intake to achieve more than 2 liters of urine output daily. In addition, there should be no changes in calcium consumption, and patients, in general, should consume the recommended daily allowance of dietary calcium. Dietary levels of sodium, foods high in oxalate, and animal protein should be reduced as each of these can affect urinary oxalate and citrate levels. Pharmacologic therapy is typically based on three different agents—thiazide diuretics, potassium citrate, and allopurinol—each of which has separate effects on calcium urine levels and calcium stone formation. Patients with uric acid stones are treated with drug therapy.[29] There are no dietary recommendations other than to increase fluid intake to raise urine output to 2 liters per day. Pharmacologic therapy in this group consists of potassium citrate and allopurinol. Many uric acid stones can be dissolved by raising urinary pH levels with use of alkalinizing agents.

Elective Surgical Management

Patients who have large stone burdens or continue to have symptomatic stones require surgical treatment of their calculous disease. Surgical treatment of renal and ureteral calculi varies from completely noninvasive, shock wave lithotripsy (SWL), to minimally invasive, percutaneous nephrolithotomy (PCNL). SWL is a transcutaneous procedure using generated shock waves to fragment stones. Shock waves create positive and negative pressure components that are focused on the stone and create fractures in the targeted stones, ultimately resulting in stone fragmentation.[30] The progress of stone fragmentation is monitored during SWL, typically with fluoroscopy, to direct treatment length and location. Nonradiopaque stones, stones larger than 2 cm, and certain ureteral calculi should not be treated with this method. Complications from SWL include renal injury, steinstrasse (street of stones), hypertension, and chronic kidney disease.[30]

Smaller renal stones and ureteral calculi can be managed in an endoscopic fashion using ureteroscopes (Fig. 72-9). As previously mentioned, ureteroscopes are both semirigid and flexible, allowing full upper tract collecting system access. Through the working channel of ureteroscopes, a variety of working instruments can be placed to fragment or to remove stones. The most common stone treatment is laser lithotripsy to completely fragment the symptomatic calculus. Smaller fragments can be removed using different basket and grasping systems to render the patient stone free. Complications of ureteroscopy include acute ureteral perforation or avulsion, UTI, and late ureteral stricture formation.

For larger renal stones or select proximal ureteral stones, PCNL is preferred because of the larger working endoscopes and better instrumentation for stone fragmentation. The basic steps of PCNL are percutaneous renal access, dilation of the nephrostomy track, placement of the working sheath for stone fragmentation and extraction, and postoperative renal drainage. The advantage of PCNL is that numerous intracorporeal lithotripsy devices are available, and large stones can be rapidly fragmented. Flexible nephroscopes can be used as well in this setting. Complications of PCNL are most significant because of the more invasive nature of the procedure; these include sepsis, renal hemorrhage, renal

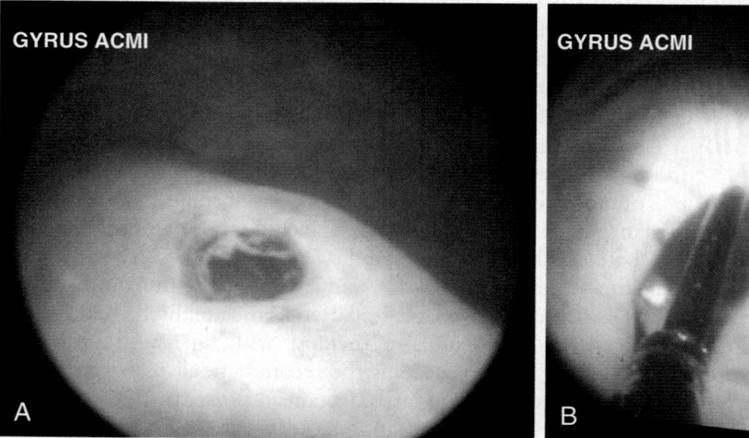

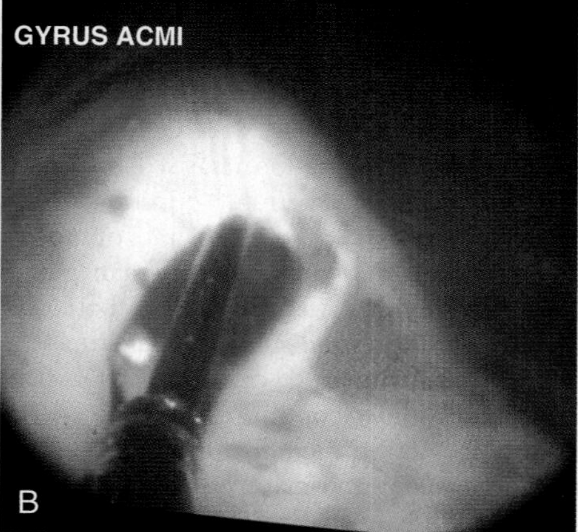

FIGURE 72-9 Ureteral Stone. A, An obstructing calculus is shown crowning within the right ureteral orifice. **B,** Cystoscopic extraction performed with a grasping forceps.

collecting system injury, and damage to adjacent organs and viscera. PCNL may result in hydrothorax or pneumothorax from transpleural or peripleural access tracks that requires evacuation. With the refinement of PCNL, open stone surgery is rarely indicated even for the most complex intrarenal calculi. Laparoscopic and robotic procedures for specific renal calculi have been described.

UROLOGIC TRAUMA

Urologic injury is present in approximately 15% of all abdominal and pelvic trauma patients regardless of mechanism, blunt or penetrating.[31] Renal injuries, for example, are reported to occur in 0.3% to 1.2% of all trauma patients; however, the kidneys are the second most common visceral organ injured, accounting for approximately 24% of injuries.[31] In many trauma centers, injuries are typically initially assessed by an emergency physician or general surgeon and may be addressed without urologic consultation, although, for complex urologic injuries, the input of a urologist can be essential. For example, high-grade, nonreconstructible renal injury can be managed with an expeditious nephrectomy; however, most renal injuries, such as an extensive parenchymal and collecting system laceration, should be repaired with renorrhaphy. Management of trauma patients is the greatest overlap between urology and general surgery and allows numerous areas for collaboration; urologic expertise can enhance the quality of care provided for all urologic injuries, whether they are managed operatively or nonoperatively.

The focus of the following section on urologic trauma is the practical management of a variety of acute urologic injuries and the optimal interaction between the urologist and general trauma surgeon. The management of common injuries throughout the urinary tract, the optimal timing of such interventions, and the role of damage control techniques are discussed.

Core Guideline and Consensus Statements for Urologic Trauma Management

The Organ Injury Scaling system of the American Association for the Surgery of Trauma describes an objective grading system for urologic injuries (Table 72-1 and Fig. 72-10).[32] The staging system for renal trauma has become well established in the urologic literature and has been externally validated. The Organ Injury Scaling system also describes staging for other urologic injuries; however, the subjective criteria applied to these divisions do not practically affect management decisions and treatment (Fig. 72-10).

In 2002, a consensus conference for the diagnosis and treatment of urologic injuries was convened by the World Health Organization and the Société Internationale d'Urologie. The resulting consensus statements were divided by organ site: kidney, ureter, bladder, urethra, and external genitalia.[33-37] These reports still constitute the centerpiece of urologic trauma management. Management guidelines have subsequently been produced by the European Association of Urology and the AUA to create core documents to guide the management of urologic injuries.[38]

Renal Injuries

The majority of renal injuries are the result of blunt trauma (80%); the remainder are the result of penetrating injury (20%).[33] Approximately 70% of all patients who sustain renal injury are male, and most of these patients are younger than 50 years. As discussed in the retroperitoneal anatomy section, the kidneys are well protected in the retroperitoneum but are close to intraperitoneal structures. The key points in evaluation, as with any trauma patient, are the ABCs: airway, breathing, and circulation. In patients with a history of blunt trauma, key findings include location of impact, flank ecchymosis, and gross or microscopic hematuria. Other relevant historical information is concomitant injury and mechanism of injury. Close attention to the entry and exit points in penetrating injuries are also important to estimate the trajectory of the missile.

TABLE 72-1 Organ Injury Scaling System: Kidney

GRADE	INJURY DESCRIPTION		AIS-90
I	Contusion	Microscopic or gross hematuria, urologic studies normal	2
	Hematoma	Subcapsular, nonexpanding, without parenchymal laceration	2
II	Hematoma	Nonexpanding perirenal hematoma confined to renal retroperitoneum	2
	Laceration	<1 cm parenchymal depth of renal cortex without urinary extravasation	2
III	Laceration	>1 cm depth of renal cortex, without collecting system rupture or urinary extravasation	3
IV	Laceration	Parenchymal laceration extending through the renal cortex, medulla, and collecting system	4
	Vascular	Main renal artery or vein injury, with contained hemorrhage	5
V	Laceration	Completely shattered kidney	5
	Vascular	Avulsion of renal hilum, which devascularizes kidney	5

Adapted from Moore EE, Shackford SR, Pachter HL, et al: Organ injury scaling: Spleen, liver, and kidney. *J Trauma* 29:1664–1666, 1989.

Imaging

There are many well-established indications for renal imaging after blunt or penetrating injury. In patients with blunt trauma, the criteria for imaging include gross hematuria, hemodynamic instability (systolic blood pressure < 90 mm Hg), microscopic hematuria (>5 red blood cells/high-power field), a traumatic mechanism, and suspicion of injury on screening radiographs (Fig. 72-11). In patients with penetrating injury who are hemodynamically stable, imaging is indicated for any degree of hematuria, microscopic or gross (Fig. 72-12).[38] The relevance of imaging to detect and to stage urinary tract injury before abdominal trauma surgery has been debated in the general surgical and urologic literature. Cross-sectional imaging, specifically contrast-enhanced CT scan, is the preferred study to evaluate the renal injuries. Proper imaging should include arteriovenous phases with delayed imaging to evaluate the urinary collecting structures. In those patients who proceed directly to surgery, the "one-shot" intravenous urogram (intravenous administration of 2 mL/kg contrast material followed by a single abdominal radiograph) can provide information concerning the presence or absence of a contralateral kidney. Ultrasound, intravenous urography, and magnetic resonance imaging (MRI) have a limited role in renal imaging for injury staging.

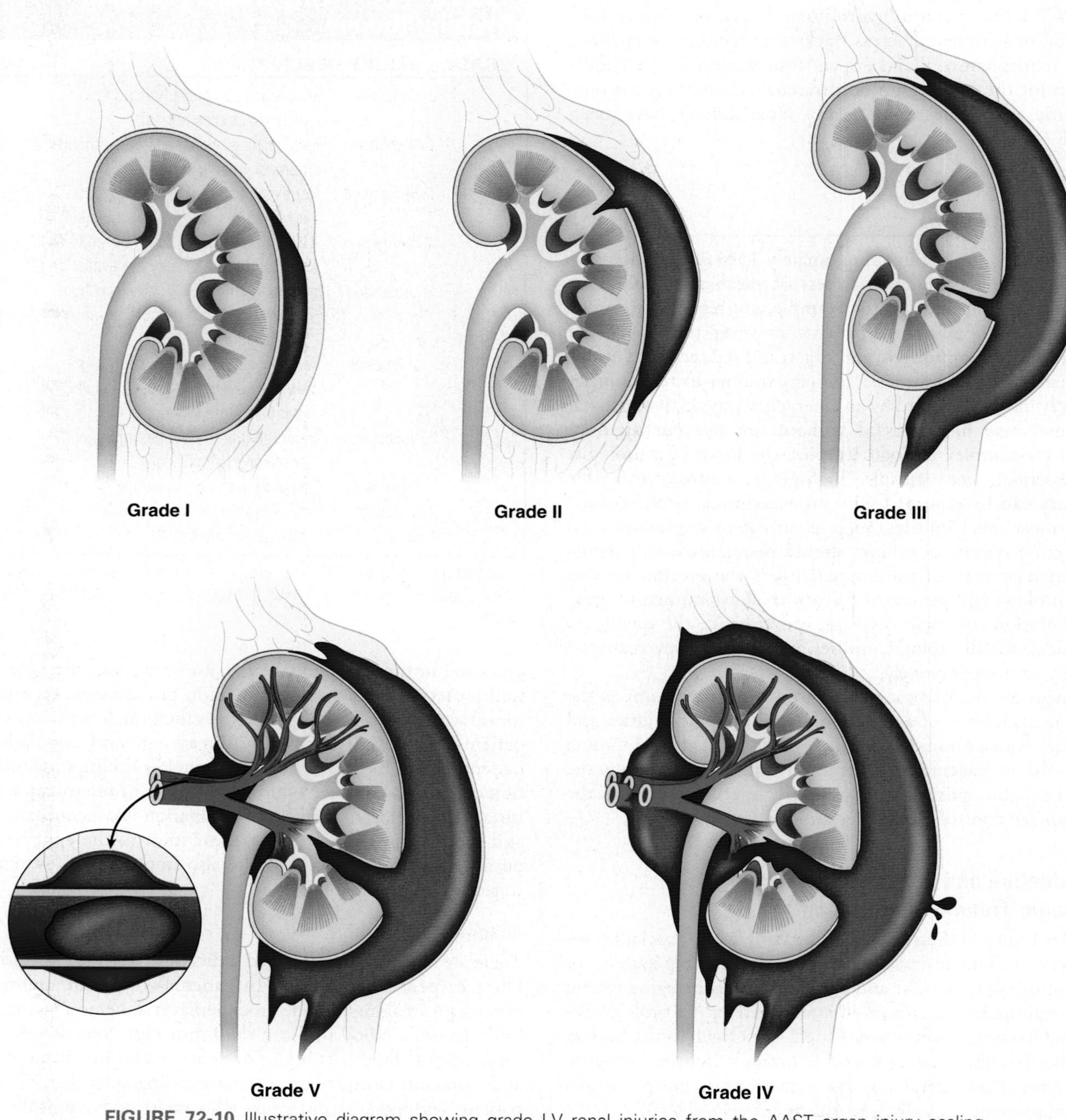

FIGURE 72-10 Illustrative diagram showing grade I-V renal injuries from the AAST organ injury scaling system. (From Moore EE, Shackford SR, Pachter HL, et al: Organ injury scaling: Spleen, liver, and kidney. *J Trauma* 29:1664–1666, 1989.)

Management: Operative versus Nonoperative

With better staging of renal injury, management paradigms have changed over time (Figs. 72-11 and 72-12). Furthermore, as urologists learned more from general trauma surgeons in the management of solid organ injury, nonoperative management of renal injuries has become more commonplace. The basis of nonoperative management centers around a properly staged injury with contrast-enhanced cross-sectional imaging (Fig. 72-13). In general, lower grade injuries, grades I to III, in hemodynamically stable patients are managed nonoperatively. Grade IV injuries are more controversial, and many are managed nonoperatively. High-grade injuries, grades IV and V, particularly in patients with concomitant intraperitoneal injuries, may undergo surgical exploration.

In hemodynamically unstable patients who proceed directly to the operating room, there are absolute and relative criteria for operative exploration. The absolute criteria for exploration are expanding hematoma, pulsatile hematoma, and persistent renal bleeding. Any of these findings are concerning for possible renal pedicle injury.[39] The relative criteria for renal exploration include persistent urinary extravasation, nonviable renal parenchyma, arterial injury, and incomplete renal staging.[39] In the absence of

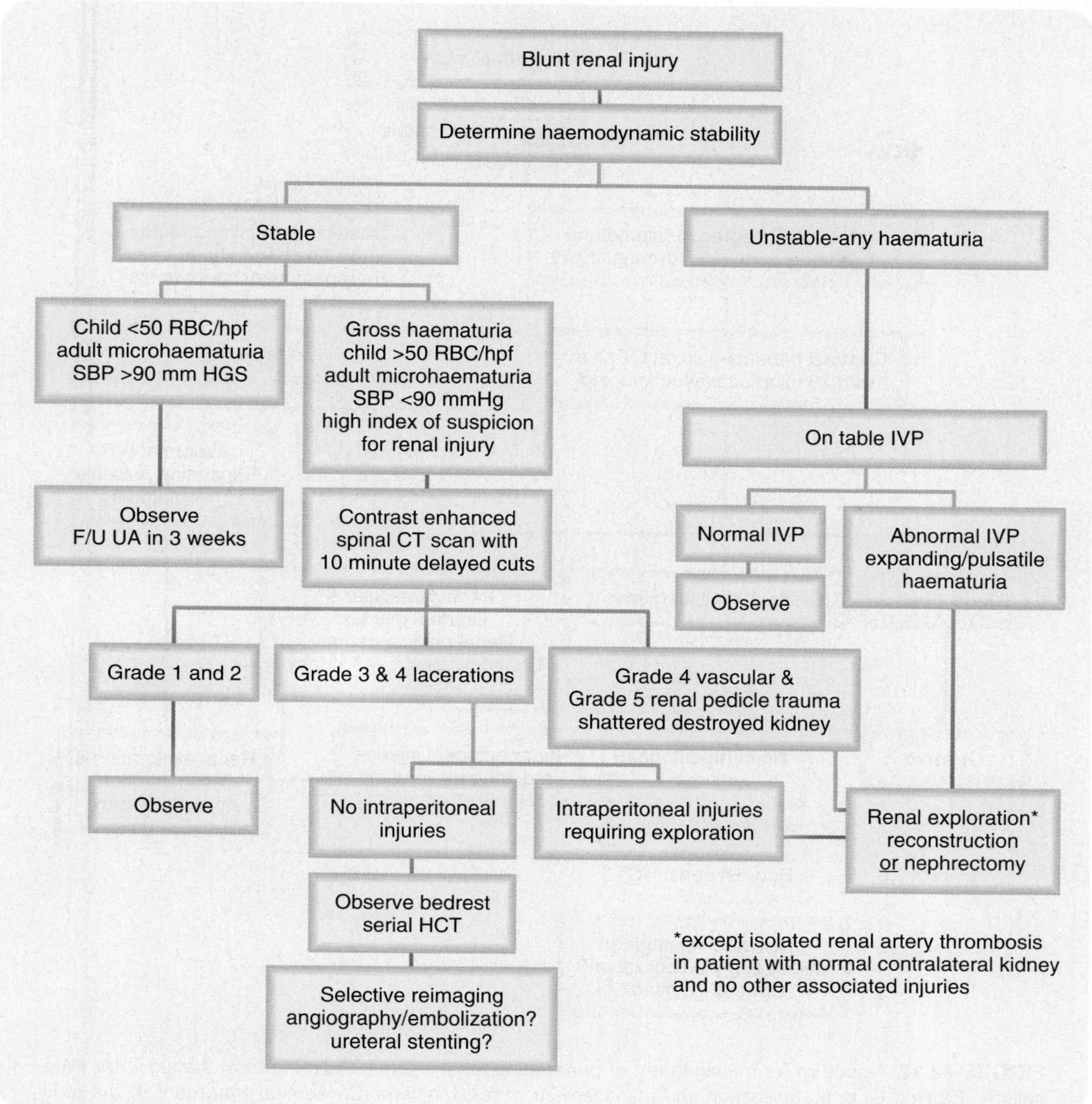

FIGURE 72-11 Algorithm for management of blunt renal injuries. (Adapted from Santucci RA, Wessells H, Bartsch G, et al: Evaluation and management of renal injuries: Consensus statement of the renal trauma subcommittee. *BJU Int* 93:937–954, 2004.)

such findings or in patients in whom a damage control approach is to be implemented, exploration may be avoided if the surgeon is uncomfortable with the potential requirements for reconstructive renal surgery.

Renal vascular injury is uncommon, and the radiologic presentation is variable. On CT imaging, these patients may have either large perinephric hematomas with intravascular extravasation of contrast material (indicating possible renal pedicle injury) or absent renal perfusion (indicating renal artery thrombosis). Segmental renal vascular injuries are usually the result of blunt renal trauma and appear as wedge-shaped defects in the renal parenchyma. These injuries rarely require intervention.

With an increase in nonoperative management of renal injuries, renal arteriography and selective angioembolization have been used with increasing frequency in management of renal trauma (Fig. 72-14). However, only select patients have been shown to benefit from this intervention: those with intravascular extravasation of contrast material, perirenal hematoma rim distance of more than 25 mm, and medial hematomas.[40] In addition, patients who are assigned to a nonoperative management protocol and have received more than 2 units of red blood cell transfusion should undergo angiography.

Surgical Exploration and Operative Approach

Strict criteria exist for renal exploration. In those patients who proceed directly to the operating room, renal exploration is indicated with an expanding, pulsatile, uncontrolled retroperitoneal hematoma or renal pedicle avulsion. Patients with persistent renal bleeding but who require damage control management may require nephrectomy for hemodynamic stability. Patients with certain intraperitoneal injuries require surgical exploration and repair of renal injuries, including patients with concomitant bowel or pancreatic injury. Patients with renal pelvic laceration or persistent urinary extravasation of contrast material may require

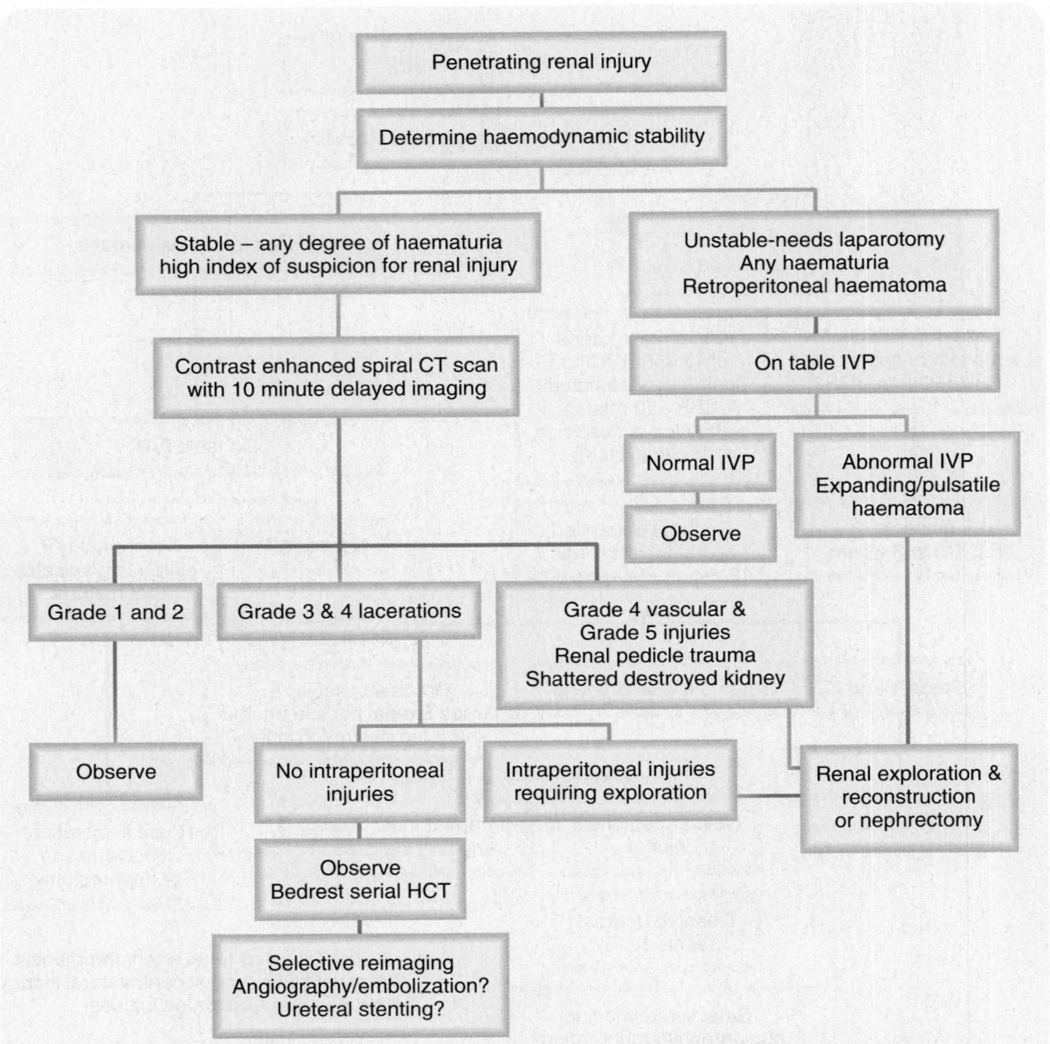

FIGURE 72-12 Algorithm for management of penetrating renal injuries. (Adapted from Santucci RA, Wessells H, Bartsch G, et al: Evaluation and management of renal injuries: Consensus statement of the renal trauma subcommittee. *BJU Int* 93:937–954, 2004.)

surgical repair of the collecting system. Patients with large segments of devitalized renal parenchyma and urinary extravasation may need early partial or total nephrectomy to prevent long-term complications. Trauma patients who have continued urinary extravasation despite percutaneous or endoscopic urinary diversion may require renal exploration and repair, although this may result in nephrectomy.

There are conflicting data concerning early vascular control before renal exploration, although the guidelines recommend vascular control.[33] Urologists are typically trained to approach the injured kidney anteriorly through a midline incision and to obtain vascular control of the renal vessels, before opening Gerota fascia and exposing the kidney, to avoid severe renal bleeding that may necessitate an urgent nephrectomy. In significant anatomic distortion, which may occur in the trauma setting, renal pedicle control can be obtained by bluntly creating a window medial to the lower pole of the kidney and lateral to the aorta (left) or vena cava (right), down to the psoas muscle fascia, which allows a vascular pedicle clamp to be placed if bleeding is encountered on renal exposure (Fig. 72-15). Once vascular access is achieved, the kidney is exposed through an anterior vertical incision in Gerota fascia, which extends from the upper to the lower pole of the kidney. If there is parenchymal injury, care must be taken to identify the renal capsule in exposing and mobilizing the kidney to avoid stripping the entire capsule from the renal parenchyma and affecting kidney closure after renal reconstruction. The entire kidney should be exposed to reveal any lacerations, to evacuate hematoma, and to facilitate full mobility for repair. In general, if half the kidney can be preserved, renal reconstruction has benefit; however, if there is extensive destruction of the hilar region, successful reconstruction is unlikely. The preferred surgical management is renorrhaphy with suture ligation of bleeding vessels and closure of the collecting system with fine absorbable suture followed by parenchyma and capsular approximation with absorbable suture. For renal reconstruction in the trauma setting, pedicle clamping with a warm ischemia time of less than 30 minutes generally will not have a permanent adverse impact on renal function. The use of hemostatic agents and tissue sealants may aid in the reconstructive effort, and

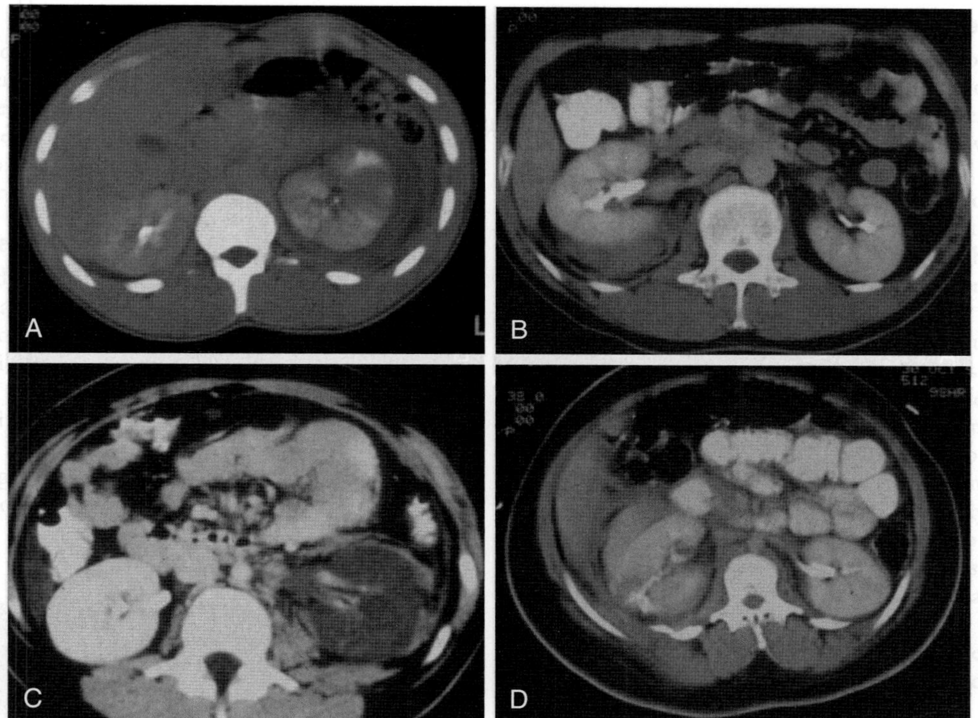

FIGURE 72-13 CT Scans Depicting Renal Trauma. **A,** Left renal contusion with heterogeneous contrast enhancement. **B,** Small right posterior pericapsular renal hematoma. **C,** Nonperfused left kidney after deceleration trauma and intimal disruption, with thrombosis of the renal artery. Vessel cutoff sign and some pericapsular enhancement are demonstrated. **D,** Grade IV laceration to the posterolateral right kidney, with posterolateral extravasation of contrast material.

closed suction drainage is beneficial in the instance of a collecting system injury or significant bleeding.

Ureteral Injuries

Ureteral injuries are uncommon (1% to 2.5% of all urologic injuries) and are rarely life-threatening but occur in the context of complex polytrauma.[39] Ureteral injuries due to external violence are most often the result of penetrating injuries; blunt injuries are the result of injuries with high-energy transfer, such as motor vehicle collision. Up to 5% to 10% of penetrating abdominal or pelvic injuries have ureteral involvement.[39] Management of ureteral injuries is dependent on mechanism of injury, anatomic location, and overall condition of the patient. The ureter is infrequently injured because of its mobility and location in the retroperitoneum protected by large muscle groups and the spine and bony pelvis. Ureteral injuries do not present with specific signs and symptoms, and their diagnosis requires heightened suspicion for injury based on mechanism and injury location.[38] Evaluation of ureteral injuries should be performed in the context of evaluation for more serious or life-threatening injuries.

Imaging

Ureteral imaging should be performed with contrast-enhanced, cross-sectional imaging, preferably CT scan, and must include delayed imaging to evaluate urinary excretion.[38] Findings suggesting ureteral injury include extravasation of contrast material, absence of contrast material distal to the suspected injury, and ipsilateral hydronephrosis. Other forms of imaging, including retrograde pyelography and intravenous urography, are difficult in the acute setting and often of lower quality.

Management

As a general principle, injuries to the ureter are best managed by surgical repair. Endoscopic ureteral stents or percutaneous diversion is generally reserved for missed injuries and for patients for whom reoperation is prohibitively morbid or the timing would make a successful repair unlikely. Ureteral contusions from adjacent penetrating trauma may benefit from ureteral stent placement to reduce progressive edema, occlusion, and ischemia and potentially to diminish the risk of delayed urinary extravasation.

Surgical Exploration and Operative Approach

When a ureteral injury is suspected, the ureter should be identified and directly inspected. The ureter can be approached surgically at any level by finding an area of normal anatomy and proceeding expeditiously to the areas in question. While dissecting around the ureter and mobilizing it from surrounding tissues, it is important to avoid stripping the periureteral tissue, causing devascularization. Ureteral injuries should be managed at the time of initial injury to decrease the chance of complication, such as urinoma, fistula, ureteral obstruction, and renal failure.[34] Repair usually involves minimal débridement of viable tissue. Lacerations are closed perpendicular to the axis of incision and transections with a spatulated, tension-free anastomosis. Injuries of the distal ureter often require reimplantation into the bladder. Gunshot wounds represent a particular concern as the viability of the ureteral stump may be compromised because of local tissue injury from the blast effect of the missile.[34] Fine absorbable suture is used in a running or interrupted fashion. Stent placement is desirable to allow low-pressure drainage, to minimize postoperative urinary extravasation, and to prevent angulation of the healing ureter.

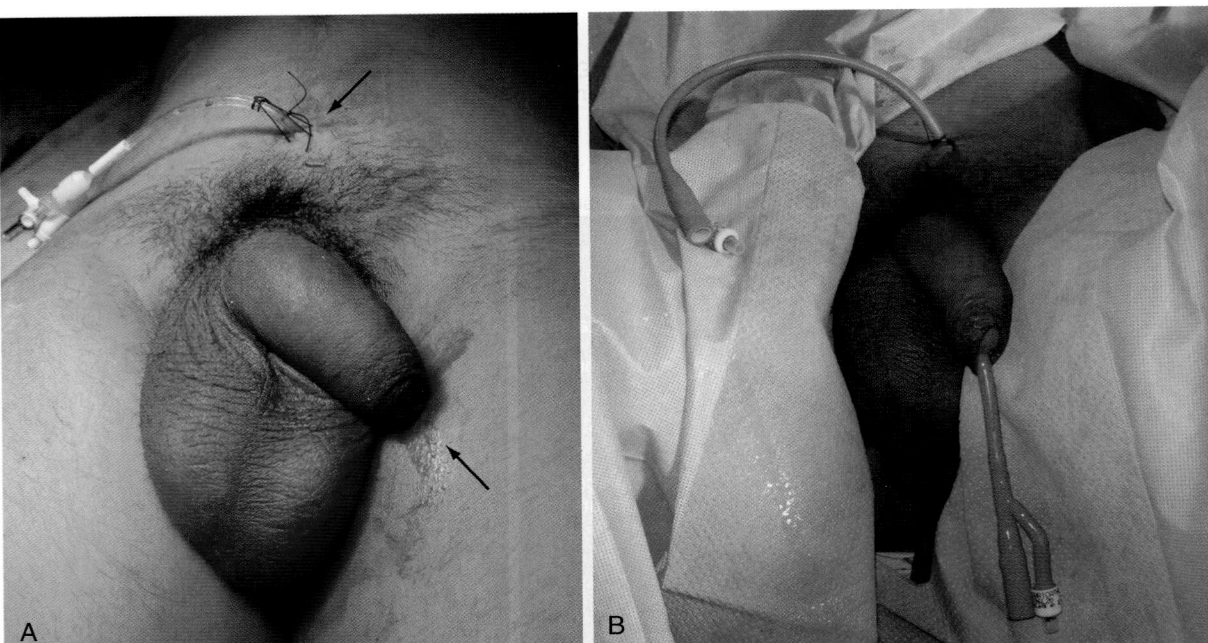

FIGURE 72-22 Posterior Urethral Disruption Injury. A, Patient with blood visible at penile meatus, managed with percutaneously placed suprapubic cystostomy tube. **B,** Patient initially managed similarly has undergone an endoscopic, fluoroscopically guided realignment procedure, with placement of urethral and suprapubic Foley catheters.

activity, penile ultrasound can demonstrate interruption of the corpora cavernosa. For blunt scrotal injuries, scrotal ultrasound may be helpful in determining whether the testis is ruptured. Key findings on ultrasound indicating testicular injury are loss of testicular contour of the tunica albuginea and heterogeneous echotexture of the testicular parenchyma.[38,42] Retrograde urethrography can be performed if there is concern for concomitant urethral injury.

Management

Because of the normal flaccid nature of the penis, the only injury that can occur is fracture of the erect penis. Management of these injuries involves surgical exploration of the penis and identification of the defect in the corporal body.[38,42] This is closed with slowly absorbing suture in a running fashion (Fig. 72-23). Blunt testicular injuries should be explored if ultrasound confirms testicular rupture. Repair of the injury is performed by limited débridement of the seminiferous tubules and closure of the tunica albuginea (Fig. 72-24). Orchiectomy is reserved for those injuries that thoroughly destroy the blood supply to the testis or those parenchymal injuries in which there is no viable parenchyma available to salvage.

Penetrating injuries to the external genitalia warrant surgical exploration in most cases. Functional and structural outcomes are greatly improved by early exploration and repair for penetrating penile, scrotal, and testicular injuries. For penile injuries, the goal is to remove foreign material, to cleanse the wound, to obtain hemostasis, to identify any defects in the tunica albuginea or urethra, and to proceed with appropriate repair while exercising caution not to be excessively aggressive with débridement of tissues of uncertain viability. For testicular injuries, débridement of devitalized parenchyma, closure of the capsule (tunica albuginea of the testis), and repair of the scrotum are key tasks.

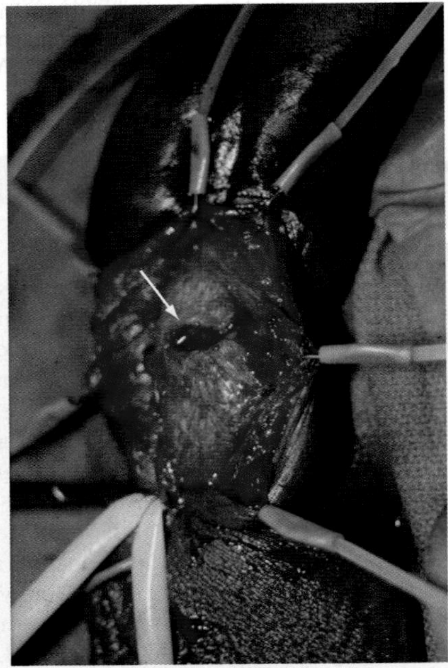

FIGURE 72-23 Penile Fracture. This patient was undergoing surgical exploration for a suspected penile fracture injury sustained during sexual activity. A ventral midline penoscrotal incision is used to expose the transverse laceration in the ventral right tunica albuginea of the corpus cavernosum, shown centrally. The Penrose drain at the bottom was used briefly as a tourniquet to control bleeding during suture repair of the injury. The hook and ring retractor system shown is useful for genital surgery.

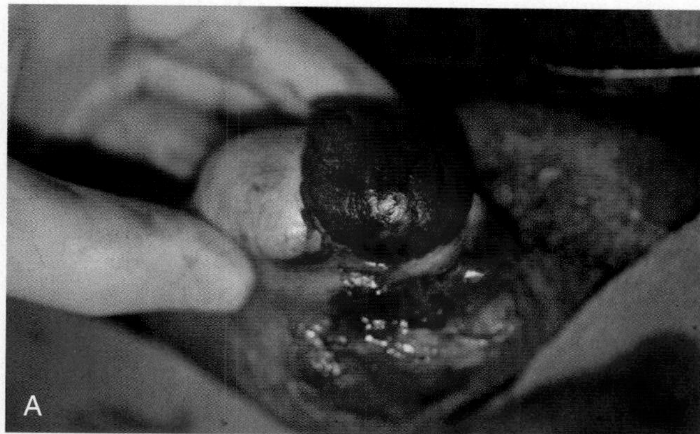

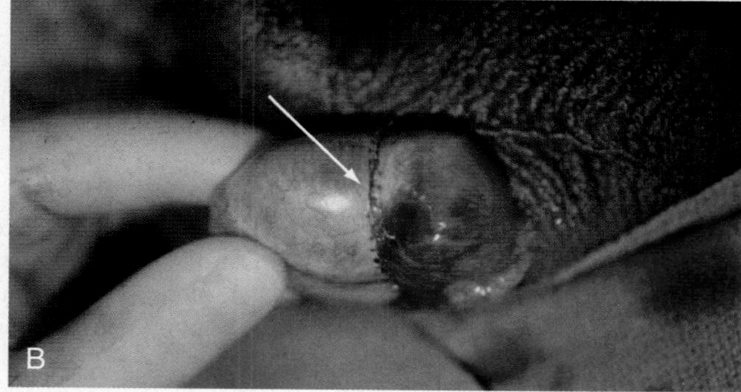

FIGURE 72-24 Testicular Rupture from Blunt Trauma. A, Intact tunica albuginea with a large transverse laceration *(left);* the extruded testicular parenchyma from the upper portion of the testis is also shown *(right).* **B,** Appearance after repair with running absorbable sutures.

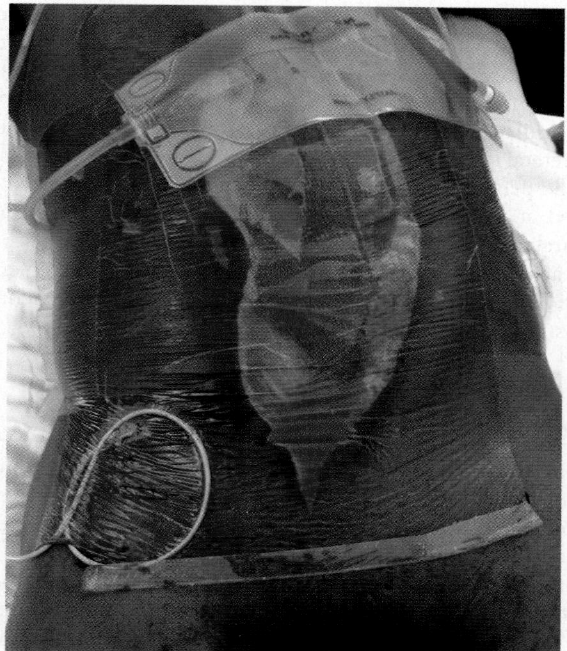

FIGURE 72-25 Damage control management of gunshot wound to right ureter. A diversion stent has been secured into the right ureter and externalized to gravity drainage.

Damage Control Techniques for Urologic Injuries

Many urologic injuries are amenable to initial management by applying damage control strategies. Damage control surgery refers to the concept of limiting the initial operative interventions, in the unstable trauma patient, to those maneuvers that are immediately lifesaving (e.g., control of surgical hemorrhage, control of continued fecal contamination). More time-consuming, definitive reconstructive efforts are delayed until later, after resuscitation, when the patient is more stable and can tolerate such reconstructive efforts. The physiologic rationale for damage control surgery relates to the metabolic consequences of extensive blood loss and blood and fluid replacement. These patients develop progressive hypothermia, acidosis, and coagulopathy (the so-called lethal triad), which can be corrected only when the patient can be brought to the intensive care unit with appropriate warming, fluid resuscitation, and other critical care interventions performed.[41]

Initially described in the military trauma literature, then applied to civilian penetrating abdominal trauma, these principles have now been successfully applied to a wide range of penetrating and blunt injuries. Extensive studies now support the view that appropriately selected patients managed by damage control strategies demonstrate improved survival compared with patients who undergo prolonged surgical efforts during the initial operative period. With the exception of patients with severe renal or bladder bleeding, urinary tract injuries do not directly result in early mortality. In the surgeon's judgment, when the patient would not tolerate the extended reconstructive effort needed to deal definitively with a urologic injury at initial laparotomy—because of pattern of injury, hypothermia, acidosis, coagulopathy, or other parameters that mandate a damage control approach—certain temporary solutions may be used. The complexity of patient selection for damage control surgery requires a multidisciplinary interaction, with the trauma surgeon and surgical specialists involved, to determine which injuries must be addressed initially and which can be definitively handled in a delayed fashion. Earlier selection of damage control surgery candidates, based on patterns of injury and response to initial resuscitative efforts, results in improved survival when the initial operative procedure can be concluded before significant metabolic deterioration occurs.[41]

Renal injuries that are incompletely staged or unstaged may be approached with delayed assessment and exploration, as long as a determination is made that life-threatening bleeding from the injury is unlikely to occur. In the absence of significant bleeding from the renal fossa into the peritoneal cavity, a large midline hematoma, or an expanding or pulsatile renal hematoma, one can elect to leave the perinephric hematoma undisturbed and fully resuscitate the patient.[41] Appropriate staging studies can be performed and delayed exploration and reconstruction completed at the time of a second-look procedure. If a major reconstructive effort is still needed in the unstable patient, packing the kidney and returning for reconstructive interventions later is also an option.

Ureteral injuries may be managed initially with externalized stents, ligation, or simple local drainage. Of these options, externalized stents are preferred as they allow control of the urinary output, minimize ongoing urinary extravasation, and can be maintained until the patient is stable enough to return to surgery for definitive reconstruction. Any number of medical tubes or catheters can be used, but the ideal solution is a 7 Fr or 8.5 Fr single-J urinary diversion stent placed into the ureter through the injury site, advanced proximally into the kidney, and then externalized through the abdominal wall (Fig. 72-25). The catheter should be tied to the very end of the injured ureter at the injury site so as not to lose ureteral length by ligating it more proximally and making later reconstruction more challenging. The distal ureteral limb is best left undisturbed; ligating it requires subsequent débridement and causes further tissue loss.

A similar approach can be used for extensive bladder injuries; the ureteral orifices can be catheterized, the catheters externalized, and the pelvis packed, leaving bladder reconstruction to be performed at a more suitable time, after appropriate resuscitation. Urethral and genital injuries are also amenable to damage control approaches, generally involving tube diversion, placement of moistened dressings, and tissue preservation until definitive reconstruction after appropriate resuscitation.

NONTRAUMATIC UROLOGIC EMERGENCIES

Within the field of urology are several emergent conditions, although not due to external violence, that represent true emergencies, some of which are life-threatening. These urologic emergencies include obstructed upper tract UTI, hematuria with urinary retention due to blood clots, and the acute scrotum—specifically testicular torsion, priapism, and Fournier gangrene. Some of these conditions have been discussed in other sections of this chapter (Fournier gangrene and obstructed upper tract UTI); the remainder are covered in this discussion.

Testicular Torsion

The most urgent cause of the acute scrotum is testicular torsion. Testicular torsion occurs when arterial blood supply is compromised by a twist of the spermatic cord, creating occlusion of the spermatic cord and loss of vascular supply. In the normal anatomic arrangement, the inferior aspect of the testicle is attached to the scrotum by the gubernaculum, preventing rotation of the testicle within the scrotum. When torsion occurs, the testicle is subjected to warm ischemia; without reversal of the occluded blood supply, irreversible damage begins as soon as 4 hours and is complete by 8 to 12 hours. Although testicular torsion is most common in adolescent males, it may occur in any age group from neonate to adult men. As many other conditions may result in the so-called acute scrotum, a high index of suspicion is necessary on the part of the treating physician to ensure rapid diagnosis and treatment. Differential diagnosis includes trauma, epididymitis, incarcerated hernia, and torsion of the appendix testis or appendix epididymis. Diagnosis is strongly suspected on the basis of history and physical examination. Classic historical findings include sudden onset of intense unilateral scrotal pain, unrelated to trauma, that may be associated with nausea and vomiting. The most consistent physical examination finding is loss of the cremasteric reflex of the testicle; however, in an acute setting, this may be difficult to elicit. The best confirmatory radiologic study is color Doppler ultrasound of the scrotum, which shows absence of arterial flow to the testis in torsion. In patients with suspected testicular torsion, there is no need to delay scrotal exploration to obtain imaging or further laboratory evaluation.

Treatment of testicular torsion involves surgical exploration through a midline or transverse scrotal incision with inspection of the testis with detorsion, if present, of the spermatic cord (Fig. 72-26). For testes that are deemed to be viable, suture orchiopexy or fixation to the interior scrotal wall is performed, followed by a similar orchiopexy on the contralateral side at the same setting to prevent contralateral torsion. Because of the important medicolegal considerations in these cases, urgent exploration is still indicated even in patients who present with a suspected late torsion (e.g., several days of fixed swelling, firmness). Many times, it is difficult to know exactly how long complete ischemia has been present and whether there is still a potentially viable testicle.

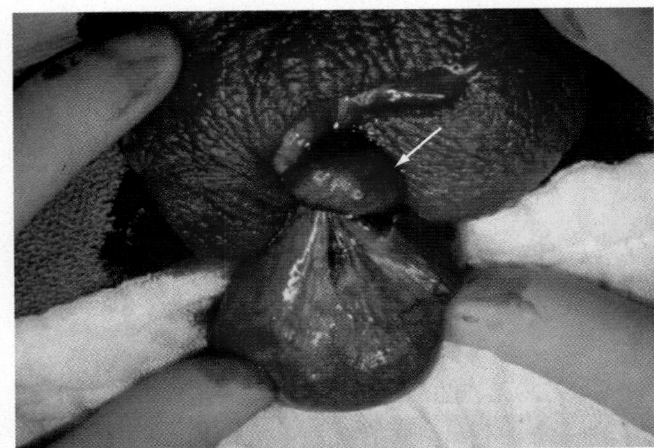

FIGURE 72-26 Testicular Torsion. Exploration through a transverse scrotal incision demonstrates the twisted cord *(top)*. Note the degree of edema, erythema, and ecchymosis present after several hours of torsion.

Gross Hematuria With Urinary Retention from Blood Clots

Most patients who have hematuria present with either microscopic hematuria or episodic gross hematuria. However, in a subset of patients, onset of gross hematuria is rapid with significant blood loss and development of blood clots within the bladder. This problem is exacerbated in patients who are receiving chronic anticoagulation for underlying cardiovascular disease processes. The blood clots are organized into larger masses; the patient may not be able to expel the clot, leading to urinary retention and a potential surgical emergency (Fig. 72-27). Other causes of significant vesical hemorrhage include postoperative bleeding after TURP or transurethral resection of bladder tumor (TURBT), radiation cystitis, pelvic trauma, upper tract arteriovenous fistula, and iliac arterial fistula to the ureter.

It is difficult to judge the amount of blood that is being lost from the urinary tract with gross hematuria because only a small amount of blood mixed with urine will darken the bladder efflux. If, however, copious amounts of clot are evacuated from the bladder, one should suspect at least moderate blood loss and monitor the patient with vital signs and hemoglobin measurements. If bleeding from these events causes symptomatic anemia, the patient may require multiple urgent blood transfusions. In the patient with a significant amount of blood clot in the bladder, it will be necessary to place a large-bore irrigation catheter (in the adult, often 20 Fr to 26 Fr) and adequately irrigate the clots from the bladder using normal saline irrigation. Special hematuria catheters are designed to allow large-volume irrigation and clot removal, but if this is unsuccessful, the patient may require urgent operative cystoscopy to evacuate the clot and to identify and fulgurate any bleeding source. Typically, this involves rigid cystoscopy with a large working sheath or resectoscope sheath and irrigation performed with a piston syringe or special evacuation devices (Ellik evacuator). After clot evacuation and fulguration, a

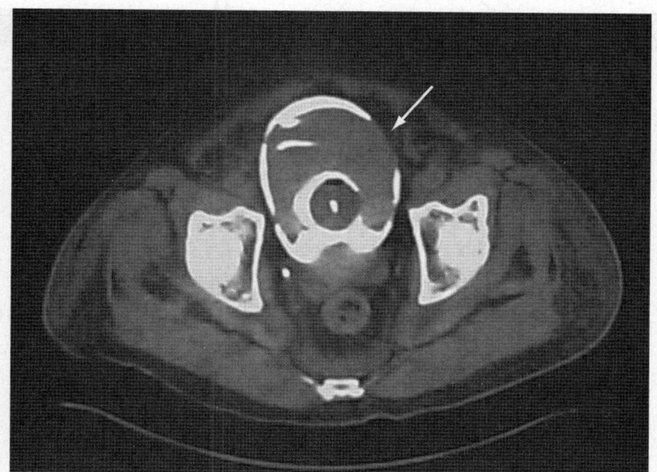

FIGURE 72-27 CT scan of the pelvis with cystography in a patient with urinary clot retention caused by chronic hemorrhagic cystitis after radiation therapy for prostate cancer. A clot may be seen surrounding the Foley catheter balloon, with instilled contrast material outlining the balloon and intact bladder wall.

large three-way catheter is left in place to run continuous irrigation to prevent a recurrent episode of clot retention. Upper tract clot formation may produce a so-called clot colic, with renal pain similar to that experienced from passage of a renal calculus. Supportive care and, in some cases, stent insertion may be helpful to address the underlying problem. If unexplained, significant, gross hematuria occurs after minor trauma, one should suspect an underlying abnormality of the urinary tract, such as a neoplasm, congenital anomaly, or arteriovenous malformation.

Priapism

Priapism is a prolonged, painful penile erection that occurs in the absence of sexual arousal or stimulation. Priapism is typically divided into ischemic and nonischemic priapism. Important causes of ischemic priapism include sickle cell disease or other blood dyscrasias and certain types of drug or medication use, especially drugs for penile erection and hematologic malignant disease. Nonischemic priapism is the pelvic or genital trauma that results in arteriovenous fistula of the penile circulation. Priapism may resolve spontaneously, but if it persists longer than 4 hours, measures should be taken to reverse the process in most cases. Patients with priapism that lasts longer than 12 hours may develop irreversible damage to the penile vascular structure and long-term ED.

Evaluation in cases of ischemic priapism is centered on detailed history for risk factors, corporal blood gas analysis, and color Doppler ultrasound of the corpora cavernosa. Nonischemic priapism is evaluated similarly; however, aspirated blood has an arterial appearance and arterial blood gas parameters.

Ischemic priapism is managed with initial needle aspiration of the corpora cavernosa and irrigation with saline. In patients who do not respond to this step, needle aspiration is repeated with the injection of small, dilute doses of an α-adrenergic agonist substance, such as dilute phenylephrine. For patients who fail to respond to these measures, various shunting procedures can be performed to create shunts between the corpus cavernosum and other vascular structures, like the corpus spongiosum, to induce blood flow. For priapism related to sickle cell disease, medical treatment of the sickle crisis (e.g., hydration, oxygenation, pain management, and addressing hemoglobin and transfusion status) with hematology support is a mainstay of therapy to resolve priapism. For nonischemic priapism, there is no role for aspiration or irrigation of the erection as this is the result of an abnormality of the vascular system. Compression of the perineum or other injury site can be performed as an initial maneuver. If this fails, the next treatment step is usually superselective angioembolization to occlude the arteriovenous fistula with reversible agents, such as autologous blood clots or Gelfoam. It is important that the general surgeon consult with the urologist about treatment because corporal fibrosis and loss of erectile function are risks that increase with significant delays in therapy.

UROLOGIC ONCOLOGY

Urologic malignant neoplasms account for a significant disease burden in adults in the United States. Cancers of the genitourinary system encompass the full spectrum of malignant neoplasms and are of some of the most common (prostate) and rare (penile) cancers in the United States. Of the 12 most common cancers diagnosed annually in the United States, three are urologic in origin: prostate, bladder, and kidney. Low-stage cancers are typically managed with extirpative surgery or therapeutic radiation. Urologic cancers may involve adjacent viscera, vasculature, and soft tissue and body wall structures so that additional surgical expertise is necessary to complete the extirpative surgery and to support reconstructive efforts. As is the case with other malignant neoplasms, cancers of the genitourinary system are often managed with a multidisciplinary approach. The major anatomic types of urologic cancers are discussed in this section, with a focus on the essential basic background knowledge, the fundamental therapeutic approaches for various stages of cancer presentation, and the basic outcomes for different tumor types.

Renal Tumors

Renal cell carcinoma, the most common type of renal malignant disease, accounts for 2% to 3% of all adult malignant neoplasms.[44] The majority of renal malignant neoplasms are now diagnosed incidentally by cross-sectional imaging or ultrasound evaluation of other nonspecific complaints. Historically, renal cell carcinoma was diagnosed only at an advanced stage because of its location within the retroperitoneum. The classic triad of renal cell carcinoma (flank pain, gross hematuria, and palpable abdominal mass) is now seen in less than 10% of patients. Despite this increase in asymptomatic diagnoses, 30% of patients present with metastatic disease.[45] Other symptoms on advanced presentation include hemorrhage, paraneoplastic syndrome, and symptoms of metastasis, such as pathologic fracture. Paraneoplastic syndromes are present in 20% of patients at diagnosis and include Stauffer syndrome (reversible hepatitis without liver metastasis), constitutional symptoms, polycythemia, and elevated inflammatory markers (erythrocyte sedimentation rate and C-reactive protein).[45] Renal cell carcinoma typically presents in the sixth to eighth decade of life and is more common in men. Risk factors for renal cell carcinoma include smoking, hypertension, obesity, acquired renal cystic disease (in patients with end-stage renal disease), and occupational exposures (aromatic hydrocarbons, asbestos, cadmium, and chemical and rubber industries).[44] These tumors typically arise in the proximal convoluted tubule or collecting duct within the renal parenchyma.[44]

Renal cell carcinoma is classified as follows: clear cell carcinoma, papillary renal cell carcinoma, chromophobe renal cell carcinoma, collecting duct carcinoma, and renal medullary carcinoma; this classification is based on microscopic appearance and cell of origin.[45] The genetics of these malignant neoplasms is fairly well described. The most common tumor, clear cell carcinoma, is the result of chromosome 3 abnormalities; papillary carcinoma is the result of aberrations of chromosome 7, 17, or Y.[45] In addition, clear cell carcinoma and papillary carcinoma are responsible for the two most common familial cancer syndromes, von Hippel–Lindau and hereditary papillary renal cell carcinoma, respectively. Most renal masses are malignant, and only 15% to 20% are benign; the two most common benign masses are oncocytoma and angiomyolipoma.[45]

A final consideration with renal neoplasms is cystic renal masses, which present diagnostic challenges. Depending on specific characteristics of renal cystic lesions, the risk of these lesions representing cystic malignant neoplasms must be considered. The Bosniak classification system describes cystic renal masses according to their malignant risk and CT appearance, ranging from category I (simple cysts) to category IV (cysts associated with enhancing or solid elements).[45] Category III and IV cysts are usually treated as representing cystic renal cell carcinomas.

Staging

Outcomes in renal cell carcinoma are directly tied to clinical stage at time of diagnosis. Evaluation and staging for renal cell carcinoma include history, physical examination, and laboratory testing. Evaluation for renal masses includes imaging of the primary tumor, usually with a contrast-enhanced CT scan or MRI study of the abdomen and pelvis, as well as chest imaging, typically chest radiography. Also, based on clinical suspicion or abnormal results of laboratory studies, bone and brain imaging is performed. A key aspect of abdominal CT or MRI is evaluation of the renal vein and inferior vena cava as renal cell carcinoma commonly forms tumor thrombus in these structures, and this finding is not necessarily correlated with tumor stage. The TNM staging system is listed in Table 72-2. Histologic grading is based on the Fuhrman nuclear grading system on a scale of I to IV.

TABLE 72-2 Staging of Kidney Cancer

Primary Tumor (T)	
TX	Primary tumor cannot be assessed
T0	No evidence of primary tumor
T1	Tumor 7 cm or less in greatest dimension, limited to the kidney
T1a	Tumor 4 cm or less in greatest dimension, limited to the kidney
T1b	Tumor more than 4 cm but not more than 7 cm in greatest dimension, limited to the kidney
T2	Tumor >7 cm in greatest dimension, limited to the kidney
T2a	Tumor >7 cm and ≤10 cm in greatest dimension, limited to the kidney
T2b	Tumor >10 cm in greatest dimension, limited to the kidney
T3	Tumor extends into major veins or perinephric tissues but not into the ipsilateral adrenal gland and not beyond Gerota fascia
T3a	Tumor grossly extends into the renal vein or its segmental (muscle-containing) branches, or tumor invades perirenal and/or renal sinus fat but not beyond Gerota fascia
T3b	Tumor grossly extends into the vena cava below the diaphragm
T3c	Tumor grossly extends into the vena cava above the diaphragm or invades the wall of the vena cava
T4	Tumor invades beyond Gerota fascia (including contiguous extension into the ipsilateral adrenal gland)
Regional Lymph Nodes (N)	
NX	Regional lymph nodes cannot be assessed
N0	No regional lymph node metastasis
N1	Metastasis in regional lymph node(s)
Distant Metastasis (M)	
M0	No distant metastasis
M1	Distant metastasis
Stage Grouping	
Stage I	T1 N0 M0
Stage II	T2 N0 M0
Stage III	T1 or T2 N1 M0, T3 N0 or N1 M0
Stage IV	T4 Any N M0

Management

The management of renal cell carcinoma has evolved in recent years. Historically, renal cell carcinoma was a surgical disease, and patients diagnosed with any renal mass underwent total radical nephrectomy. Now, select patients may undergo renal biopsy and active surveillance protocols. In the past, renal biopsies were fraught with high false-negative rates and low accuracy. Contemporary series show an accuracy rate of more than 90% in experienced centers with low complications.[45] Those patients who are appropriate for renal biopsy are patients considered for either active surveillance or renal ablation therapy. Active surveillance protocols have been developed for patients with incidentally diagnosed, small (<3 cm) renal masses and those patients who would not tolerate extirpative or ablative therapy.[45] The natural history of renal masses is a tendency to grow slowly, on average 0.5 cm/yr, and they do not metastasize. Patients assigned to surveillance protocols undergo imaging every 3 to 6 months; once mass size stability is observed, this interval is extended to 6 to 12 months.[45] Small renal masses (<5 cm) can be considered for percutaneous, laparoscopic, or open ablation using cryotherapy or radiofrequency energy.[44] This treatment should be considered more for patients with significant medical comorbidities and less often in healthy patients.

For renal tumors that are diagnosed in the absence of metastases or for those with a solitary metastasis, extirpative surgery is the standard approach. Resection of solitary synchronous metastatic disease is performed when it is technically feasible. Renal surgery has undergone a significant transformation in the past 10 years, and most renal surgery, both nephron sparing and radical excision, is now performed through either a laparoscopic or robotically assisted approach. The trend in extirpative surgery is to perform nephron sparing or partial nephrectomy for most T1 tumors. Partial nephrectomy is equivalent to radical nephrectomy in this tumor stage and should be considered for all patients with a T1a tumor and most with T1b tumors. Partial nephrectomy surgery may be straightforward in dealing with small, well-encapsulated, superficial, exophytic lesions or complex in dealing with larger, central lesions that involve the renal hilar structures. For partial nephrectomy, a negative margin should be obtained with the parenchymal resection, and only a few millimeters of normal parenchyma around the tumor are considered necessary. The general principles for partial nephrectomy include achievement of a negative surgical margin, identification and suturing of significant segmental renal vessel branches, and collecting system repair when the collecting system is entered or partially resected.

To assist with blood loss, atraumatic vascular clamping of the renal artery and surface cooling of the kidney with iced saline slush are effective. When laparoscopic or robotic approaches are used for partial nephrectomy, local hypothermia is more cumbersome, and rapid tumor resection and clamp times of less than 30 minutes are employed. Tissue sealants, hemostatic agents, and absorbable mesh reconstruction of the kidney are all useful techniques to aid in hemostasis of a partial nephrectomy in the open surgical, laparoscopic, or robotic setting.

Radical nephrectomy is performed in patients with large tumors and those patients in whom a partial nephrectomy is not technically feasible. The primary long-term risk in this surgery is chronic kidney disease and loss of renal function. In comparison to partial nephrectomy, radical nephrectomy has a lower rate of complications. The adrenal gland is no longer removed with radical nephrectomy except in cases of obvious tumor involvement as the rate of synchronous involvement is less than 10%. Typically, radical nephrectomy is performed by either a laparoscopic or open approach. Standard incisions for radical nephrectomy include anterior subcostal, flank, chevron, and midline, although the midline incision has the most difficult vascular access. Regardless of approach, dissection of the renal pedicle with ligation of a renal artery must precede vein ligation to prevent swelling and dangerous bleeding from the kidney. The entire Gerota fascial envelope, containing the perinephric fat as a margin around the kidney parenchyma and tumor, is excised intact. The ureter is ligated and divided where convenient. A regional lymph node dissection is often performed with a radical nephrectomy, although, on the basis of most evidence, it is more helpful as a staging and prognostic procedure than as a therapeutic one. For patients with locally advanced or metastatic disease, immunotherapy and targeted therapy (drugs with action on vascular endothelial growth factor and mammalian target of rapamycin) are used in a neoadjuvant or adjuvant setting. Overall organ-confined disease has an 80% to 100% 5-year survival in T1 tumors and a 50% to 80% 5-year survival in T2 disease.[45] Advanced disease has grim prognosis of 0% to 20% 5-year survival.[45]

Bladder Cancer

Urothelial malignant disease can arise anywhere in the upper or lower collecting system, but the most common site is the bladder. The entire upper and lower urinary tracts, renal collecting system through the prostatic urethra, are lined with surface epithelium called urothelium. The urothelium has a variable thickness of three to six cell layers, and transitional cell carcinoma arises from the basal cell layer. Bladder cancer is the fifth most common adult malignant neoplasm diagnosed in the United States and is more common in men than in women.[46] The tumor arises most frequently in the eighth decade of life, and men older than 70 years have a 3.7% probability for development of bladder cancer.[46] The multiple risk factors for development of bladder cancer include tobacco smoke, arsenic, chronic infections and inflammatory conditions (e.g., schistosomiasis), and occupational exposures (such as arylamines and aromatic hydrocarbons). The most common presenting symptom in bladder cancer is hematuria, microscopic in 1% to 11% and gross in 13% to 35%.[46] The other presenting symptom is irritative voiding—frequency, urgency, and dysuria. Bladder cancer can be divided into non–muscle invasive and muscle invasive, which have different treatments and outcomes. TNM staging is included in Table 72-3; the T stage at diagnosis, specifically non–muscle invasive (T1 or less) or muscle invasive (T2 or greater), is highly predictive of long-term outcome and survival. Ta disease refers to papillary tumors, with involvement of only the mucosa. T1 tumors involve the lamina propria, and T2 disease involves the detrusor muscle. Higher stages of the local tumor reflect involvement of perivesical fat or adjacent organs. Tumors are graded on the basis of histologic appearance from papilloma to high grade.

TABLE 72-3 Staging of Urothelial Cancer

Primary Tumor (T)	
TX	Primary tumor cannot be assessed
T0	No evidence of primary tumor
Ta	Noninvasive papillary carcinoma
Tis	Carcinoma in situ: "flat tumor"
T1	Tumor invades subepithelial connective tissue
T2	Tumor invades muscularis propria
pT2a	Tumor invades superficial muscularis propria (inner half)
pT2b	Tumor invades deep muscularis propria (outer half)
T3	Tumor invades perivesical tissue:
pT3a	Microscopically
pT3b	Macroscopically (extravesical mass)
T4	Tumor invades any of the following: prostatic stroma, seminal vesicles, uterus, vagina, pelvic wall, abdominal wall
T4a	Tumor invades prostatic stroma, uterus, vagina
T4b	Tumor invades pelvic wall, abdominal wall
Regional Lymph Nodes (N)	
Regional lymph nodes include both primary and secondary drainage regions. All other nodes above the aortic bifurcation are considered distant lymph nodes.	
NX	Lymph nodes cannot be assessed
N0	No lymph node metastasis
N1	Single regional lymph node metastasis in the true pelvis (hypogastric, obturator, external iliac, or presacral lymph node)
N2	Multiple regional lymph node metastasis in the true pelvis (hypogastric, obturator, external iliac, or presacral lymph node metastasis)
N3	Lymph node metastasis to the common iliac lymph nodes
Distant Metastasis (M)	
M0	No distant metastasis
M1	Distant metastasis

Non–Muscle Invasive Bladder Cancer

Urothelial tumors that have not invaded the detrusor muscle are termed non–muscle invasive bladder cancers (NMIBCs). Approximately 70% of patients who present with bladder cancer will be diagnosed with NMBIC, which includes T stages Tis (carcinoma in situ), Ta, and T1.[46] Patients who are suspected of having bladder cancer should undergo a thorough evaluation, which includes history, physical examination, basic laboratory tests, upper urinary tract imaging (preferably contrast-enhanced cross-sectional imaging), and office cystoscopy. If bladder cancer is present, characteristic flat, papillary, or bizarre, aggressive-appearing masses will be present on the urothelial surface of the bladder. NMIBCs typically appear as flat (carcinoma in situ) or papillary (Ta or T1) lesions. An adjunct test for equivocal findings is urine cytology, which is either as voided or bladder wash at the time of cystoscopy. Urine cytology is most sensitive for high-grade tumors and can be equivocal or nondiagnostic in the setting of low-grade NMIBCs. Adjunct urine tumor markers exist but are not recommended on consensus guidelines because of cost and low specificity.

Any tumor identified in the bladder should be fully resected by TURBT. TURBT allows pathologic analysis, tumor staging but identification (if present) of muscle invasion, and treatment of noninvasive, low-grade disease. TURBT is performed through a surgical endoscope, called a resectoscope, and uses either monopolar or bipolar energy to shave the tumor from the bladder wall. At the time of TURBT, patients should undergo a bimanual examination of the bladder to identify extravesical extension of disease and palpable mass. Any patient identified with high-grade T1 tumors or absence of muscle in the initial resection should undergo repeated TURBT. All patients who undergo TURBT should receive immediate intravesical chemotherapy within 6 hours of surgery; this treatment has been shown to reduce the tumor recurrence rate by 35%.[46] The agent most commonly used for this purpose is mitomycin C. Six weeks after TURBT, patients with carcinoma in situ or NMIBC with high risk for progression or recurrence should receive intravesical therapy with either immunotherapy or chemotherapeutic agents. Standard immunotherapy for NMIBC consists of serial bacille Calmette-Guérin (BCG) intravesical instillations for induction and periodic maintenance therapy. Intravesical BCG significantly decreases the invasion and progression rate for NMIBCs, compared with transurethral resection alone. Patients with recurrent NMIBC may require regimens of BCG plus interferon for salvage therapy. Maintenance BCG instillations reduce the risk of recurrence and progression and are given at variable intervals for periods of 1 to 3 years. Other salvage intravesical treatments include chemotherapeutic agents such as mitomycin C and gemcitabine. Visual surveillance by office cystoscopy is mandatory in these patients as 15% to 80% of these tumors recur, and in higher grade tumors, 25% to 50% progress to higher stage or muscle invasive tumors.[46]

Muscle Invasive Bladder Cancer

Muscle invasive bladder cancer (MIBC) includes stage T2 or greater bladder cancer at diagnosis. The majority of patients who present with MIBC have invasive disease at diagnosis; approximately 15% to 20% of patients who present with NMIBC progress to MIBC.[46] MIBC is typically urothelial cell carcinoma, but other histopathologic types occur, including squamous cell carcinoma, adenocarcinoma, and small cell carcinoma. The last two have the worst prognostic outcomes. MIBC should be staged in a similar fashion to NMIBC, with cross-sectional imaging of the abdomen and pelvis, but consideration should be given to chest CT rather than plain radiography. Despite adequate staging, 40% of patients are understaged at diagnosis and have extravesical disease on the final pathologic specimen.

Management. Standard management of MIBC is radical cystoprostatectomy. In the male patient, radical cystectomy involves the removal of the entire urinary bladder en bloc with the perivesical fat, prostate, seminal vesicles, and pelvic lymph nodes. In the female patient, radical cystectomy typically involves en bloc removal of the female pelvic viscera, although salvage of these structures may at times be considered, depending on the details of the case. Extended lymph node dissection is performed at the same setting and includes removal of the external and internal iliac lymph nodes, common iliac lymph nodes to the aortic bifurcation, and presacral lymph nodes. Improved survival is associated with extended pelvic lymph node dissection at the time of radical cystectomy. Perioperative complication rates are high, and more than 60% of patients undergoing radical cystectomy and extended pelvic lymph node dissection have at least one complication within 90 days of surgery.[46] Because of the high rate of extravesical extension at the time of radical cystectomy, many patients are treated with neoadjuvant chemotherapy. Typical regimens for neoadjuvant chemotherapy include MVAC (methotrexate, vinblastine, doxorubicin [Adriamycin], and cisplatin) and GC (gemcitabine and cisplatin). The use of neoadjuvant chemotherapy improves overall survival by 5% to 7%.[46]

The selection of the type of urinary diversion after radical cystectomy must take into account any history of pelvic irradiation, presence of renal insufficiency, liver function abnormalities, and mechanical tasks for which the patient will be responsible. There are various options for urinary diversion, including ileal conduit, orthotopic bladder substitution with anastomosis to the native urethra, and more complex forms of cutaneous catheterizable reservoirs with continence mechanisms. No randomized study has shown one type of urinary diversion to be superior to any other, and the decision is usually directed by the patient's preference or the surgeon's choice. There is an extensive and complex history involving the use of intestinal segments in the urinary tract for urinary diversion after cystectomy and in other reconstructive settings. The surgeon should be familiar with the metabolic, mechanical, and other risk factors associated with the use of intestinal segments in the reconstructed urinary tract, including electrolyte abnormalities, bone demineralization, mucus production, stone formation, chronic infection, diarrhea, vitamin B_{12} deficiency, and increased cancer risk. Patients with organ-confined, node-negative disease have the best overall disease-specific survival at 5 and 10 years at 60% to 85%.[46]

Prostate Cancer

Prostate cancer is the most common cancer diagnosed in men and the third most common cancer diagnosed in the United States, behind breast and lung, with approximately 220,000 men diagnosed annually.[47] Prostate cancer is an adenocarcinoma and arises from the glandular structures within the prostatic parenchyma. Most new prostate cancer cases are diagnosed in men 60 years of age and older, are low grade and low stage, and are diagnosed by routine screening.[48] Screening for prostate cancer is performed with the blood test PSA, a serine protease, and DRE. The most controversial aspect of prostate cancer is screening and determining which patients require treatment. The goal of prostate cancer screening is to detect potentially lethal cancer at an early, treatable stage and to intervene with intent to cure. Because of the controversy surrounding the recent U.S. Preventive Services Task Force recommendation against screening for prostate cancer in 2012, the AUA released its own guidelines for screening in 2013.[49] These recommendations are for screening in men aged 55 to 69 years to be a joint decision between the physician and the patient, with recognition that the mortality of prostate cancer is 1 in 1000 men screened per decade, and a routine screening interval to occur every 2 years.[49] Routine screening is not routinely recommended in men aged 40 to 54 years and in men older than 70 years or younger than 40 years.[49] Furthermore, screening should not be performed in men with a life expectancy of less than 10 to 15 years.

Evaluation

Patients who have either an elevated total PSA level or abnormal findings on DRE or both undergo TRUS-guided biopsy of the prostate. In equivocal cases, other testing, including determination of free PSA level or calculation of PSA velocity, can help guide the decision for biopsy or further evaluation. The standard biopsy template involves 12 cores with a spring-loaded biopsy instrument; tissue is obtained from the base, mid, and apex regions, medially and laterally from the left and right sides. Prophylactic antibiotics are routinely administered, and cleansing enemas are advised. When feasible, patients are asked to stop anticoagulants to help prevent bleeding complications. Common adverse events that follow TRUS biopsy include rectal bleeding, gross hematuria, and hematospermia, all of which are usually self-limited. Fever and urinary infection and retention occur in less than 5% of patients; bacteremia occurs, but it is a rare occurrence in less than 1% of patients.

Prostate cancer is diagnosed histologically by the Gleason grading system, which evaluates the level of abnormality in the patterns of the glandular architecture of the prostate in comparison to normal. The grading system is based on a scale of 1 to 5, with 1 being the most differentiated and 5 being the least differentiated. Most prostate cancers have a Gleason grade of 3 with a sum of 6 or 7. Patients diagnosed with prostate cancer are risk stratified on the basis of PSA level at time of diagnosis, clinical stage based on DRE, and Gleason sum score on the prostate biopsy. Patients with high-risk cancers should undergo cancer staging, which in prostate cancer may include radionuclide bone scan to evaluate for bone metastasis and cross-sectional imaging of the abdomen and pelvis to evaluate for nodal metastasis (Table 72-4).

TABLE 72-4 Staging of Prostate Cancer

Primary Tumor (T)	
TX	Primary tumor cannot be assessed
T0	No evidence of primary tumor
T1	Clinically inapparent tumor neither palpable nor visible by imaging
T1a	Tumor incidental histologic finding in 5% or less of tissue resected
T1b	Tumor incidental histologic finding in more than 5% of tissue resected
T1c	Tumor identified by needle biopsy (for example, because of elevated PSA)
T2	Tumor confined within prostate
T2a	Tumor involves one-half of one lobe or less
T2b	Tumor involves more than one-half of one lobe but not both lobes
T2c	Tumor involves both lobes
T3	Tumor extends through the prostate capsule
T3a	Extracapsular extension (unilateral or bilateral)
T3b	Tumor invades seminal vesicle(s)
T4	Tumor is fixed or invades adjacent structures other than seminal vesicles, such as external sphincter, rectum, bladder, levator muscles, and/or pelvic wall
Lymph Nodes (N)	
NX	Regional lymph nodes were not assessed
N0	No regional lymph node metastasis
N1	Metastasis in regional lymph node(s)
Distant Metastasis (M)	
M0	No distant metastasis
M1	Distant metastasis
M1a	Nonregional lymph node(s)
M1b	Bone(s)
M1c	Other site(s) with or without bone disease

Treatment

The treatment of prostate cancer has changed significantly during the past several years. As most prostate cancer, at diagnosis, is low risk, many patients are now treated with active surveillance rather than with active therapy. In general, men with cancer of low clinical stage (T1c), low grade (Gleason sum ≤ 6), and low volume on biopsy are candidates for active surveillance.[48] Patients assigned to active surveillance protocols undergo DRE and PSA monitoring every 3 to 6 months, with repeated TRUS-guided prostate biopsies every 1 to 3 years.[48] Patients with increase in Gleason sum or increase in tumor volume on biopsy typically shift to an active treatment plan.

Prostate cancer can be treated with either radical surgical excision or definitive radiation therapy. Radical prostatectomy involves the surgical removal of the entire prostate and seminal vesicles with anastomosis of the urethral stump to the bladder neck. Pelvic lymph node dissection is controversial in the management of prostate cancer; some protocols recommend no lymph node dissection for low-risk disease, and others recommend extended pelvic lymph node dissection. For prostate cancer Gleason sum 7 or higher, at a minimum, the external iliac and obturator lymph nodes should be removed. Radical prostatectomy can be performed with an open, laparoscopic, or robotically assisted laparoscopic approach. The majority of radical prostatectomies in the United States are now performed by a robotically assisted laparoscopic prostatectomy (RALP).[47] The advantages of RALP appear to be decreased blood loss, shorter hospital stay, and quicker return to work. When it is technically feasible and oncologically appropriate, a nerve-sparing approach is used, which avoids injury to the cavernous nerves that run posterolateral along the prostate in the neurovascular bundle and mediate penile erection. Important landmarks for radical prostatectomy are the dorsal venous plexus anteriorly, bladder neck cephalad, prostatomembranous urethral junction distally, and rectal wall posteriorly. The correct plane of posterior dissection in radical prostatectomy is just posterior to the Denonvilliers fascia. The primary long-term risks of radical prostatectomy are urinary incontinence and ED. Because of the recent introduction and adaptation of RALP, most long-term survival series are based on historical open radical prostatectomy data. Ten-year cancer progression-free survival is approximately 85% for patients with organ-confined disease, approximately 60% to 70% for extracapsular extension, and approximately 50% for patients with positive surgical margins.

Patients who do not desire surgical extirpation may undergo local therapy with either intensity-modulated radiation therapy (IMRT) or brachytherapy. The typical treatment dose for IMRT-based prostate cancer therapy is 76 to 86 Gy. The most common form of brachytherapy is low-dose ultrasound-guided placement of iodine-125 or palladium-103 radioisotope sources into the prostate. Both treatments are commonly used for low-risk prostate cancer. Intermediate- and high-risk prostate cancer is typically treated with IMRT coupled with androgen deprivation therapy for up to 2 years. Low- and intermediate-risk prostate cancers have outcomes after radiation-based therapy similar to those of radical prostatectomy.[47] In advanced prostate cancer, androgen deprivation therapy may become ineffective, with clinical or PSA progression observed in spite of appropriate hormonal therapy. In these cases, second-line treatment includes antiandrogens, chemotherapy, and investigational agents. Other forms of treatment that can be considered for local treatment of prostate cancer include cryotherapy and proton beam therapy, although long-term results for these modalities are still being reported.

After prostate cancer therapy, patients are monitored for post-treatment morbidities (e.g., continence, erectile function, voiding adequacy) and possible cancer recurrence. The latter involves PSA testing and potentially repeated metastatic evaluation, when indicated. Long-term follow-up for prostate cancer patients should continue at least 10 years, if not permanently, because very late recurrences can occur. If the PSA level becomes significantly detectable or is rising after definitive treatment, it may be appropriate to consider repeated TRUS of the anastomotic region, possibly with biopsy, and repeated metastatic evaluation to decide whether to proceed with local radiation therapy, androgen deprivation therapy, or observation.

Testicular Cancer

Testicular cancer is an uncommon malignant neoplasm; in the United States, the incidence is 5/100,000 men.[50] Most cases of primary testicular cancer are germ cell origin (95%); the remainder are predominantly stromal (Leydig cell) or sex cord (Sertoli cell) tumors.[50] Any solid intratesticular mass is likely to represent a malignant germ cell tumor and is typically treated as such unless there is a strong suspicion to the contrary. Risk factors for testicular tumors include cryptorchidism, family history of testicular cancer, and intratubular germ cell neoplasia.

Germ cell–derived testicular tumors can be broadly divided into seminoma and nonseminoma germ cell tumors (NSGCTs); the division is approximately 50% for each. The majority of seminomas are classic (85%); the remainder are either anaplastic or spermatocytic seminoma.[50] NSGCTs can be divided into numerous histologic types: embryonal carcinoma, yolk sac or endodermal sinus tumors, choriocarcinoma, teratoma, and mixed germ cell tumors. Testicular malignant neoplasms are the most common tumors in men between the ages of 20 and 40 years.[50] Seminomas, however, present in the fourth or fifth decade of life, and spermatocytic seminomas may present in men older than 50 years.[50] The most common presenting complaint in men with testicular cancer is a painless testicular mass; however, it is not uncommon for men to present with symptoms of metastatic disease, including palpable abdominal mass, shortness of breath, and hemoptysis. In patients who present with a painless testicular mass, scrotal ultrasonography is the diagnostic study of choice. In addition to history, physical examination, and ultrasonography, patients with testicular tumors should have determination of specific tumor markers: α-fetoprotein, β-human chorionic gonadotropin, and lactate dehydrogenase. After treatment, these markers have a characteristic half-life, and appropriate clearance has important prognostic significance.

Treatment

Initial treatment of suspected testicular tumor is radical inguinal orchiectomy, which involves removal of the testicle and spermatic cord at the level of the inguinal ring (Fig. 72-28). Because of the characteristic and well-described lymph drainage of the testicle, there is no role for trans-scrotal biopsy or orchiectomy. If the intrascrotal tissue planes are violated during orchiectomy, the lymphatic drainage can be altered, affecting future treatment. After radical inguinal orchiectomy, the patient should undergo disease staging, including cross-sectional, contrast-enhanced imaging of the abdomen and pelvis and chest imaging, either chest radiography in low-risk patients or cross-sectional chest imaging in patients with high-risk disease.

Clinical staging for testicular cancer includes primary tumor pathology, lymph and metastatic staging on imaging, and postorchiectomy serum tumor markers (Tables 72-5 and 72-6). The half-life of β-human chorionic gonadotropin is 24 to 36 hours,

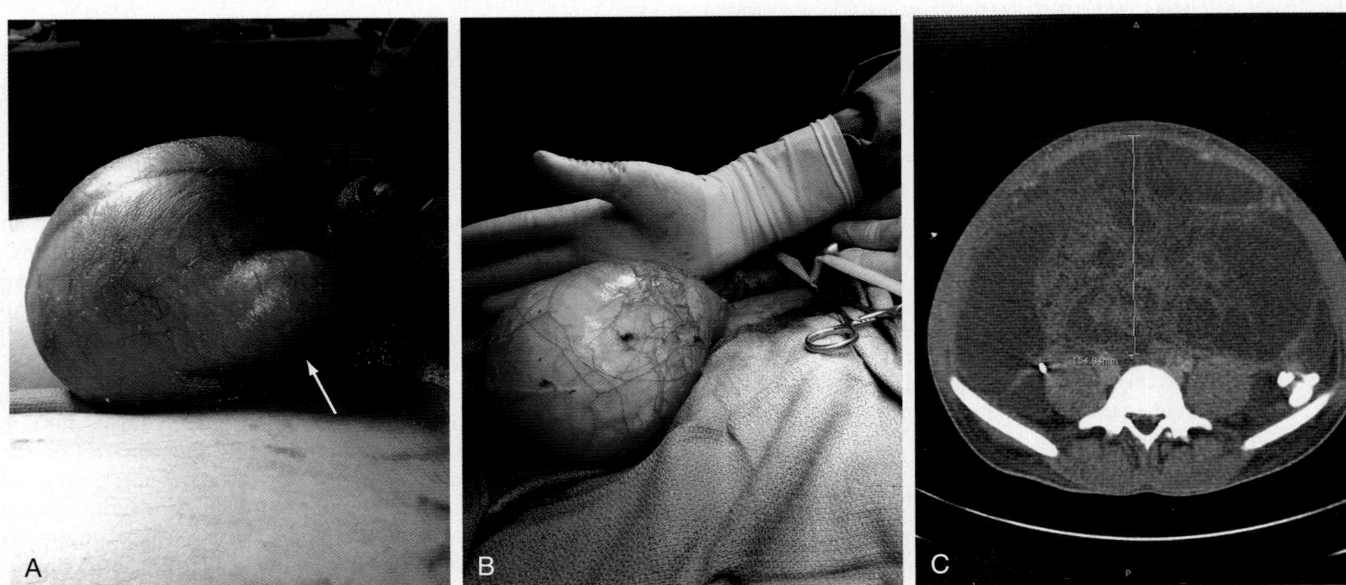

FIGURE 72-28 **Advanced Testicular Carcinoma. A,** Preoperative appearance of the scrotum in a patient with a large right testis tumor. The normal left testis is seen pushed cephalad by the right-sided mass. **B,** Surgical exploration through right inguinal incision, showing the right testis that has been dissected from the scrotum in an extravaginal plane, still attached by the spermatic cord pedicle to the right. **C,** Massive retroperitoneal lymphadenopathy in the same patient. Note that the descending colon is opacified with contrast material, but all other viscera are pushed cephalad so that no small intestine is seen in this image. The patient was managed with primary chemotherapy followed by retroperitoneal lymphadenectomy for the residual mass.

TABLE 72-5 Staging of Testicular Cancer

Primary Tumor (T)	
pTX	Primary tumor cannot be assessed
pT0	No evidence of primary tumor
pTis	Intratubular germ cell neoplasia
pT1	Tumor limited to the testis and epididymis without lymphovascular invasion, may invade tunica albuginea but not tunica vaginalis
pT2	Tumor limited to the testis and epididymis with lymphovascular invasion or tumor involving the tunica vaginalis
pT3	Tumor invades the spermatic cord with or without lymphovascular invasion
pT4	Tumor invades the scrotum with or without lymphovascular invasion
Regional Lymph Nodes (Clinical) (N)	
NX	Regional lymph nodes cannot be assessed
N0	No regional lymph node metastasis
N1	Metastasis within one or more lymph nodes less than 2 cm in size
N2	Metastasis within one or more lymph nodes greater than 2 cm but less the 5 cm in size
N3	Metastasis within one or more lymph nodes greater than 5 cm in size
Regional Lymph Nodes (Pathologic) (N)	
NX	Regional lymph nodes cannot be assessed
N0	No regional lymph node metastasis
N1	Metastasis within 1-5 lymph nodes; all node masses less than 2 cm in size
N2	Metastasis within a lymph node greater than 2 cm but not greater than 5 cm in size, or more than 5 lymph nodes involved, none greater than 5 cm and none demonstrating extranodal extension of tumor
N3	Metastasis within one or more lymph nodes greater than 5 cm in size
Distant Metastasis (M)	
MX	Distant metastasis cannot be assessed
M0	No distant metastasis
M1	Distant metastasis
M1a	Nonregional nodal or pulmonary metastasis
M1b	Distant metastasis at site other than nonregional lymph nodes or lung
Serum Tumor Markers (S)	
SX	Tumor markers not available or performed
S0	Tumor markers within normal limits
S1	LDH <1.5× normal, hCG <5000 IU/L, AFP <1000 ng/mL
S2	LDH 1.5-10× normal, hCG 5000-50,000 IU/L, AFP 1000-10,000 ng/mL
S3	LDH >10× normal, hCG >50,000 IU/L, AFP >10,000 ng/mL

AFP, α-fetoprotein; *hCG,* human chorionic gonadotropin; *LDH,* lactate dehydrogenase.

and the half-life of α-fetoprotein is 5 to 7 days; these levels should normalize in the absence of metastatic disease. Metastatic disease from testicular cancer typically follows a predictable retroperitoneal lymphatic path, although choriocarcinoma is notorious for hematogenous spread early to distant sites. From the right testis, initial lymph node metastasis is to the infrarenal interaortocaval nodes, paracaval nodes, and para-aortic nodes; on the left, the para-aortic nodes and then interaortocaval nodes. Retroperitoneal lymph nodes are the primary metastatic site in more than 70% of patients with metastatic testicular cancer.[50] If the patient has had prior groin or pelvic surgery, the natural lymphatic

TABLE 72-6 Clinical Staging of Testicular Cancer

STAGE	T	N	M	S
Stage I	pT1-4	N0	M0	SX
IA	pT1	N0	M0	S0
IB	pT2	N0	M0	S0
	pT3	N0	M0	S0
	pT4	N0	M0	S0
IS	Any pT	N0	M0	S1-3
Stage II	Any pT	N1-3	M0	SX
IIA	Any pT	N1	M0	S0-1
IIB	Any pT	N2	M0	S0-1
IIC	Any pT	N3	M0	S0-1
Stage III	Any pT	Any N	M1	SX
IIIA	Any pT	Any N	M1a	S0-1
IIIB	Any pT	N1-3	M0	S2
	Any pT	Any N	M1a	S2
IIIC	Any pT	N1-3	M0	S3
	Any pT	Any N	M1a	S3
	Any pT	Any N	M1b	Any S

distributions may be altered and the metastatic pattern may be unpredictable, potentially leading to involvement of the inguinal or pelvic nodes. Distant metastases are typically seen to the lung, liver, brain, bone, kidney, and adrenal gland.

Second-line treatment is directed by tumor histology and lymph node staging. Further treatment may consist of regular surveillance, retroperitoneal radiation therapy, retroperitoneal lymph node dissection (RPLND), systemic chemotherapy, or a multimodal therapy approach. The treatment decisions are complex, often at the direction of an institutional tumor board, but several general principles apply:

- For seminoma stage IA and IB disease, treatment options include surveillance, radiotherapy to the regional lymph nodes (20 Gy), and one or two cycles of carboplatin-based chemotherapy.[50]
- For seminoma stage IIA and IIB, radiotherapy of the retroperitoneal lymph nodes is standard therapy; for stage IIC or III, platinum-based chemotherapy is standard therapy.[50]
- For NSGCT stage I disease, the options include surveillance, RPLND, and cisplatin-based chemotherapy.[50]
- For NSGCT stage IIA, either primary RPLND (in patients with normal levels of tumor markers) or three or four cycles of cisplatin-based chemotherapy is standard; for stage IIB, three or four cycles of cisplatin-based chemotherapy is standard, followed by RPLND or surveillance.[50]

RPLND involves removal of all lymph nodes in the retroperitoneum from the renal vessels to the aortic bifurcation. An appropriate RPLND should include the lymph tissue surrounding the great vessels and division of the appropriate lumbar vessel to ensure thorough dissection, the split-and-roll technique. The most challenging RPLNDs are after chemotherapy, when the retroperitoneal tissues may be fibrotic or desmoplastic and adherent to the inferior vena cava, aorta, bowel, and mesentery. RPLND is template driven, and the appropriate levels and location of tissue excision are well described. Following the appropriate templates, the sympathetic nerve chain should be uninjured, allowing antegrade ejaculation.

Many patients undergoing RPLND will have been exposed to bleomycin chemotherapy, which requires meticulous intraoperative anesthetic management because of the exquisite sensitivity of these patients to elevated oxygen exposure; often, the anesthetic is run essentially on room air ventilation in these cases.

After orchiectomy and before any additional therapy for testicular cancer, consideration should be given to preservation of fertility. Patients should be made aware of the potential impact of radiation, chemotherapy, or RPLND on the ability to ejaculate and on spermatogenesis. It is essential that patients be offered sperm cryopreservation before therapies that could adversely affect their reproductive potential. In addition, patients should be made aware that radiation has the potential morbidity of delayed secondary malignant disease as high as 15% within 25 years of treatment.[50]

Curative treatment of testicular cancer is one of the great success stories of modern oncology. Overall, long-term survival for testicular cancer ranges from 98% to 99% for stage I seminoma or NSGCT.[50] In patients with stage II seminoma, radiotherapy yields survival of up to 100%, and stage II NSGCT standard treatments yield survival of 90% to 95%.[50] Even advanced disease, stage III seminoma, has an expected survival of more than 90%, and NSGCTs have long-term survivals of 80% to 90%.[50]

SELECTED REFERENCES

Bhasin S, Cunningham GR, Hayes FJ, et al: Testosterone therapy in men with androgen deficiency syndromes: An Endocrine Society clinical practice guideline. *J Clin Endocrinol Metab* 95:2536–2559, 2010.

The most current reference on the management of male testosterone deficiency. Broad-based consensus statement on evaluation, management, and therapy options.

Brandes S, Coburn M, Armenakas N, et al: Diagnosis and management of ureteric injury: An evidence-based analysis. *BJU Int* 94:277–289, 2004.

This article is a classic reference from the first consensus panel discussing evaluation and management of ureteral injuries.

Carter HB, Albertsen PC, Barry MJ, et al: Early detection of prostate cancer: AUA guideline. *J Urol* 190:419–426, 2013.

The evidence-based response to the U.S. Preventive Services Task Force recommendation to no longer screen men for prostate cancer. This article is a systematic critique of the literature used by the U.S. Preventive Services Task Force to give a grade D to the regular screening of prostate cancer.

Chapple C, Barbagli G, Jordan G, et al: Consensus statement on urethral trauma. *BJU Int* 93:1195–1202, 2004.

This article is a classic reference from the first consensus panel discussing evaluation and management of urethral injuries.

Gomez RG, Ceballos L, Coburn M, et al: Consensus statement on bladder injuries. *BJU Int* 94:27–32, 2004.

This article is a classic reference from the first consensus panel discussing evaluation and management of bladder injuries.

Gupta K, Hooton TM, Naber KG, et al: International clinical practice guidelines for the treatment of acute uncomplicated cystitis and pyelonephritis in women: A 2010 update by the Infectious Diseases Society of America and the European Society for Microbiology and Infectious Diseases. *Clin Infect Dis* 52:e103–e120, 2011.

This document represents the most current guideline for the diagnosis and treatment of outpatient or uncomplicated urinary tract infection in women.

Haylen BT, de Ridder D, Freeman RM, et al: An International Urogynecological Association (IUGA)/International Continence Society (ICS) joint report on the terminology for female pelvic floor dysfunction. *Neurourol Urodyn* 29:4–20, 2010.

This article is the most recent consensus guideline to standardize terminology, diagnosis, and management of pelvic floor dysfunction and incontinence.

Jarow J, Sigman M, Kolettis P, et al: The optimal evaluation of the infertile male. AUA Best Practice Statement, 2010, pp 1–39.

This article represents the best recommendations for evaluation and diagnosis of the infertile male. The AUA recommendations regarding specific aspects of the infertile male workup are highlighted throughout this manuscript, making it easily searchable.

Moore EE, Shackford SR, Pachter HL, et al: Organ injury scaling: Spleen, liver, and kidney. *J Trauma* 29:1664–1666, 1989.

This classic article describes injury grading in the urologic system.

Morey AF, Brandes S, Dugi DD, 3rd, et al: Urotrauma: AUA guideline. *J Urol* 192:327–335, 2014.

The first edition of the urologic trauma guidelines by the American Urological Association provides the best evidence-based recommendations for the management of traumatic urologic injuries.

Morey AF, Metro MJ, Carney KJ, et al: Consensus on genitourinary trauma: External genitalia. *BJU Int* 94:507–515, 2004.

This article is a classic reference from the first consensus panel discussing evaluation and management of genital injuries.

Santucci RA, Wessells H, Bartsch G, et al: Evaluation and management of renal injuries: Consensus statement of the renal trauma subcommittee. *BJU Int* 93:937–954, 2004.

This article is a classic reference from the first consensus panel discussing evaluation and management of renal injuries.

Smith TG, 3rd, Coburn M: Damage control maneuvers for urologic trauma. *Urol Clin North Am* 40:343–350, 2013.

This reference represents the only literature on management of traumatic urologic injuries using damage control principles and organized by urologic organ systems.

REFERENCES

1. Anderson JK, Cadeddu JA: Surgical anatomy of the retroperitoneum, adrenals, kidneys, and ureters. In Wein AJ, Kavoussi LR, Campbell MF, et al, editors: *Campbell-Walsh urology*, ed 10, Philadelphia, 2012, Elsevier Saunders.
2. McNeil BK: Kidney, adrenal, ureter. <https://www.auanet.org/university/core_topic.cfm?coreid=59>. Accessed August 7, 2015.
3. Kim IY, Clayton RV: Surgical renal anatomy. *AUA Update Series* 25:361–368, 2006.
4. Webster GD, Anoia E: Principles of ureteral reconstruction. In Smith JA, Howards SS, Preminger GM, et al, editors: *Hinman's atlas of urologic surgery*, ed 3, Philadelphia, 2012, Elsevier/Saunders.
5. Chung BI, Sommer G, Brooks JD: Anatomy of the lower urinary tract and male genitalia. In Wein AJ, Kavoussi LR, Campbell MF, et al, editors: *Campbell-Walsh urology*, ed 10, Philadelphia, 2012, Elsevier Saunders.
6. Smith PP: Lower urinary tract. American Urological Association. <https://www.auanet.org/university/core_topic.cfm?coreid=131>. Accessed December 18, 2014.
7. Walz J, Graefen M, Huland H: Basic principles of anatomy for optimal surgical treatment of prostate cancer. *World J Urol* 25:31–38, 2007.
8. Duffey B, Monga M: Principles of endoscopy. In Wein AJ, Kavoussi LR, Campbell MF, et al, editors: *Campbell-Walsh urology*, ed 10, Philadelphia, 2012, Elsevier Saunders.
9. Urinary tract infection. In Litwin M, Saigal C, editors: *Urologic diseases in America. U.S. Department of Health and Human Services, Public Health Service, National Institutes of Health, National Institute of Diabetes and Digestive and Kidney Diseases*, Washington, DC, 2012, U.S. Government Printing Office, pp 366–404. NIH Publication No. 12-7865.
10. Gupta K, Hooton TM, Naber KG, et al: International clinical practice guidelines for the treatment of acute uncomplicated cystitis and pyelonephritis in women: A 2010 update by the Infectious Diseases Society of America and the European Society for Microbiology and Infectious Diseases. *Clin Infect Dis* 52:e103–e120, 2011.
11. Lin WR, Chen M, Hsu JM, et al: Emphysematous pyelonephritis: Patient characteristics and management approach. *Urol Int* 93:29–33, 2014.
12. Sorensen MD, Krieger JN, Rivara FP, et al: Fournier's gangrene: Management and mortality predictors in a population based study. *J Urol* 182:2742–2747, 2009.
13. Clemens JQ: Basic bladder neurophysiology. *Urol Clin North Am* 37:487–494, 2010.
14. Gormley A, Stoffel J, Kielb S: Neurogenic bladder. American Urological Association. <https://www.auanet.org/university/core_topic.cfm?coreid=144>. Accessed August 7, 2015.
15. Haylen BT, de Ridder D, Freeman RM, et al: An International Urogynecological Association (IUGA)/International Continence Society (ICS) joint report on the terminology for female pelvic floor dysfunction. *Neurourol Urodyn* 29:4–20, 2010.
16. Irwin DE, Kopp ZS, Agatep B, et al: Worldwide prevalence estimates of lower urinary tract symptoms, overactive bladder, urinary incontinence and bladder outlet obstruction. *BJU Int* 108:1132–1138, 2011.
17. Gormley EA, Lightner DJ, Burgio KL, et al: Diagnosis and treatment of overactive bladder (non-neurogenic) in adults: AUA/SUFU guideline. *J Urol* 188:2455–2463, 2012.
18. Dooley Y, Kenton K, Cao G, et al: Urinary incontinence prevalence: Results from the National Health and Nutrition Examination Survey. *J Urol* 179:656–661, 2008.
19. Ford AA, Rogerson L, Cody JD, et al: Mid-urethral sling operations for stress urinary incontinence in women. *Cochrane Database Syst Rev* (7):CD006375, 2015.
20. McVary KT, Roehrborn CG, Avins AL, et al: Update on AUA guideline on the management of benign prostatic hyperplasia. *J Urol* 185:1793–1803, 2011.
21. Jarow J, Sigman M, Kolettis P, et al: The optimal evaluation of the infertile male. AUA Best Practice Statement, 2010, pp 1–39.
22. Jarow J, Sigman M, Kolettis P, et al: The evaluation of the azoospermic male. AUA Best Practice Statement Revised, 2010, pp 1–25.
23. Bacon CG, Mittleman MA, Kawachi I, et al: A prospective study of risk factors for erectile dysfunction. *J Urol* 176:217–221, 2006.
24. Crawford ED, Barqawi AB, O'Donnell C, et al: The association of time of day and serum testosterone concentration in a large screening population. *BJU Int* 100:509–513, 2007.
25. Bhasin S, Cunningham GR, Hayes FJ, et al: Testosterone therapy in men with androgen deficiency syndromes: An Endocrine Society clinical practice guideline. *J Clin Endocrinol Metab* 95:2536–2559, 2010.
26. Scales CD, Jr, Smith AC, Hanley JM, et al: Prevalence of kidney stones in the United States. *Eur Urol* 62:160–165, 2012.
27. Miller NL, Evan AP, Lingeman JE: Pathogenesis of renal calculi. *Urol Clin North Am* 34:295–313, 2007.
28. Preminger GM, Tiselius HG, Assimos DG, et al: 2007 guideline for the management of ureteral calculi. EAU/AUA Nephrolithiasis Guideline Panel. *J Urol* 178:2418–2434, 2007.
29. Lange JN, Mufarrij PW, Wood KD, et al: Metabolic evaluation and medical management of the calcium stone former. *AUA Update Series* 31, 2012.
30. Weizer AZ, Zhong P, Preminger GM: Shock wave lithotripsy: Current technology and evolving concepts. *AUA Update Series* 24, 2005.
31. Hotaling JM, Wang J, Sorensen MD, et al: A national study of trauma level designation and renal trauma outcomes. *J Urol* 187:536–541, 2012.
32. Moore EE, Shackford SR, Pachter HL, et al: Organ injury scaling: Spleen, liver, and kidney. *J Trauma* 29:1664–1666, 1989.
33. Santucci RA, Wessells H, Bartsch G, et al: Evaluation and management of renal injuries: Consensus statement of the renal trauma subcommittee. *BJU Int* 93:937–954, 2004.
34. Brandes S, Coburn M, Armenakas N, et al: Diagnosis and management of ureteric injury: An evidence-based analysis. *BJU Int* 94:277–289, 2004.

35. Gomez RG, Ceballos L, Coburn M, et al: Consensus statement on bladder injuries. *BJU Int* 94:27–32, 2004.
36. Chapple C, Barbagli G, Jordan G, et al: Consensus statement on urethral trauma. *BJU Int* 93:1195–1202, 2004.
37. Morey AF, Metro MJ, Carney KJ, et al: Consensus on genitourinary trauma: External genitalia. *BJU Int* 94:507–515, 2004.
38. Morey AF, Brandes S, Dugi DD, 3rd, et al: Urotrauma: AUA guideline. *J Urol* 192:327–335, 2014.
39. Voelzke BB, Hudak SJ, Coburn M: Renal, ureter trauma. American Urological Association. <https://www.auanet.org/university/core_topic.cfm?coreid=87>. Accessed August 7, 2015.
40. Charbit J, Manzanera J, Millet I, et al: What are the specific computed tomography scan criteria that can predict or exclude the need for renal angioembolization after high-grade renal trauma in a conservative management strategy? *J Trauma* 70:1219–1227, 2011.
41. Smith TG, 3rd, Coburn M: Damage control maneuvers for urologic trauma. *Urol Clin North Am* 40:343–350, 2013.
42. Myers J, Smith TG, III, Coburn M: Bladder, urethra, genitalia trauma. American Urological Association. <https://www.auanet.org/university/core_topic.cfm?coreid=88>. Accessed August 7, 2015.
43. McGeady JB, Breyer BN: Current epidemiology of genitourinary trauma. *Urol Clin North Am* 40:323–334, 2013.
44. Campbell SC, Novick AC, Belldegrun A, et al: Guideline for management of the clinical T1 renal mass. *J Urol* 182:1271–1279, 2009.
45. Raman JD, Smaldone M, Thompson RH, et al: Renal neoplasms. American Urological Association. <https://www.auanet.org/university/core_topic.cfm?coreid=75>. Accessed August 7, 2015.
46. Inman BA, Lotan Y, Daneshmand S, et al: Bladder neoplasm. American Urological Association. <https://www.auanet.org/university/core_topic.cfm?coreid=76>. Accessed August 7, 2015.
47. Meeks JJ, Lowrance WT, McBride S, et al: Prostate cancer. American Urological Association. <https://www.auanet.org/university/core_topic.cfm?coreid=74>. Accessed August 7, 2015.
48. Thompson I, Thrasher JB, Aus G, et al: Guideline for the management of clinically localized prostate cancer: 2007 update. *J Urol* 177:2106–2131, 2007.
49. Carter HB, Albertsen PC, Barry MJ, et al: Early detection of prostate cancer: AUA guideline. *J Urol* 190:419–426, 2013.
50. Woods M, Castle EP, Stroup SP, et al: Testis neoplasms. American Urological Association. <https://www.auanet.org/university/core_topic.cfm?coreid=77>. Accessed August 7, 2015.

INDEX

Page numbers followed by "*f*" indicate figures, "*b*" indicate boxes, and "*t*" indicate tables.

D

H

Q

R

S

T

U

V

W